SABISTON

TEXTBOOK *of*
SURGERY

The Biological Basis of Modern Surgical Practice

22ND EDITION

SABISTON
TEXTBOOK *of*
SURGERY

The Biological Basis of Modern Surgical Practice

EDITOR

Douglas S. Tyler, MD, MSHCT
Professor of Surgery
Associate Chair of Community Operations and Strategy
Department of Surgery
The University of North Carolina at Chapel Hill
Chapel Hill, North Carolina

ASSOCIATE EDITORS

Andrea Hayes-Dixon, MD
Dean, Vice President of Clinical Affairs
College of Medicine
Howard University College of Medicine
Washington, DC

O. Joe Hines, MD
Professor and Chair
Department of Surgery
David Geffen School of Medicine
    at University of California, Los Angeles
Los Angeles, California

Rachel R. Kelz, MD, MSCE, MBA
William Maul Measey Professor of Surgery
Department of Surgery
University of Pennsylvania
Philadelphia, Pennsylvania

Melina R. Kibbe, MD
Dean
School of Medicine
University of Virginia
Charlottesville, Virginia

Christine L. Lau, MD, MBA
Buxton Professor and Chair
Department of Surgery
University of Maryland
Baltimore, Maryland

Mayur B. Patel, MD, MPH
Chief and Professor
Division of Acute Care Surgery, Vanderbilt
    Department of Surgery, Section of Surgical
    Sciences
Vanderbilt University Medical Center
Nashville, Tennessee

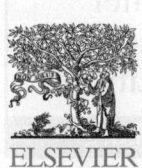

ELSEVIER

Elsevier
1600 John F. Kennedy Blvd.
Ste 1800
Philadelphia, PA 19103-2899

SABISTON TEXTBOOK OF SURGERY: THE BIOLOGICAL BASIS
OF MODERN SURGICAL PRACTICE, TWENTY-SECOND EDITION

ISBN: 978-0-443-12434-1

INTERNATIONAL EDITION

ISBN: 978-0-443-37916-1

Content Strategist: Jessica McCool
Senior Content Development Specialist: Joanie Milnes
Publishing Services Manager: Catherine Jackson
Book Production Specialist: Kristine Feeherty
Design Direction: Margaret Reid

Printed in India

Last digit is the print number: 9 8 7 6 5 4 3 2 1

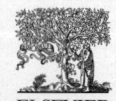
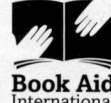

This textbook is dedicated to the patients we serve and the healthcare professionals, trainees, and students learning the art of surgery. We are grateful to our families and friends for their support in completing this project.

Mohammad Abbass, MD
Northwestern University Feinberg School of Medicine
Chicago, Illinois

Fariba Abbassi, MD
Research Fellow
Department of Abdominal Surgery and Transplantation
University Hospital Zurich;
Research Fellow
Epidemiology, Biostatistics and Prevention Institute
University of Zurich
Zurich, Switzerland

Abdurrahman T. Abdelzaher, MD
Surgical Oncology Postdoctoral Research Fellow
Surgery
Alvin J. Siteman Comprehensive Cancer Center at Washington
    University School of Medicine, Department of Surgery,
    Section of Surgical Oncology
St. Louis, Missouri

Rachael C. Acker, MD
General Surgery Resident
Department of Surgery
University of Pennsylvania
Philadelphia, Pennsylvania

Andrew Adams, MD, PhD
Professor
Department of Surgery
University of Minnesota
Minneapolis, Minnesota

Reid B. Adams, MD
Claude A Jessup Professor
Department of Surgery
University of Virginia School of Medicine;
Chief Medical Officer
University of Virginia
Charlottesville, Virginia

Divyansh Agarwal, MD, PhD
Clinical Fellow in Surgery
Harvard Medical School
Massachusetts General Hospital
Boston, Massachusetts

Alexandra Z. Agathis, MD
Resident
Department of Surgery
Icahn School of Medicine at Mount Sinai
New York, New York

Vanita Ahuja, MD, MPH, MBA
Associate Chief of Staff - Education
Minneapolis Veterans Affairs Healthcare System
Minneapolis, Minnesota

Yewande Alimi, MD, MHS
Assistant Professor of Surgery
Surgery
Georgetown University School of Medicine
Washington, District of Columbia

John C. Alverdy, MD, FACS, FSIS
Sara and Harold Lincoln Thompson Professor of Surgery,
    Executive Vice Chair
Department of Surgery
Pritzker School of Medicine
University of Chicago
Chicago, Illinois

Seema Anandalwar, MD, MPH
Clinical Instructor in Surgery
Surgery
R Adams Cowley Shock Trauma Center
Baltimore, Maryland

Peter Angelos, MD, PhD, FACS, MAMSE, HEC-C
Linda Kohler Anderson Professor of Surgery
    and Surgical Ethics
Department of Surgery
Chief, Endocrine Surgery
Director, MacLean Center for Clinical Medical Ethics
University of Chicago
Chicago, Illinois

Mark Antkowiak, MD
Resident Physician
Department of Surgery
University of California San Diego
San Diego, California

Imran J. Anwar, MD
General Surgery Resident
Department of Surgery
Duke University
Durham, North Carolina

Rachel D. Appelbaum, MD, FACS
Assistant Professor
Department of Surgery
Vanderbilt University Medical Center
Nashville, Tennessee

Shipra Arya, MD, SM
Professor
Department of Surgery
Stanford University School of Medicine
Stanford, California

Anthony Atala, MD
Director
Wake Forest Institute for Regenerative Medicine
William H. Boyce Professor and Chair
Department of Urology
Wake Forest School of Medicine
Winston-Salem, North Carolina

Andrew Nagy Atia, MD, MBA
Department of Surgery
Division of Plastic, Maxillofacial, and Oral Surgery
Duke University Hospital
Durham, North Carolina

Jason M. Aubrey, MD
Surgical Resident
General Surgery
Corewell Health - Michigan State University
Grand Rapids, Michigan

Mary T. Austin, MD, MPH
Professor
Surgical Oncology
University of Texas MD Anderson Cancer Center
Houston, Texas

Reed I. Ayabe, MD
Assistant Professor of Surgery
Department of Surgery
University of California Irvine
Irvine, California

Hassan Aziz, MD, FACS
Assistant Professor of Surgery
Department of Surgery
University of Iowa
Iowa City, Iowa

Idelberto Raul Badell, MD
Associate Professor
Department of Surgery
Emory University School of Medicine
Atlanta, Georgia

Andrew Patrick Bain, MD
Surgery Resident
Department of Surgery
UT Southwestern Medical Center
Dallas, Texas

Aditi Balakrishna, MD
Assistant Professor
Anesthesiology, Division of Critical Care
Vanderbilt University Medical Center
Nashville, Tennessee

Elise Bardawil, MD
Assistant Professor Division of Minimally Invasive Gynecologic Surgery
Obstetrics and Gynecology
Washington University in St. Louis
St. Louis, Missouri

Edward M. Barksdale, Jr., MD
Department of Orthopaedic Surgery
Washington University School of Medicine
St. Louis, Missouri

Georgia Beasley, MD, MHSc
Associate Professor of Surgery With Tenure
Department of Surgery
Duke University
Durham, North Carolina

Igor Belyansky, MD
Chief of General Surgery
Director of Abdominal Wall Reconstruction Program
General Surgery
Anne Arundel Medical Center
Annapolis, Maryland

Cherisse Berry, MD, FACS
Professor of Surgery
Vice Chair of Academic Affairs,
    Department of Surgery
Rutgers Health, New Jersey School of Medicine
Newark, New Jersey

Tina Bharani, MD
Fellow
Department of Surgery
University of Iowa Hospitals and Clinics
Iowa City, Iowa

Vijay Bhoj, MD, PhD
Assistant Professor
Department of Pathology and Laboratory Medicine
University of Pennsylvania
Philadelphia, Pennsylvania

Monica Bhutiani, MD, MEd
Assistant Professor
Anesthesiology
Vanderbilt University Medical Center
Nashville, Tennessee

Letitia Bible, MD, FACS
Assistant Professor
Trauma and Acute Care Surgery
University of Florida
Gainesville, Florida

Karl Y. Bilimoria, MD, MS
Director of Surgical Outcomes and Quality Improvement
    Center (SOQIC)
Chair, Department of Surgery
Indiana University
Indianapolis, Indiana

Dan Blazer III, MD, FACS
Professor of Surgery
Department of Surgery
Duke University
Durham, North Carolina

Joshua I.S. Bleier, MD, FACS, FASCRS
Professor of Clinical Surgery
Department of Surgery
University of Pennsylvania, Perelman School of Medicine
Philadelphia, Pennsylvania

Rachel Bluebond-Langner, MD
Associate Professor
Department of Plastic Surgery
New York University Langone Health
New York, New York

Mary E. Bokenkamp, MD
Chief Resident
Department of Surgery
Dell Medical School at the University of Texas at Austin
Austin, Texas

Genevieve Boland, MD, PhD
Vice Chair of Research
Department of Surgery
Massachusetts General Hospital
Boston, Massachusetts

Brian A. Boone, MD
Associate Professor
Department of Surgery, Division of Surgical Oncology
West Virginia University
Morgantown, West Virginia

Edmond W. Box III, MD
T32 Surgical Oncology Research Fellow
Department of Surgery
University of Miami
Miami, Florida

Ludwik Krzysztof Branski, MD, MMS
Associate Professor of Surgery
Department of Surgery
University of Texas Medical Branch;
Staff Surgeon
Shriners Hospital for Children
Galveston, Texas

Benjamin N. Breyer, MD, MAS
Chair, Department of Urology
Professor of Urology
University of California, San Francisco
San Francisco, California

Meaghan Broderick, MD
Instructor
Surgical Critical Care and Acute Care Surgery
R Adams Cowley Shock Trauma Center
Baltimore, Maryland

Ryan C. Broderick, MD
Associate Professor
Department of Surgery, Division of Minimally Invasive Surgery
University of California San Diego
La Jolla, California

Benjamin Sands Brooke, MD, PhD, FACS, DFSVS
Professor
Chief, Division of Vascular Surgery
Department of Surgery
Adjunct Professor
Department of Population Health Sciences
University of Utah
Salt Lake City, Utah

Carlos V.R. Brown, MD
Chief, Division of Acute Care Surgery
Department of Surgery
Dell Medical School at the University of Texas at Austin
Austin, Texas

Paul R. Burchard, MD
Resident
General Surgery
University of Rochester Medical Center
Rochester, New York

Clay Cothren Burlew, MD
Professor of Surgery
Department of Surgery
University of Colorado Anschutz Medical Campus
Aurora, Colorado

Ruth L. Bush, MD, JD, MPH
Professor
Associate Dean, Educational Affairs
Professor of Surgery
Department of Surgery
John Sealy School of Medicine
University of Texas Medical Branch
Galveston, Texas

Alfredo Maximiliano Carbonell II, DO
Co-Director Hernia Center
Department of Surgery
Prisma Health – Upstate;
Professor
Department of Surgery
University of South Carolina School of Medicine,
   Greenville
Greenville, South Carolina

Leandro Totti Cavazzola, MD, MSc, PhD, FACS
Associate Professor
Department of Surgery
Universidade Federal do Rio Grande do Sul,
   Porto Alegre;
Associate Professor
Department of Surgery
Hospital de Clínicas de Porto Alegre
Rio Grande do Sul, Brazil

Paul Cederna, MD
Chief of Plastic Surgery
Department of Surgery
University of Michigan
Ann Arbor, Michigan

Hani Chanbour, MD
Resident
Neurosurgery
Vanderbilt University
Nashville, Tennessee

William C. Chapman, Sr., MD
Professor of Surgery
Department of Surgery
Washington University in St. Louis
St. Louis, Missouri

Anthony Charles, MD, MPH
Professor of Surgery
Department of Surgery
University of Vermont
Burlington, Vermont

Genevieve Chartrand, MSc, MD, FRCSC
Surgeon
Chirurgie Digestive
Centre Hospitalier de l'Université de Montréal
Montreal, Quebec, Canada

Mihir Chaudhary, MD, MPH
Surgical Fellow
Department of Surgery
Emory University
Atlanta, Georgia

Michael Lee Cheatham, MD, FACS, FCCM
Trauma Surgeon
Department of Surgical Education
Orlando Regional Medical Center
Orlando, Florida

Edward P. Chen, MD
Professor of Surgery
Department of Surgery
Duke University
Durham, North Carolina

Herbert Chen, MD
Chair and Fay Fletcher Kerner Chair
Surgery
University of Alabama at Birmingham
Surgeon-in-Chief
University of Alabama at Birmingham Health System
Senior Associate Dean
University of Alabama at Birmingham Heersink School of Medicine
Birmingham, Alabama

Karan R. Chhabra, MD, MSc
Assistant Professor
Departments of Surgery and Population Health
New York University Grossman School of Medicine;
Assistant Professor
Division of Bariatric and General Surgery
NYC Health + Hospitals/Bellevue
New York, New York

Ifeanyi David Chinedozi, MD
Surgery Resident
Department of Surgery
Johns Hopkins University
Baltimore, Maryland

Perry S. Choi, MD
Resident Physician
Department of Cardiothoracic Surgery
Stanford University
Palo Alto, California

Konstantinos Chouliaras, MD
Surgical Oncologist
Division of Surgery
Baptist MD Anderson
Jacksonville, Florida

Ngoc-Quynh Chu, MD
Clinical Fellow
Thoracic Surgery
Memorial Sloan Kettering Cancer Center
New York, New York

Yun Shin Chun, MD, FACS
Professor
Surgical Oncology
University of Texas MD Anderson Cancer Center
Houston, Texas

Dai H. Chung, MD, MBA
Professor
Strauss Endowed Chair in Pediatric Surgery
Department of Surgery
UT Southwestern Medical Center;
Chief Medical Executive
Children's Health;
Chief Medical Officer
Joint Pediatric Enterprise
Dallas, Texas

Bryan M. Clary, MD, MBA
Professor and Chair
Department of Surgery
University of California San Diego
San Diego, California

Pierre-Alain Clavien, MD, PhD
Professor and Chairman
University of Zurich
Swiss Medical Network
Zurich, Switzerland

Thomas West Clements, MD, FRCSC
Assistant Professor
Department of Surgery
The University of Texas Health Science
    Center at Houston
Houston, Texas

Orly M. Coblens, MD, FACS
Associate Professor
Otolaryngology - Head and Neck Surgery
University of Texas Medical Branch
Galveston, Texas

Dawn Marie Coleman, MD
Division Chief, Vascular and Endovascular Surgery
Department of Surgery
Duke University
Durham, North Carolina

Jesse A. Columbo, MD, MS
Assistant Professor of Surgery
Section of Vascular Surgery
Dartmouth Hitchcock Medical Center
Lebanon, New Hampshire

Seth J. Concors, MD
Assistant Professor
Department of Surgery
Emory University
Atlanta, Georgia

Daniel Counihan, MD, MA
House Officer
Department of Surgery
Boston Medical Center
Boston, Massachusetts

Mitchell W. Cox, MD
Chief, Division of Vascular Surgery
Professor of Surgery
Department of Surgery
University of Texas Medical Branch
Galveston, Texas

Joshua L. Crapps, MD
Resident Physician
Department of Surgery and Perioperative Care
University of Texas at Austin Dell Medical School
Austin, Texas

Joseph G. Crompton, MD, PhD
Assistant Professor
Department of Surgery
University of California, Los Angeles
Los Angeles, California

Andi Jean Cummins, MD
Resident Physician
Plastic Surgery
University of Texas Medical Branch
Galveston, Texas

Carrie Elizabeth Cunningham, MD, MPH
Associate Professor
Department of Surgery
Massachusetts General Hospital
Boston, Massachusetts

Thomas A. D'Amico, MD
Gary Hock Endowed Professor
Department of Surgery
Duke University Medical Center;
Director
Thoracic Oncology Program
Chief
General Thoracic Surgery
Duke Cancer Institute
Durham, North Carolina

Michael I. D'Angelica, MD, FACS
Enid Haupt Endowed Chair in Surgery
Department of Surgery
Memorial Sloan Kettering Cancer Center;
Professor of Surgery
Department of Surgery
Weill Cornell School of Medicine
New York, New York

Jorge Daes, MD, FACS
Director
Minimally Invasive Surgery
Clinica Bautista
Barranquilla, Atlantico, Colombia

Brian J. Daley, MD, MBA, FACS
Vice Chair
Department of Surgery
University of Tennessee Medical Center at Knoxville
Knoxville, Tennessee

Alan Dardik, MD, PhD
Professor
Surgery and Interventional Radiology
Icahn School of Medicine at Mount Sinai
New York, New York;
Emeritus Professor
Surgery and Cellular and Molecular Physiology
Yale School of Medicine
New Haven, Connecticut

Giana H. Davidson, MD, MPH
Professor
Surgery, Health Services and Population Health
University of Washington
Seattle, Washington

Alexis N. Davis, MD
Vascular Surgery Resident
Department of Surgery, Division of Vascular Surgery,
    John Sealy School of Medicine
University of Texas Medical Branch
Galveston, Texas

Kimberly A. Davis, MD, MBA
Professor
Department of Surgery
Yale School of Medicine
New Haven, Connecticut

Hans D. de Boer, MD, PhD
Anesthesiology, Pain Medicine and Procedural Sedation and Analgesia
Martini General Hospital Groningen
Groningen, Netherlands

Marc de Moya, MD
Professor and Chief of Trauma/ACS
Department of Surgery
Medical College of Wisconsin
Milwaukee, Wisconsin

Abelardo DeAnda, Jr., MD
Professor and Chief
Division of Cardiovascular and Thoracic Surgery
University of Texas Medical Branch
Galveston, Texas

Ronald Dematteo, MD
John Rhea Barton and Chair
Department of Surgery
University of Pennsylvania
Philadelphia, Pennsylvania

Bradley M. Dennis, MD
Professor
Division of Acute Care Surgery
Vanderbilt University Medical Center
Nashville, Tennessee

Daniel L. Dent, MD
Vice Chair for Education
Department of Surgery
Chair
Department of Medical Education
UT Health San Antonio Long School of Medicine
Associate Director for Workforce Development
Mays Cancer Center
UT Health San Antonio
San Antonio, Texas

Michael P. DeWane, MD
Assistant Professor
Department of Surgery
Massachusetts General Hospital
Boston, Massachusetts

Jose J. Diaz, MD, CPE, CNS, FACS, FCCM
Professor of Surgery
Vice Chair of Faculty Affairs and Development Chief, Division Acute
    Care Surgery: Trauma, Emergency General Surgery, and Surgical
    Critical Care
University of South Florida Morsani College of Medicine;
Chief, Department of Surgery
Medical Director Acute Care Surgery Institute: Regional Trauma
    Program, Surgical/Trauma ICU, and Surgical Step-Down Unit
Tampa General Hospital
Tampa, Florida

Gerard M. Doherty, MD
Moseley Professor of Surgery
Surgery
Harvard Medical School;
Crowley Family Chair and Surgeon-in-Chief
Brigham and Women's Hospital;
Surgeon-in-Chief
Mass General Brigham Cancer Institute
Boston, Massachusetts

Timothy R. Donahue, MD
Professor
Department of Surgery
David Geffen School of Medicine at UCLA
Los Angeles, California

Daniel Donato, MD
Assistant Professor
Department of Surgery
Division of Plastic Surgery
University of Texas Medical Branch
Galveston, Texas

Anthony Douglas II, MD
Resident Physician
Department of Surgery
University of Chicago
Chicago, Illinois

Majella Doyle, MD, MBA, FRCSI, FACS
Professor of Surgery
Department of Surgery
Washington University in St. Louis
St. Louis, Missouri

Sophie Dream, MD, MPH
Associate Professor
Department of Surgery
Medical College of Wisconsin
Milwaukee, Wisconsin

Joseph DuBose, MD
Professor of Surgery
Anesthesia and Perioperative Care
Dell Medical School
Austin, Texas

Matthew J. Eagleton, MD
System Chief
Vascular and Endovascular Surgery
Massachusetts General Brigham
Professor
Surgery
Harvard Medical School
Boston, Massachusetts;
Surgeon-in-Chief
University of Alabama at Birmingham Health System
Senior Associate Dean
University of Alabama at Birmingham Heersink School of Medicine
Birmingham, Alabama

James Steven Economou, MD, PhD
Distinguished Professor
Surgery, Molecular Genetics, Molecular Pharmacology
Division of Surgical Oncology
Department of Surgery
University of California, Los Angeles
Los Angeles, California

Michael E. Egger, MD, MPH
Associate Professor
Hiram C Polk Jr, MD, Department of Surgery
University of Louisville
Louisville, Kentucky

Anne P. Ehlers, MD, MPH
Assistant Professor
Department of Surgery
University of Michigan
Ann Arbor, Michigan

Sameh Hany Emile, MBBCh, MSc, MD, FACS
Project Specialist
Colorectal Surgery Department
Digestive Disease Center, Cleveland Clinic Florida
Weston, Florida;
Associate Professor of Surgery
Colorectal Surgery
Mansoura University Faculty of Medicine
Mansoura, Egypt

Samuel J. Enumah, MD, MBA
Assistant Professor
Department of Surgery
University of Rochester
Rochester, New York

Stephanie Eosten Joyce, MD
Assistant Professor of Surgery
General Surgery, Trauma and Surgical Critical Care
Yale School of Medicine
New Haven, Connecticut

Detlev Erdmann, MD, PhD, MHSc
Professor With Tenure
Department of Surgery
Duke University Health
Durham, North Carolina

Yana Etkin, MD
Associate Professor of Surgery
Surgery
Zucker School of Medicine
Hofstra Northwell University
Hempstead, New York

Douglas B. Evans, MD
Donald C. Ausman Family Foundation Professor and Chair
Department of Surgery
Medical College of Wisconsin
Milwaukee, Wisconsin

B. Mark Evers, MD
Director, University of Kentucky Markey Cancer Center
Associate Vice President for Oncology Research and Strategic
    Development
Professor, Department of Surgery
Markey Cancer Foundation Endowed Chair
Physician-in-Chief, Oncology Service Line
Lexington, Kentucky

Aldo Fafaj, MD
Assistant Professor
General Surgery
UT Medical Center Knoxville
Knoxville, Ohio

Alik Farber, MD, MBA
James Utley Professor and Chair
Department of Surgery
Boston University Chobanian and Avedisian
    School of Medicine;
Surgeon-in-Chief
Boston Medical Center;
Chief of Surgery
Boston Medical Center Health System
Boston, Massachusetts

Orly Nadell Farber, MD
Resident
Department of Surgery
Brigham and Women's Hospital
Boston, Massachusetts

Paige Farley, MD, MS, MPH, MBA
Resident Physician
Department of Surgery
Oregon Health & Science University
Portland, Oregon

Diana Farmer, MD, FACS, FRCS
Chair and Professor
Department of Surgery
University of California Davis Health
Sacramento, California

Oluwadamilola Motunrayo Fayanju, MD, MA, MPHS, FACS
The Helen O. Dickens Presidential Associate Professor
    and Chief, Division of Breast Surgery
Department of Surgery
University of Pennsylvania Perelman School of Medicine;
Surgical Director
Rena Rowan Breast Center
Abramson Cancer Center, Penn Medicine
Philadelphia, Pennsylvania

Ryan C. Fields, MD, FACS
Chair, Department of Surgery
Seymour L. Schwartz Professor of Surgery
University of Rochester School of Medicine and Dentistry;
Surgeon-in-Chief, Strong Memorial Hospital
Director of Translational Research, J.P. Wilmont Cancer Institute
Rochester, New York

Emily Finlayson, MD, MS
Professor in Residence
Surgery, Division of General Surgery
University of California, San Francisco
San Francisco, California

Yuman Fong, MD
Sangiacomo Chair and Chairman
Department of Surgery
City of Hope National Medical Center
Duarte, California

Camila Franco, MD
Resident
General Surgery Department
University of Texas Medical Branch
Galveston, Texas

Charles D. Fraser, Jr., MD, FACS, FACC
Chair
Department of Cardiovascular and Thoracic Surgery
The University of Texas at Austin - Dell Medical School;
Executive Director
Texas Center for Pediatric and Congenital Heart Disease
Austin, Texas

Vivian Gahtan, MD
Chair
Department of Surgery
Stritch School of Medicine
Loyola University Medical Center;
Staff Physician
Surgery
Edward Hines Jr. VA Hospital
Maywood, Illinois

Katherine Gallagher, MD
Professor of Surgery
Department of Surgery
University of Michigan
Ann Arbor, Michigan

Jason M. Gauthier, MD
Fellow
Cardiothoracic Surgery
Washington University in St. Louis
St. Louis, Missouri

Joshua T. Geiger, MD, MS
Vascular Surgery Integrated Resident
Department of Surgery
Division of Vascular Surgery
University of Rochester
Rochester, New York

Rondi Gelbard, MD, FACS
Associate Professor of Surgery
Surgery
University of Alabama at Birmingham
Birmingham, Alabama

Philip George, MD, FACS
Assistant Professor
Department of Surgery
Columbia University
New York, New York

Andrea Gillis, MD, MSPH
Assistant Professor
Department of Surgery
University of Alabama at Birmingham
Birmingham, Alabama

S. Peter P. Goedegebuure, PhD
Associate Professor
Department of Surgery
Washington University School of Medicine
St. Louis, Missouri

Teodor Grantcharov, MD, PhD, FACS
Professor of Surgery
Department of Surgery
Stanford University
Palo Alto, California

Jacob Greenberg, MD, EdM
Associate Professor
Department of Surgery
Duke University
Durham, North Carolina

Rachel A. Greenup, MD, MPH
Associate Professor
Department of Surgery
Yale School of Medicine
Madison, Connecticut

Elizabeth Gardner Grubbs, MD, MS
Professor
Department of Surgical Oncology
Executive Director, Faculty Academic Career Development
Office of Chief Academic Officer
University of Texas MD Anderson Cancer Center
Houston, Texas

Oliver L. Gunter, MD, MPH
Professor and Director of Emergency General Surgery
Division of Trauma and Surgical Critical Care
Vanderbilt University Medical Center
Nashville, Tennessee

Ehab Hanna, MD
Professor and Director of Skull Base Surgery
Vice Chairman
Department of Head and Neck Surgery
University of Texas MD Anderson Cancer Center
Houston, Texas

Mariam N. Hantouli, MD
Research Assistant Professor
Department of Surgery
University of Washington
Seattle, Washington

Melike Harfouche, MD, MPH
Assistant Professor
Department of Surgery
University of Maryland School of Medicine;
Surgeon
R Adams Cowley Shock Trauma Center
University of Maryland Medical Center
Baltimore, Maryland

David Harpole, MD
Professor of Surgery and Pathology
Department of Surgery
Duke University;
Chief of Cardiothoracic Surgery
Durham Veterans Affairs Medical Center
Durham, North Carolina

Daniel Alejandro Hashimoto, MD, FACS
Assistant Professor
Department of Surgery, Division of Gastrointestinal Surgery
University of Pennsylvania Perelman School of Medicine
Philadelphia, Pennsylvania

Justin Hatchimonji, MD, MBE, MSCE
Fellow, Trauma and Acute Care Surgery
Division of Traumatology, Emergency Surgery, and Surgical Critical Care
University of Pennsylvania
Philadelphia, Pennsylvania

Christina J. Hayhurst, MD, FCCM
Associate Professor of Anesthesiology
Anesthesiology and Critical Care Medicine
Vanderbilt University Medical Center
Nashville, Tennessee

Alex Bernard Haynes, MD, MPH, FACS
Associate Chair for Investigation and Discovery
Surgery and Perioperative Care
University of Texas Austin Dell Medical School
Austin, Texas

Sarah Hays, MD
Resident Physician
Department of Surgery
University of Chicago
Chicago, Illinois

Sharon Henry, MD
Professor of Trauma Surgery
Department of Surgery
University of Maryland School of Medicine;
Director of Wound Healing and Metabolism
Program in Trauma
R Adams Cowley Shock Trauma Center
Baltimore, Maryland

Fernando A. Herbella, MD
Associate Professor
Department of Surgery
Federal University of Sao Paulo
Sao Paulo, Brazil

Paul Tarver Hernandez, MD
Assistant Professor
Colorectal Surgery
Hospital of the University of Pennsylvania
Philadelphia, Pennsylvania

John Herndon, BA
Staff Scientist
Department of Surgery
Washington University School of Medicine
St. Louis, Missouri

Jill R. Higgins, ACNP
Nurse Practitioner
Cardiothoracic Surgery
University of California San Diego
San Diego, California

Robert S.D. Higgins, MD, MSHA
President and Chief Academic Officer
Rush University
Chicago, Illinois

Vanessa P. Ho, MD, PhD, MPH
Associate Professor
Surgery
MetroHealth Medical Center;
Associate Professor
Population and Quantitative Health Sciences
Case Western Reserve University School of Medicine
Cleveland, Ohio

Melissa E. Hogg, MD, MS
Division Chief, General Surgery
Clinical Professor
Department of Surgery
NorthShore
Chicago, Illinois

Julie L. Holihan, MD, MS
Assistant Professor of Surgery
Surgery
McGovern Medical School
Houston, Texas

Rachel C. Hooper, MD
Clinical Assistant Professor of Surgery
Department of Surgery
University of Michigan
Ann Arbor, Michigan

Nir Horesh, MD
Colorectal Surgeon
Colorectal Surgery
Cleveland Clinic Florida
Weston, Florida

James R. Howe V, MD
Director, Division of Surgical Oncology and Endocrine Surgery
Department of Surgery
University of Iowa Carver College of Medicine
Iowa City, Iowa

Yinin Hu, MD, FACS
Assistant Professor
Department of Surgery
University of Maryland School of Medicine
Baltimore, Maryland

Lioba Huelsboemer, MD
Postdoctoral Research Fellow
Plastic Surgery
Yale University
New Haven, Connecticut

Tasha Hughes, MD, MPH
Clinical Associate Professor
Department of Surgery
University of Michigan
Ann Arbor, Michigan

Kelly K. Hunt, MD
Professor and Chair
Breast Surgical Oncology
University of Texas MD Anderson Cancer Center
Houston, Texas

Matthew M. Hutter, MD, MBA, MPH
Professor of Surgery
Surgery
Harvard Medical School;
Director, Codman Center for Clinical Effectiveness in Surgery
Department of Surgery
Massachusetts General Hospital
Boston, Massachusetts

Michelle Huyser, MD
Surgical Oncologist
Surgery
Phoenix Indian Medical Center;
Surgical Oncologist
Surgery
Mayo Clinic Arizona
Phoenix, Arizona

Colby John Hyland, MD
Resident Physician
Surgery
Mass General Brigham
Boston, Massachusetts

Brian P. Jacob, MD
Associate Professor of Surgery
Department of Surgery
Icahn School of Medicine at Mount Sinai
New York, New York

Kathleen Jarrell, MD, MPH
Resident Physician
Department of Surgery
Thomas Jefferson University Hospital;
Research Resident
Department of Breast Surgery
University of Pennsylvania
Philadelphia, Pennsylvania

Sudha Jayaraman, MD, MSc, FACS
Professor of Surgery
Department of Surgery
University of Utah
Salt Lake City, Utah

Whitney Jenson, MD, MPH
Assistant Professor
Department of Surgery
University of Colorado
Aurora, Colorado

Maria F. Jimenez, MD
Professor of Surgery
Surgery
Hospital Universitario Mayor Méderi
Bogota, Colombia

Joseph P. Johnson, MD
Associate Professor
Orthopedic Surgery
University of Alabama at Birmingham
Birmingham, Alabama

William Roberson Johnston, MD
Resident Physician
Department of Surgery
Hospital of the University of Pennsylvania
Philadelphia, Pennsylvania

Andrew Jones, PhD
Chief Assessment Officer
American Board of Surgery
Philadelphia, Pennsylvania

Daniel B. Jones, MD, MS
Benjamin Rush Endowed Chair of Surgery
Department of Surgery
Assistant Dean of Simulation
Rutgers New Jersey Medical School;
Surgery Chief of Service
University Hospital
Newark, New Jersey

Soren Jonzzon, MD
Resident Physician
Department of Neurological Surgery
Vanderbilt University Medical Center
Nashville, Tennessee

Mary Junak, MD
General Surgery Resident
Department of Surgery
University of Wisconsin
Madison, Wisconsin

Gregory Jurkovich, MD
Distinguished Professor and Vice Chairman
Department of Surgery
University of California, Davis
Sacramento, California

Haytham M.A. Kaafarani, MD, MPH, FACS
Professor of Surgery
Surgery
Harvard Medical School;
Trauma Medical Director
Surgery
Hospital Director of Safety and Quality
Massachusetts General Hospital
Boston, Massachusetts

Puja Kachroo, MS, MD
Associate Professor of Cardiac Surgery
Department of Surgery
Washington University in St. Louis
St. Louis, Missouri

Steven Kahn, MD, FACS, FABA
Professor of Surgery, Chief of Burn Surgery
Department of Surgery
Medical University of South Carolina
Charleston, South Carolina

Kristen N. Kaiser, MD
Resident
General Surgery
Indiana University
Indianapolis, Indiana

Matthew F. Kalady, MD, FASCRS, FACS
Professor of Surgery
Department of Surgery
Director, Division of Colon and Rectal Surgery
The Ohio State University Wexner Medical Center;
Medical Director, Clinical Cancer Genetics
Director, The James Colorectal Cancer Center
Columbus, Ohio

Elishama N. Kanu, MD, MA
Resident Physician
Department of Surgery
Duke University Medical Center
Durham, North Carolina

Lillian S. Kao, MD, MBA
Professor
Department of Surgery
McGovern Medical School at the University of Texas Health Science
    Center at Houston
Houston, Texas

Sahil Kapur, MD
Department of Plastic and Reconstructive Surgery
University of Texas MD Anderson Cancer Center
Houston, Texas

Giorgos C. Karakousis, MD
Professor of Surgery
Department of Surgery
University of Pennsylvania
Philadelphia, Pennsylvania

Jeffrey Edward Keenan, MD
Assistant Professor
Department of Surgery
Duke University Medical Center
Durham, North Carolina

Rachel R. Kelz, MD, MSCE, MBA
William Maul Measey Professor of Surgery
Department of Surgery
University of Pennsylvania
Philadelphia, Pennsylvania

Robert Keskey, MD, PhD
Surgical Critical Care Fellow
Department of Surgery
University of Chicago
Chicago, Illinois

Dineo Khabele, MD
Professor and Chair
Obstetrics and Gynecology
Washington University School of Medicine
St. Louis, Missouri

Jina Kim, MD
Endocrine Surgeon
Department of Surgery
Inova Health System
Falls Church, Virginia

Paul Taehoon Kim, MD
General/MIS Surgeon
General Surgery
Luminis Health
Annapolis, Maryland

Elizabeth Gherardi King, MD
Assistant Professor
Division of Vascular and Endovascular Surgery
Boston University Chobanian and Avedisian School of Medicine
Boston, Massachusetts

William H. Kitchens, Jr., MD, PhD, FACS, FAST
Associate Professor
Department of Surgery
Emory University School of Medicine
Atlanta, Georgia

V. Suzanne Klimberg, MD, PhD
Professor and Courtney M Townsend, Jr, MD Distinguished Chair in
    General Surgery
Department of Surgery
University of Texas Medical Branch
Galveston, Texas;
Clinical Director of the University of Texas Medical Branch
    Cancer Center
Adjunct Professor
Department of Breast Surgical of Oncology
University of Texas MD Anderson Cancer Center
Houston, Texas

Meera Kotagal, MD, MPH
Assistant Professor
Division of Pediatric General and Thoracic Surgery
Cincinnati Children's Hospital Medical Center;
Assistant Professor
Department of Surgery
University of Cincinnati College of Medicine
Cincinnati, Ohio

Benjamin D. Kozower, MD, MPH
Professor
Department of Surgery
Washington University School of Medicine
St. Louis, Missouri

Daniel Kreisel, MD, PhD
Professor of Surgery, Pathology and Immunology,
    G. Alexander Patterson MD/Mid-America Transplant
    Endowed Distinguished Chair in Lung Transplantation
Department of Surgery
Washington University School of Medicine
St. Louis, Missouri

Alexander Sasha Krupnick, MD
Chief of Thoracic Surgery
Department of Surgery
University of Maryland
Baltimore, Maryland

Kevin P. Labadie, MD
Complex General Surgical Oncology Fellow
Department of Surgery
City of Hope
Duarte, California

Mitchell R. Ladd, MD, PhD
Assistant Professor
General Surgery, Division of Pediatric Surgery
Assistant Professor
Wake Forest Institute for Regenerative Medicine
Assistant Professor
Biomedical Engineering
Assistant Professor
Pediatrics
Wake Forest University School of Medicine
Winston-Salem, North Carolina

Jennifer LaFemina, MD
Associate Professor
Program Director of General Surgery Residency
Department of Surgery
University of Massachusetts Chan Medical School
Worcester, Massachusetts

Sandhya A. Lagoo-Deenadayalan, MD, PhD, FACS
Professor of Surgery
Duke University
Durham, North Carolina

Geeta Lal, MD, MSc, FRCS(C), FACS
Professor
Department of Surgery, Division of Surgical Oncology and Endocrine
    Surgery
University of Iowa
Iowa City, Iowa

Christine L. Lau, MD, MBA
Buxton Professor and Chair
Department of Surgery
University of Maryland
Baltimore, Maryland

Jennifer Lawton, MD
Chief of Cardiac Surgery
Professor
Johns Hopkins Division of Cardiac Surgery
Baltimore, Maryland

Anson Michael Lee, MD
Assistant Professor
Cardiothoracic Surgery
Stanford University
Stanford, California

Jani J. Lee, MD, RPVI
Assistant Professor
Department of Surgery
University of Texas Medical Branch
Galveston, Texas

Jason T. Lee, MD
Chief of Vascular Surgery
Division of Vascular Surgery
Stanford University Medical Center
Palo Alto, California

Z-Hye Lee, MD
Assistant Professor
Department of Plastic Surgery
University of Texas MD Anderson Cancer Center
Houston, Texas

Joshua Leinwand, MD, MSE
Surgical Oncology Fellow
Department of Surgery
Memorial Sloan Kettering Cancer Center
New York, New York

L. Scott Levin, MD, FACS
Chairman
Orthopaedic Surgery
Professor of Surgery
Division of Plastic Surgery
University of Pennsylvania Health System
Philadelphia, Pennsylvania

Edward A. Levine, MD
Professor of Surgery
Surgery
Wake Forest University
Winston-Salem, North Carolina

Elizabeth J. Lilley, MD, MPH
Associate Surgeon
Department of Surgery, Division of Surgical Oncology
Brigham and Women's Hospital;
Associate Surgeon
Center for Sarcoma and Bone Oncology, Center for Melanoma
    Oncology
Affiliate Faculty
Department of Supportive Oncology
Dana-Farber Cancer Institute;
Assistant Professor
Department of Surgery
Harvard Medical School
Boston, Massachusetts

Ines C. Lin, MD, MSEd, FACS
Associate Professor
Surgery (Plastic Surgery); Orthopaedic Surgery (Secondary)
Program Director, Hand Surgery Fellowship
Orthopaedic Surgery
University of Pennsylvania
Philadelphia, Pennsylvania

Brenessa Lindeman, MD, MEHP
Associate Professor
Surgery
University of Alabama at Birmingham
Birmingham, Alabama

David C. Linehan, MD
CEO
University of Rochester Medical Center
Dean
School of Medicine and Dentistry
Senior Vice President
Health Sciences
University of Rochester
Rochester, New York

David Liska, MD, FACS, FASCRS
Chair
Colorectal Surgery, Digestive Disease Institute
Cleveland Clinic;
Associate Professor
Surgery
Cleveland Clinic Lerner College of Medicine at Case Western Reserve
    University
Cleveland, Ohio

Chengyang Liu, MD
Perelman School of Medicine
University of Pennsylvania
Philadelphia, Pennsylvania

Mengyuan Liu, MD
Assistant Attending
Department of Surgery
Memorial Sloan Kettering Cancer Center
New York, New York

Olle Ljungqvist, MD PhD
Professor Emeritus Surgery
Department of Surgery
School of Medical Sciences
Örebro University
Örebro, Sweden;
Professor Emeritus Surgery, Metabolism, and Nutrition
Molecular Medicine and Surgery
Karolinska Institutet
Stockholm, Sweden

Jayme E. Locke, MD, MPH
Vice President of Medical Development for Xenotransplantation
United Therapeutics
Adjunct Professor of Surgery
NYU Langone Health
New York, New York

Sarah Loh, MS, MD
Physician
Vascular Surgery
Yale New Haven Hospital
New Haven, Connecticut

David J. Lourié, MD, FACS
Director
Minimally Invasive Surgery
Huntington Hospital
Pasadena, California

Lea Lowenfeld, MD
Assistant Professor
Department of Surgery
Weill Cornell Medicine - New York Presbyterian Hospital
New York, New York

Richard Lu, MD, FACS
Associate Professor
Department of Surgery
University of Texas Medical Branch
Galveston, Texas

Heather G. Lyu, MD, MBI
Assistant Professor
Surgical Oncology
University of Texas MD Anderson Cancer Center
Houston, Texas

Michael M. Madani, MD
Professor and Chief
Cardiovascular and Thoracic Surgery
UC San Diego School of Medicine
La Jolla, California

David A. "Sasha" Mahvi, MD
Assistant Professor of Surgery
Beth Israel Deaconess Medical Center
Boston, Massachusetts

David M. Mahvi, MD
Distinguished University Professor, Department of Surgery
Medical University of South Carolina
Charleston, South Carolina

Amelia W. Maiga, MD, MPH
Assistant Professor of Surgery
Department of Surgery
Vanderbilt University Medical Center
Nashville, Tennessee

Mahmoud B. Malas, MD, MHS, RPVI, FACS
Professor of Surgery
Chief, Division of Vascular and Endovascular Surgery
Vice Chair of Surgery for Research
University of California San Diego
La Jolla, California;
Professor of Epidemiology
Johns Hopkins Bloomberg School of Public Health
Baltimore, Maryland

Flavio Malcher, MD, MSc
System Chief
Abdominal Core Health
Northwell Health
New York, New York;
Associate Professor
Donald and Barbara Zucker School of Medicine at Hofstra/Northwell
Hempstead, New York

James F. Markmann, MD, PhD
Vice President, Penn Transplant Institute
Vice Chair Transplant, Department of Surgery
William Maul Measey Professor in Surgical Research
University of Pennsylvania School of Medicine
Philadelphia, Pennsylvania;
Claude E. Welch Professor Emeritus
Harvard Medical School
Boston, Massachusetts

Colin Martin, MD
Professor of Surgery
Department of Surgery
Washington University in St. Louis
St. Louis, Missouri

Niels Douglas Martin, MD
Associate Professor
Department of Surgery
University of Pennsylvania
Philadelphia, Pennsylvania

Meredith C. Mason, MD
Assistant Professor
Department of Surgery
Emory University School of Medicine
Atlanta, Georgia

Sergio Mazzola Poli de Figueredo, MD
Assistant Professor
Department of Surgery
The University of North Carolina at Chapel Hill
Chapel Hill, North Carolina

Katharine L. McGinigle, MD, MPH
Associate Professor
Department of Surgery
The University of North Carolina at Chapel Hill
Chapel Hill, North Carolina

C. Lindsay McKnight, MD, FACS, CNSC
Associate Professor
Surgical Critical Care Fellowship Program Director
General Surgery Residency Associate Program Director
Department of Surgery
University of Tennessee Graduate School of Medicine
Knoxville, Tennessee

Kelly McMasters, MD, PhD
Ben A. Reid, Sr., MD Professor and Chair
The Hiram C. Polk, Jr., MD Department of Surgery
University of Louisville School of Medicine
Louisville, Kentucky

Robert Alexander Meguid, MD, MPH, FACS
Professor of Surgery
Department of Surgery
University of Colorado School of Medicine
Aurora, Colorado

John D. Mellinger, MD, FACS
Vice President
Executive
American Board of Surgery
Philadelphia, Pennsylvania;
Professor Emeritus
Department of Surgery
Southern Illinois University School of Medicine
Springfield, Illinois

Laleh G. Melstrom, MD, MSCI
Associate Professor and Chief of Surgical Oncology
Department of Surgery
City of Hope National Medical Center
Duarte, California

Nipun B. Merchant, MD
Professor of Surgery
Department of Surgery
University of Miami
Associate Director of Translational Research
Sylvester Comprehensive Cancer Center
Miami, Florida

Ryan Merkow, MD, MS
Associate Professor of Surgery
Department of Surgery
University of Chicago
Chicago, Illinois

Carmelo A. Milano, MD
Professor of Surgery
Cardiothoracic Surgery
Duke University Medical Center
Durham, North Carolina

Anna Miller, MD, FACS
Jerome J. Gilden Distinguished Professor and Vice Chair
    of Faculty Affairs
Orthopaedic Surgery
Washington University in St. Louis
St. Louis, Missouri

John Miura, MD
Assistant Professor of Surgery
Department of Surgery
University of Pennsylvania
Philadelphia, Pennsylvania

Jennifer M. Moffett, MD, MS, FACS
Assistant Professor
Department of Surgery
University of Texas Medical Branch
Galveston, Texas

Alicia Mohr, MD, FACS, FCCM
Professor of Surgery
Department of Surgery
University of Florida
Gainesville, Florida

Daniela Molena, MD
Surgical Director of Esophageal Cancer Surgery Program
Thoracic Surgery
Memorial Sloan Kettering Cancer Center
New York, New York

Chioma Moneme, MD, MBA
Resident
Department of Surgery
University of Virginia
Charlottesville, North Carolina

Jadie Yoonjoo Moon, BA
PhD Candidate
Graduate Program in Immunology
University of Michigan
Ann Arbor, Michigan

Marc R. Moon, MD
Denton A. Cooley, MD Chair in Cardiac Surgery
Division of Cardiothoracic Surgery
Michael E. DeBakey Department of Surgery
Baylor College of Medicine
Houston, Texas

Dimitrios Moris, MD, MSc, PhD
Surgeon
Department of Surgery
Duke University
Durham, North Carolina

David John Morrell, MD
Staff Surgeon
Surgery
Intermountain Health;
Adjunct Assistant Professor
Department of Surgery
University of Utah School of Medicine
Salt Lake City, Utah

Blake E. Murphy, MD
Vascular Surgical Resident
Division of Vascular Surgery
University of Washington
Seattle, Washington

Gary W. Nace, MD
Associate Professor
Division of Pediatric General, Thoracic, and Fetal Surgery
Children's Hospital of Philadelphia
Philadelphia, Pennsylvania

Bindi Naik-Mathuria, MD, MPH
Professor of Pediatric Surgery
Department of Surgery
University of Texas Medical Branch
Galveston, Texas

Ali Naji, MD, PhD
Professor of Surgery
Department of Surgery
University of Pennsylvania
Philadelphia, Pennsylvania

Tsukasa Nakamura, MD, PhD
Assistant Professor
Division of Transplant Surgery
the University of Arkansas for Medical Sciences
Little Rock, Arkansas

Michael L. Nance, MD
Chief, Division of Pediatric General, Thoracic, and Fetal Surgery
Department of Surgery
Children's Hospital of Philadelphia;
John M. Templeton Professor
Department of Surgery
Perelman School of Medicine at the University of Pennsylvania
Philadelphia, Pennsylvania

Matthew A. Nehs, MD
Associate Professor of Surgery
Department of Surgery
Brigham and Women's Hospital/Harvard Medical School
Boston, Massachusetts

Gregg Nelson, MD, PhD, FRCSC
Professor
Oncology
University of Calgary
Calgary, Alberta, Canada

Tim Nelson, MD
Chair
Department of Surgery
University of Oklahoma School of Community Medicine
Tulsa, Oklahoma

Hiroko Nemoto, MD, PhD
Visiting Scholar
Cardiovascular and Thoracic Surgery
University of California San Diego
La Jolla, California;
Scholar
Surgery
Yokohama City University
Yokohama, Japan

Yuri Novitsky, MD
Professor of Surgery
Department of Surgery
Columbia University Medical Center
New York, New York

Devin O'Brien Coon, MD, MSE
Associate Professor
Surgery
Harvard Medical School/Mass General Brigham
Boston, Massachusetts

Neil O'Kelly, MD
Microsurgery Fellow
Plastic Surgery
Johns Hopkins
Baltimore, Maryland

Kathleen O'Neill, MD, MSTR
Assistant Professor
Obstetrics and Gynecology
University of Pennsylvania
Philadelphia, Pennsylvania

Mitchel R. Obey, MD
Assistant Professor
Orthopaedic Surgery
Washington University in St. Louis
St. Louis, Missouri

Jon S. Odorico, MD
Professor of Surgery
Department of Surgery, Division of Transplantation
University of Wisconsin-Madison School of Medicine and Public Health;
Director, Pancreas and Islet Transplantation
Director, UW Islet Core
Surgery
University of Wisconsin Health Transplant Center
Madison, Wisconsin

John A. Olson, Jr., MD, PhD
William K. Bixby Professor and Chairman
Department of Surgery
Washington University School of Medicine;
Surgeon-in-Chief
Barnes-Jewish Hospital
St. Louis, Missouri

Franklin Olumba, MD, MPHS
Research Fellow
Department of Surgery
Washington University School of Medicine
St. Louis, Missouri

Philip Omotosho, MD
Jack Fraser Smith Professor of Surgery
Chief, Division of Minimally Invasive and Bariatric Surgery
Vice Chair, Quality and Clinical Effectiveness
Department of Surgery
Rush University
Chicago, Illinois

Mark W. Onaitis, MD
Professor of Surgery
Department of Surgery
University of California San Diego
San Diego, California

Theodore N. Pappas, MD
Professor
Department of Surgery
Duke University
Durham, North Carolina

Chetan Pasrija, MD
Johns Hopkins Hospital
Baltimore, Maryland

Hiren V. Patel, MD, PhD
Assistant Professor
Department of Urology
The Ohio State University Wexner Medical Center
Columbus, Ohio

Mayur B. Patel, MD, MPH
Chief and Professor
Division of Acute Care Surgery, Vanderbilt Department of Surgery, Section of Surgical Sciences
Vanderbilt University Medical Center
Nashville, Tennessee

Rohini Patel, MD, MPH
Resident Physician
Department of Surgery
University of California San Diego
La Jolla, California

Shalin S. Patel, MD
Assistant Professor
Orthopaedic Oncology
University of Texas MD Anderson Cancer Center
Houston, Texas

Marco G. Patti, MD
Professor
Department of Surgery
University of Virginia
Charlottesville, Virginia

Alexander Perez, MD, MSHCT, FACS
Professor of Surgery
Assistant Dean, Vice Chair, and Director for Surgical Simulation
Micheal E. DeBakey Department of Surgery
Baylor College of Medicine
Houston, Texas

Ashley A. Peters, MD, MS
Resident Physician
Department of Surgery
Loyola University Medical Center
Maywood, Illinois

Linda G. Phillips, MD, FACS
Truman G. Blocker Distinguished Professor
Chief, Division of Plastic Surgery
Department of Surgery
University of Texas Medical Branch
Galveston, Texas

Roy Phitayakorn, MD, MHPE, MAMSE, FACS
Vice Chair of Education
General and Endocrine Surgery
Massachusetts General Hospital;
Chair of Surgery Education Committee
Surgery
Harvard Medical School
Boston, Massachusetts

Iraklis I. Pipinos, MD, PhD
Professor
Department of Surgery
University of Nebraska Medical Center;
Chief
Vascular Surgery
VA Nebraska and Western Iowa Medical Center
Omaha, Nebraska

Dina Podolsky, MD
Assistant Professor of Surgery
Department of Surgery
Columbia University Medical Center
New York, New York

Bohdan Pomahac, MD
Chief
Reconstructive and Plastic Surgery
Yale School of Medicine
New Haven, Connecticut

Benjamin K. Poulose, MD, MPH
Robert M. Zollinger Lecrone-Baxter Chair
Department of Surgery
Co-Director, Center for Abdominal Core Health
The Ohio State University Wexner Medical Center
Columbus, Ohio

Alykhan M. Premji, MD
Resident Physician
Department of Surgery
University of California, Los Angeles
Los Angeles, California

Aurora D. Pryor, MD, MBA
J Murray Beardsley Professor and Chair
Department of Surgery
Warren Alpert School of Medicine, Brown University;
Surgeon-in-Chief
Department of Surgery
Brown Health
Providence, Rhode Island

Carla M. Pugh, MD, PhD
Thomas Krummel Professor of Surgery
Department of Surgery
Stanford Medicine
Stanford, California

Milo A. Puhan, MD, PhD
Professor
Epidemiology
University of Zurich;
President
Swiss School of Public Health
Zurich, Switzerland

Gretchen Purcell Jackson, MD, PhD, FACS, FACMI, FAMIA
Associate Professor, Vanderbilt University Medical Center
Vice President, Scientific Medical Officer, Intuitive Surgical
Nashville, Tennessee

Andrea L. Pusic, MD
Chief
Plastic and Reconstructive Surgery
Brigham and Women's Hospital
Boston, Massachusetts

Muhammad Umaid Rabbani, MD, FACS
Assistant Professor
Department of Surgery
University of Alabama at Birmingham
Birmingham, Alabama

Joseph Rabin, MD
Associate Professor
Department of Surgery
University of Maryland School of Medicine
Baltimore, Maryland

Ravi S. Radhakrishnan, MD, MBA
Pediatric Surgeon-in-Chief
Department of Surgery
Program Director, Pediatric Surgery Fellowship
Department of Surgery
Professor (Tenured)
Departments of Surgery and Pediatrics
University of Texas Medical Branch
Galveston, Texas

Vinay Rao, MD, MPH
Assistant Professor
Department of Plastic Surgery
Brown University
Providence, Rhode Island

Chandrajit P. Raut, MD, MSc
Chief, Division of Surgical Oncology
Department of Surgery
Brigham and Women's Hospital;
Surgeon-in-Chief and Chair
Surgery
Surgery Director
Center for Sarcoma and Bone Oncology
Dana-Farber Cancer Institute;
Professor
Surgery
Harvard Medical School
Boston, Massachusetts

Kevin M. Reavis, MD
Foregut and Bariatric Surgeon
Foregut Surgery
The Oregon Clinic;
Medical Director
Foregut Surgery
Providence Portland Medical Center
Portland, Oregon

Richard James Redett, MD
Professor and Chair
Plastic and Reconstructive Surgery
Vice Dean for Clinical Affairs
Johns Hopkins School of Medicine;
Physician-in-Chief
Johns Hopkins Medicine
Baltimore, Maryland

Caroline E. Reinke, MD, MSHP
Clinical Associate Professor
Department of Surgery
Atrium Health, Wake Forest School of Medicine
Charlotte, North Carolina

Benjamin Rejowski, MD
Assistant Professor of Clinical Surgery
Department of Surgery
Southern Illinois University School of Medicine
Springfield, Illinois

Taylor Sohn Riall, MD, PhD
Professor
Department of Surgery
Associate Director
University of Arizona Cancer Center;
Division Chief, Surgical Oncology
Department of Surgery
University of Arizona
Tucson, Arizona

William O. Richards, MD
Professor and Chair
Department of Surgery
University of South Alabama College of Medicine
Mobile, Alabama

Kaitlin Ritter, MD
Assistant Professor of Surgery
Department of Surgery
MetroHealth Medical Center
Cleveland, Ohio

Christina L. Roland, MD, MS
Associate Professor
Chief, Sarcoma Surgery
Vice Chair, Research
University of Texas MD Anderson Cancer Center
Houston, Texas

Deborah M. Rooney, PhD
Associate Professor
Learning Health Sciences
University of Michigan
Ann Arbor, Michigan

Claire Rosen, MD, MSME
Resident Physician in General Surgery
Department of Surgery
Hospital of the University of Pennsylvania
Philadelphia, Pennsylvania

Michael Rosen, MD
Professor of Surgery
Chief, Division of Gastrointestinal Surgery
Northwestern University
Chicago, Illinois

Todd Kenneth Rosengart, MD
Professor and Chairman
Michael E. DeBakey Department of Surgery
Vice President for Hospital Operations and Quality Improvement
Baylor College of Medicine;
Professor
Texas Heart Institute
Houston, Texas

Joshua Alexandr Roshal, MD
General Surgery Resident
Department of Surgery
Brigham and Women's Hospital
Boston, Massachusetts;
Surgical Simulation and Education Research Fellow
Department of Surgery
University of Texas Medical Branch
Galveston, Texas

Nikki E. Rossetti, MD, MS
Resident Physician
Surgery
Research Fellow
Cardiothoracic Surgery
Washington University School of Medicine
St. Louis, Missouri

Margaret S. Roubaud, MD
Associate Professor
Department of Plastic and Reconstructive Surgery
University of Texas MD Anderson Cancer Center
Houston, Texas

Eva Roy, MD
Resident Physician
Plastic Surgery
Brigham and Women's Hospital
Boston, Massachusetts

Nobhojit Roy, MD, MPH, PhD
Senior Fellow
Surgery
The George Institute for Global Health India
New Delhi, India;
Formerly, Professor and Chief of Surgical Services
Department of Surgery
BARC Hospital
Anushakti Nagar, Mumbai, India;
Technical Officer
Surgery and Anaesthesia (Operative Care)
WHO Headquarters
Geneva, Switzerland

Rachel M. Russo, MD
Assistant Professor
Department of Surgery
University of California, Davis
Sacramento, California;
Assistant Professor
Surgery
Uniformed Services University of the Health Sciences
Bethesda, Maryland

Reid Sakamoto, MD
Clinical Assistant Professor
Department of Surgery
University of Hawaii John A. Burns School of Medicine
Honolulu, Hawaii

Sabrina E. Sanchez, MD, MPH
Associate Professor
Surgery
Boston Medical Center/Boston University Chobanian and Avedisian
    School of Medicine
Boston, Massachusetts

Uriel Sanchez-Rangel, MD
Resident Physician
Division of Plastic and Reconstructive Surgery
Brigham and Women's Hospital
Boston, Massachusetts

Warren Sandberg, MD, PhD
Professor and Chair
Department of Anesthesiology
Chief of Staff, Vanderbilt University Hospital
Vanderbilt University Medical Center
Nashville, Tennessee

Candice A.M. Sauder, MD, MEd
Associate Professor
Department of Surgery
Division of Surgical Oncology
University of California, Davis
Sacramento, California

John E. Scarborough, MD
Associate Professor
Department of Surgery
University of Wisconsin School of Medicine and Public Health
Madison, Wisconsin

August B. Schaeffer, MD
Resident in General Surgery
Department of Surgery
University of Texas Medical Branch
Galveston, Texas

Martin Allan Schreiber, MD
Professor of Surgery and Chief, Division of Trauma, Critical Care and
    Acute Care Surgery
Department of Surgery
Oregon Health & Science University
Portland, Oregon

Paul Schroder, MD, PhD
Clinical Instructor
Department of Surgery
University of Wisconsin School of Medicine and Public Health
Madison, Wisconsin

Richard D. Schulick, MD, MBA, FACS
Professor and Chair
Department of Surgery
University of Colorado School of Medicine
Director
University of Colorado Cancer Center
University of Colorado School of Medicine
Aurora, Colorado

Daniel Joseph Scott, MD
Professor of Surgery and Assistant Dean of Simulation
Department of Surgery and UT Southwestern Simulation Center
UT Southwestern Medical Center
Dallas, Texas

Sepehr Shabani, MD
Assistant Professor
Otolaryngology-Head and Neck Surgery
City of Hope National Medical Center
Duarte, California

Aakash Shah, MD
Cardiothoracic Resident
Department of Surgery
University of Maryland School of Medicine
Baltimore, Maryland

Ashish Shah, MD
Professor of Cardiac Surgery
Cardiac Surgery
Vanderbilt University Medical Center
Nashville, Tennessee

Paras Shah, MD
Assistant Professor
Department of Urology
Mayo Clinic
Rochester, Minnesota

Shimul A. Shah, MD, MHCM
Physician
Department of Surgery
University of Cincinnati Medical Center
Cincinnati, Ohio

Vidit Sharma, MD, MS
Assistant Professor
Department of Urology
Mayo Clinic
Rochester, Minnesota

Scott K. Sherman, MD
Clinical Assistant Professor
Department of Surgery
University of Iowa Carver College of Medicine;
Staff Surgeon
Surgery
Iowa City VA Medical Center
Iowa City, Iowa

Christine L. Shokrzadeh, MD, FACS
Assistant Professor
Department of Surgery
University of Texas Medical Branch
Galveston, Texas

Jason K. Sicklick, MD, FACS
Professor
Departments of Surgery and Pharmacology
University of California San Diego Health
San Diego, California

Nicholas J. Skertich, MD
Department of Surgery
Rush University Medical Center
Chicago, Illinois

Jeffrey M. Smith, MD, PCC
Orthopaedic Traumatologist
President
Orthopaedic Trauma and Fracture Specialists;
CEO
SurgeonMasters LLC
San Diego, California

Sawyer G. Smith, MD, MBA
Assistant Professor
Department of Surgery
University of California, Davis
Sacramento, California

Andrew Sobel, MD
Assistant Professor of Clinical Orthopaedic Surgery
Department of Orthopaedic Surgery
University of Pennsylvania
Philadelphia, Pennsylvania

Sabina M. Sorondo, MD
Vascular Surgery Resident
Division of Vascular Surgery
Post-Doctorate Fellow
Stanford Cardiovascular Institute
Stanford University
Palo Alto, California

Julie Ann Sosa, MD, MA, FACS, FSSO
Leon Goldman, MD Distinguished Professor and Chair
Department of Surgery
Professor
Department of Medicine
Affiliated Faculty
Philip R. Lee Institute for Health Policy Studies
University of California, San Francisco
San Francisco, California

Jason Sperry, MD, MPH
Professor
Trauma and General Surgery Section Chief
Andrew B. Peitzman Professor of Surgery
Department of Surgery
University of Pittsburgh
Pittsburgh, Pennsylvania

Maie St. John, MD, PhD
Professor and Chair
Head and Neck Surgery
David Geffen School of Medicine at UCLA
Los Angeles, California

Benjamin W. Starnes, MD
Chief, Vascular Surgery Division
Department of Surgery
University of Washington
Seattle, Washington

Deborah M. Stein, MD, MPH
Professor of Surgery
R Adams Cowley Shock Trauma Center
University of Maryland School of Medicine
Baltimore, Maryland

Melissa Stewart, MD, FACS
Assistant Professor
Department of Surgery
The University of Texas Health Science Center at Houston
Houston, Texas

David H. Stone, MD
Professor of Surgery
Section of Vascular Surgery
Dartmouth-Hitchcock Medical Center
Lebanon, New Hampshire

Michael Stoner, MD
Chief, Division of Vascular Surgery
Vascular Surgery
University of Rochester
Rochester, New York

Erin Alyse Strong, MD, MBA, MPH
Clinical Fellow
Surgical Oncology
Moffitt Cancer Center
Tampa, Florida

Vivian E. Strong, MD
Attending Surgeon/Professor of Surgery
Department of Surgery
Memorial Sloan Kettering Cancer Center;
Professor of Surgery
Department of Surgery
Weill Medical College of Cornell University
New York, New York

Christina M. Stuart, MD
Physician
Department of Surgery
Division of Cardiothoracic Surgery
University of Colorado Anschutz Medical Campus
Aurora, Colorado

Debra Sudan, MD
Professor of Surgery
Department of Surgery
Duke University Medical Center
Durham, North Carolina

John P. Sutyak, MD, EdM, MAMSE
Emeritus Professor
Department of Surgery
Southern Illinois University School of Medicine
Springfield, Illinois;
Chair ATLS
Committee on Trauma
American College of Surgeons
Chicago, Illinois

Luciano Guilherme Tastaldi, MD
Clinical Associate
Center for Abdominal Core Health, Digestive Disease and Surgery
    Institute
Cleveland Clinic Foundation
Cleveland, Ohio

Erin M. Taylor, MD
Associate Surgeon
Department of Surgery
Division of Plastic Surgery
Brigham and Women's Hospital/Harvard Medical School
Boston, Massachusetts

Pedro G. Teixeira, MD
Professor
Division Chief, Vascular Surgery
Cardiovascular and Thoracic Surgery
University of Texas at Austin
Austin, Texas

Jonathan Robert Thompson, MD, RPVI, FACS
Associate Professor of Surgery
Department of Surgery
University of Nebraska Medical Center
Omaha, Nebraska

Steven Tohmasi, MD, MPHS
General Surgery Resident
Department of Surgery
Washington University School of Medicine
St. Louis, Missouri

Betty Caroline Tong, MD, MHS
Associate Professor
Division of Cardiovascular and Thoracic Surgery
Duke University Medical Center
Durham, North Carolina

Alfonso Torquati, MD, MSCI
Helen Shedd Keith Professor and Chairman
Department of Surgery
Rush University
Chicago, Illinois

Grant B. Torres, MS
Predoctoral Research Fellow
Plastic Surgery
University of Texas Medical Branch
Galveston, Texas

Douglas Tran, MD
Cardiothoracic Surgery Resident
Cardiac Surgery
University of Maryland
Baltimore, Maryland

Susan Tsai, MD, MHS
Professor
Department of Surgery
Ohio State University
Columbus, Ohio

Allan Tsung, MD
Chair
Department of Surgery
University of Virginia
Charlottesville, Virginia

Ayaka Tsutsumi, MD
Research Affiliate
Colon and Rectal Surgery
Yale University
New Haven, Connecticut

Michael Turturro, MD
Physician
Department of Surgery
Columbia University Medical Center
New York, New York

Douglas S. Tyler, MD, MSHCT
Professor of Surgery
Associate Chair of Community Operations and Strategy
Department of Surgery
The University of North Carolina at Chapel Hill
Chapel Hill, North Carolina

Rindi Uhlich, MD, MSPH
Medical Director, TICU
Surgery
Chippenham Hospital
Richmond, Virginia

Timothy Ullmann, MD
Assistant Professor
Surgery
Albany Medical College
Albany, New York

Raj Vaghjiani, MD
Assistant Professor of Surgery
Surgical Oncology
University of Texas Medical Branch
Galveston, Texas

Konstantinos Votanopoulos, MD, PhD
Associate Professor
Surgery
Wake Forest University
Winston Salem, North Carolina

Heather Wachtel, MD
Associate Professor
Department of Surgery
University of Pennsylvania
Philadelphia, Pennsylvania

John Patrick Walker, MD
Professor
Department of Surgery
University of Texas Medical Branch
Galveston, Texas

Claire Watkins, MD, MS
Clinical Assistant Professor
Cardiothoracic Surgery
Stanford University
Stanford, California

Ronald J. Weigel, MD, PhD, MBA
EA Crowell Jr. Professor and Chair
Department of Surgery
University of Iowa
Iowa City, Iowa;
Medical Director
Cancer Programs
American College of Surgeons
Chicago, Illinois

Roi Weiser, MD
Assistant Professor
Department of Surgical Oncology
Assistant Professor
Department of Breast Surgical Oncology
University of Texas MD Anderson Cancer Center
Houston, Texas

Andrew Well, MD, MPH, MSHCT
Assistant Professor
Surgery and Perioperative Care
Dell Medical School at The University of Texas at Austin;
Assistant Director for Health Transformation and Patient Experience
Texas Center for Pediatric and Congenital Heart Disease;
Faculty
Value Institute for Health and Care
McCombs School of Business and Dell Medical School at The
     University of Texas at Austin
Austin, Texas

Lindsay Welton, MD
Resident Physician
Department of Surgery
University of Minnesota
Minneapolis, Minnesota

Steven D. Wexner, MD, PhD (Hon), FACS, FRCS(Eng), FRCS(ED), FRCSI(Hon), Hon FRCS(Glasg)
Emeritus Chair
Colorectal Surgery
Director
Ellen Leifer Shulman and Steven Shulman Digestive Disease Center
Cleveland Clinic Florida
Weston, Florida;
Clinical Affiliate Professor
Division of Surgery
Charles E. Schmidt College of Medicine, Florida Atlantic University
Boca Raton, Florida;
Clinical Professor
Herbert Wertheim College of Medicine, Florida International University
Miami, Florida

Rebekah R. White, MD, FACS
Professor
Department of Surgery
University of California San Diego
San Diego, California

Brandt Whitehurst, MD, MS
Clinical Assistant Professor of Surgery
Department of Surgery
Southern Illinois University School of Medicine
Springfield, Illinois

Jenna N. Whitrock, MD, MS
Resident Physician
Surgery
University of Cincinnati
Cincinnati, Ohio

Elizabeth C. Wick, MD
Professor
Division of Surgical Oncology
University of California, San Francisco
San Francisco, California

Stephen Bentley Williams, MD, MBA, MS, FACS, FACHE
Associate Chief Medical Officer, Medical Director for
    High Value Care, Professor and Chief of Urology
Department of Surgery
University of Texas Medical Branch
Galveston, Texas

Joshua Winer, MD
Associate Professor
Department of Surgery
Division of Surgical Oncology
Emory University;
Director of Surgical Clerkship
Emory University School of Medicine
Atlanta, Georgia

Steven Eric Wolf, MD
Professor and Vice Chair, Strategic Planning
Department of Surgery
University of Texas Medical Branch
League City, Texas;
Division Chief - Trauma, Burns, and Acute Care Surgery
Department of Surgery
University of Texas Medical Branch
Galveston, Texas

Karen Woo, MD, PhD
Professor of Surgery
Department of Surgery
Division of Vascular Surgery
David Geffen School of Medicine at UCLA;
Professor
Department of Health Policy and Management
UCLA Fielding School of Public Health
Los Angeles, California

Y. Joseph Woo, MD
Norman E. Shumway Professor and Chair
Department of Cardiothoracic Surgery
Professor of Bioengineering (By Courtesy)
Stanford University
Stanford, California

Sara Wood, MD, MHPE
Associate Professor and Division Chief, Urogynecology and
    Reconstructive Pelvic Surgery
Department of Obstetrics and Gynecology
Washington University in St. Louis
St. Louis, Missouri

James C. Yang, MD
Senior Investigator
Surgery Branch
National Cancer Institute
Bethesda, Maryland

Sam Sunghyun Yoon, MD
Chief, Division of Surgical Oncology
Department of Surgery
Columbia University Irving Medical Center
New York, New York

Iyan Younus, MD
Resident
Neurological Surgery
Vanderbilt University Medical Center
Nashville, Tennessee

Alice Yu, MD
Resident Physician
Otolaryngology - Head and Neck Surgery
University of California, Los Angeles
Los Angeles, California

Tanya Liv Zakrison, MD, MPH, FRCSC, FACS
Professor of Surgery
Department of Surgery
Section of Trauma and Acute Care Surgery
University of Chicago
Chicago, Illinois

Victor M. Zaydfudim, MD, MPH
Associate Professor of Surgery
Department of Surgery
University of Virginia
Charlottesville, Virginia

Herbert Zeh, MD
Professor and Chair of Surgery
Department of Surgery
UT Southwestern Medical Center
Dallas, Texas

Jennifer Zhang, MD
Breast Surgeon
Department of Surgery
University of Pennsylvania
Philadelphia, Pennsylvania

Feibi Zheng, MD, MBA
Assistant Professor of Surgery
Michael E. DeBakey Department of Surgery
Baylor College of Medicine
Houston, Texas

David Zonies, MD, MBA, MPH
Professor of Surgery
Department of Surgery
University of Washington;
Chief Medical Officer
Harborview Medical Center
Seattle, Washington

Scott L. Zuckerman, MD, MPH
Assistant Professor
Neurosurgeon
Vanderbilt University Medical Center
Nashville, Tennessee

PREFACE

I am deeply honored to have been appointed as the Editor-in-Chief for the 22nd edition of the *Sabiston Textbook of Surgery.* This textbook has played a pivotal role in my surgical education since my entry into medical school, much like it has for countless surgeons around the globe. When I entered the Duke General Surgery Training program in 1985, Dr. Sabiston had recently completed his work on the 13th edition. During my residency, I had the opportunity to contribute a chapter titled "Surgical Aspects of the Acquired Immunodeficiency Syndrome" to the 14th edition, drawing from my expertise gained during 2 years (1987–1989) in the department's Surgical Virology research lab, where I studied the newly identified human immunodeficiency virus. As I transitioned to a junior faculty position at Duke, I continued my involvement with the textbook by contributing another chapter on the surgical aspects of the acquired immunodeficiency syndrome for the 15th edition.

When the editorship passed from Dr. Sabiston to Dr. Courtney Townsend in 2001, I could not have imagined that I would eventually follow in Dr. Townsend's footsteps as Chairman of the Department of Surgery at the University of Texas Medical Branch (UTMB). Upon my transition to UTMB in 2014, Dr. Townsend had just finalized the 20th edition. While at UTMB, I contributed to the 21st edition by co-authoring a chapter on melanoma and cutaneous malignancies.

As I take on the role of Editor-in-Chief for the 22nd edition, I am excited to guide a text that has significantly influenced my surgical career. In an era characterized by rapidly advancing technologies and swift information dissemination, producing a textbook that remains relevant and current poses a challenge. We have endeavored to uphold the tradition of delivering a core, evidence-based text authored by leading surgical experts. Our approach involved engaging multiple authorities from various institutions to provide diverse perspectives on contentious issues. Additionally, we significantly expanded sections that focus on patient outcomes, including chapters on healthcare disparities, global surgery, quality measurement, competence definition, and surgical simulation.

Recognizing the increasing specialization within the field of surgery, this edition emphasizes the vital role of genetic and genomic information in managing disease processes, evolving from strategies solely based on histologic pathology. Most areas of patient care necessitate a multidisciplinary approach, involving collaboration among surgeons, anesthesiologists, medical specialists, pathologists, and radiologists, which we have highlighted throughout this edition. Furthermore, new technical advancements have introduced innovative methods for performing procedures—whether through open, laparoscopic, robotic, or endovascular techniques—all of which are thoroughly reviewed both individually and in the context of their relevant chapters. We are also collaborating with experts to produce podcasts, allowing readers to glean valuable insights from various chapters. Our objective is to furnish a comprehensive, evidence-based resource that serves not only students and trainees but also established surgeons seeking surgical perspectives on clinical challenges.

Douglas S. Tyler, MD, MSHCT

First published as the *Textbook of Surgery*, edited by Dr. Frederick Christopher, in 1936, the textbook underwent four editions over the next 14 years. In 1956, the textbook was published as *Christopher's Textbook of Surgery*, edited by Dr. Loyal Davis, with three editions under the same title. In 1972, the tenth edition of the textbook was published as the *Davis-Christopher Textbook of Surgery*, edited by Dr. David C. Sabiston, Jr. The tenth edition represented an increase in volume by one-third, expanding from 40 to 57 chapters.[1] New chapters were included in the areas of cardiovascular surgery and transplantation, with more than twice the number of authors from the United States, Canada, England, and Australia. The subtitle of the tenth edition was "The Biologic Basis of Modern Surgical Practice," which stressed the biologic principles underlying surgical practice, with "voluminous" references for each chapter. The focus on biologic principles backed up by extensive references remained a defining feature of the subsequent editions with Dr. Sabiston as editor. A review by Dr. Claude E. Welch of the 11th edition published in 1977 noted that the textbook stressed the scientific basis of modern surgical practice but added, "However, a word to prospective customers is this: buy the two-volume edition if you plan to use it for bedtime reading."[2] Beginning with the 13th edition published in 1986, the textbook became known as the *Sabiston Textbook of Surgery*. In 2001, the 16th edition of the *Sabiston Textbook of Surgery* was published with editor Dr. Courtney M. Townsend and his co-editors Drs. R. Daniel Beauchamp, Kenneth L. Mattox, and B. Mark Evers. They published five subsequent editions of the *Sabiston Textbook of Surgery*, with the 21st edition being published in 2021.

Welcome to the 22nd edition of the *Sabiston Textbook of Surgery*, edited by Dr. Douglas S. Tyler. The 22nd edition continues the tradition of the *Sabiston Textbook of Surgery* being the most comprehensive and authoritative reference for the modern practice of the evolving field of general surgery. The text follows a clear and logical progression of sections that begin by covering Surgical Training and Quality Control and continuing with Perioperative Management, followed by sections on specific disease processes including Trauma and Critical Care, Transplantation and Immunology, Surgical Oncology, Endocrine Disorders, Abdominal Wall Hernias, Alimentary Tract, Vascular Surgery, Cardiothoracic Surgery, and ending with a section on Specialties in Surgery: Subspecialty Considerations Relevant for the General Surgeon that includes Pediatric Surgery, Maternal-Fetal Surgery, Hand Surgery, Gynecology Surgery, and Urologic Surgery. Authors of each chapter are individuals who are recognized leaders in their specialty in surgery and who have made seminal contributions to advance the care of surgical patients in their area of expertise. Many new chapters have been added since the last edition, which reflects the rapid evolution and expanding knowledge content in general surgery. Several new chapters related to surgical training, surgical simulation, training in innovative procedures involving minimally invasive techniques, and surgical certification provide important information on the rapidly expanding field of surgical education and maintenance of technical competence. New chapters have been added that address health disparities and focus on access to care and improving equity in surgical care; these include the chapters of "Social Determinants of Health and Their Impact on Surgical Outcomes," "Surgical Quality Improvement Programs," "Patient Reported Outcomes," "Telehealth in Surgery," "Global Surgery," and "Surgical Considerations in the Transgender Patient." Two new chapters have been added that focus on "Surgeon Health and Well-Being" and the rapidly evolving field of Surgeon Health: Ergonomics. Major new updates have been provided in chapters that focus on The evolving role of the microbiome in surgical practice, surgical considerations in palliative care, soft tissue infections, management of urologic trauma, management of pediatric trauma, management of chronic wounds, lung transplantation, GI stromal tumors, peritoneal malignancies and HIPEC, lymphadenopathy, carcinoid tumors, percutaneous heart procedures, and ECMO. Each chapter is beautifully illustrated with figures and intraoperative photographs. The *Sabiston Textbook of Surgery* is a critical reference for medical students and general surgery residents in training, providing key insight and in-depth information for the care of the surgical patient. All of these highly comprehensive chapters include extensive references to support the evidence-based literature that provides the biologic basis for current surgical practice.

The 22nd Edition of *Sabiston's Textbook of Surgery* is available in print and eBook format, providing an enhanced learning experience with text, figures, videos, and references.

Ronald J. Weigel, MD, PhD
EA Crowell Jr. Professor and Chair
Department of Surgery
University of Iowa
Iowa City, Iowa;
Medical Director for Cancer Programs
American College of Surgeons
Chicago, Illinois

REFERENCES

1. Hughes CW. Davis-Christopher Textbook of Surgery. 10th ed. *Arch Intern Med.* 1974;133(1):162-163.
2. Welch CE. Davis-Christopher Textbook of Surgery. 11th ed. *Annals of Surgery.* 1979;190(1):128.

ACKNOWLEDGMENTS

We would like to express our gratitude to Kristine Feeherty, Joanie Milnes, and Jessica McCool for their invaluable editing and administrative support, which have greatly enhanced the quality of this textbook. Additionally, we extend our heartfelt appreciation to all the chapter authors who, despite their demanding schedules, have collaborated with us to impart their knowledge and insights. Lastly, we wish to acknowledge the contributions of Drs. Joshua Rochal and Pat Walker for their role in launching a podcast companion series for this textbook.

CONTENTS

xxxiii

EXPERT INSIGHTS: THE SABISTON PODCAST

PODCAST EDITORS

Douglas Tyler, MD, MSHCT
Professor of Surgery
Associate Chair of Community Operations and Strategy
Department of Surgery
The University of North Carolina at Chapel Hill
Chapel Hill, North Carolina

Joshua A. Roshal, MD
General Surgery Resident
Department of Surgery
Brigham and Women's Hospital
Boston, Massachusetts;
Surgical Simulation and Education Research Fellow
Department of Surgery
University of Texas Medical Branch
Galveston, Texas

J. Patrick Walker, MD, FACS
Professor of Surgery
University of Texas Medical Branch
Galveston, Texas

CONTENTS

To access this title's podcasts, please scan the QR code with a mobile device.

Perioperative Management

The following chapters appear only on Elsevier eBooks+:

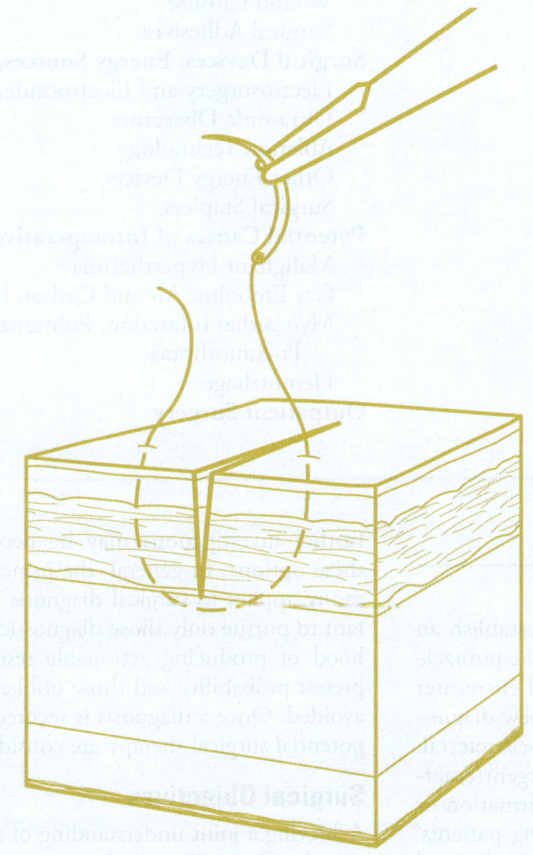

Principles of Preoperative and Operative Surgery

Chioma Moneme, Allan Tsung, Reid B. Adams, and Victor M. Zaydfudim

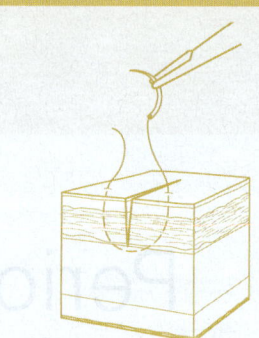

PRINCIPLES OF SURGICAL EVALUATION

Patient-Surgeon Relationship

Clear, precise, and unambiguous communication to establish an understanding of mutual expectations and trust is at the pinnacle of the patient-surgeon relationship. A surgeon's initial encounter with a patient most commonly is in the context of a new diagnosis and is initiated by either a professional referral or self-referral. A history and physical examination, whether in an urgent/emergent or elective setting, should initially focus on confirmation or rebuttal of the suspected diagnosis. Inquiries regarding patients' personal interests and relationships with their community and society help create a common bond between the patient and surgeon. In addition to direct communication with the patient, knowledge of their situation is augmented by a thorough review of relevant diagnostic laboratory and imaging results. Through this process, an experienced surgeon effectively re-creates the clinical context of a patient's situation during the period preceding evaluation for the illness in question.

Further patient management is directed by the differential diagnosis generated during the initial evaluation. If the differential diagnosis contains items of equipoise that require distinct treatments, further investigations may be necessary to distinguish between these options. In general, the principle of Occam's razor or parsimony applies to surgical diagnosis and management; it is important to pursue only those diagnostic studies that have a high likelihood of producing actionable results. Tests with a near-perfect pretest probability and those unlikely to alter treatment should be avoided. Once a diagnosis is secured, the objective and urgency of potential surgical therapy are considered.

Surgical Objectives

Achieving a joint understanding of surgical objectives and expectations between patient and surgeon is paramount to improve patient satisfaction and outcomes. There are three broad potential objectives of surgical intervention: disease prevention, disease control, and symptom palliation. Examples of operations aimed at disease prevention include prophylactic mastectomy, colectomy, pancreatectomy or thyroidectomy for heritable cancer syndromes, endarterectomy for asymptomatic carotid stenosis, or appendectomy in the setting of Ladd's procedure for intestinal malrotation. These operations are aimed at preempting a disease process. Operations for disease control address a process that is ongoing. Examples include resections for malignancy, cholecystectomy for acute cholecystitis, enterolysis for bowel obstruction, bypass for vascular occlusive disease, or knee replacement for arthritis. With these operations, patients may expect partial or complete resolution of the targeted disease process. Finally, palliative operations are aimed at improving quality of life rather than curing a disease. Examples include proximal decompression for malignant bowel obstruction or gastrojejunostomy for unresectable pancreatic cancer with gastric outlet obstruction. Inadequate communication of an operation's objectives precludes informed consent and can have dramatic, negative implications for a patient's perioperative decision-making.

Elective, Urgent, and Emergent Indications

Appropriate triage of surgical therapy is important for patient outcomes and resource distribution. Accurate categorization of surgical urgency also has implications for quality reporting. The American College of Surgeons (ACS) National Surgical Quality Improvement Program (NSQIP) differentiates between emergency and elective operations and reports different levels of accuracy for patient risk estimates, with emergency cases having both superior predictive accuracy for mortality and significantly higher observed-to-expected ratios. Within ACS NSQIP, emergency surgery is characterized by an ongoing acute process that can result in rapid deterioration in a patient's condition, for which unnecessary delay can potentially threaten the clinical outcome. On the other hand, elective operations generally involve a patient who has completed preoperative surgical evaluation during a separate patient-surgeon encounter and is subsequently scheduled for an operation. Inpatients, referrals from the emergency department, and direct transfers from the clinic are excluded from elective patient categorization. Urgent operations are a relatively ill-defined category and have an acuity level in between those of elective and emergent cases. The World Society of Emergency Surgery created the Timing of Acute Care Surgery (TACS) classification in 2013, which subdivides urgent cases into those with an ideal time to surgery falling between immediate and within 48 hours from diagnosis. In 2023, this same group sought to improve the TACS classification and validate the new classification using the Delphi method. The new TACS provides more clarity in the process of classifying patient disease severity and classifies urgent cases into an ideal time to surgery between immediate and within 4 days after diagnosis. Recognition of urgency should be one of the first steps of the preoperative surgical evaluation because it affects subsequent patient decision-making, counseling, investigatory testing, and perioperative management.

Risk Assessment

Perioperative risk assessment has an impact on all aspects of surgical planning, including the decision to operate, choice of operation, perioperative management, and goals-of-care discussions. Communication with patients regarding the risks of a proposed operation must be coupled with a thorough review of patient comorbidities and functional status. Hence, patients with prohibitively high operative risk can be protected from inappropriate operations, whereas those with borderline risk can be medically optimized preoperatively. From the viewpoint of perioperative management, appropriate risk stratification facilitates resource allocation, including intraoperative monitoring, use of intensive care unit services after the operation, and potential use of medical consultation. Finally, transparent categorization of patient risk factors improves institutional reporting and allows for multi-institutional comparisons of risk-adjusted patient outcomes.

Risk assessment begins by considering the nature of the disease and patient comorbidities while weighing the risks of possible surgical interventions. For a number of diagnoses, multiple surgical approaches may be available, each with advantages and disadvantages in terms of the morbidity profile, quality outcomes, and durability of the therapy. These must be weighed carefully in the context of each patient's presenting condition and baseline level of health. The American Society of Anesthesiologists (ASA) physical status (PS) categorization has frequently served as a simple, initial rubric to summarize baseline patient comorbidity. Patient categorization into ASA I–VI (Table 19.1) helps stratify patients as low

TABLE 19.1	American Society of Anesthesiologists Classification of Physical Status (ASA PS)	
ASA PS CLASSIFICATION	**DEFINITION**	**ADULT EXAMPLES, INCLUDING BUT NOT LIMITED TO**
ASA I	A normal healthy patient	Healthy, nonsmoking, no or minimal alcohol use.
ASA II	A patient with mild systemic disease	Mild diseases only without substantive functional limitations. Current smoker, social alcohol drinker, pregnancy, obesity (BMI between 30 and 40), well-controlled DM/HTN, mild lung disease.
ASA III	A patient with severe systemic disease	Substantive functional limitations; one or more moderate to. severe diseases. Poorly controlled DM or HTN, COPD, morbid obesity (BMI >40), active hepatitis, alcohol dependence or abuse, implanted pacemaker, moderate reduction of ejection fraction, ESRD undergoing regularly scheduled dialysis, history (>3 months) of MI, CVA, TIA, or CAD/stents.
ASA IV	A patient with severe systemic disease that is a constant threat to life	Recent (<3 months) MI, CVA, TIA, or CAD/stents; ongoing cardiac ischemia or severe valve dysfunction; severe reduction of ejection fraction; shock; sepsis; DIC; ESRD not undergoing regularly scheduled dialysis.
ASA V	A moribund patient who is not expected to survive without the operation	Ruptured abdominal/thoracic aneurysm, massive trauma, intracranial bleed with mass effect, ischemic bowel in the face of significant cardiac pathology or multiple organ/system dysfunction.
ASA VI	A declared brain-dead patient whose organs are being removed for donor purposes	

The addition of "E" denotes emergency surgery. An emergency is defined as existing when delay in treatment of the patient would lead to a significant increase in the threat to life or body part.

BMI, Body mass index; *CAD,* coronary artery disease; *COPD,* chronic obstructive pulmonary disease; *CVA,* cerebrovascular accident; *DIC,* disseminated intravascular coagulation; *DM,* diabetes mellitus; *ESRD,* end-stage renal disease; *HTN,* hypertension; *MI,* myocardial infarction; *TIA,* transient ischemic attack.

Adapted from https://www.asahq.org/standards-and-practice-parameters/statement-on-asa-physical-status-classification-system.

TABLE 19.2	**Risks of Cardiac Events Depending on the Type of Operation**	
LOW RISK: <1%	**INTERMEDIATE RISK: 1%–5%**	**HIGH RISK: >5%**

• Superficial surgery
• Breast
• Dental
• Endocrine: thyroid
• Eye
• Reconstructive
• Carotid asymptomatic
  (CEA or CAS)
• Gynecology: minor
• Orthopedic: minor (meniscectomy)
• Urologic: minor (transurethral
  resection of the prostate)
	• Intraperitoneal: splenectomy, hiatal hernia
	  repair, cholecystectomy
	• Carotid symptomatic (CEA or CAS)
	• Peripheral arterial angioplasty
	• Endovascular aneurysm repair
	• Head and neck surgery
	• Neurologic or orthopedic: major (hip and
	  spine surgery)
	• Urologic or gynecologic: major
	• Renal transplant
	• Intrathoracic: nonmajor
		• Aortic and major vascular surgery
		• Open lower limb revascularization or amputation
		  or thromboembolectomy
		• Duodenopancreatic surgery
		• Liver resection, bile duct surgery
		• Esophagectomy
		• Repair of perforated bowel
		• Adrenal resection
		• Total cystectomy
		• Pneumonectomy
		• Pulmonary or liver transplant

CAS, Carotid artery stenting; *CEA,* carotid endarterectomy.

Adapted from Kristensen SD, Knuuti J, Saraste A, et al. 2014 ESC/ESA guidelines on non-cardiac surgery: cardiovascular assessment and management. *Eur J Anaesthesiol.* 2014;31:517-573.

risk,[1,2] intermediate risk,[3] high risk,[4,5] and brain dead.[6] The addition of "E" designation signifies emergent operation, hence indicating a higher risk. First introduced in 1941, increasing ASA class was shown in a number of landmark studies to be associated with early postoperative mortality. This relationship remains true in the modern era for both emergent and elective operations, with class VE associated with a nearly 20% likelihood of early postoperative mortality.

Next, operations can be categorized into low-, intermediate-, and high-risk groups. This categorization is most commonly approached through expert opinion and consensus guidelines, such as those proposed by the European Society of Cardiology and European Society of Anesthesiology, which stratifies patients based on estimated 30-day risk of cardiac events (Table 19.2). Combination surgical risk models, including patient comorbidity and operative risk, have been developed using logistic regression, with mortality or major complication as the dependent variable.[5] For very low-risk outpatient procedures, the risk of death is less than 1 in 50,000; conversely, high-risk operations performed for life-threatening conditions in critically ill patients can have expected mortality rates routinely exceeding 20% (Fig. 19.1).

A wide variety of tools can help quantify operative risk in the preoperative setting. These tools can predict risks of broad outcomes, such as death or length of stay, or specific events, such as reoperation, intraoperative blood loss, or specific surgical complications. From a methodology standpoint, these tools can be grouped into categorical scales, risk scores, or prediction models. Categorical scales are easy to calculate and frequently subjective. The most classic example of a categorical scale is the ASA PS classification frequently used in preoperative risk estimation. Surgical risk scores combine several predictors, usually chosen using multivariable predictive modeling, to estimate risk of a specific outcome. An example of a risk score is the Model for End-Stage Liver Disease (MELD) score used to predict short-term prognosis in patients with end-stage liver disease.[6] More recently, the adoption of advanced statistics to analyze large, multi-institutional datasets has created numerous risk prediction models that account for patient-level risk factors to generate estimated likelihoods of multiple surgical outcomes. The most commonly used and cited example of a surgical risk score is the ACS NSQIP Surgical Risk Calculator (SRC).

The ACS NSQIP universal SRC was developed in 2013 using standardized clinical data from more than 500 NSQIP participant hospitals.[7] This online tool predicts adverse postoperative outcomes based on 20 preoperative patient-level characteristics, including demographics and comorbidities (Table 19.3). Risks associated with procedure type are incorporated using Current Procedural Terminology (CPT) codes. Three of the outcomes are associated with specific CPT codes related to vascular procedures, proctectomy, and pancreatectomy. Those outcomes are designated in the calculator with "T." Recalibrated in 2016, the database more accurately predicts outcomes for lowest- to highest-risk patients.[8] It currently contains data from more than 5 million cases across 874 hospitals and is publicly accessible at http://riskcalculator.facs.org. Originally designed to predict 8 postoperative adverse outcomes, the tool has evolved to currently report likelihoods of 18 specific or composite outcomes within 30 days of surgery:
- Serious complication (e.g., cardiac arrest, myocardial infarction [MI], pneumonia)
- Any complication (surgical site infections [SSIs], pulmonary embolus [PE], ventilator >48 hours)
- Pneumonia
- Cardiac complication
- Surgical site infection

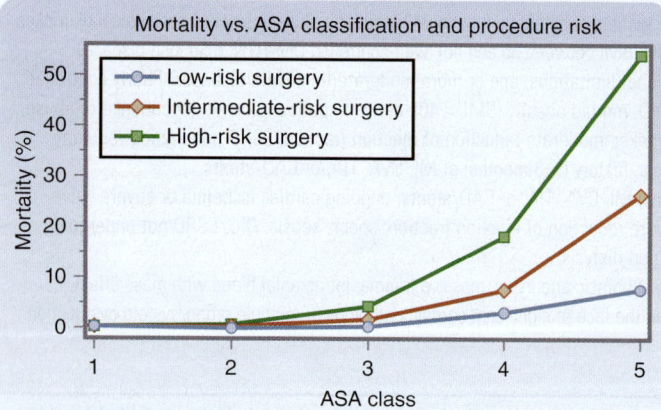

FIGURE 19.1 The observed mortality rate as a function of the American Society of Anesthesiologists *(ASA)* physical status and surgery-specific risk. (Adapted from Glance LG, Lustik SJ, Hannan EL, et al. The surgical mortality probability model: derivation and validation of a simple risk prediction rule for noncardiac surgery. *Ann Surg.* 2012;255:696-702.)

TABLE 19.3 ACS NSQIP Variables Used in the Colon-Specific and the Universal Surgical Risk Calculator

VARIABLE	CATEGORIES	COLON SPECIFIC	UNIVERSAL
Age group, years	<65, 65–74, 75–84, ≥85	✓	✓
Sex	Male, female	✓	✓
Functional status	Independent, partially dependent, totally dependent	✓	✓
Emergency case	Yes, no	✓	✓
ASA class	I or II, III, IV, or V	✓	✓
Steroid use for chronic condition	Yes, no	✓	✓
Ascites within 30 days preoperatively	Yes, no	✓	✓
System sepsis within 48 h preoperatively	None, SIRS, sepsis, septic shock	✓	✓
Ventilator dependent	Yes, no	✓	✓
Disseminated cancer	Yes, no	✓	✓
Diabetes	No, oral, insulin	✓	✓
Hypertension requiring medication	Yes, no	✓	✓
Previous cardiac event	Yes, no	✓	✓
Congestive heart failure in 30 days preoperatively	Yes, no	✓	✓
Dyspnea	Yes, no	✓	✓
Current smoker within 1 year	Yes, no	✓	✓
History of COPD	Yes, no	✓	✓
Dialysis	Yes, no	✓	✓
Acute renal failure	Yes, no	✓	✓
BMI class	Underweight, normal, overweight, severity of obesity: class 1, class 2, severe class 3	✓	✓
Colon surgery group (colectomy)	Partial lap with anastomosis, partial lap with ostomy, partial open with anastomosis, partial open with ostomy, total lap with ostomy, total open with ostomy	✓	
Indication for colon surgery	Diverticulitis, enteritis/colitis, hemorrhage, neoplasm, obstruction/perforation, vascular insufficiency, volvulus, other	✓	
CPT-specific linear risk	2805 values		✓

ACS NSQIP, American College of Surgeons National Surgical Quality Improvement Program; *BMI,* body mass index; *COPD,* chronic obstructive pulmonary disease; *CPT,* Current Procedural Terminology; *lap,* laparotomy; *SIRS,* systemic inflammatory response syndrome.
Adapted from Bilimoria KY, Liu Y, Paruch JL, et al. Development and evaluation of the universal ACS NSQIP surgical risk calculator: a decision aid and informed consent tool for patients and Surgeons. *J Am Coll Surg.* 2013;217:833-842.

- Urinary tract infection
- Venous thromboembolism (VTE)
- Renal failure
- Colon ileus (conditionally displayed based on the selected procedure)
- Colon anastomotic leak (conditionally displayed based on the selected procedure)
- Readmission
- Return to the operating room
- Death
- Discharge to nursing or rehab facility
- Predicted length of hospital stay
- Vascular lower extremity open wound
- Pancreatectomy delayed gastric
- Proctectomy ileus

Levels of discrimination for these outcomes are generally strong, with c-statistics higher than 0.75 for all predicted outcomes. In particular, discrimination for 30-day postoperative mortality is excellent, with c-statistics exceeding 0.9.[8] Recent investigations have evaluated combining ACS NSQIP SRC models with preoperative biologic markers, such as hypoalbuminemia,[9] or with organ-specific metrics, such as chronic liver disease in patients selected for liver resection.[10] The SRC model has also been adapted for the pediatric population. The Pediatric Surgical

Risk Calculator incorporates nearly 200,000 cases across 67 hospitals and accounts for 382 CPT codes; it has demonstrated excellent predictive accuracy for mortality and morbidity after operations in children. The ACS NSQIP SRC is specifically designed to facilitate patient counseling and consent before surgery; as such, it does not take into account intraoperative findings. Despite its excellent calibration within the broad ACS NSQIP dataset, studies have identified lapses in predictive accuracy within smaller homogenous patient populations.[11] Therefore, it cannot replace familiarity with institution- and surgeon-specific performance.

Informed Consent

Surgeons have an ethical obligation to discuss and pursue informed consent with any patient considering an operation. Comprehensive, transparent, and clear communication of perioperative risks and potential benefits is mandatory. A critical component of informed consent is discussing and understanding the patient's goals of care and placing these in context with the benefits and risks of the proposed procedure, thereby ensuring shared decision-making with the patient and their family. To successfully guide the patient through the consent process, a surgeon must possess a thorough technical understanding of the proposed operation, the most probable perioperative course, and potential pitfalls and complications. Clear and precise communication of risks and expectations is paramount; technical jargon should be avoided. The consent process must take into account all of the preceding facets of surgical objectives, urgency, and patient risk assessment. Systematic reviews indicate that common components of a consent discussion should include (1) the disease diagnosis, (2) the proposed procedure, (3) procedure-related risks, (4) likelihood of success of the procedure, (5) mental capacity of the patient, and (6) alternative treatment options.[12] One of the most challenging impediments to informed consent is the knowledge gap between surgeon and patient. To overcome this, consent processes can be augmented for specific diseases and procedures using decision aids, visual materials, specialized written materials, and previously discussed risk calculators. In general, these supplementary instruments have been shown to improve patient knowledge and satisfaction with decision-making.[13]

ASSESSMENT OF GERIATRIC SURGICAL PATIENTS

The population of the United States continues to age. The number of adults over the age of 65 years old is expected to increase from 13% of the total population to a staggering 23% by 2030. Geriatric patients account for more than 40% of hospital days, one-third of all inpatient procedures, and incur nearly half of all inpatient hospital charges. The geriatric population presents unique surgical challenges. Tailoring the preoperative workup to the unique needs of these patients can help surgeons address age-related functional challenges and comorbidities. To ensure that decision-making is appropriately aligned between provider and patient, the patient and their family must clearly understand operative risks, potential effects of surgery-related complications on quality of life, and likely outcomes. Conversely, the surgeon must appreciate, value, and incorporate the patient's personal goals of care in any decision-making process and final assessment.

Comprehensive Geriatric Assessment

Chronologic demarcation of the "geriatric" patient is elusive. A combination of advanced age, comorbidities, and functional and/or cognitive decline contribute to the definition of a geriatric patient. Because of the clinical and social complexities of the geriatric population, an appropriate preoperative evaluation is multifaceted. Collaboration between the ACS NSQIP and the American Geriatrics Society (AGS) produced a set of guidelines for the multidomain assessment of geriatric patients.[14] This approach was not novel; the concept of a comprehensive geriatric assessment (CGA) was first implemented in the 1980s and 1990s in medical inpatient and long-term outpatient settings. Geriatric assessments were shown to improve independent living, physical function, and long-term mortality. Studies reporting the implementation of CGA within surgical populations are rare; a recent systematic review found positive impacts of CGA use on procedural cancellation rate, surgical complications, and length of stay.[15] Importantly, historic data demonstrate that the most effective CGA programs are those that affect direct medical care recommendations. The CGA is composed of medical, mental health, functional capacity, social, and environmental domains. The ACS NSQIP/AGS collaborative framework (Table 19.4) refocuses the CGA toward themes more relevant to operative and perioperative care. Although all aspects of the framework are vital, several are more pertinent within the geriatric population considered for surgery.

Cognitive Impairment and Delirium

Nearly one in five elderly patients have dementia or cognitive impairment. The ACS NSQIP/AGS framework recommends

TABLE 19.4   ACS NSQIP/AGS Collaborative Checklist for Preoperative Assessment of Geriatric Surgical Patient

In addition to conducting a complete history and physical examination of the patient, the following assessments are strongly recommended:

- Assess the patient's **cognitive ability** and **capacity** to understand the anticipated surgery.
- Screen the patient for **depression**.
- Identify the patient's risk factors for developing postoperative **delirium**.
- Screen for **alcohol** and other **substance abuse/dependence**.
- Perform a preoperative **cardiac** evaluation according to the American College of Cardiology/American Heart Association algorithm for patients undergoing noncardiac surgery.
- Identify the patient's risk factors for postoperative **pulmonary** complications and implement appropriate strategies for prevention.
- Document **functional status** and history of **falls**.
- Determine baseline **frailty** score.
- Assess patient's **nutritional status** and consider preoperative interventions if the patient is at severe nutritional risk.
- Take an accurate and detailed **medication history** and consider appropriate perioperative adjustments. Monitor for **polypharmacy**.
- Determine the patient's **treatment goals** and **expectations** in the context of the possible treatment outcomes.
- Determine patient's **family** and **social support system**.
- Order appropriate preoperative **diagnostic tests** focused on elderly patients.

ACS, American College of Surgeons; AGS, American Geriatrics Society; NSQIP, National Surgical Quality Improvement Program. Adapted from Chow WB, Rosenthal RA, Merkow RP, et al. Optimal preoperative assessment of the geriatric surgical patient: a best practice guideline from the American College of Surgeons National Surgical Quality Improvement Program and the American Geriatrics Society. J Am Coll Surg. 2012;215:453-466.

routine neurocognitive assessment for these patients in the preoperative setting. Specifically, the guidelines recommend cognitive evaluation for any geriatric patient without a preexisting diagnosis of cognitive impairment. Methods include cognitive assessments such as the Mini-Cog (Fig. 19.2) and/or interviews with the patient's support structure (spouse or family) or affiliated healthcare providers.[16] The Mini-Cog's advantages include the large body of evidence supporting its usefulness, ease of implementation (3 minutes to complete), and focus on attention and executive function. Any findings suggestive of cognitive impairment should prompt referral to a primary care, mental health, or geriatric specialist. Establishing cognitive impairment early in the preoperative setting has direct implications for patient-physician communication, decision-making capacity, and informed consent.

In the postoperative setting, cognitive impairment strongly predicts delirium, which has an incidence of nearly 50% among geriatric patients. Documentation of preexisting cognitive impairment improves interpretation of perioperative mental status and encourages avoidance of medications that may precipitate delirium. In the geriatric population, postoperative delirium has a profound impact on hospital length of stay, long-term postoperative cognition, cost of care, and mortality.[17] Because evidence-based treatments for delirium are few, the majority of studies focus on the identification of risk factors and prevention. The AGS best practice guidelines for delirium recommend preoperative risk

Table 2. Cognitive Assessment with the Mini-Cog: 3 Item Recall and Clock Draw[9]

1. GET THE PATIENT'S ATTENTION, THEN SAY: "I am going to say three words that I want you to remember now and later. The words are: *banana, sunrise, chair.* Please say them for me now." Give the patient 3 tries to repeat the words. If unable after 3 tries, go to next item.
2. SAY ALL THE FOLLOWING PHRASES IN THE ORDER INDICATED: "Please draw a clock in the space below. Start by drawing a large circle. Put all the numbers in the circle and set the hands to show 11:10 (10 past 11)." If subject has not finished clock drawing in 3 minutes, discontinue and ask for recall items.
3. SAY: "What were the three words I asked you to remember?"

A

Table 3. Interpretation of the Mini-Cog[9]

SCORING: 3 item recall (0 to 3 points): Clock draw (0 or 2 points):	1 point for each correct word 0 points for abnormal clock 2 points for normal clock

A NORMAL CLOCK HAS ALL OF THE FOLLOWING ELEMENTS: All numbers 1 to 12, each only once, are present in the correct order and direction (clockwise) inside the circle. Two hands are present, one pointing to 11 and one pointing to 2.
ANY CLOCK MISSING ANY OF THESE ELEMENTS IS SCORED ABNORMAL. REFUSAL TO DRAW A CLOCK IS SCORED ABNORMAL.
Total score of 0, 1, or 2 suggests possible impairment. Total score of 3, 4, or 5 suggests no impairment.

B

FIGURE 19.2 (A–B) Cognitive assessment with the Mini-Cog and Interpretation of the Mini-Cog. (Adapted from Chow WB, Rosenthal RA, Merkow RP, et al. Optimal preoperative assessment of the geriatric surgical patient: a best practice guideline from the American College of Surgeons National Surgical Quality Improvement Program and the American Geriatrics Society. *J Am Coll Surg.* 2012;215:453-466. *Copyright from S Borson included in JACS publication.*)

factor screening for all geriatric surgical patients[18] (Table 19.5). Identification of these risk factors should raise awareness to avoid second-hit insults (such as high-risk medication administration and sleep cycle disturbance) and to implement simple measures that improve the patient's orientation. Such measures include holding high-risk medications preoperatively, providing hearing aids, encouraging sleep hygiene with preservation of day/night cycle, and employing the help of the patient's family for reorientation during postoperative in-hospital recovery.

Depression

Increased comorbidity and medical burden, conditions highly prevalent in the geriatric population, can exacerbate depressive symptoms. Additional risk factors include female sex, prior diagnosis of depression, sleep disturbance, low functional status, disability, and living alone.[19] Elderly patients with preoperative depressive symptoms can experience postoperative delirium at a significantly higher rate and for a longer duration. Depression also may lower the threshold for pain and is a predictor of chronic postoperative pain. In the intensive care setting, depression is associated with increased mortality and reduced quality of life after

TABLE 19.5 Risk Factors for Postoperative Delirium
Age greater than 65 years
Cognitive impairment
Severe illness or comorbidity burden
Hearing or vision impairment
Current hip fracture
Presence of infection
Inadequately controlled pain
Depression
Alcohol use
Sleep deprivation or disturbance
Renal insufficiency
Anemia
Hypoxia or hypercarbia
Poor nutrition
Dehydration
Electrolyte abnormalities (hypernatremia or hyponatremia)
Poor functional status
Immobilization or limited mobility
Polypharmacy and use of psychotropic medications (benzodiazepines, anticholinergics, antihistamines, antipsychotics)
Risk of urinary retention or constipation
Presence of urinary catheter
Aortic procedures

Adapted from American Geriatrics Society Expert Panel on Postoperative Delirium in Older Adults. Postoperative delirium in older adults: best practice statement from the American Geriatrics Society. *J Am Coll Surg.* 2015;220:136-148.

discharge. After cardiac surgery, depression and anxiety may increase the likelihood of coronary disease recurrence and mortality after coronary artery bypass graft (CABG). The ACS NSQIP/AGS guidelines recommend the Patient Health Questionnaire-2 (PHQ-2) as a pragmatic preoperative screening tool for elderly patients; positive findings should be followed by appropriate referral. Optimal management of depression requires a multidisciplinary approach frequently involving both psychiatric medications and cognitive behavioral therapy.

Medication Management

The ACS NSQIP/AGS framework emphasizes the importance of obtaining a comprehensive medication history for all older patients, including over-the-counter medications, eye drops, vitamins, and herbal products. Adverse drug reactions, inappropriate dosing, and polypharmacy can be avoided by considering potential changes in drug metabolism and clearance in the perioperative setting.

The American College of Cardiology (ACC) and American Heart Association (AHA) guidelines for perioperative β-blockade supports the continued administration of β-blockers for patients already on this medication. Patients undergoing intermediate-risk surgery with known coronary artery disease or risk factors for ischemic heart disease may be candidates for perioperative β-blockade. If initiation of β-blockers is indicated in the preoperative setting, treatment ideally should start weeks before elective surgery and should be titrated to a target heart rate of 60 to 80 beats/minute. Adverse effects of β-blocker initiation too close to the time of surgery include the risk of stroke, hypotension, and death. For patients with limited cardiac risk factors, rapid initiation of β-blockers in the acute preoperative setting is not indicated.

The AGS Beers Criteria for Potentially Inappropriate Medication Use is particularly relevant to elderly patients at risk for polypharmacy. The latest guidelines (updated in 2015) serve as a reference to check for medications with high-risk adverse effect profiles, common drug-drug interactions, impaired renal and/or hepatic clearance, perioperative sedation, and a predisposition to delirium.[20] Some of the medications, such as benzodiazepines, are categorically contraindicated because they have been demonstrated to increase risk of cognitive impairment, delirium, falls, and other adverse outcomes in older adults.

Functional Status and Frailty

Elderly patients can be impaired in their performance of tasks necessary for independent living. These functional limitations are associated with perioperative complications, failure to rescue, increased length of stay, discharge to facilities other than home, and increased postoperative mortality even after procedures considered to be minor.[21,22] The association between functional dependence and postoperative mortality is present in patients over 60 but is magnified in patients over 80.[23] A simple way to obtain a broad sense of functional dependence is to inquire about a history of falls or to use the widely recognized and validated operational definition based on patient shrinkage, weakness, exhaustion, low physical activity, and walking slowness. More detailed instruments for scoring functional status include the Activities of Daily Living and Instrumental Activities of Daily Living, which describe the ability to perform basic and higher-level functions, respectively (Table 19.6).

The social and family support systems surrounding the patient are intimately interwoven with the functional level of the geriatric patient. The living situation of the patient—independent, with family, in assisted living, or with a neighboring support structure—has far-reaching implications not only for their overall health but also as indicators of postoperative disposition and recovery. Identification and incorporation of the patients' living situation and support system into perioperative decision-making are vital to successful patient-centered recovery processes and management of expectations as well as establishing goals of care and any associated limits.

Series reporting on surgical outcomes of octogenarians and nonagenarians have shown that age is often an inaccurate independent marker for surgical risk. A more accurate predictor is frailty. Although no single definition of frailty exists, the AGS suggests that frailty is a syndrome composed of decreased physiologic reserve and a combination of weakness, fatigue, weight loss, decreased balance, low physical activity, slowed motor processing, social withdrawal, cognitive changes, and vulnerability to stressors. The impact of frailty on postoperative outcomes cannot be overstated. Frailty is associated with major complications and early postoperative mortality for cardiothoracic, orthopedic, otolaryngologic, and elective cancer operations. In a large ACS NSQIP study, the preoperative frailty index was more strongly associated with postoperative cardiac arrest and death than ASA class or history of MI.[24]

Frailty can be measured using exhaustive, multidimensional scales such as the CGA or more pragmatic tests such as the Timed Up & Go (TUG) test, which measures functional mobility.[25] In a comparison of four frailty scales to predict postoperative outcomes of cardiac surgery, gait speed outperformed several more extensive scales in predicting mortality or major morbidity.[26] As the most pervasive gait speed measure, TUG is calculated by measuring the time it takes for a patient to rise from a chair, walk 3 meters, turn, and return to a sitting position in the same chair (Fig. 19.3). In a multi-institutional study of patients undergoing minor and major elective operations for solid malignancies, TUG time >20 seconds was associated with a 50% risk of major complications among patients older than 70, compared with 14% for patients with TUG ≤20 seconds.[27]

Although the physical function domain of frailty may be the easiest and most objective to measure, more comprehensive scales such as CGA may produce more actionable results that can improve optimization in the preoperative setting for elective procedures.

Patient Counseling

Integrated into the process of informed consent is clear communication between physician and patient regarding the patient's individualized goals of treatment. The patient must have clear and

---

TABLE 19.6 **Functional Assessments for Activities of Daily Living**

Activities of Daily Living
- Bathing
- Dressing
- Toileting
- Transferring
- Continence
- Feeding

Instrumental Activities of Daily Living
- Telephone ability
- Shopping
- Food preparation
- Housekeeping
- Laundry
- Transportation
- Medication management
- Handling finances

Other
- Muscle strength
- Balance
- Gait
- Walking speed
- Transfer ability

Adapted from Knittel JG, Wildes TS. Preoperative assessment of geriatric patients. *Anesthesiol Clin.* 2016;34:171-183.

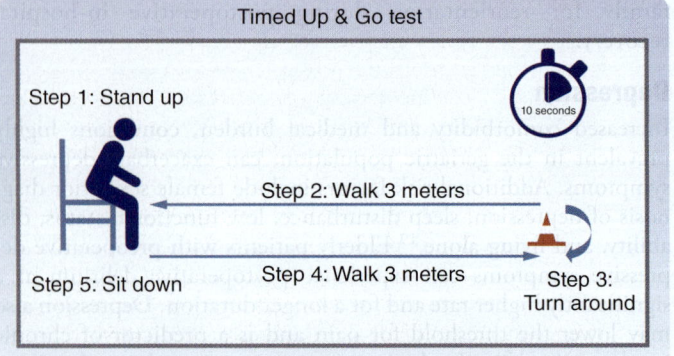

FIGURE 19.3 Timed Up & Go test. (Adapted from www.frailtytoolkit.org.)

realistic expectations regarding the likely treatment course and any potential complications. In the case of older patients, conducting this discussion in the presence of the patient's anticipated postoperative support system—including spouse, adult children, or home nurse—can help ensure that both the patient and the support system are informed regarding necessary postoperative care. This is even more vital if the patient has any cognitive impairment. Regardless of baseline cognitive or functional state, it is strongly recommended that older patients anticipating elective surgery arrange for an advance directive and designate a healthcare proxy or surrogate decision-maker. These documents should be prominently featured in the medical chart.

SYSTEMS APPROACH TO PREOPERATIVE EVALUATION

Cardiovascular System

As the US population continues to age, patients with heart disease undergoing elective, noncardiac surgery will increase. Perioperative cardiac complications are associated with morbidity, mortality, and cost. However, preoperative cardiac intervention to reduce the risk of noncardiac surgery is rarely needed, except when such an intervention is indicated for the management of a patient's baseline condition. In the preoperative setting, the goal of cardiology evaluation (if indicated) is not to provide medical "clearance," but rather to provide information regarding the patient's cardiac risk profile and the management options for this risk. The overarching principle of preoperative cardiovascular evaluation is to obtain supplemental testing only when these tests have a reasonable likelihood of changing management. These changes may involve delaying the operation, preoperative revascularization, medical optimization, modifying perioperative monitoring, or referral to a specialty care center.

The ACC and AHA published updated collaborative guidelines regarding perioperative cardiac risk in 2014.[28] In general, for patients with a low risk (<1%) of major adverse cardiac events (MACEs), there is no need for additional testing.

1. High risk category: Associated with cardiac morbidity rates greater than 5%. Examples include aortic and peripheral vascular surgery. Endovascular surgery is included in this category.
2. Intermediate-risk surgery: Cardiac morbidity rates range from 1% to 5%. Examples include abdominal and thoracic procedures, carotid endarterectomy, orthopedic surgery, and head and neck surgery.
3. Low-risk surgery: Cardiac morbidity rates are generally less than 1%. Examples include endoscopic, superficial soft tissue, cataract, breast, and ambulatory operations.

Risk Prediction Scales/Indices

Numerous published tools measure patients' risk of perioperative cardiac morbidity. The most pervasive—and the instrument cited by the 2014 ACC/AHA Guideline on Perioperative Cardiovascular Evaluation and Management of Patients Undergoing Noncardiac Surgery—is the Revised Cardiac Risk Index (RCRI). Originally published in 1999 by Lee and colleagues, the RCRI assigns 1 point to each of the six preoperative risk factors[29] (Table 19.7). Patients with zero, one, two, or more factors are assigned to classes I, II, III, or IV, respectively. The RCRI has moderate discriminatory power between patients at low versus high risk for cardiac complications; its primary advantage is its ease of implementation and relatively objective criteria. The ACC/AHA guidelines also

TABLE 19.7 Revised Cardiac Risk Index
1. High-risk type of surgery
2. Ischemic heart disease
3. History of congestive heart failure
4. History of cerebrovascular disease
5. Insulin therapy for diabetes
6. Preoperative risk factors

Adapted from Lee TH, Marcantonio ER, Mangione CM, et al. Derivation and prospective validation of a simple index for prediction of cardiac risk of major noncardiac surgery. *Circulation.* 1999;100:1043-1049.

endorse using the ACS NSQIP risk calculator as an alternative or supplement to the RCRI.

Preoperative Testing (Electrocardiogram, Echocardiogram, Stress Test, Angiography)

For patients at low risk for perioperative cardiac complications based on surgical and clinical risk factors, no further testing is indicated before surgery. For patients with known risk factors for coronary artery disease, the ACC/AHA 2014 guidelines provide a useful stepwise approach to further preoperative testing[28] (Fig. 19.4). First, the surgeon determines the urgency of the operation and identifies patient cardiac risk factors or known coronary artery disease. Any emergent operation should proceed, using patient risk factors to guide perioperative monitoring and management. Second, in cases of urgent or elective surgery, the patient should be assessed for acute coronary syndrome and, if suspected, referred for cardiology evaluation as appropriate. An important component of this assessment is an estimation of patient functional capacity, classically measured in metabolic equivalents (METs). An extensive collection of METs for common activities has been compiled by Ainsworth and colleagues.[30] Representative examples are listed in Table 19.8. ACC/ACH guidelines recommend that patients with METs ≥4 without symptoms of cardiac disease proceed with elective or urgent operation. Third, in the absence of acute coronary syndrome, additional testing is pursued based on the combined clinical and surgical risk factors listed earlier, taking into account baseline functional capacity. Any patient undergoing a low-risk operation—regardless of clinical risk factors even with functional capacity <4 METs—has a low risk for cardiac complication and does not require further testing.

For patients undergoing an operation that is not low risk, a 12-lead electrocardiogram (ECG) is indicated for patients with known coronary disease, arrhythmia, peripheral artery disease, and cerebrovascular disease. Even for asymptomatic patients, electrocardiogram may be considered, except for those undergoing a low-risk operation. Assessment of left ventricular function through echocardiography is reasonable for patients with dyspnea of unknown origin or progressive heart failure. For patients with known left ventricular dysfunction, preoperative echocardiogram should be considered if there has not been an assessment within 1 year preceding surgery or they have a decrement in functional status or change in symptoms. Exercise testing with cardiac imaging may be indicated for patients with elevated risk and poor (<4 METs) or unknown functional capacity if patients have three or more risk factors. Patients fitting these criteria who are unable to complete exercise testing may be referred for pharmacologic stress testing, either through dobutamine stress echocardiography or stress myocardial perfusion imaging.[28] Importantly, all of the

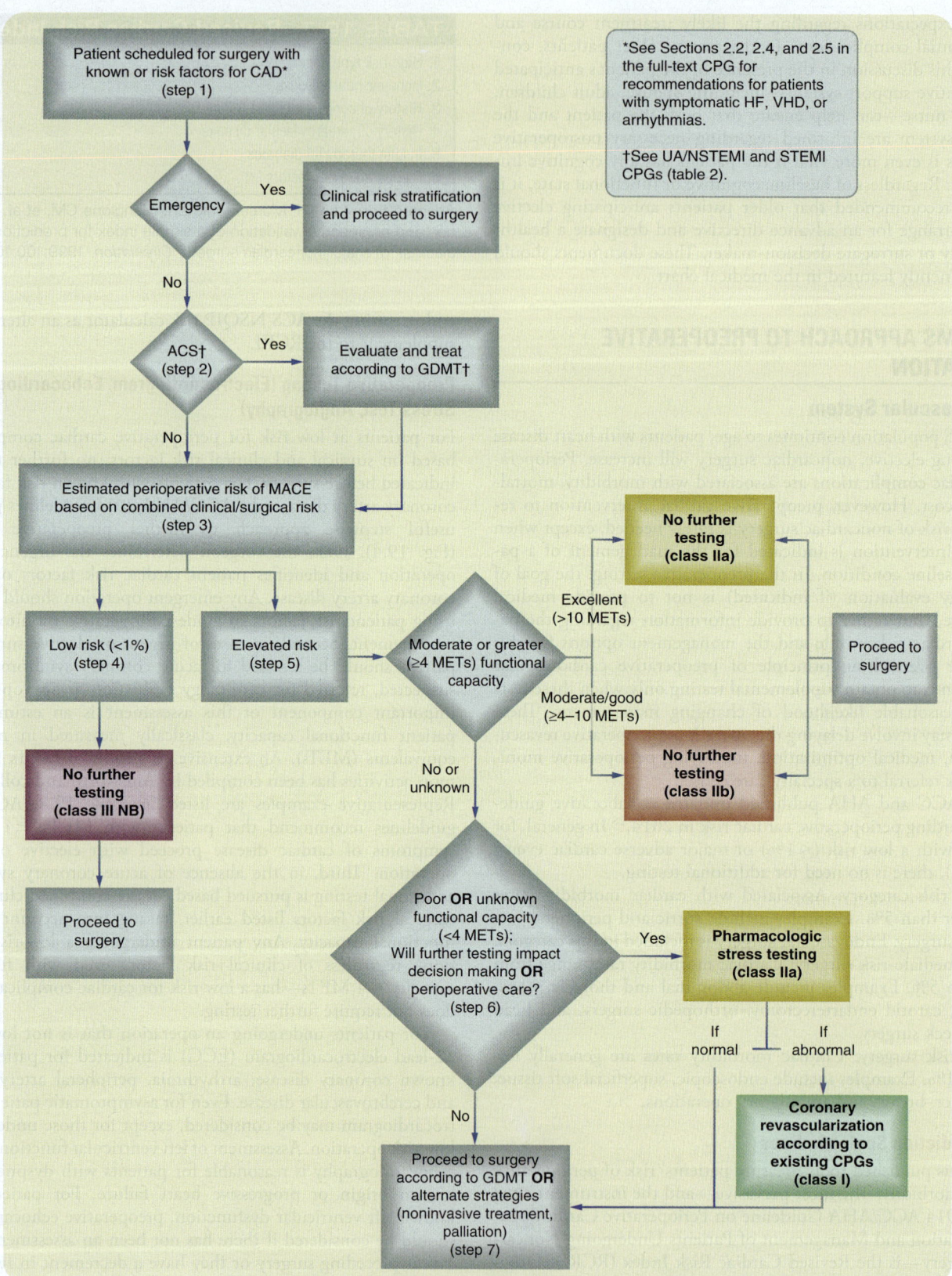

FIGURE 19.4 Stepwise approach to perioperative cardiac assessment for coronary artery disease. *ACS*, American College of Surgeons; *CAD*, coronary artery disease; *CPG*, clinical practice guideline; *GDMT*, guideline-directed medical therapy; *HF*, heart failure; *MACE*, major adverse cardiac event; *METs*, metabolic equivalents; *STEMI*, ST-elevation myocardial infarction; *NSTEMI*, non-ST-elevation myocardial infarction; *UA*, unstable angina; *VHD*, valvular heart disease. (Adapted from Fleisher LA, Fleischmann KE, Auerbach AD, et al. 2014 ACC/AHA guideline on perioperative cardiovascular evaluation and management of patients undergoing noncardiac surgery. *J Am Coll Cardiol.* 2014;64:e77-e137.)

TABLE 19.8	Estimated MET Requirements for Various Activities			
	CAN YOU...		**CAN YOU...**	
1 MET	Take care of yourself?	4 METs	Climb a flight of stairs or walk up a hill?
↓	Eat, dress, or use the toilet?	↓	Walk on level ground at 4 mph (6.4 kph)?
4 METs	Walk indoors around the house?	Greater than 10 METs	Run a short distance?
	Walk a block or two on level ground at 2–3 mph (3.2–4.8 kph)?		Do heavy work around the house like scrubbing floors or lifting or moving heavy furniture?
	Do light work around the house like dusting or washing dishes?		Participate in moderate recreational activities like golf, bowling, dancing, doubles tennis, or throwing a baseball or football?
			Participate in strenuous sports like swimming, singles tennis, football, basketball, or skiing?

kph, Kilometers per hour; *METs,* metabolic equivalents; *mph,* miles per hour.
Adapted from Fleisher LA, Beckman JA, Brown KA, et al. ACC/AHA 2007 guidelines on perioperative cardiovascular evaluation and care for noncardiac surgery: executive summary. *Circulation.* 2007;116:1971-1996.

aforementioned tests should be pursued only if there is a realistic likelihood that the obtained data could change management.

Surgery After Coronary Revascularization

In general, coronary revascularization for the exclusive purpose of reducing perioperative cardiac risk is not indicated. Revascularization is only indicated before noncardiac surgery if it is recommended by baseline clinical practice guidelines. If percutaneous coronary intervention (PCI) is indicated in the preoperative setting, balloon angioplasty, bare-metal stent (BMS) implantation, or drug-eluting stent(s) (DES) revascularization may be considered based on preoperative stress imaging and coronary angiographic findings. For patients considering elective noncardiac surgery after recent coronary revascularization, surgery should be delayed a minimum of 14 days after balloon angioplasty and 30 days after BMS implantation.[28] Ideally, elective surgery should be delayed for 6 months after implantation of DESs because of the need for dual antiplatelet therapy. An operation with interruption of dual antiplatelet therapy can be considered after 90 days following DES placement if risk of further surgical delay exceeds the risk of stent thrombosis and ischemia. As with any high-risk patient care situation, direct communication between a surgeon and medical subspecialist—in this instance a cardiologist—is imperative.

Other High-Risk Cardiac Patients

Patients with moderate to severe left-sided heart failure, right-sided heart failure and/or significant pulmonary hypertension (pulmonary artery pressure >25 mm Hg), or severe aortic stenosis (aortic valve area <1 cm^2) are at significantly increased risk of death. Elective or urgent operations in patients with these cardiac comorbidities require a multidisciplinary approach and risk-benefit discussion. Although optimization with medical management (e.g., diuretics) or preoperative valve replacement (traditional or transcatheter) might be feasible in some patients, the risk of elective operations in patients for whom cardiac function cannot be improved can exceed the potential benefit of the operation, and nonoperative management strategies should be considered.

Perioperative Cardiovascular Medications

Robust evidence supports the use of perioperative β-blockade to reduce cardiac events; however, there is a paucity of data indicating improvement in surgical mortality. Conversely, β-blockers are associated with bradycardia, hypotension, and stroke. As such, the ACC/AHA guidelines recommend that β-blockers be continued in the perioperative setting for patients for whom it is an established preoperative medication. For patients with intermediate- or high-risk myocardial ischemia and for patients with three or more RCRI risk factors, perioperative β-blockers can be initiated. However, it is important to start treatment more than 1 day before surgery.[28] Patients taking statins at baseline should continue therapy in the perioperative setting. Those who do not take statins but are about to undergo high-risk surgery—including vascular surgery—should start statin treatment.

Management of antiplatelet therapy in the early period after coronary revascularization should be determined by consensus between the surgeon, the anesthesiologist, and the cardiologist. In general, perioperative use of aspirin monotherapy is safe in the vast majority of patients who require general and cardiovascular operations. Unless surgical bleeding risk outweighs the risk of stent thrombosis, dual antiplatelet therapy should be continued within the first 4 weeks after BMS and 6 months after DES placement. If discontinuation of a $P2Y_{12}$ inhibitor (clopidogrel, prasugrel, ticagrelor) is necessary to prevent surgical bleeding, it is recommended that aspirin be continued if possible and that the $P2Y_{12}$ inhibitor be restarted as soon as possible after the operation.

Pulmonary System

Postoperative pulmonary complications occur in approximately 6% of patients after major abdominal operations and are associated with increased mortality, ICU admission, and a greater length of stay. This risk is increased in patients diagnosed with COVID-19 within 4 weeks of an operation. This increased risk decreases significantly between 4 and 8 weeks after diagnosis, and after 8 weeks the risk is equivalent to patients without COVID.[31] Although the exact definition of pulmonary complication varies, the major categories include pneumonia/infection, respiratory failure requiring prolonged ventilation, exacerbation of chronic obstructive pulmonary disease (COPD), and lobar/parenchymal collapse with or without associated effusion. The American College of Physicians (ACP) provided guidelines for pulmonary complication risk assessment in 2006 based on a systematic review of patient- and procedure-related preoperative risk factors.[32] The Assess Respiratory Risk in Surgical Patients in Catalonia (ARISCAT) study, one of the largest prospective multi-institutional studies on pulmonary complications, supplemented these guidelines in 2010 and proposed an objective scale for risk stratification[33] (Table 19.9).

Broadly, the ACP guidelines indicate that patient-related risk factors for postoperative pulmonary complications include age >50 years, ASA class II or above, functional dependence,

TABLE 19.9 ARISCAT Risk Score System (top) and Associated Postoperative Pulmonary Complication Rate by Intervals (bottom)

	MULTIVARIATE ANALYSIS OR (95% CL) N = 1624[a]	β COEFFICIENT	RISK SCORE[b]
Age, years			
≤50	1		
51–80	1.4 (0.6–3.3)	0.331	3
>80	5.1 (1.9–13.3)	1.619	16
Preoperative SpO$_2$, %			
≥96	1		
91–95	2.2 (1.2–4.2)	0.802	8
≤90	10.7 (4.1–28.1)	2.375	24
Respiratory infection in the last month	5.5 (2.6–11.5)	1.698	17
Preoperative anemia (≤10 g/dL)	3.0 (1.4–6.5)	1.105	11
Surgical incision			
Peripheral	1		
Upper abdominal	4.4 (2.3–8.5)	1.480	15
Intrathoracic	11.4 (4.9–26.0)	2.431	24
Duration of surgery (hours)			
≤2	1		
>2–3	4.9 (2.4–10.1)	1.593	16
>3	9.7 (4.7–19.9)	2.268	23
	2.2 (1.0–4.5)	0.768	8

		RISK SCORE INTERVALS[c]	
EMERGENCY PROCEDURE	LOW RISK <26 POINTS	INTERMEDIATE RISK 26–44 POINTS	HIGH RISK ≥45 POINTS
Development subsample, no. (%) of patients[d]	1238 (76.2)	288 (17.7)	98 (6.0)
Validation subsample, no. (%) of patients	645 (77.1)	135 (16.1)	57 (6.8)
PPC rate, development subsample, % (95% CI)	0.7 (0.2–1.2)	6.3 (3.5–9.1)	44.9 (35.1–54.7)
PPC rate, validation subsample, % (95% CI)	1.6 (0.6–2.6)	13.3 (7.6–19.0)	42.1 (29.3–54.9)

[a]Because of a missing value for some variables, three patients were excluded. Logistic regression model constructed with the development, subsample, c-index = 0.90; Hosmer-Lemeshow chi-square test = 7.862; P = 0.447.
[b]The simplified risk score was the sum of each β logistic regression coefficient multiplied by 10, after rounding off its value.
[c]Risk intervals were based on division of the development subsample into optimal risk intervals according to the simplified risk score and applying the minimum description length principle.
[d]Three patients were excluded because of a missing value in some variable.
ARISCAT, Assess Respiratory Risk in Surgical Patients in Catalonia; CI, confidence interval; OR, odds ratio; PPC, postoperative pulmonary complication.
Adapted from Canet J, Gallart L, Gomar C, et al. Prediction of postoperative pulmonary complications in population-based surgical cohort. Anesthesiology. 2010;113:1338-1350.

hypoalbuminemia (<3.5 g/dL), COPD, and heart failure. Although COPD is consistently associated with postoperative morbidity, there is no specific level of preoperative pulmonary impairment that precludes nonthoracic surgery. In fact, congestive heart failure—especially when associated with pulmonary hypertension—is a considerably stronger predictor of postoperative pulmonary complications than severe COPD. Active smoking is associated with a moderate increase in risk of postoperative complications, and smoking cessation at least 4 weeks before the operation reduces the risk of complications. Although there is no clear evidence supporting an association between obesity and pulmonary complications per se, both obstructive sleep apnea (OSA) and obesity hypoventilation syndrome—which often complement overweight, metabolic syndrome, and morbid obesity—are associated with pulmonary complications and death.

Procedure-related risk factors that increase the risk of pulmonary complications include vascular surgery, thoracic surgery, abdominal surgery, neurosurgery, general anesthesia, head and neck surgery, procedure duration (>3 hours), and emergency surgery. Pulmonary complications increase in likelihood the closer the surgical incision is in relation to the diaphragm. Because general anesthesia conveys a higher risk of clinically relevant pulmonary complications than regional anesthesia, the latter should be considered when possible for patients with multiple patient-related risk factors.

Appropriate preoperative pulmonary evaluation begins with a thorough history and physical examination focusing on potential patient-related risk factors. Spirometry is indicated for physiologic assessment and residual lung volume estimation preceding pulmonary resection and for patients suspected of having undiagnosed COPD. Spirometry and chest radiography should be considered in patients with a preexisting diagnosis of COPD or asthma if history and physical examination cannot determine whether the patient is at their optimal baseline physiology. However, these tests should not be used in routine screening for low-risk patients or if the results of tests will not affect clinical decision-making. There is no prohibitive spirometric threshold below which nonthoracic surgery is strictly contraindicated. Routine chest radiography may be indicated in patients >50 years of age who are undergoing high-risk surgery. Chest radiography is used in some patients for preoperative staging in preparation for resection of abdominal and gastrointestinal neoplasms, though computed tomography (CT) has supplanted x-ray in many instances as the imaging modality of choice for staging most malignancies. Pulse oxygen saturation is a risk factor within the ARISCAT index, and its low resource utilization allows for routine screening.

There are numerous predictive indices for pulmonary complications. The most frequently cited include the Arozullah index, the ARISCAT index, and the Gupta respiratory failure calculators. The ARISCAT index is the simplest to use, featuring seven readily available preoperative predictors in a simple scoring system[33] (see Table 19.9). The disadvantage of the ARISCAT index is that it may overestimate postoperative complication rate because its complication definition includes minor morbidities such as small radiographic effusions and bronchospasm/wheezing, and the current calibration of the model may not be optimal for use in homogeneous populations and may require recalibration.[34] The Arozullah index, derived from a veteran population, specifically targets postoperative respiratory failure. More cumbersome for routine implementation, it includes more than 12 risk factors, some of which may not be routinely available. More recently, Gupta and colleagues developed risk calculators using the ACS NSQIP dataset with primary outcomes of postoperative respiratory failure and pneumonia[35]; these calculators are available on the web or as a downloadable mobile app.

OSA and obesity hypoventilation syndrome deserve additional consideration. Older age, obesity, and male sex are associated with a higher prevalence of OSA. A simple STOP-BANG questionnaire has been developed to screen patients for OSA and stratify patients into risk categories based on the presence of symptoms. The eight-question scoring tool includes yes/no responses to (1) snoring, (2) daytime tiredness, (3) observation of stopped breathing or interrupted breathing during sleep, (4) high blood pressure, (5) body mass index (BMI) >35, (6) age >50, (7) neck diameter >40 cm, and (8) male sex.[36] Patients with five or more risk factors are considered at high risk for moderate to severe OSA. If an elective operation is planned, these patients should be considered for a sleep study. If positive, they should have preoperative continuous positive airway pressure (CPAP) machine fitting and optimization. Patients requiring urgent or emergent operations are managed for OSA in the postoperative setting.

Obesity hypoventilation syndrome is defined as a combination of BMI >30 with awake $PaCO_2$ >45 mm Hg indicative of hypercapnia not primarily related to other causes such as primary lung disease, medication use, or a neurologic disorder. There are no strict guidelines for arterial gas measurements in obese patients, although the highest risk for hypoventilation is in patients with a BMI exceeding 50. The problem of hypoventilation can be exacerbated in these patients during the perioperative period by general anesthesia and opioids. Consideration for postoperative capnography and adherence to OSA screening and postoperative CPAP use can decrease the risk of respiratory failure and death.

Renal System

Patients with chronic renal insufficiency—particularly those on hemodialysis—experience substantially greater perioperative morbidity and mortality than the general population. Patients on dialysis have greater pressor requirements, longer periods of mechanical ventilation, and longer ICU and overall hospital stay. The cause of this elevated risk is a high rate of concurrent cardiac disease, perioperative fluid and electrolyte disturbance, uremia-mediated bleeding diathesis, and poor perioperative blood pressure management. Preoperative measures to accommodate patients with chronic renal insufficiency primarily focus on a thorough assessment of comorbidities, optimizing fluid and electrolyte status, and securing adequate resources for perioperative care.

Chronic kidney disease (CKD) is a consistent predictor of death and cardiac arrest in the perioperative patient. Assessment of associated cardiac risk begins with a thorough history and physical examination, with attention to predictive indices such as the RCRI (see earlier). Because renal insufficiency is a risk factor within the RCRI, preoperative testing for patients with renal insufficiency broadly follows the guidelines put forth by the ACC/AHA. Patients with stage 1 to 2 chronic renal insufficiency and functional capacity >4 METs who are undergoing low- or intermediate-risk surgery do not require additional preoperative studies. Patients who have stage 3 to 5 renal insufficiency or are undergoing high-risk surgery should receive additional cardiac evaluation, including electrocardiogram, complete blood count, blood chemistry and electrolytes, and urinalysis. Echocardiography should be done in patients with volume overload despite optimal CKD management to evaluate for concomitant cardiac dysfunction.

For patients on dialysis, preoperative management focuses on fluid and electrolyte optimization and preservation of hemodynamic stability. The ideal timing of preoperative dialysis is the day before the operation or the day of surgery. Dialysis goals should include the achievement of near-normal electrolyte levels and euvolemia, making the patient close to dry weight. Hyperkalemia is a life-threatening complication of renal disease and must be considered preoperatively in all patients with renal insufficiency and addressed during all perioperative stages. A normal potassium level is a prerequisite for patients with CKD being considered for an elective or urgent operation, as intraoperative medications to counteract hyperkalemia are limited, and hyperkalemia can result in intraoperative death. Although some experts recommend increasing the amount of peritoneal dialysis for 1 week before surgery, objective data do not exist regarding this practice. Patients who have recently initiated dialysis may possess residual renal function. This function is critical for solute clearance and fluid balance during the first year on dialysis and confers a long-term survival benefit for dialysis patients. Thus, its preservation during the perioperative period is critical. Although evidence-based research remains inconclusive, holding diuretics, angiotensin-converting enzyme inhibitors, and angiotensin receptor blockers in the perioperative period should be considered because these medications can result in variable hemodynamic changes during and after surgery.[37] Once the patient is stable after the operation, these medications should be resumed early in the postoperative period because they may be associated with long-term preservation of residual glomerular filtration rate.

Chronic renal insufficiency affects hematologic function as well, and chronic anemia is common in this population. After addressing the various etiologies for chronic anemia, erythropoietin or darbepoetin may be started for preoperative optimization.

If the hemoglobin remains below target, the patient may require iron studies and investigation into possible erythropoiesis-stimulating agent (ESA) resistance. Although chronic renal insufficiency does not affect platelet count, uremic platelet dysfunction is common. Desmopressin should be readily available and administered if medical bleeding from platelet dysfunction is encountered. Cryoprecipitate and platelet transfusion can be used if necessary. Intraoperative and postoperative medications must undergo diligent dose adjustment, and nephrotoxic agents—including nonsteroidal antiinflammatory drugs (NSAIDs), aminoglycosides, amphotericin B, and contrast dye—should be avoided if possible in patients with residual renal function.

For all patients with CKD, avoidance of secondary renal insults is vital to the preservation of any residual renal function. Maintenance of adequate intravascular volume and avoidance of hypotension in the intraoperative and early postoperative periods are particularly important. For patients without residual renal function and on dialysis, the use of nephrotoxic medications and agents can be considered.

Hepatobiliary System

Patients with impaired liver function are at elevated risk for surgical- and anesthesia-related complications. A thorough preoperative history and physical examination provide cues in terms of hepatic dysfunction. Acute hepatitis of any etiology (e.g., viral, medication induced, autoimmune, obesity related) requires appropriate diagnosis, evaluation, and management. Chronic liver disease, including fibrosis and cirrhosis, can have a significant impact on patients' operative planning and postoperative outcomes. Risk factors for chronic liver disease evident on history can include social behaviors (e.g., injectable drug use, significant alcohol use, tattoos, history of multiple sexually transmitted diseases), long-term obesity, and familial chronic liver disease. Many of the findings on the review of symptoms (pruritus and other manifestations such as jaundice, ascites, and gynecomastia) and physical examination features (spider telangiectasias, caput medusae, icterus, splenomegaly, and fluid wave) are usually found in patients with long-standing cirrhosis. For patients without evidence of liver dysfunction on history and physical examination, routine preoperative testing for liver function in the setting of nonhepatobiliary surgery has low predictive value and is not recommended.

Surgical risk in patients with hepatic disease may be stratified by clinical scenarios and objective measures. Contraindications to elective surgery include acute or fulminant hepatitis and alcoholic hepatitis. Patients with fibrosis without cirrhosis can usually tolerate elective surgery with low morbidity; however, anesthetic agent modifications might be necessary. Common anesthetics, such as propofol, ketamine, etomidate, benzodiazepines, and opioids, undergo hepatic metabolism. Nondepolarizing neuromuscular blockers also pose a pharmacodynamic challenge because patients with liver disease frequently have greater volume of distribution but a slower drug elimination rate. Cirrhosis is associated with increased mortality across all types of major elective surgery. But this risk may vary depending on the type of procedure, with odds ratios ranging from 3.4 for cholecystectomy to 8.0 for CABG.[38]

The three most common objective measures of surgical risk in patients with cirrhosis are the Child-Turcotte-Pugh (CTP) score, the MELD score, and residual liver volume. The CTP classification (Table 19.10) of cirrhosis was popularized in the 1980s, given the ease of calculation and correlation with perioperative mortality after abdominal surgery. Originally proposed by Child and Turcotte, this score estimated the procedural risk for

TABLE 19.10 Modified Child-Turcotte-Pugh Scoring System With Historical Associated Survival Statistics

VARIABLES	POINTS		
	1	2	3
Encephalopathy	None	Grade 1–2	Grade 3–4
Ascites	Absent	Slight	Moderate
Serum albumin (g/L)	>3.5	2.8–3.5	<2.8
International normalized ratio	<1.7	1.7–2.3	>2.3
Total bilirubin (mg/dL)	<2	2–3	>3
or total bilirubin (mg/dL) in patients with PBC/PSC	<4	4–10	>10
	CLASS A	CLASS B	CLASS C
Total points	5–6	7–9	10–15
Historical 1-year survival	100%	80%	45%
Historical 2-year survival	85%	60%	35%

PBC, Primary biliary cirrhosis; *PSC,* primary sclerosing cholangitis.

portosystemic shunting for variceal bleeding. Later, the score was modified by Pugh and colleagues to include prothrombin time (PT) and exclude nutritional status. A CTP score of 5 to 6 is considered class A (well compensated), 7 to 9 is considered class B (significant compromise), and 10 to 15 is considered class C (decompensated). As surgical technique and perioperative care improved over recent years—particularly with the popularization of laparoscopic and robotic surgery—mortality rates for each CTP class have decreased. Although outcomes vary by type of procedure, broad estimates of mortality for abdominal operations are 10%, 20%, and 60% for CTP A, B, and C, respectively.[39]

The MELD score is predictive of disease severity and mortality risk in patients with cirrhosis and was originally developed primarily for transplant allocation. The MELD score has gradually supplanted CTP classification for both liver-directed operations and nonhepatic surgical risk stratification. Unlike CTP score, which includes equally weighted subjective components such as encephalopathy and ascites, the MELD score is composed only of objective measures: total bilirubin (mg/dL), creatinine (mg/dL), and international normalized ratio (INR, %) (Table 19.11). Thirty-day mortality ranges relatively linearly with MELD score, with MELD <8 associated with 6% mortality, and MELD >20 associated with a greater than 50% mortality.[40] Despite the creation of a more objective score, the MELD score is unable to accurately predict the risk of mortality in about 15% to 20% of patients with cirrhosis. In 2008, the MELD score was adapted to include the serum sodium to more accurately predict mortality in this patient population. In 2016, the United Network for Organ Sharing (UNOS) adopted the MELD-Na score for deceased donor liver transplant organ allocation. This new policy also accounts for the following MELD exceptions:
- Hepatocellular carcinoma (HCC)
- Hepatopulmonary syndrome
- Portopulmonary hypertension
- Familial amyloid polyneuropathy
- Primary hyperoxaluria
- Cystic fibrosis

TABLE 19.11 MELD-Na Scoring System With Associated Survival Statistics

MELD-Na = MELD + 1.32* (137-Na) - [0.033*MELD * (137-Na)]	
MELD SCORE	**3-MONTH MORTALITY RISK**
<17	<2%
17–20	3%–4%
21–22	7%–10%
23–26	14%–15%
27–31	27%–32%
>32	65%–66%

Note that sodium values less than 125 mmol/L are set to 125, and values greater than 137 mmol/L are set to 137.
MELD, Model for End-stage Liver Disease; *Na,* sodium.
Adapted from Organ Procurement & Transplantation Network. MELD Calculator. https://optn.transplant.hrsa.gov/resources/allocation-calculators/meld-calculator.

- Hilar/perihilar cholangiocarcinoma
- Hepatic artery thrombosis occurring within the initial 14 days after liver transplant

Overall, the predictive utility of both MELD and CTP scores may be greater for urgent than for elective operations. More importantly, appropriate preoperative patient selection and optimization are paramount in patients with cirrhosis selected for an elective surgical procedure.

Common general surgical problems encountered in patients with cirrhosis include abdominal wall hernias and biliary tract disease. Significant and poorly controlled ascites predisposes to hernia development through congenital abdominal wall defects. Emergency hernia repair (for repair of a transabdominal defect with leaking ascites) is associated with higher morbidity and mortality. As such, preoperative management and control or reduction of ascites is paramount for successful hernia repair, long-term durability, and perioperative safety. When hernia repair is pursued, abdominal wall closure with suture (without mesh) is both feasible and safe. Numerous studies demonstrated better outcomes after a laparoscopic approach to cholecystectomy when compared with an open approach in patients with cirrhosis. For all patients with cirrhosis, operative risk increases with higher CPT (B, C) and higher MELD (>18 20). Multidisciplinary risk-benefit analysis is vital in these patients. Patients with decompensated cirrhosis (CPT C; high MELD) awaiting liver transplantation would benefit from hernia repair after transplantation and/or delaying cholecystectomy to the time of liver transplantation.

When considering hepatic resection, residual liver volume is predictive of postoperative morbidity, particularly posthepatectomy liver failure (PHLF). Generally defined as PT >50% of normal (INR >1.7) and serum bilirubin >2.9 mg/dL (50 μmol/L) on postoperative day 5—often referred to as the *50-50 criteria*—PHLF is associated with up to 50% mortality rate.[41] For patients without cirrhosis undergoing hepatic resection, a residual liver volume of 20% is generally considered adequate. This minimum is estimated at 40% for patients with compensated cirrhosis. Residual liver volume is most commonly estimated by CT or MRI volumetry using integrated software, taking into account the proposed resected liver volume and the patient's body surface area.[42] Recently, several equations have been proposed using metrics such as total liver volume, thoracic width, liver height, sex, and patient body weight.

Patients with chronic liver disease should be medically optimized before surgery. Synthetic function should be evaluated through assessment of PT, albumin, and fibrinogen levels. Creatinine and total bilirubin are necessary to complete preoperative MELD risk assessment. However, it is important to note that PT does not directly correlate with bleeding risk in patients with cirrhosis. In fact, patients with cirrhosis and elevated PT/INR can have hypercoagulability.[43] By treating ascites with preoperative diuresis or paracentesis, surgeons may reduce the risk for dehiscence or herniation. Renal function is particularly important in patients with cirrhosis. Clinicians must be mindful that the impaired synthetic function of these patients may artificially lower urea and creatinine synthesis. Finally, malnutrition is common among patients with cirrhosis and is associated with poor perioperative outcomes. Preoperative nutritional supplementation—including replacement of fat-soluble vitamins as indicated—may be indicated for patients with evidence of recent weight loss or hypoalbuminemia.

Hematologic System

Bleeding and thromboembolism are among the most worrisome, and preventable, operative complications. As such, a thorough hematologic history and physical examination are indicated for every patient considered for an operation. This includes evaluation for symptoms of anemia (fatigue, pallor, hematochezia, dyspnea, palpitations), coagulopathy (petechiae, bleeding diathesis, medications), and hypercoagulability (thrombosis, edema). Physical examination should assess for vital signs, hepatomegaly and splenomegaly, lymphadenopathy, skin tone, extremity edema, and rectal bleeding. A thorough reconciliation of baseline medications is critical because antithrombotic medications require careful management in the preoperative setting. Information regarding liver and kidney function also affects risk assessment for bleeding and perioperative VTE prophylaxis.

Anemia

Chronic anemia is one of the most common findings on routine preoperative evaluation. Causes are frequently multimodal, including nutritional deficiency, cancer, renal disease, inflammatory disease, infection, and heritable disorders. The vast majority of blood-borne oxygen is delivered via hemoglobin within red blood cells; therefore, anemia can result in significant compromise in tissue oxygenation. However, given the reserve in oxygen delivery compared with tissue utilization, hemoglobin levels considerably below normal ranges are generally well tolerated by healthy patients. Over time, treatment of chronic and perioperative anemia has gravitated from liberal transfusion protocols to restrictive strategies. This is because of a lack of supporting evidence for liberal blood transfusion practice and the measurable risks associated with blood transfusion (Table 19.12).

Triggers for blood transfusion in the setting of anemia should be individualized based on patient and clinical factors; however, general guidelines can help promote institutional consistency. Based on data from more than 12,000 patients across 31 trials, the AABB (formerly the American Association of Blood Banks) provided updated transfusion guidelines in 2016. For most hemodynamically stable, asymptomatic hospitalized patients, transfusion is not indicated until hemoglobin level is ≤7 g/dL. This includes the critically ill patient population. These recommendations are supported by the Transfusion Requirements in Critical Care (TRICC) trial, which demonstrated no difference in 30-day mortality between restrictive and liberal transfusion protocols in critically ill, euvolemic patients

TABLE 19.12 Approximate Risk per Unit Transfusion of Red Blood Cells (RBCs)

ADVERSE EVENT	APPROXIMATE RISK PER UNIT TRANSFUSION OF RBCS
Febrile reaction	1:60[a]
Transfusion-associated circulatory overload	1:100[b]
Allergic reaction	1:250
Transfusion-related acute lung injury	1:12,000
Hepatitis C virus infection	1:1,149,000
Hepatitis B virus infection	1:1,208,000 to 1:843,000[c]
Human immunodeficiency virus infection	1:1,467,000
Fatal hemolysis	1:1,972,000

[a]Estimated to be 1:91 with prestorage leukoreduction and 1:46 with poststorage leukoreduction.

[b]Estimated risk per recipient rather than unit.

[c]The estimate is variable depending on the length of the infectious period.

Adapted from Carson JL, Guyatt G, Heddle NM, et al. Clinical practice guidelines from the AABB red blood cell transfusion thresholds and storage. *JAMA*. 2016;316:2025-2035.

with anemia in the intensive care setting. Findings from the TRICC trial were recently corroborated by the Transfusion Requirements in Septic Shock (TRISS) trial in patients with septic shock.[44] Among patients with gastrointestinal bleeding, a restrictive transfusion system is associated with lower 30-day mortality.

Potential exceptions to the 7 g/dL transfusion threshold include patients with cardiovascular disease and those undergoing cardiac surgery, for whom a transfusion threshold of 8 g/dL could be considered. The recent Transfusion Requirements in Cardiac Surgery III (TRICS III) trial found no difference in death, MI, stroke, or renal failure between transfusion thresholds of 7.5 g/dL and 8.5 to 9.5 g/dL in patients undergoing cardiac surgery.[45] For asymptomatic patients with baseline cardiovascular disease, the Functional Outcomes in Cardiovascular Patients Undergoing Surgical Hip Fracture (FOCUS) trial suggests that a transfusion threshold of 8 g/dL is not associated with worse postoperative outcomes when compared with a threshold of 10 g/dL.

Anemia in a patient who is acutely bleeding represents a fundamentally different clinical scenario. In these patients, anemia is more closely associated with hypovolemic shock, and rapid hemodynamic instability often makes laboratory-based transfusion protocols unrealistic. For hemodynamically stable patients, a restrictive transfusion system may be reasonable. However, for patients with ongoing bleeding, hemodynamic instability, or massive trauma, empiric blood transfusion and institutional massive transfusion protocols may be lifesaving.

Inherited Coagulopathy

Routine preoperative laboratory screening for bleeding diatheses is discouraged; workup should be guided by questions that assess bleeding risk. The surgeon should elicit a history of frequent nosebleeds, menorrhagia, intraarticular bleeding, and hereditary diseases. Common comorbid conditions that increase bleeding risk include chronic renal or hepatic insufficiency. Prior experiences with invasive procedures and current anticoagulation and antiplatelet medications should be assessed. On physical examination, epistaxis, gingival bleeding, and cutaneous petechiae are suggestive

of platelet or collagen disorders. Hemarthrosis, deep hematomas, and large, palpable ecchymoses may indicate factor deficiency. Because of the relatively low incidence of major bleeding in common general surgery operations, studies addressing the value of routine preoperative hemostatic testing are often inadequately powered. If a patient's history and physical examination indicate an increased risk for bleeding, initial laboratory tests should include a complete blood count comprising platelet count, PT with INR, activated partial thromboplastin time (aPTT), creatinine, and hepatic function panel. Patients with signs of hereditary bleeding disorders should be referred for preoperative hematologic consultation.

When considering the diagnostic approach to hereditary bleeding disorders, the first separation is between disorders of coagulation and those of platelets and vascular integrity. If the workup includes a normal PT/INR and aPTT, thrombocytopenia or platelet dysfunction should be suspected. Spontaneous bleeding generally does not occur unless the platelet count is below 30,000/μL. Inherited disorders in platelet function or storage include von Willebrand disease (vWD; the most common), Bernard-Soulier syndrome, and Glanzmann thrombasthenia. Acquired causes of platelet dysfunction include cirrhosis, myelodysplastic syndromes, uremia, and pharmacologic impacts of aspirin, $P2Y_{12}$ inhibitors, and NSAIDs. A normal PT/INR and aPTT do not rule out coagulopathies outside the measured pathways of these two tests (i.e., factor XIII deficiency) or vascular disorders (inherited and acquired connective tissue disorders, small vessel vasculitis).

Causes of isolated prolongation of aPTT include deficiencies in factors VIII (hemophilia A), IX (hemophilia B), and XI. Hemophilia A and B are by far the most common, and both are X-linked recessive disorders. Isolated prolonged PT, in the absence of pharmacologic contributors or cirrhosis, is indicative of the relatively rare factor VII deficiency. Abnormal results on both PT and aPTT usually indicate a defect in the common coagulation pathway, composed of factors II (prothrombin), V, and X and fibrinogen. Inherited disorders of the common pathway are rare; an extensive investigation into acquired causes is likely to indicate contributors such as vitamin K deficiency, supratherapeutic warfarin, hepatic insufficiency, or disseminated intravascular coagulation. A broad summary of the screening approach to bleeding disorders is provided in Fig. 19.5.

Institutional protocols for perioperative management in patients with inherited bleeding disorders should be a collaboration between hematologists, anesthesiologists, and surgeons. These protocols vary widely because of differences in available laboratory resources and treatments. However, a few guiding principles are relevant in all scenarios. Elective operations for patients with bleeding disorders should be planned with multidisciplinary input to ensure the availability of all laboratory and therapeutic resources in the postoperative period. Multiple avenues of intraoperative venous access should be available for accurate blood sampling away from infusion sites. Perioperative analgesia should not include medications with antiplatelet effects such as aspirin and NSAIDs.

Preoperative treatment for hemophilia A depends on disease severity. Mild phenotypes (factor VIII >5%) respond well to Desmopressin (DDAVP) given the day of surgery, which will raise factor VIII levels up to fivefold within 90 minutes. After administration, factor VIII levels should be measured in the preoperative and postoperative setting, and DDAVP may be redosed on a daily or twice-daily basis as needed. Appropriate attention should be paid

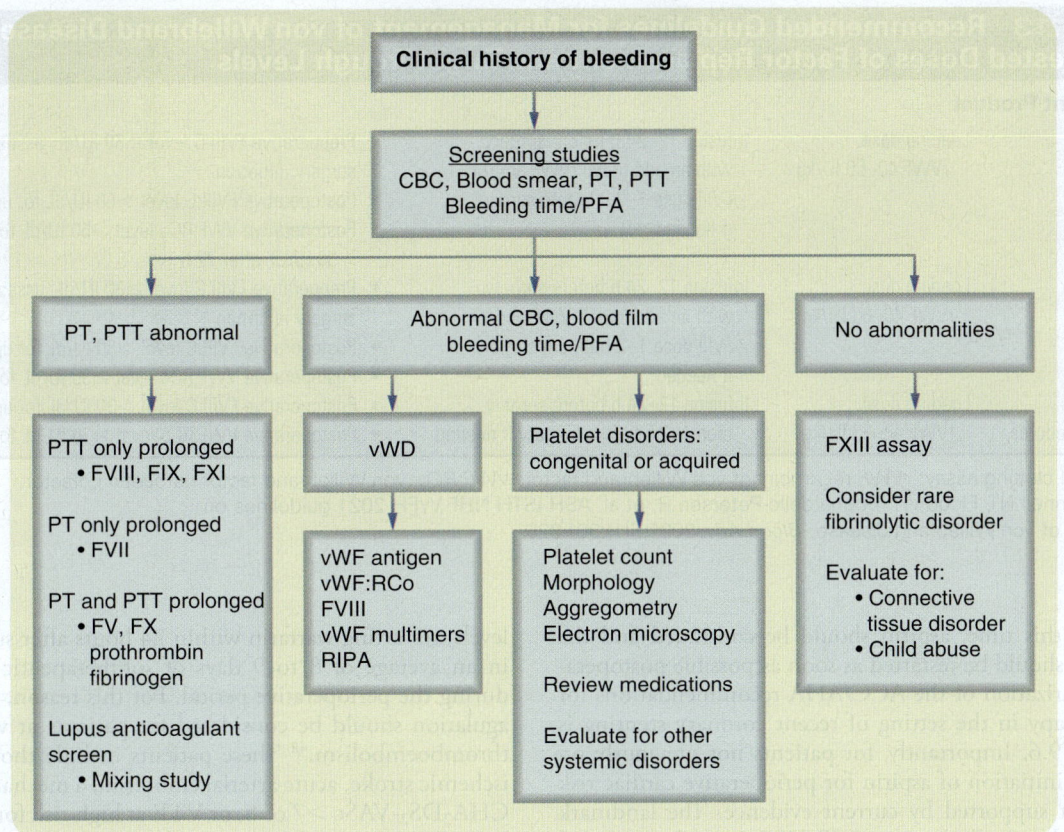

FIGURE 19.5 Laboratory evaluation of bleeding disorders. *CBC,* Complete blood count; *PFA,* platelet function assay; *PT,* prothrombin time; *PTT,* partial thromboplastin time; *RCo,* ristocetin cofactor; *RIPA,* ristocetin-induced platelet aggregation; *vWD,* von Willebrand disease; *vWF,* von Willebrand factor. (Adapted from Sharanthkumar AJ, Pipe SW. Bleeding disorders. *Pediatr Rev.* 2008;29:121-129.)

to fluid retention because hyponatremia can be a serious complication of DDAVP, particularly in elderly patients. Because factor IX does not respond to DDAVP, even mild forms of hemophilia B require factor replacement both before and after major surgery to maintain appropriate levels. For both disorders, severe phenotypes should be treated with administration of factor concentrates in the immediate preoperative setting, within 10 to 20 minutes of incision.[46] Reducing the need for repeat dosing of factor concentrates minimizes the likelihood of inhibitor development. Up to 25% of patients with severe hemophilia A will ultimately develop inhibiting antibodies to factor VIII. Inhibitors reduce effectiveness of factor replacement therapy. For patients who have had multiple prior treatments with factor replacement, preoperative inhibitor screening should be performed a week before surgery. The presence of inhibitors indicates the need for procoagulant agents that can bypass the intrinsic pathway, such as activated recombinant factor VII or activated prothrombin complex concentrate.

Von Willebrand factor (vWF) mediates platelet adhesion to collagen and other platelets. It is the carrier protein for factor VIII. vWD, a disorder of vWF, is subdivided into three broad types. Type 1 is a partial deficiency of vWF. It is the most common version and responds well to DDAVP administered 1 hour before incision. Because vWF is an acute-phase reactant, levels generally remain elevated postoperatively. Type 2 vWD comprises a variety of qualitative defects in vWF that can result in decreased binding of factor VIII and disorders in platelet function (2A, 2B, and 2M). Although DDAVP may induce a partial response in patients with

types 2A and 2M vWD, it is contraindicated in type 2B because it may cause thrombocytopenia.[46] Type 3 vWD is a complete or near-complete deficiency in vWF and universally does not respond to DDAVP. For all patients with type 3 vWD and most patients with type 2 disease, vWF concentrate is the treatment of choice. Preoperative measurement of factor levels should be obtained before elective surgery, and minimum target trough levels should be tailored to the type of surgery (Table 19.13).

Antiplatelet Therapies

The 2016 ACC/AHA guidelines recommend an individualized approach to weighing risks of surgical bleeding and cardiac risk among patients on chronic antiplatelet therapy.[28] Patients who are on chronic low-dose aspirin therapy but who have not previously undergone coronary stenting should continue aspirin in the perioperative setting if the bleeding risk is low. In general, perioperative use of aspirin antiplatelet monotherapy is safe in most patients who require general and cardiovascular operations. Elective operations that require discontinuation of dual antiplatelet therapy (e.g., aspirin and clopidogrel) should be avoided within 30 days after BMS implantation or within 6 months after DES implantation. Surgical delay after DES implantation may be reduced to 3 months if the risk of delay is greater than the risk of stent thrombosis. For urgent operations within 4 weeks after BMS or DES implantation, dual antiplatelet therapy should be continued unless there is a significant risk for life-threatening surgical bleeding. If there is a surgical need to discontinue $P2Y_{12}$ inhibitor

TABLE 19.13   Recommended Guidelines for Management of von Willebrand Disease With Suggested Doses of Factor Replacement and Target Trough Levels

A Recombinant Product			
Major surgery	Loading dose: rVWF 40–60 IU/kg	Infusion 12–24 h before surgery with an additional rVWF and/or FVIII dose 1–2 h before surgery if needed	• Preoperative FVIII:C level ≥60 IU/dL, assessed within 3 h of surgery initiation • Postoperative FVIII:C level >50 IU/dL for up to 72 h • Postoperative VWF:RCo level >50 IU/dL for up to 72 h, then >30 IU/dL after 72 h
Minor surgery	Loading dose: rVWF 40–60 IU/kg	Infusion 12–24 h before surgery with an additional rVWF and/or FVIII dose 1–2 h before surgery if needed	• Preoperative FVIII:C level ≥30 IU/dL, assessed within 3 h of surgery initiation • Postoperative FVIII:C level >30 IU/dL for up to 72 h • Postoperative VWF:RCo level ≥30 IU/dL for up to 72 h
Dental extractions or invasive procedures	Loading dose: rVWF 40–60 IU/kg	Infusion 12–24 h before surgery, then 1–2 h before surgery if needed	• Postoperative FVIII:C level >30 IU/dL for up to 72 h • Postoperative VWF:RCo level ≥30 IU/dL for up to 72 h

FVIII:C, Factor VIII clotting assay; *rVWF,* recombinant von Willebrand factor; *VWF:RCo,* von Willebrand factor ristocetin cofactor.
Adapted from Connell NT, Flood VH, Brignardello-Petersen R, et al. ASH ISTH NHF WFH 2021 guidelines on the management of von Willebrand disease. *Blood Adv.* 2021;5(1):301-325.

therapy during this time, aspirin should be continued and the $P2Y_{12}$ inhibitor should be restarted as soon as possible postoperatively. A summarization of the ACC/AHA recommendations for antiplatelet therapy in the setting of recent coronary stenting is shown in Fig. 19.6. Importantly, for patients not previously on aspirin therapy, initiation of aspirin for perioperative cardiac risk reduction is not supported by current evidence. The landmark Perioperative Ischemic Evaluation 2 (POISE-2) trial concluded that administration of aspirin in the perioperative setting has no impact on death or MI and increases the risk of major bleeding.[47]

Anticoagulation

Consideration of perioperative management of anticoagulants balances the risk of bleeding against that of thromboembolic complications. In addition to determining the duration of anticoagulant interruption, clinicians must decide whether a bridging agent is indicated. Patients at exceptionally high risk for thromboembolic complications (i.e., recent ischemic stroke, inadequate anticoagulation in the setting of atrial fibrillation with CHA_2DS_2-VASc >1 for males and >2 for females) should not undergo elective operations until the clotting risk is optimized. Operations with low risk of bleeding—such as many cutaneous operations—can proceed without interruption of chronic anticoagulation. In the case of cardiac interventions for arrhythmia, it may be undesirable to interrupt anticoagulation even in the perioperative setting. The American College of Chest Physicians Evidence-Based Clinical Practice Guidelines (2012) represent the most widely accepted recommendations for perioperative antithrombotic management.[48]

Clinicians should consider the pharmacokinetics of anticoagulants to keep interruptions in chronic anticoagulation as short as possible. Warfarin, with a half-life of 36 to 42 hours, should be discontinued 5 days before elective operations, which eliminates the need for any additional preoperative PT/INR evaluation. A preoperative INR done 1 to 2 days before the day of surgery is reasonable for a patient who discontinued warfarin <5 days before their procedure or if their recent INR is >4.5. If the INR remains above 1.5, oral vitamin K or fresh frozen plasma (FFP) can be administered preoperatively depending on the extent of coagulopathy and operative planning. Because it usually takes 4 to 5 days for warfarin to attain therapeutic anticoagulation

levels, restarting warfarin within 24 hours after surgery will result in an average of 8 to 9 days of subtherapeutic anticoagulation during the perioperative period. For this reason, bridging anticoagulation should be considered for patients at very high risk of thromboembolism.[48] These patients include those with a recent ischemic stroke, acute arterial embolism, a mechanical heart valve, CHA_2DS_2-VASc >7 or 8, or VTE at high risk for thromboembolism. Previous guidelines recommended bridging for high-risk atrial fibrillation as well. However, results from the double-blind placebo-controlled BRIDGE trial concluded that forgoing bridging with low-molecular-weight heparin (LMWH) in this setting does not increase risk for arterial thromboembolism and decreases the risk of major bleeding.[49] When used in the setting of bridging treatment, unfractionated heparin should be stopped 4 to 6 hours before surgery, whereas LMWH should be stopped 24 hours before surgery. For operations with high bleeding risk, therapeutic-dose LMWH should be resumed 48 to 72 hours postoperatively; for minor operations with a low bleeding risk, LMWH can usually be resumed after 24 hours postoperatively.

Oral Direct Thrombin and Factor Xa Inhibitors

Modern oral anticoagulant agents include the direct thrombin inhibitor dabigatran (Pradaxa) and direct factor Xa inhibitors rivaroxaban (Xarelto), apixaban (Eliquis), and edoxaban (Savaysa). These agents possess several advantages over the traditional inhibitor of vitamin K–dependent coagulation factors: warfarin. Namely, they offer more rapid onset (less than 4 hours) and shorter half-life, allowing a shorter period of interruption in the perioperative setting. Routine long-term laboratory testing for drug levels is not required. However, perioperative management of these agents requires knowledge of basic pharmacokinetics and options for reversal.[50] A summary of common oral anticoagulants is provided in Table 19.14.

The 2020 PAUSE trial evaluated a standardized approach to direct oral anticoagulant (DOAC) management for high-risk and low-risk procedures.[51] Dabigatran was approved by the US Food and Drug Administration (FDA) for stroke prevention in atrial fibrillation in 2010. Its clearance is renal, with a half-life of 12 to 17 hours. For patients with normal renal function who are anticipating major surgery or with impaired kidney function, dabigatran should be held for 48 hours before surgery and resumed

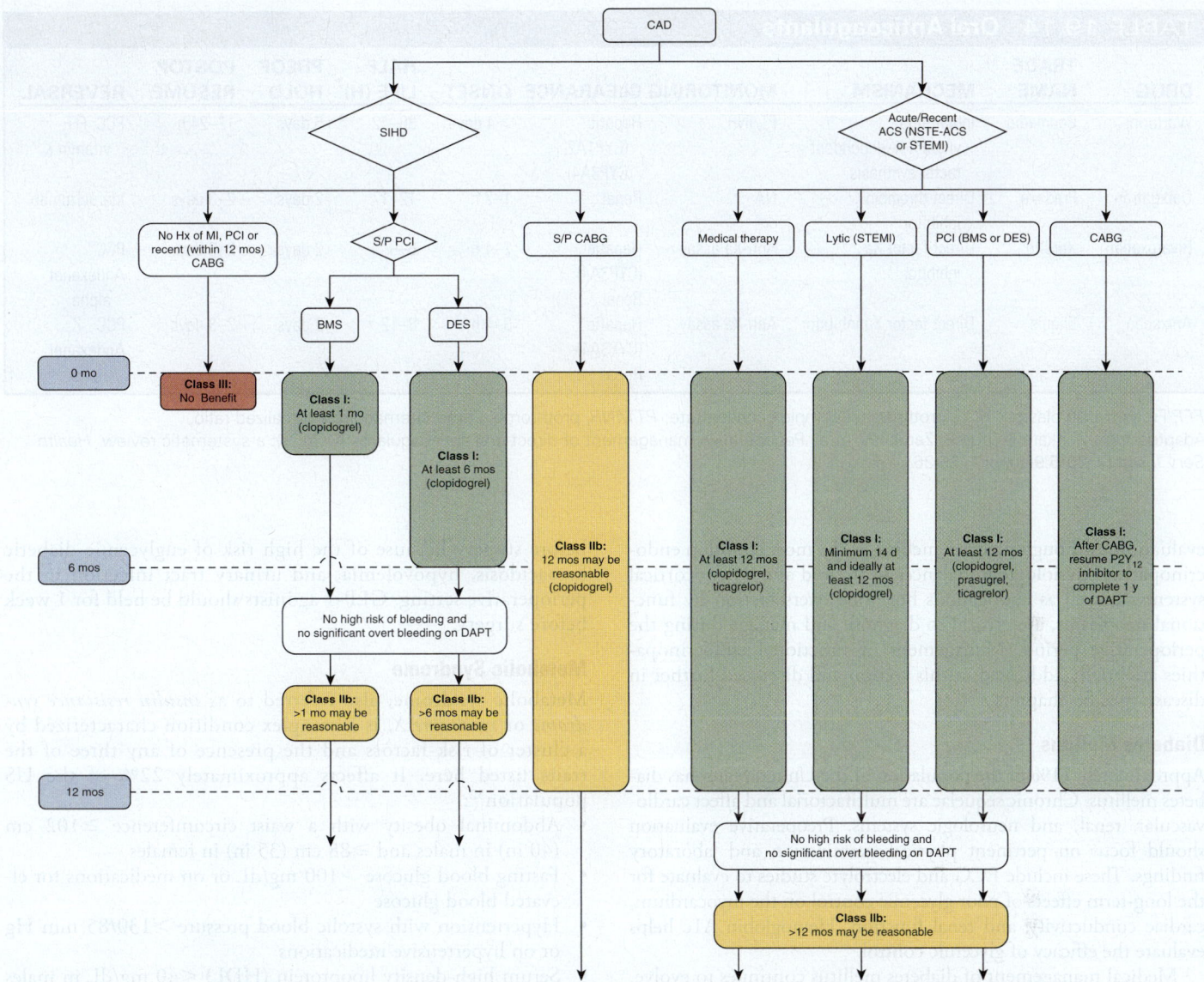

FIGURE 19.6 Management of antiplatelet agents in patients with endovascular coronary stent and noncardiac surgery. *ACS,* Acute coronary syndrome; *BMS,* bare-metal stent; *CABG,* coronary artery bypass graft surgery; *CAD,* coronary artery disease; *DAPT,* dual antiplatelet therapy; *DES,* drug-eluting stent; *Hx,* history; *lytic,* fibrinolytic therapy; *MI,* myocardial infarction; *NSTE-ACS,* non–ST-elevation acute coronary syndrome; *PCI,* percutaneous coronary intervention; *SIHD,* stable ischemic heart disease; *S/P,* status post; *STEMI,* ST-elevation myocardial infarction. (Adapted from 2016 ACC/AHA Guideline Focused Update on Duration of Dual Antiplatelet Therapy in Patients With Coronary Artery Disease. *Circulation.* 2016;134;e123-e155.)

the day after surgery for low-risk procedures and 2 days after for high-risk procedures or for patients with impaired kidney function. Dabigatran can be monitored using dilute thrombin time or liquid chromatography–mass spectrometry (LC-MS/MS) drug level. In 2015, the FDA approved idarucizumab (Praxbind) as a specific reversal agent for dabigatran. Rapid reversal is achieved with a single 5-g IV dose.

Rivaroxaban, apixaban, and edoxaban are direct factor Xa inhibitors; they can be monitored using a chromogenic anti-Xa assay or LC-MS/MS. Clearance includes renal excretion in urine and hepatic metabolism via CYP3A4. As such, drug interactions are common with cytochrome P450 inhibitors (e.g., ketoconazole, amiodarone, selective serotonin reuptake inhibitors [SSRIs], cimetidine) and inducers (e.g., carbamazepine, phenytoin, rifampin). In addition, factor Xa inhibitors are substrates of

P-glycoprotein efflux transporters. Therefore, drugs that inhibit both CYP3A4 and P-glycoprotein—the classic example is ketoconazole—can cause profound amplification of anticoagulation effects. Oral Xa inhibitors have rapid onset (2–4 hours) and relatively short half-lives, allowing for short periods of interruption perioperatively. They should be stopped 48 hours before surgery for high-risk operations and 24 hours before surgery for low-risk operations and resumed 1 to 2 days postoperatively.[51] In 2018, the FDA approved andexanet alpha (Andexxa) as a targeted reversal agent for oral factor Xa inhibitors. Administration involves an initial bolus of 400 to 800 mg, followed by a continuous infusion.

Endocrine System

Endocrine comorbidities can significantly influence perioperative physiology and are important to consider during preoperative

TABLE 19.14   Oral Anticoagulants

DRUG	TRADE NAME	MECHANISM	MONITORING	CLEARANCE	ONSET	HALF-LIFE (H)	PREOP HOLD	POSTOP RESUME	REVERSAL
Warfarin	Coumadin	Inhibitor of vitamin K–dependent factor synthesis	PT/INR	Hepatic (CYP1A2, CYP3A4)	>4 days	36–42	5 days	12–24 h	PCC, FFP, vitamin K
Dabigatran	Pradaxa	Direct thrombin inhibitor	NA	Renal	1–2 h	12–17	2 days	2–3 days	Idarucizumab
Rivaroxaban	Xarelto	Direct factor Xa inhibitor	Anti-Xa assay	Hepatic (CYP3A4) Renal	2–4 h	5–9	2 days	2–3 days	PCC Andexanet alpha
Apixaban	Eliquis	Direct factor Xa inhibitor	Anti-Xa assay	Hepatic (CYP3A4) Renal	3–4 h	8–12	2 days	2–3 days	PCC Andexanet alpha

FFP, Fresh frozen plasma; *PCC,* prothrombin complex concentrate; *PTT/INR,* prothrombin time/international normalized ratio.
Adapted from Sunkara T, Ofori E, Zarubin V, et al. Perioperative management of direct oral anticoagulants (DOACs): a systematic review. *Health Serv Insights.* 2016;9(suppl 1):25-36.

evaluation. Although diabetes mellitus is the most common endocrinopathy, physiologic imbalances of thyroid and adrenocortical systems, as well as endogenous hormone oversecretion by functional neoplasms, are critical to diagnose and manage during the perioperative period. Management of functional endocrinopathies are briefly addressed in this section and discussed further in disease-specific chapters.

Diabetes Mellitus

Approximately 11% of the population of the United States has diabetes mellitus. Chronic sequelae are multifactorial and affect cardiovascular, renal, and neurologic systems. Preoperative evaluation should focus on pertinent physical examination and laboratory findings. These include ECG and electrolyte studies to evaluate for the long-term effects of poor glycemic control on the myocardium, cardiac conductivity, and renal function. Hemoglobin A1c helps evaluate the efficacy of glycemic control.

Medical management of diabetes mellitus continues to evolve. A number of short-, intermediate-, and long-acting insulin formulations are commercially available. In general, long-acting insulin (glargine or detemir) should be administered as scheduled during the perioperative period. Intermediate-acting insulin (NPH, zinc insulin, extended zinc insulin) should be administered at half the dose on the morning of surgery and resumed at the normal dose once a normal diet has been resumed. Short-acting insulins (regular, lispro, glulisine, and aspart) are generally held and not administered during the morning of surgery. Premixed or proportional combinations of intermediate-acting with short-acting insulins such as 70/30 or 50/50 should generally be reduced by 20% the night before and by 50% on the morning of surgery. Insulin pumps should be set to the basal infusion rate and reprogrammed to regular settings once a normal diet has been established. Inpatient endocrinology consultation is frequently helpful in the management of patients with complex insulin regimens or poor glycemic control.

Perioperative management of oral hypoglycemics has also evolved. In general, sulfonylureas (e.g., glyburide, glipizide, glimepiride, and other single-agent or combination sulfonylureas) and metformin are withheld the day of surgery. DPP-4 inhibitors (gliptins) typically are administered the morning of surgery. SGLT2 inhibitors should typically be held 3 to 4 days before surgery because of the high risk of euglycemic diabetic ketoacidosis, hypovolemia, and urinary tract infection in the perioperative setting. GLP-1 agonists should be held for 1 week before surgery.

Metabolic Syndrome

Metabolic syndrome, also referred to as *insulin resistance syndrome* or *syndrome X,* is a complex condition characterized by a cluster of risk factors and the presence of any three of the traits listed here. It affects approximately 22% of the US population[52]:

- Abdominal obesity with a waist circumference ≥102 cm (40 in) in males and ≥88 cm (35 in) in females
- Fasting blood glucose >100 mg/dL or on medications for elevated blood glucose
- Hypertension with systolic blood pressure >130/85 mm Hg or on hypertensive medications
- Serum high-density lipoprotein (HDL) <40 mg/dL in males or <50 mg/dL in females
- Serum triglycerides >150 mg/dL or use of a statin for elevated triglycerides

Individuals with metabolic syndrome are at increased perioperative risk, such as delayed wound healing, postoperative infections, and cardiovascular complications. These patients require perioperative assessment involving meticulous blood pressure control and glycemic management.

Thyroid Disease

Thyroid function panel and measurement of thyroid-stimulating hormone readily identify patients with thyroid-related endocrinopathies. Patients with hyperthyroidism typically are suppressed preoperatively before thyroid surgery. Nonthyroid elective operations should be delayed until hyperthyroidism is addressed. Hypothyroidism is an indolent chronic disease, and patients with asymptomatic hypothyroidism can be started on thyroid replacement hormone at any time during perioperative care. Symptomatic hypothyroidism is manifested by a decrease in metabolism (e.g., fatigue, weight gain, heat dysregulation). Symptomatic hypothyroidism can affect electrolyte regulation, coagulation, myocardial conduction, and other metabolic pathways; elective operations in patients with symptomatic hypothyroidism should be delayed until hypothyroidism is medically corrected.

Adrenocortical System

Patients with functional adrenal neoplasms, including pheochromocytoma and functional adrenocortical carcinoma, as well as patients with functional paraganglioma, have an overproduction of catecholamines, which can be life threatening during the perioperative period. The possibility of hormone production should be tested in all patients with adrenal neoplasms, and medical management, including α- and β-adrenergic blockade, should be accomplished before the date of planned operation for those with catecholamine production. Urgent operations without sufficient adrenergic blockade should be avoided given the high risk of morbidity and mortality.

Patients with adrenal insufficiency are treated with glucocorticoid replacement. In addition, approximately 1% of the population of the United States uses glucocorticoids for a multitude of medical conditions including pulmonary, joint, inflammatory, and other diseases. Traditionally, perioperative high-dose steroid replacement has been used in patients using steroids at baseline. However, recent data suggest that additional (high-dose) steroid administration is not necessary in all patients. Patients with low-dose steroid use (prednisone 5 mg/day or dose equivalent) can continue baseline steroid dosing. Patients with higher daily doses of glucocorticoids for 3 weeks or longer can be tested for suppression of the hypothalamic-pituitary axis with a morning cortisol test. Levels below 5 mcg/dL require steroid replacement, and levels >10 mcg/dL can continue their normal dose. Patients with levels between 5 and 10 mcg/dL require further evaluation with a low-dose adrenocorticotropic hormone stimulation test. Lack of adrenal response to exogenous adrenocorticotropic hormone administration is diagnostic for adrenal insufficiency, and administration of a physiologic replacement dose of glucocorticoids is indicated. In lieu of stimulation testing for all patients using >5 mg prednisone (or dose equivalent), consensus guidelines recommend glucocorticoid replacement dependent on the extent of the planned operation (Fig. 19.7).

Neoplastic Endocrinopathies

Several solid organ neoplasms secrete endogenous hormones. Functional pancreatic neoplasms can secrete excess gastrin, insulin, glucagon, vasoactive intestinal peptide, and other rare peptides. Patients with pancreatic neuroendocrine neoplasms and symptoms concerning for endocrinopathy should complete a preoperative evaluation to establish whether they have a functional tumor. Patients with primary pancreatic, bowel, or lung carcinoid can develop serotonin hypersecretion. In general, clinically significant serotonin production by a primary tumor is rare, and symptoms typically develop primarily in patients with liver metastases.

Carcinoid liver metastases can result in significant hypersecretion of serotonin, histamine, prostaglandins, and other metabolites. Common symptoms of carcinoid syndrome are flushing and diarrhea. Urinary excretion of 5-hydroxyindoleacetic acid (5-HIAA) can be diagnostic. Patients with symptomatic clinical and/or pathologic diagnosis of carcinoid liver metastases or nonmetastatic but symptomatic (flushing/diarrhea) neuroendocrine neoplasms should be managed with a somatostatin-analogue (e.g., octreotide, octreotide long-acting repeatable [LAR], lanreotide) to suppress the activity of the endogenous hormone before pursuing any operative intervention. Patients with long-standing carcinoid symptoms should be evaluated for valvular heart disease because they can develop tricuspid regurgitation, pulmonic stenosis, and/or regurgitation. After somatostatin receptor blockade, clinically significant carcinoid heart disease should be operatively addressed before pursuing tumor-directed surgery.

Regimen	Degree of surgical stress	Glucocorticoid regimen
Patients currently on glucocorticoids	Grade I Minor	• Continue daily dose of glucocorticoid • 25 mg of IV hydrocortisone at induction if not able to tolerate PO • Resume oral daily preoperative glucocorticoid regimen
	Grade II Moderate	• Continue daily dose of glucocorticoid • 25-50 mg of hydrocortisone IV at induction • 15-25 mg hydrocortisone every 6 hours until PO is tolerated and hemodynamically stable[a] • Resume oral daily preoperative glucocorticoid regimen
	Grade III Major	• Continue daily dose of glucocorticoid • 50 mg of hydrocortisone IV at induction • 25 mg of hydrocortisone IV every 6 hours on day 1 and until hemodynamically stable, then 15 mg IV every 6 hours until PO is tolerated[a] • Resume oral daily preoperative glucocorticoid regimen
Patients who stopped or plan to stop glucocorticoids before surgery		• Assess HPA axis in patients with intermediate to high risk (see Table 4) • The closer the date of discontinuing glucocorticoids before surgery, the higher the risk of AI • Treat based on the degree of surgical stress in those who have abnormal HPA axis
Adrenal crisis		• 100 mg of hydrocortisone IV (IM if no IV access) • 50 mg every 6 hours until hemodynamically stable and then taper[a] • Taper depending on clinical response-Intravenous fluids (normal saline), dextrose 5% if hypoglycemia

FIGURE 19.7 Perioperative steroid supplementation. Note: These recommendations include the authors' personalized approach to perioperative management in patients with glucocorticoid-induced AI. *AI,* Adrenal insufficiency; *HPA,* hypothalamic-pituitary-adrenal; *IM,* intramuscular; *IV,* intravenous; *PO,* by mouth. [a]Some experts favor continuous glucocorticoid infusion. (From Chen Cardenas SM, Santhanam P, Morris-Wiseman L, Salvatori R, Hamrahian AH. Perioperative evaluation and management of patients on glucocorticoids. *J Endocr Soc.* 2023;7[2]:bvac185.)

Appropriate perioperative octreotide administration is imperative. This typically takes the form of preoperative admission for octreotide infusion or large-dose octreotide administration before anesthetic induction. Intraoperative cardiovascular instability can occur, requiring ongoing high-dose octreotide administration. Intraoperative octreotide infusion is typically weaned in the postoperative period.

Endogenous hypersecretion of antidiuretic hormone causing syndrome of inappropriate secretion of antidiuretic hormone (SIADH) is a rare manifestation of small cell lung cancer and other lung neoplasms. SIADH can also result from neurosurgery (e.g., pituitary surgery) or trauma. Management requires maintenance of euvolemia and appropriate correction of serum sodium.

Nutrition and Obesity

Establishing a patient's nutritional status is a vital component of surgical planning. Physiologic stress from surgery or trauma results in a transient catabolic state, with rapid consumption of energy and protein. Malnutrition in the perioperative setting can have severe consequences, including impaired wound healing, increased likelihood of infection, electrolyte abnormalities, and organ dysfunction. Optimizing perioperative nutrition counterbalances the effects of systemic stress to minimize these negative effects.

Preoperative Nutrition Assessment

During preoperative evaluation, indicators of malnutrition include a history of weight loss and chronic illness. A dietary history should be gathered, including use of nutritional supplements. On physical examination, relevant findings include BMI, temporal wasting, peripheral edema, muscle mass, skin turgor, and presence of petechiae, ecchymoses, or pressure ulcers. Among the many screening tools for malnutrition, the most used is the Nutritional Risk Screen tool (NRS-2002) (Table 19.15). Multiple studies have described associations between greater nutritional risk score as measured by NRS-2002 and postoperative complications, including prolonged hospital length of stay.

Because systemic protein stores are vital for postoperative wound healing, protein status has been a particular focus of preoperative assessment. The most commonly cited serum indicators of protein status are albumin, prealbumin, and transferrin. In a large Veterans Affairs study of noncardiac operations, albumin <3.5 was a strong predictor of early postoperative morbidity and mortality. Given its long half-life (20 days), albumin is generally referenced as an indicator of chronic nutritional status. Prealbumin has a much shorter half-life of 2 days and therefore may reflect more recent nutrition. Importantly, prealbumin and albumin are both negative acute-phase proteins. During acute

TABLE 19.15	**Nutritional Risk Screen (NRS-2002) Tool**			
	IMPAIRED NUTRITIONAL STATUS		**SEVERITY OF DISEASE (% INCREASE IN REQUIREMENTS)**	
Absent **Score 0**	Normal nutritional status		Absent **Score 0**	Normal nutritional requirements
Mild **Score 1**	Weight loss >5% in 3 months or food intake below 50%–75% of normal requirement in preceding week		Mild **Score 1**	Hip fracture[a] Chronic patients, in particular with acute complications: cirrhosis[a], COPD[a] *Chronic hemodialysis, diabetes, oncology*
Moderate **Score 2**	Weight loss >5% in 2 months or BMI 18.5–20.5 + impaired general condition or food intake 25%–60% of normal requirement in preceding week		Moderate **Score 2**	Major abdominal surgery[a], stroke[a] *Severe pneumonia, hematologic malignancy*
Severe **Score 3**	Weight loss >5% in 1 month (>15% in 3 months) or BMI <18.5 + impaired general condition or food intake 0%–25% of normal requirement in preceding week		Severe **Score 3**	Head injury[a] Bone marrow transplantation[a] *Intensive care patients (APACHE .10)*
Score: Age	+ if >70 years: add 1 to total score above		**Score: Age-adjusted total score**	= **Total score**

Score >3: The patient is nutritionally at risk, and a nutritional care plan should be initiated.
Score <3: Weekly rescreening of the patient. If the patient is scheduled for a major operation, for example, a preventive nutritional care plan is considered to avoid the associated risk status.
NRS-2002 is based on an interpretation of available randomized clinical trials.
[a]Indicates that a trial directly supports the categorization of patients with that diagnosis. Diagnoses shown in *italics* are based on the prototypes given below.
Nutritional risk is defined by the present **nutritional status** and risk of impairment of present status due to **increased requirements** caused by stress metabolism of the clinical condition.
A **nutritional care plan** is indicated in all patients who are:
(1) severely undernourished (score = 3), (2) severely ill (score = 3), (3) moderately undernourished + mildly ill (score 2 + 1), or (4) mildly undernourished + moderately ill (score 1 + 2).
Prototypes for severity of disease. Score = 1: a patient with chronic disease admitted to hospital due to complications. The patient is weak but out of bed regularly. Protein requirement is increased but can be covered by oral diet or supplements in most cases. **Score = 2:** a patient confined to bed due to illness (e.g., following major abdominal surgery). Protein requirement is substantially increased but can be covered, although artificial feeding is required in many cases. **Score = 3:** a patient in intensive care with assisted ventilation, etc. Protein requirement is increased and cannot be covered even by artificial feeding. Protein breakdown and nitrogen loss can be significantly attenuated.
APACHE, Acute physiology and chronic health evaluation; *BMI,* body mass index; *COPD,* chronic obstructive pulmonary disease.
Adapted from Kondrup J, Allison SP, Elia M, Vellas B, Plauth M. ESPEN guidelines for nutrition screening 2002. *Clin Nutr.* 2003;22(4):415-451.

stress and inflammation, increased production of acute-phase proteins results in decreased levels of both albumin and prealbumin, making them less reliable in the perioperative setting. Transferrin has a half-life of 8 to 9 days. In addition to being a negative acute-phase protein, transferrin levels must also take into account serum iron levels.

Nutrition Supplementation

Supplementation of nutrition in the perioperative setting is available via enteral or parental routes. The enteral route offers several advantages and is preferred in most situations. Parenteral nutrition requires special venous access that may be prone to infection. It also confers increased risks of hyperglycemia. Parenteral nutrition frequently lacks immune-bolstering glutamine and omega-3 fatty acids, which support the gastrointestinal tract's important immunologic functions. The intestinal mucosa acts as a physical barrier against infection and produces targeted antibodies including intraluminal immunoglobulin A. During starvation, the mucosa becomes more susceptible to bacterial translocation; enteral feeding helps maintain a healthy intestinal mucosa barrier, decreasing untoward immunologic and translocation effects.

Nutritional prehabilitation before surgery has been the subject of investigation for decades. In 1991, the Veterans Affairs TPN Cooperative randomized patients to preoperative total parenteral nutrition (TPN) or no treatment before noncardiac surgery. The TPN group had more infectious complications overall. However, severely malnourished patients receiving TPN experienced fewer noninfectious complications than controls, suggesting TPN prehabilitation may have a role in select patients.[53] More recent data suggest adopting NRS-2002 as a screening tool and considering parenteral or enteral prehabilitation for patients with severe malnutrition. For patients who are only mildly malnourished, surgery should not be delayed for preoperative nutritional supplementation.

In the postoperative setting, enteral feeding should be initiated early. True contraindications to enteric feeding are few: obstruction, intestinal ischemia, bowel discontinuity, high-output fistulas, and severe malabsorption.[54] Importantly, mechanical ventilation, vasopressor support, and an open abdomen are not strict contraindications to enteral nutrition. Early enteral nutrition (within 24 hours of surgery) is a key component of most enhanced recovery after surgery (ERAS) protocols and may be associated with a reduction in postoperative complications. Awaiting objective signs of bowel function before enteral feeding is not necessary. Among patients undergoing upper gastrointestinal tract resection and reconstruction, early enteral feeding is associated with fewer infections and a shorter hospital length of stay. Only when there is an expectation for more than 7 days of a nonfunctional gastrointestinal tract or longer than 5 to 7 days since the patient demonstrated preoperative malnutrition should a patient be considered for postoperative parenteral nutrition.

Obesity

Obesity is classified as a BMI >30 kg/m² and can be further subcategorized into class I with BMI of 30 to 34.9 kg/m², class II with BMI of 35 to 39.9 kg/m², and class III with BMI >40 kg/m². All three classes have varying degrees of surgical complexity and potential complications. These complications include pulmonary, cardiovascular, thromboembolic, and infectious complications. Obese patients experience longer operative times and greater hospital lengths of stay. Many of these outcomes are attributable to comorbidities associated with obesity, including cardiovascular

disease, OSA, obesity hypoventilation syndrome, metabolic syndrome, essential hypertension, and diabetes. Consequently, the AHA recommends a preoperative ECG and chest radiography for all patients with BMI >40 who have a risk factor for heart failure or poor exercise tolerance. The STOP-BANG questionnaire is a sensitive screening test for OSA.[36] Routine implementation of this eight-question survey in the obese population can help direct formal polysomnography testing and anticipate difficult airway problems.

PREOPERATIVE CONSIDERATIONS AND CARE PROTOCOLS

Evaluation of the patient in the preoperative setting on the day of surgery provides the surgeon a final opportunity to assess readiness for the operation. Interval changes in clinical condition since the preceding consultation visit should be queried. A reevaluation of preexisting medications, including the timing of the most recent doses, is performed. Appropriate management of baseline anticoagulant and antiplatelet agents, including timing of the last dose, is confirmed. Informed consent is verified again with the patient to ensure that there is an accurate and appropriate understanding of the procedure's objectives and risks. Orders relevant to the immediate perioperative setting are reviewed with the surgery and anesthesiology teams. Important to every operation is a review of the indications for antibiotic prophylaxis and VTE prophylaxis. Perioperative care protocols, such as ERAS protocols and similarly designed pathways, facilitate the standardization of patient care, including preoperative expectations, intraoperative management, and postoperative recovery.

Patient Recovery Pathways

A number of patient recovery pathways have been designed and implemented to standardize perioperative care. The enhanced recovery/ERAS protocols are the best studied and supported in the literature. Initially introduced in the late 1990s and early 2000s, these pathways were initially implemented in colorectal surgery. Strengths include standardization of care in the preoperative setting (e.g., patient education, management of concurrent health conditions, minimizing extended perioperative fasting, routine antiemetic prophylaxis, use of opioid-sparing analgesic techniques), intraoperative setting (e.g., maintenance of normothermia, lung-protective mechanical ventilation, antibiotic prophylaxis, avoidance of volume overload), and postoperative setting (e.g., early ambulation, early enteral feeding, opioid-sparing analgesia, and VTE prophylaxis).[55]

There has been a proliferation of ERAS-type protocols across abdominal general surgery, thoracic surgery, gynecologic surgery, orthopedics, and other surgical subspecialties. The protocols themselves are quite granular, typically enumerating the specific timing of preoperative, intraoperative, and postoperative medications and patient expectations.[56] Patient buy-in and acceptance by multidisciplinary staff, including surgeons, anesthesiologists, and nursing staff, are vital for the success of these patient care pathways. Although pathway implementation frequently demonstrates early improvements in postoperative metrics (e.g., infections, pain scores, length of stay, and others), demonstration of long-term sustained effects have been elusive in some studies. Standardized reporting of compliance and outcomes of such postoperative care protocols has been recommended to understand which elements and/or pathways are best supported by data.

Antibiotic Prophylaxis

SSIs are among the most common causes of nosocomial infection and are associated with increased mortality and postoperative length of stay. SSIs are classified as superficial (involving only the skin or subcutaneous tissue), deep incisional (involving fascia or muscle), and organ space infections. Risk factors for SSI are numerous, including age, obesity, smoking, malnourishment, diabetes, immunosuppression, radiation, and others. Although many risk factors are not modifiable in the immediate perioperative setting, two of the simplest actionable measures that reduce the risk of SSI are the appropriate selection of perioperative antibiotics and the administration of these antibiotics within 1 hour of incision.

The Centers for Disease Control and Prevention (CDC) categorizes wounds into four classes: clean, clean-contaminated, contaminated, and dirty-infected (Table 19.16). Although useful from the standpoint of academic inquiry, recent research has reported limited utility of wound classification as a risk factor for postoperative complications as well as frequent misclassification of surgical incisions.[57]

The Clinical Practice Guidelines for Antimicrobial Prophylaxis in Surgery, a collaborative rubric developed in 2013, provides surgery-specific recommendations for antibiotic prophylaxis[58] (Table 19.17). Selection of appropriate prophylaxis is guided by a few core principles. First, an antimicrobial agent is chosen to target common surgical site pathogens. Clean procedures encounter primarily skin flora, predominantly *Staphylococcus aureus* and coagulase-negative *Staphylococcus*. Coverage for gram-negative rods and enterococci should be added for clean-contaminated cases involving abdominal viscera, the biliary tract, and the heart. Commonly used FDA-approved agents include cefazolin, cefoxitin, cefotetan, and vancomycin. For most operations, cefazolin is an appropriate choice given its low cost, antimicrobial spectrum, and duration of activity. For patients colonized with methicillin-resistant *S. aureus* (MRSA), vancomycin may be an appropriate alternative.

The second consideration in antimicrobial prophylaxis is timing of the first dose. Historical data from the early 1990s suggested that the lowest rate of surgical wound infection was associated with antibiotic administration within 2 hours before incision compared with earlier or postoperative administration. However, the more recent Trial to Reduce Antimicrobial Prophylaxis Errors, a prospective, multicenter trial comparing antimicrobial timing before a variety of operations, reported the lowest infection risk when antibiotics were administered within 30 minutes of incision or between 31 and 60 minutes before incision.[59] As such, current data support administration of the first dose of prophylactic antibiotics within 60 minutes before surgical incision. For antibiotics that require longer infusion times (vancomycin, fluoroquinolones), administration may begin within 120 minutes before incision. Redosing of antibiotics should be performed to maintain therapeutic serum levels, generally after every two half-lives or if there is blood loss greater than 1500 mL (Table 19.18).

Duration of antimicrobial administration should be limited to the minimal effective length appropriate for each procedure. Most clean and clean-contaminated operations do not require postoperative antimicrobial administration; when indicated, postoperative antimicrobials should be limited to less than 24 hours. The evidence for short-duration or single-dose prophylaxis in cardiothoracic surgery has been inconsistent, and optimal antimicrobial duration after these operations remains contentious. Although the Society of Thoracic Surgeons recognizes risks for resistance and superinfection with *Clostridioides difficile* with prolonged antibiotic administration, there is evidence that antibiotic duration up to 48 hours reduces the risk of a sternal wound infection. Thus, the Surgical Infection Society and the Society of Thoracic Surgeons both recommend consideration of antimicrobial prophylaxis for up to 48 hours after cardiothoracic surgery.

Review of Medications

Management of home medications on the day of surgery should be tailored to the patient and the operation. The objective is to minimize disruption of baseline homeostasis while limiting risks of surgical bleeding and drug-drug interactions with anesthetic medications. A preoperative review of medications is mandatory, with attention to cardiac, psychiatric, neurologic, and diabetic medications as well as anticoagulants and antiplatelet agents. In general, cardiac drugs and inhalers should be continued on the morning of surgery. In the postoperative setting, parenteral substitutes should be administered as indicated to minimize therapeutic lapse and avoid withdrawal symptoms such as rebound hypertension. Drugs that affect perioperative bleeding risk should be discontinued preoperatively based on the drug's half-life. Institutional guidelines regarding timing for withholding antiplatelets and anticoagulants before local analgesic procedures such as epidural placement or spinal/regional blockade should be reviewed with the patient during the preoperative clinic visit.

TABLE 19.16	Wound Classification
WOUND CLASSIFICATION	**DEFINITION**
Clean	An uninfected operative wound in which no inflammation is encountered and the respiratory, alimentary, genital, or uninfected urinary tracts are not entered.
Clean-contaminated	Operative wounds in which the respiratory, alimentary, genital, or urinary tracts are entered under controlled conditions and without unusual contamination. Specifically, operations involving the biliary tract, appendix, vagina, and oropharynx, provided no evidence of infection or major break in technique is encountered.
Contaminated	Open, fresh, accidental wounds. In addition, operations with major breaks in sterile technique or gross spillage from the gastrointestinal tract and incisions in which acute, nonpurulent inflammation is encountered, including necrotic tissue without evidence of purulent drainage.
Dirty-infected	Old traumatic wounds with retained devitalized tissue and those that involve existing clinical infection or perforated viscera. Organisms causing postoperative infection were present in the operative field before the operation.

Adapted from www.cdc.gov.

TABLE 19.17 Recommendations for Surgical Antimicrobial Prophylaxis

TYPE OF PROCEDURE	RECOMMENDED AGENTS[a,b]	ALTERNATIVE AGENTS IN PATIENTS WITH β-LACTAM ALLERGY	STRENGTH OF EVIDENCE[c]
Cardiac coronary artery bypass	Cefazolin, cefuroxime	Clindamycin,[d] vancomycin[d]	A
Cardiac device insertion procedures (e.g., pacemaker implantation)	Cefazolin, cefuroxime	Clindamycin, vancomycin	A
Ventricular assist devices	Cefazolin, cefuroxime	Clindamycin, vancomycin	C
Thoracic noncardiac procedures, including lobectomy, pneumonectomy, lung resection, and thoracotomy	Cefazolin. ampicillin-sulbactam	Clindamycin,[d] vancomycin[d]	A
Video-assisted thoracoscopic surgery	Cefazolin. ampicillin-sulbactam	Clindamycin,[d] vancomycin[d]	C
Gastroduodenal[e] procedures involving entry into lumen of gastrointestinal tract (bariatric, pancreaticoduodenectomy[f])	Cefazolin	Clindamycin or vancomycin + aminoglycoside[g] or aztreonam or fluoroquinolone[h-j]	A
Procedures without entry into gastrointestinal tract (antireflux, highly selective vagotomy) for high-risk patients	Cefazolin	Clindamycin or vancomycin + aminoglycoside[g] or aztreonam or fluoroquinolone[h-j]	A
Biliary tract open procedure	Piperacillin-tazobactam, cefazolin, cefoxitin, cefotetan, ceftriaxone,[k] ampicillin-sulbactam[h]	Clindamycin or vancomycin + aminoglycoside[g] or aztreonam or fluoroquinolone,[h-j] metronidazole + aminoglycoside[g] or fluoroquinolone[h-j]	A
Laparoscopic procedure			
Elective, low-risk[l]	None	None	A
Elective, high-risk[l]	Cefazolin, cefoxitin, cefotetan, ceftriaxone,[k] ampicillin-sulbactam[h]	Clindamycin or vancomycin + aminoglycoside[g] or aztreonam or fluoroquinolone,[h-j] metronidazole + aminoglycosid[g] or fluoroquinolone[h-j]	A
Appendectomy for uncomplicated appendicitis	Cefoxitin, cefotetan, cefazolin + metronidazole	Clindamycin + aminoglycoside[g] or aztreonam or fluoroquinolone,[h-j] metronidazole + aminoglycoside[g] or fluoroquinolone[h-j]	A
Small intestine			
Nonobstructed	Cefazolin	Clindamycin + aminoglycoside[g] or aztreonam or fluoroquinolone[h-j]	C
Obstructed	Cefazolin + metronidazole, cefoxitin, cefotetan	Metronidazole + aminoglycoside[g] or fluoroquinolone[h-j]	C
Hernia repair (hernioplasty and herniorrhaphy)	Cefazolin	Clindamycin, vancomycin	A
Colorectal[m]	Cefazolin + metronidazole, cefoxitin, cefotetan, ampicillin-sulbactam,[h] ceftriaxone	metronidazole,[n] ertapenem	Clindamycin + aminoglycoside[g] or aztreonam or fluoroquinolone,[h-j] metronidazole + aminoglycoside[s] or fluoroquinolon[h-j]	A
Head and neck clean	None	None	B
Clean with placement of prosthesis (excludes tympanostomy tubes)	Cefazolin, cefuroxime	Clindamycin[d]	C
Clean-contaminated cancer surgery	Cefazolin + metronidazole, cefuroxime + metronidazole, ampicillin-sulbactam	Clindamycin[d]	A
Other clean-contaminated procedures with the exception of tonsillectomy and functional endoscopic sinus procedures	Cefazolin + metronidazole, cefuroxime + metronidazole, ampicillin-sulbactam	Clindamycin[d]	0
Neurosurgery elective craniotomy and cerebrospinal fluid-shunting procedures	Cefazolin	Clindamycin,[d] vancomycin[d]	A
Implantation of intrathecal pumps	Cefazolin	Clindamyci,[d] vancomycin[d]	C
Cesarean delivery	Cefazolin	Clindamycin + aminoglycoside[g]	A

Continued

TABLE 19.17   Recommendations for Surgical Antimicrobial Prophylaxis—cont'd

TYPE OF PROCEDURE	RECOMMENDED AGENTS[a,b]	ALTERNATIVE AGENTS IN PATIENTS WITH β-LACTAM ALLERGY	STRENGTH OF EVIDENCE[c]
Hysterectomy (vaginal or abdominal)	Cefazolin. cefotetan, cefoxitin, ampicillin-sulbactam[h]	Clindamycin or vancomycin + aminoglycoside[g] or aztreonam or fluoroquinolone,[h-j] metronidazole + aminoglycoside[g] or fluoroquinolone[h-j]	A
Ophthalmic	Topical neomycin-polymyxin B-gramicidin or fourth-generation topical fluoroquinolones (gatifloxacin or moxifloxacin) given as 1 drop every 5–15 minutes for 5 doses.[o] Addition of cefazolin 100 mg by subconjunctival injection or intracameral cefazolin 1–2.5 mg or cefuroxime 1 mg at the end of procedure is optional.	None	0
Orthopedic clean operations involving hand, knee, or foot and not involving implantation of foreign materials	None	None	C
Spinal procedures with and without instrumentation	Cefazolin	Clindamycin,[d] vancomycin[d]	A
Hip fracture repair	Cefazolin	Clindamycin,[d] vancomycin[d]	A
Implantation of internal fixation devices (e.g., nails, screws, plates, wires)	Cefazolin	Clindamycin,[0] vancomycin[3]	C
Total joint replacement	Cefazolin	Clindamycin,[d] vancomycin[d]	A
Urologic lower tract instrumentation with risk factors for infection (includes transrectal prostate biopsy)	Fluoroquinolone,[h-j] trimethoprim-sulfamethoxazole, cefazolin	Aminoglycoside[g] with or without clindamycin	A
Clean without entry into urinary tract	Cefazolin (addition of a single dose of an aminoglycoside may be recommended for placement of prosthetic material [e.g., penile prosthesis])	Clindamycin,[d] vancomycin[d]	A
Involving implanted prosthesis	Cefazolin ± aminoglycoside, cefazolin ± aztreonam, ampicillin-sulbactam	Clindamycin ± aminoglycoside or aztreonam, vancomycin ± aminoglycoside or aztreonam	A
Clean with entry into urinary tract	Cefazolin (addition of a single dose of an aminoglycoside may be recommended for placement of prosthetic material [e.g., penile prosthesis])	Fluoroquinolone,[h-j] aminoglycoside[g] ± clindamycin	A
Clean-contaminated	Cefazolin + metronidazole, cefoxitin	Fluoroquinolone,[h-j] aminoglycoside[g] + metronidazole or clindamycin	A
Vascula[p]	Cefazolin	Clindamycin,[d] vancomycin[d]	A
Heart, lung, heart-lung transplantation[q]; heart transplantation[r]	Cefazolin	Clindamycin,[d] vancomycin[d]	A (based on cardiac procedures)
Lung and heart-lung transplantation[r,s]	Cefazolin	Clindamycin,[d] vancomycin[d]	A (based on cardiac procedures)
Liver transplantation[q,t]	Piperacillin-tazobactam, cefotaxime + ampicillin	Clindamycin or vancomycin + aminoglycoside[g] or aztreonam or fluoroquinolone[h-j]	0
Pancreas and pancreas-kidney transplantation[r]	Piperacillin-tazobactam, cefazolin, fluconazole (for patients at high risk of fungal infection [e.g., patients with enteric drainage of the pancreas])	Clindamycin or vancomycin + aminoglycoside[g] or aztreonam or fluoroquinolone[h-j]	A
	Cefazolin	Clindamycin or vancomycin + aminoglycoside[g] or aztreonam or fluoroquinolone[h-j]	A

TABLE 19.17   Recommendations for Surgical Antimicrobial Prophylaxis—cont'd

TYPE OF PROCEDURE	RECOMMENDED AGENTS[a,b]	ALTERNATIVE AGENTS IN PATIENTS WITH β-LACTAM ALLERGY	STRENGTH OF EVIDENCE[c]
Plastic surgery clean with risk factors or clean-contaminated	Cefazolin, ampicillin-sulbactam	Clindamycin,[d] vancomycin[d]	C

[a]The antimicrobial agent should be started within 60 minutes before surgical incision (120 minutes for vancomycin or fluoroquinolones). Although single-dose prophylaxis is usually sufficient, the duration of prophylaxis for all procedures should be <24 hours. If an agent with a short half-life is used (e.g., cefazolin, cefoxitin), it should be readministered if the procedure duration exceeds the recommended redosing interval (from the time of initiation of the preoperative dose). Readministration may also be warranted if prolonged or excessive bleeding occurs or if there are other factors that may shorten the half-life of the prophylactic agent (e.g., extensive burns). Readministration may not be warranted in patients in whom the half-life of the agent may be prolonged (e.g., patients with renal insufficiency or renal failure).

[b]For patients known to be colonized with methicillin-resistant *Staphylococcus aureus,* it is reasonable to add a single preoperative dose of vancomycin to the recommended agents.

[c]Strength of evidence that supports the use or nonuse of prophylaxis is classified as A (levels I–III), B (levels IV–VI), or C (level VII). Level I evidence is from large, well-conducted, randomized controlled clinical trials. Level II evidence is from small, well-conducted, randomized controlled clinical trials. Level III evidence is from well-conducted cohort studies. Level IV evidence is from well-conducted case-control studies. Level V evidence is from uncontrolled studies that were not well conducted. Level VI evidence is conflicting evidence that tends to favor the recommendation. Level VII evidence is expert opinion.

[d]For procedures in which pathogens other than staphylococci and streptococci are likely, an additional agent with activity against those pathogens could be considered. For example, if there are surveillance data showing that gram-negative organisms are a cause of surgical site infections for the procedure, practitioners may consider combining clindamycin or vancomycin with another agent (cefazolin if the patient is not allergic to β-lactam antibiotics; aztreonam, gentamicin, or single-dose fluoroquinolone if the patient is allergic to β-lactam antibiotics).

[e]Prophylaxis should be considered for patients at highest risk for postoperative gastroduodenal infections, such as patients with increased gastric pH (e.g., patients receiving histamine H2 receptor antagonists or proton pump inhibitors), gastroduodenal perforation, decreased gastric motility, gastric outlet obstruction, gastric bleeding, morbid obesity, or cancer. Antimicrobial prophylaxis may not be needed when the lumen of the intestinal tract is not entered.

[f]Consider additional antimicrobial coverage with infected biliary tract.

[g]Gentamicin or tobramycin.

[h]Because of increasing resistance of *Escherichia coli* to fluoroquinolones and ampicillin-sulbactam, local population susceptibility profiles should be reviewed before use.

[i]Ciprofloxacin or levofloxacin.

[j]Fluoroquinolones are associated with an increased risk of tendinitis and tendon rupture in patients of all ages. However, this risk would be expected to be quite small with single-dose antibiotic prophylaxis. Although the use of fluoroquinolones may be necessary for surgical antibiotic prophylaxis in some children, they are not first-choice drugs in pediatric patients because of an increased incidence of adverse events compared with control subjects in some clinical trials.

[k]Ceftriaxone use should be limited to patients requiring antimicrobial treatment for acute cholecystitis or acute biliary tract infections that may not be determined before incision; ceftriaxone should not be used in patients undergoing cholecystectomy for noninfected biliary conditions, including biliary colic or dyskinesia without infection.

[l]Factors that indicate a high risk of infectious complications in laparoscopic cholecystectomy include emergency procedures, diabetes, long procedure duration, intraoperative gallbladder rupture, age >70 years, conversion from laparoscopic to open cholecystectomy, American Society of Anesthesiologists classification of ≥3, episode of colic within 30 days before the procedure, reintervention in <1 month for noninfectious complication, acute cholecystitis, bile spillage, jaundice, pregnancy, nonfunctioning gallbladder, immunosuppression, and insertion of prosthetic device. Because many of these risk factors are impossible to determine before surgical intervention, it may be reasonable to give a single dose of antimicrobial prophylaxis to all patients undergoing laparoscopic cholecystectomy.

[m]For most patients, a mechanical bowel preparation combined with oral neomycin sulfate plus oral erythromycin base or with oral neomycin sulfate plus oral metronidazole should be given in addition to IV prophylaxis.

[n]In cases in which there is increasing resistance to first-generation and second-generation cephalosporins among gram-negative isolates from surgical site infections, a single dose of ceftriaxone plus metronidazole may be preferred over the routine use of carbapenems.

[o]The necessity of continuing topical antimicrobials postoperatively has not been established.

[p]Prophylaxis is not routinely indicated for brachiocephalic procedures. Although there are no data to support it, patients undergoing brachiocephalic procedures involving vascular prostheses or patch implantation (e.g., carotid endarterectomy) may benefit from prophylaxis.

[q]These guidelines reflect recommendations for perioperative antibiotic prophylaxis to prevent surgical site infections and do not provide recommendations for prevention of opportunistic infections in immunosuppressed transplantation patients (e.g., for antifungal or antiviral medications).

[r]Patients who have left ventricular assist devices as a bridge and who experience chronic infection might also benefit from coverage of the infecting microorganism.

[s]The prophylactic regimen may need to be modified to provide coverage against any potential pathogens, including gram-negative (e.g. *Pseudomonas aeruginosa*) or fungal organisms, isolated from the donor lung or the recipient before transplantation. Patients undergoing lung transplantation with negative cultures before transplantation should receive antimicrobial prophylaxis as appropriate for other types of cardiothoracic surgeries. Patients undergoing lung transplantation for cystic fibrosis should receive 7–14 days of treatment with antimicrobials selected according to culture before transplantation and susceptibility results. This treatment may include additional antibacterial or antifungal agents.

[t]The prophylactic regimen may need to be modified to provide coverage against any potential pathogens, including vancomycin-resistant enterococci, isolated from the recipient before transplantation.

Originally from Bratzler DW, Patchen Dellinger E, Olsen KM, et al. Clinical practice guidelines for antimicrobial prophylaxis in surgery. *Surg Infections (Larchmt).* 2013;14(1):73-156.

TABLE 19.18 Clinical Practice Guidelines for Antimicrobial Prophylaxis in Surgery

ANTIMICROBIAL	RECOMMENDED DOSE ADULTS[a]	CHILDREN[b]	HALF-LIFE IN ADULTS WITH NORMAL RENAL FUNCTION (H)[58]	RECOMMENDED REDOSING INTERVAL (FROM INITIATION OF PREOPERATIVE DOSE) (H)[c]
Ampicillin-sulbactam	3 g (ampicillin 2 g/sulbactam 1 g)	50 mg/kg of ampicillin component	0.8–1.3	2
Ampicillin	2 g	50 mg/kg	1–1.9	2
Aztreonam	2 g	30 mg/kg	1.3–2.4	4
Cefazolin	2 g, 3 g for patients weighing ≥120 kg	30 mg/kg	1.2–2.2	4
Cefuroxime	1.5 g	50 mg/kg	1–2	4
Cefotaxime	1 g[d]	50 mg/kg	0.9–1.7	3
Cefoxitin	2 g	40 mg/kg	0.7–1.1	2
Cefotetan	2 g	40 mg/kg	2.8–4.6	6
Ceftriaxone	2 g[e]	50–75 mg/kg	5.4–10.9	NA
Ciprofloxaci[f]	400 mg	10 mg/kg	3–7	NA
Clindamycin	900 mg	10 mg/kg	2–4	6
Ertapenem	1 g	15 mg/kg	3–5	NA
Fluconazole	400 mg	6 mg/kg	30	NA
Gentamicin[g]	5 mg/kg based on dosing weight (single dose)	2.5 mg/kg based on dosing weight	2–3	NA
Levofloxacin[f]	500 mg	10 mg/kg	6–8	NA
Metronidazole	500 mg	15 mg/kg; neonates weighing <1200 g should receive a single 7.5-mg/kg dose	6–8	NA
Moxifloxacin[f]	400 mg	10 mg/kg	8–15	NA
Piperacillin-tazobactam	3.375 g	Infants 2–9 months: 80 mg/kg of piperacillin component. Children >9 months and ≤40 kg: 100 mg/kg of piperacillin component	0.7–1.2	2
Vancomycin	15 mg/kg	15 mg/kg	4–8	NA
Oral Antibiotics for Colorectal Surgery Prophylaxis (Used in Conjunction With Mechanical Bowel Preparation)				
Erythromycin base	1 g	20 mg/kg	0.8–3	NA
Metronidazole	1 g	15 mg/kg	6–10	NA
Neomycin	1 g	15 mg/kg	2–3 (3% absorbed under normal gastrointestinal conditions)	NA

[a]Adult doses are obtained from different studies.

[b]The maximum pediatric dose should not exceed the usual adult dose.

[c]For antimicrobials with a short half-life (e.g., cefazolin, cefoxitin) used before long procedures, redosing in the operating room is recommended at an interval of approximately two times the half-life of the agent in patients with normal renal function. Recommended redosing intervals marked as NA are based on typical case length; for unusually long procedures, redosing may be needed.

[d]Although Food and Drug Administration–approved package insert labeling indicates 1 g, experts recommend 2 g for obese patients.

[e]When used as a single dose in combination with metronidazole for colorectal procedures.

[f]Although fluoroquinolones have been associated with an increased risk of tendinitis or tendon rupture in patients of all ages, use of these agents for single-dose prophylaxis is generally safe.

[g]In general, gentamicin for surgical antibiotic prophylaxis should be limited to a single dose given preoperatively. Dosing is based on the patient's actual body weight. If the patient's actual weight is more than 20% above ideal body weight (IBW), the dosing weight (DW) can be determined as follows: DW = IBW + 0.4 (actual weight − IBW).

NA, Not applicable.

Originally from Bratzler DW, Patchen Dellinger E, Olsen KM, et al. Clinical practice guidelines for antimicrobial prophylaxis in surgery. *Surg Infections (Larchmt).* 2013;14(1):73-156.

Herbal supplements, vitamins, oral contraceptives, and hormonal therapies are often underreported. Estrogen and tamoxifen should be held for 4 weeks preoperatively because of thromboembolic risk. Many herbal medicines can affect perioperative physiology and should be stopped days to weeks before surgery (Table 19.19).

Preoperative Fasting

Bronchopulmonary aspiration can be a life-threatening complication in the perioperative setting. Limiting preoperative oral intake is intended to reduce gastric volume during induction to minimize aspiration risk. There is growing evidence, however, that the traditional protocol of fasting before surgery is not required for aspiration risk reduction. The ASA provided updated practice guidelines for preoperative fasting in 2023. Broadly, clear liquids—with carbohydrate supplementation—are permissible up to 2 hours before elective procedures requiring general anesthesia or procedural sedation. Breast milk may be ingested up to 4 hours before elective procedures. To date, evidence for a specific duration of solid food fasting is lacking. Current guidelines indicate that a light meal may be permissible for up to 6 hours before elective procedures; however, this interval may be lengthened for heavier meals and patients at higher risk for aspiration

(Table 19.20). The ASA does not recommend routine administration of gastrointestinal stimulants, antacids, antiemetics, or anticholinergics to reduce aspiration risk or shorten the recommended preoperative fasting period.

OPERATING ROOM

Adequate preparation of the operating room—to ensure the availability and functionality of systems-based resources (e.g., videoendoscopic accessibility, anesthesia team, blood products) and surgical equipment (e.g., instrument sets, stapler and/or energy devices)—is as critical to a successful operation as appropriate patient selection and preoperative evaluation. Systems-based resources include operating room particulars such as temperature control, presurgical cleaning, and availability of anesthesia, pathology, and consultative services. Appropriate preoperative communication with the anesthesia team is imperative, especially when specific perioperative challenges are anticipated. Examples include patients with high-risk cardiac disease, those with significant underlying liver and/or kidney disease, or patients scheduled for high-risk operations where appropriate intraoperative hemodynamic and volume management is imperative. Recent implementation of patient recovery pathways has standardized many aspects

TABLE 19.19   Perioperative Concerns and Recommendations for Herbal Medicines

COMMON NAME OF HERB	PERIOPERATIVE CONCERNS	RELEVANT PHARMACOLOGIC EFFECT	PREOPERATIVE RECOMMENDATIONS
Echinacea	Allergic reactions, decreased effectiveness of immunosuppressants; potential for immunosuppression with long-term use	Activation of cell-mediated immunity	
Ephedra	Risk for myocardial ischemia and stroke from tachycardia and hypertension; ventricular arrhythmias with halothane: long-term use depletes endogenous catecholamines and may cause intraoperative hemodynamic instability; life-threatening interaction with monoamine oxidase inhibitors	Increased heart rate and blood pressure through direct and indirect sympathomimetic effects	Discontinue at least 24 h before surgery
Garlic	Potential to increase risk for bleeding, especially when combined with other medications that inhibit platelet aggregation	Inhibition of platelet aggregation (may be irreversible); increased fibrinolysis; equivocal hypertensive activity	Discontinue at least 7 days before surgery
Ginkgo	Potential to increase risk for bleeding, especially when combined with other medications that inhibit platelet aggregation	Inhibition of platelet-activating factor	Discontinue at least 36 h before surgery
Ginseng	Hypoglycemia; potential to increase risk for bleeding; potential to decrease anticoagulative effect of warfarin	Lowers blood glucose; inhibition of platelet aggregation (may be irreversible); increased PT/PTT in animals	Discontinue at least 7 days before surgery
Kava	Potential to increase sedative effect of anesthetics; potential for addiction, tolerance, and withdrawal after abstinence unstudied	Sedation, anxiolysis	Discontinue at least 24 h before surgery
St. John's wort	Induction of cytochrome P450 enzymes, with effect on cyclosporine, warfarin, steroids, and protease inhibitors and possibly benzodiazepines, calcium channel blockers, and many other drugs; decreased serum digoxin levels	Inhibition of neurotransmitter uptake, monoamine oxidase inhibition is unlikely	Discontinue at least 5 days before surgery
Valerian	Potential to increase sedative effect of anesthetics; benzodiazepine-like acute withdrawal; potential to increase anesthetic requirements with long-term use	Sedation	No data

PT, Prothrombin time; PTT, partial thromboplastin time.
Originally adapted from Ang-Lee MK, Moss J, Yuan CS. Herbal medicines and perioperative care. *JAMA.* 2001;286(2):208-219.

TABLE 19.20   Recommended Minimum Fasting Periods Between Oral Intake and General Anesthesia for Elective Operations

INGESTED MATERIAL	MINIMUM FASTING PERIOD
Clear liquids	2 hours
Breast milk	4 hours
Infant formula	6 hours
Nonhuman milk	6 hours
Light meal	6 hours
Fried foods and meat	8+ hours

Adapted from Practice Guidelines for Preoperative Fasting and the Use of Pharmacologic Agents to Reduce the Risk of Pulmonary Aspiration: Application to Healthy Patients Undergoing Elective Procedures: An Updated Report by the American Society of Anesthesiologists Task Force on Preoperative Fasting and the Use of Pharmacologic Agents to Reduce the Risk of Pulmonary Aspiration. *Anesthesiology.* 2017; 126(3):376-393.

of anesthetic care; however, active communication between the surgery and anesthesiology teams remains important to ensure the most appropriate intraoperative management. Additional system-based resources include medications and products necessary in the immediate perioperative period such as analgesics, fluids, blood products, antibiotics, anticoagulants, and vasoactive drugs. Also important is the presence of appropriate surgical assistance and backup. Despite diligent preoperative planning, complex operations frequently encounter unforeseen and potentially life-threatening intraoperative challenges. Immediate availability of experienced surgeon partners and consultative services should be verified before every operation.

Although the specific assembly of surgical instruments will always depend on the operation at hand, common equipment should be available for any operation. Expected equipment includes appropriate lighting, a properly functioning operating table, surgical instruments, monitors to display preoperative imaging, a suction mechanism, and coagulation instrumentation. For minimally invasive operations, insufflation equipment, trocars, a camera, video monitors, laparoscopic and/or robotic instruments, and resources should be clearly communicated and verified. Progress in robotic-assisted laparoscopy has delivered significant benefits in the realm of minimally invasive surgery, offering superior visualization, enhanced mechanical capabilities, improved surgeon ergonomics, and complete instrument articulation in comparison to conventional laparoscopy. Robotic surgery, despite its numerous advantages, is not without some limitations. One notable constraint is the high cost of acquiring and maintaining robotic systems. Additionally, the setup and preparation for robotic procedures can be time consuming, leading to longer anesthesia times. Surgeons also require specialized training to operate the systems effectively. Furthermore, there is a lack of tactile feedback in robotic surgery, which may affect the surgeon's ability to sense tissue characteristics.[60]

The patient should be positioned securely while minimizing pressure points to prevent neuromuscular injury. For obese patients and patients in lithotomy position, the risk for extremity compartment syndrome, peripheral nerve injuries, and deep soft tissue injury (i.e., pressure ulcers) should be acknowledged and minimized, particularly for long operations. Fluid-impermeable drapes and gowns should be used to create a sterile barrier between the operative field and the ambient environment.

The importance of communication between the surgery team, anesthesiology team, and operating room nursing staff cannot be overemphasized. Clear dialogue is necessary to improve focus, eliminate or reduce confusion, and enable anticipation. A preoperative time-out process has been implemented in most institutions (Fig. 19.8); it standardizes immediate preoperative preparation of the "surgical team." Continually updating all parties in the operating room regarding key steps of the operation is vital to minimize risk to the patient and reduce delays because of equipment unavailability. Finally, best practice uses closed-loop communication techniques to ensure communication is heard, understood, and acknowledged by all parties.

Maintenance of Normothermia

Thermoregulation is based on systemic input integrated by the central nervous system, primarily the hypothalamus and spinal cord. Under normal conditions, autonomic control regulates core temperature consistently to between 36°C and 38°C. General anesthesia lowers the cold-response threshold of the body. Volatile and intravenous anesthetics impair thermoregulation, paralytics prevent the body's shivering response to hypothermia, and compensatory vasoconstriction is downregulated. Regional neuroaxial anesthesia (e.g., epidural and spinal) further blunts thermoregulatory control by reducing thermal discomfort and blocking efferent nervous control of vasoconstriction and shivering. The effects of general and regional anesthesia are roughly additive[61]; this factor is particularly relevant because of an increase in usage of regional anesthesia as a component of modern ERAS pathways. An additional factor is large-volume cavity exposure (abdominal or thoracic) that significantly contributes to heat loss. Risk of hypothermia is increased in the elderly, females, and the malnourished during long operations.

Consequences of intraoperative hypothermia are myriad. Platelet aggregation and the coagulation cascade are impaired, resulting in an association between hypothermia and nearly a 20% increased operative blood loss. Because of vasoconstriction and the consequent decreased oxygenation of surgical incisions, hypothermia has been associated with an increased rate of wound infection. Finally, hypothermia alters drug actions/metabolism such that the duration of action of many anesthetics is prolonged and correction of acidosis and electrolyte disarray is impaired. Close monitoring of core body temperature throughout the operation is mandatory. The best and most pragmatic monitoring site is the distal esophagus for intubated patients. Sublingual, axillary, and bladder temperatures also correlate well with core body temperature. Conversely, skin, forehead, external aural canal, and rectal temperatures correlate poorly with core temperature.[61]

Hypothermia is most drastic within the first hour after induction because of the rapid effect of anesthesia-induced vasodilation. Therefore, it is during this period that rewarming techniques are most critical. Rewarming can take the form of passive or active methods. Passive insulation (e.g., blankets, sheets) can reduce cutaneous heat loss by roughly 30%. Increasing ambient room temperature can passively mitigate heat loss but is impractical for raising core body temperature. Active warming with forced air is frequently effective during induction and throughout the operation to compensate for rapid thermal dysregulation. Forced air is the most common approach because of its ease of use, effectiveness, and low cost. Contrary to popular belief, intravenous fluid warming is relatively ineffective because infused fluid temperatures cannot significantly exceed the body's core temperature. However, patients can be *cooled* by infusion of ambient-temperature

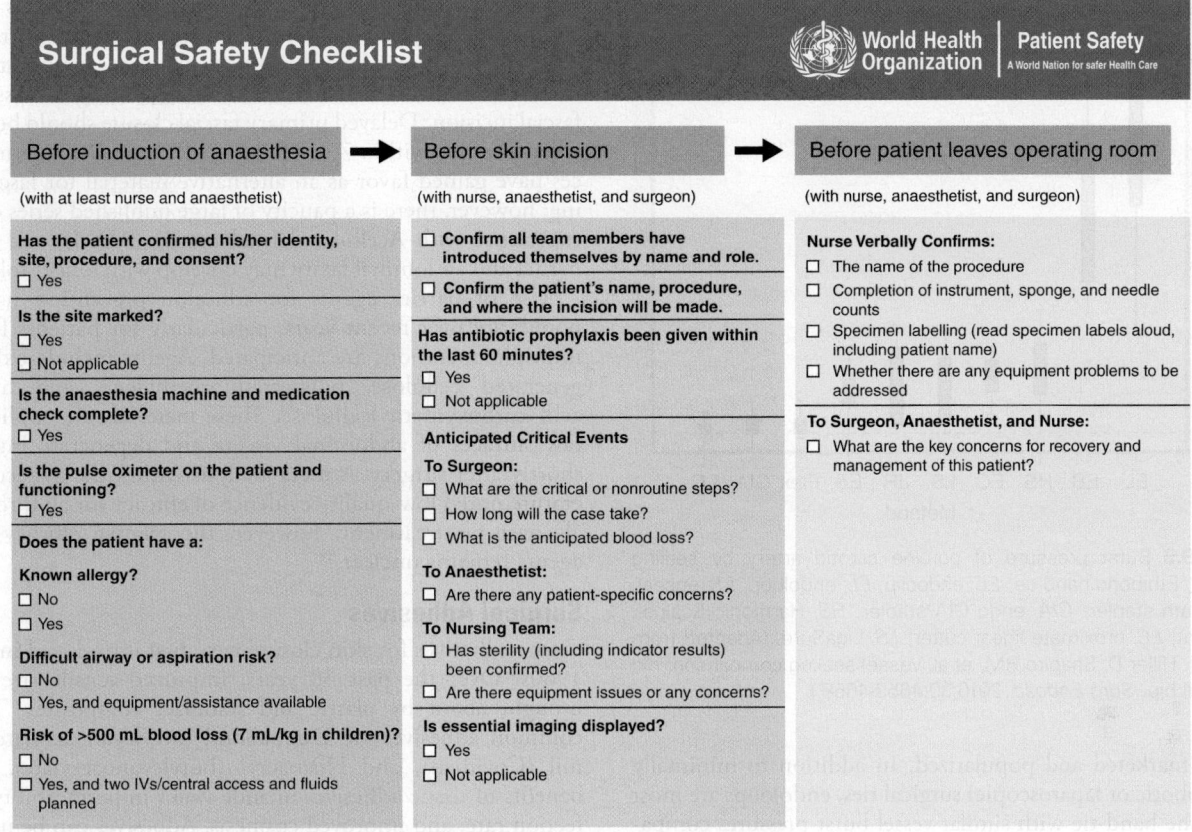

Surgical Safety Checklist

World Health Organization | Patient Safety
A World Nation for safer Health Care

Before induction of anaesthesia ➡ **Before skin incision** ➡ **Before patient leaves operating room**

(with at least nurse and anaesthetist) | (with nurse, anaesthetist, and surgeon) | (with nurse, anaesthetist, and surgeon)

Has the patient confirmed his/her identity, site, procedure, and consent?
☐ Yes

Is the site marked?
☐ Yes
☐ Not applicable

Is the anaesthesia machine and medication check complete?
☐ Yes

Is the pulse oximeter on the patient and functioning?
☐ Yes

Does the patient have a:

Known allergy?
☐ No
☐ Yes

Difficult airway or aspiration risk?
☐ No
☐ Yes, and equipment/assistance available

Risk of >500 mL blood loss (7 mL/kg in children)?
☐ No
☐ Yes, and two IVs/central access and fluids planned

☐ **Confirm all team members have introduced themselves by name and role.**

☐ **Confirm the patient's name, procedure, and where the incision will be made.**

Has antibiotic prophylaxis been given within the last 60 minutes?
☐ Yes
☐ Not applicable

Anticipated Critical Events

To Surgeon:
☐ What are the critical or nonroutine steps?
☐ How long will the case take?
☐ What is the anticipated blood loss?

To Anaesthetist:
☐ Are there any patient-specific concerns?

To Nursing Team:
☐ Has sterility (including indicator results) been confirmed?
☐ Are there equipment issues or any concerns?

Is essential imaging displayed?
☐ Yes
☐ Not applicable

Nurse Verbally Confirms:
☐ The name of the procedure
☐ Completion of instrument, sponge, and needle counts
☐ Specimen labelling (read specimen labels aloud, including patient name)
☐ Whether there are any equipment problems to be addressed

To Surgeon, Anaesthetist, and Nurse:
☐ What are the key concerns for recovery and management of this patient?

FIGURE 19.8 Surgical safety checklist published by the World Health Organization. (From https://www.who.int/patientsafety/safesurgery/checklist/en/.)

fluids, thereby exacerbating anesthesia-induced hypothermia. Therefore, any intraoperative infusion of >1 L/h should be prewarmed.

Preoperative Skin Preparation

SSIs comprise more than 20% of all hospital-acquired infections and are associated with increased length of stay, mortality, and cost.[62] Commensal skin bacteria (e.g., staphylococci, *Pseudomonas*) are responsible for the majority of superficial SSIs. Preoperative antiseptic skin preparation reduces the number of transient and commensal microorganisms. The CDC guidelines recommend the following techniques for application: (1) a wide area to include any potential incision sites, (2) concentric circle motion, (3) use of a dedicated application instrument, and (4) adequate time to allow the solution to dry. Hair removal before incision can improve exposure and allow skin marking. However, hair should only be removed with a clipper because shaving is associated with increased SSI risk.

The benefits of skin preparation depend on the antiseptic solution used. Common solutions include povidone-iodine scrub and paint (Betadine), chlorhexidine-alcohol scrub (ChloraPrep), and iodine povacrylex with isopropyl alcohol (DuraPrep). Alcohol-containing solutions should be avoided for mucosal surfaces. The optimal choice of antiseptic for intact skin remains controversial. Most randomized trials in the past comparing antiseptic solutions are underpowered. A Cochrane review in 2015 indicated that alcohol-containing products have the greatest probability of being effective but noted the overall low quality of evidence.[63] A multi-institutional randomized comparison of chlorhexidine-alcohol versus povidone-iodine scrub and paint for clean-contaminated surgeries found a lower rate of SSI in the chlorhexidine-alcohol group (9.5% vs. 16.1%).[64] Recently, a single-institution randomized trial of colorectal operations failed to conclude noninferiority of DuraPrep compared with ChloraPrep, with SSI rates of 18.7% versus 15.9%, respectively. Therefore, based on these data, a skin preparation that contains an alcohol-based agent as part of the preparation appears optimal.

Hemostasis

Meticulous dissection and intimate knowledge of surgical anatomy are mandatory for minimization of intraoperative blood loss. Surgical bleeding obscures the operative field, prolongs operating time, increases hemodynamic stress, induces coagulopathy, and makes postoperative resuscitation more challenging. For certain cancers, perioperative blood transfusion has consistently been associated with an increased risk of recurrence and a decrease in survival.

Although capillaries and small veins can be controlled and divided with monopolar electrocautery alone, vessels >1 mm in diameter—including all named vessels—are best controlled with ties, clips, staples, bipolar electrocautery, or ultrasonic devices. To prevent dislodgement of ties or clips, larger vessels may be controlled by suture ligation. Traditionally, vascular structures are ligated with permanent suture material, though use of absorbable sutures has not been associated with increased risk of bleeding or reoperation. With the rapid expansion of minimally invasive operations and the associated explosion in manufactured surgical devices, numerous alternatives to the traditional hand-tied ligation

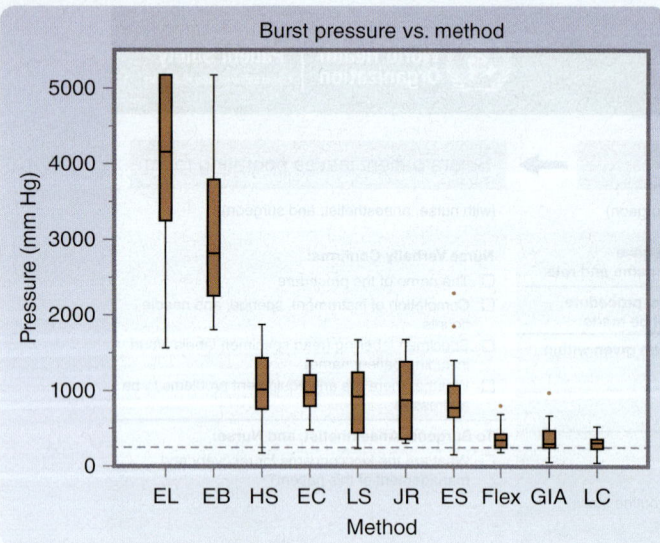

FIGURE 19.9 Burst pressure of porcine carotid artery by sealing method. *EB*, Ethibond hand-tie; *EC*, endoclip; *EL*, endoloop; *ES*, enseal; *Flex*, endopath stapler; *GIA*, endo GIA stapler; *HS*, Harmonic Scalpel; *JR*, JustRight; *LC*, proximate linear cutter; *LS*, LigaSure. (Adapted from Tharakan SJ, Hiller D, Shapiro RM, et al. Vessel sealing comparison: old school is still hip. *Surg Endosc.* 2016;30:4653-4658.)

have been marketed and popularized. In addition to minimally invasive (robotic or laparoscopic) surgical ties, endoloops are most similar to the hand-tie with similar vessel burst pressures comparable to hand-ties.[65] On the other end of the spectrum, stapling devices armed with vascular staple loads tolerate lower—but still supraphysiologic—burst pressures (Fig. 19.9).

Wound Closure

In general, incisions for clean and clean-contaminated operations can be closed primarily. Primary fascial closure can use permanent or dissolvable sutures using running or interrupted techniques. Permanent sutures are best suited for malnourished, debilitated patients and for scenarios in which early outpatient follow-up is anticipated. Dissolvable sutures, particularly when used in the subcuticular layer, can often create a cosmetically appealing closure that does not require suture removal. When an incision is anticipated to be under significant tension, vertical mattress sutures distribute tension over two levels of depth at every longitudinal point and approximate the dermal layers effectively. Running suture techniques—especially when used across multiple layers—are more effective at controlling ascites, and interrupted sutures allow intermittent wound packing for incisions at high risk for superficial SSI.

Delayed primary closure may be suitable for carefully selected patients after contaminated operations. Delayed closure is commonly attempted between 2 and 5 days after the index operation. Although there is some evidence that delayed primary closure is associated with a reduction in SSI compared with primary closure, there is substantial heterogeneity across existing trials.[66] Heavily contaminated dirty surgical wounds should be left open, allowing for healing by secondary intent with serial packing. Management of open wounds during the outpatient recovery period can often be facilitated by applying a negative pressure vacuum device.

Although covered in depth elsewhere (Chapter 37), temporary closure of abdominal incisions is useful when a short-interval second-look laparotomy is anticipated, when there is threat of compartment syndrome, and when monitoring of intraabdominal contents is prudent. In almost all cases, temporary closure involves a nonadherent material used as a bridge across an open fascial incision. Delayed primary fascial closure should be achieved when possible within 7 to 10 days.[67] Bioprosthetic dermal matrices have gained favor as an alternative material for fascial bridging; however, there is a paucity of large published series capturing experience with Acellular dermal matrix (ADM), and recurrent hernia and abdominal laxity may develop with longer follow-up.[68]

Use of barrier agents for adhesion prevention has gained popularity over recent years, particularly for patients for whom multiple operations are anticipated. Agents include oxidized regenerated cellulose, polytetrafluoroethylene, and hyaluronic acid–carboxymethylcellulose. These materials are applied to the raw surfaces of abdominal viscera and degenerate into gelatin shortly after surgery. A meta-analysis within the gynecologic literature noted low-quality evidence of efficacy for all three materials over no treatment; however, the relative efficacy between agents remains unclear.[69]

Surgical Adhesives

Tissue adhesives for skin closure were first introduced in the early 1960s. Over the past 30 years, improved tensile strength was brought about by plastic and stabilizer composites. The most common adhesives are Dermabond (octylcyanoacrylate), Indermil (Covidien), and Histoacryl (butylcyanoacrylate). Inherent benefits of tissue adhesives include water impermeability, low infection rate, and improved cosmesis. Adhesives can be used without skin sutures for small incisions and are commonly adopted in this manner in the emergency room or outpatient setting. For larger incisions, tissue adhesives are more commonly used to provide a watertight barrier after subcuticular or dermal closure with absorbable suture. A recent meta-analysis found no significant difference between tissue adhesives and sutures in terms of dehiscence, infection, and surgeon-rated cosmesis.[70]

Fibrin sealant confers both adhesive and hemostatic functions. Blood bank–derived fibrin sealant functions by combining thrombin and fibrinogen to replicate the final step in the clotting cascade. Because the agent contains all necessary components for this reaction, it forms a clot regardless of a patient's intrinsic pathway status. Randomized trials have found the addition of fibrin sealant to be superior to manual compression alone in controlling anastomotic hemorrhage after placement of polytetrafluoroethylene vascular grafts.[71] Although fibrin sealant has also been approved as an adjunct for gastrointestinal anastomoses, application for this purpose has not gained widespread popularity, and there are conflicting results in the literature as to a clinical benefit.[72] Fibrin agents have been adopted for a variety of other clinical applications. For perianal fistulae, fibrin glue avoids an adverse impact on continence; however, it exhibits inferior durability compared with conventional surgical treatment. Fibrin glue has been used to treat bronchopleural fistulae, either as a direct injection of fibrinogen followed by topical thrombin or as a diluted pleurodesis agent.

SURGICAL DEVICES, ENERGY SOURCES, AND STAPLERS

Technologic advances in energy devices and tissue stapling have revolutionized the way surgeons approach dissection, division, hemostasis, and reconstruction. As a whole, energy devices direct focused energy to the target tissue with the purpose of dissection and division, coagulation, or ablation and cytotoxicity. Stapling devices are traditionally used for alimentary tract division and anastomosis but can also be used for vascular and tissue transection. This section focuses on some of the common energy and stapling devices encountered in the operating room.

Electrosurgery and Electrocautery

Although use of electricity to induce thermal cauterization and tissue division has been reported since the mid-1800s, modern electrosurgery as we know it was introduced between 1914 and 1927 by William T Bovie. Diathermy—first described by Karl Franz in 1909—uses high-frequency electric currents to generate heat and penetrate tissues. Bovie developed a commercially available alternating current cautery device between 1914 and 1927, and Harvey Cushing popularized it with a 1928 report of 500 neurosurgical procedures.

Monopolar Electrosurgery

In strict terms, electrocautery implies thermal conduction via a probe heated by a direct electrical current. In modern surgery, this technology most commonly is seen with portable, pen-type cautery devices that function like a soldering iron. Electrosurgery, on the other hand, indicates conduction of an alternating radiofrequency current through a circuit that is completed by the patient's tissue. However, these two terms are often used interchangeably. Classically, monopolar electrosurgery is performed using a current generator, a handheld electrode that delivers current to the patient, and a second large electrode (the "pad") that returns current to complete the circuit. The application electrode has a small area of contact, resulting in focused thermal conversion, while the returning electrode has a large surface area to dissipate energy. With a continuous waveform ("cut" mode), the monopolar device cuts through tissue with little thermal spread and minimal coagulation. With an intermittent waveform ("coagulation" mode), current is delivered over less than 10% of the time that the device is activated and is interspersed with short periods of inactivity. The result is lower thermal energy and greater thermal spread, resulting in tissue dehydration and vessel thrombosis. Many surgeons adopt a blended waveform setting ("blend" mode), which replaces the pure cutting function with small periods of current inactivity to achieve a partial coagulative effect.

Bipolar Electrosurgery

Bipolar devices place the delivering and returning electrodes in close proximity in a single device. In this way, the tissue in between the two electrodes completes the electric circuit. A grounding pad is unnecessary, and thermal spread beyond the tissue between the two electrodes is minimal. By compressing vascularized tissue using bipolar forceps, blood is excluded from the circuit, improving heat delivery to the compressed tissue. Bipolar devices are most useful when precise coagulation is necessary in close proximity to vital structures. Because current is only delivered across tissue between the two handheld electrodes, bipolar devices are safe to use when a patient has an implanted electronic device that may otherwise be affected by the delivery of monopolar current.

Bipolar Fusion Devices

An adaptation of bipolar electrosurgery is the bipolar fusion device such as LigaSure and Enseal. Similar to conventional bipolar electrosurgery, these tissue dissection and division devices transmit current between two adjacent electrodes, causing tissue coagulation. By applying uniform compression of the target tissue and monitoring tissue impedance between the jaws of the instrument, these devices adjust energy delivery during the activation process to minimize thermal spread and seal larger vessels (up to 7 mm). Denaturation followed by cross-linking of collagen and elastin results in a natural tissue sealant. A blade within the instrument then divides the sealed tissue.

Saline-Cooled Radiofrequency Dissectors

A commonly encountered problem when using radiofrequency electrosurgery within highly vascularized parenchyma is the formation of dense eschar that limits coagulation and may result in delayed hemorrhage. Eschar formation occurs when temperature at the contact surface of the target tissue exceeds what is necessary for protein denaturation and vessel sealing. Saline-cooled radiofrequency dissectors (i.e., TissueLink, Aquamantys) overcome this issue by directing a steady irrigation stream of saline to the tissue contact point, thereby maintaining surface temperature <105°C. These devices are used mostly during dissection of solid organ parenchyma such as the liver or kidney. Initial division of the organ capsule is necessary (often by traditional Bovie electrosurgery) to prevent steam buildup beneath the capsule. Constant pressure with the saline-linked device is then used to achieve a constant depth of coagulation before sharp transection of the denatured tissue or clipping of larger vessels within the treatment zone.

Ultrasonic Dissectors

A distinction should be made between the use of high-frequency oscillation instruments and true ultrasonic energy technology. The classic example of therapeutic ultrasound is extracorporeal shock wave lithotripsy, through which high-energy acoustic shock waves are directed at pathologic stones to shatter material and facilitate passage. Although lithotripsy has historically been applied to symptomatic cholelithiasis, current applications are primarily focused on urologic stones and pancreatic duct stones. Shock wave lithotripsy is effective primarily for smaller stones (<2 cm) with lower radiographic density.

Harmonic Scalpel

The Harmonic Scalpel transduces high-frequency ultrasonic energy through a metallic jaw to generate mechanical vibration. When in contact with tissue, the vibration of a single blade against a static blade results in vaporization and coagulation. The coagulation effect is increased by compressing the target tissue between the two jaws of the instrument. The energy transduced through the metallic jaw is modifiable; high energy settings result in rapid cutting, whereas low energy promotes coagulation. Because the mechanism for the scalpel is vibration, the instrument divides tissue without the need for a separate cutting blade.

Cavitron Ultrasound Surgical Aspirator

The cavitron ultrasound surgical aspirator (CUSA) uses ultrasonic frequency vibration to selectively dissect parenchymal tissue. The device directs ultrasonic frequency along a hollow titanium tip that vibrates longitudinally to fragment target tissue. Hepatocytes are particularly susceptible to oscillatory fragmentation because of their high-water content, whereas endothelium and epithelium (blood vessels, bile ducts) are selectively spared because of low water content. The CUSA provides a precise dissection plane through this fragmentation process but does not itself confer any vessel-sealing capability. The CUSA tip can be connected to a monopolar electrocautery circuit for tissue ablation and is generally used in conjunction with adjunct methods of hemostasis.

Ablation Technology

Radiofrequency Ablation

Radiofrequency energy delivered via a narrow probe is termed *radiofrequency ablation (RFA)*. Applications include esophageal dysplasia, atrial fibrillation, and tumors found within solid organ parenchyma. The RFA probe can be directed toward target tissue via a percutaneous approach or during open or laparoscopic surgery. The electrode at the probe tip transmits high-frequency alternating current to the surrounding tissue, which is converted to kinetic and thermal energy and results in denaturation and coagulation. Because RFA has a similar mechanism as electrosurgery, a grounding pad is necessary, and the presence of implantable electronic devices or metallic surgical clips may be a contraindication. Tissue eschar formation surrounding the electrode has an insulator effect and limits the effective radius of RFA. When performed near a blood vessel, thermal energy is dispersed rapidly from the target tissue, creating a "heat sink" and limiting efficacy. Typically, tumors up to 3 cm can be effectively ablated by RFA; an additional margin of 0.5 cm of healthy parenchyma beyond the target lesion should be ablated to ensure complete ablation of the tumor.

Microwave Ablation

Microwave energy lies between infrared and radio waves in terms of frequency. The impact between microwave energy radiation and polar molecules such as water result in oscillation and frictional heat. Applied to target tissue, the outcome is cell death through coagulative necrosis. Like RFA, microwave ablation (MWA) can be performed percutaneously or during open or minimally invasive surgery and is generally image guided via ultrasound or CT. Advantages over RFA include a larger, more homogeneous zone of ablation, an attenuated heat-sink effect, and less time needed to complete ablation. Because the mechanism of microwave ablation does not involve transmission of electric current, a grounding pad is unnecessary, and use in the presence of metallic clips and implants is safe. Given advantages over RFA without proven disadvantages, MWA is rising in popularity as the preferred technology for tumor ablation in solid organs, including the liver and kidney.

Other Energy Devices

Argon Beam Coagulator

Argon beam coagulation (ABC) was introduced in 1989. Despite its name, ABC is not a laser device, but rather an adaptation of monopolar electrosurgery. A focused beam of argon gas—a strong conductor of electricity—is directed at target tissue. Radiofrequency current is transported from a monopolar electrode to the tissue across this pathway of argon gas. Advantages of ABC over conventional electrosurgery include more rapid activity, shallower penetration, and faster heat dispersion.[73] Moreover, the focused jet of argon gas physically disperses blood from the target tissue, providing a dry environment to promote coagulation and reduce eschar formation. For these reasons, ABC is most suitable for achieving hemostasis over surfaces of solid organ parenchyma, such as the spleen, liver, kidney, lung, and peritoneum. Because of its low depth of penetration, ABC is ineffective for control of larger blood vessels. Moreover, the focused jet of argon gas is insoluble in blood, and direct targeting of central veins can result

in cardiac arrest caused by air (argon) embolism. To minimize this risk, surgeons should keep the flow rate of argon gas low, use an angled approach toward the tissue, and avoid direct argon gas deployment into large veins in direct communication with right atrium.

Surgical Staplers

The surgical stapling device was invented in 1907–08 in Budapest, Austria-Hungary. After initial modifications to decrease weight and complexity in the 1920s, surgical staplers were further modified and popularized for use in alimentary tract surgery in the Soviet Union between the 1940s and 1950s. In 1958, a Soviet model of the surgical stapler was brought to the United States. These initial staplers were hand-made with noninterchangeable parts and required loading of individual staples by hand. Development and commercialization of surgical staplers occurred in the United States in the 1960s and 1970s. Designs were optimized for mass production, including interchangeable and disposable stapler cartridges of various staple heights.

At present, a multitude of different surgical staplers can facilitate tissue closure, division, and reconstruction during open, laparoscopic, and robotic operations. Linear cutting staplers (gastrointestinal anastomosis [GIA]) vary in length and staple height to accommodate closure, transection, and reconstruction of variable-thickness tissues. Similarly, linear noncutting staplers (thoracoabdominal [TA]) allow tissue closure without division. Circular cutting staplers (end-to-end anastomosis [EEA]) allow luminal anastomosis and transection of hollow viscera of variable diameters. In terms of staple height, smaller staples (open: 2 mm; closed: 1 mm) are best suited for vascular closure and/or transection, whereas large staples (open: 4.5 mm; closed: 2 mm) are well suited for closure and/or transection of thicker tissues such as the stomach or pancreas. Several in-between staple heights are commercially available for use in intermediate tissue types.

POTENTIAL CAUSES OF INTRAOPERATIVE INSTABILITY

With appropriate patient selection and perioperative preparation, untoward events in the operating room should be rare. Management of rare events, however, requires preparation and anticipation. This section addresses common and potentially deadly causes of intraoperative instability including etiology and management strategies.

Malignant Hyperthermia

Malignant hyperthermia (MH) is an acute episode of hypermetabolism in response to volatile halogenated anesthetic gases (e.g., sevoflurane, isoflurane, and others) and the depolarizing paralytic succinylcholine. Symptoms of MH can occur at any time during general anesthesia or up to 60 minutes after cessation of anesthesia. Intraoperative and/or postoperative manifestations can include fever/hyperthermia, tachycardia, tachypnea, increase in exhaled carbon dioxide, rhabdomyolysis, and metabolic disarray, including hyperkalemia and acidosis. An increase in end-tidal carbon dioxide despite an increase in minute ventilation is one of the earliest intraoperative harbingers of MH. The prevalence of MH has been reported to range from 1 in 10,000 to 1 in 250,000 anesthetic cases. However, prevalence among susceptible individuals with "at-risk" genetic abnormalities is considerably higher. Several genetic mutations that predispose patients to MH have been described (most commonly, a mutation in the *RYR1* gene); the majority of these mutations are autosomal dominant with incomplete penetrance.

When suspected, MH is treated by immediate discontinuation of volatile gases, intravenous administration of dantrolene in doses of 2.5 mg/kg, and body cooling using any available routes. Dantrolene can be redosed every 10 to 15 minutes for ongoing fever, acidosis, and muscle rigidity. Other supportive measures include therapy for arrhythmias, hyperkalemia, and acidosis. Typically, management and observation in the ICU are warranted. With current advances, mortality with MH has decreased from 60% to 80% a few decades ago to less than 5%.

Gas Embolus: Air and Carbon Dioxide

Air embolus is a potentially fatal complication of vascular operations. Similarly, CO_2 embolus can be a fatal complication of minimally invasive laparoscopic or robotic operations. Both are a result of air or CO_2 entering the systemic, most often venous, circulation. In cases of air embolus, air access to the venous system can occur via a planned venotomy during vascular access cases or during repair of great vessels. In contrast, CO_2 embolus occurs more commonly as an unplanned insufflation of gas into the systemic venous circulation. In both cases, an abrupt decrease in end-tidal CO_2 and cardiovascular collapse are the first manifestations, and rapid recognition of symptoms and institution of resuscitative measures are indicated.

In cases of intraoperative cardiovascular collapse because of air or CO_2 embolus, maneuvers allowing access between gas and the vascular system must be terminated. Additionally, cardiopulmonary resuscitation, including pharmacologic agents and mechanical cardiopulmonary resuscitation, have the best chance to achieve return of spontaneous circulation. Intraoperative transesophageal echocardiography can help confirm the diagnosis and measure the amount of gas trapped within the right heart. If there is appropriate vascular access in the right heart, air aspiration can be attempted. Although the Trendelenburg position may be helpful, placing the patient in left lateral decubitus position should only be used in the absence of cardiovascular collapse, as meaningful chest compressions cannot be performed in patients who are not supine. Patients with a patent foramen ovale are at risk for collapse of left ventricular function as well as gas-mediated cerebral embolus. Mortality in patients with gas embolus is approximately 20%.

Myocardial Infarction, Pulmonary Embolus, and Pneumothorax

With appropriate preoperative evaluation, both intraoperative MI and intraoperative PE are rare complications among patients selected for elective general surgery operations. Incidences of both are higher in urgent/emergent operations and operations for traumatic injury. Intraoperative monitoring can demonstrate signs of hemodynamic instability (e.g., tachycardia, hypotension). ECG changes and dysrhythmias are frequently harbingers of cardiac ischemia and/or infarction. Classic ECG changes (e.g., new profound ST elevation) are diagnostic; serum troponin levels can be used to corroborate the diagnosis in hemodynamically stable patients. In the event of a suspected MI and hemodynamic instability, nonemergent operations should be aborted.

PE is rarely suspected when hemodynamic instability is absent. In most cases, for the diagnosis to be considered, intraoperative symptoms include significant tachycardia, hypotension, hypoxia despite high oxygen fraction, and/or cardiovascular collapse.

Transesophageal echocardiography can be rapidly used to evaluate for presence of right ventricular dilatation/failure and "right heart strain." In the absence of right heart strain, a clinically significant PE is less likely; with clinically significant right heart strain, right heart failure resulting from MI, PE, and pneumothorax should be under consideration. Treatment of intraoperative PE (systemic anticoagulation vs. directed pharmacologic or mechanical thrombolysis) depends on the clinical symptoms; however, in the presence of hemodynamic instability, elective operations should be terminated.

The etiology of an intraoperative pneumothorax is multifactorial. Interventions leading to pneumothorax include central venous access resulting in iatrogenic lung injury; high ventilator volume/pressure, particularly in patients with mainstem bronchial intubation; diaphragmatic injury; and high insufflation pressures during laparoscopy. For patients with large amounts of intrapleural air, hemodynamic instability may be present when sufficient tension is present that increases mediastinal pressures that impede central venous return. The diagnosis can be made by chest auscultation and/or intraabdominal inspection of the diaphragm. In patients without breath sounds and/or a bulging diaphragm, tube thoracostomy is indicated and should lead to symptomatic improvement. If symptoms have resolved and clinical signs of pneumothorax have been reversed, a surgeon may consider completing the ongoing elective operation.

Hemorrhage

When major vascular injuries occur, rapid blood loss into the operative field can be life threatening and difficult to control. Exposure is immediately compromised, and the next surgical steps should focus on vascular control. If arterial injury is suspected, direct compression and proximal control are frequently the best first steps. Control can often be achieved by compression, proximal vascular isolation and clamping, or a combination of these maneuvers with subsequent vascular repair.

When compression is not possible and/or the major artery cannot be readily dissected, proximal control with supraceliac aortic compression can be achieved quickly by caudal retraction of the stomach, brief mobilization of the left lobe of the liver, division of the gastrohepatic ligament, and compression of the aorta (located just to the left of the esophagus) against the vertebrae. Hands-free control can then be applied by incising the peritoneum, separating the limbs of the right diaphragmatic crus to expose the thoracic aorta, and applying an aortic clamp. These measures facilitate exposure of the vascular injury under a controlled environment and allow anesthesiology colleagues to catch up with resuscitation. Endovascular balloon occlusion of the aorta is also an option for patients with femoral arterial access, and those familiar with this technology often use it in trauma and vascular operations.

In patients with major venous injury, compression of the venotomy combined with direct suture repair is frequently possible. In cases where significant bleeding precludes sufficient visualization of the venotomy, venous compression proximal and distal to the site of injury will help with visualization. Adequate intraoperative exposure and retraction are paramount in any operation. The best preparation for management of vascular injury is sufficient dissection and exposure to allow for management of a vascular injury before hemorrhage and exsanguination.

Under some circumstances, particularly in trauma surgery, multiple sites of bleeding, coagulopathy (from hypothermia, prolonged bleeding, sepsis, or acidosis), and hemodynamic instability can create a scenario in which definitive control of all sites of bleeding may be impossible or impractical. Resuscitation with blood and blood products has been well established in trauma resuscitation[74] and should be used in nontrauma patients with intraoperative hemorrhage; crystalloid should not be used. These patients with intraoperative hemorrhage, clinical instability, and coagulopathy are best served with blood product resuscitation and temporary abdominal packing, followed by ongoing resuscitation in an intensive care setting. Delayed definitive hemostasis can then be achieved under more controlled conditions, either with a return to the operating room or through angiographic embolization.

OUTPATIENT SURGERY

Over recent decades, the volume of operations performed in the outpatient setting has increased dramatically. Driving forces behind this change include improvements in risk assessment and perioperative management, cost differences between outpatient/ambulatory and inpatient/hospital-based care, patient satisfaction, and increased use of ambulatory surgery centers. Ambulatory surgery centers have expanded access to outpatient surgery for patients with suitable operative criteria without associated increases in postoperative mortality or unanticipated admission. Nevertheless, surgeons should determine indications for surgery independent of the operative setting and resist physician-induced demand.[75] Implemented appropriately, outpatient surgery can reduce time away from work and improve patient perception of the postoperative recovery process. However, surgeons and consulting services must exercise caution when selecting patients and cases for the outpatient setting.

The process of preoperative assessment for outpatient surgery should be tailored to the patient and type of operation. In general, only low-risk and some intermediate-risk operations are appropriate in the outpatient setting. Examples include elective orthopedic and plastic operations in patients who will not require postoperative hospitalization, inguinal herniorrhaphy, elective cholecystectomy, superficial excisions, and several head-and-neck and orthopedic operations. Patient risk factors should be assessed preoperatively. For patients with ASA status I to II undergoing low-risk operations, assessments may take place on the day before surgery or even the morning of surgery. Higher-risk patients should undergo assessment in a dedicated preoperative anesthesia clinic, and sufficient time between assessment and day of surgery should be allocated to allow for additional testing, if necessary.

The goals of preoperative evaluation for outpatient surgery are (1) assessment of appropriateness for the outpatient setting, (2) use of direct preoperative testing and risk stratification, and (3) reduction in cancellations on the day of surgery. Preoperative assessment can be performed by a physician, advanced practice provider (NP/PA), nurse, or via standardized questionnaires. Although physician assessments are reliable and comprehensive, they are also the costliest. Conversely, questionnaire assessments are inexpensive but rely on the patient's own perception of health. When nurse- or questionnaire-based assessments are used, reassessment on the day of surgery by either a surgeon or anesthesiologist is advisable. Risk factors associated with unplanned admission or early postoperative mortality in patients selected for an outpatient operation include advanced age, prior recent hospitalization, and invasiveness of the operation.[28]

Certain populations require additional considerations when assessing appropriateness for outpatient surgery. In general, patients with significant cardiopulmonary comorbidity in whom system-specific or other comorbid conditions have not been optimized are not suitable for outpatient surgery. Obese and morbidly obese patients are at increased risk for bronchospasm, hypoventilation, and obstructive airway, but are not strictly prohibited from outpatient operations; however, severe class III obesity with BMI >60 kg/m^2 can be considered an absolute exclusion. Organ system–specific exclusion criteria may include cardiac (unstable angina, at-risk myocardium, cardiomyopathy, moderate to severe heart failure, severe pulmonary hypertension or valvular disease); pulmonary (noncompliant OSA, STOP-BANG ≥5 with anticipation for postoperative opioids, severe and poorly controlled asthma, cystic fibrosis, or home oxygen use); hematologic (coagulation disorders requiring postoperative infusion of clotting factors and/or procoagulants); renal (end-stage renal disease and additional organ system dysfunction, too long or too short of an interval between dialysis and operation, uncertain serum potassium or serum potassium >5.5); pregnancy-specific exclusions (complicated pregnancy, fetus >21 weeks' gestation); and other high-risk patient comorbidities (muscular dystrophy, highly contagious airborne infections, e.g., tuberculosis, high risk for hemorrhage, and others). Patients with chronic reflux, difficult airway, or poorly controlled diabetes are at heightened risk of anesthesia-related complications and should be considered for outpatient surgery only at centers with capabilities for postoperative admission.

Patients considered for outpatient surgery should have adequate supportive resources after discharge. After sedation, a patient should not be responsible for transportation home and should have an adult to take them home and be available overnight to provide help if needed. Ideally, emergency care facilities should be readily accessible near the patient's residence should unforeseen complications arise. Absence of these outpatient resources should prompt consideration of elective postoperative hospitalization for observation.

SELECTED REFERENCES

Bilimoria KY, Liu Y, Paruch JL, et al. Development and evaluation of the universal ACS NSQIP surgical risk calculator: a decision aid and informed consent tool for patients and surgeons. *J Am Coll Surg*. 2013;217(5):833-842.e1.

> Study summarizing development and implementation of the American College of Surgeons National Surgical Quality Improvement Surgical Risk Calculator. The risk calculator is available online to estimate patient-specific postoperative risk of selected morbidities and mortality: https://riskcalculator.facs.org/RiskCalculator/about.html.

Canet J, Gallart L, Gomar C, et al. Prediction of postoperative pulmonary complications in a population-based surgical cohort. *Anesthesiology*. 2010;113(6):1338-1350.

> A large prospective study summarizing risk factors associated with postoperative pulmonary complications.

Chow WB, Rosenthal RA, Merkow RP, et al. Optimal preoperative assessment of the geriatric surgical patient: a best practices guideline from the American College of Surgeons National Surgical Quality Improvement Program and the American Geriatrics Society. *J Am Coll Surg*. 2012;215(4):453-466.

Summary of the best practice management guidelines for geriatric surgical patients developed in collaboration between the American Geriatrics Society and American College of Surgeons National Surgical Quality Improvement Program.

Devereaux PJ, Mrkobrada M, Sessler DI, et al. Aspirin in patients undergoing noncardiac surgery. *N Engl J Med*. 2014;370(16): 1494-1503.

A randomized controlled trial demonstrating no significant protective effect of aspirin on 30-day mortality or nonfatal myocardial infarction in patients undergoing perioperative noncardiac surgery.

Douketis JD, Spyropoulos AC, Kaatz S, et al. Perioperative bridging anticoagulation in patients with atrial fibrillation. *N Engl J Med*. 2015;373(9):823-833.

A randomized controlled trial establishing the safety of foregoing bridging anticoagulation for patients with atrial fibrillation requiring temporary interruption of chronic anticoagulation for an elective invasive procedure or operation.

Douketis JD, Spyropoulos AC, Spencer FA, et al. Perioperative management of antithrombotic therapy: Antithrombotic Therapy and Prevention of Thrombosis, 9th ed: American College of Chest Physicians Evidence-Based Clinical Practice Guidelines. *Chest*. 2012;141(suppl 2):e326S-e350S.

Summary of the best practice guidelines for management of antithrombotic medications in prevention of venous thromboembolism.

Fleisher LA, Fleischmann KE, Auerbach AD, et al. 2014 ACC/AHA guideline on perioperative cardiovascular evaluation and management of patients undergoing noncardiac surgery: a report of the American College of Cardiology/American Heart Association Task Force on practice guidelines. *J Am Coll Cardiol*. 2014;64(22):e77-e137.

Summary of the best practice management guidelines for preoperative cardiovascular evaluation and management developed in collaboration between the American College of Cardiology and American Heart Association Task Force.

Holst LB, Haase N, Wetterslev J, et al. Lower versus higher hemoglobin threshold for transfusion in septic shock. *N Engl J Med*. 2014;371(15):1381-1391.

A randomized controlled trial demonstrating safety of lower packed red blood cell transfusion threshold (7 g/dL) among critically ill patients with septic shock.

Lee TH, Marcantonio ER, Mangione CM, et al. Derivation and prospective validation of a simple index for prediction of cardiac risk of major noncardiac surgery. *Circulation*. 1999;100(10):1043-1049.

Study summarizing development and validation of the Revised Cardiac Risk Index, which has served as a backbone for study and risk stratification of patients considered for elective operation.

Steinberg JP, Braun BI, Hellinger WC, et al. Timing of antimicrobial prophylaxis and the risk of surgical site infections: results from the Trial to Reduce Antimicrobial Prophylaxis Errors. *Ann Surg*. 2009;250(1):10-16.

Study summarizing association between timing of administration of antimicrobial prophylaxis and postoperative surgical site infection.

The full reference list appears on Elsevier eBooks+.

Anesthesiology Principles, Pain Management, and Sedation

Aditi Balakrishna, Monica Bhutiani, and Christina J. Hayhurst

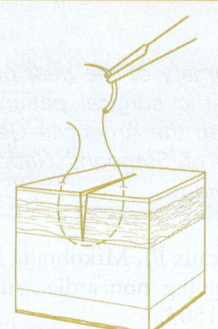

OUTLINE

INTRODUCTION OF ANESTHESIOLOGY PRINCIPLES

In 1846, the first public surgery with ether anesthetic heralded the era of modern anesthesiology. Over the next century, the risk of anesthesia-related mortality and morbidity was unacceptably high due to primitive equipment, complication-prone drugs, and lack of adequate monitors.

In recent decades, however, rapid pharmacologic and technologic advances have resulted in the ability to safely provide anesthesia for complex surgical procedures, even in patients with severe underlying disease. Pharmacologic advances include shorter-acting drugs with fewer deleterious side effects. From an equipment standpoint, anesthesia machines now have safety mechanisms to prevent delivery of hypoxic gas mixtures, and their associated ventilators can provide precise and sophisticated respiratory support. Vaporizers for inhalational anesthetics can now

deliver reliably accurate doses of these medications. Advanced airway devices can facilitate ventilation and intubation in difficult airway scenarios. Improvements in ultrasound have facilitated the safe and effective execution of peripheral nerve blocks, as well as difficult venous and arterial access, and have shepherded in the use of point-of-care ultrasound for diagnosis and monitoring in the perioperative environment. Other significant improvements in monitoring devices include in-circuit oxygen analyzers, capnometers to assess exhaled carbon dioxide (CO_2), pulse oximeters, and anesthetic vapor-specific analyzers.

This chapter begins with a discussion of foundational anesthetic topics (i.e., the drugs, equipment, and monitors requisite for safe practice) followed by discussion of preanesthetic assessment and preparation for anesthesia, selection of anesthetic techniques and drugs, airway management, conscious sedation, postanesthetic care, and management of acute postoperative pain.

PHARMACOLOGIC PRINCIPLES

Early anesthetic strategy used single drugs—such as ether or chloroform—to achieve all anesthetic end points, including hypnosis, cessation of movement, amnesia, and analgesia. The modern approach is more balanced, using medications along with techniques such as neuraxial or regional anesthesia to achieve anesthetic goals while minimizing the side-effect burden of each intervention. Most anesthesiologists initiate anesthesia with intravenous (IV) medications and maintain it with either inhalational or IV agents supplemented by pain management adjuncts, anxiolytics, and paralytic medications. The high-level benefits and drawbacks to the most used medications in these classes will be explored below.

Inhalational Agents

Inhalational anesthetics pass into the patient's bloodstream at the alveolar-capillary interface and exert their effects on receptors in the central nervous system (CNS). The exact mechanisms are unknown. Volatile anesthetics are liquids at room temperature but can evaporate easily to be delivered in gaseous form. The original volatile anesthetics—ether and chloroform, and nitrous oxide—had important limitations. Ether was characterized by notoriously slow onset and equally delayed emergence but could produce unconsciousness, amnesia, analgesia, and lack of movement without the addition of other agents. Chloroform was associated with hepatic toxicity and, occasionally, fatal cardiac arrhythmias and thus fell out of use.

Subsequent drug development created nontoxic inhalational agents that allow for rapid induction and emergence called *fluorinated ether anesthetics.* Common modern drugs are isoflurane, sevoflurane, and desflurane; halothane and enflurane were commonly used in the past but have largely fallen out of favor in the past one to two decades due to side effects and undesirable pharmacologic properties. The important properties of each volatile anesthetic can be summarized in terms of key clinical attributes (Table 20.1). Of note, in vulnerable patients, volatile anesthetics are triggering agents for the condition malignant hyperthermia (MH), in which sustained skeletal muscle contraction leads to hypermetabolic crisis due to activation of abnormal receptors in the skeletal muscle of vulnerable patients. This condition can lead to severe metabolic acidosis, hyperthermia, rhabdomyolysis, and multisystem organ failure.

Two important measures of inhalational anesthetics are the blood/gas solubility coefficient and the minimum alveolar concentration (MAC). The blood/gas solubility coefficient is a measure of the uptake of an agent by blood. In general, less soluble agents—those with lower blood/gas solubility coefficients—are associated with more rapid induction of and emergence from anesthesia, which include nitrous oxide and desflurane. Agents with high solubility in blood, such as halothane, are associated with relatively slow induction and emergence. Isoflurane and sevoflurane have intermediate rates of induction and emergence. MAC measures the dose of an inhaled anesthetic and is defined as the volume percentage of vaporized agent at which 50% of patients do not move in response to surgical stimulus at normal atmospheric pressure. A higher MAC represents a less potent volatile anesthetic. Among modern volatile agents, halothane is the most potent, with a MAC of 0.75%, whereas desflurane, the least potent of the hydrocarbon-based volatile agents, has a MAC of 6%.

The pungency of anesthetic agents also has practical implications. Agents with low pungency, such as halothane and sevoflurane, do not cause significant airway irritation when delivered at commonly used concentrations and are useful for inhalational induction of anesthesia. This type of induction can allow a patient to maintain spontaneous respiration, which can be beneficial in the case of certain airway and cardiac lesions, and it can be accomplished without IV access, making it a common strategy in pediatric anesthesia. Desflurane is highly irritating to the airways and is not useful for this type of induction. These drugs are all vasodilating, and they can cause dose-dependent myocardial depression.

All inhaled anesthetics can have deleterious effects on the environment. Each can act as a greenhouse gas with direct toxic effects on the ozone layer.[1] Accordingly, judicious use of these agents is advocated during anesthetic management. When exposed to desiccated CO_2 absorbent, the volatile anesthetics are all partially converted to carbon monoxide.[2,3] Because continued gas flow in an unused machine will desiccate the CO_2 absorbent, turning gas flow off in anesthesia machines when they are not in use can reduce carbon monoxide production.

Isoflurane

Approved by the US Food and Drug Administration (FDA) in 1979, isoflurane rapidly replaced halothane as the most used potent inhalational agent. Despite the subsequent release of sevoflurane and desflurane, isoflurane remains commonly used in modern operating rooms, in part because the cost of the now-generic compound is well below that of the newer agents. Its pungent odor virtually precludes use for inhalational induction. Compared with older agents, it causes less reduction in cardiac output, less sensitization to the arrhythmogenic effects of catecholamines, and minimal metabolism (Tables 20.1 and 20.2), but it does cause vasodilation and hypotension in many patients. Isoflurane-induced tachycardia, a variable response, can increase myocardial oxygen consumption. When it is used in patients with coronary artery disease, careful observation

TABLE 20.1 Important Characteristics of Inhalational Agents

ANESTHETIC	POTENCY	SPEED OF INDUCTION AND EMERGENCE	SUITABILITY FOR INHALATIONAL INDUCTION	SENSITIZATION TO CATECHOLAMINES	METABOLIZED (%)
Nitrous oxide	Weak	Fast	Insufficient alone	None	Minimal
Isoflurane	Potent	Medium	Not suitable	Minimal	<2
Sevoflurane	Potent	Rapid	Suitable	Minimal	<5
Desflurane	Potent	Rapid	Not suitable	Minimal	0.02
Halothane	Potent	Medium	Suitable	High	≥20
Enflurane	Potent	Medium	Not suitable	Medium	<10
Diethyl ether	Potent	Very slow	Suitable	None	10

TABLE 20.2   Cardiopulmonary Effects of Inhalational Anesthetics

INHALA-TIONAL AGENT	BLOOD PRESSURE	HEART RATE	CARDIAC OUTPUT	SENSITIZATION TO CATECHOLAMINES	VENTILATORY DEPRESSION	BRONCHODILA-TION
Nitrous oxide	Little effect	Little effect	Little effect	No	Minimal	No
Isoflurane	Moderate dose-dependent decrease	Variable increase	Minimal decrease	Minimal	Marked dose-dependent decrease	Moderate
Sevoflurane	Moderate dose-dependent decrease	Little effect	Moderate dose-dependent decrease	Minimal	Moderate dose-dependent decrease	Moderate
Desflurane	Minimal decrease	Variable; marked increase with rapid increase in concentration	Minimal decrease	Minimal	Marked dose-dependent decrease	Moderate
Halothane	Marked dose-dependent decrease	Moderate decrease	Marked dose-dependent decrease	Marked	Moderate dose-dependent decrease	Moderate
Enflurane	Marked dose-dependent decrease	Moderate decrease	Moderate dose-dependent decrease	Moderate	Moderate dose-dependent decrease	Minimal

and management of the heart rate are necessary. Isoflurane also causes cerebral vasodilation, increasing cerebral blood flow (CBF) and intracranial pressure (ICP); it also depresses cerebral metabolic rate (CMRO$_2$).[4]

Sevoflurane

Sevoflurane's relatively low blood solubility facilitates rapid induction and relatively rapid emergence. Unlike isoflurane, sevoflurane is pleasant to inhale, making it suitable for inhalational induction. It is also a potent bronchodilator, making it useful in maintenance of anesthesia in patients with bronchospastic disease. It, too, causes peripheral vasodilation and thus hypotension, but the cardiac function or conduction effects are not usually clinically significant. Like isoflurane, it can cause cerebral vasodilation and consequent increases in CBF and ICP and decreases in CMRO$_2$.[5]

An often discussed theoretical concern with the use of sevoflurane is the production of compound A, a metabolite produced via the drug's interaction with certain chemicals in the CO$_2$ absorber of the anesthesia ventilator (i.e., soda lime or Baralyme). Compound A was found to be nephrotoxic in experimental animals. However, there has never been shown to be a clinically significant difference in renal function with use of sevoflurane, so this concern appears to be theoretical. On an animal study level, β-lyase, the enzyme responsible for the formation of compound A, has 8 to 30 times greater activity in rat kidney tissue than in human kidney tissue. Furthermore, many modern CO$_2$ absorbers do not use soda lime or Baralyme and thus do not produce compound A.[6]

Desflurane

Desflurane is very insoluble and therefore has very quick onset and elimination; there is some evidence that it leads to readier emergence when compared with isoflurane.[7] It has a vapor pressure that makes its boiling point very close to room temperature, so it must be administered through a special vaporizer that heats and pressurizes it to ensure consistent dose delivery. Its pungent odor precludes inhalational induction. Of note, desflurane is associated with tachycardia and hypertension if the inspired concentration is increased too rapidly, but it can also produce dose-dependent vasodilation and hypotension.

Nitrous Oxide

Nitrous oxide is not a volatile anesthetic, as it exists as a gas at normal barometric pressure, but it is administered via inhalation. It has been used for anesthetic purposes for over 150 years and remains popular to this day. It is not a triggering agent for MH. It minimally influences respiration and hemodynamics, and it has a low solubility in blood, giving it rapid onset and emergence properties. However, nitrous has a MAC of 104% at sea level, meaning that it cannot be used alone for maintenance of general anesthesia (it is impossible not to create a hypoxic, or anoxic, gas mixture when approaching a MAC of nitrous). Therefore, it is often combined with one of the potent volatile agents, as MACs of inhaled anesthetics are additive in effect (i.e., 0.5 MAC nitrous + 0.5 MAC sevoflurane = 1 MAC anesthetic) to permit a lower dose of the potent volatile agent, thereby limiting side effects, reducing cost, and facilitating rapid induction and emergence. Although its mechanism is not completely elucidated, it has some N-methyl-D-aspartate (NMDA) antagonism and thus some analgesic properties; it is in this context that it is used by laboring parturients.

The most important clinical problem with nitrous oxide is that it is 30 times more soluble than nitrogen and diffuses into closed gas spaces faster than nitrogen diffuses out, thus increasing gas volume and pressure within the closed space. Because of this characteristic, nitrous oxide is contraindicated in the presence of closed gas spaces such as pneumothorax, small bowel obstruction, or middle ear surgery, as well as in retinal surgery in which an intraocular gas bubble is created. It may also be avoided by some anesthesiologists in procedures at risk for venous or arterial air embolism. Because nitrous oxide gradually accumulates in the pneumoperitoneum, some clinicians prefer to avoid its use during laparoscopic procedures. However, periodic venting can prevent gas accumulation.[8]

The Evaluation of Nitrous Oxide in the Gas Mixture for Anesthesia (ENIGMA) Trial, reported in 2007, indicated that patients having major surgical procedures lasting more than 2 hours had a higher incidence of postoperative complications and severe postoperative nausea and vomiting (PONV) if they received 70% nitrous oxide as part of their anesthetic regimen compared with patients randomized to not receive nitrous oxide.[9] However, the more recent ENIGMA II Trial, published in 2014, reported that use of nitrous oxide was not associated with an increased incidence of death, cardiovascular complications, or wound infection in high-risk surgical patients. Although the incidence of severe PONV was higher (15% vs. 11%) in patients receiving nitrous oxide compared with controls, the occurrence of PONV in the nitrous oxide group was effectively controlled by antiemetic prophylaxis,[10] and a subsequent subanalysis demonstrated that there was no difference in PONV rate if exposure was under 1 hour.[11] A 1-year follow-up of ENIGMA II patients did not show an increase in long-term morbidity and mortality with nitrous oxide administration.[12]

Intravenous Agents

IV agents have become an indispensable component of modern anesthetic practice. IV agents are used primarily for induction of anesthesia and as part of multidrug combinations to produce total IV anesthesia (TIVA). IV induction is rapid, pleasant, and safe for most patients; however, there are situations in which IV induction introduces hazards given the properties of available medications. Although several agents can be used for IV induction of anesthesia, propofol is the most widely used agent in the United States. Other agents are summarized in Table 20.3, and the most commonly used agents will be discussed in the following sections.

Propofol

Propofol is a short-acting induction agent that is associated with smooth, nausea-free emergence. The mechanism of action is not fully elucidated but likely involves agonism of γ-aminobutyric acid (GABA) receptors. Small doses are also useful for short-term sedation during brief procedures such as retrobulbar or peribulbar eye blocks, and it is commonly used as a continuous infusion during TIVA and for sedation during less invasive procedures such as gastrointestinal endoscopy or in an intensive care setting.

TIVA generally uses propofol as its mainstay. This anesthetic choice is popular in patients with a history of severe PONV because there is evidence that propofol either as a primary agent or as an adjunct at subhypnotic doses can attenuate PONV, particularly when combined with other antiemetic prophylaxis.[13] Propofol is also a potent bronchodilator. It decreases ICP and $CMRO_2$, so it is often favored in anesthetics for head injury, and it has anticonvulsant properties that may be leveraged when patients are seizing. The primary limitations of propofol are pain on injection, blood pressure reduction, and respiratory depression. Propofol should therefore be used with caution in patients who may be hypovolemic or who may tolerate hypotension poorly, such as those with severe coronary artery disease or severe valvular lesions, and only by individuals trained in airway management in patients without a protected airway. Uncommon side effects include hypertriglyceridemia and pancreatitis with prolonged use as well as the extremely rare but potentially fatal propofol infusion syndrome, which is associated with mitochondrial dysfunction and metabolic acidosis with circulatory collapse.[14]

Ketamine

Ketamine, which produces a dissociative state of anesthesia via NMDA receptor antagonism, is the only IV induction agent that increases blood pressure and heart rate via sympathetic stimulation. Of note, it can also be given as an intramuscular (IM) medication at higher doses to produce similar effects in patients who are acutely agitated or otherwise cannot have IV access established before sedation.

Though cardioexcitatory effects generally dominate, ketamine causes direct cardiac depression that may become evident if given to patients with exhausted sympathetic tone (e.g., hemorrhagic shock). In such a scenario, it may still be used in combination with other induction agents to reduce requirements, and thus the side effects, of any one drug. It is also an excellent bronchodilator. Of the IV induction agents, ketamine causes the least respiratory depression and preserves airway reflexes, which allows for

TABLE 20.3 Clinical Characteristics of Intravenous (IV) Induction Agents

IV INDUCTION AGENT	DOSE (MG/KG)	COMMENTS	SIDE EFFECTS	SITUATIONS REQUIRING CAUTION	RELATIVE INDICATIONS
Ketamine	1–2	Psychotropic side effects controllable with benzodiazepines; good bronchodilator; potent analgesic at subinduction doses	Hypertension; tachycardia	Coronary disease; severe hypovolemia	Rapid-sequence induction of asthmatics; patients in shock (reduced doses)
Propofol	1–2	Burns on injection; good bronchodilator; associated with low incidence of postoperative nausea and vomiting	Hypotension	Coronary artery disease; hypovolemia	Induction of outpatients; induction of asthmatics
Etomidate	0.1–0.3	Cardiovascularly stable; burns on injection; spontaneous movement during induction	Adrenal suppression	Hypovolemia	Induction of patients with cardiac contractile dysfunction; induction of patients in shock (reduced doses)
Midazolam	0.15–0.3	Relatively stable hemodynamics; potent amnesia	Synergistic ventilatory depression with opioids	Hypovolemia	Induction of patients with cardiac contractile dysfunction (usually in combination with opioids)

spontaneous breathing even while a patient is fully anesthetized. The drug can, however, induce the production of copious oropharyngeal secretions, so an antimuscarinic agent like glycopyrrolate may be coadministered. Ketamine can theoretically increase ICP, as it increases CBF, so it has been classically avoided in patients with intracranial hemorrhage, although recent data indicate this is of limited functional impact, and ketamine is often used even in patients with traumatic brain injury.

Given its NMDA activity, ketamine is able to produce significant analgesia. It can be used as a sole anesthetic for brief, superficial cases, and it can be a useful adjunct in a balanced anesthetic when given in bolus doses or as an infusion perioperatively. Some patients experience significant dysphoria and nightmares with ketamine, which can be attenuated with a short-acting benzodiazepine given before ketamine administration.

Etomidate

Etomidate is an imidazole compound that produces minimal hemodynamic changes. Because it preserves blood pressure in most patients, etomidate is often chosen as an alternative for induction of patients with cardiovascular disease or severe hypovolemia. It has rapid onset and recovery and does not induce apnea. It also decreases ICP and $CMRO_2$, making it an appropriate choice in head injury. Major drawbacks include burning pain on injection, a high incidence of PONV, abnormal muscular movements (myoclonus), and adrenal suppression via inhibition of 11β-hydroxylase in the cortisol synthesis pathway.[15] There is concern that this adrenal suppression can worsen mortality in critically ill patients when used as an induction agent in that population,[16] but the answer remains unclear, and it remains the subject of significant research. It is unlikely to have deleterious effects when used in a single dose in healthy patients.

Midazolam

Midazolam is a short-acting benzodiazepine that is generally used as an adjunct before induction of general anesthesia given its significant anxiolytic and amnestic properties. It has the potential to cause respiratory depression, particularly when given in conjunction with an opioid, and can occasionally cause paradoxical agitation. In significantly large doses (0.25–0.35 mg/kg) it can be used as an induction agent given its relative cardiovascular stability, but it can lead to prolonged effects. However, its use as an induction agent is rare in modern practice given the superiority of other agents.

Methohexital

Methohexital is an oxybarbiturate that agonizes GABA receptors and inhibits excitatory neurotransmitters with rapid onset and redistribution. It can activate seizure foci, which makes it a preferred induction agent for electroconvulsive therapy. Like many of the other IV agents, it causes vasodilation and respiratory depression, pain on injection, and myoclonus.

Opioids

Opioids are administered to the majority of patients undergoing general anesthesia and to many patients receiving regional or local anesthesia. As a component of a multifaceted anesthetic, opioids produce profound analgesia through agonism of μ receptors as well as minimal cardiac depression. Their disadvantages include ventilatory depression and inconsistent hypnosis and amnesia, which must usually be provided by other agents.

Several reasons explain the popularity of opioids in anesthetic management. First, they provide effective analgesia that can extend through the early postoperative period and can facilitate smoother awakening from anesthesia. Second, they reduce the MAC of potent inhalational agents (i.e., the amount of volatile anesthetic required to prevent a response to surgical stimulus). Third, opioids blunt the hypertension and tachycardia associated with stimulating interventions like endotracheal intubation and surgical incision. Fourth, when administered in doses 10 to 20 times the usual analgesic dose, opioids can act as complete anesthetics in many patients by providing not only analgesia but also hypnosis and amnesia. This characteristic has prompted their use in cardiac surgery patients, rarely as sole anesthetic agents, and much more often as a major component of a multimodal anesthetic. Finally, they are often added to local anesthetic solutions in epidural and intrathecal blocks to improve the quality of analgesia.

Fentanyl is a short-acting synthetic opioid that is commonly used during induction and maintenance of anesthesia. Hydromorphone and morphine are inexpensive, intermediate-acting agents that are commonly used both for maintenance and for postoperative analgesia. There are several other synthetic opioids that are popular intraoperatively. Sufentanil and alfentanil are both potent and lend themselves well to use as infusions during maintenance; their metabolism is relatively rapid but allows enough accumulation to provide short-term postoperative analgesia. Remifentanil, an opioid metabolized by serum esterases, is particularly short acting and does not accumulate during prolonged infusion, making it a useful part of IV anesthetic strategies. There is, however, concern that its use can contribute to hyperalgesia. Methadone is a long-acting opioid that not only acts as a potent μ-opioid receptor agonist but also interacts with NMDA receptors and alters the reuptake of serotonin and norepinephrine in the brain. It has been shown to be an effective and safe option in large, painful procedures like posterior spinal fusion and is gaining popularity in other surgical populations as well,[17] though concerns remain about its prolonged duration of action and variable kinetics in patients with comorbidities that may affect respiratory drive and drug metabolism.

Opioids are not without drawbacks, including PONV, decreased gastric motility, pruritus, the risk for dependence when used in a prolonged manner, and the development of hyperalgesia. Accordingly, there is much ongoing research to determine whether opioid-sparing or even opioid-free anesthetics may have preferable safety profiles while maintaining efficacy in addressing perioperative pain (described further in the following sections). However, a recent 61,249-patient cohort study demonstrated that increased fentanyl and hydromorphone use intraoperatively was associated with less pain and opioid requirement in the postanesthesia care unit (PACU) as well as decreased new chronic pain diagnoses at 3 months, decreased opioid prescriptions at 30/60/180 days, and decreased new persistent use of opioids. It has not yet been elucidated whether this type of effect requires an opioid versus any effective intraoperative analgesic strategy that prevents priming of pain receptors that may contribute to chronic pain.[18]

Neuromuscular Blockers

Paralytic medications allow for a still operating field and improved ability to manipulate muscular tissue to establish satisfactory operating conditions. During intubation, paralysis opens the vocal cords, allowing smooth passage of an endotracheal tube into the trachea. Before the advent of modern neuromuscular blocking drugs, these conditions were approximated by significantly increasing the dose of volatile anesthetic past what was necessary just to provide hypnosis and amnesia, leading to an increased risk of hypotension and other deleterious anesthetic side effects.

The two categories of neuromuscular blockers in clinical use are depolarizing (noncompetitive) and nondepolarizing (competitive) agents. The depolarizing agents exert agonistic effects at the cholinergic receptors of the neuromuscular junction, initially causing contractions evident as fasciculations followed by an interval of profound relaxation. The nondepolarizing class of drugs competes for receptor sites with acetylcholine in the neuromuscular junction and prevents depolarization, with the magnitude of block dependent on the availability of acetylcholine, the concentration of neuromuscular blocker in the neuromuscular junction, and the affinity of the agent for the receptor.

Succinylcholine, the only depolarizing agent still in clinical use, remains popular for endotracheal intubation because of its rapid onset and short duration of action when given as a bolus dose. The drug is rapidly metabolized by plasma pseudocholinesterase, except in a small fraction of patients with atypical or absent pseudocholinesterase. At intubating doses, onset of muscle relaxation is rapid (45–60 seconds), which facilitates intubation in patients at risk for aspiration. Because neuromuscular function begins to recover after about 3 minutes, a patient who cannot be successfully intubated can be ventilated by mask for a short time until spontaneous respiration resumes. However, a patient who cannot be ventilated by mask after succinylcholine administration will likely not resume spontaneous breathing before the onset of life-threatening hypoxemia. Of note, succinylcholine can also be given IM, which may be required if a patient has laryngospasm (involuntary closure of the vocal cords that can lead to severe hypoxemia) during inhalational induction or other situations in which IV access is not present or functional. Succinylcholine is not suitable for longer-term muscle relaxation during surgery, as very high cumulative doses can lead to prolonged paralysis that is not predictable in duration or reversibility and is known as phase II blockade, the mechanism of which is outside the scope of this chapter. If this occurs, the patient must be monitored and kept sedated pending recovery of strength.

Although it is extremely useful, succinylcholine is also associated with serious hazards in a small proportion of patients. It can result in severe, life-threatening hyperkalemia in patients with burns, paraplegia, and quadriplegia, as these patients express abnormal extrajunctional acetylcholine receptors that release large amounts of intracellular potassium when activated by the drug. When given alone or when combined with a volatile agent, it is also implicated in triggering MH in susceptible individuals. Therefore, it is best avoided in patients at risk for MH, including those with muscular dystrophy or a family history of MH. It can also cause severe bradycardia, particularly in children, via stimulation of muscarinic receptors at the sinus node. Because succinylcholine causes visible muscle fasciculations, it has been implicated in causing postoperative myalgias. There is ongoing investigation as to whether or not pretreatment with a small dose of a nondepolarizing agent (a "defasciculating" dose) can reduce this side effect.

Several nondepolarizing neuromuscular blockers are currently available, each with advantages and disadvantages. These drugs can be used for intubation and for intraoperative maintenance of muscle relaxation. The choice of drug is generally related to desired kinetics and clearance, with attention to side effects, especially if older drugs are used. Doses required to provide satisfactory operating conditions are summarized in Table 20.4. Rocuronium is an intermediate-acting drug (30–45 minutes effect for a standard dose) that produces intubating conditions within 3 minutes when administered at the appropriate dose. It is cleared primarily by biliary excretion, with a small amount of renal clearance as well. When the intubation dose is doubled, intubating conditions can be reached within 45 seconds, allowing for a rapid sequence intubation without the drawbacks of succinylcholine. This does increase the duration of effect significantly, which can pose difficulties in a cannot intubate–cannot ventilate situation. Vecuronium has similar characteristics to rocuronium but a longer onset time and higher potency. Cisatracurium is another intermediate-acting drug. Its major advantage is that it is eliminated via enzymatic degradation in the plasma, also known as Hofmann elimination, making its kinetics extremely predictable, even when given as an infusion or in patients with hepatic or renal dysfunction.

Dosing of nondepolarizing agents requires knowledge of several important characteristics. First, the use of neuromuscular blockers prevents movement in response to noxious stimuli. Therefore, chemical paralysis can mask the signs of inadequate anesthesia intraoperatively. Medicolegal claims of intraoperative awareness during general anesthesia are more than twice as frequent in patients receiving intraoperative muscle relaxants. Second, higher doses are required to provide satisfactory conditions for intubation than for surgical relaxation. Therefore, if a nondepolarizer is used only after intubation, smaller doses are required. Third, other anesthetic drugs potentiate the actions of nondepolarizing agents. Succinylcholine used for intubation decreases subsequent requirements for nondepolarizers. Potent inhalational

TABLE 20.4 Dose-Response Relationships of Nondepolarizing Neuromuscular Blocking Drugs in Humans				
DRUG	DURATION	ED$_{50}$ (MG/KG)	ED$_{95}$ (MG/KG)	INTUBATING DOSE (MG/KG)
Rocuronium	Intermediate	0.147 (0.069–0.220)	0.305 (0.257–0.521)	0.6–1.0
Cisatracurium	Intermediate	0.026 (0.15–0.31)	0.04 (0.32–0.55)	0.15–0.2
Vecuronium	Intermediate	0.027 (0.015–0.031)	0.043 (0.037–0.059)	0.1–0.2
Mivacurium	Short	0.039 (0.027–0.052)	0.067 (0.045–0.081)	0.15–0.2
Pancuronium	Long	0.036 (0.022–0.042)	0.067 (0.059–0.080)	0.08–0.12
Tubocurarine	Long	0.23 (0.16–0.26)	0.48 (0.34–0.56)	0.5–0.6

Data are mean (95% confidence limits). Somewhat larger doses are required to facilitate endotracheal intubation.
ED$_{50}$, Dose effective for surgical relaxation in 50% of patients; ED$_{95}$, dose effective for surgical relaxation in 95% of patients.
Modified from Naguib M, Lien CA. Pharmacology of muscle relaxants and their antagonists. In: Miller RD, Fleisher LA, Johns RA, et al, eds. *Miller's Anesthesia.* 6th ed. Philadelphia: Churchill Livingstone; 2005:481-572.

agents dose dependently potentiate the effects of competitive neuromuscular blockers. The newer inhalational agent desflurane potentiates the effects of vecuronium approximately 20% more than isoflurane. Fourth, individual responses to muscle relaxants vary widely, with patients demonstrating both markedly increased and markedly decreased neuromuscular blockade compared with expected levels.

Fifth, and most important, subtle blockade can be difficult to detect and can be associated with postoperative complications. The importance of subtle residual paralysis has recently been quantified using the train-of-four (TOF) fade ratio, a semiquantitative monitoring technique that can assess the depth of neuromuscular blockade and the adequacy of pharmacologic reversal. To determine this ratio, four electrical pulses are delivered to a nerve at 0.5-second intervals, and a muscle twitch is monitored to determine the strength of contraction with each stimulus. The gold standard monitoring location is the ulnar nerve, with expected response at the adductor pollicis muscle. When a patient is fully paralyzed, there are no twitches elicited with stimulation, as the acetylcholine receptors are saturated with drug, so acetylcholine cannot bind. As the drug is metabolized and/or cleared, twitches return. The TOF quantifies the magnitude of the fourth twitch compared with the first twitch. At the conclusion of anesthesia, a TOF ratio greater than 0.90 has been considered adequate return of neuromuscular function. Residual neuromuscular blockade results in an increased incidence of postoperative pulmonary complications, with severity ranging from mild hypoxia to reintubation and ICU admission. Of note, clinical signs of strength such as head lift and hand grip are inferior to quantitative monitoring in assessing function, and normal tidal volumes can be achieved by an intubated patient even with significant levels of neuromuscular blockade due to recovery of diaphragm function before recovery of other muscle groups required to protect the airway after extubation.[19]

Return of neuromuscular function can be prompted by administration of reversal agents. Historically, nondepolarizing relaxants are pharmacologically reversed with an anticholinesterase (neostigmine or edrophonium) accompanied by atropine or glycopyrrolate to counteract the muscarinic effects of the anticholinesterase (bradycardia, gastrointestinal effects). This makes additional acetylcholine available to compete to agonize the receptor. The ability to achieve effective competition depends on the depth of neuromuscular blockade at the time of reversal and on the dose of reversal administered. If blockade is too dense, the patient cannot be reversed in this manner, and the anesthesiologist has to wait until twitches return. Peak reversal can take up to 15 minutes even when appropriately dosed. Complete reversal must be assessed by quantitative TOF to safely extubate.

The development of sugammadex has overcome many of the problems associated with using anticholinesterases to reverse neuromuscular blockade. Sugammadex is a cyclodextrin that directly binds nondepolarizing steroidal neuromuscular blocking agents such as rocuronium and vecuronium (i.e., it cannot reverse cisatracurium). Sugammadex rapidly reverses neuromuscular blockade and avoids the muscarinic side effects associated with use of anticholinesterases. Dosing of sugammadex is based on the depth of neuromuscular blockade. Therefore, monitoring of blockade depth with a twitch monitor is required for optimal reversal of neuromuscular blockade even with sugammadex. Nevertheless, a comparison of sugammadex to neostigmine for reversal of neuromuscular blockade in patients undergoing abdominal surgery showed that sugammadex administration eliminated residual neuromuscular blockade in the PACU and shortened the time of readiness for discharge from the operating room.[20]

ANESTHESIA MACHINE

Anesthesia equipment has undergone rapid development in recent decades. The central piece of equipment for delivery of anesthesia is the modern anesthesia machine. The anesthesia machine functions primarily to deliver respiratory support and volatile anesthetics to the patient. In addition, modern anesthesia machines have sophisticated ventilators that allow for effective respiratory support and have integrated monitors that accurately measure oxygen delivery, inspired and end-tidal gas concentrations, airway pressures, minute ventilation, and fresh gas flows.

The essential elements of an anesthesia machine are gas sources (oxygen, nitrous oxide, and air), flow meters, and a flow-proportioning device. In most cases, gases are delivered to the anesthesia machine from a bank of large H cylinders housed in a central area within the hospital. A backup system of E cylinders is attached directly to the anesthesia machine and provides a source of gases, particularly oxygen, if the central gas source becomes unavailable. The flow meters allow independent administration of individual gases. To minimize the chance of delivering a hypoxic gas mixture, anesthesia machines feature so-called fail-safe valves that require pressurization of the oxygen line before nitrous oxide can be delivered and flow-proportioning devices that automatically reduce the flow of nitrous oxide if the flow of oxygen is reduced below a safe concentration. The measurement of inspired oxygen concentration provides a further safeguard against delivering hypoxic gas mixtures.

The anesthesia machine also integrates vaporizers that are able to deliver exact doses of volatile anesthetic as specified by the anesthesia provider. The aforementioned monitoring equipment also allows for close tracking of inhaled and expired concentrations of these gasses so that depth of anesthesia can be gauged.

PATIENT MONITORING DURING AND AFTER ANESTHESIA

Effective monitoring is a critical aspect of anesthesia care. The essential components of monitoring include observation and vigilance, instrumentation, data analysis, and institution of corrective measures, if indicated. The goal of patient monitoring is to provide optimal anesthetic management and to detect physiologic abnormalities early in their course so that corrective measures can be instituted before serious or irreversible injury occurs. Although it is difficult to directly relate improved patient outcomes with specific monitors, the reduction in anesthesia-related morbidity and mortality has paralleled the institution of current monitoring practices.

The indications as well as risks and benefits associated with the use of noninvasive and invasive electronic monitors must be assessed for each individual patient (Box 20.1). These decisions are guided by the patient's medical condition, the type of surgery, and the potential complications associated with invasive monitoring. However, the proliferation of electronic monitoring devices does not circumvent the need for clinical skills such as observation, inspection, auscultation, and palpation. The American Society of Anesthesiologists (ASA) has established standards for basic anesthetic monitoring that were most recently updated in 2020.[21] These standards are designed to integrate clinical skills and electronic monitoring with the goal of enhancing patient safety.

BOX 20.1 Routine and Specialized Electronic Monitors Used in Anesthetic Practice and Their Indications

Routine Monitors

- Pulse oximetry
  - Blood oxygen saturation
  - Heart rate
  - Tissue perfusion (via plethysmography)
- Automated blood pressure cuff
  - Blood pressure
- Electrocardiogram (ECG)
  - Heart rhythm
  - Heart rate
  - Monitor of myocardial ischemia
- Capnography
  - Adequacy of ventilation
  - Intratracheal placement of endotracheal tube
  - Pulmonary perfusion
- Oxygen analyzer
  - Monitoring of delivered oxygen concentration
- Ventilator pressure monitor
  - Ventilator disconnection during general anesthesia
  - Monitoring of airway pressure
- Temperature monitoring

Specialized Monitors

- Monitoring of urine output (Foley catheter)
  - Gross indicator of intravascular volume status and renal perfusion
- Arterial catheter
  - Continuous measurement of arterial blood pressure

- Sampling of arterial blood
- Central venous catheter
  - Continuous measurement of central venous pressure
  - Delivery of centrally acting drugs
  - Rapid administration of fluids and blood
- Pulmonary artery catheter
  - Measurement of pulmonary artery pressure
  - Measurement of left ventricular pressure
  - Measurement of cardiac output
  - Measurement of mixed venous oxygenation
- Precordial Doppler
  - Detection of air embolism
- Transesophageal echocardiography
  - Evaluation of myocardial performance
  - Assessment of heart valve function
  - Assessment of intravascular volume
  - Detection of air embolism
- Esophageal Doppler
  - Assessment of descending aortic blood flow
  - Assessment of cardiac preload
- Transpulmonary indicator dilution
  - Measurement of cardiac output
  - Measurement of preload
- Esophageal and precordial stethoscope
  - Auscultation of breathing and heart sounds
- Processed electroencephalogram (EEG; SedLine or bispectral index [BIS])
  - Depth of anesthesia

Standard I asserts that a qualified anesthesia care provider must be continuously present in the operating room during the administration of anesthesia. The practitioner must continuously monitor the status of the patient and alter anesthesia care based on the patient's response to the dynamic changes associated with anesthesia and surgery.

Standard II mandates continual assessment of oxygenation, ventilation, circulation, and temperature during all anesthetics. Specific requirements include the following:

- Oxygenation:
  - The use of an oxygen analyzer with a low-oxygen–concentration alarm during general anesthesia
  - Employment of quantitative assessment of blood oxygenation, such as by pulse oximetry
- Ventilation:
  - Continual clinical evaluation to assess the adequacy of ventilation, with quantitative monitoring of expired CO_2 when procedural or patient factors allow
  - Verification of endotracheal tube/laryngeal mask placement by both clinical assessment and monitors that identify the presence of CO_2 in expired gases
  - A device capable of detecting disconnection of breathing system components during mechanical ventilation that can give an audible signal when its alarm threshold is exceeded
- Circulation:
  - Electrocardiogram (ECG) monitoring from induction until departure from the anesthetizing location
  - Heart rate and blood pressure evaluation at least every 5 minutes
  - Another means of assessing circulatory function, including pulse plethysmography or oximetry, palpation, continuously monitored electronic means, or auscultation

- Temperature:
  - Ready availability of means of temperature evaluation during periods of intended or expected changes in body temperature

Oxygenation Monitoring

Monitoring the fractional concentration of oxygen in inspired gas (FiO_2) and hemoglobin oxygen saturation is a standard of care during all general anesthetics. Modern anesthesia machines are equipped with oxygen analyzers that detect the delivered oxygen concentration (FiO_2). This monitor, in combination with fail-safe devices, low-oxygen delivery alarms, and oxygen ratio monitors, greatly decreases the chance of delivering a hypoxic gas mixture during anesthesia.

Pulse oximetry capitalizes upon the fact that oxygenated and deoxygenated blood absorb and reflect different amounts of red and infrared light. Pulse oximeters send signals of both wavelengths through the patient's tissue, and a receiver determines the absorbed and reflected amounts and determines a percent saturation. These devices are fairly accurate over a saturation of 80%, but one has to be aware of a number of common sources of artifact and inaccuracy. Dark skin colors, dense nail polish, bright ambient light (e.g., operating room lights), and poor perfusion to the digit can all impact the accuracy of the monitor.

Ventilation Monitoring

The sedative hypnotic and analgesic agents used for deep sedation and/or general anesthesia can depress or abolish spontaneous ventilation, necessitating intraoperative ventilatory support. Several means are available to assess the adequacy of ventilation, among which are physical assessment of chest expansion, auscultation of breath sounds, and evaluation for evidence of upper airway obstruction and stridor. Precordial and esophageal stethoscopes provide continuous input regarding air movement and the development of wheezing. During mechanical ventilation, monitors of airway pressure and minute ventilation alert the anesthesiologist to conditions that can impair ventilation, such as disconnection of the ventilatory circuit, dislodgement of the endotracheal tube, obstruction of the gas delivery system, and changes in airway resistance or compliance, or both. These are gross assessments, however, and tools exist to be more exact.

The advent of end-tidal CO_2 ($ETCO_2$) monitoring has greatly enhanced precision and accuracy of this assessment. $ETCO_2$ can be monitored via specialized nasal cannula in patients who are spontaneously breathing and via expired gas analysis in those who are intubated or have a laryngeal mask airway (LMA) in place. In patients with normal cardiopulmonary physiology, the difference between $ETCO_2$ in and $PaCO_2$ is 2 to 5 mm Hg in a closed system. The gradient between end-tidal and arterial CO_2 reflects dead space ventilation, which is increased in cases of decreased pulmonary blood flow, such as pulmonary air embolism or thromboembolism and decreased cardiac output. Therefore, $ETCO_2$ monitoring can also provide important information regarding systemic perfusion. Specifically, $ETCO_2$ will decrease during periods of decreased cardiac output and pulmonary perfusion.

Blood Pressure Monitoring

Blood pressure monitoring is required during all anesthetics. Noninvasive blood pressure monitoring is appropriate for the majority of surgical cases, and most modern operating rooms are equipped with automated oscillometric blood pressure analyzers. Indications for invasive blood pressure monitoring with arterial catheters include anticipation of wide perioperative blood pressure swings, the need for multiple blood gas analyses or other labs, the need for continuous blood pressure monitoring in patients with significant end-organ dysfunction or those having high-risk surgical procedures, and the inadequacy of noninvasive blood pressure measurements (e.g., morbidly obese patients with irregularly shaped limbs or patients with left ventricular assist devices who lack a pulse).

Several sites for arterial cannulation are available, each with inherent advantages and potential for complications. The radial artery is most commonly cannulated because of its superficial location, relative ease of access, and in most patients, adequate collateral flow from the ulnar artery. Other potential sites for percutaneous arterial cannulation include the femoral, brachial, axillary, ulnar, dorsalis pedis, and posterior tibial arteries. Possible complications of intraarterial monitoring include hematoma, neurologic injury, arterial thrombus, limb ischemia, infection, and inadvertent intraarterial injection of drugs. Intraarterial catheters are not placed in extremities with potential vascular insufficiency. However, with proper patient selection, the complication rate associated with intraarterial cannulation is low and its benefits can be important.

Electrocardiography

ECG monitoring is a standard of care during the administration of anesthesia. Information regarding dysrhythmias and cardiac ischemia can be readily obtained from ECG data. Analysis of ECG tracings is also the cornerstone of cardiopulmonary resuscitation protocols.

Temperature Monitoring

Temperature is monitored in all patients undergoing general anesthesia. The site of measurement is dependent on the surgical procedure and the physical characteristics of the patient. Esophageal temperature is most commonly measured during general anesthesia, as it reflects core temperature. Other common sites of temperature monitoring include nasopharynx, bladder (via Foley catheter), axillary, cutaneous, rectal, tympanic membrane, and, in patients with pulmonary artery catheters (PACs), the pulmonary artery. Because of the potential morbidity associated with hypothermia and hyperthermia, it is important to monitor body temperature and institute measures to maintain temperature as close to normal as possible.

Neuromuscular Blockade Monitoring

Because of variability in sensitivity to and metabolism of neuromuscular blockers, it is essential to monitor neuromuscular function in patients receiving paralytics. The most common sites of monitoring are at the ulnar or facial nerves, with the former being the gold standard. The basis of neuromuscular monitoring is assessment of muscle activity after proximal nerve stimulation (Box 20.2), as previously described. This evaluation gives an indication of acetylcholine receptor blockade at the neuromuscular junction. The degree of neuromuscular blockade is indicated by a decreased evoked response to twitch stimulation. As noted earlier in this chapter, it is essential to monitor neuromuscular blockade and to assure resolution of blockade at the end of anesthesia to minimize the incidence of postoperative complications related to residual neuromuscular blockade.

BOX 20.2 Techniques for Assessing Neuromuscular Blockade

Train-of-Four: Four Successive 200-μs Stimuli Over a 2-second Period
- Twitch height progressively fades with increasing blockade.
  - Loss of the fourth twitch indicates 75% receptor blockade.
  - Loss of the third twitch indicates 80% blockade.
  - Loss of the second twitch indicates 90% blockade.
  - Loss of the first twitch indicates 100% blockade.
  - Clinical relaxation requires 75% to 95% blockade.
- Presence of four twitches without fade suggests adequate reversal of neuromuscular blockade.
- Use of accelerometry provides a quantitative comparison of the first and fourth twitches of the train-of-four (TOF) and generates a TOF (ratio of the fourth twitch over the first twitch), with a TOF <0.9 signifying clinically significant residual blockade.

Double-Burst Stimulation: Two Successive Sets of 50-Hz Bursts (Three Stimuli/Burst) Separated by 750 ms (Appears as Two Twitches)
- Easier to detect fade visually with this technique than with TOF.
- Loss of the second twitch indicates 80% receptor blockade.
- Presence of two twitches without fade suggests adequate reversal of neuromuscular blockade.

Tetany: Sustained 50-Hz or 100-Hz Burst
- Duration of sustained contraction fades with increasing blockade.
- Sustained contraction for 5 seconds suggests adequate reversal of neuromuscular blockade.

Central Nervous System Monitoring

Awareness during anesthesia is an uncommon, but disturbing, complication that occurs when a patient is not adequately anesthetized for the level of stimulus. The risk is highest in procedures during which significant hemodynamic instability or urgency may preclude appropriate dosing of anesthetics (i.e., traumas, cardiac surgery, emergency cesarean sections) or when TIVA is used because the dose-response curve is less consistent than that of inhaled anesthetics, and it is possible to have an unrecognized loss of IV access during a procedure. Lack of cortical arousal cannot be ensured by hemodynamic monitoring, as there can be a discordance between sympathetic response to stimulus and awareness of that stimulus. It also cannot be definitively determined by assessing movement, as a patient may have reflexive movements without cortical function (spinal reflexes are not necessarily extinguished by hypnotic agents), and in patients who are paralyzed, movement cannot be used as a sign.

Processed electroencephalogram (EEG) can directly help anesthesiologists characterize the intraoperative cortical function. There are two commercially available systems in use: SedLine, which analyzes the spatial and temporal gradients of EEG frequency bands, and the bispectral index (BIS), which analyzes the phase and power of EEG bands via a proprietary algorithm. Both produce an indexed number between 0 and 100 that is a surrogate for the depth of sedation, with a lower number representing suppression of brain activity and 100 representing an awake patient. These monitors function well to represent the depth of anesthesia.[22] Compared with end-tidal MAC monitoring when volatile anesthetics are used, these monitors have not been shown to be superior in preventing awareness,[23] but they have shown to be beneficial in preventing awareness in TIVA.[24] Processed EEG can also help prevent anesthetic overdose by allowing clinicians to decrease sedation when cortical activity is completely suppressed and address other physiologic changes directly. There is ongoing work to determine whether this type of adjustment has the potential to decrease postoperative cognitive dysfunction (POCD) and delirium. Although burst suppression on EEG under anesthesia does correlate with delirium,[25] it remains unclear if avoiding burst suppression prevents the development of POCD or delirium postoperatively.[26,27]

Advanced Hemodynamic Monitoring

Measuring cardiac output during surgical procedures can be necessary in critically ill patients or patients with severe comorbid conditions. There exist numerous modern noninvasive cardiac output monitors that use pulse wave analysis of the arterial waveform[28] and several that use finger cuffs to calculate these quantities.[29] The gold standard for these measurements remains thermodilution with a PAC. PACs and even central venous pressure monitoring via central venous catheter are no longer ubiquitous in the operating room, as numerous studies failed to demonstrate an advantage to their use, and some even suggested adverse outcomes.[30] However, in patients with heart failure or pulmonary hypertension, many anesthesiologists and surgeons still find these devices useful. Transesophageal echocardiography (TEE) plays a major role in cardiac surgery, both for monitoring and diagnostic purposes. It has found its role outside the cardiac operating rooms as well in helping to identify occult pathology and as an aid in the rescue and guidance of management for patients in shock.[31]

Point-of-Care Ultrasound

Emergency medicine physicians and trauma surgeons have been early adopters of point-of-care ultrasound with the implementation of focused assessment with sonography in trauma (FAST). Anesthesiologists have also adopted the use of point-of-care ultrasound throughout the perioperative space. The use of ultrasound in the preoperative clinic and just before surgery led to a significant impact to avoid delays for further workup and, in remote cases, identification of occult pathology that changed the trajectory of management for these patients.[32] The use of ultrasound in the operating room has found a niche for multiple facets in the care of surgical patients to include confirmation of the airway, assessment of the cardiac[33] and pulmonary systems,[34] and identification of gastric contents before surgery.[35] In some cases, the use of ultrasound has also had an impact on survival for those in septic shock.[36]

ANESTHESIOLOGY PERSPECTIVES ON PREOPERATIVE EVALUATION

The ASA has established basic standards for preanesthetic care: an anesthesiologist is required to evaluate the medical status of the patient, derive a plan for anesthetic care, and discuss the plan with the patient. The Joint Commission requires that all patients receiving anesthesia undergo a preanesthetic evaluation. Traditionally, these preanesthetic evaluations occurred in close proximity to surgical intervention as a means of identifying medical conditions necessitating special consideration when prescribing the anesthetic plan. However, over the past few decades, technologic advancements in both the surgical and anesthetic spheres have allowed surgical operations to be offered to patients with increasing medical complexity. Additionally, the understanding of factors associated with increased perioperative risk has significantly increased to include healthcare, patient, and socioeconomic characteristics. This combination has spurred a rise in preoperative clinics as a means of identifying high-risk patients, intervening upon modifiable risk factors, and optimizing medical comorbidities to improve perioperative outcomes and decrease healthcare costs. Optimally, preoperative clinics need to stratify patients into low and high-risk categories and provide efficient, predictable, and thorough evaluations for both groups. Although high-risk patients may require these visits to occur in person, possibly weeks in advance of their operations to allow for optimization, low-risk patients without complicated medical problems who are scheduled for elective, low-risk procedures may be interviewed by telephone or virtually before surgery and given preoperative instructions.

The anesthesia preoperative evaluation serves multiple purposes. First, it allows the patient an opportunity to speak to an anesthesiologist and discuss the expected impact of anesthesia, including the patient's fears and concerns regarding anesthesia and postoperative pain management. Second, the preanesthetic interview focuses on the type of surgery, the underlying conditions necessitating surgery, any history of previous anesthetics, and the presence of coexisting diseases. The preoperative interview allows evaluation of the patient's medical status to determine whether additional medical evaluation or treatment is needed before surgery. This process requires a focused history, physical examination, and, if indicated, laboratory evaluation. Current medications must be reviewed to anticipate potential drug interactions and manage medical problems during the perioperative period. Instructions regarding oral intake, changes in medication use, and other important issues that need to be addressed before surgery are communicated to the patient during the preoperative interview.

A well-focused history allows the practitioner to perform targeted physical and laboratory examinations. Laboratory testing should be tailored toward patient- and surgery-specific conditions. Healthy patients undergoing elective procedures may not need preoperative laboratory testing. The use of routine preoperative testing, especially in asymptomatic healthy patients, is costly with poor yield in both diagnostic and prognostic information. False-positive tests can cause needless delays in surgery and could require follow-up, increasing costs and potentially leading to harm or injury associated with further tests and procedures. However, targeted testing based on results of the history and physical exam can significantly improve overall patient care.

Investigation of conditions associated with increased perioperative morbidity is important for reducing the risks related to anesthesia and surgery. Coexisting conditions that must be carefully evaluated include intravascular volume status, airway abnormalities, cardiovascular disease, pulmonary disease, neurologic disease, renal and hepatic disease, and disorders of nutrition, endocrinology, and metabolism. Preoperative pregnancy testing is controversial. The rationale for performing preoperative pregnancy testing is the potential for spontaneous abortion and birth anomalies associated with surgery and anesthesia. Currently, anesthetic agents used in standard clinical dosing and duration have not been shown to have any teratogenic effects in humans, and a paucity of literature exists regarding adverse neurodevelopmental effects of anesthetic agents on the fetus.[37] A clear sexual history and documentation of the last menstrual cycle are obtained in females of childbearing age. In ambiguous situations, a preoperative pregnancy test is indicated; however, informed consent for preprocedural pregnancy testing including risks, benefits, and alternatives should be obtained.

Airway Examination

Assessing the airway is a crucial step in developing an anesthetic plan. Even if regional anesthesia is planned, general anesthesia and the need to maintain a patent airway could be necessary in the advent of failed block, surgical needs, or complications. The goal of the airway examination is to identify characteristics that could hinder assisted mask ventilation or tracheal intubation. A history of diseases or conditions that are associated with airway closure or difficult laryngoscopy will alert the practitioner to potential airway difficulties. Review of previous anesthetic records can provide invaluable information regarding previous airway management. The airway examination is completed by systematic inspection of the mouth opening, thyromental distance, neck mobility, ability to protrude the jaw (should be able to bite upper vermillion border with bottom teeth), and the size of the tongue in relation to the oral cavity (Box 20.3). The patient is observed in both frontal and profile views because many airway abnormalities, such as a recessed mandible, will not be evident from a frontal view. The size of the tongue in relation to the oral cavity can be graded by using the Mallampati classification (Fig. 20.1). The Mallampati examination is performed with the patient sitting and the head in a neutral position, the mouth opened as wide as possible, and the tongue protruded maximally. The observer views the oral and pharyngeal structures that are evident. In general, a patient in whom the uvula, tonsillar pillars, and soft palate are visible (class I) will be easy to mask ventilate and intubate. Patients in whom only the hard palate is visible, a class IV airway, have a higher likelihood of being difficult to mask ventilate and intubate. However, the Mallampati classification is only one component of the airway examination and must be used in conjunction

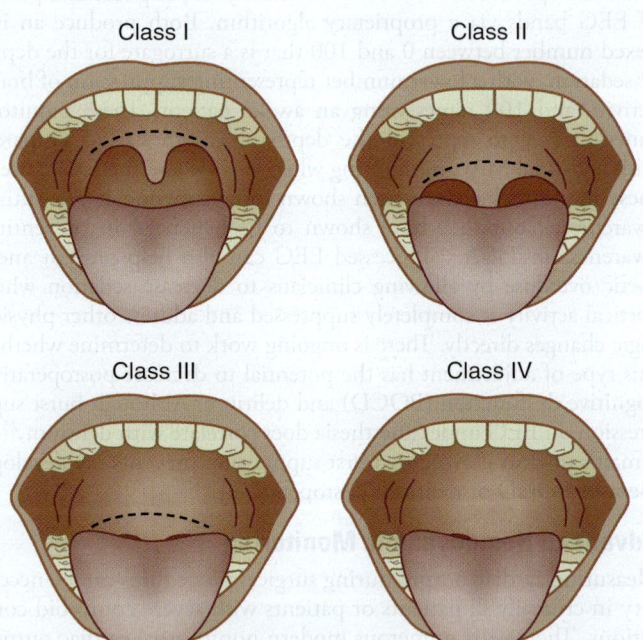

FIGURE 20.1 The Mallampati classification relates tongue size to pharyngeal size. This test is performed with the patient in the sitting position, the head held in a neutral position, the mouth wide open, and the tongue protruding to the maximum. The subsequent classification is assigned according to the pharyngeal structures that are visible: class I, visualization of the soft palate, fauces, uvula, and anterior and posterior pillars; class II, visualization of the soft palate, fauces, and uvula; class III, visualization of the soft palate and the base of the uvula; and class IV, soft palate not visible at all. (From Mallampati SR, Gatt SP, Gugino LD, et al. A clinical sign to predict difficult tracheal intubation: a prospective study. *Can Anaesth Soc J.* 1985;32:429-434.)

with other aspects of the airway examination and the patient's history to provide a complete airway assessment. Other physical factors that are associated with uncomplicated airway management are adequate mouth opening, neck extension, and thyromental distance. In a meta-analysis examining more than 30,000 patients, Detsky and coauthors[38] reported that while clinical findings are useful predictors for a higher likelihood of difficult intubation, clinical findings alone cannot reliably exclude a difficult intubation. However, inability to bite the upper lip with the lower teeth most significantly increases the probability of difficult intubation.

Cardiovascular Disease

The risk for perioperative myocardial ischemia and infarction and the risk for cardiac death have become important issues as surgery is offered to patients with increasingly severe systemic disease and as more children with congenital cardiac anomalies are surviving later into adulthood. As reviewed in Chapter 19, the American College of Cardiology (ACC) and American Heart Association (AHA) have published guidelines for perioperative cardiovascular evaluation and management of patients undergoing noncardiac surgery that were most recently revised in 2014.[39]

Functional status is a reliable predictor of perioperative and long-term cardiovascular risk. Historically, in the absence of recent exercise testing, a patient's functional status was assessed based on determination of ability to perform common activities and functional capacity is commonly expressed in terms of metabolic equivalents of the task (METs), where 1 MET is the resting or basal oxygen consumption of a 40-year-old, 70-kg male. Perioperative cardiac and long-term risks are increased in patients unable to perform 4 METs of work during daily activities, which correlates to being able to climb a flight of stairs or walking up a hill. Although functional capacity had traditionally been determined on a subjective basis during the perioperative interview, assessment tools such as the Duke Activity Status Index (DASI) have been found to be superior to subjective assessment in predicting postoperative mortality and myocardial infarction within 30 days.[40] This tool has a maximum score of 58.2, with different levels of activity conferring different points (e.g., walking one to two blocks on level ground is 2.75 points, whereas strenuous physical activities such as singles tennis is 7.5 points). With this scale, a score less than 34 signifies a patient at increased risk for cardiac morbidity and mortality in the perioperative period, and a score less than 25 represents the highest risk of major adverse cardiac events and moderate to severe postoperative complications.[41] The clinician must consider the urgency of surgery, the patient's functional capacity, and type of surgery, giving these factors appropriate weight. Since publication of the perioperative cardiovascular evaluation guidelines in 2002 and the revisions in 2007 and 2014, several new randomized trials and cohort studies have suggested modifications to the algorithm, particularly around the utilization of the DASI versus METs assessment.

The need for specific testing is dependent on the patient's exercise tolerance, comorbidities, and the type of surgery proposed. Box 20.4 defines current recommendations on specific perioperative testing including preoperative electrocardiography, echocardiography, stress testing, radionuclide perfusion scans, and coronary angiography. It is recommended that practitioners refer to the most recent ACC/AHA guidelines for detailed recommendations and level of evidence to support the guidelines.[39]

Perioperative medical management is guided by the patient's cardiovascular status, current drug regimen, and the type of surgery proposed. The need for preoperative coronary revascularization is limited to patients who are candidates for emergency or urgent revascularization under any circumstances. Such patients include those with unstable angina, active myocardial infarction, or arrhythmias caused by active ischemia. Elective coronary revascularization to decrease perioperative cardiovascular complications

---

BOX 20.4 Summary of Recommendations for Supplemental Preoperative Evaluation

The 12-Lead ECG
- Preoperative resting 12-lead ECG is reasonable for patients with known coronary heart disease or other significant structural heart disease, except for low-risk surgery.
- Preoperative resting 12-lead ECG may be considered for asymptomatic patients, except for low-risk surgery.
- Routine preoperative resting 12-lead ECG is not useful for asymptomatic patients undergoing low-risk surgical procedures.

Assessment of LV Function
- It is reasonable for patients with dyspnea of unknown origin to undergo preoperative evaluation of LV function.
- It is reasonable for patients with heart failure with worsening dyspnea or other change in clinical status to undergo preoperative evaluation of LV function.
- Reassessment of LV function in clinically stable patients may be considered.
- Routine preoperative evaluation of LV function is not recommended.
- Exercise stress testing for myocardial ischemia and functional capacity.
- For patients with elevated risk and excellent functional capacity, it is reasonable to forgo further exercise testing and proceed to surgery.
- For patients with elevated risk and unknown functional capacity, it may be reasonable to perform exercise testing to assess for functional capacity if it will change management.
- For patients with elevated risk and moderate to good functional capacity, it may be reasonable to forgo further exercise testing and proceed to surgery.
- For patients with elevated risk and poor or unknown functional capacity, it may be reasonable to perform exercise testing with cardiac imaging to assess for myocardial ischemia.
- Routine screening with noninvasive stress testing is not useful for low-risk noncardiac surgery.

Cardiopulmonary Exercise Testing
- Cardiopulmonary exercise testing may be considered for patients undergoing elevated risk procedures.

Noninvasive Pharmacologic Stress Testing Before Noncardiac Surgery
- It is reasonable for patients at elevated risk for noncardiac surgery with poor functional capacity to undergo either DSE or MPI if it will change management.
- Routine screening with noninvasive stress testing is not useful for low-risk noncardiac surgery.

Preoperative Coronary Angiography
- Routine preoperative coronary angiography is not recommended.

DSE, Dopamine stress echocardiography; *ECG,* electrocardiogram; *LV,* left ventricular; *MPI,* myocardial perfusion imaging.
Adapted from Fleisher LA, Fleischmann KE, Auerbach AD, et al. 2014 ACC/AHA guideline on perioperative cardiovascular evaluation and management of patients undergoing noncardiac surgery: a report of the American College of Cardiology/American Heart Association Task Force on practice guidelines. *J Am Coll Cardiol.* 2014;64:e77-e137.

---

in most patients undergoing noncardiac surgery is not supported by current evidence. Recommendations for management of patients who have undergone recent coronary revascularization are presented in Fig. 20.2.

Currently, the ACC/AHA recommends continuation of β-blocker therapy in those patients who are on chronic β-blocker therapy.[21] In β-blocker–naïve patients, perioperative β-blocker

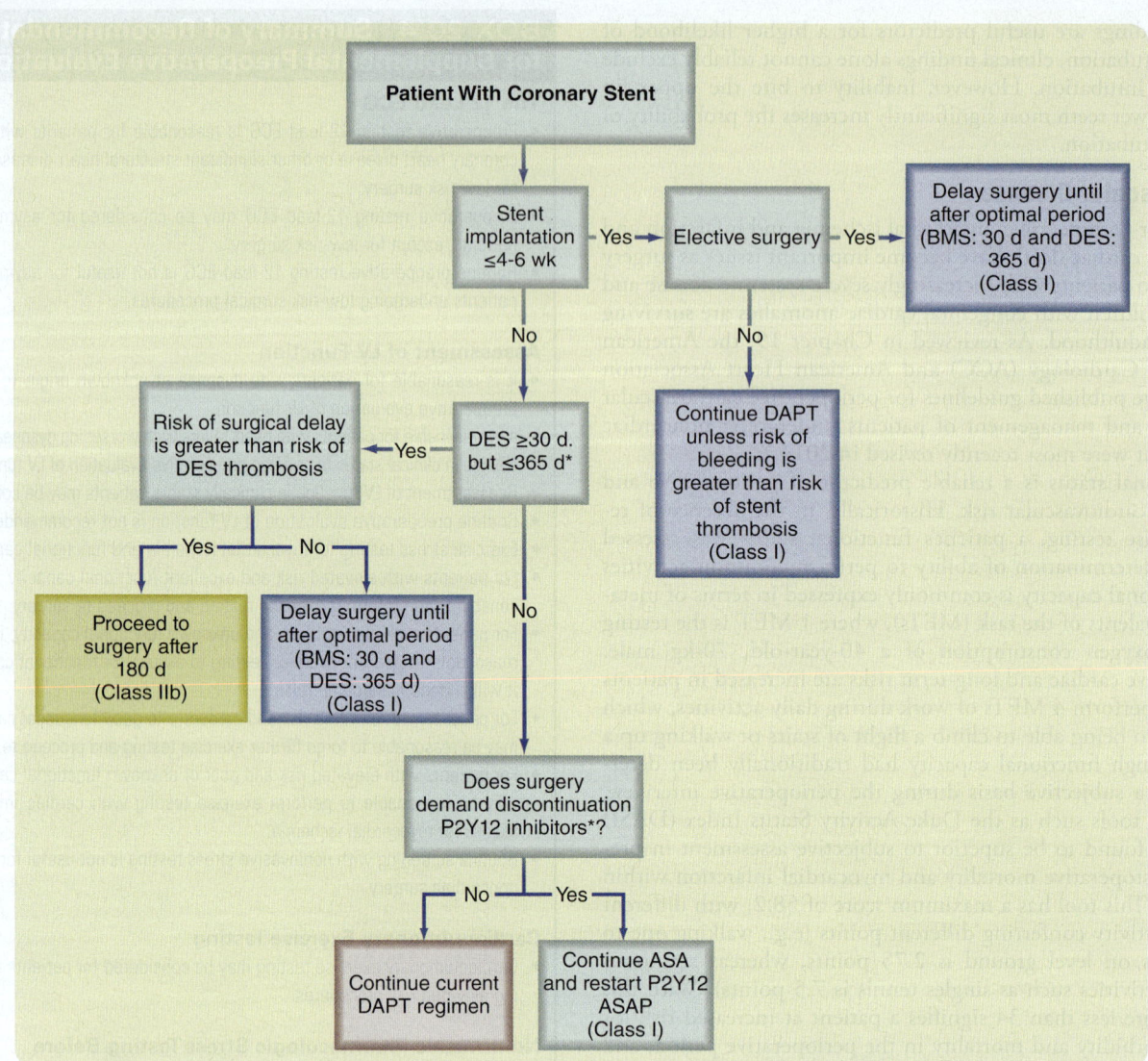

FIGURE 20.2 Stepwise approach to patients who have received recent coronary stenting and present for surgery. *ASA,* Acetylsalicylic acid; *ASAP,* as soon as possible; *BMS,* bare metal stent; *DAPT,* dual antiplatelet therapy; *DES,* drug eluting stent; *,* assuming patient currently on DAPT. (From Fleisher LA, Fleischmann KE, Auerbach AD, et al. 2014 ACC/AHA guideline on perioperative cardiovascular evaluation and management of patients undergoing noncardiac surgery: a report of the American College of Cardiology/American Heart Association Task Force on practice guidelines. *J Am Coll Cardiol.* 2014;64:e77-e137.)

therapy should be initiated with caution and based on clinical judgment. However, recent studies show that new initiation of β-blockade within 60 days of surgery may not carry an increased risk of perioperative stroke as was previously thought.[42] Similarly, the perioperative use of calcium channel blockers should be based on patient comorbidities and clinical judgment. Statins should be continued in patients on chronic statin therapy. Perioperative initiation of statin therapy should be considered in patients undergoing vascular surgery and patients at risk for cardiovascular disease who are undergoing high risk procedures. The use of α2-agonists for prevention of cardiac events is not recommended, based on the current literature. Some controversy exists around whether to hold angiotensin-converting enzyme inhibitors and angiotensin receptor antagonists 24 hours before surgery. A prospective cohort trial by Roshanov and colleagues (VISION study) demonstrated withholding these medications before surgery was associated with a lower risk of death and postoperative vascular

events.[43] However, Hollmann et al. in their subsequent meta-analysis did not confirm this observation, although they did confirm the increased incidence of intraoperative hypotension with continuing these drugs throughout the perioperative period.[44] An overview of recommendations for perioperative medical management is provided in Box 20.5.

Endocarditis Prophylaxis

Some patients with congenital or valvular heart disease are at increased risk for infective endocarditis (IE). Previous guidelines that recommended prophylactic antibiotics for at-risk patients undergoing dental, urinary, gastrointestinal, or respiratory surgical procedures were significantly scaled back by the AHA in 2007[39] when it was determined that IE was more attributable to intermittent bacteremia caused by daily activities (e.g., toothbrushing) than by dental and surgical procedures. This guidance was confirmed in a recent review by Wilson and colleagues[45];

BOX 20.5 Summary of Recommendations for Perioperative Medical Management

Coronary Revascularization Before Noncardiac Surgery
- Revascularization before noncardiac surgery is recommended when indicated by existing clinical practice guidelines.
- Coronary revascularization is not recommended before noncardiac surgery exclusively to reduce perioperative cardiac events.

Timing of Elective Noncardiac Surgery in Patients With Previous PCI
- Noncardiac surgery should be delayed after PCI, 14 days after balloon angioplasty and 30 days after BMS implantation.
- Noncardiac surgery should be delayed 365 days after DES implantation.
- A consensus decision as to the relative risks of discontinuation or continuation of antiplatelet therapy can be useful.
- Elective noncardiac surgery after DES implantation may be considered after 180 days, though some newer stents may allow a shorter interval.
- Elective noncardiac surgery should not be performed in patients in whom DAPT would need to be discontinued perioperatively within 30 days after BMS implantation or within 12 months after DES implantation, though some newer stents may allow a shorter interval.
- Elective noncardiac surgery should not be performed within 14 days of balloon angioplasty in patients in whom aspirin will need to be discontinued perioperatively.

Perioperative β-Blocker Therapy
- β-Blockers should be continued in patients who are on long-term β-blocker therapy.
- Management of β-blockers after surgery should be guided by clinical circumstances.
- In patients with intermediate-risk or high-risk preoperative test results, it may be reasonable to begin β-blocker therapy.
- In patients with three or more RCRI factors, it may be reasonable to begin β-blockers before surgery.
- Initiating β-blockers in the perioperative setting as an approach to reduce perioperative risk is of uncertain benefit in those with a long-term indication but no other RCRI risk factors.
- It may be reasonable to begin perioperative β-blockers long enough in advance to assess safety and tolerability, preferably >1 day before surgery.
- β-Blocker therapy should not be started on the day of surgery.

Perioperative Statin Therapy
- Continue statins in patients currently taking statins.
- Perioperative initiation of statin use is reasonable in patients undergoing vascular surgery.
- Perioperative initiation of statins may be considered in patients with a clinical risk factor who are undergoing elevated-risk procedures.

α₂-Agonists
- α₂-Agonists are not recommended for prevention of cardiac events.

Angiotensin-Converting Enzyme (ACE) Inhibitors
- Continuation of ACE inhibitors or angiotensin receptor blockers (ARBs) is reasonable perioperatively.
- If ACE inhibitors or ARBs are held before surgery, it is reasonable to restart as soon as clinically feasible postoperatively.

Antiplatelet Agents
- DAPT is continued in patients undergoing urgent noncardiac surgery in the first 4–6 weeks after BMS or DES implantation, unless the risk of bleeding outweighs the benefit of stent thrombosis prevention.
- In patients with stents undergoing surgery that requires discontinuation P2Y12 inhibitors, continue aspirin and restart the P2Y12 platelet receptor-inhibitor as soon as possible after surgery.
- Management of perioperative antiplatelet therapy should be determined by consensus of treating clinicians and the patient.
- In patients undergoing nonemergency/nonurgent noncardiac surgery without prior coronary stenting, it may be reasonable to continue aspirin when the risk of increased cardiac events outweighs the risk of increased bleeding.
- Initiation or continuation of aspirin is not beneficial in patients undergoing elective noncardiac noncarotid surgery who have not had a previous coronary stent.

Perioperative Management of Patients With CIEDs
- Patients with ICDs should be on a cardiac monitor continuously during the entire period of inactivation, and external defibrillation equipment should be available. Ensure that ICDs are reprogrammed to active therapy.

BMS, Bare metal stent; *CIED,* cardiac implantable electrical device; *DAPT,* dual antiplatelet therapy; *DES,* drug-eluting stent; *ICD,* implantable cardioverter-defibrillator; *PCI,* percutaneous coronary intervention; *RCRI,* revised cardiac risk index.
Adapted from Fleisher LA, Fleischmann KE, Auerbach AD, et al. 2014 ACC/AHA guideline on perioperative cardiovascular evaluation and management of patients undergoing noncardiac surgery: a report of the American College of Cardiology/American Heart Association Task Force on practice guidelines. *J Am Coll Cardiol.* 2014;64:e77-e137.

therefore, antibiotic prophylaxis is recommended for only four categories of patients thought to have the highest risk of adverse outcomes (Box 20.6). In these patients, the AHA panel states that antibiotic prophylaxis is recommended for dental procedures that involve manipulation of gingival tissues, periapical region of teeth, or perforation of oral mucosa as well as respiratory tract procedures or procedures that manipulate infected skin or musculoskeletal structures. Antibiotics for IE prophylaxis are no longer recommended for genitourinary or gastrointestinal tract procedures. Oral amoxicillin is the drug of choice, and alternative drugs and routes are recommended for patients who are unable to take oral medications or those with penicillin allergy (Table 20.5).

Pulmonary Disease

Many surgical patients have obstructive or restrictive pulmonary disease. The preoperative history focuses on functional status, exercise tolerance, severity of respiratory disease, and current medications. The recent trajectory of symptoms must be closely evaluated. A thorough chest physical examination must be performed. These factors guide preoperative testing, which may include chest radiography, arterial blood gas analysis, and pulmonary function testing. The goal of preoperative evaluation is to detect and treat reversible pulmonary pathology, optimize medical management, and allow planning for postoperative ventilatory support, if indicated.

The perioperative risk associated with preexisting pulmonary disease has been extensively studied. As described in Chapter 19, the most commonly used and validated tool in predicting postoperative pulmonary complications is the Assess Respiratory Risk in Surgical Patients in Catalonia (ARISCAT) score. Obstructive sleep apnea (OSA) is an increasingly common condition in surgical patients that also requires preoperative evaluation and optimization.

BOX 20.6 Cardiac Conditions Associated With the Highest Risk of Adverse Outcome From Endocarditis for Which Prophylaxis With Dental Procedures is Reasonable

- Prosthetic cardiac valve or prosthetic material used for cardiac valve repair
- Previous, relapsed, or recurrent infective endocarditis (IE)
- Congenital heart disease (CHD)[a]
  - Unrepaired cyanotic CHD, including palliative shunts and conduits
  - Completely repaired congenital heart defect with prosthetic material or device, whether placed by surgery or by catheter intervention, during the first 6 months after the procedure[b]
  - Repaired CHD with residual defects at the site or adjacent to the site of a prosthetic patch or prosthetic device (which inhibit endothelialization)
- Cardiac transplantation recipients who develop cardiac valvulopathy

[a]Except for the conditions listed above, antibiotic prophylaxis is no longer recommended for any other form of CHD.
[b]Prophylaxis is reasonable because endothelialization of prosthetic material occurs within 6 months after the procedure.

The ASA, Society for Ambulatory Anesthesia, and Society of Anesthesia and Sleep Medicine have released practice guidelines for the management of patients with OSA.[46–48] These guidelines emphasize the importance of preoperative identification of patients at increased risk from OSA, which can be accomplished with the use of validated screening tools such as the STOP-BANG questionnaire and the ASA checklist.[49] Currently, in the absence of concomitant uncontrolled systemic comorbidities such as cardiopulmonary disease, delay of surgical procedures for further investigation and diagnosis is not recommended. Finally, these guidelines emphasize the development of protocols to optimize perioperative care of patients with OSA that may include minimizing sedating medications and instituting postoperative use of positive airway pressure devices, particularly in the immediate postoperative period.

Patients with asthma or chronic obstructive pulmonary disease should be examined and evaluated for bronchodilator and steroid use, number and severity of recent respiratory exacerbations, history of previous intubation, and precipitating factors. Preoperative optimization is driven by patient symptomatology and encompasses smoking cessation, optimization of pharmacologic therapies including inhaled β_2-agonists, anticholinergics, and steroids, and treating other existing comorbidities such as malnutrition. The choice of anesthetic agents and technique is dependent on patient condition and type of surgery. In patients with active disease, elective surgery should be postponed until the patient is adequately treated.

Pulmonary function testing in the preoperative period remains controversial, except in patients undergoing major lung resection or who are found to have new, unexplained dyspnea. Pulmonary function testing has variable predictive value, cannot define a threshold above which the risk associated with surgery is prohibitive, and cannot identify patients at risk who do not already have clinical evidence of pulmonary disease. Arterial blood gas analysis also does not identify a group for whom the risk of surgery is prohibitive, but it may provide an informative baseline of a patient's overall respiratory status and accelerative intraoperative and postoperative decisions and comfort for extubation of patients with baseline chronic hypoxia and/or chronic hypercarbia. Spirometry may be helpful in a patient who has unexplained cough, dyspnea, or exercise intolerance, or if there is a question regarding optimal improvement of airflow obstruction.

Renal and Hepatic Disease

Patients with acute renal or hepatic insufficiency should not undergo elective surgery until these conditions can be adequately characterized and stabilized.

Chronic renal insufficiency (CRI) provides many perioperative management challenges, including acid-base abnormalities, electrolyte disturbances, and coagulation disorders. Current daily urinary output in patients making urine and the type/frequency of dialysis, dialysis access, and any related complications should be established. Physical examination should evaluate volume status as well as evaluate for CRI-complications, including coagulopathy, anemia, pericardial effusion, and encephalopathy. Laboratory evaluation includes assessment of anemia, electrolyte abnormalities (particularly hyperkalemia and acidemia), and coagulopathy. Dialysis ideally should be performed 18 to 24 hours before surgery to avoid the fluid and electrolyte shifts that occur immediately after dialysis.

Chronic liver disease poses many perioperative challenges, with increasing risk conferred by severity of dysfunction. Liver disease can alter drug metabolism, and hypoalbuminemia increases the free fraction of many drugs, impacting pharmacokinetics and dynamics of anesthetics. Altered synthetic function can also lead to coagulopathy and hypercoagulability. Patients with elevated portal pressures may

TABLE 20.5 Antibiotic Regimens for Dental Procedures

SITUATION	AGENT	REGIMEN (SINGLE DOSE ADMINISTERED 30–60 MIN BEFORE THE PROCEDURE)	
		ADULTS	CHILDREN
Able to take oral medication	Amoxicillin	2 g	50 mg/kg
Unable to take oral medication	Ampicillin	2 g IM or IV	50 mg/kg IM or IV
	Cefazolin or ceftriaxone	1 g IM or IV	50 mg/kg IM or IV
Allergic to penicillin or ampicillin	Cephalexin	2 g	50 mg/kg
	Clindamycin	600 mg	20 mg/kg
	Azithromycin or clarithromycin	500 mg	15 mg/kg
Allergic to penicillin or ampicillin and unable to take oral medication	Cefazolin or ceftriaxone	1 g IM or IV	50 mg/kg IM or IV
	Clindamycin	600 mg IM or IV	20 mg/kg IM or IV

Cephalosporins should not be used in an individual with a history of anaphylaxis, angioedema, or urticaria with penicillins or ampicillin.
IM, Intramuscular; *IV*, intravenous.

also have encephalopathy and ascites, which can impact medication doses and increase risk for aspiration, respectively.

Endocrinology, Metabolism, and Nutrition

Diabetes mellitus is prevalent in the surgical population, and there is a clear association between hyperglycemia and adverse clinical outcomes. Preanesthetic evaluation should include the type of diabetes, the current medication regimen, and any sequelae of disease, including autonomic dysfunction, cardiovascular disease, renal insufficiency, retinopathy, and neurologic complications. Patients with poorly controlled diabetes are at high risk for delayed gastric emptying and gastroesophageal reflux, which can predispose aspiration. Perioperative management of glucose requires careful attention, given the risks of both hypoglycemia and hyperglycemia. Over the long term, there is compelling evidence of a correlation between hyperglycemia and increased perioperative complications and decreased long-term survival. An A1c <8% is a commonly accepted target before elective surgeries. During a surgical encounter, there is evidence that treating hyperglycemia (>180 mg/dL) reduces complications and mortality.[50] In diabetic patients undergoing surgery, several principles of management are generally accepted. Current recommendations for diabetes medication management are as follows:

1. Insulin pumps should be continued at sleep basal rates.
2. Provide a reduced dose of intermediate-acting or long-acting insulin and hold short-acting insulin on the morning of surgery.
3. Once a diabetic who is receiving nothing by mouth is given insulin, provide glucose in IV fluids or closely monitor plasma glucose concentrations.
4. Plasma glucose concentrations should be checked before surgery and before discharge as a minimum.
5. In patients with type 2 diabetes, most authors suggest holding oral antidiabetic medications and noninsulin injectables on the day of surgery. Metformin is usually stopped because of a slight risk for perioperative drug-induced lactic acidosis.
6. Perioperative insulin requirements vary depending on body weight, liver disease, steroid therapy, infection, and the use of cardiopulmonary bypass.

As described in Chapter 19 (Figure 19.7), Patients who are receiving systemic glucocorticoids at a dose equivalent of 5 mg of prednisone daily for at least 2 weeks during the month before surgery may have adrenal insufficiency and be unable to respond adequately to surgical stress without glucocorticoid supplementation. Appropriate dosing is based on the duration of therapy and the type of surgery.

Malnutrition affects a large portion of patients undergoing major surgery and is associated with multiple adverse outcomes including postoperative morbidity, mortality, infection, poor wound healing, prolonged hospitalization, and delirium. Malnutrition risk should be evaluated in patients preoperatively using a validated malnutrition screening tool such as the perioperative nutrition screen (PONS), and patients should be supplemented with oral protein where appropriate.[51]

Fasting Before Surgery

Pulmonary aspiration of gastric contents during anesthesia is an uncommon, but serious, complication. To minimize the risk of large volume aspiration, nil per os (NPO; nothing by mouth) guidelines have been developed. Traditionally, orders for "NPO after midnight" forbade any intake of liquids and solids starting at midnight of the day of surgery. However, applying the same guidelines for clear liquids (gastric emptying time of 1–2 hours)

TABLE 20.6 Summary of Preoperative Fasting Recommendations to Reduce the Risk of Pulmonary Aspiration[a]

INGESTED MATERIAL	MINIMUM FASTING PERIOD (HOURS)
Clear liquids[b]	2
Breast milk	4
Infant formula	6
Nonhuman milk	6
Light, nonfatty solid food	6
All other food	8

[a]Applies to healthy patients undergoing elective procedures.
[b]Examples of clear liquids are water, fruit juices without pulp, black coffee, clear tea, and carbonated beverages.
Adapted from Practice guidelines for preoperative fasting and the use of pharmacologic agents to reduce the risk of pulmonary aspiration: application to healthy patients undergoing elective procedures: a report by the American Society of Anesthesiologist Task Force on Preoperative Fasting. *Anesthesiology.* 1999;90:896-905.

and solids (gastric emptying time of 6 hours) has been questioned. The ASA guidelines (first adopted in 1998 and most recently updated in 2017) recommend a minimum fasting period of 2 hours after the ingestion of clear liquids; 4 hours after the ingestion of breast milk; 6 hours for light, nonfatty solids (e.g., toast) and nonclear liquids such as infant formula, milk, or orange juice; and 8 hours for heavier foods (Table 20.6). *Clear liquids* are defined as liquids that one can see through that do not contain solids or particulates. The routine use of gastrointestinal stimulants, gastric acid secretion blockers, antacids, and antiemetics is not recommended. However, many patients have medical conditions or take medications that cause decreased gastric emptying, which may warrant use of promotility or antacid medications. When these guidelines cannot be met during emergency procedures, other precautions such as rapid sequence intubation are utilized to decrease the risk of aspiration.

The reported incidence of aspiration during general anesthesia is 1 in every 2000 to 3000 cases. A higher incidence has been noted during emergency surgery and in patients with disease processes that slow gastric emptying. Of note, some reports suggest that aspiration is at least as common during emergence from anesthesia as during the induction phase. Of patients in whom aspiration is suspected, fewer than half exhibit evidence of pulmonary injury. In one study, approximately one-third of patients with suspected aspiration during anesthesia required postoperative intubation and ventilation. Most of these patients were extubated within 6 hours of surgery. About 10% of patients required intubation and ventilation for 24 hours or longer. Approximately half the patients requiring ventilation for longer than 24 hours after aspiration of gastric contents died of pulmonary complications.

Assessment of Physical Status

As covered in Chapter 19 (Table 19.1), the ASA has developed a graded, descriptive scale to categorize preoperative comorbidity. The classification is independent of operative procedure and serves as a standardized method of communicating patient physical status to anesthesiologists and other healthcare providers.

Selection of Anesthetic Techniques and Drugs

Patient factors (e.g., comorbidities and home medications) and surgical factors both influence choice of anesthetic technique and choice of drugs. For example, operative site, positioning, and surgical duration are surgical factors that impact airway management and medication management. Expected disposition (home vs. admission) may influence factors such as appropriateness of neuraxial analgesia or choice of opioid. After completing the preanesthetic evaluation and understanding surgical needs, the anesthesiologist discusses various options regarding anesthetic care with the patient, and, ideally, a joint decision is made about approach if multiple options exist.

The major categories of anesthetic approach include monitored anesthesia care (sometimes abbreviated as MAC, to be distinguished from the identical abbreviation for minimum alveolar concentration), regional anesthesia with or without additional sedation (including regional upper and lower extremity blocks, subarachnoid blocks, and epidural anesthesia), and general anesthesia. MAC generally requires that analgesia be provided via local anesthetic delivered by the surgeon or via regional techniques performed by the anesthesia team, as sedation must be light enough that patients are able to maintain spontaneous ventilation. The target depth of sedation—be it anxiolysis alone with a responsive patient or a patient who is sedated enough to require repeated or painful stimulation to respond purposefully—should be determined intentionally based on the needs of the patient and surgical procedure. Regional techniques can allow for a fully awake patient (e.g., parturient during cesarean section under spinal, or a carotid endarterectomy under superficial and deep cervical plexus blocks) or can be supplemented with MAC or even a general anesthetic should the block be intended primarily for postoperative analgesia. The ability to convert a lighter anesthetic to a general anesthetic should procedural or patient factors require doing so must be anticipated. These approaches will be discussed at greater length in the following sections.

Risk of Anesthesia

Patients often desire information regarding the risk of death or major complications associated with anesthesia. Because perioperative death and major complications have become relatively uncommon, the risk associated with anesthesia is difficult to quantify. An estimated 313 million surgical cases occur worldwide each year. In developed nations, surgical mortality is estimated to be 0.4% to 3.7%, with morbidity rates of 6.7% to 13.8%.[52] The risk for cardiac arrest attributable to anesthesia appears to be less than 1 in 10,000 cases.[53] The American College of Surgeons National Surgical Quality Improvement Program (ACS NSQIP) risk calculator (http://www.surgicalriskcalculator.com) is a validated tool that can be used to predict patient-specific risks and help inform surgical and anesthetic decision-making and informed consent.[54] The ACS NSQIP risk calculator incorporates 20 patient predictors including age, sex, functional status, ASA physical status class, body mass index, chronic medical conditions, surgical procedure, and urgency of the procedure to predict the likelihood of 18 different outcomes within 30 days following surgery. However, this tool does not consider anesthetic technique, which may modify the overall risk.

Because so many surgical procedures are now performed without admission to the hospital, understanding the risk associated with ambulatory anesthesia is particularly important. Large studies have repeatedly demonstrated low rates of morbidity and mortality after ambulatory surgery. Patient and procedure selection as well as social factors (e.g., availability of a responsible individual to take the patient home) are important in determining the safety of outpatient anesthesia and surgical procedures.[55]

AIRWAY MANAGEMENT

Airway management is perhaps one of the most critical skills in anesthesiology. As previously discussed, the preoperative evaluation focuses on recognition of patients who may be difficult to mask ventilate or intubate. Knowledge of and skill with various techniques for establishing an airway are central to the safe practice of anesthesiology. Fortunately, the incidence of difficult intubations is low. Difficult direct laryngoscopy occurs in 1.5% to 8.5% of general anesthetics, and failed intubation occurs in 0.13% to 0.3% of general anesthetics. The LMA, the lighted stylet, and an array of video laryngoscopes are recent developments that make ventilation and intubation possible in many patients who would have failed intubation with a conventional laryngoscope. The fiberoptic bronchoscope is an additional tool for the management of a difficult airway.

Given the importance of a prompt, effective response to difficult intubation, the ASA has developed guidelines for managing difficult airways (Fig. 20.3). A key factor is the recognition of the patient with a potentially difficult airway. If the practitioner suspects that mask ventilation and tracheal intubation will be difficult, it is recommended that spontaneous ventilation be preserved. Approaches to these patients include awake intubation or the use of anesthetic techniques that preserve spontaneous ventilation. In some cases, establishment of a surgical airway in an awake patient under local anesthesia may be indicated. However, some patients are found to have a difficult airway only after anesthesia and muscle relaxation have been induced. This is an emergency situation that must be addressed quickly to avoid hypoxemia, brain injury, or death. A variety of airway adjuncts are available to preserve ventilation and facilitate tracheal intubation under emergency conditions. The practitioner should call for assistance in these situations to optimize patient safety and consider reestablishment of spontaneous ventilation. It is essential to have alternate means for securing the airway available for all patients in the event of an unanticipated difficult airway.

GENERAL ANESTHESIA

General anesthesia is a reversible state of unconsciousness. Although the mechanism of general anesthetics remains speculative and controversial, the four components of general anesthesia (i.e., amnesia, analgesia, inhibition of noxious reflexes, and skeletal muscle relaxation) are usually achieved in modern anesthesia by a combination of IV anesthetics and analgesics, inhalational anesthetics, and, frequently, muscle relaxants. Because the drugs that produce these components cause both desirable and undesirable physiologic changes, the pharmacologic effects of the agents must be matched to the pathophysiology of the patient's comorbidities. The major adverse changes associated with anesthetic drugs are respiratory depression, cardiovascular depression, and loss of airway maintenance and protection. Important complications of general anesthesia include hypoxemia with possible CNS damage; hypotension; cardiac arrest; and aspiration of acidic gastric contents, which can lead to severe pulmonary damage. Dental damage is more frequent but not life-threatening. General anesthesia can be maintained by inhalation of volatile agents or by infusion of IV agents. Both techniques can have advantages under certain conditions, and individual patient factors should be considered. Discussion of specific agents occurred earlier in this chapter (see the section "Pharmacologic Principles"). General anesthesia is required for major intraabdominal and thoracic

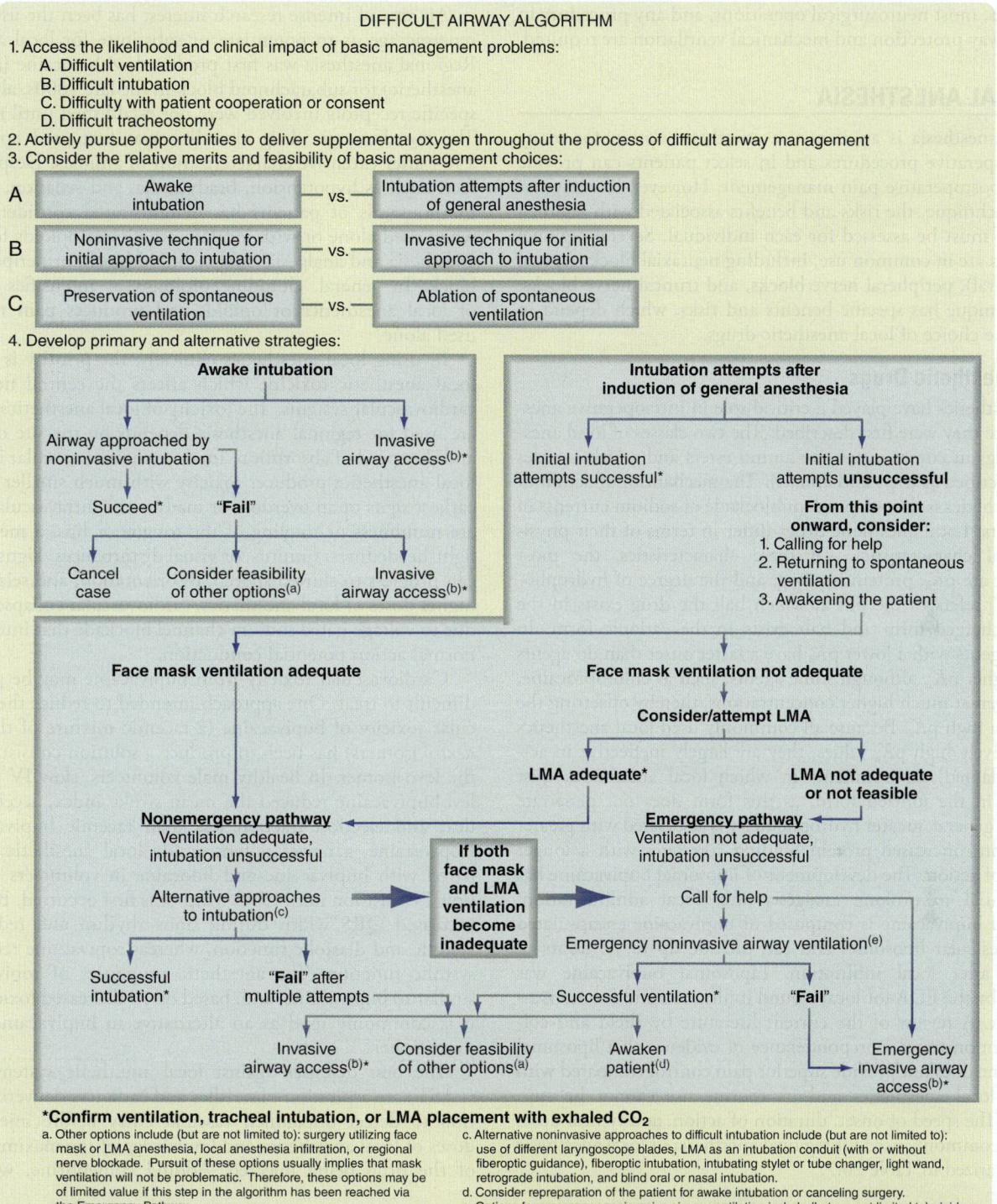

DIFFICULT AIRWAY ALGORITHM

1. Access the likelihood and clinical impact of basic management problems:
   A. Difficult ventilation
   B. Difficult intubation
   C. Difficulty with patient cooperation or consent
   D. Difficult tracheostomy
2. Actively pursue opportunities to deliver supplemental oxygen throughout the process of difficult airway management
3. Consider the relative merits and feasibility of basic management choices:

A. Awake intubation vs. Intubation attempts after induction of general anesthesia

B. Noninvasive technique for initial approach to intubation vs. Invasive technique for initial approach to intubation

C. Preservation of spontaneous ventilation vs. Ablation of spontaneous ventilation

4. Develop primary and alternative strategies:

Awake intubation
- Airway approached by noninvasive intubation
  - Succeed*
  - "Fail"
    - Cancel case
    - Consider feasibility of other options[a]
    - Invasive airway access[b]*
- Invasive airway access[b]*

Intubation attempts after induction of general anesthesia
- Initial intubation attempts successful*
- Initial intubation attempts **unsuccessful**
  - **From this point onward, consider:**
    1. Calling for help
    2. Returning to spontaneous ventilation
    3. Awakening the patient

Face mask ventilation adequate

Face mask ventilation not adequate
- **Consider/attempt LMA**
  - LMA adequate*
  - **LMA not adequate or not feasible**

Nonemergency pathway
Ventilation adequate, intubation unsuccessful
- Alternative approaches to intubation[c]
  - Successful intubation*
  - "Fail" after multiple attempts

If both face mask and LMA ventilation become inadequate

Emergency pathway
Ventilation not adequate, intubation unsuccessful
- Call for help
- Emergency noninvasive airway ventilation[e]
  - Successful ventilation*
  - "Fail"

- Invasive airway access[b]*
- Consider feasibility of other options[a]
- Awaken patient[d]
- Emergency invasive airway access[b]*

*Confirm ventilation, tracheal intubation, or LMA placement with exhaled CO$_2$

a. Other options include (but are not limited to): surgery utilizing face mask or LMA anesthesia, local anesthesia infiltration, or regional nerve blockade. Pursuit of these options usually implies that mask ventilation will not be problematic. Therefore, these options may be of limited value if this step in the algorithm has been reached via the Emergency Pathway.
b. Invasive airway access includes surgical or percutaneous tracheostomy or cricothyrotomy.
c. Alternative noninvasive approaches to difficult intubation include (but are not limited to): use of different laryngoscope blades, LMA as an intubation conduit (with or without fiberoptic guidance), fiberoptic intubation, intubating stylet or tube changer, light wand, retrograde intubation, and blind oral or nasal intubation.
d. Consider repreparation of the patient for awake intubation or canceling surgery.
e. Options for emergency noninvasive airway ventilation include (but are not limited to): rigid bronchoscope, esophageal-tracheal combitube ventilation, or transtracheal jet ventilation.

FIGURE 20.3 American Society of Anesthesiologists difficult airway algorithm. The likelihood and clinical impact of basic management problems such as difficult intubation, difficult mask ventilation, and difficulty with patient cooperation or consent should be assessed in all patients in whom airway management is being contemplated. The clinician should consider the relative merits and feasibility of basic management choices, including the use of awake intubation techniques, preservation of spontaneous ventilation, and the use of surgical approaches to establish a secure airway. Primary and alternative strategies should be considered: (a) other options include, but are not limited to, surgery under mask anesthesia, surgery under local infiltration or nerve block, and intubation attempts after induction of general anesthesia; (b) alternative approaches include the use of different laryngoscope blades, awake intubation, blind oral or nasal intubation, fiberoptic intubation, an intubating stylet or tube changer, light wand, retrograde intubation, and surgical airway access; (c) see awake intubation; (d) options for an emergency nonsurgical airway include transtracheal jet ventilation, laryngeal mask airway *(LMA)*, and Combitube. (From Practice guidelines for management of the difficult airway. A report by the American Society of Anesthesiologists Task Force on Management of the Difficult Airway. *Anesthesiology.* 1993;78:597-602.)

procedures, most neurosurgical operations, and any procedure in which airway protection and mechanical ventilation are required.

REGIONAL ANESTHESIA

Regional anesthesia is an attractive anesthetic option for many types of operative procedures and in select patients can provide excellent postoperative pain management. However, like any anesthetic technique, the risks and benefits associated with regional anesthesia must be assessed for each individual. Several regional techniques are in common use, including neuraxial blocks (spinal and epidural), peripheral nerve blocks, and truncal nerve blocks. Each technique has specific benefits and risks, which depend in part on the choice of local anesthetic drugs.

Local Anesthetic Drugs

Local anesthetics have played a critical role in intraoperative anesthesia since they were first described. The two classes of local anesthetic drugs in common use are amino esters and amino amides (often described as *esters* and *amides*). The mechanism of action of local anesthetics is dose-dependent blockade of sodium currents in nerve fibers. Local anesthetic drugs differ in terms of their physicochemical characteristics. Of these characteristics, the most important are pK_a, protein binding, and the degree of hydrophobicity; pK_a refers to the pH at which half the drug exists in the basic, uncharged form and half exists in the cationic form. In general, agents with a lower pK_a have a faster onset than do agents with a higher pK_a, although some agents, such as chloroprocaine, can be given at much higher concentrations, thereby offsetting the effects of a high pK_a. Because all commonly used local anesthetics have relatively high pK_a values, they are largely ineffective in acidotic (inflamed) environments in which local anesthetics exist primarily in the ionized form, as this form does not penetrate nerves. In general, greater hydrophobicity is associated with greater potency, and increased protein binding correlates with a longer duration of action. The development of liposomal bupivacaine has the potential to prolong analgesia after local administration. Liposomal bupivacaine is composed of bupivacaine encapsulated in multivesicular liposomes and can provide up to 72 hours of analgesia after local infiltration. Liposomal bupivacaine was approved by the FDA for local wound infiltration and for interscalene block. A review of the current literature by Ilfeld and colleagues demonstrates a preponderance of evidence that liposomal bupivacaine does not provide superior pain control compared with standard local anesthetics and its routine use cannot be supported.[56] The speed of onset, duration of action, and typical doses of agents commonly used for regional anesthesia or local anesthesia are summarized in Table 20.7.

An area of intense research interest has been the use of α_2-adrenergic agents to potentiate or substitute for local anesthetics. Regional anesthesia was first produced with cocaine (also a local anesthetic) for subarachnoid block in the late 1800s, although the specific receptors involved were not established until much later. The α_2-adrenergic drug clonidine was first used epidurally in 1984 after extensive characterization in animals. Despite side effects such as hypotension, bradycardia, and sedation, experience in thousands of patients has demonstrated considerable safety when used alone or with local anesthetics or opioids for epidural anesthesia and analgesia, subarachnoid block, or peripheral nerve block. In general, clonidine prolongs or intensifies the effects of local anesthetics or opioids and produces pain relief when used alone.

In using local anesthetics clinically, the priority is to prevent local anesthetic toxicity, which affects the central nervous and cardiovascular systems. The toxicity of local anesthetics when they are used for regional anesthesia depends on the site of injection and the speed of absorption. Inadvertent intravascular injection of local anesthetics produces toxicity with much smaller doses. The earliest signs of an overdose or inadvertent intravascular injection are numbness or tingling of the tongue or lips, a metallic taste, light-headedness, tinnitus, or visual disturbances. Signs of toxicity can progress to slurred speech, disorientation, and seizures. With higher doses of local anesthetics, cardiovascular collapse will ensue due to voltage-gated sodium channel blockade that interferes with normal action potential conduction.

Cardiovascular toxicity from bupivacaine may be particularly difficult to treat. One approach intended to reduce the cardiovascular toxicity of bupivacaine (a racemic mixture of the *levo* and *dextro* isomers) has been to produce a solution consisting of only the levo isomer. In healthy male volunteers, slow IV infusion of levobupivacaine reduced the mean stroke index, acceleration index, and ejection fraction less than racemic bupivacaine did. Ropivacaine, a newer potent amide local anesthetic, was compared with bupivacaine and lidocaine in volunteers receiving a slow IV infusion until CNS symptoms first occurred. Bupivacaine increased QRS width during sinus rhythm and reduced both systolic and diastolic function, whereas ropivacaine reduced only systolic function. The anesthetic properties of ropivacaine are similar to bupivacaine, and, based on its decreased toxicity profile, it is commonly used as an alternative to bupivacaine by many practitioners.

The best defenses against local anesthetic systemic toxicity (LAST) are aspiration of needles and catheters delivering medication to detect unplanned vascular entry before injecting large doses of local anesthetics and knowledge of the maximal safe dose of the drug being injected. Adding epinephrine, which slows

TABLE 20.7   Important Characteristics of Local Anesthetics for Major Nerve Blocks

LOCAL ANESTHETIC	AMINOAMIDE OR AMINO ESTER	SPEED OF ONSET (MIN)	DURATION OF ACTION (MIN)	MAXIMAL DOSE[a] (AXILLARY BLOCK)
Lidocaine	Amino amide	10–20	60–180	5 mg/kg
Mepivacaine	Amino amide	10–20	60–180	5 mg/kg
Bupivacaine	Amino amide	15–30	180–360	3 mg/kg
Ropivacaine	Amino amide	15–30	180–360	3 mg/kg
Chloroprocaine	Amino ester	10–20	30–50	Not generally used

[a]Maximal dose without epinephrine; doses of lidocaine and mepivacaine can be increased to 7 to 8 mg/kg if epinephrine is added. Lower doses may be toxic if infiltrated subcutaneously, as for intercostal nerve blocks; larger doses of lidocaine and mepivacaine may be tolerated if given by epidural injection.

absorption, also decreases the likelihood of a toxic response secondary to rapid absorption. The primary treatments of LAST are cessation of local anesthetic administration, airway management, seizure treatment with benzodiazepines, and cardiovascular support. Current guidelines from the American Society of Regional Anesthesia (ASRA) Pain Medicine recommend administration of a 1.5 mL/kg bolus of 20% lipid emulsion (calculated using lean body mass) over 2 to 3 minutes with a subsequent infusion of 0.25 mL/kg/min until stable (maximum dose 12 mL/kg ideal body weight). Additionally, if cardiovascular collapse occurs, several alterations to the advanced cardiac life support algorithm must be considered. Epinephrine dosing should be reduced to boluses of 1 µg/kg and all local anesthetic antiarrhythmics, β-blockers, calcium channel blockers, and vasopressin should be avoided.[57]

Spinal Anesthesia

Spinal anesthesia or subarachnoid block has many applications for urologic, lower abdominal, perineal, and lower extremity surgery. Spinal anesthesia is induced by the injection of local anesthetic, with or without opiates, into the subarachnoid space. A well-performed subarachnoid block provides excellent sensory and motor blockade below the level of the block. The block generally has a relatively rapid and predictable onset. Several factors determine the level, speed of onset, and duration of spinal blockade.

1. Local anesthetic agent. Local anesthetics have varying potencies, durations of action, and speeds of onset after subarachnoid administration. Typical doses and durations of action are shown in Table 20.8. Bupivacaine and ropivacaine have significantly longer durations of action than lidocaine or chloroprocaine. These properties are determined by the lipid solubility, protein binding, and pK_a of each agent.
2. Volume and dose of the local anesthetic. Increasing the dose will generally increase the extent of cephalad spread and duration of subarachnoid blockade. Rapidly injecting local anesthetic solutions leads to turbulent flow and unpredictable spread.
3. Patient position and local anesthetic baricity. Local anesthetic solutions can be prepared as hypobaric, isobaric, and hyperbaric solutions, as compared with cerebrospinal fluid (CSF). A solution that is hypobaric relative to CSF will ascend relative to injection site, whereas a hyperbaric solution will sink. The level of block will be determined by the baricity of the local anesthetic solution and the physical position of the patient from the time of injection until the local anesthetic firmly binds to nervous tissue. For example, administration of hyperbaric bupivacaine at the low lumbar level to a patient in the sitting position will result in intense lumbosacral blockade. The longer the patient remains in the sitting position, the less the cephalad spread of the block.

4. Vasoconstrictors. The addition of epinephrine or phenylephrine, particularly to short-acting local anesthetics, will increase the duration of action.
5. Addition of opioids. The addition of small doses of fentanyl (e.g., 20 µg) or morphine (e.g., 0.25 mg) will prolong the duration of analgesia and increase the duration of analgesia and tolerance for tourniquet pain.
6. Anatomic and physiologic factors. A higher than expected level of spinal anesthesia can result from anatomic factors that decrease the relative volume of the subarachnoid space, such as obesity, pregnancy, increased intraabdominal pressure, previous spine surgery, and abnormal spinal curvature. Elderly patients tend to be more sensitive to intrathecally injected local anesthetics.

Spinal anesthesia provides the advantage of avoiding manipulation of the airway and the potential complication of tracheal intubation, as well as the potential side effects of general anesthetics such as nausea, vomiting, and prolonged emergence or drowsiness. Spinal anesthesia also provides advantages for several types of surgery, including endoscopic urologic procedures, particularly transurethral resection of the prostate, in which an awake patient provides a valuable monitor for assessment of hyponatremia or bladder perforation. Previously, regional anesthesia for hip fracture surgery was thought to decrease postoperative delirium and confusion compared with general anesthesia. However, a recent study by Li and colleagues found no difference in rates of postoperative delirium in patients who had undergone regional anesthesia without sedation versus those who had general anesthesia.[58] Intrathecal opiate administration can provide high-quality postoperative analgesia for patients undergoing abdominal, lower extremity, urologic, and gynecologic procedures.

In most cases, spinal anesthesia is administered as a single bolus injection. Therefore, the block is of limited duration and is not suitable for prolonged procedures. The practice of continuous spinal anesthesia with the use of small-bore catheters has largely been abandoned because of neurologic complications associated with LAST. However, continuous spinal anesthesia with relatively large-bore epidural catheters can provide the advantages of incremental titration and the ability to administer additional doses in selected elderly patients. Unfortunately, in young patients this technique has a high likelihood of inducing a postdural puncture headache.

Complications of subarachnoid block include hypotension (sometimes refractory), bradycardia, postdural puncture headache, transient radicular neuropathy, backache, urinary retention, infection, epidural hematoma, and excessive cephalad spread resulting in cardiorespiratory compromise. Frank neurologic injury, although recently described with continuous techniques using small-bore catheters, is quite rare. Hypotension, which occurs

TABLE 20.8	Local Anesthetics Used for Subarachnoid Block				
DRUG	**USUAL CONCENTRATION (%)**	**TOTAL DOSE (MG)**	**BARICITY**	**GLUCOSE CONCENTRATION (%)**	**USUAL DURATION (MIN)**
Lidocaine	1.5, 5.0	30–100	Hyperbaric	7.5	30–60
Bupivacaine	0.5	10–20	Isobaric	0	75–200
	0.75	7.5–22.5	Hyperbaric	8.25	75–200
Chloroprocaine	3	30–60	Isobaric	0	40–80
Mepivacaine	1.5	30–80	Isobaric	0	120–180
Ropivacaine	0.5–1	12–25	Isobaric	0	80–210

From Berde CB, Strichartz GR. Local anesthetics. In: Miller RD, ed. *Anesthesia*. 5th ed. Philadelphia: Churchill Livingstone; 2000:491–522.

because of sympathectomy, usually responds readily to fluids and small doses of pressors such as ephedrine and phenylephrine. Although preloading or coloading with crystalloid versus colloid to decrease severity of arterial hypotension has been a controversial topic in the past, current evidence suggests that crystalloid coloading with an adequate speed of administration (over 5–10 minutes) is equally efficacious as coloading or preloading with colloid solutions, with lower overall risk of adverse reactions.[59]

Postdural puncture headache occurs after a small proportion of subarachnoid blocks; it is a result of traction on the meninges caused by loss of CSF through a dural hole. Factors that increase its incidence include female sex, younger age, and larger needles. Epidural analgesia would appear to avoid the complication, but if the dura is inadvertently punctured, it leaves a much larger hole, as epidural needles are much larger. Compared with epidural anesthesia, spinal anesthesia has a quicker onset, is more predictably satisfactory for surgery, and is less frequently associated with backache. Transient radicular neuropathy, a painful but usually self-limited condition, may occur with use of lidocaine for spinal anesthesia.

When cardiac arrest results from excessive cephalad spread of subarachnoid block or protracted hypotension, cardiopulmonary resuscitation is notoriously difficult. Patients who suffer cardiac arrest during subarachnoid block have poor survival, possibly because the profound sympathectomy causes difficulty in generating adequate coronary perfusion pressure. Relatively large doses of epinephrine may be necessary to achieve adequate perfusion pressure during cardiopulmonary resuscitation after spinal anesthesia. Absolute contraindications to spinal anesthesia include sepsis, bacteremia, infection at the site of injection, severe hypovolemia, coagulopathy, therapeutic anticoagulation, increased ICP (there is a theoretical risk of herniation if CSF is lost caudally), and patient refusal.

Epidural Anesthesia

Epidural block can be applied in a wide variety of abdominal, thoracic, and lower extremity procedures. Induction of epidural anesthesia or analgesia results from injection of local anesthetics, with or without opiates, into the lumbar or thoracic epidural space. Generally, a catheter is inserted once the epidural space has been located with a needle. The presence of the catheter provides several advantages. First, local anesthetic can be added in a controlled fashion so that the time to onset of the block can be well controlled. Second, the catheter can be used for repeated dosing so that anesthesia can be provided for the duration of lengthy procedures. Third, local anesthetics or opiates can be administered for several days to provide postoperative analgesia.

Epidural anesthesia using low concentrations of local anesthetics in conjunction with epidural opiates has several advantages over traditional parenteral opiates for analgesia in the postoperative period. It provides superior pain control, less sedation, better pulmonary function, earlier ambulation and less postoperative ileus after abdominal surgery, and decreased duration of mechanical ventilation. Additionally, epidural anesthesia has been shown to decrease blood loss and deep venous thrombosis during total joint arthroplasty.

Thoracic epidural anesthesia, but not lumbar epidural anesthesia, appears to be associated with more rapid recovery of gastrointestinal function after major abdominal surgery. However, postoperative IV lidocaine also resulted in more rapid return of bowel function (flatus and bowel movement) and decreased postoperative pain in both open abdominal and laparoscopic procedures. Thus, circulating systemic lidocaine may account for at

least some of the effects of epidural anesthesia on postoperative bowel function and may be as efficacious as epidural analgesia in some circumstances. However, effectiveness of IV lidocaine may vary by surgical procedure.[60] A continuing controversy relates to whether epidural or subarachnoid analgesia reduces subsequent analgesic requirements after the block has resolved (so-called preemptive analgesia).

The complications and contraindications associated with epidural anesthesia are similar to those for spinal anesthesia. A special cautionary note is indicated regarding neuraxial anesthesia and anticoagulation. Because of the risk of epidural hematoma that can result in cord compression, spinal anesthetics as well as placement and removal of epidural catheters in patients receiving oral or parenteral anticoagulation must follow certain guidelines governing interval between medication and intervention. The advent of low-molecular-weight heparin (LMWH) for prophylaxis of deep venous thrombosis and the advent of increasingly potent antithrombotic medications have increased the risk of epidural hematomas associated with the removal or placement of epidural catheters. Although LMWH is effective as prophylaxis against venous thromboembolism, spinal hematomas have occurred in association with perioperative use of LMWH in patients given neuraxial analgesia. The timing of catheter placement and removal in the setting of LMWH and other antithrombotic agent use is critical to avoiding this rare but catastrophic complication. Current consensus guidelines from ASRA Pain Medicine in conjunction with the European Society of Anaesthesiology and Intensive Care outline recommendations for anticoagulation administration before neuraxial insertion, during neuraxial catheter maintenance, and after procedure termination or catheter removal.[61] Timing of appropriate neuraxial placement varies greatly depending on the anticoagulation type and dose administered. Additionally, almost all anticoagulants except for unfractionated heparin are contraindicated when a neuraxial catheter is in place. Therefore, minimizing risk of epidural hematomas in the setting of neuraxial analgesia requires close consultation with anesthesia colleagues and utilization of the ASRA Pain Medicine guidelines to develop optimal anticoagulation plans for patients.

A high index of suspicion of epidural hematoma must be maintained in patients undergoing neuraxial blockade who have received or will receive anticoagulation. All persons involved in the care of patients receiving continuous epidural analgesia must be aware of the signs of epidural hematoma, including back pain, lower extremity sensory and motor dysfunction, and bladder and bowel abnormalities. Epidural abscess, a final rare complication, should be considered in patients in whom back pain develops after epidural injection; magnetic resonance imaging is an effective diagnostic tool in such patients.

Peripheral Nerve Blocks

Blockade of the brachial plexus, lumbar plexus, and specific peripheral nerves is an effective means of providing surgical anesthesia and postoperative analgesia for many surgical procedures involving the upper and lower extremities. When used as the primary anesthetic, peripheral nerve blocks can allow for avoidance of the downsides of general anesthesia, including airway manipulation, and compared with spinal or epidural anesthesia, they avoid sympathectomy and consequent physiologic derangements. This strategy requires a cooperative patient, an anesthesiologist skilled in peripheral nerve blocks, and a surgeon who is accustomed to operating on awake patients. All patients undergoing peripheral nerve block receive full preoperative evaluation under the assumption that general anesthesia could be used if the block is inadequate. Most often, blocks are used as part of a larger strategy that includes sedation or even a general anesthetic and have their benefit postoperatively.

Improvements in nerve block equipment and methodology, as well as the availability of a wide range of local anesthetics, have greatly improved the effectiveness and safety of peripheral nerve blocks. In addition to providing surgical anesthesia, peripheral nerve blocks and the placement of indwelling catheters for a prolonged nerve block provide excellent analgesia for many types of upper extremity surgery and trauma. An additional application of indwelling catheters is enhancement of blood flow after reattachment of amputated limbs and in patients with peripheral vascular disease. Each particular block has specific associated risks and benefits, but general complications include LAST, nerve injury, inadvertent neuraxial block, and intravascular injection of local anesthetics.

Abdominal Wall Blocks

The use of anterior abdominal wall blocks has increased over the past decade due to the adoption of minimally invasive and laparoscopic surgical procedures and can provide somatic pain relief in the targeted nerve distribution. Transversus abdominis plane and rectus sheath blocks are relatively easy to place under ultrasound guidance and are generally safe and effective when applied in the proper clinical context. Other abdominal wall blocks include ilioinguinal-iliohypogastric and quadratus lumborum blocks. Prospective clinical trials and meta-analyses have generally shown that abdominal wall blocks confer some analgesic benefit in adult and pediatric patients undergoing minimally invasive or laparoscopic intraabdominal procedures. Variability in results likely stems from differing approaches to performing these blocks.[62] Abdominal wall blocks also have the potential to provide analgesic benefit in patients undergoing open intraabdominal surgery who have contraindications to epidural analgesia.

Enhanced Recovery After Surgery Pathways

As patients become more complex and available treatment options expand, increasing variability has been noted in clinical management.[63] Enhanced Recovery After Surgery (ERAS) pathways have been applied to standardize perioperative management of surgical patients, with the goal of optimizing patient outcomes and improving healthcare efficiency. ERAS protocols include guidance for fluid management, pain control, temperature regulation, minimally invasive surgical approach, removal of tubes and drains, and early mobilization. They originated in the colorectal surgery space but have been applied to numerous other surgical populations.[64-66] These protocols are ideally built in a multidisciplinary fashion using an evidence-based approach that features continuous auditing, reporting, and adjustment.[67] Although these pathways do not replace clinical judgment or suggest a retreat from patient-centered care, they strive to streamline systems operations and routinely connect patients with the most up-to-date, evidence-based practices relevant to their care.

CONSCIOUS SEDATION

When anesthesiologists participate in the sedation of patients undergoing surgical procedures, the anesthetic is termed *monitored anesthesia care*, or MAC. MAC encompasses a wide range of depths of sedation ranging from anxiolysis (minimal) to deep sedation. Minimal sedation indicates that the patient has normal responses to verbal stimulation with no impairment of airway patency, ventilation, or cardiovascular function. Moderate sedation, often termed *conscious sedation* by nonanesthesiologists, indicates that the patient has purposeful responses to verbal or tactile stimulation, has a patent airway requiring no intervention, demonstrates adequate spontaneous ventilation, and has maintained cardiovascular function. There is a narrow margin between minimal sedation, which may be inadequate for surgery, and deep sedation, which may result in airway compromise as well as cardiovascular and respiratory depression. Although relatively rare in this setting, a closed claim analysis showed that hypoventilation and hypoxemia were the most common major complications of moderate sedation.[68] Because of the risks associated with moderate sedation, The Joint Commission requires that patients be managed with precautions similar to what they would receive if an anesthesiologist was managing the sedation. This includes the necessity for preprocedural evaluation, including an airway assessment, continuous presence of a trained monitoring assistant who has no other responsibilities throughout the procedure, immediate availability of airway and resuscitation equipment, monitoring after the procedure until the effects of sedation have resolved, and specific written postoperative instructions. Physicians who perform procedures under conscious sedation are granted privileges in line with their training and experience in the appropriate resuscitative procedures. Deep sedation and general anesthesia can only be administered by a licensed anesthesia provider or medical staff with privileges to administer deep sedation or general anesthesia, in accordance with hospital policy and state scope of practice laws.[69]

Drugs used for moderate sedation usually consist of an opioid such as fentanyl combined with an anxiolytic such as midazolam. Medications such as dexmedetomidine and ketamine can be useful nonopioid adjuncts. Titration of these agents requires careful assessment of a patient's level of pain or anxiety and the requirements for the surgical procedure. Induction agents such as propofol can be used for moderate sedation outside of the operating room, and while generally safe when used under proper conditions, this introduces an added element of risk due to potentially rapid progression to deep sedation or general anesthesia. Most hospitals now have specific policies and procedures governing moderate sedation. Those who use moderate sedation outside hospitals (e.g., in office-based surgical practices) need to follow the same precautions as practiced in the hospital environment.

POSTANESTHESIA CARE

The PACU is the area designated for the care of patients recovering from the immediate physiologic and pharmacologic consequences associated with anesthesia and surgery. The PACU ideally is located close to the operating rooms. Monitors for the assessment of ventilation, oxygenation, and circulation must be available for all recovering patients. Care also includes periodic assessment of neuromuscular function, mental status, temperature, pain, fluid status, urine output, nausea and vomiting, and bleeding and drainage. The extent of monitoring depends on the condition of the patient. The ASA has established standards for postanesthesia care.[70] Recovery from anesthesia is usually uneventful and routine. Most patients stay in the PACU for 30 to 60 minutes until they are fully reactive and can move to a second-stage recovery area (for ambulatory patients who are returning home that day) or to a bed on a surgical floor. However, several criteria need to be met before the patient can be safely discharged from the PACU.

Patients must be awake and oriented (if they were before anesthesia) and have stable vital signs. Patients must be breathing without difficulty, able to protect their airways, and oxygenating appropriately. Pain, shivering, nausea, and vomiting must be adequately controlled. Patients receiving neuraxial anesthesia must be observed for resolution of the block. Surgical complications such as postoperative bleeding or unacceptable drain output must be addressed before discharge from the PACU. Several types of anesthesia-related complications can be encountered in the PACU and must be promptly recognized and treated to prevent serious injury.

Postoperative Agitation, Delirium, and Cognitive Decline

Pain and anxiety often manifest as postoperative agitation, but agitation may also signal serious physiologic disturbances such as hypoxemia, hypercapnia, acidosis, hypotension, hypoglycemia, surgical complications, overdistended bladder, or adverse drug reactions. Serious underlying conditions must be excluded as the cause of agitation before empirically treating patients with pain medications, sedatives, or physical restraints.

Postoperative delirium is a common complication of surgery and anesthesia that occurs in 5% to 10% of low-risk patients and up to 40% of high-risk patients, such as those older than 60 undergoing major procedures like cardiac surgery.[71] Development of postoperative delirium in the elderly is associated with increased mortality, persistent cognitive decline, and prolongation of in-hospital care. Factors contributing to postoperative delirium are multifactorial and include preoperative cognitive function, extent of surgery, and the need for postoperative intensive care. Approaches to minimizing postoperative delirium are under investigation and include avoidance of perioperative benzodiazepines and careful titration of anesthetic depth.[71] In a recent study, there was no benefit to using regional anesthesia without sedation over general anesthesia on rates of postoperative delirium in hip fractures.[58]

Respiratory Complications

Respiratory complications occur frequently in the PACU. Airway obstruction is most commonly due to obstruction of the oropharynx by the tongue or oropharyngeal soft tissues as a result of the residual effects of general anesthetics, pain medications, or muscle relaxants, often in combination with existing OSA. Other causes of airway obstruction include laryngospasm; blood, vomitus, or debris in the airway; glottic edema; vocal cord paralysis; and external compression of the airway by a hematoma, dressing, or cervical collar. Oxygen must be administered to a patient with airway obstruction as measures are taken to relieve the obstruction. The characteristic physical signs of airway obstruction are sonorous respiratory sounds and paradoxical chest/abdomen movement.

Many obstructions created by the tongue and soft tissue can be relieved by simply applying a head-tilt and jaw-thrust maneuver with or without placement of an oral or nasopharyngeal airway. Use of quantitative neuromuscular monitoring devices intraoperatively reduce in the incidence of postoperative respiratory complications such as obstruction and hypoxia caused by residual neuromuscular blockade.[19] In cases of laryngospasm, continuous positive airway pressure is applied. If this is not successful in breaking the spasm, low doses of propofol—or in severe cases, succinylcholine—can be administered. If the laryngospasm does not resolve promptly, a patient may require mask ventilation and endotracheal intubation. In children, glottic edema or postextubation croup can result in airway obstruction. Mild cases are treated with humidified oxygen. Refractory obstruction may require the administration of systemic steroids and nebulized racemic epinephrine. Reintubation may be required.

Hypoxemia is a surprisingly common problem, and administration of supplemental oxygen during transportation to the PACU and during the immediate postoperative period decreases the incidence and severity of hypoxemia. Hypoxemia can result from inadequate alveolar recruitment, hypoventilation, ventilation-perfusion mismatching, or right-to-left intrapulmonary shunting. Reluctance to inspire deeply after abdominal or thoracic surgery may also result in hypoxemia. Clinically, hypoxemia must be suspected as an underlying problem in patients exhibiting restlessness, tachycardia, or cardiac irritability. Bradycardia, hypotension, and cardiac arrest are late signs. Hypoxemia in the PACU is frequently secondary to atelectasis, which may respond to incentive spirometry and encouragement to cough. Treatment of hypoxemia requires the administration of oxygen, assurance of adequate ventilation, and treatment of the underlying causes. Patients with sleep apnea may benefit from use of positive pressure support.

Hypoventilation resulting in hypercapnia can result from airway obstruction; central respiratory depression caused by anesthetic agents and/or opioids, hypothermia, CNS injury; or restriction of ventilation secondary to muscle relaxants, abdominal distension, and electrolyte abnormalities. Signs can include prolonged somnolence, a slow (or rapid but shallow) respiratory rate, airway obstruction, tachycardia, and arrhythmias. Severe hypoventilation can result in hypoxemia, although augmented inspired oxygen will limit the severity of hypoventilation-induced hypoxemia. Treatment is aimed at identification and treatment of the underlying problem. Naloxone can be used to rapidly reverse hypoventilation caused by opioids. In all cases, ventilation must be supported until corrective measures are instituted. Obtundation, circulatory depression, and severe respiratory acidosis are indications for endotracheal intubation and ventilatory support.

Postoperative Nausea and Vomiting

One of the most common problems in the PACU is PONV. Risk factors include female sex, postoperative opioid administration, nonsmoking status, a history of PONV or motion sickness, young patient age, longer duration of anesthesia, exposure to volatile anesthetics, and the type of surgery. A Cochrane review found aprepitant, ramosetron, granisetron, dexamethasone, and ondansetron reduce postoperative vomiting, with NK_1 receptor antagonists such as aprepitant being the most effective.[72] Fosaprepitant and droperidol probably reduce vomiting compared with placebo but were less effective than the other drugs. A combination of medications to prevent PONV is more efficacious than a single medication (Table 20.9). Due to its ability to prolong the QTc interval, droperidol was given a black box warning by the FDA, recommending ECG monitoring before and after administration of the drug.

The mechanisms that cause nausea and vomiting should guide the approach to PONV prophylaxis and treatment. Areas in the brainstem that control nausea and vomiting reflexes, such as the chemoreceptor trigger zone, contain receptors for dopamine, acetylcholine, histamine, and serotonin. Activating these receptors may precipitate nausea, vomiting, or both. Effective pharmacologic approaches to the treatment of PONV include the use of 5-HT$_3$ receptor antagonists, D_2 receptor antagonists, NK_1 receptor antagonists, corticosteroids, and antihistamines. The use of any particular agent is based on efficacy, potential side effects, and cost. In patients at high risk of PONV or in those with a history of PONV, it is often effective to employ a multimodal approach, including the avoidance of volatile anesthetics.

TABLE 20.9 **Commonly Used Antiemetic Agents**	
DRUG CLASS	**COMMON SIDE EFFECTS**
Dopamine Receptor Antagonists (D$_2$)	
Phenothiazines	
Chlorpromazine	Sedation
Prochlorperazine	
Butyrophenones	Dissociation
Haloperidol	
Droperidol	Extrapyramidal effects
Metoclopramide	
Antihistamines (H$_1$)	
Diphenhydramine	Sedation
Promethazine	Dry mouth
Anticholinergics	
Scopolamine	Sedation
Atropine	Dry mouth, tachycardia
Serotonin Receptor Antagonists	
Ondansetron	Headache, constipation
Aprepitant	
Corticosteroids	
Dexamethasone	Glucose intolerance
Methylprednisolone	Altered wound healing
Hydrocortisone	Immunosuppression, renal effects

Hypothermia

Hypothermia has been extensively studied as a perioperative complication. Hypothermia can increase oxygen consumption postoperatively due to shivering, alter drug metabolism, affect blood coagulation, and increase the rate of surgical infections. Increased oxygen consumption can be a particular problem in patients with coronary artery disease in whom shivering can trigger myocardial ischemia. Risks associated with mild hypothermia have not been well defined in otherwise healthy patients. Nevertheless, the Centers for Medicare and Medicaid Services has designated perioperative normothermia as a quality indicator and Pay for Performance issue. Hospitals and medical centers receive financial incentives if they report on and achieve perioperative normothermia (a measured temperature of 35.5°C [95.9°F] within the 30 minutes immediately before or the 15 minutes immediately after anesthesia end time for procedures lasting for more than 1 hour).

General anesthesia has profound effects on thermoregulatory mechanisms, and active intraoperative warming is required to maintain normothermia (core temperature >36°C) under most conditions. Anesthetic-induced vasodilation redistributes blood from the core to the periphery, where heat is rapidly lost via radiation to the surrounding environment. Heat is also lost via conduction, convection, and evaporation. Forced air and circulating water warmers are the most effective techniques for providing active intraoperative warming, each having advantages under different conditions. IV fluid warmers and airway warming devices can also be useful for minimizing heat loss but do not allow for active warming. Preoperative warming can minimize core hypothermia in patients undergoing procedures lasting less than an hour. Prophylactic warming decreases the incidence of postoperative hypothermia and need for intervention in the outpatient surgical setting, though time to PACU discharge and patient satisfaction are not affected. The use of prophylactic warming is associated with a significant increase in cost. Therefore, guidelines for temperature management during short, outpatient surgical procedures remain to be fully implemented.

Circulatory Complications

Hypotension in the PACU is most commonly due to hypovolemia. Other causes include residual anesthetic effect, cardiac dysfunction, arrhythmias, anaphylaxis, transfusion reactions, cardiac tamponade, pulmonary emboli, adverse drug reactions, adrenal insufficiency, and hypoxemia. Treatment involves supporting the circulation with fluids, vasoactive medications, the Trendelenburg position, and delivery of oxygen until the underlying cause is diagnosed and treated.

Hypertension is also a common finding in the PACU. Common causes include pain, anxiety, and inadequately managed essential hypertension. Hypercapnia should be ruled out. Other less common causes include hypoglycemia, drug reactions, diseases such as hyperthyroidism, pheochromocytoma, or MH, and bladder distention. The fundamental goal in control of postoperative hypertension is to identify and correct the underlying cause.

Postoperative Visual Loss

Postoperative visual loss is a rare but devastating complication that occurs most commonly in patients undergoing prolonged surgery in the prone position (spine surgery) or cardiac surgery. The overall incidence is reported as 0.03% to 0.2%. Causes include central retinal artery occlusion, cortical blindness, and ischemic optic neuropathy. Risk factors for the development of postoperative visual loss are not completely understood but include obesity, prolonged length of surgery, high intraoperative blood loss, and lower colloid to crystalloid ratio during resuscitation.[73] Because of the seriousness of the complication, the ASA has released practice advisory on postoperative visual loss.[74]

ACUTE PAIN MANAGEMENT

Pain, one of the most common and significant symptoms experienced by surgical patients, has historically been poorly evaluated and frequently undertreated. There have been massive shifts in medical care with respect to pain management, starting with a clarion call in 1990 for improved focus on pain assessment and treatment, to the declaration of pain as the fifth vital sign by The Joint Commission in 2001, through the opioid epidemic that has ensued. With increased focus on pain management, institutions have established protocols and procedures for pain management, the subspecialty of pain medicine was developed, and there has been increased interest from governmental and third-party payers. Medical personnel must continue to increase their knowledge of pain control options and their commitment to provide optimal analgesia as a key component of patient care, while avoiding the overprescribing practices that sparked a national opioid epidemic. Surveys demonstrate that continued improvement is necessary to reduce the high incidence of moderate to severe acute postoperative pain.

Acute pain occurs frequently in the setting of surgery and trauma. The pain experience may be part of the symptom complex that prompts the patient to seek medical care, or it may be caused by tissue injury sustained as a result of surgery or trauma. The term *acute pain* refers to pain that is expected to be of relatively short duration and that should resolve with tissue healing or withdrawal of the noxious stimulus. Acute pain generally resolves within minutes, hours, or days. *Chronic pain*, or persistent surgical pain, is defined as pain that persists for at least 3 months beyond the usual course of an acute disease or beyond a reasonable time in which an injury would be expected to heal.[75] The acute stress response associated with acute pain serves a useful function, although undertreatment may result in harmful pathophysiologic changes. Chronic pain serves no useful function and is now recognized as a disease itself.

Mechanisms of Acute Pain

The International Association for the Study of Pain defines pain as "an unpleasant sensory and emotional experience associated with, or resembling that associated with, actual or potential tissue damage." This definition emphasizes not only the sensory experience but also the affective component of pain. The tissue injury results in a process called nociception, which has four steps: transduction, transmission, modulation, and perception. With transduction, the noxious stimulus is converted into an electrical signal at free nerve endings, which are also known as nociceptors. Nociceptors are widely distributed throughout the body in both somatic and visceral tissues. With transmission,

the electrical signal is sent via nerve pathways toward the CNS. Nerve pathways include primary sensory afferents (primarily Aδ and C fibers) that project to the spinal cord, ascending tracts (including the spinothalamic tract) that project to the brainstem and thalamus, and thalamocortical pathways that project to the cortex. Modulation, the process that either enhances or suppresses the pain signal, occurs primarily in the dorsal horn of the spinal cord, specifically the substantia gelatinosa. Perception, the final step in the nociceptive process, occurs when the pain signal reaches the cerebral cortex. Multiple things can affect the perception of pain, making the experience extremely subjective and widely variable. The first three steps in nociception are important for the sensory and discriminative aspects of pain. The fourth step, perception, is integral to the subjective and emotional experience.

Methods of Analgesia

Multiple agents, routes of administration, and modalities are available for effective management of acute pain (Fig. 20.4). Analgesic agents can be chosen based on the type of pain

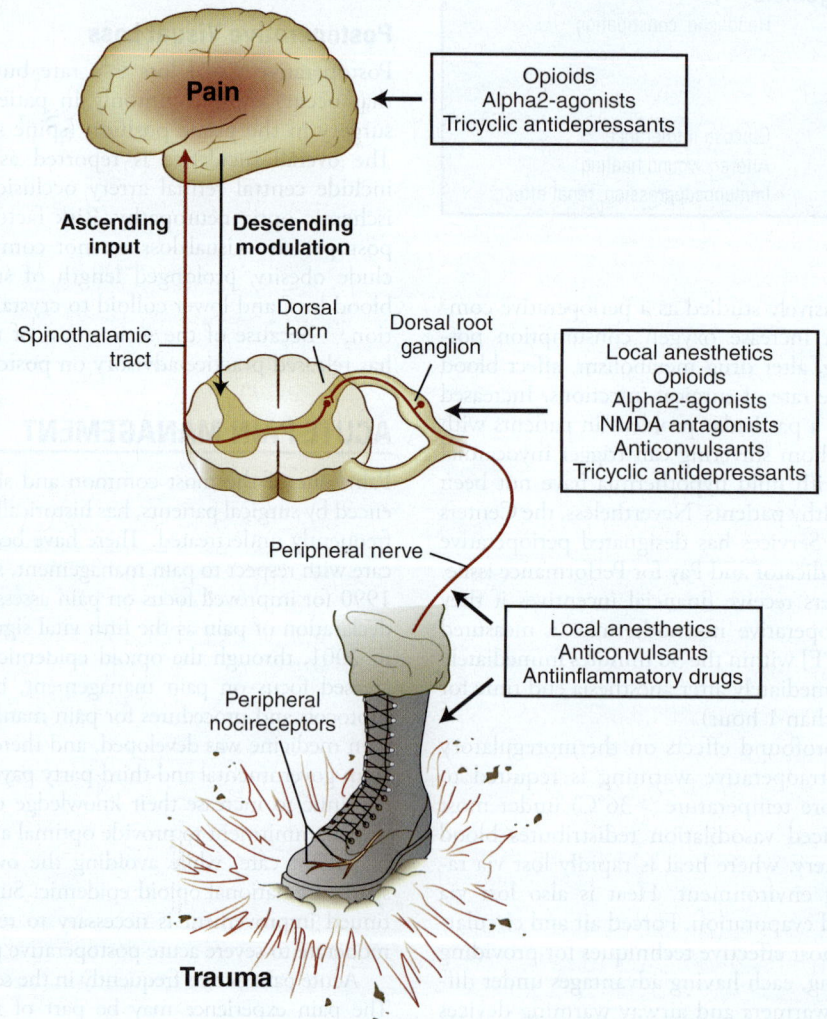

FIGURE 20.4 Schematic diagram outlining the nociceptive pathway for transmission of painful stimuli. Interventions that prevent nociceptive transmission are shown at the points in the pathway that are thought to be their sites of action. *NMDA,* N-methyl-D-aspartate. (From Buckenmaier CC III, Bleckner LL, eds. *Military Advanced Regional Anesthesia and Analgesia.* Washington, DC: Borden Institute, Walter Reed Army Medical Center; 2008.)

(somatic versus neuropathic) and include opioids, nonsteroidal anti-inflammatory drugs (NSAIDs), acetaminophen, gabapentinoids, muscle relaxants, NMDA receptor antagonists, α_2-agonists, and local anesthetics. Opioid agonist/antagonists such as buprenorphine are now routinely used for treatment of pain as well as for opioid use disorder. Routes of administration include oral, parenteral, epidural, and intrathecal routes. Patients experiencing mild to moderate acute pain can obtain effective analgesia with oral analgesics. Parenteral administration is preferred for patients experiencing moderate to severe pain, patients who require rapid control of pain, and those who cannot receive agents through the gastrointestinal tract. The IV route is preferred over IM and subcutaneous injections when the parenteral route is indicated. IM injections are painful, result in erratic absorption, and lead to variable blood levels of the administered agent.

Opioids

Opioids are potent analgesic agents that have been used for centuries but come with potentially harmful side effects. By binding to opioid receptors in the CNS, opioids modulate the nociceptive process. The best-characterized opioid receptors are μ_1, μ_2, δ, and κ receptors. The μ_1 receptors are involved in supraspinal analgesia. The δ and κ receptors are involved in spinal analgesia. Opioids can be administered via oral, parenteral, neuraxial, rectal, and transdermal routes.

Opioids have varying degrees of potency. Strong opioids are ideal for moderate to severe pain and for pain that is constant in frequency. Weak opioid agents are suitable for mild to moderate pain that is intermittent in frequency. Morphine is the prototypical strong opioid. It is broken down into to the active metabolites morphine-3-glucoronide and morphine-6-glucoronide, which can accumulate in patients who have renal impairment and cause significant respiratory depression. Other commonly used strong opioids include hydromorphone, fentanyl, methadone, and meperidine. For moderate to severe pain in patients with renal dysfunction, fentanyl and hydromorphone are more suitable agents. Meperidine is an opioid that also has anticholinergic, local anesthetic, serotonergic, and noradrenergic properties. Its use has declined because meperidine is metabolized to normeperidine, a unique toxic metabolite that can accumulate and cause seizure-like activity. Patients who are particularly vulnerable to this side effect include the elderly, patients who are dehydrated, and those with renal impairment. Methadone is a long-acting opioid with NMDA antagonist properties, making it useful for major surgery in opioid tolerant patients.

Weak opioid agents, such as oxycodone, hydrocodone, and codeine, are commonly used in conjunction with acetaminophen for a multimodal pain regimen postoperatively. Tramadol is a weak opioid analgesic that weakly inhibits serotonin/norepinephrine reuptake. It is a centrally acting agent that is administered orally and can be used for mild to moderate pain. Common opioid-related side effects include nausea, pruritus, sedation, mental clouding, decreased gastric motility, urinary retention, and respiratory depression. Appropriate selection of agents, along with the use of a multimodal regimen and appropriate monitoring, can prevent or ameliorate these side effects.

When using opioids, it is important to recognize their importance in analgesic regimens, but also their significant side effects, including the possibility of tolerance, opioid-induced hyperalgesia, and in severe cases, the development of opioid use disorder, the

diagnostic criteria of which are defined in The *Diagnostic and Statistical Manual of Mental Disorders*, 5th Edition. Key terms to understand include *tolerance, addiction* (psychological dependence), and *physical dependence*. Tolerance occurs when a previously effective opioid dose fails to provide adequate analgesia. It is a normal physiologic effect. Tolerance develops to the analgesic effect of opioids but not to most opioid-related side effects, including respiratory depression and constipation. The duration of opioid exposure also plays a role in the development of tolerance. In patients manifesting tolerance, an increased dose is required to achieve effective analgesia. Opioid-induced hyperalgesia, usually seen with prolonged exposure or high doses of opioids, can reduce the baseline pain threshold, thereby making it seem as if the patient requires higher than average doses of opioids for the same analgesic effect. Addiction or psychological dependence is a compulsive disorder manifested by preoccupation with obtaining and inappropriate use of a substance, and continued use despite harm and decreased quality of life. Psychological dependence should not be confused with physical dependence, which is a normal physiologic process. Physical dependence is manifested by the occurrence of a withdrawal syndrome when use of a drug is stopped suddenly or when an antagonist is given. The duration of opioid treatment is a factor in the development of physical dependence. The short-term use of opioids in the perioperative period rarely results in physical dependence. Short courses of opioids generally preclude withdrawal symptoms.

Nonsteroidal Anti-inflammatory Drugs

NSAIDs can reduce pain and can decrease opioid consumption when used as part of a multimodal analgesic approach. Their mechanism of action is achieved through inhibition of cyclooxygenase (COX) enzyme activity, which results in decreased production of prostaglandins. Prostaglandins are potent mediators of pain that act directly at nociceptors and increase nociceptor sensitivity. Inhibition of prostaglandin production results in analgesia but can also lead to side effects such as gastric ulceration, bleeding, and renal injury. These side effects have limited the use of NSAIDs in the perioperative period.

There is a wide range of compounds in this analgesic class, with differing chemical structures. Most of these agents are orally administered, but ketorolac is available for parenteral administration. Ketorolac, like all NSAIDs, is avoided in patients with a history of gastropathy, platelet dysfunction, or thrombocytopenia; in those with a history of allergy to the agent; and in patients with renal impairment or hypovolemia. It should be used with caution in elderly patients. An optional loading dose of 30 mg IV followed by 15 mg IV every 6 hours for a short course (5 days maximum) can provide effective analgesia for mild to moderate pain or can be a useful adjunct for moderate to severe pain when combined with opioids or other analgesic techniques.

There are at least two subtypes of the COX enzyme: COX-1 (constitutive) and COX-2 (inducible). Traditional NSAIDs are nonselective inhibitors of COX. COX-2 selective medications showed promise by targeting pain with reduced risk of gastrointestinal bleeding, bleeding diathesis, and renal compromise. Celecoxib is the only COX-2 inhibitor available in the United States. This subclass of NSAIDs have mostly been studied and used clinically in the management of arthritis-related pain. In a study by Huang and colleagues,[76] the COX-2 selective inhibitor celecoxib was administered to patients undergoing total knee arthroplasty under subarachnoid blockade. Celecoxib 200 mg was administered 1 hour before surgery and every 12 hours thereafter for 5 days. Morphine use by patient-controlled analgesia (PCA) was lower in the celecoxib group (15.1 mg) versus placebo (19.7 mg). Celecoxib use was associated with a lower pain score during the first postoperative 48 hours as well as increased knee range of motion during the first three postoperative days. Morphine-related adverse effects (nausea and vomiting) did not differ between groups in this study. Concerns about the use of these selective NSAIDs include the risk for cardiovascular events and their effects on bone healing. The FDA has placed a black box warning on all NSAIDs after the COX-2 inhibitor rofecoxib was associated with increased risk of myocardial infarction and stroke.

NMDA Antagonists

NMDA antagonists may play a role in preventing central sensitization of the CNS, a proposed pathway in the development of chronic pain. Accordingly, this class of agent has reemerged in popularity for the treatment of acute perioperative pain. Ketamine has long been recognized as a powerful induction agent with strong analgesic properties, albeit at the expense of psychotropic adverse effects, including dysphoria and even psychosis at higher doses of the drug. A Cochrane review[77] of perioperative ketamine found that in a variety of surgeries, bolus dosing and/or infusion of 2 to 5 µg/kg/min reduced pain scores and improved morphine consumption at 24 and 48 hours. Results were consistent in different operation types and varied timing of ketamine administration, with larger and smaller studies, and by higher and lower pain intensity. CNS adverse events were similar with ketamine or control.[77] Ketamine reduced the area of postoperative hyperalgesia by 7 cm² (95% CI −11.9 to −2.2; negative values indicating reduction in area), but this was low-quality evidence. A study by Rémérand and colleagues[78] demonstrated that perioperative ketamine was associated with 6-month reduction in chronic pain, with chronic pain incidence of 8% in the ketamine group compared with 21% in the placebo. As previously discussed, ketamine can cause hypertension and tachycardia when used in higher bolus doses, due to its sympathomimetic effects, and it does not cause significant respiratory depression. Memantine is an oral NMDA antagonist that has been used in the pain context as well[79]; the data for it are not clear, though research is ongoing.[80] Magnesium also antagonizes the NMDA receptor and has been shown to decrease postoperative pain scores in multiple surgical settings without a significant increase in adverse events,[81,82] but research remains ongoing to elucidate its long-term analgesic effects.[83]

α₂-Adrenergic Agonists

There is a high density of α₂-adrenergic receptors in the substantia gelatinosa of the dorsal horn of the spinal cord, where it is believed that α₂-adrenergic agonists impair the transmission of pain signals. Clonidine, due to its potent antihypertensive properties, is of limited use in the perioperative setting. Dexmedetomidine, an α₂-adrenergic agonist mainly used as a sedative in the ICU, is becoming more popular in the perioperative context. When administered for acute pain after abdominal surgery in adults, dexmedetomidine seems to have some opioid-sparing effect but no important differences in postoperative pain when compared with placebo.[84] A randomized controlled trial of opioid-free anesthesia using dexmedetomidine (versus remifentanil) was stopped early due to several episodes of clinically significant bradycardia in the dexmedetomidine group. They found no differences in pain postoperatively, but there was a reduction in morphine consumption and PONV at 48 hours.[85] Aside from analgesic

benefits, dexmedetomidine seems to have other perioperative advantages. Ji and colleagues[86] evaluated the long-term effects of dexmedetomidine in cardiac surgery patients. This study began an infusion upon weaning from cardiopulmonary bypass and continued it into the ICU for less than 24 hours. They noted a reduction in in-hospital, 30-day, and 1-year mortality and a reduction in overall complications, including delirium. Pain scores were not described by the authors. Guanfacine is an orally administered α₂-adrenergic agonist gaining attention for delirium treatment and as a pain management adjunct, though further study is needed to assess its efficacy in the perioperative setting. It has minimal cardiovascular side effects.

Gabapentinoids

Gabapentin and pregabalin are used for the treatment of chronic neuropathic pain, and there has been significant attention to including them in perioperative multimodal analgesic regimens. Current guidelines from the American Pain Society and European Society of Regional Anesthesia and Pain Therapy offer conflicting recommendations for the use of gabapentinoids in the perioperative period. Although there have been studies suggesting an analgesic benefit, the doses of gabapentin needed to realize those benefits were 900 or 1200 mg. For example, a study by Khan et al.[87] found decreased morphine use in the first 24 hours after lumbar laminectomy as well as lower pain scores and side effects when 900 or 1200 mg of gabapentin was administered either preoperatively or postoperatively. However, recent analyses have raised doubts about the benefit of these drugs as well as concerns about the potential harm they may cause. A meta-analysis of 281 trials found no clinically significant analgesic effect of perioperative gabapentinoids, and while PONV occurred at a slightly lower rate, dizziness and visual disturbance were more common in the gabapentinoid group.[88] A cohort study of 967,547 patients over 65 years of age demonstrated an increased risk of delirium, new antipsychotic use, and pneumonia with use of gabapentin after major surgery.[89]

Local Anesthetics for the Management of Acute Pain

Local anesthetics work by blocking sodium channels, thus inhibiting conduction in nerve fibers, and can be used as IV adjuncts for blockade of nerves as part of regional anesthetics, and as neuraxial agents. Several of these indications are described at length in other portions of the chapter. Continuous infusions of lidocaine may improve pain scores, but data are mixed due to variable study design and quality.[90] There is mixed evidence for use of local anesthetic infiltration at incision sites, with some studies suggesting no change in postoperative pain scores or opioid use[91,92] and others demonstrating improvement in pain with infiltration.[93] Topical local anesthetics—such as eutectic mixture of local anesthetics (EMLA) cream (containing prilocaine and lidocaine)—can be used for superficial procedures, but they must be applied significantly in advance.

Multimodal Analgesic Therapy

Combining agents from multiple analgesic classes can have synergistic effects, potentiating benefits and reducing required doses of each agent, therefore decreasing side-effect burdens. Common combinations include opioids, NSAIDs, acetaminophen, gabapentinoids, and local anesthetics in an analgesic regimen. The choice of agent and technique depends on factors such as the patient's medical history, the patient's preference, the extent of surgery, the expected degree of postoperative pain, the experience of the staff providing care for the patient, and the postoperative setting in which the patient will recover.

Neuraxial Analgesia

Neuraxial routes of administration include the epidural and intrathecal (subarachnoid) routes. These modes of administration require consultation from acute pain specialists, usually anesthesiologists who receive specialized training in use of the neuraxial route for the administration of anesthesia and analgesia. Neuraxial agents are delivered by a single injection into the epidural or subarachnoid space, by intermittent injections through an indwelling epidural catheter, by continuous infusion through an indwelling epidural catheter, or by patient-controlled epidural analgesia through an indwelling catheter. Indwelling subarachnoid catheters are rarely used for acute pain. An important consideration in selecting patients for neuraxial analgesia is the presence of abnormal coagulation, including concurrent use of antiplatelet and anticoagulant agents. Knowledge of such coagulation issues is important to minimize the risk for intraspinal bleeding and spinal hematoma formation, which can lead to severe neurologic injury. The neuraxial route requires education of the medical and nursing staff and the use of protocols and guidelines. In general, patients can be managed on surgical floors with these analgesic techniques. However, monitoring standards need to be in place to minimize the development of common side effects, such as hypotension.

Common agents used neuraxially include opioids and local anesthetics. Opioids, when delivered by the neuraxial route, act at opioid receptors in the dorsal horn of the spinal cord and can be given in much smaller doses than when administered systemically. A drug's lipid solubility has significant impact on pharmacokinetics and dynamics when it is administered epidurally. A hydrophilic opioid, when delivered into the epidural or subarachnoid space, remains in the CSF longer than a lipophilic opioid. Such a drug can travel rostrally to the brain and influence the respiratory centers hours after initial delivery. Morphine is hydrophilic, which accounts for its slow onset of analgesia, long duration of action, ability to provide analgesia over a wide dermatomal distribution, and the risk for late respiratory depression. Fentanyl is lipophilic, which accounts for its fast onset and short duration of action, ability to provide segmental analgesia, and limited risk for late respiratory depression.

Local anesthetics, when used for neuraxial analgesia, provide analgesia by blocking nerve conduction. To achieve neuraxial analgesia, local anesthetics are delivered in smaller doses and weaker concentrations than those required to achieve surgical anesthesia. This resulting sensory blockade is sufficient to provide analgesia but not sufficiently profound to interfere with motor function and mask complications. Analgesic concentrations of local anesthetics also cause less impairment of sympathetic tone. Bupivacaine and ropivacaine are the most commonly used local anesthetics for epidural analgesia. They affect sensory fibers more than motor fibers (known as *differential blockade*) and have a lower incidence of tachyphylaxis (tolerance to local anesthetic action).

Neuraxial analgesia for acute pain commonly combines opioids and local anesthetics, thus reaping the benefits of both while limiting required doses and thus side effects. A meta-analysis of the efficacy of postoperative epidural analgesia concluded that epidural analgesia, regardless of agent, location of catheter placement, and type of pain assessment provided analgesia superior to that of parenteral opioids.[94]

Intravenous Patient-Controlled Analgesia

IV PCA minimizes the steps in the delivery of analgesia and increases patient autonomy and control. Opioids are the agent of choice for IV PCA. In comparing IV PCA with conventional intermittent nurse-administered opioid delivery, patients obtain prompt analgesia, receive smaller doses of opioids at more frequent intervals, can maintain blood concentration of drug in the analgesic range, and have a lower incidence of drug-related side effects. Candidates for IV PCA are patients who can understand the basic steps involved in use of the device who are willing to assume control of their analgesia, and who are physically capable of activating the device. Such patients include children as young as 4 years of age and most adults, including geriatric patients.

The preferred agents for IV PCA are opioids, with hydromorphone being the most frequently chosen and with morphine and fentanyl as common options. Orders for IV PCA must specify the drug, drug concentration, loading dose, bolus dose, continuous infusion rate (basal rate), lockout interval, and dose limits. Selection of these parameters is based on the patient's age, medical status, and level of pain. The routine use of a continuous basal infusion rate with IV PCA is not recommended because it is associated with increased risk of respiratory depression without improved pain control. It is safest to restrict the use of basal infusions to patients in special categories, including those with severe pain from extensive surgery or trauma and patients who are tolerant because of chronic opioid use.

The use of structured protocols and guidelines is encouraged for facilities using IV PCA. The medical and nursing staff need to receive training in the care of patients using this modality. There is an increased risk for complications if staff members are not trained to understand the concept of IV PCA; to perform appropriate patient selection, education, and assessment; to use appropriate drug and dose selection; and to establish appropriate monitoring requirements and protocols for management of side effects.

SPECIFIC TYPES OF ACUTE PAIN PATIENTS

Patients With a History of Chronic Pain

Pain that persists for 3 months beyond the expected time for recovery or initial onset is considered evidence of a chronic pain syndrome. Chronic pain can be somatic or neuropathic. Neuropathic pain syndromes occur when there has been injury to the nervous system (central, peripheral, or both). Central sensitization—an increase in nociceptive signaling in the CNS leading to hypersensitivity—is believed to underlie the development of neuropathic pain. Factors that may increase the risk for chronic pain include infection at the surgical site, intraoperative trauma to nerves, diabetes mellitus, and nerve entrapment by cancer.

Because chronic pain syndromes can be difficult to diagnose in the early postoperative period, it is important for physicians to perform appropriate pain assessment during postoperative follow-up. For instance, after amputation, patients might consider it strange to continue to feel sensation and pain in the location of an amputated limb and might be reluctant to volunteer information. In such circumstances, appropriate questioning may elicit the complaint and result in patient reassurance and appropriate treatment. Referral to a pain medicine consultant is appropriate when the diagnosis of a chronic postoperative pain syndrome is made. Treatment modalities include the use of adjuvant medications such as antidepressants and anticonvulsants, nerve blocks, physical therapy, and psychological techniques.

Patients who have a history of chronic pain may experience acute pain as a result of surgery or trauma differently from patients without such history. Their pharmacologic management may impact medication choices perioperatively as well. If on chronic opioid therapy, these patients may manifest tolerance as well as hyperalgesia, resulting in higher reported pain scores and doses of analgesics. Steps to achieving effective analgesia include obtaining a pain history preoperatively, choosing anesthetic and surgical techniques to minimize tissue trauma and the response to trauma, and appropriate planning for postoperative analgesia.

Patients on Buprenorphine

Patients can take buprenorphine, the opioid agonist/antagonist, for treatment of pain or for opioid use disorder. It is recommended to continue this medication[95] at a reduced dose throughout the perioperative period, but patients will then require usually larger doses of opioids to overcome the antagonist effect.[96] The most effective opioids in this setting are hydromorphone and fentanyl. Standard PO medications such as oxycodone and hydrocodone will not be effective. Administering buprenorphine acutely to a patient who requires opioids can trigger withdrawal.

Patients With a History of Substance Use Disorder

Patients with a history of substance abuse are frequently undertreated for acute pain. The following factors contribute to undertreatment in this patient population: stigma associated with drug use, misunderstanding on the part of healthcare providers, and inappropriate pain behavior (e.g., exaggerated expression of pain that is out of proportion to what a provider may expect). Effective analgesia can be obtained with strict guidelines, patient education, and appropriate use of consultants and modalities such as regional analgesia.

Pediatric Patients

Pediatric patients experience similar severity of acute postoperative and posttraumatic pain as adults. A major historical myth that has been refuted is the belief that neonates, infants, and children do not perceive pain like adults. Effective analgesia for a pediatric patient can be achieved with pain assessment tools that are tailored for this population and the use of modalities and agents similar to those used for adults. Dosage selection in a pediatric patient must be guided by patient weight. With neonates, nurse-controlled analgesia is standard. Older children can effectively use IV PCA. Regional anesthesia is increasingly being used for pediatric surgery. Epidural analgesia or that provided via a caudally placed catheter (or single shot injection) can provide effective analgesia. Placement of a peripheral catheter for infusion of local anesthetics can also be used. Topical anesthesia with local anesthetics such as the application of EMLA cream can likewise minimize pain from IV catheter placement and other superficial procedures.

Elderly Patients

As the general population ages, a growing percentage of geriatric patients are undergoing surgery or being treated for trauma. These patients will require pain assessment and evaluation tailored to their mental status and cognitive abilities. The modalities and agents used to manage acute pain in this population must take into consideration underlying disease states, side effects of common analgesics that are not recommended for the elderly, and decreased organ function.

CONCLUSIONS

Modern anesthesia is safe and effective for the vast majority of patients, in large part because of important advances in anesthesia equipment, monitors, and drugs. With a wide variety of specific techniques to choose from, selection of anesthetic and postoperative pain regimens for each patient can be based on the requirements of the surgical procedure, the patient's preferences, and the experience and expertise of the anesthesiologist. Over time, patients with more significant comorbidities are receiving surgical care. Anesthesia practice is evolving to provide adequate risk assessment and risk adjustment and to optimize the care of the surgical patient.

SELECTED REFERENCES

Avidan MS, Jacobsohn E, Glick D, et al. Prevention of intraoperative awareness in a high-risk surgical population. *N Engl J Med.* 2011;365:591-600.

> Intraoperative awareness prevention is possible using processed electroencephalogram, but it is not superior to following known dosing guidelines for volatile anesthetics in healthy patients.

Fleisher LA, Fleischmann KE, Auerbach AD, et al. 2014 ACC/AHA guideline on perioperative cardiovascular evaluation and management of patients undergoing noncardiac surgery: a report of the American College of Cardiology/American Heart Association task force on practice guidelines. *J Am Coll Cardiol.* 2014; 64:e77-e137.

> In this extensive review, a joint task force of the American College of Cardiology and the American Heart Association reports guidelines for evaluation of patients with cardiovascular disease who are scheduled for noncardiac surgery. They thoroughly examine the importance of the history, physical findings, functional status, and the influence of various types of surgery as well as current recommendations on the perioperative use of β-blockers, statins, and other medications. The value of preoperative testing is also evaluated. This is a valuable update of a consensus approach to this topic.

Gan TJ, Belani KG, Bergese S, et al. Fourth consensus guidelines for the management of postoperative nausea and vomiting. *Anesth Analg.* 2020;131:411-448.

> This consensus statement provides evidence-based guidelines for the management of PONV in the adult and pediatric populations. It discusses mechanisms of action as well as strength of data supporting available antiemetics.

Li T, Li J, Yuan L, et al. Effect of regional vs general anesthesia on incidence of postoperative delirium in older patients undergoing hip fracture surgery: the RAGA randomized trial. *JAMA.* 2022; 327:50-58.

> Although there may be other benefits to neuraxial anesthetic techniques, avoiding general anesthesia did not impact the rate of postoperative delirium in elderly patients undergoing hip fracture surgery.

Myles PS, Leslie K, Chan MT, et al. The safety of addition of nitrous oxide to general anaesthesia in at-risk patients having major non-cardiac surgery (ENIGMA-II): a randomised, single-blind trial. *Lancet.* 2014;384:1446-1454.

In contrast to previous trials, the Evaluation of Nitrous Oxide in the Gas Mixture for Anaesthesia (ENIGMA) II Trial reported that use of nitrous oxide was not associated with an increased incidence of death, cardiovascular complications, or wound infection in high-risk surgical patients. Although the incidence of severe postoperative nausea and vomiting (PONV) was higher (15% vs. 11%) in patients receiving nitrous oxide compared with controls, the occurrence of PONV in the nitrous oxide group was effectively controlled by antiemetic prophylaxis.

American Society of Anesthesiologists Task Force on Perioperative Management of Patients with Obstructive Sleep Apnea. Practice guidelines for the perioperative management of patients with obstructive sleep apnea: an updated report by the American Society of Anesthesiologists Task Force on Perioperative Management of Patients with Obstructive Sleep Apnea. *Anesthesiology.* 2014;120: 268-286.

Guidelines for the preoperative assessment, perioperative management, and postoperative disposition of patients with obstructive sleep apnea.

Radtke FM, Franck M, Lendner J, Krüger S, Wernecke KD, Spies CD. Monitoring depth of anaesthesia in a randomized trial decreases the rate of postoperative delirium but not postoperative cognitive dysfunction. *Br J Anaesth.* 2013;110:i98-i105.

Processed electroencephalogram can help guide anesthetic dosing in a manner that can potentially reduce risk for delirium postoperatively but cannot prevent postoperative cognitive dysfunction.

Santa Cruz Mercado LA, Liu R, Bharadwaj KM, et al. Association of intraoperative opioid administration with postoperative pain and opioid use. *JAMA Surg.* 2023;158:854-864.

Recent cohort study of >60,000 surgical patients that demonstrated an improvement in postoperative pain control and a decrease in chronic pain with higher intraoperative opioid administration. This makes a different argument in the current largely opioid-sparing culture.

The full reference list appears on Elsevier eBooks+.

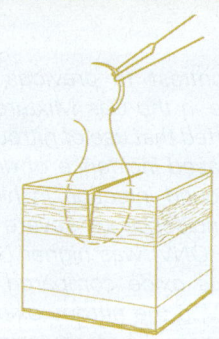

21 | CHAPTER

Optimizing Surgical Outcomes: Prehabilitation and Rehabilitation

Lindsay Welton, Emily Finlayson, and Elizabeth Wick

OUTLINE

BACKGROUND

As the field of medicine has advanced, the average surgical patient's age, comorbidities, medications, and body mass index (BMI) have all increased. As a result, surgeons are completing more challenging operations on more complex patients. It is established that preoperative multimorbidity is a strong prognostic indicator of postoperative function, morbidity, and mortality.[1] Additionally, in the last decade, the role of the surgeon and surgical practice has increased in the preoperative phase of care. Specifically, the focus on enhanced recovery after surgery (ERAS) pathways brought to light the importance of preoperative education and management of comorbidities. Most pathways include some elements of preoperative assessment and/or optimization as well as patient education. Ultimately, with the intent of proactive management of medical and functional status to ensure optimal surgical and patient-reported outcomes, the terms *prehabilitation* and *rehabilitation* have gained traction.

Prehabilitation and rehabilitation are multidimensional approaches that aim to take a holistic view of the surgical episode from the point the decision for surgery is made until the patient is back in their home environment. The preoperative period is a natural time to engage patients regarding healthy lifestyle choices because this time is generally paired with a newly diagnosed chronic illness or cancer. Therefore, the focus of prehabilitation is on engaging a patient in behavior modification for optimization, as opposed to the traditional preoperative practice of simply assessing and risk-stratifying patients. In contrast, rehabilitation focuses on restoring both physical and mental functional capacity as well as quality of life in the postoperative setting. Collectively, prehabilitation plus rehabilitation aims to deliver goal-concordant care and ensure that functional status is restored to the best level possible after major surgery. Some prehabilitation components even specifically target preparing for rehabilitation exercises the patient may participate in, such as the use of incentive spirometry or

logrolling to sit up after major abdominal surgery. Studies on surgical patients have shown an additive and synergistic effect of prehabilitation when paired with rehabilitation on functional capacity, fitness, hospital length of stay, and complication rates.[2] Additionally, prehabilitation and rehabilitation interventions together can modify frailty, which can improve functional status and mitigate morbidity and mortality.[3,4]

PREHABILITATION

Although conceptually exciting, the evidence for prehabilitation is evolving. Broadly, studies discuss prehabilitation as the idea of training and prepping for surgery, giving patients a sense of control. Studies are largely heterogeneous and highly selective regarding patient populations, interventions, and outcome measures, which makes the results difficult to generalize to surgical patients at large and across diverse health systems outside of the controlled research setting. Another challenge with studies around prehabilitation has been measuring the impact on meaningful clinical outcomes. The evidence is mixed with regard to the role of prehabilitation in reducing traditional 30-day surgical complications, but it may be that the correct outcomes are not being assessed, and, instead, rehabilitation is aimed at improving patient-reported and functional outcomes after surgery and promoting the delivery of goal-concordant care—all outcomes that are far harder to measure than traditional 30-day surgical outcomes like surgical site infection and urinary tract infections but are likely far more meaningful to patients and their loved ones.

Prehabilitation protocols can be unimodal or multimodal, and the vast majority include one or more of the following interventions: nutrition, exercise, and/or mood. Studies suggest multimodal interventions are superior given the synergistic effects, and protocols incorporating exercise, diet, and psychological interventions can improve functional outcomes both before and after surgery.[5,6] Duration and timing of intervention are also debated, especially in the setting of resource-heavy interventions. However, Ploussard et al. suggested that even a single-day prehabilitation intervention before robotic radical prostatectomies can have positive results.[7] This study intervention was a one-day "PreHab" workshop, which included nutritional advice and exercise recommendations, and was paired with an ERAS protocol. They found that the ERAS + PreHab protocol worked synergistically to significantly shorten length of stay and lessen intraoperative blood loss and operative time. Additionally, ERAS + PreHab improved costs compared with ERAS alone, and it showed improvement by 22% when compared with no intervention.[7] At the other extreme of interventions, PREHAB, an international, multicenter, randomized controlled trial (RCT) showed that a supervised 4-week, in-hospital prehabilitation program that included high-intensity exercise three times per week, nutritional and psychological intervention, and all smoking cessation (if applicable) showed a reduction of severe complications by 50% in the prehabilitation group and improved postoperative functional capacity.[8]

Keeping the many limitations in mind, studies have shown positive outcomes with prehabilitation improving functional capacity and fitness, reduced hospital length of stay, lower complication rates, and cost savings.[2,9] Howard et al. found an average savings of $21,946 per patient and recommended prehabilitation consideration for all patients.[9] Trépanier et al. pooled data from three prehabilitation studies and found in the setting of stage III colorectal cancer that prehabilitation was associated with an improved 5-year survival.[10] Additionally, in the wake of the COVID-19 pandemic, patients faced delays in care, limited resources, and added COVID-19–related morbidities. Authors have argued prehabilitation protocols can help mitigate these additional burdens that COVID-19 has placed on both individual patients and the healthcare system[11] and use the delay in surgical timing for positive interventions.

Successful efforts to systematize the preoperative period and implement prehabilitation on a larger scale can be seen in the Peri Operative Programme Péri-Opératoire (POP) at McGill, Strong for Surgery by the American College of Surgeons (ACS), and Michigan Surgical & Health Optimization Program (MSHOP). In 2007 McGill University Health Centre initiated prehabilitation efforts, and in 2011 it incorporated a not-for-profit organization, POP, to continue their robust research efforts. Research from McGill has in many ways laid the foundation for our current working definition of prehabilitation with their most recent contribution of the PREHAB randomized clinical trial previously mentioned. Current research focuses on implementation barriers and suggests a paradigm shift in the preanesthesia care structure.

Strong for Surgery is a dedicated effort by the ACS to improve preoperative comprehensive screening and risk stratification and to guide necessary referrals. This initiative encourages providers and healthcare systems to implement routine screening checklists preoperatively. They include eight targeted areas, one of which is prehabilitation. Their prehabilitation protocol recommends screening all patients older than 65 for physical limitations and frailty, suggesting baseline assessments with grip strength or the Timed Up & Go test and possible referral to a geriatrician. They also recommend consideration of preoperative consultation with a cardiologist in the setting of unstable cardiac disease, pulmonology referral in the setting of unstable pulmonary disease, and physical therapy with a daily walking program composed of two to three walks per day in patient populations with poor mobility or diminished endurance.[12] The other areas of focus in Strong for Surgery are nutrition, glycemic control, medication management,

smoking cessation, pain management, delirium, and patient directives,[13] which are all components critical for preoperative optimization whether they are included in a prehabilitation bundle or other preoperative optimization bundle or pathway.

MSHOP is a statewide comprehensive surgical preparation and training program that was developed at the University of Michigan. It shows effectiveness and generalizability of prehabilitation across diverse patient populations, hospital systems, and practices. They conducted a prospective multicenter cohort study across 21 Michigan hospitals assessing the impact of a prehabilitation program that included a home-based walking program with daily reminders and education on nutrition, smoking cessation, stress management, care planning, and incentive spirometry instruction.[14,15] Their program is an example of a scalable model of prehabilitation that decreases hospital length of stay and lowers total episode payments for Medicare beneficiaries. Their model is now standard practice for major inpatient general and thoracic surgery at the University of Michigan, and in a pilot setting, Blue Cross Blue Shield of Michigan has started a reimbursement process.

PREHABILITATION COMPONENTS

As hospital systems develop and deploy prehabilitation programs, they will inherently be variable and constructed to best fit each unique healthcare system and patient's needs. Some components may be tied into preexisting perioperative bundles or ERAS pathways. However, other prehabilitation programs will encompass all necessary preoperative patient optimization components. The evidence of the synergistic effects of multicomponent prehabilitation programs and prehabilitation programs + ERAS pathways suggests the following components should be considered for inclusion: nutrition, glycemic control, medication management, tobacco cessation, pain management, delirium prevention, exercise, and psychological optimization with a focus on anxiety and depression. Other important areas that can be considered preoperatively for optimization but are not discussed in this chapter specifically are anemia, weight loss, and completing patient directives.

Nutrition

Appropriate nutrition, especially in critically ill and malnourished patients, decreases rates of infection, hospital and intensive care unit (ICU) length of stay, and duration on the ventilator.[16] Therefore, nutritional optimization is a key area of focus in the elective surgery preoperative setting. It is key to assess nutrition multidimensionally. The ACS Nutrition Screening checklist is an example of what aspects can be important in screening for malnutrition. They recommend any patient who is not receiving established nutrition therapy to get a referral to a registered dietician if they have a BMI less than 19, over 8 pounds of unintentional weight loss in the past 3 months, a poor appetite as defined by eating less than half of their meals or fewer than two meals per day, or are unable to tolerate oral intake. They also recommend a routine serum albumin check if the patient is scheduled for an inpatient procedure and immune modulating supplementation if the patient is having "complex" surgery. However, it is important to note, and emphasized in the American Society for Parenteral and Enteral Nutrition (ASPEN) guidelines, that albumin and prealbumin should not be used in isolation for assessment of preoperative nutritional status because they are markers of inflammatory metabolism,[17] and using these laboratory values in isolation can over diagnose malnutrition. Nutrition is identified as a critical piece of optimization for surgery, and the vast majority of prehabilitation protocols incorporate a nutrition intervention.

Addressing nutrition proactively before surgery can assist in the body's ability to respond to the additional insult of surgery. Early optimization and focus on nutritional supplements, protein, complex carbohydrate intake, and proper hydration are key to prepping our patients for surgery and mitigating loss of muscle, strength, and functional capacity.[18–20] Specifically, providing nutritional guidance for patients undergoing gastrointestinal or cancer surgery is associated with improved morbidity.[21] Preoperative carbohydrate-loading nutrition drinks are a component of many preoperative pathways. A recent systematic review and network meta-analysis of phase II and III RCTs suggest that preoperative carbohydrate drinks are associated with shorter lengths of stay, improvements in insulin resistance and sensitivity, and improved C-reactive protein (CRP) values. However, carbohydrate drinks and water had equal improvements compared with fasting in regard to improvements in postoperative nausea and vomiting and overall lower morbidity.[22] Studies have also found that diet modification, especially through engagement with a dietician, can even significantly improve pain scores and quality of life in chronic pain patients, and referral to a dietician should be considered.[23–25]

Glycemic Control

Glycemic control in the perioperative period is paramount across all surgical patients, and focus on control should not be limited to the known diabetic population. Hyperglycemia is a well-established risk factor for increased rates of infection, poor wound healing, longer hospital length of stay, and increased mortality.[21,26] Despite the known negative impacts, studies show blood glucose levels greater than 140 mg/dL occur in up to 40% of general surgery patients and 90% of cardiac surgery patients.[26] In the prehospital setting providers can screen for risk factors predisposing patients to difficulty with perioperative glycemic control. One suggested way for the screening proposed is that all patients with a prior diagnosis of diabetes, age over 45, or BMI greater than 30 have their fasting blood sugar checked before entering the operating room. Hemoglobin A1c >7.0% or a fingerstick over 200 mg/dL in the prior 2 weeks warrants a referral for diabetes management.[27]

Medication Management

Obtaining an accurate medication history—including over-the-counter medications, herbal supplements, and doses—is essential in the preoperative setting. A particular focus should be placed on identifying polypharmacy and patients taking antiplatelets, anticoagulants, β-blockers, or steroids as well as those receiving immunotherapy. One should note indications and duration of use and contact the prescribing provider, if necessary, to discuss risks and benefits of holding the medication perioperatively. When safe, the ACS recommends holding anticoagulants, including Coumadin, Plavix, and others, for 1 week before surgery. Evidence is evolving, but aspirin used for preventative purposes only may be discontinued preoperatively. The American Heart Association (AHA) and American College of Cardiology (ACC) recommend that patients on chronic β-blockade undergoing noncardiac surgery should continue treatment through the perioperative period.[28] Medication management emphasizes the importance of comprehensive clinical care and multidisciplinary teams in the weeks leading up to surgery. Patients with an intermediate or high risk of myocardial ischemia or those with three or more Revised Cardiac Risk Index risk factors—such as diabetes, heart failure, coronary artery disease, renal insufficiency, or cerebrovascular accident—can be started on β-blockade preoperatively. However, the timing of initiation is critical, as is

management with a multidisciplinary team.[28] According to the AHA/ACC guidelines for preoperative management of hypertension, medical management can continue up until the planned elective procedure, and the discontinuation of angiotensin-converting enzyme (ACE) and angiotensin receptor blockers (ARBs) is considered. Additionally, it is reasonable to reschedule elective surgery for systolic blood pressures 180 mm Hg or higher and diastolic blood pressures 110 mm Hg or higher.[28,29]

All over-the-counter medications and herbal supplements that may increase risks of bleeding, such as NSAIDS, echinacea, garlic, gingko, ginseng, kava, saw palmetto, St. John's wort, and valerian, should be held 2 weeks before surgery.[30] The American Geriatrics Society Beers Criteria (AGS Beers Criteria) for Potentially Inappropriate Medication (PIM) Use in Older Adults is an essential resource for clinicians in assessing safety of medications for the geriatric population.[31] It should be used in the preoperative setting to assess what medications should be held for surgery or, in collaboration with their primary care provider, discontinued altogether.

Tobacco Cessation

Encouraging tobacco cessation preoperatively is well established as routine practice. Many institutions have incorporated cessation as part of their preoperative pathways and ERAS protocols, with some surgical subspecialties mandating it preoperatively for elective surgery, even testing for nicotine levels given the known negative effects. For institutions that have not done this, it should be strongly considered as part of a prehabilitation protocol. Tobacco smokers are at significantly higher risk of infection, poor wound and bone healing, and impaired cardiopulmonary function in the postoperative setting compared with nonusers. A subset of negative effects including prolonged recovery and adverse respiratory outcomes extends to people exposed to secondhand smoke, especially children.[32] The World Health Organization completed a review of RCTs that showed interventions to support cessation significantly reduced the incidence of any postoperative complication, surgical site infections, and morbidity. Additional observational studies show an association between tobacco use and all complications, infections, neurologic and pulmonary complications, ICU admission, wound infection, delay in healing, dehiscence, and hernia occurrence.[21,32,33] All surgical patients benefit from smoking cessation; however, the gastrointestinal tract is particularly sensitive to the toxic effects of smoking, and patients undergoing bowel resection benefit from cessation to a greater extent than other patients.[32–34] The most profound benefits are consistently seen after 3 weeks of cessation, and some studies show that each week past 4 weeks of cessation confer 19% of additional reduction of morbidity. The best evidence is for behavioral interventions with weekly check-ins, nicotine replacement therapy, and cessation programs.[32] Support in the preoperative period should be as early as possible to maximize these potential benefits, which would support early initiation of prehabilitation protocols.

Pain Management

Multimodal pain control should be considered as part of prehabilitation protocols if not already incorporated into the established care model through ERAS pathways. Up-front conversations about pain medications to set expectations and discuss strategies for safe multimodal pain control after surgery can be helpful. Additionally, referral to a pain service for patients with a 3-month or longer history of opioid use before surgery is recommended.[35] To reduce opiate use postoperatively, it is important to integrate multimodal, nonopioid agents and pain management strategies throughout the entire perioperative and operative experience.[36] Preoperative physical activity, nutrition optimization, and engagement with online platforms aiding in opioid cessation can significantly reduce postoperative opioid use and expedite opioid cessation.[24,37]

Delirium Prevention

Postoperative delirium is the rapid onset of confusion. Causes of delirium can be multifactorial. It is a problem that disproportionately affects the elderly population and up to 50% of patients undergoing high-risk procedures.[38] Delirium can be either hypoactive or hyperactive and can last days to weeks, with some patients never appearing to fully recover. Furthermore, it is associated with cognitive and functional decline, loss of autonomy, longer hospitalization, more ICU admissions, greater healthcare costs, and higher rates of mortality.[38,39] The ACS recommends screening for risk factors for delirium in the preoperative setting assessing patients over 65 years old and those with cognitive deficits, poor functional status or a history of falls, and underlying severe illnesses or infection; vision or hearing loss should also be noted. If the patient meets any of these criteria, consideration of further evaluation is necessary. Optimization to prevent delirium includes removing medications that are associated with delirium; performing sleep hygiene preoperatively; ensuring assist devices such as hearing aids, dentures, and glasses are packed for the hospital and used while an inpatient; including sign-up sheets for family and friends at bedside; checking orientation frequently; and providing large-faced clocks and visible dates in the room. It is also important to screen for metabolic and electrolyte abnormalities as well as delirium-causing medications preoperatively with enough time for safe correction and cessation. Some current study protocols are focused on the possible effects of home-based exercises, dietary management, and iron infusions on postoperative delirium.[38]

Exercise

Exercise is a critical aspect of prehabilitation protocols and has been found to significantly reduce postoperative pulmonary complications, overall morbidity, disability, and pain.[40-44] A systematic review of studies examining exercise prehabilitation in patients undergoing bowel resection found it significantly improves postoperative functional capacity.[45] Minnella et al. completed a single-center single-blinded RCT that evaluated high-intensity interval training (HIIT) versus moderate-intensity continuous training (MICT) and determined that both improved preoperative functional capacity without a significant difference between the two.[46] This suggests room for customization of prehabilitation protocols allowing for specific interventions to fit what patients will engage with most. Programs can be further individualized to meet specific populations' needs, with tailored programs for orthopedic patients versus vascular patients or programs focused on specific body parts such as the operative limb. Other studies have shown significant reduction in postoperative complications in patients who engage in community-based exercise programs or when patients are provided educational pamphlets on exercise interventions.[47,48] The significant results across exercise interventions suggest that engagement in exercise preoperatively is essential.

Psychological Health: Anxiety and Depression

Surgery is a stress to every system in the body that requires both physical and psychological reserve. Studies have shown that anxiety negatively effects outcomes and impacts length of stay, immune function, ability to heal wounds, and return to function. Additionally, it impacts patient engagement and motivation.[21] It is estimated that 50% or more of patients experience perioperative anxiety. Perioperative anxiety is associated with increased anesthetic use, which can negatively impact recovery and increase rates of nausea, emesis, and cardiopulmonary symptoms.[49] Wada et al. found that anxiety in cancer patients is a strong predictor of postoperative delirium, and Ramirez et al. found an association between depression and nonhome discharges postoperatively.[50,51] Understanding our patients' propensity for anxiety and depression in the perioperative period and improving coping mechanisms through standardized preoperative prehabilitation pathways can improve surgical outcomes. Numerous methods for stress reduction and anxiety mitigation strategies have proven effective ranging from music, meditation, guided imagery, acupuncture, cognitive behavioral therapy, and others,[52] which allows for customization to hospital resources and/or patients.

AT-RISK POPULATIONS

As discussed previously, there is no standardized time frame for prehabilitation interventions, and groups studied are heterogeneous, which makes it difficult to generalize recommendations. In an era of limited resources, it can be argued that efforts should be focused on the most at-risk populations initially. The most notable populations that targeted efforts could support are frail patients with preexisting limited physical reserve, surgical oncology patients, and other at-risk populations such as substance use disorder patients.

FRAIL PATIENTS/DECREASED PHYSICAL RESERVE

First and foremost, understanding our patients' goals in the setting of elective surgery is critical. Zattoni et al. noted that frailty is the most important prognostic factor for postoperative complications, increased length of stay, and functional and cognitive decline.[53] Frailty is also associated with increased mortality, regardless of the operative stress of the procedure,[54] morbidity, and cost.[55] Functional preservation is paramount, especially in the geriatric population where functional loss is quite difficult to regain and is often "more feared than death."[53] McLennan et al. found that patients unable to climb two flights of stairs were over four times more likely to have a postoperative complication and prolonged length of stay.[56] Poor preoperative functional status is also correlated to nonhome discharges,[57] and improved functional capacity is associated with fewer severe postoperative complications.[5] Frailty is a modifiable risk factor. Functional performance can improve with prehabilitation and rehabilitation, which can mitigate morbidity and mortality.[3,4] McIsaac and colleagues are currently completing the PREPARE trial, a multicenter RCT on a frailty-specific prehabilitation protocol that focuses on postoperative complications and disability as outcomes.[58] Healthcare providers can capitalize on frailty as a predictor of postoperative outcomes, act to improve preoperative functional status through prehabilitation measures, and work to streamline discharges for patients seeking preapproval for acute rehabilitation and care facilities. In contrast, Carli et al. completed a randomized clinical trial that assessed 30-day postoperative complications for frail patients after prehabilitation and colorectal resection, which showed no improvement in outcomes compared with rehabilitation.[59] This supports the need for continued research to assess best optimization for this population because they may benefit most from the synergistic effects of prehabilitation plus rehabilitation or evaluation at later end points such as 90 days.

SURGICAL ONCOLOGY PATIENTS

Prehabilitation in surgical oncology patients has been found to have positive effects on postoperative functional status, maintenance of lean muscle mass, shortened hospital stay, improved complication rates, and quality of life. Recent studies support that improving nutrition, functional capacity, and psychology in the time of neoadjuvant treatment for surgical oncology patients can further bolster these results.[2,60] Although delaying surgery for prehabilitation alone, particularly in cancer patients, is debated, the expanding role of neoadjuvant therapy across diseases could offer a built-in time for prehabilitation protocols to be implemented.[42] There is evidence for the use of both unimodal and multimodal prehabilitation protocols in cancer patients, with additional unique findings in oncologic subpopulations such as reduced number of days requiring chest tubes in thoracic postoperative patients who engage in prehabilitation protocols.[61] Multiphasic prehabilitation has also been suggested for cancer patients where prehabilitation is assessed for and implemented multiple times preoperatively through the course of neoadjuvant therapy.[2]

SUBSTANCE USE PATIENTS

The risks of smoking are well established and discussed previously in this chapter. Alcohol use disorder is also linked with worse surgical outcomes.[62] Over two alcoholic drinks per day is associated with increased postoperative infections, pulmonary complications, greater length of stay, and increased need for ICU care. Fernandez et al. noted additive negative effects when alcohol and smoking are combined preoperatively, and they found when the substances are used in conjunction, there are significant synergistic deleterious effects resulting in increased complications, readmissions, and reoperations.[62] Tang et al. found higher levels of opioid use in the preoperative phase was associated with higher rates of readmission,[63] highlighting the need for preoperative substance use screening and strategies for intervention for substances known to affect health and surgical outcomes. These unique considerations and complications for this population suggest that they could benefit from screening, intervention, and additional support preoperatively. A systematic review and meta-analysis of preoperative interventions for alcohol and other recreational substance use found that preoperative interventions can reduce substance use, but interventions do not reduce hospital length of stay, morbidity, or mortality.[64] Future studies could assess whether incorporation into a comprehensive prehabilitation protocol can be impactful.

IMPLEMENTATION CONSIDERATIONS

As with any novel intervention, models for achieving optimal perioperative care will vary based on existing resources and system structure. One solution trialed at the University of California San Francisco lead by Dr. Finlayson focused efforts on the at-risk geriatric population by establishing a Geriatric Optimization Clinic. Finlayson et al. found that although the prehabilitation clinic was valuable, it was challenging to support the specialists' time to participate (nutrition, physical therapy, geriatrics, and anesthesia), and, ultimately, the clinic was closed.[65] Carli et al. suggested integrating

prehabilitation into the perioperative clinic but with a paradigm shift, noting the importance of moving the intervention forward in time to enable a longer intervention period because presently traditional preanesthesia clinic visits are quite close to the time of surgery.[66,67] The cost of providing care may be partially recaptured through the clinic billing as a preoperative visit rather than the primary care provider. Cost savings in the setting of prehabilitation would be realized by the system through decreased length of stay, fewer complications, and fewer readmissions. These improvements have reputational impact by increasing referrals and improving payer compensation. MSHOP shows promise for this cost savings and the potential for insurance reimbursement.

It is possible that as payment reform is pursued in the United States, incentives will shift, and it will "make sense" financially for providers and health systems to support more robust prehabilitation programs. One example is the Centers for Medicare and Medicaid Services Bundled Payments for Care Improvement initiative. In this program, hospitals are incentivized to ensure optimal outcomes because they are paid a set amount of money per episode (usually 90 days of care, initiated by a surgical encounter), and in the event the total cost of care is lower than the payment, they share in the savings; if total cost of care exceeds the payment, they incur financial penalty. Therefore, if indeed prehabilitation can improve postoperative outcomes and reduce costs for the episode, hospitals will engage. The model is imperfect, and uptake has largely been optional, but it is anticipated that other models will be released in the next few years. This will likely continue to push the adoption of prehabilitation and rehabilitation.

REHABILITATION

Before the conception and implementation of prehabilitation, perioperative care was mainly focused on postoperative rehabilitation. Rehabilitation after surgery is most developed in the fields of orthopedic and cardiothoracic surgery and has been shown to decrease pulmonary complications, length of stay, and hospital costs.[68] Multifaceted and multidisciplinary rehabilitation programs focusing on nutrition, strength, balance, and cardiorespiratory fitness have also proven efficacious in improving outcomes in thoracic and abdominal surgery populations.[65] Rehabilitation targeted at specific patient population needs has also proven to be efficacious. Postoperative exercise programs including those studied in the PROSPER trial resulted in reduced upper limb disability after breast cancer surgery,[69] and pulmonary rehabilitation after lung resection was found to significantly impact postoperative exercise tolerance.[70]

Efficacy of rehabilitation has been proven in a variety of settings including outpatient and inpatient physiotherapy, rehabilitation centers, clinics, and at home.[68] In critically ill patients receiving ICU-level care, early inpatient rehabilitation while in the ICU setting is associated with less ICU-acquired weakness.[71] Most recently there is a trend of assessing efficacy and satisfaction with rehabilitation via online platforms including phone-based applications, telerehabilitation, Xbox 360, and using artificial intelligence.[72-77] Some studies show equivalent or even better rehabilitation results using augmented reality compared with standard rehabilitation.[74-76] Application-based rehabilitation allows patients the flexibility to train at home,[72] and smartphone app–based postoperative monitoring has been shown to have improved quality of recovery and satisfaction compared with in-person follow-up.[78,79] Given the importance of rehabilitation, continuing to explore novel modalities to engage in rehabilitation and improve patient participation and satisfaction is essential.

CONCLUSIONS

Optimizing surgical outcomes requires multifaceted and multidisciplinary approaches that span the entire perioperative period. The preoperative phase is an opportunity for the provider and the patient to work together to take control of the patient's health and capitalize on a teachable moment in which healthy habits are established, maintained, and improved upon. Postoperatively, multifaceted rehabilitation strategies can lead to improved surgical outcomes. The perioperative time is an opportunity for preventative care bundles that standardize approaches to patient care and help facilitate comprehensive assessment and treatment. Care maps can help coordinate prehabilitation and rehabilitation and streamline care across clinical sites. Routine screening in these pathways can identify at-risk populations that require additional tailored care, whereas others may progress seamlessly through standardized prehabilitation and rehabilitation protocols.

SELECTED REFERENCES

Englesbe MJ, Grenda DR, Sullivan JA, et al. The Michigan Surgical Home and Optimization Program is a scalable model to improve care and reduce costs. *Surgery.* 2017;161(6):1659-1666.

> *Englesbe et al. present their scalable home-based prehabilitation program, which decreased hospital length of stay and total episode payments for Medicare beneficiaries.*

Howard R, Yin YS, McCandless L, Wang S, Englesbe M, Machado-Aranda D. Taking control of your surgery: impact of a prehabilitation program on major abdominal surgery. *J Am Coll Surg.* 2019;228(1):72-80.

> *The Michigan Surgical and Health Optimization Program, a multimodal prehabilitation program including physical activity, pulmonary rehabilitation, nutritional optimization, and stress reduction, showed patients completing prehabilitation before colectomy had improved physiology, fewer complications, and significant cost savings per patient.*

Hung YC, Wolf JH, D'Adamo CR, Demos J, Katlic MR, Svoboda S. Preoperative functional status is associated with discharge to nonhome in geriatric individuals. *J Am Geriatr Soc.* 2021;69(7):1856-1864.

> *Discharge to rehabilitation facilities is associated with morbidity and mortality, and functional status and frailty are modifiable risk factors. A retrospective study using the American College of Surgeons National Surgical Quality Improvement Program showed better functional status preoperatively is associated with discharge home in older adults, suggesting preserving or improving preoperative functional status could alter discharge disposition.*

Kovoor JG, Nann SD, Barot DD, et al. Prehabilitation for general surgery: a systematic review of randomized controlled trials. *ANZ J Surg.* 2023;93(10):2411-2425.

> *Kovoor et al. highlight the mixed evidence of prehabilitation in randomized controlled trials and conclude there is insufficient evidence to support systemwide changes; however, they emphasize the potential benefits, discuss the noninferiority compared with current standard of care, and suggest case-by-case consideration.*

Temple-Oberle C, Yakaback S, Webb C, Assadzadeh GE, Nelson G. Effect of smartphone app postoperative home monitoring after oncologic surgery on quality of recovery: a randomized clinical trial. *JAMA Surg.* 2023;158(7):693.

The full reference list appears on Elsevier eBooks+.

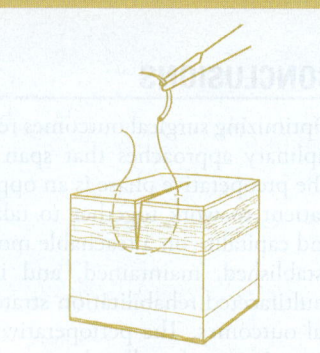

22 CHAPTER

Enhanced Recovery After Surgery (ERAS): Evidence-Based Perioperative Pathways to Optimize Outcomes

Olle Ljungqvist, Hans D. de Boer, and Gregg Nelson

OUTLINE

Introduction
    History of Enhanced Recovery After Surgery
    What Makes Enhanced Recovery After Surgery Work?
Enhanced Recovery After Surgery Society Guidelines
Enhanced Recovery After Surgery Components
    Preadmission Optimization and Prehabilitation
    Preoperative Care Elements
    Intraoperative Care Elements
    Postoperative Care Elements

    Early Mobilization
    Discharge and Follow-Up
Enhanced Recovery After Surgery Implementation Program
    Audit
    Enhanced Recovery After Surgery Team
Enhanced Recovery After Surgery Outcomes
    Roles and benefits for Enhanced Recovery After Surgery
      practitioners
Conclusion

INTRODUCTION

Enhanced Recovery After Surgery (ERAS) is a program for perioperative care based on the best available evidence in medical literature. Employing the principles of ERAS has revolutionized surgery and surgical care and has yielded marked improvements in outcomes for patients reducing recovery time and suffering from complications, while freeing up hospital resources and reducing cost. In this chapter all important aspects of ERAS will be presented.

History of Enhanced Recovery After Surgery

To understand why and how ERAS has become what it is today, it is important to understand how it developed over the past decades. In more recent times, the idea of bundling care elements to a care protocol was first presented by Engelman and coworkers for cardiac surgery patients.[1] They reported case series employing a care bundle consisting of fluid management and pain control and showed that they could "Fast Track" patients through recovery in the intensive care unit (ICU) and in the hospital with this program. Shortly thereafter Henrik Kehlet, a surgeon from Denmark, reported that his Fast Track program combined with laparoscopic surgery in eight elderly patients (ages 71–88 years old) undergoing segmental colonic resections resulted in recovery and discharge from the hospital 2 days after the operation.[2] This was a sensation at the time when length of stay for the average patient was 2 weeks for this type of operation. He later expanded his thoughts in a review paper in which he described his ideas of a multimodal approach to recovery after major surgery. The key elements included were preoperative information, attenuation of stress, pain relief, exercise, enteral nutrition, and growth factors.

In a larger case series of colonic resections, now performed with open surgery, he confirmed his earlier results by having more than half the patients discharged 2 days after surgery.[3]

These results inspired Ken Fearon (United Kingdom) and Olle Ljungqvist (Sweden) to gather a group of surgeons to form a group to study this remarkable approach further. Joined by Arthur Revhaug (Norway), Martin von Meyenfeldt (Netherlands), Cornelius DeJong (Netherlands), and Henrik Kehlet (Denmark), they initiated the Enhanced Recovery After Surgery Group in 2001.[4] It was felt that rather than aiming for *fast*, the target should be *recovery*, and that was the birth of "ERAS."

Building on the principles of a multimodal approach, but not selecting just a few care elements, the group set off to search for all elements of care that had data in support of enhancing recovery to form a care protocol. Involving younger colleagues from all units, the team scanned the literature and published the first ever evidence-based guide for perioperative care in colonic resection in 2005.[5] The elements included are shown in Fig. 22.1 and included additional items on top of the ones proposed by Kehlet.

During this early period the group made several key discoveries that helped form ERAS. Having built the first ERAS protocol, the members realized that none of them were employing all elements they had found in the literature. Second, they also saw that they had different missing items; thus, the care delivered was very different between units. They set out to change practices to align with the newly produced guideline and see if this would improve their outcomes. Before embarking on this, clinical teams had length of stay at the upper end of what was average at the time, and hence, far from the 2 days that Kehlet's group had presented. The group

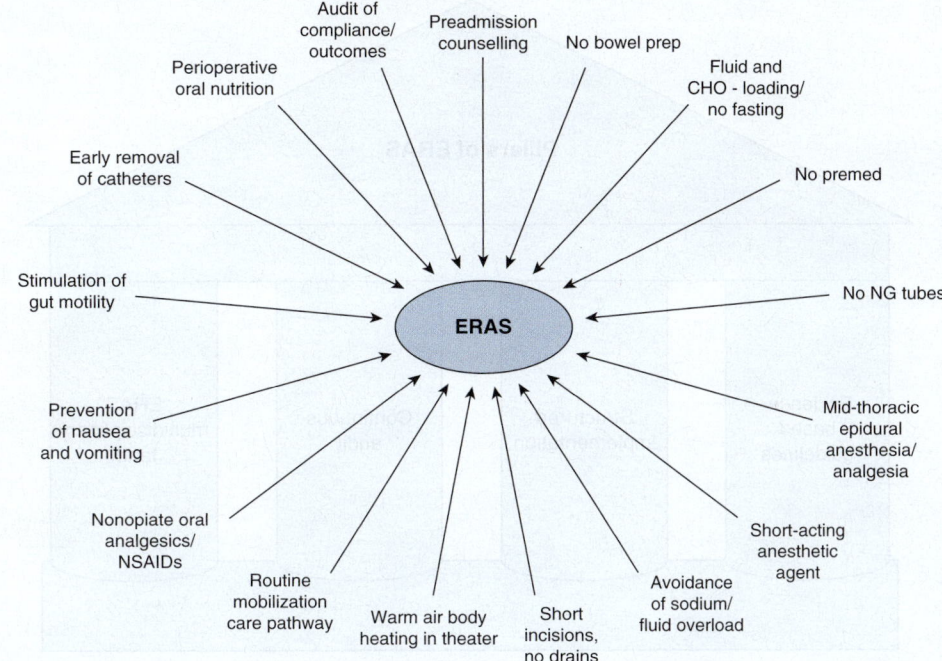

FIGURE 22.1 Main elements of the initial Enhanced Recovery After Surgery (ERAS) Consensus protocol. *CHO,* Carbohydrate; *NG,* nasogastric. (From Fearon KC, Ljungqvist O, Von Meyenfeldt M, et al. Enhanced recovery after surgery: a consensus review of clinical care for patients undergoing colonic resection. *Clin Nutr.* 2005;24[3]:466-477.)

also started to include rectal surgery to widen the scope. When setting off this project, a database was formed to capture all relevant data that could affect outcomes, including demographics, key comorbidities, all care items of the ERAS protocol, key surgical and anesthesia elements, and outcomes. All items in the database were thoroughly defined. Once reviewing the data after having collected several hundred patients, two important discoveries were made. All units found that they were wrong about their own practice. The review performed for compliance to the ERAS protocol done before the audit was very different from what the real-life data revealed. Problems existed where things were believed to be running well and vice versa. All units found elements of care that needed to be put in place, and several of them were completely unexpected by the teams. It was obvious that the only way to be able to test the guideline and its use was to continuously audit all processes and feedback continuously to those responsible for the care on the surgical floor to ensure that all elements of care were being used. Without this audit, focus would have been directed the wrong way and the important changes needed never addressed.

The group also found that the protocol was not going be sufficient to implement ERAS, a structural change in how the work was led and run was also needed (Fig. 22.2).[6] Audit is one key, but building the team to run the audit and lead the changes and ERAS on the floor was another key to success. The team had to employ representatives of all professions and disciplines involved in the care of the patient, and every station the patient passes during the care journey needs to be represented. The team needs to work in parallel and together and make sure that every ERAS care element is delivered at the right time to make the entire journey flow at its best.

These ideas were further tested in the Netherlands where Dutch colleagues teamed up with the Dutch Institute for Healthcare Improvement. They employed a structured method for implementation of the ERAS protocol and could train more than 30 hospitals

in ERAS across the Netherlands. In less than a year, length of stay averaged a 30% to 50% reduction, which showed it was possible to make marked improvements with this care in a short time.[7]

Around the same time two important studies were published that caused the interest in ERAS to boom. Dileep Lobo and the ERAS group reported that not only was length of stay reduced with ERAS, but complications were markedly reduced.[8] This was a breakthrough later confirmed many times over. Gustafsson et al. showed a clear relationship between better compliance to the elements of the care pathway for open colorectal cancer surgery and reduced complications.[9] A 5-year follow-up study reported that with higher ERAS compliance and fewer complications, survival was improved.[10]

With the insights of knowing that (1) the literature could help lead the way to better care when all elements were assembled in an evidence-based fashion, (2) structured implementation required a multidisciplinary multiprofessional ERAS team, and (3) continuous audit that captured care processes and outcomes together was needed, the ERAS Study group decided to start a nonprofit medical society. The first nonprofit enhanced recovery society was formed and named the ERAS® Society (www.erassociety.org) in 2010[4] with the mission to develop perioperative care and to improve recovery through education, research, audit, and implementation of evidence-based practice.

To be able to support the implementation with an information technology (IT) system and administration of the implementation program, the group decided that a for-profit company should be started to be contracted to the Society. This partnership has run the implementation of ERAS in more than 30 countries worldwide, where all the knowledge and medical content come from the ERAS® Society network supported by the IT systems harboring the guidelines. In this endeavor, the ERAS® Society has developed a network of hospitals around the world that work together to help units to implement ERAS (Fig. 22.3).[11] In many of these

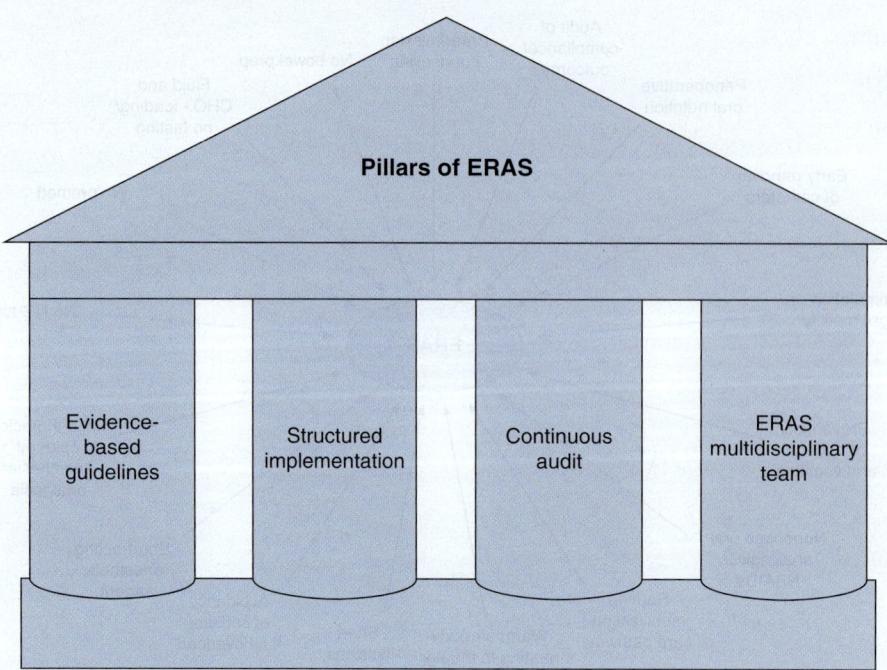

FIGURE 22.2 Pillars of Enhanced Recovery After Surgery *(ERAS)*.

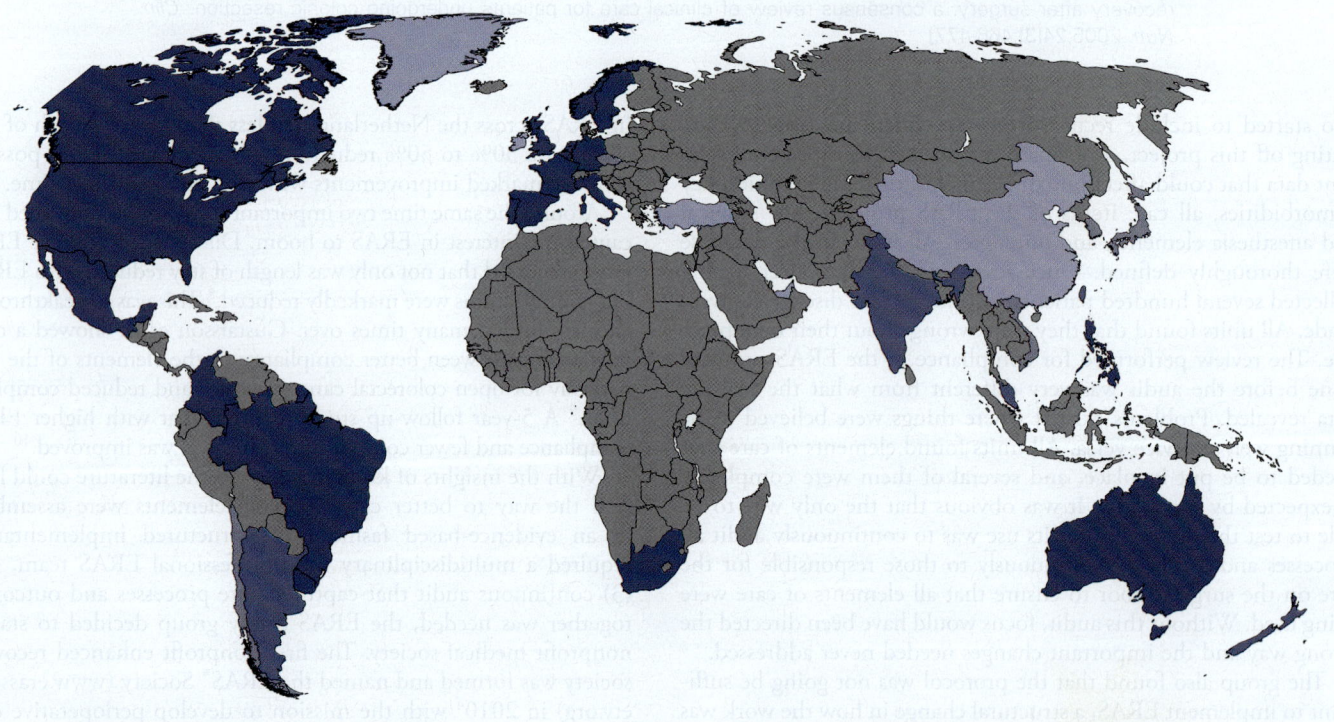

- ■ More than one implementation program
- ■ Implementation program running/announced
- ■ ERAS® center in place
- ■ ERAS® center in training
- ■ ERAS® center discussions

FIGURE 22.3 ERAS Society Global Network. (Updated September 5, 2023/O Ljungqvist.) Map lines delineate study areas and do not necessarily depict accepted national boundaries.

countries, national or regional ERAS Societies have been established, all connected to the main Society (see www.erassociety.org for details and updates). In Latin America, there is a joint Society ERAS LatAm, and countries in North America, Europe, and Asia have national societies such as ERAS USA, ERAS UK, and the newly formed ERAS Japan to mention a few. In addition to these regional and national ERAS Societies, there are also some specialty societies formed and connected to the ERAS Society, including ERAS Cardiac and ERAS Gynecologic Surgery. The same methodology has been used throughout the world for ERAS implementation, and units collect data on the same audit system. This allows for joint research to be performed in a unique way. Several research papers have been published based on data collected jointly in the ERAS® Interactive Audit System, several of them as national and international multicentric efforts.

What Makes Enhanced Recovery After Surgery Work?

Stress Reactions to Surgery

The body reacts very quickly to any type of injury, including surgery.[12] The degree to which these reactions occur are related to the extent of the injury and which body part is affected. The human body reacts to tissue injury via afferent nociceptive pathways to activate the hypothalamus, the sympathetic nervous system, the

endocrine systems (in particular the adrenals and the pancreas), and, finally, by also activating the immune system (Fig. 22.4). This stress reaction sets off a rapid release of several stress hormones including catecholamines, cortisol, glucagon, and growth hormone. In parallel, the immune systems react by releasing cytokines creating a state of inflammation. These reactions together cause an almost immediate change in body metabolism leading to a state of catabolism.

Liver glycogen is mobilized to release glucose. This is further augmented by gluconeogenesis where the building blocks come from muscle glycogen, fat depots where lipolysis is initiated, and amino acids from protein breakdown occurring in muscle. At the same time glucose uptake is hampered in muscle because of the resistance to insulin caused by the release of stress hormones. This net effect is a marked rise in glucose levels. Acute phase proteins are synthesized in the liver from amino acids released from muscle. Body temperature rises, and hypermetabolism sets in.

Central in this change is the development of insulin resistance, a pseudodiabetic state of metabolism that develops to some degree in all patients after major surgery. The purpose of these reactions is to manage the injury, protect the body from further harm, allow mobilization of energy for "fight or flight," and to prepare for a healing process. However, when exaggerated, these reactions can also cause harm. As a result of the stress

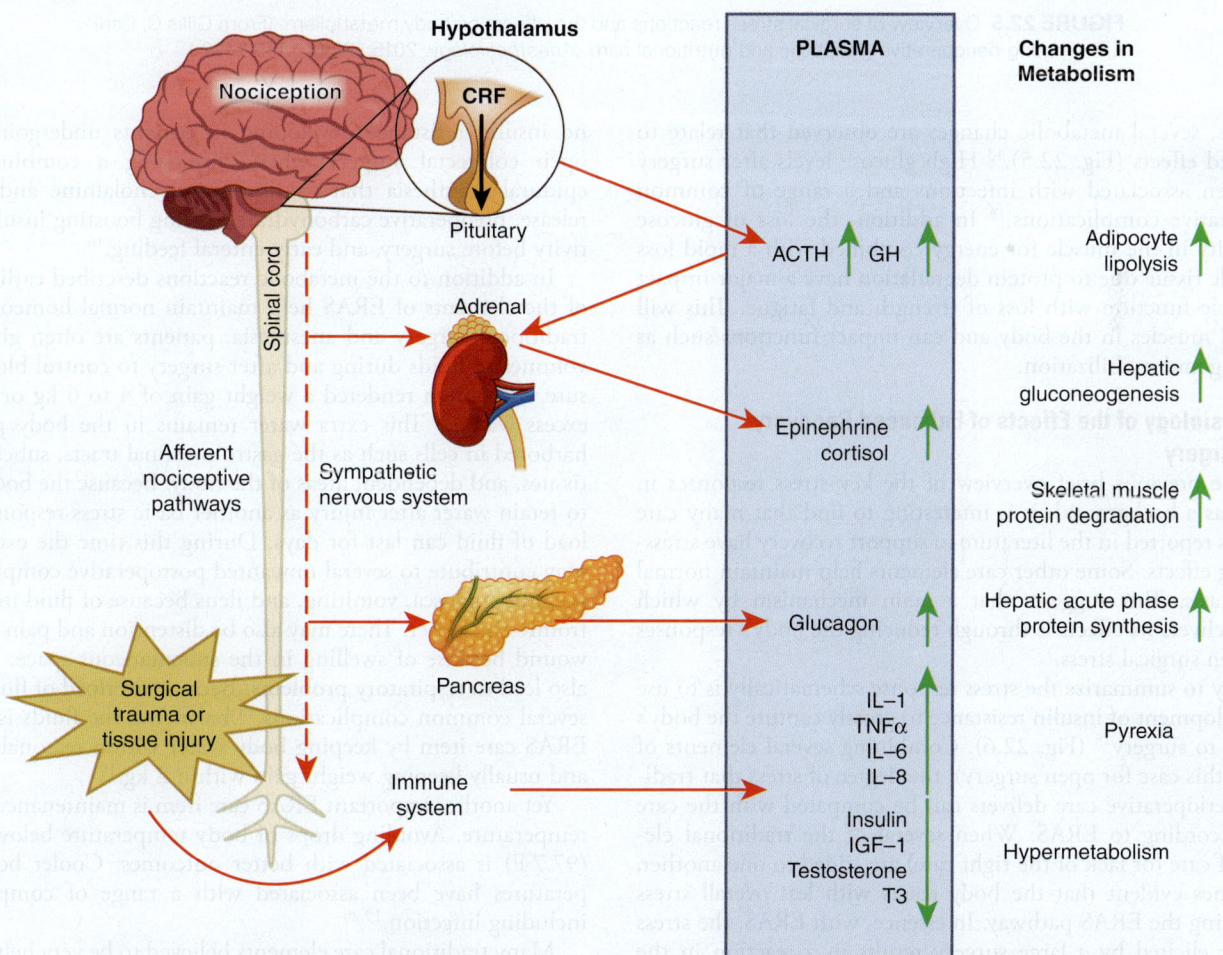

FIGURE 22.4 Overview of the surgical stress response. *ACTH*, Adrenocorticotropic hormone; *CRF*, corticotropin-releasing factor; *GH*, growth hormone; *IGF*, insulin-like growth factor; *IL*, interleukin; *TNFα*, tumor necrosis factor alpha; *T3*, triiodothyronine.

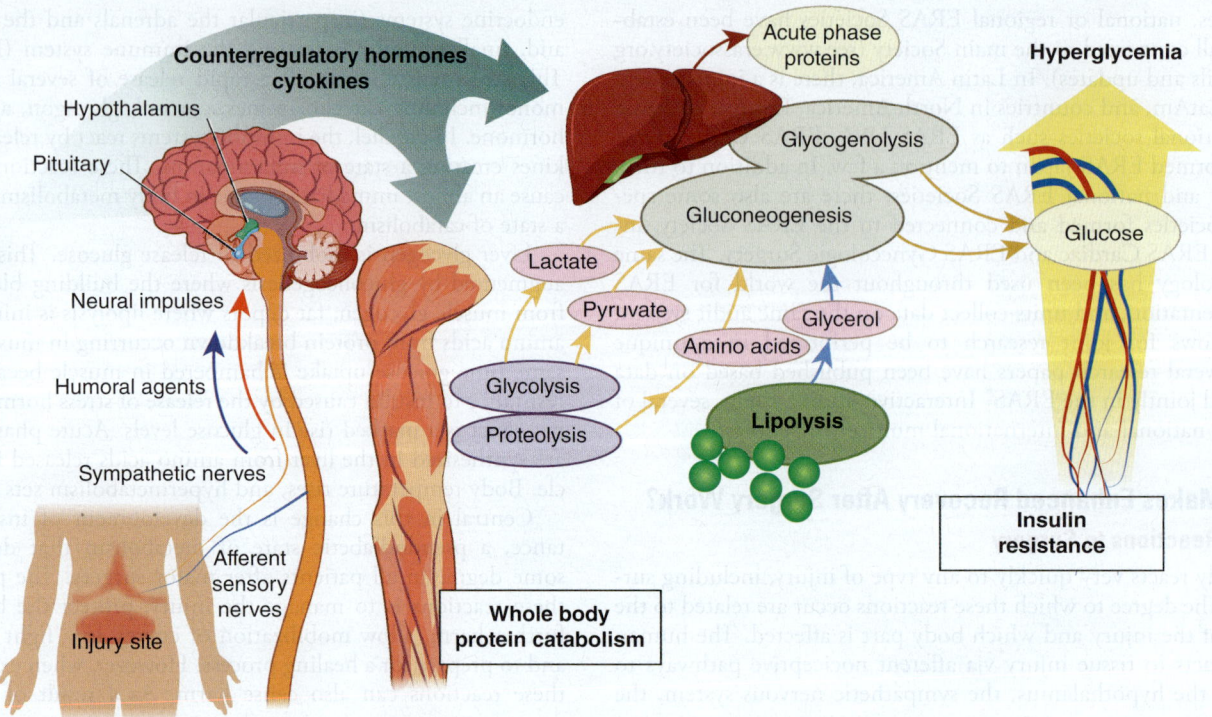

FIGURE 22.5 Overview of surgical stress reactions and the effects on body metabolism. (From Gillis C, Carli F. Promoting perioperative metabolic and nutritional care. *Anesthesiology*. 2015;123[6]:1455-1472.)

reactions, several metabolic changes are observed that relate to unwanted effects (Fig. 22.5).[13] High glucose levels after surgery have been associated with infections and a range of common postoperative complications.[14] In addition, the loss of glucose availability in the muscle for energy combined with a rapid loss of muscle tissue due to protein degradation have a major impact on muscle function with loss of strength and fatigue. This will affect all muscles in the body and can impact functions such as breathing and mobilization.

The Physiology of the Effects of Enhanced Recovery After Surgery

With the previous brief overview of the key stress responses in surgery as a background, it is interesting to find that many care elements reported in the literature to support recovery have stress-reducing effects. Some other care elements help maintain normal homeostasis. This suggests that a main mechanism by which ERAS delivers its effects is through reducing the body's responses to a given surgical stress.

A way to summarize the stress response schematically is to use the development of insulin resistance to grossly capture the body's reaction to surgery[15] (Fig. 22.6). Combining several elements of care (in this case for open surgery), the degree of stress that traditional perioperative care delivers can be compared with the care given according to ERAS. When several of the traditional elements of care (or lack of the right care) are added to one another, it becomes evident that the body reacts with less overall stress when using the ERAS pathway. In essence, with ERAS, the stress response elicited by a large surgery results in a reaction in the patient as if a much smaller surgery had been performed. This may explain why the patient feels less affected and recovers quicker and with fewer complications. One study reported almost no insulin resistance developing in patients undergoing major open colorectal surgery when employing a combination of epidural anesthesia that minimizes catecholamine and cortisol release, preoperative carbohydrate loading boosting insulin sensitivity before surgery, and early enteral feeding.[16]

In addition to the metabolic reactions described earlier, many of the elements of ERAS help maintain normal homeostasis. In traditional surgery and anesthesia, patients are often given high volumes of fluids during and after surgery to control blood pressure. This often rendered a weight gain of 4 to 6 kg or more of excess water.[17] This extra water remains in the body primarily harbored in cells such as the gastrointestinal tracts, subcutaneous tissues, and dependent areas of the body. Because the body strives to retain water after injury as another basic stress response, overload of fluid can last for days. During this time the excess fluid may contribute to several unwanted postoperative complications, including nausea, vomiting, and ileus because of fluid in the gastrointestinal tract. There may also be distention and pain from the wound because of swelling in the subcutaneous space. This can also lead to respiratory problems. Because overload of fluid causes several common complications,[18] balancing the fluids is another ERAS care item by keeping body water within reasonable limits and usually keeping weight gain within 2 kg.[19]

Yet another important ERAS care item is maintenance of body temperature. Avoiding drops of body temperature below 36.5°C (97.7°F) is associated with better outcomes. Cooler body temperatures have been associated with a range of complications including infection.[19,20]

Many traditional care elements believed to be very helpful have been shown to be either completely unnecessary or even harmful for most patients. The use of most tubes and drains to detect anastomotic leaks or bleeding have been found to be unreliable

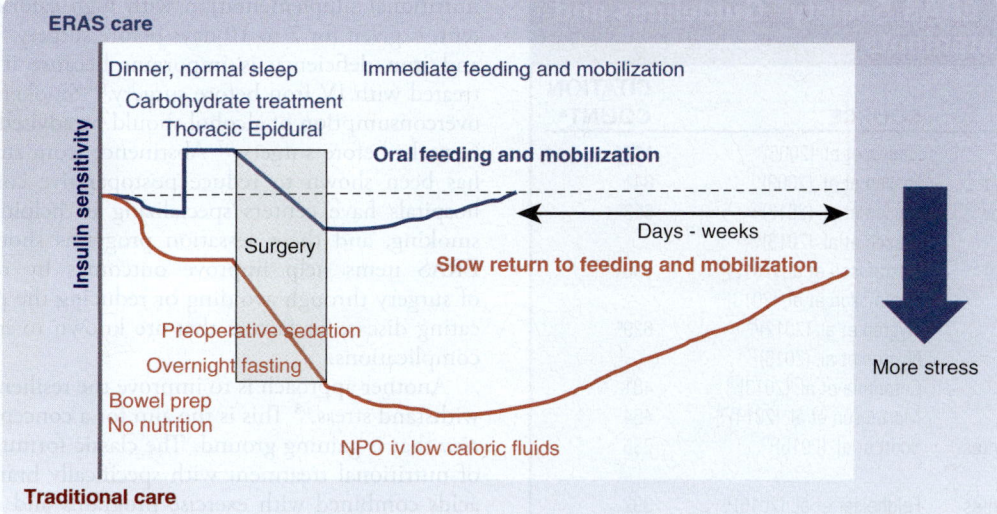

FIGURE 22.6 Schematic development of insulin resistance perioperatively in traditional and Enhanced Recovery After Surgery (ERAS) care. *NPO*, Nothing by mouth; *iv*, intravenous. (From Ljungqvist O. Jonathan E. Rhoads lecture 2011: Insulin resistance and enhanced recovery after surgery. *JPEN J Parenter Enteral Nutr.* 2012 Jul;36(4):389-98. doi: 10.1177/0148607112445580.)

and therefore only a hindrance for patients to mobilize. Nasogastric (NG) tubes have been reported to cause more harm than good when in routine use by causing pulmonary infections. These should be used only selectively. Urinary catheters were often kept in for several days, but modern studies show that they can be removed the day after surgery in most cases, if used at all on a routine basis. Finally, many studies have shown that patients can drink and eat very quickly after most surgeries. Although there is still hesitation for early oral feeding after upper gastrointestinal surgery and some ear, nose, and throat (ENT) operations, in most other operations drinking should be allowed when the patient is out of anesthesia and oral food given later the same day. This means the intravenous (IV) fluids can and should be removed, at the latest, in the morning the day after surgery and the patient allowed to eat and drink freely.[19] Although it has been reported that normal food intake often does not cover the needs of energy and protein, many patients benefit from additional oral nutritional supplements for a few days.

ENHANCED RECOVERY AFTER SURGERY® SOCIETY GUIDELINES

In 2005, the ERAS® Society published its first consensus statement, which provided evidence-based recommendations for the management of colonic resection during the preoperative, intraoperative, and postoperative phases of care. This was a turning point in the field of perioperative care globally, as demonstrated over the past two decades, with the ERAS® Society publishing guidelines now in more than 20 specialties. (Table 22.1).[5,19,21–62] The list continues to expand including the development of guidelines tailored to low- and middle-income countries. The ERAS® Society guidelines, collectively, have been cited more than 11,000 times and downloaded more than 700,000 times. A rigorous methodology and framework by which ERAS® Society guidelines are produced have developed over the years and have been published to maintain uniformity of guidelines and to ensure they do not contradict each other.[45] The quality of evidence and recommendations are evaluated according to the Grading of Recommendations Assessment, Development and Evaluation (GRADE) system whereby recommendations are given as either strong (desirable effects of adherence to a recommendation outweigh the undesirable effects) or weak (desirable effects of adherence to a recommendation probably outweigh the undesirable effects, but the panel is less confident). Quality of evidence is also included and rated as high, moderate, low, and very low.

Testing of ERAS® Society guidelines has also been conducted in several specialties with a dose-response relationship demonstrated. This was first studied in colorectal surgery patients, and the main finding was that increasing ERAS compliance was associated with fewer complications and shorter length of stay.[9] A similar relationship was identified by Wijk et al. in a study of over 2000 patients from 10 centers across North America and Europe that showed that every unit increase in ERAS guideline score was associated with an 8% to 12% decrease in days in hospital.[63]

ENHANCED RECOVERY AFTER SURGERY COMPONENTS

Preadmission Optimization and Prehabilitation

For many patients, there is a time gap from the decision to operate to the time of admission for the operation. For many cancer patients, preoperative chemoradiotherapy is indicated for several weeks. This time before surgery can and should be used to ensure that the patient is in the best possible condition to manage the stress of surgery. This involves managing the patients' comorbidities to be in the best possible control. Common medical issues are diabetes, cardiovascular problems, frailty, and poor nutritional status. Many patients with cancer suffer from iron deficiency and anemia, and many patients are sarcopenic even if their BMI may be high. Identifying and managing these medical problems can make a major difference for the outcomes of these patients.

The ERAS protocol has traditionally focused on detecting malnutrition and ensuring treatment to optimize the metabolic and nutritional status before the operation for those in need.[64] Typically, preoperative nutritional support, most often as oral

TABLE 22.1   ERAS Society® Guidelines and Consensus Statements

SPECIALTY	SOURCE	CITATION COUNT[a]
Colonic resection	Fearon et al. (2005)[5]	1111
Colorectal surgery (update)	Lassen et al. (2009)[21]	841
Pancreatoduodenectomy	Lassen et al. (2012)[22]	653[b]
	Lassen et al. (2013)[23]	
Colonic surgery (update)	Gustafsson et al. (2012)[24]	1381[b]
	Gustafsson et al. (2013)[25]	
Rectal/pelvic surgery	Nygren et al. (2012)[26]	629[b]
	Nygren et al. (2013)[27]	
Radical cystectomy	Cerantola et al. (2013)[28]	481
Gastrectomy	Mortensen et al. (2014)[29]	454
Anesthesia for Gastrointestinal Surgery Part 1	Scott et al. (2015)[30]	235
Anesthesia for Gastrointestinal Surgery Part 2	Feldheiser et al. (2016)[31]	392
Bariatric surgery	Thorell et al. (2016)[32]	373
Liver surgery	Melloul et al. (2016)[33]	365
Gynecologic Oncology Part 1	Nelson et al. (2016)[34]	305
Gynecologic Oncology Part 2	Nelson et al. (2016)[35]	292
Breast reconstruction	Temple-Oberle et al. (2017)[36]	180
Head and neck cancer	Dort et al. (2017)[37]	274
Cesarean Delivery Part 1	Wilson et al. (2018)[38]	135
Cesarean Delivery Part 2	Caughey et al. (2018)[39]	130
Cesarean Delivery Part 3	Macones et al. (2019)[40]	49
Esophagectomy	Low et al. (2019)[41]	287
Colorectal surgery (update)	Gustafsson et al. (2019)[19]	888
Lung surgery	Batchelor et al. (2019)[42]	567
Gynecologic oncology (update)	Nelson et al. (2019)[43]	362
Cardiac surgery	Engelman et al. (2019)[44]	458
Guidelines for ERAS guidelines	Brindle et al. (2020)[45]	30
Pancreatoduodenectomy (update)	Melloul et al. (2020)[46]	178
Neonatal intestinal surgery	Brindle et al. (2020)[47]	59
Cytoreduction/HIPEC Part 1	Hübner et al. (2020)[48]	71
Cytoreduction/HIPEC Part 2	Hübner et al. (2020)[49]	58
Hip/knee replacement	Wainwright et al. (2020)[50]	247
Vulvar/vaginal surgery	Altman et al. (2020)[51]	28
Spine	Debono et al. (2021)[52]	99
Bariatric surgery (update)	Stenberg et al. (2021)[53]	72
Emergency Laparotomy Part 1	Peden et al. (2021)[54]	45
Emergency Laparotomy Part 2	Scott et al. (2023)[55]	1
Emergency Laparotomy Part 3	Peden et al. (2023)[56]	1
Vascular Surgery Open aortic	McGinigle et al. (2022)[57]	14
Vascular Surgery Lower extremity	McGinigle et al. (2023)[58]	1
General surgery (LMIC)	Oodit et al. (2022)[59]	8
Liver transplant	Brustia et al. (2022)[60]	39
Gynecologic oncology (update)	Nelson et al. (2023)[61]	3
Liver surgery (update)	Joliat et al. (2023)[62]	17

[a]SCOPUS; data correct as of September 13, 2023.
[b]Published simultaneously in *Clinical Nutrition* and *World Journal of Surgery* (combined citation count for both journals).
ERAS, Enhanced Recovery After Surgery; *HIPEC*, hyperthermic intraperitoneal chemotherapy; *LMIC*, low- and middle-income countries.

nutritional supplementation with high caloric and protein content, is given for 7 to 10 days before surgery.[65] Detecting anemia and iron deficiency is important because it can be effectively treated with IV iron before surgery.[66] Smokers and patients with overconsumption of alcohol should be advised to stop, preferably 6 weeks before surgery.[67] Abstinence from smoking and alcohol has been shown to reduce postoperative complications. Many hospitals have centers specializing in helping patients to stop smoking, and these cessation programs should be used. These ERAS items help improve outcomes by reducing the stress of surgery through avoiding or reducing the presence of complicating disease or factors that are known to increase the risk for complications.

Another approach is to improve the resilience of the patient to withstand stress.[68] This is the aim for a concept called *prehabilitation* that is gaining ground. The classic formula is a combination of nutritional treatment with specifically branched chain amino acids combined with exercise programs and mental preparation for 4 to 6 weeks preoperatively. A growing number of studies support faster recovery and potentially improved clinical outcomes. Prehabilitation follows the same type of logic as ERAS by addressing the stress of surgery and should be seen as a complementary action to ERAS.[68] Prehabilitation increases the resilience of the patient to withstand the stress of surgery, while ERAS reduces the stress imposed on the patient surgery.

Preoperative Care Elements

Many patients arrive at the hospital in the early morning the day of their operation, whereas some arrive the evening before. In either case it is important to ensure that some treatments are given within the last few hours before the operation. This important part of the ERAS pathway is called the *preoperative phase*.

The immediate preoperative care items in a typical ERAS protocol are used to avoid disturbing patients' fluid homeostasis. This is achieved by avoiding unnecessary oral bowel preparation and prolonged fasting (to set body metabolism in a fed state instead of fasted at the onset of surgery), giving a carbohydrate drink, and prophylactic medications (to minimize the risk for infections, thrombosis, and pain).

In many operations it has been the tradition to treat patients with oral bowel preparation. These treatments consist of hyperosmotic fluids that are taken orally to rinse feces from the bowel. Because of their osmotic properties, these treatments attract water into the gastrointestinal tract and cause dehydration. When this treatment is used in combination with historical fasting guidelines (stopping all oral fluid intake from midnight), a state of dehydration is instituted before the operation. This will aggravate hypotension when the patient is given anesthesia. This hypotension is typically treated with IV fluids, and often this results in excess fluids given during surgery. This is a typical example of how ERAS avoids problems to be passed on from one caregiver to another by doing things right from the start. In ERAS protocols, selective oral bowel preparation is recommended, and if used, an oral antibiotic should be given in addition to the IV antibiotics to minimize the risk of infection.[19,69]

Overnight fasting allowing the patient nothing to eat or drink from midnight before elective surgery is probably one of the best known traditional medical rules worldwide.[70] The rationale for its use was that it would avoid dangerous aspiration of gastric contents during anesthesia. This belief, however, has no support in medical literature. In fact, it is perfectly safe to drink clear fluids up until 2 hours before surgery and to eat 6 hours before surgery, and guidelines from anesthesia societies worldwide have updated their recommendations.

Instead of allowing only clear fluids before surgery, ERAS protocols recommend the use of a specifically designed carbohydrate drink. The drink should be tailored for preoperative use, it should pass the stomach quickly enough to be safe, and it should elicit an insulin response to change the metabolic setting from an overnight fasted state to a fed state. Not just any drink containing carbohydrates can be used; for instance, sports drinks do not elicit the correct insulin response. It is the activation of insulin just before surgery that has postoperative effects by minimizing the development of insulin resistance after surgery. This in turn leads to better glucose control and improved protein balance.[71,72]

Two additional key components in the ERAS preoperative phase are (1) the administration of IV antibiotics within 1 hour of skin incision to reduce the risk of postoperative infections and (2) the administration of thromboprophylaxis, typically given before the induction of anesthesia.

Finally, in open surgery, the use of epidural or spinal anesthesia is recommended to be placed before the onset of major abdominal and thoracic surgery.[73] These methods have several effects. If placed to cover the dermatome T10, they will reduce the release of two key stress hormones from the adrenals, adrenaline and cortisol, and reduce insulin resistance.[74] In addition, they have excellent pain-relieving effects and minimize the need for opioids. A well-placed epidural with a catheter for continuous use postoperatively can be a very effective way of (1) achieving perfect pain management while avoiding opioids and (2) supporting the return of bowel function after major open surgery. The drawback is that epidurals can cause or aggravate hypotension, and they have been reported to have failure rates as high as 30%.

Intraoperative Care Elements

Surgical Technique

The choice of surgical technique should be based on the patient's pathology, the surgeon's skills with the techniques available, and overall resources. Although minimally invasive techniques are becoming more of the standard of care in most developed countries for the majority of surgeries of any magnitude, in the less developed part of the world open surgery still prevails. It is good to know that ERAS protocols work very well regardless of which surgical technique is used, but the combination of ERAS and minimally invasive surgery gives the best results.[75] It is also well established that for just about all major operations, the use of minimally invasive techniques has several advantages over open surgery. If available and affordable, minimally invasive techniques should be the method of choice as part of an ERAS program. In particular, the surgical technique affects the inflammatory response, and lower levels of inflammatory mediators are reported after minimally invasive surgery.[76] The patient will benefit from the lesser trauma by having a faster recovery of just about all normal functions such as eating, bowel movements, mobilization, and better pain control. To date, there is little evidence that shows any difference between the different minimally invasive techniques (laparoscopic or robotic) when it comes to their use in ERAS settings.[77,78]

Anesthetic Drugs

Modern multimodal anesthesia techniques consist of (1) the use of short-acting drugs, (2) are opioid sparing, and (3) use drugs that modulate different receptors to reduce the stress response to major surgery.[79,80] Propofol for induction in combination with short-acting

opioids—such as fentanyl, remifentanil, alfentanil, or sufentanil infusions—are used to minimize long-lasting residual effects postoperatively.[80,81] Maintenance of anesthesia can either be performed by anesthetic gases or total IV anesthesia (TIVA) with propofol infusions. The latter reduces the risk for postoperative nausea and vomiting, and data exist suggesting beneficial effects of propofol on oncologic outcomes.[80,81] In modern anesthesia, along with sedative drugs and opioids, additional antinociceptive strategies—such as neuraxial blockade, locoregional techniques, and several nonopioid drugs—are available to mitigate the effects of stress response and pain after major surgery. Antinociceptive drugs for multimodal analgesia strategies include paracetamol, NSAIDs, opioids, ketamine, magnesium, lidocaine, β-blockers, dexmedetomidine/clonidine, and dexamethasone.[81] Monitoring the depth of anesthesia is recommended by using cerebral functioning monitoring. This is particularly important for elderly patients in whom postoperative inflammatory changes in the brain lead to postoperative cognitive dysfunction and delirium.[82]

Neuromuscular Blockade Management

Muscle relaxation during anesthesia and surgery is important and instituted through the use of neuromuscular blockade. Modern neuromuscular management includes choosing an appropriate neuromuscular drug, neuromuscular monitoring, and reversal of the neuromuscular blockade at the end of the operation. Neuromuscular drugs are available to induce muscle relaxation for intubation of the trachea to secure the airway and ventilate the lungs. Choice of drug in this context depends on its pharmacologic profile and reversibility.[83–85] The steroidal neuromuscular blocking drug rocuronium is regarded as the best possible choice due to its positive safety profile and the possibility to reverse the neuromuscular blockade quickly, safely, and efficiently.[83–85] Laparoscopic and robotic surgery requires insufflation of the peritoneum to create optimal surgical conditions and may require deeper levels of neuromuscular blockade. Moreover, deeper levels of neuromuscular blockade allow surgery to be performed using low-pressure pneumoperitoneum (8–12 mm Hg). Lower intraabdominal pressure during surgery has several positive physiologic effects including a reduction in cardiac afterload, lower ventilator pressures, improvement of renal blood flow, and a reduction in the release of stress-induced immunologic factors such as interleukin (IL)-6.[86] A serious risk using neuromuscular blockade is related to any residual effects of the blocking drug that can result in postoperative pulmonary complications and increased morbidity and even mortality. Therefore, careful monitoring of the effects of these drugs should be performed by quantitative neuromuscular monitors to determine sufficient reversal of the neuromuscular blockade. Reversal of neuromuscular blockade can be achieved with a drug called sugammadex, which encapsulates the rocuronium molecules responsible for muscle relaxation. Sugammadex causes complete reversal of the neuromuscular blockade and is associated with less pain and reduced morbidity postoperatively.[84] Neostigmine is an alternative to rocuronium and is still in use in some places, but it is not as efficient and has more unwanted cholinergic side effects.[84]

Intraoperative Fluid Therapy

Fluid management is one of the key elements in ERAS programs. The aim is to optimize intravascular volume, preserve cardiac output and function, and ensure proper tissue perfusion.[87] Traditionally, fluids (often 0.9% saline) were used to manage hypotension during anesthesia and surgery. This resulted in an overload of fluids and salt that caused a multitude of complications[88] and delays in return of gastrointestinal function and ileus.[89] Instead of using fluids to manage hypotension, in ERAS, vasoactive drugs are used and fluid administration controlled to strive for a near-zero whole-body water balance for maintenance to avoid excess overload of fluids (weight gain kept at <2 kg). Additional fluids can be added to replace blood loss. It is important to keep body fluids as balanced as possible. Excessive intraoperative fluid administration results in the release of natriuretic peptides, damage to the glycocalyx, and intravascular pressure, leading to impaired gastrointestinal function and increased postoperative morbidity and mortality.[87] Similarly, too little fluid administration is also bad for the patient and leads to hypoperfusion, mucosal acidosis, increased rates of anastomotic leakage, impaired gastrointestinal function, and postoperative morbidity.[87,89] Optimal intraoperative fluid therapy should be managed to fit the patient and the type of surgery. For low-risk patients, common monitoring of fluids using balanced salt solutions for maintenance and vasoactive drugs to manage hypotension is sufficient to keep water balanced. Weighing the patient before and after surgery will give a good approximation of the total water balance. For the high-risk patient, a more sophisticated method—goal-directed fluid therapy—may be warranted.[90] In goal-directed fluid therapy, a fluid bolus up to 250 mL is administered repeatedly to optimize the patient's stroke volume according to the Frank-Starling curve.[89,90]

The optimal choice of fluid administered intraoperatively is extensively researched. Increasing evidence shows that bolus administration of colloids has no significant benefits over balanced crystalloid solutions, and the latter should be used.[91,92]

Prevention of Intraoperative Hypothermia

The maintenance of normothermia is essential in physiologic processes and homeostasis. Under normal circumstances the body's thermoregulatory mechanisms keep body temperature between 36.5°C and 37.5°C.[20] During surgery, hypothermia (defined as core temperature <36°C) may be identified at any point in the perioperative pathway, but most often it is identified in the intraoperative phase when the body is exposed to general, and sometimes neuraxial, anesthesia that impairs the finely tuned temperature regulation system in the central nervous system (hypothalamus).[20,93] Both general and neuraxial anesthesia impair vasoconstriction and cause shivering. This causes a temperature redistribution from the core to the periphery, leading to heat loss in excess of heat production.[93] Furthermore, exposure of the patient's skin and internal organs during the surgery increases heat loss even more, as does the use of cool IV and irrigation fluids.[94] Intraoperative hypothermia has been associated with several adverse events including increased blood loss, increased blood transfusion rate, increased afterload, myocardial ischemia, cardiac arrhythmias, and reduction in splanchnic blood flow. Hypothermia is also associated with longer recovery, shivering, delayed healing, longer hospital stay, unanticipated admission to high-dependency units, and reduced patient satisfaction.[95] Thus, prevention of hypothermia is essential for the patient undergoing surgery.

Maintaining normothermia should be based on temperature monitoring and management and should start preoperatively.[95] Core temperature measurement can be done in many ways, but it is best carried out by performing a nasopharyngeal measurement, with the probe inserted 10 to 20 cm.[95] Induction of anesthesia should not be started if the patient's temperature is <36°C. There are many ways to help prevent intraoperative hypothermia including ensuring that the ambient temperature is at least 21°C, using active warming of IV and irrigation fluids, warming and humidification of anesthetic gases, and, most importantly, using forced-air warming devices to cover the patient as best possible.[20,94–95] Forced-air body-warming devices can safely and efficiently transfer heat to the body and reduce heat losses in large surface areas of the skin. Other types of body-warming devices include resistive heating, circulating water mattresses, and negative pressure water-warming devices, all of which improve skin perfusion.[95] In addition, prevention of hypothermia can be achieved by forced, warmed, and humidified CO_2 used for pneumoperitoneum for patients undergoing laparoscopic surgery.[94–95]

Management of Drain and Tubes

For many years NG decompression was routinely used in most major abdominal surgery with the aim to prevent gastric distention, postoperative nausea and vomiting, and ileus. A Cochrane review proved the opposite and reported that not using NG tubes resulted in earlier return of bowel function and decreased pulmonary complications.[96–100] Moreover, with no routine use of NG tubes there was a trend toward lower risk of wound infection and ventral hernia, no difference in the rate of anastomotic leakage, and the length of hospital stay was shorter. However, critical evaluation of the benefits of the use of NG tubes in specific circumstances of different surgical scenarios is important. In the setting of esophagectomy, the use of NG tubes is still under debate. Fluid accumulation and gastric distention might increase the risk of pulmonary aspiration and anastomotic leaks when the gastric conduit is not routinely decompressed postoperatively. Recent literature shows that early removal of NG tubes in these specific settings is feasible.[96–100] In gastric surgery, routine NG decompression is not necessary for gastric cancer, irrespective of the type of digestive reconstruction and the extent of resection. In hepatic surgery, pulmonary complications are common, and the value of NG tubes is under debate. However, recent literature shows that NG decompression after elective hepatectomy does not appear to have any benefits.[100] Routine drainage of surgical cavities in abdominal and pelvic surgery was common practice for many years to allow continuous drainage from the surgical area to evacuate blood and serum and to detect signs of leaks from anastomosis. In abdominal and pelvic surgery, multiple randomized trials have studied the benefits of the use of prophylactic abdominal drains.[96–100] These studies report no significant difference or benefit from the use of routine drainage with respect to anastomotic leakage, wound infection, reoperation rates, and mortality. In fact, several studies showed a higher rate of postoperative complications and perioperative morbidity. Moreover, the use of abdominal drains resulted in a decrease in patient satisfaction and quality of life. Therefore, the routine use of drains in colorectal and pelvic surgery should be avoided when implementing ERAS pathways.

Postoperative Care Elements

The historical practice of withholding solid food from patients postoperatively until passage of flatus is not evidence based and is associated with patient dissatisfaction. Physiologically, ERAS pathway components promote gastrointestinal function sooner compared with traditional care. Introducing solid food to a patient who has undergone bowel surgery as early as 4 hours postoperatively has been shown to be safe.[9] In fact, delay in resumption of a normal diet has been shown to be associated with increased rates of infection and prolongation of recovery in major abdominal surgery.[101]

A central tenet of ERAS is multimodal opioid-sparing postoperative analgesia. Historically, opioids were the cornerstone of pain management in the postoperative period; however, there are growing concerns related to the risk of patients developing dependence on opioids during the postoperative period and ultimately becoming chronic users.[102] Surgeons prescribing opioids inappropriately have contributed to the North American opioid crisis with 50% of patients reporting not filling their opioid prescriptions after surgery.[103] Multimodal postoperative analgesic regimens are typically based on two or more analgesic classes with different mechanisms of action (e.g., combination of NSAIDs and acetaminophen). Synergism among different analgesics can allow for more sparing use of opioids, leading to less opioid consumption and its associated untoward side effects.

Early Mobilization

ERAS aims to have the patient back to their normal activities as soon as possible. For most patients this involves getting out of the hospital bed and walking around or sitting upright. Controlled mobilization can be initiated safely as early as within 30 minutes of arrival to the postanesthesia care unit (PACU)[104] and is recommended to start within a few hours after the operation once the patient is lucid. The meal taken later the day of surgery should be served sitting at a table and not in bed. From then on, all food should be served at a normal dinner table, and patients should strive to remain out of bed for 6 hours daily starting the day after surgery, even after major colorectal resection.[19]

Discharge and Follow-Up

As soon as the patient is back to normal activities of daily living (ADLs), the gut is functioning, pain is managed on oral analgesics, and there is no complication or other need for specialized in-hospital care, the patient should be discharged. At discharge, a follow-up visit should be planned for approximately 30 days after surgery to ensure that return to normality has occurred and to audit for any complications that may have arisen and were managed outside the hospital. Many cancer patients have outpatient follow-up planned for final diagnosis and any additional treatment that may be needed, and this could be a good time for the checkup. Because patients in ERAS programs leave the hospital quickly, it is also recommended to have a quick consultation line open to the ward and staff who cared for the patient in case there are questions or problems. Having the team caring for the patient see them for postoperative issues, instead of the emergency department, saves everyone a lot of unnecessary work and resources, and the patient feels more secure. Modern technology can be useful to assist with postdischarge recovery.[105]

ENHANCED RECOVERY AFTER SURGERY IMPLEMENTATION PROGRAM

There has been widespread interest in ERAS® Society guidelines; however, many clinicians are still challenged with how to initiate their ERAS® Implementation Program (EIP). A formal EIP is composed of three elements: (1) an ERAS protocol (see example in Table 22.2),[106] (2) an audit system to review protocol compliance and clinical outcomes (at minimum length of stay and complications), and (3) an ERAS team that iterates toward improved compliance and outcomes.

Audit

The only way to keep control over the care that is delivered is to audit the care processes. The same is true for outcomes, as audit of outcomes should be part of all surgeries performed. Sadly, this is far from what is happening today worldwide. Only a limited number of countries have mandatory reporting to national quality registries for their most common operations. These reports are typically available in northern Europe, with all surgical units benchmarking most outcomes on an annual basis. The American College of Surgeons National Surgical Quality Improvement Program (NSQIP) is the closest to a national quality registry, but it is not mandatory, and it does not cover all operations—only a selection of them. Most countries have no registries of outcomes.

A cornerstone in getting control of care and implementation of enhanced recovery programs is to start collecting data and audit both processes and outcomes in a systematic way. For full control, the audit system should ideally cover all aspects of care that impact outcomes. This includes key patient factors such as demographics, comorbidities, and care actions taken preadmission, in the hospital, and during and after the operation. The audit should cover surgical and anesthetic techniques and the elements of care that make up the ERAS guideline or the protocol chosen to audit. Finally, the system should have a robust outcomes section with standardized definitions. Some organizations have developed audit tools, including NSQIP (US),[107] Groupe francophone de Réhabilitation Améliorée après Chirurgie (GRACE [France]),[108] and others. The ERAS® Society has developed a tool that covers these needs and that can be used for auditing on demand anytime (https://erassociety. org/interactive-audit/).[109,110] The combination of processes and outcomes makes it possible to track and understand why certain complications may occur. This is very useful when implementing ERAS but also to retain and sustain good clinical results. The audit should be run by the ERAS team (see the following section), but it should also be open to anyone who is a stakeholder in the care of the patients. It should be used to provide feedback to everyone involved in the care of the patients. This helps everyone to better understand their unique role in the flow of care for patients.

Enhanced Recovery After Surgery Team

The ERAS team is a critical component of the EIP. This group of individuals is usually multidisciplinary in nature and is tasked with reviewing ERAS protocol element compliance and iterating toward improved perioperative outcomes. This is not the time to include naysayers, but rather those individuals who are passionate about surgical quality improvement. At a minimum, the following members should be included in the ERAS team:

- Surgeon
- Anesthesiologist
- Nursing (representatives from the preoperative clinic, operating room, inpatient ward)
- Pharmacy
- Dietitian
- Physiotherapy
- Occupational Therapy
- Manager/Administrator

ENHANCED RECOVERY AFTER SURGERY OUTCOMES

ERAS has gained its popularity and reputation because of its marked improvements in outcomes. Although Fast Track proved to be able to reduce length of stay, ERAS added dimensions that

TABLE 22.2   Recommendations for Creation of an ERAS Protocol

Preoperative

Bowel preparation	• Selective bowel preparation
	• If using oral antibiotic preparation: neomycin 1 g PO + metronidazole 500 mg PO at 1:00 PM, 2:00 PM, and 10:00 PM day before surgery
Modern fasting guidelines	• Light snack (dry toast and fruit) allowed up to 6 h before procedure
	• May ingest clear fluids up to 2 h before procedure
Carbohydrate loading	• Complex carbohydrate (e.g., maltodextrin) drink designed for surgery 2 h before surgery
Preoperative medications	• Acetaminophen 1000 mg PO once
	• Celecoxib or ibuprofen 400 mg PO once
	• Aprepitant 40 mg PO
VTE prophylaxis	• Heparin 5000 U SC given preoperatively or after induction
	• Sequential compression devices placed before induction of anesthesia
Antimicrobial prophylaxis	• Bathe or shower with soap the night before surgery
	• Chlorhexidine-alcohol for skin cleansing
	• Cefazolin 2 g IV before incision (3 g for weight >120 kg)
	• If bowel resection anticipated: cefazolin 2 g IV before incision + metronidazole 500 mg IV

Intraoperative

Nausea and vomiting prophylaxis (antiemetics to choose from)	• Droperidol 0.625–1.25 mg IV end of surgery
	• Ondansetron 4 mg IV end of surgery
	• Promethazine 6.25–12.5 mg IV end of surgery
Anesthesia	• Short-acting anesthetic agents (e.g., sevoflurane, desflurane) should be used
	Opioid-sparing multimodal analgesia techniques (options):
	• Bupivacaine 0.25% with epinephrine at incision site
	• Liposomal bupivacaine 266 mg (20 mL) diluted to at least 180 mL of sterile saline injected at incision site
	• Transversus abdominis plane (TAP) block using bupivacaine 0.25% with epinephrine
Best surgical practices	• Avoidance of peritoneal drains and nasogastric tubes
Maintenance of normothermia	• Use of active warming device and warmed fluids
Fluid therapy	• Use of lactated Ringer solution as opposed to normal saline
	• Aim for euvolemia (very restrictive or liberal fluid regimes to be avoided)
	• Use of goal-directed fluid therapy where available and in high-risk cases

Postoperative

Diet	• Solid diet started postoperative day (POD) 0
	• Chewing gum after meals three times per day starting on POD 0
	• Oral nutritional supplement on POD 0 and continue until discharge
Analgesia	• Acetaminophen 1000 mg PO q6h (should not exceed 4000 mg/24 h from all sources) (start POD 0)
	• Ibuprofen 400–800 mg PO q6h (start POD 1)
	If scheduled acetaminophen/ibuprofen ineffective (or if contraindications):
	• Oxycodone 5–10 mg PO q4h prn
	• Tramadol 100 mg PO q4–6h prn
	• Opioid IV (e.g., hydromorphone 0.5 mg IV q30 min prn) only if PO opioid medications ineffective within 30 min
	• Patient-controlled analgesia (PCA) started only if patient requires two doses or more of IV opioids in 24-h period
Nausea and vomiting prophylaxis	• Ondansetron 4 mg PO q6h prn nausea
	• Prochlorperazine 10 mg IV q6h breakthrough nausea after 30 min Ondansetron
Fluid therapy	• Fluids at 40 mL/h postoperatively (typical duration 8–12 h)
	• Fluid bolus of 250–500 mL for urine output <20 mL/h
	• Peripheral lock IV when patient has 600 mL oral intake
Urinary catheter removal	• Remove urinary catheters on the day of surgery for MIS, and no later than POD 1 for laparotomy, unless contraindications exist (e.g., bladder reconstruction)
VTE prophylaxis	• Low-molecular-weight heparin (e.g., dalteparin 5000 U SC daily or equivalent) starting POD 1
	• Extended prophylaxis for 28 days for all patients undergoing laparotomy for cancer
	• Sequential compression devices while in bed in hospital
Active mobilization program	• Ambulate 8×/day, meals in chair, out of bed 8 h/day
Bowel Routine (choose one or more of the following)	• Polyethylene glycol (PEG) 3350 17 g PO daily
	• Senna 1–2 tabs PO qhs
	• Magnesium hydroxide 25 mL PO qhs
	• Lactulose 15–30 mL PO TID
	• Psyllium mucilloid powder 1–2 packets PO daily

MIS, Minimally invasive surgery; *PO,* per os; *prn,* as needed; *q4h,* every 4 hours; *q6h,* every 6 hours; *qhs,* at bedtime; *SC,* subcutaneously.
Adapted from Nelson G, Dowdy SC, Lasala et al. Enhanced recovery after surgery (ERAS®) in gynecologic oncology - Practical considerations for program development. *Gynecol Oncol.* 2017 Dec;147(3):617-620.

were more interesting for clinicians, patients, and organizations delivering care (e.g., hospitals, hospital organizations, government-run providers). ERAS has repeatedly been reported to reduce complication rates, reoperations, and readmissions and has been associated with improved long-term survival after cancer surgery. The ERAS® Society guidelines most relevant to general surgery include those for colorectal resection,[19] hepatectomy,[62] gastrectomy,[29] pancreaticoduodenectomy,[46] esophagectomy,[41] and bariatric surgery.[53]

In a meta-analysis of randomized trials of patients undergoing colorectal surgery, Varadhan and colleagues showed that complication rates were reduced by up to 50% when ERAS principles were followed.[8] In a single institution study of almost 1000 consecutive patients undergoing colorectal resection, Gustafsson et al. demonstrated that improved compliance resulted in fewer complications, faster recovery, shorter length of stay, and fewer readmissions.[9] An association between increased compliance and a 42% improved survival was found in a 5-year follow-up of these patients.[10] Others have confirmed this relationship both in nationwide studies[111] and international collaborations.[112]

Although the weight of evidence in the literature for benefit of ERAS is in colorectal surgery, there is increasing evidence across other disciplines. In liver surgery, a meta-analysis of randomized controlled trials found significantly reduced overall morbidity rates, accelerated functional recovery, and decreased length of stay in favor of ERAS.[113] In patients undergoing surgery for pancreatic cancer, ERAS protocol compliance >80% was associated with significant reductions in mortality, major complications, and length of stay.[114] Similar outcomes favoring ERAS have been found in esophageal surgery,[115] gastric surgery,[116] and bariatric surgery.[117]

ERAS has a major impact on health system savings, and, as such, ERAS is considered value-based surgery.[118] Reports indicate cost savings ranging from $1000 to $8700 depending on surgery type as well as the country and financing of healthcare.[118,119] Systemwide economic analyses from Alberta, Canada, have shown return on investment ratios associated with implementation of ERAS ranging from 3.8 to 7.3.[120,121]

Roles and Benefits for Enhanced Recovery After Surgery Practitioners

Surgeon

The surgeon has an obvious key role in the ERAS team. It is the surgeon that is ultimately responsible for the patient, and it is "her/his/their" patient. The surgeon makes the decision to operate, decides many of the preadmission and preoperative care elements, chooses the surgical technique, decides on many postoperative care items, and is the only person who sees the patient from preoperative to postoperative phases. The surgeon has a responsibility to decide about all surgical decisions and the surgical parts of a local ERAS protocol.

Being ultimately responsible for the patient, the surgeon has a great deal to benefit from being part of or leading an ERAS Team. In most cases the surgeon is the medical leader of a local ERAS team. ERAS has proven to enhance the recovery of the patient and to avoid complications, reoperations, ICU care, and readmissions. These outcome benefits alone should be sufficient for all surgeons to get involved and start an ERAS program for their patients, but there are other aspects as well.

Being part of an ERAS team allows for exchange of knowledge and understanding of the parts of the care outside the surgeon's normal domain where usually someone else in charge (e.g., anesthesia, nursing, physiotherapy, nutritional care). Being part of a team and developing a protocol that works best for the patients gives insights and knowledge that helps the surgeon to become a better doctor. By having others relate some potential negative consequences of a routine or decision taken by the surgeon, it may help the surgeon make better choices to facilitate for others and ultimately help avoid unnecessary problems for the patient. With better understanding of the entire chain of events and all processes, the parts played by any individual becomes much more obvious. The key to a successful ERAS team is to understand the role and impact of every care decision along the care path for the patient to secure the best possible overall flow.

Anesthesiologist

The anesthesiologist is the other main medical specialist that is key to the success of an ERAS team. Like the surgeon, this person has the responsibility to decide on the details of the medical care in the local ERAS program. This person oversees the care of the vital functions of the patient while being operated on and plays a role in the preparation of the patient and the after care in many aspects. The anesthesiologist sees the patient ahead of anesthesia and ensures that the protocol is followed when it comes to fasting routines, that carbohydrate loading is given to the right patients, and that sedation is done appropriately and selectively. In many open cases, pain management and anesthesia are initiated ahead of the operation by institution of spinals and epidurals, and in some institutions blocks are placed by the anesthetist. In the postoperative care phase, the anesthetists are often responsible at the PACU, and in many countries the same specialist also manages intensive care. Pain management is commonly done by pain specialists from anesthesia.

There are important benefits for anesthesiologists to be part of an ERAS program. First and foremost, they will become an equal medical partner to the surgeon in the care of the patient. Without a partnering anesthesiologist, the surgeon will not be able to set up a functional ERAS program, and vice versa.

Nurse

The nurses have many key roles on an ERAS team.[122] Many units choose a nurse to be the coordinator and driver of an ERAS team, and for good reason. Nurses and nurse's aides work the closest to the patient's bedside. They carry out many of the treatments ordered by doctors. They motivate and support the patient in their preparation for surgery by giving detailed information and being available for questions from patients and their accompanying persons. The preoperative information is a key part of ERAS in which the patient is given a role in the care pathway and expectations and roles are explained. This information is often carried out by the nurses at the outpatient clinic. Nurses working in other parts of the patient journey have different roles; anesthesia nurses and PACU nurses keep control over vital functions for the patient during a crucial period of the care. Similarly, operating room nurses are key for the success of the surgery. These nurses have specific roles while the patient is recovering after surgery—a time when the patient is unconscious or sleepy. Still, they must understand how their work plays into the entire care delivered to the patient in order to contribute to the best possible outcome. Ward nurses have a more extended mission on the ERAS team. It is during the stay at the ward that most of the key initial postoperative care elements in ERAS are activated. If a proper ERAS program has been executed during the previous phases of care, it is now possible to put the last pieces in place to have the patient start to recover in an optimal way as soon as possible. This involves drinking fluids, beginning to eat food, and getting out of bed on the day of surgery. This is followed by a supporting role for nurses during the next days when mobilization and gut function are key to returning the patient to normality and the functional capacity they had before the operation. This is usually accomplished by teamwork between nurses, nurse's aides, physiotherapists, and nutritionists. In this team it is essential for the nurses leading this work to also involve the patient in the team. In many institutions both patients and staff are given the same checklist with tasks that are to be fulfilled day by day—patients have some assignments, and the staff have others.

The benefits for nursing with ERAS are severalfold. First and foremost, ERAS allows everyone on the nursing team to deliver better care, resulting in patients recovering faster and better. This is probably the most important reward for everyone—seeing the improvement and knowing that they are all delivering quality care for the benefit of the patient. It also has implications for the work itself. Reports show that the workload for nursing goes down with better compliance to ERAS protocols.[123] This allows for more time with the patient. Instead of changing IV fluids or emptying drainage bags and managing pain and nausea the traditional way, the nurse is now spending time supporting the patient in getting back to normal by aiding mobilization and getting the gut to recover without causing pain or nausea for the patient.

Allied Health Professionals

There are other key specialists that should be involved in the care of the patient. The physiotherapist is a specialist that has special competencies in the mobilization of the patient.[124] In frail patients and those with some disabilities, this specialist knowledge is particularly useful. Also, when moving to very early mobilization, their support and insights are invaluable.

The other key recovery aspects that ERAS emphasizes are the return to normal food as soon as possible and to ensure proper intake of calories and protein. For this, the nutritionist or dietitian is the person to involve and have join the team. Many patients have particular needs in regard to allergies or nutritional problems such as sarcopenia, obesity, or both. But almost all patients need to have nutritional supplementation orally on top of the hospital food because they rarely eat enough to fulfill their needs. The choices of supplements are many, and flavors vary as does composition; this is where the nutritional expertise is of high value.

The Manager

When ERAS is introduced to a hospital or a department, the previously mentioned outcomes of reduced hospital stay, fewer complications, less need for ICU care, and fewer readmissions translates into several important gains for those responsible for the hospital finances. Substantial savings are made, and the return on the investment ratio has been reported to be between four and seven times.[120,121] It frees up beds to increase capacity, and better results can be used to market the hospital. But to get things going, there is a need for an investment in time, and this decision must be made from management. It is therefore important that the manager is involved from the start and also in the continuation of the program so that insights and successes can be transferred to other specialties in the hospital for the benefit of many more patients. It is also important to realize that if the program is stopped, it is likely to result in worse outcomes when control is lost.[125] For sustainability and continued input of resources, the manager remains critically important.

CONCLUSION

ERAS care has revolutionized outcomes for patients in just about every domain of surgery and similarly throughout the world. Experience has shown that the ERAS hypothesis that evidence-based perioperative care can lead the way to better care holds true. Combining all the ERAS elements of care and ensuring their use appropriately are the keys to success. This creates a new way of collaborating by building a team around the ERAS pathway in every department of surgery or specialty. Change of habits is slow in medicine, and this is true for surgery as well. Although the key improvements from ERAS were established 20 years or more ago, information from national registries and similar programs (where available) show that the length of stay is much too long, indicating that ERAS is not in use in these countries. Still, progress is being made daily, and more units are adopting ERAS or ERAS-like methods to improve outcomes. At the same time, ERAS itself is evolving as new knowledge is emerging to change guidelines to improve care even more. To keep ERAS improving and spreading, it is essential that the young surgeon continues to dare to challenge current practice just like the people who started ERAS did and many followers after them.

SELECTED REFERENCES

Brindle M, Nelson G, Lobo DN, Ljungqvist O, Gustafsson UO. Recommendations from the ERAS® Society for standards for the development of enhanced recovery after surgery guidelines. *BJS Open.* 2020;4(1):157-163.

Important paper providing detailed description of required steps for development of ERAS Society guidelines.

Fearon KC, Ljungqvist O, Von Meyenfeldt M, et al. Enhanced recovery after surgery: a consensus review of clinical care for patients undergoing colonic resection. *Clin Nutr.* 2005;24(3):466-477.

Important historical reference—the very first ERAS Society guideline.

Gustafsson UO, Hausel J, Thorell A, et al. Adherence to the enhanced recovery after surgery protocol and outcomes after colorectal cancer surgery. *Arch Surg.* 2011;146(5):571-577.

First study in the literature showing that increased ERAS compliance is associated with decreased length of stay and complications.

Hübner M, Addor V, Slieker J, Griesser AC, Lécureux E, Blanc C, Demartines N. The impact of an enhanced recovery pathway on nursing workload: a retrospective cohort study. *Int J Surg.* 2015;24(Pt A):45-50.

Important study demonstrating that as ERAS compliance increases, nursing workload decreases.

Ljungqvist O, de Boer HD, Balfour A, et al. Opportunities and challenges for the next phase of enhanced recovery after surgery: a review. *JAMA Surg.* 2021;156(8):775-784.

> *This paper, written by the leadership of the ERAS Society, describes priorities for increasing uptake of ERAS globally.*

Ljungqvist O, Scott M, Fearon KC. Enhanced recovery after surgery: a review. *JAMA Surg.* 2017;152(3):292-298.

> *Definitive review of ERAS, covering all aspects of the global surgical quality improvement initiative.*

Temple-Oberle C, Yakaback S, Webb C, Assadzadeh GE, Nelson G. Effect of smartphone app postoperative home monitoring after oncologic surgery on quality of recovery: a randomized clinical trial. *JAMA Surg.* 2023;158(7):693-699.

> *Important paper showing improved quality of recovery with smartphone app–based follow-up.*

Thanh N, Nelson A, Wang X, et al. Return on investment of the Enhanced Recovery After Surgery (ERAS) multiguideline, multisite implementation in Alberta, Canada. *Can J Surg.* 2020; 63(6):E542-E550.

> *Important health economic paper demonstrating that return on investment (ROI) ratio for ERAS is as high as 7.3.*

Wijk L, Udumyan R, Pache B, et al. International validation of Enhanced Recovery After Surgery Society guidelines on enhanced recovery for gynecologic surgery. *Am J Obstet Gynecol.* 2019;221(3):237.e1-237.e11.

> *Important study showing that increased ERAS compliance is associated with decreased length of stay and complications.*

The full reference list appears on Elsevier eBooks+.

23 | CHAPTER

Wound Healing

Jadie Y. Moon and Katherine A. Gallagher

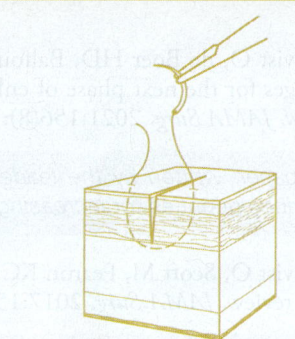

OUTLINE

TISSUE INJURY AND RESPONSE

Attempts to restore homeostasis, to repair barriers to fluid loss and infection, and to reestablish normal blood and lymphatic flow patterns are essential after injury. All healthy wounds undergo the same basic steps of repair. Orderly and timely movement through the phases of healing is needed for coordinated repair.

WOUND-HEALING PHASES

The four phases of wound healing are hemostasis, inflammation, proliferation, and maturation. For example, in a large surgical wound such as a pressure sore, the eschar or fibrinous exudate reflects the inflammatory phase, the granulation tissue is part of the proliferative phase, and the contracting or advancing edge is part of the maturational phase. All four phases may occur simultaneously, and the phases may overlap (Fig. 23.1). If orderly repair does not occur (as in diabetes or other chronic conditions), wounds can exist in a phase indefinitely and not advance along the cascade.

Hemostasis

After tissue injury, hemostasis occurs quickly and is rapidly followed by inflammation. This phase represents an attempt to limit damage by stopping bleeding; sealing the wound surface; and removing necrotic tissue, foreign debris, and bacteria. This is primarily mediated by platelets and other coagulating factors.

Inflammatory Phase

The inflammatory phase is characterized by increased vascular permeability, migration of cells into the wound by chemotaxis, secretion of cytokines and growth factors into the wound, and activation of the migrating cells.

Blood vessel injury results in intense local arteriolar and capillary vasoconstriction followed by vasodilatation and increased vascular permeability (Fig. 23.2). Erythrocytes and platelets adhere to the damaged capillary endothelium, resulting in plugging of capillaries and leading to cessation of hemorrhage. Platelet adhesion to the endothelium is primarily mediated through the interaction between high-affinity glycoprotein receptors and the integrin receptor GPIIb-IIIa ($\alpha_{IIb}\beta_3$). Platelets also express other integrin receptors that mediate direct binding to collagen ($\alpha_2\beta_1$) and laminin ($\alpha_6\beta_1$) or indirect binding to subendothelial matrix-bound fibronectin ($\alpha_5\beta_1$), vitronectin ($\alpha_v\beta_3$), and other ligands. Platelet activation occurs by binding to exposed type IV and type V collagen from the damaged endothelium, resulting in platelet aggregation. The initial contact between platelets and collagen requires von Willebrand factor VIII, a heterodimeric protein synthesized by megakaryocytes and endothelial cells.

Platelet binding results in conformational changes in platelets that trigger intracellular signal transduction pathways that lead to platelet activation and the release of biologically active proteins. Platelets release factors from two different sources: alpha granules and dense bodies. Platelet alpha granules are storage organelles that contain platelet-derived growth factor (PDGF), transforming growth factor-β (TGF-β), insulin-like growth factor 1 (IGF-1), fibronectin, fibrinogen, thrombospondin, and von Willebrand factor. The dense bodies contain vasoactive amines, such as serotonin, that cause vasodilatation and increased vascular permeability. Mast cells adherent to the endothelial surface release histamine and serotonin, resulting in increased permeability of endothelial cells and causing leakage of plasma from the intravascular space to the extracellular compartment.

The platelets become activated, and the membrane phospholipids bind factor V, which allows interaction with factor X. Membrane-bound prothrombinase activity is generated and potentiates thrombin

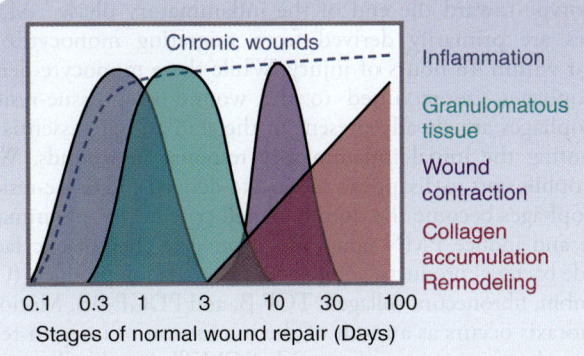

FIGURE 23.1 Stages of normal and chronic wound repair.

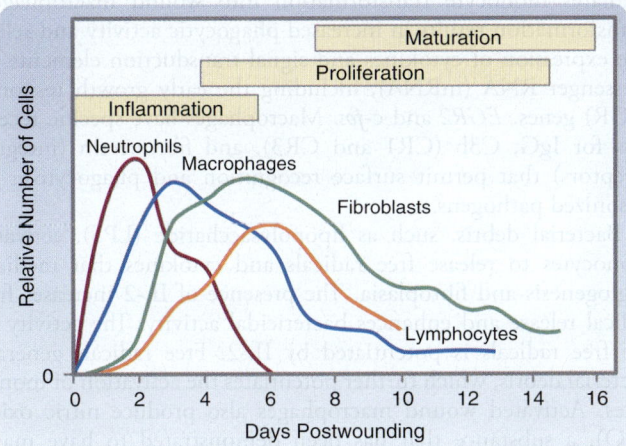

FIGURE 23.2 Time course of the appearance of different cells in the wound during healing. Macrophages and neutrophils are predominant during the inflammatory phase (peak at days 3 and 2, respectively). Lymphocytes appear later and peak at day 7. Fibroblasts are the predominant cells during the proliferative phase. (Adapted from Witte MB, Barbul A. General principles of wound healing. *Surg Clin North Am.* 1997;77:509-528.)

production exponentially. The thrombin itself activates platelets and catalyzes the conversion of fibrinogen to fibrin. The fibrin strands trap red blood cells to form the clot and seal the wound. The resulting lattice framework is the scaffold for endothelial cells, inflammatory cells, and fibroblasts to repair the damaged vessel.

Thromboxane A2 and prostaglandin F2α, formed from the degradation of cell membranes in the arachidonic acid cascade, also assist in platelet aggregation and vasoconstriction. Although these activities serve to limit the amount of injury, they can also cause localized ischemia, resulting in further damage to cell membranes and the release of more prostaglandin F2α and thromboxane A2.

Chemokines

Chemokines stimulate the migration of different cell types, particularly inflammatory cells, into the wound and are active participants in the regulation of the different phases of wound healing. The CXC, CC, and C ligand families bind to G protein–coupled surface receptors called CXC receptors and CC receptors.

Macrophage chemoattractant protein (MCP-1 or CCL2) is induced in keratinocytes after injury. It is a potent chemoattractant for monocytes/macrophages, T lymphocytes, and mast cells.

Expression of this chemokine is sustained in chronic wounds and results in the prolonged presence of polymorphonuclear cells (PMNs) and macrophages, leading to the prolonged inflammatory response. Chemokine (C-X-C motif) ligand 1 (CXCL1; previously called GRO-α) is a potent PMN chemotactic regulator and is increased in acute wounds. It is also involved in reepithelialization. Interleukin-8 (IL-8; also known as *CXCL8*) expression is increased in acute and chronic wounds. It is involved in reepithelialization and induces the leukocyte expression of matrix metalloproteinases (MMPs), which stimulates remodeling. It is also a strong chemoattractant for PMNs and participates in inflammation. Relatively low levels of IL-8 are found in fetal wounds and may be why fetal wounds have decreased inflammation and heal without scars. Expression of the keratinocyte-produced CXCL10 is elevated in acute wounds and chronic inflammatory conditions in response to interferon-γ (IFN-γ). It impairs wound healing by increasing inflammation and recruiting lymphocytes to the wound. It also inhibits proliferation by decreasing reepithelialization and angiogenesis and preventing fibroblast migration. Stromal cell–derived factor-1 (SDF-1, also known as *CXCL12*) is expressed by endothelial cells, myofibroblasts, and keratinocytes and is involved in inflammation by recruiting lymphocytes to the wound and promoting angiogenesis. It is a potent chemoattractant for endothelial cells and bone marrow progenitors from the circulation to peripheral tissues. It also enhances keratinocyte proliferation, resulting in reepithelialization.

Cells Involved in the Inflammatory Phase
Polymorphonuclear Cells/Neutrophils

The release of histamine and serotonin leads to vascular permeability of the capillary bed. Complement factors such as C5a and leukotriene B4 promote neutrophil adherence and chemoattraction. In the presence of thrombin, endothelial cells exposed to leukotriene C4 and D4 release platelet-aggregating factor, which further enhances neutrophil adhesion. Monocytes and endothelial cells produce the inflammatory mediators IL-1 and tumor necrosis factor-α (TNF-α), and these mediators further promote endothelial-neutrophil adherence. Increased capillary permeability and chemotactic factors facilitate diapedesis of neutrophils into the inflammatory site. As the neutrophils begin their migration, they release the contents of their lysosomes and enzymes such as elastase and other proteases into the extracellular matrix (ECM), which further facilitates neutrophil migration. The combination of intense vasodilatation and increased vascular permeability leads to clinical findings of inflammation, rubor (redness), tumor (swelling), calor (heat), and dolor (pain). Local tissue swelling is further promoted by the deposition of fibrin, a protein end product of coagulation that becomes entrapped in lymphatic vessels.

Evidence suggests that the migration of PMNs requires sequential adhesive and deadhesive interactions between β$_1$ and β$_2$ integrins and ECM components. Integrin molecules are a family of cell surface receptors expressed on both structural and immune cells that are closely coupled with the cell's cytoskeleton. These molecules interact with components of the ECM, such as fibronectin, to provide adhesion and to transduce signals to the interior of the cell. Not all cell types express the same composition of integrins, and some integrins have specialized roles in adhesion, whereas others contribute to migration.

Integrins are crucial for cell motility and are required in inflammation and normal wound healing as well as in embryonic development and tumor metastases. After extravasation, PMNs, attracted by chemotaxins, migrate through the ECM via transient interactions between integrin receptors and their ligands. Four phases of integrin-mediated cell motility have been described: adhesion, spreading, contractility or traction, and retraction. Activation of specific integrins through ligand binding has been shown to increase cell adhesion and activate reorganization of the cell's actin cytoskeleton. Spreading is characterized by the development of lamellipodia and filopodia. Traction at the leading edge of the cell develops through binding of integrin followed by translocation of the cell over the adherent segment of the plasma membrane. The integrin is shifted to the rear of the cell and releases its substrate, permitting cell advancement. Regulation of integrin function by adhesive substrates offers a mechanism for local control of migrant cells. Within the assembled framework of the ECM, binding sites for integrins have been identified on collagen, laminin, and fibronectin. The chemotactic agent mediates the PMN response through signal transduction as the chemotaxin binds to receptors on the cell surface. Bacterial products such as N-formyl-methionyl-leucyl-phenylalanine bind to induce cyclic adenosine monophosphate (AMP), but if there is maximal receptor occupancy, superoxide is produced at peak rates. Neutrophils also possess receptors for immunoglobulin G (IgG; Fc receptor) and the complement proteins C3b and C3bi. As the complement cascade is released and bacteria are opsonized, binding of these proteins to cell receptors on neutrophils allows recognition by the neutrophils and phagocytosis of the bacteria. When neutrophils are stimulated, they express more CR1 and CR3 receptors, permitting more efficient binding and phagocytosis of these bacteria.

Functional activation occurs after migration of PMNs into the wound site, which may induce new cell surface antigen expression, increased cytotoxicity, or enhanced production and release of cytokines. These activated neutrophils scavenge for necrotic debris, foreign material, and bacteria and generate free oxygen radicals with electrons donated by the reduced form of nicotinamide adenine dinucleotide phosphate. The electrons are transported across the membrane into lysosomes, where superoxide anion (O_2^-) is formed. Superoxide dismutase catalyzes the formation of hydrogen peroxide (H_2O_2), which is then degraded by myeloperoxidase in the azurophilic granules of neutrophils. This interaction oxidizes halides with the formation of by products such as hypochlorous acid. The iron-catalyzed reaction between H_2O_2 and O_2^- forms hydroxyl radicals (OH·). This potent free radical is bactericidal and toxic to neutrophils and surrounding viable tissues.

Migration of PMNs stops after several days or when wound contamination has been controlled. Individual PMNs survive no longer than 24 hours and are replaced predominantly by mononuclear cells (macrophages). Continuing wound contamination or secondary infection causes complement system activation that provides a steady supply of chemotactic factors and a sustained influx of PMNs into the wound. A prolonged inflammatory phase delays wound healing, destroys normal tissue, and results in abscess formation and possibly systemic infection. PMNs are not essential for wound healing because their phagocytosis and antimicrobial role can be taken over by macrophages. Sterile incisions heal normally without the presence of PMNs.

Macrophages

Macrophages are critical for wound healing by orchestrating the release of cytokines and stimulating many subsequent processes in wound healing (Fig. 23.3). They exist in multiple phenotypes in the wound, but broadly start the inflammatory phase in the inflammatory phenotype and then transition to a reparative phenotype toward the end of the inflammatory phase.[1] Macrophages are primarily derived from migrating monocytes and appear within 48 hours of injury. While these monocyte-derived macrophages are recruited to the wound site, tissue-resident macrophages are already present in the skin and are essential for promoting the initial inflammatory response in wounds. When neutrophils start to disappear, monocyte-derived and tissue-resident macrophages become the dominant cell type in the inflammatory phase and induce PMN apoptosis. Monocyte chemotactic factors include bacterial products, complement degradation products (C5a), thrombin, fibronectin, collagen, TGF-β, and PDGF-BB. Monocyte chemotaxis occurs as a result of the interaction of integrin receptors on the monocyte surface with ECM fibrin and fibronectin. The β integrin receptor also transduces the signal to initiate macrophage phagocytic activity. Activated integrin expression mediates monocyte transformation into wound macrophages. Transformation results in increased phagocytic activity and selective expression of cytokines and signal transduction elements by messenger RNA (mRNA), including the early growth response (EGR) genes, *EGR2* and *c-fos*. Macrophages have specific receptors for IgG, C3b (CR1 and CR3), and fibronectin (integrin receptors) that permit surface recognition and phagocytosis of opsonized pathogens.

Bacterial debris, such as lipopolysaccharide (LPS), activates monocytes to release free radicals and cytokines that mediate angiogenesis and fibroplasia. The presence of IL-2 increases free radical release and enhances bactericidal activity. The activity of the free radicals is potentiated by IL-2. Free radicals generate bacterial debris, which further potentiates the activation of monocytes. Activated wound macrophages also produce nitric oxide (NO), a substance that has been demonstrated to have many functions other than antimicrobial properties.

As the monocyte or macrophage is activated, phospholipase is induced, cell membrane phospholipids are enzymatically degraded, and thromboxane A2 and prostaglandin F2α are released. The macrophage also releases leukotrienes B4 and C4 and 15-hydroxyeicosatetraenoic acid and 5-hydroxyeicosatetraenoic acid. Leukotriene B4 is a potent chemotaxin for neutrophils and increases their adherence to endothelial cells.

Wound macrophages release proteinases, including MMPs (MMP-1, MMP-2, MMP-3, and MMP-9), which degrade the ECM and are crucial for removing foreign material, promoting cell movement through tissue spaces, and regulating ECM turnover. This activity is dependent on the cyclic AMP pathway and can be blocked by nonsteroidal antiinflammatory drugs or glucocorticoid drugs. Colchicine and retinoic acid appear to decrease collagenase production as well.

Macrophages secrete numerous cytokines and growth factors. IL-1, a proinflammatory cytokine, is an acute-phase response cytokine. It directly affects hemostasis by inducing the release of vasodilators and stimulating coagulation. Its effect is further amplified as endothelial cells produce it in the presence of TNF-α and endotoxin. IL-1 has numerous effects, such as enhancement of collagenase production, stimulation of cartilage degradation and bone reabsorption, activation of neutrophils, regulation of adhesion molecules, and promotion of chemotaxis. It stimulates other cells to secrete proinflammatory cytokines. Its effects extend into the proliferative phase during which it increases fibroblast and keratinocyte growth and collagen synthesis. Studies have demonstrated increased levels of IL-1 in chronic nonhealing wounds, suggesting its role in the pathogenesis of poor wound healing. The early beneficial responses of IL-1 in wound healing

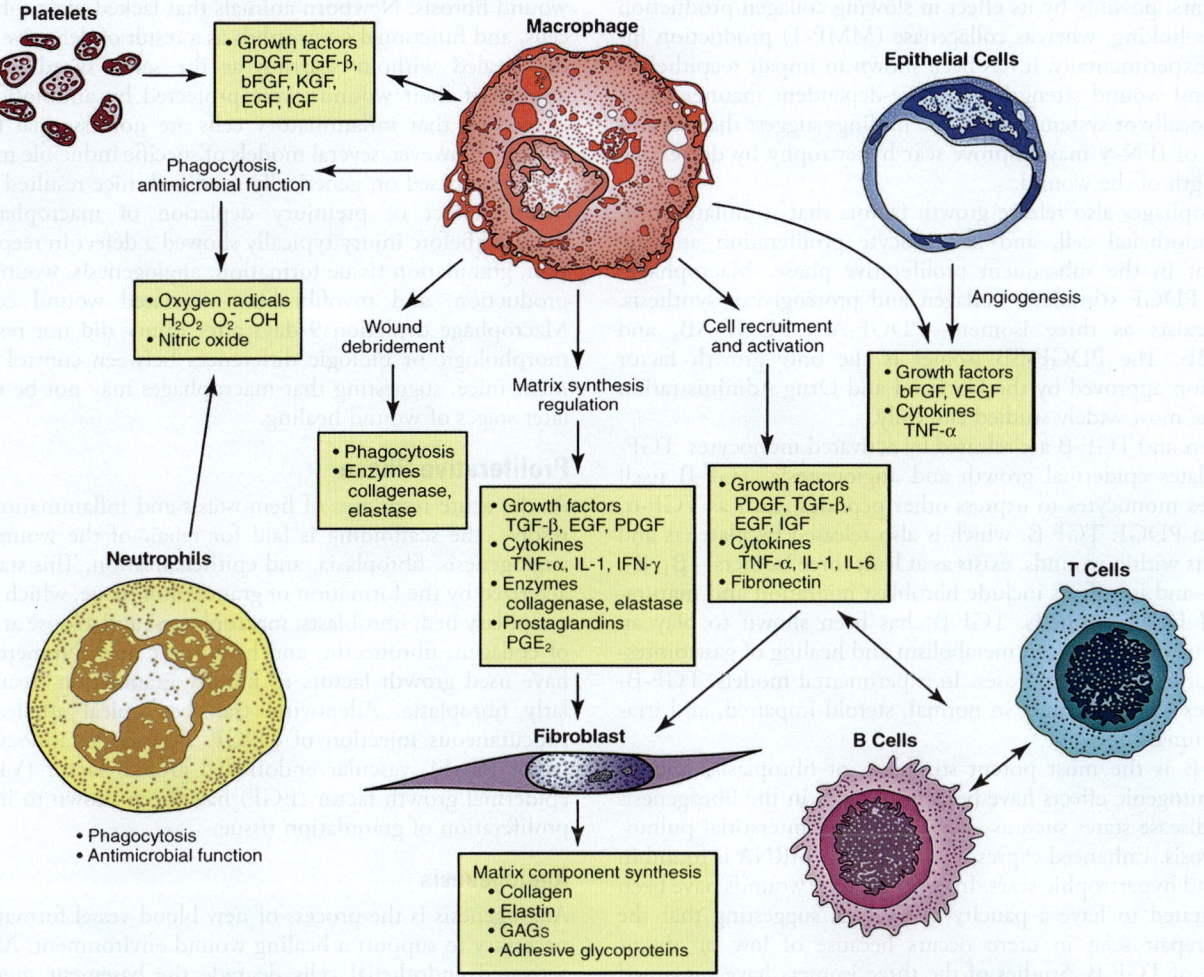

FIGURE 23.3 Interaction of cellular and humoral factors in wound healing. Note the key role of the macrophage. *bFGF,* Basic fibroblast growth factor; *EGF,* epidermal growth factor; *GAGs,* glycosaminoglycans; H_2O_2, hydrogen peroxide; *IFN-γ,* interferon-γ; *IGF,* insulin-like growth factor; *IL-1,* interleukin-1; *IL-6,* interleukin-6; *KGF,* keratinocyte growth factor; O_2^-, superoxide; $-OH$, hydroxyl radical; *PDGF,* platelet-derived growth factor; *PGE₂,* prostaglandin E2; *TGF-β,* transforming growth factor-β; *TNF-α,* tumor necrosis factor-α; *VEGF,* vascular endothelial growth factor. (Adapted from Witte MB, Barbul A. General principles of wound healing. *Surg Clin North Am.* 1997;77:509-528.)

appear to be maladaptive if elevated levels last beyond the first week after injury.

Microbial by products induce macrophages to release TNF. TNF-α is crucial in initiating the response to injury or bacteria. It upregulates cell surface adhesion molecules that promote the interaction of immune cells and endothelium. TNF-α is detected in a wound within 12 hours and peaks after 72 hours. Its effects include hemostasis, increased vascular permeability, and enhanced endothelial proliferation. Similar to IL-1, TNF-α induces fever, increased collagenase production, resorption of cartilage and bone, and release of PDGF as well as the production of more IL-1. However, excessive production of TNF-α has been associated with multisystem organ failure and increased morbidity and mortality in inflammatory disease states, partly through its effects on activating macrophages and neutrophils. Studies have noted elevated levels of TNF-α in nonhealing versus healing chronic venous ulcers. As in the case of IL-1, TNF-α appears to be essential in the early inflammatory response required for wound healing, but local and systemic persistence of this cytokine may lead to impaired wound maturation.

IL-6, which is produced by monocytes and macrophages, is involved in stem cell growth, activation of B cells and T cells, and regulation of the synthesis of hepatic acute-phase proteins. Within acute wounds, IL-6 is also secreted by PMNs and fibroblasts; an increase in IL-6 parallels the increase in the PMN count locally. IL-6 is detectable within 12 hours of experimental wounding and may persist at high concentrations for longer than 1 week. It also works synergistically with IL-1, TNF-α, and endotoxins. It is a potent stimulator of fibroblast proliferation and is decreased in aging fibroblasts and fetal wounds.

IL-8 is secreted primarily by macrophages and fibroblasts in the acute wound, with peak expression within the first 24 hours. Its major effects have already been discussed and include increased PMN and monocyte chemotaxis, PMN degranulation, and expression of endothelial cell adhesion molecules.

IFN-γ, another proinflammatory cytokine, is secreted by T lymphocytes and macrophages. Its major effects are macrophage and PMN activation and increased cytotoxicity. It has also been shown to reduce local wound contraction and aid in tissue remodeling. IFN-γ has been used in the treatment of hypertrophic and keloid scars, possibly by its effect in slowing collagen production and cross-linking, whereas collagenase (MMP-1) production increases. Experimentally, it has been shown to impair reepithelialization and wound strength in a dose-dependent manner when applied locally or systemically. These findings suggest that administration of IFN-γ may improve scar hypertrophy by decreasing the strength of the wound.

Macrophages also release growth factors that stimulate fibroblast, endothelial cell, and keratinocyte proliferation and are important in the subsequent proliferative phase. Macrophage-secreted PDGF stimulates collagen and proteoglycan synthesis. PDGF exists as three isomers—PDGF-AA, PDGF-AB, and PDGF-BB. The PDGF-BB isomer is the only growth factor preparation approved by the US Food and Drug Administration and is the most widely studied clinically.

TGF-α and TGF-β are released by activated monocytes. TGF-α stimulates epidermal growth and angiogenesis. TGF-β itself stimulates monocytes to express other peptides, such as TGF-α, IL-1, and PDGF. TGF-β, which is also released by platelets and fibroblasts within wounds, exists as at least three isomers—β$_1$, β$_2$, and β$_3$—and its effects include fibroblast migration and maturation and ECM synthesis. TGF-β$_1$ has been shown to play an important role in collagen metabolism and healing of gastrointestinal injuries and anastomoses. In experimental models, TGF-β$_1$ accelerates wound healing in normal, steroid-impaired, and irradiated animals.

TGF-β is the most potent stimulant of fibroplasia, and its strong mitogenic effects have been implicated in the fibrogenesis seen in disease states such as scleroderma and interstitial pulmonary fibrosis. Enhanced expression of TGF-β$_1$ mRNA is found in keloid and hypertrophic scars. In contrast, fetal wounds have been demonstrated to have a paucity of TGF-β, suggesting that the scarless repair seen in utero occurs because of low or absent amounts of TGF-β. Studies of the three isomers have suggested that although TGF-β$_1$ and TGF-β$_2$ play an important role in tissue fibrosis and postinjury scarring, TGF-β$_3$ may limit scarring. As the concentration of TGF-β increases in the inflammatory site, fibroblasts are directly stimulated to produce collagen and fibronectin, leading to the proliferative phase.

Wound macrophages exhibit different functional phenotypes—M1 (classically activated) and M2 (alternatively activated)—that are at the extremes of a continuum of macrophage function. LPS and IFN-γ stimulate the differentiation into M1 macrophages that release TNF-α, NO, and IL-6. These mediators are responsible for host defense but at the expense of significant collateral tissue damage. M2 macrophages are activated by IL-4 and IL-13; suppress inflammatory reactions and adaptive immune responses; and play an important role in wound healing, angiogenesis, and defense against parasitic infections. However, despite their beneficial functions, M2 macrophages can also be involved in different diseases, such as allergy, asthma, and fibrosis, which is the result of a helper T-cell (Th2) response predominated by IL-4 or IL-10. Both phenotypes are important when correctly balanced during the different phases of wound healing. In the inflammatory phase, greater M1 macrophage activity is required for macrophage debris scavenging and invading pathogen destruction. In the proliferative phase, M2 macrophages predominate. The balance between M1 and M2 macrophages is likely disturbed during abnormal wound-healing responses.

Several studies have demonstrated the importance of macrophages in wound healing by macrophage depletion. Macrophage depletion delays wound infiltration by fibroblasts and decreased wound fibrosis. Newborn animals that lacked macrophages, mast cells, and functional neutrophils as a result of defective myelopoiesis healed without scarring at the same speed as wild-type animals if their wounds were protected by antibiotic coverage, suggesting that inflammatory cells are not essential for wound closure. However, several models of specific inducible macrophage depletion based on genetically modified mice resulted in a detrimental effect of preinjury depletion of macrophages. Mice depleted before injury typically showed a defect in reepithelialization, granulation tissue formation, angiogenesis, wound cytokine production, and myofibroblast-associated wound contraction. Macrophage depletion 9 days after injury did not result in any morphologic or biologic differences between control and treatment mice, suggesting that macrophages may not be required at later stages of wound healing.

Proliferative Phase

As the acute responses of hemostasis and inflammation begin to resolve, the scaffolding is laid for repair of the wound through angiogenesis, fibroplasia, and epithelialization. This stage is characterized by the formation of granulation tissue, which consists of a capillary bed; fibroblasts; macrophages; and a loose arrangement of collagen, fibronectin, and hyaluronic acid. Numerous studies have used growth factors to modify granulation tissue, particularly fibroplasia. Adenoviral transfer, topical application, and subcutaneous injection of PDGF, TGF-β, keratinocyte growth factor (KGF), vascular endothelial growth factor (VEGF), and epidermal growth factor (EGF) have been shown to increase the proliferation of granulation tissue.

Angiogenesis

Angiogenesis is the process of new blood vessel formation and is necessary to support a healing wound environment. After injury, activated endothelial cells degrade the basement membrane of postcapillary venules, allowing the migration of cells through this gap. Division of these migrating endothelial cells results in tubule or lumen formation. Eventually, deposition of the basement membrane occurs and results in capillary maturation.

After injury, the endothelium is exposed to numerous soluble factors and comes in contact with adhering blood cells. These interactions result in upregulation of the expression of cell surface adhesion molecules, such as vascular cell surface adhesion molecule-1. Matrix-degrading enzymes, such as plasmin and the MMPs, are released and activated and degrade the endothelial basement membrane. Fragmentation of the basement membrane allows migration of endothelial cells into the wound, promoted by fibroblast growth factor (FGF), PDGF, and TGF-β. Injured endothelial cells express adhesion molecules, such as the integrin α$_v$β$_3$, which facilitates attachment to fibrin, fibronectin, and fibrinogen and facilitates endothelial cell migration along the provisional matrix scaffold. Platelet endothelial cell adhesion molecule-1 (PECAM-1), also found on endothelial cells, modulates their interaction with each other as they migrate into the wound.

Capillary tube formation is a complex process that involves cell-cell and cell-matrix interactions, modulated by adhesion molecules on endothelial cell surfaces. PECAM-1 has been observed to mediate cell-cell contact, whereas β$_1$ integrin receptors may aid in stabilizing these contacts and forming tight junctions between endothelial cells. Some of the new capillaries differentiate into arterioles and venules, whereas others undergo involution and apoptosis, with subsequent ingestion by macrophages. Regulation of endothelial apoptosis is not well understood.

Angiogenesis appears to be stimulated and manipulated by various cytokines predominantly produced by macrophages and platelets. As the macrophage produces TNF-α, it orchestrates angiogenesis during the inflammatory phase. Heparin, which can stimulate the migration of capillary endothelial cells, binds with high affinity to a group of angiogenic factors.

VEGF, a member of the PDGF family of growth factors, has potent angiogenic activity. It is produced in large amounts by keratinocytes, macrophages, endothelial cells, platelets, and fibroblasts during wound healing. Cell disruption and hypoxia, hallmarks of tissue injury, appear to be strong initial inducers of potent angiogenic factors at the wound site, such as VEGF and its receptor. VEGF family members include VEGF-A, VEGF-B, VEGF-C, VEGF-D, VEGF-E, and placental growth factor. VEGF-A promotes early events in angiogenesis and subsequently is crucial to wound healing. It binds to tyrosine kinase surface receptors Flt-1 (VEGF receptor-1) and kinase insert domain receptor (VEGF receptor-2). Flt-1 is required for blood vessel organization, whereas kinase insert domain receptor is important for endothelial cell chemotaxis, proliferation, and differentiation. Animal studies have shown that VEGF-A administration restores impaired angiogenesis found in diabetic ischemic limbs; however, other studies have shown that exogenous VEGF results in vascular leakage and disorganized blood vessel formation. VEGF-C, which is also elevated during wound healing, is primarily released by macrophages and is important during the inflammatory phase. Although it works primarily through VEGF receptor-3, which is expressed in macrophages and lymphatic endothelium, it can also activate VEGF receptor-2, increasing vascular permeability. In vivo administration of VEGF-C to genetically diabetic mice in an animal model using an adenoviral vector resulted in accelerated healing. Placental growth factor is another proangiogenic factor that is elevated after wounding. It is involved in inflammation and expressed by keratinocytes and endothelial cells. It is believed to work synergistically with VEGF, potentiating its proangiogenic function.

Both acidic and basic FGFs (FGF-1 and FGF-2) are released from disrupted parenchymal cells and are early stimulants of angiogenesis. FGF-2 provides the initial angiogenic stimulus within the first 3 days of wound repair followed by a subsequent prolonged stimulus mediated by VEGF from day 4 through day 7. There is a dose-dependent effect of VEGF and FGF-2 on angiogenesis. Both TGF-α and EGF stimulate endothelial cell proliferation. TNF-α is chemotactic for endothelial cells; it promotes formation of the capillary tube and may mediate angiogenesis through its induction of hypoxia-inducible factor 1 (HIF-1). It regulates the expression of other hypoxia-responsive genes, including inducible NO synthase and VEGF. HIF-1α mRNA is prominently present in wound inflammatory cells during the initial 24 hours, and HIF-1α protein is present in cells isolated from the wound 1 and 5 days after injury in vitro. Data also suggest that there is a positive interaction between endogenous NO and VEGF, with endogenous NO enhancing VEGF synthesis. Similarly, VEGF has been shown to promote NO synthesis in angiogenesis, suggesting that NO mediates aspects of VEGF signaling required for endothelial cell proliferation and organization.

TGF-β is a chemoattractant for fibroblasts and probably assists in angiogenesis by signaling the fibroblast to produce FGFs. Other factors that have been shown to induce angiogenesis include angiogenin, IL-8, and lactic acid. Several of the matrix materials, such as fibronectin and hyaluronic acid from the wound site, are angiogenic. Fibronectin and fibrin are produced by macrophages and damaged endothelial cells. Collagen appears to interact by causing the tubular formation of endothelial cells in vitro. Angiogenesis results from the complex interaction of ECM material and cytokines.

Cells Involved in the Proliferative Phase

Lymphocytes

Small numbers of T lymphocytes appear by day 5 after injury and peak on day 7. B lymphocytes appear to be principally involved in downregulating inflammation as the wound closes. Lymphocytes stimulate fibroblasts with cytokines (IL-2 and fibroblast-activating factor). Lymphocytes also secrete inhibitory cytokines (TGF-β, TNF-α, and IFN-γ). Antigen-presenting macrophages present bacterial "debris" or enzymatically degraded host proteins to lymphocytes, stimulating lymphocyte proliferation and cytokine release. T cells produce IFN-γ, which stimulates the macrophage to release TNF-α and IL-1. IFN-γ decreases prostaglandin synthesis, enhancing the effect of inflammatory mediators, suppressing collagen synthesis, and inhibiting macrophage exodus. IFN-γ appears to be an important mediator of chronic nonhealing wounds, and its presence suggests that T lymphocytes are primarily involved in chronic wound healing.

For example, drugs that suppress T-lymphocyte function and proliferation (steroids, cyclosporine, and tacrolimus) result in impaired wound healing in experimental wound models, possibly by inhibiting the proliferative phase.

Fibroblasts

Fibroblasts are specialized cells that differentiate from resting mesenchymal cells in connective tissue; they do not arrive in the wound cleft by diapedesis from circulating cells. After injury, the normally quiescent and sparse fibroblasts are chemoattracted to the inflammatory site; they divide and produce the components of the ECM. After stimulation by macrophage-derived and platelet-derived cytokines and growth factors, the fibroblast, which is normally arrested in the G_0 phase, undergoes replication and proliferation. Platelet-derived TGF-β stimulates fibroblast proliferation indirectly by releasing PDGF. The fibroblast can also stimulate replication in an autocrine manner by releasing FGF-2. To continue proliferating, fibroblasts require further stimulation by factors such as EGF or IGF-1. Although fibroblasts require growth factors for proliferation, they do not need growth factors to survive. Fibroblasts can live quiescently in growth factor–free media in monolayers or three-dimensional cultures.

The primary function of fibroblasts is to synthesize collagen, which they begin to produce during the cellular phase of inflammation. The time required for undifferentiated mesenchymal cells to differentiate into highly specialized fibroblasts accounts for the delay between injury and the appearance of collagen in a healing wound. This period, generally 3 to 5 days depending on the type of tissue injured, is termed the *lag phase* of wound healing. Fibroblasts begin to migrate in response to chemotactic substances such as growth factors (PDGF, TGF-β), C5 fragments, thrombin, TNF-α, eicosanoids, elastin fragments, leukotriene B4, and fragments of collagen and fibronectin.

The rate of collagen synthesis declines after 4 weeks and eventually balances the rate of collagen destruction by collagenase (MMP-1). At this point, the wound enters a phase of collagen maturation. The maturation phase continues for months or years. Glycoprotein and mucopolysaccharide levels decrease during the maturation phase, and new capillaries regress and disappear.

These changes alter the appearance of the wound and increase its strength.

Keratinocytes

In addition to being primarily responsible for reepithelialization and serving as a physical barrier in the skin, keratinocytes are integral to driving and regulating cutaneous immunity (Fig. 23.4). Previously, keratinocytes were thought to be passive cells; however, keratinocytes are highly active cells that are conditioned to respond to environmental stimuli, as they express a range of pattern recognition receptors (PRRs) and cytokine receptors. They can detect pathogen-associated molecular patterns (PAMPs) such as bacterial or fungal cell wall components (e.g., LPS) and single- and double-stranded RNA and DNA present on viral species through their PRRs.[2] In response, keratinocytes can initiate immune responses via activation of signaling pathways and secrete various antimicrobial peptides (AMPs) and cytokine mediators.[2,3] These factors contribute to host-pathogen defense and regulation of immune cell function and phenotypes. After cutaneous injury, keratinocytes secrete type I IFNs such as IFN-α, IFN-β, and IFN-κ.[2,4] Previous understanding of the role of type I IFNs was limited to transduction of antiviral signaling pathways. However, IFN-κ has been shown to be a critical cytokine for tissue repair by initiating early inflammation upon injury. IFN-κ polarizes wound macrophages toward an inflammatory (M1) phenotype, initiating early and acute inflammation. Keratinocytes also release proinflammatory cytokines such as IL-1, IL-6, IL-8, and TNF-α to activate immune cells and recruit them to the wound site.[4] Keratinocytes produce IL-7 and IL-15, which are important growth factors for T lymphocytes of the adaptive immune system that aid in the resolution of wounds.[2,5] Additionally, keratinocytes secrete chemokine factors that promote migration of distinct leukocytes to the wound site. In response to mechanical injury, keratinocytes secrete CXCL1 and CXCL5, which play an important role in recruiting neutrophils and macrophages that are the major players during early phases of wound repair.[2,3] Keratinocytes also produce CCL20 that recruits cells of the adaptive immune system

that are associated with wound healing.[6] These dynamic interactions between keratinocytes and immune cells can drive inflammatory responses that are necessary for protection against pathogens and proper tissue repair. However, overproduction of these factors can result in dysregulated inflammation and poor wound healing, as seen in diabetic wounds.

Additionally, keratinocytes can communicate with other cell types by delivering cargo such as protein, lipids, DNA, and RNA via extracellular vesicles (EVs).[7] Keratinocyte secretion of EVs promotes cutaneous wound healing, as it allows direct cell-cell communication with wound-associated cells.[8,9] Keratinocytes release exosomes, which is a class of EVs, containing miRNA to influence macrophage plasticity.[7,8] In vivo inhibition of keratinocyte-secreted exosomes has been shown to cause a significant increase of macrophages of a proinflammatory (M1) phenotype rather than a proresolution phenotype (M2).[8] Keratinocytes can actively control the fate and function of macrophages in the wound, demonstrating that bidirectional cell-cell communication between structural and immune cells is necessary for efficient wound healing.

Skin Barrier Function

The epidermis serves as a physical barrier to prevent fluid loss and bacterial invasion. Tight cell junctions within the epithelium contribute to its impermeability, and the basement membrane zone gives structural support and provides attachment between the epidermis and the dermis. The basement membrane zone consists of several layers that secure the epidermodermal interface and connect the lamina densa to the dermis: (1) lamina lucida (electron clear), consisting of laminin and heparan sulfate; (2) lamina densa (electron dense), containing type IV collagen; and (3) anchoring fibrils, consisting of type IV collagen.

The basal layer of the epidermis attaches to the basement membrane zone by hemidesmosomes. Reepithelialization of wounds begins within hours after injury. Initially, the wound is rapidly sealed by clot formation and then by epithelial (epidermal) cell migration across the defect. Keratinocytes located at the

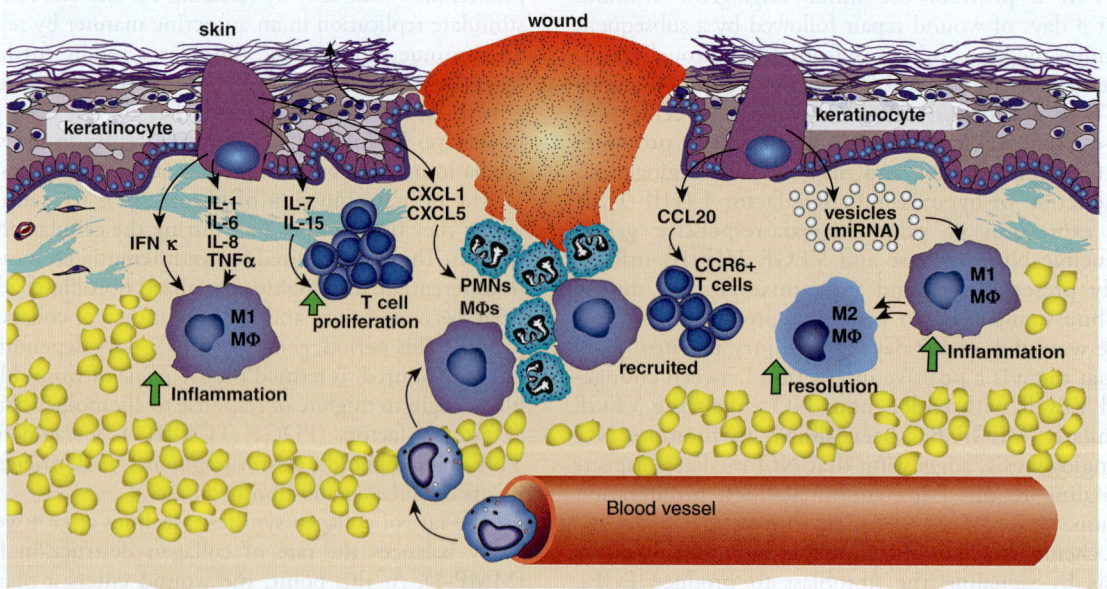

FIGURE 23.4 Keratinocyte functions in wound healing. Keratinocytes produce cytokines, chemokines, and extracellular vesicles in response to external stimuli in the wound environment to recruit immune cells or alter their functions and phenotypes.

basal layer of the residual epidermis or in the depths of epithelium-lined dermal appendages migrate to resurface the wound. Epithelialization involves a sequence of changes in wound keratinocytes—detachment, migration, proliferation, differentiation, and stratification. If the basement membrane zone is intact, epithelialization proceeds more rapidly. The cells are stimulated to migrate. Attachments to neighboring and adjoining cells and to the dermis are loosened, as demonstrated by intracellular tonofilament retraction, dissolution of intercellular desmosomes and hemidesmosomes linking the epidermis to the basement membrane, and formation of cytoplasmic actin filaments.

Epidermal cells express integrin receptors that allow them to interact with ECM proteins such as fibronectin. The migrating cells dissect the wound by separating the desiccated eschar from viable tissue. This path of dissection is determined by the integrins that the epidermal cells express on their cell membranes. Degradation of the ECM, required if epidermal cells are to migrate between the collagenous dermis and fibrin eschar, is driven by epidermal cell production of collagenase (MMP-1) and plasminogen activator, which activates collagenase and plasmin. The migrating cells are also phagocytic and remove debris in their path. Cells behind the leading edge of migrating cells begin to proliferate. The epithelial cells move in a leapfrog and tumbling fashion until the edges establish contact. If the basement membrane zone is not intact, it will be repaired first. The absence of neighboring cells at the wound margin may be a signal for the migration and proliferation of epidermal cells. Local release of EGF, TGF-α, and KGF and increased expression of their receptors may also stimulate these processes. Topical application of KGF-2 in young and aged animals accelerates reepithelialization. Basement membrane proteins, such as laminin, reappear in a highly ordered sequence from the margin of the wound inward. After the wound is completely reepithelialized, the cells become columnar and stratified again while firmly attaching to the reestablished basement membrane and underlying dermis.

Maturational/Remodeling Phase

The ECM exists as a scaffold to stabilize the physical structure of tissues, but it also plays an active and complex role by regulating the behavior of cells that contact it. Cells within it produce the macromolecular constituents, including (1) glycosaminoglycans (GAGs), or polysaccharide chains, usually found covalently linked to protein in the form of proteoglycans and (2) fibrous proteins such as collagen, elastin, fibronectin, and laminin.

In connective tissue, proteoglycan molecules form a gel-like ground substance. This highly hydrated gel allows the matrix to withstand compressive force while permitting rapid diffusion of nutrients, metabolites, and hormones between blood and tissue cells. Collagen fibers within the matrix serve to organize and strengthen the matrix, whereas elastin fibers give it resilience (matrix proteins have adhesive functions).

The wound matrix accumulates and changes in composition as healing progresses, balanced between new deposition and degradation (Fig. 23.5). The provisional matrix is a scaffold for cellular migration and is composed of fibrin, fibrinogen, fibronectin, and vitronectin. GAGs and proteoglycans are synthesized next and support further matrix deposition and remodeling. Collagens, which are the predominant scar proteins, are the end result. Attachment proteins, such as fibrin and fibronectin, provide linkage to the ECM through binding to cell surface integrin receptors.

Stimulation of fibroblasts by growth factors induces upregulated expression of integrin receptors, facilitating cell-matrix interactions.

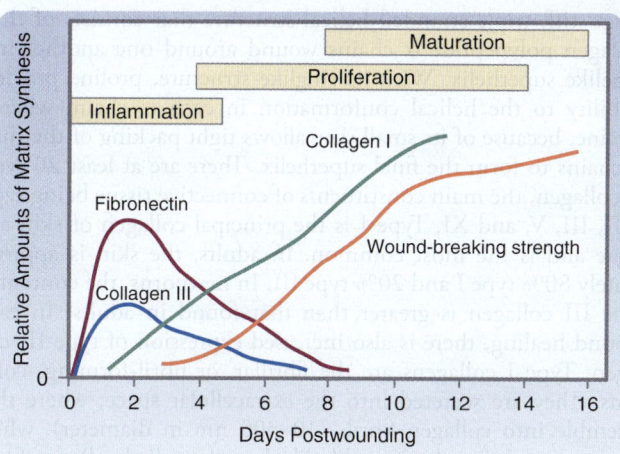

FIGURE 23.5 Wound matrix deposition over time. Fibronectin and type III collagen constitute the early matrix. Type I collagen accumulates later and corresponds to the increase in wound-breaking strength. (Adapted from Witte MB, Barbul A. General principles of wound healing. *Surg Clin North Am.* 1997;77:509-528.)

Ligand binding induces clustering of integrin into focal adhesion sites. Regulation of integrin-mediated cell signaling by the extracellular divalent cations Mg^{2+}, Mn^{2+}, and Ca^{2+} perhaps is caused by induction of conformational changes in the integrins.

A dynamic and reciprocal relationship exists between fibroblasts and the ECM. Cytokine regulation of fibroblast responses is altered by variations in the composition of the ECM. For example, expression of matrix-degrading enzymes, such as the MMPs, is upregulated after cytokine stimulation of fibroblasts. Collagenolytic MMP-1 is induced by IL-1 and downregulated by TGF-β. Activation of plasminogen to plasmin by plasminogen activator and procollagenase to collagenase by plasmin results in matrix degradation and facilitates cell migration. Modulation of these processes provides additional mechanisms whereby the cell-matrix interaction can be regulated during wound healing. Matrix modulation is also seen in tumor metastasis. Neoplastic cells lose their dependence on anchorage, mediated mainly by integrins; this is probably caused by decreased production of fibronectin and subsequent decreased adhesion, and, as a result, these cells can break away from the primary tumor and metastasize.

An example of the necessary dynamic interactions occurring in the provisional matrix during wound healing is the effect of TGF-β on incisional wounds sealed with fibrin sealant. Fibrin sealant is a derivative of plasma components that mimics the last step in the coagulation cascade. Commercially available fibrin sealant has an approximately tenfold greater concentration of fibrin than plasma and consequently provides a more airtight, waterproof seal. Fibrin sealant may serve as a mechanical barrier to the early cell-mediated events occurring in wound healing. Supplementation of fibrin sealant with TGF-β has been demonstrated to reverse the inhibitory effects of fibrin sealant on wound healing and increase tensile strength compared with sutured wounds. The increased tensile strength may be a result of improved cell migration into the wound site, more rapid clearance of fibrin sealant, suppression of gelatinase (MMP-9), and enhancement of ECM synthesis in TGF-β–supplemented wounds.

Collagens are found in all multicellular animals and are secreted by various cell types. They are a major component of skin and bone and constitute 25% of the total protein mass in mammals. The proline-rich and glycine-rich collagen molecule is a long, stiff, triple-stranded helical structure that consists of three collagen polypeptide α chains wound around one another in a ropelike superhelix. With its ringlike structure, proline provides stability to the helical conformation in each α chain, whereas glycine, because of its small size, allows tight packing of the three α chains to form the final superhelix. There are at least 20 types of collagen, the main constituents of connective tissue being types I, II, III, V, and XI. Type I is the principal collagen of skin and bone and is the most common. In adults, the skin is approximately 80% type I and 20% type III. In newborns, the content of type III collagen is greater than that found in adults. In early wound healing, there is also increased expression of type III collagen. Type I collagens are the fibrillar, or fibril-forming, collagens. They are secreted into the extracellular space, where they assemble into collagen fibrils (10–300 nm in diameter), which then aggregate into larger, cable-like bundles called collagen fibers (several micrometers in diameter).

Other types of collagens include types IX and XII (fibril-associated collagens) and types IV and VII (network-forming collagens). Types IX and XII are found on the surface of collagen fibrils and serve to link the fibrils to one another and to other components in the ECM. Type IV molecules assemble into a meshlike pattern and are a major part of the mature basal lamina. Dimers of type VII form anchoring fibrils that help attach the basal lamina to the underlying connective tissue and are especially abundant in the skin.

Type XVII and type XVIII collagens are two of a number of collagen-like proteins. Type XVII has a transmembrane domain and is found in hemidesmosomes. Type XVIII is located in the basal laminae of blood vessels. The peptide endostatin, which inhibits angiogenesis and shows promise as an anticancer drug, is formed by cleavage of the C-terminal domain of type XVIII collagen.

Collagen Synthesis

Collagen polypeptide chains are synthesized on membrane-bound ribosomes and enter the endoplasmic reticulum lumen as pro-α chains (Fig. 23.6). These precursors have amino-terminal signal peptides to direct them to the endoplasmic reticulum and propeptides at the N-terminal and C-terminal ends. Within the lumen of the endoplasmic reticulum, some of the prolines and lysines undergo hydroxylation to form hydroxyproline and hydroxylysine. Hydroxylation results in the stable triple-stranded helix through the formation of interchain hydrogen bonds. The pro-α chain then combines with two others to form procollagen, a hydrogen-bonded, triple-stranded helical molecule. In conditions such as vitamin C (ascorbic acid) deficiency (scurvy), proline hydroxylation is prevented, resulting in the formation of unstable triple helices secondary to the synthesis of defective pro-α chains. Vitamin C deficiency is characterized by the gradual loss of preexisting normal collagen, which leads to fragile blood vessels and loose teeth.

After secretion into the ECM, specific proteases cleave the propeptides of the procollagen molecules to form collagen monomers. These monomers assemble to form collagen fibrils in the ECM, driven by the tendency of collagen to self-assemble. Covalent cross-linking of the lysine residues provides tensile strength. The extent and type of cross-linking vary from tissue to tissue. In tissues such as tendons in which tensile strength is crucial, collagen cross-linking is extremely high. In mammalian skin, the fibrils are organized in a basketweave pattern to resist multidirectional tensile stress. In tendons, fibrils are in parallel bundles aligned along the major axis of tension.

Numerous factors can affect collagen synthesis. Vitamin C (ascorbic acid), TGF-β, IGF-1, and IGF-2 increase collagen synthesis. IFN-γ decreases type I procollagen mRNA synthesis, and glucocorticoids inhibit procollagen gene transcription, leading to decreased collagen synthesis.

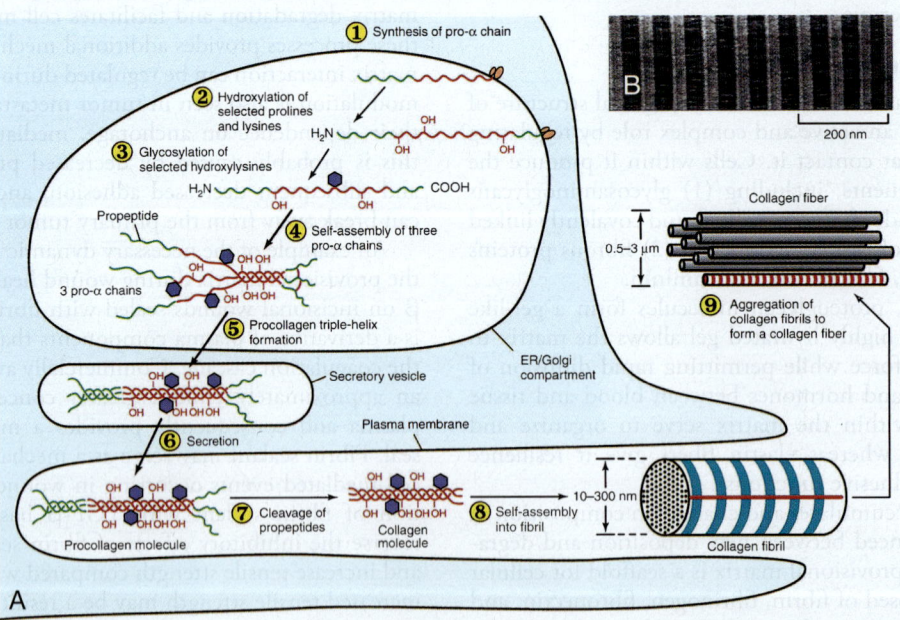

FIGURE 23.6 Intracellular and extracellular events in the formation of a collagen fibril. (A) Collagen fibrils are shown assembling in the extracellular space contained within a large infolding in the plasma membrane. As one example of how collagen fibrils can form ordered arrays in the extracellular space, they are shown further assembling into large collagen fibers, which are visible with a light microscope. The covalent cross-links that stabilize the extracellular assemblies are not shown. (B) Electron micrograph of a negatively stained collagen fibril revealing its typical striated appearance. *ER,* Endoplasmic reticulum. (A, From Alberts B, Johnson A, Lewis J, et al., eds. *Molecular Biology of the Cell.* 4th ed. Garland; 2002:1100; B, Courtesy Robert Horne.)

Several genetic disorders are caused by abnormalities in collagen fibril formation. In osteogenesis imperfecta, deletion of one procollagen α_1 allele results in weak, easily fractured bones. Ehlers-Danlos syndrome is a result of mutations affecting type III collagen and is characterized by fragile skin and blood vessels and hypermobile joints.

Elastic Fibers

Tissues such as skin, blood vessels, and lungs require strength and elasticity to function. Elastic fibers in the ECM of these tissues provide the resilience to allow recoil after transient stretching.

Elastic fibers are predominantly composed of elastin, a highly hydrophobic protein (~750 amino acids long). Soluble tropoelastin is secreted into the extracellular space, where it forms lysine cross-links to other tropoelastin molecules to generate a large network of elastin fibers and sheets. Elastin is composed of hydrophobic and alanine-rich and lysine-rich α-helical segments that alternate along the polypeptide chain. The hydrophobic segments are responsible for the elastic properties of the molecule. The alanine-rich and lysine-rich α-helical segments form cross-links between adjacent molecules. Although the proposed conformation of elastin molecules is controversial, the predominant theory is that the elastin polypeptide chain adopts a random coil conformation that allows the network to stretch and recoil like a rubber band. Elastic fibers consist of an elastin core covered by a sheath of microfibrils, which are composed of several distinct glycoproteins such as fibrillin. Elastin-binding fibrillin is essential for the integrity of the elastic fibers.

Microfibrils appear before elastin in developing tissues and seem to form a scaffold on which the secreted elastin molecules are deposited. Elastin is produced early in life, stabilizes, and does not undergo much further synthesis or degradation, with a turnover that approaches the life span. Age-related modification is a result of progressive degradation as the elastic fibers gradually become tortuous, frayed, and porous. Scanning electron microscopy shows that, in humans, the elastic meshwork grows largely undistorted during postnatal growth, during which fibers seem to enlarge in synchrony with growth of the tissue. In circumstances not involving a wound, there is little elastin degradation, probably because of the hydrophobic nature of elastin, which makes the interior of this highly folded protein inaccessible. As a result of this high degree of three-dimensionality and extensive cross-linking, cleavage must be considerable before there is much loss of elasticity. IGF-1 and TGF-β stimulate the production of elastin. Glucocorticoids and basic FGF reduce the production of elastin in adult skin cells.

Mutations causing a deficiency of elastin protein result in arterial narrowing as a consequence of excessive smooth muscle cell proliferation in the arterial wall (intimal hyperplasia). These findings suggest that the normal elasticity of an artery is needed to prevent the proliferation of these cells. Gene mutations in fibrillin result in Marfan syndrome; severely affected individuals are prone to aortic rupture.

Glycosaminoglycans and Proteoglycans

GAGs are unbranched polysaccharide chains composed of repeating disaccharide units, a sulfated amino sugar (N-acetylglucosamine or N-acetylgalactosamine), and uronic acid (glucuronic or iduronic). GAGs are highly negatively charged because of the sulfate or carboxyl groups on most of their sugars. Four types of GAGs exist: (1) hyaluronan, (2) chondroitin sulfate and dermatan sulfate, (3) heparan sulfate, and (4) keratan sulfate.

GAGs in connective tissue usually constitute less than 10% of the weight of fibrous proteins. Their highly negative charge attracts osmotically active cations, such as Na^+, which causes large amounts of water to be incorporated into the matrix. This results in porous hydrated gels and is responsible for the turgor that enables the matrix to withstand compressive force.

Hyaluronan is the simplest GAG. It is composed of repeating nonsulfated disaccharide units and is found in adult tissues, but it is especially prevalent in fetal tissues. Its abundance in fetal wounds is believed to be a factor in the scarless wound healing seen in fetal tissues. In contrast to the other GAGs, hyaluronan is not covalently attached to any protein and is synthesized directly from the cell surface by an enzyme complex embedded in the plasma membrane.

Hyaluronan plays several different roles because of its large hydration shell. It is produced in large quantities during wound healing, during which it facilitates cell migration by physically expanding the ECM and allowing cells additional space for migration; it also reduces the strength of adhesion of migrating cells to matrix fibers. Hyaluronan synthesized from the basal side of epithelium creates a cell-free space for cell migration, such as during embryogenesis and formation of the heart and other organs. When cell migration is finished, the excess hyaluronan is degraded by hyaluronidase. Studies using hyaluronic acid derivative have suggested that these derivatives can accelerate wound healing in burns, surgical wounds, and chronic wounds.

Proteoglycans are a diverse group of glycoproteins with functions mediated by their core proteins and GAG chains. The number and types of GAGs attached to the core protein can vary greatly, and the GAGs themselves can be modified by sulfonation. Because of their GAGs, proteoglycans provide hydrated space around and between cells. They also form gels of different pore size and charge density to regulate the movement of cells and molecules. Perlecan, a heparan sulfate proteoglycan, plays this role in the basal lamina of the kidney glomerulus. Decreased levels of perlecan are believed to play a role in diabetic albuminuria.

Proteoglycans function in chemical signaling by binding various secreted signal molecules, such as growth factors, and modulating their signaling activity. Proteoglycans also can bind other secreted proteins, such as proteases and protease inhibitors. This binding allows proteoglycans to regulate proteins by (1) immobilizing the protein and restricting its range of action, (2) providing a reservoir of the protein for delayed release, (3) altering the protein to allow more effective presentation to cell surface receptors, (4) prolonging the action of the protein by protecting it from degradation, or (5) blocking the activity of the protein.

Proteoglycans can be components of plasma membranes and have a transmembrane core protein or are attached to the lipid bilayer by a glycosylphosphatidylinositol anchor. These proteoglycans act as coreceptors that work with other cell surface receptor proteins in binding cells to the ECM and initiating the response of cells to extracellular signaling proteins. For example, the syndecans are transmembrane proteoglycans located on the surface of many cells, including fibroblasts and epithelial cells. In fibroblasts, syndecans are found in focal adhesions, where they interact with fibronectin on the cell surface and with cytoskeletal and signaling proteins inside the cell. Mutations leading to inactivation of these coreceptor proteoglycans result in severe developmental defects.

The ECM has other noncollagen proteins, such as the fibronectins, that have multiple domains and can bind to other matrix macromolecules and cell surface receptors. These interactions help organize the matrix and facilitate cell attachment.

Fibronectin exists as soluble and fibrillar isoforms. Soluble plasma fibronectin circulates in various body fluids and enhances blood clotting, wound healing, and phagocytosis. The highly insoluble fibrillar forms assemble on cell surfaces and are deposited in the ECM. The fibronectin fibrils that form on the surface of fibroblasts are usually coupled with neighboring intracellular actin stress fibers. The actin filaments promote assembly of the fibronectin fibril and influence fibril orientation. Integrin transmembrane adhesion proteins mediate these interactions. The contractile actin and myosin cytoskeleton pulls on the fibronectin matrix and generates tension.

Basal Lamina

Basal laminae are flexible, thin (40–120 nm) mats of specialized ECM that separate cells and epithelia from the underlying or surrounding connective tissue. In skin, the basal lamina is tethered to the underlying connective tissue by specialized anchoring fibrils. This composite of basal lamina and collagen is the basement membrane.

The basal lamina acts in numerous ways: (1) as a molecular filter to prevent the passage of macromolecules (i.e., in the kidney glomerulus); (2) as a selective barrier to certain cells (i.e., the lamina beneath the epithelium prevents fibroblasts from contacting epithelial cells but does not stop macrophages or lymphocytes); (3) as a scaffold for regenerating cells to migrate; and (4) as an important element in tissue regeneration in locations where the basal lamina survives.

Although composition may vary from tissue to tissue, most mature basal laminae contain type IV collagen, perlecan, and the glycoproteins laminin and nidogen. Type IV collagen has a more flexible structure than the fibrillar collagens; its triple-stranded helix is interrupted, allowing multiple bends.

Laminins generally consist of three long polypeptide chains (α, β, and γ). Mice lacking the laminin γ_1 chain die during embryogenesis because they cannot make a basal lamina. The laminin in basement membranes consists of several domains that bind to perlecan, nidogen, and laminin receptor proteins found on cell surfaces. The type IV collagen and laminin networks are connected by nidogen and perlecan, which act as stabilizing bridges. Many of the cell surface receptors for type IV collagen and laminin are members of the integrin family. Another important type of laminin receptor is dystroglycan, a transmembrane protein that, together with integrins, may organize assembly of the basal lamina.

Degradation of the Extracellular Matrix

Regulated turnover of the ECM is crucial to many biologic processes. ECM degradation occurs during metastasis when neoplastic cells migrate from their site of origin to distant organs via the bloodstream or lymphatics. In injury or infection, localized degradation of the ECM occurs so that cells can migrate across the basal lamina to reach the site of injury or infection. Locally secreted cellular proteases, such as MMPs or serine proteases, degrade the ECM components. Matrix proteolysis helps the cell migrate by (1) clearing a path through the matrix; (2) exposing binding sites, promoting cell binding or migration; (3) facilitating cell detachment so that a cell can move forward; and (4) releasing signal proteins that promote cell migration.

Proteolysis is tightly regulated. Many proteases are secreted as inactive precursors that are activated when required. In addition, cell surface receptors bind these proteases to ensure that they act only on sites where they are needed. Finally, protease inhibitors, such as tissue inhibitors of metalloproteinase (TIMP), can bind these enzymes and block their activity.

Wound contraction. Wound contraction occurs by centripetal movement of the whole thickness of the surrounding skin and reduces the amount of disorganized scar. In contrast, wound contracture is a physical constriction or limitation of function and is a result of the process of wound contraction. Contractures occur when excessive scar exceeds normal wound contraction, and it results in a functional disability. Examples of contractures are scars that traverse joints and prevent extension and scars that involve the eyelid or mouth and cause an ectropion.

Numerous studies have shown that fibroblasts in a contracting wound undergo change to stimulated cells, termed *myofibroblasts*. These cells have function and structure in common with fibroblasts and smooth muscle cells and express alpha smooth muscle actin in bundles termed *stress fibers*. The actin appears at day 6 after wounding, persists at high levels for 15 days, and is gone by 4 weeks, when the cell undergoes apoptosis. It appears that a stimulated fibroblast develops contractile ability related to the formation of cytoplasmic actin-myosin complexes. When this stimulated cell is placed in the fibroblast-populated collagen lattice, contraction occurs even more quickly. The tension that is exerted by the fibroblasts' attempt at contraction appears to stimulate the actin-myosin structures in their cytoplasm. If colchicine, which inhibits microtubules, or cytochalasin D, which inhibits microfilaments, is added to the tissue culture, the result is minimal contraction of the collagen gels. Fibroblasts develop a linear arrangement in the line of tension that, when removed, causes the cells to round up.

Stimulated fibroblasts, or myofibroblasts, are found to be a constant feature present in abundance in diseases involving excessive fibrosis, including hepatic cirrhosis, renal and pulmonary fibrosis, Dupuytren contracture, and desmoplastic reactions induced by neoplasia. The actin microfilaments are arranged linearly along the long axis of the fibroblast. They are associated with dense bodies that allow attachment to the surrounding ECM. Fibronexus is the attachment entity that connects the cytoskeleton to the ECM and spans the cell membrane in doing so.

As the fibroblast population decreases, the dense capillary network regresses. Wound strength increases rapidly within 1 to 6 weeks and then appears to plateau up to 1 year after the injury (see Fig. 23.6). Compared with nonwounded skin, tensile strength is only 30% in the scar. An increase in breaking strength occurs after approximately 21 days, mostly as a result of cross-linking. Although collagen cross-linking causes further wound contraction and an increase in strength, it also results in a scar that is more brittle and less elastic than normal skin. In contrast to normal skin, the epidermodermal interface in a healed wound is devoid of rete pegs, the undulating projections of epidermis that penetrate into the papillary dermis. Loss of this anchorage results in increased fragility and predisposes the neoepidermis to avulsion after minor trauma.

ABNORMAL WOUND HEALING

In such a complex series of interweaving events as wound healing, many factors can impede proper tissue repair (Box 23.1). Intrinsic factors such as age, diabetes, chemotherapeutic agents, atherosclerosis, obesity, smoking status, as well as others all affect wound healing.

Hypertrophic Scars and Keloids

Hypertrophic scars and keloids are proliferative scars characterized by excessive net collagen deposition (Fig. 23.7). Hypertrophic scars are raised scars within the confines of the original wound and frequently regress spontaneously. Keloids, by definition, grow

BOX 23.1 Factors That Inhibit Wound Healing

Infection
Ischemia
   Circulation
   Respiration
   Local tension
Diabetes mellitus
Ionizing radiation
Advanced age
Malnutrition
Vitamin deficiencies
   Vitamin C
   Vitamin A
Mineral deficiencies
   Zinc
   Iron
Exogenous drugs
   Doxorubicin (Adriamycin)
   Glucocorticosteroids

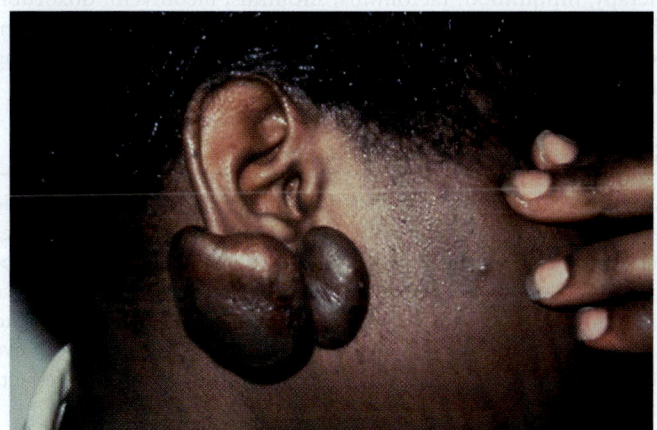

FIGURE 23.7 Keloids caused by ear piercing.

beyond the borders of the original wounds and rarely regress with time; they are more prevalent in darkly pigmented skin, developing in 15% to 20% of Blacks, Asians, and Hispanics. There is strong evidence suggesting a genetic susceptibility, including familial heritability, common occurrence in twins, and high prevalence in certain ethnic populations. Recent studies have suggested a strong multigenetic disposition to keloid formation and differential expression with a varied inheritance. Proposed pathways include apoptosis, endocytosis, cytokine–cytokine receptor interaction, mitogen-activated protein kinase signaling pathway, tenascin C, jun proto-oncogene, and growth factors such as TGF-β and VEGF.[10,11]

Keloids often occur above the clavicles, on the trunk, on the upper extremities, and on the face. Their occurrence cannot be predicted and are frequently refractory to medical and surgical intervention. To date, there is no known effective prevention method for keloid formation. Zhang and colleagues[11] have identified potential molecular and genetic targets that could allow for prevention of keloids and scarring, such as Fos proto-oncogene (FOS) and EGR1 transcriptional factors.

Keloids and hypertrophic scars differ histologically from normal scars. Hypertrophic scars primarily contain well-organized type III collagen, whereas keloids contain disorganized type I and type III collagen bundles. Keloids and hypertrophic scars have stretched collagen bundles aligned in the same plane as the epidermis, whereas collagen bundles are randomly arrayed and relaxed in normal scars. Keloid scars have thicker, abundant collagen bundles that form acellular nodelike structures in the deep dermis with a paucity of cells centrally. Hypertrophic scars, in contrast, contain islands composed of aggregates of fibroblasts, small vessels, and collagen fibers throughout the dermis.

Hypertrophic scars are often preventable. Prolonged inflammation and insufficient resurfacing (e.g., burn wounds) promote hypertrophic scarring. Scars perpendicular to the underlying muscle fibers tend to be flatter and narrower, with less collagen formation than when they are parallel to the underlying muscle fibers. Tension appears to signal the formation of activated fibroblasts resulting in excessive collagen deposition. The position of an elective scar can be chosen to induce a narrower, less obvious healed scar. As muscle fibers contract, the wound edges become reapproximated when they are perpendicular to the underlying muscle and tend to gape if placed parallel to it, leading to greater wound tension and scar formation.

Hypertrophic scars represent a reversible hyperproliferative scar phenotype that tends to regress when the original stimuli (skin tension, stimulatory growth factors) are removed. Keloids appear to be genetically predisposed and switched on irreversibly by factors such as TGF-β. In addition, in these scars, collagen synthesis is elevated, whereas collagen degradation is low. MMPs are also affected in these scars: MMP-1 (collagenase) and MMP-9 (gelatinase, early tissue repair) are decreased, whereas MMP-2 (gelatinase, late tissue remodeling) is significantly elevated. Blocking TGF-β activity with antibodies decreases scar fibrosis. Barnes and colleagues[12] demonstrated that increased mechanical stress at the wound bed promotes hypertrophic scaring by activating mechanotransduction pathways. Targeting these pathways may reduce excessive scarring and fibrosis, and new prevention therapies at the molecular and genetic level may soon be available.[12]

Prevention of Hypertrophic or Keloid Scars

The three strategies that reduce adverse scarring immediately after wound closure are tension relief, hydration/occlusion, and use of taping/pressure garments. Wounds with greater tension (perpendicular to Langer lines), wounds with excessive tension on closure, and wounds in certain anatomic locations (deltoid and sternal) are at a higher risk of adverse scarring. Scarring can be reduced by postsurgical taping of the wound for 3 months. Moisturizing lotions and moisture-retentive dressings (silicone sheets and gels) can reduce the thickness, discomfort, and itching and improve the appearance of the scar. After wound healing, water still evaporates more rapidly through scar tissue and may take more than a year to recover to preinjury levels. Silicone products may ameliorate evaporative losses and assist hydration of the stratum corneum. These strategies need to be employed soon after initial wound healing. Pressure garments should be used prophylactically in wounds that are wide (e.g., burns); these wounds may take more than 2 or 3 weeks to heal. Garments should be applied as soon as the wound is closed and the patient can tolerate the pressure.[13] Tejiram and colleagues[13] noted a significant decrease in collagen I and III levels as early as 1 week after initiation of pressure treatment. Avoidance of sun exposure and use of SPF 50+ sunscreens for 1 year postoperatively reduce scar hyperpigmentation and improve clinical appearance.

Treatment for Hypertrophic Scars

Early linear scar hypertrophy (e.g., after trauma or surgery) at 6 weeks to 3 months should be treated with pressure therapy. After 6 months, silicone therapy should be continued for as long as necessary if there is further scar maturation. Ongoing hypertrophy may be treated with intralesional corticosteroids (triamcinolone acetonide 10–40 mg/mL) injected into the papillary dermis every 2 to 4 weeks until flat. This is the only noninvasive management option that has enough supporting evidence to be recommended in evidence-based guidelines. Approximately 50% to 100% of patients respond, and up to 50% experience recurrence. Adverse steroid effects include skin atrophy, hypopigmentation, telangiectasias, and excessive pain during injections. Injections should be limited to the scar itself to minimize adjacent fat atrophy.

Surgical scar revision may be considered for permanent linear hypertrophic scars present after 1 year. Simple resection and primary closure may be combined with adjacent tissue undermining, subcutaneous sutures, adjunctive Z-plasty, and postsurgical taping and silicone therapy.

Hypertrophic scars also can be seen in conjunction with a scar contracture. Scar contractures are abnormal shortening of non-matured scars resulting in functional impairment, particularly if the scar is across a joint. Correction of a scar contracture generally requires surgery with Z-plasty, skin graft, or flap to release tension in the scar to restore function and reduce scar hypertrophy.

Severe burns, mechanical trauma, necrotizing infections, wounds requiring more than 2 to 3 weeks to heal, or wounds healed with skin grafting require early application of silicone and compression therapy.[13] This therapy should be initiated as soon as the wound is closed and the patient can tolerate the pressure.

The mechanism of action of pressure therapy is poorly understood but may involve reduction of wound oxygen tension by occlusion of small blood vessels, resulting in a decrease in myofibroblast proliferation and collagen synthesis. Pressure therapy is believed to act on cellular mechanoreceptors that are involved in cellular apoptosis and linked to the ECM. The increased pressure regulates apoptosis of dermal fibroblasts and diminishes hypertrophic scarring. In addition, sensory nerve cells transduce mechanical pressure into intracellular biochemical and gene expression, synthesizing and releasing different cytokines involved in the physiopathogenesis of proliferative scarring.[11,13]

Pressure and silicone therapy should be continued or intensified and combined with selective localized corticosteroid injections in resistant areas. Bleomycin, 5-fluorouracil (5-FU), and verapamil have been used as adjuncts to corticosteroid therapy. In a small pilot study, Losartan ointment (5%) was found to significantly decrease vascularity and pliability and improve scar quality after 3 months of treatment, with no recurrences in a 6-month follow-up.[14] More therapies are being investigated alone or in combination with conventional modalities.

Laser therapy, although invasive, is another useful adjunct to reduce scar thickness; resurface scar texture; and treat residual redness, telangiectasias, or hyperpigmentation. Hultman and colleagues[15] performed the first large-scale prospective study demonstrating remarkable improvement in signs and symptoms of hypertrophic burn scars after treatment with pulsed dye laser and CO_2 laser.

Early surgery is indicated for functional impairment. Burn scar contracture release procedures in the neck and axilla are best performed with flaps to improve functional and cosmetic outcomes further that may not be achievable with skin grafts. Widespread large hypertrophic scars may require serial excision or tissue expansion.

Treatment for Keloids

First-line treatments include intralesional corticosteroid injections in combination with silicone dressings and pressure therapy. Intralesional 5-FU, bleomycin, and verapamil should be used in accordance with established treatment protocols. One study showed improved results when intralesional triamcinolone acetonide and 5-FU were used in combination compared with individual treatments.[16] Refractory cases after 12 months of therapy should be considered for surgical excision in combination with adjuvant therapy. Excision alone results in a high recurrence rate of 50% to 100% and potential enlargement of the keloid. Immediate postoperative electron beam irradiation or brachytherapy reduces recurrence rates by 50% to 95%. Hypothetically, it may be associated with radiation damage to adjacent tissues or induction of malignancy; however, the literature has failed to prove significant association. Shin and colleagues[17] compared surgical excision with triamcinolone versus radiation therapy, and recurrence rates were found to be 15.4% and 14%, respectively. Another study demonstrated that surgical excision combined with intraoperative autologous platelet-rich plasma and postoperative radiation therapy lead to effective treatment of ear keloids with 6% recurrence rates.[18] Other potential therapies include cryotherapy, imiquimod, tacrolimus, sirolimus, bleomycin, doxorubicin, TGF-β, EGF, losartan,[14] verapamil, retinoic acid, tamoxifen, botulinum toxin A, onion extract, and skin tension-offloading devices, with limited evidence to date.

SUMMARY

Although existing strategies for the management of hypertrophic scars and keloids are broadly similar, the histologic differences between the two scars suggest that, in the future, therapeutic approaches could be developed that are specifically tailored for these different types of scars. However, at the present time, there is no single proven best therapy for the management of these excessive healing scars, and the large number of treatment options reflects this (Table 23.1).

Chronic Nonhealing Wounds

By definition, chronic wounds are wounds that have failed to proceed through an orderly and timely reparative process to produce anatomic and functional integrity over a period of 3 months. In the United States, it is estimated that 3 to 4 million patients per year are at risk of developing diabetic ulcers, up to 2 million patients per year develop chronic leg ulcers secondary to venous insufficiency, and 2 to 3 million patients per year develop pressure ulcers secondary to immobility. These numbers have been increasing as a result of an aging population and the rising incidence of risk factors for atherosclerotic disease, such as diabetes mellitus and smoking. These wounds are a significant challenge to healthcare professionals and an immense burden on healthcare systems and the economy. Patients also report reduced quality of life and social isolation.

Numerous common factors promote adverse wound healing conditions. Systemic factors, such as malnutrition, aging, tissue hypoxia, and diabetes, contribute significantly to the pathogenesis of chronic wounds. A combination of systemic and localized adverse wound factors collectively overwhelms the normal healing processes, resulting in a hostile wound-healing environment (Fig. 23.8).

Chronic wounds have derangements in the various stages of wound healing and have unusually elevated or depressed levels of cytokines, growth factors, or proteinases. Chronic wound fluid, in

TABLE 23.1 Prevention and Treatment Options for Keloids and Hypertrophic Scars

MODALITY OR TREATMENT OPTION	RESPONSE RATE (%)	RECURRENCE RATE (%)	COMMENTS	STUDY DESIGN
Prevention				
Preventive silicone sheeting (postsurgery)	0–75	25–36	Multiple preparations available; tolerated by children; expensive; avoid on open wounds; poor study design	Review of multiple case studies
Postsurgical intralesional corticosteroid injection (triamcinolone acetonide [Kenalog] 10–40 mg/mL at 6-week intervals)	NA	0–100 (mean, 50)	Patient acceptance and safety; may cause hypopigmentation, skin atrophy, telangiectasia	Review of multiple case studies
Postsurgical topical imiquimod, 5% cream (Aldara)	NA	28	May cause hyperpigmentation, irritation	Case study
Postsurgical fluorouracil, triamcinolone acetonide, and pulsed dye lasers (best outcomes)	70 at 12 weeks	NA	Effective; may cause hyperpigmentation, wound ulceration	Clinical trial
First-Line Treatment				
Cryotherapy	50–76	NA	Useful on small lesions; easy to perform; may cause hypopigmentation, pain	Review of multiple case studies
Intralesional corticosteroid injection (triamcinolone acetonide [Kenalog] 10–40 mg/mL at 6-week intervals)	50–100	9–50	Inexpensive, requires multiple injections; may cause discomfort, skin atrophy, telangiectasia	Review of multiple case studies
Silicone elastomer sheeting	50–100	NA	Multiple preparations available; tolerated by children; expensive; poor study design	Review of multiple case studies
Pressure dressing (24–30 mm Hg) worn for 6–12 months	90–100	NA	Inexpensive; difficult schedule; poor adherence	Review of multiple case studies
Surgical excision	NA	50–100	Z-plasty option for burns; immediate postsurgical treatment needed to prevent regrowth	Review of multiple case studies
Combined cryotherapy and intralesional corticosteroid injection	84	NA	See benefits of individual treatments; may cause hypopigmentation	Case study
Triple-keloid therapy (surgery, corticosteroids, silicone sheeting)	88 at 13 months	12.5 at 13 months	Tedious; time-intensive; expensive	Case study
Pulsed dye laser	NA	NA	Specialist referral needed; expensive; variable results depending on trial (controversial)	Case studies
Second-Line and Alternative Treatment				
Verapamil 2.5 mg/mL intralesional injection combined with perilesional excision and silicone sheeting	54 at 18 months	NA	Repeated injections; limited experience; may cause discomfort	Clinical trial
Fluorouracil 50 mg/mL intralesional injection two to three times a week	88	0	Effective; may cause hyperpigmentation, wound ulceration	Review of multiple case studies
Bleomycin tattooing 1.5 IU/mL	92, 88	NA	Effective; may cause pulmonary fibrosis, cutaneous reactions	Review of case study; control trial
Postsurgical interferon-α2b 1.5 million IU, intralesional injection bid for 4 days	30–50	8–19	Expensive; may cause pruritus, altered pigmentation, pain	Review of multiple case studies
Radiation therapy alone	56 (mean)	NA	Local growth inhibition; may cause cancer, hyperpigmentation, paresthesias	Review of multiple case studies
Postsurgical radiation therapy	76	NA	Local growth inhibition; may cause cancer	Review of multiple case studies
Onion extract topical gels (Mederma)	NA	NA	Limited effect alone, better in combination with silicone sheeting	Prospective case study

bid, Twice daily; NA, not available.
Adapted from Juckett G, Hartman-Adams H. Management of keloids and hypertrophic scars. *Am Fam Physician*. 2009;80:253-260.

contrast to acute wound fluid, has been shown to have greater levels of IL-1, IL-6, and TNF-α; levels of these proinflammatory cytokines decreased as the wound healed. An inverse relationship between TNF-α and essential growth factors, such as EGF and PDGF, has been demonstrated.

Chronic wounds typically exhibit powerful proinflammatory stimuli, including bacterial colonization, necrotic tissue, foreign bodies, and localized tissue hypoxia. Tissue edema is significant, and the distance between capillaries is increased, reducing oxygen diffusion to individual cells. Chronic wounds typically have high

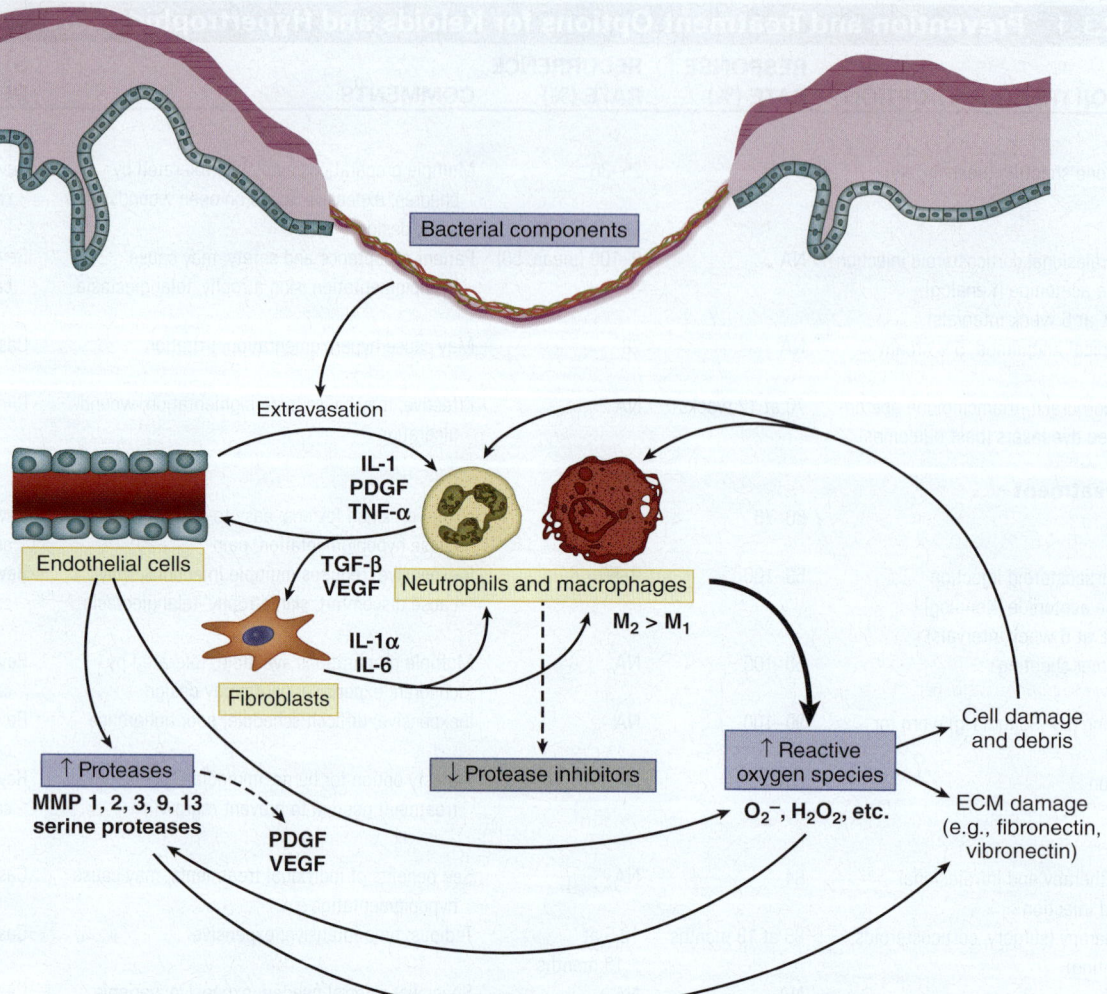

FIGURE 23.8 Mechanisms involved in the development and persistence of chronic wounds. Chronic wounds do not adequately complete the "normal" phases of wound healing. A state of chronic inflammation develops, as many of the cells recruited to the wound in the proliferative phase of healing adopt a proinflammatory secretory profile. Inflammatory cells, particularly neutrophils and macrophages (M1 phenotype > M2 phenotype), persist in the wound, creating a highly pro-oxidant, protease-rich environment with an abundance of proinflammatory cytokines such as interleukin-1 *(IL-1)*, interleukin-6 *(IL-6)*, and tumor necrosis factor-α *(TNF-α)*. The result is a hostile environment with downregulation of protease inhibitors and direct damage to extracellular matrix *(ECM)*, cellular components, and protective growth factors such as platelet-derived growth factor *(PDGF)* and vascular endothelial growth factor *(VEGF)*. Reactive oxygen species and proteases, such as matrix metalloproteinases *(MMP-1, -2, -3, -9, -13)*, are the most significant deleterious influences. *Solid lines* indicate upregulation, and *dashed lines* indicate downregulation. Width of the line is proportional to the effect of the influence. H_2O_2, Hydrogen peroxide; O_2^-, superoxide; *TGF-β*, transforming growth factor-β. (From Greaves NS, Iqbal SA, Baguneid M, et al. The role of skin substitutes in the management of chronic cutaneous wounds. *Wound Repair Regen.* 2013;21:194-210.)

bacterial counts, which stimulates an inflammatory host response, with PMNs expressing reactive oxygen species and proteases, resulting in a highly pro-oxidant environment. Disturbed oxidant balance is the likely key factor in the amplification and persistence of the inflammatory state in chronic wounds. In addition to direct cell membrane and ECM protein damage, PMN-derived reactive oxygen species, such as superoxide, hydroxyl radicals, and hydrogen peroxide, can selectively activate signaling pathways leading to the activation of transcription factors that control the expression of proinflammatory chemokines and cytokines such as IL-1, IL-6, and TNF-α and proteolytic enzymes such as MMPs and serine proteases. Bacterial components, including formyl methionyl

peptides and extracellular adherence proteins, may also contribute to the upregulation of the inflammatory response.

The amount of normal wound ECM is determined by a dynamic balance among overall matrix synthesis, deposition, and degradation. A defining feature of chronic wounds is unbalanced activity that overwhelms tissue protective mechanisms. Although activated keratinocytes, fibroblasts, and endothelial cells have been shown to increase the expression of proteases, incoming neutrophils and macrophages are considered to be the source of proteases, particularly cathepsin G, urokinase-type plasminogen activator, and neutrophil elastase. The expression and activity of gelatinases (MMP-2, MMP-9), collagenases (MMP-1, MMP-8), stromelysins (MMP-3, MMP-10, MMP-11), and membrane-type MMP (MT1-MMP) are upregulated in chronic venous ulcers.

Proinflammatory cytokines are potent inducers of MMP expression in chronic wounds, also reducing TIMP expression, resulting in a relative excess of MMP activity. For example, α_1-proteinase inhibitor, α_2-macroglobulin, and components of the ECM, such as fibronectin and vitronectin, are downgraded or inactivated within chronic wounds. Growth factors, such as PDGF and VEGF, are also targeted when there is excess protease activity.

Other proposed causes for wound chronicity include keratinocyte hyperproliferation at the periphery resulting in inhibition of fibroblast and keratinocyte migration and apoptosis. Fibroblasts have altered morphologies, slower rates of proliferation, and less responsiveness to applied growth factors. The CD4/CD8 cell ratio is significantly lower in chronic wounds and is likely to be important in the pathogenesis of diabetic ulcers. Finally, chronic wounds have reduced levels of important growth factors (FGF, EGF, and TGF-β), likely secondary to degradation by excessive proteases or trapping by ECM molecules.

Chronically inflamed wounds are susceptible to neoplastic transformation. Squamous cell carcinoma (Fig. 23.9) was originally reported in chronic burn scars by Marjolin. Chronic osteomyelitis, pressure sores, venous stasis ulcers, and hidradenitis may also develop neoplastic change. Biopsies should be performed in cases of chronic wounds that appear clinically atypical. Cutaneous wounds may first exhibit pseudoepitheliomatous hyperplasia—a premalignant condition. Such a diagnosis on biopsy should prompt additional biopsies to exclude squamous cell carcinoma, which may already be present in other areas of the wound.

Nonhealing Diabetic Wounds

Diabetes mellitus impairs wound healing in several ways.[19] Diabetes-associated large vessel occlusion and end-organ microangiopathy each lead to tissue ischemia and infection. Diabetic sensory neuropathy leads to repeated trauma and unrelieved wound pressure. Tissue hypoxia can be demonstrated by reduced dorsal foot transcutaneous oxygen tension. The thickened capillary basement membrane decreases perfusion in the microenvironment, and elevated perivascular localization of albumin suggests increased capillary leak.[20] VEGF upregulation in patients with diabetes is also impaired. Hypoxia is normally a potent upregulator of VEGF, but cells from patients with diabetes do not upregulate VEGF expression in response to hypoxia.

Sensory neuropathy in patients with diabetes predisposes them to repeated trauma. They are susceptible to infection because of an attenuated inflammatory response, impaired chemotaxis, and inefficient bacterial killing. Infection further increases local tissue metabolism, placing an additional burden on the tenuous blood supply, amplifying the risk for tissue necrosis. Lymphocyte and leukocyte function are impaired. Collagen degradation is increased, whereas collagen deposition is impaired. Collagen is brittle secondary to glycosylation in the ECM. In addition, collagen glycation diminishes focal adhesion formation between fibroblast and matrix, resulting in decreased fibroblast migration.

Hyperglycemia causes increased advanced glycation end-products, which induce the production of inflammatory molecules (TNF-α, IL-1) and interfere with collagen synthesis. High glucose exposure also results in changes in cellular morphology, decreased proliferation, and abnormal differentiation of keratinocytes. Decreased chemotaxis, phagocytosis, bacterial killing, and reduced heat shock protein expression impair the early phase of wound healing in patients with diabetes. Altered leukocyte infiltration and wound fluid IL-6 characterize the late inflammatory phases of wound healing in these patients. Growth factors are abnormally expressed and degraded rapidly in wound fluids as a result of increased insulin-degrading enzyme activity. Insulin-degrading enzyme activity in wound fluid is positively correlated with hemoglobin A1c levels. Elevated MMP and reduced TIMP levels are seen in diabetic wounds in a pattern similar to chronic wounds. Finally, there is increasing evidence that resident cells in chronic wounds undergo phenotypic changes that render them senescent and impair their capacity for proliferation and movement.

Recent literature suggests genetic pathways that may play a role in the pathophysiology of diabetic ulcers and chronic nonhealing wounds.[20] Epigenetic alterations, including micro-RNA expression patterns, impair normal inflammatory mediator release; modulate macrophage, monocyte, and fibroblast function; and derange inflammatory response in diabetic wounds.[20]

Other Causes of Abnormal Wound Healing
Hypoxia

Molecular oxygen is essential for collagen formation. Ischemia secondary to cardiac failure, arterial disease, or simple wound tension prevents adequate local tissue perfusion. Under hypoxic conditions, energy derived from glycolysis may be sufficient to initiate collagen synthesis, but the presence of molecular oxygen is critical for posttranslational hydroxylation of the prolyl and lysyl residues required for triple-helix formation and cross-linking of collagen fibrils. Although mild hypoxia stimulates angiogenesis, this essential step in collagen fibril assembly proceeds poorly when partial pressure of oxygen (po_2) becomes less than 40 mm Hg. Optimal po_2 for collagen synthesis may be present at the periphery of the wound, but the center may remain hypoxic.

Smoking and consumption of tobacco products cause peripheral vasoconstriction and a 30% to 40% reduction in wound blood flow. Elevated levels of serum carbon monoxide inhibit enzyme systems necessary for oxidative cellular metabolism. Nicotine also inhibits platelet prostacyclin, promoting platelet adhesiveness, thrombotic microvascular occlusion, and tissue ischemia. Tobacco use inhibits endothelial cell and fibroblast function, NO synthase activity, VEGF production, fibroblast proliferation, collagen synthesis, and vitamin C levels. Studies in animals suggested that nicotine cessation for 14 days before flap surgery resulted in similar outcomes to controls, although most clinicians recommend

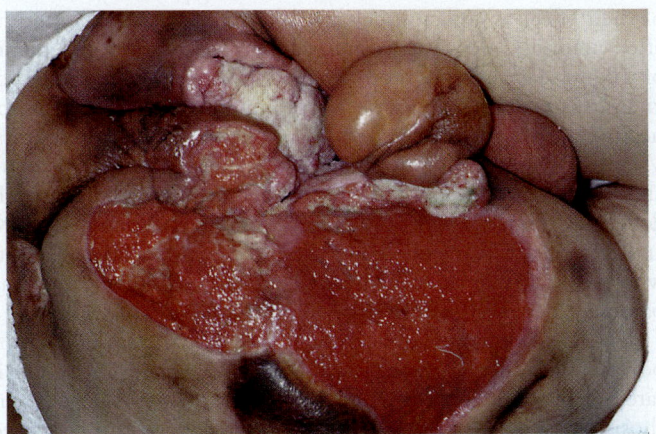

FIGURE 23.9 Squamous cell carcinoma in a chronic pressure sore.

complete smoking cessation in human patients for 4 to 6 weeks before elective procedures.

Ionizing Radiation

Ionizing radiation has its greatest effect on rapidly dividing cells in phases G_2 through M of the cell cycle. Injury to keratinocytes and fibroblasts impairs epithelialization and formation of granulation tissue during wound healing. Radiation injury in endothelial cells results in endarteritis, atrophy, fibrosis, and delayed tissue repair. Repetitive radiation injury results in repetitive inflammatory responses and ongoing cellular regeneration. Early side effects include erythema, dry desquamation, skin hyperpigmentation, and local hair loss. Late effects include skin atrophy, dryness, telangiectasia, dyschromia, dyspigmentation, fibrosis, and ulceration.[21–23] The inflammatory and proliferative phases may be disrupted by the early effects of radiation. Affected factors include TGF-β, VEGF, TNF-α, IFN-γ, and cytokines such as IL-1 and IL-8. These cytokines are overexpressed after the radiation injury, leading to uncontrolled matrix accumulation and fibrosis. NO, which induces collagen deposition, is decreased in irradiated wounds; this may explain the impaired wound strength seen in irradiated wounds. Decreased MMP-1 may contribute to inadequate soft tissue reconstitution (Table 23.2).

Keratinocytes, which are crucial for wound epithelialization, demonstrate a shift in expression from the high-molecular keratins 1 and 10 to the low-molecular keratins 5 and 14 after radiation injury. In nonhealing ulcers, these cells display decreased expression of TGF-α, TGF-β$_1$ FGF-1, FGF-2, KGF, VEGF, and hepatocyte growth factor (HGF). Expression of MMP-2, MMP-12, and MMP-13 has been shown to be elevated in irradiated human keratinocytes and fibroblasts. Fibroblasts play a central role in wound healing through deposition and remodeling of collagen fibers. However, in irradiated tissue, fibroblasts generate disorganized collagen bundles from dysregulation of MMP and TIMP. Because TGF-β regulates MMPs and TIMP, it may be of particular relevance to radiogenic ulcers (see Table 23.2).

Strategies for treating problematic radiogenic ulcers include standard wound care, negative-pressure wound therapy, nutritional optimization, and optimized blood and oxygen delivery. Hyperbaric oxygen (HBO) therapy may improve tissue oxygen partial pressure in the treatment of osteoradionecrosis via increased capillary density and more complete neovascularization.[21,24,25] HBO therapy is used clinically in patients with chronic diabetic ulcers and wound-healing complications after radiotherapy, and randomized clinical trials have demonstrated efficacy when HBO therapy was used in conjunction with standard wound care in cases of recalcitrant, diabetic, and potentially radiation-induced wounds.[25,26] In recent years, we have seen further investigation in this area. For example, Wu and colleagues[23] demonstrated improved wound healing with injection of adipose-derived stem cells, centrifuged adipose cells, and other products extracted from adipose matrix in an irradiated mouse model.

Aging

Older patients are more likely to experience delayed healing and surgical wound dehiscence. The aging epidermis has fewer Langerhans cells and melanocytes and flattening of the dermal-epidermal junction. Keratinocyte proliferation is reduced, and the turnover time is increased by 50%. The dermis has fewer fibroblasts, macrophages, and mast cells; reduced vascularity; and less collagen and fewer GAGs. There is a quantitative imbalance between collagen production and degradation and a qualitative alteration of the remaining collagen, which has fewer ropelike bundles and shows greater disorganization. Skin elasticity is decreased because of altered elastin morphology. Diminished light touch and pressure-reduced nociceptive receptors together with dermal atrophy increase susceptibility to injury by mechanical forces. Immunosenescence (reduced Langerhans cells and fibroblast activity) impairs wound healing and increases the likelihood of chronic wounds. Microvascular disturbances predispose to ischemic ulcers. Finally, there is reduced sebum secretion and vitamin D$_3$ production.

Dysregulation of ECM components, including MMPs, decreased reepithelialization, depressed collagen synthesis, impaired angiogenesis, and decreased growth factors (especially proangiogenic FGF-2 and VEGF) have been seen in elderly animal studies. Impaired macrophage activity (reduced phagocytosis and delayed infiltration) and impaired B-lymphocyte activity also have been demonstrated in animal studies. Zhao and colleagues[27] recently demonstrated the potential benefit in chronic application of antiaging agents, including metformin and resveratrol, via activation of the AMP-activated protein kinase pathway in an elderly animal study.

Malnutrition

Protein catabolism delays wound healing and promotes wound dehiscence, particularly when serum albumin levels are less than 2.0 g/dL. Protein supplements can reverse this deficiency.

Vitamin deficiencies affect wound healing primarily as a result of their effect as cofactors. Delayed healing can occur 3 months after vitamin C deprivation and can be reversed by supplements of 10 mg/day and no more than 2000 mg/day. Deficiency of vitamin A impedes monocyte activation and deposition of fibronectin, affecting cellular adhesion, and impairs TGF-β receptors. Vitamin A contributes to lysosomal membrane destabilization and directly counteracts the effect of glucocorticoids. Vitamin K deficiency limits the synthesis of prothrombin and factors VII, IX, and X. Vitamin K metabolism is impeded by antibiotics; patients who have chronic or recurrent infections need to have clotting parameters checked before surgical procedures are performed.

Zinc is a necessary cofactor for RNA polymerase and DNA polymerase. Zinc deficiency impairs early wound healing, but it is rare except with large burns, severe polytrauma, and hepatic cirrhosis. Iron deficiency anemia is a debatable cause of delayed wound healing. Although ferrous ion is a cofactor needed to

---

TABLE 23.2 Possible Key Wound-Healing Factors Affected by Radiotherapy With Respect to the Phases of Wound Healing

PHASE OF WOUND HEALING	FACTORS AFFECTED BY RADIATION THERAPY
Inflammation	TGF-β, VEGF, IL-1, IL-8, TNF-α, IFN-γ
Proliferation	TGF-β, VEGF, EGF, FGF, PDGF, NO
Remodeling	MMP-1, MMP-2, MMP-12, MMP-13, TIMP

EGF, Epidermal growth factor; *FGF,* fibroblast growth factor; *IFN-γ,* interferon-γ; *IL-1, -8,* interleukin-1, -8; *MMP-1, -2, -12, -13,* matrix metalloproteinase-1, -2, -12, -13; *NO,* nitric oxide; *PDGF,* platelet-derived growth factor; *TGF-β,* transforming growth factor-β; *TIMP,* tissue inhibitors of metalloproteinase; *TNF-α,* tumor necrosis factor-α; *VEGF,* vascular endothelial growth factor.

From Haubner F, Ohmann E, Pohl F, et al. Wound healing after radiation therapy: review of the literature. *Radiat Oncol.* 2012;7:162.

convert proline to hydroxyproline, reports are conflicting regarding the effects of acute and chronic anemia on wound healing. In general, patients should have a well-rounded diet consisting of adequate protein intake and caloric value plus vitamin and mineral supplementation.

Drugs

Some exogenously administered drugs directly impair wound healing. Chemotherapeutic agents, such as doxorubicin (Adriamycin), nitrogen mustard, cyclophosphamide, methotrexate, and bischloroethylnitrosourea, are potent wound inhibitors in animal models and interfere with uncomplicated wound healing clinically. They reduce mesenchymal cell proliferation, platelet and inflammatory cell counts, and availability of growth factors, particularly if given preoperatively. Tamoxifen, an antiestrogen, decreases cellular proliferation, with a decrease in wound-breaking strength that is dose dependent and may be secondary to decreased TGF-β production. Glucocorticosteroids impair fibroblast proliferation and collagen synthesis, resulting in decreased granulation tissue formation. Furthermore, steroids stabilize lysosomal membranes. More recently, Jozic and colleagues[28] demonstrated that steroids inhibit keratinocyte migration and proper wound healing by activating a Wnt-like phospholipase/protein kinase C signaling cascade, which is present in several types of cells, including the skin. This mechanism may shed more light on stress-induced cellular dysfunction and impaired wound healing, providing potential for future targeted therapies.

Administration of vitamin A can reverse this particular effect. Diminished wound-breaking strength caused by exogenous steroids is time and dose related. High doses of nonsteroidal antiinflammatory drugs have been reported to delay healing, but doses in the therapeutic range are unlikely to have an effect.

Treatment of Chronic Wounds and Future Areas of Research

The management of a chronic wound depends on its etiology.[29,30] Currently available therapies are slow, labor-intensive, and expensive without any guarantee of healing if all local and systemic factors are not addressed. Wound-healing research identified key structural proteins and molecules in normal and disordered wound healing as possible targets for future interventions. This research led to the application of topical growth factors to chronic wounds, which, although initially promising, almost universally failed to produce clinically significant improvements in wound healing. The reason for the failure is presumed to be a result of degradation of the growth factors by proteases in the wound fluid. This failure highlighted the complex nature of wound healing in which simply replacing one element is not enough.

Skin substitutes (discussed later) provide multiple factors that may alter the nature of the wound microenvironment in favor of and allowing healing to occur. Split-thickness skin grafting is the surgical substitution of native epidermis and partial dermis to assist wound closure, and it has a strong evidence base from treatment of acute burn wounds and chronic nonhealing wounds. Skin is harvested from the patient and transferred to an adequately prepared wound bed. The graft provides wound coverage by providing a favorable healing environment through exclusion of pathogenic bacteria and provision of ECM, cells (keratinocytes and fibroblasts), and bioactive molecules (cytokines, chemokines, and growth factors) that facilitate wound repair through a process of "dynamic reciprocity" (Fig. 23.10). However, autologous skin grafts occasionally are limited or unavailable. Biologic skin substitutes

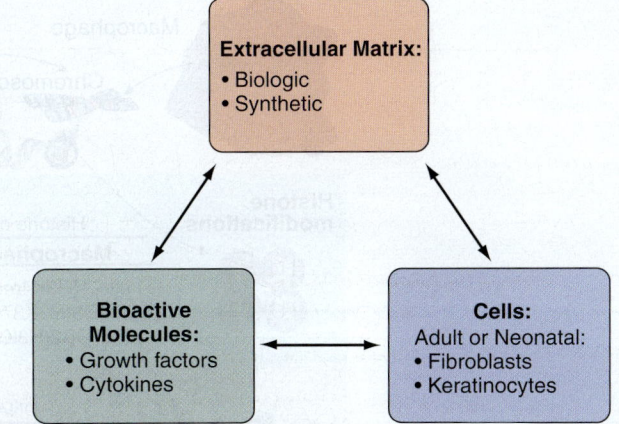

FIGURE 23.10 The "dynamic reciprocity" model of wound healing. Interactions are dynamic, as they vary with time and location within the wound site. Products of any one element influence the actions of the others. Inappropriate downregulation of any one element can result in conversion from an acute to a chronic wound. (From Greaves NS, Iqbal SA, Baguneid M, et al. The role of skin substitutes in the management of chronic cutaneous wounds. *Wound Repair Regen.* 2013;21:194-210.)

have been used for many years and include cadaveric skin allografts and porcine and bovine xenografts. These grafts are not durable because they do not integrate into the host, and they are associated with rejection and disease transfer. However, they provide adequate temporary wound cover, limiting complications until autologous grafts or other definitive management strategies are available.

Epigenetic Regulation of Cell Plasticity in Wounds

Different cell types can exhibit specific gene expression profiles leading to distinct functions and phenotypes caused by epigenetic modifications that control downstream protein expression patterns. Epigenetics is defined as heritable changes in gene transcription that are not caused by mutations or permanent changes in the genetic code. This is caused by modifications to chromatin that can lead to activation or silencing of genes. In steady-state conditions, genes are stably regulated, whether they are repressed or activated in a cell- or tissue-specific manner. However, under disease conditions, the epigenetic machinery can become dysregulated. Changes in the external stimuli, including toxic chemicals, environmental pollutants, diet, and others, can also contribute to epigenetic modifications.

There are three main types of epigenetic modifications: histone modification, DNA modification, and adenosine triphosphate (ATP)–dependent remodeling. The former two have been well studied in the context of wound healing.[31,32] Cell plasticity during tissue repair is partly regulated epigenetically and determines downstream reparative functions. Histone methylation and demethylation play critical roles in macrophage polarization during wound healing (Fig. 23.11). Methylation of a histone activates or represses transcription, depending on the number of methyl groups added and their location on the histone tail, and chromatin-modifying enzymes (CMEs) are responsible for this process. For example, methyltransferase mixed lineage leukemia-1 (MLL1) adds methyl groups to the histone 3 lysine 4 (H3K4) site, resulting in an open chromatin structure, promoting transcription of proinflammatory cytokines in macrophages.[33] In contrast, Setdb2 is a methyltransferase that adds a trimethyl group on the histone 3 lysine 9 (H3K9) site and renders the promoter region inaccessible

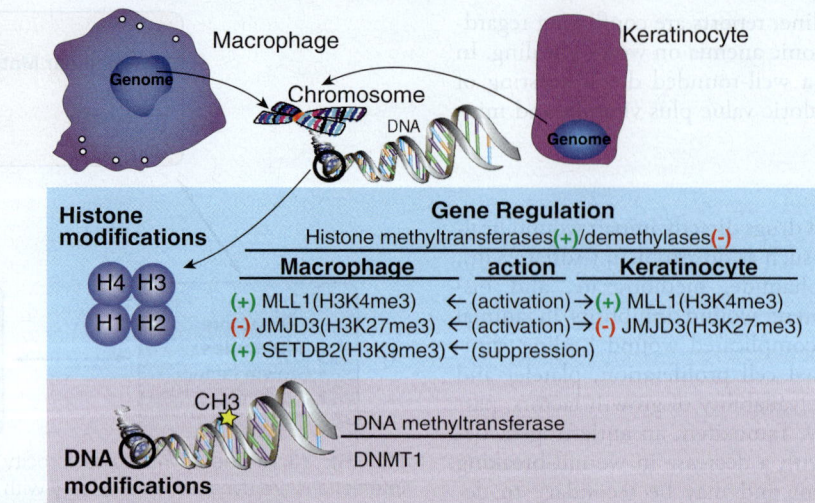

FIGURE 23.11 Epigenetic modifications that alter cells in wounds. Histone modifications associated with influencing macrophage and keratinocyte phenotypes. DNA modifications associated with influencing macrophage plasticity. Jumonji domain-containing protein *(JMJD)*; mixed-lineage leukemia *(MLL)*; SET domain bifurcated *(SETDB)*; DNA methyltransferases *(DNMT)*. (Adapted from Wolf SJ, Melvin WJ, Gallagher K. Macrophage-mediated inflammation in diabetic wound repair. *Semin Cell Dev Biol.* 2021;119:111-118.)

for transcription factor binding, silencing inflammatory gene transcription in macrophages.[1] Another CME that regulates macrophage inflammatory phenotype is histone demethylase Jumonji domain-containing protein D3 (JMJD3) that removes the repressive trimethyl group on the histone 3 lysine 27 (H3K27) site, resulting in opening of chromatin and increasing IL-6, TNF-α, and IL-1β transcription.[34] Expression and activity of these CMEs can be altered in a dysregulated state such as diabetic wound healing, leading to impaired transition of inflammatory macrophage (M1) phenotype to an immunoregulatory phenotype (M2).

Histone modifications also occur in structural cells like keratinocytes. JMJD3 regulates differentiation, proinflammatory cytokine, MMP, and growth factor gene expression in keratinocytes during early phases of wound healing.[35] Additionally, MLL1 activity in keratinocytes is critical for production of IFN-κ that induces early inflammation during tissue repair by polarizing macrophages toward an M1 phenotype.[4]

DNA methylation is predominantly associated with transcriptional repression and is regulated by DNA methyltransferases (DNMTs) that transfer a methyl group to the cytosine ring of DNA (see Fig. 23.11).[36] The methylation occurs at clusters of CpG islands in gene promoter regions, directly impeding transcription factor binding. DNMT1 and DNMT3b can activate macrophages and bone marrow progenitor cells to become inflammatory (M1), although their exact role in wound healing is unclear.[37,38]

Further investigation into specific upstream pathways of epigenetic regulation of wound-associated cells and their downstream functions may lead to development of cell-specific targeted therapies for pathologic wound healing.

WOUND DRESSINGS

Wound dressings—present since antiquity—evolved very little for many years until 1867, when Lister introduced antiseptic dressings by soaking lint and gauze in carbolic acid. Since then, numerous more sophisticated products have become available; however, certain characteristics in wound dressings should be considered in

---

BOX 23.2 Characteristics of an Ideal Dressing

Creates a moist environment
Removes excess exudate
Prevents desiccation
Allows for gaseous exchange
Impermeable to microorganisms
Thermally insulating
Prevents particulate contamination
Nontoxic to beneficial host cells
Provides mechanical protection
Nontraumatic
Easy to use
Cost-effective

Adapted from Morin RJ, Tomaselli NL. Interactive dressings and topical agents. *Clin Plast Surg.* 2007;34:643-658.

the nonsurgical treatment of a wound (Box 23.2). Wound healing is most successful in a moist, clean, and warm environment. Not all dressings can provide all of these characteristics, and not all wounds require all of them; hence, the choice of dressing should match the prevailing wound conditions.[29,30]

Two concepts that are critical when selecting appropriate dressings for wounds are occlusion and absorption. Studies have demonstrated that the rate of epithelialization under a moist occlusive dressing is twice that of a wound that is left uncovered and allowed to dry. An occlusive dressing provides a mildly acidic pH and low oxygen tension on the wound surface, which is conducive for fibroblast proliferation and formation of granulation tissue. However, wounds that produce significant amounts of exudate or have high bacterial counts require a dressing that is absorptive and prevents maceration of the surrounding skin. These dressings also need to reduce the bacterial load while absorbing the exudate produced. Placement of a pure occlusive dressing without bactericidal properties would allow bacterial overgrowth and worsen the infection.

Dressings can be categorized into four classes: (1) nonadherent fabrics; (2) occlusive dressings; (3) absorptive dressings; and (4) creams, ointments, and solutions (Table 23.3). Briefly, nonadherent fabrics are fine-mesh gauze supplemented with a substance to augment their occlusive properties or antibacterial abilities, such as scarlet red, a relatively nonocclusive dressing that is impregnated with *O*-tolylazo-*O*-tolylazo-β-naphthol that is used on skin graft harvest sites in burn care. Xeroform is a relatively occlusive, hydrophobic dressing containing 3% bismuth tribromophenate in a petrolatum base, which helps mask wound odors and has antimicrobial activity against *Staphylococcus aureus* and *Escherichia coli*.

Occlusive dressings provide moisture retention, mechanical protection, and a barrier to bacteria. These dressings can be divided into biologic and nonbiologic dressings. Examples of biologic dressings are allograft, xenograft, amnion, and skin substitutes. An allograft is a graft transplanted between genetically unique

TABLE 23.3 Types of Dressings

CATEGORY	COMPOSITION AND CHARACTERISTICS	FUNCTION	EXAMPLES	COMMENTS
Nonadherent fabrics	Fine mesh gauze with supplement to augment occlusive and nonadherent properties, healing-facilitating capabilities, and antibacterial characteristics	Protection, moist environment	Scarlet red, Vaseline gauze, Xeroform, Xeroflo, Mepitel, Adaptic, Telfa	Scarlet red, Xeroform, Telfa, Vaseline gauze—hydrophobic, more occlusive; Xeroflo, Mepitel, Adaptic—less occlusive, allow drainage of fluid into overlying dressing layers
Absorptive				
Gauze	Wide mesh gauze	Removal of exudates, prevention of maceration	Wide mesh gauze	Not effective when saturated; can be used for wound debridement if in contact with wound
Foams	Hydrophobic polyurethane sheets	Protection, absorption of exudate	Lyofoam, Allevyn, Curafoam, Flexzan, VigiFOAM	Advantages—comfortable, can expand and conform to wound, easily removed for cleansing Disadvantages—need to be replaced as wounds heal, custom shapes are labor-intensive to make, limited protection from bacteria, cannot be used while bathing
Occlusive				
Nonbiologic		Insulation, moisture retention, protective barrier acts against bacteria		
Films	Clear polyurethane membranes with acrylic adhesive on one side	See above	Tegaderm, Mefilm, Carrafilm, Bioclusive, Transeal, Opsite	Waterproof; permeable to oxygen, carbon dioxide, and water vapor; do not interfere with patient function; allow visualization of wound; nonabsorptive, can leak; require intact skin around wound area; wound contraction may be slowed; removal may disrupt new epithelium
Hydrocolloids	Hydrocolloid matrix (gelatin, pectin, carboxymethylcellulose)	As above; absorbs water from wound exudates, swells, liquefies to form moist gel	DuoDERM, Nu-Derm, Comfeel, Hydrocol, Cutinova, Tegasorb	Available as adhesive wafers, paste, powders; similar features as films, but bulkier; more protection, but may interfere more with function
Alginates	Cellulose-like polysaccharide fibers derived from calcium salt of alginate (seaweed)	As above; calcium alginate conversion to soluble sodium salt after contact with wound exudates results in hydrophilic gel	AlgiDerm, Algosteril, Kaltostat, Curasorb, CarraSorb, Melgisorb, SeaSorb, Kalginate, Sorbsan	Occlusive environment; various forms—ropes, ribbons, pads
Hydrogels	Polyethylene oxide or carboxymethylcellulose polymer and water (80%)	As above; rehydrating agents for dry wounds; little water absorption (high water content)	Vigilon, Nu-gel, Tegagel, FlexiGel, Curagel, Flexderm	Available as gels, sheets, impregnated gauze; occlusive environment
Biologic		Similar to nonbiologics		
Homograft	Derived from genetically unique humans		Cadaver skin	Temporary dressing; is rejected if left on wound for extended period
Xenograft	Interspecies graft (e.g., pig)		Pigskin	Same as above
Amnion	Human placenta			Good biologic dressing

Continued

TABLE 23.3   Types of Dressings—cont'd

CATEGORY	COMPOSITION AND CHARACTERISTICS	FUNCTION	EXAMPLES	COMMENTS
Skin substitutes	Different compositions		Integra, AlloDerm, Apligraf, Bio-brane, TransCyte	Integra—bilayered membrane skin substitute; AlloDerm—acellular cadaveric dermis; Apligraf—living, bilayered, biologic dressing composed of neonatal dermal fibroblasts on collagen matrix

Creams, Ointments, and Solutions

CATEGORY	COMPOSITION AND CHARACTERISTICS	FUNCTION	EXAMPLES	COMMENTS
Antibacterial	Different compositions	Used to treat infected wounds	Acetic acid (gram-negative, *Pseudomonas*); Dakin's solution (broad antibacterial spectrum); iodine-containing antibacterials (Iodosorb, Iodoflex, Betadine; broad antibacterial and antifungal spectrum); silver nitrate (broad antibacterial spectrum); mafenide acetate (Sulfamylon; broad antibacterial spectrum); silver sulfadiazine (Silvadene; broad antibacterial, antifungal, and antiviral spectrum); Acticoat (broad antibacterial spectrum)	Acetic acid—impairs wound healing; Dakin's—toxic to fibroblasts; iodine-containing solutions—toxic to fibroblasts, impairs wound healing; silver nitrate—treats burns, slows epithelialization, hyponatremia, stains clothes black; mafenide acetate—penetrates eschar, painful application, inhibits reepithelialization, carbonic anhydrase inhibitor; silver sulfadiazine—transient neutropenia, accelerates epithelialization of partial-thickness burns, neovascularization, commonly used for burns; Acticoat—silver-impregnated occlusive dressing, antibacterial activity lasts 3 days
Antibacterial ointments	Different compositions	Used to treat infected wounds; soothing to apply; lubricates wound surface; occlusive; antibacterial activity lasts 12 hours	Bacitracin (gram-positive cocci and bacilli); neomycin (gram-negative); polymyxin B sulfate (gram-negative); Polysporin (polymyxin B, bacitracin); Neosporin (polymyxin B, bacitracin, neomycin); triple-antibiotic ointment (polymyxin B, bacitracin, neomycin)	Neosporin—increased reepithelialization in experimental wounds by 25% compared with wounds with no dressing
Enzymatic	Different compositions; uses naturally occurring enzymes	Removal of necrotic tissue	Sutilains (derived from *Bacillus subtilis*); collagenase (Santyl; derived from *Clostridium histolyticum*); papain (derived from vegetable pepsin)	Sutilains—digests denatured collagen; collagenase—digests denatured and native collagen; papain—effective against collagen in presence of cofactor containing sulfhydryl group; addition of urea doubles enzymatic action of papain
Other	Normal saline wet to dry gauze dressing	Removal of necrotic tissue		Nondiscriminating—necrotic and newly formed granulation tissue and epithelium removed; can be painful

Adapted from Lionelli GT, Lawrence WT. Wound dressings. *Surg Clin North Am.* 2003;83:617-638.

humans, whereas a xenograft is a graft, such as pigskin, transplanted between species. Allografts and xenografts are temporary dressings; both will be rejected if left on a wound for an extended period. Amnion is derived from human placentas and is another effective biologic wound dressing. Initially, these dressings were most often used in the treatment of burn wounds; however, they can be used as a temporary measure in other wounds.

Absorptive dressings are useful for wounds with a significant amount of exudate. Leg ulcers can produce 12 g/10 cm^2/24 hours of exudate. Examples include wide-mesh gauze, the oldest of this type of dressing, which loses its effectiveness when saturated and newer materials such as foam dressings, which provide absorbent qualities for removing large quantities of exudate and have a non-adherent quality to prevent disruption of newly formed granulation

tissue on removal. Examples include Lyofoam (ConvaTec, Skillman, NJ), Allevyn (Smith & Nephew, Largo, FL), and Curafoam (Kendall Company, Mansfield, MA). Wound healing beneath absorptive dressings appears to be slower than under occlusive dressings, possibly because of wicking of cytokines from the wound bed or decreased keratinocyte migration.

The final class of wound dressings consists of creams, ointments, and solutions. This is a broad category that extends from traditional materials such as zinc oxide paste to preparations containing growth factors. Various categories include dressings with antibacterial properties such as acetic acid, Dakin solution, silver nitrate, mafenide (Sulfamylon), silver sulfadiazine (Silvadene), iodine-containing ointments (Iodosorb), and bacitracin. Application of these products is indicated when clinical signs of infection are present or if quantitative culture demonstrates more than 10^5 organisms per gram of tissue.

The number of available wound products is constantly growing so that the surgeon must have information about available dressings to allow effective wound management (Box 23.3).

OTHER THERAPIES

Hyperbaric Oxygen Therapy

Wound ischemia is the most common cause of wound-healing failure. HBO therapy uses oxygen as a drug and the hyperbaric chamber as a delivery system to increase po_2 at the target area. HBO therapy is used for myriad disease processes, including bacterial infections, decompression sickness, improvement of split-thickness skin graft take, flap survival and salvage, acute thermal burns, necrotizing fasciitis, chronic wounds, hypoxic wounds, osteoradionecrosis, and radiation injuries. There is evidence for treatment of chronic diabetic ulcers and radiation-induced wounds.[29,30] Ischemia or tissue hypoxia (po_2 <30 mm Hg) significantly impairs normal metabolic activity and decreases wound healing by impairing fibroblast proliferation, collagen synthesis, and epithelialization. HBO therapy involves inhalation of 100% oxygen at 1.9 to 2.5 atmospheres (atm), which can increase tissue po_2 10 times higher than usual. A higher Pao_2 is sufficient to supply the tissue with all its metabolic requirements, even in the absence of hemoglobin; this elevated level lasts for 2 to 4 hours after termination of HBO therapy and induces synthesis of endothelial cell NO synthase as well as angiogenesis. Oxygen has been reported to stimulate angiogenesis, enhance fibroblast and leukocyte function, and normalize cutaneous microvascular reflexes.

A recent animal study analyzed the effects of HBO therapy on rodent cell metabolism, angiogenesis, and wound healing in diabetic wounds.[39] Experiments showed increased proliferation of stem cells, upregulated angiogenesis, and improved wound healing capacity. Additionally, this study demonstrates that a combination of HBO treatment and stem cell therapy has a synergistic effect and may open new horizons in treatment of nonhealing wounds.[39]

Evaluation of the vascular supply to the target area is essential, and revascularization before HBO therapy is an essential prerequisite. Patients will likely benefit from adjuvant HBO therapy if improvement in tissue oxygenation can be demonstrated in a hypoxic wound while breathing oxygen under hyperbaric conditions. Transcutaneous oxygen pressure ($tcpO_2$) is used to assess wound perfusion and oxygenation. A wound $tcpO_2$ less than 35 mm Hg in room air indicates a hypoxic wound. An in-chamber $tcpO_2$ of 200 mm Hg or more suggests potential benefit from HBO therapy.

HBO treatments for hypoxic wounds are usually delivered at 1.9 to 2.5 atm for sessions of 90 to 120 minutes each, with the patient breathing 100% oxygen during the treatment. Treatments are given once daily, five to six times per week, and should be given as an adjunct to surgical or medical therapies. Clinical evidence of wound improvement should be noted after 15 to 20 treatments.

Complications of HBO therapy are caused by changes in atmospheric pressure and elevated po_2. Middle ear barotrauma, ranging from tympanic membrane hyperemia to eardrum perforation, is the most common complication. Pneumothorax (particularly tension pneumothorax) is far less common but potentially life threatening. Other complications associated with increased po_2 include brain oxygen toxicity, manifested by convulsions resembling grand mal seizures; oxygen lung toxicity, resulting from damage from oxygen free radicals to lung parenchyma and airways and ranging from tracheobronchitis to full-blown respiratory distress syndrome; and transient myopia. Absolute contraindications to HBO therapy are (1) uncontrolled pneumothorax, (2) current or recent treatment with bleomycin or doxorubicin (potential aggravation of cardiac and pulmonary toxicity), and (3) treatment with disulfiram (increases risk of developing oxygen toxicity).

Older small-scale randomized clinical trials had demonstrated that HBO is a useful adjunctive therapy for diabetic ischemic foot ulcers and reduces the rate of extremity amputation. Thistlethwaite and colleagues[40] performed a double-blinded randomized study in patients with chronic venous ulcers that demonstrated that HBO therapy can improve refractory healing but that patient selection is important. Patients with hypoxic periwound margins should have 4 weeks of high-quality wound care to achieve a healthy wound bed and establish their wound healing trajectory.[40] A more recent multicenter randomized clinical trial (DAMO-2CLES study) in Europe showed improved rates of limb salvage and wound healing 12 months after initiation of treatment and amputation-free survival, but the results were not statistically significant.[41] A systematic review of the Cochrane Database in 2016 reviewed HBO therapy for chronic irradiated wounds and concluded that HBO therapy improves outcomes in patients who had undergone radiation in the head, neck, and anus and rectum area and reduces rates of osteoradionecrosis after teeth extractions.[25] However, the recommendations were based on small, underpowered studies, and further randomized studies were greatly needed to clarify the benefits of this costly therapy. These results, which concluded that HBO therapy may have promising results in chronic radiation-induced wounds, are consistent with a different systematic review by Borab and colleagues.[26] However, further evidence is required.

In 2016, the European Consensus Conference on Hyperbaric Medicine reviewed the available evidence on the effects of HBO therapy and concluded that it is indicated in open fractures with crush injury, prevention or treatment of osteoradionecrosis of the mandible, soft tissue radionecrosis (cystitis, proctitis), diabetic foot ulcers, and femoral head necrosis.[42] Additionally, the consensus agreed that there is weak evidence supporting the beneficial effects of HBO therapy in compromised skin grafts and flaps, ischemic ulcers, refractory osteomyelitis, extensive second-degree burns, and osteoradionecrosis to bones other than the mandible.[42]

Despite evidence suggesting potential benefit of HBO therapy on healing chronic wounds, its cost is high. Patients often travel long distances for daily treatments at great cost to themselves and their families. Although reported protocols for treatment of ischemic limb ulcers vary significantly, most involve a total cost of $15,000 to $40,000. HBO therapy is not recommended as a primary treatment for patients with uncomplicated diabetic or ischemic ulcers; however, in selected more complicated cases, HBO therapy may have a role.

Negative-Pressure–Assisted Wound Therapy

One of the most significant discoveries in wound management in recent decades was the improvement in wounds with negative-pressure–assisted wound therapy (NPWT) (Fig. 23.12). With this technology, the surgeon has options in addition to immediate closure of wounds (i.e., adjunctive therapy before or after surgery or an alternative to surgery in extremely ill patients).

Argenta and associates[43] originally described the use of negative pressure to assist in wound closure in 1997. By applying subatmospheric pressure to wounds, they demonstrated removal of chronic edema, an increase in local blood flow, and stimulation of granulation tissue. This technique may be used on acute, subacute, and chronic wounds. Additional studies demonstrated significant improvement in wound depth in chronic wounds treated with NPWT compared with wounds treated with saline wet-to-moist dressings. In addition, treatment with negative pressure results in faster healing times with fewer associated complications.[20,21,27]

The exact mechanism of the improvement in healing with NPWT has yet to be determined. Many investigators initially believed that the reason for increased wound healing is the removal of wound exudates while keeping the wound moist. As originally hypothesized by Argenta and associates,[43] with NPWT, there is a fivefold increase in blood flow to cutaneous tissues. Further studies showed an increase in capillary caliber and stimulated endothelial proliferation and angiogenesis. It is well known that increased bacterial loads result in slowed wound healing; however, despite increased wound healing with NPWT, it has been shown to result in increased bacterial counts. Other studies suggested that NPWT produces three-dimensional stress within the cells (microstrain) and across the whole area of the wound (macrostrain), resulting in changes such as increased cellular

proliferation and higher microvessel density. Evidence suggests that NPWT alters wound fluid composition by removing potentially deleterious proteinases and inflammatory cytokines, such as MMP-1, MMP-2, MMP-9, and TNF-α.[44]

Clinical benefits of NPWT have been demonstrated in randomized controlled trials and include a decrease in wound volume or size, accelerated wound bed preparation and granulation tissue formation, accelerated wound healing, improved rate of graft take, decreased drainage time for acute wounds, reduction of complications, enhancement of response to first-line treatment, increased patient survival, and decreased cost. More recent data have demonstrated improved outcomes in patients with diabetic wounds; ischemic ulcers; and complex vascular, abdominal, gynecologic, and other oncologic surgical wounds with or without contamination. Karam and colleagues[44] performed a randomized controlled trial including a total of 40 patients with diabetic nonhealing ulcers. Pretreatment and posttreatment biopsies were obtained after 10 days of continuous therapy, and molecular analysis was performed. Results demonstrated that NPWT led to significant downregulation of IL-1β, TNF-α, MMP-1, and MMP-9 and significant upregulation of VEGF, TGF-β1, and TIMP-1 compared with advanced wound care with dressing changes. The authors concluded that NPWT significantly increased growth factors, decreased inflammatory cytokines, and normalized MMP activity, enhancing wound healing.

In addition to the improved outcomes, this treatment represents a significant improvement in cost-effectiveness and has decreased length of stay after acute and chronic wounds. There have been reports of a 78% decrease in hospital stay and a 76% decrease in cost with NPWT. This cost decrease and effectiveness of wound treatment with NPWT have translated to home healthcare treatment of Medicare patients.

NPWT with instillation has been another recent development. Evolution of the technology of this novel treatment method has allowed for creation and use of open-cell foam sponge that allows for periodic instillation of the wound bed with sterile fluid, facilitating removal of thick exudate and infectious products. The duration and time interval between each instillation can be adjusted based on the requirements of the wound. Different solutions have been used for instillation, including normal saline and dilute Dakin solution. Kim and colleagues[45] performed a prospective randomized study and concluded that there was no difference in the effectiveness of normal saline and an antiseptic solution (0.1% polyhexanide plus 0.1% betaine) in the treatment of infected wounds. Another technologic improvement is the implementation of portable wound vacuum-assisted closure devices that are suitable for outpatient treatment. Additionally, the utilization of one-use disposable devices has become more popular recently. These devices do not require replacement of the dressing, typically last for a few days, and are particularly useful in the setting of incisional NPWT or treatment of relatively superficial wounds with low exudative fluid output.

FETAL WOUND HEALING

Fetal skin wounds heal rapidly without the scarring and inflammation characteristic of adult skin wounds. In adult cutaneous healing, dermal appendages (hair follicles, sweat and sebaceous glands) fail to regenerate. In addition, healed adult wounds have densely packed collagen bundles oriented perpendicularly to the wound surface, whereas collagen in uninjured and fetal skin retains a reticular pattern. Fetal wounds reepithelialize faster, with

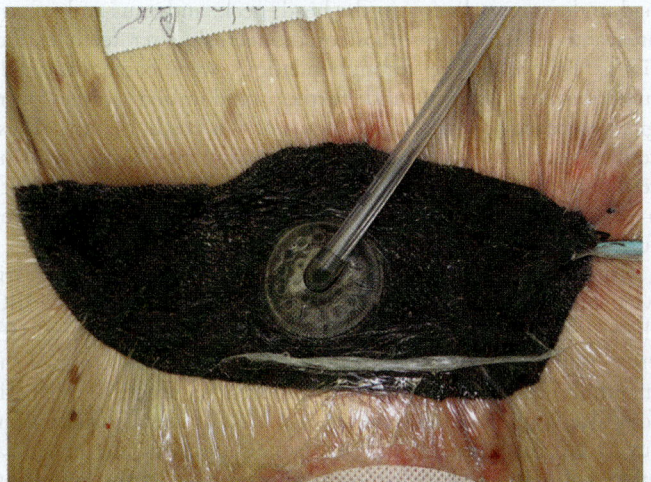

FIGURE 23.12 Negative-pressure–assisted wound closure sponge in place on a patient's abdomen.

less neovascularization and a faster increase in strength. Fetal wounds differ in inflammatory responses, ECM components, growth factor expression, and biologic responses to growth factor expression. It was thought that fetal wound healing represented ideal tissue repair and that understanding fetal wound healing would provide surgeons the tools to regulate and control the different steps in adult wound healing.[46,47]

Fetal repair depends on gestational age and wound size. The wound size threshold (diameter of excised skin at which 50% of wounds heal without scarring at a given gestational age) appears to be 6 to 10 mm for 60-day-gestation and 70-day-gestation animals and 4 to 6 mm for 80-day-gestation and 90-day-gestation animals. Larger wounds may extend the time to healing and expose wound tissue to a different ECM and growth factor profile. Larger excisional wounds may also stimulate the formation of myofibroblasts, resulting in scar formation. The transition from scarless to scarring repair occurs at the beginning of the third trimester. Wounds heal faster in a fetus than in a neonate, and they heal more slowly in adults compared with neonates.

Skin appendages are formed when dermal fibroblasts induce the epithelium to form hair follicles or glands. Wounds created early in gestation heal without scarring and with dermal appendages, suggesting tissue regeneration versus repair. In contrast, late-gestation wounds heal with scarring and without dermal appendages. The transition from scarless healing to healing without dermal appendages suggests that fetal fibroblasts lose their ability to induce the epithelium to form dermal appendages with advancing gestational age.

Extrinsic (amniotic fluid environment) and intrinsic (i.e., oxygen tension of the human fetus, differences in cellular receptor and growth hormone expression) properties between fetal and adult wound healing explain the difference in wound healing and scar formation.[47]

The fetal environment, an extrinsic difference between fetal and adult wounds, is characterized by a sterile hyaluronic acid–rich amniotic fluid with concomitant decreased inflammatory response. Additionally, the increased number of hyaluronic acid receptors and increased amount of hyaluronic acid may create a permissive environment in which fibroblast movement is facilitated, resulting in the increased rate and efficiency of fetal healing.

Much of fetal wound-healing research has recently focused on fetal fibroblasts and other intrinsic factors that are thought to play a more critical role. Fetal fibroblasts appear to have characteristics quite different from adult fibroblasts. Proline hydroxylation is a rate-limiting step in collagen synthesis by dermal cells. Early-gestation fetal human fibroblasts have increased prolyl hydroxylase activity that gradually decreases to adult levels after 20 weeks' gestation. Collagen types I, III, V, and VI appear earlier, and the ratio of type III to type I is greater in fetal wounds, which is consistent with the higher prevalence of type III collagen in normal fetal tissue. Fetal fibroblasts in vitro have higher collagen production than their adult counterparts. This higher collagen production may be secondary to the unique regulatory mechanism for prolyl hydroxylase and may explain why there is higher fibroblast activity in fetuses younger than 20 weeks' gestation.

Collagen synthesis decreases to adult levels after 20 weeks' gestation, and collagen degradation increases with gestational age. Increased gene expression of MMP-1, MMP-3, and MMP-9 correlates with the onset of scar formation in nonwounded fetal skin. These findings suggest that late-gestation fetal rat skin undergoes an adult type of tissue remodeling after wounding that leads to the scarring seen in adult skin.

There are also differences in the components of the ECM of fetal and adult wounds. After injury, fibronectin levels are similar in adults and fetuses, but tenascin, an inhibitor of fibronectin, increases earlier and returns to normal more rapidly in the fetus. Larger amounts of fibronectin in fetal wounds stimulate immediate cell attachment, whereas the more rapid deposition of tenascin in the fetus allows cells to migrate and fully epithelialize the wound more rapidly and decrease wound-healing time.

Hyaluronic acid is persistently elevated in fetal wounds. During gestation, decreasing levels of hyaluronic acid correlate with increasing scarring potential. The unique ECM composition of fetal tissues may influence collagen fibril deposition by facilitating cell mobility and migration, leading to the loose collagen pattern seen in healed fetal wounds as opposed to the dense collagenous pattern seen in adult scars. However, few studies have examined the effect of modifying the ECM components.

In addition, the fetus exhibits a reduced inflammatory response with a lack of neutrophil infiltration and decreased infiltration of endogenous immunoglobulins. The paucity of macrophages and a difference in the temporal appearance of macrophages in fetal wounds may explain differences in growth factor profiles and the reduced inflammatory response. These studies cite a direct correlation between increased macrophage recruitment in older fetuses and the development of increased scarring.

Fetal wounds have decreased levels of TGF-β and FGF-2. TGF-β is the growth factor that has been most extensively studied in fetal wound repair. Its production may be blunted in hypoxemic conditions, leading to the theory that the decreased oxygen tension in the fetal environment inhibits TGF-β production and results in decreased scar formation. It has been suggested that differential expression of the different TGF-β isoforms, rather than the presence of TGF-β, may be important in explaining the differences in repair.

Wnt signaling plays a significant role in embryogenesis and in multiple phases of wound healing.[46] This pathway is involved in tissue remodeling and repair, leading to scarring when dysfunctional. Several studies have also identified a link between Wnt signaling and TGF-β expression and function. Further insight into its mechanism of action and interaction with other pathways involved in wound healing may allow for therapeutic interventions toward decreased scarring and fibrosis.[46]

PDGF also disappears more rapidly in fetal wounds. The paucity of growth factors may be explained by decreased inflammatory cell recruitment. Normal inflammatory (adult-type) wound healing may have evolved to reduce the risk of infection at the expense of healing quality. Growth factor manipulation to make wounds more fetal-like has failed to result in completely scarless healing and has failed to regenerate dermal appendages. Other growth factors and cytokines have been proposed to play a role in fetal healing, including IGF, EGF, migration stimulation factor, TNF-α, and IL-1β.

The presence of myofibroblasts and concurrent scar formation suggests that a transition in fibroblast phenotype may contribute to scarring. Excisional wounds in 75-day-gestation fetal lambs showed an absence of scar formation and alpha smooth muscle actin expression. Alpha smooth muscle actin appears after 100 days of gestation along with scar formation.

Additional recent findings have highlighted the role of multiple pluripotent stem cells, such as epithelial stem cells, mesenchymal stem cells (MSCs), and "small dot" cells, in fetal wound healing. The slowly proliferating epithelial stem cells, which are interspersed throughout the basal layers, are surrounded by more quickly proliferating basal cells and their suprabasal progeny to form epidermal proliferative units. Epithelial stem cells are also found within the bulge area of hair follicles and are believed to migrate to the epidermis after injury and differentiate into dermal, vascular, and neural components.

MSCs play a role in regenerative healing, including immunomodulation, antifibrosis, antiapoptosis, and angiogenesis, and in preventing excessive inflammation. They immunoregulate through multiple independent pathways, including the induction of IL-10 secretion by macrophages. "Small dot" cells also have been identified to play a role in fetal wound healing. There is a twentyfold greater increase of these cells in fetal blood than in postnatal blood. Fluorescence-labeled "small dot" cells transplanted into a postnatal murine incisional wound model migrated to the wound bed and decreased scarring. Further investigations should help to elucidate the importance of these stem cell populations in fetal wound healing and in treating abnormal wound healing.

Finally, it has been shown that cells may lose their ability to replicate after certain stimuli, such as multiple cycles of duplication and exposure to subcytotoxic doses of exogenous stresses (e.g., ionizing radiation, oxidative agents, chemotherapeutic drugs, inflammatory cytokines), even though they remain metabolically active. This phenomenon is described as *cellular senescence*. Even though its role was initially identified to contribute to delayed wound healing in venous or diabetic ulcers, it is now believed that it may influence wound healing and tissue remodeling and potentially explain the differences between fetal and adult wound healing.[47]

Further investigations should help to elucidate the importance of these mechanisms and pathways in fetal wound healing and will allow for clinical application aiming to improve wound healing with decreased scarring (Table 23.4).[46,47]

TISSUE ENGINEERING

In 1987, the National Science Foundation bioengineering panel defined tissue engineering as "the application of the principles and methods of engineering and the life sciences toward the development of biologic substitutes to restore, maintain, or improve function." These principles and methods have been used in the creation of skin products made of cells, ECM components, or combinations of the two. This tissue-engineered skin has developed and progressed rapidly over the past 25 years, mainly driven by the limitations associated with autografts, and may function by providing the cellular or matrix components that could be necessary for wounds to heal. These new skin substitutes more accurately mimic native tissues to promote sustained healing without rejection. The use of biologic dressings, scaffolds, stem cell therapy, and gene therapy is an example of tissue engineering in which new tissues are created rather than transferred.

Bioengineered skin substitutes can potentially save millions of dollars a year in healthcare delivery services through reduced spending on dressings and treatment of wound-induced complications, particularly in the treatment of venous, diabetic, and pressure ulcers that form 90% of all chronic wounds. Bioengineered skin substitutes act as protective dressings by limiting bacterial colonization and fluid loss, but they also stimulate healing (Fig. 23.13).

TABLE 23.4	**Comparison of Fetal Regenerative Wound Healing Profile With Postnatal Wound Healing**					
	FETAL	**POSTNATAL**			**FETAL**	**POSTNATAL**
Phenotype	Regenerative	Scar formation		Type III collagen	High levels	Low levels
				Deposition	Immediate	Delayed
Growth Factors				Cross-linking	Low levels	High levels
bFGF	Lower	Higher		TGF-β$_1$–stimulated deposition	Absent	Present
PDGF	Lower	Higher				
VEGF	Higher	Lower		*Hyaluronan*		
TGF-β				Expression	High levels	Low levels
TGF-β$_1$	Low levels	High levels			Persistent expression	Transient expression
TGF-β$_2$	Low levels	High levels				
TGF-β$_3$	High levels	Low levels		Molecular weight	High	Low
				HA receptors (fibroblast)	High levels	Low levels
Inflammatory Response						
Inflammatory cell	Minimal	High levels leukocytes, macrophages, mast cells infiltrate		*Mechanical Force*		
				Myofibroblast (day 14)	Absent	Present
				Stem Cells		
Cytokines				MSC	High levels	Lower levels
Proinflammatory: IL-6, IL-8	Low levels	High levels		Dot cells	Present	Absent
Antiinflammatory: IL-10	High levels	Low levels				
Extracellular Matrix						
Collagen						
Histology	Fine, reticular weave	Thick, ropelike bundles				

bFGF, Basic fibroblast growth factor; *HA,* hyaluronan; *IL-6, -8, -10,* interleukin-6, -8, -10; *MSC,* mesenchymal stem cell; *PDGF,* platelet-derived growth factor; *TGF-β,* transforming growth factor-β; *VEGF,* vascular endothelial growth factor.
From Leung A, Crombleholme TM, Keswani SG. Fetal wound healing: implications for minimal scar formation. *Curr Opin Pediatr.* 2012;24:371-378.

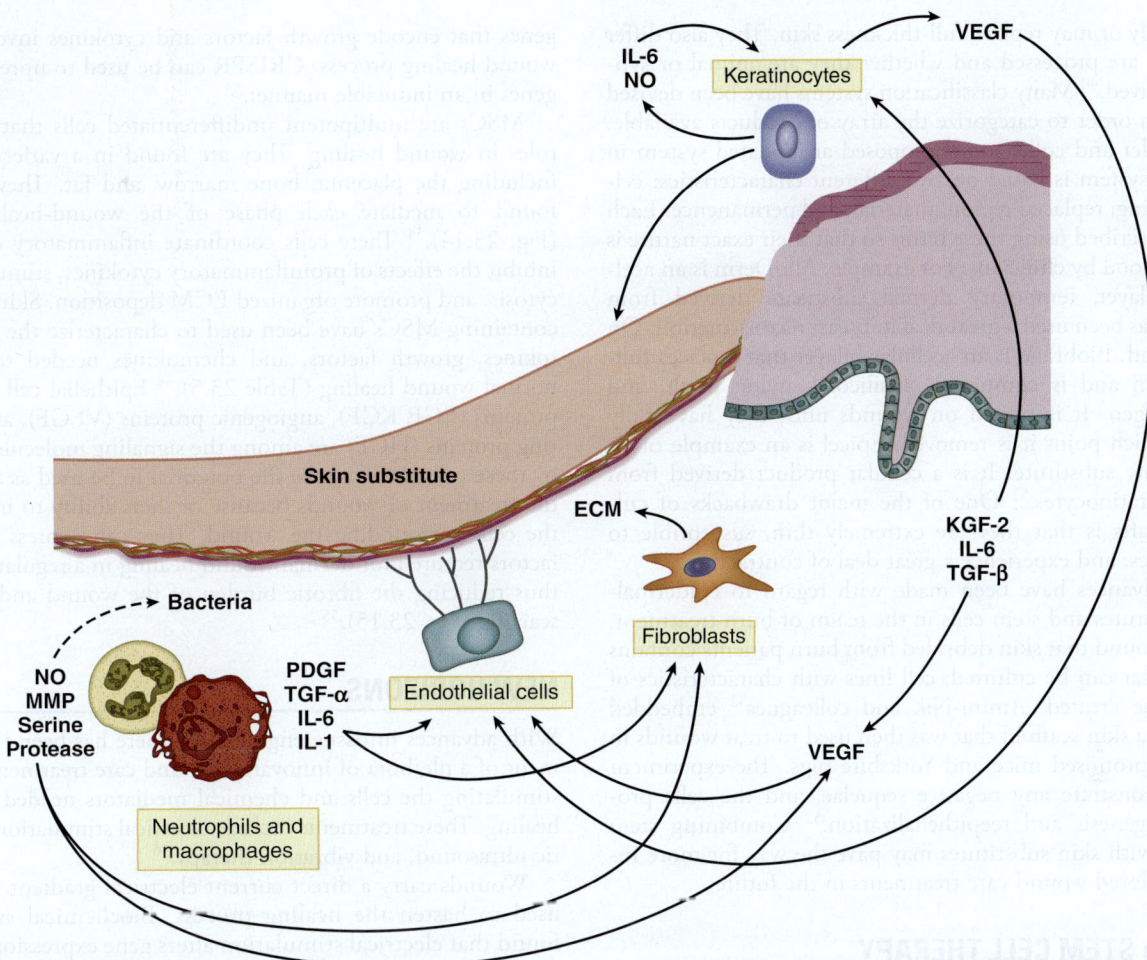

FIGURE 23.13 The effect of skin substitutes in the wound bed. Skin substitutes have variable structures and cellular content. They may be cellular or acellular, but both forms induce the influx of endogenous cells, including fibroblasts, keratinocytes, endothelial cells, macrophages, and neutrophils into the wound bed. These cells secrete various cytokines and growth factors that stimulate angiogenesis, extracellular matrix (ECM) deposition, and reepithelialization via the process of dynamic reciprocity. The skin substitute is replaced by native tissues, eventually resulting in a healed wound. *Solid lines* indicate upregulation, and *dashed lines* indicate downregulation. *IL-1,* Interleukin-1; *IL-6,* interleukin-6; *KGF-2,* keratinocyte growth factor-2; *MMP,* matrix metalloproteinase; *NO,* nitric oxide; *PDGF,* platelet-derived growth factor; *TGF-α,* transforming growth factor-α; *TGF-β,* transforming growth factor-β; *VEGF,* vascular endothelial growth factor. (From Greaves NS, Iqbal SA, Baguneid M, et al. The role of skin substitutes in the management of chronic cutaneous wounds. *Wound Repair Regen.* 2013;21:194-210.)

Their design is variable and dependent on the layer of skin they are designed to replace.

There are epidermal, dermal, and bilayer skin substitutes. Epidermal replacements are created by expansion of patient-derived keratinocytes in the laboratory.[48] These are fragile constructs that are attached to a carrier material to facilitate application to the wound. Dermal substitutes are based on a structural three-dimensional matrix material that behaves similar to ECM and may incorporate cells or bioactive molecules. Provision of these key factors to the wound bed may provide the necessary stimulus to rebalance the wound microenvironment in favor of healing. Bilayer materials represent a combination of features seen in epidermal and dermal models.

Skin substitutes can be used in the treatment of both acute and chronic wounds. This wide array of products has advantages and disadvantages. Some, such as Apligraf, are temporary, whereas others offer permanent wound coverage. However, like any medical device, a high cost is often involved. There is no one ideal skin substitute, making this an active realm of research.[48,49]

Although skin grafts can provide adequate permanent wound coverage, donor site morbidity, pain, scarring, and limitations in donor site locations have pushed researchers into the development of skin substitutes. One of the first major breakthroughs in tissue engineering for wound coverage was the development of Integra. Integra is a bilayer substitute containing a silicone outer layer and a deeper layer consisting of bovine cartilage and GAGs. The outer layer can be removed after 2 to 3 weeks of application, and a split-thickness skin graft can be applied over the dermal component. It can be used for burn wound coverage and can be directly applied to tendon and bone.[49]

Regenerative medicine is playing a key role in new advances in wound care and has provided for the development of many other skin substitutes; these products have been found to advance reconstructive outcomes. These substitutes may be epidermal only or dermal only or may replace full-thickness skin. They also differ on how they are processed and whether they are animal or synthetically derived.[50] Many classification systems have been devised in the past in order to categorize the array of products available. Davison-Kotler and colleagues[51] proposed an updated system in 2018. Their system is based on five different characteristics: cellularity, layering, replaced region, material, and permanence. Each product is described using these terms so that their exact nature is easily understood by clinicians. For example, AlloDerm is an acellular, single-layer, temporary dermal substitute derived from cadavers; it has been used a great deal in breast reconstruction. On the other hand, Biobrane is an acellular bilayer that replaces full-thickness skin and is composed of silicone, nylon mesh, and porcine collagen. It is placed on wounds until they have fully healed, at which point it is removed. Epicel is an example of an epidermal-only substitute. It is a cellular product derived from autogenic keratinocytes.[51] One of the major drawbacks of cultured autografts is that they are extremely thin, susceptible to shearing forces, and experience a great deal of contraction.

Recent advances have been made with regard to epidermal-dermal substitutes and stem cells in the realm of burn treatment. Researchers found that skin debrided from burn patients contains living cells that can be cultured; cell lines with characteristics of MSCs can be created. Amini-Nik and colleagues[52] embedded these cells in a skin scaffold that was then used to treat wounds in immunocompromised mice and Yorkshire pigs. The experiment did not demonstrate any negative sequelae, and the cells promoted angiogenesis and reepithelialization.[52] Combining stem cell therapy with skin substitutes may pave the way for more individually tailored wound care treatments in the future

GENE AND STEM CELL THERAPY

Gene therapy has applications in wound healing as well. The clustered regularly interspersed short palindromic repeats (CRISPR) system is used for gene editing. Originally a prokaryotic cell defense mechanism, this system has the potential to target human

genes that encode growth factors and cytokines involved in the wound healing process. CRISPR can be used to upregulate these genes in an inducible manner.[53]

MSCs are multipotent undifferentiated cells that play major roles in wound healing. They are found in a variety of tissues, including the placenta, bone marrow, and fat. They have been found to mediate each phase of the wound-healing process (Fig. 23.14).[54] These cells coordinate inflammatory cell activity, inhibit the effects of proinflammatory cytokines, stimulate phagocytosis, and promote organized ECM deposition. Skin substitutes containing MSCs have been used to characterize the array of cytokines, growth factors, and chemokines needed to carry out normal wound healing (Table 23.5).[54] Epithelial cell stimulatory proteins (EGF, KGF), angiogenic proteins (VEGF), and antiscarring proteins (HGF) are among the signaling molecules produced by these cells. MSCs have the potential to be used as a therapy in the treatment of wounds because of their ability to interact with the cells surrounding the wound. They can express the trophic factors required for dermal wound healing in a regulated manner, thus reducing the fibrotic burden of the wound and improving scarring (Fig. 23.15).[55]

NEW HORIZONS

With advances in tissue engineering, there has been the development of a plethora of innovative wound care treatments aimed at stimulating the cells and chemical mediators needed for wound healing. These treatments include electrical stimulation, therapeutic ultrasound, and vibration therapy.[56]

Wounds carry a direct current electrical gradient that can be used to hasten the healing process. Biochemical studies have found that electrical stimulation alters gene expression; this then affects the production of chemokines, cytokines, and collagen, promoting an environment favorable for healing.[56] Pathways activated by electrical energy include those of intracellular polyamines, the PI3K/PTEN pathway, and the KCNJ15/Kir4.2 membrane channel.[57] Nguyen and colleagues[58] found that

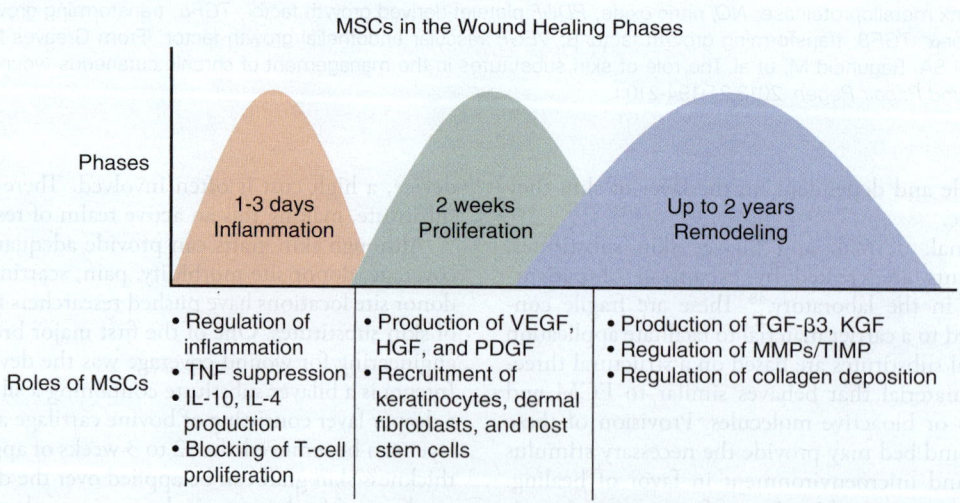

FIGURE 23.14 Mesenchymal stem cell *(MSC)* roles in each phase of the wound-healing process. *HGF,* Hepatocyte growth factor; *IL-4,* interleukin-4; *IL-10,* interleukin-10; *KGF,* keratinocyte growth factor; *MMPs,* matrix metalloproteinases; *PDGF,* platelet-derived growth factor; *TGF-β3,* transforming growth factor-β3; *TIMP,* tissue inhibitors of metalloproteinase; *TNF,* tumor necrosis factor; *VEGF,* vascular endothelial growth factor. (From Maxson S, Lopez EA, Yoo D, et al. Concise review: role of mesenchymal stem cells in wound repair. *Stem Cells Transl Med.* 2012;1:142-149.)

TABLE 23.5 Functional Classes of Wound-Healing Proteins in Human Mesenchymal Stem Cell–Containing Skin Substitutes

SPECIFIC PROTEINS	PRIMARY FUNCTION
MMP-1, MMP-2, MMP-3, MMP-7, MMP-8, MMP-9, MMP-10, MMP-13	Matrix and growth factor degradation, facilitate cell migration
TIMP-1 and TIMP-2	Inhibit activity of MMPs, angiogenic
Ang-2, HB-EGF, EGF, FGF-7 (also known as KGF), PIGF, PEDF, TPO, TGF-α, IGF	Stimulate growth and migration
bFGF, PDGF-AA, PDGF-AB, PDGF-BB, VEGF, VEGF-C, VEGF-D	Promote angiogenesis, also proliferative and migration stimulatory effects
TGF-β₃, HGF	Inhibit scar and contracture formation
IFN-α2	Prevent fibrosis by decreasing TGF-β₁ and TGF-β₂
α₂-Macroglobulin	Inhibit protease activity, coordinate growth factor bioavailability
Acrp-30	Regulate growth and activity of keratinocytes
IL-1Ra	Antiinflammatory
N-GAL	Antibacterial
LIF	Support of angiogenic growth factors
SDF-1β	Recruit cells to site of tissue damage
IGFBP-1, IGFBP-2, IGFBP-3	Regulate IGF and its proliferative effects

Acrp-30, Adiponectin; *Ang-2*, angiotensin-2; *bFGF*, basic fibroblast growth factor; *EGF*, epidermal growth factor; *FGF-7*, fibroblast growth factor-7; *HB-EGF*, heparin-bound epidermal growth factor; *HGF*, hepatocyte growth factor; *IFN-α2*, interferon-α2; *IGF*, insulin-like growth factor; *IGFBP-1, -2, -3*, insulin-like growth factor binding protein-1, -2, -3; *IL-1Ra*, interleukin-1 receptor antagonist; *KGF*, keratinocyte growth factor; *LIF*, leukemia inhibitory factor; *MMP-1, -2, -3, -7, -8, -9, 10, -13*, matrix metalloproteinase-1, -2, -3, -7, -8, -9, 10, -13; *N-GAL*, neutrophil gelatinase–associated lipocalin; *PDGF*, platelet-derived growth factor; *PEDF*, pigment epithelium-derived factor; *PIGF*, placenta growth factor; *SDF-1β*, stromal cell–derived factor-1β; *TGFα*, transforming growth factor-α; *TIMP-1, -2*, tissue inhibitors of matrix metalloproteinase-1, -2; *TPO*, thrombopoietin; *VEGF*, vascular endothelial growth factor.
From Maxson S, Lopez EA, Yoo D, et al. Concise review: role of mesenchymal stem cells in wound repair. *Stem Cells Transl Med.* 2012;1:142-149.

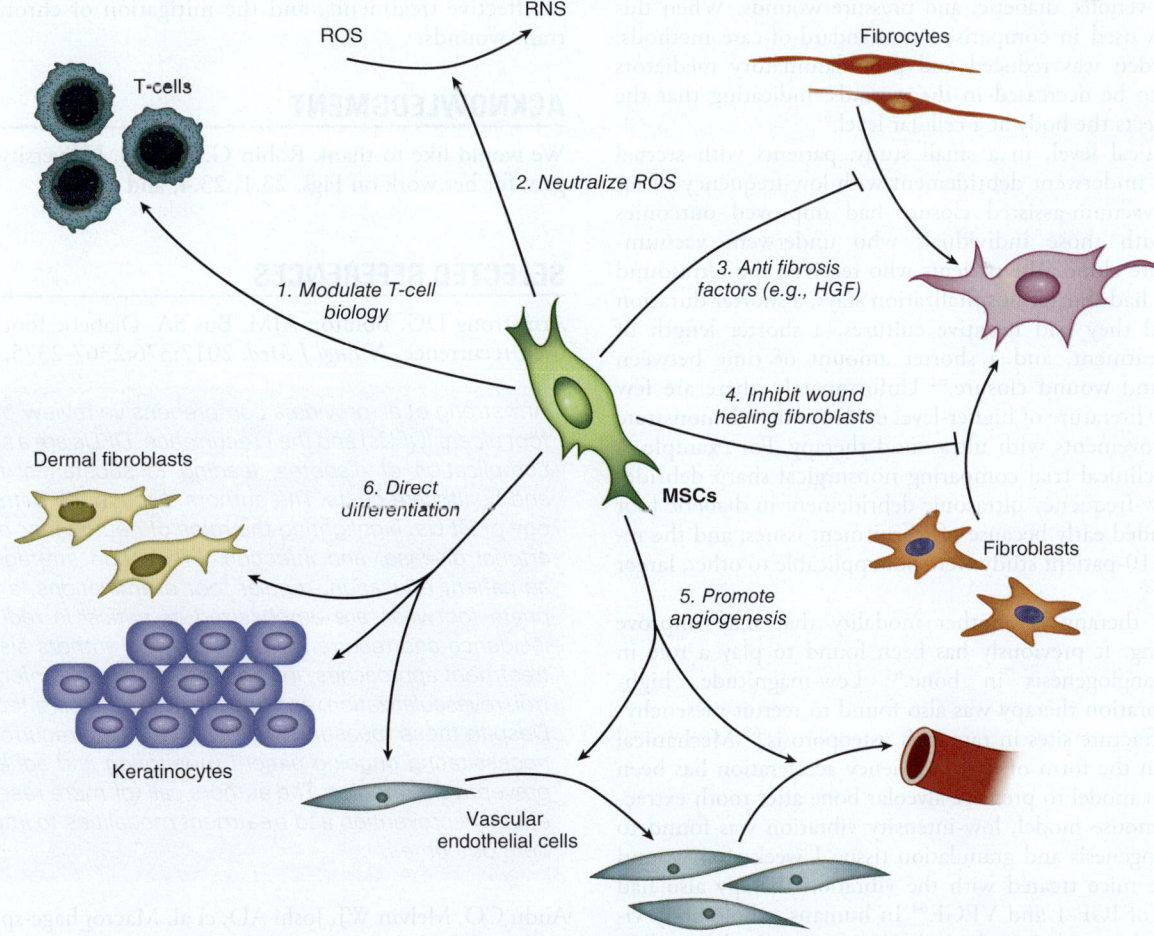

FIGURE 23.15 Mesenchymal stem cells *(MSCs)* can influence cutaneous regeneration by multiple distinct mechanisms acting on multiple cell types. *HGF,* Hepatocyte growth factor; *RNS,* reactive nitrogen species; *ROS,* reactive oxygen species. (From Jackson WM, Nesti LJ, Tuan RS. Mesenchymal stem cell therapy for attenuation of scar formation during wound healing. *Stem Cell Res Ther.* 2012;3:20.)

when human dermal fibroblasts are stimulated with electrical current in a bioreactor, collagen and MMP-1 levels increase within the cells.

Studies in humans have found that monophasic and biphasic pulsed currents have been effective, but microcurrents impregnated in dressings have not.[56] A pilot study conducted in a small sample of older adults with lower extremity pressure wounds found that patients treated with transcutaneous electrical nerve stimulation treatment plus standard wound care had significant improvements in pain and wound size, among other outcome measures, than standard wound care alone.[59] It is likely that electrical stimulation affects gene expression. When healthy volunteers were exposed to electrical stimulation via a small medical device over 2 days, the levels of expression of 105 genes were found to be changed; the majority had decreased protein production compared with before the treatment.[60]

Ultrasound, particularly kilohertz ultrasound, causes microstreaming and cavitation, which produces mechanical energy and alters the cell membrane through conformational changes in proteins and activation of signaling pathways in cells. It is believed that ultrasound therapy affects the proliferative phase of wound healing; among other effects, it increases macrophage activity and increases collagen production. Low-frequency ultrasound has been shown to decrease venous leg ulcer size in 4 weeks.[56]

Noncontact low-frequency ultrasound has been used in the treatment of venous, diabetic, and pressure wounds. When this modality was used in comparison to standard-of-care methods, bacterial burden was reduced and proinflammatory mediators were found to be decreased in the wounds, indicating that the treatment affects the body at a cellular level.[61]

On a clinical level, in a small study, patients with sternal wounds who underwent debridement with low-frequency ultrasound and vacuum-assisted closure had improved outcomes compared with those individuals who underwent vacuum-assisted closure alone. The patients who received the ultrasound debridement had shorter hospitalization stays, a shorter duration of time until they had negative cultures, a shorter length of antibiotic treatment, and a shorter amount of time between eradication and wound closure.[62] Unfortunately, there are few studies in the literature of higher-level evidence that demonstrate clinical improvements with ultrasound therapy. For example, a randomized clinical trial comparing nonsurgical sharp debridement and low-frequency ultrasonic debridement in diabetic foot ulcers was ended early because of recruitment issues, and the results of their 10-patient study were not applicable to other, larger populations.[63]

Vibration therapy is another modality that may improve wound healing. It previously has been found to play a role in promoting angiogenesis in bone.[64] Low-magnitude, high-frequency vibration therapy was also found to recruit mesenchymal cells to fracture sites in rats with osteoporosis.[65] Mechanical stimulation in the form of high-frequency acceleration has been found in a rat model to preserve alveolar bone after tooth extraction.[66] In a mouse model, low-intensity vibration was found to increase angiogenesis and granulation tissue 1 week after wound creation. The mice treated with the vibration therapy also had higher levels of IGF-1 and VEGF.[64] In humans, whole body vibration may play a role in reducing pain of extremity burns. Ray and colleagues[67] conducted a randomized pilot study in which patients with 1% or greater burns to at least one extremity were randomized to receive whole body vibration therapy or standard-of-care treatment during rehabilitation. The researchers found that patients who received the therapy had less pain during and after their therapy sessions.[67] Although this study did not demonstrate an impact of vibration therapy on wound healing directly, it did demonstrate a potential benefit in the overall well-being of patients with burn wounds. Whole body vibration therapy was also found in a small randomized study to mitigate bone loss in pediatric burn patients.[68]

In 2016, Ennis and colleagues[56] published a review of the current literature regarding these treatment modalities and found that most studies were underpowered and inconclusive. There is a paucity of Level I data for electrical stimulation and ultrasound-guided therapy. However, the strongest evidence exists for the use of electrical stimulation therapy. It is often used as an alternative treatment once others fail, but the evidence is mounting to indicate its use more readily. Much more work needs to be done regarding the efficaciousness of these treatments and how to use them in clinical practice, but this is an area of active research.[56]

As the 21st century continues to unfold, wound healing will continue to be a major area of innovation and discovery. The field provides for the intersection of genetics, molecular biology, stem cell therapy, bioengineering, and complementary/alternative medicine modalities. Advances in these fields will ultimately translate to improved patient outcomes, a wider array of effective treatments, and the mitigation of chronic, recalcitrant wounds.

ACKNOWLEDGMENT

We would like to thank Robin G. Kunkel, University of Michigan, for her work on Figs. 23.1, 23.4, and 23.11.

SELECTED REFERENCES

Armstrong DG, Boulton AJM, Bus SA. Diabetic foot ulcers and their recurrence. *N Engl J Med.* 2017;376:2367-2375.

Armstrong et al. provide a comprehensive review of diabetic foot ulcers (DFUs) and their recurrence. DFUs are a significant complication of diabetes, leading to substantial morbidity and healthcare costs. The authors discuss the pathophysiology of DFUs, highlighting the roles of neuropathy, peripheral arterial disease, and infection. Prevention strategies, such as patient education, regular foot examinations, and appropriate footwear, are emphasized as critical in reducing the incidence and recurrence of DFUs. The authors also outline treatment approaches, including debridement, infection control, revascularization, and advanced wound care techniques. Despite these measures, DFUs have a high recurrence rate, necessitating ongoing patient monitoring and adherence to preventive strategies. The authors call for more research into effective prevention and treatment modalities to improve patient outcomes.

Audu CO, Melvin WJ, Joshi AD, et al. Macrophage-specific inhibition of the histone demethylase JMJD3 decreases STING and pathologic inflammation in diabetic wound repair. *Cell Mol Immunol.* 2022;19(11):1251-1262.

Audu et al. explore the role of the histone demethylase JMJD3 (Jumonji domain-containing protein 3) in macrophage-mediated inflammation and its impact on diabetic wound healing. The activation of the STING (stimulator of interferon genes) pathway is responsible for production of type I interferons and other inflammatory mediators. STING is associated with chronic inflammation and is elevated in T2D wounds. The authors reveal that JMJD3 is crucial in regulating STING-mediated inflammation in macrophages by activating the expression of proinflammatory genes. JMJD3 removes the repressive trimethyl group around the histone 3 lysine 27 site of gene promoters, leading to increased gene transcription. However, JMJD3 expression is increased in the diabetic setting during late phases of healing, contributing to prolonged inflammation. Macrophage-specific inhibition of JMJD3 via treatment with macrophage-targeting lipid nanoparticles results in reduced pathologic inflammation in murine diabetic wounds and improved in vivo wound repair, supporting the therapeutic potential of targeting JMJD3 in diabetic wound healing.

Jiang Y, Tsoi LC, Billi AC, et al. Cytokinocytes: the diverse contribution of keratinocytes to immune responses in skin. *JCI Insight*. 2020;5(20):e142067.

This review by Jiang et al. explores the multifaceted roles of keratinocytes, termed cytokinocytes, in modulating immune responses in the skin. The authors provide a comprehensive overview of how keratinocytes contribute to both innate and adaptive immunity, highlighting their significance beyond their traditional structural role. Keratinocytes are described as active participants in the skin's immune system, capable of producing a wide range of cytokines and chemokines. These cells play a crucial role in initiating and regulating immune responses to pathogens, injury, and inflammatory stimuli. The study outlines the various ways keratinocytes contribute to immune responses, including antimicrobial defense, modulation of inflammatory processes, and interaction with other immune cells. Keratinocytes can influence the behavior of dendritic cells, T cells, and macrophages, thereby shaping the overall immune environment of the skin. The authors discuss the involvement of keratinocytes in the pathogenesis of various skin diseases, such as psoriasis, atopic dermatitis, and skin cancer. Dysregulation of keratinocyte-derived cytokines and chemokines can lead to chronic inflammation and immune dysfunction, contributing to disease progression. Understanding the immune functions of keratinocytes opens new avenues for therapeutic interventions in skin diseases. Targeting keratinocyte-specific pathways may offer novel strategies for modulating immune responses and treating inflammatory and autoimmune skin conditions.

Kimball AS, Davis FM, denDekker A, et al. The histone methyltransferase Setdb2 modulates macrophage phenotype and uric acid production in diabetic wound repair. *Immunity*. 2019;51(2):258-271.

Kimball et al. investigate the role of the histone methyltransferase Setdb2 in the regulation of macrophage phenotype and uric acid production during type 2 diabetic (T2D) wound healing. The authors explore how Setdb2 influences the inflammatory response and tissue repair mechanisms in the context of diabetes, a condition that significantly impairs wound healing. Setdb2 promotes the transition of macrophages from an inflammatory to an antiinflammatory phenotype, which is critical for resolution of inflammation and proper healing. Setdb2 regulates gene expression by adding methyl groups to the histone 3 lysine 9 (H3K9me3) site, which leads to condensed chromatin structure and decreased gene transcription. Kimball et al. reveal that Setdb2 is regulated via an upstream type I interferon/JAK/STAT mechanism in macrophages. In diabetic macrophages, type I interferons are decreased, leading to decreased Setdb2 expression, which increases inflammatory gene expression. Further, the authors demonstrate that Setdb2 plays a critical role in modulating production of uric acid, which is known to be elevated in T2D and associated with impaired healing. Therefore, the findings suggest that targeting Setdb2 could be a potential therapeutic strategy to improve wound healing in patients with diabetes. Modulating Setdb2 activity may help in reprogramming macrophages to enhance tissue repair and reduce chronic inflammation.

Na J, Lee K, Na W, et al. Histone H3K27 demethylase JMJD3 in cooperation with NF-κB regulates keratinocyte wound healing. *J Invest Dermatol*. 2016;136(4):847-858.

Na et al. investigate the role of the histone H3K27 demethylase JMJD3 in regulating keratinocyte-mediated wound healing, focusing on its interaction with the NF-κB signaling pathway. JMJD3 is identified as a crucial regulator of keratinocyte activity during the wound healing process. The authors revealed that JMJD3 cooperates with NF-κB to enhance keratinocyte functions in wound healing by regulating the expression of genes involved in inflammation, proliferation, and migration. Modulating JMJD3 activity affects the speed and quality of the wound healing process. Targeting JMJD3 or its regulatory pathways could offer new therapeutic approaches for enhancing wound healing, particularly in conditions where wound repair is compromised.

The full reference list appears on Elsevier eBooks+.

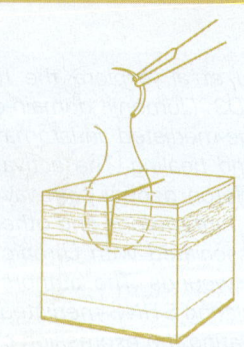

Surgical Site Infections

Melissa K. Stewart and Lillian S. Kao

INTRODUCTION

Surgical site infections (SSIs) are responsible for marked perioperative patient morbidity and mortality as well as increased healthcare utilization and cost. Generically speaking, an SSI refers to an infection related to an operation that occurs at or near an incisional site. SSIs are among the most prevalent of all healthcare-acquired infections, occurring in 0.5% to 3% of patients undergoing surgical procedures, and are the leading cause of readmission to the hospital after surgery.[1,2] It is noted that the presence of an SSI is associated with a twofold to elevenfold increase in the risk of mortality, with 75% of SSI-associated deaths directly attributable to the SSI.[3,4] SSIs are also the most costly of all hospital-acquired infections, with an estimated annual cost of $3.3 billion.[4,5] Given the impact of SSIs on patients and healthcare systems alike, SSI prevention is a high-priority goal. In fact, The Joint Commission includes SSI prevention guidelines as one of its National Patient Safety Goals, and the Centers for Medicare and Medicaid Services require hospitals to report SSI rates, which are publicly disseminated.

This chapter reviews epidemiology, pathophysiology, risk factors, preventive strategies, diagnosis, and management of SSIs.

DEFINITIONS AND EPIDEMIOLOGY

The Centers for Disease Control and Prevention (CDC) National Healthcare Safety Network (NHSN) and the National Surgical Quality Improvement Program (NSQIP) provide specific SSI definitions to allow for complete and accurate surveillance and epidemiologic assessment. The CDC definition of an SSI, which is also used by NSQIP, is an infection related to an operative procedure that occurs at or near the surgical incision within 30 days of a procedure, or within 90 days if prosthetic material is implanted at the time of surgery. Both the CDC NHSN and NSQIP classify SSIs into three groups based on the depth or tissue layer involved: superficial incisional, deep incisional, and organ/space deep to the incision. *Superficial incisional* refers to an infection involving the skin or subcutaneous tissue layers of the incision. Deep incisional infections involve the muscle or connective tissue layers of the incision. Lastly, organs/deep space infection describes an infection underlying the incision that involves tissue deep to the muscle or connective tissue layer that is opened or manipulated during the operative procedure (Fig. 25.1). Broadly summarizing, to be considered a superficial or deep incisional SSI, the site of infection must meet one of the following criteria: exhibit purulence, have positive cultures, or be deliberately opened or aspirated by a practitioner secondary to local signs of infection. To diagnose an organ/deep space infection, the patient must meet one of the following criteria: exhibit purulence from a drain within the organs/deep space, have positive cultures from fluid/tissue within the space, or have evidence of abscess or infection involving the organs/deep space on anatomic, histopathologic, or radiographic examination. Additionally, the infectious process must meet at least one criterion for specific organ/space infection as defined by the NHSN. The granular details outlining the criteria for diagnosis can be found in Table 25.1.[6]

As previously noted, SSIs are a significant source of patient and hospital-system morbidity. Although an incidence rate of 0.5% to 3% may not seem staggering, when accounting for the large number of operations performed annually in the United States, this quickly becomes a burdensome problem. Recent data would estimate that over 110,000 SSIs occur in the United States each year.[7] SSIs account for 20% of all hospital-acquired infections and are responsible for extending hospital length of stay by 9.7 days. This increased length of stay, in conjunction with additional required interventions, increases the cost of hospitalization by $20,000 per admission. This issue and the subsequent need for surveillance and intervention have been recognized by multiple national and international organizations. The CDC published surveillance and prevention guidelines for hospital-acquired infections in 1999, which were reviewed and updated based on recent evidence in 2017.[1,8] Similarly, the World Health Organization (WHO)

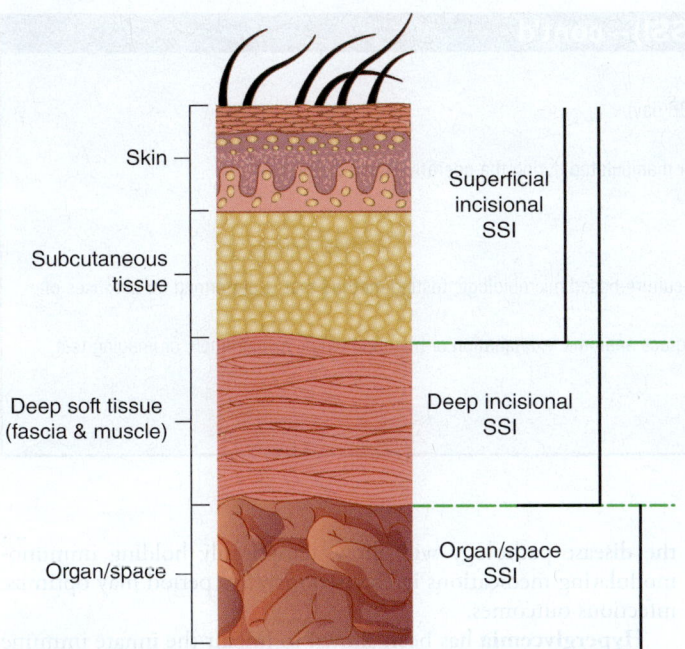

Skin

Subcutaneous tissue

Deep soft tissue (fascia & muscle)

Organ/space

Superficial incisional SSI

Deep incisional SSI

Organ/space SSI

FIGURE 25.1 Schematic of anatomic classification of surgical site infection *(SSI)*. (From Young PY, Khadaroo RG. Surgical site infections. *Surg Clin North Am.* 2014;94:1245-1264.)

published international guidelines for the prevention of SSIs in 2016, with updates published in 2018.[9] Additionally, the National Institute for Health and Care Excellence (NICE) published guidelines in 2019 predicated on the prevention and treatment of SSIs.[10] Despite these concerted global efforts to improve the incidence of SSIs, SSIs remain prevalent. In fact, because of their prevalence and importance, SSI data emerged as the leading publicly reported surgical outcome, and SSIs are tied to payment determinations.[11] As outlined earlier, the vital importance of understanding the intricacies of SSIs to allow for the optimization of patient care and the healthcare economy is evident.

RISK FACTORS AND PREVENTIVE STRATEGIES

Most simply stated, the acquisition of an SSI is dependent on bacterial exposure via an operative incision and the host response to control this bacterial contamination. Although this concept appears straightforward, the actual acquisition of an SSI is quite nuanced and is dependent on many factors, factors both specific to the patient and those related to the operative process.

Patient-Related Factors

Many host-specific factors have shown association with SSIs (Table 25.2). Identified factors include obesity, presence of immunosuppression, hyperglycemia, tobacco use, malnutrition, and

---

TABLE 25.1 Criteria for Surgical Site Infection (SSI)

Superficial Incisional:

Date of event occurs within 30 days after the operative procedure (day 1 = operating room [OR] date).

AND

Involves only skin and subcutaneous tissue of the incision.

AND

Patient has at least *one* of the following:
- Purulent drainage from the superficial incision.
- Organism(s) identified from an aseptically-obtained specimen from the superficial incision or subcutaneous tissue by a culture or non–culture-based microbiologic testing method that is performed for the purpose of clinical diagnosis or treatment.
- A superficial incision that is deliberately opened by a surgeon, physician, or physician designee, and culture or non–culture-based testing of the superficial incision or subcutaneous tissue is not performed.

AND

Patient has at least one of the following signs or symptoms: localized pain or tenderness, localized swelling, erythema, or heat.
- Diagnosis of a superficial incisional SSI by a physician or physician designee.

Deep Incisional:

Date of event occurs within 30 (or 90) days after the operative procedure (day 1 = OR day).

AND

Involves deep soft tissues of the incision (e.g., fascial and muscle layers).

AND

Patient has at least *one* of the following:
- Purulent drainage from the deep incision.
- A deep incision that is deliberately opened or aspirated by a surgeon, physician, or physician designee or spontaneously dehisces.

AND

- Organism(s) identified from the deep soft tissues of the incision by a culture or non–culture-based microbiologic testing method that is performed for purposes
of clinical diagnosis or treatment.

AND

- Patient has at least *one* of the following signs or symptoms: fever (>38°C), localized pain, or tenderness.
- An abscess or other evidence of infection involving the deep incision detected on gross anatomic examination, histopathologic examination, or imaging test.

TABLE 25.1 Criteria for Surgical Site Infection (SSI)—cont'd

Organ/Deep Space:

Date of event occurs within 30 (or 90) days after the operative procedure (day 1 = OR day).

AND

Involves any part of the body deeper than the fascial/muscle layers that is opened or manipulated during the operative procedure.

AND

Patient has at least **one** of the following:

- Purulent drainage from a drain placed into the organ/space.
- Organism(s) identified from fluid or tissue in the organ/space by a culture or non–culture-based microbiologic testing method that is performed for purposes of clinical diagnosis or treatment.
- An abscess or other evidence of infection involving the organ/space detected on gross anatomic examination or histopathologic examination, or imaging test evidence definitive or equivocal for infection.

AND

- Meets at least one criterion for a specific organ/space infection site.

TABLE 25.2 Patient-Related Factors Associated With Surgical Site Infection

Obesity[12]
Immunosuppression[13,14]
Hyperglycemia[15,16]
Tobacco use[18,19]
Malnutrition[20–23]
Staphylococcal colonization[26]

staphylococcal colonization. Knowledge of these factors is of utmost importance, for many are modifiable.

Obesity is thought to increase the risk of infection secondary to decreased delivery of oxygen, nutrients, and antibiotics through poorly vascularized adipose tissue. This pathophysiologic concept is clinically revealed in a myriad of studies across a multitude of surgical specialties. The data consistently show that rates of SSIs are positively correlated with increasing body mass index in a nearly dose-dependent fashion.[12] As such, regardless of operation type, it is prudent to discuss the expected effect of obesity on postoperative infectious complications. Further, if the case is elective and the disease pathology will allow, the patient may be better served by attempts at weight optimization before operative intervention.

Immunosuppression is postulated to lead to a dysregulated immune response that diminishes the inflammatory phase of wound healing, thereby inhibiting incisional healing and increasing the risk of infection postoperatively.[13] In the clinical realm, *immunocompromised* refers to a heterogeneous group of patients, including those with congenital conditions (T- or B-cell defect, macrophage dysfunction) and those with acquired conditions. Acquired conditions encompass the following pathologies: human immunodeficiency virus and acquired immunodeficiency syndrome; hematologic malignancy; and immune conditions, transplantation, or malignancy requiring the assumption of immunomodulatory drugs or chemotherapy. It is also well established that aging leads to immunosuppression secondary to remodeling and immunosenescence. Numerous clinical studies have established that the immunocompromised patient population has an increased risk of SSIs across most specialties.[14] Given the association, it is prudent to weigh and discuss the role of immunosuppression in postoperative infectious complications. Additionally, if

the disease pathology will allow, temporarily holding immuno-modulating medications in the perioperative period may optimize infectious outcomes.

Hyperglycemia has been shown to impair the innate immune response, thereby compromising wound healing. Thus, limiting perioperative hyperglycemia, in both diabetics and nondiabetics, is of utmost importance to promote healing and prevent SSI occurrences. Recent literature across a multitude of specialties demonstrates that patients who suffer from intraoperative and postoperative hyperglycemia are more likely to develop SSIs than those with normoglycemia.[15] Additionally, data support that it is more difficult to control perioperative blood glucose levels in diabetic patients who have poor blood glucose control preoperatively.[16] As such, it is likely prudent to optimize glucose management perioperatively to reduce the risk of SSI.

Tobacco use and abuse are associated with numerous postoperative complications, including SSI. Within the United States, >50 million adults use tobacco products.[17] The nicotine within the tobacco limits blood flow, thereby decreasing nutrient and oxygen delivery to the tissue. Moreover, tobacco limits the inflammatory response and alters collagen metabolism, both of which negatively affect wound healing and increase infection risk. Recent literature across varying surgical specialties confirms previously reported randomized controlled trials (RCTs) and concludes that tobacco use increases the odds of experiencing an SSI.[18] Despite this knowledge, it is unclear what duration of cessation is needed to neutralize the effect of tobacco on SSI. Frequently, 1 month of tobacco abstinence is recommended to mitigate the risk of tobacco use, primarily based on an RCT in 2003 that showed that the rate of SSI in smokers was double the rate of both nonsmokers and smokers who abstained from tobacco use for 4 weeks preoperatively.[19]

Malnutrition is also a known risk factor for complications and adverse outcomes after operative intervention, including SSIs. Surgery creates a state of insulin resistance, contributing to both hyperglycemia and protein catabolism. Patients with preoperative malnutrition are ill-equipped to fight catabolism and promote anabolism, a process that is vital to healing.[20] Much has been studied and written in this realm, not only detailing the increased risk of SSIs after operative intervention in malnourished patients but also the ability to improve outcomes in malnourished patients with nutritional intervention.[21–23] Given our knowledge, it is vital that patients are screened for malnutrition and available means are used to address malnutrition preoperatively.

Staphylococcal colonization before surgery is also thought to increase the risk of SSI, and nearly one-third of the population is colonized with *Staphylococcus aureus*. When reviewing microbial data, *S. aureus* is the leading cause of SSIs.[24,25] Many methods have been proposed for decolonization, including various intranasal antimicrobials and skin antiseptic agents. Although the literature is conflicting, decolonization has most convincingly been shown to lower the rates of SSIs caused by gram-positive bacteria in the orthopedic and cardiovascular realms.[26] As such, SSIs may be mitigated by screening and treating staphylococcal colonization in the preoperative time frame.

Procedure-Related Factors

Equally important as host factors, many procedure-specific factors have been shown to play a role in the development of SSIs (Table 25.3). Such factors include wound classification, perioperative antibiotics, skin preparation, intraoperative hypothermia, bowel preparation, surgical attire, oxygenation, blood loss or blood transfusion, preoperative hair removal, barrier device use, wound protector use, irrigation, wound closure method, fascial suture choice, and use of closing instrument. Like intrinsic factors, many of the noted extrinsic factors are modifiable and provide opportunities for intervention and subsequent improvement in clinical and economic outcomes.

Wound classification refers to the degree of contamination of the surgical wound at the time of the operation. The CDC and NSQIP stratify operative wound contamination into four groups: clean, clean-contaminated, contaminated, and dirty-infected (Table 25.4).[27] The classification of the wound is pertinent because it correlates with the risk of postoperative SSI. Clean wounds confer the lowest risk, approximating 1% to 5%. The risk increases with increasing contamination: clean-contaminated, 3% to 11%; contaminated, 10% to 17%; and dirty-infected, >27%.[8] Interestingly, 70% to 95% of all SSIs are found to be caused by the patient's endogenous flora.[28]

Antibiotic prophylaxis is recommended in all SSI prevention guidelines.[1,9,10] Such recommendations are supported by a scoping review that showed a decreased risk of SSI across all procedural wound classifications.[29] Antibiotics should be tailored to the skin- and viscus-specific organisms that will be encountered at the time of surgery. Comprehensive guidelines to guide antibiotic selection are provided by many medical and surgical societies, including the Infectious Disease Society of America.[30] Guideline

TABLE 25.3 Procedure-Related Factors Associated With Surgical Site Infection

Wound classification[8,27]

Antibiotic prophylaxis[29–32]

Skin preparation[33]

Thermoregulation[35–37]

Bowel preparation[38,39]

Operating room attire[40–43]

Oxygenation[44,45]

Blood loss/transfusion[46]

Hair removal[47]

Operative drapes/barriers[48]

Wound protectors[49–51]

Wound closure technique, suture, irrigation, tray change, and glove change[53–55]

TABLE 25.4 Operative Wound Contamination Stratification

Clean	Atraumatic
	No inflammation or infection encountered
	No break in sterile technique
	No entry into gastrointestinal, genitourinary, or respiratory tracts
Clean-contaminated	Controlled entry into gastrointestinal, genitourinary, or respiratory tracts without unusual contamination
Contaminated	Open, fresh, accidental wounds
	Major breaks in sterile technique
	Acute, nonpurulent, inflammation encountered
Dirty-infected	Old, traumatic wounds with retained devitalized tissue
	Existing clinical infection or perforated viscera

consensus is that antibiotics should be given within 60 minutes of the incision to optimize the concentration of the antibiotic within the tissue. Multiple studies have evaluated further narrowing the antibiotics window, but none has found a significant advantage to early or late antibiotic prophylaxis.[31] Additionally, it is recommended that antibiotic dosing be weight based and redosed at appropriate intervals to maximize effect. Guidelines globally recommend cessation of antibiotic prophylaxis when the wound is closed, which is primarily based on literature suggesting that additional doses of antibiotics do not mitigate SSI risk but do increase the risk of adverse events from antimicrobial therapy.[32]

Preparation of the skin overlying the operative site has also shown importance in limiting SSIs. Topical alcohol is favorable, given that it is highly bactericidal. Its activity, however, is limited in duration. As such, it is recommended that a combination of alcohol plus another antiseptic be used for operative site antisepsis. The two options that presently exist are chlorhexidine gluconate and povidone-iodine. Recent substantial evidence indicates that the risk of SSI is decreased when the surgical site is prepared with chlorhexidine gluconate rather than povidone-iodine.[33] As such, it is now standard that chlorhexidine + alcohol preparation be used for surgical site antisepsis unless contraindicated based on allergy, open skin, or exposed mucosa within the surgical site.

Intraoperative **thermoregulation,** specifically, prevention of hypothermia, has also long been implicated in SSI acquisition. It is thought that perioperative hypothermia results in vasoconstriction at the local tissue level, resulting in impaired tissue perfusion and decreased immune and inflammatory activity.[34] Studies across multiple surgical specialties have shown variable results in this realm. However, a recent meta-analysis showed that hypothermia, defined as temperature <36°C, is associated with an increase in SSIs.[35] Thus, further investigation has been ongoing regarding the best means to attain normothermia. Prewarming—that is, the act of using warming devices in the preoperative realm—shows promise in reduction of SSI.[36] The ideal methodology for intraoperative warming has also been studied. A recent systematic review and meta-analysis concludes that forced-air warming systems outperformed passive insulation. Further, an underbody forced-air warming system outperformed upper body and lower body forced-air warming systems.[37]

Bowel preparation in elective colorectal surgery has also been thoroughly questioned and studied. Although the data are mixed, recent large studies have shown its value. As such, many surgical society clinical guidelines recommend the use of bowel preparation when colorectal intervention is planned. Data would suggest that combining mechanical and enteral antibiotic bowel preparation results in fewer SSIs in comparison with no bowel preparation. Interestingly, mechanical bowel preparation alone has been shown to increase SSI.[38] On the contrary, enteral antibiotic bowel preparation alone is protective against SSI.[39] In sum, it seems that enteral antibiotic prophylaxis ± mechanical bowel preparation offers benefit to colorectal surgery patients in regard to postoperative infection risk.

The **attire** of the surgeon and accompanying medical staff within the operating room has long been thought to not only provide safety to the staff but also play an active role in operating room sterility and patient infectious outcomes. Surgical attire (e.g., scrub, surgical cap, beard cover) is felt to provide a barrier to microorganisms shed from healthcare workers' skin and hair, thereby protecting the patient from exogenous contamination and possible infection. Despite this long-held belief, there are limited data to support this argument. The Association of Perioperative Registered Nurses (AORN) Guidelines for Perioperative Practice outline recommendations for surgical attire. Notably, the Occupational Safety and Health Administration requires that grossly contaminated scrubs be removed immediately or as soon as possible and replaced with clean attire.[40] It is further recommended that reusable surgical attire be laundered within the healthcare facility to ensure the optimal temperature (>140°C) is met to kill many pathogenic organisms. Also of interest, the AORN conditionally recommends use of arm coverage when performing preoperative skin antisepsis. Although there is no evidence that associates SSIs with bare arms during skin antisepsis, there is evidence that squames shed from skin are aerosolized and settle on operative surfaces. As such, it is hypothesized that wearing long sleeves during high-risk tasks, such as skin antisepsis, may mitigate shedding and transfer of contamination.[41] Lastly, the AORN recommends that personnel cover the scalp, hair, and beard while in the operating room because moderate-quality data suggest hair carries bacteria. No recommendation regarding the type of head covers to be worn is given because no evidence indicates that the type of head covering or extent of hair covered is associated with SSIs.[42,43]

Surgical wounds are known to be poorly oxygenated, and low oxygen tension has been shown to be associated with SSI. Use of perioperative **hyperoxia** as a means to increase oxygen delivery and oxygen tension has been thoroughly studied. Hyperoxia has been broadly defined as 0.80 FiO_2. The data regarding the efficacy of hyperoxia on surgical infectious outcomes have been mixed; however, the most recent data suggest a protective effect of hyperoxia on SSIs in patients undergoing general anesthesia with tracheal intubation.[44] Importantly, the safety of hyperoxia has been studied, with the conclusion that use of hyperoxia is safe.[45] Based on its safety and likely contribution to SSI mitigation, current WHO and CDC guidelines support its use.[1,9]

Blood loss and need for allogenic blood product **transfusion** are also associated with SSI. Intraoperative blood loss without consideration of transfusion has shown an association with increased surgical infection risk. Is it postulated that blood loss leads to an increased risk of infection secondary to loss of circulating antibiotics within the serum, which become even further diluted by subsequent volume and blood product resuscitation. Perioperative transfusions are also thought to play a role in postoperative infections secondary to immunomodulating effects.

Clinical data would support these conclusions. Data reveal that red blood cell (RBC) transfusion is associated with increased risk of SSI in a dose-response relationship, with escalating risk of SSI with increasing transfusion need.[46] This knowledge undoubtedly informs perioperative care of patients and expectations regarding risk of SSI.

Removal of **hair** from the operative field has been a long-established practice of preoperative surgical preparation. If hair removal is necessary, data indicate that clippers should be used to remove hair from the site of operation. SSI risk is shown to be elevated if a razor or depilatory cream is used in place of clippers.[47]

Operative drapes or **barriers** are routinely used in surgery to isolate the operative field after skin preparation. It is thought that drapes and barriers protect the incision site from possible external contamination, hence limiting the opportunity for SSI. The type of barrier used—specifically, the use of plastic adhesive drapes with or without iodine or antimicrobial impregnation—has been evaluated in the literature. Although data on the topic are limited and show variable results,[48] national guidelines continue to recommend use of an iodophor-impregnated drape if a plastic adhesive is required and not otherwise contraindicated.[10] The use of **wound protectors** to exclude the abdominal wall and subcutaneous tissue from intraoperative contamination has also been studied. Data indicate improved infectious outcome with use of wound protectors across a multitude of studied patient populations.[49-51] Thus, use of a wound protector in intraabdominal surgery, specifically in clean-contaminated or contaminated fields, is likely useful in decreasing SSI risk.

The effect of **irrigation** and **wound closure** method on SSI rates has also been questioned and thoroughly researched. Specific questions of interest relate to the type of **irrigation**, **suture**, and **dressing** used. Additionally, the use and benefit of **closing trays** and **glove and gown change** before closure have been evaluated. Despite the existing research, there still exists much heterogeneity between providers on the best means to close an incision based on operation, contamination status, and clinical stability.[52] In regard to **wound closure,** there has been increasing interest in use of negative-pressure wound therapy (NPWT) overlying a closed incision. Recent sound data across most surgical specialties conclude that the use of prophylactic NPWT over a closed incision improved infectious outcomes across all contamination statuses.[53] Although not yet currently included in SSI prevention guidelines, NPWT over closed wounds should be seriously considered. In regard to **suture** type, much has been studied about the use of triclosan-coated sutures, that is, Vicryl or Polydioxanone suture coated with triclosan, an antimicrobial. Although the evidence is mixed,[54] multiple SSI prevention guidelines include the use of triclosan-coated suture. The use and type of **irrigation** and association with SSI have also been well studied. Intraoperative wound irrigation is thought to remove tissue debris, metabolic waste, and tissue exudate. Multiple meta-analyses in the past have shown reduction of SSI with irrigation; hence, irrigation is the standard of care. Many studies have subsequently evaluated the type of irrigant used and the effect on SSI. Much attention has specifically been paid to the efficacy of aqueous povidone-iodine as an irrigant. In fact, multiple guidelines recommend its use.[1,9] Despite these recommendations, the most recent evidence from both meta-analysis and RCTs has failed to prove its effectiveness.[55,56] The effect of **changing gown and gloves** before closing and the use of **clean instruments for closure** have also been well studied. A recent

RCT showed efficacy in routine sterile glove and instrument change at time of abdominal wall closure in clean-contaminated and contaminated cases.[57]

Enhanced Recovery After Surgery Protocols and Surgical Site Infections

Enhanced Recovery After Surgery (ERAS) protocols are multidisciplinary, multiphase pathways that have been developed to optimize patient outcomes based on available evidence. Although introduced over 30 years ago, the concept continues to gain momentum as the breadth of procedural protocols developed and studied continues to increase. ERAS protocols often combine preoperative, operative, and postoperative components, many of the very same components discussed within this chapter as factors associated with SSIs. Although many advantages of ERAS protocolization have been studied, one of the benefits is that of SSI reduction.

Many surgical specialties have trialed ERAS protocolization and have shown reduction in SSI rates. Colorectal surgery was among the first specialties to embrace ERAS pathways and study their efficacy. Many studies within the colorectal realm have shown benefit, and a comprehensive recent systematic review and meta-analysis similarly concluded that ERAS significantly reduced the incidence of SSI.[58] A plethora of additional studies in non–colorectal surgery patients—encompassing general surgery, obstetrics/gynecology, surgical oncology, orthopedics, thoracic surgery, and urology—have similarly concluded that ERAS use is associated with a decreased risk of SSI.[59–63]

Although the benefits appear to be clear, ERAS protocolization remains challenging to implement. The development, implementation, and data collection and analysis require significant resources. Additionally, protocolization often requires standardization among multiple providers and specialties, which often proves challenging secondary to resistance to change.

Surgical Site Infection Bundles

Before the energy and excitement around ERAS protocolization for improved perioperative outcomes, including infectious and noninfectious measures, much attention had been given to the idea of "bundling" interventions to mitigate risk of infectious complications. Like ERAS protocols, SSI bundles often combine multiple preoperative, operative, and postoperative interventions that have been proven or suggested to decrease infectious risk. SSI bundles continue to be used at facility and institutional levels in an effort to reduce infectious postoperative complications. Data have shown that implementation of SSI bundles decreases infectious risks, particularly when a high proportion of the components are evidence based.[64] However, like any quality improvement initiative, actualized improved outcomes are highly variable and dependent on buy-in and effective, widespread utilization.[65,66]

Safety Culture

Safety culture refers to shared perceptions of safety policies and practices within a team, unit, or healthcare institution. Per the Agency for Healthcare Research and Quality, a culture of safety encompasses acknowledgment of the high-risk nature of an organization's activities and the determination to achieve consistently safe operation, a blame-free environment where individuals are able to report errors or near misses without fear or reprimand or punishment, encouragement of collaboration across ranks and disciplines to seek solutions to patient safety problems, and organizational commitment of resources to address safety concerns.[67] Although it is logically assumed that a safety climate is predictive of safe outcomes, effects in the healthcare realm, specifically in relation to healthcare-associated infections, remain unclear.[68] Understanding how safety culture—that is, the reliable performance of evidence-based prevention practices—relates to successful infection prevention is of utmost importance because the data and evidence are only as meaningful as their implementation. A recently published analysis of 55 articles supports a positive relationship between safety culture, improvement in infection prevention and control processes, and decreased healthcare-acquired infections.[69] As such, it seems that the effort and resources spent on building and maintaining a culture of safety will likely lead to improved rates of SSIs.

DIAGNOSIS AND TREATMENT OF SURGICAL SITE INFECTIONS

SSIs tend to present like most other infections; that is, patients seek medical care secondary to experiencing symptoms of local infection: redness, warmth, swelling, wound drainage, pain, and/or wound-healing concerns. Additionally, patients may endorse symptoms consistent with systemic infection—namely, lethargy, fevers, chills, and night sweats. Lastly, patients may present with symptoms related to the body cavity, deep space, or organ space associated with the operation. For example, an intraabdominal/pelvic infection after laparotomy for a cecal volvulus may present with enteral intolerance or dysuria. Alternatively, a mediastinal infection after ascending aortic arch repair via sternotomy may present with heart palpitations, chest pain, or pain with inspiration.

The timing of onset and diagnosis of an SSI are variable and dependent on the operation type as well as the many perioperative factors previously discussed. Some patients may be diagnosed while still hospitalized from the index operation, whereas others will be diagnosed after discharge. Data suggest that patients undergoing laparotomy will present with an associated SSI at a median of 10 days postsurgery, with greater than 60% presenting postdischarge.[64,70] Thus, the use of technology to diagnose SSIs has been studied so as to potentially ease the patient burden of physically traveling to a care facility. Use of telemedicine only—that is, verbal communication without pictorial assessment—appears to be a feasible option across most locales and settings. However, data suggest that telemedicine-only postoperative assessment may lead to underreporting of SSIs and possible patient harm.[71] As a result, the use of remote assessment via patient-taken wound images and/or patient-generated health data has gained attention. Not only does this technology ease patient burden, but it allows for increased frequency of patient assessment. Increased oversight may lead to more timely identification of SSIs, thereby decreasing SSI-associated morbidity and healthcare use. Moreover, in the future, artificial intelligence will likely allow for automated patient assessment and diagnosis.[72]

If an SSI is suspected based on clinical history, a comprehensive physical examination is warranted. To allow for complete assessment, all surgical dressings should be removed. The incisional site should then be examined for objective features of local infection, such as rubor, calor, purulent drainage, and tissue necrosis. Additionally, the patient should be evaluated for evidence of systemic infection, primarily via vital sign assessment of temperature, heart rate, blood pressure, and respiratory rate. Lastly, the deep space associated with the operation should be evaluated. For example, a patient presenting with concern for an infection of their laparotomy incision after a sigmoidectomy for perforated diverticulitis warrants an examination of the abdomen, pelvis, and anorectum. Alternatively, a patient who underwent debridement of the right superficial posterior compartment of the lower leg with subsequent closure warrants a thorough examination of the lower extremity.

Based on the previously described examination, if concern exists only for superficial SSI, the incision will be often opened and drained, with microbiologic assessment of drainage via aerobic and anaerobic culture of the fluid. If the patient is exhibiting symptoms or signs of systemic and/or deep space infection, further investigation is often warranted via biochemical and radiographic studies. Pertinent laboratory evaluation often includes a complete blood count because an elevated white blood cell count may be indicative of infection. Inflammatory markers, C-reactive protein, and erythrocyte sedimentation rate are often elevated in the setting of infection and can be helpful diagnostically. If there is suspicion of deep-seated infection, ultrasound or cross-sectional imaging (CT scan/MRI) may yield diagnostic benefit.

The treatment of SSIs must be tailored to the type and severity of infection. Most SSIs will require initiation of antimicrobial therapy. Initiation of empiric antimicrobial therapy should be based on the likely causative organism. Both endogenous flora (the microbial makeup of the patient's skin, mucous membranes, and viscera) and exogenous flora (contamination via the operating room via air, instrument, materials, and staff) can be the causative source organism. The most common endogenous organisms implicated in SSIs are *S. aureus,* coagulase-negative staphylococci, *Enterococcus,* and *Escherichia coli.* The expected causative organism depends greatly on the procedure performed. In abdomino-pelvic operations, gram-negative bacilli and anaerobes are more common, whereas in orthopedic, cardiac, and vascular surgeries, the most common pathogens are *S. aureus* and coagulase-negative staphylococci. Additionally, when choosing empiric antibiotic therapy, it is also crucial to understand the local antibiotic resistance patterns as well as the patient's allergies, prior antibiotic exposure, and medical comorbidities. Once culture and sensitivity data return, the antibiotics should then be deescalated and tailored to the specific pathogen and its susceptibility profile. The duration of antimicrobial therapy is dependent on the source of the infection, the ability to attain adequate source control, and clinical response.

In addition to antimicrobial therapy, the management of SSIs often requires procedural intervention to attain source control. For superficial infections, removing sutures, staples, or topical glue is often required to allow for adequate drainage of the infection. Additionally, if devitalized or necrotic tissue is noted within the incisional wound, excisional debridement to healthy tissue is required. For deep incisional or organ space infection, drainage is often required via percutaneous or operative drainage with or without debridement. Regardless of modality chosen, the intention to liberate infection from a closed space is the same. If the superficial or deep space infection is noted to be in continuity with a foreign body (mesh, implant, metal), removal of that material, given concern for biofilm formation and

inability to clear infection, must be entertained. Lastly, in patients with signs and symptoms of systemic infection, the tenets of therapy for the management of sepsis and septic shock should be followed.

NOVEL EXPLANATION OF SURGICAL SITE INFECTION PATHOGENESIS AND THE MICROBIOME

As previously noted, it has long been postulated that SSI pathogenesis is secondary to direct incisional contamination in the perioperative period. Despite this widely held belief, the supportive evidence is weak. For instance, most pathogens that are causative of postoperative SSIs do not match cultures of the wound taken intraoperatively at the end of the case. As such, clinicians and researchers continue to explore alternative means of SSI pathogenesis. One such explanation is the Trojan horse hypothesis. This hypothesis is rooted in the idea that sterile postoperative wounds can become inoculated by a pathogen originating from a site remote from the operative wound. For example, pathogens from a site distant from the SSI location—such as teeth, gums, or gastrointestinal tract—can be taken up by immune cells, traverse to the operative site, and express virulence in parallel with inflammatory mediators (Fig. 25.2).[73] This hypothesis may provide clarity to the incongruency between operative incisional wound cultures and SSI causative organism as well as the emergence of SSIs at a time removed from the operation.

Given increased acceptance of the Trojan horse mechanism for SSI pathogenesis, the role of the microbiome in SSI acquisition is gaining attention. The microbiome is defined as all of the commensal and pathogenic bacteria, viruses, and fungi and their genes, gene products, community structure, and environment. The skin microbiome has always been implicated, studied, and discussed in the realm of SSIs because the skin microbiome is deemed responsible for local contamination of an incision perioperatively. Increasing interest is being paid to the impact of the intestinal and oral microbiome on distant incisional infections. It is now conceptualized and understood that the intestinal microbiome provides health-promoting influence beyond the intestine via intestinal epithelial receptors that communicate via dendritic cells with elements of the systemic immune system. As such, although not fully elucidated in the literature, it is postulated that the ability to predict infectious outcomes may be tied to the ability of the microbiome to refaunate and direct a recovery immune response. Many perioperative stressors have been shown to negatively affect the intestinal microbiome, for instance, surgical stress, lack of enteral nutrition, exposure to antibiotics, and use of opioids. As such, the quest to understand the molecular details and mechanisms behind SSIs and the potential association with the intestinal microbiome must continue. Similarly, it is thought that pathogenic strains of bacteria within the oral cavity can possibly be causative of the development of distant incisional infections. Similar to the gut, it is described that oral pathogens camouflaged within gum crypts can travel to the site of stress (i.e., operative incision) and release their infectious payload jointly with immune mediators needed for healing. Clinically, poor oral hygiene has been linked to an increased risk of SSI. Investigation continues to better understand the molecular mechanisms underlying this association.[74]

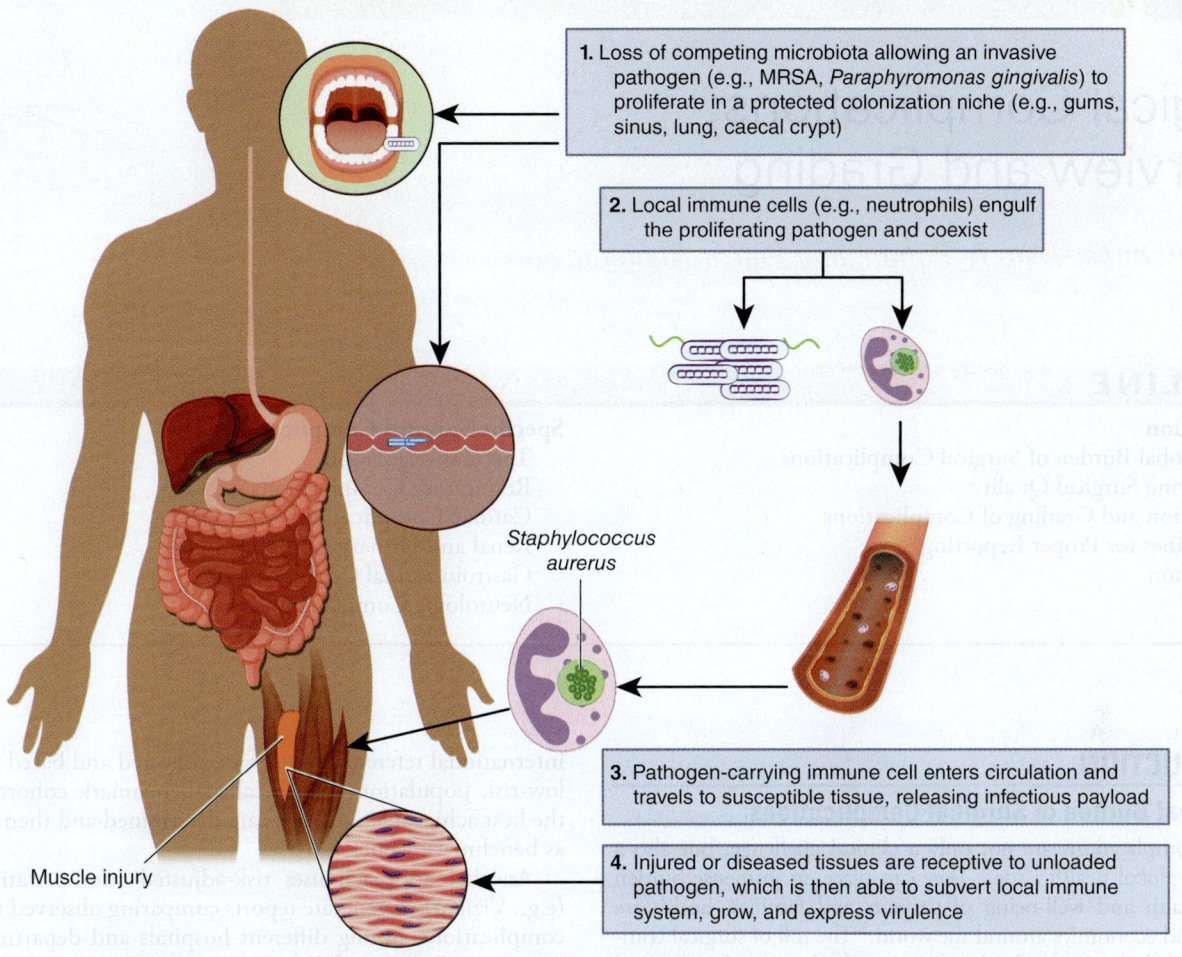

1. Loss of competing microbiota allowing an invasive pathogen (e.g., MRSA, *Paraphyromonas gingivalis*) to proliferate in a protected colonization niche (e.g., gums, sinus, lung, caecal crypt)

2. Local immune cells (e.g., neutrophils) engulf the proliferating pathogen and coexist

3. Pathogen-carrying immune cell enters circulation and travels to susceptible tissue, releasing infectious payload

4. Injured or diseased tissues are receptive to unloaded pathogen, which is then able to subvert local immune system, grow, and express virulence

Staphylococcus aurerus

Muscle injury

FIGURE 25.2 Trojan horse hypothesis. *MRSA,* Methicillin-resistant *Staphylococcus aureus.* (From Alverdy JC, Hyman N, Gilbert J. Re-examining causes of surgical site infections following elective surgery in the era of asepsis. *Lancet Infect Dis.* 2020;20:e38-e43.)

SELECTED REFERENCES

Berrios-Torres SI, Umscheid CA, Bratzler DW, et al. Centers for Disease Control and Prevention guideline for the prevention of surgical site infection, 2017. *JAMA Surg.* 2017;152:784-791.

This citation is the Centers for Disease Control and Prevention guidelines for the prevention of surgical site infections, which were published in 2017.

CDC. *National Healthcare Safety Network: Surgical Site Infection Event.* 2023. https://www.cdc.gov/nhsn/pdfs/pscmanual/9pscssicurrent.pdf

This citation is the most up-to-date Center for Disease Control National Healthcare Safety Network surgical site infection event protocol. It serves to describe and define surgical site infections as well as delineate the necessary surveillance and other aspects.

Agency for Healthcare Research and Quality, US Department of Health and Human Services. *Culture of Safety.* PSNet [Internet]. Rockville, MD: Agency for Healthcare Research and Quality; 2019 [Online]. Available from: https://psnet.ahrq.gov/primer/culture-safety

This citation is the National Institute for Health and Care Excellence guidelines for the prevention and treatment of surgical site infections, which were published in 2020.

Leaper DJ, Edmiston CE. World Health Organization: global guidelines for the prevention of surgical site infection. *J Hosp Infect.* 2017;95:135-136.

This citation is the World Health Organization global guidelines for the prevention of surgical site infections, which were published in 2017.

Seidelman JL, Mantyh CR, Anderson DJ. Surgical site infection prevention: a review. *JAMA.* 2023;329:244-252.

This citation is an updated analysis of surgical site infection prevention that amasses and reviews the available literature on associated patient and procedural factors.

The full reference list appears on Elsevier eBooks+.

Surgical Complications: Overview and Grading

Fariba Abbassi, Milo A. Puhan, and Pierre-Alain Clavien

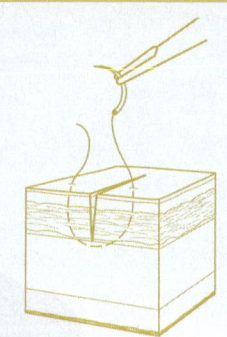

INTRODUCTION

The Global Burden of Surgical Complications

Surgical complications are not only a clinical challenge, but also a significant global health issue.[1] They can place an immense burden on the health and well-being of patients and families, healthcare systems, and economies around the world.[2] The toll of surgical complications includes not only the direct medical costs of prolonged hospital stays, additional treatments, and increased healthcare utilization, but also the indirect costs associated with lost productivity, increased caregiver burden, and long-term disability.

In high-income countries such as the United States, the additional health costs each year are estimated to be in the billions of dollars. In low- and middle-income countries, the burden of surgical complications is compounded by limited access to healthcare resources and infrastructure. Complications that may be preventable in well-resourced settings can have disastrous consequences in areas with fewer medical facilities and trained health workers.

Improving Surgical Quality

The awareness for cost and quality of surgical care has risen in recent years. The strong association between financial risks and complications may incentivize healthcare providers to select patients low risk of complications, also referred to as *cherry-picking*.[3] Consequently, comparison of quality indicators between centers should always be adjusted for the case mix of patients (i.e., the proportion of low-risk vs. high-risk cases), otherwise there is a danger of risk aversion, as providers may adopt avoidance strategies toward high-risk or complex cases.[4,5] To mitigate this risk, recently a novel approach called *benchmarking* was proposed to estimate the best achievable outcomes for a given surgical procedure.[6–8] Originally, benchmarking comes from the economic practice, and its concept appeals to most surgeons, which is striving for the highest possible level of performance, not just the average. The aim of benchmarking is to determine the best achievable outcome of a surgical procedure. For this purpose, data from international reference centers are collected and based on an ideal low-risk population, the so-called benchmark cohort, in which the best achievable outcomes are determined and then considered as benchmark values.

Another approach uses risk-adjusted administrative datasets (e.g., Vizient) to generate reports comparing observed to expected complications among different hospitals and departments.[9] The American College of Surgeons National Surgical Quality Improvement Program (NSQIP) collects individual patient data and reports institution-specific, risk-adjusted surgical outcomes.

Definition and Grading of Complications

The need for enhancing healthcare delivery has been on the rise, prompting the need for a standardized approach to assess and compare outcome quality across different institutions over time.[10] In the scientific literature, the incidence of postoperative complications was and still is one of the most commonly used parameters for the quality of surgery. However, the definition of surgical complications lacked a standard definition until the early 1990s. In 1992, Clavien and colleagues began to coin the term *adverse outcome* based on complications, failure to cure, and sequelae.[11]

Postoperative adverse events can be categorized into three groups. First, there is "failure to cure," signifying the intended outcome of an intervention was not achieved (such as the absence of curative resection for a malignant tumor). Second, there are "sequelae," where the unfavorable event is inherent to the procedure (for instance, amputation unavoidably leading to disability). Last, there are "complications," encompassing all other incidents.

A major barrier to reduce the burden of surgical interventions is the lack of standardized data on which to act, and even when available, data on postoperative outcomes are often of poor quality. The lack of consistent reporting is well documented in the medical literature.[1,12] Even the best surgical journals often fail to provide adequate information on postoperative events, for example, in defining the severity of complications or providing sufficient follow-up beyond hospitalization for a thorough evaluation.

TABLE 26.1 The Clavien-Dindo Classification

GRADES	DEFINITION
Grade I	Any deviation from the normal postoperative course without the need for pharmacological treatment or surgical, endoscopic, and radiological interventions. Allowed therapeutic regimens are drugs as antiemetics, antipyretics, analgesics, diuretics and electrolytes, and physiotherapy. This grade also includes wound infections opened at the bedside.
Grade II	Requiring pharmacological treatment with drugs other than such allowed for grade I complications. Blood transfusions and total parenteral nutrition are also included.
Grade III	Requiring surgical, endoscopic, or radiological intervention
IIIa	Intervention not under general anesthesia
IIIb	Intervention under general anesthesia
Grade IV	Life-threatening complication (including CNS complications)[a] requiring IC/ICU management.
IVa	Single organ dysfunction (including dialysis)
IVb	Multiorgan dysfunction
Grade V	Death of a patient

[a]Brain hemorrhage, ischemic stroke, subarachnoid bleeding, but excluding transient ischemic attacks.
IC, Intermediate care; ICU, intensive care unit.
From Dindo D, Demartines N, Clavien PA. Classification of surgical complications: a new proposal with evaluation in a cohort of 6336 patients and results of a survey. Ann Surg. 2004;240(2):205-213.

TABLE 26.2 The Accordion Severity Grading System

Expanded GRADES	DEFINITION
1 Mild complication	Requires only minor invasive procedures that can be done at the bedside, such as insertion of intravenous lines, urinary catheters, and nasogastric tubes, and drainage of wound infections. Physiotherapy and the following drugs are allowed: antiemetics, antipyretics, analgesics, diuretics, electrolytes, and physiotherapy.
2 Moderate complication	Requires pharmacologic treatment with drugs other than those allowed for minor complications (e.g., antibiotics). Blood transfusions and total parenteral nutrition are also included.
3 Severe: invasive procedures without general anesthesia	Requires management by an endoscopic, interventional procedure, or reoperation without general anesthesia.
4 Severe: operation under general anesthesia	Requires management by an operation under general anesthesia.
5 Severe: organ system failure	Organ system failure (i.e., ≥1 organ failure).
6 Death	Postoperative death (i.e., 100-day and in-hospital death).

Contracted GRADES	DEFINITION
1 Mild complication	Requires only minor invasive procedures that can be done at the bedside, such as insertion of intravenous lines, urinary catheters, and nasogastric tubes, and drainage of wound infections. Physiotherapy and the following drugs are allowed: antiemetics, antipyretics, analgesics, diuretics, electrolytes, and physiotherapy.
2 Moderate complication	Requires pharmacologic treatment with drugs other than those allowed for minor complications (e.g., antibiotics). Blood transfusions and total parenteral nutrition are also included.
3 Severe complication	All complications requiring endoscopic or interventional radiologic procedures or reoperation and complications resulting in failure of one or more organ systems.
4 Death	Postoperative death.

Adopted from Strasberg SM, Linehan DC, Hawkins WG. The accordion severity grading system of surgical complications. Ann Surg. 2009; 250(2):177-186.

To prevent harmful events after an intervention and allow for credible comparisons of competing therapies or care providers, standardized tools assessing both the positive and negative outcomes of a procedure are essential. Such tools must be relevant for patients and healthcare providers, as well as all other stakeholders within society, and must be widely accepted among various healthcare systems and cultures.

Efforts were made to categorize surgical complications before 1990, yet none of these gained widespread acceptance or popularity. In 1992, Clavien et al. not only defined the term *complication* but also introduced a standardized method to grade them. This so-called T92 classification system determines the severity of morbidity according to the therapeutic treatment used for complication management.[11] In 2004, Clavien and Dindo revised the fundamental T92 model, leading to the "Clavien-Dindo Classification," which consisted of five grades, two of which are each subdivided into two subgroups (Table 26.1).[13] Five years later the pioneers reevaluated this Clavien-Dindo Classification. Surgeons from seven international centers graded clinical complication scenarios according to the Clavien-Dindo Classification and achieved >90% agreement.[14]

In 2009 Strasberg et al. introduced the Accordion Severity Grading System for surgical complications.[15] This more complex grading system has the ability to cover a wider range of postoperative complications and exists in a contracted and expanded version. The main difference between the two is that the severe group gets split into three subgroups so that the contracted version has four levels, whereas the expanded version has six levels and is used for complex procedures like pancreatic or esophageal resections (Table 26.2). In addition, the proposed time frame for recording complications has been extended to 100 days after surgery.

Another classification system is the Memorial Sloan Kettering Cancer Center (MSKCC) Surgical Secondary Events System, which defines complications by organ systems and for oncologic-specific procedures.[16] It represents a modification of the Clavien-Dindo Classification with a focus on five tiered grades. The key distinction between the Clavien-Dindo Classification and the classification of the MSKCC lies in the criteria for grade IV. In 2004, Clavien's initial 4-grade classification was altered into a 5-grade system, introducing "Life-threatening complication requiring ICU management" as grade IV. In contrast, the modification of the MSKCC in 2001 included chronic disability as a grade IV criterion.

In 2011, the Japan Clinical Oncology Group (JCOG) challenged representatives from nine different surgical specialties to establish detailed criteria for the grading of each complication, consistent with the overarching principles of Clavien-Dindo Classification.[17] The resulting JCOG Postoperative Criteria (JCOG PC) includes a comprehensive set of 72 surgical adverse events commonly encountered in surgical practice. This specification and listing allow for straightforward classification.

A disadvantage of all these classification systems is that they require extensive tabulation of complication details, making it difficult to compare outcomes. In addition, many studies tend to focus only on the most severe complications, omitting those of lesser severity.[18] In response to this limitation, the Comprehensive Complication Index® (CCI®), based on the Clavien-Dindo Classification, was developed to assess the overall morbidity burden by including all complications experienced by an individual patient.[19,20] The creation of the CCI® explicitly took into account the patient's perspective by allowing the patient to assign weights to the respective complications. The CCI® provides a single measure, normalized on a scale from 0 (no complication) to 100 (death), that captures both the number and severity of complications. The validity of the CCI® has been confirmed by evaluation in several independent patient groups,[21,22] shows a strong correlation with costs,[23,24] and serves as a highly sensitive end point for randomized trials.[25,26] To facilitate the calculation

of the CCI®, a web application is available (https://www.cci-calculator.com). For illustration, some clinical scenarios are described in Box 26.1. The severity of the complication is indicated by the Clavien-Dindo Classification and the overall morbidity by the CCI®. The Clavien-Dindo Classification and the CCI® have become well-established metrics in surgery, widely adopted across various surgical disciplines globally. Both metrics have undergone various refinements and validations to enhance the quality of surgical outcome reporting. In 2024, the most significant refinement to date was performed. Based on an extensive comprehensive literature review and a survey among international surgeons, a core group of experts developed detailed recommendations on how to count and rate complications in scenarios that proved challenging over the years.[1]

Guidelines for Proper Reporting

The quality of patient care depends on the availability and use of standardized outcome measures, particularly when comparing competing treatment options or different care providers. The absence of standardized and universally accepted surgical end points has resulted in inconsistent, arbitrary, and frequently clinically inconsequential outcome assessments. This situation has paved the way for biased interpretations and has also impeded the improvement of healthcare quality.[18,27] In 2022 a major international effort brought different stakeholders such as patients, payers, and policymakers

---

BOX 26.1   Illustration of the Clavien-Dindo Classification and the Comprehensive Complication Index® With Clinical Scenarios

SCENARIOS	CD CLASSIFICATION	CCI®
A 45-year-old female presented with abdominal pain 24 hours after a cholecystectomy. The liver function tests were found to be abnormal with elevated levels of pancreatic enzymes. An ERCP was performed, and a gallstone was removed from the common bile duct.	Grade IIIa for choledocholithiasis	26.2
A 25-year-old female underwent appendectomy for perforated appendicitis. Postoperatively a deep vein thrombosis in the left leg was proven by phlebography, and full anticoagulation therapy was initiated on the ward. In addition, there was a severe paralytic ileus, which required prokinetic medication and parenteral nutrition.	Garde II for deep vein thrombosis, and grade II for paralytic ileus	29.6
A sigmoid resection was performed in a 56-year-old patient for acute diverticulitis. The patient developed fever and abdominal pain four days after surgery. A CT scan revealed an intraabdominal abscess, which was treated by relaparotomy. The patient was discharged 2 weeks after surgery without further complications.	Grade IIIb for abscess	33.7
A 63-year-old male underwent a right hemi-liver resection for a hepatocellular carcinoma. The patient complained about right upper quadrant pain and developed a fever on postoperative day 4. A CT scan revealed an infected biloma in the right upper quadrant, which was drained percutaneously. After successful drainage of the biloma, the patient became acutely dyspneic due to a significant pneumothorax. A thorax drain was inserted to treat the pneumothorax. Finally, a subcutaneous seroma in the area of the abdominal wound had to be relieved bedside.	Grade IIIa for biloma, grade IIIa for pneumo-thorax, and grade I for wound seroma	38.1
A 62-year-old patient developed severe liver failure following a right hemihepatectomy. The patient became encephalopathic and hemodynamically unstable and was transferred to the ICU. He developed transient kidney failure requiring dialysis. A urinary tract infection was treated by antibiotics. The patient fully recovered after 3 weeks in the ICU.	Grade IVb for multiorgan failure, and grade II for urinary tract infection	50.7
A 47-year-old patient underwent a Whipple's procedure for a pancreatic cancer. The postoperative observation at the ICU was uneventful and the patient was moved to the ward on postoperative day 1. After 4 days the fluid from a drain changed its color from serous to yellow. The fluid chemistry revealed a bilirubin of 500 μmol/L. The patient underwent a relaparotomy confirming the diagnosis of an anastomotic leak of the hepaticojejunostomy. The bile duct was reconstructed. The next day, the patient developed significant ascites and developed anuric kidney failure. For this reason, the patient was readmitted to ICU for hemofiltration. Due to increasing amount of ascites, a bedside ultrasound was performed, demonstrating absence of flow in the portal vein. A CT scan confirmed a portal vein thrombosis. The patient was treated with therapeutic anticoagulation, and the amount of ascites subsequently decreased and stopped. Finally, the drains could be removed. After 3 weeks' stay on the ICU the patient could be moved to the floor with restored kidney function.	Grade IIIb for relaparotomy, grade IVa for anuric kidney failure, and grade II for portal vein thrombosis	58.1

CD, Clavien-Dindo; *CCI®*, Comprehensive Complication Index®; *ERCP*, endoscopic retrograde cholangiopancreatography; *ICU*, intensive care unit.
From Dindo D, Demartines N, Clavien PA. Classification of surgical complications: a new proposal with evaluation in a cohort of 6336 patients and results of a survey. *Ann Surg.* 2004;240(2):205-213 and Slankamenac K, Graf R, Barkun J, Puhan MA, Clavien PA. The comprehensive complication index: a novel continuous scale to measure surgical morbidity. *Ann Surg.* 2013;258(1):1-7.

together with the aim of developing guidelines for standardized and improved surgical outcome reporting, considering developments made over the past decades. Based on extensive literature reviews and expert input, an independent jury offered a framework for outcome assessment and quality improvement after surgical procedures.[28] The core document, published in the journal *Nature Medicine,* recommends (1) the collection of outcome parameters at multiple, standardized time points perioperatively and postoperatively; (2) the routine use of patient-reported outcomes; (3) the assessment of global and individual morbidity using the Clavien-Dindo Classification and the CCI®; (4) defining benchmarks and comparing results between centers and over time; (5) appointing a "data quality guarantor" at each institution; and (6) following the TRACK principle of transparency, respect, accountability, continuity, and kindness in the event of unwarranted results. In the same year the Consolidated Standards for Reporting of Trials (CONSORT) statement published a CONSORT-Outcomes 2022 Extension,[29] which integrates outcome-reporting standards for clinical trials.

Reporting guidelines such as the CONSORT statement for randomized controlled trials (RCTs)[30] or the Preferred Reporting Items for Systematic Reviews and Meta-Analyses (PRISMA) statement[31,32] can greatly improve the reporting if the scientific community and journals adopt and, to some extent, enforce their use, as was already demonstrated.[33-38] A similar effort is now needed for outcome reporting after surgical interventions.

Education

In addition to developing and implementing our own evidence-based surgical practices, we must educate the next generation of surgeons on best practices and quality improvement to reduce complication rates in our patients. With this in mind, the Accreditation Council for Graduate Medical Education developed the Continuous Learning Environment Review program designed to provide teaching hospitals with feedback on their graduate medical education environment as it relates to patient safety, healthcare quality, care transitions, supervision, duty hours, and fatigue management and professionalism. In addition, the American College of Surgeons developed the Quality In-Training Initiative, which provides a detailed curriculum on quality improvement for surgical residents. These and other initiatives like the Milestones project that require resident involvement and engagement in the Improvement of Care practice domain should help trainees to develop the skills required to improve quality and reduce complications.

Surgical complication is an extensive topic. In this chapter we would like to give an overview of the most important postoperative complications, focusing in each case on the cause, diagnosis, and treatment.

SPECIFIC SURGICAL COMPLICATIONS

Thermal Regulation

Hypothermia

Maintenance of normothermia is important as even modest deviations in core body temperature contribute to metabolic alterations, resulting in cellular and tissue dysfunction. Hypothermia is a common complication in surgical patients and is defined as core body temperature below 35°C. It can be classified by severity into three categories: mild (32°C–35°C), moderate (28°C–32°C), and severe (<28°C). Vasoconstriction and shivering are the body's major thermoregulatory protective mechanisms, both of which may be impaired in the perioperative period. Risk factors for heat loss and perioperative hypothermia include elderly patients, burn injuries, open surgical procedures, cool operating rooms, prolonged surgeries (>4 hours), infusion of room-temperature fluids, cutaneous vasodilatation from anesthetic agents, and increased evaporative losses from serosal surfaces. Hypothermia can develop during any stage of surgery. Preoperatively, the use of muscle relaxants impairs shivering. Intraoperatively, heat loss occurs from large, exposed operative areas, anesthetic effects on heat production, cool room temperatures, vasoconstriction, and shivering.

Hypothermia impairs the function of many organ systems. Cardiovascular manifestations of hypothermia include cardiac depression, myocardial ischemia, dysrhythmias, peripheral vasoconstriction, impaired tissue oxygen delivery, blunted response to catecholamines, and hypotension. When the core temperature falls below 32°C, significant reductions in blood pressure and cardiac output occur. The characteristic electrocardiogram finding of J point elevation, and Osborn wave (notch and deflection at the QST-ST junction) are considered pathognomonic of hypothermia.

Mild core hypothermia results in immune dysfunction by impeding granulocyte chemotaxis and phagocytosis, macrophage function, and antibody production. These changes in immune function, in combination with decreased tissue oxygen tension, abnormal collagen deposition, and poor wound healing, increase susceptibility to infection.

Hypothermia also induces coagulopathy by attenuating hemostatic enzyme function and platelet sequestration, resulting in an increased risk of bleeding.

Patients at risk for hypothermia should be monitored frequently and every attempt should be made to maintain normal central core temperature. Continuous temperature monitoring and maintaining normothermia are essential during surgery as anesthesia, cool operating room environment, and significant evaporative cooling occurs during skin preparation making most surgical patients susceptible to hypothermia. Increasing the ambient room temperature, administering warmed IV fluids, covering patients with blankets, and using forced-air warming devices are commonly used techniques to prevent intraoperative hypothermia.

Postoperative Fever

Fever refers to an increase in the body's normal core temperature. Postoperative fevers can be broadly divided into infectious and noninfectious (systemic inflammatory response syndrome [SIRS]) causes (Table 26.3). Fevers are most often transient increases in temperature caused by the systemic inflammatory stimuli as a normal response to injury (including surgery). However, fever can also be an early sign of potentially life-threatening infection.

The timing of fever onset provides an important diagnostic clue. Immediate postoperative fever occurring within the first 48 hours after surgery is most likely due to proinflammatory mediators. They cause a cascade of systemic effects that induce a febrile inflammatory response, also known as SIRS.[39]

A fever that develops 72 hours or more after surgery is more likely to be due to infection. Hence, it can sometimes be clinically challenging to delineate the precise etiology of these fevers because they can result from infectious and/or noninfectious causes.

In the postoperative period, the most common infectious causes are wound infections, urinary tract infections (UTIs), and pneumonia. Prolonged IV access, bladder catheterization, or endotracheal intubation presents ongoing risks of infection.

Catheter-related bloodstream infection (CRBSI) is the most common cause of nosocomial bacteremia and septicemia. As such, early diagnosis and treatment are vital to reduce the morbidity and mortality involved. The mode of contamination for

TABLE 26.3	Causes of Postoperative Fever
INFECTIOUS	**NONINFECTIOUS**
Abscess	Acute hepatic necrosis
Acalculous cholecystitis	Adrenal insufficiency
Bacteremia	Allergic reaction
Decubitus ulcers	Atelectasis
Device-related infections	Dehydration
Empyema	Drug reaction
Endocarditis	Head injury
Fungal sepsis	Hepatoma
Hepatitis	Hyperthyroidism
Meningitis	Lymphoma
Osteomyelitis	Myocardial infarction
Pseudomembranous colitis	Pancreatitis
Parotitis	Pheochromocytoma
Perineal infections	Pulmonary embolus
Peritonitis	Retroperitoneal hematoma
Pharyngitis	Solid organ hematoma
Pneumonia	Subarachnoid hemorrhage
Retained foreign body	Systemic inflammatory response
Sinusitis	syndrome
Soft tissue infection	Thrombophlebitis
Tracheobronchitis	Transfusion reaction
Urinary tract infection	Withdrawal syndromes
	Wound infection

CRBSI varies with the duration of catheterization (short vs. long). Short-term CRBSIs (<10 days) are extraluminal and are preventable as they result from contamination by normal resident flora of the skin at the insertion site. In contrast, the source of infection is endoluminal if it propagates the infection in long-term CRBSI (>10 days) that results in sepsis with multiorgan failure. The organisms most commonly involved in CRBSI are Staphylococci (both *Staphylococcus aureus* and the coagulase-negative staphylococci), enterococci, aerobic gram-negative bacilli, and fungal species (e.g., *Candida albicans*). The diagnosis of CRBSI requires at least one positive blood culture obtained from a peripheral vein, clinical manifestations of infection (e.g., fever, chills, and/or hypotension), and no apparent source for the bloodstream infection (BSI) except the catheter. Antibiotic therapy is often initiated empirically. Factors responsible for recurrent bacteremia despite parenteral therapy include antibiotic administration through retained catheter and biofilm formation. Severe sepsis and metastatic infectious complications (e.g., infective endocarditis) prolong the course of CRBSI. Catheters should be removed from patients with CRBSI associated with any local or systemic inflammation or immunocompromised condition.

Respiratory Complications
General Considerations
Surgical interventions (especially thoracic and abdominal) and anesthesia impact pulmonary physiology by decreasing functional residual capacity (FRC). In most patients, this is well tolerated, but patients with underlying pulmonary disease (e.g., chronic obstructive pulmonary disease, emphysema, cigarette smokers) may be prone to develop pulmonary complications. Identifying "high-risk" patients before surgery can be helpful and preoperative pulmonary function testing, tobacco cessation, or sleep studies may help the surgical team reduce the risk of complications by optimizing the patient's condition before surgery (e.g., preoperative

bilevel positive airway pressure ventilation, bronchodilator therapy). More recently, standard patient care protocols (e.g., ICOUGH) have been developed to decrease the risk of pulmonary complications, which include incentive spirometry, coughing and deep breathing, oral care (brushing teeth and using mouthwash), elevating the head of bed, and getting out of bed three times a day. Multimodal pain control and judicious use of regional analgesia (e.g., thoracic epidurals) may also help to prevent pulmonary complications in surgical patients.

Atelectasis
Atelectasis due to partial or complete collapse of alveoli is the most common respiratory complication in the postoperative patient. Predisposing factors for atelectasis include general anesthesia and upper abdominal or thoracic surgery with stimulation of gastrointestinal (GI) viscera, which can alter diaphragmatic function for several days. The mechanisms include decreased lung compliance (due to reduced FRC), along with accumulated endobronchial secretions, resulting in V/Q mismatch and shunt, which directly correlates with the degree of atelectasis. Anesthesia, cigarettes, morbid obesity, and preexisting pulmonary disease also impair mucociliary clearance and decrease the patient's ability to cough and clear secretions, contributing to an increased risk of atelectasis.

Atelectasis is the most common cause of postoperative fever in the early postoperative period. It may also present with tachypnea, decreased oxygen saturation ± accessory muscle use. On physical examination, breath sounds may be absent or reduced, or "bronchial" in nature. The chest radiograph may reveal loss of the left hemidiaphragm, air bronchograms, or decreased lung volume with tracheal deviation toward the collapsed side in severe cases. Atelectasis can be reversed in the first 24 to 48 hours with early mobilization, deep breathing (five sequential breaths held for 5–6 seconds), incentive spirometry, coughing, chest physiotherapy, bronchodilator therapy, hydration, and tracheal suctioning. Multimodal pain control using acetaminophen, nonsteroidal antiinflammatory agents, and opioids as needed or regional blocks represent the most commonly effective approach for optimal perioperative pain control.

Aspiration Pneumonitis and Aspiration Pneumonia
Aspiration of gastric contents in the perioperative period is associated with significant pulmonary morbidity and mortality. Aspiration pneumonitis (Mendelson syndrome) refers to an acute inflammatory injury of the lung parenchyma resulting from aspiration of usually sterile acidic gastric contents (critical pH is 2.5), whereas aspiration pneumonia is a common infectious complication of enteral nutrition usually resulting either from contamination of the initial aspirate or secondarily from aspiration of colonized oropharyngeal secretions. Although the underlying patient characteristics that predispose to these conditions are similar, the distinction between the two entities is important since aspiration pneumonia requires antibiotic treatment and aspiration pneumonitis is managed supportively.

The factors that predispose an individual to increase risk of aspiration include emergency surgery, chronic debilitating disease, oropharyngeal or airway instrumentation, small bowel obstruction, autonomic neuropathy with delayed gastric emptying (DGE), impaired consciousness (e.g., from general anesthesia, epileptic seizure, trauma, alcohol, drug overdose, or cerebrovascular accident), and medications that lead to DGE (e.g., glucagon-like peptide-1 [GLP-1] receptor agonists).

GLP-1 receptor agonists are used to improve glycemic control in people with type 2 diabetes mellitus and for weight loss. They are associated with adverse GI effects such as vomiting, nausea, and DGE. In theory, GLP-1 receptor agonists could delay gastric emptying enough to pose a threat to perioperative patients by increasing the risk of pulmonary aspiration of regurgitated gastric contents. This potentially harmful effect during the perioperative period is why the American Society of Anesthesiologists (ASA) Task Force on preoperative fasting has provided some guidance on GLP-1 receptor agonist use before surgery, advising that daily medications should be held a day before surgery, and weekly medications should be held a week before surgery. If a patient has not held their GLP-1 receptor agonist, it is recommended that they be treated using "full-stomach" precautions.[40]

Older patients are at increased risk of oropharyngeal aspiration secondary due to the combination of pharyngeal dysmotility, gastroesophageal reflux, and poor oral hygiene in this population. The common infectious organisms in aspiration pneumonia are *Escherichia coli*, *Klebsiella*, *Staphylococcus*, *Pseudomonas*, and *Bacteroides* species.

The pathogenesis and outcomes of gastric aspiration depend on the nature of aspirated matter, volume and pH of gastric acid, and immunologic status of the patient. The more acidic (e.g., pH <2.5) and voluminous (>20 mL) the aspirate, the greater the severity of pulmonary damage. The initial parenchymal inflammatory changes (airspace edema, hemorrhage, hyaline membrane) in Mendelson syndrome are similar to acute respiratory distress syndrome (ARDS) and attributed to neutrophil activation and recruitment and inflammatory cytokine release.

The risk-benefit ratio for using prophylactic H_2 receptor antagonists or proton pump inhibitors (PPIs) to reduce the gastric acid pH is favorable in high-risk patients. However, none of these drugs are absolutely reliable in preventing the risk of aspiration pneumonitis.

Gastric aspiration may cause mild, subclinical pneumonitis, or more severe progressive respiratory failure with significant morbidity and mortality. After an aspiration event, the clinical and radiographic changes begin to appear within the next 24 to 36 hours. Common signs and symptoms of gastric aspiration include fever, cough, rales, diminished breath sounds, wheezing, and infiltrates on chest radiograph. Hypoxia is the earliest and most reliable sign.

Aspiration pneumonitis differs from other aspiration sequelae because it frequently has a rapid onset, is self-limiting, and most radiographic changes of simple toxic aspiration usually clear within 48 hours. In contrast, the persistence of symptoms and associated signs of bacterial infection should raise concerns about the possibility of aspiration pneumonia.

The risk of aspiration is decreased by reducing the volume of gastric contents, minimizing regurgitation, and protecting the airway. Patients should be NPO (nothing by mouth) for 2 or more hours before elective procedures requiring general or regional anesthesia or deep levels of conscious sedation. In intubated patents with suspected or increased risk of aspiration, extubation can be delayed until the patient is fully awake and has protective airway reflexes. Gastric decompression and rapid sequence induction of anesthesia with cricoid pressure has been advocated as the most effective way to prevent aspiration during intubation in high-risk patents, but it is not 100% effective.[41]

When aspiration occurs, the treatment is usually supportive with supplemental oxygen. The airway should be suctioned, the stomach decompressed, and bronchoscopy should be considered for retrieval of aspirated particulate matter. In more severe cases, the patient requires mechanical ventilation and positive end-expiratory pressure.

Antibiotics are not required in most cases because aspirated gastric content is usually sterile. However, in certain cases (e.g., feculent small bowel contents with intestinal obstruction), antibiotics should be administered. Empiric antibiotics (fluoroquinolones, piperacillin/tazobactam, or ceftriaxone) are recommended in patients with small bowel obstruction or ileus and for pneumonitis that fails to resolve within 48 hours.

Venous Thromboembolism

Venous thromboembolism (VTE) includes deep vein thrombosis (DVT) and pulmonary embolism (PE). DVT describes a blood clot in the deep venous system of the upper or lower extremities. Newly formed thrombi are not firmly attached to the vessel wall and can detach and embolize through the venous system, ending up in the pulmonary vasculature. These pulmonary emboli are subsequently coated with fibrin and platelets, causing mechanical obstruction of the pulmonary blood flow, pulmonary hypertension, and acute right ventricular (RV) strain.

VTE is associated with increased postoperative morbidity and mortality in surgery patients but is less significant when detected early and properly treated. Conditions related to the Virchow triad increase the risk of clot formation and VTE development, including long-distance travel (>4 hours), increased age, obesity, frailty, malignancy, nephrotic syndrome, varicose veins, inflammatory bowel disease, prolonged immobilization, history of VTE, inherited hypercoagulation conditions, pregnancy, use of contraceptive medication, trauma, and indwelling venous catheters.

The clinical symptoms of VTE are variable, and patients can be asymptomatic if the clot is small or nonobstructing. However, many patients with DVT have significant symptoms, including unilateral or bilateral swelling of the extremities, warmth, and localized tenderness.

In patients with an acute PE, the most common symptoms are dyspnea or shortness of breath. However, there can be significant variability in PE symptomatology depending on the size of the clot, its location in the pulmonary vasculature, and the patient's underlying cardiac and pulmonary function. Massive PEs can cause obstruction of pulmonary blood flow and acute right heart strain, leading to hemodynamic compromise. Consequently, patients with massive PE can present with life-threatening symptoms of severe hypotension, unconsciousness, and/or cardiac arrest. Other PE-related symptoms include dyspnea, anxiety, cough, pleuritic or dull chest pain, hemoptysis, and syncope. Physical examination may show tachycardia, low-grade fever, loud P2, or poor perfusion.

Because clinical findings can be variable, a number of scoring systems have been developed and validated to determine the probability of VTE before diagnostic imaging. For example, the Wells criteria categorize patients into likely or unlikely groups. D-dimer is a product of fibrin breakdown, which is increased in VTE but is also elevated in many other conditions and is not useful in patients with recent surgery or trauma. Although these scoring systems and D-dimer level are sensitive screening tools, they are not specific, and the diagnosis of VTE should not be made based on these factors alone. In patients where VTE is suspected, imaging studies should be used to confirm or exclude the diagnosis.

Venous duplex ultrasonography is the imaging of choice for DVT showing cross-sectional vein incompressibility, direct thrombus with vein enlargement, abnormal spectral Doppler, and color Doppler flow, which provides useful information regarding clot location and size.

CT pulmonary angiography has become the diagnostic imaging procedure of choice for PE due to the routine availability of the CT scan at most institutions.

Many surgery patients are at increased risk of VTE and should be risk stratified for prophylactic therapy. Although pharmacologic DVT prophylaxis is generally considered to be "low risk" for bleeding complications, certain situations are considered "high risk." Patients with active GI bleeding, intracranial hemorrhage, liver disease, bleeding disorder, thrombocytopenia, recent head trauma, or spinal injury/surgery should be carefully assessed for risk-benefit ratio before initiating pharmacologic VTE prophylaxis.

VTE prophylaxis modalities include pharmacologic prophylaxis with low-molecular-weight heparin (LMWH), unfractionated heparin (UFH), fondaparinux, and mechanical prophylaxis with intermittent pneumatic compression, foot pumps, and graduated compression stockings. Decisions regarding VTE prophylaxis modalities are based on assessment of VTE and bleeding risk in the specific patient or population.

In suspected PE patients, the management depends on severity and mortality risk assessed by patient conditions. Patients with hypotension, RV failure by echocardiography or CT, elevated cardiac biomarkers, and PE severity index score of class III or higher are considered high risk for mortality. The first priority is to maintain hemodynamics and ventilation, and the patient care team should be prepared for cardiac life support in case of cardiac arrest. Patients may need intubation, mechanical ventilation, and vasopressors to maintain blood pressure and cardiac output. IV fluids should be administered carefully in patients with PE as increased vascular volume can worsen right heart failure. Patients should be cared for in an ICU setting, parenteral anticoagulation should be initiated immediately unless strongly contraindicated, and echocardiography should be considered when patients are hemodynamically unstable. Levophed is commonly used as the vasopressor of choice in this situation and interventions to treat obstructing PE causing severe pulmonary hypertension and RV failure should be considered. These include fibrinolytic drugs like streptokinase, urokinase, recombinant tissue plasminogen activator (rTPA) or catheter-directed therapy, and surgical embolectomy. Extracorporeal membrane oxygenation can both provide hemodynamic support and improve oxygenation and is considered in potentially reversible patients for stabilization before embolectomy. However, the majority of PE cases are less severe and hemodynamically stable, and the management is similar to DVT with therapeutic anticoagulation and transition to long-term anticoagulants for usually 6 months. The routine use of fibrinolytic medication for PE outweighs the benefits in most patients and should be reserved for hemodynamically unstable patients with clinical deterioration despite anticoagulation and aggressive supportive care.

Cardiac Complications
Perioperative Myocardial Ischemia and Infarction
Perioperative myocardial ischemia and infarction (PMI) are important and potentially severe complications in noncardiac surgery. Normally, acute myocardial infarction is diagnosed by an elevation of cardiac enzymes with either ischemic symptoms, electrocardiographic changes attributable to myocardial ischemia, infarction, or imaging findings. However, 65% of patients with PMI do not experience ischemic symptoms, according to the Perioperative Ischemia Evaluation (POISE) trial.[42]

The cause of PMI is from two main mechanisms. The first is the classic theory of plaque rupture and thrombosis of coronary vessels occluding the blood supply to the myocardium. The second cause is the imbalance between oxygen demand and supply during the perioperative period and postoperative care. Therefore, patients at

risk for cardiac complications are those who have underlying coronary artery disease, recent myocardial infarction or stenting, recent stroke, and other risk factors for coronary disease, including peripheral arterial disease, diabetes, hyperlipidemia, smoking, family history, or hypertension. Other risk factors are the types of surgery and perioperative events contributing to alteration of oxygen demand and supply. Major surgeries are more stressful to the patient and can impact normal homeostasis by causing inflammation, hypercoagulability, platelet activation, tachycardia, or high blood pressure, which exert stress on coronary vessels, leading to preexisting plaque rupture. Furthermore, the stress response to surgery activates the sympathetic nervous system, resulting in elevated catecholamines, which can lead to coronary vasoconstriction and increased myocardial oxygen demand.

During the perioperative period, alterations in hemodynamics, oxygenation, and ventilation related to surgery can affect coronary blood flow and cause imbalance of myocardial oxygen demand and supply. Examples include hypoxia, hypothermia, hypotension, hypertension, tachycardia, bleeding, and anemia.

Most patients have perioperative ischemia or infarction within 48 hours after surgery. Symptomatic patients may develop substernal chest pain or pressure radiating to the left shoulder or neck. They may also experience arrhythmia, tachycardia, sweating, dyspnea, or signs of heart failure, hypoxia, acidosis, cardiogenic shock, and cardiac arrest. When these symptoms occur, cardiac biomarkers should be measured and electrocardiography should be performed. Changes in electrocardiography are another indication of cardiac ischemia and range from ST-segment elevation, ST depression, T-wave inversion, or Q waves. However, most patients with perioperative ischemia or infarction are asymptomatic, and there are still no standardized diagnostic criteria for this group. Cardiac biomarkers are associated with perioperative ischemia and infarction and may be the only abnormality detected.

Identification of patients with increased risk of developing PMI allows their physicians to evaluate their cardiac risks more carefully before surgery. Several methods for cardiac risk stratification are available, and the most commonly used today is the revised cardiac risk index (RCRI). Patients with at least two risk factors are at increased risk for major cardiac complications (Box 26.2).

Electrocardiography should be done within 3 months before surgery, and patients with unknown dyspnea or change in functional class should have left ventricular function examined.

Perioperative β-blockers have been shown to reduce the risk of myocardial infarction. Therefore, β-blockers should be continued

---

BOX 26.2 **Six Independent Risk Predictors for the Revised Cardiac Risk Index**

Patients with two or more risk factors are considered elevated risk.

High-risk type of surgery (intraperitoneal, intrathoracic, suprainguinal vascular surgery)

History of ischemic heart disease

History of congestive heart failure

History of cerebrovascular disease

Insulin therapy for diabetes

Preoperative serum creatinine >2 mg/dL

From Lee TH, Marcantonio ER, Mangione CM, et al. Derivation and prospective validation of a simple index for prediction of cardiac risk of major noncardiac surgery. *Circulation.* 1999;100:1043-1049.

in patients who already take them and initiation of β-blockers should be considered in high-risk patients (≥3 RCRI) several days before surgery. Aspirin and statins are two commonly used medications in patients with coronary disease and should also be continued perioperatively.

Patients with coronary disease who have been treated with percutaneous coronary intervention (PCI) ± stents are placed on dual antiplatelet therapy (DAPT) with aspirin and a P2Y12 receptor inhibitor to prevent thrombosis. Thrombotic risk is considered low 4 weeks after balloon angiography, 6 months after bare metal stents, and 1 year after drug-eluting stents. Elective surgery for PCI patients should be postponed if possible during the high-thrombotic risk periods described earlier. Perioperative management of DAPT for noncardiac surgery patients should consider the risk of thrombosis and the risk of hemorrhage. Specific guidelines are available to guide perioperative antiplatelet therapy, but surgeon judgment is required to optimize care for individual patients. Anemia should be corrected to optimize oxygen delivery during operation.

Once myocardial tissue has been damaged, the median time from PMI to death is approximately 12 days.[43] The challenge in management comes in determining the pathophysiology of PMI between plaque rupture/thrombosis (type I) or imbalance of oxygen demand and supply (type II). Patients with suspected type I injury should receive aggressive aspirin therapy, with caution exerted for bleeding risk, and statin therapy with consideration of angiography. Secondary prevention using β-blockers and angiotensin-converting enzyme (ACE) inhibitors should be given when feasible. Patients suspected of type II injury should have optimal hemodynamics and oxygenation therapy with possible angiography during follow-up after surgery.

The consequences of severe myocardial infarction can be life-threatening and include cardiogenic shock or cardiac arrest. Life-threatening complications of severe myocardial infarction include free rupture of the cardiac wall or septum, acute mitral valve regurgitation from rupture of chordae tendineae, and complete heart block. Aggressive management is required to prevent death and includes hemodynamic and oxygenation support in case of cardiogenic shock and cardiopulmonary resuscitation in cardiac arrest. However, the mortality in this group is as high as 70%.

Postoperative Arrhythmias

Arrhythmias are alterations of cardiac electrical impulse including conduction (reentry, delay or blocking) and initiation (premature impulse, change in automaticity). Dysrhythmia-induced changes in heart rate (HR) or rhythm can cause abnormal beating or myocardial contraction of the heart, resulting in increased or decreased HR and possibly cardiac output. Postoperative arrhythmias or dysrhythmias can happen due to direct disturbance of the heart or in patients with underlying structural heart abnormalities like valvular heart disease, ischemia, or scarring. Dysrhythmias may occur after noncardiac surgery due to surgical stress, anesthesia, or complications from surgery. Patients with postoperative arrhythmias tend to have a longer hospital stay and higher mortality. Risk factors include increasing age, male sex, history of arrhythmias, valvular heart disease, hypertension, history of stroke, chronic lung disease, and obesity. In the postoperative period, arrhythmias can be triggered by acid-base and electrolyte abnormalities, inflammatory or surgical stress caused by pain, PMI, heart failure, hypoxia, infections, bacteremia, or sepsis; medications can also trigger arrhythmias. Withdrawing β-blockers can result in a surge of catecholamines and lead to arrhythmias.

Most dysrhythmias after surgery are transient and cause no hemodynamic compromise. Patients may feel nothing or just palpitations. If the dysrhythmias are persistent or severe, they can cause hemodynamic alterations, including signs and symptoms of low cardiac output like chest pain, pulmonary edema, confusion, desaturation, hypotension, low urine output, or even cardiac arrest. Tachydysrhythmias may reduce diastolic time and coronary flow, potentially triggering myocardial ischemia or infarction. Patients with postoperative arrhythmias should be examined with 12-lead electrocardiography and have their hemodynamic status monitored. The two most common arrhythmias after surgery are atrial fibrillation and atrial flutter, which commonly develop within 3 days of surgery.

Management of postoperative atrial fibrillation is similar to new-onset atrial fibrillation. In hemodynamically normal patients, initial treatment involves control of the ventricular rate with β-blockers, calcium channel blockers, or digoxin. Chemical cardioversion may be considered to decrease the risk of thromboembolism when the atrial arrhythmia is less than 48 hours' duration. However, if the onset is more than 48 hours or unknown, anticoagulation therapy is recommended because the risks of atrial clot formation increase over time. The decision to start anticoagulation for postoperative atrial fibrillation must balance the risks of thromboembolism with the risks of bleeding after surgery. The most commonly used thromboembolic risk stratification tool is the CHA_2DS_2-VASc risk score, which recommends routine anticoagulation if the score is ≥2.[44] Antiarrhythmic drugs commonly used to convert atrial fibrillation are amiodarone, flecainide, dofetilide, propafenone, or ibutilide. In most cases, rate control is indicated before initiating chemical conversion. Electrical cardioversion ± anticoagulation should be considered in patients with rapid atrial fibrillation and hemodynamic compromise. In addition, physicians should simultaneously treat and correct potentially precipitating problems, including infection, sepsis, acid-base and electrolyte abnormalities, and anemia. If patients fail to convert to sinus rhythm, long-term anticoagulation should be considered based on the individual patient's risk factors.

Narrow complex supraventricular tachycardia (e.g., from electrical reentry of atrioventricular nodal conduction) can be treated with vagal maneuvers such as carotid sinus massage (in patients with no risk of stroke from carotid artery disease), with IV adenosine, or cardioversion in case of hemodynamic compromise. Bradyarrhythmias include sinus bradycardia, which is the most common, and different grades of atrioventricular blocks. Medications used to treat symptomatic bradycardias include atropine, aminophylline, or cardiac pacing in patients with sustained symptomatic bradyarrhythmias.

Renal and Urinary Complications
Acute Kidney Injury

Acute kidney injury (AKI), formerly known as acute renal failure, is a rapid decline in the ability of the kidney to clear waste products. AKI is a common postoperative complication that increases morbidity and mortality, especially after major surgical procedures. The standardized criteria for diagnosing AKI were established by the risk, injury, failure, loss, and end-stage kidney disease (RIFLE) criteria in 2004 and were modified to the Acute Kidney Injury Network (AKIN) criteria in 2007 using the serum creatinine level and urine output as indicators of kidney function. The most recent consensus statement on the diagnosis of AKI are the 2012 Kidney Disease: Improving Global Outcomes (KDIGO) criteria (Table 26.4), which classifies AKI into stages based on severity.

TABLE 26.4   The 2012 KDIGO Clinical Practice Guidelines for Acute Kidney Injury

Definition of Acute Kidney Injury

Increase in serum creatinine by ≥0.3 mg/dL within 48 hours

OR

Increase in serum creatinine to ≥1.5 times baseline, which is known or presumed to have occurred within the prior 7 days

OR

Urine volume <0.5 mL/kg/h for 6 hours.

Staging of Acute Kidney Injury

SERUM CREATININE	URINE OUTPUT
Stage 1	
1.5–1.9 times baseline OR ≥0.3 mg/dL increase	<0.5 mL/kg/h for 6–12 hours
Stage 2	
2.0–2.9 times baseline	<0.5 mL/kg/h for ≥12 hours
Stage 3	
3 times baseline OR Increase in serum creatinine to ≥4.0 mg/dL OR Initiation of renal replacement therapy OR In patients <18 years, decrease in eGFR to <35 mL/min/1.73 m²	<0.3 mL/kg/h for ≥24 hours OR Anuria for ≥12 hours

eGFR, Estimated glomerular filtration rate; *KDIGO*, Kidney Disease: Improving Global Outcomes.

The higher stages are associated with worse outcomes, mortality, and need for renal replacement therapy (RRT).

The pathophysiology of AKI can be characterized as either prerenal, renal, or postrenal. Prerenal AKI or renal hypoperfusion, an important cause of kidney injury in surgical patients, is caused by loss of intravascular volume from bleeding or dehydration, medications that affect regulation of the renin-angiotensin-aldosterone system (RAAS) or impair the normal regulatory mechanisms of afferent and efferent arterioles, vasodilatation from inflammation, sepsis, or anesthetic agents. Renal etiologies of AKI include medications or chemicals that are directly toxic to the kidney such as nonsteroidal antiinflammatory drugs (NSAIDs), aminoglycosides, and amphotericin B. Trauma patients with crush injuries or impaired blood supply to the extremities may develop rhabdomyolysis. The release of myoglobin from injured muscle in patients with rhabdomyolysis may cause kidney injury by several mechanisms,

including renal vasoconstriction, the formation of tubular casts caused by myoglobin precipitation, and most importantly the injury of tubular cell by free oxygen radicals. The use of contrast media in radiographic imaging is one of the most common causes of AKI in surgical patients.

It is important to monitor urine output and serum creatinine in patients at risk for AKI. Urine output is easy to measure and can be monitored continuously using indwelling bladder catheters. An acute reduction in urine output (<0.5 mL/kg/h) is an important and useful tool in the diagnosis and prevention of AKI. Despite its utility, reductions in urine output are of limited use in predicting AKI in certain conditions, including hyperglycemia, osmotic diuresis, nonoliguric AKI, and postrenal obstruction.

The signs and symptoms of renal insufficiency present in the later stages as nitrogen waste products accumulate and patients become fluid overloaded. Signs and symptoms of more advanced renal failure can include nausea, vomiting, fatigue, confusion from uremia, asterixis, pericardial rub from uremic pericarditis, and abnormal bleeding. In cases of volume overload, peripheral edema, shortness of breath, and increased pulmonary infiltration on chest x-ray could be noted and are suggestive of congestive heart failure. Laboratory tests that help to discriminate prerenal, renal, and postrenal causes of AKI are summarized in Table 26.5.

The optimal management strategy for AKI is the identification of high-risk patients and preventively managing their care to minimize the risk of developing AKI. Risk factors for perioperative AKI include age, obesity, high ASA class, preexisting renal disease, diabetes, and hypertension. Preventive strategies to reduce perioperative AKI include attention to volume status and hemoglobin levels before surgery, which can reduce the risk of intraoperative renal hypoperfusion and hypoxia. Patients with vomiting, diarrhea, anorexia, preoperative bowel preparation, or bleeding are at increased risk for hypovolemia/prerenal AKI and need to be aggressively resuscitated. Patients with a history of chronic kidney disease or previous episodes of AKI are at risk for postoperative AKI, and the adjustment of nephrotoxic medications should be considered before the operation. During the perioperative period, the goal is to maintain adequate renal perfusion; a mean arterial pressure lower than 60 mm Hg is associated with a higher risk of postoperative AKI. Therefore, during anesthesia, the mean arterial pressure should be maintained above 65 mm Hg or 75 to 80 mm Hg in patients with hypertension. Invasive hemodynamic monitoring (e.g., central venous catheter or arterial line) should be considered in certain cases. Intraoperative urine output should be maintained at ≥0.5 mL/kg/h in the perioperative period if possible.

Once AKI has developed, there is no specific treatment to regain kidney function. The goal is to maintain adequate renal perfusion and to avoid further kidney injury, allowing the return of renal function. Repeated episodes of AKI can lead to permanent deterioration of renal function and chronic renal insufficiency, increasing the risk of long-term RRT. Volume assessment

TABLE 26.5   Diagnostic Evaluation of Acute Renal Failure

PARAMETER	PRERENAL	RENAL	POSTRENAL
Urine osmolality	>500 mOsm/L	= Plasma	Variable
Urinary sodium	<20 mOsm/L	>50 mOsm/L	>50 mOsm/L
Fractional excretion of sodium	<1%	>3%	Variable
Urine, plasma creatinine level	>40	<20	<20
Urine, plasma urea level	>8	<3	Variable
Urine, plasma osmolality	<1.5	>1.5	Variable

is critical and can be challenging, especially for patients with heart failure or underlying renal insufficiency. Because hypovolemia can cause prerenal AKI and too much volume can reduce renal blood flow by increasing abdominal pressure and causing renal congestion, the evaluation of volume status and whether the patient is volume responsive is critical and can determine the direction of management. Diuretics should be used primarily to prevent volume overload; however, they should not delay RRT if indicated. Further, vasopressors should be used to maintain blood pressure in AKI patients as needed.

Contrast-induced AKI is another important cause of AKI, especially in patients with underlying renal insufficiency. Several strategies have been used to prevent contrast-induced AKI, such as reducing reactive oxygen species by acetylcysteine, vitamin C, or bicarbonate or using diuretic drugs to dilute contrast and reduce exposure time in the renal tubules. Unfortunately, these preventive strategies are still controversial. However, volume expansion appears to be the most beneficial intervention possibly by suppression of vasopressin, inhibition of RAAS, and dilution of contrast. IV fluids of choice include isotonic normal saline or sodium bicarbonate solution and should be started 6 to 12 hours before the procedure and for 4 to 12 hours after the procedure in patients at risk of AKI.

In cases of severe AKI, RRT prevents mortality from volume overload, electrolyte imbalance, and uremia. The indication and timing of RRT is still varied, and there are no standard criteria of RRT initiation.

Urinary Retention

Postoperative urinary retention has no standardized definition. However, it is a common postoperative complication and refers to the inability to spontaneously empty the urinary bladder after surgery. The urinary bladder has a capacity of approximately 500 mL. Overstretching the bladder wall will cause muscular ischemia and reduce sensation and contractility; thus, factors that interfere with the micturition reflex, over distend the bladder, or compromise the outflow of the urinary tract can result in urinary retention. Risk factors of urinary retention are shown in Table 26.6.

Patients usually complain of lower abdominal fullness, suprapubic pain, or discomfort. Although uncommon, the massively distended bladder can stimulate the vasovagal reflex causing cardiovascular symptoms, including bradycardia, arrhythmia, hypotension, or asystole. Physical examination may demonstrate

a palpable bladder at the lower abdomen. However, some patients show no signs or symptoms of bladder distention and present with overflow incontinence. If left untreated, urinary retention can result in a UTI, which may lengthen hospital stay and increase morbidity. Chronic retention could permanently damage the detrusor muscle and cause long-term complications such as bladder stone, hydronephrosis, incontinence, or renal insufficiency.

Prevention of urinary retention starts with careful evaluation of patient risk factors, minimizing damage during surgery, pain control, fluid administration, and monitoring postoperative urination. Most patients should void within 6 to 8 hours after surgery. When postoperative urinary retention is suspected, ultrasound should be used to estimate the bladder volume. Bladder volumes of 500 mL or more require intervention, most commonly urinary catheterization, and suprapubic tube placement in cases of urethral stricture or trauma.

Gastrointestinal Complications
Postoperative Ileus

After abdominal surgery, there is a normal time course and pattern for return of intestinal motility. The small bowel usually develops contractile activity within several hours, the stomach requires 24 to 48 hours, and the colon recovers 3 to 5 days after surgery. Postoperative ileus is considered as intolerance of oral intake due to disruption of the normal coordinated propulsive motor activity of the GI tract following abdominal or nonabdominal surgery, without any mechanical element and can be classified as physiologic or paralytic ileus depending on the etiology, timing, and involvement of the GI tract. The duration of ileus generally correlates with the type of surgery and degree of surgical trauma. Advances in surgical techniques such as minimally invasive surgery minimize surgical stress response and help to maintain normal physiology throughout the perioperative period. This, in turn, ultimately results in a reduced risk of postoperative ileus.

The pathophysiology of postoperative ileus is complex and multifactorial in nature. Neurogenic (enteric nervous system and CNS), inflammatory, enteric hormones and neuropeptides, perioperative electrolyte disturbances, and opioids are all contributing factors.[45] The combination of these factors results in impaired local neuromuscular function, impaired contractility, motility, relative hypoxemia, and bowel edema.

Delayed bowel movement or passage of flatus is the hallmark of postoperative ileus. Common symptoms include abdominal distension, bloating, diffuse, persistent pain, nausea, vomiting, inability to pass flatus, and intolerance to an oral diet. Physical exam findings are also typically nonspecific, but often patients can have distended, tympanic abdomens on exam associated with absent or sluggish bowel sounds. Tenderness or rebound tenderness should be further investigated for other more serious causes.

Postoperative physiologic ileus is usually self-limiting and can be managed conservatively. In the case of paralytic ileus, treatment of the underlying etiology, such as treatment of electrolyte abnormalities and an associated intraabdominal process (e.g., pancreatitis), will hasten the return of bowel function. Further measures include IV fluid replacement, early ambulation, and often nasogastric (NG) tube placement.

Postoperative Bowel Obstruction

Early postoperative mechanical bowel obstruction is defined as occurring within the first 6 weeks of surgery. Adhesions are

TABLE 26.6	Risk Factors for Urinary Retention
Age	Degeneration of neurons in micturition reflex and narrowing of urinary passage
Sex	Narrower outflow
Anesthetic choice	Spinal, epidural anesthesia can affect micturition reflex
Intraoperative IV fluid and operation time	Increased total fluid intake and rapid filling of bladder
Medication	Anticholinergic, opioid
Patient comorbidities	BPH, neurologic bladder, DM, neurologic disorders
Types of surgery	Colorectal surgery, spine surgery, hernia

BPH, Benign prostatic hyperplasia; *DM*, diabetes mellitus.

responsible for the majority of early postoperative bowel obstructions (>90%), with internal herniation, intraabdominal abscess, intramural hematoma, intussusception, and anastomotic edema or leak as less likely causes. Postoperative adhesions may occur after any intraabdominal surgery but are more likely to cause bowel obstructions after pelvic surgery, especially colorectal and gynecologic procedures. Ideally, early postoperative mechanical bowel obstruction could be prevented with meticulous surgical technique (e.g., minimally invasive surgery). Minimizing tissue trauma by handling tissues gently, constant bathing of the tissues with saline, avoiding ischemia and desiccation, maintaining hemostasis, and avoiding contamination and infection are conceptually associated with fewer adhesions, but their impact is difficult to quantify.

Postoperative mechanical bowel obstruction can be classified as either intrinsic or extrinsic; partial or complete; or proximal (pylorus to proximal jejunum), intermediate (mid-jejunum to mid-ileum), or distal (distal ileum to ileocecal valve) in location. With a partial obstruction, luminal contents pass distally despite slow transit time, whereas with complete obstruction, the lumen is totally occluded. Complete obstruction can be described as simple, closed-loop, or strangulated in nature.

The classical presentation of mechanical bowel obstruction includes intermittent or colicky abdominal pain, distention, acute obstipation, nausea, and vomiting. The presence of severe constant or localized pain may indicate strangulation (especially if subjective pain is disproportional to exam findings). Mechanical proximal bowel obstruction typically presents with severe, crampy visceral pain, occurring in short recurrent paroxysms (30 seconds to 2 minutes) in a crescendo/decrescendo pattern. In contrast, with distal mechanical obstruction, the episodes are usually spaced farther apart in time and tend to last longer (minutes rather than seconds). Complete obstruction often presents earlier and with more acute findings than partial obstruction. The more proximal the obstruction, the earlier and more prominent the symptoms of nausea and vomiting (bilious), whereas vomiting with distal bowel obstruction is typically delayed in presentation and feculent in nature. Findings concerning for strangulation include fever, tachycardia, and leukocytosis. Closed-loop obstruction may be caused by incarcerated bowel in a hernia sac or intestinal torsion and is associated with increased risk of vascular compromise and irreversible intestinal ischemia. Closed-loop obstruction presents more rapidly with acute symptoms compared with partial or "open-loop" obstruction.

Bowel sounds are frequently high pitched with metallic "rushes" and "groans" in patients with partial small bowel obstruction.

Postoperative mechanical obstruction is usually characterized by dilated small and large bowel. CT imaging can help to identify the presence or absence of a focal site of obstruction. The presence of a dilated proximal small bowel with decompressed distal bowel is concerning, but usually, a clearly defined transition point is seen with mechanical obstruction. CT imaging may also help diagnose the cause of obstruction (hernia, solid mass, inflammatory lesion, or intussusception), the presence of closed-loop obstruction, and a mesenteric swirl is frequently seen with internal hernias. The use of IV contrast helps to identify vascular patency, and decreased bowel wall enhancement may indicate ischemic bowel. The use of enteral contrast with the CT scan is helpful to differentiate between partial and complete bowel obstruction.

Initial management of mechanical obstruction requires appropriate fluid resuscitation, opioid discontinuation, and NG decompression of the obstructed bowel as intraluminal distension results in mucosal ischemia. Patient-controlled epidural analgesia or NSAIDs are alternative choices, instead of opioids, for postoperative pain control.

An initial trial of nonoperative management is appropriate for most cases of partial mechanical obstruction in the early postoperative period in the absence of clinical deterioration and when the patient shows signs of improvement during the first 12 to 24 hours. Nonoperative management begins with aggressive fluid resuscitation and correction of any electrolyte disorders. Several centers recommend algorithm-based treatment of small bowel obstruction. NG decompression is followed by water-soluble contrast administration down the NG tube with follow-up abdominal plain films to assess contrast in the cecum at 8 and 24 hours. If the contrast reaches the cecum in 8 hours, the NG tube can be removed and liquids started. If the contrast does not reach the cecum in 24 hours, early surgical intervention is recommended. Contraindications to nonoperative management include suspected ischemia, closed-loop obstruction, strangulated hernia, and perforation. Patients with complete or high-grade partial obstruction and presence of fever, tachycardia, worsening leukocytosis, peritonitis, bowel perforation, or strangulation require immediate surgery.

Simple or open-loop obstruction is characterized by no vascular compromise and can be decompressed proximally via emesis or NG tube. If a large segment of bowel appears to be threatened, or if bowel viability cannot be clearly established, the surgeon can leave the abdomen open with plans to return to the operating room in 24 to 48 hours for a repeat assessment.

Postoperative Gastrointestinal Bleeding

Postoperative GI bleeding encompasses many clinical scenarios, including primary intestinal disease, stress-related, and/or surgical complications with varying locations and severities. Depending upon the etiology and presentation, GI bleeding is commonly categorized as either upper GI bleeding (UGIB) or lower GI bleeding (LGIB). UGIB is defined as hemorrhage proximal to the ligament of Treitz and is commonly caused by peptic ulcer disease, stress erosions, Mallory-Weiss tear, and gastric varices. LGIB is anatomically located distal to the ligament and is caused by arteriovenous malformations, diverticulosis, or postpolypectomy/colectomy in the colon. LGIB from the small bowel is less common and includes arteriovenous malformations, ulcerated small bowel tumors, and Meckel diverticula in the differential diagnosis.

Postoperative GI bleeding is associated with significant morbidity; therefore, it is imperative to recognize risk factors before operation, as persistent hemorrhage necessitates reoperation in 2% to 5% of patients. Stress gastritis is more commonly seen in critically ill patients. Prophylaxis with PPIs, H_2 blockers, or sucralfate should be considered in these patients.

When evaluating patients with a GI bleed, the patient's medical history provides important diagnostic clues and may help guide management decisions. Despite the increased use of PPIs and understanding of *Helicobacter pylori*, peptic ulcer disease remains the most common cause of nonvariceal UGIB. Mallory-Weiss tears are mucosal lacerations at the gastroesophageal junction caused by forceful emesis and more commonly seen in alcoholic patients. A history of liver disease, cirrhosis, or the stigmata of portal hypertension on examination suggests variceal etiology of UGIB. The most common sources of LGIB are diverticular and postpolypectomy bleeding. In patients with recent intestinal surgery, the anastomotic site should be considered as a potential source of bleeding. In a patient with previous intraabdominal aortic surgery, aortoenteric fistula should be considered. Additionally, coagulopathies due to liver disease, NSAIDs, antiplatelet agents, or anticoagulation therapies increase the risk of bleeding.

Hematemesis, melena, or hematochezia are common manifestations of GI bleeding. UGIB typically presents with hematemesis or melena, but brisk UGIB can also present with hematochezia; the redder the blood, the more rapid is the bleed. Flexible endoscopy is the standard of care for localization and control of GI bleeding in the stable patient when UGIB suspicion is high. Also, in evaluation of LGIB, upper endoscopy or gastric aspiration should be considered to exclude UGIB sources. Tachycardia, hypoxemia, or hypotension suggest the need for immediate resuscitation.

The basic principles of management of postoperative GI bleeding include the following: fluid resuscitation and restoration of intravascular volume, monitoring clotting parameters and correcting abnormalities, identification and treatment of aggravating factors, transfusion of blood products, and identification and treatment of the source of the bleeding.

Stress ulcers are superficial mucosal lesions that are usually confined to the mucosa of the stomach and proximal duodenum. These lesions typically heal without any sequelae, but, rarely, deep penetration or perforation can cause peritonitis. Intraluminal pH should be maintained above 3.5, and prophylaxis with H_2 blockers, PPIs, sucralfate, and anticholinergics decreases bleeding. However, in patients with uncontrolled bleeding, endoscopic therapy using electrocautery or heater probe hemostasis or angiographic injection of vasopressin or Gelfoam may be required. Surgery is occasionally needed and may include gastrostomy with oversewing of focal areas of active bleeding, subtotal gastric resection, or total gastrectomy in intractable cases.

Aggressive resuscitation with correction of hemodynamics, hemoglobin, and coagulopathy can reduce mortality in patients with postoperative GI bleeding. Serial blood counts and coagulation studies (prothrombin time, partial thromboplastin time, and bleeding time) should be performed every 6 hours and corrected with appropriate transfusion therapy.

After initial workup, based on the clinical status of the patient (stable or unstable), the localization of the bleeding source to either the upper or lower GI tract aids in determining the appropriate diagnostic and treatment options. The major goals of treatment are to stop active bleeding and prevent recurrent bleeding. Endoscopy is the major diagnostic tool for localization and treatment of UGIB and is indicated for control of active bleeding. Therapeutic interventions include the combination of thermal coagulation, hemoclips, and/or endoscopic band ligation, with or without epinephrine injection. Recurrent bleeding after endoscopic control is seen in 15% to 20% of patients, and the common risk factors include older adults (>65), malignancy, and use of NSAIDs. Repeat endoscopy can control long-term bleeding and has fewer complications when compared with surgery for recurrent bleed. Patients with repeat bleeding after second endoscopic therapy should be considered for angiography with transarterial embolization. Surgical control of the bleeding may be required in patients who failed angiographic therapy.

Localization of LGIB requires a combination of CT angiography, tagged red blood cell (RBC) scintigraphy, video capsule endoscopy, and colonoscopy. Upper GI endoscopy should be considered to exclude UGIB sources. Patients who are stable and can tolerate bowel preparation are commonly assessed with colonoscopy. CT angiography is useful in patients with active bleeding, whereas video capsule endoscopy is commonly used for initial evaluation of suspected small bowel bleeding. The advantage of

tagged RBC scintigraphy is that it is highly accurate (75%) in localization even in cases of intermittent and delayed bleeding (>48 hours). Angiography with selective embolization may be used to treat active LGIB and is successful in >90% of cases with a relatively low (<8%) risk of bowel ischemia. Anoscopy or rigid proctoscopy can be used to localize bleeding from a colorectal, coloanal, or ileoanal anastomosis. Bleeding from diverticular and postpolypectomy bleeding can be successfully localized with colonoscopy and treated with epinephrine injection and hemostatic clip placement.

Acute variceal bleeding, especially in patients with decompensated liver cirrhosis (with ascites or hepatic encephalopathy), is associated with a high mortality rate. Correction of hypovolemia, rapid hemostasis, prevention of early rebleeding and complications related to bleeding, and restoration of liver function are most important components in the management. Furthermore, in contrast to patients with nonvariceal bleeding, aggressive fluid administration may result in increased portal venous pressure complicated by pulmonary edema or ascites. Treatment with vasopressors (octreotide and vasopressin) to decrease the portal pressure should be initiated. Hemoglobin level >8 g/dL, systolic blood pressure (>90–100 mm Hg), HR <100/min, and central venous pressure (1–5 mm Hg) are required to achieve hemodynamic stability. In stable patients, endoscopic hemostasis can be achieved either by performing endoscopic variceal ligation or injection of sclerotherapy; transjugular intrahepatic portosystemic shunt (TIPS) can be lifesaving when ligation fails. Use of nonselective β-blockers prevents long-term rebleeding. Also, repeat endoscopic banding is recommended every 10 to 14 days for complete eradication of varices.

Bleeding from Mallory-Weiss tears is usually self-limited and does not usually require endoscopic hemostasis. Likewise, bleeding from an intestinal anastomosis during the early postoperative period also resolves spontaneously. However, when bleeding does not spontaneously cease, transfusion with 4 to 6 units of blood and repair of the leak should be done in the operating room either by oversewing or resection of the anastomosis and recreation of an anastomosis or end stoma. Hemorrhage from a low colorectal anastomosis can be managed with transanal suture ligation.

Clostridioides difficile Colitis

Clostridioides difficile (C. difficile), formerly known as *Clostridium difficile,* is a gram-positive, anaerobic, toxin-producing, spore-forming bacillus. The spores are resistant to heat, acid, and antibiotics and can be transmitted through the fecal-oral route. Normally, the indigenous microbiota of the intestine inhibits the growth of *C. difficile* and prevents its proliferation. *C. difficile* infection (CDI) can occur when normal gut flora are disrupted by antibiotic usage or when spores germinate resulting in *C. difficile* overgrowth in the colon.

C. difficile colitis is caused by the production of enterotoxin A and cytotoxin B, which damage intestinal epithelia, impair cell function, and promote local inflammation. Some strains of *C. difficile* have mutations in the toxin-producing gene, leading to increased toxin secretion and virulence. CDI is the most common cause of nosocomial diarrhea, although not all patients colonized with *C. difficile* will develop symptoms.

The risk factors of CDI are antibiotic exposure, increased age (>65 years), hospitalization, inflammatory bowel disease, GI surgery, immunosuppressive medication, or an immunologically compromised host. Nearly all antibiotics are associated with CDI, including the ones used to treat the disease (vancomycin, metronidazole). The risk of CDI is increased by a prolonged course of antibiotic treatment or the administration of multiple antibiotics. Surgery patients are at risk for CDI because they are usually elderly and hospitalized, have associated comorbidities, and are relatively immunosuppressed.

CDI symptoms range from asymptomatic, mild to moderate diarrhea, or life-threatening fulminant colitis. The distal colon is most commonly affected, but CDI can present as localized colitis in any part of the colon or as diffuse colitis. Most patients develop watery diarrhea during antibiotic therapy or shortly after a course of antibiotics but can also present weeks later. Other symptoms of CDI include abdominal pain, fever, weakness, loss of appetite, nausea, and vomiting. Severe cases of CDI may present with significant dehydration, abdominal distension, ileus, toxic megacolon, bowel ischemia, colonic perforation, peritonitis, renal failure, sepsis, shock, and death. Patients with fulminant CDI present with hypotension, shock, ileus, and toxic megacolon, which is associated with a higher mortality.

Stool testing for *C. difficile* is commonly performed in patients who have three or more episodes of unexplained loose or watery stools within 24 hours. Laboratory testing can detect either free toxin (toxin A, toxin B) by enzyme immunoassay or the presence of *C. difficile* by detecting common antigen, toxin genes, cells, or spores. Fresh stool should be collected and sent to the laboratory as soon as possible. Flexible or rigid proctoscopy can be performed at the bedside in critically ill patients when urgent surgical intervention is necessary. Patients with CDI demonstrate white to yellow pseudomembranes about 2 cm in size separated by normal mucosa. Abdominal x-rays may show dilated, edematous colon or toxic megacolon in severe cases. An abdominal CT scan with oral contrast can evaluate toxic megacolon (cecal diameter >12 cm, colon >6 cm) or bowel perforation. Blood tests frequently demonstrate a significant leukocytosis, metabolic acidosis, high lactate, AKI, and hypoalbuminemia in severe cases. Presence of hypotension, shock, ileus, and toxic megacolon is seen with fulminant CDI.

Transmission of *C. difficile* is prevented by contact precaution. Patients with CDI are usually placed in a single room on "isolation precautions" with a separate toilet or on "contact isolation precautions." Patients should be encouraged to wash hands and take regular showers if possible to reduce the risk of spore transmission. All healthcare providers should wear gowns and gloves and wash hands with soap and water before and after they are in contact with CDI patients because the spores are resistive to alcohol-based solutions. Visitors should also be advised to follow these precautions as well. Sporicidal solutions should be used for cleaning the room to facilitate decontamination after discharge.

Treatment of CDI starts by discontinuing the patient's inciting antibiotics as soon as possible and administering IV fluids to prevent or correct dehydration. Only symptomatic patients with CDI should be treated. The drugs of choice for CDI are vancomycin or fidaxomicin. When the clinical suspicion of CDI is high, laboratory testing should not delay the treatment. For the initial episode of CDI, vancomycin 125 mg is given orally four times per day or fidaxomicin 200 mg orally two times per day for 10 days.[39] In less severe cases of CDI, metronidazole (500 mg orally three times per day for 10 days) is an alternative if vancomycin and fidaxomicin are not available. In fulminant CDI, vancomycin (500 mg orally four times per day) is given with additional metronidazole (500 mg IV three times per day), and the use of vancomycin enemas (500 mg in 100 mL normal saline enema) is also recommended. Surgical intervention is considered in patients with peritonitis, colonic perforation, bowel ischemia,

abdominal compartment syndrome (ACS), worsening acidosis, sepsis, and shock despite appropriate resuscitation, and worsening clinical presentation of CDI despite adequate medical management. For many years, total abdominal colectomy with ileostomy was viewed as the procedure of choice for life-threatening CDI. More recently, laparoscopic loop ileostomy and colonic lavage with 8 L of polyethylene glycol (PEG 350) and antegrade vancomycin flushes (500 mg in 500 mL lactated Ringer solution every 8 hours) and IV metronidazole for 10 days has been adopted at many centers. Colectomy may still be required in refractory cases of CDI but is more commonly used for salvage of nonresponders to the fecal diversion and colonic lavage protocol.

Anastomotic Leak

Intestinal anastomoses are commonly performed in emergency and elective general surgery. Successful intestinal anastomoses require a combination of meticulous surgical technique, good blood supply, and no tension at the anastomosis.

Numerous factors have been implicated in the failure of anastomotic healing and are summarized in Table 26.7. While anastomotic integrity depends on the complex interplay of patient factors and underlying disease processes, the surgeon must ensure these factors are considered and the anastomotic technique is appropriate for the clinical situation. Technical factors contributing to early leakage include gaps in the suture line, misplacement of sutures, stapler misfiring, enterotomy, or tear near the suture line.

When elective intestinal surgery is performed, there are opportunities to optimize patient-related risk factors to decrease the risk of anastomotic leak. These include smoking cessation, nutritional optimization to correct protein malnutrition, and replacement of deficient essential nutrients (e.g., protein, zinc, and copper) and vitamins (e.g., A, C, and E). Patients with significant cardiac or pulmonary disease should be risk stratified and optimized if possible.

The signs and symptoms of anastomotic leak are variable depending on the intestinal location, the size of the leak, the degree and spread of contamination, and the timing of presentation

TABLE 26.7	Risk Factors Associated With Anastomotic Leak
DEFINITIVE FACTORS	**IMPLICATED FACTORS**
Technical aspects	Mechanical bowel preparation
Blood supply	Drains
Tension on suture line	Advanced malignancy
Airtight and watertight anastomosis	Shock and coagulopathy
	Emergency surgery
Location in gastrointestinal tract	Blood transfusion
Pancreaticoenteric	Malnutrition
Colorectal	Obesity
Above peritoneal reflection	Sex
Below peritoneal reflection	Smoking
Local factors	Steroid therapy
Septic environment	Neoadjuvant therapy
Fluid collection	Vitamin C, iron, zinc, and cysteine deficiency
Bowel-related factors	
Radiotherapy	Stapler-related factors
Compromised distal lumen	Forceful extraction of stapler
Crohn disease	Tears caused by anvil or gun insertion
	Failure of stapler to close

(early vs. late). Fever, tachycardia, increasing abdominal pain, elevated white blood cell (WBC) count, decreased urine output, and shortness of breath are commonly seen with intraabdominal leaks. Leaks may present early with severe symptoms, sepsis, and multiorgan failure if intestinal contents are disseminated throughout the peritoneal cavity. Patients may also present in a more delayed and subtle fashion with vague abdominal pain, prolonged ileus, or delayed return of bowel function if they present late or the abscess has been "walled off" by omentum or other viscera. Anastomotic leaks may also present as drainage of intestinal contents from intraabdominal drains or as surgical site infections (SSIs) with enterocutaneous fistulas (ECFs) draining from the skin incision. Many symptoms of anastomotic leak are nonspecific and may overlap with other complications or delays in postoperative recovery. The surgical team should have a high index of suspicion and aggressively investigate unexpected symptoms in patients with recent intestinal anastomoses because delays in diagnosis and treatment of anastomotic leaks are associated with worse outcomes.

Laboratory tests like complete blood test, C-reactive protein, and procalcitonin may be elevated with anastomotic leak but are considered relatively nonspecific. The most common imaging techniques to assess for anastomotic leak are water-soluble contrast studies and CT scans. Fluoroscopic contrast studies are most useful for proximal GI or distal colorectal anastomoses. Abdominopelvic CT scans with oral or rectal contrast are used to assess for anastomotic leaks but do not routinely demonstrate contrast leakage from the site of the leak. Signs of local inflammation like stranding and thickened bowel, and large amounts of fluid (>300 mL) around the anastomosis ÷ free air should raise concern for a leak. Interventional radiology sampling or drainage of the fluid may be used to confirm and, in some instances, treat a small or contained leak.

Depending on the clinical condition of the patient, management of an anastomotic leak ranges from drainage, bowel rest, and antibiotic therapy to exploratory laparotomy with repair, resection, proximal diversion, or ostomies. When the diagnosis of anastomotic leak is clinically obvious and the patient has peritonitis or severe sepsis, many surgeons will proceed with immediate exploratory laparotomy or diagnostic laparoscopy. Asymptomatic, radiographic-discovered leaks may require no treatment. In patients with localized abscesses who are not toxic, successful management may include abscess drainage, broad-spectrum antibiotics, and/or bowel rest. A contained leak, along with an abdominal or pelvic abscess and clinical signs of sepsis, requires drainage of the abscess with broad-spectrum antibiotic coverage. Surgical intervention is required in the absence of clinical improvement or deterioration, sepsis, or diffuse peritonitis. The surgical treatment of anastomotic leaks is determined by the patient's medical condition and intraoperative findings; small leaks (<1 cm) can be managed with simple repair and drainage when there are healthy tissues and minimal inflammation. When severe peritonitis, bowel edema and inflammation, and systemic sepsis are present, a diverting stoma should be considered. Small leaks with localized inflammation from a low colorectal anastomosis can be managed with pelvic drains and a diverting loop ileostomy. The use of protective stomas is not just limited to rectal surgery but is applicable to all anastomoses. Although a proximal diverting stoma does not prevent an anastomotic leak, it will mitigate the clinical impact of anastomotic failure by diverting the fecal stream away from the newly created anastomosis. Anastomotic breakdown in the pelvis is commonly caused by ischemia and frequently results in peritoneal contamination. In this situation, takedown of the anastomosis is required with complete fecal diversion using a colostomy or ileostomy.

Intestinal Fistulas

A fistula is defined as an abnormal communication between two epithelialized surfaces. Fistulas in the GI tract originate from the intestinal wall or biliary or pancreatic ducts and communicate with adjacent organs or intestine (internal fistulas) or externally with the abdominal wall (external fistula). Most GI fistulas (75%–85%) are iatrogenic or traumatic and caused by faulty operative technique, injury to the intestine during handling, lysis of adhesions, abdominal fascial closure, or percutaneous drainage.

Intestinal fistulas are classified as internal, external, or mixed. Mixed fistulas involve two or more hollow viscera with a cutaneous connection and are almost always associated with an abscess. External intestinal fistulas, or ECFs, are the most common type and are usually the result of complications from previous abdominal surgery (e.g., anastomotic leak, bowel injury, iatrogenic injury, or from bowel exposure to large abdominal defects or prosthetic mesh). The ileum is the most common site for an ECF. Proximal ECFs (e.g., small bowel) are usually high output, whereas distal ones (e.g., colon) tend to be low output. Colocutaneous fistulas may also be seen with diverticulitis, cancer, inflammatory bowel disease, and appendicitis or radiation therapy. Aortoenteric fistulas occur due to erosion of prosthetic aortic grafts into the surrounding viscera, usually the duodenum.

The fistula output over a 24-hour period is the most important determinant of its physiologic impact (on fluid and electrolyte status) on the patient and guides management.

Medical treatment of fistulas commonly include wound management, pharmacologic (e.g., H_2 blockers), nutrition, fluid, and electrolyte management. Fistula closure is considered spontaneous in the absence of radiologic or surgical intervention. Anatomic characteristics associated with nonhealing fistulas include large adjacent abscess, fistula tract <2 cm in length, enteral defects >1 cm, and fistulas arising from certain bowel segments (e.g., stomach, lateral duodenum, ligament of Treitz, and ileum). Furthermore, fistulas associated with concurrent pancreatic fistulas, presence of malnutrition, or adjacent infection have a low rate of spontaneous closure.

Patients with ECFs can present with a wide range of symptoms. They may demonstrate delayed return of bowel function and controlled drainage of enteric contents from an intraabdominal drain with minimal signs of infection. However, sepsis is the most common complication seen in patients with an ECF. With this presentation, patients may demonstrate fever, tachycardia, elevated WBC count, leakage of purulent material, and finally enteric contents draining from their surgical incision. The diagnosis of ECFs is usually straightforward because the drainage of enteric contents through the skin (enterocutaneous) or vagina (enterovaginal) is clinically obvious. ECFs may also present with severe abdominal wall infections caused by bacterial invasion and chemical erosion that facilitates extension of infectious process through fascial planes, subcutaneous tissue, and muscle. In contrast, internal fistulas (e.g., colovesical) may present more subtly and require imaging or endoscopy to diagnose.

CT scans of the abdomen and pelvis are commonly obtained in patients with postoperative sepsis and concerning intraabdominal fluid collections are drained with radiographic guidance to treat infected fluid collections. When oral contrast leaks from the GI tract or enteric contents are drained, the diagnosis is made.

Other commonly used methods of diagnosing small bowel fistulas include a fistulogram for external fistulas or upper and lower GI series (internal fistulas). Fistulograms provide information about the length and origin of the fistula, which can help in determining whether the fistula might close spontaneously.

Prevention of fistulas is facilitated by the use of healthy bowel for anastomosis, preoperative mechanical bowel preparation, preoperative intraluminal or systemic antibiotics, anastomotic techniques, and preoperative optimization of the nutritional status.

The overall treatment goals in managing ECFs include control of sepsis, prevention of fluid/electrolyte depletion, management the fistula drainage, prevention of skin damage, and enhancement of healing by optimizing the patient's nutritional status with total parenteral nutrition (TPN) and enteral feeding as tolerated.[46] Once sepsis is controlled, initial management includes NPO status, NG decompression, and/or pharmacologic measures (e.g., PPIs or H_2 blockers) to decrease gastric secretions. The use of somatostatin analogues (e.g., octreotide) may lead to decreased fistula output, and reduced fistula healing time. Infliximab (monoclonal antibody to tumor necrosis factor-alpha [TNF-α]) may help with fistula closure in patients with Crohn disease.

After the basal fistula output is measured, enteral feeding can be initiated to see how this impacts fistula output. If enteral feeding causes a significant increase in fistula output, the patient should be made NPO and started on TPN with an appropriate volume and electrolyte composition to replace fistula losses.[47] For low-output and colonic fistulas, the use of enteral nutrition facilitates early fistula closure, reduced pneumonia rate, improved intestinal barrier function, and decreased rate of fistula recurrence. However, enteral nutrition usually requires at least 122 cm of bowel. In many patients with high output fistulas and complex intraabdominal pathology, long-term TPN is necessary to provide nutritional support, maintain normovolemia, and prevent electrolyte disorders.

Wound management is a major consideration in all patients with ECFs, and nurses with experience in wound/ostomy management are critical for this. Spillage of enteral contents causes severe local skin excoriation at the site of an ECF. Fistula output >500 mL/day usually requires a pouch system, whereas output <50 mL/day can be managed with dressing and skin barrier treatment. Various techniques are available to manage these frequently complex wounds, including protective substances (stomahesives, fibrin sealants), wound management systems, and negative pressure wound therapy.

Once the sepsis is controlled, the patient's fluid and nutrition status is improving, and the wound is managed, the probability of spontaneous closure and timing of surgical intervention needs to be considered. Medical therapy should be continued as long as the patient is continuing to improve. The majority of fistulas that close spontaneously do so in the first 4 weeks. Therefore, in most cases, patients should be given at least 8 weeks for the fistula to heal spontaneously before surgery is considered. Surgical therapy is inevitable in many cases. Indications for surgical management of ECFs include persistent drainage, sepsis, or abscess. However, the timing of surgical intervention requires an assessment of the risk-benefit ratio for the individual patient. Surgical intervention for ECFs should be delayed until both the intraabdominal and systemic conditions have been optimized. In many cases, there is a dense peritoneal reaction caused by abdominal sepsis and ECF that peaks around 10 to 21 days and lasts at least 6 to 8 weeks before subsiding. In some cases, delaying surgery even longer (e.g., 3–6 months) may allow peritoneal inflammation to significantly subside and allow the patient to be nutritionally and physiologically optimized before subjecting them to major surgery with its associated complications.

Surgery for ECFs is technically challenging and time consuming. Many patients with ECFs have large abdominal wall defects that need to be repaired in conjunction with the fistula surgery. In most cases, the fistulous tract and the surrounding skin will be completely resected, an extensive adhesiolysis is usually required, and the entire bowel is examined to exclude distal pathology or obstruction. The fistula is usually resected, followed by an end-to-end intestinal anastomosis. In some cases (e.g., low rectal fistulas), diverting ostomies may be used to decrease the risk of pelvis sepsis. Many patients require abdominal wall reconstruction procedures with component separation, use of bioabsorbable mesh, and/or acellular dermal prostheses.

Postoperative Pancreatic Fistula

Postoperative pancreatic fistula (POPF) occurs after pancreatic surgery such as pancreaticoduodenectomy (10%–15%), and mid and distal pancreatectomy (20%–30%), but also after percutaneous drainage (especially for ductal disconnection syndrome), left renal or adrenal surgery, splenic surgery, and splenic flexure mobilization.

POPF is a particularly serious complication as it can cause a cascade of secondary injuries, including delayed gastric emptying, abdominal infections, false aneurysms, and abdominal bleeding. Among these complications, postoperative pancreatic hemorrhage (PPH) is the most fatal, occurring in 3% to 20% of patients, with associated mortality rates as high as 20% to 50%. To establish a standardized definition of pancreatic fistula in different regions, the International Study Group on Pancreatic Fistula (ISGPF) has published objective definitions.[48] Grade A POPF denotes a biochemical leak with no discernible clinical impact on the typical postoperative course. Clinically significant POPFs fall into the categories of grade B and grade C. Grade B has a clinical impact and requires a change in management to include therapeutic agents and less invasive treatments or percutaneous, endoscopic, or angiographic interventional procedures. Finally, grade C fistulas are those that lead to reoperation, single or multiple organ failure, or even death.

The risk factor consistently identified as predictive of grade C POPF after pancreatic surgery is soft glandular texture. Other factors, such as male sex, small pancreatic duct diameter (<3 mm), BMI ≥25.0 kg/m², preoperative serum albumin <3.0 g/mL, high intraoperative blood loss, and operative time ≥480 minutes, have also been reported.

In addition, anastomotic techniques are critical in pancreatic surgery. More than 50 methods of pancreaticojejunostomy (PJ) have been developed, including end-to-end and end-to-side anastomosis, coating, binding, and duct-to-mucosa. The incidence of pancreatic fistula varies between these techniques. Currently, the most widely used clinical anastomosis techniques are end-to-end invagination PJ and end-to-side duct-to-mucosa PJ. The latter involves anastomosis of the pancreatic duct and jejunal mucosa, which is challenging in narrow ducts and soft pancreas. End-to-end invagination PJ is a simpler procedure in which the intact pancreatic stump is inserted into the jejunum, often as a single or double anastomosis.[49]

Recent studies have found a superiority of the Blumgart anastomosis (BA) developed by L.H. Blumgart in 2000. Combining duct-to-mucosa anastomosis with the end-to-side invagination technique, BA shows superiority over traditional PJ in reducing major complications, including grade C POPF, reoperation rates, and 90-day mortality.

Stent placement in PJ anastomosis is also controversial, as is whether the stent should be an external or internal stent.

The choice of treatment for POPF is determined by its grade, with conservative measures usually sufficient for grades A and B. Conservative treatment includes nutritional support, somatostatin analogues, and adequate drainage. However, grade B and C POPF may require interventional therapies such as endoscopic or percutaneous procedures, and some cases may require reoperation. Adequate drainage is fundamental to the management of POPF and can be effectively managed by routine abdominal drainage, percutaneous peritoneal drainage under CT or ultrasound guidance, and internal drainage using endoscopic ultrasound with pancreatic duct stenting. Combined with nutritional support, antibiotic therapy and inhibition of pancreatic secretion, most patients can recover from POPF without complications.

Following nonsurgical management, patients with persistent pancreatic fistula, abdominal bleeding, abdominal abscess, sepsis, or other critical conditions require further surgical intervention. Surgical approaches may include debridement and open drainage, completion pancreatectomy, the revision of the pancreatic anastomosis, Roux-en-Y fistula tract-jejunostomy, and the bridge stent technique.[50]

Bile Duct Injuries

Bile duct injury (BDI) is the most common severe and problematic complication associated with gallbladder surgery. The likelihood of sustaining a major BDI during cholecystectomy is relatively low (e.g., 3/1000 procedures). However, these potentially preventable injuries can be devastating and are associated with significant morbidity and mortality.

The incidence and consequences of these injuries vary between different surgical techniques. Overall, BDIs are less common in open cholecystectomy, with a rate below 0.2%. However, in the laparoscopic approach, the incidence is slightly higher, ranging between 0.2% and 0.8%.[51]

Iatrogenic BDI most commonly occurs by misidentifying the common bile duct (CBD) for the cystic duct during laparoscopic cholecystectomy. Risk factors associated with BDI can be characterized as patient factors, local factors, and learning curve effect. The biliary tree and relationship of the cystic duct and its insertion onto the common hepatic duct is noted to have variable and anomalous anatomy. Aberrant or distorted anatomy due to inflammation; a short, wide cystic duct; or when the cystic duct runs parallel to the common hepatic duct results in close approximation of the cystic and CBD. A number of other contributing factors have been recognized, such as excessive cephalad retraction on the gallbladder fundus, excessive use of cautery, tenting of the common duct from excessive lateral retraction on the infundibulum resulting in a tear, and aberrant biliary anatomy. Patients who are severely obese and have prior hepatobiliary surgery or underlying liver disease can impair visualization and increase the risk of injury. The presence of any of these risk factors should alert the surgeon to the increased possibility of encountering a potentially dangerous situation during laparoscopic cholecystectomy. Most surgeons prefer the "critical view of safety" technique, and intraoperative cholangiography can help surgeons better identify the anatomy of the biliary tract to avoid biliary tract injury. In recent years, the application of near-infrared fluorescence imaging for intraoperative navigation has received increasing attention from clinicians. By using indocyanine green fluorescence imaging

during laparoscopic cholecystectomy, components of the biliary tract system can be visualized in real-time helping surgeons to promptly grasp the situation.[52,53]

Less than one-third of iatrogenic BDIs are detected at the time of laparoscopic cholecystectomy. If a BDI or leak is identified intraoperatively, the surgeon must decide whether they have adequate training, staff, and resources to assess and manage the injury appropriately. If the surgeon decides to proceed, cholangiography must be performed to delineate the anatomy and plan treatment. If the surgeon feels they cannot safely repair the injury, no further dissection or conversion to laparotomy should be performed and the patient should be drained and transferred to a facility with experienced surgeons. If a cholangiogram catheter can be easily placed into the injury, this may help the next team to identify the injury and perform a cholangiogram promptly.

Most biliary injuries are diagnosed in a delayed fashion. Recognition and proper diagnosis of BDIs are advantageous in preventing serious complications. Patients often present with nonspecific symptoms, such as vague abdominal pain, nausea and vomiting, and low-grade fever, usually resulting from uncontrolled bile leakage into the peritoneal cavity. Some patients may present with sepsis from severe bile peritonitis, jaundice, or intraabdominal abscess. Patients who have ligation or early stricture formation may also present with cholangitis and jaundice. Also, excessive use of cautery or laser in the region of the common duct results in biliary strictures that manifest as recurrent cholangitis, obstructive jaundice, or secondary biliary cirrhosis. Cholangiography is considered the gold standard for evaluating BDIs, but the hepatobiliary iminodiacetic acid scan is frequently used to screen for bile leaks. Ultrasound and CT are capable of detecting intraabdominal fluid collections and ductal dilatations.

Biliary injuries are best avoided by understanding the circumstances in which biliary injuries are likely to occur and how to avoid injury in these situations. Strasberg and colleagues proposed a classification system that encompassed injuries commonly incurred during laparoscopic cholecystectomies (Table 26.8).[54]

Treatment for BDIs varies based on the severity and complexity of injury. It can range from simple drainage procedures to the

TABLE 26.8   Strasberg Classification of Bile Duct Injury

TYPE	DEFINITION
Type A	Leak from the cystic duct or small ducts in the gallbladder or liver bed
Type B	Occlusion of an aberrant right hepatic duct
Type C	Transection without ligation of an aberrant right hepatic duct with subsequent leakage
Type D	Injury to the lateral bile duct involving less than 50% of the duct circumference
Type E	Strictures of the common hepatic duct Subdivided as follows depending on the proximal extent:
Type E1	Strictures have a common duct stump of >2 cm
Type E2	Strictures have a common duct stump of <2 cm
Type E3	Strictures occur at the confluence
Type E4	Strictures indicate a separation of the right and left hepatic ducts due to the destruction of the confluence
Type E5	Stricture is due to the injury of an aberrant right hepatic duct with concomitant stricture of the common hepatic duct

Reprinted with permission from the *Journal of the American College of Surgeons,* formerly *Surgery Gynecology & Obstetrics.*

reconstruction of the biliary system. Regardless of when the injury is identified (immediately or after a delay), it is advisable to refer all cases to specialized centers with appropriate clinicians and resources for optimal care.

The Strasberg classification is used to guide treatment decisions. In Strasberg type A injuries, monitoring the output of a previously placed drain can help assess for spontaneous closure of the leak. Endoscopic stenting across the lesion may help to seal the leak and promote biliary drainage by reducing pressure. If peritonitis or worsening intraabdominal sepsis is present, exploration for washout may be required.

Strasberg type B injuries, characterized by minimal pain and mildly elevated liver function tests, can be managed conservatively and monitored. If cholangitis occurs due to obstruction, drainage of the affected segment may be required by percutaneous transhepatic cholangiogram with placement of a biliary drainage tube or hepaticojejunostomy. Segmental resection may be necessary if there is significant atrophy.

Treatment options for Strasberg type C injuries are similar, including percutaneous drainage to promote spontaneous closure and prevent biliary peritonitis. Hepaticojejunostomy or hepatectomy may be required in rare cases.

Strasberg type D injuries involve partial injury to the CBD. Small injuries without devascularization can be closed with a drain left in place, together with endoscopic sphincterotomy and stent placement. If devascularization is present, repair with a drain left in place is recommended in anticipation of bile leakage. Endoscopic stenting with interventional radiologic drain placement is an alternative, especially in postoperative injuries.

Strasberg type E injuries identified at the time of injury can be repaired end to end with a T-tube draining externally or a Y-tube draining into the duodenum. If a tension-free anastomosis is not possible, a Roux-en-Y hepaticojejunostomy is the preferred reconstruction option. In cases of friable tissue or dense adhesions where a hepaticojejunostomy is not feasible, a pedicled omental patch may be used as a temporary repair pending definitive reconstruction.

Neurologic Complications
Postoperative Delirium

Delirium refers to a state of mental dysfunction that presents with a wide range of neuropsychiatric symptoms. Delirium is characterized by disturbance of consciousness and change in cognition (memory deficit, disorientation, language, and perceptual disturbance) that develops in a short period of time, fluctuates during the day, and is not explained by preexisting dementia or neurodegenerative disorders. Delirium is especially common in elderly patients and its causes are multifactorial. The incidence of postoperative delirium (POD) varies from 15% to 53% in elderly surgical patients and represents a significant cause of morbidity.

There are many hypotheses regarding the pathogenesis of POD, including neuroinflammation from infection or stress of surgery, alterations in blood-brain barrier permeability, poor cerebral perfusion, imbalances in neuroendocrine and neurotransmitter activity (especially cholinergic), cerebral atrophy, and reduction of cognitive reserve in elderly. The risk factors for POD include patient-related risk factors, illness-related factors, and interventions triggering POD. Patient-related factors for POD include advanced age (>65 years), multiple medical comorbidities, malnutrition, polypharmacy, history of cerebral infarction, chronic renal or hepatic disease, depression, and anxiety. The hospital environment (noise, sleep disturbance due to light/dark cycle and

waking patients for vital signs and medication administration, the ICU) and medical/surgical interventions (NG tubes, drains, Foley catheters, endotracheal intubation) are also associated with an increased risk for POD. Other factors that contribute to developing POD include pain, infection, hypoxia, dehydration, anemia, emotional and physical stress, sleep deprivation, medication such as anticholinergics and benzodiazepines, and physical restraints.

POD mostly presents within 5 days postoperatively. The symptoms of POD are acute, fluctuate over 24 hours, and are often reversible. These include sleep alteration, such as daytime drowsiness, nighttime insomnia, and psychomotor alteration with lucid intervals. POD symptoms can be hyperactive, hypoactive, or both. Hyperactive symptoms include agitation, anger, restlessness, verbal and physical aggression, or mood lability. Hypoactive symptoms are more common and present as lethargy, inattention, flat mood, somnolence, and decreased response to stimuli. For this reason, patients with hypoactive POD are less likely to be diagnosed.

Although certain risk factors for POD cannot be changed (e.g., patient age, type of operation, anesthetic choice), many predisposing POD factors can and should be modified in the perioperative period. Nutritional status, anemia, volume status, and hydration should be corrected before surgery. In addition, anticholinergic and benzodiazepine medications should be avoided unless the patient is "high risk" for alcohol withdrawal or severe anxiety. Prevention of deep sedation by monitoring anesthesia depth during surgery with electroencephalogram (EEG) monitoring or by using dexmedetomidine for light sedation during ICU care reduces the incidence of POD. In surgical and trauma patients, pain control should be adequate with multimodal analgesia using additional nonopioid medication if possible. Surgical patients should have physical restraints such as Foley catheters, endotracheal tubes, and drains removed and be transferred out of the ICU as soon as possible. Physicians and teams should routinely check for responsiveness and arouse patients during rounds (especially elderly patients) to screen for hypoactive symptoms. Sleep disturbance should be avoided if possible, and the room environment should be adjusted to enhance patient comfort with access to outside windows for maintenance of circadian rhythms. Family members can be involved in taking care of patients to support daily care and early mobilization is recommended.

Once delirium is detected, the caregiving team should consider safety of the patients and staff and perform a comprehensive assessment (physical examination, laboratory tests, etc.) to identify possible causes, including myocardial infarction, stroke, seizure, electrolyte imbalance, hypoxia, hypothermia, hypoglycemia, and acidosis. In the absence of treatable medical causes for POD nonpharmacologic interventions—including cognitive reorientation, decreasing sleep disturbance, optimizing nutrition, fluid and oxygenation, providing hearing and vision aids, and more—are preferable. Pharmacologic intervention should be reserved for patients who are not responsive to nonpharmacologic methods or for hyperactive patients who are at risk of harming themselves, other patients, or caregivers. Antipsychotics (e.g., haloperidol, olanzapine, and quetiapine) are commonly used to treat hyperactive POD. Gabapentin is used to prevent alcohol withdrawal and benzodiazepines are used to treat alcohol and benzodiazepine withdrawal. In most instances, POD is treated using a small dose of medication and titrating the dose as needed and for the shortest duration possible. POD patients should be closely monitored during treatment and receive follow-up after discharge to assess cognitive function.

SELECTED REFERENCES

Afshari A, Ageno W, Ahmed A, et al. European Guidelines on perioperative venous thromboembolism prophylaxis: executive summary. *Eur J Anaesthesiol.* 2018;35:77-83.

> *This is a comprehensive summary of European guidelines for perioperative venous thromboembolism prophylaxis.*

Dino D, Demartines N, Clavien PA. Classification of surgical complications: a new proposal with evaluation in a cohort of 6336 patients and results of a survey. *Ann Surg.* 2004;240(2): 205-213.

> *Surgical article with over 27,000 citations that provides a classification system for complications. It is based on the type of therapy required to correct the complication.*

Domenghino A, Walbert C, Birrer DL, et al. Consensus recommendations on how to assess the quality of surgical interventions. *Nat Med.* 2023;29(4):811-822.

> *An independent jury provides guidance for standardized and improved outcome reporting of surgical procedures, based on extensive literature reviews and expert input.*

Halvorsen S, Mehilli J, Cassese S, et al. 2022 ESC Guidelines on cardiovascular assessment and management of patients undergoing non-cardiac surgery. *Eur Heart J.* 2022;43:3826-3924.

> *This article describes the assessment and perioperative management of cardiac conditions that are potential sources of complications during noncardiac surgery.*

Slankamenac K, Graf R, Barkun J, et al. The comprehensive complication index: a novel continuous scale to measure surgical morbidity. *Ann Surg.* 2013;258(1):1-7.

> *This article presents the Comprehensive Complication Index (CCI®), which is based on the Clavien-Dindo Classification, and assesses the overall morbidity burden by including all complications experienced by an individual patient.*

Abbassi F, Pfister M, Lucas KL, et al. Outcome Reporting Group. Milestones in Surgical Complication Reporting. Clavien-Dindo Classification 20 Years and Comprehensive Complication Index 10 Years. *Ann Surg.* 2024;280(5):763–771.

> *This article provides improved guidance for the consistent application of the Clavien-Dindo classification (CDC) and Comprehensive Complication Index (CCI®) in challenging clinical scenarios.*

The full reference list appears on Elsevier eBooks+.

27 CHAPTER

Surgery in the Geriatric Patient

Vanita Ahuja, Ayaka Tsutsumi, and Sandhya A. Lagoo-Deenadayalan

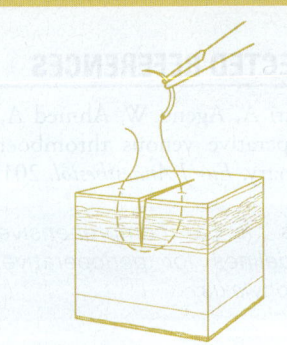

OUTLINE

INTRODUCTION

Life expectancy has increased dramatically in the past several decades. An average 65-year-old female today can expect to live an additional 20.6 years, nearly twice as long as her counterpart in 1900. An average 80-year-old female can expect to live nearly 9.8 more years (Table 27.1).[1] With this increase in life expectancy comes a growth in the number of people living into old age with diseases and chronic conditions that would have caused death in past decades. At present, more than 75% of adults older than age 65 years have at least one chronic condition, with five or more present in 20% of the Medicare population. Many of these diseases, which include cancer, degenerative joint disease, coronary artery disease, and visual impairment, have a surgical option as part of the treatment algorithm. Currently, 15% of the population age 65 years old and older accounts for 40% of the surgical procedures in the United States.

OUTCOMES OF SURGERY IN OLDER ADULTS

There appears to be worse outcomes after surgery with increasing age.[2] Mortality from high-risk operations such as esophagectomy can be two and three times the mortality for similar procedures in younger adults.[3] Multiple studies, however, now confirm that the age of the patient alone is not the major predictor of poor outcome, but rather how successfully the patient has aged.[4] It is now generally accepted that frailty, rather than chronologic age, is the most important predictor of traditional surgical outcomes. Studies have shown significant mortality in older patients within 1 year of undergoing surgery, and poor function, cognition, and psychological well-being were associated with mortality. This has led to a concentrated effort in measuring function, cognition, and psychological well-being at the time of

preoperative assessment to enhance surgical decision-making and patient counseling.[2]

Most studies of surgical outcomes in older and younger adults focus on 30-day mortality and 30-day complications, such as pneumonia and surgical site infections. The American College of Surgeons National Surgical Quality Improvement Program (ACS NSQIP) Surgical Risk Calculator is an extremely useful tool in predicting the likelihood of these outcomes.[5] Preoperatively, individual patient and procedural risk factors can be entered into the NSQIP model, and rates of various traditional outcomes for that individual are calculated. This information can be used to help inform shared decision-making. However, other outcomes that are more relevant to older adults, such as cognitive decline, functional decline, and loss of independence, are rarely, if ever, measured. In one study exploring the treatment preferences of seriously ill adults, patients were much more willing to take a treatment if there was a possibility of death than they were if there was a possibility of cognitive or functional decline (Fig. 27.1).[6]

Unfortunately, because few data are collected on the cognitive or functional outcomes of surgery, it is difficult to advise older adults about the likelihood of these outcomes. In response to the need to provide such data, in 2014, the NSQIP began a new geriatric pilot with 23 volunteer hospitals collecting new risk and outcome variables more relevant to older adults.[7] These variables covered the areas of goals of care, cognition, mobility, and function (Fig. 27.2). These data were also used to develop a Geriatric Risk Calculator for older adults for postoperative outcomes with some information on the likelihood of the outcomes that are more relevant to them.[8]

In addition to the differences discussed in outcomes in older adults, there is great variability in surgical mortality rates in Medicare patients linked to the hospital in which they receive treatment. Mortality rates can vary as much as threefold between the best-performing hospitals and the worst performers. There is also

TABLE 27.1 Life Expectancy of Older Persons at Various Ages		
	ALL RACES	
AGE (IN YEARS)	**MALE**	**FEMALE**
65	17.9	20.6
70	14.4	16.6
75	11.2	12.9
80	8.3	9.8
85	5.9	7.0
90	4.1	4.8
95	2.8	3.3
100	2.0	2.3

From Life Expectancy of Older Persons at Various Ages in the United States, 1900-2010, by Robert L. Brown and Steven G. Prus. This is a journal article published in *the Journal of Population Ageing* in 2017. It provides data and analysis on the life expectancy of older Americans from 1900 to 2010, based on the Human Mortality Database and the Social Security Administration.

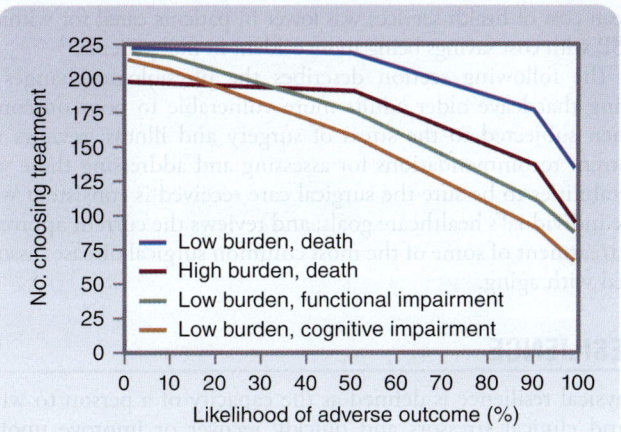

FIGURE 27.1 Many patients are willing to undertake high- or low-burden treatments, even if the risk of death is high (up to 50%). However, when there is even a small risk of cognitive or functional decline, the number of patients willing to undergo even a low-burden treatment sharply declines. (From Fried TR, Bradley EH, Towle VR, et al. Understanding the treatment preferences of seriously ill patients. *N Engl J Med.* 2002;346:1061-1066.)

great variability in the rates at which surgical care is provided in older adults. In a study looking at the rates of surgery in patients near the end of life, 31.9% of decedents had surgery in the last year and 18.3% in the last month.

In response to the need to provide more standardization in the surgical care of older adults, ACS partnered with the John A. Hartford Foundation to form the Coalition for Quality in Geriatric Surgery. The coalition was composed of nearly 60 major national and regional organizations representing patients and family advocacy groups, regulators and insurers, surgeons in many specialties, geriatricians and other medical specialists, nurses, social workers, and other health professionals. Over a 4-year period the coalition developed a set of 30 evidence- and consensus-based standards that form the basis for the ACS Geriatric Surgery Verification program.

This ACS Quality program, like those in trauma, bariatrics, cancer, and pediatrics, hopes to improve the outcomes for surgical care in older adults by providing a consistent framework for care that is patient centered, interdisciplinary, and embedded in the function of the hospital at https://www.facs.org/quality-programs/geriatric-surgery.[9–11]

Preliminary data demonstrate that the Geriatric Surgery Verification program reduces postoperative length of stay.[9] Additionally, implementation of a geriatric surgery pathway (GSP) has led to improved geriatric-specific surgical outcomes with decreased loss of independence and decreased incidence of major complications.[10] The total

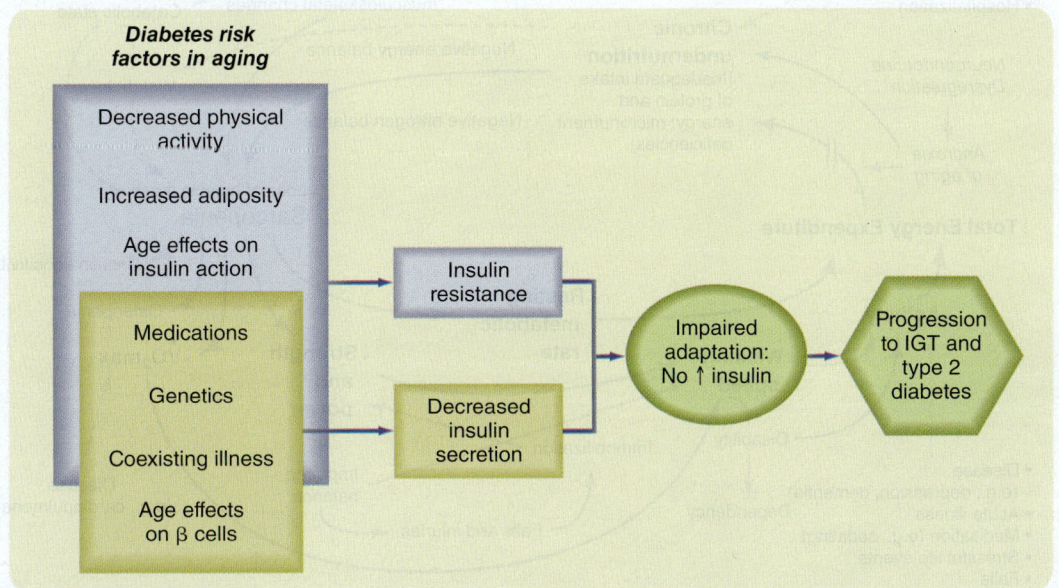

FIGURE 27.2 The normal response to hyperglycemia is for the β cell to adapt and secrete sufficient insulin to restore euglycemia. In aging, there is a decrease in insulin secretion and a probable increase in insulin resistance, which, when combined with comorbid illness, genetic factors, and medications, leads to a failure of this glucoregulatory process. *IGT*, Impaired glucose tolerance. (From Chang AM, Halter JB. Aging and insulin secretion. *Am J Physiol Endocrinol Metab.* 2003;284:E7-E12.)

mean cost of health services was lower in patients cared for within a GSP, with cost savings being more evident in frail patients.[11]

The following section describes the physiologic changes of aging that leave older adults more vulnerable to poor outcomes when subjected to the stress of surgery and illness; reviews the current recommendations for assessing and addressing these vulnerabilities to be sure the surgical care received is consistent with the individual's healthcare goals; and reviews the current approach to treatment of some of the most common surgical diseases associated with aging.

RESILIENCE

Physical resilience is defined as the capacity of a person to withstand clinical stressors and quickly recover or improve upon a baseline functional level.[12] The three domains of resilience include physical, cognitive, and psychosocial. Stressors in one area can lead to effects in other domains. Studies exploring resilience phenotypes and surrogate measures of resilience can help us to devise strategies to improve resilience in older adults undergoing surgery.

FRAILTY AND PHYSIOLOGIC DECLINE

With aging, there is a decline in physiologic function in all organ systems, but the significance of this decline is variable among organs and individuals. Attempts have been made to define the specific changes in organ function that are directly attributable to aging; however, this remains difficult because aging is also accompanied by increased vulnerability to disease. It is often difficult to determine whether an observed decline in function is secondary to aging or the associated disease. The overall effect, however, is still the same—a much smaller margin for error in the care of older patients.

Frailty

Frailty is defined as "a biologic syndrome of decreased reserve and resistance to stressors, resulting from cumulative declines across multiple physiologic systems causing vulnerability to adverse outcomes." The actual mechanism of frailty is complex and thus beyond the scope of this chapter; however, a conceptual model is shared to show that the frail state is characterized by loss of muscle mass (sarcopenia), chronic undernutrition, weakness, and decreased exercise tolerance (Fig. 27.3). The manifestation of frailty is linked with many poor health outcomes, such as falls, disability, hospitalization, and death as well as worse outcomes from any healthcare intervention, including surgery. The impact of frailty on surgical outcomes has been the subject of many studies over the past decade. These studies are complicated by the many different methods used to define the characteristics of the frail individual; however, the conclusion that frailty is associated with worse outcomes is common to all of them.[13]

The Fried frailty phenotype[14] is the most widely used method to describe frailty. It defines the frail phenotype by five characteristics: weight loss, weak grip strength, self-reported exhaustion, slow walking speed, and low energy expenditure. Using this definition, frail patients undergoing elective surgery were found to have more postoperative complications, longer lengths of stay, and more frequent discharge to a location other than home.

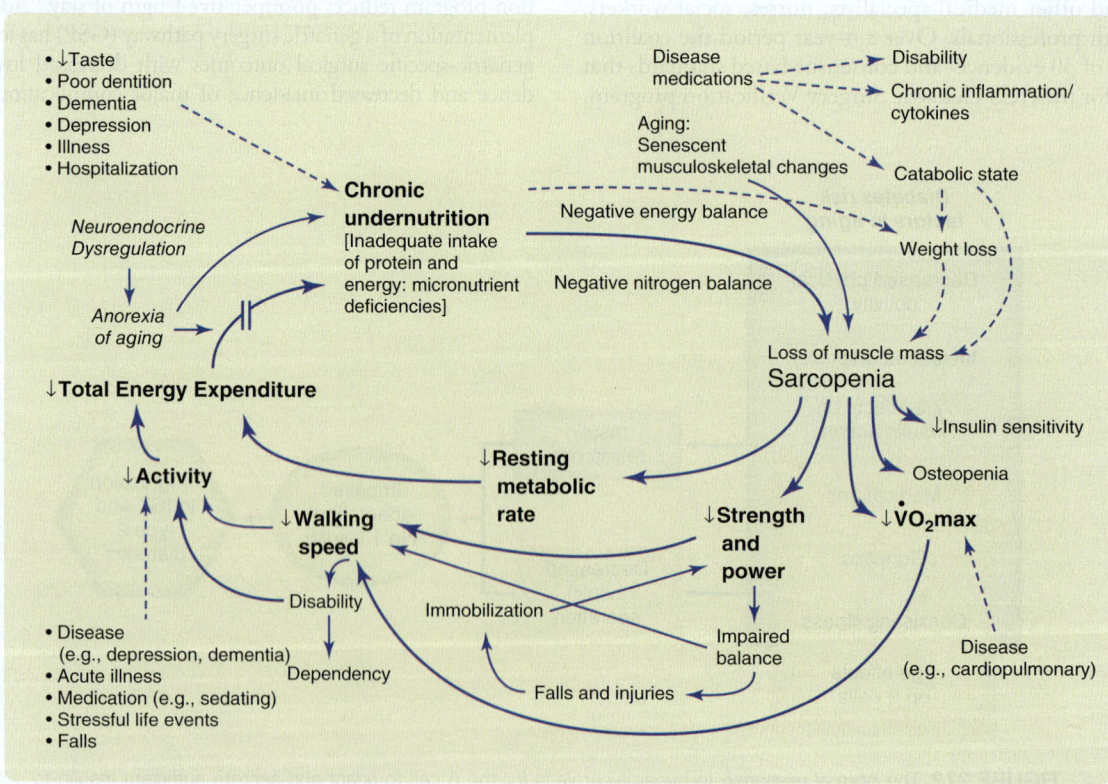

FIGURE 27.3 The cycle of frailty is characterized by chronic undernutrition, loss of lean muscle mass (sarcopenia), and decreased exercise tolerance. (From Fried LP, Walston J. Frailty and failure to thrive. In: Hazzard WR, Blass JP, Ettinger WH Jr, Halter JB, Ouslander JG, eds. *Principles of Geriatric Medicine and Gerontology.* 4th ed. New York, NY: McGraw Hill; 1998:1387-1402.)

Another method of describing frailty is the multidomain model that includes measures of cognition and mood, function, malnutrition, chronic disease, and geriatric syndromes.[15] Using elements of this model (cognition, activities of daily living [ADLs], low serum albumin, anemia, comorbidity, and falls), frail patients undergoing surgery that required an intensive care unit (ICU) stay were found to have higher rates of mortality at 6 months after surgery.

There are many tools to measure frailty, such as the Timed Up & Go Test, measurement of gait speed, and the simplified frailty index, which includes weight loss, low energy level, and the inability to rise from a chair five times in succession without using the arms. Other methods for measuring frailty based on data from large datasets include the Risk Analysis Index and several other administrative claims-based tools.[16]

Regardless of the method used to identify frailty, the presence of this geriatric syndrome is now widely recognized as a significant risk factor for poor surgical outcomes. Although frailty cannot be reversed in preparation for surgery, recognition of the increased risk caused by the various components of frailty, such as chronic undernutrition and impaired mobility, can help direct a preoperative preparation program and a postoperative management program that may help mitigate the risk.

Organ-Specific Decline

Cardiovascular System

Cardiovascular disease is a major cause of death in the United States in both sexes. Of these deaths, about 80% occurred in persons older than 65 years in 2021 according to the CDC.[17] In surgery, cardiac events account for a significant portion of the complications in older adults in the postoperative period. The prevalence is attributable to cardiac function and structural changes secondary to aging (Box 27.1). A knowledge of cardiac aging is important in directing the postoperative management of older adults.

As one ages, morphologic changes take place in the great vessels as well as the heart itself such as myocardium, conducting pathways, valves, and vasculature of the heart. Myocytes are replaced by collagen and elastin, resulting in myocardium fibrosis and an overall decline in ventricular compliance. Conducting systems are also affected by aging. Almost 90% of the autonomic tissue is replaced by fat and connective tissue in the sinus node, affecting the conduction in the intranodal tracts and bundle of His. These changes influence the high incidence of sick sinus syndrome, atrial arrhythmia, and bundle branch block in the elderly population. Progressive dilation of all four valvular annuli

---

BOX 27.1 Major Cardiovascular Changes With Age

- Decreased number of myocytes
- Fibrosis of conducting pathways with increased arrhythmias
- Decrease in ventricular and arterial compliance (increased afterload)
- Decreased β-adrenergic responsiveness
- Increased dependence on preload (including atrial kick)
- Increased diastolic dysfunction
- Increased silent ischemia

From Ahuja V, Rosenthal RA. Surgery in the geriatric patient. In: Townsend CM Jr, Beauchamp RD, Evers BM, Mattox KL, eds. *Sabiston Textbook of Surgery: The Biological Basis of Modern Surgical Practice.* Philadelphia: Elsevier; 2021:284-314.

BOX 27.2 Major Renal Changes With Age

- Decrease in the number of functional nephrons
- Decrease in the number of tubular cells
- Decreased renal blood flow
- Decreased glomerular filtration rate
- Decline in creatinine clearance despite normal serum creatinine level
- Decline in tubular function (loss of concentrating ability)
- Increased susceptibility to dehydration
- Decreased clearance of certain drugs
- Increase in lower urinary tract dysfunction and infection

From Ahuja V, Rosenthal RA. Surgery in the geriatric patient. In: Townsend CM Jr, Beauchamp RD, Evers BM, Mattox KL, eds. *Sabiston Textbook of Surgery: The Biological Basis of Modern Surgical Practice.* Philadelphia: Elsevier; 2021:284-314.

---

is likely the cause for the multivalvular regurgitation demonstrated in healthy older persons. Finally, there is a gradual increase in rigidity and decrease in distensibility of the coronary arteries and great vessels. Changes in the peripheral vasculature are likely related to increased systolic blood pressure, increased resistance to ventricular emptying, and compensatory loss of myocytes, with ventricular hypertrophy.[18]

Renal System

Approximately 25% of all Americans 70 years and older have moderately or severely decreased kidney function (Box 27.2). With increasing age, there is a gradual decrease in the renal cortex. Over time, approximately 40% of the nephrons become sclerotic, with the residual functional units becoming hypertrophic in a compensatory manner. Additionally, there is atrophy of the afferent and efferent arterioles and decrease in renal tubular cell number. Renal blood flow also falls by approximately 50%. Functionally, the changes lead to a decline in the glomerular filtration rate of approximately 45% by age 80 years.

Renal tubular function also declines with advancing age, and this results in decreased ability to conserve sodium and excrete hydrogen ions, with diminished capacity to regulate fluid and acid-base balance. Dehydration becomes an issue because losses of sodium and water from nonrenal causes are not compensated for by the usual mechanisms. The inability to retain sodium is assumed to be caused by a decline in the activity of the renin-angiotensin system. The increasing inability to concentrate the urine is caused by a decline in end-organ responsiveness to antidiuretic hormone. The observed decline in the subjective feeling of thirst is also well documented but not well understood. Alterations of osmoreceptor function in the hypothalamus may be responsible for the failure to recognize thirst despite significant elevations in serum osmolality.[18]

Circulating levels of erythropoietin (EPO) are higher in the healthy elderly as compared with younger individuals. Increased EPO production in the elderly is interpreted as a counterregulatory mechanism aimed at preserving normal red blood cell mass in response to a higher turnover as well as to EPO resistance. However, EPO levels are reduced in anemic elderly individuals, suggesting an impaired counterregulatory response to low hemoglobin levels. Elderly people may develop vitamin D deficiency due to the impaired capacity of the aging kidney to convert 25-hydroxyvitamin-D to 1,25 dihydroxy vitamin-D, but extrarenal factors (i.e., 25-OH-vitamin D availability) are at least equally responsible for vitamin D insufficiency in this age group.[19]

Acute kidney injury (AKI) is defined as a 0.3 mg/dL or 50% or higher change in the serum creatinine level from baseline or a reduction in urine output of less than 0.5 mL/kg/hour over a 6-hour interval within a 48-hour period after adequate volume resuscitation. AKI is a common occurrence after major surgery and can affect up to 7.5% of patients with a normal preoperative serum creatinine level. AKI is correlated with increased short-term morbidity and mortality as well as increased long-term mortality.

Risk factors for the development of postoperative AKI are age, emergency surgery, ischemic heart disease, and congestive heart failure. Also, older patients with already compromised renal function are at increased risk of postoperative AKI. The keys to avoiding postoperative AKI are to recognize that older patients are at increased risk and to take steps to avoid unnecessary hypovolemia and to make sure proper dosing of drugs that are cleared by the kidney and of drugs that are nephrotoxic.

The bladder in an older patient has increased collagen content, leading to limited distensibility and impaired emptying with age. Overactivity of the detrusor muscle secondary to neurologic disorders or idiopathic causes is also identified. In females, decreased circulating levels of estrogen and decreased tissue responsiveness to this hormone cause changes in the urethral sphincter that leads to urinary incontinence. In males, prostatic hypertrophy impairs bladder emptying. Both of these factors lead to urinary incontinence in 10% to 15% of older persons living in the community and 50% of those in nursing homes.[20] There is also an increased prevalence of asymptomatic bacteriuria with age, which varies from 10% to 50% depending on sex, level of activity, underlying disorders, and place of residence. Urinary tract infections alone account for 30% to 50% of all cases of bacteremia in older patients.

Hepatobiliary System

Overall, hepatic function is well preserved with aging. However, there is an increase in liver disease and in liver disease–related mortality in persons between the ages of 45 and 85 years. Morphologic changes include a reduction in overall liver weight, size, and volume. Hepatocyte size and the number of binucleated cells increase, and the number of mitochondria decreases.[18,21] Functionally, hepatic blood flow decreases by 20% to 40%.

The synthetic capacity of the liver, as measured by standard tests of liver function, remains unchanged (Box 27.3). However, the metabolism of and sensitivity to specific types of drugs is changed. Drugs requiring microsomal oxidation (phase I reactions) before conjugation (phase II reactions) may be metabolized more slowly, whereas those requiring only conjugation may be cleared at a normal rate. Drugs that act directly on hepatocytes, such as warfarin (Coumadin), may have the desired therapeutic

---

> ### BOX 27.3 Major Hepatobiliary Changes With Age
>
> - Decrease in the number of hepatocytes
> - Decrease in hepatic blood flow
> - Synthetic capacity remains unchanged
> - Increased sensitivity to and decreased clearance of certain drugs
> - Increased incidence gallstones and gallstone-related diseases
>
> From Ahuja V, Rosenthal RA. Surgery in the geriatric patient. In: Townsend CM Jr, Beauchamp RD, Evers BM, Mattox KL, eds. *Sabiston Textbook of Surgery: The Biological Basis of Modern Surgical Practice*. Philadelphia: Elsevier; 2021:284-314.

---

effects at lower doses in older adults because of an increased sensitivity of cells to these agents. Recent evidence has also proposed that aging may be linked with a decline in the ability of the liver to protect against the effects of oxidative stress.

The most significant correlation of altered hepatobiliary function in older adults is the increased incidence of gallstones and gallstone-related complications. Gallstone prevalence rises steadily with age depending on the population, where stones have been shown in as many as 80% of nursing home residents older than 90 years. Biliary tract disease is the single most common cause for abdominal surgery in older adults.[22]

Glucose Homeostasis

Data from the National Health and Nutrition Examination Survey have shown an increase in the prevalence of glucose homeostasis disorders with age; more than 20% of persons older than 60 years have type 2 diabetes mellitus. An additional 20% have glucose intolerance described by normal fasting glucose and a postchallenge glucose level higher than 140 mg/dL but less than 200 mg/dL. This glucose intolerance may be caused by a decrease in insulin secretion, increase in insulin resistance, or both (see Fig. 27.2).[21]

These factors, along with comorbid illness, medications, and genetic predisposition, put older surgical patients at particularly high risk for uncontrolled hyperglycemia when exposed to the usual insulin resistance that accompanies the physiologic stress of surgery. Both the endogenous glucose response to traumatic stress and glycemic response to an exogenous glucose load are amplified in injured older patients.

Although most of the data on glucose control and surgical outcomes are in the cardiac surgery literature, recent evidence showed that uncontrolled hyperglycemia in the immediate perioperative period is related with an increase in infections in almost all types of surgery. The ideal level of glucose control, however, is still controversial. Earlier prospective studies indicated that tight control of blood sugar (80–110 mg/dL), achieved by continuous infusion of insulin, improved some outcomes, including mortality, in critically ill patients in the surgical ICU, but more recent data have cast some doubt on the benefits of such strict control. In general, maintenance of the blood glucose level below 180 mg/dL in the perioperative period is now widely accepted as an appropriate target, even in older patients.[23–25]

SURGICAL DECISION-MAKING

The first and perhaps the most important consideration in the preoperative assessment is being sure the patient and their family understand the ramifications of the care that is being suggested and that this care is concordant with the patient's goals for that care and for their overall health.

Surgeons traditionally measure surgical success in terms of 30-day mortality and morbidity. For older patients, however, the definition of good outcome is more complex. Although we are now able to perform even the most complicated surgery on our oldest patients with traditional surgical success, the quality of the outcome in the patient's view is more likely to depend on whether they can continue to function as before the surgery. For some older patients, losing functional independence because of a major surgical intervention may be a far worse outcome than living with, or even dying of, the disease for which surgery is offered. In a study of older patients with limited life expectancy because of serious chronic disease, Fried and colleagues examined the impact of treatment burden (low, minor interventions, such as intravenous

[IV] antibiotics; high, major interventions, such as surgery) and expected outcome (desirable vs. undesirable) on patient preferences for treatment. Results indicated that more than 70% of older patients would not want even a low-burden treatment if severe functional impairment or cognitive impairment were the expected outcome. The concern for functional and cognitive impairment was more dramatic than the fear of death (see Fig. 27.1).

In another study of preferences for permanent nursing home placement in seriously ill hospitalized patients, 56% of patients were very unwilling or would rather die than live permanently in a nursing home. The correlation between the patient's wishes and both the surrogate's and physician's opinion of the patient's wishes was poor.

Therefore, it is fundamental that the older patient be given a realistic estimate of the overall functional outcome of the planned surgical treatment in addition to the likelihood of control or cure of the particular disease. It is also essential that the surgeon realizes the patient's preferences in the context of this broader view of surgical success. Patients' overall goals of care and postoperative quality of life are often overlooked. As mentioned earlier, the new NSQIP Geriatric Surgical Calculator can be used to help older adults understand the risk of postoperative delirium and functional decline and better inform the shared decision-making.

Outcomes after emergency surgery are known to be worse than outcomes after elective surgery. In older adults, frailty is associated with significant mortality in those undergoing emergency surgical procedures, even in patients undergoing low-risk procedures. Preoperative assessment of frailty or assessment in the immediate postoperative period, even in patients undergoing emergency surgery, can help to set expectations, guide decision-making, and individualize perioperative care, discharge planning, and postoperative follow-up.

Several tools have been developed to help surgeons communicate more effectively with the older patient and their family in the acute setting. The "Best Case/Worst Case" model provides a structured way of discussing what the postoperative period will look like for the patient and has been shown to improve the quality of these difficult discussions. Another model provides a structured framework for the discussion that puts the decision-making in the context of the patient's overall health and healthcare goals (Box 27.4A).[26]

Advance Directives

All patients should be encouraged to make a formal advance directive and identify a surrogate decision-maker should the need

arise. Providers should be sure to discuss the patient's preferences directly with the patient, as discussions of these issues are not always easy and surrogates may not be fully aware of the patient's preferences. Tools, such as "PREPARE" (https://prepareforyourcare. org) and the "Five Wishes" (https://fivewishes.org) are available to help patients and families have these discussions and create advance care plans (ACPs). Providers should also be sure when advance directives do exist that they are clearly documented and easily accessible in the patient's medical record. Studies have found that less than 15% of older patients (age ≥65 years) undergoing inpatient elective surgery had ACP documentation, and only 19.5% of patients who were admitted to the ICU had this documentation. Disparities in eliciting ACP highlight healthcare inequities, with a decreased ACP in males, individuals with a non-English–preferred language, and those without Medicare insurance coverage.[27] Other reports show that even when done, almost three-quarters of ACP documentations were uploaded on the day of surgery and were often elicited by nonsurgical healthcare professionals, indicating several golden but missed opportunities for the surgical team to enhance the provision of goal-concordant care.[28]

Palliative Care

Honoring a patient's preferences for treatment at the end of life is a necessary component of quality healthcare. Studies have documented that the extent of burden plays a role in a patient's decisions to choose aggressive care, and often, if the risk and benefits are appropriately discussed, aging patients may choose less aggressive treatment. An inpatient do not resuscitate (DNR) order is associated with risk of death or hospice transition within 30 days of surgery, independent of traditional markers of poor surgical outcomes.[29] Further research is necessary to understand factors leading to a DNR order that may aid early recognition of high-risk older adults who would benefit from early palliative care consultation.

For patients with a poor prognosis, discussions regarding palliative care should happen early in the treatment conversation and do not preclude treatment of the disease or symptoms. Patients and their family members should be encouraged to complete and discuss their advance directives, which have been shown to make decisions for care at the end of life easier for patients and their families and more in line with patient wishes. Early palliative care has been shown to lead to substantial improvements in quality of life and mood and in some studies has even been shown to have increased survival.[30] As there has been an increased focus on the quality of care, physicians and surgeons have come to understand that treatment is not only about curing disease but also about quality of life and alleviating suffering in patients.

Screening to Identify High-Risk Characteristics

To ensure the best surgical decision-making and the best surgical outcome for the individual older patient, the preoperative assessment must be thorough and must address all the relevant concerns. With this in mind, the ACS and the American Geriatric Society worked together to define a set of best practice guidelines for the preoperative assessment of the geriatric patient. These guidelines provide a 13-item checklist of cognitive, comorbid, functional, and psychosocial factors that have all been shown to have an impact on the outcome of care for older surgical patients (Fig. 27.4). Based on preoperative assessment findings, providers can recommend targeted prehabilitation, rehabilitation, medication management, care coordination, and/or delirium prevention interventions to improve postoperative outcomes for older surgical patients.[31] Structured goals-of-care discussions using the question

---

BOX 27.4A Goals of Structured Communication

- Place the patient's acute surgical condition in the context of the patient's underlying illness.
- Elicit the patient's goals, priorities, and what is acceptable regarding life-prolonging and comfort-focused care.
- Describe treatment options—including palliative approaches—in the context of the patient's goals and priorities.
- Direct treatment to achieve these outcomes and encourage the use of time-limited trials in circumstance of clinical uncertainty.
- Affirm continued commitment to the patient's care.

From Cooper Z, Koritsansky LA, Cauley CE, et al. Recommendations for best communication practices to facilitate goal-concordant care for seriously ill older patients with emergency surgical conditions. *Ann Surg.* 2016;263:1-6.

ACS NSQIP©/AGS BEST PRACTICE GUIDELINES:
Optimal Preoperative Assessment of the Geriatric Surgical Patient

Preoperative Assessment

In addition to conducting a complete and thorough history and physical examination of the patient, the following assessments are strongly recommended:

☐ Assess the patient's **cognitive ability** and **capacity** to understand the anticipated surgery (see Section I.A, Section I.B, and Appendix I).

☐ Screen the patient for **depression** (see Section I.C).

☐ Identify the patient's risk factors for developing postoperative **delirium** (see Section I.D).

☐ Screen for **alcohol** and other **substance abuse/dependence** (see Section I.E).

☐ Perform a preoperative **cardiac** evaluation according to the American College of Cardiology/American Heart Association (ACC/AHA) algorithm for patients undergoing noncardiac surgery (see Section II and Appendix II).

☐ Identify the patient's risk factors for postoperative **pulmonary** complications, and implement appropriate strategies for prevention (see Section III).

☐ Document **functional status** and history of **falls** (see Section IV).

☐ Determine baseline **frailty** score (see Section V and Appendix III).

☐ Assess patient's **nutritional status**, and consider preoperative interventions if the patient is at severe nutritional risk (see Section VI and Appendix IV).

☐ Take an accurate and detailed **medication history,** and consider appropriate perioperative adjustments. Monitor for **polypharmacy** (see Section VII, Appendix V, Appendix VI, and Appendix VII).

☐ Determine the patient's **treatment goals** and **expectations** in the context of the possible treatment outcomes (see Section VIII).

☐ Determine patient's **family** and **social support system** (see Section VIII).

☐ Order appropriate preoperative **diagnostic tests** focused on elderly patients (see Section IX).

FIGURE 27.4 Best practice guidelines checklist. *ACS,* American College of Surgeons; *AGS,* American Geriatrics Society; *NSQIP,* National Surgical Quality Improvement Program. (From Chow WB, Rosenthal RA, Merkow RP, et al. Optimal preoperative assessment of the geriatric surgical patient: a best practices guideline from the American College of Surgeons National Surgical Quality Improvement Program and the American Geriatrics Society. *J Am Coll Surg.* 2012;215:453-466.)

prompt list ensure that older patients have a realistic understanding of their surgery, risks, and recovery. This preoperative workup, combined with engaging with family members and interdisciplinary teams, can improve postoperative outcomes.[32]

Cognitive Assessment

Preoperative cognitive status as a risk factor for negative postoperative outcomes in older patients is often not assessed. However, preoperative cognitive deficits are common; the prevalence of dementia is approximately 1.5% at age 65 years and approximately doubles with every 5 additional years of life. More than one-third of people older than age 70 years have some cognitive impairment or dementia. Preexisting cognitive dysfunction can impair a patient's capacity to give informed consent and can have significant short- and long-term consequences in the postoperative period. A history of dementia before surgery has been associated with increased rates of mortality and serious morbidity. Dementia is also the single greatest risk factor for postoperative delirium.

Although there are several methods to assess baseline cognitive status, the Mini-Cog[33] is an accurate test for cognitive impairment that is easy to perform in a busy clinic setting. The Mini-Cog test combines a three-item word learning and recall task (0–3 points; each correctly recalled word, 1 point), with a simple clock-drawing task (abnormal clock, 0 points; normal clock, 2 points, used as a distraction before word recall). Total possible Mini-Cog scores range from 0 to 5 points, with 0 to 2 suggesting a high likelihood and 3 to 5 suggesting a low likelihood of cognitive impairment. Another test is the Montreal Cognitive Assessment (MoCA). The MoCA[34] was developed by Dr. Ziad Nasreddine in Montreal, Canada, in 1995 for the detection of mild cognitive impairment (MCI) by health professionals. MCI is a syndrome defined as cognitive decline greater than expected for an individual's age and education level but that does not interfere with ADLs. The prevalence of MCI in population-based epidemiologic studies ranges from 3% to 19% in adults older than 65 years, and more than half progress to dementia within 5 years. The MoCA may be useful in the occupational health setting for detecting MCI or early dementia, especially as the workforce ages. A comprehensive website provides the test, instructions, normative data, references, frequently asked questions, and permissions and updates.

Capacity

To give informed consent, a patient must have decision-making capacity. The essentials of decision-making capacity are well described. In essence, the patients must be able to understand the nature of their illness, the risks and benefits of the treatment recommended, and the risks and benefits of the treatment alternatives. To be considered competent to give consent, the patient must be able to:

1. Clearly indicate a treatment choice
2. Understand the relevant information given
3. Appreciate the medical condition and the consequences of treatments
4. Reason about the treatment options

Capacity assessments can be outlined in a framework to understand the next steps in care or a patient's ability to live independently. These assessments should include contribution from a multidisciplinary team, including social workers and physical and occupational therapists, who can provide information on the ability to manage self-care and optimize support structures. Patients who scored 19 or less on the MoCA were at highest risk for incapacity, suggesting that the MoCA can be useful to identify older adults undergoing surgery who are at the highest risk of incapacity.[35] It may be prudent in such cases to identify a surrogate decision-maker who can represent the patient.

Delirium Risk

Delirium is defined as an acute disorder of cognition and attention and is among the most common and potentially devastating complications seen in older surgical patients. Delirium occurs in from 5% to over 50% of older surgical patients and is associated with longer hospital stays, increased rates of mortality and morbidity, poor functional recovery, and more discharges to locations other than home. Both cognitive dysfunction and depression are risk factors for delirium; however, other factors must also be assessed. Risk factors for delirium are divided into two groups: the preoperative or predisposing factors and the precipitating factors or those that occur in the postoperative period (Table 27.2). Delirium risk can be evaluated using a predictive rule that considers the patient's age, comorbidities, and type of surgery. It can also be assessed using the DEAR tool or ACS NSQIP Geriatric Surgical Risk Calculator described previously.[36]

Depression

Depression is present in approximately 11% of persons older than age 71 years. Unrecognized depression in the postoperative period

TABLE 27.2 Risk Factors and Precipitating Factors for Delirium

RISK (PREDISPOSING) FACTORS	PRECIPITATING FACTORS
Advanced age	Infection
Cognitive impairment	Medications
Functional impairment	Hypoxemia
Poor nutrition	Electrolyte abnormalities
Comorbidity	Undertreated/overtreated pain
Alcohol abuse	Neurologic events
Psychotropic medications	Dehydration
Sensory impairment	Sensory deprivation
Type of surgery	Sleep disruption
Severe illness	Use of bladder catheters
	Unfamiliar environment
	Use of physical restraints

may explain poor oral intake, lack of participation in the postoperative treatment plan, and higher requirements for analgesics. Depression also has been associated with higher mortality and longer hospital stays in patients undergoing cardiac surgery. Screening for depression is easily accomplished using the Patient Health Questionnaire-2, which requires the patient to answer two questions:

1. In the past 12 months, have you ever had a time when you felt sad, blue, depressed, or down for most of the time for at least 2 weeks?
2. In the past 12 months, have you ever had a time, lasting at least 2 weeks, when you did not care about the things that you usually care about or when you did not enjoy the things that you usually enjoy?

Functional Assessment

There are several ways to evaluate function in the preoperative period. Each has value in predicting outcomes of surgery.

Activities of daily living. For older adults, the ability to perform ADLs (e.g., feeding, continence, transferring, toileting, dressing, bathing) and instrumental ADLs (IADLs, e.g., telephone use, transportation, meal preparation, shopping, housework, medication management, managing finances) has been shown to correlate with postoperative mortality and morbidity. In a study of patients over 80 years old, function (defined as independent, partially dependent, or totally dependent in ADLs) was a better predictor of mortality than age. More importantly, evaluating ADLs and IADLs preoperatively is essential for perioperative and discharge planning.[37]

American Society of Anesthesiologists classification. The physical status classification of the American Society of Anesthesiologists (ASA) has been used effectively to stratify operative risk. This classification ranks patients according to the functional limitations affected by coexisting disease. When curves for mortality versus ASA class are examined regarding age, there is little difference between younger and older patients, which indicates that mortality is a function of frailty and coexisting disease rather than chronologic age. ASA classification has been shown to predict postoperative mortality accurately, even in patients older than 80 years old.

Exercise tolerance. In older adults, exercise tolerance is the most sensitive predictor of postoperative cardiac and pulmonary complications. The metabolic requirements for many routine activities have been determined and are quantitated as metabolic equivalents of the task (METs). One MET, defined as 3.5 mL/kg/

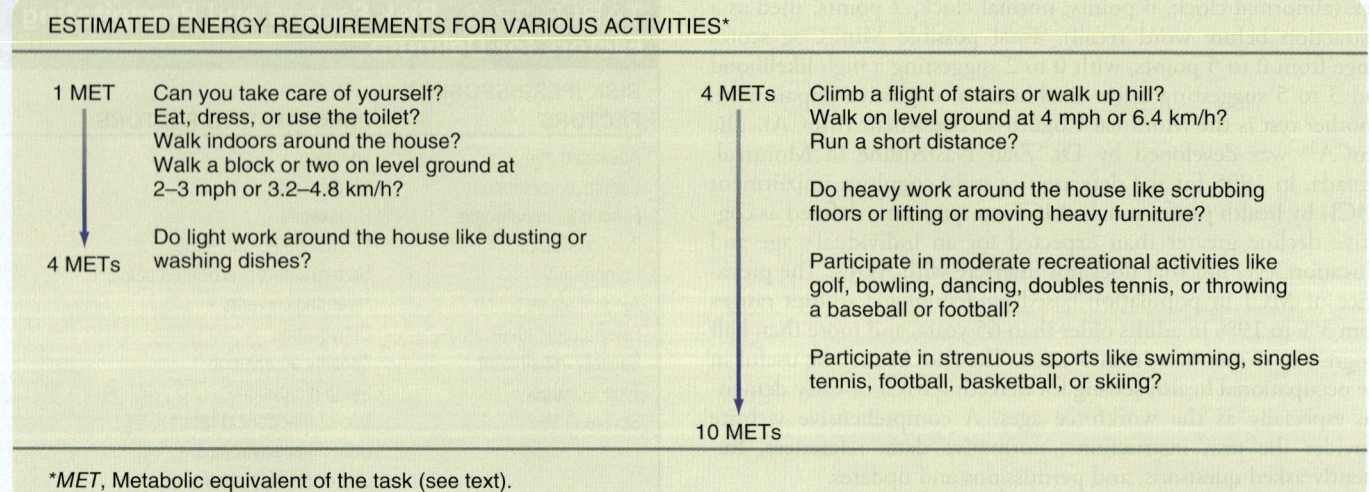

ESTIMATED ENERGY REQUIREMENTS FOR VARIOUS ACTIVITIES*

1 MET	Can you take care of yourself?	4 METs	Climb a flight of stairs or walk up hill?
	Eat, dress, or use the toilet?		Walk on level ground at 4 mph or 6.4 km/h?
	Walk indoors around the house?		Run a short distance?
	Walk a block or two on level ground at 2–3 mph or 3.2–4.8 km/h?		
			Do heavy work around the house like scrubbing floors or lifting or moving heavy furniture?
4 METs	Do light work around the house like dusting or washing dishes?		Participate in moderate recreational activities like golf, bowling, dancing, doubles tennis, or throwing a baseball or football?
			Participate in strenuous sports like swimming, singles tennis, football, basketball, or skiing?
		10 METs	

*MET, Metabolic equivalent of the task (see text).

FIGURE 27.5 Estimated energy requirements for various activities. With increasing activity, the number of metabolic equivalents of the task (METs) increases. An inability to function above 4 METs has been associated with increased perioperative cardiac events and long-term risk. (From Eagle KA, Berger PB, Calkins H, et al. ACC/AHA guideline update for perioperative cardiovascular evaluation for noncardiac surgery—executive summary: a report of the American College of Cardiology/American Heart Association Task Force on Practice Guidelines [Committee to Update the 1996 Guidelines on Perioperative Cardiovascular Evaluation for Noncardiac Surgery]. *Circulation.* 2002;105:1257-1267.)

minute, represents the basal oxygen consumption of a 70-kg, 40-year-old male at rest. Estimated energy requirements for various activities are shown in Fig. 27.5. An inability to function above 4 METs has been associated with increased perioperative cardiac events and long-term risk.[38] By asking appropriate questions about the level of activity, functional capacity can be accurately determined.

Studies incorporating prehabilitation strategies in patients undergoing laparoscopic- or robotic-assisted colorectal cancer surgery showed that the number of severe complications was significantly lower favoring prehabilitation compared with standard care. Secondary parameters of functional capacity in the postoperative period generally favored prehabilitation compared with standard care.[39]

Mobility/Fall Risk Assessment

Falls, considered one of the geriatric syndromes, are a leading cause of injury in older adults and are associated with declining overall health. A fall in the hospital is considered a never event. Recent evidence also suggests that a fall in the preoperative period may predict negative postoperative outcomes. Every older patient should be asked about a history of falls and should be assessed for gait and mobility factors that may predispose to a fall. A simple way to assess gait and mobility impairment is the Timed Up & Go Test,[40] which can easily be accomplished in the office setting. The patient is asked to rise from a chair without using the armrests, walk a measured 10 feet, turn and return to the chair, and sit back down. The inability to rise from the chair without the armrests or a test time of more than 15 seconds is considered an indication of a high fall risk. Patients identified as high risk for fall should be considered for preoperative gait and balance training if time allows and should have physical therapy assist with early mobilization in the postoperative period.

Nutritional Status

The impact of poor nutrition has long been recognized as a risk factor for perioperative mortality and morbidity such as pneumonia

and poor wound healing. Psychosocial issues and comorbid conditions familiar to older adults place this population at high risk for nutritional deficits. Malnutrition is estimated to be present in approximately 0% to 15% of community-dwelling older persons, 35% to 65% of older patients in acute care hospitals, and 25% to 60% of institutionalized older adults. Factors that lead to inadequate intake and uptake of nutrients in this population include the ability to obtain food (e.g., financial constraints, availability of food, limited mobility), desire to eat food (e.g., living situation, mental status, chronic illness), ability to eat and absorb food (e.g., poor dentition, chronic gastrointestinal disorders such as gastroesophageal reflux disease [GERD] or diarrhea), and medications that interfere with appetite or nutrient metabolism (see Box 27.4B).

In the frail older adult, several factors influence neuroendocrine dysregulation of the signals that control appetite and satiety and lead to what is termed the *anorexia of aging.* Although the anorexia of aging is the result of multifactorial events, the result is chronic undernutrition and loss of muscle mass (sarcopenia). Malnutrition has been linked with increased risk of falls and hospital admission.

Measurement of nutritional status in older adults is difficult. Standard anthropomorphic measures do not consider the changes in body composition and structure that accompany aging. Immune measures of nutrition are influenced by age-related changes in the immune system in general. Complicated markers and indices of malnutrition exist but are not required in the routine surgical setting. Subjective assessment by history and physical examination, in which risk factors and physical evidence of malnutrition are examined, has been shown to be as effective as objective measures of nutritional status.

Several screening tools may be used, including the Subjective Global Assessment (SGA) and Mini Nutritional Assessment (MNA). The SGA is a relatively simple, reproducible tool for assessing nutritional status from history and physical examination. SGA ratings are most strongly influenced by loss of subcutaneous tissue, muscle wasting, and weight loss. The SGA has been validated in

BOX 27.4B Factors Associated With Increased Risk of Malnutrition

Recent weight loss
Limited ability to obtain food
  Immobility
  Poverty
Disinterest in eating
  Depression
  Isolation
  Cognitive impairment
  Decreased appetite
  Decreased taste
Difficulty eating
  Poor dentition
  Swallowing disorder
  GERD
Increased gastrointestinal losses
  Diarrhea
  Malabsorption
Systemic diseases
  Chronic lung
  Liver
  Cardiac
  Renal
  Cancer
Drugs and medication
  Alcohol
  Suppressed appetite
  Block nutrient metabolism

GERD, Gastroesophageal reflux disease.
From Ahuja V, Rosenthal RA. Surgery in the geriatric patient. In: Townsend CM Jr, Beauchamp RD, Evers BM, Mattox KL, eds. *Sabiston Textbook of Surgery: The Biological Basis of Modern Surgical Practice.* Philadelphia: Elsevier; 2021:284-314.

older and critically ill patients and has been related to the development of postoperative complications.[41–44] The MNA, which measures 18 factors, including body mass index (BMI), weight history, cognition, mobility, dietary history, and self-assessment, is also a reliable method for assessing nutritional status. Nutritional status, as determined by the SGA and MNA, has been shown to predict outcomes in outpatient and hospitalized geriatric medical patients.

Severe nutritional deficits can be identified by measuring the BMI (weight in kilograms/height in meters squared) and serum albumin and inquiring about unintentional weight loss. BMI <18.5 kg/m^2, albumin <3.0 g/dL, and unintentional weight loss $>10\%$ to 15% within 6 months identify patients at high risk for nutritional-related complications. For these patients, a course of preoperative nutritional supplementation may be reasonable, even if surgery needs to be delayed for several weeks.

Medication Management

Physiologic changes, such as decreased lean muscle mass and decline in renal function (see "Renal System" section), affect the distribution and elimination of many drugs. Older patients are at increased risk for adverse events related to inappropriate drugs or inappropriate dosing of drugs. The Beer's list is a comprehensive list of medications that should be avoided or used with caution in the older adult.[42] The most common drugs to be avoided include all benzodiazepines, the analgesic meperidine (Demerol), and the antihistamine diphenhydramine (Benadryl).

Multiple medication use also poses a risk to older patients in the perioperative period. In a random sample of older adults living in the community, over 80% were found to take at least one prescription medication, with 68% taking an over-the-counter drug or supplement as well. More than 50% of persons over age 60 take five or more medications and supplements, many of which are unnecessary or inappropriately prescribed. Therefore, a thorough review of all medications should be conducted before surgery. All nonessential medications should be stopped, including all supplements, as the content of these is frequently unclear.

Other medications, such as those with potential for withdrawal, including β-blockers, should be continued in the perioperative period. For patients with significant cardiac or vascular disease not currently on β-blockers or statin therapy, consideration should be given to starting these medications.

INTRAOPERATIVE AND POSTOPERATIVE MANAGEMENT

Frail older adults benefit from interdisciplinary care but remain vulnerable and at high risk for poor functional outcomes after surgery unless systemic changes are incorporated across the entire clinical continuum for all older adults undergoing either elective or unplanned surgeries. To eliminate the great variability seen in current surgical outcomes in older adults, perioperative processes should be standardized to address the common problems that older adults experience when subjected to the stress of surgery, illness, and hospitalization. Electronic health records (EHRs) are an invaluable asset in modern healthcare. To facilitate standardized geriatric surgical care, it is necessary to engage clinicians in the initial stages of EHR implementation and during evaluation and optimization of EHR usability.[43]

Multimodality Pain Control

Older adults are much more sensitive than are younger adults to the adverse effects of many drugs, including the analgesics, antiemetics, and anxiolytics commonly used in the intraoperative and postoperative periods. It is important to minimize opioids, as they are associated with cognitive impairment, delirium, falls, and constipation. Pain undertreatment is also common in older adults and associated with delirium.[44]

Structured protocols, such as the Enhanced Recovery After Surgery (ERAS) program, formalize the use of multimodality, opioid-sparing postoperative treatment regimens for pain. Although not designed specifically for older adults, ERAS protocols have been used successfully to improve outcomes in this population.[44] The new ACS Geriatric Surgery Verification Program has a standard devoted to multimodality postoperative pain management. Components of this standard are found in Box 27.5.[45]

Postoperative Delirium

Delirium incidence depends on the type of procedure and the individual risk factors, which were discussed in the screening section (see Table 27.2). Although delirium is common in older patients after surgery, the diagnosis may be missed. Agitation and confusion are usually recognized, but depressed levels of consciousness may also be exhibited. The Confusion Assessment Model (CAM) developed by Wei and colleagues[46] is a simple, well-validated tool to diagnose delirium. A positive CAM requires the following: (1) acute onset with waxing and waning course and

TABLE 27.3 Organ System Effects of Bed Rest

SYSTEM	EFFECT
Cardiovascular	↓ Stroke volume, ↓ cardiac output, orthostatic hypotension
Respiratory	↓ Respiratory excursion, ↓ oxygen uptake, ↑ potential for atelectasis
Muscles	↓ Muscle strength, ↓ muscle blood flow
Bone	↑ Bone loss, ↓ bone density
Gastrointestinal	Malnutrition, anorexia, constipation
Genitourinary	Incontinence
Skin	Shearing force, potential for skin breakdown
Psychological	Social isolation, anxiety, depression, disorientation

(2) inattention with (3) disordered thinking or (4) altered level of consciousness.

The best treatment for delirium remains prevention. Strategies that center on maintaining orientation (e.g., family at the bedside, sensory devices available), encouraging mobility, maintaining normal sleep-wake cycles (no medications during sleep hours), and avoiding dehydration and inappropriate medications may aid to decrease the number and duration of episodes of delirium in hospitalized patients. Pharmacologic prevention trials have not been linked to positive results.

Once delirium is diagnosed, a search for causative factors such as infections, hypoxia, metabolic disturbances, inappropriate medications, and undertreated pain should be conducted. Invasive devices and catheters should be removed as soon as possible, and restraints should be avoided. A complete review of the history should also be conducted and the family inquired about possible predisposing factors, such as unrecognized alcohol consumption. The use of antipsychotic medications, such as very-low-dose haloperidol, should be reserved only for those patients whose behavior presents a danger to themselves or others.

Aspiration

Aspiration is a common reason for morbidity and mortality in older patients in the postoperative period. The incidence of postoperative aspiration pneumonia increases dramatically with increasing age. Hence, aspiration risk should be evaluated preoperatively in all older patients with risk factors for aspiration and in those with any report of a swallowing abnormality. Aspiration precautions should be ordered for any patient at risk. These include 30- to 45-degree upright positioning, careful evaluation of gastrointestinal function before starting an oral diet and, frequently thereafter, careful monitoring of gastric residuals in patients with feeding tubes, and upright position during meals and for 30 to 45 minutes after meals in those on an oral diet. Before feeding patients at risk for aspiration, swallowing function can be assessed by a 3-ounce bedside swallow test. Passing this test is a good indication of the ability to tolerate thin liquids.[47]

Signs suggestive of aspiration are often observed in older adults. Aspiration is a precursor to aspiration pneumonia and can suggest swallowing dysfunction. In adults aged 60 years and older, the male sex and feeding and mobility dependence are suggestive of likely aspiration during oral intake. Older adults who regularly show signs of aspiration demonstrate a distinct profile that is in line with frailty. Speech-language pathology involvement is recommended for older adults who receive rehabilitation therapy even if they are not exhibiting explicit signs of swallowing difficulties.[48]

Deconditioning

In older patients, the prolonged period of immobility due to hospitalization for a major surgical procedure often results in functional decline and overall deconditioning. Functional decline has been seen after even 2 days of immobility. Deconditioning is a distinct clinical entity, characterized by specific changes in function of many organ systems (Table 27.3). Deconditioned individuals have ongoing functional limitations, despite improvement in the original acute illness. The period for functional recovery may be as much as three times longer than the period of immobility. Older adult surgical patients who develop functional decline while in the hospital are also at greater risk of readmission, complications, and death within 300 days after discharge.[49]

A major risk factor for deconditioning during hospitalization is a prior functional limitation. For example, patients needing ambulation assist devices such as canes or walkers before hospitalization are more likely to suffer significant further functional decline. There are other functional limitations, such as the inability to perform activities and walking up a flight of steps carrying a bag of groceries (4 METs), which are also associated with higher rates of postoperative complications and greater chances of functional decline. Other risk factors include two or more comorbidities, five or more medications, and a hospitalization or emergency room visit in the preceding year. Patients who develop delirium while in the hospital are also at greater risk of developing serious functional decline and may need placement in short-term rehabilitation or long-term care facilities.

Assessment of functional capacity is a necessary part of the preoperative assessment. In patients identified at risk for functional decline, a plan for early directed methods to promote mobility, including early physical therapy consultation, should be established before surgery. The "out of bed" order may be the most important of all postoperative orders.

Structured models for the in-hospital care of geriatric patients have been developed. Adaptation of these models for surgery patients could lead to improvements in functional and cognitive status. Preoperative conditioning to improve function before surgery, termed *prehabilitation* or *prehab*, has theoretical merit, although evidence is still lacking in its usefulness.

Transition of Care

Discharge planning for older adults should begin on the day the decision is made to proceed with surgery. High-quality discharge summaries can mitigate this risk through improved provider communication.[50] Functional and cognitive deficits present on admission are exacerbated by the stress of surgery and constraints of hospitalization and immobilization, even if the surgery itself is uncomplicated. Not surprisingly, the need for postacute care is higher in older adults, as are the rates of readmission after surgical discharge. Unfortunately, a quarter of these readmissions are to facilities other than the initial treating hospital and with the possibility that the providers lacking knowledge of the events of the surgery and perioperative period are at a great disadvantage when caring for complex older adults. The outcome for these readmissions is much worse than readmissions to the initial treating institution.

Starting early in the perioperative period, it is important to set expectations for both patients and their families regarding length of stay, likelihood of the need for postacute nursing or rehabilitation placement, or the need for special services or equipment in the home. In addition, expectations regarding functional outcomes should be discussed. There may be specific requirements for patients coming from a nursing home to be able to keep their place in the facility. Obviously, in an emergency setting, this is not possible, but as soon as needs are realized, case management should be involved in the care.

Important factors in discharge planning include assessment of family involvement, home readiness (i.e., does the patient have stairs, what will they need to be able to do functionally to return to their home), a physical and occupational therapy evaluation, and an open discussion with the patient about the surgeons' and the physicians' expectations for return of function. Studies have shown that advance discharge planning, with involved case management, can improve patient outcomes and patient satisfaction and decrease readmission, even improving cost of care.[51] And although it may be resource intensive, in these high-risk patients, there is some evidence that a more intensive follow-up by nursing staff aimed at looking for early warning signs (such as dehydration) may promote earlier treatment and decrease rates of readmission.

A comprehensive discharge discussion and documentation are essential for a patient's postoperative success because there may be new medications, new functional limitations, and new wounds to care for. Add to that the preexisting functional and cognitive challenges, the effects of immobility and deconditioning, and the long list of prior medications so common in vulnerable older adults, and it is not surprising that serious problems can and do occur. A carefully documented discharge summary that recognizes the individual's vulnerabilities (as identified on the preoperative screens) and gives clear information to the caregivers about how to deal with predictable problems is essential. This, combined with a thorough verbal review of the major concerns described in the summary with the patient and the caregivers, can help avoid some of the more common problems.

Discharge communications should also occur with the postacute care facility when the patient requires nursing home care or postoperative rehabilitation. Clear, frequent, and two-way communication, starting with the thorough discharge summary and a discussion of it (or warm hand-off), will help focus the postoperative care on the individual patient's vulnerabilities.[22]

SELECTED REFERENCES

Finlayson E, Wang L, Landefeld CS, et al. Major abdominal surgery in nursing home residents: a national study. *Ann Surg.* 2011; 254:921-926.

> *This study analyzed Medicare beneficiaries aged 65 and older who underwent surgery for benign conditions between 1999 and 2006, including bleeding duodenal ulcer, colectomy, cholecystectomy, and appendectomy. Between 1999 and 2006, 70,719 nursing home residents and 1,060,389 non-institutionalized Medicare beneficiaries underwent surgery. Nursing home residents had significantly higher operative mortality: 11% vs. 3% for cholecystectomy (adjusted odds ratio [AOR] 2.65), 12% vs. 2% for appendectomy (AOR 3.27), 32% vs. 13% for colectomy (AOR 2.06), and 42% vs. 26% for duodenal ulcer surgery (AOR 1.79). Secondary invasive interventions were also more frequent among nursing home residents, with rates ranging from 18% for cholecystectomy to 55% for duodenal ulcer surgery. Life-sustaining interventions such as mechanical ventilation was higher for nursing home residents (13% vs. 10% for duodenal ulcer surgery, 9% vs. 4% for colectomy), and feeding tube placement was more common in nursing home residents, particularly for duodenal ulcer surgery (18% vs. 12%) and colectomy (9% vs. 3%). These findings highlight the substantially higher morbidity and mortality associated with surgery in nursing home residents compared to the general Medicare population.*

Fried TR, Bradley EH, Towle VR, et al. Understanding the treatment preferences of seriously ill patients. *N Engl J Med.* 2002; 346:1061-1066.

> *This study investigated treatment preferences among 226 older adults with limited life expectancy due to cancer, heart failure, or chronic obstructive pulmonary disease. Participants were presented with hypothetical treatment scenarios involving varying levels of burden and potential outcomes. Results showed that most participants prioritized quality of life over quantity, with a significant decline in treatment preference as the likelihood of severe functional or cognitive impairment increased. Notably, even when a high-burden treatment offered a certain return to health, a substantial number of participants opted against it. These findings highlight the importance of understanding patients' values and preferences in end-of-life care.*

Lederle FA, Freischlag JA, Kyriakides TC, et al. Long-Term Comparison of Endovascular and Open Repair of Abdominal Aortic Aneurysm. *N Engl J Med.* 2012;367(21):1988-1997.

> *This randomized controlled trial compared open surgical repair and endovascular repair for abdominal aortic aneurysms (AAA) in 881 patients. While no significant difference in overall long-term mortality was observed, endovascular repair demonstrated better survival in younger patients (hazard ratio: 0.65) and a lower perioperative mortality rate (0.5% vs. 3.0%). However, endovascular repair was associated with a higher risk of aneurysm rupture (6 vs. 0) and required more secondary procedures (148 vs. 105).*

Pastorino U, Silva M, Sestini S, et al. Prolonged lung cancer screening reduced 10-year mortality in the MILD trial: new confirmation of lung cancer screening efficacy. *Ann Oncol.* 2019; 30(7):1162-1169.

The MILD study, a randomized controlled trial, examined the effectiveness of low-dose CT (LDCT) screening for lung cancer for up to 10 years in high-risk smokers (n = 4,099). While the study demonstrated an increase in early-stage lung cancer detection and a trend towards reduced lung cancer mortality, a definitive reduction in overall mortality at 10 years was not observed. However, a landmark analysis revealed a significant decrease in overall mortality for the screening group beyond 5 years, which was 32% (95%CI 6% to 51%). These findings suggest that LDCT screening may offer potential benefits for early detection and improved outcomes in lung cancer, but further research is needed to confirm long-term survival advantages.

Tang VL, Jing B, Boscardin J, et al. Association of functional, cognitive, and psychological measures with 1-year mortality in patients undergoing major surgery. *JAMA Surg.* 2020;155(5): 412-418.

A study of 1,341 older adults (average age 76) from Health and Retirement Study (HRS) who underwent major surgery found that geriatric risk factors, including functional impairment, cognitive impairment, and psychological factors (e.g., depression), were significantly associated with increased mortality within one year of surgery. Even after accounting for traditional medical risk factors like comorbidity and age, these geriatric factors remained strong predictors of mortality.

The full reference list appears on Elsevier eBooks+.

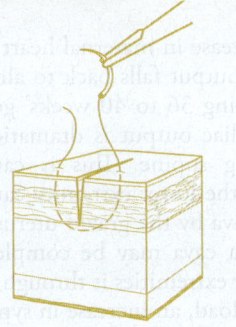

CHAPTER 28

Surgery in the Pregnant Patient

Rachel M. Russo, Gregory J. Jurkovich,
Diana L. Farmer, and Candice A.M. Sauder

OUTLINE

The pregnant patient presents a unique clinical challenge for the general surgeon. About 7% of pregnancies are complicated by nonobstetric surgical problems, and an estimated 1 in 500 pregnancies will need an operation for nonpregnancy-related issues. Table 28.1 is adapted from a 10-year review of the hospital episode statistics of all admissions to English National Health Services (NHS) hospitals. Of 6.5 million pregnancies, 47,600 nonobstetric surgeries occurred, and 12,500 were abdominal of any kind. In a review of 44 papers and 12,452 patients, the effects of nonobstetric surgical procedures on maternal and fetal outcomes were studied; a maternal death rate of 0.006% and a miscarriage rate of 5.8% were reported. Most indications for surgical intervention are common for the patient's age group and unrelated to pregnancy, such as acute appendicitis, symptomatic cholelithiasis, perianal, soft tissue, breast masses, or trauma.[1]

Changes in maternal anatomy and physiology and safety of the fetus are among the issues of which the surgeon must be cognizant. The presentation of surgical diseases in the pregnant patient may be atypical or may mimic signs and symptoms of a normal pregnancy.[2] A standard evaluation may be unreliable because of pregnancy-associated changes in diagnostic tests or laboratory test results. Finally, many physicians may be more hesitant to employ diagnostic evaluation and treatment. Any of these factors may result in a delay in diagnosis and treatment, adversely affecting maternal and fetal outcome. The fundamental principle of managing a pregnant patient with a nonobstetric surgical problem is to not penalize the patient, and her care, for being pregnant. There are two patients to be sure, but the baby's health is dependent on the mother's. Although consultation with an obstetrician is ideal when caring for a pregnant patient, the surgeon needs to be aware of this fundamental principle when this resource is unavailable. This chapter discusses key points when caring for the pregnant patient who presents with nonobstetric surgical disorders.

PHYSIOLOGIC CHANGES OF PREGNANCY

Progesterone and estrogen, two of the principal hormones of pregnancy, mediate many of the maternal physiologic changes in pregnancy. Normal laboratory values differ in the gravid compared with the nonpregnant patient. The diaphragm can be elevated in pregnancy up to 4 cm, and the lower chest wall can widen up to 7 cm.[3] These changes may also mimic similar pathophysiology that occurs in nonpregnant patients who have cardiac or liver disease. Elevated progesterone levels as well as decreased serum motilin result in smooth muscle relaxation, producing multiple effects on several organ systems. In the stomach, this decreased smooth muscle tone results in diminished gastric tone and motility. The lower esophageal sphincter tone is also decreased and, when combined with increased intraabdominal pressure, results in an increase in the incidence of gastroesophageal

TABLE 28.1 Operations Performed Out of 6.5 Million Pregnancies in the United Kingdom From 2002–12

	NUMBER OF OPERATIONS (%)
Abdominal, any kind	12,493 (26.2)
Appendectomy	3062 (6.4)
Cholecystectomy	1306 (2.7)
Dental	5365 (11.3)
Skin, nail	4762 (10.0)
Orthopedic	4563 (9.6)
ENT	3060 (6.4)
Perianal	2977 (6.2)
Breast	1884 (4.0)
Cancer	710 (1.5)

ENT, Ear, nose, and throat.
Adapted from Balinskaite V, Bottle A, Sodhi V, et al. The risk of adverse pregnancy outcomes following nonobstetric surgery during pregnancy: estimates from a retrospective cohort study of 6.5 million pregnancies. *Ann Surg.* 2017;266:260-266.

reflux. Small bowel motility is reduced, increasing small bowel transit time. Absorption of nutrients, however, remains unchanged, with the exception of iron absorption, which is increased because of increased iron requirements. In the colon, pregnancy-related changes usually manifest as constipation. This is caused by a combination of increased colonic sodium and water absorption, decreased motility, and mechanical obstruction by the gravid uterus. An increase in portal venous pressure, and therefore an increase in the pressure in the collateral venous circulation, results in dilation of the veins at the gastroesophageal junction. This is of importance only if the patient had esophageal varices before becoming pregnant. The most common result of the increased portal venous pressure is dilation of the hemorrhoidal veins, leading to the well-known complaint of hemorrhoids.

In addition to alterations in smooth muscle tone and motility, other notable changes occur in the gastrointestinal tract. The function of the gallbladder is altered, as is the chemical composition of bile. During the second and third trimesters, the volume of the gallbladder may be twice that found in the nonpregnant state, and gallbladder emptying is markedly slower. Up to 4% of pregnant patients have gallstones on routine obstetric ultrasound. Still, only 1 of every 1000 pregnant patients develops symptoms. It is unknown whether the increased biliary stasis, changes in bile composition, or combination of these two factors results in an increased risk for gallstone formation, but the risk for developing gallstones increases with multiparity. However, the incidence of symptomatic cholelithiasis during pregnancy is similar to the incidence in age-related nonpregnant females.

Some of the changes of pregnancy closely resemble those of liver disease. These include spider angiomas and palmar erythema from elevated serum estrogen levels. Hypoalbuminemia is also seen along with elevated serum cholesterol, alkaline phosphatase, and fibrinogen levels. Serum bilirubin and hepatic transaminase levels remain unchanged during pregnancy.

In the cardiovascular system, peripheral vascular resistance is decreased as a consequence of diminished vascular smooth muscle tone. Cardiac output increases by as much as 50% during the first trimester of pregnancy. Initially, this is caused by an increased stroke volume resulting from an increase in plasma volume and

red blood cell mass, but a gradual increase in maternal heart rate also is a contributing factor. Cardiac output falls back to almost normal late in pregnancy, usually during 36 to 40 weeks' gestation. During the third trimester, cardiac output is dramatically decreased when the mother is lying supine. This is caused by compromised venous return from the lower extremity caused by compression of the inferior vena cava by the gravid uterus. In the supine position, the inferior vena cava may be completely occluded; venous drainage of the lower extremities is through collateral channels. With this drop in preload, an increase in sympathetic tone usually maintains peripheral vascular resistance and blood pressure. However, up to 10% of patients may experience supine hypotensive syndrome in which the sympathetic response is not adequate to maintain blood pressure. During anesthesia induction in the operating room, anesthetic agents may inhibit the compensatory sympathetic response, causing a more precipitous fall in blood pressure. This finding is of particular importance in evaluating the pregnant trauma patient, who must be rolled onto the left side in the lateral decubitus position to accurately assess blood pressure. The pregnant patient should always be placed in the left lateral decubitus position during any procedures performed during the third trimester, relieving caval compression caused by the enlarged uterus.

Inguinal swelling secondary to varicosities of the round ligament is also a phenomenon that occurs during pregnancy. The increase in swelling is a result of hormonal and mechanical changes. It is often mistaken for an inguinal or femoral hernia. Appropriate treatment includes careful physical examination and ultrasound if needed. The varicosities generally resolve postpartum.

Oxygen consumption increases during pregnancy. Minute ventilation increases by 50% because of an increase in tidal volume, which appears to be a result of an elevated serum progesterone level.[3] Progesterone not only increases the sensitivity of the respiratory centers to carbon dioxide (CO_2) but also acts as a direct stimulant to the respiratory centers. As a consequence of the increased minute ventilation, the maternal partial arterial oxygen tension (PaO_2) level during late pregnancy ranges from 104 to 108 mm Hg and the maternal partial arterial CO_2 ($PaCO_2$) level ranges from 27 to 32 mm Hg. Renal compensation maintains a normal maternal pH. The decreased $PaCO_2$ level increases the CO_2 gradient from the fetus to the mother, facilitating CO_2 transfer from the fetus to the mother. These findings are critical in managing the ventilator-dependent pregnant patient during and after surgery. The oxygen-hemoglobin dissociation curve of maternal blood is shifted to the right; this, coupled with the increased affinity of fetal hemoglobin for oxygen, results in increased oxygen transfer to the fetus. Elevation of the diaphragm by as much as 4 cm results in a decrease in total lung volume by 5%. Diminished expiratory reserve volume and residual volume result in a functional residual capacity that is 20% lower than that in the nonpregnant patient. Vital capacity and inspiratory reserve volume remain stable.

In the kidney, there is an increase in the glomerular filtration rate by 50% that accompanies a 75% increase in renal plasma flow. Urinary glucose excretion increases as a direct consequence of the increased glomerular filtration rate. The blood urea nitrogen level decreases by 25% during the first trimester and is maintained at that level for the remainder of the pregnancy. The serum creatinine level also decreases by the end of the first trimester from a nonpregnant value of 0.8 to 0.7 mg/dL and may be as low as 0.5 mg/dL by term. A five- to tenfold increase in the serum renin level occurs with a subsequent four- to fivefold increase in the angiotensin level. Although the pregnant patient is apparently less sensitive to the hypertensive effects of the increased angiotensin, elevated aldosterone levels result in an increase in sodium reabsorption, overcoming the natriuresis produced by elevated progesterone levels. Serum sodium levels are decreased, however, because the increase in sodium reabsorption is less than the increase in plasma volume. Serum osmolality is decreased to 270 to 280 mOsm/kg.[3]

The increase in plasma volume and red blood cell mass is accompanied by a progressive rise in the leukocyte count during pregnancy, an important consideration when evaluating for systemic signs of infection. During the first trimester, the white blood cell count ranges from 3000 to 15,000 cells/mm^3, increasing to a range of 6000 to 16,000 cells/mm^3 during the second and third trimesters.[3] The platelet count progressively declines throughout pregnancy, whereas the mean platelet volume tends to increase after 28 weeks' gestation.

Increasing platelet counts together with high levels of circulating estrogen, increasing procoagulants, and progressive venous stasis generate a hypercoagulable state during normal pregnancy.[4] Plasma fibrinogen; von Willebrand factor; and factors II, V, VII, VIII, IX, X, and XII increase, whereas protein S and the response to activated protein C decrease.[4] Serum plasminogen activator inhibitor 1 (PAI1) and placental PAI2 increase, decreasing the body's response to intrinsic tissue plasminogen activator (tPA), resulting in a decrease in fibrinolysis. Increasing pressure from the gravid uterus on the inferior vena cava together with decreased venous tone contribute to venous stasis that progresses with increasing pregnancy. The end result is a fivefold increase in the risk of venous thromboembolism during pregnancy that increases to more than twentyfold during the puerperium. In females with inherited hypercoagulable mutations, the risk of thrombosis increases further still. Despite these alterations in the coagulation cascade and platelet count, bleeding and clotting times are unchanged.

RADIOLOGIC CONCERNS

Radiographic studies remain useful diagnostic tools for the pregnant patient. The greatest concern with radiation exposure is the risk to the fetus. The accepted maximum dose of ionizing radiation during the entire pregnancy is 5 cGy. The fetus is at the highest risk from radiation exposure from the preimplantation period to approximately 15 weeks' gestation. Primary organogenesis occurs during this time and the teratogenic effects of radiation, particularly to the developing central nervous system, are at their highest. Perinatal radiation exposure has also been associated with childhood leukemia and certain childhood malignancies. The radiation dose that has been associated with congenital malformation is higher than 10 cGy. As shown in Table 28.2, radiation exposure to the fetus with the doses from the more common radiology procedures is well below that threshold. Nonetheless, prudence on the part of the clinician is required to avoid unnecessary fetal exposure to ionizing radiation, especially during the first and early second trimesters, when the risk from exposure is greatest.

Magnetic resonance imaging (MRI) avoids exposure to ionizing radiation but poses an unknown risk to the fetus. Animal studies have shown no teratogenic effect or increased incidence of fetal death or congenital malformations from the electromagnetic radiation, static magnetic field, radiofrequency magnetic fields, or intravenous (IV) contrast agents used during MRI. Theoretically,

TABLE 28.2 Fetal Radiation Exposure With Radiographic Imaging

EXAMINATION TYPE	ESTIMATED FETAL RADIATION EXPOSURE (CGY)
Two-view chest radiography	0.00007
Cervical spine radiography	0.002
Pelvis radiography	0.04
Head CT	<0.050
Abdomen CT	2.60
Upper GI series	0.056
Barium enema	3.986
HIDA scanning	0.150

CT, Computed tomography; GI, gastrointestinal; HIDA, hepatobiliary iminodiacetic acid.

the gradient magnetic fields may produce electric currents in the patient, and the high-frequency currents induced by radiofrequency fields may cause local generation of heat. The long-term effect of exposure is not known.[5] The National Radiological Protection Board has advised against the use of MRI during the first trimester of pregnancy. MRI has become the diagnostic modality of choice, however, in the workup of complex fetal anomalies in the second and third trimester.

Contrast media may be administered with various techniques of body imaging. If computed tomography (CT) has been performed during pregnancy with iodide contrast, neonatal thyroid function should be checked during the first week after delivery. No effect on the fetus has been observed after the use of gadolinium contrast medium with MRI.

Ultrasonography is routinely used by obstetricians during pregnancy. Although tissue heating and cavitation are theoretical effects of ultrasound exposure, such effects have never been reported. Ultrasound may be a helpful alternative diagnostic tool when trying to avoid exposure to ionizing radiation but does have some limitations. Deeper structures are difficult to visualize and may be obscured by superficial structures that are more echo dense. Ultrasound imaging has a limited field of view and is highly operator dependent. Despite these limitations, certain disease processes, such as a palpable breast mass or suspected appendicitis, may be evaluated effectively and safely. Importantly, a pregnant patient should never be denied or encouraged to delay necessary medical treatment, to include diagnostic imaging and surgery, regardless of trimester. Such delays can adversely affect the health of the female and her fetus.

MEDICATION CONCERNS

The surgeon will, on occasion, need to prescribe medications to treat the pregnant patient with surgical disease. In this section, we provide an overview of medications the surgeon may commonly prescribe. The list is by no means comprehensive, and before using any medication, consultation with the patient's obstetrician is necessary. It is noteworthy that over 50% of pregnant patients take at least 1 medication, with an average of 2.6 medications, and the use of 4 or more medications in the first trimester has tripled (9.9%–27.6%) over the past three decades.[6]

In 1979, the US Food and Drug Administration (FDA) established five letter risk categories (i.e., A, B, C, D, X) to indicate the potential fetal risk if used during pregnancy. In 2015, the FDA developed a new labeling system known as the *Pregnancy and Lactation Labeling Rule (PLLR)* in an effort to provide more relevant information for better provider decision-making and patient-specific counseling. As of 2020, this new classification system removes the pregnancy risk category lettering system and provides information in a narrative form in order to more accurately describe the risks involved with using medications in pregnancy.[7,8] One limitation of PLLR is medications (both prescription and over the counter) approved before June 1, 2001, do not have to provide a narrative summary, potentially making it more difficult for providers to locate information on pregnancy risk.

Despite this new classification system, the five pregnancy risk categories are most commonly referenced and used.

Category A: These drugs have been tested and found to be safe during pregnancy. Category A includes drugs such as folic acid, vitamin B_6, and some thyroid medicines in prescribed doses.

Category B: These drugs are frequently used during pregnancy and do not appear to cause major birth defects or other problems. Category B includes some antibiotics, prednisone, insulin, acetaminophen (Tylenol), aspartame (Equal, NutraSweet), famotidine (Pepcid), and ibuprofen (Advil, Motrin) before the third trimester. Pregnant patients should not take ibuprofen during the last 3 months of pregnancy.

The FDA offers the following classifications for prescription drugs that should not be taken during pregnancy:

Category C: These are drugs that are more likely to cause problems for the mother or fetus and drugs for which safety studies have not been finished. Most of these drugs do not have safety studies in progress. These drugs often come with a warning that they should be used only if the benefits of taking them outweigh the risks. This is something the surgeon would need to discuss with the patient's obstetrician. These drugs include prochlorperazine (Compazine), pseudoephedrine (Sudafed), fluconazole (Diflucan), and ciprofloxacin (Cipro). Some antidepressants are also included in this group.

Category D: These include drugs that have clear health risks for the fetus and include alcohol, lithium, phenytoin (Dilantin), and except for select circumstances, most forms of chemotherapy.

Category X: These drugs have been shown to cause birth defects and should never be taken during pregnancy. These include drugs to treat skin conditions such as cystic acne (isotretinoin [Accutane]) and psoriasis (etretinate [Tegison], acitretin [Soriatane]), thalidomide (sedative), and diethylstilbestrol (DES; prevents miscarriage) that was used up until 1971 in the United States and until 1983 in Europe.

Analgesics

Over-the-Counter Medications

Acetaminophen, the active ingredient in Tylenol, is considered safe during pregnancy. Well researched by scientists, acetaminophen is used primarily for headaches, fever, aches, pains, and sore throat. It can be used during all three trimesters of pregnancy.

Nonsteroidal antiinflammatory drugs (NSAIDs) include aspirin, ibuprofen (Advil, Motrin), and naproxen (Aleve). Aspirin, which contains salicylic acid as its active ingredient, should generally be avoided by expectant mothers because it can pose risks for the mother and fetus. Generally, aspirin is not recommended

during pregnancy; the exception is for pregnant patients with recurrent pregnancy loss, clotting disorders, and preeclampsia.[9,10]

The use of higher doses of aspirin poses various risks depending on the stage of pregnancy. During the first trimester, use of higher doses of aspirin poses a concern for pregnancy loss and congenital defects. Taking higher doses of aspirin during the third trimester increases the risk of the premature closure of a vessel in the fetus's heart. Use of high-dose aspirin for long periods in pregnancy also increases the risk of bleeding in the brain of premature infants.

Ibuprofen and naproxen are safer options, but both should be used with caution during pregnancy. The use of NSAIDs immediately before and during early pregnancy has been associated with an increased risk of miscarriages. Use after 32 weeks' gestation increases the risk of premature closure of the ductus arteriosus, similar to aspirin. Additionally, NSAIDS should be avoided in the final 3 months of pregnancy because they can increase bleeding during delivery. Indomethacin may be an alternative during the third trimester. It is occasionally used short-term for preterm labor treatment. However, long-term use can lead to decreased amniotic fluid volume, is associated with necrotizing enterocolitis, and may cause increased bleeding at delivery.

Prescription Medications

Prescription analgesics are available in several different forms and brand names, including codeine, tramadol, hydrocodone and acetaminophen (Vicodin, Norco, Lortab), oxycodone (OxyContin), oxycodone and acetaminophen (Percocet), morphine (MS Contin), meperidine (Demerol), and fentanyl (Duragesic, Sublimaze). These drugs may be used occasionally in pregnant patients when the benefits of the drug outweigh the potential risks. Opioids such as methadone (Dolophine) and buprenorphine (Butrans) are often used in pregnant patients with opioid use disorder to prevent withdrawal or the nonmedical use of opioids.[6,11]

However, there is no known safe level of narcotic use during pregnancy. Risks to the fetus include poor fetal growth, stillbirth, preterm delivery, and a very low risk of birth defects.[11] Chronic use of opioids during pregnancy can lead to neonatal abstinence syndrome. Used late in pregnancy and close to delivery, a neonate is at increased risk of withdrawal symptoms and respiratory depression.

Antibiotics

Antibiotics may be necessary to treat various surgery-related infections in pregnancy. The common antibiotics used are listed by class.[12]

Aminoglycosides

In general, aminoglycosides, including gentamicin, tobramycin, and amikacin, are determined to be low risk to the fetus and are used commonly in pregnancy and surrounding labor and delivery.[13] The only well-known risk seen with other aminoglycosides (i.e., kanamycin and streptomycin) when used during pregnancy is fetal auditory nerve damage to the eighth cranial nerve causing deafness. No epidemiologic studies have demonstrated congenital anomalies in infants whose mothers were treated with aminoglycosides during pregnancy. Only one case report exists of gentamicin use in pregnancy where congenital defects were exhibited. Nephrotoxicity has been observed in many patients receiving aminoglycosides, which raises the concern of whether fetal kidney damage may occur with maternal treatment. Although fetal renal damage after maternal gentamicin treatment has not been documented, there have been cases of severe neonatal nephropathy after therapy with this drug.

Tetracyclines

With the use of tetracyclines, including doxycycline, tetracycline, and minocycline, accumulation of the drugs occurs in developing teeth and long tubular bones. Ingestion during the second or third trimester of pregnancy can cause irreversible dental staining in childhood.[13] Depression of bone growth (especially of the fibula in preterm pregnancies) can occur after in utero exposure to tetracyclines. Acute fatty metamorphosis of the liver in pregnancy after tetracycline therapy has been described and is often fatal. Epidemiologic studies have not demonstrated a clear link between exposure to tetracyclines and congenital abnormalities. Therefore, a small risk cannot be excluded, but there is no indication of increased risk of malformations in children of females treated with this agent during pregnancy. Although data on the specific safety of doxycycline use during pregnancy are limited, it is assumed that the risks of dental staining and depression of bone growth by tetracyclines in general also pertain to doxycycline use during the second and third trimesters.

Metronidazole

Rare reports and studies have shown no consistent pattern of congenital malformations in infants exposed to metronidazole in utero, making its use in pregnancy controversial. Given the limited information available and no conclusive human studies, the risk of birth defects caused by exposure to metronidazole during pregnancy appears to be low, and it is recommended by the Centers for Disease Control and Prevention (CDC) for the treatment of certain infections during pregnancy. It should be noted, however, that the use of metronidazole in the first trimester for the treatment of vaginal trichomoniasis or bacterial vaginosis is contraindicated by the manufacturer.

Penicillins

Penicillins are a widely used group of antibiotics that include ampicillin, amoxicillin, nafcillin, penicillin G, penicillin V, and piperacillin. Although penicillins accumulate in amniotic fluid in large amounts during maternal ingestion, no adverse fetal effects have been associated with this group of medications. It must be noted that all penicillins may produce anaphylaxis during pregnancy or immediately after delivery. If anaphylaxis is severe and uncontrolled, it could result in compromising placental circulation and cause fetal damage or death. However, in general, the penicillins have not been shown to be teratogenic, and there have been no recognized adverse effects caused by exposure to this antibiotic class.[13] One point to note: Drug elimination may be enhanced for some of the penicillins during pregnancy; thus, a higher dose or more frequent administration may be needed to achieve optimal concentrations.

Cephalosporins

Cephalosporins are the most widely used class of antibiotics that include cefazolin, cephalexin, cefotetan, cefuroxime, cefoxitin, cefdinir, cefotaxime, cefpodoxime, ceftriaxone, cefepime, and ceftaroline. Based on their spectrum of activity against gram-positive and gram-negative bacteria, they are classified into five generations. Many of the first- and second-generation cephalosporins have been studied extensively in pregnant patients. It is thought that most of them are not associated with any known or suspected teratogenic effects and are assumed safe for use during pregnancy. The third-, fourth-, and fifth-generation cephalosporins, however, have not been used extensively during pregnancy, and therefore, little information is known about their effects, but they are assumed to be safe to use in pregnancy.[13]

Lincosamide (Clindamycin)

The teratogenic risk of the use of lincosamide antibiotics during pregnancy is undetermined, and there are limited data. Clindamycin, the most widely used antibiotic in this category, is considered in the same pregnancy risk class (FDA Pregnancy Category B) as amoxicillin, penicillin, and vancomycin. The drug has been safely used in the second trimester as an effective treatment of bacterial vaginosis and abnormal vaginal flora.[14]

Macrolides (Azithromycin)

Many reports describing the use of azithromycin in pregnancy have been published. Overall, no increase in the frequency of congenital anomalies was observed among infants of females treated with azithromycin at any time during pregnancy, and it is considered safe to use.

Sulfonamide Derivatives

Trimethoprim/sulfamethoxazole is used during pregnancy but is often avoided in the first and late third trimesters because of potential risks to the fetus. These agents have been associated with increased risk of congenital malformations, namely neural tube defects, cardiovascular malformations, urinary tract defects, oral clefts, and clubfoot. This is mainly due to the trimethoprim component of the antibiotic. Because of trimethoprim being a dihydrofolate reductase inhibitor, it is thought that folic acid supplementation can reduce the risk of congenital defects if they are administered before conception or concurrently with the antibiotic. Although there has been some concern over kernicterus with sulfonamide use, this concern has not been borne out in clinical practice even with high doses of trimethoprim/sulfamethoxazole in the second and early third trimesters.

Fluoroquinolones

The use of fluoroquinolones (i.e., ciprofloxacin, levofloxacin, moxifloxacin, gemifloxacin) during pregnancy remains controversial. Although there are many reports of birth defects displayed in infants when fluoroquinolones were ingested during pregnancy, no pattern in these malformations has been identified.[13] However, animal studies of the fluoroquinolones have suggested some malformation risk, including fetal cartilage damage, and thus, their risk cannot be excluded. In general, it is accepted that fluoroquinolones should be avoided if a safer alternative is available to use.[7]

Other Gram-Positive Agents

Vancomycin and clindamycin are commonly used for multidrug-resistant gram-positive infections or for penicillin-allergic patients. No studies or reports have attributed congenital malformations or other adverse events to their use; thus, they are considered safe to use in pregnancy.[7]

Summary of Antibiotic Use

Although antibiotics are commonly prescribed to pregnant patients, details relating to the effects of many of these drugs remain poorly understood. If an antibiotic must be prescribed, it is important to be aware of the effects these drugs can have on pregnancies and to prescribe the most suitable agent with the least risk.

Antithrombotic Agents

Anticoagulants

Pregnant patients undergoing nonobstetric surgery should be screened for venous thromboembolism and should have appropriate perioperative chemoprophylaxis.

Heparin. The recommended therapeutic agent used in pregnancy for the prevention and treatment of venous thromboemboli is low-molecular-weight heparin (Category B), which has largely replaced standard, unfractionated heparin (Category C). Neither of these agents cross the placenta and are safe in pregnancy; however, unfractionated heparin may be associated with increased maternal bone loss.[4]

Danaparoid. Danaparoid is a low-molecular-weight heparinoid with both anti-Xa and antithrombin effects.[15] This agent was removed from the US market by the manufacturer in 2002 because of a shortage of substrate. However, it remains available elsewhere around the world. Danaparoid neither crosses the placenta nor is secreted in breast milk and thus is theoretically safe in pregnancy.[16,17] A review of the literature from 1981 and 2004 by Lindhoff-Last and colleagues[16] reported use of danaparoid in 51 pregnancies with heparin intolerance with no adverse pregnancy effects. As it is a heparinoid, there remains the (remote) possibility of heparin-induced thrombocytopenia. However, it remains the anticoagulant of choice for use in pregnancy when heparin-induced thrombocytopenia has occurred.

Coumadin. Although vitamin K antagonists such as warfarin are well-established and highly effective anticoagulants, they are contraindicated in pregnancy. Vitamin K antagonists cross the placenta and anticoagulate the fetus (Category D). Warfarin use during pregnancy has been associated with miscarriage, prematurity, lower birth weight, neurodevelopmental problems, and fetal bleeding as well as a risk of major birth defects with first trimester exposure.[17] In select circumstances, warfarin has been used in pregnant patients with newer mechanical aortic valves, targeting a lower international normalized ratio (INR) of 1.5 to 2.0 without complications for the mother or fetus. However, this use of warfarin is still investigational. In the postnatal period, however, warfarin is a suitable alternative to parenteral anticoagulants such as heparin. This transition usually takes place when risk of obstetric hemorrhage is low, commonly about days 5 to 7 after the delivery of the baby. It is not contraindicated in breastfeeding.

Factor Xa and direct thrombin inhibitors. The novel anticoagulants include direct factor Xa inhibitors and direct thrombin inhibitors. At present, very limited data are available regarding the safety of these agents in pregnancy. The literature consists primarily of case reports and small retrospective series.

Although the new oral factor Xa inhibitors are more attractive than parenteral preparations for long-term use, these may cross the placenta and pose problems for the fetus. Such concern may explain the lack of data on their use in pregnancy, as the risks to the developing and maturing fetus in utero are unknown.

In situations of severe reactions to heparin and danaparoid, the American College of Chest Physicians recommends that direct thrombin inhibitors be used.[4] Fondaparinux is the agent of choice, as it does not cross the placenta and is an FDA Class B medication/Australian Category C. The manufacturers of

fondaparinux have collected information on 120 females who used fondaparinux around the time of pregnancy, and it has shown no adverse outcomes. Direct thrombin inhibitors, including hirudin, lepirudin, and argatroban, are not licensed for use in pregnancy because tvane is currently limited evidence of their safety.[18]

Antiplatelet Agents

Aspirin

Aspirin is the leading antiplatelet drug used for a variety of indications, including cardiovascular disease and vascular injury. In pregnant patients, however, aspirin may cause teratogenicity and fetal toxicity. Premature closure of the ductus arteriosus and increased perinatal mortality have been reported in animal studies with higher doses of aspirin. Therefore, aspirin is typically avoided in early pregnancy. However, the FDA has assigned Pregnancy Category C at lower doses (60–100 mg),[10] indicating treatment is relatively safe at these levels.[19] Low-dose aspirin once daily is recommended by the American Heart Association for pregnant patients with either a mechanical prosthesis or bioprosthesis in the second and third trimesters. In our practice, we keep females on low-dose aspirin through the first trimester as well. In cases of pre-eclampsia prevention, beginning higher doses (up to 162 mg) as early as the first trimester has also been recommended.

Clopidogrel

Clopidogrel has shown no adverse pregnancy effects when studied in animal models, earning it a category B designation from the FDA.[13] Limited data are available on the use of clopidogrel in human pregnancy. From the available literature, there is no evidence that clopidogrel increases placental abruption or other antepartum obstetric bleeding events. Additionally, thus far, there are no reports of fetal hemorrhagic events or excessive neonatal bleeding from the manufacturer's safety data. However, it is generally recommended to hold clopidogrel for 7 days before an elective delivery or administration of epidural anesthesia; thus, caution should be used when delivery may be unplanned.

Thrombolytic Agents

Extremely limited data are available on the effect of thrombolytic therapy during pregnancy; therefore, it is classified as a Category C drug. Thrombolytics may be considered when benefits of administration outweigh the risk of hemorrhage. In the case of acute venous thrombosis, including May-Thurner syndrome, mechanical thrombolysis is recommended over thrombolytics. However, in the case of acute arterial thrombosis, including stroke, the timely administration of recombinant tPA has been associated with significant improvements in morbidity and mortality. In general, intraarterial tPA with or without mechanical thrombectomy is preferred to systemic tPA administration. Insufficient data are available on other thrombolytic agents, including streptokinase, anisoylated plasminogen streptokinase activator complex, and urokinase, to draw any reasonable conclusions.

Sedatives

Benzodiazepines

Diazepam. The use of benzodiazepines, specifically diazepam, was previously thought to be associated with an increased frequency of cleft lip and/or palate; this finding has not been supported by most recent studies. Although the balance of evidence from human studies of the benzodiazepines (chiefly diazepam) does not show first-trimester usage to be teratogenic, the surgeon should check with the patient's obstetrician before administering this class of drugs.

Midazolam. Midazolam is generally considered unsafe for use during pregnancy. Midazolam was given a Pregnancy Category D rating by the FDA because it is a benzodiazepine and other benzodiazepines have been shown to cause birth defects and other problems. However, studies of midazolam in pregnant rabbits and rats did not show any problems.

ANESTHESIA CONCERNS

Anesthesia concerns during pregnancy include the safety of the mother and fetus.[20] The fetus may be affected by exposure to teratogenic effects of anesthetic agents, risk for preterm labor, and risk from changes in maternal physiology as a consequence of anesthesia. Changes in uterine blood flow and maternal acid-base status may cause hypoxemia or asphyxia in the fetus. These can be a result of maternal hypotension or hypoxia, maternal hyperventilation, or placental passage of anesthetic agents that affect the fetal central nervous system or cardiovascular system.

The effects of anesthesia during pregnancy can be divided into direct, or active, and indirect, or passive, effects. The direct effects relate to the possible teratogenic or embryotoxic properties of the drugs used for anesthesia, some of which cross the placenta. The indirect effects are those mechanisms whereby an anesthetic agent or surgical procedure may interfere with maternal or fetal physiology and, in doing so, harm the fetus. For the most part, the fetus experiences indirect effects as a consequence of anesthetic agents administered to the mother and hemodynamic changes in the mother from blood loss or anesthetic agents. The most profound effects on the fetus are related to decreased uterine blood flow or decreased oxygen content of uterine blood. Unlike circulation to other vital organs, most notably the brain, the uterine circulation is not autoregulated. During the third trimester, uterine circulation represents almost 10% of cardiac output. When treating maternal hypotension, vasopressors such as dopamine and epinephrine, although increasing the maternal systemic pressure, have little or no effect on uterine circulation. Phenylephrine and metaraminol are α-agonists that are effective in maintaining maternal blood pressure and preventing fetal acidosis. Other maneuvers, such as fluid bolus, Trendelenburg position, compression stockings, and leg elevation, have a larger impact on increasing uterine blood flow.

In addition to the risks related to maternal hypoxia or hypotension, the risk for spontaneous abortion and teratogenesis related to anesthetic agents is of major concern. Many nonhuman studies have demonstrated different teratogenic effects with similar agents but have not led to definitive conclusions regarding their teratogenic potential in humans. For a congenital defect to result, exposure to the teratogen must occur during the vulnerable differentiation stage of the affected organ system. As noted, differentiation of the major organ systems occurs during the first trimester of human embryonic development. Therefore, delaying semielective surgical procedures until after the first trimester may reduce the risk for teratogenicity. However, large survey studies have demonstrated an increased risk for spontaneous abortions, intrauterine growth retardation, and low-birth-weight neonates in females who require surgery during pregnancy. These studies lacked information on the indications for nonobstetric surgical procedures and failed to elucidate the etiology of this association. At present, the degree to which fetal development may be affected by anesthetic exposure, surgical stress, or the underlying disease state that prompted surgery remains unclear. Fetal surgery during the second and third trimesters has not been demonstrated to have specific adverse effects on fetal neurodevelopment, but long-term studies are lacking. Despite a black box warning from the FDA regarding anesthesia in young children, the PANDA trial failed to demonstrate significant long-term adverse effects from a single anesthetic before 36 months of age in matched sibling pairs.[21]

Elective surgical procedures are delayed until at least 6 weeks after delivery, when maternal physiology has returned to the nonpregnant state and when the impact on the fetus is no longer a concern.[20] When emergent procedures are required, obviously the life of the mother takes priority, although an experienced anesthesiologist will be able to modify the anesthesia used according to maternal physiology and fetal well-being. For semielective surgical procedures, attempts are made to delay surgery until after the first trimester whenever possible. This needs to be determined on an individual basis because continued exposure to the underlying disease process may be more harmful than the operative risk to the mother and fetus. During the second trimester, after organ system differentiation has occurred, there is almost no risk for anesthetic-induced malformation or spontaneous abortion. Later in pregnancy, during the third trimester, the risk for preterm delivery is at its highest.

When the pregnant patient requires surgical intervention, consultation with the obstetrician and possibly a perinatologist is essential. The specialist is helpful in determining the optimum technique to monitor fetal status and can assist with perioperative management and diagnose and manage preterm labor. Typically, when emergent surgery occurs during the first or early second trimester, fetal heart tones are monitored before and after anesthesia exposure. During the late second and third trimesters, when the fetus is of viable age, continuous intraoperative monitoring is performed when possible. Transvaginal ultrasound can be used when the surgical field involves the abdomen. Continuous monitoring is used if significant blood loss is possible or anticipated to assess fetal well-being. Checking the fetal heart rate for fetal status and tocometer monitoring for uterine activity are done before and after the procedure, even if intraoperative monitoring is not believed necessary or is unavailable.

Postoperative pain control in the pregnant patient needs to be monitored closely. NSAIDs are not used in pregnancy because of the risk for premature closure of the ductus arteriosus. The newly available IV acetaminophen, morphine, and fentanyl are good choices postoperatively when oral analgesics are insufficient or cannot be used. Morphine has a higher associated incidence of nausea and vomiting, but most surgeons have extensive experience with it. A patient-controlled analgesia pump after surgery may be the best choice because of the associated low incidence of maternal respiratory depression and drug transfer to the fetus.

Postoperative oral narcotic use is generally considered safe in pregnancy. Narcotic analgesics have not been found to cause birth defects in humans in normal dosages. Oxycodone, hydrocodone, and codeine are commonly used narcotics and can be safely used in moderation. Chronic use of narcotics during pregnancy may cause fetal dependency. It is recommended that the pregnant postsurgical patient be weaned off narcotic use as soon as possible.

PREVENTION OF PRETERM LABOR

The incidence of preterm labor associated with nonobstetric surgery is related to gestational age and the indication for surgery. Studies have suggested that the rate of premature labor induced by nonobstetric surgical intervention is 3.5%. Gestational age at treatment and severity of the underlying disease are the most predictive indicators of patients at risk for preterm labor. The later in gestation the patient is, the higher the risk for preterm contractions or preterm labor. Intraperitoneal surgeries and disease processes with intraperitoneal inflammation are the most likely to have a postoperative course complicated by preterm contractions and preterm labor. In a number of studies, a significant difference was found in the number of patients with preterm contractions based on the average time from onset of symptoms to operative intervention. A delay in treatment appears to increase the chance of preterm labor, likely related to the primary disease process. Laparoscopic and open techniques have an equal associated incidence of preterm labor.

There is no general consensus on the use of prophylactic tocolytics after nonobstetric surgery during pregnancy. Tocolytic use varies widely among centers and physicians. Most studies have suggested that tocolytics only be used if contractions are noted during postoperative monitoring or are appreciated by the patient. Tocolytics used as needed are generally successful at preventing preterm labor and preterm delivery when postoperative contractions are detected. Terbutaline, magnesium, and indomethacin (Indocin) have been used in different studies, with equivalent results. Almost 100% of patients with postoperative contractions were successfully given tocolytics and delivered at term. In general, for patients with postoperative contractions before 32 weeks, indomethacin would be a reasonable treatment, whereas terbutaline could be used as first-line treatment for patients at more than 32 weeks' gestation. The use of prophylactic tocolysis is individualized, depending on the patient's gestational age and underlying disease process.

SURGERY FOR DISEASES IN PREGNANCY

Abdominal Pain and the Acute Abdomen in Pregnancy

When the pregnant patient presents with abdominal pain, it may be difficult to distinguish a pathophysiologic cause from normal pregnancy-associated symptoms. Changes in the position and orientation of abdominal viscera from the enlarging uterus and the alterations in physiology already described may modify the perception or manifestation of an intraabdominal process. If it is early in the pregnancy, the patient may not know that she is pregnant. Also, some intraabdominal processes are exclusive to pregnancy, such as ectopic pregnancy; hemolysis, elevated liver enzymes, and low platelets (HELLP) syndrome; or acute fatty liver of pregnancy. Both patient and physician may attribute the patient's complaints to normal pregnancy, resulting in a delay in evaluation and treatment. These delays in diagnosis and definitive intervention are the most serious adverse events affecting maternal and fetal outcome. It is usually not the treatment but the delay in diagnosis and severity of the primary disease process that affects outcomes poorly. Box 28.1 lists the more common causes of abdominal pain in the pregnant patient, classified according to location.

BOX 28.1 Common Causes of Abdominal Pain in Pregnant Patients

Right Upper Quadrant
Gastroesophageal reflux
Peptic ulcer disease
Acute cholecystitis
Biliary colic
Acute pancreatitis
Hepatitis
Acute fatty liver of pregnancy
HELLP syndrome
Preeclampsia
Pneumothorax
Pneumonia
Acute appendicitis
Hepatic adenoma
Hemangioma

Right Lower Quadrant
Acute appendicitis
Ectopic pregnancy
Renal or ureteral colic
Pelvic inflammatory disease
Tuboovarian abscess
Endometriosis
Adnexal torsion
Ruptured ovarian cyst
Ruptured corpus luteum

Lower Abdomen
Threatened, incomplete, or complete abortion
Abruptio placentae
Preterm labor
Pelvic inflammatory disease
Tuboovarian abscess
Inflammatory bowel disease
Irritable bowel syndrome
Pyelonephritis

Flank
Pyelonephritis
Hydronephrosis of pregnancy
Acute appendicitis (retrocecal appendix)

Diffuse Abdominal Pain
Early acute appendicitis
Small bowel obstruction
Acute intermittent porphyria
Sickle cell crisis

HELLP, Hemolysis, elevated liver enzymes, and low platelets syndrome.

Minimally Invasive Surgery in Pregnancy

When laparoscopic techniques were initially described, pregnancy was considered to be a contraindication. Effects of CO_2 pneumoperitoneum on venous return and cardiac output, uterine perfusion, and fetal acid-base status were unknown. Laparoscopy was safely used in several series to evaluate pregnant patients for ectopic pregnancy.[22] Patients with an intrauterine pregnancy had no increase in fetal loss or observed negative effect on long-term outcome.[23] When comparing laparoscopic and open techniques in nonpregnant patients, patients who underwent laparoscopic procedures had decreased pain, shorter hospital stays, and a quicker return to normal activity.

Major concerns of laparoscopy during pregnancy include injury to the uterus, decreased uterine blood flow, fetal acidosis, and preterm labor from increased intraabdominal pressure. During the second trimester, the uterus is no longer contained within the pelvis. The open technique for abdominal access can reduce the risk for injury. Using a Veress needle for insufflation or optical trocar can be done safely if the site of initial abdominal access is adjusted according to fundal height and the abdominal wall is elevated. Decreased uterine blood flow from pneumoperitoneum remains a theoretical concern because significant changes in intraabdominal pressure occur normally during pregnancy with maternal Valsalva maneuvers. The risk for pneumoperitoneum may also be less than the risk for direct uterine manipulation that occurs with laparotomy. Fetal respiratory acidosis with subsequent fetal hypertension and tachycardia have been observed in a pregnant ewe model but were reversed by maintaining maternal respiratory alkalosis.[24] Also, in the largest series comparing laparoscopy and open techniques, no significant differences in preterm labor or delivery-related side effects were observed.[23] Box 28.2 illustrates the general comparison between laparoscopic and open technique.

The Society of American Gastrointestinal and Endoscopic Surgeons (SAGES) recommends the following guidelines for laparoscopic surgery during pregnancy based on a literature review of 154 articles from 2011 to 2016, with a four-tiered system of quality of evidence (very low [+], low [++], moderate [+++], or high [++++]) and a two-tiered system for strength of recommendation (weak or strong). Updated SAGES guidelines for laparoscopic surgery are as follows[25,26]:

1. Obstetric consultation is obtained preoperatively.
2. When possible, operative intervention is deferred until the second trimester, when fetal risk is lowest, but laparoscopy can be safely performed during any trimester of pregnancy when the operation is indicated (++++; strong).
3. Pneumoperitoneum enhances lower extremity venous stasis already present in the gravid patient, and pregnancy induces a hypercoagulable state. Therefore, pneumatic compression devices are used whenever possible, and beyond the first trimester, gravid

patients should be placed in the left lateral decubitus position or partial left lateral decubitus position to minimize compression of the vena cava (++; strong).
4. Fetal and uterine status as well as maternal end-tidal CO_2 and arterial blood gas levels need to be monitored (+++; strong).
5. The uterus needs to be protected with a lead shield if intraoperative cholangiography is a possibility. Fluoroscopy is used selectively (++; strong).
6. Initial abdominal access can be safely accomplished with an open (Hasson), Veress needle, or optical trocar technique by surgeons experienced with these techniques if the location is adjusted according to fundal height (++; weak).
7. Pneumoperitoneum CO_2 pressures of 10 to 15 mm Hg can be safely used for laparoscopy in the pregnant patient. The level of insufflation should be adjusted to the patient's physiology (+++; strong).

According to SAGES guidelines, safe abdominal access for laparoscopy can be accomplished using either an open or closed technique, when used appropriately.[25,26] Of course, this is in the hands of experienced laparoscopic surgeons writing for this professional organization. The concern for use of closed access techniques (Veress needle or optical entry) has largely been based on the concern for higher risk of injury to the uterus or other intraabdominal organs. Because the intraabdominal domain is altered as the uterus grows, trocar placement should be altered from the standard configuration to supraumbilical or subcostal (Fig. 28.1). An angled endoscope may aid in viewing over or around the uterus. If the site of initial abdominal access is adjusted according to fundal height and the abdominal wall is elevated during insertion, both the Hassan technique and Veress needle have been safely and effectively used.[24-26] Ultrasound-guided trocar placement has been described in the literature as an additional safeguard to avoid uterine injury. Regardless of technique, the uterus should be manipulated as little as possible. Should an inadvertent entry into the uterus occur during a laparoscopic procedure, simple closure of the defect with an absorbable suture followed by monitoring and possible indomethacin tocolysis are usually adequate to prevent preterm delivery. If any concern exists regarding potential damage to the fetus or placenta, then obstetric consultation with ultrasound examination of the fetus is indicated.

BOX 28.2 Advantages and Disadvantages of Laparoscopy Instead of Laparotomy in Pregnancy

Advantages
Decreased fetal depression secondary to decreased narcotic requirement
Lower rates of wound infections and incisional hernias
Diminished postoperative maternal hypoventilation
Decreased manipulation of the uterus
Faster recovery with early return to normal function
Decreased risk of ileus

Disadvantages
Possible uterine injury during trocar placement
Decreased uterine blood flow
Preterm labor risk secondary to increased intraabdominal pressure
Increased risk of fetal acidosis and unknown effects of CO_2 pneumoperitoneum
Decreased visualization with gravid uterus

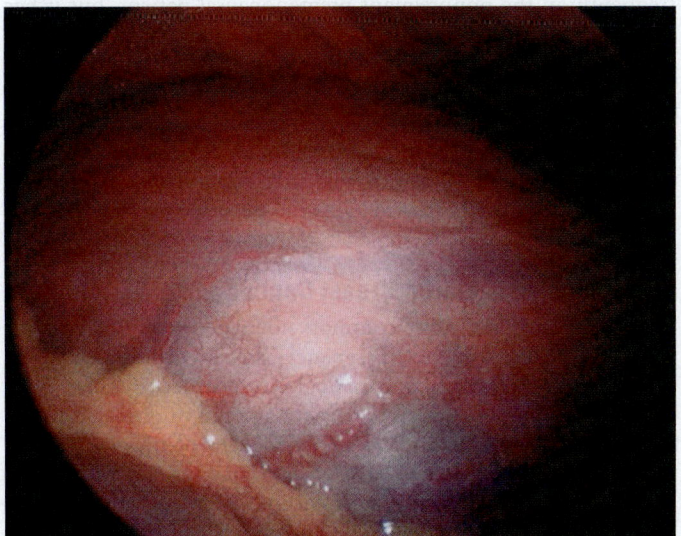

FIGURE 28.1 Intraoperative image of a 24-week gravid uterus taken with a 5-mm, 30-degree high-definition camera.

BREAST MASSES IN PREGNANCY

During pregnancy and lactation, a female's breasts physiologically change with reorganization and specialization of the breast tissue. These changes can be attributed to the various hormones that are induced with the start of embryo implantation, therefore making the interpretation of physical and radiologic examinations difficult. Especially because diagnosis can be challenging, it is important to note that most breast lesions during pregnancy and lactation are benign; however, the differential diagnosis does still include breast cancer.[27] Pregnancy-associated breast cancer is defined as breast cancer diagnosed during pregnancy, within 1 year after pregnancy, or anytime during lactation. Overall, pregnancy-associated breast cancer has been reported to occur in 15 to 35 per 100,000 pregnancies, with the largest incidence in the postpartum period.[28] As more patients delay childbearing until much later in life, the likelihood of breast cancer increases, but still only represents 7% of all breast cancers diagnosed in females under 45 years old.[28,29]

Physiologic changes of breast engorgement, rapid cellular proliferation, and increased vascularity make a reliable physical examination difficult; masses of similar size that would be easily palpable in the nonpregnant state may be obscured, or palpable masses may be attributed to normal pregnancy-related changes. Benign breast lesions such as galactoceles, mastitis, abscesses, lipomas, fibroadenomas, and lactational adenomas account for 80% of breast masses that occur during pregnancy or lactation. However, any palpable mass or skin change that persists for 4 weeks or longer needs to be evaluated.[29]

Imaging and Biopsy During Pregnancy

Because of the changes in the breast tissue with pregnancy, imaging modality findings may be difficult to interpret. Breast parenchyma proliferates, increasing in size and density, therefore increasing the mammographic parenchymal density. If used with appropriate shielding, mammography carries a limited risk to the fetus during both pregnancy and lactation with a radiation dose of <0.03 microGy to the uterus.[30] Ultrasonography can safely be performed as an initial evaluation or in conjunction with mammography. Ultrasound is very sensitive, with some data reporting a 100% negative predictive value.[29,30] MRI of the breast is used frequently in the nonpregnant premenopausal patient, but it has limited use in pregnant patients because of increased breast vascularity leading to increased background enhancement and concerns of gadolinium exposure for the fetus. Gadolinium contrast is listed as a Pregnancy Category C drug and has been associated with fetal abnormalities in rats. With other reliable imaging modalities available, MRI is not currently recommended for pregnant patients. Core biopsy remains the most appropriate method of tissue diagnosis in pregnancy.

Pregnancy-Associated Breast Cancer

Breast cancer is the most common nongynecologic malignancy associated with pregnancy. Pregnancy-associated breast cancer is thought to be clinically and biologically distinct. Because most pregnant females are under 40 years of age and thus not undergoing breast imaging, as well as the challenges of imaging during pregnancy, pregnancy-associated breast cancer usually presents as a painless palpable mass, with or without nipple discharge. As is true for nonpregnant patients, ductal carcinoma is the most common histology, with the triple-negative phenotype accounting for approximately 50% to 60% of breast cancers in pregnant patients.

Unfortunately, pregnancy-associated cancers are often larger in size and lymph node positive.

Although the initial reports of pregnancy-associated breast cancer more than 100 years ago proposed a dismal prognosis, more recent literature has suggested that this is because of a more advanced stage at the time of diagnosis.[29] When compared with age-matched nonpregnant controls, females with pregnancy-associated breast cancer present with a larger primary tumor and higher risk for positive axillary lymph nodes. Patients with pregnancy-associated breast cancer have a similar stage-related prognosis compared with nonpregnant controls. Overall, these patients bear a worse prognosis because of the more advanced disease at presentation, not the pregnancy itself. Pregnancy is a hyperestrogenic state and may correlate with rapid tumor proliferation and axillary lymph node metastases, although pregnant females and nonpregnant young females have a higher percentage of estrogen receptor–negative cancers than older females.[31] This higher incidence of estrogen receptor–negative cancer is likely caused by a downregulation of estrogen receptors during pregnancy. In a recent case control study, young females with pregnancy-associated triple-negative breast cancer were compared with their nonpregnant counterparts; no difference was seen in either disease-free or overall survival.[32]

Tissue diagnosis is essential. Core-needle biopsy, with or without ultrasound guidance, is a safe and reliable method for obtaining tissue. The major risks are hematoma formation and milk fistula development. The risk for milk fistula is as small as 1.4% and may be reduced by emptying the breast of milk just before the procedure.[33] Even if a milk fistula develops, cessation of breastfeeding is not mandatory, and the milk fistula should still close with consistent breast emptying. Fine-needle aspiration may be a reliable alternative to core-needle or open biopsy in the correct situation. It can be performed safely with ultrasound guidance under local anesthesia without exposing the patient and fetus to the risks involved with general anesthesia, but its accuracy is dependent on the pathologist's experience in distinguishing the proliferative changes of pregnancy from those of cancer.

Therapy for pregnancy-associated breast cancer, as it is with most other nonmetastatic breast cancer, needs to be decided in a multidisciplinary manner involving surgical oncologists, medical oncologists, radiation oncologists, and, in this case, high-risk obstetricians. Traditionally modified radical mastectomy was considered the appropriate choice for local control; however, this paradigm is changing. Data have suggested that the combination of local control and adjuvant therapy may be tailored to the patient according to the stage of pregnancy as well as the stage of the cancer.[31] Surgical intervention is considered safe throughout pregnancy and should follow nonpregnant recommendations when possible. However, trimester should be considered when evaluating patients for mastectomy or breast conservation, as radiation is not considered safe at any point during pregnancy and a delay of more than 8 to 12 weeks without undergoing chemotherapy leads to an increase of in-breast recurrence.[28,34] Therefore, typically if surgery is considered before 24 weeks and chemotherapy is not expected, mastectomy is often the preference. Reconstruction in these situations is often delayed until after surgery because of difficulty in achieving symmetry and concerns for extended operation time. However, recent data in some small retrospective datasets have shown no major fetal or obstetric complications.[35] Sentinel node biopsy using radiolabeled sulfur colloid is thought to be safe during pregnancy even though there are only small series looking at its safety.[36] Unlike sulfur colloid, blue dye is considered contraindicated. However, the procedure should be considered on a case-by-case basis because there are no prospective trials.

Chemotherapy has many complex indications in pregnant patients, as it does in the nonpregnant patient, and similar treatment regimens should be followed with a few exceptions. Most current chemotherapeutic regimens are safe after the first trimester, when there is a large teratogenic risk. In the second and third trimester, there are no differences in the risk of fetal malformation that that seen in a nonexposed population. The increased plasma volume, hypoalbuminemia, and change in glomerular filtration rate change drug pharmacokinetics and make accurate dosing difficult but should be based on current body surface area.[37] Antimetabolites such as methotrexate are avoided because of the high risk for spontaneous abortion, even after the first trimester. Anthracyclines and alkylating agents such as cyclophosphamide have been shown to be safe in pregnant patients for many years. In one study, 24 patients with pregnancy-associated breast cancer were given a chemotherapeutic regimen during the second and third trimesters that included fluorouracil, cyclophosphamide, and doxorubicin. None of the infants had congenital malformations; the median age at delivery was 38 weeks.[37] Cyclophosphamide and doxorubicin can enter breast milk; breastfeeding is contraindicated during chemotherapy. The safety data for the use of platinum derivatives and taxane-based therapeutics during pregnancy are still unknown. Anti-HER2 therapeutics and immunotherapy are considered contraindicated because there are only case reports of their use in pregnancy with multiple fetal complications. Endocrine therapy is also considered a teratogen.

Radiation is thought to be contraindicated during pregnancy because of its teratogenic risk and risk for induction of childhood malignancies. The risk is directly related to dose and developmental stage. During the preimplantation stage and continuing to 15 weeks after conception, during organogenesis, the rapidly proliferating cells of the fetus are most sensitive to radiation, and exposure greater than 0.2 Gy in utero can lead to malformations.[28] The standard therapeutic course of 40 to 50 Gy results in varying exposure to the fetus, depending on the gestational age and proximity of the gravid uterus to the radiation bed. Even with abdominal shielding, the greatest fetal exposure is caused by scatter. Although there have been several case reports of healthy infants born after maternal radiation exposure, radiation is not recommended during pregnancy because of the risks for radiation-induced microcephaly, intrauterine growth retardation, and spontaneous abortion.

Elective termination of the pregnancy to receive appropriate therapy without the risk for fetal malformation is no longer routinely recommended because no improvement in survival has been demonstrated. With the treatment options available to the pregnant patient with breast cancer, a combined approach among the patient, surgical oncologist, medical oncologist, and maternal-fetal medicine specialist ensures optimal treatment of the disease while minimizing risk to the patient and fetus.

HEPATOBILIARY DISEASE

Liver Disorders

Liver abnormalities during pregnancy can be classified as occurring exclusively during pregnancy as a direct result of conditions during pregnancy, occurring simultaneously but not exclusively during pregnancy, or developing before the pregnancy. Examples of liver disorders unique to pregnancy include acute fatty liver of pregnancy,

intrahepatic cholestasis of pregnancy, and liver disease related to preeclampsia or eclampsia, specifically HELLP syndrome and spontaneous hepatic hemorrhage or rupture. Preexisting liver disorders that may manifest with complications during pregnancy include hepatic adenoma and hepatocellular carcinoma.

The cause of acute fatty liver of pregnancy is unknown, although it is more common in first pregnancies, twin pregnancies, and females who are pregnant with a male fetus. Although it has been diagnosed as early as 26 weeks' gestation, it usually occurs during the third trimester, typically around 35 weeks' gestation. Acute fatty liver of pregnancy carries a 20% maternal and fetal mortality rate. Initial nonspecific symptoms such as malaise, nausea, vomiting, and right upper quadrant pain are followed by signs of significant liver dysfunction within 2 weeks of onset of symptoms. Progression to fulminant hepatic failure quickly leads to preterm labor and an increased risk for fetal mortality. Although there is no specific treatment for acute fatty liver of pregnancy, prompt delivery after diagnosis may prevent progression to fulminant hepatic failure and reduce the risk for fetal death. Liver function typically returns to normal after delivery.

Approximately 10% of females with preeclampsia or eclampsia have associated liver involvement,[38] ranging from severe elevation of hepatic enzyme levels, to HELLP syndrome, to hepatic rupture. Hepatic hemorrhage or rupture occurs primarily during the third trimester or can develop up to 48 hours after delivery. Right upper quadrant pain is the initial manifestation, followed by hepatic tenderness, peritonitis, chest and right shoulder pain, or the development of hemodynamic instability within a few hours. The diagnosis is suspected in a pregnant patient with preeclampsia who develops right upper quadrant pain. A CT scan of the abdomen is highly sensitive and specific in diagnosis; ultrasonography findings are usually nonspecific and have a higher incidence of false-negative studies. The diagnosis may also be made during cesarean section. Management depends on a suspicion of ongoing intraperitoneal hemorrhage or vascular instability. Hepatic hematomas without evidence of ongoing bleeding in hemodynamically stable patients may be managed nonoperatively with serial imaging and close monitoring, and these lesions typically heal without intervention. If there is evidence or suspicion of rupture, immediate intervention is required because maternal and fetal mortality rates from hepatic hemorrhage are 60% and 85%, respectively. Immediate laparotomy with abdominal packing or hepatic artery ligation reduces maternal and fetal mortality. Coagulopathy must be corrected aggressively. If the patient is relatively stable or abdominal packing has been unsuccessful in controlling hemorrhage, angiography with selective embolization may be performed. Angiography is most useful when the diagnosis is made postpartum.

Hepatic adenomas are uncommon benign lesions usually associated with oral contraceptive use in young females.[39] Hepatic adenomas are also associated with glycogen storage disease, diabetes, exogenous steroids, and pregnancy. They are usually solitary lesions that have a low potential for malignant transformation. Although the specific cause is unknown, it has been hypothesized that a change in hormone levels, specifically of the sex steroids, leads to hepatotoxicity or exposes a hereditary defect in carbohydrate metabolism that results in hepatocyte hyperplasia and adenoma formation. The observation that adenomas may resolve after cessation of exogenous steroid or oral contraceptive use supports this hypothesis. The association of hepatic adenomas with pregnancy also supports the hypothesis that elevated levels of endogenous hormones may contribute to adenoma formation, although no data have shown regression of a hepatic adenoma after pregnancy. Similarly, the actual incidence of hepatic adenomas during pregnancy is unknown. Again, diagnosis is best done with CT or MRI of the liver.

The major risk of a hepatic adenoma during pregnancy is spontaneous rupture, which carries a mortality rate of approximately 60% for mother and fetus, even with operative intervention. When spontaneous rupture does occur, the presentation may be similar to that described for hepatic hemorrhage associated with preeclampsia—right upper quadrant pain with referred right shoulder pain and progression to shock. Immediate laparotomy is performed with cesarean birth, control of hemorrhage, and resection of the adenoma, if possible.

Because of the high mortality associated with the rupture of a hepatic adenoma, elective resection may be performed. Resection during the second trimester minimizes the operative risk to the mother and fetus and does not interfere with the remainder of the pregnancy or subsequent pregnancies. Because of the unknown recurrence risk, however, subsequent pregnancy and oral contraceptive use may be discouraged in these patients.

Cavernous hemangiomas are the most common benign tumors of the liver and are found in approximately 2% of autopsy patients. The vast majority of these tumors are small and asymptomatic; however, there have been a few reported cases in which these lesions led to spontaneous fatal hemorrhage. Although liver hemangiomas occur in both sexes, most studies have indicated to a female predominance; one study reported a ratio of female predominance of 4.5:1. It has been suggested that estrogen may be associated with the growth of liver hemangiomas, but the incidence of these lesions in pregnancy and the effects of increased estrogen levels during pregnancy on them are unknown. Symptomatic liver hemangiomas have been treated by steroids, radiation therapy, surgical resection, and recently embolization, but surgeons may sometimes be confronted with intraabdominal hemorrhage originating from the rupture of asymptomatic liver hemangiomas. A case of an incidental intraabdominal hemorrhage originating from a liver hemangioma in a 36-week twin pregnancy being delivered emergently by cesarean section because of fetal distress has been reported.

Cholelithiasis

Cholecystectomy for symptomatic cholelithiasis is second to appendectomy as the most common nonobstetric surgical procedure performed during pregnancy. As noted, pregnancy is associated with an increased incidence of cholelithiasis. Most pregnant patients are asymptomatic. Although an estimated 2% to 5% of pregnant females may be found to have gallstones by ultrasound, only 0.05% to 0.1% of them will be symptomatic. Biliary cholesterol concentrations in gallbladder bile increase gradually from the first to the third trimester, along with a progressive increase in gallbladder volume and delayed emptying, leading to increased biliary sludge. Pregnancy hormonal changes of elevated estradiol and estrone also increase lithogenicity. The symptoms of biliary colic are the same in pregnant and nonpregnant patients. In patients with symptoms consistent with cholelithiasis, ultrasound is the diagnostic examination of choice. In pregnant patients, ultrasound is as accurate in identifying gallstones and signs of inflammation as in nonpregnant patients.

Historically, before laparoscopic techniques, pregnant patients with a clear operative indication, such as obstructive jaundice, gallstone pancreatitis, and choledocholithiasis, underwent cholecystectomy regardless of gestational age. Patients with recurrent

biliary colic or acute cholecystitis who responded to medical management were treated expectantly until after delivery, at which time they underwent cholecystectomy. However, laparoscopic cholecystectomy during pregnancy is associated with shorter length of stay, shorter operative times, and fewer complications compared with open cholecystectomy.[40] A recent literature meta-analysis of 11 studies and over 10,000 patients demonstrated that the laparoscopic approach was associated with decreased risks for fetal (odds ratio [OR] 0.42, 95% confidence interval [CI] 0.28–0.63, $P < 0.001$), maternal (OR 0.42, 95% CI 0.33–0.53, $P < 0.001$), and surgical (OR 0.45, 95% CI 0.25–0.82, $P = 0.01$) complications. The average length of hospital stay was 3.2 days in the laparoscopic approach versus 6.0 days after open cholecystectomy ($P = 0.02$). The conversion rate from laparoscopic cholecystectomy to open cholecystectomy was 3.8%. Of note, 91% of the patients in this study had their cholecystectomy performed in the first or second trimester, and the author acknowledge gestational age may be a confounding factor.[41] Fetal demise is rare to nonexistent after laparoscopic cholecystectomy performed during the first and second trimesters.[42] Furthermore, decreased rates of spontaneous abortion and preterm labor are noted after laparoscopic cholecystectomy when compared with open cholecystectomy.[43] These data argue for the performance of laparoscopic cholecystectomy for symptomatic biliary colic in the first or second trimester and not waiting for the third trimester or postpartum. Further arguing for early cholecystectomy is the finding that symptomatic cholelithiasis may resolve, but there is a 92% recurrence of symptoms if the initial presentation was in the first trimester, 64% in the second trimester, and 44% in the third trimester.[44]

As it became understood that adverse maternal and fetal outcomes are related more to the disease process and not to the surgical intervention, management patterns have changed. Also, complications from nonoperative management of gallstone disease result in an increase in maternal and fetal mortality. With gallstone pancreatitis during pregnancy, a maternal mortality rate of 15% and a fetal mortality rate of 60% have been reported. In a study of 63 patients who were admitted with symptomatic cholelithiasis, surgical management reduced the need for labor induction, rate of preterm deliveries, and fetal mortality.[45] Therefore, surgical intervention is considered the primary treatment of gallstones in pregnancy.

The timing of cholecystectomy for biliary colic depends on the gestational age and severity of symptoms. A spontaneous abortion rate of 12% with open cholecystectomy during the first trimester falls to 5.6% and 0% during the second and third trimesters, respectively. The risk for preterm labor is almost 0% during the second trimester and 40% during the third trimester. The optimum time for cholecystectomy is the second trimester, when the risks for spontaneous abortion and preterm labor are the lowest, unless the patient develops a complication of cholelithiasis. In a study of 122 patients who were admitted with biliary colic, 69 (56.5%) underwent minimally invasive intervention. Eight patients were treated during the first, 54 during the second, and 7 during the last trimester. There was no fetal morbidity or mortality and only minor maternal morbidity, with no mortality.[42]

Laparoscopic cholecystectomy is safest during the second trimester. The gravid uterus is not large enough at this gestational age to interfere with visualization; the uterus also is less likely to be inadvertently instrumented at this size. The open technique using the Hasson trocar is recommended for obtaining access to the abdomen. If intraoperative cholangiography or endoscopic retrograde cholangiopancreatography is indicated for choledocholithiasis, the uterus needs to be protected with appropriate shielding. If the severity of symptoms prevents delaying surgical intervention until after delivery, laparoscopic cholecystectomy can be safely performed during the third trimester, although the risk for preterm labor is substantially increased. In several small series of patients, preterm labor was successfully managed with tocolytics, and the patients delivered healthy term infants.

Endocrine Disease

Adrenal Disease

Pheochromocytomas originate from chromaffin cells in the adrenal medulla or from extramedullary paraganglion cells. They are hormonally active tumors, secreting the catecholamines norepinephrine, epinephrine, and, less commonly, dopamine. Pheochromocytomas are usually described by the rule of 10, which states that 10% of pheochromocytomas are extraadrenal, 10% are bilateral, 10% are malignant, and 10% are familial. These tumors can occur sporadically or as part of a syndrome, such as multiple endocrine neoplasia (MEN) type 2A (MEN2A), MEN2B, or von Hippel-Lindau disease.

Although pheochromocytomas are uncommon in pregnancy, they have devastating effects on the mother and fetus. Pheochromocytomas that remain undiagnosed during pregnancy have a postpartum maternal mortality as high as 55%, with fetal mortality also exceeding 50%. The greatest risk occurs from the onset of labor to 48 hours after delivery. The index of suspicion must be high in any patient with preeclampsia, paroxysmal hypertension, or unexplained fever after delivery. With diagnosis and appropriate treatment, the maternal mortality rate is reduced to almost 0% and the fetal mortality rate is decreased to 15%. Diagnosis is made by elevated urine catecholamine levels; urinary catecholamine levels in the pregnant patient without a pheochromocytoma are the same as in the nonpregnant patient. Lack of proteinuria also helps eliminate preeclampsia as a cause of hypertension. Metaiodobenzylguanidine-I131 (MIBG) imaging is not recommended during pregnancy because the small molecule may cross the placenta; however, the use of MIBG imaging has not been evaluated in pregnancy.

Surgical resection needs to be performed before 20 weeks' gestation, when spontaneous abortion is less likely and the size of the gravid uterus does not interfere with the procedure. If the diagnosis is made late in the second trimester or during the third trimester, medical management followed by combined cesarean birth and resection of the pheochromocytoma may be an option. It is unknown whether the standard preoperative management with α-blockade or calcium channel blockade followed by perioperative β-blockade in nonpregnant patients is safe during pregnancy. The long-term effects of the α-blocker phenoxybenzamine on the fetus have not been determined, although calcium channel blockers are safe to use during pregnancy. β-Blockers are frequently used during pregnancy with close monitoring for intrauterine growth retardation. Consultation with a maternal-fetal medicine specialist is essential to determine the preoperative management that will ensure the optimal postoperative result for the patient and fetus. In nonpregnant patients, the method of approach depends on suspected malignancy, unilateral versus bilateral tumors, extraadrenal location, size of the tumor, and surgeon's preference and experience. In all series comparing the different approaches, including open versus laparoscopic technique, pregnant patients were not included.

Recent studies have indicated the safety of the laparoscopic approach in pregnancy.

Thyroid Disease

Thyroid disease during pregnancy can be categorized into three groups: hypothyroidism, hyperthyroidism, and thyroid cancer. Hypothyroidism is found in 2.5% of pregnancies. Of these, only 20% to 30% of patients develop symptoms. The first step is to obtain a serum thyroid-stimulating hormone (TSH) concentration. This will help categorize primary hypothyroidism versus hypothyroidism resulting from pituitary or hypothalamic causes.[46]

Current guidelines from LeBeau and Mandel for the treatment of hypothyroidism during pregnancy are as follows:
1. Check serum TSH level.
2. Initial levothyroxine dosage is based on severity of symptoms. Levothyroxine is started at 1 to 2 μg/kg/day. If TSH is less than 10 mU/L, the dose is adjusted to 0.1 mg/day.
3. For previously diagnosed hypothyroidism, monitor TSH level every 3 to 4 weeks.
4. Goal TSH level is less than 2.5 mU/L.
5. Monitor serum TSH and total TSH every 3 to 4 weeks with each dose change.

Hyperthyroidism during pregnancy has an incidence of 0.1% to 0.4%.[47] Gestational thyrotoxicosis is a multifactorial phenomenon. High serum concentrations of human chorionic gonadotropin during pregnancy activate the TSH receptors. Elevated serum-free thyroxine (T_4) and low serum TSH levels are seen with this form of thyrotoxicosis. Gestational thyrotoxicosis is usually self-limited and spontaneously resolves by 20 weeks' gestation, when the human chorionic gonadotropin level declines. Repeat evaluation is warranted if thyrotoxicosis persists. Most cases of hyperthyroidism are a result of Graves disease. After the diagnosis is made, medical treatment with thionamides (e.g., propylthiouracil, methimazole) is the mainstay of treatment. Iodides are avoided, except in patients preparing for thyroidectomy during pregnancy. Subtotal thyroidectomy for Graves disease is reserved for patients who are taking high-dose propylthiouracil (>600 mg/day) or methimazole (>40 mg/day), are allergic to thionamides, are noncompliant, or have compressive symptoms because of goiter size. Surgery is performed during the second trimester before 24 weeks' gestation to minimize the risk for miscarriage. A 2-week course of a β-adrenergic agent, along with potassium iodide, is implemented before surgery to minimize perioperative complications. Radioactive iodine therapy is contraindicated during pregnancy.

Because of hormonal changes, thyroid nodules may have a higher prevalence during pregnancy, but thyroid cancers do not. Thyroid cancers are worked up in the traditional fashion during pregnancy. Fine-needle aspiration, along with ultrasonic evaluation, remain the cornerstone of diagnosis. If cytology shows thyroid cancer, surgery is recommended during the second trimester, before 24 weeks' gestation. If thyroid cancer is found after the second half of pregnancy, surgery can be performed after delivery. This statement is supported by a recent study in which 201 pregnant females underwent thyroid ($N = 165$) and parathyroid ($N = 36$) procedures. Of these patients, 46% had thyroid cancer. When compared with nonpregnant patients ($N = 31$), the pregnant patients had a higher rate of endocrine (15.9% vs. 8.1%; $P < 0.001$) and general complications (11.4% vs. 3.6%; $P < 0.001$) and longer unadjusted lengths of stay (2 days vs. 1 day; $P < 0.001$). The fetal and maternal complication rates were 5.5% and 4.5%, respectively.[48] Postoperative radioactive iodine therapy also needs to be delayed until after delivery.

Small Bowel Disease

Intestinal obstruction is the third most common nonobstetric abdominal surgical issue in pregnancy, after acute appendicitis and acute cholecystitis. The incidence of small bowel obstruction during pregnancy has been reported to be between 1 in 1500 and 17,000 pregnancies. Small bowel obstructions usually occur during the second and third trimesters. Adhesions resulting from prior abdominal and pelvic surgeries are the most frequent causes of intestinal obstruction in pregnancy, accounting for 53% to 59% of cases. Other causes of small bowel obstruction in the pregnant patient include volvulus, intussusception, malignancy, and hernia, although the displacement of the small bowel out of the pelvis by the enlarging uterus makes this a rare cause.

The symptoms of an obstruction are identical to those in the nonpregnant patient and consist of the triad of abdominal pain, vomiting, and obstipation. Pain, present in 85% to 98% of cases, is usually colicky in nature and located in the midabdomen, although the character and duration are highly variable. Nausea and vomiting are seen in 80% of pregnant patients with small bowel obstruction; however, nausea and vomiting are not uncommon during the first trimester of normal pregnancy. Nausea and vomiting that persist or begin later in pregnancy should arouse suspicion and be evaluated. Bowel distention may be marked but difficult to assess because of the gravid uterus. Diagnosis is made by serial examination and plain abdominal radiography.

Treatment for small bowel obstruction in pregnancy is identical to that in the nonpregnant patient. Therapy consists of nasogastric decompression and IV fluids. However, a lower threshold for operative management is necessary. If, after 6 to 8 hours of nonoperative treatment, there is no satisfactory patient response, a laparotomy/laparoscopy is performed before perforation or bowel necrosis occurs. Maternal mortality ranges from 6% to 20% because of sepsis and multisystem organ failure, and fetal loss is as high as 26% to 50%. To avoid the risk to the mother and fetus, a more aggressive approach is used.

Midgut volvulus remains a dreaded diagnosis during the postpartum period. It is usually more common in the pregnant patient if she has undergone previous abdominal surgery; however, spontaneous midgut volvulus may occur. A case report of maternal death caused by midgut volvulus after bariatric surgery has been reported.[49] The key is increased vigilance for all those involved in the patient's care. Early exploration is warranted if the diagnosis is unclear.

Appendix, Colon, and Rectal Disease

Acute appendicitis is the most common nonobstetric abdominal surgical problem in the pregnant patient, occurring in 1 in 1000 to 1500 pregnancies.[50] The incidence is fairly evenly distributed among the trimesters of pregnancy, with a slight predominance during the second trimester. Timely and accurate diagnosis is challenging because the typical clinical findings of nausea, vomiting, abdominal pain, and mild leukocytosis may be seen in a normal pregnancy. Delay in diagnosis results in an increased perforation rate of 10%, which has significant consequences for the patient and fetus. Fetal mortality increases from 1.5% in acute appendicitis to 35% in perforated appendicitis; preterm labor and premature delivery rates are as high as 40% in perforated appendicitis[51] compared with a 13% rate of preterm labor and 4% rate of premature delivery in uncomplicated appendicitis.[52]

In 1932, Baer et al. studied 78 healthy pregnant females with radiographic studies at regular intervals from the second month of pregnancy to 10 days postpartum. As the uterus enlarges, the appendix is driven upward with a counterclockwise rotation. Baer concluded that early in pregnancy, pain is low and that as the gestation progresses, pain is located higher in the abdomen.[53] A review of 45 pregnant patients with acute appendicitis demonstrated that pain in the right lower quadrant is the most common symptom, regardless of gestational age (first trimester, 86%; second trimester, 83%; third trimester, 85%).[52] Despite the inconsistency, acute appendicitis needs to be included in the differential diagnosis of every pregnant female who presents with right-sided abdominal pain. Treatment of suspected acute appendicitis in the pregnant patient is emergent appendectomy. Although helical CT scans have demonstrated higher than 90% sensitivity and specificity in the diagnosis of acute appendicitis, few data are available in pregnant patients. In nonpregnant patients, a 10% to 15% negative laparotomy rate is considered acceptable. Because of the increased risk to mother and fetus with appendiceal perforation, a negative rate of 30% to 33% has been widely accepted until recently, when it was reported that even negative appendectomy may be associated with an increased risk of fetal loss. In a series of 3133 patients, the rates of fetal loss and preterm delivery in complicated appendicitis were 6% and 11%, respectively, in comparison to the rates of fetal loss and preterm delivery of 4% and 10%, respectively, in patients who underwent negative appendectomy.[54] It was concluded that improvement in fetal outcomes would result from improvement in diagnostic accuracy and reduction of the rate of negative appendectomy. In a small series of 47 patients, a positive ultrasound was considered to be diagnostic for appendicitis, with MRI without gadolinium or CT being used to confirm or exclude the diagnosis in a negative or nondiagnostic ultrasound diagnosis of appendicitis in pregnancy.[55] The debate is then for an open or laparoscopic technique. The argument for open appendectomy is that the laparoscopic approach exposes the fetus to risks for pneumoperitoneum and trocar placement without the benefit of a significantly smaller incision. The laparoscopic technique enables examination of a larger portion of the abdomen with less uterine manipulation and allows locating the appendix, as it is pushed into the right upper quadrant by the enlarging uterus.

The SAGES guidelines for the use of laparoscopy during pregnancy currently state that laparoscopy appendectomy may be performed safely in pregnant patients with acute appendicitis and rate the data supporting this stance moderately strong but acknowledge that the data supporting it as the procedure of choice are weak.[26]

The preponderance of studies demonstrate that laparoscopic appendectomy is safe and effective, with low rates of preterm labor and no fetal demise. We agree that there is no role for nonoperative management of uncomplicated acute appendicitis in pregnant patients because of a higher rate of peritonitis, fetal demise, shock, and venous thromboembolism as compared with operative management. Recent evidence for the use of antibiotics alone for treating acute appendicitis has not been extended to the gravid patient.

Because of concern and weak evidence suggesting a negative laparoscopy for appendicitis is associated with adverse maternal and fetal outcome, accurate diagnosis of appendicitis in the pregnant patient should be assured. When the diagnosis remains uncertain with clinical findings and ultrasound, MRI is the preferred adjunct to establish an accurate diagnosis. CT scan may be used when MRI is unavailable, but the risks of ionizing radiation exposure must be considered.

Port placement in the pregnant patient is determined by uterine size. The peritoneal cavity is first entered in the supraumbilical midline in patients operated on during the first trimester of pregnancy. After the third month of pregnancy, the trocar is inserted progressively higher, about 3 to 4 cm above the uterine fundus, located by palpation. Fig. 28.2 shows the routine positioning of the working trocars and the recommended displacement lines in relation to uterine size.

Colonic pseudoobstruction, or Ogilvie syndrome, is a functional obstruction, or adynamic ileus, without a mechanical cause. Of all cases of Ogilvie syndrome, 10% occur in postpartum patients. It is characterized by massive abdominal distention with cecal dilation. Although neostigmine is effective first-line therapy in nonpregnant patients, its safety in pregnancy is unknown. It can be used safely in the postpartum period. Colonoscopic decompression has been described in postpartum patients, with laparotomy indicated only in suspected perforation.

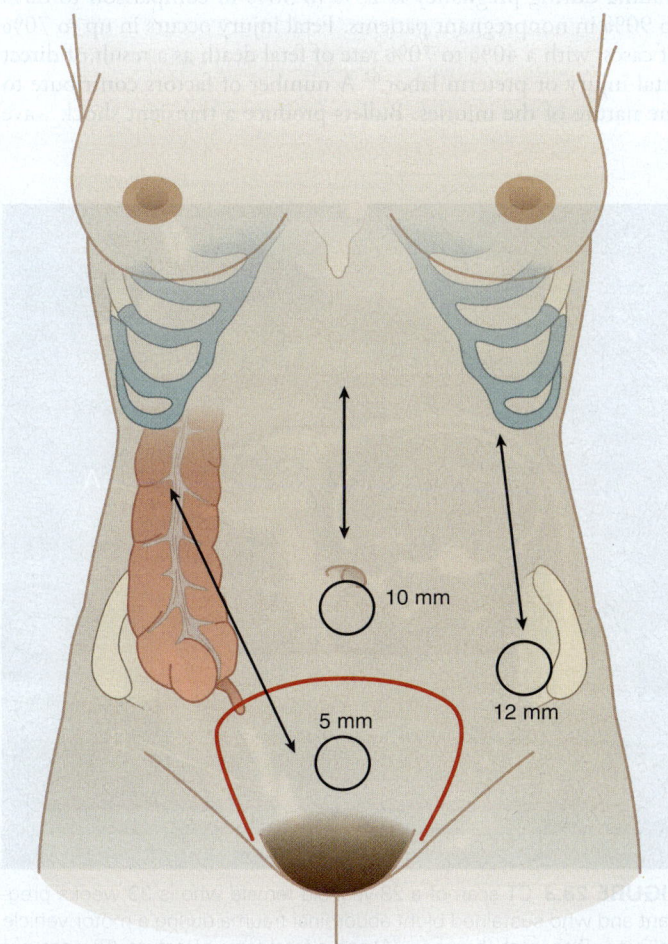

FIGURE 28.2 Configuration of laparoscopic port sites for laparoscopic appendectomy at various stages of pregnancy. (Adapted from Moreno-Sanz C, Pascual-Pedreno A, Picazo-Yeste JS, et al. Laparoscopic appendectomy during pregnancy: between personal experiences and scientific evidence. *J Am Coll Surg.* 2007;205:37-42.)

Labels in figure: 10 mm, 12 mm, 5 mm

Vascular Disease

Of more than 400 cases of ruptured splenic artery aneurysms in the literature, approximately 100 cases during pregnancy have been reported, with only 12 cases of maternal and fetal survival.[56] Rupture occurred during the third trimester in two-thirds of cases and was typically misdiagnosed as splenic rupture or uterine rupture. The maternal mortality rate was 75%, with a fetal mortality rate of 95%. Increased portal pressures, high splenic artery flow caused by distal aortic compression, and progressive arterial wall weakening are contributing factors. Multiparity may increase the risk; 78% of patients with ruptured splenic artery aneurysms have been in their third pregnancy. Survival is most likely related to a two-stage rupture, in which the lesser sac temporarily tamponades the bleeding aneurysm.

When treated electively in nonpregnant patients, the mortality rate is only 0.5% to 1.3%. When the diagnosis is made in a female of childbearing age or in a pregnant patient, a splenic artery aneurysm of 2 cm or larger is treated electively because of the increased risk for rupture during pregnancy.[56]

Acute iliofemoral venous thrombosis is six times more frequent in pregnant than nonpregnant patients. Pregnancy may increase the risk for thrombosis via a number of factors, including mechanical obstruction of venous drainage by the enlarging uterus, decreased activity in late pregnancy and at time of delivery, intimal injury from vascular distention or surgical manipulation during cesarean section, and abnormal levels of coagulation factors (see the section entitled "Physiologic Changes of Pregnancy"). Also, a wide spectrum of pathologic abnormalities, such as the presence of lupus anticoagulant antibodies and deficiencies of proteins C and S, may further increase the risk for thrombotic disease. Protein S serves as a cofactor for activated protein C, which has anticoagulant activity. Therefore, a deficiency of protein S leads to spontaneous, recurrent thromboembolic complications in nonpregnant adults. Even in normal individuals, protein S levels are substantially reduced during pregnancy.

The management of acute iliofemoral venous thrombosis during pregnancy is controversial because thrombolytic therapy poses hazards to the fetus. The risk for pulmonary thromboembolism with manipulation of the clot during thrombectomy would have catastrophic effects on both the patient and fetus. Techniques that have been described include interruption of the inferior vena cava through a right retroperitoneal approach or interruption of the inferior vena cava by passage of a Fogarty catheter through the unaffected contralateral femoral vein. The disadvantage of the retroperitoneal approach is that an extensive dissection is required. The disadvantages of the Fogarty catheter are that the catheter may still dislodge clots that have extended into the vena cava and that once the catheter is removed, an inferior vena cava filter must still be placed. However, the most effective technique is filter placement in the inferior vena cava either through the internal jugular vein or femoral vein using ultrasound guidance, followed by thrombectomy. Caval filters have been successfully placed in all trimesters of pregnancy; however, changes in approach or patient positioning (left lateral decubitus) to offload uterine compression of the cava may be necessary.[57] Unlike in the nonpregnant patient, caval filters placed in pregnancy should be positioned in the suprarenal cava to reduce the risk of compression by or erosion into the growing uterus or damage to the cava or filter during contractions.[58] Suprarenal location additionally protects against thrombus generated in the dilated ovarian veins. The increased caval flow in this position may also improve lysis of clots trapped in the filter. There is a hypothetical risk of renal injury if a suprarenal caval filter becomes completely occluded; however, this concern has not been borne out in the literature.[59] Providers should remain vigilant through close follow-up and prompt filter removal when no longer clinically necessary.

TRAUMA IN PREGNANCY

Trauma is the leading nonobstetric cause of maternal mortality and occurs in approximately 5% of pregnancies. The most common mechanisms of injury are from falls or from motor vehicle accidents. When compared with age-matched pregnant controls, pregnant patients who sustained trauma had a higher incidence of spontaneous abortion, preterm labor, fetomaternal hemorrhage, abruptio placentae, and uterine rupture.[60] A number of studies have attempted to identify risk factors that predict morbidity and mortality in the pregnant trauma patient. The maternal injury severity score, mechanism of injury, and physical findings are unable to adequately predict adverse outcomes, such as abruptio placentae and fetal loss. Pregnant patients with severe head, abdominal, thoracic, or lower extremity injuries are at high risk for pregnancy loss.[61] Early involvement of an available obstetrician is important to evaluate maternal and fetal well-being.

In the treatment of the pregnant trauma patient, the critical point is that resuscitation of the fetus is accomplished by resuscitation of the mother. Therefore, the initial evaluation and treatment of the injured pregnant patient is identical to that of the injured nonpregnant patient. Rapid assessment of the maternal airway, breathing, and circulation as well as ensuring an adequate airway avoids maternal and fetal hypoxia. In the later stages of pregnancy, as described earlier, uterine compression of the vena cava may result in hypotension from diminished venous return; thus, the pregnant trauma patient needs to be placed in a left lateral decubitus position. If spinal cord injury is suspected, the patient may be secured to a backboard and then tilted to the left.

The increased blood volume associated with pregnancy has important implications in the trauma patient. Signs of blood loss such as maternal tachycardia and hypotension may be delayed until the patient loses almost 30% of her blood volume. As a result, the fetus may be experiencing hypoperfusion long before the mother manifests any signs. Early and rapid fluid resuscitation should be initiated, even in the pregnant patient who is normotensive.

As with the primary survey, the secondary survey proceeds in a fashion similar to that in the nonpregnant patient. Special attention is given to the abdominal examination. The uterus remains protected by the pelvis until approximately 12 weeks' gestation and is relatively well sheltered from abdominal injury until then. As the uterus grows, it becomes more prominent and more vulnerable to injury. Measurement of fundal height provides a rapid approximation of gestational age. At 20 weeks' gestation, it is at the level of the umbilicus and is approximately 1 cm per week of gestation. Intrauterine hemorrhage or uterine rupture may result in a discrepancy in measurement. A pelvic examination is performed, by an obstetrician if possible, to evaluate for vaginal bleeding, ruptured membranes, or a bulging perineum. Vaginal bleeding may indicate abruptio placentae, placenta previa, or preterm labor. Rupture of the amniotic membrane may result in umbilical cord prolapse, which compresses the umbilical vessels and compromises fetal blood flow. This requires immediate cesarean section. If cloudy white or greenish fluid is seen from the cervical os or perineum, the presence of amniotic fluid is confirmed

by testing with nitrazine paper, which indicates pH and changes from green to blue.

The Kleihauer-Betke test for the assessment of fetomaternal transfusion is useful after maternal trauma and is ordered with the initial laboratory studies, which include typing and crossmatching. Because of the sensitivity of the Kleihauer-Betke test, a small amount of fetomaternal transfusion may be undetected. Therefore, all Rh-negative pregnant trauma patients are considered for Rh immunoglobulin (RhoGAM) therapy.

The most common cause of fetal death after blunt injury is abruptio placentae. Deceleration of the fetal heart rate may be the earliest sign of abruption. The uterus needs to be evaluated for contractions, rupture, and abruptio placentae. Early initiation of cardiotocographic fetal monitoring adequately warns of deterioration in the condition of the fetus. Because fetal survival is most greatly affected by maternal hemodynamics, early identification and prompt treatment of maternal injuries are paramount. When clinically indicated, x-rays, CT scans, and operative intervention should be completed without hesitation. Although the survival of the mother always takes precedence, injuries to the fetus necessitating additional follow-up may be identified (Fig. 28.3).

Penetrating trauma results in maternal death in less than 5% of cases. Penetrating trauma is primarily from gunshot wounds and knife wounds. The incidence of visceral injury with penetrating trauma during pregnancy is 16% to 38% in comparison to 80% to 90% in nonpregnant patients. Fetal injury occurs in up to 70% of cases, with a 40% to 70% rate of fetal death as a result of direct fetal injury or preterm labor.[62] A number of factors contribute to the nature of the injuries. Bullets produce a transient shock wave

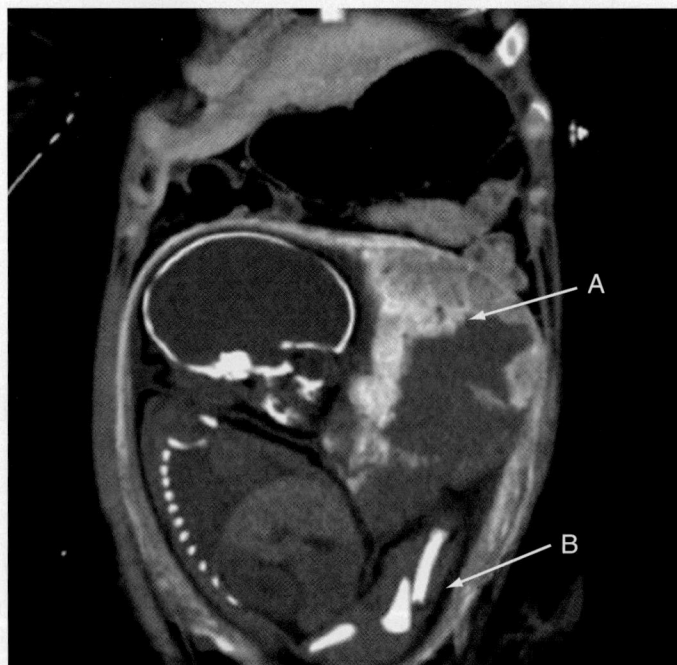

FIGURE 28.3 CT scan of a 23-year-old female who is 33 weeks pregnant and who sustained blunt abdominal trauma during a motor vehicle collision. Placental abruption *(A)* and a fetal femur fracture *(B)* were not detected on initial ultrasound but were evident on computed tomography. (From Romanowski KS, Struve I, McCracken B, et al. Fetal injuries and placental abruption detected on CT scan not observed on ultrasound, paper #6. 45th Western Trauma Association Annual Meeting; March 2, 2015; Telluride, CO, p. 47.)

and cavitation as they transmit kinetic energy to body tissues. The density of the tissue, such as the thick density of the uterus during early pregnancy, may rapidly dissipate the lower amount of kinetic energy from a low-velocity projectile, protecting the fetus from significant injury. Higher-velocity projectiles may produce more serious injuries to mother and fetus. As pregnancy progresses and the growing uterus displaces the abdominal viscera, location of the injury becomes crucial in determining which of the maternal viscera are injured and whether the fetus has sustained a direct injury. Management of penetrating injuries during pregnancy is similar to that for nonpregnant patients. It should be individualized, with early involvement by an obstetrician. Diagnostic and treatment options include surgical exploration, supraumbilical diagnostic peritoneal lavage, diagnostic laparoscopy, CT, local wound exploration, and observation. Emergency cesarean section may be indicated in maternal arrest after 4 minutes of unsuccessful resuscitation, fetal compromise with a stable mother if the fetus is of viable gestational age, obvious impending maternal death, or when the gravid uterus interferes with trauma-related surgical intervention. Also, emergent cesarean section may also improve chances of maternal survival by removing aortocaval compression and increasing cardiac output. Maternal and fetal survival rates as high as 72% and 45%, respectively, have been reported after emergency cesarean section at more than 25 weeks' gestational age. No fetal survival has been documented when fetal heart tones were absent before emergent delivery, but a 75% chance of fetal survival has been reported when fetal heart tones were present and gestational age was at least 26 weeks.[63] The best chance for fetal survival with an intact infant is when cesarean section occurs within 5 minutes of maternal death. Four minutes of resuscitation followed by a 1-minute cesarean section offers the best chance for infant survival. In a review of 61 infants born by perimortem cesarean section between 1900 and 1985, 70% of the infants survived who were delivered within 5 minutes of maternal death, and all of the survivors were neurologically intact.[64]

CONTROL OF MAJOR HEMORRHAGE

General and emergency surgeons may be called upon to support the obstetric team in response to massive hemorrhage or when planning obstetric operations in this high-risk patient population. Obstetric hemorrhage is the leading cause of maternal morbidity and mortality worldwide and has been increasing in incidence in the United States. The increasing incidence of abnormal placentation, otherwise known as *placenta accreta spectrum (PAS)*, has been implicated as the cause of increasing maternal mortality. PAS describes penetration of the chorionic villi into and, in some cases, through the uterine wall, substantially increasing the risk of massive obstetric hemorrhage. In the United States alone, the incidence of PAS doubled over the last 6 years. The most severe form, placenta percreta, in which chorionic villi penetrate through the uterine wall and into adjacent organs, has increased fiftyfold in the last 50 years. The end result is an increasing need for multidisciplinary approaches to maternal hemorrhage control.[65]

Mechanical Hemorrhage Control
Surgical Ligation
Traditional methods of intraoperative hemorrhage control include hypogastric artery ligation, uterine artery ligation, and rapid hysterectomy. Ligation of the hypogastric arteries theoretically reduces pulse pressure to the uterus; however, it is successful in reducing operative blood loss in less than 50% of cases.

Furthermore, ligation is estimated to be even less useful in PAS involving the bladder. These disparate findings are most likely explained by the persistent proximal collateral circulation to the uterus, which contributes to retrograde hemorrhage and venous bleeding during surgery. Temporary aortic cross-clamping can aid in hemorrhage control when hypogastric artery occlusion is insufficient or technically difficult to achieve in the presence of the gravid uterus.

Resuscitative Endovascular Balloon Occlusion of the Aorta
Resuscitative endovascular balloon occlusion of the aorta (REBOA) is a minimally invasive technique to control noncompressible hemorrhage. Although initially developed for the management of traumatic hemorrhage, REBOA has been adopted for the control of nontraumatic hemorrhage. REBOA for temporizing obstetric hemorrhage has been successful at decreasing blood loss and salvaging mothers in extremis from uterine rupture, placental abruption, and uncontrolled hemorrhage during cesarean hysterectomy for PAS. When used prophylactically before high-risk obstetric surgery, REBOA reduces blood loss, improves maternal outcomes, and decreases rates of hysterectomy compared with traditional techniques of uterine balloon tamponade and hypogastric or uterine artery occlusion. In cases of emergent obstetric hemorrhage, REBOA use has demonstrated lower transfusion volumes than other occlusion techniques, including internal iliac artery ligation, uterine artery ligation, or transvaginal intrauterine balloon occlusion.[66] This may be because REBOA insertion, positioning, and inflation can be completed in approximately 2 to 3 minutes by a trained provider, which is particularly helpful when placental blood loss approaches 700 mL/min. Furthermore, the current wireless catheters (ER-REBOA Plus and P-REBOA-Pro, Prytime Medical, Boerne, TX; Cobra-OS, Frontline Medical Technologies, London, Ontario, Canada) are modified to allow placement without fluoroscopy, which leads to little or no fetal radiation exposure.

Positioning a REBOA catheter in a pregnant patient may not be straightforward. Catheter measurements based on anatomic landmarks can serve as a basis for positioning of the balloon within the aorta; however, the effect of a gravid abdomen on the accuracy of these external landmarks has not been established. Placement based on catheter length has now supplanted measurements of external anatomic landmarks. Anatomic studies demonstrate that inserting the balloon 46 cm from the insertion site achieves a zone 1 (supraceliac) position in 99% of the population, and zone 3, the infrarenal aorta, is reached at 28 cm for 95% of the population. These population-based studies have been validated across the United States and Europe and hold true during pregnancy. Length markings have been incorporated on some of the newer catheters including the ER-REBOA plus and the P-REBOA-Pro (Prytime Medical).

Other methods of placement have been reported for pregnant patients undergoing REBOA. If preoperative imaging is available, target distances can be measured in advance. If the abdomen is open, the balloon may be palpated within the aorta. Image-guided placement can be used when time allows. Confirming catheter position with an x-ray is quick and easy and limits radiation exposure to the fetus compared with the use of fluoroscopy. Recently, modification of balloon positioning within the intrarenal aorta distal to the inferior mesenteric artery has been shown to further reduce blood lost from collateral circulation (Fig. 28.4).[67] This position corresponded accurately to localization of balloon markers at the level of the L2 vertebra on x-ray. Fluoroscopy-guided

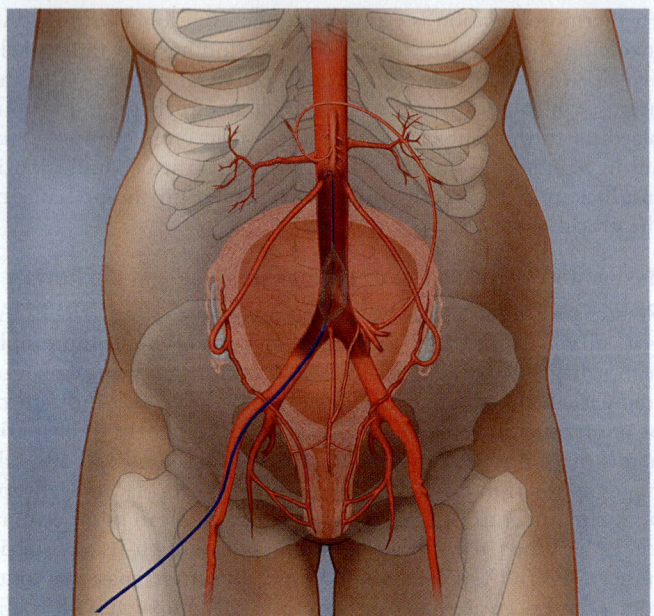

FIGURE 28.4 Blood supply to the gravid uterus is robust with numerous collaterals. Positioning of resuscitative endovascular balloon occlusion of the aorta (REBOA) distal to the inferior mesenteric artery (zone 3B) optimally occludes pelvic collaterals. This position can be achieved without fluoroscopy by aligning the radiopaque markers on the ER-REBOA or P-REBOA-Pro (Prytime Medical Devices, Inc; Boerne, TX) over the second lumbar vertebra on x-ray. Alternatively, infrarenal positioning (zone 3A) can be achieved without image guidance by inserting the catheter to 28 cm, which will also provide a significant reduction in pelvic bleeding.

balloon occlusion is a well-described technique in the obstetric population and is thought to pose little risk to the fetus from the short duration of radiation exposure.[68] Any of these positioning methods can be performed in a standard operating room with a standard table. Intraoperatively, the catheter can be inflated, deflated, and repositioned as needed throughout the case without needing to move the patient or obtain additional imaging if attention is paid to correlating catheter markings with anatomic measurements at the initial placement. REBOA requires a dedicated provider to secure against catheter migration, manage inflation and deflation, and faithfully monitor the ipsilateral lower extremity for ischemia.

The risks and limitations of REBOA for obstetric hemorrhage are still being described, and the relative incidence of each is not yet known. The majority of data published on this topic describes the application of REBOA in the trauma population that consists largely of male patients with concomitant hemorrhagic shock. Potential complications from REBOA include those related to arterial access, balloon positioning and inflation, and the physiologic changes that result from inflation and deflation of the device. From the trauma literature, access site complications are similar to those encountered during other forms of arterial puncture, but may be severe, including limb ischemia requiring amputation. Balloon malposition into an aortic branch vessel or migration into a higher or lower position within the aorta has also been described, sometimes resulting in uncontrolled arterial rupture and death.[69]

Complete occlusion of the supraceliac (zone 1) aorta for more than 30 minutes is not advised because of the increased ischemic burden conferred by occluding blood flow in the abdominal viscera and the increased aortic afterload conferred by more proximal occlusion. Infrarenal (zone 3) aortic occlusion is better tolerated for longer periods with fewer complications and has been shown to improve survival in trauma patients.[70] The incidence of these complications in the obstetric population, in whom zone 3 occlusion is preferred almost exclusively, is low. International studies from Japan and Europe indicate planned obstetric surgeries in which REBOA is used as an adjunct to reduce operative blood loss is quite safe, whereas REBOA placed emergently for a parturient in extremis carries a higher risk of access site complications, thrombosis, and arterial dissection.[71,72]

As might be expected with a small femoral vessel diameter and increased thrombogenicity in the pregnant female, the most common complication is nonocclusive arterial thrombosis at the sheath site. It would therefore be important to select the smallest sheath that will accommodate the available REBOA catheter and have a low threshold for postprocedural arteriography. Low-profile, 7-Fr common femoral arterial sheaths placed with ultrasound guidance have fewer access site complications than larger 12-Fr sheaths. Additionally, distal thrombosis is rare with 7-Fr sheaths, and limb ischemia requiring amputation has not been reported. Frequent monitoring of distal pulses in the ipsilateral extremity should be maintained after reperfusion and for 24 hours after sheath removal. Continuous Doppler may be a helpful adjunct to aid in early detection of arterial access complications.

The robust collateral circulation that exists in the gravid uterus, particularly in the case of PAS, may lead to incomplete hemorrhage control from aortic occlusion alone. Retrograde flow and venous hemorrhage may result in liters of additional blood loss despite aortic occlusion; thus, additional adjuncts to hemorrhage control may be necessary. The potential for severe complications exists, and providers performing the procedure should be aware of these risks to improve patient management and the informed consent process. Risks of REBOA use can be reduced with multidisciplinary expertise, proper training, and adherence to good techniques.

Intrauterine Balloon Tamponade

Emergency surgeons may be called upon to support obstetricians in the event of uncontrolled postpartum hemorrhage. The most common cause of massive hemorrhage after delivery is uterine atony; up to 80% of the cases result from suboptimal contraction of the myometrium after placental separation. Other etiologies may include retained placenta, uterine rupture, pubic trauma, uterine inversion, and coagulopathy. The management of acute postpartum hemorrhage refractory to medical management may require invasive therapies already described, including arterial ligation, occlusion or embolization, uterine suture compression, or, ultimately, hysterectomy. These interventions are highly invasive and resource intense. Intrauterine balloon tamponade has gained popularity as a minimally invasive adjunct with similar efficacy and less morbidity. Several balloon types have been used effectively, including Bakri balloon, balloon tamponade catheter, Foley catheters, Rusch balloon, condom catheters, and the Sengstaken-Blakemore tube. The American College of Obstetricians and Gynecologists specifically recommended the Bakri postpartum balloon for its specially tailored design that enables nonoperative management of uterine bleeding in cases of uterine atony and other causes of postpartum hemorrhage.[73] The Bakri balloon has proven an effective means of controlling postpartum hemorrhage, with success rates ranging from 57% after cesarean section to 100% after vaginal delivery.[74]

Adjuncts for Major Hemorrhage

Cell Salvage

Cell salvage has become an important component of operative hemorrhage management for high-risk patients. However, there are important limitations of cell salvage to consider when it comes to the pregnant patient. Cell salvage can only use blood collected into the canister, must have a minimum of 500 mL of blood before the cells can be washed, and returns at most 50% of the washed blood volume back to the patient. This technique does not allow for easy collection of vaginal blood loss and therefore has limited utility in many obstetric hemorrhage cases. Intermixing of fetal blood, amniotic fluid, or bacteria with salvaged blood is a contraindication to autologous transfusion. However, safe use of the cell-saver has been demonstrated in obstetric patients, particularly when no future pregnancy is planned. The presence of leukocyte depletion filters and cell washing may reduce the presence of these contaminants and produce a product similar to maternal blood, with the exception of not fully eliminating fetal hemoglobin. Anti-D immune globulin, also known as *RhoGAM,* is used to prevent isoimmunization and should be administered to any Rh-negative mother who receives cell salvage blood that may contain fetal hemoglobin from an Rh-positive infant. Support for the use of cell salvage in obstetric hemorrhage is now provided by 1100 published cases in which blood contaminated with amniotic fluid has been washed and readministered without complication.[75]

Damage Control Techniques

Once surgical hemostasis has been maximized, damage control techniques such as packing and temporary abdominal closure may be useful in cases of disseminated intravascular coagulation. Damage control surgery in the pregnant patient mirrors the principles and management strategies used in the nonpregnant patient. Avoiding excessive manipulation of the uterus when placing packs and temporary abdominal closures can reduce the impact on the fetus. Delayed abdominal closure may lead to intraabdominal hypertension. Additional fetal monitoring may be necessary during closure attempts to detect signs of fetal distress that may result from increased intraabdominal pressure. Cesarean section may be considered when clinically appropriate for maternal or fetal indications.

PREGNANCY AFTER MAJOR ABDOMINAL SURGERY

Not infrequently, the surgeon will be asked about pregnancy after treatment of surgical disease. Each case should be individualized. The conditions can be divided into those involving benign disease and those involving malignant disease.

BENIGN DISEASES

After most abdominal procedures for benign disease, there is no contraindication for pregnancy. Special circumstances include bariatric surgery and total colectomy with ileal pouch–anal anastomosis.

Bariatric Surgery

Bariatric surgery is rapidly becoming one of the most common procedures done in the United States. With approximately 160,000 females undergoing weight loss surgery in 2009, pregnancy after bariatric surgery is a common occurrence. There is an improvement in fertility and pregnancy outcomes after weight loss surgery.[76] There is also a decreased incidence of maternal complications in patients who have undergone bariatric surgery, particularly complications related to diabetes mellitus, hypertensive disorders, and fetal macrosomia, as compared with their morbidly obese counterparts. Currently, the consensus of studies supports a delay in planned pregnancy for up to 2 years after bariatric surgery. Outcomes in maternal or fetal health do not differ whether a patient has had a Roux-en-Y gastric bypass or restrictive procedure (e.g., verticalbanded gastroplasty, laparoscopic adjustable gastric banding).[77] Current recommendations for females who become pregnant after bariatric surgery are to continue with a prenatal multivitamin, vitamin B_{12}, iron, and folate supplement. Protein supplementation may also be necessary for patients who have undergone malabsorptive operations. For patients who have undergone adjustable gastric band placement, deflation of the band is recommended to aid in optimal nutrition.

Ileal Pouch–Anal Anastomosis

Ulcerative colitis can be a debilitating disease that might eventually require a total colectomy with an ileal pouch–anal anastomosis. Long-term outcomes of pregnancy after this procedure have been generally positive. In a study of 37 females who became pregnant before and after ileal pouch–anal anastomosis, there were no differences in birth weight, duration of labor, complications, and unplanned cesarean sections.[78] Another study comparing patients who underwent cesarean section versus vaginal delivery after ileal pouch–anal anastomosis has demonstrated that the vaginal delivery patients have a significant higher incidence of anterior sphincter defect (13% vs. 50%) and worse quality of life evaluated by the time tradeoff method.[79]

MALIGNANT DISEASE

This discussion will be limited to breast cancer because it is the most likely oncologic disease seen in females of reproductive age in comparison to many other oncologic diseases treated by the general surgeon or surgical oncologist that present at much older ages. Because of the age demographic, these patients will need advice on some unique areas including (1) maintenance of fertility, (2) the impact of pregnancy on disease treatment, (3) the timing of pregnancy relative to the diagnosis of breast cancer, and (4) pregnancy outcome.

Although breast cancer treatment often yields excellent outcomes, treatments can affect future reproductive options. Cytotoxic chemotherapy is used for many aggressive breast cancer subtype treatments, including triple-negative and HER2–positive breast cancers that are more common in premenopausal females, leading to treatment-related amenorrhea. Many patients regain menses after completion of treatment, but ultimately, the rate of premature ovarian insufficiency is thought to be approximately 30%.[80] At diagnosis of breast cancer in patients of reproductive age who are interested in having children after treatment, the surgeon or medical oncologist may consider referral to a reproductive endocrinologist to explore methods of fertility preservation. The best-established method of fertility preservation is embryo cryopreservation. This involves ovarian stimulation to retrieve oocytes for in vitro fertilization before freezing; this is still the best option for females with breast cancer whose risk of fertility may be compromised by adjuvant chemotherapy. However, little is known about the impact, if any, of ovarian stimulation on disease progression. Additionally, if situationally fertility preservation though a reproductive endocrinologist is not accessible, patients can consider ovarian suppression during treatment. This involves injections of a gonadotropin-releasing hormone (GnRH) agonist usually starting 1 to 2 weeks before chemotherapy and continues thought the treatment.

For patients with hormone receptor–positive breast cancer, endocrine therapy (tamoxifen) is of great importance for 5 to 10 years after initial therapy to decrease recurrence. However, endocrine therapy also necessitates a delay in pregnancy, as it is a teratogen. Among females with hormone receptor–positive breast cancers as well as all cancers, subsequent pregnancies have been considered to possibly increase breast cancer recurrence. As such, some recommend that patients wait at least 2 years from the time of diagnosis, but this is controversial. Partridge et al. looked at a temporary interruption of endocrine therapy for pregnancy after 18 to 30 months. They found that the 3-year incidence of a breast cancer event was no different from that of the control cohort.[81]

There is no evidence that pregnancy influences recurrence rate or survival in patients treated for breast cancer. This fact holds true for those who have had a mastectomy as well as those who have opted for breast-conserving therapy. The odds of survival was related to initial breast cancer stage and was not affected by hormonal receptor status or pregnancy.[35] Many premenopausal females wish to consider future pregnancy after treatment for their breast cancer, which currently is considered safe. The optimal timing of pregnancy varies with the treatment protocol and should occur after a reassessment for recurrent disease.

SUMMARY

Pregnant patients are susceptible to the same surgical diseases as nonpregnant patients of similar age. Maternal physiologic changes as well as the enlarging uterus may result in atypical presentation of surgical disease, or symptoms may be attributed to normal pregnancy. A delay in diagnosis and treatment of surgical illnesses in pregnancy poses a greater risk to maternal and fetal well-being than the risks of anesthesia or surgical intervention. Early consultation with an obstetrician, maternal-fetal medicine specialist, and perinatologist can ensure optimal outcomes and avoid pitfalls. Laparoscopy is becoming increasingly accepted in the pregnant patient, and future advances should make it even safer. Preterm labor prevention needs to be individualized, given the patient's gestational age and underlying disease process.

SELECTED REFERENCES

ACOG Committee Opinion No. 775: Nonobstetric surgery during pregnancy. *Obstet Gynecol.* 2019;133(4):e285-e286.

Reaffirmed in 2021, the American Congress of Obstetricians and Gynecologists' Committee on Obstetric Practice together with the American Society of Anesthesiologists published this updated opinion to guide clinical decision-making when nonobstetric surgery is required during pregnancy. Because there is limited evidence in the form of head-to-head randomized controlled trials, most guidance is based on expert consensus.

Bates SM, Greer IA, Middeldorp S, et al. VTE, thrombophilia, antithrombotic therapy, and pregnancy: antithrombotic therapy and prevention of thrombosis, 9th ed: American College of Chest Physicians Evidence-Based Clinical Practice Guidelines. *Chest.* 2012;141:e691S-e736S.

The use of anticoagulant therapy during pregnancy is challenging because of the potential for fetal and maternal complications. This guideline was developed as part of the Antithrombotic Therapy and Prevention of Thrombosis Guidelines 9th edition by the American College of Chest Physicians. It focuses on the management of venous thromboembolisms (VTEs) and thrombophilia as well as the use of anticoagulants during pregnancy.

Bookstaver, PB, Bland CM, Griffin B, et al. A review of antibiotic use in pregnancy. *Pharmacotherapy.* 2015;35(11):1052-1062.

Antibiotics account for the majority of medications prescribed to pregnant patients; however, few medications have sufficient safety data that are inclusive of parturients and their unborn children. This review outlines what is known and what remains unknown to help guide the use of antibiotics during pregnancy.

Pearl JP, Price RR, Tonkin AE, Richardson WS, Stefanidis D. *Guidelines for the Use of Laparoscopy During Pregnancy.* Society of American Gastrointestinal and Endoscopic Surgeons; 2022.

These are current guidelines for laparoscopy in pregnancy.

Stewart MK, Terhune KP. Management of pregnant patients undergoing general surgical procedures. *Surg Clin North Am.* 2015;95(2):429-442.

This 2015 article outlines diagnostic, physiologic, medication, and technical considerations for performing general surgical procedures on pregnant females. In 2023 it was highlighted as a key review for the practice of comprehensive general surgery by the American Board of Surgery.

The full reference list appears on Elsevier eBooks+.

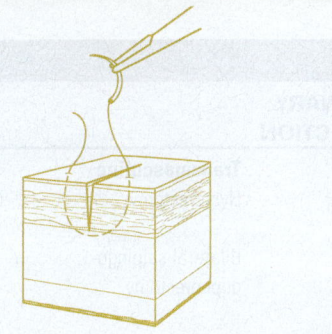

CHAPTER 29

Surgical Considerations in the Transgender Patient

Uriel Sanchez-Rangel, Rachel Bluebond-Langner, and Devin O'Brien Coon

INTRODUCTION

Although gender-affirming surgery has garnered increased attention in recent years, this branch of surgery is not new. The earliest documented case of an individual undergoing genital masculinization for the purpose of gender affirmation may be attributed to Lawrence Michael Dillon, a British physician who underwent a series of phalloplasty surgeries performed by Sir Harold Gillies in 1946.[1] The origins of facial gender-affirming surgery can be attributed to Douglas Ousterhout's anatomic distinction between the skeletal architecture of the forehead in males and females, which took place in 1987.[1] Dr. Ousterhout developed the surgical feminization of the forehead, formulated through an extensive investigation of numerous skulls obtained from the University of the Pacific School of Dentistry in San Francisco.[2] However, despite the historical nature of these developments, significant research, clinical, and societal attention has only recently been devoted to gender-affirming treatments. This chapter is meant to serve as an overview of the care of transgender patients and introduction to the breadth of gender-affirming procedures (Table 29.1).

Transgender identity encompasses a diverse group of individuals whose gender does not align with the sex they were assigned at birth.[3] Within this community, there is a wide range of gender identities and expressions. Some individuals identify within the traditional male-female binary and use terms like *trans man* or *trans woman* to reflect a gender identity opposite of

TABLE 29.1   Overview of Gender-Affirming Procedures[a]

FACIAL RECONSTRUCTION		CHEST RECONSTRUCTION		GENITO-URINARY RECONSTRUCTION	
Transfeminine	Transmasculine	Transfeminine	Transmasculine	Transfeminine	Transmasculine
Hairline Advancement	Rhinoplasty	Implant Based	Mastectomy: Periareolar	Orchiectomy Penectomy	Hysterectomy
Brow lift	Genioplasty	Breast augmentation	Mastectomy: Infra-areolar	Inversion	Bilateral salpingo- oophorectomy
	Jaw augmentation	Lipofilling		Vaginoplasty	
	Forehead/orbital augmentation	Procedures			
Frontonasal-orbital Contouring			Mastectomy: Double incision with free nipple grafts	Minimal depth Vaginoplasty	Metoidioplasty
Fat grafting/malar implant placement				Sigmoid intestinal Vaginoplasty	Phalloplasty: Radial forearm free flap
Zygomatic				Vulvoplasty	Phalloplasty:
Osteotomies				Clitoroplasty	Anterior lateral thigh free flap
Rhinoplasty					
Mandibular contouring					
Genioplasty					
Laryngoplasty					
Phonosurgery					

[a]Gender-affirming procedures are a broad range of surgical interventions. These are summarized here according to feminine and masculine genital reconstruction surgery, chest surgery, and facial surgery. The specific procedures available and their suitability depend on individual goals and anatomy. Not listed are the broad range of nonsurgical interventions to include hair removal or transplantation, voice training, and medical tattooing.

their assigned sex, whereas others identify outside binary notions of gender.

It is important to note that most transgender patients seen by surgical providers will be presenting for medical concerns *unrelated* to the treatment of gender dysphoria. These patients are often worried about the stigma and challenges of being identified as transgender.[4] Similarly, they are often concerned that excess focus is placed on their gender-affirming interventions (e.g., relating symptoms to effects of hormone therapy) at the expense of typical diagnostic approaches and considerations.

The clash between one's self-identity and society's perception can have profound effects on overall well-being, potentially leading to psychological distress. According to the *Diagnostic and Statistical Manual of Mental Disorders, Fifth Edition* (DSM-5), this persistent psychological and emotional distress is known as *gender incongruence* or *dysphoria*.[5] Gender dysphoria is diagnosed in 2 to 3 out of every 1000 individuals assigned female at birth and 5 to 14 out of every 1000 individuals assigned male at birth.[6] Recent studies indicate that these numbers may be underestimated.[6] Regardless of prevalence, it is important to note that the severity of dysphoria can vary greatly. *Gender incongruence* is a more recent term that attempts to acknowledge that some individuals may have a discrepancy between body and psychological gender that they seek to change without experiencing distress per se.[7,8] This highlights the need for personalized treatment decisions and avoiding tendencies to center all of a patient's care around their gender identity.

Ideally, a team of mental health professionals, endocrinologists, surgeons, and medical specialists conducts a thorough evaluation and provides multidisciplinary support for people who are experiencing gender dysphoria. Before initiating surgical interventions, a mental health or medical professional with expertise in working with transgender patients and diagnosing gender dysphoria typically completes a psychosocial assessment.[7] This assessment considers the potential presence of medical or mental health comorbidities and determines readiness and suitability for treatment. Although

many transgender people seeking to align their identities during the transition process choose not to pursue surgical intervention, demand for such procedures has been steadily rising nationwide.[9]

Gender-affirming surgeries encompass a variety of surgical procedures designed to modify bodily features, with the goal of reducing gender incongruence and alleviating dysphoria (see Table 29.1). Because of the well-organized and often well-informed nature of this patient community, colloquial terminology is commonly adopted by healthcare providers for the sake of effective communication. *Bottom surgery* includes procedures such as phalloplasty, metoidioplasty, and vaginoplasty. Conversely, *top surgery* refers to gender-affirming procedures that aim to masculinize or feminize the chest, including mastectomy or breast augmentation.[3]

WORLD PROFESSIONAL ASSOCIATION FOR TRANSGENDER HEALTH STANDARDS AND INSURANCE COVERAGE

The World Professional Association for Transgender Health (WPATH) has developed a set of clinical guidelines known as the *Standards of Care (SOC)* that aim to provide healthcare professionals with evidence-based summaries to aid with decisions in gender-affirming care.[9] SOC 7, published in 2012, was a key reference for private and government insurance providers.[10] It suggested that patients meet SOC criteria in order to be good candidates for gender-affirming surgeries and stipulated that two letters of referral from qualified mental health professionals were necessary before undergoing genital surgeries.[10] Key court decisions relating to Section 1557 of the Affordable Care Act were significant milestones in legislation to forbid gender-based discrimination in healthcare coverage and greatly expanded access to gender-affirming surgeries in the 2013–15 period, allowing a large pool of preexisting patients who had long been financially unable to obtain surgery to access it for the first time.[11]

The eighth version of the SOC from 2022 changed criteria for genital gender-affirming surgeries, including the elimination of the requirement to spend 12 consecutive months in the identified gender, reducing the hormone treatment duration required, and proposing one mental health evaluation instead of two. This revision proposed expansion of the pool of evaluating professionals beyond solely mental health experts, acknowledging that a large amount of transgender care is delivered by primary care specialists with extensive experience in this population.[7] It is crucial to note that the SOC functions only as a reference point. Ultimately, it is the surgeon's prerogative to use professional discretion in assessing whether a patient is an appropriate candidate for surgery.

HORMONE THERAPY: WOUND HEALING, HYPERCOAGULABILITY RISK, AND ERYTHROCYTOSIS

In the period surrounding surgery, there has traditionally been caution in administering gender-affirming hormone therapy (GAHT) because of concerns about the occurrence of venous thromboembolism (VTE) (with estrogen) or the potential risks of hematoma or thrombocytosis-induced thrombosis (with testosterone supplementation).[12] The skin has been shown to be a steroidogenic tissue containing the full cytochrome P450 system required for the de novo production of sex steroids, and bioactive hormones may play a role in surgical healing.[12]

ESTROGEN

Estradiol (E2) is the primary hormone used in gender-affirming therapy for direct feminizing effects. E2 can be administered orally, intramuscularly, or transdermally. It promotes breast growth and fat redistribution but does not intrinsically suppress testosterone levels, so it is often paired with an androgen blocker (e.g., spironolactone), which helps suppress testosterone's secondary sex characteristics.[13]

E2 has been well studied from postmenopausal hormone replacement and oral contraceptives. Exogenous estrogen has potential prothrombotic effects and an increased risk of thromboembolic disease. The route of E2 administration affects the degree of risk, with transdermal administration being associated with a lower risk compared with oral administration due to first-pass effects.[12] Regarding transfeminine individuals, studies have shown an increased risk of arterial and venous thrombosis compared with cisgender women. Some data found a significantly higher risk of myocardial infarction and stroke.[14] There is a higher prevalence of VTE significantly associated with older age and a longer length of E2 therapy. However, it is important to note that estrogen management used in gender-affirming therapy has changed, with the use of E2 and transdermal administration resulting in much lower thrombosis rates compared with previous studies that involved ethinyl E2.[14]

Estrogen is a steroidal hormone that plays a key role in numerous physiologic processes and functions, including wound healing. Exogenous estrogen has been shown to be able to reverse delayed cutaneous healing in postmenopausal women.[14] Estrogen stops skin from thinning by modifying keratinocyte function, increasing the skin's ability to hold water, increasing sebum production, and increasing the number of properly aligned elastin fibers. Similarly, estrogen may accelerate the healing process by reducing inflammation, accelerating reepithelialization and granulation, and improving keratinocyte proteinolysis efficiency.[15]

Within this context, management of patients on E2 therapy before gender-affirming surgery is still debated, and there is no consensus on whether E2 should be halted or for how long before surgery. However, the risk of thrombosis with gender-affirming surgery is generally low. E2 cessation is also not without negatives: Patients can experience cessation effects with similarities to perimenopausal symptoms—potentially including sweating, hot flashes, and labile emotions—and often report it to be a psychologically distressing experience. As a result, continuing E2 therapy through surgery has become more popular recently, in some cases using reduced doses and coupled with appropriate thrombosis prophylaxis based on risk assessment.[16]

TESTOSTERONE

Gender-affirming therapy for transmasculine individuals aims to halt menses and induce masculine effects like fat redistribution and body hair growth. Testosterone levels are typically monitored to ensure they are within the normal range for cisgender men. Unlike E2, testosterone suppresses luteinizing hormone (LH) and follicle-stimulating hormone (FSH) secretion, and therefore, an estrogen blocker is generally not required to reduce E2 levels. Testosterone therapy does not consistently elevate the risk of arterial disease and may even be protective for those with existing heart conditions.[17] Venous thrombosis risk also does not appear to be increased.[18] Exogenous testosterone elevates hematocrit and can enhance iron absorption. Monitoring cardiovascular risk factors and blood cell counts is important because of the potential development of erythrocytosis over time.[19] Extreme erythrocytosis is rare, and dose adjustments can decrease hematocrit levels.

In the surgical context, increased testosterone levels are associated with delayed wound healing in elderly males, and blocking androgen receptors has been demonstrated in animal studies to accelerate wound healing.[20] However, the role of testosterone in wound repair is complex; variability exists by type of wound and the concentration of testosterone. In rodent models, surgical, pharmacologic, and genetic approaches targeting androgen actions in the skin have shown that androgens increase interleukin-6 and tumor necrosis factor production and reduce wound reepithelialization and matrix deposition, delaying cutaneous wound healing.[21] However, in major burn injuries, which trigger not only local wound-healing processes but also systemic hyperinflammation, a synthetic androgen (oxandrolone) has been shown to increase protein synthesis, improve lean body mass, and shorten the length of hospital stay in burn injuries.[22] As such, androgens appear to play a complex role in wound repair, but the biologic effects are still being elucidated.

Similar to E2, testosterone cessation can induce negative psychological effects. Management of perioperative testosterone is thus a balancing decision made in conjunction between the surgeon and patient. Factors such as the patient's overall health, age, and specific surgical needs should be taken into consideration when determining management of testosterone therapy.

FACIAL SURGERY

Facial appearance plays a dominant role in conveying gender. Sexually dimorphic facial properties can be categorized as primary/structural (i.e., the bony skeleton) or secondary/nonstructural. Testosterone enables irreversible growth of facial structures (e.g., the frontal sinus) during puberty. Because this growth cannot be reversed through medical interventions, primary sex characteristics are typically treated through surgery. Conversely, hormone therapy is a more successful strategy for changing nonstructural sexual traits. Exogenous hormone therapy is particularly important in changing a variety of facial factors, including hair density, facial hair, skin texture, and the amount and distribution of facial fat.[23,24]

It is ideal to start hormone therapy at least 12 months before having surgery so the soft tissue envelope is stable at the time of surgery. Skeletal contouring procedures, such as forehead, mandible, zygoma, and major rhinoplasty, should be performed before any soft tissue or skin tightening procedures (e.g., lip lift, face/neck lift, midface lift, blepharoplasty, and fat grafting) to facilitate the readaptation of soft tissue to the new bone surface, as postsurgical contraction alone generates adequate tightening for some patients.[25]

ANATOMY

Among the key gender-defining areas, the forehead, brow, and frontonasal-orbital complex are particularly important. In terms of structural differences, the craniomaxillofacial skeletal and soft tissue envelopes in males tend to be larger compared with females. Male individuals typically exhibit frontal bossing, prominent supraorbital ridges, lower eyebrows, an M-shaped hairline, and male pattern baldness. On the other hand, female individuals often have a more obtuse nasofrontal angle, a gradual curve of the frontal bone, arched eyebrows, and a round or ovoid hairline.[24]

In the middle third of the face, males tend to have a wider bizygomatic distance and greater malar bone volume. In contrast, females exhibit a greater concentration of malar fat, resulting in prominent and round feminine cheeks. Differences in nasal characteristics are also apparent. Females typically have a slightly lower radix, a narrower nasal width, curved dorsal aesthetic lines, less projection, greater cephalic tip rotation, a wider nasolabial angle, a narrower alar base, and a shorter upper lip.[24]

In the lower third of the face, males often have a squarer jaw and a more acute gonial angle. In comparison, females tend to display a more trapezoidal jaw shape and softer chin features. It is worth noting that the laryngeal prominence, commonly referred to as the *Adam's apple,* is a testosterone-sensitive structure that enlarges during puberty and does not respond to cross-gender hormones.[24,25]

UPPER THIRD

Frontonasal-Orbital Contouring

Most surgeons use osteotomies and setback of the frontal sinuses, along with frontonasal-orbital complex burring, to feminize the forehead and brow. This approach allows for proper modification of the nasoglabellar transition, ensuring harmonious facial proportions and a natural appearance. Isolated burring without setback increases the risk of perforating the anterior table and does not provide adequate nasoglabellar transition modification. Forehead feminization surgery is a safe and effective procedure, accompanied by a low complication rate. However, complications such as alopecia, bone malunion, infection, and cerebrospinal fluid (CSF) rhinorrhea can occur.[26]

Brow Lift and Hairline-Redefining

Simultaneous brow lifts and hairline-redefining procedures are commonly used in conjunction with burring and set-back procedures. Careful consideration of the hairline format, height, and density is crucial for achieving optimal results. Centers differ in their thresholds

for using a coronal approach with hair transplantation versus a pretrichial approach with hairline lowering. Factors such as patient preference and the potential need for future hair transplantation need to be considered when deciding on the most suitable approach.

Middle Third

In the midface, various procedures, including fat grafting, malar onlay implants, and zygomatic osteotomies, are commonly employed. The evaluation of the midface presents challenges due to limited data on dimorphic malar structure in humans. This limitation hinders the use of absolute measurements within the craniofacial skeleton as a guide for surgical management. Nevertheless, in the context of facial gender surgery (FGS), the overarching goal of malar alteration is to achieve round and well-projected cheeks with subtle lateral prominence. It is vital that the modified cheeks appear natural when compared with the projection of the forehead as well as the bitemporal and bigonial widths. Achieving harmonious facial proportions while maintaining a feminine aesthetic is paramount in midface procedures.[25-27]

Malar Implants

Malar hypoplasia in facial feminization surgery (FFS) patients can be effectively addressed using malar implants or fat grafting. The choice between these options depends on the severity and underlying cause of the hypoplasia. Different alloplastic materials like polyetheretherketone (PEEK), porous polyethylene (Medpor), and titanium implants offer contrasting advantages and disadvantages. Careful selection and consideration of these options are crucial to ensuring optimal malar projection outcomes.[28]

Zygomatic Osteotomies

Zygomatic osteotomies can be used to reduce excessive bizygomatic width in FFS patients. These osteotomies can alter the position and projection of the malar area by rotating, translating, or reducing the mobilized zygomatic segment (Fig. 29.1). An L-shaped osteotomy, extending from the medial edge of the zygoma to the inferior orbital rim and out diagonally to the junction of the lateral orbital rim and zygoma, is commonly employed.[28] Precise planning with patient-specific cutting and drill guides created through computer-aided design/computer-aided manufacturing (CAD/CAM) and virtual surgical planning (VSP) technology can be used to improve the accuracy and predictability of zygomatic osteotomies.[29] Accurate diagnosis of midface deformities is important. For instance, performing malar augmentation to hide a wide face can result in an unbalanced appearance and a top-heavy look. Jaw feminization and reducing the lower third width can worsen this problem, as discussed later. Complications of zygomatic osteotomies include asymmetry, nonunion or malunion, and facial nerve injury.[29,30]

Autologous Fat Grafting

Autologous fat grafting is a versatile technique used in most FFS cases to soften masculine regions. Fat can be harvested from various donor sites, and the harvested fat is transferred to the malar region.[28,29]

Rhinoplasty

Feminizing rhinoplasty aims to create a more feminine appearance by altering the size and shape of the nose. Although the techniques used in feminization rhinoplasty are not fundamentally different

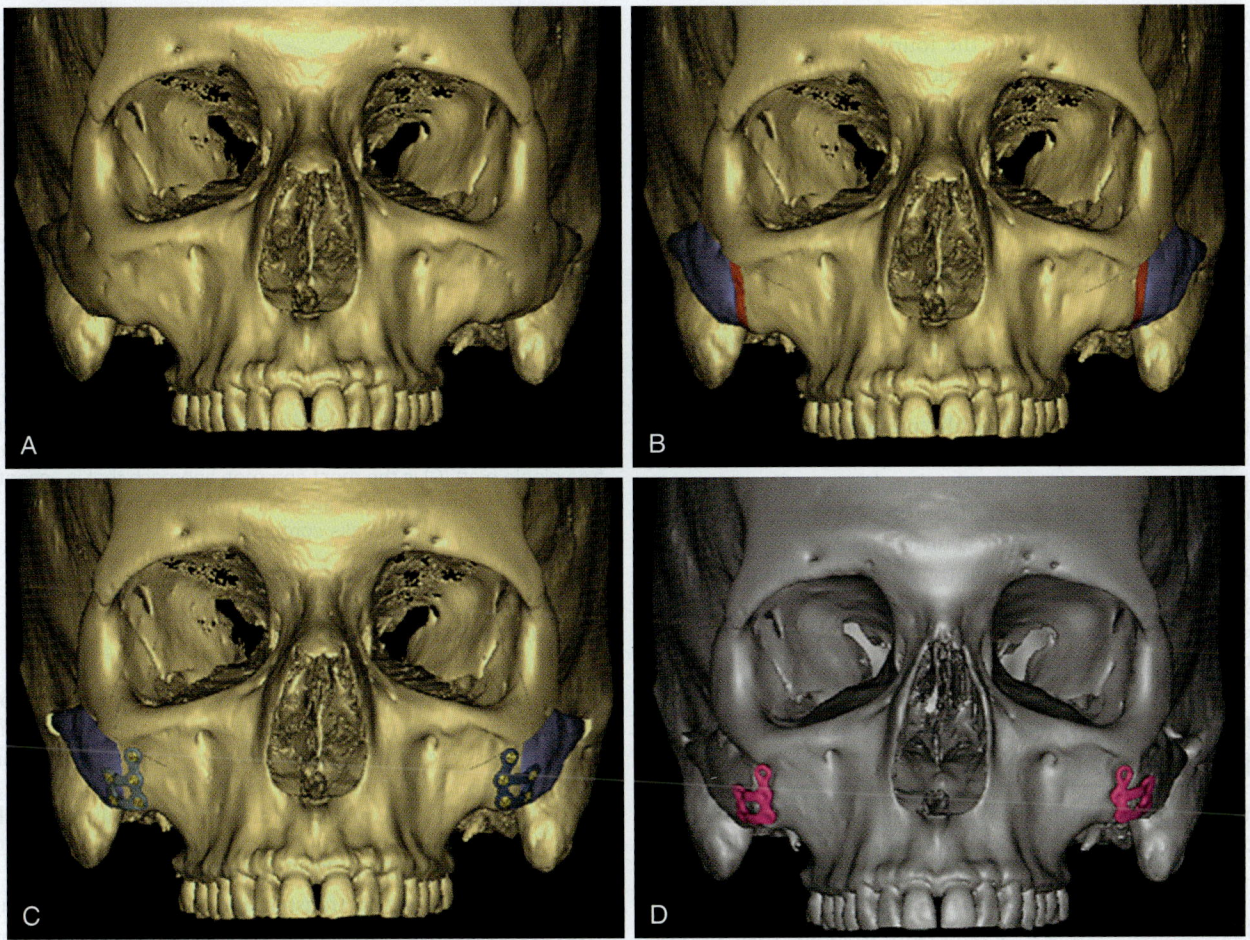

FIGURE 29.1 Zygomatic osteotomies can be used to achieve feminization of the midface and reduction of bi-zygomatic width by rotating or translating the malar bone. Computer-aided design is used to create custom guides and plates to improve accuracy. (A) Preoperative 3D CT reconstruction; (B) planned resection of bone *(red)* and zygomatic movement *(blue)*; (C) planned final result; (D) actual postoperative result on 3D CT reconstruction.

compared with those in standard rhinoplasty, the manner and degree to which these techniques are applied to patients seeking facial gender confirmation surgery distinguishes it from traditional rhinoplasty.

Anatomy

The female nose has certain distinguishing features, including a wider nasofrontal angle, a lower radix (located just above the pupil), narrower nasal width, curved dorsal aesthetic lines, less projection, greater cephalic tip rotation, wider nasolabial angle, narrower alar base, and a shorter upper lip. These features contribute to the overall feminine appearance of the face. When performing rhinoplasty in the context of FGS, there are three goals to accomplish. First, a nose that appears feminine needs to be created with the previously described points. Second, harmony between the nose, forehead, and maxillomandibular complex should be maintained. Finally, an aesthetically pleasing result that accounts for individual differences such as ethnicity and age must be achieved.[31]

LOWER THIRD

Lower jaw recontouring in FGS involves techniques such as gonial angle reduction, mandibular body projection reduction, and

genioplasty. Gonial angle and body reduction can help achieve a more feminine trapezoidal shape. The chin also plays a role, with softer features and a narrow tapering being perceived as more feminine.[32] Cutting guides are often employed to ensure consistent results in difficult-to-visualize areas like the gonial angle.[33]

VOCAL CORDS

Addressing the voice is an important aspect of FGS. Speech therapy helps most patients achieve their desired goals. However, for those who do not, phonosurgery is highly successful in increasing the natural vocal pitch.[34] There are three main techniques: vocal cord shortening, increasing vocal cord tension, and reducing vocal cord mass. Vocal cord shortening yields the greatest increase in pitch. Vocal cord shortening procedures involve altering the vocal cords to create a new anterior commissure.[34]

CHEST RECONSTRUCTION: MASCULINIZATION

Chest contouring aims to create a male chest appearance in trans men. The procedure involves the removal of breast tissue, reduction in size, relocation of the nipple-areola complex (NAC), and potentially excision of excess skin. In creating a more male-appearing chest, one must consider the location and shape of the

NAC, which is generally smaller and more ovoid in males as well as being more lateral, located at the fourth or fifth rib over the pectoralis. Individual patient evaluation ideally factors in preoperative parameters such as breast volume, excess skin, and skin elasticity. The goal of the surgeon should be to contour to a flat chest with minimization of scars as well as optimal placement of scars. Many transmasculine patients may desire greater pectoral definition, or a "pectoral shadow," which may be achieved by proper inferiorly based placement of incisions and scars during the double incision technique described next.[35]

DIFFERENCES FROM GYNECOMASTIA TREATMENT

Chest contouring in trans men differs significantly from gynecomastia treatment. Trans men typically present with larger breast volume, excess skin, and ptosis when compared with individuals with gynecomastia. In some cases, the distribution of breast tissue may extend to the tail of Spence, requiring further excision and consideration of final contour.[36] Furthermore, the practice of breast binding, often employed by trans men to minimize chest visibility, can lead to increased skin elasticity. Consequently, reduction of the skin envelope through direct excision becomes necessary.[36]

DIFFERENCES FROM MASTECTOMY FOR CANCER PROPHYLAXIS OR TREATMENT

Chest surgery in trans men differs from a mastectomy performed for cancer prophylaxis or treatment. To mitigate contour deformities, relatively thick adipocutaneous flaps are used, requiring a distinct dissection plane. Given the potential technical difficulties in conducting mammography postoperatively, trans men should continue appropriate breast cancer screening based on their personal and familial risk factors.[37]

TECHNIQUES FOR CHEST CONTOURING IN TRANS MEN (FIG. 29.2)

Double-Incision Technique

The double-incision technique is appropriate for patients with significant breast parenchyma or skin necessitating excision. The name simply refers to the fact that there is a sizable incision on each side of the chest, unlike periareolar techniques. It involves a long inferior/midpole skin crescent excision that emulates the contour of the pectoralis major muscle. This technique provides maximum control over the skin envelope and nipple-areola positioning and is by far the most commonly used technique. However, it results in the most visible scarring, although effective camouflage along the pectoralis major can be achieved.[37]

Infraareolar Approach

This approach is suitable for patients with small breasts, acceptable skin elasticity, and expected postoperative skin contraction. It involves a semicircular infraareolar incision that preserves tissue just beneath the NAC, known colloquially to patients as the *keyhole*. Adjunct suction lipectomy may be employed to access peripheral parenchymal tissue. Skin excision is not performed, and there may be residual skin excess and wrinkling. Areolar position cannot be changed to a more masculine location.[36,37]

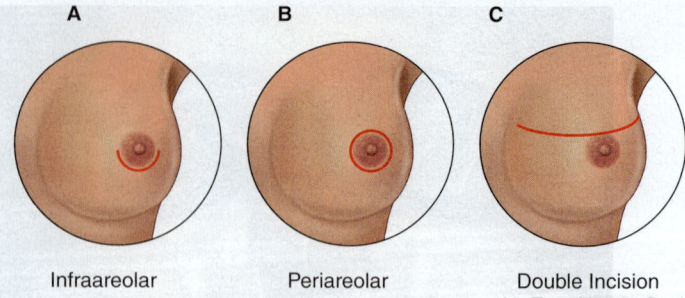

Infraareolar   Periareolar   Double Incision with Free Nipple Graft

FIGURE 29.2 Comparison of gender-affirming mastectomy incision designs. Infraareolar incisions (A) and periareolar (B) incisions are reserved for patients with a limited amount of breast tissue and high-quality skin elasticity. These incisions benefit from minimal scarring and preservation of nipple-areola complex sensation. Double incision with free nipple graft (C) is the most common approach that is acceptable for most breast sizes and has an easily hidden inferior scar that can be used to define the pectoralis contour.

Circumareolar Incision

Suitable for patients with excess skin and/or a large NAC, the circumareolar incision technique involves reducing the areolar and surrounding skin through a circumareolar incision. An inferior, full-thickness access incision is necessary to achieve the parenchymal reduction. Although the NAC can be repositioned, severe ptosis may not be adequately addressed using this approach.[36]

Chest Reconstruction: Feminization

Breast reconstruction in transfeminine patients shares similarities with breast reconstruction and augmentation in cisgender women. Successful outcomes require careful consideration of various factors, including the effects of feminizing hormones, chest wall anatomy, and incision choice.

ANATOMIC CONSIDERATIONS

Transfeminine patients commonly undergo hormone therapy to achieve feminization. Transdermal E2 is an effective hormone for enlarging breasts and increasing subcutaneous fat within the initial 2 years of administration.[16] However, the final size and shape of the breasts remain unpredictable. Some patients may choose to complement their hormone therapy with progesterone therapy to optimize breast development and achieve a more feminine appearance, though data on this are lacking. Tender breast buds typically form within 3 to 6 months of hormone therapy, with the maximum development of breast tissue reaching 18 to 24 months.[38] However, hormone therapy effects may vary among patients, resulting in inadequate breast development in some cases.

BREAST IMAGING AND SCREENING GUIDELINES

Transfeminine individuals should adhere to national breast cancer screening guidelines. For women aged 50 to 74, screening mammograms are typically recommended every other year. The American College of Radiology (ACR) suggests annual screening mammograms starting at age 40, including trans women. However, patients require screening modalities tailored to their specific characteristics, such as age, hormone use, surgical history, and genetic predisposition. Transfeminine individuals who are over 40 years old with at least 5 years of hormone use should undergo annual screening through digital breast tomosynthesis (DBT) or mammography.[39,62] Additionally, those aged 25 to 30 with higher-than-average risk factors and at least 5 years of hormone use should also receive annual screening.[39] Average-risk patients with no hormone use or fewer than 5 years of hormone use do not require breast imaging. Patients with silicone implants should undergo magnetic resonance imaging (MRI) surveillance 3 years after surgery and every 2 years thereafter.[39]

IMPLANT TYPES

In the past, textured implants were designed to reduce the risks of malposition and capsular contracture. However, because of concerns about breast implant–associated anaplastic large cell lymphoma (BIA-ALCL), the use of textured implants has declined.[38] Surgeons should engage in discussions with patients regarding choices between silicone and saline options. Saline implants can be inserted through smaller incisions and allow for easy detection of deflation. However, they are more prone to skin rippling. Silicone implants, on the other hand, require longer incisions but offer a more natural feel and are nearly always our preferred choice. Because of limited breast tissue and a wider chest in transfeminine patients, larger implants are frequently necessary. It is essential to inform patients about size limitations based on their specific anatomy and soft tissue coverage.[38]

TECHNIQUES FOR CHEST AUGMENTATION IN TRANS WOMEN

Although the administration of exogenous E2 typically leads to breast growth, it is typically constrained in its extent. Gender-affirming chest feminization is a surgical procedure that aims to treat the lack of breast tissue and the presence of masculine chest characteristics, such as a wider and longer chest wall, variations in fat distribution, and changes in NAC size and position. Males typically have small, lateralized nipples, hypertrophied pectoralis major muscles, wide sternums, and a shorter distance between the nipple and inframammary fold (IMF). Breast augmentation can stretch the skin and increase nipple size to some extent but may not fully feminize the appearance of the nipples. Achieving maximal cleavage while maintaining a centralized nipple position requires a delicate balance. However, overall, rates of complications are low and satisfaction is high.[38]

BOTTOM SURGERY

Phalloplasty

Phalloplasty's goal is to create an aesthetic-appearing penis but also to enable urination, provide sensory pleasure, support a prosthetic device, and withstand the physical demands of intercourse. Although there are numerous techniques for phalloplasty, the radial forearm free flap (RFF; Fig. 29.3) has been the historic gold standard and will be used as the primary example, though other donor sites (thigh, abdomen, back) are also viable. To determine the suitability of an RFF procedure, Allen's test is recommended. Donor site morbidity should be discussed preoperatively to aid in the decision-making process.[40]

Staging

Whereas early phalloplasty procedures involved multiple stages and random-pattern tube flaps, the RFF technique was originally performed as a combined procedure encompassing the creation of the phallus, perineal masculinization, vaginectomy, scrotoplasty, and clitoral burying. High complication rates led to the rise in popularity of "staged approaches," where the phalloplasty flap stage and the perineal/pelvic stage are performed separately. Currently, some centers use the "staged approach" (Fig. 29.4), with a perineal masculinization stage following the initial phalloplasty flap stage, whereas others prefer the "combined approach." However, even in the latter case, it is generally recognized that immediate glansplasty tends to flatten, leading combined-approach centers to include an additional smaller stage for glansplasty. Furthermore, testicular and penile prostheses are always placed in a separate stage once all components have sufficiently healed. Thus, the use of terms like *single-stage phalloplasty* is inaccurate and discouraged. Generally, the combined approach offers the advantage of avoiding an extra surgery but comes with the drawback of increased complexity, longer surgical time, and potentially more difficult complication management.[41]

Urologic Considerations

Among individuals undergoing phalloplasty, the majority express a desire for urethral lengthening (UL). Some patients may opt for "shaft-only phalloplasty" if standing micturition is not their priority to avoid potential complications or to preserve the vagina.[41]

UL involves two anatomic components: the creation of a neo-urethra within the phallus (the penile urethra or pars pendulans)

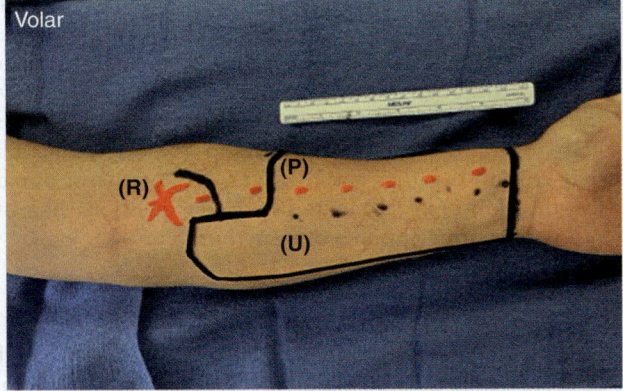
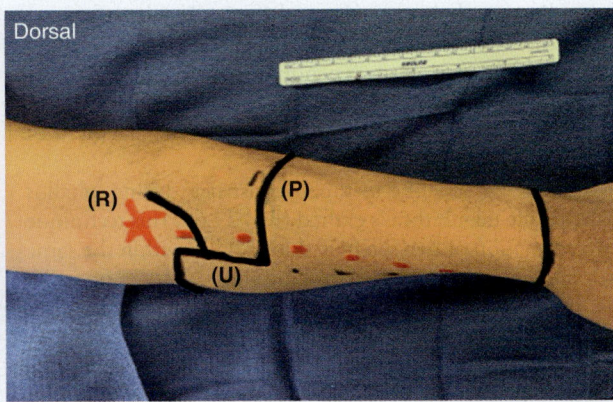

FIGURE 29.3 Markings for a radial forearm phalloplasty, indicating the penile area *(P)*, ulnar area *(U)*, and radial artery *(R)*.

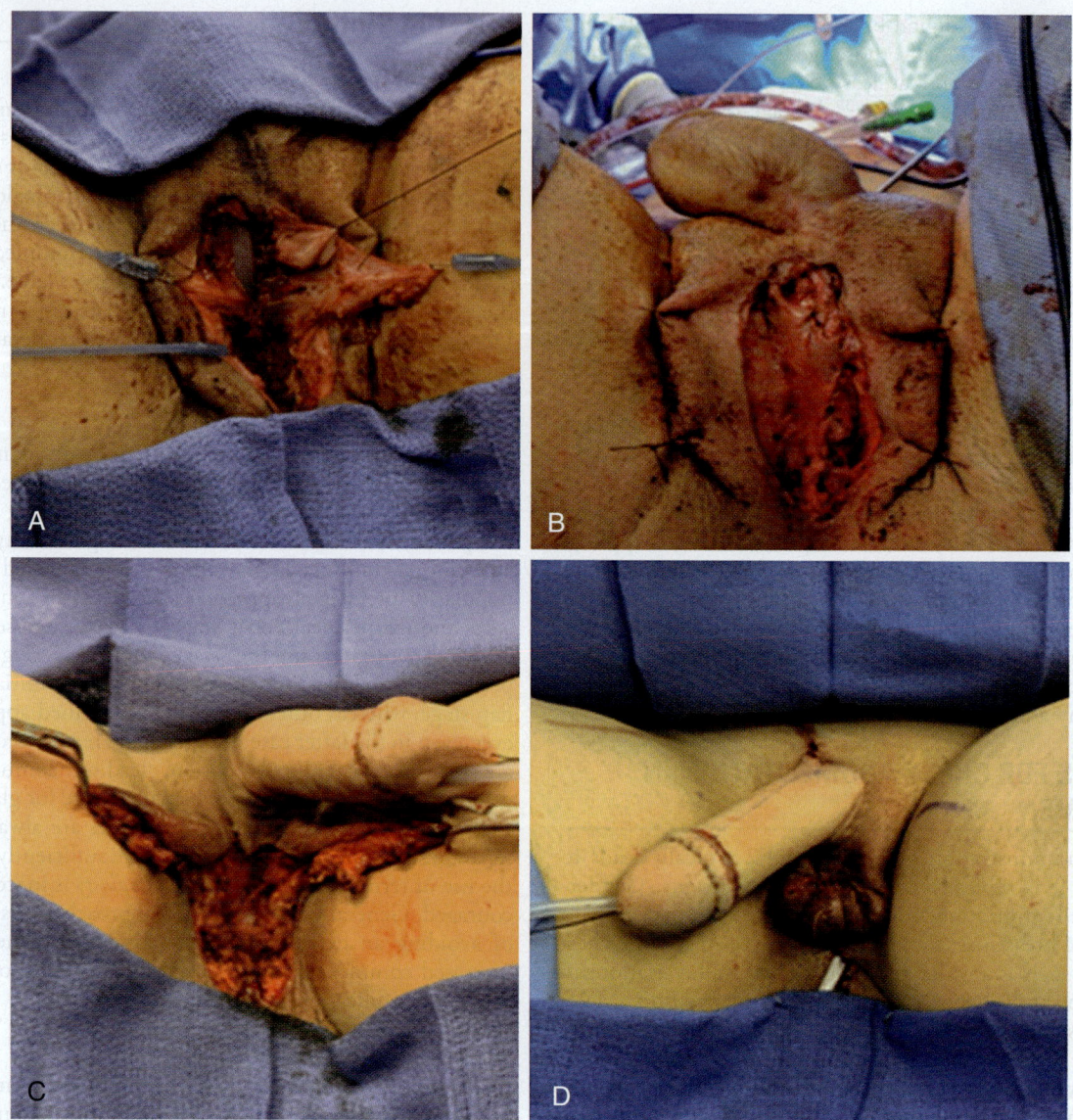

FIGURE 29.4 The perineal masculinization stage of phalloplasty typically includes glansplasty and scrotoplasty. As depicted in images A–D, the labia majora are reelevated and used to create a neoscrotum.

and the perineal urethra (pars fixa) that connects the natal urethra to the penile urethra (Fig. 29.5). Both urologic and plastic surgeons, depending on their expertise and institutional preference, may perform each step in the construction of the perineal urethra (pars fixa) and penile urethra (pars pendulans). Surgeons performing UL should possess experience and proficiency in cystoscopy, suprapubic (SP) tube placement, and the surgical management of urethral complications.[42]

When employing a "tube-in-tube" construct during phallus creation, the penile neourethra is crafted (Fig. 29.6). This technique involves the formation of two separate skin paddles within the same flap, which are then tubularized. By rolling the paddles in opposite directions, an inner tube (the pars pendulans urethra) and an outer tube (the penile skin) are created.

Composite Flaps

In cases where the tube-in-tube method is not feasible, two alternative approaches can be considered. The first involves using a composite flap, where the urethral tube and the outer skin tube are derived from separate donor sites. Although this technique adds complexity and has high complication rates, it remains a viable option for atypical cases.[41]

Another strategy involves using tissue grafts to create the penile urethra. Although various graft types have been employed, the most effective from the perspective of the senior author is a skin graft, as it offers the most reliable and practical results. However, it is crucial to gather more data on the long-term durability of lengthy skin graft segments to address questions like infection resistance during episodes of bacteriuria.[41]

Perineal Urethra

To create the pars fixa, flaps of vulvar mucosa and/or labia minora mucosa are tubularized, connecting the natal meatus to the constructed penile urethra. Traditionally, pedicled vaginectomy tissue flaps or labial ring flaps have been used for constructing the dorsal bulb portion of the perineal urethra. The tubularization process

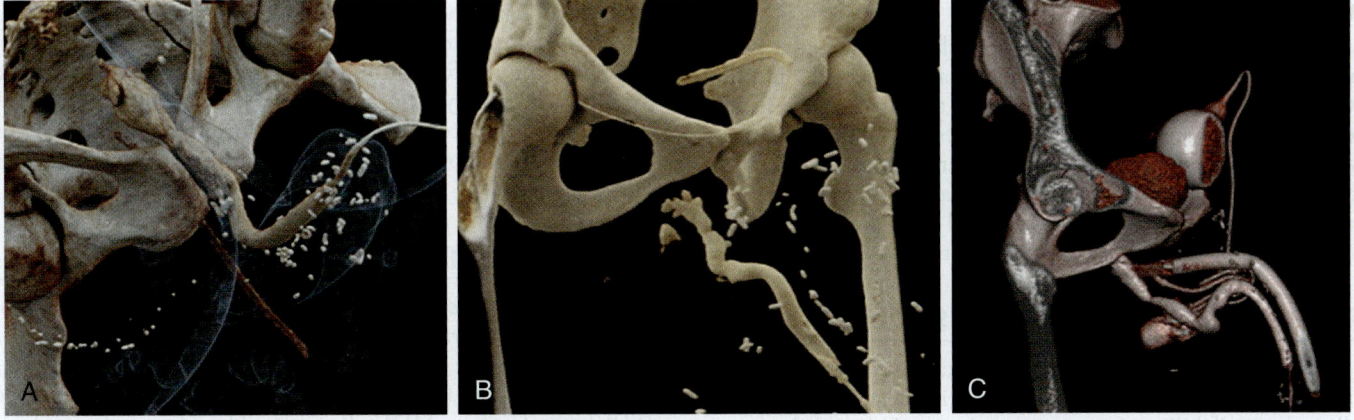

FIGURE 29.5 Additional procedures may be performed to provide functionality. These include urethral lengthening (A–B) to bring the neourethra into continuity and allow for urination while standing and penile implants (C) for penetrative intercourse.

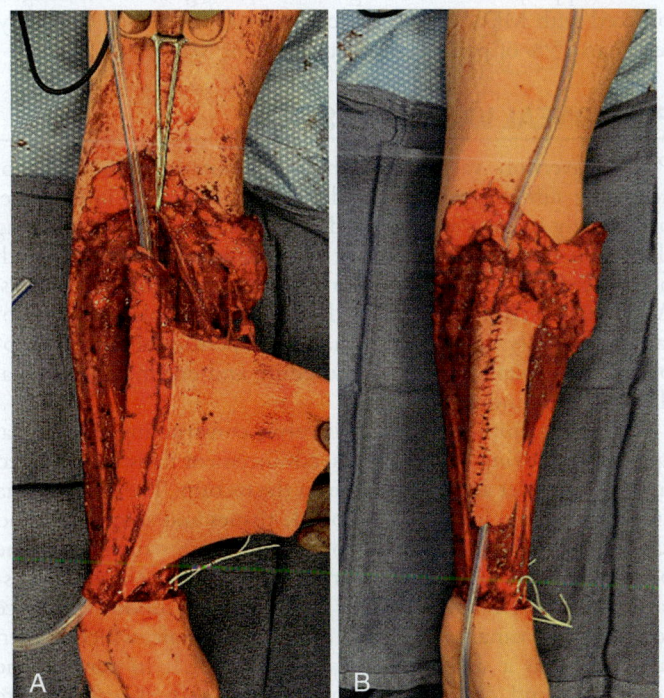

FIGURE 29.6 Creation of a neourethra by creating a tube-within-a-tube construct from the ulnar, neourethral, portion (A) of the radial forearm and the external radial portion encompassing this tube (B).

may vary depending on whether it is staged with the penile urethra or performed concurrently.[42]

Postprocedure Care

A penile Foley catheter is placed in the lengthened urethra, while a SP catheter is inserted to divert urine away from the repair site. After a period of 10 to 14 days, the penile Foley catheter is removed. At 2 to 4 weeks, a series of voiding trials commence with the SP catheter clamped. Retrograde urethrograms (RUGs) or low-dose 3D CT urethrogram protocols offer anatomic assessment to identify any postoperative issues.[43]

Gynecologic Considerations

Fertility preservation is an important consideration within gender-affirming surgery. There is a substantial impact on a patient's ability to conceive in the future when surgical interventions are undertaken to modify reproductive anatomy. Although it is customary to address the risk of infertility and explore fertility preservation options during the informed consent process for hormone therapy, these discussions can also occur before surgery as well.[7]

Gynecologists typically perform hysterectomy and salpingo-oophorectomy in a surgical procedure preceding phalloplasty. Vaginectomy is another component, involving mucosal ablation and colpocleisis, which may be done during the UL stage or during hysterectomy. Vaginectomy should generally be accompanied by hysterectomy because proper surveillance of the cervix will no longer be possible. Additionally, in most phalloplasty centers, vaginectomy is a prerequisite for phalloplasty with UL because the presence of an open vaginal canal can hinder healing in the short term, and in the long term, an open vaginal vault posteriorly may lead to urethral and bladder complications like diverticulum, prolapse, or pelvic floor dysfunction.[42]

RADIAL FOREARM FREE FLAP

The RFF is the most commonly used flap in phalloplasty because of its consistent vascular pedicle, pliability, and excellent sensory innervation.[40,41] However, the flap used for phalloplasty is larger than the traditionally described RFF (see Fig. 29.6). Several lateral, medial, and posterior antebrachial cutaneous nerve branches may also be harvested, which are then coapted to one dorsal clitoral nerve (while preserving the other intact) and the ilioinguinal nerve.[40] For recipient vessels there are two primary options: end-to-side into the superficial femoral artery (SFA) and great saphenous vein (GSV) or end-to-end use of the deep inferior epigastric vessels along with GSV. The deep inferior epigastric artery (DIEA) is generally preferred, and the SFA can often be employed in revisions and unique patient-specific cases. Combined staging centers often prefer the SFA because it allows for a more efficient distribution of surgical time when performing urethral work simultaneously.[41]

Vaginoplasty

Vaginoplasty involves the creation of both a vagina and a vulva. The primary objectives include achieving an aesthetically pleasing external appearance, enabling the patient to urinate while sitting, preserving erogenous sensation, and, if desired by the patient, allowing for penetrative intercourse. Several techniques are employed in performing vaginoplasty, such as penile inversion with penoscrotal flaps and grafts, extragenital skin grafts, peritoneal flaps and grafts, and the use of intestinal tissue.[44]

PREOPERATIVE CONSIDERATIONS

In cases where patients undergo an orchiectomy, it is important to consider any history of inguinal hernia, with or without repair, as well as the availability of penoscrotal tissues. Although hormone treatments during puberty have psychological benefits for trans women, they can also result in penoscrotal hypoplasia that makes traditional penile inversion vaginoplasty techniques difficult. In some instances, patients who have not undergone hormone treatments can also exhibit significant hypoplasia.

PENILE INVERSION VAGINOPLASTY

Penile inversion vaginoplasty is generally acknowledged as the standard technique and preserves the skin envelope of the penis as a pedicled skin flap. The flap is inverted and used to line the introitus and a newly formed vaginal cavity between the rectum and the urethra or bladder. To ensure sufficient depth in the canal, the inverted skin flap is usually extended with a full-thickness skin graft. Although the scrotum is a common donor site for this graft, alternative sites like the groin or buttock crease may be used if the scrotal skin is inadequate.[45] The harvested scrotal skin is thinned and tubularized around the end of a vaginal dilator on a separate work surface.[45]

After scrotectomy, orchiectomy is performed, followed by exposing the pelvic floor musculature and then dissecting the vaginal canal. This dissection takes place through the central tendon, progressing toward the prostate capsule, where the rectum is closest and the risk of rectal injury is highest. Sharp dissection is carried out around the prostate and through the posterior aspect of the capsule, allowing entry into the plane defined by the Denonvilliers fascia. From there, blunt dissection is carried back to the peritoneal reflection. The difficulty of this dissection is highly variable; in some cases, androgen blockade–induced atrophy of the prostate can make identification of the gland and capsule difficult. Next, the penis is degloved beneath the Dartos fascia to preserve vascularity in the skin flap.[45]

The proximal portion of the glans penis is used to fashion the clitoris while carefully separating it from the underlying corpora cavernosa and preserving the dorsal neurovascular bundle (NVB). The dissection for this can be performed either deep or superficial to the tunica albuginea. Subsequently, the corpus spongiosum and urethra are separated from the corpora cavernosa, which are then resected at the base. To control bleeding from the cavernosal arteries, the stumps of the corpora cavernosa are ligated. The urethra is trimmed and spatulated, positioning the neoclitoris at its anterior end to construct the vulvar plate.

The inverted tubularized scrotal skin graft is inserted at the distal part of the inverted penile skin flap over the dilator, and the entire structure is advanced into the vaginal canal. An incision is made at the midline of the penile skin flap to externalize the meatus, vulvar plate, and neoclitoris. Before attaching the posteriorly based perineal flap, the penile skin flap is split posteriorly to prevent excessive tension. This precaution is essential in preventing the formation of a posterior fourchette web (skin bridge), which may require additional surgical intervention.[45]

The procedure concludes with the formation of the labia majora and labia minora using the surrounding skin and subcutaneous tissues.[45]

MINIMAL-DEPTH VAGINOPLASTY

In certain instances, individuals who have previously undergone pelvic surgeries or radiation therapy or those who do not wish to engage in receptive penetrative intercourse may opt for minimal-depth vaginoplasty (MDV), also known as *short-depth vaginoplasty (SDV)* or *vulvoplasty*. MDV offers several benefits, such as reducing the duration of the surgical procedure, eliminating the need for dilation, a quicker recovery period, avoiding epilation, and significantly lowering the risk of rectal injury. The main drawback of MDV is the lack of a functional vaginal canal. Although patients may find this acceptable in certain clinical contexts, it is crucial to provide appropriate counseling before the surgery, as choosing to proceed with MDV is typically considered irreversible. Generally, less than 15% of patients ultimately opt for MDV.[45]

PERITONEAL VAGINOPLASTY

Penile inversion vaginoplasty has its limitations in terms of achieving sufficient neovaginal depth for penetrative intercourse, particularly in cases with limited natal tissue. Vaginoplasty using the colon has largely fallen out of favor because of issues with odor, need for colonoscopic surveillance, and other drawbacks. Alternative methods have been developed, particularly the use of laparoscopically or robotically harvested peritoneal flaps to supplement the penile inversion procedure and enhance neovaginal depth at the fundus.[44,45]

The most employed variant involves constructing the vaginal apex by employing two peritoneal advancement flaps: one sourced from the bladder and the other from the rectum. The distal vagina and introitus are formed using penile tissues and skin grafts, and careful suturing is performed to connect these structures to the peritoneal flaps, which are in turn connected to each other to establish the vaginal apex. Another technique uses robotic assistance to dissect the canal and acquire a peritoneal graft, which is then tubularized as a substitute for a scrotal graft.[45] In general, the advantages and disadvantages of this approach in cases where there is no shortage of scrotal skin are still being defined.

POSTOPERATIVE CARE

The success of vaginoplasty is dependent on the management of the postoperative period. Vaginal packing is inserted to promote graft or flap adherence and is usually maintained for approximately 4 to 6 days after surgery. During this time, a urinary catheter is kept in place and may be removed at 5 to 14 days postoperatively. After the removal of the packing, dilation of the vaginal canal is initiated, and it is generally recommended to continue lifelong dilation.[46]

Because the neovagina does not possess the ability to clean itself, most surgeons advise patients to follow a routine of intravaginal washing to assist in the removal of lubrication and debris. Pelvic physical therapy can offer both physical and psychological support, aiding in postoperative vaginal dilation.[46]

COMPLICATIONS

Complications after vaginoplasty are common, although many are minor and self-resolving. Wound dehiscence, particularly at the posterior fourchette, can occur in a significant number of patients because of excessive moisture, skin maceration, high bioburden, and tensile forces experienced during walking. However, these usually respond well to local wound care and resolve through conservative management. Other complications that may arise include canal stenosis, introital stenosis, issues with the direction or spray of the urinary stream, and urinary retention necessitating catheter placement. Major complications, such as skin flap necrosis, loss of clitoral sensation, or clitoral necrosis, are rare. Clitoral sensation rates are estimated to be approximately 84%.[45,46] Among the various complications, rectovaginal fistula (RVF) is probably the most important. Fortunately, RVF is uncommon, occurring in approximately 0.5% to 4% of cases in a large series.[46] The management of rectal injuries and subsequent RVF can vary, traditionally involving a low-residue diet, delayed dilation, and colostomy diversion. Overall, the long-term outcomes of vaginoplasty are generally positive, and patients report exceedingly high levels of satisfaction, both functionally and aesthetically, with very low regret rates.[5,7,46]

GENERAL SURGERY CONSIDERATIONS FOR THE POSTOPERATIVE GENDER SURGERY PATIENT

Foley Placement

The placement of a Foley catheter is an important aspect of surgical care. The specific approach to Foley catheter placement depends on the type of surgery performed. In the case of postphalloplasty with UL, an initial gentle attempt may be made without guidance. However, if this proves unsuccessful, the next step is to involve a urologist who may perform cystoscopy to aid in catheter placement. If no urologist is available or cystoscopy is unsuccessful, the next alternative is an ultrasound or fluoroscopic-guided SP tube placement, typically by interventional radiology.

If UL has not been performed as part of phalloplasty, typically a perineal urethrostomy on the perineum serves as the new urethral meatus, which, once identified, is typically straightforward to catheterize.

For metoidioplasty with UL, the preferred method for catheter placement involves initially attempting a 12-French (Fr) catheter. If this attempt is unsuccessful, the next step is to involve a urologist who can use a guidewire or pediatric cystoscope to aid in catheter placement. Again, if Foley catheterization is unsuccessful, SP placement will be needed.

In contrast, a Foley catheter in the postvaginoplasty patient is inserted in a standard fashion and typically does not require a specialist. Careful inspection of the neoanatomy, attention to sterile technique, and note of the sensitivity of the procedure should be considered.

URINARY TRACT INFECTION IN PHALLOPLASTY PATIENTS

Urine analysis and culture post-phalloplasty often show colonization because the neourethra is primarily composed of skin tissue, and natural flora present on skin can be found in urine samples. It is important to note that colonization of the urine does not necessarily indicate a urinary tract infection (UTI) that requires antibiotic treatment before or after surgery. It is essential for healthcare professionals to properly interpret the results of urine analysis and culture in the context of postphalloplasty patients, understanding that colonization is a common occurrence rather than an indicator of a UTI requiring antibiotic treatment.[43] Symptomatic report by the patient as to whether they are experiencing significant urinary symptoms compared with baseline is an important data point in decision-making.

Pelvic and Abdominal Incision Placement

For surgical incision placement, knowledge of prior surgical procedures is important. This is particularly true when dealing with phalloplasty, where the immediate area around the phalloplasty should be avoided. Evidence of femoral vessel or DIEA vessel exposure scars are important references, as crossing the region between this area and the pubis with incisions or undermining can result in transection of the pedicle and complete loss of the neophallus. Unlike most other free flaps, phalloplasties generally remain pedicle-dependent for life. Additionally, it is crucial to consider the presence of a penile prosthesis or testicular implant. Subsequent surgeries in the scrotum or pelvis after the placement of these prosthetics pose a risk of exposing the implants, which can lead to implant infection and potential loss, and are ideally avoided when possible.

CANCER SURVEILLANCE

For transmasculine individuals, those who are at average risk for breast cancer and have not undergone mastectomy may consider DBT or digital mammography screening after the age of 40. However, for those with an intermediate risk, it is recommended to have annual DBT or mammography after the age of 30, or an MRI if there is a previous history of breast cancer. It is worth noting that for transmasculine individuals who have undergone bilateral masculinizing mastectomy, the risk of breast cancer is very low.[37,47] Surveillance in such patients, when warranted, generally requires MRI.

In terms of cervical cancer screening, transmasculine individuals who have not undergone hysterectomy should follow standardized recommendations for all persons with a cervix. This includes adhering to the recommended screening intervals and initiating and ending screening at the appropriate ages. The American Cancer Society (ACS) recommends cervical cancer screening with a human papilloma virus (HPV) test every 5 years for everyone from age 25 until age 65.[47]

With regard to breast cancer screening, the ACR recommends that transfeminine individuals undergo a risk assessment at the age of 30 to determine whether screening before the age of 40 is necessary.[48] Concurrently, it is advised that patients undergo screening 5 years after starting E2 therapy if applicable, regardless of age.[48]

In terms of testicular cancer screening, routine screening is not recommended for cisgender men, and in parallel there is currently no evidence to support the need for screening in transfeminine patients. If a prostate examination is indicated, patients who have undergone vaginoplasty have the prostate located anterior to the vaginal wall, making a digital neovaginal examination relatively straightforward. Some data suggest that when prostate-specific antigen (PSA) testing is performed in transfeminine patients with low testosterone levels, it may be appropriate to adjust the upper limit of normal.[48]

INTUBATION POST–VOCAL CORD SURGERY

After gender-affirming vocal cord surgery, the size of the glottis is often reduced.[49] This can mean that a smaller tube diameter may be required for successful tube passage and intubation. However, the exact size can vary depending on the individual's anatomy. Use of a GlideScope along with a smaller-than-usual endotracheal (ET) tube is often helpful, with fiberoptic intubation as a backup option.

CONCLUSION

Gender-affirming surgery has life-changing impacts for individuals seeking alignment between their gender identity and physical presentation. We have addressed various aspects of this transformative process, which encompass the medical, surgical, and social dimensions of gender-affirming care. These procedures not only offer physical changes but also pave the way for improved mental well-being and an enhanced quality of life for patients. As surgeons and healthcare professionals, it is essential to continue advocating for accessibility, inclusivity, and respect for diverse gender identities, ensuring that all patients can access the healthcare they need.

SELECTED REFERENCES

Asa ER, Walter PB, George RB, Annelou LDV, Madeine BD, ttner et al. "Standards of care for the health of transgender and gender diverse people, version 8 (2022) International Journal of Transgender Health 23 no.

The WPATH Standards of Care are the most commonly referenced multi-specialty guidelines on the management of gender incongruence and gender-affirming care.

Oles N, Darrach H, Landford W, Garza M, Twose C, Park CS, Tran P, Schechter LS, Lau B, Coon D (2021) Gender Affirming Surgery: A Comprehensive, Systematic Review of All Peer-reviewed Literature and Methods of Assessing Patient-centered Outcomes (Part 2: Genital Reconstruction). Annals of Surgery 275:e67–e74

This study presents the first aggregated systemic review of cohort studies across all types of gender-affirming surgery to provide a succinct summary of extant surgical data.

Arrington-Sanders R, Connell NT, Coon D, Dowshen N, Goldman AL, Goldstein Z, Grimstad F, Javier NM, Kim E, Murphy M, Poteat T, Radix A, Schwartz A, St Amand C, Streed CG Jr, Tangpricha V, Toribio M, Goldstein RH. Assessing and Addressing the Risk of Venous Thromboembolism Across the Spectrum of Gender Affirming Care: A Review. Endocr Pract. 2023 Apr;29(4):272-278. doi: 10.1016/j.eprac.2022.12.008. Epub 2022 Dec 17. PMID: 36539066; PMCID: PMC10081942.

Management of gender-affirming hormone therapy, especially in the perioperative period, is one of the most widely discussed topics in the field and this multi-specialty consensus paper organized by the North American Thrombosis Forum presents an overview of key questions and data.

Coon D, Morrison SD, Morris MP, et al (2023) Gender-Affirming Vaginoplasty: A Comparison of Algorithms, Surgical Techniques and Management Practices across 17 High-volume Centers in North America and Europe. Plastic and Reconstructive Surgery - Global Open 11:e5033

Vaginoplasty is a procedure with remarkable variance between surgeons in technique and perioperative management, and this study that includes the leading US/European centers identifies the many areas of both agreement and divergence.

Morrison SD, Vyas KS, Motakef S, Gast KM, Chung MT, Rashidi V, Satterwhite T, Kuzon W, Cederna PS (2016) Facial Feminization: Systematic Review of the Literature. Plastic & Reconstructive Surgery 137:1759–1770.

Facial feminization remains the gender-affirming procedure with the greatest barriers to recognition that it is medically necessary; this systematic review attempts to summarize the key data for these procedures.

The full reference list appears on Elsevier eBooks+.

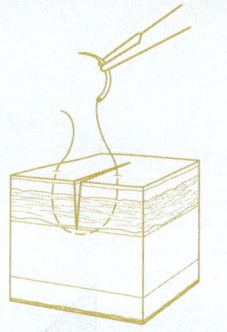

CHAPTER 30

Surgical Palliative Care

Orly N. Farber, Erin A. Strong, and Elizabeth J. Lilley

OUTLINE

BACKGROUND

Historically, surgeons have helped define and shape palliative care—both as a concept and as a formalized field. Today, surgical care and palliative care are interwoven: Modern palliation encompasses a range of operative procedures, and surgical patients have a host of palliative needs. Surgical palliative care—defined as palliative care as it is applied to patients with surgical conditions—has become a significant area of clinical and research activity, warranting a dive into its origins, principles, and future directions. In this chapter we will review the history of surgical palliative care, discuss the basics of its practice and communication principles, and describe the evidence to date. Surgical palliative care is a relatively new focus within surgery, with anticipated changes in its practice as the field evolves and as surgical patient demographics shift over time.

A Brief History

Although the care of patients with advanced illness is not a new concept, the history of palliative medicine as a specialty is fairly new. The field originated with the work of Cicely Saunders. Originally trained as a nurse and social worker, she cared for patients with terminal diseases in the years after World War II and observed that patients and their families were "devastated by unrelieved pain."[1] Thoracic surgeon Norman Barrett encouraged her to pursue a medical degree to deepen her understanding of her patients' suffering and gain authority in addressing it. After obtaining her degree, Saunders established the first modern inpatient hospice, St. Christopher's, in London in 1967, born out of the concept of "total pain," which Saunders used to denote the multifaceted nature of pain as it relates not only to the physical but also to emotional, social, and spiritual elements of suffering. Nearly a decade after Saunders paved the way for modern hospice, the urologic surgical oncologist Balfour Mount coined the term *palliative care* to distinguish it from care directed primarily toward

the dying.[2] Instead, palliative care, as recognized by the World Health Organization in 1990, is considered an approach focused on improving quality of life for patients and their family members with life-threatening illness.[3]

Surgical palliative care then developed in the 1990s alongside other subspecialties as a result of the understanding that different patient populations have different needs (Fig. 30.1). Surgical palliative care is, at its broadest, the practice of palliative care in surgical patient populations. Around that time, the American College of Surgeons (ACS) began advocating for palliative care for patients undergoing surgery[4] and, recognizing an educational gap in surgical training, they formed the Surgeons Palliative Care Workgroup in 2001. By 2006, the American Board of Surgery sponsored certificates in hospice and palliative medicine.[2] Today, the Surgical Palliative Care Society, founded in 2021,[5] works to educate surgeons on the principles of palliative care and the continued need for incorporating it into surgical practice.

Who Needs Palliative Care?

Palliative care is often mistakenly conflated with hospice. Hospice is symptom-focused interdisciplinary care for terminally ill patients nearing the end of life. Although hospice benefit criteria vary slightly among insurance providers, generally to qualify for hospice care, patients must have an estimated survival of 6 months or fewer and choose to forego further attempts at disease-directed treatment (Box 30.1).[6] In contrast, palliative care is intended for patients with serious illness at all phases of their disease course. This includes seriously ill surgical patients who are receiving potentially curative therapies. Recognizing the breadth of palliative care, the ACS Task Force on Surgical Palliative Care released a statement on its principles in 2005 (Box 30.2), noting that palliative care includes "the life-affirming quality of active, symptomatic efforts to relieve the pain and suffering of individuals with chronic illness and injury."[7] Importantly, they recognized that palliative care is not just for patients nearing the end of life and may be appropriate for many

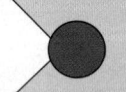

1843
The word hospice is used to describe a place to care for the terminally ill in Lyon, France.

1976
Balfour Mount creates the first Palliative Care Unit at the Royal Victoria Hospital in Montreal, comprised of an inpatient unit, consultation service, and home care.

2005
The ACS Surgical Palliative Care Workgroup publishes a Statement of the Principles of Palliative Care.

2016
The National Institutes of Health, The National Institute on Aging and National Palliative Care Research Center hold a workshop on subspecialty palliative care research priorities. Research priorities are developed and published for surgical practice.

1967
Cicely Saunders establishes St. Christopher's Hospice in London and introduces the idea of total pain.

2001
The American College of Surgeons (ACS) forms a Surgical Palliative Care Workgroup.

2009
The ACS and Cuniff-Dixon Foundation publish *Surgical Palliative Care: A Resident's Guide.*

2021
The Surgical Palliative Care Society is founded.

FIGURE 30.1 Major milestones in surgical palliative care. Palliative medicine is a relatively young specialty in medicine. This timeline depicts major milestones in its short history, including the recent development of subspecialty surgical palliative care, defined as palliative care as it is applied to patients with surgical conditions.

BOX 30.1   Medicare Hospice Benefit: Eligibility and Coverage as of 2023

Hospice Eligibility
- Enrolled in Medicare Part A
- Patient's hospice doctor and another physician certify status of terminal illness with life expectancy of 6 months or less
- Patient accepts focus on comfort care rather than further attempts at curative treatments
- Patient agrees to choose hospice care rather than other Medicare-covered treatments for the terminal illness and related conditions

Covered Services
- Physician, nursing, and other medical services
- Medical equipment and supplies (e.g., hospital bed, home oxygen, wound care needs)
- Medications prescribed for symptom control (copayment ≤$5)
- Hospice aide and homemaker services
- Physical therapy, occupational therapy, and speech-language pathology services if appropriate
- Social services
- Dietary counseling

- Spiritual and grief counseling
- Short-term inpatient care for pain and symptom management
- Short-term inpatient respite care in nursing home, hospice inpatient facility, or hospital for up to 5 days each time to allow caregiver to rest (5% copay of the Medicare-approved amount for inpatient respite care, not to exceed the annual inpatient hospital deductible)
- Any other Medicare-covered services recommended by hospice team for pain and symptoms related to terminal illness (may include treatments for symptom relief)

Services Not Covered by Hospice
- Treatments or prescription drugs intended to cure the terminal illness or related conditions
- Hospice care from clinicians that are not part of the chosen hospice provider team
- Room and board
- Hospital outpatient (e.g., emergency room) or inpatient care unless it is arranged by the hospice provider or it is unrelated to the terminal illness
- Ambulance transportation unless it is arranged by the hospice provider or it is unrelated to the terminal illness

Whereas palliative care is appropriate for all patients with serious illness, hospice is specialized care for patients nearing the end of life. The 2023 Medicare hospice benefit eligibility criteria and coverage are listed here. Private insurance hospice eligibility and benefits may differ. Adapted from Centers for Medicare and Medicaid Services. *Hospice Care.* https://www.medicare.gov/coverage/hospice-care. Accessed September 28, 2023.

---

patients treated by surgeons. As depicted in the enhanced model of palliative care delivery (Fig. 30.2), palliative care should be delivered from diagnosis until death. Its role begins alongside disease-directed treatments and may take different forms as patients' needs change along the disease continuum.

As the population ages and surgical innovation makes major operations a viable option for increasingly old, frail, and medically complex patients, surgical patients' demographics are changing. Consequently, surgeons must be competent and comfortable with attending to their patients' palliative needs.

Who Provides Palliative Care?

The aging population has led to growing demand for palliative care. However, workforce shortages in palliative care have led to staffing issues for hospitals, outpatient clinics, and hospices that are projected to worsen in the coming years (Fig. 30.3).[8,9] As a result, overreliance on specialists to meet all palliative care needs of surgical patients is unsustainable and will further strain a limited resource. Recognizing this, the National Academy of Medicine stated that all clinicians who care for seriously ill patients must know how to address their palliative needs.[10] Therefore, to ensure

---

BOX 30.2   Statement on the Principles of Palliative Care Released in 2005

- Respect the dignity and autonomy of patients, patients' surrogates, and caregivers.
- Honor the right of the competent patient or surrogate to choose among treatments, including those that may or may not prolong life.
- Communicate effectively and empathically with patients, their families, and caregivers.
- Identify the primary goals of care from the patient's perspective, and address how the surgeon's care can achieve the patient's objectives.
- Strive to alleviate pain and other burdensome physical and nonphysical symptoms.
- Recognize, assess, discuss, and offer access to services for psychological, social, and spiritual issues.

- Provide access to therapeutic support, encompassing the spectrum from life-prolonging treatments through hospice care, when they can realistically be expected to improve the quality of life as perceived by the patient.
- Recognize the physician's responsibility to discourage treatments that are unlikely to achieve the patient's goals, and encourage patients and families to consider hospice care when the prognosis for survival is likely to be less than a half-year.
- Arrange for continuity of care by the patient's primary and/or specialist physician, alleviating the sense of abandonment patients may feel when "curative" therapies are no longer useful.
- Maintain a collegial and supportive attitude toward others entrusted with care of the patient.

The Statement on the Principles of Palliative Care from the American College of Surgeons Task Force on Surgical Palliative Care specified its role in the management of seriously ill surgical patients alongside disease-directed care.
Adapted from Task Force on Surgical Palliative Care. Statement of principles of palliative care. *Bull Am Coll Surg.* 2005;90(8):34-35. Reprinted with permission, American College of Surgeons.

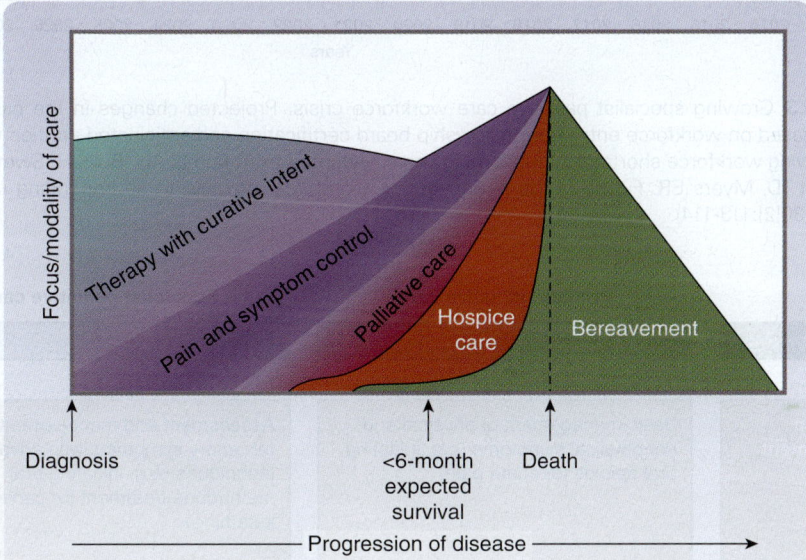

FIGURE 30.2 The enhanced model of palliative care. Palliative care should be delivered alongside potentially curative treatments from the time of diagnosis until death. During different phases of the disease course, patients' palliative needs will change. (Adapted from Perone JA, Riall TS, Olino K. Palliative care for pancreatic and periampullary cancer. *Surg Clin North Am.* 2016;96[6]:1415-1430).

that patients receive high-quality care, it is imperative that surgeons possess basic skills in palliative care.

To address the workforce crisis, Quill and Abernethy offered a model of palliative care delivery whereby basic palliative needs were met by the patient's care team, and more advanced needs could then be addressed by specialists.[11] Nonspecialist delivery of palliative care services is termed *primary palliative care.* Key components of a primary palliative care assessment include screening for physical or psychological symptoms and distress, identifying spiritual or existential concerns, determining the patient's understanding of their illness and its likely trajectory, eliciting goals of care, and anticipating postdischarge care needs. Nonspecialists, including surgeons, providing care to seriously ill patients should be equipped to address the basic needs that might arise from these inquiries. For more advanced care needs such as management of advanced or refractory symptoms, complex communication, and end-of-life care, consultation with specialist palliative care teams is indicated (Fig. 30.4).

Although surgeons are responsible for meeting their patients' basic palliative needs, few receive formal training in communication about goals of care and management of nonpain symptoms.[12] In the next sections, we provide an overview of basic symptom management principles and communication techniques. For further study, we recommend *Surgical Palliative Care: A Resident's Guide,*[13] a free resource for surgical trainees from the ACS and *Surgical Palliative Care: Integrating Palliative Care,*[14] a comprehensive textbook on surgical palliative care.

BASICS OF SYMPTOM MANAGEMENT

Surgeons encounter a wide range of symptoms and must have a basic understanding of the principles of symptom management. Some patients may have preexisting symptom burdens from chronic ailments or related to the condition they are presenting for. Others will experience acute symptoms after the operative

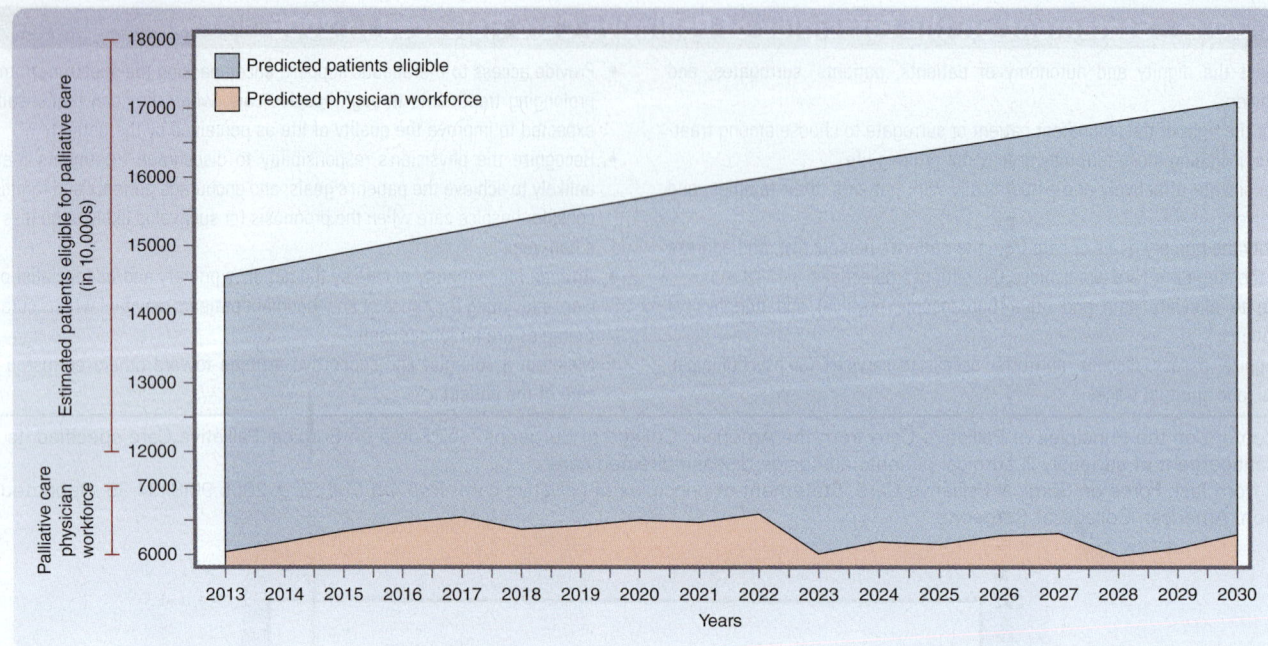

FIGURE 30.3 Growing specialist palliative care workforce crisis. Projected changes in the palliative care workgroup based on workforce entry from fellowship board certification and anticipated attrition will contribute to a growing workforce shortage in the coming years. (Adapted from Kamal AH, Bull JH, Swetz KM, Wolf SP, Shanafelt TD, Myers ER. Future of the palliative care workforce: preview to an impending crisis. *Am J Med.* 2017;130[2]:113-114).

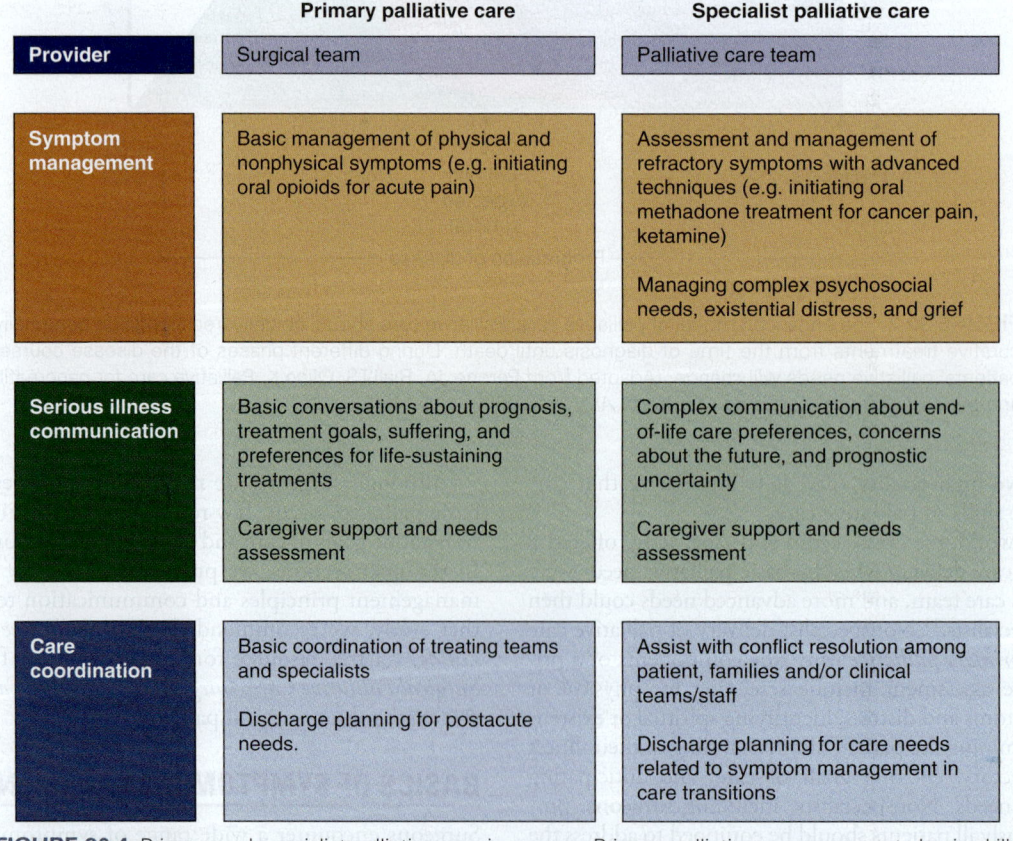

FIGURE 30.4 Primary and specialist palliative care in surgery. Primary palliative care represents basic skills for treatment of physical or psychological symptoms, spiritual concerns, communications about serious illness, and care coordination that can be provided by all members of the patient's care team. Specialist palliative care is management of advanced or refractory symptoms, complex communication, and end-of-life care that is provided by interdisciplinary clinicians with advanced palliative medicine training.

intervention. This section provides a brief overview of how to assess and treat common symptoms.

Symptom Assessment

Measuring symptoms is a critical component of patient care. Many symptoms that are experienced by surgical patients may go undetected by surgeons and/or underreported by patients. Several symptom assessment instruments exist to help clinicians gather information on patients' symptom burden and severity and the impact of those symptoms on their quality of life. Initial symptom assessment can help clinicians identify patterns or clusters that may provide insight to their etiology. Performing repeated symptom assessments over time can help gauge the effectiveness of various interventions. Examples of validated symptom assessment tools can be found in Table 30.1.

Physical Symptoms: Pain, Nausea, and Fatigue

A thorough assessment of pain is needed to identify its source and develop a tailored approach to treatment. The acronym OPQRSTU can be helpful in obtaining a pain history (Box 30.3). Responses to these questions—addressing factors such as the pain's quality, location, severity—provide clues to the type of pain and its likely etiology, and they can help to guide management (Table 30.2).

The three main categories of pain are nociceptive, neuropathic, and nociplastic. Nociceptive, or inflammatory pain, is caused by damage to a body tissue. It is a normal response to noxious stimulation. Neuropathic pain is caused by damage to a nerve or group of nerves. It can result from trauma or impingement, diseases like diabetes or multiple sclerosis, or as an adverse drug effect. Neuropathic pain is a pathologic process caused by ectopic activity of the damaged nerves rather than a normal response to noxious stimuli. Nociplastic pain is a newer concept and is used to describe conditions in which nociception occurs in the absence of actual or threatened damage to tissues. Nociplastic pain is experienced as a result of alterations in the nervous system's processing of pain. It is often associated with fatigue, anxiety, depression, and other nonphysical symptoms.

BOX 30.3 OPQRSTU: An Acronym for Pain Assessment

- **O**nset – What were you doing when the pain started? Did it start suddenly or gradually get worse?
- **P**rovokes/ **P**alliates – What makes the pain worse? What makes the pain better? What medicines or nonmedicines have been helpful? Were they and are they still effective?
- **Q**uality – How does the pain feel? What words can you use to describe the pain (sharp, stabbing, burning, shooting, dull, achy, throbbing, crampy)?
- **R**egion/ **R**adiates – Where is your pain primarily located? Does it travel anywhere?
- **S**everity – What is the present and past intensity of the pain, at its worst and at its best? (See scales later.)
- **T**ime – How often does it occur? Is it constant or intermittent?
- **U** – How is this pain affecting YOU and your life?

This simple acronym can help ensure a thorough pain history is taken, which allows the provider to determine what type of pain the patient is experiencing (e.g., nociceptive vs. neuropathic) and select an appropriate treatment plan.

The goal of pain management is not necessarily to eliminate pain completely, but rather to maximize patients' function and enhance their quality and enjoyment of life. Nonpharmacologic therapies, including exercise, physical therapy, and alternative treatments (e.g., acupuncture or therapeutic massage), should be considered. Multimodal pain management should begin with nonopioids, nonpharmacologic interventions, treatment of underlying syndromes that contribute to pain (e.g., depression and anxiety), and interventional pain therapies such as nerve blocks. Short-acting opioid medications are appropriate for managing acute pain. Severe pain may require long-acting opioids. A full description of specific medications is beyond the scope of this chapter. We recommend the Dana-Farber Cancer Institute/ Brigham and Women's Hospital Pink Book,[15] a pocket-reference resource that includes opioid conversion tables, medication charts, and other clinical pearls for pain management.

TABLE 30.1 Symptom Assessment Instruments Used in Surgical Populations

SYMPTOM	TOOL	BRIEF DESCRIPTION
Health-related quality of life	Short-Form 36-item survey	36-item survey measuring 8 concepts divided into mental and physical component scores.
	Euro-QOL 5 Dimension Questionnaire	5-item survey, assessing mobility, self-care, usual activities, discomfort, and anxiety/depression.
Pain	Brief Pain Inventory Short-Form	9-item survey measures average, least, worst, and current pain intensity.
	Short-Form McGill Pain Questionnaire	Contains 2 subscales, 11 sensory items, and 4 affective. Includes present pain intensity index and visual analog scale.
Fatigue	Functional Assessment of Chronic Illness Therapy Fatigue Scale	13-item survey measuring fatigue during usual activities over the past week.
	Fatigue Severity Scale	9-item survey measuring severity of fatigue and impact on life.
Psychological well-being	Hospital Anxiety and Depression Scale	14-item survey with 7 items assessing depression and 7 items assessing anxiety.
	Patient Health Questionnaire-9	9-item instrument to assess severity of depressive symptoms.
	Beck Depression Inventory II	21 items measuring severity of depression in the past 2 weeks.
Other	MD Anderson Symptom Inventory	Multisymptom assessment for patients with cancer, with 13 core items and additional disease-specific modules.
	Edmonton Symptom Assessment Scale	9-item scale assessing symptoms in patients receiving palliative care.
	Integrated Palliative Care Outcome Scale	10-item scale assessing physical, emotional, psychological, spiritual, and provision of information and support dimensions.

TABLE 30.2 Classification and Characteristics of Pain

CLASSIFICATION	TYPES	DESCRIPTION	EXAMPLES	TREATMENTS
Nociceptive or Inflammatory Caused by injury or inflammation	Somatic	Well-localized, dull, aching, throbbing	Incisional pain, bone fracture, cellulitis, arthritis	Antiinflammatory, muscle relaxants, opioids
	Visceral	Poorly localized, aching, can be referred to dermatomal sites	Early appendicitis, intestinal obstruction, liver metastases, diaphragmatic irritation referred to shoulder	
Neuropathic Caused by nerve damage, impingement, or irritation	Peripheral	Shooting and stabbing pain with background of aching and burning	Sciatica, nerve entrapment, diabetic neuropathy	Tricyclic antidepressants, anticonvulsants, weak opioids (second line), botulinum toxin A (third line), nerve blocks
	Central		Brain injury, Parkinson disease, stroke	
Nociplastic Caused by altered nociception in the absence of tissue damage		Widespread, intense pain often associated with tiredness, difficulty with memory, insomnia, and mood	Fibromyalgia, complex regional pain syndrome, depression	Tricyclic antidepressants, serotonin and norepinephrine reuptake inhibitors, gabapentinoids

Nausea is another physical symptom that is commonly experienced by surgical patients, who may develop nausea because of alterations in normal gastrointestinal function, including ileus or obstruction, and from frequently used medications such as opioids, anesthetics, and antibiotics. Pharmacotherapy targets different mechanisms involved in the sensation of nausea (Fig. 30.5), and certain treatments may be better or worse depending on the source of nausea (Fig. 30.6). For example, nausea can be mediated by central mechanisms or via the periphery, with some drugs targeting central signals to suppress nausea and vomiting and others targeting peripheral signals to modulate gastrointestinal motility (see Fig. 30.5). Because the sensation of nausea is complex and can involve different parts of the nervous system, using a multimodal approach is helpful for treating refractory nausea.

Although pain and nausea are within the surgeon's scope of practice, other physical symptoms that surgical patients frequently encounter may go unrecognized and, therefore, unaddressed. For example, postoperative fatigue is experienced as an unpleasant lack of energy that may occur because of the body's increased metabolic demands when healing from surgery coupled with sleep disturbances and altered energy consumption if appetite is slow to return postoperatively. Typically, fatigue gradually improves after surgery, but it may take weeks to resolve and can be distressing to patients in the interim. Inquiring about fatigue can help normalize it and reassure patients that it is an expected part of recovery. Furthermore, surgeons can encourage sleep hygiene and recommend recovery-appropriate exercises to reduce fatigue. Insomnia and depression can contribute to fatigue and should be addressed if present. Short-term use of stimulants, such as methylphenidate, can also be considered in cases of severe fatigue that limits daily function.

Nonphysical Symptoms: Anxiety, Depression, and Surgical Fear

Since Cicely Saunders's pioneering work on total pain recognized different dimensions of pain and the need for a holistic approach to pain management, there has been a growing acceptance that nonphysical symptoms such as anxiety and depression contribute to suffering in patients with advanced illness.

Anxiety and depression are a common symptom cluster in patients with cancers and other life-limiting chronic diseases. Unaddressed anxiety and depression contribute to poor quality of

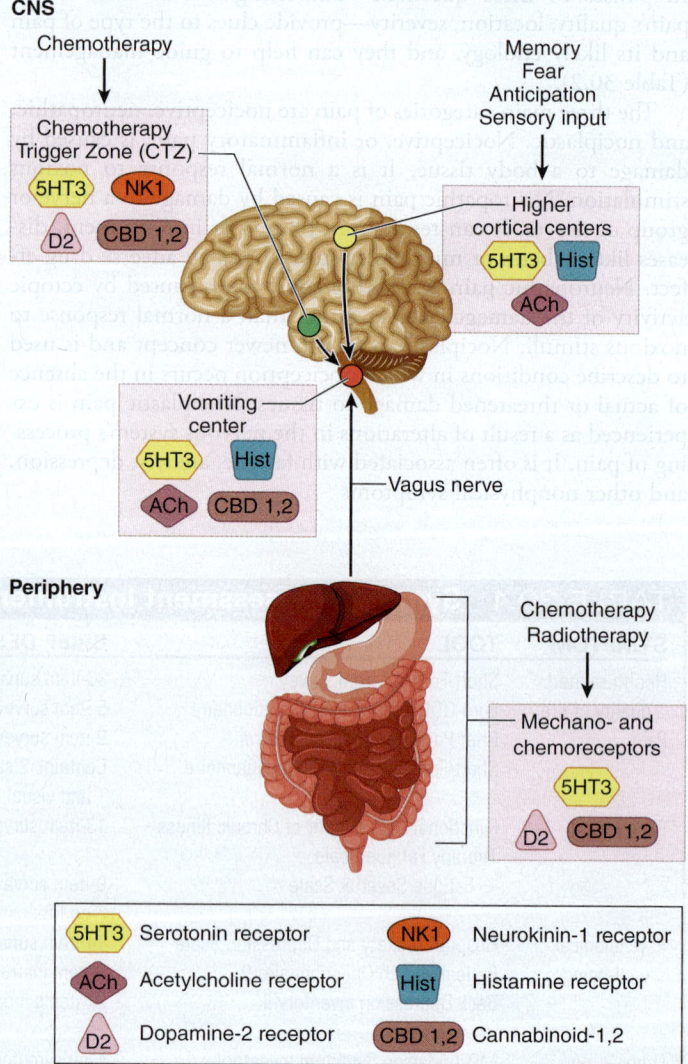

FIGURE 30.5 Antiemetic targets. There are central and peripheral contributors to the sensation of nausea, which can be targeted to reduce symptom severity. (From Suliman I, Phantumvanit V, Rostamnjad L, et al. *Adult Guidelines for Assessment and Management of Nausea and Vomiting.* Dana-Farber Cancer Institute; 2023. Pinkbook.dfci.org.)

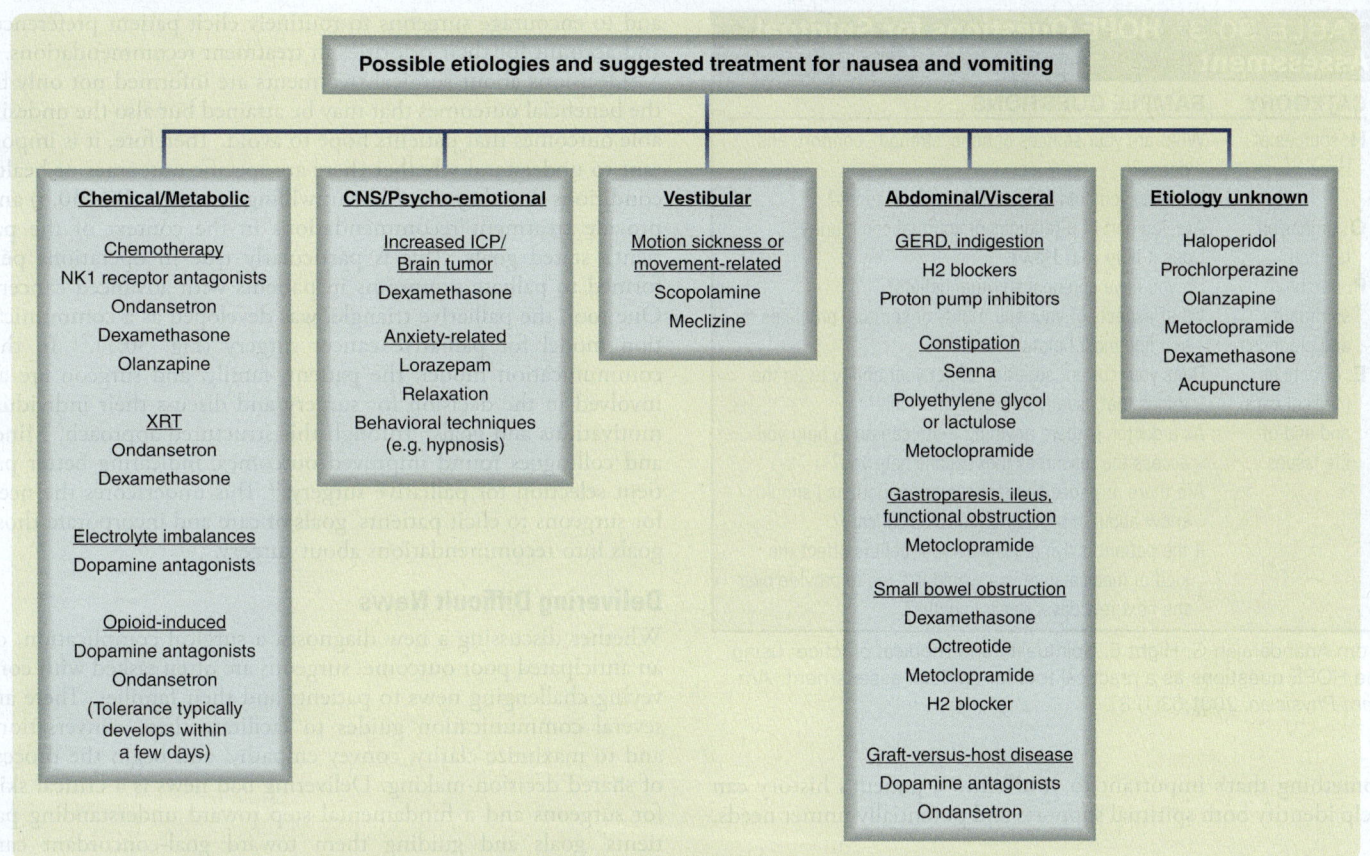

FIGURE 30.6 Antiemetic drugs based on common etiologies. The choice of antiemetic drug depends on the etiology of nausea and vomiting. This diagram provides recommendations for common etiologies of nausea. *CNS,* Central nervous system; *GERD,* gastroesophageal reflux disease; *H2 blockers,* histamine H2 receptor blocker; *ICP,* intracranial pressure; *NK1 receptor,* neurokinin-1; *XRT,* radiation therapy. (Adapted from Suliman I, Phantumvanit V, Rostamnjad L, et al. *Adult Guidelines for Assessment and Management of Nausea and Vomiting.* Dana-Farber Cancer Institute; 2023. Pinkbook.dfci.org.)

life and are associated with both increased complication rates and worse surgical outcomes. Patients can struggle to recognize these symptoms as anxiety and depression and may experience physical manifestations. The associations between depression, fatigue, and pain are long established, as is the relationship between anxiety and nausea. Because of these interactions, anxiety and depression should be assessed in patients with physical symptoms that are refractory to treatment.

Fear also plays a role in the care of surgical patients. Surgical fear is defined as fear that patients have in the perioperative setting over multiple dimensions of the surgical experience. This can lead to negative outcomes including higher pain levels, increased administration of anesthesia and analgesia, delayed wound healing, poorer adherence to prescribed treatment plans, prolonged hospital length of stay, reduced physical functioning, and aggravated mental health.[16] Recognizing surgical fear in the lived experience of patients may allow for interventions such as consultation with appropriate clinicians (e.g., social work, psychology, spiritual care) to help mitigate poor outcomes.[16] However, surgeons are rarely formally taught how to identify, discuss, and ameliorate surgical fear.

Existential and Spiritual Distress

Although the demographics around religion and spirituality in the United States are changing, many patients and family members explicitly or implicitly incorporate their religious or spiritual beliefs into their conceptions of their disease, clinical care, and approach to decisions. Life-threatening illness forces patients to reflect on their lives and confront thoughts of death. In doing so, patients can experience existential or spiritual distress, which is suffering related to difficulty experiencing meaning in one's connections to self, others, or superior beings.[17] It can be typified by loss of hope, meaning, or pleasure. Unaddressed spiritual needs can manifest in physical and psychosocial ways that impede optimal care.

Recognizing spiritual and existential distress is a primary palliative care skill, but this does not mean that surgeons must be equipped to manage spiritual and existential distress themselves. Multidisciplinary team involvement can be of use in addressing spiritual or existential suffering. Chaplains are trained to attend to patients' spiritual needs, regardless of whether they are rooted in religion. Formalized spiritual services engagement is associated with increased spiritual well-being of patients and families as well as increased satisfaction with care in general and with shared decision-making.[18] However, for patients to access chaplain services, surgeons and other care team members need to inquire about and recognize spiritual needs. There are several assessment tools for taking a spiritual history, including the HOPE acronym (Table 30.3). Incorporating questions like "What do you hold on to during difficult times?" or "Is spirituality, faith, or religion

TABLE 30.3   HOPE Questions for Spiritual Assessment

CATEGORY	SAMPLE QUESTIONS
H: sources of hope	What are your sources of hope, strength, comfort, and peace? What do you hold on to during difficult times?
O: organized religion	Are you part of a religious or spiritual community? Does it help you? How?
P: personal spirituality and practices	Do you have personal spiritual beliefs? What aspects of your spirituality or spiritual practices do you find most helpful?
E: effects on medical care and end-of-life issues	Does your current situation affect your ability to do the things that usually help you spiritually? As a doctor, is there anything that I can do to help you access the resources that usually help you? Are there any specific practices or restrictions I should know about in providing your medical care? If the patient is dying: How do your beliefs affect the kind of medical care you would like me to provide over the next few days/weeks/months?

From Anandarajah G, Hight E. Spirituality and medical practice: using the HOPE questions as a practical tool for spiritual assessment. *Am Fam Physician.* 2001;63(1):87.

something that's important to you?" into a patient's history can help identify both spiritual supports and potentially unmet needs.

COMMUNICATION

Like any other technical skill that surgeons gain during years of training, communication can be taught, practiced, and improved. This section provides information on a shared approach to decision-making as well as communication guides for decision-making, delivering bad news, and eliciting goals of care.

Decision-Making in Surgery

In the past, decision-making in medicine was often paternalistic, whereby the physician's recommendation for clinical care was accepted with little scrutiny or discussion. The culture of medicine, and surgery along with it, has trended toward increasing patient autonomy, and therefore, decision-making is viewed as a collaborative, dynamic process between patient and provider. High-quality shared decision-making may be especially important for patients considering operations that pose a high risk of morbidity or mortality, whether because of the extent of surgery itself or the individual patient's baseline poor health status.

Research examining patient and surgeon engagement in shared decision-making reveals limitations in mechanisms to increase patient engagement and variability in surgeon performance. A multi-institutional randomized clinical trial analyzed recorded conversations at surgical consultation visits.[19] In the intervention arm, before meeting with their surgeons, patients received a question prompt list to facilitate their engagement in decision-making conversations. The research team found no differences in patient engagement or well-being relative to usual care. In a secondary qualitative analysis, they found that use of shared decision-making was highly variable.[20] Notably, decisions were perceived as shared more often when the surgeon expressed a reluctance to operate. These findings suggest that to promote shared decision-making, strategies are needed both to support patient engagement

and to encourage surgeons to routinely elicit patient preferences and account for their priorities in treatment recommendations.

Decisions about surgical treatments are informed not only by the beneficial outcomes that may be attained but also the undesirable outcomes that patients hope to avoid. Therefore, it is important to understand whether there are specific outcomes or health conditions that they would be unwilling to accept (Box 30.4) and provide treatment recommendations in the context of the patient's stated goals. This is particularly true in operations performed to palliate symptoms in patients with advanced cancers. One tool, the palliative triangle, was developed as a communication model for palliative cancer surgery (Fig. 30.7).[21] In this communication model, the patient, family, and surgeon are all involved in the decision for surgery and discuss their individual motivations and goals. Through this structured approach, Miner and colleagues found improved outcomes, indicating better patient selection for palliative surgery.[22] This underscores the need for surgeons to elicit patients' goals of care and incorporate those goals into recommendations about surgery.

Delivering Difficult News

Whether discussing a new diagnosis, a surgical complication, or an anticipated poor outcome, surgeons are often tasked with conveying challenging news to patients and their families. There are several communication guides to facilitate these conversations and to maximize clarity, convey empathy, and begin the process of shared decision-making. Delivering bad news is a critical skill for surgeons and a fundamental step toward understanding patients' goals and guiding them toward goal-concordant care choices.

In approaching difficult conversations, it is important to begin by gathering any necessary information in order to avoid discordant messages from different teams, which can lead to patient frustration and distrust. Speaking with other members of the patient's care team helps ensure that you are providing accurate

BOX 30.4   Postoperative Outcomes Where Treatment Burdens May Outweigh the Benefits

- Permanent nursing home residence
- Prolonged hospitalization or ICU course
- Dependence on life-sustaining therapies
  - Mechanical ventilation
  - Hemodialysis
  - Feeding tubes
  - Total parenteral nutrition
- Severe cognitive impairment
- Complete functional dependence
- Burden to family or loved ones
- Intractable pain
- No time to get affairs in order
- Inability to enjoy a personal milestone (birthday, wedding, anniversary)
- Death away from home

ICU, Intensive care unit.
Patient may have limitations on what functional and quality-of-life outcomes they deem acceptable after surgery. These examples of potential poor outcomes should be discussed with frail or seriously ill patients before surgery.
From Table 2 in Cooper Z, Courtwright A, Karlage A, Gawande A, Block S. Pitfalls in communication that lead to nonbeneficial emergency surgery in elderly patients with serious illness: description of the problem and elements of a solution. *Ann Surg.* 2014;260(6):949-957.

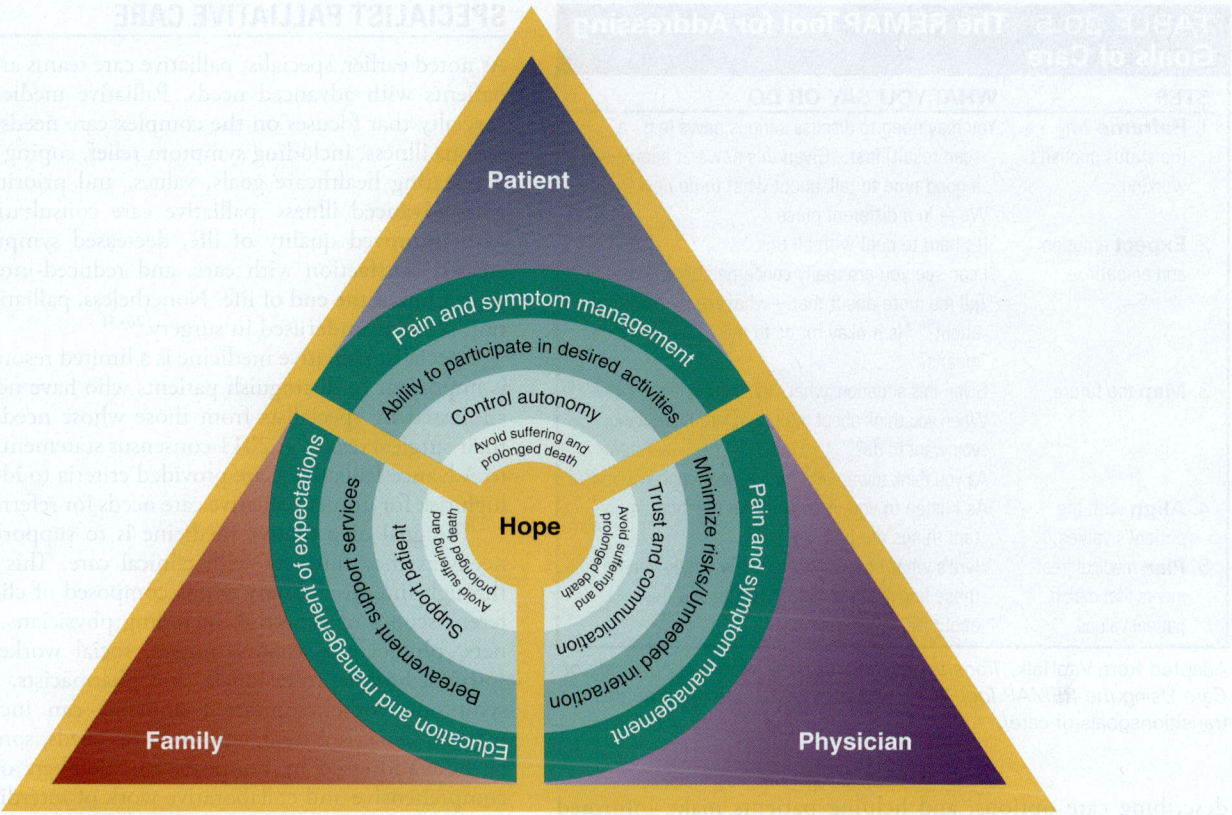

FIGURE 30.7 The palliative triangle. This communication model was developed by Thomas Miner and colleagues[21,22] to assist in decisions about palliative surgery for patients with cancer through the involvement of the patient, family, and surgeon. Treatment decisions are guided by the goals and desires of each person, with hope as a central tenet of the process. (From Perone JA, Riall TS, Olino K. Palliative care for pancreatic and periampullary cancer. *Surg Clin North Am.* 2016;96[6]:1415-1430).

information based on a shared understanding of the disease, prognosis, and treatment options. Achieving this prognostic alignment between all care teams allows for direct communication and goal-concordant care planning. Similarly, eliciting the patient's illness understanding at the beginning of the conversation allows surgeons to address any discrepancies. Additionally, this avoids starting the conversation with an unnecessary recitation of facts.

When sharing difficult information, it is helpful to give a warning shot to prepare the patient ("unfortunately, I have some difficult news to share") and then deliver the information as a clear headline (e.g., "the CT scan showed that the tumor is unresectable") followed by a pause. In this pause, you await the patient's response. If they respond with emotion, as is often the case, the emotion should be acknowledged and addressed before moving forward. This can be accomplished using the NURSE mnemonic statements (Table 30.4). A common misconception is that attending to patients' emotions is prohibitively time intensive, but moving forward in a conversation without addressing their emotions is ultimately inefficient because patients are unlikely to absorb information and may have more questions or may not feel prepared to discuss treatment options. Furthermore, failing to address the emotions that arise is a missed opportunity to provide support and empathy, establish trust and rapport, and ensure that the patient feels heard and understood.

Clear and empathic delivery of difficult news lays the foundation for the work that follows: eliciting patients' goals,

TABLE 30.4 NURSE Statements for Responding to Emotion

	EXAMPLE	NOTES
Naming	"It sounds like you are frustrated"	In general, turn down the intensity a notch when you name the emotion.
Understanding	"This helps me understand what you are thinking"	Think of this as another kind of acknowledgment but stop short of suggesting you understand everything (you don't).
Respecting	"I can see you have really been trying to follow our instructions"	Remember that praise also fits in here (e.g., "I think you have done a great job with this").
Supporting	"I will do my best to make sure you have what you need"	Making this kind of commitment is a powerful statement.
Exploring	"Could you say more about what you mean when you say that . . ."	Asking a focused question prevents this from seeming too obvious.

Adapted from VitalTalk. *Responding to Emotion: Respecting.* 2019. https://www.vitaltalk.org/guides/responding-to-emotion-respecting/.

TABLE 30.5   The REMAP Tool for Addressing Goals of Care

STEP	WHAT YOU SAY OR DO
1. **Reframe** why the status quo isn't working.	You may need to discuss serious news (e.g., a scan result) first. "Given this news, it seems like a good time to talk about what to do now." "We're in a different place."
2. **Expect** emotion and empathize.	"It's hard to deal with all this." "I can see you are really concerned about [x]." "Tell me more about that—what are you worried about?" "Is it okay for us to talk about what this means?"
3. **Map** the future.	"Given this situation, what's most important for you?" "When you think about the future, are there things you want to do?" "As you think toward the future, what concerns you?"
4. **Align** with the patient's values.	"As I listen to you, it sounds like the most important things are [x, y, z]."
5. **Plan** medical treatments that match patient values.	"Here's what I can do now that will help you do those important things. What do you think about it?"

Adapted from VitalTalk. *Transitions/Goals of Care: Addressing Goals of Care Using the REMAP Tool.* 2019. https://www.vitaltalk.org/guides/transitionsgoals-of-care/.

describing care options, and helping patients make informed treatment decisions that align with their goals. One communication tool, the REMAP communication guide, was developed to provide a framework for goals-of-care conversations for patients with advanced cancers.[23,24] This conversation map (Table 30.5) picks up after difficult news has been shared. It begins with reframing the clinical picture in light of the bad news (for example, "Given the scan results, we're in a different place"). It encourages providers to help patients map out their futures, align themselves with their patients' priorities, and plan treatments that are consistent with patients' goals. The REMAP proposed questions and statements help to elicit patients' goals of care in the context of new information, all while continuing to address emotion.

Miracle Statements

Many surgeons have heard a patient or their family member—amid a difficult clinical situation—express hope for a miracle. In most cases, surgical training has not explicitly prepared surgeons to interpret or address these hopes and wishes. Surgeons may misinterpret what these hopes mean in regard to the patient's or family's prognostic understanding and their willingness to consider difficult choices or undesirable outcomes. In a 2018 paper, Shinall and colleagues suggest a framework to delineate the different patterns of hopes for a miracle that patients and their families might express, along with suggestions for physician responses that can promote dialogue, rapport, trust, and shared decision-making.[25] They noted four types of hope: innocuous (object of hope is plausible but an unlikely outcome), shaken (patient is expressing anger or sadness that a miracle has not happened), integrated (hope stems from a religious perspective), and strategic (adversarial assertion of rights and unwillingness to discuss the grounds of hope). Each type merits a different response, which can help clinicians engage in treatment discussions effectively and compassionately.

SPECIALIST PALLIATIVE CARE

As noted earlier, specialist palliative care teams are appropriate for patients with advanced needs. Palliative medicine is a medical specialty that focuses on the complex care needs of patients with serious illness, including symptom relief, coping with illness, and delineating healthcare goals, values, and priorities. For patients with advanced illness, palliative care consultation is associated with improved quality of life, decreased symptom burden, increased satisfaction with care, and reduced-intensity healthcare utilization at the end of life. Nonetheless, palliative care consultation remains underused in surgery.[26–31]

Specialist palliative medicine is a limited resource. Therefore, it is important to distinguish patients who have needs that are best addressed by specialists from those whose needs can be met by their surgical teams. A 2011 consensus statement from the Center to Advance Palliative Care provided criteria to identify patients at high risk for unmet palliative care needs for referral (Table 30.6).[32]

The goal of palliative medicine is to support patients' broad needs as they intersect with clinical care. This is accomplished through interdisciplinary teams composed of clinicians with different scopes of expertise, including physicians, nurse practitioners, physician assistants, nurses, social workers, chaplains or spiritual health professionals, and pharmacists. Beyond physical symptoms, other supported domains can include emotional, mental, social, spiritual, and financial needs, some of which may be best addressed by nonphysician members of the team. The comprehensive and collaborative work of interdisciplinary palliative care teams is associated with higher-quality care and improved patient outcomes.[33]

EVIDENCE FOR SURGICAL PALLIATIVE CARE

In the past 20 years, the evidence for palliative care in surgery has continued to grow. Still, much work remains to be done. To characterize the state of the science, a 2015 systematic review examined palliative care interventions for surgical patient populations.[29] The 25 included articles provided evidence that palliative care reduces healthcare utilization and improves advance care planning in surgical patient populations without increasing mortality. There was a paucity of research on how to align surgical decisions with patients' goals of care and how to integrate palliative care principles into surgical culture. Furthermore, heterogeneous outcomes, small sample sizes, single-center studies, and inadequate follow-up all limited the scope and generalizability of the available findings. In 2016, the National Institutes of Health, the National Institute on Aging, and the National Palliative Care Research Center held a workshop on subspecialty palliative care research priorities. This culminated in a national research agenda for surgical palliative care.[34] The identified priority areas for research included defining outcomes that matter to patients, communication and decision-making, and delivery of palliative care to surgical patients. An updated systematic review was recently published and included 22 articles published from 2016 to 2022.[30] The authors found that although some progress was made, particularly in studying mechanisms of palliative care delivery, major knowledge gaps persist.

In the setting of a growing body of evidence for early integration of palliative care in cancer care, two large, randomized trials examined the role of perioperative specialist palliative care for patients undergoing major oncologic resections with curative intent. The SCOPE trial was performed at a single tertiary academic

TABLE 30.6	Referral Criteria for Specialty Palliative Care
General referral criteria *Presence of a serious illness and one or more of the following:*	• New diagnosis of life-limiting illness for symptom control, patient/family support • Declining ability to complete activities of daily living • Weight loss • Progressive metastatic cancer • Admission from long-term care facility (nursing home or assisted living) • Two or more hospitalizations for illness within 3 months • Difficult-to-control physical or emotional symptoms • Patient, family, or physician uncertainty regarding prognosis • Patient, family, or physician uncertainty regarding appropriateness of treatment options • Patient or family requests for futile care • DNR order conflicts • Conflicts or uncertainty regarding the use of nonoral feeding/hydration in cognitively impaired, seriously ill, or dying patients • Limited social support in setting of a serious illness (e.g., homeless, no family or friends, chronic mental illness, overwhelmed family caregivers) • Patient, family, or physician request for information regarding hospice appropriateness • Patient or family psychological or spiritual/existential distress
Intensive care unit criteria *Presence of a serious illness, any of the above, and one or more of the following:*	• Admission from a nursing home • Two or more ICU admissions within the same hospitalization • Prolonged or failed attempt to wean from ventilator • Multiorgan failure • Consideration of ventilator withdrawal with expected death • Metastatic cancer • Anoxic encephalopathy • Consideration of patient transfer to a long-term ventilator facility • Family distress impairing surrogate decision-making
Cancer criteria *Presence of any of the above and/or:*	• Metastatic or locally advanced cancer progressing despite systemic treatments • Karnofsky score <50 or ECOG performance status >3 • Brain metastases, spinal cord compression, or neoplastic meningitis • Malignant hypercalcemia • Progressive pleural/peritoneal or pericardial effusions
Neurologic criteria *Presence of any of the above and/or:*	• Folstein Mini Mental score <20 • Feeding tube is being considered for any neurologic condition • Status epilepticus >24 h • ALS or other neuromuscular disease considering mechanical ventilation • Any recurrent brain neoplasm • Parkinson disease with poor functional status or dementia • Advanced dementia with dependence in all activities of daily living

ALS, Amyotrophic lateral sclerosis.; *ECOG*, Eastern Cooperative Oncology Group; *ICU*, intensive care unit.
Adapted from CAPC. *Policies and Tools for Hospital Palliative Care Programs.* 45. https://media.capc.org/filer_public/88/06/8806cedd-f78a-4d14-a90e-aca688147a18/nqfcrosswalk.pdf.

cancer center,[35] whereas the PERIOP-PC trial was a multisite study at five cancer centers.[36] In both studies, patients were randomized to usual care or specialist palliative care consultation before surgery. Neither study found an association between specialist palliative care and quality of life. These findings indicate that surgeons are meeting the palliative needs of this patient group, and they would not benefit from routine involvement of specialist palliative care. More work is needed to identify patient populations who derive the greatest benefit from early palliative care involvement.

LOOKING TO THE FUTURE OF SURGICAL PALLIATIVE CARE

Since its recent beginnings, the field of surgical palliative care has expanded at a rapid pace. The creation of palliative care interest groups within surgery and anesthesiology societies is a testament to the growing recognition of seriously ill surgical patients' palliative needs. Researchers and educators have made great strides in promoting palliative care integration into surgical practice. In addition, a new wave of surgeons has attained training and board certification in palliative care and is establishing and refining new pathways for palliative care implementation in surgery. And yet, much work is still needed to help understand how to best integrate palliative care principles into the care of seriously ill surgical patients.

SELECTED REFERENCES

Aslakson RA, Rickerson E, Fahy B, et al. Effect of perioperative palliative care on health-related quality of life among patients undergoing surgery for cancer: a randomized clinical trial. *JAMA Netw Open.* 2023;6(5):e2314660.

This randomized control trial builds on the literature demonstrating a benefit of early palliative care interventions for medical oncology patients and explores whether surgeon–palliative care team comanagement of patients undergoing curative-intent surgery for upper gastrointestinal cancers improved patient-reported perioperative outcomes. Their findings did not suggest palliative care–associated improvements in patient-reported outcomes in this patient group.

Kopecky KE, Florissi IS, Greer JB, Johnston FM. Palliative care interventions for surgical patients: a narrative review. *Ann Palliat Med.* 2022;11(11):3530-3541.

This narrative review explores the literature in the field of palliative care interventions published after the systematic review by Lilley et al.

Lilley EJ, Cooper Z, Schwarze ML, Mosenthal AC. Palliative care in surgery: defining the research priorities. *Ann Surg.* 2018; 267(1):66-72.

This paper reviews the existing science of palliative care in surgery within three priority areas and exposes gaps in the field to define future research priorities.

Lilley EJ, Khan KT, Johnston FM, et al. Palliative care interventions for surgical patients: a systematic review. *JAMA Surg.* 2016;151(2):172-183.

This systematic review characterizes the content, design, and results of a multitude of interventions intended to improve access to palliative care or the quality of palliative care for surgical patients.

Miner TJ, Cohen J, Charpentier K, McPhillips J, Marvell L, Cioffi WG. The palliative triangle: improved patient selection and outcomes associated with palliative operations. *Arch Surg.* 2011;146(5):517-522.

The palliative triangle, a model that can aid in difficult decision-making around palliative surgical procedures, was used to select patients for palliative operations. These carefully selected patients demonstrated significantly better symptom resolution and fewer postoperative complications.

Mosenthal AC, Dunn GP. *Surgical Palliative Care. Integrating Palliative Care.* Oxford University Press; 2019:xii, 367.

This seminal textbook describes core palliative skills and knowledge needed to care for patients with serious illness undergoing surgery.

The full reference list appears on Elsevier eBooks+.

Trauma and Critical Care

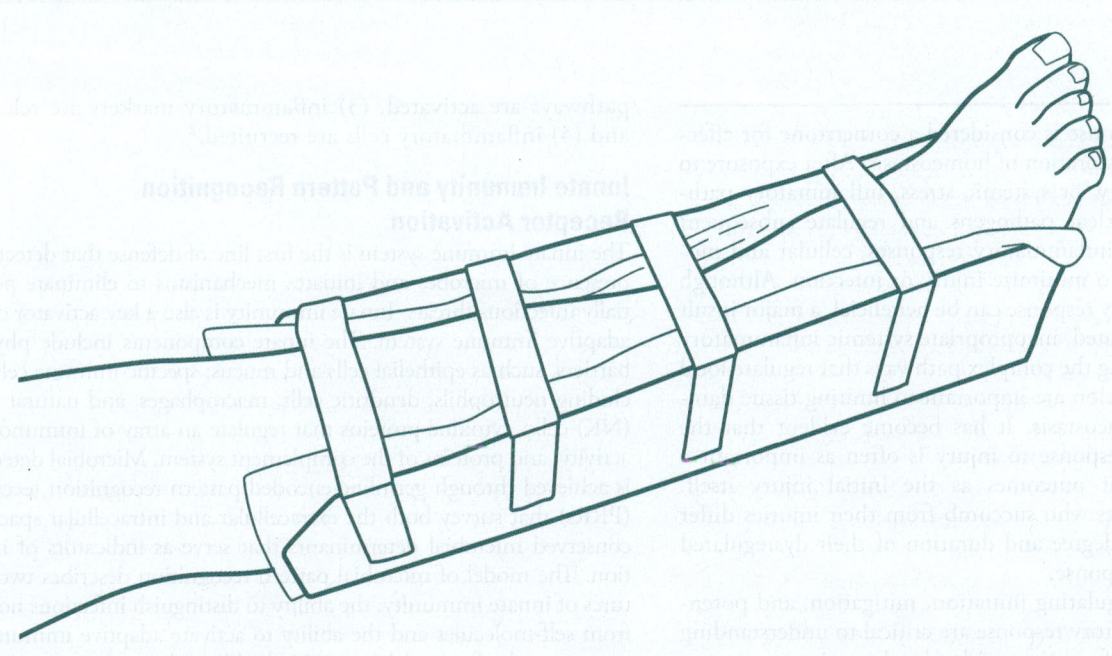

32 CHAPTER

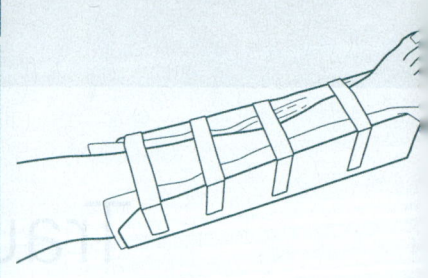

The Inflammatory Response

Letitia E. Bible and Alicia M. Mohr

OUTLINE

Introduction
Inflammatory Response Mechanisms
   Innate Immunity and Pattern Recognition Receptor
     Activation
   Activation of Inflammatory Pathways
   Inflammatory Markers
   Cellular Components
   Microbiome
   Extracellular Vesicles

Stress Response and Inflammation
   The Nervous System and Immunity
   The Inflammatory Reflex
   Chronic Inflammatory Response
Inflammation and the Critically Ill
   Expected and Pathologic Courses of Inflammation
   Interventions

INTRODUCTION

The inflammatory response is considered a cornerstone for effective tissue repair and restoration of homeostasis. After exposure to foreign microbes, injury, or systemic stress, inflammatory pathways are initiated to clear pathogens and regulate subsequent healing. During acute inflammatory responses, cellular and molecular events interact to minimize injury or infection. Although a localized inflammatory response can be beneficial, a major insult can result in a dysregulated, inappropriate systemic inflammatory response. Understanding the complex pathways that regulate local and systemic inflammation are important to limiting tissue damage and restoring homeostasis. It has become evident that the body's inflammatory response to injury is often as important a determinant in patient outcomes as the initial injury itself. Severely injured patients who succumb from their injuries differ from survivors in the degree and duration of their dysregulated acute inflammatory response.[1]

The mechanisms regulating initiation, mitigation, and potentiation of the inflammatory response are critical to understanding the many phenotypes of a patient with a local reaction to surgery, systemic inflammatory response syndrome (SIRS), multiple organ failure, and chronic critical illness (CCI).

INFLAMMATORY RESPONSE MECHANISMS

At the tissue level, inflammation is characterized by redness, swelling, heat, pain, and loss of tissue function, which result from immune, vascular, and inflammatory cell responses. The inflammatory response is the coordinated activation of signaling pathways that regulate inflammatory cells from the blood and inflammatory mediators in resident tissue cells. Inflammatory response processes depend on the nature of the stimulus and its location in the body, but they all share common mechanisms: (1) cell surface pattern receptors recognize stimuli, (2) inflammatory

pathways are activated, (3) inflammatory markers are released, and (4) inflammatory cells are recruited.[2]

Innate Immunity and Pattern Recognition Receptor Activation

The innate immune system is the first line of defense that detects the presence of microbes and initiates mechanisms to eliminate potentially infectious threats. Innate immunity is also a key activator of the adaptive immune system. The innate components include physical barriers, such as epithelial cells and mucus; specific immune cells including neutrophils, dendritic cells, macrophages, and natural killer (NK) cells; cytokine proteins that regulate an array of immunologic activity; and proteins of the complement system. Microbial detection is achieved through germline-encoded pattern recognition receptors (PRRs) that survey both the extracellular and intracellular space for conserved microbial determinants that serve as indicators of infection. The model of microbial pattern recognition describes two features of innate immunity: the ability to distinguish infectious nonself from self-molecules and the ability to activate adaptive immune responses to the former.[3] Many microbial ligands, ranging from structural components of bacteria, fungi, and viruses to biosynthetic molecules such as nucleic acids, activate PRRs and induce the innate immune responses that protect us from infectious threats.[3]

Microbial structures known as *pathogen-associated molecular patterns (PAMPs)* can trigger the inflammatory response through activation of PRRs. Some PRRs also recognize various endogenous signals activated during tissue or cell damage and are known as *danger-associated molecular patterns (DAMPs),* also termed *alarmins* (Fig. 32.1). DAMPs are host biomolecules that can initiate and perpetuate a noninfectious inflammatory response. DAMPs have several characteristics: (1) they are rapidly released following nonprogrammed cell death; (2) cells of the immune system also can be induced to produce and release DAMPs without dying; (3) they recruit and activate receptor-expressing cells of

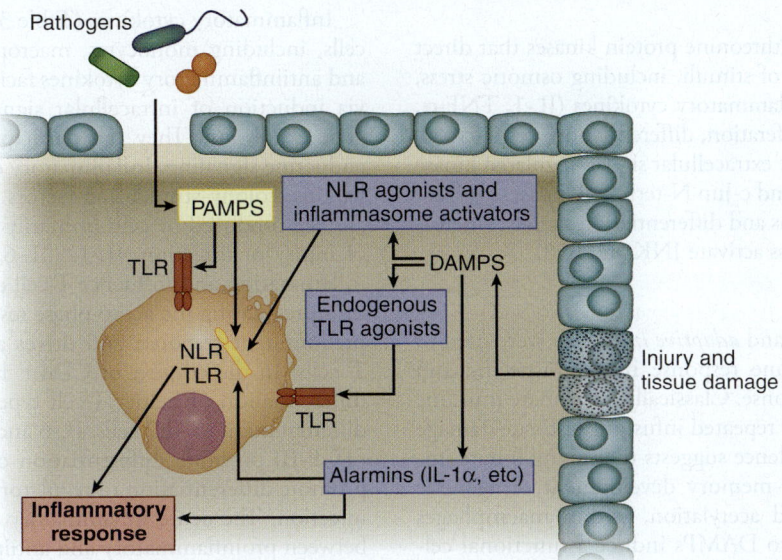

FIGURE 32.1 Pathogen-associated molecular patterns *(PAMPs)* present on foreign invaders and danger-associated molecular patterns *(DAMPs)* prompted by cellular damage trigger multiple cellular signaling pathways via toll-like receptors *(TLRs)* and nucleotide-binding and oligomerization domain–like receptors *(NLRs)*. The result is the production of pro- and antiinflammatory cytokines and the propagation of the inflammatory response. *IL*, Interleukin.

the innate immune system, including dendritic cells, and thus directly or indirectly also promote adaptive immunity responses; and (4) they restore homeostasis by promoting the reconstruction of the tissue that was destroyed either because of the direct insult or the secondary effects of inflammation.

DAMPs are recognized by PRRs that are found either on the cell surface or intracellularly. Classes of PRR families include toll-like receptors (TLRs), C-type lectin receptors (CLRs), retinoic acid–inducible gene (RIG)-I-receptors, AIM2-like receptors, and leucine-rich repeat (LRR)–containing (or NOD-like) receptors. TLRs are the most well studied of the known PRRs. Signaling through TLRs activates an intracellular signaling cascade that leads to nuclear translocation of transcription factors, such as nuclear factor kappa-B (NF-κB) or interferon regulatory factor 3 (IRF3). These transcription factors bind to regulatory elements in promoters of target genes that include interferon (IFN)-α and tumor necrosis factor (TNF). DAMPs and PAMPs share receptors, such as TLR4, suggesting similarities between infectious and noninfectious responses. TLR signaling is controlled at multiple levels, both post transcriptionally via ubiquitination, phosphorylation, and microRNA actions, and by the localization of the TLRs and their signaling complexes within the cell. Ten human TLRs have been identified that trigger a variety of downstream cellular responses. TLR4 plays a key role in recognition of bacterial lipopolysaccharide (LPS), and TLR1, TLR2, and TLR6 recognize other common bacterial lipoproteins. TLR4 additionally plays a role in recognition of high-mobility group box protein 1 (HMGB1) and heat shock protein 70, two common DAMPs, as well as mediation of sterile inflammation in the setting of ischemia-reperfusion injury. TLR3 recognizes double-stranded ribonucleic acid (RNA), and TLR7 and TLR8 recognize single-stranded RNA specific to viral invaders.[4]

Another well-characterized family of PRRs is the NLR family. NLRs are assembled in the cytoplasm to form a key intracellular structure known as the *inflammasome*, an essential intracellular PRR. NLRs complex with apoptosis-associated specklike protein containing a caspase recruitment domain to form the inflammasome.[5] The inflammasome plays an essential role in regulating sterile inflammation via recognition of endogenous alarmins, as well as activating the innate immune response via recognition of foreign PAMPs. The best-studied NLR is NLRP3. Once an NLRP3 inflammasome has been primed, it activates protease caspase 1. Caspase 1 is essential in the cleaving and subsequent secretion of proinflammatory cytokines interleukin (IL)-1β and IL-18 by macrophages in addition to the proinflammatory alarmin, HMGB1. The inflammasome plays a key role in the sterile inflammatory process that accompanies metabolic diseases, atherosclerosis, and neuroinflammatory disorders. Emerging evidence suggests that the NLRP3 inflammasome also plays a role in cardiomyopathy associated with sepsis.[6]

Activation of Inflammatory Pathways

Inflammatory pathways involve common inflammatory mediators and regulatory pathways. Primary inflammatory stimuli, including microbial products and cytokines such as IL-1β and IL-6 and TNF-α, mediate inflammation through interaction with TLRs, IL-1 receptor, IL-6 receptor, and TNF receptor. Receptor activation triggers important intracellular signaling pathways, including mitogen-activated protein kinase (MAPK), NF-κB, and Janus kinase (JAK) signal transducer and activator of transcription (STAT) pathways.

NF-κB Pathway

The NF-κB transcription factor plays important roles in inflammation and the immune response as well as apoptosis. NF-κB activity is induced by a range of stimuli, including pathogen-derived substances, inflammatory cytokines, and many enzymes. LPS interacts with TLR4, leading to the release of NF-κB, allowing its transport into the nucleus and upregulating the transcription of many genes involved in cytokine production. IκB proteins in the cytoplasm inhibit NF-κB transcription factor. This pathway regulates proinflammatory cytokine production and inflammatory cell recruitment.

MAPK Pathway

MAPKs are a family of serine/threonine protein kinases that direct cellular responses to a variety of stimuli, including osmotic stress, mitogens, heat shock, and inflammatory cytokines (IL-1, TNF-α, IL-6), which regulate cell proliferation, differentiation, cell survival, and apoptosis. MAPKs include extracellular signal–regulated kinase (ERK1/2), p38 MAP kinase, and c-Jun N-terminal kinases (JNKs). ERKs are activated by mitogens and differentiation signals, whereas inflammatory stimuli and stress activate JNK and p38.

Adaptive Immunity

Historically, the terms *innate* and *adaptive immunity* were used to broadly categorize the immune response into nonspecific and specific phases of cellular response. Classically, the innate immune response responds the same to repeated infusions of tissue damage or infection. More recent evidence suggests that many innate immune cells have capacity for memory development. Epigenetic changes, via methylation and acetylation, within macrophages and NK cells after exposure to DAMPs induce a functional cellular reprogramming. Therefore, the line between innate and adaptive immunity has become less distinct.[7,8]

Adaptive immunity is characterized by a targeted immune response to an invading pathogen and the subsequent development of memory cells. If the pathogen is encountered again, memory cells induce a vigorous, specific immune response. The adaptive immune system retains one critical, unique function, that is, the ability to undergo clonal expansion and the clonal expression of highly diversified antigen receptors, including T-cell receptors (TCRs) and immunoglobulins (Igs).[7]

Adaptive immunity is further categorized into the humoral immune response and the cell-mediated immune response. The cell-mediated immune response is driven by activated T lymphocytes; the effects of T cells are driven by cytokines. The humoral immune response is directed by activated B cells; Igs and cytokines carry out the end effects of the humoral immune system. In cellular immunity, when the TCR recognizes its corresponding antigen–major histocompatibility class (MHC) complex, the T cell undergoes maturation and differentiation. Essential in this process is IL-2, a potent T-cell growth factor. IL-2 is produced by CD4+ helper T cells and results in accelerated T-lymphocyte differentiation and clonal expansion. IL-2 also promotes survival of regulatory T cells. In a secondary response to a repeat provocation of the immune system, IL-2 can be produced by CD8+ cytotoxic T cells directly. This drives rapid CD8+ cytotoxic T-cell expansion and activation, rather than CD8+ cells depending on CD4+ cells for stimulation by IL-2.[9] The humoral immune response is driven by activated B lymphocytes. In contrast to T cells, which require the presence of MHC molecules to recognize an antigen, B cells can recognize lone soluble and membrane-bound antigens via the B-cell receptor. Once an antigen is recognized, the B cell requires costimulatory signals for full activation. The costimulatory signals are provided by CD4+ helper T cells. The result is B-cell maturation; class switching to IgG, IgA, and IgE production; and B-cell clonal expansion.

Inflammatory Markers

Inflammatory markers are predictive of inflammatory diseases and correlate with the consequences of various inflammatory diseases, such as infection, endothelial dysfunction, and cardiovascular diseases. Inflammatory cytokines and proteins can potentially serve as biomarkers for disease diagnosis, prognosis, and therapeutic decisions.

Inflammatory cytokines (Table 32.1) are released from immune cells, including monocytes, macrophages, and lymphocytes. Pro- and antiinflammatory cytokines facilitate and inhibit inflammation via induction of intracellular signaling pathways that influence gene expression. They can participate in autocrine, paracrine, or endocrine signaling. Inflammatory cytokines are classified as interleukins, colony-stimulating factors (CSFs), IFN, and chemokines and are produced by cells primarily to recruit leukocytes to the site of injury or infection. IL-12, IL-6, and TNF-α potentiate acute inflammation and influence T-cell differentiation. IL-1 is essential for upregulating the acute-phase response. IFN drives an antiviral-predominant response and drives activation of CD8+ cytotoxic T cells. In the context of CD4+ helper T cells, IL-12 promotes differentiation of helper T-cell type 1 (Th1) cells. IL-4 promotes differentiation to Th2 cells. IL-6 and transforming growth factor-β (TGF-β) promote differentiation of Th17 cells. TGF-β can also promote differentiation to regulatory-type T cells in the absence of infection. The acute inflammatory response is a complex balance between proinflammatory and antiinflammatory mediators. Excessive inflammatory cytokine production can lead to tissue damage, hemodynamic changes, organ failure, and death. Proinflammatory cytokines are also intricately involved in the procoagulant state seen in trauma and infection.

Key cytokines involved in the acute proinflammatory response include TNF-α, IL-1, IL-6, IL-8, IL-12, and IFN-γ.[10,11] TNF-α and IL-1β are considered hyperacute mediators of the acute inflammatory response, exhibiting effects within 1 to 2 hours of injury, whereas IL-6 and IL-8 function in a subacute fashion between 1 and 4 hours with a more sustained plasma concentration. Neither TNF-α nor IL-1β have been proven to be a valuable prognosticator for injury severity or predict organ dysfunction because of their short half-life. Both TNF-α and IL-1 mediate the fever response and are thus pyrogens. In addition to being secreted by macrophages, TNF-α and IL-1 act on macrophages in an autocrine and paracrine fashion to promote increased macrophage production, activity, and survival. Both TNF-α and IL-1, and the various cytokines they induce, also activate the hypothalamic-pituitary-adrenal (HPA) axis and increase cortisol production.

IL-6 is considered a secondary cytokine, induced by TNF-α, IL-1, and bacterial endotoxin. IL-6 is secreted from multiple cell types, primarily macrophages, dendritic cells, lymphocytes, endothelial cells, fibroblasts, and smooth muscle cells. The key function of IL-6 is to mediate the acute-phase response, an early stage of the inflammatory cascade characterized by fever, leukocytosis, and an increase in acute-phase reactants. In trauma patients with sepsis and multiple organ dysfunction, IL-6 is considered an accurate prognosticator of outcome, and sustained increases of IL-6 correlate with a poor prognosis.[10,11] IL-6 not only influences the innate immune response, but it also has direct influence on the adaptive immune response by facilitating the activation and differentiation of T and B cells. Of note, IL-6 also has antiinflammatory effects. IL-6 inhibits the subsequent release of TNF-α and IL-1 and stimulates the release of IL-10 and TGF-β. Prostaglandin E2, a potent endogenous immunosuppressant, is released from macrophages after IL-6 signaling.

The antiinflammatory cytokine IL-4 is secreted by innate immune cells common to the inflammatory response directed against extracellular pathogens, including mast cells, basophils, and eosinophils, as well as the adaptive immunity Th2 cell. It can act in both autocrine and paracrine pathways to increase release of IL-4, TGF-β, and IL-10. The most well-characterized role of IL-4 is the promotion of Th2-cell differentiation and simultaneous

TABLE 32.1 Cytokines: Cellular Sources and Immunologic Effects

CYTOKINE	SOURCE	EFFECT
IL-1	Macrophages, neutrophils, epithelial cells, endothelial cells, fibroblasts	Induces fever, increases ACTH secretion, and glucocorticoids
IL-2	Th1 cells	Promotes differentiation of T cells, promotes proliferation of activated B cells, increases cytotoxicity of NK cells
IL-3	T cells, NK cells	Stimulates differentiation of hematopoietic stem cells
IL-4	Th2 cells, mast cells, macrophages	Promotes growth and differentiation of B cells, mediates allergic and antiinflammatory responses
IL-5	Th2 cells, mast cells, eosinophils	Increases secretion of immunoglobulins, activates eosinophils
IL-6	Macrophages, Th2 cells, B cells, fibroblasts	Increases hepatic acute-phase proteins, promotes B-cell maturation and differentiation, stimulates HPA axis, induces fever
IL-7	Dendritic cells, fibroblasts	Promotes development of B and T cells
IL-8	Macrophages	Stimulates chemotaxis by neutrophils, stimulates oxidative burst by neutrophils
IL-9	Th2 cells	Promotes proliferation of activated T cells, prevents apoptosis
IL-10	Th2 cells, B cells, monocytes	Antiinflammatory
IL-11	Dendritic cells, bone marrow	Increases production of platelets, inhibits proliferation of fibroblasts
IL-12	Macrophages, B cells, Langerhans cells	Antiangiogenesis, stimulates differentiation of T cells
IL-23	Macrophages, dendritic cells	With TGF-β, promotes differentiation of naïve T cells into Th17 cells
IL-27	Macrophages, dendritic cells	Suppresses effector functions of lymphocytes and macrophages
IFN-α	Leukocytes	Increases expression of cell surface class I MHC molecules; inhibits viral replication
IFN-γ	Th1 cells	Activates macrophages, promotes differentiation of CD4+ T cells into Th1 cells, inhibits differentiation of CD4+ T cells into Th2 cells
TNF-α	Macrophages, T cells, fibroblasts	Induces cachexia, increases expression of adhesion molecules, activates neutrophils and macrophages
GM-CSF	Macrophages, T cells, fibroblasts, endothelial cells	Stimulates granulocyte and monocyte production
G-CSF	Macrophages, fibroblasts	Enhances production of granulocytes by bone marrow
TGF-β	Macrophages, neutrophils	Antiinflammatory

ACTH, Adrenocorticotropic hormone; *G-CSF,* granulocyte colony-stimulating factor; *GM-CSF,* granulocyte-macrophage colony-stimulating factor; *HPA,* hypothalamic-pituitary-adrenal; *IFN,* interferon; *IL,* interleukin; *MHC,* major histocompatibility class; *NK,* natural killer; *Th1/Th2,* T helper cell type 1/type 2; *TGF-β,* transforming growth factor beta; *TNF-α,* tumor necrosis factor alpha.

inhibition of Th1-cell differentiation. Thus, IL-4 promotes the humoral, B-cell–mediated immune response and antagonizes the cell-mediated cytotoxic immune response.[10]

IL-10 is produced by cells of the innate and adaptive immune systems, including monocytes, macrophages, NK cells, and lymphocytes. IL-10 downregulates the expression of proinflammatory TNF-α, IL-1, IL-6, and IFN-γ while simultaneously upregulating the expression of proinflammatory cytokine modulators to neutralize circulating TNF-α and IL-1. IL-10 impairs phagocytosis and prevents efficient antigen presentation among antigen-presenting cells (APCs).

TGF-β is a cytokine with an array of functions that overall exert an antiinflammatory effect. It has three isoforms—TGF-β₁, -β₂, and -β₃—that exhibit overlapping functions. TGF-β₁ is found within the bone, cartilage, and skin; TGF-β₂ is expressed in neurons and astroglial cells; and TGF-β₃ is localized to the palate and lung tissue. TGF-β regulates the epithelial-to-mesenchymal transition, a process essential for embryonic development, tissue remodeling, and wound repair. TGF-β upregulates vascular endothelial growth factor (VEGF) on endothelial cells and is intricately involved in angiogenesis. It also inhibits various T-cell functions, including IL-2 secretion and T-cell proliferation; the presence of TGF-β promotes the development of immunosuppressive regulatory T cells. Proinflammatory mediators from monocytes and macrophages, including IL-1, TNF-α, and HMGB1, are suppressed by TGF-β, whereas the immunosuppressive soluble TNF receptor and IL-1 receptor antagonist are upregulated by TGF-β.[10]

Inflammatory proteins in the blood, including C-reactive protein (CRP), haptoglobin, HMGB1, heat shock proteins, and α₁-acid glycoprotein, help restore homeostasis and reduce microbial growth. HMGB1 is an endogenous DAMP that mediates many downstream effects within the inflammatory cascade. Within the nucleus, HMGB1 plays a role in the regulation of gene transcription. Extracellular HMGB1 stimulates release of proinflammatory cytokines TNF-α, IL-1, IL-6, and IL-18 and macrophage inflammatory protein 1 (MIP-1). It also serves as a chemoattractant for macrophages and neutrophils. HMGB1 is a rapidly growing target of molecular and clinical research, both as a predictor of morbidity and mortality and an immunologic therapeutic target.[12] It has clinical implications in many acute conditions, including sepsis and hemorrhagic shock, as well as conditions of chronic inflammation, such as atherosclerosis and inflammatory bowel disease, and displays a key role in both pathogen-associated immune response and sterile immunity.[12]

In addition to inflammatory proteins, there is also abnormal activation of certain enzymes during inflammation and oxidative stress. These include superoxide dismutase (SOD), NADPH oxidase (NOX), inducible nitric oxide synthase (iNOS), and cyclooxygenase (COX)-2. Antioxidant defense systems, including antioxidant enzymes, influence oxidative stress. Elevated oxidative stress can induce production of reactive oxygen species (ROS), malondialdehyde (MDA), and isoprostanes, each of which activates various transcription factors. Nitric oxide is another inflammatory mediator that functions at the level of the microvasculature. In response to hypoxia, cellular injury, and endotoxin, the endothelium generates nitric oxide, which causes vasodilation and a reduction of platelet aggregation. Upregulation of iNOS results in a large quantity of nitric oxide, which contributes to excessive vasodilation seen in a dysregulated inflammatory response such as septic shock. Oxidative stress is associated with the pathogenesis of multiple diseases, such as cardiovascular disease, cancer, diabetes, hypertension, aging, and atherosclerosis.

Cellular Components

Endothelial Cells

Damaged endothelial cells release factors that trigger the inflammatory cascade. Endothelial cells also regulate leukocyte access to the tissues. During acute or chronic inflammatory responses, leukocytes exit the circulation and enter the tissues via postcapillary venules. After activation, endothelial cells undergo structural and functional changes that lead to the extravasation of fluid. Selectin, adhesion molecules, and chemokines are expressed and released. Finally, the release of proinflammatory chemokines is abrogated, and the endothelial barrier and vascular function is restored. During the entire process of acute, resolving inflammation, the endothelial cell serves as a gatekeeper, controlling which cell type enters the site of inflammation.

Neutrophils

The neutrophil, a type of polymorphonuclear (PMN) leukocyte, is a potent mediator of acute inflammation and is often the first cell type recruited in response to injury. Neutrophils are produced in the bone marrow in response to granulocyte colony-stimulating factor (G-CSF), and their production is regulated by IL-17 from T cells and by IL-23 from macrophages. The neutrophil undergoes a process of tethering, rolling, adhesion, crawling, and transmigration to move from the bloodstream to the tissue (Fig. 32.2). Neutrophils contain three types of proinflammatory granules: azurophilic (primary) granules, specific (secondary) granules, and gelatinase (tertiary) granules. Proteolytic contents of

these granules can be released extracellularly or into the intracellular phagosome to aid elimination of invading microbes. Neutrophils also release a fiber meshwork to which histones, proteins, and enzymes adhere; this is the neutrophil extracellular trap (NET). Extracellular pathogens are trapped within the NET to prevent spread of the pathogen and aid phagocytosis.[13] Neutrophils program APCs to activate T cells and release factors to attract monocytes and dendritic cells.

Although classically considered a key mediator of the initial inflammatory response, the functions of the neutrophil have been shown to extend beyond the acute inflammatory period. The neutrophil granules contain a number of proteases that are essential for tissue remodeling and wound healing. They directly stimulate angiogenesis via the release of VEGF. In addition, neutrophils display plasticity, and, although typically proinflammatory, antiinflammatory subsets of neutrophils have been identified in certain pathologic states.[13]

Macrophages

Monocytes, the precursor to the macrophage, differentiate into macrophages in response to infection and injury. The macrophage is the key player in innate immunity and a key component of the phagocyte system. During inflammation, macrophages present antigens, undergo phagocytosis, and modulate the immune response by producing cytokines and growth factors. In inflammation, macrophages play a role in initiation, maintenance, and resolution.

In response to PRR stimulation, macrophages neutralize invading pathogens via phagocytosis and lysosomal degradation; they additionally secrete proinflammatory mediators, including IL-1β and TNF-α, that recruit other immune cells to the damaged tissue. Macrophages also process antigenic substances and present them on their surface to help stimulate the differentiation of helper T cells. Macrophages demonstrate plasticity and phenotypic variance depending on environment. M1 macrophages express proinflammatory cytokines and proteolytic substances; they

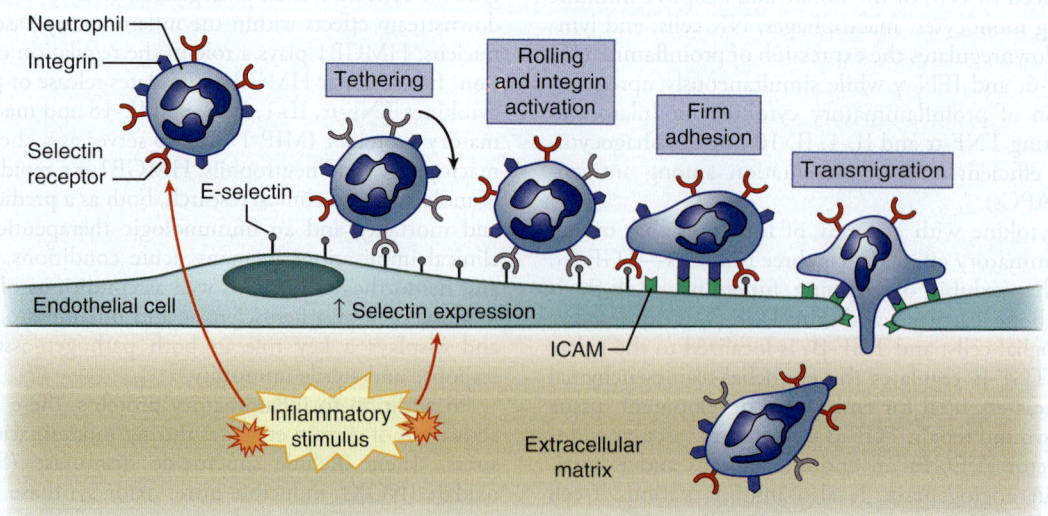

FIGURE 32.2 Neutrophil recruitment and migration from the blood to the peripheral tissue. Once activated by an inflammatory signal, endothelial cells upregulate expression of adhesion molecules or selections. Neutrophils bind selectins and roll along the endothelial cell. Integrins on the neutrophil surface interact tightly with intracellular adhesion molecules (*ICAMs*) on the endothelial cell. Expression of molecules such as cadherin and platelet endothelial cell adhesion molecule facilitate transmigration into the periphery. (Adapted from Ouellete Y. *Pediatric Critical Care*. Philadelphia: Elsevier; 2017.)

predominate in viral and bacterial infection. M1 macrophages also stimulate proinflammatory helper T cells. Although M1 macrophage products facilitate a beneficial inflammatory response against invading microbes, they can result in a dangerous inflammatory state for the human host. High concentrations of M1-type cytokines correlate with mortality in sepsis models. M2 macrophages are essential for tissue remodeling and wound healing; they express a variety of antiinflammatory markers, including IL-10.[14] Macrophages are abundant throughout the body. Their functions vary depending on the tissue in which they reside. For example, Kupffer cells of the liver and microglia of the central nervous system are macrophages.

Dendritic Cells

Dendritic cells bridge the innate and adaptive immune response as the major APC. Upon encountering foreign material, the dendritic cell will engulf and degrade pathogen-derived proteins. These antigenic proteins are loaded onto an MHC complex class I or class II molecule. The antigen-MHC complex is transported to the surface of the dendritic cell, and the dendritic cell travels from the tissue to the lymphoid organs, primarily the lymph nodes, and the spleen. Within the lymphoid organs, it stimulates naïve, resting T cells to differentiate into either cytotoxic T cells or helper T cells.[15] Extracellular proteins are processed within the dendritic cell lysosome, and they are presented in conjunction with the MHC class II molecule to activate CD4+ helper T cells. In contrast, intracellular proteins are processed within the cytosol by the proteasome, and they are presented via the MHC class I molecule to CD8+ cytotoxic T cells. Certain subsets of dendritic cells process extracellular proteins through a process called cross-presentation and allow for presentation of these molecules via MHC class I. Through the process of MHC-antigen presentation, the adaptive immune response is initiated.[7] As a result of its many costimulatory mechanisms, dendritic cells are highly efficient at provoking the adaptive immune response. Although macrophages and B cells are also considered APCs, they do not function at this level of efficiency for adaptive immune stimulation.

Dendritic cells also process self-antigens and nonpathogenic antigens. Presentation of this antigen type to a naïve T cell induces the regulatory T cell, an immunosuppressive cell type, essential for tolerance and immune homeostasis. Disorders of this pathway result in autoimmunity to self-antigens and allergy response against nonpathogenic environmental material. The fact that dendritic cells use similar machinery to induce both an active immune response to foreign pathogens and a tolerant response toward self-antigens is an interesting paradox and an area of interest in cancer immunobiology. Tumor cells can be considered master evaders of the immune system.

T Cells (T Lymphocytes)

T and B lymphocytes are the primary effector cells of the adaptive immune system; T cells are the primary effector cells of the cellular immune response, whereas B cells primarily mediate the humoral immune response. T and B cells are unique in their ability to recognize specific antigens and rapidly respond through clonal expansion. They are essential for the development of immune memory.

T-cell activation is a complex, multifaceted process. It can be simplified to three key steps, while keeping in mind that activation of the immune system is not a linear process, and there are many branch points within the pathway that influence the ultimate outcome. Once transported to the lymphoid organs, mature dendritic cells present antigen-MHC complexes to naïve T cells. Antigens derived from cytosolic proteins are presented via the MHC class I molecule; the antigen-MHC class I complex activates CD8+ cytotoxic T cells. Antigens derived from extracellular proteins are presented via the MHC class II molecule; the antigen-MHC class II complex activates CD4+ helper T cells. Whereas MHC class I molecules can be found on all nucleated cells, MHC class II is confined to APCs. Although consistent with classic teaching, emerging research indicates that the formation of antigen-MHC complexes is not so straightforward. Activation of certain PRRs can alter whether a protein is loaded onto an MHC class I or MHC class II receptor after uptake. For example, activation of TLR4 at the cell surface transiently results in an increase in cross-presentation and thus an increase in loading of antigenic peptides onto MHC class I molecules with activation of CD8+ cytotoxic T cells. However, once engulfed within the endosome, TLR4 switches to promote loading of antigenic peptides onto MHC class II molecules; this ultimately promotes a CD4+ helper T-cell–predominant immune response.[16]

As self-antigens and benign environmental antigens can be loaded on to MHC molecules, presentation of the antigen-MHC complex alone is not sufficient to activate the adaptive immune pathway. Costimulatory molecules are additionally necessary for full T-cell activation, most notably, CD80 and CD86, located on the activated dendritic cell and its interaction with CD28 upon T cells (Fig. 32.3). Stimulation of CD28 pathways results in a lower threshold for T-cell activation and production of IL-2.[16]

Cytokines are essential for full T-cell activation, and the innate cytokine milieu varies based on the type of PRR that has been stimulated. Each activated T cell produces a unique profile of cytokines to elicit a variety of downstream effects. Of the CD4+ helper T-cell lineage, the best-characterized cells are Th1, Th2, and Th17 cells. Regarding infection, Th1 cells primarily fight intracellular pathogens and do so via upregulation of IFN-γ and propagation of the inflammatory response. Th2 cells function to clear extracellular pathogens and mediate the allergic response through production of IL-4, IL-5, and IL-13. A growing body of research indicates that a healthy immune response is heavily influenced by the proportional response of Th1 and Th2 cells.[17]

Th17 cells differentiate in response to extracellular pathogens and fungi; they are frequently implicated in autoimmune disorders, and Th17 cells can acquire the characteristic of Th1 cells in chronic inflammatory states. Th17 cells drive production of IL-17. Regulatory T cells, another class of CD4+ helper T cells, are essential for the development of memory and tolerance to self-antigens; they produce potent antiinflammatory cytokines such as IL-10 and TGF-β. CD8+ cytotoxic T cells target cells that have been infected with a virus for destruction, and they produce the potent proinflammatory cytokine IFN-γ.[17] In summary, T-cell activation is achieved by three key steps: presentation of an antigen-MHC complex to a naïve T cell by a mature dendritic cell, costimulation of the T cell by surface molecules located on the dendritic cell, and the presence of cytokines produced by cells of the innate immune system.[16]

B Cells (B Lymphocytes)

B cells are the primary effector cells of the humoral immune response and produce antibodies or Igs and function as APCs. B cells initially develop in the bone marrow, where their cellular maturation can be correlated to the rearrangement of the Ig gene segments. B cells have the capacity to recognize more than 5×10^{13} different antibodies. Surface-bound IgM marks the entrance of

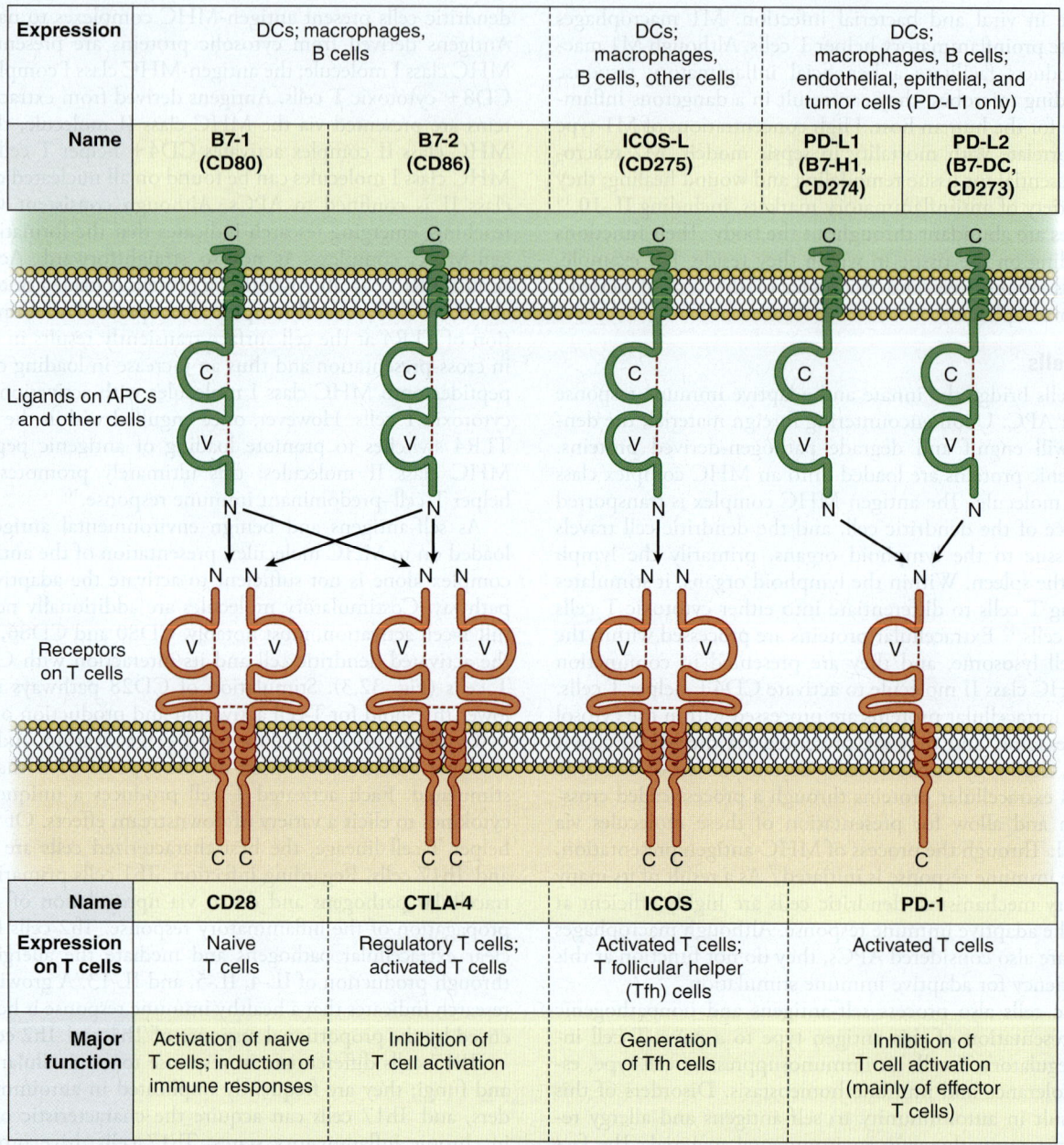

Expression	DCs; macrophages, B cells		DCs; macrophages, B cells, other cells	DCs; macrophages, B cells; endothelial, epithelial, and tumor cells (PD-L1 only)	
Name	B7-1 (CD80)	B7-2 (CD86)	ICOS-L (CD275)	PD-L1 (B7-H1, CD274)	PD-L2 (B7-DC, CD273)

Ligands on APCs and other cells

Receptors on T cells

Name	CD28	CTLA-4	ICOS	PD-1
Expression on T cells	Naïve T cells	Regulatory T cells; activated T cells	Activated T cells; T follicular helper (Tfh) cells	Activated T cells
Major function	Activation of naive T cells; induction of immune responses	Inhibition of T cell activation	Generation of Tfh cells	Inhibition of T cell activation (mainly of effector T cells)

FIGURE 32.3 Costimulatory molecules of the B7 family, including CD80/CD86, are expressed on antigen-presenting cells *(APCs)*. CD28 receptors are expressed primarily on naïve T cells. The ligand-receptor binding produces a different effect depending on the type of T cells being stimulated. *CTLA-4,* Cytotoxic T-lympho-cyte–associated protein 4; *DCs,* dendridic cells; *ICOS,* inducible T-cell costimulator; *ICOS-L,* Inducible T Cell Costimulatot ligand; *PD-1,* programmed cell death 1; *PD-L1,* programmed cell death ligand 1. (Adapted from Abbas AK, Lichtman AH, Pillai S. *Cellular and Molecular Immunology.* Philadelphia: Elsevier; 2018.)

the B cell into the immature B-cell state; it is at this point that it leaves the bone marrow and migrates to the spleen. Within the spleen, immature B cells will become naïve follicular or marginal zone B cells.[18]

Marginal zone B cells function in the spleen as the first line of defense against blood-borne invaders. These B cells can rapidly produce soluble IgM during the early stages of infection, which is T cell independent. Naïve follicular B cells can be found within the lymph nodes or as circulating B cells. Their activation is T cell dependent. Activation of follicular B cells results in a process termed *class switching* in which B cells transition from the produc-tion of IgM antibodies to the production of other classes of Ig,

primarily IgG, IgA, and IgE, during times of infection. Memory B cells are maintained after an immune response. These memory cells retain the capacity to produce high-affinity Igs toward a cer-tain antigen, and should that antigen ever be introduced again, these B cells can rapidly mount a robust immunologic response.[18]

Natural Killer Cells

NK cells are an innate immune cell type with unique features. They are lymphoid cells that do not express antigen-specific recep-tors derived from exposure to specific antigens, such as T-cell recep-tors or surface Ig on B cells. NK cells are recognized not only for their ability to kill infected cells but also for mediating cytotoxicity against a range of normal immune cells. They thereby play an important physiologic role in controlling immune responses and maintaining homeostasis. NK cells can also alter their behavior based on prior exposure to particular antigens, including after viral infection, by a mechanism that is different from that of T and B cells. In humans, NK cells represent 8% to 20% of circulating lymphocytes. They function in an antigen-independent manner that does not give rise to immunologic memory or long-term protective immunity.

Microbiome

The microbiome, the collection of bacteria, fungi, and viruses that live in and on the body, may also be considered a component of the innate immune system because it profoundly affects mechanisms of host defense.[19,20] The body's microbial composition directly influences the maturation of the immune response and its continued effectiveness, protects against pathogen overgrowth, and modulates the balance between inflammation and immune homeostasis.[19,20] For example, skin microbes interact with the immune system to promote wound healing. Nonpathogenic coagulase-negative staphylococci on the skin produce an antimicrobial peptide that can inhibit growth of pathogenic *Staphylococcus aureus*. Oral microbiota can form symbiotic biofilms that balance pH levels and suppress pathogen growth in the mouth. There are now convincing data that the gut microbiome influences the nervous system, and there are efforts to determine the mechanism and to develop therapeutics capable of acting on the brain.[21]

The term *dysbiosis* refers to an underlying impairment of the functions that regulate gut homeostasis, reflected as a change in the composition, diversity, or metabolites of the microbiome from a healthy pattern to a pattern associated with disease or a predisposition to disease. Antibiotic use is the classic cause of dysbiosis, and *Clostridioides difficile* infection is a common, serious sequelae. Dysbiosis is believed to play a role in obesity, type 2 diabetes,

coronary artery disease, food allergy, asthma, and atopic dermatitis.[22] Because of its role as an orchestrator of biologic processes, the microbiome offers an attractive target for therapeutic intervention. Manipulation of the gut microbiome through dietary change has been used with some success to treat type 2 diabetes.[23] The microbiome-derived metabolite trimethylamine N-oxide promotes immune activation and boosts immune checkpoint blockade in pancreatic cancer.

Extracellular Vesicles

Recently, a new mechanism of intercellular communication has emerged in the form of small extracellular vesicles (EVs). EVs can be divided into apoptotic bodies, microvesicles, and exosomes based on size (Fig. 32.4). Apoptotic bodies are 1 to 5 μm in diameter. Microvesicles, which range in size from 50 to 1000 nm, are produced by the direct germination and division of the plasma membrane into the extracellular space. Exosomes are bilayer, phospholipid membrane vesicles formed by the fusion of polyvesicles and plasma membranes, with a diameter of 30 to 100 nm, and appear as double concave disc-shaped or cup-shaped vesicles when observed under an electron microscope. EVs are involved in several homeostatic processes, including the rapid removal of unnecessary molecules from cells, enabling cell maturation and quick adaptation to environmental changes, and activation of blood clotting. In addition, they modulate the functions of other cells by delivering intercellular signals.[24] As signaling units, EVs affect the functions of other cells through their surface proteins, encapsulated cargo molecules (such as proteins and RNAs), and conveyed lipids and glycans.

All the immune cell types that participate in inflammation can secrete EVs, which in turn have multiple roles in inflammatory processes. EVs have been shown to have both proinflammatory and antiinflammatory roles.[25] The effects of EVs depend on the donor cell type and the phase of inflammation in which the EVs

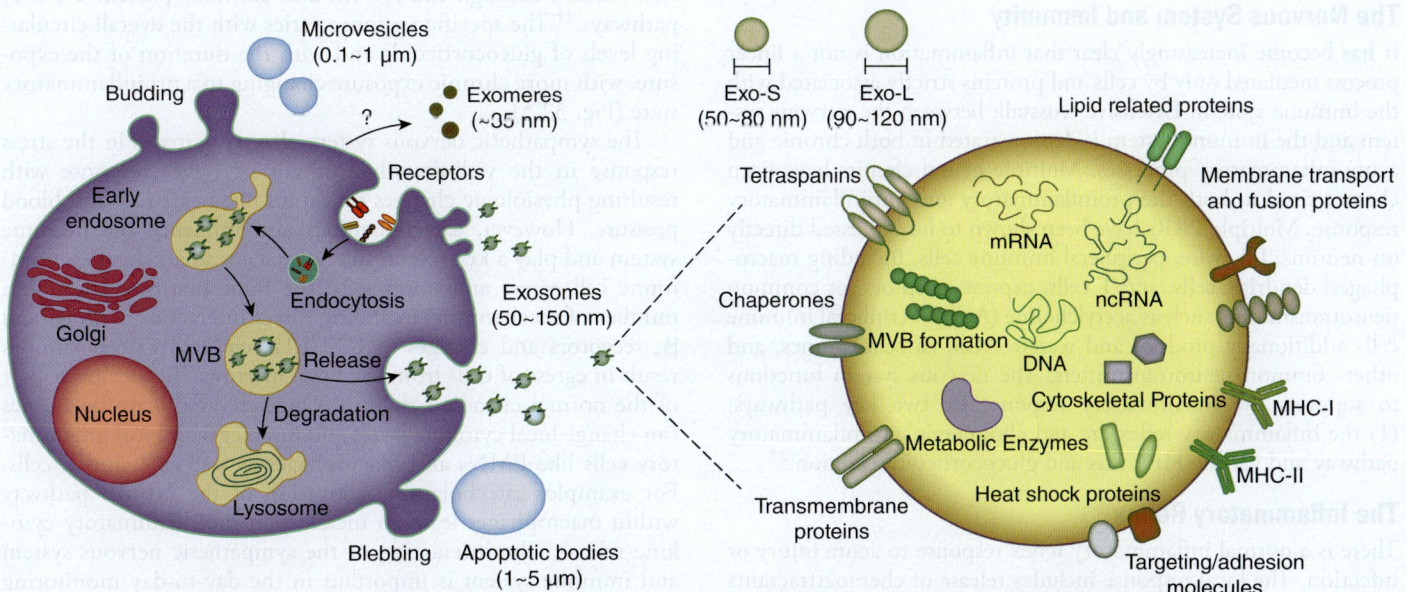

FIGURE 32.4 Exosome biogenesis and composition. Exosomes originate not only from intraluminal vesicles *(ILVs)* in multivesicular bodies *(MVBs)* but also from plasma membrane budding. Microvesicles are generated by budding from the cytomembrane. Apoptotic bodies are generated during programmed cell death *(left)*. Exosomes have spherical structures consisting of a lipid bilayer and contain complex contents, including proteins, mRNA, miRNA, ncRNA, and DNA *(right)*. (Adapted from Zhou X, Xie F, Wang L, et al. The function and clinical application of extracellular vesicles in innate immune regulation. *Cell Mol Immunol.* 2020;17[4]:323-334.)

are analyzed. The proinflammatory effects are related to EV-associated cytokines and DAMPs, which induce macrophage polarization to an M1-type phenotype and cytokine secretion, T helper cell differentiation from naïve T cells, and leukocyte chemotaxis. By contrast, certain EVs have antiinflammatory effects, which include downregulation of complement factors and acute-phase signaling, reduction of leukocyte chemotaxis, reduction in serum proinflammatory cytokine levels, and reduction in the expression of adhesion molecules on endothelial cells. In addition, EVs also play a role in adaptive immunity. EVs play a role in T-cell and B-cell development, antigen presentation to lymphocytes, and the immune synapses formed by lymphocytes.

Numerous molecules known to participate in immune regulation have been identified on the surface of EVs. These include the immune-checkpoint molecules cytotoxic T lymphocyte antigen 4 and programmed cell death ligand 1 (PD-L1), the apoptosis-inducing ligand FASL (also known as *CD95L*), and the ectoenzymes CD39 and CD73, which generate immunosuppressive adenosine from adenosine triphosphate.[26] Regulatory T cells release EVs that contribute to the immunosuppressive activity of these cells by various mechanisms such as by surface expression of CD73. Of note, the activity of T regulatory cell–derived EVs is also mediated by EV-associated microRNAs (such as miR155, Let7b, and Let7d).

Recently, wide attention has been given to the therapeutic potential of EVs. They can serve as the cargo to transfer the bioactive molecules that can be applied as the drug delivery system for treatment of various human diseases. However, this is a complex area of study because EVs are derived from different sources/cell types, and EVs from different conditions and treatments have different cargo compositions and properties. Large-scale prospective clinical trials will be required to investigate the specific therapeutic effects and adverse events of the exogenous EVs before they can be widely used clinically.

STRESS RESPONSE AND INFLAMMATION

The Nervous System and Immunity

It has become increasingly clear that inflammation is not a linear process mediated only by cells and proteins strictly associated with the immune system. Extensive crosstalk between the nervous system and the immune system is demonstrated in both chronic and acute inflammatory processes. Multiple neural circuits have been characterized in both the proinflammatory and antiinflammatory response. Multiple PRRs have been shown to be expressed directly on neurons. Likewise, peripheral immune cells, including macrophages, dendritic cells, and T cells, express receptors for common neurotransmitters such as acetylcholine (ACh). Peripheral immune cells additionally produce and secrete ACh, catecholamines, and other common neurotransmitters. The nervous system functions to suppress the inflammatory response by two key pathways: (1) the inflammatory reflex arc and cholinergic antiinflammatory pathway and (2) the HPA axis and glucocorticoid secretion.[27]

The Inflammatory Reflex

There is a normal inflammatory reflex response to acute injury or infection. The local response includes release of chemoattractants from the tissues and platelets, attracting macrophages and neutrophils. These cells work in conjunction with factors released from the tissues systemically to alert the body to the insult. Inherent to this process is a concomitant reaction to keep the response localized. This essential balance has been studied extensively but has yet to be fully elucidated.

First is the local tissue response to injury or inflammation, which is initiated with the activation of the coagulation cascade and complement cascade. Platelets degranulate, releasing TGF-β, platelet-derived growth factor (PDGF), platelet activating factors, and fibronectin, in addition to local tissue factors that, in reference to inflammation, attract PMNs. PMNs increase endothelial permeability and prostaglandin release and release additional chemoattractants IL-1, TNF-α, and TGF-β, which stimulate neutrophil migration. Macrophages subsequently arrive, increasing ROS and nitric oxide synthase and also releasing TGF-β, VEGF, insulin-like growth factor, and epithelial growth factors. In the standard healing of injured tissues, the T cells arrive and mark the bridge from the inflammatory stage of healing to the proliferative stage. This symphony should be familiar from discussions on the early phase of healing from direct tissue injury. Although these events occur at the local tissue level, many of the factors are released systemically and can activate a systemic response both perpetuating the inflammatory response and inducing an antiinflammatory response.

Systemically, there is a neuroendocrine response to injury, infection, and inflammation in general, through the HPA axis and the sympathetic and parasympathetic nervous system. These systems can be either activated in response to a local injury or infection or primarily activated systemically in response to a stressor. The HPA axis responds to stress signals, like TNF-α, by releasing glucocorticoids, like cortisol. Glucocorticoids have variable and wide-reaching reactions depending on the cell they are interacting with and the local environment of the cell. Steroids are frequently prescribed for their antiinflammatory properties, and elevated glucocorticoids can suppress both IL-1 and TNF with delayed wound healing. They also directly interact with immune cells, changing their receptors and influencing their demargination and homing. After the glucocorticoid binds to the glucocorticoid receptor, the complex translocates to the nucleus and downregulates transcription of proinflammatory genes, most well studied through the NF-κB and activator protein 1 (AP1) pathways.[28] The specific response varies with the overall circulating levels of glucocorticoids and with the duration of the exposure, with more chronic exposure changing to a proinflammatory state (Fig. 32.5).

The sympathetic nervous system also participates in the stress response in the well-described "flight or fight" response with resulting physiologic changes on things like heart rate and blood pressure. However, catecholamines also influence the immune system and play a key role in the normal circadian changes in immune cell egress and homing to the bone marrow. Through a number of mechanisms, including direct interaction with β$_2$ and β$_3$ receptors and changes in CXCL12, elevated catecholamines result in egress of cells from the bone marrow. This occurs as part of the normal circadian rhythm. Once elevated, catecholamines can change local cytokine levels and interact with local inflammatory cells like PMNs and macrophages as well as T and B cells. For example, catecholamine activation of the NF-κB pathway within macrophages leads to increases in proinflammatory cytokine release. The interaction of the sympathetic nervous system and immune system is important in the day-to-day monitoring and is part of the acute inflammatory response. However, like cortisol, the sympathetic system can convert to a more chronic activation of the inflammation pathways. The pathways to chronic inflammation will be reviewed later in this chapter. To balance the local and systemic activation, an antiinflammatory response is modulated through feedback loops (Fig. 32.6).

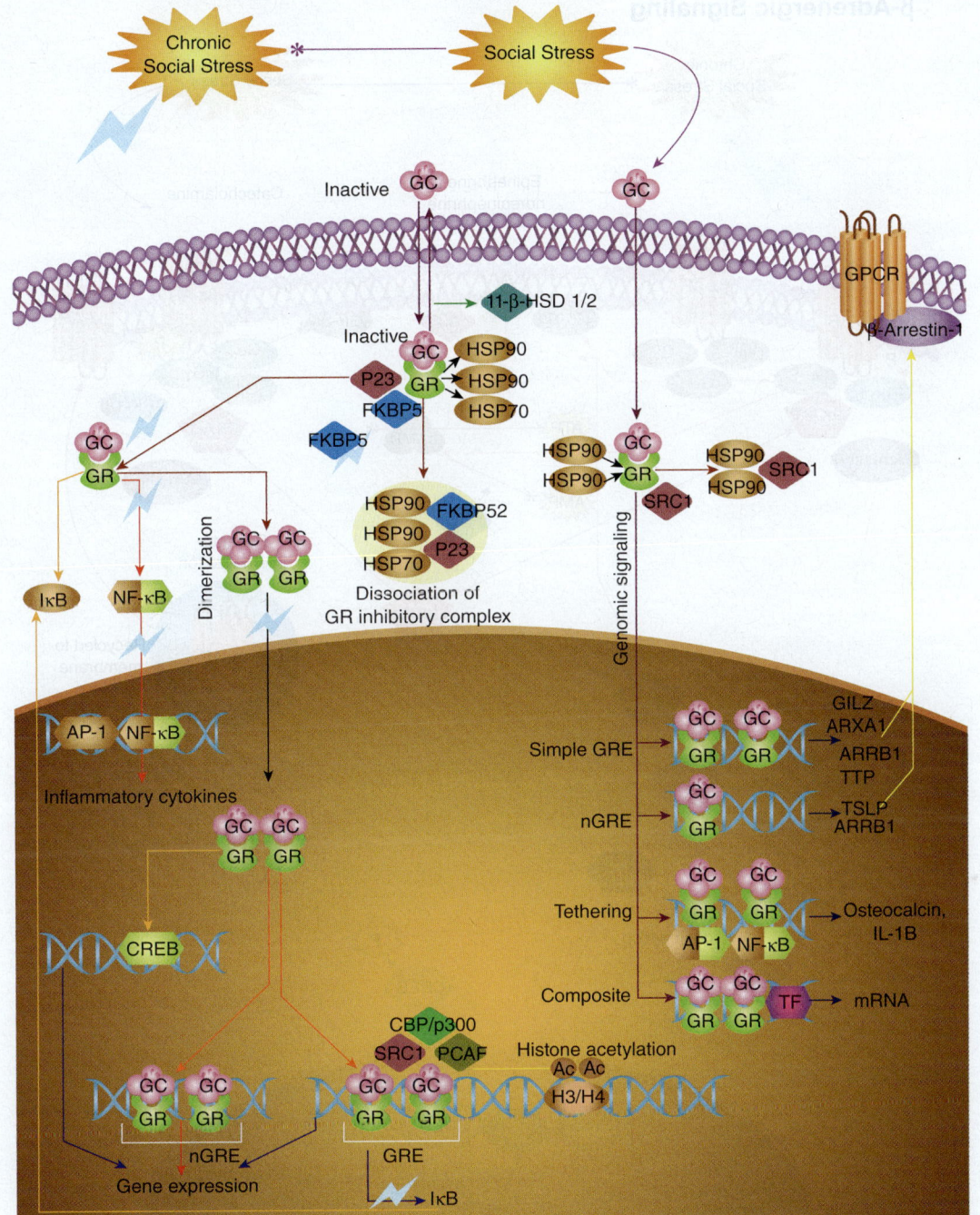

FIGURE 32.5 Chronic stress and intracellular glucocorticoid signaling within an immune cell. *11-β-HSD-1/2,* Enzyme that converts GC from an active to inactive form in the cytoplasm; *AC,* acetylation; *AP-1/NFκB,* activator protein-1/nuclear factor kappa-light-chain-enhancer of activated B cells, proinflammatory transcription factors; *CBP/p300,* CREB-binding protein, a transcription coactivator; *composite,* a GR transcription mechanism in which two GRs dimerize together with another transcription factor (TF); *CREB,* cyclic adenosine monophosphate (cAMP) response element–binding protein, a transcription factor important in immune signaling; *DNA,* deoxyribonucleic acid; *GC,* glucocorticoid; *GR,* glucocorticoid receptor; *GRE/simple GRE,* GR response element, promotes gene transcription; *histone acetylation,* a dynamic gene regulation mechanism that allows transcription factors access to gene transcripts that are tightly packed within structural units; *HSP70/90, FKBP5, P23,* proteins that reduce binding affinity to GCs when associated with the GR; *IκB,* inhibitory protein that sequesters NF-κB in the cytoplasm; *lightning bolt,* alterations in GR signaling as a consequence of chronic stress; *mRNA,* messenger ribonucleic acid, the genetic message to encode proteins; *nGRE,* negatively regulated GRE, largely inhibits gene transcription; *PCAF,* a histone acetyltransferase, promotes transcriptional activation; *SRC1,* steroid receptor coactivator protein; *tethering,* a GR transcription mechanism in which two GRs dimerize. (Adapted from Walsh CP, Bovbjerg DH, Marsland AL. Glucocorticoid resistance and β2-adrenergic receptor signaling pathways promote peripheral pro-inflammatory conditions associated with chronic psychological stress: a systematic review across species. *Neurosci Biobehav Rev.* 2021;128:117-135.)

β-Adrenergic Signaling

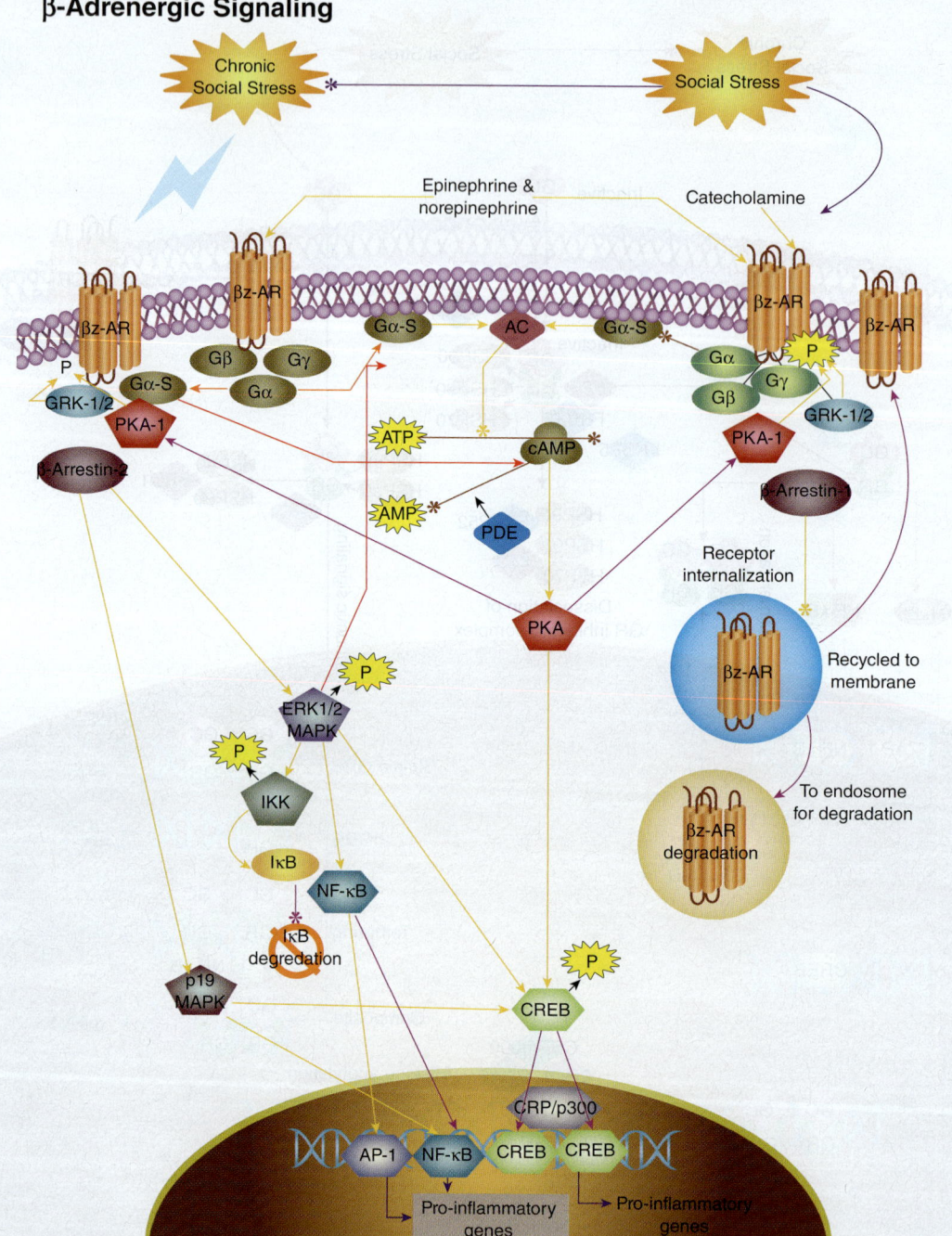

FIGURE 32.6 Chronic stress and intracellular β-adrenergic signaling. *AC,* Adenylate cyclase, enzyme that catalyzes the conversion of ATP to cyclic AMP; *AMP,* adenosine monophosphate; *ATP,* adenosine triphosphate; *AP-1/NF-κB,* activator protein-1/nuclear factor kappa-light-chain-enhancer of activated B cells, proinflammatory transcription factors; *β2-AR,* β2-adrenergic receptor; *β-arrestin,* a scaffolding protein that changes the conformation of the GPCR, can mediate intracellular signaling independent of the β2-AR; *cAMP,* cyclic adenosine monophosphate; *CBP/p300,* CREB-binding protein, a transcription coactivator; *CREB,* cAMP response element–binding protein; *ERK1/2,* extracellular signal-regulated kinase, a conventional MAPK signaling pathway (typically: Ras-Raf-MEK-ERK chain of proteins); *Gα, Gγ, Gβ,* G-proteins that dissociate from the β2-AR on catecholamine binding, mediating downstream signaling; *GαS,* G-protein-alpha-S, dissociation from GPCR activates AC, initiating canonical signaling pathway; *Gαl,* G-protein-alpha-l, recruitment inhibits signaling through canonical pathway; *GPCR,* G-protein coupled receptor; *GRK,* G-protein–coupled receptor kinase; *IκB,* inhibitory protein that sequesters NF-κB in the cytoplasm; *IKK,* IκB kinase, enzyme important in dissociation of IκB from NF-κB, allowing NF-κB to move into the cytoplasm; *MAPK,* mitogen-activated protein kinase, a family of intracellular signaling proteins; *p38,* a conventional MAPK signaling pathway; *PDE,* phosphodiesterase, an enzyme that converts cAMP to AMP; *PKA,* protein kinase A. (Adapted from Walsh CP, Bovbjerg DH, Marsland AL. Glucocorticoid resistance and β2-adrenergic receptor signaling pathways promote peripheral pro-inflammatory conditions associated with chronic psychological stress: a systematic review across species. *Neurosci Biobehav Rev.* 2021;128:117-135.)

Although this can appear counterintuitive, the antiinflammatory response is needed to prevent pathologic inflammation and allow the inflammatory response to localize at the area of insult. The exact mechanism of this response continues to be investigated, with the two major theories being a parasympathetic response through the vagus nerve or direct modulation of the catecholamine response. Like much of medicine, it is a less linear response with multiple pathways and redundancies.

The cholinergic antiinflammatory pathway can modulate the inflammatory response through the vagus nerve. Preclinical models of sepsis and injury have modulated the vagus nerve, resulting in changes in the inflammatory response, with deactivation of the vagus having increased inflammation and reinstituting vagal stimulation returning the antiinflammatory response. Preclinical models of endotoxemia where the vagus nerve has been transected resulted in increased TNF-α and an earlier onset of shock. Within peripheral tissues, the vagus releases ACh, and some subtypes of ACh receptors—the most frequently studied is alpha 7 nicotinic (α7nAChR)—when activated, are associated with inhibition of proinflammatory cytokine production. With activation there is downregulation of TLR4 expression and changes in intracellular signaling pathways through suppression of NF-κB nuclear translocation, which is a known instigator of proinflammatory cytokine production. This nicotinic receptor is found on many immune cells and on the endothelium[29] (Fig. 32.7). Additional studies identified T cells with both choline acetyltransferase (ChAT) and β-adrenergic receptors as an important mediator of the vagus response, especially in tissues without ACh receptors, as found in the spleen.[30] Although further research is ongoing, activation of the vagus nerve alters cell receptor expressions, and through activation of intracellular signaling, there are changes in cytokine production. The vagus nerve also receives information through its afferent fibers. Low levels of circulating IL-1 will activate the vagus to initiate a fever response. If circulating levels are high enough, even with a transected vagus, the same changes will occur. The implication is that the vagus provides extremely sensitive feedback, but if divided, there is a failsafe. Other molecules can interact with the vagus beyond the visceral nerve endings, allowing for feedback at its various synapses. Alternatively, or in conjunction, the catecholamine elevation associated with injury and infection leads to direct activation of immune cells and alters end organs. Adrenergic receptors within the bone marrow play a role in demarginating progenitor and immune cells and as receptors on some of the individual immune cells. There is conflicting evidence involving activation of the antiinflammatory reflex through the splanchnic nerve activation from the sympathetic chain rather than directly through the vagus nerve; in animal models, no activation potential is seen in the splenic nerve from vagus activation.[30,31] Additionally, there is evidence that the ChAT lymphocytes may be activated through upregulation of chemokine CXCL13 after sympathetic activation.[32]

The activation overlap of the proinflammatory and antiinflammatory systems at the local level allows for the eventual return to homeostasis and progression of the normal healing pathway. There are many places where this delicate equilibrium can be tilted, leading to a chronic and more detrimental response.

Chronic Inflammatory Response

The pathway to chronic proinflammatory activation is thought to be from an inability of the antiinflammatory pathways to appropriately downregulate the proinflammatory state or from continued excessive activation or a combination and is thought to be

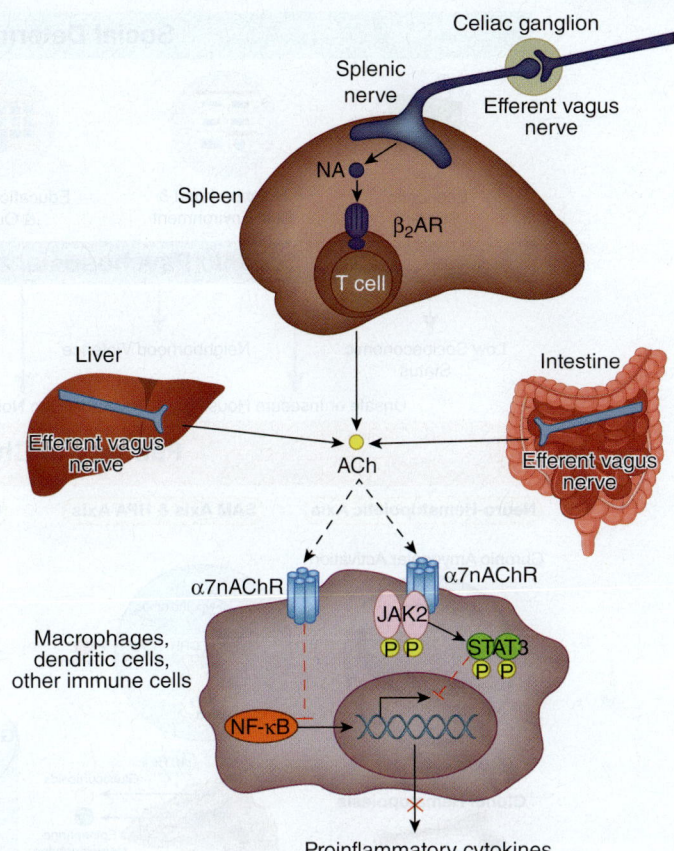

FIGURE 32.7 Molecular mechanisms of cholinergic control of inflammation. Efferent vagus nerve activity is translated into catecholamine-mediated activation of T cell–derived acetylcholine release in the spleen and into direct acetylcholine release from efferent vagus nerve endings in other organs. Inhibition of NF-κB nuclear translocation and activation of a JAK2–STAT3-mediated signaling cascade in macrophages and other immune cells are implicated in cholinergic α7nAChR-mediated control of proinflammatory cytokine production. *α7nAChR*, α7 nicotinic acetylcholine receptor; *ACh*, acetylcholine; *β2AR*, β2 adrenergic receptor; *JAK2*, Janus kinase 2; *NA*, noradrenaline; *NF-κB*, nuclear factor κB; *STAT3*, signal transducer and activator of transcription 3. (Adapted from Pavlov VA, Tracey KJ. The vagus nerve and the inflammatory reflex – linking immunity and metabolism. *Nat Rev Endocrinol.* 2012;8[12]:743-754.)

mediated by changes in the immune system, frequently referred to as *reprogramming scars*. Through the aberrant activation, changes in the pathways occur, leading to new activation thresholds. These changes can include everything from epigenetic changes to microbiome changes and can occur throughout the patients' lifetime (Fig. 32.8). For example, in the adaptive immune system, this can take the form of immune exhaustion from chronic activation, as with chronic viral infections and some cancers. Within innate immune memory cells, the chromatin packaging can change, which alters the accessibility of the genes encoding proinflammatory molecules, thus lowering the barriers to activating the proinflammatory state. In addition to further understanding the pathways, the permanence and reversibility of these changes are being actively investigated. Some studies have shown continued changes in T-cell responses in patients with chronic hepatitis C even after cure, implying ongoing immune system changes despite removal of the source of chronic inflammation. In setting of chronic social stress in human and animal

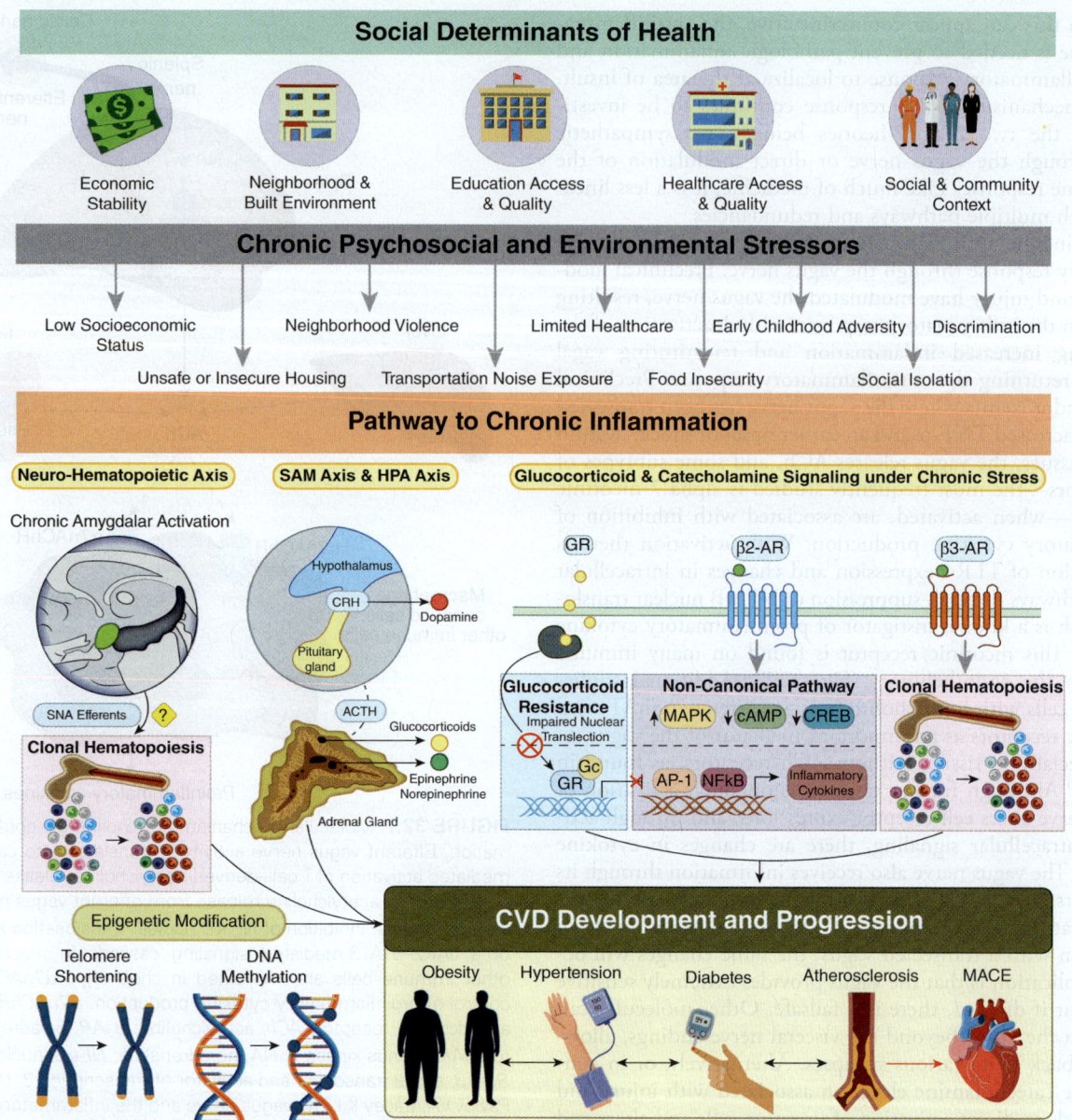

FIGURE 32.8 The social determinants of health and the biology of adversity. Social determinants of health encompass an individual's economic stability, neighborhood and built environment, education access, healthcare access, and social and community relationships. These areas can be sources of chronic psychosocial stressors to individuals who suffer from low socioeconomic status, unsafe housing, neighborhood violence, limited access to healthcare, early childhood adversity, discrimination, increased noise exposure, food insecurity, and decreased sleep quality, among others. Pathway to chronic inflammation: Biologic consequences of adversity promote pathways to chronic inflammation. Sympathoadrenomedullary (SAM) axis and hypothalamic-pituitary-adrenal (HPA) axis: The SAM axis and the HPA axis are activated by psychosocial stress and regulate the production of catecholamines (dopamine, norepinephrine, and epinephrine) and glucocorticoids, respectively. Glucocorticoid and catecholamine signaling under chronic stress: (1) Glucocorticoid receptor (GR) shows impaired nuclear translocation and decreased antiinflammatory gene transcription in chronic stress. (2) β-Adrenergic receptors (ARs) have been found to alter their gene signaling to a noncanonical pathway (via β-arrestin 2 scaffolding) that increases production of inflammatory cytokines, which also upregulate NLRP3 (NLR family pyrin domain-containing 3) inflammasome activity. β₃ receptors have also been found to play a role in clonal hematopoiesis, which may contribute to atherosclerotic plaque formation. Neurohematopoietic axis: Chronic amygdala activation has been linked to clonal hematopoiesis, possibly by direct sympathetic nervous system (SNS) innervation of the bone marrow; stress-induced leukopoiesis has been directly linked to atherosclerotic plaques. All of these inflammatory processes lead to increased cardiovascular disease (CVD) risk factors, such as obesity, hypertension, diabetes, and atherosclerosis, ultimately contributing to major adverse cardiac events (MACE) and CVD mortality. ACTH, Adrenocorticotropic hormone; AP-1, activating protein-1; CREB, cAMP response element–binding protein; CRH, corticotropin-releasing hormone; MAPK, mitogen-activated protein kinases; NFκB, nuclear factor κ-light-chain-enhancer of activated B cells; SNS, sympathetic nervous system. [Created with BioRender.com.] (Adapted with permission from Powell-Wiley TM, Baumer Y, Baah FO, et al. Social determinants of cardiovascular disease. *Circ Res.* 2022;130[5]:782-799.)

models, there is evidence of increased circulating early monocytes with proinflammatory gene expression.[33,34] This persistent inflammatory state is associated with poor health outcomes after surgery like increased infections, aberrant healing, and prolonged intensive care unit (ICU) course.

Chronic elevated glucocorticoid levels can result in decreased receptor sensitivity with subsequent reduced antiinflammatory effects. The exact mechanism of the reduction continues to be investigated, but the result is an increase in inflammation either to reduced transcription of antiinflammatory genes or reduced inhibition of proinflammatory genes. Studies examining changes in inflammatory markers and circulating immune cell populations in people with various degrees of chronic stress have been mixed and inconsistent. However, studies specifically looking at the transcription of proinflammatory genes in peripheral immune cells in people with chronic social stress showed increased transcription in proinflammatory genes.[28] There is evidence that ongoing exposure to elevated glucocorticoids can cause epigenetic changes in these cells. The type of epigenetic changes induced appear to depend on the chronicity of exposure, the intensity, and the developmental stage when the exposure occurs. These epigenetic changes appear to alter access to genes involved in the inflammatory reflex, but the clinical significance of these changes continues to be investigated.[35] The sympathetic response also alters in the setting of chronic activation, although this is less well studied. Like the glucocorticoid response, there is decreased receptor sensitivity from internalizing the receptors or a change in the receptor conformation through phosphorylation. However, in the setting of ongoing exposure, the cells can change from the usual activation pathway to a noncanonical pathway—MAPK—which results in continued proinflammatory gene transcription.

Although there are changes in the receptors and signaling in chronic inflammation and stress, there have been no consistency in studies evaluating the plasma levels of cortisol or catecholamines, leaving a gap in our understanding of the pathways. With newer investigations in distinct genomic phenotypes, it is possible that rather than the circulating hormone levels, the individual cellular response to hormones may play a more significant role in determining the ongoing inflammatory response.

In addition to ongoing systemic release of inflammatory factors from actual injury or illness, the body can respond similarly to conditions like stress, which can be viewed as preparatory for an expected injury or insult. Not all stress leads to the same response, and which stressors elicit a stress response depends on the individual. Understanding the individualized stress responses is important to postoperative recovery because surgery and many postoperative events, like an ICU stay, can be significant stressors. Stress is often categorized based on the timescale of the stress and the severity and duration. Additionally, individuals' response to similar stressors is highly variable, creating difficulty in researching stress exposure and the intensity of the stress response. It is easy to consider a traumatic injury or surgery as an acute stressor with the expected stress response. For these conditions, patients have expected clinical courses, which most follow. However, when stress changes from being acute to more chronic, the clinical course can change. When this change occurs and how it is internalized is an area of highly active investigation.

Although the mechanism is not completely understood, chronic activation of inflammatory pathways plays a profound role in many disease processes and has been linked to worse health outcomes. Social determinants of health (SDoH), "conditions in the environment where people are born, live, learn, work, play, worship, and age that affect a wide range of health, functioning, and quality of life outcomes and risks," have been robustly linked to inflammation and subsequent worse health outcomes in a number of medical diseases like cardiovascular disease and asthma[36] and less well-studied postsurgical health outcomes. For example, neighborhood social environment changes the incidence of stroke, heart disease, and hypertension, whereas perceived discrimination increases cardiovascular disease events. Specific to postoperative patients, increased social vulnerability is associated with increased complications and readmissions in procedures as varied as elective brain[37] and hepatobiliary[38] surgery. After brain tumor resections, individuals with more disparities in their SDoH experienced a 1.5-day increased postoperative length of stay and 2.1 increased odds of 90-day mortality.[37] This finding was mirrored in individuals undergoing pancreatic or hepatic resections; those with more SDoH have worse postoperative outcomes, including mortality (7.5% in low SDoH compared with 9.9% in high SDoH; $p < 0.001$) and increased postoperative complications (23.4% in low SDoH compared with 26.7% in high SDoH; $p < 0.001$).[38] Preexisting stressors can change health outcomes.

Chronic inflammation affects all ages; it can be particularly taxing on patients as they age. Chronic inflammation is part of the proposed mechanism behind inflammaging, described as a chronic low-grade inflammation that contributes to diseases related to aging. Part of this is normal cellular senescence during which proinflammatory cytokines are released; the byproducts of senescence can cause inflammation if not cleared. The body's reduced ability to respond to antigens and to eliminate senescence is called *immunosenescence*.[39] Some of these changes are secondary to diminished capacity for renewal from hematopoietic stem cells, but some are from changes to the immune cells themselves. For example, NK cells from older donors expand less robustly in response to appropriate cytokines compared with younger donors. In T cells, some costimulatory molecules are less frequently displayed.[40] The inability of the immune system to appropriately dissipate the byproducts of cellular senescence is hypothesized to lead to the chronic inflammation that is a hallmark of inflammaging and to the clinical outcomes seen in older patients such as difficulty in recovering from a major complication.

Continued stress and inflammation after an acute stressor also alter the normal healing and inflammatory reflex. Within wound beds, there fails to be progression to normal functional macrophages; instead, the wound bed continues to have active lingering PMNs and changes in macrophage subtype.[41] Chronic stress associated with being a caregiver lengthens healing time by 24%, and in these caregivers there is robust cytokine release in response to LPS, which should prompt an immune response.[42] Chronic stress alters the duration of neutrophil infiltration at the site of injury and alters the phenotype of the macrophage and its ability to perform necessary phagocytosis.[43] Chronic elevation of catecholamines alters neutrophil trafficking to injured tissues using the IL-6–mediated pathway with resulting impaired wound healing.[41]

INFLAMMATION AND THE CRITICALLY ILL

The range and extent of the host response to inflammation and stress depend not only on the type of insult but also various host factors. As local tissue inflammation becomes more extensive, a systemic response ensues. Systemic responses occur secondary to several factors, including neurohormonal input and release of bioactive molecules from damaged tissue or infectious organisms. An uncontrolled or inappropriate inflammatory response can result in hemodynamic instability and multiple organ dysfunction syndrome. As critical care continues to improve, there is an increase in patient survival associated with prolonged ICU stays.

Expected and Pathologic Courses of Inflammation

The understanding of the severity of immune response and progression to recovery has been investigated, and a bimodal incidence of multiorgan failure (MOF) was identified (Fig. 32.9). The first peak was described as SIRS and is defined as an exaggerated inflammatory response to a stressor. The clinical criteria for SIRS in adults from the Society of Critical Care Medicine and Surviving Sepsis Campaign require two of the following: (1) temperature >38°C or <36°C, (2) heart rate >90 beats/min, (3) respiratory rate >20 breaths/min or CO_2 <32 mm Hg, and (4) leukocyte count >12,000 or <4000 per mL. Implied in the criteria is sterility, for if there is an infectious insult causing these physiologic derangements, the patient would meet the criteria for sepsis. The immune response in SIRS is similar to the local response for healing. There is an early proinflammatory immune response in conjunction with the systemic stress response involving the HPA and catecholamines.

Eventually, a compensatory antiinflammatory response syndrome (CARS) was identified and is defined by the overactivation of the antiinflammatory response tasked with modulating the proinflammatory response, leading to a relative immunosuppressed state. Within CARS, there are alterations to APCs, reducing their human leukocyte antigen (HLA) receptors and reducing proinflammatory cytokine production. Additionally, there appears to be an increase in apoptosis of immune cells, which is associated with the downstream induction of antiinflammatory cytokine release, like IL-10 and TGF-β. This correlates with findings of leukopenia and peripheral apoptosis seen in patients with sepsis.

Originally CARS was thought to contribute to the second mortality peak, whereas SIRS contributed to the first, as though they were independent and sequential processes. However, this is not as linear as once thought, and as care for the critically ill and injured has improved, these peaks have become less pronounced. Now, often patients who do not recover early languish in the ICU with persistent low-level organ dysfunction. Individuals with persistent end-organ dysfunction and an ICU stay over 10 to 14 days meet criteria for CCI.[44] These patients have prolonged immune dysfunction with simultaneous ongoing inflammation and immunosuppression. CCI has a profound impact on recovery after an ICU stay. After ICU admission for surgical sepsis, patients with CCI demonstrated worse quality-of-life metrics and worse physical function compared with those who recovered rapidly from their critical illness. In addition, only 10% of

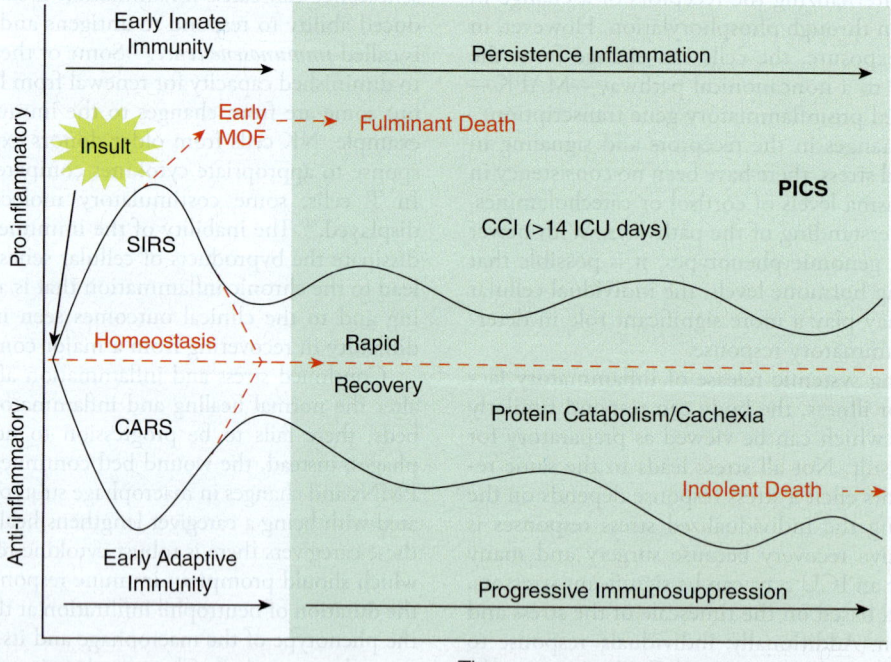

FIGURE 32.9 Persistent inflammation, immunosuppression, and catabolism syndrome (PICS) paradigm. After a major inflammatory insult (e.g., trauma, sepsis, burns, acute pancreatitis), there is a simultaneous inflammatory and immunosuppressive response. Early deaths from acute multiorgan *failure (MOF)* are now rare because of early recognition of shock and rapid implementation of supportive care through effective application of evidence-based medicine *(EBM)* and standard operating procedures *(SOPs)*. Survivors may progress through two pathways: (1) patients readily return to immune homeostasis and achieve a rapid recovery or (2) patients smolder in the intensive care unit *(ICU)* with chronic critical illness *(CCI)* and develop chronic inflammation, suppression of adaptive immunity, and ongoing protein catabolism with cachectic wasting and have recurrent nosocomial infections. These patients often have PICS, many of whom fail to achieve functional independence, are discharged to long-term acute care facilities, have an extremely poor quality of life, and ultimately die an indolent death. (Adapted from Gentile LF, Cuenca AG, Efron PA, et al. Persistent inflammation and immunosuppression: a common syndrome and new horizon for surgical intensive care. *J Trauma Acute Care Surg.* 2012;72[6]:1491-501.)

patients with CCI will be alive without functional dependency a year after discharge.[44]

A subset of the chronically critically ill will progress to persistent inflammation, immunosuppression, and catabolism syndrome (PICS—not to be confused with post–intensive care syndrome using the same acronym). PICS describes the clinical phenotype of patients with a prolonged ICU course experiencing continued organ dysfunction, recurrent infections, and a general inability to survive outside the ICU (Fig. 32.10). This group of patients will have even longer ICU stays than patients with CCI, more infections, more bouts of sepsis, more ventilator days, and more procedures.[45] The current proposed mechanism, and most supported, of PICS revolves around changes in the immune system resulting in ongoing emergency myelopoiesis.[46] During inflammation, granulocytes demarginate from the bone marrow, and depending on the signals received, the bone marrow can continue to make new myeloid innate immune effector cells at high rates. This diverts the bone marrow from creating new erythrocytes and lymphocytes. Emergency myelopoiesis can be beneficial in the initial stages by regulating the initial inflammatory response and keeping it from becoming too vigorous. Additionally, emergency myelopoiesis expands immature myeloid cells, called *myeloid-derived suppressor cells (MDSCs)*. These cells have a number of

subsets and overall are immunomodulatory. MDSCs and their impact on recovery from a prolonged ICU stay is an area of active research. Early excessive enhancement of MDSCs was associated with early mortality and persistent expansion associated with prolonged stays in the ICU. MDSCs appear to create an immunosuppressive environment through a number of mechanisms, including regulating arginase and nitric oxide synthase, increasing IL-10, and initiating T regulatory expansion.

After an ICU hospitalization, many patients experience some degree of post–intensive care syndrome, and although the etiology of these issues is multifactorial and the exact mechanisms still being researched, one of the leading theories revolves around aberrant inflammation and immune response during CCI leading to maladaptive repair. In patients with ICU-acquired weakness, the atrophy from prolonged immobility is important and can be ameliorated by early mobilization; however, even after patients recover their muscle mass, they remain weak, implying a more complicated pathway leading to ICU-acquired weakness.[47] ICU-acquired weakness includes both critical illness polyneuropathy and critical illness myopathy, which together occur in almost half of patients with sepsis or MOF.[48,49] Supporting the hypothesis of aberrant inflammation and healing is the finding of increased inflammatory gene expression in patients' muscles 6 months after an ICU stay.[50]

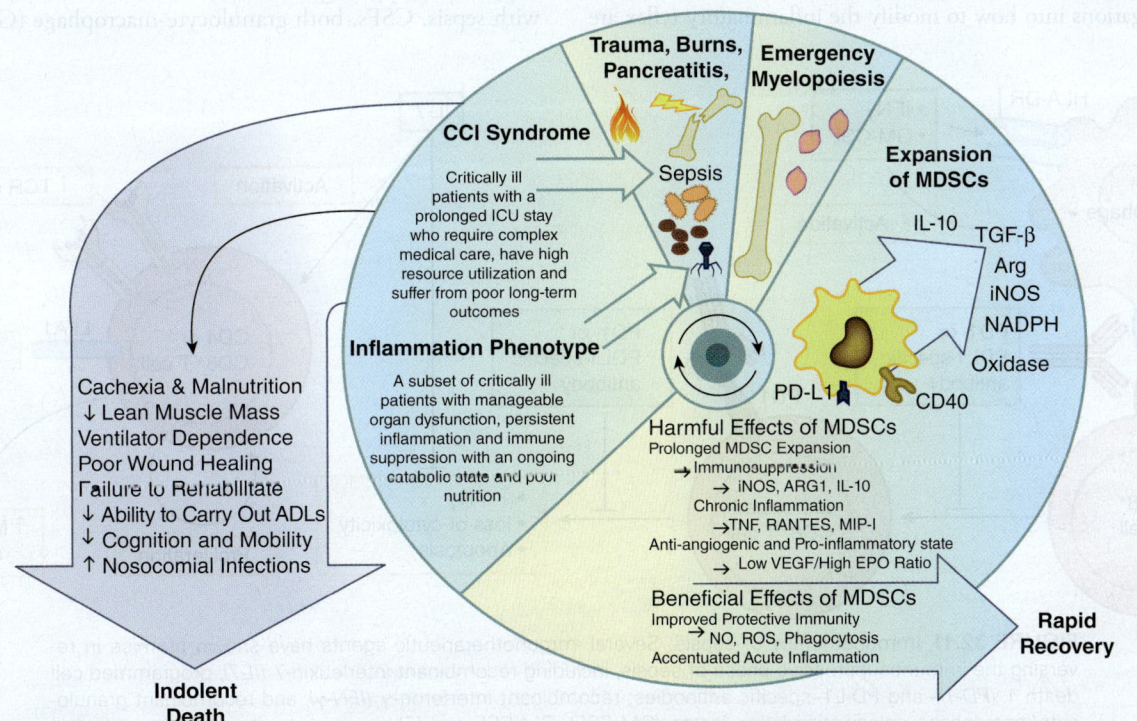

FIGURE 32.10 The persistent inflammation, immunosuppression, and catabolism syndrome (PICS) cycle. PICS can be represented as a recurring, vicious cycle. First, the inciting inflammatory event stimulates an emergency myelopoietic response. Although the ensuing expansion of myeloid-derived suppressor cells (*MDSCs*) can be protective, prolonged expansion promotes suppression of adaptive immunity and chronic inflammation. After this initial response, patients may convalesce or progress to chronic critical illness (*CCI*). In a subset of patients with CCI, PICS develops and is characterized by manageable organ dysfunction, ongoing inflammation and immune suppression, protein catabolism, muscle wasting, and unmet nutritional needs. This state predisposes patients for recurrent infections and recidivism of this cycle. *ADLs*, Activities of daily living; *Arg*, arginase; *EPO*, erythropoietin; *iNOS*, inducible NO synthase; *NADPH*, nicotinamide adenine dinucleotide phosphate; *TGFβ*, transforming growth factor β; *VEGF*, vascular endothelial growth factor. (Adapted from Mira JC, Gentile LF, Mathias BJ, et al. Sepsis pathophysiology, chronic critical illness, and persistent inflammation-immunosuppression and catabolism syndrome. *Crit Care Med*. 2017;45[2]:253-262.)

Similar hypotheses have been suggested to explain persistent renal and pulmonary dysfunctions. During acute kidney injury, there is a local proinflammatory state within the kidney with apoptosis, cytokine release, and macrophage infiltration. This can lead to fibrosis during healing, which puts patients at risk for progression to chronic kidney disease, with a hazard ratio of 8.8.[51]

Post–intensive care syndrome is a consensus term describing new or worsening impairments in physical, cognitive, or mental health domains after critical illness that persist beyond the acute hospitalization.[52] In one study of five US hospitals enrolling adults admitted with shock or acute respiratory distress syndrome (ARDS), they found that 3 months after discharge, 64% of patients had post–intensive care syndrome and 20% included multiple domains.[53] At 12 months this improved slightly to 56%, demonstrating the frequency of these chronic issues after a hospitalization requiring intensive care.[53] Although multifactorial in the cause, the sequelae of CCI and its prolonged ICU course are significant.

Interventions

Although at the moment, there are few well-supported interventions to change these immune system disturbances, identifying which patients are at risk for this transition to PICS and subsequent interventions is currently at the forefront of sepsis and critical care research. Many of these efforts revolve around altering the immune and inflammatory response.

Given the number of diseases attributed to excessive inflammation, investigations into how to modify the inflammatory reflex are extensive. Vagal nerve stimulation has been shown in preclinical models and some small clinical trials to improve joint damage, symptoms, and systemic markers of inflammation (CRP, erythrocyte sedimentation rate [ESR]). TNF-α biologics are actively used in treatment of inflammatory bowel disease. Centrally acting ACh inhibitors, such as galantamine, were found to lower TNF and leptin, elevate IL-10, and improve insulin resistance in patients with metabolic syndrome, many of whose symptoms were associated with an abnormal proinflammatory state.[54,55] Some of these interventions have been evaluated in sepsis without improvement, emphasizing the complexity of inflammation in the patient with sepsis.[56]

In the setting of postoperative ICU immune dysfunction, one of the large barriers to effective novel treatments is the overlap with essential pathways. Multiple studies of immunotherapies in the setting of sepsis have failed to show improvement in clinical trials, despite promising results in preclinical studies. One of the better-remembered examples is protein C in sepsis, which despite promising preclinical studies, did not improve mortality and resulted in increased bleeding risks.[57] The extremely complex balance of the inflammatory response in terms of recovery from the significant insults often experienced by the surgical patient makes it clear that ongoing research is needed to better understand these pathways and to eventually find areas to manipulate them to benefit recovery. Newer research is attempting to restore a more normal immune response (Fig. 32.11). Some of these immunotherapy targets have started to be evaluated in patients with sepsis. CSFs, both granulocyte-macrophage (GM)-CSF and

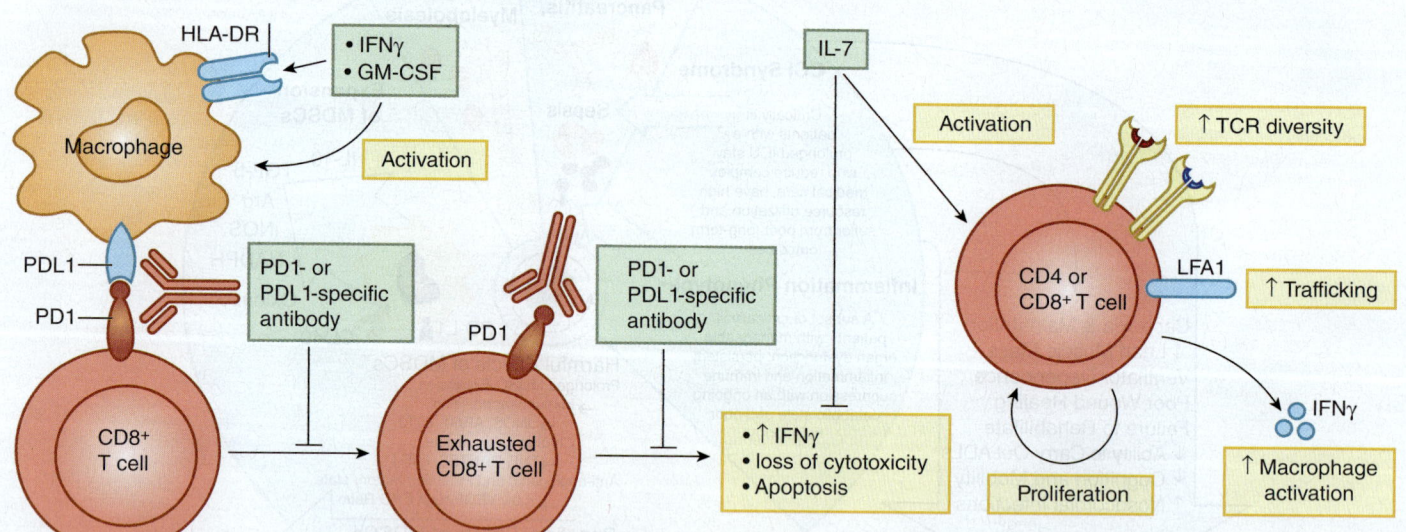

FIGURE 32.11 Immunotherapy of sepsis. Several immunotherapeutic agents have shown promise in reversing the immunosuppressive phase of sepsis, including recombinant interleukin-7 (*IL-7*), programmed cell death 1 (*PD-1*)– and PD-L1–specific antibodies; recombinant interferon-γ (*IFN-γ*); and recombinant granulocyte/macrophage colony-stimulating factor (*GM-CSF*). GM-CSF and IFN-γ act primarily on monocytes and macrophages to increase HLA-DR expression and induce activation. IL-7 and PD-1–specific antibodies have the advantage of targeting CD4+ and CD8+ T cells to restore the function of the adaptive immune system. By reengaging CD4+ T cells, both recombinant IL-7 and PD-1–specific antibodies will have effects not only on adaptive immune cells but indirectly on monocytes and macrophages. PD-1– and PD-L1–specific antibodies will prevent and/or reverse T-cell exhaustion. Thus, the net effects of these antibodies will be to prevent decreased IFN-γ production, T-cell apoptosis and decreased CD8+ T-cell cytotoxicity. IL-7 will block T-cell apoptosis, induce T-cell proliferation, increase IFN-γ production by T cells, increase T-cell receptor (*TCR*) diversity, and increase T-cell trafficking by increasing the expression of cell integrins such as lymphocyte function–associated antigen 1 (*LFA1*). The application of immunotherapeutic agents will depend on the use of various biomarkers or tests of immune function to document that patients have entered the immunosuppressive phase of sepsis. (Adapted from Hotchkiss RS, Monneret G, Payen D. Sepsis-induced immunosuppression: from cellular dysfunctions to immunotherapy. *Nat Rev Immunol.* 2013;13[12]:862-874.)

G-CSF, have been evaluated in patients with sepsis but with mixed results. In one study of 38 patients with sepsis, there were improved biochemical markers of immunosuppression, reduced length of stay, and fewer ventilator days.[58] However, a large study of 700 patients with sepsis failed to show a difference in ventilator days, length of stay, mortality, or organ dysfunction.[59] A meta-analysis of 12 randomized control studies in sepsis showed improvement in resolution of infection but without a mortality benefit.[60] IL-7 was evaluated in 27 patients with sepsis with lymphopenia and found an improvement in absolute lymphocyte cell count and improved T-cell proliferation and activation, although further studies are needed to evaluate the clinical impact of these apparent immune system improvements.[61] Similarly, IFN-γ has been recently evaluated in 18 patients with sepsis, with resulting improved sequential organ failure assessment (SOFA) scores and cytokine profiles.[62] In sepsis, the programmed cell death 1 (PD-1) is upregulated and is associated with secondary infections. The PD-1/PD-L1 interaction limits CD8+ T-cell proliferation and increases lymphocyte apoptosis.[63] In preclinical models, inhibiting this interaction improved viral clearance and reduced lymphocyte depletion. An inhibitor acting on PD-L1 improved organ dysfunction and lymphopenia without increasing cytokines.[64] Despite success in patients with cancer, preclinical studies modulating MDSC in sepsis have been mixed. In a preclinical model of burns, decreasing MDSC with gemcitabine resulted in improved outcomes after LPS but was worse after *Pseudomonas* infection.[65] In a preclinical model of sepsis, reduced MDSC resulted in worsened mortality, which was improved with reintroduction of MDSC.[66] There are a number of areas in the immune response to sepsis that are potential areas for intervention but need more research before incorporation into standard of care.

Additional investigations are ongoing into the epigenetic modifications that occur in the setting of chronic inflammation and if these are either modifiable or can be used as a biomarker to identify at-risk patients. Exposure to infectious agents can cause epigenetic modifications within immune cells to help avoid detection. LPS alters histone methylation, resulting in upregulation of proinflammatory genes.[67] Additionally, after infection, immune cells undergo epigenetic changes, making it easier to access proinflammatory genes and allowing for an excessive inflammatory response to the next immune challenge.[68] This is only partially reversed after resolution of the infection and is one of the ways of training immunity. Evidence is accumulating that for some people these epigenetic changes are associated with increased inflammation and inflammatory diseases like atherosclerosis.[69] In sepsis, there are known modifications that appear to change depending on the model.[70] Another interesting area of epigenetic investigation is in inflammaging and cell senescence. It is known that older cells are hypermethylated, changing what portions of the genome are accessible. During and after sepsis, immune cells need to repopulate, and in older cells there is evidence that DNA methylation changes can lead to the decline in progenitor cells' regenerative ability.[39] Epigenetics and the role it plays in chronic inflammation and sepsis continues to be investigated and holds the possibility of personalized therapeutics once better understood.

During sepsis, EVs are associated with organ failure and mortality and appear to exacerbate the proinflammatory state.[71–73] Currently they are being investigated as both a biomarker of diseases and for therapeutics.[74] Particular cargo has been associated with sepsis survival and disease progression.[75–77] For example, patients with EV cargo, including a protein involved in sphingolipid metabolism, had improved fevers and CRP.[77] EVs from mesenchymal stem cells have shown promise in improving acute lung injury in various preclinical models.[78–81] In preclinical models, EVs have been used as a drug delivery system to improve acute lung injury.[82,83] EVs are also being evaluated for treatment of diseases with a large inflammatory component.[84] In a clinical trial, EVs were found to improve serum creatinine and blood urea nitrogen in patients with stage 3 and 4 kidney disease.[85] EVs are a broad category of molecules with varying cargos that require continued investigation; however, they hold promise for improved therapeutics for wide range of inflammatory disease and biomarkers of diseases.

The intestinal microbiome is now understood to play a significant role in inflammation and changes in response to stress and illness, often resulting in a pathobiome. Research into whether modifying the microbiome can improve outcomes is ongoing. For many diseases, researchers are still investigating exactly what changes in the microbiome occur and if and how those changes affect the disease progression. Fecal microbiota transplant (FMT) is best known for successfully treating refractory or recurrent *C. difficile* infections. It is being investigated for use in inflammatory bowel disease and was found to have improved remission rates and symptom improvement.[86] In preclinical models of sepsis, FMT improved intestinal barrier integrity and reduced mortality.[87] In addition, there have been case studies and series documenting benefit in critically ill patients.[88–90] Further research is needed, especially in the setting of critical illness, as there have been reports of iatrogenic colitis after FMT with enteropathogenic *Escherichia coli* and Shiga toxin–producing *E. coli*.[91]

Given the complexity of the inflammatory pathways and the individualized response to insults like stress and infection, there is increasing interest in evaluating and modifying the individual response through precision medicine. Success will require improved understanding of the inflammatory pathways and which markers insinuate prolonged inflammation.

SELECTED REFERENCES

Buzas EI. The roles of extracellular vesicles in the immune system. *Nat Rev Immunol.* 2023;23(4):236-250.

Extracellular vesicles play an active role in both the inflammatory and immune responses and are actively being investigated for therapeutics, which is reviewed here.

Cross D, Drury R, Hill J, Pollard AJ. Epigenetics in sepsis: understanding its role in endothelial dysfunction, immunosuppression, and potential therapeutics. *Front Immunol.* 2019;10:1363.

Inflammation and infection alter the immune system through epigenetic modifications altering subsequent immune activations. This article discusses epigenetic changes and the relationship to persistent inflammation, immunosuppression, and catabolism syndrome.

Darden DB, Kelly LS, Fenner BP, Moldawer LL, Mohr AM, Efron PA. Dysregulated immunity and immunotherapy after sepsis. *J Clin Med.* 2021;10(8):1742.

Persistent inflammation, immunosuppression, and catabolism syndrome is associated with significant healthcare burden. The dysfunctional immune system and persistent inflammation and areas for possible interventions are discussed.

Gershon MD, Margolis KG. The gut, its microbiome, and the brain: connections and communications. *J Clin Invest.* 2021;131(18): e143768.

Bidirectional communication between the intestinal microbiome and the brain plays an important role in homeostasis. The pathways and role played in immune activation and inflammation are explored in this article.

Margraf A, Ludwig N, Zarbock A, Rossaint J. Systemic inflammatory response syndrome after surgery: mechanisms and protection. *Anesth Analg.* 2020;131(6):1693-1707.

This article discusses the necessary systemic inflammatory response after surgery and the damage caused by its dysregulation as well as possible interventions.

The full reference list appears on Elsevier eBooks+.

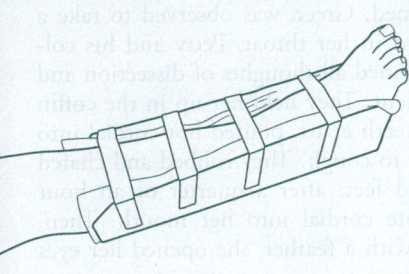

CHAPTER 33

Shock, Electrolytes, and Fluid

Paige Farley, Sawyer G. Smith, Jason L. Sperry, and Martin Allan Schreiber

INTRODUCTION

Surgeons are the masters of fluids because they need to be. They care for patients who cannot eat or drink for various reasons; for example, they have bled, undergone surgery, or lost fluids from tubes, drains, or wounds. Surgeons are obligated to know how to care for these patients, who put their lives in their hands. This topic might appear simple only for those who do not understand the complexities of the human body and its ability to regulate and compensate fluids. In reality, the task of managing patients' blood volume is one of the most challenging burdens surgeons face, often requiring complete control of the intake and output of fluids and electrolytes and often in the presence of blood loss. Given the nature of the profession, they have studied those topics and dealt with patients who bleed and sometimes exsanguinate. Historically, wartime experience has always helped them move ahead in their knowledge of the management of fluids and how to better resuscitate. The recent wars in Iraq and Afghanistan are no exception; we have learned much from these wars.

Constant attention to and titration of fluid loss therapy is required because the human body is dynamic. The key to treatment is to realize what an individual patient's initial condition is and to understand that their fluid status is constantly changing. Bleeding, sepsis, neuroendocrine disturbances, and dysfunctional regulatory systems can all affect patients who are undergoing the dynamic changes of illness and healing. The correct management of blood volume is highly time dependent. If it is managed well, surgeons are afforded the chance to manage other aspects of surgery, such as nutrition, administration of antibiotics, drainage of abscesses, relief of obstruction and incarceration, treatment of ischemia, and resection of tumors. Knowing the difference between dehydration, anemia, hemorrhage, and overresuscitation is vital.

The human body is predominantly water, which resides in the intravascular, intracellular, and interstitial (or third) space. Water movement between these spaces is dependent on many variables. This chapter focuses on the management of the intravascular space because it is the only space surgeons have direct access to, and managing the intravascular space is the only way to affect the other two fluid compartments.

This chapter also examines historical aspects of shock, fluids, and electrolytes—not just to note interesting facts or pay tribute to deserving physicians but also to try to understand how knowledge evolved over time. Doing so is vital to understanding past changes in management as well as to accept future changes. We are often awed at the discoveries of the past yet also astounded by how wrong we often were and why. Certainly, in turn, future surgeons will look back at our current body of knowledge and be amazed at how little we knew and how frequently we were wrong. A consequence of not studying the past is to repeat its errors.

After the historical highlights, this chapter discusses various fluids that are now used, along with potential fluids under development. Finally, caring for perioperative patients is explored from a daily requirements perspective.

HISTORY

History is disliked by those who are in a hurry to just learn the bottom line. Learning from the past, however, is essential to know which treatments have worked and which have not. Dogma must always be challenged and questioned. Are the current treatments based on science? Studying the history of shock is important for at least three reasons. First, physicians and physiologists have been fascinated with blood loss out of necessity. Second, we need to assess what experiments have or have not been done. Third, we need to know more because our current understanding of shock is elementary.

Resuscitation

One of the earliest authenticated resuscitations in the medical literature is the "miraculous deliverance of Anne Green," who was executed by hanging on December 14, 1650.[1] Green was executed in the customary way by "being turned off a ladder to hang by the neck." She hanged for half an hour, during which time some of her friends pulled "with all their weight upon her legs, sometimes lifting her up, and then pulling her down again with a sudden jerk, thereby the sooner to dispatch her out of her pain" (Fig. 33.1). When everyone thought she was dead, the body was taken down, put in a coffin, and taken to the private house of Dr. William Petty, who, by the king's orders, was allowed to perform autopsies on the bodies of all persons who had been executed.

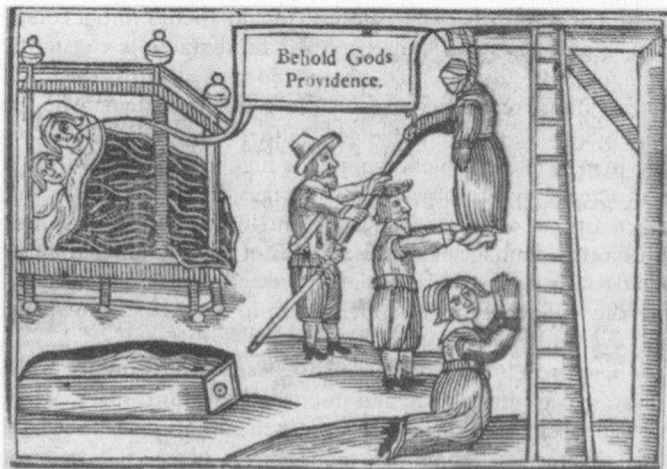

FIGURE 33.1 Miraculous deliverance of Anne Green, who was executed in 1650. (From Hughes JT. Miraculous deliverance of Anne Green: an Oxford case of resuscitation in the seventeenth century. *Br Med J [Clin Res Ed].* 1982;285:1792-1793; by kind permission of the Bodleian Library, Oxford.)

When the coffin was opened, Green was observed to take a breath, and a rattle was heard in her throat. Petty and his colleague, Thomas Willis, abandoned all thoughts of dissection and proceeded to revive their patient. They held her up in the coffin and then, by wrenching her teeth apart, poured hot cordial into her mouth, which caused her to cough. They rubbed and chafed her fingers, hands, arms, and feet; after a quarter of an hour of such effort, they put more cordial into her mouth. Then, after they tickled her throat with a feather, she opened her eyes momentarily.

At that stage, they opened a vein and bled her of 5 ounces of blood. They continued administering the cordial and rubbing her arms and legs. Next, they applied compressing bandages to her arms and legs. Heating plasters were put to her chest, and another plaster was inserted as an enema "to give heat and warmth to her bowels." They then placed Green in a warm bed with another female to lie with her to keep her warm. After 12 hours, Green began to speak; 24 hours after her revival, she was answering questions freely. At 2 days, her memory was normal, apart from her recollection of her execution and the resuscitation.

Shock

Hemorrhagic shock has been extensively studied and written about for many centuries. Injuries, whether intentional or not, have occurred so frequently that much of the understanding of shock has been learned by surgeons taking care of the injured.

What is shock? The current widely accepted definition is inadequate perfusion of tissue. However, many subtleties lie behind this statement. Nutrients for cells are required, but the specific nutrients are not currently well defined. Undoubtedly, the most critical nutrient is oxygen, but concentrating on just oxygenation alone probably represents very elemental thinking. Blood is highly complex and carries countless nutrients, buffers, cells, antibodies, hormones, chemicals, electrolytes, and antitoxins. Even if we think in an elemental fashion and try to optimize the perfusion of tissue, the delivery side of the equation is affected by blood volume, anemia, and cardiac output (CO). Moreover, the use of nutrients is affected by infection and drugs. The vascular tone plays a role as well; for example, in neurogenic shock, the sympathetic tone is lost, and in sepsis, systemic vascular resistance decreases because of a broken homeostatic process or possibly because of evolutionary factors.

The term *shock* appears to have been first employed in 1743 in a translation of the French treatise of Henri Francois Le Dran regarding battlefield wounds. He used the term to designate the act of impact or collision rather than the resulting functional and physiologic damage. However, the term can be found in the book *Gunshot Wounds of the Extremities*, published in 1815 by Guthrie, who used it to describe physiologic instability.

Humoral theories persisted until the late 19th century, but in 1830, Herman provided one of the first clear descriptions of intravenous (IV) fluid therapy. In response to a cholera epidemic, he attempted to rehydrate patients by injecting 6 ounces of water into the vein. In 1831, O'Shaughnessy also treated cholera patients by administering large volumes of salt solutions intravenously and published his results in *Lancet*.[2] Those were the first documented attempts to replace and maintain the extracellular internal environment or the intravascular volume. Note, however, that the treatment of cholera and dehydration is not the ideal treatment of hemorrhagic shock.

In 1872, Gross defined shock as "a manifestation of the rude unhinging of the machinery of life." His definition, given its accuracy and descriptiveness, has been repeatedly quoted in the literature. Theories on the cause of shock persisted through the late 19th century; although it was unexplainable, it was often observed. George Washington Crile concluded that the lowering of the central venous pressure in the shock state in animal experiments was due to a failure of the autonomic nervous system.[3] Surgeons witnessed a marked change in ideas about shock between 1888 and 1918. In the late 1880s, there were no all-encompassing theories, but most surgeons accepted the generalization that shock resulted from a malfunctioning of some part of the nervous system. Such a malfunctioning has now been shown to *not* be the main reason— but surgeons are still perplexed by the mechanisms of hemorrhagic shock, especially regarding the complete breakdown of the circulatory system that occurs in the later stages of shock.

In 1899, using contemporary advances with sphygmomanometers, Crile proposed that a profound decline in blood pressure (BP) could account for all symptoms of shock. He also helped alter the way physicians diagnosed shock and followed its course. Before Crile, most surgeons relied on respiration, pulse, or a declining mental status when evaluating the condition of patients. After Crile's first books were published, many surgeons began measuring BP. In addition to changing how surgeons thought about shock, Crile was a part of the therapeutic revolution. His theories remained generally accepted for nearly two decades, predominantly in surgical circles. Crile's work persuaded Harvey Cushing to measure BP in all operations, which in part led to the general acceptance of BP measurement in clinical medicine. Crile also concluded that shock was not a process of dying but rather a marshaling of the body's defenses in patients struggling to live. He later deduced that the reduced volume of circulating blood, rather than the diminished BP, was the most critical factor in shock.

Crile's theories evolved as he continued his experimentations; in 1913, he proposed the kinetic system theory. He was interested in thyroid hormone and its response to wounds but realized that epinephrine was a key component of the response to shock. He relied on experiments by Walter B. Cannon, who found that epinephrine was released in response to pain or emotion, shifting blood from the intestines to the brain and extremities. Epinephrine release also stimulated the liver to convert glycogen to sugar for release into the circulation. Cannon argued that all the actions of epinephrine aided the animal in its effort to defend itself.[4]

Crile incorporated Cannon's study into his theory. He proposed that impulses from the brain after injury stimulated glands to secrete their hormones, which, in turn, effected sweeping changes throughout the body. Crile's kinetic system included a complex interrelationship among the brain, heart, lungs, blood vessels, muscles, thyroid gland, and liver. He also noted that if the body received too much stress, the adrenal glands would run out of epinephrine, the liver of glycogen, the thyroid of its hormone, and the brain itself of energy, accounting for autonomic changes. Once the kinetic system ran out of energy, BP would fall, and the organism would go into shock.

Henderson recognized the importance of decreased venous return and its effect on CO and arterial pressure. His work was aided by advances in techniques that allowed careful recording of the volume curves of the ventricles. Fat embolism also led to a shocklike state, but its possible contribution was questioned because study results were difficult to reproduce. The vasomotor center and its contributions to shock were heavily studied in the early 1900s. In 1914, Mann noted that unilaterally innervated vessels of the tongues of dogs, ears of rabbits, and paws of kittens appeared constricted during shock compared with contralaterally denervated vessels.

Battlefield experiences continued to intensify research on shock. During the World War I era, Cannon used clinical data from the war as well as data from animal experiments to examine the shock state carefully. He theorized that toxins and acidosis contributed to the previously described lowering of vascular tone. He and others then focused on acidosis and the role of alkali in preventing and prolonging shock. The adrenal gland and the effect of cortical extracts on adrenalectomized animals were of fascination during this period.

Then, in the 1930s, a unique set of experiments by Blalock[5] determined that almost all acute injuries are associated with changes in fluid and electrolyte metabolism. Such changes were primarily the result of reductions in the effective circulating blood volume. Blalock showed that those reductions after injury could be the result of several mechanisms (Box 33.1). He clearly showed that fluid loss in injured tissues was loss of extracellular fluid (ECF) that was unavailable to the intravascular space for maintaining circulation. The original concept of a "third space," in which fluid is sequestered and therefore unavailable to the intravascular space, evolved from Blalock's studies.

Carl John Wiggers first described the concept of "irreversible shock."[6] His 1950 textbook, *Physiology of Shock,* represented the attitudes toward shock at that time. In an exceptionally brilliant summation, Wiggers assembled the various signs and symptoms of shock from various authors in that textbook (Fig. 33.2), along with his own findings.

His experiments used what is now known as the *Wiggers prep*. In his most common experiments, he used previously splenectomized dogs and cannulated the arterial system. He took advantage of an evolving technology that allowed him to measure the pressure within the arterial system, and he studied the effects of lowering BP through controlled hemorrhage. After removing the dogs' blood to an arbitrary set point (typically, 40 mm Hg), he noted that their BP soon spontaneously rose as fluid was spontaneously recruited into the intravascular space.

To keep the dogs' BP at 40 mm Hg, Wiggers had to continually withdraw additional blood. During this compensated phase of shock, the dogs could use their reserves to survive. Water was recruited from the intracellular compartment as well as from the extracellular space. The body tried to maintain the vascular flow necessary to survive. However, after a certain period, he found that to keep the dogs' BP at the arbitrary set point of 40 mm Hg, he had to reinfuse shed blood; he termed this phase *uncompensated,* or *irreversible, shock.* Eventually, after a period of irreversible shock, the dogs died.

BOX 33.1   Causes of Shock, According to Blalock in 1930

- Hematogenic (oligemia)
- Neurogenic (caused primarily by nervous influences)
- Vasogenic (initially decreased vascular resistance and increased vascular capacity, as in sepsis)
- Cardiogenic (failure of the heart as a pump as in cardiac tamponade or myocardial infarction)
- Large-volume loss (extracellular fluid, as occurs in patients with diarrhea, vomiting, and fistula drainage)

Data from Blalock A. *Principles of Surgical Care: Shock and Other Problems.* St. Louis: CV Mosby; 1940.

SYMPTOM COMPLEX OF SHOCK

General appearance and reactions	Skin and mucous membranes	Circulation and blood
Mental state	*Skin*	*Superficial veins*
Apathy	Pale, livid, ashen	Collapsed and
Delayed responses	gray	invisible
Depressed cerebration	Slightly cyanotic	Failure to fill
Weak voice	Moist, clammy	on compression
Listless or	Mottling of	or massage
restlessness	dependent parts	Inconspicuous
	Loose, dry,	jugular
Countenance	inelastic, cold	pulsations
Drawn–anxious		
Lusterless eyes	*Mucous membranes*	*Heart*
Sunken eyeballs	Pale, livid,	Apex sounds feeble
Ptosis of upper lids	slightly cyanotic	Rate usually rapid
(slight)		
Upward rotation of	*Conjunctiva*	*Radial pulse*
eyeballs (slight)	Glazed, lusterless	Usually rapid
		Small volume
Neuromuscular state	*Tongue*	"feeble,"
Hypotonia	Dry, pale, parched,	"thready"
Muscular weakness	shriveled	
Tremors and		*Brachial blood*
twitchings		*pressures*
Involuntary muscular	*Respiration and*	Lowered
movements	*metabolism*	Pulse pressure
Difficulty in		small
swallowing		
	Respiration	*Retinal vessels*
Neuromuscular tests	Variable but not	Narrowed
Depressed tendon	dyspneic	
reflexes	Usually increased	*Blood volume*
Depressed sensibilities	rate	Reduced
Depressed visual	Variable depth	
and auditory	Occasional deep	*Blood chemistry*
reflexes	sighs	Hemoconcentration
	Sometimes irregular	or hemodilution
General but variable	or phasic	Venous O_2
symptoms		decreased
Thirst	*Temperature*	A-V O_2 difference
Vomiting	Subnormal, normal,	increased
Diarrhea	supernormal	Arterial CO_2
Oliguria		reduced
Visible or occult	*Basal metabolic rate*	Alkali reserve
blood in vomitus	reduced (?)	reduced
and stools		

FIGURE 33.2 Wiggers' description of symptom complex of shock. (From Wiggers CJ. The present status of shock problem. *Physiol Rev.* 1942;22:74-123.)

The ideal model is uncontrolled hemorrhage, but its main problem is that the volume of hemorrhage is uncontrolled by the nature of the experiment. Variability is the highest in this model, even though it is the most realistic. Computer-assisted pressure models that mimic the pressures during uncontrolled shock can be used to reduce the artificiality of the pressure-controlled model. Smith and colleagues[7] developed a hybrid model of controlled, uncontrolled hemorrhage whereby a standardized grade V liver laceration is made in swine. The swine bleed to either a specified pressure or fixed volume, and bleeding is controlled with packing. This removes the variability classically associated with uncontrolled hemorrhage.[7]

Fluids

How did the commonly used IV fluids, such as normal saline, enter medical practice? It is often taken for granted, given the vast body of knowledge in medicine, that they were adopted through a rigorous scientific process, but that was not the case.

Normal saline has a long track record and is extremely useful, but we now know that it also can be harmful. Hartog Jakob Hamburger, in his in vitro studies of red cell lysis in 1882, incorrectly suggested that 0.9% saline was the concentration of salt in human blood. He chose 0.9% saline because it has the same freezing point as human serum. This fluid is often referred to as *physiologic* or *normal saline*, but it is neither physiologic nor normal. In 1831, O'Shaughnessy described his experience in the treatment of cholera:

Universal stagnation of the venous system, and rapid cessation of the arterialization of the blood, are the earliest, as well as the most characteristic effects. Hence the skin becomes blue—hence animal heat is no longer generated—hence the secretions are suspended; the arteries contain black blood, no carbonic acid is evolved from the lungs, and the returned air of expiration is cold as when it enters these organs.[8]

O'Shaughnessy wrote those words at the age of 22, having just graduated from Edinburgh Medical School. He tested his new method of infusing IV fluids on a dog and observed no ill effects. Eventually, he reported that the aim of his method was to restore blood to its natural specific gravity and to restore its deficient saline matters. His experience with human cholera patients taught him that the practice of bloodletting, then highly common, was good for "diminishing the venous congestion" and that nitrous oxide (laughing gas) was not useful for oxygenation.

In 1832, Robert Lewins reported that he witnessed Thomas Latta injecting extraordinary quantities of saline into veins, with the immediate effects of "restoring the natural current in the veins and arteries, of improving the color of the blood, and [of] recovering the functions of the lungs." Lewins described Latta's saline solution as consisting of "two drachms of muriate, and two scruples of carbonate, of soda, to sixty ounces of water." Later, however, Latta's solution was found to equate to having 134 mmol/L of Na^+, 118 mmol/L of Cl^-, and 16 mmol/L of bicarbonate (HCO_3^-).

During the next 50 years, many reports cited various recipes used to treat cholera, but none resembled 0.9% saline. In 1883, Sydney Ringer reported on the influence exerted by the constituents of the blood on the contractions of the ventricle (Fig. 33.3). Studying an isolated heart model from frogs, he used 0.75% saline and a blood mixture made from dried bullocks' blood.[9] In his attempts to identify which aspect of blood caused better results, he found that a "small quantity of white of egg completely obviates the changes occurring with saline solution." He concluded that the benefit of "white of egg" was because of the albumin or the potassium chloride. To show what worked and what did not, he described endless experiments with alterations of multiple variables.

However, Ringer later published another article stating that his previously reported findings could not be repeated; through careful study, he realized that the water used in his first article was actually not distilled water, as reported, but rather tap water from the New River Water Company. It turned out that his laboratory technician, who was paid to distill the water, took shortcuts and used tap water instead. Ringer analyzed the water and found that it contained many trace minerals (Fig. 33.4). Through careful and diligent experimentation, he found that calcium bicarbonate or calcium chloride—in doses even smaller than in blood—restored good contractions of the frog ventricles. The third component that he found essential to good contractions was sodium bicarbonate. Thus, the three ingredients that he found essential were potassium, calcium, and bicarbonate. Ringer solution soon became ubiquitous in physiologic laboratory experiments.

In the early 20th century, fluid therapy by injection under the skin (hypodermoclysis) and infusion into the rectum (proctoclysis) became routine. Hartwell and Hoguet reported its use in intestinal obstruction in dogs, laying the foundation for saline therapy in human patients with intestinal obstruction.

As IV crystalloid solutions were developed, Ringer solution was modified, most notably by pediatrician Alexis Hartmann. In 1932, wanting to develop an alkalinizing solution to administer to his acidotic patients, Hartmann modified Ringer solution by adding sodium lactate. The result was lactated Ringer (LR) or Hartmann solution. He used sodium lactate (instead of sodium bicarbonate); the conversion of lactate into sodium bicarbonate was sufficiently slow to lessen the danger posed by sodium bicarbonate, which could rapidly shift patients from compensated acidosis to uncompensated alkalosis.

In 1924, Rudolph Matas, regarded as the originator of modern fluid treatment, introduced the concept of the continued IV drip but also warned of potential dangers of saline infusions. He stated, "Normal saline has continued to gain popularity but the problems with metabolic derangements have been repeatedly shown but seem to have fallen on deaf ears." In healthy volunteers, modern-day experiments have shown that normal saline can cause abdominal discomfort and pain, nausea, drowsiness, and decreased mental capacity to perform complex tasks.

The point is that normal saline and LR solution have been formulated for conditions other than the replacement of blood, and the reasons for the formulation are archaic. Such solutions have been useful for dehydration; when they are used in relatively small volumes (1–3 L/day), they are well tolerated and relatively harmless; they provide water, and the human body can tolerate

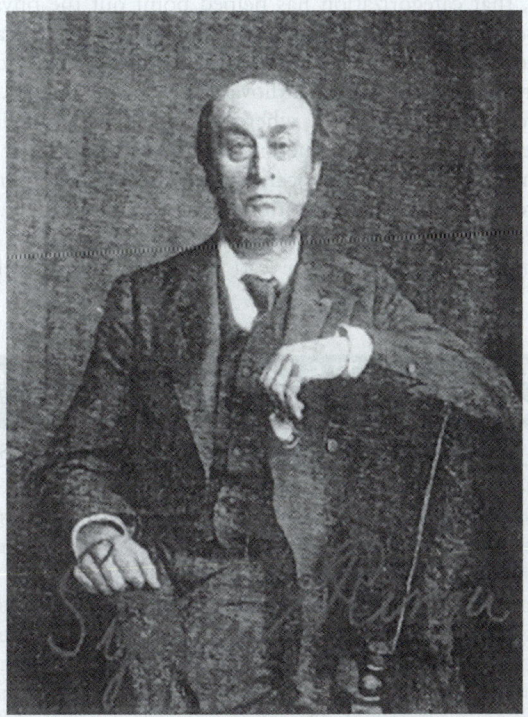

FIGURE 33.3 Sydney Ringer, credited for the development of lactated Ringer solution. (From Baskett TF. Sydney Ringer and lactated Ringer's solution. *Resuscitation.* 2003;58:5-7.)

They consist of:		
Calcium	38.3	per million.
Magnesium	4.5	"
Sodium	23.3	"
Potassium	7.1	"
Combined carbonic acid	78.2	"
Sulfuric acid	55.8	"
Chlorine	15	"
Silicates	7.1	"
Free carbonic acid	54.2	"

FIGURE 33.4 Sidney Ringer's report of contents in water from the New River Water Company. (From Baskett TF. Sydney Ringer and lactated Ringer's solution. *Resuscitation.* 2003;58:5-7.)

the amounts of electrolytes they contain. Over the years, LR solution has attained widespread use for treatment of hemorrhagic shock. However, normal saline and LR solution are mostly permeable through the vascular membrane, but they are poorly retained in the vascular space. After a few hours, only about 175 to 200 mL of a 1-L infusion remains in the intravascular space. In countries other than the United States, LR solution is often referred to as *Hartmann solution,* and normal saline is referred to as *physiologic* (sometimes even spelled *fisiologic*) solution. With the advances in science in the past 50 years, it is difficult to understand why advances in resuscitation fluids have not been made.

Blood Transfusions

Concerned about the blood that injured patients lost, Crile began to experiment with blood transfusions. As he stated, "After many accidents, profuse hemorrhage often led to shock before the patient reached the hospital. Saline solutions, adrenaline, and precise surgical technique could substitute only up to a point for the lost blood." At the turn of the 19th century, transfusions were seldom used. Their use waxed and waned in popularity because of transfusion reactions and difficulties in preventing clotting in donated blood. Through his experiments in dogs, Crile showed that blood was interchangeable: He transfused blood without blood group matching. Alexis Carrel was able to sew blood vessels together with his triangulation technique, using it to connect blood vessels from one person to another for the purpose of transfusions. However, Crile found Carrel's technique too slow and cumbersome in humans, so he developed a short cannula to facilitate transfusions.

By the time World War II occurred, shock was recognized as the single most common cause of treatable morbidity and mortality. At the time of the Japanese attack on Pearl Harbor on December 7, 1941, no blood banks or effectual blood transfusion facilities were available. Most military locations had no stocks of dried pooled plasma. Although the wounded of that era were evacuated quickly to a hospital, the mortality rate was still high. IV fluids of any kind were essentially unavailable, except for a few liters of saline manufactured by means of a still in the operating room. IV fluid was usually administered by an old Salvesen flask and a reused rubber tube. Often, a severe febrile reaction resulted from the use of that tubing.

The first written documentation of resuscitation in World War II patients was 1 year after Pearl Harbor, in December 1942, in notes from the 77th Evacuation Hospital in North Africa. E. D. Churchill stated, "The wounded in action had for the most part either succumbed or recovered from any existing shock before we saw them. However, later cases came to us in shock, and some of the early cases were found to be in need of whole blood transfusion. There was plenty of reconstituted blood plasma available. However, some cases were in dire need of whole blood. We had no transfusion sets, although such are available in the United States: no sodium citrate; no sterile distilled water; and no blood donors."

The initial decision to rely on plasma rather than on blood appears to have been based in part on the view held in the Office of the Surgeon General of the Army and in part on the opinion of the civilian investigators of the National Research Council. Those civilian investigators thought that in shock, the blood was thick and the hematocrit level was high. On April 8, 1943, the surgeon general stated that no blood would be sent to the combat zone. Seven months later, he again refused to send blood overseas because of the following: (1) his observation of overseas theaters

had convinced him that plasma was adequate for resuscitation of wounded soldiers; (2) from a logistics standpoint, it was impractical to make locally collected blood available farther forward than general hospitals in the combat zone; and (3) shipping space was too sparse. Vasoconstricting drugs such as epinephrine were condemned because they were thought to decrease blood flow and tissue perfusion as they dammed the blood in the arterial portion of the circulatory system.

During World War II, out of necessity, efforts to make blood transfusions available heightened and led to the institution of blood banking for transfusions. A better understanding of hypovolemia and inadequate circulation led to the use of plasma as a favored resuscitative solution, in addition to whole blood replacement. Thus, the treatment of traumatic shock greatly improved. The administration of whole blood was thought to be extremely effective, so it was widely used. Mixing whole blood with sodium citrate in a 6:1 ratio to bind the calcium in the blood, which prevented clotting, worked well.

However, no matter what solution was used—blood, colloids, or crystalloids—the blood volume seemed to increase by only a fraction of what was lost. In the Korean War era, it was recognized that more blood had to be infused for the blood volume lost to be adequately regained. The reason for the need for more blood was unclear, but it was thought to be due to hemolysis, pooling of blood in certain capillary beds, and loss of fluid into tissues. Considerable attention was given to elevating the feet of patients in shock.

PHYSIOLOGY OF SHOCK

Bleeding

Research and experience have both taught us much about the physiologic responses to bleeding. The Advanced Trauma Life Support (ATLS) course defines four classes of shock (Table 33.1). In general, that categorization has helped point out the physiologic responses to hemorrhagic shock, emphasizing the identification of blood loss and guiding treatment. Conceptually, shock occurs in three anatomic areas of the cardiovascular system (Fig. 33.5). The first level occurs in the heart, where cardiogenic abnormalities can be either extrinsic (tension pneumothorax, hemothorax, or cardiac tamponade) or intrinsic (myocardial infarction causing pump failure, cardiac contusion or laceration, or cardiac failure). The second level occurs at the large- or medium-vessel level, in which hemorrhage and loss of blood volume lead to shock. The last level occurs

TABLE 33.1	**ATLS Classes of Hemorrhagic Shock**			
	CLASS I	**CLASS II**	**CLASS III**	**CLASS IV**
Blood loss (%)	0–15	15–30	30–40	>40
Central nervous system	Slightly anxious	Mildly anxious	Anxious or confused	Confused or lethargic
Pulse (beats/min)	<100	>100	>120	>140
Blood pressure	Normal	Normal	Decreased	Decreased
Pulse pressure	Normal	Decreased	Decreased	Decreased
Respiratory rate	14–20/min	20–30/min	30–40/min	>35/min
Urine (mL/h)	>30	20–30	5–15	Negligible
Fluid	Crystalloid	Crystalloid	Crystalloid + blood	Crystalloid + blood

ATLS, Advanced Trauma Life Support.

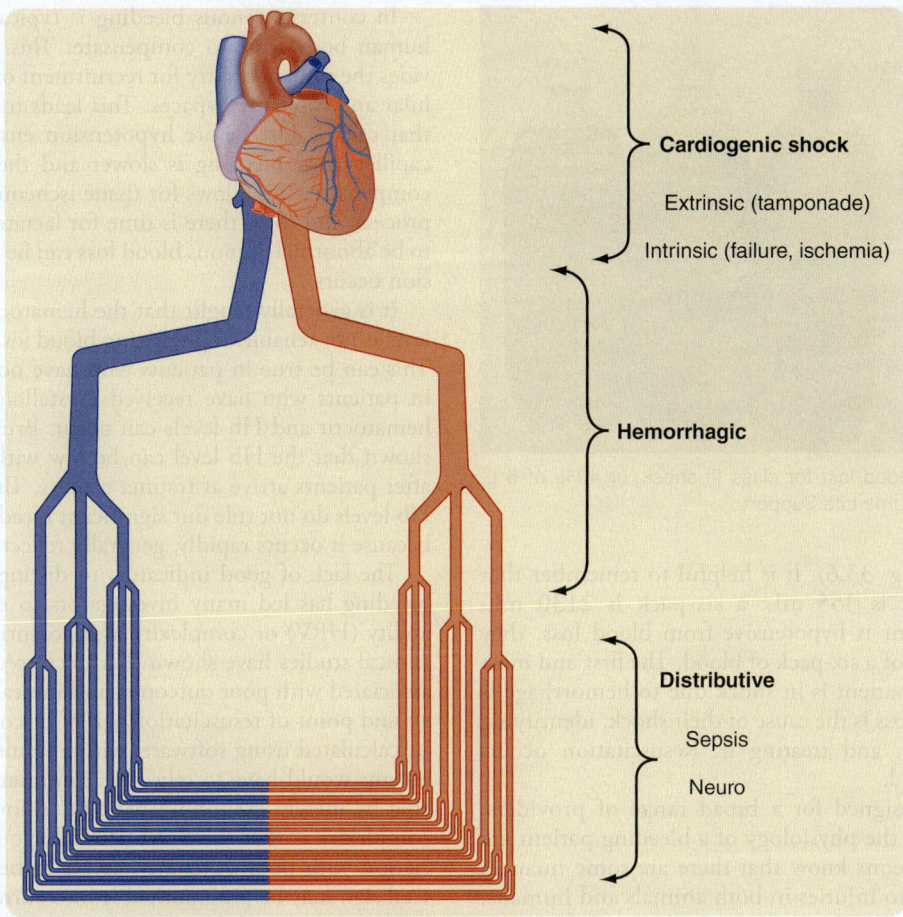

FIGURE 33.5 Types of shock.

with the small vessels, in which either neurologic dysfunction or sepsis leads to vasodilatation and maldistribution of the blood volume, leading to shock.

The four classes of shock, according to the ATLS course, are problematic because they were not rigorously tested or proven and were admittedly arbitrarily generated. Patients often do not exhibit all of the physiologic changes described by this table, particularly those at age extremes. Because of the higher water composition of their bodies, children are able to compensate with large volumes of blood loss, often exhibiting only tachycardia until they reach a tipping point where they are no longer able to compensate, at which point they have a rapid clinical decline. Elderly patients show almost an opposite physiology because they are less equipped to compensate for blood loss and will show signs of a higher level of shock at a lower volume of blood loss. This is due to a reduced cardiac compensation capability and fluid reserve recruitment.

The problem with the signs and symptoms classically taught in ATLS is that in reality, the manifestations of shock can be confusing and difficult to assess, particularly in trauma patients. For example, changes in mental status can be caused by blood loss, traumatic brain injury (TBI), pain, or illicit drugs. The same dilemma applies to respiratory rate and skin changes. Are alterations in a patient's respiratory rate or skin color caused by pneumothorax, rib fracture pain, or inhalation injury?

Although there are various methods that have been developed for monitoring patients in shock, BP continues to be the most clinically useful measure. When caring for a patient in shock, goals of resuscitation need to be established, remembering that baseline BP and blood volume are extremely variable and often unknown while initiating treatment. Although there is no single universally applicable end point of resuscitation, a combination of normalization of serum lactate, base deficit, pH, and hemorrhage control, if applicable, are markers that can be considered along with the rest of the patient's overall clinical status.

Clinical symptoms are relatively few in patients who are in class I shock, with the exception of anxiety. Is the anxiety after injury from blood loss, pain, trauma, or drug intoxication? A heart rate higher than 100 beats/min has been used as a physical sign of bleeding, but evidence of its significance is minimal. Brasel and colleagues[10] have shown that heart rate was neither sensitive nor specific in determining the need for emergent intervention, the need for packed red blood cell (PRBC) transfusions in the first 2 hours after an injury, or the severity of the injury. Heart rate was not altered by the presence of hypotension (systolic BP [SBP] <90 mm Hg).

In patients who are in class II shock, ATLS teaches that heart rate is increased, but as previously mentioned, this is a highly unreliable marker; pain and anxiety can also increase heart rate. The change in pulse pressure, the difference between systolic and diastolic pressure, is also difficult to identify because the baseline BP of patients is not always known. The change in pulse pressure is thought to be caused by an epinephrine response constricting vessels, resulting in higher diastolic pressures.

Not until patients are in class III shock does BP theoretically decrease. At this stage, patients have lost 30% to 40% of their blood volume; for an average male weighing 75 kg, this equates

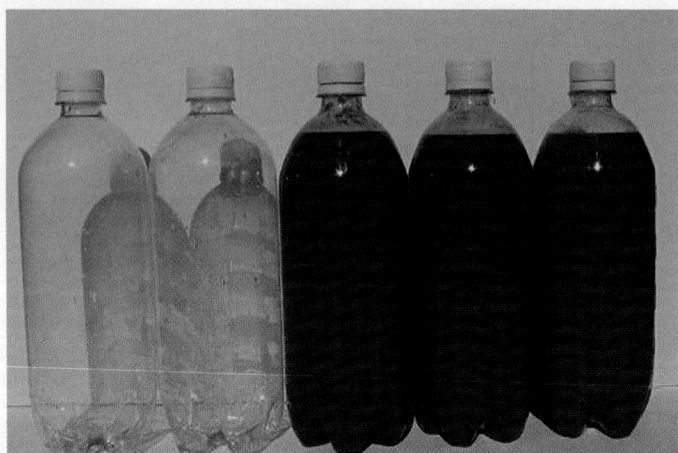

FIGURE 33.6 Liters of blood lost for class III shock, or 40% of 5 L, according to Advanced Trauma Life Support.

to 2 L of blood loss (Fig. 33.6). It is helpful to remember that a can of soda or beer is 355 mL; a six-pack is 2130 mL. Theoretically, if a patient is hypotensive from blood loss, they have lost the equivalent of a six-pack of blood. The first and most important key when a patient is in shock due to hemorrhage is recognizing that blood loss is the cause of their shock, identifying the source of bleeding, and treating it. Resuscitation occurs simultaneously as needed.

Because ATLS is designed for a broad range of providers, many subtleties around the physiology of a bleeding patient are missing. However, surgeons know that there are some nuances in the varied responses to injuries in both animals and humans. In the case of arterial hemorrhage, for example, animals do not necessarily manifest tachycardia as their first response when bleeding, but they actually become bradycardic. It is speculated that this is a teleologic mechanism because a bradycardic response reduces CO and minimizes uncontrolled exsanguination. A bradycardic response to bleeding is not consistently shown in all animals, including humans. Some evidence shows that this response, termed *relative bradycardia,* does occur in humans. Relative bradycardia is defined as a heart rate of less than 100 beats/min while simultaneously having an SBP below 90 mm Hg. When bleeding patients have relative bradycardia, their mortality rate is lower. Up to 44% of hypotensive patients who are not bleeding have relative bradycardia. However, this lower heart rate is only protective to a certain level because patients with a heart rate below 60 beats/min are usually moribund. Bleeding patients with a heart rate of 60 to 90 beats/min have the highest survival rate compared with patients with tachycardia (a heart rate of more than 90 beats/min).[11]

The physiologic response to bleeding also subtly differs according to whether the source of bleeding is arterial or venous. Arterial bleeding is an obvious problem, but it often stops temporarily on its own; the human body has evolved to trap the blood loss in adventitial tissues, and the transected artery will spasm and thrombose. A lacerated artery can actually bleed more than a transected artery because the spasm of the lacerated artery can enlarge the hole in the vessel. Thrombosis of the artery sometimes does *not* occur in transected or lacerated vessels. Also, because the arterial system does not have valves, the recorded BP can drop early, even before large-volume blood loss has occurred. In patients with arterial bleeding, hypotension may occur before tissue ischemia, so lactate and base deficit may be normal.

In contrast, venous bleeding is typically slower, allowing the human body time to compensate. This slower progression provides the time necessary for recruitment of fluid from the intracellular and interstitial spaces. This leads to large volumes of blood that can be lost before hypotension ensues. Because venous or capillary bed bleeding is slower and the body has a chance to compensate, this allows for tissue ischemia to develop during the process, and thus, there is time for lactate and base deficit results to be abnormal. Venous blood loss can be massive before hypotension occurs.

It is generally taught that the hematocrit or hemoglobin (Hb) level is not reliable in predicting blood loss on initial presentation. This can be true in patients who have not been resuscitated, but in patients who have received crystalloids, a rapid drop in the hematocrit and Hb levels can occur. Bruns and associates[12] have shown that the Hb level can be low within the first 30 minutes after patients arrive at trauma centers. Therefore, high or normal Hb levels do not rule out significant bleeding. But a low Hb level, because it occurs rapidly, generally reflects severe blood loss.

The lack of good indicators to distinguish which patients are bleeding has led many investigators to examine heart rate variability (HRV) or complexity as a potential new vital sign. Many clinical studies have shown that decreased HRV or complexity is associated with poor outcome, and increased HRV can be used as an end point of resuscitation. HRV or complexity would have to be calculated using software, with a resulting index on which clinicians would have to rely. This information would not be available by merely examining patients. Another issue with HRV or complexity is that the exact physiologic mechanism for its association with poor outcome has yet to be elucidated.[13] This new vital sign may be programmable into currently used monitors and has been marketed, but its usefulness has yet to be confirmed.

Compensatory reserve measurement (CRM), based on arterial pulse waveform, is another measurement that may be more specific and sensitive than HRV for determining degree of hemorrhagic shock. This method measures early compensatory mechanisms in the arterial system protecting against low delivery of oxygen to identify patients in need of resuscitation earlier. Software is currently being developed to integrate CRM into standard pulse oximeter hardware.[14,15]

Hypotension has been traditionally set, arbitrarily, at 90 mm Hg and below. But this level can be variable from patient to patient, especially depending on age. It has been suggested that hypotension be redefined as below 110 mm Hg. In 2008, Bruns and colleagues[16] confirmed the concept, showing that a prehospital BP below 110 mm Hg was associated with an inflection point in mortality and that 15% of patients with a prehospital BP below 110 mm Hg would eventually die in the hospital. As a result, they recommended redefining prehospital trauma triage criteria. In older patients, normal vital signs may miss occult hypoperfusion because geriatric patients are often hypertensive at baseline.

Shock Index

Because heart rate and SBP individually are not accurate at identifying hemorrhagic shock and because the traditionally taught combination of tachycardia and decreased SBP does not always occur together, the shock index (SI), which uses these two variables together, was developed. SI is defined as heart rate divided by SBP. It has been shown to be a better marker for assessing severity of shock than heart rate and BP alone. It has utility not only in trauma patients, who are often in hemorrhagic shock, but also in patients who are in shock from other causes, such as sepsis, obstetrics, myocardial infarction, stroke, and other acute illnesses. In the trauma population, SI has been shown to be more useful than heart rate and BP alone, and it has also been shown to be of benefit specifically in the pediatric and geriatric populations. It has been correlated with need for interventions such as blood transfusion and invasive procedures, including operations. SI is known as a *hemodynamic stability indicator*. However, SI does not consider the diastolic BP (DBP), and thus, a modified SI (MSI) was created. MSI is defined as heart rate divided by mean arterial pressure. As MSI rises, this indicates a low stroke volume and low systemic vascular resistance, a sign of hypodynamic circulation. In contrast, low MSI indicates a hyperdynamic state. MSI has been considered a better marker than SI for mortality rate prediction. Although SI or MSI is better than heart rate and SBP alone, the combination of one of these variables with heart rate and SBP will undoubtedly be more useful. There are additional studies showing that more complex calculations with more variables are more useful than simpler ones. For example, taking into account patient age, mechanism of injury, Glasgow Coma Scale (GCS) score, lactate levels, Hb levels, and other physiologic parameters will result in statistically better prediction than with one individual vital sign. It is intuitive that the addition of variables would be more predictive of outcome. That is why the presence of an experienced surgeon is critical; in a few seconds, the astute clinician will quickly consider multiple variables, including sex, age, GCS score, mechanism of injury, and other parameters. Whereas SI and MSI are statistically more accurate than one individual parameter, there is no substitute for the experienced clinician at the bedside. This may be the reason that SI and MSI have not been widely adopted.

Other risk assessment scores have been developed in recent years in an attempt to identify patients who will require a massive transfusion, including the Assessment of Blood Consumption (ABC) score and the Trauma ALgorithm Examining the Risk of massive Transfusion (ALERT) score. The ABC score uses mechanism of injury, SBP, heart rate, and the focused assessment with sonography in trauma (FAST) examination to predict which patients will require a massive transfusion. This score may be less sensitive than the SI, with more variables to use.[17] Interestingly, the ALERT score was stratified by prehospital and admission in an attempt to predict massive transfusion in both settings with the data available at each time interval—namely, SBP, DBP, heart rate, respiratory rate, SpO_2, motor GCS score, and penetrating mechanism for the prehospital setting and admission SBP, heart rate, respiratory rate, GCS score, temperature, the FAST examination result, and prehospital SBP and DBP on admission. Both accurately predict massive transfusion, with the admission score outperforming the scene score.[18]

There may be utility in the future for automatically accounting for these variables in the electronic health record (EHR) in an hour-by-hour format using artificial intelligence. One study by Park et al. was able to program the Parkland Trauma Index of Mortality, which accounts for 23 variables, including GCS, vital signs, and laboratory data, into their EHR with hourly predictions of mortality that then assisted with decision-making and timing of interventions.[19]

Lactate and Base Deficit

Lactate has stood the test of time as an associated marker of injury and possibly ischemia.[20] However, new data question the etiology and role of lactate. The emerging information is confusing; it suggests that we may not understand lactate for what it truly implies.

Lactate has long been thought to be a byproduct of anaerobic metabolism and is routinely perceived to be an end waste product that is completely unfavorable. Physiologists are now questioning this paradigm and have found that lactate behaves more advantageously than not. An analogy would be that firefighters are associated with fires, but that does not mean that firefighters are bad, nor does it mean that they caused the fires.

Research has shown that lactate increases in muscle and blood during exercise. It is at its highest level at or just after exhaustion, which led to the assumption that lactate was a waste product. In addition, we also know that lactic acid appears in response to muscle contraction and continues in the absence of oxygen. Furthermore, accumulated lactate disappears when an adequate supply of oxygen is present in tissues.

Recent evidence indicates that lactate is an active metabolite, capable of moving between cells, tissues, and organs, where it may be oxidized as fuel or reconverted to form pyruvate or glucose. It now appears that increased lactate production and concentration, as a result of anoxia or dysoxia, are often the exception rather than the rule. Lactate seems to be a shuttle for energy; the lactate shuttle is now the subject of much debate. The end product of glycolysis is pyruvic acid. Lack of oxygen is thought to convert pyruvate into lactate. However, lactate formation may allow carbohydrate metabolism to continue through glycolysis. It is postulated that lactate is transferred from its site of production in the cytosol to neighboring cells and to a variety of organs (e.g., heart, liver, and kidney), where its oxidation and continued metabolism can occur.

Lactate is also being studied as a pseudohormone because it seems to regulate the cellular redox state through exchange and conversion into pyruvate and through its effects on the ratio of nicotinamide adenine dinucleotide to nicotinamide adenine dinucleotide (reduced)—the $NAD^+/NADH$ ratio, a key measure of cellular redox state. It is released into the systemic circulation and taken up by distal tissues and organs, where it also affects the redox state in those cells.[21] Further evidence has shown that it affects wound regeneration with promotion of increased collagen deposition and neovascularization. Lactate may also induce vasodilatation and catecholamine release and stimulate fat and carbohydrate oxidation.

Lactate levels in blood are highly dependent on the equilibrium between production and elimination from the bloodstream. The liver is predominantly responsible for metabolizing lactate, and liver disease affects lactate levels. Lactate was always thought to be produced from anaerobic tissues, but it now seems that a variety of tissue beds that are not undergoing anaerobic metabolism produce lactate when they are signaled with distress.

In canine muscle, lactate is produced by moderate-intensity exercise when the oxygen supply is ample. A high adrenergic stimulus also causes a rise in lactate as the body prepares for or responds to stress. A study of climbers of Mount Everest showed that the resting PO_2 on the summit was about 28 mm Hg and decreased even more during exercise. The blood lactate level in those climbers was essentially the same as at sea level, even though they were in a state of hypoxia.[22] These facts have led us to question what we believed we knew about lactate and its true role.

In humans, lactate may be the preferred fuel in the brain and heart; in these tissues, infused lactate is used before glucose at rest and during exercise. Because lactate is glucose sparing, it allows glucose and glycogen levels to be maintained. Lactate's role in TBI remains unclear, but there appear to be reliable metabolic patterns, with high lactate being associated with elderly patients who have a degree of insulin resistance and younger patients with a degree of systemic shock at play.[23] The level of lactate, whether it is a waste product or a source of energy, seems to signify tissue distress, whether it is from anaerobic conditions or other factors. During times of stress, there is a release of epinephrine and other catecholamines, which also causes a release of lactate.

Base deficit, a measure of the number of millimoles of base required to correct the pH of a liter of whole blood to 7.4, seems to correlate well with lactate level, at least in the first 24 hours after a physiologic insult. Rutherford, in 1992, showed that a base deficit of 8 was associated with a 25% mortality rate in patients older than 55 years without a head injury or in patients younger than 55 years with a head injury. When base deficit remains elevated, most clinicians believe that it is an indication of ongoing shock.[24] Recent literature suggests the time to correction of base deficit is an important factor in all-cause mortality after trauma, namely, a return to physiologically normal levels within 48 hours.[25] One problem with base deficit is that it is commonly influenced by the chloride in various resuscitation fluids, resulting in a hyperchloremic nonanion-gap metabolic acidosis. In patients with renal failure, base deficit can also be a poor predictor of outcome; in the acute stage of renal failure, a base deficit of greater than 6 mmol/L is associated with poor outcome.[26] With the use of hypertonic saline (HTS), which has three to eight times the sodium chloride concentration of normal saline, the hyperchloremic acidosis has been shown to be relatively harmless. However, when HTS is used, base deficit should be interpreted with caution.

Compensatory Mechanisms

When shock occurs, blood flow is diverted from less critical to more critical tissues. The earliest compensatory mechanism in response to a decrease in intravascular volume is an increase in sympathetic activity. Such an increase is mediated by pressure receptors or baroreceptors in the aortic arch, atria, and carotid bodies. A decrease in pressure inhibits parasympathetic discharge while norepinephrine and epinephrine are liberated and cause adrenergic receptors in the myocardium and vascular smooth muscle to be activated. Heart rate, contractility, and peripheral vascular resistance are increased, resulting in increased BP. However, the various tissue beds are not affected equally; blood is shunted from less critical organs (e.g., skin, skeletal muscle, and splanchnic circulation) to more critical organs (e.g., brain, liver, and kidneys).

The juxtaglomerular apparatus in the kidney, in response to the vasoconstriction and decrease in blood flow, produces the enzyme renin, which leads to the generation of angiotensin I. The angiotensin-converting enzyme located on the endothelial cells of the pulmonary arteries converts angiotensin I to angiotensin II. In turn, angiotensin II stimulates an increased sympathetic drive at the level of the nerve terminal by releasing hormones from the adrenal medulla. In response, the adrenal medulla affects intravascular volume during shock by secreting catechol hormones—epinephrine, norepinephrine, and dopamine—which are all produced from phenylalanine and tyrosine. They are called *catecholamines* because they contain a catechol group derived from the amino acid tyrosine. The release of catecholamines is thought to be responsible for the elevated glucose level in hemorrhagic shock. Although hyperglycemia is thought to be a normal part of the physiologic stress response to trauma, persistent hyperglycemia after injury is deleterious, which has been demonstrated by multiple studies.[27] Elevated glucose in the prehospital setting may be an early indicator of impending hemodynamic instability.[28]

However, when lactate and therefore degree of shock are considered simultaneously with hyperglycemia, the association with mortality may be more tenuous.[29] Cortisol, also released from the adrenal cortex, plays a major role in fluid equilibrium. In the adrenal cortex, the zona glomerulosa produces aldosterone in response to stimulation by angiotensin II. Aldosterone is a mineralocorticoid that modulates renal function by increasing recovery of sodium and excretion of potassium. Angiotensin II also causes the reabsorption of sodium through a direct action on the renal tubules. Sodium is the primary osmotic ion in the human body in the regulation of water balance, with the reabsorption of sodium leading to the reabsorption of water, which subsequently leads to intravascular volume expansion in response to shock. One problem is that the release of these hormones is not infinite, and thus, the supply can be exhausted in a state of ongoing shock.

This regulation of intravascular fluid status is further affected by the carotid baroreceptors and the atrial natriuretic peptides. Signals are sent to the supraoptic and paraventricular nuclei in the brain. Antidiuretic hormone (ADH) is released from the pituitary, causing retention of free water at the level of the kidney. Simultaneously, volume is recruited from the extravascular and cellular spaces. A shift of water occurs as hydrostatic pressures fall in the intravascular compartment. At the capillary level, hydrostatic pressures are also reduced because the precapillary sphincters are vasoconstricted more than the postcapillary sphincters.

Lethal Triad: Acidosis, Hypothermia, and Coagulopathy

The lethal triad of acidosis, hypothermia, and coagulopathy is common in resuscitated patients who are bleeding or in shock from various factors. Our basic understanding is that inadequate tissue perfusion results in acidosis caused by lactate production. In the shock state, the delivery of nutrients to the cells is thought to be inadequate, leading to a decrease in the body's main energy storage molecule, adenosine triphosphate (ATP). The human body relies on ATP production to maintain homeostatic temperatures, like all homeothermic (warm-blooded) animals do. Thus, if ATP production is inadequate to maintain body temperature, the body will trend toward the ambient temperature. For most human patients, this is 22°C (72°F), the temperature inside typical hospitals. The resulting hypothermia and acidosis then affect the efficiency of enzymes, which work best at 37°C and a pH of 7.4. For surgeons, the critical issue with hypothermia is the coagulation cascade's dependence on enzymes that are affected by hypothermia. If enzymes are not functioning optimally as a result of hypothermia, coagulopathy worsens, which can contribute to uncontrolled bleeding from injuries or surgery. Further bleeding continues to fuel the triad. The optimal method to break the "vicious circle of death" is to stop the bleeding and the causes of hypothermia. In most typical scenarios, hypothermia is not spontaneous from ischemia but is induced because of use of room-temperature fluid or cold blood products.

Acidosis

Bleeding causes a host of responses. During the resuscitative phase, the lethal triad (acidosis, hypothermia, and coagulopathy) is frequent in severely bleeding patients, most likely because of two major factors. First, decreased perfusion causes lactic acidosis and consumptive coagulopathy. Second, room-temperature and large-volume fluids lead to worsening hypothermia and dilutional coagulopathy, creating a resuscitation injury. Some believe that the acidotic state is not necessarily undesirable because the body tolerates acidosis better than alkalosis. Oxygen is more easily offloaded from Hb in the acidotic environment. Basic scientists who try to preserve tissue ex vivo find that cells live longer in an acidotic environment. Correcting acidosis with sodium bicarbonate has classically been avoided because it is treating a laboratory value or symptom. The focus should be on correcting the cause of the acidosis. Treating the pH alone has shown no benefit, but it can lead to complacency. It is also argued that rapidly injecting sodium bicarbonate can worsen intracellular acidosis from the diffusion of the converted CO_2 into the cells.

The best fundamental approach to metabolic acidosis from shock is to treat the underlying cause of shock. In the surgeon's case, this is due to blood loss or ischemic tissue. However, some clinicians believe that treating the pH has advantages because the enzymes necessary for clotting function better at an optimal temperature and optimal pH. Coagulopathy can contribute to uncontrolled bleeding, so some have recommended treating acidosis with bicarbonate infusion for patients in dire scenarios. Treating acidosis with sodium bicarbonate may have a benefit in an unintended and unrecognized way. Rapid infusion of bicarbonate is usually accompanied by a rise in BP in hypotensive patients. This rise is usually attributed to correcting the pH; however, sodium bicarbonate, in most urgent scenarios, is given in ampules. The 50-mL ampule of sodium bicarbonate has 1 mEq/mL—in essence, similar to giving a hypertonic concentration of sodium, which quickly draws fluid into the vascular space. Given its high sodium concentration, a 50-mL bolus of sodium bicarbonate has physiologic results similar to 325 mL of normal saline or 385 mL of LR solution. Essentially, it is like giving small doses of HTS. Sodium bicarbonate quickly increases CO_2 levels by its conversion in the liver, so if the minute ventilation is not increased, respiratory acidosis can result.

Tromethamine; tris[hydroxymethyl] aminomethane (THAM) is a biologically inert amino alcohol of low toxicity that buffers CO_2 and acids. It is sodium-free and limits the generation of CO_2 in the process of buffering. At 37°C, the pK_a of THAM is 7.8, making it a more effective buffer than sodium bicarbonate in the physiologic range of blood pH. In vivo, THAM supplements the buffering capacity of the blood bicarbonate system by generating sodium bicarbonate and decreasing the partial pressure of CO_2. It rapidly distributes to the extracellular space and slowly penetrates the intracellular space, except in the case of erythrocytes and hepatocytes, and it is excreted by the kidney. Unlike sodium bicarbonate, which requires an open system to eliminate CO_2 to exert its buffering effect, THAM is effective in a closed or semiclosed system, and it maintains its buffering ability during hypothermia. THAM acetate (0.3 M, pH 8.6) is well tolerated, does not cause tissue or venous irritation, and is the only formulation available in the United States. THAM may induce respiratory depression and hypoglycemia, which may require ventilatory assistance and the administration of glucose.

The initial loading dose of THAM acetate (0.3 M) for the treatment of acidemia may be estimated as follows:

THAM (in milliliters of 0.3M solution) = Lean body eight (in kilograms) × Base deficit (in millimoles per liter)

The maximal daily dose is 15 mmol/kg/day for an adult (3.5 L of a 0.3-M solution in a patient weighing 70 kg). It is indicated in the treatment of respiratory failure (acute respiratory distress syndrome [ARDS] and infant respiratory distress syndrome) and has been associated with the use of hypothermia and permissive hypercapnia (controlled hypoventilation). Other indications are diabetic and renal acidosis, salicylate and barbiturate intoxication, and increased intracranial pressure (ICP) associated with brain trauma. It is used in cardioplegic solutions and during liver transplantation. Despite these attributes, THAM has not been documented clinically to be more efficacious than sodium bicarbonate.

Hypothermia

Hypothermia can be both beneficial and detrimental. A fundamental knowledge of hypothermia is of vital importance in the care of surgical patients. The beneficial aspects of hypothermia are mainly a result of decreased metabolism. Injury sites are often iced, creating vasoconstriction and decreasing inflammation through decreased metabolism. This concept of cooling to slow metabolism is also the rationale behind using hypothermia to decrease ischemia during cardiac, transplant, pediatric, and neurologic surgery. Also, amputated extremities are iced before reimplantation. Cold water near-drowning victims have higher survival rates, thanks to preservation of the brain and other vital organs. Also, there has been waxing and waning data supporting cooling (to 32°C–36°C for 12–24 hours) of unconscious adults who have a return of spontaneous circulation after out-of-hospital cardiac arrest. Induced hypothermia is vastly different from spontaneous hypothermia, which is typically from shock, inadequate tissue perfusion, or cold fluid infusion.

Medical or accidental hypothermia is vastly different from trauma-associated hypothermia (Table 33.2). The survival rates after accidental hypothermia range from about 12% to 39%. The average temperature drop is to about 30°C (range, 13.7°C–35.0°C). That lowest recorded temperature in a survivor of accidental hypothermia (13.7°C, or 56.7°F) was in an extreme skier in Norway; she was trapped under the ice and eventually fully recovered neurologically.

The data in patients with trauma-associated hypothermia differ. Their survival rate falls dramatically with their core temperature, reaching 100% mortality when it reaches 32°C at any point—whether it is in the emergency department, operating room, or intensive care unit (ICU). In trauma patients, hypothermia is due to shock, and it perpetuates uncontrolled bleeding because of the associated coagulopathy. Trauma patients with a postoperative core temperature below 35°C have a fourfold increase in death; below 33°C, they have a sevenfold increase in death. Hypothermic trauma patients tend to be more severely injured, older, and have increased blood loss requiring an increased number of transfusions.[30] Surprisingly, in a study using the National Trauma Data Base, Shafi and colleagues showed that hypothermia and its associated poor outcome were not related to the state of shock. It was previously thought that a core temperature below 32°C was uniformly fatal in trauma patients who have the additional insult of tissue injury and bleeding. However, a small number of trauma patients have now survived despite a recorded core temperature below 32°C. Beilman and coworkers demonstrated that hypothermia was associated with more severe injuries, bleeding, and a higher rate of multiple-organ dysfunction in the ICU, but not with death, on multivariate analysis.[31]

To understand hypothermia, we have to remember that humans are homeothermic (warm-blooded) animals, in contrast to poikilothermic (cold-blooded) animals such as snakes and fish.

TABLE 33.2	**Classification of Hypothermia**	
	TRAUMA	**ACCIDENTAL**
Mild	36°C–34°C	35°C–32°C
Moderate	34°C–32°C	32°C–28°C
Severe	<32°C	<28°C

To maintain a body temperature of 37°C, the hypothalamus uses a variety of mechanisms to tightly control core body temperature. We use oxygen as the key ingredient or fuel to generate heat in the mitochondria in the form of ATP. When ATP production is below its lowest threshold, one of the side effects is the lowering of body temperature to the ambient temperature, which typically is less than core body temperature. In contrast, during exercise, we use more oxygen as more ATP is required, and we produce excess heat. In an attempt to modulate core temperature, we start perspiring to use the cooling properties of evaporation.

Hypothermia, although potentially beneficial, is detrimental in trauma patients mainly because it causes coagulopathy. Cold affects the coagulation cascade by decreasing enzyme activity, enhancing fibrinolytic activity, and causing platelet dysfunction. Platelets are affected by the inhibition of thromboxane B_2 production, resulting in decreased aggregation. A heparin-like substance is released, causing diffuse intravascular coagulation–like syndrome. Hageman factor and thromboplastin are some of the enzymes most affected. Even a drop in core temperature of just a few degrees results in 40% inefficiency in some of the enzymes.

Heat affects the coagulation cascade so much that when blood is drawn in cold patients and sent to the laboratory, the sample is heated to 37°C because even 1 or 2 degrees of cold delays clotting and renders test results inaccurate. Thus, in a cold and coagulopathic patient, if the coagulation profile obtained from the laboratory shows an abnormality, the result represents the level of coagulopathy if the patient (and not just the sample) had been warmed to 37°C. Therefore, a cold patient is always more coagulopathic than indicated by the coagulation profile. A normal coagulation profile does not necessarily represent what is going on in the body.

Heat is measured in calories. One calorie is the amount of energy required to raise the temperature of 1 mL of water (which has, by definition, a specific heat of 1.0). It takes 1 kcal to raise the temperature of 1 L of water by 1°C. If an average male (weight, 75 kg) consisted of pure water, it would take 75 kcal to raise his temperature by 1°C. However, we are not made of pure water, and blood has a specific heat coefficient of 0.87. The human body as a whole has a specific heat coefficient of 0.83. Therefore, it actually takes 62.25 kcal (75 kg × 0.83) to raise body temperature by 1°C. If a patient were to lose 62.25 kcal, body temperature would drop by 1°C. This basic science is important in choosing methods to retain heat or treat hypothermia or hyperthermia. It allows one to compare the efficacy of one method with another.

The normal basal metabolic heat generation is about 70 kcal/h. Shivering can increase this to 250 kcal/h. Heat is transferred to and from the body by contact or conduction (as in a frying pan and Jacuzzi), air or convection (as in an oven and sauna), radiation, and evaporation. Convection is an extremely inefficient way to transfer heat because the air molecules are so far apart compared with liquids and solids. Conduction and radiation are the most efficient ways to transfer heat. However, heating the patient with radiation is fraught with inconsistencies and technical challenges, and thus it is difficult to apply clinically, so we are left with conduction to transfer energy efficiently.

Warming or cooling through manipulation of the temperature of IV fluids is useful because it uses conduction to transfer heat. Although IV fluids can be warmed, the US Food and Drug Administration (FDA) allows fluid warmers to be set at a maximum of 40°C. Therefore, the differential between a cold trauma patient (34°C) and warmed fluid is only 6°C. Thus, 1 L of warmed fluids

can transfer only 6 kcal to the patient. As previously calculated, one needs about 62 kcal to raise the core temperature by 1°C. Therefore, we need 10.4 L of warmed fluids to raise the core temperature by 1°C to 35°C. Once that has been achieved, the differential is now only 5°C between the patient and the warmed fluid, so it actually takes 12.5 L of warmed fluids to raise the patient from 35°C to 36°C. A cold patient at 32°C needs to be given 311 kcal (75 kg × 0.83) to be warmed to 37°C. Note that a liter of fluid must be given at the highest rate possible because if the infusion rate is slow, it cools to room temperature as the IV line is exposed to ambient room temperature. To avoid IV-line cooling, devices that warm fluids up to the point of insertion into the body should be used.

Warming of patients by infusion of warmed fluids is difficult, but fluid warmers are still critically important; the main reason to warm fluids is to prevent patients from being cooled further. Cold fluids can cool patients quickly. The fluids that are typically infused are at either room temperature (22°C) or 4°C if the fluids were refrigerated. The internal temperature of a refrigerator is 4°C, and this is where PRBCs are stored. Therefore, it takes 5 L of 22°C fluid or 2 L of cold blood products to cool a patient by 1°C. Again, the main reason for using fluid warmers is not necessarily to warm patients but to prevent cooling them during resuscitation.

Rewarming techniques are classified as passive or active. Active warming is further classified as external or internal (Table 33.3). Passive warming involves *preventing* heat loss. Examples of passive warming include drying the patient to minimize evaporative cooling, giving warm fluids to prevent cooling, or covering the patient so that the ambient air temperature immediately around the patient can be higher than the room temperature. Covering the patient's head helps reduce a tremendous amount of heat loss. Aluminum-lined head covers are preferred; they reflect back the heat that is normally lost through the scalp. Warming of the room technically helps reduce the heat loss gradient, but the surgical staff is usually unable to work in a humidified room of 37°C. Preventing evaporative heat loss also includes closing an open body cavity, such as the chest or abdomen. The most important way to prevent heat loss is to treat hemorrhagic shock by controlling bleeding. Once shock has been treated, metabolism will heat the patient from their core.

Active warming is the act of transferring calories to the patient, either externally through the skin or internally. Skin and fat are designed to be highly efficient in preventing heat transfer. Although fat is insulating against loss of heat, it is also the reason that transfer of heat past the skin is difficult. Active external warming is thus inefficient because of our built-in insulation compared with internal warming. The first and most important step for active rewarming is to remove any wet clothes or bedding that is present and dry the patient before starting any active

TABLE 33.3	Classification of Warming Techniques	
PASSIVE	**ACTIVE EXTERNAL**	**ACTIVE INTERNAL**
Dry the patient	Bair hugger	Warmed fluids
Warm fluids	Heated warmers	Heat ventilator
Warm blankets and sheets	Lamps	Cavity lavage, chest tube, abdomen, bladder
Provide head covers	Radiant warmers	Continuous arterial or venous rewarming
Warm the room	Clinitron bed	Full or partial bypass

warming technique. Without this step, the efficiency of all methods will drop dramatically, and the importance of this step cannot be overstated. External active warming with forced-air heating, such as with the Bair Hugger temperature management therapy (Arizant Healthcare Inc., Eden Prairie, MN), is technically classified as active warming, but because air is an inefficient medium, few calories are provided to patients. Forced-air heating increases only the patient's ambient temperature, but it can actually cool the patient initially because it increases evaporative heat loss if the patient is wet from blood, fluids, clothes, or sweat. Warming the skin may feel good to the patient and the surgeon, but it actually decreases shivering (a highly efficient method of internal warming that tricks the thermoregulatory nerve input on the skin). Because forced-air heating uses convection, the actual amount of active warming is estimated to be only 10 kcal/h.

Active external warming is more efficiently performed by placing patients on heating pads, which use conduction to transfer heat. Beds are available that can warm patients faster, such as the Clinitron bed (Hill-Rom, Batesville, IN), which uses heated air-fluidized beads. Such beds are not practical in the operating room but are applicable in the ICU. Another option is the use of heating pads, which use heated water for countercurrent heat exchange. These can be placed under the patient during surgery and can be effective in minimizing mild hypothermia. The number of kilocalories per hour depends on the extent of dilatation or vasoconstriction of the blood vessels in the skin. This countercurrent heat exchange system can also be used to cool the patient if necessary.

The best method to warm patients is to deliver calories internally (Table 33.4). Heating the air used for ventilators is technically a form of internal active warming, but again, it is an inefficient method because this transfers heat via convection. The surface area of the lungs is massive, but the energy is mainly transferred through humidified water droplets, mostly by convection and not conduction. The amount of heat transferred through warmed humidified air is also minimal in comparison to methods that use conduction. One method by which this can be done is the lavage of warmed fluids into body cavities via nasogastric tubes, Foley catheters, chest tubes, or lavage of the peritoneal cavity. If gastric lavage is desired, one method is continuous lavage by infusion of warmed fluids through the sump port while the fluid is sucked out of the main tube. Instruments to warm the hand through conduction show much promise but are not yet readily available.

A method that can actively rewarm a patient and also assist in the treatment of shock is extracorporeal membrane oxygenation (ECMO). With ECMO, the patient's blood is pumped through an artificial lung and then back into the bloodstream, which can support either a failing pulmonary or cardiac system. Along with oxygenation in the artificial lung, the blood can also be warmed

and then returned to the patient. Recent literature also shows promise in using ECMO for rewarming after accidental hypothermia. A retrospective cohort analysis of 44 hypothermic patients demonstrated greater survival (71% vs. 29%) in patients who experienced cardiac arrest in the ECMO group relative to the conventional rewarming group.[32] Cardiopulmonary bypass can also be used because it delivers heated blood at a rate of more than 5 L/min to every place in the body where there are capillaries. If full cardiopulmonary bypass is not available or not desired, alternatives include continuous venous or arterial rewarming. Venous-venous rewarming can also be accomplished using the roller pump of a dialysis machine (which is often more available to the average surgeon). A prospective study showed arterial-venous rewarming to be highly effective. It can warm patients to 37°C in about 39 minutes compared with an average warming time of 3.2 hours with standard techniques. Special Gentilello arterial-warming catheters are inserted into the femoral artery, and a second line is inserted into the opposite femoral vein. The pressure from the artery produces flow, which is then directed to a fluid warmer and back into the vein. This method depends highly on the patient's BP because flow is directly related to BP. There are also commercially available central line catheters that directly heat the blood; a countercurrent exchange system heats the tip of the catheter with warmed fluids, and as blood passes over this warmed catheter, heat is directly transferred.

During recent decades, with the changes in resuscitation methods, the incidence of hypothermia has decreased. Dilutional coagulopathy also occurs less frequently because the volume of crystalloids has been minimized and particular attention has been paid to ensure that all resuscitation fluids and blood are warmed before infusion.

Coagulopathy

Coagulopathy in surgical patients is multifactorial. In addition to acidosis and hypothermia, systemic inflammation exacerbates coagulation derangements such as platelet dysfunction, endothelial activation, fibrinolysis, clotting factor consumption, increased tissue plasminogen activator (tPA), and dysregulation of activated protein C. The dysregulation can be secondary to consumption, dilution (from infused fluids devoid of clotting factors), and genetic (hemophilia) factors.[33]

Coagulopathy often needs to be corrected. The most used tests for coagulopathy are prothrombin time, partial thromboplastin time, and international normalized ratio. However, these tests have been shown to be inaccurate in detecting coagulopathy in surgical patients. One of the major reasons is that coagulopathy is a dynamic state that evolves through different stages of hypocoagulability, hypercoagulability, and fibrinolysis. The traditional tests of blood clotting lack the ability to detect the evolution of coagulopathy through these stages because they only depict the coagulation state at a snapshot in time. Moreover, the traditional tests are performed at normal pH and temperature, so they do not consider the effects of hypothermia and acidosis on coagulation. These traditional tests are also performed on serum and not on whole blood and do not have the ability to measure the interaction of coagulation factors and platelets.

More recently, thromboelastography (TEG) and rotational thromboelastometry have emerged as dynamic measures of coagulation that provide a more sensitive and accurate measure of the coagulation changes seen in surgical patients. TEG and thromboelastometry are based on similar principles of detecting clot strength, which is the final product of the coagulation cascade.

TABLE 33.4	Calories Delivered By Active Warming	
METHOD	**KCAL/H**
Airway from vent	9
Overhead radiant warmers	17
Heating blankets	20
Convective warmers	15–26
Body cavity lavages	35
Continuous arteriovenous rewarming	92–140
Cardiopulmonary bypass	710

They are also performed on whole blood, so they consider the functional interaction of coagulation factors and platelets.

TEG parameters include R-time, or reaction time; α, or alpha angle; and MA, or maximum amplitud; and K-time, or coagulation time. The R-time reflects the latent time until fibrin formation begins. An increase in this time may result from either decreased activity or deficiencies of coagulation factors, whereas a decrease in R-time reflects a hypercoagulable state. The steepness of the α-angle reflects the rate of fibrin formation and cross-linking, with a sharper angle indicating increased fibrin formation and a flatter angle indicating slower formation. The measure of clot strength is MA, which reflects clot elasticity. The value of MA is a measure of the strength of interaction between the coagulation factors, fibrin, and platelets. Qualitative or quantitative defects in either of these would result in decreased MA. The K-time measures the time until a clot reaches a fixed firmness, which relies on fibrinogen. TEG provides the additional ability to measure the fibrinolytic arm of the coagulation cascade. LY30 and LY60 indices provide a measure of the fibrinolysis rate by calculating the decrease in clot strength at 30 and 60 minutes, respectively. A large lysis index reflects rapid fibrinolysis and may help guide the use of antifibrinolytic therapy, which has been shown to reduce mortality if it is used within 3 hours of injury. Components of a TEG can help guide treatment of a bleeding patient because they can give the surgeon information regarding what part of the clotting cascade is defective. These tests are commonly used in cardiac surgery, trauma and liver transplant surgery, and other surgical disciplines in the form of point-of-care testing or in the central lab (Fig. 33.7).

The methods to define and treat coagulopathy are still varied. As discussed earlier, stopping the lethal triad is the most important step to stop the vicious cycle of hemorrhage. Prothrombin complex concentrate (PCC) has become popular for the treatment of surgical coagulopathy. PCC actually has many factors (factors II, VII, IX, X) in it, including variable amounts of factor VIIa, depending on the brand of PCC used. For patients taking warfarin, PCC is the recommended treatment of choice because this treatment replaces the factors inhibited with warfarin. This is of particular benefit in elderly patients with TBI, in whom treatment with fresh frozen plasma (FFP) can potentially be a problem if the patient has comorbid cardiac disease and could induce cardiac heart failure from volume overload. An additional benefit of using PCC is that the time to reversal of coagulopathy is shorter than when FFP is used. The use of blood-based component therapy is paramount in treating coagulopathy (see later, "Evolution of Modern Resuscitation"). A recent multicenter randomized trial demonstrated that PCC administration in trauma patients at risk for massive transfusion was not associated with reduced blood product administration and was associated with increased thromboembolic

events.[34] This was a relatively small study using a PCC comprising fewer anticoagulant factors, and all thromboses, including superficial thrombosis, were included. Other randomized trauma trials with different PCCs are ongoing. If there was a drug that would stop or reduce bleeding, treat coagulopathy at a low cost, and not cause serious complications, it would be a landmark contribution to medicine. Again, the problem is that current candidates are expensive, and the adverse events from administering such drugs are still not fully elucidated.

Another target of the coagulation cascade for medications is modulating the fibrinolytic pathways. Tranexamic acid (TXA) is a synthetic analogue of the amino acid lysine and is an antifibrinolytic medication that competitively inhibits the activation of plasminogen to plasmin. It prevents degradation of fibrin, which is a protein that forms the framework of blood clots. TXA has about eight times the antifibrinolytic activity of an older analogue, ε-aminocaproic acid. It is used to treat or prevent excessive blood loss during cardiac, liver, vascular, and orthopedic surgical procedures. It seems that topical TXA is effective and safe after total knee and hip replacement surgery, along with mucosal oropharyngeal bleeding in patients who are thrombocytopenic, reducing bleeding and the need for blood transfusions. Studies have shown similar results in children undergoing craniofacial surgery, spinal surgery, and others. It is even used for heavy menstrual bleeding in oral tablet form and in dentistry as a 5% mouthwash. It has been advocated for use in trauma. It seems to be effective in reducing rebleeding in spontaneous intracranial bleeding. A small double-blinded placebo-controlled randomized study of 238 patients showed a reduction in progression of intracranial bleeding after trauma, but because of the small sample size, it was not statistically significant. TXA is used to treat primary fibrinolysis, which is integral in the pathogenesis of the acute coagulopathy of trauma.

The Clinical Randomization of an Antifibrinolytic in Significant Hemorrhage (CRASH-2) trial, a multicenter randomized controlled civilian trial of 20,211 patients, showed that TXA reduced all-cause mortality versus placebo (14.5% vs. 16.0%).[35] The risk of death caused by bleeding was also reduced (4.9% vs. 5.7%). CRASH-2 also suggested that TXA was less effective and could even be harmful if treatment was delayed more than 3 hours after admission. This was confirmed in the retrospective Military Application of Tranexamic Acid in Trauma Emergency Resuscitation (MATTER) study and rapidly incorporated into military practice guidelines and subsequently for civilians worldwide.[36] The PED-TRAX study demonstrated that in children treated at a military hospital in Afghanistan, TXA administration to 66 of the 766 children was independently associated with decreased mortality and improved neurologic and pulmonary outcomes. Although the CRASH-2 trial was a randomized study with placebo, the critics of the study point out that it was performed in 270 hospitals in 40 countries, and the large sample size may result in a beta 1 error, meaning that the study was statistically significant because of the large number of patients in the study, but the small differences in outcome may not necessarily be clinically relevant. The absolute risk reduction was approximately 1.5%, with an estimated number needed to treat of 68.

The effects of TXA on death, disability, vascular occlusive events, and other morbidities in patients with acute TBI were investigated in a randomized placebo-controlled trial (CRASH-3) that assessed the effect of TXA on the risk of death or disability in patients with TBI. Patients were randomized in the field by emergency medical services (EMS) or in the hospital by providers—study arm patients received a 1-g loading dose and a 1-g dose delivered over 8 hours. Patients with a GCS of 12 or less or evidence

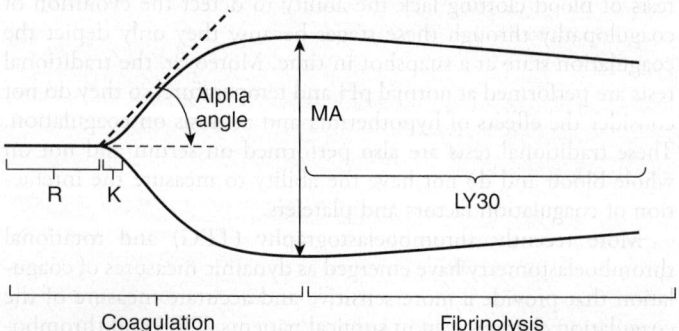

FIGURE 33.7 Coagulation and fibrinolysis testing. *K,* K-Time (coagulation time); *MA,* maximum amplitude; *R,* R-Time (reaction time).

of bleeding on head CT ($n = 12,737$) were studied, demonstrating a head injury–related risk of death of 12.5% in the study group and 14% in the placebo group. Of note, these results were significant for the group with mild to moderate head injuries, but there was no statistically significant difference in the severely injured. The protocol initially included patients within 8 hours of injury but was amended to include patients within 3 hours of injury in 2016. These data would suggest that TXA is useful within 3 hours in patients with mild to moderate TBI.[37] The TXA in TBI trial was another randomized trial in patients with moderate to severe TBI. Patients were randomized to a 2-g bolus in the field and a placebo infusion in the hospital, 1 g in the field and 1 g in the hospital, or placebo in the field and in the hospital. Patients with intracranial hemorrhage who received a TXA did not have improved neurologic outcomes by the extended Glasgow outcome scale. Despite some of the limited supporting data, TXA remains attractive because it is inexpensive and easy to use, with minimal side effects reported in randomized trials.[38]

Oxygen Delivery

The definition of shock is inadequate tissue perfusion, but many clinicians have incorrectly simplified it to inadequate tissue oxygenation. Much of what we know about oxygen delivery and consumption started with a physiologist named Archibald V. Hill. He was an avid runner who measured the oxygen consumption of four runners running around an 88-m grass track (Fig. 33.8). In the process of his work, Hill defined the terms *maximum O2 intake, O2 requirement,* and *O2 debt*. He is mostly known for his work with Otto Meyerhof, who unraveled the distinction between aerobic and anaerobic metabolism, for which they were awarded the Nobel Prize in 1922.

Blood delivers oxygen by red cells, which contain Hb. The simple calculation of oxygen delivery (DO_2) is the CO multiplied by the content of oxygen carried by a volume of blood: (CaO_2): $DO_2 = CO \times CaO_2$. The average Hb molecule carries 1.34 mL of oxygen per gram, depending on the arterial Hb oxygen saturation (SaO_2) of the red cell. In addition, a minor amount of oxygen is dissolved in plasma. This amount is calculated by multiplying the solubility constant 0.003 times the partial pressure of oxygen in the arterial blood (PaO_2). The CaO_2 of arterial blood is calculated as follows: $CaO_2 = (1.34 \times Hb \times SaO_2) + (0.003 \times PaO_2)$, where Hb is in grams per deciliter. CO is heart rate multiplied by the stroke volume. In a normal state, the stroke volume can be increased by shunting blood from one tissue bed to the central vasculature, but most of the change in CO is due to increased heart rate. In states of hemorrhage and resuscitation, the stroke volume is affected by infusion of fluids. As blood volume is decreased, it will ultimately affect stroke volume and is compensated by an increase in heart rate.

Oxygen consumption (VO_2) by cells is calculated by subtracting the content of oxygen in the venous system (CVO_2) from delivered oxygen content in the arterial blood (CaO_2): $VO_2 = CO \times (CaO_2 - CVO_2)$. After simplifying the terms and converting the units, the result is as follows: $VO_2 = CO \times 1.34 \times Hb \times (SaO_2 - SVO_2)$. The most conventional method of sampling the venous oxygen content is by drawing blood from the most distal port of a pulmonary artery catheter. The sample is taken from the pulmonary artery because venous blood is mixed there from all parts of the body. Oxygen content in the inferior vena cava is typically higher than in the superior vena cava, which is higher than in the coronary sinus. The average mixed venous sample is 75% saturated, so the oxygen consumption is thought to be, on average, 25% of the oxygen delivered (Fig. 33.9). Thus, teleologically, there is an ample reserve of oxygen delivered.

With advancements in technology, catheters are now available that can continuously measure the venous saturation in the pulmonary artery. These use technology similar to the pulse oximeter built into the tip of a pulmonary artery catheter, which uses near-infrared (NIR) light waves to measure the oxygen saturation state of Hb. These advanced catheters can also provide CO continuously. In the past, CO was inferred by measuring the rate of change in temperature in the heart at the distal aspect of a pulmonary artery catheter by infusing a standard volume of iced or room-temperature water into the proximal port and measuring the change in temperature. In recent years, pulmonary artery catheters are no longer commonly used. Venous oxygenation can still be measured from central lines, but these assessments are no longer mixed venous in nature.

CO and oxygen delivery are also affected by the end-diastolic volume of the left ventricle. As described by Starling in 1915, CO increases when the ventricular fibers increase in length. There is a maximum filling point, after which CO no longer increases (Fig. 33.10). Left ventricular end-diastolic (LVED) volume can be inferred by using a pulmonary artery catheter and measuring the wedge pressure, which represents preload. This reflects the pressure in the left ventricle because the vessels from the pulmonary artery to the left ventricle have no valves. Alternative approaches can help optimize the filling volume in the left ventricle. Pulmonary artery catheters for calculating the right ventricular end-diastolic volume are available but are rarely used. Echocardiography using transthoracic or esophageal probes can

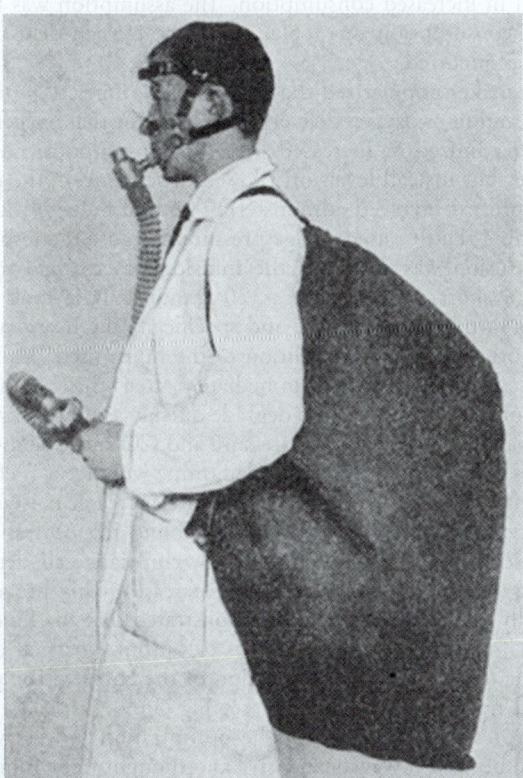

FIGURE 33.8 Bag with side tube, low on the left-hand side, for use while running. The tap is carried in the left hand. (From Hill AV, Lupton H. Muscular exercise, lactic acid, and the supply and utilization of oxygen. *Q J Med.* 1923;16:135-171.)

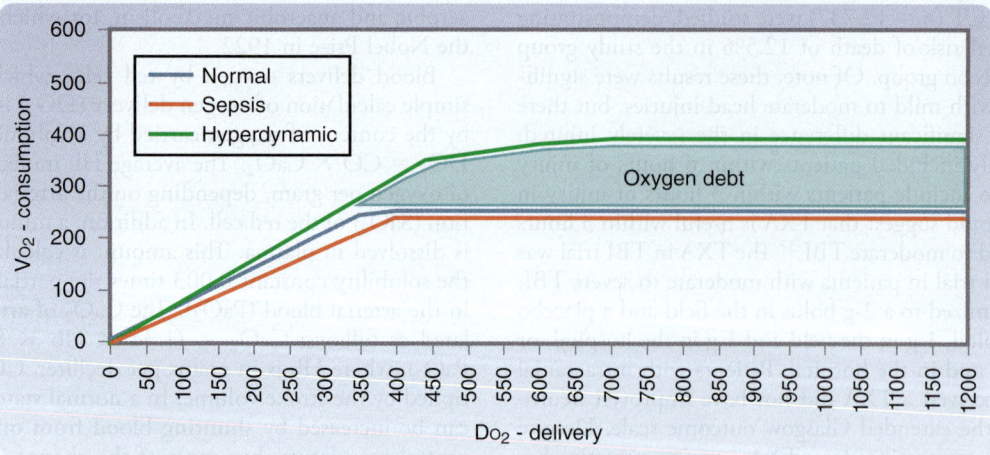

FIGURE 33.9 Oxygen delivery *(DO₂)* and consumption *(VO₂)*. During normal states, oxygen delivery is approximately 1000 mL/min of O₂. The oxygen consumption in a normal state is 25% of delivery and is approximately 250 mL/min. At very low oxygen delivery, it is believed that consumption is delivery dependent and occurs in shock. There is oxygen debt during shock and during recovery, and there is a hyperdynamic stage during which the circulatory system is paying back its oxygen debt.

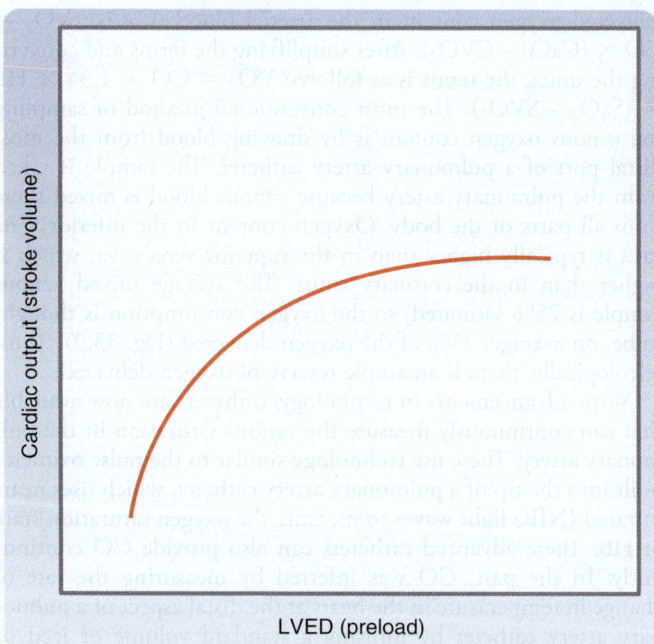

FIGURE 33.10 Starling curve. As left ventricular end-diastolic *(LVED)* pressure is increased, the fibers of the heart muscle are lengthened, resulting in increased contraction and increased cardiac output. This occurs up to a certain point, after which increases in volume and length do not result in increases in cardiac output.

directly estimate filling volumes in the heart. However, variations in volume and heart size can distort results. Heart size is also affected by medical conditions that can stress and dilate the heart. The interpretation of heart size and adequate resuscitation data is thus subjective.

Optimization

During the late 1980s, surgical critical care evolved into a specialty, focusing heavily on ventilator support and optimizing oxygen delivery to tissues. One of the pioneers of modern surgical critical care, William Shoemaker, theorized that during shock,

because of a lack of oxygen delivery, there was anaerobic metabolism and an oxygen debt that needed to be repaid. He showed that after volume loading, if oxygen delivery increased, consumption would also increase—until a certain point, when an additional increase in oxygen delivery did not result in increased consumption. This increased oxygen consumption was thought to be the process of paying back the oxygen debt that occurred during ischemia throughout the body. Patients in shock were found to have a hyperdynamic stage in which increased oxygen delivery resulted in increased consumption. The assumption was that increased consumption was replenishing the oxygen debt that the body had incurred.

Shoemaker popularized the concept of optimization or supernormalization of oxygen delivery, which means that oxygen delivery is maximized or increased until its consumption no longer increases but instead levels off (flow independence). The optimization process involved administering a rapid bolus of fluid and confirming that it raised wedge pressure. Because the response to fluid infusion was dynamic, the infusion process had to occur during a short period, such as 20 minutes. If it took longer, changes in the vascular space and specifically the heart might be due to other variables in addition to the fluids used. Also, if the response was not measured immediately after infusion, the effect of the infusion was known to degrade quickly as fluids moved out of the vascular space. Wedge pressure and CO must be measured minutes before fluid infusion to determine whether it is effective. If CO increases with the wedge pressure increase, it is assumed that oxygen delivery increases. By sampling the central venous oxygen content when measuring CO, clinicians can determine whether oxygen consumption also increases. This process was originally repeated until it was demonstrated that the fluid bolus did not increase CO. The goal was to optimize oxygen delivery from the delivery-dependent portion of the curve to the portion that was not delivery dependent (see Fig. 33.9).

The preferred fluid during the optimization process was LR solution because it was inexpensive and thought to be innocuous. Once the Starling curve was optimized, in that LVED volume could no longer be increased with increases in wedge pressure (preload), wedge pressure would be kept at that maximal level. Further increases in wedge pressure without increasing

LVED volume meant that patients might suffer from unnecessary pulmonary edema.

Once fluid infusion maximized CO and oxygen delivery, an inotropic agent would be added to further push CO to a higher level. The agent recommended at that time was dobutamine. The dose was increased, and its effect on CO was documented. With each maneuver, oxygen consumption was measured, and CO was "optimized" to meet the consumption demands. This optimizing process maximized oxygen delivery to ensure that all tissue beds were adequately perfused. Shoemaker's earlier clinical trials had shown that patients resuscitated in this manner had a lower incidence of multiple-organ dysfunction syndrome (MODS) and death. During this optimizing era, ARDS and MODS were the leading causes of late death in trauma patients.

However, subsequent clinical studies failed to repeat Shoemaker's success. Randomized prospective trials showed that the optimization of oxygen delivery and consumption did not improve outcome. In general, patients who responded to the optimization process did well, but those who could not have their oxygen delivery augmented to a higher level did poorly. Thus, although response to optimization was prognostic of outcome, the process itself did not seem to change outcome. One of the reasons that the earlier studies succeeded may have been because the control patients were not adequately resuscitated. With the later trials, when patients were adequately resuscitated, the optimization process did not improve outcome. In fact, the aggressive use of fluids to achieve supranormal oxygen delivery could cause increased multiple-organ failure, abdominal compartment syndrome, and increased mortality from excessive crystalloid infusions.[39] Over time, the widely used pulmonary artery catheter fell out of favor. Studies have shown that the discontinued use of the pulmonary artery catheter has not adversely affected outcome. Because of the invasive nature of the pulmonary artery catheter and concern that the data derived from the catheter were often misinterpreted, its use has virtually disappeared from the modern-day surgical ICU, aside from its use in cardiac surgery patients.

Moreover, oxygen delivery in hyperdynamic patients could not be driven to a point at which consumption seemed to level off. One theory was that as the heart was being pushed with the supernormalization process, the heart's metabolism increased such that it was the major organ seemingly consuming all of the excess oxygen being delivered. The harder the heart worked to deliver the oxygen, the more it had to use. Normal CO for an average human is about 5 L/min, yet patients were often driven to a CO of 15 L/min or more for prolonged periods.

The critics of the optimization process asserted that there was a point during oxygen delivery when it was flow dependent, but the coupling of consumption and delivery made it seem like increased delivery was the factor that increased consumption. Furthermore, optimization advocates neglected the fact that the body was usually already at the flat part of the oxygen consumption curve. Rarely was oxygen delivered when it was critical or when the body was consuming all that was being delivered. The result of the optimization process usually meant that patients were flooded with fluids. The hyperdynamic response and MODS may have resulted from the fluids used, which may have caused an inflammatory response at excessive volumes.

The concept of oxygen debt, introduced by the physiologist Archibald Hill almost 100 years ago, may have some vital flaws in it. His original work on aerobic and anaerobic metabolism in just four patients has now been propagated for a century. However, modern exercise physiology studies have shown that oxygen debt is repaid over a short period; it does not take days. In contrast, the optimization process showed oxygen debt for long periods.

During massive hemorrhage, ischemia to some tissues is theoretically possible. However, in acute hemorrhage, when the BP falls to 40 mm Hg, CO and thus oxygen delivery are typically reduced by only 50%. Before resuscitation with acellular fluids, the Hb level does not fall significantly. In this state, oxygen delivery is cut by only half, and the body is designed to have plenty of reserves (cells consume only 25% of the delivered oxygen in the normal state). Whether any ongoing anaerobic metabolism is actually occurring is questionable because the oxygen delivery has to fall to 25% of baseline to theoretically be anaerobic. When resuscitation takes place without blood to restore the intravascular volume, the Hb level theoretically may fall by 50%, but CO is generally restored to the original state. Again, oxygen delivery is only halved, with plenty of oxygen still being delivered to avoid ongoing anaerobic metabolism. It is difficult to reduce CO and Hb level to a level at which oxygen delivery is reduced by 75%, that is, to below the anaerobic threshold.

In hypovolemic shock states, it was thought that even though global oxygen delivery may be adequate, regional hypoxia is ongoing. Different organs and tissue beds are not similar in their oxygen needs or consumption. Hypoxic insult may be experienced by the critical organs, whose flow is usually preserved, whereas nonessential organs are sacrificed in terms of oxygen delivery. Yet such patients are not actively moving, and their oxygen demand is minimal. Thus, the theory of oxygen debt is in question. In exercise states, even if there is oxygen debt, it is paid back quickly and does not take days.

To optimize oxygen delivery, one of the most efficient ways, according to past calculations, was to add Hb. If the Hb level increased from 8.0 to 10 g/dL by transfusing 2 units of blood, oxygen delivery would increase by 25%. Blood transfusions were part of the optimization process because they also increased wedge pressure and LVED volume and thus CO, but it was rarely noted that transfusions placed patients on the flat part of the consumption curve (see Fig. 33.9).

Decades ago, it was also thought that an increased hematocrit would reduce flow in the capillaries, so clinicians had reservations about transfusing too much blood. Studies in the 1950s demonstrated better flow at the capillary level with diluted blood. However, the small amount of decreased flow with the higher viscosity was in the range of a few percentage points and did not compare to the 25% increase in oxygen delivery with a transfusion of a couple of units of PRBCs. Blood transfusions by calculations would be the most efficient way of increasing oxygen delivery if that were the goal.

Current exercise physiology studies have shown that professional athletes perform better when their Hb levels are above normal. Athletes who blood dope, by undergoing autologous blood transfusions or by taking red cell production enhancers such as erythropoietin or testosterone, are now banned for illegal performance enhancement. Such athletes have COs of more than 20 to 50 L/min. They do not seem to have any problems with blood sludging from the higher flow and more viscous blood than normal. The argument against this analogy of athletes and their capability to deliver oxygen despite a high hematocrit level is that injured patients have capillaries that are not vasodilated and are often plugged with white and red cells.

Global Perfusion Versus Regional Perfusion

Gaining the ability to measure BP was revolutionary. However, because the main functions of the vascular system are to deliver needed nutrients and carry out excreted substances from the cells, clinicians constantly ask whether BP or flow is more important. During sepsis, systemic vascular resistance is low. A malfunction somewhere in the autoregulatory system is assumed.

A teleologic explanation, however, is possible. Lower systemic vascular resistance could be a way our bodies evolved so that CO can be easily increased as afterload is reduced. Some shunting is believed to occur at the capillary level; however, an important question is, "Should BP be augmented with exogenous administration of pressor agents, normalizing BP at the expense of capillary flow?" High doses of pressor agents most likely worsen flow because lactate levels rise if the pressor dose is too high. That rise in lactate levels could be caused by a stress response because catecholamines are known to increase lactate levels, or it could also be caused by decreased flow at the capillary bed.

Purists would prefer to have lower pressure as long as flow is adequate, but some organs are somewhat sensitive to pressure. For example, the brain and kidneys are traditionally thought to be pressure dependent; however, when early experiments were done, it was difficult to isolate flow from pressure because of the interrelation of those two values. With the concept that flow might be more important than just pressure, technology developed to focus on measuring flow of nutrients rather than pressure.

Septic Shock

In 2001, Rivers and colleagues reported that among patients with severe sepsis or septic shock in a single urban emergency department, mortality was significantly lower among those who were treated according to a 6-hour protocol of early goal-directed therapy than among those who were given standard therapy (30.5% vs. 46.5%). The premise was that usual care was not aggressive or timely. Early goal-directed therapy addressed this by calling for central venous catheterization to monitor central venous pressure and central venous oxygen saturation, which were used to guide the use of IV fluids, vasopressors, PRBC transfusions, and dobutamine to achieve prespecified physiologic targets. Based on this type of research, the Surviving Sepsis Campaign clinical guidelines were initially published in 2004 and subsequently updated in 2008, 2014, 2016, and 2021.[40] The various methods of therapy were graded by a panel of international experts.[41] A randomized prospective study has now shown that protocol-based care for early septic shock does not improve outcome.[42] The newer study was not identical to the original Rivers

study because the survival rates were much higher, but this study may just show that the usual therapy may have already adopted many of the principles of early goal-directed therapy, and thus the difference is negligible. This study also found no significant benefit of the mandated use of central venous catheterization and central hemodynamic monitoring in all patients.

In the 2016 update of the Surviving Sepsis campaign clinical guidelines, there was a major transition in the way that sepsis was defined. Previous iterations of the campaign used systemic inflammatory response syndrome (SIRS) criteria (Table 33.5) to define sepsis, in which the patient needed to have two out of four of the criteria present and a source of infection to be deemed to have sepsis. This definition was fraught with problems because any noninfectious process that activated the inflammatory cascade could lead to a similar physiologic picture. Instead of using SIRS criteria, sepsis was then defined as an increase in a patient's sequential organ failure assessment (SOFA) score by 2 points from baseline (Table 33.6). Because the SOFA score can be cumbersome to calculate at the bedside and requires laboratory test results, a simpler version was developed. The quick SOFA (qSOFA) (Table 33.7) can be calculated at patient's bedside by identifying tachypnea, altered mental status, and hypotension. If the patient meets two of these criteria and they are at risk for sepsis, further workup for an infectious source should be conducted. In the most recent guidelines from 2021, the recommendation is against using qSOFA compared with SIRS, National Early Warning Score (NEWS), or Modified Early Warning Score (MEWS) as a single screening tool for sepsis or septic shock. MEWS is a simplified screening tool based on respiratory rate, SBP, heart rate, level of consciousness, and body temperature. NEWS is a scoring system based on routinely recorded bedside measurements. It measures respiratory frequency, oxygen saturation, SBP, pulse

TABLE 33.5   SIRS Criteria

Body temperature	>38°C or <36°C
Heart rate	>90 beats/min
Tachypnea	Respiratory rate >20/min or $PaCO_2$ <32 mm Hg
White blood cell count	>12,000/mm³, <4000/mm³, or >10% immature neutrophils

SIRS, Systemic inflammatory response syndrome.

TABLE 33.6   Sequential Organ Failure Assessment (SOFA) Score

SYSTEM		SCORE				
		0	1	2	3	4
Respiratory	PaO_2/FiO_2, mm Hg	≥400	<400	<300	<200 With respiratory support	<100 With respiratory support
Coagulation	Platelets, ×10 > 3/μL	≥150	<150	<100	<50	<20
Liver	Bilirubin, mg/dL	<1.2	1.2–1.9	2.0–5.9	6.0–11.9	>12.0
Cardiovascular		MAP ≥70 mm Hg	MAP <70 mm Hg	Dopamine <5 or dobutamine (any dose)	Dopamine 5.1–15 or epinephrine ≤0.1 or norepinephrine ≤0.1	Dopamine >15 or epinephrine >0.1 or norepinephrine >0.1
Central nervous system	Glasgow Coma Scale score	15	13–14	10–12	6–9	<6
Renal	Creatinine, mg/dL	<1.2	1.2–1.9	2.0–3.4	3.5–4.9	>5.0
	Urine output, mL/day				<500	<200

FiO₂, Percentage of inspired oxygen; *MAP,* mean arterial pressure; *PaO₂,* partial pressure of arterial oxygen.

TABLE 33.7 **Quick Sequential Organ Failure Assessment**
Respiratory rate ≥22
Altered mental status
Systolic blood pressure ≤100 mm Hg

TABLE 33.8 **Mortality Rates**		
	KILLED IN ACTION (%)	DIED OF WOUNDS (%)
Civil War	16.0	13.0
Russo-Japanese War	20.0	9.0
World War I	19.6	8.1
World War II	19.8	3.0
Korean War	19.5	2.4
Vietnam War	20.2	3.5

rate, neurologic level of consciousness, and body temperature, with scores ranging from 0 to 3.

PROBLEMS WITH RESUSCITATION

Lessons learned from the Korean War showed that resuscitation with blood and blood products was useful. Throughout that war, the concept prevailed that a limited amount of salt and water should be given to patients after injuries. By the time of the Vietnam War, volume resuscitation in excess of replacement of shed blood became an acceptable practice. That practice may have been influenced by studies of hemorrhagic shock performed by Tom Shires. In his classic study, Shires used the Wiggers model and bled 30 dogs to a mean BP of 50 mm Hg for 90 minutes. He then infused LR solution (5% of body weight) followed by blood in 10 dogs, plasma (10 mL/kg) followed by blood in another 10 dogs, and shed blood alone in the remaining 10 dogs. The dogs that received LR solution had the best survival rate. Shires concluded that although the replacement of lost blood with whole blood remains the primary treatment of shock, adjunctive replacement of the coexisting functional volume deficit in the interstitium with a balanced salt solution appears to be beneficial. Shires concluded that resuscitation with LR solution should be initiated while whole blood transfusions are being mobilized.

The surgical community soon went from being judicious with crystalloid solutions to being aggressive. Surgeons returning from the Vietnam War advocated the use of crystalloids, a seemingly cheap and easy method of resuscitating patients, touting that it saved lives. However, what evolved from this method of resuscitation was the so-called Da Nang lung (named after the US Navy field hospital in Da Nang, Vietnam), also known as *shock lung* and eventually *ARDS*. The explanation for the evolution of the new condition was that battlefield patients were now living long enough to develop ARDS because their lives were saved with aggressive resuscitation and better critical care, including a greater capability to treat renal failure.

However, that explanation had no supporting evidence. The killed-in-action rate (the number of wounded patients who died before reaching a facility that had a surgeon) had not changed for more than a century (Table 33.8). The died-of-wounds rate (the number of wounded patients who died after reaching a facility that had a physician) had decreased during World War II, thanks to the use of antibiotics, but it was slightly higher during the Vietnam War. The perceived reason for slightly higher died-of-wounds rates was that patients in Vietnam were transported to medical facilities much more quickly by helicopters. Transport times did indeed decrease from an average of 4 hours to 40 minutes, but if the sicker patients who would have normally died in the field were transported more quickly to die in the medical facility, then the killed-in-action rate should have fallen—and it did not.

Moreover, the renal failure rate and the cause of renal failure did not significantly change between the Korean War and the Vietnam War. Another false argument was that the wounds seen during the Vietnam War were worse because of the enemy's high-velocity

AK-47 rifles. Actually, the rounds or bullets used by the AK-47 were similar to those used by the enemy in the Russo-Japanese War, World War I, and World War II. The 7.62-mm round used in the AK-47 rifle was invented by the Japanese in the 1890s.

In the early 1970s, the prehospital system in the United States started to evolve. Previously, ambulances were usually hearses driven by morticians. That is why the early ambulances had a station wagon configuration. As the career paths of emergency medical technicians and paramedics grew, they started resuscitation in the field and continued it to the hospital. In 1978, the first ATLS course was given. To prevent shock, the ATLS course recommended that all trauma patients have two large-bore IV lines placed and receive 2 L of LR solution. The actual recommendation in the ATLS text specifically stated that patients in class III shock should receive 2 L of LR solution *followed by blood products*. However, clinicians learned that crystalloid solutions seemed innocuous and improved BP in hypotensive patients. Later versions of ATLS advocate for transfusion.

In the 1980s and early 1990s, aggressive resuscitation was taught and endorsed. The two large-bore IV lines started in the field were converted to larger IV lines through a wire-guided exchange system. Central venous lines were placed early for aggressive fluid resuscitation. In fact, some trauma centers routinely performed cut-downs on the saphenous vein at the ankle to place IV tubing directly into the vein and thereby maximize flow during resuscitation.

Technology soon caught up, and machines were built to rapidly infuse crystalloid solutions. The literature was filled with data showing that ischemia to tissues resulted in disturbances of all types. Optimization of oxygen delivery was the goal. As a result, massive volumes of crystalloids were infused into patients. Residents were encouraged to "pound" patients with fluids. If trauma patients did not develop ARDS, it was taught that the patients were not adequately resuscitated, but many clinical trials eventually showed that prehospital fluids did not improve outcome (Table 33.9).

Bleeding

One of the most influential studies on hemorrhagic shock was performed by Ken Mattox, and in 1994, the results were reported by Bickell and coworkers.[43] The aim of Mattox's study, a prospective clinical trial, was to determine whether withholding of prehospital fluids affected outcomes in hypotensive patients after a penetrating torso injury. IV lines were started in patients with penetrating torso trauma with BP lower than 90 mm Hg. On alternating days, patients received standard fluid therapy in the field or had fluids withheld until hemorrhage control was achieved. Withholding of prehospital fluids conferred a statistically significant survival advantage—a revolutionary, counterintuitive finding that shocked surgeons.

That 1994 article popularized the concept of permissive hypotension, that is, allowing hypotension during uncontrolled

TABLE 33.9 **Prehospital Fluid Studies in Trauma Patients**

ARTICLE	SUMMARY OF FINDINGS
Aprahamian C, Thompson BM, Towne JB, et al. The effect of a paramedic system on mortality of major open intraabdominal vascular trauma. *J Trauma.* 1983;23:687-690.	Paramedic system Open intraabdominal vascular trauma
Kaweski SM, Sise MJ, Virgilio RW. The effect of prehospital fluids on survival in trauma patients. *J Trauma.* 1990;30:1215-1218.	Prehospital fluids Trauma patients
Bickell WH, Wall MJ Jr, Pepe PE, et al. Immediate versus delayed fluid resuscitation for hypotensive patients with penetrating torso injuries. *N Engl J Med.* 1994;331:1105-1109.	Presurgery fluids Hypotensive penetrating torso injuries
Turner J, Nicholl J, Webber L, et al. A randomised controlled trial of prehospital intravenous fluid replacement therapy in serious trauma. *Health Technol Assess.* 2000;4:1-57.	Prehospital 1309 Serious trauma patients
Kwan I, Bunn F, Roberts I. Timing and volume of fluid administration for patients with bleeding following trauma. *Cochrane Database Syst Rev.* 2001;1:CD002245.	Prehospital Bleeding trauma patients
Dula DJ, Wood GC, Rejmer AR, et al. Use of prehospital fluids in hypotensive blunt trauma patients. *Prehosp Emerg Care.* 2002;6:417-420.	Prehospital Hypotensive blunt trauma patients
Greaves I, Porter KM, Revell MP. Fluid resuscitation in pre-hospital trauma care: a consensus view. *J R Coll Surg Edinb.* 2002;47:451-457.	Prehospital A consensus view
Dutton RP, Mackenzie CF, Scalea TM. Hypotensive resuscitation during active hemorrhage: impact on in-hospital mortality. *J Trauma.* 2002;52:1141-1146.	Presurgery fluids Hypotensive active hemorrhage

hemorrhage. The fundamental rationale for permissive hypotension was that restoration of BP with fluids would increase bleeding from uncontrolled sources. In fact, Cannon, in 1918, had stated that "inaccessible or uncontrolled sources of blood loss should not be treated with IV fluids until the time of surgical control."

Animal studies have validated the idea of permissive hypotension. Burris and colleagues have shown that moderate resuscitation results in a better outcome compared with no resuscitation or aggressive resuscitation. In a swine model of uncontrolled hemorrhage, Sondeen showed that raising BP with either fluids or pressors could lead to increased bleeding. The theory was that increasing BP would dislodge the clot that had formed. The study also found that the pressure that would cause rebleeding was a mean arterial pressure of 64 ± 2 mm Hg, with an SBP of 94 ± 3 mm Hg and diastolic pressure of 45 ± 2 mm Hg. Other animal studies have confirmed these concepts.

The next question was whether the continued strategy of permissive hypotension in the operating room would result in improved survival. Dutton and associates randomized one group of patients to a target SBP of higher than 100 mm Hg and another group to a target SBP of 70 mm Hg. Fluid therapy was titrated until definitive hemorrhage control was achieved. However, despite attempts to maintain BP at 70 mm Hg, the average BP was 100 mm Hg in the low-pressure group and 114 mm Hg in the high-pressure group. Patients' BP rose spontaneously. Titrating patients' BP to the low target was difficult, even with less use of fluids. The survival rate did not differ between the two groups.

Despite the level 1 evidence from Houston, animal data, and the theoretical benefit, permissive hypotension was not rapidly instituted. The argument against allowing anything besides aggressive resuscitation was dismissed. Critics continued to emphasize that the Mattox trial focused only on penetrating injuries and should not be extrapolated to blunt trauma. Clinicians feared that patients with traumatic blunt head injuries would be harmed without a normalized BP. However, Shafi and Gentilello examined the National Trauma Data Bank and found that hypotension was an independent risk factor for death, but it was not associated with an increased mortality rate in patients with TBIs any more than in patients without TBIs. The risk of death quadrupled in patients with hypotension in both the TBI group (odds ratio, 4.1;

95% confidence interval, 3.5–4.9) and the non-TBI group (odds ratio, 4.6; 95% confidence interval, 3.4–6.0). Furthermore, in 2006, Plurad and coworkers showed that emergency department hypotension was not an independent risk factor for acute renal dysfunction or failure.

Trauma Immunology and Inflammation

The 1990s witnessed an explosion of information regarding alterations of homeostasis and cellular physiochemistry during shock. The scientific investigations of Shires, Carrico, Baue, and countless others shed light on the basic mechanisms underlying resuscitation of patients in shock. The pathophysiologic process has been identified as having an aberrant inflammatory status, resulting in the body's immune system damaging the endothelial tissues and, ultimately, the end organ. This inflammatory state leads to a spectrum of conditions, including fluid sequestration, which leads to edema and progresses to acute lung injury, SIRS, ARDS, and MODS. Such conditions were seen in every surgical ICU. Attention focused on biochemical perturbations and altered mediators as sites for possible interventions. The fundamental cause was thought to be that ischemia and reperfusion, as shown in animal models, would create a state of damage to the capillary endothelium and subsequent changes to the end organ. It was generally accepted that the reason for the reperfusion injury was mediated by activated neutrophils that emitted deleterious cytokines and released free oxygen radicals. The animal models used to study these concepts were actually ischemia-reperfusion models in which the superior mesenteric artery that supplied blood to the intestines was clamped for a prolonged time before the clamp was removed. Later it was thought that this was not an appropriate model to study hemorrhagic shock. It was found that there was a difference in pathophysiologic mechanisms between ischemia-reperfusion injury and resuscitation injury.

Death after traumatic injury was traditionally described by Trunkey as trimodal. Some patients died almost immediately after injury, some died in the hospital within a few days, and many died late in the hospital course. However, a more recent trauma trial revealed that there is a high incidence of death immediately after injury, with 74% of deaths occurring within the first 72 hours and 26% of deaths occurring at a slow, steady rate over the next

174 days. One reason for the initial trimodal distribution was that patients who died after 24 hours were labeled under late deaths, and the others were lumped together as immediate or early. Another factor may be advances in trauma and critical care in concert with adoption of damage control surgical principles.[44]

According to the traditional trimodal pattern, the patients who typically died first could be aided by a better prehospital system and, more importantly, by injury prevention because these patients generally have devastating injuries. For the second group of patients, better resuscitation and hemorrhage control were thought to be a potentially lifesaving intervention. For the third group (the late deaths), immunomodulation was considered to be integral to survival. The cause was thought to be the inflammatory adaptive aberrancy after successful resuscitation. When there is prolonged end-arteriole cessation of flow, producing tissue ischemia for a prolonged period, followed by reperfusion, it is termed *reperfusion injury*. For example, with an injury to the femoral artery that requires 4 to 6 hours for circulation to be restored, muscle cells undergo ischemia and reperfusion, during which the cells will start to swell, which can result in compartment syndrome. Such ischemia and reperfusion were thought to occur after a period of hypotension. However, it is now known that the pathophysiologic change is contributed by resuscitation injury in addition to reperfusion injury.

With improved technology, the immunologic response after trauma was heavily researched. In the past, we were limited to studying physiology. A theory started to evolve that shock caused an aberrant inflammatory response that then needed to be modulated and suppressed. Many studies during this era showed that the inflammatory system was upregulated or activated after shock. The white cells in the blood became activated. Neutrophils were identified as the relevant mediators in the acute phase of shock, whereas lymphocytes are typically more important in chronic diseases (e.g., cancer and viral infections). Shock, caused by various mechanisms, was thought to induce ischemia to tissues and, after reperfusion, to set off an inflammatory response, which primarily affected the microcirculation and caused leaks (Fig. 33.11).

Typically, neutrophils are rapidly transported through capillaries. However, when they are signaled by chemokines, neutrophils will start to roll, firmly adhere to the endothelium, and migrate out of the capillaries to combat foreign substances and initiate healing. Early researchers thought that neutrophils killed bacteria through phagocytic activity and the release of oxygen free radicals; this was thought to be the reason for the leak in the capillary system (Fig. 33.12). Because neutrophils can be primed to have an enhanced response, a massive search took place to identify causes of neutrophil priming and downregulation. The many cytokines targeted included interleukin types 1 through 18, tumor necrosis factor (TNF), and adhesion molecules, such as intercellular adhesion molecules, vascular cell adhesion molecules, E-selectin, L-selectin, P-selectin, and platelet-activating factor.

That research had much overlap with the research being performed in the arenas of reimplantation, vascular ischemia, and reperfusion. Clinically, it was already known that the implantation of severed extremities would have pathophysiologic results similar to those from ischemia, reperfusion, and swelling caused by permeable capillaries. The immune response was described as bimodal. The first response was the priming by trauma or shock, followed by an exaggerated response to a second insult, such as sepsis.

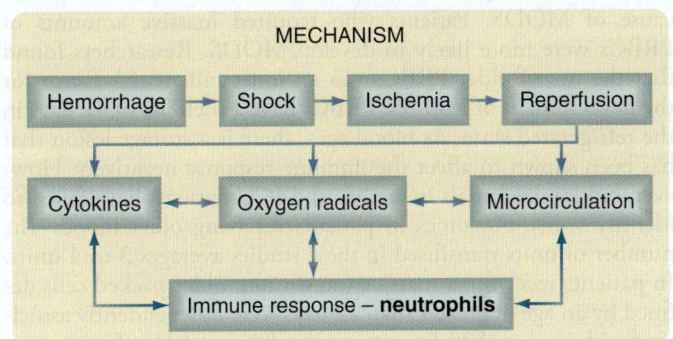

FIGURE 33.11 Hemorrhage causing neutrophil activation.

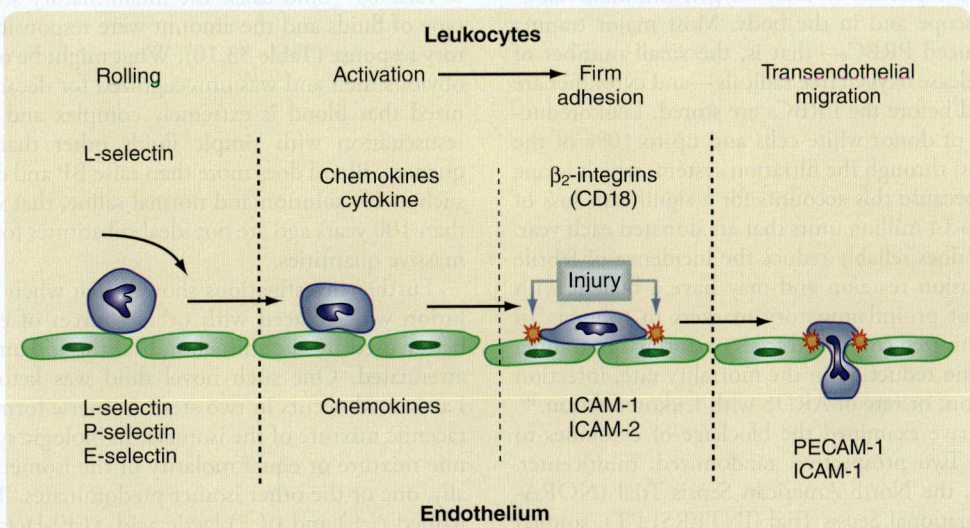

FIGURE 33.12 Intravascular neutrophils that are activated will adhere and roll until another set of mechanisms causes firm adherence and transendothelial migration out of the vascular system occurs. It is believed that this transmigration process injures the endothelium with the release of an oxygen free radical. This could result in fluid leaks out of the vascular system. *ICAM,* Intercellular adhesion molecules; *PECAM,* platelet–endothelial cell adhesion molecule.

In the late 1990s, other researchers focused on the role of the alimentary tract. They knew that the splanchnic circulation was shunted of blood by vasoconstriction during hemorrhagic shock, so the gut suffers the most ischemia during shock and is the most susceptible to reperfusion injury. The animal model most often used to study the gut's role in inflammation was a rat model of superior mesenteric artery occlusion and reperfusion. Because SIRS is a sterile phenomenon, the gut was implicated as a potential mediator in the development of MODS. Animals were shown to have a translocation of bacteria into the portal system, and this initiation of the inflammatory cascade was investigated as the source of MODS. Investigators also knew that *Escherichia coli* bacteria in the blood released endotoxins that further initiated release of cytokines (e.g., TNF, cachectin). However, studies in humans failed to demonstrate translocation of bacteria in intraoperative samples of the portal vein during resuscitation. The problem was that although complete occlusion of the superior mesenteric artery for hours followed by reperfusion does result in swollen, necrotic, injured bowel, these findings were extrapolated to humans undergoing hemorrhagic shock. Again, during hemorrhagic shock, the superior mesenteric artery is not occluded, and even in severe states, there is some flow of blood to the splanchnic organs.

Because patients who are in shock bleed and receive blood transfusions, transfusion of PRBCs was also implicated as the cause of MODS. Patients who required massive amounts of PRBCs were more likely to develop MODS. Researchers found that the use of older PRBCs was an independent risk factor for the development of MODS. PRBCs have a shelf life of 42 days in the refrigerated state. As blood ages, there is a storage lesion that has been shown to affect the immune response negatively. However, randomized trials in cardiac and ICU patients have failed to identify worse outcomes in patients receiving older blood. The number of units transfused in these studies averages 3 to 4 units. In patients receiving a massive transfusion, older packed cells defined by an age of greater than 22 days were independently associated with increased 24-hour mortality; however, the effect was not replicated for those receiving under 10 units.[45]

In the past, when technology was limited, PRBCs were mainly tested for the red cells' capability to carry oxygen and their viability under the microscope and in the body. Most major trauma centers use leukoreduced PRBCs—that is, the small number of white cells that can release oxygen free radicals—and cytokines are now routinely filtered before the PRBCs are stored. Leukoreduction removes 99.9% of donor white cells and up to 10% of the red blood cells (RBCs) through the filtration system, which is one potential drawback because this accounts for a significant loss of volume over the 12 to 14 million units that are donated each year. Leukocyte reduction does reliably reduce the incidence of febrile nonhemolytic transfusion reaction and may have a benefit with regard to reduction of proinflammatory markers in trauma. To date, four small randomized controlled trials performed in trauma patients have shown no reduction in the mortality rate, infection rate, organ dysfunction, or rate of ARDS with leukoreduction.[46]

Numerous trials have examined the blockage of cytokines to treat septic patients. Two prospective, randomized, multicenter, double-blinded trials, the North American Sepsis Trial (NORASEPT) and the International Sepsis Trial (INTERSEPT), studied the 28-day mortality rate of critically ill patients who received anti-TNF antibody. Neither trial showed benefit. Trials testing other potential cytokines were disappointing as well. The cytokines tested included CD11/CD18,[47] anti–interleukin-1 receptor, antiendotoxin antibodies, bradykinin antagonists, and platelet-activating factor receptor antagonists. The search continues for one key mediator that could be manipulated to solve the "toxemia" of shock. However, such attempts to simplify the complex mechanisms and find one solution may be the main problem because there is no simple solution. The answer may lie in cocktails of substances. The humoral and endocrine systems, which are always mediated by blood, are exceedingly complex. Shock has many causes and mechanisms, so solutions to the treatment of shock may also be complex.

EVOLUTION OF MODERN RESUSCITATION

Detrimental Impact of Fluids

As early as 1996, the US Navy used a swine model to study the effects of fluids on neutrophil activation after hemorrhagic shock and resuscitation. It was shown that neutrophils are activated after a hemorrhage of 40% blood volume when followed by resuscitation with LR solution. That finding was not surprising. What was enlightening was that the level of neutrophil activation was similar in control animals that did not undergo hemorrhagic shock but merely received LR solution (Fig. 33.13). In other control animals that did not receive LR solution but instead were resuscitated with shed blood or HTS after hemorrhagic shock, the neutrophils were not activated. The implication was that the inflammatory process was not caused by shock and resuscitation but by LR solution itself.

Those findings were repeated over several years in a series of experiments using human blood as well as in experiments in small and large animal models of hemorrhagic shock. When the blood was diluted with various resuscitation fluids, the inflammatory changes depended on the fluid used; despite similar physiologic results in vivo, the immunologic results were different (Fig. 33.14). The response was ubiquitous throughout the entire inflammatory response system, including at the levels of deoxyribonucleic acid (DNA) and ribonucleic acid (RNA) expression.

Ultimately, it was recognized that the inflammatory response was due to the various resuscitation fluids. The type and amount of fluids directly caused inflammation. All the artificial fluids used to raise BP could cause the inflammatory sequelae of shock. The type of fluids and the amount were responsible for the inflammatory response (Table 33.10). What might be obvious today was not obvious then and was unrecognized for decades. It was not recognized that blood is extremely complex and that replacement or resuscitation with simple fluids other than blood had consequences. Blood does more than raise BP and carry red cells. Fluids, such as LR solution and normal saline, that were developed more than 100 years ago are not ideal substitutes for blood when used in massive quantities.

Further investigations showed that when the lactate in LR solution was replaced with other sources of energy that could be better used by the mitochondria, the inflammatory aspects were attenuated. One such novel fluid was ketone Ringer solution. Lactic acid occurs in two stereoisomeric forms as well as in a true racemic mixture of the isomers. In biologic systems, the true racemic mixture or equal molarity of the isomers rarely occurs. Usually, one or the other isomer predominates. The stereoisomers are named L(+) and D(−) lactic acid. L(+)-lactate is a normal intermediary of mammalian metabolism. The isomer D(−)-lactate is produced when tissue glyoxalase converts methylglyoxal into a lactic acid of the D form, such as in lactose-fermenting bacteria. L(+)-lactate has low toxicity as a consequence of the rapid metabolism. D(−)-lactate, however, has a higher toxic potential.

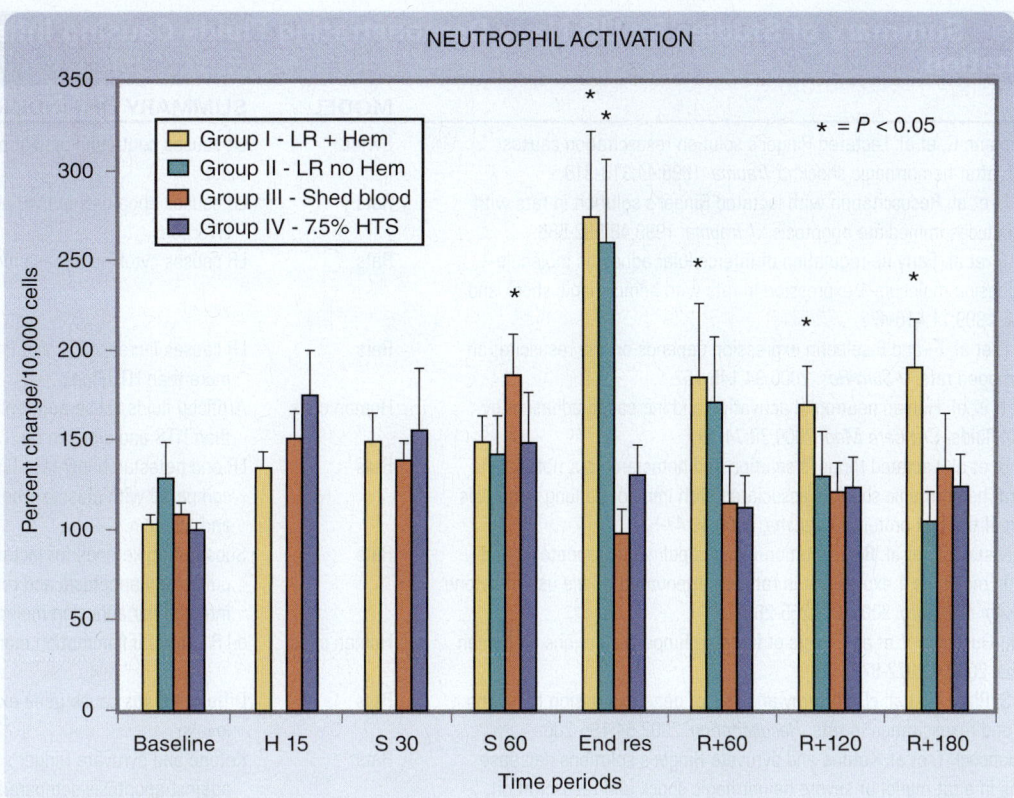

FIGURE 33.13 Neutrophil activation in whole blood of swine measured by flow cytometry. The highest neutrophil activation followed hemorrhagic shock *(Hem)* and resuscitation *(res)* using lactated Ringer *(LR)* solution. Similar neutrophil activation occurred when the animal was not resuscitated but was infused with LR solution. No activation occurred when shocked animals were resuscitated with whole blood or 7.5% hypertonic saline *(HTS)*. (From Rhee P, Burris D, Kaufmann C, et al. Lactated Ringer's resuscitation causes neutrophil activation after hemorrhagic shock. *J Trauma.* 1998;44:313-319.)

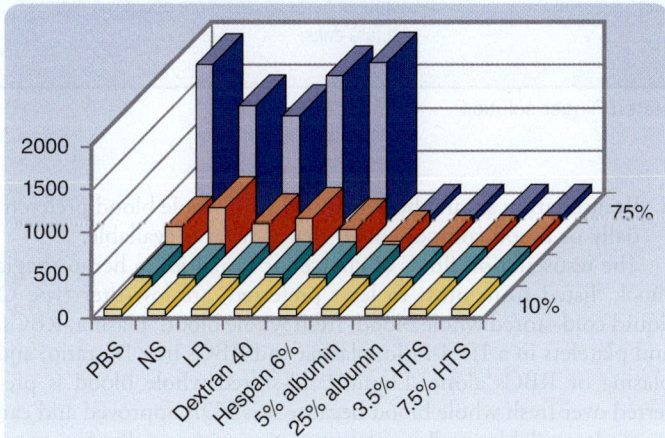

FIGURE 33.14 Human neutrophil activation using whole blood diluted with various resuscitation fluids, as measured by flow cytometry. Phosphate-buffered saline *(PBS)* was used because it has a pH of 7.4. *HTS,* Hypertonic saline; *LT,* lactated Ringer; *NS,* normal saline. (From Rhee P, Wang D, Ruff P, et al. Human neutrophil activation and increased adhesion by various resuscitation fluids. *Crit Care Med.* 2000;28:74-78.)

Psychoneurotic disturbances have been described with pure D(−)-lactate. Increasing evidence has indicated a connection between high plasma concentration of racemic lactate and anxiety and panic disorders. Racemic dialysis fluids have reportedly been associated with clinical cases of D-lactate toxicity. Experiments with the isomers have shown that D(−)-lactate causes significant inflammatory changes in rats and swine, as well as activation of human neutrophils.

In 1999, with the new information implicating LR solution as the cause of ARDS and MODS, the US Navy contracted with the Institute of Medicine to review the topic of the optimal resuscitation fluid.[48] The report made many recommendations; key recommendations were that LR solution be manufactured with only the L(+) isomer of lactate and that researchers continue to search for alternative resuscitation fluids that do not contain lactate but rather other nutrients, such as ketones. It stated that the optimal resuscitation fluid is 7.5% HTS because of the decreased inflammation associated with it as well as its logistic advantage in terms of weight and size. Although the Institute of Medicine had been asked to make recommendations for the military, the report's authors thought that the evidence was applicable to civilian injuries as well. The US military also requested Baxter, among other manufacturers of LR solution, to eliminate D(−)-lactate in LR solution, which it has done. The LR solution from Baxter currently contains only the L(+)-lactate isomer.

HTS has a long record of research and development. It has been used in humans for decades and has been consistently shown to be less inflammatory than LR solution. This represented a paradigm shift in recognizing that LR solution and normal saline may be detrimental. Again, blood is complex, and the fluids used in the past were a poor replacement.

TABLE 33.10   Summary of Studies By US Navy Demonstrating Fluids Causing Inflammation After Resuscitation

ARTICLE	MODEL	SUMMARY OF FINDINGS
Rhee P, Burris D, Kaufmann C, et al. Lactated Ringer's solution resuscitation causes neutrophil activation after hemorrhagic shock. *J Trauma.* 1998;44:313-319.	Swine	LR causes neutrophil activation; blood HTS does not.
Deb S, Martin B, Sun L, et al. Resuscitation with lactated Ringer's solution in rats with hemorrhagic shock induces immediate apoptosis. *J Trauma.* 1999;46:582-588.	Rats	LR causes apoptosis in liver and gut more than HTS does.
Sun LL, Ruff P, Austin B, et al. Early up-regulation of intercellular adhesion molecule-1 and vascular cell adhesion molecule-1 expression in rats with hemorrhagic shock and resuscitation. *Shock.* 1999;11:416-422.	Rats	LR causes cytokine release more than HTS does.
Alam HB, Sun L, Ruff P, et al. E- and P-selectin expression depends on the resuscitation fluid used in hemorrhaged rats. *J Surg Res.* 2000;94:145-152.	Rats	LR causes increased E- and P-selectin expression more than HTS does.
Rhee P, Wang D, Ruff P, et al. Human neutrophil activation and increased adhesion by various resuscitation fluids. *Crit Care Med.* 2000;28:74-78.	Human cells	Artificial fluids cause neutrophil activation more than HTS and albumin do.
Deb S, Sun L, Martin B, et al. Lactated Ringer's solution and hetastarch but not plasma resuscitation after rat hemorrhagic shock is associated with immediate lung apoptosis by the up-regulation of the Bax protein. *J Trauma.* 2000;49:47-53.	Rats	LR and hetastarch increase lung apoptosis compared with plasma whole blood, plasma, and albumin.
Alam HB, Austin B, Koustova E, et al. Resuscitation-induced pulmonary apoptosis and intracellular adhesion molecule-1 expression in rats are attenuated by the use of ketone Ringer's solution. *J Am Coll Surg.* 2001;193:255-263.	Rats	Substituting ketones for lactate reduces pulmonary apoptosis and release of intercellular adhesion molecules.
Koustova E, Stanton K, Gushchin V, et al. Effects of lactated Ringer's solutions on human leukocytes. *J Trauma.* 2002;52:872-878.	Human cells	D-LR causes inflammation more than L-LR does.
Alam HB, Stegalkina S, Rhee P, et al. cDNA array analysis of gene expression following hemorrhagic shock and resuscitation in rats. *Resuscitation.* 2002;54:195-206.	Rats	Different fluids cause gene expression at different levels.
Koustova E, Rhee P, Hancock T, et al. Ketone and pyruvate Ringer's solutions decrease pulmonary apoptosis in a rat model of severe hemorrhagic shock and resuscitation. *Surgery.* 2003;134:267-274.	Rats	Ketone and pyruvate Ringer solutions protect against apoptosis compared with LR.
Stanton K, Alam HB, Rhee P, et al. Human polymorphonuclear cell death after exposure to resuscitation fluids in vitro: apoptosis versus necrosis. *J Trauma.* 2003;54:1065-1074.	Human cells	Artificial fluids cause apoptosis and necrosis.
Gushchin V, Alam HB, Rhee P, et al. cDNA profiling in leukocytes exposed to hypertonic resuscitation fluids. *J Am Coll Surg.* 2003;197:426-432.	Human cells	LR causes more cytokine release by gene expression than HTS does.
Alam HB, Stanton K, Koustova E, et al. Effect of different resuscitation strategies on neutrophil activation in a swine model of hemorrhagic shock. *Resuscitation.* 2004;60:91-99.	Swine	Artificial fluids cause neutrophil activation despite resuscitation rates.
Jaskille A, Alam HB, Rhee P, et al. D-Lactate increases pulmonary apoptosis by restricting phosphorylation of bad and eNOS in a rat model of hemorrhagic shock. *J Trauma.* 2004;57:262-269.	Rats	D-Lactate in fluids causes more apoptosis than L-lactate does.

cDNA, Complementary deoxyribonucleic acid; *HTS,* hypertonic saline; *LR,* lactated Ringer solution.

It was also being recognized that PRBCs are different from whole blood and a poor replacement of whole blood lost during hemorrhage. PRBCs are separated by centrifuge, washed, and then filtered. Much of the plasma and its content is removed. Clotting factors, glucose, hormones, and cytokines crucial for signaling are not in PRBCs or in most of the fluids formerly used for resuscitation. Evidence that the fluid type affects the inflammatory response is now growing and has been confirmed in a number of studies.[49]

The Committee on Tactical Combat Casualty Care was formed in 2000 by a joint military force and now represents the Joint Trauma System's policy on the prehospital management of combat casualties. Its recommendations and algorithm for resuscitation were revolutionary compared with the civilian recommendations (Fig. 33.15). The algorithm was formed with the following points in mind:

1. Most combat casualties do not require fluid resuscitation.
2. Oral hydration is an underused option because most combat casualties require resuscitation.
3. Aggressive crystalloid resuscitation has not been shown to be beneficial in civilian victims of penetrating trauma.

4. Resuscitation should be performed with whole blood preferentially or blood components if that is what is available.

The resuscitation fluids of choice for casualties in hemorrhagic shock, listed from most to least preferred, are low-titer type O liquid cold-stored whole blood; fresh whole blood, plasma, RBCs, and platelets in a 1:1:1 ratio; plasma and RBCs in a 1:1 ratio; and plasma or RBCs alone. Liquid cold-stored whole blood is preferred over fresh whole blood because it is FDA approved and can be made available in all combat scenarios without affecting combat readiness because donating blood in a firefight may not be feasible.

Damage Control Resuscitation

Once crystalloid solutions were recognized as being contributors to the inflammatory process after traumatic hemorrhagic shock and exacerbating the lethal triad, efforts were made to exclude their use on the battlefield. Abdominal compartment syndrome (Fig. 33.16), which had been described after aggressive resuscitation, was also found to be directly associated with the volume of crystalloid infused. Thus, the concept of damage control resuscitation or hemostatic resuscitation was developed.[50] It involved

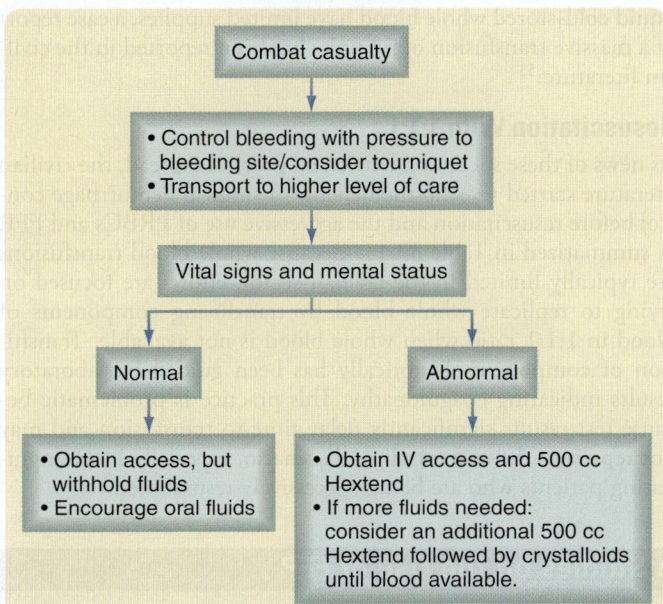

FIGURE 33.15 Recommendation for fluid resuscitation from the US military by the Committee on Tactical Combat Casualty Care. (From Rhee P, Koustova E, Alam H. Searching for the optimal resuscitation method: recommendations for the initial fluid resuscitation in combat casualties. *J Trauma.* 2003;54:S52-S62.)

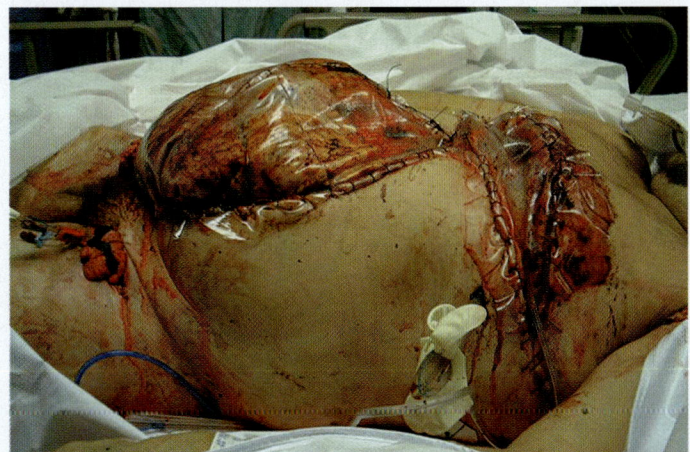

FIGURE 33.16 Patient after damage control surgery with abdominal and thoracic compartment syndrome caused by massive fluid resuscitation. (Courtesy Dr. Demetri Demetriades, Trauma Recovery Surgical Critical Care Program, USC University Hospital, Los Angeles.)

> **BOX 33.2** **Components of Damage Control or Hemostatic Resuscitation**
>
> - Permissive hypotension until definitive surgical control
> - Minimize crystalloid use
> - Initial use of 5% hypertonic saline
> - Early use of blood products (PRBCs, FFP, platelets, cryoprecipitates)
> - Consider drugs to treat coagulopathy (rFVIIa, prothrombin complex concentrate, TXA)

FFP, Fresh frozen plasma; *PRBCs,* packed red blood cells; *rFVIIa,* recombinant factor VIIa; *TXA,* tranexamic acid.
From Dellinger RP, Levy MM, Carlet JM, et al. Surviving Sepsis Campaign: international guidelines for management of severe sepsis and septic shock: 2008. *Crit Care Med.* 2008;36:296-327.

empirically for massively bleeding patients with ongoing uncontrolled hemorrhage. Mental status was also used, and the presence and quality of the radial pulse were used to determine who needed resuscitation.

With the promotion of damage control resuscitation, clinical studies indicated that aggressive early use of blood products, such as PRBCs and FFP, actually reduced the total volume of PRBCs used by 25%.[51] These studies also used permissive hypotension and focused on surgical control of hemorrhage rather than on resuscitation first. Other studies have shown that with damage control resuscitation, the incidence of ARDS, MODS, extremity and abdominal compartment syndromes, and mortality have decreased in severely injured trauma patients.[52] ARDS now occurs in patients with pulmonary contusion, long bone fractures, pneumonia, or sepsis, but *ARDS is no longer a common complication in trauma patients who undergo damage control resuscitation.*

Whole Blood Resuscitation

Damage control resuscitation was developed because surgeons in the wars in Iraq and Afghanistan recognized that fresh whole blood was associated with improved survival in massively bleeding warfighters. Returning military surgeons repeatedly noted that patients resuscitated with whole blood did not seem to have the coagulation or pulmonary problems seen previously. After operative procedures, even patients who underwent several blood volume replacement procedures were warm, not acidotic, and not coagulopathic. The knowledge from the battlefield concerning damage control resuscitation was translated into civilian practice. Because it was only recently recognized that the use of excessive fluids had an impact on outcome, they had not yet had a chance to develop the optimal resuscitation fluid to replace blood. As a result, military surgeons advocated the aggressive use of FFP, not because it was ideal but because it was likely better than crystalloid or colloidal solutions.

The military has a logistical advantage that the civilian sector does not yet have. When casualties arrive, military surgeons activate the walking blood bank, resulting in warfighters reporting to donate their blood. Given the relative safety of these donors from an infectious aspect because they were all prescreened and they had been previously blood typed, fresh whole blood is readily available. Donated blood undergoes rapid testing for human immunodeficiency virus (HIV) and hepatitis C. These tests are around 85% sensitive. Bleeding patients are transfused with PRBCs and plasma in a 1:1 ratio until fresh whole blood is available, usually within 60 minutes of activating the walking blood bank. Aliquots of donated blood are sent for formal transfusion-associated infectious

concentrating on rapid control of bleeding as the highest priority; using permissive hypotension because this would minimize potential disruption of natural clot formation; excluding all clear fluids; using blood products early; and considering the use of drugs, such as PCC and TXA, to stop bleeding and reduce coagulopathy (Box 33.2). The rationale for the early use of blood products was that large volumes of crystalloids were detrimental; if whole blood is available, this should be used first, followed by component therapy with PRBCs, thawed plasma, and platelets in a 1:1:1 ratio that would approximate whole blood and stop acellular fluids. Component therapy is not as ideal compared with fresh whole blood, but because of logistical problems, it was not always readily available, and component therapy was used

disease testing, so surviving recipients can be followed and potentially treated in the rare event of infected whole blood being transfused.

Retrospective studies performed by Nessen and Spinella showed that in combat scenarios controlling for injury severity, transfusion of fresh whole blood is associated with improved survival. With the ending of the conflicts in Iraq and Afghanistan, austere surgical teams that provide care at the site of injury have been developed for existing conflicts around the world. These teams use liquid cold-stored whole blood. The whole blood is stored at 4°C in citrate-phosphate-dextrose-adenosine for up to 35 days. These teams also use cold-stored platelets that can be stored for up to 21 days and lyophilized plasma. An increasing number of centers in the United States are now using liquid cold-stored whole blood for resuscitation, and this has been extended to the prehospital setting. Type O whole blood with low antibody titers to A and B antigens is used. Although most sites that use liquid cold-stored whole blood have limited supplies, a case report of a massive transfusion of 38 units has been reported in the civilian literature.[53]

Resuscitation With 1:1:1

As news of these successful battlefield practices spread, the civilian literature started to echo the benefits of surgical hemorrhage control before resuscitation and the aggressive use of PRBCs and FFP, as summarized in Table 33.11. Because whole blood transfusions are typically limited in the civilian sector, efforts are focused on trying to replicate whole blood by transfusing components of blood in 1:1:1 ratio when whole blood is not available. Transfusion of components historically has been guided by laboratory results indicating coagulopathy. This practice is problematic because test results significantly delay time to transfusion and may not represent the current clinical scenario, especially in exsanguinating patients who are being aggressively resuscitated.

TABLE 33.11   Summaries of Recent Retrospective Studies on the Use of FFP

ARTICLE	SUMMARY OF FINDINGS
Borgman MA, Spinella PC, Perkins JG, et al. The ratio of blood products transfused affects mortality in patients receiving massive transfusions at a combat support hospital. *J Trauma*. 2007;63:805-813.	Retrospective study of 246 patients; PRBC:FFP ratio group of 1:1.4 had better survival rates.
Gonzalez EA, Moore FA, Holcomb JB, et al. Fresh frozen plasma should be given earlier to patients requiring massive transfusion. *J Trauma*. 2007;62:112-119.	Retrospective study of 97 patients; they recommended early use of FFP before ICU admission.
Kashuk JL, Moore EE, Johnson JL, et al. Postinjury life threatening coagulopathy: is 1:1 fresh frozen plasma:packed red blood cells the answer? *J Trauma*. 2008;65:261-270.	Retrospective study of 133 patients; logistic regression showed improved coagulopathy but no improvement in survival.
Gunter OL, Jr, Au BK, Isbell JM, et al. Optimizing outcomes in damage control resuscitation: identifying blood product ratios associated with improved survival. *J Trauma*. 2008;65:527-534.	Retrospective study of 259 patients; increased use of FFP and platelets improved survival after major trauma.
Holcomb JB, Wade CE, Michalek JE, et al. Increased plasma and platelet to red blood cell ratios improves outcome in 466 massively transfused civilian trauma patients. *Ann Surg*. 2008;248:447-458.	Retrospective study of 467 patients undergoing transfusion of 10 units of PRBCs or more; survival was better with increased use of FFP and platelets.
Spinella PC, Perkins JG, Grathwohl KW, et al. Effect of plasma and red blood cell transfusions on survival in patients with combat-related traumatic injuries. *J Trauma*. 2008;66:S69-S77.	Study of 708 patients undergoing transfusion showed that FFP use was associated with improved survival.
Maegele M, Lefering R, Paffrath T, et al. Red-blood-cell to plasma ratios transfused during massive transfusion are associated with mortality in severe multiple injury: a retrospective analysis from the Trauma Registry of the Deutsche Gesellschaft für Unfallchirurgie. *Vox Sang*. 2008;95:112-119.	Retrospective study of 713 patients showed improved survival with increased aggressive use of FFP in patients undergoing massive transfusion.
Duchesne JC, Hunt JP, Wahl G, et al. Review of current blood transfusions strategies in a mature level I trauma center: were we wrong for the last 60 years? *J Trauma*. 2008;65:272-276.	Retrospective study of 135 patients with massive transfusions who had better outcome with 1:1.
Sperry JL, Ochoa JB, Gunn SR, et al. An FFP:PRBC transfusion ratio ≥1:1.5 is associated with a lower risk of mortality after massive transfusion. *J Trauma*. 2008;65:986-993.	Multicenter prospective cohort study with 415 patients showed that higher FFP use was associated with less mortality.
Moore FA, Nelson T, McKinley BA, et al. Is there a role for aggressive use of fresh frozen plasma in massive transfusion of civilian trauma patients? *Am J Surg*. 2008;196:948-958.	Retrospective study of 93 patients; concluded that damage control resuscitation with FFP may have a role in civilian trauma.
Teixeira PG, Inaba K, Shulman I, et al. Impact of plasma transfusion in massively transfused trauma patients. *J Trauma*. 2009;66:693-697.	Retrospective study of 383 patients showing that high FFP use was associated with better survival.
Duchesne JC, Islam TM, Stuke L, et al. Hemostatic resuscitation during surgery improves survival in patients with traumatic-induced coagulopathy. *J Trauma*. 2009;67:33-37.	Seven-year retrospective study with 435 patients showed survival advantage in patients receiving FFP:RBC ratio of 1:1 compared with 1:4.
Snyder CW, Weinberg JA, McGwin G Jr, et al. The relationship of blood product ratio to mortality: survival benefit or survival bias? *J Trauma*. 2009;66:358-362.	Retrospective study of 134 patients showed improved survival with higher use of FFP, but the advantage was not persistent when adjusted for survival bias.
Watson GA, Sperry JL, Rosengart MR, et al. Fresh frozen plasma is independently associated with a higher risk of multiple organ failure and acute respiratory distress syndrome. *J Trauma*. 2009;67:221-227.	Prospective multicenter cohort study of blunt trauma patients showed that FFP was associated with an increased risk of multiple-organ failure and ARDS.

TABLE 33.11 Summaries of Recent Retrospective Studies on the Use of FFP—cont'd

ARTICLE	SUMMARY OF FINDINGS
Zink KA, Sambasivan CN, Holcomb JB, et al. A high ratio of plasma and platelets to packed red blood cells in the first 6 hours of massive transfusion improves outcomes in a large multicenter study. *Am J Surg.* 2009;197:565-570.	Retrospective multicenter (16) study with 466 patients who had lower mortality if FFP and platelets were used early and as 1:1.
Riskin DJ, Tsai TC, Riskin L, et al. Massive transfusion protocols: the role of aggressive resuscitation versus product ratio in mortality reduction. *J Am Coll Surg.* 2009;209:198-205.	Retrospective study of 77 patients; concluded that massive transfusion protocol was associated with improved survival.
Ohbe H, Tagami T, Endo A, Miyata S, Matsui H, Fushimi K, Kushimoto S, Yasunaga H. Trends in massive transfusion practice for trauma in Japan from 2011 to 2020: a nationwide inpatient database study. *J Intensive Care.* 2023;11(1):46.	Retrospective study of 5247 patients over 9-year period; found that massive transfusions with lower FFP-to-RBC ratio and platelets-to-RBC ratio were associated with increased mortality.

ARDS, Acute respiratory distress syndrome; *FFP,* fresh frozen plasma; *ICU,* intensive care unit; *PRBC,* packed red blood cell; *RBC,* red blood cell.

In a retrospective review of combat casualties, Borgman and colleagues showed an association between high transfusion ratios of plasma:platelets:RBCs and improved survival. In a civilian setting, Maegele and colleagues have reported that the aggressive use of FFP also resulted in improved outcome. Similar findings were reported by Duchesne and associates, who showed that aggressive resuscitation with FFP is associated with reduced mortality and coagulopathy.

Teixeira and coworkers have shown that although a ratio-based approach to transfusion is associated with better outcomes, the ratio of 1 unit of FFP to 2 units of RBCs may be equivalent. The previous studies had a tendency to place patients with a 1:2 ratio into the aggressive group and could not clearly distinguish among 1:1 versus 1:2 versus 1:3. Other studies also failed to find a survival benefit with FFP but showed that it reduces coagulopathy. Aggressive use of platelets[54] and fibrinogen[55] have also been associated with improved outcome. In a six-center retrospective study, Zink and associates[56] showed that early administration of a high ratio of FFP and platelets improved survival and decreased overall need for RBCs in massively transfused patients. The largest difference in mortality occurred during the first 6 hours after admission, suggesting that the early administration of FFP and platelets is critical. Most hospitals use apheresis platelets, which are pooled platelets; 1 unit is equivalent to what was previously called a *six-pack* of platelets. *Hence, to achieve a 1:1:1 transfusion ratio, 1 unit of apheresis platelets should be given for every 6 units of PRBCs and FFP.*

There have been multiple studies using large databases and prospective studies trying to determine if aggressive use of FFP and platelets can lead to improved outcome. It was argued that the studies showing an advantage were flawed in that they suffered from selection bias, whereby early survivors lived long enough to achieve high ratios. The Prospective, Observational, Multicenter, Major Trauma Transfusion (PROMMTT) study demonstrated that clinicians were transfusing patients with a blood product ratio of 1:1:1 or 1:1:2 and that early transfusion of plasma was associated with improved 6-hour survival.[57]

To settle this debate, the Pragmatic, Randomized Optimal Platelet and Plasma Ratios (PROPPR) trial was designed. This study was a prospective, randomized, multicenter clinical trial designed as an effectiveness and safety study in severely bleeding trauma patients comparing plasma, platelets, and RBCs transfused in a 1:1:1 ratio to a 1:1:2 ratio. The primary outcomes were 24-hour and 30-day all-cause mortality. The results showed that there was no significant difference in mortality at 24 hours ($P = 0.12$) or at 30 days ($P = 0.26$). However, more patients in the 1:1:1 group achieved hemostasis, and fewer experienced death by exsanguination at 24 hours.

Significantly more patients in the 1:1:1 group were alive at 3 hours. There were no safety differences between the two groups. The 1:1:1 group received more blood products but did not experience high rates of ARDS or MODS, infection, venous thromboembolism, or sepsis. Holcomb and colleagues suggested that clinicians should consider using a 1:1:1 transfusion protocol, starting with the initial units transfused while patients are actively bleeding and then transitioning to laboratory-guided treatment once hemorrhage control is achieved. The authors also noted that the 1:1:2 group approached a cumulative ratio of 1:1:1 after the initial ratio-driven protocol ended and they used laboratory-guided treatment, which caused them to catch up to the 1:1:1 group.[58] The delivery of increased clotting factors to exsanguinating patients may explain part of the benefit of a high-ratio approach in massive transfusion. Plasma is composed of over a thousand proteins, some of which may have beneficial effects. Trauma and shock result in degradation of the vascular glycocalyx and increased endothelial permeability, which is known as the *endotheliopathy of trauma*. Resuscitation with LR solution exacerbates this process, whereas resuscitation with plasma rebuilds the glycocalyx and reduces vascular permeability.[59] This phenomenon likely explains the development of ARDS and abdominal compartment syndrome that occurs with massive crystalloid reduction and the reduction in multiple-organ dysfunction that has occurred as crystalloid resuscitation after trauma has been deemphasized.

Massive Transfusion Protocol

Studies have led to the development of the massive transfusion protocol (MTP), which calls for the aggressive use of liquid cold-stored, low-titer O whole blood (LTOWB) or components given in a high ratio when whole blood is not available. The protocol was designed to enable a hospital's blood bank to improve logistical systems for the empirical use of blood components. A number of studies have shown that implementing an MTP improves survival in trauma patients.[60] To qualify as a trauma center, the American College of Surgeons Verification Review Committee requires that all trauma centers have an MTP in place and have a system for reviewing the adequacy of these resuscitations.

An example of an MTP directive is that for severely injured patients, the blood bank should provide a cooler containing 5 units of LTOWB or 4 units of type O RBCs and 4 units of AB or A plasma. If possible, a patient's blood sample should be drawn before the uncrossmatched blood is transfused; even 1 unit of RBCs can sometimes interfere with crossmatching. O-negative blood is reserved for transfusing females of childbearing age when their blood type is unknown or when they are known to be Rh−. If the initial cooler of blood is used, the blood bank sends additional coolers containing LTOWB or plasma, platelets, and RBCs in a 1:1:1 ratio.

CURRENT STATUS OF FLUID TYPES

Crystalloids

The unit of *milliequivalents per liter* (mEq/L) refers to the number of electrical charges; *milliosmoles per liter* (mOsm/L) refers to the number of osmotically active particles or ions. A milliequivalent in a solution must be precisely balanced by the same number of milliequivalents of a cation and anion. The balance affects the direction of water as it equilibrates. The *osmotic pressure* of a solution refers to the actual number of osmotically active particles present in the solution, but it does not depend on the chemical-combining capacities of the substances. For example, sodium chloride dissociates to 2 mOsm, whereas sodium sulfate (Na_2SO_4) dissociates into three particles: 2 mOsm of sodium and 1 mOsm of sulfate. However, 1 mOsm of an un-ionized substance such as glucose is equal to 1 mOsm of the substance.

Large-volume normal saline resuscitation produces acidosis by dilution of serum HCO_3^-. Normally, chloride and bicarbonate ions are reciprocated up or down with each other, maintaining electrical neutrality. Often, the result of massive normal saline infusion is a hyperchloremic non–anion-gap metabolic acidosis. At extreme levels, acidosis can impair cardiac performance, decrease responsiveness to cardiac inotropic drugs, affect cellular metabolism, change enzyme activity, and alter the coagulation cascade. Many would argue that for cellular protection, the human body offloads oxygen more easily from Hb in the acidotic state and that acidosis, at least to a degree, is actually better for a patient than alkalosis. Normal saline is an ideal solution for the resuscitation of vomiting patients who develop a contraction alkalosis.

Surgeons with experience using HTS sometimes encounter induced metabolic acidosis but have found it to be of minimal clinical consequence. Induced metabolic hyperchloremic acidosis is different from spontaneous metabolic acidosis and from hypovolemic lactic acidosis. No evidence exists that hyperchloremic acidosis does anything more than confuse the interpretation of the metabolic state. Given the lack of any significant proven benefit of one crystalloid over another, many trauma systems use normal saline in the prehospital setting. This is because stocking just one form of fluid is convenient. Another reason is that when transfusion is required, the LR solution has

to be switched to normal saline because LR solution contains calcium, which binds citrate, theoretically producing clotting. This is a regulatory policy even though studies have shown that the use of LR solution as a carrier in the same IV line as blood has no relevant side effects.

Plasma-Lyte (Baxter, Deerfield, IL), a balanced crystalloid solution, was developed more than 20 years ago and contains additional electrolytes, such as acetate and gluconate. The overall chloride level is also lower. Plasma-Lyte also contains magnesium, so this should be considered in patients with renal failure. It may also affect peripheral vascular resistance and heart rate, and it may worsen organ ischemia. It is similar to other crystalloids in that it can cause lung edema and increase ICP and generalized edema. Numerous reports of its use have addressed its safety during the priming of extracorporeal circulation pumps and its use in cold ischemia, circulatory arrest, organ transplantation, and organ preservation.

In a study examining the use of HTS with dextran, patients were randomized to receive 7.5% HTS with dextran or Plasma-Lyte A. The 2-hour sodium, bicarbonate, CO_2, and pH values were comparable. The HTS with dextran group required less crystalloid. However, the volumes infused were also different. In a study by McFarlane, 30 patients undergoing hepatobiliary or pancreatic surgery were randomized to 0.9% normal saline or Plasma-Lyte 148 at 15 mL/kg/h. During surgery, Plasma-Lyte was found to be more efficacious, also producing less hyperchloremia and acidosis. However, no significant difference in sodium, potassium, or blood lactate levels was found. In a kidney transplantation study, Plasma-Lyte A did not increase lactate levels (like LR solution) and did not cause acidosis (like normal saline); the best metabolic profile was maintained in patients receiving Plasma-Lyte. Plasma-Lyte is also favored in various cell preparations and as a storage medium for platelets. A randomized trial by Young and colleagues[61] showed that compared with normal saline, patients resuscitated with Plasma-Lyte A had improved acid-base status and less hyperchloremia at 24 hours after injury. The components of the various crystalloids are shown in Table 33.12. In summary, there are advantages and disadvantages for various crystalloids. Plasma-Lyte has the advantage in that it has magnesium, and studies have shown that this reduces the need for magnesium replacement, although there are concerns about infusing large volumes of Plasma-Lyte because of too much magnesium. From the chloride point of view, LR solution may be better than Plasma-Lyte, which may be better than normal saline. In a large volume, there may be an advantage of resuscitating with LR solution because it has the

TABLE 33.12 Commercially Available Crystalloids and Their Composition

	NORMAL SALINE	LACTATED RINGER	PLASMA-LYTE A	NORMOSOL	PLASMA
Positive Ions					
Sodium	154	130	140	140	134–145
Potassium		4	5	5	3.4–5
Calcium		3			2.25–2.65
Magnesium			3	3	0.7–1.1
Negative Ions					
Chloride	154	109	98	98	98–108
Lactate		28	27	27	
Bicarbonate					22–32
Gluconate			23	23	
pH	5.4–7.0	6.5	7.4	7.4	7.4
Osmolarity	308	273	294	295	280–295

least amount of chloride. In short-term hemorrhagic shock studies in swine using large volumes of crystalloids, LR solution was shown to be better than normal saline and Plasma-Lyte solution. In most institutions, the cost of normal saline and LR and Plasma-Lyte solutions is similar, about $3.00/L. In a pragmatic, randomized trial of 15,802 ICU patients, LR and Plasma-Lyte solutions were compared with normal saline as primary resuscitation fluids. Patients who received balanced crystalloids had a lower rate of the composite outcome of death, new renal replacement therapy, and persistent renal dysfunction compared with patients who received normal saline.[62]

Hypertonic Saline

HTS has been extensively studied. In summary, the studies have shown that sodium is the main electrolyte that controls intravascular volume. Investigators who have worked with HTS in bleeding animals have learned that resuscitation goals can be achieved with much smaller volumes as long as the sodium load is the same. For example, in an animal model of hemorrhagic shock, if 1 L of normal saline is required to achieve a BP of 120 mm Hg, the same result can be obtained with an infusion of 120 mL of 7.5% normal saline. For 5% HTS, only 182 mL would be needed. In animal studies, HTS draws water into the intravascular space from the intracellular and interstitial spaces.

HTS has consistently been shown to reduce the inflammatory response and is thus considered to be immunomodulatory (Fig. 33.17). Immunosuppression from HTS may thus be beneficial and detrimental, depending on when and how it is used. In randomized prospective studies with HTS alone or with a colloid such as hetastarch or dextran, results show that HTS is equivalent to crystalloid solutions in terms of mortality. The concentration that has been studied the most is 7.5% HTS. From 1995 to 2005, when inflammation was being extensively studied, the theoretical advantages of HTS were a decrease in the inflammatory response and potentially a reduction in ARDS and MODS. Thus, it was thought to be potentially the ideal fluid of choice in hemorrhagic shock resuscitation. One of the main problems with 7.5% HTS is that there is no manufacturer that makes and sells it. This is because it is extremely difficult and expensive to obtain FDA approval, and there is little profit in selling salt water. In Europe, 7.5% HTS with dextran is available.

The Resuscitation Outcomes Consortium (ROC), which was composed of 10 trauma centers in the United States and Canada, was funded to participate in trauma and emergency medicine trials. ROC is a federally funded organization with the aim of examining potential prehospital interventions. The first trauma trial by ROC examined HTS. This prospective randomized trial enrolled hypotensive patients with blunt or penetrating trauma, with and without traumatic head injury. Patients were randomized into one of three arms by dose and fluid: (1) 250-mL bolus of normal saline, (2) 250-mL bolus of 7.5% HTS, and (3) 250-mL of 7.5% HTS with 6% dextran 70. The HTS trial enrolled 2221 patients using exception from informed consent. There were two studies in this trial. The hemorrhagic shock study enrolled 894 patients, and 1327 patients were enrolled in the TBI study. The TBI trial enrolled patients with or without hypotension; the main enrollment criterion was a GCS score of 8 or less.

The HTS shock trial showed that patients receiving HTS had only a mild elevation in their sodium level (147 mEq/L vs. 140 mEq/L in the normal saline group) because the infusion volume was small and only in the prehospital setting. The admission Hb level was also significantly lower. The patients who

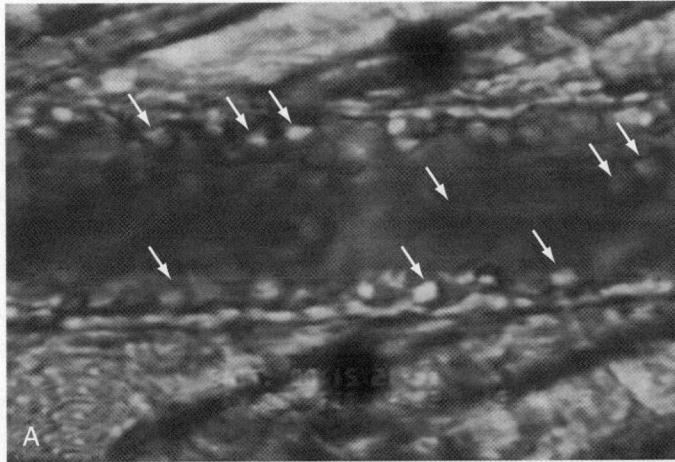
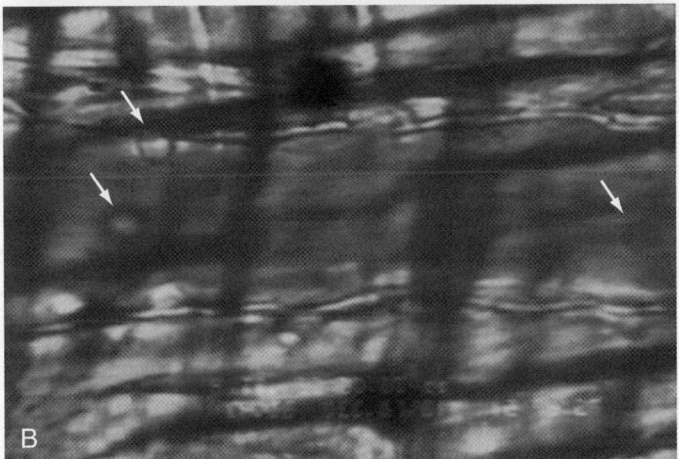

FIGURE 33.17 (A–B) Immunologic response from hypertonic resuscitation is less than that after lactated Ringer solution has been given. (From Pascual JL, Khwaja KA, Ferri LE, et al. Hypertonic saline resuscitation attenuates neutrophil lung sequestration and transmigration by diminishing leukocyte-endothelial interactions in a two-hit model of hemorrhagic shock and infection. *J Trauma.* 2003;54:121-132.)

received HTS with or without dextran had a Hb level of 10.2 g/dL compared with 11.1 g/dL in the normal saline group. This may reflect the amount of intravascular resuscitation from HTS versus normal saline. The overall 28-day survival rates were almost identical: HTS patients, 73%; HTS with dextran patients, 74.5%; and normal saline patients, 74.4% ($P = 0.91$).

However, the HTS trial was stopped before the end of its planned enrollment by the Data Safety and Monitoring Board for two main reasons. First, interim analysis showed futility because the outcomes were so similar. Second, a detailed subgroup analysis found a potential for harm in a subgroup of patients who did not receive RBC transfusion in the first 24 hours. For unexplained reasons, their mortality rate was significantly higher if they received HTS or HTS with dextran. Patients in the HTS and HTS with dextran groups who received more than 10 units of RBCs within the first 24 hours had a lower mortality rate, although the difference was not statistically significant.[63]

The main criticism of this study was that it allowed only a small dose in the prehospital phase, and HTS infusion did not continue in the hospital. Additional resuscitation was not regulated in this study, and all patients received about the same amount of prehospital fluid. Also, the sodium level was raised to only 147 mEq/L, signifying that not enough HTS was used to affect the immunomodulatory capability of HTS because some feel that the sodium level needs to be much higher to achieve that effect. In hypotensive patients, 250 mL of normal saline is clinically irrelevant, but because 250 mL of HTS with dextran 0 or HTS is approximately equivalent to 2 L of normal saline, individuals in the group of patients who received HTS were being resuscitated more, whereas the normal saline group was not. Thus, the trial seemed to compare 250 mL of normal saline to the equivalent of 2 L of normal saline. Support for this theory is that the Hb level was lower in the group of patients who received HTS. The trial of HTS in patients with TBI was also halted; the interim analysis also showed futility, meaning that the primary outcome was almost identical between the normal saline and HTS groups. Such an outcome can also be interpreted as showing that HTS is safe, but technically, the trial was not powered to show noninferiority.

HTS was studied in TBI because preliminary studies had shown promise. HTS infusion is highly effective in decreasing ICP and can do this while increasing blood volume, BP, and blood flow to the brain. Compared with mannitol, which is customarily used for lowering ICP, HTS might do this without dehydrating patients or putting them at further risk for secondary brain injury caused by hypotension or renal failure from mannitol. Patients receiving high-dose mannitol drips are also susceptible to pulmonary insufficiency, causing longer ICU stays. Infusion of mannitol requires high daily volumes. Mannitol is safe if it is used carefully in patients with isolated TBIs, but in hypotensive polytrauma patients, it can be detrimental and might exacerbate hypotension.

Commercially, HTS comes in 23%, 5%, and 3% concentrations in the United States. Curiously, all the human studies used 7.5% HTS, but this formulation is not commercially available. This could be the main strategic mistake of the HTS studies. Most animal and human studies have used 7.5% HTS, an arbitrary concentration because 10% HTS was found to be highly irritating to peripheral veins. HTS injected rapidly into human volunteers causes pain at the infusion site. Thus, the preferred route is through a central vein. In animal studies, if 7.5% HTS is given through the interosseous route, osteomyonecrosis and compartment syndrome can ensue. Some nontrauma studies have used 3% and 23% concentrations, but minimal clinical experience has been reported with 5%. There are two studies reporting their experience using 5% HTS in trauma patients, with or without TBI, and it has been found to be safe.[64] This finding is logical because the 7.5% HTS studies have also shown safety. Using 5% HTS may be the best strategy to recruit intravascular volume compared with crystalloid resuscitation. The method used in trauma patients is to give 5% HTS in 250-mL infusions and, if more than 500 mL is needed, to check sodium levels. The sodium content of 250 mL of 5% HTS is equivalent to 1645 mL of LR solution. Thus, a bolus can be given quickly, without having to use hypotonic solutions such as LR solution.

Colloids

Human albumin (4%–5%) in saline is considered to be the reference colloidal solution. It is fractionated from blood and heat treated to prevent transmission of viruses. It has many theoretical advantages, especially in animal studies, but clinical studies have not shown outcome differences. Its main theoretical advantage is that compared with crystalloids, it is less inflammatory. This may be because it is a natural molecule. Other than its dilutional effect, albumin is associated with minimal coagulopathy. No clinical

evidence has shown that albumin is better than other colloids, but the Saline Versus Albumin Fluid Evaluation (SAFE) study in Australia has shown 4% albumin to be safe, compared with normal saline, in ICU patients.[65] The SAFE study, whose main intent was to show equivalency, found no difference in the primary outcome (28-day mortality rate) or in any secondary outcome. The adoption of damage control or hemostatic resuscitation has been thought to result in improved outcome, decreased blood use, and decreased incidence of ARDS. ARDS and MODS still occur, but at a much lower rate than previously seen.

There are still other advantages of 25% albumin over artificial colloids. Albumin has a proven immunologic antiinflammatory effect and five times less volume than current artificial colloids. Unlike artificial colloids, it does not potentially lead to coagulopathic side effects. It has been proven to be safe from infectious and clinical standpoints. The volume of fluid that has to be carried is obviously much less (Fig. 33.18). Albumin costs approximately 30 times more than crystalloids and 3 times more than dextran or Hextend, but those comparisons were made against 5% human albumin. The cost of 100 mL of 25% albumin, compared with 500 mL of Hextend on a physiologic basis, is only approximately 3 times as much. During the Vietnam War, 25% albumin was first made available, and it seemed to have worked well. It was packaged in a green can that could be transported without damage, had a long shelf life, and was easy to use.

The commonly used synthetic colloids are plasma, albumin, dextran, gelatin, and starch-based colloids. Hetastarch solutions are produced from amylopectin obtained from sorghum, maize, or potatoes. Extensive randomized controlled trials have examined the safety and efficacy of 5% albumin, 6% hetastarch, and 6% dextran.

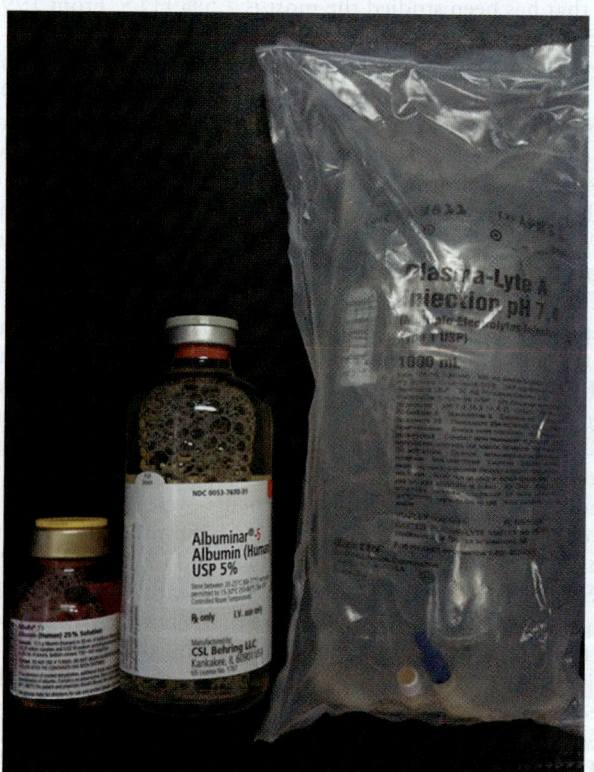

FIGURE 33.18 Comparison of container sizes: 50 mL of 25% albumin, 500 mL of 5% albumin, and 1 L of lactated Ringer solution. The 50 mL of 25% albumin is physiologically equivalent to approximately 2000 to 2500 mL of crystalloids.

However, no evidence has shown that one colloid is superior to another or that colloids are better or worse than crystalloids.[66] Colloids such as hetastarch can have proinflammatory effects similar to those of crystalloids. In some cases, colloids will do more harm in large volumes than crystalloids, but not all colloids should be considered the same. It is well known that artificial colloids can perpetuate coagulopathy; dextran is used specifically to help prevent clotting after vascular surgery. The inflammatory system is tightly interwoven with the coagulation process. Hetastarch, particularly the high–molecular-weight preparations, is associated with alterations in coagulation, specifically resulting in changes in the viscoelastic measurements and fibrinolysis. Studies have questioned the safety of concentrated (10%) hetastarch solutions with a molecular weight of more than 200 and a molar substitution ratio of more than 0.5 in patients with severe sepsis, citing increased rates of death, acute kidney injury, and use of renal replacement therapy. To prolong intravascular expansion, a high degree of substitution on glucose molecules protects against hydrolysis by nonspecific amylases in the blood. However, this results in accumulation in reticuloendothelial tissues such as the skin, liver, and kidneys. Because of the potential for accumulation in tissues, the recommended maximal daily dose of hetastarch is 33 to 55 mL/kg/day. Studies in trauma patients have shown an association between acute kidney injury and death after blunt trauma. Patients with severe sepsis assigned to fluid resuscitation with hydroxyethyl starch 130/0.4 had an increased risk of death at day 90 and were more likely to require renal replacement therapy compared with those receiving Ringer acetate. In animal models, albumin seems to be better for preventing inflammation, whereas hetastarch and dextran, in high doses, appear to cause inflammation and coagulopathy.

FUTURE RESUSCITATION RESEARCH

Blood Substitutes

In contrast to volume expanders, blood substitutes are fluids that can carry oxygen. Each year in the United States, 15 million units of RBCs are transfused. Methods to decrease the need for blood transfusions include preoperative autologous donation, intraoperative blood retrieval with reinfusion, and isovolemic hemodilution. Such methods allow withdrawing of a patient's blood at the start of surgery, replacing it with volume expanders, and then, at the end of surgery, retransfusing the patient with their donated blood. Because of blood supply limitations, infectious and transfusion complications, and storage limitations, the need for blood substitutes remains. The ideal blood substitute would do the following:

- Deliver oxygen
- Be compatible with all blood types
- Have few side effects
- Have prolonged storage capabilities
- Persist in the circulation
- Be cost-effective

Currently, blood substitutes are either Hb based or nonHb based. Research on Hb-based fluids dates back to the 1920s when the stroma of the cells was lysed to obtain Hb. Purification and sterilization were hurdles that took decades to overcome, but it was soon realized that free Hb had toxic effects (because of the breakdown products). Problems with free Hb include osmotic diuretic effects, renal toxicity, coagulation abnormalities, short half-life, and vasoconstrictive effects (which are known to be caused by Hb solutions scavenging nitric oxide).

During the next three decades (the 1930s, 1940s, and 1950s), efforts concentrated on stabilizing the Hb molecule to increase its persistence in the circulation and prevent toxic effects. Such strategies included cross-linking the molecule between the tetramer subunits, polymerizing it, encapsulating it in an artificial red cell or in liposomes, and using microsphere technology to form a million stable micromolecules. Development of some Hb substitutes advanced to clinical trials.

Blood substitutes are referred to as *hemoglobin oxygen carriers* (HBOCs). Current second-generation HBOCs are pasteurized and thus free of communicable pathogens; they also have no ABO/Rh or other blood antigens. They are universally compatible and require no blood banking. They can be easily administered without special training or expertise. The problems of a short half-life and renal toxicity have now been overcome, but some troublesome side effects remain: free radical generation and exacerbation of reperfusion injury, methemoglobin production, and immunologic effects (including immunosuppression and potentiation of endotoxin-related pathogenicity).

The Hb for blood substitutes comes from a variety of sources, such as outdated donated human blood, bovine or swine blood, and transgenic *E. coli*. Each source has its benefits (availability, cost) as well as its side effects (infections, other complications). Human Hb has the advantage of being a naturally occurring product that has been extensively studied, but its obvious disadvantage is lack of availability. About 2 units of discarded blood are required to make 1 unit of the HBOC. Even if we were to capture all of the discarded human blood, the numbers of units made would only be half of what was discarded.

The potential advantages of animals as a source of Hb are tremendous; they are a relatively cheap source, and their supply is unlimited. Yet despite efforts at controlling a herd, problems such as bovine spongiform encephalitis and other infectious diseases will inevitably surface. Recombinant Hb has problems as well. Volumes of bacterial culture and the stringent processing methods are costly. It is estimated that only 0.1 g of Hb can be generated from 1 L of *E. coli* culture. This equates to 750 L to make 1 unit. Production of 3 million units would require more than 1.125 billion liters of culture.

One of the first HBOC products tested was manufactured by Baxter in 1999. Diaspirin cross-linked Hb (DCLHb), known as *HemAssist*, was tested. This chemically modified human Hb solution was used in a highly publicized trial in patients with traumatic hemorrhagic shock, one of the first trials to use exception from informed consent (instead of individual patient consent). Baxter terminated the trial early because the patients who received the test product had a higher 28-day mortality rate (47%) than those who received normal saline (25%) ($P < 0.015$). A recent analysis compared data from the Baxter trial with the 17 US emergency departments and the parallel 27 European Union prehospital systems now using DCLHb. This analysis did not show any difference in outcome. The authors reported that neither mean BP readings nor elevated BP readings correlated with DCLHb treatment of traumatic hemorrhagic shock patients. As such, no clinically demonstrable DCLHb pressor effect could be directly related to the adverse mortality outcome observed in the Baxter trial.

Two other products currently have potential for clinical use. Both are polymerized rather than tetramerized. Polymerization is thought to be better because the molecular masses are higher (130 kDa) than with tetramerization (65 kDa), resulting in longer intravascular presence. Some investigators have proposed that polymerization avoids contact with nitric oxide, attenuating the vasoconstriction seen with previous products.

One of those products is HBOC-201 (Hemopure; Biopure Corporation), made from bovine blood. It is universally compatible and is stable at room temperature for up to 3 years. Animal studies showed great promise. Human trials involving orthopedic patients also showed promise, but safety issues were a concern; patients who received Hemopure had an increased number of serious adverse events. The vasoconstrictive properties of Hemopure may have caused myocardial infarction in susceptible patients. Biopure Corporation went bankrupt and was taken over by OPK Biotech, which has a product called *Oxyglobin* (HBOC-301) for veterinary use. OPK Biotech has continued to develop Hemopure for human use; the US Navy is supporting research for potential use in the military setting. Studies have been proposed to coinfuse a nitric oxide donor, such as nitroglycerin, in a fixed ratio, in a single-bag compound, or as separate infusions. However, there is little likelihood that surgeons will accept a product to treat shock that requires coinfusion of a vasodilator. A recent study in the April 2019 issue of *Nature* found that Hemopure could potentially restore brain circulation and cellular function up to 4 hours after death in animal models. Hemopure is approved for clinical use in Russia and South Africa. Hemopure is available for compassionate use in the United States under investigational protocols.

HemO2life is a polymerized extracellular Hb with a molecular weight about 50 times that of human Hb and the ability to bind 156 molecules of oxygen relative to 4 derived from the polychaete *Arenicola marina* and developed by the French company Hemarina. It has been approved by the European Union for donor organ preservation before transplantation and has been studied to improve oxygenation in COVID-19 patients and minimize tracheal intubation.

A meta-analysis of 16 HBOC trials, including 4 trauma trials involving HemAssist or PolyHeme, showed that HBOC patients had a significantly increased risk of myocardial infarctions and death compared with controls. The problem of vasoconstriction remains. Vasodilators can be added to mitigate vasoconstriction, but whether enthusiasm for HBOCs persists remains to be seen. Without doubt, however, they have a real potential benefit for patients who do not have access to RBCs, such as in rural areas or austere combat conditions, or patients who refuse blood transfusions.[67]

Third-generation Hb substitutes have begun to address the deficiencies of earlier formulations. The encapsulation of Hb in liposomes is an innovation, but efforts to optimize these continue. The mixing of phospholipids and cholesterol in the presence of free Hb forms a sphere with Hb in the center. These liposomes have oxygen dissociation curves similar to those of red cells, and administration can transiently achieve high circulating levels of Hb and oxygen delivery. Research is still in the preclinical testing stage; progress in prolonging the half-life and elucidating the effects on the immune system, particularly reticuloendothelial sequestration, is crucial before clinical testing can begin.

Perfluorocarbons

Perfluorocarbons (PFCs) are completely inert biologically and similar to Teflon or Gore-Tex. Altering the molecule (by fluoridating the ring structure) lowers the melting point and thus makes it a liquid at room temperature. PFCs captured the imagination of many in 1966, when photographs were introduced of a mouse completely submerged in the liquid form but breathing and surviving in it (Fig. 33.19). PFCs dissolve larger quantities of oxygen and CO_2 than plasma. They have yet to find a purpose in liquid form, but enthusiasm has increased for their

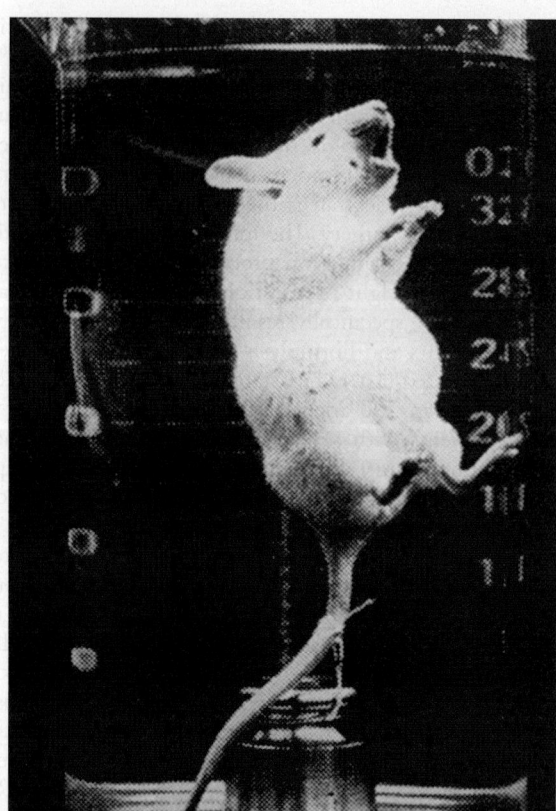

FIGURE 33.19 Mouse surviving while submerged in perfluorocarbons. (From Shaffer TH, Wolfson MR. Liquid ventilation. In: Polin RA, Fox WW, Abman SH, eds. *Fetal and Neonatal Physiology*. 3rd ed. Philadelphia: WB Saunders; 2003.)

use in partial liquid ventilation. Trials in adults with ARDS have shown no benefit, but trials are still ongoing in children with hyaline membrane disease.

PFCs have two challenges to overcome for use as blood substitutes. The first is that the liquid form is immiscible in water; thus, PFCs must be suspended as microdroplets with the use of emulsifying agents. The second is that unlike Hb, the oxygen that is dissolved in PFCs has a linear relationship to the PO_2, whereas Hb has a sigmoidal disassociation curve favoring full loading at normal atmospheric oxygen levels. Thus, the percentage of inspired oxygen (FiO_2) that is required to be applied for PFCs is high.

Second-generation PFCs have been formulated to allow more oxygen-carrying capacity, with alterations in the emulsion properties. Such new compounds can also be stored at 4°C, whereas previous solutions had to be frozen. Oxygent (Alliance Pharmaceutical Corp./Baxter Healthcare Corp.) is a 60% perflubron emulsion with a median particle diameter of less than 0.2 μm. The use of lecithin as an emulsifier eliminated the adverse effects of complement activation observed in earlier studies of PFCs. Possible current scenarios for its use include cardiopulmonary bypass with normovolemic hemodilution and balloon angioplasty (to provide oxygenated blood past the catheter while it is inflated). In a phase III study, Oxygent was shown to reduce the need for RBC transfusion in patients undergoing noncardiac surgery (16%, Oxygent group; 26%, control group; $P < 0.05$). Oxygent patients, however, had more serious adverse events (32% in the Oxygent group vs. 21% in the control group; $P < 0.05$). In another phase III study, in patients undergoing cardiac bypass,

Oxygent possibly increased the incidence of strokes. All further studies were halted.

Two other PFC products have been introduced. In early-phase clinical trials, OxyFluor (HemaGen) produced mild thrombocytopenia and influenza-like symptoms in healthy volunteers. Baxter International has withdrawn support for further development. Phase II trials of Oxycyte (Synthetic Blood International) have been suspended; it has been taken over by Oxygen Biotherapeutics, Inc., and is being sold over the counter as a cosmetic product known as Dermacyte, an oxygen concentrate gel for wound healing. Dermacyte is also being investigated for the treatment of cancer during chemotherapy or radiation therapy because oxygen free radicals are thought to kill cancer cells. PFCs are not free of side effects and are not efficacious for oxygen delivery and use.[68]

Novel Fluids

The recognition that currently available fluids are not a replacement for blood and that they, in fact, can be harmful if used in large amounts to expand blood volume has initiated exciting research for better fluids. Blood is so highly complex that the ultimate goal is to develop artificial whole blood, but doing so will take much time. The ideal method would be to manufacture whole blood with a bioreactor using stem cells, but the development of this would take decades. The permutations of future fluid development are endless. Novel crystalloids are being tested, as are hypertonic solutions with and without oxygen carriers, hypertonic colloids, freeze-dried plasma (FDP), and drug therapy.

The Institute of Medicine in 1999 recommended research to eliminate lactate in LR solution and investigate the use of alternative energy substrates in resuscitation fluids. It recognized that although reperfusion injury can occur in shock resuscitation, a separate entity called *resuscitation injury* is a result of the method of resuscitation and the fluids used.

Two substances have since been identified that may alter the inflammatory response after resuscitation. In small and large animal models, studies found that simply replacing the lactate in LR solution with either ketones or pyruvate reduced the inflammatory response after hemorrhagic shock resuscitation. Other investigators have concentrated on various forms of pyruvate to minimize resuscitation injury; ethyl pyruvate seems promising. Studies in animals show that pyruvate Ringer solution corrects lactic acidosis and prolongs survival during hemorrhagic shock in rats. At the cellular level, a combination of antiinflammatory constituents in fluids seems more efficacious.

Studies of the mechanisms behind such improved results found that monocarboxylate-supplemented resuscitation provides energy substrates, with minimal alteration in the conventionally used fluids such as LR solution. Replacing the lactate in LR solution with either pyruvate or ketones protected the brain and other tissues after shock. That finding led to research on the reasons for this protective effect and on the potential of using drugs alone to treat hemorrhagic shock.

Dried Plasma

Dried plasma was used during World War II, when the US Army initially believed that plasma was adequate to resuscitate hemorrhagic shock (Fig. 33.20). Dried plasma used in WWII came from multiple donors and was not screened for viral pathogens. Hepatitis transmission in injured warfighters was common. There has been no dried plasma product available in the United States since WWII. However, the capability of removing potential infectious agents, along with the improved technology for manufacturing of dried

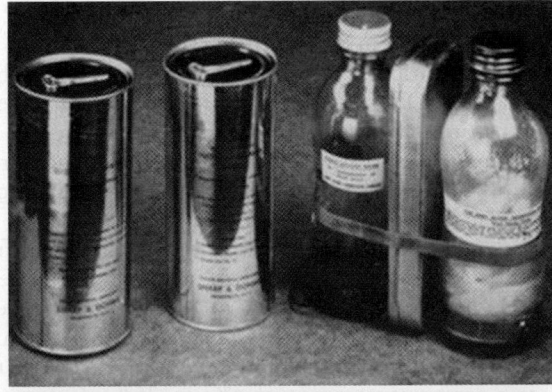
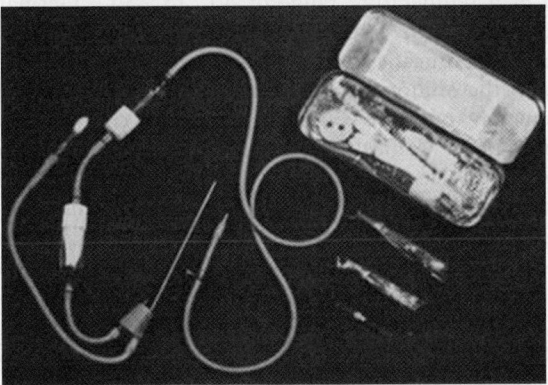

FIGURE 33.20 Freeze-dried plasma used during World War II. (Courtesy Office of Medical History, US Army Medical Department, Center of History and Heritage, Washington, DC.)

plasma, resurrected research in this field. Dried plasma is prepared in one of two ways. It can be FDP or lyophilized with a combination of low-temperature, low-pressure, and low-moisture circulating air. It can also be spray dried in a high-temperature chamber, where it is aerosolized. The product can be stored in either of these forms with minimal protein degradation until it is reconstituted, pH adjusted, and then administered. The advantages of dried plasma are the long shelf life and that it does not need refrigeration and tight temperature control. It avoids the difficult logistics of storing fresh frozen products and the preparation time of thawing FFP. Modern-day dried plasma has been pathogen reduced so that the historical concerns of transmitting viruses are minimized.

Through funding by the US military, plasma separated from fresh porcine blood was lyophilized to produce FDP and then compared with FFP. After a 60% blood volume hemorrhage, pigs were resuscitated with reconstituted FDP, which was just as efficacious as thawed plasma and had an identical coagulation profile. A multi-institutional polytrauma animal trial found that FDP was better than Hextend (which led to anemia and coagulopathy).[62] Currently, this area of research and development is exciting and promising. FDP is currently available in Europe, the Middle East, and Africa but not in the United States.

The French army has been using freeze-dried and secured plasma (FDSP) since 1994. It is made from fresh leukodepleted blood of up to 10 volunteers. Blood type selection allows the dilution and neutralization of natural anti-A and anti-B hemagglutinins. This FDSP is thus compatible with any blood type. It is also shelf stable in ambient temperatures for 2 years and is easily rehydrated with 200 mL of water for use in less than 3 minutes. FDSP contains all clotting factors and proteins. The fibrinogen and clotting factor levels of FDSP are equivalent to those of FFP. Early reports of using FDSP in 87 battlefield casualties show that it was effective for preventing or treating coagulopathy in a French ICU in Afghanistan. FDSP has been studied in the civilian setting, revealing that it is effective compared with FFP and results in increased fibrinogen levels early after trauma. This French product is carried by US Special Forces medics for use in austere conditions under an institutional review board (IRB) protocol.

Germany also has FDP (LyoPlas N-w), which comes from a single donor screened for bloodborne pathogens. Unlike FFP, LyoPlas N-w undergoes filtration to further remove cellular remnants to reduce the risk of infection or transfusion immune reactions. It remains effective for 12 months when it is maintained at a temperature range of 4°C to 25°C. Germany has fielded more than 500,000 units of LyoPlas N-w without unusual or significant adverse effects compared with FFP. In addition to the ability to prevent or treat coagulopathy, it is an excellent way to restore volume because it is a colloid. The Israeli Defense Forces Medical Corps policy is that plasma is the fluid of choice for selected severely wounded patients, and thus, it included LyoPlasN-w as part of its armamentarium for use at the point of injury by advanced lifesavers across the entire military. Several companies are developing dried plasma in the United States, but to date, there is no FDA-approved product.

There has been research to develop freeze-dried RBCs, but the challenge has been to overcome the freezing, drying, and rehydration process without stressful injury to the RBCs. Although freeze-dried RBCs have been shown to have acceptable viscoelastic deformability properties, with storage times of about 1 week by adding trehalose, a sugar molecule, this product is still in the very early stages of development. Freeze-dried platelets and platelet-derived particles are also being developed. Frozen platelets are cryopreserved in 6% dimethyl sulfoxide and can be stored for up to 10 years at −80°C. Freeze-dried platelets have been in development for more than 50 years, but preserving functionality has been a challenge. Modern preparations, which are treated with 1.8% paraformaldehyde, frozen in 5% albumin, and then lyophilized, have been more encouraging. Once rehydrated, they seem structurally intact, contain most of the glycoproteins, and are capable of supporting thrombin generation and fibrin deposition. However, in vivo testing shows that the duration of hemostatic activity is brief, approximately 4 to 6 hours, and sometimes limited to 15 minutes. Recent studies of human freeze-dried platelets in a swine liver injury model have demonstrated improved survival and reduced blood loss, but 13% of the surviving animals were found to have thrombotic complications. The idea of FDP, RBCs, and platelets would mean potentially reconstitutable whole blood.

Pharmacologic Agents

Resuscitation fluids simply replace the lost intravascular volume but have no inherent prosurvival properties. Therefore, a body of work is investigating whether it would be logical to design therapies promoting a prosurvival phenotype. Among patients resuscitated from hemorrhagic shock, a wide spectrum of responses is observed. Although some patients recover without any complications, others develop multiple-organ failure. This unpredictable response is not caused by a widespread variation in the human genome. Since the decoding of the human genome, it has become apparent that only 20,000 to 35,000 protein-coding genes are responsible for millions of different phenotypes. The rapidly expanding field of epigenetics focuses on mechanisms and phenomena that affect the phenotype of a cell or an organism without affecting the genotype. Over the years, many pharmacologic agents have been tested as possible adjuncts (or substitutes) to conventional fluid resuscitation. These drugs cover a wide spectrum, including neuroendocrine agents, calcium channel blockers, ATP pathway modifiers, prostaglandins, sex steroids, antioxidants, antiinflammatory agents, and immune modulators. Although there is strong laboratory evidence of their beneficial effects on tissue perfusion, myocardial contractility, reticuloendothelial function, cell survival, oxidative injury, and immune activation, most of these agents are not yet in clinical use as resuscitative agents.

This area of work is an example of translational research that is novel and could be revolutionary. DNA transcription is regulated, in part, by acetylation of nuclear histones that are controlled by two groups of enzymes: histone deacetylases (HDACs) and histone acetyltransferases. Animal experiments showed that hemorrhagic shock and resuscitation were associated with HDAC/histone acetyltransferase activity misbalance and that the acetylation status of cardiac histones is influenced by the choice of resuscitation strategy. Shock-induced changes can be reversed through the infusion of a pharmacologic HDAC inhibitor, even when it is administered for only a limited period after the insult. Animal experiments have shown tremendous promise in elucidating mechanisms behind the success of using an HDAC inhibitor to prolong life after shock.[69]

Alam and colleagues have been investigating the role of HDAC inhibitors, such as valproic acid (VPA; an anticonvulsant) and suberoylanilide hydroxamic acid. They hypothesized that these may be useful in the treatment of shock through restoration of normal cellular acetylation. In their experiments, large swine subjected to trauma (femur and liver injury) and to severe hemorrhage (60% blood loss) were randomized into one of three groups: no treatment (control group), treatment with fresh whole blood, or treatment with VPA (400 mg/kg) without resuscitation. The early survival rate was 100% in the fresh whole blood group, 86% in the VPA group, and 25% in the control group.[70] Impressively, this survival improvement was achieved without conventional fluid resuscitation or blood transfusion, which makes this approach appealing for the logistically constrained prehospital and battlefield environments. It appears that HDAC inhibitors rapidly activate nuclear histones as well as numerous cellular proteins to create a prosurvival phenotype in hemorrhagic and septic shock. This group has also reported that VPA is neuroprotective and is promising for the treatment of TBI. It has also been shown to be beneficial in sepsis. A number of these HDAC inhibitors are being tested in phase I and II clinical trials (nontraumatic situations).

Given concerns that inflammation after trauma might be a pathologic event, another unique approach is to use estrogen and progesterone to treat patients after traumatic hemorrhagic shock. A number of independent laboratory studies have pointed to the use of estrogen and progesterone as a promising method to reduce secondary injury in hemorrhagic shock and other similar processes. Those studies have shown that the early administration of estrogen (a strong antioxidant, antiinflammatory, and mitochondrial stabilizer as well as an antiapoptotic agent) significantly decreased the severity of injury caused by early, devastating cell death. The use of estrogen and its derivative has now been tested in 60 clinical trials, mostly in the fields of prostate cancer, uremic bleeding, liver transplantation, spine surgery, cardiology, cardiac surgery, and TBI. Its safety record is good. Large-scale randomized clinical trials in TBI have failed to show any efficacy of these compounds.

PERIOPERATIVE FLUID MANAGEMENT

Body Water

Humans are made predominantly of water (50%–70% of body weight). The precise percentage is affected by sex, body fat, and age, with an increase in water percentage in males, in those with increased lean body mass, and extremes of age. The human body can do without many things for long periods, but water is not one of them. In the body, water resides in three compartments or spaces: (1) intracellular, (2) intravascular, and (3) interstitial. The intracellular compartment has the largest volume of water, constituting about 30% to 40% of body weight (two-thirds of the body's total water). The intravascular volume is usually calculated as 5% to 7% of body weight (one-sixth of the body's total water). Water shifts rapidly between the three compartments. Large resources of water can be pulled from the intracellular compartment into the intravascular compartment; large volumes of water can be stored in the interstitial compartment. Water in the interstitial compartment is recirculated by the lymphatics and eventually returns to the intravascular compartment. A fixed amount of water is in bones and dense connective tissue, but this water is relatively stable and not considered to be in circulation. Water is secreted by various cells in the skin and cerebrospinal fluid and in the intraocular, synovial, renal, and GI systems; this water is also not considered to be in circulation.

Clinical tools are available to accurately measure the volume of water in the body. One method is bioimpedance spectroscopy, which measures electrical current impedance that is imperceptible to the person to estimate total body water. The method is best used to calculate body fat.

Methods to measure intravascular volume are also commercially available. They usually involve injecting a known concentration of tagged molecules (such as potassium-40 or albumin) that remain intravascular for a known time period. Potassium is predominantly an intracellular solute, and albumin is predominantly extracellular. Sampling the blood and calculating the volume based on the decreased concentration of the injected tracer is fairly accurate. This method has not caught on for clinical use because the baseline volume is not known; even if it were known, the intravascular volume is contractible and expandable, so the desired intravascular target volume is not yet known. During injuries and illnesses, when homeostasis has not been maintained, normal values may not be applicable or desirable during resuscitation. The practicality of measuring these spaces has not been identified, yet research has shown that a person's extracellular volume can be expanded even if they are dehydrated intracellularly.

The main intracellular electrolytes are potassium and magnesium. Intracellularly, they are the principal cations; phosphates and proteins are the principal anions. Extracellularly, in contrast, sodium is the predominant cation; chloride and bicarbonate are the predominant anions. In plasma (given its higher protein content, which is due to organic anions), the total concentrations of cations are higher, whereas the concentrations of inorganic anions are lower than in the interstitial fluids. The Gibbs-Donnan equilibrium equation states that the product of the concentrations of any pair of diffusible cations and anions on one side of a semipermeable membrane will equal the product of the same pair of ions on the other side. Cell walls are semipermeable membranes; the flow of water is determined by the osmotically active particles (about 290–310 mOsm). The effective osmotic pressure depends on those substances that fail to pass through the pores of the semipermeable membrane.

The dissolved proteins in the plasma are responsible for the effective osmotic pressure between the plasma and the interstitial fluid, frequently referred to as the *colloid osmotic pressure*. Sodium is pumped outside the cell, and potassium is pumped inside the cell. Thus, sodium is the major electrolyte responsible for the osmotic pressure, but glucose and urea (which do not easily penetrate the cell membrane) also increase the effective osmotic pressure. Water passes across the cell membrane freely, so sodium has a highly important impact on the movement of water. However, the concentration of sodium is not necessarily related to the volume status of ECF. A severe extracellular volume deficit can occur with a low or high sodium concentration over time.

The osmotic gradient is also important in controlling water. The number of osmotic particles is the key. The size of the osmotic particle does not matter. For example, transfusion of PRBCs will actually cause water to pass from the intravascular space to the interstitial space. Immediately after transfusion of PRBCs, hydrostatic pressure increases inside the vascular space, and water is pushed out. Although the hematocrit level of PRBCs is 60% to 70%, the red cells act as one osmotic particle. Because of the size difference between red cells and proteins in the blood, fewer osmotic particles are in a given volume of PRBCs compared with whole blood. Therefore, the osmotic pressure intravascularly is actually reduced after transfusion of PRBCs.

The size difference between a red cell and albumin is large (like a soccer ball versus a grain of sand), but each will act as one osmotic particle. The number of soccer balls that can fit into a stadium is limited, but the number of grains of sand that can fit is many orders of magnitude higher. Similarly, with a transfusion of PRBCs, water is pushed out of the intravascular space into either the interstitial or the intercellular space because of the decrease in the number of osmotic particles per volume.

Maintenance Fluids

In surgical patients, assessing the intravascular status is a pivotal task but also one of the most difficult. Surgical patients have blood loss from trauma, operations, and diseases. In addition, volume deficits occur from losses of GI fluids because of vomiting, diarrhea, nasogastric suctioning, fistulas, and drains. Fluid also shifts out of the intravascular space because of burns, inflammation (as in pancreatitis), intestinal obstruction, infection, and sepsis.

Nonetheless, the main daily task of perioperative patient care is assessing the intravascular status. Is it where it needs to be? It is safer for surgeons to assume that a patient is hypovolemic or hypervolemic than normal; the normovolemic band is very small. The maintenance fluid should constantly be adjusted, depending on the individual patient's current status. Surgeons must pay attention to each patient's fluid status and body needs rather than infuse maintenance fluid at a fixed rate.

For the routine preoperative care of patients about to undergo elective surgery, the customary approach is to start a maintenance drip of crystalloids. Note, however, that patients who undergo same-day surgery have little need for preoperative fluids. All preoperative patients are asked not to take in any fluids by mouth starting the night before surgery, a directive that typically does not result in any problems. Remember that all of us (whether or not we are surgical patients) are NPO (Latin for *nil per os* or nothing by mouth) when we go to sleep; we do not normally wake up hypotensive or in renal failure. Thus, for patients about to undergo major surgery requiring inpatient hospitalization after surgery, IV fluids the night before are not necessary; they typically will receive plenty of fluids from the anesthesiologist during the operation.

In patients who underwent a colectomy, a small prospective randomized study showed that minimizing crystalloids during surgery led to a better outcome; such patients had less nausea and vomiting, decreased hospital length of stay, and faster return of GI function. However, starting such patients on a maintenance fluid is safe, mainly to provide water (Box 33.3). In adult patients weighing more than 40 kg, the simple rule for calculating the fluid rate in milliliters per hour is 40 plus the weight in kilograms; that is, a 73-kg patient's maintenance rate would be 113 mL/h (73 + 40).

Maintenance fluids have not been rigorously tested, so the ideal fluid is unknown. The current standard is to use 5% dextrose in half-normal saline with 20 mEq/L of potassium. The source of the standard's formulation remains unclear. For a 70-kg NPO male, it would provide sodium and potassium, yet it is not what the average person requires (Table 33.13). The average 70-kg male's requirements are listed in Table 33.14.

The average salt intake per day in American males has been difficult to assess; the median is an estimated 7.8 to 11.8 g/day. Because that range does not include salt added at the table, it is probably an underestimate. The US Department of Agriculture recommends a salt intake of less than 2.3 g/day. Normal saline contains 9 g of sodium chloride in 1 L of water. The amount of fluids and electrolytes infused into patients with the standard formulation is highly inaccurate. The decision to give 5% dextrose in maintenance fluid is thought to derive from fasting studies of Harvard medical students in the 1920s. Those studies found that providing about 100 g of glucose decreased protein spillage in the urine. The rationale for the use of half-normal saline and 20 mEq/L of potassium is unknown. A survey of critical care intensivists showed that most did not know the daily recommended intake of sodium or potassium.

Surgeons fear that an insufficient volume of fluid will lead to renal failure. Oliguria in a 70-kg male is defined by less than 400 mL of urine produced and excreted in a 24-hour period. That is the minimum volume required to maintain normal serum blood urea nitrogen (BUN) and creatinine levels so that the kidney is able to function maximally. That volume equates to 0.24 mL/kg/h. Historically, surgical residents were mandated to give patients enough IV maintenance fluid to produce 0.5 mL/kg/h, probably

TABLE 33.13   Contents of Maintenance Solution[a]

	TOTAL IN 24 HOURS
Water	2760 mL
Dextrose	132 g
Sodium	11.8 g (203 mEq)
Potassium	1.9 g (53 mEq)

[a]With 5% dextrose in half-normal saline with 40 mEq/L of potassium in a 70-kg patient for 24 hours.

TABLE 33.14   Normal Needs for a 70-kg Male Per Day

	TOTAL IN 24 HOURS
Water	2000 mL
Urine	1500 mL
Sodium	2–4 g
Potassium	100 mEq

to build in a safety margin to ensure enough volume. Today, it is not uncommon to see residents give patients a 1-L fluid bolus of crystalloids for urine output of less than 0.5 mL/kg/h, a practice that will usually lead to overhydration. The kidneys are marvelous at protecting the body from physicians who have not studied physiology. In general, overhydration has not been typically seen as a problem, and hypervolemia has been seen as harmless; however, that view is inaccurate because it can lead to issues such as pulmonary edema and intraabdominal hypertension.

Postoperatively, patients are more often hypervolemic initially as a result of higher-than-necessary IV fluid infusions. Because of bleeding from surgery and the need for IV infusion, patients often receive too much blood and fluid during surgery due to fears of hypotension. Giving a few liters of blood and fluid is probably inconsequential. For patients who have lost liters of blood, however, accurate measurement is impossible; inferences have to be made as to what the volume status is. Patients who have lost a minimal amount of blood during elective surgery, who have received liters of crystalloids, and who have adequate urine output do not necessarily need IV maintenance fluids. For typical patients on the surgical ward, normal functioning kidneys will generally make up for any errors in the amount of blood and fluid given. However, for ICU patients on a ventilator who have severe traumatic injuries, sepsis, other comorbid conditions, or blood loss, there is less room for error.

For ICU patients, maintaining an isovolemic state can be critical to good outcomes. Pulmonary failure has an associated mortality rate of 20% to 25%, whereas renal failure has an associated mortality rate of 48%. Surgical patients are often intravascularly depleted, despite being total body fluid overloaded. This is due to the combination of the inflammatory response of surgery and crystalloid resuscitation that leads to increased permeability of the vasculature, also known as *endotheliopathy*, and increasing fluid in the interstitial space. The total daily water input in such patients may be elevated, but determining the intravascular volume is vital to predict volume status over time as the water shifts from the interstitial space to the intravascular space.

Especially for ICU patients, the same maintenance rate over days can be a problem. Again, determining their fluid status is

BOX 33.3   Maintenance Fluid Calculation

Maintenance Intravenous Fluid Calculation
- 4 mL/kg/h for first 10 kg
- 2 mL/kg/h for next 10 kg
- 1 mL/kg/h for every kilogram over 20 kg

Sample Calculation for 45-kg Patient
- 10 kg × 4 mL/kg/h = 40 mL/h
- 10 kg × 2 mL/kg/h = 20 mL/h
- 25 kg × 1 mL/kg/h = 25 mL/h
- Maintenance rate = 85 mL/h

Sample Calculation for 73-kg Patient
- 10 kg × 4 mL/kg/h = 40 mL/h
- 10 kg × 2 mL/kg/h = 20 mL/h
- 53 kg × 1 mL/kg/h = 53 mL/h
- Maintenance rate = 113 mL/h

difficult. Surgeons need to gather as much information as possible to estimate what the IV maintenance rate should be. Knowing the ratio of BUN to creatinine is helpful. A ratio higher than 20 is generally thought to be prerenal; a ratio lower than 10 suggests a volume-replete state. Such generalizations are true only for patients with normal renal function. Urine output is an excellent way to determine volume states. High output generally mean that the body is trying to rid itself of water; surgeons should assist it by decreasing the maintenance fluid rate. Anasarca is another helpful clue, as are the customary vital signs.

In older patients with heart failure or sepsis who are intravascularly hypovolemic, anasarca can be profound. Many such patients will need more IV fluids despite having anasarca. To help estimate vascular volume, central venous pressure and other volume measurement adjuncts can be helpful. However, caution should be taken in interpreting heart rate. Heart rate is affected by many known and unknown variables, including pain, anxiety, hormone levels, and temperature.

For patients with arterial blood gases, the ratio of PaO_2 to FiO_2 (P/F) is extremely helpful. The P/F ratio is the arterial oxygen concentration divided by the inspired percentage of oxygen. In a healthy young patient without heart disease, the arterial oxygen content is about 100; because room air is 21% oxygen, the P/F ratio is about 500 (100/0.21). If that same patient is placed on 100% oxygen, arterial oxygen content would be 500 with a P/F ratio of 500. In a healthy patient who does not have pneumonia, sepsis, or pulmonary contusion, the P/F ratio can reflect interstitial or lung water status; it will help direct fluid management.

Low urine output postoperatively means that there is deceased renal blood flow from insufficient effective intravascular volume. When blood flow to the kidneys is decreased, the kidneys sense inadequate intravascular volume; therefore, the renin-angiotensin system, ADH, atrial natriuretic peptide, carotid baroreceptors, and other mechanisms function in an effort to preserve water. This hormonal milieu can also occur after trauma or surgery, creating low urine output despite adequate intravascular volume. If furosemide is injected in a hypovolemic oliguric patient as a bolus, it prevents the distal Henle loop from reabsorbing water, thus increasing urine output. Increased urine output in patients with an intravascular volume deficit can be harmful. The costs of monitoring and replacing electrolytes can be significant. Normal saline is problematic because of the chloride load, and balanced fluids like Plasma-Lyte reduce the need for frequent replacement of electrolytes such as calcium, potassium, and magnesium. None of the crystalloids is truly balanced, and they all have some advantages and disadvantages. These solutions can also be problematic when the patient is in renal failure. High doses of magnesium are also a potential issue in certain circumstances. Because surgical patients often require blood transfusions, purists will urge the use of crystalloids as carriers without calcium because there is fear that calcium will cause blood to clot in the IV lines. Whole blood or PRBCs mixed with an equal volume of LR solution have not increased clot formation in vitro compared with saline reconstitution. These are tools in the armamentarium, and there are times for all of them. For daily maintenance needs of a few liters a day in a patient without renal failure, Plasma-Lyte or Normosol may be better than LR or saline solutions.

Adrenal Gland

The adrenal medulla affects intravascular volume during shock by secreting catechol hormones. They are called catecholamines because they contain a catechol group derived from the amino acid tyrosine. The most abundant catecholamines are epinephrine, norepinephrine, and dopamine, all of which are produced from phenylalanine and tyrosine. Cortisol is also released from the adrenal cortex and plays a major role in controlling fluid equilibrium. From the adrenal cortex and the zona glomerulosa, aldosterone is produced in response to stimulation by angiotensin II and hyperkalemia. Aldosterone is a mineralocorticoid that modulates renal function by increasing recovery of sodium and excretion of potassium.

Many other organs are involved in the control of hormones, including the hypothalamic-pituitary interface, which leads to the release of adrenocorticotropic hormone from the anterior pituitary gland. This system is affected by a variety of circumstances, including intravascular pressure, intravascular volume, and electrolytes such as sodium. The juxtaglomerular apparatus of the kidney produces the enzyme renin, which generates angiotensin I. Angiotensin I is converted to angiotensin II by the angiotensin-converting enzyme located on the endothelial cells of the pulmonary arteries. This regulation of intravascular fluid status is further affected by the carotid baroreceptors and the atrial natriuretic peptides. To infuse any of these hormones or block them leads to compensatory mechanisms and perturbations within this complicated system.

The system is also affected by many other factors that we have recently discovered—and is likely affected by others that have yet to elucidated. For example, TBI has been shown to affect the hypothalamic-pituitary interface directly by mechanical trauma or by elevated ICP. For such patients, treatment becomes difficult to control because they go through a wide range of physiologic responses. Patients undergoing brain herniation will go from a bradycardic hypertensive state to a profoundly tachycardic and hypotensive state. This produces a rapidly changing state where urine output is also affected, and diabetes insipidus (DI) or syndrome of inappropriate ADH (SIADH) can occur. Most likely, the human body has teleologically evolved to try to reduce brain edema at all costs; high-volume urine output often results, requiring vasopressin infusions. Patients whose regulatory system is malfunctioning or whose adrenal glands have been exhausted also have a need for high-dose pressors. However, studies have shown that the infusion of cortisol and thyroid hormone in drip form can decrease such instability and minimize the need for fluid infusion and pressors. Patients undergoing brain herniation illustrate how complex the regulatory system is; surgeons must be cognizant of the minute-to-minute changes that can occur.

Adrenal glucocorticoid insufficiency, but not complete failure, occurs in patients with impaired function of the hypothalamic-pituitary-adrenal axis. Such patients produce limited amounts of corticosteroids. Clinical problems develop when patients are stressed by hypovolemia from hemorrhage, onset of an infection, fear, or hypothermia. In evaluating patients during a surgical emergency, chronic adrenal insufficiency may be initially diagnosed after intractable hypotension is found. Pathologic causes of chronic adrenal insufficiency include autoimmune destruction of the adrenal gland, in which cytotoxic lymphocytes gradually destroy cortisol-synthesizing cells in the adrenal cortex. Patients can also develop adrenalitis, where symptoms of fatigue, inanition, weight loss, and postural dizziness occur gradually. Their chief complaint may be vague cramping abdominal pain, nausea, and a change in bowel habits. Laboratory findings suggesting adrenal insufficiency are hyperkalemia, acidemia, hyponatremia, and elevated serum creatinine levels resulting from a deficiency in aldosterone. The diagnosis of adrenal insufficiency secondary to end-organ failure is established by disproportionately elevated adrenocorticotropic hormone levels (compared with cortisol levels).

Clinical findings in patients with sudden acute adrenal insufficiency can be nonspecific. If plasma cortisol levels precipitously decline to nil, patients will have abdominal pain syndrome, vomiting, and a tender abdomen and then will progress to prostration, coma, and hypotension unresponsive to catecholamine infusion. Signs and symptoms of a gradual reduction in cortisol function include malaise, fatigue, and hyponatremia with hyperkalemia. Patients with a complete loss of circulating glucocorticoids can die within hours after irreversible hypotension.

In critically ill patients, quickly establishing the diagnosis of adrenal insufficiency is difficult. Laboratory tests can confirm that plasma levels of the hormones are depressed, but test results take hours to obtain. Pending the laboratory test results, surgeons treat such patients empirically with hormone replacement therapy. Treatment of glucocorticoid deficiency in adults consists of an IV infusion of dexamethasone, methylprednisolone, or hydrocortisone. Using dexamethasone is preferred if sending simultaneous laboratory tests to confirm the diagnosis of acute hypercortisolism because this medication does not interfere with the cosyntropin test. Once test results have returned, the exogenous steroids can be rapidly tapered during the subsequent days as the patient's condition stabilizes.

Methylprednisolone has an antiinflammatory milligram-per-milligram potency of 5; dexamethasone has a potency of 25 (relative to 1.0 for hydrocortisone). Patients whose adrenal glands are nonfunctional may also require replacement of mineralocorticoids. Patients with primary adrenal failure should be treated with 50 to 200 μg/day of fludrocortisone for mineralocorticoid replacement.

Antidiuretic Hormone and Water

ADH causes water to be reabsorbed and thus reduces urine output. Synthesized in the hypothalamic region, ADH is stored in the pituitary from where it is released into the circulation. Excess production or release of ADH causes overhydration; water is retained, and thus sodium levels are lowered. Because serum osmolality is predominantly related to sodium, it will be lower than normal (285 mmol/kg) with excess ADH.

One example of overhydration is SIADH. Despite being overhydrated due to excess ADH production, the kidneys are signaled to retain water. Therefore, urine osmolality will be high (>300 mmol/kg) even though serum osmolality is low.

Yet if ADH is not synthesized or released, such as in patients with TBI, urine output will increase pathologically; urine osmolality will be as low as 100 mmol/kg. The resulting dehydration will lead to elevated serum sodium levels. In patients with TBI, the development of DI is associated with significant brain injury and poor prognosis. In patients with DI or SIADH, close attention needs to be paid to maintain isovolemia. Treatment of patients with DI should include desmopressin (1-desamino-8-D-arginine vasopressin, or DDAVP); treatment of patients with SIADH should include water restriction.

ELECTROLYTES

Sodium

Sodium is vital for homeostasis and the action potential in the body. It is the predominant molecule that controls water movement in and out of the vascular system. The normal range of serum sodium concentration is 135 to 145 mEq/L. Hyponatremia and hypernatremia, heavily controlled by ADH, are common problems in surgical patients. In general, mild forms of hyponatremia and hypernatremia are not a problem, but hyponatremia is more concerning than hypernatremia. Of the many signs and symptoms associated with each, none of them is specific; none of the signs or symptoms alone would lead a clinician to diagnose a sodium abnormality. A blood test is always required.

Hyponatremia

Hyponatremia can be mild (130–138 mEq/L), moderate (120–130 mEq/L), or severe (<120 mEq/L). Both mild hyponatremia and moderate hyponatremia are common but only rarely symptomatic. Severe hyponatremia, however, can cause headaches and lethargy; patients can even become comatose or have seizures. Typically, acute hyponatremia is symptomatic, whereas chronic severe hyponatremia can often be asymptomatic. Hyponatremia is a problem when cells swell as a result of the body's decreased ability to maintain homeostatic osmolality. The most common reason for hyponatremia is iatrogenic, with excess water given via IV fluids, but it can also be commonly caused by pathologic processes in the brain or lungs resulting in hormonal imbalances.

Assessing the cause of hyponatremia is important because patients are usually classified on the basis of their volume status. Patients with hyponatremia are usually hypotonic; on occasion, they may be hypertonic, with high serum glucose or mannitol levels. In severe hyperglycemia, osmolality of the ECF rises and exceeds that of the intracellular fluid. Glucose penetrates cell membranes slowly when insulin is absent, so hyperglycemia draws water out of the cells and into the ECF. Serum sodium concentrations fall in proportion to the dilution caused by hyperglycemia. The measured sodium level is lowered by 1.6 mEq/L for every 100 mg/dL of glucose above 100. That phenomenon is referred to as *transitional hyponatremia* because no net change in body water occurs. No specific therapy is required other than treating the hyperglycemia; artificially lowered sodium concentrations will return to normal once the plasma glucose level is normalized. The most common formulas for sodium are shown in Box 33.4.

The patient's fluid volume status is critical in assessing hyponatremia. In general, hyponatremia is thought of as either renal or extrarenal. Impaired excretion of sodium by the kidneys is due to

---

BOX 33.4 Sodium Equations for Clinical Use

Sodium Deficit
Sodium deficit (mEq) = ([Na] goal − [Na] plasma) × TBW
TBW = (Weight × 60%)

Free Water Deficit
Free water deficit = (([Na]/140) − 1) × TBW

Corrected Sodium
Corrected sodium = [Na] + 0.016 × (Glucose − 100)

Serum Osmolality (Calculated)
2 × [Na] + BUN/2.8 + Glucose/18

Fractional Excretion of Sodium
FeNa = [Na] urine + Creatinine plasma /[Na] plasma + Creatinine urine
<1% = ?Prerenal (hypovolemia)
>2% = Intrinsic renal disorder

BUN, Blood urea nitrogen; *TBW,* total body weight.

renal failure, problems with ADH, or diuretics. Extrarenal causes include sodium loss due to wounds, burns, sweating, congestive heart failure, cirrhosis, hypothyroidism, GI losses, and cerebral salt-wasting syndrome. Acute hyponatremia can also occur if dehydrated patients are infused with fluids free of sodium. In patients who have bled or who are intravascularly depleted (e.g., because of vomiting, diarrhea, pancreatitis, or burns), IV infusion of 5% dextrose in water can rapidly cause hyponatremia. Because the normal response to hyponatremia is the suppression of ADH release in the pituitary, leading to the secretion of water to increase the sodium concentration in the serum, the problem is exacerbated in hypovolemic patients because the hypothalamus is secreting ADH in an effort to preserve water. Thus, hyponatremic patients should have undetectable levels of ADH. However, ADH release can be stimulated both by elevated ECF osmolality and by reduced ECF volume. ADH secretion commonly occurs transiently after trauma or burns and even in the early postoperative period, causing euvolemic hyponatremia. In hypovolemic patients, baroreceptors also stimulate the hypothalamus to retain water through ADH release because the homeostatic mechanism for maintaining intravascular volume is stronger than that for maintaining proper sodium concentration.

Diuresis with furosemide or mannitol, in addition to causing intravascular fluid loss, can cause hyponatremia. It also increases sodium loss by the kidneys and increases ADH release as the body tries to counteract the rapid fluid loss by preserving water. Hyperglycemia, if it is high enough to cause glucosuria, will also induce an osmotic diuresis that depletes extracellular water and also leads to hyponatremia. Along with diuresis, hyperglycemia can lead to a variety of electrolyte imbalances (many regulatory mechanisms are involved) and can cause significant hormonal swings and imbalances.

Renal loss of sodium can lead to hyponatremia and excessive release of natriuretic peptides related to brain injury or disease. One particularly difficult condition to treat is cerebral salt-wasting syndrome. Even when such patients are treated with salt, the regulatory mechanisms cause high urine output (up to 4–6 L/day) with consequent urine sodium losses. Those losses correlate with elevated brain natriuretic peptide levels in plasma. The lost sodium must be replaced either through an IV line or by enteral intake.

In patients with a brain injury, hyponatremia that is normally well tolerated may be devastating; it is thought to cause cerebral intracellular swelling as osmolality is reduced. In such patients, infusion of HTS may be required. Depending on the electrolyte imbalances, salt infusions can take a variety of forms; sodium can be provided as sodium chloride, sodium acetate, or sodium bicarbonate or in combinations. If urologic or gynecologic surgery is performed with hypoosmotic irrigation, acute hyponatremia can occur. During endometrial resection and in transurethral resection of the prostate, acute water intoxication has been reported as a complication.

In surgical ICU patients, a frequent cause of hyponatremia is SIADH. This syndrome can be acute or chronic. In hypovolemic patients, the body's natural response is to release ADH; however, if the body is euvolemic and yet releases ADH inappropriately, the diagnosis of SIADH can be made. Therefore, the diagnosis of SIADH should be made only in euvolemic patients. In addition, the urine osmolarity is usually above 150 mmol/kg, and the urine sodium is above 20 mmol/L. Given the aberrant release of ADH, the serum osmolality is often less than 270 mmol, and yet the kidneys still excrete concentrated urine. It is usually managed with fluid restrictions. Furthermore, it is important to differentiate SIADH from adrenal insufficiency, in which hypokalemia also occurs.

A hyponatremic patient with a urine osmolality of 350 mmol is producing ADH, and the kidneys are concentrating it; the source of hyponatremia is usually extrarenal. ADH-secreting tumors (such as carcinoid tumors or small cell carcinomas of the lung) can cause chronic SIADH. These lung tumors usually cause euvolemic hyponatremia. Up to 35% of patients with active acquired immunodeficiency syndrome (AIDS) who are admitted for hospitalization have SIADH. Hyponatremia can also be caused by renal dysfunction in patients with conditions that impair the capability to retain sodium, such as medullary cystic disease, polycystic kidney disease, analgesic nephropathy, chronic pyelonephritis, and obstructive uropathy after decompression syndrome.

Hypernatremia

Hypernatremia is usually defined as serum sodium concentration above 145 mEq/L. Moderate hypernatremia (146–159 mEq/L) is fairly well tolerated, whereas severe hypernatremia (>160 mEq/L) can be detrimental. Hypernatremia is associated with muscle weakness, restlessness, lethargy, insomnia, and in severe cases, central pontine myelinolysis or coma. The common causes of hypernatremia include endocrine syndromes (in which ADH synthesis or release fails), failure of renal tubular cells to respond to ADH, increased salt intake or infusion, and loss of water. Hypernatremia can be a problem because osmosis will cause cellular dehydration; the primary concern is that it is thought to contract the cerebral cells. However, recent experience with HTS has shown that acutely elevated sodium levels are relatively safe. HTS is used to contract cerebral intracellular volume in patients with TBI to reduce the total brain volume when intracranial swelling or mass effect is a factor. The normal response to hypernatremia is for the kidneys to generate hyperosmolar urine and retain water. Renal correction of hypernatremia depends on the patient having access to water.

Hypernatremia is associated with hypertonicity and should be classified in the context of hypovolemia, euvolemia, or hypervolemia. Hypovolemic hypernatremia commonly occurs in dehydrated patients with low water intake and high fluid losses, such as through vomiting, nasogastric tube loss, or diarrhea. Euvolemic hypernatremia is seen in patients with DI (nephrogenic or neurogenic) because of excess loss of urinary free water. Hypervolemic hypernatremia is usually iatrogenic, caused by resuscitation with hypertonic solutions, or a result of excess mineralocorticoids in Conn or Cushing syndrome.

Hypernatremia (like hyponatremia) is thought of as either renal or extrarenal. Renal fluid losses are due to diuretics, the polyuric phase of acute tubular necrosis, or postobstructive diuresis of the kidney. After decompression of a chronically obstructed ureter, renal tubular cells seem to respond less to ADH. *Nephrogenic DI* is defined as an impaired capacity of the renal tubules to respond to ADH and to concentrate urine. Moderate hypernatremia develops in patients with nephrogenic DI when they lose water in dilute urine, despite elevated plasma levels of ADH. If an infusion of ADH does not increase urine osmolality, nephrogenic DI is the likely diagnosis. Drugs such as lithium, glyburide, demeclocycline, and amphotericin B can induce DI. The treatment for patients with lithium-induced nephrogenic DI is amiloride (5–10 mg daily).

Hypercalcemia or severe hypokalemia also impairs the capacity of renal tubular cells to absorb sodium. Patients with end-stage renal dysfunction and low glomerular filtration rates may produce a fixed volume of 2 to 4 L/day of isosmotic urine. In hot and arid environments, such patients are particularly susceptible to dehydration and hypernatremia.

The extrarenal causes of hypernatremia include loss of water from vomiting, diarrhea, nasogastric tube suctioning, burns, sweating, fever, or problems with insufficient ADH levels. Infusion of sodium (like HTS) can also cause hypernatremia; the duration depends on the volume of crystalloids infused for resuscitation during 24 hours. A study on the use of 5% HTS in trauma patients showed that sodium levels rose above 150 mEq/L and stayed elevated for days. In contrast, previous studies on the use of 7.5% HTS infusions found that the hypernatremia was brief. The transient hypernatremia was probably caused by aggressive use of other crystalloids for resuscitation after the HTS infusion, which quickly diluted the hypernatremia.

In dealing with hypernatremia, it is again important to first assess volume status. In hypovolemic patients, offsetting the volume deficit with isotonic fluids is sufficient. However, nonhypovolemic patients need free water replacement with hypotonic solutions. In hypervolemic patients, diuretics may be used—carefully. In general, in asymptomatic patients, sodium levels should not be corrected too rapidly; doing so could cause cerebral edema. In patients with acute hypernatremia, the rate is usually no more than 1 to 2 mEq/h; with chronic hypernatremia, the rate is no more than 0.5 mEq/h. Sodium levels should not be corrected at a rate of more than 8 mEq/day. Careful and frequent sodium monitoring is often required.

Patients with DI are producing dilute urine at rates of hundreds of milliliters per hour. They should be treated with desmopressin (DDAVP), a synthetic analogue of ADH that has a half-life of several hours. DDAVP increases water movement out of the collecting duct, but it does not have the vasoconstrictive properties of ADH. Patients with mild DI can be treated with intranasal DDAVP and water intake. DDAVP can be administered orally, intranasally, subcutaneously, or intravenously. The intranasal dose is 10 μg once or twice daily. In ICU patients, IV administration is preferred for control and accuracy.

Potassium

Potassium is the main intracellular ion; sodium is the main extracellular ion. The normal potassium concentration in serum is 4.5 mmol/L. Small changes in serum reflect large intracellular changes that may cause significant morbidity and mortality. The daily average intake of potassium is 50 to 100 mmol/day. The kidneys control the daily excretion, which ranges widely from 20 to 400 mmol. The renin-angiotensin-aldosterone hormone axis is the key regulator of potassium clearance. As aldosterone increases in plasma, so does potassium excretion.

Hypokalemia

Patients with hypokalemia have a [K$^+$] lower than 3.5 mmol/L. Hypokalemia is commonly a result of hyperpolarization of the resting potential of the cell. Hyperpolarization interferes with neuromuscular function. Hypokalemia is associated with generalized fatigue and weakness, ileus, atrial arrhythmia, and acute renal insufficiency. On occasion, rhabdomyolysis occurs in patients whose [K$^+$] drops below 2.5 mmol/L. Flaccid paralysis with respiratory compromise can occur as [K$^+$] decreases to less than 2 mmol/L.

Hypokalemia is caused by renal losses, extrarenal losses, intracellular shifts from medications, or hyperthyroidism. Extrarenal losses can be caused by persistent vomiting, gastric tubes, diarrhea, alkalosis, catecholamine secretion, insulin administration, or high-output enteric or pancreatic fistulas. Hypokalemia is a common problem in patients with congestive heart failure who are receiving multiple drugs. It can also develop in patients treated with diuretics that force renal function to excrete urine with an elevated potassium concentration. Long-term diuretic therapy can produce a sustained negative potassium balance. Patients with a chronic potassium deficiency can develop a cardiac rhythm disturbance. The electrocardiogram of patients with hypokalemia will show depressed T waves and development of U waves. Hypokalemia leads to cardiac arrhythmia, particularly atrial tachycardia with or without block, atrioventricular dissociation, ventricular tachycardia, and ventricular fibrillation. The risk for hypokalemia-associated arrhythmia is higher in patients treated with digoxin, even when potassium concentrations are in the low-normal range. Hypokalemia not caused by diuretics may be due to a rare endocrine disorder, including primary hyperaldosteronism and renin-secreting tumors. Hypokalemia is also frequently associated with hypomagnesemia and acidemia.

Hypokalemic patients require potassium replacement, which can be achieved by oral or IV routes. Oral supplementation is generally 40 to 100 mEq/day, in two to four doses. The IV rate is 10 to 20 mEq/h; if potassium is infused at rates of more than 10 mEq/h, cardiac monitoring is required. In emergency situations, the rate can be as high as 40 mEq/h, but it should be infused through a central vein; high concentrations of potassium in IV fluids can be irritating to peripheral veins. Notably, for every 10 mEq of IV potassium, there is typically a diluent of 100 mL of fluid; thus, when repleting potassium in the setting of intentional forced diuresis for hypervolemia, oral repletion is preferred if possible to avoid conflicting volume status goals. In patients with renal dysfunction, whose potassium excretion is reduced, both the IV rate of potassium replacement and the total dose should be lower.

After treatment, frequent monitoring of potassium levels is necessary. Because hypokalemia represents large intracellular deficits, replenishing total body levels may take days. Potassium therapy is given as the chloride salt because hypokalemia is commonly associated with a contraction in the extracellular water, in which chloride is the predominant anion. Potassium in foods is linked to phosphate. Potassium phosphate salts may need to be given by the IV route, particularly when expansion of intracellular water is anticipated. To reduce the risk of serious cardiac arrhythmia with cardiac disease or after cardiac surgery in patients who have a serum value below 3.5 mmol/L, serum [K$^+$] should be promptly corrected to a level higher than 4.0 mmol/L. Patients with substantial and continuing GI loss of potassium require extraordinary potassium replacement to achieve correction of hypokalemia.

Magnesium levels should be concomitantly monitored; hypomagnesemia can produce refractory hypokalemia. Magnesium is an important cofactor for potassium uptake and for maintenance of intracellular potassium levels, and magnesium levels must be replete before repletion of potassium. In addition, supplemental magnesium reduces the risk of arrhythmia.

Hypokalemic patients with concurrent acidemia are treated with potassium replacement before their pH is corrected by bicarbonate administration. Diabetic patients with ketoacidosis may initially have normal [K$^+$], but hypokalemia rapidly develops as insulin is administered and as glucose shifts into cells; for such patients, potassium supplements should be added to the resuscitation fluid once the physician is confident that renal function is adequate. If hypokalemia develops while patients are undergoing diuretic therapy, additional drugs can reduce the renal loss of potassium. For example, triamterene or spironolactone blocks the effect of aldosterone and reduces potassium loss in urine.

Hyperkalemia

Hyperkalemia is defined as $[K^+]$ of more than 5.0 mmol/L. If levels exceed 6 mmol/L, perturbations in the resting cell membrane potential occur, and normal depolarization and repolarization are impaired. The most common cause of hyperkalemia is renal failure in hospitalized patients. The transport of potassium is passive, but the transport of sodium requires energy. This difference across the cell is maintained by Na^+, K^+-adenosine triphosphatase (ATPase) activity, which requires energy. This energy is supplied in the form of cellular ATP. Its levels are highly variable in different stages of shock when nutrients are not available (whether carbohydrates or oxygen). When cellular ATP levels fall, the sodium pump is impaired. If either sodium or potassium levels are severely high or low, the membrane potential will be affected. Eventually, without energy, cell death occurs, and the sodium-potassium gradient cannot be maintained; the sodium gradient is needed to maintain the membrane potential.

The primary clinical problem with hyperkalemia is cardiac arrhythmia, which can be lethal. Hyperkalemia is associated with peaked T waves; dangerous hyperkalemia (6–7 mmol/L) is indicated by T waves higher than R waves (Fig. 33.21).

The most common cause of hyperkalemia is acute onset of renal dysfunction or failure. Cellular injury (such as sepsis or ischemia-reperfusion) can also release potassium from its intracellular source, which can overwhelm the kidneys' ability to clear potassium. At least 20% of normal renal function is required to respond to aldosterone and maintain normal potassium levels. The reperfusion of ischemic tissues resulting in rhabdomyolysis causes high potassium levels; to prevent cardiac arrest, a bolus of IV sodium bicarbonate may be of some benefit. The bicarbonate shifts potassium intracellularly.

Drugs can have a direct effect on the renal tubules and on potassium excretion; examples include triamterene, spironolactone, β-blockers, cyclosporine, and tacrolimus. They are usually a contributing factor but not a primary cause. Succinylcholine, a depolarizing paralytic agent, is used in patients with muscle atrophy from disuse, prolonged bed rest, neurologic denervation syndromes, severe burns, direct muscle trauma, or rhabdomyolysis; it can cause severe hyperkalemia, resulting in cardiac arrest. When drawing blood samples from patients, clinicians must recognize that sample hemolysis can release potassium, so laboratory test results could be spurious. If the sample or test results are

suspect, another sample should be taken before drastic efforts are made to treat hyperkalemia.

In addition, ischemia-reperfusion injury is associated with hyperkalemia. Revascularization after an ischemic injury may cause severe hyperkalemia based on duration of the ischemic episode, ranging from 4 to 6 hours. As a result, it is usually recommended to administer bicarbonate before reperfusion.

In patients at risk for development of cardiac arrhythmia from hyperkalemia, several interventions are useful. Calcium administered via IV can immediately reduce the risk of arrhythmia, and this should be the first therapy administered; it antagonizes the depolarization effect of elevated $[K^+]$. Sodium bicarbonate infusion buffers extracellular protons and allows net transfer of cytosolic protons across the cell membrane through carbonic acid. The shift of protons out of the cell is associated with a shift of potassium into the cells. Bicarbonate therapy is most effective in hyperkalemic patients with metabolic acidemia. Insulin and glucose infusions prompt an increase in Na^+, K^+-ATPase activity and a decline in extracellular water potassium concentration as the extracellular water potassium is driven into the cell.

In patients with both aldosterone deficiency and hyperkalemia, a mineralocorticoid drug such as 9α-fludrocortisone will increase renal excretion of potassium. In patients with acute renal failure, hemodialysis is the most reliable method to control hyperkalemia. Continuous filtration methods clear potassium at a slower rate than hemodialysis does. Chronic hyperkalemia associated with renal dysfunction can be managed by oral or rectal administration of sodium polystyrene sulfonate, a cation exchange resin that binds potassium in the gut lumen. Rectally administered binding resins are particularly effective because the colonic mucosa can excrete mucus with large amounts of potassium. Surgeons should clearly establish a process for managing hyperkalemia because rapidly escalating potassium levels pose an immediate threat and require prompt therapy (Box 33.5). Dysfunctional renal handling of potassium from mineralocorticoid deficiency or

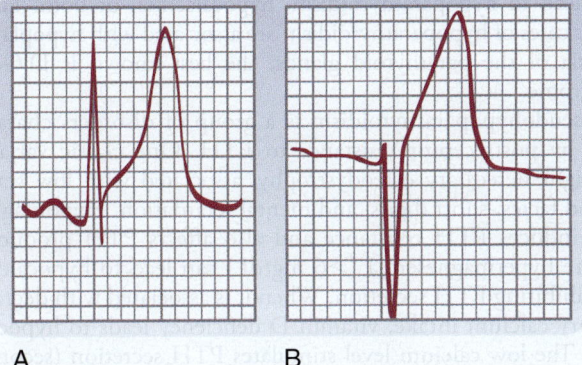

FIGURE 33.21 Electrocardiographic changes. (A) Indicating hyperkalemia. The T wave is tall, narrow, and symmetric. (B) Indicating acute myocardial infarction. The T wave is tall but broad based and asymmetric. (From Somers MP, Brady WJ, Perron AD, et al. The prominent T wave: electrocardiographic differential diagnosis. *Am J Emerg Med.* 2002;20:243-251.)

BOX 33.5 Guidelines for Treatment of Adult Patients With Hyperkalemia

First: Stop all infusion of potassium.

Electrocardiographic Evidence of Pending Arrest

Loss of P wave and broad slurring of QRS; immediate effective therapy indicated
1. Intravenous (IV) infusion of calcium salts
   10 mL of 10% calcium chloride during a 10-minute period *or* 10 mL of 10% calcium gluconate during a 3- to 5-minute period
2. IV infusion of sodium bicarbonate
   50–100 mEq during a 10- to 20-minute period; benefit proportional to extent of pretherapy acidemia

Electrocardiographic Evidence of Potassium Effect

Peaked T waves; prompt therapy needed
1. Glucose and insulin infusion
   IV infusion of 50 mL of $D_{50}W$ and 10 units of regular insulin; monitor glucose
2. Immediate hemodialysis

Biochemical Evidence of Hyperkalemia and No Electrocardiographic Changes

Effective therapy needed within hours
1. Potassium-binding resins into the gastrointestinal tract with 20% sorbitol
2. Promotion of renal kaliuresis by loop diuretic

resistance leads to hyperkalemia. Renal failure is commonly associated with tubular defects and potassium management problems, along with hyperaldosteronism. However, in patients with normal renal function, assessing levels of aldosterone, renin, and cortisol can help differentiate between mineralocorticoid deficiency and resistance. In patients with aldosterone deficiency, fludrocortisone is useful.

Calcium

Calcium, a divalent cation, is a critical component of many extracellular and intracellular reactions. It is the most abundant electrolyte in the body overall. About 99% of it is found in the bones; the remaining 1% circulates in the blood. For surgeons, it is of particular interest; it is an essential cofactor in the coagulation cascade, and intracellular ionized calcium (iCa^{2+}) participates in the regulation of neuronal, hormonal, muscular, and renal cellular function. Total serum calcium concentration (normally, 8.5–10.5 mg/dL) is present in three molecular forms: protein-bound calcium, diffusible calcium bound to anions (bicarbonate, phosphate, and acetate), and freely diffusible calcium as iCa^{2+}.

The biochemically active species is iCa^{2+}, which constitutes about 45% of total serum calcium. More than 80% of protein-bound calcium is attached to albumin, so the total calcium concentration in serum will decrease in patients with hypoalbuminemia. Physiologically, the total plasma calcium level must be corrected relative to the albumin level. Normal calcium levels may range from 8.5 to 10.5 mg/day, assuming an albumin level of 4.5 g/dL. The calcium concentration [Ca] usually changes by 0.8 mg/dL for every change of 1.0 g/dL in plasma albumin concentration. This formula estimates the actual total plasma calcium level:

$$iCa^{2+}_{Corrected} = Total\ [Ca] + (0.8 \times [4 - serum\ albumin\ level])$$

Acidosis decreases the amount of calcium bound to albumin, whereas alkalosis increases the bound fraction of calcium. A small amount of calcium (about 6%) is bound to anions such as citrate and sulfate. The remainder is iCa^{2+} that is biologically active.

The increase in iCa^{2+} is controlled by cell membrane enzymes that transport calcium out of the cell. In muscle cells, iCa^{2+} is stored in the sarcoplasmic reticulum. It can be quickly released into intracellular fluid, in which it has a key role in the molecular events that cause muscle contraction. Tight control of iCa^{2+} in ECF is essential. The serum calcium concentration is controlled by the interaction of parathyroid hormone (PTH), calcitonin, and vitamin D. PTH and calcitonin are hormones subject to regulatory release by endocrine cells, whereas vitamin D is either consumed in the diet or formed in the skin as cholecalciferol in response to ultraviolet irradiation. Bone contains an enormous reservoir of calcium in the form of a matrix of calcium and other molecules. Turnover of calcium salts in bone is constant and integral to maintaining a stable iCa^{2+} in ECF. Receptors in the membranes of parathyroid cells release PTH when iCa^{2+} in ECF declines. PTH activates osteoclasts in bones, which release calcium from the structural matrix of bone. PTH stimulates tubule cells in the proximal nephron both to absorb calcium from the filtrate and to excrete phosphates. PTH with vitamin D enhances calcium absorption from the lumen of the gut.

Calcitonin has the opposite effects on calcium metabolism (compared with PTH). As calcitonin levels in the ECF increase because of its excretion from type C cells of the thyroid, iCa^{2+} declines, and more calcium becomes bound to the bone matrix. Vitamin D

circulating in blood is converted in the liver to 25-hydroxycholecalciferol. Then, 25-hydroxycholecalciferol circulating in blood encounters kidney cells that further hydroxylate the sterol to 1,25-dihydroxycholecalciferol, which is the most potent calcium-modulating hormone. Next, 1,25-dihydroxycholecalciferol increases the transport of calcium and phosphate from the lumen of the bowel into the ECF of the intestine. Furthermore, in conjunction with PTH, 1,25-dihydroxycholecalciferol increases bone resorption, increasing the calcium concentration in ECF. In summary, multiple hormonal mechanisms produce a balance of influences on the concentration of calcium in ECF.

Hypocalcemia

Hypocalcemia is defined as total serum concentration below 8.4 mg/dL or ionized calcium concentration below 4.5 mg/dL. It varies from an asymptomatic biochemical abnormality to a life-threatening disorder, depending on its duration, severity, and rapidity of development. It is caused by loss of calcium from the circulation or by insufficient entry of calcium into the circulation.

Acute hypocalcemia can be life threatening. It impairs transmembrane depolarization; $[iCa^{2+}]$ below 0.8 mEq/L can lead to central nervous system dysfunction. Hypocalcemic patients can have paresthesias, muscle spasms (including tetany), and seizures. If patients hyperventilate, a respiratory alkalosis may exacerbate their condition and further reduce $[iCa^{2+}]$. Cardiac dysfunction is also common. Patients with low $[iCa^{2+}]$ may require IV infusion of calcium to restore cardiac function. Hypocalcemic patients have a prolonged QT interval on electrocardiograms that may progress to complete heart block or ventricular fibrillation.

Hypoparathyroidism, the most common cause of hypocalcemia, often develops because of surgery in the central neck, such as radical resection of head and neck cancers or incidentally after thyroidectomy. Hypocalcemia develops in 1% to 2% of patients after a total thyroidectomy. The hypocalcemia may be transient, permanent, or intermittent, as with vitamin D deficiency during the winter. Autoimmune hypoparathyroidism can be an isolated defect or part of polyglandular autoimmune syndrome type I in association with adrenal insufficiency and mucocutaneous candidiasis; most of these patients have autoantibodies directed against the calcium-sensing receptor. Congenital causes of hypocalcemia include activation of mutations of the calcium-sensing receptor, which resets the calcium-PTH relation to a lower serum calcium level. Mutations affecting intracellular processing of the pre-pro-PTH molecule can lead to hypoparathyroidism, hypocalcemia, or both. Finally, some cases of hypoparathyroidism are associated with hypoplasia or aplasia of the parathyroid glands; the best known is DiGeorge syndrome.

Pseudohypoparathyroidism is a group of disorders characterized by postreceptor resistance to PTH. One classic variant is Albright hereditary osteodystrophy, associated with low stature, round facies, short digits, and mental retardation. Hypomagnesemia induces PTH resistance and also affects PTH production. Severe hypermagnesemia (>6 mg/dL) can lead to hypocalcemia by inhibiting PTH secretion. When it is associated with decreased dietary calcium intake, vitamin D deficiency leads to hypocalcemia. The low calcium level stimulates PTH secretion (secondary hyperparathyroidism), leading to hypophosphatemia.

Rhabdomyolysis and tumor lysis syndrome cause loss of calcium from the circulation when large amounts of intracellular phosphate are released, thereby increasing calcium levels in bone and extraskeletal tissues. A similar mechanism causes hypocalcemia with phosphate administration.

Acute pancreatitis results in calcium sequestration in the abdomen, causing hypocalcemia. After surgery for hyperparathyroidism, patients with severe prolonged disease (such as those with secondary or tertiary hyperparathyroidism who are in renal failure) can develop a form of hypocalcemia known as *hungry bone syndrome,* in which serum calcium is rapidly deposited into the bone. The syndrome is also rarely seen after correction of long-standing metabolic acidosis or after thyroidectomy for hyperthyroidism.

Several medications (such as ethylenediaminetetraacetic acid [EDTA], citrate present in transfused blood, lactate, and foscarnet) chelate calcium in the circulation, sometimes producing hypocalcemia in which the iCa^{2+} level is decreased even though the total calcium level may be normal. Acute hypocalcemia in the postoperative period can occur in response to rapid blood transfusions. In the past, stored blood contained a higher concentration of citrate, which binds to and chelates serum calcium. Now that citrate has been eliminated from blood-banking techniques, this is rarely seen. Extensive osteoblastic skeletal metastases (such as from prostate and breast cancers) may also cause hypocalcemia. Chemotherapy, including cisplatin, 5-fluorouracil, and leucovorin, causes hypocalcemia mediated through hypomagnesemia. In patients with sepsis, hypocalcemia is usually associated with hypoalbuminemia.

Tumor lysis syndrome is a constellation of electrolyte abnormalities that include hypocalcemia, hyperphosphatemia, hyperuricemia, and hyperkalemia. Such abnormalities occur when antineoplastic therapy causes a sudden surge in tumor cell death and a release of cytosolic contents. Solid tumors and lymphomas have been implicated. Acute renal failure occurs in patients with tumor lysis syndrome and prevents spontaneous correction of the electrolyte abnormalities; emergency dialysis may be the only way to comprehensively correct the abnormalities.

Acute hypocalcemia is frequent after resuscitation from shock. In a study of patients in burn shock, Wray and associates hypothesized that a major factor contributing to the development of hypocalcemia was depressed levels of 1,25-dihydroxycholecalciferol, perhaps caused by a sudden lack of vitamin D in the diet. In patients with severe pancreatitis, the fall in calcium is speculated to be the consequence of ionized extracellular calcium becoming linked to fats in the peripancreatic inflammatory phlegmon. Rapid infusion of a citrate load during the transfusion of blood products (particularly platelet concentrates and FFP) may also lead to acute severe hypocalcemia ($[iCa^{2+}] < 0.62$ mmol/L) and hypotension. Rapid increases in serum phosphate can occur after improper administration or excessive dosing of phosphate-containing cathartics; as the phosphate concentration increases, severe hypocalcemia ensues.

Patients with acute symptomatic hypocalcemia (calcium level <7.0 mg/dL, iCa^{2+} level <0.8 mmol/L) should be treated promptly with an IV calcium infusion. Calcium may be given orally or intravenously in the form of calcium gluconate or calcium chloride. Calcium gluconate is preferred to calcium chloride because it causes less tissue necrosis if it extravasates. The first 100 to 200 mg of elemental calcium (1–2 g calcium gluconate) should be given over 10 to 20 minutes. Faster administration may result in cardiac dysfunction and even arrest. Those first 100 to 200 mg should then be followed by a slow calcium infusion at 0.5 to 1.5 mg/kg/h. Calcium infusion should continue until the patient is receiving effective doses of oral calcium and vitamin D. Calcium for infusion should be diluted in saline or dextrose solution to avoid vein irritation. The infusion should not contain bicarbonate or phosphate, either of which can form an insoluble calcium salt. If bicarbonate or phosphate administration is necessary, a separate IV line should be used.

Coexisting hypomagnesemia should be corrected in every patient. Care should be taken in patients with renal insufficiency because they cannot excrete excess magnesium. Magnesium is given by infusion, initiated with 2 g of magnesium sulfate over 10 to 15 minutes, followed by 1 g/h. In patients with severe hyperphosphatemia (such as those with tumor lysis syndrome, rhabdomyolysis, or chronic renal failure), treatment is focused on correcting the hyperphosphatemia.

Acute hyperphosphatemia usually resolves in patients with intact renal function. Phosphate excretion may be aided by saline infusion (this can lead to worsening of hypocalcemia); in addition, acetazolamide, a carbonic anhydrase inhibitor, can be given at 10 to 15 mg/kg every 3 to 4 hours. Hemodialysis may be necessary for patients with symptomatic hypocalcemia and hyperphosphatemia, especially if renal function is impaired. Chronic hyperphosphatemia is managed by a low-phosphate diet and use of phosphate binders with meals.

Chronic hypocalcemia (hypoparathyroidism) is treated by oral calcium administration and, if that is insufficient, vitamin D supplementation. The serum calcium level should be targeted to about 8.0 mg/dL. Most patients will be entirely asymptomatic at that level. Further elevation will lead to hypercalciuria because of the lack of PTH effect on the renal tubules. Chronic hypercalciuria carries the risks of nephrocalcinosis, nephrolithiasis, and renal impairment.

Several oral calcium preparations are available. Calcium carbonate is the cheapest form, but it may be poorly absorbed, especially in older patients and those with achlorhydria. Similarly, various forms of vitamin D are available. If oral calcium preparations cannot achieve adequate calcium repletion, vitamin D should be added. The usual initial daily dose is 50,000 IU of 25-hydroxyvitamin D (or 0.25–0.5 mg of 1,25-hydroxyvitamin D). Calcium and vitamin D doses are established by gradual titration. When adequate calcium levels are achieved, urinary calcium excretion is measured. If hypercalciuria is detected, a thiazide diuretic may be added to diminish calciuria and further increase the serum calcium level. If the phosphorus level is higher than 6.0 mg/dL when the calcium level is satisfactory, an unabsorbable phosphate binder should be added. Once calcium and phosphorus levels are controlled, the patient should be monitored every 3 to 6 months for both levels and for urinary calcium excretion.

Special consideration is necessary for the treatment of females with hypoparathyroidism who are pregnant or nursing. During pregnancy, vitamin D requirements gradually increase, up to three times as high as the prepregnancy requirements. Supplementary doses of vitamin D should be titrated, using frequent serum calcium level measurements. After delivery, if the baby is to be bottle-fed, the dose should be decreased to the prepregnancy dose. If the baby is to be nursed, the dose of calcitriol should be decreased to 50% of the prepregnancy dose because endogenous calcitriol production is stimulated by prolactin and by increased production of PTH-related peptide (PTHrP), which is also stimulated by prolactin.

Several reports have described successful control of hypocalcemia with synthetic PTH (1,34-PTH, teriparatide) by twice-daily subcutaneous administration, with a lower risk of hypercalciuria.

Hypercalcemia

Mild hypercalcemia is suspected when total serum calcium levels are in the range of 10.5 to 12 mg/dL. Patients with a serum calcium concentration of 12 to 14.5 mg/dL have moderate hypercalcemia. Patients with transient hypercalcemia are generally asymptomatic. Those with sustained elevations in renal calcium excretion are susceptible to the development of renal lithiasis, abdominal pain, and bone pain. Patients have severe hypercalcemia when serum calcium levels exceed 15 mg/dL; such patients have symptoms of weakness, stupor, and central nervous system dysfunction. In hypercalcemic patients, a renal concentrating defect also occurs, leading to polyuria and loss of sodium and water. Indeed, many hypercalcemic patients are dehydrated. Hypercalcemic crisis is a syndrome in which total serum calcium levels exceed 17 mg/dL; such patients are subject to life-threatening cardiac tachyarrhythmia, coma, acute renal failure, and ileus with abdominal distention.

The most common cause of hypercalcemia (in fact, in 90% of all patients) is primary hyperparathyroidism; other causes include unregulated PTH secretion and malignant disease. It occurs most commonly with malignant diseases in hospitalized patients and with hyperparathyroidism in the general population. Breast cancer is the most common malignant cause. Other rare causes include thyrotoxicosis, vitamin A and D overdose, granulomatous diseases, and commonly used drugs like thiazide diuretics and lithium. Another rare cause of hypercalcemia is familial hypocalciuric hypercalcemia, which is due to an autosomal dominant mutation in the calcium-sensing receptor causing increased calcium and magnesium retention by the kidneys. Signs and symptoms of hypercalcemia are nonspecific and include nausea, vomiting, altered mental status, constipation, depression, lethargy, myalgias, arthralgias, polyuria, headache, abdominal and flank pain (renal stones), and coma. They are sometimes described as abdominal groans, psychic moans, and renal stones. However, most of these symptoms are manifested after chronic hypercalcemia and not after acute hypercalcemia. Usually, a patient's clinical presentation is recognized as related to hypercalcemia only after it has been diagnosed by blood test results. It is extremely difficult to diagnose hypercalcemia by a patient's history alone.

Bone demineralization is found in patients with severe and prolonged hyperparathyroidism. The majority (85%) of such patients have a solitary hyperfunctioning adenoma in one parathyroid gland; the remaining 15% have excessive PTH release as a result of hyperplasia of all four glands. PTH induces phosphaturia and depresses serum phosphate concentrations; such a laboratory finding corroborates the diagnosis of primary hyperparathyroidism. Secondary hyperparathyroidism, an endocrine disease characterized by hyperplasia of the parathyroid glands, develops in patients with chronic renal failure. Decreased renal function results in impaired synthesis of 1,25-dihydroxycholecalciferol. Although patients have low serum calcium levels, their osteomalacia indicates excessive PTH secretion. To control elevated PTH levels in patients with secondary hyperparathyroidism, surgical removal of most of the parathyroid tissue may be required.

Humoral hypercalcemia of malignancy (HHM) is a clinical syndrome in which elevated calcium levels are caused by synthesis of the humoral factor by the tumoral process. Usually, HHM is applied to patients with excessive tumoral production of PTHrP. However, rare cases characterized by excessive production of PTH and calcitriol have also been described. Patients with HHM constitute about 80% of all patients with hypercalcemia associated with malignant disease. PTHrP and PTH share the same receptor, but the clinical presentation differs. HHM patients have a markedly larger degree of renal calcium excretion; PTH potently stimulates tubular calcium resorption, and hypercalciuria is less pronounced. HHM is usually associated with low serum calcitriol levels; PTH

stimulates calcitriol production, and its level is usually elevated. PTHrP stimulates only bone resorption, with very low osteoblastic activity and therefore usually normal alkaline phosphatase levels; PTH stimulates bone resorption and formation.

HHM patients usually have a clinically obvious malignant disease and a poor prognosis. The only exceptions to this rule are patients with small, well-differentiated endocrine tumors (such as pheochromocytomas or islet cell tumors). However, such tumors constitute a minority of cases. HHM is most commonly seen with squamous cell carcinomas (e.g., of the lung, esophagus, cervix, or head and neck) and with renal, bladder, and ovarian cancers. Treatment of HHM patients is aimed at reducing the tumor burden, reducing osteoclastic resorption of the bone, and increasing calcium excretion through the urine.

Most cases of hypercalcemia are associated with Hodgkin disease. The other third of cases are associated with non-Hodgkin lymphoma and are caused by increased production of calcitriol by the malignant cells. Hypercalcemia usually responds well to treatment with corticosteroids. Multiple myeloma, lymphoma, and solid tumors metastatic to bone (particularly breast, lung, and prostate cancer) cause hypercalcemia by excessive osteoclastic activity. Drugs can also cause hypercalcemia, including theophylline, lithium, thiazide diuretics, and extraordinarily high doses of vitamins A and D. In addition, hypercalcemia can develop in young, normally active patients with high bone turnover rates who are suddenly forced into immobility, such as during forced bed rest after injury or major illness. This hypercalcemia of immobilization resolves with return to normal activity.

Another cause of hypercalcemia is milk-alkali syndrome, a rare condition caused by ingestion of large amounts of calcium together with sodium bicarbonate. It is currently associated with ingestion of calcium carbonate in over-the-counter antacid preparations and in drugs used to prevent and treat osteoporosis. Features of the syndrome include hypercalcemia, renal failure, and metabolic alkalosis. The exact pathophysiologic mechanism is unknown. In rare cases, the amount of calcium ingested may be as low as 2000 to 3000 mg/day, but in most patients, the amount is between 6000 and 15,000 mg/day. Treatment consists of rehydration, diuresis, and cessation of calcium and antacid ingestion. If diuresis is impossible because of renal failure, dialysis using a dialysate with a low calcium concentration is effective. Renal failure usually resolves in patients with short-term hypercalcemia but may persist in those with chronic hypercalcemia.

Definitive management of hypercalcemia depends on correction of the primary problem. Thus, patients with hyperparathyroidism secondary to a parathyroid adenoma or hyperplasia are cured of hypercalcemia by excision of the diseased parathyroid tissue. Hypercalcemic patients taking thiazide drugs should be converted to alternative therapies. Patients with a malignant neoplasm and hypercalcemia may respond to surgical excision, radiation therapy, or chemotherapy. Symptomatic patients with severe hypercalcemia related to malignant disease can be quickly and effectively treated by saline infusion to expand intravascular volume, followed by the administration of a loop diuretic (e.g., furosemide) to induce saline diuresis with associated urinary calcium clearance. Patients with severe hypercalcemia frequently have a contracted extracellular volume, so isotonic saline infusion is essential. Hypercalcemic patients in renal failure who cannot benefit from drug-induced diuresis can be treated by hemodialysis.

Severe hypercalcemia, referred to as *hypercalcemic crisis,* occurs with serum calcium concentrations above 14 mg/dL and is related to release of calcium from bone by tumor; it can be managed by administration of bisphosphonates. Such drugs have a potent capacity to reduce osteoclast-mediated release of calcium from bone. Several formulations of bisphosphonates are available (in order of preference, zoledronic acid, pamidronate disodium, and etidronate disodium), all of which produce a slow decline in [iCa²⁺] over several days. In patients with metastatic breast cancer, bisphosphonates given as long-term prophylactic agents at a regular dosage have been shown to effectively prevent hypercalcemia.

Administration of exogenous calcitonin is often initially effective in patients with hypercalcemia. Calcitonin (4 U/kg subcutaneously every 12 hours) inhibits bone resorption and decreases renal tubular resorption of calcium, with a shorter onset of action than bisphosphonates; therefore, it is the better choice for short-term control of calcium. However, long-term treatment frequently leads to tachyphylaxis, possibly related to the development of antibodies to the exogenous calcitonin. Chelating agents (EDTA or phosphate salts) that bind and neutralize [iCa²⁺] are rarely indicated. Such agents are associated with the complications of metastatic calcification and acute renal failure, as well as the risk of depressing [iCa²⁺] to hypocalcemic levels.

Magnesium

Magnesium, an essential cation in the cell, is the second most prevalent cation. It is a critical cofactor in any reaction powered by ATP, so deficiencies can affect metabolism. It also acts as a calcium channel antagonist and plays a key role in the modulation of any activity involving calcium, such as muscle contraction and insulin release. The normal concentration of magnesium [Mg^{2+}] in plasma ranges between 1.5 and 2.0 mEq/L. Like calcium, it exists in three states: protein bound (30%, bound mostly to albumin), bound to anions (10%), and ionized (60%).

Magnesium is primarily intracellular, with less than 1% of body stores in the ECF. Measured plasma magnesium levels often do not reflect total body magnesium content. Clinical sequelae of altered magnesium content depend more on tissue magnesium levels than on the blood magnesium concentration. Consequently, it is often difficult to consistently correlate symptoms to specific plasma magnesium levels. One method to infer the tissue magnesium level is a physiologic test that measures the renal response to a magnesium load. Patients who retain more than 30% of an 800-mg load of magnesium via IV are thought to be magnesium depleted, whereas those who retain less than 20% are said to be magnesium replete.

The kidneys are responsible for maintaining magnesium balance by excreting the absorbed magnesium. The ionized and bound forms of magnesium are freely filtered by the glomerulus. The distal tubule resorbs 10% of the filtered magnesium and plays an important role in calcium-independent magnesium homeostasis. The hormonal regulation of magnesium homeostasis has not been completely determined. PTH, glucagon, and ADH increase the resorption of magnesium in the Henle loop. In the distal convoluted tubule, aldosterone, ADH, and glucagon are thought to increase magnesium resorption. To maintain magnesium homeostasis, renal resorption of magnesium varies widely. Fractional resorption of filtered magnesium can decline to nearly zero in the presence of hypermagnesemia or reduced glomerular filtration rate. In contrast, in response to magnesium depletion or decreased intake, the fractional resorption of magnesium can rise to 99.5% to minimize urinary losses.

Hypomagnesemia

In ICU patients, the prevalence of hypomagnesemia ranges from 11% to 65%, but it is usually asymptomatic. Some studies have shown little significance to hypomagnesemia; other studies have shown an association with mortality. Any association with mortality is not necessarily causal, of course, and may merely reflect the patient's state of health. Symptoms of hypomagnesemia have been reported at modest degrees of depletion, but in general, symptoms become more common as the serum magnesium level falls below 1.2 mg/dL. Associating specific symptoms with hypomagnesemia is difficult. However, severe hypomagnesemia in postsurgical patients can lead to life-threatening ventricular arrhythmias such as torsades de pointes.

Hypokalemia is commonly associated with hypomagnesemia and reportedly occurs in 40% of patients with hypomagnesemia. The converse is also true; 60% of patients with hypokalemia have concurrent hypomagnesemia. The causes of hypomagnesemia are multiple, including renal, GI, and skin losses as well as hungry bone syndrome. Skin losses can be due to burns or toxic epidermal necrolysis. Renal losses can be due to a long list of drugs, but the most common are diuretics.

Hypomagnesemia also causes a specific disorder of renal potassium wasting that is refractory to potassium supplementation until magnesium is adequately repleted. Recently, the mechanism whereby magnesium depletion results in renal potassium loss has been elucidated. Decreased intracellular magnesium slows ATP production. Throughout the body, such slowed ATP production has a negative effect on Na^+, K^+-ATPase activity. The result is loss of intracellular potassium, which flows down its concentration gradient into the tubule and is lost in the urine.

Hypocalcemia, hyponatremia, and hypophosphatemia are also common in patients with hypomagnesemia. Intracellular hypomagnesemia can develop in patients with chronic diarrhea or in those who undergo prolonged aggressive diuretic therapy. Magnesium deficiency is also common in patients with heavy ethanol intake. Diabetic patients with persistent osmotic diuresis from glycosuria commonly have hypomagnesemia.

Patients with mild hypomagnesemia can be treated with oral replacement; symptomatic hypomagnesemia should be treated with an IV magnesium infusion. The most common formulation is magnesium sulfate; 1 g of magnesium sulfate contains 0.1 g of elemental magnesium. No trials have been done to determine the optimal regimen for magnesium replacement, but consensus statements suggest 8 to 12 g of magnesium sulfate in the first 24 hours followed by 4 to 6 g/day for 3 or 4 days to replete body stores. IV magnesium therapy is advocated in some acutely ill patients without documented magnesium depletion. The American College of Cardiology and the American Heart Association recommend 1 to 2 g of magnesium sulfate as an IV bolus over 5 minutes for torsades de pointes therapy. Emerging data have suggested that magnesium may also play a role in reducing reperfusion injury and decreasing infarct size in patients with acute myocardial infarction. Currently, the American Heart Association recommends 2 g of magnesium sulfate for 15 minutes, followed by 18 g over 24 hours in patients with suspected myocardial infarction who have hypomagnesemia.

Magnesium replacement should be done cautiously in patients with renal insufficiency, and recommendations call for dose reductions of 50% to 75% of baseline. During infusions, patients should be monitored closely for decreased deep tendon reflexes. Magnesium levels should be checked at regular intervals. Oral supplementation has been shown to successfully correct increased magnesium retention. Potassium-sparing diuretics may be helpful in patients with chronic renal magnesium wasting. Diuretics that block the sodium channel in the distal convoluted tubule, such as amiloride and triamterene, reduce magnesium wasting in some patients. Severe hypomagnesemia (<1.0 mEq/L) requires sustained therapy because of the slow equilibration of extracellular magnesium with intracellular stores. Correction of hypomagnesemia can also reduce the risk of cardiac arrhythmia. The magnitude of magnesium deficiency frequently parallels the magnitude of hypocalcemia. Hypocalcemia in patients with magnesium deficiency is resistant to calcium replacement alone, so such patients should receive magnesium concurrently.

Hypermagnesemia

Hypermagnesemia is a common abnormality in patients with renal failure but is otherwise uncommon among other patients. Theophylline toxicity, now rare, was associated with hypermagnesemia in the past. Hypermagnesemia can be exacerbated by the ingestion of magnesium-containing drugs, particularly antacids; Epsom salts also contain magnesium, as does magnesium citrate, which is often used in surgical care. High levels of magnesium seem to be tolerated well and, in general, without sequelae. In one report, a patient in diabetic ketoacidosis with hypomagnesemia received 50 g of magnesium sulfate for 6 hours rather than the intended 2 g. Despite a documented magnesium level of 24 mg/dL and significant short-term morbidity, the patient completely recovered.

Magnesium overdoses given via IV may be better tolerated than oral overdoses. Hypermagnesemia due to oral ingestion of magnesium is unusual in the absence of renal insufficiency. A fatal case of hypermagnesemia was documented in a developmentally disabled child who was given magnesium to relieve constipation. Despite calcium infusions and dialysis, the child died. The chronic ingestion of magnesium likely made the child's condition refractory to treatment, perhaps because of a greater total body magnesium burden from chronic overload. Hypermagnesemia has also been repeatedly reported after the use of magnesium-containing enemas. In postsurgical patients who are oliguric, hypermagnesemia may occur because of magnesium retention, particularly if the patient is acidotic.

Magnesium can block synaptic transmission of nerve impulses. It also causes the initial loss of deep tendon reflexes and may lead to flaccid paralysis and apnea. Neuromuscular toxicity also affects smooth muscle, resulting in ileus and urinary retention. In cases of oral intoxication, the development of ileus can slow intestinal transit times, further increasing absorption of magnesium. Hypermagnesemia has also been reported to cause a parasympathetic blockade that results in fixed and dilated pupils, mimicking brainstem herniation. Other neurologic signs include lethargy, confusion, and coma.

Magnesium blocks the shift of calcium into myocardial cells and can act as a calcium channel blocker. In cardiac tissue, it also blocks potassium channels needed for repolarization. Patients with severe hypermagnesemia can show evidence of heart failure. Other cardiac manifestations of hypermagnesemia, at least initially, include bradycardia and hypotension. Higher magnesium levels cause a prolonged PR interval, increased QRS duration, and prolonged QT interval. Extreme cases can result in complete heart block or cardiac arrest.

Metabolic disturbances due to hypermagnesemia have been less recognized than those due to hypomagnesemia. Hypocalcemia can occur, although it is typically mild and asymptomatic. Symptomatic hypermagnesemia (despite normal renal function) has been reported with magnesium infusions, typically during treatment of patients who are in preterm labor or who have preeclampsia or eclampsia. Routine magnesium measurements are often not performed, although the infusion protocols (a load of 4–6 g, followed by 1–2 g/h) result in serum magnesium levels of 4 to 8 mg/dL. Obstetric patients who experience accidental overdoses of magnesium usually have good outcomes despite magnesium levels as high as 19 mg/dL.

The principles for treatment of hypermagnesemia are similar to those for treatment of hypercalcemia. Calcium is given to stabilize the heart, normal saline is given for fluid expansion, and diuretics are given to hasten renal excretion. In patients with hypermagnesemia and intact renal function, stopping the infusion or supply of magnesium will allow them to recover. Severe hypermagnesemia is treated with calcium gluconate 10% (10–20 mL for 10 minutes) administered via IV. Patients are typically given 100 to 200 mg IV of elemental calcium over 5 to 10 minutes. To speed the renal clearance of magnesium, loop diuretics and saline diuresis are intuitive options, but no literature explicitly supports this use.

In critically ill patients, disorders of magnesium homeostasis can have dramatic effects. Yet such disorders often go unrecognized. In ICU patients, hypomagnesemia is common and associated with poor outcomes, so measurement of serum magnesium should be routine. Unlike magnesium depletion, hypermagnesemia is a rare but frequently iatrogenic and fatal problem.

In patients with renal insufficiency, dialysis rapidly corrects hypermagnesemia and is the only way to acutely lower magnesium levels. Aggressive use of dialysis may improve survival. In patients with severe renal dysfunction, dialysis offers a way to rapidly clear magnesium. Both peritoneal dialysis and hemodialysis are effective at lowering magnesium levels. Intermittent hemodialysis corrects hypermagnesemia more rapidly than peritoneal dialysis or continuous renal replacement therapy.

Phosphate

Phosphate is a predominantly intracellular anion important for energy metabolism and skeletal mineralization. Normal serum phosphate concentrations range from 2.5 to 4.5 mg/dL. Hypophosphatemia is defined as a serum phosphate value less than 2.5 mg/dL, and hyperphosphatemia is defined as a serum phosphate value higher than 4.5 mg/dL.

Hypophosphatemia

Hypophosphatemia is seen frequently in critical illness, and the effects are primarily related to the impairment of cellular energy metabolism. This can be caused by impaired intestinal absorption, increased renal losses (acidosis, diuretics, steroids), or redistribution into the intracellular space, which can be affected by respiratory alkalosis, serum catecholamine levels, and glucose or insulin. Impaired oxygen delivery to peripheral tissue occurs with hypophosphatemia due to the left shift of the oxyhemoglobin dissociation curve caused by 2,3-DPG depletion.

Hypophosphatemia can lead to diaphragm dysfunction, which can cause respiratory failure and prolonged ventilator weaning. In postoperative patients, particularly in major hepatic resection, hypophosphatemia can occur due to consumption of phosphate secondary to regeneration. In patients with trauma or thermal injury, hypophosphatemia is common and may be related to the extracellular shifts, LR resuscitation causing a metabolic alkalosis, or a hypermetabolic state. Refeeding syndrome is a constellation of electrolyte abnormalities that can occur in patients with prolonged nutritional deficiency. The hallmark feature is hypophosphatemia, but other disturbances, such as hypomagnesemia, hypokalemia, thiamine deficiency, fluid balance irregularities, and abnormal glucose metabolism, are common. Timely recognition is important in preventing death from cardiac failure, muscle weakness, and immune system dysfunction in these patients, as are slow refeeding and careful electrolyte repletion.

Repletion of severe hypophosphatemia (<1.0 mg/dL) can be accomplished with IV phosphate doses up to 45 mmol (up to 20 mmol/h). There is a danger of precipitation with calcium with too-rapid administration. Sodium phosphate versus potassium phosphate should be selected depending on potassium level. Moderate hypophosphatemia can be treated with oral supplementation; up to triple normal intake in divided doses is appropriate. Patients with refeeding syndrome will require additional supplementation and more frequent electrolyte checks.

Hyperphosphatemia

The symptoms of hyperphosphatemia are usually related to the underlying cause, such as renal failure. In the acute setting, the symptoms of severe hyperphosphatemia include hypotension or signs of hypocalcemia. Hyperphosphatemia in critically ill patients is commonly due to exogenous causes, such as excess intake of phosphate-based laxatives or enemas or high-dose fosphenytoin; endogenous sources, such as rhabdomyolysis or tumor lysis or extracellular shift (in patients with normal renal function); or acute or chronic renal dysfunction (elevated BUN, creatinine). Acute hyperphosphatemia may induce significant hypocalcemia, which should not be corrected until elevated phosphorus levels are addressed.

Hyperphosphatemia will quickly resolve if renal function is normal. Treatments include crystalloid administration to encourage renal excretion, although this may worsen the accompanying hypocalcemia, which requires monitoring or the use of loop diuretics to promote diuresis. Hemodialysis may be used in patients with significant renal dysfunction.

SELECTED REFERENCES

Bickell WH, Wall Jr MJ, Pepe PE, et al. Immediate versus delayed fluid resuscitation for hypotensive patients with penetrating torso injuries. *N Engl J Med.* 1994;331:1105-1109.

Classic study, probably the most referenced article in trauma, showing that despite these patients being hypotensive in the field after penetrating torso injury, treating these patients with crystalloid solutions resulted in worse outcomes, and not infusing fluids improved outcomes.

Bouzat P, Charbit J, Payen JF, et al. Efficacy and safety of early administration of 4-factor prothrombin complex concentrate in patients with trauma at risk of massive transfusion: the PROCOAG randomized clinical trial. *JAMA.* 2023;329(16):1367-1375.

Demonstrates the lack of utility and possible harm in PCC use in trauma patients at risk for massive transfusion.

Committee on Fluid Resuscitation for Combat Casualties. *Fluid Resuscitation: State of the Science for Treating Combat Casualties and Civilian Injuries. Report of the Institute of Medicine.* Washington, DC: National Academy Press; 1999.

Considered a white paper by the Institute of Medicine, it was seen as radical in that it did not recommend lactated Ringer solution as the fluid of choice for civilians and the military. It recommended hypertonic saline and additional research to eliminate d-isomer lactate from lactated Ringer solution and to investigate other metabolites, such as ketones, as an alternative.

CRASH-3 Trial Collaborators. Effects of tranexamic acid on death, disability, vascular occlusive events and other morbidities in patients with acute traumatic brain injury (CRASH-3): a randomised, placebo-controlled trial [published correction appears in *Lancet.* 2019;394(10210):1712]. *Lancet.* 2019; 394(10210):1713-1723.

Shows the safety and TBI-related mortality benefit of TXA use in mild to moderate TBI patients.

Evans L, Rhodes A, Levy M, et al. Surviving sepsis campaign: international guidelines for management of sepsis and septic shock 2021. *Intensive Care Med.* 2021;47(11):1181-1247.

Most recent update on conscious guidelines on the definition, diagnosis, and management of patients in sepsis and septic shock.

Finfer S, Bellomo R, Boyce N, et al. A comparison of albumin and saline for fluid resuscitation in the intensive care unit. *N Engl J Med.* 2004;350:2247-2256.

Prospective multicenter study designed to show that albumin is safe in the intensive care unit. However, it used 4% albumin and showed that the outcome was no different.

Fluid resuscitation of combat casualties: conference proceedings. June 2001 and October 2001. *J Trauma.* 2003;54(suppl): S1-S234.

This entire supplement summarizes the rationale for the changes recommended for the treatment of combat casualties.

Holcomb JB, Jenkins D, Rhee P, et al. Damage control resuscitation: directly addressing the early coagulopathy of trauma. *J Trauma.* 2007;62:307-310.

This article describes the evolution of damage control resuscitation and rationale behind the recommendation of permissive hypotension, reduction of crystalloid use, use of hypertonic saline, and aggressive use of blood products early and often for best results.

Holcomb JB, Tilley BC, Baraniuk S, et al. Transfusion of plasma, platelets, and red blood cells in a 1:1:1 vs a 1:1:2 ratio and mortality in patients with severe trauma: the PROPPR randomized clinical trial. *JAMA.* 2015;313:471-482.

This article demonstrates a benefit in time to hemostasis with a 1:1:1 transfusion ratio and a decreased rate of exsanguination at 24 hours.

Moore EE, Moore FA, Fabian TC, et al. PolyHeme study group: human polymerized hemoglobin for the treatment of hemorrhagic shock when blood is unavailable: the USA Multicenter trial. *J Am Coll Surg.* 2009;208:1-13.

Study showing that artificial hemoglobin made from expired human blood could be used safely and as a replacement for blood in the field and in the hospital.

Plurad D, Martin M, Green D, et al. The decreasing incidence of late post-traumatic acute respiratory distress syndrome: the potential role of lung protective ventilation and conservative transfusion practice. *J Trauma.* 2007;63:1-7.

This article shows the decreasing incidence of ARDS in trauma and its association with decreased crystalloid use.

Spinella PC, Perkins JG, Grathwohl KW, et al. Warm fresh whole blood is independently associated with improved survival for patients with combat-related traumatic injuries. *J Trauma.* 2009;66:S69-S76.

Describes the usefulness of whole blood transfusion practice founded by the military.

The full reference list appears on Elsevier eBooks+.

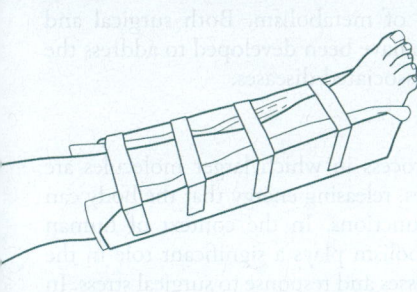

CHAPTER 34

Metabolism and Nutrition in Surgical Patients

Catherine L. McKnight, Stephanie Eosten Joyce, Brian J. Daley, and Kimberly A. Davis

OUTLINE

▶ **Please access Elsevier eBooks+ to view the videos for this chapter.**

INTRODUCTION

The Importance of Metabolism and Nutrition in Surgery

Metabolism constitutes an intricate web of biochemical and biophysical reactions that take place inside the cells of all living organisms when responding to changes in their surroundings.[1,2] This complex system consists of a series of interconnected chemical reactions that cooperate to sustain life. To gain a comprehensive understanding of these metabolic processes in surgical patients, one must delve into the intersection of chemistry, physics, and biology.[2] These processes are conceptually organized into pathways where enzymes and substrates interact in a sequential manner to produce vital outputs for life.[2] These pathways are intertwined and mutually influenced, meaning that the outcome of one pathway can either serve as input or act as a regulator for another pathway.[2] Consequently, metabolic pathways possess the capacity to both exert influence and be influenced by one another.[2] These pathways are categorized as either catabolic, responsible for breaking down components of the organism, or anabolic, dedicated to building and nurturing the organism.[1,2] Both of these categories of processes collaborate under strict regulation to accomplish the primary objectives of metabolism: maintaining life's balance by ensuring energy equilibrium, structural development, and the proper management of waste production and elimination.[1,3]

Nutrition and metabolism are inextricably linked. Nutrition is the repletion of our bodies through the intake of food and nutrients. This intake provides the raw materials that fuel our metabolic processes. Nutrients include carbohydrates, proteins, fats, vitamins, minerals, and water, which have specific roles in supporting metabolism, maintaining bodily functions, and preventing disease. The intricate relationship between metabolism and nutrition is a central theme in the broader field of medicine. Nutrition influences energy levels, body composition, and susceptibility to chronic diseases, such as diabetes, heart disease, and obesity. These can have consequences on health and quality of life, directly affecting the outcomes of surgical patients.

The objectives of this chapter are to describe the basic science of cellular metabolism and nutrition, understand the principles of perioperative nutritional assessment and repletion, focus on routes of nutritional replacement in the perioperative period, and describe the complications related to alimentation.

METABOLISM

The History of Metabolism

The origins of nutrition can be traced back to ancient civilizations. Neanderthals determined their diets based on the availability of food. Greek philosophers like Empedocles and Aristotle contemplated the nature of life processes and speculated about the presence of a "vital force" responsible for these processes. The term *metabolism* finds its roots in the Greek word *metabole*, which means "change." Around 300 BCE, Aristotle proposed the idea that food was transformed into heat as a byproduct as well as urine, bile, and feces as waste products.[4] Nevertheless, it was the Roman physician Galen who made substantial contributions to early concepts of metabolism. Galen introduced the notion of natural faculties governing bodily functions, including digestion and metabolism.

A pivotal moment in the study of metabolism occurred during the 17th and 18th centuries with the advent of the scientific method and the chemical revolution. Prominent figures such as Robert Boule and Antoine-Laurent de Lavoisier achieved groundbreaking insights into chemical reactions and the role of oxygen in combustion. In 1614, Santorio published the book *Ars de Statica Medicina* in which he observed that a significant portion of food was lost through "insensible perspiration," which he discovered by measuring his weight before and after various daily activities.[5] In the late 1700s, formal research into metabolism commenced in the laboratory of the French chemist Antoine-Laurent de Lavoisier, who was often referred to as the "Father of Modern Chemistry."[2,3] He not only coined the term *metabolism* but also demonstrated that respiration involved the consumption of oxygen and the production of carbon dioxide, paving the way for crucial studies on the chemical composition of food. Additionally, during this period, British naval physician James Lind discovered scurvy and its association with vitamin deficiency. After his work, Kanehiro Takaki, a Japanese naval officer, used an epidemiologic approach to identify the cause of beriberi as a nutritional deficiency.

The 19th century witnessed a heated debate between vitalists, who believed that living organisms possessed a unique, life-giving force, and mechanists, who sought to explain biologic processes in terms of chemistry and physics. The discovery of enzymes, catalysts that facilitate biochemical reactions within living organisms, played a pivotal role in resolving this debate. Scientists like Justus von Liebig and Eduard Buchner provided evidence that enzymes were responsible for metabolic reactions, supporting the mechanistic perspective.

In the 20th century there were tremendous advancements in biochemistry, which significantly contributed to our understanding of metabolism. The elucidation of the Krebs cycle (citric acid cycle) by Hans Krebs and the discovery of adenosine triphosphate (ATP) as the primary energy currency of cells by Fritz Lipmann were landmark achievements. By the 1930s, David Cuthbertson had described the phenomenon of negative nitrogen balance after tissue trauma and argued that the losses were mostly due to muscle wasting.[6] These breakthroughs laid the foundation for understanding how energy is generated and used in metabolic pathways.

Advances in molecular biology and genetics have propelled our understanding of metabolism to unprecedented levels. The Human Genome Project and subsequent technologies have revealed the intricate network of genes, proteins, and metabolites that govern metabolism. Research into metabolic diseases, such as diabetes and obesity, has also expanded, leading to innovative therapies and preventative strategies.

Today, the study of metabolism is a multidisciplinary field that encompasses biochemistry, physiology, genetics, and systems biology. Researchers continue to uncover new metabolic pathways, regulatory mechanisms, and metabolic adaptations in response to various physiologic and environmental challenges. The integration of metabolic research with medical science has yielded invaluable insights into health and disease, opening the door to personalized medicine and novel therapeutic interventions, along with the creation of medical and surgical subspecialties whose primary focus is on diseases of metabolism. Both surgical and pharmacologic breakthroughs have been developed to address the management of obesity and associated diseases.

Catabolism

Catabolism is the biologic process in which larger molecules are broken down into smaller ones, releasing energy that the body can use for various physiologic functions. In the context of human metabolism and surgery, catabolism plays a significant role in the body's natural metabolic processes and response to surgical stress. In the absence of surgical stress, the body's catabolic processes continually operate to uphold its energy equilibrium and guarantee the presence of crucial molecules. This process involves the breakdown of macronutrients like carbohydrates, fats, and proteins into simpler compounds or essential molecules, such as glucose and fatty acids, which are used for generating energy and preserving cellular health (Table 34.1). The decomposition of ingested proteins is particularly crucial because it provides essential amino acids that the human body cannot produce but are essential for various biosynthetic processes.[7] This ongoing catabolic activity plays a pivotal role in rejuvenating and repairing tissues, allowing the body to replace aging or damaged cells with new ones, thus ensuring optimal organ function and overall well-being. Beyond cellular turnover, the body also requires energy to sustain fundamental life functions like respiration, temperature regulation, and the continuous operation of the heart. This fundamental energy expenditure is referred to as *basal metabolic rate* (BMR).

Surgical interventions, no matter how intricate or precise, elicit a physiologic stress reaction within the body. This stress response initiates a sequence of hormonal and metabolic adjustments, primarily intended to supply the required energy and materials for facilitating tissue recovery and recuperation. Stress-related hormones, such as cortisol, catecholamines, growth hormones, and prolactin, are released during the perioperative phase. This series of events can result in the breakdown of muscle proteins into amino acids. Although this process is essential at the time, sustained use of muscle tissue as an energy source can lead to muscle atrophy and postoperative weakness, particularly in cases of extended immobilization.

It is evident that tissue damage resulting from surgical procedures or injuries triggers a catabolic condition driven by stress signals, as depicted in Fig. 34.1.[2,3,5] This stress response affects the patient at various levels, from individual cells to the entire body, leading to significant reactions to stress.[4] Consequently, a knowledgeable surgeon is well informed about the metabolic effects of injuries and illnesses, and the surgeon is also skilled in employing strategies to mitigate these disruptions for the well-being of their patients.[4]

Inflammatory responses, in addition to modifying macronutrients, bring about shifts in micronutrients (comprising vitamins and minerals) from their normal physiologic levels, as indicated in Table 34.2.[8,9] The most notable of these alterations is the development of anemia, attributed to the action of interleukin (IL)-1 and tumor necrosis factor (TNF), which reduce the levels of iron and zinc in the bloodstream. It is believed that these abrupt reductions in serum concentrations of iron and zinc are part of the body's defense mechanisms against invading microorganisms because many microorganisms require these elements for growth.[8,10,11] Moreover, although these elements decrease in serum levels, they are not expelled from the body; instead, they are stored in the liver and can be reused for the host's cellular metabolism once the infection is resolved. Simultaneously, whereas zinc and iron concentrations decrease in the serum, plasma copper levels increase due

TABLE 34.1 Proteinogenic Amino Acids

CATEGORY	NAME
Essential amino acids	Histidine
	Isoleucine
	Leucine
	Lysine
	Methionine
	Phenylalanine
	Threonine
	Tryptophan
	Valine
Conditionally essential amino acids	Arginine
	Cysteine
	Glutamine
	Glycine
	Proline
	Tyrosine
Nonessential amino acids	Alanine
	Asparagine
	Aspartate
	Glutamate
	Selenocysteine
	Serine

to a notable rise in ceruloplasmin, an additional acute-phase protein.[8,10,11] Although serum concentrations of both zinc and iron decrease, plasma copper concentrations rise because of the significant increase in ceruloplasmin, an additional acute-phase protein.[8,10,11] Additionally, deficiencies in water-soluble vitamins may become apparent as diuresis commences during the resolution of the acute phase of stress.[8,9,11]

The most prominent change during critical illness involves the breakdown of proteins found in lean body mass.[12,13] Unlike fats and carbohydrates, the body lacks a mechanism for long-term storage of free amino acids; therefore, it releases them from structural proteins, particularly within skeletal muscle.[3] The extent of protein turnover can be understood in its most basic form by assessing the daily nitrogen balance:

Daily Nitrogen Balance = Total Protein Intake (grams)/6.25 − (Urinary Urea Nitrogen + 4 grams)

After the depletion of glycogen stores in the liver due to starvation, the body undergoes a shift toward using fatty acids as its primary energy source, leading to the production of ketone bodies.[3] This metabolic transition occurs as the body moves from a well-fed state to a starved state. Initially, proteolysis facilitates gluconeogenesis until essential tissues can predominantly rely on ketone bodies for energy.[3] Even in the early stages of starvation, an average adult's body breaks down around 75 g of muscle

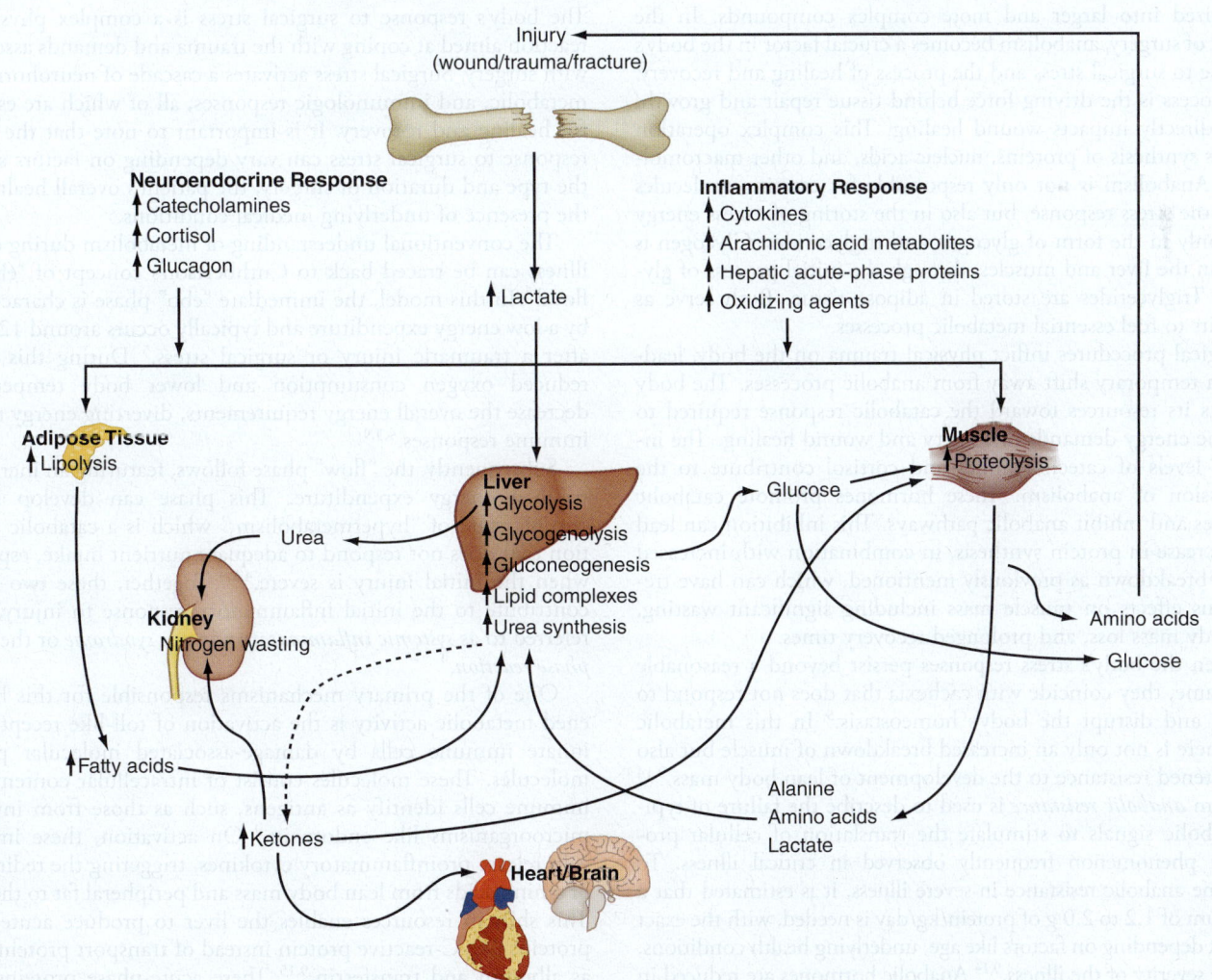

FIGURE 34.1 Metabolic pathways—basic version.

TABLE 34.2   Micronutrients

MICRONUTRIENT	FUNCTION	DEFICIENCY	RELEVANCE
Vitamin A	Cofactor in collagen synthesis and cross-linking; antioxidant; immune stimulation; macrophage extravasation; mucosal integrity; regulation of glycoprotein synthesis	Dermatitis; night blindness; xerophthalmia; respiratory ailments (pneumonia, bronchopulmonary dysplasia); impaired gut epithelial integrity	Wound healing and epithelial regeneration; deficiency can result in diminished activity of helper T cells, impaired mucous secretion; retinol-binding protein sensitive to nutritional status of individuals
Vitamin D	Promotes absorption of calcium and phosphorus (by intestine and kidney), bone growth, and bone remodeling (by osteoblasts and osteoclasts); regulates synthesis of several structural proteins, including type I collagen	Bone demineralization	Deficiency and impairment causing bone demineralization and osteopenia

Adapted from Norbury WB, Situ E, Herndon DN. Nutritional support in the critically ill. In: Cameron JL, ed. *Current Surgical Therapy.* 9th ed. Philadelphia: Mosby; 2007:1234-1245.

protein daily.[3,8,14] This breakdown is primarily driven by hormones like glucagon, catecholamines, and glucocorticoids and contributes to the observed loss of muscle mass in critically ill individuals.[3,8,14]

Anabolism

Anabolism, the counterpart of catabolism, refers to the constructive processes within the body in which smaller molecules are synthesized into larger and more complex compounds. In the context of surgery, anabolism becomes a crucial factor in the body's response to surgical stress and the process of healing and recovery. This process is the driving force behind tissue repair and growth, which directly impacts wound healing. This complex operation involves synthesis of proteins, nucleic acids, and other macromolecules. Anabolism is not only responsible for creating molecules during the stress response, but also in the storing of excess energy commonly in the form of glycogen and triglycerides. Glycogen is stored in the liver and muscles, through the initial process of glycolysis. Triglycerides are stored in adipose tissue. Both serve as reservoirs to fuel essential metabolic processes.

Surgical procedures inflict physical trauma on the body, leading to a temporary shift away from anabolic processes. The body redirects its resources toward the catabolic response required to meet the energy demands of surgery and wound healing. The increased levels of catecholamines and cortisol contribute to the suppression of anabolism. These hormones promote catabolic processes and inhibit anabolic pathways. This inhibition can lead to a decrease in protein synthesis, in combination with increased muscle breakdown as previously mentioned, which can have tremendous effects on muscle mass including significant wasting, lean body mass loss, and prolonged recovery times.

When the body's stress responses persist beyond a reasonable time frame, they coincide with cachexia that does not respond to feeding and disrupt the body's homeostasis.[9] In this metabolic state, there is not only an increased breakdown of muscle but also a heightened resistance to the development of lean body mass.[9,14] The term *anabolic resistance* is used to describe the failure of typical anabolic signals to stimulate the translation of cellular proteins, a phenomenon frequently observed in critical illness. To overcome anabolic resistance in severe illness, it is estimated that a minimum of 1.2 to 2.0 g of protein/kg/day is needed, with the exact amount depending on factors like age, underlying health conditions, and the severity of the illness.[9,14] Anabolic hormones are reduced in cases of severe stress, and patients are often immobile, both of which

contribute to anabolic resistance.[9,14] However, it is worth noting that immobility-induced anabolic resistance may be reversible, as early mobilization and physical therapy have been linked to shorter stays in the intensive care unit (ICU) and the hospital.[9,14]

THE METABOLIC RESPONSE TO SURGICAL STRESS AND CRITICAL ILLNESS

The body's response to surgical stress is a complex physiologic reaction aimed at coping with the trauma and demands associated with surgery. Surgical stress activates a cascade of neurohormonal, metabolic, and immunologic responses, all of which are essential for healing and recovery. It is important to note that the body's response to surgical stress can vary depending on factors such as the type and duration of surgery, the patient's overall health, and the presence of underlying medical conditions.

The conventional understanding of metabolism during critical illness can be traced back to Cuthbertson's concept of "ebb and flow."[5] In this model, the immediate "ebb" phase is characterized by a low energy expenditure and typically occurs around 12 hours after a traumatic injury or surgical stress.[5] During this phase, reduced oxygen consumption and lower body temperatures decrease the overall energy requirements, diverting energy toward immune responses.[4,5,9]

Subsequently, the "flow" phase follows, featuring an increase in baseline energy expenditure. This phase can develop into a chronic state of "hypermetabolism," which is a catabolic condition that does not respond to adequate nutrient intake, especially when the initial injury is severe.[4,5,9] Together, these two phases contribute to the initial inflammatory response to injury, often referred to as *systemic inflammatory response syndrome* or the *acute-phase reaction.*[9]

One of the primary mechanisms responsible for this heightened metabolic activity is the activation of toll-like receptors on innate immune cells by damage-associated molecular pattern molecules. These molecules consist of intracellular contents that immune cells identify as antigens, such as those from invading microorganisms like endotoxin.[9] On activation, these immune cells release proinflammatory cytokines, triggering the redirection of amino acids from lean body mass and peripheral fat to the liver. This shift in resources enables the liver to produce acute-phase proteins like C-reactive protein instead of transport proteins such as albumin and transferrin.[9,15] These acute-phase proteins serve various functions, including acting as antiproteases, opsonins, coagulation factors, and structural components for wound healing.[9,15] Although a variety of amino acids can be used to produce acute-phase proteins, glutamine becomes the preferred energy source for immune cells because it is used in the synthesis of the antioxidant glutathione.[9,14]

Even though the immune system possesses numerous self-regulatory mechanisms to dampen inflammation, in cases of severe initial injuries, these regulatory responses can become excessive, leading to a state of immunosuppression. This condition is referred to as *compensatory antiinflammatory response syndrome*, or "CARS."[16] Although the hyperimmune and immunosuppressive responses are essential for maintaining a delicate balance between combating infections and limiting harm to the host, they can result in chronic immunosuppression.[9,16] As more patients survive their initial injuries, a condition known as *persistent inflammation, immunosuppression, and catabolism syndrome* has become well documented. This syndrome affects 30% to 50% of patients who survive extended stays in the ICU with organ dysfunction.[16] Managing this catabolic state is particularly challenging because it does not respond well to nutritional interventions.[16] This deficiency of essential nutrients contributes to a widespread weakening of the host's immune and sympathetic responses because there is less fuel available to support these protective mechanisms.[9,16]

Efforts to mitigate the "flow" phase by targeting inflammatory cytokines like TNF-α, IL-1, and IL-6 have not yielded positive results in clinical trials involving ICU patients.[12,17] Similarly, medications designed to reduce overstimulated stress responses by blocking β-adrenergic receptors (β-ARs) have demonstrated benefits but are only effective in specific patient populations, such as severely burned individuals.[18]

Furthermore, attempts to enhance immune function using antioxidants and amino acid supplementation, including substances like glutamine and arginine, have been made, but many of these interventions have not led to improved outcomes and, in some cases, have even had adverse effects on ICU patients.[12,19–21] These challenges underscore the intricate ways in which alterations in metabolism can bring about complex changes in the immune system.

The Metabolic Response

Surgical stress induces a state of hypermetabolism, characterized by increased energy expenditure. The body's energy needs surge to support wound healing, tissue repair, and immune responses. Liver glycogen stores are broken down into glucose through glycogenolysis to provide immediate glucose release. This helps maintain blood glucose levels and is in part caused by increased levels of glucagon. In the absence of adequate glucose, the liver initiates gluconeogenesis increasing production by as much as 50%, synthesizing glucose from the breakdown of amino acids from muscle protein and glycerol. Critically ill patients frequently develop insulin resistance, leading to impaired glucose utilization. This can result in hyperglycemia associated with increased morbidity and mortality in critically ill patients. It is essential that blood glucose levels are closely monitored and controlled with insulin therapy when necessary.

Fats stored in adipose tissue are broken down into fatty acids and glycerol, which are used for energy production. This is related to increased circulating catecholamines. This shift can lead to the production of ketone bodies, which may serve as an alternative energy source for some tissues, particularly the brain. Septic patients have difficulty converting fatty acids to ketones efficiently in the liver, potentiating the effect of proteolysis.

Muscle protein catabolism increases, leading to muscle wasting. This is partly due to the release of catabolic hormones in response to stress and periods of immobility. The amino acids released are used for glucose production and acute-phase proteins. Extended proteolysis is associated with increased glutamine metabolism, which potentially causes the breakdown of the gut mucosal barrier resulting in microbial translocation and increasing the inflammatory response and risk of infection.

The Neuroendocrine Response

Surgical stress activates the hypothalamic-pituitary-adrenal axis, leading to adrenocorticotropic hormone release. This results in increased circulating levels of cortisol, which can remain elevated for 24 to 48 hours after surgery. Cortisol has widespread effects on tissue catabolism and mobilizes amino acids from skeletal muscle to supply the substrates necessary for healing. It also increases circulating blood glucose levels.

Surgical stress also activates the sympathetic nervous system, resulting in the release of catecholamines from the adrenal medulla stimulating the circulatory system by increasing heart rate and blood pressure; alertness is also increased, preparing the body for the physiologic demands of surgery. Aldosterone and antidiuretic hormone are released in response to anesthesia and surgical stress, altering the salt and water excretion along with serum osmolarity. This can be associated with water retention, weight gain, and potential edema in the perioperative period; water excretion is restricted during this time.

The Immunologic Response

Surgical stress triggers an inflammatory response, involving the release of cytokines and other immune mediators. Inflammation is a critical component of tissue repair and defense against infection. The body mobilizes immune cells, such as neutrophils and macrophages, to the surgical site to clear debris and combat potential infections. Inflammatory cytokines, such as IL-6 and TNF-α, contribute to insulin resistance and metabolic alterations. Prolonged or severe surgical stress can lead to a temporary suppression of the immune system, making the patient more vulnerable to infections.

SURGICAL NUTRITION

Nutritional Status Assessment

Nutrient availability plays an important role in determining the likelihood of successful recovery from an operation, making the assessment of nutritional status one of the quintessential aspects of care for the surgical patient.[8] Patients with surgical needs can present anywhere on the spectrum of nutritional status, from underfed to overfed, and both can cause serious detriment to patients, as evidenced by increases in surgical morbidity and mortality.[8,14] The appropriate assessment and diagnosis of malnutrition is important for normalizing outcomes and should be noted in the medical record according to the following sections.

Clinical Evaluation

History and physical examination. In the initial assessment, the healthcare provider must first investigate potential historical factors that could impact the patient's present nutritional condition. This includes looking into potential causes of insufficient food intake, malabsorption problems, or issues with nutrient utilization. Common factors to consider encompass socioeconomic status, previous gastrointestinal (GI) surgeries, substance abuse, and congenital or pathologic malabsorption conditions.[8]

The next step is to determine the specific type of malnutrition the patient is experiencing, whether it is related to protein deficiency, micronutrient deficiencies, and overall calorie deficit, or another cause.[13,15] Categorization can then be made based on the underlying pathology, whether it is associated with starvation, a specific disease, or an injury.[8,10,15] In pediatric patients, acute malnutrition might manifest as observable signs such as pitting edema, sunken eyes, and reduced skin turgor. Chronic malnutrition, on the other hand, could lead to symptoms like signs of kwashiorkor and impaired growth.[8,10,15] For adults, obtaining a timeline from the patient or their family is often more informative. This is because severe conditions like cancer or malabsorption syndromes can result in rapid or gradual weight loss, even though both scenarios might present similar physical appearances within weeks or years.[8,10,15] It is also crucial to recognize that outward physical changes can be misleading. Even in cases where patients are overweight, they may still be malnourished due to factors like hormonal resistance and insufficient lean body mass.[22]

Serum markers. Although serum markers such as albumin, prealbumin, retinol binding protein, and transferrin were once considered reliable indicators of nutritional status, their effectiveness has been called into question.[9,15] In a recent meta-analysis involving otherwise healthy individuals with nutrient deficiencies, it was found that albumin and prealbumin levels remained within the normal range until severe malnutrition had already set in, typically with a body mass index (BMI) below 12 or after 6 weeks of starvation.[15] Furthermore, in case of inflammatory stress, the body may divert amino acids toward the production of inflammatory proteins, leading to reduced levels of these nutritional markers even when the patient is adequately nourished.[9,23] Specifically, the fractional synthesis of albumin remains unchanged after procedures like abdominal surgery and other inflammatory processes, while the leakage of albumin into the capillaries positively correlates with inflammation, resulting in a net decrease in intravascular albumin and prealbumin.[15,24]

The connection between low albumin levels and patient outcomes is unlikely to be causal because multiple clinical studies have revealed that administering albumin to address low serum concentrations did not lead to improved clinical outcomes.[25] Despite these limitations related to the use of nutritional serum markers in the postoperative context, studies have demonstrated a strong or excellent correlation between preoperative albumin serum concentrations and patient outcomes, as illustrated in Table 34.3.[10,24] Therefore, serum markers can be considered useful as preoperative prognostic factors may not serve as reliable

indicators of a patient's nutritional status.[10,25] Although none of the previously mentioned assessment methods are perfect, the combination of screening to identify "at-risk" patients and a recognition of phenotypic and etiologic factors can reliably establish a patient's nutritional risk stratification.

Functional status. A functional assessment provides insights into the patient's functional capabilities and their ability to perform activities of daily living. Evaluating frailty and conducting a preoperative physical therapy assessment are valuable in gauging risk and shedding light on potential malnutrition. It is essential to consider additional patient-specific risk factors, such as age, underlying health conditions, the type of surgical procedure, expected fasting duration before surgery, and any preoperative chemotherapy.

A collaborative approach involving a multidisciplinary team, consisting of surgeons, dietitians, nurses, physical therapists, and other healthcare professionals, is crucial for assessing and addressing the nutritional requirements of surgical patients. Based on the findings from the nutritional assessment, tailored interventions can be implemented to address each patient's specific needs. These interventions may encompass nutritional counseling, adjustments to the diet, support through enteral or parenteral nutrition, and perioperative nutritional optimization to enhance the patient's nutritional status before undergoing surgery.

Imaging. Imaging techniques can be adjuncts to the information obtained from medical history and physical examinations, providing valuable insights into changes in lean body mass, bone mineral density, and adiposity over time. This proves particularly helpful in long-term nutritional assessments.[8,9]

Among these imaging methods, dual-energy x-ray absorptiometry (DXA) scans are widely regarded as the gold standard.[8,26,27] They offer highly accurate measurements of both bone and soft tissues by using low-dose ionizing radiation at two different energy levels to distinguish between these tissue types.[8,26,27] DXA calculates the density of each tissue type, enabling the determination of body fat, lean body mass, and bone mineral density or content.[8,26,27] However, it is crucial to note that the precision and reproducibility of DXA scans may decline whether a standardized protocol is not consistently followed across measurements.[8,27,28] Variables like clothing, nasogastric tubes, or prosthetics have the potential to influence the results.[8,26,27]

Ultrasound, on the other hand, has emerged as a quick and dependable method for assessing muscle mass, especially when patient age and sex are factored in.[8,26,27] In contrast to DXA, ultrasound offers radiation-free assessment that can be performed at the bedside, allowing individual muscle measurements.[8,26,27] Additionally, it provides both quantitative and qualitative evaluations of muscle mass by combining muscle dimensions with muscular density.[8,27,28] Recent studies have demonstrated a good correlation between ultrasound measurements and DXA scans. Nevertheless, standardized measurement protocols are essential due to the operator-dependent nature of ultrasound examinations.[8,26,27] A-mode ultrasound measurements can be taken at the midpoint of the femur between the anterior iliac spine and the upper lateral epicondyle of the femur to determine the cross-sectional dimensions of the rectus femoris.[8,27,28]

Computed tomography (CT) scans can also be used to calculate lean body mass with the assistance of computer algorithms. For example, at the L3 vertebrae, psoas muscles can be employed to estimate whole-body lean mass.[8,26,27] CT scans offer the additional advantage of measuring Hounsfield density units, which can serve as an indicator of muscle quality in addition to quantitative

TABLE 34.3 Association Between Preoperative Serum Albumin and Surgical Outcome

SERUM ALBUMIN (g/dL)	30-DAY MORTALITY RATE (%)	30-DAY MORBIDITY RATE (%)
>4.5	≤1	≤10
3.5	5	25
3	9	35
2.5	15	45
<2.1	≈30	65

Adapted from Gibbs J, Cull W, Henderson W, et al. Preoperative serum albumin level as a predictor of operative mortality and morbidity: results from the National VA Surgical Risk Study. *Arch Surg.* 1999; 134:36-42.

muscle size measurements.[8,26,27] However, it is important to note that CT scanning has limitations, including its high cost and exposure to ionizing radiation. Therefore, the measurement of lean mass using CT scans should be reserved for preexisting imaging data.[8,26,27]

Anthropometric assessment. Anthropometry encompasses all physical measurements of the human body. In medicine, regardless of the specific anthropometric measurement employed, whether for clinical applications or research, the critical factor is consistent standardization of measurement techniques across different assessments. To ensure this standardization, the Centers for Disease Control and Prevention (CDC) has issued the National Health and Nutrition Examination Survey (NHANES) anthropometry procedures manual, which is aimed at promoting uniformity in anthropometric measurements on a national scale. Standardization is of paramount importance for reliable and consistent data collection.[28]

Weight. Accurate and precise weight measurements are essential for hospitalized patients because they contribute to better fluid resuscitation and enable more effective monitoring of a patient's nutritional status.[8,10] In the intensive care setting, daily weight assessments serve as a valuable tool for tracking both long-term trends and smaller fluctuations that can result from nutrient or fluid boluses.[8,10] Body weight increase early in a patient's ICU stay, likely due to fluid overload, is associated with an increased risk of mortality, making close monitoring of body weight a vital component of ICU care.[8,10] It is worth noting that a remarkable increase in body weight early in a patient's ICU stay, often attributed to fluid overload, has been linked to a higher risk of mortality. Therefore, the meticulous monitoring of body weight plays a crucial role in ICU patient care.[8,10]

To assess fluid overload, healthcare professionals should consider the difference between the patient's current weight and their historical dry weight while also taking into account intake and output records and physical examination findings.[8,10] Determining dry weight is typically based on clinical judgment, involving the patient's initial admission weight or extrapolation from documented height and wight data from their medical records before admission.

Like the approach for nutritional assessment, evaluating a patient's fluid status is most effectively done by considering a combination of factors, allowing for a comprehensive clinical assessment.

For patients who fall into the extreme ends of the body-size spectrum, determining their ideal body weight (IBW) through calculation is often more clinically relevant than relying solely on their measured weight. One commonly employed calculation method is as follows:

$$\text{IBW for males} = 50 \text{ kg} + 2.3 \text{ kg for every inch over 5 feet for height}$$

$$\text{IBW for females} = 45.5 \text{ kg} + 2.3 \text{ kg for every inch over 5 feet for height}$$

However, it is important to realize that this method has limitations because it applies only to patients taller than 5 feet and tends to underestimate the IBW for females. In such cases, an alternative approach is to use the BMI method. This involves taking the patient's height and calculating the ideal weight range based on a BMI value within the range of 10 to 21 or 21 to 23 for females.[8,10] For obese patients, an adjusted body weight can be a more suitable consideration. This adjusted body weight is calculated as follows[29,30]:

$$\text{Adjusted Body Weight} = \text{IBW} + 0.4 \text{ (Actual Body Weight - IBW)}$$

Nutritionists frequently use the adjusted body weight when preforming energy calculations, particularly in the context of bariatric surgery.[29,30]

Height. Typically, the patient's height remains relatively stable during their hospitalization, so an initial height measurement is usually adequate for medical purposes, except in cases of pediatric patients with prolonged hospital stays.[4,8,10] However, it is important to be aware that height measurement in intensive care and infant patients are often taken while they are supine, whereas outpatient measurements are taken with the patient standing. This difference in measurement positions can potentially result in incorrect assessments of growth impairment in pediatric patients, emphasizing the need for caution when interpreting such measurements.[4,8,10]

Body mass index. BMI is computed by dividing a person's weight in kilograms by the square of their height in meters. Although it serves as reasonable approximation of body size, BMI has its limitations because it cannot distinguish the proportions of fat, muscle, and bone that constitute the total body mass.[10] Hence, relying solely on BMI to gauge health or nutritional status can be deceptive.[20,31]

Lean body mass. Assessing total lean body mass can be a valuable supplement to BMI. The reduction in lean body mass resulting from catabolic conditions seen in critical illness and following surgery is believed to be a factor in poorer outcomes, such as elevated mortality rates, prolonged time on mechanical ventilation, and extended stays in the ICU.[9,11,12]

In summary, anthropometric measurements provide valuable information about a person's health, growth, and nutritional status, and BMI is the most common anthropometric measurement used. While not a perfect measure, it can provide an initial assessment of nutritional status. An increased risk of morbidity and mortality are noted at either end of the BMI index. Advanced tools like DXA or bioelectrical impedance analysis can help assess body fat and lean body mass. Obese individuals are at significant risk of nutritional deficiencies. Vitamin D, folate, B_{12}, and iron deficiencies are present in this population. Early supplementation of vitamins and minerals, optimization of eating behaviors, and increased physical activity are recommended before undergoing elective surgery. Obese patients also have a history of restrictive diets, which may contribute to lean body mass depletion and impaired muscle function. Sarcopenia and osteopenia are also common, increasing perioperative morbidity and mortality.

Laboratory studies may assist in nutritional assessments. Although not a highly specific marker, low serum albumin levels may indicate chronic malnutrition or inflammation. It has limited value in short-term nutrition assessments given its long half-life of 3 weeks. Low serum albumin is a reliable prognostic indicator of morbidity and mortality. Prealbumin has a shorter half-life (2 days) than albumin and may be a more sensitive indicator of short-term changes in nutritional status. It can be a better index of visceral protein stores in the acute states, but levels can be falsely elevated in renal dysfunction. Anemia can be related to nutritional deficiencies or chronic disease. Low serum transferrin levels may indicate iron deficiency, although they can also be influenced by inflammation. Abnormally high or low levels can indicate protein malnutrition or excess protein intake. These biochemical markers, when used with clinical and dietary assessments, provide a full picture of a patient's nutritional status. It is important to note that no single marker is sufficient on its own, and healthcare professionals consider multiple markers and patient-specific factors to make accurate nutritional assessments and recommendations.

Nutritional Assessment Scores

There are validated nutritional assessment tools that also can be used to identify patients at risk of complications related to malnutrition. The Nutritional Risk Screening (NRS) is a validated tool used to identify patients at risk of malnutrition. It assesses factors such as weight loss, BMI, and severity of disease. The Subjective Global Assessment involves a comprehensive clinical evaluation of nutritional status, including weight loss, dietary intake, GI symptoms, and functional capacity. The Mini Nutritional Assessment is designed for older adults and assesses various aspects of nutritional status, including anthropometric measurements, dietary intake, and psychosocial factors.

Several nutritional assessment scores have been developed to complement the patient's medical history and physical examination. Of these scores, the NRS and the Nutrition Risk in Critically Ill (NUTRIC; Table 34.4), are the only two that consider the severity of the patient's disease and nutritional factors.[8,10,14] In contrast, other scores like the Malnutrition Universal Screening Tool (MUST), the Mini Nutritional Assessment, and the more recent perioperative nutrition screen, illustrated in Fig. 34.2, solely focus on the patient's current nutritional status.[8,10,14]

Due to the ineffectiveness of serum markers in accurately assessing the risk of malnutrition postoperatively, especially considering the acute stress response, it is recommended that all patients admitted to the ICU, as well as those with suspected malnutrition risk, should undergo at least a general assessment.[8,10,14] In cases

TABLE 34.4   The Nutrition Risk in Critically Ill (NUTRIC) Score

VARIABLE	CRITERIA	POINTS
Age	<50 years	0
	50 to <70 years	1
	≥75 years	2
APACHE II	<15 points	0
	15 to <20 points	1
	20–28 points	2
	≥28 points	3
SOFA	<6 points	0
	6 to <10 points	1
	≥10 points	2
Number of comorbidities	0–1	0
	≥2	1
Days from hospital admission to ICU admit	0 to <1	0
	≥1	1
Total	0–4	Low malnutrition risk
	5–9	High malnutrition risk, need nutritional plan

A score of 5 or greater signifies a high risk of malnutrition. The NUTRIC score can also include IL-6 concentrations, with ≥400 adding 1 point. If IL-6 concentrations are obtained, a score of 6 or greater is then considered high risk.
APACHE II, Acute Physiology and Chronic Health Evaluation; *ICU,* intensive care unit; *IL-6,* interleukin-6; *SOFA,* sequential organ failure assessment.
Adapted from Heyland DK, Dhaliwal R, Jiang X, et al. Identifying critically ill patients who benefit the most from nutrition therapy: the development and initial validation of a novel risk assessment tool. *Crit Care.* 2011;15:R268.

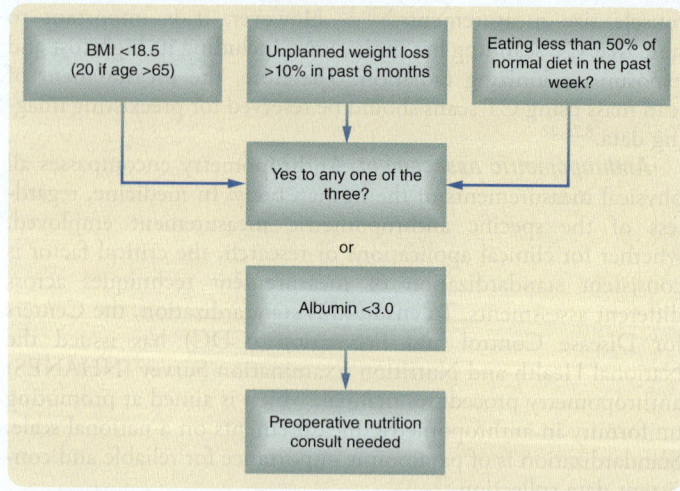

FIGURE 34.2 The perioperative nutrition screen is a simple tool to assess the need for dietician/nutrition consultation to optimize preoperative nutritional status. *BMI,* Body mass index. (Adapted from Nygren J, Thacker J, Carli F, et al. Guidelines for perioperative care in elective rectal/pelvic surgery: Enhanced Recovery After Surgery (ERAS®) Society recommendations. *World J Surg.* 2013;37:285-305.)

where malnutrition is a concern, it is advisable to employ a nutrition risk score as well.[8,10,14]

Nutritional Requirements
Predicted Nutritional Needs

Once the clinical risk of malnutrition in the patient has been evaluated, the consideration shifts to determining the appropriate nutritional supplementation. It is not just the quantity of calories that matters, but also the composition of these calories.[32] For instance, burn patients are believed to gain advantages from diets rich in protein and carbohydrates but low in fat.[18,27] In general, critically ill adult patients are believed to benefit from high protein diets. However, this approach is not suitable for patients with renal failure, as they require low-protein diets with high concentration to prevent urea toxicity and fluid overload.[9,33]

Energy expenditure. Accurately estimating a patient's energy needs remains a significant challenge in clinical practice. Indirect calorimetry is considered the gold standard for estimating resting energy expenditure (REE), but there is a notable degree of variation when REE is measured in clinical settings.[20,26] Errors between two tests conducted on the same day can be as high as 13%, and within the same week, they can be up to 23%.[20,26] Additionally, studies have shown that supplementing caloric goals with REE measurements does not significantly improve patient outcomes.[20,26] Therefore, when indirect calorimetry is used, it is crucial to have strict protocols in place to standardize the measurements.[20,26] In cases where an indirect calorimeter is not available, REE can be estimated using equations like the Harris-Benedict formula:

$$BMR \text{ for males} = (10 \times \text{weight in kg}) + (6.25 \times \text{height in cm}) - (5 \times \text{age in years}) + 5$$

$$BMR \text{ for females} = (10 \times \text{weight in kg}) + (6.25 \times \text{height in cm}) - (5 \times \text{age in years}) - 161$$

Various equations fore estimating energy expenditure exist, including the Korth and World Health Organization equations, which are more accurate for normal-weight patients, and the Harris-Benedict equation, which performs better for obese

TABLE 34.5 Harris-Benedict Energy Expenditure Multipliers

SCENARIO	ENERGY EXPENDITURE MULTIPLIER
Resting (AF)	1.1
Confined to bed (AF)	1.2
Out of bed (AF)	1.3
Minor operation (IF)	1.2
Skeletal trauma (IF)	1.35
Cancer cachexia (IF)	1.3–1.5
Major sepsis (IF)	1.6
Severe thermal injury (IF)	2.1
Febrile (IF)	1 + 0.09 per 0.5°C >38.5

AF, Activity factor; *IF*, injury factor.
Adapted from Long CL, Schaffel N, Geiger JW, et al. Metabolic response to injury and illness: estimation of energy and protein needs from indirect calorimetry and nitrogen balance. *JPEN J Parenter Enteral Nutr.* 1979;3:452-456; and Reeves MM, Capra S. Predicting energy requirements in the clinical setting: are current methods evidence based? *Nutr Rev.* 2003;61:143-151.

patients.[10,22] It is essential to understand that REE is calculated for a patient at rest, but critically ill and postsurgical patient have elevated metabolic rates.[26,24] To account for this, stress and activity factor multipliers, which range from 1.2 for light activity to 2 for thermal injury, should be applied to adjust for the clinical context, providing an estimate of the total energy expenditure (Table 34.5).[18,20,26] Using a combination of parameters is crucial to ensure that patients are neither underfed nor overfed, as single assessment methods can consistently underestimate or overestimate caloric requirements.[26,34] Underfeeding to less than 70% of the true REE can increase mortality, while overfeeding can lead to a higher mortality rate, longer duration on ventilators, and extended hospital stays.[10,35–37]

Additionally, it is important to consider factors like fluid and protein losses due to the patient's clinical condition. For instance, burn patients require 1.5 to 2.5 g of protein per kilogram of body weight per day to compensate for increased protein losses.[10,18] Similarly, critically ill surgical patients with open abdominal wounds have protein requirements similar to patients with 40% total body surface area burns, necessitating approximately 15 to 30 g of extra protein for each liter of intraperitoneal fluid lost to compensate for protein losses.[8,10,18]

Nutritional Support of the Surgical Patient
Preoperative Nutrition Optimization

Identifying malnourished or at-risk patients allows for targeted interventions to optimize their nutritional status before surgery. Malnourished patients are three times more likely to suffer complications and five times more likely to die.[38] A systematic review published in *Journal of Clinical Nutrition* in 2019 emphasized the importance of nutritional assessment in surgical patients.[39] Preoperative supplementation with energy and protein-rich diets or oral nutritional supplements can enhance muscle mass, immune function, and overall nutritional status. A systematic review and meta-analysis in the *Annals of Surgery* in 2019 showed that preoperative nutritional supplementation reduced the risk of postoperative complications in GI surgical patients.[40]

Carbohydrate loading before surgery can help reduce insulin resistance, improve glucose control, and enhance muscle glycogen stores, potentially reducing the risk of postoperative complications. A Cochrane review in 2014 found that preoperative carbohydrate loading was associated with improved outcomes and reduced length of hospital stay in surgical patients.[41] An adequate intake of vitamins and minerals, such as vitamin D, vitamin C, and zinc, is essential for wound healing and immune function. An article in the *Journal of Parenteral and Enteral Nutrition* in 2019 highlighted the role of micronutrients in surgical recovery and emphasized the importance of assessing and correcting deficiencies before surgery.[42]

Achieving and maintaining a healthy BMI before surgery can reduce the risk of complications and improve surgical outcomes. Preoperative weight loss in obese patients improves surgical outcomes and reduces the risk of postoperative complications. Adequate hydration and fluid balance are essential for maintaining organ function and preventing dehydration-related complications. Guidelines from surgical and anesthesia societies emphasize the importance of preoperative hydration and appropriate fasting guidelines to optimize fluid status.

In summary, evidence-based preoperative nutrition involves a comprehensive assessment of nutritional status and targeted interventions to optimize nutritional status before surgery. These interventions can include energy and protein supplementation, carbohydrate loading, micronutrient optimization, lifestyle modifications, and a multidisciplinary approach. Individualized care plans based on patient-specific needs and surgical procedures are crucial to achieving the best possible surgical outcomes.

Evaluating a patient's nutritional status before surgery is of utmost importance to identify those at risk of malnutrition and implement necessary interventions aimed at optimizing their nutritional condition before the procedure. This not only reduces the likelihood of postoperative complications but also promotes tissue healing and enhances overall surgical outcomes. The assessment should encompass a review of the patient's typical dietary patterns and any recent weight fluctuations.

Notably, changes in weight, particularly unintended weight loss, can be indicative of malnutrition and serve as a red flag for healthcare providers. Recognizing such weight shifts can aid clinicians in uncovering underlying medical conditions, such as diabetes, GI disorders, metabolic diseases, or cancer, which all have a significant impact on nutritional status. A weight loss exceeding 5% within the past month or 10% over a 6-month period is suggestive of nutritional risk, and it is associated with increased morbidity and mortality.

Furthermore, the physical examination plays a valuable role in assessing a patient's nutritional status. Observations related to the condition of the hair, skin, nails, and the oral cavity can provide insights into potential vitamin and mineral deficiencies (Table 34.6).

In chronically ill patients, preoperative nutrition is pivotal in enhancing postoperative outcomes. Key elements shown to be beneficial for underweight surgical patients are omega-3 fatty acids and arginine. Each of these components has individually demonstrated the ability to reduce hospital stays and infection rates following surgery.[12,19] Omega-3 fatty acids offer a valuable antiinflammatory effect by competing with proinflammatory omega-6 fatty acids. This competition helps mitigate the inflammatory response triggered by surgery by diverting arachidonic acid away from the production of inflammatory prostaglandins and leukotrienes, specifically PGE2 and LTB2, and instead directing it toward PGE3 and LTB5. Furthermore, omega-3 fatty acids may contribute to reducing local inflammation by preventing the movement of neutorphils.[12,19]

During the stress response, there is a decrease in arginine synthesis and reduced arginine uptake, leading to an overall deficiency

TABLE 34.6	Common Findings of Nutritional Deficiencies	
SYSTEM	**FINDINGS**	**DEFICIENT NUTRIENT**
General	Weight loss, edema, poor growth, anemia	Calories/protein, vitamin A, iron
Skin	Poor wound healing, xerosis, hair loss, excessive bleeding, petechiae, red swollen skin lesions	Vitamin A, niacin, zinc, vitamin C, zinc, vitamin K
Nails	Koilonychia, ridging of nail bed plate, splinter hemorrhages	Vitamins A and C, iron
Hair	Dyspigmentation and corkscrew hair	Copper
Face	Facial paresthesias	Calcium
Eyes	Conjunctival xerosis, keratomalacia, angular palpebritis	Vitamin A, niacin/riboflavin, pyridoxine
Lips	Cheilosis, angular stomatitis	Niacin, riboflavin, iron
Tongue	Atrophic filiform papillae, glossitis	Niacin, vitamin B_{12}
Teeth	Caries	Vitamin C
Gums	Bleeding, spongy, receding	Vitamin C
Neck	Enlarged thyroid	Iodine
Thorax	Decreased muscle mass and strength, dyspnea	Protein/calories
Cardiac	Heart failure	Thiamine
Gastrointestinal	Poor wound healing, hepatomegaly	Protein
Musculoskeletal	Osteomalacia, persistently open fontanelle (infants), epiphyseal enlargement, swollen joints	Vitamin D, vitamin C, thiamine
Nervous system	Mental confusion, weakness, paresthesias, depressed reflexes, sensory loss, tetany	Thiamine, vitamin B_6, niacin, vitamin B_{12}, calcium/magnesium

of arginine. This situation suggests that supplementation could help restore arginine levels to normal concentrations, resulting in improved T-cell function and enhanced collagen synthesis.[12,13]

For surgical patients, the most beneficial results have been observed when omega-3 and omega-6 fatty acids are administered in a 1:1 ratio, often referred to as an *immune-neutral* balance. It is important to note that while various formulations and ratios have been studied, meta-analyses have not shown any formulation or ratio to be consistently superior to others.[12,19] In cases where oral administration is not feasible, parenteral supplementation can be considered as an alternative approach.[43]

Conversely, in adult ICU settings, just under 50% of patients are obese, while approximately 19% of pediatric patients fall into the obese category.[22] It is crucial to distinguish obese patients from those with normal body size because their nutrition requirements differ significantly.[22] Even when the signs of malnutrition may not be as apparent as in underweight patients, obese individuals are at a substantial risk of malnutrition. In fact, patients with a BMI exceeding 30 are 1.5 times more likely to be malnourished compared with those with a normal BMI.[22] Obese patients experience inherent difficulties in nutrient mobilization, making it challenging for their bodies to respond adequately to the stress of surgery.[22]

For obese surgical patients, it is recommended to provide them with high-protein, low-fat, low-carbohydrate diets to best preserve lean body mass and reduce unnecessary triglyceride storage.[22] In such cases, caloric intake should be adjusted toward their IBW by using 65% to 70% of their REE or 11 to 14 kcal/kg of actual body weight per day.[22] Additionally, it is essential to maintain a protein intake of 2.0 to 2.5 g/kg of IDW per day to prevent the catabolism of lean body mass, as outlined in Table 34.7.[22] Furthermore, obese patients face an elevated risk of complications, including hyperlipidemia, and hyperglycemia due to increased gluconeogenesis, among others. Therefore, they should be closely monitored during their hospital stay to address complications related to both overfeeding and underfeeding.

Enhanced recovery after surgery (ERAS) protocols, which encompass preoperative and postoperative nutritional considerations, have demonstrated their effectiveness in improving surgical

TABLE 34.7	Varying Caloric Needs Based on BMI Classification	
BMI	**CLASSIFICATION**	**BASELINE DAILY CALORIC INTAKE**
<18.5	Underweight	30–40 kcal/kg actual body weight
18.5–24.9	Normal weight	25–30 kcal/kg actual body weight
25.0–29.9	Overweight	11–14 kcal/kg actual body weight
30.0–34.9	Obesity class I	11–14 kcal/kg actual body weight
35.0–39.9	Obesity class II	11–14 kcal/kg actual body weight
≥40.0	Obesity class III	11–14 kcal/kg actual body weight
>50	Obesity class III[a]	22–25 kcal/kg ideal body weight

[a]Subdivision created solely for caloric intake; obesity class III consists of any BMI greater than 40.0.
Adapted from Dickerson RN, Boschert KJ, Kudsk KA, et al. Hypocaloric enteral tube feeding in critically ill obese patients. *Nutrition.* 2002;18:241-246; Dickerson RN. Hypocaloric, high-protein nutrition therapy for critically ill patients with obesity. *Nutr Clin Pract.* 2014;29:786-791; and Choban PS, Burge JC, Scales D, et al. Hypoenergetic nutrition support in hospitalized obese patients: a simplified method for clinical application. *Am J Clin Nutr.* 1997;66:546-550.

outcomes.[44] Before surgery, these protocols often involve ensuring proper nutrition up to the day before the procedure and carbohydrate loading with clear liquids up to 2 hours before surgery.[44] After surgery, ERAS protocols aim to reduce the use of opioid medication, which can slow down gastric and intestinal movement, while ensuring adequate pain control. Additionally, they promote initiating a regular diet as soon as the patient is awake enough to swallow after the surgery, rather than waiting for clear signs of restored bowel function.[44] These recommendations have the potential to both shorten the length of hospital stay and enhance the overall results of the surgical procedure.[44]

Preoperative fasting guidelines. Preoperative fasting is a crucial aspect of ensuring patient safety during surgical procedures and anesthesia administration. Guidelines typically recommend fasting from solids for at least 6 to 8 hours and clear liquids for 2 hours before elective surgery and anesthesia to reduce the risk of aspiration, which can lead to severe pulmonary complications.[45] Furthermore, there is no need to postpone elective procedures for adult patients who chew gum, but it is important for healthcare providers to ensure that any gum is removed before administering anesthesia. However, specific fasting instructions may vary depending on factors like age, underlying medical conditions, and the type of procedure.[45] The goal is to strike a balance between minimizing the risk of aspiration and maintaining the patient's comfort and well-being.[45]

Individualized nutrition plans. An individualized preoperative nutrition plan is a tailored dietary strategy crafted to meet the unique needs of a patient before surgery. These plans are designed with a deep understanding of the patient's specific health conditions, nutritional status, and the type of surgical procedure they will undergo. Collaboratively developed by the patient's healthcare team, which may include the surgeon, anesthesiologist, and registered dietitian, these plans aim to optimize the patient's nutritional intake and overall well-being before the surgery. They may involve dietary modifications, supplementation, or other nutritional interventions, such as correcting deficiencies in vitamins and minerals. The goal of such a plan is to enhance the patient's immune function, reduce the risk of complications during and after surgery, and promote a swifter recovery. By addressing the individual needs of the patient, these personalized preoperative nutrition plans play a vital role in improving surgical outcomes and ensuring the patient's health and safety throughout the perioperative period.

Perioperative Nutrition

Enteral versus parenteral nutrition. The current American Society for Parenteral and Enteral Nutrition (ASPEN) guidelines recommend enteral feeding as the preferred option over parenteral nutrition based on the best available evidence.[8] Recent meta-analyses have indicated that there are no significant differences in mortality rates between early enteral nutrition (EN) and early parenteral nutrition.[36] However, the EN group has shown benefits such as reduced infectious complications, including catheter-related bloodstream infections, and shorter hospital stays.[37,46,47]

In the perioperative period, most patients will be able to take enough calories by mouth to prevent the malnutrition associated with surgical stress. However, in the more critically ill patients, and those with underlying comorbidities, nutritional repletion may be required. Enteral and parenteral nutrition are two routes used to provide nutrition to individuals who are unable to meet their nutritional goals orally. Each method has its own set of risks and benefits, and the choice between them depends on the patient's condition, medical requirements, and the clinical context. Patients who are unable to meet at least 60% of their total caloric goals through the oral route need enteral feeding, and patients who are unable meet at least 60% of their total caloric goals through the enteral route need total parenteral nutrition (TPN).

Enteral nutrition helps maintain the integrity and function of the GI tract, as it delivers nutrients directly into the digestive system. This supports the mucosal lining of the gut, reduces the risk of bacterial translocation, and maintains gut motility. EN is associated with fewer infections compared with parenteral nutrition.[47,48] Critically ill patients receiving EN have lower infection rates and improved outcomes compared with those on parenteral nutrition. EN is less expensive than parenteral nutrition, making it cost-effective. Some patients may experience GI intolerance, leading to diarrhea, bloating, and vomiting. This can limit the amount of nutrition delivered and may require adjustments to the feeding regimen.

Tube feeds can be administered through different routes, including nasogastric, nasoenteric, orogastric (in intubated patients), or via a surgically placed gastrostomy or jejunostomy tube. Before use, the tube's correct placement must be confirmed. After nasogastric or nasoenteric placement, an x-ray can confirm placement. After the surgical feeding tubes are placed, they are usually confirmed from direct visualization during the procedure, but if there is any doubt, a contrasted study of the tube with x-ray can confirm placement. Tube feedings are initiated at a slow rate such as 10 or 20 cc/h and increased to goal as tolerated. The head of the bed should be elevated 30 to 45 degrees. The tubes should be cared for, including regular flushing with water, securing the tube, and assessing the tube site for signs of infection or leakage.

Once feedings are tolerated by the patient there are several options to continue. Bolus feeding involves the delivery of larger amounts of formula over shorter periods of time and is the most physiologic method, but this can only be done with gastric feeding. Patients should exhibit adequate gastric emptying before initiation. This is an excellent choice for patients in the outpatient setting. Intermittent feedings involve infusing formula over 20- to 30-minute periods and can be done by both gastric and enteral routes. Continuous feeds are mostly used for inpatients and tend to be the best tolerated among patients.

Contraindications to EN include bowel discontinuity (as in the case of damage control surgery), bowel obstruction, severe GI bleeding, GI perforation, intractable vomiting and diarrhea, severe hemodynamic instability, bowel ischemia, severe acute pancreatitis causing shock, short bowel syndrome (SBS), intestinal malabsorption, and feeding intolerance.

Complications of EN include aspiration pneumonia, tube displacement or malposition, GI disturbances, tube occlusion, and refeeding syndrome. Aspiration pneumonia occurs when gastric contents enter the respiratory tract, leading to inflammation and potential secondary infection. Proper head-of-bed elevation during feeding can help reduce the risk of aspiration. Tube displacement can lead to complications. Tube placement verification, including radiographic confirmation, is essential. Diarrhea, constipation, abdominal cramps, and bloating can occur with enteral feeding. Adjusting the formula composition, fiber content, and rate of administration can help manage these issues. Feeding tube occlusion can hinder the delivery of nutrition. Flushing the tube before and after feeding as well as with medication administration helps prevent clogs. Refeeding syndrome is characterized by electrolyte imbalances, with the hallmark being hypophosphatemia, and fluid shifts in malnourished patients who are aggressively fed. Gradual advancement of enteral feeding rates and monitoring electrolytes can decrease the risk.

Parenteral nutrition should be considered when patients are unable to meet their nutritional needs orally and EN is not feasible or contraindicated. The indications for postoperative parenteral nutrition may vary depending on the patient's clinical condition, surgical procedure, and ability to tolerate oral or enteral feeding. If unable to tolerate at least 60% of total caloric goals enterally, then parenteral nutrition should be considered. Guidelines from the ASPEN emphasize the use of parenteral nutrition when enteral intake is insufficient to meet energy and protein requirements.

Parenteral nutrition provides complete nutritional support, making it suitable for patients with severe malabsorption, bowel obstruction, or impaired GI function. Patients with a high-output GI fistula, defined by an output of 400 mL every 24 hours, may lose significant amounts of nutrients and fluids through the fistula output, necessitating parenteral nutrition to support nutritional needs and fluid balance.[49] Patients with severe GI dysfunction, such as SBS, intestinal failure, or intractable vomiting, may require postoperative parenteral nutrition to ensure adequate nutrient absorption. It is important to note that the decision to use postoperative parenteral nutrition should be made on a case-by-case basis, considering the patient's clinical condition, nutritional status, and the feasibility of other routes of nutrition. Postoperative parenteral nutrition carries risks and should be used judiciously, with ongoing monitoring and assessment to ensure appropriate nutrition support. A multidisciplinary team, including dietitians and clinicians, should be involved in making decisions regarding parenteral nutrition.

Parenteral nutrition is delivered into the central venous system, predisposing patients to all the risks associated with the use of central venous lines. Patients have a risk of catheter line–associated bloodstream infections,[50] highlighting the importance of strict aseptic techniques to minimize infection risk.[50] Complications of parenteral nutrition include catheter-related infections, catheter-related thrombosis, metabolic complications, liver dysfunction, hyperglycemia, and fluid and electrolyte imbalances. Parenteral nutrition can increase the risk of catheter-related thrombosis. Periodic assessment for catheter-related thrombosis and implementing anticoagulation measures when indicated can help mitigate this risk. Metabolic complications of parenteral nutrition include hyperglycemia, hypertriglyceridemia, and electrolyte imbalances. Regular monitoring and adjustment of parenteral nutrition components can prevent these issues. Parenteral nutrition–associated liver disease (PNALD) is a concern, particularly in long-term parenteral nutrition. Strategies to minimize PNALD include optimizing lipid composition and providing EN when feasible.[51] Hyperglycemia is common in patients receiving parenteral nutrition. Tight glycemic control with insulin therapy and appropriate monitoring can manage hyperglycemia.

In summary, the preferred choice will be EN over parenteral, unless there is a hard contraindication, such as bowel obstruction, high-output fistula, severe malabsorption, or long-term impaired GI disfunction. EN should be started as soon as possible through the most natural route the patient's condition allows.

Postoperative Nutritional Care

Safe initiation of postoperative nutrition.
Proper postoperative nutrition depends on the specific clinical circumstances, which may involve factors like a patient's ability to swallow, intestinal continuity, and more.[52] If there are no absolute contraindications to enteral feeding, such as a lack of intestinal continuity, EN can safely commence within the first 24 hours after surgery.[43,52] Early postoperative nutrition has been shown to reduce mortality compared with relying solely on intravenous fluids and may also help alleviate issues like nausea and vomiting.[37,43]

Traditionally, it has been customary practice to initiate oral feeding with a clear liquid diet after surgery, but there is no evidence to support this over starting with a regular, solid diet.[39] When no contraindications to solid food exists, clear liquid diets have demonstrated no physiologic advantage over solid foods.[39,53] Immediate postoperative nutrition of the appropriate consistency has proven beneficial in various surgical contexts, such as after colorectal anastomosis and esophagectomy, where it has led to reduced hospital stays and fewer postoperative complications.[37,43]

According to the ASPEN guidelines, early EN is recommended, even if the patient's bowel function is not yet fully restored.[8] Lack of bowel function could result from mucosal atrophy and immune barrier dysfunction and initiating enteral feeds may help improve postoperative GI dysfunction and reduce the occurrence of ileus.[10]

In the case of surgical patients, either enteral or parenteral nutrition should continue until they can meet at least 60% of their caloric needs though oral intake.[10] Lastly, it is crucial to emphasize that nutritional supplementation for patients should not cease upon discharge as those with malnutrition are twice as likely to be readmitted.[10] Therefore, patients should receive necessary instruction and prescriptions and maintain close follow-up appointments.[10]

When considering nutritional support planning, it is crucial to acknowledge the disparities between the recommended feeding regimen and the actual feeding administration.[9] In the case of surgical patients, interruptions in their feeding regimen can account for approximately 12% to 20% of their total feeding time.[52] Notably, a significant portion of these interruptions is due to preventable factors rather than feeding intolerance. Therefore, it is advisable for hospitals to establish rigorous protocols to minimize instances where feedings are halted. Recent research suggests that up to 65% of the missed feeding time can be prevented through proper planning. To meet the anticipated nutritional requirements, one potential solution involves implementing nurse-directed feeding with 24-hour objectives rather than hourly rates.[43,52]

Macronutrients and micronutrients.
As mentioned earlier, surgical stress and critical illness can make patients more prone to a catabolic and hypermetabolic state, which can be counteracted through adequate nutritional replenishment during the postoperative period. Typically, surgical patients need about 25 to 30 calories/kg and 1.2 to 2 g of protein per kilogram each day, with protein requirements varying depending on the extent of the surgical procedure.

Carbohydrates play a vital role as the body's primary energy source. They are converted into glucose, providing rapid energy for cellular processes, including the healing of wounds. Surgical patients require carbohydrates in amounts that align with their daily energy requirements. Sufficient carbohydrate intake helps prevent the breakdown of muscle protein for energy. Proteins are essential for tissue repair, immune function, and the preservation of lean body mass. Postsurgery, protein is particularly critical for wound healing and reducing muscle loss. Surgical patients may have increased protein requirements due to the demands of the healing process. Fats serve as a source of stored energy, support cell structure, and are involved in the absorption of fat-soluble vitamins. There are no specific recommendations for fat intake in surgical patients, except for the inclusion of healthy fats like omega-3 instead of omega-6.

Vitamin supplementation can also be important in the postoperative period. Vitamin A supports wound healing, vitamin C is required for collagen synthesis, and vitamin E acts as an antioxidant and supports tissue repair. Immune function is enhanced by vitamins A, C, and D. Vitamin K is essential for blood clotting, whereas the B vitamins play various roles in metabolism, energy production, and cell function.

Fluids and electrolytes.
The human body is primarily composed of water, accounting for approximately 60% of total body weight in adults. Body fluids are distributed in various compartments, including intracellular fluid and extracellular fluid. Extracellular fluid further consists of interstitial fluid and plasma. These fluids contain dissolved solutes, including electrolytes and non-electrolytes.

Types of formulas. Enteral nutrition is available in various formulations tailored to address specific clinical requirements. Although most patients typically respond favorably to standard EN formulas, which are not only cost-effective but also suitable for widespread use, there are instances where specialized formulations may be necessary. *It is worth noting that many of these specialized formulas lack extensive clinical trials validating their superiority over standard formulations.*[32] For instance, there are modified formulas designed for patients with allergies, including those allergic to gluten, eggs, lactose, whey, casein, and soy, which cater to their specific dietary needs.[32]

Fiber. The use of fiber can enhance enteral feeding in many ways, depending on the type of fiber employed. A patient's daily total fiber intake should be 25–30 grams. There are two types of fiber: soluble and insoluble. For instance, soluble fiber can undergo fermentation by gut bacteria, leading to slower digestion, particularly in cases of diarrhea.[32] Despite this theoretical benefit, there have been limited studies demonstrating a reduced incidence of diarrhea, especially among critically ill individuals, when using soluble fiber. Soluble fiber also serves as an energy source for colon cells through bacterial fermentation of disaccharides and oligosaccharides, producing short-chain fatty acids like butyrate, propionate, and acetate.[8,10,32]

In contrast, insoluble fiber promotes the movement of nutrients through the digestive system by increasing peristalsis and fecal bulk.[8,32] Typical recommendations for fiber intake is 10 grams per day in healthy individuals experiencing unexplained diarrhea.[8,32] Additionally, prebiotics, which are fibers digested exclusively in the colon following bacterial fermentation, have been demonstrated to positively influence the composition of gut microbiota. Fiber can augment enteral feeding in numerous ways depending on the type of fiber used.[10,32]

Trophic feeds. Trophic feeding is recommended when a patient may be unable to tolerate full feeding. The advantage of trophic feeding in such cases lies in its potential to support intestinal health while minimizing the risks associated with feeding intolerance.[37,43] Nevertheless, numerous multicenter trials have compared full feeding to trophic feeding and found no significant disparities in critical outcomes like mortality, infection rates, and the number of days a patient requires ventilation.[8,10,51]

Continuous versus bolus feeding. In many hospitals across the United States, continuous feeding methods are still commonly employed.[37,43] For a patient, an hourly or daily feeding rate is typically estimated, with the goal of maintaining this rate consistently throughout the day.[37,43] To evaluate a patient's tolerance, hospitals frequently continue to rely on assessing gastric residuals, even though this practice has been shown to be an inadequate predictor of complications.[53] Several randomized controlled trials have indicated that increasing the threshold for gastric residuals from 50 to 150 mL to 250 to 500 mL does not lead to a higher incidence of aspiration.[37,43,53]

As an alternative, hospital protocols should include measures to screen for and prevent aspiration, such as adjusting the patient's bed to an elevated position. Additionally, a physical examination should be conducted to check for signs of distention or abdominal pain in the patient. Prokinetic agents like erythromycin (30–50 mg/kg/day) or metoclopramide (10 mg four times daily) can be used, although there is no demonstrated change in clinical outcomes associated with these therapies.[37,43]

Bolus feeding is theoretically advantageous as it mimics the more typical eating pattern, although at present, there is insufficient evidence to determine whether continuous or bolus feeding is superior.[37,43] When employing bolus feeding, it is recommended

to use formulas with higher caloric density to minimize the risk of fluid overload. In situations where hydration is needed between feeds, water, half-normal saline, or normal saline boluses may be administered via the enteral tube, depending on the patient's sodium levels.[37,43]

Caloric concentration. The formula's concentration can be adjusted based on the patient's age and the cause of their hospitalization.[32] Some medical conditions that might necessitate using more concentrated formulas include renal failure, congestive heart failure, liver failure, and the syndrome of inappropriate antidiuretic hormone (SIADH) secretion.[32] It is crucial to recognize that raising the caloric concentration does not necessarily result in an equivalent change in volume.[10,32]

Gastrointestinal anastomoses. Previously, there was a belief that patients should be kept nil per os (NPO) for several days following intestinal anastomosis due to concerns about the risk of perforation.[10,51] However, recent research has shown that EN is actually beneficial for the healing of anastomoses.[8,10] Alternatively, in cases where oral intake is genuinely not possible and the insertion of a nasogastric feeding tube could lead to perforation, parenteral nutrition is recommended after 5 to 7 days for low-risk patients, and even earlier for high-risk patients if it is anticipated that they will require it for a period of 7 days or longer.[10,51] The greatest benefits were observed in patients who began receiving parenteral nutrition 7 days before surgery, highlighting the importance of preoperative planning when postoperative enteral feeding may not be feasible.[10,43,51]

The timing of nutritional repletion. Early postoperative feeding is associated with reduced catabolism, preservation of lean body mass, and improved wound healing. Guidelines from surgical societies, such as ERAS guidelines, recommend initiating oral or enteral feeding within 24 to 48 hours after surgery, when tolerated. ERAS is a multidisciplinary approach that includes evidence-based strategies to optimize preoperative, intraoperative, and postoperative care, including nutrition, to enhance recovery and reduce complications. Research has demonstrated that ERAS protocols lead to shorter hospital stays, decreased postoperative complications, and improved patient outcomes in various surgical specialties.

Early EN in critically ill patients was associated with a significant reduction in muscle wasting compared with delayed nutrition.[54–57] Early feeding provides essential nutrients and energy, which can promote tissue repair, wound healing, and overall recovery, and may lead to faster recovery and reduced length of hospital stay compared with delayed nutrition.[54–57] Early feeding can support the immune system, potentially reducing the risk of infections and complications.[58,59] Early feeding helps maintain gut function and integrity, preventing gut atrophy and bacterial translocation, but early parenteral nutrition in critically ill patients has been associated with gut mucosal atrophy, whereas early EN has been associated with preserved gut integrity.[60,61] Early feeding can help prevent malnutrition, which is associated with poor outcomes and increased healthcare costs. The literature supports the importance of early nutrition in reducing the risk of malnutrition and improving clinical outcomes in hospitalized patients.[54–57] Starting nutrition early can lead to better tolerance to enteral or oral feeding, reducing the risk of complications like aspiration pneumonia.[62] In 2017, the European Society of Intensive Care Medicine (ESICM) published an updated clinical practice guideline for early EN in critically ill patients. They addressed several different critical illnesses including traumatic brain injury, severe acute pancreatitis, abdominal trauma, and general ICU populations.[63] Early feeding can help prevent postoperative complications, including anastomotic leak after GI surgery.

In summary, evidence-based postoperative nutrition focuses on early initiation of feeding, appropriate nutritional support, and adherence to ERAS principles when applicable. The goal is to optimize recovery, reduce complications, and improve patient outcomes by addressing individual patient needs and surgical requirements. The use of feeding tubes is indicated in specific cases where oral intake is not possible, and EN is preferred over parenteral nutrition whenever feasible due to its associated benefits.

Nutrition in the Critically Ill

For critically ill patients with a baseline of malnutrition, TPN may be beneficial. According to the Society of Critical Care Medicine guidelines, early TPN is recommended for any patient with an NRS 2002 or NUTRIC score of 5 or higher or severe malnutrition who cannot tolerate enteral nutrition. Biochemically, patients with good nutritional status, indicated by low-risk nutrition scores (NRS <3 or NUTRIC score <5), can endure starvation for up to 7 days without significant detrimental effects, provided that clinical improvement and the resumption of nutrition support are anticipated within this period.[9]

Enteral nutrition has been found to enhance intestinal blood flow, trigger the release of bile salts and gastrin, and help maintain the integrity of tight junctions in the gut.[33,43] Failure to provide enteral feeding can lead to gut microbiome dysbiosis, enabling bacteria to breach the intestinal wall, resulting in sepsis and multiorgan failure.[43,61] The overall impact of enteral feeding on gut and immune response is still a topic of ongoing debate. The literature contains both supporting and opposing viewpoints. The beneficial perspective points to improved intestinal villi and structural integrity, whereas the opposing perspective highlights that enteral feeding can provide precursors for leukotrienes and prostaglandins, potentially worsening the inflammatory response.[20,61]

Regarding the choice of location for enteral feeding, studies have demonstrated no differences in pneumonia rates, length of hospital stay, and mortality.[37,43,47] Some studies have suggested improved nutrient delivery with small bowel feeding compared with gastric feeding.[51] Present evidence indicates that gastric feeding is safe, except in cases with an elevated risk of aspiration. In such cases, postpyloric feeding can help reduce the risk of aspiration and pneumonia. Patients at elevated risk of aspiration include those with conditions like gastroparesis.

Hemodynamic Instability/Vasopressor Support

In cases of hemodynamic instability and the initiation or escalation of vasopressor support, EN should be temporarily halted due to inadequate blood flow to the gut and the potential risk of nonocclusive mesenteric ischemia.[10] However, if a patient is showing signs of improvement and vasopressor support is being gradually reduced, enteral feeding may be considered.[8,10] If early EN during vasopressor withdrawal is being contemplated, close monitoring for potential intestinal ischemia should be carried out.[10]

Nutritional Support of Refeeding Syndrome

Refeeding syndrome is a potentially life-threatening condition that can occur in individuals who have endured prolonged periods of starvation.[8,10,14] When nutritional support is initiated, whether through enteral or parenteral means, patients may undergo significant fluid and electrolyte shifts in the early stages, or they may experience episodes of low blood sugar later.[8,10,14] This syndrome is characterized by hypophosphatemia, and often includes other

features like a cachectic appearance, thiamine deficiency, hypomagnesemia, and hypokalemia.[8,10,14]

As phosphate is redirected into the intracellular compartment for ATP production, there is a substantial decrease in extracellular phosphate levels.[8,10,14] Hypophosphatemia can lead to cardiac arrhythmias, infarctions, and even cardiac arrest.[10,14] Before starting nutritional support for severely malnourished patients, any electrolyte imbalances or deficiencies must be identified and corrected.[8] In cases where refeeding syndrome is anticipated, it is advisable to administer high-potency B vitamins and daily vitamin supplementation before beginning enteral nutrition.[8]

Feeding should commence at a rate of 10 calories/kg/day, with gradual increases over 4 to 7 days. Rehydration should progress with the replacement of potassium, phosphate, calcium, and magnesium, and this process should be monitored until the patient's body condition returns to a healthy state.[10]

Burn Injury Metabolic Response and Nutritional Support

A severe burn is not just a physical injury; it is also a profound metabolic challenge. After any significant trauma, the body initiates inflammatory and hormonal reactions that affect how macronutrients are used.[18] Among all types of trauma, burned tissue stands out as an exceptionally potent trigger of the body's overall immune response.[18] Consequently, the metabolic reaction to burn injuries offers valuable lessons about how the body responds to stress and trauma.[18] Studying the process of recovery after thermal injuries has provided valuable insights into the broader realm of surgical nutrition.

Burn injuries exemplify the extreme impact of stress on metabolic processes. The stress response triggered by thermal injuries sets off a range of physiologic reactions aimed at adapting to altered nutritional demands and restoring balance.[27] These responses affect nutrient intake, absorption, and substrate use. Although they may have short-term advantages in the context of the immediate fight-or-flight reaction to injury, in the setting of prolonged critical illness, these changes are often magnified and prolonged.[18]

The metabolic disruption associated with extensive thermal injuries directly contributes to clinical complications, delays in recovery, and increased mortality.[4] The inflammatory and hormonal mechanisms at the root of this response are intricate, involving a sustained elevation in circulating catecholamines, glucocorticoids, and glucagon levels.[18,26] This leads to increased rates of gluconeogenesis, glycogenolysis, and protein breakdown.[18,26] Other notable changes in macronutrient use encompass insulin resistance and heightened peripheral fat breakdown.[4]

Predicting nutrient requirements becomes more challenging, and additional enteral or parenteral feeding is often necessary to address significant deficits.[18] Even with aggressive nutritional support, significant loss of lean body mass is inevitable during acute burn treatment, following the current standard of care.[18] Beyond the acute phase of burn injury, pediatric survivors of extensive thermal injuries continue to experience aspects of catabolic pathology.[4] Negative nitrogen balance, insulin resistance, fat breakdown, and protein loss may persist for up to 2 years after severe injuries, leading to substantial delays in rehabilitation.[4] Researchers are actively pursuing therapies capable of halting or even reversing this protein breakdown in burn patients.[4]

An examination of the progress in burn center nutrition literature offers a glimpse into the evolving field of surgical nutrition. During the pre-early excision era, studies involving burn patients provided some of the earliest empirical evidence showcasing a surge in catecholamines and increased REE in response to trauma.[4] After the establishment of the idea that there is a proportional metabolic reaction to traumatic injuries, the field of burn nutrition played a pivotal role in recognizing the variability of this response among different patients.[4]

Burn surgery played a pioneering role in shifting away from blanket calorie recommendations. It revealed that even in a population with similar injuries, particularly when controlling for burn size, none of the commonly employed equations for predicting calorie requirements could accurately forecast a patient's REE.[4] Furthermore, the burn literature significantly contributed to affirming the importance and safety of initiating enteral feeding at an early stage for critically ill burn patients.[18] Several key principles of modern surgical nutrition have their origins in burn research. These include the understanding of enteric bacterial translocation, the significance of trophic feeding, the safety of uninterrupted postpyloric feeding in the perioperative period, and the recognition of inflammatory side effects associated with high-fat nutrition therapy.[4]

One of the most crucial contributions of burn nutrition research is its role in a fundamental change in surgical nutrition. Through both animal models and human studies of thermal injuries, it was demonstrated that the stubborn deficits in protein and calorie intake associated with such injuries were directly linked to the fundamental connections between systemic inflammation and catabolic processes.[4,38] Moreover, through meticulous examination of the impact of different nutritional approaches on body mass and composition in burn patients, Hart and colleagues established that once a certain threshold was reached, increasing calorie intake for severely burned patients ultimately led to an accumulation of fat rather than the restoration of muscle mass.[27] Collectively, these findings laid the foundation for a pivotal transformation in contemporary surgical nutrition—a shift in perspective from malnutrition being perceived solely as a condition of starvation to understanding it as a comprehensive state of metabolic dysfunction.[4]

Burn surgery has played a foundational role in the development of therapies aimed at addressing the heightened energy expenditure in acutely stressed surgical patients. Patients with thermal injuries have been the focal point for testing numerous interventions designed to alleviate the catabolic response to trauma.[4] In terms of pharmaceutical approaches, various treatments such as recombinant human growth hormone in children, oxandrolone, insulin, insulin-like growth factor (IGF-1), and β-AR blockers like propranolol have been employed to mitigate the excessive catabolic response to thermal injury.[4] Among these, propranolol and oxandrolone have demonstrated the most significant impact, although the latter has been withdrawn from US markets for safety concerns.

Propranolol, a nonselective β-AR antagonist, has been proven to reduce thermogenesis, tachycardia, and REE in burn patients. It also appears to diminish the prolipolytic effects of excessive circulating catecholamines and reduces fatty infiltration in the liver.[4] These findings have encouraged researchers in other fields to explore β-blockade as a strategy to counteract the metabolic repercussions of distinct types of injuries, including brain injury, mechanical trauma, and sepsis.

Of all the measures employed to alleviate the stress-related response to thermal injuries, the early removal of burn eschar stands out as the most effective in terms of reducing the overall energy demand.[4] Although burn excision is most relevant to patients with thermal injuries, there is a broader lesson to be learned that

applies to other surgical patients. The favorable outcomes observed when burn patients undergo early excision emphasize the importance of "source control" in handling the inflammatory response to trauma.[4] We have long recognized the value of early surgical intervention in preventing the harmful consequences of cancers and infections.[4] In the past 25 years, a generation of burn surgeons has shown that the same principle of early, aggressive management of the inflammatory focus in acutely injured patients is, ultimately, our most effective approach to addressing the physiologic imbalances associated with traumatic conditions.[4]

Studies involving burn injuries were among the pioneers in uncovering the molecular mechanisms that underlie enhanced immune responses resulting from dietary modifications.[4] In a particular animal model of severe burn injury, modifying nutrition was observed to lead to reductions in the release of cytokines.[4] In human studies, the REE decreased when early enteral feeding was initiated, as opposed to delayed enteral feeding.[20]

However, the incorporation of immunonutrients, such as glutamine and omega-3 fatty acids, has not demonstrated significant advantages in this patient population.[18] The established guidelines for the care of severely burned patients encompass principles like initiating feeding as early as possible; providing high-protein, high-carbohydrate, and low-fat feeds to counteract hypermetabolism; promoting gut feeding whenever feasible; and supplementing micronutrients even if deficiencies have not been identified.[18] Although it is evident that early nutrition is vital, there are currently insufficient data to endorse specific feeding formulas or nutritional supplements for this patient group.[18]

Nutrition Support in Sepsis

Managing septic patients begins with prevention. Many tools at the disposal of critical care physicians, such as blood transfusions and the use of invasive catheters in veins, arteries, or the urinary tract, have been linked to an increased risk of infections.[12] To prevent infections, it is essential to minimize the use of these interventions and optimize infection prevention. Additionally, these preventive measures can be complemented by early mobilization and prophylaxis against deep vein thrombosis to prevent clot formation and other factors associated with critical illness that can contribute to immune suppression and secondary sepsis.[11,12]

In contrast to the clear benefits of preventive measures, there is ongoing debate about the nutritional support of patients who have developed sepsis. Although some advocate for the immediate and aggressive provision of nutritional support, more commonly, trophic EN is recommended.[37,43,47] EN is believed to be advantageous for septic patients as it helps maintain the integrity of the gut's epithelial lining, thus preventing the translocation of bacteria and additional microbial burden. The recommended protein intake for septic patients during acute resuscitation is approximately 1.2–2.0 g/kg/day, and the recommended nonprotein calorie intake is around 20 calories/kg/day.[37,43,47]

Furthermore, it is not advisable to use immunonutrition with glutamine or arginine, as studies have revealed adverse effects, particularly in ICU patients with preexisting infections.[12,64] The general approach to nutritional support in septic patients still involves closely observing the patient's ability to tolerate or not tolerate feeds during the initial stages of critical illness while providing extended protein calorie support (exceeding 1.5 g/kg/day) during the recovery phase of care.[37,43,47]

During severe sepsis, the body's oxygen consumption can increase significantly, often reaching 50% to 60% above the baseline level.[12] In cases where a septic patient experiences impaired lung function due to conditions like edema, pneumonia, or weakened respiratory muscles, they may struggle to meet the body's oxygen requirements. This situation can be exacerbated by certain dietary choices.[11,12]

The respiratory quotient (RQ) is a measure of the ratio of carbon dioxide produced to oxygen consumed (VCO_2/VO_2) during the metabolic breakdown of fuel substrates.[11,12] Different RQ values are associated with the use of fats and carbohydrates. Pure carbohydrate consumption results in an RQ of 1.0, whereas lipid consumption results in an RQ of 0.7.[11,12] Normally, the pulmonary reserve is substantial enough to effectively eliminate carbon dioxide, irrespective of dietary composition. However, in critically ill patients, overfeeding with carbohydrates can worsen this issue, making it more challenging for patients to be weaned off ventilator support.[32] Nevertheless, the reduction of carbohydrate intake should be approached with caution, considering studies suggesting a potential risk of lung injury with diets that are high in fat, particularly those containing omega-6 fatty acids.[12,19] Tailoring the appropriate balance of macronutrients and addressing micronutrient deficiencies may help enhance survival and aid in the return to daily activities after an acute stay in the ICU and healing of chronic wounds. Nevertheless, further research in this patient population is necessary.[8]

Nutrition Support in Hepatic Insufficiency

To manifest clinical signs of cirrhosis, such as ascites, caput medusa, or jaundice, a significant degree of liver damage is necessary, typically involving the destruction of up to 90% of hepatocytes. When assessing patients with liver insufficiency, their laboratory results will often show elevated levels of alanine aminotransferase and aspartate aminotransferase, along with decreased levels of albumin and a prolonged prothrombin time. It is worth noting that the liver is responsible for producing all coagulation factors except von Willebrand factor (vWF)/factor VIII, which is produced by the endothelium.[65] Consequently, the most consistent indicators of reduced intrinsic liver function are a prolonged prothrombin time and hypoalbuminemia.[65] While partial thromboplastin time tends to remain within the normal range in cases of hepatic insufficiency, bleeding time may either be prolonged or remain normal.[65]

In the absence of the usual glycemic regulation provided by the liver, which includes processes like glycogenesis, glycogenolysis, and gluconeogenesis, the glycogen stores in muscle are swiftly depleted, leading to the development of insulin resistance.[65] This shift forces proteins and lipids to serve as sources of energy, resulting in a decrease in peripheral reserves.[65] This state resembles a catabolic condition seen in conditions like burn hypermetabolism or sepsis, where elevated levels of inflammatory markers like TNF-α, IL-1, and IL-6 have been identified and are considered as potential mechanisms contributing to protein-calorie malnutrition.[65] While there have been suggestions to mitigate protein wastage by including diets rich in branched-chain amino acids, these strategies lack robust scientific validation.[65] Patients with hepatic insufficiency often exhibit concurrent nutrient deficiencies, which may necessitate supplementation, such as addressing low serum levels of potassium, magnesium, and zinc.[65]

The management of patients with hepatic insufficiency revolves around achieving the necessary caloric intake to preserve lean body mass while concurrently limiting fluid intake.[65] However, there is limited research regarding the optimization of specific dietary plans, timing, and methods of supplementation for this patient group.[65] Strategies to enhance oral intake include approaches focused on improving the sensory appeal of meals, promoting uninterrupted meal consumption, increasing meal frequency, reducing meal portion sizes, fortifying meals with high-protein or high-calorie components, and providing greater assistance from healthcare personnel.[65] Even though encephalopathy is a consequence of elevated ammonia levels, it is no longer advisable to restrict protein due to risk of malnutrition. Protein should be 1.2–1.5 mg/kg/day.[65] In cases where ascites is present, treatment entails reducing sodium intake and implementing diuretic therapy or paracentesis when necessary.[65]

SPECIAL CONSIDERATIONS FOR SPECIFIC SURGICAL PROCEDURES

Bariatric Surgery

After undergoing weight loss surgery, such as Roux-en-Y gastric bypass (RYGB) or gastric sleeve, patients may require specialized postoperative diets to prevent deficiencies. Preoperative nutritional evaluation and optimization is standard. Most patients will then follow the stage 1 to 5 diet, advancing from clear liquid diet for 1 to 2 weeks, depending on surgeon preference and advancing to the solid diet set forth by nutrition over several weeks after surgery. Most patients will require multivitamin supplementation including B_{12} injections.

Given the widespread prevalence of obesity, interventions for obese patients are common. Among these interventions, surgical procedures provide the most effective means of alleviating obesity-related metabolic syndromes.[66] The management of nutrition in obese patients starts before surgery and involves efforts to minimize the impact of the metabolic syndrome, enhance blood sugar regulation, and address deficiencies in both macronutrients and micronutrients. It is important to assess vitamin and mineral levels, with a particular focus on fat-soluble vitamins for malabsorptive procedures, necessitating preoperative repletion. A comprehensive understanding of how changes in intake, absorption, and use affect outcomes is crucial for achieving successful results and reducing complications.

Vitamins A, B_1 (thiamine), B_6 (pyridoxine), B_9 (folate), B_{12} (cobalamin), D, E, K, along with minerals such as calcium, iron, zinc, copper, and selenium, are assessed before and after the surgery, and any deficiencies are corrected through established supplementation protocols. For procedures that affect nutrient absorption, there is a greater need for protein and fat-soluble vitamins, with a strong emphasis on vitamin D and calcium. Patients who have undergone bariatric surgery need ongoing nutritional support during the initial phase of weight loss, typically the first year after the surgery, and continuous monitoring to address and prevent any persisting deficiencies.[67]

Nutrient Deficiencies in Bariatric Patients

Extensive research has been dedicated to unraveling the mechanisms that govern appetite and finding ways to address excessive appetite. When an individual consumes fewer calories as part of a planned diet or experiences undesired starvation, the primary hormone responsible for stimulating appetite, ghrelin, is released. It is believed that one of the factors contributing to the success of bariatric surgery in reducing appetite is the removal of stomach sections that are major sources of ghrelin secretion, thereby diminishing hunger signals.[22,29,30]

Operative techniques designed to induce weight loss can be broadly categorized into two groups: restrictive and malabsorptive procedures. Restrictive procedures work by reducing the volume of the stomach, leading to neurohumoral responses of satiety with smaller meal sizes. Examples of restrictive procedures include banding techniques, vertical banded gastroplasty, and sleeve gastrectomy. In contrast, malabsorptive procedures involve altering the normal nutrient absorption route, often involving the removal of a significant portion of the intestine to reduce nutrient absorption and induce weight loss. Malabsorptive procedures encompass jejunoileal bypass (JIB), biliopancreatic diversion (BPD), BPD with duodenal switch (BPD-DS), and RYGB. Among these, JIB operates exclusively through a malabsorptive mechanism, while BPD/BPD-DS and RYGB include the resection of portions of the stomach, providing both a restrictive and malabsorptive mechanism to maximize weight loss. It is important to note that each procedure comes with predictable postoperative complications, including specific nutrient deficiencies.

Despite a well-established awareness of the risks associated with nutrient deficiencies following each surgical procedure, the prevalence of such deficiencies among bariatric patients continues to be notably high.[30] Among macronutrients, the primary concern is the development of protein deficiency, stemming from patients' inability to fulfill their daily protein requirements due to reduced overall food intake.[30] The occurrence of dietary deficiencies in postoperative bariatric patients is believed to arise from a combination of factors, including suboptimal compliance with prescribed dietary supplementation and undiagnosed preoperative deficiencies.[30] For instance, it is worth noting that before undergoing bariatric surgery, 44% of adults were found to have iron deficiency, rendering it one of the most frequently encountered deficiencies in bariatric patients.[29] Additionally, it is important to recognize that most studies on bariatric procedures only track patients for a brief period, typically 1 to 2 years after the surgery, leaving the long-term metabolic consequences unknown.

Adjustable Gastric Band

The adjustable gastric band procedure commonly leads to iron deficiency as the primary nutrient deficiency, prompting clinicians to maintain a vigilant approach in investigating iron-deficiency anemia.[30] Among all bariatric procedures, the lap band demonstrates the lowest incidence of nutrient deficiencies, but it also exhibits the highest rates of reoperation and weight loss failure.[30]

Gastric Sleeve

In the case of sleeve gastrectomy, the fundus of the stomach is the primary site of intrinsic factor production, a cofactor essential for vitamin B_{12} absorption in the ileum.[29] When the greater curvature is stapled or resected during a sleeve gastrectomy, the production of intrinsic factor diminishes, resulting in reduced vitamin B_{12} absorption in the ileum.[29] Consequently, vitamin B_{12} deficiency is the most prevalent nutrient deficiency associated with sleeve gastrectomy. Clinically, this deficiency becomes apparent through symptoms like pallor, fatigue, and megaloblastic anemia as observed in blood smears.[29]

Roux-en-Y Gastric Bypass Surgery

Open RYGB surgery, laparoscopic RYGB, and laparoscopic sleeve gastrectomy have all demonstrated significant effectiveness in achieving weight loss, surpassing the outcomes of adjustable gastric banding.[30] RYGB stands out for its ability to maintain long-term weight loss results, a feature not typically observed in restrictive procedures, while simultaneously avoiding the severe complications associated with other malabsorptive procedures.[22] Following RYGB, patients experience heightened levels of

glucagon-like peptide-1 (GLP-1), also referred to as *incretin*, which has been shown to contribute to reduced appetite. Furthermore, patients enjoy lasting improvements in conditions such as obstructive sleep apnea, diabetes, hypertension, and other aspects of metabolic syndrome.[22]

RYGB is most associated with iron-deficiency anemia, as it carries the risk of incomplete protein digestion and the malabsorption of protein-bound nutrients like iron, intrinsic factor, and vitamin B_{12} when parts of the stomach are bypassed or resected.[29] Additionally, when the proximal small bowel is bypassed, a scenario seen in procedures like JIB, BPD, BPD-DS, and RYGB, there is an increased susceptibility to deficiencies in nutrients primarily absorbed early in the small bowel, especially iron, vitamin D, copper, and calcium.[29] The extent of small bowel bypass is directly proportional to the risk of nutrient deficiencies, with JIB and BPD posing the greatest risk.[29]

Biliopancreatic Diversion With/Without Duodenal Switch

BPD and BPD-DS are only considered after an extremely thorough patient evaluation because they have the highest prevalence of nutritional deficiencies.[29] In these procedures, protein malnutrition, reflected by hypoalbuminemia, is the most prevalent deficiency, occurring in 3% to 11% of cases.[29] Iron-deficiency anemia is also frequent, affecting approximately 5% of cases but potentially reaching up to 12% to 47%.[29] Long-term follow-up of patients who have undergone these procedures has revealed deficiencies in various vitamins and minerals, with a notable focus on calcium and zinc.[29] Furthermore, these procedures result in a 70% reduction in fat absorption and are associated with elevated rates of deficiencies in fat-soluble vitamins.[29]

General Recommendations for Nutritional Optimization in Bariatric Patients

Patients who have undergone bariatric surgery can exhibit a wide spectrum of changes in nutrient levels and utilization, varying from mild to life threatening.[29] Furthermore, postoperative complications can pose significant challenges in helping these patients recover from the effects of the surgery or nutrient imbalances.[29] In general, nutritional counseling should commence several months before bariatric or other reconstructive surgeries. Many healthcare providers use a preoperative weight loss period to assess whether patients can adhere to dietary restrictions similar to those following surgery.[30] Even a 10% reduction in body weight for severely obese patients can offer significant benefits, aiding surgical visualization by reducing the size of the liver, omentum, and peritoneal fat.[29] This preoperative weight loss also contributes to lower rates of postoperative complications related to the heart, lungs, and blood vessels.[68]

These patients necessitate frequent follow-up in outpatient clinic settings. It is advisable for all patients who have undergone bariatric procedures to take daily multivitamins, along with additional supplementation of iron and vitamin B_{12} to prevent anemia after restrictive-malabsorptive procedures.[29] The American Society for Metabolic and Bariatric Surgery offers comprehensive guidance on recommended screening procedures and specific supplement recommendations based on the type of bariatric surgery to address the increased risk of nutrient deficiencies.[29]

Bowel Resection

Patients may experience malabsorption issues. The amount of small bowel required to prevent malabsorption is between 75 and 125 cm depending on the presence of the ileocecal valve. Despite having adequate length, some patients will have diarrhea that requires intervention to promote adequate fluid and nutrient absorption. Often diarrhea can be managed with motility agents to improve intestinal absorption. Common vitamin losses include the B vitamins and interruption of the bile salt absorption affecting fat and fat-soluble vitamin absorption, and loss of the ileum contributes to loose bowel movements even with an intact colon.

Colon resection often leads to the development of diarrhea, while rectal resections, especially in smokers, are more likely to result in loose stools.[69–71] Interestingly, the specific resected segment does not seem to make a difference in this regard, and patients do not report a noticeable decrease in postoperative bowel movement frequency due to colon adaptation.[72]

Patients with ileostomies should receive counseling regarding the signs and symptoms of high output and how to address them, as dehydration is a common cause for readmission.[73,74] Moreover, it is advisable for them to consume provocative foods and beverages in moderation, including alcohol, coffee, and raw fruits, as excessive intake may lead to frequent readmissions with acute kidney injuries and metabolic imbalances.[75] It is crucial for ileostomy output to be around 1000 mL/day or less before the initial discharge.

Short Bowel Syndrome

Short bowel results when the length of the remaining small intestine is insufficient to provide absorption of nutrients. Malabsorption affects energy sources as well as fluid and electrolytes, vitamins, minerals, and drugs. Although most will say less than 200 cm of remaining small intestine results in SBS, there are also other anatomic factors that may or may not allow the absorption of enteral nutrition. The remaining ileocecal valve, length of colon, resection location, and intrinsic disease will affect how the patient will respond to feeding and maintaining fluids and electrolytes.

The ileal brake is a GLP-1-mediated suppression of proximal gastric secretion and emptying, which increases the time for digestion and absorption. If this is missing it may lead to unabated proximal secretions, maldigestion, and lack of satiety.[76] Loss of the ileum also results in B_{12} and bile salt malabsorption with resulting deficiencies, contributing to diarrhea. New therapies for SBS beyond parenteral support and enteral supplementation include antacid medications such as proton pump inhibitors, histamine 2 receptor blockers, and antidiarrheal agents. Novel therapies with GLP-2 agonists act to improve fluid absorption and intestinal and portal blood flow as well as to reduce gastric secretions. Additional benefits are improving intestinal barrier function and inducing growth factors promoting intestinal hypertrophy. As with any disease process, adaptation of the gut can occur, and frequent alterations are necessary to promote the best metabolic state of the patient; therefore, long-term follow-up is needed.

After the resection of the small bowel, the endothelial lining of the remaining bowel undergoes hypertrophy within 48 hours, allowing for sufficient nutrient absorption despite the substantial resection.[10,12] However, in cases where gut resection lacks hypertrophy or a significant amount of gut is removed (typically less than 100 cm of gut remaining without the ileocecal valve or 50 to 75 cm with the ileocecal valve), chronic nutrient deficiencies may develop.[10,12] Crohn disease is the most common cause of SBS in adults, followed by mesenteric thrombosis and gut volvulus.[10,12,77] In children, necrotizing enterocolitis is the primary cause of SBS.[58] The recommended treatment approach for SBS revolves around providing aggressive enteral support to stimulate villi hypertrophy.[77]

In the most extreme cases, the treatment of choice is home TPN, which has demonstrated the potential to extend life expectancy by a significant margin, generally ranging from 10 to 20 years, thereby enhancing overall survival.[10] Moreover, a combination of growth hormone, glutamine, and dietary adjustments has been explored in clinical trials involving individuals with SBS.[64] These trials have shown promise in reducing the quantity of TPN required or even obviating the need for TPN altogether.

Growth hormone has displayed positive effects on weight gain and the absorption of energy. However, it is worth noting that most of these trials have been short, and patients often return to their baseline state of undernourishment after discontinuing the treatment.[77] As of now, the evidence regarding the use of human growth hormone and glutamine in patients with SBS remains inconclusive.[77] Furthermore, there are suggestions that fiber supplementation and elemental feeds may play a role in optimizing nutrient uptake, although the available evidence supporting these practices is weak.[32]

Gastric Resection

Although gastric resections were previously a common treatment for peptic ulcer disease, they are now primarily performed for cancer. Recovery after gastric resection is a lengthy process, with patients typically regaining approximately 75% of their preoperative meal capacity within 2 years. Patients experience a 10% weight loss and tend to stabilize just below this 10% loss after about 3 years. Notably, the outcomes are not influenced by the remaining stomach volume, and increased meal volumes are primarily due to improved digestion and transit. These data enable healthcare providers to better inform patients about the expected weight loss, changes in eating habits, and the recovery timeline.

Transplant Patients

The number of transplant surgeries is on the rise, thanks to improvements in donor systems and hospital capabilities in managing chronic, treatment-resistant diseases. Advances in surgical methods and immunosuppressive drugs have significantly increased survival rates. Transplant patients tend to have elevated REEs for up to a year after the transplant, which can exacerbate nutritional deficiencies caused by the stress of surgery and inflammation.[65] Additionally, the side effects of immunosuppressive medications, including symptoms like nausea, vomiting, dyspepsia, pancreatitis, and diarrhea, often lead to reduced food intake.[65]

After the surgery, providing proper nutrition becomes crucial in preventing protein-calorie malnutrition. This condition can develop due to several factors, including the adverse effects of immunomodulatory medications, the inflammatory response triggered by surgical stress, or immune responses to the transplanted organ.[65] Because of this, the current guidelines recommend a daily caloric intake of 30 to 35 calories/kg and a protein intake of 1.5 to 2.0 g/kg in the acute phase. Calories and protein can be 25 to 30 per kg and 1.3 to 1.5 g/kg respectively in the chronic phase.[65]

Opportunistic infections pose a significant threat to the survival of patients who have undergone major organ transplants.[20,65] Nutritional optimization plays a crucial role in mitigating the immune system suppression that makes these infections more likely. The physiologic effects of organ transplantation differ depending on the organ being transplanted; therefore, specific nutritional guidelines vary based on the type of organ system involved.

For individuals assessed for kidney transplantation, end-stage renal disease leads to changes in protein metabolism, with some patients accumulating harmful ammonia-containing compounds, necessitating dietary protein restriction.[65] Similarly, patients undergoing hepatic transplantation experience a hypermetabolic response similar to that observed in severe burns or cancer. Because the liver is responsible for producing most of the body's circulating proteins, its failure can disrupt critical physiologic processes like blood clotting and glucose regulation, increasing the demand for dietary protein.[65]

In summary, transplant patients present a broad spectrum of metabolic challenges before surgery and experience various patterns of immunosuppression after it. Although detailed regimens tailored to specific transplant types and the nutritional challenges posed by immunosuppressive drug regimens go beyond the scope of this chapter, additional resources for in-depth study can be found through the American Society of Transplantation (www.myast.org) and The Transplantation Society (www.tts.org).

Inflammatory Bowel Disease

Individuals with inflammatory bowel disease, encompassing conditions like Crohn disease and ulcerative colitis, frequently contend with symptoms such as abdominal pain, diarrhea, and constipation. These issues can stem from either reduced caloric intake or the autoimmune disease's damage to the absorptive mucosal lining. Consequently, these patients are at risk of developing protein-calorie malnutrition and deficiencies in essential micronutrients.[77]

Typical instances include deficits in selenium and glutathione, and osteoporosis triggered by vitamin D deficiency, which is especially prevalent among children and the elderly. This type of malnutrition, coupled with the tissue damage inflicted by the autoimmune disease itself, can lead to a vicious cycle of protein depletion and tissue damage. This, in turn, can result in complications such as GI bleeding, the formation of fistulas, and steatorrhea.[58]

The microbial imbalance in the gut brought about by these conditions is characterized by reduced bacterial diversity and increased levels of more harmful strains such as *Escherichia coli*, *Bacteroides* species, and *Mycobacterium avium* subspecies.[77] This can further exacerbate the malabsorption of nutrients. Current approaches focus on rectifying the unhealthy gut microbiome through dietary modifications. Other strategies being explored include prebiotics (foods rich in fiber used to rebalance the gut microbiome), probiotics (foods or supplements containing live microorganisms), antibiotics, and fecal transplantation.[77]

The most effective dietary plans to enhance oral food intake in individuals with inflammatory bowel disease involve high-protein, low-fat, low-carbohydrate diets.[77] Diets that are rich in sucrose, refined carbohydrates, and omega-6 fatty acids, and low in fruits and vegetables, are linked to an increased risk of developing inflammatory bowel disease, particularly Crohn disease. It remains uncertain whether symptoms are a result of heightened consumption of simple sugars or if individuals turn to these sugars to alleviate their symptoms, as restricting these foods has shown limited improvements.[77] To identify specific trigger foods, fasting for a week followed by a gradual reintroduction of individual items while assessing symptom improvement or worsening with each food can be employed. These dietary adjustments can lead to substantial long-term symptom improvement.[77] It is worth noting that diets high in meat and alcohol raise the likelihood of ulcerative colitis relapse. As many dietary plans tend to be highly individualized, efforts related to single-nucleotide polymorphism genotyping may offer a way to enhance symptom management with personalized medical approaches.[77]

Enterocutaneous Fistula

For individuals dealing with primary or iatrogenic enterocutaneous fistulas, TPN is the preferred approach[10] because of its association with increasing the spontaneous closure rate of fistulas without causing a rise in mortality rates.[10,79] Additionally, advancements in surgical techniques and the safety of parenteral nutrition have significantly reduced mortality in this patient population.

In cases involving patients with irradiated bowel or other types of fistulas with a low likelihood of closure, aggressive surgical treatment should be considered only after achieving preoperative control of sepsis, conducting diagnostic studies to determine the path of the fistula, and providing aggressive TPN support.[10,12] An exception to this guideline is when a fistula is located in the distal bowel or has very low output (less than 200 mL/day). In such situations, EN can be attempted with careful monitoring for any increases in fistula output. The administration of parenteral nutrition should be kept as brief as possible and can be complemented with antibiotics, such as ciprofloxacin, metronidazole, or rifaximin, which offer coverage of both aerobic and anaerobic gut flora when administered as home therapy.[10,12]

Acute and Chronic Pancreatitis

In the past, patients dealing with complicated pancreatitis were typically advised to fast until the inflammatory episode subsided.[79] However, a meta-analysis of clinical trials has provided evidence that low-fat diets initiated within 48 hours of hospital admission are safe for individuals with severe acute pancreatitis or those at risk of developing it.[79] Such early dietary intervention has been shown to reduce the incidence of multiorgan failure, although it does not have a significant impact on mortality when compared with EN that commences after the initial 48-hour window.[79]

For optimal enteral feeding, healthcare providers often recommend peptide-based formulas, low in long-chain fatty acids, enriched with medium-chain fatty acids, and hypertonic solutions administered directly into the jejunum.[79] If patients struggle with enteral feedings, parenteral options are available, including crystalline amino acids and hypertonic glucose-containing solutions, containing just enough lipid to meet essential fatty acid requirements.[79]

The management of patients with chronic pancreatitis can be particularly complex. Symptoms of exocrine pancreatic failure, like steatorrhea, typically become evident only when approximately 80% to 90% of exocrine tissue is lost.[79] These patients tend to respond best to diets that are low in fat, low in carbohydrates, and high in protein (usually 1.0–1.5 g/kg/day).[79] In many cases, dietary optimization, which includes a reduction in fat intake and pancreatic enzyme supplementation, proves sufficient for treating malnutrition induced by chronic pancreatitis, offering a viable treatment approach for around 80% of affected patients.[79]

If dietary modifications do not succeed in reinstating proper nutritional levels, alternative approaches to enteral feeding should be explored (as illustrated in Fig. 34.3 and Table 34.8).[79] One option is to attempt nasojejunal tube feeding with a low-fat formula, and if this method is well-tolerated, the consideration of a jejunostomy for home EN becomes viable.[79] Employing jejunal EN may help enhance nutritional status without exacerbating abdominal pain, potentially allowing the postponement of definitive surgery until nutritional health improves. In some cases, this can even lead to the avoidance of surgery altogether.[79] Furthermore, the recommendation is to supplement with calcium, vitamin B, and fat-soluble vitamins due to the common deficiencies

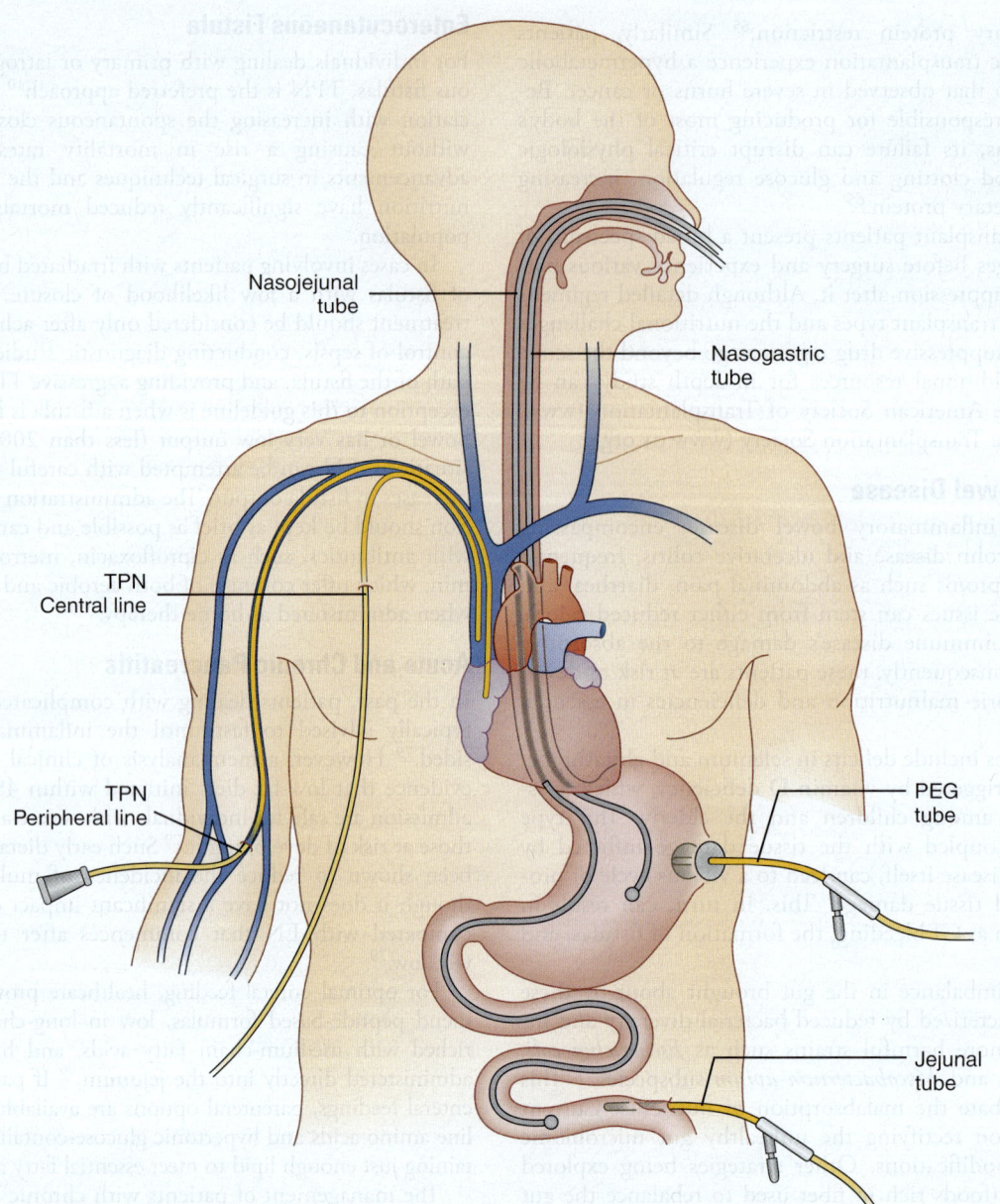

Nasojejunal
tube

Nasogastric
tube

TPN
Central line

TPN
Peripheral line

PEG
tube

Jejunal
tube

FIGURE 34.3 Nasogastric and nasojejunal tube positions. *PEG,* Percutaneous endoscopic gastrostomy; *TPN,* total parenteral nutrition. (From Norbury WB, Herndon DN. Modulation of the hypermetabolic response after burn injury. In: Herndon DN, ed. *Total Burn Care.* 3rd ed. Edinburgh: Saunders; 2007:423.)

of these micronutrients.[79] Various pancreatic enzyme supplements have been suggested as a means of restoring exocrine function to the gut. However, it is worth noting that no studies have provided sufficiently reliable evidence to routinely recommend their use for patients dealing with acute or chronic pancreatitis.[79] Finally, there is evidence to support prolonged preoperative nutritional supplementation aimed at raising albumin levels to over 1.5 g/dL, as this has been associated with decreased mortality rates and fewer infectious complications after surgery for chronic pancreatitis.[79]

Malignancy

Cancer resection patients may encounter alterations in their appetite, taste, and digestive processes. Ensuring proper nutrition is essential for preparing patients to cope with the side effects of cancer treatments. This is significant for individuals who have undergone neoad-

juvant chemoradiation therapy and those with partially obstructing GI tumors. Additionally, patients often experience malnutrition due to the heightened metabolic state that malignancy can induce.

Considerable debate exists regarding the most effective use of nutritional support to enhance outcomes in cancer patients and those with compromised immune systems.[8,9,12] Low-protein diets have been associated with lower cancer rates due to their ability to hinder tumor growth through the engagement of molecular pathways like mammalian target of rapamycin (mTOR) and IGF-1 as well as fibroblast growth factor-21. Several nutritional interventions have shown promise in patients, including omega-3 fish oil supplements, high-dose vitamin D, increased dietary fiber, and coffee, all of which have been found to reduce the risk of colorectal cancer recurrence, extend survival, and decrease mortality. Omega-3 fatty acid supplements have demonstrated effectiveness

TABLE 34.8   Routes for Tube Feeding

ROUTE	SUITABILITY	INSERTION METHOD, CONFIRMATION	ADVANTAGES	DISADVANTAGES
Nasogastric	Short term: functional GI tract	Blind at bedside; fluoroscopy guided	Easy to insert, replace; can monitor gastric pH and residual volume; capable of bolus feeding	Misplacement complications, sinusitis, epistaxis, nasal necrosis, esophageal strictures, erosive esophagitis
Nasoduodenal, nasojejunal	Short term: functional GI tract but poor gastric emptying, reflux, aspiration risk; begin feed only when volume resuscitated and hemodynamically stable	Blind at bedside; fluoroscopy guided; endoscopy guided	Reduced aspiration risk; some tubes enable decompression of stomach while feeding into jejunum	Easily clogged or displaced, aspiration risk, misplacement complications, displacement and reflux into stomach, sinusitis, epistaxis, nasal necrosis; requires continuous infusion; cannot check gastric residuals except with specialized gastric port
Gastrostomy	Long term: good gastric emptying; avoid if significant reflux or aspiration problem	Surgical, percutaneous, endoscopic, radiologic	Bolus feeding; large-bore tube less likely to block	Procedure risks include bleeding, perforation, aspiration risk, dislodgment with peritoneal contamination, wound site infection, granulation
Jejunostomy	Long term: functional GI tract but poor gastric emptying, reflux, aspiration risk, gastroparesis, gastric dysfunction	Surgical, percutaneous, endoscopic, radiologic	Theoretical reduced aspiration risk	Bleeding, infection, perforation, migration, aspiration, dislodgment and leakage into peritoneal cavity, occlusion, pneumatosis, intestinal ischemia or infarction, bowel obstruction; difficult to replace; cannot check residuals; requires continuous infusion

GI, Gastrointestinal.
Adapted from Al-Mousawi A, Branski LK, Andel HL, et al. Ernährungstherapie bei brandverletzten. In: Kamolz LP, Herndon DN, Jeschke MG, eds. *Verbrennungen: Diagnose, Therapie und Rehabilitation des Thermischen Traumas.* New York: Springer-Verlag; 2009:183-194.

in alleviating cancer cachexia, particularly in cases of bile duct and pancreatic cancer.[12,19]

Acquired Immunodeficiency Syndrome

The quest to uncover the underlying cause of protein wasting that does not respond to nutritional supplementation has led to the identification of TNF-α, also known as *cachexin*.[10,16] Subsequently, it was discovered that this cytokine plays a role in promoting cachexia not only in cases of acute inflammation, like sepsis, but also in various other health conditions.[10,16] Cachexia in cancer closely resembles the cachexia observed in individuals with acquired immunodeficiency syndrome (AIDS).[10,16] This similarity arises from the shared mechanisms of chronic inflammation and similar cytokine profiles characterized by elevated levels of proinflammatory cytokines such as TNF-α, IL-1, and IL-6.[10,16] These cytokines can be released either by the host's immune system or directly from the tumor itself.[16] Regardless of the trigger (a virus or chemotherapy), both patient groups can experience profound immunosuppression alongside severe cachexia.[16]

Individuals with AIDS often confront opportunistic infections that affect the upper digestive and respiratory systems, leading to issues like *Candida* overgrowth or viral ulcers.[16] Furthermore, the side effects associated with highly active antiretroviral therapy or chemotherapy frequently result in digestive problems that hinder a patient's ability to maintain proper nourishment.[16] Whether these issues stem from the primary cancer itself or ulcerative lesions, many patients experience nutrient deficiencies due to complications in the oral cavity, esophagus, or the neuromuscular aspects of the swallowing process.[16] In managing these complex health conditions, a general approach to optimize nutritional support involves delivering nutrients through enteral or parenteral methods when the disease symptoms or medication side effects impede the patient's ability to consume sufficient nutrients.[16,32] If

caloric restriction is due to partial obstructions in the oropharynx or esophagus, alternative solutions like high-nutrient liquid or puree drinks can be prepared as substitutes for enteral feeding when the obstruction is not complete.[31]

TPN plays a vital role in treating malnutrition stemming from abdominal or pelvic radiation and the accompanying epithelial inflammation that hinders nutrient absorption.[8,52] It is a useful intervention until enteritis resolves, allowing for the resumption of enteral feeding. In many cases, dysgeusia can develop because of underlying mineral deficiencies like iron, zinc, and B vitamins.[8] Correcting these deficiencies can contribute to restoring regular nutritional intake.[8] Additionally, medications designed to alleviate nausea or enhance gut motility can be valuable in addressing concurrent symptoms like nausea, constipation, or diarrhea, which can further dampen appetite.[8]

There have been experimental approaches aimed at mitigating the immune response underlying cachexia.[9,12,38] These include treatments with nonsteroidal antiinflammatory drugs, anticytokine medications, amino acids, and omega-3 fatty acid supplements. Furthermore, factors like concurrent depression or pain can lead to appetite suppression and are linked to inflammation resulting from the stress response.[10]

LONG-TERM NUTRITIONAL CARE FOR SURGICAL PATIENTS

The goal of surgery is to restore the individual's ability to function independently, which requires energy and building blocks necessary for healing and activity. This requires the ability to take in nutrients and energy sources and have the anatomic and physiologic capabilities to process them. Surgical nutrition does not end after hospitalization and requires continued problem-solving for the surgeon, as every surgical intervention poses some risk to normal physiology.

When one thinks of long-term nutritional support several interventions require constant management. SBS, bariatric surgery, and recovery from resection of any part of the GI tract mandate ongoing therapeutic interventions. Even a common operation such as cholecystectomy can result in sufficient alterations in digestion that must be addressed. Follow-up is paramount in good surgical care.

FUTURE DIRECTIONS AND RESEARCH

Surgical nutrition is undergoing constant evolution. New fields of research emerge as nascent technologies and pharmaceuticals are developed. One such trend that requires further research is the new class of weight loss medications, the GLP-1s. Their popularity is surging with notable effects on weight loss. However, their long-term effectiveness and effects on the perioperative period require further study. Medical weight loss programs are becoming integrated into the preoperative preparation for patients with large ventral hernias in attempts to reduce infection risks and recurrence rates.

The development of prehabilitation programs focusing on physical therapy and nutrition will continue to develop more robust support as their effectiveness is evaluated. Cardiac surgery research is looking at preoperative nutrition optimization and their effects on surgical outcomes. Surgical oncology continues to focus on this, and the European Society of Parenteral and Enteral Nutrition (ESPEN) and ASPEN guidelines continue to be updated to reflect such changes.

CONCLUSIONS

An understanding of nutrition and metabolism in surgical patients is essential for all clinicians. Nutritional optimization and support have constantly been shown to improve outcomes and reduce complications in patients. It is one of the most important, and at times overlooked, interventions we can provide for our patients. The understanding of nutrition's effects on physiology, biochemistry, and immunology continues to be revealed through ongoing research. Nutritional support has advanced beyond just the provision of calories in the surgical patient. It is a therapeutic tool for both elective and critically ill patients. We can now focus on preoperative nutritional optimization, early enteral feeding, and the use of specific substrates (e.g., fatty acids, glutamine) as an integrated approach to nutrition in surgical patients. As our understanding evolves, one can expect even more tailored approaches to nutritional supplementation in patients based on genetics, pathology, and other factors.

Surgeons with extensive experience are well acquainted with the causes and repercussions of disrupted metabolism, especially in the most severe cases encountered by medical experts. Consequently, these knowledgeable surgeons possess a deep understanding of the intricate connections among metabolic processes and how to manipulate them to benefit their patients. As the field of bioenergetics continues to advance, it is likely that we will uncover improved therapies that can enhance the body's metabolic responses to diseases and injuries, whether inside or outside the operating room. Nutritional disorders have become increasingly complex, and dedicated surgeon-scientists will persist in making significant contributions to groundbreaking solutions addressing these challenges.

SELECTED REFERENCES

Elke G, van Zanten AR, Lemieux M, et al. Enteral versus parenteral nutrition in critically ill patients: an updated systematic review and meta-analysis of randomized controlled trials. *Crit Care*. 2016;20:117.

A high-quality systematic review and meta-analysis of the literature's most relevant randomized clinical trials in enteral against parenteral nutrition in the critically ill patients.

McClave SA, Taylor BE, Martindale RG, et al. Guidelines for the provision and assessment of nutrition support therapy in the adult critically Ill patient: Society of Critical Care Medicine (SCCM) and American Society for Parenteral and Enteral Nutrition (A.S.P.E.N.). *JPEN J Parenter Enteral Nutr*. 2016;40:159-211.

An all-inclusive overview of the most recent guidelines for nutrition support in the critically ill patient.

Reignier J, Boisrame-Helms J, Brisard L, et al. Enteral versus parenteral early nutrition in ventilated adults with shock: a randomised, controlled, multicentre, open-label, parallel-group study (NUTRIREA-2). *Lancet*. 2018;391:133-143.

A large-scale multicenter randomized controlled trial comparing early enteral versus parenteral nutrition in a severe critically ill patient population.

Reintam Blaser A, Starkopf J, Alhazzani W, et al. Early enteral nutrition in critically ill patients: ESICM clinical practice guidelines. *Intensive Care Med*. 2017;43(3):380-398.

This clinical practice guidance by the European Society of Intensive Care Medicine includes 17 recommendations and encompasses five meta-analyses that address topics such as traumatic brain injury (TBI), severe acute pancreatitis, gastrointestinal procedures, abdominal trauma, and the broader ICU patient population.

Wischmeyer P, Carli F, Evans DC, et al. American Society for Enhanced Recovery and Perioperative Quality Initiative Joint Consensus Statement on Nutrition Screening and Therapy Within a Surgical Enhanced Recovery Pathway. *Anesth Analg*. 2018;126(6):1883-1895.

Discusses Enhanced Recovery After Surgery Protocol, which includes nutrition aiming to shorten length of stay, improved time on return of bowel function, decrease overall complications, and increase patient satisfaction.

The full reference list appears on Elsevier eBooks+.

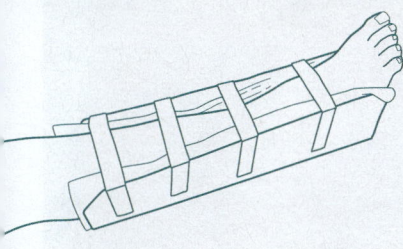

CHAPTER 35

Primary Soft Tissue Infections

Rondi B. Gelbard and Rindi Uhlich

OUTLINE

INTRODUCTION

Skin and soft tissue infections (SSTIs) are a heterogeneous group of conditions affecting the epidermis, dermis, subcutaneous tissue, and fascia. They range from cellulitis or simple abscesses that can be treated with drainage or oral antibiotics alone to polymicrobial deep soft tissue infections requiring surgical intervention. Complicated SSTIs, which also include necrotizing and burn wound infections, large or deep space abscesses, and infected pressure ulcers, account for significant morbidity, mortality, and hospital costs, frequently entailing prolonged intensive care unit (ICU) stays and complex therapies. Without early recognition and effective source control, they may lead to sepsis and life-threatening organ dysfunction due to dysregulated host-response to infection.[1] SSTIs that lead to disseminated infection can become a serious clinical problem with extensive diagnostic and therapeutic challenges.

Various classification systems exist to describe SSTIs based on depth of infection, anatomic location, or severity of clinical presentation. In the past, SSTIs were broadly categorized into uncomplicated and complicated infections. More recently, the US Food and Drug Administration (FDA) introduced the new terminology, "acute bacterial skin and skin structure infections (ABSSSI)," to describe cellulitis, erysipelas, wound infection, and major cutaneous abscesses. In 2018, the World Society of Emergency Surgery (WSES) and the Surgical Infection Society–Europe (SIS-E) recommended a classification approach based on anatomic location, presence or absence of purulence and necrotizing tissue, and clinical condition of the patient.[2] Given the complex nature of SSTIs, these two societies, along with the Global Alliance for Infections in Surgery (GAIS), World Surgical Infection Society (WSIS), and the American Association for the Surgery of Trauma (AAST) joined forces in 2022 to generate a document guiding management and promoting global standards of care for SSTIs.[2] Given the vast differences in management and clinical outcomes, this chapter will mainly focus on necrotizing and non-necrotizing SSTIs, in addition to a few important soft tissue infections in unique patient populations.

NONNECROTIZING SOFT TISSUE INFECTIONS

Nonnecrotizing SSTIs affect approximately 10% of patients admitted to the hospital and are a common problem encountered by general surgeons.[2] Such infections are typically limited to the level of the subcutaneous tissues and include erysipelas, impetigo, folliculitis, and simple and complex abscesses. Our skin, normally colonized by multiple different strains of bacteria, is the primary physical barrier preventing microbial invasion of the dermis and deeper tissue layers. Although SSTIs can occur via the hematogenous spread of infection, more often it is a compromised skin barrier (due to trauma, surgery, pressure, etc.), along with the host's weakened defenses (e.g., diabetes, steroids, immunosuppressants), that ultimately leads to infection.[3,4]

Diagnostic Workup of Nonnecrotizing Soft Tissue Infection

The diagnosis of nonnecrotizing infections is predominantly made clinically. However, imaging can be a useful adjunct depending on the patient's clinical condition and available resources.[5] It is important to note that obtaining diagnostic imaging should never delay operative intervention, especially in the acutely ill patient. Options include plain radiographs, ultrasound, computed tomography (CT) scan, and magnetic resonance imaging (MRI). Ultrasound is a cost-effective, readily available method of determining whether an SSTI has a deeper component or associated abscess. It is more sensitive than plain radiographs and can help to avoid unnecessary incision and debridement of indurated wounds where an underlying fluid collection cannot be ruled out definitively on physical examination alone.[6] The Surgical Infection Society (SIS) recommends performing point-of-care ultrasound (POCUS), as it changes management in up to 10% of cases.[7,8] However, this imaging modality does have several limitations, including the inability to evaluate deeper structures and potential underestimation of the extent of infection.

A CT scan has multiple advantages including fast acquisition time, availability, and interpretability. This modality also allows for evaluation of deeper structures than ultrasound.[5,9] Findings on contrasted CT scans may include skin thickening, fat stranding, edema, presence or absence of gas, and potentially a thickened fascial layer. If an abscess is present, it will appear as a ring-enhancing collection of fluid. MRI is a superior modality for evaluation of the soft tissues and has a greater sensitivity than CT for detecting inflammation, fasciitis, myositis, and areas of necrosis.[5] When used in the investigation of SSTIs, IV gadolinium–based contrast should be administered. Unfortunately, obtaining an MRI can be quite time intensive and costly and may not be readily available in some centers.

It can be difficult to determine exactly when detailed culture data will be required in the treatment of nonnecrotizing SSTIs. In the setting of a recurrent abscess, any foreign material should be identified and removed, and bacterial cultures should be obtained for species identification and determining antibiotic susceptibility. Conversely, routine cultures, tissue aspirates, or skin biopsies of cellulitis or erysipelas are not warranted, unless the patient is immunocompromised or other signs of systemic illness are present.[8] This is because blood cultures are positive in less than 5% of cellulitis cases and are therefore very low yield. Similarly, biopsy specimens may yield organisms in up to 30% of cases, but bacterial concentrations are often very low. As with necrotizing soft tissue infections (NSTIs), appropriate antibiotic therapy and source control, when necessary, are the tenets of successful management.

Types and Treatment of Nonnecrotizing Soft Tissue Infection

Erysipelas

Erysipelas presents as a painful, erythematous area of induration. It is distinguished from cellulitis by its involvement of the upper dermis, clearly demarcated borders, and raised areas of skin. Erysipelas is most commonly caused by group A β-hemolytic streptococci (GAS; *Streptococcus pyogenes*) or another *Streptococcus* species. Although few studies have demonstrated the superiority of any one antibiotic over another,[10] for routine outpatient management, the choice of oral antibiotics includes amoxicillin-clavulanate or cephalexin.[2] Among patients at risk for community-acquired (CA) methicillin-resistant *Staphylococcus aureus* (MRSA; i.e., immunocompromised, contact with MRSA infection, colonization within the past year, 5 or more days of antibiotics within the past 90 days, or no response to first-line treatment), trimethoprim and sulfamethoxazole (TMP-SMZ), minocycline, or doxycycline are reasonable options, although they are not active against group A and B streptococci so combination therapy might be required.[2] In case of severe β-lactam allergy (i.e., anaphylaxis), clindamycin may be substituted for this regimen, although resistance to this antibiotic is becoming more common. In the inpatient setting, antibiotic choices include cefazolin or amoxicillin-clavulanate.

For patients exhibiting signs of systemic illness, IV antibiotics targeting both *S. aureus* and streptococci should be initiated immediately, and coverage for MRSA with vancomycin or linezolid should be considered based on the previously mentioned risk factors, although CA-MRSA in this setting is very rare.[2,8] Linezolid has the advantage of high bioavailability even in its oral preparation and is capable of protein synthesis inhibition (i.e., toxin production). Daptomycin is another agent that has rapid bactericidal effect and is active against gram-positive bacteria including MRSA. Five days of antibiotics will resolve most episodes of erysipelas; however, if symptoms persist, therapy may be continued for up to 10 days.[8]

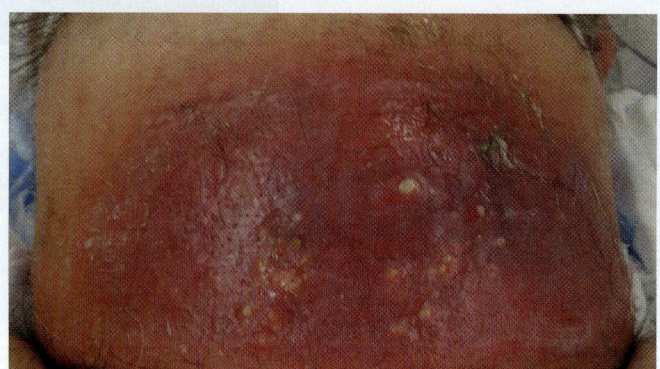

FIGURE 35.1 Carbuncle on the nape of the neck. (From Henry S, Strong BL. Soft tissue infections. In: Asensio JA, Meredith WJ, eds. *Current Therapy of Trauma and Surgical Critical Care*. 3rd ed. Elsevier Inc.; 2024:669.e46-669.e59.)

Furuncles and Carbuncles

Furuncles or "boils" are pus-filled collections involving hair follicles, where suppuration extends through the dermis into the subcutaneous tissue. Furuncles are most commonly caused by *S. aureus*. A carbuncle occurs when the infection involves multiple adjacent follicles causing a coalescent inflammatory lesion with purulent drainage. These often develop on the back of the neck (Fig. 35.1). Treatment for both of these superficial infections is incision and drainage, and antibiotics are not routinely required, unless there is extensive surrounding cellulitis. In the case of recurrent furunculosis, eradicating staphylococcal carriage is the best way to control further outbreaks. Application of mupirocin ointment in the anterior nares for patients with nasal colonization reduces recurrence by 50%. Daily clindamycin use is also helpful for decreasing subsequent infections.

Cutaneous Abscesses

A cutaneous abscess is a collection of pus located in the dermis that may involve the deeper soft tissue. They tend to be painful with fluctuant red nodules surrounded by swelling and erythema. A simple abscess can usually be distinguished from a more complex infection on physical examination. Characteristics of a simple abscess include localized erythema and induration without deep tissue extension, and a single cavity without the presence of multiloculated areas. Simple abscesses in immunocompetent patients are typically treated with incision and drainage without packing.[2,8] Ultrasound-guided aspiration alone is likely to fail. Antibiotics are indicated for immunocompromised patients; multiple abscesses or those larger than 5 cm; abscesses in the face, hand, genitalia or other areas that are difficult to drain; and those that fail to improve with incision and drainage.[2] In such cases, amoxicillin-clavulanate, cephalexin, doxycycline, TMP-SMZ, clindamycin for 5 days (extended up to 10 days if symptoms fail to resolve) is recommended for simple abscesses after drainage.[2] For deeper, more severe purulent infections, vancomycin, linezolid, tigecycline, daptomycin, ceftaroline, or telavancin are appropriate options.[11] The addition of anti-MRSA therapy may minimize recurrence, although the data supporting this are limited.

Cellulitis

Typical cellulitis is a simple infection involving the deeper dermal layer of skin as well as the subcutaneous fat. It occurs when bacteria enter through a disrupted cutaneous barrier, so patients with less effective host defenses (i.e., obesity, diabetes), fragile skin, or

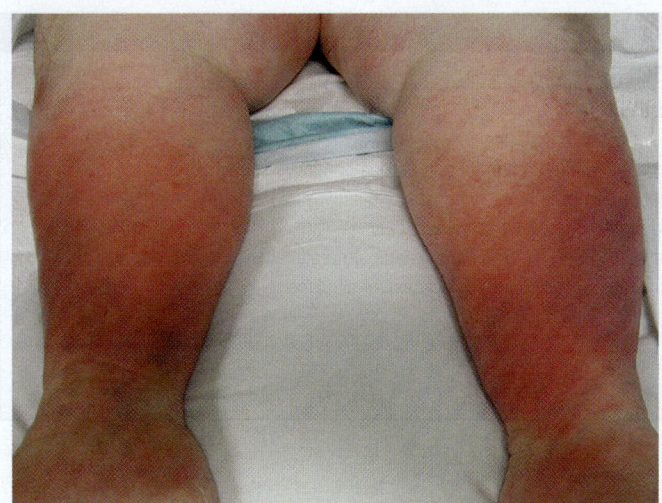

FIGURE 35.2 Cellulitis involving the lower leg in a patient with obesity and lymphedema. (From Henry S, Strong BL. Soft tissue infections. In: Asensio JA, Meredith WJ, eds. *Current Therapy of Trauma and Surgical Critical Care*. 3rd ed. Elsevier Inc.; 2024:669.e46-669.e59.)

preexisting skin conditions are more susceptible. Cellulitis occurs most frequently in the lower extremities and typically causes local signs of inflammation including erythema, warmth, lymphangitis, and pain at the affected site. The most frequently involved pathogens are streptococci and *S. aureus*, although *S. aureus* alone is responsible for the majority of purulent cellulitis cases (Fig. 35.2).

Although there is no evidence of differences in clinical response rates for antibiotic route or duration,[11,12] typical cellulitis is usually treated with oral amoxicillin-clavulanate or a narrow-spectrum β-lactam antibiotic effective against streptococci for no more than 5 days (although this can be extended up to 10 days for persistent symptoms). Purulent cellulitis, on the other hand, requires incision and drainage. For severe infections requiring inpatient therapy, cefazolin is appropriate, whereas a course of piperacillin/tazobactam should be initiated for immunocompromised patients at risk for gram-negative infections.[2] Clindamycin is a reasonable alternative for patients with β-lactam allergy. Although MRSA coverage is not routinely required for typical cellulitis in average-risk patients, antimicrobials affective against CA-MRSA should be considered in cases of purulent cellulitis.[2]

In terms of other antibiotic regimens for nonnecrotizing infections, fluoroquinolones are no longer recommended due to their safety profile and risk of severe and potentially irreversible side effects such as tendinitis and tendon rupture, peripheral neuropathy, and central nervous system effects.[8] Tetracycline derivatives such as omadacycline have been shown to be noninferior to linezolid for treatment of SSTIs but are typically reserved for multidrug-resistant pathogens and are not recommended as first-line agents.[13] Duration of antimicrobial therapy for cellulitis varies based on patient-specific characteristics, including the etiology and clinical severity of infection, patient comorbidities, and adequacy of source control. In general, there are no data supporting antibiotic courses exceeding 5 days for improved efficacy, although therapy can be extended if needed, depending on individual patient response.[14] In addition to treating macerated skin and keeping skin well hydrated, limb elevation and compression stockings should be used to reduce edema and minimize recurrent episodes.

NECROTIZING SOFT TISSUE INFECTIONS

Necrotizing soft tissue infection (NSTI) is an all-inclusive term describing any rapidly progressing soft tissue infection involving any or all layers of the soft tissue compartment, including the dermis, subcutaneous tissue, superficial and deep fascia, and muscle. Unlike nonnecrotizing infections, NSTIs are characterized by thrombosis of venules and arterioles leading to ischemia and necrosis of the tissue that typically extends beyond the subcutaneous tissue layer. Although the nomenclature and classification of NSTI differs across the literature, it may include necrotizing cellulitis, necrotizing fasciitis, necrotizing myositis, Fournier gangrene, Meleney streptococcal gangrene, and clostridial myonecrosis. NSTI is most commonly seen in the extremities and abdominal wall, although any part of the body can be affected. Fournier gangrene, for example, is a fulminant form of NSTI that involves the perineal, genital, or perianal regions. Regardless of the affected body region or tissue layer, NSTIs are all characterized by rapid progression, tissue necrosis, and high rates of sepsis and mortality. They require rapid surgical intervention and adjunctive therapies to mitigate poor outcomes.

Establishing an early diagnosis depends on a high index of suspicion. The problem lies in the fact that this is a relatively rare diagnosis and there is a lack of familiarity with NSTIs. In terms of the incidence of NSTIs in the United States, estimates range from 1000 to 1500 cases annually in the literature. However, these numbers likely underestimate its occurrence because many of these numbers are extrapolated from CDC surveillance data for GAS infections, which only constitute a percentage of NSTIs. A more recent analysis of the National Inpatient Sample estimated an annual incidence of 33,600 cases in 2018, or 10.3 per 100,000.[15] Although the number of NSTI cases appears to be increasing, it is unclear whether this is due to an increased awareness of the diagnosis, aging of the population, or improved survival of immunosuppressed individuals.

Clinical Manifestations of Necrotizing Soft Tissue Infection

It is thought that up to 71% of NSTIs are misdiagnosed on initial evaluation.[16] This often results in inadequate treatment and delayed surgical source control, which contributes to higher mortality. One of the reasons for misdiagnosis is that the presentation of NSTI can be very heterogeneous. NSTIs due to GAS, *Clostridium,* and *Vibrio* species are more likely to present with rapid onset, rapid progression of symptoms (e.g., pain out of proportion to examination, cutaneous findings), and severe systemic toxicity resulting in sepsis. In these critically ill patients with classic signs and symptoms of disease, the diagnosis is more clear and definitive treatment will likely be initiated rapidly without further testing. In contrast, polymicrobial NSTIs may present in an indolent fashion with ambiguous symptoms and no signs of systemic toxicity. In this scenario, patients may not seek medical attention right away, and when they do, unnecessary imaging and testing may result in further delays in care, resulting in worse outcomes.[16]

Types of Necrotizing Soft Tissue Infection

Although the cause of varying severity of presentations is unknown, patient demographics likely play a role, as do the different microorganisms involved. Three distinct categories of NSTI are typically described. Type I is the most common; is caused by polymicrobial gram-positive, gram-negative, and anaerobic organisms; and typically affects immunocompromised patients, or those with multiple comorbidities such as diabetes, renal failure, and peripheral vascular disease. The microbial synergy of the contributing microorganisms is thought to lead to a more insidious presentation. In contrast, type II is

TABLE 35.1   Bacterial Toxins and Effects

ORGANISM	TOXIC SUBSTANCE	EFFECTS
Clostridia	Alpha toxin	• Tissue necrosis • Cardiovascular collapse
Streptococci and staphylococci	• M-1 and M-3 proteins • Exotoxins A, B, and C • Streptolysin O • Superantigen	• Increased ability to adhere and escape phagocytosis • Damage endothelium, cause loss of microvascular integrity and tissue edema and impair blood flow at the capillary • Stimulate CD4 cells and macrophages to produce TNF-α, IL-1, and IL-6 • Stimulate T cells to produce excessive cytokine • Emesis
Vibrio vulnificus	• Hemolysin • Cytolysin • LPS	• Iron release; vascular permeability, apoptosis of endothelium; hypotension • Cytokine release TNF-α

IL, Interleukin; *LPS,* lipopolysaccharide; *TNF,* tumor necrosis factor.

monomicrobial, with GAS (especially the toxin-producing strains of *S. Pyogenes*) as the most frequently isolated microbe, although MRSA is seen in parts of the United States. These isolated organisms produce exotoxins that trigger T-cell activation and a cytokine cascade that can lead to fulminant systemic toxicity, without the need for synergy (Table 35.1). Compared with type I, patients with type II NSTIs tend to be younger and healthier and may report a history of trauma, surgery, or IV drug use as an inciting event. Type III is typically described as consisting of *Vibrio vulnificus* or *Clostridium* species, although some consider these to also fall into the type I category.[16] Classic clostridial myonecrosis has become relatively uncommon, although the prevalence of gram-negative and multidrug-resistant infections are reportedly increasing.[17] Regardless of the type or causative pathogen, all have the potential to cause severe infection, necessitating immediate surgical intervention.

Diagnosis of Necrotizing Soft Tissue Infection

In most cases, superficial cutaneous findings are underwhelming and mask the extent of deeper soft tissue necrosis. Although erythema, warmth, and pain are common, these are also seen in milder infections including cellulitis. Findings more specific to NSTI, such as crepitus, skin necrosis, and bullae, are present less than 40% of the time, so they cannot be relied upon for diagnosis. Although signs and symptoms of systemic illness (i.e., fever, hypotension, organ failure) should raise suspicion for NSTI, the lack of obvious necrosis should not delay further investigation, including local wound exploration, if necessary. Over the years, multiple risk calculators, including the Fournier Gangrene Severity Index (FGSI), Uludag Fournier Gangrene Severity Index (UFGSI), and the Laboratory Risk Indicator for Necrotizing Fasciitis (LRINEC; Table 35.2) score, have been created to facilitate earlier diagnosis and predict outcomes of NSTI. Although the LRINEC score is among the most widely used, studies have shown that it lacks sensitivity for ruling out NSTI and does not accurately predict NSTI outcomes.[18–20]

With regard to imaging, various modalities have been studied for their efficacy in diagnosing NSTI, including plain radiographs, CT, MRI, and ultrasound. Gas in the soft tissues is seen in less than half of plain radiographs done for NSTI but is detected more readily on CT scan. Inflammatory changes, abnormal signal intensity, fluid collections, or lack of fascial enhancement can help establish a diagnosis of NSTI, especially when clinical findings are absent or ambiguous. However, adjunctive imaging should not be obtained if it will delay definitive management, especially in unstable patients. Moreover, an absence of imaging findings does not definitively rule out a diagnosis of NSTI.

TABLE 35.2   Laboratory Risk Indicator for Necrotizing Fasciitis Scoring System

VARIABLE	UNITS	SCORE
C-reactive protein	≥150 mg/L	4 points
White blood cell count (per mm)	15–25	1 point
	>25	2 points
Hemoglobin	11.0–13.5 g/dL	1 point
	<11 g/dL	2 points
Serum sodium	≥135 mmol/L	1 point
	<135 mmol/L	2 points
Serum creatinine	>1.6 mg/dL (or >141 pmol/L)	2 points
Serum glucose	>180 mg/dL (or >10 mmol/L)	1 point

RISK CATEGORY	LRINEC SCORE, POINTS	PROBABILITY OF NSTI (%)
Low	≤5	<50
Intermediate	6–7	50–75
High	≥8	>75

LRINEC, Laboratory Risk Indicator for Necrotizing Fasciitis; *NSTI,* necrotizing soft tissue infection.
From Santos A, Onkendi E, Dissanaike S. Surgical infections and antibiotic use. In: Townsend CM, ed. *Sabiston Textbook of Surgery: The Biological Basis of Modern Surgical Practice.* 21st ed. Dokumen PUB; 2021:226.

When the diagnosis is not entirely clear based on clinical examination or imaging alone, local exploration with a 2-cm full-thickness elliptical excision of the soft tissue (including skin, subcutaneous tissue, fascia, and muscle) can be performed. Depending on the anatomic location of the infection, this can either be done at the bedside with local anesthesia or in the operating room. The excised tissue is carefully inspected for gross tissue necrosis, purulent fluid, grayish discoloration, or noncontractile muscle, although these pathognomonic findings are only seen in approximately 50% of cases.[16] For patients with equivocal findings on macroscopic evaluation, a full-thickness biopsy with fresh frozen section and Gram stain may be helpful, although care must be taken to avoid performing a smaller, superficial incision that will lead to partial evaluation of the tissue layers or false-negatives due to sampling error.

If pathology or fresh frozen biopsy is not readily available, the "push" or "finger" test, in which the surgeon applies blunt finger pressure to the subcutaneous tissue at the margins of the incision, can be performed. If the tissue is easily dissected without any resistance, this is suggestive of NSTI and wide excisional debridement is indicated.[21] Collection of superficial samples should be avoided, but blood cultures, as well as fluid and deep tissue cultures from the wound, can help guide antimicrobial therapy. Metagenomic next-generation sequencing is an emerging method for rapidly detecting broader ranges of pathogens (including anaerobic bacteria, yeasts, viruses) compared with routine microbiologic testing. Although this has the potential to eventually change how we diagnose infections, especially those caused by organisms that are difficult to culture, these tools are not yet ready for widespread use.[22]

Treatment of Necrotizing Soft Tissue Infection
Surgical Debridement

Surgical debridement remains the mainstay of treatment for NSTI. Early and complete debridement has been shown to significantly impact outcome with the most aggressive strategies associated with lower mortality.[23] One study found that surgery within 6 hours of diagnosis lowered mortality by 50%.[23] A generous incision is performed and macroscopic findings are used to help guide the extent of the debridement. Incisions must be extended as needed to enable complete visualization and removal of all infected or necrotic tissue. Even questionable tissue should be sharply removed during the initial debridement, and some surgeons will even excise a 1- to 2-cm rim of normal-appearing tissue to ensure negative margins (Figs. 35.3–35.4). Skin-sparing approaches may have better cosmetic and functional reconstructive outcomes, but should only be used if the skin is completely uninvolved, and wide undermining must still be performed to remove all underlying necrotic tissue. Some studies have classified the degrees of skin viability into zones to help guide debridement. For NSTI of the extremities, limb amputation may be necessary to achieve healthy margins. Although several scoring tools such as the amputation in necrotizing fasciitis (ANF) risk score have been evaluated for their ability to predict the need for amputation, they should not replace clinical judgement, and intraoperative findings will often dictate when amputation is necessary.[24]

After the initial debridement, patients are usually managed in the ICU and interval debridements are performed until no further necrosis or infected tissue is encountered. There is no high-level evidence to guide the timing or frequency of re-debridement.

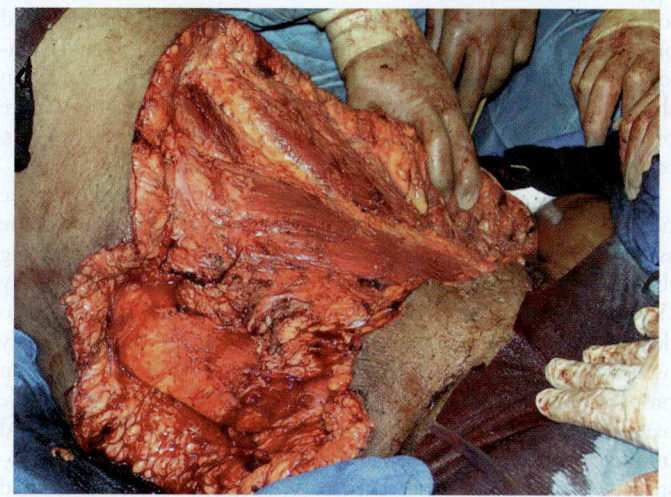

FIGURE 35.3 Surgical debridement of necrotizing soft tissue infection.

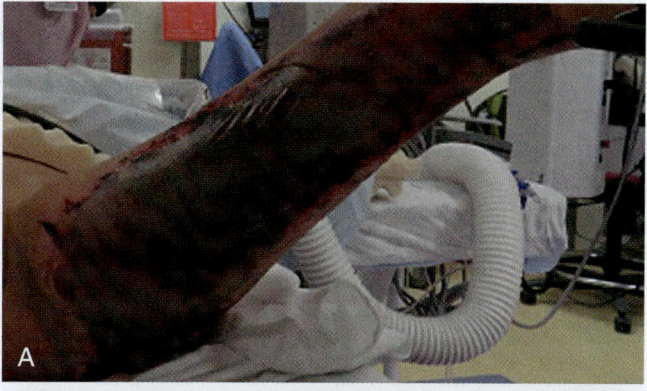

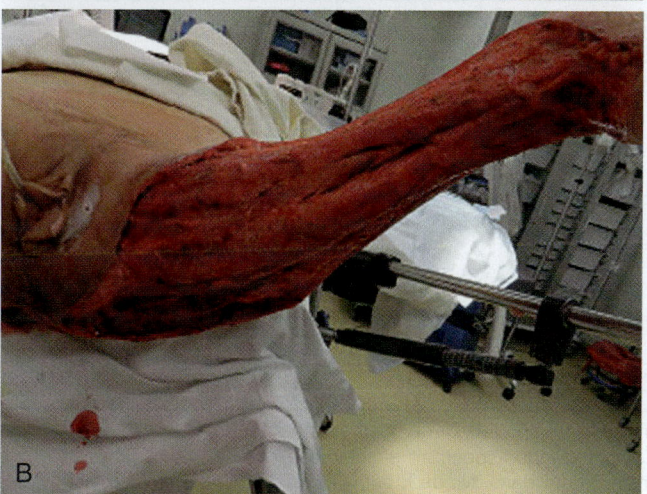

FIGURE 35.4 (A) Necrotic posterior thigh necrotizing soft tissue infection before debridement. (B) After debridement to viable muscle. Fascia, subcutaneous fat, and necrotic skin removed. (Taken from Henry S, Strong BL. Soft tissue infections. In: Asensio JA, Meredith WJ, eds. *Current Therapy of Trauma and Surgical Critical Care.* 3rd ed. Elsevier Inc.; 2024:669.e46-669.e59.)

Older studies have found that short interval re-debridement is associated with improved outcomes, while more recent findings suggest that a single debridement is sufficient if all necrotic tissue is removed at the index operation, and bedside wound checks allow for thorough evaluation of the wound.[25] In the authors' experience, patient physiology and signs of ongoing tissue ischemia should determine the need for ongoing debridements.

Antimicrobial Treatment

Broad-spectrum antibiotics effective against gram-positive, gram-negative, and anaerobic organisms as well as MRSA should be initiated as soon as the diagnosis is suspected (Table 35.3). There are really no data to support one antibiotic regimen over another. In general, empiric treatment with a broad-spectrum β-lactam (i.e., piperacillin-tazobactam) and anti-MRSA agent (i.e., vancomycin, linezolid or daptomycin) is recommended. Clindamycin is typically added to the regimen for its toxin-neutralizing properties against streptococcal and clostridial species. The SIS and Infectious Disease Society of America (IDSA) guidelines strongly recommend combination therapy with penicillin and clindamycin for NSTI due to GAS (with or without toxic shock syndrome).[8] The use of carbapenems for covering resistant gram-negative bacilli should be guided by local antibiograms and individual patient risk factors including recent β-lactam exposure, hospital-acquired infection,

TABLE 35.3	Antibiotic Options for Necrotizing Soft Tissue Infections	
BACTERIA ISOLATED	**ANTIMICROBIAL AGENTS**	**ADULT RECOMMENDED DOSAGE**
Polymicrobial (streptococci, *Staphylococcus aureus, Escherichia coli, Bacteroides* spp.)	Piperacillin/tazobactam	4.5 g every 6 h
	Or meropenem	1–2 g every 8 h
	Or ceftriaxone + metronidazole	2 g once daily + 0.5 g every 8 h
	Or cefotaxime + metronidazole	1–2 g every 6–8 h + 0.5 g every 8 h
	All with clindamycin	600–900 mg every 6–8 h
Monomicrobial group A *Streptococcus (Streptococcus pyogenes)*	Penicillin G	2×10^6–4×10^6 units every 4–6 h
	Or ampicillin	1–2 g every 4–6 h
	All with clindamycin	600–900 mg every 8 h
Clostridium spp.	Penicillin G	2×10^6 to 4×10^6 units every 4–6 h
	Or ampicillin	1–2 g every 4–6 h
	All with clindamycin	600–900 mg every 8 h
Aeromonas hydrophila	Doxycycline	100 mg every 12 h
	Plus ciprofloxacin	500 mg every 12 h
	Or ceftriaxone	1–2 g once daily
Vibrio vulnificus	Doxycycline	100 mg every 12 h
	Plus cefotaxime	1–2 g every 8 h
	Or ceftriaxone	1–2 g once daily
Methicillin-resistant *S. aureus*	Linezolid	600 mg every 12 h
	Or clindamycin (if susceptible)	600–900 mg every 8 h
	Or vancomycin	1 g every 12 h, trough level adjustment (15–25 µg/mL) or 20–25 mg/kg bolus followed by 25–35 mg/kg/24 h in continuous infusion
ESBL-producing Enterobacterales *(E. coli, Klebsiella pneumoniae)*	Meropenem	1–2 g every 8 h
	Tigecycline[a]	50–100 mg every 12 h

[a]Tigecycline should not be used as monotherapy.
ESBL, Extended-spectrum β-lactamase.
From Peetermans, M, de Prost N, Eckmann C, et al. Necrotizing skin and soft-tissue infections in the intensive care unit. *Clin Microbiol Infect.* 2020; 26(1): 8-17.

and a history of extended-spectrum β-lactamase (ESBL) infection.[26] In fact, multidrug-resistant organisms including ESBL-producing *Escherichia coli* or *Klebsiella* species are emerging in different parts of the world and anaerobic bacteria are often underappreciated in Fournier gangrene. These factors should be taken into consideration when initiating antimicrobial therapy.[27,28]

It is important to keep in mind that the delivery of antibiotics to the affected tissue in NSTIs may be impaired by tissue necrosis and altered tissue perfusion from microvascular thrombosis, although most available data on antibiotic diffusion are derived from non-NSTI patient populations. In addition, vasodilation, capillary leak, and extravasation of fluid into the interstitial space is a common phenomenon among patients with septic shock. This "third spacing" may lead to low plasma levels of hydrophilic antibiotics and, therefore, inadequate antibiotic distribution to the target tissues.[29] This is true for antibiotics including β-lactams, glycopeptides, and aminoglycosides, which selectively distribute into the extracellular space.[2] β-Lactams demonstrate time-dependent activity, so treatment efficacy is impacted by the amount of time that unbound plasma drug concentrations remain above the minimum inhibitory concentration (MIC). As a result of these pharmacokinetic alterations, prolonged or continuous infusions, higher frequency dosing, and therapeutic drug monitoring may be required to achieve desired concentrations for optimal bactericidal activity.[29]

Antibiotics must be deescalated once the patient is clinically improving and culture results are available. In terms of duration of antimicrobial therapy, some studies suggest continuing antibiotic therapy until no further debridement is needed and the patient has clinically stabilized for at least 48 hours.[30,31] In 2021 SIS published

updated guidelines for the management of complicated SSTIs stating that "…shorter course antimicrobial therapy (<7 days) appears equivalent to longer therapy and should be considered."[8] Multicenter observational studies are underway in this area to help determine the optimal duration of antibiotics (Fig. 35.5).

Adjuvant Therapy

In addition to source control and antibiotics, early goal-directed resuscitation with fluids and vasopressor support is often required throughout the perioperative period, especially for patients exhibiting signs of sepsis or septic shock. Close monitoring in an ICU is essential for early detection and management of clinical decompensation and organ failure. Of note, while fluid resuscitation and reversal of coagulopathy should be initiated immediately for those presenting in shock, it is not necessary to fully correct all abnormalities before proceeding to surgery. *Without achieving adequate source control first, complete reversal of metabolic derangements is unlikely.*

Intravenous immunoglobulin (IVIG) is thought to mitigate the superantigen-mediated cytokine cascade and toxic shock syndrome associated with streptococcal or staphylococcal NSTI by neutralizing the exotoxin produced superantigens. Although the results of early IVIG studies were promising, subsequent randomized trials failed to demonstrate a clinical, functional, or survival benefit; thus, it is rarely used today.[28] The use of hyperbaric oxygen (HBO) has also been proposed as an adjunctive treatment for NSTI, as it may increase oxygen delivery to hypoxic tissues, killing anaerobic bacteria and improving leukocyte activity (Table 35.4). Although several retrospective studies found that hyperbaric oxygenation was associated with lower mortality rates and a decreased number of debridements

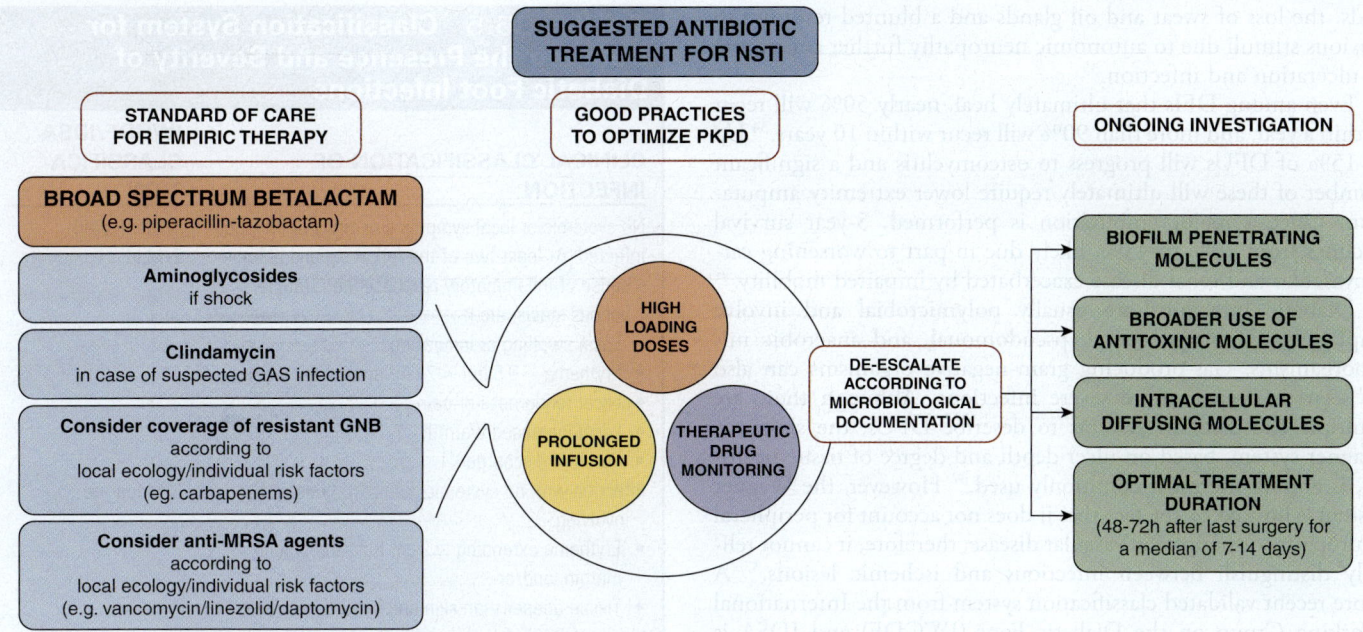

FIGURE 35.5 Suggested antibiotic treatment for necrotizing soft tissue infection. *GAS,* Group A β-hemolytic streptococci; *GNB,* gram negative bacteria; *MRSA,* methicillin-resistant *Staphylococcus aureus; PKPD,* pharmacokinetic–pharmacodynamic. (From Urbina T, Razazi K, Ourghanlian C, et al. Antibiotics in necrotizing soft tissue infections. *Antibiotics [Basel].* 2021;10[9]:1104.)

TABLE 35.4 Proposed Beneficial Effects of Hyperbaric Oxygen

Inhibits growth of anaerobic organisms

Reduces the production of clostridial toxin

Improves leukocyte bacterial killing

Bactericidal and bacteriostatic effects on a variety of organisms

Enhances efficacy of certain antibiotics

Modulates cytokine levels

Decreases tissue edema

Increases collagen formation

to achieve source control, others found no significant mortality difference.[28,32] In addition, it is not readily available in most centers, and there is insufficient evidence at this time to recommend its routine use. Other immune modulators, such as reltecimod, a CD28 T-lymphocyte receptor mimetic, may also improve Sequential Organ Failure Assessment scores, but it does not have widespread clinical acceptance or penetrance currently given the lack of clinical benefit or change in hospital resource usage.[33]

Wound Care and Reconstruction

Wounds can be managed with wet-to-dry gauze dressings that are changed once or twice daily. Depending on the affected area, dressing changes can be quite cumbersome and painful and may initially require additional analgesia or sedation. For perineal NSTIs, it may be necessary to divert the fecal stream with a loop colostomy to prevent further contamination of the wounds. Once the acute infection is resolved and no further debridement is needed, negative pressure vacuum dressings can be used for several weeks to assist with dermotraction and preparation of the wound bed for autografting or placement of dermal matrix. Negative pressure (with or without continuous instillation of irrigation solutions) can also augment tissue perfusion and blood supply, decrease edema and bacterial bioburden, and accelerate the wound healing process. Extensive reconstruction for coverage of any resulting soft tissue defects should be delayed until patients have recovered from the acute episode.

Long-term management of NSTI requires a multidisciplinary approach that extends beyond the operative period. Patients with NSTI often have significant morbidity due to the infection itself, including chronic pain and poor functional outcomes, which significantly impact quality of life. They can also develop complications associated with critical illness, including ventilator-associated pneumonia and other nosocomial infections, acute kidney injury, and thromboembolic events. As such, they are best managed at centers with critical care, wound care, nutrition, and physical and occupational therapy capabilities to help achieve the best long-term outcomes. Early transfer to a facility with these resources should be considered.

OTHER TYPES OF SKIN AND SOFT TISSUE INFECTIONS

Diabetic Foot Infections

Diabetes is associated with a high incidence of foot complications, which are a leading cause of disability worldwide. Up to one-third of people with diabetes will develop a foot ulcer in their lifetime, and over half of these will become infected, contributing to even higher morbidity, mortality, and poor quality of life. In fact, diabetic foot ulcers (DFUs) are an independent risk factor for premature death.[34] DFUs usually begin with a break in the skin as the inciting event. Preexisting comorbid conditions such as cardiovascular and renal disease, as well as microvascular injury and malnutrition, all predispose to the development of diabetic foot infections (DFIs), which range in severity from cellulitis to gangrene. In addition to shunting of blood around capillary beds, the loss of sweat and oil glands and a blunted response to noxious stimuli due to autonomic neuropathy further contribute to ulceration and infection.[35]

Even among DFIs that ultimately heal, nearly 50% will recur within a year, and more than 90% will recur within 10 years.[34] Up to 15% of DFUs will progress to osteomyelitis and a significant number of these will ultimately require lower extremity amputation. Once a major amputation is performed, 5-year survival declines from 70% to 43%, likely due in part to worsening cardiovascular and renal disease exacerbated by impaired mobility.[36]

Diabetic infections are usually polymicrobial and involve staphylococcal, streptococcal, pseudomonal, and anaerobic microorganisms. Gas-producing gram-negative organisms can also be seen in deeper, more severe infections. Although there are multiple classification systems to describe DFUs, the six-grade Wagner system, based on ulcer depth and degree of tissue necrosis, is among the most commonly used.[37] However, the Wagner system is limited by the fact that it does not account for peripheral neuropathy or peripheral vascular disease; therefore, it cannot reliably distinguish between infectious and ischemic lesions.[37] A more recent validated classification system from the International Working Group on the Diabetic Foot (IWGDF) and IDSA is shown in Table 35.5.

DFIs are typically diagnosed clinically with a thorough physical examination. Unfortunately, there is no isolated lab value that can definitively diagnose or rule out an infected diabetic foot lesion, although elevated levels of inflammatory biomarkers such as C-reactive protein (CRP) and erythrocyte sedimentation rate (ESR) may help support the diagnosis of infection in equivocal cases.[38] Microbial analysis for determining bacterial colony counts is unreliable for differentiating infected from noninfected DFUs because there is no consistent value that defines an infection in the literature.[39] Similar to other SSTIs, plain radiographs can help detect foreign bodies and gas within the soft tissue, although bone erosion and other findings of osteomyelitis may not be visible in the acute period. CT scans can identify deeper abscesses, whereas MRI will enable earlier diagnosis of osteomyelitis. If cultures are performed, samples should be taken from the deeper soft tissue rather than a superficial swab to avoid detecting clinically insignificant colonization. In cases of suspected osteomyelitis, bone cultures can help confirm the diagnosis and guide antimicrobial selection. Although newer technologies such as hyperspectral imaging devices or infrared thermography may facilitate earlier detection and treatment of DFUs, they are not yet available for widespread use.[40]

In addition to maintaining euglycemia, treatment of DFIs includes keeping a moist wound environment, treating cellulitis and osteomyelitis with systemic antibiotics, debriding necrotic tissue, and offloading the affected area with orthotic devices. Debridement of calluses should be performed to lower peak plantar pressure, thereby reducing the risk of ulcer formation.[41] Urgent surgical debridement is required for severe or necrotizing foot infections, deep abscess, compartment syndrome, or limb ischemia. For necrotizing infections, all diseased soft tissue, muscle, and bone must be resected back to healthy margins. Early debridement is associated with lower rates of major lower extremity amputation and improved wound healing.[42]

Antibiotics targeting aerobic gram-positive organisms including β-hemolytic *Streptococcus* and *Staphylococcus* species (Table 35.6) should be initiated and continued for 1 to 2 weeks, although this can be extended if the infection persists. Because blood flow is often compromised in diabetic patients with DFIs, antibiotics may not reach the affected tissue easily, and longer courses of

TABLE 35.5 Classification System for Defining the Presence and Severity of Diabetic Foot Infections

CLINICAL CLASSIFICATION OF INFECTION	IWGDF/IDSA CLASSIFICATION
No systemic or local symptoms or signs of infection	1/Uninfected
Infected: At least two of the following and no other cause of inflammatory response (i.e., trauma, venous stasis, etc.): • Local swelling or induration • Erythema >0.5 but <2 cm[b] around the wound • Local tenderness or pain • Local increased warmth • Purulent discharge	2/Mild
Infection with no systemic manifestations and involving: • Erythema extending ≥2 cm from the wound margin, and/or • Tissue deeper than skin and subcutaneous tissues (e.g., tendon, muscle, joint, bone)[a]	3/Moderate
• Infection involving bone (osteomyelitis):	Add "(0)"
Any foot infection with associated systemic manifestations (of the systemic inflammatory response syndrome [SIRS]), as manifested by ≥2 of the following: • Temperature, >38°C or <36°C • Heart rate, >90 beats/min • Respiratory rate, >20 breaths/min, *or* $PaCO_2$ <4.3 kPa (32 mm Hg) • White blood cell count >12,000/mm³, *or* <4 g/L, *or* >10% immature (band) forms	4/Severe
• Infection involving bone (osteomyelitis):	Add "(0)"

[a]If osteomyelitis is demonstrated in the absence of two or more signs/symptoms of local or systemic inflammation, classify the foot as either grade 3(O) (if less than two SIRS criteria) or grade 4(O) if greater than or equal to two SIRS criteria; see text.
[b]In any direction, from the rim of the wound.
IWGDF, International Working Group on the Diabetic Foot; *IDSA,* Infectious Disease Society of America.
Modified from Senneville E, Albalawi Z, van Asten SA, et al. IWGDF/IDSA Guidelines on the Diagnosis and Treatment of Diabetes-related Foot Infections (IWGDF/IDSA 2023). *Clin Infects Dis.* 2023;ciad527.

antimicrobial therapy are often required, especially for moderate to severe infections.[42] A 6-week course of antibiotics is typically required for osteomyelitis if bone resection or amputation is not performed.[42] If the underlying conditions predisposing the patient to osteomyelitis are not addressed, a new infection may occur at the same site. Patients require long-term follow-up (i.e., at least 1 year) before determining whether or not an infection is in remission. If the infection persists after an extended period of time, alternative diagnoses should be considered.

Although surgical debridement and antimicrobial therapy are the mainstay of treatment, improving blood flow to the affected limb and optimizing oxygen delivery to the tissues may facilitate healing. Transcutaneous oxygen measurements (TCOMs) can be used to risk stratify patients with DFUs. Because a transcutaneous oxygen tension of at least 40 mm Hg is needed for normal wound healing, patients with DFUs and an oxygen tension below this threshold may benefit from HBO therapy.[43] Although HBO

TABLE 35.6			Type and Duration of Antibiotic Therapy for Diabetic Foot Infections	
SKIN AND SOFT TISSUE				
Class 2: Mild	Oral	GPC, MRSA	Oxacillin, cephalexin[a]; clindamycin, trimethoprim-sulfamethoxazole, doxycycline,[b,c] amoxicillin/clavulanate or ampicillin/sulbactam[c]; linezolid[d]	1–2 weeks[e]
Class 3/4: Moderate/severe	Oral/initially IV	GPC ± GNR, Pseudomonas, anaerobes, MRSA, ESBL	Amoxicillin/clavulanate or ampicillin/sulbactam, cefuroxime, cefotaxime, ceftriaxone[a]; ticarcillin/clavulanate, piperacillin/tazobactam, carbapenem[f]; vancomycin, linezolid, daptomycin, trimethoprim-sulfamethoxazole[g]; fluoroquinolone, aminoglycoside[h]	2–4 weeks
Bone/joint				
Resected	Oral/initially IV			2–5 days
Debrided (soft tissue infection)	Oral/initially IV			1–2 weeks
Positive culture or histology of bone margins after bone resection	Oral/initially IV			3 weeks
No surgery or dead bone	Oral/initially IV			6 weeks

[a]If no complicating features.
[b]If high risk of MRSA.
[c]β-lactam allergy of intolerance.
[d]If recent antibiotic exposure.
[e]Ten days following surgical debridement.
[f]If recent antibiotics, macerated ulcer or warm climate, or ischemic limb/necrosis/gas forming.
[g]Add or substitute if MRSA risk factors.
[h]Add if risk factors for resistant GNR.
ESBL, Extended-spectrum β-lactamase; *GNR*, gram-negative rod; *GPC*, Gram-positive cocci; *MRSA*, methicillin-resistant *Staphylococcus aureus*.

treatment has been studied for its ability to accelerate DFU healing and lower the risk of amputation, its potential role in controlling infection is unknown. Therefore, the use of HBO for the management of diabetic soft tissue or bone infection is currently not recommended.[42] Among patients with peripheral vascular disease, revascularization of the affected limb may also be necessary to improve chances of successful wound healing, although these surgical bypasses often fail over time.

Given the complex nature of DFIs, an interdisciplinary approach consisting of daily wound care; surgical intervention; antibiotics; frequent follow-up visits; and input from endocrinologists, general and vascular surgeons, podiatrists, pharmacists, dieticians, and infectious disease and wound care specialists is essential for avoiding treatment failure and achieving the best possible long term outcomes.

Infected Deep Tissue and Pressure Injuries

Pressure ulcers, also known as bedsores, decubitus ulcers, and pressure injuries, are localized areas of tissue necrosis developing when soft tissue is compressed between a bony prominence (e.g., sacrum, heels, greater trochanters) and an external surface for a prolonged period of time. This impedes blood flow to the capillary network and deprives the tissue of oxygen and nutrients, resulting in local ischemia and tissue damage. Limited mobility, poor nutrition, and unrelieved pressure or friction are all predisposing factors. Pressure ulcers provide an ideal environment for microbial colonization, especially those that are exposed to bacterial contamination from fecal material.

Once the tissue becomes necrotic, this further promotes bacterial growth and impedes wound healing as it acts as a barrier for reepithelialization. Treatment entails drainage of abscesses and sharp excisional debridement of all devitalized tissue until granulation tissue is present. For noninfected wounds, enzymatic, mechanical (e.g.,

hydrotherapy, high-pressure irrigation, wet-to-dry dressings), and autolytic debridement can be implemented, although these methods may take longer to be effective. Autolytic debridement utilizes agents that maintain a moist environment, allowing endogenous enzymes from the wound to "auto-digest" nonviable tissue.

The choice of dressing depends on the type of wound being treated. Transparent films, hydrogels, alginates, and hydrocolloids are equally effective and can be used alone or in combination.[2] Hydrogels are best for deeper wounds with minimal exudate, whereas alginates and foams are useful for wounds with heavier exudate given their absorptive capacity. Hydrocolloids retain moisture and are effective for autolytic debridement. Any open pressure ulcer is superficially contaminated with environmental flora. However, it is important to prevent added contamination if the wound is near the fecal stream as in ischial or sacral pressure ulcers. Systemic antibiotics should be administered only when there is clinical evidence of infection, including cellulitis, underlying osteomyelitis, or sepsis.

Fungal Skin and Soft Tissue Infections

Fungal SSTIs are a complex and often underappreciated cause of morbidity and mortality. Although primary fungal SSTIs can occur in immunocompetent patients, especially after traumatic injury, secondary opportunistic fungal SSTIs usually affect patients with some type of immunodeficiency and are associated with higher mortality. Patients with autoimmune or rheumatologic conditions, on hemodialysis, or undergoing chemotherapy for malignancy or immunosuppression for organ or stem cell transplantation are most susceptible to invasive fungal infections, although total parenteral nutrition, critical illness, prolonged mechanical ventilation, and chronic indwelling catheters are also risk factors.

Fungal SSTIs are composed of a number of pathologic conditions that vary widely depending on the site of infection, route of acquisition, and virulence of the involved pathogen. They are typically classified according to their invasiveness, ranging from local cutaneous mycoses involving the epidermis, to deep subcutaneous mycoses that penetrate the dermis, to disseminated fungal infections with multiorgan involvement.[44]

Diagnosis of Fungal Skin and Soft Tissue Infections

Early diagnosis and accurate identification of the causal pathogen is crucial for initiating targeted antifungal therapy, as resistance patterns are a growing problem worldwide. If a fungal SSTI is suspected, a thorough history including exposures, travel history, and past medical history must be obtained. A complete physical examination noting the morphology of the lesion is also helpful for narrowing down the diagnosis. Sterile punch biopsies (6-mm punch excision) of the skin and soft tissue enable direct mycologic identification and are considered the gold standard for identifying the causative pathogen, although molecular-based tests (i.e., real-time nucleic-acid polymerase chain reaction [PCR]) are increasingly being used to more rapidly identify fungal species.[45] Microscopic histopathology can provide a presumptive diagnosis while culture results are pending, and fungal antigen tests such as galactomannan (for *Aspergillus*) and 1-3 β-D-glucan (for *Candida* and *Aspergillus*) are sometimes used to support the diagnosis. Imaging and biopsies of noncutaneous anatomic sites may be necessary in the setting of systemic infection.

Treatment of Fungal Skin and Soft Tissue Infections

Candida species normally colonize the gastrointestinal tract, but when a disturbance in the competing bacterial flora occurs, the yeast can proliferate, causing superficial mucous membrane infection among immunocompetent hosts, or disseminated candidiasis among neutropenic patients. Initial treatment is often with an echinocandin class antifungal (i.e., caspofungin, micafungin, or anidulafungin), with deescalation to an azole agent (i.e., fluconazole) when possible. Amphotericin B can be used in the setting of azole and echinocandin intolerance or resistance but is often limited by toxicity. In rare cases, *Candida* can cause necrotizing SSTIs that must be aggressively debrided for source control in addition to antifungal therapy. Treatment duration is generally 2 weeks after the infection has cleared, based on negative blood cultures.

Cryptococcus species are encapsulated yeasts that cause opportunistic infections in immunocompromised hosts through inhalation of spores that disseminate from the lungs to the central nervous system and secondarily infect the skin. Primary cutaneous cryptococcal infections are less common but can usually be treated with fluconazole, while disseminated infection requires systemic therapy.

Aspergillus species are a common cause of opportunistic infections in immunocompromised patients. When cutaneous aspergillosis occurs, this is usually a result of secondary infection from hematogenous spread or direct skin invasion. Primary cutaneous aspergillosis can affect immunocompetent hosts, however, and usually occurs in the setting of severe burns or traumatic injury. Both treatment with

voriconazole (for up to 12 weeks) and aggressive surgical debridement are often required for treatment of aspergillosis.

Mucormycosis is a less common fungal infection transmitted via direct contact with soil and decaying vegetation, or through inhalation of spores. Although rhino-orbito-cerebral and pulmonary infection are more common manifestations, cutaneous mucormycosis occurs in up to 22% of infected individuals, particularly those with poorly controlled diabetes, neutropenia, or trauma.[44] Treatment involves antifungals and expeditious and aggressive debridement of infected tissue.

SELECTED REFERENCES

Cross ELA, Jordan H, Godfrey R, et al. Route and duration of antibiotic therapy in acute cellulitis: a systematic review and meta-analysis of the effectiveness and harms of antibiotic treatment. *J Infect.* 2020;81(4):521-531.

A systematic review and meta-analysis highlighting the fact that antibiotics tend to be overused for treating cellulitis.

Fernando SM, Tran A, Cheng W, et al. Necrotizing soft tissue infection: diagnostic accuracy of physical examination, imaging, and LRINEC score: a systematic review and meta-analysis. *Ann Surg.* 2019;269:58-65.

This article showed the poor sensitivity of the laboratory risk indicator for necrotizing fasciitis score, physical examination, and plain radiography in diagnosing necrotizing soft tissue infection; it affirmed that high clinical suspicion warrants immediate surgical consultation.

Peghin M, Ruiz-Camps I. Recent concepts in fungal involvement in skin and soft tissue infections. *Curr Opin Infect Dis.* 2022; 35(2):103-111.

Given the increasing frequency of fungal SSTIs and their significant morbidity and mortality, this paper provides a comprehensive overview of these complex pathologic conditions

Sartelli M, Coccolini F, Kluger Y, et al. WSES/GAIS/WSIS/SIS-E/AAST global clinical pathways for patients with skin and soft tissue infections. *World J Emerg Surg.* 2022;17(1):3.

Updated and comprehensive international consensus on the diagnosis and management of skin and soft tissue infections.

The full reference list appears on Elsevier eBooks+.

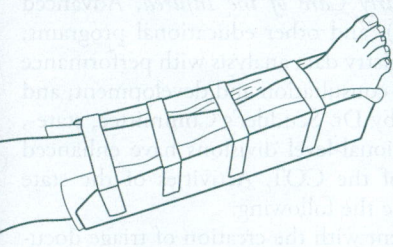

CHAPTER 36

Management of Acute Trauma

*Sharon M. Henry, Melike Harfouche, Meaghan Broderick,
Benjamin Rejowski, Brandt Whitehurst, and John P. Sutyak*

OVERVIEW, MAGNITUDE OF DISEASE BURDEN, HISTORY

Throughout medical history and continuing to the present, coordination of care and management of acute injuries remain the responsibility of a surgeon. The treatment of trauma necessitates mastery of diverse cognitive and psychomotor skills spanning all areas of anatomy, physiology, and pathophysiology. The socioeconomic impact of trauma is immense. Despite a recent global pandemic, trauma remained the overall fourth leading cause of mortality in the United States, behind cardiac disease, malignancy, and COVID-19 and ahead of cerebrovascular disease and chronic lung disease. As of 2021 Centers for Disease Control and Prevention (CDC) statistics,[1] unintentional injury remains the leading cause of death from ages 1 to 44, is the fourth leading cause for ages 45 to 65, and persists in the top 10 beyond age 65.

Deaths due to unintentional injury in ages 45 and greater rose more than threefold from 1980 to 2021, and the rate for ages 1 to 44 rose 50%, indicating a relatively rising burden of injury in the more senior population. Suicides have doubled overall, with a more than threefold increase in those >44 years of age over the same time. To place the magnitude of death due to injury in perspective, during 2020 and 2021, deaths due to injury were 58-fold higher than deaths due to HIV and equal to approximately 75% of the deaths due to COVID-19. Thus, from a purely mathematical standpoint, injury mortality is similar to a COVID-19–severity epidemic every 16 months. Strikingly, since 2018, firearm injuries have surpassed motor vehicle traffic injuries as a cause of death in ages 1 to 25 in the United States.[1]

Because injury is prevalent in younger age groups, the economic impact is immense. For 2019, the US estimated total lifetime cost for medical care, lost productivity, lost quality of life, and loss of life was $4.2 trillion.[2] This represents a staggering 19% of the US gross national product for 2019. For perspective, the entire US government budget for 2023 was $7.6 trillion.[3] Thus, the cost for injury is close to the combined amount the US government budgeted for Medicare, Social Security, defense, and health in 2023!

Because of the great injury burden sustained in conflict, care for the trauma patient has advanced profoundly during wartime. "He who wishes to be a surgeon should go to war" has been attributed to Hippocrates (460–377 BCE). Military-based research programs and funding continue to influence and improve care provided in austere and civilian environments. Box 36.1 lists some major contributions to trauma care that were developed during US military conflicts. Common themes over time include improvements in wound management, resuscitation, and trauma systems. Likewise, advancements in civilian care have had a reciprocal effect within the military. Military-civilian partnerships, including training of military providers, and continued clinical research on hemostasis, resuscitation, and damage control techniques have saved the lives of countless personnel across the globe.

Traumatology has matured over the last century into a distinct surgical field with a multiorganizational infrastructure. The American College of Surgeons (ACS) was founded in 1913. The early leadership of

BOX 36.1   Advances and Discoveries in Trauma Care During War

French and Indian War (1754–63)
Wound contraction during healing
Primary and secondary healing
Description of granulation tissue and epithelialization

American Revolutionary War (1775–83)
Exhaustive therapy (bleeding, diarrhea, vomiting, salivation, sweating)
Centralization of medical care
Establishment of first medical school

American Civil War (1861–65)
Primary amputation (vs. secondary)
Use of topical antiseptic agents
Whole blood transfusion
Development of specialty hospitals (eye/ear, orthopedics, hernia)
Extremity traction splinting
Battlefield ambulance transport
Creation of first trauma manual

World War I (1914–18)
Laparotomy for penetrating abdominal trauma
Wound debridement and delayed closure
Early use of plasma and crystalloid
First blood bank
12 to 18 h from injury to treatment

World War II (1939–45)
Guillotine amputation with delayed primary closure
Exteriorization of colon injuries
Mobile surgical teams
Organ dysfunction after injury described
6 to 12 h from injury to treatment

Korean War (1950–53)
Vascular surgery for limb salvage
Hypovolemic shock recognition
Mobile Army Surgical Hospital (MASH) units
Rapid transport, 2 to 4 h from injury to treatment

Vietnam War (1955–64)
Improved aeromedical transfer (helicopter)
Sulfamylon for burn care
Recognition of acute respiratory distress syndrome (Da Nang lung)

Operation Enduring Freedom and War in Afghanistan (Middle East, 2001 to 2021)
Damage control resuscitation
Balanced and whole blood resuscitation
Highly efficient staged-care trauma systems
Tactical Combat Casualty Care (TCCC)
Revival of and refined protocols for tourniquet use
Rapid data analysis and targeted quality improvement

the ACS recognized the unique field of injury management. In 1922, the ACS designated its first disease-specific committee, the Committee on Fractures. Charles L. Scudder was appointed as the founding chair. As the scope of this committee expanded, in 1949 it was redesignated the Committee on Trauma (COT).

The COT has been instrumental in advancing trauma care throughout the United States and the world via initiatives such as the 1972 first edition of *Early Care of the Injured*, Advanced Trauma Life Support (ATLS), and other educational programs; trauma center verification; registry data analysis with performance improvement; trauma system consultation and development; and political advocacy. Designed by Dr. Scudder's Committee, state-, region-, and (eventually) national-level divisions have enhanced the grassroots effectiveness of the COT. Activities of the state committees frequently include the following:

1. Trauma system development with the creation of triage documents, maximizing local prehospital and hospital resources
2. Injury prevention initiatives
3. Maintenance of statewide trauma registries
4. Advancement of performance improvement endeavors
5. Delivery of educational programs
6. Coordinated advocacy efforts

Several other exceptional professional organizations are dedicated to promoting research and improving trauma care. The American Association for the Surgery of Trauma (AAST) originated in 1938.[4] It is the oldest and largest of all trauma professional organizations. The inclusion of emergency general surgery in the scientific proceedings at the Annual Meeting of the AAST and Clinical Congress of Acute Care Surgery reflected the maturation of the discipline of acute care surgery beyond trauma. The AAST was the central organization leading to the 2008 initiation of an acute care surgery training fellowship, with a curriculum involving advanced education in trauma, emergency general surgery, and surgical critical care. As of late 2023, there are 32 approved acute care surgery fellowship centers.[5]

The Eastern Association for the Surgery of Trauma (EAST) and the Western Trauma Association (WTA) promote the exchange of scientific knowledge in trauma care. Both groups contain active multi-institutional trial committees and, along with the AAST, have developed evidence-based practice management guidelines, which are available electronically.[6] The American Trauma Society (ATS), founded in 1968, has been instrumental in injury prevention and trauma systems development by advocating for the injured patient and promoting trauma-related legislation. The Orthopedic Trauma Association (OTA) and the American Association of Neurological Surgeons (AANS) are surgical organizations actively involved in improving trauma care. Outside of the surgical disciplines, the Society of Trauma Nurses (STN), the American College of Emergency Physicians (ACEP), the National Association of EMS Physicians (NAEMSP), the National Association of Emergency Medical Technicians (NAEMT), and many other outstanding professional organizations represent members who are part of the multidisciplinary injury management team and are essential to improving the care of the injured patient. All organizations mentioned previously maintain active interorganizational communication and have collaborated on numerous projects, consensus statements, educational programs, military-civilian partnerships, and advocacy efforts, including those aimed at a national trauma system.

TRAUMA CENTERS AND SYSTEMS

"Accidental Death and Disability: The Neglected Disease of Modern Society" was a landmark report by the National Academy of Sciences (NAS) in 1966 that identified trauma as a "neglected epidemic." Congressional legislation (National Highway Safety Act of 1966) was subsequently passed to allocate funding for care of motor vehicle crash victims. The first hospitals with programs dedicated to trauma care appeared the same year. Maryland,

Illinois, and Florida implemented state trauma infrastructures, with resultant demonstrable reductions in mortality.

Recognizing that not all hospitals have the resources to provide ideal care for all injured patients, the primary goal of a trauma system is to seamlessly (from the patient's perspective) transport the right patient to the right place at the right time. Outcomes in trauma are highly dependent on the geography of injury, reflecting rapid access to care. A trauma system is an organized approach to maximizing survival and meaningful recovery. The ideal trauma system comprises the entire continuum of care, including injury prevention, lay public and provider education, prehospital care, acute hospital services, postinjury rehabilitation, registry data analysis, performance improvement, and research.[7]

To disseminate and promote consensus-derived recommendations for structures, processes, and outcomes at trauma centers, the COT created the first edition of *Resources for Optimal Care of the Injured Patient* in 1976. The seventh edition (2022 Standards) of this reference manual is accessible on the ACS website.[8] In 1997, the COT introduced the National Trauma Data Bank (NTDB). The NTDB remains the largest database related to trauma ever assembled. The Trauma Quality Improvement Project (TQIP) was developed out of the NTDB. As of late 2023, 14.2 million records exist in the databases, with participation of 901 trauma centers across all TQIP programs.[9] Data from the NTDB and TQIP are included in approximately 2000 publications.

A follow-up to the 1966 NAS report, "Injury in America: A Continuing Public Health Problem," was published in 1985. Inadequate, poorly coordinated care for the injured persisted at the national level. Congress legislated the Trauma Care Systems Planning and Development Act of 1990, which formally addressed the need and funding of new or revised state trauma systems. Further advancement occurred in 1992, when the National Center for Injury Prevention and Control was installed within the CDC. The Health Resources and Services Administration (HRSA) released the "Model Trauma Care System Plan," intending to provide each state with a template for systems development. Revised in 2006 and renamed "Model Trauma System Planning and Evaluation," this work applied a public health disease-based approach to trauma and identified three critical functions:

1. Epidemiologic assessment
2. Policy development and implementation
3. Assurance of high-quality, well-regulated care[10]

As the American healthcare system developed, trauma care was naturally centered on the large, academic hospital with seemingly infinite resources. All patients were transported to a small number of major teaching trauma centers, generally located in large urban areas, regardless of the degree of injury and resources for transport. Although this "exclusive" trauma system was beneficial to the severely injured, with documented improved survival, it resulted in the transfer of a significant number of minimally injured patients and failed to develop local resources. Surgeons who were trained in the larger centers were unable to use their expertise when practicing in smaller suburban and rural hospitals. Data emerged revealing similar outcomes and improved measures of efficiency in patients who were managed outside of Level 1 trauma centers at hospitals with resources appropriate for a lower severity of injury.

Thus, the trauma system paradigm was adjusted to include all hospitals, regardless of trauma designation, to address the needs of all injured patients. These inclusive trauma systems identify roles

---

BOX 36.2 Components of Comprehensive Inclusive Trauma System

Injury prevention/violence intervention efforts
Prehospital care
Triage protocols
Multiple-casualty protocols
Communication
Transportation
Tiered acute care facilities
Trauma center designation and verification
Post–acute care and rehabilitation
Performance improvement
Education and outreach
Legislative advocacy

---

for facilities as a continuum, from critical access and newly defined Level 3 and 4 hospitals to the larger Level 1 and Level 2 trauma centers. Guided by prehospital triage protocols and transfer agreements, injured patients are transported to the appropriate facility as indicated by the severity and specificity of injury. Box 36.2 lists the common components of a coordinated, effective, inclusive trauma system. The benefits of the inclusive approach include preservation of limited medical resources, preservation of practitioner skill, and provision of appropriate care within the patient's community. Fig. 36.1 illustrates the core functions and essential services of a trauma system optimally integrated with public health agencies.

Evidence for the mortality benefit of trauma system care is provided by two seminal publications. In 2006, the National Study on Costs and Outcomes of Trauma (NSCOT) was performed to evaluate variations in the care provided between trauma centers and non–trauma center hospitals. Supported by the National Center for Injury Prevention and Control of the CDC, NSCOT represents one of the largest epidemiologic studies ever to evaluate the care of the injured patient. Including more than 5000 patients from 69 hospitals, NSCOT established that patient outcomes are improved when care is provided at a trauma center versus a non–trauma center. After correction for injury severity, care at a trauma center was associated with a 20% in-hospital mortality reduction and a 25% reduction in 1-year mortality.[11] At the system level, Nathens and colleagues demonstrated the value of a coordinated response to injury after studying 400,000 patients during a 17-year period. The study spanned 1979–95, during which trauma systems were established and optimized. After accounting for many possible contributors to improved outcomes, the development of a trauma system resulted in an 8% reduction in mortality during a 15-year period.[12]

Although progress has been made in national trauma care, there is no "one-size-fits-all" approach, and systems implementation must be tailored to locations ranging from rural to urban geographies. In 2015, the COT developed the Needs-Based Assessment of Trauma Systems (NBATS) tool to assist with designation or creation of new trauma centers within a region. Criteria for the tool include point values assigned to six categories within a trauma service area:

1. Population
2. Median transport time
3. Community support for a trauma center

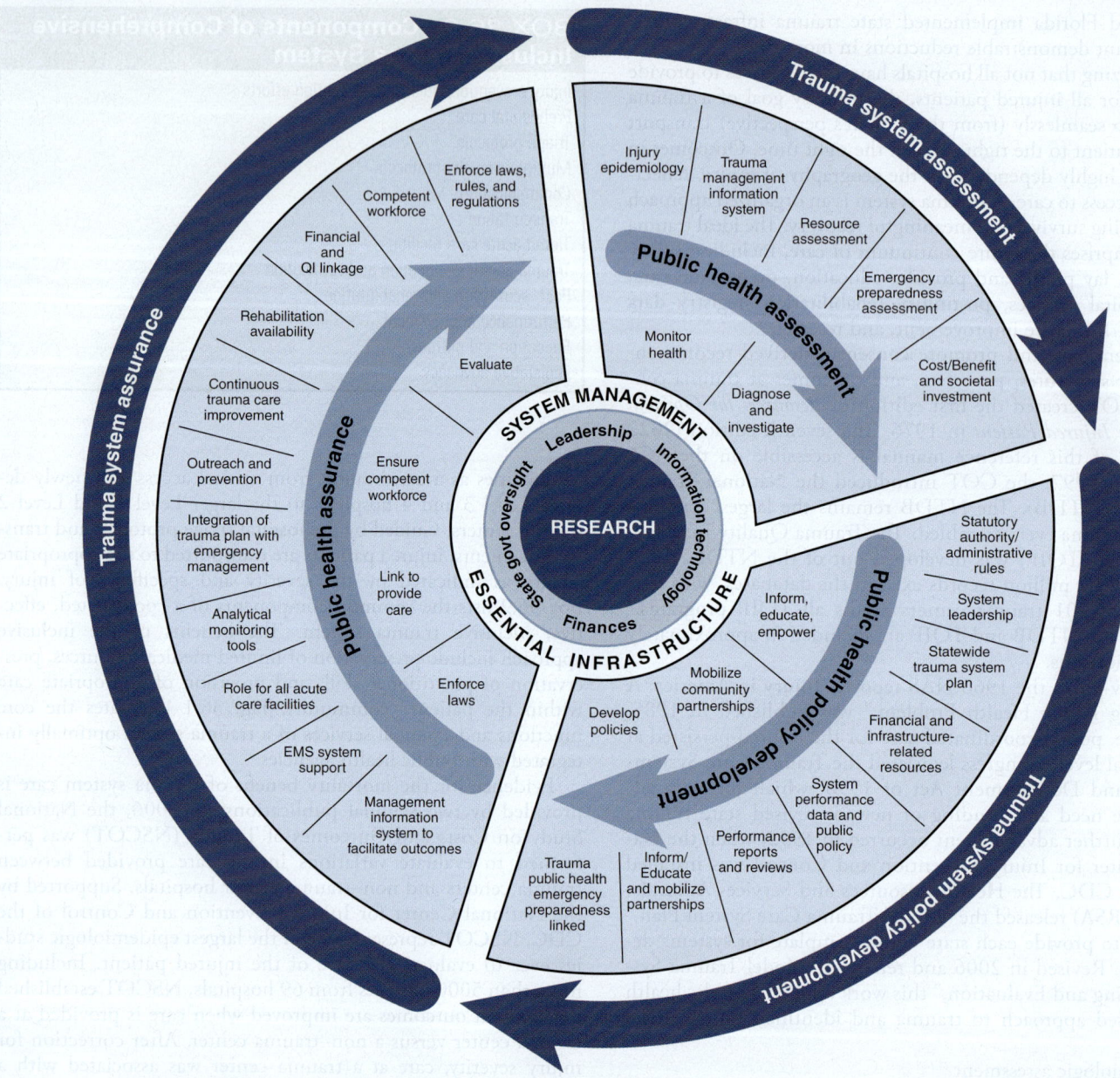

FIGURE 36.1 Structure of an integrated trauma system. Core functions and essential services of the trauma system integrated with public health. Research is at the center as a core component that drives system evolution. *EMS,* Emergency medical services; *QI,* quality improvement. (From Health Resources and Services Administration. *Model Trauma System Planning and Evaluation.* Rockville: Health Resources and Services Administration; 2006:18; American College of Surgeons. *Regional Trauma Systems: Optimal Elements, Integration, and Assessment. Systems Consultation Guide.* Chicago: American College of Surgeons; 2008:ix.)

4. Number of severely injured patients (Injury Severity Score [ISS] >15) discharged from nontrauma acute care facilities
5. Number of Level 1 trauma centers
6. Number of severely injured patients evaluated at trauma centers already in the trauma service area[13]

Analysis of the NBATS revealed it overestimated trauma centers required in rural areas and underestimated centers existent in urban areas.[14] Therefore, a second version (NBATS-2) was created to incorporate predictive geospatial modeling.[15] Benefits of this update include assessment of how established center volumes and payer mixes would be affected by the addition of a new trauma center. As the current understanding of trauma systems continues

to evolve, tools like these will provide valuable insight into structure and organization unique to each region of the country.

Despite more than five decades of studies and legislative actions, large disparities in access to optimal care for the injured remain throughout the country, from economically challenged urban areas to sparsely served rural regions with dramatic transport distances. Despite documented improved survival with trauma center care and National Highway Traffic Safety Administration (NHTSA) Fatality Analysis Reporting System (FARS) data reflecting that 40% of fatalities were alive when first responders arrived, more than one-third of seriously injured victims are not transported to a Level 1 or Level 2 trauma center.[16] In 2016, the National Academy of Sciences, Engineering, and Medicine released "A National Trauma System. Integrating Military and Civilian Trauma Systems to Achieve Zero Preventable Deaths," concluding that 20% of trauma deaths are preventable with optimal emergency and trauma care.[17] This report remains the rallying force for trauma surgeons, the COT, and many other organizations to advocate for funding of a national trauma system.

INJURY SCORING

Concurrent with the development of trauma systems has been the need for a reliable method of comparing the magnitude of injury. Scoring systems are typically based on either injury anatomy or postinjury physiology. First described in 1971, the Abbreviated Injury Scale (AIS) has been the most used anatomic system of injury classification. Injuries are coded with a six-digit taxonomy that includes the body region, type of anatomic structure, and specific anatomic detail of the injury. Table 36.1 demonstrates the body regions and the associated first-digit code within the AIS lexicon. The AIS severity code (frequently described as the postdot code) adds a seventh digit to describe severity and potential risk of death for each injury. Postdot codes range from 1 (minimal severity) to 6 (fatal) and are frequently used to cohort injuries and compare outcomes. The Association for the Advancement of Automotive Medicine frequently embarks on a rigorous process to refine the AIS to maintain accurate characterization of injury.

AIS is the foundation for other scoring systems that attempt to account for the severity of multiple injuries. In 1974, Baker and colleagues presented the ISS, calculated by summing the squares of the highest AIS severity score from each of the three most severely injured body regions, with only one score used per body region. The ISS ranges from 1 to 75, with severity groupings defined as minor injury (ISS <9), moderate injury (ISS 9–14), serious injury (ISS 16–25), and severe injury (ISS >25). Although the ISS has inherent statistical challenges, it has been commonly used throughout the literature to quantify the overall burden of injury sustained by a patient. The AAST Organ Injury Scale (OIS) has been incorporated into more recent versions of the AIS. By introducing the concept of injury grades, the OIS has enhanced anatomic detail for specific organs and better delineated organ injury severity. An example of the OIS for lung with related AIS and *International Classification of Diseases* (ICD) codes is listed in Table 36.2. OIS severity has been validated with the NTDB to optimize the associated risk of morbidity and mortality.[18] The New ISS (NISS) is calculated by summing the squares for the three most severe injuries regardless of body region.[19] The NISS significantly improves mortality prediction, particularly in penetrating injury, and is

TABLE 36.1 Abbreviated Injury Scale (AIS) Body Regions

AIS FIRST DIGIT	BODY REGION
1	Head
2	Face
3	Neck
4	Thorax
5	Abdomen
6	Spine
7	Upper extremity
8	Lower extremity
9	Unspecified

TABLE 36.2 Lung Organ Injury Scale

GRADE[a]	INJURY TYPE	DESCRIPTION OF INJURY	ICD-9	AIS
I	Contusion	Unilateral, <1 lobe	861.12 861.31	3
II	Contusion	Unilateral, single lobe	861.20 861.30	3
	Laceration	Simple pneumothorax	860.0/1	3
III	Contusion	Unilateral, >1 lobe	861.20 861.30	3
	Laceration	Persistent (>72 h) air leak from distal airway	860.0/1 860.4/5 862.0	3–4
	Hematoma	Nonexpanding intraparenchymal	861.30	
IV	Laceration	Major (segmental or lobar) air leak	862.21 861.31	4–5
	Hematoma	Expanding intraparenchymal		
	Vascular	Primary branch intrapulmonary vessel disruption	901.40	3–5
V	Vascular	Hilar vessel disruption	901.41 901.42	4
VI	Vascular	Total uncontained transection of pulmonary hilum	901.41 901.42	4

[a]Advance one grade for bilateral injuries up to grade III. Hemothorax is scored under thoracic vascular injury scale.
AIS, Abbreviated Injury Scale; *ICD-9*, *International Classification Diseases*, 9th revision.
From Moore EE, Malangoni MA, Cogbill TH, et al. Organ injury scaling. IV: thoracic vascular, lung, cardiac, and diaphragm. *J Trauma.* 1994;36(3):299-300.

more predictive of hospital resource use and complications.[20] More recent anatomic models based on ICD coding, such as the Trauma Mortality Prediction Model (TMPM), provide improved predictions using more common coding systems.[21]

In addition to anatomic scoring systems, other scales have been developed that incorporate physiologic status after injury. These physiologic scoring systems stratify the patient's overall condition and can guide real-time decision-making. The Glasgow Coma Scale (GCS) score is a commonly used calculation that reflects level of consciousness. With scores ranging from 3 to 15, the GCS score is composed of three assessments: eye opening, verbal response, and motor function. The motor component provides most of the statistical power of GCS score to predict survival after traumatic brain injury (TBI).[22] The Revised Trauma Score is another well-studied physiologic scoring system that characterizes the condition of the injured patient by incorporating coded values of the GCS score, systolic blood pressure (SBP), and respiratory rate (RR). The New Trauma Score (NTS) incorporates the actual GCS score, along with coded values of SBP and pulse oximetry (SpO$_2$). These scoring systems have been used for triage decisions, quality improvement, resource allocation, and research purposes.

TABLE 36.3 Revised Trauma Score (RTS) and New Trauma Score (NTS)

	RTS		NTS	
Glasgow Coma Scale score	13–15	4	3–15	Actual value
	9–12	3		
	6–8	2		
	4–5	1		
	3	0		
Systolic blood pressure (mm Hg)	>89	4	110–149	4
	76–89	3	>150	3
	50–75	2	90–109	2
	1–49	1	70–89	1
	0	0	<70	0
Respiratory (RTS—rate breaths/min; NTS—SpO$_2$)	10–29	4	≥94	4
	>29	3	80–93	3
	6–9	2	60–79	2
	1–5	1	40–59	1
	0	0	<40	0
Total score		0–12		3–23

Table 36.3 summarizes the calculation of the Revised Trauma Score (RTS) versus the NTS.

PREHOSPITAL TRAUMA CARE

Overview

The prehospital phase of care begins immediately after injury. Optimal trauma care is time dependent, and the prehospital team (including public bystanders) plays an integral role. The importance of prehospital care and transportation of the injured was emphasized in the landmark 1966 NAS report "Accidental Death and Disability." Approximately one-half of preventable deaths from exsanguination occur before hospital arrival.[23] An analysis of more than 40,000 cases of torso hemorrhage in the NTBD documented an increase in mortality with longer time to hemorrhage control, with the highest risk within 30 minutes.[24] Another review of firearm injuries, excluding isolated extremity wounds, demonstrated that trauma patients with prehospital hypotension (<90 mm Hg) and GCS of ≤8 have higher mortality with increasing prehospital time.[25] In a TQIP analysis of over 43,000 penetrating injuries, scene time (increased by 1% per minute) and prehospital time (2% per minute) were independently associated with mortality.[26] As opposed to the benefit of rapid transport for hemorrhaging patients, a distinct relationship between transport time and mortality for undifferentiated and nonhypotensive patients with varying etiologies of trauma was not present in a systemic review. However, more recently, in a heterogeneous group of patients in a Netherlands multicenter study focusing on moderately and severely injured patients (ISS >8), increased scene time was associated with increased 24-hour and 30-day mortality. Transport time alone was not associated with an increased risk of mortality.[27]

Rapid transport must be balanced with the risks of ground and air ambulance travel. Several decision support tools, such as the Air Medical Prehospital Triage (AMPT) score, have been developed to help identify those patients who are more likely to benefit from helicopter emergency medical services (EMS) transport.[28] In 2021, there were 39 fatalities after ground ambulance crashes. Thirty-one

(80%) of these mortalities were ambulance personnel.[29] Overall, more than 2500 crashes involving emergency vehicles are estimated to occur annually, with many injuries to EMS providers. Use of lights and sirens (L&S) has been associated with emergency vehicle crashes.[30] Confirming this risk, the NAEMSP released a position statement in 2022: "L&S response increases the chance of an EMS vehicle crash by 50% and almost triples the chance of crash during patient transport."[29] EMS providers tending to a patient are at a high risk of injury due to a low compliance with mechanical restraints while providing patient care.[31] An effective prehospital system will initiate medical care while providing safe and rapid patient transport to a location capable of providing definitive injury management.

In the prehospital setting, there are four key priorities in the initial approach to an injured patient:
1. Evaluate the scene.
2. Perform an initial patient assessment.
3. Determine optimal triage and transport.
4. Initiate critical interventions while providing safe transport.

Assessing and maintaining scene safety are critical to protect the prehospital providers and bystanders. Proximity to continual vehicular traffic, potential ongoing violence, fires, toxic chemicals, aerosolized agents (unintentional and intentional), and booby traps designed to injure first responders are all risks faced by these dedicated individuals.

Field Assessment: x Control of Hemorrhage

Rapid initial patient assessment consists of a systematic approach designed to identify and mitigate life-threatening conditions. The NAEMT Prehospital Trauma Life Support (PHTLS) course is the global standard for prehospital civilian trauma education. The NAEMT and COT maintain close collaborations to facilitate communication and congruency between prehospital and in-hospital teams. Exsanguinating hemorrhage control is a key component of the military Tactical Combat Casualty Care (TCCC) system, which uses MARCH (**M**assive hemorrhage, **A**irway, **R**espiration, **C**irculation, **H**ypothermia) as a management algorithm. Because this system saved lives on the battlefield, the 10th edition of PHTLS and the 11th edition of ATLS have adapted the battlefield approach to civilian trauma.[32,89] The xABCDE mnemonic reflects initial management: e**x**sanguinating e**x**ternal hemorrhage, **A**irway, **B**reathing, **C**irculation, **D**isability (neurologic status), and **E**xposure (examine the entire patient)/**E**nvironment (avoid hypothermia; evaluate thermal, chemical, extremity, and other injuries).

Emergent interventions in the field can be lifesaving. Massive external hemorrhage, such as occurs with extremity and other open wounds, is immediately controlled. Direct pressure and wound packing are the initial maneuvers.[33] A bandage material containing hemostatic agents may be employed. Scene tourniquet application has demonstrated improved survival and other outcomes in combat experiences.[34] In civilian practice, the incidence of tourniquet use has increased with improved outcomes and no increase in complications.[35,36] The xABC protocol has recently demonstrated improved survival over the ABC protocol in a prehospital study.[37]

After the Sandy Hook tragedy in 2012, a meeting of trauma leaders (the Hartford Consensus) developed and released a lay public bleeding control education program. This COT program is called STOP THE BLEED. Over 2.6 million civilians of primary school age and older in 138 countries have been trained

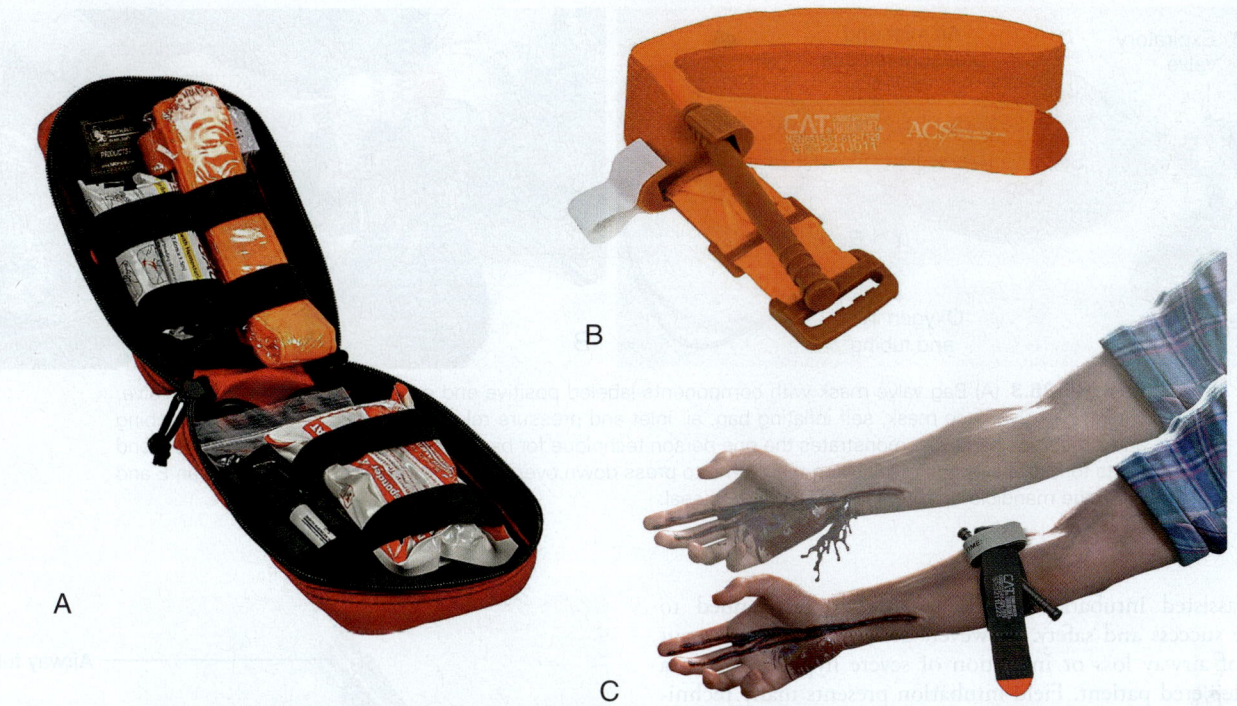

FIGURE 36.2 (A) Bleeding control kit. Kit contains tourniquet, gauze (plain and/or hemostatic), gloves, scissors, a pen and instructions. (B) Tourniquet is applied when pressure and/or packing fail to control hemorrhage. The stick (windless) allows it to be tightened to exceed systolic blood pressure. The white tab is used to note the time of placement. (C) An extremity tourniquet should be applied 2 to 3 inches (5–8 cm) proximal to the bleeding site on the skin, not over clothing, and not over a joint. Bleeding should be controlled once adequately tightened. (A and B, From https://www.bleedingkits.org/all-products.html and https://www.aed-cpr.com/images/arm-tourniquet.png. C, North American Rescue, LLC.)

through in-person, online, and interactive courses.[38] Part of the bleeding control public health campaign has been the installation of bleeding control kits in many schools, government buildings, and other public locations. These kits will frequently contain tourniquets and gauze. Fig. 36.2 is an example of a bleeding control kit and tourniquet that may be in public areas and an appropriate tourniquet application, which is also described later in this chapter.

Field Assessment: Airway

After control of massive hemorrhage, the prehospital provider opens and maintains the airway while simultaneously protecting the spine from excess motion. Several trauma mechanisms (e.g., vehicle crashes, falls from height, ground-level falls in frail patients) have a reasonable risk of unstable spine injury. Providing spinal motion restriction during airway maintenance maneuvers for these patients is important. If hemorrhagic shock is present, airway maneuvers are performed concurrently with initiation of resuscitation (preferentially with blood products; see later) and rapid preparation for transport.

As EMS providers rapidly assess the airway, they consider the available resources, their scope of practice, and the time for transport to select the best intervention to maintain ventilation and oxygenation. Appropriate airway management is critically important in the prehospital setting. Airway management failures account for 8% to 15% of potentially preventable trauma deaths.[39] The initial maneuver to open the airway is a chin lift/jaw thrust

followed by manual clearance or aspiration of secretions, blood, and foreign bodies. For a spontaneously breathing patient, this is often the only maneuver required. An oropharyngeal airway may be inserted in an obtunded patient. However, tolerance of an oropharyngeal airway indicates a blunted or absent gag response and a high potential for airway loss. More advanced techniques, supraglottic or endotracheal airways, will likely be necessary. Nasopharyngeal airways are tolerated in more alert patients. Nasopharyngeal airways are contraindicated in the presence of facial trauma because of the risk of facial and base-of-skull fractures. After application of these "basic" airway maneuvers, ventilation may be assisted with a bag-valve-mask (BVM) device. Fig. 36.3 illustrates a BVM device. A proper seal of the face mask and maintenance of an open airway may be challenging due to lacerations, bleeding, emesis, fractures, an unstable face and/or mandible, intraoral injury, burns, facial hair, body habitus, and many other reasons. Frequently, multiple personnel are needed to maintain an open airway, adequate face mask seal for BVM, ventilation, and spinal motion restriction. In situations where an inadequate number of EMS providers are available to maintain an open airway and ventilation, more advanced and invasive techniques may be employed. Whether via the BVM, a mask, or a cannula, supplemental oxygen is administered.

The most secure airway for a severely injured patient remains a tube with a cuff sealing the trachea distal to the vocal cords. The most frequently practiced technique in civilian practice is endotracheal intubation. Frequently, rapid-sequence intubation (RSI)

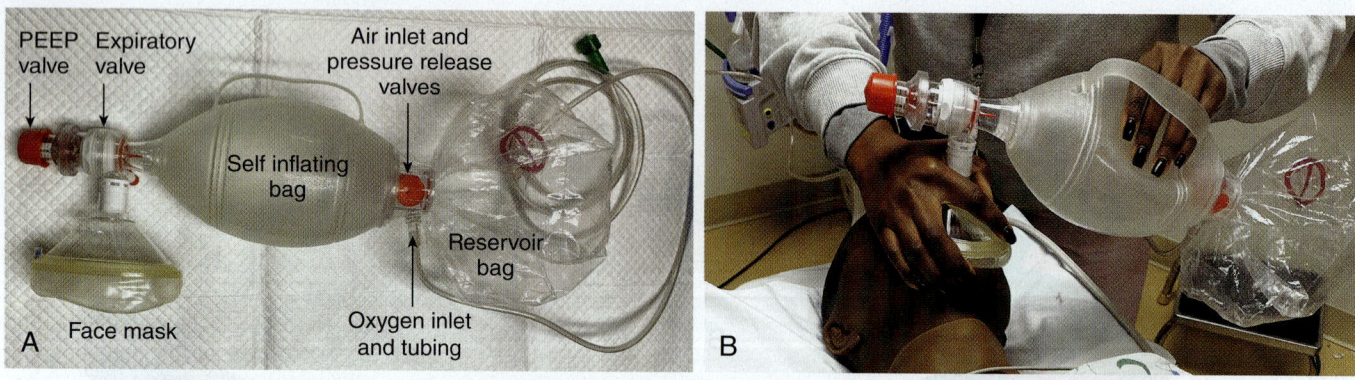

FIGURE 36.3 (A) Bag valve mask with components labeled positive end expiratory pressure (PEEP) valve, expiratory valve, face mask, self inflating bag, air inlet and pressure release valves, oxygen inlet and tubing and a reservoir bag (B) demonstrates the one person technique for bag mask ventilation. The first and second digits form a C over the mask using the thumb to press down over the nose. The 3-5th fingers form an E and bring the mandible up to the mask to create a seal.

or drug-assisted intubation (DAI) techniques are applied to maximize success and safety. However, these techniques present the risk of airway loss or induction of severe hypotension in a volume-depleted patient. Field intubation presents many technical obstacles to success, such as inadequate visualization, glare from the sun and traffic lights, and suboptimal ergonomics (patient and provider). Because medical staffing challenges affect the prehospital system as well as hospitals, the skills and experience of available prehospital providers vary widely, from advanced medics with high-volume intubation exposure and remarkable success rates to basic life support crews with no to minimal intubation training and practice. Multiple intubation attempts increase scene time, which may be detrimental.[40] Increased availability of video laryngoscopy has improved first-pass success rates.[41,42] After decades of study, routine prehospital intubation remains controversial.[43–46] High success rates are possible by facile providers, and patient benefit is clear in specific populations (e.g., inhalation injuries, airway edema).

Supraglottic airway devices have improved technically and add great value as a bridge to intubation in a patient with an absent gag reflex. These devices are placed without laryngoscopic guidance ("blind insertion"). A supraglottic laryngeal mask airway (LMA) is placed by guiding the device manually over the tongue and into the hypopharynx. The mask cuff seals the anterior airway and may be inflatable or filled with a polymer gel. The LMA does not protect against aspiration. Some supraglottic LMAs allow for the passage of a tube for gastric decompression and potential reduction of aspiration risk. Fig. 36.4 illustrates one type of LMA. Various other blind insertion devices generally have two lumens and two balloons. These devices are designed to pass a tube into the esophagus. One balloon blocks air passage into the esophagus. The second balloon is inflated in the posterior oropharyngeal region, isolating the airway between the balloons. Ventilation is performed through openings between the balloons (Fig. 36.5). The optimal method for prehospital airway management is not yet determined, and studies are ongoing, for example, the Prehospital Airway Control in Trauma (PACT) trial (NCT04100564).[47]

Field Assessment: Breathing

Once the airway has been opened or obtained, adequacy of pulmonary gas exchange is assessed. Effective breathing includes adequate

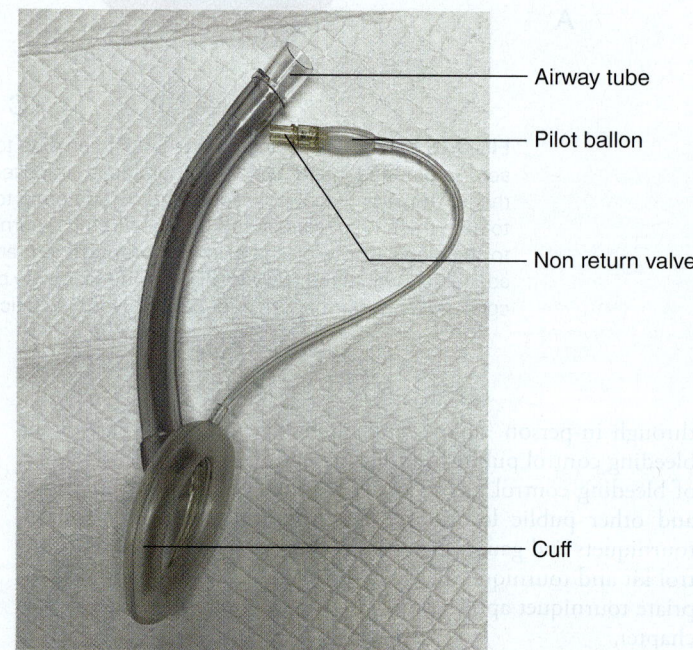

Airway tube

Pilot ballon

Non return valve

Cuff

FIGURE 36.4 Supraglottic laryngeal mask airway.

ventilation and oxygenation. SpO_2 and end-tidal carbon dioxide ($ETCO_2$) are monitored. $ETCO_2$ evaluation, capnography, is recommended in the PHTLS course.[32] $ETCO_2$ is recognized as the optimal method for confirming appropriate placement of prehospital advanced airways, both supraglottic and endotracheal. A normal reading is between 30 and 40 mm Hg. Increased mortality and a higher likelihood of blood transfusion have been documented for trauma patients with low prehospital $ETCO_2$ values.[48–52] In a 2023 prospective, observational, multicenter study of trauma patients with either nasal cannula or in-line ventilator circuit (for intubated patients) monitoring, $ETCO_2$ significantly predicted mortality and had a higher area under the curve than both SBP and shock index (SI).[53] These findings are supported when initial readings are obtained in the emergency department (ED).[54]

Breath sounds are auscultated, and the chest is examined for open injury, asymmetric movements, tracheal deviation at the

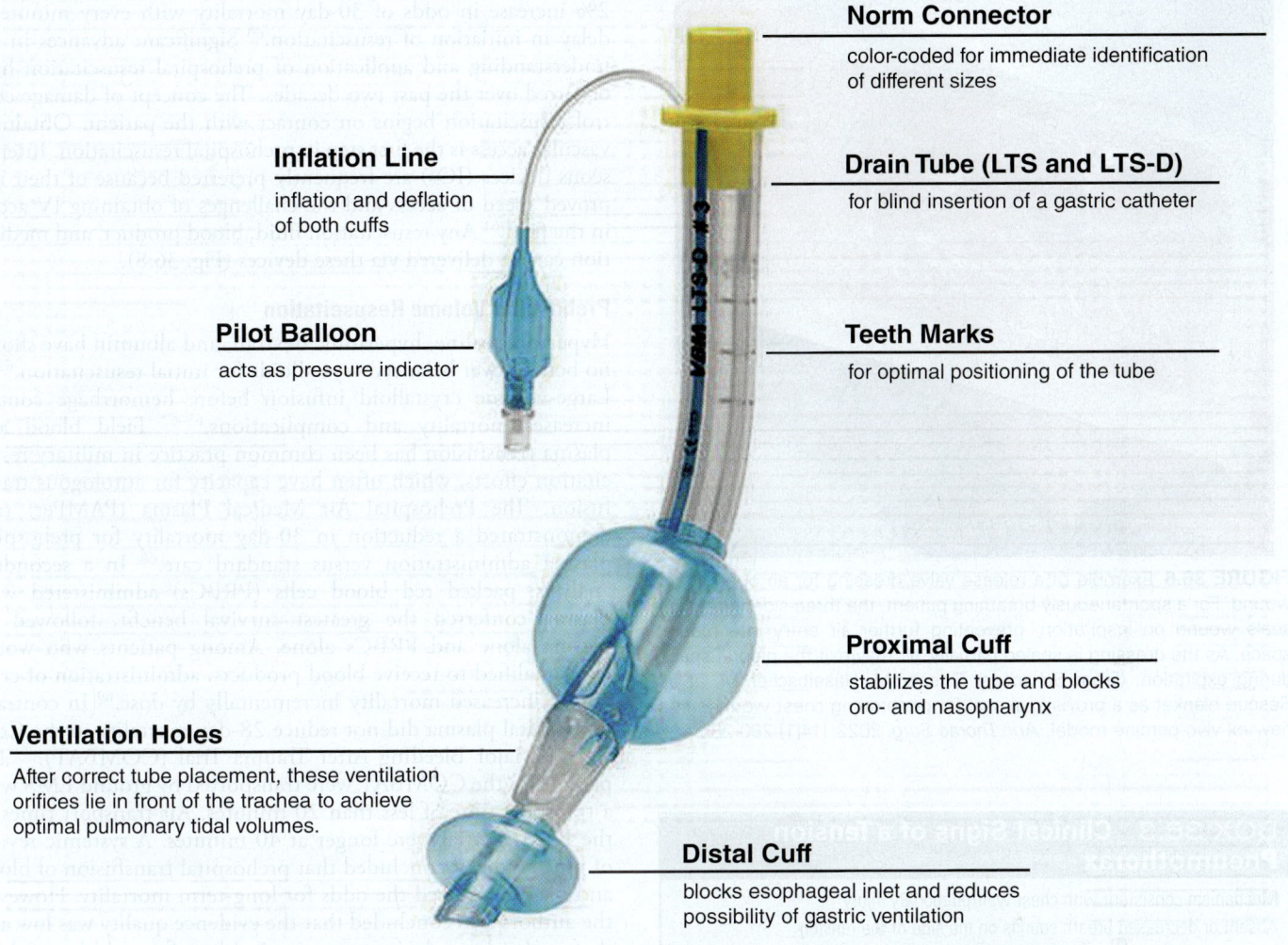

Norm Connector

color-coded for immediate identification
of different sizes

Inflation Line

inflation and deflation
of both cuffs

Drain Tube (LTS and LTS-D)

for blind insertion of a gastric catheter

Pilot Balloon

acts as pressure indicator

Teeth Marks

for optimal positioning of the tube

Proximal Cuff

stabilizes the tube and blocks
oro- and nasopharynx

Ventilation Holes

After correct tube placement, these ventilation
orifices lie in front of the trachea to achieve
optimal pulmonary tidal volumes.

Distal Cuff

blocks esophageal inlet and reduces
possibility of gastric ventilation

FIGURE 36.5 Dual-balloon supraglottic airway. One balloon blocks air passage into the esophagus. The second balloon is inflated in the posterior oropharyngeal region, isolating the airway between the balloons. Ventilation is performed through openings between the balloons. (From Singh K. Second generation supraglottic airway [SGA] devices. In: Nabil AS, ed. *Special Considerations in Human Airway Management.* IntechOpen; 2020.)

sternal notch, and palpable deformities. Open wounds associated with air release and/or visible lung are dressed using a system that allows periodic release of intrathoracic air (Fig. 36.6). Air release is required to avoid transition of a simple pneumothorax to a tension pneumothorax, a cause of rapid and potentially preventable trauma mortality. A tension pneumothorax is associated with several clinical findings summarized in Box 36.3.

If a tension pneumothorax is suspected based on clinical signs, emergent field treatment is dependent on the scope of practice of the prehospital provider. However, most are trained and proficient in placement of a percutaneous 10- to 16-gauge IV catheter at the fifth intercostal space (at or superior to the inframammary fold), either at the anterior axillary line or between the anterior axillary and midaxillary lines. Placement on the anterior chest at the second intercostal space and midclavicular line is an option for patients with a higher BMI or when the lateral approach is not available. These locations are suggested for ease of access and to avoid injury to the great vessels, heart, and intraabdominal structures.

Field Assessment: Circulation, Transport Considerations, and Care During Transport

After initial scene and patient assessments, optimal outcomes additionally depend on rapid, effective triage and transport decisions. Using the "load-and-go" approach, many essential resuscitative interventions are provided while the patient is being transported to a trauma center. Although rapid departure from the scene is important, identifying where to go and the best method of transport is also critical to optimal recovery. Well-defined protocols promote consistent field triage. The 2021 Field Triage Decision Guidelines (Fig. 36.7) were developed by a multidisciplinary panel led by the COT, with support from the NHTSA, the HRSA's Maternal and Child Health Bureau, and the EMS for Children Program.[55] Injury patterns, physiologic status, mechanism of injury, and EMS judgment are combined to determine risk for serious injury and which patients might benefit from care at a trauma center. Most prehospital agencies attempt to assess a patient rapidly, initiating the transport process while minimizing scene time to less than 15 minutes.

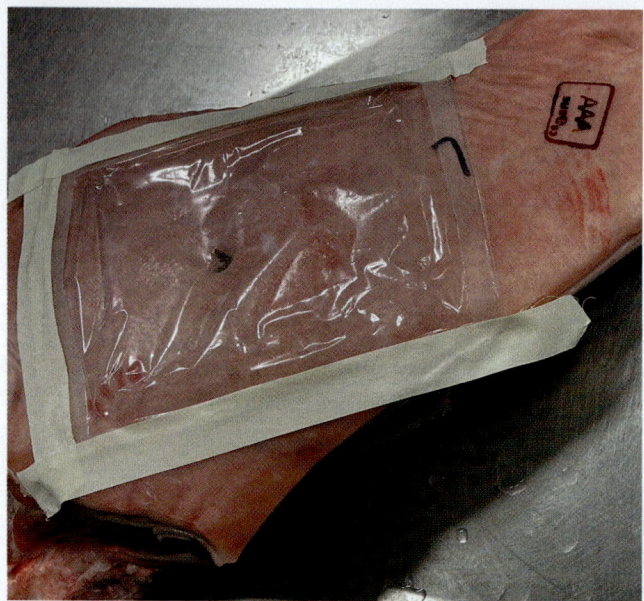

FIGURE 36.6 Example of a release valve dressing for an open chest wound. For a spontaneously breathing patient, the three-sided dressing seals wound on inspiration, preventing further air entry into pleural space. As the dressing is sealed partially, air may exit the pleural space during expiration. (From Schachner T, Isser M, Haselbacher M, et al. Rescue blanket as a provisional seal for penetrating chest wounds in a new ex vivo porcine model. *Ann Thorac Surg.* 2022;114[1]:280-285.)

BOX 36.3   Clinical Signs of a Tension Pneumothorax

Mechanism consistent with chest wall/pulmonary injury

Absent or decreased breath sounds on the side of the tension

Hypotension (due to inadequate venous return to the heart)

High ventilatory pressure (if receiving positive pressure ventilation)

Distended neck veins (difficult to visualize)

Subcutaneous emphysema

Deviation of the trachea away from the side of tension (often subtle and detected at the sternal notch)

Monitoring of blood pressure, pulse, oxygen saturation, and ETCO$_2$ during transport is the standard of care. SI is defined as heart rate divided by SBP. A normal SI is ≤0.7. An SI ≥1 is correlated with higher mortality.[56] In battlefield situations, SI ≥0.8 is correlated with need for massive transfusion and emergent surgical therapy.[57] In a review of TQIP data, SI was correlated with 24-hour and in-hospital mortality, blood product transfusions, and intensive care unit (ICU) and hospital lengths of stay.[58] Modifications of SI, such as rSIG (reversed SI multiplied by GCS score), may provide improved prehospital identification of patients who will benefit from rapid interventions.[59] Thus, SI and its derivatives are potentially very valuable prehospital and ED triage tools for recognition of patients who will most likely benefit from the resources available at higher-level trauma centers.

Prehospital identification of shock and initiation of resuscitation, concurrent with efforts toward temporary hemorrhage control and airway maintenance, are vital. The time to initiation of hemodynamic resuscitation is related to mortality, with up to a 2% increase in odds of 30-day mortality with every minute of delay in initiation of resuscitation.[60] Significant advances in the understanding and application of prehospital resuscitation have occurred over the past two decades. The concept of damage control resuscitation begins on contact with the patient. Obtaining vascular access is the first step in prehospital resuscitation. Interosseous devices (IOs) are frequently preferred because of their improved speed of access and the challenges of obtaining IV access in the field.[61] Any resuscitation fluid, blood product, and medication can be delivered via these devices (Fig. 36.8).

Prehospital Volume Resuscitation

Hypertonic saline, hypertonic dextran, and albumin have shown no benefit over balanced crystalloids for initial resuscitation.[62–64] Large-volume crystalloid infusion before hemorrhage control increases mortality and complications.[65–67] Field blood and plasma transfusion has been common practice in military resuscitation efforts, which often have capacity for autologous transfusion. The Prehospital Air Medical Plasma (PAMPer) trial demonstrated a reduction in 30-day mortality for prehospital plasma administration versus standard care.[68] In a secondary analysis, packed red blood cells (PRBCs) administered with plasma conferred the greatest survival benefit, followed by plasma alone and PRBCs alone. Among patients who would have qualified to receive blood products, administration of crystalloid increased mortality incrementally by dose.[69] In contrast, prehospital plasma did not reduce 28-day mortality in the Control of Major Bleeding After Trauma Trial (COMBAT).[70] The patients in the COMBAT were transported by ground EMS with a transport time of less than 20 minutes. Air transport times in the PAMPer trial were longer at 40 minutes. A systemic review of nine studies[71] concluded that prehospital transfusion of blood and plasma reduced the odds for long-term mortality. However, the authors also concluded that the evidence quality was low and that no hard conclusion on a survival benefit could be made at the time of publication.

Since that systemic review, several other studies have been published in attempts to clarify the value of prehospital transfusion. A subgroup analysis of PAMPer revealed that the mortality-reducing effect was not seen in patients who went on to receive ongoing massive transfusion (>10 units PRBCs in initial 24 hours) but in patients who received 4 to 7 units of blood within the first 24 hours.[72] The Resuscitation With Pre-Hospital Blood Products Study (RePHILL) also demonstrated no survival benefit for prehospital blood and plasma (2 units of each). Ground transport was used for 62% of the patients in this UK-based study, which was halted before achieving the goal enrollment due to the COVID-19 pandemic.[73] A retrospective review of prehospital whole blood transfusions from two Level 1 centers showed a greater improvement in SI and decreased use of massive transfusion protocols versus no prehospital blood. Regretfully, the study was underpowered to detect a mortality difference.[74] Clearly, the ideal prehospital resuscitative scheme has yet to be identified, particularly the position of blood product transfusion, and several studies are in process. Many of the challenges limiting prehospital transfusion are logistical (i.e., supply, storage, cost). As a result, many prehospital agencies provide mixed crystalloid and product-based resuscitation practices based on local resources.[75]

Another prehospital therapy is tranexamic acid (TXA), a synthetic analog of lysine that functions as a competitive reversible inhibitor of plasminogen conversion to plasmin. Thus, TXA reduces fibrinolysis and promotes more rapid and stable clot

National guideline for the field triage of injured patients
RED CRITERIA
High risk for serious injury

Injury patterns	Mental status and vital signs
• Penetrating injuries to head, neck, torso, and proximal extremities • Skull deformity, suspected skull fracture • Suspected spinal injury with new motor or sensory loss • Chest wall instability, deformity, or suspected flail chest • Suspected pelvic fracture • Suspected fracture of two or more proximal long bones • Crushed, degloved, mangled, or pulseless extremity • Amputation proximal to wrist or ankle • Active bleeding requiring a tourniquet or wound packing with continuous pressure	**All Patients** • Unable to follow commands (motor GCS <6) • RR <10 or >29 breaths/min • Respiratory distress or need for respiratory support • Room-air pulse oximetry <90% **Age 0–9 years** • SBP <70 mm Hg + (2 × age in years) **Age 10–64 years** • SBP <90 mm Hg or • HR > SBP **Age ≥65 years** • SBP <110 mm Hg or • HR > SBP

Patients meeting any one of the above RED criteria should be transported to the highest-level trauma center available within the geographic constraints of the regional trauma system

YELLOW CRITERIA
Moderate risk for serious injury

Mechanism of injury	EMS judgment

• High-risk auto crash
  – Partial or complete ejection
  – Significant intrusion (including roof)
    • >12 inches occupant site OR
    • >18 inches any site OR
    • Need for extrication for entrapped patient
  – Death in passenger compartment
  – Child (age 0–9 years) unrestrained or in unsecured child safety seat
  – Vehicle telemetry data consistent with severe injury
• Rider separated from transport vehicle with significant impact (e.g., motorcycle, ATV, horse, etc.)
• Pedestrian/bicycle rider thrown, run over, or with significant impact
• Fall from height >10 feet (all ages)
	Consider risk factors, including:
	• Low-level falls in young children (age ≤5 years) or older adults (age ≥65 years) with significant head impact
	• Anticoagulant use
	• Suspicion of child abuse
	• Special, high-resource healthcare needs
	• Pregnancy >20 weeks
	• Burns in conjunction with trauma
	• Children should be triaged preferentially to pediatric capable centers
	
	If concerned, take to a trauma center

Patients meeting any one of the YELLOW CRITERIA WHO DO NOT MEET RED CRITERIA should be preferentially transported to a trauma center, as available within the geographic constraints of the regional trauma system (need not be the highest-level trauma center)

FIGURE 36.7 National guideline (2021) for the field triage of injured patients. For the red criteria transport recommendations, patients in extremis (e.g., unstable airway, severe shock, or traumatic arrest) may require transport to the closest hospital for initial stabilization before transport to a Level 1 or 2 trauma center for definitive care. Pediatric patients meeting the red criteria should be preferentially triaged to pediatric-capable trauma centers. The EMS Judgment criteria should be considered in the context of resources available in the regional trauma system, including consideration of online medical control for further direction. Examples of patients with special, high-resource healthcare needs include tracheostomy with ventilator dependence and cardiac assist devices, among others. Patients with combined burns and trauma should be preferentially transported to a trauma center with burn care capability. If not available, then a trauma center takes precedence over a burn center. Specific age used to define "children" is based on local system resources and practice patterns. *ATV,* All-terrain vehicle; *GCS,* Glasgow Coma Scale score; *HR,* heart rate; *RR,* respiratory rate; *SBP,* systolic blood pressure. (From Newgard CD, Fischer PE, Gestring M, et al. National guideline for the field triage of injured patients: recommendations of the National Expert Panel on Field Triage, 2021. *J Trauma Acute Care Surg.* 2022;93[2]:e49-e60.)

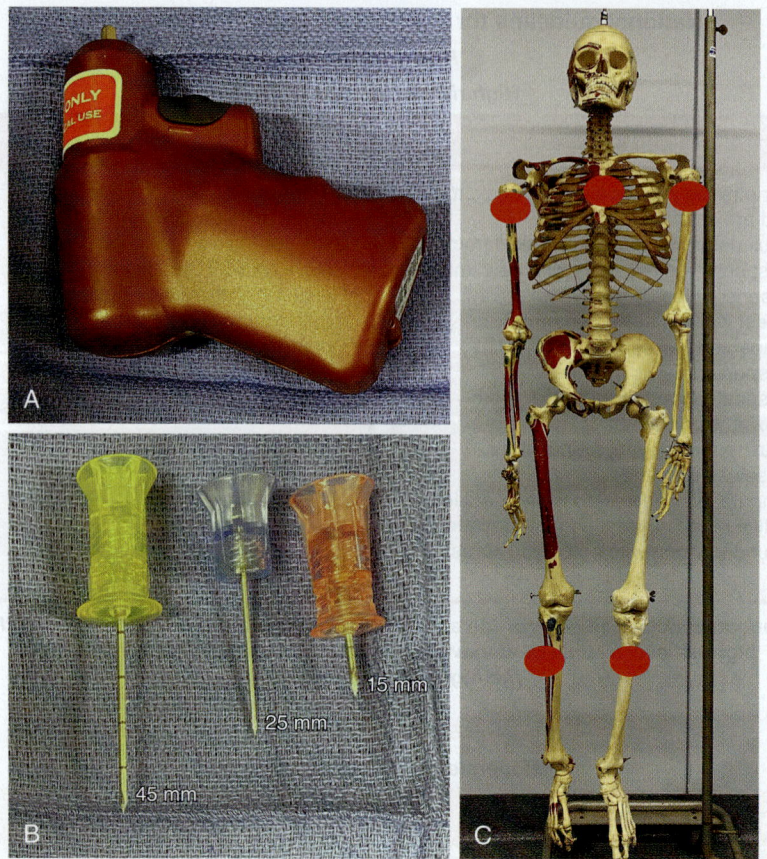

FIGURE 36.8 (A) Interosseous insertion battery powered device (B) Various needles (would change colors as numbers they are indistinct) options yellow 45 mm used to access the humerus blue 25 mm used for tibial access and pink 15 mm used for pediatric access (C) Potential sites of IO access represented on skeleton. Most commonly used are humerus at the greater tubercle and tibia 2–3 cm distal to the tibial tuberosity or 2 cm proximal to the medial malleolus. Humerus allows for higher flows with less discomfort, tibia is easier to access. Sternal access requires specialized device not shown here.

formation. The Clinical Randomization of an Antifibrinolytic in Significant Hemorrhage 2 (CRASH-2) trial was published in 2010. Although TXA was administered in-hospital, this study of more than 20,000 patients in 274 hospitals spread over 20 countries demonstrated that TXA reduced all-cause mortality and death from hemorrhage.[76] Further analysis demonstrated that the mortality benefit in hemorrhage was present only when TXA was administered within 3 hours of injury.[77] Because of the heterogeneous nature of trauma systems and resources in the participating institutions, the applicability of the results of CRASH-2 to the US trauma systems was questioned. A subsequent retrospective military medicine study of wounded warriors who received at least 1 unit of blood, the Military Application of Tranexamic Acid in Trauma Resuscitation study (MATTERs), was published in 2012.[78] This study concluded that TXA improved survival and coagulopathy, particularly in patients for whom a massive transfusion protocol was activated, and that TXA should be included in wartime injury resuscitation. A double-blind, placebo-controlled randomized trial with 927 patients demonstrated what may be the current understanding of prehospital TXA in the civilian US population. An overall 30-day mortality difference was not present. However, a mortality benefit was present for patients with severe shock (SBP ≤70 mm Hg) when TXA was administered within 1 hour.[79] Other studies have concluded that TXA is beneficial in reducing hemorrhage in TBI.[80,81] However, the recent randomized placebo

Pre-hospital Antifibrinolytics for Traumatic Coagulopathy and Hemorrhage (PATCH-Trauma) trial, which enrolled 1310 patients transported by 15 EMS systems in Australia, New Zealand, and Germany, found no difference in survival with a favorable functional outcome after prehospital TXA.[82] However, there were more survivors with severe disability in the TXA group.

Because TXA improves clot formation and stability, a major concern regarding the early administration of TXA is thrombotic complications. Early study results on this topic were mixed. Some[83,84] report higher risks of thrombosis and seizures. Others[80,82,85,86] report no differences in adverse events. The PATCH-Trauma trial confirmed the absence of increased vascular occlusive events. A 2024 publication harmonized the results of two prior large studies, concluding that prehospital TXA was not associated with a higher risk of thrombosis or seizure and was associated with reduced transfusion and mortality across a wide range of injured patients.[87] Although the precise indications for prehospital TXA in the civilian population are continuing areas of study, prehospital administration of 2 g IV, administered within 3 hours of injury, is likely safe and efficacious, particularly in patients with hemorrhagic shock.

Several other therapies designed to reduce time to hemorrhage control are under evaluation. These include prehospital retrograde balloon occlusion of the aorta (REBOA), external compression devices, focused abdominal ultrasound for trauma (FAST), and even administration of vasopressin.[88]

INITIAL ASSESSMENT AND MANAGEMENT AT HEALTHCARE FACILITY

Witnessing the suffering of a trauma victim and facing complex care decisions are stressful and daunting, even panic-producing situations. However, knowledge, training, and practice instill the skills and confidence to manage emotions and save lives. Globally, the standard course that defines and instructs the initial approach to the injured patient is ATLS. Like many advances in trauma care, it was born out of tragedy.[89] Since the first course in Nebraska in 1978, ATLS has been rapidly adopted throughout the United States and quickly promulgated throughout the world. More than 1 million students globally, at a rate of more than 60,000/year in more than 80 countries, have received training. The course presents a structured approach, derived from global literature review and consensus opinion, that is based on rapid identification and simultaneous management of life-threatening conditions. ATLS presents "one safe way" to manage an injured patient. Globally, specific injuries, training, resources, practice environments, and a multitude of other factors differ for an individual resuscitation. ATLS recognizes that modifications of protocols are necessary to meet these patient-unique variables and provide optimal outcomes. Three important concepts greatly enhance the ability to manage injured patients, regardless of the environment where care is provided:

1. Treat the greatest threat to life first.
2. The lack of a definitive diagnosis should not delay the application of urgent treatment.
3. An initial, detailed history is not essential to begin the evaluation and treatment of a patient with acute injuries.

To be applicable in a global environment and assist inexperienced providers, ATLS follows a defined order of evaluation, recognizing that experienced traumatologists will frequently use the steps as a mnemonic rather than an unwavering sequence. This initial assessment, or primary survey, is paused immediately to treat life-threatening conditions as they are identified. Based on data supporting the need for immediate control of massive external hemorrhage, for the first time in its more than 45-year history, the 11th edition (2025 planned release) of ATLS has modified the primary survey sequence from ABCDE to xABCDE.

As noted earlier, xABCDE stands for the following:

e**X**sanguinating e**x**ternal hemorrhage control
Airway maintenance with cervical spine protection
Breathing
Circulation
Disability/neurologic assessment
Exposure and **E**nvironmental control

The primary survey is repeated after a therapeutic intervention and a change in patient condition. Despite its simple design, the primary survey offers a proven tool that the surgeon can trust to structure trauma resuscitation (Fig. 36.9).

Team Factors and Preparation

Team Dynamics and Communication

Initial assessment and management of a severely injured patient is one of the most intense and challenging activities in healthcare. A team approach is necessary to provide simultaneous critical interventions for life-threatening problems. Trauma teams are frequently formed on an ad hoc basis—that is, whoever is available, on call, or on shift. These multidisciplinary teams include surgeons, emergency physicians, advanced practice providers, nurses, respiratory therapists, radiology technicians, and a plethora of other specially

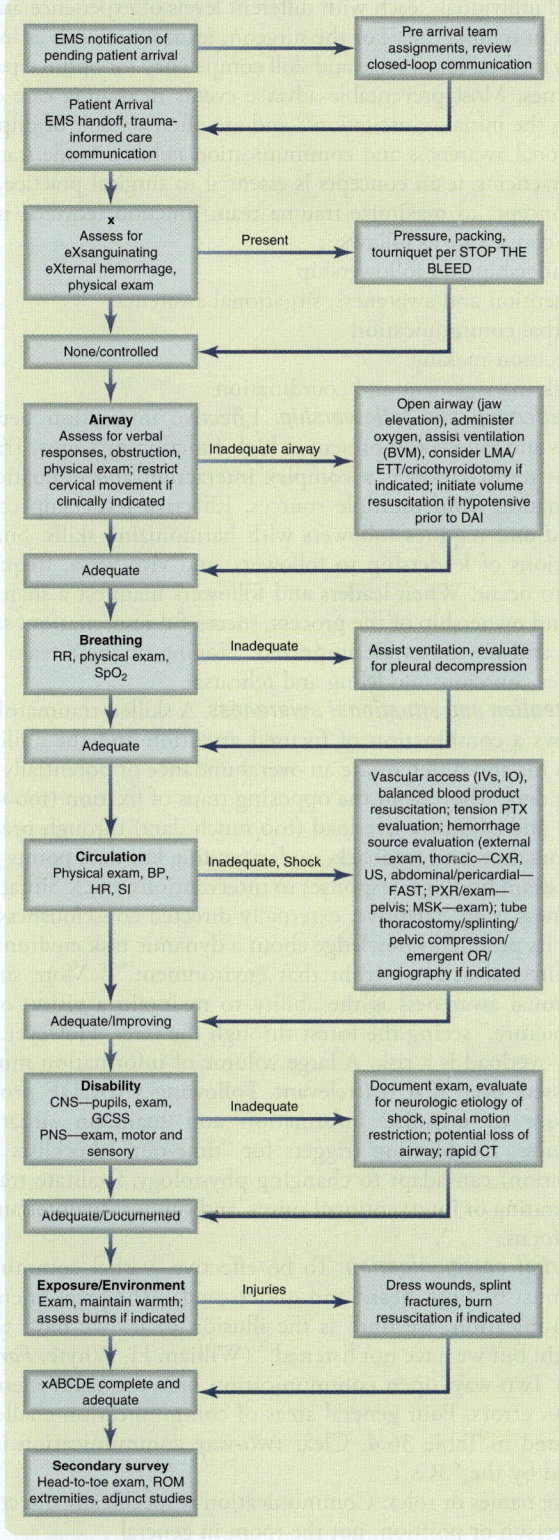

FIGURE 36.9 Overview algorithm for initial assessment of the injured patient. *BP,* Blood pressure; *BVM,* bag valve mask; *CNS,* central nervous system; *CT,* computed tomography; *CXR,* chest radiograph; *DAI,* drug-assisted intubation; *EMS,* emergency medical services; *ETT,* endotracheal intubation; *FAST,* focused abdominal sonography in trauma; *GCSS,* Glasgow Coma Scale score; *HR,* heart rate; *IO,* intraosseous; *IV,* intravenous catheter; *LMA,* laryngeal mask airway; *MSK,* musculoskeletal; *OR,* operation; *PNS,* peripheral nervous system; *PTX,* pneumothorax; *PXR,* pelvis radiograph; *ROM,* range of motion; *RR,* respiratory rate; *SI,* shock index; *Spo₂,* pulse oximetry; *US,* ultrasound.

trained individuals, each with different levels of experience and expertise in trauma care. For the surgeon, team function is as important as medical knowledge and skill competency for optimal patient outcomes. Most preventable adverse events in trauma care occur during the initial resuscitation[90] and are often a result of impaired situational awareness and communication failures. Understanding and practicing team concepts is essential to surgical practice. Five key concepts to maximize trauma team function (covered in the ATLS course) are as follows[89]:

1. Leadership and followership
2. Attention and awareness, situational awareness
3. Verbal communication
4. Decision-making
5. Task management and coordination

Leadership and followership. Effective interaction between leaders and followers is present in high-functioning teams. Trauma patient resuscitation is a complex interaction and evaluation of information from multiple sources. Effective leadership can be learned and requires followers with harmonizing skills. Smooth transitions of leadership to followers, and vice versa, frequently need to occur. When leaders and followers manifest a shared vision and ownership of the process, successful resuscitation, saving a life, and outcomes are improved. Honing of these team skills requires conscious modeling and rehearsal.

Attention and situational awareness. A skilled traumatologist employs a combination of focused attention and the ability to search for and differentiate an overabundance of potentially confusing data. They avoid the opposing traps of fixation (too much focus) and cognitive overload (too much data) through preparation, practice, and feedback, understanding key data points (vital signs, exam findings, responses to interventions, etc.). Situational awareness is an "adaptive, externally directed consciousness that has as its products knowledge about a dynamic task environment and directed action within that environment."[91] More simply, situational awareness is the ability to maintain a vision of the "big picture," seeing the forest through the trees. However, cognitive overload is a risk. A large volume of information must be processed, even if it is irrelevant. Following xABCDE provides structure to organize information and maintain situational awareness. Establishing triggers for "time-out" checklists (e.g., intubation) can adapt to changing physiology, facilitate transfer to operating or interventional suites, and support maintenance of team focus.

Verbal communication. To be effective, verbal communication must be both heard and understood. "The great enemy of communication, we find, is the illusion of it. We have talked enough; but we have not listened." (William H. Whyte, *Fortune,* 1950) Two-way, open communication between team members reduces errors. Four general areas of communication challenges are listed in Table 36.4. Clear two-way communication is enhanced by the "3Cs":

1. Cite names or roles: Communication is specifically directed to a person or position, not the room in general.
2. Clear instructions: Use precise and concise wording—for example, "Respiratory, we are going to intubate the patient now."
3. Close the loop: Instructions and their completion are repeated back to the sender.[92]

Decision-making. Educational psychology demonstrates that humans can manage approximately 7 to 10 discrete pieces of information at a time in working memory (a phone number). This is reduced when more cognitive processes are activated to manage the information. Through practice and experience,

TABLE 36.4	**Areas of Communication Challenges**	
AREA	**DEFINITION**	**MITIGATION**
What is meant is not said	Passive word choice, not speaking up	Team leader "thinking out loud." Reduce hierarchical barriers.
What is said is not heard	Vague wording, lack of assertiveness, room noise	Control room noise, 5-step advocacy method: Get attention, state concern, state problem as seen, state solution, and obtain agreement.
What is heard is not understood	Reception altered by aggressive or passive communication	Maintain focus on patient activity, what is right versus who is right.
What is understood is not performed	Task completion, provider distraction, unclear assignments	"3Cs" of verbal exchanges

experts develop more efficient neuropathways that clear working memory for new tasks. Clinical intuition is the pattern recognition resulting from this acquired knowledge and experience. Thus, effective and efficient decision-making may be developed through simulations and practice.

Task management and coordination. Maintaining team shared mental models and situational awareness is crucial for task management and coordination. Active sharing of information is needed during trauma resuscitation. Larger teams will simultaneously be involved in several discrete endeavors. Even critical access hospital "teams" composed of two to three people will perform some tasks simultaneously. Task coordination can be either explicit or implicit. A prearrival huddle establishes an implicit model, which is a sign of a high-functioning team.[89,93] Because of the ad hoc nature of trauma teams, a standardized and consistent prebrief allows the entire team to understand member capabilities and experience, resource challenges, and patient status. Specific tasks are assigned. When a member faces a challenge, reassignment and adjustments are facilitated. Development of protocols for procedures, assessments, communications, and other activities will likewise increase efficiency and improve outcomes.

Education and training build shared mental models and are accomplished through institutional or standardized courses such as ATLS, PHTLS, Advanced Trauma Care for Nurses (ATCN), and Trauma Nurse Specialist (TNS). Examples of effective team skills training courses are the Simulated Trauma and Resuscitative Team Training (STARTT) Course, Trauma Team Dynamics: A Trauma Crisis Resource Management Manual, and TEAMStepps. Situation-specific multidisciplinary team simulations conducted regularly boost team coordination, confidence, and competency. Training and simulation are mandatory for optimal response after human-origin and natural mass casualty events. Multiple programs are available through the Federal Emergency Management Agency (FEMA), the Department of Homeland Security, the ACS COT, and others. Practice and experience allow explicit coordination to evolve into an implicit pattern through shared understanding of roles.[94]

Team dynamics and communication during trauma evaluation and resuscitation can be organized into six phases:

1. Hospital planning
2. Prearrival huddle
3. Arrival handover
4. Resuscitation

5. Departure handover

6. Event debrief

Hospital planning. Effective participation in a trauma system involves purposeful hospital commitment to resources, protocols, performance improvement, and transfer agreements. These must be developed before patient arrival. Some practical parts include triage and declaration criteria (pre- and within hospital, diversion processes), designated recipient of prehospital call, designated responding personnel at patient arrival, blood product availability, availability of other medical services (orthopedics, neurosurgery, anesthesia, operating room [OR] staff, radiology, and others), and method (air, ground) and destination of transfer if needed.

Prearrival huddle. When adequate notification time is available, a prearrival huddle should be performed to discuss patient status, potential injuries, potential for external transfer, staff roles, designation of team leader, potential procedures and task assignments, and equipment availability (e.g., intubation box, fluids, blood, trays [thoracostomy, open chest, tracheostomy], IVs, intraosseous catheters, pelvic immobilization device).

Arrival handover. A key moment in patient care occurs as primary responsibility transfers from the prehospital providers to the hospital team. The verbal transfer of information is succinct, structured, and limited to the data essential to immediate treatment.[95] Local practices influence the specific handover protocol that is employed. However, a standardized approach is most effective. One example from ATLS is the clinical handover protocol between prehospital and hospital staff (Box 36.4). The prehospital provider receives the active attention of the trauma team, particularly the leader, and is permitted to report without interruption before the patient is transferred to the hospital bed. When critical care is being delivered or immediately required, for example, chest compressions or respiratory distress, the report is delivered in an abbreviated fashion while care is delivered. Brief questions can be addressed with a thorough review after the trauma team performs initial assessment and life-preserving therapies. Notably, this is an example of a handoff and its position in the resuscitation sequence, which may be optimized for local context. For example, some institutions position the handoff after the initial assessment and key life-preserving therapies and may subtly stratify handoff timing based on blunt versus penetrating mechanism.

Resuscitation. Provider assignments and locations are well summarized in the ATLS manual.[89] Frequently, the provider assigned to airway assessment and management is located at the head of the bed. If adequate team members are present, the team leader stands at the foot of the bed or to one side to maintain a

---

BOX 36.5 S-ABC BAR Departure Handover

S—Situation: Identify patient (name, alias, and other factors to avoid error) and mechanism. State receiving provider, facility, and transfer indication if indicated.

A, B, C: Summarize resuscitation using xABCDE structure.

B—Background: AMPLE (**A**llergies, **M**edications, **P**ast medical history, **L**ast meal, **E**vents not mentioned in situation step) history, imaging, fluids/blood products, procedures performed, and so forth.

A—Assessment: Current medical status, response to interventions, continuing treatments.

R—Recommendations: During transport (internal and external)—mode, estimated time of departure/arrival, interventions to be continued during transport.

---

global view of resuscitation. This assists the leader in maintaining situational awareness. Based on the architecture of the resuscitation area, team members are deployed to the sides of the patient to perform various tasks. The 3Cs of communication are followed. Communication is directed by and to the team leader. Confirmation of task instruction and completion is repeated to the team leader. All non–patient-centered noise and verbal communication is minimized and preferably avoided.

A time-out led by the leader is proven to promote united mental models and team situational awareness.[91] Time-out analyses are useful at care transition points, such as at completion of the primary survey, completion of procedures, and transport to radiology or the OR. These reviews help to ensure all members are functioning in a coordinated fashion, provide an opportunity for further information delivery, and define a time to ask questions. One intraresuscitation and departure time-out method is the SMARTT Stepback, which stands for **S**ituation review, **M**anagement delivered, **A**ctivities to be performed, **R**apidity of the activities, **T**roubleshooting, and **T**alk to me.[96] The last two portions of SMARTT empower team members to speak and clarify the plan.

Departure handover. At the time of patient disposition from the resuscitation area or transfer to definitive care, a departure handover is performed to the receiving team. ATLS supports the S-ABC BAR method covering **S**ituation, **ABC**s of resuscitation, **B**ackground, **A**ssessment, and **R**ecommendations during transport (Box 36.5).

Debrief. As part of general performance improvement processes, after disposition of the patient, scheduled structured debriefing sessions aid leaders and followers in professional development. Focus of these sessions is on team factors and must avoid personal accusations.

Pathogen Protection

Exposure to blood-borne and aerosolized pathogens is a modifiable risk for the team delivering care to a trauma patient. Before entry to the trauma bay, all providers can reduce the risk of acquiring hepatitis, HIV, COVID-19, and other diseases by wearing a head covering, surgical grade mask, eye protection, gloves, shoe covers, and a gown. These items should be replaced if saturated or damaged during patient care. Radiologic protective devices are recommended for centers that use imaging during the primary survey.

Patient-Centered Care

A trauma resuscitation is stressful for the staff and extremely emotionally challenging to the patient. The principles and practice of

---

BOX 36.4 IMIST-AMBO Protocol for Prehospital to Trauma Bay Handover

I—Identify patient's name and age

M—State the mechanism of injury

I—Provide assessment of likely injuries

S—Signs, most recent observations

T—Treatments provided and trends in patient's condition

A—Allergies

M—Medication

B—Background history

O—Other information

Modified from Shah Y, Alinier G, Pillay Y. Clinical handover between paramedics and emergency department staff: SBAR and IMIST-AMBO acronyms. *Int Paramed Pract.* 2016;6(2):37-44.

recognizing the impact of medical interventions from the patient's perspective has been termed *trauma-informed care*. Even if the patient appears unconscious, anxiety, fear, and psychological trauma can be reduced by speaking to the patient, explaining procedures, maintaining modesty, providing reassurance, administering anesthetic agents for procedures, providing pain relief when safe, and respecting the patient's personhood. These interventions are followed despite any member of the care team's opinion regarding the patient's responsibility for injury etiology. Patients who appear unconscious may have recall and develop postinjury stress. Preventing emotional injury improves long-term functional outcomes and may potentially restore faith in the medical system within disenfranchised communities. Further education on trauma-informed care is available online and in the ATLS manual.[89]

x Control of Exsanguinating External Hemorrhage

Traumatic hemorrhage can be divided into compressible and noncompressible types. Compressible hemorrhage may be defined as bleeding that is visible and potentially controlled with nonincision procedures such as pressure, packing, and tourniquet application. Compressible hemorrhage may be due to an extremity injury or a massively bleeding nonextremity wound. Both are included in the "x" stage of assessment. If bleeding was not controlled by prehospital providers, active significant compressible external hemorrhage is immediately controlled upon patient arrival to the resuscitation area. The process is identical to that described in the "Prehospital Trauma Care" section of this chapter and follows consensus statement[38] and STOP THE BLEED principles.

The area of exsanguination is completely exposed. All clothing is removed around the injury and proximally. Direct pressure and wound packing are performed. Tourniquet application is recommended if extremity bleeding is not rapidly controlled with pressure, if "spurting" arterial hemorrhage is visualized, or if a complete or near-complete amputation is present. Bleeding control interventions are lifesaving, take seconds to initiate, and are provided while other team members simultaneously proceed to airway assessment and management. From the standpoint of initial patient assessment in the hospital environment, hemorrhage within the chest, abdomen, and pelvis cavities and at junctional locations (i.e., too proximal on an extremity for tourniquet application) is considered noncompressible. Junctional tourniquets are available and are being evaluated for efficacy. Recommendations for junctional bleeding control devices cannot be made at the time of publication due to inadequate clinical experience and data. Control of pelvic hemorrhage by application of external pelvic devices is covered in the "Circulation" and "Injuries to the Pelvis" sections of this chapter.

Tourniquet use was recognized as an effective method to control hemorrhage during World Wars I and II. However, prolonged tourniquet application led to increased complications, such as amputations of potentially viable limbs, rhabdomyolysis, and neuropathies. Thus, through the latter half of the 20th century, tourniquet use almost disappeared from both military and civilian practice. Military experiences during conflicts of the 1990s and early 21st century changed practice. During these conflicts, tourniquets were initially recommended for Special Operations activities.[97] By 2011, tourniquet application was adopted throughout the US military, with a resultant 85% decrease (from 23.3 to 3.5) in deaths per year due to extremity hemorrhage.[98] Civilian prehospital tourniquet use lagged military adoption. The Sandy

Hook tragedy and the Hartford consensus occurred at the same time as the success of military tourniquets was confirmed. The Bleeding Control Basic (B-CON) course was released in 2014 for a lay audience. B-CON was successful beyond expectations and was transitioned to the STOP THE BLEED program. Subsequently, tourniquets became a standard component of law enforcement, EMS, and civilian first-aid equipment. Bleeding control kits are frequently located next to automatic defibrillators in public areas. Several studies have documented a lower rate of mortality, blood transfusion, and complications after tourniquet application, without an increased rate of amputations and tourniquet-related adverse events if duration is less than 2 hours.[34,99,100]

An extremity tourniquet should be applied 2 to 3 inches (5–8 cm) proximal to the bleeding site on skin, not over clothing, and not over a joint (see Fig. 36.2).[101] The tourniquet must be tightened sufficiently to overcome SBP. Thus, a pulse should not be palpated distal to the tourniquet, and bleeding should cease. The tourniquet is frequently painful. If bleeding continues, a second tourniquet is placed 2 to 3 inches proximal to the first device. Of extreme importance, time of application is recorded on the device.

After completion of the primary survey and adequate resuscitation, assessment for tourniquet conversion is performed. Tourniquet conversion is the deliberate process of exchanging a tourniquet for another method of hemorrhage control. Complications of a tourniquet are minimized when the device is removed within 2 hours. Prolonged tourniquet application results in unacceptable rates of amputation, rhabdomyolysis, neuropathy, and other complications. After completion of an initial xABCDE assessment, hemorrhage control may be successfully obtained by other, less potentially morbid methods. Approximately 50% of military and civilian tourniquet applications were not indicated on retrospective reviews.[102] Conversion should be considered in the following scenarios[101]:

1. Potential transport time to surgical support is >2 hours.
2. Shock has resolved.
3. Continuous injury monitoring is available, including during transport.
4. Injury is *not* a complete or near-complete amputation.
5. Tourniquet application was <6 hours before assessment.

The process of tourniquet conversion is diagrammed in Fig. 36.10.

Airway

Assessment and management of an airway are fundamental skills for care of the trauma patient. Planning, practice, performance, and debriefing are essential to optimal outcomes because even skilled providers may experience challenges and complications. An adequate airway is necessary for ample ventilation and oxygenation. Just a few minutes of hypoxia can have drastic, unfortunate consequences.

Simultaneously with immediate control of exsanguinating external hemorrhage, the status of the airway should be evaluated upon patient arrival to the trauma bay. A rapid, simple, and accurate method to assess the airway is to talk to the patient. "What is your name?" will elicit a verbal response and provide meaningful information. The ability to speak usually indicates adequate airway protection. Patients who have disordered speech have either mental status depression and/or obstruction to airflow, both of which are indications for urgent airway management. Further indicators of airway compromise include patient agitation (potential hypoxemia, sensation of doom); noisy breathing; history of inhalation exposure (smoke, cyanide from burning furniture, toxic fumes); and visible facial trauma, such as unstable mandibular fractures,

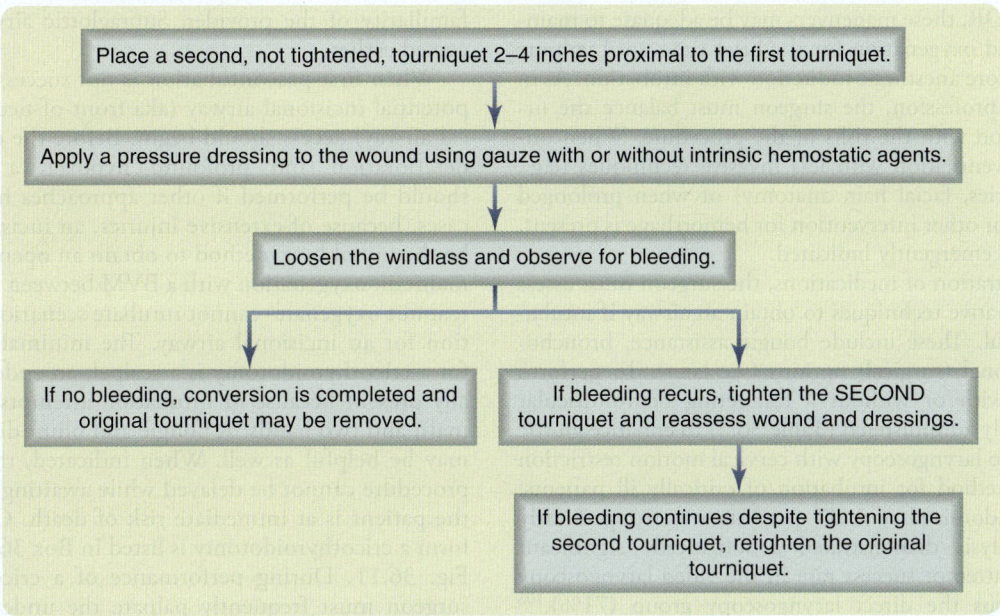

Place a second, not tightened, tourniquet 2–4 inches proximal to the first tourniquet.

Apply a pressure dressing to the wound using gauze with or without intrinsic hemostatic agents.

Loosen the windlass and observe for bleeding.

If no bleeding, conversion is completed and original tourniquet may be removed.

If bleeding recurs, tighten the SECOND tourniquet and reassess wound and dressings.

If bleeding continues despite tightening the second tourniquet, retighten the original tourniquet.

FIGURE 36.10 Process for tourniquet conversion.

burns, penetrating injury, and oropharyngeal blood or foreign bodies. EMS report of dyspnea, change in consciousness, hypoxia (low SpO_2), and alterations in $ETCO_2$ provides indication for airway interventions to improve ventilation and oxygenation. If the initial airway is adequate, frequent reassessment for deterioration and the development of airway compromise is vital.

Patients may present with significant mandibular, facial, and/or open neck injuries yet be alert and able to maintain adequate ventilation. These patients may manage secretions and blood when in a sitting position, perhaps with addition of oral suctioning, and should be allowed to remain in that position. Medication administration for intubation may convert a passable airway into an emergent airway, with a potentially disastrous result. An adequate airway is better than no airway. Thus, these patients are often best treated by urgent consultation with anesthesia and surgical airway experts before attempts at intubation. Supplemental oxygen is administered. Awake intubation and preparation for surgical airway in an OR are two techniques that may facilitate care in these challenging clinical situations.

Manipulation of the head and neck occurs while the airway is managed. During initial assessment, an unstable cervical spine injury should be assumed in all patients who have experienced an appropriate mechanism, such as a vehicular crash, fall, or direct force (e.g., diving injury), or who demonstrate extremity paralysis. Cervical spine motion restriction should be maintained using a hard cervical collar, manually, or with other techniques. The anterior portion of the cervical collar may be removed to optimize exposure and assessment. When the collar is removed, manual stabilization from an assistant should be provided.

When assessed as inadequate, an airway must be established. Similar to prehospital management, the precise technique is determined by the injuries, anatomy, physiology, provider expertise, and available resources (e.g., video laryngoscopy, supraglottic devices, bougies). Preparation is important. An emergency airway kit with laryngoscopes, various tubes, tracheal guides, and surgical airway equipment must be present in every emergency area. These materials are vigilantly inspected and restocked. The time to search for equipment is not during the emergency.

The definitive in-hospital airway of choice for most injured patients remains oral endotracheal intubation via a medication-assisted technique. However, evidence is accumulating that mortality is increased for hypotensive hemorrhaging patients who receive endotracheal intubation before volume resuscitation and before exsanguinating hemorrhage is controlled. Elevated SI may indicate patients at risk of cardiovascular collapse during intubation. A review of four studies comparing ABC (airway, breathing, circulation) versus CAB (circulation, airway, breathing) approaches reported a significantly reduced mortality (50% vs. 78%, $p < 0.001$) when blood transfusion was initiated before intubation in hypotensive patients.[103] An AAST multicenter retrospective trial found that delaying intubation until resuscitation was initiated and bleeding control was imminent was not inferior to intubation first.[104] In these studies, the airway was not ignored. Management was continued but without early intubation. Medications frequently induce hypotension through vasodilation. Positive pressure ventilation may decrease cardiac output through decreased preload. Both effects may precipitate lethal hypotension.

Therefore, the concept of damage control airway maneuvers (DCAM) has been proposed.[105] As intubation equipment and personnel are organized, volume resuscitation is initiated, preferably with blood products. The airway is opened and maintained by nonintubation techniques. Cervical spine motion restriction is maintained if indicated. When a prehospital supraglottic airway, is present, it is assessed for adequacy by measuring $ETCO_2$ and SpO_2. Depending on the type of supraglottic device, a gastric tube may be passed. For patients without a prehospital supraglottic airway, a chin lift or jaw thrust is performed, followed by manual clearance or aspiration of secretions, blood, and/or foreign bodies. Supplemental oxygen is administered. For an adequately ventilating and spontaneously breathing patient, other maneuvers may not be required until the physiologic status improves or operative intervention is initiated.

For an obtunded patient, an oropharyngeal airway may be inserted, with ventilation assisted by a BVM device. Tolerance of an oral airway indicates a blunted or absent gag response and high potential for airway loss and aspiration. For a hypotensive patient proceeding to the OR, these maneuvers may be adequate to maintain ventilation and oxygenation for the brief time until volume is administered before anesthetic induction with intubation. As in any aspect of the profession, the surgeon must balance the urgency for intubation with the risks of the procedure. When unable to maintain ventilation with less invasive techniques (e.g., due to facial injuries, facial hair, anatomy) or when prolonged time to operation or other intervention for hemorrhage is present, intubation may be emergently indicated.

Before administration of medications, the surgeon must assess and plan for alternative techniques to obtain an airway if intubation is unsuccessful. These include bougie assistance, bronchoscopic, and incisional (surgical) options (see later). To perform DAI, a sedative with or without a fast-acting neuromuscular blocker is frequently administered (Table 36.5) to enhance glottic visualization. Video laryngoscopy with cervical motion restriction is the preferred method for intubation of critically ill patients. A multicenter randomized of 1417 patients was stopped early after interim analysis demonstrated a statistically significant ($p < 0.001$) first-attempt success rate in the video laryngoscopy group (85%) versus the direct laryngoscopy group (71%).[106] Rates of severe complications, esophageal intubation, injury to teeth, and aspiration were similar between the groups. ETCO$_2$ is the best method to confirm appropriate position of the tube in the trachea.[107] Chest and abdomen auscultation with a chest radiograph are also performed, although these maneuvers are insufficiently accurate for this high-stake procedure.

An adequate airway is frequently challenging to obtain in a trauma patient. The surgeon must prepare and be facile with multiple methods other than endotracheal intubation to rapidly secure adequate ventilation and oxygenation. Common adjuncts in a difficult intubation scenario include a tracheal tube introducer (gum elastic bougie) and supraglottic devices. When the normal view of the glottis is obscured, the bougie may be placed with a limited view of the vocal cords. A characteristic "click" sensation is appreciated as the device passes over tracheal cartilage. An endotracheal tube is subsequently passed over the guide. Studies and meta-analyses regarding routine use of a tracheal guide have reported mixed results. Some suggested improvement in success rates of first-pass emergency intubation with a bougie compared with standard stylets.[108,109] Others have found no benefit.[110-112] The tracheal guide remains a useful adjunct in management of a difficult airway, with value dependent on the skill and familiarity of the provider. Supraglottic airway devices are discussed earlier.

When first-pass intubation is not successful, preparation for potential incisional airway (aka front-of-neck airway and surgical airway) access should begin. Before the onset of physiologic deterioration and profound hypoxia, a cricothyroidotomy should be performed if other approaches have failed. In some cases, because of extensive injuries, an incisional approach may be the initial best method to obtain an open airway. Inability to maintain oxygenation with a BVM between intubation attempts (cannot oxygenate–cannot intubate scenarios) is another indication for an incisional airway. The minimal equipment needed for a cricothyroidotomy is a scalpel, an endotracheal tube (usually present because of intubation attempts; a #6 tube is optimal), and two hands. A bougie and blunt dissection instrument may be helpful as well. When indicated, the incisional airway procedure cannot be delayed while awaiting equipment because the patient is at immediate risk of death. One method to perform a cricothyroidotomy is listed in Box 36.6 and illustrated in Fig. 36.11. During performance of a cricothyroidotomy, the surgeon must frequently palpate the underlying structures to maintain midline dissection and avoid injury to the lateral structures of the neck. The complication of mainstem intubation is frequent and may be avoided by attention to the depth of tube insertion. Regardless of the method in which an airway is obtained, frequent and diligent reassessment is necessary. Common causes of postintubation hypoxia and/or clinical deterioration may be recalled through the "DOPE" mnemonic: related to **D**isplacement, **O**bstruction, **P**neumothorax, or **E**quipment failure (Box 36.7).

Breathing

Limited respiratory effort, hypoxemia, and/or dyspnea are treated with oxygen, support of ventilation, and further assessment for etiology. After the upper airway is assessed and managed, diagnosis and treatment of thoracic injuries that affect oxygen delivery, ventilation, and blood pressure are performed. The surgeon visualizes chest movement for paradoxical motion and muscle retractions, auscultates breath sounds, palpates and inspects the entire thorax for instability and wounds (including the posterior chest via a log roll or other technique that limits spine mobility), visualizes the neck veins, evaluates tracheal position at the sternal notch for deviation off midline, inspects nail beds and lips for cyanosis, and

TABLE 36.5	Some Medications Used During Drug-Assisted Intubation		
MEDICATION	**ACTION**	**DOSING**	**COMMENTS**
Ketamine	Dissociative anesthetic	0.5–1 mg/kg, repeated if necessary	May induce airway/respiratory collapse. Cardiac depression with higher doses (>1 mg/kg) during shock as a result of catecholamine depletion.
Etomidate	Anesthetic, sedative-hypnotic	0.15–0.3 mg/kg	Short acting, rapid onset, relative few cardiac effects, less respiratory depression
Propofol	Anesthetic	0.5–2 mg/kg	Cause or exacerbate hypotension. Do not administer with shock.
Midazolam	Benzodiazepine	0.2–0.3 mg/kg	Amnestic effects, dose-related myocardial depression
Fentanyl	Narcotic	0.5–1 mcg/kg	Pain relief. May exacerbate hypotension with shock. Respiratory depression.
Rocuronium	Nondepolarizing neuromuscular blocker	1 mg/kg	No hemodynamic effects. Prolonged paralysis. Administer sedative and pain relief to avoid awake paralysis.
Succinylcholine	Depolarizing neuromuscular blocker	1–2 mg/kg	Use another agent if hyperkalemia, renal failure, burn, spine injury, myopathy, open globe, malignant hyperthermia, or pseudocholinesterase deficiency.
Phenylephrine	Vasopressor	50-mcg (or 1-mcg/kg) boluses	Treat intubation-associated hypotension.
Ephedrine	Vasopressor	6-mg (or 0.5-mg/kg) boluses	

BOX 36.6 Technique of Cricothyroidotomy

1. An assistant maintains manual cervical motion restriction. The front of the cervical collar is removed (if present).
2. The nondominant hand identifies the thyroid cartilage, spreads and retracts the tissues overlying the cricothyroid space, and stabilizes the larynx. An assistant may be helpful if a large amount of tissue is present. Continuous retraction accomplished by not releasing the nondominant hand facilitates visualization.
3. Maintaining lateral tension on the tissues with the nondominant hand to stretch the skin, a vertical incision is made in the midline from the thyroid cartilage superiorly to the cricoid cartilage inferiorly. The vertical incision minimizes potential to encounter larger vessels.
4. Blunt or sharp dissection is used to identify the cricothyroid membrane, which is palpated with the dominant hand and is located between the thyroid cartilage and cricoid ring.
5. The cricothyroid membrane is incised transversely. The scalpel is rotated so that the blade is facing away from the patient. The back (blunt) end of the scalpel handle is inserted partially into the trachea and rotated several times to dilate the cricothyroidotomy. Using the blunt end of the scalpel reduces the risk of laceration to the posterior wall of the trachea.
6. Insertion of the fifth digit of the dominant hand will confirm entry into a hollow rigid tube. A bougie (if immediately available) may be passed into the trachea.
7. A 6-0 endotracheal tube is inserted directly (or over the bougie) through the cricothyroidotomy into the trachea. The precise size of the tube is not critical. The tube needs to be small enough for easy insertion and large enough for adequate air passage.
8. The tube should be passed only until the balloon is within the trachea to avoid mainstem intubation.
9. The endotracheal tube balloon is inflated. The bougie is removed if present. Assisted ventilation is performed. Appropriate location is verified with $ETCO_2$ detection and auscultation of bilateral breath sounds.
10. The tube is secured with sutures to the skin after ensuring a tracheal location without mainstem placement.

reviews oxygen saturation and capnography. In some centers, a chest radiograph is often able to be obtained simultaneously without disrupting or delaying other aspects of the primary survey.

Focused ultrasound is increasingly available and functions as an extension of physical exam. The extended focused assessment with sonography for trauma (eFAST) technique has demonstrated value. Training and practice in critical trauma ultrasound techniques are recommended. Ventilatory problems may be secondary to pain from thoracic cage injuries such as pneumothorax (simple, tension, open), hemothorax, flail chest, and/or pulmonary contusion. Discussion in this section is limited to emergent management during the primary survey.

Retractions, paradoxical chest wall movements (movement of a portion of the chest wall "in" with inspiration and "out" with expiration), hypoxia, and cyanosis indicate potential imminent respiratory collapse. Rapid intervention is essential. Decreased breath sounds are consistent with pneumothorax, hemothorax, pulmonary contusion, bronchial injury, bronchial obstruction (foreign body), diaphragm rupture with viscerothorax, and mainstem intubation. Palpated instability, asymmetric chest motion, and a flail (paradoxical) segment indicate thoracic cage fractures, frequently associated with pulmonary contusion. The pain related to chest fractures may quickly lead to respiratory fatigue. A wound with communication to the pleural cavity diagnoses an open pneumothorax. Spontaneous negative-pressure breathing is

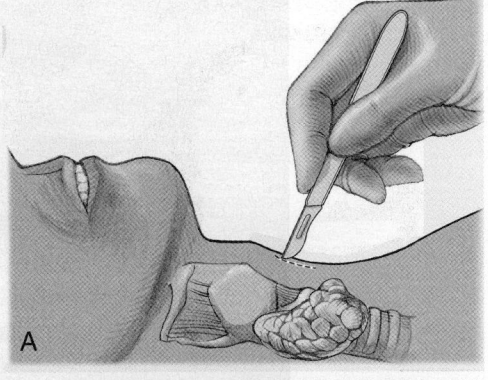
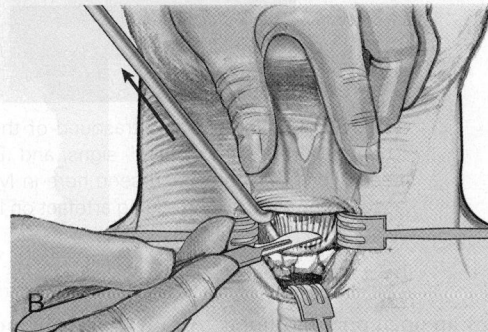
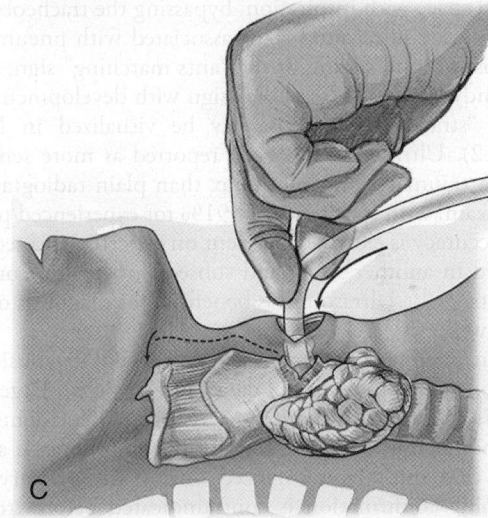

FIGURE 36.11 Technique of cricothyroidotomy. The cricothyroid membrane is identified by palpation, and a longitudinal incision is made along the trachea centered on the membrane (A). The incision and dissection are continued through the cricothyroid membrane in transverse fashion, and the cricothyroidotomy is spread (B), allowing the passage of a tracheal tube (C). (From Katos MG, Goldenberg D. Emergency cricothyrotomy. *Oper Tech Otolaryngol Head Neck Surg.* 2007;18[2]:110-114.)

BOX 36.7 DOPE Mnemonic

Displacement: Endotracheal tube displacement (right mainstem) or dislodgement.
Obstruction: Mucous plug, kink in ventilator tubing.
Pneumothorax: Simple or tension, increased due to positive pressure ventilation.
Equipment failure: Disconnect from ventilator and perform manual ventilation.

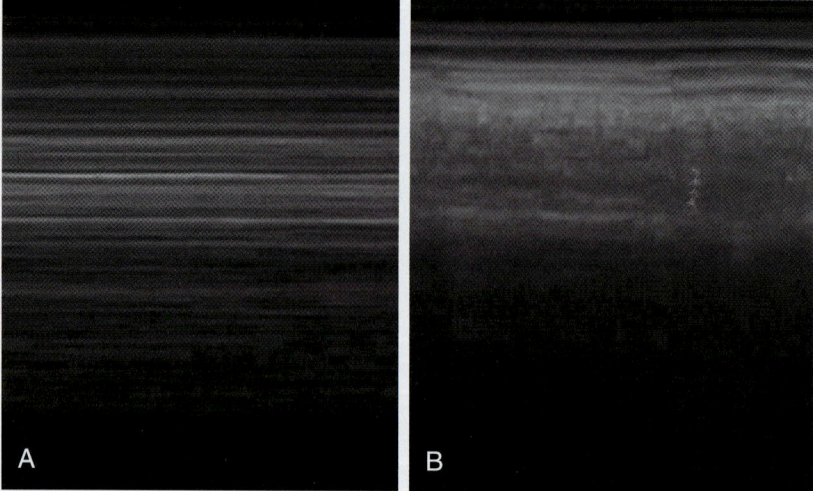

FIGURE 36.12 M-mode ultrasound of the lung. (A) Positive for pneumothorax (absent lung sliding), with "bar code" or "stratosphere" signs, and (B) negative or normal findings (lung sliding present), with "sandy beach" or "seashore" sign seen here in M-mode ultrasound. (From VanBerlo B, Wu D, Li B, et al. Accurate assessment of the lung sliding artefact on lung ultrasonography using a deep learning approach. *Comput Biol Med*. 2022;148:105953.)

impaired by an open pneumothorax. Air preferentially moves into the pleural space with inspiration, bypassing the tracheobronchial system. B-mode ultrasound signs associated with pneumothorax include loss of lung sliding or the "ants marching" sign. Absence of the "sandy beach" or "seashore" sign with development of "bar code" or "stratosphere" signs may be visualized in M-mode (Fig. 36.12). Ultrasound has been reported as more sensitive to diagnose a traumatic pneumothorax than plain radiography and physical exam, with specificities of 91% for experienced practitioners.[113] Accuracy is clearly dependent on expertise and technique, as outlined in another study and subsequent replies, comments, and reports.[114–117] Ultrasound is beneficial for diagnosis of hemothorax as well.

Tension pneumothorax represents a specific diagnosis with a defined constellation of clinical data (see Box 36.3). Urgent management is indicated to reduce the risk of patient demise from rapid hemodynamic collapse. Tension pneumothorax is a clinical diagnosis that must be recognized during the primary survey. Radiographic confirmation is contraindicated before treatment. Clinical findings include hypotension (due to decreased cardiac venous return), unilateral absent or reduced breath sounds, pneumothorax by eFAST, deviation of the trachea at the sternal notch, and potential cervical venous distention. As described earlier, emergent chest decompression is indicated without further diagnostic study. The optimal site for needle location is debated, with some studies reporting thinner chest wall tissue at the anterior axillary line and another reporting less tissue (particularly in higher-BMI patients) on the anterior chest. Thus, decompression may be performed via needle catheter thoracostomy at the fifth intercostal space (at or superior to the inframammary fold) and either at the axillary line or between the anterior and midaxillary lines. An alternative location is on the anterior chest at the second intercostal space and midclavicular line (Fig. 36.13). These locations are recommended to avoid injury to the great vessels, heart, and intraabdominal structures. A "finger thoracostomy" incision at the fifth intercostal space and between the anterior axillary and midaxillary lines permits finger entry into the pleural cavity for more reliable decompression with subsequent tube placement.

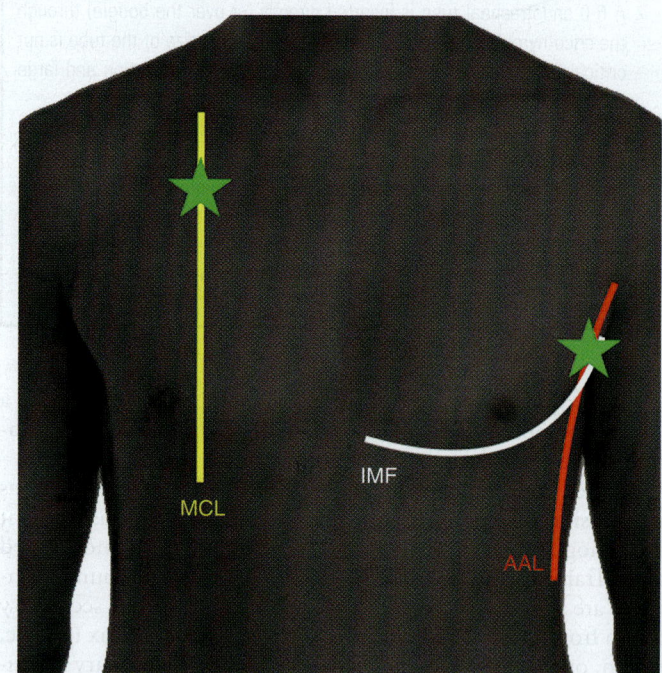

FIGURE 36.13 Locations for needle chest decompression. *Stars* denote approximate locations for emergent pleural decompression. *AAL*, Anterior axillary line; *IMF*, inframammary fold; *MCL*, midclavicular line.

The procedure of finger thoracostomy is identical to open chest tube placement until tube insertion. Creating a more cephalad incision reduces the chance of abdominal entry and misplacement of the tube into the liver, spleen, or other abdominal structure.

Despite a plethora of potential diagnoses, initial management of chest injuries involves a limited number of interventions. Delivery of supplemental oxygen with potential ventilatory support (manual or mechanical) is indicated for hypoxia, hypercarbia, and/or respiratory fatigue secondary to pulmonary contusion, chest cage fractures, and severe chest pain. The respiratory abnormalities related to an open pneumothorax may be treated with chest tube placement followed by an airtight dressing. Depending on the clinical situation, positive pressure ventilation via an endotracheal tube to improve aeration may be performed initially. A dressing and chest tube are placed after initiation of positive pressure ventilation to prevent expansion of a pneumothorax and development of tension physiology. Tube thoracostomy, even if needle decompression has been successful, is the initial treatment for most chest injuries because the procedure allows thoracic decompression, evacuation of air and blood, and expansion of the lung. Tube size is no longer considered critical.[118] Smaller chest tubes (12–20 Fr) are effective. Percutaneous kits are available. However, time to chest decompression is important, and an open technique may be best for the patient in extremis. For tracheobronchial injuries, a large air leak may be present, and ventilation may be ineffective. Advanced airway skills with fiberoptic-assisted advancement of the endotracheal tube to place it distal to the injury or selective intubation of the unaffected bronchus may be beneficial.

Circulation

The primary goal of a cardiovascular assessment is determining the presence or absence of shock. During initial assessment of the trauma patient, shock is defined as clinical evidence of end-organ hypoperfusion. Clinical signs of shock are demonstrated in Box 36.8. Although hypotension is a clear indicator of cardiovascular decompensation, shock may be present before the onset of hypotension due to the efficiency of physiologic compensatory mechanisms, particularly in fit individuals. Shock may be unappreciated in patients with preinjury hypertension. As mentioned previously, an SI of >0.8 and $ETCO_2$ <30 mm Hg are associated with mortality and massive blood transfusion. The most common cause of shock in the injured patient is hemorrhage. Acute blood loss must be evaluated before other etiologies of shock are assumed.

The study of hemorrhagic shock and resuscitation has produced rapid advances and changes in therapy over the past decade. These changes may be summarized with the term *DCR*.[67] Time to hemodynamic resuscitation is related to mortality.[60] DCR combines the use of exsanguinating hemorrhage control (e.g., wound packing, tourniquets), whole blood or balanced blood product transfusions, minimal crystalloid administration, minimal viable blood pressure resuscitation (systolic approximately 90 mm Hg) until definitive hemorrhage control, and correction of metabolic and coagulation abnormalities. Definitive hemorrhage control must be accomplished in a timely fashion.

Upon recognizing the potential of shock, circulatory access with two short-length, large-bore (16-g and larger) peripheral IV catheters, an intraosseous (IO) device, and/or a large-bore central venous catheter (CVC) is obtained. An EAST multicenter trauma video study of 1410 venous access attempts demonstrated that IO devices (tibial and humeral) can be placed more rapidly than CVCs and are more often successful than peripheral IVs.[119] IO devices have become widely used for trauma and code-related resuscitations as a reasonable alternative to failed IV access attempts in severe hypovolemic shock.[61] Resuscitation fluids are connected to a rapid volume warming device to improve speed of administration and decrease development of iatrogenic hypothermia.

Although advocated and practiced for decades, crystalloid volume resuscitation worsens acidosis, creates coagulopathy, and is associated with the development of acute respiratory distress syndrome (ARDS).[120,121] Because crystalloids are frequently not warmed to body temperature, the "lethal triad" of coagulopathy, acidosis, and hypothermia is accelerated.[120] Volume resuscitation with whole blood or blood products in a balanced (1:1:1 or 1:1:2, plasma: platelets: red cells) fashion is recommended. This treatment has demonstrated improved survival for patients with hemorrhagic shock in military and, subsequently, civilian practice.[122,123] Current studies are evaluating the relative efficacy of whole blood compared with balanced component therapy.[123] To facilitate appropriate transfusion ratios, massive transfusion protocols (MTPs; or massive hemorrhage protocols [MHPs]) are a standard in most hospitals. Although blood product resuscitation is preferred, ATLS recognizes that adequate volumes and types of products may not be available in all practice environments. In these situations, the surgeon uses the available materials, attempting to minimize crystalloid while maintaining adequate perfusion until blood is available.

Trauma-induced coagulopathy (TIC) is a postinjury inflammatory state associated with acidemia, hypothermia, and disruption of coagulation. TIC occurs in approximately 25% of trauma patients.[124] Several treatments are available to support the coagulation cascade. For patients using preinjury anticoagulant medication, vitamin K, cryoprecipitate, and/or prothrombin precipitate complex (PCC) may be administered depending on the specific anticoagulant, injuries, and laboratory results. Thromboelastography (TEG) and rotational thromboelastometry (ROTEM) are viscoelastic hemostatic assays (VHAs) that are used to provide targeted maintenance of the coagulation system. Clot formation is assessed based on a small quantity of whole blood. A real-time graphic is produced, providing a dynamic representation of clot generation. Component deficiencies are illustrated as morphologic changes (Fig. 36.14).

Hyperfibrinolysis occurs in a subset of bleeding patients and has been associated with poor outcomes.[125] TXA is a synthetic reversible competitive inhibitor to the lysine receptor on plasminogen. TXA prevents plasmin from binding to fibrin, thus reducing fibrinolysis and stabilizing a fibrin clot. When administered within 3 hours of injury, TXA has demonstrated a decrease in mortality in specific high-risk hypotensive bleeding populations.[77] Initially, the recommended dosing was a 1-g TXA bolus within 3 hours from injury followed by a second 1-g infusion over 8 hours. However, a single dose of 2 g used in a study of patients with TBI and/or hemorrhagic shock is also safe and simpler.[126,127]

While volume resuscitation is performed, a rapid evaluation is initiated to elucidate the source of blood loss and initiate mitigation therapies. A quick mnemonic for potential sources is "Four and the Floor." This corresponds to five major locations in which

---

BOX 36.8 Indicators of Shock in the Injured Patient

Agitation or confusion
Tachycardia
Tachypnea
Diaphoresis
Cool, mottled extremities
Weak distal pulses
Decreased pulse pressure
Decreased urine output
Hypotension
Elevated shock index (SI)

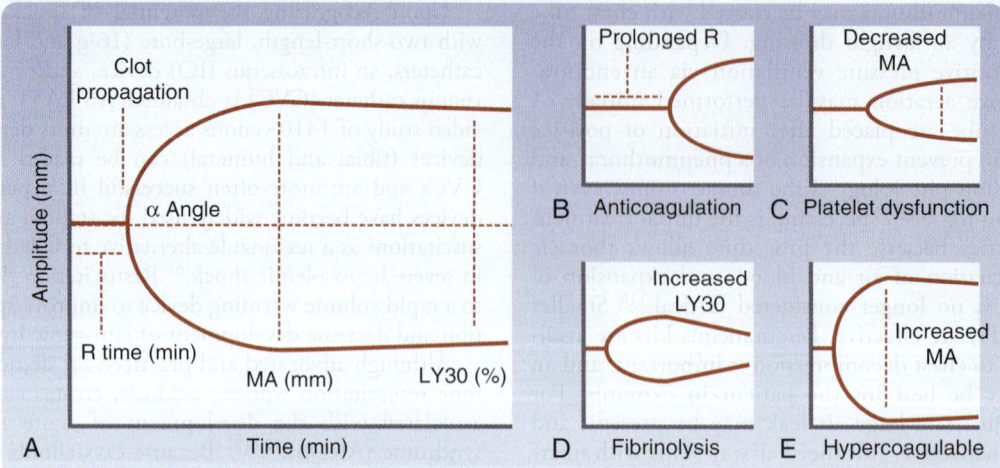

FIGURE 36.14 Thromboelastogram (TEG) with standard parameters and pathologies. (A) Normal TEG. (B) Delayed clot formation with prolonged R time, treated with plasma transfusion. (C) Decreased maximum amplitude with low platelet function, treated with platelet transfusion. (D) Elevated LY30 representing fibrinolysis, treated with tranexamic acid. (E) Decreased R time and elevated MA representing hypercoagulable state. α *Angle*, Clot formation/polymerization; *LY30*, percent amplitude decrease at 30 minutes, index of clot breakdown (lysis); *MA*, maximum amplitude, clot strength; *R time*, time to clot formation.

exsanguination may occur: four noncompressible compartments (chest cavity, abdominal cavity, retroperitoneum/pelvis, and intramuscular from long bone fractures and tissue injury) and compressible external wounds (onto the floor). Evaluation under the "x" portion will locate and treat external hemorrhage. Chest radiography, pelvis radiography, and ultrasound are employed to assist with identification of the location of hemorrhage and allow quick cavitary triage. A chest radiograph and eFAST will diagnose a large hemothorax, which is initially managed by drainage with chest tube placement. A pelvic radiograph will identify fractures, which are frequently the etiology of retroperitoneal hemorrhage. An "open-book" or displaced pelvic fracture is managed by placement of an external pelvic binder, either a commercial device or a bed sheet, which closes a widened pelvic inlet, reduces the potential pelvic space, and promotes tamponade of venous bleeding. FAST is the most common initial method to detect intraperitoneal fluid. FAST visualizes the hepatorenal, splenorenal, and pelvic spaces. This fluid is presumed to be blood in the clinical scenario of trauma. FAST can be performed rapidly in the trauma bay and repeated if necessary. An example of blood in the hepatorenal space on FAST scan is demonstrated in Fig. 36.15.

Patients who respond to therapy by developing a normalizing physiology may subsequently receive comprehensive evaluation to diagnose all injuries more precisely. A common pitfall is continued administration of volume at a high rate that may mask ongoing blood loss. Failure to respond to initial volume resuscitation indicates continued bleeding, necessitating immediate intervention. Ongoing intrathoracic bleeding after chest tube placement may require thoracotomy. Intraabdominal bleeding in the hemodynamically nonresponding patient warrants emergent laparotomy. After application of an external binder, continued hemorrhage due to pelvic fractures is managed by either emergent operative packing or catheter-based embolization.

Although hemorrhagic shock is common, trauma patients may present with other etiologies for impaired hemodynamics. The surgeon must be aware of these potential diagnoses and be prepared to intervene. Table 36.6 lists alternative etiologies of shock in the trauma patient, the associated clinical features, potential

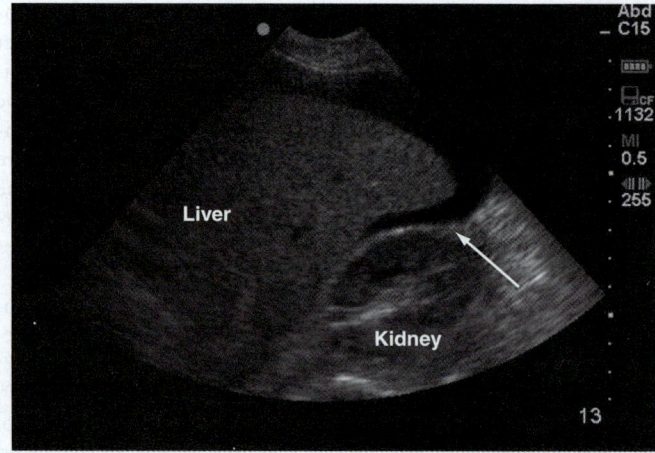

FIGURE 36.15 Focused abdominal sonography in trauma (FAST) scan. This FAST shows fluid in the hepatorenal space (Morison pouch), suggestive of new hemorrhage. The *arrow* identifies fluid (potential blood) between the liver and the right kidney.

diagnostic modalities, and treatments. In all cases, secure, reliable venous access is important. Etiologies may be combined or have an additive component of hemorrhagic or hypovolemic shock. Fluid resuscitation frequently remains a component of therapy. Concomitant acute nontrauma diagnoses may be present, including myocardial infarction, stroke, pulmonary embolus, and preinjury sepsis. These diagnoses may be the etiology of injury.

Traditional teaching states that vasoactive medications have no role in hemorrhagic shock. However, recent experience supports vasopressor administration for temporary adjunctive management of hypotension during intubation. In addition, refractory vasodilatation is prevalent in the final phase of all types of decompensated shock. Hemorrhagic shock can alter neurohormonal function. A vasopressin-depleted state occurs even with continued blood product resuscitation. In a randomized study of 100 patients, the addition of vasopressin (4-U bolus followed by 48-h infusion at

TABLE 36.6 Etiologies Nonhemorrhagic Shock in Trauma Patient

ETIOLOGY	CLINICAL FEATURES	DIAGNOSIS	TREATMENT
Tension pneumothorax	Hypotension, absent breath sounds on side of injury, tracheal deviation away from side of injury, distended neck veins	Clinical, pneumothorax by eFAST	Pleural decompression
Neurogenic, spinal injury	Hypotension, bradycardia, fall/diving/motor vehicle/penetrating injury to spine	Limb paralysis, radiographs	Volume support, pressor agent(s)
Cardiac tamponade	Hypotension, distended neck veins, penetrating chest wound	Clinical, eFAST	Pericardiocentesis (ultrasound guided), resuscitative thoracotomy if in extremis
Cardiac contusion	Hypotension, arrhythmias, motor vehicle/blunt force to chest	ECG, eFAST, echocardiogram, troponin levels	Pressors, support oxygenation, antiarrhythmics
Sepsis	Prolonged time from injury to evaluation, vehicle crash/penetrating injury, peritoneal exam, cellulitis	Clinical, CT scan	Volume resuscitation, pressors, source control
Nontraumatic	History of collapse before injury	ECG, CT imaging	Treatment per primary etiology, volume support, pressor

CT, Computed tomography; *ECG,* electrocardiogram; *eFAST,* extended focused assessment with sonography for trauma.

≤0.04 U/min with goal mean arterial pressure [MAP] ≥65) to initial resuscitation decreased total blood products transfused without an increase in mortality or complications. Rates of deep venous thrombosis were reduced despite theoretical enhanced platelet function.[128] Data regarding adjunctive vasopressin during modern blood product–based trauma resuscitation is extremely limited.

Disability and Exposure

After assessment and critical management of circulatory status, rapid determination of global neurologic function is the next step in the primary survey. The surgeon performs a focused neurologic assessment to detect abnormalities in brain and spinal cord function. Early diagnosis and management of TBIs and avoidance of exacerbating a spinal cord injury (SCI) through conversion of a partial to a complete defect are important to maximize functional recovery. Conclusions regarding neurologic function are made based on responses to the questions, "What is your name?" and "Move your arms and legs." Appropriate response demonstrates cognitive and spinal function.

The GCS score (see Table 36.3) and pupil reactivity should be documented before administration of sedation and/or intubation medications. Severe head injury is assumed at a GCS score of ≤8. The spinal cord is grossly assessed by visualizing movement of the extremities. Neurogenic shock should be considered if hypotension and lack of extremity movement are present. However, the provider must be careful in attributing shock solely to an SCI because concomitant hemorrhage is frequently present. The incidence of neurogenic shock with spinal injuries is difficult to determine because of the heterogenicity of studies. Rates of 20% to 29% have been reported in patients with cervical injuries. Neurogenic shock is much rarer with injuries below the sixth thoracic vertebra.[129,130]

All clothing is removed from the patient to permit complete examination, core body temperature measurement, and other indicated interventions. Maintaining patient dignity and modesty is a priority during this process. Patient belongings are collected and secured per institution policy. Hypothermia will aggravate shock and coagulopathy. Therefore, warmed blankets, heating elements (i.e., Bair Hugger), elevated room temperature, and warmed resuscitative fluids are of critical importance. Once the primary survey is completed and all aspects (xABCDE) demonstrate adequate physiologic response, the secondary survey is initiated.

Resuscitative Thoracotomy and Endovascular Aortic Occlusion

After critical injury, select patients who experience cardiac arrest may benefit from resuscitative thoracotomy (RT) in the ED. First formally described by Cooley and Debakey over 50 years ago for penetrating cardiovascular trauma, RT provides opportunity for four therapeutic maneuvers: release of cardiac tamponade, temporary repair of cardiac injury, cross-clamping of the distal thoracic aorta, and management of intrathoracic bleeding. Because of risks to healthcare providers performing the procedure and overall low rates of salvage, multiple studies have attempted to define what groups of patients should be candidates for the procedure on the basis of injury mechanism and physiology at the time of presentation. Patients with the best outcomes after RT are those with penetrating thoracic injuries and signs of life (reactive pupils, spontaneous ventilation, carotid pulse, measurable or palpable blood pressure, extremity movement, or cardiac electrical activity) upon reaching the ED. Seamon and colleagues reviewed 72 studies with 10,238 patients, concluding that patients presenting after penetrating chest mechanism, with and without signs of life, survived at 21.3% and 8.3%, respectively. Conversely, blunt trauma patients presenting with and without signs of life revealed 4.6% and 0.7% survival from RT, respectively.[131] Moreover, an NTDB review of 11,380 patients undergoing RT revealed a 100% mortality in both blunt and penetrating mechanisms for patients above the age of 57.[132] In these circumstances, thoracostomy tubes, as indicated with conservative transfusion measures, are likely more appropriate.

These research studies and others form the basis of the 2015 EAST recommendation against RT after blunt traumatic injury without signs of life and in favor of RT in penetrating trauma with and without signs of life.[131] An alternative guideline for performance of RT was proposed by the WTA in 2012, which endorsed a time-based approach for injured patients undergoing cardiopulmonary resuscitation (CPR). They advocate for RT for prehospital CPR time of <15 minutes in penetrating torso injury, <10 minutes in blunt trauma, and <5 minutes in penetrating neck and extremity injury.[133] Regardless of which algorithm is followed, RT should only be performed in locations with readily available surgical support for definitive repair of thoracic injuries if return of spontaneous circulation is achieved.

REBOA has emerged over the past decade as an alternative method of obtaining temporary hemorrhage control in the decompensating trauma patient. Although traditionally employed in the setting of abdominal aortic aneurysm repair, application for combat casualty care in noncompressible truncal hemorrhage was first described during the Korean War. With the evolution of this technology for rapid deployment in both military and civilian sectors, REBOA is now being used in over 50 domestic trauma centers in the setting of advanced shock and imminent cardiac arrest. Depending on the zone of trauma, REBOA is introduced through the common femoral artery, advanced proximal to level of injury, and inflated, effectively shunting blood to the heart and brain while also decreasing hemorrhage. Whereas the original ER-REBOA device is inserted through a 7-Fr sheath and produces complete aortic occlusion, newer devices are being developed that can be placed through smaller sheaths and/or achieve partial aortic occlusion.

Currently, there is no high-grade evidence to support indications for or the superiority of REBOA beyond standard care, and a comparison of technique to RT introduces both survival and indication biases. In October 2023 the first randomized clinical trial evaluating REBOA versus standard resuscitation measures across UK trauma centers was published, which was halted early due to worse outcomes in the REBOA group. Ninety patients were randomized, and mortality at 3, 6, and 24 hours was significantly higher in the REBOA group.[134] Inclusion criteria were very broad, and only 19 of the 46 in the REBOA treatment arm received the treatment. These findings underscore the need for more clinical trials evaluating the technology in subsets of trauma patients for whom it may have potential benefit. At present, protocols for utility are developed by multidisciplinary committee and vary by institution. Deployment of this technology should only take place within a trauma system capable of managing definitive surgical hemostasis and the multiple possible complications of placement (i.e., vascular injury, extremity ischemia, spinal cord ischemia).[135]

SECONDARY SURVEY

Although the primary survey identifies immediate life-threatening conditions, many significant injuries may remain undetected. The secondary survey serves to uncover these injuries through a comprehensive head-to-toe physical examination, coupled with a detailed medical history and an account of the injury's circumstances. ATLS emphasizes the importance of obtaining AMPLE information: **A**llergies, **M**edications, **P**ast illnesses and pregnancy, **L**ast meal, and **E**vents/**E**nvironment related to the injury.[89]

The secondary survey commences after the primary survey is completed in hemodynamically normal patients and once unstable patients respond to resuscitation. Reevaluation of vital signs is critical at this stage. Throughout evaluation, respect and preservation of personhood, modesty, and autonomy are paramount. The surgeon must inform the patient regarding all steps and request permission to examine. Documentation of exam findings is optimal if a scribe can record findings, positive and negative, as the surgeon performs the assessments.

The examination begins with the head, palpating for less obvious lacerations requiring attention, hidden in the hair or beneath hematomas. Because bruising and swelling may intensify over time, these areas warrant careful examination. The facial examination includes reassessment of the pupils, evaluation of the conjunctiva and sclera for hemorrhage or lacerations, and a basic vision assessment. Inquiries about diplopia, eye pain, or foreign body sensation are vital, along with evaluation for proptosis or enophthalmos. Ocular movements are assessed, with the removal of contact lenses if present. Limitations in eye motion might suggest cranial nerve injury, muscular entrapment, orbital fractures, or retrobulbar hemorrhage. Palpation of the facial bones can reveal tenderness, crepitus, or step-offs. The nose is examined for septal hematomas requiring treatment, and the mouth is examined for external and intraoral lacerations, broken teeth, or alveolar fractures.

Neck examination follows, necessitating an assistant to limit motion if a cervical collar is present. The posterior neck is assessed for tenderness, deformities, or step-offs, along with the presence of hematomas, lacerations, crepitus, and bruit. Changes in voice quality may signify swelling and potential airway compromise. The carotid pulse and presence of a thrill are palpated, with careful auscultation for bruits.

The chest examination includes inspection for ecchymosis, swelling, or lacerations, particularly in patients with crush injuries to the thorax or abdomen. Observation of breathing patterns helps identify paradoxical breathing or flail segments. Lung sounds are examined, with attention to the possibility of increasing pneumothorax or hemothorax. Palpation over the clavicle, sternum, and ribs is performed to detect tenderness and crepitus, with percussion identifying areas of dullness or hyperresonance, suggestive of hemo- or pneumothorax.

Abdominal assessment starts with inspection for distention, bruising, hematomas, and wounds, specifically searching for seat-belt signs after motor vehicle collisions. Bowel sounds are auscultated, and the abdomen is palpated to discern peritonitis or localized tenderness, distinguishing soft tissue injury from intraabdominal damage. The pelvis is reevaluated for bruising, swelling, or hematoma formation. The perineum is assessed for injury, with particular attention to scrotal hematoma and blood at the meatus, indicative of urethral injury. Vaginal inspection is important in unconscious patients who menstruate to avoid prolonged presence of devices, which may lead to toxic shock syndrome. Vaginal inspection for blood in appropriate clinical scenarios (e.g., severe pelvic fracture, penetrating injury) is indicated. Appropriate modesty, permission, and chaperone presence are to be maintained.

In cases where SCI is a possibility, the patient is turned using a modified log roll technique, employing at least four people: one controlling the head and neck, two rotating the torso, and one performing the examination. This procedure is synchronized, led by the person at the head. The backboard, if present, is ideally removed at this time to prevent discomfort and skin breakdown. A rectal examination is performed if indicated to assess rectal tone or bleeding.

The extremity and vascular examinations include looking for deformities, swelling, and bruising, followed by palpation for tenderness. Joint mobility and muscle strength are assessed, as is pulse strength. In the absence of palpable pulses, a Doppler is used. An injured extremity index, akin to the ankle-brachial index, is evaluated in injured extremities to determine the need for further vascular evaluation. Extremities with fractures or crush injuries are at risk for compartment syndrome, necessitating assessment of muscle compartments for swelling and pain on passive stretch.

A neurologic examination concludes the physical assessment. The GCS score is calculated based on eye opening, verbal responses, and motor responses. Orientation and memory are assessed, along with cranial nerves, sensation, and motor strength. Detailed sensory examination and assessment of muscle strength should be performed. This will characterize the injury level in spinal cord trauma and identify nerve injury associated with fractures and dislocations.

In patients with penetrating injuries, vigilance is essential to account for all wounds. Skin folds, the axilla, perineum, scalp, and buttock folds are thoroughly examined. Marking wounds with radiopaque indicators before imaging is often beneficial. Identified injuries are further evaluated with imaging, including eFAST examinations and chest, abdomen, and pelvic radiographs to identify fractures, pneumo- and hemothoraces, and the position of foreign bodies. Plain radiographs are obtained for extremity injuries to localize foreign bodies and identify fractures. Fractures and dislocations might necessitate computed tomography (CT) evaluation.

After physical examination, necessary laboratory and imaging tests are obtained. These include blood type and cross-matching, hemoglobin/hematocrit levels, lactate, base deficits, metabolic profiles, and coagulation profiles (TEG and ROTEM) for patients at high risk for coagulopathy or on anticoagulants. Alcohol and drug testing may aid in identifying etiologies of mental status abnormalities and candidates for substance use disorder treatment. Urinalysis should be obtained. Hematuria occurs with genitourinary injury. FAST and eFAST are valuable examinations and can be repeated as needed. Diagnostic peritoneal lavage has been supplanted by FAST and eFAST because ultrasound examinations are noninvasive and easily performed in the trauma bay. FAST is often used as a screening tool. CT is commonly used for comprehensive injury identification within the head, face, neck, chest, abdomen, and pelvis. Multiple CT scans are routinely performed in adult patients with significant blunt injury. Electrocardiograms are performed for patients with chest trauma or those potentially suffering from new or exacerbated medical conditions. Magnetic resonance imaging may be beneficial to further characterize neurologic or musculoskeletal injuries. Contrast studies such as retrograde urethrograms, cystograms, and esophagrams may be useful to characterize specific injuries. Bronchoscopy, esophagogastroduodenoscopy, and endoscopic retrograde pancreatography may be employed for specific diagnostic purposes.

Repeated evaluations reduce the risk of missed or delayed injury diagnoses because missed injuries may occur in 1% to 40% of trauma patients as a result of various factors, including patient complexity, altered consciousness, emergency surgery, and distracting injuries. Between 15% and 22% of these injuries are clinically significant.[136] Consultants are engaged as necessary. The tertiary survey, conducted the day after admission and once altered consciousness resolves, follows the secondary survey pattern, including imaging and laboratory review, to uncover overlooked findings or identify symptom progression.

MANAGEMENT OF SPECIFIC INJURIES

Damage Control Principles

The concept of damage control arose from critical review of the traditional approach of definitive injury repair at index operation. A portion of definitive repair patients would develop progressive intraoperative physiologic derangement with lethal triad exacerbation: hypothermia, coagulopathy, and metabolic acidosis. Damage control emerged as a method of halting this rapid deterioration through expeditious hemostasis (including abdominal packing), management of gastrointestinal (GI) contamination

with repair or resection, and temporary abdominal closure. The patient was subsequently transported to the ICU for continued resuscitation. Definitive reconstruction was delayed until physiologic improvement. Rotondo and associates first coined the term *"damage control"* surgery (DCS) to describe this approach to management in a series of 46 patients operated for penetrating abdominal injury. Although actual survival rates were similar between damage control and definitive laparotomy groups (55% vs. 58%, respectively), a significant improvement in survival was noted in a subset of patients with major vascular injury and two or more visceral injuries (77% vs. 11%, $P < 0.02$).[137] Although DCS began as a method to manage severe injuries in the abdomen, it is now used in the chest, pelvis, and extremities.

Damage control approaches in the chest employ similar principles to the abdomen, with control of major vascular and lung injury followed by temporary closure. Temporary closure in the chest can be constructed with placement of chest tubes and a clear drape or Esmarch bandage over the lung, followed by towels, nasogastric tubes, and a large Ioban dressing. Damage control orthopedics consists of temporary stabilization of fractures, such as use of an external fixator or C-clamp for the pelvis and external fixators for the extremities. Damage control vascular surgery involves placement of a vascular shunt using the largest shunt available that will fit the injured vessel to temporize bleeding and restore distal perfusion. Patients return to the OR no more than 48 hours after the index operation, at which time packs are removed and a definitive operation is performed.

Although an abbreviated operation may be beneficial in the setting of massive hemorrhage, hemodynamic instability, and the resultant lethal triad, it does carry risks that must be weighed against the benefits. Overuse of DCS can lead to additional surgeries, development of ventral hernias, enteroatmospheric fistula, prolonged ventilation, and delay in initiation of enteral nutrition, which can cause significant morbidity. It is important to be judicious when applying DCS so as not to put patients at risk for further morbidity.[138]

Functioning in tandem with DCS, MTPs or MHPs have emerged from military experience demonstrating improved survival with transfusion of 1:1:1 blood component ratios (plasma:platelets:PRBC) to approximate whole blood. This approach to the severely injured patient is termed *damage control resuscitation* and is defined by permissive hypotension, facilitation of rapid hemostasis with early balanced transfusion, treatment of coagulopathy, and minimization of crystalloid.[67] To inform initiation of MTP, the Assessment of Blood Consumption score provides a 4-point metric (penetrating mechanism, positive FAST, arrival SBP 90 mm Hg, and arrival pulse >120 bpm) whereby clinicians may request product coolers based on prehospital (if available) or initial vital signs. A score of at least 2 was predictive of MTP need (75% sensitivity, 86% specificity), and a delay in initiation is associated with a 5% increase in mortality per minute.[139,140] Many trauma centers have adopted this strategy and now have well-defined MTPs.

TEG provides adjunctive guidance to ongoing MTP and is a rapidly obtainable point-of-care metric. Originally developed approximately 70 years ago for assessment of inherited bleeding disorders, TEG has historically been employed in liver transplant and cardiac surgery. In traditional analyzers, clot formation is assessed based on resistance transduced from a pin in a small quantity (360 μL) of whole blood. As the blood oscillates, a real-time graphic is produced, providing a dynamic representation of clot generation. Newer generations of analyzers use nonmechanical methods. Component deficiencies are illustrated as morphologic changes to the clot cylinder (see Fig. 36.14). Potential advantages to use of TEG-based resuscitation include rapid results for individualized component transfusion, overall conservation of blood products, and a survival benefit with fewer deaths due to hemorrhagic shock in the first 6 hours after injury.[141]

An additional treatment adjunct to MTP in damage control resuscitation is TXA. TXA is a synthetic derivative of lysine with high affinity for lysine-binding sites on plasminogen, thus inhibiting fibrinolysis via antagonism of plasmin binding to fibrin surfaces. Administration of 2 g TXA is often used in initial resuscitation within many prehospital systems and some trauma centers.

Management of the Open Abdomen

Damage control laparotomy introduces potential additional morbidity for the patient, including formation of complex ventral hernias and enteroatmospheric fistulae. Management of the abdominal wall is focused on achieving primary closure as soon as safely possible or on reducing the expectant hernia to a more modest size. Several major trauma and emergency surgery societies publish and update guidelines regarding the management of the open abdomen.[142,143] Return to the OR for additional management of specific injuries typically commences at 24 to 48 hours from the index laparotomy but may proceed sooner if the patient's physiologic state improves as indicated by decreasing transfusions, improving lactate level, and resolving pressor use.

Injuries to the Brain
Traumatic Brain Injury Management

Several stakeholder organizations have endeavored to create guidelines based on the best available evidence or best practices as determined by experts in the field to ensure patients receive care that is likely to result in the best possible outcome. See Chapter 41 on several TBI practice management guidelines (PMGs). The care provided at the time of injury can have a substantial impact on a patient's recovery. The primary goal of TBI management is to prevent secondary brain injury, or treatment of recoverable cells (penumbra) around the traumatic focus. Because the primary brain injury process cannot be reversed or corrected, outcomes after TBI are dictated by how well secondary injury is prevented. The management of patients with TBI is to minimize all secondary brain injury, recognizing that many patients with severe brain injury will have nonneurologic injuries and organ dysfunction that can influence the goals and strategies of treatment. Raised intracranial pressure (ICP), decreased cerebral perfusion pressure (CPP), hypoxia, hypotension, hypertension, impaired cerebral autoregulation, systemic inflammatory response, seizures, and hyperpyrexia all have adverse effects on neurologic recovery. Thus, the mainstay of preventing secondary brain injury is standardized ATLS-based resuscitative efforts to facilitate normative brain physiology as quickly as possible. Control of severe uncontrolled hemorrhage, airway control, and ventilatory support are critical immediately after TBI. Hypotension and hypoxia must be prevented to ensure the best chance of survival with a good neurologic outcome. Resuscitation blood pressure goals sometimes target higher MAP than in the absence of TBI.

Injuries to the Spinal Cord and the Vertebral Column

Prehospital practice has evolved such that all patients with a potential mechanism to produce spinal injury are no longer systematically immobilized on long spine boards with cervical collars, neck blocks, and straps. This practice was thought to immobilize the spine and thereby prevent further damage to an injured spine during extrication and transport. This ingrained practice was questioned because of a lack of data supporting the purported benefits.[144] The detriments of ubiquitous use of this equipment have been validated. Cervical collars, particularly when ill-fitting, may increase intracranial pressure. About 5% of patients with TBI have a spine injury, and 25% of patients with a spine injury have at least a mild TBI.[145] Other concerns include reduced mouth opening and alteration of pharyngeal mechanics that can impede airway management. Cervical collars are uncomfortable, can cause pressure-related skin injury, can obscure wounds in patients with penetrating mechanisms, and can impede swallowing and increase the risk of aspiration. Similarly, long spine boards are uncomfortable and can result in pressure-related skin injury.[146]

However, excessive motion of the spine in a patient with an SCI can produce further damage. Data from the German trauma registry identified several factors that, in addition to pain, are most strongly associated with SCI and merit spinal motion restriction (SMR) until appropriate imaging can be performed: falls from greater than 3 m, age greater than 65, serious trauma injury, and TBI.[147] Expansion of cord ischemia can worsen the primary injury. High cervical SCI (C3–C5) may have immediate respiratory suppression requiring airway management and ventilatory support as a result of paresis of the phrenic nerves. Early ventilatory support may be indicated for patients with lower levels of spinal injury because of loss of abdominal and thoracic support for breathing, which produces atelectasis and potential progressive respiratory failure. Injuries to descending sympathetic pathways (T6 and above, intermediolateral column) may affect vasomotor tone, resulting in unopposed parasympathetic vagal outflow and neurogenic shock. Such patients may benefit from intravascular volume expansion and vasopressor support. A gross assessment of spinal cord function occurs during the primary survey by observing extremity movement.

Tenderness over the injured vertebrae or the presence of a vertebral column deformity is indicative of an associated acute fracture. Back examination may be performed using a log roll maneuver, with extreme attention to procedural details by at least three people (excluding the examiner) who turn the patient. One person supports the neck and shoulders at the head of the patient, and two people rotate the torso in synchrony. A fourth person performs the examination of the back and performs a digital rectal examination, which is indicated if spinal injury is suspected. If a backboard was previously placed, it is often removed at this time. The firm surface of a stretcher is adequate support. Patients with SCI have difficulty maintaining core temperature, and hypothermia may rapidly develop. Therefore, it is important to prevent heat loss by keeping the patient covered. Frequent reassessment is critical to detect a new or progressing deficit. The involvement of a spine surgeon upon injury diagnosis will guide further evaluation and expedite operative intervention when it is indicated. Immediate arrangements should be made for transfer when spine surgery services are not available. To avoid delays, subsequent imaging should be avoided unless the results will have an immediate impact on the care provided. See Chapter 41 for additional details on spine trauma.

Injuries to the Maxillofacial Region

It is estimated that more than 3 million facial injuries occur annually in the United States, and 25% of injuries reported to the

NTDB involve the face.[148,149] These injuries range from simple lacerations to complex facial fractures. Injury can result from blunt or penetrating mechanisms. The incidence of facial injury has decreased with the use of seat belts, the use of helmets, the establishment of stricter laws against drunk driving, graduated licenses for youth, restrictions regarding the use of mobile phones while driving, and increases in the use of passive safety devices such as airbags and safety glass. However, common mechanisms of injury continue to include motor vehicle and motorcycle crashes, falls, assaults, and sports-related injuries.[150] Maxillofacial trauma can be life threatening when associated with hemorrhage or airway obstruction. TBI frequently occurs in combination with facial fracture. Of those with a facial fracture, 20% to 80% will also have a head injury. Cervical fractures are seen in 4.9% to 8%.[151] In addition, long-term complications may produce deficits in vision, olfaction, hearing, and taste. Soft tissue and nerve injury can permanently impair appearance, with scarring and loss of facial expression. Bony injury can have a lasting impact on occlusion and speech.[152]

Immediate Management

Maxillofacial trauma can result in life-threatening hemorrhage, which is complicated by a threatened airway. There is a rich vascular supply to the midface, with multiple anastomoses between the internal and external carotid arteries. Approximately 1 in 10 patients with complex facial fractures will bleed significantly. In unconscious or altered patients, controlling hemorrhage, initiating blood product resuscitation, and providing a definitive airway are crucial early steps in treatment.[153] Compression, packing, and suture repair of lacerations are the initial steps in hemorrhage control of facial injuries. Topical hemostatic agents and hemostatic-impregnated packing materials are useful tools. Catheter or open approaches to identification and control of bleeding may be needed. Fracture stabilization can limit bleeding. Patients who are neurologically normal without spinal injury may benefit from sitting upright and leaning forward to prevent aspiration of blood during the resuscitation. Even without hemorrhage, airway compromise subsequent to maxillofacial injury may develop. There are six potential mechanisms for airway compromise with facial trauma: posterior displacement of maxillary fractures that block the nasal passages; loss of the anterior insertion point of the tongue with a mandible fracture, resulting in blockage of the oropharynx; fragments of teeth or soft tissue obstructing the airway; naso- or oropharyngeal bleeding; soft tissue swelling; and injury to the larynx or trachea.[154] Soft tissue swelling, alteration of the bony alignment of the face, hematoma, increased secretions, inability to manage secretions and blood, and nausea with vomiting can also lead to airway compromise. Early intubation may be lifesaving if there is potential for an unstable airway. Blood or debris in the oropharynx can greatly complicate intubation, and the application of backup airway options, including a surgical approach, should be anticipated and may be necessary. Standard approaches to airway management can be challenging in patients with maxillofacial trauma. Supine positioning predisposes to aspiration with vomiting, bleeding, and aspiration of foreign bodies. The face may be deformed and painful, hampering successful BVM ventilation. The jaw thrust maneuver may not be possible in the patient with a comminuted mandible fracture. Staff experienced in complex airway management should be present before administration of medications in an awake, neurologically normal patient. These medications may hamper the patient's ability to cough and clear secretions. It is better to tolerate an adequate, imperfect airway until assistance arrives than to create an airway emergency with inability to ventilate and inability to intubate. Cervical SMR is frequently needed during airway management, increasing the challenge of managing an already difficult airway. Frequently, bleeding from the face is exacerbated by hypothermia and coagulopathy, which should be uncompromisingly prevented or treated.

Evaluation

Facial injuries are identified on physical examination, during which the extent of soft tissue involvement is determined. The eyes are grossly examined for diplopia and subjective changes in visual acuity. The condition of the globe and the surrounding orbit requires careful evaluation for rupture or extraocular muscle entrapment, which requires urgent treatment. The external ear is examined, and drainage from the ear canal is identified when present. Midface and mandibular stability, proper dental occlusion, and quality of the dentition are assessed. Forehead and midface deformities are indicative of underlying frontal and maxillary bone fractures, respectively. When fractures or soft tissue injuries are identified, the motor function of the face should be assessed to evaluate facial nerve function.

Injuries to the face often benefit from three-dimensional imaging with thin-cut CT to visualize the facial bones. Sagittal, coronal, and three-dimensional reconstructions can aid in thorough structural assessment and evaluation of deep soft tissue. CT is indicated when severe external injury is identified on secondary survey or when facial abnormality is identified on cranial CT. Orbital views should be included when there is potential retrobulbar hemorrhage. Clinical signs of significant retrobulbar hemorrhage include subconjunctival hemorrhage, proptosis, and increased ocular pressure.[155] Lateral canthotomy and cantholysis can be sight-saving interventions. Imaging of the face should be performed only after life-threatening injuries have been addressed.

The facial skeleton is supported by four paired vertical and four horizontal buttresses (Fig. 36.16). Several patterns of facial fractures can occur. Frontal sinus fractures can include anterior wall, posterior wall, or both. The posterior wall separates the sinus from the cranium and may be associated with cerebrospinal fluid (CSF) leak. The floor of the frontal sinus creates the medial orbital roof, and injuries can involve the nasofrontal duct. Zygomaticomaxillary complex (ZMC) fractures involve the temporal bone laterally, the sphenoid bone posteriorly, the maxilla medially, and the frontal bone superiorly. When these fractures are identified, the orbital wall laterally and inferiorly can be disrupted. Enophthalmos can result from injury. Operation to restore anatomic alignment is usually recommended. Nasal fractures can involve the frontal bone superiorly, the medial orbital wall laterally, the ethmoid sinus posteriorly, and the maxilla laterally. Injury at the medial orbit can involve the attachment of the medial canthal tendon or damage to the lacrimal drainage pathway.[156] Le Fort fractures involve the midface, disrupt the facial buttresses, and can result in cosmetic and functional alterations (Fig. 36.17). Le Fort I is characterized by a transverse fracture through the maxilla above the teeth. It may be bilateral and may produce dental malocclusion. Le Fort II fractures involve the nasal bridge, maxilla, orbital floor, and rim. Le Fort III fractures are also termed *craniofacial dissociation* because they produce a discontinuity between the skull and the face. They extend from the nasal bridge to the medial wall and floor of the orbit and then laterally to the zygomatic arch. Posteriorly, they extend to the base of the sphenoid and can be associated with CSF leak. These fractures result from significant

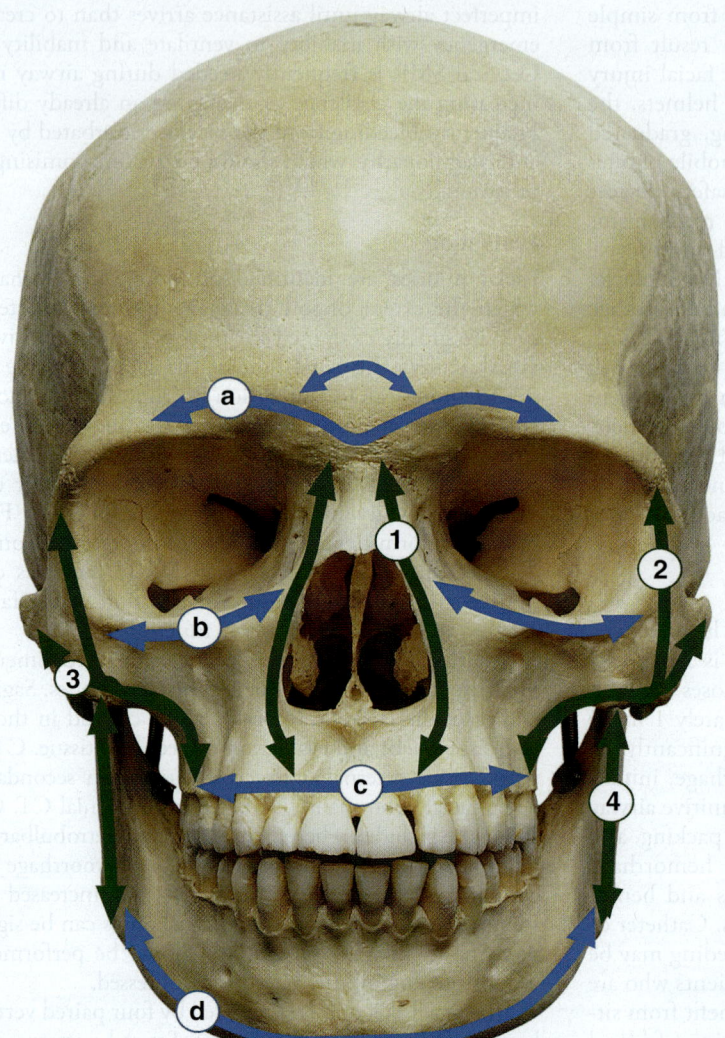

FIGURE 36.16 Buttresses of the facial skeleton. (From Ghosh SK, Narayan RK. Fractures involving bony orbit: a comprehensive review of relevant clinical anatomy. *Transl Res Anat.* 2021;24:100125.)

Horizontal Buttresses
a. Frontal bar
b. Infraorbital rim
c. Hard palate
d. Horizontal mandible

Vertical Buttresses
1. Nasomaxillary
2. Zygomaticomaxillary
3. Pterygomaxillary
4. Vertical mandible

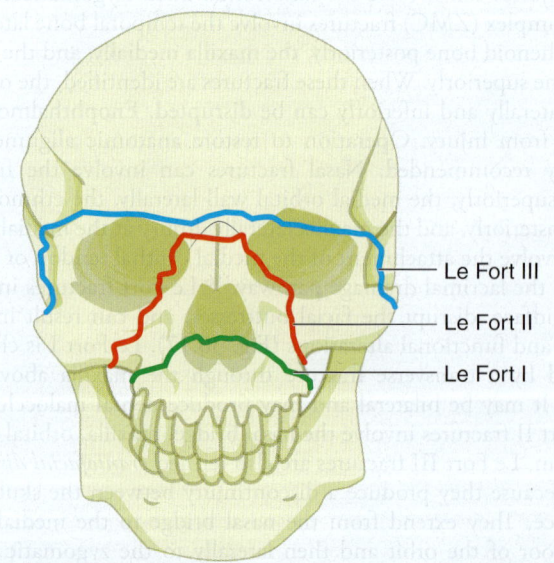

FIGURE 36.17 Le Fort fracture patterns. Le Fort I—*green line;* Le Fort II—*red line;* Le Fort III—*blue line.*

force and can occur in combination with fractures to other areas of the face, including the hard palate, dentoalveolar units, and the mandible. Orbital fractures can produce ocular injury that can threaten sight. Careful evaluation for signs of injury is required to avoid missing a timely diagnosis. Diplopia, painful eye movement, limited ocular mobility, bradycardia, nausea, and vomiting may indicate eye injury. Urgent evaluation by an ophthalmologist is required.[149] Goals of facial trauma management include restoration of anatomic deformity, restoration of dental occlusion to allow mastication, restoration of nasal airflow, and restoration of ocular function while minimizing morbidity and allowing early functional recovery.[157]

Management

Management of facial fractures and severe soft tissue injury often benefits from the involvement of a maxillofacial surgical consultant. As previously described, airway management and bleeding are the immediate priorities. Direct pressure and wound closure are often effective in controlling facial bleeding. In severe cases, angiography with embolization may be employed. Before wound closure, jagged or nonviable skin edges should be debrided, followed by irrigation of the wound with sterile fluid. Lacerations can frequently be closed with local anesthesia, using deep absorbable sutures followed by closure of the skin with 5-0 or 6-0 interrupted or running sutures. Lacerations to the lip, nose, ear, and orbit are more complex in nature, and closure requires special consideration to facilitate optimal wound healing.

The urgency of management of facial injuries varies. The management of facial fractures can often be deferred until after other injuries are addressed. Severely depressed facial bone fractures are an exception because these may involve the underlying brain and require urgent reduction. Those injuries associated with injury to the airway, those associated with severe hemorrhage, those that involve the cranium or eye, and those with severe soft tissue involvement that include the lacrimal ducts require immediate interventions. Soft tissue and contaminated wound closure can be delayed but should be addressed within a few hours. Most other injuries can be addressed in a delayed manner.[158] Most facial fractures are repaired after time allows for reduction in the associated soft tissue edema. Large open wounds and fractures involving sinuses or the aerodigestive tract may benefit from antibiotics shortly after admission, but overextending antibiotic duration should be avoided. When repair is appropriate, fractures often benefit from open reduction and internal fixation, typically with screws and plates. Reconstructive efforts are aimed at optimizing functional and cosmetic outcomes. These include the preservation of normal extraocular motor function by addressing orbital fractures with rectus muscle involvement. Mandibular fractures can be treated with maxillary-mandibular fixation, although significant fracture displacement may best be managed with internal fixation with plating.

Injuries to the Neck

The neck contains multiple vital structures in close proximity, complicating diagnosis, exposure, and treatment in the setting of injury. Nevertheless, as with other areas of the body, management is possible by implementing an organized approach. Trauma to the neck is relatively uncommon but results in the highest mortality of all body regions (17% mortality for AIS ≥3 injuries in the NTDB).[159] Penetrating injuries from gunshot and stab wounds are the most common mechanisms. At first glance the wound may appear superficial. However, thorough evaluation is imperative to ensure deeper injury hasn't occurred. Penetrating injuries can directly lacerate vascular and aerodigestive structures, resulting in substantial bleeding or contamination, respectively. Excluding injury to the cervical spine, a primarily blunt mechanism is present in only 5% of all neck trauma.[160] Blunt forces can cause sudden compression, with subsequent fracture of the larynx or trachea. Blunt pharyngeal or esophageal injuries are even less common but can result in tissue devitalization, with leakage into the surrounding soft tissues and consequent abscess or mediastinitis. Blunt force to the neck may also cause injury to the carotid or vertebral arteries, termed *blunt cerebrovascular injuries* (BCVIs).

Immediate Management

Rapid intervention is frequently indicated due to the vulnerability of contained vital cervical structures. In keeping with ATLS highest-priority concerns, initial focus is on identifying and controlling life-threatening hemorrhage and establishing a secure airway. Massive hemorrhage causes 50% of the mortality from penetrating neck injury.[161] Deterioration can occur rapidly, necessitating timely recognition and definitive care. Surgical control is frequently the optimal treatment for injury to the carotid sheath vasculature, with MTP-based resuscitation rapidly and concurrently initiated when

needed. Direct pressure with either a finger or Foley balloon effectively tamponades most bleeding from the neck during transport to the OR. Airway management is optimally performed in the OR immediately before operation for hemorrhage. Expanding neck hematomas quickly compress the upper airway, leading to airway obstruction or inadequate ventilation. Immediate intubation should occur in the setting of an expanding neck hematoma or if there is potential impending airway compromise.

Direct injury to the larynx or trachea can present one of the most challenging circumstances for airway management. Importantly, some patients with a threatened airway who are spontaneously maintaining their own airway should have a planned approach to airway management that may include awake intubation or tracheostomy in the OR. Rapid-sequence medications and intubation attempts can worsen a tenuous airway and should not be performed without a well-developed backup plan. A loss of airway requires emergent intervention, including performance of a cricothyroidotomy or tracheotomy. The surgical airway of choice for an upper airway injury is a tracheotomy because injury to the larynx may make cricothyroidotomy ineffective.

Neurologic abnormalities may be an indication of cerebral blood flow disruption. Decreased level of consciousness, hemiparesis, and facial asymmetry are indications of carotid artery injury. Cervical spine injury can be the result of either a blunt or penetrating mechanism. It is extremely rare that penetrating neck injury leads to cervical spinal instability, even when cervical spine injury is present. Empiric placement of a cervical collar is not needed for penetrating neck injury. When a cervical collar is present, it is important to open the collar and completely evaluate the neck to avoid missing injuries that may be hidden by the collar.[162]

Evaluation

The neck contains vital structures that are positioned in a relatively small anatomic area. It is, for the most part, protected only by soft tissue. Penetrating injuries to the neck are usually described by the anatomic zone in which they appear (Fig. 36.18).

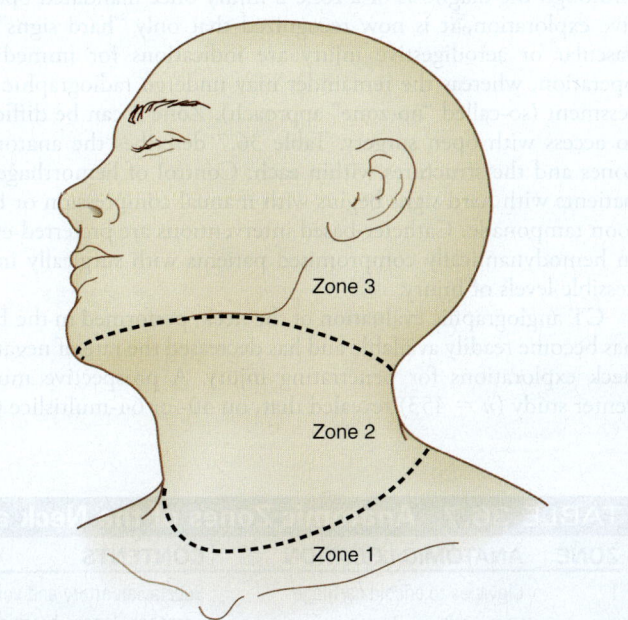

FIGURE 36.18 Anatomic zones of the neck. *Zone 1* extends from the thoracic inlet to the cricoid cartilage. *Zone 2* is between the cricoid cartilage and the angle of the mandible. *Zone 3* extends from the angle of the mandible to the skull base.

Zone 1 is defined as the area between clavicles and cricoid cartilage. Zone 2 represents the most surgically accessible anatomic region and extends from the cricoid cartilage to the angle of the mandible. Zone 3 is the most difficult area to access surgically and is the area that lies between the angle of the mandible and the skull base. Projectiles may begin in one zone and come to rest or exit in another. Clinical findings will dictate evaluation and management.

Patients with hemodynamic instability and/or "hard signs" of vascular or aerodigestive injury (i.e., airway compromise, massive subcutaneous emphysema, air bubbles necessitating through wound, expanding or pulsatile hematoma, active bleeding, neurologic deficit, hematemesis) should be immediately transported to the OR for surgical exploration.[163] Projectiles can extend from the neck into the chest, causing injury to thoracic structures. Thus, rapid bedside chest x-ray and eFAST may be beneficial to evaluate for thoracic involvement. Hemodynamically adequate patients with adequate respiratory function may undergo further evaluation for neck injury with thin-slice multidetector CT angiography (MDCTA) imaging. Patients with crepitus, odynophagia, hematemesis, or air in the neck soft tissues may have aerodigestive injury, and contrast study with Gastrografin or thin barium will detect injury with 57% to 80% accuracy. Esophagoscopy can be added to contrast evaluation to improve diagnostic accuracy for aerodigestive injury to 100%.[164] Laryngoscopy or bronchoscopy examinations in patients with stridor, hoarseness, hemoptysis, or paratracheal or mediastinal air on imaging can diagnose laryngeal or tracheal injuries.

Penetrating injuries to the neck have classically been managed based on anatomic location and surgical accessibility. Exploration of zone 1 injuries, although they are surgically approachable, can require a variety of incisions, depending on the injury. Zone 2 injuries are more easily exposed through a standard oblique cervical incision anterior to the sternocleidomastoid muscle. The common and internal carotid arteries, jugular vein, cervical esophagus, larynx, and trachea can be explored using this incision. Although the diagnosis of a zone 2 injury once mandated operative exploration, it is now recognized that only "hard signs" of vascular or aerodigestive injury are indications for immediate operation, whereas the remainder may undergo radiographic assessment (so-called "no-zone" approach). Zone 3 can be difficult to access with open surgery. Table 36.7 describes the anatomic zones and the structures within each. Control of hemorrhage in patients with hard signs begins with manual compression or balloon tamponade. Catheter-based interventions are preferred even in hemodynamically compromised patients with surgically inaccessible levels of injury.

CT angiographic evaluation of the neck, performed in the ED, has become readily available and has decreased the rate of negative neck explorations for penetrating injury. A prospective multicenter study ($n = 453$) revealed that, on 40- or 64-multislice CT

scanners, the sensitivity and specificity for penetrating vascular or aerodigestive injuries were 100% and 97.5%, respectively. Specificity was depreciated by two patients with falsely positive vascular imaging, resulting in a negative exploration and catheter angiography, and three patients with air tracking had potential aerodigestive injury subsequently excluded endoscopically. Compared with evaluation of the neck by anatomic zones, MDCTA, in appropriate patients, allows evaluation of the neck as a unit and obviates, in many cases, the need for additional invasive testing (i.e., bronchoscopy, rigid/flexible endoscopy, esophagram, digital subtraction angiography [DSA]). Patients with equivocal MDCTA, as may occur with a retained ballistic, may benefit from additional selective diagnostics. Standard DSA images are not degraded by scatter from metal fragments and may provide added information in this setting.[165]

Blunt trauma to the neck is often manifested by BCVI. The improved technology of MDCTA has cast light on this entity, which is now recognized as a major source of morbidity. BCVIs result from seat-belt compression or stretching flexion-extension mechanisms. BCVI severity ranges from intimal tears (grade I), with or without thrombosis, to full-thickness injury with pseudoaneurysm formation (grade III) and transection (grade V) (see Chapter 38) The morbidity associated with BCVI is predominantly due to ischemic stroke from acute thromboembolic phenomenon. Initially considered uncommon, the emergence of high-risk screening criteria and improved detection have led to a significant increase in the diagnosis of BCVI. Criteria have evolved to determine which patients require screening for BCVI. The list is ever enlarging (Table 36.8). The emergence and evolution of MDCTA have replaced DSA as the study of choice for diagnosis of BCVI, and recent studies report an incidence of approximately 2% to 3% in all blunt trauma patients. Contemporary screening criteria liberally prompt the evaluator toward MDCTA in the setting of (1) any injury above the clavicle, regardless of mechanism; (2) neurologic examination not explained by brain imaging; and (3) Horner syndrome.[166] Because blunt aerodigestive injury is exceedingly rare, diagnostics will likely favor a tailored approach with selected application of MDCTA, esophagoscopy, esophagography, and/or bronchoscopy.

Management

As previously mentioned, "hard signs" of vascular or aerodigestive injury are indications for immediate neck exploration, as outlined in the WTA 2013 guidelines (Fig. 36.19). Most commonly, structures of the neck are exposed by an incision along the anterior border of the sternocleidomastoid on the side of injury. A collar incision may be more versatile, especially if a bilateral neck exploration is indicated. The platysma is divided to expose the anterior border of the sternocleidomastoid, which is dissected from the underlying tissue to expose the carotid sheath (common carotid artery, vagus nerve, internal jugular vein). An injured internal

TABLE 36.7	Anatomic Zones of the Neck and Associated Structures	
ZONE	**ANATOMIC LOCATION**	**CONTENTS**
1	Clavicles to cricoid cartilage	Subclavian artery and veins, thoracic duct, proximal vertebral and carotid arteries and veins, esophagus, proximal trachea, larynx, brachial plexus, pleura
2	Cricoid cartilage to angle of the mandible	Carotid artery, jugular veins, vertebral arteries, trachea, larynx, esophagus, spinal cord, thyroid and parathyroid glands, cranial nerves
3	Angle of the mandible to base of the skull	Distal vertebral and carotid arteries, pharynx, parotid gland, and spinal cord

TABLE 36.8 Screening Criteria for BCVI

SCREEN	CLINICAL SIGNS	RISK FACTORS
Expanded Denver Criteria	Arterial hemorrhage from neck, nose, or mouth	High-energy mechanism of injury with Le Fort II or III fracture
	Cervical bruit <50 years	Basilar skull fracture involving the carotid canal
	Expanding cervical hematoma	Cervical vertebral body or transverse foramen fracture, subluxation, or ligamentous injury at any level of any fracture at C1–C3
	Focal neurologic deficit (i.e., TIA, hemiparesis, vertebrobasilar symptoms, Horner syndrome)	Closed head injury consistent with DAI and GCS <6
	Neurologic deficit incongruous with head CT	Near hanging with anoxia
	Degloving scalp injury	Clothesline-type injury or seat-belt abrasion with significant swelling, pain, or AMS
		CT or MRI evidence of stroke
		TBI with thoracic injuries
Modified Memphis Criteria	Neurologic examination not explained by imaging	Cervical spine fracture
	Horner syndrome	LeFort II or III facial fractures
	Midface instability	Skull base fractures involving the foramen lacerum
	Potential head or skull injury: loss of consciousness, AMS, signs of basilar skull fracture	
	Cervical paralysis or step-off	

AMS, Altered mental status; BCVI, blunt cerebrovascular injury; CT, computed tomography; DAI, drug-assisted intubation; GCS, Glasgow Coma Scale; MRI, magnetic resonance imaging; TIA, transient ischemic attack; TBI, traumatic brain injury.
Chatterjee AR, Malhotra A, Curl P, et al. Universal screening for blunt cerebrovascular injury. J Trauma Acute Care Surg. 2021;90(2):224-231.

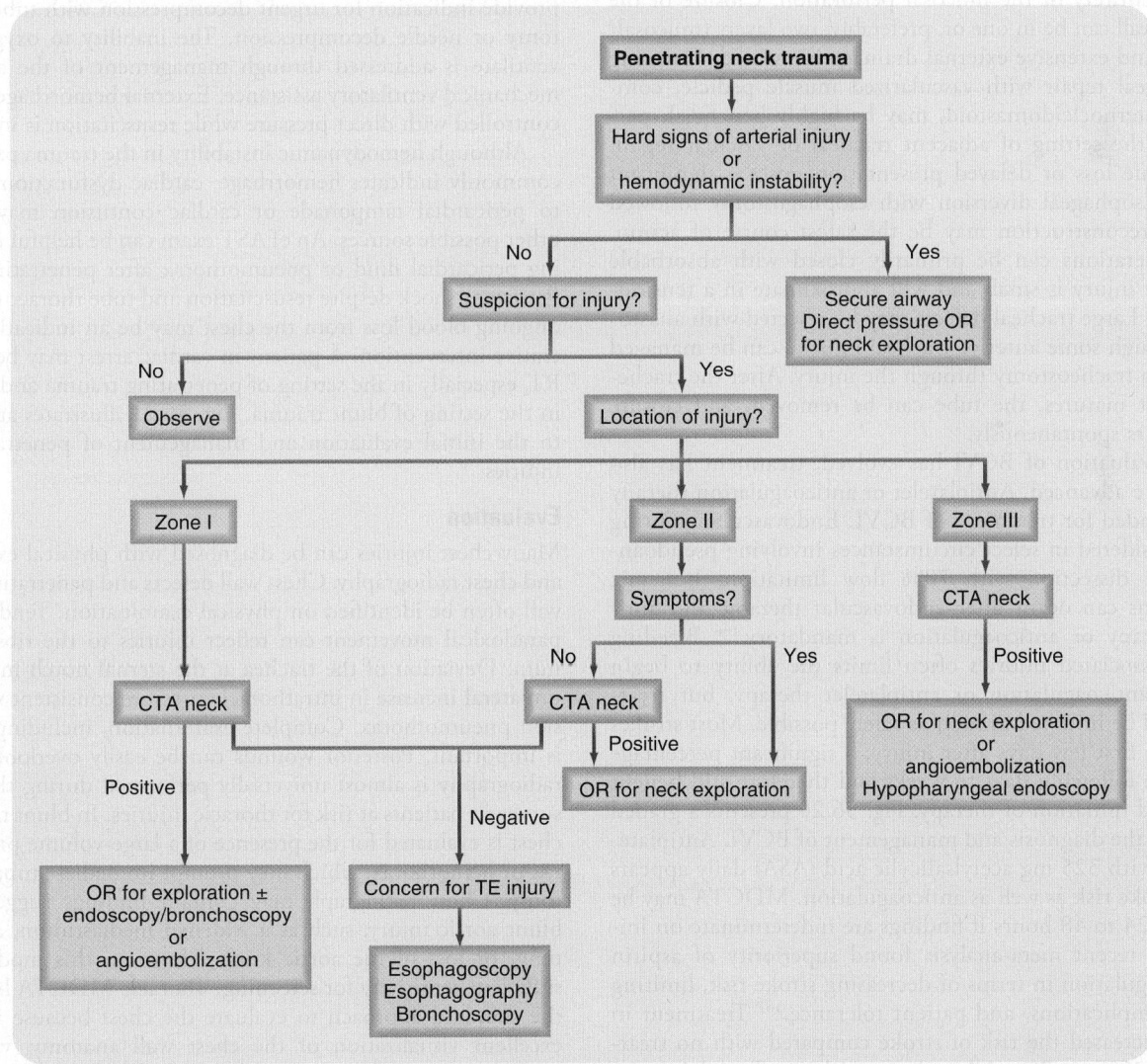

FIGURE 36.19 Algorithm for the management of penetrating neck injuries. Hard signs of vascular or aerodigestive injury include airway compromise, massive subcutaneous emphysema, air bubbles necessitating through wound, expanding or pulsatile hematoma, active bleeding, neurologic deficit, and hematemesis. CTA, Computed tomography angiography; OR, operating room; TE, tracheoesophageal. (Modified from Sperry JL, Moore EE, Coimbra R, et al. Western Trauma Association critical decisions in trauma: penetrating neck trauma. J Trauma Acute Care Surg. 2013;75:936-940.)

jugular vein may be directly repaired with monofilament suture or ligated if closure is not possible. The facial vein is identified entering the anterior surface of the internal jugular vein. Ligation and division of the facial vein allow the deep structures of the vascular compartment to be exposed. With the internal jugular vein retracted laterally, the carotid artery and vagus nerves are exposed. If necessary, the carotid artery may be controlled proximally and distally. Care is taken to avoid injury to either the vagus or hypoglossal nerves, which lie adjacent to and superiorly crossing the carotid artery, respectively. Short-segment carotid artery injuries may be repaired with either simple closure or end-to-end anastomosis. More extensive injuries are addressed by reconstruction with a synthetic graft or autologous vein. In damage control situations, the carotid artery can be shunted or ligated in extreme circumstances, although cerebral blood flow may be compromised.

Exploration of the trachea and esophagus is achieved via lateral retraction of the carotid artery. Dissection is continued medially, and the esophagus is identified immediately anterior to the cervical vertebral bodies; detection may be aided by nasogastric tube placement. Injuries to the esophagus are debrided to expose the entirety of the mucosal perforation. Closure of the esophageal wall can be in one or, preferably, two layers (mucosal/muscular), and extensive external drainage is ensured. Covering the esophageal repair with vascularized muscle pedicle, commonly the sternocleidomastoid, may be highly beneficial, particularly in the setting of adjacent tracheal or vascular repair. Massive tissue loss or delayed presentation poses a significant challenge. Esophageal diversion with esophagostomy followed by delayed reconstruction may be the safest course of action. Tracheal lacerations can be primarily closed with absorbable suture if the injury is small and will approximate in a tension-free fashion. Large tracheal defects may be resected with anastomosis, although some anterior tracheal injuries can be managed by creating a tracheostomy through the injury. After the tracheostomy tract matures, the tube can be removed, and closure usually occurs spontaneously.

As the evaluation of BCVI has evolved, treatment has also become more advanced. Antiplatelet or anticoagulation therapy is recommended for treatment of BCVI. Endovascular stenting may be considered in select circumstances involving pseudoaneurysm and dissection with 70% flow limitation. Ischemic complications can occur after endovascular therapy, and antiplatelet therapy or anticoagulation is mandatory.[166] Bleeding risk from associated injuries often limits the ability to begin immediate anticoagulation or antiplatelet therapy, but treatment should be initiated as soon as safely possible. Most strokes occur in the first few days after injury; a significant percentage occur in the following days to weeks and therefore still benefit from delayed initiation of therapy. Fig. 36.20 presents a graded approach to the diagnosis and management of BCVI. Antiplatelet therapy with 325 mg acetylsalicylic acid (ASA) daily appears to lower stroke risk as well as anticoagulation. MDCTA may be repeated in 24 to 48 hours if findings are indeterminate on initial scan. A recent meta-analysis found superiority of aspirin over anticoagulation in terms of decreasing stroke risk, limiting bleeding complications, and patient tolerance.[167] Treatment in any form decreased the risk of stroke compared with no treatment from 25% to 3%. All patients with confirmed injuries should undergo repeat imaging at 7 to 10 days to evaluate for progression or resolution and subsequent discontinuation of therapy. Persistent injury should receive antiplatelet treatment for 3 months with serial outpatient MDCTA.

Injuries to the Chest

Blunt and penetrating injuries to the chest are common, with significant morbidity and mortality. A significant proportion of multiply injured patients will have a major chest injury. Falls and motor vehicle collisions are etiologies in many blunt chest trauma cases because transmission of high-energy forces damages the chest wall and underlying structures. The relative prominence of the chest makes it particularly vulnerable to penetrating mechanisms as well. Both blunt and penetrating trauma can cause contusions to the lung parenchyma. Despite the potentially serious nature of these injuries, isolated chest injury is rarely an indication for urgent operative management, although the rate of operation is higher in penetrating trauma than blunt trauma.

Immediate Management

Thoracic injuries frequently receive immediate intervention during the primary survey. Pulmonary compromise and physiologic derangement necessitate immediate evaluation for a pneumothorax or tension pneumothorax. Physical exam findings such as decreased breath sounds and poor pulmonary compliance may provide indication for urgent decompression with tube thoracostomy or needle decompression. The inability to oxygenate and ventilate is addressed through management of the airway and mechanical ventilatory assistance. External hemorrhage should be controlled with direct pressure while resuscitation is initiated.

Although hemodynamic instability in the trauma patient most commonly indicates hemorrhage, cardiac dysfunction secondary to pericardial tamponade or cardiac contusion may represent other possible sources. An eFAST exam can be helpful in identifying pericardial fluid or pneumothorax after penetrating trauma. Persistent shock despite resuscitation and tube thoracostomy with ongoing blood loss from the chest may be an indication for operative intervention. A patient in cardiac arrest may benefit from RT, especially in the setting of penetrating trauma and selectively in the setting of blunt trauma. Fig. 36.21 illustrates an approach to the initial evaluation and management of penetrating chest injuries.

Evaluation

Many chest injuries can be diagnosed with physical examination and chest radiography. Chest wall defects and penetrating wounds will often be identified on physical examination. Tenderness and paradoxical movement can reflect injuries to the ribs and sternum. Deviation of the trachea at the sternal notch may reveal a unilateral increase in intrathoracic pressure consistent with a tension pneumothorax. Complete examination, including the back, is important. Posterior wounds can be easily overlooked. Chest radiography is almost universally performed during the primary survey in patients at risk for thoracic injuries. In blunt trauma, the chest is evaluated for the presence of a large-volume pneumothorax or hemothorax, which may prompt immediate tube thoracostomy. Chest radiograph may contain findings suggestive of a blunt aortic injury, such as a widened mediastinum, apical capping, or loss of the aortic knob. However, this modality lacks sufficient sensitivity for screening. Thoracic MDCTA has become the standard approach to evaluate the chest because it provides excellent visualization of the chest wall anatomy, vasculature, pleural spaces, and lung parenchyma. CT angiography (CTA) has replaced standard angiography of the chest in trauma because of its speed, accuracy, availability, and noninvasive nature. Ultrasound represents an additional modality for rapid repeatable bedside thoracic imaging, although accuracy is dependent on user

The protocol below could be used as an example of treatment and follow up by grade.
R Adams Shock Trauma Center Blunt Cerebrovascular Injury (BCVI) Management Protocol

Blunt Cerebrovascular Injury (BCVI)
These injuries can present with or lead to a devastating stroke and largely arise from flexion-extension injuries. Some injuries are time dependent, and STC has a dedicated vascular trauma service to support the trauma service with management of these patients. This protocol presents the management of BCVI and when to consult with vascular trauma.

Criteria for Screening[1]
Pan CT scan
If no Pan CT scan done: Denver Criteria

Imaging and Imaging Schedule
Follow-up imaging should consist of a CTA head and CTA neck
Imaging schedule: 48–72 hours; 2–4 weeks; 3 months; 12 months

Antiplatelet
Low ASA: Aspirin 81 mg qD
ASA: Aspirin 325 mg qD
Plavix: Clopidogrel 75 mg qD

Carotid or Vertebral Artery Injury

Grade	Description	High Risk Features*	Management[2,3]	Follow-Up[2]
I	Luminal irregularity or dissection with <25% luminal stenosis	Progression of lesion grade on rpt CTA	**Initial therapy:** Start low ASA **Resolved:** Stop ASA when resolved on imaging **Stable:** Stop ASA after 3 months **High-risk features only: Urgent** vascular trauma consult	Follow imaging schedule for 3 months unless resolved sooner Stop therapy if stable/resolved at 3 months
IIa	Dissection with 25%–50% stenosis			
IIb	Dissection with >50% stenosis	Progression of lesion grade on rpt CTA. Multiple injured arteries (grade IIb or higher)	**Initial therapy:** Start ASA **Resolved:** Stop ASA when resolved on imaging **Stable:** Switch to low ASA at 3 months **High-risk features only: Urgent** vascular trauma consult	Follow imaging schedule for 12 months unless resolved sooner Continue low ASA for life
III	Pseudoaneurysm	Progression of lesion on rpt CTA. Multiple injured arteries (grade IIb or higher); pseudoaneurysm >5 mm size; associated stenosis >50%	**Initial therapy:** Start ASA and Plavix **Resolved:** Stop all therapy when resolved on imaging **Stable:** Switch to low ASA at 3 months **High-risk features only: Urgent** vascular trauma consult	Follow up in Trauma Vascular Clinic Follow imaging schedule for 12 months unless resolved sooner Continue low ASA for life
IV	Vessel occlusion	Progression of lesion on rpt CTA. Multiple injured arteries (grade IIb or higher)	**Initial therapy:** Start ASA and Plavix; **urgent** endovascular trauma consult **Resolved:** Stop all therapy when resolved on imaging **Stable:** Switch to low ASA at 3 months **High-risk features only: Emergent** vascular trauma service consult	Follow up in Trauma Vascular Clinic Follow imaging schedule for 12 months unless resolved sooner Continue low ASA for life
V	Vessel transection	All transections are high risk	**Emergent vascular trauma service consult**	Lesion specific, per vascular trauma service

*All symptomatic lesions are considered high risk, and Trauma Vascular should be consulted emergently.
[2]If a patient undergoes stent placement, treatment will be dictated by Trauma Vascular.
[3]If recommended therapy cannot be initiated, Trauma Vascular should be consulted.

Intervention
Intervention for BCVI is infrequent and consists of a wide range of treatment modalities designed to balance the need for cerebral perfusion, reduction of thromboembolic stroke risk, and minimize bleeding complications. Moreover, the patient's larger injury profile must be taken into account. Intervention can therefore only occur as a result of close collaboration between multiple services.

Tailored Management
A single pathway of medical management that applies to all trauma patients is impractical. Although the above provides indications for antiplatelet/anticoagulation therapy, other injuries may make such treatment contraindicated. Discussion with the vascular trauma service regarding other pathways for diagnosis, management, and surveillance of these patients is welcomed.

[1]**Denver Criteria for Screening**
For patients who do not undergo Shan scan (i.e. transfers from outside hospitals who come with imaging already complete), please use the following list of criteria when considering the need for dedicated CTA Head/Neck to rule out BCVI:
- *Arterial hemorrhage*
- *Cervical bruit*
- *Expanding cervical hematoma*
- *Focal neurologic deficit*
- *Neurologic examination incongruous with head CT scan findings*
- *Stroke on secondary CT scan*
- *High energy transfer mechanism with:*
  - *Le-Fort II or III fracture*
  - *Cervical spine fracture patterns: subluxation, fractures extending into the transverse foramen, and fractures of C1-3*
  - *Basilar skull fracture with carotid canal involvement*
  - *Petrous bone fracture*
  - *Diffuse axonal injury*
  - *Near hanging with anoxic brain injury*
  - *Suspected cervical spine fracture any level*
  - *All head-on MVC*

FIGURE 36.20 Protocol for the management of blunt cerebrovascular injury. *ASA,* Acetylsalicylic acid (aspirin); *BCVI,* blunt cerebrovascular injury; *CTA,* computed tomography angiography; *MVC,* motor vehicle collision; *rpt,* repeat; Shan scan, pan CT scan (under Denver Criteria for Screening); *STC,* shock trauma center.

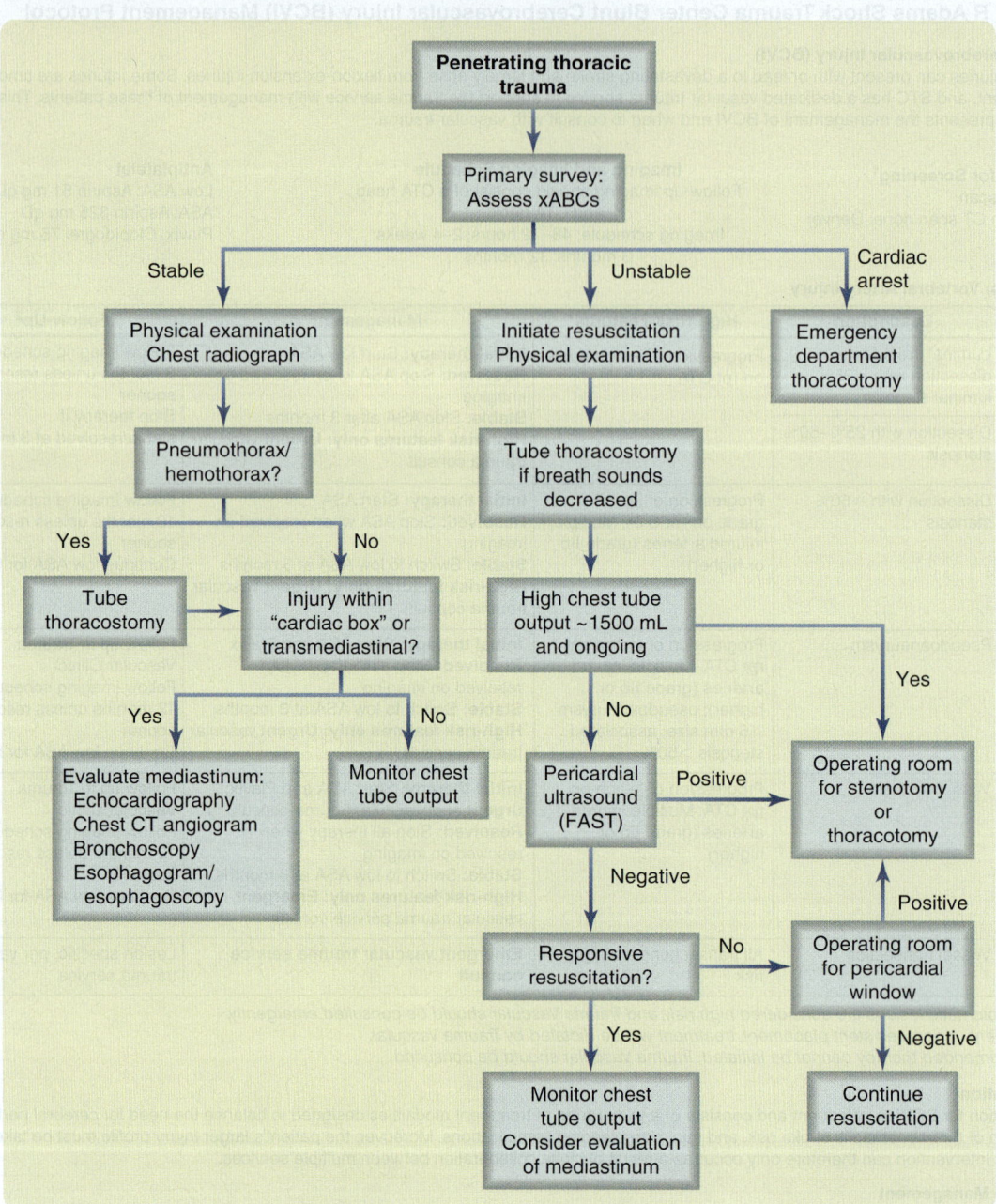

FIGURE 36.21 Algorithm for the management of penetrating thoracic injuries. *CT,* Computed tomography; *FAST,* focused abdominal sonography in trauma.

experience. Ultrasound may diagnose pneumothoraces, hemothoraces, and pericardial tamponade. Cardiac motion and volume status may be assessed as well.

Penetrating trauma to the chest should be identified rapidly on physical exam. Injuries that involve or cross the mediastinum mandate further evaluation. Wounds within the area defined by the sternal notch superiorly, the costal margin inferiorly, and the nipples bilaterally ("the cardiac box") constitute high-risk injuries. Immediate ultrasound is performed to evaluate the pericardium for effusion, although decompression into a hemothorax through traumatic pericardiotomy may yield false-negative results.[168] The great vessels are evaluated for injury with MDCTA, although standard catheter-based angiography or DSA may be employed if artifact-producing foreign bodies are present. Depending on the trajectory of the penetrating object, the trachea and proximal

airways may be evaluated with bronchoscopy. Visualization of the esophagus for injury is accomplished via a combination of esophagoscopy and contrast esophagography. The sensitivity of diagnosis approaches 100% when multiple complementary studies are performed.[164]

Management

Thoracic injuries are often straightforward to manage, with the majority successfully treated with single tube thoracostomy. When emergent insertion is indicated, an open technique is safe and rapidly completed. Sterile procedure should be followed. The skin is cleaned with chlorhexidine and draped with sterile towels. External landmarks for reliable placement are defined by a "triangle of safety," which is bordered by the level of the nipple or inframammary fold inferiorly, midaxillary line posteriorly, and the lateral edge of the pectoralis major medially. After infusion of local analgesia into the skin, subcutaneous tissues, and chest wall, an approximately 2-cm skin incision is made within the triangle at or just superior to the level of the inframammary fold at the fourth to fifth intercostal spaces. This location protects against intraabdominal placement or injury to the diaphragm. A subcutaneous tunnel is created in a superior direction over the rib to avoid the inferiorly located neurovascular structures. The thoracic cavity is entered bluntly at an interspace above the skin incision. The lung is digitally palpated to confirm chest entry, release a pneumothorax/tension (finger thoracotomy), and evaluate for intrathoracic adhesions. The track of the subcutaneous tunnel naturally directs the chest tube toward an apical position. The size of chest tube for trauma has traditionally ranged from 32 to 36 Fr. However, current evidence suggests equivalent success and decreased morbidity of hemothorax drainage with 14-Fr percutaneous catheters.[169] The technique for percutaneous placement varies slightly depending on the specific manufacturer of the device. Ultrasound may be used for assistance during insertion. Because percutaneous placement frequently takes more time than an open technique, the open procedure is preferred for patients in extremis. Regardless of technique, the tube is secured to the skin with a nonabsorbable suture and connected to a chest drainage device providing −20 cm H_2O suction.

The traditional indications for emergent thoracotomy to treat hemorrhage have included more than 1500 mL of blood drained on chest tube insertion, 200 mL/h of drainage for 4 consecutive hours, or persistent hemodynamic instability with ongoing transfusion requirement.[170] However, these indications are based on Vietnam War–era data from patients who died from chest injury rather than contemporary trials. There are no absolute tube output volumes that mandate operation. The surgeon determines clinically if chest tube output represents continued bleeding or drainage of accumulated blood from injuries that have ceased bleeding. Like other zones of injury, physiology and response to resuscitation guide the decision for operative intervention. Other indications to consider thoracotomy include a massive air leak with associated pneumothorax and drainage of esophageal or gastric contents from the chest tube.

When thoracotomy is performed, the choice of surgical approach is dependent on the suspected injury. Access to the lungs, pulmonary vasculature, and hemidiaphragm is achieved through a posterolateral thoracotomy that is performed through the fifth interspace. On the right, this incision exposes the proximal and midesophagus as well as the trachea and bilateral mainstem bronchi. The distal esophagus, left lung, left ventricle, descending aorta, and left subclavian artery are best approached through a left thoracotomy. A median sternotomy can be a highly versatile approach, providing exposure to the right side of the heart, ascending aorta, aortic arch with right-sided arch vessels, and pulmonary vasculature.

Chest Wall and Pleural Space Injuries

Chest wall injuries are the most common thoracic injury, with approximately 10% of trauma admissions sustaining at least one rib fracture. Rib fractures occur frequently in cases of ballistic chest trauma. Rib fractures are a marker of other severe injury; nearly 50% of multiply injured patients will have a rib fracture. The mortality rate of the multiply injured with chest wall injuries is approximately 6% to 12%.[171,172] Rib fractures typically occur secondary to compression of the thoracic cage in an anteroposterior or lateral direction due to a sudden high-energy transfer, such

as in a motor vehicle collision or fall from height. During motor vehicle crashes, the steering wheel and seat belt are commonly the cause of chest wall deformation. Large amounts of energy transferred to the chest wall can result in a flail segment, which includes two or more adjacent ribs fractured in two or more locations. Clinically, a flail segment results in a portion of the chest wall that moves independently and paradoxically to the remainder of the chest. The magnitude of forces needed to create a flail segment often results in a significant pulmonary contusion, which causes great physiologic insult and may ultimately be the indication for the supportive interventions. Pneumothorax and hemothorax are commonly associated with chest wall injury, owing to compressive forces upon the lung or penetrating mechanisms resulting in parenchymal damage.

Injuries involving the chest wall or pleural space can frequently be identified on chest radiographs, in which a pneumothorax appears as a lucency peripheral to the standard lung markings (Fig. 36.22) and a hemothorax as a dependent opacification. Chest CT is a valuable evaluation methodology that identifies injuries with a greater degree of sensitivity and specificity. CT can diagnose chest wall deformities, such as flail segment, displaced ribs, and sternal fractures. An occult pneumothorax is defined by identification on chest CT without evidence on plain radiography.

All pneumothoraces and hemothoraces visible on a chest radiograph should be considered for tube thoracostomy. In the absence of hemodynamic instability and respiratory compromise, studies suggest that observation may be safe for blunt and penetrating pneumothoraces with a CT radial diameter of up to 35 mm.[173] Asymptomatic pneumothoraces not accompanied by respiratory compromise can be managed with observation and a repeated chest radiograph in 12 to 24 hours to demonstrate stability.

Hemothoraces visible on upright chest x-ray represent an approximate volume of 400 to 500 mL, and evacuation with tube thoracostomy is recommended. Retained hemothorax increases morbidity, and adequate, successful drainage is important.[174] Recent trials document reduced incidence of retained hemothorax and video-assisted thoracoscopic surgery (VATS) interventions if the thoracic cavity is irrigated immediately after tube insertion

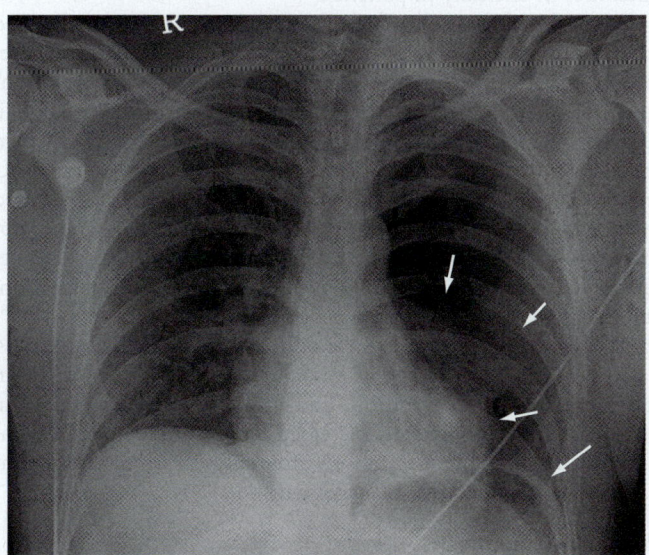

FIGURE 36.22 Large left-sided pneumothorax on chest radiograph. The *arrows* identify the lateral border of the collapsed lung.

until the effluent returns clear.[175] Residual hemothorax that does not resolve after insertion of a chest tube should be considered for VATS for hematoma evacuation to prevent development of a trapped lung and empyema. This approach has been shown to result in shorter duration of chest tube drainage, shorter hospital length of stay, lower hospital costs, and prevention of a subsequent surgical procedure when compared with the placement of a second chest tube. Retained hemothorax after chest tube placement has been associated with a 33% risk of empyema. VATS intervention is best undertaken in days 3 to 7 of hospitalization to reduce the risk of conversion to thoracotomy.[170,176] Chest tubes may be safely removed after demonstrated pleural space evacuation, on underwater seal, and with <300-mL output over the prior 24 hours.

The impact of rib fractures on patient physiology varies greatly, depending on the morphology of injury and patient characteristics. A great challenge is inadequate performance of pulmonary hygiene due to pain, with subsequent development of respiratory compromise and pneumonia. Institutional protocols often involve multimodal narcotic-sparing pain regimens, with the assistance of an acute pain service and consideration of extradural catheterization. Adequate analgesia allows for optimal pulmonary hygiene. Elderly patients are particularly susceptible to complications from rib fractures and have an increased incidence of infectious complications. Fractures to upper ribs (#1–3) are associated with concomitant thoracic vascular injuries or BCVIs. Appropriate diagnostic studies, such as MDCTA, are recommended. Lower rib fractures (#9–12) have a higher incidence of associated intraabdominal organ injury.

Several scoring systems have been developed to help quantify the degree of injury. The RibScore assigns 1 point to each of six objective radiographic measures related to rib fracture pattern, including the number of fractures, presence of a flail segment, laterality of fractures, and location.[177] It has been shown to be predictive of adverse pulmonary outcomes and may be useful in determining initial patient disposition to ICU, intermediate care, or general status. The Sequential Clinical Assessment of Respiratory Function (SCARF) score is another model that uses repeated clinical measurements and assigns 1 point for incentive spirometry <50% predicted, RR >20, numeric pain score ≥5, and inadequate cough. SCARF has been demonstrated to predict adverse outcomes in critically ill patients.[178]

Surgical stabilization of rib fractures is an increasingly used adjunct over the past two decades. Although routine use has remained controversial, increasing numbers of studies have demonstrated benefit, especially in patients with a documented flail segment. Reported outcomes in selected patients include pain relief with decreased duration of mechanical ventilation, ICU length of stay, and overall hospital length of stay and decreased incidence of pneumonia. Both open and thoracoscopic approaches have been described. Wound complications; device-related complications, including malalignment and migration; and infections may occur and must be balanced with benefits.[179–181] Patient selection is critical. A randomized controlled study of 84 patients with radiologic flail without clinical flail, more than four consecutive rib fractures, and any fracture with bicortical displacement demonstrated increased length of stay without improved quality of life at 1 month after surgical rib fixation compared with nonoperative management.[182]

Pulmonary Injuries

Trauma to the lung is caused by direct or indirect energy transfer through the chest wall to the pulmonary parenchyma, resulting in

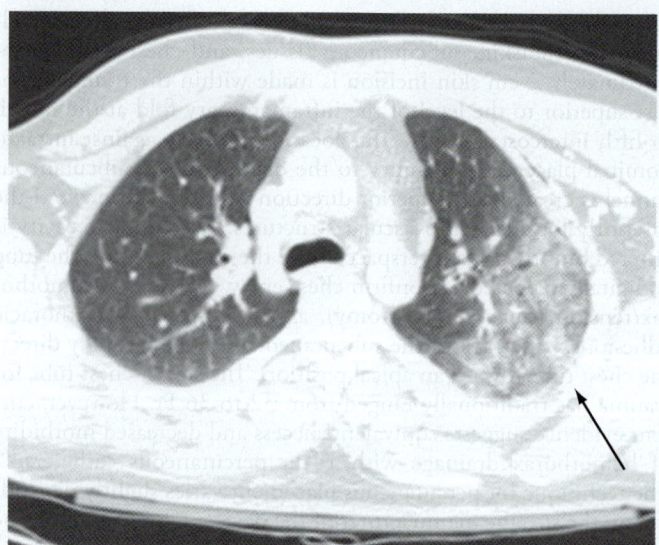

FIGURE 36.23 Left pulmonary contusion on thoracic computed tomography scan. The *arrow* identifies contused lung, which appears as higher-density tissue because of air space hemorrhage and associated edema.

tissue damage and hemorrhage into the alveolar and interstitial spaces. Mortality and morbidity after pulmonary contusion are predominately a result of respiratory failure from ARDS or pneumonia. The tissue damage causes a physiologic shunt with hypoxemia. Pulmonary contusions often occur in combination with rib fractures and are often more clinically significant than the rib fractures themselves. Beyond clinical suspicion, chest radiographs may be the first indication of pulmonary injury. Lung contusions may be present on the initial chest radiograph but typically become more apparent after 24 to 48 hours. Pulmonary contusions that are identified on initial chest x-ray are frequently severe and rapidly progressive to respiratory failure. CT is sensitive for the identification of pulmonary contusion (Fig. 36.23) and may diagnose clinically inconsequential contusions as well. Differentiating contusion from atelectasis can be difficult. However, atelectasis does not cross pulmonary fissures, whereas contusions are not limited by ventilatory segments.

Pulmonary contusions are typically managed with supportive care, including pulmonary hygiene and a multimodal approach to pain control. Patients are monitored for signs of respiratory decompensation, including hypoxemia, increased work of breathing, and agitation. The progressive nature of severe pulmonary contusions may prompt application of mechanical ventilatory support or extracorporeal membrane oxygenation (ECMO). Lung-protective ventilation strategies should be used. The clinical severity of a pulmonary contusion does not always correlate with the imaging findings. The Murray Lung Injury Score classifies the clinical severity of acute lung injury in mechanically ventilated patients and can help predict the need for ECMO.[183] A large analysis of the Extracorporeal Life Support Organization (ELSO) registry focused on trauma patients found that survival to discharge was 61% in trauma patients undergoing ECMO cannulation.[184]

Nonoperative measures and tube thoracostomy manage the majority of thoracic trauma. In most cases, tube thoracostomy with lung expansion adequately manages low-pressure lung bleeding and small air leaks. Continued bloody output from the chest tube indicates the potential of a more central or high-pressure source. Intervention for control of hemorrhage may be indicated.

At institutions with interventional radiology support, embolization of bleeding vessels within the pulmonary vasculature may be a less morbid alternative to surgery. In penetrating trauma, stapled tractotomy and wedge resection are more commonly performed than in blunt trauma. Conversely, anatomic lobectomy and pneumonectomy are more commonly performed if resection is indicated after blunt etiologies. If significant bleeding is encountered upon entry into the chest, rapid control may be obtained via hilar control with either a clamp or "hilar twist" maneuver (Fig. 36.24).[185] Bleeding from pulmonary parenchyma is controlled through suture (3-0 polypropylene) ligation of bleeding vessels. Stapled tractotomy may expose injured vessels and bronchi for ligation. Trauma pneumonectomy is extremely morbid, with mortality rates exceeding 50%, and should only be performed for a patient in extremis. Damage control principles may also be applied to the chest with laparotomy sponges and

temporary closure over chest tubes.[186] As opposed to abdominal packing, packs in the chest should occupy minimal space and be constructed to allow maximal lung expansion.

Cardiac Injuries

Despite being uncommon, cardiac injuries are some of the most severe injuries sustained by patients after penetrating and blunt trauma. Penetrating injury to the heart occurs in <1% patients with penetrating trauma and in less than 10% of the subset with penetrating chest trauma alone. These statistics likely underestimate the true incidence of penetrating cardiac injuries because >90% of injuries are immediately lethal and never present to a hospital. Mortality among patients arriving to a trauma center with a penetrating cardiac injury ranges from 17% to 58% and has been increasing along with the percentage with a ballistic etiology.[187,188]

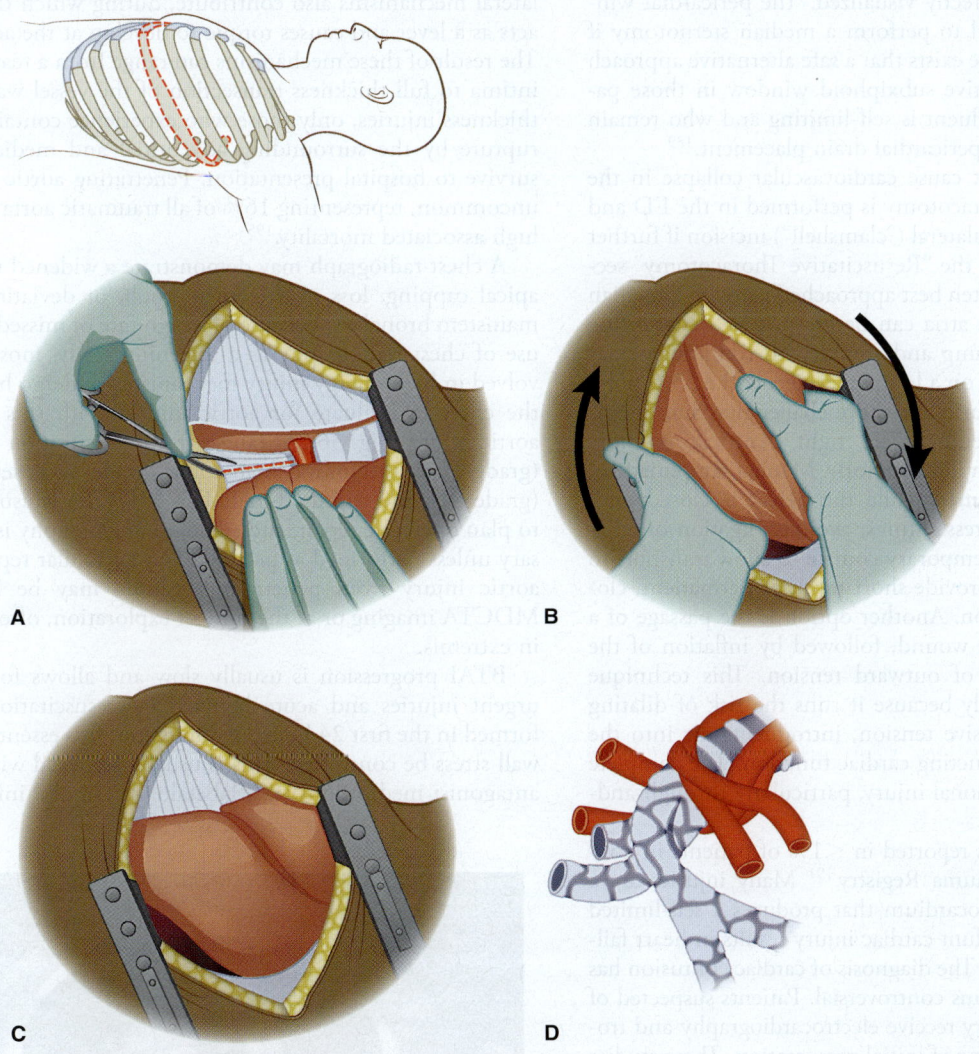

FIGURE 36.24 Hilar twist maneuver. (A) Sharply divide the inferior pulmonary ligament. The ligament should be divided to the level of the inferior pulmonary vein. (B) Place one hand on the anterior aspect of the upper lobe and the other hand on the posterior aspect of the lower lobe. Rotate the lower lobe anteriorly and the upper lobe posteriorly 180 degrees. (C) Once twisted, the apex of the lung will rest along the diaphragm. To maintain this position, place laparotomy packs at the apex, base, and around the hilum. (D) The vascular structures will be twisted around the bronchus with effective occlusion. (From Wilson A, Wall MJ Jr, Maxson R, Mattox K. The pulmonary hilum twist as a thoracic damage control procedure. *Am J Surg*. 2003;186[1]:49-52.)

The location of penetrating injury on initial examination will often be suggestive of cardiac injury (i.e., within the "cardiac box"). Patients may present in extremis with pericardial tamponade or bleeding into one of the pleural spaces. Those who require immediate RT in the ED may have a cardiac injury identified during that procedure. In others, indicators of pericardial tamponade may be present. Beck's triad of hypotension, jugular venous distention, and muffled heart sounds may be present, although sensitivity is very low. Ultrasound is an excellent method for quickly assessing the pericardium for fluid and should be performed in all patients with hemodynamic instability or an injury in a high-risk location. When the results of ultrasound are inconclusive or potentially falsely negative, as in the setting of left or right hemothorax, and the patient cannot receive further studies such as a CT scan, an operative subxiphoid pericardial window may be performed to evaluate for the presence of blood in the pericardium. On making a small opening in the pericardium, the pericardial space can be directly visualized. The pericardial window may then be extended to perform a median sternotomy if blood is visualized. Evidence exists that a safe alternative approach to sternotomy after a positive subxiphoid window in those patients for whom bloody effluent is self-limiting and who remain hemodynamically stable is pericardial drain placement.[189]

For cardiac injuries that cause cardiovascular collapse in the ED, a left anterolateral thoracotomy is performed in the ED and may be extended to a contralateral ("clamshell") incision if further visualization is needed. See the "Resuscitative Thoracotomy" section. Cardiac injuries are often best approached through a median sternotomy. Injuries to the atria can be grasped in a side-biting fashion with a Satinsky clamp and closed with running permanent monofilament sutures on a long taper needle (i.e., 3-0 polypropylene). Ventricular injuries are more challenging and associated with significant bleeding. The right ventricle is more frequently injured because it lies anteriorly. Manual tamponade of a laceration can be performed while the defect is closed with horizontal pledgetted mattress sutures, avoiding ligation of adjacent coronary vessels. For temporary control to allow transport to the OR, skin staples may provide short-term, or permanent, closure of the cardiac laceration. Another option is the passage of a Foley catheter through the wound, followed by inflation of the balloon and maintenance of outward tension. This technique must be performed carefully because it runs the risk of dilating the cardiotomy with excessive tension, introducing air into the cardiac chamber, and obstructing cardiac function. The complete heart is inspected for additional injury, particularly through-and-through penetration.[190]

Blunt cardiac injury was reported in <1% of patients in a review of the Oklahoma Trauma Registry.[191] Many injuries are a likely contusion of the myocardium that produces a self-limited arrhythmia. In rare cases, blunt cardiac injury results in heart failure with cardiogenic shock. The diagnosis of cardiac contusion has been well studied but remains controversial. Patients suspected of having a blunt cardiac injury receive electrocardiography and troponin I evaluation at the time of initial presentation. These studies exclude significant blunt cardiac injury if both are negative.[192] A new abnormality on the electrocardiogram (ECG), most commonly tachyarrhythmia, is an indication for further continuous ECG monitoring. Clinical findings of cardiac contusion that are absent on admission are unlikely to develop and, in their continued absence, require no further evaluation. The presence of ECG abnormalities, elevated troponin I, Trand/or hemodynamic instability with evidence of heart failure prompts echocardiography to

assess cardiac wall and septal motion as well as valvular function. Cardiogenic shock may be treated with inotropic support and right ventricular afterload reduction because the right ventricular is more anterior and more frequently affected. Patients who demonstrate structural abnormalities, such as valvular incompetence, may require urgent operation for repair.

Thoracic Aortic Injuries

Thoracic aortic injuries are fortunately uncommon but are associated with poor outcomes. Approximately 80% of trauma patients with blunt traumatic aortic injury (BTAI) die before they reach a hospital, and 50% of those surviving to the hospital die within 24 hours.[193,194] As with other severe injuries, the described incidence of these injuries underestimates the actual frequency because the denominator is unknown. BTAIs are believed to be a result of rapid deceleration, which tears the aortic wall in the vicinity of the ligamentum arteriosum. Other theories suggest that lateral mechanisms also contribute, during which the aortic arch acts as a lever and causes torque to develop at the aortic isthmus. The result of these mechanisms can range from a tear in the aortic intima to full-thickness transection of the vessel wall. With full-thickness injuries, only those who experience containment of the rupture by the surrounding adventitial and mediastinal tissues survive to hospital presentation. Penetrating aortic injury is also uncommon, representing 16% of all traumatic aorta injuries, with high associated mortality.[195]

A chest radiograph may demonstrate a widened mediastinum, apical capping, loss of the aortic knob, or deviation of the left mainstem bronchus. Because of a high rate of missed injuries with use of chest radiography as a screening study, most patients involved in high-energy injury mechanisms undergo helical CTA of the chest to evaluate for aortic injury. With this modality, an aortic injury (Fig. 36.25) ranges from a disruption in the intima (grade I) to intramural hematoma (grade II), pseudoaneurysm (grade III), and rupture (grade IV). MDCTA is usually sufficient to plan operative repair, and standard angiography is rarely necessary unless performed as part of an endovascular repair. Similarly, aortic injury from penetrating trauma may be identified on MDCTA imaging or at the time of exploration, often in a patient in extremis.

BTAI progression is usually slow and allows for other more urgent injuries and acute hemorrhage resuscitation to be performed in the first 24 hours of admission. It is essential that aortic wall stress be controlled. This is usually achieved with β-receptor antagonist medications (i.e., labetalol or esmolol infusions), with

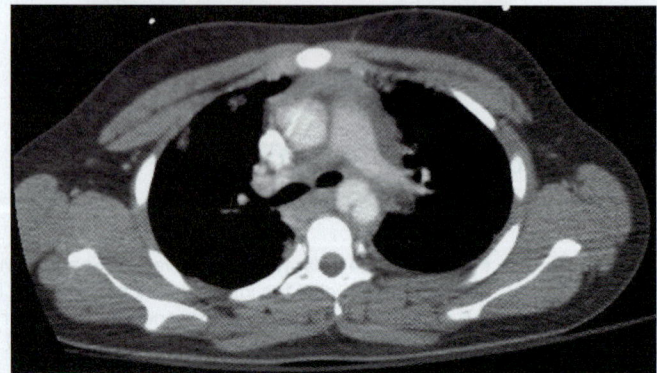

FIGURE 36.25 Aortic dissection on thoracic computed tomography. Image demonstrates a large traumatic dissection of the thoracic aorta.

a goal of SBP of less than 100 mm Hg and heart rate less than 100 in non–head injury patients.[196] Treatment is based on injury grade (see Chapter 38).[197] Grade I injuries are managed medically, as are many grade II injuries.[198] Endovascular approaches are the most predominant technique for aortic repair of higher-grade injuries. Medical and endovascular treatment have evolved and demonstrate equivalent mortality to open repair. The rapid progression of catheter-based technology has made endovascular repair the treatment of choice at most trauma centers. Access to the thoracic aorta is through the groin, and the stent graft is placed under fluoroscopic guidance. On occasion, the graft will cover the ostia of the left subclavian artery, at which time a carotid-to-subclavian bypass may also be required if extremity symptoms develop. Patients are treated with β-blocker therapy and receive follow-up imaging to ensure the absence of expansion and, ultimately, the resolution of the injury.

When open surgical repair is performed, the aorta is exposed through a left thoracotomy. Large penetrating injuries and blunt transection require replacement of a segment of the aorta with a prosthetic graft. Cardiopulmonary bypass through a femoral-femoral approach or with a centrifugal pump and left-sided heart bypass is frequently employed. The use of cardiopulmonary bypass has been associated with a decreased incidence of paraplegia, which can result from cessation of aortic blood flow during a "clamp-and-sew" technique if adequate spinal collaterals are not present.

Tracheobronchial Injuries

Tracheobronchial tree injuries are uncommon but associated with significant morbidity and mortality. Penetrating mechanisms are the most common etiology, although these injuries historically represent rare occurrences. Blunt injury to the tracheobronchial tree can occur but is similarly uncommon, resulting from the application of a large amount of energy to the anterior chest. These forces pull the lungs laterally and avulse the bronchi from the fixed carina. A tracheal rupture may occur when lungs and airways are rapidly compressed against a closed glottis, perforating the trachea along the membranous portion. Penetrating tracheobronchial injuries are predominantly a result of gunshot wounds that cause direct laceration of the tracheobronchial tree.

The location of the airway disruption dictates clinical presentation and the method of injury identification. Injuries that involve the thoracic trachea and proximal bronchi may result in large amounts of pneumomediastinum identified by chest radiography or CT imaging. More distal airway injuries will typically cause a pneumothorax treated initially by performance of a tube thoracostomy. A continuous chest tube air leak with persistent pneumothorax is highly suggestive of an injury to a bronchus or large bronchiole. Significant subcutaneous air may also be present on physical examination. Diagnosis is made with either rigid or flexible bronchoscopy, depending on the location of the injury and the ability to manipulate the neck. Bronchoscopy allows the identification of the injury and a detailed characterization, such as the location and severity of the disruption.

The management of tracheobronchial injuries begins with thoughtful assessment and control of the airway. With the placement of any airway, avoidance of further disruption is vital. Bronchoscopic guidance and direct visualization may be beneficial. Bronchial injuries that occupy less than one-third of the luminal circumference may be considered for nonoperative management if lung expansion with a chest tube results in resolution of the pneumothorax and associated air leak. Management

includes humidified oxygen, gentle suctioning, and observation, monitoring for the development of infectious sequelae. Operative management of the trachea, right airways, and proximal left mainstem bronchus is best approached through a right posterolateral thoracotomy. Distal left injuries are repaired through a left thoracotomy. A vascularized intercostal muscle flap is mobilized and carefully preserved during creation of the thoracotomy. Inappropriate placement of a retractor will prevent harvest of this valuable tissue coverage. Devitalized tissue is debrided, and injuries are closed with absorbable monofilament suture. Large injuries may require segmental resection with anastomosis. Coverage of the repair with a tissue pedicle, such as an intercostal muscle flap, may improve healing. If possible, patients who require sustained mechanical ventilation should have the endotracheal tube advanced so that the end of the tube is distal to the repair, protecting the repair from positive pressure. Other ventilatory options include dual-lung ventilation and extracorporeal life support during the immediate postoperative period. As with other injuries, minimally invasive and nonoperative techniques may be employed for tracheobronchial injuries. In selected cases, placement of intraluminal stents may be adequate. Because the incidence of these injuries is quite low, high-grade evidence for recommendations is currently not present.

Esophageal Injuries

Like the tracheobronchial tree, the thoracic esophagus is uncommonly injured by either blunt or penetrating mechanisms. However, penetrating injury is more common. Most penetrating injuries are caused by gunshot wounds (GSWs), followed by stab wounds. The mortality associated with penetrating esophageal injuries is 20% to 44% as a result of mediastinal sepsis and injury to adjacent vital structures.[199,200] Mortality is augmented by challenges with timely diagnosis and treatment. Whereas penetrating injury causes direct tissue laceration, blunt esophageal injury is likely caused by rapid intraluminal pressure elevation during compression of the chest or abdomen. An impact to the upper abdomen can compress the distended stomach, leading to transmission of an air and fluid pressure wave into the esophagus and resulting in a perforation, usually in the distal segment.

The location of penetrating injuries and the presumed trajectory through the mediastinum are often suggestive of esophageal injury. The esophagus is best evaluated through a combination of contrast esophagography (water-soluble first, followed by thin barium) and esophagoscopy. Together, these two modalities result in a sensitivity of almost 100% for esophageal injury.[201] Diagnostic studies may reveal leak of contrast material from the esophageal lumen or a disruption of the mucosa visualized during endoscopy. Helical CT esophagography may be a reasonable alternative to a fluoroscopic esophagram, obviating the need for patient participation (i.e., intubated patients) and radiologist administration of the study. In the absence of contrast, chest CT reveals air adjacent to the esophagus but outside the lumen, with surrounding soft tissue inflammation. High-resolution CT imaging may demonstrate an esophageal wall defect. The location of the injury should be determined to assist in operative planning.

Prompt diagnosis and control of esophageal injuries with associated mediastinal contamination is critical because delays are associated with worse outcomes. The goals of operative repair are to close the defect, ideally in two layers (mucosal/muscular), and provide adequate drainage. Management of injuries to the cervical esophagus is described earlier. The upper and midthoracic esophagus is best approached through a right posterolateral thoracotomy through the fourth or fifth interspace, whereas the lower esophagus is exposed from the left through the sixth or seventh interspace. As with tracheobronchial injuries, creation of a vascularized intercostal muscle flap on entry into the chest permits coverage of the repair with a vascularized patch. Alternatives to the intercostal muscle flap include pleura, pericardium, or diaphragm. The entire circumference of the esophagus is inspected to detect additional injuries.

An injury at the gastroesophageal junction may best be approached through a laparotomy. The injury is entirely exposed, which usually requires opening of the esophageal muscle layer superiorly and inferiorly to reveal the extent of the mucosal defect, which is commonly larger than the muscle disruption. The esophageal injury is closed in one or two layers, frequently with an absorbable mucosal suture followed by interrupted muscle sutures of a permanent material. Coverage of the repair with a muscle flap or adjacent tissue may help reduce the high risk of leak. Esophageal repairs at the gastroesophageal junction can be covered with a fundoplication of gastric tissue. Wide drainage of the mediastinum and chest is extremely important to control any leak that may develop postoperatively. Decompression of the stomach and distal feeding access are necessary, whether through nasoenteral tube placement or surgical gastrostomy and feeding jejunostomy. After repair, an esophagram may be performed to confirm healing and initiation of oral intake.

Inflammation within the mediastinum develops quickly, and primary repair of injuries that are identified late may not be possible. Salvage techniques to be considered in these circumstances include repair of the defect over a T-tube for creation of a controlled fistula, esophageal diversion through a cervical incision, or esophageal stenting. Esophagectomy, followed by planned elective reconstruction, is rarely necessary in trauma cases. However, it may be the only option to allow recovery. Like airway stents, esophageal stents are a minimally evaluated option.[201]

Diaphragmatic Injuries

Traumatic diaphragmatic injuries have a relatively low incidence, with a study of the NTDB revealing an overall incidence of 0.46%. Penetrating trauma accounted for 67% of the injuries, with motor vehicle injuries being the most common mechanism for blunt diaphragmatic injury.[202] Higher mortality was identified among blunt over penetrating trauma (19.8% vs. 8.8%), likely because of the high energy needed for blunt diaphragmatic injury, causing severe concomitant injuries. Isolated diaphragmatic injuries are usually of limited immediate threat to life. As opposed to direct laceration of the tissue by a missile, blunt diaphragmatic injuries are believed to be a result of a rapid increase in intraabdominal pressure, resulting in a blow-out of the diaphragmatic tissue. The left diaphragm is injured in approximately 75% of the cases because the liver protects the right hemidiaphragm. Morbidity related to diaphragmatic injuries is occasionally identified months to years after injury when a giant diaphragm hernia is diagnosed. When untreated, the natural history of these injuries is progressive enlargement with herniation of abdominal viscera into the chest. Diaphragmatic injuries can be categorized by the AAST grading system, which assesses the size of the wound and tissue loss for higher-grade injuries.

Injuries to the diaphragm can be a diagnostic challenge. A high index of suspicion is beneficial for their detection. If the injury is large and located on the left, chest radiograph may show intraabdominal viscera in the chest (Fig. 36.26). CT scans may demonstrate the presence of abdominal viscera in the chest

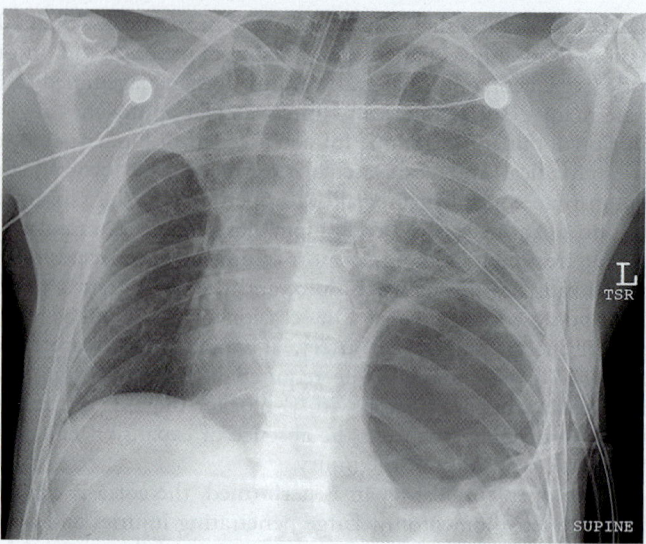

FIGURE 36.26 Left diaphragm injury on chest radiograph. The gas-filled stomach can be visualized on the left side of the chest because of herniation through a large diaphragmatic laceration.

or an abnormality of the diaphragm itself, such as thickening, elevation, or defect. Studies have shown CT to have overall sensitivities of up to 78% and specificities of 72% to 100% for detecting diaphragmatic injuries. However, diagnosis remains a challenge, particularly in cases of stab wound injury.[203]

Laparoscopy is a recommended diagnostic and therapeutic procedure.[204] Penetrating diaphragmatic injuries are usually diagnosed on operative exploration of the chest or abdomen. During exploration, following the trajectory of the injury will usually allow identification of the diaphragmatic defect. In the hemodynamically adequate patient without peritonitis, laparoscopy is recommended over CT scanning alone to decrease the incidence of missed traumatic diaphragmatic injuries after penetrating injury. Because right hemidiaphragm injuries rarely present in a delayed fashion, penetrating thoracoabdominal trauma to the right thoracoabdominal region may be considered for nonoperative management. In the absence of radiographic stigmata, blunt injuries are more elusive, and laparoscopic evaluation is beneficial when imaging is suggestive. The application of VATS has been reported as an alternative means of visualizing the diaphragm, although no demonstrable superiority exists compared with laparoscopy.

Diaphragmatic injuries are repaired by debriding nonviable tissue at the site of injury and closing the defect. Because of the redundancy and pliability of the diaphragm, most defects can be approximated primarily. Closure is typically achieved with a single layer of nonabsorbable suture incorporating the full thickness of the diaphragm. These injuries can bleed significantly from branches of the phrenic artery at the edges of the tear. Large areas of tissue loss precluding primary closure are rare in traumatic rupture, but when present, reconstruction with a prosthetic mesh may be considered. Nonabsorbable synthetic materials can be used to reconstruct the diaphragm in clean surgical fields but should be avoided if contamination is present. A peripheral detachment of the diaphragm from the wall of the torso can be repaired by reinserting the injured tissue one or two interspaces superior. During open procedures on the posterior diaphragm when access is challenging, laparoscopic-length instruments may facilitate repair.

Injuries to the Abdomen

The abdomen is a commonly injured body region and frequently requires the care of a surgeon for definitive management. Within the 2016 NTDB, 11.7% of all patients sustained abdominal injuries, with an associated case fatality rate of 12.9%.[159] The vital nature of the organs contained within the abdomen makes evaluation and management a priority. The predominant sources of morbidity and mortality are bleeding and visceral perforation with associated sepsis. In the setting of blunt trauma, solid organs often sustain contusion or laceration, causing bleeding that may require surgical management. Furthermore, blunt forces can cause rupture of hollow viscera due to rapid compression of a segment of intestine containing fluid and air. Penetrating mechanisms directly lacerate solid and hollow viscera, resulting in bleeding and intraabdominal contamination that often require operative repair.

As described for other cavities, the initial evaluation of the abdominally injured patient varies based on mechanism, although a common priority is rapidly determining the presence or absence of ongoing hemorrhage. Patients who respond to resuscitation and maintain appropriate hemodynamics are termed *responders*. This population is considered likely to "have bled" rather than suffering persistent bleeding. On the contrary, patients who do not respond to resuscitation with persistent physiologic instability are considered *nonresponders* and likely require immediate intervention. *Transient responders* are those in whom there is an initial response to resuscitation but return to instability within a short time period. In the trauma bay, ATLS surveys are designed for expeditious identification of cavitary hemorrhage after assessment of airway and breathing.

Blunt Abdominal Trauma Evaluation

Ultrasound has become a nearly ubiquitous technology in EDs internationally and has found routine application in the assessment of intraabdominal hemorrhage after blunt trauma. It is considered an adjunct to the primary survey in ATLS and has the advantage of being rapidly performed at the bedside.[89] Ultrasound for trauma evaluates the pericardium, hepatorenal fossa, splenorenal fossa, and retrovesicular space (pouch of Douglas). Fig. 36.15 depicts fluid in the hepatorenal space. An extended FAST, or eFAST, also includes views of the lung looking for hemo- or pneumothorax. These exams are advantageous because they can be repeated, particularly in patients with physiologic decline. Abdominal exploration is classically indicated in blunt trauma patients who fail to respond or are transient responders in the presence of intraabdominal fluid on FAST. If FAST examination capabilities are unavailable, diagnostic peritoneal lavage can be used. The peritoneal cavity is accessed through open, semi-open, or percutaneous technique, and a catheter is inserted. Immediate aspiration of blood or bile is considered positive. Absent these findings, 1 L of isotonic fluid can be instilled into the abdomen, with 250 mL collected and sent to the laboratory for analysis. Results demonstrating >100,000 red blood cells/mL or >500 white blood cells/mL are considered positive. In the modern area, the diagnostic peritoneal lavage (DPL) has been largely replaced by a diagnostic peritoneal aspirate (DPA) alone, which itself is almost never performed. Peritoneal aspiration revealing GI contents, bile, or more than 10 mL of gross blood suggests intraabdominal trauma that mandates operative intervention. Notably, neither technique of rapid assessment is flawless. FAST is limited by operator familiarity, body habitus, and subcutaneous emphysema/bowel gas. DPA is very rarely performed, associated with iatrogenic injury, relatively contraindicated in obesity, and suffers from low specificity. Both techniques are unable to evaluate the retroperitoneum, which may represent a considerable source of hemorrhage.

Technologic advancements and increased availability of CT over the past two decades have made it the primary method for comprehensive evaluation of the blunt trauma patient. This evolution has supported the development of nonoperative management strategies for many solid abdominal organ injuries. Abdominal CT for trauma is typically performed with administration of IV contrast agent timed to capture the arterial and portal venous phases, which best demonstrates the perfusion of the solid abdominal organs. This technique provides the necessary visualization of the solid organs to allow the determination of injury severity, including the presence of active bleeding. Imaging findings prompt management decisions, such as the need for operative, nonoperative, or angiographic therapy. Historically, blood within the abdomen mandated laparotomy, although commonly, the bleeding from solid organs was self-limited by the time of exploration. Subsequently, surgeons recognized that the physiologic state was more indicative of the need for laparotomy than the presence of injury alone. Thus, consideration of nonoperative management in the presence of hemoperitoneum with stable vital signs became an accepted pathway. As practice continues to evolve with the proximity and speed of CT scanning in the ED, damage control resuscitation under trauma team management can continue throughout the ever-shortening diagnostic window. The multiple potential sources of shock often germane to the blunt trauma patient have led some contemporary practices to advocate whole body CT scanning even in the presence of hypotension (systolic <90). The resultant information from rapidly obtained CT scanning may lead the surgeon down vastly different treatment algorithms (i.e., operative, endovascular, or continued resuscitation). The key term in these cases is "rapid" and requires the capability to continue resuscitative measures in the CT scanner. At most centers, obtaining a whole body CT scan can take anywhere from 10 to >30 minutes, time that can be better spent obtaining definitive hemorrhage control. The decision to proceed to CT with a hemodynamically unstable patient must be made cautiously. A repeat FAST and x-rays must be obtained to identify evolving injuries that should be addressed.

Despite being sensitive for solid organ injury, CT is less capable of detecting injuries to the hollow viscera. As CT technology evolves, its sensitivity has improved, although there are still significant limitations. Injury to the GI tract is suggested by bowel wall thickening, inflammation in the surrounding adipose tissue (stranding), or the presence of free intraperitoneal fluid. Unexplained free fluid must be carefully considered, given the high risk for associated bowel injury. In a significant percentage of cases, unexplained free fluid represents blood from a mesenteric tear that is no longer bleeding. Clinical findings such as the presence of an abdominal seat-belt mark or tenderness on examination raise concern for bowel injury in the presence of these CT findings. Serial examinations of the abdomen to monitor for worsening tenderness and peritoneal irritation are required for those patients who are not taken directly for exploration. Alternatively, laparoscopy may be a safe and feasible alternative to open exploration in patients without shock or other indications for surgery. A representative flow diagram of blunt abdominal trauma evaluation is depicted in Fig. 36.27.

Penetrating Abdominal Trauma Evaluation

The evaluation of penetrating abdominal trauma requires an approach unique from that for blunt mechanisms. In the setting of

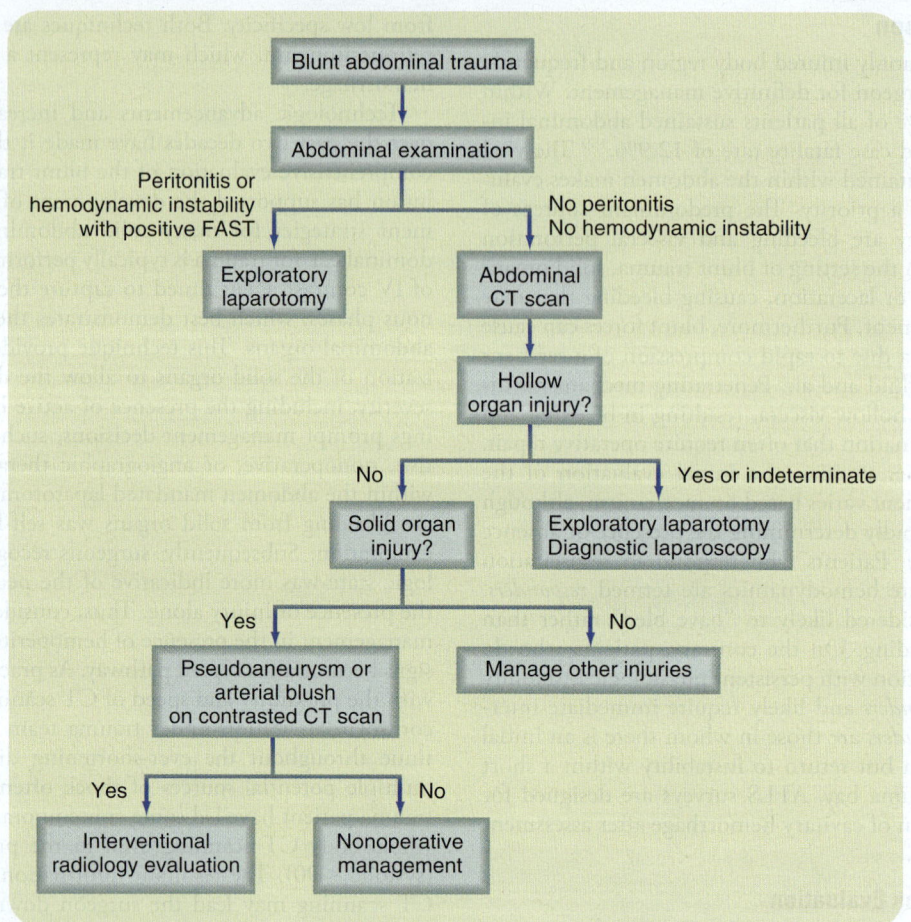

FIGURE 36.27 Algorithm for the evaluation and management of blunt abdominal trauma. *CT,* Computed tomography; *FAST,* focused abdominal sonography in trauma.

GSWs, injuries should be identified with radiopaque markers and plain radiographs obtained to establish possible trajectory and pneumoperitoneum. These radiographs should be obtained "skin to skin," ensuring that the image also encompasses the soft tissue. The role of FAST in abdominal GSWs is of controversial utility. When positive, it may support the need for abdominal exploration but is insufficient to rule out major hemorrhage or other operative trauma. The number of missiles and skin wounds should add up to an even number, or a more intense search for either retained bullets or wounds is required. Patients in extremis who are protecting their airway should be resuscitated before intubation in the trauma bay or in the OR. In the presence of normal physiology, abdominal GSW patients may proceed to CT scan for further delineation of their injuries. GSWs involving the thoracoabdomen may also require evaluation of the chest for mediastinal, pleural, or pulmonary injuries.[205]

Similar to patients with GSWs, patients with abdominal stab wounds and hemodynamic instability, peritonitis, or evisceration require immediate laparotomy. In patients who are not examinable, evaluation for peritoneal violation may be conducted via local wound exploration, CT, or diagnostic laparoscopy. All others can be managed by one of several pathways depending on the location of the wound. For stab wounds to the flank or back, CT imaging with IV contrast (± rectal contrast) should be undertaken to identify signs of operative injury. If solid organ injury is identified with active extravasation, angioembolization can be considered. Anterior

stab wounds allow for discretion of the attending surgeon. Local wound exploration to determine fascial violation, serial clinical exams, or diagnostic imaging for the hemodynamically appropriate patient represent equivalent pathways to safe management. Patients without any fascial penetration can be considered for discharge. If the local wound exploration reveals any evidence of possible fascial penetration, patients should be monitored with serial abdominal examinations, undergo CT imaging, or be considered for diagnostic laparoscopy. Diagnostic laparoscopy is highly accurate for the identification of peritoneal violation. Once peritoneal violation is identified, the decision to evaluate the peritoneal cavity via laparoscopic or open approach is based on surgeon skillset.

The development of peritonitis, hemodynamic instability, significant decreases in hemoglobin level, or leukocytosis should prompt further evaluation, usually with laparotomy. Patients without clinical change after 24 hours can have a diet instituted and be considered for discharge. However, this approach requires the presence of an infrastructure that allows close surveillance of these patients, which may not be available in all facilities. Thoracoabdominal stab wounds should employ a chest x-ray to evaluate for pneumothorax and pericardial ultrasound for effusion. Stab wounds to the left upper quadrant will likely require laparoscopy for diaphragmatic assessment. This is optional in right upper quadrant injuries because of the presence of the liver.[206] A suggested abdominal stab wound algorithm is demonstrated in Fig. 36.28.

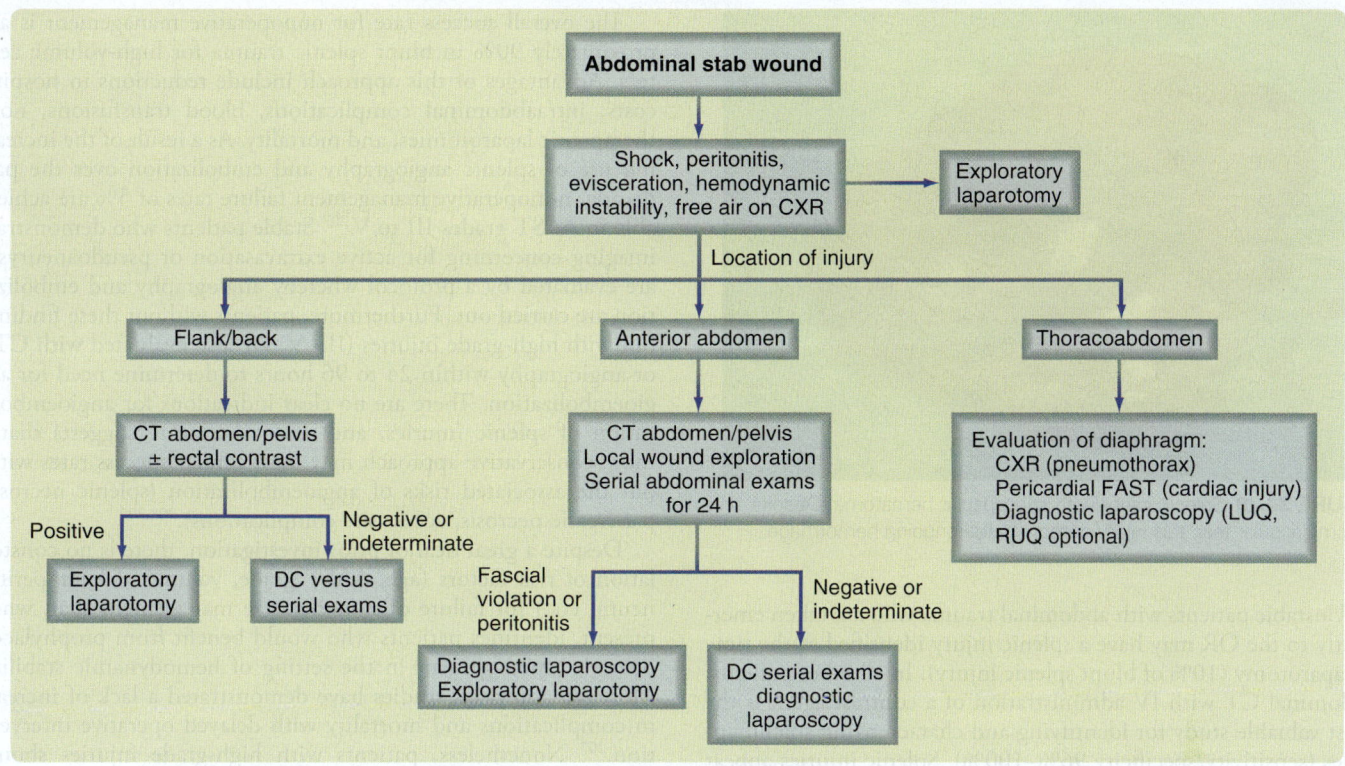

FIGURE 36.28 Algorithm for the evaluation and management of anterior abdominal stab wounds. *CT,* Computed tomography; *CXR,* chest x-ray; *DC,* discharge; *FAST,* focused abdominal sonography in trauma; *LUQ,* left upper quadrant; *RUQ,* right upper quadrant. (Adapted from Martin MJ, Brown CVR, Shatz DV, et al. Evaluation and management of abdominal stab wounds. *J Trauma Acute Care Surg.* 2018;85[5]:1007-1015.)

Management

A laparotomy is performed to explore the abdomen and repair injuries that are identified. It is important that the exploration of the abdomen be performed systematically to avoid missing injuries that may be subtle. As described in the setting of damage control, this approach may require abbreviation when physiologic deterioration occurs. The abdomen is opened from the xiphoid process to the pubic symphysis to provide adequate exposure. The falciform ligament is divided to separate the liver from the abdominal wall to prevent injury from retraction and to facilitate perihepatic packing. In cases where hemorrhage is minimal or the source of hemorrhage is known (due to either preoperative imaging or trajectory assessment), the surgeon may choose to approach the area directly, evacuate blood, and control the bleeding without antecedent packing. Alternatively, or in cases where the source of hemorrhage is unknown, blood can be quickly evacuated from all four quadrants of the abdomen and laparotomy sponges placed to provide temporary hemostasis. A fixed retractor is useful to facilitate optimal exposure. Sponges placed in the four quadrants are systematically removed to identify and address bleeding. They can be replaced if damage control is needed. Once bleeding is controlled, the entire GI tract is carefully evaluated, from the gastroesophageal junction to the proximal rectum at the peritoneal reflection. The lesser sac is also entered to visualize the posterior stomach and the pancreas. When injuries are identified, they are repaired, as detailed in subsequent sections. The development of physiologic compromise prompts the need to abbreviate the operation and proceed with damage control methods, including temporary abdominal closure. Effective two-way communication between the surgical and anesthesia teams facilitates determination of the need for damage

control use. If the operation can be completed without conversion to damage control, the abdominal fascia is closed, and the subcutaneous wound is addressed as dictated by the level of intraabdominal contamination.

Splenic Injuries

The spleen and liver are the most commonly injured abdominal organs. Isolated splenic injury comprises approximately 42% of abdominal injuries.[207] The frequency of these injuries requires the surgeon to possess a sound understanding of management strategies in splenic injury. Treatment is based on patient physiology and injury grade.

In blunt trauma, direct compression of the spleen with parenchymal fracture is a common pathophysiologic mechanism at the tissue level. Additionally, injury can be secondary to rapid deceleration that tears the splenic capsule and/or parenchyma where it is fixed to the retroperitoneum. This mechanism can create a subcapsular hematoma, which is demonstrated in Fig. 36.29. Penetrating splenic trauma is less common but represented 8.5% of all penetrating abdominal injuries in the 2012 NTDB. Hemorrhage from a splenic injury can be ongoing, with instability at the time of presentation or, more commonly, will have resolved spontaneously. As with other abdominal injuries, patients who are resuscitation nonresponders with intraabdominal fluid on FAST require exploration. Patients who respond to resuscitation with normalized physiology can often be managed nonoperatively, although this group is at risk for delayed hemorrhage (majority <72 hours). Over the past several decades, rates of nonoperative management in splenic trauma have increased from roughly 40% to 70%, with coincident decreases in mortality among the higher grades of injury.[207]

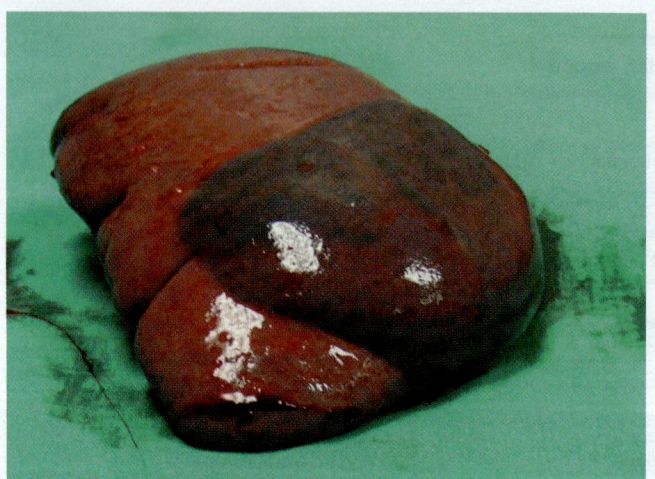

FIGURE 36.29 Splenic injury with subcapsular hematoma. Despite only a 1-cm capsular tear, this injury demonstrated ongoing hemorrhage.

Unstable patients with abdominal trauma who are taken emergently to the OR may have a splenic injury identified at the time of laparotomy (10% of blunt splenic injury). In all other patients, abdominal CT with IV administration of a contrast agent is the most valuable study for identifying and characterizing splenic injuries (sensitivity/specificity 96%–100%). Splenic injuries appear as disruptions in the normal splenic parenchyma, frequently with surrounding hematoma and free intraabdominal blood. Active bleeding can be identified by visualizing extravasation of contrast material (i.e., high-density blush or accumulation of contrast-laden blood). At times, this extravasation will be free into the peritoneal space or contained within an intraparenchymal pseudoaneurysm. A splenic injury with active extravasation into a pseudoaneurysm is demonstrated in Fig. 36.30. Other types of splenic injury can include a hematoma confined to the subcapsular space and even complete devascularization of the organ caused by injury of the hilar vessels. Spleen injuries are characterized by the AAST Injury Scoring Scale, which grades injuries on the basis of parenchymal or subcapsular abnormality and the presence of vascular involvement (Table 36.9).

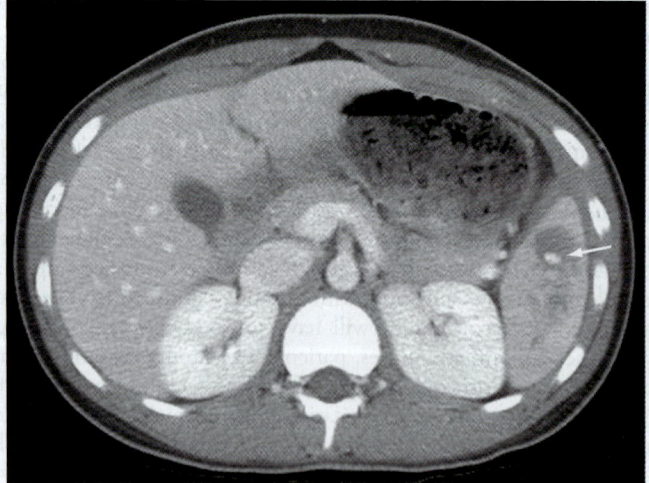

FIGURE 36.30 Grade III splenic laceration on abdominal computed tomography. Note the focus of active extravasation of contrast material within the injured splenic parenchyma as identified by the *arrow.*

The overall success rate for nonoperative management is approximately 90% in blunt splenic trauma for high-volume centers. Advantages of this approach include reductions in hospital costs, intraabdominal complications, blood transfusions, nontherapeutic laparotomies, and mortality. As a result of the increasing use of splenic angiography and embolization over the past decade, nonoperative management failure rates of 5% are achievable in AAST grades III to V.[207] Stable patients who demonstrate imaging concerning for active extravasation or pseudoaneurysm are evaluated by a protocol whereby angiography and embolization are carried out. Furthermore, patients without these findings but with high-grade injuries (III–V) are also evaluated with CTA or angiography within 24 to 96 hours to determine need for angioembolization. There are no clear indications for angioembolization of splenic injuries, and recent literature suggests that a more conservative approach may have similar success rates without the associated risks of angioembolization (splenic necrosis, pancreatic necrosis, access site complications).[208,209]

Despite a great deal of prior investigation, there is no constellation of risk factors (age, AAST grade, volume of hemoperitoneum, etc.) for failure of nonoperative management that, when present, identifies patients who would benefit from prophylactic operative management in the setting of hemodynamic stability. Moreover, previous studies have demonstrated a lack of increase in complications and mortality with delayed operative intervention.[207] Nonetheless, patients with high-grade injuries should undergo intensive care monitoring on admission, maintaining a low threshold for surgical management in the setting of decline.

Operative management of splenic injuries may be required in the setting of instability at the time of admission or after failed nonoperative management. Surgical approach is through a midline incision, which can allow for assessment of the entire peritoneal cavity if needed. A fixed retractor can improve exposure, and any packs placed in the left upper quadrant are removed to expose the injured spleen. To mobilize the spleen, retract it posteromedially to expose the retroperitoneal attachments. The white line of Toldt (splenocolic ligament) is divided, and the dissection continues superiorly until the short gastric vessels are encountered. A blunt plane is created posterior to the spleen in a medial direction, extending behind the tail of the pancreas. This maneuver mobilizes the entire spleen and distal pancreas, allowing the spleen to be delivered up into the wound. While avoiding the greater curve of the stomach, the short gastric vessels are ligated and divided. Finally, the spleen is removed after the hilar vessels are clamped and ligated, taking care not to injure the tail of the pancreas. A drain should be placed only if there is concern that the tail of the pancreas was injured. Postsplenectomy vaccines must be provided to ensure protection from encapsulated bacteria (*Streptococcus pneumoniae, Neisseria meningitidis,* and *Haemophilus influenzae*) and prevention of overwhelming postsplenectomy sepsis (incidence 0.5%–2%, mortality 30%–70%). Although splenic salvage techniques are well described, their utility is limited in the era of highly effective nonoperative management and endovascular approaches to splenic trauma.

Hepatic Injuries

Liver injuries are extremely common after blunt trauma, at a rate of 22.2% within the 2012 NTDB. Similarly, the liver is the most injured abdominal organ after penetrating trauma, present in 26.1% of cases. Mechanisms of blunt hepatic trauma include compression with direct parenchymal damage and shearing forces, which tear hepatic tissue and disrupt vascular and ligamentous

TABLE 36.9   AAST Spleen Injury Scale (2018 Revision)

GRADE	AIS SEVERITY	IMAGING CRITERIA (CT FINDINGS)	OPERATIVE CRITERIA	PATHOLOGIC CRITERIA
I	2	Subcapsular hematoma <10% surface area	Subcapsular hematoma <10% surface area	Subcapsular hematoma <10% surface area
		Parenchymal laceration <1 cm in depth	Parenchymal laceration <1 cm in depth	Parenchymal laceration <1 cm in depth
		Capsular tear	Capsular tear	Capsular tear
II	2	Subcapsular hematoma 10%–50% surface area	Subcapsular hematoma 10%–50% surface area	Subcapsular hematoma 10%–50% surface area
		Intraparenchymal hematoma <5 cm	Intraparenchymal hematoma <5 cm	Intraparenchymal hematoma <5 cm
		Parenchymal laceration 1–3 cm	Parenchymal laceration 1–3 cm	Parenchymal laceration 1–3 cm
III	3	Subcapsular hematoma >50% surface area	Subcapsular hematoma >50% surface area or expanding	Subcapsular hematoma >50% surface area
		Ruptured subcapsular or intraparenchymal hematoma ≥5 cm	Ruptured subcapsular or intraparenchymal hematoma ≥5 cm	Ruptured subcapsular or intraparenchymal hematoma ≥5 cm
		Parenchymal laceration >3 cm depth	Parenchymal laceration >3 cm depth	Parenchymal laceration >3 cm depth
IV	4	Any injury in the presence of a splenic vascular injury or active bleeding confined within the splenic capsule	Parenchymal laceration involving segmental or hilar vessels producing >25% devascularization	Parenchymal laceration involving segmental or hilar vessels producing >25% devascularization
		Parenchymal laceration involving segmental or hilar vessels producing >25% devascularization		
V	5	Any injury in the presence of a splenic vascular injury with active bleeding extending beyond the spleen into the peritoneum	Hilar vascular injury, which devascularizes the spleen	Hilar vascular injury which devascularizes the spleen
		Shattered spleen	Shattered spleen	Shattered spleen

AAST, American Association for the Surgery of Trauma; *AIS,* Abbreviated Injury Scale; *CT,* computed tomography.

attachments. The liver is partially protected by the thoracic cage, although the ribs provide little support during high-energy mechanisms. Penetrating mechanisms directly lacerate the hepatic parenchyma while also causing adjacent tissue contusion. Mortality from liver injury, not unlike the management of other abdominal solid organs, has decreased over time as practices have evolved from primarily operative to nonoperative management with endovascular and endoscopic treatments. Associated morbidity from liver injury includes bleeding, biliary, fistula (i.e., hemobilia, biliary fistula), infection, and hepatic necrosis.

Like other abdominal organs, liver injuries are often first diagnosed on entering the abdomen in the unstable patient explored for free fluid on FAST examination. Those who do not require immediate operation should be imaged with abdominal CT enhanced with IV administration of a contrast agent. CT can provide excellent anatomic detail that allows highly accurate characterization of injuries. Timing of contrast for delineation of hepatic injury occurs in three phases (noncontrast, arterial, portal venous), giving insight into the hemorrhage type. Common findings on CT indicative of liver injury include disruption of the hepatic parenchyma with perihepatic blood or hematoma and hemoperitoneum. Bleeding from the liver can be seen on CT as extravasation of contrast material, either within the liver parenchyma or into the peritoneal space, as seen in Fig. 36.31. The characteristics of the liver injury on CT can be used to categorize the injury with the AAST OIS, which accounts for parenchymal involvement and the presence of vascular injury (Table 36.10).

Treatment of liver trauma has progressed over prior decades from aggressive operative to largely nonoperative care, coinciding with decreased in-hospital mortality. As described by Peitzman

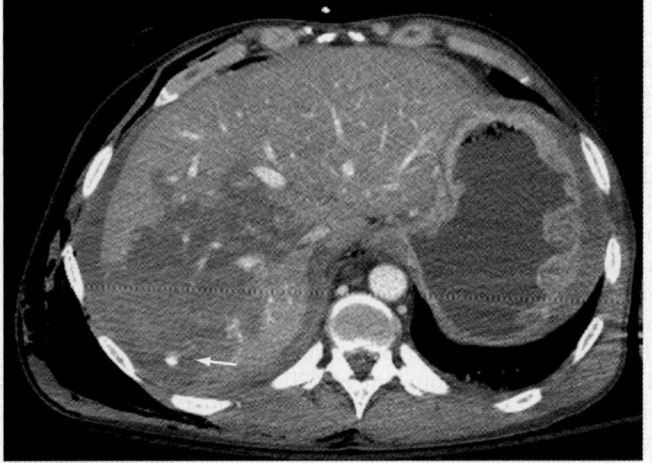

FIGURE 36.31 Grade IV liver laceration involving the right hepatic lobe on abdominal computed tomography. Note the focus of active extravasation of contrast material within the injured liver parenchyma at the periphery of the injury, as identified by the *arrow.*

and Richardson, the period of 1960–75 presented multiple series of patients who underwent resectional management, hepatic artery ligation, and T-tube choledochostomy for liver injury. At that time, morbidity and mortality, ranging from 27% to 65%, were suspected to arise from biliary/septic complications rather than hemorrhage. In 1976, Lucas and Ledgerwood shifted the focus of care to prioritize bleeding management in hepatic trauma, with a subsequent decrease in mortality to 22%. Furthermore, the

TABLE 36.10   AAST Liver Injury Scale (2018 Revision)

GRADE	AIS SEVERITY	IMAGING CRITERIA (CT FINDINGS)	OPERATIVE CRITERIA	PATHOLOGIC CRITERIA
I	2	Subcapsular hematoma <10% surface area	Subcapsular hematoma <10% surface area	Subcapsular hematoma <10% surface area
		Parenchymal laceration <1 cm depth	Parenchymal laceration <1 cm depth	Parenchymal laceration <1 cm depth
		Capsular tear	Capsular tear	Capsular tear
II	2	Subcapsular hematoma 10%–50% surface area	Subcapsular hematoma 10%–50% surface area	Subcapsular hematoma 10%–50% surface area
		Intraparenchymal hematoma <10 cm in diameter	Intraparenchymal hematoma <10 cm in diameter	Intraparenchymal hematoma <10 cm in diameter
		Laceration 1–3 cm in depth and ≤10 cm in length	Laceration 1–3 cm in depth and ≤10 cm in length	Laceration 1–3 cm in depth and ≤10 cm in length
III	3	Subcapsular hematoma >50% surface area	Subcapsular hematoma >50% surface area	Subcapsular hematoma >50% surface area
		Ruptured subcapsular or parenchymal hematoma	Ruptured subcapsular or parenchymal hematoma	Ruptured subcapsular or parenchymal hematoma
		Intraparenchymal laceration >10 cm, laceration >3 m in depth	Intraparenchymal laceration >10 cm, laceration >3 m in depth	Intraparenchymal laceration >10 cm, laceration >3 m in depth
		Any injury in the presence of a liver vascular injury or active bleeding contained within liver parenchyma		
IV	4	Parenchymal disruption involving 25%–75% of a hepatic lobe	Parenchymal disruption involving 25%–75% of a hepatic lobe	Parenchymal disruption involving 25%–75% of a hepatic lobe
		Active bleeding extending beyond the liver parenchyma into the peritoneum		
V	5	Parenchymal disruption >75% of a hepatic lobe	Parenchymal disruption >75% of a hepatic lobe	Parenchymal disruption >75% of a hepatic lobe
		Juxtahepatic venous injury to include retrohepatic vena cava and central major hepatic veins	Juxtahepatic venous injury to include retrohepatic vena cava and central major hepatic veins	Juxtahepatic venous injury to include retrohepatic vena cava and central major hepatic veins

AAST, American Association for the Surgery of Trauma; *AIS,* Abbreviated Injury Scale; *CT,* computed tomography.

partners described the use of temporary abdominal packing for control of liver bleeding. This approach was later promoted by Feliciano, Mattox, and Jordan for critically ill patients in whom surgical solutions for bleeding had failed. After these practice-changing reports, the AAST OIS for liver, spleen, and kidney was first described in 1989 and remains a consistent scheme for defining solid abdominal organ injury. As data began to accumulate for a nonoperative management option in blunt liver trauma, a review of the literature by Pachter and Hofstetter concluded that nonoperative management should be the approach of choice for the hemodynamically stable patient, regardless of AAST grade. The continued development of CT technology in tandem with endovascular/endoscopic support has resulted in the majority of patients with grades I to III injuries being successfully managed nonoperatively, whereas two-thirds of grades IV and V require surgical care. Polanco and colleagues, in a review of resectional management for complex blunt and penetrating liver trauma, report a mortality rate from liver injury of 9%. They attribute the improved mortality within their series to early decision for major operation, intraoperative resuscitation technique, and senior surgical/subspecialty assistance.[210]

Patients who are hemodynamically stable in the setting of blunt and penetrating liver trauma should be considered primarily for nonoperative management. Parenchymal bleeding or pseudoaneurysm on cross-sectional imaging should prompt consideration of angiography. The natural history of hepatic pseudoaneurysms is not entirely elucidated, but it is believed that they may be associated with an increased risk of delayed bleeding, especially when associated with

hepatic arterial branches. In appropriately selected patients, the use of angioembolization has improved the rate of successful nonoperative management, with a reduction in conversion to surgical treatment. Aggressive embolization of all vascular lesions, however, is associated with increased rates of hepatic necrosis and abscess formation. The decision to perform angioembolization should not be made reflexively and should be preceded by a conversation between the trauma surgeon and the interventionalist.[211,212]

Even successful nonoperative management may require the treatment of complications (12%–14%), such as bile leaks with biloma formation, hemobilia, and development of liver abscesses.[210] Frequently, these are suggested by the development of abdominal symptoms with, at times, the addition of systemic infection or inflammation. CT or ultrasound imaging can be valuable in evaluating for abscess and biloma; these can usually be managed with percutaneous drainage guided by CT or ultrasound. Endoscopic retrograde cholangiopancreatography (ERCP) with stent placement is occasionally required to decompress the biliary tree and promote healing of a bile leak. Biliary ascites not amenable to percutaneous drainage may require laparoscopy or laparotomy for adequate drainage to be obtained. Hemobilia is managed with angiography, which includes embolization of the hepatic vessel that is communicating with the biliary tree.

Although there have been great advances in the nonoperative management of liver injuries, it should not be overlooked that unstable patients require operative management of bleeding. In blunt trauma, a recent systematic review reported a pooled nonoperative management failure rate of 9.5%, predictive factors including signs of shock and peritoneal signs on presentation, high ISS, and associated intraabdominal trauma.[210] Similarly, an analysis from LA county demonstrates failure of selective nonoperative management in approximately 5% of patients suffering GSWs to the liver.[213] Polanco and colleagues, in a review of resectional management for complex blunt and penetrating liver trauma, report a mortality rate from liver injury of 9%. The surgical approach to hepatic injuries as developed by the WTA is presented in Fig. 36.32. When operative management is required, a midline laparotomy is the most versatile approach for managing any liver injury that might be encountered. The falciform ligament is divided, and perihepatic sponges are placed to temporarily manage bleeding from the liver. A fixed retractor can be placed to improve exposure of the right upper quadrant structures. When needed, perihepatic packing and manual compression can temporize bleeding to provide the opportunity to catch up with the resuscitation. Once the patient is reasonably stable, the packs are removed, and the injuries to the liver are evaluated. Mild injuries with minimal ongoing bleeding may be managed with further compression, topical hemostatic agents, or suture hepatorrhaphy. Management of liver injuries may be facilitated by dividing the triangular ligaments to mobilize the right or left hepatic lobes. This will allow injuries to be better exposed for repair but may also allow more effective packing by optimizing anterior-to-posterior compression. Any mobilization of the liver must be

carefully considered if there is any chance that the attachments of the liver are providing lifesaving tamponade of retrohepatic bleeding. Most liver injuries will require only superficial techniques for hemostasis to be obtained.

When more severe bleeding from the liver is present, a Pringle maneuver is a valuable adjunct to slow blood flow enough to visualize the injury. The hepatoduodenal ligament is encircled with a vessel loop or vascular clamp to occlude hepatic blood flow from the hepatic artery and portal vein. This maneuver helps distinguish hepatic arterial and portal venous bleeding from hepatic vein bleeding, which will persist with the hepatoduodenal ligament clamped. In many cases, the liver laceration can then be explored, and any actively bleeding vessels may be controlled with suture ligation. Hepatic parenchyma that appears to be devitalized should be debrided and drains placed when injuries appear to be at risk for a bile leak. A vascularized pedicle of omentum may reduce parenchymal bleeding and promote healing of the laceration when it is packed within the liver injury.

Liver injuries in the vicinity of the retrohepatic vena cava that are not actively bleeding should be packed and not explored. There are many heroic techniques described in the literature that outline the repair of retrohepatic vena cava injuries, but the approach with the greatest likelihood of success is preserving the natural tamponade of this low-pressure region when feasible. An atriocaval (Shrock) shunt is one method that includes isolation of

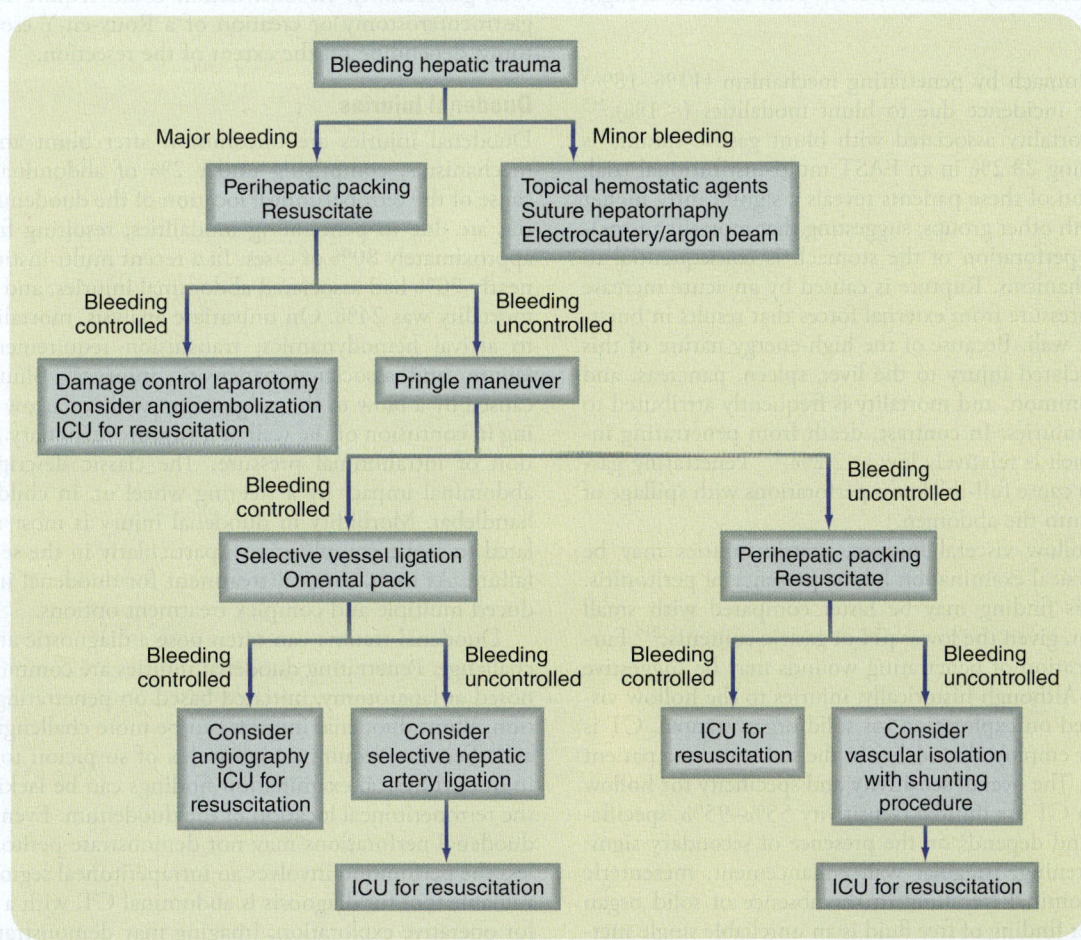

FIGURE 36.32 Algorithm for the operative management of hepatic injuries. *ICU,* Intensive care unit. (Modified from Kozar RA, Feliciano DV, Moore EE, et al. Western Trauma Association/critical decisions in trauma: Operative management of adult blunt hepatic trauma. *J Trauma.* 2011;71:1-5.)

the retrohepatic vena cava by placing an intravascular shunt between the right atrium and infrahepatic vena cava. Isolation of the liver with an atriocaval shunt with the addition of a Pringle maneuver theoretically allows repair of the vena cava or hepatic veins with less ongoing blood loss. Alternatives to the Shrock shunt include total hepatic vascular isolation with veno-venous extracorporeal membrane oxygen (V-V ECMO) and the Bridge balloon. The Bridge balloon is an endovascular venous occlusion balloon that was originally used to control bleeding at the time of pacemaker lead extraction. It can be placed via femoral venous access using a 12-Fr sheath and guided either via manual palpation or fluoroscopically into the retrohepatic cava.[214]

Damage control techniques are often required because many patients who require operative intervention for liver injuries have already deteriorated physiologically. Control of surgical bleeding is obtained, and the liver is packed, followed by temporary abdominal closure. It is inappropriate to leave surgical bleeding in the hope that packing alone will provide adequate control. Conversely, diffuse liver bleeding due to coagulopathy will not respond to repeated attempts at placement of suture. Instead, this should be treated with reversal of physiologic derangements. Patients are then resuscitated in the ICU until hypothermia, coagulopathy, and acidosis resolve, at which time the abdomen can be reexplored and packs removed. After damage control, angiography with embolization may provide additional assistance with management of ongoing bleeding from hepatic artery branches. Nonetheless, the mortality in this cohort of patients remains high.

Gastric Injuries

Injuries to the stomach by penetrating mechanism (11%–18%) far outweigh the incidence due to blunt modalities (<1%).[215] However, the mortality associated with blunt gastric trauma is significant, reaching 28.2% in an EAST multi-institutional trial. A closer evaluation of these patients reveals a significantly higher ISS compared with other groups, suggesting that mortality associated with blunt perforation of the stomach is consequential to high-energy mechanisms. Rupture is caused by an acute increase in intraluminal pressure from external forces that results in bursting of the gastric wall. Because of the high-energy nature of this mechanism, associated injury to the liver, spleen, pancreas, and small bowel is common, and mortality is frequently attributed to these associated injuries. In contrast, death from penetrating injury to the stomach is relatively low at 2.2%.[215] Penetrating gastric injuries often cause full-thickness perforations with spillage of gastric contents into the abdomen.

Like other hollow visceral injuries, gastric injuries may be identified on physical examination by the presence of peritonitis. The onset of this finding may be faster compared with small bowel perforation, given the lower pH of gastric contents.[215] Furthermore, the location of penetrating wounds may be suggestive of gastric injury. Although historically, injuries to the hollow viscus were identified on exploration for solid organ trauma, CT is now a commonly employed modality in the stable trauma patient before operation. The overall sensitivity and specificity for hollow visceral injury on CT are limited (sensitivity 55%–95%, specificity 48%–92%) and depends on the presence of secondary signs: bowel wall thickening, irregular wall enhancement, mesenteric defects, and abdominal free fluid in the absence of solid organ trauma. The latter finding of free fluid is an unreliable single metric for operation, in the setting of which therapeutic laparotomy ranges from 27% to 54%. Similarly, isolated pneumoperitoneum in blunt trauma may also be an untrustworthy indicator for

hollow viscus injury.[215] As described previously, the algorithmic evaluation of blunt or penetrating abdominal trauma may include a period of observation, whereby injury to the hollow viscus becomes clinically apparent. Importantly, if suspicion is high based on multiple metrics, the decision to explore should be expeditiously made because mortality increases proportional to surgical delay.

A full evaluation of the stomach includes visualization of the anterior and posterior walls, requiring entry into the lesser sac. Failure to accomplish this may lead to missed injuries with subsequent morbidity. The approach to repair is based on the amount of tissue loss and the injury location. Hematomas within the gastric wall should be evacuated to ensure the absence of perforation. This is followed by control of bleeding and closure of the seromusculature with nonabsorbable suture. Injuries that are full thickness should have all nonviable tissue debrided; the gastric wall is then closed in one or two layers. A common approach is to close the perforation with absorbable suture and then invert the suture line with nonabsorbable seromuscular stitches. A stapler can also be used to close a perforation because of the redundancy of gastric tissue and the unlikelihood of overly decreasing the volume of the stomach lumen. Injuries involving the gastroesophageal junction, lesser curve, fundus, and posterior wall may be more challenging to approach and require better exposure of the upper abdomen. Rarely, highly destructive injuries that cause the loss of large portions of the stomach will require partial or even total gastrectomy. Reconstruction could require Billroth I or II gastroenterostomy or creation of a Roux-en-Y esophagojejunostomy, depending on the extent of the resection.

Duodenal Injuries

Duodenal injuries are uncommon after blunt and penetrating mechanisms, comprising under 2% of abdominal trauma. Because of the retroperitoneal location of the duodenum, most injuries are due to penetrating modalities, resulting from GSWs in approximately 80% of cases. In a recent multi-institutional series, nearly 70% had associated abdominal injuries, and the associated mortality was 24%. On univariate analysis, mortality was related to arrival hemodynamics, transfusion requirement, ISS, renal failure, and associated pancreatic injury.[216] Blunt injuries are caused by a blow to the epigastrium with a narrow object, resulting in contusion of the wall or a rupture secondary to acute elevation of intraluminal pressure. The classic description includes abdominal impact by a steering wheel or, in children, a bicycle handlebar. Morbidity in duodenal injury is most commonly related to septic complications, particularly in the setting of repair failure. As such, surgical treatment for duodenal injury has produced multiple and complex treatment options.

Duodenal trauma can often pose a diagnostic and therapeutic challenge. Penetrating duodenal injuries are commonly first diagnosed at laparotomy, initiated based on penetrating wound location. Blunt duodenal injuries can be more challenging to identify and therefore require a high index of suspicion to avoid missed injuries. Physical examination findings can be lacking because of the retroperitoneal location of the duodenum. Even full-thickness duodenal perforations may not demonstrate peritoneal signs unless the perforation involves an intraperitoneal segment. The most valuable tool for diagnosis is abdominal CT, with a low threshold for operative exploration. Imaging may demonstrate a thickened duodenal wall with periduodenal air and fluid. Low-grade injuries, such as a duodenal hematoma, may also be identified by CT. If initial emergent imaging in hemodynamically stable patients is suggestive of duodenal trauma, repeat imaging in the form of oral contrast-enhanced CT, timed for duodenal transit, or upper GI fluoroscopy should be performed. Any evidence of duodenal perforation on imaging requires immediate operative intervention. Findings may be subtle, but a low threshold for exploration must be maintained because of the potential for false-negative abdominal CT results.

The approach to management of duodenal injuries depends on the location of the injury and the amount of tissue destruction. Hematomas of the duodenal wall will often resolve without intervention and are an issue only if they cause a gastric outlet obstruction. Treatment of obstructing hematomas consists of gastric decompression, initiation of total parenteral nutrition, and re-evaluation of gastric emptying with a contrast study after 5 to 7 days. If the duodenal obstruction persists after approximately 14 days, operative exploration is warranted to evacuate hematoma and evaluate for perforation, stricture, or associated pancreatic injury. Hematomas will frequently decompress spontaneously during mobilization of the duodenum, and the intestinal wall should then be evaluated for injury. Duodenal hematomas identified incidentally during laparotomy should not be intentionally opened unless there is a concern for full-thickness injury.

A retrospective study from the Panamerican Trauma Society found that 98% of patients with operative duodenal injury were amenable to primary repair, inclusive of all AAST grades.[216] Duodenal wall perforations can be repaired by a single- or double-layer approach after debridement of devitalized tissue. Complete mobilization of the duodenum with a wide Kocher maneuver is required to provide necessary exposure and ensure a tension-free repair. Larger amounts of tissue loss or duodenal transection can be managed with resection and primary anastomosis if the ampulla is not involved and the injured segment is short. Longer segments of duodenal injury or areas adjacent to the ampulla may require enteric bypass with a Billroth II or Roux-en-Y reconstruction. If possible, a healthy piece of omentum should be placed over any repair for reinforcement. Additional maneuvers for protection of suture lines from enteric contents (i.e., duodenal diverticulization, pyloric exclusion with gastrojejunostomy, tube duodenostomy) have been questioned in previous reviews and should be individualized to select cases. Similarly, drain placement after definitive repair is not mandatory, although a potential benefit may be controlled fistula creation if leak occurs. In the damage control setting, the use of resection with wide drainage and temporary discontinuity is highly effective for controlling contamination.

Pancreatic Injuries

Pancreatic injuries commonly occur in association with injury to the duodenum because of their proximity. However, the overall incidence in abdominal trauma is relatively low (0.2%–12%).[217] A penetrating mechanism is more commonly the cause, with 4.4% of patients with penetrating abdominal trauma sustaining a pancreatic injury. True pancreatic trauma–related mortality is difficult to identify because deaths are often attributable to associated pathology. Nonetheless, morbidity and mortality are noted to increase with AAST grade (up to 40% in grade V injury), along with delays in diagnosis and management.[217] Pancreatic enzymes are caustic; thus, ductal injury with leak (≥grade III) is the most significant contributor to organ-specific morbidity and mortality. Pancreas tissue injury can result from direct laceration of the organ or through the transmission of blunt force energy to the retroperitoneum. A common mechanism of blunt pancreatic injury involves crushing of the body of the pancreas between a rigid

structure, such as a steering wheel or seat belt, and the vertebral column. The impact to the pancreas causes injury that ranges from mild contusion to complete transection with ductal disruption.

The identification of pancreas injuries can be challenging, particularly because available imaging modalities are not highly effective. As with the duodenum, the retroperitoneal location of the pancreas makes physical examination findings less helpful for diagnosis. Three-dimensional imaging with IV contrast-enhanced abdominal CT provides the best view of the pancreas and associated injury. Despite this, sensitivity and specificity for the detection of parenchymal injury (sensitivity 47%–79%) and the presence of ductal involvement (sensitivity 52%–54%, specificity 90%–95%) remain inconsistently reported in the literature, potentially reflecting variations in radiologic interpretation between centers.[217] CT alone may not be satisfactory to rule out a clinically significant pancreatic injury, and a high index of suspicion must be maintained. On abdominal CT, findings suggestive of pancreatic injuries include malperfusion of the pancreatic parenchyma, surrounding fluid, or hematoma and stranding in the adjacent soft tissue. An injury involving the neck of the pancreas on CT is demonstrated in Fig. 36.33.

The identification of clinically significant pancreatic injuries may require the use of other diagnostic studies. Reported incidence of missed pancreatic trauma on CT approximates 15%.[217] Repeated CT imaging may suggest a pancreatic injury that required time to develop inflammation in the patient who remains persistently unwell. When obtained more than 3 hours after injury occurrence, an elevated serum amylase level may reflect pancreatic trauma. Used in this way, serum amylase levels are reasonably sensitive but lacking in specificity and are of limited value. Imaging of the pancreatic ducts with ERCP or magnetic resonance cholangiopancreatography may increase diagnostic yield, especially for those patients who have a suggestion of pancreatic injury. These additional modalities continue to be studied and may occasionally be valuable in planning therapy and the operative approach.

The gold standard for management of pancreatic injuries that involve the main pancreatic duct is operative exploration.

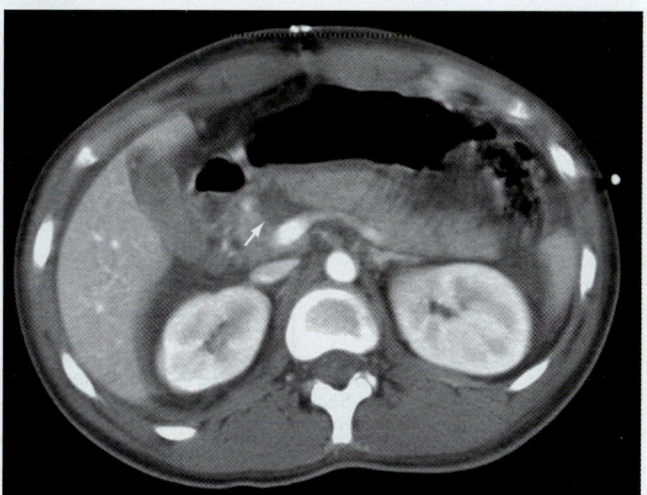

FIGURE 36.33 Pancreatic injury on abdominal computed tomography. The injury involves the pancreatic neck and appears as a 2-cm segment of nonperfused pancreas tissue with surrounding edema, as identified by the *arrow*.

Exposure of the entire pancreas is required to evaluate for injury and develop an effective surgical plan. This exposure includes mobilization of the hepatic flexure and division of the gastrocolic ligament, allowing retraction of the transverse and mesocolon inferiorly. A Kocher maneuver will mobilize the pancreatic head and facilitate visualization. Assessment of the pancreas includes determining the amount of parenchymal involvement, location of the injury, and presence of ductal trauma. Pancreatic ductal injuries to the left of the superior mesenteric vessels are managed with a distal pancreatectomy. The proximal pancreatic stump can be managed by individually ligating the duct, then oversewing the parenchyma or using a stapling device. Healing of the retained pancreas may be enhanced by coverage with a piece of healthy omentum. A closed suction drain should be placed to manage any pancreatic enzyme leak.

Treating injuries of the ductal system within the head of the pancreas can be more challenging. When tissue destruction is limited, managing these injuries with drainage alone often diverts the leakage of pancreatic fluid externally, creating a controlled fistula that will frequently close spontaneously. The closure of a fistula may be facilitated by biliary decompression through the placement of stents by ERCP. Massive destruction of the pancreatic head with devitalized parenchyma (grade V) or combined pancreatic and duodenal injuries may require a

pancreaticoduodenectomy (Whipple procedure). This presents the patient with a large surgical burden and is associated with a high postoperative complication rate. Only patients with normalized physiology should be considered candidates for pancreaticoduodenectomy; others undergo an abbreviated operation with later reconstruction. Damage control for pancreatic injury includes hemorrhage control, external drainage, and temporary abdominal closure with plans for reexploration.

Effective external drainage is an important component in the management of pancreatic injuries, the value of which cannot be overstated. Pancreatic enzyme diversion is required to prevent retroperitoneal exposure to caustic enzymes, which will provoke a massive inflammatory response and progressive organ dysfunction. Less severe pancreatic injuries identified at the time of operative intervention that do not involve the pancreatic duct (grades I and II), including hematomas, parenchymal contusions, and lacerations of the capsule or superficial parenchyma, should be managed with external drainage. Closed suction systems are associated with a reduced rate of abscess development compared with open-style drains.[217] Routine operative exploration for grade I or II pancreatic injury is not required. Distal feeding access may be valuable to provide early enteral nutrition, depending on the overall clinical picture. Fig. 36.34 demonstrates an approach to the operative management of pancreatic injuries.

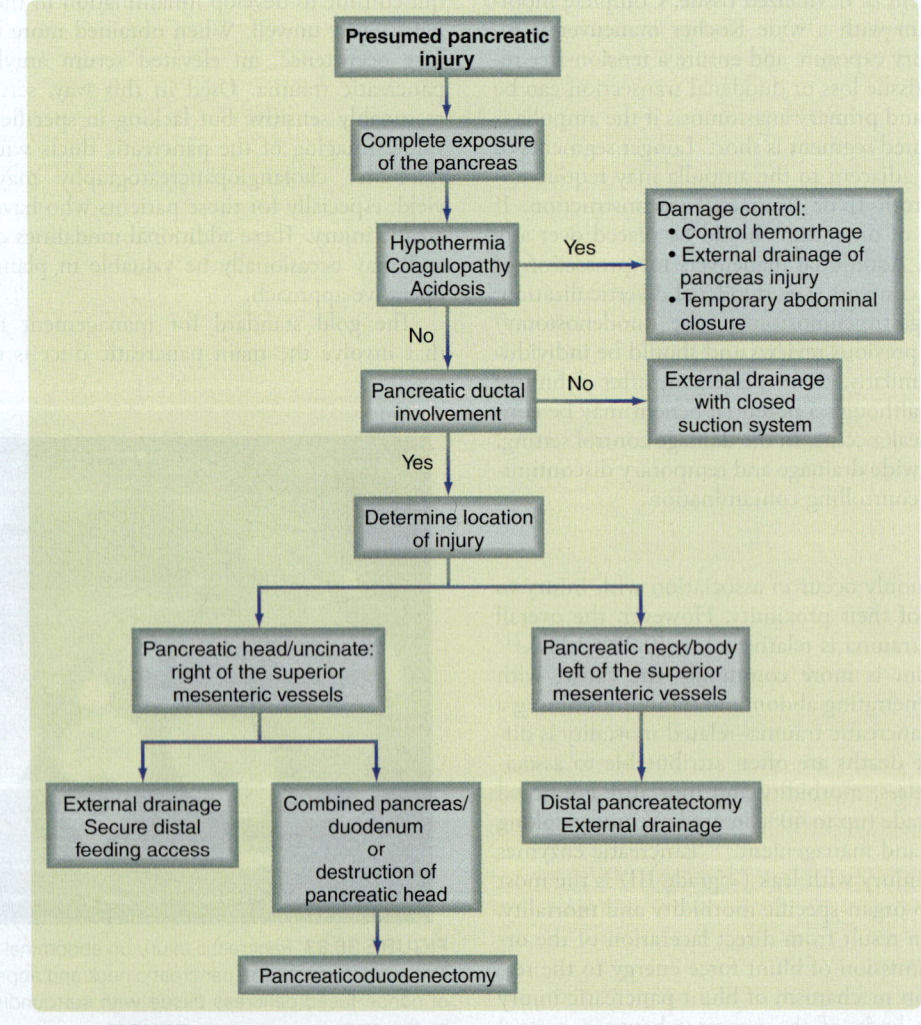

FIGURE 36.34 Algorithm for the operative management of pancreatic injury.

Small Bowel Injuries

Although the small intestine is one of the more frequently injured organs after penetrating abdominal trauma, it is a rarely injured entity by blunt mechanism (0.3%). Mortality rates range from 15% to 20%, with most caused by associated vascular injuries.[215] At the tissue level, injury can be secondary to crushing, rupture, and shearing mechanisms. Penetrating injuries can range from tiny perforations to large destructive injuries that devitalize circumferential segments of small bowel. Direct blunt tissue injury can occur when the small bowel is crushed between the steering wheel or seat belt and a rigid structure, such as the vertebral column. Small bowel rupture occurs when the intraluminal pressure rapidly increases, causing a blow-out along the antimesenteric border. Deceleration mechanisms can result in a shearing of the serosa or muscularis throughout a segment of small bowel. Injuries to the small bowel mesentery can result in devascularization and subsequent intestinal necrosis without direct tissue injury.

In the setting of penetrating mechanisms, small bowel injuries are often identified at the time of abdominal exploration. Patients may have peritonitis on presenting examination, or their abdominal findings may worsen in the hours after arrival. As with other hollow abdominal viscera, the evaluation can be challenging and is similar to the evaluation of the stomach and duodenum, as described earlier. Abdominal CT imaging has significant limitations, and a high index of suspicion must exist to avoid a missed injury.

The repair of small bowel injuries depends on the amount of intestinal wall destruction in relation to the overall luminal circumference. Injuries to the intestinal serosa can be reinforced with interrupted nonabsorbable suture, which imbricates the injury. Small perforations can be repaired primarily with one or two layers after debridement of devitalized tissue. Care must be taken to avoid overly compromising the size of the intestinal lumen. In the setting of multiple perforations, primary repair can still be safely performed as long as the injuries are not so close as to result in narrowing of the bowel lumen when closed. Despite this, many surgeons choose to perform a resection with anastomosis when multiple perforations are present within a segment of bowel. When injuries involve more than 50% of the intestinal wall circumference, bowel resection with anastomosis should be performed. There has been no difference in leak rates demonstrated between stapled and hand-sewn anastomoses after resection. Selection of the anastomosis technique should be based on the preference of the surgeon and the amount of experience with the chosen technique. Hand-sewn anastomoses are frequently constructed in two layers, but single-layer methods are equally efficacious. *Bucket-handle* is used to describe injuries to the bowel mesentery, which can be of variable size and lead to devascularization of the small intestine. The decision to resect the small bowel should be made based on the size of the mesenteric defect and/or appearance of the affected intestine. Even in the setting of small (<5-cm) defects, a resection should be performed if there is any evidence of malperfusion.

Damage control for small bowel injuries includes rapid closure of perforations to control contamination with resection when large injuries are present. Patients in shock may benefit from resection without immediate anastomosis because of a higher risk of anastomotic dehiscence and the need for an abbreviated operation. The abdomen is temporarily closed, and the patient is resuscitated to correct physiologic derangements. After resuscitation, intestinal continuity can be reestablished on return to the OR.

Colon and Rectal Injuries

Colon and rectal injuries occur most commonly after penetrating abdominal trauma and rarely after blunt mechanisms. Similar to other hollow visceral injuries, trauma to the colon and rectum takes place in only 0.3% of bluntly injured patients, the majority being hematomas and serosal tears.[215] Historical data reveal a 22% to 35% mortality rate during World War II, at which time colostomy creation for colon trauma was mandatory. Contemporary reports of mortality related to colon injury are as low as 1%.[218] In the literature, colonic trauma is commonly classified as either *destructive* or *nondestructive*. Destructive injury in penetrating trauma is defined by wounds more than 50% of the colonic circumference, complete transection, and the presence of devascularized segments. In blunt injury, serosal tears more than 50% colon circumference, full-thickness perforation, and mesenteric devascularization are considered destructive. These pathologies in blunt trauma are produced by direct crush or rupture when the rate of compression results in a rapid elevation in intraluminal pressure. Importantly, depending on the involved colonic segment, colon injury with perforation can occur into the retroperitoneum. Most commonly seen in the retroperitoneal portions, shearing forces can cause a separation of the serosa or muscularis from the underlying mucosa over a long segment. The results of this injury mechanism are evident in Fig. 36.35. In addition to GSWs, injury to the rectum may also occur when severe pelvic fractures with sharp bone fragments cause a laceration.

From an examination standpoint, patients may present with a wide range of physiology. Peritonitis may be present on exam in the setting of free perforation, yet the retroperitoneal location of the right and left colon may obscure this finding. Furthermore, colonic injuries may first be identified at the time of laparotomy prompted by hemodynamic instability or a suggestive penetrating mechanism. For the physiologically stable patient, the evaluation of the colon is similar to that of previously described hollow viscus injury. Abdominal CT is limited in capability, although it may demonstrate colonic wall thickening with surrounding stranding or fluid. Imaging may identify the track of a penetrating mechanism, allowing the surgeon to assess proximity to the colon. Finally, care must be taken to adequately assess the segments of the colon that are retroperitoneal in location. This has led some authors to advocate

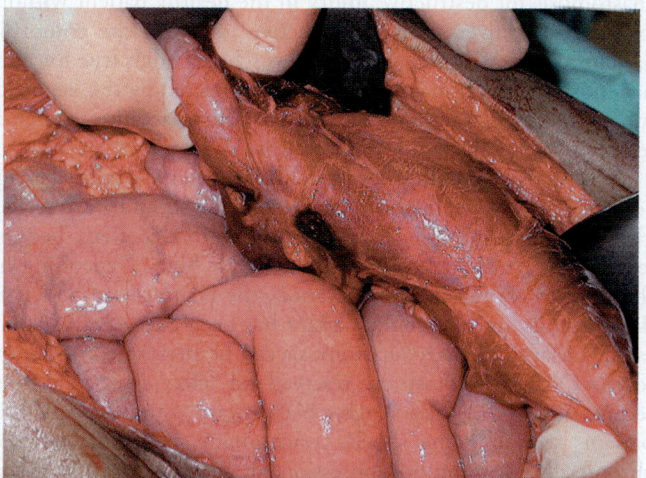

FIGURE 36.35 Blunt left-sided colon injury at the time of laparotomy. The injury mechanism resulted in a deserosalizing-type injury that involved a segment of colon several centimeters long.

for routine utility of enteral contrast ("triple contrast": oral, rectal, and IV) to increase CT diagnostic yield in identification of operative injuries after penetrating trauma. Others contend equivalent results without these adjunctive measures, leading recent guidelines to allow for attending surgical discretion.[206]

Evaluation of the rectum may require a slightly different approach. Although the absence of blood identified on digital rectal examination may be adequate to rule out injury, its presence does not confirm it. Nonetheless, positive digital rectal examination for gross blood or a penetrating pelvic trajectory requires further evaluation with imaging. Should the CT be negative for injury, clinically relevant trauma is much less likely. However, if the imaging results are indeterminate or there is clinical concern, an exam under anesthesia with rigid proctosigmoidoscopy can be valuable in providing visualization of the rectum and distal sigmoid colon. Findings on endoscopy may include a mucosal injury to the rectum, hematoma in the rectal wall, or a large amount of blood in the rectal vault. Characterization of the injury (destructive rectal [>25% circumference] vs. nondestructive) and location relative to the peritoneum will be valuable for planning surgical management. Upper rectal injuries, especially those on the anterior or lateral surfaces, may be first identified during visualization of the pelvic structures at the time of laparotomy.

The approach to operative repair depends on the presence or absence of destructive injury and the overall physiology of the patient. Historically, the approach to all colon injuries included resection with the creation of a colostomy because of fear of anastomotic dehiscence and intraabdominal sepsis. Subsequent experience questioned the need for mandatory proximal fecal diversion to manage colonic perforations. Stone and Fabian first prospectively described primary repair of colon injury versus colostomy creation in 1979, observing a lower incidence of intraabdominal infection with primary repair. Since that time, extensive investigation from Memphis has led to conceptually divergent management of colon injuries based on the identification of a destructive injury. Destructive wounds in the face of significant resuscitation (>6 units PRBCs) and medical comorbidity were noted to experience anastomotic leak at 42% versus 3% in otherwise healthy, minimally transfused patients after resection. This led to the development of surgical stratification for optimal outcomes in operative colon injury, recommending primary repair (one or two layers) in all nondestructive injuries, resection, and anastomosis for destructive injury in the healthy patient without extremis and diversion for destructive injury in the comorbid patient requiring resuscitation.[218] This schema holds true for both penetrating and blunt injury and is not affected by the degree of intraabdominal contamination. Distal injuries require segmental resection with colocolonic anastomosis.

Destructive colon injuries that are encountered during damage control laparotomy in the unstable patient should be resected. Historically, an anastomosis was avoided in these patients because leak rates were thought to be prohibitively high. Depending on the need to abbreviate the operation, the GI tract can be left in discontinuity until after the patient has been adequately resuscitated. Delayed primary anastomosis can be performed on return to the OR, with colostomy reserved for select cases. The most recent WTA guidelines suggest bias toward ostomy creation in patients with ongoing shock, concomitant abdominal injuries, chronic illness, immunosuppression, or inability to close fascia. The 2019 EAST guidelines, however, recommend primary anastomosis even in the setting of damage control laparotomy.[219] A question that remains unanswered is whether a diverting loop ileostomy after colonic anastomosis would serve the same function in this population as it has in other inflammatory states.

Extraperitoneal rectal injuries that result in perforation can cause significant contamination, leading to pelvic sepsis. For this reason, operative management is often required. Destructive rectal injuries (>25% circumference) are predominantly managed with fecal diversion (loop ileostomy or colostomy) and consideration of presacral drainage until healing has occurred. Routine presacral drainage is not advised because it adds significant morbidity to the procedure. More recent evidence suggests that extraperitoneal rectal injuries may be managed without drainage and with diversion alone.[218] A rectal contrast enema as early as 6 weeks after injury will serve to define wound resolution with subsequent ostomy reversal. If a rectal injury is visualized at laparotomy, management should convert to treatment of intraperitoneal colon trauma.

Abdominal Great Vessel Injuries

The major blood vessels of the abdomen are predominantly located within the retroperitoneum, with some larger vessels also in the intestinal mesenteries. Because of massive associated blood loss, visualization of the vessels can be compromised, making management of these injuries challenging. Most commonly, major abdominal vascular injuries are secondary to penetrating mechanisms. In the setting of blunt trauma, hematomas within the retroperitoneum are often secondary to pelvic fractures with bleeding from pelvic blood vessels that dissect superiorly.

Abdominal vascular injuries are often first recognized at the time of laparotomy being performed for penetrating abdominal trauma. These injuries are frequently associated with significant ongoing blood loss and hemodynamic instability. The specific vascular injury is better delineated after exploration and exposure of the retroperitoneal structures. Penetrating injuries to the back in hemodynamically stable individuals frequently benefit from three-dimensional imaging, given that most do not enter the peritoneal cavity. CT is often used to identify the path of the injury and therefore suggest possible involvement of adjacent structures. Similarly, evaluation of the abdominal vasculature after blunt trauma is best achieved with contrast-enhanced CT if the individual's hemodynamics allow.

During laparotomy, the location of retroperitoneal hematoma guides surgical decision-making. As seen in Fig. 36.36, the retroperitoneum can conceptually be divided into three zones. For both blunt and penetrating injuries, zone 1 hematomas require exploration because these frequently involve the aorta, proximal visceral vessels, or inferior vena cava. A hematoma in the region of zone 2, which predominantly contains the kidneys, should be explored for penetrating injury and only if it appears that the hematoma is expanding for blunt injury. Finally, a hematoma in zone 3 should be explored in penetrating injury but can be left alone for blunt injury because it is usually secondary to pelvic fracture bleeding and should not be explored unless exsanguinating hemorrhage is obvious.

Although the details of repairs for retroperitoneal vascular injury are discussed elsewhere, knowledge of the basic exposure of these structures is important. Hematomas of the infrarenal vasculature or the right renal hilum are exposed with a right medial visceral mobilization, also known as the *Cattell-Braasch maneuver*. A wide Kocher maneuver is performed, and the peritoneal dissection is continued inferiorly to mobilize the right colon. The dissection continues around the cecum and superiorly up the mesenteric root. Retraction of the abdominal viscera superior and to the left will expose the

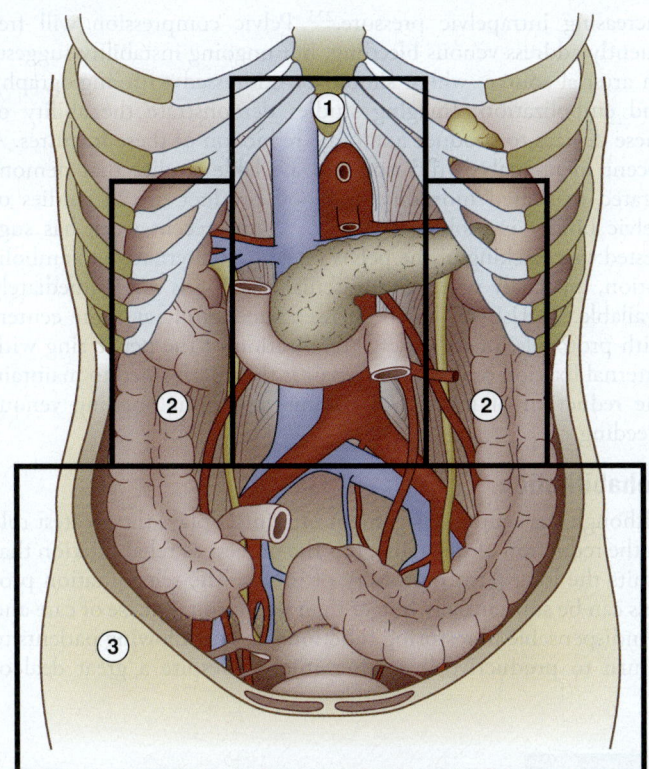

FIGURE 36.36 Zones of the retroperitoneum visualized at the time of laparotomy. *Zone 1* includes the central vascular structures, such as the aorta and vena cava. *Zone 2* includes the kidneys and adjacent adrenal glands. *Zone 3* describes the retroperitoneum associated with the pelvic vasculature.

lower midline vascular structures (right colon should eviscerate to lay upon the chest). Basic tenets of vascular repair, including proximal and distal control of the injured vessel, are achieved when possible. Injuries to the suprarenal great vessels or the left renal hilum are exposed by performing a left medial visceral mobilization (the Mattox maneuver). This is achieved by dividing the peritoneum along the entire left side of the abdomen, from above the spleen down to the distal left colon. The plane posterior to the colonic mesentery and the pancreas is developed, and the abdominal viscera are retracted to the right to expose the superior retroperitoneal vasculature. Although penetrating injuries almost always mandate exploration and repair, blunt abdominal vascular injuries in hemodynamically stable individuals may be considered for endovascular therapy, depending on the nature of the injury. See Chapter 38 for additional context on vascular trauma.

Genitourinary Injuries

The genitourinary organs include the kidneys, ureters, bladder, and urethra, all of which are contained within the retroperitoneum. Bleeding and extravasation of urine are the major concerns with injuries to these structures. Blunt mechanisms can result in renal laceration or bladder rupture, which can occur into the peritoneal space or the soft tissue of the pelvis. The typical mechanism for bladder injuries is the transmission of significant energy to the urine-filled bladder, resulting in wall rupture. This is almost universally associated with some amount of pelvic fracture. All genitourinary structures are vulnerable to penetrating mechanisms, many of which cause urine extravasation. See Chapter 39 for additional details on management of genitourinary trauma.

Injuries to the Pelvis and Extremities

Most injuries sustained by trauma patients involve the musculoskeletal system. Orthopedic injuries constituted the greatest number of cases in the 2016 NTDB report, with 31.66% of patients having upper extremity and 40.09% having lower extremity trauma. Although the mortality is low for each group (approximately 4%–5%), the long-term morbidity and functional implications can be significant.[159] Various physical mechanisms are responsible for orthopedic injuries, with falls and motor vehicle crashes being the most common causes. See Chapter 40 for additional details on management.

Fractures can be associated with soft tissue injury that can be closed or open. Morel-Lavallee lesions result from closed degloving tissue injury that shears skin and subcutaneous fat from the underlying muscular fascia. Hemorrhage and fluid sequestration can lead to early and late wound complications. Fig. 36.37 shows the evolution of skin changes in the leg of a patient involved in a pedestrian–motor vehicle crash and the subsequent result after debridement of the nonviable tissue completely disconnected from the underlying fascia. Tissue necrosis and infection are potential sequelae. Compression, drainage, and debridement are strategies used to treat and/or prevent complications from this injury. Open fractures require the administration of appropriate antibiotics and tetanus prophylaxis. Early washout is also recommended.

Clinical evidence of vascular injury requires further evaluation, either via imaging or direct exploration. CTA has replaced conventional angiography for the initial evaluation of peripheral vascular injury. However, conventional angiography may be

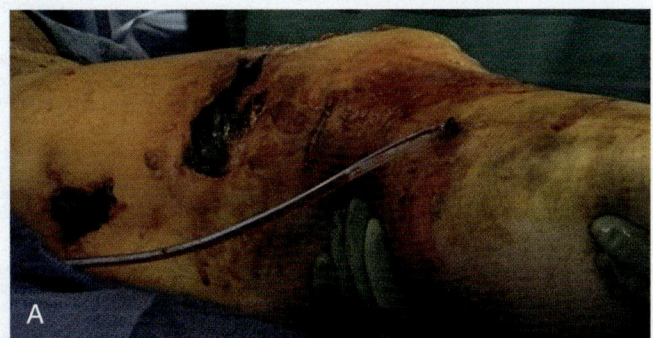

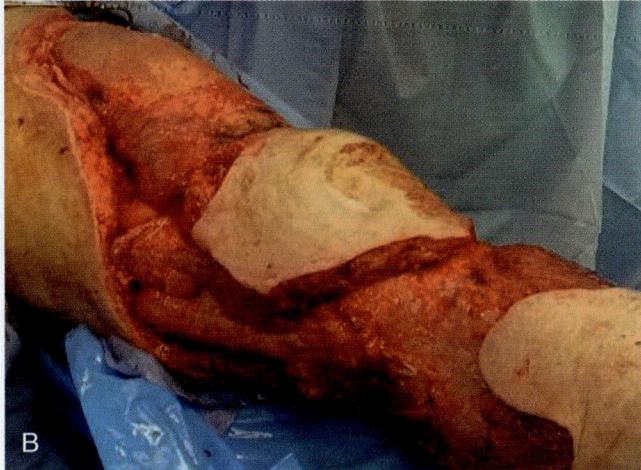

FIGURE 36.37 (A) Appearance of a lower extremity wound with a Morel-Lavallee injury after attempted drainage and compression. Note the areas of skin necrosis. (B) Appearance of the leg after operative debridement. Nonviable tissue has been removed.

indicated if an injury is identified.[220] Damage control principles may be required to manage fractures in multisystem-injured patients, especially those with moderate or severe TBI.

Bleeding from complex pelvic fractures presents a unique challenge. A multidisciplinary approach to management is required, involving trauma surgery, orthopedic surgery, and a team with endovascular capabilities, either vascular surgery or interventional radiology.[221] These injuries result from serious mechanisms, including motor vehicle crashes, motorcycle crashes, pedestrians struck by vehicles, and falls from heights. Mortality can reach over 50% in patients who present with shock.[222] As depicted in Fig. 36.38, hemodynamically unstable patients should have a prompt pelvic radiograph for fracture evaluation. Although some fracture patterns are associated with a higher risk of hemodynamically significant bleeding, it is important to note that any fracture is capable of bleeding and should be addressed in unstable patients.

Pelvic fractures that demonstrate an increase in pelvic volume, so-called open-book fractures, should be compressed with a commercial pelvic binder or sheet applied at the level of the greater trochanters to reduce the space available for hematoma formation. These immobilizing devices are typically placed prehospital but can be placed in the ED as well. The lower extremities should also be bound together to aid in decreasing the pelvic volume and increasing intrapelvic pressure.[223] Pelvic compression will frequently address venous bleeding, but ongoing instability suggests an arterial source, which should be addressed with angiography and embolization. Imaging studies demonstrate the ability of these devices to produce anatomic reduction of these fractures. A recent meta-analysis did not find available studies that demonstrated decreased mortality or blood product use in studies of pelvic binder immobilization.[224,225] Some recent work has suggested that packing of the pelvis may be an alternative to embolization, especially when endovascular therapy is not immediately available.[226] REBOA has been used successfully at some centers with protocols for its use.[227] Stabilization of the pelvic ring with external fixation or definitive repair is then performed to maintain the reduction of the pelvic volume and limit ongoing venous bleeding.

Rehabilitation

Although the acute management of injuries plays the greatest role in the reduction of mortality, it is the process of rehabilitation that limits the long-term morbidity of injury. The rehabilitation process can be substantially longer than the hospital phase of care and is indispensable in restoring functionality and allowing patients to return to productive lives after injury. Despite a great deal of

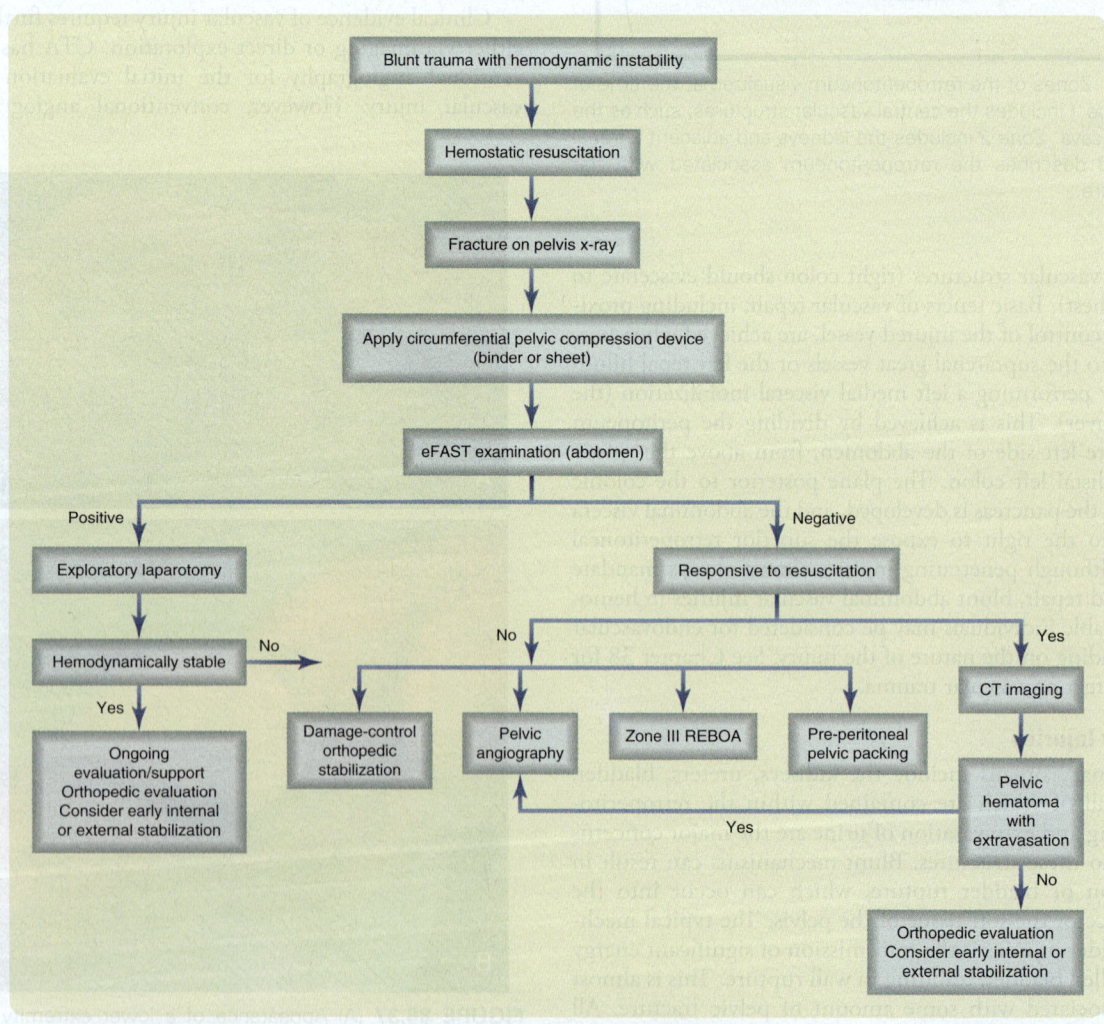

FIGURE 36.38 Pelvic fracture management algorithm. Algorithm for the evaluation and management of pelvic fractures with associated hemorrhage. *CT,* Computed tomography; *FAST,* focused abdominal sonography in trauma; *REBOA,* retrograde balloon occlusion of the aorta.

emphasis being placed on trauma-related fatalities, there were approximately 31 million nonfatal injuries in 2013, many of which required rehabilitative services.

The rehabilitation process begins immediately after the acute needs of the injured patient have been met. Early mobilization is extremely important to circumvent deconditioning. Physical and occupational therapists frequently begin the process by initiating therapy and determining what resources may be required when the patient leaves the hospital. With these recommendations available, case managers and social workers can begin identifying the inpatient or outpatient resources required to address the unique rehabilitation needs of the patient. Early engagement by the rehabilitation team can expedite referrals and transfer to appropriate facilities. Select populations of patients may benefit from rehabilitation centers that focus on the recovery from specific conditions, such as TBIs and SCIs. These two patient cohorts have specific needs that are best addressed at centers with specialized expertise. Health systems committed to trauma care must place a high priority on supporting the rehabilitation process, given that this is one of the most important aspects of a patient's long-term recovery.

SELECTED REFERENCES

Guyette FX, Brown JB, Zenati MS, et al. Tranexamic acid during prehospital transport in patients at risk for hemorrhage after injury: a double-blind, placebo-controlled, randomized clinical trial. *JAMA Surg.* 2021;156(1):11-20.

In this pragmatic, phase III, multicenter, double-blind, placebo-controlled, superiority randomized clinical trial of injured patients at risk for hemorrhage, TXA administered before hospitalization did not result in significantly lower 30-day mortality but also did not increase rates of thromboembolism.

Jansen JO, Hudson J, Cochran C, et al. Emergency department resuscitative endovascular balloon occlusion of the aorta in trauma patients with exsanguinating hemorrhage: the UK-REBOA randomized clinical trial. *JAMA.* 2023;330(19):1862-1871.

This pragmatic, Bayesian, randomized clinical trial of trauma patients with exsanguinating hemorrhage in UK emergency departments compared a strategy of REBOA and standard care to standard of care alone. REBOA with standard of care did not reduce, and may increase, mortality compared with standard care alone.

Meyer DE, Harvin JA, Vincent L, et al. Randomized controlled trial of surgical rib fixation to nonoperative management in severe chest wall injury. *Ann Surg.* 2023;278(3):357-365.

This single-center randomized controlled trial compared surgical rib fixation to nonoperative management in severe chest wall injury. Rib fixation increased hospital length of stay (primary outcome) and did not provide any quality of life benefit for up to 6 months.

Moore HB, Moore EE, Chapman MP, et al. Plasma-first resuscitation to treat haemorrhagic shock during emergency ground transportation in an urban area: a randomised trial. *Lancet.* 2018;392:283-291.

This pragmatic, single-center randomized clinical trial showed that during rapid ground transport of trauma patients in hemorrhagic shock, the use of prehospital plasma was not associated with survival benefit.

Prekker ME, Driver BE, Trent SA, et al. Video versus direct laryngoscopy for tracheal intubation of critically Ill adults. *N Engl J Med.* 2023;389(5):418-429.

This multicenter, randomized trial of critically ill adults undergoing tracheal intubation involved assignment to a video-laryngoscope intervention or a direct-laryngoscope intervention. The trial was stopped for efficacy because the use of a video laryngoscope resulted in a higher incidence of successful intubation on the first attempt.

Sperry JL, Guyette FX, Brown JB, et al. Prehospital plasma during air medical transport in trauma patients at risk for hemorrhagic shock. *N Engl J Med.* 2018;379(4):315-326.

This pragmatic, multicenter, cluster-randomized, phase III superiority trial compared the administration of thawed plasma with standard-care resuscitation during air medical transport of patients at risk for hemorrhagic shock. This trial showed that the prehospital administration of plasma was safe and resulted in lower 30-day mortality.

The full reference list appears on Elsevier eBooks+.

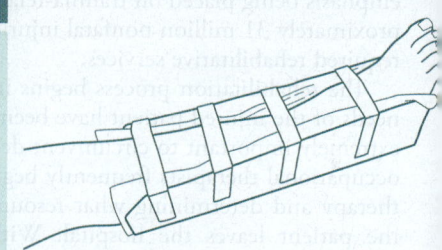

37 CHAPTER

The Difficult Abdominal Wall

Whitney R. Jenson, Oliver L. Gunter, and Clay Cothren Burlew

▶ **Please access Elsevier eBooks+ to view the video for this chapter**.

In damage control laparotomies for trauma, vascular surgery, and/or emergency general surgery, primary fascial closure can ultimately be achieved in 60% to 90% of the cases. Patients for whom the abdomen cannot be closed at initial laparotomy comprise the category of those with a difficult abdominal wall. The causes of the difficult abdominal wall share common features: loss of abdominal domain, risk of the development of intraabdominal hypertension (IAH) and/or abdominal compartment syndrome (ACS), potential infectious complications or enterocutaneous fistula (ECF), systemic inflammatory response syndrome, and a higher than 50% risk of hernia formation. When temporary coverage of the abdomen is necessary, the technique should be easy to apply, tension free, atraumatic, inexpensive, and should ultimately facilitate delayed primary fascial closure. The goal of this chapter is to illustrate techniques of both temporary and final closure, as well as perioperative considerations, of the difficult abdominal wall.

MAJOR ETIOLOGIES OF THE DIFFICULT ABDOMINAL WALL

Damage Control Surgery

Damage control surgery (DCS) developed in the 1970s to 1990s as the surgical community recognized that definitive surgical intervention became futile once the patient developed irreversible metabolic failure. This physiologic dysfunction, also known as the *lethal triad*,

is characterized by hypothermia, acidosis, and coagulopathy. A reduction in mortality and morbidity was seen by abbreviating the laparotomy, performing only necessary surgical intervention (halt hemorrhage, control succus, and restore vascular continuity with shunts if required) followed by resuscitation and correction of physiologic derangements in the intensive care unit (ICU). Definitive surgical intervention (e.g., restoring bowel continuity, placement of vascular grafts) was delayed to a second laparotomy. With the recognition that DCS improves outcomes in severely injured patients, the practice was expanded to include critically ill patients with intraabdominal sepsis and nontraumatic hemorrhage.

The basic tenets of DCS include hemorrhage control, reestablishing vascular continuity if necessary via shunting, control of contamination from gastrointestinal sources, and temporary abdominal closure (TAC); this operation is followed by correction of physiologic derangements in the ICU.[1] Hemorrhage control is achieved by ligation or repair of bleeding vessels, resection of nonsalvageable organs (e.g., splenectomy, nephrectomy), and the use of intraabdominal or preperitoneal packing. Once bleeding has been controlled, attention is turned to management of gastrointestinal contamination. This is accomplished by primary repair of hollow viscus perforations or, if primary repair is not a feasible option, resection of the injured, perforated, or ischemic segment of bowel. The bowel is left in discontinuity to allow for rapid completion of the operation. The abdomen should be irrigated to limit ongoing contamination. Options for TAC and the ICU care of the patient with an open abdomen will be addressed later in this chapter.

A period of overutilization of DCS resulted in unnecessary complications for patients who were appropriate for definitive

---

BOX 37.1 Indications for Damage Control Surgery

Traumatic and Nontraumatic Hemorrhage
- Systolic blood pressure <90 mm Hg
- Hypothermia <34°C
- Acidosis: pH <7.2 or lactate >4 mmol/L
- INR, PTT, or PT >1.5 time normal
- Clinically observed coagulopathy
- >10 units PRBCs transfused during the preoperative or intraoperative period
- Need for intraabdominal packing
- Time required for surgery >90 minutes
- Estimated blood loss >4 L

Emergency General Surgery
- Preoperative severe sepsis/septic shock
- Lactate ≥3 mmol/L
- pH ≤7.25
- ≥70 years of age
- Male sex
- Multiple comorbidities

INR, International normalized ratio; *PT,* prothrombin time; *PTT,* partial thromboplastin time; *PRBCs,* packed red blood cells.

BOX 37.2 World Society of Abdominal Compartment Syndrome Consensus Definitions

Intraabdominal Hypertension
- Grade I: IAP 12–15 mm Hg
- Grade II: IAP 16–20 mm Hg
- Grade III: IAP 21–25 mm Hg
- Grade IV: IAP >25 mm Hg

Abdominal Compartment Syndrome
- Sustained IAP >20 mm Hg (with or without APP <60 mm Hg) that is associated with new-onset organ dysfunction or failure

APP, Abdominal perfusion pressure; *IAP,* intraabdominal pressure.

---

management at the index operation. Several studies have helped define the indications for DCS in both trauma and emergency general surgery (Box 37.1).[2,3] In general, DCS should be considered in patients who are more likely to succumb to the physiologic effects of shock than the inability to perform a definitive operation. Although patients who are treated with DCS have a significant reduction in the observed to expected mortality rate, they have more complications than those who undergo definitive management at the initial laparotomy.[4] These complications include difficult abdominal wall closure, surgical site infections (SSIs), intraabdominal abscesses, enteroatmospheric fistulas (EAFs), and ventral hernias. Faster time to fascial closure has been shown to reduce the rates of complications associated with the open abdomen.[4,5]

Abdominal Compartment Syndrome

ACS is the pathologic end point of the spectrum of IAH. It is defined as a sustained intraabdominal pressure (IAP) >20 mm Hg with accompanying new-onset organ dysfunction or failure (Box 37.2).[6] IAH impedes venous return resulting in decreased preload and cardiac output. Clinically, ACS manifests as abdominal distention with hypotension, increased airway pressures with resultant hypoventilation and shunting, and renal failure with decreased urine output. Although the rates of postinjury ACS are declining, primarily due to advances in damage control resuscitation, IAH remains a significant source of morbidity and mortality among critically ill and injured patients.

IAH and ACS occur when the intraabdominal contents exceed the compliance of the abdominal wall and diaphragm resulting in a rapid increase in IAP. Iatrogenic and pathologic processes that increase intraabdominal volume and decrease abdominal wall compliance place the patient at risk for developing ACS. These include intraabdominal packing, visceral and retroperitoneal edema (e.g., acute pancreatitis, large-volume resuscitation), hematoma, ascites, severe ileus, severe burns with >60% total body surface area (TBSA) involvement, or abdominal wall reconstruction for hernias with significant loss of domain. Many of the indications for DCS are also risk factors for ACS; therefore, patients who receive >10 units of packed red blood cells (PRBCs) or >15 L of crystalloid resuscitation likely should be managed with an open abdomen if an exploratory laparotomy is performed.[7]

In critically ill patients who are at risk for ACS, bladder pressure should be measured every 4 hours to monitor for IAH. Bladder pressures should be measured when the abdominal wall muscles are relaxed and at the end-expiratory phase of respiration. If the patient is agitated or dyspneic, sedation or chemical paralysis may be required to obtain an accurate bladder pressure. It is important to note that the bladder pressure may not be reliable with certain disease processes (e.g., bladder hematoma, severe pelvic fracture with retroperitoneal hematoma, preperitoneal packing for hemorrhage, prior bladder surgery). Once the patient has had a bladder pressure <12 mm Hg for several hours and is improving clinically, serial IAP measurements can be stopped.

The World Society of Abdominal Compartment Syndrome recommends initiating nonoperative management of IAH once the IAP is 12 mm Hg or higher (grade I IAH) with the goal of maintaining IAP ≤15 mm Hg.[6] Evacuation of intraluminal contents has a theoretical benefit for reducing IAP; however, there are no prospective trials that have investigated the impact of these maneuvers. Options for removal of intestinal contents include nasogastric tube suction, rectal tube placement, enemas, or colonoscopic decompression. Elimination of abdominal space-occupying lesions such as ascites or excessive intraabdominal packs left during DCS may also decrease IAP. Paracentesis or placement of an intraabdominal catheter with evacuation of >1 L of ascites has been shown to significantly decrease IAP; however, drainage of <1 L of ascites or a decrease in IAP of <9 mm Hg in the first 4 hours is predictive of failure of this nonoperative intervention.[6,8,9] Efforts to improve abdominal wall compliance may reduce IAP. Options to improve compliance include administration of adequate analgesia and sedation, removal of constrictive dressings, escharotomies, and neuromuscular blockade. Though neuromuscular blockade will decrease IAP, this is a temporary effect, and it should only be used to temporize the patient until a more definitive procedure, such as drainage of large-volume ascites or decompressive laparotomy, can be performed. Optimizing fluid balance is also imperative to the prevention of ACS and nonoperative treatment of IAH. This may be achieved by avoiding excessive crystalloid resuscitation, diuresis once the patient is hemodynamically stable, or even hemodialysis or ultrafiltration. There is evidence to support the benefit of fluid removal with diuresis or ultrafiltration after resuscitation; however, the benefit is less well defined than the benefits of primarily preventing volume overload. If nonoperative management for IAH fails and the patient develops end-organ dysfunction defining ACS, the patient should undergo decompressive laparotomy with TAC. One must remain vigilant even after a decompressive laparotomy is performed as up to 20% of patients may develop recurrent ACS despite an open abdomen.

Mesh Failure

The use of synthetic prosthetic mesh is well established as the surgical treatment of choice for repair of ventral incisional hernias and, in most cases, can provide a long-lasting repair with low recurrence rates. The development of synthetic mesh material was a major advancement in hernia surgery, and its advantages include decreased recurrence rates, ease of use, and a low cost compared with biologic mesh. This has resulted in synthetic mesh being the most used prosthetic for reinforcement for initial incisional and recurrent hernia repairs. Although the application of synthetic mesh has resulted in a significant improvement in failure and recurrence rates, the use of these mesh materials may result in specific complications that range from minor to potentially life-threatening. Synthetic mesh may variably become infected dependent on the degree of contamination of the wound and the nature of the prosthetic material used.

Infections should be eradicated before considering any major repair, and measures should be taken to heal open wounds, as the bacterial colonization may be significant even in the absence of a frank infection. In the case of mesh infection, this often requires removal of the infected mesh material or anchoring sutures, drainage of any abscesses, and debridement of the wound. Lighter-weight, macroporous meshes carry a lower risk of infection compared with the heavier microporous meshes such as extended polytetrafluoroethylene (ePTFE).[10] Any mesh that is not incorporated should be excised completely from the edge of the wound to healthy tissues. If the wound has a large amount of contamination, requires major debridement, or necessitates a bowel resection or ECF takedown, a multistage approach may be required to achieve a clean wound before definitive abdominal wall reconstruction is entertained. Challenges to hernia repair in an infected field are multiple.

When there is insufficient autologous tissue for layered closure, often the case after emergent surgery in the setting of peritonitis, the surgeon is then faced with several challenges that must be addressed in a prioritized fashion. After the infection is eradicated, bowel resection performed, and necrotic tissue debrided, the visceral contents must then be contained. In this scenario, it is generally not advisable to create large skin flaps or perform myofascial component separations during this acute phase of management. After source control and treatment of infections, preparation of the wound for definitive repair should not interfere with possible reconstruction options in the future. Tissue repair during this period is an anabolic process, and malnourished or actively catabolic patients have impaired healing. Additionally, the open abdomen creates an environment that is conducive to the development of ECFs and can represent a significant source of protein calorie malnutrition.

It may be necessary to rely on TAC and fascial bridging techniques to develop a clean wound for later definitive repair. Determining the proper way to deal with this residual defect is still a source of controversy. Negative-pressure devices have been used to help in this situation, first to eradicate all infection and then to cover a biologic mesh bridged repair (Fig. 37.1).

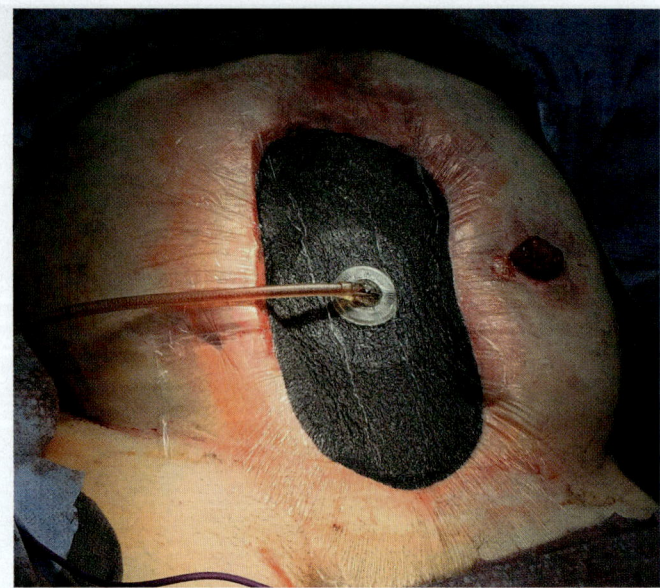

FIGURE 37.1 Negative-pressure wound therapy over a bridged repair.

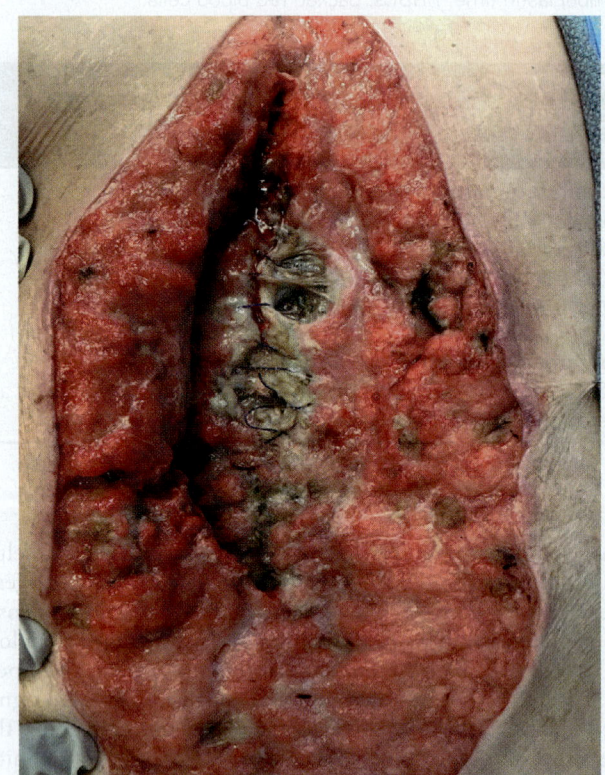

FIGURE 37.2 Fascial dehiscence.

Abdominal Fascial Dehiscence

The incidence of fascial dehiscence has been reported in the literature to be between 3% and 3.5% after major abdominal surgery and is associated with significant morbidity and mortality. Acute fascial dehiscence may be heralded by increased serosanguinous drainage from the laparotomy wound and often can be confirmed on physical exam, especially after wound opening (Fig. 37.2). Patient risk factors and disease/surgical risk factors for abdominal

BOX 37.3   Patient Risk Factors for Abdominal Wall Suture Complications

- Age >70
- Obesity
- Cigarette use/chronic obstructive pulmonary disease
- Steroid use
- Diabetes mellitus
- Malnutrition
- Ascites
- Previous laparotomies

BOX 37.4   Disease: Surgical Risk Factors for Abdominal Wall Suture Complications

- Abdominal trauma
- Ruptured abdominal aortic aneurysm
- Retroperitoneal hematoma
- Pancreatitis
- Peritonitis/sepsis
- Bowel occlusion surgery with resection or suture
- Wound infection
- Wound class III (contaminated) or class IV (dirty)
- Presence of enterocutaneous fistula
- Synthetic mesh infection
- Necrotizing fasciitis
- Abdominal wall defect >10 cm in width

wall suture complications are illustrated in Boxes 37.3 and 37.4. Several different multifactor scoring systems predictive of abdominal wall suture complications have been described in the literature, including the Veterans Affairs Medical Center score and the Rotterdam score.[11]

Surgical management of acute dehiscence is based on the underlying cause, with SSI and intraabdominal abscess being the most common.[12] The technical causes of acute fascial dehiscence are knot or suture material failure and fascial damage related to tension or ischemia. The usual time frame for fascial dehiscence is within the first 7 days after primary closure, although the risk of fascial dehiscence may persist beyond 3 weeks postoperatively.

The decision to proceed with immediate reoperation versus local drainage and wound care depends on the etiology, the extent of the dehiscence, and the accessibility of the peritoneal cavity. In the setting of acute postoperative wound complication such as seroma, fascial integrity must be examined, even if this requires further opening of the wound and removal of wound adjuncts (incisional wound vac, dressings, etc.). In the immediate postoperative period, urgent return to the operating room should be considered default treatment to minimize treatment delay and to avoid further complications such as evisceration or bowel injury. Identification of the etiology of dehiscence is critical to prevent recurrence and to help define options for surgical management. Etiology is usually determined intraoperatively, although in select cases, cross-sectional imaging may be useful, especially in the setting of delayed dehiscence.

If the abdominal viscera are contained and/or the degree of postoperative peritoneal sclerosis precludes safe reentry to the abdominal cavity, local wound care can be employed with care to prevent desiccation of bowel, which could lead to development of perforation and ECF, a dreaded complication of fascial dehiscence. The wound should then be managed as a planned ventral

incisional hernia, with reconstruction in a delayed fashion once the acute physiologic process has dissipated.

TEMPORARY ABDOMINAL CLOSURE

Techniques in DCS have become standard adjuncts in trauma, general surgery, and subspecialty surgical procedures. With up to 36% of patients undergoing an emergent laparotomy requiring a damage control procedure during the index operation, and thus requiring a method of TAC, this is an important tool in any surgeon's repertoire.[13] Indications for TAC are shown in Box 37.5, and current options for TACs are illustrated in Table 37.1.

TAC techniques should (1) minimize damage to the abdominal contents; (2) minimize adherence of the viscera to the anterior abdominal wall; (3) prevent fascial retraction; (4) maintain a viable, minimally traumatized fascial midline edge for suturing; and (5) ultimately promote reduction of visceral contents. Current options for TAC include a tension-free, atraumatic abdominal visceral coverage using the vacuum-pack technique popularized by Barker and colleagues,[14] or simple modifications of this technique (Fig. 37.3A). This TAC option is best used at the initial operation, permits inspection of the viscera, and is compatible with the use of direct peritoneal resuscitation (DPR; Fig. 37.3B). Another option for TAC at the index operation is a negative-pressure wound therapy (NPWT) vacuum system (VAC or AbThera, 3M, Beirut, Lebanon). In either of these techniques, placement of a plastic barrier such as a fenestrated 1010 drape or the AbThera drape prevents the abdominal viscera from adhering to the undersurface of the abdominal wall (Fig. 37.3C). This, in turn, permits sliding of the abdominal wall forward over the viscera at the second laparotomy during attempts at fascial closure. The goal of preventing fascial retraction should happen at the second laparotomy if the abdomen cannot be primarily closed. Options used to keep the fascia under tension and closer to midline include sutures (over NPWT sponges to prevent bowel injury), synthetic mesh (Fig. 37.3D), and silicone elastomers (TAWT, StarSurgical, or ABRA System, Southmedic Inc., Almonte, Ontario, Canada). Each of these "fascial tension" options has variable impact on the fascia, which may impact future fascial viability for final closure.

NPWT has gained wide acceptance for its use in a variety of complex abdominal wall circumstances (Fig. 37.4). In a contaminated

BOX 37.5   Indications for Temporary Abdominal Closure

- Damage Control Surgery
  - Severe hemorrhage
  - Hypothermia <34°C
  - Acidosis: pH <7.2 or lactate >4 mmol/L
  - INR, PTT, or PT >1.5 time normal
  - Clinically observed coagulopathy
  - Need for intraabdominal packing
- Intraabdominal hypertension/impending abdominal compartment syndrome
- Visceral and/or retroperitoneal tissue edema
- Planned second look operation (questionable bowel viability)
- DPR for severe intraabdominal sepsis
- Triage purposes (transfer of patient to higher level of care, temporize patient until expertise available for more definitive surgery)

DPR, Direct peritoneal resuscitation; *INR,* International normalized ratio; *PT,* prothrombin time; *PTT,* partial thromboplastin time.

TABLE 37.1 **Current Techniques for Temporary Abdominal Closure**

TECHNIQUE	DESCRIPTION
Initial Laparotomy Closure	
Vacuum pack: (Barker vacuum pack or 1010 Ioban closure)	Perforated polyethylene sheet placed under the fascia, covering the viscera. Two surgical drains placed along the fascial edge over the sheet, covered with adhesive plastic drape. Drains placed to continuous suction.
Vacuum-assisted closure (VAC)	Perforated polyethylene sheet placed under the fascia, covering the viscera. Sponge placed over the drape up to the edges of the wound. Entire open wound plus adjacent abdominal wall skin covered with adhesive plastic drape. VAC suction via standard mechanism.
Negative-pressure wound therapy (AbThera)	Unique capsulated foam extension system incorporated into polyethylene sheet placed over abdominal viscera. Sponge placed over the drape up to the edges of the wound. Entire open wound plus adjacent abdominal wall skin covered with adhesive plastic drape. VAC suction via standard mechanism.
Repeat Laparotomy	
Sequential fascial closure	After the superior and inferior aspects of incisions of the fascia are closed primarily as possible, NPWT is placed over the viscera. Options to keep the fascia under tension toward midline include sutures, synthetic mesh, or silicone elastomers. These "fascial tension" options are placed over VAC sponges or the AbThera sponge. A second sponge is placed over the drape up to the edges of the wound. Entire open wound plus adjacent abdominal wall skin covered with adhesive plastic drape. VAC suction via standard mechanism.

NPWT, Negative-pressure wound therapy.

environment, NPWT techniques have been used to promote wound healing and minimize infectious complications. The use of NPWT for open abdomen management improves the primary closure rate, lowers mortality, and lowers the incidence of ECF formation.[15] Combining NPWT with suture techniques to prevent lateral fascial retraction (termed sequential fascial closure) has demonstrated delayed primary fascial closure rates of over 90% (Fig. 37.5A–D). This technique extends beyond the 8-day benchmark, with low complications rates in several series.[15–18]

Our five-stage management algorithm has helped minimize variability in patients with an open abdomen, with the goal to successfully close the abdominal fascia during stage 3 of this algorithm (Fig. 37.6). Staging of abdominal reconstruction serves several vital functions: ICU resuscitation and optimization, reduction of contamination and control of intraabdominal sepsis, debridement of devitalized or contaminated tissue, and allowance for decisions on subsequent reconstruction. The goal of delayed primary fascial closure (i.e., closure at subsequent laparotomy during the acute hospital stay) is to have the fascia closed as soon as possible, ideally within the first 8 days, to minimize complications related to the open abdomen. However, the risk for development of IAH and ACS from an ongoing inflammatory response, visceral edema, retraction of abdominal wall musculature/fascia (loss of domain), lack of source control, intraabdominal abscess, or ECF may complicate primary closure. In this setting, there should be ongoing attempts to close the fascia with sequential fascial closure techniques following the placement of abdominal drains or fecal diversion as needed (stage 4). Ultimately, the surgeon may have to accept a planned delayed abdominal wall reconstruction and use alternative means of visceral coverage (stage 5).

MANAGEMENT OF THE OPEN ABDOMEN AND ASSESSING READINESS FOR ABDOMINAL CLOSURE

Intensive Care Unit Optimization

In the ICU, the primary goal in the initial resuscitation of the patient with an open abdomen is correction of hypothermia, acidosis, and coagulopathy. This physiologic restoration can usually be accomplished within 24 to 36 hours. To correct hypothermia, the ambient temperature in the room is increased, convection blankets are applied to the patient, and the ventilator circuit is warmed. The goal is to raise the patient's core temperature to 37°C within 4 hours of arrival in the ICU.[8] Acidosis resolves as circulating blood volume is replenished and perfusion is restored. Massive transfusion protocols and minimizing crystalloid infusions during this period have been shown to improve rates of primary fascial closure at reoperation and to reduce rates of ACS.[8] If ongoing resuscitation is required, blood products are transfused in a 1:1:1 ratio of PRBCs:fresh frozen plasma (FFP):platelets until the results of thromboelastography (TEG) are available[19] and goal-directed treatment is initiated.

One of the most important goals for ICU care of the patient with an open abdomen is to avoid fluid overload. Hypervolemia results in significant visceral and retroperitoneal edema, and rates of fascial closure fall from 60% to 91% to 39%.[8] Multiple studies have aimed to identify methods to decrease visceral edema after resuscitation, thereby improving fascial closure rates. These studies have investigated the use of diuretics, colloid, and hypertonic saline. No significant benefit in fascial closure rates was seen with these systemically administered adjuncts.[2,20] DPR, however, has shown promise for improving fascial closure rates. Infusion of hypertonic glucose-based peritoneal dialysis fluid into the peritoneal cavity helps to correct several of the physiologic derangements that lead to organ dysfunction by improving visceral perfusion and reducing inflammatory mediators. Published reports of DPR have demonstrated more rapid and higher rates of fascial closure as well as reduced intraabdominal complications.[21]

Early enteral nutrition (EN) in the patient with an open abdomen should be strongly considered in all patients with a viable gastrointestinal tract that is in continuity. EN should be started once the resuscitation is complete, ideally within the first 24 to 48 hours. Multiple studies have shown the benefits of EN in increasing abdominal fascial closure rates, decreased complication rates, and decreasing mortality.[22]

Patients managed with open abdomens who are being resuscitated in the ICU remain mechanically ventilated until their

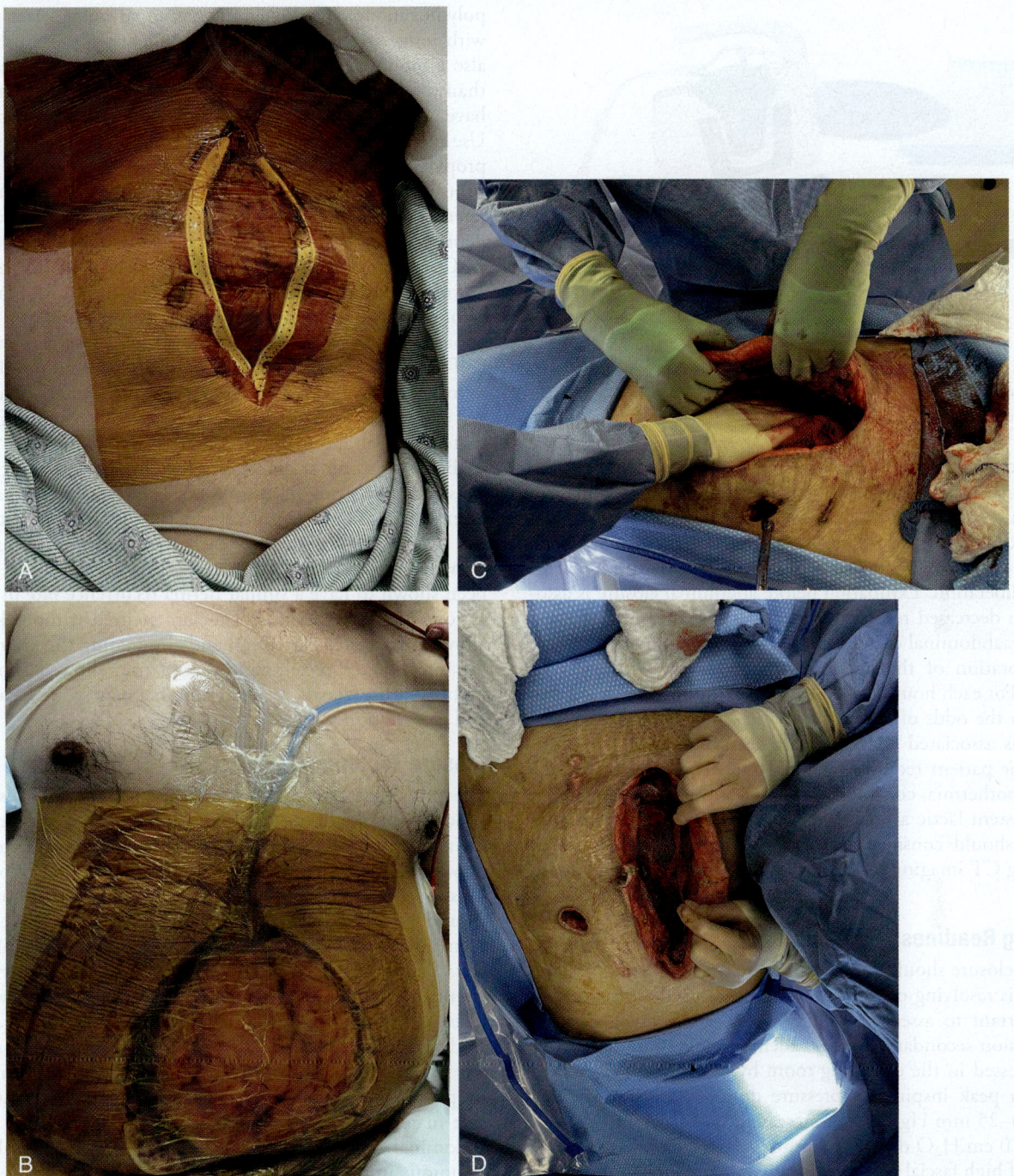

FIGURE 37.3 (A) Modified Barker vac-pack technique. This temporary closure uses a fenestrated drape over the viscera to separate them from the undersurface of the abdominal wall followed by placement of two Jackson-Pratt (JP) drains exiting cephalad; an occlusive loban covering is placed over the middle viscera and adjacent abdominal wall circumferentially. This closure is locally known as the "1010 (ten-ten) loban closure." (B) Using the 1010 loban closure, a 19-French round Blake drain can be placed under the occlusive loban directed into the pelvis to instill the peritoneal dialysate. The JP drains on the anterior surface of the viscera then evacuate this fluid after it bathes the intestines and retroperitoneal tissues. (C) Both of the temporary closure techniques (1010 loban or AbThera) incorporate a plastic barrier that prevents the abdominal viscera from adhering to the undersurface of the abdominal wall. This is seen at a second laparotomy with a large potential space between the viscera and the abdominal wall. (D) One option to keep the fascia under tension and closer to midline includes suturing mesh to the fascia that is then sequentially tightened at each repeat laparotomy to bring the fascial edges closer together for eventual final closure.

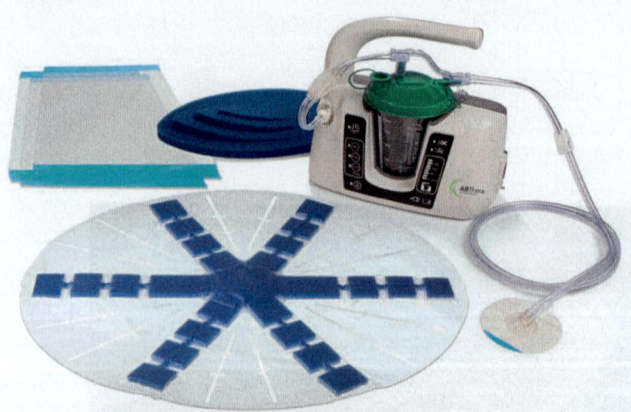

FIGURE 37.4 Negative-pressure wound therapy system.

physiologic derangements are corrected. Lung-protective ventilation strategies using with lower tidal volumes and limited plateau pressures are employed. Because multiple operations may be required before fascial closure may be achieved, patients with open abdomens can be extubated once they meet standard criteria for ventilator liberation. Extubation before abdominal closure is associated with decreased respiratory complications and no increased risk of intraabdominal complications.[23]

Reexploration of the abdomen should occur within 24 to 48 hours. For each hour delayed beyond 24 hours there is a 1.1% decrease in the odds of primary fascial closure and delay beyond 48 hours is associated with increased intraabdominal complications. If the patient requires ongoing transfusion despite correction of hypothermia, coagulopathy, and acidosis, or if the patient has a persistent lactic acidosis that is not responsive to resuscitation, one should consider returning to the operating room or performing CT imaging to identify sources of bleeding or missed injuries.

Assessing Readiness for Closure

Definitive closure should only be attempted when the underlying condition is resolving or resolved. During surgical reexploration, it is important to assess the ability to close the fascia without undue tension secondary to tissue edema or loss of domain. This can be assessed in the operating room by measuring IAP and/or changes in peak inspiratory pressure during closure. Sustained IAH (>20–25 mm Hg) and an increase in peak inspiratory pressure of >10 cm H_2O during attempts at fascial closure are warning signs of high fascial tension with the potential for compromise to the abdominal wall, underlying viscera, renal function, and ventilation. Delayed closure of the fascia, or, if this is not possible, a planned ventral hernia, may be prudent for this subgroup of critically ill patients with an open abdomen.

DEFINITIVE CLOSURE OF THE ABDOMINAL WALL

Suture Material

Abdominal wall closure has changed over time in large part due to improvements in suture materials and characteristics. The ideal suture material for abdominal wall closure is one that resists infection, provides adequate tensile strength to prevent abdominal wall disruption, minimizes tissue damage, and is absorbable. In current practice, a significant percentage of abdominal wall incisions are closed with slow-absorbing monofilament sutures such as

polydioxanone. Polydioxanone has an advantage over polyglactin with longer strength retention profile and absorption time; it is also a monofilament that may resist infection to a greater degree than the braided suture. Fast absorbing suture has been shown to have an increased rate of ventral incisional hernia formation.[24] Use of nonabsorbable sutures for abdominal closure (e.g., polypropylene) has been associated with increased patient pain and sinus tract formation, and their use has shown no significant difference in the incidence of incisional hernia formation, wound dehiscence, or SSI compared with that of absorbable suture.[25]

Characteristics of abdominal fascial healing suggest that fast absorbing suture has an insufficient half-life to support early development of facial tensile strength. Polyglactin has a half-life of approximately 3 weeks, whereas polydioxanone has an estimated half-life of 6 weeks. A large meta-analysis found no difference in hernia formation between these two suture materials, and a number of surgical societies advocate for use of slow absorbing suture material for abdominal wall closure.[26]

Barbed sutures are increasingly being used for fascial closure. This suture has tiny barbs in a helical arrangement that allow an even distribution of tension across the incision rather than just at the knots. In a porcine model, barbed and smooth sutures were shown to have similar burst strength.[27] Barbed sutures have also been shown to have a similar hernia recurrence rate in fascial plication for rectus diastasis. They are secured without knots, thus allowing for faster placement and eliminating the knot as a nidus for infection. A recent randomized trial showed superiority of barbed suture versus regular monofilament with regards to SSI and evisceration.[28]

Closure Technique

The principles of wound closure applied for the closure of the abdominal wall are essentially the same for closure of any surgical incision. Minimization of tissue damage is imperative, and this may be done by limiting the incorporation of the abdominal wall musculature in the closure. Historically, a 4:1 ratio of suture to wound length had been advocated with 2-cm tissue bites and 1-cm advancement. Recent evidence in elective surgical cases suggests that a strategy of taking smaller (5-mm) bites with smaller (5-mm) space between them is associated with a lower rate of incisional hernia.[29] Layered closure of the abdominal wall to include separate layered closure of the peritoneum and subcutaneous tissues in addition to the skin and fascia is discouraged, and simple closure is preferred. A continuous suture of slowly absorbable material is the recommended method of closure in elective abdominal surgery; there is little evidence to alter this closure technique in the emergency setting.[25,30]

Although retention sutures are intended to prevent evisceration, there is no consensus on the ideal adjunct to standard techniques of abdominal wall closure. Internal retention sutures are typically used in an interrupted fashion in the fascia, placed 4 to 6 cm back from the fascial edge, and spaced 5 to 7 cm apart from each other to prevent evisceration. External retention sutures incorporate a full-thickness closure of the entire abdominal wall (skin, subcutaneous tissue, fascia) with external prosthetics or "bolsters" placed to minimize pressure ulceration of the skin. Retention sutures have been associated with increased pain, wound inflammation, and wound complications as well as skin breakdown and problems with ostomy appliance placement. Thus, routine use of retention sutures, while theoretically advantageous, is not without potential complications and routine use is not advocated.

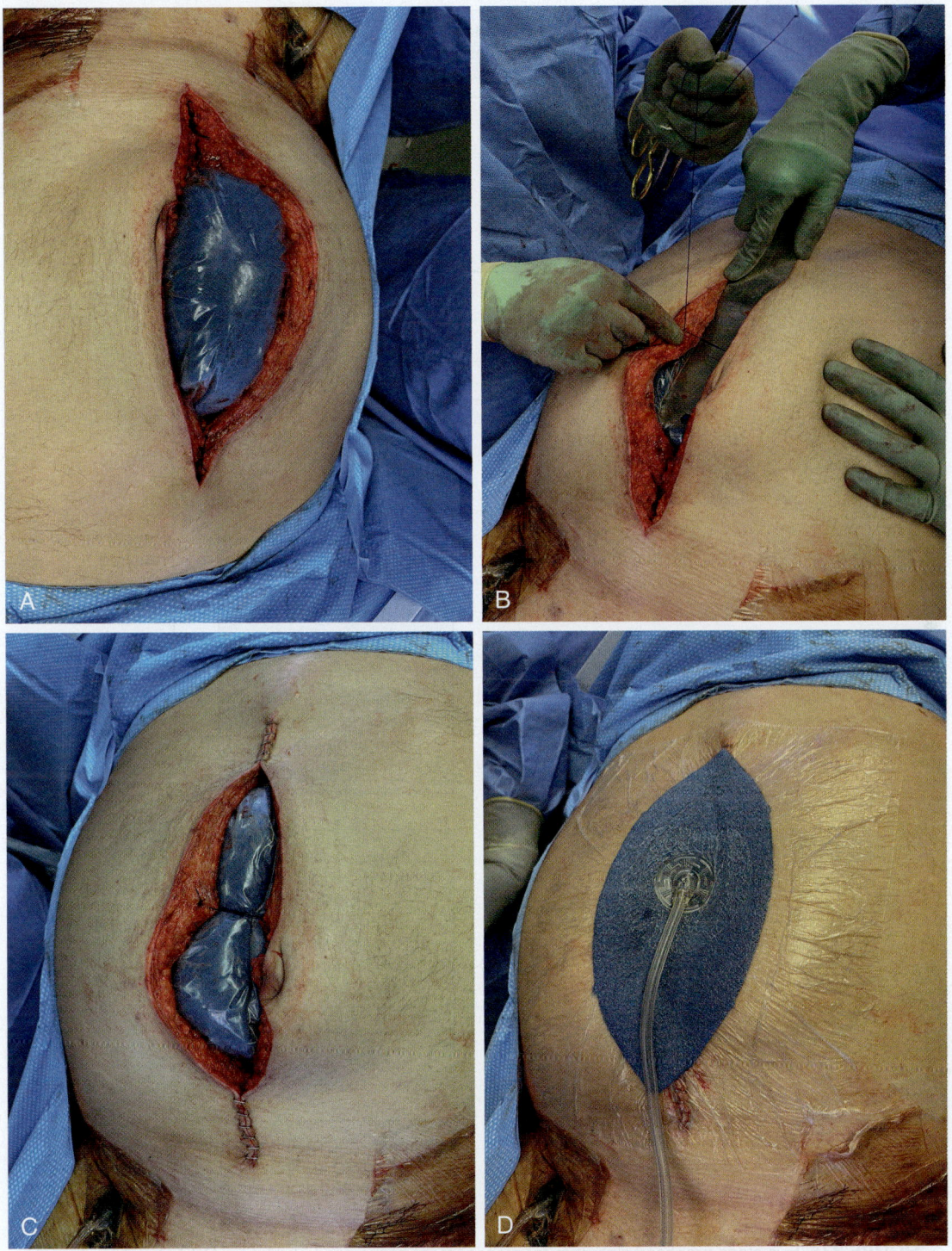

FIGURE 37.5 (A) The sequential fascial closure technique created in Denver first elucidated the five temporary abdominal closure techniques. The AbThera silastic drape, or alternatively negative-pressure wound therapy (NPWT) white sponges, is placed over the viscera to minimize damage to the abdominal contents (principle 1) and minimize adherence of the viscera to the anterior abdominal wall (principle 2). (B) Spaced fascial sutures to hold tension toward the midline are placed over either NPWT white sponges or the AbThera silastic drape (principle 3). (C) Because these are simple facial sutures of #1 PDS and they are spaced 5 to 6 cm apart from superior to inferior along the fascia, there is minimal trauma to the fascial edge (principle 4). (D) A second sponge, either a black NPWT sponge or the blue AbThera "football" sponge, is placed over the sutures and the first sponge; this sponge sandwich promotes abdominal closure and reduction of the visceral contents (principle 5).

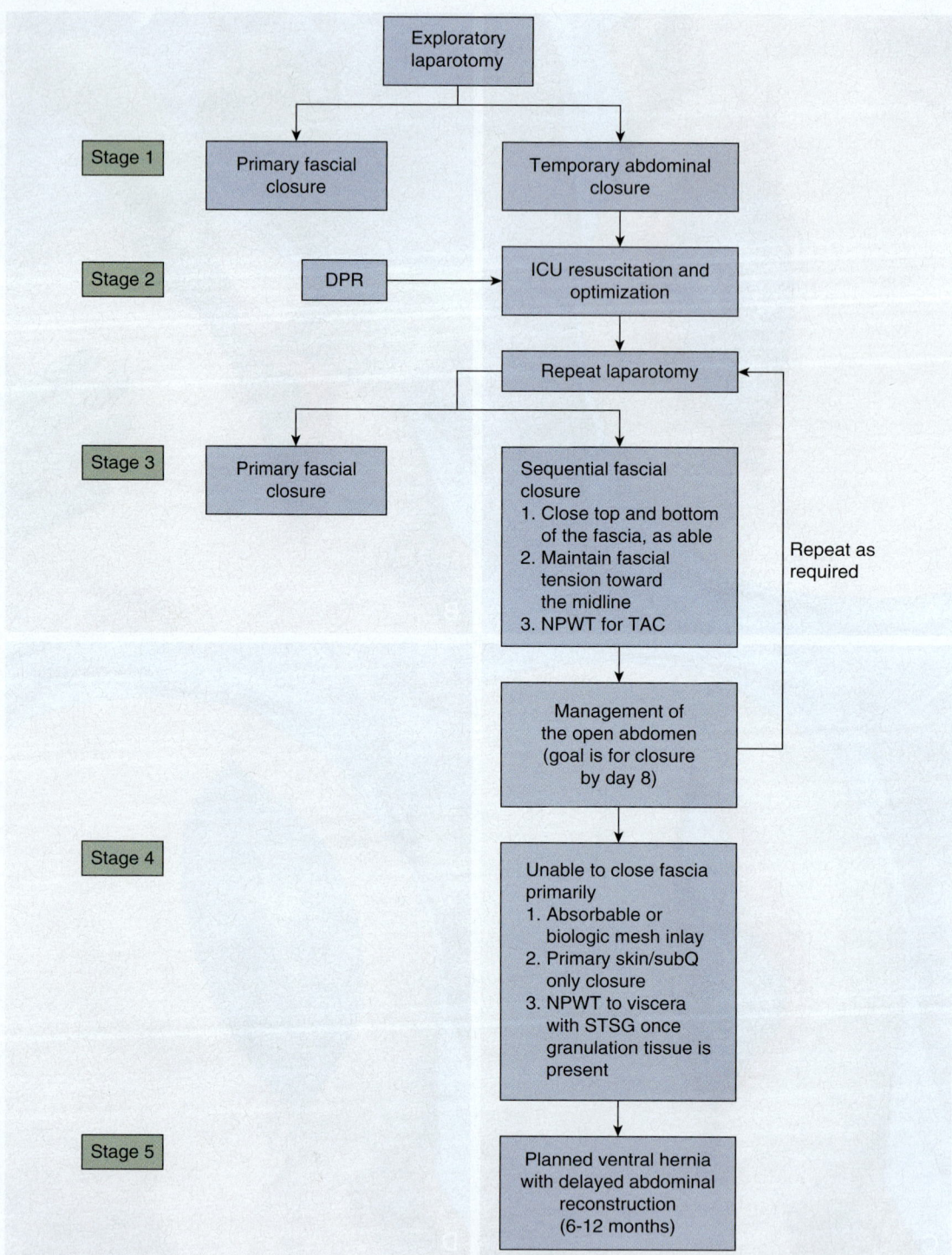

FIGURE 37.6 Five-stage proposed algorithm for management of the open abdomen. *DPR*, Direct peritoneal resuscitation; *NPWT*, negative-pressure wound therapy; *STSG*, split-thickness skin graft; *TAC*, temporary abdominal closure.

Patients at high risk of acute fascial dehiscence may benefit from some method of evisceration prophylaxis, and some surgeons have promoted the use of synthetic mesh in high-risk abdominal wall closures. Identification of the patient who is at higher risk of abdominal wall dehiscence may alter surgical technique of abdominal wall closure tand should be considered in any abdominal operation.[11]

Prophylactic Mesh

With incisional hernia rates after midline laparotomy in high-risk groups of 30% or more in some series, placement of prophylactic mesh at the index laparotomy for high-risk patients has drawn a large interest. Both the onlay and sublay positions have been used for this purpose. In multiple studies, there is a decrease in incisional hernia rates when a mesh is used, with no increase in surgical site occurrence (SSO) rates. Additionally, prophylactic mesh placement has been shown to be cost-effective.[31,32] There is an increase in postoperative seroma rates in patients that undergo mesh placement, particularly in the onlay position.

Considerations for Delayed Abdominal Wall Closure

Ideal conditions for optimal abdominal wall closure include source control and minimizing visceral edema as well as abdominal hypertension to allow for a tension-free closure. Mass closure of healthy fascia in an uncontaminated field is not encountered as often in the setting of emergency general surgery operations. Determination of abdominal fascial tension is subjective; closure with excessive tension increases the risk of dehiscence, evisceration, or late development of ventral incisional hernia. If the abdominal wall is unable to be closed primarily with the usual suture techniques, the better option may be to close the abdominal wall in such a way that future optimal reconstruction options are not lost. Component separation techniques are possible in the emergency setting; however, given the lack of optimal anatomic and physiologic conditions, these should be reserved for elective settings when possible. The use of incisional negative-pressure wound devices may be used in high-risk cases to minimize postoperative SSI, although clear evidence of their effectiveness is limited.[33] Additionally, placement of diverting stomas as lateral as possible (i.e., not through the rectus sheath) will preserve this critical fascial component for future reconstruction.

Challenges in the Contaminated Field

There are many challenges to hernia repair in an infected field. After an infection is eradicated, bowel resection performed, and necrotic tissue debrided, the visceral sac must then be contained. In this scenario, we advise against creating large skin flaps or performing myofascial component separation during the acute phase of management. After source control and treatment of infections, preparation of the wound for definitive repair should not interfere with possible reconstruction options in the future. Tissue repair during this time is an anabolic process, and malnourished or actively catabolic patients may have significantly impaired wound healing response and catabolic state.

Although less than ideal, it may be necessary to rely on TAC and fascial bridge techniques first to reduce the bacterial burden and then to develop a clean wound for later definitive repair. The most efficacious management strategy of a ventral hernia in a contaminated wound continues to be debated and includes methods of staging the repair with the use of negative-pressure devices, primary fascial closure alone, the use of permanent or absorbable synthetic mesh, or biologic mesh.

Biologic mesh was developed and promoted primarily for use in contaminated fields in which synthetic mesh use was contraindicated. A variety of biologic mesh material currently used includes sources from human, porcine, and bovine species with variable amounts of elastin and collagen and may or may not be cross-linked. The donor sites include dermis, intestinal mucosa, and pericardium. The processing of these materials removes all cellular elements, microbes, and epitopes responsible for rejection, leaving only the extracellular matrix and vascular channels intact. The theoretical benefits of biologic mesh over synthetic mesh include revascularization and incorporation into the host tissues, thus causing less of an inflammatory reaction, less adhesion formation, and improvement of bacterial clearance in a contaminated wound. There still are many unanswered questions

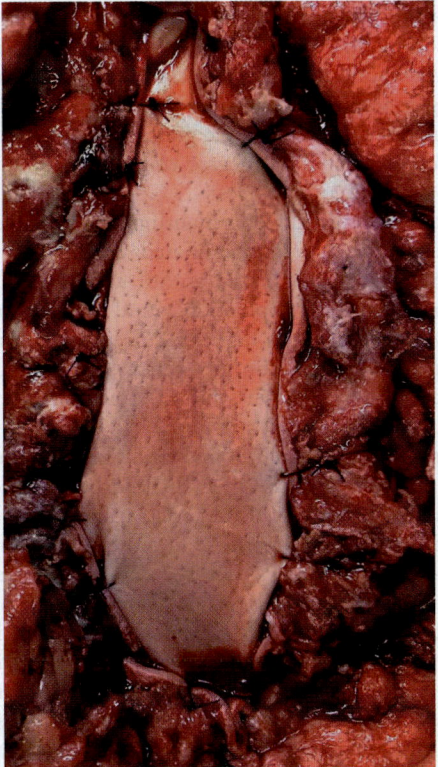

FIGURE 37.7 Bridged repair with biologic mesh.

about the ideal source material, processing methods, and most appropriate placement techniques.

In the case of sepsis and/or a prolonged inflammatory process with a large abdominal wound defect or major fascial dehiscence, use of a non–cross-linked biologic mesh as an inlay bridge protects and maintains abdominal domain[34] (Fig. 37.7). This method can help protect the abdominal viscera from desiccation and fistula formation. Local wound care with healing by secondary intention technique and skin coverage over drains are accepted maneuvers in this circumstance. Delayed ventral hernia repair can then be performed once the patient has recovered and their protein calorie malnutrition has been repleted.

This biologic bridge technique is useful for patients with significant comorbidities, for the acutely ill, and in cases in which definitive reconstruction is a prohibitive risk. There is clear evidence that when the biologic mesh is used as a bridge repair, the result is a high recurrence rate because of stretching of the biologic mesh over time, causing laxity and bulging, or an actual recurrence within a year.[35] Thus, the bridge repair should not be thought of as a definitive reconstruction alternative, but more as a biologic mesh covering of the peritoneal cavity that prevents desiccation and ECF formation. Complications related to biologic mesh use include seroma and hematoma formation, SSO, graft degradation, and desiccation. Ensuring ongoing hydration of the biologic mesh with the use of hydrating gels, enzymatic debriding agents, and overlying skin or vacuum-assisted closure (VAC) therapy can reduce these complications.

Since the introduction of these bioprosthetic materials, there has been an ever-expanding market of both new biologic, biosynthetic, and lightweight macroporous synthetic materials that claim superiority in the contaminated field. Few of these materials have been subjected to critical evaluation of their outcomes in humans for complex abdominal wall reconstruction. The Ventral

Hernia Working Group and a recent systematic review and meta-analysis recommend consideration of biologic mesh in contaminated or dirty wounds (class III and class IV). The primary benefits when biologic mesh is used in contaminated cases are less need for removal compared with synthetic grafts, and their 30-day SSI is not increased based on the degree of wound contamination in contrast to synthetic mesh.[36]

A multicenter prospective study using a porcine biologic mesh for repair of infected or contaminated ventral hernias demonstrated an SSO rate of 66% and an SSI rate of 30%.[37] A 5-year follow-up of this patient population found a 50% recurrence rate at 3 years with a two times higher recurrence when the biologic mesh was placed intraperitoneally versus retrorectus. The mean fascial defect size was 236 cm² with 80% ability of complete fascial closure over the biologic mesh.

A large multicenter, longitudinal study for contaminated ventral hernia repair (Complex Open Bioabsorbable Reconstruction of the Abdominal Wall [COBRA] trial) using biosynthetic mesh (biologic with absorbable synthetic mesh) found at 24 months an SSO rate of 28%, an SSI rate of 18%, and a recurrence rate of 17%. This is less than the Repair of Infected or Contaminated Ventral Incisional Hernias (RICH) study,[37] but critical reviews comparing the two studies stated that they were different patient populations and mean hernia size in the COBRA study was significantly less (137 cm²) with a compete fascial closure rate of 100%.[38] Multiple studies now clearly demonstrate that a bridged repair is a significant predictor of hernia recurrence.

Other potential options for abdominal wall reconstruction include the use of absorbable synthetic mesh. Polyglactin mesh can be used to maintain the visceral sac but has disadvantages of limited half-life and porosity that can allow for bowel desiccation if used in conjunction with NPWT devices. Poly-4-hydroxybutyrate (Phasix) is another option that has longer half-life compared with polyglactin; its use is being studied in complex abdominal wall hernia reconstruction and contaminated fields, but long-term biologic behavior in direct contact with viscera remains unclear.[39]

Recent literature now suggests that lightweight permanent synthetic mesh may be an option to biologic mesh in the contaminated environment with comparable risk of SSO and need for mesh removal. Carbonell and colleagues challenged the fact that permanent mesh is contraindicated in contaminated fields, reviewing 100 patients with clean-contaminated or contaminated ventral hernia repairs using lightweight polypropylene mesh. SSO was 26.2% in clean-contaminated wounds and 34% in contaminated wounds. The recurrence rate was 7% with a mean follow-up of 10.8 months.[40] Use of prosthetic mesh in these settings would be considered off-label and should only be considered on a case-by-case basis in the absence of other alternatives.

COMPLICATIONS OF ABDOMINAL CLOSURE

Seroma and Skin Necrosis

Seroma and skin necrosis are frequent complications related to major abdominal wall reconstruction (Fig. 37.8). Seromas occur especially in cases with wide subcutaneous dissection or with premature drain dislodgement or clogging. Release of fascial planes or creation of large tissue flaps creates a potential space that can fill with exudate that exceeds the capacity to be reabsorbed. To reduce seroma formation, closed suction drains should be placed in the subcutaneous and/or retrorectus space. Retrorectus drains have been associated with decreased rates of noninfectious SSO and no increase in rates of SSI.[41] These drains should be stripped

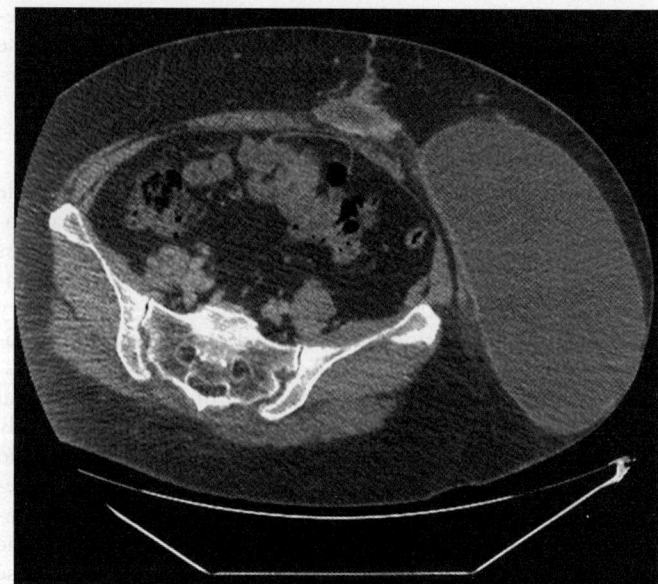

FIGURE 37.8 Seroma after skin flap creation.

regularly during the early postoperative period and are typically removed when less than 25 to 30 mL in a 24-hour period has been recorded. In addition, external compression with abdominal binders may aid in the abdominal wall and skin flap adherence and may hinder fluid collection formation.

Methods that have been described in the literature to decrease seroma formation include quilting stiches, talc application, or, most recently, surgical tissue adhesive application under skin flaps or over mesh application in the retrorectus space. However, there are no large studies to definitively show the benefit of these methods, and they should be considered on a case-by-case basis. If the seroma is asymptomatic and small, it will often resorb without any invasive intervention. Aspiration or reoperative drainage may be required if the seroma enlarges or shows signs of infection.[42] For seromas that fail to resolve with aspiration or catheter drainage, catheter-directed chemical sclerotherapy (e.g., talc tetracycline, doxycycline, ethanol, erythromycin, fibrin glue) or mechanical sclerotherapy (endoscopic argon beam ablation) may be considered.[43]

The blood supply to the skin is primarily distributed through the subcutaneous fat and perforators originating from the deep inferior epigastric artery. Intraoperative methods for optimizing and preserving the circulation to the skin and preventing postoperative skin necrosis are essential. In creating any skin flap, dissection should be in the plane between the subcutaneous layer and the underlying fascia. Techniques to preserve the perforators are well described in the literature. The perforators' density is highest around the periumbilical area; thus, it is important to spare a circular distance of about 3 cm around the umbilicus area during dissection.

Impending skin necrosis can be manifested as duskiness, blistering, and blanching redness that can progress to definitive necrotic tissue. Management varies by the depth and the total area of necrosis. Superficial skin necrosis can be treated locally with hydrating gels or enzymatic debriding agents. These products reduce the bacterial and necrotic tissue burden and maintain a moist environment for healing. Full-thickness wounds require skin and subcutaneous sharp debridement. Negative-pressure wound management systems can aid in sterile wound coverage and epithelialization for this complication.

Management of Mesh Infection

Prosthetic mesh infection is a dreaded complication of abdominal wall hernia repair and reconstruction. Heavyweight microporous mesh may develop material biofilms and local abdominal wall infections that often require explantation of the prosthetic. Lightweight, macroporous mesh has the advantage of earlier tissue incorporation and greater resistance to microbial biofilms. Ideal positioning of a prosthetic implant is in the retromuscular plane. This confers additional microbial resistance secondary to the well-vascularized muscle tissue and is well demonstrated in reconstructive surgery using muscle flaps in other body regions for the purposes of infection control and wound healing.

Management of established mesh prosthetic infections is based on degree of incorporation, associated soft tissue defects, symptoms, and long-term reconstructive plans. Although biologic mesh is generally accepted for use in contaminated fields, it rapidly loses its integrity when exposed to succus and may be completely lost in the setting of an anastomotic disruption or development of acute ECF. This setting may force debridement of the remaining biologic mesh and planned open abdomen management with complex wound care challenges. PTFE (Gore-Tex) mesh is considered heavyweight microporous and diminishes its ability to incorporate into body tissues, increasing its risk of developing biofilms. Infections involving this type of prosthetic typically involve full explantation. Lightweight and midweight macroporous mesh may be salvaged to some degree. Management of infections of these implants involves debridement of unincorporated mesh and local wound care to optimize rapid granulation and healing. Rarely, these mesh infections may result in long-term sinus tracts that would typically be managed with incision and drainage, prosthetic debridement as needed, and antimicrobial therapy. Fully incorporated mesh typically does not require routine removal. Like management of other soft tissue and deep infections, source control and optimal wound management are key.

Enteroatmospheric and Enterocutaneous Fistulas

Prevention of EAFs and ECFs is a critical component of managing the open abdomen. Prompt abdominal wall closure (before 8 days), use of plastic sheeting and omentum to protect the bowel from contact with temporary closure devices (especially when using NPWT), and covering enteric anastomoses with other loops of bowel all help with EAF prevention.[43] Once an EAF/ECF has formed, care is focused on nutritional optimization and wound healing.

Early initiation of EN improves outcomes for patients with EAF/ECF. EN, however, may result in increased fistula output and difficulty managing wound contamination and metabolic derangements (e.g., dehydration, electrolyte imbalances, and acid-base abnormalities). Contraindications to EN for patients with EAF/ECF include bowel discontinuity, ileus, and inability to tolerate EN due to metabolic and wound concerns. Patients who are unable to tolerate EN or are unable to meet nutritional goals with EN alone should be managed with parenteral nutrition. By optimizing nutrition, wound healing is maximized, and mortality rates are reduced.[44]

The mainstay of wound care for ECF/EAF is isolating the fistula effluent from the surrounding tissues to allow for wound healing and potentially spontaneous closure. Application of an ostomy appliance around the ECF is generally sufficient for ECF care. As opposed to ECF, wound management of EAF can be challenging due to lack of epithelialization around the wound. A combination of NPWT with commercially available devices (Wound Crown, 3M, Beirut, Lebanon) to isolate the EAF effluent allow for the formation

of granulation tissue around the fistula and eventual reepithelialization or skin grafting, thereby converting an EAF into an ECF. If spontaneous fistula closure does not occur after nutritional support and wound care, nonoperative and operative interventions should be considered. Options for nonoperative closure include fibrin glue, endoscopic clipping, and extracellular matrix plug. These minimally invasive options result in successful fistula closure in 44% to 100% of patients, but data regarding these approaches remains scant.[45] Surgical intervention for persistent ECF should not be performed for at least 6 months and only once the wound has healed and the patient has fully recovered.

DELAYED ABDOMINAL WALL RECONSTRUCTION

Preparation for Abdominal Wall Reconstruction

The goal of definitive reconstruction is first to optimize the patient's condition and then to restore the structure and functional continuity of the musculofascial system to provide stable and durable wound coverage to minimize additional complications. Once the decision has been made to operate, preoperative risk factors must be carefully evaluated and optimized before an elective complex abdominal wall reconstruction is performed. Understanding preoperative risk factors during the process of patient and procedure selection is essential to minimize adverse postoperative occurrences.

Minimizing risk in abdominal wall reconstruction surgery is a multidisciplinary effort aimed at tobacco cessation, clearing active infections, controlling diabetes, and normalizing BMI. Other risk factors associated with wound complications are less controllable and include enterotomy or stoma and previous ventral hernia repair. Every effort should be made to control diabetes by targeting a hemoglobin A1c less than 7, to maximize protein-calorie repletion, and to optimize cardiopulmonary status. Mandatory cigarette smoking cessation is required for at least 4 to 6 weeks before repair and urine cotinine screening can help document patient compliance. In patients with a previous methicillin-resistant *Staphylococcus aureus* infection, consideration should be given to decolonizing the patient or suppressing methicillin-resistant *S. aureus* carriers preoperatively and using vancomycin prophylaxis perioperatively.

Definitive Repair: Creating a Dynamic Abdominal Wall

Even with a great deal of preoperative planning, there is still no single approach that will solve all the needs for the reconstruction of a complex abdominal wall defect. It is essential that the surgeon review all prior operative reports and have a clear understanding of what remains in the wound and in what location. A preoperative CT scan of the abdominal wall is essential before any consideration of major reconstruction.

Various techniques for mobilization of the fascia medially with the component separation provide a tension-free repair of the rectus fascia and subsequent protection from infection from the overlying subcutaneous fat and skin. The classically described Ramirez technique for component separation requires large subcutaneous flaps to gain access to the lateral abdominal wall and release the external oblique fascia.[46] This technique has high wound morbidity and is, in general, not recommended for high-risk patients. Recently developed endoscopic methods to perform component separation release of the external oblique aponeurosis by using an endoscopic camera and avoiding division of the perforators have recently been described.[47]

The appreciation of abdominal wall function to create a dynamic abdominal wall unit has popularized two ideal reconstruction

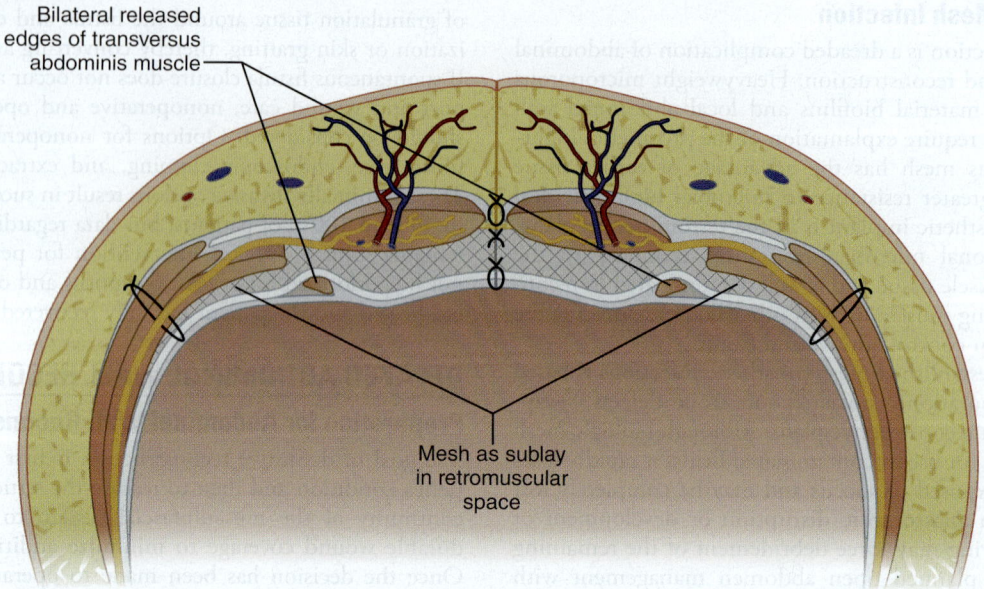

FIGURE 37.9 Retrorectus positioning of mesh after Rives-Stoppa-Wantz repair.

techniques: the Rives-Stoppa-Wantz repair and the transversus abdominis release. Both use a retromuscular placement of mesh and are widely considered procedures of choice in abdominal wall reconstruction. Both techniques use a posterior component separation and the placement of lightweight macroporous synthetic mesh in the retrorectus space and outside of the peritoneal cavity. These techniques serve as optimal protection of the bowel from the mesh provided by the posterior rectus sheath, peritoneum, and omentum.

Rives-Stoppa-Wantz and Transversus Abdominis Release Techniques

In this technique, the posterior rectus sheath is incised approximately one-half of a centimeter from the fascial edge of the defect. The retrorectus plane is then developed to the lateral extent of the dissection, which is the linea semilunaris.[48] If this dissection is insufficient to close the posterior rectus fascia, an extension of this technique includes release of the transversus abdominis. In this technique, the transversus abdominis muscle is divided, which then allows entrance into the space between the transversalis fascia and the lateral edge of this divided transversus abdominis muscle. This allows the creation of a wide lateral dissection plane with substantial posterior and anterior fascial advancement. Both procedures avoid a major subcutaneous dissection and preserve the neurovascular bundle (Figs. 37.9 and 37.10).

Perioperative Considerations

Reconstruction of large abdominal defects can markedly change the physiology of respiration and alter the function of the diaphragm and respiratory musculature. Many surgeons have advocated the use of plateau pressure as an intraoperative method for gauging the effects of hernia repair on pulmonary function. Postoperative respiratory complications have been found to be significantly increased when the plateau pressure was raised above 6 mm Hg, and patients were nine times more likely to have complications with this finding.[49] Additionally, intraoperative and postoperative monitoring of abdominal pressures indirectly using bladder

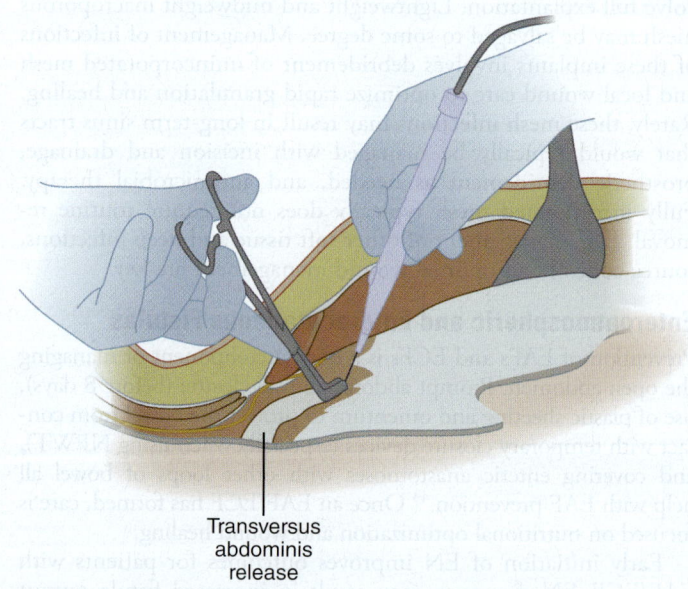

FIGURE 37.10 Transversus abdominis release.

pressure measurements is routinely recommended when the abdominal wall defect is more than 600 cm^2.[49]

Pain management is essential in this patient population, and the use of epidural catheters and transversus abdominis plane blocks substantially improves pain relief. These reduce narcotic use within the postoperative phase and decrease costs and postoperative morbidity. Both techniques increase early mobilization, thus reducing additional complications related to this extensive surgery. Long-acting injectable bupivacaine medication can provide prolonged relief of pain and reduce the use of narcotics.[50] Abdominal binders can also improve patient ambulation, pain control, and comfort.

Finally, a thorough understanding of the determinants of outcomes may be the most important factor in reducing complications and even death in this patient population. Nonoperative close observation strategies for asymptomatic large incisional hernias may be prudent in certain patient populations. Currently, there is no study evaluating patients with known incisional hernias who are managed nonoperatively.

SUMMARY

Patients with a difficult abdominal wall comprise a variety of etiologies and physiologic conditions. The now routine use of DCS for both trauma and emergency general surgery conditions results in an open abdomen, mandating surgeon knowledge of temporary closure techniques and also comfort with ICU optimization. After normalization of adverse physiology, abdominal reexploration is performed with either primary fascial closure or a plan for attempts at sequential closure of the abdomen. Efforts during these critical early postoperative days are paramount as inability to close the abdomen by 8 days is associated with a significant increase in complications, including EAFs. Coordinated efforts between surgeons and intensivists will ensure patients attain the best possible closure, whether this is eventual primary facial closure via multiple trips to the operating room, making the decision to place bridging biologic mesh to protect the abdominal viscera followed by subcutaneous tissue/skin closure or directed skin grafting, or the last option of a planned ventral hernia with subcutaneous tissue/skin repair closure. Careful monitoring of these patients for postoperative complications is paramount as they are common in this complex and critically ill patient population.

SELECTED REFERENCES

Atema JJ, Gans SL, Boermeester MA. Systematic review and meta-analysis of the open abdomen and temporary abdominal closure techniques in non-trauma patients. *World J Surg.* 2015; 39(4):912-925.

> This systematic review explores the indications for and the complications of temporary abdominal closure in the nontrauma population.

Carbonell AM, Criss CN, Cobb WS, Novitsky YW, Rosen MJ. Outcomes of synthetic mesh in contaminated ventral hernia repairs. *J Am Coll Surg.* 2013;217(6):991-998.

> Contamination of the surgical field has long been thought to be an absolute contraindication to the use of prosthetic mesh for hernia repair. There is growing evidence that synthetic materials may be safely used despite the presence of contamination, potentially resulting in improved long-term outcomes of hernia repair.

Chabot E, Nirula R. Open abdomen critical care management principles: resuscitation, fluid balance, nutrition, and ventilator management. *Trauma Surg Acute Care Open.* 2017;2(1):e000063.

> This is a review article that discusses the physiologic impacts of temporary abdominal closure and optimal critical care for patients with open abdomens.

Roberts DJ, Bobrovitz N, Zygun DA, et al. Evidence for use of damage control surgery and damage control interventions in civilian trauma patients: a systematic review. *World J Emerg Surg.* 2021;16(1):10.

> This is a systematic review of studies that investigated the use of damage control surgery in civilian populations. It is aimed at identifying indications for abbreviated surgical intervention followed by definitive intervention after normalizing patient's physiology.

Wouters D, Cavallaro G, Jensen KK, et al. The European Hernia Society Prehabilitation Project: a systematic review of intraoperative prevention strategies for surgical site occurrences in ventral hernia surgery. *Front Surg.* 2022;9:847279.

> This systematic review examines preventive strategies for reducing the incidence of surgical site infections and occurrences in ventral hernia repairs.

The full reference list appears on Elsevier eBooks+.

38 | CHAPTER

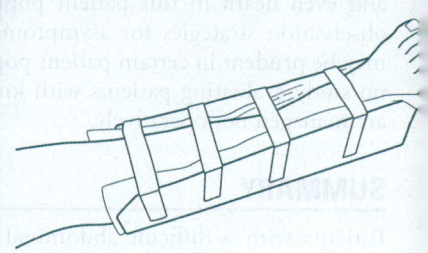

Management of Vascular Trauma

Mary Bokenkamp, Joshua Crapps, Joseph DuBose,
Pedro G. Teixeira, and Carlos V.R. Brown

EPIDEMIOLOGY

Although trauma as a whole has been well characterized on local and international scales, the epidemiology of vascular injury specifically is relatively undefined. Epidemiology is dependent on accurate data, and there is a lack of large-scale data on vascular injury. This is because of the heterogeneity of the injuries, mechanisms, circumstances, and consequences of vascular injury.[1] The rate and impact of vascular injury are more well understood in individual populations. For example, in the most recent military engagements in Iraq and Afghanistan, the rate of vascular injury was as high as 12%.[2] Military vascular injuries tend to result more from extremity trauma, whereas civilians experience more torso wounds. The overall incidence is certainly lower in the civilian setting, yet exact numbers are hard to define. Iatrogenic trauma has also become a significant contributor, with endovascular techniques becoming standard practice in many instances. These have yet to be fully characterized. For the trauma and vascular surgeon, an understanding of the local factors contributing to the incidence and consequences of vascular trauma is vital to treatment and outcomes.

DIAGNOSIS

The prompt recognition and rapid and effective surgical management of vascular trauma remain challenging despite major advances in access to care produced by trauma systems development.

The risk to life and limb remains significant, and the margin for error in both diagnosis and treatment of these injuries is very thin. Either delay in recognition of or failure in adequate management of vascular injuries remains alarmingly common in trauma centers. An organized approach with well-planned and implemented practice guidelines is essential to convert an error-prone process into one of timely diagnosis and safe and effective treatment.

Vascular injuries have a broad spectrum of clinical manifestations, varying from profound hemorrhagic shock to subtle findings, such as an asymptomatic bruit.[3] Because such a broad spectrum of clinical findings is associated with vascular trauma, it is best to assume that vascular injury is present until proven otherwise in all patients with hemorrhagic shock and all patients with extremity fractures.[3] Vascular injury can produce systemic symptoms of hypotension, tachycardia, and altered mental status due to hemorrhagic shock. As a result, vascular injury can be life threatening, and attention must initially be directed to the primary survey using the principles of Advanced Trauma Life Support (ATLS).[3] The airway must be assessed, adequate oxygenation and ventilation ensured, and intravenous access achieved. Once this is completed and resuscitation is under way, the secondary survey is undertaken. A thorough history and careful physical examination are then performed. This examination must include a careful inspection of the injured sites and wounds, a complete sensory and motor assessment, and a pulse examination of each extremity. The presence of a hematoma, bruit, or thrill must be noted.

The workup and diagnosis of vascular injuries should be based on three contiguous phases: physical examination, bedside diagnostic modalities, and targeted imaging or operative exploration. Initial history and physical examination are of the utmost importance, with specific attention to hemorrhagic or ischemic signs. Hemorrhagic signs, including an active external hemorrhage, large or expanding hematoma, pulsatile mass or palpable thrill, and hypotension or shock, indicate disruption of major blood vessels, arterial or venous, at the site of injury. Regardless of anatomic location, these signs should prompt expeditious attempts at hemorrhage control, requiring either further imaging localization or direct operative management.[4]

Hemorrhage management can be broken into five anatomic areas, each with specific considerations. In the head and neck, external hemorrhage is required for vascular injuries to result in shock. Relatively small and tightly organized tissue planes preclude significant internal hemorrhage. In the chest, each hemithorax can accommodate lethal amounts of hemorrhage from cardiac, pulmonary, or great vessel arterial and venous injuries. Abdominal and pelvic vascular injuries can also result in lethal hemorrhage, particularly from the aorta and iliac arteries. As in the head and neck, extremity vascular injuries generally cause hemorrhagic shock only if there is significant external hemorrhage. The patient with hypotension and a lack of chest, abdomen, and pelvic findings may have what appears to be a trivial neck or extremity laceration that initially communicated with a major vessel injury. A hemorrhage sufficient to produce hypotension can be followed by thrombosis. It is therefore necessary to obtain a history from the prehospital personnel about the amount of blood at the scene or the initial presence of severe wound hemorrhage. It is also necessary to thoroughly examine the patient for additional wounds and carefully assess each of them.[3]

Extremity vascular trauma may be immediately apparent on presentation because of external hemorrhage, hematoma, or obvious limb ischemia. A history of penetrating trauma associated with hypotension, pulsatile bleeding, or a large quantity of blood at the scene suggests vascular injury. Blunt trauma is also capable of causing significant vascular injury that can be overlooked when serious head, chest, or abdominal injuries are present. Extremity fractures may result in vascular injury. Supracondylar humerus fracture can be associated with brachial artery injury, and knee dislocation carries a significant risk of popliteal artery injury.[5] Crush injuries of the extremity without fracture may also result in vascular injury.

Some vascular injuries are manifested in a delayed fashion without initial findings. These consist of thrombosis of a previously partially disrupted but initially patent vessel, distal emboli from an intimal tear of the arterial wall with formation of platelet debris, and least commonly, rupture or expansion of a pseudoaneurysm that was initially small and contained by the outer arterial wall and local tissue. Ischemic signs, such as limb malperfusion, end-organ dysfunction, and various embolic phenomena, can be subtle or masked by various physiologic disturbances in trauma; therefore, careful evaluation is paramount. Ischemic signs manifest as loss of flow distal to the lesion, whether this be diminished or absent extremity pulses, neurologic or strokelike symptomatology, or abdominal pain and physiologic findings of hollow viscus and solid organ malperfusion. Although ischemic symptoms present distal to a suspected injury, it is not possible to fully localize or characterize these lesions based on history and physical examination alone. Further diagnostic modalities are therefore necessary in these instances to guide therapy.[4]

If distal pulses are diminished or absent, ankle or wrist systolic blood pressure should be determined with a continuous-wave Doppler device and compared with the uninjured side. A significant difference in systolic blood pressure (10 mm Hg) between extremities may be an indication of vascular injury. Doppler waveforms may also aid in determining presence of a vascular injury, with monophasic waveforms indicating limited proximal flow. If anything other than strong biphasic or triphasic waveforms is obtained, the contralateral limb should also be evaluated in comparison. Doppler may also be used to calculate an Injured Extremity Index (IEI), the ratio of systolic blood pressure in the injury limb to that in the unaffected limb. Any IEI less than 1.0 is considered abnormal and representative of limited arterial flow in the injured extremity.

In addition to Doppler, focused assessment with sonography in trauma (FAST) should be routinely performed to evaluate for free intraabdominal, pelvic, pericardial, and thoracic fluid indicative of hemorrhage. Although nonspecific, findings on this examination may help guide further management of hemorrhage.

X-ray is another imaging modality that can be quickly performed at bedside to guide evaluation of vascular injury. Although vascular injuries cannot be directly imaged with radiographs, both plain chest and pelvic radiographs may contain findings suggestive of major vascular injury, such as massive hemothorax or an unstable pelvic fracture.

It is well established that patients with "hard" findings of vascular injury (Table 38.1) should be taken directly to the operating room. However, in patients with "soft" findings (see Table 38.1), vascular imaging can be used to rule out the need for operation. In addition, patients with hard findings but with multilevel injuries in the same extremity may also need imaging. Catheter arteriography is both sensitive and specific in the diagnosis of extremity vascular injuries. However, computed tomography angiography (CTA) with the latest generation scanners is readily available and highly accurate and obviates the delay caused by mobilizing the angiography suite for catheter angiography.[6] Although this imaging technique requires an infusion of contrast material, it does not require arterial catheterization, is easily performed, and is less costly and less time consuming than conventional angiography.[6] In patients with suspected vascular injury, CTA has become the standard imaging modality for diagnosis and intervention planning. CT has the added benefit of evaluating surrounding soft tissue and bony injury, which may aid in surgical planning or

TABLE 38.1 History and Physical Examination Findings of Vascular Injury

Hard Findings

Indicate need for immediate intervention for vascular injury
- Pulsatile bleeding
- Expanding or pulsatile hematoma
- Palpable thrill or audible bruit
- Absent pulse
- Hypotension

Soft Findings

Consider further imaging and evaluation for vascular injury
- History of moderate hemorrhage
- Proximity fracture, dislocation, or penetrating wound
- Diminished but palpable pulse
- Level of peripheral nerve deficit in proximity to major vessel

prognostication. A downside to CT, which can often be seen in firearm trauma, is the presence of imaging artifact (Fig. 38.1) resulting from the presence of metallic fragments (e.g., bullets, pellets, shrapnel).[7]

Although CT and CTA imaging modalities have become commonplace in the modern trauma patient's workup, formal angiography remains the gold standard for evaluation of vascular luminal characteristics. It is able to provide dynamic information regarding flow characteristics within the injured vessel and has the potential to aid both diagnosis and treatment (if amenable to endovascular repair). This modality, however, requires specialized equipment and training that may not be readily available at some trauma centers.[8]

Severely injured patients who must be taken to the operating room for treatment of life-threatening associated injuries, such as penetrating thoracic injury or ruptured spleen, may not be able to undergo CTA. In such cases, it is not prudent to delay operative therapy to obtain formal vascular imaging. An on-table arteriogram can be obtained in the operating room by cannulating the artery proximal to the suspected vascular injury, injecting 20 to 25 mL of a full-strength radiographic contrast agent, and taking a radiograph or using fluoroscopy. This may be helpful in both initial diagnosis of injury and subsequent evaluation of a vascular repair or bypass before leaving the operating room.

If doubt remains about the presence of a vascular injury and the imaging studies and other diagnostic tests are inconclusive, there is a role for operative exploration and direct assessment of the artery. Routine operative exploration in the stable patient with soft signs, however, has a 5% to 30% incidence of morbidity, occasional mortality, and low diagnostic yield.[9] These patients are better served with formal vascular imaging.

Duplex color flow imaging is not used for the acute assessment of vascular injury. Wounds, swelling, air in the tissue, and dressings or splints impair the ability to obtain satisfactory images. Duplex imaging does have a role in the follow-up of treated lesions (e.g., to assess patency of bypass grafts or to detect luminal stenosis at an anastomosis) and in the follow-up of nonoperative management of minimal vascular injury, such as small pseudoaneurysms or arteriovenous fistulas.

PRINCIPLES OF OPEN MANAGEMENT

Preparation for Operative Management

Operative procedures to manage vascular injuries should be limited to those surgeons who are capable, experienced, and qualified. Board certification in vascular surgery is not enough to qualify a surgeon as capable of handling these injuries, just as the lack of certification does not necessarily disqualify a surgeon. Many surgeons who perform elective vascular surgery are not sufficiently experienced in the management of vascular trauma. Conversely, there are many trauma surgeons who are very skilled in vascular technique by virtue of their interest and experience. The results of major open vascular repairs are dependent on the skill level of the vascular trauma–capable surgeon, independent of board preparation. In a multicenter review of close to 700 major extremity vascular injuries, board-certified general surgeons and board-certified vascular surgeons had nearly identical high limb salvage rates for major vascular surgical repairs.[10] Every trauma center needs to develop a call panel of surgeons with the skill and knowledge to perform the full spectrum of vascular trauma repairs.

Successful operative management of vascular injuries requires a systematic approach with careful preparation. This begins with airway control, adequate intravenous access, and availability of blood products. The administration of these blood products, however, should not begin before obtaining control of hemorrhage unless the patient is profoundly hypotensive.[3] If the blood pressure is below 80 to 90 mm Hg, the goal should be to provide adequate volume restoration with whole blood or balanced resuscitation (1:1:1) to support transport to the operating room for definitive hemorrhage control without delay. Volume infusion that raises the blood pressure above a systolic pressure of 90 to 100 mm Hg may increase bleeding and have a negative impact on outcome, particularly if the infusion delays transport to the operating room.[3]

The most commonly omitted step in preparation is a failure to document preoperative extremity neurologic status. The presence of a neurologic deficit after operative vascular repair without knowing the preoperative status presents a difficult management

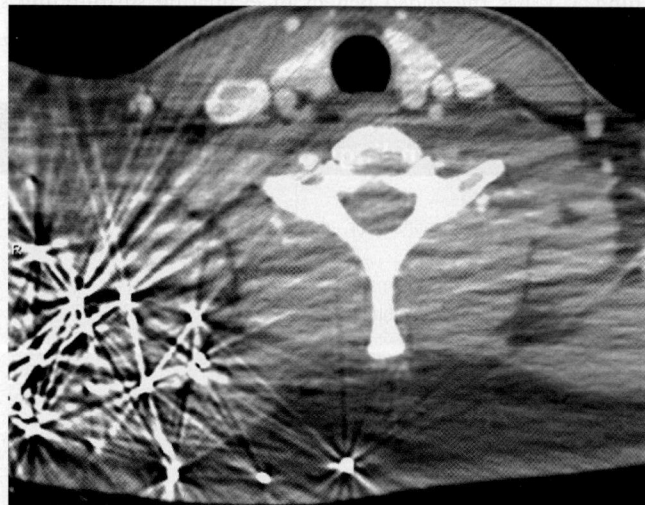
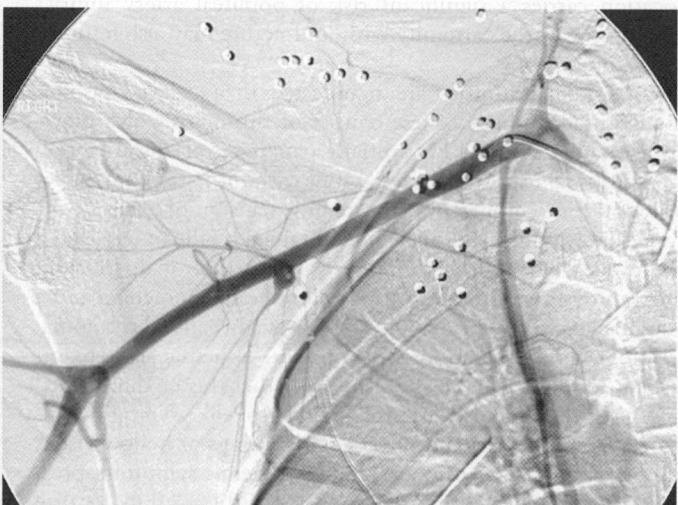

FIGURE 38.1 CT with contrast imaging of gunshot wound to the right shoulder. Metallic scatter obscures adequate visualization of the arterial structures to exclude injury. The image on the *right* shows the subsequent traditional angiogram, which afforded multiplanar views that subsequently confirmed the absence of arterial injury.

challenge. A new neurologic deficit after vascular repair merits investigation and, possibly, reoperation. Therefore, a thorough preoperative neurologic examination and careful documentation are essential to effective management.

After the decision is made to proceed with open management, the operating room and staff should be properly prepared for potential needs within the case. Ideally, a radiolucent operating table should be used in anticipation of performing an on-table angiogram if needed. The patient should be positioned supine with arms abducted and should have skin preparation in usual trauma fashion from chin to midthighs and to the table bilaterally. Depending on the site of suspected vascular injury, the upper or lower extremities should be prepped circumferentially to aid in vascular exposure or allow for harvest of greater saphenous vein for use as a graft. If an upper extremity peripheral vascular injury is suspected, an arm board should also be added to aid in positioning and exposure.[4]

Broad-spectrum preoperative antibiotics (and tetanus toxoid, if it is a penetrating wound) should be administered, and if there is an isolated extremity injury without other significant systemic sources of hemorrhage, a bolus of 100 to 150 units/kg of heparin or a fixed dose of 5000 units may also be given intravenously. Systemic heparinization should be avoided in patients with torso injuries, head injuries, or multiple extremity injuries.[11] Although this is common in elective vascular surgery, systemic heparinization is debated in trauma. A safe alternative to this may be to regionally instill heparinized saline at the site of repair to prevent thrombosis.[11] Ultimately, its use should be determined by the operative surgical team.

The operative management of extremity vascular injuries must be carefully orchestrated with the overall care of the patient. The choice between definitive repair and damage control should be made as soon as possible in patients with life-threatening torso injuries or severe head injuries. This includes coordinating two surgical teams, if possible, to work simultaneously to care for the torso injury and the extremity vascular injury at the same time. Associated injuries to the soft tissue and bone require a coordinated assessment and treatment with orthopedic and plastic surgery consultants. These specialists should be involved as early as possible to facilitate any additional imaging or diagnostic procedures before proceeding to the operating room. The conduct of the operation should also be discussed with these colleagues. For example, the use of damage control procedures with shunt placement, followed by orthopedic stabilization, can remove the sense of urgency to definitively repair the vasculature. Extensive soft tissue injuries may compromise the proper coverage of vascular repairs and fracture fixation. The advice and assistance of a plastic and reconstructive surgeon can be helpful in obtaining coverage of exposed grafts and fractures.

Vascular Exposure and Control

Proximal control is the first priority in the exposure of vascular injuries. In the torso, chest injuries with life-threatening hemorrhage are best approached through a fourth intercostal space left anterolateral thoracotomy that can be extended across the sternum into the third intercostal space of the right side of the chest to create a "clamshell" incision. Thoracic outlet and proximal neck vascular injuries may require median sternotomy with extension above the clavicle up along the ipsilateral sternocleidomastoid muscle.

Retrograde endovascular balloon occlusion of the aorta (REBOA) with the 7-French (Fr) catheter via common femoral access should be considered for patients with suspected abdominal or pelvic injury (Fig. 38.2).[12] In unstable patients, it can be advanced to the descending aorta in the chest and inflated. In stable patients in whom difficulty with proximal control is

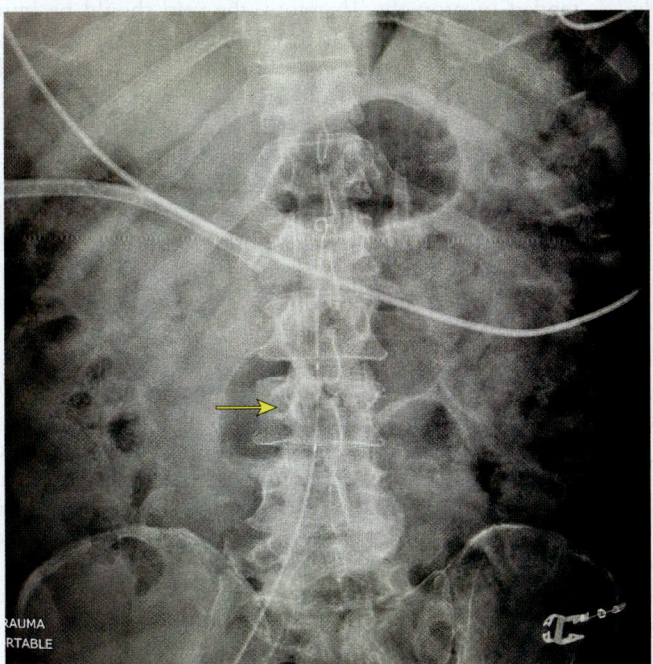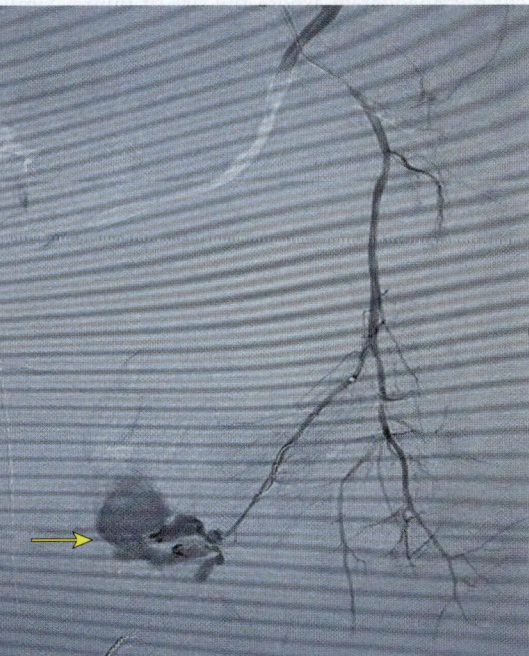

FIGURE 38.2 Plain film on the *left* demonstrates positioning of a resuscitative endovascular occlusion of the aorta balloon *(arrow)* placed in the emergency department for a hypotensive patient with pelvic hemorrhage not responding to a binder and transfusion. The patient was subsequently taken emergently to the hybrid suite for embolization of significant hemorrhage from his left internal iliac artery *(right image and arrow)*.

anticipated, it can be similarly positioned but left uninflated. For abdominal vascular injury, a generous xiphoid-to-pubis incision is needed for adequate exposure.[13] Proximal control for abdominal aortic injuries should be obtained just below the aortic hiatus of the diaphragm or may require a left anterolateral thoracotomy to clamp the distal thoracic aorta. If REBOA or intrathoracic aortic clamping is used, it should be converted to a clamp low on the aorta while providing proximal control as possible to allow visceral artery perfusion to prevent ischemic injury.

In proximal extremity injuries with active hemorrhage, the first incision site is chosen to give the fastest exposure of inflow vessels for clamping. For proximal upper extremity injuries, this may include incisions over the infraclavicular region of the chest to expose the axillary artery. For injuries in the groin, prepare to enter the lower quadrant of the abdomen for access to the external iliac vessels. In mid- and distal extremity vascular injuries associated with active hemorrhage, tourniquets can rapidly obtain control in the trauma resuscitation room. In the operating room, have one team member precisely compress the bleeding site with a gloved hand and a sponge, remove the tourniquet, and prepare the extremity. A heparin bolus is then given, if appropriate, the extremity is prepared and draped, and a sterile tourniquet is placed proximal to the wound and inflated. The injury site can then be explored in a controlled fashion, with clamps or vessel loops placed above and below the vascular injury. In certain injuries, distal arterial occlusion and retrograde intraluminal insertion of a Fogarty catheter with a stopcock to maintain balloon inflation will provide rapid hemorrhage control.[5]

Incisions used to manage vascular injuries are often the same as those used to manage elective cases but are generally more generous. The use of smaller incisions may lead to errors in identifying the extent of vascular injury, adequately controlling branch vessel hemorrhage, and identifying associated venous lacerations. This is particularly true for popliteal artery and vein injuries. A limited approach with separate medial above- and below-knee incisions will not adequately expose the site of injury. Similarly, the posterior approach with the patient prone is not recommended because of the difficulty in obtaining adequate proximal and distal exposure for both vascular repair and bleeding control of associated venous injuries. A medial incision from the proximal popliteal space to the distal popliteal space with division of the medial head of the gastrocnemius muscle and the semimembranosus and semitendinosus muscles with full exposure of the popliteal artery and vein and the tibial nerve provides adequate exposure. This ensures adequate vascular control and the opportunity for successful repair. Closure of the wound to include approximation of the divided muscles yields an excellent functional result. Dividing the inguinal ligament in the groin, dividing the pectoralis major in the axilla, and removing the midclavicle may rarely be necessary. In each of these areas, rapid endovascular balloon occlusion offers an excellent adjunct to proximal control. In the presence of life-threatening hemorrhage that cannot be controlled by any other approach, these structures should not stand in the way of adequate exposure and control.

Once both proximal and distal control of the vessel has been achieved, careful dissection can then be carried out to identify the site of injury. The injury can typically be found within a hematoma extending into surrounding soft tissue. Once the injury is identified and characterized, the decision is made regarding definitive repair or damage control with a temporary shunt. This is mainly based on the patient's physiology. Unstable patients should undergo damage control management, whereas stable patients may proceed with definitive repair. Damage control of vascular injuries is discussed in a later section.

Choice of Repair and Vascular Conduits

In preparation for definitive repair, the injured vessel should be debrided back to healthy tissue in all layers, including intima, media, and adventitia. This may require resection of a large portion of vessel; however, this is vital to ensure a healthy repair without further complications such as pseudoaneurysm, thrombosis, or intimal dissection flap. The options for definitive repair of vascular injury include primary closure, patch angioplasty, primary end-to-end anastomosis, or repair with interposition graft. The choice of repair is dictated by the injury type identified. Primary repair of an artery or vein can include direct suturing of a vessel wall injury or an end-to-end repair of two vessel segments that are less than 2 cm apart. The lack of anastomoses and prosthetic material is advantageous; however, there is a risk of dehiscence if under too much tension or luminal narrowing or stenosis.[11]

Vessel injuries that cannot be repaired by primary repair or end-to-end anastomosis will require an interposition graft. The most desirable graft is autologous great saphenous vein harvested from an uninjured leg.[5] Native vein graft is preferable because it has elastic properties that make it compliant with the normal pulsatile flow of an artery; it has a diameter that approximates that of an extremity artery, producing an adequate size match for grafting in the arm and leg; it is not thrombogenic; and it has superior long-term patency in elective vascular surgery compared with prosthetic material when it is used with smaller vessels (popliteal and tibial). The cephalic vein and lesser saphenous vein have been suggested as suitable second choices, but the cephalic vein is less muscular than the greater saphenous and, like the lesser saphenous, may present problems with harvesting in a trauma patient.[5] Also, upper extremity venous access becomes compromised when the cephalic vein is used. It is imperative to remember, however, that venous valves may impair or fully occlude flow if not attended to properly. Therefore, the vein should be implanted in reverse orientation, or if this is not possible, a valvulotomy may be performed. Venous side branches should also be ligated to prevent extravasation from the repair and should be done in a fashion that avoids venous stenosis or kinking.[14]

The saphenous vein may not be suitable in all instances because of inadequate size or because it has been traumatized or harvested previously. In such cases, a prosthetic conduit may be needed. Initial experiences with the use of prosthetic material (e.g., Dacron) in traumatic vascular injuries were not good. Rich and Hughes reported a complication rate of 77% (infection and thrombosis were the most common) in 26 patients.[15] However, more recent experience with newer graft material (polytetrafluoroethylene [PTFE]) has shown improved patency (70%–90% short term) and rare infection (even in contaminated wounds).[16] Early rates of patency with PTFE grafts are equivalent to those with vein for injuries proximal to the popliteal artery and in the brachial artery. Distal to these levels, PTFE is inferior to vein for popliteal and more distal vessels and in the arm and leg. PTFE grafts of less than 6 mm should not be used.[16] PTFE and vein grafts must be covered, or there is a significant risk of hemorrhage from desiccation of the vein, with subsequent autolysis or breakdown of the anastomosis.[12,16]

Intraoperative Imaging and Noninvasive Evaluation

The successful management of vascular injury requires precisely knowing the status of blood flow in the area of the vessel injury.

Preoperative imaging with catheter angiography or CTA is not always possible. In addition, when a vascular repair has been completed, the presence of thrombus, kinking, or unexpected technical problems may cause early failure. Intraoperative imaging is therefore an important part of assessing the injured vessels and the repair site.[5] Either single-injection radiography or fluoroscopy is effective in providing images in the operating room. Intraoperative duplex scanning is also effective but requires significant training and experience for it to be performed adequately. Handheld continuous-wave Doppler interrogation can be helpful but requires considerable experience to be used effectively. Measurements of ankle or wrist pressure may be misleading because of regional vasospasm in the proximal injured extremity, resulting in a reduced distal pressure compared with the uninjured leg. Intraoperative radiographic imaging remains the most accurate and useful method to detect technical problems with a vascular repair or determine the presence of thrombus in the runoff vessels distal to a repair. Routine completion arteriography after vascular repairs will yield findings of clinical importance in approximately 10% of patients.[5] All postrepair assessments should be accurately documented and communicated among the care team. The first 24 to 48 hours after a vascular repair are the most critical for identifying potential complications, and patients should ideally be admitted to an intensive care unit (ICU) for frequent hourly neurovascular monitoring.[17]

Role of Tissue Coverage

All vascular repairs must be covered to prevent desiccation and disruption. In crushed or badly mangled extremities, this can be a difficult challenge. Rotation of regional muscle or skin flaps may be required. The early involvement of a plastic and reconstructive surgeon is essential to obtain tissue coverage when there is extensive soft tissue injury or loss. Local muscle can be advanced into the wound at the initial operation. If there is a large, contaminated wound and local muscle viability is questionable, early reexploration and preparation for a free flap should be considered. On occasion, tissue loss may be so extensive that an extraanatomic course for an interposition graft may be required. Attention to coverage is also essential in damage control procedures to avoid shunt dislodgment during dressing changes.

Common Errors and Pitfalls

The management of vascular injuries is challenging. An organized approach is necessary to avoid the common errors and pitfalls. One of the most common errors is the lack of recognition of an extremity vascular injury in a patient with multiple torso injuries. Failure to recognize and adequately treat compartment syndrome is another error that is all too common and has devastating consequences. In torso injuries to the great vessels, failure to adequately expose and control the injured site can lead to a rapid death from exsanguination. Finally, failure to recognize the need for damage control techniques and a rapid completion of the operation in an unstable patient can also be deadly. The condition of the patient determines the timing of definitive vascular repair after damage control. Hemorrhage must be controlled, coagulopathy and acidosis corrected, and temperature normalized. An organized approach to the trauma patient mitigates errors.

PRINCIPLES OF ENDOVASCULAR MANAGEMENT

Minimal Vascular Injury and Nonoperative Management

The widespread application of CTA in the evaluation of injured vessels results in the detection of clinically insignificant lesions.[18]

There is now an extensive body of experience with lesions that are not limb or life threatening. These minimal vascular injuries include intimal irregularity, small nonocclusive intimal flaps, focal spasm with minimal narrowing, and small pseudoaneurysms. They are often asymptomatic and usually do not progress.[5,18]

A small, nonocclusive intimal flap is the most commonly encountered clinically insignificant minimal vascular injury. The likelihood that it will progress to cause either occlusion or distal embolization is approximately 10% or less.[5,18] This progression, if it occurs, will be early in the postinjury course. Spasm is another common minimal vascular injury. This finding should resolve promptly after initial discovery. Failure of the return of normal extremity perfusion pressure indicates that a more serious vascular injury is present, and intervention is needed. Small pseudoaneurysms are more likely to progress to the point of needing repair and must be actively observed with duplex color flow imaging. Arteriovenous fistulas always enlarge over time and should be promptly repaired.

There is extensive evidence supporting nonoperative therapy for many asymptomatic lesions. However, successful nonoperative therapy requires continuous surveillance for subsequent progression, occlusion, or hemorrhage. Operative therapy is required for thrombosis, symptoms of chronic ischemia, and failure of small pseudoaneurysms to resolve.[18]

Endovascular Management

Endovascular repair of vascular injuries is increasingly common.[19,20] This approach has become particularly effective in stable large-vessel injuries and in areas difficult to expose for direct repair. However, despite advances in endovascular techniques and devices, this approach has not supplanted open surgery in the management of most peripheral vascular injuries. Endovascular therapy for atherosclerotic arterial disease has become the first choice in management. Endoluminal stent deployment for occlusive lesions and stent graft for aortic aneurysms have become widely accepted. However, there is a strong tendency to generalize from this elective experience in elderly patients with atherosclerosis to the treatment of younger patients with acute vascular injuries. The evidence to support these approaches in preference to traditional open techniques in peripheral arterial injuries is yet to be demonstrated, and there have been problems.[5,20] The striking decrease in open vascular surgical experience among general surgeons and vascular surgeons trained in the 21st century creates a lack of comfort and competence in performing open vascular repairs.[21] A balanced approach using each of these techniques where they best apply, supported by clinical evidence, is essential to good outcomes in patients with vascular trauma.

Endovascular Operating Rooms

There is a widespread proliferation of "hybrid" operating rooms. These high-technology suites have both advanced imaging capability and traditional operating room properties. They require a major commitment of resources and personnel to be effective. They are ideal for complex elective endovascular cases. Not all trauma centers have hybrid operating rooms, or if they do, they may not be able to staff them on an emergency basis for the often-after-hours management of vascular trauma.

Many centers do, however, have highly functional hybrid rooms with high-resolution digital subtraction C-arm fluoroscopy equipment, mobile cabinets with the appropriate catheters and stent grafts, and on-call technical staff. They can create hybrid suite capabilities in an operating room large enough for the C-arm and the rolling cabinets with a standard orthopedic surgery operating table that accommodates fluoroscopy. An unstable trauma patient taken directly to the operating room with a major vascular injury or solid organ hemorrhage can be placed on a radiolucent surgery table and then be managed with all the functionality of a dedicated hybrid operating room. Many trauma centers already provide these mobile capabilities to their vascular surgeons performing elective endovascular abdominal aortic aneurysm repair. All trauma centers need to develop this capacity for their trauma patients. Rooms such as these allow for the expedient treatment of the subset of trauma patients who may require and benefit from simultaneous endovascular and open surgical interventions.

Vascular Access

Once the choice for endovascular approach is made, arterial and/or venous access options must be considered. After open cutdown, nearly any adequately sized vessel may be cannulated, including the common carotid, iliac, and aorta, if necessary. Percutaneous access may also be achieved at numerous sites, including venous access at the basilic, cephalic, subclavian, internal jugular, saphenous, popliteal, and common femoral veins and arterial access at the common femoral, popliteal, radial, brachial, axillary, and pedal arteries. When considering access site, one must consider the feasibility of endovascular methods from this site, the ability to maintain hemostasis after sheath removal or convert to open cutdown if necessary, and what downstream tissue may be affected by either partial or complete flow occlusion during sheath placement.[22]

Although numerous access sites exist, the majority of percutaneous interventions may be achieved through retrograde access to the common femoral artery.[22] This site should ideally be accessed below the inguinal ligament, demarcated by the line between the anterior-superior iliac spine and the pubic tubercle, to decrease the risk of retroperitoneal hemorrhage. Access may be obtained through palpation and use of anatomic landmarks alone; however, ultrasound guidance greatly facilitates safe and successful cannulation if available. Ideally, a standard 18-G or micropuncture 21-G access needle should be passed through a noncalcified portion of the common femoral artery overlying the femoral head, to allow for compression for hemostasis, and 1 cm proximal to the bifurcation into the superficial femoral and profunda arteries. Once percutaneous access is achieved, a guidewire may be advanced through the access needle, and the needle may be then exchanged for a sheath. The sheath should then be flushed with heparinized saline, and placement should be confirmed with fluoroscopy.

Upon completion of the endovascular procedure, hemostasis should be achieved after removal of the sheath to prevent hematoma or pseudoaneurysm formation. Sheaths up to 7 Fr may be safely removed with only manual pressure to the access site. Commonly, pressure is held immediately proximal to the puncture site for 3 minutes per French size in sheath diameter (e.g., 21 minutes for a 7-Fr sheath). Additionally, various percutaneous arteriotomy closure devices are currently available on today's market. Broadly, these devices either place an extravascular plug onto the artery or place a percutaneous suture through the arteriotomy for closure.[22] Both types of closure devices should be managed only by those trained to do so because misuse carries the risk of complications such as arterial thrombosis, distal emboli, dissection, hemorrhage, and infection.

Endovascular Management of Torso Vascular Injuries

Endovascular techniques offer a variety of options for hemorrhage control in the torso. Intraarterial catheter-directed embolization has become a mainstay of the management of solid organ hemorrhage in the abdomen. Whether it is used as the sole treatment or in combination with open procedures, this approach has been effective in liver, spleen, and kidney injuries. Less commonly used intraarterial balloon occlusion for proximal control is a promising adjunct to open repair.[12,23] The availability of REBOA is growing, and in many institutions, it has become common practice in the same clinical setting of exsanguinating abdominal hemorrhage in which an aortic cross-clamp in the chest is needed. In trauma centers with appropriately trained surgeons and proper equipment, these techniques are quick, accurate, and easily performed. The reluctance to adopt new and promising technology must be avoided, and trauma surgeons need to either add surgeons or radiologists with endovascular capabilities to their specialty physician call panels or obtain the training themselves.

The early use of catheter-directed control of hemorrhage associated with pelvic fracture is an effective method of limiting blood loss and improving outcome.[24] This approach is well tolerated and has proved superior to open attempts at hemorrhage control by packing in most patients. Unstable patients benefit from an immediate trip to the operating room. If intraoperative endovascular capability is present, a combined approach may offer the best results.

Endovascular stent graft placement for the management of select great vessel injuries has become the procedure of choice (Fig. 38.3).[25,26] New devices with better proximal fixation seem to be preventing many of the early catastrophic graft failures of older devices. A comparison of the relative degree of risk of endovascular techniques to open repair reveals why this newer approach has gained widespread application.[26,27] Lifelong CT imaging is necessary because of the possibility of delayed endoleak and the possible loss of device fixation as the aorta enlarges over time. There is a definite role for covered stents in proximal branches of the aorta in both the thorax and abdomen. In stable injuries at risk for delayed hemorrhage or thrombosis, carefully placed stents have the potential to lower morbidity compared with open procedures that require extensive operative dissection for exposure and control. Endoluminal management with stent grafts appears most effective in those torso injuries that are surgically inaccessible with the potential for significant hemorrhage in stable patients. These techniques should be used only in centers with an active elective endovascular practice that has experience in treating trauma patients.

Endovascular Management of Cerebrovascular Vascular Injuries

Endovascular techniques offer advantages in anatomic regions where direct operative control is difficult or impossible. For example, hemorrhage from a penetrating injury at the base of the skull is extremely difficult to control. Catheter-directed placement of coils, balloons, or hemostatic agents in the injured carotid or vertebral artery could be lifesaving. The use of balloon occlusion to achieve proximal control may negate the need for a larger operation with increased morbidity, such as a sternotomy for zone I neck injuries. Care must be taken, however, to choose the correct balloon size for occlusion, given the risk of rupture.

Embolization is another tool that may be safely and selectively used in cerebrovascular injury (Fig. 38.4). The external carotid and its branches may be safely embolized, and embolization has

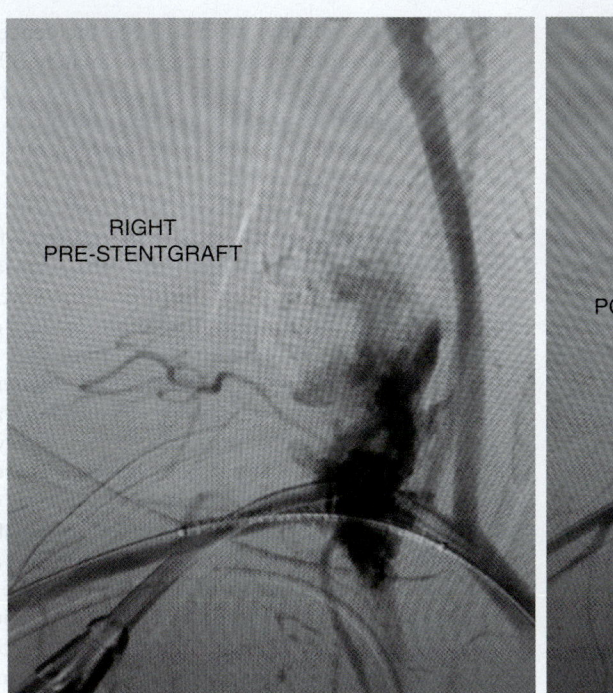
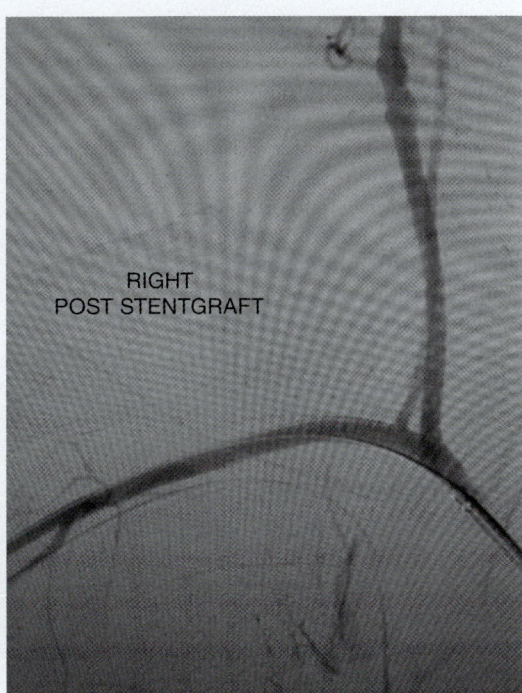

FIGURE 38.3 Right subclavian artery injury with demonstrated active extravasation on angiogram *(left panel)*. Subsequent endovascular stent graft deployment and repair of the injury with completion angiogram *(right panel)*.

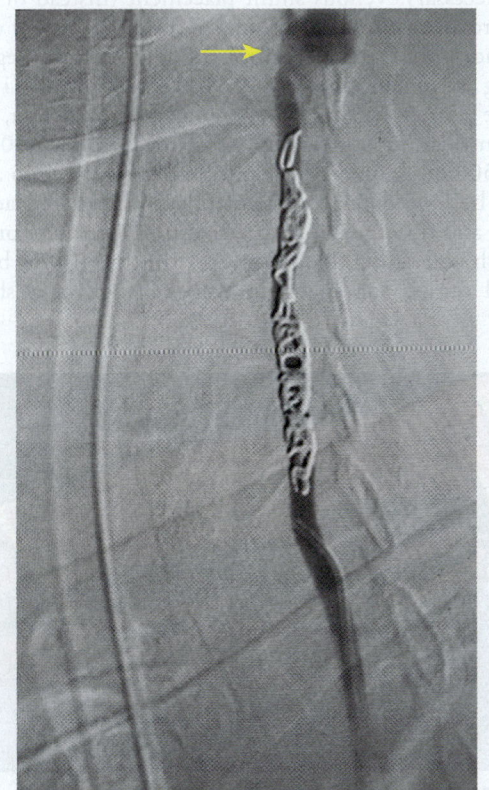

FIGURE 38.4 Penetrating vertebral artery injury managed with coil embolization. *Yellow arrow* points to point of injury with extravasation of contrast.

become the preferred management in stable patients with isolated injuries. Proximal embolization of a nondominant vertebral artery may also be used in select patients, with good outcomes.[4]

Stent placement initially appeared less effective than anticoagulation in partially occluded injuries without associated hemorrhage.[28] However, the role of stents in cerebrovascular trauma continues to evolve, and stents may prove to be safe.[29,30] For internal carotid artery injuries in zone III, which are technically difficult to access through an open approach, bare-metal stents have become a safe and useful management strategy. This use of endoluminal cerebrovascular interventions requires significant expertise and experience. If such experience does not exist at the receiving hospital, consideration should be given to transferring the patient to a medical center with experience in this mode of therapy.

Endovascular Management of Extremity Vascular Injuries

The use of stent grafts in extremity vascular injuries is becoming more common.[19,20] The long-term results, however, have not been documented, and caution should be used in considering this type of treatment. In hemodynamically stable patients with contained hemorrhage, difficult-to-access proximal subclavian or iliac arterial injuries may be effectively treated with covered stents. In the extremities distal to these areas, autologous vein interposition grafts have excellent long-term patency rates and remain the gold standard for vascular repairs.

The loss of open vascular surgery experience in general surgery residencies and vascular fellowships has resulted in many trauma and vascular surgeons resorting to endovascular repair in the extremities. This trend is particularly dangerous in the popliteal artery, where there is a high risk of stent or endograft thrombosis and subsequent limb-threatening ischemia. Early patency of endovascular repairs can be, unfortunately, followed by delayed thrombosis, with an extremely high rate of severe distal ischemia. Open repair with suitable saphenous vein interposition graft placement is the best approach, and the results of all other techniques need to be compared with this traditional standard treatment.

Catheter-directed therapies for controlling hemorrhage from large branch vessels in the extremities are often effective and sufficient to manage these injuries. Endoluminal treatment is used sparingly for pseudoaneurysms of extremity arteries. Small pseudoaneurysms are likely to resolve without any intervention, and large pseudoaneurysms are best treated with open techniques because the risk of arterial thrombosis or distal embolization is high with this endovascular intervention.

Who Should Perform Endovascular Repairs?

Successful management of vascular injuries requires that the most qualified person do the indicated intervention in the appropriate patient in the appropriate place at the appropriate time. Endovascular surgery is an operative procedure and, like all operations, should be performed by readily available trained clinicians who not only are cognizant of the technical aspects of a procedure but also are knowledgeable about the disease for which the procedure is being performed. In many centers, this person is the interventional radiologist. Other centers have catheter-trained vascular surgeons, and a few others have trauma surgeons who are capable of performing endovascular procedures. Catheter skills training is being integrated into many surgical critical care fellowships and may subsequently become more available in the near future at many trauma centers.

Endoluminal management of vascular trauma does not require a full endovascular hybrid operating room, as explained before. Planning and preparation, however, are essential for the endovascular capability, which, more often than not, is needed in the middle of the night. Preparing a team that can perform these techniques and can organize the appropriate equipment with brief notice requires commitment, dedication, collaboration, and training.

PRINCIPLES OF DAMAGE CONTROL

Vascular Damage Control

Damage control has gained wide acceptance in trauma surgery and is directed at rapid control of hemorrhage and closure of enteric wounds so that the patient can be warmed and resuscitated. The choice between definitive, time-consuming vascular repair and temporary measures that achieve control must be made early in care of patients with vascular injury and hypovolemic shock. This is particularly important when an extremity vascular injury is associated with major torso injuries. Damage control strategies in vascular surgery focus on rapid hemorrhage control and restoration of end-organ perfusion. Hemorrhage control mainstays include tourniquet and ligation and, in extreme instances, amputation. Temporary restoration of blood flow is accomplished using intraluminal shunts, with the addition of fasciotomy as needed. Intraaortic balloon tamponade with REBOA has also emerged as a temporary method of hemorrhage control while simultaneously improving end-organ perfusion.

Hemorrhage Control

Field tourniquet use was repopularized during recent US military conflicts and was a large success.[31] The associated morbidity in

combat was overall low, with a 1.5% incidence of nerve palsy, 0.4% risk of amputation, and approximately 30% rate of fasciotomy in those left for greater than 2 hours.[32] Similarly, tourniquet use in civilian practice has been found to be effective for prehospital control of extremity hemorrhage and has been associated with improved survival.[24]

Ligation should be reserved for vessels with adequate distal collateral flow in patients who are too unstable for definitive repair. In the torso, this includes the subclavian and innominate arteries, the celiac artery, and the inferior mesenteric artery. In the upper extremity, proximal injuries of the axillary artery and distal injuries to either the radial or ulnar artery may be ligated, provided there is evidence of adequate distal collateral flow assessed by either physical examination or continuous-wave Doppler interrogation. In the groin, profunda femoris artery injuries can be ligated if the common and superficial femoral arteries (SFAs) are intact. Similarly, in the lower extremity, ligation of a single tibial artery or the peroneal artery can be performed after a similar assessment. If distal perfusion is compromised, an intraluminal shunt should be inserted rather than ligating the vessel. Superior mesenteric artery (SMA) ligation is associated with a high risk of bowel necrosis, and damage control is best accomplished with placement of an intraluminal shunt. In the extremities, ligation of the brachial, external iliac, superficial femoral, or popliteal artery has a high likelihood of producing limb-threatening ischemia and should be avoided, if possible.

Temporary Restoration of Blood Flow

A variety of commercially available shunts can be used for damage control (Fig. 38.5). If these are not available, sterile intravenous tubing is of adequate size to "shunt" both the artery and the vein, if necessary. Venous shunt placement (instead of ligation) may improve extremity perfusion and lower the risk of compartment syndrome. Damage control shunt placement begins with obtaining adequate proximal and distal control. Thrombus should be cleared with a Fogarty embolectomy catheter, followed by the instillation of regional heparinized saline (5000 units heparin/500 mL saline). The shunt should be placed in a straight line and be long enough to remain safely held in place in the proximal and distal vessel with a tied umbilical tape or 2-0 silk tie at each end. Long, looped shunts run the risk of becoming dislodged during subsequent dressing changes and should be

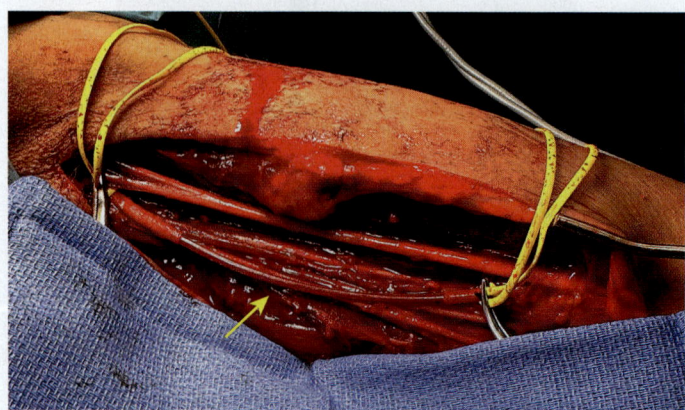

FIGURE 38.5 Brachial artery injury with large missing segment from penetrating injury. A temporary vascular shunt *(arrow)* was used to restore perfusion while the patient was resuscitated, and saphenous vein harvest was undertaken for interposition repair.

avoided. The ties securing the shunt cause intimal damage, and those portions of the artery must be resected at the time of definitive vascular repair.

Role of Fasciotomy

Failure to perform an adequate fasciotomy after revascularization of an acutely ischemic limb is the most common cause of preventable limb loss.[5] Calf compartment syndrome is the most common indication for fasciotomy. Forearm and thigh compartment syndromes are less common. Any muscle group can develop compartment syndrome, including those in the hands and feet.

Compartment syndrome may be manifested immediately or delayed to 12 to 24 hours after reperfusion. If it is not promptly diagnosed and treated, the risk of limb loss or limb dysfunction is high. Calf compartment syndrome most commonly results from prolonged ischemia or a crush injury. Frequent physical examinations augmented with compartment pressure measurements are necessary to detect this complication in its early stage. The first clinical findings are pain and loss of light-touch sensation in the distribution of the nerve in the compartment. The diagnosis of compartment syndrome should be suspected in any patient complaining of increasing pain after injury. Other physical findings include a tense compartment, pain on passive range of motion, progressive loss of sensation, and weakness. The loss of arterial pulses is a late finding, which usually indicates a poor prognosis. Neurologic signs and symptoms, although helpful, are neither sensitive nor specific in the upper extremity after arterial injury because associated peripheral nerve injury often exists. A high index of suspicion is especially needed in patients who are intubated and sedated, and measurement of compartment pressures can be especially useful in such cases. The normal tissue compartment pressure ranges from 0 to 9 mm Hg. Much controversy exists about what constitutes a pathologic elevation. However, the safest approach is to perform fasciotomy when compartment pressure exceeds 25 mm Hg.[5,33]

A compartment syndrome can also develop in either the upper arm (triceps, deltoid, or along the axillary sheath) or the forearm. The forearm compartment syndrome is more common. Increased tissue pressure can follow either blunt or penetrating trauma because of hematoma, posttraumatic transudation of serum into the interstitial space, venous thrombosis, or reperfusion after ischemia.[33] The possibility of a compartment syndrome must always be a consideration in a patient who has been injured, particularly one with prolonged ischemia before reperfusion.

Role of Immediate Amputation

A very limited role for primary amputation exists in the management of complex extremity vascular injuries. Patients with extensive soft tissue loss, neurologic deficit, extensive fractures, and vascular injuries should be evaluated collaboratively with orthopedic, neurosurgical, and plastic and reconstructive surgery colleagues to determine if primary amputation is the best initial management. Scoring systems to predict the need for amputation have not been useful.[34] Because of the emotional impact of amputation and because marginally viable tissue often takes hours to demarcate or declare, it may be best to proceed with initial intraoperative evaluation and documentation (pictures, radiographs, and consultation), damage control using intravascular shunts for the vascular injuries, and a second look in 24 hours. The interval of time allows communication with the patient and the family and a more planned approach. Immediate amputation should also be considered in patients

with extensive soft tissue, bone, and neurovascular disruption who have life-threatening torso injuries, as mentioned earlier in the discussion of damage control techniques. If immediate amputation is required, extensive documentation of the extremity injury, with photographs (Fig. 38.6) placed in the medical record, will be helpful in later explaining the decision to the patient and family and will help with their acceptance of this drastic surgical procedure.

Resuscitative Endovascular Balloon Occlusion of the Aorta

Intraaortic balloon tamponade for trauma was first described during the Korean War and has made a comeback in recent years.[35] REBOA consists of a catheter with an inflatable balloon near the tip that is inserted via the common femoral artery into the aorta as a minimally invasive alternative to open thoracotomy and cross-clamping of the aorta to control hemorrhage below the diaphragm. This has been shown to improve overall survival, mainly in patients not requiring cardiopulmonary resuscitation.[36,37]

Although its minimally invasive nature and simple design are attractive, the use of REBOA remains a polarizing topic in trauma as the precise indications continue to be elucidated. The generally agreed-upon indication is for obtaining temporary hemorrhage control from abdominal, pelvic, and junctional injuries for patients in extremis.[38] There are three zones of occlusion where REBOA can be placed, which is determined by the suspected location of injury. Zone I is the descending thoracic aorta from the left subclavian to celiac trunk, zone II is the aorta between the celiac trunk to the lowest renal artery ("zone of nonocclusion"), and zone III encompasses the abdominal aorta from the lowest renal artery to the aortic bifurcation. REBOA simultaneously controls noncompressible torso hemorrhage and augments central and cerebral perfusion during aortic occlusion.

The outcomes of REBOA hinge on rapid arterial access and minimal occlusion time, meaning time to definitive hemorrhage control is of utmost importance. These patients are still hemodynamically unstable, and REBOA is a bridge to emergent

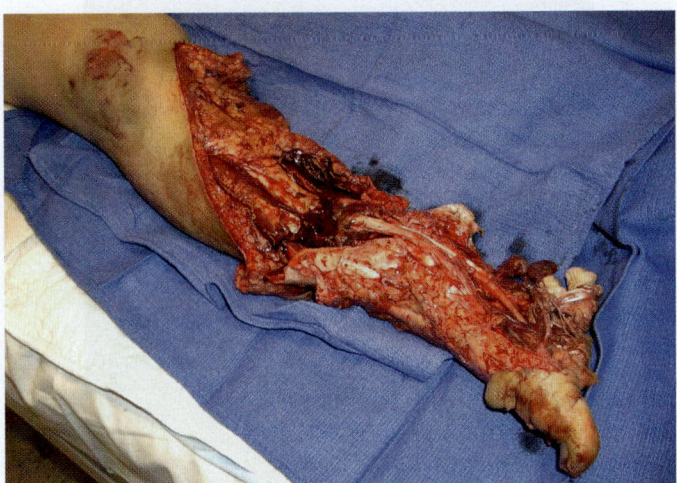

FIGURE 38.6 Major disruption of tissues in a mangled extremity after an auto-versus-pedestrian accident. After consultation with both the patient and their family regarding the severity of nerve, vascular, and soft tissue loss, a collaborative team performed an amputation.

operation. The general steps for placement include (1) determination of appropriate balloon insertion length, (2) femoral artery access below the inguinal ligament (ultrasound guided or cutdown), (3) placement of a 7-Fr sheath, (4) REBOA insertion, (5) REBOA inflation, and (6) REBOA management.[4] Occlusion time should be limited to 30 minutes in zone I and 60 minutes in zone III. Once definitive hemorrhage control has been achieved, the balloon should be deflated gradually over 5 minutes. The catheter and sheath should be removed.

Complications from REBOA include access site hematoma, pseudoaneurysm, thromboembolism, arteriovenous fistula, compartment syndrome, and vessel rupture resulting from inappropriate positioning (Fig. 38.7). These patients are also at high risk for systemic responses secondary to occlusion of the aorta in combination with massive resuscitation, including acute respiratory distress syndrome (ARDS), ischemia-reperfusion injury, acute kidney injury, and multisystem organ failure.[4] A recent analysis of the American College of Surgeons Trauma Quality Improvement Program (TQIP) database found an increased incidence of kidney injury, lower extremity amputation, and mortality in a matched analysis between patients who received REBOA versus those who did not.[39] Furthermore, the recently published UK-REBOA Randomized Clinical Trial compared REBOA to standard care and concluded that in the emergency department, REBOA does not reduce, and may increase, mortality compared with standard care alone.[40] It is imperative for surgeons who use REBOA to be proficient in technical placement and management and optimize patient selection to mitigate complications and improve outcomes in this subset of patients.

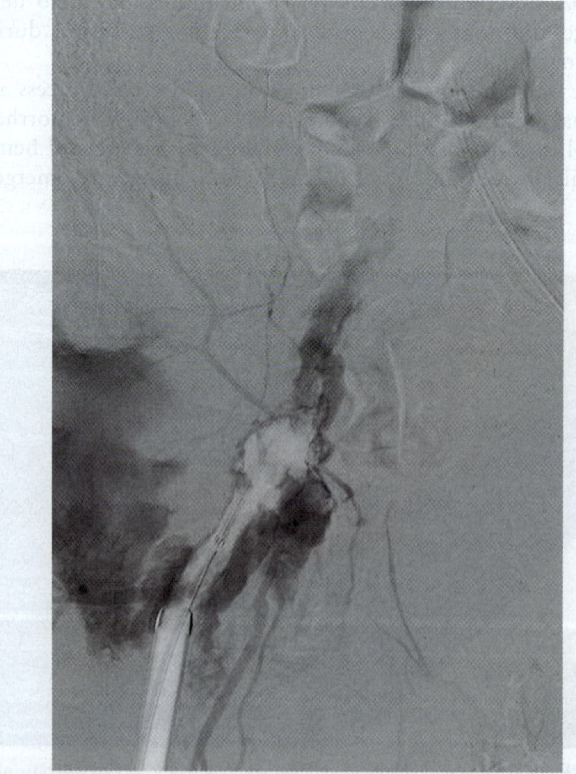

FIGURE 38.7 Angiogram images demonstrating massive extravasation from a right iliac artery rupture after resuscitative endovascular occlusion of the aorta balloon inflation in the iliac artery.

MANAGEMENT OF SPECIFIC INJURIES

Neck Injuries

Vascular injuries of the head, neck, and thoracic outlet are often challenging to manage. Penetrating trauma can injure large vessels, such as the innominate and subclavian arteries, which can lead to exsanguination. Blunt trauma to the carotid and vertebral arteries, collectively known as *blunt cerebrovascular injuries,* is often occult and, if not diagnosed and treated rapidly, can lead to cerebral ischemia, infarction, and possibly death.

Penetrating

The management of penetrating neck trauma has historically been based on the location of the injury relative to the three zones of the neck: zone I, inferior to the cricoid cartilage; zone II, cricoid cartilage to the angle of the mandible; and zone III, cephalad from the angle of the mandible. This anatomic classification required exploration for any zone II injury. This resulted in a high rate of negative neck explorations, with up to 50% being nontherapeutic.[4] The management has since evolved to be more selective, and the paradigm has shifted to a "no-zone" approach. Patients with penetrating neck trauma and hard signs of vascular injury should undergo immediate exploration, regardless of zone. Patients who are hemodynamically stable and without hard signs of vascular injury should be evaluated with physical examination and CTA. The classic zones of neck injury are still helpful in describing the anatomic location, locating potential injured structures, and planning for intervention.

In a stable patient with a suspected vascular injury in either zone I or zone III, vascular imaging is mandatory to confirm the suspicion of vascular injury and plan proximal and distal control.[41] Vascular imaging is also recommended for stable patients with penetrating trauma in zone II, but exploration should be undertaken expeditiously for patients with an expanding hematoma or impending airway compromise (manifested by hoarseness and tracheal deviation).[41] In the unstable patient, a Foley urinary catheter with the balloon inflated can be inserted into the wound to achieve temporary tamponade of injuries in these regions. Conventional angiography can have a dual role for injuries in zone I or zone III. It not only can provide the diagnosis but also may provide a venue for endoluminal management—coiling of bleeding vessels or pseudoaneurysms in zone III or placement of covered stents in zone I.

Vascular injuries of the thoracic outlet are challenging because they involve large-caliber vessels that can be difficult to expose and control. Unstable patients with vascular injury in the region of the thoracic outlet must be expeditiously taken to the operating room. Stable patients should have preoperative imaging with catheter angiography or CTA to locate the injury and determine its extent. This will allow planning for endoluminal treatment or open exposure. Operative control may require a simple supraclavicular incision, a sternotomy, or a combination of the two incisions, depending on the location and extent of the injury. Clamp application on the proximal subclavian and carotid arteries must be precise to avoid injury to the vagus, phrenic, or recurrent laryngeal nerves, all of which reside in this anatomic region. Sternotomy is frequently used for proximal innominate, proximal right subclavian, and proximal right carotid arterial injuries. Left subclavian artery proximal control may be difficult through sternotomy alone and may require concomitant clavicular incision or third intercostal space anterolateral thoracotomy. Distal control of the carotid arteries is obtained by extending the median sternotomy superiorly along the border of the ipsilateral sternocleidomastoid muscle. Distal subclavian arterial control is obtained through a clavicular incision. Resection of the clavicle results in little or no morbidity and can be performed quickly to control hemorrhage if needed. Suturing of the subclavian and axillary arteries must be done with extreme caution. Undue tension or traction will result in a tear of these fragile vessels. Endovascular balloon occlusion, when it is rapidly available, is an excellent adjunctive measure for proximal control.

Blunt Cerebrovascular Injury

Blunt cerebrovascular injuries (BCVIs) are often occult and asymptomatic. Therefore, rapid diagnostic screening is essential and provides the underpinning of successful management.[29,30] Initially, BCVIs were thought to be rare, occurring in about 0.1% of patients, but with use of the screening criteria developed by the group at Denver General Hospital, the incidence is actually 10 to 20 times that.[29] Factors associated with these injuries include displaced midface fractures, basilar skull fracture with carotid canal involvement, cervical spine fracture, closed head injury consistent with diffuse axonal injury and Glasgow Coma Scale score below 6, and blunt neck trauma from hanging or seat-belt injuries. Both carotid and vertebral artery injuries occur from stretching or tearing of the intima of the vessels produced by rapid extreme extension or flexion of the neck or by direct blunt-force injury. The carotid artery is particularly vulnerable where it lies close to the second and sixth cervical transverse processes. The vertebral artery is also vulnerable to stretch injuries and fractures of the transverse process of the cervical vertebrae that involve the foramen transversarium. Cerebrovascular injuries vary from minor intimal irregularities to arterial rupture and severe hemorrhage.[29] The grading of these injuries is detailed in Table 38.2.

Patients who fulfill the Denver criteria should undergo CTA of the neck.[7,29] The treatment of blunt carotid and vertebral artery injuries is antiplatelet or anticoagulation in patients who do not have a contraindication.[28] Antiplatelet agents like aspirin are often the only alternative in patients who cannot be systemically anticoagulated. The use of endovascular techniques has a very limited role, as discussed earlier. However, in patients with carotid injuries at the base of the skull or injuries of the vertebral artery, covered stents or embolization offers the best results.

Chest Injuries

Great Vessels

Penetrating injuries of the intrathoracic great vessels (aorta, superior and inferior venae cava, pulmonary arteries and veins) usually cause death at the time of injury from exsanguination. The small number of patients with penetrating injuries of the intrathoracic great vessels who arrive to the trauma center alive often present with hemodynamic instability and require emergent operative

intervention. Repair of intrathoracic great vessel injuries may be achieved through sternotomy, left or right anterolateral thoracotomy, or in many cases, bilateral (or clamshell) anterolateral thoracotomy.[42] Although many of these structures are exposed through a posterolateral thoracotomy in the elective setting, patients who present in hemorrhagic shock and without a distinct diagnosis should be managed with more versatile incisions, such as median sternotomy and anterolateral thoracotomy.

Injuries to the ascending aorta and the superior or inferior vena cava are best exposed and treated through a median sternotomy.[42] These injuries should be controlled with digital pressure and then placement of a side-biting clamp to allow suture repair of the injury, and they may require cardiopulmonary bypass to achieve repair. Injuries of the descending aorta are ideally approached through a left posterolateral thoracotomy. However, most of these injuries will be discovered during emergent left anterolateral thoracotomy and will need to be quickly repaired. Injuries of the pulmonary arteries and veins can be approached through a sternotomy or anterolateral thoracotomy, depending on their proximity to the heart.[42] If possible, these injuries should be repaired primarily. However, destructive injuries to the pulmonary arteries and veins may necessitate pneumonectomy for definitive control.

As endovascular techniques continue to develop, their role in management of great vessel injury has increased greatly in recent years. The decision for this approach should take into consideration the mechanism of injury, hemodynamic stability, and ease of arterial access. Although, as previously noted, penetrating injuries to this location often lead to expiration in the prehospital setting or severe instability upon initial presentation, blunt injuries may often present in a much more stable manner. These injuries are increasingly being managed with the use of endovascular stents, such as thoracic endovascular aortic repair (TEVAR).[26]

Blunt Thoracic Aortic Injury

Blunt injuries to the intrathoracic great vessels consist primarily of blunt thoracic aortic injury (BTAI). BTAI occurs as a result of high-energy blunt trauma. The most common mechanisms of injury resulting in BTAI are high-speed motor vehicle crashes and falls from a height. The aorta is typically injured in a location where it is relatively fixed (root of the aorta, ligamentum arteriosum, diaphragmatic hiatus), and the majority (85%–90%) of patients die at the scene. Patients with BTAI who arrive at the hospital alive have typically sustained multisystem associated injuries. BTAI must be ruled out when there is a high-energy mechanism of injury or a chest radiograph shows a widened mediastinum. Traditionally, such findings on chest x-ray as widened mediastinum or loss of the aortopulmonary window were thought to be diagnostic for BTAI. However, recent literature has shown these classically taught findings to be unreliable and present in approximately 58% of all patients with BTAI.[43] Definitive diagnosis of BTAI is established with a high-resolution CT scan of the chest. Injuries vary from an intimal injury to pseudoaneurysm or a contained periaortic hematoma just distal to the left subclavian artery.[6]

Once the diagnosis of BTAI is confirmed, the initial management is focused on blood pressure control while addressing associated immediately life-threatening injuries, followed by endovascular repair of higher-grade injuries.[44] Blood pressure is best controlled with a short-acting intravenous β-blocker (e.g., esmolol) that can be titrated to a systolic blood pressure of less than 110 mm Hg while also keeping heart rate below 100 beats/min,

TABLE 38.2	**Grading Scale for Blunt Cerebrovascular Injury (BCVI)**
Grade I	Irregularity of the vessel wall or a dissection/intramural hematoma with ≤25% luminal stenosis
Grade II	Intraluminal thrombus or raised intimal flap is visualized, or dissection/intramural hematoma with >25% luminal narrowing
Grade III	Pseudoaneurysm
Grade IV	Vessel occlusion
Grade V	Vessel transection

should baseline comorbidities and injury burden allow this.[42] If β-blockade does not achieve blood pressure goals, other intravenous agents, such as calcium channel blockers, nitroglycerin, and nitroprusside, may be used. Lower-grade injuries (grade I [intimal tear], grade II [intramural hematoma]) can generally be managed without intervention and only require blood pressure control and repeat imaging (Table 38.3). Grade III injuries (pseudoaneurysm) should be repaired in a delayed fashion after stabilizing other life-threatening injuries. The most severe injuries (grade IV [rupture]) should be managed urgently to prevent exsanguination.

Open repair of BTAI was the mainstay of treatment for decades. Open repair is achieved through a left posterolateral thoracotomy, cardiopulmonary bypass, and placement of a synthetic aortic interposition graft. However, TEVAR has become the standard of care for the surgical management of BTAI. The advent of new and improved stent grafts and the widespread adoption of endovascular techniques have made this approach the first choice at most centers. Although there are no prospective, randomized trials comparing open versus endovascular management of BTAI, there have been two multicenter American Association for the Surgery of Trauma trials showing lower morbidity (spinal

cord ischemia, stroke) and mortality with the endovascular approach.[26,27] However, patients who undergo endovascular repair require lifelong surveillance because there is no information about long-term sequelae of endovascular grafts in the aortic position in young patients. In addition, some young patients may not have favorable anatomy for endovascular repair and still require the open approach.

Abdominal Injuries

Aortoiliac Injuries

Abdominal vascular injuries most often result from penetrating trauma, and all are treated through a generous midline laparotomy.[13] Many of these injuries will require supraceliac control of the aorta to achieve adequate visualization to complete exposure and repair. Penetrating injuries to the abdominal aorta are best exposed and repaired with a left medial visceral rotation that exposes the aorta from the diaphragmatic hiatus to the iliac bifurcation (Fig. 38.8). The injury can typically be controlled with direct digital pressure, which allows time for placement of vascular clamps proximal and distal to the site of injury.[13] Abdominal aortic injuries may be repaired primarily after stab wounds, but gunshot wounds will often require a patch repair or interposition graft. Uncommonly, patients will sustain a blunt abdominal aortic injury without life-threatening hemorrhage, and these injuries are best repaired by endovascular techniques (Fig. 38.9).

The right common, external, and internal iliac arteries are best exposed by widely mobilizing the cecum, whereas injuries to the left iliac arteries are exposed by completely mobilizing the sigmoid colon.[13] Keep in mind the course of the ureter on both sides as it crosses the iliac vessels. Injuries to the common and external

TABLE 38.3	**Grading Scale for Blunt Thoracic Aortic Injury (BTAI)**
Grade I	Intimal tear
Grade II	Intramural hematoma
Grade III	Pseudoaneurysm
Grade IV	Rupture

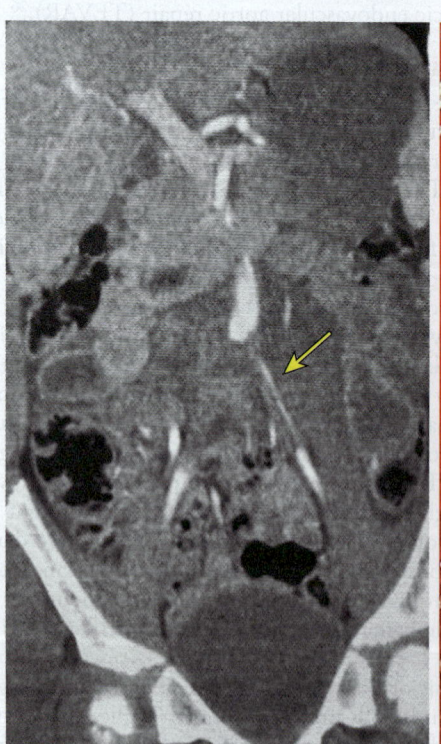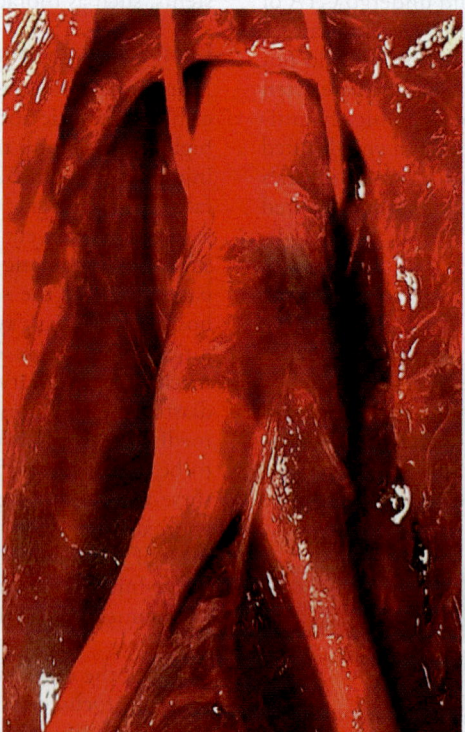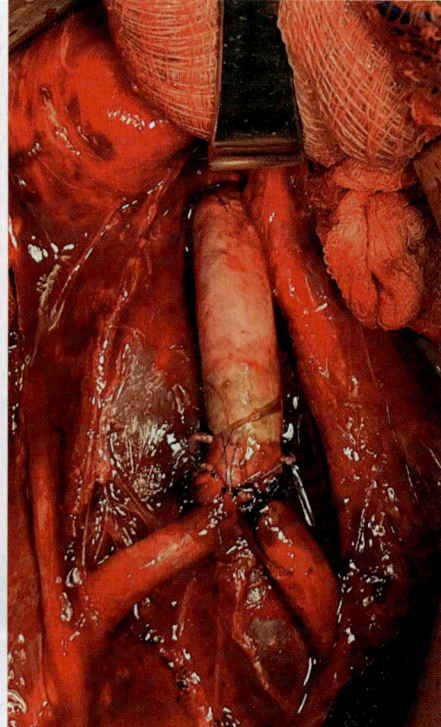

FIGURE 38.8 Pediatric seat-belt injury to the abdominal aorta with aortoiliac occlusion demonstrated on CT *(arrow, left panel)*. Open exposure revealed a contused aorta, and after vascular control and vessel entry, devastating dissection was observed. *Right panel* demonstrates interposition repair and iliac bifurcation reconstruction with cadaveric iliac artery in this very young patient.

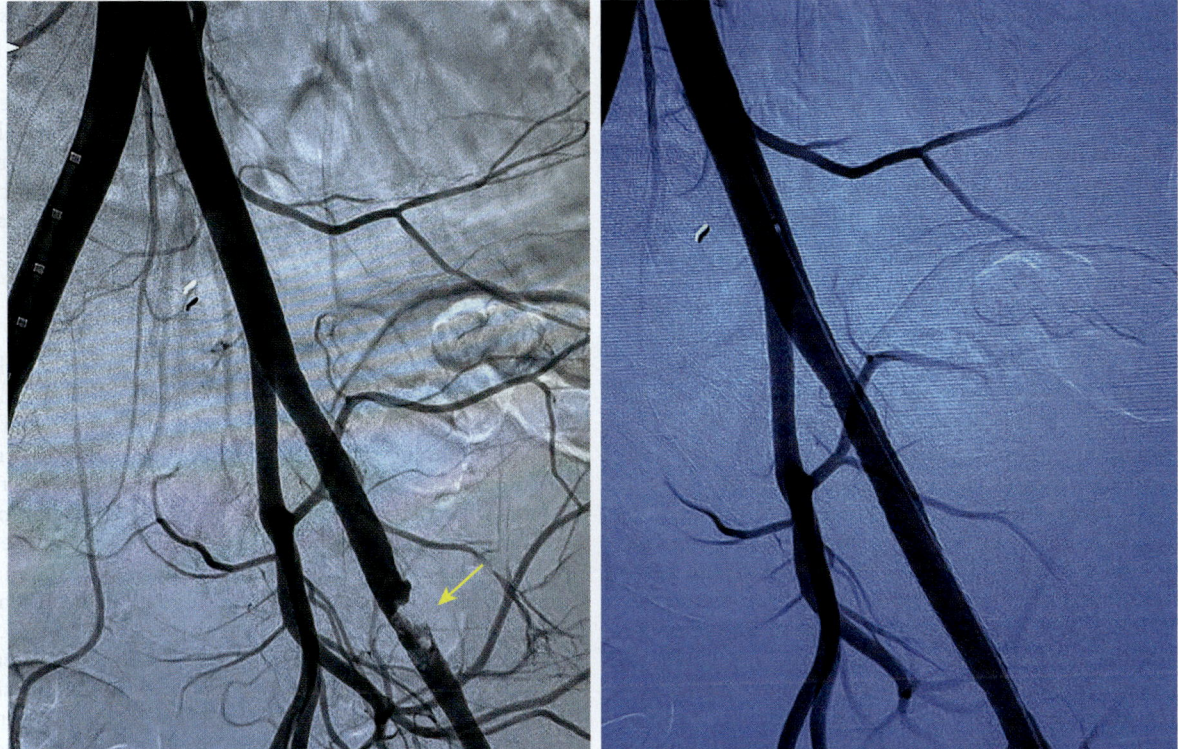

FIGURE 38.9 Blunt left external iliac artery injury *(arrow)*. Angiogram after endovascular repair is demonstrated on the *right*.

iliac arteries are initially controlled with digital pressure to allow proximal and distal control with vascular clamps or vessel loops. Injuries to the common and external iliac arteries may be repaired primarily but will often require a synthetic interposition graft. The common and external iliac arteries should never be ligated; if a patient is hemodynamically unstable, these injuries should be shunted and repaired in a delayed fashion. However, injuries to the internal iliac artery can be routinely ligated.[13]

Mesenteric and Renal Arterial Injuries

Injuries to the mesenteric vessels are some of the most challenging injuries to expose and repair. In the elective setting, the celiac trunk is often approached through the lesser sac, but in the setting of trauma, this may prove difficult because of a large lesser sac hematoma that obscures the usual landmarks. In the setting of trauma, the celiac trunk is best exposed through a wide left medial visceral rotation that mobilizes the spleen and tail of the pancreas but leaves the left kidney in situ.[13] Once exposed, most injuries to the celiac trunk should be ligated because repair is difficult, and ligation is well tolerated in the majority of patients. Although the SMA and celiac trunk take off from the aorta within 1 to 2 cm of each other, the exposure and treatment algorithm for SMA injuries is different. Management of SMA injuries will depend on location based on the Fullen classification: zone I, beneath the pancreas; zone II, between the pancreaticoduodenal and middle colic branches; zone III, beyond the middle colic branch; zone IV, enteric branches. Injuries that present with a large contained central hematoma at the root of the mesentery are best approached with a left medial visceral rotation. Active hemorrhage is controlled by manual compression, followed by left medial visceral rotation.[13] This will allow exposure and control of the aorta proximal and distal to the SMA or direct clamping of the SMA as

it comes off the aorta. Once this control has been achieved, attention is turned anteriorly for definitive exposure and repair of the SMA injury.

Zone I and zone II SMA injuries can be exposed and repaired through the lesser sac by dividing the gastrocolic ligament. The pancreas will need to be retracted inferiorly to expose the origin of the SMA or superiorly to expose the proximal SMA. Uncommonly, in active bleed SMA injuries behind the pancreas, it may need to be divided to completely visualize and control that segment of the SMA. Zone III and zone IV injuries should be approached by reflecting the transverse colon and its mesentery superiorly with or without taking down the ligament of Treitz. All zones of SMA injuries (except distal zone IV injuries) should always be repaired with a primary repair, end-to-end anastomosis, or interposition graft of reversed saphenous vein.[13] If the patient is in extremis, the SMA may be shunted, with a plan for delayed repair.

Penetrating renal vascular injuries are easily exposed on either side after medial visceral rotation. Gerota's fascia is opened, and the kidney is bluntly mobilized into the wound. Once the kidney is mobilized, the vascular injury can be controlled with direct manual pressure while proximal and distal control is obtained with vessel loops. Renal artery injuries can be managed with primary repair, end-to-end anastomosis, vein patch, interposition graft, or nephrectomy (after confirming a normal contralateral kidney by palpation). Treatment of renal artery injuries is based on complexity of the injury and physiologic status of the patient. Combined injuries to the renal artery and vein should be treated with nephrectomy in unstable patients. Renal artery injuries rarely occur after blunt trauma. These injuries may be managed nonoperatively, with expected involution of the affected kidney or nephrectomy. It is uncommon to successfully salvage renal function with vascular reconstruction of complete blunt renal artery occlusion. Management must consider several factors, including overall status of the patient, warm ischemia time, and need for laparotomy for associated intraabdominal injuries.

Abdominal Venous Injuries

The inferior vena cava is exposed with a right medial visceral rotation that exposes the vena cava from the iliac vein confluence to the inferior edge of the liver.[13] Injury to the vena cava is best controlled with direct digital pressure, with subsequent proximal and distal control using sponge sticks or vessel loops. Lumbar tributaries and renal veins may also need to be controlled to clearly visualize and repair the injury. Injuries to the anterior or lateral surfaces of the vena cava can most often be repaired primarily as long as the repair does not narrow the lumen more than 50%. Penetrating injuries to the vena cava may be through-and-through injuries and require repair of a posterior injury as well. Injuries to the posterior vena cava may be repaired through the anterior injury, or the vena cava may be mobilized after ligating and dividing lumbar veins. Complex injuries may require patch repair, interposition graft, shunting with delayed reconstruction, or ligation.[13] The complexity of repair will depend on the physiologic status of the patient and the location of the injury. Hemodynamically unstable patients with ongoing hemorrhage are not candidates for complex repairs and should have the vena cava ligated or shunted. Hemodynamically stable patients with injuries at or above the level of the renal veins may be candidates for complex reconstruction, but ligation is still an option for the exsanguinating patient.[13]

Iliac veins are exposed in the same manner as iliac arteries. Exposure is made more challenging by the location of the confluence of the iliac veins with the inferior vena cava directly posterior to the right common iliac artery. It will need to be widely mobilized to allow access to the confluence of the iliac veins. However, we do not advocate division of the right iliac artery to achieve exposure of the iliac vein confluence. Once the common, external, and internal iliac veins are exposed, the injury is best controlled with direct digital pressure; then proximal and distal control may be achieved with vessel loops. If possible, simple injuries to the iliac veins should be repaired with primary venorrhaphy. However, complex repairs of destructive injuries to the iliac veins should not be attempted, and these injuries should be ligated.[13]

The superior mesenteric vein (SMV) can be exposed in the same fashion as the SMA. SMV injuries should be repaired or reconstructed when possible, although shunting with delayed repair is also an option. The SMV may be ligated for patients in extremis who would otherwise exsanguinate. Injuries to the inferior mesenteric artery may be ligated if there is adequate collateral flow from the middle colic branch of the SMA and the inferior and middle hemorrhoidal branches of the internal iliac arteries. The inferior mesenteric vein may be safely ligated if required.

The portal vein runs close to the inferior vena cava and is the most posterior structure within the portal triad, closely associated with the common bile duct and hepatic artery. Portal vein injuries are initially controlled with direct manual pressure. A right medial visceral rotation, including a generous Kocher maneuver, is performed to expose and visualize the lateral and inferior portal vein. The common bile duct and hepatic artery will need to be mobilized to expose the anterior surface of the portal vein. Similar to SMA and SMV exposure, the neck of the pancreas may need to be divided to visualize the entirety of the portal vein.[13] These injuries should be managed in the same fashion as SMV injuries,

with repair or reconstruction in the majority of cases, shunting and delayed repair if necessary, and ligation only for patients in extremis who would otherwise exsanguinate.

Renal vein injuries can be repaired with primary venorrhaphy or ligation. On the right, ligation of the renal vein will require a nephrectomy, and patch angioplasty or interposition graft may be considered in stable patients. The left renal vein may be safely ligated near the inferior vena cava because of collateral flow through the left adrenal, gonadal, and lumbar veins.[13]

Extremity Injuries

Upper Extremity

Penetrating injury often presents with a history of either arterial hemorrhage or ongoing bleeding. Blunt injury usually causes thrombosis and the signs of acute arterial occlusion with resultant ischemia. Significant neurologic injury, usually involving the median nerve, is present in 60% of patients with upper extremity arterial injury.[5,45] Concomitant venous injury is common. In the setting of multisystem injury, arterial occlusion in the upper extremity is easily missed. Delay in diagnosis resulting in prolonged ischemia is an important contributing factor to preventable limb loss or long-term disability from irreversible ischemic nerve injury. All significant vascular injuries of the upper extremity result in clinical findings that are apparent on thorough physical examination. Unfortunately, associated severe torso or lower extremity injuries distract the trauma team from the injured and ischemic upper extremity. Delays in diagnosis and treatment are common in collected series of patients with upper extremity arterial injury and are more common after blunt-force trauma.[5,45]

The diagnosis of upper extremity arterial injury is often made on physical examination alone, particularly in penetrating injuries. Noninvasive evaluation of the injured upper extremity adds little to a thorough history and physical examination. Patients with obvious arterial or venous lacerations from penetrating trauma or those with blunt trauma and hard findings should be taken directly to the operating room. The arterial bed of the upper extremity is extremely reactive to vasoconstriction produced by hypovolemic shock, pain, and drugs, including cocaine and methamphetamine. Absent pulses in the presence of complex fractures or crush injuries of the upper extremity need to be assessed with imaging (either multidetector CT or conventional angiography) if normal perfusion does not return after resuscitation and the administration of adequate pain medications.

There is currently not a role for endovascular therapy in the brachial artery and forearm vessels. Traditional operative exposure, catheter thrombectomy, and repair remain the best approaches to optimize results.[5,45] In patients unstable from associated torso injuries, damage control with arterial shunt placement followed by repair when the patient is hemodynamically stable is the best management option. Vascular injuries in the upper extremity are often associated with significant musculoskeletal, neurologic, and soft tissue injuries. When this occurs, a multidisciplinary approach is often required with orthopedics, neurosurgery, and plastic surgery. Venous injuries of the upper extremity can be ligated unless there is extensive soft tissue injury and loss of venous collaterals. In that setting, some form of venous reconstruction should be considered.

On occasion, bleeding from a partially transected arm or forearm vessel can be significant. The surgeon should make certain that adequate control is obtained and maintained during resuscitation, transportation to the operating room, and surgical preparation and draping. Tourniquets have proved lifesaving in the field for management of hemorrhage from extremities, and they have a role in the trauma bay for obtaining hemorrhage control during resuscitation and a timely, thorough evaluation for other injuries. Tourniquets from the field or applied in the trauma bay should be carefully monitored for both adequacy of compression and duration of application by the senior surgeon present.

The patient should be widely prepared and draped with generous inclusion of the entire upper extremity, the shoulder, and the anterior-superior aspect of the chest to allow incisions for proximal control.[5] An uninjured leg should also be prepared and draped from the inguinal region to the toes to allow saphenous vein harvest. Adjunctive measures, such as bolus intravenous systemic heparinization, administration of a continuous infusion of low-molecular-weight dextran, and administration of intravenous antibiotics, should be considered and used where appropriate. In patients with multisystem injuries, especially head injury, local or regional infusion of heparin should be used in place of systemic administration. Loupe magnification and coaxial lighting ("headlight") are technical adjuncts that may be useful in suturing small blood vessel with fine suture.

Surgical exposure requires generous incisions placed to maximize exposure and provide appropriate options for further exploration and repair. The brachial artery is best exposed through a longitudinal incision along the medial aspect of the upper arm over the groove between the triceps and biceps muscles. The incision can be extended distally with an S-shaped extension across the antecubital fossa from the ulnar to radial aspect and onto the forearm to expose the origins of the forearm vessels.[5,45] Proximal brachial artery injuries may require control of the infraclavicular axillary artery. Vascular repair requires attention to detail in all phases. Balloon catheter thrombectomy and flushing with heparinized saline followed by debridement of damaged arterial wall are essential to successful repair. Lacerated veins should be ligated. If the duration of arterial occlusion and ischemia is a concern, temporary intraluminal shunts may be placed in the artery. Primary arterial repair of undamaged ends of vessels (end-to-end anastomosis) should be performed only if the repair is tension free. Saphenous vein interposition should be chosen whenever vessel injury is extensive or if primary tension-free repair is not possible. PTFE needs to remain a second choice to autologous vein in the management of injuries of the brachial artery and forearm vessels.[2,5,45] Forearm fasciotomy, particularly in the setting of prolonged ischemia, should be considered before completion of the operation, and patients should be followed closely for the development of postoperative compartment syndrome.

There is a limited but important role for "primary" or early amputation in the management of upper extremity vascular injuries. Patients with extensive soft tissue loss or with scapulothoracic dissociation who have severe neurologic deficits, extensive fractures, and vascular injuries should be evaluated collaboratively with orthopedic, neurosurgery, and plastic surgery colleagues to determine whether early amputation is appropriate. The best approach is intraoperative, multidisciplinary assessment; damage control; and a plan for reoperative assessment in 24 to 48 hours. This will allow discussions with the patient and family and a second look.

Combined ulnar and radial artery injury in the forearm requires repair of at least one vessel. The ulnar artery is usually larger in the proximal forearm and is a better target for direct repair or saphenous vein bypass. Distally, the vessel repair should be performed in whichever vessel is largest or amenable to simple repair.[5,45]

Isolated ulnar or radial artery injuries can be managed with simple ligation only if there is absolute certainty that flow through the remaining vessel is adequate. Close inspection of the forearm and hand with palpation of pulses augmented by continuous-wave (handheld) Doppler interrogation is essential.[5]

Lower Extremity

Vascular injuries in the legs are more common in military settings (30%–40%) than in civilian practice (20%).[46] Although penetrating injuries are more common, blunt vascular trauma in the lower extremity remains a significant challenge. In the thigh and the leg, fractures and dislocations can be associated with vascular injuries. The popliteal artery is at particularly high risk of injury after dislocation of the knee.[46]

Findings at presentation vary from significant hemorrhage from a wound (i.e., open fracture, stab, or gunshot) to occult arterial occlusion from blunt injury. A systematic approach with a thorough extremity vascular examination is essential to avoid errors in recognition and delays in treatment.

Exposure is obtained with incisions used for elective surgical procedures. The common femoral artery is best exposed through a longitudinal incision overlying its course from the inguinal ligament inferiorly for 8 to 12 cm. Proximal control may require exposure of the external iliac artery, best accomplished through an oblique muscle-splitting lower-quadrant abdominal incision carried into retroperitoneum, where the artery and vein can be controlled. SFA injuries are best exposed through a longitudinal groin incision similar to that used for femoral bifurcation exposure for the proximal portion. The mid-SFA is approached through an oblique incision over the sartorius muscle. The junction of the SFA and popliteal can be exposed by extending this incision, dividing the adductor tendon.

Popliteal injuries are exposed through a generous medial incision. Exposure of the artery in the area at the knee joint requires division of the medial head of the gastrocnemius muscle and the semimembranosus and semitendinosus muscles. The distal popliteal artery is exposed with an incision along the posterior margin of the tibia.

Repair of lower extremity vascular injuries usually requires an interposition graft (Fig. 38.10). This is particularly true in the popliteal artery. Reverse saphenous vein from the contralateral extremity is the first choice for interposition grafts. In the common femoral artery, PTFE is an acceptable choice for interposition if the saphenous vein is not of sufficient size. However, saphenous vein remains the best graft for repair of the superficial femoral, popliteal, and tibial vessels.[16] Similar to the upper extremity, fasciotomy of the lower leg should be considered before completion of the operation, particularly with prolonged ischemia, and patients should be followed closely for the development of postoperative compartment syndrome.

Injuries below the popliteal artery at the level of the tibial vessels are best managed by ligation if two of the three calf vessels are patent and there is adequate collateral flow. In the presence of both anterior and posterior tibial vessel occlusion, the peroneal artery is usually not sufficiently connected to the distal arterial bed by collaterals, and repair of one of the injured vessels should be performed. The choice of which vessel to repair is based on both the extent of associated soft tissue injury and the patency of the distal segments of those vessels.

Damage control techniques with arterial and venous shunt placement with delayed definitive repair are an important part of managing lower extremity vascular injury associated with major torso

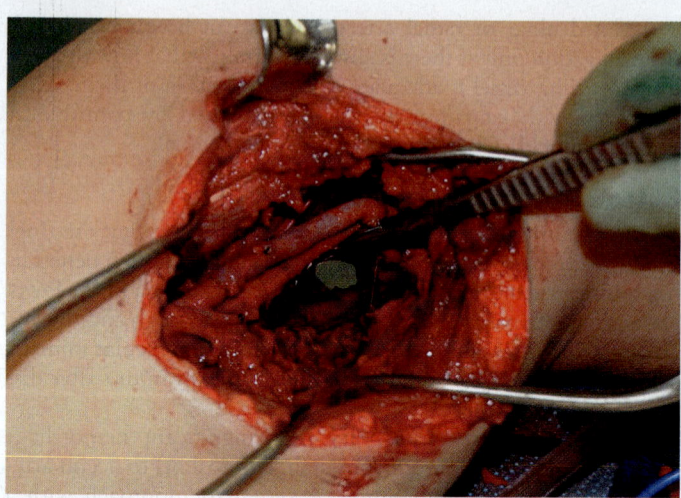

FIGURE 38.10 Interposition repairs of left distal femoral artery and vein using greater saphenous vein. The injury location corresponded well with a traditional medial vascular exposure. The bullet wound tract after debridement can be seen extending through to the other side of the leg.

injuries and hemodynamic instability. All efforts should be made early postoperatively to achieve adequate stability as rapidly as possible to allow a timely return to the operating room for definitive vascular repair before shunt thrombosis and prolonged ischemia.

COMPLICATIONS

Despite advances in modern trauma care, morbidity and mortality after vascular trauma remain significant. The anatomic location and mechanism of the injury heavily influence the outcomes in this patient population. Emergent vascular repair also carries higher rates of morbidity and mortality compared with elective vascular surgery populations.

Cerebrovascular injury carries the risk of both mortality and debilitating stroke. The most important factor in decreasing morbidity in this injury pattern lies in initial recognition and diagnosis. Early initiation of antithrombotic therapy with either heparin or aspirin is extremely important in reducing stroke rates. Although the majority of BCVIs may initially be managed nonoperatively in this manner, close follow-up imaging and neurologic monitoring are paramount. In those managed with antithrombotic therapy, hemorrhage also carries a significant risk if the patient has concomitant injuries. Careful risk and benefit assessment should occur before initiation.[47]

Local complications such as infection, nerve injury, and lymphatic injury can also occur with vascular repair. Lymphatic injury may result in lymphedema, lymphocele formation, chylothorax, or chylous ascites. Management may include simple drainage of the lymphocele or mechanical massage to the affected area to promote lymphatic drainage. Lymphatic bypass may also be an option in select patients. Chylothorax and chylous ascites are decidedly rare, although management may include drainage, dietary modification with limited long-chain fatty acid intake or total parenteral nutrition (TPN) initiation, and identification of the source. Nerve injury often occurs at the time of the index injury, not during vascular repair. However, care must be taken during repair to identify adjacent nerve bundles and avoid further trauma. If a nerve injury is identified, early repair has been associated with improved outcomes. If this is not possible at the

time of initial operation, tagging the nerve is useful for future identification and repair. Traumatic vascular injuries, particularly those repaired with nonautologous grafts, are at high risk of infection. These injuries often coexist with local soft tissue or bony injury as well as other factors like hypotension, hypothermia, and metabolic abnormalities, all of which may impair proper wound healing. It is therefore of the utmost importance to use prophylactic preoperative antibiotics, such as a second-generation cephalosporin, and sterile technique whenever possible. Surgical site infections should be managed with the attempt to separate vascular repair from infection. If a graft or repair becomes infected, risk of vascular anastomotic blowout increases. Antibiotics should be broadened, and cultures should be obtained if able. Decision-making should then become focused on either excision and revision or attempted salvage, although this is often nuanced and patient dependent.[4]

Aside from local complications, repairs themselves are associated with their own complications, including anastomotic complications, bypass thrombosis, fistula formation, endoleaks, and dissection. Anastomotic disruption, stricture, and pseudoaneurysm are all potentially devastating occurrences. Care must be taken to provide a durable and fully patent anastomosis during repair. The use of on-table angiography or a hybrid suite can be useful in evaluating the adequacy of a repair before leaving the operating room. Bypass thrombosis has many factors but can threaten life and limb. Attention must be given to conduit material, wound bed preparation, adequate inflow and outflow, and anastomotic sites. Aortoenteric fistulas, although rare, may be heralded by gastrointestinal bleed, abdominal pain, systemic septic characteristics, and graft thrombosis. Principles of management include resuscitation, use of broad-spectrum antibiotics, graft explanation, and revascularization. Endoleaks, or persistent arterial flow around an endovascular stent graft, are defined as types 1 through 5. Type 1 involves flow around the proximal or distal extent of the stent, and these leaks often require further intervention for repair. Type 2 results from back-bleeding from a branch vessel covered by the stent. These leaks often have a benign course and may self-resolve without need for intervention. Type 3 occurs with leakage at stent junctions, often where there is inadequate overlap of stents. This also often requires repair. Types 4 and 5 occur from graft porosity or the theoretical phenomenon of endotension. As stent graft technology has progressed, type 4 and 5 endoleaks have become rare within the elective setting and exceedingly so after vascular trauma repair.[48]

SELECTED REFERENCES

Brown CVR, de Moya M, Brasel KJ, et al. Blunt thoracic aortic injury: a Western Trauma Association critical decisions algorithm. *J Trauma Acute Care Surg.* 2023;94(1):113-116.

This practice recommendation from the Western Trauma Association gives an evidence-based approach to the evaluation and management of blunt thoracic aortic injuries.

Feliciano DV. For the patient—evolution in the management of vascular trauma. *J Trauma Acute Care Surg.* 2017;83:1205-1212.

This excellent review traces the evolution of surgical management for the last 100 years. The advances in surgical science, imaging, antibiotics, anticoagulation, and graft materials are thoughtfully discussed. This is a unique and valuable contribution to the literature.

Jansen JO, Hudson J, Cochran C, et al. Emergency department resuscitative endovascular balloon occlusion of the aorta in trauma patients with exsanguinating hemorrhage: the UK-REBOA Randomized Clinical Trial. *JAMA.* 2023;330(19):1862-1871.

This multicenter, randomized clinical trial from the United Kingdom examined the effect of REBOA when used in the emergency department along with standard care versus standard care alone on mortality in exsanguinating trauma patients. The researchers found that this may increase mortality.

Kim DY, Biffl W, Bokhari F, et al. Evaluation and management of blunt cerebrovascular injury: a practice management guideline from the Eastern Association for the Surgery of Trauma. *J Trauma Acute Care Surg.* 2020;88(6):875-887.

This practice recommendation from the Eastern Association for the Surgery of Trauma offers an evidence-based approach to the diagnosis of blunt cerebrovascular injuries.

Patterson BO, Holt PJ, Cleanthis M, et al. Imaging vascular trauma. *Br J Surg.* 2012;99:494-505.

This systematic review involved literature relating to radiologic diagnosis of vascular trauma from 2000 to 2010. This excellent review conclusively established the superiority of CTA for the diagnosis of vascular injuries.

Shackford SR, Dunne CE, Karmy-Jones R, et al. The evolution of care improves outcome in blunt thoracic aortic injury: a Western Trauma Association multicenter study. *J Trauma Acute Care Surg.* 2017;83(6):1006-1013.

The full reference list appears on Elsevier eBooks+.

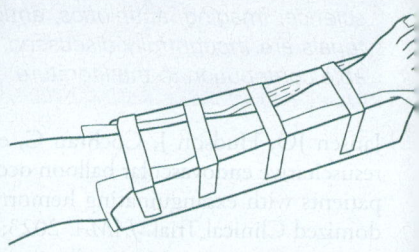

39 | CHAPTER

Management of Urologic Trauma

Hiren V. Patel and Benjamin N. Breyer

OUTLINE

Background on Urologic Trauma
Guidelines for Urologic Trauma Management
Renal Trauma
  Imaging for Renal Trauma
  Management of Renal Trauma
  Surgical Exploration and Operative Approach for Renal Trauma
Ureteral Trauma
  Imaging for Ureteral Trauma
  Management of Ureteral Trauma
  Surgical Exploration and Operative Approach for Ureteral Trauma
Bladder Trauma
  Imaging for Bladder Trauma

Management of Bladder Trauma
Surgical Exploration and Operative Approach for Bladder Trauma
Urethral Trauma
  Imaging for Urethral Trauma
  Management of Urethral Trauma
  Surgical Exploration and Operative Approach for Urethral Trauma
Genital Trauma
  Imaging for Genital Trauma
  Management of Genital Trauma
  Surgical Exploration and Operative Approach for Genital Trauma
Damage Control Situations

BACKGROUND ON UROLOGIC TRAUMA

Approximately 10% to 15% of all abdominal and pelvic trauma involve the genitourinary system. Isolated urologic injuries are uncommon because the genitourinary tract is well sheltered within the abdominal cavity. Often these injuries can be subtle, yet their prompt diagnosis is essential to avoid serious complications. Initial management should include obtaining hemodynamic stability and determining the mechanism of injury because visceral organ injury patterns can vary based on mechanism of injury. A thorough physical examination can provide insight into possible injuries to deeper organs within the retroperitoneum or pelvis. Patients who are deemed to be hemodynamically stable and without life-threatening injuries should have advanced imaging to evaluate and stage abdominal and pelvic injuries.

Although initial assessment and management are typically done by emergency physicians or general surgeons, early collaboration with urologists can be critical. For example, as management of renal injuries has evolved, conservative approaches with observation, embolization, or renorrhaphy can aid in preserving renal function. Urologic expertise can augment the care of urologic trauma. Early consultation can help guide imaging and management strategies in conjunction with the emergency and surgery teams.

GUIDELINES FOR UROLOGIC TRAUMA MANAGEMENT

The Organ Injury Scaling system of the American Association for the Surgery of Trauma (AAST) has developed a long-standing

grading system for different types of organ injuries. Trauma guidelines from the European Association of Urology and the American Urological Association (AUA) were developed by integrating these scaling systems into the management algorithms. The AUA initially created a urologic trauma guideline in 2014 and recently updated the guidelines in 2020.[1,2]

RENAL TRAUMA

Approximately 80% of renal trauma is the result of blunt trauma, and the remainder are penetrating injuries. Physical examination should focus on identifying the location of impact, assessing the flank, and examining the urine for microscopic or gross hematuria. For penetrating injuries, it is important to identify entry and exit points.

In evaluating renal injuries, it is important to note that the AAST recently updated the long-standing renal injury scale to reflect contemporary data on diagnosis and management of renal trauma (Table 39.1).[3,4] The original grading system that was devised in 1989 was based on anatomic findings, largely found during surgical exploration, and was used to standardize research efforts. The revised staging system has incorporated current data regarding management of high-grade renal trauma and radiologic findings.

Recent research from the Multi-institutional Genito-Urinary Trauma Study (MiGUTS) has shed light on potential additional changes that can be addressed in future revisions of the renal trauma injury scale.[5–14] Some changes in the updated renal injury scale remain controversial because of ambiguity and upstaging of certain injuries.[15,16] Particularly, segmental vascular injuries to the

TABLE 39.1 Organ Injury Scaling System: Kidney

GRADE	DESCRIPTION	AIS SEVERITY
I	• Subcapsular hematoma or parenchymal contusion without laceration	2
II	• Perirenal hematoma confined to Gerota fascia	2
	• Renal laceration ≤1 cm depth without urinary extravasation	
III	• Renal laceration >1 cm depth without urinary extravasation	3
	• Any injury in the presence of a kidney vascular injury or active bleeding contained within Gerota fascia	
IV	• Parenchymal laceration with urinary extravasation	4
	• Renal pelvis laceration and/or ureteropelvic junction disruption	
	• Active bleeding beyond Gerota fascia into retroperitoneum or peritoneum	
	• Segmental or complete kidney infarction caused by vessel thrombosis without active bleeding	
V	• Main renal artery or vein laceration or avulsion of hilum	5
	• Devascularized kidney with active bleeding	
	• Shattered kidney with loss of identifiable parenchymal renal anatomy	

AIS, Abbreviated Injury Scale.

Adapted from Kozar RA, Crandall M, Shanmuganathan K, et al. Organ injury scaling 2018 update: spleen, liver, kidney. *J Trauma Acute Care Surg*. 2018;85:1119-1122.

kidney have remained a point of confusion.[16] Based on the recent staging systems, it is unclear if segmental vascular injury refers to the renal segmental arteries or just a segment of the kidney that is injured. Consequently, about a third of grade III injuries are upgraded to grade IV injuries, which increases the heterogeneity among grade IV renal injuries.[10] Importantly, the revised grading system did not outperform the 1989 grading system in predicting intervention for renal hemorrhage. Therefore, ongoing efforts are underway to propose additional changes to the kidney organ injury scale.

Imaging for Renal Trauma

Diagnostic imaging should be performed on hemodynamically stable patients when there is suspicion of renal injury based on physical examination finding or mechanism of injury. Patients with stable blunt trauma with gross or microscopic hematuria should have contrast-enhanced computed tomography (CT) of abdomen and pelvis with delayed images. Optimal delay for detection of urinary extravasation is 9 minutes.[8] In many centers, if there are no signs of kidney trauma in the contrast phase, a delayed view is not obtained; however, to limit diagnostic delay if kidney trauma is recognized by the trauma team during the contrast phase, a delayed phase is preferably pursued while the patient remains on the table. If patients are unable to have CT scans because of hemodynamic instability or require immediate intervention, a "one-shot" intravenous pyelogram (IVP) can be performed

by administering 2 mL/kg contrast followed by a single abdominal radiograph, which can inform the surgeon about the presence of the contralateral kidney before considering renal exploration or nephrectomy. Several critical CT findings are important predictors for requiring intervention. Every centimeter increase in perinephric hematoma size is associated with 66% increased likelihood of requiring intervention. Additionally intravascular contrast extravasation is associated with a threefold increase in odds of requiring interventions for hemorrhage.[9,11,14]

Management of Renal Trauma

Advances in imaging, and thus staging, of renal injury have led to the evolution of the management paradigms for renal injuries (Fig. 39.1). In hemodynamically stable patients, noninvasive management, such as serial hematocrit monitoring, should be used; however, historical adjuncts such as bed rest have fallen out of favor and usefulness. Patients who are hemodynamically unstable require immediate intervention, which includes surgery or angioembolization in select patients.[17] Unstable patients with critical CT findings such as perirenal hematoma >4 cm and/or intravascular contrast extravasation should have immediate intervention. High-grade renal trauma—grade IV and V—may undergo exploration, but nephrectomy in this setting is associated with higher mortality.[6] Recent data have demonstrated that in a subset of grade V renal injuries, nonoperative management is a viable option and does not increase the length of stay for patients.[5,18,19]

Kidneys injured because of blunt trauma can often be managed conservatively, even in conditions where urinary extravasation or nonviable tissue is present. Penetrating injuries will require intervention more often when the retroperitoneum is violated based on the extent of the injury (Fig. 39.2). Nevertheless, in select cases where injuries are isolated to the kidney without abdominal involvement, conservative management should be used. After initial imaging, patients with high-grade renal trauma (AAST grade IV–V) should have repeat CT imaging to assess for urinoma, hematoma, or abscess formation. Additionally, patients with signs of complications such as fever, worsening flank pain, ongoing blood loss, and abdominal distention should be reassessed using CT imaging. Asymptomatic low-grade injuries do not require interval imaging. When a large or expanding urinoma is present, urinary drainage should be performed using a ureteral stent, and additional percutaneous drains can be added to augment drainage and promote healing.[20,21]

Surgical Exploration and Operative Approach for Renal Trauma

Absolute indications for intervention with either renal exploration or expedient angioembolization are (1) expanding, pulsatile retroperitoneal hematoma or renal pedicle avulsion, (2) hemodynamic instability that is not responsive to resuscitation, (3) suspected renal vascular pedicle avulsion, and (4) ureteropelvic junction avulsion. Relative indications for intervention are (1) urinary extravasation in a devascularized renal unit, (2) renal injury with concomitant colon or pancreatic injury, and (3) urinary extravasation from parenchymal injury.

Renal exploration should be performed through a transabdominal approach, which allows complete inspection of the viscera.[22] Renal vessels are isolated to provide vascular control if massive hemorrhage is present when Gerota fascia is opened. The small bowel is lifted out of the abdomen, and an incision is made medial to the inferior mesenteric vein and extended to the ligament of Treitz, which provides a window over the aorta at the

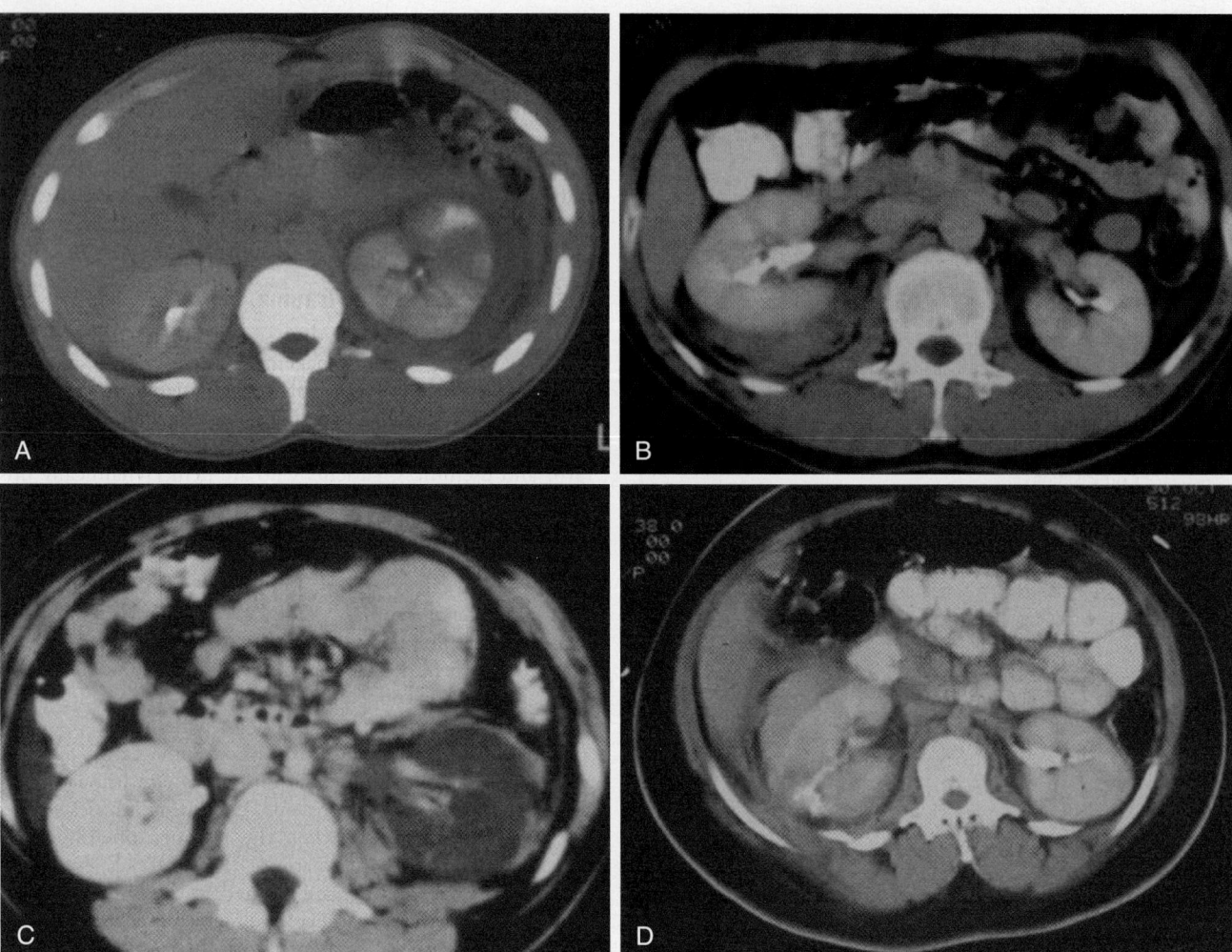

FIGURE 39.1 Computed tomography scans depicting renal trauma. (A) Grade I kidney injury with left renal contusion with heterogeneous contrast enhancement. (B) Small right posterior perirenal hematoma consistent with grade II kidney injury. (C) Grade IV renal infarction caused by left renal artery thrombosis without active bleeding. (D) Grade IV laceration to the posterolateral right kidney with posterolateral extravasation of contrast material.

level of the renal arteries. Renal vessels are controlled with individual vessel loops. Renal veins must be retracted cephalad to identify the left and right renal arteries, which run below the renal veins. If a large hematoma obscures landmarks, this approach will require dissecting through hematoma before approaching the anterior surface of the aorta. The kidney can be exposed by incising the white line of Toldt to lateralize the colon, followed by dissecting off Gerota fascia. The splenic attachments (for left) or hepatic attachments (for right) must be freed to allow mobility of the kidney.

Whenever possible, renal preservation should be a consideration, especially if urology specialists are available. Renal reconstruction requires complete exposure of the kidney, temporary vascular control, debridement of nonviable tissue, hemostasis, and closure of collecting system if needed and reapproximation of parenchymal defect. Renorrhaphy can be performed with 3-0 Vicryl suture to reapproximate the capsule over a bolster with absorbable hemostatic agent (Surgicel or Nu-Knit). If a partial nephrectomy is necessary, the collecting system should be closed, and hemostatic agents can be applied over this repair. If possible, this repair should be covered with a flap of omentum or Gerota fascia to aid with healing. A closed suction drain should be

placed around the site of repair to help monitor the repair site postoperatively.

URETERAL TRAUMA

Although ureteral injuries account for 1% to 2.5% of all urologic injuries, 95% of these injuries are the result of penetrating injuries and 5% are blunt injuries. A high clinical suspicion for ureteral injury is needed based on mechanism and injury location. Because penetrating injuries, such as bullets, impart large energy transfer through a small area, damage can be as little as 2 cm away from the point of transection. Unrecognized ureteral injury is associated with significant morbidity such as urinoma, abscess, fistula formation, and possible nonfunctional renal unit. Therefore, ureters should be evaluated when evaluating other injuries.

Imaging for Ureteral Trauma

CT imaging with contrast must include delayed views to evaluate the ureter in stable patients. Extravasation of contrast, lack of contrast distal to suspected injury, or hydronephrosis can be critical findings suggestive of ureteral injury. Other imaging modalities,

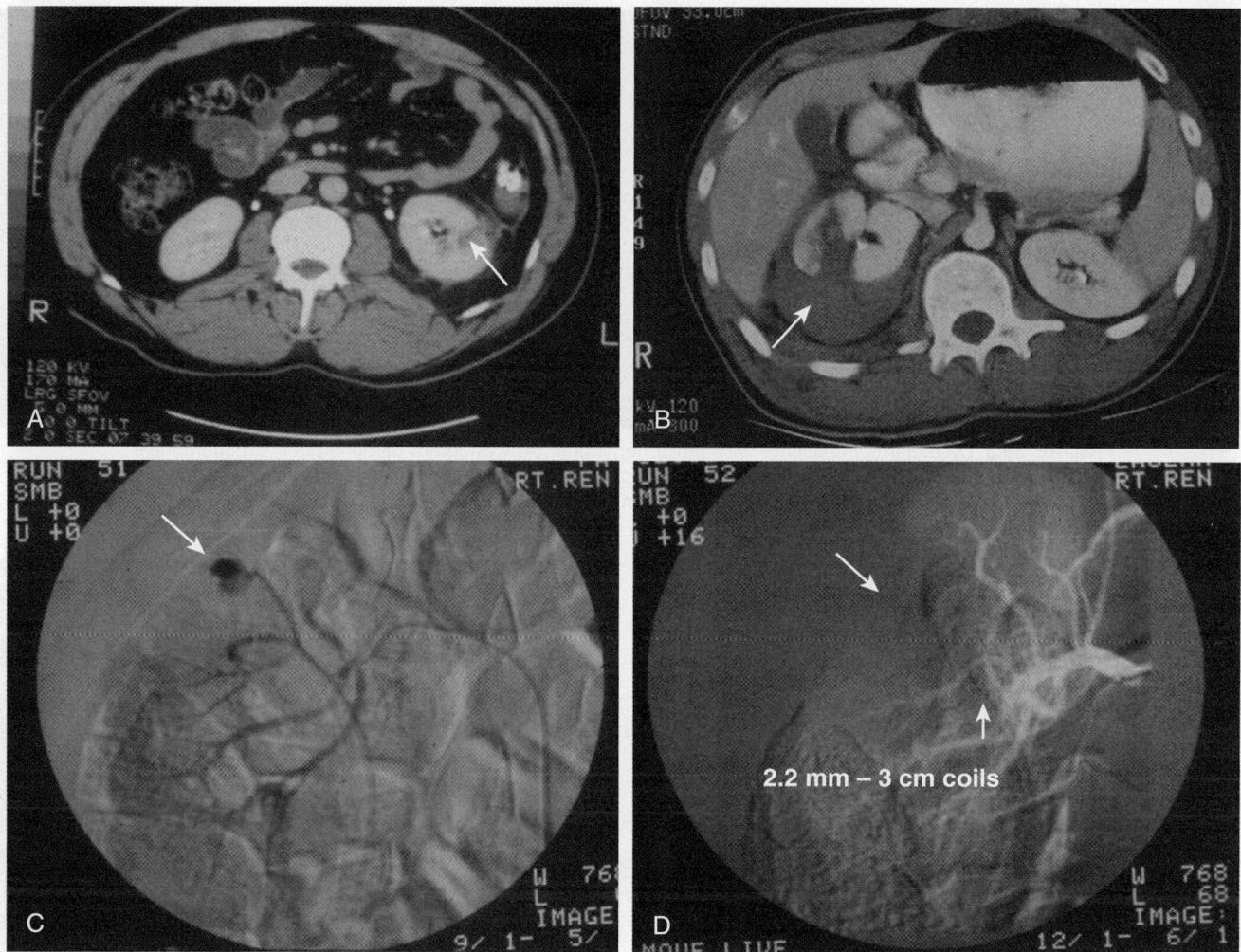

FIGURE 39.2 Penetrating renal injury on computed tomography scans. (A) Stab wound caused a superficial laceration *(arrow)* to the lateral left kidney. Small hematoma and location of posterior descending colon are notable. (B) Right kidney with deep laceration and large hematoma *(arrow)* in proximity to the renal hilum after stab injury. (C) Pseudoaneurysm *(arrow)* on renal angiography for significant hematuria and hemodynamic instability postinjury. (D) Successful embolization results in wedge-shaped defect *(arrow)* in the right kidney.

such as MRI or IVP, are not reliable in this setting. Retrograde pyelography is useful and the most sensitive radiographic test, but it is cumbersome and not a time-sensitive study in an acute setting.

Management of Ureteral Trauma

Injuries to the ureters are best managed with direct inspection and surgical repair. Specifically, when suspicion for ureteral injury remains high or in patients who have not undergone preoperative imaging, direct inspection of the ureters at time of laparotomy is critical. Intraoperative administration of methylene blue or other intravascular dye excreted in the urinary system can aid in the identification of ureteral injuries. Traumatic injuries should be repaired in hemodynamically stable patients, whereas in unstable patients, simple intraoperative tagging of the ureter with subsequent nephrostomy tube placement and delayed definitive repair can be planned. In general, nonviable tissue should be excised before reconstructing ureter. Intact ureters with minor contusion can be managed with ureteral stenting.[23] When ureteral stenting fails, patients can be managed with percutaneous nephrostomy with delayed repair.

Surgical Exploration and Operative Approach for Ureteral Trauma

Whenever possible, the injured ureter should be repaired at the same time as the initial laparotomy in stable conditions, but this may not always be possible. The ureters should be mobilized carefully, taking care to avoid stripping the adventitia to prevent further devascularization. The ureters can be debrided, albeit minimally and until bleeding edge is identified. The ureter should be spatulated and anastomosed in a tension-free fashion using fine absorbable sutures. The type of ureteral repair depends on the location of the injury. Injuries that are located proximal to the iliac vessels can be repaired primarily over a ureteral stent, and injuries distal to the iliac vessels can be reimplanted into the bladder or repaired primarily over a ureteral stent. A drain should be placed to help with postoperative management.

BLADDER TRAUMA

Approximately 1% to 2% of patients with blunt abdominal trauma have associated bladder injuries. The bladder is well insulated

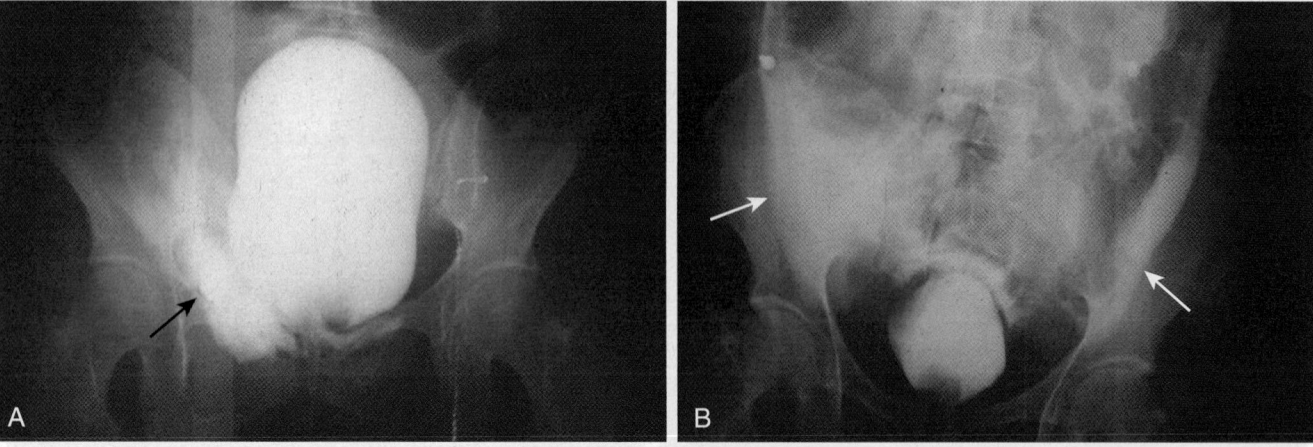

FIGURE 39.3 Cystograms in patients with gross hematuria. (A) Cystogram demonstrates extraperitoneal injury *(black arrow)*. (B) Cystogram demonstrates intraperitoneal extravasation of contrast with contrast in the colic gutters *(white arrows)* and within the peritoneum.

behind the pubic bone and within the pelvis, but significant acceleration-deceleration injuries can lead to disruption of fascial attachments, and bone fragments can directly injure the bladder. In fact, pelvic fracture is associated with 83% to 95% of bladder injuries, whereas bladder injury was associated with only 5% to 10% of pelvic fractures.[24–26] Clinical findings such as suprapubic pain or tenderness, free fluid on CT or ultrasound, low urine output, clots in urine or in bladder on CT, scrotal ecchymosis, and abdominal distention can indicate bladder injury. Nevertheless, gross hematuria is present in 75% to 100% of injuries.[25] Clinicians should have a high index of suspicion for bladder injury in patients with blunt trauma and alcohol intoxication.[27]

Imaging for Bladder Trauma

Retrograde cystography is the gold standard imaging technique to diagnose bladder injury. Given similar specificity and sensitivity, plain film or CT cystography can be performed.[28,29] Clinicians can decide on modality based on resource availability, patient stability, and ease. Antegrade distention by clamping the urethral catheter after CT with delayed imaging is not adequate for diagnosing rupture because of the lack of distention and should not be performed.[30–32] A retrograde cystography allows for (1) adequate retrograde filling with a minimum of 300 mL of contrast or until patient reaches tolerance, (2) imaging at maximal fill, and (3) imaging after bladder drainage. Retrograde cystography is important in differentiating between extraperitoneal and intraperitoneal bladder injuries. Extraperitoneal injuries are confined outside of the peritoneal cavity, whereas intraperitoneal injuries are within the peritoneal cavity (Figs. 39.3 and 39.4).

Management of Bladder Trauma

Bladder rupture does not happen as an isolated event in normal adults. Approximately 30% of patients with a bladder injury will present with gross hematuria and pelvic fracture; therefore, retrograde cystography must be performed.[33] Patients with pubic symphysis diastasis and obturator ring fracture with clinical findings suggestive of bladder injury should have retrograde cystography.[25,34]

In general, intraperitoneal bladder injuries, regardless of mechanism, should be surgically repaired. The bladder neck and ureteral orifices should be assessed for additional injuries at time of repair. Intravenous administration of indigo carmine, methylene blue, fluorescein green, or retrograde passage of a ureteral catheter

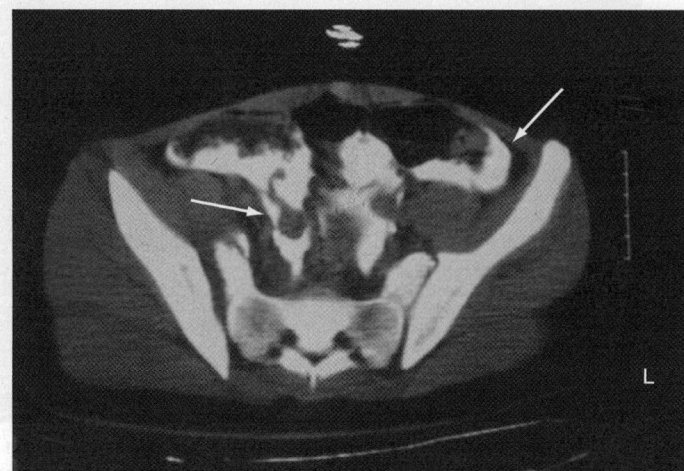

FIGURE 39.4 Computed tomography cystogram showing intraperitoneal bladder rupture. Contrast is seen in the colic gutters and around the ovaries *(arrows)*.

TABLE 39.2   **Indications for Repair of Bladder Injury**
• Intraperitoneal injury from blunt or penetrating trauma
• Inadequate bladder drainage or clots in urine
• Concomitant bladder neck, rectal or vaginal injury
• Open pelvic fracture
• Pelvic fracture requiring open reduction and internal fixation
• Bone fragments protruding into the bladder
• Stable patients that are undergoing laparotomy

can be used to assess the ureters. Extraperitoneal bladder injuries can be managed with catheter drainage for 2 to 3 weeks. Follow-up cystography should be performed to assess the injury before catheter removal. If the injury has not healed after 4 weeks of catheter drainage, open repair should be considered. There are several scenarios where immediate repair is indicated for an extraperitoneal bladder injury (Table 39.2) to reduce complications such as fistula formation, failure to heal, orthopedic hardware infection, and sepsis.[35,36]

Surgical Exploration and Operative Approach for Bladder Trauma

The anterior bladder wall can be identified in the midline, often by extending a laparotomy incision. Intraperitoneal injuries are often apparent and should be extended to examine the integrity of the bladder neck and ureteral orifices. The cystotomy can then be repaired in two layers using absorbable 2-0 Vicryl through 4-0 Vicryl sutures to achieve a watertight closure. Extraperitoneal injury can be closed intravesically using absorbable 2-0 Vicryl suture by entering through the anterior bladder wall. If possible, pelvic hematoma should not be disturbed. A catheter should be left to promote drainage, and a suprapubic tube is rarely needed; however, cases with complex bladder lacerations or concurrent spinal cord injury and paralysis may benefit from a suprapubic tube. If concomitant pelvic injuries are present, tissue interposition flaps should be used to separate suture lines.

URETHRAL TRAUMA

Injuries to the urethra occur in the posterior urethra (prostatic urethra, membranous urethra) or the anterior urethra (penile and bulbar urethra). Posterior urethral injuries are almost solely associated with pelvic fractures, occurring in 1.5% to 10% of pelvic fractures.[35,37] These injuries can be associated with bladder injuries 15% of the time.[38] The anterior urethra is most commonly injured at the bulbar urethra, which accounts for 85% of all urethral injuries. Blood at the meatus is present in 37% to 93% of patients with urethral injury, but patients can present with inability to void and a distended bladder.[25,33] A "butterfly" hematoma may also be present in the perineum because of rupture in Buck fascia, leading to spread of hematoma into the scrotum and along layers of the dartos and Scarpa fascia (Fig. 39.5).

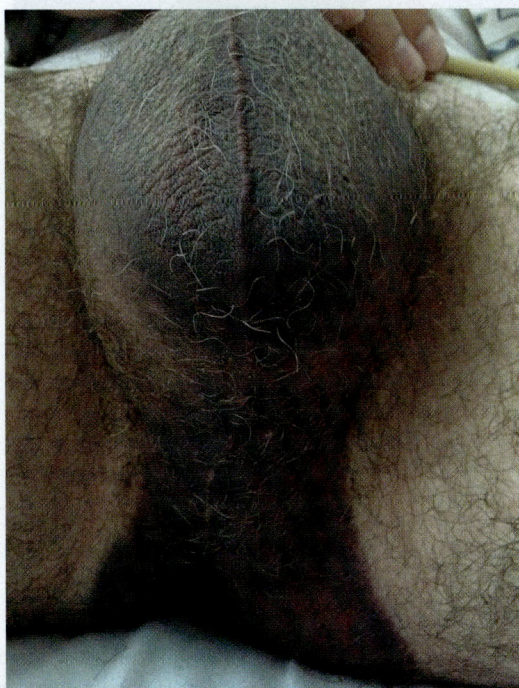

FIGURE 39.5 Rupture of Buck fascia results in butterfly hematoma after urethral injury.

Imaging for Urethral Trauma

Retrograde urethrography should be performed when blood is present at the urethral meatus after pelvic trauma (Fig. 39.6). Blind passage of a urethral catheter should be avoided. The study is performed by placing the patient obliquely on their side and filling the entire urethra with contrast such that it passes into the bladder. The penis should be placed on gentle stretch to help visualize the entire urethra. Extravasation can be visualized when contour of the urethra is lost because of partial or complete disruption. If a catheter has been placed before evaluation and urethral injury is suspected, pericatheter retrograde urethrography can be performed by injecting contrast with a 3-Fr catheter held at the urethral meatus to prevent contrast leakage.

Management of Urethral Trauma

Prompt drainage of the bladder is critical when urethral injury is present. Percutaneous or open suprapubic tube placement can provide a fast and efficient method for draining the bladder (Fig. 39.7). The placement of a suprapubic tube with delayed urethroplasty is likely superior to endoscopic primary realignment in the initial management of the ruptured posterior urethra due to pelvic fracture (see Fig. 39.7).[37] When endoscopic primary realignment is employed, prolonged attempts at realignment should be avoided because they can worsen injury severity. These patients are at a high risk of stricture formation, erectile dysfunction, and incontinence; thus, they should be followed for at least 1 year after urethral injury.[37,39-41] Straddle injuries to the bulbar urethra require prompt urinary drainage; most can be fixed primarily, although if there is extensive local tissue damage, suprapubic urinary drainage and delayed repair are preferred. Stricture formation is increased among these patients and requires follow-up surveillance with uroflowmetry, retrograde urethrogram, and/or cystoscopy. Patients with uncomplicated penetrating trauma of the anterior urethra should be repaired primarily.

Surgical Exploration and Operative Approach for Urethral Trauma

In patients who are hemodynamically stable, anterior urethral injuries caused by penetrating trauma should be explored and repaired primarily. Urethra should be examined, minimally debrided, and spatulated before primary repair. Repair should be performed over a catheter using fine absorbable suture.

Other injuries to the anterior and posterior urethra can be managed with suprapubic tube placement. If bladder is palpable and patient does not have a history of abdominal surgery, it can be placed in a percutaneous fashion. In patients with abdominal surgery, bladder ultrasound can be used to identify a safe window to place a suprapubic tube in an open fashion. A cut-down can be performed to safely identify the bladder, and a cystotomy can be created under vision. A catheter is placed in the bladder through cystostomy, and a purse-string closure is performed around the catheter. Skin closure is performed, and a suprapubic tube is secured to the skin.

GENITAL TRAUMA

Genital trauma is a diverse set of injuries caused by various mechanisms, such as blunt and penetrating injuries; amputation; bites; burns; or avulsion injuries to penis, scrotum, testicles, or vulva. As a result, the mechanism and organ that is injured should dictate how to stabilize and manage the patient. Approximately

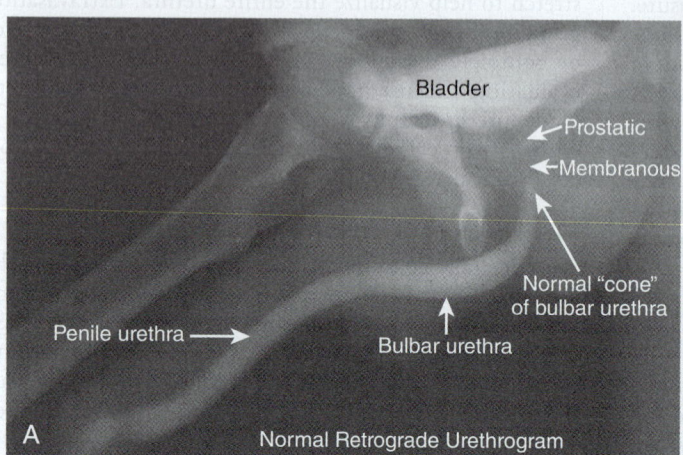
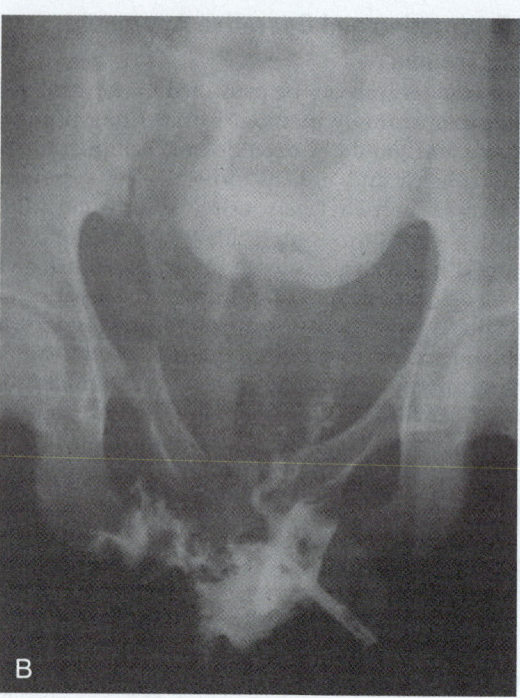

FIGURE 39.6 Retrograde urethrogram highlights urethral patency or defects. (A) With patient in an oblique position, contrast material opacifies the anterior and posterior urethra. (B) Displaced pelvic fracture results in a posterior urethral disruption. Contrast is seen above and below the urogenital diaphragm with the bladder displaced cephalad. This demonstrates the classic "pie-in-the-sky" bladder, which is caused by a pelvic hematoma that displaces the bladder cephalad and urethra caudally.

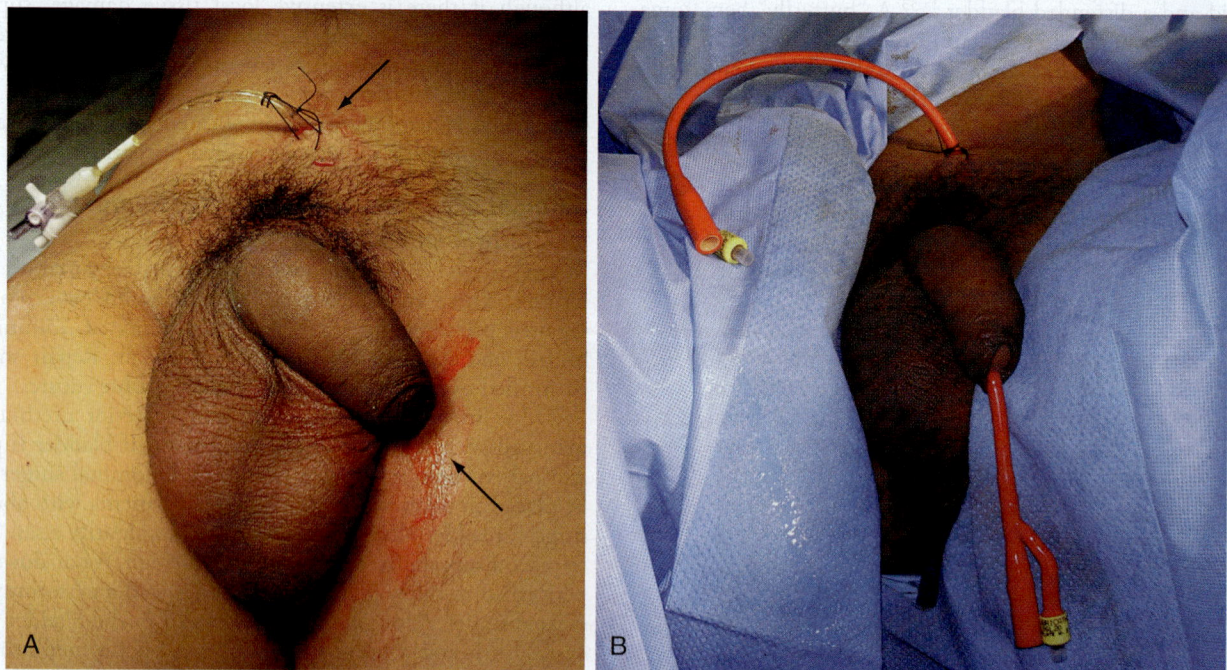

FIGURE 39.7 Posterior urethral disruption injury. (A) Blood at the urethral meatus is visible *(bottom arrow)*. Suprapubic cystotomy tube was placed percutaneously *(top arrow)*. (B) Patient underwent endoscopic realignment procedure with placement of urethral and suprapubic catheter.

50% to 66% of all penetrating genitourinary injuries involve the external genitalia.[42] Penetrating penile injuries can have concomitant urethral injuries in 11% to 29% of cases, and testicular rupture can be present in over 50% of cases of penetrating scrotal injuries.[42]

Imaging for Genital Trauma

With a high degree of clinical suspicion from the history and physical examination, the diagnosis can often be made without additional imaging. Penile swelling and ecchymosis are associated with penile fracture. Most often patients will report a snapping sound followed by immediate detumescence. Penile fracture can often be a clinical diagnosis; however, an equivocal sign may undergo penile ultrasound or penile MRI. Because penile fractures are associated with urethral injuries in 10% to 22% of cases, it is important to evaluate the urethra either by retrograde urethrography or cystoscopy.[43]

Scrotal ultrasonography should be performed for blunt scrotal trauma because it can accurately diagnose testicular rupture. A normal testicle will have a clear tunica albuginea surrounding the testicle, which is lost with rupture resulting in heterogenous echotexture. However, scrotal ultrasonography should not be performed with penetrating scrotal injuries, as its utility in evaluating testicular injury is limited.

Management of Genital Trauma

A thorough history and physical examination are vital for diagnosing penile fracture. Evaluating the urethra for blood and asking about urinary symptoms can help understand if the urethra is involved. Penile fractures should be promptly explored and surgically repaired to aid in faster recovery and decreased rates of penile curvature and erectile dysfunction.

For testicular injuries that require scrotal exploration, early repair of the testes is associated with increased testicular salvage and preservation of fertility and hormonal function. Additionally surrounding structures such as the spermatic cord and vas deferens can be inspected, given 7% to 9% of gunshot wounds to the scrotum injure the vas deferens.

Animal or human bites of the genitals can translocate bacteria to the wound, and therefore, copious irrigation and debridement are necessary. Immediate primary closures can be performed after animal bites with appropriate antibiotic coverage and immunization. However, human bites produce contaminated wounds that should not be closed primarily because patients often present in a delayed fashion with infected wounds.

Genital skin loss can occur from mechanical devices such as industrial machinery or from burns caused by explosive injuries. In most cases, the genitalia should be examined carefully, and healthy tissue should be preserved. Placement of a suprapubic tube early can be beneficial for wound care and avoid prolonged catheterization. Burn injuries to the genitalia should be managed like other burn injuries. Eschars should be resected early, and skin grafts should be applied when appropriate.

Surgical Exploration and Operative Approach for Genital Trauma

When penile fracture is suspected, surgical exploration should be performed regardless of equivocal imaging. Often the urethra is examined using flexible cystoscopy. Most fractures occur ventrally or laterally, and a penoscrotal incision is usually made to gain exposure over the fracture. Alternatively, an incision can be made over the area directly or a distal circumcising incision can be made to gain exposure to the corporal bodies and urethra (Fig. 39.8). Once a tunical defect is identified, a 2-0 or 3-0 absorbable suture is used to close the defect in an interrupted fashion. Debridement and ligating vessels are avoided in order to preserve erectile tissue. Similarly for penetrating trauma to the penis, the wound should be explored immediately, irrigated, any foreign body removed, and surgical closure should be performed. Urethra should also be considered to rule out any concomitant urethral injury. If a urethral injury is present, it should be closed using standard urethroplasty techniques.

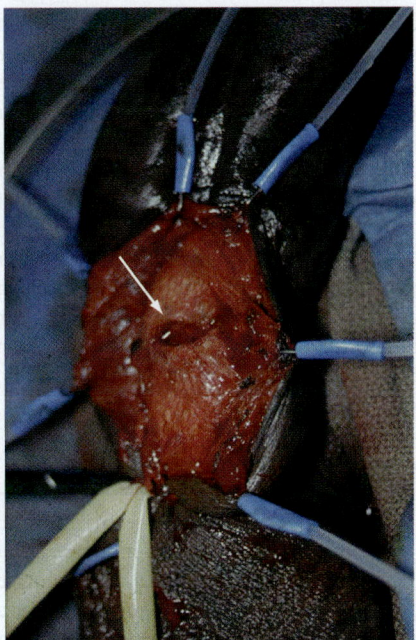

FIGURE 39.8 Surgical exploration of penile fracture demonstrates a disruption of the tunica albuginea of the corpora cavernosum *(white arrow)*. Tourniquet with a Penrose drain can help control the bleeding during repair.

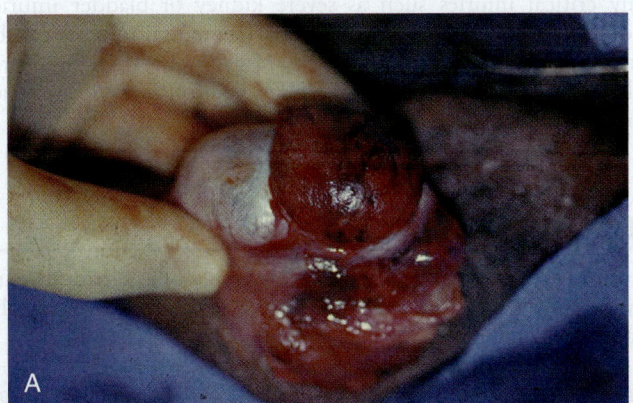
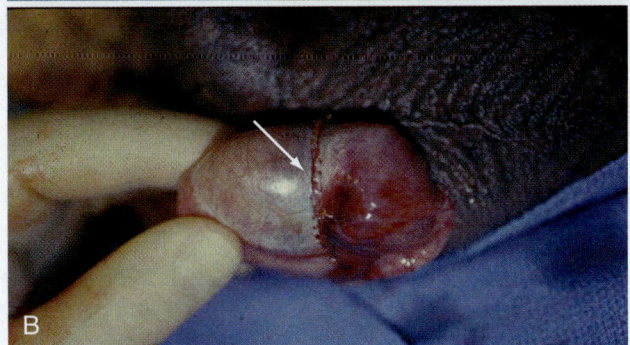

FIGURE 39.9 Scrotal exploration for testicular rupture. (A) Tunica albuginea of the testicle is disrupted with extruded testicular contents. (B) Tunica vaginalis is used to repair defect *(white arrow)*.

When testicular rupture is suspected/present or there is penetrating trauma to the scrotum, a scrotal exploration is prudent (Fig. 39.9). A transverse or vertical incision can be made on the scrotum, and the testicle should be delivered. The tunica vaginalis should be carefully dissected because it can serve as a flap to cover possible large defects in the tunica albuginea. Necrotic seminiferous tubules should be debrided, and tunica albuginea should be closed using a fine absorbable suture. Sometimes because of the degree of trauma, the testicle cannot be closed and tunica vaginalis flap can be used to cover the defect.

For patients with extensive genitalia skin loss, a split-thickness skin graft should be performed. A thick (0.012- to 0.015-inch), nonmeshed, split-thickness graft should be used for penile reconstruction. A thick, meshed, split-thickness graft should be used for scrotal reconstruction. This is most often performed in a delayed fashion. If scrotal skin is present, it can be mobilized to cover both testicles. Eventually over 6 to 12 months the neoscrotum will become more pliable and the testicles will take a more dependent position.

DAMAGE CONTROL SITUATIONS

As with any multidisciplinary surgical team, communication is a vital part of the care during traumatic injuries. Urologic injuries usually require coordinated care between the urologist, the trauma surgeon, and potentially other surgical specialists. Often when the patient is unstable, genitourinary reconstructive procedures can be deferred and temporizing measures can be taken instead. When conditions of extensive blood loss occur, significant blood and fluid replacement can occur, which can cause worsening hypothermia, acidosis, and coagulopathy. In these circumstances, only critical injuries such as severe kidney or bladder injuries should be addressed, whereas ureteral or urethral injuries can be temporized with stents or catheters, respectively. Therefore, careful patient selection is necessary when genitourinary reconstruction is undertaken.

SELECTED REFERENCES

Bjurlin MA, Fantus RJ, Mellett MM, Goble SM. Genitourinary injuries in pelvic fracture morbidity and mortality using the National Trauma Data Bank. *J Trauma.* 2009;67:1033.

> *This study provides a compendium of genitourinary injuries and associated healthcare use after traumatic pelvic fracture.*

Keihani S, Rogers DM, Putbrese BE, et al. The American Association for the Surgery of Trauma renal injury grading scale: implications of the 2018 revisions for injury reclassification and predicting bleeding interventions. *J Trauma Acute Care Surg.* 2020;88:357.

> *This seminal study demonstrates that current renal injury scaling does not outperform the original renal injury scaling system in determining the need for hemostatic intervention. It is the foundation for proposed revisions to the renal injury scale.*

McAninch JW, Carroll PR. Renal trauma: kidney preservation through improved vascular control – a refined approach. *J Trauma.* 1982;22:285.

> *This seminal work highlights that prompt hilar control before renal exploration increased the rates of renal salvage and reduced nephrectomy rates at the time of exploration.*

McCormick BJ, Keihani S, Hagedorn J, et al. A multicenter prospective cohort study of endoscopic urethral realignment versus suprapubic cystostomy after complete pelvic fracture urethral injury. *J Trauma Acute Care Surg.* 2023;94:344.

> *This prospective multicenter study provided evidence that endoscopic urethral realignment after pelvic fracture urethral injury did not improve rates of urethral obstruction or need for urethroplasty compared with initial suprapubic catheter placement, providing evidence that suprapubic tube placement should be the first initial treatment.*

Moore EE, Shackford SR, Pachter HL, et al. Organ injury scaling. *J Trauma.* 1989;29:1664.

> *This landmark paper was the first to provide a scaling system for organ injury in the trauma setting, which has been instrumental in understanding the impact of various traumatic injuries in a clinical and research setting.*

The full reference list appears on Elsevier eBooks+.

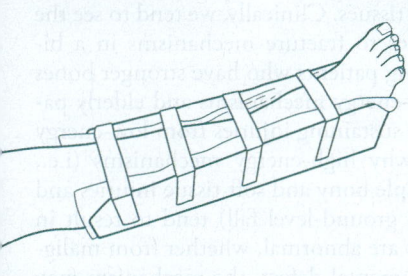

CHAPTER 40

Emergency Care of Musculoskeletal Injuries

Anna N. Miller and Mitchel R. Obey

EPIDEMIOLOGY OF ORTHOPEDIC INJURIES

Musculoskeletal (MSK) injuries are a leading cause of pain and disability and account for nearly 20% of all emergency department and primary care visits annually in the United States.[1] In 2004, MSK complaints comprised more than 57 million healthcare encounters in the United States, which represented approximately 60% of all injury treatment encounters in diverse care settings.[2] In 2006, the Centers for Disease Control and Prevention (CDC) reported that over 40 million encounters in the emergency department and primary care settings were the result of MSK complaints. Furthermore, previous authors have estimated that 8% of all emergency department encounters in the United States and Canada are due to MSK complaints,[3] whereas more recent studies have estimated it could be as high as 30% of all visits. The economic burden of MSK injuries on the healthcare system is significant and comprises both the direct costs associated with healthcare services and the indirect costs that occur due to

lost work productivity. In 2014, the annual costs for medical treatment and lost wages due to MSK complaints in the United States were estimated at $980 billion, which accounted for 5.76% of the gross domestic product.[4] Patients who are 65 years of age and older are disproportionately affected compared with younger populations, and the rate is expected to continue to increase as the population ages. The utilization of the emergency department and urgent care services is also higher among older adults, with MSK complaints accounting for 31.4% of all encounters in that age group in the United States. As such, it is crucial to understand how to evaluate and identify these injuries because improper management of patients with MSK injuries can lead to poor outcomes and increased morbidity.

In the United States, it has been estimated that 46% of patients sustaining a traumatic injury have an orthopedic injury, and between 13% and 25% of these patients require an orthopedic traumatologist. At the national and global levels, substantial improvements in transportation safety and delivery of medical care have helped address this growing pandemic. Seat belt and helmet laws, enforcement of drunk driving laws, mandates for improved safety features in automobiles, rapid deployment of emergency medical teams, and establishment of trauma centers have decreased the number of accident scene fatalities. As an increasing number of patients are surviving motor vehicle collisions (MVCs) that may have been fatal in the past, emergency medicine providers and first responders will be challenged with managing more complex fractures and soft tissue wounds. These realities demand that trauma teams be aware of the frequency and consequences of MSK injuries in every trauma patient. In particular, the immediate assessment and determination of severity are of the utmost importance, as this facilitates the correct triage of patients. Furthermore, an appreciation for the unique features of skeletal injury in patients who may also have severe head, thoracic, or intraabdominal trauma is essential. In this way, a cohesive, integrated approach to the diagnosis and treatment of MSK injuries may be used in the care of the multiply injured patient.

FRACTURE BIOMECHANICS

The human skeleton provides a rigid framework for our muscles to attach, which allows for the power of movement through the contraction of those muscles on the skeleton. Movement is dependent on the integrity of the skeletal system, and if it becomes fractured or diseased, then function will become decreased. The mechanical and structural properties of bone vary throughout different locations in the body, and as a result the amount of deformation that occurs during physiologic loading and loads that cause failure differ. The strength of a particular bone is gained by the bone mineral density and the characteristics of the trabecular component (i.e., thickness and connectivity) of the bone. Also, the structure of bone affects its material characteristics and strength, and normal bone typically comes in two different forms: cortical or cancellous. Cortical bone is typically quite strong, lines the outer surface of long bones, and provides load-bearing support. Cancellous, or trabecular, bone is more porous in structure, is less strong than cortical bone, and is typically found within the metaphysis of long bones. The density of trabecular varies greatly depending on the location in the body, function, and age of the patient.

Fractures usually result when the applied load to the bone exceeds its load-bearing capacity, or when the skeleton is placed in an unaccustomed position, or is struck by an outside load. Generally, fracture patterns occur because of separate and specific types of loading, and understanding the loading pattern that caused the fracture can assist in maneuvers to reduce the fracture and/or dislocation to its reduced or nondisplaced state. Examples of these traumatic loading conditions include axial, bending, torsion, and crush, and they can also be categorized as blunt or penetrating. In the case of bending, the bone is subjected to high tensile stresses on the convex side of the bone, whereas high compressive stresses develop on the concave side. These result in a predictable fracture pattern that is composed of a transverse fracture on the tension side and a "butterfly" or "wedge" fragment found on the compressive side. The patient's age and the mechanism of injury are both strong determinants of the fracture pattern as well as the soft tissue injury that occurs simultaneously with the fracture. In the setting of an MVC, physics states that kinetic energy equals $(1/2)$ (mass)(velocity^2), and therefore, the greater the velocity, the higher the amount of energy stored within a system. This energy is absorbed by the body and the MSK system, which results in

fracture and injury to the soft tissues. Clinically, we tend to see the concept of energy as it relates to fracture mechanisms in a bimodal distribution, with young patients who have stronger bones sustaining injuries from high-energy mechanisms and elderly patients with osteoporotic bone sustaining injuries from low-energy mechanisms. This explains why high-energy mechanisms (i.e., MVC) tend to result in multiple bony and soft tissue injuries and low-energy mechanisms (i.e., ground-level fall) tend to result in isolated injuries. When bones are abnormal, whether from malignancy, infection, or a developmental defect, the mechanism may not "match" the fracture pattern, and in such cases the provider should recognize this and complete a further workup of the patient.

TERMINOLOGY

A key component of fracture care, specifically in the emergency setting, is the ability to communicate fracture characteristics effectively and concisely among providers. When initial radiographs are obtained in the emergency department, an understanding of general fracture descriptors and terminology by providers can be helpful when discussing injuries with consulting services. Fractures occur in a wide variety of anatomic locations throughout the body, involve different aspects of the bone itself, and may also be accompanied by soft tissue injuries that may or may not communicate directly with the fracture. As will be discussed later, it is important to have a general understanding of fracture terminology and the potential implications for acute treatment of various fracture types depending on their location and associated soft tissue injuries. The most practical and universally understood terminology of fractures is simply one that includes basic anatomic and mechanical descriptors, which ensures concise communication among providers. Table 40.1 includes a list of common fracture descriptors.

Fracture Types

Fractures can be classified as acute, subacute, or chronic (i.e., nonunion). Subacute and chronic fractures, although frequently needing treatment, can often be managed on an ambulatory basis and do not require emergent care. Rather, they can often be braced or splinted for comfort and treated with protected weight-bearing if indicated until further outpatient evaluation by a specialist. Radiographically, acute fractures can be differentiated from older fractures by the identification of sharp, well-defined edges of the fracture fragments and an injury mechanism to explain the injury. Subacute fractures will display evidence of callus formation and/or softening and blunting of the fracture edges and may or may not display signs of instability on physical examination. Fracture nonunions are typically at least 6 months old and radiographically can appear in a diverse variety of ways. In these cases, obtaining a detailed history from the patient will often identify the chronic nature of the injury (Fig. 40.1).

Pediatric patients experience fractures that are often different from those of adults, and this is because their bones are less dense and have increased plasticity, thicker periosteum, and open physes (Fig. 40.2). *Plastic deformity* of a long bone in a pediatric patient describes deformation of the bone without complete disruption of the cortex, and this is commonly observed in pediatric forearm fractures. The bone will show signs of angulation in one or more planes but may not have any visible fracture lines present, such as is seen with the ulna in Fig. 40.2A. In such cases, radiographs of the contralateral extremity can be quite helpful in the diagnosis by

TABLE 40.1	Fracture Terminology and Descriptors.
TERM	**MEANING**
General Terms	
Skeletal Maturity	Open versus closed physes (e.g., growth plates)
Pathologic	Fracture involving an area of abnormal bone
Insufficiency, fragility	Osteoporotic bone
Open	Fracture communicates with outside environment
Closed	Fracture does not communicate with outside environment
Children	
• Greenstick	Incomplete cortical disruption, plastic deformation
• Physeal	Involvement of the physis
• Buckle, torus	Axial crush with buckling of cortex
Location	
• Diaphysis	Shaft of long bone, thick cortical bone
• Metaphysis	Flare between the shaft and the joint surface, thin outer cortical bone
• Epiphysis	End of bone that forms joint surface
• Supracondylar	Proximal to the epicondyles (e.g., humerus and femur)
• Intercondylar	Extension between the articular condyles (e.g., humerus and femur)
• Intraarticular	Extension into the articular surface
Pattern	
• Transverse	Perpendicular to the long axis of the bone
• Oblique	Angular to the long axis of the bone
• Spiral	Torsional
• Butterfly	Separate fracture fragment at the fracture
• Comminuted	Multiple fracture fragments
Displacement	
• Translation	Percent displacement of the distal fragment relative to the proximal fragment
• Angulation	Apex volar or dorsal, apex valgus or varus
• Length	Shortened or distracted
• Rotation	Relative to the proximal fragment

confirming asymmetry between limbs. *Buckle fracture* describes an injury that occurs with axial loading of a long bone, such as a fall on an outstretched hand, leading to buckling of one or more cortices and with or without a visible fracture line. This is commonly seen in pediatric distal radius fractures (see Fig. 40.2B). *Greenstick fracture* describes an incomplete disruption of a bony cortex and usually consists of a complete cortical disruption on one side of the bone, with a buckle fracture or plastic deformation on the opposite side (see Fig. 40.2C). The dense overlying periosteum can contribute stability to many of these pediatric fracture types if the layer remains intact, which is why many are treated successfully with closed reduction and splinting. Not uncommonly, a pediatric patient will present with pain or refusal to use an extremity, yet radiographs will appear normal. In those cases, radiographs of the contralateral extremity can be obtained to assess for deformity; however, care must also be taken to not miss an injury to nonossified, cartilaginous physis (i.e., growth plate). *Physeal fractures* are unique to pediatric patients and may present in six different types, as described by the Salter-Harris classification system (Fig. 40.3A). The physis of a bone is typically located

at the ends of bones at the metaphyseal-epiphyseal junction, represent the center of longitudinal bony growth, and ossify at different points throughout a child's life. Fracture through or disruption of one of these "ossification centers" can alter the future growth of the affected bone, leading to length discrepancies and/or angular deformities. Especially in younger patients whose skeleton is largely not ossified, these injuries can be difficult to diagnose, and therefore, providers should maintain a high level of clinical suspicion when radiographs appear normal.

When a bone fails through an area weakened by preexisting disease, it is termed a *pathologic fracture*. Common causes of this may include weakness from primary bone tumors, metastatic lesions, infection, metabolic disease, skeletal dysplasia, and injury through an old fracture site. Although they are not commonly referred to in this way, fractures in osteoporotic bone may be considered pathologic. The term *insufficiency* or *fragility fracture* is more commonly used to describe these injuries. In contradistinction to acute fractures in healthy bone, fragility fractures result from an injury mechanism with much lower energy, such as a fall from standing height. Hip fractures, distal radius fractures, and compression fractures of the vertebral bodies in older adults are common examples. When diagnosed, in addition to providing appropriate acute treatment of these injuries, it is also important to ensure these patients receive a referral to a bone health specialist for further evaluation and treatment to help prevent future fragility fractures.

A fracture is considered *open* when an open wound communicates with the fracture site, which may often display evidence of fracture hematoma draining through the wound. Wounds that communicate with the fracture may not always directly overly the fracture site, and therefore, a thorough physical examination and inspection of the wound are critical in the diagnosis. It is extremely important that open fractures are not missed because their presence has implications for immediate treatment in the emergency department (i.e., prophylactic antibiotics), treatment in the operating room, and the long-term outcomes. Open fractures present on a spectrum, ranging from small (<1 cm, "poke-hole") wounds to severe soft tissue wounds with extensive stripping and degloving of the underlying tissues. The Gustilo-Anderson classification is most widely used to classify the open fractures. In practice, it can be dichotomized into *high energy* and *low energy* injuries, leading to a more consistent determination of treatment. High-energy fracture patterns indicate that the soft tissues and the bones have experienced a much greater degree of energy and forces. Although a skin laceration may be the most evident component found on physical examination, the energy of the fracture, degree of contamination, and soft tissue injury must all be taken into account in evaluating the severity of the injury. For example, a highly comminuted distal femur fracture with a 10-cm open wound after a high-speed MVC would most appropriately be classified as a type III open fracture because of extensive soft tissue damage that often occurs in these fractures. This communicates the severity of injury to the surgical team and also initiates appropriate antibiotic prophylaxis in the emergency department. Finally, the true classification of open fractures occurs only in the operating room, after thorough debridement and evaluation of the soft tissue envelope.

A fracture that extends into a joint is termed *intraarticular*. These injuries may result from an axial load across the joint (i.e., tibia plateau or tibia plafond fractures) or from a variety of other mechanisms. The articular surface must remain congruent to ensure proper function and articulation, so displaced intraarticular fractures generally require open anatomic reduction to restore the

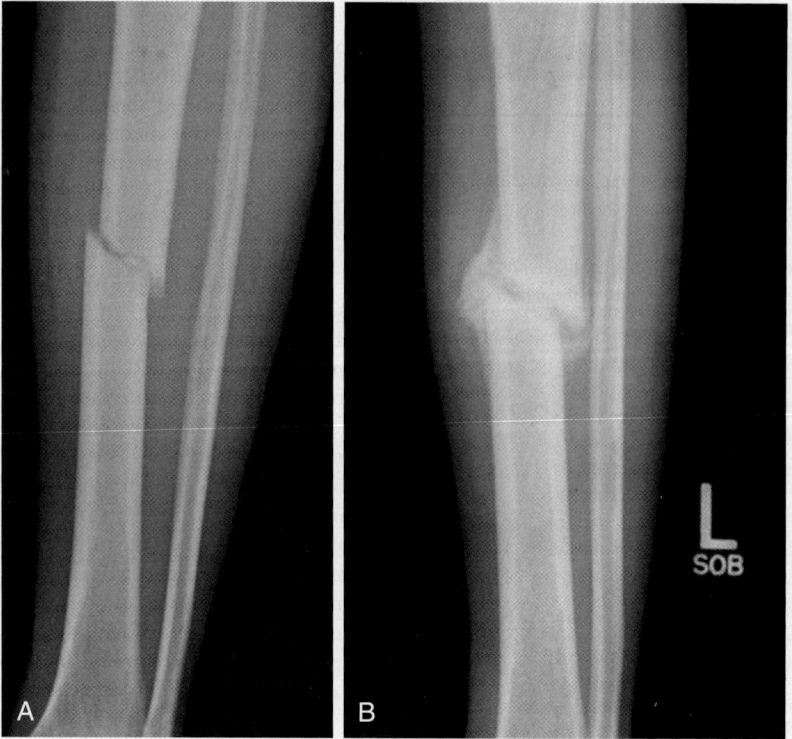

FIGURE 40.1 (A) Acute fracture. Note the sharp, well-defined edges. (B) Nonunion. Six months later, the fracture line is still clearly visible, the edges of this fracture are blunted, and the bone ends are sclerotic with callus formation. There was still motion at the fracture site on clinical examination, and the patient had significant chronic pain.

articular surface and are stabilized with rigid internal fixation to minimize the risk of posttraumatic arthritis. This is distinctly different from a fracture of the diaphysis (shaft) of a long bone, such as the femur, which can be treated with a closed reduction to restore length, alignment, and rotation. If the bone heals imperfectly from a radiographic appearance but the mechanical axis has been restored, the patient will likely experience a good outcome.

Long bone fractures are characterized by the anatomic location of the fracture (see Fig. 40.3B). The epiphysis comprises the area between the physis, or physeal scar, and articular surface. The metaphysis is located between the epiphysis and diaphysis and includes the growth plate. The diaphysis encompasses the shaft of the bone between the proximal and distal metaphyses. The diaphysis is composed of dense cortical bone that surrounds a medullary canal, and the metaphysis generally has thinner cortical bone that surrounds a core of cancellous bone. The diaphysis has relatively less vascularity than the soft cancellous bone of the metaphysis, and this difference in vascularity affects the rate at which the bone heals. Long bone fractures can also be described according to their location along the bone—proximal, middle, or distal third, and this classification is known as the *AO/OTA (Arbeitsgemeinschaft für Osteosynthesefragen/Orthopedic Trauma Association) Classification scheme.* Because long bones are important for movement and have several soft tissue attachments, such as those from muscles and tendons, fracture displacement is often a product of the deforming forces from those soft tissue attachments, and knowledge of their insertions can aid in achieving a successful reduction.

Metaphyseal fractures of the distal humerus and femur are referred to as *supracondylar* and may or may not be accompanied by intercondylar extension if there is involvement of the articular surface. The condyles are the medial and lateral bony prominences to which the stabilizing ligaments and muscles of the elbow and knee are attached. Presence of articular surface involvement, such as an intercondylar distal humerus fracture, is an important distinction to make when considering treatment because, as stated earlier, the articular surface requires an anatomic reduction to restore joint congruity.

After properly identifying the location of a fracture, the actual fracture pattern should be described (Fig. 40.4). The orientation of the primary fracture line may be transverse, oblique, or spiral. Bones are generally weakest in torsion, and spiral fractures result from torsional forces. Transverse and oblique patterns result from forces that occur perpendicularly or at an angle to the anatomic axis of the bone. However, there is often a combination of these forces, which results in a pattern that is a summation of the forces. Fracture comminution can occur in the form of a wedge or "butterfly" fragment. When a bending moment is applied to a bone, the concave side experiences a compressive force while the reciprocal convex side experiences a tensile force. Bone initially fails on the tension side, and as the fracture propagates toward the concave side, the fracture exits proximal and distal to compressed bone, creating a wedge-shaped fragment, or "butterfly." *Comminution* refers to the presence of multiple fragments within an individual fracture site and usually indicates a higher-energy injury or weakened bone in an older patient. Segmental patterns are composed of fractures at multiple locations along the same bone, with at least one intercalary segment of bone that is intact between the fractures. These also represent a higher-energy fracture pattern.

Displacement, if present, is described through a combination of principles. Deformities may occur in any plane,

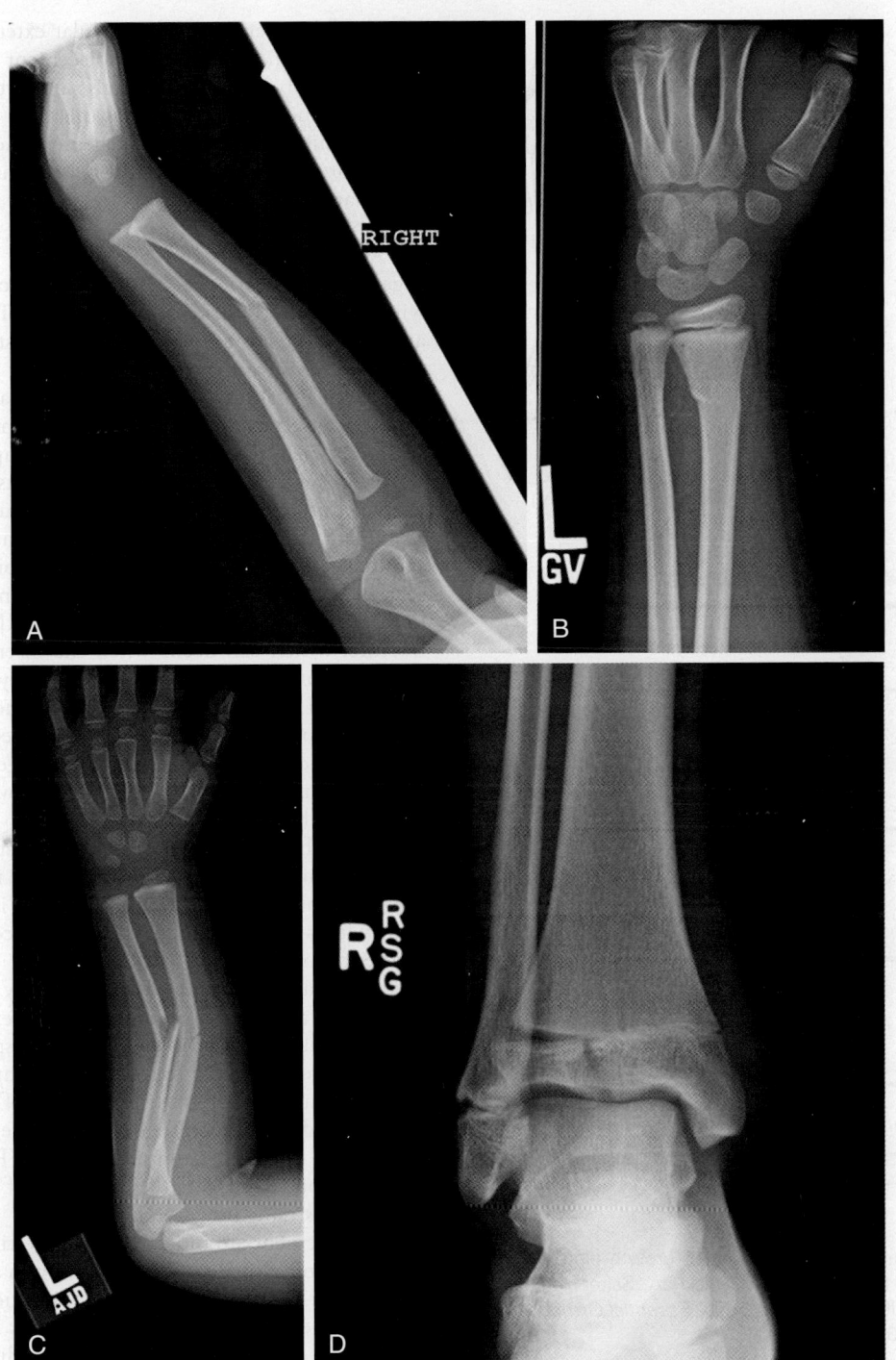

FIGURE 40.2 (A) Plastic deformity. Note the bowing of the ulna. (B) Buckle fracture. The cortex of the distal radius is deformed but intact. (C) Greenstick fracture. Disruption of radial cortices, without disruption of the ulnar cortices, in this forearm fracture in both bones. (D) Physeal fracture. Note the gapping of the lateral tibial physis.

including the coronal, sagittal, and axial planes. When viewed on plain orthogonal radiographs, fractures can be described by their coronal or sagittal displacement. However, the true displacement is a summation of all three planes. As such, fractures can be further described by their degree of translation, angulation, rotation, and shortening. Translation is the relationship of the distal fracture fragment to the proximal segment and is described in units of length (i.e., centimeters)

or a percentage of the bone's width at that level. Angulation is simply the angle created by the two ends of the fracture and is conventionally described in two ways. The first is by the direction of displacement of the distal segment relative to the proximal segment, and the second is by the direction of the apex of the fracture. For example, the fracture shown in Fig. 40.5 may be described as dorsal angulation of the articular surface or apex volar angulation at the fracture site.

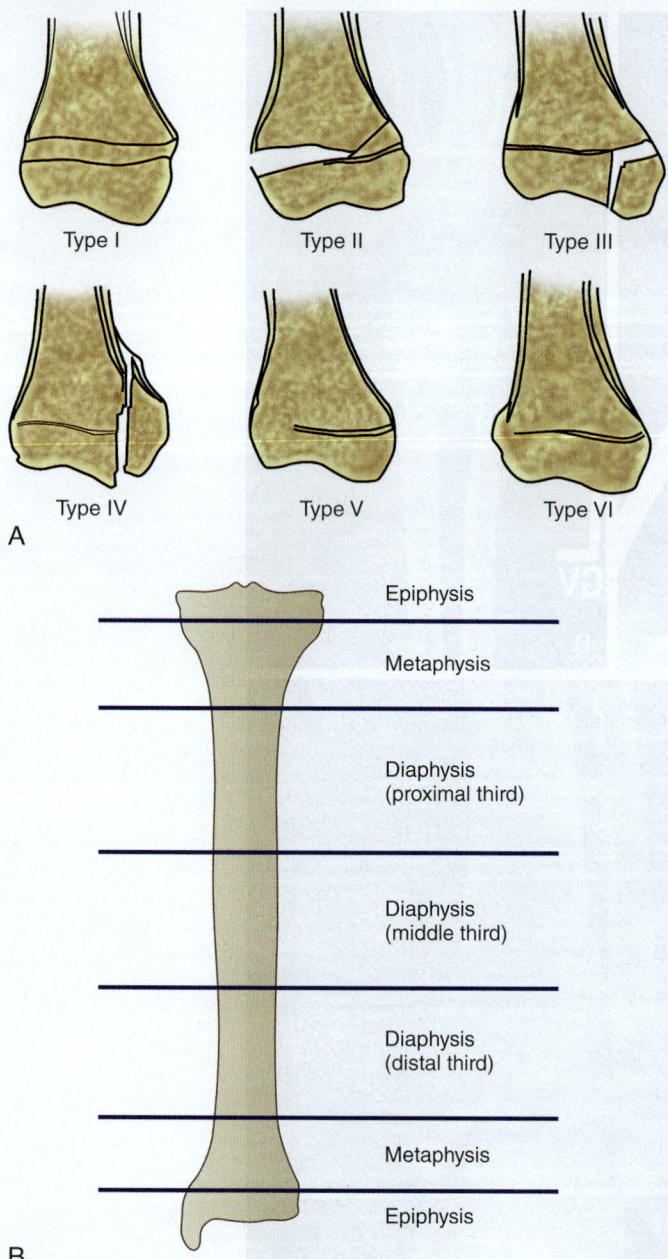

Type I   Type II   Type III

Type IV   Type V   Type VI

A

Epiphysis

Metaphysis

Diaphysis
(proximal third)

Diaphysis
(middle third)

Diaphysis
(distal third)

Metaphysis

Epiphysis

B

FIGURE 40.3 (A) Salter-Harris classification of growth plate injuries. (B) Anatomic regions of the tibia. (From Janicki JA. Salter-Harris fractures. In: Miller M, Hart JF, MacNight JM, eds. *Essential Orthopaedics.* Saunders Elsevier; 2010;939-943.)

Rotational deformity can be difficult to determine on radiographs, and full-length films of the limb segment involved, including the joints above and below, must be imaged to determine rotation. Advanced imaging, such as a computed tomography (CT) scan, viewed in the axial plane can also give information on rotation. Alternatively, rotational deformity may be assessed clinically by comparing the injured limb with the contralateral side.

Once a fracture has been identified, it must be described in a consistent, systematic manner. All descriptions begin with whether the fracture is open or closed, and if open, the degree of soft tissue injury must be communicated. Next, fracture laterality, location of the fracture along the bone involved, and fracture pattern are

stated. The presence of intraarticular extension, if visible, should be noted. Then the general displacement pattern of the fracture can be described. Finally, it is also important to indicate any associated nonorthopedic injuries that may alter the timing of any planned initial orthopedic management. Adherence to this scheme allows for comprehensive and concise communication of the fracture characteristics.

Other Injuries

Ligamentous injuries are commonly encountered in association with traumatic injuries to bones and joints. When a ligament attached to a joint is damaged but is still in continuity, it is termed a *sprain* and can range in severity from minor injuries to significant instability about the joint. Grade I ligamentous injuries are caused by stretching of a ligament or ligament complex without causing instability, and an example of this would be a simple ankle sprain. Grade II ligamentous injuries are caused by partial ruptures of ligaments and can result in minor instability. Complete ruptures, or grade III ligamentous injuries, result in significant instability of the associated joint and are commonly seen in the setting of multiligamentous injuries after a knee dislocation. Another example of a grade III injury is an avulsion fracture, which can occur when the insertion of a ligamentous structure completely avulses from its bony insertion, resulting in instability. Ligamentous injuries should not be overlooked when evaluating patients with MSK injuries because they can lead to significant joint instability, which endangers the cartilage surface and surrounding soft tissue and neurovascular structures. As such, a full neurovascular examination should be performed whenever there is suspicion of joint instability or dislocation. Although many ligamentous injuries do not require urgent orthopedic management, stabilization or immobilization of the joint with a splint or brace is usually recommended to prevent further injury.

In contrast, a *strain* describes an injury to a muscle or tendon that is not attached to a joint, and therefore does not as commonly result in joint instability. Like sprains (noted earlier), strains range from mild to severe and commonly are the result of an overuse injury pattern. In the setting of injury, further loading of the already weakened tendon or muscle can worsen the injury and lead to partial or complete rupture. Rest, ice, compression, and elevation (RICE) are the mainstays of treatment for a muscle or tendon strain; however, more urgent orthopedic evaluation and management are indicated in the setting of rupture. Tendon ruptures can be treated nonoperatively in some cases, and therefore, proper positioning and immobilization of the joint are important to ensure that the tendon scars down in a functional position. If operative management is indicated, prompt evaluation by an orthopedic provider should occur to direct further treatment and prevent scarring of the tendon and contracture of the muscle that may complicate the operative reparative or reconstructive procedure.

Joint injuries without fracture such as articular contusions or bone bruises are common in axial loading mechanisms and may present with significant pain and inability to bear weight. Treatment is typically nonoperative with a period of rest and protected weight-bearing; however, cartilaginous injury from the axial load can lead to late degenerative changes in the joint. An osteochondral fracture or defect can result when a piece of articular cartilage and its underlying subchondral bone become separated from the surrounding joint surface. Small osteochondral defects can be asymptomatic, but, in other cases, the patient

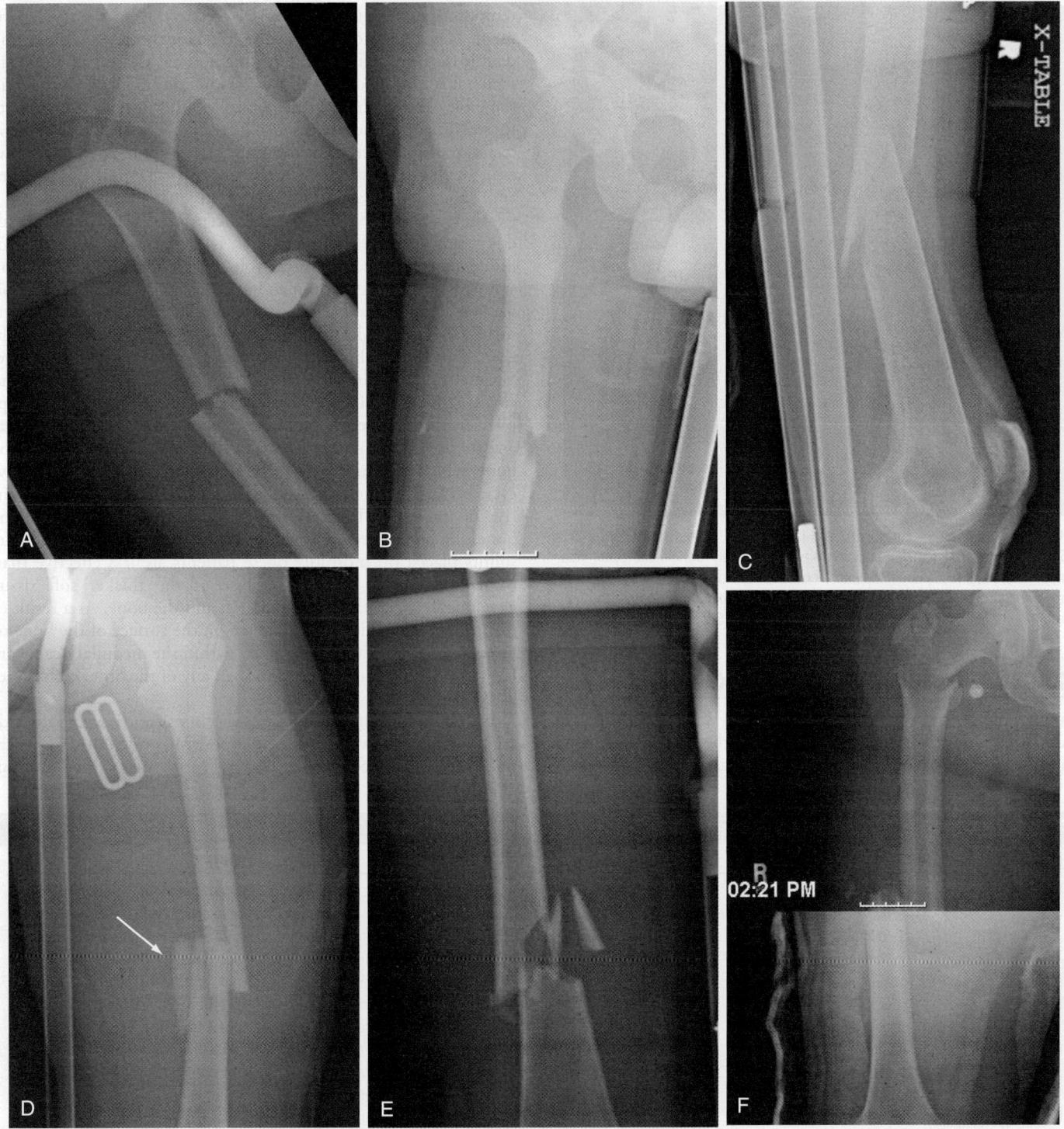

FIGURE 40.4 Femur fracture patterns. (A) Transverse. (B) Oblique. (C) Spiral. (D) Butterfly fragment *(arrow)*. (E) Comminuted. (F) Segmental.

may report mechanical symptoms such as locking/catching with joint range of motion. If missed during evaluation, these injuries can lead to chronic pain and joint degeneration. In some injuries, the osteochondral fragment will be large enough to be diagnosed on plain radiographs. When recognized, it is important to immobilize the joint to minimize further joint injury from the fragment and direct further evaluation to an orthopedic provider. Other commonly injured joints are the intervertebral discs in the spine. These discs are made up of a viscoelastic nucleus pulposus surrounded by a dense, fibrous anulus fibrosus. With a large enough axial load, the nucleus pulposus can herniate through the anulus, resulting in a disc herniation. This disc bulge can impinge on nerve roots, causing back and radicular pain, and most often these injuries do not require acute intervention. Very rarely, severe disc bulge in the lumbar spine can cause significant impingement on the cauda equina, resulting in cauda equina syndrome. This is a surgical emergency and is discussed in more detail later in the chapter.

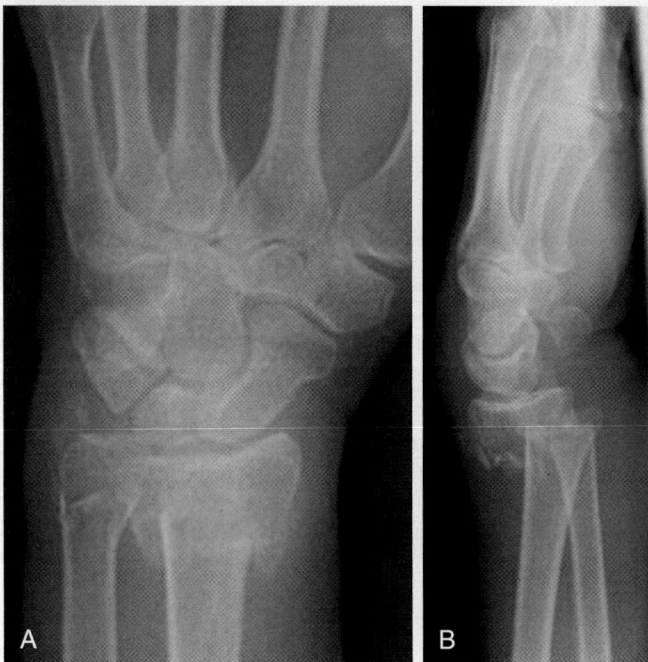

FIGURE 40.5 Posteroanterior (A) and lateral (B) left wrist radiographs of a 75-year-old patient who fell and sustained a dorsally translated, apex volar angulated, distal radius fracture and a comminuted displaced distal ulna fracture. (From Foster B, Bindra R. Intrafocal pin plate fixation of distal ulna fractures associated with distal radius fractures. *J Hand Surg.* 2012;137:356-350.)

FRACTURE STABILIZATION AND FIXATION

In the emergency setting, there are several ways to stabilize an injured extremity, varying in how effective they are in stabilizing the fracture and/or joint. Table 40.2 summarizes the methods of

temporary stabilization that can be used in the emergency department as well as more invasive methods of both temporary and definitive fracture fixation. Each method has clinical situations in which it is indicated, and those general indications are outlined in the table. The methods are arranged in order of increasing ability to stabilize the fracture and/or joint. For completeness, several techniques for fracture fixation are listed within the table; however, further discussion of the principles of fixation and implant application fall outside the scope of this chapter.

There are a couple important concepts to discuss when considering each of these methods. First, is the bone being directly or indirectly controlled? Splinting (plaster/fiberglass/boot or traction splint) is the most common and least invasive form of limb stabilization. Splints are commonly applied in the emergency department setting and do not directly contact the bone. As a result, their ability to stabilize a fracture and/or joint is less effective. Skeletal traction, and in some institutions external fixation and closed reduction with percutaneous pinning (CRPP), may be applied in the emergency department under light sedation or local anesthesia. These modalities of stabilization directly involve the bone, which can improve stabilization of the fracture/joint; however, because of their invasive nature, they do have an inherent risk of infection. The closer an implant can be applied to the bone, the more effective it will be at stabilization. As an example, splints placed on morbidly obese patients are less effective than those on thinner patients because of the thicker soft tissue envelope between the splint material and the bone. As a result of this principle, application of a plate on the surface of the bone or insertion of an intramedullary nail within the medullary canal are far more effective at stabilization than any of the other techniques listed in the table.

Second, one must always consider infection risk when deciding on treatment, whether it be temporizing or definitive. Skeletal traction, percutaneous pins, and all forms of external fixation

TABLE 40.2	Methods of Skeletal Stabilization and Fixation			
METHOD	**DETAILS**	**COMMON INDICATIONS**	**PROS**	**CONS**
Splinting	Plaster, fiberglass, fracture boot	Temporary stabilization of acute extremity injuries	Accommodates soft tissue swelling	Indirect control of the bone; not length stable
Traction splint	Commercially produced device	Temporary stabilization of femoral shaft fractures	Helps control pain and bleeding; maintains length	Indirect control of the bone; may produce pressure ulcers at the ischial tuberosity and ankle
Skeletal traction	Transosseous pin, traction bow, and weight	Temporary stabilization of femur and pelvis fractures	Helps control pain and bleeding; maintains length	Indirect control of the bone; does not allow for patient mobilization
External fixation (pins/bars)	Multiple transosseous pins with attached external bars	Temporary stabilization of acute extremity injuries	Improved control of the bones and thus improved soft tissue control; length stable	May allow too much motion for most fractures to heal
Closed reduction and percutaneous pins (CRPP)	Transosseous pins across a fracture site	Small bone fixation; pediatric fixation	Limited soft tissue disruption; removed once fracture healed	Risk of pin-site infection; indirect reduction of fracture
External fixation (pins/wires, rings)	Multiple transosseous pins/wires with attached external rings	Definitive fixation with the ability to manipulate the bones	Can be used for complex deformity correction and fractures	Risk of pin-site infection; indirect reduction of fracture
Intramedullary nailing (IMN)	Nail placed within the medullary canal of the bone	Long bone fracture treatment	Limited soft tissue disruption; relative stability	Indirect reduction of fracture; limited utility in treating articular fractures
Open reduction and internal fixation (ORIF)	Plates and screws	Articular fractures; upper extremity long bone fractures; ankle fractures	Direct anatomic reduction and absolute stability	Larger soft tissue disruption; biomechanically less strong than nails because of location of implant relative to mechanical axis

involve placement of an implant that communicates between the bone and the outside environment. This does carry a risk of infection; however, pin-site infections are common and often respond well to pin-site care and oral antibiotics. In the event of a more severe pin-site infection, removal of the pin or wire usually facilitates eradication of the infection.

Finally, does the surgeon have direct visualization of the fracture? Apart from displaced intraarticular fractures or fracture dislocations, not all other fractures necessarily require an open anatomic reduction. An important risk of the surgical exposure, fracture cleaning, and reduction to keep in mind is the stripping of the soft tissue attachments from the bone. This leads to decreased vascularity at the fracture site, increasing the risk of delayed or nonunion and possibly infection. When considering fixation of long bones, fractures in specific bones such as the radial shaft may benefit more from open reduction and internal fixation, whereas a femoral shaft fracture can be treated with an intramedullary nail through closed reduction and no direct visualization of the fracture site; in this case, the primary objective of the surgery is to restore length, alignment, and rotation of the mechanical axis. Overall, each method of fracture stabilization and fixation has its own set of indications and advantages and disadvantages. The choice of the most appropriate method of fracture stabilization (whether it is temporary or definitive) depends on the clinical situation, the resources available, and the surgeon's capabilities.

PATIENT EVALUATION

History

Obtaining a detailed history from patients with MSK injuries is essential for accurate diagnosis and treatment. At times this can be quite challenging depending on the clinical status of the patient. It is not uncommon for trauma patients to arrive intubated, intoxicated, or delirious. In these cases, an account of the mechanism of injury and patient history should be obtained from family members, emergency medical response crew members, or other witnesses to the accident. Descriptions from the injury scene can be helpful when deciding on acute treatment because common injury patterns often occur from specific mechanisms (Table 40.3).

A general history that includes demographic information, past medical history, past surgical history, and social history should be obtained. Knowledge of allergies, current medications, and time since last oral intake is important in guiding treatment. Each patient should be kept from eating or drinking anything until a full evaluation is performed by all pertinent services. Information about the position of the limb before and after the injury and the direction of the deforming force can help predict injuries and potentially associated injuries. Ambulatory status before the injury helps determine realistic goals for functional recovery, and it can also drive treatment decisions. For example, if an elderly patient presents with a femoral neck fracture, it is helpful to know if they previously ambulated in the community or primarily within their household because it may indicate one surgery over another. Any transient neurologic symptoms, such as loss of consciousness, numbness, dysesthesias, and spasm, must be documented. Loss of bowel or bladder control in patients with back or neck pain must also be noted. Finally, the time elapsed since injury becomes critical information in patients with an ischemic limb secondary to a vascular injury, an open wound with gross contamination, or a joint dislocation.

TABLE 40.3 Common Injury Mechanisms and Associated Injuries

INJURY PATTERN OR MECHANISM	ASSOCIATED INJURIES
Fall from a height	• Calcaneus fracture • Tibia plateau fracture • Tibia plafond fracture • Fractures around the hip (proximal femur, acetabulum) • Pelvic ring or sacral fracture, including vertical shear injuries • Vertebral body fracture

Fall onto outstretched hand	• Distal radius fracture
	• Elbow dislocation
	• Pediatric
	  • Both-bone forearm fracture
	  • Supracondylar humerus fracture

Fall onto shoulder	• Clavicle fracture • Acromioclavicular (AC) joint separation • Proximal humerus fracture
Ejection from vehicle	• Closed head injury • Spine fracture
T-bone motor vehicle crash	• Lateral compression–type pelvic ring injury • Closed head injury • Thoracic injury

Head-on motor vehicle crash	• Abdominal visceral injury
	• Retroperitoneal bleeding
	• Injuries caused by floor board intrusion
	  • Calcaneus fracture
	  • Tibia plateau fracture
	  • Posterior hip dislocation

Motorcycle crash	• Anterior-posterior compression-type pelvic ring injury • Mangled limb
Posterior knee dislocation	• Popliteal artery or vein injury • Common peroneal nerve injury • Multiligamentous knee injury
Supracondylar humerus fracture	• Brachial artery injury • Nerve injury (median or radial)
Anterior shoulder dislocation	• Axillary nerve injury
Posterior hip dislocation	• Sciatic (peroneal division) nerve injury • Posterior wall acetabulum fracture

Trauma Evaluation

Although beyond the scope of this chapter, examination of a multiply injured patient must adhere to Advanced Trauma Life Support (ATLS) protocols in a systematic fashion and must be accompanied by appropriate treatment. The concept of life before limb dictates the rapid initial evaluation of the injured patient. Hemodynamically unstable patients are assumed to be in hemorrhagic shock until proven otherwise. Historically, there has been debate about whether the anteroposterior (AP) pelvis radiograph, which has traditionally been considered part of the standard trauma radiographic series, is justified with the advent of newer CT scanners. However, many interdisciplinary trauma programs still obtain an AP pelvis radiograph at the time of the initial survey, especially for those in hemorrhagic shock, because it can be done quickly and will provide immediate information regarding the presence of a hip dislocation, acetabulum fracture, or pelvic ring injury. Additionally, it will serve as a baseline radiograph for comparison before any acute intervention that is provided, such as reduction of a hip dislocation or application of a pelvic binder in a patient with a volume-expanding pelvic ring injury. It is essential that if an institution enacts a protocol that skips the AP pelvis x-ray in favor of CT that the patient is expedited to intravenous contrasted CT in a timely fashion so that these potentially life-threatening findings are not missed.

In the initial care of MSK injuries, open fractures, those with vascular injury or compromise, or those developing compartment syndrome take precedence over lesser MSK diagnoses. In the setting of an open fracture, one of the most important treatment decisions a provider can make is prompt administration of appropriate prophylactic antibiotics and tetanus prophylaxis as soon as possible. Delayed administration of antibiotic prophylaxis has been shown in multiple studies to markedly increase the risk of infection.[5,6] In a recent review of 276 recommendations with regard to systemic antibiotic administration, all authors recommended administration within 3 hours of injury, and half of those recommended administration immediately after injury and/or on presentation to the emergency department.[5] Authors generally recommend coverage for gram-positive bacteria (i.e., cefazolin) in type I and II injuries and the addition of gram-negative and organic material contamination coverage (i.e., vancomycin) in more severe type III injuries.[5,6] When possible, providers should also consider an initial splinting and sterile dressing wound coverage in the emergency department to bridge the patient reaching an orthopedic assessment and ultimately the operating room.

Generally, examination and management of the extremities are deferred to the secondary survey after the airway has been controlled and hemodynamic stability has been obtained, especially because open extremity wounds can be distracting to the team. One caveat is the conscious patient who is able to follow commands but will need intubation to protect the airway. In this case, a quick neurologic examination of the extremity motor and sensory function can be performed before sedation or intubation, which provides valuable information and takes only seconds to carry out.

Unstable pelvic fractures are typically addressed in the primary survey, and stabilization with a pelvic binder/sheet in volume-expanding injury patterns can limit further hemodynamic deterioration. Evidence of large flank or buttock contusions and swelling may also indicate underlying pelvic bleeding or more superficial soft tissue injuries. A Morel-Lavallée lesion is commonly present in patients with pelvic or lower extremity trauma and represents a subcutaneous degloving injury from the underlying muscle and fascia. Blood at the urethral meatus, signifying injury to the genitourinary tract, may be a sign of an underlying pelvic fracture as well. Palpation of the symphysis pubis can help determine the presence of disruption of this joint; however, this will generally be discovered on the AP pelvis radiograph or CT scan. Gentle lateral compression through the iliac crests can assess for instability of the pelvic ring. Rectal and vaginal examinations are performed, noting the presence of gross blood, lacerations, bone fragments, hematomas, or masses. Wounds and palpable bone fragments found on either of these examinations are diagnostic of an open pelvic fracture and should be promptly treated as such. Rectal examination can also reveal a high-riding prostate gland (i.e., longer distance from the anal verge or nonpalpable), which is another suggestion of injury to the genitourinary tract after a pelvic fracture.

Examination of the extremities in either a patient with an isolated injury or a multiply injured patient should follow a simple, systematic, and reproducible algorithm. Even when an isolated extremity injury is the primary reason for evaluation, the entire skeleton must be examined. The examiner must not be distracted by other obvious or more severe injuries. Deformity, edema, ecchymosis, crepitus, tenderness, and pain with motion are the cardinal signs of an acute fracture or joint injury. Each aspect of each extremity needs to be examined for lacerations and the signs of trauma described earlier. All joints are put through passive range of motion, at a minimum, and active range of motion is tested whenever possible. Joint effusions may indicate intraarticular disease (i.e., ligamentous or intraarticular fracture). The joints are manually stressed to assess the integrity of the ligamentous structures. A neurovascular examination is performed and documented for each extremity. Pulses are recorded and compared with the opposite uninvolved extremity when possible. Doppler signals are obtained when palpable pulses are not present or are weak. Measuring the ankle-brachial index (ABI) is important when vascular injury is suspected or could be present (i.e., tibia plateau fracture dislocation). Motor function and sensation must be documented for the extremity dermatomes in all patients. A high suspicion for compartment syndrome should be maintained at all times, including patients with increased pain or abnormally tense compartments. This should raise suspicion for acute compartment syndrome and prompt further evaluation, with fasciotomies performed emergently if diagnosed. Realignment and immobilization of long bone fractures should be done expeditiously, as these maneuvers help prevent further damage to underlying soft tissues, facilitate clot formation, reduce patient discomfort, facilitate transportation, and may prevent embolization of intramedullary contents.

Diagnostic Imaging

As a general rule, when imaging a specific MSK injury (e.g., tibia shaft fracture), radiographs of the joints above (e.g., knee) and below (e.g., ankle) the level of injury should also be obtained. Similarly, when an injury to a joint is suspected (e.g., knee), the bones above (e.g., femur) and below (e.g., tibia) should be imaged in addition to the dedicated radiographs of the injured joint. Adhering to this protocol not only helps to obtain multiple views of the injured segment, which in turn provides more information about the injury, but will also decrease the odds of missed injuries in adjacent bones and joints.

Another important tenet of MSK imaging is obtaining high-quality orthogonal images of each bone of interest. In many cases, the extremity will have deformity secondary to the injury, but it is important that standard radiographs are obtained in order to best evaluate the anatomy. This will not only allow for effective detection of injuries but will also provide information on the overall deformity pattern, including the displacement, angulation, and length. As an example, a fracture may appear minimally or nondisplaced in one plane but in another view will be significantly displaced (Fig. 40.6). If at any point a reduction of a fracture or dislocated joint is performed, imaging should be obtained after the reduction to verify and document improvement in fracture alignment or joint congruency.

Some patients will have anatomic variants or congenital deformities. In those cases, if there is a question regarding the presence of an injury, imaging of the contralateral, uninjured side can be very useful in determining what is normal for that individual patient. When finer detail is necessary—such as in the assessment of

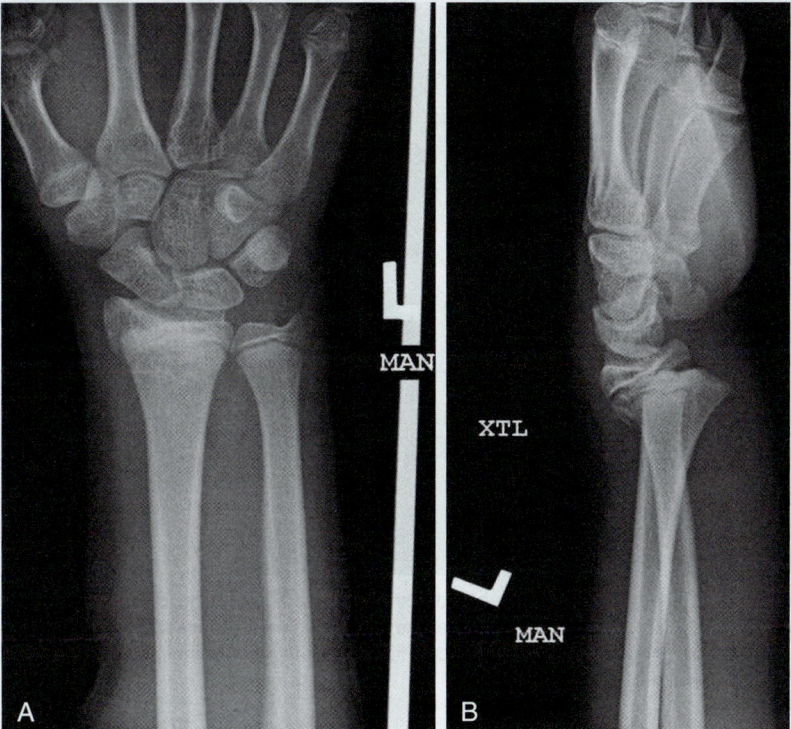

FIGURE 40.6 (A) Anteroposterior radiograph of the wrist showing disruption of the distal radial physis but adequate alignment. (B) Lateral view showing complete physeal separation with 50% dorsal displacement and significant angulation.

an intraarticular injury or to confirm the findings of an equivocal radiograph—a CT scan should be considered. Magnetic resonance imaging (MRI) has also become a particularly useful imaging modality as it has become easier to obtain for some institutions. It provides a more detailed evaluation of soft tissues (i.e., tendon or muscle injury), acute nondisplaced fractures, stress fractures (e.g.., femoral neck), spinal cord injuries, and intraarticular pathology (e.g., ligamentous injury). Its role in the trauma setting continues to expand, providing detailed information on spinal cord injuries and occult femoral neck fractures. It some situations in which plain radiographs are normal but high suspicion for an occult fracture remains, an MRI can be considered for further evaluation.

Shoulder

Multiple radiographic views of the shoulder can be obtained, and each helps to better evaluate specific anatomic structures of the shoulder girdle. In general, it is recommended to obtain a four-view series of the shoulder, which includes an AP, true AP ("Grashey view"), axillary lateral, and scapular "Y" view of the shoulder (Fig. 40.7). The most important lateral view is the axillary lateral because this will confirm a diagnosis of an anterior or posterior shoulder dislocation (Fig. 40.8). To obtain this image, the tube is angled cephalad, with the plate on the superior aspect of the abducted shoulder. This view is often difficult to obtain because of pain or instability of the shoulder in the setting of trauma. In those cases, a Velpeau view, which is a modified axillary view, can be obtained and provides orthogonally equivalent images. To obtain this image, the patient leans backward approximately 30 degrees over the cassette on the table. The x-ray tube is positioned cranial to the shoulder, and the beam is projected vertically down through the shoulder onto the cassette

(Fig. 40.9). This allows the radiograph to be taken with the shoulder adducted and, in a sling, allows acquisition of the axillary images without the pain of shoulder abduction. Another useful radiographic view is the scapula "Y" view, and this is an image of the scapula down its long axis (Fig. 40.10).

Elbow

AP and lateral views of the elbow provide visualization of most of the bony anatomy. Internal and external oblique views are included in a complete elbow series and allow better visualization of the medial and lateral epicondyles. On the lateral view, it is important to look for the fat pad sign, or "sail sign," which can be indicative of a joint effusion from an occult fracture. The "sail sign" is produced when hemarthrosis from an intraarticular fracture displaces the anterior and posterior fat pads out of the coronoid and olecranon fossae, respectively. On radiography, the visualized fat pads resemble a sail (Fig. 40.11). Although the anterior fat pad can be visualized in a normal elbow, the presence of a posterior fat pad sign is strongly suggestive of an occult fracture and, if clinically appropriate, warrants a CT scan and consideration for an MRI in pediatric patients. In patients with a supracondylar distal humerus fracture, a CT scan is often ordered to assess for intraarticular extension and for preoperative planning. A traction view of the elbow may also be obtained in cases of comminuted distal humerus fractures to better understand the fracture pattern.

Forearm and Wrist

The forearm should be imaged entirely on a single x-ray cassette in both the AP and lateral planes. The elbow and wrist should always be included. The radius and ulna have a complex relationship, essentially acting as a joint as the radius rotates around the

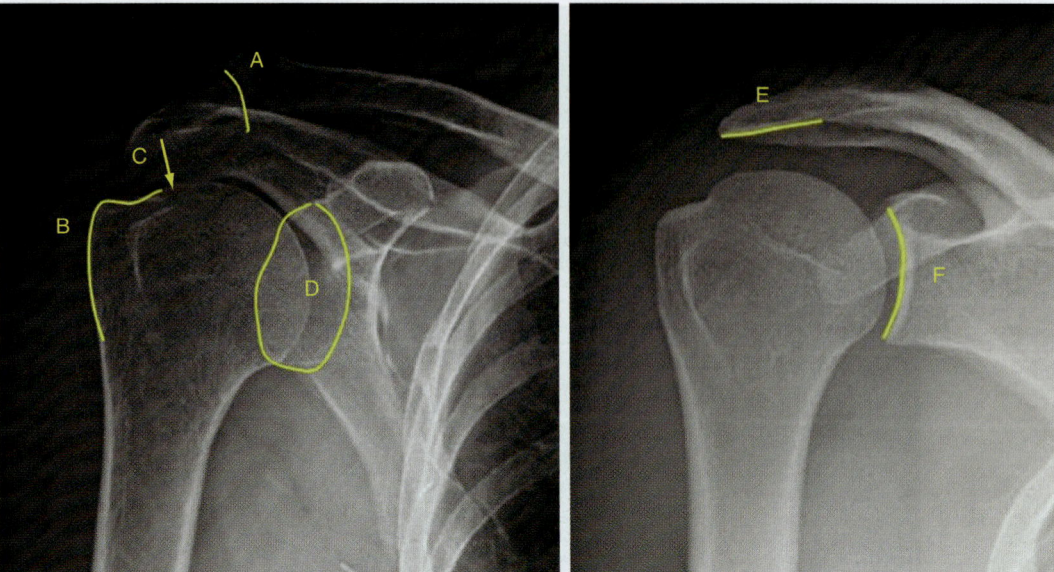

FIGURE 40.7 Anteroposterior view of the shoulder showing the acromioclavicular joint *(A)*, greater tuberosity *(B)*, acromiohumeral distance of 7 mm on average *(C)*, and glenoid fossa viewed at an angle to its face *(D)*. Grashey view of the shoulder showing the acromion down its longitudinal axis *(E)* and the glenoid fossa down its longitudinal axis *(F)*.

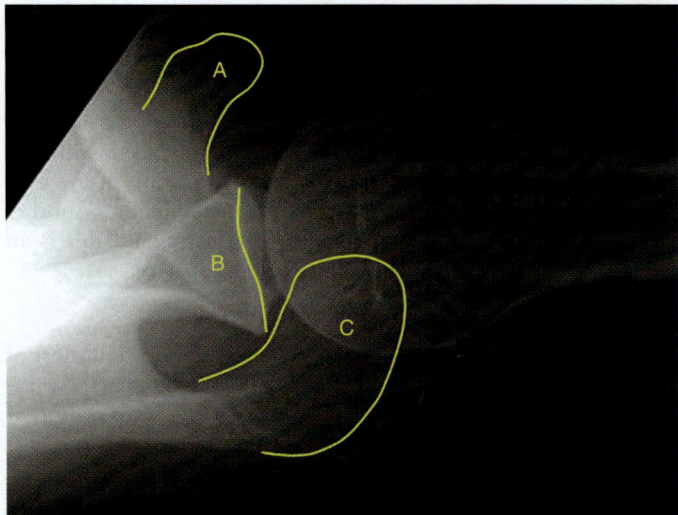

FIGURE 40.8 Axillary lateral view of the shoulder showing the cora-coid process *(A)*, glenoid fossa *(B)*, and acromion process *(C)*. This view allows for the assessment of anterior-to-posterior translation of the humeral head relative to either the glenoid fossa (dislocations) or the humeral shaft (fractures).

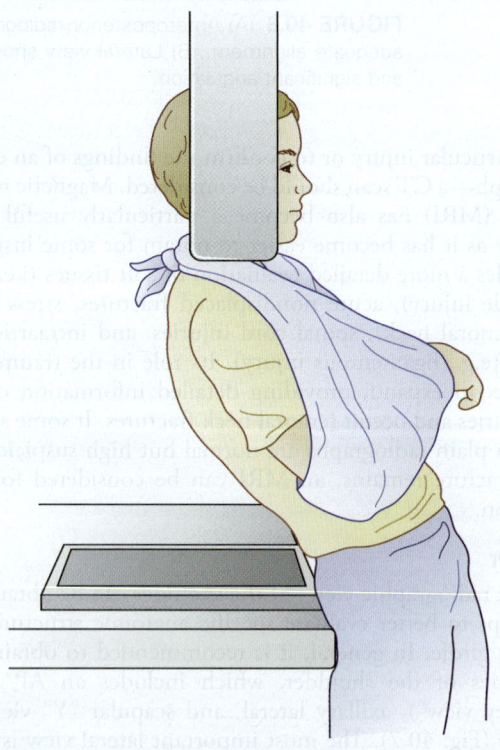

FIGURE 40.9 Velpeau or Bloom-Obata modified axillary view. (From Green A, Norris TR. Proximal humeral fractures and glenohumeral dislocations. In: Browner BD, Levine AM, Jupiter JB, et al., eds. *Skeletal Trauma: Basic Science, Management, and Reconstruction.* 4th ed. WB Saunders; 2008.)

ulna with forearm supination and pronation. Injuries may occur to each bone in isolation; however, both bones and their articulations at the elbow and wrist are often involved in some way. For example, an Essex-Lopresti injury describes a radial head fracture with an associated disruption of the forearm interosseous membrane and a dislocation of the distal radioulnar joint (DRUJ). A Monteggia fracture is another example in which the proximal ulna is fractured and a radial head dislocation also occurs as part of the injury. Finally, the wrist should be imaged in the AP, oblique, and lateral views. Do not forget that it is important that any distal radius or wrist injury that undergoes a closed reduction and splinting should have postreduction imaging as well.

Pelvis and Acetabulum

The pelvis is among the more complex three-dimensional bony structures of the human skeleton, and because of that, imaging can be difficult to evaluate by the untrained eye. CT scans ordered as part of the trauma protocol workup generally include a

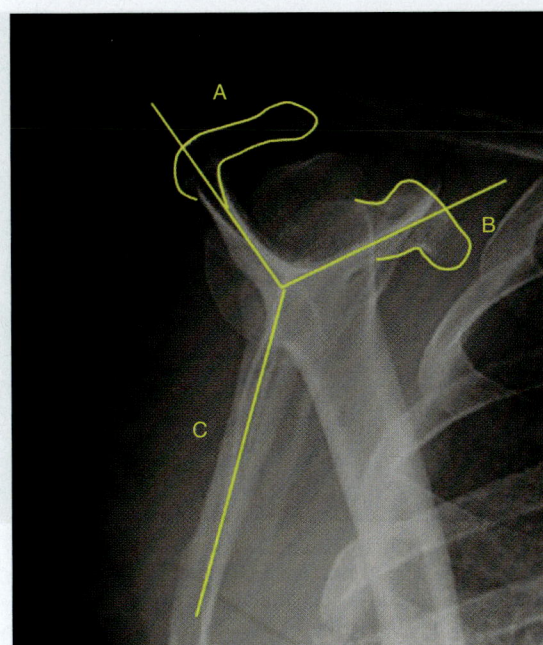

FIGURE 40.10 Scapula "Y" view showing the acromion process (A), coracoid process (B), and scapula body (C). This view allows for the assessment of anterior-to-posterior translation of the humeral head relative to either the glenoid fossa (dislocations) or the humeral shaft (fractures).

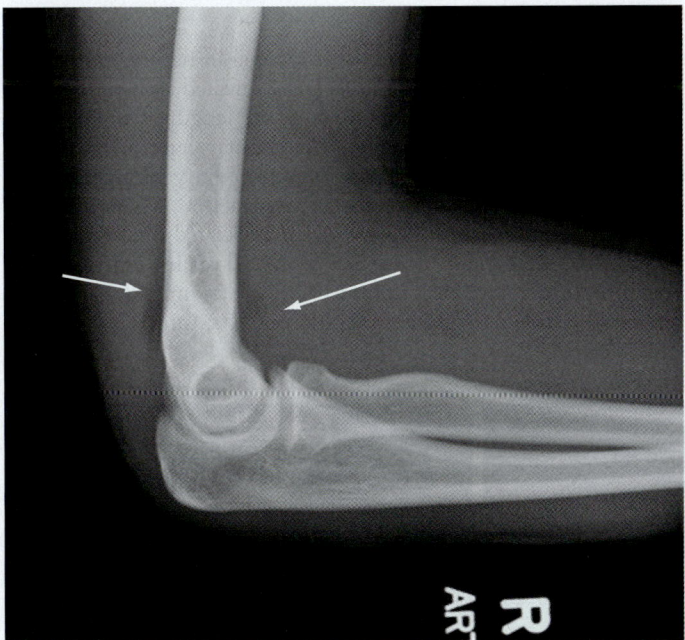

FIGURE 40.11 Positive fat pad or sail sign in a patient with a nondisplaced radial neck fracture. Note the anterior and posterior areas of radiolucency (arrows) representing the extruded fat pads.

CT scan of the pelvis, and so some may argue against the necessity of plain radiographs. However, pelvis radiographs remain important to orthopedic surgeons because they allow for the visualization of the entire pelvis in one image. The standard AP radiograph of the pelvis provides an immense amount of information on the pelvic ring, acetabulum, hip joints, and proximal femurs. If pathology is confirmed on the initial AP radiograph or suspected on

physical examination, additional views can be obtained. The first of these include the Judet views, or 45-degree oblique views, which are termed the *obturator oblique* and *iliac oblique views*. These are used to evaluate the acetabulum and give detailed information regarding specific components of the acetabulum (Fig. 40.12). It is recommended that all acetabular fractures are evaluated with an AP radiograph and both Judet views.

Inlet and outlet views of the pelvis are obtained to evaluate the pelvic ring, sacroiliac joints, and sacrum and to better characterize the deformity pattern of the pelvis. The inlet view is taken with the beam angled 25 to 40 degrees caudal to be perpendicular to the anterior cortex of the upper sacral body. Fractures of the sacrum, displacement of the sacroiliac joints, and displacement of the pubic symphysis in the AP plane are best evaluated on this view. The outlet view obtained with the beam angled 20 to 45 degrees cephalad, which views the sacrum, is pictured en face and gives information on the cranial-caudal translation of the injured pelvis.

Pelvic CT has become standard of care in many institutions for the evaluation of fractures of the pelvic ring, sacrum, and acetabulum. This provides much greater detail regarding fractures of the sacrum and acetabulum and greatly helps surgeons formulate a preoperative plan. It also allows for detailed measurement of fracture displacement, articular surface impaction, and the presence of any intraarticular fracture fragments. Finally, in patients with hemodynamic instability suspected to be caused by a pelvic or acetabular fracture, CT with IV contrast helps identify sources of hemorrhage and locations of hematomas. MRI has little role in acute, traumatic pelvic ring and acetabulum injuries; however, it is an imaging modality of choice for evaluating stress fractures, osteomyelitis, pelvic abscesses, and malignancies.

Hip

A hip series consists of AP and cross-table lateral radiographs. A plain AP pelvis radiograph should also be ordered to allow for comparison to the contralateral side. The cross-table lateral radiograph is generally recommended over the frog leg lateral in trauma patients because in the setting of a hip fracture, it will allow for less manipulation of the injured extremity. In an adult patient with acute groin pain and inability to bear weight with negative radiographs, it is critical to have a high suspicion for an occult femoral neck or intertrochanteric femur fracture, and this can be diagnosed with an MRI. Failure to identify these injuries can result in progression into a complete and displaced fracture, which can have a significantly negative impact on the patient's outcome. There is also a well-established association between a high-energy femoral shaft fracture (typically comminuted mid-to-distal shaft) and an ipsilateral femoral neck fracture. This was first described in 1953 and has since been reported to have an incidence between 2% and 9%.[7–9] Because of increased awareness, it is recommended that thin-cut high-resolution CT scan of the hip be ordered to assess for occult fracture. However, CT remains imperfect in the diagnosis, and, as such, new protocols have been developed for rapid limited-sequence MRI to diagnose occult femoral neck fractures missed on plain radiographs and thin-cut CT scans[8,9] with very positive results.

Knee

AP, lateral, and oblique (internal and/or external) radiographs will visualize most traumatic bony injuries of the knee. If possible, standing films are useful for evaluating knee alignment and joint space narrowing if there is concern for osteoarthritis; however,

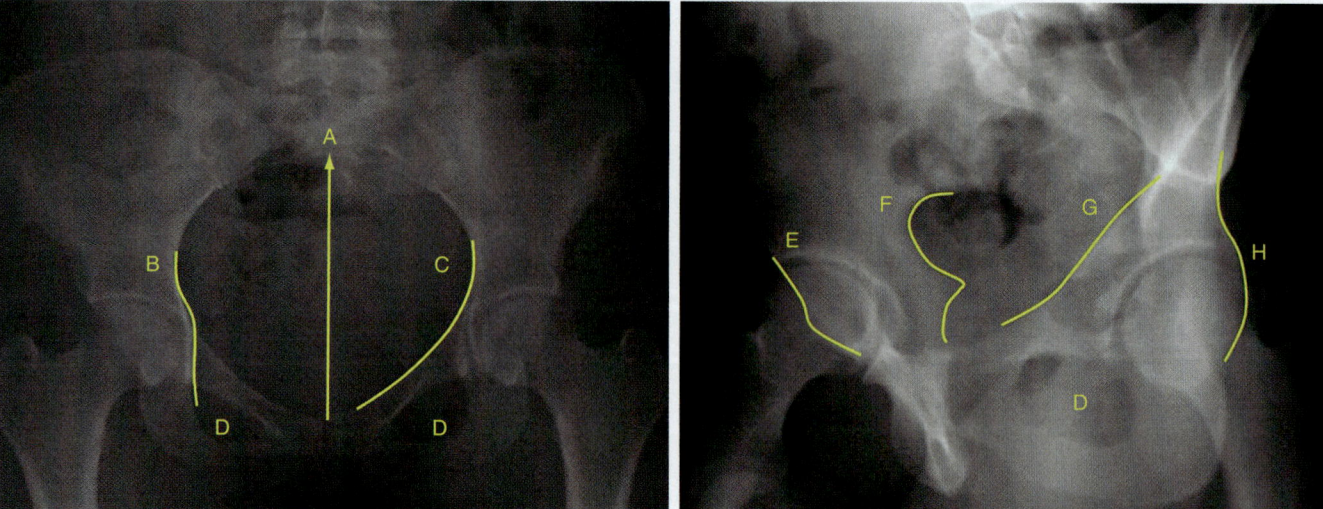

FIGURE 40.12 Anteroposterior and Judet pelvic radiographs. *(A)* The pubic symphysis should line up with the center of the sacrum to ensure no rotation. *(B)* The ilioischial line. *(C)* The iliopectineal line. *(D)* The obturator foramen are even in size and shape, ensuring no rotation. The obturator oblique is so named because the obturator foramen is visualized en face. The obturator oblique of one acetabulum is the iliac oblique of the contralateral hip in which the *(E)* anterior wall and *(F)* the posterior column are visualized. The *(G)* anterior column and *(H)* posterior wall are visualized on the obturator oblique.

most trauma patients will not be able to stand for imaging studies. Imaging both knees on a single weight-bearing AP allows for easy comparison to the contralateral side. The lateral radiograph can show an effusion, patellar fracture, posterior tibial plateau fracture, or tibial tubercle fracture. Assessment for patella baja (distal displacement) or alta (proximal displacement) can provide information if there is a suspected quadriceps tendon or patellar tendon rupture, respectively. If there is any doubt as to the degree of articular involvement, displacement, or depression, a CT scan should be ordered (Fig. 40.13). Although MRI can be helpful in the acute setting, evaluation for ligamentous, meniscal, or osteochondral injury can be performed in the outpatient setting. In the setting of a knee dislocation, there should be high suspicion for a vascular or neurologic injury. Serial measurements of the ABI in addition to assessment of distal pulses (palpation or Doppler) are

important for diagnosing vascular injury. If there is any asymmetry in vascular examination, additional imaging such as CT angiography or MR angiography should be strongly considered.

Ankle

The majority of ankle injuries are rotational in nature, and similar to the forearm, the tibia and fibula are connected by ligaments and an interosseous membrane throughout the length of the leg. As a result of this relationship, ankle injuries may have an associated proximal fibula injury as part of the same injury mechanism. An example of this would be a Maisonneuve fracture, which is a spiral fracture of the proximal fibula with an associated syndesmotic injury and a deltoid ligament rupture or medial malleolus fracture. To ensure an injury like this is not missed, it is recommended to obtain formal tibia/fibula radiographs in addition to a formal ankle series.

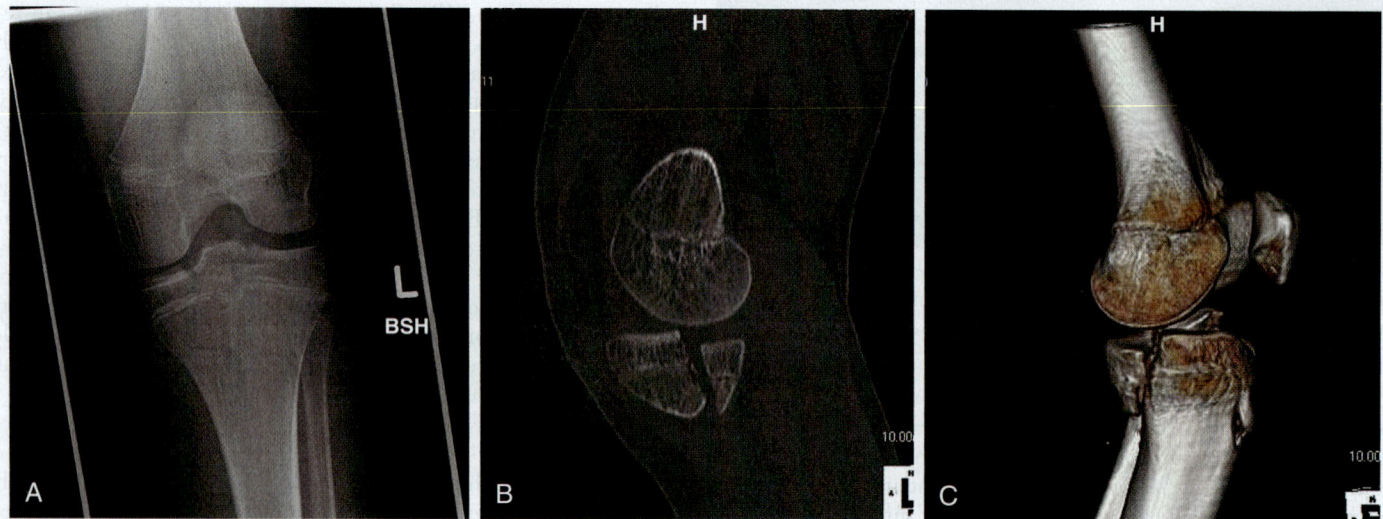

FIGURE 40.13 (A) Minimally displaced fracture of the tibial eminence. (B) Computed tomography scan of the knee shows a significant step-off of the posterior medial tibial plateau. (C) Three-dimensional reconstruction.

Assessment of ankle mortise congruency is a key tenet in the evaluation of ankle injuries, and the stability of the mortise depends on both bony and ligamentous support. It is recommended that a standard three-view series of radiographs (AP, mortise, and lateral) be obtained when evaluating any ankle injury. Most ankle fractures can be diagnosed from these three views, and, although ligamentous structures are not visualized directly, assumptions about their integrity can be made by evaluating spaces with well-established values between the tibia and fibula. Three main parameters commonly used are the tibiofibular overlap, tibiofibular clear space, and medial clear space (Fig. 40.14). The tibiofibular overlap and clear space are generally measured on the AP radiograph, and the medial clear space is best measured on the mortise radiograph. When internally rotating the ankle from the AP to the mortise view, the medial clear space and tibiofibular overlap will change, but tibiofibular clear space should remain constant.

Although bimalleolar and trimalleolar ankle fractures are usually indicated for surgery, isolated distal fibula (i.e., lateral malleolus) fractures can potentially be treated nonoperatively with a splint or fracture boot. A radiographic stress examination should be performed when evaluating any isolated lateral malleolus fracture. The ankle is stressed on the mortise radiograph and can be performed manually (neutral dorsiflexion and external rotation of the ankle) or by using gravity, and these are generally considered equivalent. The latter is performed by lying the patient on the ipsilateral side with a stack of sheets under the lateral leg. This allows the affected ankle to hang freely to the lateral side. In a positive stress examination, either or both the medial clear space and the tibia-fibula clear space will widen, indicating an unstable ankle mortise, which should be evaluated for surgical intervention.

As noted in earlier sections, articular injuries of the tibial plafond (i.e., pilon fractures) generally require a CT scan for more detailed evaluation of the injury and preoperative planning.

However, an important point to make in pilon fractures is that they commonly are initially treated in an ankle-spanning external fixator until soft tissues become amenable for definitive treatment. Therefore, orthopedic surgery specialists often recommended that a CT scan be obtained *after* application of the external fixator; the same is often true with tibial plateau fractures.

Foot (Hindfoot and Midfoot)

When foot trauma is suspected, the workup should start with a standard three-view series of AP, lateral, and oblique radiographs of the foot. The bony anatomy of the foot is a complex three-dimensional structure, and as a result, the standard series of films may not always be adequate to visualize certain bones. In the case of a calcaneus fracture, a Harris axial view should be added to evaluate the varus-valgus deformity of the tuberosity and to better visualize fractures in the sagittal plane. The Böhler angle of the calcaneus is measured on the lateral radiograph; it is the angle between a line from highest point of anterior process to highest point of posterior facet and a line tangential to superior edge of tuberosity (Fig. 40.15). The normal range for a Böhler angle is between 20 and 40 degrees, and values lower than this indicate depression of the posterior facet. The angle of Gissane may also be measured to evaluate the posterior facet, and a Broden view can be obtained to better visualize the posterior facet articular surface.

For fractures of the talus, the standard three-view foot series should be obtained. The lateral view will reveal fractures of the neck or body, and all views together should be assessed to confirm congruency of the tibiotalar, subtalar, and talonavicular joints. A Canale view is best for demonstrating talar neck fractures. If radiographs are negative or equivocal and the patient has evidence of fracture—ecchymosis, pain out of proportion to plain film findings, significant soft tissue swelling—a CT scan can be ordered to further evaluate. In general, most talus and calcaneus

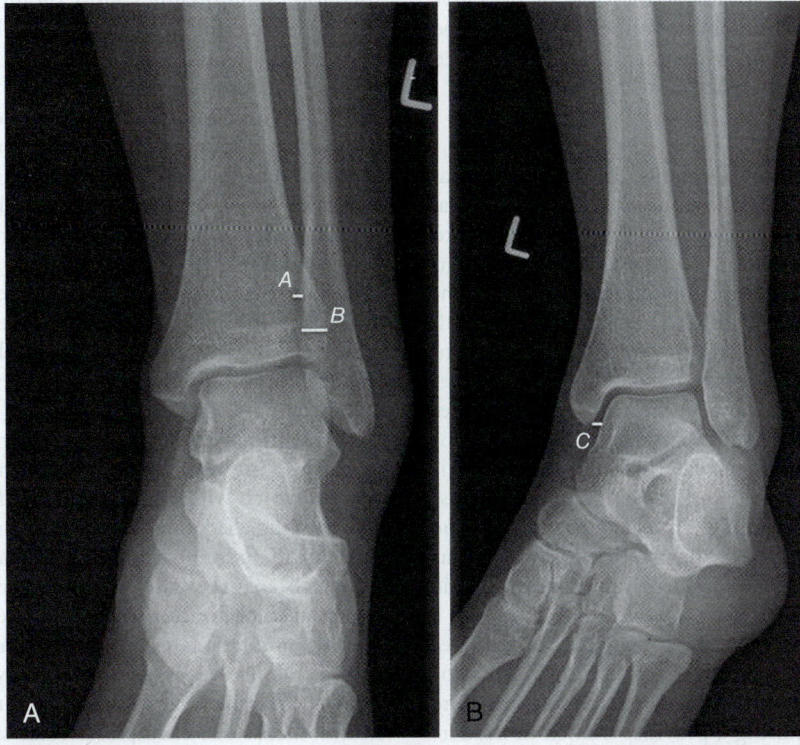

FIGURE 40.14 (A) Anteroposterior and (B) mortise radiographs of the ankle showing tibia-fibula clear space (A), tibia-fibula overlap (B), and medial clear space (C).

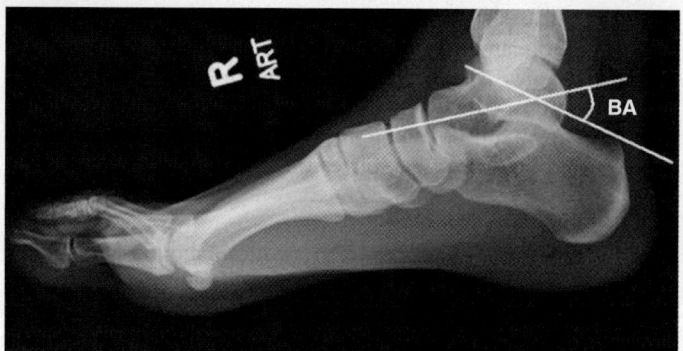

FIGURE 40.15 Lateral radiograph of the foot showing Bohler angle (BA).

fractures should have a CT scan ordered to allow the orthopedic provider to better understand the fracture pattern and determine its surgical candidacy. Finally, with the exception of suspected osteomyelitis, deep abscess, or stress fracture, MRI of the foot is rarely indicated in the emergency setting.

Wound Management

All wound dressings and splints placed in the field or at an outside hospital should be removed to evaluate the wounds for their severity and degree of contamination and to determine whether there are any open fractures. If an open fracture is suspected, tetanus prophylaxis and appropriate antibiotic prophylaxis should be given immediately to reduce the risk of infection.[5,6] Using sterile technique, wounds should then be irrigated with sterile saline to remove superficial gross contamination such as dirt, gravel, or grass in the emergency department. Soft tissue bleeding can be controlled by direct manual pressure, followed by application of sterile dry dressings. After sterile dressings are placed over the wounds in the emergency department, they should remain in place until the orthopedic specialist evaluation, ideally at the time of operative irrigation and debridement. Immobilization of the fractured extremity is then carried out in the same manner as for a closed injury to allow for soft tissue rest and hemorrhage control.

Reduction and Immobilization

All displaced fractures, fracture-dislocations, and joint dislocations should be gently and promptly reduced to restore general limb alignment. The injured extremity is then properly splinted to maintain the fracture reduction, and postreduction radiographs should be obtained to confirm acceptable reduction. Reductions generally require analgesia in the form of a hematoma block with local anesthetic, intravenous narcotics, or conscious sedation to allow for appropriate relaxation of the patient. Hip and shoulder dislocations are a good example in which muscle spasm can prevent successful reduction, and in those instances, it is important to ensure adequate sedation is achieved. If a joint reduction is unsuccessful after adequate sedation and relaxation, general anesthesia may be necessary. However, it is critical to ensure that the patient does not have an irreducible hip fracture-dislocation, as more aggressive attempts at reduction may result in iatrogenic femoral neck fracture (Fig. 40.16).

Reduction maneuvers follow the same general set of principles for all fracture and dislocation types. First, in-line traction is applied to the limb after sedation is administered and allowed time to become effective, often requiring a provider trained in moderate sedation. If the soft tissue envelope surrounding the fracture is intact, in-line traction alone may produce satisfactory alignment

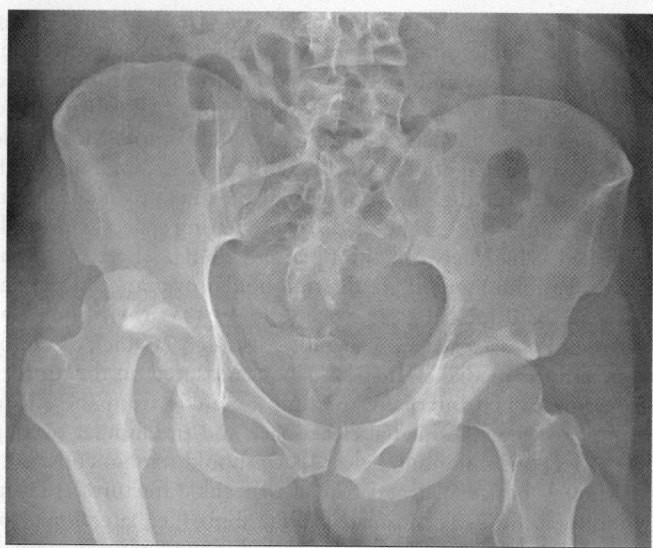

FIGURE 40.16 Anterior-posterior radiograph of irreducible hip fracture dislocation.

through ligamentotaxis. In most cases, the deformity must be recreated and exaggerated to allow for appropriate mobilization and reduction. It is important that neurovascular status is documented before and after any reduction maneuver or splint application. Once satisfactory reduction or alignment is achieved, it must be maintained by immobilization through casting, splinting, or traction. Immobilization of the joints above and below the fracture is generally recommended to ensure adequate stability and prevention of a lost reduction. Postreduction radiographs are required to confirm reduction. Nondisplaced fractures are splinted in a similar manner, but without a formal reduction maneuver. Most nondisplaced fractures do not require surgical treatment, and therefore, high-quality splints should be applied, as they may remain in place for 2 to 3 weeks. Splints are placed initially and then often exchanged to circumferential casts in the outpatient setting after the swelling subsides.

It is recommended that ligamentous injuries are immobilized with either a splint or brace depending on the injury. The joint is fully evaluated as described earlier, and a thorough neurovascular examination is performed on the limb. Frequently, joint effusions, hemarthroses, or lipohemarthroses are present, which indicate the presence of an intraarticular injury. Therapeutic aspiration of a traumatic hemarthrosis is not recommended because of the risk of iatrogenic infection in the unsterile environment of the emergency department. After a successful reduction, the joint should then be immobilized and can be reevaluated after the acute pain and swelling decrease.

The rationale for immobilization is threefold. First, a wellpadded splint applies stabilization and compression to the soft tissues, which will aid in decreasing further bleeding and soft tissue swelling. Second, providing appropriate immobilization and stability to the injured extremity may prevent further soft tissue injury to an otherwise already traumatized soft tissue envelope. Third, immobilization of the fracture reduces the patient's discomfort and facilitates transportation and radiographic evaluation of the fracture(s). There are a variety of different splinting techniques, and they vary depending on which body part is being immobilized. For example, a volar splint, ulnar gutter splint, or thumb spica split is often used for fractures of the hand. A sugar tong splint (Fig. 40.17A–D) is indicated for wrist or forearm

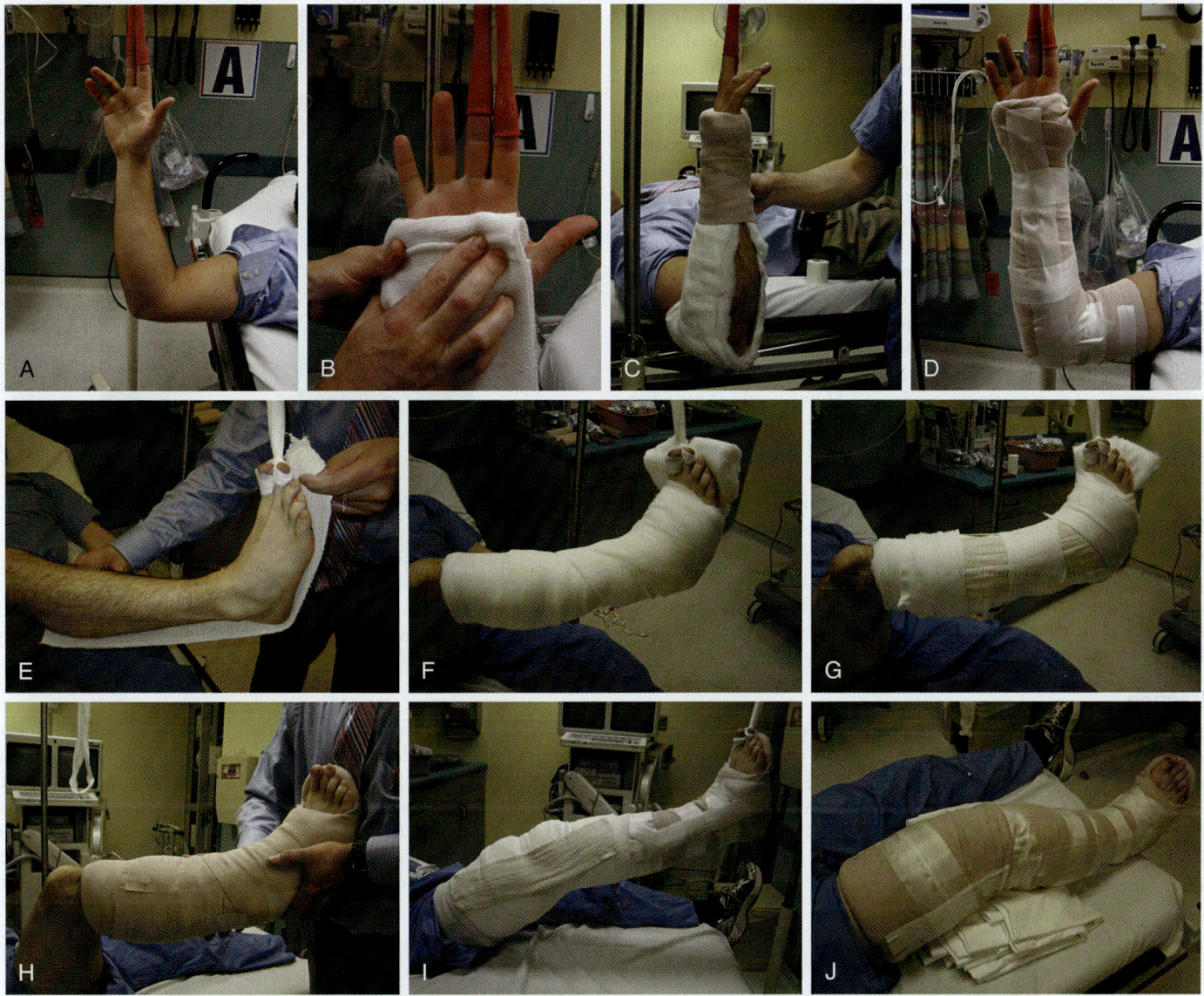

FIGURE 40.17 Application of sugar tong (A–D), short leg (E–H), and long leg (I–J) splints. (A) Finger traps are used to apply gravity traction. (B–C) A well-padded splint (plaster or fiberglass) is measured and applied to the limb. The splint should extend from the distal palmar crease volarly (B) to the metacarpophalangeal joints dorsally. This allows motion of the metacarpophalangeal joints. (D) The compressive wrap (bias bandage or elastic wrap) is applied and secured with tape. (E) Gravity traction is applied by hanging the limb by the toes in a figure-4 position across the bed. This serves two functions. First, flexion at the knee relaxes the pull of the gastrocnemius muscle across the ankle; second, the inversion produced by this position helps maintain fibular length and the reduction of the medial malleolus. Both a posterior slab and a U or stirrup component (plaster or fiberglass) are measured. (F) The limb is protected with a soft dressing (circumferential Robert Jones cotton). (G) The posterior followed by the stirrup splints are applied to the injured extremity and held in place with cast padding. (H) The compressive wrap (bias bandage or elastic wrap) is applied and secured with tape. When possible, the knee is flexed and the ankle is placed in neutral position to prevent equinus contracture. (I) The short leg splint may be extended into a long leg splint by protecting the remainder of the limb with a soft dressing and then applying medial and lateral side slabs overlapping the short leg splint and extending to the proximal thigh. (J) Again, the compressive wrap (bias bandage or elastic wrap) is applied and secured with tape.

fractures. This splint provides immobilization of the wrist and elbow, which effectively will also prevent pronation and supination of the forearm. Fractures about the elbow are placed in a posterior long arm splint. For humeral shaft fractures, a coaptation splint is used. If there is minimal swelling present with a humeral shaft fracture, a functional brace (i.e., Sarmiento brace) may be applied acutely in the emergency department. A short leg splint consisting of a posterior slab and a U or stirrup component (see Fig. 40.17E–H) is used for fractures of the foot and ankle. With the addition of side slabs crossing the knee, this splint can be extended into a long leg splint for tibial shaft plateau fractures or knee dislocations (see Fig. 40.17I–J). Once the cotton wrap and plaster have been applied, the splint can be gently wrapped with an ACE wrap or other nonconstrictive dressing.

An important concept to keep in mind when performing reductions and splinting is to appropriately mold the initial splint or cast in a way that will maintain the reduction. The natural tendency of many fractures is to displace back into their initial deformity. Molding of the splint is an important technique that should be implemented into every splint to maintain the reduction in the proper position. Common examples of this include a valgus mold for humeral shaft fractures to avoid displacement into varus deformity and a volar-directed mold for dorsally displaced distal radius fractures (Fig. 40.18).

Application of a circumferential cast is rarely indicated in the acute treatment of adult fractures, especially because soft tissues in the injured extremity will continue swell for 48 to 72 hours after injury. Thus, a circumferential cast that does not allow room for swelling can be too constrictive and could potentially lead to pressure necrosis or compartment syndrome. However, there are a few cases in which a cast will be the definitive treatment for a patient (i.e., most pediatric fractures and some nondisplaced fractures in adults). In these cases, it is recommended to "bivalve" the initial circumferential cast after it is applied, and this is done by cutting the fiberglass or plaster portion of the cast longitudinally on opposite sides to allow room for swelling. This technique remains effective in maintaining the reduction, more than an open splint, and after the soft tissues have been allowed time to rest (2–3 weeks), the cast is then overwrapped with fiberglass or plaster material at the first clinic visit.

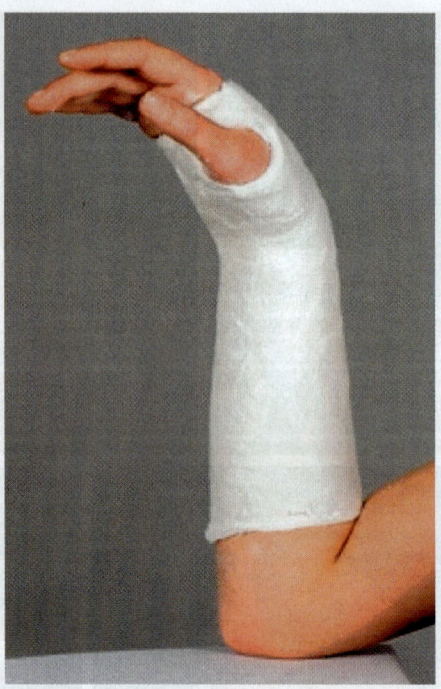

FIGURE 40.18 Distal radius mold. (From The Royal Children's Hospital, Melbourne, Australia. http://www.rch.org.au/fracture-education/management_principles/Management_Principles/.)

Traction

Immobilization of fractures in the pelvis, acetabulum, and proximal part of the femur can be difficult with traditional splinting techniques. A variety of forms of traction can be used in such situations to aid in fracture stabilization and pain control, and those include skeletal traction, skin traction, or traction splints. Skeletal traction has proved to be an effective alternative means of immobilization and may be placed through the distal femur or proximal tibia (Fig. 40.19). Common indications for its application include unstable pelvic ring and acetabular fractures, femoral shaft fractures, and injuries with intraarticular fracture fragments to offload the cartilage and prevent further joint injury from pressure necrosis. Skeletal traction is generally more effective and a safer option for patients in which the traction is intended to remain in place for a longer period of time (i.e., polytrauma patients

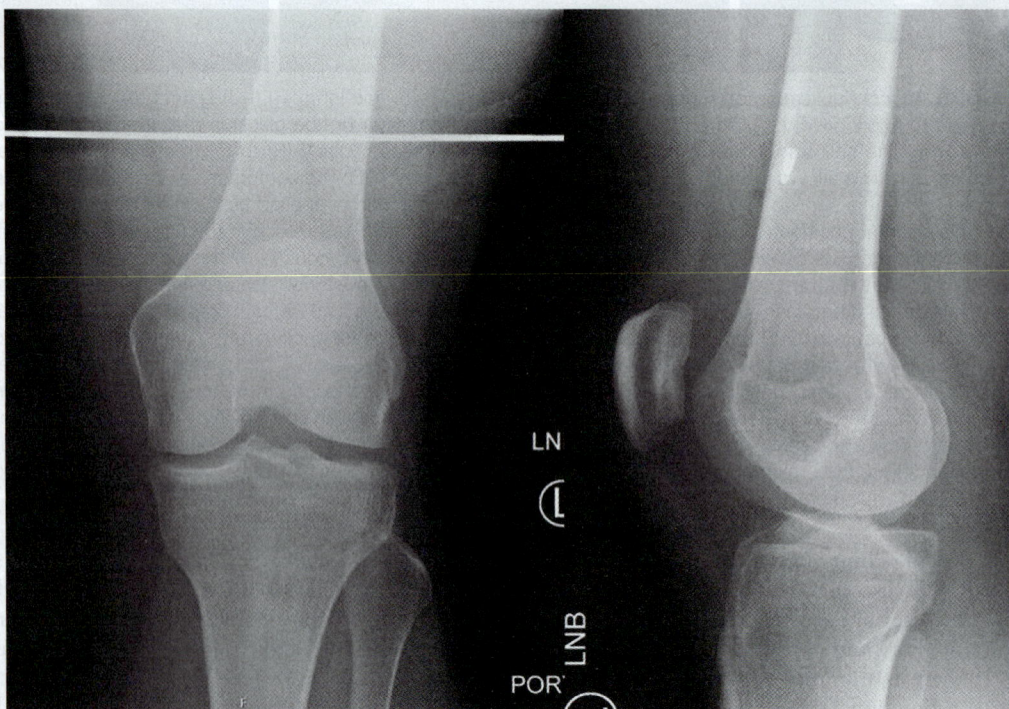

FIGURE 40.19 Distal femur skeletal traction pin.

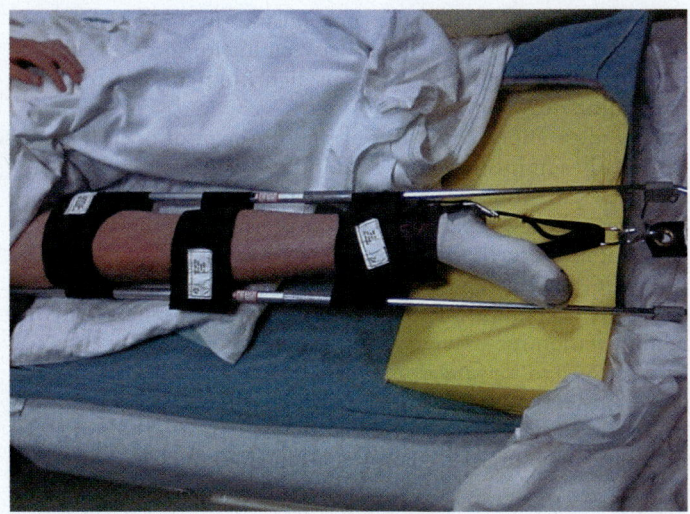

FIGURE 40.20 Hare traction splint placed at the scene of the accident to stabilize a femoral shaft fracture.

who may not be cleared for surgery). There are previously well-described techniques for placement of skeletal traction, with either a Kirschner wire or Steinmann pin, in anatomic "safe zones" to decrease the risk of complications and iatrogenic injury to local neurovascular structures. The most common complication of skeletal traction is superficial pin-site infection; however, the rate is very low (~0.6%) given that most pins are placed only for a short period of time. A recent review of placement of lower extremity skeletal traction in orthopedic trauma patients provides a detailed outline of indications, techniques for placement, and rate of complications.[10]

Skin traction (also known as *cutaneous traction* or *Buck's traction*) is similar to skeletal traction in that it imparts axial load on the limb to aid in length restoration, but it also differs in that it is noninvasive.[10] The primary complication of skin traction is local skin damage, sloughing, or necrosis, and, although this is rarely encountered, the risk must be evaluated before its use, especially in elderly patients with fragile skin. Traction splints, such as the Hare or Sager traction splint, may also be used. They use a ratchet-based form of traction that is distally docked to a frame that proximally rests against the patient's ischium and can be effective for femoral shaft fractures (Fig. 40.20). These are generally applied in the prehospital setting by emergency medical services

personnel, but it is generally recommended that they be removed upon arrival to the emergency department to prevent skin complications. Overall, each method of traction has been shown to be effective in the setting of short-term use and carries its own set of advantages, disadvantages, and complications. When choosing one form over another for your patient, it is recommended to consider patient-related factors, timing of planned surgical intervention, and provider experience.

TIME-DEPENDENT ORTHOPEDIC INJURIES

Open Fractures

Open fractures can occur in young and elderly patients and after both high- and low-energy injury mechanisms, depending on the location of the body and the soft tissue envelope in that region. The majority of open fractures result from high-energy impact to the lower extremity (e.g., MVC), which results in significant soft tissue trauma, periosteal stripping, fracture comminution, and contamination. Management of these injuries often requires a multidisciplinary approach involving orthopedic surgeons, plastic surgeons, and vascular surgeons. By definition, an open fracture communicates with the outside environment through a soft tissue wound that may be located either directly over the fracture site or several centimeters away. The mechanism may be considered "inside-out," which means that as the fracture occurred, the bone lacerated out through the soft tissues into the outside environment (e.g., tibia shaft fracture), or "outside-in," which means the bone was fractured from something that penetrated through the soft tissues (e.g., knife stabbing). Regardless of the mechanism, most open fractures require a prompt history and physical examination, stabilization, systemic antibiotics, debridement and irrigation, temporary or definitive fixation, and, if needed, soft tissue coverage and/or vascular repair.

Classification

Several classification systems have been developed and used to guide appropriate management and outcomes of open fractures. The most commonly used and recognized classification scheme is the Gustilo-Anderson classification system, which evaluates open fractures on the basis of the size of the wound, the degree of contamination, and the extent of the soft tissue injury (Table 40.4).

The primary prognostic value of this classification system is the increasing risk of infection with each successive open fracture

TABLE 40.4 Gustilo-Anderson Classification of Open Fractures

FRACTURE TYPE	DESCRIPTION	RECOMMENDED PROPHYLACTIC ANTIBIOTICS
I	Wound <1 cm, clean; most likely inside-to-outside lesion; minimal muscle contusion; simple transverse or oblique fracture	First-generation cephalosporin
II	Wound >1 cm with extensive soft tissue damage, flaps, or avulsion; minimal to moderate crushing; simple transverse or short oblique fracture with minimal comminution	First-generation cephalosporin ± aminoglycoside
III	Extensive soft tissue damage including muscle, skin, and neurovascular structures; often a high-velocity injury with a severe crushing component (barnyard injuries)	First-generation cephalosporin + aminoglycoside + penicillin G
IIIA	Extensive laceration, adequate soft tissue coverage; segmental fracture; gunshot injuries	
IIIB	Extensive soft tissue damage with periosteal stripping and bone exposure necessitating formal soft tissue coverage; usually associated with contamination	
IIIC	Any open fracture with vascular injury requiring repair	

From Gustilo R, Mendoza R, Williams DN. Problems in the management of type III (severe) open fractures. *J Trauma*. 1984;24:742-746.

type. Multiple previous studies have reported infection rates of 0% to 2% for type I, 2% to 10% for type II, and 10% to 50% for type III fractures, with type IIIC fractures exhibiting the highest rates of infection.[11–13] Overall, this classification system is a practical guide to management, but it does have limitations, such as poor interobserver reliability that has been shown to range from 42% to 94%.[14,15] This is thought to be because the system inaccurately assesses the true extent of deep soft tissue injury (i.e., soft tissue stripping), which is why true scoring can only be made at the time of surgery.

For example, in Fig. 40.21A, a clinical photo of the lateral aspect of an ankle is shown with two small, minimally contaminated soft tissue wounds. The radiograph of the underlying fracture is displayed in Fig. 40.21B. Strictly from the clinical appearance of the soft tissue injury, this would likely be classified as a type I open distal tibia and fibula fracture in most cases. However, taking the underlying fracture pattern into consideration would more appropriately classify this injury as a type IIIA open fracture. This is because the injury mechanism was a high-energy MVC, with fracture site comminution, mottling and contusion of the soft tissues, and air densities throughout the soft tissues on the radiograph suggesting a more extensive soft tissue injury. Thus, it is critical to consider all pieces of information available to you when assigning the diagnosis because it will affect your decision on acute treatment (e.g., prophylactic antibiotics) and possibly the patient's outcome. As discussed earlier, it can be helpful to categorize injuries into either *high-* or *low-*energy injuries based on the mechanism, fracture pattern, and degree of soft tissue injury. In doing so, low-energy injuries will be more appropriately classified as types I and II, and high-energy injuries will be types IIIA–C.

Initial Management

The initial management is the same as all other high-energy traumatic injuries: a thorough understanding of the injury mechanism and appropriate treatment for other injuries based on the ATLS protocol. Table 40.5 is an example of our institution's open fracture protocol, and another can be found in a recent review on antibiotic prophylaxis in open fractures.[6] Although the details may differ between institutions, it is important that each institution have an algorithm similar to this to help guide treatment.

The most important aspect of the treatment of open fractures is the early administration of antibiotics.[5,6,12] It is strongly recommended that antibiotics be administered within 1 hour of injury to the emergency department and, if possible, as soon as they arrive. Additionally, previous studies have suggested that the 1-hour time limit should begin at the time of injury, and thus, some institutions have implemented protocols for prehospital antibiotic administration for severe open fractures.[16]

The concern for infection is what motivates the use of prophylactic antibiotics, and as many previous studies have shown significant decreases in rates of infection after their administration, traumatic open injuries continue to remain responsible for up to 19% of cases of osteomyelitis.[17] The antibiotic regimen administered to each patient is generally dictated by the classification type; however, there is evidence for both seasonal and geographic variation in the organisms responsible for the infection.[18] As a result, there may be slight variation in protocols based on which organisms are more endemic to the particular region in which the institution is located. Discussion with infectious diseases specialists at your institution is recommended to ensure your chosen antibiotic protocol is providing adequate coverage.

It is recommended to provide coverage for gram-positive bacteria, such as *Staphylococcus* or *Streptococcus*, with systemic antibiotics at the time of presentation for type I and II fractures because they are the most commonly found bacteria in these injuries.[5] First-generation cephalosporins (e.g., cefazolin) have been the most common and effective agents given after open fractures, and early administration has been supported by multiple reviews.[5,6,11] In patients with a true penicillin allergy, alternative agents for coverage such as clindamycin have been recommended by the Surgical Infection Society. Additionally, in patients with a penicillin allergy presenting to hospitals with a high rate of community-acquired methicillin-resistant *Staphylococcus aureus* (MRSA), vancomycin usage has been recommended. In patients with type III

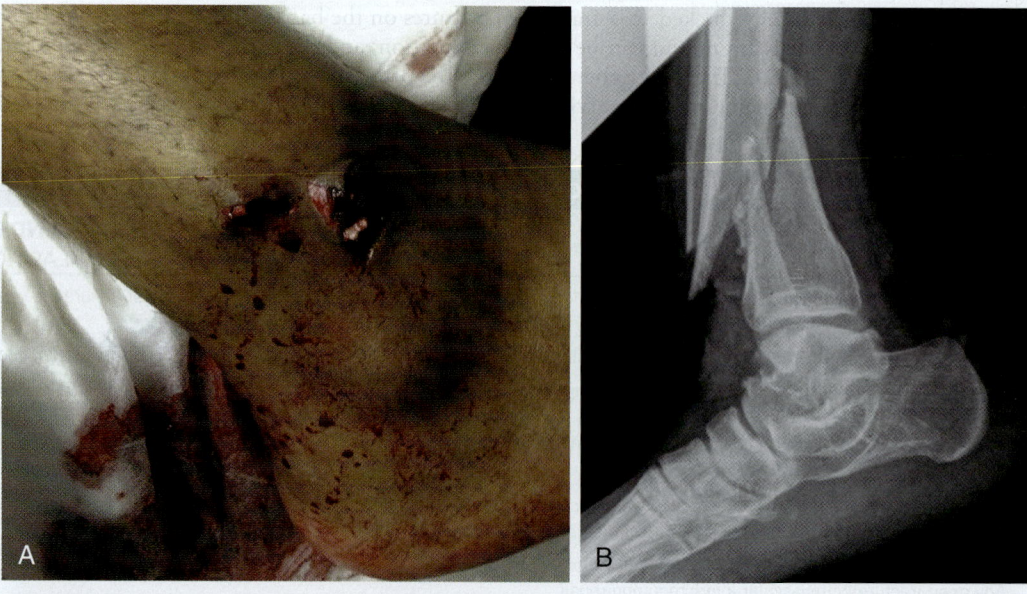

FIGURE 40.21 Two small lateral ankle lacerations (A) above a comminuted distal tibia fracture with intraarticular extension (B).

TABLE 40.5 General Guidelines for Open Fractures

Treatment Goals
- Systemic prophylactic antibiotic therapy initiated within 1 hour of arrival
- Operative debridement within 6–24 hours
- When necessary, soft tissue coverage within 7 days of injury

Prophylactic Antibiotics

Types I and II	Ancef	48 hours from presentation
		24 hours after subsequent intervention
Type IIIA–C	Ancef/tobramycin	48 hours from presentation
		24 hours after subsequent intervention
Soil contamination	Penicillin	Single dose
Marine contamination	Levaquin	Single dose
Ballistic fracture	Ancef/tobramycin	48 hours from presentation
		24 hours after subsequent intervention
Transcolonic gunshot injury to the spine or pelvis	Vancomycin/cefepime/Flagyl	7 days from presentation
		24 hours after subsequent intervention
Lawnmower injury	Unasyn	24 hours from presentation
	Augmentin	7 days postdebridement or presentation

Emergency Room Management
- Systemic prophylactic antibiotics (see earlier)
- Radiographs, bedside irrigation and removal of gross contamination from wound, fracture reduction, loose approximation of skin, dry sterile dressings, splint
- NPO, obtain acute care surgery clearance

NPO, Nothing by mouth.

open fractures, increasing severity of soft tissue injury, and soil-contaminated wounds, gram-negative coverage should be added to the antibiotic regimen, such as an aminoglycoside (e.g., gentamicin). In one series of 126 type III open fractures, the authors reported a significantly higher rate of acute kidney injury in patients treated with aminoglycosides.[19] In contrast, in a separate study of 167 patients with open fractures, the authors did not observe an association between aminoglycosides and acute kidney injury except in patients with higher injury severity scores and hypotension on presentation.[20] Nonetheless, its use has fallen out of favor in some institutions because of these reports of dose-dependent reversible nephrotoxicity and irreversible ototoxicity. Given those concerns and a lack of evidence supporting its clinical efficacy, the authors of a recent review article recommended against the use of aminoglycosides in routine prophylactic management.[6] Finally, providers should consider broader coverage in patients presenting with aquatic wounds contaminated by salt water (*Vibrio* species) and fresh water (*Aeromonas* and *Pseudomonas* species).[5,6]

Delayed administration has been shown to increase the risk of infection markedly, especially if given longer than 66 minutes after injury.[21,22] In addition to timing of administration, the duration of prophylactic antibiotic therapy should also be taken into consideration.[23,24] Prolonged antibiotic therapy past 24 hours has not demonstrated a notable decrease in infection risk, including in type III open fractures. Studies comparing infection rates in patients treated for 24 hours or 5 days of antibiotic treatment have shown no difference in infection rates, and several review articles have demonstrated similar results at cutoffs of both 24 and 72 hours.[6,23,24] A recent systematic review recommended discontinuation of prophylactic antibiotics after 24 hours of therapy in type I and II open fractures and after 72 hours or 24 hours after wound closure/coverage (whichever occurs first) in type III open fractures.[23]

The appropriate timing of surgical debridement remains a controversial topic, with much of the available evidence conflicting, yet it is generally accepted that timely surgical management is of paramount importance. Classically, the recommendation was for initial debridement to be performed within the first 6 hours after injury. However, multiples studies have since demonstrated that the historical "6-hour rule" for debridement offers little benefit over debridement performed within 24 hours of injury for type I and II open fractures.[25,26] Regarding more severe type III open fractures, a recent meta-analysis showed an increased infection risk when surgical management was delayed more than 12 hours, which led to the recommendation of operative debridement within 12 hours of injury for type III injuries.[26] Similar results were reported in a retrospective analysis of 10,651 open tibia and femur fractures in the Surgical Implant Generation Network (SIGN) surgical database, with the probability of infection increasing by 0.23% for every 6-hour delay in debridement in type III injuries and 0.13% in type I and II injuries.[27]

Local antibiotic therapy, such as intrawound powdered antibiotics or antibiotic cement spacers/beads, has experienced increasing popularity for the treatment of both open and closed fracture management and in other fields of orthopedic surgery. Soft tissue injury and vascular compromise can limit the delivery of intravenously administered antibiotics to fracture sites. Thus, the benefits of locally delivered antibiotic agents have the ability to obtain a higher concentration at the surgical site, while also limiting the potential for systemic toxic levels of the drug.[28–30] Some authors have expressed concern that administration of local antibiotics may increase the risk of developing drug-resistant organisms; however, there is a paucity of literature to support this. A recent study evaluated the species distribution and resistance patterns of organisms causing surgical site infection with and without the use of local antibiotic powder and reported no measurable increase in infections caused by antibiotic-resistant organisms.[31] Two recent reviews demonstrated similar results, reporting a potential 23% reduction in the odds of deep surgical site infection[32] and significantly decreased the overall incidence of infection in both open and closed fractures.[33]

When performing surgical debridement, it should be done in a systematic manner and one that includes meticulous handling of the soft tissues. Debridement should begin in the superficial layers and progress to deeper layers. All foreign and devitalized tissue should be removed, including any bone without soft tissue attachments. In higher-energy injuries, the zone of injury may take several days to demarcate itself, and, because of that, the wound should undergo serial debridement every 48 to 72 hours until a stable and healthy soft tissue bed is obtained. Determination of soft tissue and muscle viability during debridement is a subjective process. Evaluation of muscle viability by the "4 Cs" of color, contractility, consistency, and capacity to bleed were established tenets of debridement decades ago and have served as a general guideline for many when performing debridement. However, a recent histopathologic study found that neither the "4 Cs" nor the surgeon's impression correlate with muscle viability and suggested the possibility that surgeons may be debriding potentially viable muscle.[34]

The method of irrigation and the solution used during the irrigation have also been studied. The FLOW study sought to investigate the effects of castile soap versus normal saline solution delivered by three different irrigation pressures in 2447 patients with open fractures.[35] They reported no difference in rates of reoperation based on irrigation pressure; however, the reoperation rate was higher in the soap group than in the saline group. Earlier studies in animal models demonstrated higher rates of bacterial seeding of the intramedullary canal and myonecrosis of the soft tissues with high-pressure irrigation methods in animal models; however, this was confirmed to be clinically relevant in the FLOW study. Additional studies have investigated the effect of different irrigation solutions such as bacitracin versus castile soap solution, saline versus iodophor and hydrogen peroxide, saline versus chlorhexidine, and saline versus distilled water. Overall, no advantages were seen in using nonsaline solutions, and in some studies, more wound healing disturbances and adverse wound inflammation were seen with use of antibiotic additive and antiseptic solutions. Finally, with regard to volume of irrigation solution used, there are no reliable data to provide formal recommendations.

In situations where the wound cannot be closed primarily or there is concern for progression of soft tissue necrosis, negative-pressure wound therapy (NPWT; i.e., vacuum-assisted closure) is recommended. In theory, the device removes blood and draining fluid from the wound and may potentially increase the formation of granulation tissue. The results of a prospective randomized trial known as the "UK Wound management of open lower limb fractures (UK WOLLF)" study did not show any difference in surgical site infections or quality of life between patients treated with NPWT versus standard sterile dressings.[36] Similarly, in a recent Cochrane review, the authors concluded that it remains uncertain whether NPWT is superior to standard sterile dressings in wound infection, adverse events, or time to closure/coverage.[37] In contrast, in the 2023 American Academy of Orthopaedic Surgeons (AAOS) clinical practice guidelines for prevention of surgical site infection after major extremity trauma, the role of NPWT was considered and received a strong recommendation in both open and closed fracture situations.

The discussion of fixation and soft tissue reconstruction strategies for open fractures is well beyond the scope of this text because

the timing of both temporary and definitive fixation of open fractures is at the treating surgeon's discretion with regard to the status of the soft tissue envelope cleanliness of the fracture site. In general, after the secondary survey is completed and necessary diagnostic studies are obtained, a multiply injured patient may be quickly transferred to the operating room for intervention. In polytraumatized patients, the trauma surgeon generally serves as the primary coordinator of care, consulting with the anesthesiologist, neurosurgeon, and orthopedic surgeon to determine the most appropriate treatment algorithm for each patient. Critical procedures to address life-threatening injuries are prioritized, and timing of subsequent interventions is continuously reviewed as the patient's status evolves.

Limb Salvage Versus Primary Amputation

Although beyond the scope of this chapter, the absolute indications for primary amputation are few, and as such, the decision-making algorithm must involve evaluation and recommendation from a multidisciplinary team (if possible), with formal documentation of recommendations and detailed accounts of injury severity uploaded to the patient's medical record. In some instances, life must be chosen over limb, but, if at all possible and if the situation allows, temporary operations can be performed initially until a formal discussion can be held with the patient and their family regarding goals of treatment. The decision between primary amputation and salvage of a severely injured extremity is complex and should involve input from multiple providers in multiple disciplines (i.e., orthopedic, trauma, and vascular surgery). It can be beneficial for consulting services such as physical medicine and rehabilitation physicians or prosthetics team members to provide additional information to help reach a decision. A key tenet of limb salvage is reconstruction of a functional extremity, including motor and sensory function to some degree, in order to give the patient the best chance for a good outcome. If amputation is chosen, multidisciplinary management with prosthetic and rehabilitation teams is critical, and patients should be screened for symptoms of depression and PTSD to ensure the patient's psychological health is cared for.

Fractures Secondary to Firearm Injury

In the United States, the incidence of firearm-related injuries and fractures has continued to increase despite an overall fall in the rates worldwide.[38] There have been more than 1 million nonfatal injuries resulting in emergency department visits in the United States since 2010, and in 2020, firearm-related injuries became the third leading cause of nonfatal violence-related emergency department visits.[38] These injuries are associated with substantial healthcare costs (estimated at $2.5 billion in the first year) and significant socioeconomic consequences for both the patient and society. Historically, firearm injuries have been characterized by the type of firearm and the muzzle velocity of the firearm, which is divided into low velocity (<2000 feet per second [fps]) and high velocity (>2000 fps). The muzzle velocity directly correlates with the kinetic energy of the bullet, and therefore, the greater the kinetic energy of the bullet, the greater the energy that is imparted on the tissues upon impact.

In the United States, the majority of firearm-related fractures are caused by low-velocity weapons, and unfortunately, there is a paucity of high-level evidence in the literature regarding their management. In general, most low-velocity firearm-related fractures can be managed similarly to non–firearm-related fractures, with the goals of restoring function and decreasing the rate of complications. There are very few high-level studies to support the administration of prophylactic antibiotics in patients with nonoperatively treated injuries; however, a recent review found the majority of studies recommend a short course of prophylactic antibiotics to reduce the risk of infection, and no data suggest superiority of intravenous or oral administration.[38] Low-velocity wounds generally have minimal soft tissue injury, and routine operative debridement is not recommended unless grossly contaminated. Fixation of long bone fractures, in terms of indications and techniques, is similar to those of standard care for other fracture patterns (closed and open) and should be treated at the discretion of the attending surgeon.

Fractures caused by high-velocity firearms (muzzle velocity >2000 fps) are generally associated with a more severe and larger zone of injury to the soft tissues. The infection risk tends to be higher because of the increased amount of devitalized tissue, and because of this, it has been suggested that these injuries be treated similarly to type III open fractures.[38] Wounds often require repeat operative debridement, and in some cases, soft tissue reconstruction for coverage after the complete zone of injury has been identified. Furthermore, high-velocity firearms often produce larger areas of soft tissue cavitation with significant comminution and bone loss at the fracture site, higher rates of neurologic and vascular injuries, and, as a result, increased risk of nonunion and amputation.[38] Initial management should include administration of broad-spectrum antibiotics and tetanus prophylaxis to decrease risk of infection. Finally, depending on the overall extent of the soft tissue and bony injuries, it is at the surgeon's discretion whether to perform temporary or definitive fixation at the time of the initial debridement.

Firearm injuries with intraarticular involvement require special consideration because of a number of factors, which include periarticular fracture management, potential risk of septic arthritis, chondral damage from retained metallic fragments, and, historically, the concern for lead arthropathy. Suggested treatment algorithms have been well described in previous reviews and meta-analyses.[38] Antibiotic prophylaxis is a consideration in these injuries, and two previous meta-analyses recommended their use after reporting no significant difference in infection rates between patients treated with surgical debridement versus antibiotics alone.[38] In the case of retained intraarticular bullets or loose bodies, most studies recommend surgical removal and debridement of the joint, either through an open approach or arthroscopically. In doing so, it is thought to decrease risk of lead toxicity, septic arthritis, and further mechanical damage to the articular surface. Finally, the literature has not found a significant difference in infection rates in patients who did and did not undergo an operative debridement. However, the entire clinical picture should be taken into consideration, including the bullet characteristics, injury pattern, appearance of the wound and level of contamination, or presence of bowel contamination.

Firearm-related fractures of the hip, pelvis, and spine have high rates of associated perforated viscus and bowel injuries. Most authors have recommended surgical debridement of intraarticular fractures associated with an injury to the bowel. Several studies have assessed the rate of infection after nonoperative treatment and intravenous antibiotics alone, reporting rates ranging from 0% to 21%.[38] When an associated bowel or urinary tract injury is confirmed, it is recommended that gram-negative coverage be added to the antibiotic regimen. In the context of firearm-relative pelvic ring injuries, operative debridement and prophylactic antibiotics should be performed as indicated earlier. The decision to perform stabilization of the pelvic ring injury is controversial because the fracture pattern and resultant instability caused by a traversing bullet are often different from those caused by nonfirearm blunt trauma. A recent review of 86 patients with pelvic ballistic injuries investigated both treatment patterns and injury profiles.[39] They reported 9.3% of patients underwent a surgical debridement; however, no firearm-related pelvic fractures required surgical stabilization.

Skeletal Stabilization

Skeletal stabilization has been shown to be crucial for soft tissue healing, especially in the setting of an open fracture. Compared with casts and splints, internal and external fixation permit greater access for wound care and are more effective in controlling pain during mobilization. In general, the decision to use one mode of fixation over another is dependent on the fracture pattern and associated soft tissue injuries, the degree of contamination, and the overall clinical status of the patient at the time of surgery. If a clean soft tissue envelope can be achieved at the index operation, definitive fracture fixation through open reduction internal fixation (i.e., plating) or intramedullary nailing are both acceptable options and can result in good outcomes. However, assessment of the soft tissue envelope and its cleanliness with regard to both timing and method of definitive fixation is at the discretion of the treating surgeon.

In hemodynamically unstable patients or those with grossly contaminated wounds, standard or ringed external fixation devices can be used for both temporary stabilization and definitive fixation. External fixators can be applied relatively quickly with minimal soft tissue dissection and avoid the application of surface implants in wounds with concern for contamination or infection. They can be easily removed, replaced, and adjusted and can also be combined with other means of fixation when indicated. However, external fixators are not without their problems. The most common complication of external fixators is superficial pin tract infections, which can often be treated successfully with local pin-site care and oral antibiotics. Pin track osteomyelitis is a relatively rare complication with modern surgical techniques; however, its risk is not zero, particularly in poor hosts or settings in which the external fixator remains in place for multiple weeks or months. Their use can be effective in temporary stabilization of severe soft tissue wounds that require soft tissue coverage, but location of the pins and bars can make subsequent debridement and reconstructive procedures cumbersome. Periarticular and more extensive fracture patterns may require the application of Ilizarov circular external fixators, which can further limit access. Although effective in providing temporary skeletal stabilization during repeat debridement and soft tissue reconstruction, external fixation is not ideal for achieving fracture union, and additional surgical procedures, such as conversion to internal fixation with or without bone grafting, are often necessary.

Intramedullary nailing of open fractures at the time of the initial operation has become a standard treatment option in recent decades. Historically, open fractures (e.g., tibia shaft fractures) were initially stabilized with external fixators until a stable and clean soft tissue bed could be achieved, at which point the external fixator was removed and definitive implants were placed. Acute intramedullary nailing of open fractures has gained popularity, and multiple meta-analyses have supported their use in treating open fractures.[40] A more recent meta-analysis of 12 randomized controlled trials that included 1090 patients compared outcomes of definitive fixation of open tibia shaft fractures with external fixation versus intramedullary nailing.[41] The authors reported no difference in rates of deep infection, nonunion, delayed union, or implant failure between groups and also observed higher incidence of superficial infection, pin-tract infection, and malunion in the external fixation group. This led the authors to conclude that intramedullary nailing is advantageous and supported its use over external fixation for definitive fixation.[41] The consideration between reamed and unreamed intramedullary nailing has also been extensively studied, with most authors reporting benefit to reamed nailing with lower rates of nonunion, implant failure, and reoperations.

ACUTE COMPARTMENT SYNDROME

Acute compartment syndrome can be a devastating condition for patients, developing from a variety of injuries and medical conditions, and has become a common source of medical litigation. Early recognition and treatment of compartment syndrome is critical to decrease the risk of limb dysfunction, amputation, and in some cases death. The most common etiologies include fractures (open and closed), soft tissue injury without fracture, patients on anticoagulants or with bleeding disorders, drug overdoses, circumferential burns, vascular injuries, crush injuries, reperfusion injuries, ballistic injuries, and tight circumferential dressings or casts. Although uncommon, it can develop during surgery, including patient positioning during surgery such as the lithotomy position with prolonged flexion, elevation, and abduction of the well leg during an operation. Elevations in compartment pressures have also been reported during intramedullary nailing of tibia shaft fractures; however, the pressure changes are generally transient and eventually return to baseline.

A 19th-century German doctor, Richard von Volkmann, was among the first to describe the sequelae of postischemic contracture (known as *Volkmann ischemic contracture*), which he attributed to trauma, swelling, and tight bandaging. These contractures were often due to missed compartment syndromes. Classically, this condition was associated with a supracondylar humerus fracture leading to forearm ischemia from acute compartment syndrome. As late complications of compartment syndrome, such as Volkmann ischemic contracture, of the upper and lower extremities have been elucidated, the importance of early recognition and fasciotomy has become paramount. Missed or delayed diagnosis and prompt treatment of this condition has resulted in numerous cases of preventable morbidity and rare cases of mortality and is one of the most common causes of malpractice litigation for orthopedic surgeons. The etiologies are many, but this section will primarily address the pathogenesis, diagnosis, and management of acute compartment syndrome, specifically in the forearm and lower leg.

Pathogenesis

The pathophysiologic mechanism underlying the development of acute compartment syndrome is decreased intracompartmental space or increased intracompartmental fluid volume leading to increased pressure within the compartment. In general, compartments are separated by their own fascia, which is a thin, inelastic form of connective tissue that surrounds muscle compartments and limits its ability to expand. Increased pressure within the compartment leads to hemodynamic disruption within the compartment and reduction of venous outflow. As arterial inflow remains undisrupted, at least initially, blood continues to flow in but cannot flow out, which results in increased venous pressure

and a local arteriovenous gradient that does not allow sufficient blood flow to meet the metabolic demands of the tissue. Eventually, pressures may increase high enough to disrupt arterial inflow leading to decreased oxygenation of the tissues, ischemia, and eventual irreversible tissue necrosis. When muscle tissue is deprived of oxygen, inflammatory cytokines are released that increase capillary permeability producing additional swelling and further elevating compartment pressure. Muscle ischemia also leads to the release of myoglobin and other inflammatory and toxic metabolites into circulation, which can result in renal failure, shock, and cardiac arrhythmias. As such, this pathologic process is difficult to reverse once it has begun, and the only treatment is release of the fascial tissues to allow additional room for the swelling.

Diagnosis

The diagnosis of compartment syndrome requires a high degree of clinical suspicion; performing serial examinations in high-risk patients is essential, with well-documented changes in physical examination over time indicating compartment syndrome. Patient history and mechanism of injury are also important in identifying at-risk patients. Although general understanding of the existence and implications of compartment syndrome is common among providers, no clear definition of when it is present exists. Institutional protocols for diagnosis and management of compartment syndrome have been developed as part of a multidisciplinary collaboration, and an example is illustrated in Fig. 40.22. Historically, the clinical diagnosis included presence of the 6 Ps: pain out of proportion, pressure or firmness of the compartment, pulselessness, paralysis, paresthesia, and pallor. More commonly accepted clinical signs of compartment syndrome include those of pain that is out of proportion from what is expected from a particular injury (one of the earliest and most sensitive signs), pain with passive stretch of involved muscle groups, and paresthesia in the distribution of sensory nerves located within the compartment. However, previous studies have found the clinical signs and symptoms of compartment syndrome have low sensitivity, and furthermore, these signs can also be found in patients without compartment syndrome. Pain may even be absent in a patient with acute compartment syndrome, often as the result of a superimposed central or peripheral neurologic deficit, or in an obtunded patient who cannot provide a reliable examination.

Whenever a clinical examination is not reliable, measurement of compartment pressures is highly recommended, and this can be performed serially over time or continuously depending on the resources available to you. Some authors have recommended routine measurement of pressures in all patients, yet more recent studies have found the need for pressure monitoring to be controversial, and some have even refuted its value. This was exemplified in a previous study that closely followed compartment and blood pressure measurements in 19 patients with lower extremity fractures who did not have clinical criteria diagnostic for compartment syndrome.[42] They observed 84% of patients to have at least one compartment measurement that equated with a perfusion pressure less than 30 mm Hg, which is a diagnostic criterion and represents the difference between the measured compartment pressure and concomitant diastolic blood pressure. More recent studies have suggested that continuous pressure monitoring should be the gold standard for diagnosis and recommended using a perfusion pressure threshold of 30 mm Hg that is present over 2 consecutive hours or more, which demonstrated a 94% sensitivity for diagnosis of acute compartment syndrome.[43]

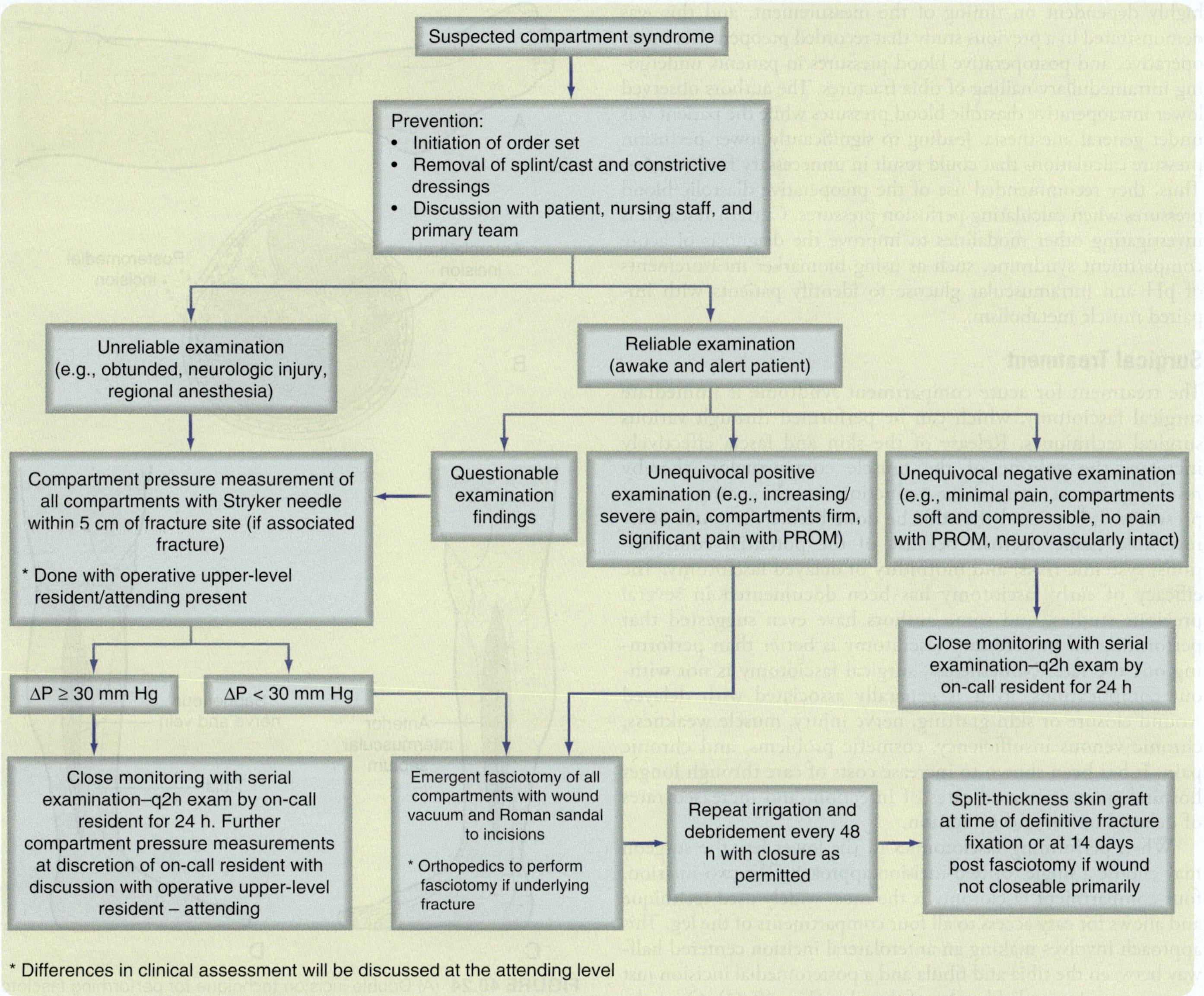

```
┌─────────────────────────────────┐
│ Suspected compartment syndrome  │
└─────────────────────────────────┘
                 │
                 ▼
┌──────────────────────────────────────────┐
│ Prevention:                                │
│  • Initiation of order set                 │
│  • Removal of splint/cast and constrictive │
│    dressings                               │
│  • Discussion with patient, nursing staff, │
│    and primary team                        │
└──────────────────────────────────────────┘
```

| Unreliable examination (e.g., obtunded, neurologic injury, regional anesthesia) | Reliable examination (awake and alert patient) |

```
Compartment pressure measurement of       Questionable       Unequivocal positive       Unequivocal negative examination
all compartments with Stryker needle       examination       examination (e.g., increasing/   (e.g., minimal pain, compartments
within 5 cm of fracture site (if associated  findings         severe pain, compartments firm,   soft and compressible, no pain
fracture)                                                     significant pain with PROM)       with PROM, neurovascularly intact)

* Done with operative upper-level
resident/attending present
```

Close monitoring with serial examination–q2h exam by on-call resident for 24 h

| ΔP ≥ 30 mm Hg | ΔP < 30 mm Hg |

Close monitoring with serial examination–q2h exam by on-call resident for 24 h. Further compartment pressure measurements at discretion of on-call resident with discussion with operative upper-level resident – attending

Emergent fasciotomy of all compartments with wound vacuum and Roman sandal to incisions

* Orthopedics to perform fasciotomy if underlying fracture

Repeat irrigation and debridement every 48 h with closure as permitted

Split-thickness skin graft at time of definitive fracture fixation or at 14 days post fasciotomy if wound not closeable primarily

* Differences in clinical assessment will be discussed at the attending level

FIGURE 40.22 Algorithm for the management of a patient with suspected compartment syndrome. *PROM,* Passive range of motion.

Potential shortcomings should be considered when using compartment pressure measurements for decision-making and diagnosis. Pressure measurements should be taken using a side-port needle and a pressure measurement system. The most common method of measurement is the Stryker Intra-Compartmental Pressure Monitor System (STIC; Stryker, Mahwah, NJ), which uses the side-port needle technique (Fig. 40.23). Alternative measurement systems include a wick or slit catheter or an arterial line setup. Slit catheters can be used in continuous monitoring systems, and although arterial line setups are widely available, they tend to artificially elevate pressure measurements. Second, the location of the pressure measurement within a given muscle compartment has been shown to affect results. Pressures obtained within 5 cm of a fracture are the highest, and pressures measured more centrally within a muscle are generally higher than those obtained peripherally. It is suggested that obtaining measurements farther away from the zone of injury is more representative of the entire compartment; however, no formal consensus of this has been established. Technique used when measuring pressures can also introduce

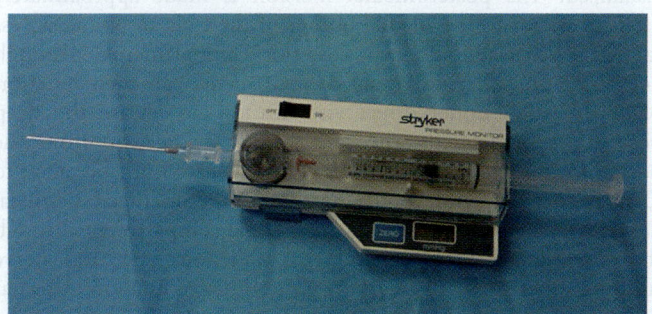

FIGURE 40.23 Stryker Intra-Compartmental Pressure Monitor System (STIC) catheter.

variability in pressure values. A previous cadaveric study demonstrated significant variability in measurement technique, and with a known compartment pressure before measurements, only 60% of measurements were within 5 mm Hg of the known compartment pressure. Finally, calculation of the perfusion pressure is highly dependent on timing of the measurement, and this was demonstrated in a previous study that recorded preoperative, intraoperative, and postoperative blood pressures in patients undergoing intramedullary nailing of tibia fractures. The authors observed lower intraoperative diastolic blood pressures while the patient was under general anesthesia, leading to significantly lower perfusion pressure calculations that could result in unnecessary fasciotomies. Thus, they recommended use of the preoperative diastolic blood pressures when calculating perfusion pressures. Current research is investigating other modalities to improve the diagnosis of acute compartment syndrome, such as using biomarker measurements of pH and intramuscular glucose to identify patients with impaired muscle metabolism.

Surgical Treatment

The treatment for acute compartment syndrome is immediate surgical fasciotomy, which can be performed through various surgical techniques. Release of the skin and fascia effectively increases the volume of the muscle compartment, thereby resulting in an immediate reduction in the compartment pressures. It is critical that this be done before the onset of irreversible tissue necrosis because of the potential complications, systemic risks, and morbidity of delayed fasciotomy. The efficacy of early fasciotomy has been documented in several previous studies, and some authors have even suggested that performing an unnecessary fasciotomy is better than performing one too late. Nonetheless, surgical fasciotomy is not without complications, as it is generally associated with delayed wound closure or skin grafting, nerve injury, muscle weakness, chronic venous insufficiency, cosmetic problems, and chronic pain. It has been shown to increase costs of care through longer hospital stays, increased rates of infection, and increased rates of delayed union and nonunion.

When performing fasciotomies in the lower leg, the surgeon may choose a single- or two-incision approach. The two-incision, four-compartment fasciotomy is the most widely used technique and allows for easy access to all four compartments of the leg. This approach involves making an anterolateral incision centered halfway between the tibia and fibula and a posteromedial incision just posterior to the medial border of the tibia (Fig. 40.24). Once the fascia is identified through the lateral incision, the intermuscular septum separating the anterior and lateral compartments can be visualized. The posteromedial incision is made approximately 2 cm posterior to the medial border of the tibia to obtain access to the superficial and deep posterior compartments. Through both incisions, the individual compartments can then be completely released under direct visualization; to release the deep posterior compartment, the soleus must be released from the posteromedial corner of the tibia. Extreme care must be taken to identify, protect, and avoid injury to the superficial peroneal nerve, which can be seen within the lateral compartment through the anterolateral incision, and the saphenous vein and nerve running superficially through the posteromedial incision. Alternatively, a single-incision, four-compartment fasciotomy can be performed through a parafibular posterolateral skin incision, and this has also been shown to provide a highly effective means of decompression of all four compartments.

It is generally recommended that incisions not be closed primarily at the time of fasciotomy because skin closure may lead to unintended reelevation of compartment pressures by allowing less space for expansion of swollen tissues. The fasciotomy wounds are generally dressed with either a negative-pressure wound vacuum

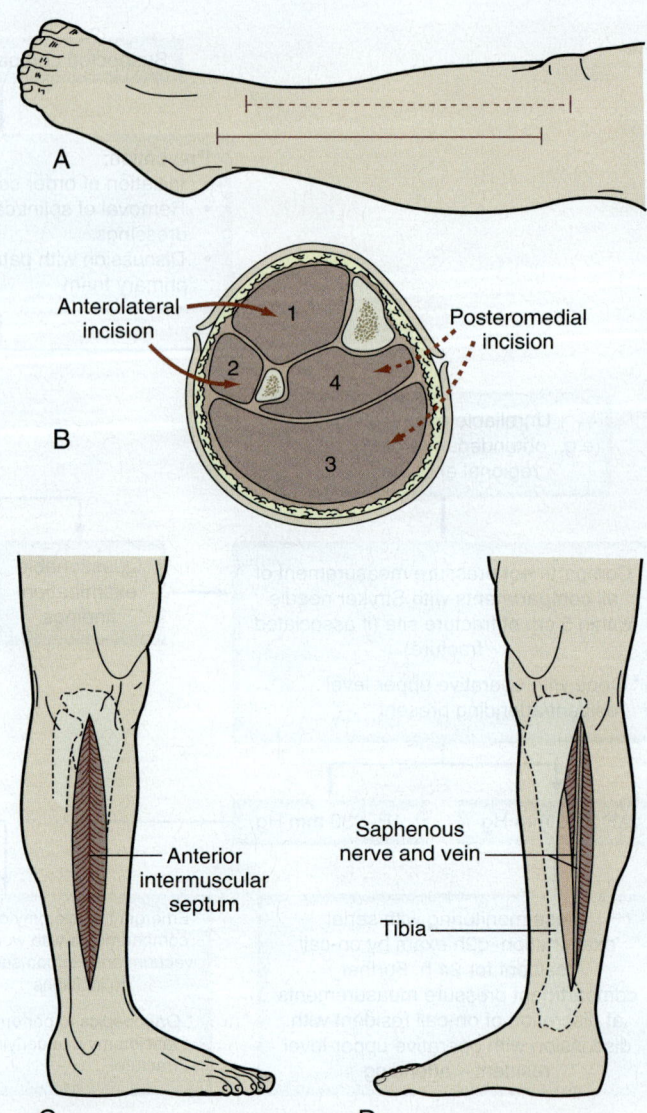

FIGURE 40.24 (A) Double-incision technique for performing fasciotomies of all four compartments of the lower extremity. (B) Cross-section of the lower extremity showing positions of anterolateral and posteromedial incisions that allow access to the anterior and lateral compartments (*1* and *2*) and the superficial and deep posterior compartments (*3* and *4*). (C) The anterior intramuscular septum should be identified in the lateral incision, as it marks the division of the anterior and lateral leg compartments. (D) The saphenous nerve and vein are identified in the medial incision and should be protected during compartment release.

or wet-to-dry dressings, depending on surgeon preference. Negative-pressure dressings reduce swelling through removal of excess fluid from the tissues, which may aid in staged primary skin closure. Repeat irrigation and debridement of the fasciotomy incisions and necrotic tissue should be performed every 2 to 3 days, and attempts at early or delayed primary skin closure can be attempted. Numerous adjunctive wound closure techniques have been described to aid in this process, including gradual suture approximation, the "shoelace technique" with tensioned vessel loops through staples at the skin edges, vacuum-assisted closure, and dynamic dermatotraction devices. If a tension-free closure is not possible, the exposed muscle can be covered with a split-thickness skin graft.

PELVIC RING INJURIES

The overall incidence of pelvic ring injuries is approximately 37 per 100,000 people per year across the United States. Pelvic ring injuries are a major cause of patient morbidity and mortality, and they may present in a wide spectrum of injury depending on patient age, bone quality, and mechanism of injury. Low-energy ground-level falls in elderly patients may simply result in a pubic ramus fracture, whereas high-energy motor vehicle accidents in younger patients may present with a significantly unstable injury pattern with life-threatening hemorrhage. It has been reported that up to 80% of these patients also have additional MSK injuries, and mortality rates vary from 15% to 25% depending on the severity and number of associated injuries. Because of the high-energy nature of these injuries, they are often associated with other non-MSK injuries, such as concomitant chest trauma, head injuries, visceral organ damage, and genitourinary injuries. Higher Injury Severity Scores (ISS) scores, shock on arrival, greater transfusion requirements, and patient age are risk factors for mortality in patients with pelvic ring fractures, and risk of mortality increases almost thirteenfold when the patient is hypotensive. In combination with a head or abdominal injury that requires surgical intervention or if the pelvis fracture is open, mortality increases to 50%. When both procedures are necessary, mortality approaches 90%. Routine ATLS protocols should be enacted in the initial workup and evaluation of these patients, and this should include a rectal/vaginal examination and assessment of open perineal wounds as part of the physical examination. Long-term disability, such as low back or pelvic pain, leg length discrepancies, dyspareunia, difficulty with childbearing, impotence, and incontinence, may result as sequelae from the injury itself and/or from nonanatomic reduction of the pelvic ring. Furthermore, even with successful restoration of the anatomy, patients can have long-term disability from the associated genitourinary and neurologic injuries affecting the lower extremity.

Classification

Pelvic ring injuries present with a wide spectrum of levels of instability. From an osseous standpoint, the pelvic ring is composed of the sacrum and bilateral innominate bones (includes an ilium, ischium, and pubis). In isolation, the bony pelvis has no inherent stability, but rather, through several strong ligamentous and soft tissue attachments, the pelvic ring is able to maintain its shape and withstand physiologic forces without deformation (Fig. 40.25). There are multiple previously described classification systems for pelvic ring injuries, and the two most common are the Tile classification and Young and Burgess classification schemes. The Tile classification categorizes injuries into three types, and each differs by its spectrum and direction of stability. Type A injuries are considered stable (e.g., avulsion injuries), type B are considered rotationally unstable but vertically stable (e.g., pubic symphysis disruption), and type C are considered rotationally and vertically unstable (e.g., vertical shear injury) (Fig. 40.26).

The Young and Burgess system classifies injuries mechanistically, with fracture patterns correlating with the direction of the applied energy at the time of the trauma. This is the most commonly used system for classification and is useful in guiding treatment decision-making. The system is composed of anterior-to-posterior compression (APC) injuries, lateral compression (LC) injuries, and vertical shear (VS) injuries (Fig. 40.27). In general, APC injuries have the greatest risk for retroperitoneal hemorrhage, and APC III patterns result in a significant increase in the intrapelvic volume and potential space for blood loss (Fig. 40.28). APC III injuries have the highest rate of mortality, blood loss, and need for transfusion among all pelvic ring injuries.

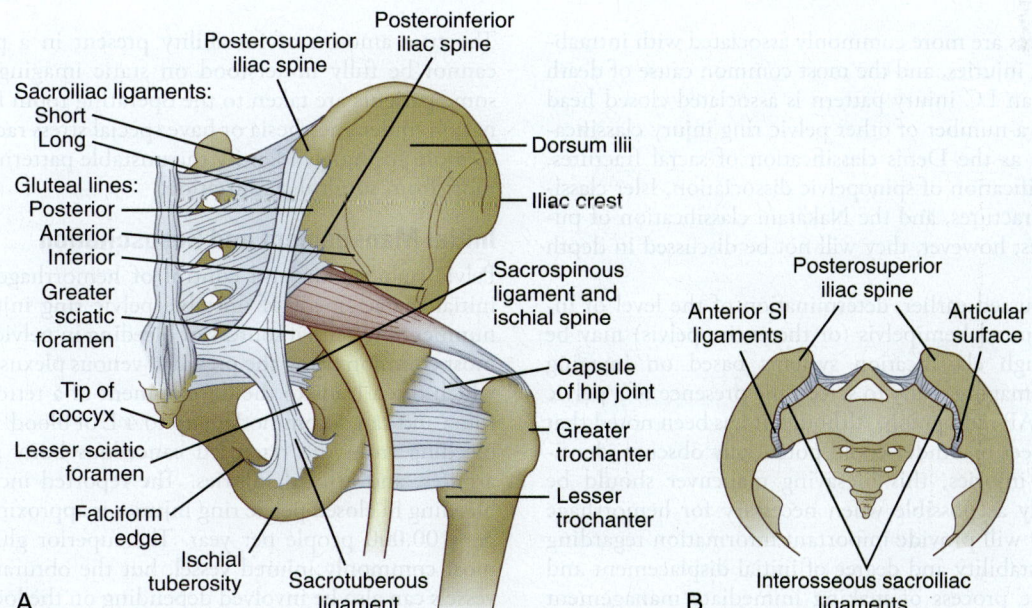

FIGURE 40.25 Ligamentous complexes of the pelvis. (A) Posteriorly, the major ligaments noted in the region of the sacroiliac (SI) joint are the posterior SI ligaments, both long and short. The long ligaments blend with the sacrospinous and sacrotuberous ligaments. (B) In cross-section, the orientation of the very thick posterior interosseous SI ligaments is noted. (From Stover MD, Mayo KA, Kellam JF. Pelvic ring disruptions. In: Browner BD, Levine AM, Jupiter JB, et al., eds. *Skeletal Trauma: Basic Science, Management, and Reconstruction.* 4th ed. WB Saunders; 2008.)

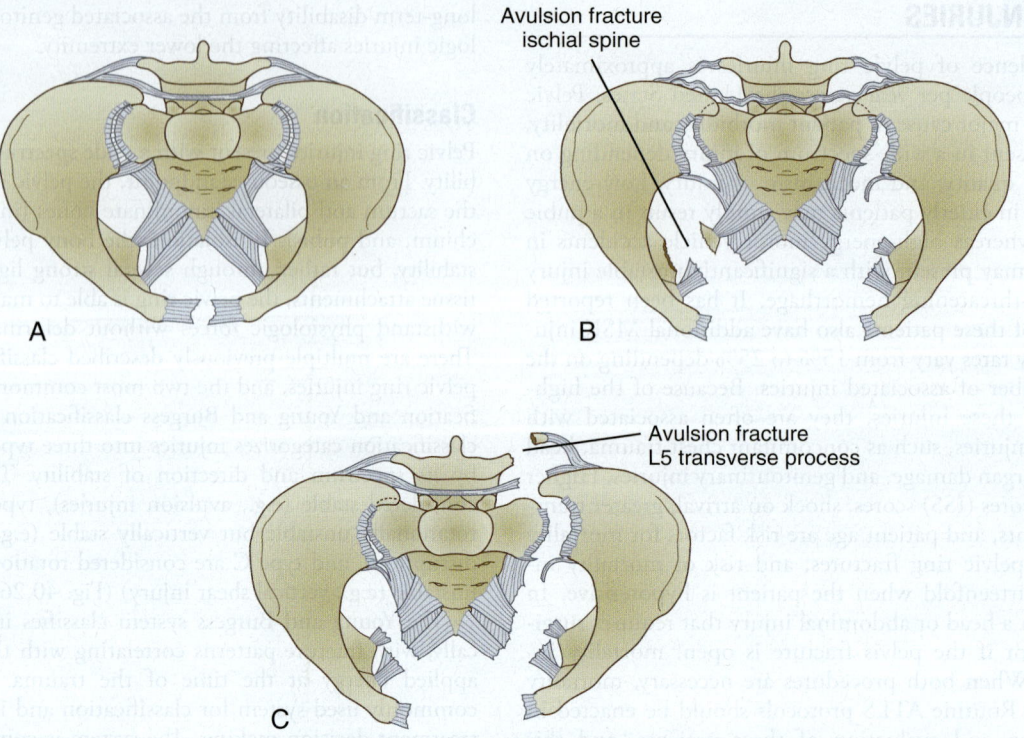

FIGURE 40.26 (A) Division of the symphysis pubis allows the pelvis to open to approximately 2.5 cm with no damage to any posterior ligamentous structures. (B) Division of the anterior sacroiliac and sacrospinous ligaments, either by direct division of their fibers *(right)* or by avulsion of the tip of the ischial spine *(left)*, allows the pelvis to rotate externally until the posterior superior iliac spines abut the sacrum. Note, however, that the posterior ligamentous structures (e.g., the posterior sacroiliac and iliolumbar ligaments) remain intact. Therefore, no displacement in the vertical plane is possible. (C) Division of the posterior band ligaments, that is, the posterior sacroiliac and the iliolumbar, causes complete instability of the hemipelvis. Note that global displacement is now possible. (From Stover MD, Mayo KA, Kellam JF. Pelvic ring disruptions. In: Browner BD, Levine AM, Jupiter JB, et al., eds. *Skeletal Trauma: Basic Science, Management, and Reconstruction.* 4th ed. WB Saunders; 2008.)

LC and VS fractures are more commonly associated with intraabdominal and head injuries, and the most common cause of death in a patient with an LC injury pattern is associated closed head trauma. There are a number of other pelvic ring injury classification systems such as the Denis classification of sacral fractures, Roy-Camille classification of spinopelvic dissociation, Isler classification of sacral fractures, and the Nakatani classification of pubic ramus fractures; however, they will not be discussed in depth here.

Finally, as discussed earlier, determination of the level of instability of the injured hemipelvis (or the entire pelvis) may be determined through classification systems based on imaging studies. The best imaging study to screen the presence of a pelvic fracture is a plain AP radiograph. Although it has been noted that placement of a sheet or binder could potentially obscure identification of these injuries, this lifesaving maneuver should be performed as early as possible when necessary for hemorrhage control. The x-ray will provide important information regarding the amount of instability and degree of initial displacement and greatly aids in the process of making immediate management decisions. The vast majority of trauma patients will undergo routine CT scans of the chest, abdomen, and pelvis as part of institutional protocols, and this will provide more detailed information on subtle injuries not appreciated on plain radiographs. If there is concern for a urethral injury or bladder injury, a retrograde urethrogram or cystogram may be obtained, respectively.

The true amount of instability present in a pelvic ring injury cannot be fully understood on static imaging, and as a result some patients are taken to the operating room for a stress examination under anesthesia or have special stress radiographs ordered to more accurately identify the unstable patterns that will benefit most from surgical stabilization.

Initial Management and Resuscitation

Pelvic stabilization and control of hemorrhage are the goals of initial management of unstable pelvic ring injuries. There are a number of potential sources of bleeding in pelvic ring injuries, the most common being the presacral venous plexus within the pelvis, which often leads to the development of a retroperitoneal hematoma and can accommodate up to 4 L of blood. Other sources are bleeding from the fractured cancellous bony surfaces, nutrient arteries, and arterial injuries. The reported incidence of arterial bleeding in closed pelvic ring injuries is approximately 1 to 2 cases per 100,000 people per year. The superior gluteal artery is the most commonly injured vessel, but the obturator and pudendal vessels can also be involved depending on the location of fractures and the injury pattern.

If patients present with hemodynamic instability, it is important to have a high suspicion for pelvic bleeding as a potential source because in approximately 60% of those patients, the pelvis is the main source of blood loss. Therefore, the temporary initial treatment of pelvic ring injuries with volume expansion is to place

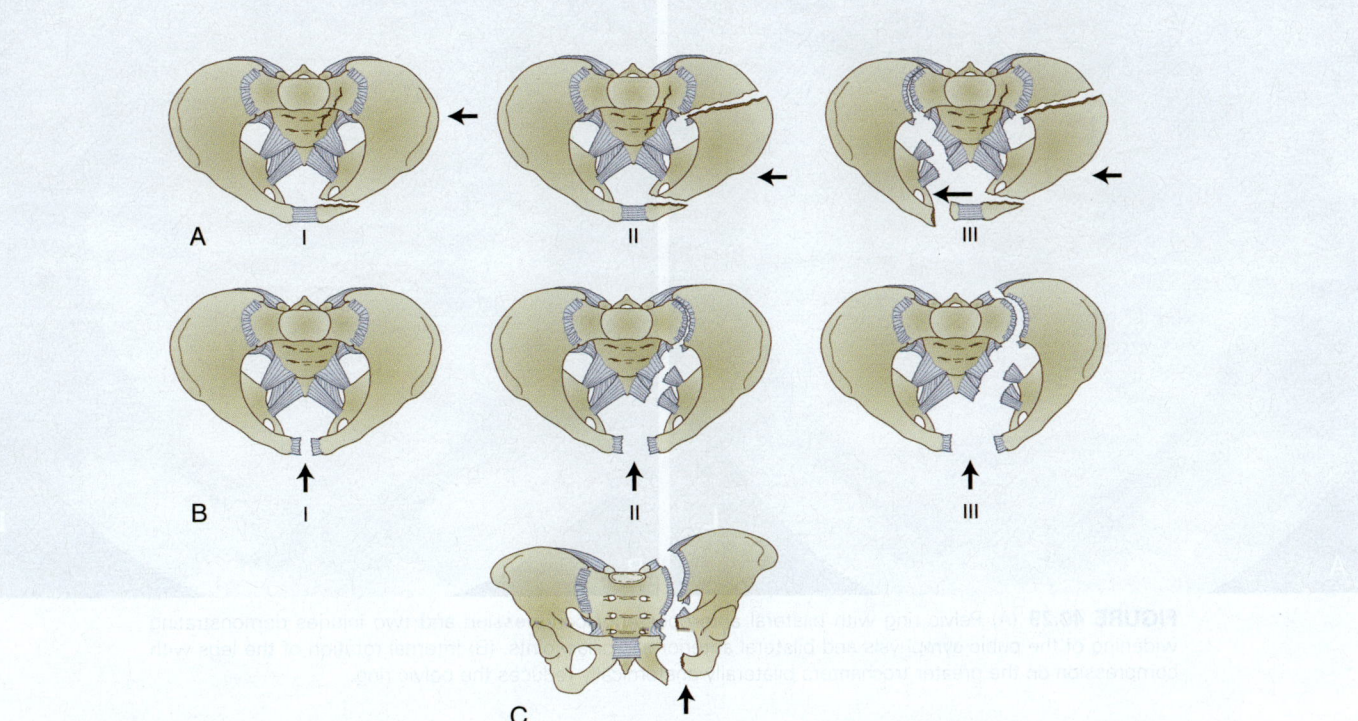

FIGURE 40.27 Young and Burgess classification. (A) Lateral compression force. Type I, a posteriorly directed force causing a sacral crushing injury and horizontal pubic ramus fractures ipsilaterally. This injury is stable. Type II, a more anteriorly directed force causing horizontal pubic ramus fractures with an anterior sacral crushing injury and either disruption of the posterior sacroiliac joints or fractures through the iliac wing. This injury is ipsilateral. Type III, an anteriorly directed force that is continued and leads to a type I or type II ipsilateral fracture with an external rotation component to the contralateral side; the sacroiliac joint is opened posteriorly, and the sacrotuberous and spinous ligaments are disrupted. (B) Anteroposterior compression fractures. Type I, an anteroposterior-directed force opening the pelvis but with the posterior ligamentous structures intact. This injury is stable. Type II, continuation of a type I fracture with disruption of the sacrospinous and potentially the sacrotuberous ligaments and an anterior sacroiliac joint opening. This fracture is rotationally unstable. Type III, a completely unstable or vertical instability pattern with complete disruption of all ligamentous supporting structures. (C) A vertically directed force at right angles to the supporting structures of the pelvis leading to vertical fractures in the rami and disruption of all the ligamentous structures. This injury is equivalent to an anteroposterior type III or a completely unstable and rotationally unstable fracture. (Adapted from Young JWR, Burgess AR. *Radiologic Management of Pelvic Ring Fractures*. Urban and Schwarzenberg; 1987.)

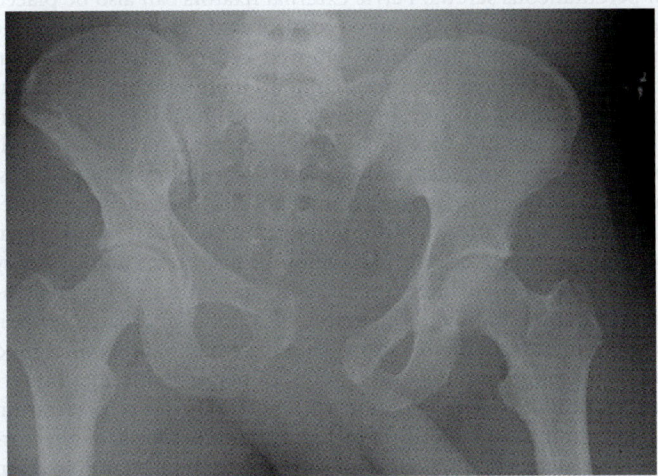

FIGURE 40.28 Anteroposterior pelvic radiograph showing the anterior-to-posterior compression (or "open-book") pelvis. Complete disruption of the anterior and posterior ligamentous structures leaves this pelvis rotationally and vertically unstable.

a circumferential binder or sheet to stabilize the pelvic ring and decrease the volume within the pelvis (Fig. 40.29). To apply properly, the binder or sheet must be centered over the greater trochanters with the legs adducted and internally rotated and tightened at the level of the trochanters. One benefit of using a sheet instead of a binder is that holes can be cut for access during angiography and placement of percutaneous screws. The added stability allows for clot formation, reapposition of anatomic surfaces, and decreased hemorrhage for all fracture patterns. Although historically there was concern that binders or sheet use could lead to skin breakdown or pressure ulcers, the current consensus is that this is not a concern unless the patient does not receive attentive and frequent turning, which patients with pelvic fractures should undergo even before fixation.

In patients who remain hemodynamically unstable despite appropriate resuscitation measures and temporary stabilization, the possibility of arterial hemorrhage should be considered. A prospective study of 143 patients with high-energy pelvic fracture showed that 10% had arterial injury, and factors predictive of arterial bleeding included a base deficit of

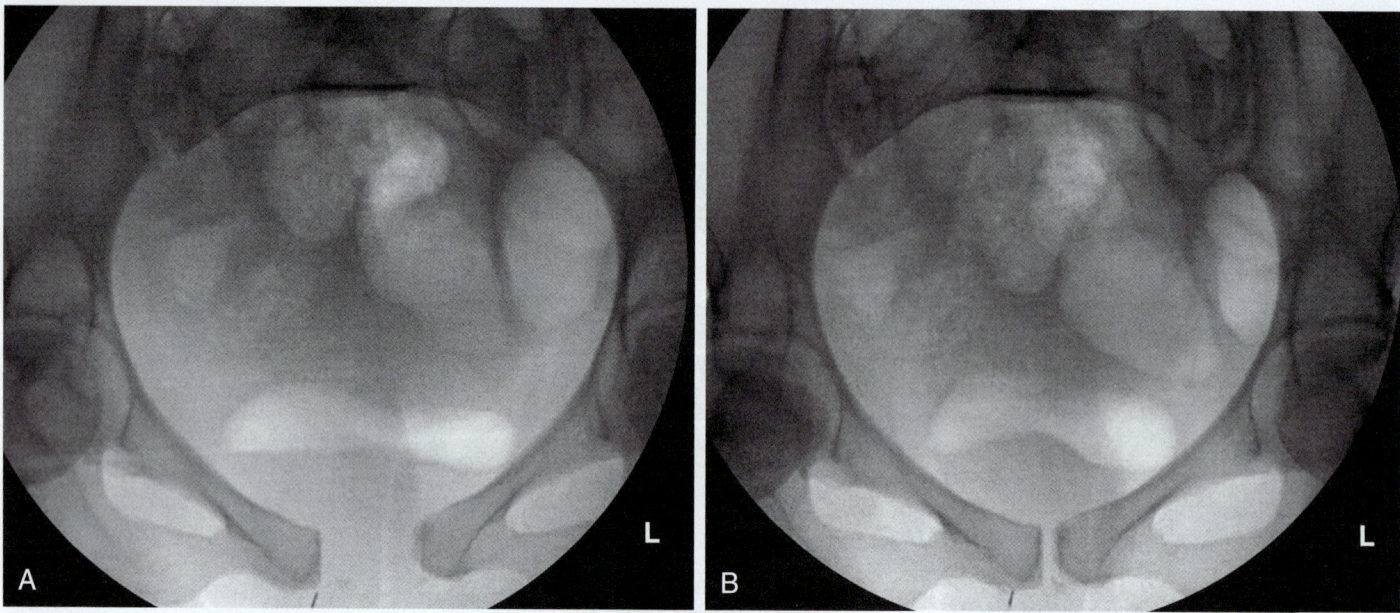

FIGURE 40.29 (A) Pelvic ring with bilateral anteroposterior compression and two injuries demonstrating widening of the pubic symphysis and bilateral anterior sacroiliac joints. (B) Internal rotation of the legs with compression on the greater trochanters bilaterally anatomically reduces the pelvic ring.

6 mmol/L, a systolic blood pressure less than 104 mm Hg, and the need for transfusion in the emergency department.[44] In many centers pelvic angiography with angioembolization is the gold standard for controlling pelvic arterial bleeding. This intervention is minimally invasive, effective, and specifically targeted to bleeding vessels. It is recommended that institutions have interventional radiologists readily available to perform these procedures when needed, no matter what time of day or night. It can be performed in either the internal iliac artery (nonselective) or distal to the internal iliac artery (selective). Although its benefit in pelvic fracture patients with hemodynamic instability is well documented, there are complication rates of 11%, including muscle necrosis, surgical wound breakdown, infection, and impotence. Complication rates are particularly high when associated with bilateral or nonselective pelvic angioembolization, which was demonstrated in one retrospective review that showed a 20% complication rate associated with nonselective angioembolization, so selective pelvic angioembolization is recommended when possible.[45]

If angioembolization is not an available resource, preperitoneal pelvic packing is an alternative technique. This may be effective in addressing venous bleeding, but it is less effective against arterial bleeding because some prior studies have reported up to 30% of patients still requiring angioembolization despite placement of packing. It also requires some degree of skeletal stabilization (pelvic external fixator or sheet/binder) in place to serve as a foundation to pack against and has higher reported rates of infection and complications. It is recommended that approximately six to nine laps are placed, starting posteriorly at the sacrum and moving anteriorly to the pubis. Packing should be removed after resuscitation in 24 to 48 hours, as delays in removal of the packing or repeat packing have been associated with increased infection rates. Ultimately, the decision to perform angioembolization versus preperitoneal pelvic packing is institutional specific, and timing of intervention requires a multidisciplinary treatment approach with the trauma surgeon, interventional radiologist, and orthopedic surgeon in order to improve outcomes, decrease time to intervention, and decrease complications.

Definitive Management

Definitive surgical stabilization of unstable pelvic ring injuries is dependent on the overall medical status and resuscitation of the patient and the planned treatment approach. Studies have demonstrated that early definitive fixation of pelvic ring injuries is both safe and effective, can be performed within 48 hours of injury, and will help to decrease complications and quicken recovery. In some cases, urgent percutaneous fixation strategies can be used to provide definitive internal fixation, such as placement of percutaneous screws. Pelvic external fixators can also be placed temporarily, usually during a concomitant surgery with the trauma team, and then later removed before definitive fixation after the patient has been resuscitated. There are certain circumstances in which an anterior pelvic external fixator is used definitively, and examples may include patients with open or contaminated anterior wounds, complex anterior ring fracture patterns, or bony anatomy that is not amenable to fixation with plates and/or screws. Patients with a large panniculus, associated open perineal wounds, or complex genitourinary tract injuries may also pose increased infection risks in the setting of internal instrumentation and would therefore be a poor candidate for open reduction and internal fixation. Patients who are otherwise good surgical candidates may undergo both open reduction and internal fixation or closed reduction with percutaneous screw fixation of their injuries at the discretion and comfort level of the surgeon. A detailed discussion of surgical approach and fixation techniques is beyond the scope of this text; however, examples of pelvic ring injuries and their definitive fixation constructs are displayed in Fig. 40.30.

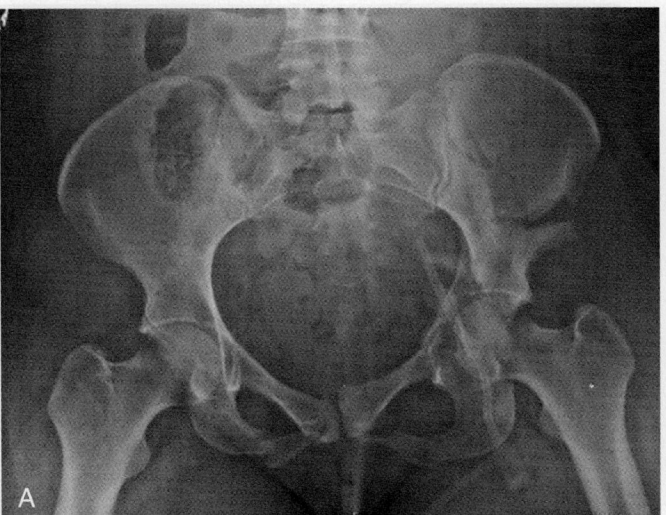
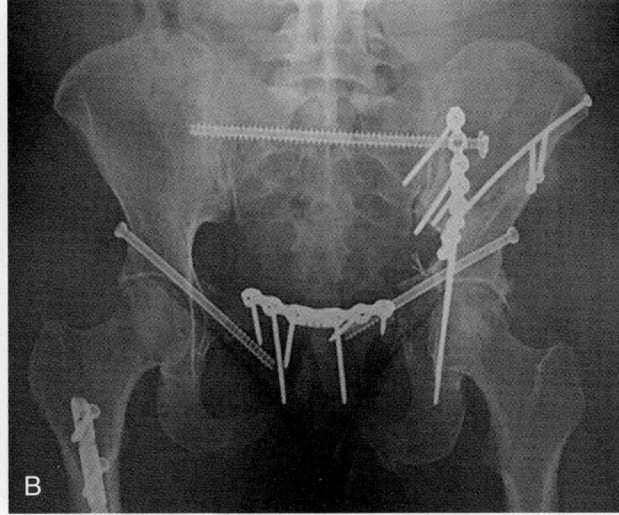

FIGURE 40.30 (A) Example of an unstable pelvic ring injury and (B) postoperative fixation construct.

DISLOCATIONS

Joint dislocations are generally considered an orthopedic emergency because of the increased risk of neurovascular injury and damage to the articular surface. Acute dislocations should be treated immediately because prolonged dislocation can lead to chondrocyte death, posttraumatic arthritis, joint ankylosis, and potentially avascular necrosis. Dislocations of major joints (e.g., shoulder, elbow, hip, knee, or ankle) are particularly concerning because of the high risk of neurovascular injury. Native joint dislocations are seen most commonly in young active patients as the result of a wide spectrum of injury mechanisms, and emergency department providers must be skilled in diagnosing and managing these injuries.

Patient Evaluation

It is important to immediately establish if this is a native versus prosthetic joint dislocation and whether it is an acute or chronic condition. A detailed patient history will help in providing information to answer those questions because some patients will have histories of recurrent dislocations or conditions that predispose them to dislocate with minimal trauma (e.g., recurrent shoulder dislocations in patients with hyperlaxity). The physical examination will include some common features across all joints, such as the joint's range of motion will be very limited and muscles surrounding the joint will be contracted. Completion of a thorough neurovascular examination is important, and certain neurovascular structures are known to be at risk with various dislocations that should be focused on (Table 40.6). Additionally, obtaining a baseline neurovascular examination before reduction will not only identify injuries present before the reduction (e.g., axillary nerve palsy in shoulder dislocation) but will also allow you to determine whether a neurovascular deficit improves after a reduction or gets worse. In some cases, a patient may not have a neurovascular deficit before a reduction but develops one afterward, and that is important to be aware of and document.

On examination the patient will commonly present with the dislocated joint in a pathognomonic position that will clue you into the most likely direction of the joint dislocation. For example, the majority of hip dislocations occur when the femoral head

TABLE 40.6 Joint Dislocations and Commonly Associated Neurovascular Injuries

JOINT	STRUCTURE AT RISK	ASSOCIATED INJURIES OR LONG-TERM CONSEQUENCES
Hip	• Sciatic nerve • Femoral artery	• Common peroneal nerve palsy • Complete sciatic nerve palsy • Avascular necrosis of the femoral head • Posttraumatic arthritis
Knee	• Popliteal artery and vein • Common peroneal nerve	• Common peroneal nerve palsy • Popliteal artery and vein injury • Multiligamentous knee injury
Shoulder	• Axillary nerve • Axillary artery • Brachial plexus	• In patients <40 years old, labral tear • In patients >40 years old, rotator cuff tear
Elbow	• Brachial artery • Radial, ulnar, and median nerves	• Chronic instability • Stiffness • Posttraumatic arthritis • Heterotopic ossification

dislocates posteriorly relative to the acetabulum, and the patient will present with their leg flexed at the hip, internally rotated, adducted, and shortened. In the shoulder, the humeral head generally dislocates anterior to the glenoid, and the patient will present with their arm in an externally rotated and abducted position. In thin patients, there may be loss of the normal contour of the deltoid, the acromion is prominent posteriorly and laterally, and the humeral head itself may be palpable anteriorly.

Radiographs should be ordered initially to confirm the diagnosis and identify associated fractures. A high percentage of posterior hip dislocations have associated acetabular fractures (e.g., posterior wall acetabular fracture), and many shoulder dislocations will have impaction injuries to the humeral head (e.g., Hill Sachs lesion) or fractures of the glenoid rim (e.g., bony Bankart lesion). Standard orthogonal views are usually enough to establish the direction of dislocation; however, as mentioned in the section on radiography, these must be true orthogonal images of the shoulder and not just internal and external rotation views of the proximal humerus.

Special Considerations for the Trauma Setting

Although all joint dislocations should be identified and reduced in a timely fashion, hip and knee dislocations require special consideration because of the potentially devastating consequences of delayed or missed diagnosis. Hip dislocations most commonly occur after high-energy motor vehicle crashes (46%–84% of reported dislocations), and this high level of energy often results in associated injuries to the femoral head, acetabulum, and soft tissues surrounding the hip. Sciatic nerve injuries are reported in 10% to 15% of posterior dislocations, with the peroneal branch most commonly affected because of the position of its fibers within the nerve and its tethering at the pelvis and fibular head. Anterior dislocations are more rare and have been associated with vascular injury to the common femoral artery and vein. Once an initial physical examination has been obtained to rule out both vascular and neurologic injury before any attempt at closed reduction is made and baseline imaging reviewed, a closed reduction under conscious sedation can be performed in an urgent manner. Previous studies have shown that delayed reduction may decrease the incidence of severity of nerve injury associated with dislocation, and additionally, delayed reduction is thought to decrease femoral head blood flow, increasing the risk of avascular necrosis. Several complications and morbidities have been reported after sustaining a hip dislocation, and those include posttraumatic arthritis (16%–24% of all hip dislocations), sciatic nerve palsy (10%–15%), avascular necrosis (6%–13%), and heterotopic ossification (2.8%–9%).[46]

Traumatic knee dislocations represent 0.02% to 0.2% of orthopedic injuries, approximately 0.5% of all major joint dislocations, and 40% to 64% are associated with vascular injuries, with the popliteal artery being the most commonly injured structure. Neurologic injuries are also associated with knee dislocations, and injury to the common peroneal nerve in particular has an incidence of 4.5% to 40% depending on the direction of the dislocation. These may present to the emergency department after having spontaneously reduced or still be dislocated. Similar to hip dislocations, they require a thorough neurovascular examination and imaging workup before reduction, but then should be reduced in an urgent fashion. They are also commonly associated with concomitant fractures of the proximal tibia, fibula, and sometimes the distal femur (Fig. 40.31). Vascular examination distal to the dislocation is critical, and pulses of the dorsal pedis and posterior tibia arteries should be assessed. This should be done through palpation, Doppler examination, and obtaining ABIs. If there are any signs of asymmetric or absent distal pulses, distal limb ischemia, or abnormal ABIs, one should have high suspicion for the presence of a vascular injury. Additional imaging in the form of CT angiography must then be considered, and if positive, vascular surgery should be consulted immediately. If the examination is otherwise negative for signs of vascular injury, patients should be braced and undergo serial examinations for up to 48 hours to monitor for an occult vascular injury.

Treatment

Once the initial physical examination and imaging workup are completed, the reduction should be urgently performed with

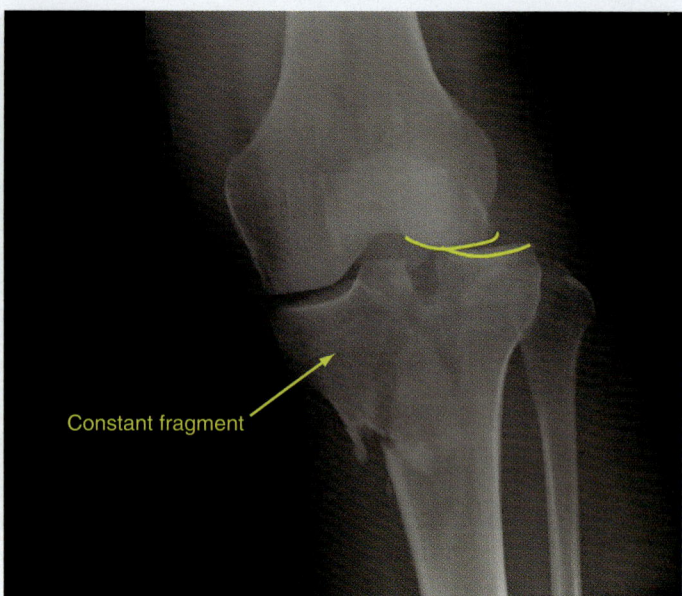

FIGURE 40.31 Medial tibial plateau fracture with a concomitant dislocation of the knee joint. Although it appears that the medial "constant fragment" is fractured off of the tibia shaft, this fractured fragment is maintaining its attachments to the distal femur. The tibia shaft is actually fractured off of the "constant fragment" and dislocated laterally. The incongruence of the lateral tibial plateau is noted.

some degree of sedation to aid in the reduction. The general reduction technique is to re-create the deforming force, apply traction, and then reverse the deforming force. For example, in a posterior hip dislocation, the position of the hip at the time of dislocation was most likely flexed, internally rotated, and adducted. When the hip dislocates, the femoral head usually rests on the posterior wall of the acetabulum, which inhibits reduction. Therefore, to reduce the joint, you must flex and internally rotate the hip and gently adduct to unhinge the femoral head from the posterior aspect of the acetabulum. Finally, axial traction will pull the femoral head anteriorly into the acetabulum and complete the reduction. Knee dislocations may be classified as medial, lateral, posterior, anterior, or rotatory, and this describes the position of the tibia relative to the distal femur. Anterior knee dislocations are the most common, with a reported incidence of approximately 40%. These can be reduced with axial traction and anterior translation of the femur. When a successful reduction is performed, the knee should be braced and a repeat neurovascular examination obtained and documented. Shoulder dislocations are treated in a similar fashion, and there are numerous well-described reduction maneuvers. The provider should choose whichever they are most comfortable with and trained in. If any joint dislocation is deemed irreducible after attempts at closed reduction with adequate sedation are made, the patient should be brought to the operating room for an attempt at closed reduction under general anesthesia and possible open reduction if indicated.

Finally, the majority of reduced joint dislocations should be immobilized using well-padded splints (e.g., elbow, wrist, and ankle) or joint-specific immobilizers (e.g., shoulder sling, knee immobilizer). All dislocations require either in-hospital or outpatient evaluation by an orthopedic surgeon.

VASCULAR AND MUSCULOSKELETAL INJURIES

Recognition

Prompt recognition of these injuries can be difficult because normal pulses are present in 5% to 15% of patients with a vascular injury, and overt hemorrhage causing obvious blood pressure changes is rare. Certain orthopedic injuries are known to be associated with vascular injuries and therefore should give the provider heightened suspicion, and these include knee dislocations and fracture dislocations, supracondylar humerus fractures, elbow dislocations, and unstable pelvic or acetabular fractures. However, certain findings on clinical examination, especially when compared with the unaffected limb, can have high sensitivity for early detection and diagnosis. These include pulselessness, pallor, paresthesia, paralysis, rapidly expanding hematomas, relative loss/decreased Doppler signals, obvious massive bleeding, and a palpable thrill or audible bruit. In lower extremity injuries, an ABI of less than 0.9 warrants further workup for vascular injury, and CT angiography is the recommended test of choice for diagnosis.

Management

A comprehensive description of surgical techniques for repair or reconstruction of vascular injuries is beyond the scope of this chapter. More relevant to this chapter are considerations specific to patients with concomitant orthopedic injuries that require skeletal stabilization either before or immediately after vascular repair. In general, skeletal stabilization should occur before vascular repair so that the manipulation performed during the reduction and skeletal stabilization does not endanger the repair. Additionally, temporary stabilization is typically recommended rather than definitive stabilization at the index procedure. Delaying vascular repair prolongs warm ischemia and tissue injury, so the patient may need a temporary shunt while the skeletal stabilization is performed before proceeding with the full vascular repair. Finally, concomitant fasciotomies (both prophylactic and postoperative therapeutic) should be considered in all patients who have had restored blood flow and have been associated with a significantly lower risk for amputation and other complications after limb revascularization.

COMMON LONG BONE FRACTURES

Femur Shaft Fractures

Epidemiology and Significance

The overall incidence of femoral shaft fractures ranges between 10 and 21 per 100,000 people per year across the world. They typically present in a bimodal distribution, with younger males (age 15–35 years) sustaining them from higher-energy injury mechanisms, and older females (age 60 years and older) sustaining them from lower-energy injury mechanisms. The most common cause is a motor vehicle crash, but they can also occur from falls from height, ground-level falls in the setting of osteoporosis, and ballistic injuries. Atypical fractures, such as those from bisphosphonate usage, occur from lower-energy mechanisms and have a reported incidence of 3.5% to 16% across studies. These trauma patients should be evaluated as part of the ATLS protocol to evaluate for other associated orthopedic injuries, in particular, ipsilateral femoral neck

fractures and bilateral femoral shaft fractures. In patients with high-energy femoral shaft fractures (typically comminuted mid-to-distal shaft), there is a reported incidence between 2% and 9% of ipsilateral femoral neck fracture.[7–9] Because of its increased awareness, it is recommended that thin-cut high-resolution CT scan of the hip be ordered to assess for occult fracture. Bilateral femoral shaft fractures account for 2% to 7% of all femur fractures, are associated with high-energy injury mechanisms, can result in significant bleeding within the thigh, and therefore require more aggressive resuscitation. Providers should have a high index of suspicion for onset of systemic complications such as fat embolism syndrome (FES) and acute respiratory distress syndrome (ARDS) in these patients.

Initial Management

It is strongly recommended that femur shaft fractures be immobilized in some way before the patient is transported from the scene of the accident, and when performed by first responders, it generally includes placement in a traction splint. Without immobilization, displaced femoral shaft fractures will continue to cause increased pain, edema, bleeding, and potentially further damage to the surrounding soft tissues. Continued motion at the fracture site can also increase the risk of FES. Proper immobilization begins with in-line traction, which grossly restores length, alignment, and rotation, thereby decreasing the diameter of the thigh compartment and reducing its volume. The soft tissues are then under tension and can tamponade bleeding and facilitate clot formation at the fracture site. For patients in extremis, a posterior splint alone provides adequate immobilization until appropriate skeletal traction can be applied.

Definitive Stabilization

The recommended timing of definitive fixation of femoral shaft fractures has followed a parabolic course over the last few decades. In the 1970s, patients with a femoral shaft fracture were often thought of as being "too sick to operate on," but this changed in the 1980s, as these patients were considered "too sick *not* to operate on." Thus, there became a movement to operate on femoral shaft fractures within 24 hours after admission, and this treatment algorithm was termed *early total care (ETC)*. In the 1990s, treatment algorithms and recommendations began to change, as pulmonary complications were shown to be more prevalent in patients who had both chest injuries and early femoral shaft fracture fixation. The reasoning behind these observations was that the systemic inflammatory system was primed after the initial injury, and the pulmonary load and subsequent inflammatory response of femoral nail insertion caused a "second-hit phenomenon" of hypoxemia and hypotension that led to the development of ARDS. This was the birth of damage control orthopedics (DCO).

DCO primarily consists of the placement of an external fixator on the femur to provide restoration of length, alignment, and rotation, as well as a closed reduction. The goals of DCO include provisional fracture fixation that allows mobilization of the patient, hemorrhage control, soft tissue management, and the prevention of the "second hit." It is generally not recommended to definitively treat femoral shaft fractures in an external fixator because of high rates of loss of reduction, malunion, nonunion, and pin-site infections. Therefore, the external fixator is generally removed and definitive fixation (e.g., intramedullary nail) is placed once the patient is medically cleared for a second surgery.

Since the 1990s, the debate of DCO versus ETC has continued as our ability to more effectively resuscitate patients has improved. Multiply injured patients in extremis still benefit from DCO, and DCO is indicated in patients with persistent hypotension, metabolic acidosis, or a severe head injury but are otherwise going to the operating room for other urgent procedures. However, as new algorithms for determining clearance for surgery have been described, definitive treatment within the first 24 hours has become standard of care. Patients who are considered to be "borderline" are generally those with both soft organ and MSK injuries. Since the 1990s, multiple studies have disputed the idea that DCO is the best first-line treatment for borderline patients. When considering the incidence of ARDS, mortality, and length of stay, these studies have found either no difference between DCO and ETC or, if there was a difference in those end points, it was almost always in favor of ETC. Furthermore, the "borderline" patient is hemodynamically transient, but that patient frequently becomes "stable" within 24 hours of admission with appropriate resuscitation measures, especially with more liberal transfusion practices. Thus, many authors continue to advocate for definitive fixation of femoral shaft fractures in these patients within the first 24 to 48 hours, as multiple studies have shown it reduces the incidence of pulmonary complications, infections, and mortality.

Tibia Shaft Fractures

Epidemiology and Significance

The incidence of tibial shaft fractures is approximately 16.9 per 100,000 people per year, and it tends to be more prevalent in males than in females (21.5 vs. 12.3 per 100,000). They generally occur in a bimodal distribution with regard to high- versus low-energy mechanism, and because of its subcutaneous location, these injuries are commonly open. High-energy mechanisms are commonly caused by direct trauma, resulting in short oblique or comminuted fractures with associated soft tissue injuries (e.g., open fracture), bone loss, compartment syndrome, and a fibula fracture at the same level. Low-energy injuries typically occur with indirect trauma or torsional forces that result in spiral fractures and often an associated fibula fracture at a different level.

Blood Supply

Tibial shaft fractures tend to be slow healing as a result of their tenuous blood supply and limited soft tissue envelope. A single nutrient artery that branches from the posterior tibial artery (distal continuation of the popliteal artery) supplies blood to the entire diaphysis. It enters the medullary canal and travels proximally and distally to anastomose with metaphyseal endosteal vessels. Although there is some contribution from the penetrating branches of the periosteal arteries that supply the outer third of the cortex, a diaphyseal fracture can easily compromise the nutrient arterial blood supply. Concomitant soft tissue stripping may leave an entire segment of tibia devascularized, and as a result, tibial shaft fractures are anatomically predisposed to impaired or prolonged healing and, with open fractures, to nonunion and infection.

Associated Soft Tissue Injuries

A comprehensive neurovascular examination should be performed to assess and document the status of the dorsal pedis and posterior tibial pulses. The soft tissues should be carefully evaluated for any signs or symptoms of compartment syndrome, open fractures, or fracture blisters. The incidence of compartment syndrome in tibial shaft fractures has been reported as high as 10%, so serial monitoring of the patient's signs and symptoms and, if necessary, compartment pressures is important. Neurovascular injury should be carefully evaluated for, as several structures traversing the lower leg may be injured by the initial trauma or subsequently became entrapped within the fracture site. Several previous case reports have documented entrapment of neurovascular and tendonous structures within fracture sites, impeding reduction, and so the provider should have a high index of suspicion for this when an appropriate reduction is unable to be achieved or if the neurovascular examination worsens after a reduction is performed.

Neurologic examination includes assessment of all five major nerves that traverse the lower leg to supply motor and sensory input to the muscles and overlying skin. The deep peroneal nerve, traveling in the anterior compartment, can be evaluated by testing first dorsal web space sensation as well as the patient's ability to extend the greater toe or dorsiflex the ankle. Testing of sensation on the dorsum of the midfoot and eversion strength will assess the superficial peroneal nerve, which travels in the lateral compartment. The tibial nerve travels in the deep posterior compartment and provides sensation to the plantar aspect of the foot and motor control of ankle and toe plantarflexion. The sural and saphenous nerves travel superficially to the fascia and are both pure sensory nerves. The sural nerve supplies sensation to the lateral aspect of the heel and midfoot, and the saphenous nerve supplies sensation to the medial ankle and hindfoot.

Management and Treatment

The definitive management of tibial shaft fractures may be operative or nonoperative. A closed fracture with minimal displacement and alignment that falls within the acceptable parameters of alignment (i.e., <5 degrees of varus/valgus, <10 degrees of anterior/posterior angulation, <1 cm of shortening, and >50% cortical apposition) can be treated by cast immobilization and later transition to functional bracing. However, the negative to nonoperative treatment is that patients must remain non–weight-bearing for an extended period of time, which is something not all patients may be able to comply with. Operative fixation with intramedullary nailing, which is the most common and preferred method of treatment, will allow the patient to begin weight-bearing immediately with therapy. Open reduction and internal fixation with plating can be considered for diaphyseal tibial fractures; however, it is more commonly used when the fracture extends proximally into the articular surface, distally into the metaphysis, or in patterns not amenable to intramedullary nailing with modern implants. To circumvent the need for large surgical incisions and soft tissue dissection around the fracture site, minimally invasive percutaneous plating techniques have been developed and lead to good outcomes. Historically, external fixation has been used as a definitive means of tibial shaft fracture fixation; however, it is more often used in patients who are too unstable for intramedullary nailing (i.e., DCO) or have severe soft tissue injuries that will require multiple debridements with possible soft tissue coverage. In these cases, the external fixation device will generally be removed and an intramedullary nail placed for definitive fixation once the patient has stabilized or when the soft tissues have stabilized and are appropriate for coverage.

Humerus Shaft Fractures

Epidemiology, Acceptable Alignment, and Associated Injuries

Fractures of the humeral shaft account for approximately 3% of all fractures and have an incidence of 13 per 100,000 people each year. They generally occur in a bimodal distribution with peak incidence in young males (age 21–30 years) after high-energy trauma and older females (age 60–80 years) after low-energy trauma. Historically, nonoperative treatment with bracing has been the treatment of choice, with studies reporting a nearly 95% rate of union and 85% return to full shoulder and elbow function after nonoperative treatment with a functional (Sarmiento) brace. If humeral shaft fractures can be maintained in acceptable alignment with nonoperative treatment, satisfactory outcomes can be achieved with minimal functional deficits. The parameters defining acceptable alignment include <20 degrees of sagittal plane deformity, <30 degrees of coronal plane deformity, and <3 cm of shortening. However, in recent years operative treatment has become more common with the advent of new operative techniques and implants, and several high-level systematic reviews have focused on the comparison of treatment methods. Overall, operative interventions have demonstrated lower rates of reoperation but higher rates of transient radial nerve palsy, whereas nonoperative treatment with functional bracing has demonstrated higher rates of nonunion and malunion requiring revision operations.

Radial nerve injuries occur in up to 6% to 18% of closed mid- and distal-third fractures at presentation (Fig. 40.32), and reported rates of postoperative radial nerve palsy range from 3% to 7%. The radial nerve is at risk of injury because of its close relationship with the humeral shaft as it travels from medial to lateral in the spiral groove, entering about 20 cm proximal to the medial epicondyle and exiting 14 cm proximal to the lateral epicondyle. In the setting of a closed fracture, treatment is generally nonoperative with observation for return of function over the subsequent months. In open fractures or ballistic injuries, the nerve is generally explored to assess whether or not it has been lacerated or transected by the initial injury, in which case the appropriate service is consulted for consideration of acute nerve repair versus delayed repair or grafting. When a radial nerve palsy is diagnosed on the initial physical examination, it is most commonly a neurapraxia and will recover spontaneously within 3 to 4 months in the majority of patients. The patient should be placed in a removable forearm splint during that time to support the wrist and fingers. If the nerve function does not return by 3 months, an electromyography can be ordered to determine if exploration is indicated. If a coaptation splint is placed and the patient develops a radial nerve palsy afterward, then the splint should be promptly removed. If the nerve function does not return after removal, then surgical exploration should be considered.

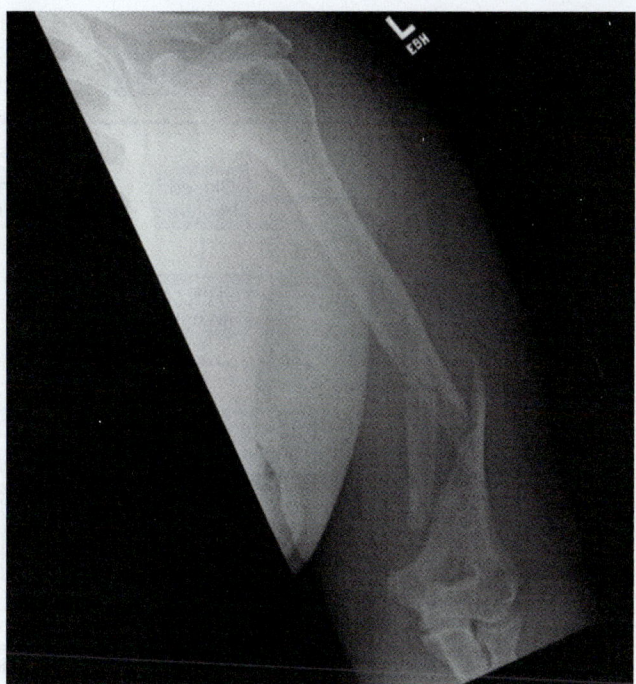

FIGURE 40.32 Holstein-Lewis fracture of the humeral shaft. This patient had no radial nerve function at presentation. At the time of surgery, the nerve was found to be intact but interposed between two fracture fragments. Full radial nerve function returned by 6 months.

Treatment

There are multiple nonoperative treatment methods: coaptation splints, hanging arm casts, "sling and swathe," and functional bracing (i.e., Sarmiento). Although there are studies showing minor benefits to each method, the most common treatment is an initial coaptation splint followed by transition to a functional brace (Sarmiento brace) at clinic follow-up once swelling has decreased (usually 3–7 days later). Functional bracing is not initiated in the acute setting because it relies on the compression of soft tissues to exert a hydraulic, stabilizing force on the fracture; that pressure in the face of an acute injury can result in significant pain. During the functional brace stage, patients are allowed free elbow flexion-extension and arm abduction to 60 degrees, as motion will generate compressive forces from muscle contraction, helping to maintain alignment. However, potential complications of bracing include skin irritation, malunion, nonunion, and failure of nonoperative management requiring transition to operative treatment.

If a patient fails closed management, has an open fracture, has unstable fracture pattern (e.g., comminution, segmental), has an ipsilateral forearm or elbow fracture, or is a polytrauma patient who could benefit from earlier mobility to rehabilitate from other injuries, operative management should be considered. The mainstay of surgical management is compression plating for a transverse fracture pattern or lag screw compression and neutralization plating, and in some instances, an intramedullary nail may be used. An algorithm for decision of treatment is displayed in Fig. 40.33.

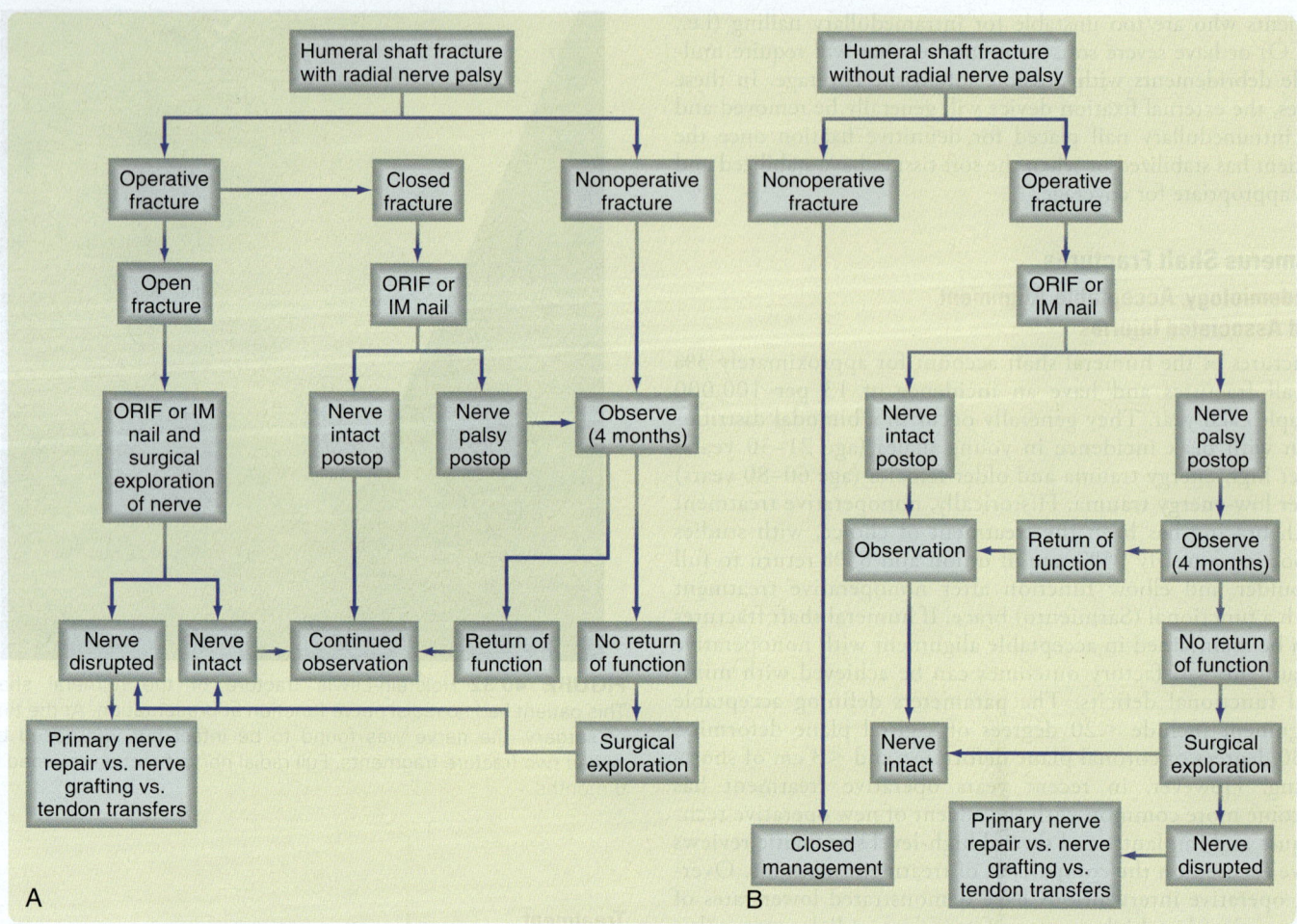

FIGURE 40.33 Algorithms for management of a patient presenting with a humeral shaft fracture with (A) and without (B) radial nerve palsy. *IM*, Intramedullary; *ORIF*, open reduction internal fixation.

CHALLENGES AND COMPLICATIONS

Missed Injuries

The incidence of missed injuries after the primary and secondary surveys in trauma patients widely varies across studies and has been reported between 0.6% and 39%. MSK injuries, specifically in the extremities, are among the most commonly missed injuries. Previous studies have identified several factors that increase the risk of a missed injury, and those include head injuries, low Glasgow Coma Scale (GCS) scores, high ISS, and mechanically ventilated patients.[47] These factors are often present in multiply injured patients, and although the primary and secondary surveys performed in the emergency department are aimed at identifying life-threatening injuries, inadequate physical examinations, deviation from routine care algorithms, and misinterpretation/lack of adequate radiographs can all contribute to missed or delayed diagnoses. The tertiary survey, which includes a comprehensive physical examination and review of imaging studies within 24 hours after the primary survey, was implemented in the 1990s and resulted in the detection of more than 50% of previously missed injuries. If possible, the tertiary survey should be completed when the patient is conscious and responsive; however, this is not always plausible in severely injured patients within 24 hours of admission.

Drug and Alcohol Use

The incidence of drug and alcohol use in patients with MSK injuries has been reported to be as high as 50%. Prescription opiate use and abuse have also become more common in recent years and is a well-documented societal problem. Orthopedic trauma patients have a higher preinjury use of opioids than the general population. In addition, one study reported that lower-income and unemployed patients are more likely to feel that their surgeon is not prescribing them enough pain medicine, use their prescribed opioid medications at higher-than-recommended doses, and use additional opioid medications in addition to those prescribed to them. Several institutions have begun to implement multimodal pain management algorithms with good success in decreasing overall opioid administration and usage in orthopedic patients. Rates of alcohol abuse disorders in hospitalized trauma patient populations have been reported to be greater than 50% in some studies. Alcohol withdrawal syndrome occurs approximately 6 to 48 hours after the cessation of alcohol consumption and may be characterized by tremor, anxiety, agitation, seizures, and delirium tremens. As such, due to the increased prevalence of alcohol abuse in trauma patients, it is important to establish alcohol withdrawal protocols, screen for histories of abuse, monitor for symptoms, and consult appropriate services such as addiction management to provide resources to the patient.

Thromboembolic Complications

Multiply injured trauma patients are at significantly higher risk of developing deep venous thrombosis (DVT) and pulmonary embolism (PE), with reported rates as high as 60% in some studies. A systematic review reported the overall incidence of venous thromboembolism to be 12% in patients who received no prophylaxis and 7% in those who received mechanical prophylaxis.[48] Higher rates are likely seen in patients with multiple severe injuries (e.g., traumatic brain and spinal injuries) and those undergoing multiple surgeries. As such, the use of thromboprophylaxis is strongly recommended in hospitalized trauma patients because even with appropriate prophylaxis, venous thromboembolism remains among the leading causes of mortality in this patient population.

Recent systematic reviews have demonstrated that both pharmacologic and mechanical prophylaxis reduces the risk of DVT in trauma patients. The decision to begin pharmacologic prophylaxis in particular should be balanced with the potential risk of bleeding related to the patient's injuries, specifically in the setting of solid organ injury, intracranial hemorrhage, and spinal injury. The American Society of Hematology (ASH) 2019 guidelines for prevention of venous thromboembolism in hospitalized surgical patients recommended pharmacologic prophylaxis over no prophylaxis for patients undergoing major surgery in general. In a more recent randomized controlled trial comparing aspirin and low-molecular-weight heparin for thromboprophylaxis after fracture, the authors reported that in patients with extremity fractures who had been treated operatively or with any pelvic or acetabular fracture, thromboprophylaxis with aspirin was noninferior to low-molecular-weight heparin in preventing death and was associated with low incidences of DVT and PE and low 90-day mortality.[49] In a study of 12,211 patients, thromboprophylaxis was administered while inpatient and then for 21 days after discharge, with reported rates of DVT and PE in both groups to be ≤2.51%. Despite these updated findings, there remains a lack of a universally accepted protocol for orthopedic trauma patients, with a wide range of protocols used across the United States. Recent reviews of general dosing guidelines, combination therapy, timing/duration of anticoagulation, and numerous societal recommendations have been published for reference. An example protocol used at the author's institution is displayed in Table 40.7.

Fat Embolism Syndrome and Acute Respiratory Distress Syndrome

Multiply injured patients are at increased risk of cardiopulmonary complications, such as FES and ARDS secondary to an already diminished respiratory reserve. FES is a known complication of long bone fractures, with a reported incidence between 2% and 5% in patients with isolated long bone fractures and as high as 19% in multiply injured patients. FES is a clinical phenomenon characterized by systemic dissemination of fat emboli within the circulation, which can deposit in and disrupt the microvasculature. It is most common in orthopedic trauma patients and may present with skin (petechiae), central nervous system (altered mental status), respiratory (hypoxemia), and eye (retinal hemorrhages) manifestations. Multiple diagnostic criteria have been proposed, and the signs and symptoms may present within hours to days after injury or surgery. The treatment of FES generally involves respiratory support and elevation to a higher level of care.

Fixation of multiple lower extremity long bone fractures with intramedullary fixation poses a significant cardiopulmonary risk

TABLE 40.7 Inpatient and Discharge Thromboembolism Prophylaxis Protocol

Isolated Upper Extremity Injury
- Preoperative: SCDs
- Postoperative: SCDs, EC ASA 81 mg PO BID
- Discharge: indication discussed with attending surgeon

Unilateral Lower Extremity Injury
- Preoperative/postoperative: SCDs, Lovenox 40 mg QHS
- Discharge: EC ASA 81 mg PO BID × 14 days to take with food

Hip/Pelvis/Acetabulum Fracture
- Preoperative/postoperative/nonoperative: SCDs, Lovenox 40 mg QHS
- Discharge: Eliquis 2.5 mg PO BID × 4 weeks

Bilateral Lower/Multiple Extremity Injuries
- Preoperative/postoperative: SCDs, Lovenox 40 mg QHS
- Discharge: Eliquis 2.5 mg PO BID × 4 weeks

Other
- Newly wheelchair-bound patients should be discharged on 4 weeks of Eliquis 2.5 mg PO BID.
- Baseline wheelchair-bound patients should be assessed case by case with the attending surgeon.
- Patients who are being discharged to return for staged orthopedic surgery should be discharged Lovenox 40 mg QHS until return to hospital.
- Patients that are at high risk for DVT (e.g., history of DVT/PE, hypercoagulable state, active cancer) require screening ultrasound to evaluate for DVT. Discharge on Eliquis for negative study, and discuss treatment with attending surgeon if positive study.

BID, Twice daily; *EC ASA,* enteric-coated aspirin; *DVT,* deep venous thrombosis; *PE,* pulmonary embolism; *PO,* by mouth; *QHS,* nightly; *SCD,* sequential compression device.

to polytraumatized patients. As the femoral or tibial medullary canal is instrumented with guidewires, reamers, and intramedullary nail implants, the marrow contents and intramedullary fat are released into circulation, causing activation of the coagulation cascade, platelet dysfunction, release of vasoactive substances and inflammatory cytokines, and subsequent neutrophil infiltration. In at-risk patients, this may result in the onset of FES, pneumonia, ARDS, multiple organ failure, and in some cases death. The increased risk of these complications after intramedullary fixation of long bone fractures has been well described, and in the setting of multiple long bone fractures, surgeons commonly opt for a staged fixation approach. However, there is a paucity of high-level data regarding actual cardiorespiratory burden with simultaneous versus staged fixation of multiple lower extremity injuries, and because of that no universal treatment guidelines exist. A recent study investigated the rate of cardiopulmonary complications in 146 patients with multiple lower extremity long bone fractures treated simultaneously or staged and found no difference in cardiopulmonary complications, which is in contrast to previous studies.[50]

ARDS is an acute respiratory failure and life-threatening condition characterized by the 2012 Berlin criteria (i.e., three strata of progressive hypoxemia, noncardiogenic cause, bilateral pulmonary infiltrates). Risk factors are many and include trauma, sepsis, crystalloid resuscitation, drug overdose, and FES. Early fixation (<24 hours) of fractures has been shown to reduce the incidence of FES and ARDS in trauma patients; however, there has been some debate about whether the method of fixation affects the incidence of FES. Additionally, separate clinical and experimental studies have suggested that the presence of chest injury, not the method of fracture fixation, is responsible for ARDS. Therefore, it is recommended that a multidisciplinary approach be taken to balance the perceived risks of surgery when deciding both treatment timing and method of fixation. In patients with severe acute chest injury and concomitant long bone fractures, it may be advisable to delay definitive fixation of the fracture with intramedullary devices until the patient's pulmonary status has stabilized. Temporary stabilization with external fixation may be warranted, which not only helps with resuscitation and pain control but also decreases the embolization of fat seen with moving fracture ends.

POSTOPERATIVE MOBILIZATION

The benefits of early fixation and mobilization of multiply injured patients have been discussed. However, a distinction between mobilization and weight-bearing is essential. Mobilization is transfer of the patient from the supine position, either under the patient's own power or with the help of nurses or therapists. This includes turning the patient every few hours by nursing staff, sitting the patient up in bed, or transferring the patient to a chair. All patients should be mobilized by the first or second postoperative day if their general condition permits; this can help prevent the development of postoperative complications.

Weight-bearing, in contrast, is transmission of a load through an extremity. In general, the goal of fracture care is to achieve an anatomic reduction with stable fixation that will restore function and allow the patient to begin motion as soon as possible. In some cases, often related to fracture site comminution or soft tissue injuries, the surgeon may choose to limit weight-bearing status to touch-down weight-bearing, partial weight-bearing, or non–weight-bearing completely. This recommendation is made while taking a variety of different patient and injury factors into consideration and also to protect the fixation construct and prevent early implant failure. It is also important to assess the patient's social, psychological, and overall mental status first to determine if a patient will be able to abide by weight-bearing restrictions. In polytraumatized patients, surgical fixation of certain injuries may be indicated in order to allow for the patient to mobilize sooner. An example of this might be treating a clavicle or humeral shaft fracture with open reduction and internal fixation so that the patient may use their upper extremities to mobilize with use of a walker. If patients are made non–weight-bearing after surgical fixation of an injury or are intubated and sedated in the intensive care unit, surgeons will still strongly recommend passive range of motion of involved joints to increase mobility and prevent stiffness. Early joint range of motion has been shown to be beneficial for joint health, as it promotes nutrition of the articular cartilage through movement of synovial fluid and has become a basic tenet of fracture care to decrease the morbidity associated with MSK injuries.

SUMMARY

In the setting of the multiply injured patient, preservation of a patient's life takes precedence over preservation of a limb. However, injuries to the axial and appendicular skeleton may be life-threatening in rare circumstances (e.g., hemorrhage or vascular injury from pelvic or long bone fractures) and must be promptly recognized and managed appropriately. MSK injuries represent a major cause of posttraumatic morbidity, as demonstrated by increased healthcare costs, lost workdays, physical disability, emotional distress, and diminished quality of life. Accordingly, it is essential that a thorough, comprehensive MSK examination be performed on every trauma patient upon presentation to identify life- or limb-threatening injuries and decrease the risk of missed or delayed diagnoses. This includes ordering and review of all appropriate imaging studies, laboratory tests, and placement of an orthopedic surgery consultation in timely fashion. Ideally, patients should not be transported from the trauma room, unless for emergent lifesaving interventions, until the orthopedic team has evaluated the patient, appropriately stabilized all injured extremities, and provided recommendations on any potentially emergent conditions. Most importantly, providing appropriate treatment of MSK injuries is truly a multidisciplinary endeavor. Only through collegial and efficient collaboration between all treating services—general surgery, vascular surgery, neurosurgery, spine surgery, plastic surgery, internal medicine, and physical therapy—are we able to ensure the best possible outcome for our patients.

SELECTED REFERENCES

de Ridder VA, Whiting PS, Balogh ZJ, Mir HR, Schultz BJ, Routt MC. Pelvic ring injuries: recent advances in diagnosis and treatment. *OTA Int.* 2023;6(suppl 3):e261.

> Pelvic ring injuries are common after high-energy injury mechanisms and are associated with higher mortality secondary to acute life-threatening hemorrhage leading to shock and metabolic derangements. Implementation of organized institutional protocols for the acute management of these injuries has been shown to decrease mortality and improve outcomes. Early management should be focused on hemorrhage control and resuscitative measures.

Garner MR, Sethuraman SA, Schade MA, Boateng H. Antibiotic prophylaxis in open fractures: evidence, evolving issues, and recommendations. *J Am Acad Orthop Surg.* 2020;28(8):309-315.

> Open fractures are commonly associated with high-energy trauma and have an increased risk of infection secondary to soft tissue damage and contamination. Early administration of appropriate antibiotic prophylaxis is one of the most important treatment interventions that can be initially performed and has been shown to drastically reduce the risk of infection and improve outcomes.

Major Extremity Trauma Research Consortium (METRC), O'Toole RV, Stein DM, et al. Aspirin or low-molecular-weight heparin for thromboprophylaxis after a fracture. *N Engl J Med.* 2023;388(3):203-213.

> Venous thromboembolism (VTE) is a potentially fatal complication after orthopedic trauma. Prophylaxis (chemical or mechanical) reduces the risk of deep vein thrombosis (DVT) by around 50%. Previous guidelines recommend use of low-molecular-weight heparin (LMWH) in cases of orthopedic trauma patients. In this study, aspirin was demonstrated to be noninferior to LMWH in preventing all-cause mortality after orthopedic trauma, and there were similar rates of pulmonary embolism and deep venous thrombosis.

Portney DA, Baker HP, Selkridge I, El Dafrawy MH, Strelzow JA. Firearm-related injuries – wound management, stabilization, and associated injuries: a critical analysis review. *JBJS Rev.* 2023;11(1):e22.00153.

As firearm-related violence and injuries begin to rise in the United States, there continues to be minimal high-level evidence to guide treatment in patients with these injuries. Assessment of commonly associated injuries, such as neurologic and vascular, is an important part of their initial evaluation. These injuries present unique challenges in treatment and are associated with high rates of complications and morbidity.

Vallier HA, Moore TA, Como JJ, et al. Teamwork in trauma: system adjustment to a protocol for the management of multiply injured patients. *J Orthop Trauma.* 2015;29(11):e446-e450.

Early resuscitation of multiply injured patients requires a comprehensive and multidisciplinary team approach. As the trend continues to move more toward early appropriate care in these patients, it is important to develop institutional protocols to determine the adequacy of resuscitation when determining timing of definitive fixation.

The full reference list appears on Elsevier eBooks+.

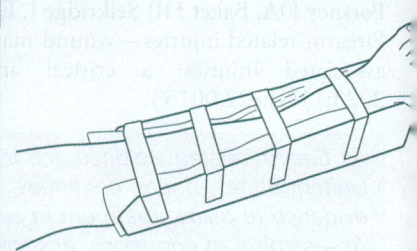

41 | CHAPTER

Emergency Care of Neurologic Injuries

*Amelia W. Maiga, Rachel Hooper, Paul Cederna, Hani Chanbour,
Iyan Younus, Soren Jonzzon, Scott L. Zuckerman, and Mayur B. Patel*

TRAUMATIC BRAIN INJURY

Introduction

The goal of this section on traumatic brain injury (TBI) is not to give a comprehensive review of TBI epidemiology, basic science research, and clinical trials, but rather to provide surgeons with a practical approach to the initial management of traumatic injuries of the brain. At most US hospitals, trauma surgeons are the primary providers responsible for hospitalized TBI patients. General surgery residency has historically involved extensive exposure to the initial evaluation, stabilization, and intensive care management of trauma patients, a sizable percentage of whom are hospitalized with and affected by TBI.

Evidence-based guidelines form the basis of many institutional protocols for physicians caring for brain-injured patients. The following section on the management of TBI is based in large part on these guidelines. As with all practice guidelines, they can and need to be modified as dictated by the experience of the treating physician and in accordance with the needs of the patient and practice setting. The protocols laid out in the Advanced Trauma Life Support (ATLS) guidelines as well as the Best Practice Guidelines in the Management of TBI, both published by the American College of Surgeons (ACS), are invaluable practical resources,[1] as is the Brain Trauma Foundation Guidelines for the Management of TBI.[2] Nevertheless, data from high-quality clinical trials on the acute management of TBI are sparse, and thus, the following represents the best available evidence, including expert consensus in some cases.

Epidemiology

Worldwide, 69 million people experience a TBI annually, with higher incidences and fatality rates in low- and middle-income countries than in high-income countries. The majority of TBIs are mild, including concussions, but it is difficult to differentiate mild TBI from moderate or severe TBI in the prehospital setting.[3] Severe TBI is a leading cause of morbidity and mortality in the United States, and there are about 3 million TBI-related emergency department (ED) visits, hospitalizations, and deaths annually. More than 5 million people are known to be living in the United States with the unmeasured long-term functional, cognitive, and psychological effects of TBI, with annual direct and indirect costs approaching $80 billion. The 2022 National Academies of Sciences, Engineering, and Medicine report on TBI highlighted the long-term consequences of TBI on individuals, families, communities, and society at large.[4] Even after a "mild" TBI, more than 50% of patients report persistent symptoms and functional impairment a year after injury.

Classically, the epidemiology of TBI has been described using patient characteristics (e.g., age, sex), injury characteristics (blunt vs. penetrating), and injury severity (mild, moderate, and severe). TBI may occur in isolation or, perhaps 50% of the time, in combination with other traumatic injuries (i.e., in the polytrauma patient). The most common mechanisms of injury leading to TBI are motor vehicle collisions (MVCs) and falls, with MVCs predominating in low- and middle-income countries. Penetrating TBI constitutes a fraction of cases and ranges from mild to moderate to catastrophic depending on the trajectory of the primary ballistic injury. TBI and criminal offenses are bidirectionally linked, with a high prevalence of self-reported history of TBI in the incarcerated population. TBI overlaps with intimate partner violence and has disproportionately worse outcomes than do other forms of intimate partner violence.

TBI injury severity is described using the Glasgow Coma Scale (GCS), with subscores for eye opening, verbal response, and motor response summing to a range of 3 to 15 points. Mild TBI corresponds to GCS 13 to 15, moderate TBI to GCS 9 to 12, and severe TBI to GCS 3 to 8. The term *traumatic brain injury* actually encompasses a heterogenous group of diseases with distinct means of primary prevention, targets for treatment, and trajectories of recovery. There is also a growing awareness of the need to better classify TBI beyond mild, moderate, and severe, incorporating neuroimaging details, TBI-specific biomarkers (e.g., GFAP and UCH-L1), and disease modifiers including social determinants of health.

Pathophysiology

A TBI occurs when a direct or indirect force to the brain disrupts normal brain function. This force may be blunt or penetrating. The primary brain injury describes the injury at the time of impact and includes (1) fractures, (2) intracranial hemorrhage, and (3) diffuse axonal injury (DAI), which can each occur in isolation or in any combination. Secondary brain injury describes subsequent injury to the brain tissue caused by cerebral hypoperfusion and ischemia, hypoxia, increased intracranial pressure (ICP), metabolic dysregulation, and temperature instability, among other factors.

Primary Brain Injury: Fractures

Fractures of the skull, including the cranial vault and the skull base, occur when a direct blunt or penetrating force is applied to the bone at the moment of impact. Fractures can be classified as open versus closed (based on violation of the overlying skin and soft tissue), depressed versus nondepressed, and linear versus comminuted (Fig. 41.1A). Skull base fractures should always prompt an assessment for associated cranial nerve injuries, cerebrovascular injuries, and even cerebrospinal fluid (CSF) fistulas because of the close anatomic relationships. Although skull fractures can occur in isolation, they often occur together with intracranial hemorrhage. This is because disruption of the bony structure is frequently associated with disruption of the underlying meningeal arteries and/or dural venous sinuses.

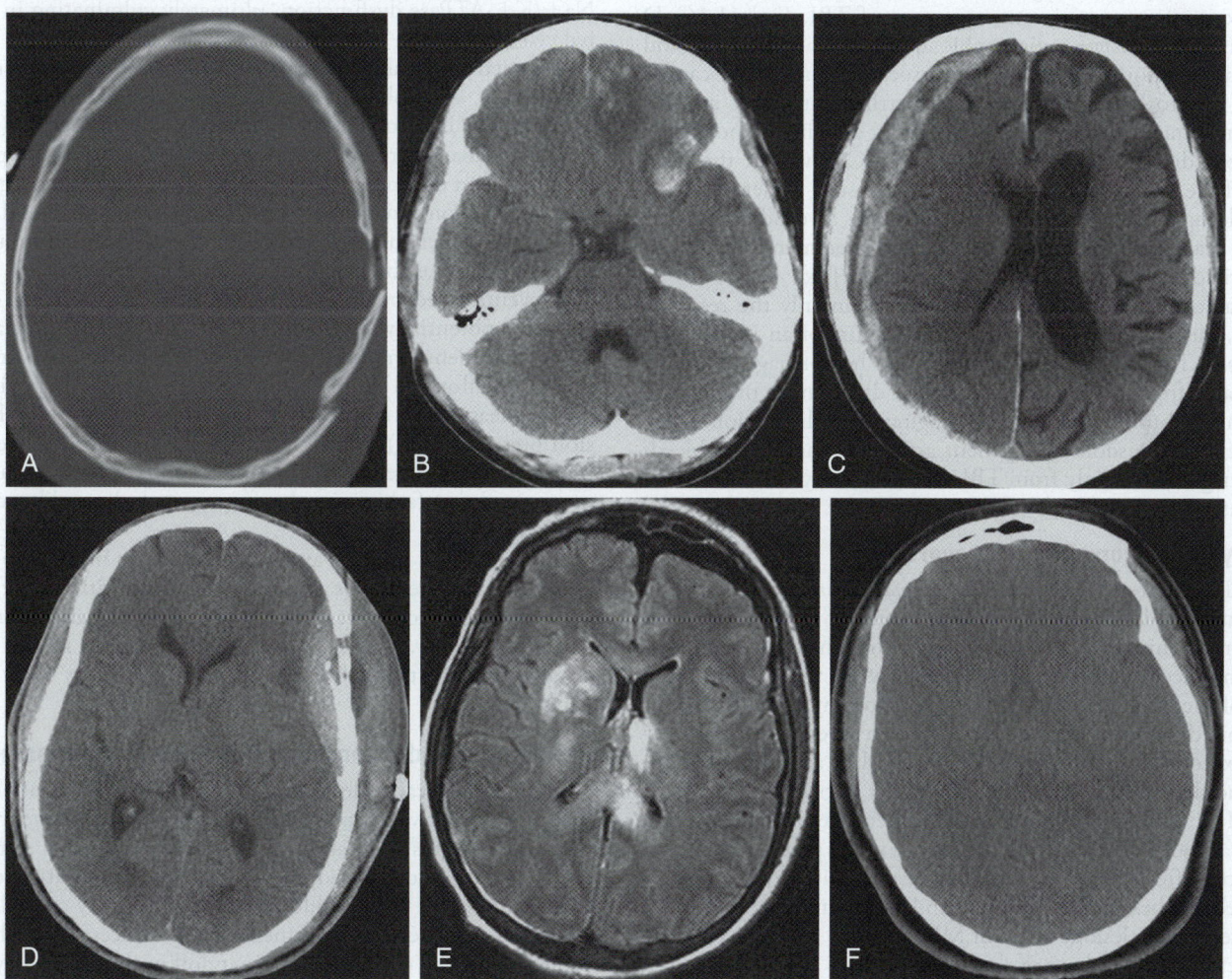

FIGURE 41.1 Typical radiographic findings in traumatic brain injury. All images are computed tomography (CT) except for (E), which is magnetic resonance imaging (MRI). (A) Comminuted, depressed skull fracture. (B) Intraparenchymal frontal lobe contusions. (C) Subdural hematoma with midline shift caused by mass effect. (D) Epidural hematoma with associated skull fracture and midline shift caused by mass effect. (E) Diffuse axonal injury on MRI. (F) Intracranial hypertension with effacement of the sulci and gray-white matter differentiation.

Primary Brain Injury: Intracranial Hemorrhage

Any bleeding within the skull is termed *intracranial hemorrhage*. Bleeding can occur in the spaces between the dura and skull (*epidural hemorrhage*, typically caused by a meningeal artery tear), between the dura and the arachnoid (*subdural hemorrhage*, caused by injury to the bridging veins between the brain and the dural venous sinuses), into the spinal fluid spaces surrounding the blood vessels feeding the cerebral cortex (*subarachnoid hemorrhage*), or into the brain parenchyma itself (*intraparenchymal or intracerebral hemorrhage*, sometimes caused by a "coup-contrecoup" mechanism). Small intraparenchymal bleeds may also be referred to as *contusions* or *bruises* to the brain parenchyma (see Fig. 41.1B). Although initially underwhelming on imaging and physical examination, these contusions can blossom and become life threatening within hours to days, earning them the label "talk and die." Blood within the cerebral ventricular system (*intraventricular hemorrhage*) may also be seen, although rarely in isolation because the blood must originate from somewhere.

Epidural and subdural hemorrhages occupy the space outside of the brain and are thus mostly likely to (1) place external pressure on the brain and put patients at risk for herniation and (2) be amenable to urgent surgical decompression, as described in the later sections on operative management of TBI. Fig. 41.1C–D highlight the different radiographic appearances of epidural and subdural hematomas as well as the associated mass effect caused by the Monro-Kelli doctrine. This doctrine states that any increase in intracranial blood (i.e., caused by ongoing hemorrhage) leads to a displacement of the brain and CSF within the fixed space of the skull. This process ultimately results in herniation as the building pressure caused by bleeding seeks an exodus by pushing the brain downward through the skull's foramen magnum or across rigid membranes like the tentorium or falx.

Subarachnoid hemorrhages are most commonly the result of trauma, but they may also occur after rupture of an intracranial aneurysm. The etiology of a subarachnoid hemorrhage is usually discernable from the patient history and distribution of bleeding on computed tomography (CT) imaging. This distinction is important to make soon after patient arrival, as aneurysmal bleeds are managed differently from TBI, but both carry risk of cerebral vasospasm.

Primary Brain Injury: Diffuse Axonal Injury

DAI, also referred to as *traumatic axonal injury* or *shear injury*, represents a radiographically insidious form of TBI that is often not seen on initial CT imaging. DAI is thought to be caused by rotational acceleration-deceleration injury to the white matter tracts of the brain, resulting in primary axotomy or functional or anatomic disruption of these pathways. In severe cases, this primary axotomy is then followed by a secondary axotomy of apoptosis and degeneration over the subsequent 6 to 12 hours.

DAI is usually diagnosed on magnetic resonance imaging (MRI) as multifocal hyperintense lesions at the gray-white matter interfaces, often graded in increasing severity with involvement of the cerebral lobes, corpus callosum, and brainstem (see Fig. 41.1E). However, visible lesions on both MRI and CT are believed to be just the tip of the iceberg of the actual primary injury. As such, it is virtually impossible to understand the true incidence and prevalence of DAI with current clinical neuroimaging.

DAI can occur with or without focal or structural TBI (i.e., intracranial hemorrhage and fractures). DAI ranges from mild TBI, akin to a concussion, to severe TBI. Mild cases of DAI may present with axonal stretching and transient neuronal dysfunction rather than complete disruption. DAI should be on the differential diagnosis of patients who fail to improve after surgical evacuation of a subdural or epidural hematoma, or in patients who remain unconscious despite the absence of intracranial hemorrhage on CT imaging, but the utility of pursuing current clinical MRI diagnostics is uncertain given its weak correlation with outcomes.

Secondary Brain Injury

Secondary brain injury refers to a cascade of events that results in additional, cumulative injury to the brain after the initial direct injury. At least half of all patients with hospitalized TBI have polytrauma or other associated traumatic injuries, which may place them at particular risk of secondary brain injury, while other competing life-threatening injuries require management. Cerebral hypoxia, or decreased oxygen delivery to the brain, is thought to be a key driver of secondary brain injury. Severe TBI can disrupt the normal physiology of cerebral blood vessel autoregulation. Adding systemic hypotension to this impaired autoregulation results in decreased cerebral blood flow and thus relative cerebral ischemia. This vicious cycle then is further exacerbated by systemic hypoxia, intracranial hypertension, and cerebral inflammation, leading to a cascade of excitotoxicity, calcium influx, and $Na+/K+$-ATPase dysfunction, ultimately culminating in neuronal cell dysfunction and neuronal cell death.

Elevated ICP, also known as *intracranial hypertension* (see Fig. 41.1F), is a global measure that may reflect multiple mechanisms at play in secondary brain injury, including edema (cellular or extracellular), cerebral venous outflow obstruction, hyperemia (engorgement of cerebral vessels caused by a loss of autoregulation and vasodilation), mass effect (expanding hematoma), and disturbances in CSF circulation. However, secondary brain injury may occur even in the absence of intracranial hypertension.

Preventing secondary brain injury is thought to be the cornerstone of potentially reversing the morbidity and mortality of TBI. At present, the management of secondary brain injury is limited to efforts to simply avoid hypotension and hypoxia while taking measures to control ICP and to maintain cerebral perfusion pressure (CPP). Multiple preclinical neuroprotective therapies are in the pipeline to prevent secondary brain injury in a more proactive fashion in the future, including glibenclamide and xenon gas.[5]

In some cases, primary and secondary brain injury also lead to persistent and irreversible neurologic deficits, with loss of neurologic function, cognitive decline, psychological alterations, and chronic disability. At least 3% of dementia cases in the general population are attributable to TBI, although this is likely an underestimate.[3]

Prehospital and Emergency Department Management

Severe TBI may cause death within the first few hours after injury as a result of airway compromise or herniation. Secondary brain injury also begins soon after injury in the prehospital setting. As such, prompt and focused prehospital care is essential to avoid hypoxia, preserve cerebral blood flow, and identify candidates for surgical decompression. Treatment begins on scene by prehospital professionals and continues until handoff in the emergency room. At present, prehospital identification of patients with possible TBI relies on physical examination, including evidence of obvious injury to the head or neck and determination of the GCS, described later, in combination with the severity of the known mechanism of injury.

Patients with suspected moderate to severe TBI (GCS ≤13) should be transported directly from the scene to the highest-level trauma center available in a defined trauma system for prompt CT neuroimaging and neurosurgical care.[1] In most cases, any patient with a suspected TBI of any type, particularly in combination with polytrauma, should be transported directly to the nearest trauma center rather than stabilized at a nontrauma center first. Transfer of patients from one hospital to a higher level of care should follow ATLS guidelines, and the transferring center should ensure a secure airway, adequate ventilation, and circulation before transfer. Vigilance and attention to detail as well as communication between the transferring and accepting teams are key to the successful management of these patients.

Avoidance of Hypoxia, Hypotension, and Hyperventilation

It is critical that emergency medical services (EMS) and other prehospital professionals anticipate, prevent, and avoid hypoxia (<90% saturation), hypotension (<100 mm Hg systolic blood pressure [SBP]), and hyperventilation (end-tidal CO_2 [$ETCO_2$] less than 35) in any patient with suspected TBI, with frequent prehospital monitoring (at least every 5 minutes, or continuously where available).[2] For example, the Excellence in Prehospital Injury Care Study implemented prevention against these three prehospital pitfalls, thus improving TBI outcomes across more than 130 EMS systems and agencies throughout the state of Arizona.[6] Ventilation of patients with altered levels of consciousness should aim for an $ETCO_2$ of 35 to 45 mm Hg. Hypothermia and hyperthermia should also be avoided.

Airway, Breathing, and Circulation

As with all trauma patients, airway, breathing, and circulation (ABC) should be the initial focus of prehospital care. Attention should be first directed to securing a patent airway, establishing adequate ventilation and oxygenation, and maintaining adequate circulation—key steps to avoid hypotension and hypoxia and thereby minimize secondary brain injury. Because of this critical need to avoid hypoxia, all patients with suspected TBI should be placed on oxygen via nasal cannula or face mask and monitored for hypoxemia (oxygen saturation <90%), which should be corrected promptly. In patients with suspected severe TBI and/or the inability to maintain an adequate airway, or if hypoxemia is not promptly corrected by supplemental oxygen and bag-valve-mask ventilation in conjunction with an oropharyngeal airway, a definitive advanced airway (e.g., endotracheal tube) should be established by a trained prehospital professional.

With regard to circulation in the prehospital setting, hypotensive patients with suspected TBI should be treated with isotonic fluids and/or blood products if available in an effort to treat and/or limit hypotension to the shortest duration possible. There is weak evidence for the use of hypertonic fluids in the prehospital setting. Table 41.1 shows the goals of treatment in the prehospital setting and beyond, as defined by the Brain Trauma Foundation and ACS Trauma Quality Improvement Program (TQIP) Best Practice Guidelines for TBI.

Neurologic Assessment With the Glasgow Coma Scale

Originally developed in 1974, the GCS is the most widely used scale to quickly assess the level of consciousness after a possible TBI. The GCS includes assessment of eye opening (up to 4 points), motor response (up to 5 points), and verbal response (up to 6 points), for a total of 3 to 15 points (Table 41.2). The GCS is a repetitive, reproducible scale that allows for ongoing neurologic

TABLE 41.1 Goals of Treatment for Traumatic Brain Injury		
PARAMETER	PREHOSPITAL AND ED[a]	INTENSIVE CARE UNIT[b]
Oxygenation (pulse oximetry)	≥90%	≥94%
Oxygenation (PaO_2)		80–100 mm Hg
Circulation (systolic blood pressure)	100–150 mm Hg	≥100 mm Hg
Ventilation (breaths per minute)	10	
Ventilation ($ETCO_2$)	35–40 mm Hg[c]	35–45 mm Hg
Ventilation ($PaCO_2$)		7.35–7.45
Acid-base status (pH)		
Intracranial pressure (ICP)		<22 mm Hg
Cerebral oxygenation ($PbtO_2$)		≥15 mm Hg
Cerebral perfusion pressure (CPP)		60–70 mm Hg[d]
Temperature	36.0°C–37.0°C	36.0°C–37.9°C
Glucose		100–180 mg/dL
Serum sodium		135–145 mEq/L[e]
Serum osmolality		300–320 mOsm
Hematologic (INR)		≤1.4
Hematologic (platelets)		≥75 × 10³/mm³
Hematologic (hemoglobin)		≥7 g/dL

[a]Based on Brain Trauma Foundation guidelines.
[b]Based on American College of Surgeons Trauma Quality Improvement Program Best Practice Guidelines for Traumatic Brain Injury.
[c]Except in cases of imminent herniation, for which a goal of 30 to 35 mm Hg is acceptable.
[d]Depending on status of cerebral autoregulation.
[e]Except when patients are undergoing tier 2 hyperosmolar therapy for intracranial hypertension.
ED, Emergency department; ETCO₂, end-tidal carbon dioxide; INR, international normalized ratio; PaCO₂, partial pressure of carbon dioxide; PbtO₂, brain tissue oxygen tension; PaO₂, partial pressure of oxygen.

assessments performed by a variety of healthcare professionals both in the prehospital and hospital environment. Of the three components, the motor score carries the most prognostic weight. Although assessment of the GCS is critical to the initial management of a patient with suspected TBI, it should only be done after stabilization of the ABC in a trauma patient. Provided that patient stability allows, the GCS should be measured before sedative or paralytic medications are administered.

The GCS score should be determined at least every 30 minutes in the prehospital setting and whenever there is an apparent change in mental status to identify improvement or deterioration over time. Often, the prehospital GCS will vary from the GCS determined on arrival to the ED or the postresuscitation GCS. An initial depressed GCS may reflect true TBI severity, but it may also reflect hemorrhagic shock with poor perfusion to the brain or the impact of hypoglycemia, seizure activity, sedatives, or other ingestions. Once one or more of these reversible conditions are addressed, the GCS may improve. Alternatively, the GCS may decrease because of an interval worsening of the actual brain injury or physiologic state. Repeat assessments are critical to identify and treat underlying TBI and other reversible causes of morbidity and mortality in the trauma population. In addition to GCS, other neurologic assessment scales in some use in the prehospital settings include the Simplified Motor Score (SMS) and the Simplified Verbal Score (SVS).

TABLE 41.2 Neurologic Assessment Using the Glasgow Coma Scale (GCS)

EYE-OPENING RESPONSE		VERBAL RESPONSE		MOTOR RESPONSE	
EYE SCORE	RESPONSE	VERBAL SCORE	RESPONSE	MOTOR SCORE	RESPONSE
4	Spontaneous	5	Oriented	6	Obeys commands
3	To speech	4	Confused	5	Localizes to painful stimulus
2	To pain	3	Inappropriate responses	4	Withdraws to painful stimulus
1	No response	2	Incomprehensive responses	3	Flexion to painful stimulus
		1	No response	2	Extension to painful stimulus
				1	No response

Summed GCS scores range from 3 to 15, with GCS 3 to 8 corresponding to severe traumatic brain injury (TBI), 9 to 12 to moderate TBI, and 13 to 15 to mild TBI. Intubated patients receive a "T" in place of the verbal response, so the best possible score for an intubated patient is GCS 11T.

Pupil Examination

The prehospital evaluation of a patient with suspected TBI should also include a thorough assessment of pupil size, symmetry, and reactivity. The pupil examination allows an understanding of the function of many different neuroanatomic pathways and, as such, adds value to the acute management and long-term prognosis of TBI. When present in combination with a depressed GCS, abnormalities of pupillary response or asymmetry may portend impending neurologic deterioration or poor long-term neurologic outcomes. The pupil examination should be done at the same time as the GCS assessment, again once the patient has been stabilized from an ABC standpoint.

The bilateral pupillary examination consists of evaluation of pupil size, symmetry, and reactivity to light. The normal light reflex requires a functioning lens, retina, optic nerve, brainstem, and oculomotor nerve. The consensual pupil response to light assesses the function of the contralateral oculomotor nerve. Infrared pupillometry may allow for more consistent pupil assessment evaluation across a range of prehospital and hospital settings but has not yet been implemented widely. An abnormal pupillary examination can be an early warning sign in the setting of TBI. Absence or asymmetry of these reflexes may indicate herniation or brainstem ischemia. New pupillary changes or anisocoria (unequal pupils with >1 mm of difference) may indicate an increase in ICP that would require reimaging and/or intervention. For example, ongoing bleeding from an epidural or subdural hematoma may be causing impending transtentorial herniation, which may be reversible with emergent surgical evacuation. A unilateral fixed and dilated pupil may represent herniation, whereas bilateral fixed and dilated pupils may reflect global anoxia and dismal prognosis.

Pupillary abnormalities in a patient with a normal GCS should also be noted and communicated to the ED team upon handoff, but these are less associated with the diagnosis and severity of TBI. In the setting of traumatic globe rupture or other ophthalmologic trauma, the pupillary examination may be unreliable. Metabolic, pharmacologic, or toxic etiologies can also cause pupillary abnormalities, as can prior ophthalmologic procedures or genetic conditions. Nevertheless, pupillary abnormalities should be presumed to indicate a primary brain injury until proven otherwise.

Prehospital Management of Intracranial Pressure

As mentioned previously, hyperventilation should be avoided in patients with suspected TBI, and in those with advanced airway monitoring, ventilation should target an ETCO$_2$ of 35 to 45 mm Hg. The exception is in patients with a prehospital GCS <9 and signs of imminent herniation, including Cushing triad

(hypertension, bradycardia, irregular breathing pattern), posturing or lateralizing findings, and unilateral or bilateral fixed, dilated pupils. In such cases, hyperventilation should temporarily target an ETCO$_2$ of 30 to 35 mm Hg. Hyperosmolar therapy (e.g., mannitol and hypertonic saline) should not be administered for the prophylactic treatment of suspected elevated ICP in the prehospital setting and has not shown benefit in large randomized clinical trials. At present, prehospital administration of tranexamic acid (TXA) is used empirically in some practice settings for clot stabilization in patients with suspected intracranial hemorrhage or elevated ICP.

Emergency Department Management

The ED management of patients with suspected TBI follows the same principles as in the prehospital setting. First, ABC should be addressed and stabilized. Next, a thorough neurologic assessment should be done, including evaluation of the GCS and pupils. Prompt neuroimaging is necessary to guide further management, including surgical decompression. While still in the ED, candidates should be identified by history for expeditious reversal of coagulopathy and/or impaired platelet function with the appropriate agents, typically prothrombin complex concentrate for anticoagulants and desmopressin for nonaspirin antiplatelet agents.

Neuroimaging

A noncontrast head CT scan is used to evaluate the presence or absence of fracture, intracranial hemorrhage, midline shift, and appearance of the basal and perimesencephalic cisterns (see Fig. 41.1). At the same time, routine scanning of the cervical spine should also be performed to rule out acute fractures or traumatic dislocations. If life-threatening injuries in the polytrauma patient mandate immediate operative exploration for hemorrhage control, CT scanning should be delayed until after patient stabilization. Should there be concern for undiagnosed intracranial injury and/or extended intraoperative time, intraoperatively placed ICP monitors can be a useful adjunct. In some clinical scenarios, if a polytrauma patient has an impaired GCS and a suspected unilateral intracranial mass lesion, as evidenced by a unilateral fixed and dilated pupil, an exploratory burr hole may be performed in the operating room concurrently with the laparotomy or thoracotomy. However, this situation should rarely occur, as CT neuroimaging is best used to guide emergent evacuation of epidural and subdural hematomas.

Operative Management

It is critical to promptly identify patients with TBI who would benefit from surgical evacuation. In general, the types of TBI most amenable to evacuation are intracranial hemorrhage outside the brain (i.e., epidural and subdural hemorrhages, termed *mass lesions*). An epidural hematoma more than 30 mL in size in association with neurologic deficits or radiographic signs of midline shift or effacement of the basal cisterns is commonly accepted as criteria for emergent craniotomy (see Fig. 41.1C–D). A subdural hematoma of at least 1 cm in size or with any midline shift in combination with a decline in neurologic examination should also prompt evacuation. Regardless of examination findings, a large mass lesion should be evacuated before neurologic deterioration develops, if in accordance with a patient's goals of care. Epidural and subdural hematomas are treated similarly with a formal craniotomy centered on the clot, rather than a burr hole. Depending on the degree of brain swelling and specific clinical scenario, the neurosurgeon may elect to leave the bone flap off (termed a *craniectomy*) to allow the brain to heal before coverage. A recent international clinical trial reached equipoise on the question of routine craniectomy versus craniotomy.[7]

ICP monitors are often placed at the time of craniotomy, particularly for patients with a preoperative GCS <8. The decision about whether to place an ICP monitor is at the operating surgeon's discretion and involves consideration of preoperative examination findings, the degree of swelling of the brain at the time of the operation, and potential risk for deterioration. Post-craniotomy patients are managed similarly to those with nonoperative TBI (see "Critical Care Management" and Table 41.1).

Decompressive craniectomy for intracranial hypertension in the absence of mass lesions is performed at some institutions as part of tier 3 management of elevated ICP, but this practice is not well supported by the literature.[8] The 2011 randomized controlled DECRA trial (Decompressive Craniectomy in Patients with Severe Traumatic Brain Injury) demonstrated that the successful reduction in ICP brought out by decompressive craniectomy was associated with worse neurologic outcomes at 6 months with similar findings in the 2016 RESCUEicp trial (Randomised Evaluation of Surgery with Craniectomy for Uncontrollable Elevation of Intracranial Pressure).

Critical Care Management

Goal-directed TBI treatment extends care from the prehospital and ED arenas to the intensive care unit (ICU) for patients with a confirmed diagnosis of moderate to severe TBI (see Table 41.1). As before, adequate oxygenation and normocapnia should be maintained. Systolic and mean arterial blood pressure should be tracked closely to avoid hypotension and to optimize CPP. Paroxysmal sympathetic hyperactivity can also occur in patients after severe TBI and is associated with elevated catecholamines resulting in hypertension and other negative effects.[10] Body temperature, glucose levels, and electrolytes should be maintained in the normal range. Hyponatremia should specifically be avoided because of the risk of cerebral edema. Coagulopathy should be reversed when apparent on laboratory testing or a history of taking anticoagulants to limit the expansion of intracranial bleeding.[9] Patients with severe TBI merit frequent monitoring of their serum sodium and osmolality levels, as they are at risk of developing diabetes insipidus or the syndrome of inappropriate antidiuretic hormone (SIADH).

Intracranial Pressure Monitoring and Management

ICP monitoring is indicated for comatose patients (GCS ≤8) with evidence of structural brain injury on CT imaging, or in patients judged to be at high risk for progression of their primary brain injury (e.g., because of large contusions or coagulopathy).

ICP monitoring may also be considered in patients with moderate TBI undergoing urgent extracranial surgery. The placement of an ICP monitor allows for continuous or intermittent measurement of CPP, defined as the mean arterial pressure (MAP) minus the ICP [CPP = MAP – ICP]. The CPP should be maintained at 60 to 70 mm Hg to optimize cerebral blood flow and to minimize secondary brain injury. ICP should be kept below 20 to 25 mm Hg, but importantly, monitoring should not replace careful, repeated neurologic assessments and prompt repeat CT imaging in cases of neurologic deterioration.

ICP monitoring can be accomplished with either an external ventricular drain (EVD) or an intraparenchymal monitor. Either type can be placed in the operating room or ICU. The advantage of an EVD over an intraparenchymal bolt is the ability to drain CSF in order to lower ICP. Monitors placed in the subdural or epidural place are also available, but these tend to be less accurate and are thus less frequently used. When available, ICP monitoring in the appropriate patient population appears to be associated with a more intensive therapeutic approach and lower short-term mortality.[10] In underresourced settings, reasonably good outcomes from severe TBI can still be obtained using institutional protocols that include empiric treatment of elevated ICP, repeat imaging, and meticulous clinical examinations.

Treatment of elevated ICP or intracranial hypertension (persistent elevation above 22 mm Hg) follows the three-tiered approach recommended by the ACS TQIP guidelines.[1] Other groups, including the Seattle International Severe Traumatic Brain Injury Consensus Conference (SIBICC), recommend a slightly different three-tiered algorithm.[11] Serial CT scans are critical throughout this treatment algorithm, and their use should be tailored to the individual clinical scenario. Tier 1 involves elevating the head of the bed to 30 degrees while keeping the head in a neutral position to use gravity to improve cerebral venous outflow, taking care to ensure that cervical spine immobilization devices do not obstruct jugular venous flow. Tier 1 also involves the use of short-acting sedation agents (e.g., propofol, fentanyl) in intubated patients to allow for frequent neurologic reassessments off sedation. When available, intermittent drainage of CSF with an EVD or ventriculostomy also decreases ICP and is considered part of tier 1 management.

If the ICP remains persistently elevated above 22 mm Hg, tier 2 management includes the use of hyperosmolar therapy with either mannitol or hypertonic saline. Serum sodium and osmolality should be monitored every 6 hours while patients are receiving hyperosmolar therapy, and treatment should be held if levels reach 160 mEq/L or 320 mOsm/L, respectively. Cerebral autoregulation should be assessed by a trained intensivist as described in the recent SIBICC guidelines.[11] Neuromuscular paralysis should be employed with a single test dose, followed by continuous infusion if the test dose is successful in reducing ICP (the infusion is considered tier 3 treatment). Hyperventilation to a $PaCO_2$ of 30 to 35 mm Hg may be considered, although brain hypoxia may occur as a side effect because of reduced cerebral blood flow. At some centers, advanced neuromonitoring, including measurement of jugular venous oxygen saturation and brain tissue oxygenation, appears to help inform management of intracranial hypertension.[9] Multiple randomized controlled trials are currently underway to assess the added benefit of brain tissue oxygenation in the management of these patients, which remains an area of active debate.

Tier 3 management of intracranial hypertension includes consideration for decompressive bilateral craniectomy (with the reservations described earlier), continuous neuromuscular blockage (if the test dose in tier 2 was successful), or barbiturate coma with continuous electroencephalogram (EEG) monitoring for titration to burst suppression. Institutional protocols may guide selection of tier 3 approaches, and high-quality data are limited. Hypothermia is not recommended for salvage treatment for intracranial hypertension.[8] In a patient who is deeply sedated with or without paralysis, providers rely on the pupillary examination and ICP measurements to determine any change in intracranial dynamics. A persistently elevated ICP and/or a new blown pupil necessitates emergent CT neuroimaging.

Other Considerations for Critical Care Management

Patients with severe TBI are known to have increased energy or caloric requirements. As such, nutritional support is critical and should begin as soon as possible after injury, ideally within 24 to 48 hours, with full nutrition by 7 days after injury at the latest. Enteral nutrition is preferred. The hypermetabolic and hypercatabolic state of TBI lasts from 1 week to several months after the injury. Steroids have no benefit in the management of TBI and should not be used. Other therapies that should be avoided in the management of TBI are listed in Table 41.3.

Prophylactic use of anticonvulsant drugs should be given to prevent early posttraumatic seizures within the first week. Once there is no evidence of ongoing intracranial hemorrhage, pharmacologic prophylaxis for venous thromboembolism (VTE) should be started as soon as 24 to 48 hours after injury in TBI patients, because of the high rates of VTE in this population. Adrenergic blockage with β-blockers is commonly used in patients with severe TBI who are deemed at risk of paroxysmal sympathetic hyperactivity, or "storming," although evidence for benefit is variable. The dopamine agonist amantadine may improve cognitive function after TBI, especially when give within the first week of injury.[12] Early tracheostomy (within the first 5–7 days) should also be considered in patients with TBI requiring mechanical ventilation to reduce risk of ventilator-associated pneumonia and other complications. Other detailed considerations for the critical

care management of patients with severe TBI are beyond the scope of this chapter and have been covered elsewhere.[13]

Prognostication and Long-Term Outcomes

This chapter focuses on the acute management of TBI and will not delve into the chronic phase of recovery and rehabilitation, which often extends for years even after a mild TBI with intracranial hemorrhage. After discharge, TBI recovery is varied and poorly understood, with predictions limited to 6 months. It is unknown at what point TBI recovery plateaus and remains fixed. In some patients, post-TBI neuroplasticity continues for multiple years. The path of recovery after TBI encompasses at least four domains: biologic, psychological, sociologic, and ecologic (including economic).[4] Patients experiencing severe or recurrent TBI may be at higher risk for long-term neurodegenerative conditions, including the development of dementia.[3]

The most commonly used outcome metrics after TBI are mortality and the Glasgow Outcome Scale-Extended (GOSE), which measures disability and functional recovery (Table 41.4). However, GOSE has its limitations, and long-term patient-centered outcomes for TBI are needed.[14] While patients are in the acute phase of recovery, other scales may be used, such as the Rancho de Los Amigos Scale or the Galveston Orientation and Amnesia Test. These scales help assess a patient's short-term progress and are used to identify patients who would benefit from specific brain-related therapies after hospital discharge.

Currently available prognostic models do not adequately predict long-term outcomes for individual patients and should be used with caution when making treatment-limiting decisions. Despite the broad acceptance of TBI prognostic models such as IMPACT and CRASH-TBI in the research arena, they are infrequently used in clinical practice and predict only 35% of the variance in patient outcomes.[3] One exception is the Baylor score for penetrating intracranial gunshot wounds, which does adequately predict mortality and functional outcomes to inform goals-of-care discussions in the acute setting.[15] However, in general, clinical fluctuations during the first 72 hours after injury may help inform prognosis and trajectory, and patients with severe TBI should receive full treatment for *at least* 72 hours unless their goals of care do not align with this trial of full treatment. There is a growing consensus in the field that premature withdrawal of life-sustaining measures (i.e., <72 hours) can lead to a self-fulfilling prophecy of fatalism or inappropriate therapeutic nihilism.[16] A substantial minority of patients with seemingly devastating TBIs can recover to independent functional status.

TABLE 41.3 Treatments Not Recommended in the Management of Severe Traumatic Brain Injury

Mannitol by non-bolus continuous infusion

Scheduled infusion of hyperosmolar therapy (e.g., every 4–6 hours)

Lumbar drainage of cerebrospinal fluid

Furosemide

Routine use of steroids

Routine use of therapeutic hypothermia to temperatures <35°C

High-dose propofol to attempt EEG burst suppression

Hyperventilation to decrease $PaCO_2$, <30 mm Hg

Routinely raising CPP >90 mm Hg

Platelet transfusions in adults on antiplatelet therapy

Antibiotic prophylaxis for external ventricular drain placement

CPP, Cerebral perfusion pressure; *EEG*, electroencephalogram; *$PaCO_2$*, partial pressure of carbon dioxide.

From Hawryluk GWJ, Aguilera S, Buki A, et al. A management algorithm for patients with intracranial pressure monitoring: the Seattle International Severe Traumatic Brain Injury Consensus Conference (SIBICC). *Intensive Care Med.* 2019;45(12):1783-1794; Moore L, Tardif PA, Lauzier F, et al. Low-value clinical practices in adult traumatic brain injury: an umbrella review. *J Neurotrauma.* 2020;37(24):2605-2615.

TABLE 41.4 Glasgow Outcome Scale-Extended (GOSE) Score for Traumatic Brain Injury Outcomes

GOSE SCORE	NEUROLOGIC FUNCTIONAL PERFORMANCE
1	Dead
2	Vegetative state
3	Lower severe disability (completely dependent on others)
4	Upper severe disability (dependent on others for some activities)
5	Lower moderate disability (unable to return to work or participate in social activities)
6	Upper moderate disability (return to work and/or social functions at reduced capacity)
7	Lower good recovery (minor social or mental deficits)
8	Upper good recovery

Ultimately, "no head injury is too severe to despair of, nor too trivial to ignore" (Hippocrates, 400 BCE). Better prognostic modeling in the future may translate to better TBI care, guiding patient and family expectations, goals of care, and best treatment. Prognostic stratification would allow us to understand which TBI subgroups benefit most from therapies in the preclinical pipeline to inform clinical trials that could change practice for TBI care. Multiple TBI therapies have failed in clinical translation because of basic challenges in patient selection and predicting TBI recovery. Until active targeted neuroprotective treatments become available for TBI, providers should adhere to the ATLS principles of ABC, with minimization of secondary brain injury and then prompt neuroimaging to identify mass lesions appropriate for neurosurgical evacuation.

PERIPHERAL NERVE INJURIES

Upper and lower extremity peripheral nerve injuries are extremely common, resulting from traumatic or iatrogenic mechanisms including crush, stretch/traction, laceration, or a combination thereof. An estimated 3% of all patients presenting to a Level 1 trauma center have a peripheral nerve injury to the upper extremity.[17] From an iatrogenic standpoint, several surgical procedures have been associated with peripheral nerve injuries including shoulder (1%–8%), hip (0.17%–7.6%), and knee (0.3%–1.3%) arthroplasties.[18]

Types of Peripheral Nerve Injuries

The two major nerve injury classification systems are Seddon and Sutherland.[17-19] The Seddon classification divides nerve injuries broadly into neuropraxia, axonotmesis, and neurotmesis (Table 41.5). Neuropraxic injuries have intact axons, with a conduction block at the site of the lesion. The associated demyelination affects the speed of nerve transmission; however, the conduction block can be improved with elimination of the insulting agent (i.e., compression). With neuropraxic injuries, there is the potential for spontaneous recovery within 3 months.

Axonotmetic injuries are characterized by damage to the continuity of axons, which can occur with crush and compression/traction injuries. In this nerve injury, the basal lamina remains intact. Lastly, neurotmetic injuries are characterized by complete nerve transection, including the basal lamina; the nerve is markedly damaged and disorganized.[20,21] During axonotmesis and neurotmesis, Wallerian degeneration occurs distal to the site of injury. With axonotmesis and neurotmesis, nerve recovery is seldom possible without surgical intervention because there is loss of axonal continuity.[17,19]

With increased clinical and basic science research, it became clear that the Seddon classification alone does not comprehensively capture the complexity and spectrum of nerve injuries. To address this, the Sutherland classification was created; this system further subdivides the Seddon classification based on the layers of the nerve that are damaged. Although the Sutherland classification is more specific, it is often difficult to determine the level of injury based on clinical examination alone. Neuropraxia is designated as a first-degree injury, and neurotmesis is a fifth-degree injury and includes damage to all structures within the nerve, including the epineurium. Axonotmesis includes second-, third-, and fourth-degree injuries with variable damage to the internal architecture of the nerve while maintaining the outer epineurium. A sixth-degree Sutherland injury refers to a mixed injury comprising conduction block and axonal loss/discontinuity.[21]

Clinical Evaluation of Patients With Nerve Injury

A careful history taking and physical examination are of paramount importance, with a focus on the mechanism and timing of the injury relative to presentation. Nerve injuries should be suspected among patients with hyperesthesia, sensory, or motor deficits attributable to a specific nerve or common procedure and/or laceration or wound directly in the path of a specific nerve. For upper extremity nerve injuries, the patient's handedness and occupation are important aspects of the history. Open wounds should be carefully cleaned and inspected for injured structures. Sensation can be assessed using a two-point discriminator, Semmes-Weinstein monofilaments, or the subjective "tens" assessment (a patient compares sensation in the region of injury to the contralateral uninjured area with a numerical value out of 10).[19,22] When percussion over the area of nerve injury produces electric shocks, or "pins and needles," or an otherwise painful stimulus in the distribution of the nerve, this is referred to as a *Tinel sign*. A Tinel sign is indicative of disrupted axons and can be used to make the diagnosis of a nerve injury as well as follow progression of nerve healing after repair.

Mechanism of the Injury

It is important to understand the time that has occurred between injury and presentation as well as associated structures that have been injured. The condition of the wound associated with a nerve injury is critical because it informs the type of operative wound management as well as the timing of definitive nerve repair. Wounds created by sharp injury (knife/scalpel) have minimal contamination and devitalized tissue; the area of tissue damage is easily defined and well delineated. Dirty wounds include open fractures or those resulting from gunshot injuries; these injuries are devastating with a large zone of injury. Penetrating, blast, crush, and stretch injuries can be associated with vascular, soft tissue, or bone injuries, which can affect the timing and outcome of nerve repair. Vascular and bony injuries should be repaired, and the extremity should be stabilized before nerve repair. In wounds with significant tissue damage, the wound or nerve injury may not be suitable for acute repair/reconstruction, and the zone of nerve injury may not be clearly delineated. For these reasons, it may not be appropriate to perform an immediate nerve repair, but instead, tag the nerve ends so that they can be easily identified later for a delayed repair.

TABLE 41.5 Seddon Classification of Nerve Injuries

Seddon and Sunderland Classification System of Peripheral Nerve Injury (Including Mackinnon and Dellon Modification)

SEDDON	SUNDERLAND	
Neuropraxia	Type 1	Focal demyelination. Axon remains intact.
Axonotmesis	Type 2	Axonal continuity lost. Endoneurium, perineurium, and epineurium remain intact.
	Type 3	Axonal continuity lost. Endoneurium disrupted. Perineurium and epineurium remain intact.
	Type 4	Axonal continuity lost. Endoneurium and perineurium disrupted. Epineurium remains intact.
Neurotmesis	Type 5	Complete disruption of nerve structures.
	Type 6	Mixed injury.

From Lin JS, Jain SA. Challenges in nerve repair and reconstruction. *Hand Clin.* 2023;39:403-415.

Nerve Conduction/Electrodiagnostic Studies

Nerve conduction studies (NCSs) provide information on the health of the axons and whether there is demyelination or continuity. Localization of nerve injuries is possible by detecting focal slowing or a conduction block on NCS. After nerve transection, conduction may be detectable for up to 72 hours until Wallerian degeneration occurs (the nerve end distal to the injury will not elicit a response upon stimulation).[21] Electromyography (EMG) measures muscle response and innervation through the detection of motor unit potentials and muscle recruitment. Denervation is heralded by fibrillations and fasciculations but can take up to 14 days to become detectable; therefore, EMG should not be ordered before this. As such, 3 weeks after closed injury is an appropriate time to order the first EMG to distinguish neuropraxic from more neurotmesis-type injuries.[23] When voluntary motor units are seen on EMG, this is suggestive of muscle recovery and reinnervation.

Ultrasonography and Magnetic Resonance Neurography

High-resolution ultrasonography (USN) is useful in the acute setting to detect nerve injury, including continuity as well as derangements in the fascicular topography. USN has several advantages, including decreased cost, dynamic evaluation, and minimal discomfort, and can be performed in the presence of implanted devices or hardware.[24] Sonographic grading of nerve injuries can be made based on the relative echogenicity of the nerve components including the epineurium, perineurium, axons, and fascicles; however, USN is not able to adequately visualize the endoneurium, and the quality of the images is dependent on the expertise of the operator.[24] Nerves that are entrapped or tethered in scar can be detected based on the appearance of an indentation and dilation proximal or distal to the affected area. A neuroma-in-continuity can be detected based on the presence of a nerve with maintained epineurium but with focal dilatation and effaced internal architecture.[24] On USN, completely transected nerves demonstrate epineurium with an intervening gap and possibly a proximal stump neuroma depending on the time after injury.[24]

Magnetic resonance neurography (MRN) is a powerful tool to detect and define the extent of peripheral nerve injuries. MRN relies on the specific properties of water in nerves and provides enhanced images, allowing for the detection of a nerve lesion. This information is incredibly helpful and accelerates surgical decision-making when the site or extent of the injury is not otherwise clear on physical examination or EMG.[17] MRN has increased spatial resolution and anatomic detail compared with USN but can be limited by the presence of hardware, although newer MRN protocols are available to accommodate the presence of metal.[18] MRN is also preferable to USN when the nerve of interest is deep, for example, in the axillary or lumbosacral space.[18] In addition to visualizing the nerve, MRN can detect muscle denervation and affords a global assessment and comparison of muscles in the area to detect changes.[18]

Timing of Repair

After a sharp laceration, if a patient presents with a nerve deficit in the zone of injury or distally, surgical exploration within the week is recommended to maximize the opportunity for primary repair; if later exploration is necessary, a discussion of nerve reconstruction with the patient is needed. Early primary repair is associated with improved outcomes. Blunt penetrating injuries in the absence of an associated vascular injury are often observed for spontaneous recovery. A baseline EMG at the time of injury is recommended. After 3 months of observation, if no recovery is noted, EMG is recommended to assess the extent of nerve injury, with a decision to proceed with surgical exploration or continued observation made based on the EMG results. Crush and compression injuries result in increased intraneural pressures and nerve dysfunction. These injuries should be observed for 3 months to identify spontaneous recovery. If there is none, an EMG should be performed. If the EMG does not demonstrate significant recovery, surgical intervention should be performed.

In summary, sharp/penetrating injuries with associated neurologic deficit corresponding to the zone of injury should be surgically explored. Compression/crush and avulsion type injuries with associated nerve deficit can be observed with serial examinations up to 3 months.[19] EMG is used to guide next steps in management including continued observation versus surgical intervention.

Goals of Repair

Axonal regeneration is estimated to occur at a rate of 1 mm/day after repair or decompression; it is prudent that muscle reinnervation occurs within 12 to 18 months to maximize return of motor function.[19] After repair or reconstruction of a nerve, there are specific goals from a sensory and motor standpoint. Sensory recovery grading includes:

S0: no sensation
S1: deep cutaneous pain
S2: superficial pain
S3: superficial pain/touch
S4: complete recovery

The goal is "protective sensation," or superficial pain/touch. Return of sensation is determined sequentially using moving and static two-point discrimination as well as Semmes-Weinstein monofilament testing. From a motor standpoint, recovery is graded as follows:

M0: no contraction
M1: perceptible contraction of proximal muscles
M2: perceptible contraction of proximal and distal muscles
M3: contraction against gravity
M4: contraction against resistance
M5: full recovery

The minimal goal of return of motor function is the ability to have antigravity strength. To achieve this goal, the location, type, and extent of nerve injury must be diagnosed as early as possible so that the appropriate repair can be performed to optimize functional outcomes.

Operative Techniques for Nerve Injuries

Direct Repair

During World War I and II, a large number of nerve injuries required surgical intervention; during this time, surgeons explored the wounds, debrided, and often repaired nerves with tension.[25] Since this time, many advancements in the understanding of nerve injuries and optimal repair have been made, including the use of an operating microscope, intraoperative nerve stimulation, and principles of tension-free repairs and/or reconstruction. At the time of exploration, the existing wound/laceration is opened with extensions. Neurolysis is performed, and the proximal and distal ends of the nerve are dissected free of surrounding tissue. If there is significant contamination, insufficient soft tissue wound bed, or the zone of injury is unclear, the nerve ends can be tagged with a suture for later identification and repair. If conditions are suitable, the nerve ends are resected to healthy fascicles and aligned in preparation for repair. An operating microscope (or loupe magnification) and microsurgical instruments are needed, and 8-0, 9-0, or 10-0 monofilament suture can be used to perform epineural repair or grouped fascicular repair depending on the size of the nerve and surgeon preference (Fig. 41.2). Epineural repair is less technically challenging but provides no axonal specificity. Additionally, with mixed nerves, there is the potential for malalignment of the nerve fascicules. The internal vasculature and the appearance of the fascicles can be used to guide orientation and alignment during the repair. Grouped fascicular repair allows for more specificity but is technically demanding and can introduce more intraneural scar with the additional dissection. With either type of repair, it is critical to avoid tension at the nerve repair site because this decreases blood flow and increases scar formation. If there is any tension, slight flexion of the extremity can be performed to relieve this; however, if there is excess tension, one should consider nerve reconstruction. Fibrin glue or nerve conduits can be used at the neurorrhaphy site; fibrin glue has been shown to decrease the number of required sutures and minimize gapping.

Nerve Reconstruction

Nerve gaps of approximately 5 mm can typically be repaired primarily after neurolysis and possible transposition of the nerves; however, larger gaps typically cannot be repaired without undue tension or significant changes in joint position. In these cases, nerve reconstruction should be considered. Nerve reconstruction is also considered when there are additional injuries or medical conditions that necessitate delayed repair as well. Nerve reconstruction should be performed as soon as possible, given the time

required for nerve elongation after repair. Reinnervation of muscle before the 12- to 18-month point is necessary to avoid irreversible muscle atrophy and fibrosis.[17] Gaps are largely divided into those <10 mm, 10 to 30 mm, or >30 mm. This distinction is used to make recommendations about the type of nerve graft used for reconstruction. For gaps <10 mm, reconstruction can be performed with any type of conduit. For gaps 10 to 30 mm, it is possible to use allograft or autograft for reconstruction; however, with gaps >30 mm, autograft is recommended.

Autograft is expendable nerve harvested from the injured patient (Fig. 41.3). Common sources include the sural nerve, medial antebrachial cutaneous nerve, lateral antebrachial cutaneous nerve, superficial radial nerve, and posterior interosseus nerve. Donor site is chosen based on the amount of length and diameter of the nerve graft needed for reconstruction; the sural nerve provides the longest and largest-diameter graft. For larger-caliber injured nerves, a single nerve graft is not large enough to support the regeneration of all axons in the proximal nerve stump to the distal nerve stump. In this case, multiple nerve grafts are used to reconstruct the gap.

The use of nerve allografts has increased in popularity related to the lack of donor site morbidity and the readily available supply. These decellularized human nerves undergo proprietary processing to remove all antigenic cells; this allows them to be used without risk of immune reaction.[26] Nerve allograft has been used in a variety of settings, including digital, sensory, motor, and mixed sensory-motor nerves.[22,26] Gaps of less than 30 mm are recommended when choosing to use allograft; however, some studies have demonstrated adequate nerve recovery and favorable outcomes[19] in larger gaps.[26] There is no conclusive evidence supporting their use for gaps greater than 30 mm in major peripheral nerves.

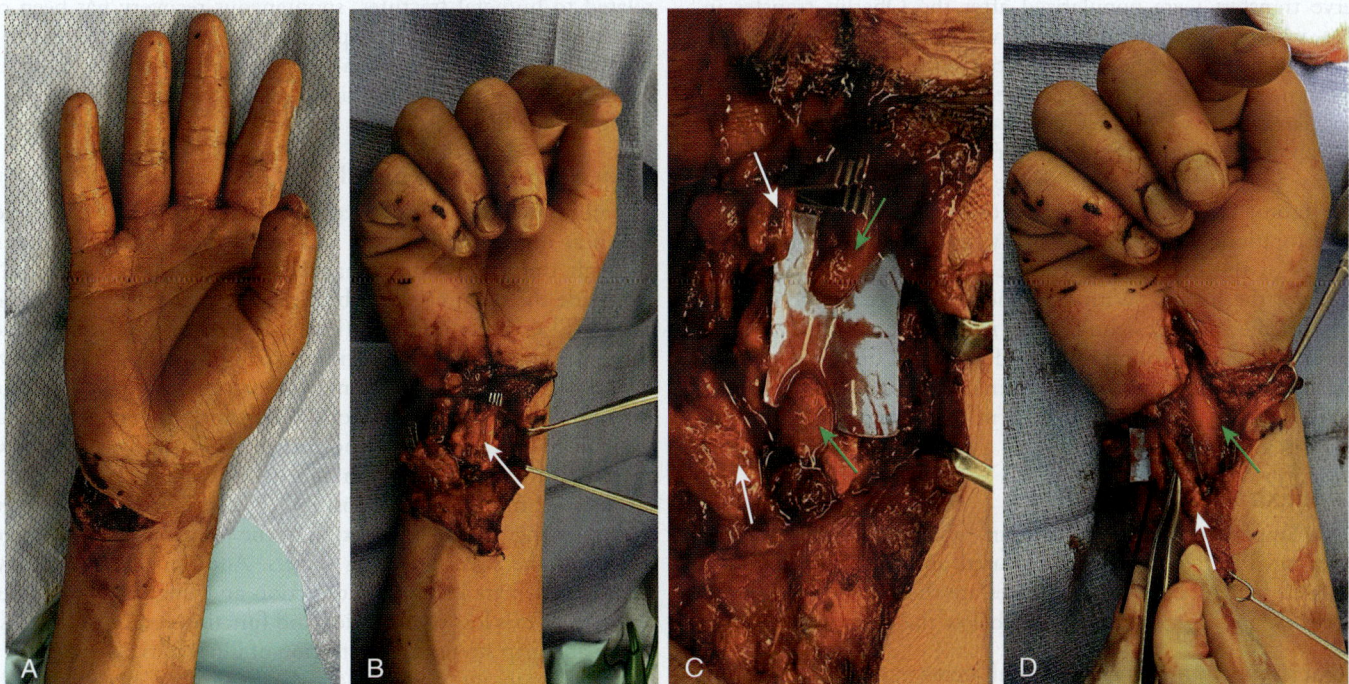

FIGURE 41.2 Combined flexor tendon, ulnar artery, and median and ulnar nerve injuries with primary repair. (A) Clean distal ulnar forearm laceration. (B) Repair of flexor tendons *(white arrow)* with restoration of finger cascade. (C) Identification of ulnar artery and nerve distal and proximal *(white arrows)*. (D) Tension-free primary repair ulnar nerve *(black arrow)*, ulnar artery *(white arrow)*, and median nerve *(green arrow)*.

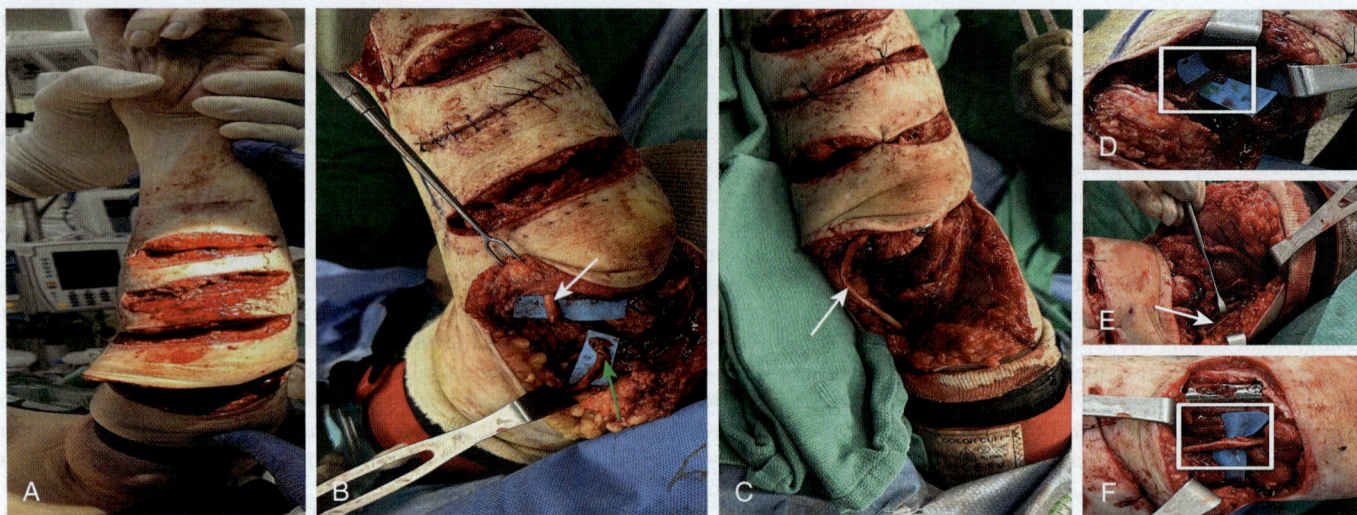

FIGURE 41.3 (A) Multilevel upper arm, elbow, and forearm sharp laceration with underlying fractures. (B) Identification of ulnar nerve injury at elbow with distal *(white arrow)* and proximal *(green arrow)* ends. (C) Reconstruction of the ulnar nerve at the elbow with graft *(white arrow)*. (D) Partial ulnar nerve injury in forearm *(white box)*. (E) Identification of medial antebrachial cutaneous (MABC) nerve donor graft *(white arrow)*. (F) Reconstruction of ulnar nerve partial injury with MABC nerve graft.

Nerve Transfer

Nerve transfers are a technique used to reconstruct a proximal injured nerve by providing distal intact axons from another expendable nerve, for expeditious reinnervation of sensory and motor end organs. Transfers should be performed distal to the site of injury. Confirmation of a functional donor nerve is necessary before transfer. Typically, the donor nerve is dissected as distal as possible to create enough length. The recipient nerve is dissected distal to the injury and close to the end muscle target. A tension-free donor-to-recipient neurorrhaphy is performed. Nerve transfers were popularized after the Oberlin transfer in 1994, whereby ulnar nerve fascicles were transferred to musculocutaneous nerve branches of the biceps to restore elbow flexion.[25] Several nerve transfers have been effective in restoring hand function, particularly when the injuries are above the elbow. Patients with above-elbow ulnar nerve injuries are candidates for distal anterior interosseus nerve (from the pronator quadratus) to the ulnar motor fascicle for restoration of intrinsic hand function.[25] For restoration of ulnar nerve sensory function, the median nerve fascicles of the third webspace can be transferred to the ulnar border of the hand.[27] With distal nerve transfers, there is a decrease in the distance required for regeneration. Another common nerve transfer to improve hand and wrist function involves transfer of the branches of the supinator nerve to the posterior interosseous in the proximal forearm to restore finger, thumb, and wrist extension.[25]

Upper Extremity Nerve Injuries

In the upper extremity, the median, ulnar, radial, and digital nerves are the most frequently injured and will be specifically discussed here. "High" nerve injuries are those that occur above the elbow, and "low" injuries occur below the elbow.

Radial Nerve: Anatomy and Clinical Assessment

The radial nerve is one of the terminal branches of the posterior cord of the brachial plexus. In the upper arm, it passes deep to the long head and between the lateral and medial heads of the triceps. In this region, it is highly susceptible to injury; 22% of all humeral fractures are associated with radial nerve injury.[23] It is a mixed motor and sensory nerve that divides into the superficial radial nerve and posterior interosseous nerve (PIN).[23] The superficial radial nerve provides sensation to the dorsoradial aspect of the hand; the radial nerve proper and PIN nerve provide motor innervation to the triceps; brachialis; brachioradialis; and extensors of the wrist, fingers, and thumb.[23] Injury is often heralded by loss of sensation in the distribution of the nerve as well as inability to actively extend the wrist, fingers, and thumb.

Among patients with closed neuropraxic radial nerve injuries related to humeral fractures, spontaneous recovery has been observed in 60% to 92% of patients; however, among humeral fractures associated with high-velocity gunshot wounds, vascular injuries, or other penetrating trauma, surgical exploration is recommended.[23]

Ulnar Nerve: Anatomy and Clinical Assessment

The ulnar nerve travels between the medial epicondyle and olecranon as it crosses the elbow and enters the medial forearm and through the flexor carpi ulnaris. It continues distally, running alongside the ulnar artery in between the flexor digitorum superficialis (FDS) and profundus (FDP). It is responsible for sensation along the volar small finger and one-half of the ring finger as well as the dorsoulnar hand. From a motor standpoint, it innervates the flexor carpi ulnaris, FDP of the ring and small fingers, adductor pollicis, and intrinsic hand muscles. Classically, patients will present with loss of sensation and hand weakness manifested by an intrinsic minus clawing position (hyperextension of the metacarpophalangeal joint and flexion of the proximal interphalangeal joints) of the small and ring fingers. Additionally, patients will also have deficits in thumb adduction and finger adduction and abduction; this loss of intrinsic hand function results in decreased pinch and grip strength.[27] Detection of ulnar nerve deficits can be challenging in the presence of Martin-Gruber anastomosis between the ulnar and median nerves in the forearm; under such circumstances, muscles normally innervated by the ulnar nerve are supplied by the median nerve, producing a heterogenous clinical picture.[27]

Median Nerve: Anatomy and Clinical Assessment

The median nerve lies deep in the proximal forearm as it runs between the heads of the pronator teres, but it becomes more superficial at the wrist, placing it at increased risk during penetrating injuries (lacerations) and blunt trauma (MVC). The median nerve is responsible for sensation of the volar thumb, index, middle, and one-half of the ring finger; it provides motor innervation to the pronator teres, flexor digitorum, flexor pollicis brevis, flexor carpi radialis, palmaris longus, and thenar musculature including the abductor pollicis brevis. The median nerve is of critical importance to hand sensation, and injury results in loss of sensation over the volar fingertips as well as decreased thumb motion, including opposition and palmar abduction. Because of its location, the median nerve is often injured in conjunction with the flexor tendons. Sharp penetrating injuries in the location of the median nerve with associated deficits should be explored within a week of injury to increase the chances of primary repair.[28]

Surgical Treatment of Median, Ulnar, and Radial Nerves

At the time of exploration, existing lacerations are extended proximal and distal to allow full exploration and neurolysis if needed. Large nerves can be repaired with loupe magnification or operating microscope using 6-0 Prolene or 8-0/9-0 nylon. Because the median, ulnar, and radial nerves are mixed motor and sensory, it is critical to use the orientation and appearance of grouped fascicles and blood vessels to align the nerve ends and perform a tension-free epineural repair (see Fig. 41.3). The ulnar nerve internal topography has been studied extensively with distinct organization of the motor and sensory components. The ulnar nerve is often injured with adjacent tendons and/or the ulnar artery. Slight wrist flexion may be used to facilitate direct repair in certain circumstances.[28] If too much tension or too much flexion is required, reconstruction with autograft or allograft is needed. The autograft of choice is the sural nerve, which is harvested from the lower extremity and cut into cables of the appropriate length to bridge the gap (Figs. 41.4 and 41.5). Concomitant arterial

injuries should be repaired with upper extremity fasciotomies performed if there is prolonged ischemia or concern for compartment syndrome.

Outcomes of Median, Ulnar, and Radial Nerve Injuries

Motor and sensory recovery are affected by the age of the patient (younger age better than older), site of injury (proximal worse than distal), and time delay to surgery.[27,28] The best possible outcomes have been achieved with direct primary repair. Among ulnar nerve injuries treated with neurolysis alone, M3 or greater motor function is achieved in 92% of cases.[27] Because intrinsic hand muscle function is difficult to restore after injury, median nerve repairs have better reported and functional outcomes compared with the ulnar nerve.[27] In a meta-analysis including 623 patients who underwent median and ulnar nerve injury repair, 43% regained S3+ sensory and 52% regained >M4 motor recovery; the authors identified that younger patients were four times more likely to recover motor function and the ulnar nerve was 70% less likely to have motor recovery compared with the median nerve.[27,29] Examination of >1000 nerve injuries at a large single-center institution demonstrated good recovery (S3/M4) among 80% to 100% of radial nerve injury patients, with poorer outcomes among ulnar nerve patients.[20] Because of the relative proximal innervation of the wrist, hand, and finger extensors, radial nerve repairs have better potential for functional recovery than do other peripheral nerves. Despite this, results are mixed; among radial nerve injuries directly repaired within 6 months of injury, good to fair results are reported in 60% of patients, whereas a series of combined radial nerve (proximal) and PIN (distal) nerve injuries (repair and reconstructions) demonstrated a 42% failure rate.[23] In all cases of failed or incomplete recovery after median, ulnar, or radial nerve injuries, tendon transfers can be performed using remaining expendable muscles to perform critical hand functions.

Digital Nerves: Anatomy, Assessment, and Treatment

Each digit has a radial and ulnar nerve along the volar aspect that is responsible for sensation. The digital nerves lie volar (palmar) to

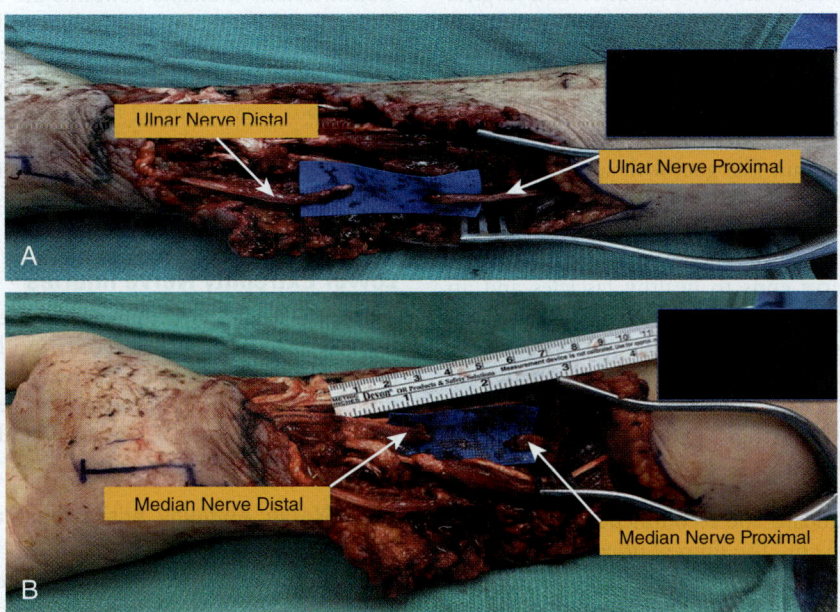

FIGURE 41.4 (A) Upper extremity median (A) and ulnar nerve (B) avulsion/laceration injuries.

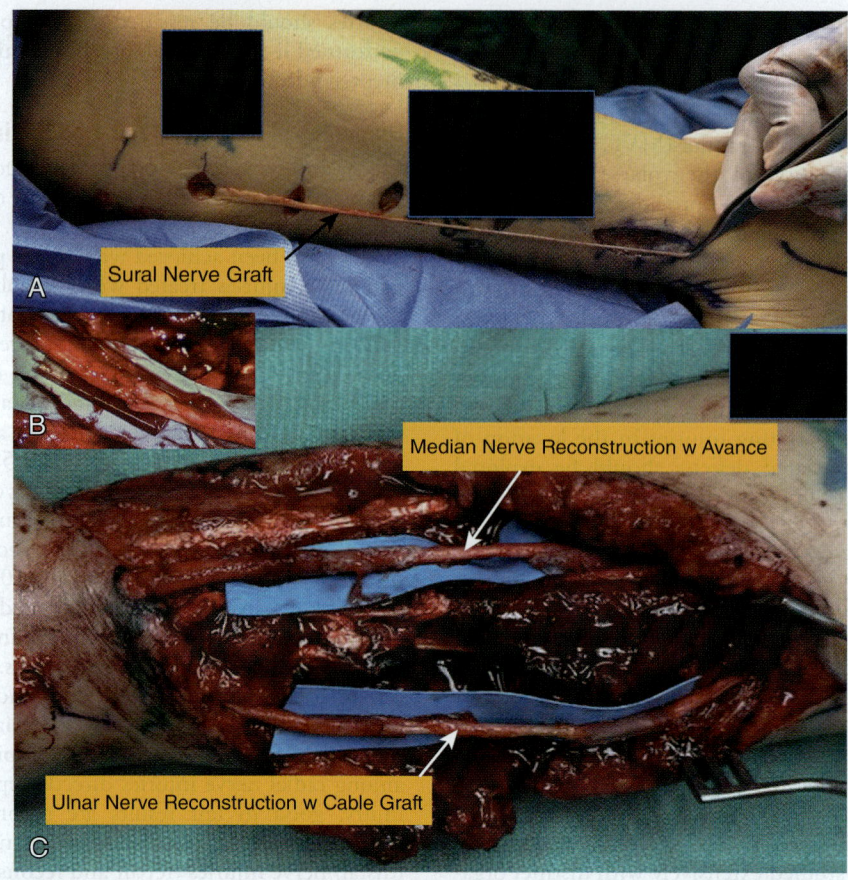

A Sural Nerve Graft

B

C Median Nerve Reconstruction w Avance

Ulnar Nerve Reconstruction w Cable Graft

FIGURE 41.5 (A) Harvest of sural nerve allograft. (B) Microscopic view of reconstruction of ulnar nerve with multiple sural nerve grafts. (C) Reconstruction of median nerve with allograft and ulnar nerve with autograft.

the digital arteries and along the flexor tendons. Digital nerves are commonly injured in conjunction with tendon and bone, with mechanisms including sharp laceration, stretch, and compression.

Careful history and physical can elucidate the presence of a digital nerve injury. Both the radial and ulnar sides of the digit or thumb should be tested individually and compared with the uninjured digits. Treatment options include observation and surgical exploration. If there is a high suspicion of complete transection, surgical exploration is recommended; however, 10% of patients at the time of exploration may not have a complete transection and may undergo neurolysis and closure.[30] Among those who choose surgery, exploration within the first week after injury provides the best opportunity for direct repair. The goal with surgical repair is to ensure axonal continuity and achieve protective sensation; in the most optimal of conditions, "normal sensation" can be obtained. A tension-free direct repair proceeds with debridement of the proximal and distal nerve ends to healthy fascicles and an epineural repair with 8-0 or 9-0 microsuture. Up to 11% of direct nerve repairs are considered "failures."[30] With concomitant tendon or bone injuries, the surgeon must consider the period of postoperative immobilization and time to initiation of the appropriate rehabilitation protocol.

If the presentation or diagnosis is delayed, nerve reconstruction with autograft, allograft, or conduits is possible. Traditionally, autograft is the gold standard and recommended for any gap size, but especially those >3 cm. The injured proximal and distal nerve ends are prepared, and a graft of appropriate size and length is chosen for reconstruction; the graft is directly sutured to the nerve ends using 8-0 or 9-0 microsuture to create a tension-free

repair. In a systematic review from 2020 including a heterogenous group of digital nerve injuries, 95% had good to excellent recovery and 28% regained normal recovery.[30] Decellularized human nerve allografts are increasingly being used for variable digital nerve injury gaps (10–70 mm) with 69% to 80% of patients reporting good or excellent recovery in a recent review.[30] Commercially available conduits are available and composed of biocompatible materials including collagen, chitosan, and polyglycolic acid. Conduits are typically used when the gap is less than 15 mm and the surgeon prefers to avoid a donor site to harvest autologous nerve. During this procedure, the proximal and distal nerve ends are intubated into the conduit using sutures.[30] The conduit provides an enclosed space for the proximal axons to grow toward the distal end and has been associated with good to excellent recovery.[30]

Lower Extremity Nerve Injuries

Injuries to the lower extremity peripheral nerves are less common than those to the upper extremity. Within the lower extremity, the peroneal, tibial, and sciatic nerves are the most injured. As with upper extremity nerve injuries, lower extremity injuries can result in chronic pain, loss of sensation, and loss of motor function of the extremity.

Tibial Nerve: Anatomy, Assessment, and Treatment

The tibial nerve is one of the terminal branches of the sciatic nerve and is responsible for sensation on the plantar aspect of the foot as well as motor function of the posterior leg compartment including the ankle and toe plantar flexors and intrinsic muscles.[31]

Surgical options after tibial nerve injury include neurolysis, nerve repair, nerve reconstruction, or nerve transfer. The sural nerve is the most used autograft. Nerve transfers using the saphenous nerve for sensation and obturator nerve for motor function have been described for tibial nerve injuries.[31]

Peroneal: Anatomy, Assessment, and Treatment

The peroneal nerve is one of the terminal branches of the sciatic nerve. It crosses lateral to the head of the fibula and gives rise to the superficial and deep peroneal nerves. The superficial peroneal nerve is a mixed motor-sensory nerve; it innervates the lateral compartment muscles (peroneus brevis and longus) and provides sensation to the lower one-third of the anterior calf and lateral dorsal foot (except the first webspace). The deep peroneal nerve is also a mixed motor-sensory nerve that innervates the muscles of the anterior compartment and provides sensation to the first dorsal webspace of the foot. Injuries to the common peroneal nerve (CPN) result in foot drop, altered gait, inability to evert the ankle, and sensory loss along the distal anterior calf and dorsal foot. Because of its position along the fibular head, the CPN is in a vulnerable position and susceptible to injury.

The CPN is the most common lower extremity nerve that is injured after trauma, representing 10% to 21% of peripheral nerve injuries.[32] Mechanisms of injury include traumatic knee dislocation/fractures, gunshot wounds, lacerations, and other crush injuries. CPN injuries are difficult to manage and are often associated with poor outcomes. Outcomes are predicated on several factors including the mechanism of injury, zone of injury, associated injuries, delay in treatment of nerve injury, length of damaged nerve, and other medical comorbidities. After CPN injuries, two-thirds of patients report difficulty walking and neuropathic pain.[32] Nonoperative treatment ranges from observation, to physical therapy, to ankle-foot orthoses. Operative intervention for transected nerves includes direct repair or reconstruction with autograft or allograft.[32] If the nerve is transected, direct repair should be performed. Functional recovery ≥M3 was achieved in (63/80) 78.8% of patients who underwent primary repair.[32] If there is a gap, peroneal nerve reconstruction with nerve grafting should be performed; however, variable outcomes have been reported.

If patients are not able to regain function of the anterior tibialis 18 months after observation or surgical intervention, a posterior tibialis tendon to anterior tibialis transfer can be performed to facilitate foot dorsiflexion. Patients stand to regain up to 42% of strength compared with the contralateral side with this transfer.[32] Some surgeons may consider performing concurrent neurolysis/nerve reconstruction and posterior tibial tendon transfer if the presentation is delayed or the nerve gap significant.

Outcomes After Tibial and Peroneal Nerve Repair and/or Reconstruction

Tibial nerve injuries that require neurolysis alone have the best outcomes.[31] Tibial nerves amenable to direct repair resulted in 89% of patients achieving a good outcome.[31] In a meta-analysis examining outcomes after nerve transfer among 30 patients, 71% achieved a good outcome.[31]

In a meta-analysis examining traumatic peroneal nerve injuries, surgical intervention was recommended if no spontaneous improvement was seen 6 months after the injury, but shorter preoperative times were associated with improved outcomes.[32] Among 465 patients who underwent peroneal nerve reconstruction, 49% achieved >M3 recovery; mean nerve graft length was 7 cm, but shorter grafts improved outcomes.[32] Nerve transfers for common peroneal injuries have been described; tibial nerve branches have been successfully transferred to the distal CPN in an end-to-end fashion yielding >M3 function for 62.9% of patients in one meta-analysis.[32]

Summary of Peripheral Nerve Injuries

Peripheral nerve injuries of the upper and lower extremities are extremely common and can have a profound impact on patient quality of life. Careful history, physical examination, and early diagnosis are key to appropriate intervention. Mechanism of injury, preoperative interval, patient age, direct repair versus reconstruction, gap length, and the use of allograft or autograft all affect outcome. Injuries associated with sharp lacerations have better outcomes than those associated with blast and gunshot wounds.[23,27,31] Delay in time between injury and repair or reconstruction is associated with poor motor recovery.[23,27,31] Nerve injuries managed by direct repair have better reported outcomes than those where reconstruction is required. Under circumstances of reconstruction, poor recovery of sensory and motor function is associated with gaps greater than 3 cm (regardless of graft material).[31] Because of the longer distance the regenerating axons must travel to get to end organs after nerve injuries, proximal nerve injuries have worse outcomes than do distal injuries.[22,26,33]

SPINE EMERGENCIES

Spinal emergencies are defined as any injury to the spinal column, spinal cord, or nerve roots that requires emergent or urgent treatment. The most common reason for spinal emergencies is some form of traumatic spinal injury, which comprises both fractures to the spinal column, where the spinal column is injured with or without damage to the spinal cord, and spinal cord injury (SCI), where the spinal cord itself is damaged. Importantly, fractures without SCI are still emergent conditions, where the spine is unstable, and without fixation, injury to the spinal cord can occur with minor movement. When the spinal cord itself is damaged, SCI can leave patients with debilitating neurologic deficits, leading to permanent disability with concomitant societal and economic effects. SCI primarily affects young adult males, with trauma being the most common etiology. According to recent demographic and epidemiologic insights, ~450,000 persons living in the United States are permanently disabled because of traumatic SCI, with ~11,000 new cases each year. Notably, the incidence in the United States exceeds that of many other countries. The pattern of injury exhibits a bimodal age distribution, with the initial peak affecting young adults and accounting for approximately 50% of new cases, whereas the second peak primarily involves individuals over the age of 60. The financial burden is substantial, with direct medical expenses ranging from $500,000 to $2 million over the lifetime of an affected individual. Remarkably, alcohol is implicated in at least 25% of traumatic SCI cases.

Certain underlying spinal conditions may predispose individuals to becoming susceptible to traumatic SCI, including cervical degeneration/spondylosis, atlantoaxial instability, congenital conditions, osteoporosis, and spinal arthropathies, such as ankylosing spondylitis (AS) or rheumatoid arthritis. After acute SCI, patients are at risk of further neurologic deterioration because of secondary injury to the spinal cord either by inadvertent manipulation of the spine in the setting of an unstable spinal column injury or failure in medical management to maintain adequate perfusion of the spine. Timely intervention in SCI is paramount. Fast and appropriate management during the early stages of injury, whether it occurs in a prehospital setting or at a healthcare facility, can help prevent further damage to the spinal cord, reduce the risk of complications, and improve the chances of functional recovery. The current guidelines advocate for surgical intervention to be performed within a 24-hour window from the time of injury. In patients with incomplete injuries with salvageable neurologic function, the urgency for surgical treatment is even greater, with some authors suggesting surgical intervention in <8 hours.

Although trauma is likely the most common cause of spinal emergencies, nontraumatic conditions can also lead to spinal emergencies. Around 372,000 persons in the United States live with nontraumatic spinal injuries. Patients with degenerative pathology can present with symptoms of spinal cord compression as a consequence of cervical spondylotic myelopathy or disc herniation. In addition, patients with spinal tumors may present with acute or subacute neurologic deterioration that requires urgent medical, surgical, or radiation therapy. Other etiologies of nontraumatic spinal emergencies include inflammatory/autoimmune conditions such as multiple sclerosis and neuromyelitis optica as well as infections such as epidural abscess. High-income countries tend to have a higher proportion of cases secondary to degenerative conditions and tumors, whereas in developing countries, infection contributes to the majority of nontraumatic spinal emergencies. Vascular disorders may also result in spinal emergencies requiring urgent management, including spontaneous hematomas, arteriovenous malformations (AVMs), and spinal cord infarction caused by thrombotic, embolic, vasoocclusive, or hemorrhagic etiologies. Other miscellaneous conditions that require emergent treatment include amyotrophic lateral sclerosis and primary lateral sclerosis as well as metabolic causes such as subacute combined degeneration caused by vitamin B_{12} deficiency.

The current chapter provides an overview of select spinal emergencies and highlights the nuances of prompt recognition and definitive management, without delving into nuances of surgical technique. It is important to clarify that the focus of this chapter is on all spinal emergencies for the targeted audience of general surgeons and acute care surgeons caring for the critically injured patient, rather than neurosurgeons or orthopedic surgeons. Herein, we describe three major areas of spinal emergencies, including (1) an overview of SCI, (2) spinal emergencies caused by traumatic events, and (3) spinal emergencies caused by nontraumatic events. Although we recognize this is not an exhaustive list of all spinal emergencies, the discussion that follows addresses common areas of spinal emergencies most relevant to the general surgeon.

Spinal Cord Injury General Management

Spinal Anatomy

The spinal cord originates at the base of the brainstem, specifically the medulla, and commences at the first cervical vertebra, just distal to the craniocervical junction. The spinal cord terminates at L1–L2 in adults and as low as L3–L4 in children, where it is called the *conus medullaris*. Extending from the apex of the conus medullaris is the filum terminale, an extension of the pia mater that attaches to the posterior surface of the coccyx. After the spinal cord terminates, the cauda equina travels from approximately L1–L2 to the sacrum, carrying lumbar and sacral nerve roots that control lower extremity, bowel/bladder, and sexual function.

The spinal cord generates 31 pairs of spinal nerves that predominantly innervate the trunk and limbs. These spinal nerves are categorized into cervical (8 pairs), thoracic (12 pairs), lumbar (5 pairs), and sacral (5 pairs each), along with one pair of coccygeal nerves. In the cervical spine there are seven vertebrae but eight nerve roots, which is why the lower-level roots exit at each level (i.e., the C5 root exits in the C4/5 foramen, the C6 root exits at the C5/6 foramen, and so on). After C7/T1, when the thoracic spine starts, the roots exit at the same level (i.e., the T1 root exits at the T1/2 foramen, the L2 root exits at the L2/3 foramen, and so on). The spinal nerves have two roots, a ventral or motor root and a dorsal or sensory root. The dorsal root has a distinctive swelling called the *dorsal nerve root ganglion,* which contains cell bodies of pseudounipolar sensory neurons. At the conus medullaris, nerve roots coming from the lower lumbar, sacral, and coccygeal nerves form a bundle of nerves known as *cauda equina.* The spinal cord is enveloped from outermost to innermost by the dura mater, arachnoid mater, and pia mater. The space situated between the dura mater and the wall of the vertebral canal is referred to as the *extradural* or *epidural space,* which is filled with copious epidural veins. The area between the dura mater and arachnoid mater is known as the *subdural space,* and the subarachnoid space lies between the arachnoid mater and pia mater, containing CSF. It is most often the epidural space that gets invaded by fracture fragments, hematoma, and tumors, which leads to epidural spinal cord compression. Occasionally, intradural pathology can also cause cord compression.

The spinal cord is nourished by one anterior spinal artery and two posterior spinal arteries. The anterior spinal artery runs along the front median fissure, whereas the two smaller posterior spinal arteries pass through the posterolateral sulcus on either side. In the cervical spine, these spinal arteries primarily branch from the vertebral arteries, which ascends from C6–C2 in the foramen transversarium, though it can enter early at C7 or later at C5 and above. Farther down the spinal cord, blood supply is provided by radicular arteries that reach both the cord and the roots of the spinal nerves. These radicular arteries branch from various sources, including the vertebral, cervical, intercostal, lumbar, and sacral arteries. The most noteworthy radicular contributor to the anterior spinal artery, known as the *artery of Adamkiewicz,* arises from the left posterior intercostal artery and is located between the T9 and T12 vertebrae. The spinal cord's venous drainage system is organized into a network consisting of six longitudinal channels: an anteromedian vein, a posteromedian vein, and a pair of anterolateral and posterolateral veins. The venous blood collected in these veins ultimately flows into the venous plexus and radicular veins, which, in turn, discharge into segmental veins.

Protecting these delicate neural elements is the spinal column, or the vertebral column, which consists of 33 vertebrae: 7 cervical, 12 thoracic, 5 lumbar, 5 sacral, and 4 coccygeal. Anteriorly, a typical vertebra consists of a solid cylindrical body attached posteriorly to two pedicles connecting to flat laminae. Extending outward are transverse processes to which muscles and ligaments attach. The spinous process projects posteriorly, often palpable along the spine. Additionally, each vertebra features superior and inferior articular processes that form facet joints, facilitating spinal movement. Adjacent vertebrae create intervertebral foramina, allowing for the passage of spinal nerves and blood vessels.

Initial Management of Spinal Cord Injury

The acute management of SCI adheres to the concept of "time is spine"—a key tenet that guides interventions.[34] Concern for a cervical or thoracic SCI should prompt immediate immobilization of the spine at the scene, which can be achieved through application of a rigid cervical collar or use of supportive blocks and straps on a backboard. Similarly, when dealing with unstable fractures, immobilization of the spine should be ensured while transferring the patient with multiple people in a "logroll" fashion. Most commonly in blunt trauma, efforts to maintain immobilization should be made, provided that it does not impede essential resuscitation efforts. These measures are meant to minimize the risk of exacerbating spinal cord damage by excess movement that cannot be supported by an unstable spinal column or damaged spinal cord.

After immobilization, ATLS guidelines should be meticulously applied to ensure the assessment and management of the injured patient. In patients with compromised airways, it is imperative to secure a definitive airway while ensuring continuous spinal immobilization during the intubation process. Additionally, cervical and thoracic injuries may impede proper innervation of vital respiratory muscles, including the diaphragm, intercostal muscles, and abdominal muscles, which can result in decreased respiratory drive, hypoxemia, and hypercarbia. Approximately one-third of patients with injuries to the cervical spine require intubation within the first day after injury.

In addition to the inflammatory response contributing to secondary SCI, spinal cord blood flow reduction can exacerbate the primary SCI. Patients with SCI in the setting of polytrauma may also suffer from dehydration, extraspinal injuries, and vasogenic shock. Maintaining adequate spinal cord flow is often recommended for nonsurgical management for an SCI, but there are no direct measurements of spinal blood flow. Knowing that flow does not equal pressure, it is often accomplished by keeping MAP above 85 mm Hg, or at least 10 points higher than their baseline, relevant for patients with known baseline uncontrolled hypertension. After ensuring euvolemia, vasopressors are sometimes needed. Furthermore, the severity of the SCI correlates with the need for vasopressors based on the extent of injury: complete cervical SCI, 90%; incomplete cervical SCI, 52%; complete thoracic SCI, 33%; and incomplete thoracic, 25%. Sometimes, vasopressors cannot be safely used because of competing clinical priorities (e.g., impulse control for aortic or cardiovascular injuries, myocardial ischemia, emergency hypertensive crisis, intracranial hemorrhage risk).

In patients with SCI in the cervical and upper thoracic regions (above T6), damage to the sympathetic tracts within the intermediolateral column can precipitate neurogenic shock. This condition is characterized by bradycardia and hypotension caused by reduced vascular tone resulting from unopposed parasympathetic vagal activity. Neurogenic shock exacerbates the ischemic burden on the already vulnerable injured spinal cord, leading to global hypoperfusion—a situation further compounded in cases of concurrent blood loss, as seen in polytrauma patients. In conjunction with crystalloid volume resuscitation, vasopressors may be considered to counteract peripheral vasodilation.

Neurologic Examination

Patients with SCI can manifest with varying degrees of severity, classified as either complete, meaning no neurologic function below the level of injury, or incomplete, with preservation of some motor and/or sensory function below the level of injury. The assessment and description of the severity of SCI often adhere to the American Spinal Injury Association (ASIA) scoring system, a universally recognized tool. This system allows for a comprehensive evaluation of the motor and sensory deficits, facilitating a standardized and effective means of characterizing the extent of the SCI. *One of the most important things for general surgeons and acute care surgeons caring for injured patient with acute SCI is to be familiar with the neurologic and spinal examination and communicate findings and future changes to the spine surgery team.*

First, the GCS (described earlier in the "Traumatic Brain Injury" section) is used to assess the level of awareness in patients with impaired consciousness and concomitant brain injury. A quick mental status examination is equally important to screen for abnormalities that may warrant further investigations, and it involves asking for orientation to time, place, and person.

The assessment of muscle strength adheres to the following muscle grading system (0–5): 0, no muscle contraction is seen or identified with palpation; 1, flicker of contraction insufficient to produce any movement; 2, active movement with gravity eliminated; 3, active movement against gravity with no resistance; 4, active movement against gravity with moderate resistance; and 5, normal muscle strength against gravity and with full resistance. Testing muscle strength should be done in an orderly manner, aiming to differentiate proximal/distal and left/right muscle weakness. Motor examination of the upper extremity includes shoulder abduction (C5), elbow flexion (C5–C6), elbow extension (C6–C7), wrist extension (C6–C7), wrist flexion (C7–C8), finger flexion (C8), finger extension (C8), and finger abduction (T1). In the lower extremity, the following movements are tested: hip flexion (L2–L3), hip extension (L4–L5), knee flexion (L5–S1), knee extension (L3–L4), ankle dorsiflexion (L4–L5), big toe extension (through extensor hallucis longus muscle, L5), and ankle plantar flexion (S1–S2).

Reflexes are then tested. The biceps and brachioradialis reflexes are mediated by C5–C6, the triceps reflex by C6–C7, knee jerk by L3–L4 (mainly L4), and the ankle jerk S1 nerve root. Reflexes are graded according to the following: 0 = absent, 1 = reduced (hypoactive), 2 = normal, 3 = increased (hyperactive), and 4 = clonus. Other reflexes include the plantar response where the sole of the patient's foot is stroked with a blunt and narrow surface object such as the handle of a reflex hammer. A normal response is whenever all toes flex, and it is called a *flexor plantar response;* an abnormal response occurs when the great toe dorsiflexes and the other toes fan out, indicating damage to the upper motor neuron pathways, and is known as the *Babinski sign.* Another indicator of upper motor neuron weakness is Hoffmann sign, elicited by flipping the fingernail of the middle finger, resulting in an involuntary flexion of the interphalangeal joint of the index finger and thumb. In some cases, the abdominal reflexes (T8–T12) and cremasteric reflex (L1–L2) are performed to localize the level of injury. Another key aspect of the spinal exam is the bulbocavernosus reflex (S2–S4), which involves monitoring of the anal sphincter contraction in response to squeezing the glans of the penis or clitoris or tugging on an indwelling Foley catheter. The absence of the bulbocavernosus reflex indicates that the patient is still in spinal shock, and the current examination cannot be interpreted as the real evaluation of neurologic function.

The sensory examination usually consists of pinprick sensation to determine the sensory level, comparing proximal with distal and right/left upper/lower extremities. In some case such as Brown-Sequard syndrome, an extensive sensory examination is required and consists of pain and temperature and vibration and proprioception. A rectal examination is similarly important to assess the sensation of the anal orifice and the contraction of the external anal sphincter. The absence of tone and volitional squeeze of the anal sphincter may indicate SCI. Although a detailed neurologic examination may take time, it localizes and assesses the severity of the SCI before surgical treatment.

The ASIA Impairment Scale categorizes SCI into five main grades: ASIA A, B, C, D, and E. ASIA A represents the most severe injury, denoting a complete injury manifesting in a total loss of motor and sensory function below the level of the injury, with no sensation in the anal and perineal regions (S4–S5). Additionally, there is an increased tendency for urinary retention and bladder distention. *Sacral sparing* is a term that applies to preservation of sacral cord function in the form of intact rectal tone or intact rectal sensation, which is associated with a better prognosis. Fig. 41.6 shows the ASIA score sheet commonly used by spine surgeons.

Incomplete SCI ranges from ASIA B to ASIA D. ASIA B signifies an incomplete injury with preserved sensory function but no motor function below the injury level, with sacral sparing. ASIA C indicates an incomplete injury but includes some motor function below the injury level, with most muscles graded less than 3 on the motor scale. ASIA D is another incomplete injury, but in this case, there is preserved motor function below the injury level, with most muscles graded at 3 or higher. Lastly, ASIA E denotes a normal neurologic status with no deficits, signifying the absence of any SCI. A mnemonic-based way to remember the scale is that ASIA E represents normal motor/sensory function, remembered with the word E = everyone, as most people do not have an SCI. Conversely, ASIA A is such that A = albatross, denoting rarity, that SCI is a rare event.

In the immediate aftermath of a severe SCI, it is important to note the presence of spinal shock, which may mean the current examination cannot be trusted. Spinal shock encompasses complete loss of motor and sensory function below the injury level, along with the absence of deep tendon reflexes and the bulbocavernosus reflex. Particularly, the absence of the bulbocavernosus reflex complicates accurate prognostication during this phase because if a bulbocavernosus reflex is not present, the patient is in shock, and a future neurologic examination may improve beyond the current state. Traditionally, return of the bulbocavernosus reflex has been regarded as an indicator marking the end of spinal

shock. Even in an ASIA A complete injury, a bulbocavernosus reflex should be present, indicating the patient is not in spinal shock.

Spinal shock is inherently transient, and its temporal progression can be delineated by the gradual return of spinal reflexes. The neurologic progress typically commences with the bulbocavernosus reflex, which may reappear as early as 1 hour after the injury. Subsequently, the anal cutaneous reflex and the plantar reflex may also gradually return. It is crucial to differentiate between spinal shock and neurogenic shock, as the latter typically occurs with injuries at cervical and high thoracic vertebral levels (above T6) and is characterized by sympathetic dysfunction, leading to hypotension, hypothermia, and bradycardia. Importantly, the occurrence of these two types of shock is not mutually exclusive, can overlap in individuals with SCI, and can also be challenging to differentiate which exact pattern of shock is present.

Various patterns of SCI can result from different mechanisms of injury. *Central cord syndrome* often occurs in older individuals suffering from hyperextension injury exacerbating preexisting cervical spondylosis or central canal stenosis caused by hypertrophied ligamentum flavum posteriorly or the presence of disc herniations and/or osteophytes anteriorly. The physical examination displays greater motor impairment in the upper extremities, especially the distal aspects, compared with the lower extremities, which aligns with the somatotopy of the arms in the spinal tracts. Central cord syndrome can also lead to bladder dysfunction and varying degrees of sensory loss in the lower body. *Anterior cord syndrome* involves damage to the anterior two-thirds of the spinal cord.[35] It can result from a vascular injury or a direct mechanical injury, such as disc or bone fragment retropulsion. Anterior cord syndrome leads to complete motor paralysis and loss of pain and temperature sensation, but preservation of tactile position and vibration sense. *Brown-Sequard syndrome* occurs because of unilateral damage to the dorsal column, corticospinal tract, and spinothalamic tract. Patients experience ipsilateral weakness and loss of vibration and proprioception, whereas contralateral loss of pain and temperature sensation occurs about two spinal levels below the injury. Common causes include ballistic and penetrating injuries. *Posterior cord syndrome* is a rare condition involving the loss

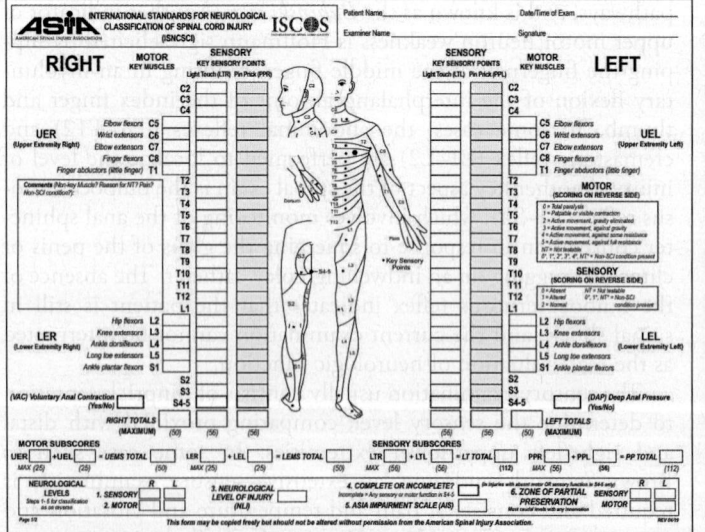

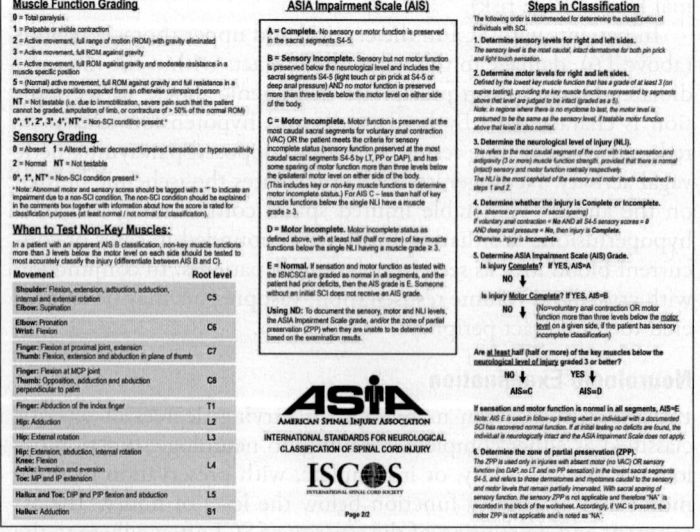

FIGURE 41.6 (A–B) ASIA score sheet.

of function in the posterior column, responsible for deep touch, proprioception, and vibration sensation. Patients can still ambulate but rely heavily on visual input for spatial orientation.

Imaging for Spinal Cord Injury

Imaging plays a pivotal role in the initial assessment of patients with suspected SCI. The selection of the appropriate imaging is contingent on the patient's clinical presentation and the accessibility of imaging resources at the trauma center. CT and MRI are currently the most used after the initial phase of the injury.[36]

CT is usually used as the primary imaging modality, which provides a detailed visualization of the osseous anatomy and associated fractures, traumatic disc herniations, and epidural/subdural hematomas in the spinal canal. CT has a sensitivity of 97% to 100% in identifying cervical spine fractures compared with standard lateral x-rays, which have a sensitivity of only 63%. In thoracolumbar trauma, CT was associated with sensitivity ranging from 78.1% to 100%; x-rays had sensitivity of 32% to 74%. However, CT imaging is not without problems. Concerns for a significant radiation exposure as well as artifacts from image acquisition in the setting of instrumentation from previous spine fusion can occur.

The gold standard of imaging in evaluating patients with SCI remains the MRI, which provides visualization of the spinal cord and neural elements. Through its multiplanar capabilities, MRI offers useful information regarding spinal cord compression, ligamentous injuries, disc herniation, spinal cord contusions, hemorrhage, swelling, and cord edema as well as injuries to the paraspinal tissues. The T2 sequence is the most often used, given the clear ability to see hyperintense CSF surrounded by a hypointense spinal cord. One downside of MRI includes time taken to acquire imaging. Constant communication of the MRI technician with the radiologist and spine surgeon is recommended to ensure the efficient acquisition of these images. MRI is also contraindicated in the presence of cardiac pacemaker and metallic foreign bodies.

Other less studied images in the setting of SCI include MRI protocols including diffusion-weighted imaging (DWI), functional MRI, and perfusion MRI, all of which were reportedly used to assess for the extent of the SCI. When MRI is unavailable, CT myelography with intrathecal soluble contrast injection can be used when a compromise of the spinal canal is suspected. In the setting of cardiac stents, shrapnel, or spinal implants with heavy artifact, an emergent CT myelogram is necessary to visualize the neural elements.

Traction

In the setting of an SCI with spinal cord compression, the primary objective is to take pressure off the cord, which can sometimes be accomplished with closed reduction and cervical traction. In hospitals without spine surgery capabilities or resource-poor settings where emergent surgery is not possible, traction can open up the spinal canal just as effectively as an open, direct surgical decompression. In most cases, surgery is still needed after successful closed reduction for stabilization reasons. Although thoracic and lumbar fractures do not typically respond to traction, patients with cervical spine subluxation through perched facets may benefit from closed reduction techniques. However, there are also some important contraindications, as traction is not safe in everyone and can also cause or worsen an SCI, such as more proximal fractures, AS, diffuse idiopathic skeletal hyperostosis (DISH), fracture patterns with retropulsed bone,

and the presence of a herniated disc. Consultation with a spine surgeon is necessary to decide if traction is safe. Importantly, the patient must be awake to comply with examinations to closely monitor any new symptoms or neurologic deficits.

Traction involves employing longitudinal forces using either skull tongs or a halo headpiece cranially to reduce a fracture or perched/locked facets. Initially, a force of 5 to 15 pounds is applied, and this force is gradually increased in 5-pound increments, with lateral radiographs taken after each increment. For dislocations located more toward the upper part of the spine, less force is used, typically around 3 to 5 pounds per vertebral level. After weight is added, the patient is assessed for a complete neurologic examination to ensure no deterioration. After each weight is incrementally added, patients should get an x-ray and serial examinations until the limit is reached. Additionally, the administration of a muscle relaxant, analgesia, and/or sedation may facilitate the reduction process. An attentive neurologic examination is the gold standard for monitoring any impediment on the spinal cord. Once reduction is achieved, weight can be decreased to maintain the reduction.

Time to Surgery and Recovery

Timely access to decompressive surgery and early rehabilitation has suggested improvement in patient outcomes. The Surgical Timing in Acute Spinal Cord Injury Study found that performing decompressive surgery within the first 24 hours after SCI was associated with improved neurologic recovery, defined as achieving at least a two-grade advancement on the ASIA scale at 6-month follow-up.[37] Whether patients have an SCI or fracture with no damage to the SCI, stabilizing unstable fractures urgently is critical to continuing their ongoing care after trauma. Although important differences exist between high- and low-income countries with regard to available resources to provide timely intervention,[38] delays in surgical intervention can give rise to various nonneurologic complications associated with immobilization, such as pressure ulcers, deep venous thrombosis, pulmonary embolism, and pneumonia.

Although some studies have not witnessed any improvement in ASIA A patients after surgical treatment, recent data show that after at least 6-months of postoperative follow-up, as many as 20% of patients tend to have gradual neurologic recovery to a less severe ASIA grade.[39] Given prior studies showing the potential for improvement in select ASIA A patients, even patients with complete SCI may be taken to the operating room urgently at our center. Though this may not be necessary for all forms of SCI, it is worth a discussion between the trauma team and the spine surgeons.

Role of Steroids in Spinal Cord Injury

Despite some of the older randomized control trials indicating benefit,[40] the use of steroids in traumatic SCI has largely fallen out of favor and phased out of practice. The risks of high-dose glucocorticoid therapy, such as pneumonia, sepsis, gastrointestinal bleeding, wound infection, and diabetic ketoacidosis, are felt to outweigh its benefit in the injured patient.

Pediatric Spinal Cord Injury

Just as in adults, SCI in pediatric patients requires timely intervention, with some subtle differences. These injuries can occur at various levels along the spine, with the cervical spine being the most prone to injury (55%), followed by the thoracic spine (15%), the thoracolumbar junction (15%), and the lumbosacral region (15%). In adults, the most common cause of SCI is traumatic injuries, whereas in children, nontraumatic causes are more common. The most common nontraumatic causes of pediatric SCIs include congenital anomalies, spinal cord tumors, infections, and vascular malformations. The primary causes of traumatic SCI in children are diverse, with blunt trauma being the most common etiology related to motor vehicle accidents, falls, and sports-related injuries.

Distinct anatomy differentiates children's from adults' spines because children's vertebrae are incompletely ossified and their ligaments are firmly attached to articular bone surfaces that are more horizontal than in adults. In particular, younger children may have incomplete ossification of the odontoid process extending from the C2 level, along with a relatively large head and weaker neck muscles, which increases the risk of spinal instability compared with adults. This unique anatomic feature increases risk of SCI, without a fracture or radiographic abnormality in children under 8 years of age, as spinal elements may shift rather than break when subjected to force. A high index of suspicion is needed, and in the setting of a high-energy mechanism without fracture, close inspection of soft tissues for prevertebral edema in the cervical spine on CT imaging can trigger an MRI. A lower threshold for MRI in kids is advised to avoid missing unstable ligamentous injuries.

Traumatic Spinal Emergencies
Craniocervical Junction, C1, and C2 Injuries

Atlantooccipital dissociation (AOD) results from disruption of the craniocervical junction from ligamentous injury. These injuries are twice as common in pediatrics compared with adults, likely owing to higher cranium-to-body ratio and increased ligamentous laxity.[41] Clinical symptoms range from minimal neurologic deficit, given the spinal canal is often wide at the craniocervical junction, to severe upper cervical cord or brainstem damage from stretch injury to the neural elements. The Traynelis classification for AOD categorizes injuries based on the occipital condyle position in relation to atlas, distinguishing between three types: type I denotes anterior displacement, type II signifies distraction or inferior displacement, and type III represents posterior displacement.[42] Type II is the most dangerous, as the spinal cord does not tolerate stretch well.

Several radiographic methodologies can be used to diagnose AOD, with CT scan measurements having higher sensitivity and specificity compared with plain radiographs. One CT measurement assesses the occipital condyle to C1 distance, which should be 1 to 2 mm in adults (Fig. 41.7).[43] This distance is measured on each side, and if it is >2 mm or if any asymmetry exists, an MRI should be obtained. Other measurements include a basiondental interval (BDI), atlantooccipital interval, and the Powers ratio. Other imaging findings like craniocervical subarachnoid hemorrhage may be a marker of concomitant craniocervical junction instability.

Initial management for a patient in which AOD is suspected is immediate immobilization of the neck with halo or sandbags. AOD is a hard contraindication for traction. Surgical treatment with occipitocervical fusion is indicated. An example of AOD is illustrated in Fig. 41.8.

Occipital condyle fractures are often diagnosed on CT and are rarely surgical in isolation. Type I occurs from axial loading and results in comminuted fractures, type II is an extension of linear basilar skull fractures, and type III is an avulsion fracture of condyle fragment resulting from traction during rotation or lateral bending mechanisms. Almost all of these fractures can be managed in rigid cervical collar and radiographic follow-up in the absence of other cervical fractures.[44]

C1 fractures, or atlas fractures, were described by Sir Geoffrey Jefferson in 1920 and most commonly occur from axial loading resulting in fractures through the C1 arches, which are the thinnest part of the C1 vertebrae. Type I Jefferson fractures involve the posterior arch alone, type II fractures involve the anterior arch alone, type III fractures involve both the anterior and posterior arch, and type IV fractures involve the lateral mass. Clinical findings can include neck pain and associated vertebral artery dissections; however, neurologic deficits are rare with isolated C1 fractures because of the large diameter of the canal at this level. Stability at this level is primarily provided by ligaments, and therefore, integrity of the transverse ligament on MRI is the most important determinant of stability in C1 fractures and suitability for rigid cervical collar and follow-up. In some cases where the C1 lateral mass is fractured, if not stabilized, a cock-robin rotational deformity can ensue, where the lateral mass collapses on one side and the occipital condyle rests on the superior facet of C2. These patients may be treated with C1 open reduction and internal fixation (ORIF). Additionally, C1/2 ligamentous injuries can also present, with or without fractures of C1. A widened C1/2 joint distance can be seen, along with a widened atlantodental interval (ADI) of >3 mm.

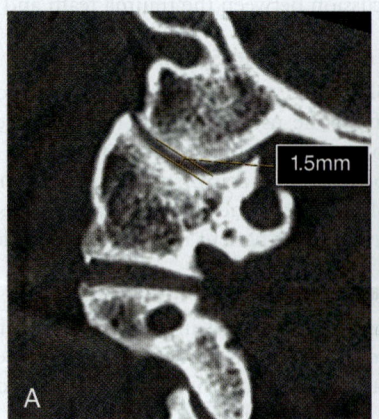
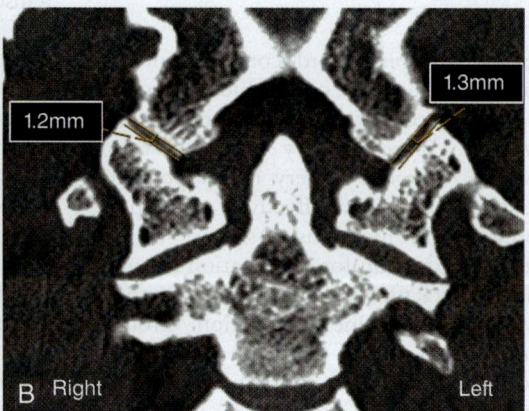

FIGURE 41.7 Example of normal occipital condyle to C1 distance <2 mm as measured on sagittal (A) and coronal (B) computed tomography scan.

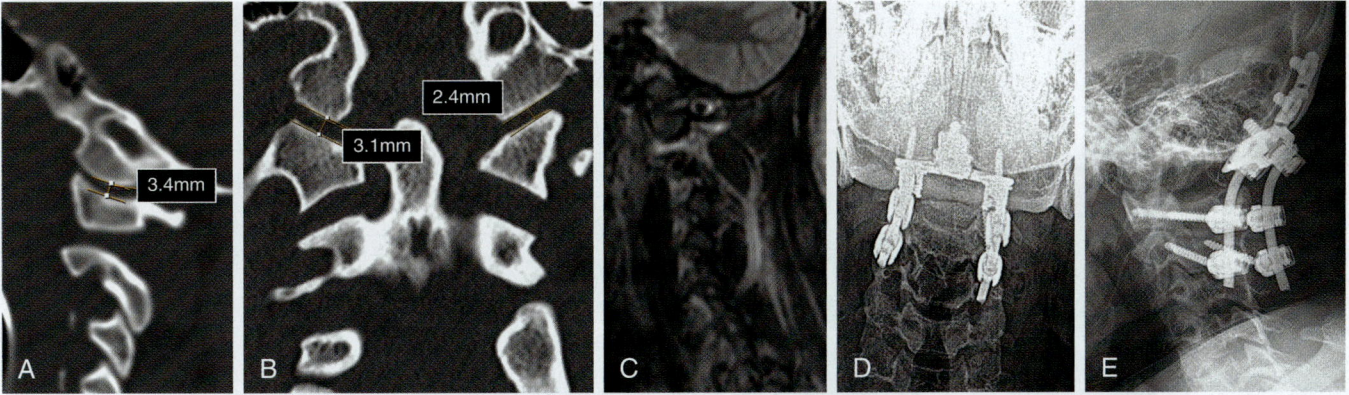

FIGURE 41.8 (A–E) Atlantooccipital dissociation on sagittal (A) and coronal (B) seen on computed tomography scan and hyperintensity within the C1–C2 facet seen on parasagittal magnetic resonance imaging (C). The patient underwent occiput-C2 fusion, seen on postoperative anteroposterior (D) and lateral x-ray (E).

C2 fractures, or axis fractures, can be classified as hangman's fractures, odontoid fractures, or a combination of both. As evident by the name, hangman's fractures occur from hyperextension and axial loading resulting in bilateral fracture though the pars interarticularis of C2. The majority of hangman's fractures can be managed with rigid cervical collar or halo immobilization. Levine and Edwards classification and the Effendi classification are commonly used to classify C2 fractures. An MRI should be obtained in cases of anterior subluxation of C2 on C3 >3 mm or severe C2 on C3 angulation, which can be a surrogate for C2–C3 disc and posterior longitudinal ligament disruption. Overall, spondylolisthesis of C2 on C3 of >6 mm, severe angulation of C2 flexed forward on top of C3 of more than 12 degrees, and damage to the C2/3 disc may warrant surgical stabilization. Odontoid fractures comprise 10% to 15% of all cervical spine fractures, and flexion is the most common mechanism of injury.[45] The Anderson and D'Alonzo classification system is the most widely used and best applied using coronal CT. Type I fractures involve the tip of the odontoid resulting from traction on the alar ligament, type II fractures involve the base of the odontoid, and type III fractures extend through the vertebral body. There is level II evidence that type II odontoid fractures in adults >50 years of age should be considered for surgical stabilization and fusion given higher rates of nonunion. The reason for higher nonunion rates in type II fractures is that the osseous dens has limited

cancellous bone and blood supply, making healing a challenge. Nondisplaced type I to III odontoid fractures are initially managed with rigid cervical collar and immobilization. Surgical fixation is typically considered for dens displacement >5 mm, comminuted fractures, or failure to achieve alignment with external immobilization. Miscellaneous C2 fractures such as those involving the spinous process, lamina, facets, and lateral mass may be treated with rigid cervical immobilization with cervical collar or halo. Examples of hangman's and dens fracture are presented in Fig. 41.9.

Overall, many fractures of the occipital-C2 region are not emergencies and can be treated with cervical collars. However, the ones that require immediate attention are AOD, C1/2 instability, and certain hangman's or odontoid fractures. Any AOD finding, hangman's fracture that meets operative criteria as mentioned earlier, and severely displaced type II odontoid fractures are the ones to be most concerned about.

Cervical Teardrop Fractures

Teardrop fractures are flexion/compression injuries to the cervical spine and often lead to retropulsion, canal compromise, and SCI. Hyperflexion injuries can also result in fracture of the anterior inferior edge of the vertebral body, which is termed a *teardrop fracture*. Ultimately, MRI is necessary to assess the integrity of the disc and posterior ligaments to differentiate teardrop fractures

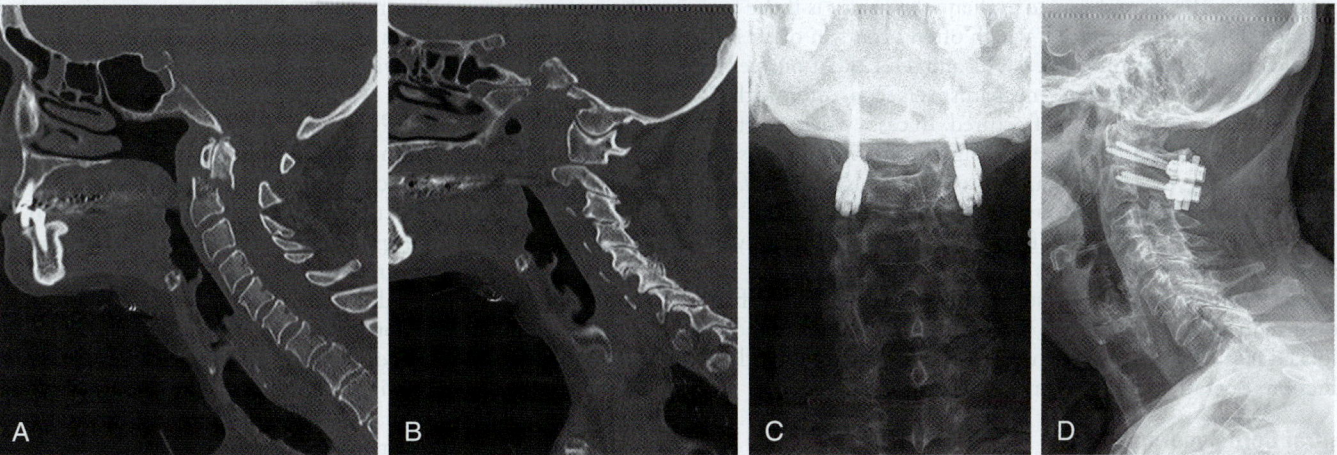

FIGURE 41.9 (A–D) Posteriorly displaced dens fracture (A) and hangman's fracture (B) on sagittal computed tomography scan. Patient underwent C1–C2 posterior fusion, as seen on postoperative anteroposterior (C) and lateral (D) x-ray.

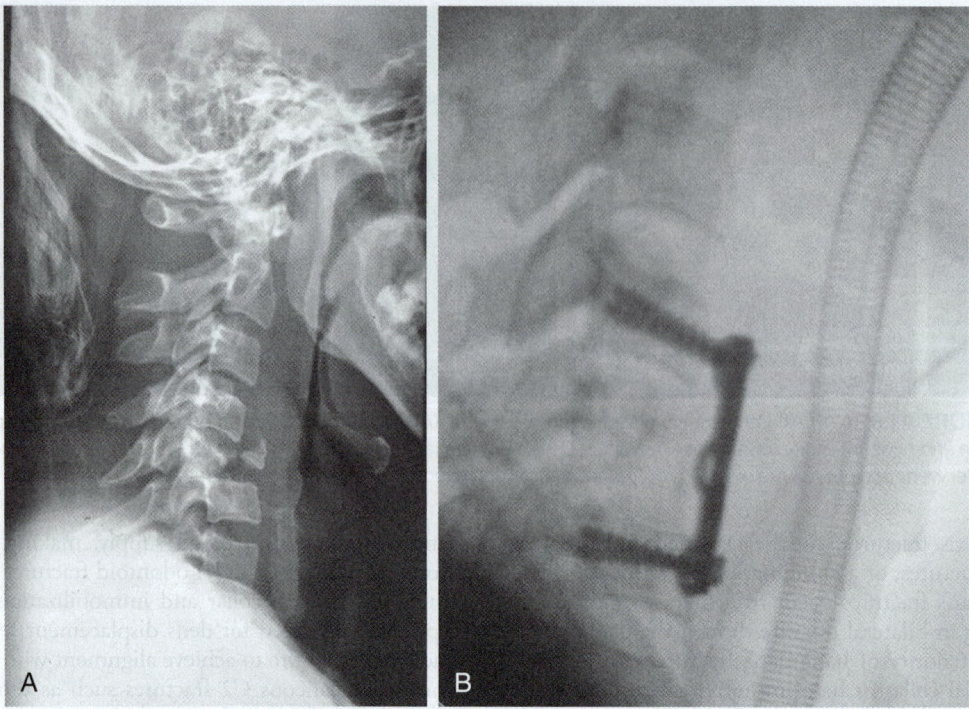

FIGURE 41.10 Teardrop fracture dislocation on lateral x-ray (A) in a resource-poor, low- to middle-income country. Although this fracture is usually treated by an anteroposterior approach, only anterior cervical corpectomy and fusion were performed using iliac crest autograft, as seen on postoperative lateral x-ray (B).

from spine avulsion fractures, the latter of which can be treated with rigid collar and repeat radiographs. Importantly, a teardrop fracture must be differentiated from an anterior osteophyte fracture. The former is a highly unstable injury, whereas an anterior osteophyte fracture is minor and only needs a collar. An example of a teardrop fracture is presented in Fig. 41.10.

Perched or Locked Cervical Facets

Severe flexion injuries can also result in locked, or "jumped," facets, which involves disruption of the facet capsule. These injuries can best be classified in two ways. First, the injury is assessed to be unilateral or bilateral. Unilateral perched/locked/fractured facets usually result in an isolated radiculopathy, whereas bilateral perched/locked/fractured facets can often lead to SCI given the canal stenosis. The second way to evaluate the injury is if the facet is perched, locked, or fractured, which often occurs in older individuals with degeneration (Figs. 41.11 and 41.12). At our center, some combination of the three mechanisms is seen, often with the superior articular process being fractured. In cases where facets are not completely locked but have had significant ligamentous disruption resulting in distraction, the term used is *perched facets*. Typically, unilateral locked facets result from flexion and rotation injury, whereas bilateral locked facets typically result from hyperflexion only, with simultaneous disruption of the posterior ligamentous complex, and may result in SCI or nerve root deficits. Closed reduction with traction is employed for closed reduction of locked facets, which also opens up the spinal canal. After closed reduction, operative stabilization is often required.

Central Cord Syndrome

Central cord syndrome was originally described by Schneider and colleagues in 1954 and is the most common type of incomplete SCI. Central cord syndrome is most commonly seen in the adult

trauma population after acute hyperextension injury in the setting of preexisting spinal stenosis from bony hypertrophy, redundant ligamentum flavum, or superimposed on congenital spinal stenosis. Injury can also be associated with cervical fracture or dislocation, acute traumatic disc herniation, or listhesis of one vertebra on another. Long tract cervical fibers passing through the cervical spinal cord are more medial and in the centermost vascular watershed zone, rendering them more susceptible to injury. Therefore, patients classically present with upper extremity weakness greater than lower extremity with varying degrees of sensory disturbances. Severe hyperesthesia, where patients are extremely sensitive to touch (allodynia and hyperalgesia) is common. MRI can detect T2 changes that may show spinal cord edema acutely. Initial management as previously described is recommended, and if there is ongoing cord compression, emergent surgery is needed. If the cord bruising is seen without significant compression, these patients can be treated without surgery.[46]

Thoracic/Lumbar Injuries and Burst Fractures

The Denis three-column model of the spine helps identify unstable thoracolumbar fractures with good predictive value. Minor injuries involve only part of a column and do not lead to acute instability and include spinous process fractures, transverse process fractures, pars fractures, and isolated laminar fractures. These minor injuries typically do not require intervention and may not require spine surgery consultation given local practice patterns and institutional protocols. However, thoracic/lumbar fractures in the setting of underlying AS and DISH may be highly unstable and warrant immediate immobilization and surgical evaluation. The thoracolumbar injury classification and severity score (TLICS) is a helpful tool for triaging when surgical intervention may be warranted and comprises three categories that include the morphology of injury (compression fracture, burst fracture,

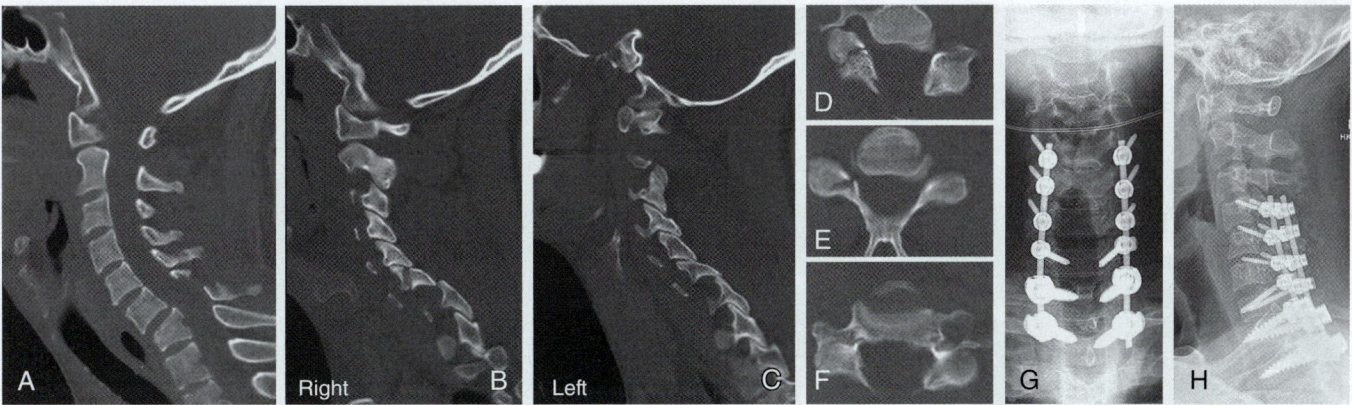

FIGURE 41.11 (A–H) C6 fracture dislocation on sagittal computed tomography (CT) (A), with right-sided jumped facet on right parasagittal CT (B), perched facet on left parasagittal CT (C), and right lateral mass fractures on axial CT scan (D–F). Patient underwent C4–T2 posterior fusion with restoration of normal alignment, as seen on postoperative anteroposterior (G) and lateral (H) x-ray.

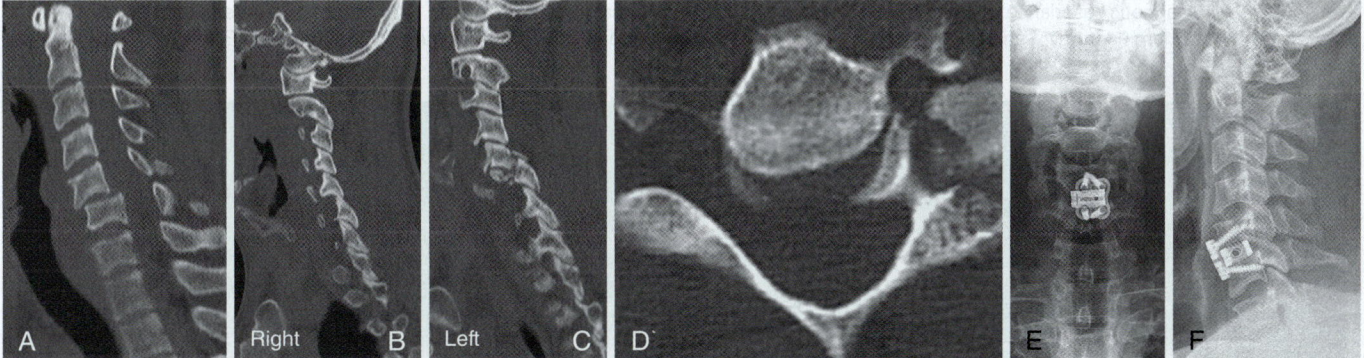

FIGURE 41.12 (A–F) C5–C6 fracture dislocation (A), with right normal alignment (B), left jumped facet on sagittal computed tomography (CT) (C), and left lateral mass fracture on axial CT (D). Patient underwent C5–C6 anterior cervical discectomy and fusion, as seen on postoperative anteroposterior (E) and lateral (F) x-ray.

distraction injury, and translational/rotational injury), neurologic status (intact, root injury, complete SCI, incomplete SCI, and cauda equina syndrome [CES]), and posterior ligamentous disruption. A TLICS of ≤3 is usually managed nonoperatively, whereas TLICS >4 is a candidate for surgery.[47]

Burst fractures typically occur because of axial loading accompanied by a bending moment resulting in an implosion of a vertebra, often causing a failure of the anterior and middle vertebral columns. Although conservative treatment can be used with bracing, close follow-up is needed to make sure the fracture is not progressing into more collapse or more kyphosis. Surgical intervention is often indicated if there is observable evidence of increasing angular deformity and the presence of spinal cord or cauda equina compression. Individuals exhibiting more than 30 degrees of angulation, greater than a 50% loss of vertebral body height, and neurologic symptoms should be considered candidates for surgical stabilization. An example of a burst fracture is illustrated in Fig. 41.13.

Chance Fractures and Flexion-Extension Injuries

Flexion-extension injuries encompass a broader range of spinal injuries resulting from sudden forward and backward movements of the spine, often in the midthoracic area where seatbelts are worn. A severe type of flexion-extension injury is represented by chance fracture, an unstable type of spine fracture. It is

characterized by a horizontal break that spans from the posterior to the anterior aspect of the spinal column, traversing the spinous process, pedicles, and vertebral body.[48] Identifying chance fractures during a clinical examination can be challenging because patients seldom exhibit neurologic deficits. As stated, a seatbelt sign is a common finding on the physical examination, and accompanying intraabdominal injuries can be present in as high as 50% of cases, such as bowel or bladder rupture.[48] Current literature predominantly supports surgical treatment given the inherently unstable nature of this fracture and the disruption of ligaments. Examples of a chance fracture and flexion-extension injury are illustrated in Fig. 41.14.

Fracture Dislocation

Dislocations of the thoracic and lumbar vertebrae typically occur as a consequence of exceptionally high-energy trauma.[49] They result from the simultaneous application of multidirectional forces, combining both distracting and compressive elements across different spinal components. Consequently, these forces lead to the development of translational and rotational instability within the spinal column, often accompanied by associated fractures. Because of the instability resulting from posterior facet dislocation, treatment is often surgical and includes an open reduction with posterior fusion.[49] An example of fracture dislocation is illustrated in Fig. 41.15.

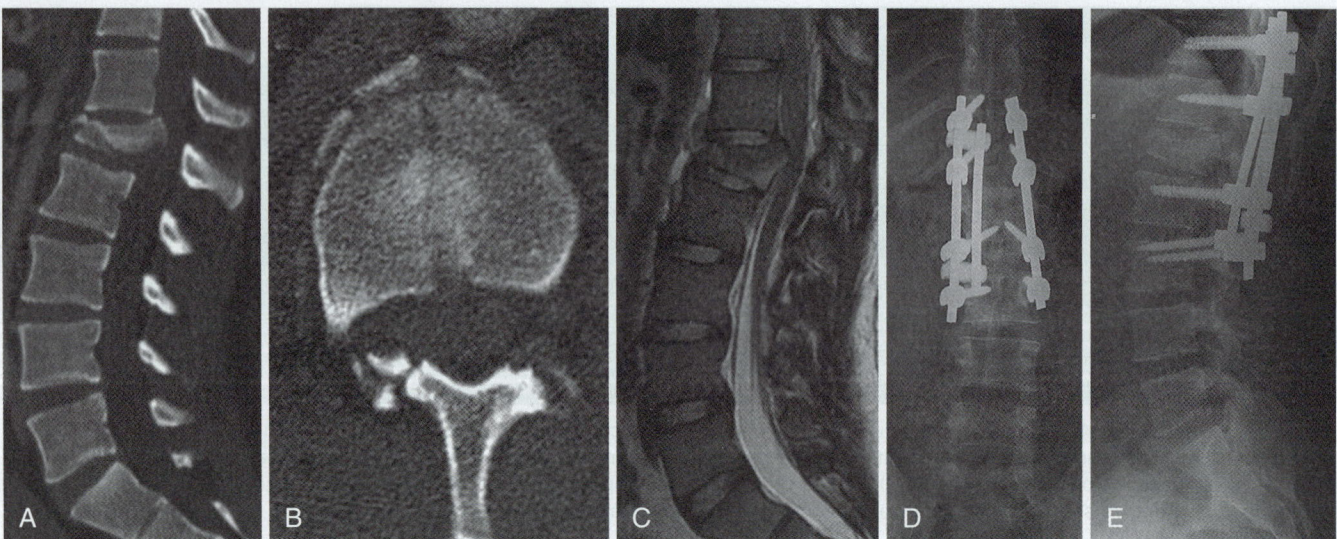

FIGURE 41.13 (A–E) Burst fracture of L1 on sagittal (A) and axial (B) seen on computed tomography scan. Magnetic resonance imaging showed canal stenosis and thecal sac compression (C). The patient underwent L1 laminectomy with T11–L3 posterior fusion, as seen on postoperative anteroposterior (D) and lateral (E) x-ray.

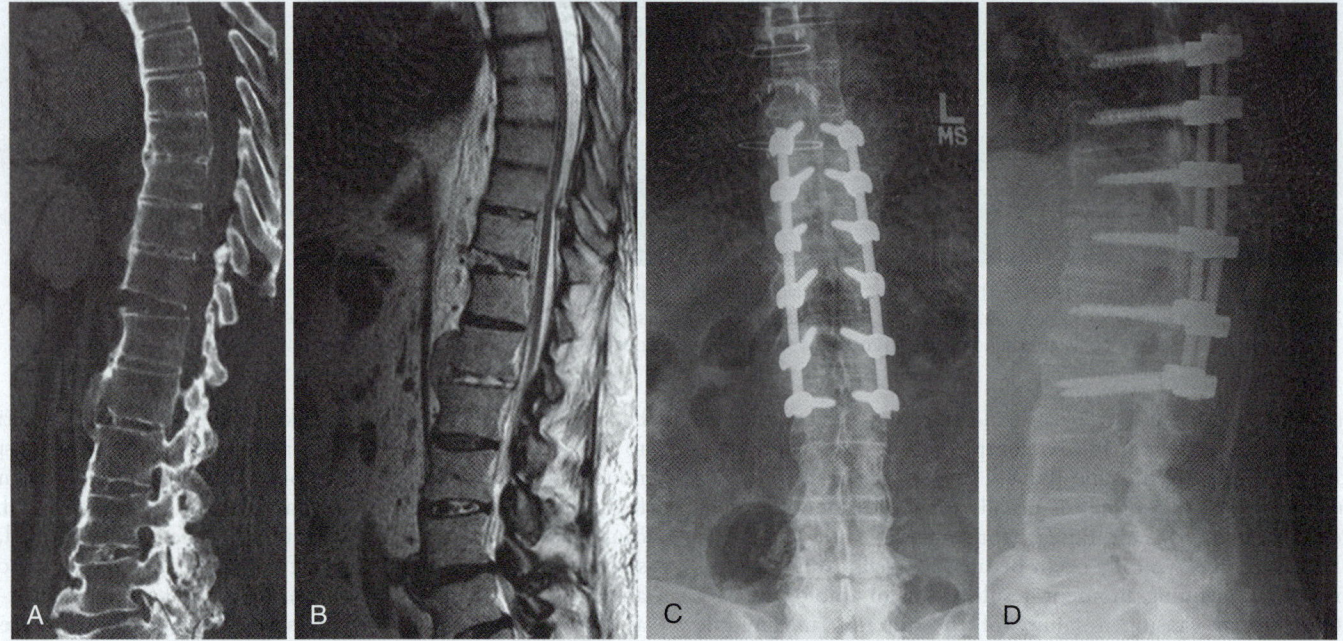

FIGURE 41.14 (A–D) Three-column T11–T12 extension injury with widening of the disc space anteriorly and extension of fracture through the posterior elements of T11 as shown on sagittal computed tomography scan (A) and T2 magnetic resonance imaging (B). The patient underwent T9–L2 posterior fusion, as seen on postoperative anteroposterior (C) and lateral (D) x-rays.

Nontraumatic Spinal Emergencies

Spinal emergencies can occur in the nontraumatic setting as well. In this section, we cover CES, spinal tumors, spinal vascular malformations, and spine infections.

Cauda Equina Syndrome

Cauda equina comes from Latin for *horse tail* because of the appearance of the nerves dangling within the thecal sac. When these nerves are compressed, a classic series of symptoms termed *cauda equina syndrome* can be seen, thought to be the result of a combination of mechanical and ischemic changes. A classic trio of symptoms includes bilateral lower extremity weakness and decreased sensation, loss of bowel/bladder function, and saddle anesthesia. It is rare to see all three symptoms at once, whereas in reality, CES presents incompletely with some symptoms, such as urinary hesitancy, groin numbness, and slight pain/weakness.

In the setting of an acute disc rupture, approximately 1% to 3% of patients will develop CES, and 45% of cauda equina cases are attributable to a lumbar disc herniation. When the cause of CES is a disc rupture, these patients are often younger with large, well-hydrated discs that can herniate, compared with an older population that suffers from lumbar stenosis. Other etiologies

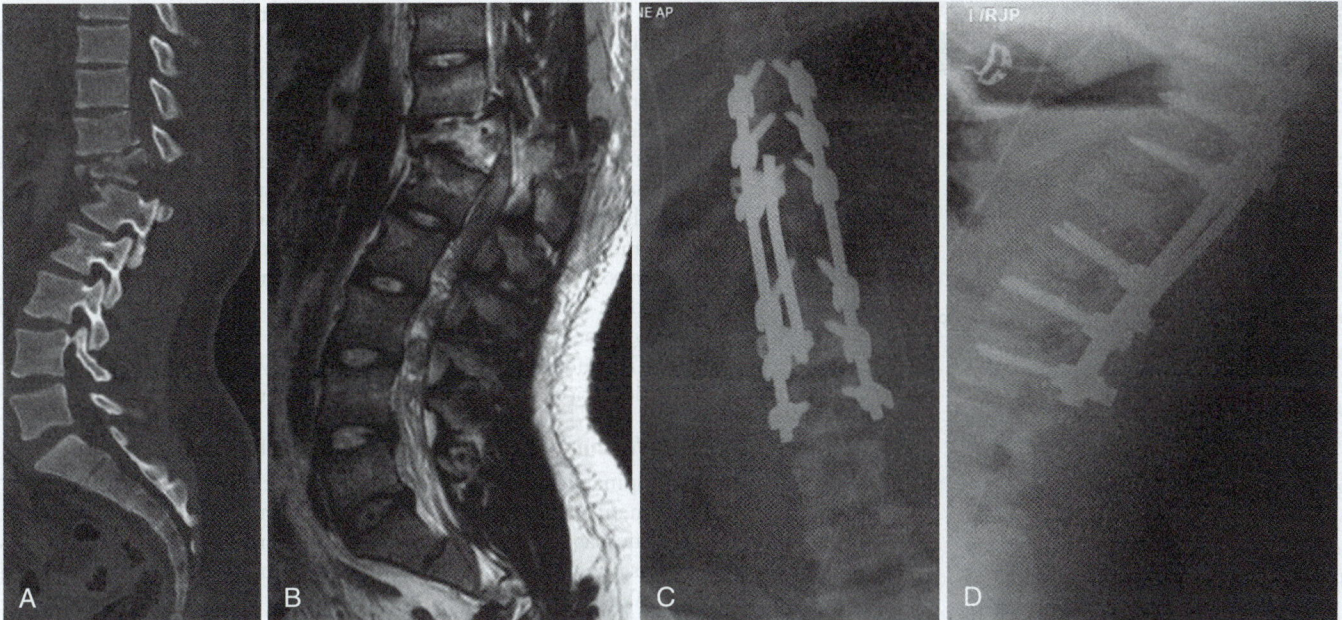

FIGURE 41.15 (A–D) Sagittal computed tomography scan showing fracture dislocation of T12 vertebra (A). Magnetic resonance imaging showed severe spinal cord compression (B). The patient underwent T9–L3 posterior fusion with a significant improvement of alignment, as seen on postoperative anteroposterior (C) and lateral (D) x-ray.

that may lead to CES include infection, symptomatic stenosis, hematoma, trauma, tumor, vascular abnormalities, or iatrogenic causes.

When evaluating a patient with concern for CES, a thorough and accurate physical examination, including a digital rectal examination, is essential. Bowel and bladder dysfunction are mainly due to disruption of the parasympathetic and sympathetic nerve function. Bilateral lower extremity weakness and saddle anesthesia also originate from compression of their corresponding nerves. Patients may also have decreased reflexes, and symptoms often start slowly but reach a critical threshold where patients become acutely symptomatic or their symptoms become progressive enough to warrant treatment. It is important to assess reflexes and muscle strength in the lower extremities, conduct a digital rectal examination to assess anal tone, and evaluate for any numbness in the perineal region. If a patient presents with these symptoms, an emergent MRI of the lumbar spine is of the utmost importance as this will drive surgical decision-making. If the patient is unable to undergo MRI because of contraindication, an emergent CT myelogram of the thoracic or lumbar spine should be obtained. To assess bladder function, an ultrasound bladder scan or catheterization should be performed to obtain a postvoid residual value. Patients may or may not have pain related to their CES depending on the acuity and severity of compression. If the MRI or CT myelogram shows evidence of compression of the cauda equina, spine surgery should be contacted immediately to determine need for emergent decompression.

Surgical management includes decompression of the cauda equina by laminectomy as well as removal of the offending lesion (e.g., disc herniation, infection). Although the quality of literature regarding timing of decompression in CES is poor, the recommendation is to take the patient to the operating room within the first 48 hours of symptom onset. Given the often unclear timeline of symptoms, emergent decompression within hours is often pursued. Studies suggest that as many as 85% of patients will return

to their previous baseline, including bowel/bladder function and motor function, within 1 year after decompression. Reiterating the importance of timing, despite loose recommendations of timing, these injuries are best dealt with immediately, within hours of presentation.

Although CES is uncommon compared with many other spinal pathologies that are seen, incorrect evaluation, diagnosis, and management can result in severe neurologic impairment and have a devastating impact on a patient's quality of life.

Spinal Tumors

Metastatic spinal lesions are the most common spinal tumors and are seen in more than 20,000 people per year in the United States. Up to 14% of all cancer patients have metastatic spinal involvement. In addition, primary spinal tumors (PSTs) affect 2.5 to 8.5 people per 100,000 per year. Metastatic tumors most commonly cause cord compression and myelopathy, leading to an indolent onset of pain, weakness, numbness, balance deficits, urinary issues, hyperreflexia, and, in severe cases, weakness.

A full discussion of spinal tumor management is outside the scope of this chapter; however, we mention several key aspects of management. As noted earlier, a detailed neurologic examination is required. Additionally, imaging of the neural elements, most often an MRI with and without contrast, is needed, in addition to CT of the chest, abdomen, and pelvis to assess for bone quality and any other primary tumor source. Additionally, lesions that affect bony or ligamentous components of the spine can lead to inherent instability of the spine, which increases risk of neurologic deficit caused by secondary injury of neural elements. A score that is used to assess stability of the spine is the Spinal Instability in Neoplastic disease Score (SINS) (Table 41.6).[50] The SINS was created for nonspine surgeons, such as oncologists and radiologists, to recognize unstable fractures, and using it can be an important tool in knowing who needs urgent/emergent evaluation. A SINS of 0 to 6 receives a

TABLE 41.6 Spinal Instability Neoplastic Score (SINS)

ELEMENTS OF SINS	SCORE
Location	
Junctional (occiput–C2, C7–T2, T11–L1, L5–S1)	3
Mobile spine (C3–C6, L2–L4)	2
Semirigid (T3–T10)	1
Rigid (S2–S5)	0
Pain Relief With Recumbency and/or Pain With Movement/Loading of the Spine	
Yes	3
No (occasional pain but not mechanical)	1
Pain-free lesion	0
Bone Lesion	
Lytic	2
Mixed (lytic/blastic)	1
Blastic	0
Radiographic Spinal Alignment	
Subluxation/translation present	4
De novo deformity (kyphosis/scoliosis)	2
Normal alignment	0
Vertebral Body Collapse	
>50% collapse	3
<50% collapse	2
No collapse with >50% body involved	1
None of the above	0
Posterolateral Involvement of the Spinal Elements (Facet, Pedicle or CV Joint Fracture, or Replacement With Tumor)	
Bilateral	3
Unilateral	1
None of the above	0

CV, Costovertebral.

"stable" designation, 7 to 12 receives an intermediate designation, and 13 to 18 is designated "unstable." Surgical consultation is recommended for patients with a SINS score of 7 or higher, which serves as a valuable tool for both surgeons and nonsurgeons to assess stability of the spine. If an unstable lesion is encountered, keep the patient in strict spine precautions until a spine surgeon can assess the patient.

From a surgical perspective, there are three main reasons to perform surgery: curative resection of a primary spinal malignancy, relieve cord compression and neurologic deficit, or stabilize an unstable spine. In patients presenting with neurologic deficits secondary to compression of neural elements, the goal of surgery is to decompress those elements and maintain normal function or allow the patient the best opportunity for return of function. In patients with spinal cord compression from spinal metastases, studies have shown that decompressing the spinal cord improves ability to walk, among other outcomes.[50] Another goal of decompressing the spinal cord allows for the creation of a margin to optimize radiosurgery planning to allow for higher doses to the entire lesion while protecting the spinal cord, known as *separation surgery*.

Intradural spinal tumors, both extramedullary and intramedullary tumors, account for less than 5% of all CNS tumors. The most common presentation is nocturnal back and leg pain, when endogenous steroids have worn off, and the presence of neurologic deficits becomes apparent. Examples of intradural extramedullary tumors include meningiomas, nerve sheath tumors, and schwannomas. Intramedullary tumors are most commonly gliomas, including ependymomas (most common in adults), astrocytomas (most common in pediatric populations), and oligodendrogliomas. When first encountered in an emergency setting with neurologic deficit, after consultation with a neurosurgeon, optimizing cord perfusion and starting steroids is the best initial management. Treatment for these lesions is typically surgical resection with consideration of radiation and chemotherapy as indicated.

Vascular Malformations and Spine Infections

Spinal vascular malformations are the result of abnormal development of blood vessels of the spine and include neoplastic lesions such as hemangioblastomas and cavernous malformations as well as benign lesions such as dural arteriovenous fistulas (dAVFs) and AVMs.

Patients will typically present in an acute manner, if there was hemorrhage, or in a chronic fashion, often secondary to venous hypertension, cord ischemia, or mass effect. Patients endorse symptoms of myelopathy including lower extremity weakness, decreased sensation, and bowel or bladder incontinence. A vascular etiology should also be suspected if the patient has a series of acute neurologic deficits after each other, consistent with a stepwise decline, which can often be seen because of episodic venous congestion and hypertension leading to hypoperfusion.

After presentation, lesions are most frequently diagnosed on MRI or magnetic resonance angiography (MRA) of the spine. Scans typically show T2 hyperintensity secondary to surrounding edema or venous congestion at the level of the lesion. CT angiography (CTA) is feasible as a diagnostic modality when MRI is not available. The gold standard of evaluation for these lesions is spinal angiography, which not only allows for characterization of the lesion itself but also an assessment of the dynamic inflow and outflow of blood within the lesion.

Treatment options include use of endovascular technology to occlude the inflow and/or outflow of the lesion, thus decreasing or obliterating the lesion. In cases planned for open surgical resection, preoperative embolization can minimize blood loss and simplify the procedure. In select patients, radiosurgical treatment may be used, but the data regarding this intervention are minimal and of poor quality.

Infection

Spine infections account for 2% to 7% of all musculoskeletal infections. The infection may involve the vertebral body or disc or create an abscess within the spinal canal. Multiple locations are often seen at the time of diagnosis as there is often a nonspecific and indolent nature to the presentation. Patients present with systemic infectious symptoms as well as back pain or neurologic deficit. Neurologic deficits are secondary to compression from an epidural abscess or a pathologic fracture.

Workup for these patients includes laboratory studies (complete blood count and basic metabolic panel, erythrocyte sedimentation rate, C-reactive protein, and blood cultures) to assess for signs of infection. Blood cultures and urine cultures should be obtained before initiation of any antibiotics to allow for possible identification of the causative microbe.

Involvement of the spine is often found by CT scan, which will show evidence of bony changes secondary to chronic inflammatory responses and osteomyelitis; however, CT scans may be negative in the setting of an isolated abscess without osteomyelitis. These patients usually undergo an MRI, which allows for further classification of the infection regarding surrounding tissues as well as the spinal canal. The most common causative agents are bacterial and fungal infections. *Staphylococcus aureus* accounts for as much as 80% of these infections. *Escherichia coli* is another common bacterium causing these infections.

In patients with no sign of instability, evidence of neurologic deficits, or spinal cord compression, a CT-guided biopsy is recommended, if safe, to narrow antibiotic coverage. If the patient presents with acute-onset neurologic deficits and is found to have a compressive epidural abscess, emergent surgical intervention is warranted to decompress the neurologic structures and optimize the patient's overall recovery. In these cases, no CT-guided biopsy is needed as intraoperative cultures can be obtained for diagnostic purposes.

Once a sample is obtained, the patient is started on broad-spectrum antibiotics until culture results finalize, including sensitivities, to allow for targeted antimicrobial therapy. Antibiotic regimen and course are guided by the causative agent. Appropriate management of this pathology typically requires a multidisciplinary team including infectious disease, interventional radiology, and spine surgery.

Summary of Spine Emergencies

Time plays a decisive role in managing traumatic SCI, and swift recognition by neurologic examination and imaging is the cornerstone to diagnosis and treatment. Furthermore, the importance of spinal cord perfusion and consideration of MAP goals on presentation is helpful in almost any type of SCI, particularly for the acute care surgeons who are the first to triage these injuries. Simply put, surgical treatment often comes in the form of decompressing compressed neural elements and stabilizing an unstable spinal column. The landscape of emergency spinal injury care is in a state of perpetual evolution, driven by dedicated researchers, healthcare professionals, and breakthrough technologic innovations.

SELECTED REFERENCES

American College of Surgeons. *ACS TQIP Best Practice Guidelines for the Management of Traumatic Brain Injury.* 2024. https://www.facs.org/media/vgfgjpfk/best-practices-guidelines-traumatic-brain-injury.pdf.

Best practice guidelines for the management of TBI.

Hawryluk GWJ, Aguilera S, Buki A, et al. A management algorithm for patients with intracranial pressure monitoring: the Seattle International Severe Traumatic Brain Injury Consensus Conference (SIBICC). *Intensive Care Med.* 2019;45(12):1783-1794.

Consensus conference guidelines on ICU management for severe TBI.

Lin JS, Jain SA. Challenges in nerve repair and reconstruction. *Hand Clin.* 2023;39(3):403-415.

Comprehensive review of nerve injuries, nerve reconstruction, and most common nerve transfers.

Lulla A, Lumba-Brown A, Totten AM, et al. Prehospital guidelines for the management of traumatic brain injury. 3rd ed. *Prehosp Emerg Care.* 2023;27(5):507-538.

Prehospital guidelines for the management of TBI.

Moore AM, Wagner IJ, Fox IK. Principles of nerve repair in complex wounds of the upper extremity. *Semin Plast Surg.* 2015;29(1):40-47.

Provides a broad overview of complex nerve injuries and management.

Okereke I, Mmerem K, Balasubramanian D. The management of cervical spine injuries – a literature review. *Orthop Res Rev.* 2021;13:151-162.

Overview of the management of cervical spine injury.

Ramakonar H, Fehlings MG. "Time is Spine": new evidence supports decompression within 24h for acute spinal cord injury. *Spinal Cord.* 2021;59(8):933-934.

Reviews the importance of early intervention (<24 hours) after spine injury.

Safa B, Shores JT, Ingari JV, et al. Recovery of motor function after mixed and motor nerve repair with processed nerve allograft. *Plast Reconstr Surg Glob Open.* 2019;7(3):e2163.

Provides a broad overview of nerve reconstruction using allograft and autograft.

Theodore N, Aarabi B, Dhall SS, et al. The diagnosis and management of traumatic atlanto-occipital dislocation injuries. *Neurosurgery.* 2013;72(suppl 2):114-126.

Overview of traumatic atlantooccipital dislocation.

The full reference list appears on Elsevier eBooks+.

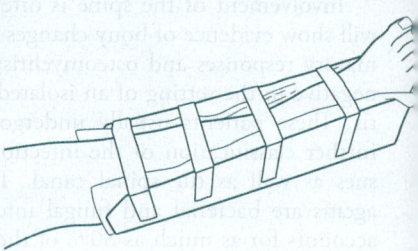

42 | CHAPTER

Management of Pediatric Trauma

William R. Johnston, Meera Kotagal, Michael L. Nance, and Gary W. Nace

INTRODUCTION

Epidemiology

Trauma is the leading cause of mortality for children and young adults aged 1 to 19 years and the third leading cause of death for infants <1 year of age.[1] Blunt injury accounts for over 90% of pediatric injuries, with falls and motor vehicle crashes (MVCs) being the most common mechanisms of injury (MOIs). MOI varies substantially with the age of the child and depends on developmental abilities and exposure to potential harms. Nonaccidental trauma (NAT) must be habitually considered at all ages, particularly for ages <2 years. The most common causes of death from *unintentional* injury per age group are suffocation for children <1 year, drowning for children 1 to 4 years, and MVCs for children older than 5 years.[1] Among all children aged ≤19 years, there were 9.0 deaths per 100,000 children in 2019 from unintentional injury, exceeding all other causes of mortality in the pediatric population. Furthermore, fatality rates differ with geography and were higher in rural settings compared with urban settings (17.8 per 100,000 vs. 6.8 per 100,000). Despite overall improvements in mortality from unintentional injury, there has been a steady increase in the number of pediatric deaths from all types of firearm injury, including homicide, suicide, and unintentional shootings. As such, firearm injury is now the leading cause of mortality for all children.[2]

Pediatric Differences

The aphorism "a child is not a small adult" is particularly pertinent when discussing pediatric trauma because injured children are frequently treated at centers that primarily care for adults. It is easy to *inappropriately* extrapolate adult-based principles and management strategies to the child. Further, within the pediatric population, there is an enormous degree of heterogeneity.[3]

Providers should be intimately familiar with anatomic and physiologic differences between age groups so that infants, young children, and adolescents can all be treated within the unique context of their physiologic and developmental stage. For example, securing a stable airway, obtaining intravenous access, and providing adequate resuscitation are very different for an infant than for an adolescent. Emotional, psychological, and social needs also differ significantly as children mature.

Despite this heterogeneity, several key tenets should remain front of mind during the trauma evaluation. First, the developing skeleton is relatively flexible and lacks the maturity of an adult skeleton. This, combined with the reduced body mass, leads to the potential for transmission of energy to internal organs. This may result in a greater degree of internal morbidity than would be suggested from the initial *external* examination, such as the development of pulmonary contusions in the absence of rib fractures or a bladder injury in the absence of a pelvic fracture. Second, children have an increased head size relative to their body, making them particularly vulnerable to head trauma. Finally, their increased surface area to mass ratio puts children at risk for hypothermia.

Prehospital Arrival

Early hospital notification allows the trauma resuscitation team to assemble in the emergency department (ED) with appropriate personal protective equipment donned, team roles assigned, and any prehospital information clearly communicated before arrival. Relevant consulting services (e.g., neurosurgery, orthopedics) can be notified in advance based on available information, and necessary equipment should be confirmed as available and properly functioning. The trauma resuscitation team will include, at a minimum, a senior team leader trained in Advanced Trauma Life Support (ATLS), a clinician responsible for the primary and secondary survey, a clinician assigned to the airway, an airway assistant or respiratory therapist, two nurses, a provider responsible for medication preparation and administration, and someone to document. Representatives from anesthesia, social work, child life, and pharmacy may also be included based on availability and the specific needs of the patient. Roles should be clearly assigned, and crowd and noise control maintained at all times.

RESUSCITATION

Primary Survey

The initial assessment of injured children mirrors that of adults, systematically addressing the "ABCDEs" using ATLS principles. However, despite similar processes, when caring for children there are unique characteristics that are important to recognize. To optimally care for injured children, providers should be familiar with the nuanced differences in anatomy, physiology, injury pattern, and psychosocial needs of injured children. Adding to this complexity of caring for children are variable size, maturity, and developmental stage. For example, the management of the neonatal airway is markedly different from that of the teenager. It is worth noting that even when an adolescent child nears physical maturity and looks "adult," their emotional, psychological, and social needs still require special attention. Regardless of age, development stage, or injury, the *primary goal of trauma resuscitation is to restore and maintain oxygen delivery, identify and manage injuries in order of greatest threat to life, and expeditiously provide appropriate disposition.*

Airway

Errors in airway management can be unforgiving and lead to preventable death.[4] Given their increased metabolic rate and decreased reserve, children have a nefarious ability to desaturate on pulse oximetry in seconds—with resultant hypoxia the most frequent cause of cardiac arrest. That being said, with thoughtful preparation and anticipation of potential pitfalls, airway complications can be avoided.

Rapid assessment of airway patency and ability to protect the airway can be accomplished by having the child phonate. A child that is speaking or crying clearly is one that has a patent airway. Hoarseness, stridor, or evidence of inhalation injury are all indicators that airway compromise may be imminent. Simultaneous with assessment of airway, the cervical spine should also be assessed to confirm cervical immobilization is *correctly* applied. Frequently the cervical collar is the wrong size, misapplied, or improvised.

Specifically related to the pediatric airway and anatomy, the child's large occiput can create relative neck flexion leading to obstruction. One solution is to place a blanket or roll under the upper back to help the neck maintain a neutral position. Other pertinent anatomic differences include a large tongue, small mouth, anteriorly displaced epiglottis, short trachea, and small diameter (which is most narrow at the level of the cricoid cartilage; Fig. 42.1). Regarding the shorter trachea, attention is needed to prevent inadvertent mainstem intubation or accidental tube dislodgement.

Despite these differences, the chin lift and jaw thrust are particularly good maneuvers to open the airway. Children can typically be maintained with these techniques and bag-valve-mask (BVM) ventilation for substantial periods while the appropriate medications, equipment, and personnel are being readied to perform intubation. The indications to intubate injured children typically mirror that of the adult trauma patient.

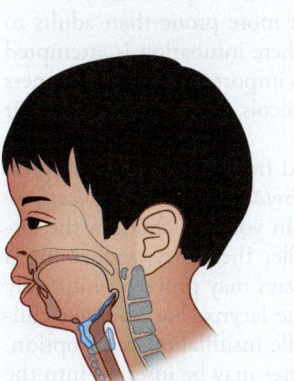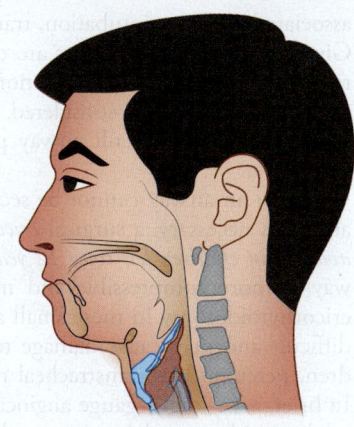

FIGURE 42.1 Differences in anatomy between the pediatric and adult airways.

Indications for endotracheal intubation in the pediatric trauma patient include:
- Airway obstruction
- Respiratory distress
- Poor respiratory effort
- Inability to protect airway
- Deteriorating mental status
- Glasgow Coma Scale (GCS) <8
- Penetrating neck trauma with possible airway compromise
- Suspicion for inhalation injury

Pediatric airway pearls:
- Infants typically will require a 3.0 to 3.5 uncuffed endotracheal tube (ETT).
- Older children can usually accommodate a cuffed ETT with size calculated as follows: (age in years/4) + 3.5.
- Alternatively, the size of ETT is roughly the diameter of the child's pinky finger or diameter of their nostril.
- Depth can by estimated by three times the ETT size.
- Size of oral airway can be estimated by the distance from central incisors to angle of mandible.
- Size of nasal airway is from nose to tragus.

Although video laryngoscopes (VLs) are becoming more widely available and can be helpful for visualization, in children with limited neck mobility, retrospective reviews have not shown that intubation using VL leads to a higher first-pass success rate.[5] Given a child's ability to rapidly decompensate, the most experienced provider should routinely be assigned to manage the airway. Yet even with the most experienced providers and teams, it is always important to have a backup plan. One scenario that can unravel the most seasoned team is the child who is able to be BVM ventilated before administration of rapid-sequence intubation (RSI) drugs but subsequently obstructs their airway after paralysis, resulting in a "can't intubate, can't ventilate" scenario. Having adjunctive measures immediately available, such as an oral airway or laryngeal mask airway (LMA) may be lifesaving. Caution is also warranted when administering RSI drugs in the setting of compensated hemorrhagic shock, where a child may have reduced sympathetic tone, and administration of RSI medications may precipitate cardiovascular collapse. If the patient needs to be managed in the operating room for hemorrhagic shock and the child still has an airway and can be oxygenated and ventilated, the operating room is frequently the safer place to obtain a definitive airway. In adults, not only does ED intubation not decrease time until definitive surgery, but it is also associated with postintubation, traumatic cardiopulmonary arrest.[6] Given that pediatric patients are even more prone than adults to rapid decompensation, the location where intubation is attempted should be thoughtfully considered. It is important that practitioners be familiar with difficult airway protocols and resources at their institution.

When an airway cannot be secured from above and a surgical airway is necessary, a surgical *cricothyroidotomy should typically be avoided in children less than 12 years*. In younger children the airway is more compressible and mobile; therefore, performing a cricothyroidotomy in these small airways may prove prohibitively difficult and may cause damage to the larynx. For younger children, percutaneous transtracheal needle insufflation is an option. In brief, a 14- or 16-gauge angiocatheter may be inserted into the trachea with a caudal trajectory, being cautious not to enter the backwall of the trachea. This is then attached to a 3-mL Luer-Lok syringe with the plunger removed. The open end of the syringe can then be attached to the hub of a 7.0 ETT and may be hooked up to high-flow oxygen (15–20 L/min). This may serve as a temporizing measure because hypoxia is the most time-sensitive physiologic determinate and hypercarbia is very well tolerated in children. Such measures can allow time for advanced airway techniques (e.g., use of fiberoptic equipment) or conversion to a formal tracheostomy for children requiring a surgical airway.

Breathing

Initial assessment of breathing is performed by inspection of the chest wall for evidence of trauma or asymmetry, auscultation bilaterally, palpating for crepitus or chest wall instability, and feeling for tracheal deviation. Respiratory distress may be indicated by grunting, nasal flaring, belly breathing, or use of accessory muscles. As assessment is ongoing, supplemental oxygen should be empirically administered and pulse oximetry monitored. When BVM ventilation is necessary, care should be taken to avoid overventilation. Typical tidal volumes range from 6 to 10 mL/kg for children, and appropriate respiratory rate will vary dependent on age. Use of BVM ventilation and the upset, crying child may both result in profound gastric distention from aerophagia, with resultant change in respiratory mechanics as the air-filled stomach pushes up on the diaphragm. Additionally, profound gastric distention may misdirect the naïve practitioner to the deduce that there is abdominal pathology (i.e., abdominal distention or rigidity, or gastric distention; see Fig. 42.4).

Breath sounds may be present bilaterally, despite significant unilateral pathology. Listening more laterally may help prevent confusing referred sounds from the contralateral chest. When breath sounds are unequal, the differential diagnosis of contusion, pneumothorax, hemothorax, or mainstem intubation should be considered. It is easy to advance the ETT into the mainstem bronchus (especially on right side), and this must be included in the differential when breath sounds are absent unilaterally in the intubated patient.

If life-threatening pathology is noted when examining the chest, just as when caring for adult trauma patients, intervention is warranted. Treatment of tension pneumothorax should be based on clinical suspicion, not radiographic confirmation. Inserting an angiocatheter into the pleural space, either in the midclavicular line at the second intercostal space or anterior axillary line at the fifth intercostal space, is an appropriate initial treatment. Alternatively, a chest tube may be placed if time permits. Although arbitrary, the indication for thoracotomy to manage massive hemothorax includes initial drainage of 20% of total blood volume or ongoing losses of ~2 mL/kg/h. As with all pediatric resuscitation and management, this threshold is weight dependent, and a 3-month-old will reach this threshold at a much lower volume of blood loss compared with a 13-year-old. However, regardless of absolute outputs, the overall clinical picture should be the primary determinant of when to pursue operative intervention for hemothorax.

Circulation

When evaluating and managing circulation in pediatric trauma, goals include:
1. Control external bleeding
2. Recognize shock
3. Quickly obtain IV access
4. Initiate resuscitation

Although these goals appear simple enough, children can present unique challenges. The smaller the child, the smaller the circulating blood volume. The overall circulating blood volume in children is ~70 cc/kg (~80 cc/kg for infants). Unlike adults in shock, children typically do not increase stroke volume in response to hypovolemia; rather, they are dependent on heart rate to maintain cardiac output along with a robust compensatory ability to increase vascular tone. Blood pressure is maintained by cardiac output (tachycardia) and increased vascular tone until late in hemorrhagic shock. In children, blood pressure may be preserved until loss of >45% of blood volume. Evidence that a child is in shock can be subtle, and an astute clinician will recognize clues in the level of consciousness, skin including capillary refill, heart rate, and blood pressure. Blood pressure has intentionally been listed last. Children may maintain their blood pressure right up until the point of cardiac collapse. Providers should be familiar with normal vital signs of different age groups (Table 42.1).

When significant external bleeding is identified, direct pressure is the preferred method of immediate control. Supplementary methods for control include pressure on the proximal arterial inflow or application of a tourniquet. If a tourniquet is not available, a blood pressure cuff can be effective, with inflation of the cuff above the arterial pressure and clamping of the tubing to keep it inflated. A tourniquet can be left in place roughly 2 hours with little risk of permanent ischemic injury. Continuous application for 6 hours or more will likely require amputation of the extremity.

If external hemorrhage is not present, assessment of circulation can begin with palpation of the central pulses, obtaining a peripheral blood pressure with an appropriately sized cuff, applying

TABLE 42.1	Normal Vital Signs of Different Age Groups			
AGE	**KG**	**RESPIRATORY RATE**	**HEART RATE**	**SYSTOLIC BLOOD PRESSURE (SBP)[a]**
Preemie	1–3	<60	<180	>60
Infant (0–6 mo)	3–5	<60	<180	>60
Infant (6–12 mo)	7	<40	<160	>70
Toddler (1–3 yr)	10–15	<35	<150	>70
Preschool (3–6 yr)	15–20	<30	<140	>75
School age (6–12 yr)	20–40	<25	<120	>80
Adolescent (≥13 yr)	40–70	<20	<100	>90

[a]SBPf >70 + (2 × age in years).

electrocardiogram (ECG) leads, and obtaining venous access. If peripheral intravenous access is difficult, ultrasound guidance should be readily available. If that remains difficult, intraosseous (IO) access at the proximal tibia, distal femur, or humerus should be used. An injured extremity should not be used for IO access. Central venous access can be considered but can be challenging and time consuming in the small child. Proximal or distal saphenous vein cut-down is a useful technique as well, although infrequently necessary. IO access should be the first approach in the child in extremis without access.

Once IV access is obtained, children typically first receive a 20 mL/kg fluid bolus. If hemorrhagic shock is present, early transfusion of O-negative blood should be pursued with consideration of activation of the massive transfusion protocol. Principles of damage control resuscitation—avoiding excess crystalloid, balanced resuscitation, early hemorrhage control—should be applied to children as in adults. Excess crystalloid administration has prospectively been evaluated and found to be associated with worse outcome, supporting use of an early transfusion approach in the resuscitation of injured children.[7] Balanced transfusion should be pursued, although a rigorous 1:1:1 balanced transfusion ratio has less support in the pediatric literature than it has in adults.[8] Additionally, evidence is growing that use of low-titer whole blood may be beneficial in the resuscitation of children in hemorrhagic shock.[9] Although tranexamic acid (TXA) is a useful adjunct to address hyperfibrinolysis in adults, its use in children remains under investigation; however, it can be administered within 3 hours of injury. When used, TXA is first given as a loading dose of 15 mg/kg (max 1 g) and then infusion of 2 mg/kg/h for 8 hours.

Transfusion volumes:
- Packed red blood cells: 10 to 20 mL/kg
- Plasma: 20 mL/kg
- Cryoprecipitate: 1 unit/10 kg
- Platelets: 15 mL/kg

While resuscitation is pursued, the potential locations of blood loss should be assessed including the chest, abdomen, pelvis, extremities, and externally. Typically, the location of hemorrhage can be ascertained via the physical examination, chest x-ray (CXR), and pelvic x-ray. The role of focused assessment with sonography for trauma (FAST) is less defined in injured children than in adults. The hemodynamically unstable child with a tender or distended abdomen will still need to be taken to the operating room regardless of findings on FAST. Conversely, a stable patient with free fluid on FAST will still require CT of the abdomen/pelvis to define the injury. In the setting of multisystem blunt injury, FAST may be helpful, provided it can be obtained quickly, can be interpreted with appropriate skepticism, and does not interfere with more pressing maneuvers. Some centers have adopted "extended" FAST (eFAST) in which the pleural space is evaluated for pneumothorax and hemothorax.

Additional points worth emphasizing when discussing circulation include that the quiet child with tachycardia and cool extremities in the trauma bay should make the practitioner very anxious—this is the child at risk of imminent cardiovascular collapse. Although tachycardia is the most consistent indicator of shock, this is not specific. Fear, anxiety, and pain are also common causes of tachycardia in the injured child. Clinical experience is important to help interpret the subtle clues to determine why a child is tachycardic. Bradycardia should also raise the practitioner's anxiety, as this may also suggest impending cardiovascular collapse.

Disability

Traumatic brain injury (TBI) is the leading cause of morbidity and mortality in pediatric trauma. The relatively large size of the child's head compared with the rest of the body predisposes them to impact of the head. Additionally, their skull is less rigid and the subarachnoid space smaller, leading to greater kinetic forces imparted to the brain parenchyma. Given the predisposition of children to TBI, careful assessment of the level of consciousness, pupillary examination, and neurologic examination is critical.

A GCS score can be quickly obtained with appropriate modification for young children (Table 42.2). Sternal rub should be avoided, and pressure to the nail bed is preferred. Infants with an open fontanelle will demonstrate bulging in the setting of elevated intracranial pressure (ICP) and are potential exceptions to the rule that intracranial bleeding cannot lead to hemorrhagic shock.

If there is concern for TBI on examination, clinicians can take immediate steps to reduce secondary insults of hypotension and hypoxia. Appropriate measures to ensure a stable airway, adequate oxygenation and ventilation, and appropriate resuscitation are prioritized, followed by additional measures to reduce ICP. The head of the bed can be elevated (15–30 degrees) and cervical collar assessed to ensure it is not overly tight and reducing venous outflow. Hypertonic 3% saline (3–5 mL/kg) is preferred, although mannitol is an acceptable alternative as long as its tendency to cause osmotic diuresis and hypotension is accounted for. In the setting of seizures, lorazepam, levetiracetam, and phenytoin are reasonable first-line agents.

In addition to disability, "D" should also trigger the provider to think of "dextrose." In pediatric patients, hypoglycemia can present with altered mental status and seizures, similar to the presentation of TBI, and should be included in the differential. Children who are severely hypoglycemic should be treated with IV bolus of 0.25 g/kg of dextrose (either 2.5 mL of 10% dextrose or 1 mL/kg of 25% dextrose) followed by maintenance fluids containing dextrose. Intoxication is less common in children but may also be considered as a cause for altered mental status in the appropriate circumstance.

TABLE 42.2 Components of Glasgow Coma Scale

RESPONSE	<2 YEARS	≥2 YEARS	SCORE
Eye	Spontaneous	Spontaneous	4
	To sound	To sound	3
	To pressure	To pressure	2
	No response	No response	1
Verbal	Babbles, coos (age appropriate)	Oriented (age appropriate)	5
	Cries but consolable	Confused (not age appropriate)	4
	Inconsolable crying		3
	Sounds, agitated, restless	Inappropriate words, irritable	2
	No response	Incomprehensible	1
		No response	
Motor	Normal spontaneous movement	Obeys commands	6
		Localizes	5
	Withdraws to touch	Withdraws	4
	Withdraws to pain	Flexion	3
	Flexion	Extension	2
	Extension	No response	1
	No response		

Exposure and Environmental Support

Complete exposure of the patient is necessary to ensure relevant injuries are rapidly noted and subtle injuries are not missed. This is particularly important in penetrating trauma as early knowledge of entry and exit wounds can help estimate trajectory and guide decision-making. Wounds can be marked with a paper clip for x-ray identification. On imaging the number of penetrating wounds and retained bullets should add up to an even number.

Children have a relatively high surface area to body mass, making them rapidly susceptible to iatrogenic hypothermia. Even mild hypothermia can impair platelet function, inhibit clotting factors, promote diuresis, and increase oxygen consumption secondary to shivering. Cold and wet clothing should be quickly removed and warm blankets provided once the patient has been turned and a full examination, including the axilla and perineum, has been performed. Use of a forced air strategy, such as a Bair Hugger, can also be invaluable in the pediatric patient. The decision to perform a rectal examination should be based on clinical suspicion and should not be performed as a matter of course.

Secondary Survey

After completion of the primary survey, the examiner will complete an organized head-to-toe examination quickly within the trauma bay. If not already obtained, adjunctive imaging such as CXR, lateral cervical spine x-ray, and pelvic x-ray may be obtained during this time. NAT, or child abuse, is common and should always remain on the differential. Subtle findings of NAT include subconjunctival scleral hemorrhage, oral trauma such as torn frenulum, unusual bruising patterns, and enlarged head circumference. When evaluating the head of infants, it is especially important to examine open fontanelles.

Adjuncts
Catheters

Orogastric or nasogastric tubes may be helpful in select patients. Nasogastric tubes are contraindicated when a basilar skull fracture or maxillofacial instability is suspected, and orogastric tubes are indicated in this scenario. It is not unusual that a child's stomach will be filled from air, either from crying or iatrogenic introduction from positive pressure ventilation, leading to abdominal competition and hypoventilation. The naïve practitioner can be misled, leading to unnecessary imaging and/or intervention. Additionally, a functional oro/nasogastric tube may also reduce the risk of aspiration from vomiting. Rarely will placement of bladder catheters be necessary while in the trauma bay.

Imaging

Most injured children are initially (if not definitively) cared for at nonpediatric trauma centers. Thus, it is important to note that imaging of the injured child requires a thoughtful approach. The adult trauma assessment with *pan-scan* should be avoided given long-term implications of ionizing radiation in children. Choice of imaging modality is heavily guided by clinical presentation, injury location, MOI, and clinical concern.

The relative risk of radiation exposure is of particular concern in children. Young, rapidly dividing tissues are more susceptible to the effects of radiation exposure. In addition, the damage that occurs results in a cumulative lifetime risk of carcinogenesis. The majority of radiation exposure in a pediatric trauma patient is a result of CT scanning that delivers the highest radiation dose of the common imaging modalities.[10] In children, there seems to be a dose-response relationship between CT-related radiation exposure and brain cancer.[11] The "as low as reasonably achievable"

(ALARA) principle can help clinicians balance the risk of radiation with the informational benefit of a given study. ALARA should guide pediatric protocols to minimize regions scanned, radiation dose, and multiphase scans and to be judicious with follow-up studies. That being said, an indicated study should not be delayed if that information is needed to guide therapy.

CXR is good at identifying thoracic pathology that requires intervention (e.g., pneumothorax, hemothorax, diaphragm rupture). CT of the chest will rarely offer clinically impactful information and should be obtained selectively.[12] However, in scenarios where there is concern for aortic injury on CXR, such as widened mediastinum, CT angiogram (CTA) of the chest is indicated. Of note, thymic tissue can masquerade as a widened mediastinum in young children.

Although FAST is a mainstay in the initial evaluation of abdominal trauma in the adult patient, it has less clinical utility in children, especially in the stable child. FAST as currently used has limited sensitivity to screen for intraabdominal injury in children sustaining blunt abdominal trauma.[13] A randomized trial of stable pediatric patients treated for blunt trauma found that FAST did not improve ED length of stay, rate of missed intraabdominal injuries, or hospital charges—leading to the conclusion that routine abdominal FAST after blunt injury in stable patients is not supported.[14] Rarely will FAST alter the management of the pediatric trauma patient, and occasionally it will misdirect or delay appropriate care. There continues to be substantial variation in the use of FAST among pediatric trauma centers.[13] Many centers use FAST in the unstable patient to rapidly assess the pericardial and abdominal cavities for sources of blood loss.

SPECIFIC INJURIES

Head Trauma

Pediatric TBI from any mechanism is the leading cause of pediatric trauma death and disability, resulting in over 60,000 hospitalizations per year.[15,16] Falls and MVCs are the most common contributors, although NAT is a major cause as well. Children <4 years of age with hypotension, low initial GCS score, and coagulopathy or hypoglycemia have particularly poor outcomes.[17] GCS can be used to categorize TBI into mild (13–15), moderate (9–12), and severe (3–8). These categories do not diagnose underlying injury, but they do provide a straightforward means of communicating neurologic status and helping providers consider immediate diagnostic and therapeutic maneuvers that should be performed.[18]

Regardless of GCS category, the overarching goal of treating TBI is preventing secondary neurologic injury that accompanies additional hypoxia and hypotension.[19–21] Preventing hypoxia requires maintaining an adequate airway to provide oxygen for gas exchange in addition to treating increases in ICP that would impair cerebral blood flow and decrease oxygen delivery. Volume resuscitation and control of bleeding are essential to maintain circulation. Sequelae of severe head injury are bound by the Monro-Kellie doctrine that recognizes the cranial vault is a rigid container and an increase in intracranial volume caused by one component (e.g., intracranial hemorrhage) must be offset by a volumetric decrease in another component (parenchyma). Displacement of cerebrospinal fluid (CSF) and venous blood can initially compensate, but once they are exhausted, ICP will increase precipitously and lead to cerebral ischemia and herniation. As such, the early manifestations of TBI—headache, irritability, vomiting—should prompt alarm because the late signs of TBI—posturing, pupillary changes, Cushing triad—can rapidly progress to significant cerebral ischemia, secondary injury, and death.

Initial Management

As with any pediatric patient presenting to the trauma bay, the initial evaluation and resuscitation should follow ATLS standards. Rapid stabilization is vital to preventing secondary brain injury from hypoxia and hypotension. After the ABCDEs of care have been addressed, neurologic status is quickly assessed by calculating GCS. A score <8 should generally prompt providers to secure a mechanical airway, initiate measures to lower ICP, and obtain a noncontrast head CT scan. In patients with mild TBI, the indications for scanning are less clear. Use of the Pediatric Emergency Care Applied Research Network (PECARN) criteria has been shown to limit the number of unnecessary head CTs by up to 60% without increasing rates of missed life-threatening injuries.[22] Importantly, all patients with loss of consciousness, skull fractures or scalp hematoma, significant MOI, and GCS <14 warrant CT without contrast. Factors such as age of the patient, loss of consciousness, and multiple injuries can be considered as well.

If there is concern for severe TBI and elevated ICP, several immediate maneuvers can be performed in the trauma bay. The head of the bed can be elevated to 30 degrees to increase venous return, and the cervical collar can be appropriately loosened to prevent outflow obstruction.[23] This is done by placing the bed in reverse Trendelenburg to allow maintenance of thoracic and lumbar spine precautions until those areas are cleared of concern. Hypercosmolar therapy with hypertonic (3%) saline will reduce intracranial edema and is preferred to mannitol, which can worsen hypotension due to its diuretic effects. Hyperventilation with $PaCO_2$ <35 should only be performed when there is concern for active herniation and is otherwise avoided given the cerebral vasoconstrictive effect of hypocarbia. Seizure activity raises the metabolic demands of the brain and should be aggressively controlled if clinically evident. Prophylactic antiepileptic therapy reduces early (<1 week) posttraumatic seizure activity and can be considered in the setting of intracranial bleeding, age <4 years, depressed skull fracture, concern for abusive head trauma, and GCS <8.

Once the patient has been hemodynamically stabilized, the primary and secondary survey completed, and seizure activity controlled, a noncontrast head CT should be performed as soon as possible if clinically indicated. Patients with ongoing intracranial processes may look well until precipitously declining, making timely transfer to the CT scanner critically important.

Medical Management of Refractory Elevated Intracranial Pressure

Regardless of the cause of injury, prevention and management of intracranial hypertension is key in the care of children with TBI. Patients with GCS <8 and a nonsurgical lesion on CT may be candidates for an ICP monitor. An external ventricular drain allows both monitoring of ICP and therapeutic drainage of CSF, while modern intraparenchymal monitors provide additional information such as cerebral oxygen saturation and temperature. The general goals of therapy are ICP <20 mm Hg and cerebral perfusion pressure >40 mm Hg. The benefits of ICP monitors must be carefully weighed against the risks of bleeding and infection associated with their use. A recent review of over 3000 patients demonstrated no survival advantage for ICP monitoring for patients with severe TBI.[24] All patients with concern for severe TBI must be admitted to the pediatric intensive care unit (PICU) for close neurologic monitoring.

If initial measures fail to adequately address ICP, sedation and analgesia should be provided to lower cerebral metabolic demand. Neuromuscular blockade can be instituted to prevent shivering and improve ventilator synchrony. Because neuromuscular blockade prevents ongoing neurologic examinations and may mask seizure activity, continuous electroencephalogram monitoring is generally recommended. Additional options include barbiturate infusion and higher levels of hyperosmolar therapy. At one of the authors' institutions, 3% hypertonic saline is given in 5 mL/kg doses (max: 500 mL/dose) with an infusion rate that can be titrated as high as 1 mL/kg/h.

Types of Injuries

Epidural hematomas (EDHs) typically result from damage to a middle meningeal artery or a venous bone bleed that leads to accumulation of blood between the skull and the dura.[25,26] Epidural blood cannot cross suture lines and classically presents with initial loss of consciousness followed by a lucid interval and subsequent rapid decline (Fig. 42.2A). An overlying temporal skull fracture

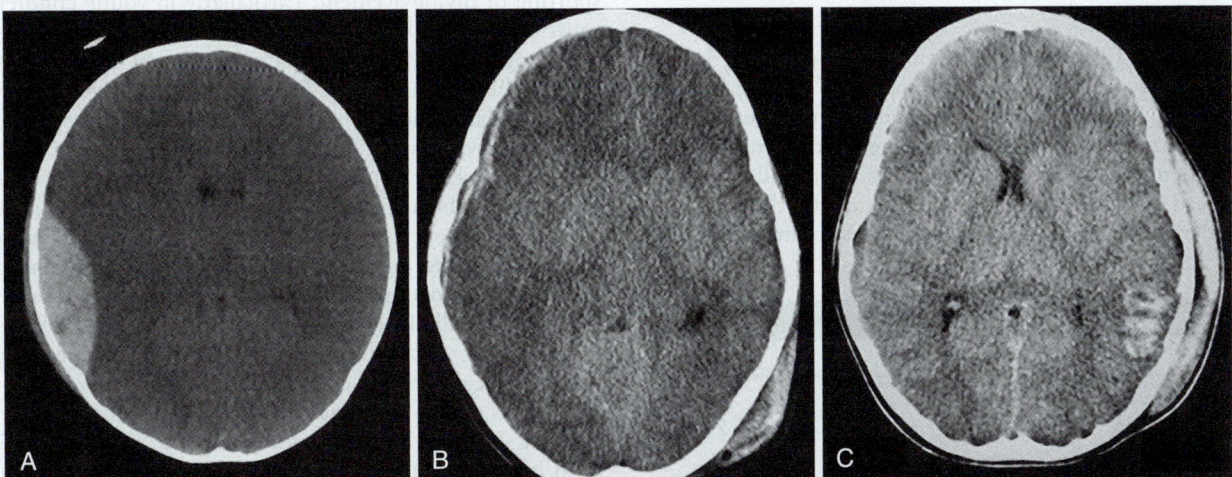

FIGURE 42.2 (A) Epidural hematoma. (B) Subdural hematoma. (C) Intraparenchymal hematoma. (From Tieves KS, Rilinger J. Traumatic brain injury. In: St. Peter S, ed. *Holcomb and Ashcraft's Pediatric Surgery.* 7th ed. Edinburgh: Elsevier; 2020:254-266; Jea A, Luerssen TG. Central nervous system injuries. In: Coran AG, Caldamone A, Adzick NS, Krummel TM, Laberge JM, Shamberge R, eds. *Pediatric Surgery.* 7th ed. Philadelphia: Elsevier Mosby; 2012:343-360.)

commonly coexists. Subdural hematomas (SDHs) are typically caused by tearing of the bridging veins that cross the subdural space. In contrast to EDH, SDHs cross suture lines and demonstrate a classic crescent moon appearance (see Fig. 42.2B). The presence of an SDH implies a substantial force imparted to the head, and patients should be closely monitored in the PICU for signs of neurologic decline that would require operative decompression. Intraparenchymal hematomas (IPHs) are acceleration-deceleration injuries that result from the brain striking the inside of the skull. IPHs tend to "blossom" in the 24 to 48 hours after the initial event, with dramatic changes often noted on interval CT scans (see Fig. 42.2C). This blossoming can worsen cerebral edema and lead to significant spikes in ICP. In the setting of significant mass effect, operative decompression will be required. Whenever an intracranial bleed is noted on CT, neurosurgery should be promptly consulted to help facilitate proper treatment.

Skull fractures are classified as linear, depressed, or basilar. Linear skull fractures are the most common but least worrisome, provided there is no underlying intracranial injury. Patients with isolated linear, nondepressed skull fractures can likely be discharged from the ED if neurologic status is normal and the patient is tolerating an enteral diet. Depressed skull fractures typically result from a more significant injury and commonly involve underlying parenchyma. Neurosurgical evaluation is mandatory, and operative intervention will likely be required in the setting of significant intracranial hematoma, neurologic deficit, or CSF leak. Basilar skull fractures involve the bones of the skull base and often coexist with injuries to surrounding structures such as the auditory canals, carotid artery, and facial nerve. If there is evidence of injury to the carotid artery, CTA of the head and neck should be considered. The McGovern score has recently been validated to further guide the evaluation for pediatric blunt cerebrovascular injury (BCVI).[27] The score incorporates physical examination and imaging findings, with a CTA recommended for all patients with a score >3. As in adults, low-grade BCVI is treated with aspirin, whereas higher grades are addressed with endovascular techniques. Before 4 years of age, the skull is relatively thin and pliable, leading to "ping-pong" fractures in which the skull is depressed inward without a clear fracture line. These injury patterns typically do not require surgery and can be monitored over time (Table 42.3).

Concussion

Concussions are TBIs that cause neurologic impairment in the absence of a gross structural injury on imaging.[28] The underlying pathophysiology involves altered permeability of cell membranes, cell rupture, axonal stretch and shearing, and disruption of synapses. Microvascular injury, vasospasm, and inflammatory responses lead to a mismatch between metabolic demand and supply. Patients may demonstrate a variety of common findings including physical, cognitive, emotional, and visual deficits. Loss of consciousness occurs with only 10% of concussions, and symptoms may take up to 24 hours to become apparent. Importantly, concussion is a diagnosis of exclusion. Patients with red flag symptoms such as persistently altered mental status, severe headache, and focal neurologic deficits must be rigorously evaluated for an underlying structural injury.

The treatment for concussion focuses on limiting metabolic demand while the brain heals.[29–31] Physical and cognitive rest for the first 24 to 48 hours after a concussion is essential to limit further cellular stress. Children should be held out of sports and restricted from activities that involve significant visual tracking such as video games and reading. Parents should be advised that concussed children may struggle with cognitive tasks they previously mastered and may require an increased need for sleep. As they recover, children will find they can tolerate increased amounts of physical and mental exertion and should be allowed to gradually increase activity with breaks as needed. Up to 80% of children demonstrate full recovery by 4 weeks, whereas others may take months to fully recover. Patients who do not recover in a predictable time frame (weeks) or have persistent symptoms are best managed by those who specialize in concussion care.

Spine

There are key differences in injury patterns, radiographic findings, and management for pediatric spinal injury compared with adults.[26,32] However, regardless of the type of injury, the first objective is to ensure cervical spine immobilization as standard ATLS assessments are underway. Subsequently, treatment focuses on addressing other injuries, particularly TBI, that may affect evaluation and treatment of a potential spinal injury.

Injury Patterns

The causes and distribution of spinal injury change with age.[33,34] In very young children, the male-to-female ratio is roughly equal, whereas in older children it is primarily male (ratio is about 4:1). Overall, about one-half of pediatric spinal injuries are caused by MVCs. Younger children are more likely to be injured after a fall, whereas older children are more likely to be injured due to a sporting or diving accident. Particularly in young children, NAT must be thoroughly considered.

Young children tend to have injuries of the upper cervical spine, whereas children older than 8 years have a distribution more similar to adults, with injuries typically occurring in the subaxial cervical spine and cervicothoracic junction.[35,36] Infants and toddlers have disproportionately large heads and weak cervical muscles, which create a greater fulcrum of motion in the cervical region. They also have greater elasticity of their posterior tension band and joint capsules with shallow facet joints and less developed uncinate processes. This allows for a greater degree of movement in all planes and transmission of energy. Consequently, 10% to 15% of spinal injuries involve "skip" injuries at multiple levels. These differences decrease linearly with age.

Injuries can be anatomically grouped into those involving the anterior, middle, and posterior columns.[33,34,37–40] Anterior column injuries are from the anterior longitudinal ligament to the midportion of the vertebral body. Middle column injuries are from the midvertebral body to the pedicles, and posterior injuries are from the pedicles to posterior tension band. Injuries can also be described as compression, burst, flexion-distraction, and fracture-dislocation. Compression fractures involve only the anterior

TABLE 42.3 **McGovern Score**	
	POINTS
Glasgow Coma Scale (GCS) ≤8	1
Focal neurologic deficit	2
Carotid canal fracture	2
Mechanism of injury	2
Petrous temporal bone fracture	3
Cerebral infarction on computed tomography	3

A score >3 indicates a high risk for blunt cerebrovascular injury (BCVI) and indicates the patient should undergo angiography.

column and do not usually have clinical deficits. Burst fractures involve the anterior and middle columns and can demonstrate neurologic deficits if a posterior portion of the vertebral body protrudes into the spinal canal. Flexion-distraction injuries involve compression of the anterior column with distraction injury of the middle and posterior columns. These injuries are commonly referred to as *chance fractures* and are often associated with a seat-belt sign and intraabdominal injury. Fracture-dislocation injuries involve all three columns with significant deformation of the spinal canal. These often result in spinal cord injury and are more likely to require operative intervention.

Initial Management and Workup

When a patient presents to the trauma bay, providers must first address the ABCDEs of trauma care before moving on to a dedicated workup of the spine. As part of the secondary survey, a more thorough examination of the spine should be performed to identify tenderness or palpable defects along the entire spine. Loss of sensation or motor function should be noted and clearly documented before the administration of any sedating or paralyzing agents. The American Spinal Injury Association (AISA) Impairment Scale can be used to help grade and characterize the extent of injury. When the mechanism is appropriate, the abdomen should be assessed for a seat-belt sign, which should heighten suspicion for a lumbar spine injury. Until spinal injury is excluded, the entire spinal axis should be immobilized and log roll precautions maintained. The disproportionately large head of young children leads to cervical flexion when they are placed on a neutral board. As such, either a specialized board or a bump placed under the torso is necessary for proper alignment. An accurately sized cervical collar is essential for both stability and patient comfort.

Imaging

The relative lack of available guidelines makes it difficult to determine when spinal imaging should be performed for pediatric patients. In the adult population, the NEXUS criteria identify patients at low risk of cervical injury who can be safely observed without imaging. The criteria include the absence of focal neurologic deficits, midline spinal tenderness, altered level of consciousness, patient intoxication, and distracting injury.[41] Given the limited ability of NEXUS to triage young children, the PEDSPINE and PEDSPINE II trials have more recently proposed easy-to-use scoring systems with high negative predictive value for cervical spinal injury in the youngest pediatric patients.[42–44] Whether plain radiograph or CT should initially be used to assess for cervical injury continues to be debated as well. The American College of Radiology recommends cervical spine radiography in children 3 to 16 years of age with at least one PECARN or NEXUS risk factor, whereas the Congress of Neurological Surgeons notes either CT or plain radiography is acceptable for initial imaging, with CT preferred for pediatric patients with suspected craniocervical junction injuries.[45,46] Atlanto-occipital dislocation (AOD) injuries are particularly devastating and can be easily missed on clinical examination. A lateral c-sine film can be useful early in the resuscitation of an obtunded patient, as identification of AOD would notably affect subsequent management.

Additionally, there are several normal radiologic findings in pediatric spines that would be considered pathologic in adults, including cervical pseudosubluxation, synchondroses, and nonvisible vertebral bodies on lateral plate studies.[47] Because of the hypermobility of the pediatric spine, up to 20% of young children have spinal cord injury without radiographic abnormality (SCIWORA), which results in neurologic deficits in the absence of vertebral anomalies.[33] MRI is a useful adjunct to detect subtle signs of injury within the cord and is superior to CT in the detection of ligamentous and soft tissue injury. MRI is most useful for obtunded or nonverbal children with suspicious injury mechanisms, equivocal radiographs or CT, or unexplained neurologic findings.[48] Experienced radiologists familiar with the pediatric spine can ensure unnecessary confusion during the trauma workup is avoided.

Management

Most pediatric fractures and dislocations can be reduced and maintained in anatomic alignment with nonoperative orthotic braces, whereas surgery is typically reserved for children with persistent deformity or ligamentous instability.[49,50] The goal of braces is to immobilize the injured segment and prevent the patient from motions that could exacerbate their injury. Early operative intervention is indicated for patients with neurologic deterioration, irreducible compression of the spinal cord, or enlarging hematoma. There are no data to support the use of corticosteroids to treat spinal cord injury. Prompt consultation with a spine surgeon when spinal injury is suspected can help ensure proper diagnostic workup and timely intervention.

Neck

An organized, rapid assessment for pediatric neck injuries is essential for initial airway stabilization and ultimate treatment of the injury.[51] Specific characteristics of pediatric anatomy can make management particularly difficult.[52,53] Compared with the adult airway, the pediatric airway is smaller and more susceptible to partial or complete obstruction from edema or hematoma. The pediatric neck is proportionally shorter with a higher, more anterior larynx and underdeveloped muscles that lead to greater transmission of forces to internal structures. Ensuring a stable, secure airway before considering imaging or therapeutic maneuvers is essential.

Initial Management

If early airway intervention is not required, providers may proceed with a focused physical examination once the initial primary survey is complete. A hematoma or bruit suggests vascular injury, whereas subcutaneous emphysema indicates aerodigestive injury. As with adult trauma, the neck is divided into three zones: zone 1 from the sternal notch to the cricoid cartilage, zone 2 from the cricoid cartilage to the base of the mandible, and zone 3 from the base of the mandible to the skull base. However, these guidelines are less reliable in children as the cricoid cartilage migrates caudally throughout childhood. As such, zone 1 injuries may be accessible through a neck incision even when below the cricoid.

Imaging

Patients with hard signs of vascular or aerodigestive injuries such as expanding hematoma, palpable thrill, and wound bubbling should proceed directly to the operating room. Selected stable patients may undergo a focused CT to assess the structures of the neck. Otherwise, patients can be considered for focused imaging based on their specific injury pattern.[54] CXR can identify concomitant pneumothorax, hemothorax, or widened mediastinum in the setting of a zone 1 injury, and cervical x-rays can help define spinal injuries. CTA of the chest and neck provides vascular detail and is most useful for stable patients with zone 1 and 3 injuries and for selected patients with a zone 2 injury. In the setting of blunt injury, the McGovern score (see Table 42.3) can be used to triage patients at high risk for BCVI and determine whether imaging is indicated.[55,56] When aerodigestive injury is suspected in stable patients, laryngoscopy, endoscopy, and esophagram can be used to identify the injured organ and facilitate operative planning.

Operative Management

Close communication with the anesthesia team is essential throughout the operation, and trauma surgeons should have a low threshold for involving a dedicated otolaryngologist. A cervical spine injury should be considered with any blunt neck trauma, and appropriate stabilization must be maintained throughout the case. If the patient is stable, a bronchoscopy and esophagoscopy should be considered before proceeding with surgical exploration. A unilateral injury can typically be accessed via an anterior incision over the sternocleidomastoid, whereas bilateral injuries are approached with a collar incision.[57] A collar incision may also be preferable in infants and toddlers because of their shorter necks. Zone 1 injuries may require sternotomy, particularly when cervical injury prevents neck extension. Zone 3 injuries are often particularly difficult to access in small children because of their relatively compressed anatomy and may require superior extension of the incision. Endovascular therapy can be used when the patient is large enough, as vessel size may be prohibitively small in younger children.[58]

Arterial injuries are addressed by first obtaining proximal and distal control of the common, external, and internal carotid. Primary repair is preferred for common carotid injuries, though extensive injuries will require repair with a patch angioplasty or interposition graft, both of which are ideally performed with a vein conduit.[59] If necessary, ligation can be considered provided there is good back-bleeding. If necessary, unilateral internal jugular vein injuries can be ligated if needed. Pediatric patients generally tolerate vascular ligation well, given the absence of underlying atherosclerosis. Esophageal injuries can be approached by retracting the carotid sheath laterally. If there is difficulty identifying the esophagus, an orogastric tube can be placed and then palpated. Devitalized tissue should be debrided, and the esophageal injury primarily repaired when possible and left. Tracheal lacerations should be repaired with a single layer of monofilament absorbable suture. More complicated airway injuries are best approached with the assistance of an otolaryngologist. A pedicled segment of strap or sternocleidomastoid muscle can be interposed between suture lines or used to buttress a repair, particularly in the setting of devitalized tissue.

Thoracic Trauma

Whereas approximately 80% of pediatric thoracic injuries result from a blunt mechanism of injury, penetrating thoracic injury is associated with a high mortality rate. Most pediatric chest injuries do not require operative intervention and need only oxygen, pain control, and possibly chest tube placement. Yet there is a subset of children whose chest injuries are life threatening and require immediate and thoughtful intervention for survival.

There are notable differences between adult and pediatric chest anatomy that warrant recognition. For one, a child's skeleton has increased compliance, allowing for the energy of impact to be transmitted to internal organs, such as pulmonary parenchyma. Whereas rib fractures are unusual in children, pulmonary contusions are common. Additionally, a simple pneumothorax may progress to a tension pneumothorax fairly quickly as the mobile mediastinum can shift rapidly, reducing venous return and compressing the contralateral lung.

Rib Fractures

As mentioned previously, given the compliance of the chest wall, rib fractures in children are relatively uncommon. When they are found, especially fractures of the first rib, a high-energy mechanism should be suspected. Flail chest is even more unusual in children. It is worth noting that rib fractures in children under 3 years old have a 95% positive predictive value (PPV) for NAT.[60] Supportive therapy is recommended for rib fractures and typically requires no other intervention.

Pulmonary Contusion

Given decreased chest wall rigidity, mechanical forces can easily be transmitted to the underlying parenchyma. Pulmonary contusions are the most frequent injury and range from asymptomatic and incidentally discovered to fatal. Although they may be identified on the CXR in the trauma bay, they may also take time to "blossom." Traumatic pneumatoceles can be associated with contusions and are relatively common. Treatment of both pulmonary contusion and pneumatoceles is supportive with judicious fluid administration. Most patients have no untoward consequence of pulmonary contusions, but there is potential to have significant V/Q mismatch and profound refractory hypoxia. Advanced ventilation strategies or even extracorporeal membrane oxygenation (ECMO) may occasionally be necessary when there are severe bilateral pulmonary contusions.

Pneumothorax and Hemothorax

The management of pneumothorax and hemothorax in the child typically mirrors that of adults. Very small and asymptomatic pneumothorax and even hemothorax may be managed expectantly without intervention. The complications of retained hemothorax, such as entrapped lung, are frequently a concern in adult trauma patients but are uncommon in children. With massive hemothorax, monitoring chest tube output is important as a large amount of blood loss ($\geq$15 mL/kg) at the time of chest tube placement or ongoing blood loss ($\geq$2–3 mL/kg/h for 3 hours) may be an indication for a thoracotomy. However, clinical parameters should primarily guide therapy.

Cardiac and Great Vessel Injury

Cardiac and great vessel injury is rare in children. Most cardiac injuries are blunt cardiac contusions occurring after high-energy mechanism (e.g., MVC). Initial evaluation may include measurement of serum cardiac enzymes and ECG. Contusions can lead to dysrhythmia and hypotension. Management is primarily supportive with continuous electrocardiography to monitor for cardiac arrhythmias. Echocardiogram is warranted if there is concern for rupture, valvular disruption, or cardiac failure.

Aortic and great vessel injuries are also rare in children. Most aortic injuries occur via blunt mechanism after high-speed MVC or fall from a significant height. CXR is a useful initial screening tool to evaluate pediatric trauma patients for aortic transection along with clinical presentation.[61] Widened mediastinum (although beware of thymus), indistinct or abnormal aortic contour, deviation of trachea or esophagus to the right, depression of left main bronchus, loss of the aortopulmonary window, left apical pleural cap, and large left hemothorax are findings on the initial CXR that may indicate thoracic aortic injury (Fig. 42.3). CTA of

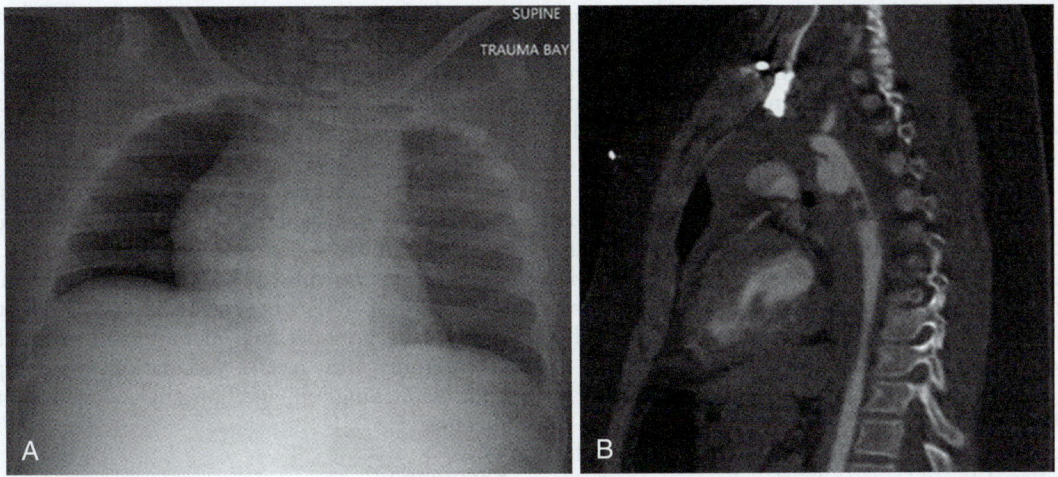

FIGURE 42.3 An 11-year-old patient after motor vehicle crash. Note chest x-ray demonstrates widening of the mediastinum suspicious for aortic injury (A) and computed tomography confirms the injury (B).

the chest is indicated if there is concern for aortic injury. Once an injury is identified, impulse control should be initiated with a β-blocker and possibly a vasodilator if needed to minimize the propagation of aortic injury with each heartbeat. Definitive management will depend on the grade of injury, age/size of patient, location and size of injured vessel, and expertise of treating center. Both endovascular and open repairs have been successful in pediatric patients.

Diaphragm Injury

Diaphragmatic injury may occur after blunt injury secondary to increased intraabdominal pressure causing rupture or after penetrating thoracoabdominal injury. After blunt injury, left-sided injuries are more common given that the liver helps to protect the right diaphragm. Classically after blunt left-sided diaphragmatic rupture a CXR will demonstrate gas-filled bowel loops or gastric bubble, possibly with a gastric tube, above the level of the diaphragm. Although most blunt diaphragmatic ruptures may occur on the left side, occasionally right-sided blunt diaphragmatic ruptures will occur after a high-energy mechanism. Right-sided diaphragmatic rupture is frequently associated with significant liver injury, and a right-sided chest tube may drain a large amount of blood from the associated liver injury (Fig. 42.4). When diagnosed acutely, diaphragmatic injury should be repaired via laparotomy given the high incidence of associated abdominal injuries. Penetrating injuries of the diaphragm may result in small, difficult-to-detect injuries and should have a high index of suspicion based on trajectory. If missed acutely, chronically there may be progressive entrapment of abdominal contents in the thoracic cavity. Chronic injuries can be repaired either through the chest or abdomen.

Asphyxia

Traumatic asphyxia occurs after a large compressive force is applied to the chest and/or upper abdomen. Venous hypertension within the superior vena cava (SVC) produces the clinical manifestations of thoraco-cervico-facial petechiae, facial edema and cyanosis, subconjunctival hemorrhage, and neurologic symptoms. Capillaries and small veins in the face, neck, and chest wall can rupture leading to petechia and conjunctival hemorrhage. The associated cerebral edema and neurologic symptoms are typically transient and will resolve with conservative measures, although

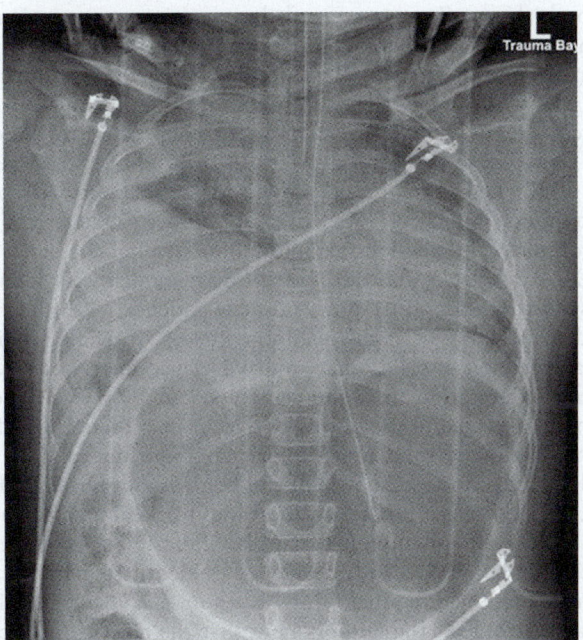

FIGURE 42.4 Right-sided diaphragmatic rupture in a 7-year-old patient after restrained-passenger motor vehicle crash. Note liver above the diaphragm and a large right hemothorax.

long-term impairment can occur depending on period of hypoxia. Therapy includes elevation of the head of the bed, supportive care, and management of associated injuries.

Abdominal Trauma

Background and Anatomic Considerations

Approximately 1 in 10,000 children sustain abdominal trauma each year.[62] Blunt trauma is responsible for up to 90% of pediatric abdominal injury and accounts for 10% of fatalities. Over half of blunt abdominal injuries occur because of MVCs, though NAT is the most common etiology in infants and toddlers.[63] Fatalities commonly occur in the setting of polytrauma, often secondary to associated TBI.

Unique anatomic and physiologic characteristics must be accounted for when evaluating pediatric abdominal trauma.[63]

Skeletal immaturity and pliability make young children more susceptible to intraabdominal injury. In particular, the spleen and kidneys are poorly protected by the less ossified lower ribcage, and the bladder rises above the protective confines of the developing pelvis. Because pediatric bones are less ossified and more pliable, significant intraabdominal injury can occur even in the absence of bony fracture. If fracture does occur, providers should suspect a high-energy mechanism and have an increased index of suspicion for concomitant intraabdominal injury. Seat belts tend ride up above the anterior superior iliac spine (ASIS) in children and transfer energy to the abdomen, increasing the risk for spine and hollow viscus injury (HVI). A "seat-belt" contusion above the ASIS should raise suspicion for intraabdominal injury.

Initial Evaluation and Diagnosis

Initial management for all patients follows standard ATLS guidelines. Once airway and breathing stability has been ensured, assessment of circulatory status is prioritized. However, significant hemorrhage in children is often masked by compensatory increases in vasomotor tone and tachycardia.[64,65] The presence of abdominal guarding or a seat-belt contusion on examination should point to the abdomen as a potential source of hemorrhage.

In the unstable patient in the trauma bay, FAST examinations may quickly help determine whether intraabdominal hemorrhage is the source of instability. However, for stable pediatric patients, FAST may have less clinical utility than in adults.[66,67] A recent trial of 975 hemodynamically stable pediatric patients with blunt torso trauma found that FAST did not improve ED length of stay, rate of missed intraabdominal injuries, or hospital charges.[68]

CT scan with IV contrast is the primary modality for identifying suspected abdominal injury in stable patients.[69] CT allows for rapid acquisition of high-resolution images, providing reliable characterization of solid organ injury. Delayed images can evaluate for extravasation from the urinary system.[70] HVI should be strongly suspected in the setting of free air or if there is free fluid in the absence of solid organ injury, although unexplained free fluid is present in at least 50% of children without bowel perforation.[71,72] Mesenteric stranding, focal wall thickening, and abnormal bowel wall enhancement may also indicate HVI.[73] A recent prediction tool was recently developed to identify patients at very low risk of intraabdominal injury in whom a CT scan can likely be safely avoided. The authors note that the absence of a complaint of abdominal pain, abnormal physical examination, abnormal pancreatic enzymes, aspartate aminotransferase (AST) >200, or abnormal CXR demonstrated a negative predictive value of over 99%.[74] From the standpoint of abdominal injury, most children with a normal CT scan can be safely discharged home from the ED.

Liver and Spleen

The liver and spleen are the most commonly injured solid organs in pediatric trauma. Injury grade alone does not dictate treatment, and nonoperative treatment strategies form the foundation of modern management protocols.[75,76] Protocols vary by institution, but for significant injury they incorporate a brief period of bed rest, serial hemoglobin laboratory draws, and ICU admission for patients with abnormal vital signs. Recent guidelines note that bed rest and serial laboratory draws are unnecessary for hemodynamically normal patients and those admitted to the regular surgical floor.[77] Patients with ongoing evidence of bleeding are monitored in the ICU with coagulopathies systematically addressed. Angiography/angioembolization can be selectively used

in both the acute setting and in a delayed fashion depending on hemodynamic stability. Although extravasation should heighten the clinician's concern, therapy is guided by hemodynamics and response to resuscitation rather than imaging findings alone. Even in the presence of high-grade injuries, routine follow-up imaging is not recommended in asymptomatic children. Operative intervention is necessary in the setting of ongoing instability that cannot be safely managed through nonoperative means. In the setting of splenic injury, every effort should be made to prevent splenectomy, given the subsequent risk of overwhelming postsplenectomy sepsis (OPSI), but splenorrhaphy is rarely successful once an injury fails nonoperative management. Patients who undergo splenectomy must receive vaccinations for encapsulated bacteria and, depending on age, prophylactic antibiotic maintenance therapy.

Pancreas

Pancreatic injuries are typically the result of blunt upper abdominal impact, of which handlebar injuries are the most common mechanism, but occasionally occur with other mechanisms such as MVC and NAT. Whereas liver and spleen injuries are treated based on hemodynamic parameters, treatment of pancreatic injury is guide by American Association for the Surgery of Trauma (AAST) injury grade.[78] Low-grade injuries without ductal involvement (grade I–II) are managed nonoperatively, whereas higher-grade injuries with ductal involvement pose more difficult management decisions. For grade III injuries with involvement of the distal pancreatic duct, early (<48 hour) spleen-preserving laparoscopic distal pancreatectomy results in faster time to full enteral diet and discharge compared with nonoperative management, but long-term data are lacking. Nonoperative management is frequently successful but is associated with higher rates of pseudocyst formation and an increased risk of readmission.[79] Grade IV and V injuries involve injury to the proximal pancreatic duct. Higher-grade injuries frequently require involvement of a multidisciplinary team, possibly with the use of adjunctive measures, such as endoscopic retrograde cholangiopancreatography (ERCP). It should be noted that the optimal management of high-grade pancreatic injuries continues to be debated, with some centers managing almost all injuries nonoperatively.

Duodenal

Similar to pancreatic injury, duodenal trauma is typically caused by handlebar injury, NAT, or MVC.[80] Retroperitoneal duodenal injuries are often difficult to detect, and high suspicion for a delayed presentation should be maintained in the appropriate clinical context. Isolated duodenal hematomas are managed nonoperatively and typically resolve within 1 to 3 weeks.[80] Total parenteral nutrition (TPN), bowel rest, and nasogastric decompression can be used until obstructive symptoms resolve and enteral feeds can be reintroduced. Duodenal perforation, which is less common, requires operative intervention, the extent of which will depend on the degree of circumferential involvement of the injury.[81]

Hollow Viscus

Patients with HVI may present with immediate evidence of free air secondary to a full-thickness perforation or may demonstrate a delayed presentation after a devascularization injury that subsequently progresses to ischemia.[82] Patients with free air, peritonitis, or instability are taken immediately to the operating room, whereas stable patients with suspicious CT findings such as unexplained free fluid, bowel wall thickening, and mesenteric stranding are closely monitored with serial abdominal examinations. When patients have worsening or otherwise unexplained abdominal pain, diagnostic laparoscopy can evaluate for occult HVI.

Penetrating Injuries

Unfortunately, penetrating injuries are increasingly common in children. Compared with blunt mechanism, penetrating injuries are more lethal, requiring thoughtful and efficient diagnosis and management. The approach to penetrating injuries in children mirrors that of adults—early identification of all wounds is critical and will guide treatment decisions. All penetrating wounds should be quickly identified with the removal of all clothing and surveying the entire body by quickly rolling the child and looking in all cracks and crevices. Typically, children do not have a large amount of subcutaneous tissue to protect underlying viscera, and penetrating wounds have high likelihood of visceral injury (Fig. 42.5). Abdominal stab wounds that penetrate fascia warrant operative exploration; whether this entails a laparoscopic or open approach is dependent on the injury, patient, and provider expertise. As a general rule, firearm injuries to the abdominal cavity universally require exploratory laparotomy.

Pelvis

Pelvic fractures are relatively rare in children, accounting for 0.3% to 4% of pediatric injuries.[83,84] The developing pelvis demonstrates greater elasticity and higher cartilaginous volume than the adult pelvis, which makes pediatric pelvic fractures dependent on high-energy forces.[84,85] Given this, children tend to have less severe fractures than adults, but mortality is similar across age groups, as the extent of associated injuries more directly correlates with overall morbidity and mortality than the pelvic fracture itself.[85,86] Pediatric pelvic fractures most commonly occur as a result of pedestrians hit by cars and are frequently associated with significant additional injuries to the brain, liver, spleen, rectum, urinary tract, and femur.

Diagnosis and Management

A standard ATLS trauma evaluation is necessary for patients with suspected pelvic fractures, which are frequently in the setting of polytrauma. After the primary survey, the pelvis is palpated for tenderness and crepitus. Pelvic stability is assessed by carefully compressing the iliac wings, although rocking of the pelvis back and forth should be avoided as it may increase hemorrhage in the setting of a fracture. Complete examination of the perineum, rectum, and urethra should be performed. The standard radiologic examination in the trauma bay is an anteroposterior pelvic radiograph. If requested by orthopedics, additional views can subsequently by performed after initial stabilization.[83] A retrograde urethrogram is performed if a urethral injury is suspected. Abdominopelvic CT is highly useful in the stable patient to assess fracture pattern, evaluate associated injuries, and plan for the operating room.

When a pelvic fracture is suspected in the setting of hemodynamic instability, a pelvic binder can be applied in the trauma bay to reduce pelvic volume and tamponade bleeding.[87] Regardless of manufacturer, a pelvic binder should be appropriately sized and centered over the greater trochanter. If a pelvic binder is unavailable, a sheet can be used instead. If there is ongoing instability despite pelvic compression, external fixation or angiography with embolization can be performed.[88]

Most pediatric pelvic fractures are treated nonoperatively and heal without complication.[83,88] Nonoperative treatment usually entails a certain period of protected weight-bearing followed by physical therapy. Very young patients with stable fractures with acetabular extension may be treated with spica cast immobilization. Operative intervention is reserved for significantly displaced and unstable fractures of the pelvic ring. Surgery is typically performed in a delayed manner as dictated by the orthopedic surgery team.

Perineal Injury

Pediatric perineal injuries range from relatively mild superficial lacerations to severe injury with involvement of the genitourinary tract, anal sphincters, and deep soft tissue compartments. Injuries occur most frequently in the setting of MVCs, bicycle accidents, impalement, sexual abuse, and straddle injuries.[89,90] Diagnosis is often challenging given the sensitive location, but a complete assessment of the injury is critical to ensure proper treatment. The lack of external findings does not preclude rectal, vaginal, or bladder injuries. Providers should not hesitate to provide conscious sedation or general anesthesia to ensure an adequate examination is performed.[91,92] An array of additional evaluations, including proctoscopy, vaginoscopy, urethrogram, and cystoscopy, may be required based on clinical suspicion.

Management of the injury is dependent on severity and specific structures involved.[91,93–95] Combined injuries are common, and early consultation with gynecology and urology can ensure proper diagnosis and eventual treatment. Superficial soft tissue lacerations can be irrigated thoroughly and repaired with suture. Injury to the anal sphincters should be repaired primarily in the operating room, whereas more complex rectal injuries or combined anorectal and urethrovaginal injuries may require placement of a colostomy. Complex urinary tract injuries may require placement of a Foley or suprapubic catheter by urology.

Nonaccidental Trauma

Tragically, NAT is a leading cause of morbidity and mortality in the United States. Young children are at particular risk, with 80% of cases occurring in children younger than 5 years and 70% of fatalities occurring in children younger than 3 years. However, all ages are affected by physical abuse, and over 1500 fatalities are attributed annually to child abuse or neglect.[96,97]

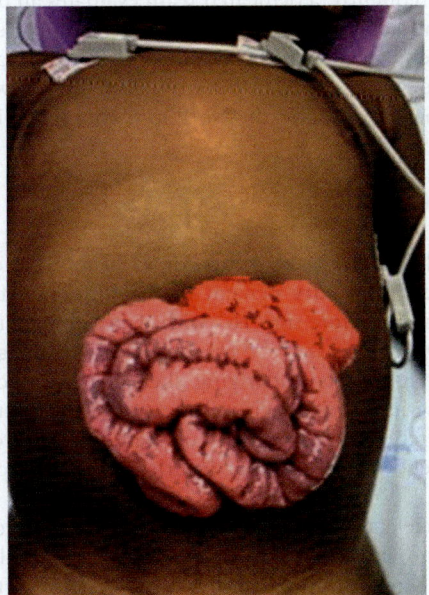

FIGURE 42.5 Infant with intestinal evisceration from abdominal stab wound.

The overarching theme in identifying child abuse is the need for a high level of suspicion and a systematic evaluation of all patients, regardless of socioeconomic status. Infants and toddlers likely will not be able to communicate a history, making it crucial to have a detailed knowledge of necessary physical examination steps, laboratory tests, and imaging studies. Regardless of injury, a multidisciplinary approach to management is necessary to address the complex immediate and long-term physical, emotional, and psychiatric needs of each patient.

Evaluation

Initial evaluation should always begin with a standard primary and secondary survey as per ATLS principles. Regardless of initial suspicions for abuse, the initial priority is stabilizing the patient. Once stable, a detailed history and physical is performed to identify any possible features suggestive of abuse. The injury itself and any other bruising are carefully documented. Even relatively minor, self-limited injuries are important potential pieces of forensic evidence. Standard trauma laboratory tests, including complete blood count (CBC), coagulation studies, electrolytes, liver function tests, and lipase/amylase, are ordered. Children younger than 2 years of age should have an x-ray skeletal survey performed to assess for fractures. A head CT should be strongly considered in children younger than 6 months in the appropriate clinical context. For children older than 2 years with a reliable examination, targeted imaging can be performed based on physical examination findings. Prior studies indicate that minority, lower health literacy, and underinsured families are more likely to be suspected of NAT, leading to higher rates of screening for abuse among these populations.[98,99] Establishing standard screening criteria and ensuring early involvement of social work and dedicated child abuse teams can minimize disparities in care.[100]

Cutaneous Injury

Bruises, bites, and burns are the most common signs of child abuse. Although isolated bruises over bony prominences are common throughout childhood, multiple bruises in different stages of healing and particularly over the buttocks, cheeks, ears, mouth, and genitalia should raise suspicions for abuse. Belt marks, hand-prints, and linear injuries are frequent patterns indicative of NAT. Additionally, nonambulatory children rarely have accidental bruising. Abusive burns most frequently result from scald injuries and often demonstrate splash marks and clear lines of demarcation. Immersion injuries of the buttock and genitalia often spare the flexor creases. Accidental burns are more likely nonuniform and have a story consistent with the burn pattern.

Head Trauma

Abusive head trauma is the leading cause of death and disability in children <2 years old. However, its presence may be difficult to detect as symptoms are often nonspecific and presentation is frequently delayed. Of children <2 years hospitalized for head injury, those with abusive head trauma were more likely to present with abnormal mental status and seizures, whereas children with accidental head injury were more likely to have scalp hematomas.[101] Patients younger than 2 years with isolated parietal skull fractures are more likely to be accidental, whereas complex skull fractures with intracranial injury are more often abusive trauma.[102] In a retrospective chart review of children with isolated, non–motor vehicle-related, skull fractures, children with a clear history of trauma, no extracranial injuries, and no social concerns were almost exclusively found to be accidental.[103]

Children younger than 6 months are particularly prone to shaken baby syndrome in which the infant is vigorously shaken, typically because of inconsolable crying by the infant. This results in direct trauma to the brain, SDH secondary to tearing of bridging veins, and shearing of axons.[104] Associated retinal hemorrhages and rib fractures are common. Overall, intracranial hemorrhage in children younger than 3 years has been associated with a 99% probability of abuse in the appropriate clinical context.

Fractures

Fractures are the second most common resultant injury of child abuse.[105] The most frequently injured long bones are the femur, humerus, and tibia, with fractures near the growth plate particularly suspicious for child abuse.[106] A systematic review of 32 studies demonstrated that fractures resulting from abuse were most common in patients younger than 3 years of age. Rib fractures were most predictive of abuse.[107] Multiple fractures should raise particular concern for abuse because the likelihood of abuse increases four- to sixfold for children with three or more fractures compared with those with only one.[108]

Abdomen

Although abdominal abusive injuries are relatively rare, they are the second most common cause of death after abusive head trauma. Solid organ injuries are the most common injury pattern, with the liver most frequently injured followed by the spleen. Pancreatic injuries are rarer and typically occur in conjunction with duodenal or other HVI. Patients often demonstrate bruising of the abdomen and may have elevations in liver function tests and pancreatic enzymes. In the setting of NAT, it is worth noting that the history is unreliable, so even without a reported mechanism concerning for abdominal trauma, the child should be considered a potential victim of assault, and the clinician should maintain appropriate concern for occult injury. When there is suspicion for injury, a CT with IV contrast is warranted.

Management

Although treatment depends on the specific injury pattern, a multidisciplinary approach will optimize short- and long-term outcomes. Frequently, a dedicated team evaluates all patients with suspected child abuse or neglect. This ensures all patients are seen by a team dedicated to ensuring a thorough history and physical is performed, all necessary laboratory tests are drawn, imaging studies are performed, and the workup is completed in a manner that minimizes bias.

Musculoskeletal
General

Musculoskeletal trauma accounts for 10% to 15% of all childhood injuries.[109,110] Fifty percent of males and 25% of females suffer a fracture before age 16, with a peak incidence in both groups at 10 to 14 years.[111,112] Fracture location varies with age in a manner that reflects underlying skeletal maturation and age-specific activities. The capacity of the pediatric skeleton to grow and rapidly remodel allows many of these fractures to be treated nonoperatively, whereas similar injuries in adults would require surgery.

Normal skeletal growth depends on the physes (growth plates) located at the ends of the long bones and vertebral body end-plates.[113] The growth plates are the weakest point of the skeleton and account for roughly 30% of long bone fractures.[109] Improper treatment can lead to deformity or cessation of development. The

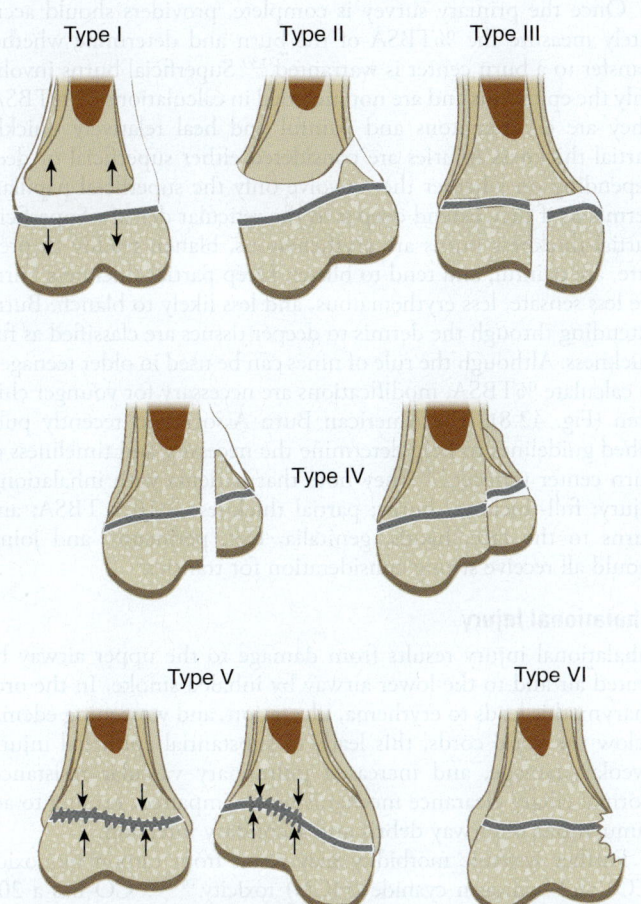

FIGURE 42.6 Salter-Harris classification system for physeal fractures. (From Leschied JR, Soliman SB. Pediatric musculoskeletal trauma: special considerations. *Semin Roentgenol.* 2021;56:70-78.)

Salter-Harris classification system is used to describe physeal injuries and predict outcomes (Fig. 42.6).[113,114]

The possibility of NAT must be accounted for in all pediatric fracture workups.[110,112] Abuse is especially common when the fracture pattern does not fit the reported history, the child is under 18 months of age, and there are fractures in different stages of healing.

Lower extremity. Femur fractures are the most common pediatric fractures requiring hospitalization.[115,116] In children younger than 1 year, up to two-thirds of femur fractures are secondary to child abuse, whereas fractures are commonly caused by falls in children aged 2 to 3 years and MVCs in older children.[117] A fracture of the femoral shaft in a nonambulatory infant should raise particularly high suspicion for child abuse, especially with transverse fracture patterns. Anteroposterior and lateral radiographs of the femur, hip, and knee are usually sufficient, although CT and MRI may be selectively used to evaluate more complex fractures or those requiring surgical management.[112] In general, young children are often treated nonoperatively with closed reduction, older children with flexible nails or plates, and adolescents more similarly to adults with solid femoral nails.[118–120]

Proximal tibial physeal injuries typically involve high-energy mechanisms and require careful vascular examination to detect injury to the popliteal artery. By contrast, nonphyseal fractures of the tibia and fibula occur as a result of lower-energy mechanisms

and are much more common. Regardless of the specific fracture location, patients should be closely monitored for the development of compartment syndrome, with a low threshold for fasciotomy given adequate clinical suspicion. Most fractures to the tibia and fibula can be treated nonoperatively, though patients with open fractures and significant malalignment will require surgery.[121,122]

Upper extremity. Clavicular fractures in pediatric patients are common, typically uncomplicated, and usually adequately treated by sling immobilization alone.[109] Injuries to the medial clavicle have the potential to compress mediastinal structures. They must be promptly evaluated by CT or MRI and will likely require open reduction with careful evaluation of deeper structures.[123–125]

Fractures of the proximal humerus are usually treated nonoperatively, as rapid growth leads to predictable remodeling in all but the most angulated fractures.[126,127] Older adolescents might require surgery if they have insufficient remaining growth potential. In the distal humerus, a supracondylar fracture is the most common injury and typically results from a fall on the outstretched hand. A thorough neurovascular examination is critical to detect impingement of the median nerve and brachial artery, which would require immediate operative reduction.[128,129] In the growing elbow there are multiple centers of ossification, which can make identification of a fracture difficult. A comparison radiograph of the contralateral elbow can help distinguish normal growth patterns from an occult fracture.

Distal forearm fractures are typically treated with closed manipulation and casting, often under conscious sedation. After reduction, the extremity is immobilized in a sugar tong splint or bivalved cast to account for early swelling. When the shaft of the radius or ulna is involved, internal fixation is often required to maintain stabilization. Generally, once the fracture is stabilized, the child should be relatively comfortably with a tolerable pain level. Pain out of proportion to the fracture should raise alarm for developing compartment syndrome.

Most hand injuries can be adequately diagnosed and treated with a careful history and physical examination alone.[130,131] The hand should be manipulated gently, with careful attention to neurovascular status. Plain films are commonly ordered to evaluate bony abnormality or foreign body. Ultrasound can assess tendons, foreign bodies, and fluid collections, whereas CT and MRI are more useful for evaluating complex injuries. Typically hand and wrist injuries can be managed nonoperatively with appropriate manipulation and casting, with exceptions for open and severely angulated fractures. In the setting of a traumatic amputation, the amputated part should be wrapped in saline-moistened gauze, placed in a container containing a slurry of ice and water, and quickly evaluated by a hand specialist for reimplantation.

Burns

Although care for burn and inhalational injuries has dramatically improved in recent decades, these injuries remain complex with the potential for substantial morbidity and mortality.[132,133] Children younger than 2 years old are at particular risk of morbidity given their relatively thin skin, which leads to more severe burns given the same thermal exposure.[134–136] Furthermore, a larger surface area to body mass ratio places young children at particularly high risk of insensible fluid losses, and their immature kidneys require larger fluid volumes for adequate resuscitation. Scald injuries, whether accidental or abusive, are the most common injury in younger children, whereas flame burns are more common in teenagers. Given the severe physiologic consequences of burns, a multidisciplinary approach is critical to ensuring initial stabilization, short-term resuscitation, and long-term rehabilitation.

Initial Evaluation

All patients with large burns (>10% total body surface area [TBSA]) should undergo initial ATLS evaluation, with special attention paid to other traumatic injuries in addition to the burn.[137] During the primary and secondary surveys, the burned area should be covered with a dry sheet and attempts at debridement deferred. Close attention should be paid to the evaluation of the airway, and a decision to intubate a tenuous patient should be made quickly.[138] The small cross-sectional area of the pediatric airway makes it susceptible to rapid collapse in the setting of worsening edema.[7] Signs such as increased respiratory effort, stridor, and hoarseness are ominous and should prompt rapid intervention. If there is uncertainty, fiberoptic bronchoscopy is the gold standard for evaluation of the airway. Whenever there is concern for inhalational injury, patients should receive 100% oxygen empirically while an arterial blood gas and carboxyhemoglobin levels are obtained. Carbon monoxide poisoning will falsely elevate pulse oximeter readings, making it necessary to review laboratory values to assess tissue oxygenation. As the airway is secured, two large-bore IVs and a Foley catheter should be placed with resuscitation promptly started. Reasonable urine output goals are 0.5 mL/kg/h for patients >30 kg and 1 mL/kg/h for patients <30 kg (Fig. 42.7).

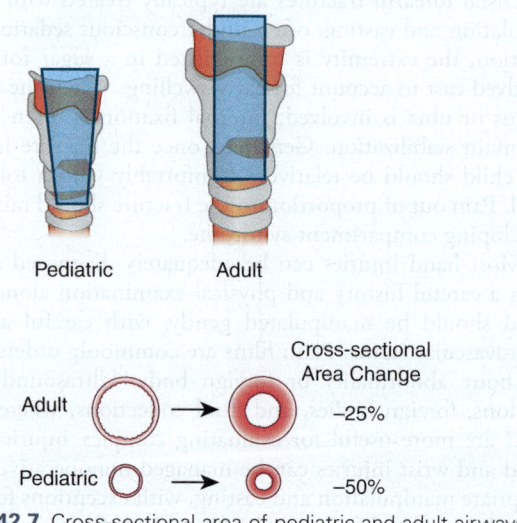

FIGURE 42.7 Cross-sectional area of pediatric and adult airways.

Once the primary survey is complete, providers should accurately measure the %TBSA of the burn and determine whether transfer to a burn center is warranted.[139] Superficial burns involve only the epidermis and are not included in calculations of %TBSA. They are erythematous and painful and heal relatively quickly. Partial-thickness injuries are considered either superficial or deep depending on whether they involve only the superficial papillary dermis or if they extend deeper to the reticular dermis. Superficial partial-thickness burns are erythematous, blanch readily to pressure, are painful, and tend to blister. Deep partial-thickness burns are less sensate, less erythematous, and less likely to blanch. Burns extending through the dermis to deeper tissues are classified as full thickness. Although the rule of nines can be used in older teenagers to calculate %TBSA, modifications are necessary for younger children (Fig. 42.8). The American Burn Association recently published guidelines to help determine the necessity and timeliness of burn center transfer.[140] They note that patients with inhalational injury; full-thickness burns; partial thickness ≥10% TBSA; and burns to the face, hands, genitalia, feet, perineum, and joints should all receive strong consideration for transfer.

Inhalational Injury

Inhalational injury results from damage to the upper airway by heated air and to the lower airway by inhaled smoke. In the oropharynx this leads to erythema, ulceration, and worsening edema. Below the vocal cords, this leads to substantial epithelial injury, alveolar damage, and increased pulmonary vascular resistance. Normal ciliary clearance mechanisms are impaired, leading to accumulations of airway debris and secondary infection.

Further systemic morbidity may result from carbon monoxide (CO) and hydrogen cyanide (HCN) toxicity.[141,142] CO has a 200 times greater affinity for hemoglobin than oxygen, causing a left shift of the oxygen dissociation curve. Patients will have a normal pulse oximeter reading but substantial deficits in tissue oxygenation. Carboxyhemoglobin (COHb) blood levels should be quickly obtained in all patients suspected of inhalational injury. At low COHb levels, patients may develop headaches, blurred vision, nausea, and vomiting. At higher levels, seizures, loss of consciousness, and impaired respirations can occur. In patients with suspected CO poisoning, initial management should be placing child on 100% humidified high-flow oxygen to decrease the half-life of COHb. HCN is released due to the combustion of synthetic household products and disrupts aerobic metabolism by binding to mitochondrial cytochrome c oxidase. Patients develop neurologic deficits, persistent acidosis, and elevated lactate levels despite appropriate resuscitation.

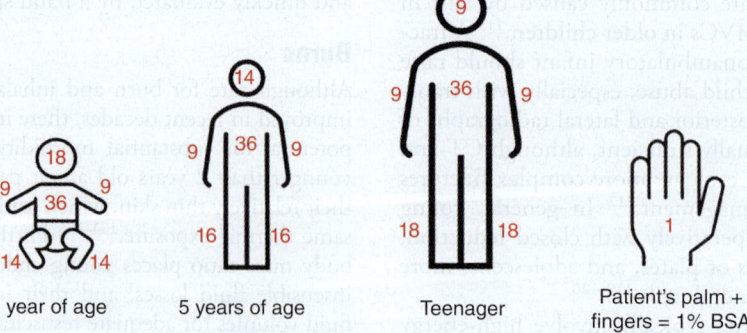

FIGURE 42.8 Percent body surface area of each body part by age. *BSA,* Body surface area. (Adapted from Duggan RP, Palackic A, Branski L. Burns. In: Mattei P, ed. *Fundamentals of Pediatric Surgery.* Cham: Springer; 2022:223-240.)

Hydroxocobalamin can be administered to bind and metabolize cyanide for excretion in the urine.

All patients with inhalational injury should receive aggressive supportive care with aggressive chest physiotherapy, clearance of secretions, and early mobilization. Inhaled heparin, acetylcysteine, and racemic epinephrine can facilitate the breakdown of fibrin plugs, improve clearance of secretions, and minimize bronchospasm. Chest wall oscillation and bronchoalveolar lavage can further assist in removing secretions and collecting microbial specimens.

Burn Resuscitation

Burns cause severe physiologic impairments secondary to substantial cellular derangements and increased capillary permeability.[143,144] Underresuscitation leads to decreased cardiac output and end-organ damage, whereas overresuscitation leads to fluid creep, pulmonary edema, and compartment syndromes.[145,146] Finding the right balance is challenging and requires constant reassessment of the patient's examination, urine output, and laboratory values. Doing so is made more difficult by the changes in total TBSA relative to overall mass as the pediatric patient develops. The Parkland formula that is used for adults tends to underresuscitate children with minor burns and substantially overresuscitate large burns. The Cincinnati and Galveston formulas better account for TBSA variability in pediatric patients (Table 42.4).[147,148] Regardless of the formula chosen, fluid resuscitation should begin even before the %TBSA burned is calculated. Two large-bore IVs are placed, resuscitative fluids started, and a Foley catheter inserted. The total fluid to be given over the next 24 hours is then calculated, with constant adjustments made based on serial assessment of vital signs, mental status, physical examination findings, and laboratory values.

Burn Wound Management

Burn wound management varies substantially depending on the depth and size of the wounds. Superficial wounds typically heal without surgical intervention within 10 to 14 days and can be managed nonoperatively with dressings and topical agents. Traditionally, antimicrobial agents such as silver sulfadiazine, mafenide acetate, and silver nitrate were used for partial-thickness wounds to create a moist environment and prevent infection of the wound. In many centers, these agents have been largely replaced by synthetic and biologic wound dressings that require less frequent changes and improve healing time.[149] Deep partial-thickness burns require excision and grafting if the surgeon does not anticipate healing within 3 weeks, although differentiating superficial and deep partial-thickness wounds can be challenging. Wound biopsy and laser Doppler imaging can help providers more reliably assess depth.[150,151] If the burn is less than 20% TBSA, it can be initially managed conservatively until depth is accurately determined. Full-thickness burns should generally be excised and grafted within the first 24 to 48 hours.

Burn wounds are typically excised tangentially, using a dermatome or VersaJet water dissector, and then grafted using autograft skin.[152] Autografts are either split or full thickness depending on the depth of tissue harvested. Full-thickness grafts have better cosmetic results and are used for facial, hand, genital, and joint burns. Full-thickness donor sites are limited to tissues that can be closed primarily such as the inguinal and postauricular regions. Split-thickness grafts are used for burns that cover a more extensive area. Grafts can be meshed to increase coverage and allow better drainage of hematomas and seromas. If donor sites are not available, burns can be temporarily covered with a dermal substitute to minimize fluid loss and reduce pain.[153] A split-thickness skin graft can be subsequently applied on top of the substitute.

Injury Prevention and Advocacy

Injury is the leading cause of death and disability in children worldwide. In fact, more than 60% of deaths among children and adolescents in the United States result from injury-related causes.[154] The most frequent MOIs include falls, MVCs, sports injuries, abuse, and firearm-related injuries. In 2020, firearm-related injuries surpassed all other causes as the most common cause of death for children in the United States.[155] Addressing these causes of injury is a key focus of trauma surgeons—in addition to the critical work of caring for injured children. This focus on injury prevention is recognized as being of such importance that it is a requirement of certification by the American College of Surgeons as a level I trauma center.

Efforts to prevent injuries must acknowledge that the burden of injuries is not borne equally by all children in the United States, with significant inequities in who is injured and how severe those injuries are. These inequities are associated with both individual and neighborhood-level social determinants of health (SDOHs).[156–158] As such, the SDOHs are key upstream targets in injury prevention efforts.

Injury prevention efforts can be divided into three primary categories: primary, secondary, and tertiary prevention.[159] Primary prevention focuses on preventing disease before it happens through modification of existing risk factors and prevention of development of risk factors. Examples of primary prevention may include provision of bike helmets, car seats, gun locks, and other home safety equipment (e.g., baby gates) to reduce the likelihood that a child is injured.[160,161] Secondary prevention addresses recovery from injury to prevent additional injury and works to modify risk factors identified after the injury that put the child at risk for future injury. This may include particular work around firearm safety after a child sustains an unintentional injury while

TABLE 42.4	Pediatric Resuscitation Formulas After Burn Injury
Cincinnati formula	Young children: • 4 mL/kg/% TBSA burn + 1500 mL/m^2 total BSA of LR. • Half over the first 8 h, half over the next 16 h. • First 8 h, 50 mEq/L of sodium bicarbonate is added. Second 8 h is LR alone. Third 8 h, albumin (12.5 g of 25% albumin per liter of crystalloid) is added. • 5% dextrose as needed. Older children: • 4 mL/kg/% TBSA burn + 1500 mL/m^2 total BSA of LR. Half of the volume in the first 8 h, followed by remainder in 16 h. • 5% dextrose as needed.
Galveston formula	LR: • 5000 mL/m^2 burn + 2000 mL/m^2 total. Half of the volume in the first 8 h, followed by remainder in 16 h. • 12.5 g of 25% albumin per liter of crystalloid. • 5% dextrose as needed.

BSA, Body surface area; *LR*, lactated Ringer; *TBSA*, total body surface area.
From Carvajal HF. A physiologic approach to fluid therapy in severely burned children. *Surg Gynecol Obstet.* 1980;150:379-384; Stevens JV, Prieto NS, Ridelman E, Klein JD, Shanti CM. Weight-based vs body area-based fluid resuscitation predictions in pediatric burn patients. *Burns.* 2023;49:120-128.

handling a loaded firearm. Tertiary prevention focuses on mitigating long-term effects from injury and may include addressing acute stress or posttraumatic stress after injury.[162]

Each of these areas is seminal in reducing and preventing the impact of injury on child health and wellness as well as the health of the family and community more broadly. Injury prevention efforts are integrally linked with advocacy by all providers who care for children. Such advocacy focuses on increasing resources allocated to injury prevention within healthcare systems as well as changing laws and regulations on the local, state, and national level to reduce risk. Examples of successful efforts include legislation for bike helmet laws and child access laws for firearm safety, among others. These legislative changes have been shown to clearly reduce injuries in children.[163] These must also be tied to efforts to improve the mental health of children, as there are clear linkages between worsening mental health and rising suicide rates among children as well.[164] Recognizing that inequities in injuries overall, and firearm injuries in particular, are rooted in long-standing structural racism, addressing such structural factors is critical to the success of injury prevention strategies. This also requires recognition that community-level violence is a complex, dynamic challenge that requires tools that acknowledge these systemic factors.[165]

Injury prevention endeavors are a key focus of trauma systems to reduce the devastating short- and long-term impact of injuries on children, their families, and their communities.

SELECTED REFERENCES

Goldstick JE, Cunningham RM, Carter PM. Current causes of death in children and adolescents in the United States. *New Engl J Med.* 2022;386(20):1955-1956.

> *Firearm injuries have now passed motor vehicle crashes as the leading cause of death among children and adolescents 1 to 19 years of age.*

Kuppermann N, Holmes JF, Dayan PS, et al. Identification of children at very low risk of clinically important brain injuries after head trauma: a prospective cohort study. *Lancet.* 2009; 374(9696):1160-1170.

> *Implementation of PECARN guidelines limits the number of unnecessary head CTs for up to 60% of emergency department TBI evaluations without increasing rates of missed life-threatening injuries.*

Luckhurst CM, Wiberg HM, Brown RL, et al. Pediatric cervical spine injury following blunt trauma in children younger than 3 years. The PEDSPINE II Study. *JAMA Surg.* 2023;158(11): 1126-1132.

> *The PEDSPINE II trial investigated whether a prediction tool could help decrease the use of imaging, aid in clinical decision-making, and decrease hospital resource use.*

Pearce MS, Salotti JA, Little MP, et al. Radiation exposure from CT scans in childhood and subsequent risk of leukemia and brain tumors: a retrospective cohort study. *Lancet.* 2012;380:499-432.

> *Childhood radiation exposure may predispose children to cancers later in life. The "as low as reasonably achievable" (ALARA) principle can help clinicians balance the risk of radiation with the informational benefit of a given study.*

Williams RH, Grewal H, Jamshidi R, et al. Updated APSA guidelines for the management of blunt liver and spleen injury. *J Pediatr Surg.* 2023;58:1411-1418.

> *Recently released guidelines for the management of blunt liver and spleen injuries present an easy-to-follow management strategy for children.*

The full reference list appears on Elsevier eBooks+.

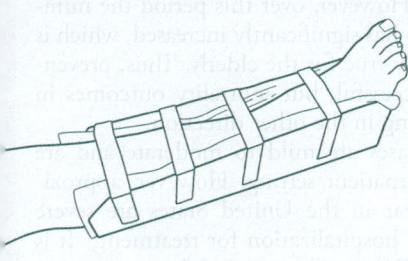

Burns

Steven A. Kahn and Steven E. Wolf

INTRODUCTION

Overall, surgery has evolved at a remarkable pace over the past three decades. The world witnessed a transition to minimally invasive approaches, moving from open procedures to laparoscopic and now robot-assisted procedures. In addition, principles of enhanced recovery are now the standard of care in many subspecialties. However, the field of burn surgery has lagged behind until just recently. Early excision, metabolic management, and dermal template advances pushed the field forward 40 to 50 years ago, but since then only a few additions such as better ventilator management and the appropriate use of renal support emerged. Importantly, new efforts for improved resuscitation techniques and novel skin replacement technologies have returned to center stage (Fig. 43.1).

Progress in our field has been somewhat limited in the marketplace of ideas by the decreasing incidence of severe burns in the developed world; unfortunately this is not the case worldwide. Disparate patterns of care remain across centers, and training has wide variability in content related to less emphasis on burns in surgery overall. Further, difficulty remains in performing high-quality prospective studies given the heterogeneity of burn wounds and unmeasured confounders in these complex patients. However, recent concerted efforts to develop agreeable clinical practice and training guidelines, expansion of regenerative medicine technologies, and a commitment to high-quality study performance

have resulted in a new push forward. For example, training guidelines for fellowships with on-site review have now been established by the American Burn Association. Further, a point-of-care autologous skin cell suspension allowing 80:1 expansion, dermis-sparing enzymatic excision of wounds, and novel bioengineered cell constructed skin substitutes now allow for earlier closure of wounds and less use of conventional skin grafts.[1] Improvements in diagnosis with new imaging technology have also come to the fore. Finally, a portfolio of positively disruptive technologies has been funded by the US Department of Defense (DoD) and Biomedical Advanced Research and Development Authority (BARDA), resulting in significant strides forward. The field continues to merge with the aim to maximize survival with a push for high-value, multidisciplinary, patient-centered care with optimal functional and cosmetic outcomes coupled with reintegration back into society. Rehabilitation is no longer considered "aftercare" and starts immediately after injury.

To review the field of burn care, both established and emerging, this chapter covers burn epidemiology, pathophysiology, burn treatment paradigms, and new technologies that are rapidly becoming standard of care.

GENERAL CONSIDERATIONS

In 2020, approximately 290,000 people were burned in the United States, 4000 of whom died (overall mortality rate 1.4%).

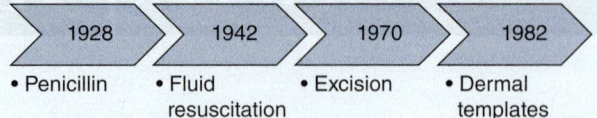

1928	1942	1970	1982
• Penicillin	• Fluid resuscitation	• Excision	• Dermal templates

FIGURE 43.1 Evolution of burn surgery.

Epidemiologic trends from 2001 to 2021 demonstrate that the US population grew from 285,000,000 to 332,000,000 people, a nominal 16% increase. Correspondingly, the incidence of burns diminished from 520,000 to 290,000, a 43% decrease. However, the number of fatal burns has increased with an inflection point in 2012, from 2500 deaths in 2001 to 4000 deaths in 2021.[2] From these data, we conclude that the number of burns has appreciably decreased per capita over this period; however, the population (aka "capita") continues to increase nominally; thus, burns remain a steady public health threat (Fig. 43.2). When separated into children (0–18 years), adults (19–65 years), and the elderly (>65 years), these trends remain, decreasing mostly in children and young adults with moderate decreases per capita in

older adults and the elderly. However, over this period the number of deaths caused by burns has significantly increased, which is of concern. This is particularly true for the elderly. Thus, prevention strategies have been successful, but mortality outcomes in those who are burned are going in the other direction.

Fortunately, most burn cases are mild to moderate and are commonly treated in the outpatient setting. However, approximately 40,000 burns per year in the United States are severe enough to undergo inpatient hospitalization for treatment.[2] It is estimated by the Centers for Disease Control and Prevention that the annual direct medical costs for burn care was $2.64 billion in 2020. What is more striking is the estimates of work loss and quality-of-life costs at $3.46 billion, for a total annual cost of $5.79 billion; the average cost of hospitalization for burns is $68,000, with ongoing costs after discharge at $89,000 per patient (total $157,000 per patient). For context, in 2020, about 7% of the US population suffered some form of injury and received recorded treatment, but few sustained fatal injuries (1.3% of those injured). For comparison, deaths in those with burns represented 1.4% of all injury fatalities, which accords with injury overall.

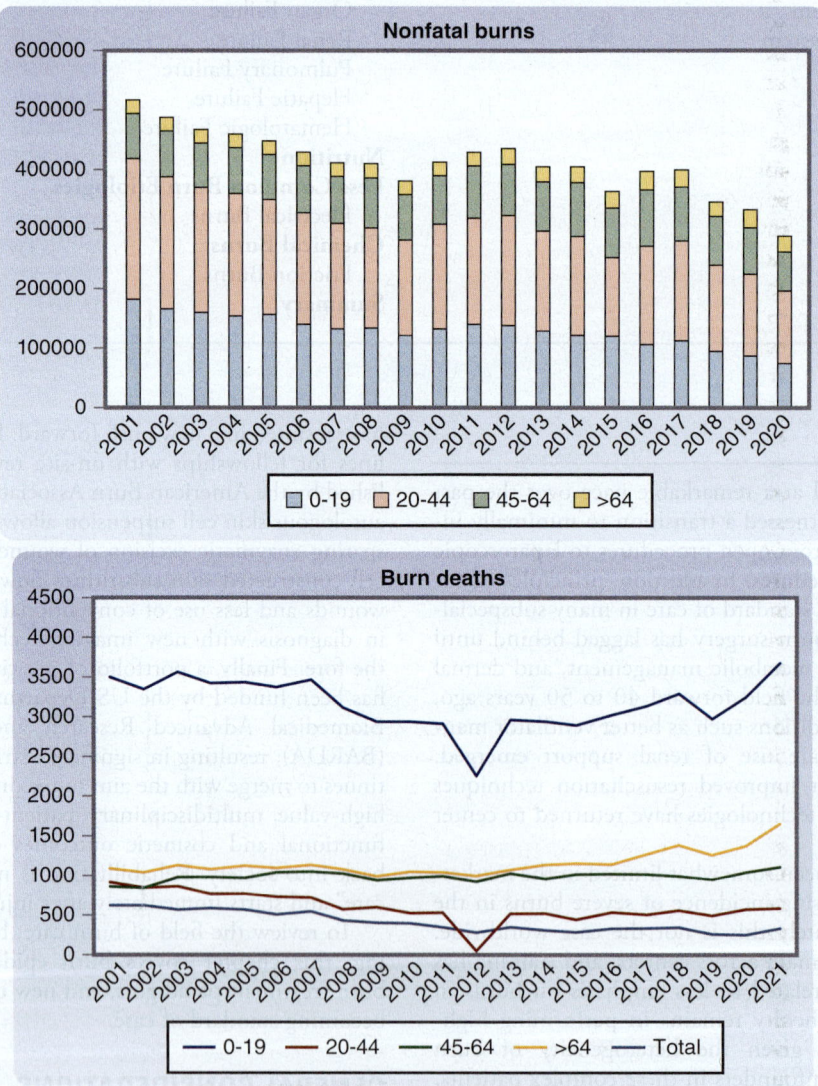

FIGURE 43.2 US burn incidence rate (2001–21). Groups are stratified by ages in the legend. (Top) Nominal numbers of burns cited in the WISQARS database from the US Centers for Disease Control and Prevention. (Bottom) Nominal number of deaths related to burns in the same database.

Burn deaths generally occur in a bimodal distribution, either immediately after the injury or weeks later as a result of multiple organ failure, a pattern similar to all trauma-related deaths and in keeping with the maxim espoused by Basil Pruitt: "burns is the universal trauma model." Therefore, burns remain a major morbid problem in the United States as a representative of high-income countries. However, it is much worse in low- and middle-income countries.[3]

Approximately 43% of burns in the United States are caused by fire and flame, 34% from scalding with hot liquid or grease burns, 9% from contact burns, 3% from chemical burns, and 4% from electrical burns.[4] Three-quarters of all burns occur at home and commonly involve children less than 10 years of age, adult males, and, increasingly, the elderly. In a 10-year average from 2011 to 2020 in the United States, 30% of burns occurred in the 0- to 19-year-old age group (children) and another 41% in the 20- to 44-year-old adult age group. The rest were in older adults aged 45 to 64 (22%) and persons over 64 years of age (7%). In terms of sex, 54% of burns in the United States occur in males, which is a more equitable sex distribution than found previously.

Seventy-five percent of all burn-related deaths occur in house fires commonly associated with food preparation or heating equipment. Interestingly, the cause of fire with the highest mortality is still from cigarette smoking, which leads to 22% of house fire–related deaths. Young adults are frequently burned with flammable liquids, whereas toddlers are often scalded by hot liquids at a proportion of 60%. A significant percentage of burns in children are the result of child abuse. Other risk factors include low socioeconomic class and unsafe environments.[5] These generalizations emphasize that most burn injuries are preventable and therefore amenable to prevention strategies.

A recent probit analysis on the overall mortality from burns regardless of age in the United States showed an LD_{50} at a 55% total body surface area (TBSA) burn; therefore, in current times, a 55% TBSA burn has a 50% probability of death. When a similar analysis was done with Baux score (age + TBSA burned) accounting for improved survival probability in younger age groups, the LD_{50} was 105 and LD_{90} was 130.[5]

Prevention strategies have decreased the number and severity of injuries. Successful approaches include legislation for fire-safe cigarettes and some cultural transition to e-cigarettes—although e-cigarettes are not without fire risk associated with battery ignition, they do decrease the rate of structure fires. Other effective events were changes in the National Electrical Code, elevation of hot water heaters from the ground, and increased smoke alarm use, which have significantly decreased fire death rates.

Burn Units

Improvements in burn care originated principally in specialized care units dedicated to burned patients, first developed in the United Kingdom during WWII by Gilles and MacIndoe. These consist of experienced personnel with dedicated resources to maximize outcome from these devastating injuries (Box 43.1). The American Burn Association currently provides a program to verify whether burn units meet a series of qualifications for personnel, space, equipment, supplies, and processes to secure best outcomes, with over 90 verified burn centers currently in the United States.[6] They also recommend that patients with the following criteria be referred to a verified burn center:

1. Partial-thickness burns greater than 10% TBSA
2. Burns involving the face, hands, feet, genitalia, perineum, or major joints

---

BOX 43.1 Burn Unit Organization and Personnel

- Experienced burn surgeons (burn unit director and qualified surgeons)
- Dedicated nursing personnel
- Physical and occupational therapists
- Social workers
- Dietitians
- Pharmacists
- Respiratory therapists
- Psychiatrists and clinical psychologists
- Prosthetists

---

3. Any full-thickness burn
4. Electrical burns, including lightning injury
5. Chemical burns
6. Inhalation injury
7. Burns in patients with preexisting medical disorders that could complicate management, prolong recovery, or affect outcome
8. Any patient with burns and concomitant trauma (such as fractures) in which the burn injury poses the greater immediate risk of morbidity and mortality. In such cases, if the trauma poses the greater immediate risk, the patient may be initially stabilized in a trauma center before being transferred to a burn unit. Physician judgment is necessary in such situations and should be in concert with the regional medical control plan and triage protocols
9. Burned children in hospitals without qualified personnel or equipment to care for children
10. Burns in patients with poorly controlled pain

PATHOPHYSIOLOGY OF BURNS

Local Changes

Thermal burns cause damage to the skin and occasionally underlying structures through abrupt temperature change exceeding biologic tolerance. Membranes disrupt, protein denatures, and necrosis results. The injury extends from the skin surface to deeper structures in a first-order logarithmic distribution depending on the temperature of the burning agent and duration of exposure. Severe burns to the skin reaching over 280°F on the surface induce a Maillard-type reaction, with changes in consistency and color common in flame full-thickness burns. Burns that induce necrosis of the surface with temperatures below 280°F, such as scald burns from hot water, have a different appearance and texture and can be mistaken for partial-thickness burns. The thermal conductivity of the causative agent for scald and contact burns also affects the depth, which is typically by conduction rather than convection or radiation common with flame burns, particularly those sustained during explosions. Thermal conductivity is the ability to transfer heat; for water, it is 0.61 W/m/°C; for hot cooking oil, it is 4.2 joule/g/°C; and for grease, it is 1.8 joule/g/°C. Therefore, with cooling being the opposite of heating, more energy is transferred more rapidly. From a public health perspective, it is important to encourage patients to keep appropriate (class A, B, and C for residential and K for commercial) fire extinguishers in the kitchen for injuries associated with hot oil and grease. Grease fires should be extinguished by putting a lid on the pan or using a fire extinguisher. Persons should never attempt to extinguish the flame with running water, and they

BOX 43.2   Burn Classifications

Causes of Injury

Flame—damage from superheated oxidized air by convection and radiation

Scald—damage from contact with hot liquids

Contact—damage from contact with hot or cold solids

Electrical—conduction of electrical current through tissues

Chemical—contact with noxious chemicals

Friction—shearing injury from moving belts or contact with the ground at velocity

Depth of Injury

Superficial—injury confined to the epidermis

Superficial partial-thickness—injury to the epidermis and papillary dermis

Deep partial-thickness—injury to the epidermis and reticular dermis

Full-thickness—injury extending through the epidermis and dermis into subcutaneous fat

should be discouraged from carrying a flaming pan of grease outside to throw it in the yard because this is how most injuries occur.

Burns are classified into six different causal categories and four depths of injury (Box 43.2). The causes include injury from flame, hot liquids (scald), contact with hot or cold objects (contact), conduction of electricity, chemical exposure, and friction. The first three induce cellular damage primarily by transfer of energy, inducing coagulative necrosis (except for cold injuries, which do not cause protein denaturation). Electricity and chemicals cause direct injury to cellular membranes in addition to the transfer of heat, and finally, friction is by direct shearing forces.

The skin provides a robust barrier to transfer of energy to deeper tissues; therefore, much of the injury is confined to this layer. Further, and as mentioned previously, transfer of energy generally follows a first-order distribution; thus, distance from the source induces logarithmic decreases in energy transmission. Time is also a key component, with direct correlation to the severity and depth of the injury. This is important to note because people often attempt to quickly remove themselves from environments where burns occur, thus limiting the severity of injury. Considering this in the history of the event is important in determining wound depth and thus optimal treatment.

After the inciting focus is removed, the response of local tissues often leads to injury in the deeper layers. The area of cutaneous injury has been divided into three zones: zone of coagulation, zone of stasis, and zone of hyperemia.[7] The necrotic area of burn where cells were directly disrupted is termed the *zone of coagulation;* this tissue is irreversibly damaged at the time of injury. The area immediately surrounding the necrotic zone has a moderate degree of initial insult that is worsened with decreased tissue perfusion. This is termed the *zone of stasis* and, depending on the wound microenvironment, can either survive or go on to coagulative necrosis. The zone of stasis is associated with vascular damage and vessel leakage. The last area is termed the *zone of hyperemia,* which is characterized by vasodilation from inflammation surrounding the burn wound. This region contains the clearly viable tissue from which the healing process begins and is generally not at risk for further necrosis. This concept, termed *the Jackson Levels,* has been questioned recently with the development of new molecular and imaging techniques for measurement of the process, although it remains the basis for the physiologic description of burn wound progression and results.[7]

Burn Depth

Burn depth depends on the initial tissue damage, classified by penetrance from the surface to the epidermis, dermis, subcutaneous fat, and underlying structures (Fig. 43.3). Superficial burns (previously termed *first-degree*) are, by definition, injury confined to the epidermis. These injuries are painful, erythematous, and blanch to the touch with an intact epidermal barrier. Examples include sunburn or a very minor scald from a kitchen incident. These do not disrupt any underlying structures and therefore do not result in scarring. Treatment is aimed at comfort with the use of topical soothing salves and oral nonsteroidal antiinflammatory agents.

Partial-thickness burns (formerly called *second-degree*) are divided into two types: superficial and deep. All partial-thickness burns have some degree of dermal damage, and the division is based on the depth of injury into this structure. Superficial partial-thickness burns are limited to the papillary dermis and are erythematous, painful, blanch to touch, and often blister. Hair follicles remain viable and intact; thus, a finding on physical examination is retention of hairs to gentle pulling. Examples include scald injuries

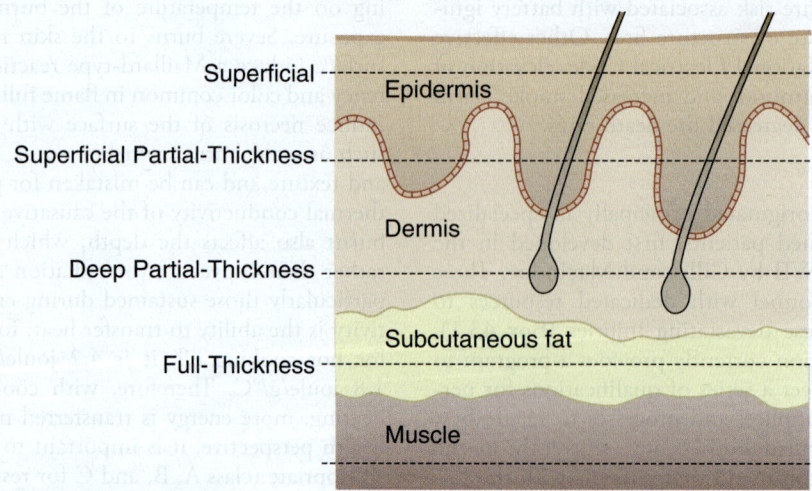

FIGURE 43.3 Depths of a burn. Superficial burns are confined to the epidermis. Superficial partial-thickness burns are limited to the epidermis and papillary dermis. Deep partial-thickness burns extend through the epidermis and reticular dermis. Full-thickness burns extend through the epidermis and dermis into subcutaneous fat and can involve injury to underlying tissue structures, such as muscle, tendons, and bone.

sustained in kitchen incidents and flash flame burns. These wounds spontaneously reepithelialize from retained epidermal structures in rete ridges and hair follicles in the follicular dermis in 7 to 14 days. After healing, these burns may have skin discoloration and textural differences without other significant scarring. Deep partial-thickness burns within the reticular dermis appear more pale and mottled, do not blanch to touch, and remain painful to pinprick. These burns heal in 15 to 21 days by reepithelialization from deep hair follicles and sweat gland keratinocytes, often with severe scarring as a result of loss of dermal integrity.

Full-thickness burns (formerly termed *third-degree*) extend through the epidermis and dermis into the underlying fat and are characterized by a hard leathery eschar that is painless and black, white, or cherry red in color depending on the temperature of the source and any associated Mailliard reaction. No epidermal or dermal keratinocytes remain; thus, these wounds must heal by reepithelialization from the wound edges. Deep dermal and full-thickness burns benefit from excision of the eschar with autologous skin grafting in order to heal in a timely fashion and to minimize contraction. Full-thickness burns can extend below the superficial fat to involve other structures, such as muscle and bone (formerly termed *fourth-degree*).

Currently, burn depth is most accurately assessed by judgment of experienced practitioners, although modern imaging technologies, such as laser Doppler flowmetry, laser speckle imaging, optical coherence, and multispectral imaging with or without artificial intelligence techniques hold the promise of improving assessment and guiding better treatment and outcomes.[8–10] Accurate assessment of depth is critical to determine optimal treatment for each affected area and ensure the best outcomes in terms of scarring and distress during treatment. Examination of the entire wound by surgeons ultimately responsible and accountable for management is the gold standard to guide treatment decisions. Imaging techniques and decision-support algorithms, some of which can be used sequentially, hold the promise to make such improvements.

Burn Size

Determination of burn size estimates the extent of injury. Burn size is traditionally assessed manually by the "rule of nines." In adults, each upper extremity and the head and neck are 9% of the TBSA, the lower extremities and the anterior and posterior trunk are 18% each, and the perineum and genitalia are assumed to be 1% of the TBSA (Fig. 43.4). Another method of estimating smaller burns is to equate the area of the open hand (including the palm and the extended fingers) of the patient as approximately 1% TBSA and then to transpose that measurement visually onto the wound for a determination of its size. This method is helpful when evaluating splash burns and other burns of disparate distribution.

Children have a relatively larger portion of the body surface area in the head and neck, which is compensated by a relatively smaller surface area in the lower extremities. Infants have 21% of the TBSA in the head and neck and 13% in each leg, which incrementally approaches adult proportions with increasing age. The Berkow formula is used to accurately determine burn size in children (Table 43.1).

SYSTEMIC CHANGES

Inflammation and Edema

Burns induce a massive increase in inflammation in response to injury in the wound first that is then generalized to all other tissues. The Glue Grant Investigators demonstrated that over 80%

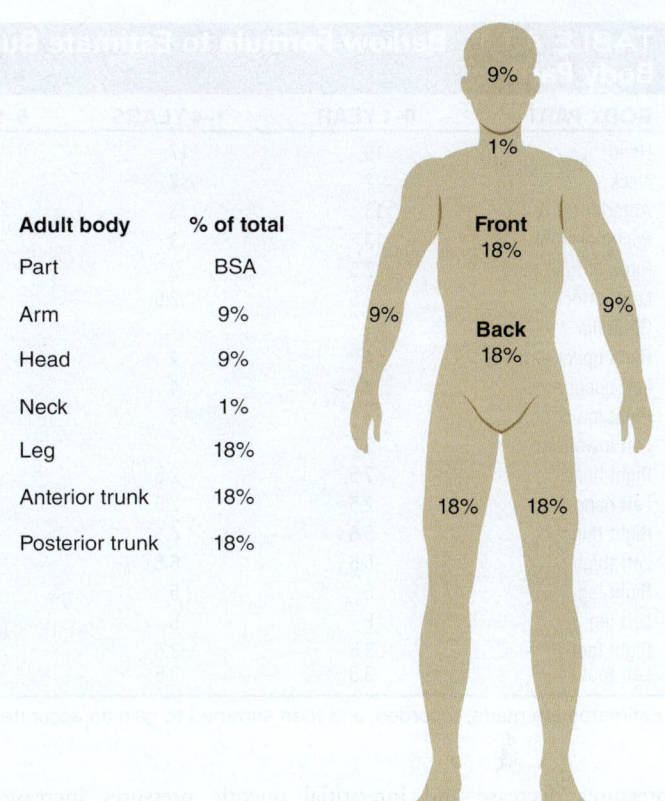

Adult body Part	% of total BSA
Arm	9%
Head	9%
Neck	1%
Leg	18%
Anterior trunk	18%
Posterior trunk	18%

FIGURE 43.4 Rule of Nines for estimation of total body surface area *(BSA)* burned.

of the genes in circulating immune cells are radically changed after severe injury, including burns.[10] The changes involve most, if not all, cellular functions and pathways and was termed a *genomic storm*. This breadth and degree of change were not anticipated by the investigators, identifying that circulating leukocytes are radically activated in response to severe injury with dramatically increased expression of genes in the inflammatory, innate immunity, and antiinflammatory spheres. They also noted a significant downregulation of genes associated with adaptive immunity. Perhaps most interestingly, they found that later complications such as infection and organ failure were not related to tangible genomic changes during the course of recovery, differing only in the magnitude and duration of the initial changes. Persons with many types of injury were included in the study, but a large proportion of them had severe burns. The investigators further found no differences in the response by injury type; therefore, these findings are clearly applicable to burned patients. In particular, it is prudent to recognize that severe burns induce massive physiologic and immune changes that are prolonged for about a year after injury.[11] Further, tracking genomic and inflammatory mediator changes along the course of treatment is not likely to be fruitful to predict complications and infections because these are already established at the time of injury.[12]

Mediators that are produced locally induce vasoconstriction and vasodilation, increased capillary permeability, and edema. The whole body response then ensues based on the extent of injury, with changes in permeability and activity of mediators causing generalized edema through Starling forces in both burned and unburned skin. Initially, the interstitial hydrostatic pressures in the burned skin decrease dramatically with an associated slight increase in nonburned skin interstitial pressures. As plasma oncotic

TABLE 43.1   **Berkow Formula to Estimate Burn Size (%) Based on Area of Burn in an Isolated Body Part[a]**

BODY PART	0–1 YEAR	1–4 YEARS	5–9 YEARS	10–14 YEARS	15–18 YEARS	ADULT
Head	19	17	13	11	9	7
Neck	2	2	2	2	2	2
Anterior trunk	13	13	13	13	13	13
Posterior trunk	13	13	13	13	13	13
Right buttock	2.5	2.5	2.5	2.5	2.5	2.5
Left buttock	2.5	2.5	2.5	2.5	2.5	2.5
Genitalia	1	1	1	1	1	1
Right upper arm	4	4	4	4	4	4
Left upper arm	4	4	4	4	4	4
Right lower arm	3	3	3	3	3	3
Left lower arm	3	3	3	3	3	3
Right hand	2.5	2.5	2.5	2.5	2.5	2.5
Left hand	2.5	2.5	2.5	2.5	2.5	2.5
Right thigh	5.5	6.5	8	8.5	9	9.5
Left thigh	5.5	6.5	8	8.5	9	9.5
Right leg	5	5	5.5	6	6.5	7
Left leg	5	5	5.5	6	6.5	7
Right foot	3.5	3.5	3.5	3.5	3.5	3.5
Left foot	3.5	3.5	3.5	3.5	3.5	3.5

[a]Estimates are made, recorded, and then summed to gain an accurate estimate of the body.

pressures decrease and interstitial oncotic pressures increase, edema forms in the burned and nonburned tissues. The edema is greater in the burned tissues because of lower interstitial pressures.

Many mediators are proposed to account for changes in permeability after burns, including histamine, bradykinin, vasoactive amines, prostaglandins, leukotrienes, activated complement, and catecholamines, among others. Recently, investigators showed that shedding glycocalyx from plasma membranes is also instrumental in the process.[13] Mast cells in burned skin release histamine in large quantities immediately after injury, eliciting a characteristic response in venules by increasing intercellular junction space formation. The use of antihistamines in the treatment of burn edema, however, has had limited success. In addition, aggregated platelets release serotonin to play a major role in edema formation. This agent acts directly to increase pulmonary vascular resistance, and it indirectly aggravates the vasoconstrictive effects of various vasoactive amines. In addition, decreases in resuscitation fluid are seen with high-dose vitamin C therapy immediately after burns, presumably because of its antiinflammatory effects, although this has been questioned recently because the doses given are likely to have an independent osmotic diuretic effect.[14]

Microvascular changes induce cardiopulmonary alterations characterized by loss of plasma volume, increased peripheral vascular resistance, and subsequent decreased cardiac output immediately after injury. Studies in efforts to sustain intravascular volume by increasing oncotic pressure with colloid solutions, such as albumin, are currently underway. Cardiac output remains depressed from decreased blood volume and increased blood viscosity as well as decreased cardiac contractility. Ventricular dysfunction in this period is attributed to a circulating myocardial depressant factor present in lymphatic fluid, although the specific factor has never been isolated. Cardiac output is completely restored with resuscitation.[15]

Only over the past 10 years have we begun to understand the glycocalyx, its role in protecting against endotheliopathy, and that its breakdown in shock states contributes to extravascular fluid

leak. The glycocalyx is a glycoprotein-polysaccharide matrix that serves as a barrier shielding the endothelium from direct blood flow, preventing vascular permeability, inhibiting coagulation, and deterring leukocyte adhesion.[16,17] Various shock and diseases states disrupt the glycocalyx, particularly a severe burn injury. Resuscitation with plasma may ameliorate this glycocalyx disruption, and research is ongoing.

Effects on the Renal System

Diminished blood volume and cardiac output result in decreased renal blood flow and glomerular filtration rate; this is mitigated somewhat by intravenous volume resuscitation. Other stress-induced hormones and mediators such as angiotensin, aldosterone, vasopressin, and thromboxane B_2 further reduce renal blood flow immediately after the injury. These effects result in oliguria, which, if left untreated, will cause acute tubular necrosis and renal failure. Before 1984, acute renal failure in burn injuries was almost always fatal. After 1984, however, techniques in intermittent dialysis became widely used to support the kidneys during recovery. Since that time, developments in continuous renal replacement therapies have radically changed outcomes related to renal failure in the severely burned. It was shown that 28-day mortality and in-hospital mortality in the severely burned with renal failure decreased by 50% and 25%, respectively, with the use of continuous venovenous hemofiltration compared with intermittent hemodialysis.[18] This is a massive improvement that has received significant attention corroborated by several other studies.[19]

Effects on the Immune System

Burns cause a global depression in immune function, which is demonstrated most prominently by prolonged allograft skin survival on burn wounds. As stated previously, after severe injury, adaptive immunity is downregulated in favor of innate immune mechanisms. Burned patients are then at great risk for a number of infectious complications, including bacterial wound infection, pneumonia, and fungal and viral infections. These susceptibilities and conditions are based on depressed cellular function in all parts of the immune system, including activation and activity of neutrophils, macrophages, T lymphocytes, and B lymphocytes. With burns of more than 20% TBSA, impairment of these immune functions is proportional to burn size.

Macrophage production after burns is relatively diminished, which is related to spontaneous elaboration of negative regulators of myeloid growth. This effect is enhanced by the presence of endotoxin and can be partially reversed with granulocyte colony-stimulating factor treatment or inhibition of prostaglandin E2.[20] Total neutrophil counts are initially increased after burn by demargination and decreased cell death by apoptosis. However, neutrophils that are present are dysfunctional in terms of diapedesis, chemotaxis, and phagocytosis; this is related to abnormalities in granulopoiesis and life span, cell trafficking, and antimicrobial effector functions. After 48 to 72 hours, neutrophil counts decrease somewhat like macrophages, with similar causes.

T-cell function is depressed after a severe burn. Until recently, T helper cells were categorized as Th1 and Th2 phenotypes, but this has been dramatically expanded to other phenotypes such as Th9, Th17, Th22, and T-regs; work on this categorization and relevant functions is ongoing. In particular, the Th17 phenotype is likely to play a significant role in the burn wound given its association with adaptive immunity on mucosal surfaces and the skin. This field continues to evolve as we examine the roles of each phenotype in response to antigens. Each is associated with typical cytokines, such as interleukin (IL)-2 for Th1 responses, IL-4 and IL-10 for Th2, and IL-17 and 22 for Th17. Burns also impair cytotoxic T-lymphocyte activity as a function of burn size, thus increasing the risk of infection, particularly from fungi and viruses. Early burn wound excision improves cytotoxic T-cell activity.[21]

Hypermetabolism

After severe burn and resuscitation, typically 3 to 4 days after injury, the condition of *hypermetabolism* develops, characterized by tachycardia, increased cardiac output, elevated energy expenditure, increased oxygen consumption, and massive proteolysis and lipolysis (Fig. 43.5). This response is seen in all major injuries but is present in its most dramatic form in severe burns. The condition is likely related to the massive inflammatory response already mentioned, but delivery of nutrition to support recovery from the wound and bed rest and immobility associated with treatment also plays a major, if not primary, role. Hypermetabolism may be sustained for months, leading to massive weight loss and decreased strength, particularly when muscle strength is needed to functionally recover from the injury. These changes in metabolic activity are caused in part by the release of catabolic hormones, such as catecholamines, glucocorticoids, and insulin/glucagon, among others. Catecholamines act directly and indirectly to increase glucose availability through hepatic gluconeogenesis and glycogenolysis and fatty acid availability through peripheral lipolysis. Effects are direct through α- and β-adrenergic receptors on myocytes, lipocytes, and hepatocytes. The indirect effects are mediated through stimulation of adrenergic receptors in endocrine tissue within the pancreas, which causes a relative increase in glucagon release compared with insulin. Normally, glucagon increases hepatic glucose production and peripheral lipolysis, whereas insulin has the opposite effects. Catecholamine stimulation of β-adrenergic receptors within the pancreas increases the release of both glucagon and insulin, but concurrent stimulation of α receptors has a greater inhibitory effect on insulin than on glucagon, resulting in a greater net release of glucagon. The effects of catecholamine-stimulated glucagon release then outweigh the

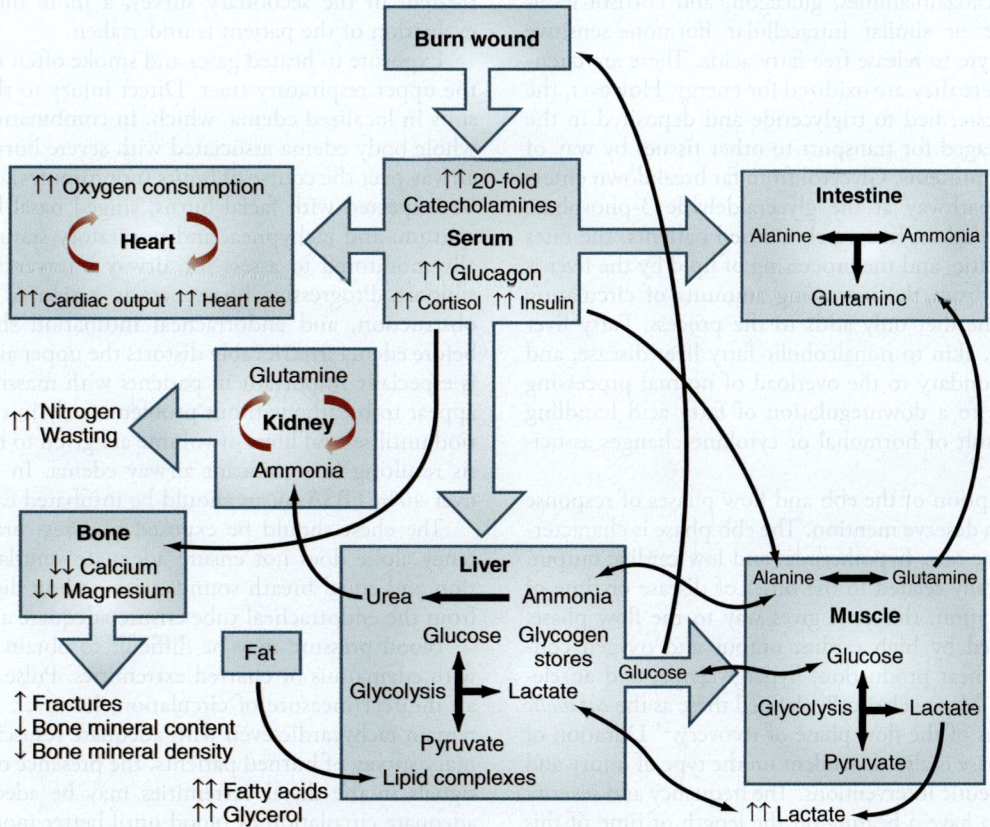

FIGURE 43.5 Metabolic effects of severe burns.

effects of insulin on glucose and fatty acid production and release. Glucocorticoid hormones, released by way of the hypothalamic-pituitary-adrenal axis, are mediated through neural stimulation. Cortisol has similar actions on energy substrates, and it induces insulin resistance, which is an additive to the hyperglycemia because of the release of liver glucose. Catecholamines, when combined with glucagon and cortisol, augment glucose release, which initially could be beneficial because glucose is the principal fuel of inflammatory cells and neural tissue.

Substrate supply for hepatic gluconeogenesis is produced through feeding (either enteral or parenteral), proteolysis of existing muscle tissue, and, to some extent, by peripheral lipolysis. Structural and constitutive proteins degraded to amino acids enter into (1) the tricarboxylic acid cycle for energy production, (2) the liver to be used as substrate for gluconeogenesis, or (3) the synthesis of acute-phase proteins. Lactate and alanine are important intermediates that are released in proportion to the extent of injury. Glutamine is also released in massive quantities, depleting muscle tissue stores to 50% of normal concentrations. After conversion to pyruvate or oxaloacetate, these amino acids form glucose with a net loss of adenosine triphosphate (ATP). Eighteen of the 20 amino acids are gluconeogenic. Increased acute-phase protein synthesis in the liver includes representative factors such as C-reactive protein, fibrinogen, α_2-macroglobulin, and complement. These are often used as proxies for the degree of hypermetabolism that is present, but, as discussed, the inflammatory response is so massive that most treatments will have little effect; perhaps the best strategy is to address the inflammatory condition of the wound through wound closure rather than untoward attention to the effects.

Peripheral lipolysis, mediated through the catabolic hormones, is another principal component of the metabolic response to severe burn. Elevation of catecholamines, glucagon, and cortisol levels stimulates the same or similar intracellular hormone-sensitive lipases in the adipocyte to release free fatty acids. These are circulated to the liver where they are oxidized for energy. However, the vast majority are reesterified to triglyceride and deposited in the liver or further packaged for transport to other tissues by way of very low-density lipoproteins. Glycerol from fat breakdown enters the gluconeogenic pathway at the glyceraldehyde 3-phosphate level after phosphorylation. In severely burned patients, the rates of lipolysis are dramatic, and the processing of lipid by the liver is often compromised from the increasing amounts of circulating fat. Adding fat in the diet only adds to the process. Fatty liver commonly develops, akin to nonalcoholic fatty liver disease, and is thought to be secondary to the overload of normal processing enzymes or perhaps to a downregulation of fatty acid handling mechanisms as a result of hormonal or cytokine changes associated with the injury.[22]

The classic description of the ebb and flow phases of response to illness and trauma deserve mention. The ebb phase is characterized by low metabolic rate, hypothermia, and low cardiac output. This is often temporally related to the onset of disease or time of injury. After resuscitation, this state gives way to the flow phase, which is characterized by high cardiac output and oxygen consumption, increased heat production, hyperglycemia, and an elevated metabolic rate. Moore classically defined these as the *catabolic* and *anabolic* portions of the flow phase of recovery.[23] Duration of the catabolic flow phase is also dependent on the type of injury and the efficacy of therapeutic interventions. The frequency and severity of complications also have a bearing on the length of time of this phase of recovery, which in critically ill patients can last for weeks

or months. The anabolic flow phase is characterized by a slow reaccumulation of protein and fat that can extend for years after the injury.

INITIAL TREATMENT OF BURNS

Prehospital

During and immediately after injury, burned patients must be removed from the source and the burning process stopped. In the prehospital setting, this should be achieved first, but care must be taken that the rescuer does not become another victim. Universal precautions include wearing gloves and protective eyewear during retrieval. Burning clothing should be extinguished and removed as soon as possible to prevent further injury. Next attention should be directed at initial resuscitation, starting with the airway. For those burned with flames, inhalation injury should always be suspected and 100% oxygen given by facemask. All rings, watches, jewelry, and belts should be removed because they retain heat and can produce a tourniquet-like effect. Room-temperature water should be copiously poured on the wound for up to 30 minutes within 3 hours of injury to decrease the depth of the wound and improve healing and scarring.[24,25] Any subsequent measures to cool the wound should be avoided to preclude hypothermia during resuscitation. Patients should be rapidly transported to a local emergency department for initial stabilization; for those who meet the American Burn Association criteria for transfer to a burn center, timely arrangements should be made for transport.[26]

Initial Assessment

As with any injured patient, the initial assessment of a burn patient is divided into the primary and secondary survey. First, immediate life-threatening conditions are quickly identified and treated; in the secondary survey, a more thorough head-to-toe evaluation of the patient is undertaken.

Exposure to heated gases and smoke often results in damage to the upper respiratory tract. Direct injury to the upper airway results in localized edema, which, in combination with generalized whole body edema associated with severe burn, may obstruct the airway over the course of hours (not minutes). Airway injury must be suspected with facial burns, singed nasal hairs, carbonaceous sputum, and tachypnea, and respiratory status must be continually monitored to assess for airway intervention and ventilatory support. Progressive hoarseness is a sign of impending airway obstruction, and endotracheal intubation should be instituted before edema irretrievably distorts the upper airway anatomy. This is especially important in patients with massive burns, who may appear to breathe without problems early in the resuscitation period until several liters of volume are given to maintain homeostasis resulting in significant airway edema. In general, those with over 40% TBSA burns should be intubated early for this reason.

The chest should be exposed to assess breathing; airway patency alone does not ensure adequate ventilation. Chest expansion and equal breath sounds with carbon dioxide (CO_2) return from the endotracheal tube ensure adequate air exchange.

Blood pressure may be difficult to obtain in burned patients with edematous or charred extremities. Pulse rate can be used as an indirect measure of circulation; however, most burn patients remain tachycardic even with adequate resuscitation. For the primary survey of burned patients, the presence of pulses or Doppler signals in the distal extremities may be adequate to determine adequate circulation of blood until better monitors, such as arterial pressure measurements and urine output, can be established.

In those who have been in an explosion or deceleration incident, a possibility exists for spinal cord injury and other fractures. Appropriate cervical spine stabilization must be accomplished by whatever means necessary, including using cervical collars to keep the head immobilized until the condition can be evaluated and excluded.

Wound Care

Prehospital care of the burn wound is basic and simple. Protection from the environment with application of a clean dry dressing or sheet to cover the involved part is sufficient after the source has been controlled; damp dressings should not be used. Irrigation to cool the wound in the first 3 hours after injury might be considered in controlled conditions, but this should be done actively and not passively with dressings. Further, the patient should be wrapped in a blanket to minimize heat loss and for temperature control during transport. The first step in diminishing pain is to cover the wounds to prevent contact with exposed nerve endings. Intramuscular or subcutaneous narcotic injections for pain should never be used because drug absorption is decreased as a result of the peripheral vasoconstriction resulting in later and unexpected release with respiratory complications. Small doses of intravenous opioids may be given after complete assessment of the patient and after it is determined to be safe by an experienced practitioner.

Although prehospital management is simple, it is often difficult to accomplish appropriately, particularly in at-risk populations. Studies showed that initial burn first-aid treatment was inadequate in many patients.[24] These authors also showed that inadequate first-aid care was clearly associated with poorer outcomes. They suggested that defined education programs targeted to at-risk populations might improve these outcomes.

Transport

Rapid, uncontrolled transport of the burn victim is not a priority except when other life-threatening conditions coexist. In most incidents involving major burns, ground transportation of victims to the receiving hospital is appropriate, with air transport of greatest use when the distance from the incident and the hospital is 30 to 150 miles. For distances greater than 150 miles, transport by fixed-wing aircraft is most appropriate. Whatever the mode of transport, it should be of appropriate size and have emergency equipment available with trained personnel on board, such as a nurse, physician, paramedics, or respiratory therapists who are familiar with polytrauma patients.

Resuscitation

Formulas are used to estimate fluid volumes for resuscitation of a burned patient, all originating from classical experimental studies on the pathophysiology of burn shock (Table 43.2). Baxter established the basis for modern fluid resuscitation protocols,[27] showing that edema fluid in burn wounds is isotonic and contains the same amount of protein as plasma and that the greatest loss of fluid is into the interstitium. Baxter used various volumes of

TABLE 43.2 Resuscitation Formulas

FORMULA	CRYSTALLOID VOLUME
Parkland	4 cc/kg/% TBSA burned
Brooke	2 cc/kg/% TBSA burned
Galveston (pediatric)	5000 cc/m² burned + 1500 cc/m² total surface area

TBSA, Total body surface area.

intravascular fluid to determine the optimal amount in terms of cardiac output and extracellular volume in a canine burn model, and this was applied to the clinical realm with the Parkland formula. Plasma volume changes were not related to the type of resuscitation fluid in the first 24 hours, but, thereafter, colloid solutions increased plasma volume by the amount infused. From these findings, the author concluded that colloid solutions should not be used in the first 24 hours until capillary permeability returned closer to normal.

Concurrently, Pruitt et al. showed the hemodynamic effects of fluid resuscitation in burns, which culminated in the Brooke formula.[28] They found that fluid resuscitation caused an obligatory 20% decrease in both extracellular fluid and plasma volume that concluded after 24 hours. In the second 24 hours, plasma volume returned to normal with the administration of colloid. Cardiac output was low in the first day despite resuscitation, but it subsequently increased to supernormal levels as the flow phase of hypermetabolism was established. Since these studies, investigators have found that much of the fluid needs are the result of "leaky" capillaries that permit passage of large molecules into the interstitial space, increasing extravascular colloid osmotic pressure. Intravascular volume follows the gradient to tissues, both into the burn wound and the nonburned tissues. Approximately 50% of fluid resuscitation given is sequestered in nonburned tissues in 50% TBSA burns.[29] Early resuscitation formulas such as the Evans and Brooke formulas aimed to administer 2 cc/kg/%TBSA, using colloid in the form of plasma. When plasma became unsafe (before the advent of modern viral screening), crystalloid and albumin became the mainstays of resuscitation. As a response to the changing paradigm, the original work done by Dr. Baxter was a crystalloid-only resuscitation, followed by an additional period of albumin after the 24-hour end point had been reached. When only lactated Ringer solution was given during the first 24 hours, most patients received 4 cc/kg/%TBSA to maintain urine output, and the Parkland formula became almost universally adopted and used for the next 40 to 50 years. When the use of colloid shifted from plasma products to simple albumin, it was thought to simply restore the oncotic gradient and also served as an antioxidant.

Recently, a small but growing body of convincing evidence suggests that administration of healthy plasma restores the damaged glycocalyx and reverses the capillary leak.[16,17] Despite advances in safety of blood products and some clinical studies circa 2000 showing reduction in resuscitation fluids, plasma was not universally readopted by the burn community. Crystalloid-based resuscitations, with some centers using rescue albumin, continue to be mainstream.

The term *fluid creep* was coined in 2000 by Basil Pruitt.[30] Literature from the 2000s demonstrated that patients were receiving almost twice the amount of fluids predicted by the Parkland formula, with the common development of complications such as abdominal compartment syndrome.[31] In the 2000s overresuscitation was a problem in many burn centers, and the etiology was multifactorial. Oversedation with opioids, surgeons moving to shift work and losing continuity of care, older patients with more comorbidities, higher incidence of obesity, and improved trauma systems allowed patients in more remote areas access to burn centers where some of the issues were implicated. Some of the patients previously considered nonsurvivable were now survivable and underwent challenging resuscitations. Since then, a concerted effort has ensued to safely reduce resuscitation fluids given.

The authors of this chapter currently use strategies to reduce fluid administration during burn shock. One author's burn center

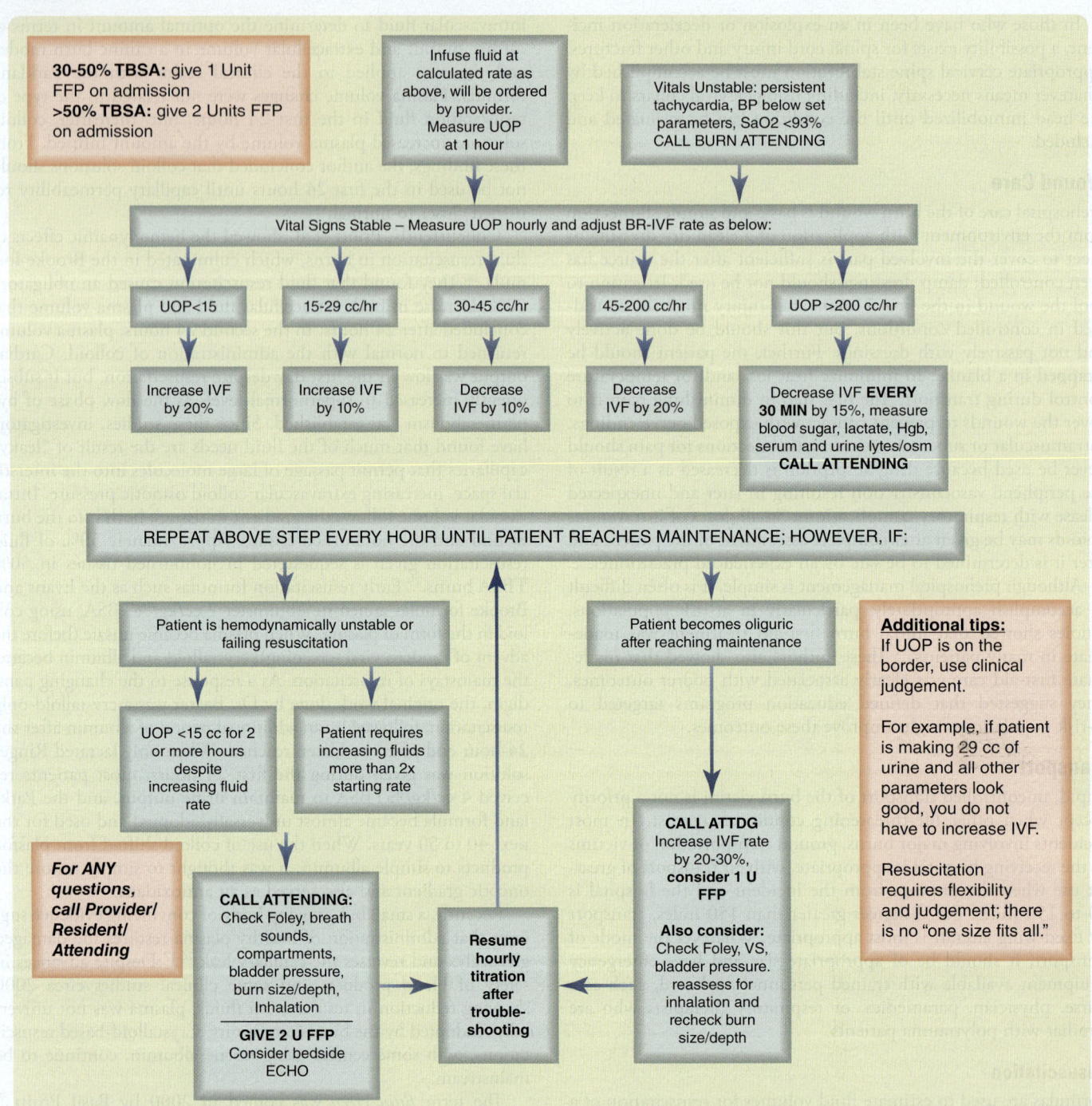

FIGURE 43.6 Severe burn resuscitation protocol-intravenous fluid. *BR-IVF*, * ; *ECHO*, * ; *FFP*, fresh frozen plasma; *TBSA*, total body surface area; *UOP*, * ; *VS*, * .

uses Burn Navigator, a computer algorithm–based decision support tool that has been shown in prospective studies to result in fluid administration of approximately 4 cc/kg/%TBSA.[32] This program has the advantage of assisting the less experienced provider who may not be as comfortable with a complex resuscitation as a career burn surgeon. The other author uses early plasma administration to address capillary leak for adjusted ideal body weight index instead of actual weight, with the addition of more plasma as indicated by clinical response. The adjusted ideal body weight index is a third of the difference between the ideal and actual body weight—an equation used to dose hydrophilic medications for obese patients receiving dialysis. The concept of resuscitating an overweight burn patient is similar, as adipose tissue does not contain the vascular supply or water content of lean tissue. In this protocol (Fig. 43.6), those with >30% TBSA receive plasma on admission and if oliguric for 2 consecutive hours during resuscitation. Initially, patients were started at 2 cc/kg/%TBSA, increasing to 3 cc/kg/%TBSA for those with extensive deep injuries *or* inhalation injury and 4 cc/kg/%TBSA if they had *both* inhalation and third-degree burns. This approach resulted in

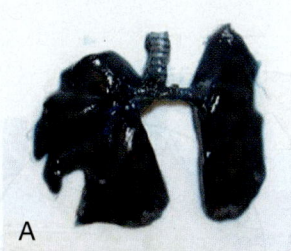
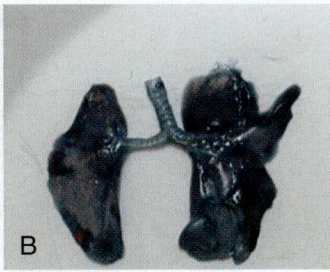
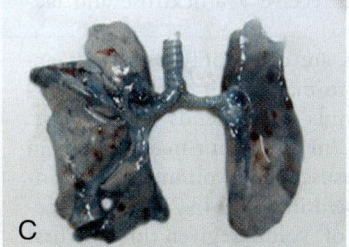
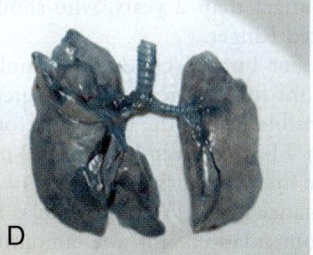

40% LR only   40% LR + Albumin   40% LR + FFP   Uninjured

FIGURE 43.7 Lungs in severely burned animals treated with lactated Ringer *(LR)* alone (A), LR with albumin (B), and LR with fresh frozen plasma (C). Uninjured lungs are controls (D). Blue coloration is from capillary leakage of dye injected during resuscitation.

reduction of fluid volumes from 4.1 to 3.3 cc/kg/%TBSA in a single burn center accompanied by significant improvements in mortality, ventilator-free days, acute kidney injury (AKI), tracheostomy, and dialysis.[33] Fluid administration was further reduced in an updated version that aimed to start almost everyone at 2 cc/kg/%TBSA unless high-grade inhalation and mostly full-thickness burn were present; the most severely injured patients are started at a rate corresponding to 3 cc/kg/%TBSA. This algorithm has resulted in a reduction of median fluid administration to 1.7 cc/kg/%TBSA, with a median of 30 ventilator-free days and an observed to expected length of stay ratio of 0.4, without an increase in mortality or significant AKI compared with the first publication.[34]

Shupp et al. elucidated the details of the mechanism of plasma utility in burn resuscitation in rodent models.[16] In Fig. 43.7, photos of a rat lung explant model depict Evans blue dye extravasation after burn injury as a marker of endotheliopathy. When glycocalyx is damaged and capillary permeability increases, blue dye extravasates in addition to other fluids. The blue staining and endotheliopathy were most striking in resuscitation with lactated Ringer alone, with the lungs completely blue. With crystalloid and colloid, a slight attenuation of the blue dye leakage and staining was found. In contrast, the appearance of the lungs treated with crystalloid and plasma have a marked improvement, very close in appearance to the uninjured lungs. This study also demonstrated a significant reduction in edema per gram of tissue when plasma was added to crystalloid, whereas the small reduction with the addition of albumin was not statistically significant. Serum markers of endotheliopathy such as SCD-1 were significantly increased in injured animals compared with controls, but plasma significantly attenuated SCD-1 levels.

Use of the Parkland and modified Brooke formulas remains within the standard of care; however, current evidence suggests reexamination. Inexperienced providers often take the formula and its application as rote, particularly the point in that it is used to calculate a starting fluid rate, which then must be titrated up or down on an hourly basis. This dynamic process demands the provider match the fluids with the evolving capillary leak over time, which often differs based on patient and injury characteristics. The best marker of a successful resuscitation is urine output. Traditional metrics tout 30 cc/h as adequate for most adults or, alternatively, 0.5 cc/kg/h, and 1 cc/kg/h for children. In analyzing the area under the curve of a Parkland formula resuscitation (fluid administered over time), most patients receive approximately half of the total 4 cc/kg/%TBSA in the first 8 hours (Fig. 43.8). The two rectangles are equivalent size and approximate the total area

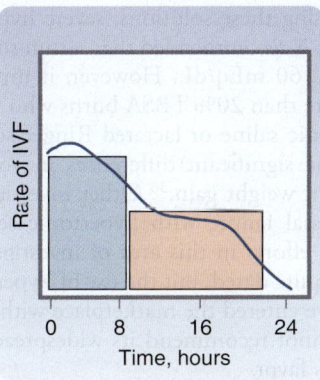

FIGURE 43.8 Typical declines in intravenous fluid administration during burn resuscitation. Colored boxes represent Parkland formula calculations, and the line represents the typical dynamics of a closely monitored resuscitation. *IVF,* Intravenous fluid.

under the curve. Hence, one approach is to divide the estimated total fluid over 24 hours (4 cc/kg/%TBSA) by 8 and then by 2, with half in the first 8 hours. Dividing the total 24-hour volume calculation by 16 eliminates a step to obtain the starting hourly fluid rate. Another approach is the "Rule of Tens," multiplying TBSA burned times 10 as an initial rate.[35] The same general concept should be used in applying the consensus formula with 2 or 3 cc/kg/%TBSA, then divide by 16 to calculate the starting fluid rate. This is usually necessary only for patients with 20% TBSA or greater, as smaller injuries rarely develop burn shock or a clinically significant endotheliopathy.

Adequate resuscitation of the burned patient involves establishing and maintaining reliable intravenous access. Increased times to beginning resuscitation of burned patients result in poorer outcomes, and delays should be minimized. Venous access is best attained through short peripheral catheters in unburned skin; however, veins in burned skin can be used and are preferable to no intravenous access. Superficial veins are often thrombosed in full-thickness injuries and are therefore not suitable for cannulation. Saphenous vein cut-downs are useful in cases of difficult access and are used in preference to central vein cannulation because of lower complication rates. Modern techniques with ultrasound imaging of veins have made this practice rare. In children younger than 6 years of age, experienced practitioners can use intramedullary (i.e., intraosseous) access in the proximal tibia until intravenous access is accomplished. Lactated Ringer solution without dextrose is the fluid of choice except in children younger than 2 years, who should receive 5% dextrose and lactated Ringer.

For burned children, formulas are commonly used that account for changes in surface area to mass ratios and baseline insensible losses. The Galveston formula recommends 5000 mL/m^2 per TBSA burn in m^2 + 1500 mL/m^2 TBSA for maintenance in the first 24 hours to account for resuscitation volumes and maintenance needs. All the formulas listed in Table 43.2 calculate recommendations for the amount of volume given in the first 24 hours after injury (not arrival to the hospital), one half of which is to be given in the first 8 hours after injury. Ongoing monitoring and adjustment are indicated.

Hypertonic saline solutions have theoretical advantages in burn resuscitation. These solutions are purported to decrease net fluid intake, decrease edema, and increase lymph flow, probably by the transfer of volume from the intracellular space to the interstitium. When using these solutions, severe hypernatremia must be avoided, and it is recommended that serum sodium concentrations not exceed 160 mEq/dL. However, it must be noted that patients with more than 20% TBSA burns who were randomized to either hypertonic saline or lactated Ringer solution resuscitation did not have significant differences in volume infused or changes in percent weight gain.[36] Other investigators also found an increase in renal failure with hypertonic solutions that has tempered further efforts in this area of investigation.[37] Many of these studies are quite dated, but the use of hypertonic saline does not appear to have entered the marketplace with any enthusiasm. Currently, we cannot recommend its widespread use unless new data emerge in its favor.

To combat any complications of aspiration, a nasogastric tube should be inserted in all patients with major burns. This is especially important for all patients being transported in aircraft at high altitudes. Additionally, all patients should be restricted from taking anything by mouth until the transfer has been completed. Decompression of the stomach is usually indicated because the apprehensive patient will swallow considerable amounts of air and distend the stomach.

Recommendations for tetanus prophylaxis are based on the condition of the wound and the patient's immunization history. All patients with burns greater than 10% TBSA should receive 0.5 mL tetanus toxoid. If prior immunization is absent or unclear, or the last booster dose was more than 10 years ago, 250 units of tetanus immunoglobulin is also given.

Escharotomies

When deep partial-thickness or full-thickness burns encompass the circumference of an extremity, peripheral circulation to the limb can be compromised. Development of generalized edema beneath a nonyielding eschar impedes venous outflow and eventually affects arterial inflow to the distal beds. This is recognized by numbness and tingling in the limb and increased pain in the digits. Arterial flow can be assessed by determination of Doppler signals in the digital arteries and the palmar and plantar arches in affected extremities; capillary refill and compartment pressures can also be assessed. Extremities at risk are identified either on clinical examination or on measurement of tissue pressures greater than 30 mm Hg. These extremities should undergo escharotomy, which releases the burn eschar only. This procedure is generally performed at the bedside by incising the lateral and medial aspects of the extremity with a scalpel or electrocautery unit. The entire constricting eschar must be incised longitudinally to completely relieve impediment to venous blood flow. For the upper extremities,

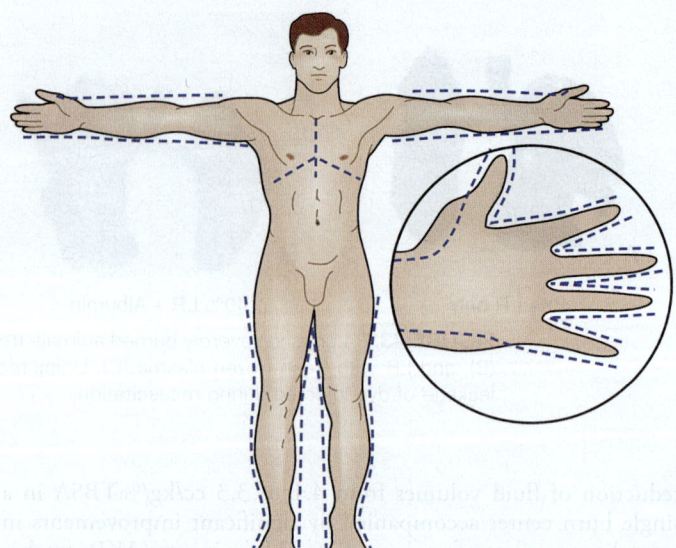

FIGURE 43.9 Recommended location for escharotomies. In limbs with escharotomies indicated, the incisions are made on the medial and lateral sides of the extremity through the eschar. In the case of the hand, incisions are made on the dorsum of the hand and thenar and hypothenar eminences.

incisions are carried down onto the thenar and hypothenar eminences if indicated. Distensible tissues in the fingers is minimal; therefore, finger escharotomies are not indicated during resuscitation in the absence of clear signs of ischemia (Fig. 43.9). If it is clear that the wound will undergo excision and grafting because of its depth, escharotomies are safest to restore perfusion to the underlying nonburned tissues until formal excision. If vascular compromise has been prolonged, reperfusion after an escharotomy may cause reactive hyperemia and further edema formation in the muscle, making continued surveillance of the distal extremities necessary. Increased muscle compartment pressures after escharotomies may then indicate fasciotomies if pressures are not released with escharotomy. The most common complications associated with these procedures are blood loss and the release of anaerobic metabolites, causing transient hypotension. If distal perfusion does not improve with these measures, central hypotension from hypovolemia should be suspected and treated.

A constricting truncal eschar can cause a similar phenomenon, except the effect is to decrease ventilation by limiting chest excursion. Any acute decrease in ventilation in a burn patient should produce inspection of the chest with appropriate escharotomies to relieve the constriction and allow adequate tidal volumes. This becomes evident for patients whose peak airway pressures increase.

Inhalation Injury

One major factor contributing to death in severe burns is the presence of inhalation injury. Smoke damage adds another inflammatory focus and impedes normal airway function for critically injured patients. Inhalation injury increases the amount of time spent on mechanical ventilation, a strong predictor of mortality. Early diagnosis and prevention of complications are of interest to decrease morbidity and mortality rates related to this condition.

With inhalation injury, damage is primarily from chemical burns associated with inhaled toxins. Heat is dispersed in the upper airways, whereas the cooled particles of smoke and toxins are carried distally into the major airways principally, and occasionally to the lower airways and the alveoli depending on the type of smoke and duration of exposure. Direct thermal damage to the lung is rarely seen because of dispersal of the heat in the pharynx. The exception is high-pressure steam inhalation, which has 4000 times the heat-carrying capacity of dry air.

The response of the airways to smoke inhalation is an immediate dramatic increase in blood flow from the bronchial arteries with edema formation and increased lung lymph flow. The lung lymph in this situation is similar to serum, indicating that permeability at the capillary level is markedly increased. The edema that results is associated with an increase in lung neutrophils, and it is postulated that these cells may be the primary mediators of pulmonary damage with this injury. Neutrophils release proteases and oxygen free radicals to produce conjugated dienes by lipid peroxidation. High concentrations are present in the lung lymph and pulmonary tissues after inhalation injury, suggesting that the increased concentration of neutrophils is active in producing cytotoxic materials. When neutrophils are depleted before injury by nitrogen mustard, increases in lung lymph flow and conjugated diene levels are markedly reduced.[38]

Another hallmark of inhalation injury is separation of the ciliated epithelial cells from the basement membrane followed by exudate formation within the airways. The exudate consists of proteins found in the lung lymph, and, eventually, it coalesces to form fibrin casts. Clinically, these fibrin casts can be difficult to clear with standard airway suction techniques. These casts also add distal barotrauma to localized areas of lung by forming a ball valve that is open with inspiration/airway dilatation and closes during expiration; the additional volume of air adds pressure that is associated with numerous complications, including pneumothorax and decreased lung compliance.

Smoke inhalation is commonly associated with a clinical history of closed-space smoke exposure, hoarseness, wheezing, and carbonaceous sputum. It may also be associated with facial burns and singed nasal hairs. Each of these findings individually has poor sensitivity and specificity; therefore, the definitive diagnosis should be further clarified by the use of bronchoscopy. Bronchoscopy reveals early inflammatory changes such as erythema, ulceration, and prominent vasculature in addition to infraglottic soot. The findings of airway erythema and ulceration alone are also nonspecific, and these findings must be placed with the entire clinical presentation to verify significant inhalation injury. Initial treatment for severe inhalation injury is institution of mechanical ventilation for airway management and lung support to maintain gas exchange. Repeated bronchoscopy often reveals continued ulceration of the airways with granulation tissue formation, exudate formation, inspissation of secretions, and focal edema. Eventually, the airway heals by replacement of the sloughed cuboidal ciliated epithelium with squamous cells and scar.

Combustion products of organic and inorganic materials found in smoke cause direct damage to the airway cells, but also have significant systemic effects. Most notably, carbon monoxide (CO) and hydrogen cyanide (HCN) can cause physiologic derangements that can lead to death if not recognized and treated appropriately. CO exposure should be presumed in all cases of suspected inhalation injury. It is impossible to detect without special equipment because of its properties of being colorless, odorless, tasteless, and nonirritating. Once inhaled, CO rapidly crosses the pulmonary capillary membrane and binds to hemoglobin with approximately 200 times the affinity of oxygen, forming carboxyhemoglobin. CO also causes a conformational change to hemoglobin that diminishes oxygen off-loading ability in peripheral tissues (left-shift in the hemoglobin dissociation curve).

Oxygen delivery is further impaired by hypoxia-induced cardiac dysfunction. Intracellularly, CO also has been shown to bind cytochrome c oxidase, disrupting the electron transport chain in mitochondria, resulting in a functional shift from aerobic to anaerobic metabolism and worsening oxidative stress. The impact of CO is most apparent in organ systems with high metabolic output such as the brain and heart; CO poisoning therefore most commonly manifests as neurologic changes such as dizziness or altered mental status and cardiovascular findings such as arrhythmias and even infarction.

Widespread use of synthetic materials in construction and home furnishings has led to production of increased levels of HCN gas during house fires. Cyanide is a potent and rapidly acting poison, which, under normal conditions, is converted into thiocyanide that is excreted through the urine. This system is easily overwhelmed in the setting of inhalation injury, leading to accumulation of circulating cyanide ions. The cyanide ion interferes with cellular energy production, leading to rapid depletion of ATP stores and the subsequent development of lactic acidosis. These events aside, debate exists as to whether HCN is truly a significant contributor to inhalation injury, in large part because of the fact that HCN has a low flash point and is therefore rapidly oxidized by the fire, thus limiting exposure. Unfortunately, the unpredictable nature of the gaseous compounds iteratively generated and consumed during a fire limits ability to study subsequent effects both systemically and as a direct pulmonary irritant.

CO poisoning is measured by carboxyhemoglobin levels, with elevations above 5% considered to have toxicity ramifications. Headaches are generally present with levels above 10%, dizziness and impaired judgment at 20%, dyspnea above 30%, and syncope, seizures, and obtundation over 40%. Initial treatment is 100% oxygen to decrease the half-life of carboxyhemoglobin from 4 hours on room air to 1 hour. For extreme conditions, hyperbaric oxygen might be considered. For cyanide toxicity, removal from the source is indicated, and hydroxocobalamin might be given intravenously; this will result in orange coloration of the urine.

The clinical course of patients with inhalation injury is divided into three stages. The first is acute pulmonary insufficiency. Patients with severe lung injuries begin to show signs of pulmonary failure from the time of injury with asphyxia, CO poisoning, bronchospasm, and upper airway obstruction. Clinical signs of parenchymal damage with hypoxia are not common during this phase. The second stage occurs from 72 to 96 hours after injury and is associated with increased extravascular lung water, hypoxia, and development of diffuse lobar infiltrates. This condition is similar clinically to adult respiratory distress syndrome (ARDS) occurring in nonburned injured and critically ill patients. In the third stage, clinical bronchopneumonia dominates and appears in up to 60% of these patients. These infections generally occur 3 to 10 days after burn injury and are associated with the expectoration of large mucous casts formed in the tracheobronchial tree. The differentiation of pneumonia from tracheobronchitis is difficult at this stage, and bronchoscopy with lavage may be of assistance. Early pneumonias are usually caused by penicillin-resistant *Staphylococcus* species, whereas after 5 to 7 days, the changing flora of the burn wound is reflected in the appearance in the lung of gram-negative species, especially *Pseudomonas* and *Klebsiella*. Ball-valve effects and ventilator-associated barotrauma are also hallmarks of this period.

Management of inhalation injury is directed at maintaining open airways and maximizing gas exchange while the lung heals. A coughing patient with a patent airway can clear secretions much more effectively than any suctioning technique (including bronchoscopy), and efforts should be made to manage patients without mechanical ventilation if possible. If respiratory failure is imminent, intubation should be instituted, with frequent chest physiotherapy and suctioning performed to maintain pulmonary toilet. Frequent bronchoscopy may be indicated to clear inspissated secretions. Mechanical ventilation should be used to provide gas exchange with as little barotrauma as possible using permissive hypercapnia and ARDS ventilation protocols. Arterial oxygen tensions of greater than 60 (or an oxygen saturation of 92%) are also tolerated to minimize oxygen toxicity to the lungs. When the clinical condition improves to the point of weaning from ventilatory support, oxygen concentration, positive end-expiratory pressure, and ventilator volumes and rate should be decreased in a graduated manner until the patient can be extubated. This may take several weeks.

Inhalation treatments have been effective in improving the clearance of tracheobronchial secretions and decreasing bronchospasm (Table 43.3). Intravenous heparin has been shown to reduce tracheobronchial cast formation, minute ventilation, and peak inspiratory pressures after smoke inhalation.[39] When heparin was administered directly to the lungs in a nebulized form, it had similar effects on casts without causing systemic coagulopathy. When N-acetylcysteine treatments are added to nebulized heparin in burned children with inhalation injury, reintubation rates and mortality rates are decreased.[40] In addition to the measures already discussed, adequate humidification and treatment of bronchospasm with β-agonists are indicated. Steroids are not of benefit in inhalation injury and should not be given unless the patient is steroid dependent before injury or if the patient has bronchospasm resistant to standard therapy. Other potential treatments are hypertonic saline to induce coughing and racemic epinephrine to reduce mucosal edema for those who are extubated.

In addition to conventional ventilator methods, novel ventilator therapies have been devised to minimize barotrauma, including high-frequency percussive ventilation. This method combines standard tidal volumes and respirations (ventilator rates 6–20/minute) with smaller high-frequency respirations (200–500/minute) and permits adequate ventilation and oxygenation in patients who failed conventional ventilation. One reason for the greater utility of this method is that it recruits alveoli at lower airway pressures. This ventilator method may also have a percussive effect that loosens inspissated secretions and improves the pulmonary toilet, although the percussive effects can lead to additional airway injury.[39]

Several clinical studies showed pulmonary edema is not prevented by fluid restriction. Indeed, fluid resuscitation appropriate for the patient's other needs results in a decrease in lung water, has no adverse effect on pulmonary histology, and improves survival rate. Although overhydration can increase pulmonary edema, inadequate hydration increases the severity of pulmonary injury by sequestration of neutrophils, leading to increased risk of death.

In both animal and clinical studies, resuscitation was adequate if normal cardiac index or urine output was maintained.

Prophylactic antibiotics for inhalation injury are not indicated but are clearly to be used for diagnosed lung infections. Empirical choices for treatment of pneumonia before culture results are returned should include coverage of methicillin-resistant *Staphylococcus aureus* and gram-negative organisms (especially *Pseudomonas*).

As patients recover from lung injury, extubation should ensue as soon as possible. Patients are able to clear their own airways through coughing more effectively than suction through an endotracheal tube. This is preferably done as soon as upper airway edema has resolved (injury day 1–2) in those who were intubated to control the airway or for burn excision. It is our experience that patients who are extubated with the same degree of inhalation injury do better than those who are intubated. Standard extubation criteria can be used, although many patients who do not meet these criteria may also do well without mechanical ventilation. If the airway is easily accessible by airway experts, a trial of extubation might be of benefit in patients with borderline weaning parameters.

Wound Care

After the airway is assessed, other injuries are addressed, and resuscitation is underway, attention must be turned to the burn wound. Treatment depends on the characteristics and size of the wound, with all treatments aimed at rapid and less painful healing. Current therapy directed specifically toward burn wounds can be divided into three stages: assessment, management, and rehabilitation. Once the extent and depth of the wounds have been assessed and the wounds thoroughly cleaned and debrided, the management phase begins. Each wound should be dressed initially with an appropriate covering that serves several functions. First, it should protect the damaged epithelium, minimize bacterial and fungal colonization, and provide splinting action to maintain the desired position of function. Second, the dressing should be reasonably occlusive to reduce evaporative heat loss and minimize cold stress. Third, the dressing should provide comfort over the painful wound.

The management of a very deep or very superficial burn wound is relatively straightforward. A large third-degree burn will likely benefit from excision of the burn eschar and wound closure with skin grafts or local flaps, if available, after initial treatment. The clearly superficial burn will heal with almost any reasonable wound care strategy (described later). The challenge in decision-making lies in management of the indeterminate burn, where a significant depth of the dermis is injured with uncertainty regarding whether it will heal spontaneously in a timely fashion without increased risk of infection. Some providers allow a period for these indeterminate-depth wounds to "declare," involving painful dressing changes, increased hospital stay, and protracted time to reintegration. As another confounder, topical antibiotic use during this period often obfuscates the wound appearance by formation of pseudoeschar, making the wound appear to be deeper than it is. Thus, treatment of burn-injured patients absolutely requires accurate wound assessment to determine appropriate interventions. Strategies are further complicated by the fact that clinical assessment of these challenging middle to deep partial-thickness burn depths, even by experts in the field, has an accuracy of only 60% to 80%. A recent study demonstrated 73% accuracy from a group of multidisciplinary burn experts in predicting whether a burn wound would be nonhealing and would ultimately receive a skin graft.[41]

TABLE 43.3 **Inhalation Treatments of Smoke Inhalation Injury**	
TREATMENT	**TIME AND DOSE**
Bronchodilators (e.g., albuterol)	q2h
Nebulized heparin	5000–10,000 units in 3 cc normal saline q4h
Nebulized acetylcysteine	20%, 3 cc q4h

q2h, Every 2 hours; *q4h,* every 4 hours.

Improving indeterminate burn wound assessment performance optimizes the use of limited resources in burn care by accurately determining wound depth with immediate implementation of timely strategies. Several older technologies designed to aid in burn depth assessment exist, but they are not the standard of care in the United States. These technologies include but are not limited to laser Doppler imaging (LDI), laser speckle imaging, thermography, video-microscopy, optical coherence, and spatial frequency domain imaging.[9] Many of these technologies can be used in conjunction with artificial intelligence (AI), and LDI is the most highly validated, but they all have significant limitations.

Some newer promising technologies have recently been developed. Preliminary data suggest that an experimental device (Deep-View Wound Imaging System, Spectral MD, Dallas, TX) using multispectral imaging combined with a convolutional neural network AI architecture may be more accurate than experienced burn providers in predicting nonhealing of burns. Early proof-of-concept data demonstrate a >90% accuracy and improved specificity, sensitivity, positive predictive value, and negative predictive values.[10] However, the device is not yet commercially available as of 2025.

Another novel method of accurate burn depth estimation is immediate enzymatic excision of burn wounds with bromelain (Nexobrid, Mediwound Ltd., Yavne, Israel). This technology removes eschar while preserving healthy dermis, allowing the provider to directly visualize and firmly assess depth of dermal injury previously obscured by eschar. Preliminary data suggest that this method results in chemical escharotomy and direct assessment of residual dermis 2.8 to 5.9 days sooner than standard of care. With early visualization and dermal preservation, patients treated with bromelain also undergo less autografting. This product was FDA approved in 2023.[42] The authors also currently use other technologies for a more selective surgical excision including the circular dermatome, dermabrasion, and water jet scalpel (Versajet, Smith & Nephew, Watford, England).

The choice of initial dressing is based on the characteristics of the treated wound. Superficial epidermal wounds are minor, with minimal loss of barrier function; thus, no dressing is indicated, with treatment by topical salves to keep the skin moist. Systemic nonsteroidal antiinflammatory agents given by mouth assist in pain control. Partial-thickness wounds are treated with daily or every-other-day dressing changes with topical antibiotics, cotton gauze, and elastic wraps or with one of the longer-lasting silicone or cloth dressings containing silver as an antimicrobial. Alternatively, the wounds can be treated with a temporary biologic or synthetic covering to close the wound that may or may not be applied in the operating room (Table 43.4). Identified deep partial-thickness or full-thickness wounds benefit from excision and grafting for sizable burns (i.e., >5 cm²), and the choice of initial dressing should be aimed at holding bacterial proliferation in check and providing occlusion until the operation is performed.

TABLE 43.4 Biologic Coverings

Xenograft	Occlusive closure of the wound, some immunologic benefits
Allograft	Occlusive closure of the wound, provides normal functions of skin, dermal elements can engraft and worsen scarring
Suprathel	Occlusive closure of the wound, decreased pH inhibiting microbial growth
StrataGraft	Occlusive closure of the wound, active allogeneic cells inhibiting infection

Antimicrobials

The timely and effective use of antimicrobials has revolutionized burn care by decreasing invasive wound infections. The untreated burn wound rapidly becomes colonized with bacteria and fungi with loss of innate skin barrier mechanisms. As the organisms proliferate to high wound counts (>10^5 organisms per gram of tissue), some may penetrate into viable tissue. Organisms then invade blood vessels, causing a systemic infection that often leads to the death of the patient. This scenario has become uncommon in most burn units because of the effective use of antibiotics and wound care techniques. The antimicrobials that are used can be divided into those given topically and systemically.

Available topical antibiotics can be divided into three classes: salves, soaks, and antimicrobial dressings. Salves are generally applied directly to the wound with cotton dressings placed over them (Table 43.5); soaks are solutions poured into cotton dressings on the wound; and antimicrobial dressings contain active agents to inhibit microbial growth, generally some form of silver ion or other antibiotic. Each of these classes of antimicrobials has advantages and disadvantages. Salves may be applied daily but may lose their effectiveness between dressing changes. Frequent dressing changes can result in shearing with loss of grafts or underlying healing cells as well as procedural pain. Soaks remain effective because antibiotic solution can be added without removing the dressing; however, the underlying skin can become macerated. Longer-term antimicrobial dressings have the advantage of less frequent painful changes, decreasing both pain and provider effort, but some of these must remain moist and thus must be monitored.

Topical antibiotic salves include 11% mafenide acetate (Sulfamylon), 1% silver sulfadiazine (Silvadene), polymyxin B, neomycin, bacitracin, mupirocin, and the antifungal agent nystatin, among others. No single agent is completely effective, and each has advantages and disadvantages. Silver sulfadiazine was commonly used before the development of newer antimicrobial dressings. It has a broad spectrum of activity because its silver and sulfa moieties are effective against gram-positive, most gram-negative, and some fungal forms. Some *Pseudomonas* species possess plasmid-mediated resistance. Silver sulfadiazine is relatively painless upon application, has high patient acceptance, and is easy to use. However, it must be changed daily, which induces significant repeated painful episodes. Occasionally, patients complain of a burning sensation after it is applied, and, in a few patients, a transient leukopenia develops 3 to 5 days after its continued use. This leukopenia is generally harmless and resolves with or without treatment cessation. Of some concern is the finding of wound healing inhibition by the agent.

Mafenide acetate is another topical agent with a broad spectrum of activity owing to its sulfa moiety. It is particularly useful against resistant *Pseudomonas* and *Enterococcus* species. It also penetrates eschar, which silver sulfadiazine does not. Disadvantages include painful application on skin, such as in second-degree wounds. It also can cause an allergic skin rash, and it has carbonic anhydrase inhibitory characteristics that can result in a metabolic acidosis when applied over large surfaces. For these reasons, mafenide sulfate is typically reserved for small full-thickness injuries.

Petroleum-based antimicrobial ointments with polymyxin B, neomycin, and bacitracin are clear on application, painless, and allow for easy wound observation. These agents are commonly used for treatment of facial burns, graft sites, healing donor sites, and small partial-thickness burns. Mupirocin is a petroleum-based ointment that has improved activity against gram-positive

TABLE 43.5   Burn Wound Dressings

DRESSING	ADVANTAGES AND DISADVANTAGES
Salves	
Silver sulfadiazine	Broad spectrum, painful daily dressing changes, does not penetrate eschar, inhibition of epithelialization
Mafenide acetate 8.5%	Broad spectrum, penetrates eschar, painful application to partial-thickness burns, painful daily dressing changes, potential for metabolic acidosis, inhibition of epithelialization
Bacitracin	Gram-positive coverage, painful daily dressing changes
Neomycin	Gram-positive coverage, painful daily dressing changes
Bactroban	Gram-positive coverage, painful daily dressing changes
Polymyxin B	Gram-negative coverage, painful daily dressing changes
Nystatin	Fungal coverage, cannot be used in combination with mafenide acetate
Solutions	
Silver nitrate 0.5%	Effective against all microbes, stains contacted areas, associated with methemoglobinemia
5% Mafenide acetate	Broad spectrum, penetrates eschar, painful application to partial-thickness burns, painful daily dressing changes, potential for metabolic acidosis, inhibition of epithelialization
Dakin's solution	0.5% sodium hypochlorite with buffers, effective against all microbes, inhibits epithelialization
Domboro solution	0.25% acetic acid with buffers, effective against most microbes particularly *Pseudomonas*, inhibits biofilm formation
Antimicrobial Dressings	
Silver-containing dressings	Broad spectrum, long-term use minimizing painful wound care, does not penetrate eschar, difficult to assess the wound

bacteria, particularly methicillin-resistant *S. aureus* and selected gram-negative bacteria. Nystatin, either in a salve or powder form, can be applied to wounds to control fungal growth. Nystatin-containing ointments can be combined with other topical agents to decrease colonization of both bacteria and fungus.

Available agents for application as a soak include 0.5% silver nitrate solution, 0.05% Dakin (sodium hypochlorite with buffers), and 0.25% Domboro (acetic acid with buffers). Mafenide acetate 5% solution was previously available but has been removed from the marketplace to the detriment of burned patients and providers. Silver nitrate has the advantage of being painless on application and having complete antimicrobial effectiveness. The disadvantages include its staining of surfaces to a dull gray or black when the solution dries. This can become problematic in deciphering wound depth during burn excisions and in keeping the patient and their surroundings clean of the black staining. The solution is hypotonic as well, and continuous use can cause electrolyte leaching, with rare methemoglobinemia as another complication. Dakin's solution, which is a dilute solution of sodium hypochlorite with added buffering agents, has effectiveness against most microbes; however, it also has cytotoxic effects on the healing cells of patients' wounds. Low concentrations of sodium hypochlorite have less cytotoxic effects while maintaining most of the antimicrobial effects. Hypochlorite ion is inactivated by contact with protein, so the solution must be continually changed. A similar compound is available to be used in the same way with hypochlorous ion rather than hypochlorite (Vashe). The same is true for acetic acid solutions, which may be more effective against *Pseudomonas*. Mafenide acetate soaks have the same characteristics of the mafenide acetate salve, except in liquid form.

Many new antimicrobial dressings containing silver ions have reached the marketplace and provide the advantages listed earlier. Most wound care companies offer a dressing with these characteristics; therefore, the choice among them is principally based on the dressing characteristics, such as a cloth or silicone, elastic or nonelastic, and so on, rather than the antimicrobial properties. The advantage is that these can be applied and left in place for several days, providing for prolonged occlusive treatment for 3 to 7 days typically, and antimicrobial activity. Monitoring of the

patient and wound is still indicated because these dressings typically do not allow direct observation of the wound.

The use of perioperative systemic antimicrobials also has a role in decreasing burn wound sepsis until the burn wound is closed. Common organisms that must be considered when choosing a perioperative regimen include *S. aureus*, *Pseudomonas* species, and *Klebsiella*, which are prevalent in burn wounds.

Synthetic and Biologic Dressings

Synthetic and biologic dressings are an alternative to antimicrobial dressings. These types of dressings provide for stable coverage without painful dressing changes, provide a barrier to evaporative losses, and decrease pain in the wounds. They do not inhibit epithelialization, which is a feature of all topical antimicrobials. These coverings include allograft (cadaver skin), xenograft (e.g., pig skin, fish skin), Biobrane, Suprathel, and dermal equivalent–like products. These should generally be applied within 72 hours of the injury before high bacterial colonization of the wound occurs. Most often, synthetic and biologic dressings are used to cover second-degree wounds while the underlying epithelium heals, or it is used to cover full-thickness wounds for which autograft is not yet available. Each type of dressing has its advantages and disadvantages.

Biologic dressings include xenografts and allografts from cadaver donors. These human skin equivalents are applied to the wounds in the manner of skin grafts, where they engraft and perform the immunologic and barrier functions of normal skin. Thus, these biologic dressings are the optimal wound coverage in the absence of normal skin. Some of these are live tissue, such as fresh or frozen human allograft, whereas other formulations are treated with glycerol to lyse any live cells, leaving the extracellular matrix and proteins intact. Eventually, these biologic dressings will be rejected by usual immune mechanisms, causing the grafts to slough. They can then be replaced, or the open wound can be covered with autograft skin from the patient. Generally, severely burned patients are immunosuppressed, and allograft biologic dressings that have adhered will not reject for several weeks. Biologic dressings can be used to cover any wound as a temporary dressing. They are particularly well suited to massive partial-thickness injuries

(>50% TBSA) to close the wound and allow for healing to take place underneath the dressing. Disadvantages include the possible transmission of viral diseases with allograft and the possibility that a residual mesh pattern will be left from engrafted cadaver dermis if meshed allograft is used.

Biobran and similar products, such as Permeaderm, consist of collagen-coated silicone manufactured into a sheet. Suprathel is another similar formulation, but it is in sheets rather than mesh. These are placed on the wound and become adherent in 24 to 48 hours with dried wound transudate. This sheet then provides a barrier to moisture loss, and it provides a relatively painless wound bed without dressing changes. When the epithelium is complete under the sheet, it is easily peeled off the wound, except for Suprathel, which dissolves. Caution must be exercised when using this product to ensure that copious exudate does not form under the sheet, which provides an optimum environment for bacterial proliferation and risk of invasive wound infection. Biobrane has no antimicrobial activities, whereas Suprathel has some effects because it has a pH of less than 5.5. These agents should be used primarily in superficial second-degree burns and split-thickness skin graft donor sites.

Dermal equivalents such as Integra and Bio-Temporising Matrix (BTM) combine a collagen matrix (dermal substitute) with a silicone sheet outside layer (epidermal substitute). The collagen matrix engrafts into the wound, and after 2 weeks, the silicone layer is removed and replaced with available autograft. The advantages of this product are that it can be used in full-thickness burns to close the wound. It also provides a dermal equivalent that has the theoretical advantage of inhibiting future scarring of the burn wound, although this has not been clinically confirmed to date. The disadvantages are similar to those of all synthetic products, in that it has no antimicrobial properties; thus, its use can be complicated by invasive wound infections. Additionally, it takes two operations for wound coverage, as the silicone layer simulating the epidermis must be replaced 2 to 3 weeks after application with autograft.

In 2021, a novel bioengineered allogeneic cellularized construct was FDA approved for the treatment of burns. This product, Strata-Graft (Stratatech, a Mallinckrodt Company, Madison, WI), consists of an immortal, nonimmunogenic, nontumorigenic, karyotypically stable line of human keratinocytes. Human dermal fibroblasts are also embedded in the collagen gel matrix that serves as a scaffold.[43,44] The skin substitute has a complete, stratified epithelial layer that reconstitutes barrier function, as it contains stratum corneum. The product can be meshed and secured to a healthy, postexcision wound bed with fibrin glue, cyanoacrylate, and/or sutures or staples. Several randomized clinical studies bioengineered allogeneic cellularized construct treated wounds, which did not undergo a donor site and had equivalent outcomes to the sites treated with autograft, which did involve a cutaneous donor site. At 3 months, bioengineered allogeneic cellularized construct DNA was not detectable in biopsies, suggesting the product turns over as it stimulates autologous healing. At the time this chapter was written, full thickness burn studies using the product as an overlay for widely meshed autografts had completed enrollment. Data regarding the study was not yet available. Although FDA approved 2 years ago, this product is approximately $40/sq. cm and has not become standard of care. Although it may play a role in reducing donor site size, more clinical data and economic analyses are indicated to drive more widespread use.

Excision and Grafting

Deep partial-thickness and full-thickness burns do not heal in a timely fashion without autografting. In fact, the practice of leaving these dead tissues only serves as a nidus for inflammation and infection that could lead to the patient's death. It leads to the maxim, "there is no advantage to unexcised eschar," as a corollary to the golden rule of burn surgery and wound surgery in general: "close the wound promptly." Early excision and grafting of these wounds, first used by Janzekovich in the 1970s, are followed by most burn surgeons because reports show benefit over serial debridement and dressing changes in terms of survival, blood loss, incidence of sepsis, and length of hospitalization.[45] The technique of early excision and grafting has made conservative management of full-thickness wounds a practice to be used only in those with very high operative risks. Attempts are made to excise tangentially to optimize cosmetic outcome. Rarely, excision to the level of fascia is necessary to remove all nonviable tissue, or it may become necessary at subsequent operations for infectious complications. These excisions can be performed with tourniquet control or with application of topical epinephrine and thrombin to minimize blood loss.

After a burn wound has been excised, the wound must be covered. This covering is ideally the patient's own skin. Wounds covering 20% to 30% TBSA can usually be closed at one operation with autograft split-thickness skin taken from the patient's available donor sites. In these operations, the skin grafts either are not meshed are meshed with a narrow ratio (2:1 or less) to maximize cosmetic outcome. In major burns, autograft skin may be limited to the extent that the wound cannot be completely closed. The availability of cadaver allograft skin has changed the course of modern burn treatment for these massive wounds. A typical method of treatment is to use widely expanded autografts (4:1 or greater) covered with cadaver allograft to completely close the wounds for which autograft is available. The 4:1 skin heals underneath the cadaver skin in approximately 21 days, and the cadaver skin separates. The portions of the wound that cannot be covered with even widely meshed autograft are covered with allograft skin in preparation for autografting when donor sites are healed. Ideally, areas with less cosmetic importance are covered with the widely meshed skin to close most of the wound before using nonmeshed grafts at later operations for the cosmetically important areas, such as the hands, forearms, and face.

Most surgeons excise the burn wound in the first week, sometimes in serial operations by removing portions of the burn wound at operations on subsequent days. Others remove the whole of the burn wound in one operative procedure; however, this can be limited by the development of hypothermia or continuing massive blood loss and experienced anesthesia support. It is our practice to perform the excision immediately after stabilization of the patient after injury because blood loss diminishes if the operation can be done early. This may be caused by the relative predominance of vasoconstrictive substances, such as thromboxane and catecholamines, and the natural edema planes that develop immediately after the injury. When the wound becomes hyperemic after 4 to 7 days, blood loss can be a considerable problem. The use of hemostatic agents, such as epinephrine, thrombin, and tourniquets, sometimes aids in this approach.

Occasionally, split-thickness skin grafts do not adhere. Loss of skin grafts is the result of one or more of the following reasons in order of frequency: inadequate excision of the wound bed with remaining necrotic tissue, shearing forces disrupting an adhered graft, presence of infection causing graft lysis, or fluid collection under the graft. With a good excision and the use of topical antimicrobial agents, infection is *not* common. Technical attention to the depth by excising to punctate bleeding, meticulous hemostasis, appropriate meshing of grafts, or "rolling" of sheet grafts or bolsters over appropriate areas minimizes fluid collections. Shearing is decreased by immobilization of the grafted area. Infection is controlled by the appropriate use of topical antimicrobials at the time of surgery.

One alternative to split-thickness autografts typically used for skin grafting is cultured keratinocytes from the patient's own skin. Keratinocytes can be cultured in sheets from full-thickness skin biopsies, which are used as autografts. This technology has been used to greatly expand the capacity of a donor site, such that most of the body can be covered with grafts from a single small full-thickness biopsy sample. Cultured epithelial autografts are of use in truly massive burns (>80% TBSA) because of their limited donor sites. The disadvantages of cultured epithelial autografts are the length of time required to grow the autografts (2–3 weeks), 50% to 75% take rate of the grafts after initial application, the low resistance to mechanical trauma over the long term, proposed increase in scarring potential associated with the lack of dermis, and the potential for squamous cell cancer. These grafts are also expensive to produce. When a group of patients with greater than 80% TBSA burns who received cultured epithelial autografts were compared with a group who received conventional treatment, the acute hospitalization length of stay and the number of subsequent reconstructive operations were lower in the conventional group. These results demonstrate that more research and experience are needed to further optimize this technique. Technologies like cultured epithelial autografts hold the promise to radically limit donor sites, and it may be the optimal closure in combination with a dermal equivalent in the future.

In this vein, recent technologic advancements in cell separation and expansion by spraying on the operating table have been tested. The RECELL Autologous Skin Cell Suspension (ASCS; RECELL System; AVITA Medical, Valencia, CA) is a point-of-care technique that facilitates a donor skin-sparing approach for burns or other soft tissue defects. In the operating room, a kit is used to prepare an autologous skin cell suspension that can be expanded to 80:1—a sharp increase in expansion from the traditional expansion of conventional grafts. A small skin graft is generally harvested between 6 and 8 one-thousandths of an inch and incubated in an enzyme well to break extracellular attachments. Next, a scalpel is used to perform mechanical delamination of the epidermis and disaggregation of the thin layer of dermis in the sample. The resulting suspension contains mostly keratinocytes, fibroblasts, and melanocytes. This can be applied to a partial-thickness wound, or a meshed autograft can be over-sprayed in the interstices to treat a full-thickness wound. The device is currently approved by the FDA and multiple other regulatory bodies worldwide.

Key evidence for the safety and efficacy of autologous skin cell suspension in burn treatment is available from two prospective, randomized, phase III clinical trials, which were funded by the BARDA.[46,47] Additional data are available from retrospective analyses of patients enrolled in expanded and continued access protocols, including pediatric patients and those with >50% TBSA full-thickness wounds.

One of the two phase III trials evaluated autologous skin cell suspension and autografting versus autografting alone among patients with mixed-depth thermal burns, including full-thickness injuries. An intrapatient control design was employed in which treatment areas were randomly assigned to control (autograft alone) or autologous skin cell suspension plus autografting. Noninferiority of the autologous skin cell suspension to autografting alone was established for wound healing at week 8 (92.3% vs. 84.6%, respectively; treatment difference, −7.7% [one-sided

97.5% CI upper bound, 6.40%]). Additionally, superiority of autologous skin cell suspension was established for relative reduction of donor site harvesting: on average, 32% less donor skin was taken with the use of autologous skin cell suspension ($p < 0.001$). The other phase III trial, which focused on deep partial-thickness burns and studies of patients treated via expanded and continued access protocols, has shown similar results. Additionally, greater overall patient satisfaction and reduced pain have also been reported with the use of autologous skin cell suspension. This product has been shown to reduce length of stay and costs in a subset of complex burn patients.[48] Many surgeons also use the product to treat autograft donor sites, and the myriad of off-label uses is expanding.

In all burned patients, every effort should be made to optimize the long-term appearance of the wound, because almost all patients will survive to bear the scars of their injury. Burn wound scarring causes both functional and cosmetic deficits associated with wound contracture. Experience has shown that full-thickness skin grafts that include the entire dermal and epidermal layer provide the best scarring outcomes, with diminished contracture and superior skin appearance, compared with split-thickness skin grafts. Split-thickness and full-thickness grafts have a complete epidermal layer; therefore, the superior function and appearance of full-thickness grafts lies in the near-complete dermal layer. The challenge to burn surgeons in terms of minimizing scarring, then, is to provide complete dermis during wound coverage. This might be addressed through using thicker split-thickness skin grafts, but our experience suggests that thicker split-thickness grafts do not always result in better scarring. Thick grafts also result in prolonged donor site healing. Therefore, it is reasonable to conclude that standard-thickness skin grafts are appropriate for acute coverage of burn wounds.

Full-thickness skin grafts to supply the dermal layer are not plentiful and cannot be used more than once. The use of tissue expanders to increase available full-thickness donor skin is conceivable, but impractical for most injuries. For these reasons, these grafts are not commonly used in acute burn wound coverage. Engrafted cadaver dermis that has the epidermis removed by dermabrasion 1 to 2 weeks after placing it on the wound has been used with some success to provide the dermal layer. Presumably, the sparse cellular component of the dermis is removed by immunologic processes, leaving the dermal matrix in place as scaffolding for the ingrowth of normal dermal cells. Some commercially available decellularized preserved dermis products are available to provide a dermal equivalent in wound coverage. As discussed earlier, the products Integra and BTM also have a dermal-equivalent component to form a neo-dermis. All of these have the potential to minimize scarring contractures and to maximize the cosmetic appearance of burn scars. The long-term results with the use of these techniques are not yet known.

Minimally Invasive Skin Grafting

When dermal-sparing excision techniques are used, the chances of spontaneous healing with an acceptable outcome are increased. Some of the novel products described in this chapter stimulate autologous healing with human cells. Autologous skin cell suspension uses the patient's own cells, and BACC is an allograft-based product. Kahn et al. published their experience using these products in combination with bromelain-based chemical escharotomy followed by treatment with autologous skin cell suspension. After an initial proof-of-concept/feasibility study, they achieved approximately a 300% reduction in donor site size in patients with a mix of deep partial-thickness and full-thickness burns.[49]

As early as 2 hours after the bromelain is removed, the areas that are clearly full thickness received meshed split-thickness skin grafts with an autologous skin cell suspension overspray, whereas deep to middepth partial-thickness injuries received cell suspension spray alone. Depending on wound and patient characteristics, this is then dressed with polylactic acid sheets (Suprathel) or high-density porous polyethylene film as a primary dressing with periodic secondary dressing changes every few days. Several burn centers across the United States use this approach successfully. The technique is in its infancy; further study and optimization are forthcoming. Many of the studies that brought these products to market were funded by the DoD/BARDA, with the goal of using them synergistically as "multiple medical countermeasures" not only for mass casualty events but also developing the products to be a routine component in both military and civilian burn care.

The idea of enhanced recovery after burn injury has not been well characterized in the literature. However, many centers already use key components of standard programs, particularly related to temperature monitoring, fluids, and nutrition. The idea of enhanced recovery after burn surgery first presented as a formal protocol in 2018, approximately 20 years after it was first described for any patient, by Henrik Kehlet.[50] In addition to the strategies noted earlier, narcotic reduction through multimodal pharmacologic approaches combined with skin substitutes and glues instead of aggressive use of staples and sutures may reduce the need for sedation and heavy narcotic use.

MINIMIZING COMPLICATIONS

Early aggressive resuscitation regimens have improved survival rates dramatically. With the advent of vigorous fluid resuscitation, irreversible burn shock has been replaced by sepsis and subsequent multiple organ failure as the leading cause of death associated with burns. What is required is an inflammatory focus, which in severe burns is the massive skin injury with associated inflammation that is required to heal.

Etiology and Pathophysiology

The progression to multiple organ failure after severe burn is not well explained, although some of the responsible mechanisms are recognized. As shown in the Glue Grant data, massive changes in the inflammatory genome are already present in those who are severely burned; development of infectious sources is not uncommon, mostly associated with the burn wound but also from other sources such as the lungs. As organisms proliferate out of control, mediators are liberated from both microbes and endogenous sources such as mitochondria. Their release is associated with a cascade of inflammatory mediators that can result, if unchecked, in further damage and progression toward organ failure.

Inflammation from the presence of necrotic tissue and open wounds can incite a similar inflammatory mediator response. It is known that a cascade of systemic events is set in motion either by invasive organisms or from open wounds that initiate massive inflammation, which may progress to multiple organ failure. Evidence from animal studies and clinical trials suggests that these events converge to a common pathway. Those circulating mediators can, if secreted in excessive amounts, damage organs distal from their site of origin. Among these mediators are endotoxin, the arachidonic acid metabolites, mitochondrial fragments, cytokines, neutrophils and their adherence molecules, nitric oxide, complement components, and oxygen free radicals.

Prevention

Because different cascade systems are involved in the pathogenesis of burn-induced multiple organ failure, it is so far impossible to pinpoint a single mediator that initiates the event. Thus, because the mechanisms of progression are not well known, prevention is currently the best solution. The current recommendations are to prevent the development of organ dysfunction and to provide optimal support to avoid conditions that promote the onset. The great reduction of mortality rate from large burns was seen with early excision and an aggressive surgical approach to deep wounds; thus, the best solution is likely early wound closure.

Removal of devitalized tissue prevents wound infections and decreases inflammation associated with the wound. In addition, it eliminates small-colonized foci, which are a frequent source of transient bacteremia. Transient bacteremia during surgical manipulations may prime immune cells to react in an exaggerated fashion to subsequent insults, leading to whole body inflammation and remote organ damage. We recommend complete early excision of clearly full-thickness wounds within 48 hours of the injury with rapid closure of the wound by autologous skin grafting or skin substitute.

Oxidative damage from reperfusion after low-flow states makes early aggressive fluid resuscitation imperative. This is particularly important during the initial phases of treatment and operative excision with its attendant blood losses. Furthermore, the volume of fluid may not be as important as the timeliness with which it is given. In a study of children with greater than 80% TBSA burns, it was found that one of the most important contributors to survival was the time to starting intravenous resuscitation, regardless of the initial volume given.

Topical and systemic antimicrobial therapy has significantly diminished the incidence of invasive burn wound sepsis. Perioperative systemic antibiotics likely benefit patients with injuries greater than 30% TBSA burns. Vigilant and scheduled replacement of intravascular devices minimizes the incidence of catheter-related sepsis. Where possible, peripheral veins should be used for cannulation, even through burned tissue. New technologies such as central access through peripheral veins also likely decreases the incidence of line sepsis.

Pneumonia, which contributes significantly to death in burned patients, should be vigilantly anticipated and aggressively treated. Every effort should be made to wean patients as early as possible from the ventilator to reduce the risk of ventilator-associated nosocomial pneumonia. Furthermore, early ambulation is an effective means of preventing respiratory complications. With sufficient analgesics, even patients on continuous ventilatory support can be out of bed and in a chair.

The most common sources of sepsis are the wounds and/or the tracheobronchial trees; efforts to identify causative agents should be concentrated there. Another potential source, however, is the gastrointestinal tract, which is a natural reservoir for bacteria. Starvation and hypovolemia shunt blood from the splanchnic bed and promote mucosal atrophy and failure of the gut barrier. Early enteral feeding reduces septic morbidity and prevents failure of the gut barrier. At our institution, patients are fed immediately through a nasogastric tube. Early enteral feedings are tolerated in burn patients and preserve mucosal integrity and likely reduce the magnitude of the hypermetabolic response to injury. Support of the gut goes along with carefully monitored hemodynamics. One other infection to consider, usually late in the course, is endocarditis with microbes associated with the cardiac valves usually late in the course of treatment. This can be detected with echocardiography and should be considered in the face of infection for which no other source is identified.

Organ Failure

Even with the best efforts at prevention, the presence of the systemic inflammatory syndrome, which is ubiquitous in burn patients, may progress to organ failure. It was found that approximately 28% of patients with greater than 20% TBSA burns develop severe multiple organ dysfunction, of which 14% also develop severe sepsis and septic shock. Around 40% of deaths after severe burn are related to organ failure, which universally involves the renal system with, on average, at least three other systems. The general development begins in the renal or pulmonary systems and can progress through the liver, gut, hematologic system, and central nervous system. The development of multiple organ failure does not accurately predict mortality but does increase risk. Therefore, efforts to support the organs until they heal are justified.

Renal Failure

With the advent of early aggressive resuscitation, the incidence of renal failure coincident with the initial phases of recovery has diminished significantly in severely burned patients. However, a second period of risk for the development of renal failure 2 to 14 days after resuscitation is still present. Renal failure is hallmarked by decreasing urine output, hypervolemia, electrolyte abnormalities including metabolic acidosis and hyperkalemia, the development of azotemia, and increased serum creatinine. Treatment is aimed at averting complications associated with these conditions.

Urine output of more than 1 mL/kg/h in children and 30 cc/h in adults is an adequate measure of renal perfusion in the absence of underlying renal disease. Decreasing the volume of fluid given alleviates volume overload in burned patients. These patients have increased insensible losses from the wounds, which can be roughly calculated at 1500 mL/m² TBSA + 3750 mL/m² TBSA burned. Decreasing the infused volume of intravenous fluids and enteral feedings to less than the expected insensate losses alleviates hypervolemia problems. Almost invariably, severely burned patients receive exogenous potassium because of the heightened aldosterone response that results in potassium wasting; therefore, hyperkalemia is rare even with some renal insufficiency.

If the problems listed earlier overwhelm the conservative measures, some form of dialysis may be indicated. The indications for dialysis are hypervolemia unresponsive to diuretics or electrolyte abnormalities not amenable to other treatments. Kidney Disease: Improving Global Outcomes (KDIGO) criteria may be used to determine utility of dialysis, and level 3 or severe acute renal failure indicates use. Hemodialysis and hemofiltration are the most common modalities, either intermittent or continuous. With the advent of relatively simple continuous renal replacement technologies, these treatments can often be managed by critical care specialists with consultation from experienced nephrologists in difficult cases. After beginning dialysis, renal function is almost certain to return, associated with the abundant regeneration properties of the kidney in the absence of preexisting disease. Therefore, patients undergoing such treatment rarely undergo lifelong dialysis.

Pulmonary Failure

Many burn patients undergo mechanical ventilation to protect the airway in the initial phases of their injury. We recommend these patients be extubated as soon as possible after the risk is diminished. A trial of extubation is often warranted in the first few days after injury, and reintubation in this setting is not a failure. Performing this technique safely, however, requires the involvement of experts in obtaining an airway. The goal is extubation as soon as possible to allow the patients to clear their own airways, because they can perform their own pulmonary toilet better than through an endotracheal tube or tracheostomy. Often, the first sign of impending pulmonary failure is a decline in oxygenation. This is best monitored with continuous oximetry, and a decrease in saturation to less than 92% is indicative of failure. Increasing concentrations of inspired oxygen are necessary, and when ventilation begins to fail, denoted by increasing respiratory rate and hypercarbia, intubation is indicated.

Some have stated that early tracheostomy (within the first week) might be indicated in those with significant burn who are likely to require long-term ventilation. A randomized study comparing those severely burned patients who underwent early tracheostomy with those who did not found some early improvements in oxygenation; however, no significant differences were found in outcome measures such as ventilator days, length of stay, incidence of pneumonia, or survival. In fact, 26% of those not undergoing tracheostomy were successfully extubated within 2 weeks of admission, implying that they would not have benefited from tracheostomy at all. Tracheostomy also has its risks, which are often overlooked, including acute loss of airway and, most importantly, lifelong risk of aspiration associated with anatomic changes in the neck. It seems that although tracheostomy may benefit some severely burned patients on ventilatory support, the advantages of early tracheostomy do not always outweigh the disadvantages.

Hepatic Failure

The development of hepatic failure in burned patients is a challenging problem without many solutions. The liver synthesizes circulating proteins, detoxifies the plasma, produces bile, and provides immunologic support. When the liver begins to fail, protein concentrations of the coagulation cascade decrease to critical levels and the patient becomes coagulopathic. Toxins are not cleared from the bloodstream, and concentrations of bilirubin increase. Complete hepatic failure is not compatible with life, but a gradation of liver failure with some decline of the function is common. Efforts to prevent hepatic failure are the only effective methods of treatment.

With the development of coagulopathies, treatment should be directed at replacement of factors II, VII, IX, and X until the liver recovers. Albumin replacement may also be indicated. Attention to obstructive causes of hyperbilirubinemia, such as acalculous cholecystitis, should be considered as well. Initial treatment of this condition should be gallbladder drainage, which can be done percutaneously in those at high risk.

Hematologic Failure

Burn patients may become coagulopathic through two mechanisms: (1) depletion and impaired synthesis of coagulation factors or (2) thrombocytopenia. Issues associated with factor depletion are through disseminated intravascular coagulation often associated with sepsis. This process is also common with coincident head injury. With breakdown of the blood-brain barrier, brain lipids are exposed to the plasma, which activates the coagulation cascade. Varying penetrance of this problem results in differing degrees of coagulopathy. Treatment of disseminated intravascular coagulation should include infusion of fresh frozen plasma and cryoprecipitate to maintain plasma levels of coagulation factors best monitored with dynamic coagulation testing with thromboelastography. Impaired synthesis of factors from liver failure is treated, as alluded to earlier.

Thrombocytopenia is common in severe burns from depletion during burn wound excision and is one of the best signs of the development of sepsis. Platelet counts of less than 50,000 are common and do not require treatment. Only when the bleeding is diffuse and is noted from the intravenous sites should consideration for exogenous platelets be given.

Paradoxically, it was found that severely burned patients are also at risk for thrombotic and embolic complications likely related to immobilization. Complications of deep venous thrombosis was associated with increasing age, weight, and TBSA burned.

NUTRITION

The response to injury known as *hypermetabolism* is dramatically exhibited after severe burn. Increases in oxygen consumption, metabolic rate, urinary nitrogen excretion, and lipolysis are directly proportional to the size of the burn. This response can be as high as 200% of the normal metabolic rate and continues unabated for 9 to 12 months after injury. Because the metabolic rate is so high, energy utilization is immense. Endogenously, these are met by mobilization of available carbohydrate, fat, and protein stores. Because the demands are prolonged, these energy stores are depleted, leading to loss of active muscle tissue and malnutrition. Immobilization for treatment further worsens the condition, leading to malnutrition. This is associated with functional impairment of many organs, delayed and abnormal wound healing, and decreased immunocompetence. Malnutrition in burns can be subverted to some extent by delivery of adequate exogenous nutritional support, but the goals of this treatment are principally to prevent nutritional complications.

Several formulas are used to calculate caloric requirements in burn patients. One multiplies the basal energy expenditure determined by the Harris-Benedict formula by 2 in burns greater than 40% TBSA, assuming a 100% increase in total energy expenditure. When total energy expenditure was measured by the doubly labeled water method, actual expenditures were found to be 1.3 times the predicted basal energy expenditure for pediatric patients with burns greater than 40% TBSA.[51] When measured during convalescence after initial hospitalization, it remained elevated at 1.1 times predicted energy expenditure.[52] These studies indicate that the calculation of 2 times the predicted basal energy expenditure might be too high.

Another commonly used calculation is the Curreri formula, which calls for 25 kcal/kg/day plus 40 kcal per percent TBSA burned per day. This formula provides for maintenance needs plus the additional caloric needs related to the burn wounds. This formula was devised as a regression from nitrogen balance data in severely burned adults. In children, formulas based on body surface area are more appropriate because of the greater body surface area per kilogram of weight. We recommend the following formulas depending on the child's age (Table 43.6). These formulas were determined to maintain body weight in severely burned children. The formulas change with age based on the body surface area alterations that occur with growth.

The composition of the nutritional supplement is also important. The optimal dietary composition contains 1 to 2 g/kg/day of protein, which provides a calorie-to-nitrogen ratio at around 100:1 with the earlier suggested caloric intakes. This amount of protein provides for the synthetic needs of the patient, thus sparing to some extent the proteolysis occurring in the active muscle tissue. Nonprotein calories can be given as either carbohydrate or fat. Carbohydrates have the advantage of stimulating endogenous insulin production, which has beneficial effects on muscle and the

TABLE 43.6 Formulas to Predict Calorie Needs in Severely Burned Children

AGE GROUP	MAINTENANCE NEEDS	BURN WOUND NEEDS
Infants (0–12 months)	2100 kcal/% TBSA burned/24 hours	1000 kcal/% TBSA burned/24 hours
Children (1–12 years)	1800 kcal/% TBSA burned/24 hours	1300 kcal/% TBSA burned/24 hours
Adolescents (12–18 years)	1500 kcal/% TBSA burned/24 hours	1500 kcal/% TBSA burned/24 hours

TBSA, Total body surface area.

burn wounds as an anabolic hormone.[53] In addition, it was shown that almost all of the fat transported in very-low-density lipoprotein after severe burn is derived from peripheral lipolysis and not from de novo synthesis of fatty acids in the liver from dietary carbohydrates.[53] Reliance on fat to deliver noncarbohydrate calories thus has little support.

The diet may be delivered in two forms: either enterally through enteric tubes or parenterally through intravenous catheters. Parenteral nutrition may be given in isotonic solutions through peripheral catheters or with hypertonic solutions in central catheters; however, the caloric demands of burn patients prohibit the use of peripheral parenteral nutrition. Total parenteral nutrition delivered centrally in burned patients has been associated with increased complications and mortality rate compared with enteral feedings. Total parenteral nutrition is reserved only for those patients who cannot tolerate enteral feedings. Enteral feeding has been associated with some complications, however, which can be disastrous. These include mechanical complications, enteral feeding intolerance, and diarrhea.

Nutritional adjunctive treatment with anabolic agents has received attention as a means to decrease lean mass losses after severe injury. Agents used include growth hormone, insulin-like growth factor, insulin, oxandrolone, testosterone, and propranolol. Studies supporting the use of each are now over 12 years old and mature. Of these oxandrolone and propranolol were the most commonly used. However, oxandrolone has been removed from the marketplace by the FDA. In combination, each of these agents has different actions to stimulate protein synthesis through an increase in protein synthetic efficiency. Put simply, the free amino acids available in the cytoplasm from protein breakdown with severe injury or illness are preferentially shunted toward protein synthesis rather than exported out of the cell.

LESS COMMON BURN ETIOLOGIES

Electrical Burns

Of all admitted burned patients, 3% to 5% are injured from electrical contact. Electrical injury is unlike other burns in that the visible areas of tissue necrosis represent only a small portion of the injured tissue. Electrical current enters a part of the body, such as the fingers or hand, and proceeds through tissues with the lowest resistance to current, generally nerves, muscles, and blood vessels. The skin has a relatively high resistance to electrical current and is therefore mostly spared. The current then leaves the body at a "grounded" area on some other part of the body. Heat generated by the transfer of electrical current and passage of the current itself then injures the tissues. During this exchange, the muscle is the major tissue through which the current flows and thus sustains the most damage. Most muscle is in close proximity to bones; therefore, that is where the most injury is evident. The bone itself does not sustain any increase in temperature or injury. Blood vessels transmitting much of the electricity initially remain patent, but they may proceed to progressive thrombosis as the cells either die or repair themselves, thus resulting in further tissue loss from ischemia that might be evident days later.

Injuries are divided into high- and low-voltage injuries. Low-voltage injury is similar to thermal burns without transmission to the deeper tissues; zones of injury from the surface extend into the tissue. Most household currents (110–220 volts) produce this type of injury, which usually causes only local damage. The worst of these injuries are those involving the edge of the mouth (oral commissure) sustained when children gnaw on household electrical cords with alternating current. Most households are on direct current; therefore, these types of injuries are now rare.

The syndrome of high-voltage injury consists of varying degrees of cutaneous burn at the entry and exit sites, combined with hidden destruction of deep tissue. Often, these patients also have cutaneous burns associated with ignition of clothing from the discharge of electrical current. In these cases, the burns on the skin are mostly thermal and not electrical and should be treated as such. Initial evaluation consists of cardiopulmonary resuscitation if ventricular fibrillation is induced. Thereafter, if the initial electrocardiogram findings are abnormal or with a history of cardiac arrest associated with the injury, continued cardiac monitoring is indicated along with pharmacologic treatment for any dysrhythmias. The most serious derangements occur in the first 24 hours after injury. If patients with electrical injuries have no cardiac dysrhythmias on initial electrocardiogram or recent history of cardiac arrest, no further monitoring is necessary.

Patients with electrical injuries are at risk for other injuries, such as being thrown from the electrical jolt or falling from heights after disengaging from the electrical current. In addition, the violent tetanic muscular contractions that result from alternating current sources may cause a variety of fractures and dislocations. These patients should be assessed as any other patient with blunt traumatic injuries.

The key to managing patients with an electrical injury lies in the treatment of the wound. The most significant injury is within the deep tissue, and subsequent edema formation can cause vascular compromise to any area distal to the injury. Assessment should include circulation to distal vascular beds, because immediate escharotomy and fasciotomy may be indicated. If the muscle compartment is extensively injured and necrotic, such that the prospects for eventual function are dismal, early amputation may be indicated. We advocate early exploration of affected muscle beds and excision of devitalized tissues with attention given to the deeper periosteous planes, because this is the area with the most muscle. Fasciotomies should be complete and may include nerve decompressions, such as carpal tunnel and Guyon canal releases. Tissue that has questionable viability should be left in place, with planned reexploration. Many such reexplorations may occur until the wound is completely controlled. Electrical damage to vessels may be delayed, and the extent of necrosis may extend after the initial procedures.

After the devitalized tissues are removed, closure of the wound becomes paramount. Although skin grafts suffice as closure for most wounds, flaps may offer a better alternative, particularly with exposed bones and tendons. Even exposed and superficially infected bones and tendons can be salvaged with coverage by vascularized tissue. Early involvement by reconstructive surgeons versed in the various methods of wound closure is optimal.

Muscle damage results in release of hemochromogens (myoglobin), which are filtered in the glomeruli and may result in obstructive nephropathy. Therefore, vigorous hydration and infusion of intravenous sodium bicarbonate (5% continuous infusion) and mannitol (25 g every 6 hours for adults) were historically used to solubilize the hemochromogens and maintain urine output if significant amounts are found in the serum, though this has been questioned. These patients also benefit from additional intravenous volumes over predicted amounts for the wound area because most of the wound is deep and cannot be assessed by physical examination.

Neurologic deficits may occur that may seem somewhat random. Serial neurologic evaluations should be performed as part of routine examination in order to detect any early or late neuropathology. Central nervous system effects such as cortical encephalopathy, hemiplegia, aphasia, and brainstem dysfunction injury have been reported up to 9 months after injury; others report delayed peripheral nerve lesions characterized by demyelination with vacuolization and reactive gliosis. Another devastating long-term effect is the development of cataracts, which can be delayed for several years. These complications may occur in up to 30% of patients with significant high-voltage injury, and patients should be made aware of this risk even with the best treatment.

CHEMICAL BURNS

Most chemical burns are incidental from mishandling of household cleaners, although some of the most dramatic presentations involve industrial exposures. Thermal burns are, in general, short-term exposures to heat, but chemical injuries may be of longer duration, even for hours in the absence of appropriate treatment. The degree of tissue damage as well as the level of toxicity are determined by the chemical nature of the agent, concentration of the agent, and the duration of skin contact. Chemicals cause their injury by protein destruction, with denaturation, oxidation, formation of protein esters, or desiccation of the tissue. In the United States, the composition of most household and industrial chemicals can be obtained from the Poison Control Center in the area, which can give suggestions for treatment.

Speed is essential in the management of chemical burns. For all chemicals, lavage with copious quantities of clean water should be done immediately after removing all clothing. Dry powders should be brushed from the affected areas before irrigation. Early irrigation dilutes the chemical, which is already in contact with the skin, and timeliness increases effectiveness of irrigation; several liters of irrigant may be used. For example, 10 mL of 98% sulfuric acid dissolved in 12 L of water decreases the pH to 5.0, a range that can still cause injury. If the chemical composition is known (acid or base), monitoring of the spent lavage solution pH gives some indication of lavage effectiveness and completion. A reasonable rule of thumb is to lavage with 15 to 20 L of tap water or more for significant chemical injuries. The lavage site should be kept drained in order to remove the earlier, more concentrated effluent. Care should be taken to drain away from uninjured areas to avoid further exposure (Fig. 43.10).

All patients must be monitored according to the severity of their injuries. They may have metabolic disturbances, usually from pH abnormalities, because of exposure to strong acids or caustics. If respiratory difficulty is apparent, oxygen therapy and mechanical ventilation must be instituted. Resuscitation should be guided by the body surface area involved (burn formulas); however, the total fluids given may be dramatically different from the calculated volumes. Some of these injuries may be more

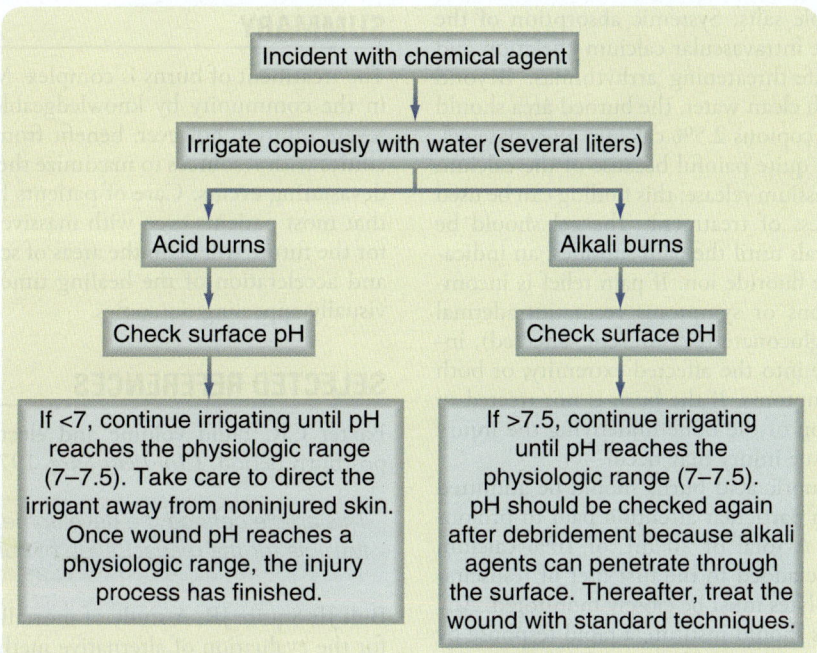

FIGURE 43.10 Treatment of acid and alkali burns.

superficial than they appear, particularly in the case of acids because of coagulative necrosis, and therefore have less resuscitation volume. Injuries from bases, however, may penetrate beyond that which is apparent on examination (liquefactive necrosis); therefore, more volume might be indicated. For this reason, patients with chemical injuries should be observed closely for signs of adequate perfusion. All patients with significant chemical injuries should be monitored with indwelling bladder catheters to accurately measure outputs.

Operative excision, if indicated by clinical assessment of wound depth, should take place as soon as the patient is stable and resuscitated. After adequate lavage and excision, burn wounds are covered with antimicrobial agents or skin substitutes. Once the wounds have stabilized with the indicated treatment, they are taken care of as with any loss of soft tissue. Skin grafting or flap coverage is performed as indicated.

For alkali burns in particular, these are often from chemicals such as lime, potassium hydroxide, bleach, and sodium hydroxide and are among the most common agents involved in chemical injury. Incidental injury frequently occurs in infants and toddlers exploring cleaning cabinets. Three factors are involved in the mechanism of alkali burns: (1) saponification of fat causes the loss of insulation of heat formed in the chemical reaction with tissue, (2) massive extraction of water from cells causes damage because of the hygroscopic nature of alkali, and (3) alkalis dissolve and unite with the proteins of the tissues to form alkaline proteinates, which are soluble and contain hydroxide ions. These ions induce further chemical reactions, penetrating deeper into the tissue. Treatment involves immediate removal of the causative agent with lavage of large volumes of fluid, usually water. Attempts to neutralize alkali agents with weak acids are not recommended because the heat released with neutralization reactions compounds the injury through the thermoplastic reaction. Particularly strong bases should be treated with lavage and consideration for the addition of wound debridement in the operating room. Tangential removal of affected areas is performed until the tissues removed are at a normal pH.

Cement (calcium oxide) burns are alkali in nature, occur commonly, and are usually work-related injuries. The critical substance responsible for the skin damage is the hydroxyl ion. Often, the agent has been in contact with the skin for prolonged periods, such as underneath the boots of a cement worker who seeks treatment hours after the exposure or after the cement penetrates clothing and, when combined with perspiration, induces an exothermic reaction. Treatment consists of removing all clothing and irrigating the affected area with water and soap until all the cement is removed and the effluent has a pH of less than 8. Injuries tend to be deep because of exposure times, and surgical excision and grafting of the resultant eschar may be indicated.

Acid injuries are treated initially like any other chemical injury, with removal of all chemicals by disrobing the affected area and copious irrigation. Acids such as sulfuric or hydrochloric acid induce protein breakdown by hydrolysis and coagulative necrosis, which results in a hard eschar that does not penetrate as deeply as the alkalis. These agents also induce thermal injury by heat generation with contact of the skin, further causing soft tissue damage.

Formic acid injuries are relatively rare, usually involving an organic acid for industrial descaling and as a hay preservative. Electrolyte abnormalities are of great concern for patients with extensive formic acid injuries, with metabolic acidosis, renal failure, intravascular hemolysis, and pulmonary complications being common. Acidemia detected by a metabolic acidosis on arterial blood gas analysis should be corrected with intravenous sodium bicarbonate. Hemodialysis may be indicated when extensive absorption of formic acid has occurred. A formic acid wound typically has a greenish appearance and is deeper than what it initially appears to be; it is best treated by surgical excision.

Hydrofluoric acid is a toxic substance used widely in both industrial and domestic settings and is the strongest known inorganic acid. Management of these burns differs from other acid burns in general. Hydrofluoric acid produces dehydration and corrosion of tissue with free hydrogen ions. In addition, the fluoride ion complexes with bivalent cations such as calcium and magnesium to form insoluble salts. Systemic absorption of the fluoride ion then can induce intravascular calcium chelation and hypocalcemia, leading to life-threatening arrhythmias. Beyond initial copious irrigation with clean water, the burned area should be treated immediately with copious 2.5% calcium gluconate gel. These wounds in general are quite painful because of the calcium chelation and associated potassium release; this finding can be used to determine the effectiveness of treatment. The gel should be changed at 15-minute intervals until the pain subsides, an indication of removal of the active fluoride ion. If pain relief is incomplete after several applications or symptoms recur, intradermal injections of 10% calcium gluconate (0.5 mL/cm^2 affected), intraarterial calcium gluconate into the affected extremity, or both may be used to alleviate symptoms. If the burn is not treated in such a fashion, decalcification of the bone underlying the injury and extension of the soft tissue injury may occur.

All patients with hydrofluoric acid burns should be admitted for cardiac monitoring, with particular attention paid to prolongation of the QT interval. A total of 20 mL of 10% calcium gluconate solution should be added to the first liter of resuscitation fluid, and serum electrolytes must be closely monitored. Any electrocardiographic changes should institute a rapid response by the treatment team with intravenous calcium chloride to maintain heart function. Several grams of calcium may be needed until the chemical response has run its course. Serum magnesium and potassium also should be closely monitored and replaced. Speed is the key to effective treatment.

The organic solvent properties of hydrocarbons promote cell membrane dissolution and skin necrosis. Symptoms include erythema and blistering, and the burns are typically superficial and heal spontaneously. If absorbed systemically, toxicity can produce respiratory depression and eventual hepatic injury thought to be associated with benzenes. Ignition of the hydrocarbons on the skin induces a deep full-thickness injury.

Friction Burns

Friction burn usually presents in two distinct forms: contact with a high-speed motorized belt such as a treadmill or "road rash." Friction burn from the ground (road rash) is a unique injury that has both thermal and mechanical components, adding significant complexity to the wound. First, the heat generated from the friction between the skin and the abrasive surface creates a thermal injury. The severity of injury is determined by the texture of the surface, velocity of the skin when it impacts, temperature of the surface (climate, ambient temperature, time of day), protection by clothing, force generated between the ground and body, and anatomic location. Injury will generally be worse in areas of thin tissue, particularly over bony prominences. Mechanically, these wounds often contain abrasions, lacerations, avulsions, and degloving injuries. Furthermore, a deeper vascular shear or direct impact and tissue death can result in hematomas and skin/fat/muscle necrosis. These patients often have other injuries such as fractures, solid organ injury, and head injury, further complicating their course. Nonviable wound edges may not be amenable to closure and often have irregular, stellate patterns. Finally, these often have significant environmental contamination and are at higher risk of infection.

Most burn centers treat friction burn similarly to other burns with dressing changes, skin substitutes, and more invasive procedures when necessary. Many of these patients benefit from an aggressive lavage with heavy sedation or general anesthesia to remove contaminants. These wounds also have the risk of tattooing the dermis with contaminating materials.

SUMMARY

The treatment of burns is complex. Minor injuries can be treated in the community by knowledgeable physicians. Moderate and severe injuries, however, benefit from treatment in dedicated facilities with resources to maximize the outcomes from these often-devastating events. Care of patients has markedly improved such that most patients even with massive injuries survive. Challenges for the future will be in the areas of scar minimization and control and acceleration of the healing time to result in functional and visually appealing outcomes.

SELECTED REFERENCES

Baxter CR. Fluid volume and electrolyte changes of the early postburn period. *Clin Plast Surg*. 1974;1:693-703.

This article defined the development and use of the Parkland formula for the resuscitation of burned patients.

Bull JP, Squire JR. A study of mortality in a burns unit: standards for the evaluation of alternative methods of treatment. *Ann Surg*. 1949;130:160-173.

This landmark article was one of the first to describe the incidence of burn mortality.

Herndon DN, Hart DW, Wolf SE, et al. Reversal of catabolism by beta-blockade after severe burns. *N Engl J Med*. 2001;345:1223-1229.

This landmark clinical trial showed that propranolol, a nonselective β-receptor antagonist, attenuates the profound hypermetabolic response and the muscle-protein catabolism after severe burn injury.

Herndon DN, Tompkins RG. Support of the metabolic response to burn injury. *Lancet*. 2004;363:1895-1902.

This review was one of the premier articles to highlight the many methods to attenuate the hypermetabolic response and to thoroughly describe the physiologic and metabolic derangements postburn.

Jeschke MG, Chinkes DL, Finnerty CC, et al. Pathophysiologic response to severe burn injury. *Ann Surg*. 2008;248:387-401.

This landmark clinical trial delineated the complexity of the hypermetabolic, hypercatabolic response to severe burn injury.

Wolf SE, Rose JK, Desai MH, et al. Mortality determinants in massive pediatric burns. An analysis of 103 children with > or = 80% TBSA burns (> or = 70% full-thickness). *Ann Surg*. 1997;225:554-565.

The treatment of severely burned pediatric patients and the major determinants of mortality are described in this article. A formula was also devised to predict those who will survive or succumb to their injuries.

The full reference list appears on Elsevier eBooks+.

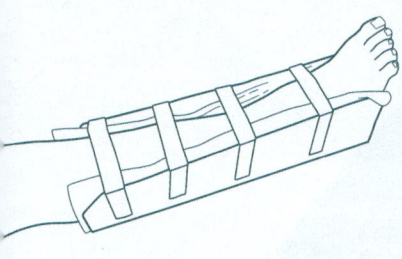

CHAPTER 45

Management of Chronic Wounds

Camila Franco-Mesa, Grant B. Torres, Ludwik K. Branski, and Linda G. Phillips

From the oldest descriptions of wound healing back in 2200 BCE to the numerous therapeutic advances nowadays, wound care has remained one of the most challenging topics in the medical field. Although the understanding of mechanisms involved in wound repair has improved over time, specific details regarding healing, especially in the setting of chronic wounds, are still lacking.

TISSUE INJURY AND RESPONSE

Wound repair refers to all attempts to restore mechanical integrity, reinstate the barriers to fluid loss and infection, and reestablish normal blood and lymphatic flow patterns. Unlike regeneration, in which perfect restoration of preexisting tissue architecture is achieved, in wound repair, flawless reconstruction is sacrificed to prioritize return to function. Regeneration is achievable only during embryonic development, in lower organisms, or in certain tissues such as bone and liver.

The path toward wound repair is universally composed of three stages: inflammation, proliferation, and maturation, which includes remodeling. Acute wounds are those that complete all three healing phases promptly. Chronic wounds stall in the inflammatory phase and fail to progress.

WOUND-HEALING

Wounds present in different stages of the wound-healing phases. For instance, in a large wound such as a pressure sore, the eschar or fibrinous exudate reflects the inflammatory phase, the granulation tissue is part of the proliferative phase, and the contracting or advancing edge is part of the maturational phase. All three phases may occur simultaneously, and the phases may overlap with their processes (Fig. 45.1).

Phases

Inflammatory

During the immediate reaction of the tissue to injury, hemostasis occurs quickly and is rapidly followed by inflammation. This phase represents an attempt to limit damage by stopping bleeding; sealing the wound surface; and removing necrotic tissue, foreign debris, and bacteria. The inflammatory phase is characterized by increased vascular permeability, migration of cells into the wound by chemotaxis, secretion of cytokines and growth factors into the wound, and activation of the migrating cells (Fig. 45.2).

Proliferative

As the acute responses of hemostasis and inflammation begin to resolve, the scaffolding is laid for the repair of the wound through angiogenesis, fibroplasia, and epithelialization. This stage is characterized by the formation of granulation tissue, which consists of a capillary bed; fibroblasts; macrophages; and a loose arrangement of collagen, fibronectin, and hyaluronic acid. Numerous studies have used growth factors to modify granulation tissue, particularly fibroplasia. Adenoviral transfer, topical application, and subcutaneous injection of platelet-derived growth factor (PDGF), transforming growth factor-β (TGF-β), keratinocyte growth factor (KGF), vascular endothelial growth factor (VEGF), and epidermal growth factor (EGF) have been shown to increase the proliferation of granulation tissue.

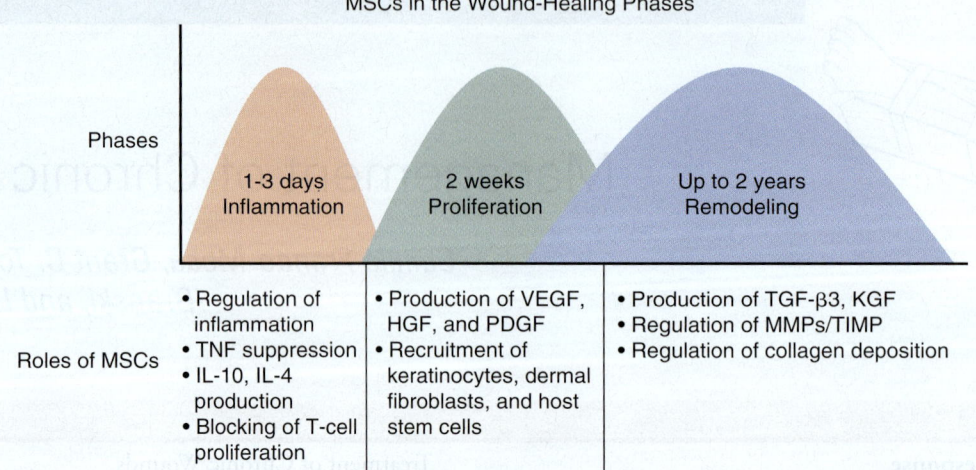

FIGURE 45.1 Mesenchymal stem cell *(MSC)* roles in each phase of the wound-healing process. *HGF,* Hepatocyte growth factor; *IL-4,* interleukin-4; *IL-10,* interleukin-10; *KGF,* keratinocyte growth factor; *MMPs,* matrix metalloproteinases; *PDGF,* platelet-derived growth factor; *TGF-β3,* transforming growth factor-β3; *TIMP,* tissue inhibitors of metalloproteinase; *TNF,* tumor necrosis factor; *VEGF,* vascular endothelial growth factor. (From Maxson S, Lopez EA, Yoo D, et al. Concise review: role of mesenchymal stem cells in wound repair. *Stem Cells Transl Med.* 2012;1:142-149.)

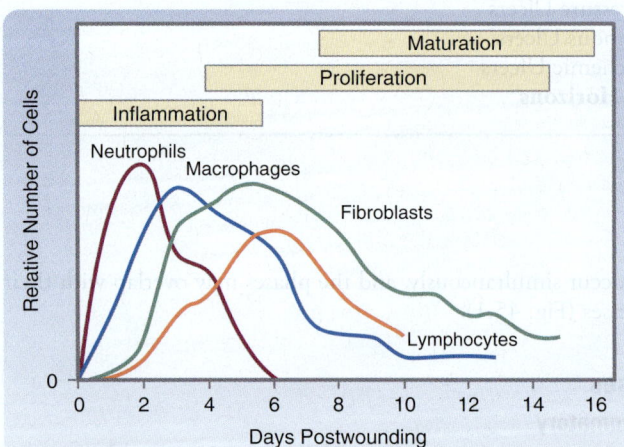

FIGURE 45.2 Time course of the appearance of different cells in the wound during healing. Macrophages and neutrophils are predominant during the inflammatory phase (peak at days 3 and 2, respectively). Lymphocytes appear later and peak at day 7. Fibroblasts are the predominant cells during the proliferative phase. (Adapted from Witte MB, Barbul A. General principles of wound healing. *Surg Clin North Am.* 1997;77:509-528.)

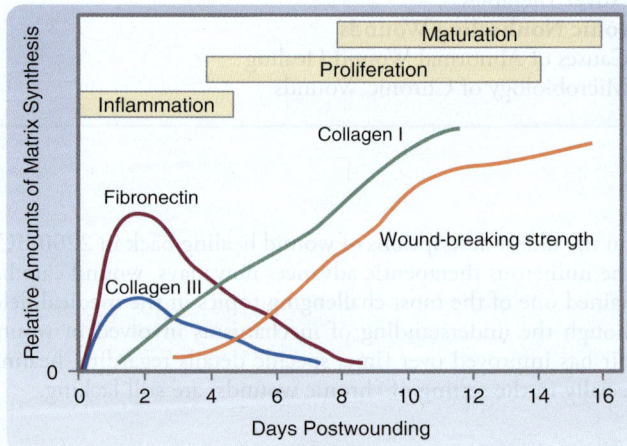

FIGURE 45.3 Wound matrix deposition over time. Fibronectin and type III collagen constitute the early matrix. Type I collagen accumulates later and corresponds to the increase in wound-breaking strength. (Adapted from Witte MB, Barbul A. General principles of wound healing. *Surg Clin North Am.* 1997;77:509-528.)

Maturational

Wound contraction occurs by centripetal movement of the whole thickness of the surrounding skin and reduces the amount of disorganized scar. Wound contraction appears to take place as a result of a complex interaction of the extracellular materials, which is addressed later, and fibroblasts that is not completely understood. Fibroblasts in a contracting wound change to stimulated cells, termed *myofibroblasts.* These cells have function and structure in common with fibroblasts and smooth muscle cells and express α-smooth muscle actin in bundles termed *stress fibers.* The actin appears on day 6 after wounding, persists at high levels for 15 days, and is gone by 4 weeks when the cell undergoes apoptosis. It appears that a stimulated fibroblast develops contractile ability related to the formation of cytoplasmic actin-myosin

complexes. When this stimulated cell is placed in the fibroblast-populated collagen lattice, contraction occurs even more quickly. The tension that is exerted by the fibroblast's attempt at contraction appears to stimulate the actin-myosin structures in its cytoplasm. If colchicine, which inhibits microtubules, or cytochalasin D, which inhibits microfilaments, is added to the tissue culture, the result is minimal contraction of the collagen gels. Fibroblasts develop a linear arrangement in the line of tension that, when removed, causes the cells to round up.

Remodeling

The fibroblast population decreases, and the dense capillary network regresses. Wound strength increases rapidly within 1 to 6 weeks and then appears to plateau up to 1 year after the injury (Fig. 45.3). Compared with nonwounded skin, tensile strength is only 30% in the scar. An increase in breaking strength occurs after approximately 21 days, mostly as a result of cross-linking. Although collagen cross-linking causes further wound contraction and an increase in strength, it also results in a scar that is more brittle and less elastic than normal skin. In contrast to normal skin, the epidermal-dermal interface in a healed wound is devoid of rete pegs, the undulating projections of the epidermis that penetrate the papillary dermis. Loss of this anchorage results in increased fragility and predisposes the neoepidermis to avulsion after minor trauma.

Extracellular Matrix

The majority of the wound-healing stages take place or have direct interaction with the extracellular matrix (ECM). The ECM exists as a scaffold to stabilize the physical structure of tissues, but it also plays an active and complex role by regulating the behavior of cells that contact it. Cells within it produce the macromolecular constituents, including (1) glycosaminoglycans (GAGs), or polysaccharide chains, usually found covalently linked to protein in the form of proteoglycans, and (2) fibrous proteins such as collagen, elastin, fibronectin, and laminin.

- GAGs and proteoglycans: GAGs are unbranched polysaccharide chains composed of repeating disaccharide units, a sulfated amino sugar (N-acetylglucosamine or N-acetylgalactosamine), and uronic acid (glucuronic or iduronic). GAGs are highly negatively charged because of the sulfate or carboxyl groups on most of their sugars. Four types of GAGs exist: hyaluronan, chondroitin sulfate and dermatan sulfate, heparan sulfate, and keratan sulfate.

  GAGs in connective tissue usually constitute less than 10% of the weight of fibrous proteins. Their highly negative charge attracts osmotically active cations, such as Na^+, which causes large amounts of water to be incorporated into the matrix. This results in porous hydrated gels and is responsible for the turgor that enables the matrix to withstand compressive force.

  Proteoglycans are a diverse group of glycoproteins with functions mediated by their core proteins and GAG chains. The number and types of GAGs attached to the core protein can vary greatly, and the GAGs themselves can be modified by sulfonation. Because of their GAGs, proteoglycans provide hydrated space around and between cells. They also form gels of different pore sizes and charge densities to regulate the movement of cells and molecules.

- Collagen: Collagens are found in all multicellular animals and are secreted by various cell types. They are a major component of skin and bone and constitute 25% of the total protein mass in mammals. There are at least 20 types of collagen, the main constituents of connective tissue being types I, II, III, V, and XI. Type I is the principal collagen of skin and bone and is the most common. In adults, the skin is approximately 80% type I and 20% type III. In newborns, the content of type III collagen is greater than that found in adults. Other types of collagens include types IX and XII (fibril-associated collagens) and types IV and VII (network-forming collagens). Type IV molecules assemble into a meshlike pattern and are a major part of the mature basal lamina.

  Numerous factors can affect collagen synthesis. Vitamin C (ascorbic acid), TGF-β, insulin-like growth factor-1 (IGF)-1, and IGF-2 increase collagen synthesis. Interferon (IFN)-γ decreases type I procollagen messenger RNA (mRNA) synthesis, and glucocorticoids inhibit procollagen gene transcription, leading to decreased collagen synthesis.

Several genetic disorders are caused by abnormalities in collagen fibril formation. In osteogenesis imperfecta, deletion of one procollagen α_1 allele results in weak, easily fractured bones. Ehlers-Danlos syndrome is a result of mutations affecting type III collagen and is characterized by fragile skin and blood vessels and hypermobile joints.

- Elastic fibers: Tissues such as skin, blood vessels, and lungs require strength and elasticity to function. Elastic fibers in the ECM of these tissues provide the resilience to allow recoil after transient stretching. Elastic fibers are predominantly composed of elastin, a highly hydrophobic protein (~750 amino acids long). Microfibrils appear before elastin in developing tissues and seem to form a scaffold on which the secreted elastin molecules are deposited. Elastin is produced early in life, stabilizes, and does not undergo much further synthesis or degradation, with a turnover that approaches the life span. Age-related modification is a result of progressive degradation as the elastic fibers gradually become tortuous, frayed, and porous.

  Mutations causing a deficiency of elastin protein result in arterial narrowing as a consequence of excessive smooth muscle cell proliferation in the arterial wall (intimal hyperplasia). These findings suggest that the normal elasticity of an artery is needed to prevent the proliferation of these cells. Gene mutations in fibrillin result in Marfan syndrome; severely affected individuals are prone to aortic rupture.

- Fibronectin: Soluble plasma fibronectin circulates in various body fluids and enhances blood clotting, wound healing, and phagocytosis. The highly insoluble fibrillar forms assemble on cell surfaces and are deposited in the ECM. The fibronectin fibrils that form on the surface of fibroblasts are usually coupled with neighboring intracellular actin stress fibers. The actin filaments promote the assembly of the fibronectin fibril and influence fibril orientation. Integrin transmembrane adhesion proteins mediate these interactions. The contractile actin and myosin cytoskeleton pull on the fibronectin matrix and generate tension.

- Laminin: Basal laminae are flexible, thin (40- to 120-nm) mats of specialized ECM that separate cells and epithelia from the underlying or surrounding connective tissue. The basal lamina acts in numerous ways: (1) as a molecular filter to prevent the passage of macromolecules (i.e., in the kidney glomerulus), (2) as a selective barrier to certain cells (i.e., the lamina beneath the epithelium prevents fibroblasts from contacting epithelial cells but does not stop macrophages or lymphocytes), (3) as a scaffold for regenerating cells to migrate, and (4) as an important element in tissue regeneration in locations where the basal lamina survives. Laminins generally consist of three long polypeptide chains (α, β, and γ). Mice lacking the laminin γ_1 chain die during embryogenesis because they cannot make a basal lamina.

In connective tissue, proteoglycan molecules form a gel-like ground substance. This highly hydrated gel allows the matrix to withstand compressive force while permitting rapid diffusion of nutrients, metabolites, and hormones between blood and tissue cells. Collagen fibers within the matrix serve to organize and strengthen the matrix, whereas elastin fibers give it resilience because matrix proteins have adhesive functions.

The wound matrix accumulates and changes in composition as healing progresses, balanced between new deposition and degradation (Fig. 45.4). The provisional matrix is a scaffold for cellular migration and is composed of fibrin, fibrinogen, fibronectin, and

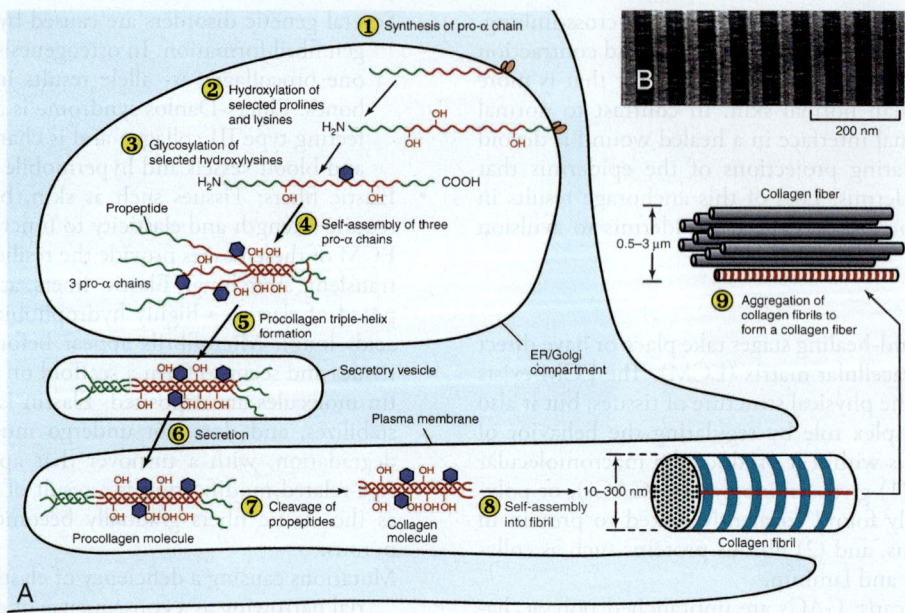

FIGURE 45.4 Intracellular and extracellular events in the formation of a collagen fibril. (A) Collagen fibrils are shown assembling in the extracellular space contained within a large infolding in the plasma membrane. As one example of how collagen fibrils can form ordered arrays in the extracellular space, they are shown further assembling into large collagen fibers, which are visible with a light microscope. The covalent cross-links that stabilize the extracellular assemblies are not shown. (B) Electron micrograph of a negatively stained collagen fibril revealing its typical striated appearance. *ER,* Endoplasmic reticulum. (From Alberts B, Johnson A, Lewis J, et al., eds. *Molecular Biology of the Cell.* 4th ed. Garland; 2002:1100; B, Courtesy Robert Horne.)

vitronectin. GAGs and proteoglycans are synthesized next and support further matrix deposition and remodeling. Collagens, which are the predominant scar proteins, are the result. Attachment proteins, such as fibrin and fibronectin, provide linkage to the ECM through binding to cell surface integrin receptors.

Stimulation of fibroblasts by growth factors induces upregulated expression of integrin receptors, facilitating cell-matrix interactions. Ligand binding induces clustering of integrin into focal adhesion sites. Regulation of integrin-mediated cell signaling by the extracellular divalent cations Mg^{2+}, Mn^{2+}, and Ca^{2+} is perhaps caused by the induction of conformational changes in the integrins.

A dynamic and reciprocal relationship exists between fibroblasts and the ECM. Cytokine regulation of fibroblast responses is altered by variations in the composition of the ECM. For example, expression of matrix-degrading enzymes, such as the matrix metalloproteinases (MMPs), is upregulated after cytokine stimulation of fibroblasts. Collagenolytic MMP-1 is induced by interleukin-1 (IL-1) and downregulated by TGF-β. Activation of plasminogen to plasmin by plasminogen activator and procollagenase to collagenase by plasmin results in matrix degradation and facilitates cell migration. Modulation of these processes provides additional mechanisms whereby the cell-matrix interaction can be regulated during wound healing. Matrix modulation is also seen in tumor metastasis. Neoplastic cells lose their dependence on anchorage, mediated mainly by integrins; this is probably caused by decreased production of fibronectin and, subsequently, decreased adhesion, and as a result, these cells can break away from the primary tumor and metastasize.

An example of the necessary dynamic interactions occurring in the provisional matrix during wound healing is the effect of TGF-β on incisional wounds sealed with fibrin sealant. Fibrin sealant is a derivative of plasma components that mimics the last step in the coagulation cascade. Commercially available fibrin sealant has an approximately tenfold greater concentration of fibrin than plasma and consequently provides a more airtight, waterproof seal. Fibrin sealant may serve as a mechanical barrier to the early cell-mediated events occurring in wound healing. Supplementation of fibrin sealant with TGF-β has been demonstrated to reverse the inhibitory effects of fibrin sealant on wound healing and increase tensile strength compared with sutured wounds. The increased tensile strength may be a result of improved cell migration into the wound site, more rapid clearance of fibrin sealant, suppression of gelatinase (MMP-9), and enhancement of ECM synthesis in TGF-β–supplemented wounds.

Regulated turnover of the ECM is crucial to many biologic processes. ECM degradation occurs during metastasis when neoplastic cells migrate from their site of origin to distant organs via the bloodstream or lymphatics. In injury or infection, localized degradation of the ECM occurs so that cells can migrate across the basal lamina to reach the site of injury or infection. Locally secreted cellular proteases, such as MMPs or serine proteases, degrade the ECM components. Matrix proteolysis helps the cell migrate by (1) clearing a path through the matrix; (2) exposing binding sites, promoting cell binding or migration; (3) facilitating cell detachment so that a cell can move forward; and (4) releasing signal proteins that promote cell migration. Proteolysis is tightly regulated. Many proteases are secreted as inactive precursors that are activated when required. In addition, cell surface receptors bind these proteases to ensure that they act only on sites where they are needed. Finally, protease inhibitors, such as tissue inhibitors of metalloproteinase (TIMP), can bind these enzymes and block their activity.

ABNORMAL WOUND HEALING

Wound healing is a complex series of intertwining events that is affected by intrinsic and extrinsic factors (Box 45.1). The amount of tissue lost or damaged, the amount of foreign material or bacterial inoculation, and the length of exposure to toxic factors can affect the time to recovery. Intrinsic factors such as age, chronic medical conditions such as atherosclerosis, cardiac or renal failure, medications, genetic factors, and anatomic location of the wound all affect wound healing. Ultimately, the efficacy of the wound-healing process will be determined by the ability to go through the stages of wound repair promptly. When the regular repair mechanisms go amiss, one of two pathways develops: dysregulated and excessive formation of scar tissue termed *hypertrophic scarring* or *keloid* or a persistent and stagnant inflammatory state represented by an ulcerative skin defect designated *chronic wound*.

HYPERTROPHIC SCARS AND KELOIDS

Hypertrophic scars and keloids are proliferative scars characterized by dysregulated and excessive net collagen deposition from increased production or decreased degradation of collagen (Fig. 45.5). Hypertrophic scars are raised scars within the confines of the original wound that frequently regress spontaneously. Keloids, by definition, grow beyond the borders of the original wounds and rarely regress with time. The latter is more prevalent in darkly pigmented skin, developing in 15% to 20% of African Americans, Asians, and Hispanics. Keloids are more likely to be present in females. There is strong evidence suggesting a genetic susceptibility, including familial heritability, common occurrence in twins, and high prevalence in certain ethnic populations.

BOX 45.1 Factors That Inhibit Wound Healing

Hypoxia
Ischemia
Diabetes
Ionizing radiation
Aging
Malnutrition
- Vitamin deficiencies: A and C
- Mineral deficiencies: Zinc and iron
Exogenous drugs
Infection

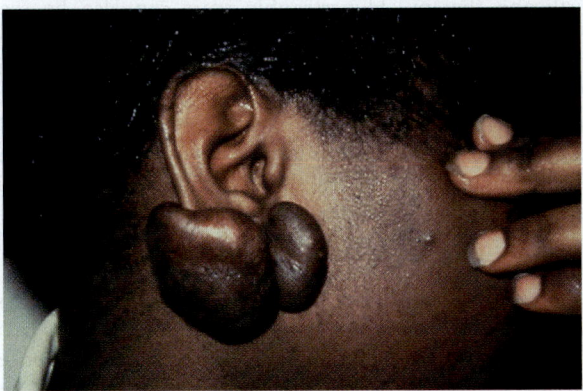

FIGURE 45.5 Keloids caused by ear piercing.

Inheritance patterns can be autosomal dominant, autosomal recessive, or even X-linked. Single-nucleotide polymorphisms, as seen in Mendelian disorders, have been associated with keloids. Proposed pathways include apoptosis, endocytosis, cytokine-cytokine receptor interaction, mitogen-activated protein kinase signaling pathway, tenascin C, jun proto-oncogene, and growth factors such as TGF-β and VEGF.[1-4]

Keloids often occur above the clavicles, on the trunk, on the upper extremities, and on the face and less frequently on the palms, soles, and genitalia. Their occurrence cannot be predicted, and it can take place spontaneously or throughout an extended time period. This type of lesion can be hyperpigmented and associated with life-limiting pruritus, which is explained by a high quantity of mast cells in the keloid's dermal layer. Keloids are frequently refractory to medical and surgical intervention. To date, there is no known effective prevention method for keloid formation.

Keloids and hypertrophic scars differ histologically from normal scars. Hypertrophic scars primarily contain well-organized type III collagen, whereas keloids contain disorganized type I and type III collagen bundles (Table 45.1). Keloids and hypertrophic scars have stretched collagen bundles aligned in the same plane as the epidermis, whereas collagen bundles are randomly arrayed and relaxed in normal scars. Keloid scars have thicker, abundant collagen bundles that form acellular nodelike structures in the deep dermis with a paucity of cells centrally. Additionally, they contain higher levels of macrophages with increased affinity for the Th2-immune chronic response pathway, which enables them to secrete transforming growth factors constantly and promote collagen deposition.[3] Hypertrophic scars, in contrast, contain islands composed of aggregates of fibroblasts, small vessels, and collagen fibers throughout the dermis.

Hypertrophic scars are often preventable. High tension, prolonged inflammation, and insufficient resurfacing (e.g., burn wounds) promote hypertrophic scarring. Scars perpendicular to the underlying muscle fibers tend to be flatter and narrower, with less collagen formation than when they are parallel to the underlying muscle fibers. Tension appears to signal the formation of activated fibroblasts, resulting in excessive collagen deposition and thus a higher risk for dysregulated collagen accumulation. The position of an elective scar can be chosen to induce a narrower, less obvious healed scar. As muscle fibers contract, the wound edges become reapproximated when they are perpendicular to the underlying muscle and tend to gape if placed parallel to it, leading to greater wound tension and scar formation.

Hypertrophic scars represent a reversible hyperproliferative scar phenotype that tends to regress when the original stimuli (skin tension, stimulatory growth factors) are removed. Keloids appear to be genetically predisposed and are switched on irreversibly by growth factors. In addition, in these scars, collagen synthesis is elevated, whereas collagen degradation is low. MMPs are also affected in these scars: MMP-1 (collagenase) and MMP-9 (gelatinase, early tissue repair) are decreased, whereas MMP-2 (gelatinase, late tissue remodeling) is significantly elevated. Blocking TGF-β activity with antibodies decreases scar fibrosis. The use of mesenchymal stem cell (MSC) therapy to regulate the inflammatory pathway of hypertrophic scarring and keloids is currently being studied in rats. Systemic and topical injected MSCs have been noted to improve the macroscopical and histologic characteristics of these lesions.

Prevention of Hypertrophic Scars and Keloids

Some of the strategies that reduce adverse scarring immediately after wound closure are tension relief, pressure therapy, hydration/

TABLE 45.1	**Characteristics of Hypertrophic Scars and Keloids**	
	HYPERTROPHIC SCARRING	**KELOIDS**
Description	Contained within the site of injury	Spread beyond the borders of the injury
Localization	Areas prone to high tension: back, chest, shoulders, elbows and other joints	Earlobes, shoulders, chest, back, cheeks, and knees
Collagen distribution	Wavy, regular pattern of type III collagen	Disorganized pattern, no distinct organization of type I and III collagen
Prognosis	Tend to regress over time and resolve completely	Persist
Response to excision	Low incidence of recurrence	High recurrence rate

occlusion, and the use of taping. Wounds with greater tension (perpendicular to Langer lines) or with excessive tension on closure and in certain anatomic locations (deltoid and sternal) are at a higher risk of adverse scarring. It is believed that greater tension results in a stronger activation of the inflammatory mechanisms, resulting in excessive scarring. Pressure therapy is used as an adjacent instrument to decrease the cytokine response and reduce collagen synthesis in scar formation, particularly in wide wounds. Pressure is applied via garments, bandages, adhesives, or specialized devices as soon as the patient can tolerate them. In general, wounds that remain hydrated tend to have less generation of static and mast cells. After wound healing, water still evaporates more rapidly through scar tissue and may take more than a year to recover to preinjury levels. Moisturizing lotions and moisture-retentive dressings can reduce the thickness, discomfort, and itching and improve the appearance of the scar. Sunscreen is a topical option that promotes hydration and protects the wound from ultraviolet light, which is known to increase pigmentation. Silicone products may ameliorate evaporative losses and assist in hydration of the stratum corneum. Silicon tape provides structural passive stabilization of the wound and decreases tension at the edges. These strategies need to be employed soon after initial wound healing.

Types of Treatments

Treatments can be divided into noninvasive, injectable, and surgical interventions. Noninvasive therapies include first-line silicone sheeting and pressure garments, as described earlier. For instance, early linear scar hypertrophy (e.g., after trauma or surgery) at 6 weeks to 3 months should be treated with pressure therapy. After 6 months, silicone therapy should be continued for as long as necessary if there is further scar maturation. Severe burns, mechanical trauma, necrotizing infections, wounds requiring more than 2 to 3 weeks to heal, or wounds healed with skin grafting require early application of silicone and compression therapy. This therapy should be initiated as soon as the wound is closed and the patient can tolerate the pressure. The mechanism of action of pressure therapy is poorly understood but may involve reduction of wound oxygen tension by occlusion of small blood vessels, resulting in a decrease in myofibroblast proliferation and collagen synthesis. Pressure therapy is believed to act on cellular mechanoreceptors that are involved in cellular apoptosis and linked to the ECM. The increased pressure regulates the apoptosis of dermal fibroblasts and diminishes hypertrophic scarring. Pressure and silicone therapy should be continued or intensified and combined with selective injections in resistant areas. Similarly, for keloids, first-line treatments include a combination of silicone dressings, pressure therapy, and injected steroids. Other noninvasive therapies include experimental medications on the market. Imiquimod, for example, has been targeted as an immune system–modulating agent when used topically as a cream, and the

calcium channel blocker verapamil has been investigated for its role in collagen degradation. Data regarding the use of these medications are conflicting; thus, further research is required before considering them a first-line safe and standard-of-care option.

In the injectable category, intralesional corticosteroids are the first-line treatment for hypertrophic scarring and keloids. Their antiinflammatory and antiproliferative properties decrease collagen synthesis and fibroblast action. Ongoing hypertrophy unresponsive to noninvasive methods may be treated with intralesional corticosteroids (triamcinolone acetonide, 10–40 mg/mL) injected into the papillary dermis every 2 to 4 weeks until flat. This is the only noninvasive management option that has enough supporting evidence to be recommended in evidence-based guidelines. Approximately 50% to 100% of patients respond, and up to 50% experience recurrence. Adverse steroid effects include skin atrophy, hypopigmentation, telangiectasias, and excessive pain during injections. Injections should be limited to the scar itself to minimize adjacent fat atrophy. Although systemic effects are rare, certain cases with multiple lesions warranting concomitant injections can result in adverse consequences. Bleomycin, 5-fluorouracil (5-FU), and verapamil have been used as adjuncts to corticosteroid therapy. The pyrimidine analogue 5-FU is known to alter the cell cycle, promoting fibroblast apoptosis when used intralesionally, whereas bleomycin has proapoptotic and antiproliferative properties. Both 5-FU and bleomycin are novel therapies that require high-power clinical studies.

Surgical interventions include cryotherapy, excision, and laser. Cryotherapy is effective for small lesions. It can be applied intralesionally or topically via spray. In general, it has proven to be a suitable option, with a regression rate of up to 75% in the second session. Adverse events include depigmentation, pain, telangiectasia, skin atrophy, and recurrence. Regarding hypertrophic scarring, surgical scar revision may be considered for permanent linear hypertrophic scars present after 1 year. Simple resection and primary closure may be combined with adjacent tissue undermining, subcutaneous sutures, adjunctive Z-plasty, and postsurgical taping and silicone therapy. Hypertrophic scars can also be seen in conjunction with a scar contracture. Scar contractures involve abnormal shortening of unmatured scars, resulting in functional impairment, particularly if the scar is across a joint. Correction of a scar contracture generally requires surgery with Z-plasty, skin graft, or flap to release tension in the scar to restore function and reduce scar hypertrophy. Early surgery is indicated for functional impairment. Burn scar contracture release procedures in the neck and axilla are best performed with flaps to improve functional and cosmetic outcomes further, which may not be achievable with skin grafts. Widespread large hypertrophic scars may require serial excision or tissue expansion. Surgical excision for keloids is a controversial therapy. Excision alone results in a high recurrence rate of 50% to 100% and potential enlargement of the keloid. However, immediate postoperative electron beam irradiation or brachytherapy reduces recurrence rates by 50% to 95%. Ogawa and associates recently published a protocol of electron beam radiation for postsurgical excision based on high-risk areas for keloid recurrence.[5] Doses of 15 Gy for 2 days were applied to high-risk regions, such as those above the chest, and doses of 8 Gy for 1 day were applied to earlobes.[5] As a result, exposure to radiation decreased, and the rate of keloid recurrence was <10%.[5] Finally, laser therapy is reserved for last after the first-line treatments fail. Commonly used machines include pulsed dye lasers, fractional CO_2 lasers, and laser Erbium-Yag (ER: YAG) resurfacing. Although this method reduces erythema, decreases the height of the keloid, and increases the pliability of the skin, further clinical trials are warranted.

Novel Therapies

New treatments for hypertrophic scarring and keloids include IFN, botulinum toxin, bleomycin, mitomycin, calcium channel blockers, MSC therapy, angiotensin-converting enzyme inhibitors, and fat grafting.

IFN—especially IFN-α and IFN-γ— has been shown to result in keloid size regression and decreased recurrence. The effect is secondary to the antiproliferative properties of these components. Although a decrease in collagen and an increase in collagenase have been seen, the rate of recurrence still remains above 50%. Thus, this therapy is better suited as an adjuvant treatment.

Regarding botulinum toxin, injecting it in the periphery of the wound will limit underlying muscle mobility and tension. This is thought to decrease the stimulus for collagen deposition, modulate fibroblastic activity, and alleviate tension at the wound site.[6] A recent literature review of intralesional botulinum toxin therapy in keloid scar management by Sohrabi and colleagues reported a reduction in keloidal volume, height, and vascularity, with outcomes comparable to those of intralesional corticosteroids.[6]

Angiotensin-converting enzyme inhibitors aid in scarring by modulating collagen production via the renin-angiotensin system because higher concentrations of angiotensin I receptors are seen in keloids. Both Captopril and Enalapril have been studied. Better outcomes are seen in recent scars rather than long-standing ones.

Mitomycin inhibits nucleic acid and protein synthesis. In humans, it decreases scar formation by inhibiting fibroblast proliferation. Mitomycin has had conflicting findings in the field of wound healing. In murine models, it has been shown to decrease the rate of scar contraction, whereas in rat models, it did not show long-term differences in wound characteristics after topical application.[7] Although mitomycin could potentially be considered as a treatment agent, further research is required.

Bleomycin inhibits the synthesis of DNA and the cross-linking of collagen fibers through the lysyl-oxidase enzyme. It is used in conjunction with injected corticosteroids (starting dose of 0.1 mL) after failure of monotherapy with the latter. When used weekly for a month by Huu and associates in a 55-patient study, 70.8% of scars had complete resolution, and the remaining had partial improvement.[4] Despite the promising results, the rate of recurrence was elevated, and side effects such as blisters, ulceration, and hyperpigmentation were reported.[4]

Calcium channel blockers, in particular verapamil, promote collagen degradation and induce fibroblast apoptosis, which results in decreased ECM component production. Intralesional verapamil use in conjunction with other therapies has been used in different plastic surgery procedures to improve and prevent abnormal scarring. Zhang and colleagues evaluated 9 randomized controlled trials involving 567 patients who underwent verapamil or triamcinolone intralesional injection for keloids and hypertrophic scars.[1] Although triamcinolone had superior results regarding reduction in height, pliability, and vascularity, verapamil had comparable long-term outcomes with a lower incidence of skin atrophy, telangiectasia, and hyperpigmentation.[1]

Stem cell therapy, especially MSCs, are known to release growth factors that hinder inflammatory response and promote antifibrotic components. Local and systemic injections of MSCs have been attempted in animal models. Bojanic and associates reviewed 11 case-control animal studies using MSCs for hypertrophic scarring ($n = 10$) and keloids ($n = 1$).[3] Improvement in the histologic and macroscopic appearance of the treated scars was noticed.[3] Despite the positive outcomes in animal models, there are no human studies currently available to evaluate the applicability of this treatment.

The idea behind fat grafting lies in the potential role of adipose-derived stem cells in regulating angiogenic growth factors and antiapoptotic proteins to decrease fibrous tissue and disorganized collagen deposition. Although there is a potential role for this therapy in scar treatment, research is extremely limited with this technique, even from the standpoint of adjuvant therapy.

Although existing strategies for the management of hypertrophic scars and keloids are broadly similar, the histologic differences between the two scars suggest that in the future, therapeutic approaches could be developed that are specifically tailored for these different types of scars. However, at present, there is no single proven best therapy for the management of these excessive healing scars, and the large number of treatment options reflects this (Table 45.2).

CHRONIC NONHEALING WOUNDS

By definition, chronic wounds are wounds that have failed to proceed through an orderly and timely reparative process to produce anatomic and functional integrity over a period of 3 months. The overall prevalence of chronic wounds worldwide is estimated to be 2.2 per 1000 population; the prevalence specifically for chronic leg ulcers is 1.51 per 1000 population.[8] In the United States, 1.6 million people are affected by diabetic foot ulcers (DFUs) per year,[9] up to 2 million patients per year develop chronic leg ulcers secondary to venous insufficiency, and 2 to 3 million patients per year develop pressure ulcers secondary to immobility. These numbers have been increasing as a result of an aging population and the rising incidence of risk factors for atherosclerotic disease, such as diabetes mellitus, cardiovascular disease, and smoking. These wounds are a significant challenge to healthcare professionals and an immense burden on healthcare systems and the economy. Patients also report reduced quality of life, psychological repercussions, and social isolation.

Different factors that promote adverse wound-healing conditions have been identified (Fig. 45.6). Systemic conditions, such as malnutrition, aging, tissue hypoxia, and diabetes, contribute significantly to the pathogenesis of chronic wounds. A combination of systemic and localized adverse wound factors collectively overwhelm the normal healing processes, resulting in a hostile wound-healing environment (Fig. 45.7).

Chronic wounds have derangements in the various stages of wound healing and have unusually elevated or depressed levels of cytokines, growth factors, or proteinases. Chronic wound fluid, in contrast to acute wound fluid, has been shown to have greater levels of IL-1, IL-6, and tumor necrosis factor-α (TNF-α); levels of these proinflammatory cytokines decreased as the wound

TABLE 45.2 **Prevention and Treatment Options for Keloids and Hypertrophic Scars**

MODALITY OR TREATMENT OPTION	RESPONSE RATE (%)	RECURRENCE RATE (%)	COMMENTS	STUDY DESIGN
Prevention				
Preventive silicone sheeting (postsurgery)	0–75	25–36	Multiple preparations available, tolerated by children, expensive, avoid on open wounds, poor study design	Review of multiple case studies
Postsurgical intralesional corticosteroid injection (triamcinolone acetonide [Kenalog], 10–40 mg/mL at 6-week intervals)	NA	0–100 (mean, 50)	Patient acceptance and safety; may cause hypopigmentation, skin atrophy, telangiectasia	Review of multiple case studies
Postsurgical topical imiquimod, 5% cream (Aldara)	NA	28	May cause hyperpigmentation, irritation	Case study
Postsurgical fluorouracil, triamcinolone acetonide, and pulsed dye lasers (best outcomes)	70 at 12 weeks	NA	Effective; may cause hyperpigmentation, wound ulceration	Clinical trial
First-Line Treatment				
Postsurgical radiation therapy	80–100	<10	Local growth inhibition	Clinical trials
Intralesional corticosteroid injection (triamcinolone acetonide [Kenalog], 10–40 mg/mL at 6-week intervals)	50–100	9–50	Inexpensive, requires multiple injections; may cause discomfort, skin atrophy, telangiectasia	Review of multiple case studies
Silicone elastomer sheeting	50–100	NA	Multiple preparations available, tolerated by children, expensive, poor study design	Review of multiple case studies
Pressure dressing (24–30 mm Hg) worn for 6–12 months	90–100	NA	Inexpensive, difficult schedule, poor adherence	Review of multiple case studies
Cryotherapy	50–76	NA	Useful on small lesions; easy to perform; may cause hypopigmentation, pain	Review of multiple case studies
Surgical excision alone	NA	50–100	Z-plasty option for burns; immediate postsurgical treatment needed to prevent regrowth	Review of multiple case studies
Combined cryotherapy and intralesional corticosteroid injection	84	NA	See benefits of individual treatments; may cause hypopigmentation	Case study
Triple-keloid therapy (surgery, corticosteroids, silicone sheeting)	88 at 13 months	12.5 at 13 months	Tedious, time intensive, expensive	Case study
Pulsed dye laser	NA	NA	Specialist referral needed, expensive, variable results depending on trial (controversial)	Case studies
Second-Line and Alternative Treatment				
Verapamil, 2.5 mg/mL, intralesional injection combined with perilesional excision and silicone sheeting	54 at 18 months	NA	Repeated injections, limited experience, may cause discomfort	Clinical trial
Fluorouracil, 50 mg/mL, intralesional injection two to three times a week	88	0	Effective; may cause hyperpigmentation, wound ulceration	Review of multiple case studies
Bleomycin tattooing, 1.5 IU/mL	92, 88	NA	Effective; may cause pulmonary fibrosis, cutaneous reactions	Review of case study, control trial
Postsurgical interferon-α2b, 1.5 million IU, intralesional injection bid for 4 days	30–50	8–19	Expensive; may cause pruritus, altered pigmentation, pain	Review of multiple case studies
Radiation therapy alone	56 (mean)	NA	Local growth inhibition; may cause cancer, hyperpigmentation, paresthesias	Review of multiple case studies
Onion extract topical gels (Mederma)	NA	NA	Limited effect alone, better in combination with silicone sheeting	Prospective case study

bid, Twice daily; *NA*, not available.

Updated from Townsend CM, Beauchamp RD, Evers BM, Mattox KL, Sabiston DC. Chapter 6: Wound healing. In: Townsend CM, ed. *Sabiston Textbook of Surgery: The Biological Basis of Modern Surgical Practice.* Elsevier; 2022; Juckett G, Hartman-Adams H. Management of keloids and hypertrophic scars. *Am Fam Physician.* 2009;80:253-260.

healed. An inverse relationship between TNF-α and essential growth factors, such as EGF and PDGF, has been demonstrated.

Chronic wounds typically exhibit powerful proinflammatory stimuli, including bacterial colonization, necrotic tissue, foreign bodies, and localized tissue hypoxia. Tissue edema is significant, and the distance between capillaries is increased, reducing oxygen diffusion to individual cells. Chronic wounds typically have high bacterial counts, which stimulates an inflammatory host response, with polymorphonuclear neutrophils (PMNs) expressing reactive oxygen species (ROS) and proteases, resulting in a highly pro-oxidant environment. Disturbed oxidant balance is the likely key factor in the amplification and persistence of the inflammatory state in chronic wounds. In addition to direct cell membrane and ECM protein damage, PMN-derived ROS, such as superoxide,

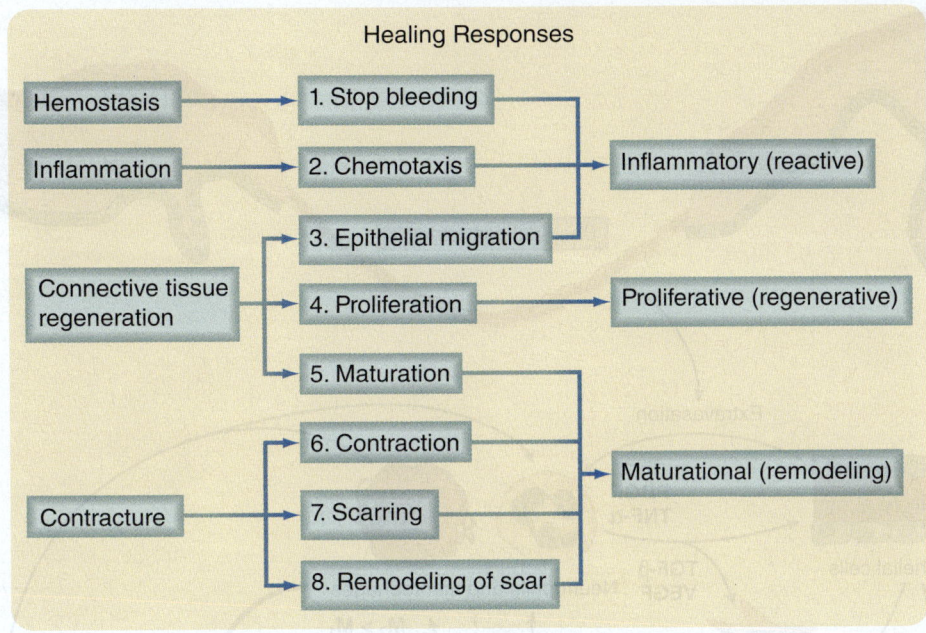

FIGURE 45.6 Schematic diagram of the wound-healing continuum.

hydroxyl radicals, and hydrogen peroxide, can selectively activate signaling pathways, leading to the activation of transcription factors that control the expression of proinflammatory chemokines and cytokines such as IL-1, IL-6, and TNF-α and proteolytic enzymes such as MMPs and serine proteases. Bacterial components, including formyl methionyl peptides and extracellular adherence proteins, may also contribute to the upregulation of the inflammatory response.

The amount of normal wound ECM is determined by a dynamic balance among overall matrix synthesis, deposition, and degradation. A defining feature of chronic wounds is the unbalanced activity that overwhelms tissue-protective mechanisms. Although activated keratinocytes, fibroblasts, and endothelial cells have been shown to increase the expression of proteases, incoming neutrophils and macrophages are considered to be the source of proteases, particularly cathepsin G, urokinase-type plasminogen activator, and neutrophil elastase. The expression and activity of gelatinases (MMP-2, MMP-9), collagenases (MMP-1, MMP-8), stromelysins (MMP-3, MMP-10, MMP-11), and membrane-type MMP (MT1-MMP) are upregulated in chronic venous ulcers.

Proinflammatory cytokines are potent inducers of MMP expression in chronic wounds, also reducing TIMP expression, resulting in a relative excess of MMP activity. For example, α_1-proteinase inhibitor, α_2-macroglobulin, and components of the ECM, such as fibronectin and vibronectin, are downgraded or inactivated within chronic wounds. Growth factors, such as PDGF and VEGF, are also targeted when there is excess protease activity.

Other proposed causes for wound chronicity include keratinocyte hyperproliferation at the periphery, resulting in inhibition of fibroblast and keratinocyte migration and apoptosis. Fibroblasts have altered morphologies, slower rates of proliferation, and less responsiveness to applied growth factors. The ratio of CD4 to CD8 cells is significantly lower in chronic wounds and is likely to be important in the pathogenesis of diabetic ulcers. Finally, chronic wounds have reduced levels of important growth factors

(fibroblast growth factor [FGF], EGF, and TGF-β), likely secondary to degradation by excessive proteases or trapping by ECM molecules.

Chronically inflamed wounds are susceptible to neoplastic transformation. Squamous cell carcinoma (Fig. 45.8) was originally reported in chronic burn scars by Jean Nicholas Marjolin. Nowadays, any chronic wound that develops malignant degeneration can be referred to as a *Marjolin ulcer*. Chronic osteomyelitis, pressure sores, venous stasis ulcers, and hidradenitis may also develop neoplastic change. Biopsies should be performed in cases of chronic wounds that appear clinically atypical. This condition is attributed to a long-standing cyclic poor wound-healing pattern based on inflammation, ulceration, and irritation. Cutaneous wounds may first exhibit pseudoepitheliomatous hyperplasia—a premalignant condition. Such a diagnosis on biopsy should prompt additional biopsies to exclude squamous cell carcinoma, which may already be present in other areas of the wound.

Causes of Abnormal Wound Healing

Hypoxia

Molecular oxygen is essential for collagen formation. Ischemia secondary to cardiac failure, arterial disease, or simple wound tension prevents adequate local tissue perfusion. Under hypoxic conditions, energy derived from glycolysis may be sufficient to initiate collagen synthesis, but the presence of molecular oxygen is critical for posttranslational hydroxylation of the prolyl and lysyl residues required for triple-helix formation and cross-linking of collagen fibrils. Although mild hypoxia stimulates angiogenesis, this essential step in collagen fibril assembly proceeds poorly when the partial pressure of oxygen (PO_2) becomes less than 40 mm Hg. Optimal PO_2 for collagen synthesis may be present at the periphery of the wound, but the center may remain hypoxic. The partial pressure of oxygen in chronic wounds tends to be decreased, ranging from 5 to 20 mm Hg compared with the 35 to 50 mm Hg found in healthy tissue. Most physiologic routes in the repair cycle are oxygen dependent; thus, several steps in the repair process are halted or decreased in hypoxic scenarios.[10]

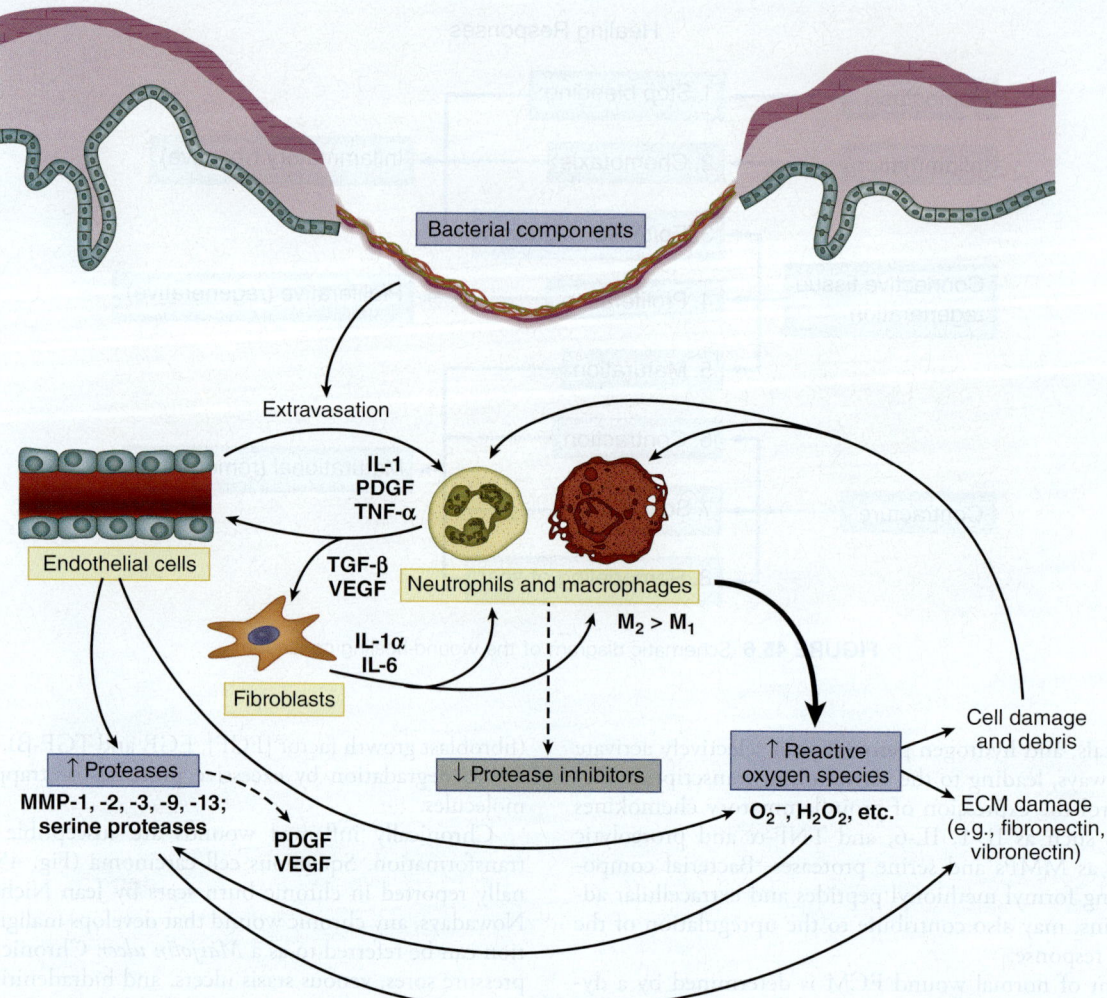

FIGURE 45.7 Mechanisms involved in the development and persistence of chronic wounds. Chronic wounds do not adequately complete the "normal" phases of wound healing. A state of chronic inflammation develops as many of the cells recruited to the wound in the proliferative phase of healing adopt a proinflammatory secretory profile. Inflammatory cells, particularly neutrophils and macrophages (M1 phenotype > M2 phenotype), persist in the wound, creating a highly pro-oxidant, protease-rich environment with an abundance of proinflammatory cytokines such as interleukin-1 *(IL-1)*, interleukin-6 *(IL-6)*, and tumor necrosis factor-α *(TNFα)*. The result is a hostile environment with downregulation of protease inhibitors and direct damage to extracellular matrix *(ECM)*, cellular components, and protective growth factors such as platelet-derived growth factor *(PDGF)* and vascular endothelial growth factor *(VEGF)*. Reactive oxygen species and proteases, such as matrix metalloproteinases *(MMP-1, -2, -3, -9, -13)*, are the most significant deleterious influences. *Solid lines* indicate upregulation, and *dashed lines* indicate downregulation. The width of the line is proportional to the effect of the influence. H_2O_2, Hydrogen peroxide; O_2^-, superoxide; *TGF-β*, transforming growth factor-β. (From Greaves NS, Iqbal SA, Baguneid M, et al. The role of skin substitutes in the management of chronic cutaneous wounds. *Wound Repair Regen.* 2013;21:194-210.)

The role of anemia in wound healing has long been attributed to be predominantly secondary to hypoperfusion. However, studies evaluating colonic anastomoses in a crystalloid-resuscitated hemorrhagic shock model demonstrated that altered histologic parameters decreased white blood cell infiltration, angiogenesis, fibroblast production, and collagen production, all contributing to delayed wound healing.

Tobacco smoking and consumption of tobacco products cause peripheral vasoconstriction and a 30% to 40% reduction in wound blood flow. Elevated levels of serum carbon monoxide inhibit enzyme systems necessary for oxidative cellular metabolism. Nicotine also inhibits platelet prostacyclin, promoting platelet adhesiveness, thrombotic microvascular occlusion, and tissue ischemia. Tobacco use inhibits endothelial cell and fibroblast function, nitric oxide (NO) synthase activity, VEGF production, fibroblast proliferation, collagen synthesis, and vitamin C levels. Studies in animals suggested that nicotine cessation for 14 days before flap surgery resulted in similar outcomes to controls, although most clinicians recommend complete smoking cessation in human patients for 4 to 6 weeks before elective procedures.

Diabetes

Diabetes mellitus impairs wound healing in several ways. Diabetes-associated large-vessel occlusion and end-organ microangiopathy

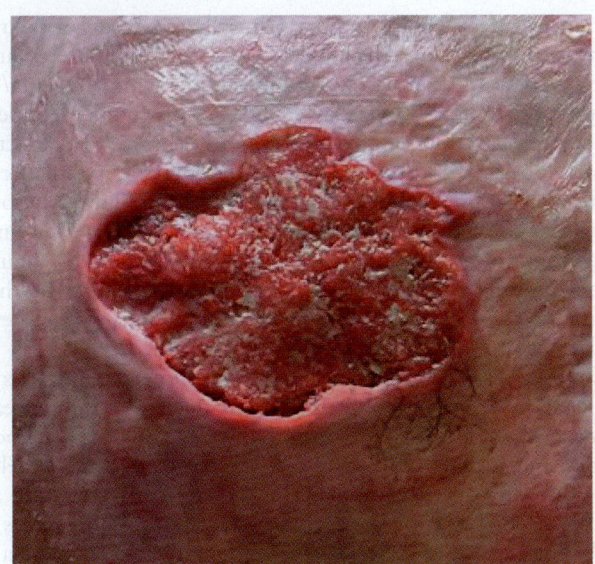

FIGURE 45.8 Squamous cell carcinoma of the back after chronic burn injury.

each lead to tissue ischemia and infection. Diabetic sensory neuropathy leads to repeated trauma and unrelieved wound pressure. Tissue hypoxia can be demonstrated by reduced dorsal foot transcutaneous oxygen tension. The thickened capillary basement membrane decreases perfusion in the microenvironment, and elevated perivascular localization of albumin suggests an increased capillary leak. VEGF upregulation in patients with diabetes is also impaired. Hypoxia is normally a potent regulator of VEGF, but cells from patients with diabetes do not upregulate VEGF expression in response to hypoxia.

Sensory neuropathy in patients with diabetes predisposes them to repeated trauma. They are susceptible to infection because of an attenuated inflammatory response, impaired chemotaxis, and inefficient bacterial killing. Infection further increases local tissue metabolism, placing an additional burden on the tenuous blood supply and amplifying the risk for tissue necrosis. Lymphocyte and leukocyte function are impaired. Collagen degradation is increased, whereas collagen deposition is impaired. Collagen is brittle secondary to glycosylation in the ECM. In addition, collagen glycation diminishes focal adhesion formation between fibroblast and matrix, resulting in decreased fibroblast migration.

Hyperglycemia causes increased advanced glycation end products, which induce the production of inflammatory molecules (TNF-α, IL-1) and interfere with collagen synthesis. High glucose exposure also results in changes in cellular morphology, decreased proliferation, and abnormal differentiation of keratinocytes. Decreased chemotaxis, phagocytosis, bacterial killing, and reduced heat shock protein expression impair the early phase of wound healing in patients with diabetes. Altered leukocyte infiltration and wound fluid IL-6 characterize the late inflammatory phases of wound healing in these patients. Growth factors are abnormally expressed and degraded rapidly in wound fluids as a result of increased insulin-degrading enzyme activity. Insulin-degrading enzyme activity in wound fluid is positively correlated with hemoglobin A1c levels. Elevated MMPs are seen in diabetic wounds in a pattern similar to chronic wounds. Finally, there is increasing evidence that resident cells in chronic wounds undergo phenotypic changes that render them senescent and impair their capacity for proliferation and movement.

Approximately 15% of patients with diabetes will develop DFU disease, which precedes over 80% of diabetes-related lower limb amputations. Recent literature reports decreased levels of IGF-1 and TGF-β in human and animal hyperglycemic models, which resulted in altered granulation and epithelialization.[11] Additionally, an abnormal relationship between VEGF caused by unstable hypoxia-inducible factor-1α (HIF-1α) in diabetic mice models was associated with dysregulated angiogenesis.[11]

Genetic pathways that may play a role in the pathophysiology of diabetic ulcers and chronic nonhealing wounds. Epigenetic alterations, including microRNA-expression patterns, impair normal inflammatory mediators release; modulate macrophage, monocyte, and fibroblast function; and derange inflammatory response in diabetic wounds.

Ionizing Radiation

Ionizing radiation has its greatest effect on rapidly dividing cells in phases G2 through M of the cell cycle. Injury to keratinocytes and fibroblasts impairs epithelialization and formation of granulation tissue during wound healing. Radiation injury in endothelial cells results in endarteritis, atrophy, fibrosis, and delayed tissue repair. Repetitive radiation injury results in repetitive inflammatory responses and ongoing cellular regeneration. Early side effects include erythema, dry desquamation, skin hyperpigmentation, and local hair loss. Late effects include skin atrophy, dryness, telangiectasia, dyschromia, hypopigmentation, fibrosis, and ulceration. The inflammatory and proliferative phases may be disrupted by the early effects of radiation. Affected factors include TGF-β, VEGF, TNF-α, IFN-γ, and cytokines such as IL-1 and IL-8. These cytokines are overexpressed after the radiation injury, leading to uncontrolled matrix accumulation and fibrosis. NO, which induces collagen deposition, is decreased in irradiated wounds; this may explain the impaired wound strength seen in irradiated wounds. Decreased MMP-1 may contribute to inadequate soft tissue reconstitution (Table 45.3).

Keratinocytes, which are crucial for wound epithelialization, demonstrate a shift in expression from the high molecular keratins 1 and 10 to the low molecular keratins 5 and 14 after radiation injury. In nonhealing ulcers, these cells display decreased expression of TGF-α, TGF-β₁ FGF-1, FGF-2, KGF, VEGF, and hepatocyte growth factor (HGF). Expression of MMP-2, MMP-12, and MMP-13 is elevated in irradiated human keratinocytes and fibroblasts. Fibroblasts play a central role in wound healing

TABLE 45.3 Possible Key Wound-Healing Factors Affected by Radiotherapy With Respect to the Phases of Wound Healing

PHASES OF WOUND HEALING	FACTORS AFFECTED BY RADIATION THERAPY
Inflammation	TGF-β, VEGF, IL-1, IL-8, TNF-α, IFN-γ
Proliferation	TGF-β, VEGF, EGF, FGF, PDGF, NO
Remodeling	MMP-1, MMP-2, MMP-12, MMP-13, TIMP

EGF, Epidermal growth factor; *FGF,* fibroblast growth factor; *IFN-γ,* interferon-γ; *IL-1, -8,* interleukin-1, -8; *MMP-1, -2, -12, -13,* matrix metalloproteinase-1, -2, -12, -13; *NO,* nitric oxide; *PDGF,* platelet-derived growth factor; *TGF-β,* transforming growth factor-β; *TIMP,* tissue inhibitors of metalloproteinase; *TNF-α,* tumor necrosis factor-α; *VEGF,* vascular endothelial growth factor.

Adapted from Haubner F, Ohmann E, Pohl F, et al. Wound healing after radiation therapy: review of the literature. *Radiat Oncol.* 2012;7:162.

through the deposition and remodeling of collagen fibers. However, in irradiated tissue, fibroblasts generate disorganized collagen bundles from dysregulation of MMPs and TIMP. Because TGF-β regulates MMPs and TIMP, it may be of particular relevance to radiogenic ulcers (see Table 45.3).

Strategies for treating problematic radiogenic ulcers include physical therapy with massage, antioxidants, topical treatments, standard wound care, negative-pressure wound therapy, and optimized blood and oxygen delivery. Hyperbaric oxygen (HBO) therapy may improve tissue oxygen partial pressure in the treatment of osteoradionecrosis via increased capillary density and more complete neovascularization. HBO therapy is used clinically in patients with chronic diabetic ulcers and wound-healing complications after radiotherapy, and randomized clinical trials have demonstrated efficacy when HBO therapy was used in conjunction with standard wound care in cases of recalcitrant, diabetic, and potentially radiation-induced wounds.[12]

Recently, autologous fat grafting (AFG) has been described as a treatment for radiation wounds. The study demonstrated improved vascularization and decreased fibrosis in tissue biopsies after grafting.[13] Likewise, irradiated animal models had decreased collagen disorders and improved skin perfusion after undergoing fat grafting.[13] Although AFG has mostly been tested in breast, head, and neck cases, it continues to be a widely studied area of radiation-induced skin fibrosis.[13]

Aging

Older patients are more likely to experience delayed healing and surgical wound dehiscence. The aging epidermis has fewer Langerhans cells and melanocytes and flattening of the dermal-epidermal junction. Keratinocyte proliferation is reduced, and the turnover time is increased by 50%. The dermis has fewer fibroblasts, macrophages, and mast cells; reduced vascularity; and less collagen and GAGs. There is a quantitative imbalance between collagen production and degradation and a qualitative alteration of the remaining collagen, which has fewer ropelike bundles and shows greater disorganization. Skin elasticity is decreased because of altered elastin morphology. Diminished light touch and pressure-reduced nociceptive receptors, together with dermal atrophy, increase susceptibility to injury by mechanical forces. Immunosenescence (reduced Langerhans cells and fibroblast activity) impairs wound healing and increases the likelihood of chronic wounds. Microvascular disturbances predispose to ischemic ulcers. Finally, there is reduced sebum secretion and vitamin D_3 production.

Dysregulation of ECM components, including MMPs, decreased reepithelialization, depressed collagen synthesis, impaired angiogenesis, and decreased growth factors (especially proangiogenic FGF-2 and VEGF), have been seen in elderly animal studies. Impaired macrophage activity (reduced phagocytosis and delayed infiltration) and impaired B-lymphocyte activity also have been demonstrated in animal studies. Treatments that target age-deficient mechanisms, such as the reduced expression of superoxide dismutase 1 in situations with high oxidative stress, and the identification of overexpressed micro-RNAs that delay epithelialization and replenishment of hormonal disbalances expected with aging are trending in the literature.[14]

Malnutrition

Protein catabolism delays wound healing and promotes wound dehiscence, particularly when serum albumin levels are less than 2.0 g/dL. Protein supplements can reverse this deficiency. Vitamin

deficiencies affect wound healing primarily as a result of their effect as cofactors. Delayed healing can occur 3 months after vitamin C deprivation and can be reversed by supplements of 10 mg/day and no more than 2000 mg/day. Deficiency of vitamin A impedes monocyte activation and deposition of fibronectin, affecting cellular adhesion, and impairs TGF-β receptors. Vitamin A contributes to lysosomal membrane destabilization and directly counteracts the effect of glucocorticoids. Vitamin K deficiency limits the synthesis of prothrombin and factors VII, IX, and X. Vitamin K metabolism is impeded by antibiotics; patients who have chronic or recurrent infections need to have clotting parameters checked before surgical procedures are performed.

Zinc is a necessary cofactor for RNA polymerase and deoxyribonucleic acid (DNA) polymerase. Zinc deficiency impairs early wound healing, but it is rare except with large burns, severe polytrauma, and hepatic cirrhosis. Iron deficiency anemia is a debatable cause of delayed wound healing. Although ferrous ion is a cofactor needed to convert proline to hydroxyproline, reports are conflicting regarding the effects of acute and chronic anemia on wound healing. Mehl and colleagues evaluated the use of an oral nutritional supplement containing arginine; proline; vitamins A, C, and E; zinc; and selenium in chronic wounds.[15] In the study, a significant reduction in the surface area of the wound was described.[15] In general, patients should have a well-rounded diet consisting of adequate protein intake and caloric value plus vitamin and mineral supplementation.

Regarding the route of nutritional supplements, a recent meta-analysis determined that the systemic route for supplementation was more effective than the topical. Nutritional supplementation was favorable as an adjunct to medical treatment, according to Ye and colleagues.[16]

Drugs

Some exogenously administered drugs directly impair wound healing. Chemotherapeutic agents, such as doxorubicin (Adriamycin), nitrogen mustard, cyclophosphamide, methotrexate, and bischloroethylnitrosourea, are potent wound inhibitors in animal models and interfere with uncomplicated wound healing clinically. They reduce mesenchymal cell proliferation, platelet and inflammatory cell counts, and availability of growth factors, particularly if given preoperatively. Tamoxifen, an antiestrogen, decreases cellular proliferation, with a decrease in wound-breaking strength that is dose dependent and may be secondary to decreased TGF-β production. Glucocorticosteroids impair fibroblast proliferation and collagen synthesis, resulting in decreased granulation tissue formation. Recently, Polcz and colleagues described the reversal of the inhibitory effects of antiinflammatory steroids by using vitamin A.[17] This component was found to promote cell turnover, promote ECM components, and enhance the role of fibroblasts.[17] Diminished wound-breaking strength caused by exogenous steroids is time and dose related. High doses of nonsteroidal antiinflammatory drugs have been reported to delay healing, but doses in the therapeutic range are unlikely to have an effect.

Microbiology of Chronic Wounds

Although microorganisms are ubiquitous, human epithelia generally prevent infections in healthy individuals, aside from injuries that disrupt the protective barrier provided by skin. However, chronic wounds tend to occur in those with impaired wound-healing mechanisms. Briefly, mechanisms that cause impaired wound healing involve dysfunction in regeneration and immunologic or physiologic responses. Thus, the burden of persisting health conditions such as type 2 diabetes and obesity as well as the aging process, provide an opportunity for infectious processes to occur. The International Wound Infection Institute functionally defined a wound infection as the invasion and proliferation of microorganisms in a wound to a degree invoking a local and/or systemic response in the host.[18] However, there is not an exact understanding as to why some wounds develop acutely, whereas others develop chronically.

At the local level, microorganisms cause tissue damage and further impede the wound-healing process. In chronically nonhealing wounds that are typically hindered by hypoxia, microbial metabolism further depletes local PO_2. Yet distinctions need to be made among microbial organisms because different phenotypes exhibit unique effects and warrant tailored treatment. When considering bacteria, they largely exist within one of two domains, either planktonic bacteria or biofilms. Planktonic bacteria are those that many tend to envision when considering bacteria—freely meandering organisms existing unicellularly as viewed under a microscope. However, bacteria exist predominantly as colonies that form biofilms. A "biofilm" is a heterogeneous collection of distinct microorganism populations existing within a matrix composed largely of exopolysaccharides. These exopolysaccharides grant adherent properties to surfaces. Biofilm formation was previously thought to follow a characteristic three-step process consisting of attachment, maturation of cell populations, and release of bacteria. More recently, researchers have described an expanded five-step process when investigating the biofilm formation of *Pseudomonas aeruginosa*.[19] They describe the cyclic, progressive formation beginning with either a reversible attachment of planktonic bacteria or an irreversible attachment that would lead to two phases of maturation. These maturation phases correspond to the formation of cell clusters (phase 1) and microcolonies (phase 2). After maturation, the complex is poised for the dispersion of cells from the surrounding matrix. Although dispersion appears to lead to the degradation of the matrix, dispersion results in the dissemination and colonization of bacteria to other locations.

Bacteria that colonize the skin largely derive from Acinetobacteria, Bacteroidetes, Firmicutes, and Proteobacteria. Interestingly, different locations on the body harbor different bacteria. For instance, anaerobic bacteria show preferential colonization in intertriginous areas such as the groin, axillae, and between digits. In chronic wound infections, bacterial colonization is typically polymicrobial. The pathogens encountered in chronic wounds are heavily influenced by an individual's clinical condition and the nature of the wound. Common pathogens found in chronic wounds include *Staphylococcus aureus,* coagulase-negative staphylococci, *Streptococcus* species, *P. aeruginosa,* and *Enterococcus faecalis,* among others.

Treatment of Chronic Wounds

The management of a chronic wound depends on its etiology. Most of the currently available therapies are slow, labor intensive, and expensive, without any guarantee of healing if all local and systemic factors are not addressed. This is especially worrisome considering the financial burden placed on both individuals and providers. To put matters into perspective, the global chronic wound care market was valued at around $13 billion in 2022, with expectations of a $21-billion increase by 2030.[20] These expected increases largely correlate with the increasing prevalence of chronic diseases such as type 2 diabetes and increased rates of obesity. As such, wound-healing research revealed key structural proteins and molecules in both normal and disordered wound healing as potential targets for future interventions. This research

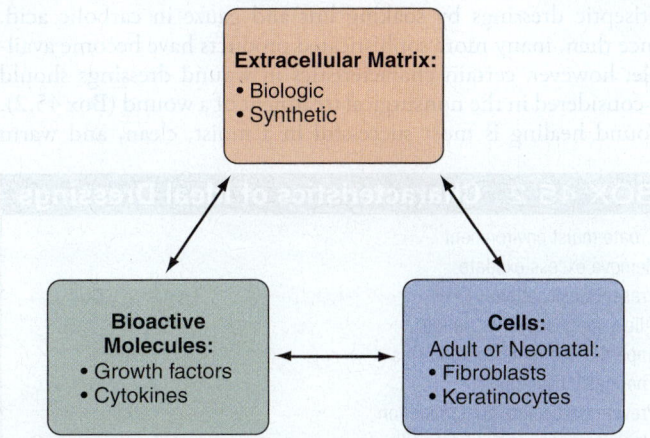

FIGURE 45.9 The "dynamic reciprocity" model of wound healing. Interactions are dynamic because they vary with time and location within the wound site. Products of any one element influence the actions of the others. Inappropriate downregulation of any one element can result in conversion from an acute to a chronic wound. (From Greaves NS, Iqbal SA, Baguneid M, et al. The role of skin substitutes in the management of chronic cutaneous wounds. *Wound Repair Regen.* 2013;21:194-210.)

led to the application of topical growth factors to chronic wounds, which, although initially promising, almost universally failed in producing clinically significant wound-healing improvements. The reason for the failure is presumed to be a result of degradation of the growth factors by proteases in the wound fluid, and other treatment options need to be explored. Importantly, this failure highlighted the complexity of wound healing—simply replacing one element is not enough. Many factors need to be synchronized to confer optimal wound-healing benefits.

Skin substitutes, which will be discussed later in the chapter, provide multiple factors that tend to alter the microenvironment of the wound to facilitate and accelerate wound healing. Comparably, split-thickness skin grafting describes the surgical substitution of cutaneous tissue, native epidermis, and partial dermis to assist wound closure. Split-thickness skin grafting has exhibited strong efficacy as a treatment option for acute burn wounds and chronic nonhealing wounds. During the procedure, skin is harvested from the patient and transferred to an adequately prepared wound bed. The graft provides wound coverage by providing a favorable healing environment through the exclusion of pathogenic bacteria and provision of ECM, wound-healing cells (such as keratinocytes and fibroblasts), and bioactive molecules (including cytokines, chemokines, and growth factors) that facilitate wound repair through a process of "dynamic reciprocity" (Fig. 45.9). However, autologous skin grafts occasionally are limited or unavailable depending on the circumstances and clinical setting. Thus, biologic skin substitutes have been used for many years and include, but are not limited to, cadaveric skin allografts and porcine and bovine xenografts; however, these grafts lack significant durability because they do not integrate into the host. As a result, these grafts are associated with rejection and occasionally disease transfer. Be that as it may, they provide an adequate temporary wound cover, limiting complications until autologous grafts or other definitive management strategies are available.

Wound Dressings

Wound dressings have been present since antiquity. They evolved very little for many years until 1867, when Lister introduced antiseptic dressings by soaking lint and gauze in carbolic acid. Since then, many more sophisticated products have become available; however, certain characteristics in wound dressings should be considered in the nonsurgical treatment of a wound (Box 45.2). Wound healing is most successful in a moist, clean, and warm environment. However, not many dressings can provide all of these characteristics simultaneously, although not all wounds require all of them; hence, the choice of dressing should match the prevailing wound conditions.

Two concepts that are critical when selecting appropriate dressings for wounds are occlusion and absorption. Studies have demonstrated that the rate of epithelialization under a moist occlusive dressing is twice that of a wound that is left uncovered and allowed to dry. An occlusive dressing provides a mildly acidic pH and low oxygen tension on the wound surface, which is conducive to fibroblast proliferation and the formation of granulation tissue. However, wounds that produce significant amounts of exudate or have high bacterial counts require a dressing that is absorptive and prevents maceration of the surrounding skin. These dressings also need to reduce the bacterial load while absorbing the exudate produced. Placement of a pure occlusive dressing without bactericidal properties would allow bacterial overgrowth and worsen the infection.

Dressings can be categorized into four classes: (1) nonadherent fabrics; (2) occlusive dressings; (3) absorptive dressings; and (4) creams, ointments, and solutions (Table 45.4). Briefly, nonadherent fabrics are fine-mesh gauze supplemented with a

---

BOX 45.2 Characteristics of Ideal Dressings

Create moist environment
Remove excess exudate
Present desiccation
Allow for gaseous exchange
Impermeable to microorganisms
Thermally insulating
Prevent particulate contamination
Nontoxic to beneficial host cells
Provide mechanical protection
Nontraumatic
Easy to use
Cost-effective

Adapted from Morin RJ, Tomaselli NL. Interactive dressings and topical agents. *Clin Plast Surg.* 2007;34:643-658.

TABLE 45.4 Types of Dressings

CATEGORY	COMPOSITION AND CHARACTERISTICS	FUNCTION	EXAMPLES	COMMENTS
Nonadherent fabrics	Fine-mesh gauze with supplement to augment occlusive and nonadherent properties, healing-facilitating capabilities, and antibacterial characteristics	Protection, moist environment	Adaptic, Mepitel, Scarlet Red, Telfa, Vaseline gauze, Xeroform, Xeroflo	Scarlet Red, Xeroform, Telfa, Vaseline gauze: hydrophobic, more occlusive; Xeroflo, Mepitel, Adaptic: less occlusive, subject to drainage of fluid into overlying dressing layers
Absorptive				
Gauze	Wide mesh gauze	Exudate removal, maceration prevention	Wide mesh gauze	Not effective when saturated; can be used for wound debridement if in contact with wound
Foams	Hydrophobic polyurethane sheets	Protection, absorb exudate	Allevyn, Curafoam, Flexzan, Lyofoam, Vigifoam	Advantages—comfortable, can expand and conform to wound, easily removed for cleansing. Disadvantages—need to be replaced as wounds heal, custom shapes are labor intensive to make, limited protection from bacteria, cannot be used while bathing
Occlusive				
Nonbiologic		Insulation, moisture retention, protective barrier acts against bacteria		
Films	Clear polyurethane membranes with acrylic adhesive on one side	As above	Bioocclusive, Hydrofilm, Mefilm, Opsite, Tegaderm, Transeal	Waterproof; permeable to oxygen, carbon dioxide, and water vapor; do not interfere with patient function; allow visualization of wound; nonabsorptive, can leak; require intact skin around wound area; wound contraction may be slowed; removal may disrupt new epithelium
Hydrocolloids	Hydrocolloid matrix (gelatin, pectin, carboxymethylcellulose)	As above; absorbs water from wound exudates, swells, liquefies to form moist gel; facilitates angiogenesis and granulation	Comfeel, Duoderm, Hydrocoll, Nu-Derm, Replicare, Tegasorb	Available as adhesive wafers, paste, powders; similar features as films, but bulkier; more protection, but may interfere more with function

TABLE 45.4 Types of Dressings—cont'd

CATEGORY	COMPOSITION AND CHARACTERISTICS	FUNCTION	EXAMPLES	COMMENTS
Alginates	Cellulose-like polysaccharide fibers derived from calcium salt of alginate (seaweed)	As above; highly absorbent, contact with wound exudates results in hydrophilic gel	Algisite, Algoderm, Kaltostat, Curasorb, Melgisorb, SeaSorb, Alginate, Sorbsan, Suprasorb	Occlusive environment, yet easily removed; hemostatic and flexible; exists in various forms (ropes, ribbons, pads)
Hydrogels	Polyethylene oxide or carboxymethylcellulose polymer and water (80%)	As above; rehydrating agents for dry wounds; little water absorption; facilitate autolytic debridement; smart hydrogels have robust functions	Curagel, FlexiGel, Flexderm, Purilon, Intrasite, Hydrosorb, Hydrotac, Tegagel	Occlusive environment; provides a soothing, cooling effect; available as gels, sheets, impregnated gauze
Biologic		Similar to nonbiologics		
Homograft	Derived from genetically unique humans		Cadaver skin	Temporary dressing; is rejected if left on wound for extended period
Xenograft	Interspecies graft (e.g., pig)		Pigskin	Same as above
Amnion	Human placenta			Good biologic dressing
Skin substitutes	Different compositions		Integra, AlloDerm, Apligraf, Biobrane, TransCyte	Integra—bilayered membrane skin substitute; AlloDerm—acellular cadaveric dermis; Apligraf—living, bilayered, biologic dressing composed of neonatal dermal fibroblasts on collagen matrix

Creams, Ointments, and Solutions

CATEGORY	COMPOSITION AND CHARACTERISTICS	FUNCTION	EXAMPLES	COMMENTS
Antibacterial	Different compositions	Used to treat infected wounds	Acetic acid (gram-negative *Pseudomonas*); Dakin's solution (broad antibacterial spectrum); iodine-containing antibacterials (Iodosorb, Iodoflex, Betadine; broad antibacterial and antifungal spectrum); silver nitrate (broad antibacterial spectrum); mafenide acetate (Sulfamylon; broad antibacterial spectrum); silver sulfadiazine (Silvadene; broad antibacterial, antifungal, and antiviral spectrum); Acticoat (broad antibacterial spectrum)	Acetic acid—impairs wound healing; Dakin's—toxic to fibroblasts; iodine-containing solutions—toxic to fibroblasts, impair wound healing; silver nitrate—treats burns, slows epithelialization, hyponatremia, stains clothes black; mafenide acetate—penetrates eschar, painful application, inhibits reepithelialization, carbonic anhydrase inhibitor; silver sulfadiazine—transient neutropenia, accelerates epithelialization of partial-thickness burns, neovascularization, commonly used for burns; Acticoat—silver-impregnated occlusive dressing, antibacterial activity lasts 3 days
Antibacterial ointments	Different compositions	Used to treat infected wounds; soothing to apply; lubricates wound surface; occlusive; antibacterial activity lasts 12 hours	Bacitracin (gram-positive cocci and bacilli); neomycin (gram-negative) polymyxin B sulfate (gram-negative); Polysporin (polymyxin B, bacitracin); Neosporin (polymyxin B, bacitracin, neomycin); triple-antibiotic ointment (polymyxin B, bacitracin, neomycin)	Neosporin—increased reepithelialization in experimental wounds by 25% compared with wounds with no dressing
Enzymatic	Different compositions; uses naturally occurring enzymes	Removal of necrotic tissue	Sutilains (derived from *Bacillus subtilis*); collagenase (Santyl; derived from *Clostridium histolyticum*); papain (derived from vegetable pepsin)	Sutilains—digests denatured collagen; collagenase—digests denatured and native collagen; papain—effective against collagen in presence of cofactor containing sulfhydryl group; addition of urea doubles enzymatic action of papain
Other	Normal saline wet-to-dry gauze dressing	Removal of necrotic tissue		Nondiscriminating necrotic and newly formed granulation tissue and epithelium removed; can be painful

Updated from Townsend CM, Beauchamp RD, Evers BM, Mattox KL, Sabiston DC. Chapter 6: Wound healing. In: Townsend CM, ed. *Sabiston Textbook of Surgery: The Biological Basis of Modern Surgical Practice*. Elsevier; 2022.

TABLE 45.5   Hydrogels

HYDROGEL APPLICATIONS	COMMON MATERIAL	FUNCTIONS
Antibiotic delivery	Polyethylene glycol	Prevent infections
Stem cell delivery	Adipose ECM, collagen derivatives, gelatin variations, etc.	Reepithelialization, neovascularization, accelerated wound closure, etc.
Bioactive agent delivery	PEG and heparin, gelatin, alginates, etc.	Accelerated wound closure, advanced granulation formation, vascularization, etc.
Skin substitution	Collagen, gelatin variations	Accelerated wound healing, angiogenesis, tissue regeneration, etc.
Stimuli responsive	Variable	Responsivity to pH, ROS, enzymes, glucose, temperature, photo or magnetic stimulation

ECM, Extracellular matrix; *PEG*, polyethylene glycol; *ROS*, reactive oxygen species.

substance to augment their occlusive properties or antibacterial abilities, such as Scarlet Red, a relatively nonocclusive dressing that is impregnated with O-tolylazo-O-tolylazo-β-naphthol that is used on skin graft harvest sites in burn care. Xeroform is a relatively occlusive, hydrophobic dressing containing 3% bismuth tribromophenate in a petrolatum base, which helps mask wound odors and has antimicrobial activity against *S. aureus* and *Escherichia coli.*

Occlusive dressings provide moisture retention, mechanical protection, and a barrier to bacteria. These dressings can be divided into biologic and nonbiologic dressings. Examples of biologic dressings are allograft, xenograft, amnion, and skin substitutes. An allograft is a graft transplanted between genetically unique humans, whereas a xenograft is a graft, such as pig skin, transplanted between species. Allografts and xenografts are temporary dressings; both will be rejected if left on a wound for an extended period. Amnion is derived from the human placenta and is another effective biologic wound dressing. Initially, these dressings were most often used in the treatment of burn wounds; however, their use has been extrapolated to all other wound etiologies.

Absorptive dressings are useful for wounds with a significant amount of exudate. Leg ulcers can produce 12 g/10 cm²/24 hours of exudate. The origination of standardized absorptive dressings came with the creation of wide mesh gauze, which, although functional and economical, loses its effectiveness when saturated. Shortly thereafter, foam dressings emerged with absorbent qualities permitting removal of large quantities of exudate while also maintaining a nonadherent quality to prevent disruption of newly formed granulation tissue upon removal. Examples include Lyofoam (ConvaTec, Skillman, NJ), Allevyn (Smith & Nephew, Largo, FL), and Curafoam (Kendall Company, Mansfield, MA). Although beneficial, wound healing beneath absorptive dressings appears to be slower than under occlusive dressings, possibly because of wicking of cytokines from the wound bed or decreased keratinocyte migration.

Hydrogels, insoluble and hydrophilic, are synthetic polymers composed of 70% to 90% water. Their properties maintain moisture and promote increased wound healing. Recent advances in stimuli-responsive hydrogels allow for the release of retained products within the hydrogel in response to particular stimuli in the wound-healing environment. Because of their biochemical and mechanical properties, hydrogels confer better efficacy in the delivery of certain ingredients compared with other creams and topical remedies.[21] With recent developments, hydrogels have been adapted to respond to physical and chemical stimuli such as temperature, pH, ROS, glucose, trand light. These advances not only promote wound care in dry chronic wounds, burns, pressure

ulcers, and necrotic wounds but also have implications in chronic diabetic wounds as well. The most significant drawback of hydrogels lies in exudate accumulation, which can damage structural integrity and ultimately lead to microbial contamination (Table 45.5).

The final class of wound dressings consists of creams, ointments, and solutions. This is a broad category that extends from traditional materials, such as zinc oxide paste, to preparations containing growth factors. Various categories include dressings with antibacterial properties, such as acetic acid, Dakin solution, silver nitrate, mafenide (Sulfamylon), silver sulfadiazine (Silvadene), iodine-containing ointments (Iodosorb), and bacitracin. Application of these products is indicated when clinical signs of infection are present or if quantitative culture demonstrates more than 10^5 organisms per gram of tissue. The number of available wound products is constantly growing; thus, surgeons must have information about available dressings to aid wound management techniques.

Hyperbaric Oxygen Therapy

HBO therapy uses oxygen as a drug and the hyperbaric chamber as a delivery system to increase PO_2 at the target area. Clinicians use HBO therapy in a myriad of disease processes, including but not limited to severe anemia, carbon monoxide and cyanide poisoning, air and gas embolism, decompression sickness, improvement of skin graft integrity, improvement of flap survival and salvage, crush injuries, traumatic brain injuries, acute thermal burns, necrotizing fasciitis, refractory osteomyelitis, osteoradionecrosis, chronic wounds, hypoxic wounds, and radiation injuries. Recent advances show further evidence for the treatment of cancer, COVID-19, and chronic diabetic ulcers as well.[22] Regardless of the circumstances being addressed, HBO therapy acts as a modulator of tissue injury and promotes tissue regeneration through the upregulation of certain processes related to cellular repair mechanisms while downregulating processes related to tissue damage. HBO therapy acts as a stabilizing force that restores physiologic balance.

When administering HBO therapy, evaluation of the vascular supply to the target is essential. Thus, revascularization before therapy is an important prerequisite to HBO therapy. Generally, the patients most likely to benefit from adjuvant HBO therapy are those who can demonstrate improvement in tissue in the setting of a hypoxic wound while breathing oxygen under the set hyperbaric conditions. The parameters measured to monitor the effects of HBO therapy mainly include transcutaneous oxygen pressure ($TcPO_2$), which assesses wound perfusion and oxygenation. Accordingly, a wound $TcPO_2$ of less than 35 mm Hg in room air indicates a hypoxic wound, whereas an in-chamber

$TcPO_2$ of 200 mm Hg or more suggests a potential benefit from HBO therapy. HBO treatments for hypoxic wounds are usually delivered at 1.9 to 3.0 atmospheric pressure (atm) for sessions of 90 to 120 minutes each, with the patient breathing 100% oxygen during the treatment. Treatments are given once daily, five to six times per week, and should be given as an adjunct to surgical or medical therapies. Clinical evidence of wound improvement should be noted after 15 to 20 treatments.

The importance of oxygen in the wound-healing process has long been a topic of discussion because wound ischemia is the most common cause of wound-healing failure. Ischemia or tissue hypoxia (PO_2 <30 mm Hg) significantly impairs normal metabolic activity and decreases wound healing by impairing fibroblast proliferation, collagen synthesis, and epithelialization. HBO therapy involves inhalation of 100% oxygen at 1.9 to 2.5 atm, which can increase tissue PO_2 10 times higher than usual and reduce complications related to ischemia or tissue hypoxia. Sustaining a high PaO_2 is sufficient to supply the tissue with all its metabolic requirements, even in the absence of hemoglobin. This degree of hyperoxygenation triggers functional and structural changes at the molecular level, yielding the therapeutic action of HBO therapy. The elevated oxygen concentrations after HBO therapy last for 2 to 4 hours after termination of the session, inducing the synthesis of endothelial cell NO synthase and other factors, stimulating angiogenesis, and encouraging granulation tissue formation as well as other beneficial cellular processes. HBO therapy also provides a bactericidal effect, with evidence of the effect shown in a study by Oley and associates that demonstrated significantly decreased bacterial growth after burn injuries.[23] From a physiologic standpoint, oxygen has been reported to stimulate angiogenesis, enhance fibroblast and leukocyte function, and normalize cutaneous microvascular reflexes.

Investigations into HBO therapy described a potential role in treating diabetic wounds. Previous experiments showed increased proliferation of stem cells, upregulated angiogenesis, and improved wound-healing capacity. This is evident in animal studies that analyzed the effects of HBO therapy on rodent cell metabolism, angiogenesis, and wound healing in diabetic wounds. Likewise, one of these investigations demonstrated a potential synergistic effect for HBO therapy when combined with stem cell therapy, paving the way for new horizons in treatment of nonhealing wounds.[24] In addition to improvement in cell metabolism, HBO therapy decreases ROSs and proinflammatory cytokines and promotes matrix synthesis during wound repair. These findings have prompted multiple clinical trials investigating HBO therapy as adjuvant therapy for the treatment of chronic DFUs and prevention of extremity amputation. Older small-scale randomized clinical trials have demonstrated that HBO is a useful adjunctive therapy for diabetic ischemic foot ulcers and reduces the rate of extremity amputation. These findings are supported by a recent systematic review and meta-analysis that investigated 20 randomized controlled trials and 1263 trials regarding the efficacy of HBO therapy on DFUs. This study noted a significantly increased healing rate, decreased healing time, and decreased incidence of major amputation when compared with conventional therapy, although no difference was seen with the incidence of minor amputation.[22] Pasek and colleagues noted similar findings regarding accelerated ulcer healing and also reported decreased intensity of perceived pain with HBO therapy.[25] When compared with other treatments that increase microperfusion in chronic DFUs such as low-intensity laser irradiation (LILI), HBO therapy was found to achieve greater rates of improvement in chronic

DFU healing.[26] HBO therapy in conjunction with standard treatment confers greater wound-healing benefits than those seen with standard therapy alone. The efficacy of HBO therapy as an adjuvant for chronic DFUs cannot be ignored, and a similar rationale has led to investigations into its potential in other ulcer types.

HBO therapy has also demonstrated beneficial effects in treating chronic venous ulcers, peripheral arterial disease, and other refractory ulcers. Lalieu and colleagues stated that HBO therapy assisted patients with nonhealing venous leg ulcers in achieving marked or complete wound healing with improvement in perceived pain and overall health scores.[27] Similarly, a systematic review and meta-analysis revealed that HBO therapy combined with surgical management reduced venous ulcer healing time and surface area as well as lowered perceived pain scores. In addition to the efficacy shown in treating chronic venous leg ulcers, HBO therapy has also displayed improved wound healing in ulcers of rare etiologies. A study investigating multiple case series and case reports involving nonhealing ulcers from vasculitis, livedoid vasculopathy, calcific uremic arteriolopathy, and pyoderma gangrenosum suggested that HBO therapy improved healing rates and pain in these cases; furthermore, the study authors recommend that HBO therapy be used in refractory wounds that are unresponsive to standard therapy.[28]

Complications of HBO therapy are caused by the changes in pressure and oxygen. More specifically, adverse effects from elevated atm and PO_2. Adverse effects from increased pressure most commonly manifest as middle ear barotrauma, ranging from tympanic membrane hyperemia to eardrum perforation. Theoretically, however, increased pressure may cause barotrauma within any enclosed, fluid-filled cavities. Adverse effects related to oxygen typically involve pulmonary, neurologic, and ophthalmologic sequelae. Pneumothorax (particularly tension pneumothorax) is far less common than barotrauma but is a potentially life-threatening condition. Other complications associated with increased PO_2 include oxygen toxicity in brain tissue, which manifests as convulsions resembling grand mal seizures. Oxygen toxicity in the lung results from damage from oxygen free radicals to lung parenchyma and airways, which can cause sequelae ranging from tracheobronchitis to full-blown respiratory distress syndrome. Within the eye, oxygen toxicity may cause transient myopia, hyperopia, and other conditions. A recent study shows that the adverse effects associated with HBO therapy tend to present themselves with chamber pressure above 2.0 atm absolute for at least 10 sessions.[29] As such, clinicians and therapists should be keenly alert for the development of adverse effects with repeated HBO therapy sessions. Zhang et al. also revealed a higher incidence of adverse effects for patients with DFUs receiving HBO therapy, documenting the importance of glucose monitoring to prevent hypoglycemic episodes. Absolute contraindications to HBO therapy are (1) uncontrolled pneumothorax, (2) current or recent treatment with bleomycin or doxorubicin (potential aggravation of cardiac and pulmonary toxicity), and (3) treatment with disulfiram (increases risk of developing oxygen toxicity).[29] Relative contraindications include lung pathologies such as obstructive lung disease, anatomic abnormalities such as blebs or bullae, and other occurrences such as recent thoracic surgery and airway or sinus infection, among others.

There have also been developments for HBO therapy in chronic irradiated wounds. Theoretically speaking, HBO therapy would act to enhance radiation therapy in hypoxic tumors, which are typically more resistant to standard radiation therapy. A systematic review of the Cochrane Database concluded that HBO therapy improved outcomes in patients who had undergone radiation in the head, neck, anus, and rectum area while also reducing rates of osteoradionecrosis after teeth extractions.[16] However, the recommendations were based on small, underpowered studies, and further randomized studies are greatly needed to clarify the benefits of this therapy. These results, which concluded that HBO therapy may have promising results in chronic radiation-induced wounds, are consistent with subsequent systematic reviews by Fernandez and colleagues.[12]

Currently, the use of HBO therapy is covered for reimbursement by the Centers for Medicare and Medicaid Services under specific circumstances. Acute conditions regarding wound care include gas gangrene, acute peripheral ischemia, crush injuries, necrotizing infections, and soft tissue radionecrosis. Chronic diagnoses that are reimbursed are preservation of skin grafts, diabetic lower extremity wounds that have failed standard care, and chronic osteomyelitis unresponsive to medical management. Similarly, the most recent European Consensus Conference on Hyperbaric Medicine reviewed the available evidence on the effects of HBO therapy and concluded that it is indicated in open fractures with crush injury, prevention or treatment of osteoradionecrosis of the mandible, soft tissue radionecrosis (e.g., cystitis, proctitis), DFUs, and femoral head necrosis. Despite evidence suggesting the potential benefit of HBO therapy in healing chronic wounds, its cost is high. Patients often travel long distances for daily treatments at great cost to themselves and their families. Although reported protocols for the treatment of ischemic limb ulcers vary significantly, most involve a total cost of $15,000 to $40,000, thus the importance of Medicare and Medicaid reimbursement services. HBO therapy is not recommended as a primary treatment for patients with uncomplicated diabetic or ischemic ulcers. However, in certain complicated cases, HBO therapy may have a role.

Negative-Pressure–Assisted Wound Therapy

One of the most significant innovations in wound management in recent decades was the improvement in negative-pressure–assisted wound therapies (NPWTs) (Fig. 45.10). The application of uniform negative pressure on wounds, along with a capacity to remove extracellular fluid, promotes accelerated healing. Thus, this technique may be used on acute, subacute, and chronic wounds. By applying subatmospheric pressure to wounds, wound vacuums (wound vacs) remove edema, increase local blood flow, and stimulate formation of granulation tissue. Studies demonstrated significant improvement in wound depth in chronic wounds treated with NPWT compared with wounds treated with saline wet-to-moist dressings.[30] In addition, treatment with negative pressure results in faster healing times with fewer associated complications. With this technology, the surgeon is not only capable of immediate wound closure but can also integrate NPWT before and after surgery or even as an alternative to surgery in extremely ill patients.

The exact mechanism of the improvement in healing with NPWT has continued to be a topic of discussion. Many investigators initially believed that the reason for accelerated wound healing chiefly involved the removal of wound exudates while maintaining moisture within the wound. As originally hypothesized by negative-pressure inception studies from the 1970s, there is a fivefold increase in blood flow to cutaneous tissues with NPWT. Afterward, studies showed an increase in capillary caliber and stimulated endothelial proliferation and angiogenesis. Normandin et al. described the most important mechanisms of NPWT: drainage of inflammatory extracellular fluid, stabilization of wound environment, macrodeformation, and microdeformation.[31] In addition to the removal of exudate for better wound perfusion, the resultant fluid flow applies shear forces and establishes an ion gradient that ultimately leads to a cellular proliferative response. *Macrodeformation* refers to the forced three-dimensional (3D) reduction of wound surface area, whereas *microdeformation* refers to the mechanical forces at the cytoskeletal level that initiate an intracellular cascade leading to gene transcription. The resulting cellular adaptations include cellular proliferation, angiogenesis, and the formation of granulation tissue, as described earlier.

Clinical benefits of NPWT have been demonstrated in randomized controlled trials and include a decrease in wound volume or size, accelerated wound bed preparation and granulation tissue formation, accelerated wound healing, improved rate of graft take, decreased drainage time for acute wounds, reduction of complications, enhancement of response to first-line treatment, increased patient survival, and decreased cost. More recent data have demonstrated improved outcomes in patients with diabetic wounds; ischemic ulcers; and complex vascular, abdominal, gynecologic, and other oncologic surgical wounds with or without contamination.

NPWT has also been directly applied to closed incisions after surgical procedures to prophylactically mitigate surgical site infections (SSIs) and wound dehiscence. Gabriel et al. further investigated this modified NPWT, dubbed *closed-incision negative-pressure therapy* (ciNTP), in preventing postoperative complications related to surgical wounds.[32] They found that NPWT significantly reduces the incidence of SSIs, although they did not find a significant difference in the incidences of dehiscence and hematoma formation. Similar findings have been seen in other recent studies, with evidence finding NPWT superior to debridement or traditional treatment.[33,34] As such, normalization of NPWT could play a vital role in reducing SSIs, which cost billions of dollars annually and lead to further complications and higher mortality rates.

In difficult-to-treat wounds, such as nonhealing diabetic ulcers, NPWT is becoming more widely used as well. Results demonstrated that NPWT led to significant downregulation of IL-1β, TNF-α, MMP-1, and MMP-9 and significant upregulation of

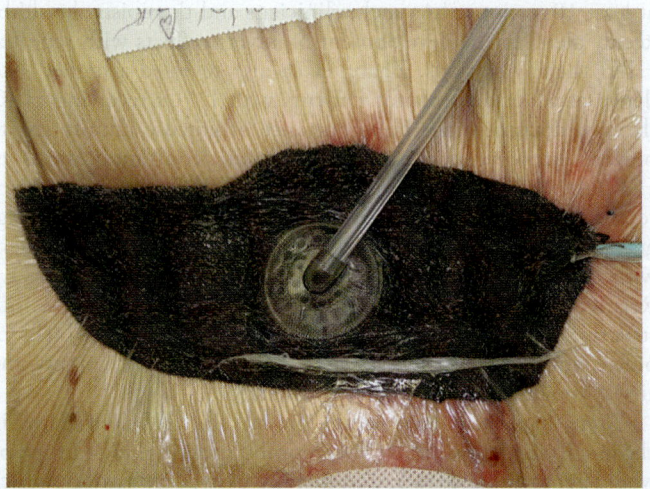

FIGURE 45.10 Negative-pressure–assisted wound closure sponge in place on a patient's abdomen.

VEGF, TGF-β₁, and TIMP-1 compared with advanced wound care with dressing changes. NPWT significantly increases growth factors, decreases inflammatory cytokines, and normalizes MMP activity, enhancing wound healing. Recent randomized control trials with DFUs displayed the proposed improvement in wound healing with NPWT, showing accelerated reduction of ulcer size with increased granulation tissue; moreover, the studies noted higher rates of complete wound healing, fewer rates of complications, and shorter hospital stays.[33,34] Chen et al. performed a systematic review and meta-analysis supporting said findings on the efficacy of NPWT in treating DFUs, stating that NPTW is equally safe as routine treatment.[35] In addition to treating DFUs, NPWT has shown promise in treating other difficult nonhealing ulcers. A meta-analysis from Song and colleagues using NPWT for stage III/IV pressure injuries noted improved rates of wound healing, shorter healing times, lowered pain scores, and hospital costs.[36]

In addition to the improved outcomes, this treatment represents a significant improvement in cost-effectiveness and has decreased the length of stay after acute and chronic wounds. As previously mentioned in the studies described earlier, NPWT displayed evidence of decreasing costs related to SSIs, chronic DFUs, and other nonhealing injuries. Other literature supports these findings, stating that NPWT offers more overall savings than standard dressings alone.[37] There have been reports of a 78% decrease in hospital stays and a 76% decrease in cost with NPWT. This is substantial, considering the annual financial burden for wound management accounts for over $10 billion in the United States alone.[38] This cost decrease, coupled with efficacy in wound healing from NPWT, has even permitted its use as an at-home treatment for Medicare patients with home healthcare.

Developments of NPWT have further bolstered its widespread use. NPWT with instillation has allowed for the creation of an open-cell foam sponge that allows for periodic installation of the wound bed with sterile fluid, facilitating removal of thick exudate and infectious products. The duration and time interval between each installation can then be adjusted based on the requirements of the wound. The specific solution applied can be variable as well—with installations compatible with normal saline and Dakin solution, among others. Another technologic improvement is the implementation of portable wound vacuum-assisted closure (VAC) devices that are suitable for outpatient treatment. Additionally, the use of one-use disposable devices has become more popular. These devices do not require replacement of the dressing, typically last for a few days, and are particularly useful in the setting of incisional NPWT or treatment of relatively superficial wounds with low exudative fluid output. Of late, there have been developments in noncommercial NPWT alternatives to further minimize costs. A study compared VACs with noncommercial NPWT devices, such as wall suction applied to a sealed gauze dressing (GSUC), Redon drains, and AquaVac.[39] Compared with the VAC, GSUC was the far cheaper option and had comparable granulation tissue formation, effects on wound size, and graft take while also being less painful and time consuming with dressing changes. The AquaVac displayed similar findings, aside from no differences between pain and time required for dressing changes.[39] With noncommercial NPWT alternatives exhibiting similar efficacy at a fraction of the costs, NPWT will be able to have a greater impact in communities lacking sufficient financial resources.

Tissue Replacements

In 1987, the National Science Foundation bioengineering panel defined *tissue engineering* as "the application of the principles and methods of engineering and the life sciences toward the development of biologic substitutes to restore, maintain, or improve function." These principles and methods have been used toward the creation of skin products made of cells, ECM components, or combinations of the two. This tissue-engineered skin has developed and progressed rapidly over the past 25 years, mainly driven by the limitations associated with autografts, and may function by providing the cellular or matrix components that could be necessary for wounds to heal. These new skin substitutes more accurately mimic native tissues to promote sustained healing without rejection. The use of biologic dressings, scaffolds, stem cell therapy, and gene therapy is an example of tissue engineering in which new tissues are created rather than transferred.

Bioengineered skin substitutes can potentially save millions of dollars a year for healthcare delivery services through reduced spending on dressings and treatment of wound-induced complications, particularly in the treatment of venous, diabetic, and pressure ulcers, which form 90% of all chronic wounds. Bioengineered skin substitutes act as protective dressings by limiting bacterial colonization and fluid loss, but they also stimulate healing (Fig. 45.11). Their design is variable and dependent on the layer of skin they are designed to replace.

Skin substitutes can be used in the treatment of both acute and chronic wounds. This wide array of products has advantages and disadvantages. Some, such as Apligraf, are temporary, whereas others offer permanent wound coverage. However, like any medical device, a high cost is often involved. There is not one ideal skin substitute, making this an active realm of research.[40]

Although skin grafts can provide adequate permanent wound coverage, donor site morbidity, pain, scarring, and limitations in donor site locations have pushed researchers into the development of skin substitutes.

Regenerative medicine is playing a key role in new advances in wound care and has provided for the development of many other skin substitutes; these products have been found to advance reconstructive outcomes. These substitutes may be epidermal only or dermal only or may replace full-thickness skin (Table 45.6). They also differ in how they are processed and whether they are animal or synthetically derived. Many classification systems have been devised in the past to categorize the array of products available. One of the most efficient categorizations is based on five different characteristics: cellularity, material, layering, replaced region, and permanence. Each product is described using these terms so that their exact nature is easily understood by clinicians.

Acellular products are, by definition, immunologically inert because they are created by removing all or almost all cellular components from sources such as animal tissue, human amnion, and cadaveric dermis. These types of skin replacements resist shelf storage and can be stored for years, which provides an advantage over cellular skin replacements. Although the production and maintenance of cellular skin grafts are more demanding than the acellular versions, it is thought that the preserved viable cells within these constructs provide unmatched benefits toward healing.

Material-wise, substitutes of human origin are termed *allografts,* whereas those derived from animals are referred to as *xenografts*. Examples of allograft precursors include placenta, amniotic membrane, foreskin, and donated human dermis. In the xenograft category, the use of bovine, porcine, ovine, and most recently, fish skin has been described.

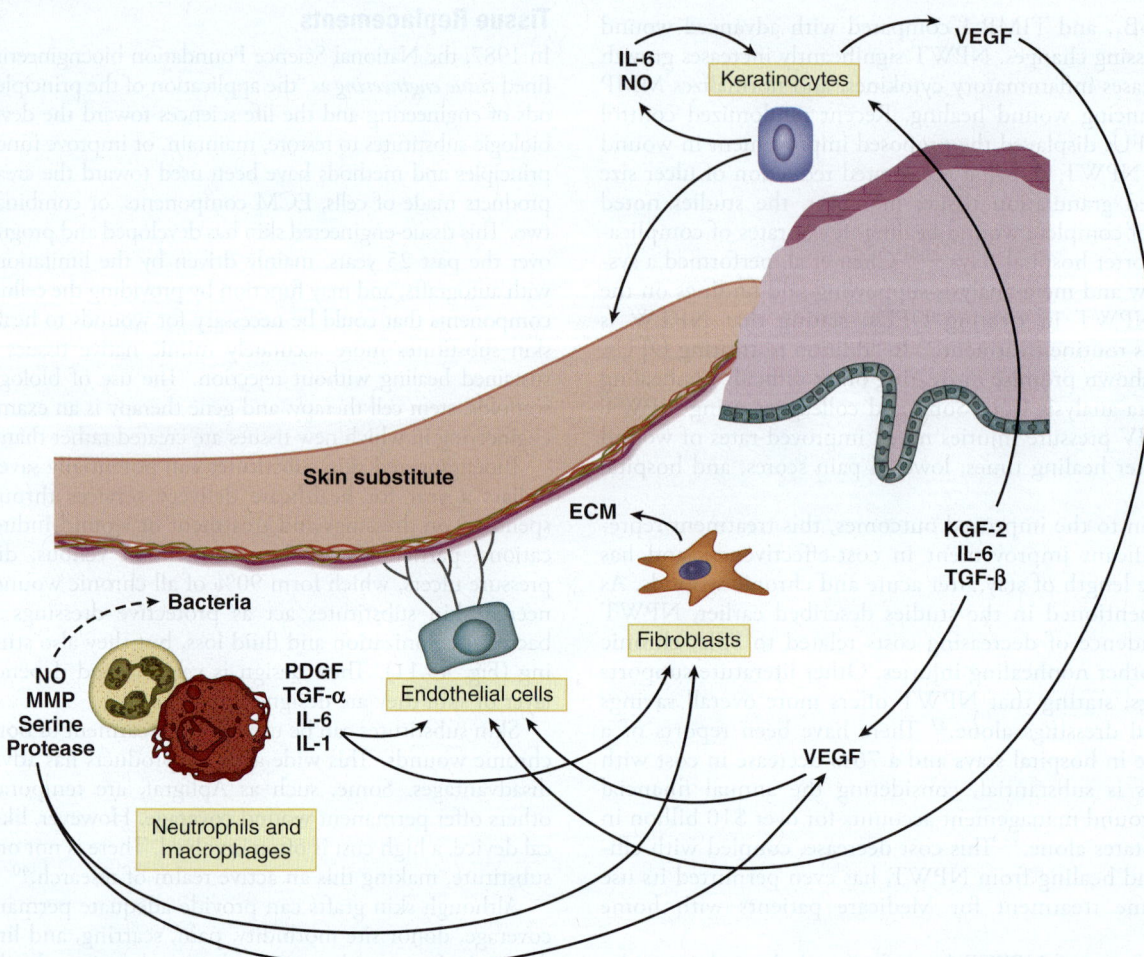

FIGURE 45.11 The effect of skin substitutes in the wound bed. Skin substitutes have variable structures and cellular content. They may be cellular or acellular, but both forms induce the influx of endogenous cells, including fibroblasts, keratinocytes, endothelial cells, macrophages, and neutrophils, into the wound bed. These cells secrete various cytokines and growth factors that stimulate angiogenesis, extracellular matrix (ECM) deposition, and reepithelialization via the process of dynamic reciprocity. The skin substitute is replaced by native tissues, eventually resulting in a healed wound. *Solid lines* indicate upregulation, and *dashed lines* indicate downregulation. *IL-1*, Interleukin-1; *IL-6*, interleukin-6; *KGF-2*, keratinocyte growth factor-2; *MMP*, matrix metalloproteinase; *NO*, nitric oxide; *PDGF*, platelet-derived growth factor; *TGFα*, transforming growth factor-α; *TGF-β*, transforming growth factor-β; *VEGF*, vascular endothelial growth factor. (From Greaves NS, Iqbal SA, Baguneid M, et al. The role of skin substitutes in the management of chronic cutaneous wounds. *Wound Repair Regen.* 2013;21:194-210.)

Regarding the replaced region, epidermal skin substitutes are created by the expansion of patient-derived keratinocytes in the laboratory. The primary role is to provide a protective barrier against microorganisms and prevent fluid loss. These are fragile constructs that promote the proliferation of keratinocytes. Given their thin nature, they are attached to a carrier material to facilitate application to the wound. One of the major drawbacks of cultured autografts is that they are extremely thin, susceptible to shearing forces, and experience a great deal of contraction; thus, not many epidermal-only skin substitutes are available on the market. Two available options are as follows:

- Epicel is one of the cultured epidermal autografts used solely as an epidermal replacement. To obtain Epicel, keratinocytes from the patient are inactivated Trauma and harvested into sheets. The layer of keratinocytes is then held together by a reinforcement-carried layer.

- MySkin is an epidermal skin substitute with a different presentation and delivery mechanism. MySkin is a solution delivered as a spray.

Dermal substitutes are based on a structural 3D matrix material that behaves similarly to ECM and may incorporate cells or bioactive molecules. Delivering these key factors to the wound bed may provide the necessary stimulus to rebalance the wound microenvironment in favor of healing. The epidermis is removed, and the dermal ECM is preserved to act like a scaffold for cell migration. Thus, these constructs provide a physiologically similar framework for healing. Most dermal substitutes are acellular and have high macroporosity to promote cell migration and revascularization. Some examples of dermal substitutes are as follows:

- AlloDerm is an allograft acellular, single-layer, temporary dermal substitute derived from cadavers; it has been used a great deal in breast reconstruction.

TABLE 45.6 Tissue Replacements: Epidermal, Dermal, and Bilayer

TYPE	DESCRIPTION	CELLULARITY AND MATERIALS	EXAMPLES
Epidermal	Protective barrier against microorganisms and prevent fluid loss. Require carrier materials and are fragile.	Cellular Human keratinocytes	Epicel, Epidex, and MySkin
Dermal	Structural three-dimensional matrix material that behaves similarly to ECM and may incorporate cells or bioactive molecules. The dermal extracellular matrix is preserved in this constructs and acts like a scaffold for cell migration. Thus, dermal replacements provide a physiologically similar framework for healing.	Acellular and cellular Human derived: dermis and amnion chorion Animal derived (*in italics*): ovine, bovine, porcine, fish Other: synthetic (<u>underlined</u>)	Affinity Human Amniotic, FloGraft Amniotic, Grafix, GrafixPL Prime, AlloWrap, AltiPlast, AmnioBand, Amnioexcel, AmnioFill, AmnioFix, Amniomatrix, Artacent, Bio-ConneKt, BioDFactor, BioDFence, Biovance, Cellesta, CollaWound, Cygnus Amnio Patch, Dermavest, EpiCord, EpiFix, FlowerAmnio Patch, Genesis, Integra BioFix, Interfyl, Neox Wound, NuShield, PalinGen, Restorigin, Revita, WoundEx, Xwrap, AlloDerm, AlloPatch, AlloSkin, Coll-e-derm, Dcell, DermACELL, DermaPure, DermaSpan, FlowerDerm, Gamma-Graft, GraftJacket, hMatrix ADM, InteguPly, Matrix HD, *Talymed*, *Excellagen, Helicoll, Integra Avagen, Integra Flowable, MatriDerm, PriMatrix, Endoform, Cyta wound, EZ Derm, Geistlich Derma, MicroMatrix* *MiroDerm, Nevelia, Oasis, Ologen, PuraPly, Theraform, Puracol, Kerecis,* Hyalograft, NovoSorb, Hyalomatrix, Restrata, Dermagraft
Bilayer	Represent a combination of features seen in epidermal and dermal models. These components are the most complex because of their physiologic resemblance to natural tissue. Strong ability to induce angiogenesis.	Acellular and cellular Human, bovine, and porcine derived	AltiPly, Apligraf,* OrCel,* SkinTE, Stratagraft, TheraSkin, *Biobrane*

All are human derived except those in *italics*, which are animal derived, and those that are underlined, which are synthetic.
*Indicates both human and animal derived.
Adapted from Bay C, Chizmar Z, Reece EM, et al. Comparison of skin substitutes for acute and chronic wound management. *Semin Plast Surg.* 2021;35(3):171-180.

- Integra is an acellular dermal substitute composed of sheets of bovine tendon and shark GAGs developed in the 1970s. Although initially developed for tissue coverage in burn patients, it is currently used for coverage of areas nonamenable to skin grafting, such as joint capsules, bone, and tendon from all etiologies.
- Kerecis is an acellular xenograft derived from North Atlantic cod fish. Unlike other skin substitutes, the molecular components and structural characteristics of nature are kept intact. Fish derivatives contain proteoglycans, glycoproteins, collagen, elastin, fibronectin, and omega-3 polyunsaturated fatty acids in a high-tensile-strength and rapidly degradable matrix; these components are thought to act synergistically in tissue repair. Recently, Yoon et al. demonstrated faster reepithelialization and cell proliferation with Kerecis compared with a bovine collagen skin graft.[41]
- In recent years, NovoSorb Biodegradable Temporizing Matrix (BTM) has become more widely used in the reconstruction of complex wounds. BTM is a synthetic dermal matrix consisting of a biodegradable polyurethane open foam cell that faces the wound surrounded by an overlying nonbiodegradable sealing membrane. The open matrix facing the wound permits the infiltration of cells and cellular products and functions as a scaffold in the formation of neodermis. The nonbiodegradable sealing membrane functionally provides a means of physiologic wound closure but also contains microfenestrations in the membrane to stave off accumulation of debris that would otherwise disrupt the integrity of the matrix. BTM application occurs in two stages. First, BTM is applied and secured to a clean wound bed, allowing cells and vascular elements to integrate and form a vascularized neodermis. This integration usually occurs over the course of a few weeks. After adequate integration and consolidation, the overlying nonbiodegradable membrane is removed and is promptly replaced with a split-thickness skin graft over the defect. The applications for NovoSorb BTM are robust. Indications include both partial- and full-thickness wounds, surgical wounds, traumatic wounds, and chronic ulcers. Recently, studies have touted BTM efficacy in reconstructing DFUs as well.[42] Contraindications for BTM application include wounds that require debridement, such as necrotic wounds or devitalized tissue as well as wounds that are infected.

Bilayer materials represent a combination of features seen in epidermal and dermal models. These components are the most complex because of their physiologic resemblance to natural tissue. In vitro studies support the use of bilayer materials over single-layer substitutes based on their strong ability to induce angiogenesis. Different constructs with cellular and acellular components have been released to the market as well as both animal and human-derived composites:

- Biobrane, for instance, is an acellular bilayer that replaces full-thickness skin and is composed of silicone, nylon mesh, and porcine collagen.
- StrataGraft is an allogenic cellularized bilayer substitute that completed a phase III multicenter trial in the burn wound care setting in 2021. This construct is composed of human fibroblasts embedded in a collagen gel. As of now, it has been shown to decrease the area of required autografting and produces results comparable to those of autografts.

Given the steep influx of research, tissue engineering is a rapidly growing and changing field. Over 70 different types of skin substitutes have been released in the market, and many more are currently being studied. Although the literature compares the characteristics of these constructs between each other, it's the distinctive qualities of the wound and the patient that determine the best fit.

Bioengineering: Gene and Stem Cell Therapy

Bioengineered skin substitutes can potentially save millions of dollars a year for healthcare delivery services through reduced spending on dressings and treatment of wound-induced complications, particularly in the treatment of venous, diabetic, and pressure ulcers, which form 90% of all chronic wounds. Bioengineered skin substitutes act as protective dressings by limiting bacterial colonization and fluid loss, but they also stimulate healing (see Fig. 45.11). Their design is variable and dependent on the layer of skin they are designed to replace.

Stem cell therapy is a widely investigated area in wound repair. Somatic cells were initially used to provide a barrier-like protective function for open wounds. Single and bilayer constructs of keratinocytes and fibroblasts were developed for skin regeneration. However, their use was cumbersome and limited to large wounds. MSCs proved to be a superior option because they can differentiate into epidermal and dermal cell lineages while promoting extensive cellular expansion. The administration of stem cells enhances wound-healing processes through direct cell differentiation and molecule-signaling mechanisms. A recent meta-analysis evaluated the efficacy of autologous stem cell therapy from bone, peripheral blood, or adipose-derived MSCs to treat lower extremity chronic wounds secondary to diabetes and peripheral arterial disease.[43] MSCs improved microvascular regeneration, especially when applied intramuscularly.

MSCs are a source of exosomes, which are responsible for transport and communication functions within cells. The majority of exosomes originate from adipose tissue, bone marrow, umbilical cord, and placental MSCs. Exosomes can regulate components in all phases of the wound-healing process. In the inflammatory phase, they act as antiinflammatory molecules, reducing the levels of TNF-α, NO, and cyclooxygenase-2 (COX-2). Their immunomodulatory properties are due to their ability to modulate microRNA in immune cells by promoting negative-feedback mechanisms. During the proliferation phase, exosomes stimulate cell proliferation and inhibit apoptotic pathways. Additionally, they upregulate different types of growth factors, including those associated with angiogenesis. Finally, exosomes endorse collagen and elastin formation and organization during matrix remodeling. Although several in vitro and in vivo studies in different animal models have described the use of exons for wound-healing purposes, data regarding human studies are scant.[44] As described by Ngoc and colleagues, very few human clinical trials have been reported in the wound care setting; other studies have targeted other conditions, such as diabetes and acute respiratory distress syndrome.[44]

Gene therapy has applications in wound healing, as well. Zinc finger nucleases, transcription activator-like effector nuclease (TALEN), and the clustered regularly interspersed short palindromic repeats (CRISPR) system are used for gene editing. Genetically engineered somatic and mesenchymal cells are used to correct gene mutations in chronic skin disorders. Autologous stem cells are genetically modified and transplanted to restore the regular functions of the skin layers. Treatment mechanisms of gene-alteration therapy have been used for cases of epidermolysis bullosa (EB) and recessive dystrophic EB (RDEB).

Electrical Therapy

With advances in tissue engineering, there has been the development of a plethora of innovative wound care treatments aimed at stimulating the cells and chemical mediators needed for wound healing. These treatments include electrical stimulation (ES), therapeutic ultrasound, and vibration therapy (VT) (Table 45.7).

Wounds carry a direct-current electrical gradient that can be used to hasten the healing process. Biochemical studies have found that ES alters gene expression; this then affects the production of chemokines, cytokines, and collagen, promoting an environment favorable for healing. Pathways activated by electrical energy include those of intracellular polyamines, the PI3K/PTEN pathway, and the KCNJ15/Kir4.2 membrane channel.

TABLE 45.7	Electrical Therapy		
TYPE	**MECHANISM**	**DETAILS**	**DEVICES**
Electric stimulation	Increased blood flow Promote cell recruitment Muscle stimulation Antibacterial properties Tailored remodeling	Unidirectional or bidirectional direct current or pulsatile current	• Battery-powered units • Challenge 8000A • BLT-5000 series • Portmax 300 electrical • Triboelectric nanogenerator (TENG) • Piezoelectric nanogenerator (PENG)
Ultrasound	Vasodilation Cavitation microstreaming Ultrasound-targeted microbubble destruction Antibiotic synergy	Low (30–40 kHz) and high (1–3 MHz) frequency Bubble size 50 nm to 10 μm	• MIST therapy system • Misonix low-frequency ultrasound • Sonic One • SONOCA device • Qoustic wound therapy system

Vibration therapy	Decrease neutrophils and TNF-α
	Increase collagen deposit
	Alters blood flow at skin level
		Low-intensity vibration at 45 Hz	• RelaWave
			  Matsuda
			  Microsonics
			  Vibrators
			• Vibrating plates

TNF-α, Tumor necrosis factor-α.

Several hypothetical mechanisms that explain the effects of ES in wound healing have been described:

- Increase blood flow: ES has been seen to increase blood delivery to tissues, thus facilitating nutrient distribution. When used in rodents, low-frequency ES promoted sensory nerve activation, resulting in vasodilation and accelerated healing.
- Cellular recruitment: ES has been shown to promote the recruitment of neutrophils, macrophages, lymphocytes, and fibroblasts during different stages of the wound-healing process. Readiness of these cells is beneficial for the formation of granulation tissue and the reepithelialization process.
- Remodeling effect: Electrical current encourages the migration of fibroblasts through the PI3K/PTEN pathway. It is also thought to enhance the structure of collagen fibers and their arrangement in the ECM.
- Antibacterial properties: ES has been noted to decrease the bacterial load in wound tissue. Although the exact mechanism is unknown, it is believed to be related to the different polarity fields in direct current. A study evaluating the load of *P. aeruginosa* in rabbits found that the negative pole had antibacterial tendencies.
- Muscle stimulation: It is thought that ES can increase blood flow to affected areas and increase the production of growth factors. In patients with neurologic involvement, ES can be used to facilitate regular muscle contractility to prevent atrophy and skin injuries.

Although there is no conclusive evidence to support any of these hypotheses, ES remains a highly researched alternative in wound healing. Current can be delivered through different methods; however, the most common is directly at the wound level. Two or more electrodes are placed on the skin and then attached to battery-like devices controlled manually. Current is applied either in a direct or pulsatile fashion, with the latter one dividing into monophasic or biphasic settings. Other factors, such as frequency, polarity, amplitude, and exact electrode placement, can be determined based on the wound characteristics. Arora and colleagues presented a meta-analysis of 20 randomized controlled clinical trials evaluating ES plus standard care versus standard care alone for pressure ulcers.[45] On average, ES was administered for 5 hours per week. They concluded with moderate certainty that ES improved the number of ulcers healed. However, the exact area of improvement and time to healing were not able to be estimated. Complications reported in the study included redness and discomfort at the application site.[45]

Different types of devices that deliver ES have been developed. Initially, large and traditional battery-powered units were used; however, these devices had limited availability, poor portability, high cost, and safety concerns. As a result, miniature devices that mimic endogenous electric fields have been the leading trend in research. Nanogenerators (NGs) are self-powered electric systems that transform mechanical energy into electrical energy. These constructs are a wearable and safe alternative to promote fibroblast proliferation and migration in animal models. Although the data regarding NGs are promising, human studies are still lacking.

Ultrasound

Ultrasound, particularly kilohertz ultrasound, causes microstreaming and cavitation as particles are displaced by the vibratory waves. The cavitation protects healthy tissue and promotes the degradation of nonviable tissue. Additionally, the mechanical energy alters the cell membrane through conformational changes in proteins and activation of signaling pathways in cells. For instance, in the proliferative phase of wound healing, it increases macrophage activity and increases collagen production.

Low-frequency (30- to 40-kHz) and high-frequency (1- to 3-MHz) ultrasound are the available types of therapies for chronic wounds. The sound waves from both raise the surface temperature of wounds between 39°C and 41°C, which results in localized vasodilation. Treatment with ultrasound usually lasts 5 to 10 minutes and is done after a topical fluid has been applied as a medium.

A recent meta-analysis compared low-frequency, high-intensity contact ultrasound to standard wound care. High-intensity ultrasound was associated with lower rates of nonhealed DFUs and a higher percentage of ulcer area reduction at 3 months.[46] On a similar note, when low-frequency, low-intensity, noncontact ultrasound was evaluated side by side with nonstandard care, ultrasound treatment was found to be associated with fewer nonhealed ulcers and reduced ulcer area.[46]

Ultrasound debridement is a rather novel term that refers to the disruption of the superficial wound layers to potentiate topical medication application and promote new tissue regeneration. Compared with standard debridement, this technique is noninvasive and moderately painless. This method has been used to treat wounds infected by biofilm by inducing gas bubbles that disrupt the structure of colonizing microorganisms. Given that the range of bubble sizes available is between 50 nm and 10 μm, the desired size must be set based on the goals of the treatment itself. Low concentrations of gas created by the ultrasound result in small bubbles referred to as *nanobubbles*.[47] Greater concentrations of gas create larger bubbles

Ultrasound-targeted microbubble destruction refers to the use of bubbles as a mechanical advantage to shed and potentialize other compounds surrounding the molecules. When used synergistically with antibiotics, this ultrasound technique has been found to decrease levels of bacteria in biofilm significantly. For instance, Darvishi and colleagues depicted how the use of targeted microbubbles, in combination with vancomycin, decreased the levels of *Staphylococcus epidermidis* found on biofilm.[47]

Vibration Therapy

VT has been relevant in orthopedic surgery by promoting bone angiogenesis and mineralization as well as an adjacent therapy to ligament repair treatments. In the wound care field, VT is a rather new concept that is slowly building strength. The benefit behind this approach relies on the tissues' neuromuscular response to vibration waves. Several studies are being carried out with different combinations of mechanical settings (frequency, amplitude, displacement, and peak acceleration) to evaluate the response in wound healing. Most of the current research targeting wound healing is in mice or rat animal models. Currently, the low-intensity vibration (LIV) setting is the most common setting described in the literature regarding tissue repair. VT sessions last 20 to 30 minutes and are carried out once a day and five to seven times per week.

Wano and colleagues evaluated the role of vertical LIV at 45 Hz on male mice with soft tissue wounds.[48] At 7 days, they found decreased neutrophil infiltration and TNF-α levels.[48] At 14 days, there were increased levels of collagen and significantly improved wound closure when compared with the control group.[48] Likewise, when Roberts and associates compared different VT mechanical settings in mice, LIV 45 Hz with a peak of 0.3 was the only setting that resulted in increased angiogenesis, reepithelialization, and granulation tissue.[42]

A recent double-blind study used local VT plantar skin in 10 healthy participants.[49] Blood flow at the level of the first metacarpal was measured after the exposure using wavelet amplitudes.[49] A significant difference in amplitudes of metabolic and neurogenic blood flow was noted in the patients exposed to VT compared with the placebo group, suggesting that local vibrations alter plantar skin blood flow.[49] In 2023, a prospective study that included 40 patients with DFUs was published.[50] VT was used at 47 Hz for 15 minutes daily after standard wound care (off-loading, debridement, and daily monitoring) for 12 weeks in these patients.[50] Syabariyah and colleagues found that participants exposed to VT had a significantly faster wound-healing rate compared with unexposed controls (25 days vs. 33 days).[50] Although the results are promising, the small sample sizes are a limitation. Further research on VT in wound care in human subjects will be required before including VT as a standard of chronic wound care.

SPECIAL CONSIDERATIONS IN ULCER MANAGEMENT

As mentioned before, chronic wounds fail to progress through the normal sequence of the tissue repair process, resulting in a prolonged healing period that impedes the restoration of normal anatomic and functional integrity. The most common types of chronic wounds are pressure ulcers, venous ulcers, and ischemic ulcers.

Pressure Ulcers

Pressure ulcers develop as a result of prolonged pressure over bony prominences such as the sacrum, ischium, and heels. They are common in the elderly and patients with impaired mobility. The prolonged weight-bearing status elevates tissue pressure above capillary perfusion pressure (32 mm Hg), which restricts oxygen delivery. Worsening factors include shear forces, friction, moisture, malnutrition, and impaired blood supply. Great effort should be placed on preventing pressure ulcers by identifying patients at risk and promptly establishing local contact and pressure precautions (e.g., turning schedule). However, if an ulcer has developed, treatment consists of diminishing modifiable detrimental factors that delay wound healing. Specifically, targeting malnutrition with adequate protein intake, decreasing immobility by remedying the underlying condition (if possible) and providing guidance with physical therapy, and correcting hypoperfusion. Once all modifiable factors have been addressed, local and regional fasciocutaneous and musculocutaneous flaps can be considered as an option for wound closure if the lesion persists.[3,8,48,51]

Venous Ulcers

Venous ulcers are the most common type of chronic leg ulcer. They result from incompetent venous valves and calf-muscle pump failure that generate capillary wall distention and leakage of macromolecules, limiting oxygen delivery. Venous ulcers are associated with tortuous varices, dermatitis, and brown pigment discoloration. Treatment is bimodal by addressing the underlying venous insufficiency and providing local wound care of the ulcers. A joint effort with a vascular specialist is required because the specialist provides guidance regarding the management of chronic venous insufficiency. Measures such as compression stockings and leg elevation can be temporizing. Regarding local wound care, the same strategies of chronic wound management apply to this type of ulcer.[3,8,27]

Ischemic Ulcers

Ischemic or arterial ulcers develop in areas where poor circulation exists, such as the toes, lateral feet, malleolus, and pretibial area, commonly affected by atherosclerotic disease. They are associated with factors such as diabetes, hypertension, advanced age, hyperlipidemia, and smoking. Clinical characteristics of these lesions include well demarcated, deep, pale color, poor granulation tissue, and ischemic borders in patients with skin atrophy, lack of hair, delayed capillary refill, and decreased ankle-brachial index (ABI). Patients with ischemic ulcers should be referred urgently to a vascular surgery specialist to determine the need for revascularization and monitor chronic limb-threatening ischemia. The severity of the lesion is determined by the grade of the wound, the level of ischemia, and whether infection is present. Multiple individual patient factors play a role in determining the type of revascularization offered and subsequent antithrombotic, lipid-lowering, and/or antihypertensive medication required. Although local wound care remains the same as that for any other chronic wound, this type of lesion is unlikely to heal properly without adequate perfusion.[3,8,11]

Unfortunately, ulcers are a common, insidious, and morbid type of chronic wound. The cornerstone treatment relies on identifying the triggering factor and addressing it as able. Additional strategies include local wound care, nutrition optimization, and reinforcement of environmental precautions. Nonetheless, these types of wounds continue to be a challenge to healthcare providers.

NEW HORIZONS

Technology has enabled multiple discoveries regarding wound care in the past decades. A greater understanding of the physiopathology of wound healing has opened the way to novel therapies. Coupled with the exponential influx of research in the area, this field is rapidly changing and adjusting to patient's needs. Some of the rising treatment topics for chronic wounds include nanotechnology in both materials and devices, 3D printing, and telemedicine.

Nanomaterials are organic or inorganic components at a nanometer size. They have specific properties and characteristics that apply to medicine, especially wound care. Organic nanomaterials are derived from natural components such as chitosan, collagen, and dendrimers, and inorganic nanomaterials are those made synthetically, for instance, silver, titanium, and copper. Given their nano size, these elements have a high ratio of surface area to volume. Their applications in wound healing rely on nanomaterials whose intrinsic characteristics are beneficial for wound healing or nanomaterials that act as vehicles to deliver medications or other therapeutically advantageous components. Their particular size allows high concentrations of localized drug delivery with fewer side effects than other methods. Nanomaterials can be biodegradable, which is an accepted alternative to other not-so-environmentally-friendly options.

Some examples include carbon nanotubules, which are inorganic biomaterial nanoparticles used to induce platelet aggregation and generate a prothrombotic stage. Carbon nanotubules have been found useful in settings where accelerated hemostatic control is required. Another example is the use of chitosan-based nanomaterials in rat models. Accelerated wound-healing times have been achieved by enhancement of both the proliferative and remodeling stages. Interestingly, chitosan-based components tend to display unique properties that are not common in the individual materials, suggesting a synergistic relationship. Regarding metallic nanomaterials, Vijayakumar and colleagues identified the antibacterial properties of silver, gold, and copper nanoparticles when applied in a polymeric matrix. These minerals are noted to inhibit bacterial growth and accelerate wound healing in diabetic rat models. In general, nanomaterials have demonstrated positive effects in in vitro and in vivo animal studies, especially when acting synergistically in combination.

Another area that is gaining momentum is 3D-printed scaffolds. Unlike premade dressings, these adjust to size, dimension, material, oxygen penetration, and medication release, thus providing a flexible coverage alternative for complex wounds. Additionally, these specialized frames can act as a means for cells, proteins, genes, and drugs to be incorporated into a wound. The layer-by-layer printing nature allows full control of the geometry and structure that best fits the patient in question, with the advantage that certain characteristics, such as porosity, degradability, degree of cell ingrowth, proliferation, or even nutrient transport, can be predetermined. 3D prints resemble autologous tissue by individualizing therapy at its maximum degree. Bioink is an essential component; *bioink* refers to the materials that provide support and structure to the newly created matrix. Common elements of bioink include collagen, polymers, and cells. 3D printing is an area with increasing potential. In combination with nanotechnology, further enhancement of each therapy's wound-healing mechanisms can be obtained. Hu and colleagues evaluated the use of a cryptogenic 3D-printed hydrogel scaffold with exosomes in diabetic wounds in Sprague-Dawley rats.[51] The matrix was composed of decellularized small intestine submucosa, mesoporous bioactive glass, and isolated exosomes.[51] After application of the scaffold, accelerated wound healing by increased angiogenesis and stimulation of organized ECM component deposition was evidenced.[51]

Since the onset of the COVID-19 pandemic, telemedicine has become more widely used in many fields of medicine because many essential healthcare services were disrupted. This is especially true for the treatment of individuals with chronic wounds, where we have seen a shift in management tactics largely as a result of resource scarcity as well as patient and provider limitations. Generally, traditional wound care practices require frequent assessments and stringent therapy regimens, which can be burdensome—especially in this patient population that generally has higher rates of comorbidities. Through the incorporation of telemedicine for wound care treatment, patients suffering from chronic wounds have more expedient access to be clinically assessed. As such, the convenience of telemedicine relieves much of the burden placed on providers, caregivers, and patients, with decreased travel time, scheduling, and costs. Moreover, telemedicine can improve outcomes because it facilitates more prompt assessments and subsequent treatment. Notably, telemedicine has also shown similar safety and efficacy when compared with conventional chronic wound care treatment. Depending on patient and/or provider preferences, telemedicine can be used in a couple of different ways. Telemedicine can function synchronously in real time or function asynchronously with image upload to electronic medical record systems. The flexibility of telemedicine has changed the way we approach wound care management, and further large-scale studies are required to identify its efficacy in other unique clinical settings.

Currently, there are a few types of telehealth models that providers implement. Typically, providers opt toward blended care models as opposed to solely virtual modalities. Blended care models involve conventional in-person care by a practitioner followed by digital monitoring with remote specialists. Purely virtual models were largely implemented due to COVID-19, when providers had to consider exposure risks for themselves and their patients, although it is a viable option if circumstances dictate. Regardless of the modality, telemedicine for wound care is founded on image assessment, phone and/or video consultations, and text-based information delivery. Text-based information is usually accompanied by an electronic medical record system, email, or text messaging. With studies emphasizing the efficacy of telemedicine in wound care, telemedicine could become inherently tethered with chronic wound care management for patients. This notion is exemplified in recent developments such as Project ECHO (Extension for Community Healthcare Outcomes), which aims to provide teleconsulting and telementoring partnerships between specialists and providers in underserved communities, including rural populations. Further evaluation and adaptation of these models are necessary; however, the adoption of telemedicine is becoming more universal.

Wound care is a dynamic area of medicine in which developments occur continuously. The challenging nature of wound care management as well as the substantial psychological and economic burden necessitates further investigation into wound pathogenesis with subsequent innovation in effective treatment options. Moving forward, developments in chronic wound care management will target even more individualized patient needs to improve their quality of life while also reducing costs.

SELECTED REFERENCES

Bai Q, Han K, Dong K, et al. Potential applications of nanomaterials and technology for diabetic wound healing. *Int J Nanomedicine*. 2020;15:9717-9743.

Thorough review that provides an extensive view of nanomaterials in the chronic wound setting.

Barone N, Safran T, Vorstenbosch J, Davison PG, Cugno S, Murphy AM. Current advances in hypertrophic scar and keloid management. *Semin Plast Surg*. 2021;35(03):145-152.

In-depth description of novel therapeutic advances in the area of hypertrophic scars and keloids.

Bay C, Chizmar Z, Reece EM, et al. Comparison of skin substitutes for acute and chronic wound management. *Semin Plast Surg*. 2021;35(3):171-180.

Comparison of the different types of skin substitutes and their application in the acute and chronic setting.

Dai C, Shih S, Khachemoune A. Skin substitutes for acute and chronic wound healing: an updated review. *J Dermatolog Treat*. 2020;31(6):639-648.

Extensive description of traditional and novel skin substitutes based on their characteristics and functions.

Naik PP. Novel targets and therapies for keloid. *Clin Exp Dermatol*. 2021;47(3):507-515.

Update on the physiopathology of keloids and new therapeutic targets for management purposes.

The full reference list appears on Elsevier eBooks+.

46 | CHAPTER

Surgical Critical Care

Justin S. Hatchimonji, Seema Anandalwar,
Niels D. Martin, and Deborah M. Stein

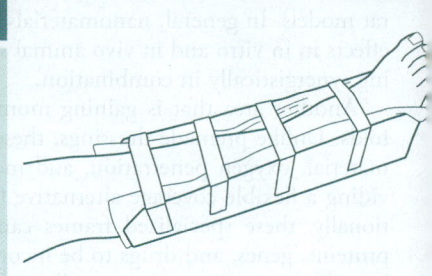

OUTLINE

INTRODUCTION

Critical care provides a systems-based algorithm for organ support during critical illness. Surgical critical care adds specific understanding of surgical pathology and its unique corresponding elements of critical illness. Expertise, therefore, allows for earlier recognition and intervention with the critically ill or injured surgical patient. Surgical disease can be further specialized into several distinct populations, including trauma, cardiac, neurologic, and "general" surgical. Surgical critical care, therefore, also has specific training pathways to develop expertise in these specific surgical areas.

Critical care is best delivered in a systems-based approach; therefore, this chapter is organized by organ system. Specific interplay between systems will be discussed where appropriate. A systems-based approach most effectively also involves a multidisciplinary team, with each component supplying critical and complementary expertise. This team commonly includes but is

not limited to pharmacy, respiratory therapy, nutritional support, advanced practice nursing, social work, and case management. Finally, although surgical intensivists have broad expertise, involvement of specific specialists with deeper knowledge in specific areas is also common and encouraged. Frequent consultants in this space include infectious diseases, nephrology, and palliative care.

NEUROLOGIC SYSTEM

Pain

The International Association for the Study of Pain (IASP) newly defined pain as "an unpleasant sensory and emotional experience associated with actual or potential tissue damage."[1] Intensive care unit (ICU) patients have multiple sources of pain, from readily recognized sources, such as procedures, endotracheal tubes, and dressing changes, to less recognized and often overlooked sources, such as suctioning, turning, and other aspects of daily care. Even immobility is a source of pain for patients because it creates musculoskeletal discomfort and neuropathies.

In addition, ICU patients experience hyperalgesia or hypernociception (heightened pain sensation). Studies have shown that proinflammatory cytokines, including interleukin-1 (IL-1) and IL-6, are released after local tissue injury and induce peripheral and central nervous system sensitization, leading to enhanced pain sensation.[2] This is true for patients in both surgical and medical ICUs.[3]

As high as 50% of patients have stated that their pain was inadequately treated in the ICU.[4,5] Inadequately treated pain results in serious clinical and psychological sequelae. It can lead to physiologic alterations, such as activation of catecholamines leading to vasoconstriction and increased myocardial oxygen demand as well as create metabolic disturbances, such as enhanced catabolic states altering glycemic control. Pain leads to inadequate coughing and deep breathing, predisposing patients to pneumonias and respiratory failure. In the short and long term, undertreated pain can lead to anxiety, lack of sleep, and posttraumatic stress disorder.[6]

ICU patients pose a unique challenge when it comes to recognition and quantification of pain. The barriers to effective pain management are numerous and from different sources. At the provider and nursing level, there is a knowledge gap in the physiologic effects of pain and the various types of medications that can be used, as well as a misconception that sedation is equivalent to analgesia. At the patient level, specifically for ICU patients, there is often an inability to report pain and a fear of being perceived as drug seeking.[6]

Numerous scales have been developed to standardize pain scores. For patients who are able to verbalize, the two primary pain scales are the numerical rating scale (NRS) and the verbal rating scale (VRS). The NRS asks patients to rate or circle a number between 0 and 10 or 0 and 100 that rates their pain, with 0 being "no pain" and the maximum number being the "worst pain they have ever experienced." The VRS asks patients to describe different levels of pain using adjectives such as *mild, moderate,* or *severe* pain.[7] Both scales have been shown to be comparable in quantifying acute pain.[8]

In patients who are unable to verbalize, there is the Wong-Baker FACES Pain Rating Scale, the Behavioral Pain Scale (BPS), and the Critical Care Pain Observation Tool (CPOT). The FACES pain scale allows the provider to determine a patient's level of pain based on a scale of facial expressions from smiling to grimacing. The BPS and CPOT scales quantify pain based on variables that have to do with compliance with the ventilator, movement/muscle tension of limbs, and facial expression to add up to a numeric score to quantify a pain level. Additionally, the use of vital sign parameters should also be considered, with tachycardia, hypertension, and tachypnea often being the most obvious signs of uncontrolled pain. Although these nonverbal behavioral scoring systems may be the only options for patients who are unable to communicate, they have several limitations, particularly in patients with dementia, cultural differences, or confounding factors that can influence any of the measured parameters. In head-to-head comparisons, self-reported pain scales have been felt more ideal than behavioral pain scores.[9]

Pain Control Medications—Opioids

Narcotic is a general term used to describe a class of drugs that produce sensory depression. Opioids are derived from the natural chemical opiate. Opioids bind to the three most recognized opioid receptors, the μ (now known as mu opioid [MOP]), δ (delta opioid [DOP]), and κ (kappa opioid [KOP]) receptors (however, up to 17 different classes of opioid receptors have been discovered). The physiologic effect of each opioid is determined by its pharmacodynamics in relation to each class of receptors.

Agonists to the MOP receptor cause analgesia and respiratory depression. Activation of MOP receptors in the midbrain activates descending inhibitory neurons and, through a series of effects, causes a reduction in the nociceptive transmission to the thalamus.[10] Agonists to the DOP receptor cause spinal analgesia and reduced gastric motility. Finally, agonists to the KOP receptor produce diuresis and dysphoria.[10] Through the same receptors, opiates produce a series of side effects, such as depressed consciousness and euphoria (leading to its addictive potential), respiratory depression, histamine release that can cause pruritus and reduction in systemic vascular resistance (SVR; hypotension), and gastrointestinal (GI) dysmotility resulting in constipation, nausea, and vomiting.

Morphine is the opioid that all other opioids are compared with. It can be given in an oral, intravenous, transdermal, or sublingual form. Morphine has low lipid solubility and slow penetration through the blood-brain barrier, making its onset of action relatively slow. In addition, half of orally ingested morphine will be metabolized through first-pass metabolism and will not reach the systemic circulation. In comparison, fentanyl and remifentanil are 600 times more lipid soluble than morphine and have a rapid onset of action with a lower risk of hypotension because they do not promote histamine release. Remifentanil offers the added benefit of being rapidly metabolized, as opposed to fentanyl, which gets stored in fat, making remifentanil the drug of choice in the operating room. Uniquely, tramadol, another opioid medication, acts on the MOP receptors and acts as a serotonin-norepinephrine reuptake inhibitor. Morphine-equivalent dosing of all commonly used opioids and their onset of action and half-lives are listed in Table 46.1.

Patients with a history of chronic narcotic use will not only build up a tolerance for opioids (a larger dose will be required to obtain the same effect), but it is now thought that they also experience opioid-induced hyperalgesia.[11] The mechanism for this

TABLE 46.1	Morphine Milligram Equivalents and Pharmacokinetics of Opioids						
	ORAL MORPHINE	IV MORPHINE	CODEINE	IV FENTANYL	ORAL HYDROMORPHONE	OXYCODONE	TRAMADOL
Equivalent dosage (mg)	1 (Ref)	0.3	7	0.003	0.2	0.67	4
Onset of action (min)	20–30	5–10	30–60	0.5	15–30	10–15	60
Peak effect (hours)	1–1.5	0.3	1–1.5	0.08–0.25	0.5–1	0.5–1	2–3
Half-life (hours)	2–4	1.5–3	3	0.5–1	2-3	3–4	6

is likely multifactorial but involves altered opioid intracellular signaling and neuronal sensitization via glial toll-like receptor 4 (TLR4) signaling, among other pathways.[11] Many patients with a history of chronic opioid use or abuse will be on methadone or buprenorphine (buprenorphine in combination with naloxone is known as *Suboxone*). Methadone is a synthetic opioid agonist that is used to both curb withdrawal symptoms and control cravings. In the ICU, the goal for these patients is to provide adequate pain control and prevent withdrawal. This may often require a multidisciplinary approach.

In the acute setting, a patient's home methadone dose should be started as soon as possible, and additional analgesia may be given for acute pain management. Methadone dosage changes should only be done in conjunction with an addiction or substance abuse specialist.[11] Similarly, patients on buprenorphine maintenance therapy should continue their standard dose (without the naloxone component) with additional analgesic medications for the management of acute pain. Previously, there was a concern that buprenorphine, a potent partial MOP receptor agonist, may act as a competitor against full MOP receptor agonists, making any additional pain control difficult. However, multiple studies have shown similar morphine-equivalent opioid requirements with either methadone or buprenorphine maintenance therapy.[12,13]

For opioid overdose or concerns with respiratory depression, naloxone can be given. Naloxone is a nonselective opioid receptor antagonist, with its highest affinity being to the MOP receptor, becoming a competitive inhibitor. When given intravenously and intranasally, its effects can be seen within 2 minutes. Repeated doses may be necessary because the half-life of naloxone is shorter than the half-life of many opioids.

Pain Control Medications—Nonopioids

Multimodal pain therapy is essential for both adequate pain control and for its opioid-sparing effects. Ibuprofen and ketorolac are nonsteroidal antiinflammatory drugs (NSAIDs) that inhibit the activity of cyclooxygenase enzymes, which inhibits the synthesis of prostaglandins (important in inflammation) and thromboxanes (important in clotting). Ketorolac has been shown to reduce the use of opioids by up to 50%.[14] Ketorolac should only be used for up to 5 days, given the risk of bleeding and kidney injury in longer durations. In addition, the dose should be reduced in elderly patients or those with a lower body mass index.

Similar to NSAIDs, acetaminophen also inhibits cyclooxygenase, without the antiinflammatory effects, and also has effects centrally, with multiple proposed mechanisms of action.[15] Regardless, it provides extremely good pain control and is an important adjunct in multimodal pain protocols. Caution should be used in patients with liver disease or when using it in addition to other drug combinations that contain acetaminophen because overdose and toxicity can lead to severe hepatic failure.

Other adjuncts include long-acting local anesthetic regional blocks for injury patterns or surgical incisions with identifiable pain distributions. Blocks have been shown to reduce opioid requirements in the first 24 to 72 hours.[16-18] A downside is that these are temporary forms of pain control that will wear off with the half-life of the anesthetic used. However, an epidural catheter can provide a continuous infusion of local anesthetic, with or without an opioid, for continuous pain relief.

For neuropathic pain, drugs like gabapentin and pregabalin can be used. Both bind to a subunit of voltage-dependent calcium channels and act as an inhibitor. It is debated whether pregabalin

has a higher affinity for the targeted ligand, but it is known to be at least two times more potent of an analgesic than gabapentin.

Agitation and Delirium
Agitation

Agitation is a "psychomotor disturbance characterized by an increase in both motor and psychological activities," often driven by anxiety, with disorganized actions and thoughts that can compromise a patient's care in the ICU.[19] To assess level of consciousness, there are several scoring systems. The Glasgow Coma Scale (GCS) provides a global assessment of a patient's level of consciousness, particularly after a brain injury. It has three components: ocular response, verbal response, and motor response. The score ranges from 3 to 15, with 3 being completely unresponsive and 15 being a normal level of responsiveness. In the ICU, the most commonly used method of assessing level of sedation and agitation is the Richmond Agitation-Sedation Scale (RASS).[20] This scale has been validated and demonstrated to have interrater reliability and consistency.[21]

The first steps for the treatment and prevention of agitation in the ICU should always be nonpharmacologic. These include providing frequent reassurance, prioritizing comfort, providing adequate pain control, encouraging family visitation, and prioritizing sleep when able.[19] Restraints can be used if a patient is harming themselves or others, but the decision to use restraints should be made with careful consideration and reassessed on a daily basis because of their potential for physical and psychological harm.

Sedation medications. Benzodiazepines bind to the gamma-aminobutyric acid-A (GABA-A) receptor to alter its configuration and increase the flow of GABA, an inhibitory neurotransmitter, causing sedation, anxiolysis, and muscle relaxation. Common uses are for alcohol withdrawal, anxiety disorders, seizures, and sedation in the ICU. Benzodiazepines are categorized into three groups: short acting (i.e., midazolam), intermediate acting (i.e., lorazepam), and long acting (i.e., diazepam). Midazolam and lorazepam are the primary benzodiazepines used for sedation in the ICU. Midazolam has high lipid solubility and therefore has rapid onset and rapid uptake by tissues, resulting in its short-acting nature. Given that it is rapidly stored in tissues, the use of midazolam infusions is typically limited to a short duration to avoid drug accumulation. The other downside of benzodiazepines is that they can promote delirium, particularly in the elderly. Given the concern for accumulation in tissues and delays in waking patients up after weaning sedation, the American College of Critical Care Medicine's (ACCM) Pain, Agitation and Delirium Clinical Practice Guidelines advise the use of nonbenzodiazepines for sedation in critically ill patients.[22] This recommendation was confirmed by studies showing decreased duration of mechanical ventilation and ICU length of stay with the use of nonbenzodiazepines for sedation.[23]

The most commonly used nonbenzodiazepine sedative in the ICU is propofol. Similarly, it acts as a potentiator of the GABA-A receptor, and at high doses, it may act as an agonist as well. Propofol does not have any analgesic effects. It can be given as boluses and often as an intravenous infusion for mechanically ventilated patients in the ICU. After discontinuing the medication, awakening occurs within 15 minutes. The adverse effects are significant respiratory depression (which is why its use is limited to monitored settings and/or mechanically ventilated patients) and systemic vasodilation leading to hypotension. Green urine may be noted from phenol metabolites. A relatively harmless side effect is the hypertriglyceridemia that can occur because of the lipid emulsion in propofol solutions. A more serious but rare side effect is propofol-related infusion syndrome (PRIS). The risk factors include high doses (>4 mg/kg/h) over a long duration (>48 hours). The syndrome is characterized by lactic acidosis, rhabdomyolysis, acute renal failure, and heart failure, with an overall mortality of up to 50%.[24] Treatment involves supportive management and discontinuing propofol.

Dexmedetomidine is an α_2-receptor agonist and produces cooperative sedation, meaning that patients have a certain level of arousal that allows them to interact but can return to their prior sedation state (similar to sleep/wake). Dexmedetomidine has sedative, amnestic, and some analgesic properties. It does not cause respiratory depression and can be used in patients who are not mechanically ventilated. Multiple randomized controlled trials have shown that sedation using dexmedetomidine was noninferior to sedation with midazolam or propofol and was associated with a shorter duration of mechanical ventilation.[25] Adverse effects, due to its potent α_2 effects, include hypotension and bradycardia, which are dose-dependent side effects. Similarly, clonidine is an oral or transdermal α_2-agonist and can be used to wean from benzodiazepines or dexmedetomidine.

Regardless of the pharmacologic agent, daily sedation holidays, defined as an interruption in sedative infusions until patients are awake, reduce the duration of mechanical ventilation and ICU length of stay. It is now standard of care for mechanically ventilated patients in the ICU to receive daily sedation holidays.

Delirium

Delirium is a disturbance in attention that is associated with impaired cognition that develops over a short period of time.[26] Up to 80% of mechanically ventilated patients develop delirium.[27] Delirium can present as hyperactive (restless, combative), hypoactive (lethargy, apathy), or mixed type (fluctuating between hyper- and hypoactive). The presence of delirium is associated with poor outcomes, including increased length of stay and higher mortality.[28] It can be difficult to identify patients suffering from early delirium, particularly those with hypoactive delirium. The Confusion Assessment Method for the Intensive Care Unit (CAM-ICU) is a commonly used, reliable, validated, and rapid instrument to assess for delirium.

There is limited high-quality evidence to suggest that any pharmacologic agent can prevent delirium. In multicenter, randomized controlled trials with placebo controls, antipsychotics, whether given prophylactically or for the treatment of delirium, failed to reduce the delirium rates or associated ICU mortality.[29,30] Dexmedetomidine has also been shown, compared with placebo, to decrease the incidence of delirium without a difference in any other clinical outcome measures.[31] Despite their common use, a 2018 Cochrane review showed that antipsychotics have no effect on delirium severity or mortality.[32] *The only conclusive preventative measure is nonpharmacologic therapies that include establishing a sleep/wake cycle and frequent reorientation.*

Delirium management is complex and involves a combination of pharmacologic and nonpharmacologic therapies. Nonpharmacologic mechanisms include treating any underlying medical conditions, managing pain, using sedation holidays, and providing frequent reorientation. Antipsychotic agents are often used to treat hyperactive delirium (i.e., agitation). Haloperidol, a first-generation (typical) antipsychotic, blocks dopamine receptors in the central nervous system. Adverse effects include extrapyramidal reactions, such as rigidity and spasmodic movements,

and neuroleptic malignant syndrome with severe muscle rigidity and rhabdomyolysis. Atypical antipsychotics work through the same dopamine mechanism but are less likely to cause extrapyramidal symptoms.

CARDIOVASCULAR SYSTEM

The cardiovascular system is integral to the perfusion of all systemic organs. Cardiovascular dysfunction can be separated broadly into three categories: cardiac arrhythmias, cardiogenic shock, and myocardial ischemia. All of these areas are affected in the setting of primary cardiac dysfunction, such as heart failure or a myocardial infarction (MI), but they may also be affected by extracardiac disease processes. For example, pulmonary embolism (PE) can lead to right heart failure, hyperthyroidism can lead to arrhythmias, and increased metabolic demand can lead to cardiac ischemia. This section begins by briefly covering normal physiology, continues on to disorders encountered in these three areas and their treatments, and concludes with invasive and noninvasive methods of monitoring the heart and fluid status.

Cardiac Physiology

The heart is a two-pump circuit in sequence. All blood that goes out of the right ventricle to the pulmonary circulation must then be pumped out of the left ventricle to the system circulation, with important exceptions that arise in the setting of congenital cardiac anomalies and a minor exception from bronchial arteries and veins. There is a vast difference in resistance between the pulmonary vascular bed faced by the right heart and the systemic vascular bed faced by the left heart, with the pulmonary pressures and resistance being significantly lower. The heart's ultimate function is to supply oxygenated blood to the tissues of the human body. This is quantified by the oxygen delivery (DO_2) equation:

$$\text{Oxygen delivery} = (\text{cardiac output [CO]})(\text{hemoglobin} \times 1.3 \times \text{oxygen saturation} + 0.003 \times \text{partial pressure of dissolved oxygen})$$

In examining this equation, one observation is evident: the primacy of the hemoglobin and oxygen saturation in determining the carrying capacity of oxygen by the blood and the relatively trivial contribution of dissolved oxygen. CO is defined as the blood flow put out by the heart per unit time, typically expressed in liters per minute. In an average-sized adult, CO is 4 to 6 L/min. A common method of normalizing the CO is the use of cardiac index (CI), which is defined as the CO per unit total body surface area (TBSA).

Vascular resistance is the collective resistance of all vessels, including arteries and veins, against the flow of blood, and there are two such resistances: the SVR faced by the left ventricle and the pulmonary vascular resistance (PVR) faced by the right. The relationship between flow, pressure, and resistance is defined by Ohm's law:

$$V = IR$$

which can be translated to any portion of the cardiovascular circuit as follows:

$$\text{Pressure gradient} = (\text{flow})(\text{resistance})$$

For example, (MAP – CVP) = CO(SVR), where MAP = mean arterial pressure, and CVP = central venous pressure, but this can likewise be applied to the pulmonary circulation.

These relationships guide decisions about fluid and vasopressor therapy, which are discussed later. The lower PVR consequently requires a smaller right heart muscle volume (lower pulmonary artery pressure) to supply the lungs with the same CO as the rest of the body. This means that the right heart is unable to maintain its CO in the face of large, acute rises in PVR, and this lack of reserve has significant consequences in situations such as trauma pneumonectomy and acute PE. In both these situations, a sudden rise in PVR, particularly in the context of a low preload, can lead to cardiovascular collapse.

The myocardium is supplied primarily by the coronary arteries. During systole, the subendocardial vessels experience retrograde flow, and thus, the heart is primarily supplied during diastole. Additionally, the aortic valve leaflets cover the coronary ostia to an extent during normal systole and aortic flow. This has important implications for cardiopulmonary resuscitation because failure to allow for full recoil of the chest may reduce blood supply to the subendocardium during resuscitation.

The heart's rhythm is controlled by pacemaker cells. The primary node is the sinoatrial node, which is influenced by sympathetic stimulation from the sympathetic trunk, mainly arising from the T1 to T4 spinal levels, which stimulates positive chronotropy. Parasympathetic stimulation results in negative chronotropy and is mediated via the vagus nerve. The heart has a series of escape pacemakers, which are, in order, the atria, the atrioventricular (AV) node, and the ventricles themselves. As long as the sinoatrial node paces above the intrinsic rate of these escape pacemakers, and as long as those impulses are transmitted through the AV node and to the ventricles, impulses from the sinoatrial node control the heart rate.

Cardiac Arrhythmias

Supraventricular Tachycardias

Atrial fibrillation. Postoperative atrial fibrillation is common, occurring in 8% of major surgery and 45% of cardiac/thoracic operations. Recent work has noted that the risk of thromboembolism after the development of atrial fibrillation after noncardiac surgery is similar to that of patients with nonvalvular atrial fibrillation. However, although the 2016 European Society of Cardiology guidelines now recommend anticoagulation for postoperative atrial fibrillation after cardiac surgery, they do not address other major surgical procedures. In general, if the rhythm persists for >48 hours after surgery, consideration should be given to initiate anticoagulation based on CHA_2DS_2VASc score, as with other, nonoperative patients, provided the surgical bleeding risk is acceptable.

For atrial fibrillation with rapid ventricular response, acute management is dependent on the hemodynamic stability of the patient. If the patient is acutely unstable, immediate synchronized electrocardioversion is mandated, as it is for any tachyarrhythmia causing acute instability. In the context of hemodynamic stability, pharmacologic methods should be employed, including amiodarone, β-blockers, and calcium channel blockers. Amiodarone is favored in the context of heart failure because calcium channel blockers are contraindicated in heart failure. That said, a recent retrospective review documented that metoprolol had the greatest success in the treatment of acute atrial fibrillation, defined by rate control without the need for a second agent. Other studies have noted more rapid rate control (without cardioversion) of atrial fibrillation with diltiazem in both the emergency department and the ICU but also noted an increased rate of hypotension with its use relative to amiodarone. Acutely, digoxin alone is not recommended owing to its slow onset and comparative lower success in controlling atrial fibrillation, although this is sometimes used in conjunction with the aforementioned agents and in the long term in the setting of refractory atrial fibrillation.

Two points of caution should be noted. Traditionally, it was held that cardioversion of an atrial rhythm into a sinus rhythm could safely occur up to 48 hours after initiation of the rhythm. Thereafter, either a transesophageal echocardiogram to verify lack of clot formation in the left atrium or 4 weeks of anticoagulation was recommended before cardioversion if done after the initial 48 hours, except in cases of acute hemodynamic compromise. However, recent work suggests that the safe period of cardioversion may be much shorter, as little as 12 hours. Although all drugs used to treat atrial fibrillation may induce cardioversion into sinus rhythm, amiodarone is especially prone to do so. Thus, it should be used with caution in patients with longer time periods of atrial fibrillation because of its higher tendency to result in a return to sinus rhythm. Second, in patients with an accessory pathway, such as Wolf-Parkinson-White syndrome, atrial fibrillation with preexcitation may develop. The use of calcium channel blockers, β-blockers, amiodarone, and digoxin is contraindicated in such instances because of the risk that after suppression of the AV node, the accessory pathway will result in an exacerbated tachycardia. In this scenario, ibutilide or procainamide is recommended by the most recent guidelines.

In summary, if the patient is hemodynamically stable, carefully review 12-lead electrocardiograms (ECGs) (both those taken during the acute episode and historical comparisons, if available) to confirm the rhythm and rule out an accessory pathway, and make aggressive attempts at prompt chemical cardioversion using β-blockade and/or amiodarone. If the rhythm persists, a transition to a rate control strategy with β-blockers or calcium channel blockers and consideration of anticoagulation may be warranted.

Multifocal atrial tachycardia. Multifocal atrial tachycardia is most commonly associated with hypomagnesemia. Pulmonary insufficiency, hypokalemia, and coronary artery disease are other known precipitating factors. An empiric push of 6 mg of IV magnesium sulfate often terminates multifocal atrial tachycardia. If correcting hypomagnesemia and hypokalemia (in that order) is not effective, then β-blockers and calcium channel blockers should be tried.

Atrial flutter. Atrial flutter is commonly caused by the same disorders that give rise to atrial fibrillation. It is also not infrequent after the treatment of atrial fibrillation with amiodarone. It is an unstable rhythm and has the potential to spontaneously degenerate into atrial fibrillation or revert to normal sinus rhythm, particularly if the underlying factors have been addressed. The management of atrial flutter is similar to that of atrial fibrillation, with rate- and rhythm-control options, but electrocardioversion is the preferred therapy. Antiarrhythmic drug therapy is also an option and may be selected for stable patients who are too high risk to undergo the sedation that would typically be required before electrocardioversion. Additionally, ibutilide is FDA approved for the conversion of atrial flutter to normal sinus rhythm and has shown superiority to amiodarone and procainamide in this setting. It should be remembered that all antiarrhythmic drugs have proarrhythmic tendencies, and ibutilide is no exception, with a significant risk of torsades de pointes. It must be used with caution in patients at high risk for torsades de pointes, and patients should be in a monitored setting after its use. IV magnesium given alongside ibutilide will enhance its ability to break atrial flutter and prevent torsades de pointes.

Atrioventricular nodal reentrant tachycardia. There are numerous other subtypes of supraventricular tachycardias, of which the most common is AV nodal reentrant tachycardia. The pathophysiology is a reentrant circuit. Although it is sometimes difficult to distinguish from sinus tachycardia and ventricular tachycardia, blocking the AV node by using vagal maneuvers can reveal the underlying rhythm. Agents acting at the AV node (adenosine, β-blockers, and calcium channel blockers) are all options to terminate these rhythms. It is important to distinguish a paroxysmal supraventricular tachycardia with a block from a ventricular tachycardia because both may present with a widened QRS. A history of heart disease or operation portends a ventricular tachycardia. Furthermore, adenosine will aid in distinguishing the rhythms because it will stop a supraventricular tachycardia but not a ventricular tachycardia. Additionally, ventricular tachycardia will not respond to β-blockers or calcium channel blockers.

Ventricular Tachycardia

Monomorphic ventricular tachycardia. Ventricular arrhythmias are rare in young patients and those without a history of heart disease. Options for treatment in stable patients include lidocaine, amiodarone, and procainamide; these are also adjuncts to consider if initial defibrillation for stable or unstable patients fails to convert a ventricular tachycardia into a sinus rhythm. Additionally, a recent study demonstrated the superiority of procainamide to amiodarone in the conversion of stable ventricular tachycardia. Because procainamide is a therapeutic option for atrial fibrillation with rapid ventricular response, supraventricular tachycardias, and ventricular tachycardias, it may be a reasonable option if one is uncertain of the rhythm. Although some patients with ventricular tachycardia may appear stable, they are at high risk for sudden deterioration and must be monitored closely and treated expeditiously.

Polymorphic ventricular tachycardia. Fundamentally, a monomorphic ventricular tachycardia indicates that ectopic beats are arising from one, often ischemic, focus in the ventricles, typically secondary to coronary artery disease. Polymorphic ventricular tachycardia indicates either multiple foci of ectopic beats or, more commonly, global dysfunction. The latter is a rhythm classically known as *torsades de pointes,* a feared rhythm for which a predisposing factor is a prolonged QT interval. This can be caused by a variety of drugs and with or without an inherited prolonged QT interval. It is imperative to note that many antiarrhythmics, including procainamide, lidocaine, and ibutilide, prolong the QT interval, as do commonly used antipsychotic drugs such as haloperidol and antiemetics such as ondansetron. The treatment is focused on aggressive administration of magnesium and unsynchronized cardioversion if unstable.

Bradycardia

Similar to the tachyarrhythmias, management of bradycardia can be broken down into pharmacologic and electrical support. In some cases, bradycardia may be physiologic or the patient's baseline (e.g., many young trauma patients). If the bradycardia is not causing any hemodynamic compromise, it may not be necessary to treat. However, sudden acute and symptomatic bradycardia may be indicative of severe underlying pathology, including acute spinal cord injury, MI, hypoxia, and various toxicologic states, as well as global dysfunction from severe sepsis. In general ICU populations, bradycardia can be a sign of profound cardiac dysfunction. Acute management includes atropine, epinephrine, and

pacing; however, these are temporary supports (apart from spinal cord injury), and the priority must be reversal of the underlying cause.

Sinus bradycardia. Sinus bradycardia may be a normal resting rhythm for many fit, young individuals, and no treatment is required. However, context is important because it may also be seen in profound shock states as a peri-arrest rhythm. Most cases of hemodynamically stable sinus bradycardia can be treated with atropine. Sinus bradycardia secondary to a spinal cord injury can occur in high (cervical) spinal cord injuries and should be treated with atropine and concomitant vasopressor therapy to treat neurogenic shock as required (an agent with additional chronotropic effects should be considered). Similarly, sinus bradycardia associated with MI, commonly seen in inferior wall infarctions as a result of involvement of the sinoatrial node, can be treated with atropine as well.

Sinus bradycardia secondary to the use of dexmedetomidine, increasingly used for sedation and anxiolysis in the ICU, requires a different mindset. If this occurs, treatment of the resultant hypotension with vasopressors is required until the drug wears off, and/or pacing may be required if the hypotension is significant and unresponsive to moderate vasopressor use. Atropine and epinephrine will be ineffective with this etiology because of the α_1-antagonist effect of dexmedetomidine.

Heart block, junctional or ventricular bradycardia. Junctional or ventricular bradycardia is a result of profound AV node dysfunction. There is no apparent atrial activity. Treatment with temporary pacing may be required if the CO falls. Atropine is not effective in this scenario because it acts on the dysfunctional AV node.

Relatedly, AV conduction blocks may result in bradycardia.[33] In a first-degree block, there is simply a delay in conduction between atria and ventricles, with a PR interval >0.2 s. In a second-degree block, beats are intermittently not conducted through the AV node. In a second-degree Mobitz I ("Wenckebach") block, there is a progressive lengthening of the PR interval until a ventricular beat is eventually dropped. The cycle then starts again. In a Mobitz II block, the PR interval is constant, but intermittent beats are dropped. In a third-degree or "complete" heart block, there is no relationship between atrial and ventricular rhythms. First-degree blocks generally do not require treatment, third-degree blocks will often require pacing, and indications for pacing in second-degree blocks are dependent on context and hemodynamic stability.

Shock

The most severe hemodynamic alteration is shock, which is a condition of circulatory failure resulting in end-organ dysfunction secondary to reduced perfusion. A shock state itself is indicated by signs of end-organ dysfunction, such as rising lactate, altered mental status, falling urine output, and liver enzyme elevation. Each form of shock demands different responses, and when different forms of shock are combined, the appropriate diagnosis and management can be challenging. Shock is classified broadly into four categories: distributive, hypovolemic, cardiogenic, and obstructive.

Distributive Shock

Neurogenic shock. Neurogenic shock occurs secondary to the loss of sympathetic tone after a spinal cord injury. The overall etiology is decreased vascular resistance; however, there are two variants based on the location of the spinal cord injury. In lower spinal cord injuries below C5, the hypotension causes an appropriate reflex tachycardia. In higher spinal cord injuries at C5 and above, the patient is often bradycardic because the heart does not respond appropriately to the increased vagal tone due to the lack of sympathetic innervation to the heart. Neurogenic shock generally results in a "warm" shock because peripheral vasculature remains dilated. Treatment consists of vasopressor support to maintain blood pressure. Although phenylephrine was previously considered the first-line pressor in neurogenic shock for the sake of peripheral vasoconstriction, norepinephrine is increasingly used, particularly in bradycardic patients.

Of note, neurogenic shock does not equate to spinal shock. Spinal shock is *not* a hemodynamic phenomenon; rather, it results in the temporary loss of reflexes after a spinal cord injury, most commonly the bulbocavernosus and cremasteric reflexes. Although these phenomena may co-present in the setting of spinal cord injury, they are to be distinguished.

Septic shock. Septic shock is one of the most common types of shock encountered in the surgical ICU and consists of a dysregulated immune response arising from inflammatory mediators released by the body in response to bacterial or fungal pathogens. In the past, sepsis was defined as a systemic inflammatory response syndrome (SIRS) accompanied by a suspected source of infection, with SIRS being defined as derangements in two or more of four parameters: white blood cell count, temperature, heart rate, and respiratory rate. Also previously, septic shock was then sepsis unresponsive to fluid resuscitation, requiring vasopressor support to maintain the blood pressure. These definitions are now considered outdated, and they have been superseded by new guidelines that base the definition of sepsis and septic shock on sequential organ failure assessment (SOFA) scores. Specifically, organ dysfunction represented by an increase in SOFA score of 2 or more represents sepsis, whereas sepsis with hypotension despite fluid resuscitation and/or a serum lactate greater than 2 despite a lack of hypovolemia represents septic shock.[34] A "quick SOFA" or "qSOFA" consists of respiratory rate, altered mentation, and low systolic blood pressure and may be used similarly, although it should be noted that the most recent Surviving Sepsis Campaign guidelines recommend against using qSOFA over SIRS or other previous criteria.[35]

Previous sepsis management guidelines included immediate lactate measurement (and other laboratory values), an empiric 2-L fluid bolus, empiric antibiotic administration after cultures being drawn, appropriate measurement and titration of fluid resuscitation to CVP and central venous oxygen saturation, and potentially a Swan-Ganz catheter to accurately capture hemodynamic variables. This was known as an *early goal-directed therapy* (EGDT).[36] Subsequent randomized controlled trials suggest little benefit to this type of "bundle"; however, some feel that the control groups were flawed in that much of EGDT has become the standard of care. If anything, these studies showed that attempting to correct every hemodynamic metric may result in overresuscitation. Currently, the underlying principles of EGDT—metric-guided hemodynamic resuscitation to goal euvolemia—are still very much accepted; what has changed are the hemodynamic measures of volume status.

What is widely accepted is that early recognition and administration of antibiotics lead to increased survival, although this must be balanced against the risk of increasing antibiotic resistance and the harms associated with administering antibiotics to patients who do not require them. Early source control of the infection is also positively associated with outcomes.

Regarding treatment, it is important to realize that the underlying pathophysiology consists of both vasodilation and leakage of fluid into the interstitial spaces resulting from an increase in vascular permeability. Consequently, increasing vasoconstriction alone will not by itself reverse the shock state. Traditionally, fluid resuscitation followed by vasopressor therapy only when fluids no longer produce an increase in blood pressure (fluid responsiveness) has been standard.

The most recent updated guidelines for the overall management of sepsis were released by the Surviving Sepsis Campaign in 2021.[35] They continue to recommend crystalloid fluid resuscitation in the form of 30 cc/kg in the first 3 hours. Less controversially, the guidelines recommend continued close monitoring, a target MAP of 65 mm Hg, and the use of lactate as a measure of tissue hypoperfusion and as a guide to resuscitation.[37] The use of CVP to guide fluid resuscitation has been largely discredited, owing to its inability to reliably predict fluid responsiveness. In its place, the guidelines recommend the use of dynamic parameters, including passive leg raise, fluid challenges, pulse pressure variation in response to mechanical ventilation, and other techniques. Many devices and techniques exist to predict fluid responsiveness, but ultimately, clinical judgment must still be used to interpret the end points of resuscitation and guide fluid resuscitation and vasopressor therapy in septic shock states.

Currently, when crystalloid fluid resuscitation is not effective at raising blood pressure, the vasopressor of choice is norepinephrine, which has been shown to be superior to the other vasopressors. Epinephrine can be substituted if norepinephrine is inadequate, particularly if a cardiogenic component of shock is suspected; however, it may lead to falsely elevated lactate concentrations and difficulty in using this as an end point for resuscitation. Phenylephrine should not be considered a first-line agent because it has been associated with higher in-hospital mortality in septic shock.

When norepinephrine requirements increase significantly (past a value of approximately 5 mcg/min), low-dose vasopressin should be added. This is based on research suggesting a relative vasopressin deficiency in inflammatory vasodilatory shock. The dose is 0.04 units/min and may decrease norepinephrine requirements to maintain the blood pressure. High-dose vasopressin is not recommended. When high doses of norepinephrine and added vasopressin are insufficient, epinephrine may then be added, with no data suggesting a clear benefit. Dobutamine may also be used to augment tissue perfusion if the CO is low.

The use of corticosteroids in septic shock has been controversial for over three decades. The current recommendation by the Surviving Sepsis Campaign is for low-dose steroids in vasopressor-dependent, volume-replete septic shock. There have been several studies investigating the use of glucocorticoids in septic shock, with mixed results. For example, the Adjunctive Glucocorticoid Therapy in Patients with Septic Shock (ADRENAL) study did not demonstrate decreased 90-day mortality, but it did demonstrate faster resolution of shock and shorter initial duration of mechanical ventilation.[38]

Other etiologies of distributive shock. Other etiologies of distributive shock include anaphylactic and endocrine shock. The former occurs in response to an allergic stimulus, with the first-line treatment being epinephrine. Optionally, adjuncts such as diphenhydramine and steroids may be used. It should be noted that diphenhydramine does not manage airway symptoms and may cause hypotension, and steroids take several hours to be effective and have never been proven to be of benefit.

Endocrine shock results from severe myxedema coma from hypothyroidism and Addisonian crisis from acquired or iatrogenic hypothalamic-pituitary-adrenal axis suppression. The diagnosis depends on an accurate history and physical examination in both cases. Often, until laboratory tests rule out coexisting Addison disease, the treatment for myxedema coma includes empiric steroids alongside levothyroxine and liothyronine.

Hypovolemic Shock

Hypovolemic shock is characterized by increased SVR and decreased CO, with the latter being secondary to decreased preload. This is a so-called "cold shock," with cold extremities secondary to vasoconstriction. For hypovolemic shock from dehydration or fluid losses, the treatment is relatively straightforward and includes fluid resuscitation with crystalloid.

Hemorrhagic Shock

In hemorrhagic shock, blood products are the resuscitative fluid of choice. Crystalloid administration leads to anemia and coagulopathy. Broadly speaking, two resuscitation strategies are possible: empiric resuscitation, often with a so-called "massive transfusion protocol" (MTP),[39] or resuscitation based on analysis of clotting via thromboelastography (TEG) or rotational thromboelastometry (ROTEM). If empiric transfusion is to be pursued, this can be done with either component therapy or using whole blood. The first strategy, administration of blood products in an empiric ratio, is commonly employed in many centers as part of an MTP to be administered until control of bleeding can be obtained and/or resuscitation end points have been met. Alongside this are adjuncts such as the administration of tranexamic acid (TXA).[40] If component therapy is used, a 1:1:1 ratio of plasma (i.e., fresh frozen plasma [FFP]) to packed red blood cells (pRBCs) to platelets should be used. Recent data suggest that, if available, whole blood may be superior to component therapy in hemorrhagic shock.[41]

Although empiric whole blood and/or component therapy is certainly a reasonable approach, if available, viscoelastic testing (TEG or ROTEM) may be beneficial. These are dynamic tests of clotting ability and strength—for example, TEG uses vibration of a blood sample at a fixed frequency, with a light detector to measure meniscus motion. The impedance of the clot is displayed graphically over time, providing guidance as to which components or adjuncts (i.e., FFP, cryoprecipitate, platelets, or TXA) may be helpful.

There is some evidence for the use of TEG to augment empiric MTPs in trauma. In general, it seems that outcomes are equivalent *until* the amount of resuscitation surpasses a certain threshold. In a study from 2013, outcomes were generally similar, but there was a mortality benefit to TEG versus empiric MTP (33.3% vs. 54.1%) in patients with a penetrating mechanism who received more than 10 units of pRBCs.[42] This suggests that, at a minimum, once transfusion requirements surpass some threshold, TEG may be helpful. This has resulted in an Eastern Association for the Surgery of Trauma (EAST) practice management guideline endorsing TEG in trauma, surgical patients, and ICU patients.[43]

Although there is minimal evidence for the use of early vasopressors in hemorrhagic shock,[44] few would disagree that this may be a necessary temporizing adjunct as blood products are administered. Furthermore, there is specific evidence for a "vasopressin-deficient" state in which vasopressin administration may be helpful.[45]

Cardiogenic Shock

Cardiogenic shock is a "cold" shock in that it is characterized by decreased CO because of intrinsic "pump failure" or cardiac heart dysfunction, with compensatory vasoconstriction. Numerous causes for heart failure resulting in cardiogenic shock exist, but the most commonly seen is the acute or long-term sequelae of coronary artery disease. This shock state has multiple variants, including diastolic versus systolic failure and left heart versus right heart failure. Valvular obstruction may also be a cause of dysfunction. Heart failure progresses through three stages. Initially, the filling pressure of the ventricle increases, but contractility is preserved at the expense of increased pressure and congestion in the lungs. Next, the stroke volume begins to fall, but an increase in heart rate preserves CO. Finally, CO begins to fall.

Right heart failure. The mainstay of right heart failure therapy is straightforward. This includes fluid boluses until clinical euvolemia is achieved, followed by inodilator therapy with dobutamine or milrinone. This being said, fluid therapy must be used judiciously because dilation of the right ventricle may cause the septum to bow out into the left ventricle, resulting in decreased left ventricular function through interventricular interdependence. Inodilators both dilate the vasculature, reducing blood pressure, and promote CO by increasing contractility. They are ideal choices when the CO is low and the SVR high, but they often are not options if systemic blood pressure is low. For this reason, inodilators in conjunction with vasopressors such as norepinephrine are a commonly pursued strategy, with the inodilator titrated to the CO and the vasopressor titrated to an appropriate systemic blood pressure. Likewise, management of systemic hypotension accompanied by right heart failure should avoid vasopressors that increase the PVR (e.g., phenylephrine) and should instead favor those that do not (e.g., vasopressin, receptors for which do not exist in the pulmonary vasculature).

Left heart failure. It is imperative to determine the patient's fluid status when managing left heart failure. Although diuretics historically have been given to almost all patients in left heart failure on the basis of the theory that such patients are past the inflection point on the Starling curve, in reality, patients who are in cardiogenic shock may be fluid overloaded, hypovolemic, or euvolemic. Determination of fluid status may be deceptively difficult. Measures to determine volume status should include weight, pedal edema, and inferior vena cava ultrasound. Newer noninvasive monitoring tools that employ proprietary arterial waveform analysis may be helpful in management of hemodynamically deranged patients, although their accuracy may be limited to specific conditions.[46]

Similarly, the heart failure patient may be hypertensive, normotensive, or hypotensive. If the patient is hypertensive, then nitroglycerin, nitroprusside, or nicardipine may be used. All three will decrease the afterload, allow for the forward flow of blood to peripheral tissues, reduce the myocardial oxygen demand, and protect the heart from ischemic damage. Nitroprusside has the risks of worsening coronary ischemia and causing cyanide toxicity, so it is less preferred compared with the other agents. If the blood pressure is normal in a state of cardiogenic shock, inodilators may be used. Vasodilators can also be used with caution as long as the blood pressure is maintained. Finally, if both the blood pressure and CO are low, epinephrine or dopamine infusions may be tried; however, because of their peripheral vasoconstriction, they can further increase the afterload and worsen the patient's condition. This state has an extremely high mortality, and if it is refractory to pharmacologic measures, mechanical circulatory support may be warranted. These options include intraaortic balloon pumps, left ventricular assist devices, and venoarterial (VA) extracorporeal membrane oxygenation (ECMO). If a facility does not have these resources in-house, the patient should be considered for transfer to a center with these capabilities, possibly by having a mobile unit from the accepting facility arrive at bedside and placing the patient on mechanical circulatory support before transfer.

Obstructive Shock

The etiologies of obstructive shock include tension pneumothorax, cardiac tamponade, constrictive pericarditis, and massive PE. In all cases, the treatment is interventional in that it requires removal of the cause of the obstructive shock. Options include a needle decompression or thoracostomy tube in the case of pneumothorax; pericardiocentesis, pericardial window, or thoracotomy/sternotomy in the case of tamponade; and heparinization and systemic or catheter-directed thrombolysis with or without thrombectomy in the case of PE. A high index of suspicion is required in making these diagnoses.

Myocardial Infarction

Both myocardial ischemia and MI are feared entities in the perioperative period, both of them portending significant morbidity and mortality. The lack of ischemic symptoms or ECG changes associated with a rise in troponins is not a sign of safety; mortality remains high. Two fundamental types of MI exist. Type 1 MI is based on atherosclerotic plaque rupture and consequent ischemia and infarction of muscle that was being supplied by that blood vessel. In contrast, type 2 MI is based on a mismatch of the supply of blood and the heart's demand for it and is also commonly referred to as *demand ischemia*. The treatments for each type of MI flow naturally from their causes: revascularization for type 1 MI and reduction of cardiac oxygen demand for type 2 MI.

Type 1 MIs can be broken down into ST-elevation MI (STEMI) and non-STEMI (NSTEMI). As its name indicates, a STEMI classically involves symptoms and elevations in cardiac enzymes as well as evidence of ST elevations on ECG, whereas an NSTEMI is similar but without ECG evidence of infarction. Unstable angina is a symptom of ischemia but without cardiac biomarker elevation indicating injury. All three together form part of the spectrum of acute coronary syndrome.

The treatment of a type 1 MI in the postoperative period focuses on a percutaneous coronary intervention, with thrombolysis as an option if timely percutaneous coronary intervention is unavailable. In NSTEMI, intervention can be delayed in some cases for up to 72 hours. However, the overall intervention decision is complicated by the added burden of deciding on the risks and benefits of full-dose systemic anticoagulation in postoperative patients. In certain populations, such as those who recently underwent neurosurgical procedures, the risks of stroke or death from hemorrhage make percutaneous coronary intervention with its attendant anticoagulation unacceptable, whereas in other patients, the risks can be accepted.

In addition to the primary intervention, the complications of an acute MI must be managed. Cardiogenic shock should be managed as previously discussed. Nitroglycerin, either sublingual or IV, can be given for hypertension and chest pain. The distinction between a right- and left-sided MI is critical because giving nitroglycerin to reduce the afterload and myocardial oxygen demand in the setting of presumed left-sided MI may reduce the preload, resulting in right-sided heart failure if in fact the patient is suffering a right-sided MI. This could have catastrophic consequences. Pain control with any IV opiate, such as morphine, can be used to control chest pain symptoms if not relieved by nitroglycerin. The patient should be given aspirin and additional anticoagulant medications as specified by local protocol and depending on the course of therapy chosen. β-blockers should be initiated if there are no signs of cardiogenic shock because these are cardioprotective. However, if the patient is hypotensive or has a decreased ejection fraction or bradycardia, these should be avoided. Above all else, a defibrillator should be immediately available for the case in which the patient degenerates into a life-threatening unstable arrhythmia.

RESPIRATORY SYSTEM

A common manifestation of critical illness is respiratory failure requiring mechanical ventilation. Acute respiratory failure is caused by an inflammatory response resulting in alveolar collapse and interstitial edema, both resulting in hypoxia. The mainstay of treatment is supportive while minimizing the complications of positive pressure ventilation itself. Mastery of both airway management and mechanical ventilation is fundamental to the practice of critical care medicine.

Respiratory Physiology

Respiratory physiology is characterized by two linked processes: oxygenation and ventilation. *Oxygenation* refers to the addition of oxygen (O_2) to the bloodstream from inspired air. The fraction of inspired oxygen (FiO_2) of room air is typically 21%. Ventilation is the clearance of carbon dioxide (CO_2) generated by cellular respiration from the bloodstream. Although it is easiest to conceptualize these processes as entirely separate, they are clearly interrelated.

Both processes rely on air coming down the oral cavity, into the trachea, through the bronchi, and into the lung parenchyma (ventilation), where blood from the pulmonary arteries and arterioles flows to meet it (perfusion) at the alveolar-capillary interface. Ventilation is commonly referred to as *V*, whereas perfusion is commonly referred to as *Q*, such that an imbalance of ventilation and perfusion is referred to as *V/Q mismatch*. At the extremes of V/Q mismatch are shunt physiology, in which there is perfusion without ventilation, and dead space physiology, in which there is ventilation without perfusion. Some amount of both of these is normal: Less than 10% of total CO does not participate in gas exchange, and 20% to 30% of total ventilation does not equilibrate with blood. Increases in shunt fraction occur secondary to asthma, distention of alveoli from pulmonary edema or pneumonia, atelectasis, or PE, where excessive CO flows through nonembolized regions. Dead space ventilation takes place when the alveolar-capillary interface is destroyed by emphysema, when the CO is low, or when air overdistends the alveoli during positive pressure ventilation. It should be noted that there is some amount of "physiologic dead space"—that is, parts of the respiratory tract that do not participate in air exchange, including the trachea and bronchi.

Oxygen Therapy

Although supplemental oxygen via nasal cannula (NC) is commonplace in the ICU, it must be emphasized that oxygen itself is a drug, with risks and benefits, and should be used only when indicated. In intubated and mechanically ventilated patients, a target FiO₂ should be less than 50% if tolerated because this setting appears to be safe and without risks of pulmonary toxicities. Although theoretically, the FiO₂ could be dropped to 21% if tolerated, this is not commonly done, with extubation often taking place at an FiO₂ of 30% to 40% (and transitioning to another mode of supplementary oxygen delivery).

Noninvasive Ventilation

Some patients in impending respiratory failure may avoid intubation with noninvasive ventilatory support via continuous or bilevel positive airway pressure (CPAP or BIPAP). As the names suggest, CPAP involves the continuous delivery of a single set level of pressure, whereas BIPAP is set to different pressures for inspiration (IPAP) and exhalation (EPAP). Both CPAP and BIPAP provide positive end-expiratory pressure (PEEP), helping to keep the alveoli open at the end of expiration; BIPAP also adds extra pressure above and beyond the PEEP. Both CPAP and BIPAP are often worn at night by many patients with sleep apnea at home and should be provided to such patients in the hospital if indicated. BIPAP in particular has been shown to significantly benefit patients with pulmonary edema from a congestive heart failure exacerbation and is well suited to providing support over CPAP in cases of hypercarbic ventilatory insufficiency.

It is important to remember the contraindications of such devices, including altered mental status and consequent inability to protect the airway. Both machines involve a mask worn over the face, and any large-volume emesis event can rapidly turn into a large-volume aspiration and cardiac arrest event. Furthermore, the use of these modalities in patients with fresh esophageal, gastric, or duodenal anastomoses is relatively contraindicated because the positive pressure can increase upper GI insufflation. Although the normal resting pressure of the lower esophageal sphincter is greater than 10 mm Hg and noninvasive positive pressure ventilation (NIPPV; including CPAP and BIPAP) would often not exceed this pressure, many conditions and patient characteristics can reduce this protective mechanism and make the use of NIPPV a riskier proposition.

High-Flow Nasal Cannula

High-flow nasal cannula (HFNC) is another noninvasive mode of ventilatory support, by which oxygen is delivered at considerably higher flow rates than is achievable by regular NC. Whereas regular NC can deliver a maximum of about 10 L/min, HFNC can deliver oxygen up to 100% FiO₂ via up to 60 L/min of flow. Although there is some thought that HFNC may provide "some" positive pressure, this seems mechanistically unlikely, and the benefit seems more likely to simply be due to the more rapid delivery of oxygen. A 2015 study randomized hypoxic patients to HFNC, NC, or NIPPV and found no difference in intubation rates, but it did find favorable results for HFNC with regard to 90-day mortality.[47] There may also be some benefit to HFNC after extubation; a randomized trial in 2016 demonstrated a lower rate of 72-hour reintubation with HFNC versus conventional NC.[48]

Intubation and Mechanical Ventilation

Broadly, the indications for intubation are (1) airway protection, (2) hypoxia, and (3) hypercarbia. "Airway protection" can be required for a variety of reasons. One is depressed mental status, which is often taught with the mnemonic "GCS less than 8,

intubate." However, this practice is not based on evidence and has been questioned in recent years.[49] Alternatively, impending loss of airway patency can be caused by edema secondary to hereditary angioedema, trauma, severe allergic reactions, or airway burns.

Hypoxia may be a result of pneumonia, pulmonary contusion, severe pulmonary edema, or acute respiratory distress syndrome (ARDS), among other causes. Hypercarbia and hypoventilation may be a result of respiratory depression secondary to opioids or other sedating medications, exhaustion and subsequent inadequate respiratory effort in the setting of increased work of breathing, or spinal cord injury, among others. Patients with a high spinal cord injury (above C5) may have a delayed presentation of ventilatory failure because there may be initial compensation by accessory muscles.

Intubation and the induction medications required to perform it are not without risk. Particularly in the patient who is already hemodynamically unstable, intubation can trigger hemodynamic collapse. The causes are multifactorial, including hemodynamic shifts induced by induction agents, temporary hypoxia during the procedure itself, and the influence of positive pressure ventilation on venous return to the heart. It is essential to resuscitate patients adequately before intubation and to use adjuncts such as vasopressors before and during intubation if indicated.

Standard Modes of Mechanical Ventilation

There are essentially four basic parameters that may be set in any ventilator mode. The first is some measure of "how big" a breath to give. In a volume-controlled mode, this would be a tidal volume; in a pressure-controlled mode, this would be an inspiratory pressure. The second is some measure of "how often" to give a breath. In a completely controlled mode, this is a respiratory rate; in other modes of partial support, this may be only intermittently controlled, with the patient triggering some to all of their own breaths. Third is PEEP. There may be some variation in how this is referred to and used, particularly in more advanced modes like "bilevel" or airway pressure release ventilation (APRV), but there will nearly always be some amount of positive pressure present in the circuit. Finally, the ICU provider can modulate the amount of oxygen in the delivered breaths by setting the FiO₂. Next, we will discuss in more detail some of the more common ventilator modes.

Assist Control

Assist control (AC) is one of the most commonly used modes of mechanical ventilation. AC can be achieved by setting either a tidal volume ("volume control," VC) or inspiratory pressure ("pressure control," PC). The former is more common. The other three parameters are set as described earlier. If the patient is not breathing spontaneously, the set respiratory rate is exactly what the patient will receive. If the patient triggers their own breaths, they will receive a "full" breath as set each time.

The choice of VC or PC is often dependent on which variable the clinician wants to control more. As stated, VC is more common because we generally desire control over the patient's minute ventilation (i.e., tidal volume multiplied by the respiratory rate) to ensure adequate CO₂ clearance. However, in the case of very poor compliance, it may be desirable to control the pressure to guard against barotrauma. With either mode, the so-called "free" variable (i.e., the peak and plateau pressures while in VC and the tidal volumes when in PC) must be carefully monitored.

Peak pressure, as measured by the ventilator, is the sum of the dynamic airway pressure (flow × resistance) and the alveolar pressure. For the most part, the component of concern is the alveolar pressure because this is where there is potential for barotrauma. When faced with elevated peak airway pressures, the first step is to rule out causes of increased airway resistance, such as a kinked tube or auto-PEEP from breath stacking, as well as other causes, such as tension pneumothorax or asthma. The airway component of this equation can be removed from the question by measuring a plateau pressure using an "inspiratory hold" or pausing the ventilator at the end of inspiration. With no flow through the airways, that term of the equation goes to zero, and the alveolar pressure is isolated. A high plateau pressure is a better reflection of the pressure seen by the alveoli and lung compliance. Keeping the plateau pressure below 30 cm H_2O is felt to be lung protective.

Pressure Support Ventilation

Another fundamental mode of mechanical ventilation is pressure support ventilation (PSV). It is directly analogous to a BIPAP machine. Every breath the patient takes is supported by a set pressure support with additional PEEP that is constant throughout the respiratory cycle. There are no mandatory breaths; every breath is triggered by the patient. This mode is an excellent tool to wean the patient from mechanical ventilation and is discussed further under extubation.

Synchronized Intermittent Mandatory Ventilation

Synchronized intermittent mandatory ventilation (SIMV) is a hybrid of AC and PSV. The primary difference between AC and SIMV involves the spontaneous breaths. In AC, every patient-initiated breath receives full support up to the set tidal volume. In SIMV, a fifth parameter is set: pressure support. This value is analogous to the inspiratory positive airway pressure setting on BIPAP and provides a set level of pressure support for all spontaneous breaths. Thus, in SIMV, spontaneous breaths above and beyond the set rate generate whatever the patient is capable of doing with the applied pressure support. Notably, if the patient is fairly deeply sedated and/or the rate is set high enough, SIMV is essentially equivalent to VC because mandatory breaths are delivered at a set volume. On the contrary, if the rate is set low enough, the mode is essentially equivalent to PSV, perhaps with a minimal number (say, 2) of sigh breaths per minute. Those who advocate for the regular use of SIMV suggest that the benefit is in the ability to gradually wean between these two. Whether AC or SIMV forms the "default" mode of mechanical ventilation in an ICU is typically practitioner and unit specific.

Advanced Modes of Mechanical Ventilation
High-Frequency Oscillatory Ventilation

High-frequency oscillatory ventilation is an infrequently used mode involving extremely low tidal volumes at a high rate. It has been used as a salvage mode and/or a bridge to ECMO in severe ARDS. Although the concept behind this mode would seem to make physiologic sense in ARDS, clinical trials have not shown benefit.[50] There may be benefit in the pediatric population, but that topic is beyond the scope of this chapter.

Airway Pressure Release Ventilation and Bilevel Positive Airway Pressure Ventilation

Both APRV and bilevel ventilation provide two levels of CPAP that allow a mixture of spontaneous and ventilator-mandated breaths. They minimize the pressures seen by the alveoli and are thus most commonly used in patients with significantly reduced lung compliance, such as patients with ARDS. Specifically, APRV consists of a high CPAP (P_H) for a greater period of time (T_H), which then falls to a lower pressure (P_L) for a shorter period of time (T_L). This may be particularly useful in patients with severely noncompliant lungs and/or a large chest wall who suffer from frequent derecruitment. Bilevel is similar, but with a longer T_L. The specifics of these settings are beyond the scope of this text, but in brief, the P_H is set at a level to ensure oxygenation, whereas P_L and T_L are set to ensure adequate ventilation but not to allow for derecruitment. Opponents of these modes maintain that they can achieve similar results by adjusting the inspiratory and expiratory times in AC with resultant inverse ratio ventilation. Although these modes are still infrequently used compared with the other modes described earlier, there may be an appropriate population for which this is beneficial. A recent meta-analysis of nearly 19 years' worth of studies in patients with acute hypoxemic respiratory failure suggested a mortality benefit to APRV as compared with more conventional modes, although there was no difference in the need for rescue maneuvers such as prone positioning or ECMO.[51]

Extracorporeal Membrane Oxygenation

In patients with entirely refractory hypoxemia, ECMO may be considered. A detailed discussion of ECMO is beyond the scope of this chapter, but briefly, ECMO may be VA or venovenous (VV); the former is often used for those with concomitant cardiac dysfunction, and the latter is most often used for those with isolated lung pathology and hypoxia. An inflow cannula carries blood from a central vein, usually a common femoral vein, to an oxygenator, which both oxygenates and removes CO_2 through a membrane. This is done by diffusion, with "sweep gas" carried on the other side of the membrane. Blood then returns to the body via an outflow cannula, either to a central vein (common femoral or internal jugular) or artery (common femoral or, in the case of "central cannulation," the aorta). The use of ECMO may be controversial in some cases, particularly in those patients whose ability to recover is questionable; the technology should be considered a "bridge" therapy. However, the landmark CESAR (Efficacy and Economic Assessment of Conventional Ventilatory Support versus Extracorporeal Membrane Oxygenation for Severe Adult Respiratory Failure) trial suggested a mortality benefit to ECMO in patients with acute hypoxemic respiratory failure, and this is now a generally accepted indication.[52]

Extubation or Tracheostomy

Unless significant hemodynamic instability or other considerations prevent it, one should always be weaning the patient from the ventilator. The details of weaning techniques may vary by provider or center, but the overall idea is to slowly reduce the amount of support received by the patient in conjunction with increasing the amount of "work" the patient must do on their own. For example, when the patient is awake enough, a volume-controlled mode might be transitioned to a pressure support (spontaneous) mode, followed by a slow weaning of the amount of pressure support being provided, such that the patient is required to provide more of the work.

The weaning process, of course, culminates with extubation. The decision to extubate a patient is based on the following concepts:
1. Is the patient's airway patent (and can they protect it)?
2. Can the patient sufficiently oxygenate and ventilate?

In assessing airway patency, a leak test is performed. After deflation of the endotracheal tube cuff, a loss of 10% to 20% of the ventilated volume should be observed. If it is not, this suggests airway swelling to the degree that extubation may be perilous. IV steroids and reassessment in 24 hours are generally employed, although in some cases (particularly if there is a persistent lack of cuff leak over multiple days), extubation may be performed anyway with adequate precautions and preparations for reintubation. The patient must also be able to protect their airway, which is evaluated by the patient's GCS score and/or their ability to follow commands. Lack of ability to follow commands is not an absolute contraindication to extubation, particularly in neurosurgical patients; however, such decisions should be made by experienced clinicians.

There are numerous means of assessing the oxygenation and ventilation capabilities of the intubated patient. The successful tolerance of a spontaneous breathing trial is the best predictor of successful extubation. A spontaneous breathing trial is performed by placing the patient on a minimal amount of PSV, the standard for which varies by institution. For example, a patient may be placed on PSV 7/+5 at 40% FiO_2. Such settings essentially only compensate for the resistance of the endotracheal tube itself; it should be noted that the amount of pressure support that is considered "minimal" may vary with the size of the endotracheal tube. The rapid shallow breathing index (RSBI) is another commonly employed measure. While the patient is on pressure support, it is calculated by dividing the respiratory rate by the tidal volume (L). A variety of cutoff values have been used, but for example, an RSBI of less than 105 may be considered predictive of a successful extubation. However, a recent meta-analysis of data using a variety of cutoffs (nearly all of which were less than 105) suggested only moderate sensitivity and poor specificity of this metric.[53] Other respiratory mechanics, such as respiratory rate <25, negative inspiratory force more negative than -20 cm H_2O, tidal volume >5 cc/kg, minute ventilation <10 L/min, and vital capacity >10 cc/kg, have been used to predict successful extubation.

If a patient is likely to remain intubated for an extended period of time, conversion to a tracheostomy should be considered. Although the data on when to perform a tracheostomy are debatable, a commonly used date for evaluation is on mechanical ventilator day 7. Advocates for early tracheostomy cite decreased sedation needs, decreased airway risks, and more expedient liberation from the mechanical ventilator as benefits.

Pulmonary Pathology

Pulmonary Embolism

Pulmonary emboli primarily cause issues by two mechanisms: (1) increase in PVR with or without right heart strain and (2) increased dead space ventilation and resultant hypoxia. Prevention is the best weapon and should include early ambulation, intermittent pneumatic compression devices, and prophylactic low-level anticoagulation in at-risk populations (which includes nearly all surgical patients). The treatment consists of supplemental oxygen, along with systemic anticoagulation (heparin infusion or weight-based low-molecular-weight heparin) to prevent clot propagation. In severe cases, intubation, catheter-directed thrombolysis, pulmonary embolectomy, or ECMO may be required.

Pneumonia

Pneumonia is diagnosed by a new infiltrate on chest radiograph together with fever, leukocytosis, and/or purulent secretions.

However, these findings are common in the ICU, and this clinical diagnosis can be much more difficult than it may seem.

Community-acquired pneumonia. The recommended treatment of community-acquired pneumonia is a β-lactam combined with a macrolide. Patients with severe disease, including those with septic shock and respiratory failure requiring mechanical ventilation, as well as those empirically treated for methicillin-resistant *Staphylococcus aureus* (MRSA) or *Pseudomonas,* should undergo sputum culture and blood culture.[54]

Ventilator-associated pneumonia. The most recent joint American Thoracic Society and Infectious Diseases Society of America clinical practice guidelines recommend abandoning the term *hospital-acquired pneumonia,* but ventilator-associated pneumonia (VAP) remains a distinct entity and is defined as pneumonia diagnosed after a patient has been mechanically ventilated for more than 48 hours.

Before initiating therapy in VAP, it is critical to send cultures (bronchoalveolar lavage). Patients with VAP are at high risk for multidrug-resistant organisms, and any patients with septic shock, ARDS, 5 or more hospitalization days, and/or renal replacement therapy should be covered with broad-spectrum antibiotics, until cultures allow targeting of therapy, for a total of 7 days. Patients without these risk factors should be treated with a single agent covering *Pseudomonas,* other gram-negative bacilli, and methicillin-sensitive *S. aureus.* However, it should be noted that local practices, formularies, and antibiotic resistance patterns vary widely throughout the United States and the world. Development of guidelines in conjunction with an ICU pharmacist will lead to improved quality of care and outcomes.

A key in managing VAPs is prevention. All patients should have the head of the bed elevated to 30 to 45 degrees. Patients on a mechanical ventilator should also have daily chlorhexidine rinses and interruptions of sedation. The ultimate prevention measure for VAP is liberation from the mechanical ventilator as early as safely possible.

Acute Respiratory Distress Syndrome

ARDS is an inflammatory response of the lung to multiple inciting factors, including blood product transfusions, sepsis, severe pancreatitis, trauma, and bleeding and/or hypotension. It is characterized by decreasing ability to oxygenate and decreased compliance ($\Delta V / \Delta P$) of the lung. The so-called Berlin definition involves bilateral infiltrates on chest radiograph or CT scan, a PaO_2-to-FiO_2 ratio of <300 (<300 is mild, <200 is moderate, and <100 is severe), a known clinical insult within 7 days before the diagnosis, and an explanation for pulmonary edema other than heart failure or fluid overload. Although the last criterion formerly required the measurement of a wedge pressure, objective assessment may now include other means (e.g., ultrasound).[55]

The management of ARDS revolves around mechanical ventilator settings. It consists of several goals:
- 6- to 8-cc/kg tidal volumes
- PaO_2 55 to 80 mm Hg or SpO_2 88% to 95%
- Plateau pressure ≤30 cm H_2O
- pH 7.30 to 7.45

There are many adjuncts to assist in meeting oxygenation requirements. Diuresis and optimization of fluid status to reduce any extrapulmonary edema are a sensible first step. Additionally, deep sedation and/or neuromuscular blockade with paralytics can be employed to ensure lack of any ventilator asynchrony, although some authorities maintain that this step is unnecessary if sedation is sufficiently deep. Finally, prone positioning is one of the few options that have been shown to reduce mortality in a randomized controlled trial.[56] However, this intervention should be used with caution and in a unit with personnel experienced in this technique. Placing a patient prone significantly reduces access, and turning a patient who has many lines and other attachments is not a risk-free endeavor. Close coordination with nursing staff and all ancillary staff is required. If this method is used, it should be used early in the course of ARDS.

ECMO serves as a final option for refractory ARDS. As noted earlier, the CESAR trial documented reduced mortality for patients with ARDS referred to ECMO centers. Notably, approximately 25% of the group of patients transferred for possible ECMO did not actually receive ECMO. The more recent Extracorporeal Membrane Oxygenation for Severe Acute Respiratory Distress Syndrome (EOLIA) trial concluded that there was no significant benefit of ECMO.[57] It should be noted that this trial was stopped early, and the benefit or lack thereof remains unclear. Adoption of standard guidelines and algorithms at the institutional level is likely to be of benefit.

Steroids, inhaled nitric oxide, inhaled epoprostenol, and high-frequency oscillatory ventilation techniques have all been shown to have no mortality benefit and are not commonly used, although they do improve hypoxia. Similarly, the alternative modes of mechanical ventilation previously discussed, as well as inverse ratio ventilation, do not have a proven mortality benefit.

GASTROINTESTINAL SYSTEM

Nutritional Requirements of the Critically Ill Patient

The energy requirements of the critically ill patient are higher than the baseline caloric demands of the average patient because of the hypermetabolic state that is induced by acute stressors. Major trauma, surgery, burns, or critical illness such as sepsis, congestive heart failure, or respiratory failure induce a catabolic state with an increase in inflammation, cytokines, and subsequent loss of weight and lean body mass. Combined with underlying comorbidities, bed rest and inactivity, and poor oral feeding, it is common for the overall metabolic demands of a patient to exceed nutritional intake and result in malnutrition, poor healing, and an increase in complications.

The most recent (2021) American Society of Parenteral and Enteral Nutrition (ASPEN) guidelines for the critically ill patient recommend feeding 12 to 25 kcal/kg/day.[58] This represents a change from prior recommendations for higher-calorie feeding and is reflective of more recent evidence suggesting, at a minimum, a lack of harm of lower-calorie feeding, including The Augmented versus Routine approach to Giving Energy Trial (TARGET) trial of energy-dense versus routine enteral feeding.[59] Compared with carbohydrates and fats, protein requirements are considered proportionally higher and vital for wound healing, maintaining lean body mass and preventing its loss, and supporting immune function. That said, there is also recent evidence to suggest that high-protein feeding may not provide any benefit over lower-protein supplementation.[60] This is again reflected in the most up-to-date ASPEN guidelines.

Given that the serum markers of albumin, transferrin, and prealbumin are negative acute-phase reactants, in the setting of significant stress or trauma, their levels will decrease as a result of increases in vascular permeability and reallocation of hepatic protein synthesis. ASPEN recommends against using such markers as proxies for nutritional status, and their values should

be interpreted in conjunction with a patient's hospital course and clinical status.

Without a single modality to reliably and accurately measure a patient's overall nutritional status, one must continue to assess the patient with a complete physical exam, use clinical judgment, and gather additional data from ancillary studies to develop an individualized and comprehensive plan for nutritional support. Further aspects of nutritional support, including enteral versus parenteral nutrition, are covered in Chapter 34.

Stress Ulcer Prophylaxis

The GI mucosa is highly sensitive to the hemodynamic alterations often experienced by the critically ill patient. Splanchnic hypoperfusion, mucosal ischemia, reperfusion injury, and decreased mucosal protection can all result in the formation of ulcerations that have the potential to bleed or cause perforation. Mechanical ventilation influences a patient's hemodynamics, especially in cases that use high PEEP and/or higher than normal tidal volumes. Increased intrathoracic pressures decrease venous return and right heart filling, thus decreasing CO. Gastric ulcerations can be found in up to 90% of patients after severe trauma or hypotension, but their consequence is not clear because only a small percentage of these patients go on to have clinically relevant GI bleeding.

Classically, patients requiring mechanical ventilation for greater than 48 hours and the development of coagulopathy have been identified as the two main risk factors associated with the formation of GI ulcerations and GI bleeding. These patients are often administered gastric acid suppressants such as proton pump inhibitors (PPIs), histamine-2 receptor antagonists, or gastric mucosa protective agents, either as prophylaxis or treatment. Additional clinical considerations for which prophylaxis may be given include patients with elevated intracranial pressures (Cushing ulcer), burns (Curling ulcer), high-dose corticosteroid use, chronic or high-dose NSAID use, and prior history of gastric ulceration or GI bleed.

PPIs and histamine-2 receptor antagonists are the main choice for prophylaxis and treatment. They are not without risk because gastric acid is a natural barrier against pathogens, and suppression is thought to lead to gastric and duodenal bacterial overgrowth, aspiration pneumonia, and increased survival rates of *Clostridioides difficile*. In a recent randomized trial comparing PPIs to histamine-2 receptor antagonists, there was no difference in mortality, hospital length of stay, or *C. difficile* infection, although there was a lower rate of clinically important upper GI bleeding with PPIs. Notably, however, there was significant crossover from the H_2-blocker group to PPIs.[61]

There is controversy regarding the necessity of near-universal GI prophylaxis in light of significantly improved ICU care and the practice of early enteral feeding for GI mucosal maintenance and protection, resulting in less frequent use. Given the paucity of evidence outside of patients on mechanical ventilation and those with coagulopathy, neurotrauma, and new use of steroids or NSAIDs, it may be reasonable to restrict prophylaxis to these groups.

The Open Abdomen

The open abdomen is increasingly common in the ICU. It results from several situations, most commonly damage-control surgery and abdominal compartment syndrome. Damage-control surgery is a technique whereby patients who are critically ill but require urgent surgery—most often in the setting of trauma—are taken to the operating room for temporization of injuries and brought to the ICU with a temporary abdominal closure for correction of coagulopathy, hypothermia, and acidosis. Once stabilized, the patient returns to the operating room, where definitive repairs are performed.

The techniques of damage control will be addressed in other chapters. The review here focuses on the critical care elements. The primary goal for these patients in the ICU should be to correct the physiology—that is, any acidosis, hypothermia, and/or coagulopathy. Historically, the majority of these patients were traumatically injured. Increasingly, the concept of leaving the abdomen open is being employed in emergency general surgery (EGS), although often for other reasons (abdominal sepsis, the desire for a "second look")—there may be less for the critical care practitioner to correct in these patients.

Outside of the correction of deranged physiology, considerations for ICU providers include fluid management. The overuse of large-volume crystalloid resuscitation may result in bowel edema that decreases the ability to close the abdomen. The judicious use of such resuscitation, in addition to being generally helpful in ICU patients, will benefit in this regard. There has been some interest in the use of hypertonic saline for resuscitation, with the idea that this "draws fluid" out of the bowel and into the vasculature, facilitating closure. This idea is largely based on a small, retrospective study without subsequent high-quality evidence. The benefit of doing this may simply be the result of lower volumes of crystalloid. Finally, an emerging area of research on this front is the use of direct peritoneal resuscitation (DPR), in which a hypertonic (peritoneal dialysate) solution is used to reduce edema and mitigate inflammatory mediators in the bowel. This DPR concept may see increased use in the coming years.

HEPATIC SYSTEM

Cirrhosis

Cirrhosis is characterized by chronic liver inflammation that replaces normal liver parenchyma with diffuse fibrosis. The most common causes are alcohol-related liver disease, nonalcoholic fatty liver disease, hepatitis B and C, and autoimmune diseases. The gold standard for assessing the presence and cause of liver fibrosis is a liver biopsy. Liver elastography and magnetic resonance imaging (MRI) can be used to determine the degree of fibrosis. The presence of symptoms is termed *decompensated cirrhosis.*

Physical exam findings indicative of cirrhosis are typically seen in patients with decompensated disease. Exam findings include scleral icterus, gynecomastia, loss of secondary sexual characteristics, ascites, spider angiomata, and caput medusae.[62] Laboratory findings include either low or high transaminases, high bilirubin (typically direct bilirubinemia), hyponatremia, coagulopathy (elevated partial thromboplastin time [PTT] and international normalized ratio [INR]), elevated creatinine, low albumin, anemia, and thrombocytopenia.

There are two main scoring systems to estimate mortality risk in patients with cirrhosis. The Child-Turcotte-Pugh score categorizes patients into A, B, or C classes based on a patient's albumin, bilirubin, INR, amount of ascites, and degree of encephalopathy. Critics of this scoring system note that there are two subjective measures (amount of ascites and degree of encephalopathy), which can make scoring inconsistent and easy

to manipulate. The 1-year survival ranges from 100% for class A to 45% for class C cirrhotic patients. Postoperative mortality after nonhepatic surgical procedures ranges from 10% for class A to 63% for class C.[63] Several studies have shown that the Acute Physiology and Chronic Health Evaluation (APACHE II) scores can be used in patients with cirrhosis to predict mortality in the ICU.[64,65] The Model for End-Stage Liver Disease (MELD) score was initially developed to predict mortality after a transjugular intrahepatic portosystemic shunt (TIPS) but has now been useful for determining surgical risk and for transplantation listing. This scoring system contains objective variables such as INR, creatinine, and bilirubin. Although not included in the original model, hyponatremia was found to be a significant predictor of 3-month waiting-list mortality and has been shown to be a predictor of ascites and renal dysfunction. Patients with cirrhosis and hyponatremia have been shown to have elevated renal artery resistances, elevated renin and aldosterone, and reduced MAP, all of which are causes of ascites and renal failure.[66,67] Subsequently, a new scoring system called *MELD-Na,* which added sodium to the model (an independent predictor of mortality in cirrhosis), is now being used for transplant organ allocation.

Portal Hypertension

There are several sequelae of decompensated cirrhosis, which all begin with the development of portal hypertension. The first step to the development of portal hypertension results from changes in hepatic architecture that create increased resistance in the portal system. In addition, the hepatic sinusoids produce less nitric oxide, a potent vasodilator, creating a shift in the balance of vasoconstrictive and vasodilatory substances and causing net vasoconstriction in the portal system. In contrast, the production of nitric oxide in the splanchnic circulation is increased (from shear stress and bacterial translocation), leading to splanchnic vasodilation, which decreases effective circulating blood volume, creating hypotension and an increase in portal flow. The combination of these factors leads to portal hypertension. The PRE-DESCI trial, a randomized, double-blind, placebo-controlled trial, showed that patients with clinically significant portal hypertension have a decreased risk of decompensation, particularly the development of ascites, with the use of β-blockers compared with placebo.[68] Further analysis has shown that carvedilol outperforms propranolol, leading to a new consensus guideline that carvedilol is the β-blocker of choice in clinically significant portal hypertension to prevent decompensation.[69] β-blockers work by both decreasing CO (β1 receptors) and causing splanchnic vasoconstriction (β2). Carvedilol has the additional benefit of having some α1 blockade effects, which also helps to reduce the hepatic venous pressure gradient.[70]

Ascites

Portal hypertension causes several pathologies, the most common being ascites. This is defined as the accumulation of fluid in the peritoneal space. This occurs because of several factors. The decrease in systemic effective circulating volume, as described earlier, causes an increase in catecholamine release and stimulates the renin-angiotensin-aldosterone system (RAAS). This promotes sodium and water retention and a subsequent increase in plasma volume. Given the splanchnic vasodilation and the portal hypertension, this volume is preferentially retained in the splanchnic system, which increases the hydrostatic pressure gradient and moves fluid from the splanchnic circulation to the peritoneal space. The degree of ascites is categorized into three grades: grade 1 is mild ascites detected on ultrasound alone; grade 2 is moderate ascites, defined as the presence of abdominal distension; and grade 3 is severe ascites, defined as a tense abdomen with a fluid wave.[71] When the cause of ascites is not obvious, a serum-ascites albumin gradient (SAAG) can be calculated (serum albumin concentration − ascites albumin concentration). A SAAG of ≥1.1 g/dL indicates portal hypertension as the etiology of the ascites. Treatment of portal hypertension–induced ascites includes a low-salt diet, sodium restriction, and diuretics. Commonly used diuretics are furosemide (to decrease sodium reabsorption in the thick ascending limb) and spironolactone (given that aldosterone plays a part in the ascites pathway). For grade 3 ascites, the immediate treatment is large-volume paracentesis followed by volume expansion with 25% albumin (6–8 g/L of fluid removed).[71] This will help to prevent postparacentesis circulatory dysfunction, which is characterized by renal failure and increased mortality.

Spontaneous Bacterial Peritonitis

An increase in bacterial translocation in the presence of extra fluid in the peritoneal cavity can lead to spontaneous bacterial peritonitis (SBP). Clinical signs can be nonspecific but generally include signs of infection with or without abdominal pain and gastrointestinal symptoms. The diagnosis is made based on ascites fluid analysis. An ascites fluid neutrophil count of >250 cells/μL is diagnostic of SBP, and initial treatment includes supportive measures along with intravenous antibiotics. The choice of antibiotics is based on the institution's resistance patterns but should cover a broad spectrum of bacteria. Indications for SBP prophylaxis (typically ciprofloxacin or trimethoprim-sulfamethoxazole) are an active GI bleed, prior history of SBP (may require lifelong prophylaxis), or ascites fluid protein <1.5 g/dL.

Varices

When portal pressures exceed 12 mm Hg, reversal of flow occurs in the portal/splanchnic circulation and creates varices (dilated veins), typically in the stomach and esophagus. If these veins rupture as a result of excess wall tension, they can cause variceal hemorrhage. Initial therapy for variceal hemorrhage should be aimed at restoring plasma volume with blood, antibiotics for 7 days to prevent secondary infections, and a somatostatin analogue (e.g., octreotide) for 3 to 5 days. Somatostatin analogues cause splanchnic vasoconstriction and a decrease in portal inflow, reducing the risk of continued hemorrhage and active bleeding. After a secure airway is established, the mainstay of therapy is to stop the hemorrhage. For a temporizing measure, balloon tamponade may be attempted with a Sengstaken-Blakemore tube. The tube is inserted through the mouth or naris until about 50 cm. The gastric balloon is insufflated with 100 cc of air, and a radiograph is used to confirm a position below the diaphragm. Once confirmed, the balloon is filled to its total amount (for a typical tube, 250 cc), and tension is placed on the tube to secure it in place at the gastroesophageal junction. For continued bleeding, the esophageal balloon is then inflated. This can be left in place for up to 24 to 48 hours, but it must be acknowledged that any amount of time that the esophageal balloon is inflated increases the risk for esophageal ischemia and perforation. The definitive treatment for variceal bleeding is esophageal band ligation

or sclerotherapy when ligation is not feasible. Prevention of variceal hemorrhage includes nonselective β-blockade and esophageal band ligation. TIPS is reserved for refractory cases or when there is a portal vein thrombus because TIPS has been associated with an increase in portal vein recanalization in those cases.[72]

Transjugular Intrahepatic Portosystemic Shunt

Patients with refractory ascites or recurrent variceal bleeding may meet the criteria for TIPS. For this procedure, access is obtained through the right internal jugular vein, a hepatic venogram is performed, the portal veins are identified, and a stent is deployed to connect the high-resistance portal system to the low-resistance hepatic/systemic system (i.e., shunting blood away from the portal circulation). Contraindications for TIPS include heart failure and advanced liver disease with a MELD of >18. TIPS has been shown to decrease mortality in patients with severe bleeding, ascites, and hepatorenal syndrome.[73] However, TIPS is associated with up to a 20% risk of new or worsened hepatic encephalopathy. Hepatic encephalopathy is a risk with all portosystemic shunts because the ammonia that is produced by the bowel gets transported directly into the systemic circulation, bypassing even the small amount of metabolism that would have been accomplished by the liver.

Hepatic Encephalopathy

Hepatic encephalopathy is defined as potentially reversible neuropsychiatric abnormalities secondary to hepatic dysfunction and/or portal shunting.[62] The accumulation of ammonia (NH_3) has been implicated as the primary factor in the development of encephalopathy. Ammonia is the byproduct of protein degradation in the bowel. The liver converts ammonia to urea using the urea cycle. When this cycle is not functioning optimally (e.g., in cirrhosis), an accumulation of ammonia occurs in the blood. Ammonia then crosses the blood-brain barrier and is converted to glutamine by astrocytes. Glutamine acts as an osmotic load and causes cellular swelling, damage, and impaired synaptic transmissions.[74] Clinical features include lethargy, disorientation, asterixis, and in more severe cases, depressed consciousness and stupor. The degree of encephalopathy is graded from grade 0 (no encephalopathy) to grade 4 (coma). Grade 2 encephalopathy or higher occurs in up to 40% of all patients with cirrhosis.[75] The treatment involves reducing the production of ammonia in the bowel to stop the accumulation at its start. Lactulose is a nonabsorbable disaccharide and is broken down by the bacteria *Lactobacillus acidophilus* and acts to acidify the bowel. This causes eradication of the gram-negative aerobic bacilli that are essential to converting protein into ammonia. Additionally, acidification of the bowel decreases the absorption of ammonia into the bloodstream.[74] The European Association for the Study of the Liver (EASL) guidelines recommend starting and titrating lactulose to 2 to 3 bowel movements per day for encephalopathy prophylaxis after an episode of overt hepatic encephalopathy.[75] Rifaximin is an antibiotic that also works to eradicate the gram-negative bacilli responsible for ammonia generation in the bowel. Guidelines recommend using rifaximin as an adjunct to lactulose for encephalopathy prophylaxis.[75]

Hepatorenal Syndrome

Hepatorenal syndrome (HRS) is defined as renal failure that occurs in patients with cirrhosis, typically after an episode of sepsis or a hyperinflammatory state. Although the mechanism is not entirely understood, it is thought to occur because of splanchnic vasodilation and reduced CO. This causes renal arterial vasoconstriction, resulting in hypoperfusion and a reduction in the glomerular filtration rate (GFR). Sepsis is also associated with splanchnic vasodilation, but a new theory suggests that proinflammatory cytokines may also play a role by inducing microvascular dysfunction in the renal tubules, indirectly causing an increase in RAAS and further lowering GFR.[71] The major criteria for the diagnosis of HRS are renal dysfunction in the setting of cirrhosis, not explained by other causes and not responsive to diuretic withdrawal and volume expansion. Although urine studies can vary, the most common findings are a urine sodium of <10 mmol/L and urine osmolality greater than plasma osmolality because tubular function is typically preserved.[76] HRS is categorized into two types: HRS–acute kidney injury (HRS-AKI) (formerly type 1) is defined as rapidly progressing deterioration of renal function (over 1–2 weeks), and HRS–nonacute kidney injury (HRS-NAKI) (formerly type 2) is characterized by more gradual renal dysfunction, resistant to diuretics, resulting from refractory ascites.[77] The management of HRS includes a splanchnic vasoconstrictor to increase renal perfusion pressures (vasopressin analogue) and a volume expander (albumin). Terlipressin is a vasopressin analogue that has recently been approved for use in the United States as first-line therapy for the treatment of HRS-AKI and is continued for up to 14 days after creatinine levels return to baseline.[77] The Multi-Center, Randomized, Placebo Controlled, Double-Blind Study to Confirm Efficacy and Safety of Terlipressin in Subjects With Hepatorenal Syndrome Type 1 (CONFIRM) trial, a phase III randomized placebo-controlled trial, compared terlipressin to placebo in patients with HRS-AKI and found an increased rate of HRS reversal in the terlipressin group when combined with albumin. However, terlipressin was associated with a risk of respiratory failure; therefore, oxygen levels should be monitored carefully.[78] Other management options for patients who do not respond to or cannot receive terlipressin are renal replacement therapy, TIPS, or liver transplant.

Portopulmonary Hypertension/Hepatopulmonary Syndrome

Portopulmonary hypertension (PPHT) should be considered in patients with portal hypertension who have right-sided heart failure from increased pulmonary artery pressures (PAPs) with normal pulmonary occlusion pressures (to rule out left-sided heart failure as the cause). PPHT is categorized as mild (mean PAP of 25–35), moderate (mean PAP of 35–45), or severe (mean PAP of ≥45).[71] Although the pathogenesis is poorly understood, the current understanding is that PPHT occurs because of pulmonary vascular vasoconstriction from increased endothelin-1 released and not metabolized by the cirrhotic liver and decreased prostacyclin from pulmonary endothelial cells. Treatment includes endothelin receptor antagonists (e.g., Bosentan), phosphodiesterase-5 inhibitors (e.g., sildenafil), and prostacyclin analogues (e.g., epoprostenol). Severe PPHT (mean PAP of ≥45) is an absolute contraindication to liver transplant because of very poor postoperative outcomes. To prevent patients from reaching that stage, MELD exception points are granted to patients with moderate PPHT. Studies have shown that up to 60% of patients who receive pre- and postoperative therapy are able to discontinue pulmonary hypertension medications over time after their liver transplant. However, compared with non-PPHT patients, PPHT MELD exception patients have worse 1-year mortality after liver transplant.[71]

RENAL

Anatomy and Physiology

The primary function of the kidney is to maintain homeostasis and metabolize toxins. The human kidneys make up less than 0.5% of the total body weight but receive 25% of the CO (~6 L/day). From anterior to posterior, the kidney is connected to the renal vein, artery, and pelvis/ureter. The kidney itself is contained in Gerota's fascia, and from superficial to deep, it contains the fibrous capsule, renal cortex, and renal medulla, which is made up of the renal pyramids and renal papilla. These lead to the minor and major calyx, which combine to form the renal pelvis and, subsequently, the ureter. The nephron, the functional unit of the kidney, contains the glomerulus and renal tubules, which span the cortex and medulla. The branch that enters the glomerulus is the afferent arteriole, and the branch that exits the glomerulus is the efferent arteriole. Blood flow is primarily directed to the cortex to optimize glomerular filtration (PO_2 in the cortex of ~50 mm Hg), making blood flow very low in the medulla in order to preserve osmotic gradients (PO_2 in the medulla of ~10–20 mm Hg). Despite wide fluctuations in renal arterial perfusion pressures (80–180 mm Hg), the renal blood flow, and therefore glomerular filtration, is closely autoregulated by the afferent and efferent arterioles.

The plasma that flows from the afferent to the efferent arterioles is filtered by the glomerulus. The GFR is determined by the rate of blood flow, the combination of hydrostatic and oncotic pressure gradients, surface area, and membrane permeability (normal GFR is ~120 mL/min). The blood flow and hydrostatic pressures are controlled by either constriction or dilation of the afferent and efferent arterioles, determined by various hormones, such as angiotensin and prostaglandins. When renal perfusion pressures fall, renin is released from the juxtaglomerular cells (in the walls of the afferent arteriole), which converts angiotensin to angiotensin I in the liver, which is then converted to angiotensin II in the lungs, which causes vasoconstriction of the efferent arteriole, increasing the hydrostatic pressure at the glomerulus to maintain GFR. Similarly, prostaglandins cause vasodilation of the afferent arteriole to increase blood flow and hydrostatic pressure at the glomerulus to increase GFR.

The proximal tubule reabsorbs almost all of the glucose and amino acids and about 65% of the sodium (Na) and water. The luminal fluid then enters the loop of Henle in the medulla, made up of the descending loop and thick ascending limb. The descending loop contains aquaporins, which are water channels that allow water to passively travel along its gradient. Water travels from low osmolality in the lumen to high osmolality in the medulla. This osmotic gradient is created by the thick ascending limb. The thick ascending limb is impermeable to water but creates an ionic gradient between the lumen and medulla and reabsorbs Na and chloride (Cl). As the solutes increase the osmolality of the medulla, more water continues to be reabsorbed from the descending limb, which then causes more reabsorption of solutes from the thick ascending limb, all of which leads to a rise in osmolality to reach a maximum of 1200 mOsm/L in the deepest areas of the medulla. This is called the *countercurrent multiplier*. This creates the corticomedullary osmotic gradient. Once fluid leaves the ascending limb, it enters the distal tubule and collecting duct. Both reabsorb ions but are only permeable to water in the presence of antidiuretic hormone (ADH). In the presence of ADH, aquaporin channels are inserted into the apical membrane of the collecting tubule, and water is reabsorbed down its osmotic gradient. Disorders and management of electrolytes, such as sodium, potassium, calcium, and magnesium, are covered in depth in Chapter 33.

Acid-Base Regulation

The body pH is tightly regulated by the respiratory and renal systems. One of the main buffer systems in the body is the carbonic acid–bicarbonate buffer system. Carbon dioxide combines with water to form carbonic acid, which then dissociates into bicarbonate and a hydrogen ion with the help of carbonic anhydrase.

The respiratory system changes the pH by regulating how much CO_2 is expired. This system can alter the pH within hours. The renal system regulates pH by reabsorbing bicarbonate and excreting hydrogen. Hydrogen is excreted in the form of hydrogen ions or in the form of ammonium. Almost all the filtered bicarbonate is reabsorbed in the proximal tubule. This mechanism changes body pH over a longer period of time, on the order of days.

The pH of the body represents the concentration of hydrogen ions in the blood. There are two broad categories of systems that are evaluated when assessing the etiology of a patient's acid-base status: metabolic and respiratory. When evaluating an acid-base disorder, there is typically a primary disorder that is driving the imbalance, and the other system attempts to compensate. The compensation will always occur in the direction of normalizing the pH. The method for determining the primary disorder is to analyze the blood gas. The blood gas contains the pH, $PaCO_2$, and HCO_3^-. The direction of the pH is the disorder (i.e., acidosis or alkalosis). If the $PaCO_2$ and the pH change in opposite directions, it is a primary respiratory disorder, and if the pH and the HCO_3^- change in the same direction, then it is a primary metabolic disorder. If both exist, then it is a mixed respiratory and metabolic disorder. Normal values are as follows: pH, 7.35 to 7.45; $PaCO_2$, 35 to 45 mm Hg; and HCO_3^-, 22 to 26 mEq/L. Equations can be used to calculate the expected compensatory response. If the expected compensatory response is different from the measured value, then there is likely a mixed acid-base disorder involving both systems.

Respiratory Acidosis

Respiratory acidosis is caused by hypoventilation, which decreases the amount of CO_2 exhaled and increases the $PaCO_2$. Metabolic compensation occurs when the kidneys increase bicarbonate reabsorption in the proximal tubules. For acute respiratory acidosis, the metabolic compensation will be very little:

$$\Delta HCO_3^- = \Delta PaCO_2 \times 0.1$$

For chronic respiratory acidosis, the metabolic compensation is as follows:

$$\Delta HCO_3^- = \Delta PaCO_2 \times 0.4$$

Respiratory Alkalosis

Respiratory alkalosis occurs in the setting of increased minute ventilation (respiratory rate and tidal volume). In acute respiratory alkalosis, the metabolic compensation is as follows:

$$\Delta HCO_3^- = \Delta PaCO_2 \times 0.2$$

In chronic respiratory alkalosis, the metabolic compensation is as follows:

$$\Delta HCO_3^- = \Delta PaCO_2 \times 0.4$$

Metabolic Acidosis

Metabolic acidosis is characterized by a primary reduction in bicarbonate (HCO_3^-) concentration. This occurs either by the addition of an acid that is buffered by HCO_3^-, loss of HCO_3^-, or addition of nonbicarbonate fluid that dilutes the bicarbonate

concentration in the plasma. When an additional acid is buffered by HCO_3^-, an organic anion is created. This creates an anion gap (AG) metabolic acidosis. When bicarbonate is lost or diluted, chloride concentrations increase to preserve electroneutrality. This creates a non-AG metabolic acidosis. The AG is calculated as follows:

$$AG = [Na^+] - [Cl^-] - [HCO_3^-]$$

A normal AG is between 3 and 11. There is an additional formula that has been suggested that corrects for hypoalbuminemia, but for simplicity, the previous formula should suffice. If the AG is higher than the normal AG, then the disorder is considered an AG metabolic acidosis. Common causes are typically remembered by the mnemonic "MUDPILES": methanol, uremia, diabetic ketoacidosis, paracetamol, isoniazid, lactic acidosis, ethanol/ethylene glycol, and salicylates. In order to determine whether there are two metabolic acid-base disorders, a delta gap (or gap-gap ratio, not listed here) can be calculated.

$$\text{Delta gap} = (\text{normal AG} - \text{calculated AG}) - (\text{normal } HCO_3^- - \text{calculated } HCO_3^-)$$

If the delta gap is significantly positive ($>+6$), then there is an associated metabolic alkalosis present, and if the delta gap is significantly negative (<-6), then there is an associated non-AG metabolic acidosis also present. This is an extremely simplified method of evaluating a very complicated buffering system in the body, and it makes several assumptions, the main one being that bicarbonate is the only buffering system in the body when in fact, there are several others, including phosphate, hemoglobin, and other plasma proteins.

Causes of non-AG metabolic acidosis include diarrhea, normal saline infusion, and renal tubular acidosis. The respiratory response to metabolic acidosis is a decrease in $PaCO_2$ by increasing the minute ventilation. The expected change in $PaCO_2$ is as follows:

$$\Delta PaCO_2 = 1.2 \times \Delta HCO_3^-$$

Initial decreases in pH are typically well tolerated and can actually assist in certain functions, such as oxygen unloading from hemoglobin. However, as the acidosis worsens, myocardial contractility is affected, and its response to catecholamines becomes blunted.[79]

Metabolic Alkalosis

Metabolic alkalosis is characterized by an increase in bicarbonate concentration in the plasma. This can occur by net loss of hydrogen ions (i.e., from the GI tract), addition of bicarbonate at a rate unable to be regulated/excreted by the kidneys, loss of fluid with low bicarbonate concentration (i.e., diuretics), or loss of fluid that leads to a contraction alkalosis. The theory behind contraction alkalosis is that a loss of plasma volume causes activation of the RAAS. Aldosterone causes an increase in bicarbonate reabsorption in the proximal tubule and an increase in hydrogen ion excretion in the distal tubule. The expected change in $PaCO_2$ in metabolic alkalosis is as follows:

$$\Delta PaCO_2 = 0.7 \times \Delta HCO_3^-$$

Acute Kidney Injury

Acute kidney injury (AKI) is defined as an increase in serum creatinine of ≥ 3 mg/dL over 48 hours, an increase in creatinine of ≥ 1.5 times baseline over 7 days, or a urine output of <0.5 cc/kg/hour over 6 hours.[80] AKI is categorized into three stages: stage 1, serum creatinine of 1.5 to 1.9 times baseline;

stage 2, serum creatinine of 2.0 to 2.9 times baseline; and stage 3, serum creatinine of 3 times baseline or initiation of renal replacement therapy (RRT).

The Kidney Disease Improving Global (KDIGO) guidelines recommend preventing AKI by ensuring adequate volume resuscitation using crystalloids rather than colloids, avoiding hypoglycemia and nephrotoxic agents, and giving intravenous fluids with contrast agents if at high risk for contrast-induced nephropathy. RRT is indicated for toxin removal or in the setting of AKI that has resulted in severe complications, including hyperkalemia, acidosis, or fluid overload. Several studies have evaluated early versus standard timing of RRT initiation. A recent multinational, randomized controlled trial in ICU patients with AKI compared patients who received RRT within hours versus when standard clinical criteria were met. They found no difference in mortality and a higher dependence on dialysis and adverse events in the early RRT group.[81]

Renal Replacement Therapy

Methods of RRT are broadly categorized into hemodialysis and peritoneal dialysis. Hemodialysis is divided into continuous versus intermittent methods. Continuous RRT (CRRT) is indicated for patients who cannot tolerate large hemodynamic changes. The basic flow of hemodialysis involves the following: Blood is removed from the patient and flows through a blood pump, then travels through a filter with a semipermeable membrane where fluid/solutes are removed (effluent), and the remainder flows back into the patient. Methods of fluid and solute removal include ultrafiltration, which is the removal of fluid across its pressure gradient as determined by the combination of hydrostatic and oncotic pressures; convection, which is the removal of solutes that get dragged with high flows of fluid ("solute drag"); and diffusion, which is the movement of solutes down their concentration gradients (this involves a dialysate on the other side of the membrane to establish a steady concentration gradient). Slow continuous ultrafiltration (SCUF) uses ultrafiltration only and is used to remove fluid from patients. The blood flow is set at a slower rate so that little to no solute drag (convection) is achieved. Continuous venovenous hemofiltration (CVVH) is similar to SCUF except that the blood flow is much higher, and this causes faster ultrafiltration of fluid and creates a convection force to drag solutes across the membrane as well. This works well for all sizes of molecules and for electrolyte/acid clearance. This mode requires that a lot of fluid be filtered out in order to achieve appropriate solute clearance, so replacement fluid is added to the circuit to give fluid back to the patient. Replacement fluid can be placed prefilter (dilutes the blood and decreases clearance but decreases filter clotting), postfilter (improved clearance but increases filter clotting), or more likely, a combination of the two. Continuous venovenous hemodialysis (CVVHD) adds a dialysate around the semipermeable membrane in the filter to clear solutes using diffusion. The amount of solute clearance is based on the concentration of each solute in the dialysate, which determines the concentration gradient. Because solutes are being filtered by diffusion and not convection, this does not require a large amount of fluid loss and therefore does not require replacement fluid to be given back. Finally, continuous venovenous hemodialysis filtration (CVVHDF) is a combination of all the different modes. Intermittent hemodialysis (iHD) uses dialysis/diffusion for removal of solutes and can also remove fluid. iHD uses much higher blood flow rates over a shorter period of time. This can cause fluctuations in hemodynamics compared with a slow, continuous blood flow rate over 24 hours, as in CRRT.

HEMATOLOGIC SYSTEM

Transfusion Strategies

Anemia is common in all ICUs, largely secondary to so-called "anemia of chronic disease" and frequent phlebotomy, but in the surgical ICU, more nefarious etiologies, such as trauma and GI bleeding, must be considered. Generally speaking, evidence supports a restrictive transfusion strategy, or transfusing to a goal hemoglobin of 7 g/dL. Some have considered a higher goal in GI bleed and traumatic brain injury (TBI) patients, although this is not supported. The one special population in which a hemoglobin goal of 8 g/dL may make sense is those with stable cardiovascular disease. It is important to note that transfusion-related complications can occur and include allergic or anaphylactic reactions, fluid overload, iron overload, transmission of blood-borne infections, transfusion-related acute lung injury, immunosuppression, hypersensitivity reactions, and life-threatening hemolysis from ABO incompatibility.

On the other hand, it is imperative to understand that a declining hemoglobin is a late manifestation of active bleeding. In trauma patients or others with reason to suspect active bleeding, transfusion should be based on other clinical parameters, such as tachycardia, hypotension, and lactate, and intervention to achieve hemostasis should be pursued. Approaches to transfusion in hemorrhagic shock are detailed further in the cardiovascular section earlier in the chapter, but component therapy should be balanced, and whole blood should be considered, if available. In massive transfusion scenarios, TEG may be beneficial.

Viscoelastic Testing

Viscoelastic testing (VET), which can be performed by either TEG or ROTEM, was devised in the 1950s to assess the clotting capability of whole blood. Despite its potential applications, its widespread use was limited by a lack of accessibility and complexity in testing, and thus, the more common and conventional coagulation tests, such as PT/INR, PTT, platelet count, and fibrinogen level, were preferred. It was not until the 1980s, when testing became more practical, quicker, and reproducible, that TEG was used to guide resuscitation during transplant and cardiac surgeries and was found to decrease the total administration of blood products and mortality.

Currently, TEG and ROTEM are used with increasing regularity in the bleeding patient. The advantage of VET over traditional coagulation tests is that VET is a real-time, detailed functional assay that provides information about clot formation, propagation, strength, and lysis.

Traditional TEG involves a pin suspended in a sample of patient blood, oscillating at a fixed frequency. As a clot forms and slows the movement of the pin, the torque is measured by a transducer and traced into the thromboelastogram. The more recent iteration of the TEG system (TEG 6s, Haemonetics) involves vibration of the blood sample itself and a light detector that measures meniscus motion as clot forms.[82] The thromboelastogram shows four key values—clot formation, clot propagation, clot strength, and thrombolysis—as shown in Fig. 46.1. ROTEM evolved from TEG technology and has slightly different parameters and reagents that can be used to evaluate various aspects of coagulation. Data on the use of TEG in EGS patients are still emerging, but data for its use in trauma patients, particularly those with massive exsanguination, continue to be promulgated. It may be most useful after hemorrhage control in the ICU, where residual clot dysfunction can be uncovered and treated. The 2020 EAST guidelines conditionally

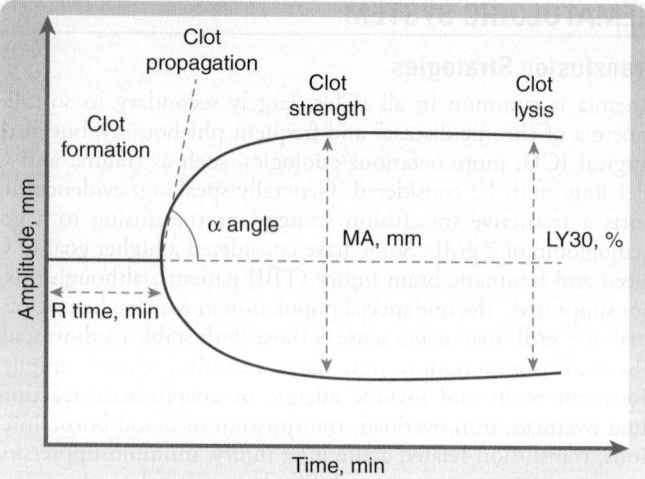

FIGURE 46.1 Thromboelastogram parameters. *R time* represents the time to clot formation; a prolonged R time may indicate a need for plasma transfusion. Clot propagation is represented by the *α angle*, with a low angle indicating a need for cryoprecipitate. The strength of the clot is shown by the maximum amplitude *(MA)*, a representation of platelet function. Lastly, the LY30, or percent decrease of tracing width at 30 minutes, measures thrombolysis and potential need for tranexamic acid.

recommend its use in bleeding trauma, surgical, and ICU patients with suspected coagulopathy.[43]

Heparin-Induced Thrombocytopenia

Heparin-induced thrombocytopenia (HIT) is a life-threatening complication that occurs in 1% to 5% of patients exposed to any of the forms of heparin.[83] The patient produces platelet-activating IgG antibodies to the complex of heparin bound to circulating platelet factor-4 (PF4). These immune complexes release additional prothrombotic molecules, thus propagating platelet consumption. The reticuloendothelial system eliminates these circulating immune complexes, leading to thrombocytopenia.

In order to make the diagnosis of HIT, the patient must exhibit the classic clinical signs of HIT in conjunction with appropriately timed heparin exposure. Thus, a description of the clinical features also serves as a description of initial diagnostic criteria. One of the most commonly used scores to diagnose HIT is the "4 Ts score," with variable points for **T**hrombocytopenia, **T**iming, **T**hrombosis and systemic events, and o**T**her causes of thrombocytopenia.

Classically, the degree of thrombocytopenia should be a reduction of >50%, although 10% of patients will have a 30% to 50% reduction. The most suspicious timing is 5 to 10 days from heparin exposure, although a more rapid onset may occur in patients previously exposed to heparin. Also, 25% to 68% of patients will have a thrombotic event, which may be apparent before the onset of thrombocytopenia. Finally, the presence of other, more plausible causes of thrombocytopenia should be considered because this may lower the pretest probability.

If the 4 Ts score indicates a low probability of HIT, heparin should be continued, and other causes of thrombocytopenia should be considered. If intermediate or high risk, heparin should be discontinued, alternative anticoagulation (often a direct thrombin inhibitor [DTI], such as argatroban or bivalirudin) should be started, and further testing should be undertaken.

Laboratory assessment for HIT generally begins with an enzyme-linked immunosorbent assay (ELISA), which is sensitive but not specific for HIT. If negative, HIT is ruled out. If positive, a confirmatory serotonin release assay should be performed. Although a serotonin release assay is considered the "gold standard," it is not as readily available and requires testing in a reference laboratory.

Over 40% of patients in the ICU develop thrombocytopenia, but HIT is rarely the cause, with an overall incidence of only 0.02% to 0.45%. However, even with treatment, mortality rates associated with HIT can be as high as 14.5% to 25%. In any patient with clinical suspicion of HIT, it is prudent to avoid all heparin exposure until a definitive diagnosis is obtained.

Venous Thromboembolism

Critically ill patients are at high risk for developing venous thromboembolism (VTE) because they have all the components of the Virchow triad to some degree: endothelial injury, venous stasis, and hypercoagulability. VTE is a preventable cause of death that is common but often undiagnosed and clinically silent. All patients admitted to the ICU should be assessed for and treated against the development of VTE as recommended by the American College of Chest Physicians Evidence-Based Clinical Practice Guidelines.[84] Most cases in which thromboprophylaxis is held are due to physician perception that the risk of bleeding outweighs the risk of VTE. However, delays of over 24 hours in initiating pharmacologic VTE prophylaxis after ICU admission are associated with a threefold increase in VTE formation after major trauma.

Absolute contraindications to chemical thromboprophylaxis include active bleeding or intracranial hemorrhage, coagulopathy, and severe thrombocytopenia. However, in patients with relative contraindications, such as recent GI bleeding, recent surgery, and moderate thrombocytopenia, the decision to initiate chemical thromboprophylaxis must be made on a case-by-case basis. At a minimum, mechanical thromboprophylaxis should be provided by means of intermittent pneumatic compression devices. Mechanical compression is used to promote venous blood flow and is thought to activate tissue plasminogen and local fibrinolysis. When no absolute contraindications are present, chemical thromboprophylaxis should be administered because it has been proven superior to mechanical compression for the prevention of deep vein thromboses (DVTs) and PEs.

Perhaps the most often-discussed contraindication to chemoprophylaxis in ICU patients is TBI, out of concern for worsening intracranial hemorrhage. However, there is evidence to suggest that in most cases, particularly in cases of mild TBI, early chemoprophylaxis (24–72 hours) is associated with decreased thromboembolic events without an increase in neurosurgical interventions or death. In the subset of patients who might be considered to have the highest risk—patients who require neurosurgical intervention on presentation—there is evidence that early chemoprophylaxis is associated with an increased risk of needing a repeat neurosurgical operation, although the same study suggested an increased risk of thromboembolic events with delays in prophylaxis in these patients.[85] Needless to say, decision-making in this context is complex and should take place after a conversation with both trauma surgeons and neurosurgeons caring for the patient.

Low-molecular-weight heparin has been shown to be more effective than unfractionated heparin for the prevention of DVTs, but it is renally excreted; this should be considered in the setting of AKI or renal failure. Despite adherence to chemical thromboprophylaxis administration, obesity and proinflammatory states such as sepsis convey higher rates of VTE prophylaxis failure. In these cases, goal-directed therapy and titration of low-molecular-weight heparin dosing based on anti-Xa levels have been proven effective. As the Xa assays become more available, ensuring target levels is becoming more mainstream in trauma patients in general. In patients in whom chemical thromboprophylaxis is contraindicated for an extended period of time, one could consider placement of an inferior vena cava filter to prevent large DVT embolization and clinically significant PEs.

ENDOCRINE SYSTEM

Glucose Control

Stress hyperglycemia, defined as hyperglycemia and insulin resistance in the setting of acute illness, occurs in up to 50% of patients in the ICU.[86] Hyperglycemia occurs because of an increase in catecholamines and cortisol, which increase gluconeogenesis in the liver, and inflammatory cytokines that create insulin resistance.[87] A certain amount of hyperglycemia may be protective by increasing the plasticity and ischemic resistance of cells, but as the glucose levels increase or become more chronic, it appears to increase morbidity and mortality.[87,88] Several studies have attempted to evaluate the benefit of tight glycemic control. The landmark study by the NICE-SUGAR investigators compared tight glycemic control (glucose 81–108 mg/dL) versus a more liberal target (glucose < 180 mg/dL) and found lower mortality with the more liberal strategy.[89] This was attributed to the higher incidence of hypoglycemia in the group with tight glycemic control. Based on the available evidence, the most important considerations in glycemic control are to prevent severe hyperglycemia, prevent hypoglycemia, and likely most importantly, prevent large fluctuations in glucose. With these considerations, the current standard practice is to employ some glucose control and to aim for a glucose of <180 mg/dL.

The next frontier of glucose control in the ICU is continuous glucose monitors. However, this method has not been shown to improve glycemic control (i.e., prevent hyperglycemia) but has been shown to decrease rates of hypoglycemia.[90,91] It was approved for emergency use during the pandemic, and with increasing implementation across hospitals, it may provide an avenue for further investigation.

Critical Illness Adrenal Insufficiency

The stress response is controlled by the hypothalamic-pituitary-adrenal axis (HPA). The hypothalamus senses stress in the body and releases corticotropin-releasing hormone (CRH), which stimulates the anterior pituitary to release adrenocorticotropic hormone (ACTH). ACTH stimulates the secretion of cortisol in the adrenal cortex.[92] In healthy patients, cortisol is released in a circadian rhythm, with its peak in the early hours of the morning and then gradually decreasing during the day. Cortisol then exerts a negative inhibitory effect on the hypothalamus and pituitary. Critical illness is marked by a loss of circadian rhythm, decreased adrenal synthesis/secretion of cortisol, decreased cortisol availability, tissue resistance to cortisol, and inhibition of ACTH synthesis through increased negative feedback mechanisms or medications.[93]

Critical illness-related corticosteroid insufficiency (CIRCI) is defined as the relative impairment of the hypothalamic-pituitary axis during critical illness.[94] Based on the low quality of evidence, guidelines recommend starting stress-dose steroids in patients in

septic shock, not responsive to fluid, and on moderate- to high-dose vasopressor therapy.[94] Patients on chronic steroids for pathology related to inadequate HPA axis should also receive stress-dose steroids because they likely cannot mount a stress response. Patients on chronic steroids for reasons other than an HPA axis deficiency should receive their home-dose equivalent steroid dose and can be given a stress dose at the provider's discretion.[95,96] Guidelines recommend using a dose course that is long and low (IV hydrocortisone <400 mg/day for ≥3 days).[94] However, studies have shown mixed results regarding whether steroids have any effect on mortality in patients with septic shock, but there is some evidence that they may shorten the duration of shock.[38,97-100] Although not typically done in practice, these guidelines recommend testing patients for adrenal insufficiency with a high-dose ACTH stimulation test.

Thyroid Dysfunction

Thyroid-stimulating hormone (TSH) is released from the pituitary gland to stimulate the thyroid gland to produce thyroxine (T_4), which converts to its activated form, triiodothyronine (T_3). Thyroid hormones exert negative feedback on TSH secretion. TSH levels are the most reliable method of checking thyroid function; however, TSH is a negative acute-phase reactant and is often falsely depressed and inaccurate in the setting of acute illness.

Hyperthyroidism is defined as excess circulating thyroid hormones. This can be primary (due to excess thyroid activity) or secondary (due to HPA axis dysfunction). Thyroid storm is a rare form of hyperthyroidism, occurring in less than 0.2% of hospitalized patients, but it carries a 40% mortality rate.[101] The most common causes include Grave disease, amiodarone-associated thyrotoxicosis, and infection. Symptoms include hyperpyrexia, agitation/delirium, tachycardia, and high-output heart failure. The treatment is β-blockers (propranolol is the drug of choice in thyroid storm) to manage the tachycardia and agitation and antithyroid drugs, such as methimazole or propylthiouracil.

Hypothyroidism is also rare in the critical illness setting. Causes include autoimmune thyroiditis, HPA axis dysfunction, and drug induced. Symptoms include fatigue, muscle cramps, and constipation. There is also an increased risk of a pericardial or pleural effusion because of increased capillary permeability. A more severe form is myxedema coma, which is hypothyroidism plus depressed mental status. Treatment includes steroids (if adrenal insufficiency is also suspected) and thyroid hormone supplementation.

INFECTIOUS DISEASES

General Principles

Around 50% to 60% of ICU patients develop a nosocomial infection, defined as an infection acquired while receiving healthcare that was not present at admission.[102] The mortality reaches up to 35%, and nosocomial infections account for almost half of hospital costs.[101] The most common routes and locations of infection are pulmonary, abdominal, genitourinary, and bloodstream. These infections are more common in ICU patients, likely because of the number of invasive procedures these patients receive in addition to the immunosuppression that accompanies critical illness. The most common organisms are gram-positive bacteria, such as *S. aureus,* and gram-negative bacteria, such as *P. aeruginosa* and *Escherichia coli.*[102] Risk factors for the development of a nosocomial infection in the ICU include ICU length of stay (the risk doubles from 1 day to 1 week in the ICU) and severe medical comorbidities.

Sepsis

Sepsis is defined as an infection with organ dysfunction. This occurs because of an unregulated immune and inflammatory response. More specifically, the new definition is the presence of infection and a change in SOFA score of >2 points.[103] Septic shock is the addition of cardiovascular dysfunction, specifically hypotension despite fluid resuscitation, and the need for vasopressors. The precise pathophysiology is not clear but likely involves activation of both pro- and antiinflammatory cytokines and mediators. There is an overwhelming proinflammatory and immunosuppression response, both occurring at the same time but at different intensities based on comorbidities or infectious etiology. This explains the increased incidence and risk of additional nosocomial infections during and after sepsis recovery. Shock occurs because of alterations in microcirculation, leaky capillaries from the inflammatory response, and vasodilation that leads to altered distribution of systemic blood flow. This creates a mismatch between tissue oxygenation needs, which are higher in patients with sepsis/critical illness, and oxygen delivery, leading to shock. The combination is termed *distributive shock.*[103] Given the high mortality, early recognition can make all the difference. Sepsis can be harder to identify in ICU patients, given that traditional objective findings may be altered from other comorbid conditions. For example, patients may not mount a white blood cell count; may not develop a fever (if on CRRT or ECMO); and may have many other reasons for respiratory failure, altered mental status, and lactic acidosis that can mislead providers. When there is concern for or proven sepsis, the most recent Surviving Sepsis Campaign guidelines recommend resuscitation with 30 cc/kg of balanced crystalloid solution targeting dynamic measures, starting antimicrobials within 1 hour of sepsis recognition, and early initiation of vasopressors.[35] Norepinephrine is first line, associated with decreased mortality and less volume resuscitation needs, followed by vasopressin.[104]

Nosocomial Infections

Ventilator-Associated Pneumonia

As discussed earlier in the section on the respiratory system, VAP is defined as a pulmonary parenchymal infection after 2 days of mechanical ventilation. Although ICU patients with VAP have high mortality, it is hard to evaluate whether the presence of a VAP is an independent predictor of mortality or, rather, a sign of overall illness and morbidity. Early-onset pneumonia is typically associated with oropharyngeal flora, and late-onset pneumonia is associated with multidrug-resistant pathogens.[105] Criteria for the diagnosis of VAP are >2 days of mechanical ventilation, worsening oxygenation, purulent secretions, and a positive culture. VAP-prevention bundles are considered the standard of care and include direct preventative measures such as head-of-bed elevation to 30 to 45 degrees, daily sedation holidays, daily spontaneous breathing trials, oral chlorhexidine wash, and subglottic suctioning. Indirect measures include peptic ulcer prophylaxis and DVT prophylaxis.[106] Implementation of VAP bundles has been shown to decrease VAP rates, reduce mortality, and reduce overall hospital costs.[107,108] Treatment for VAP is typically 1 week of antibiotic therapy, which has been shown to have comparable outcomes to the prior typical 14-day course.[109]

Central Line–Associated Bloodstream Infections

A central line–associated bloodstream infection (CLABSI) is defined as a confirmed bloodstream infection in a patient with a central line, without another source for the infection. CLABSIs occur because skin flora travels along the catheter and colonizes the catheter, making its way into the bloodstream. Tunneled catheters have a cuff that creates a barrier to bacterial migration, which makes them less prone to infection. CLABSI is associated with a 15% mortality rate.[110] This is why prevention strategies are so important and have been effective at reducing the overall rate of CLABSI around the country. Prevention strategies include aseptic technique during insertion (hand hygiene, chlorhexidine for skin preparation, and sterile draping), choice of catheter site (in order of infection risk: femoral vein > internal jugular vein > subclavian vein), the use of antibiotic-impregnated catheters, early definitive catheter removal (scheduled replacement of catheters does not reduce the CLABSI risk), and chlorhexidine-impregnated dressings.[111] Treatment includes antibiotics and prompt removal of the catheter. Catheter salvage is only acceptable in patients with very limited access sites or in the setting of long-term catheters. In these cases, antimicrobial locks are used to preserve catheters while being treated for the infection. Antibiotic duration is dependent on the organism isolated.

Catheter-Associated Urinary Tract Infection

A *catheter-associated urinary tract infection* (CAUTI) is defined as a urinary tract infection in a patient with a urinary catheter or in the setting of catheterization in the prior 48 hours. CAUTIs are the most common nosocomial infection, with the main risk factor being the duration of catheter therapy. Catheters carry risk because they provide a direct path for pathogens from the rectal flora or ambient environment to travel to the bladder, allow bacteria to bypass the urethral sphincters, eliminate the protective turbulence associated with natural voiding, and cause trauma to the urothelium that makes it susceptible to bacterial colonization and entry.[112] Prevention involves removing the catheter as soon as it is no longer necessary and the use of aseptic technique during placement. There is also a suggestion in the literature that intermittent catheterization is better than indwelling catheters in certain populations, specifically in patients with spinal cord injuries.[113] Diagnosis is made by urinalysis and urine culture, which should only be sent in the setting of symptoms. Symptoms include typical infectious symptoms, such as fevers, rigors, and malaise, and more specific urinary symptoms, such as dysuria and pain, although these are hard to assess in patients with catheters. A CAUTI is diagnosed when the urinalysis reveals either $\geq 10^3$ colony-forming units/mL based on the Infectious Diseases Society of America guidelines or $\geq 10^5$ colony-forming units/mL based on the Centers for Disease Control and Prevention guidelines. The presence of pyuria, or white blood cells in the urine, in patients with a urinary catheter does not differentiate between a CAUTI and asymptomatic bacteriuria. However, the absence of pyuria makes CAUTI highly unlikely. Treatment includes removal or exchange of the urinary catheter, typically before initiating antibiotic therapy, and antibiotics. Antibiotic duration can range from 7 days for patients who are prompt responders to 14 days in delayed responders.

Clostridioides difficile

C. difficile is a gram-positive anaerobic organism that proliferates in the bowel when the microbiome is altered, particularly during and after antibiotic use. It is transmitted via the fecal-oral route and, in the hospital setting, typically spread via hospital personnel. *C. difficile* releases toxins that lead to inflammation of the bowel wall and create raised mucosal plaques called *pseudomembranes.* This is usually only seen in severe disease. Risk factors for a *C. difficile* infection include antibiotic exposure, hospitalization, and gastric acid suppression (e.g., PPIs). The primary symptom is watery diarrhea, which can develop, as the disease progresses, into shock, multiorgan failure, and toxic megacolon, noted by a very dilated colon on imaging. Diagnosis is made by sending a stool sample. Most institutions test for both the presence of the bacteria in the stool and the presence of the cytotoxin.

C. difficile infection is categorized into three severity levels: *nonsevere disease,* defined as white blood cell count <15,000 cells/mL and creatinine <1.5 mg/dL; *severe disease,* defined as white blood cell count ≥15,000 cells/mL and creatinine >1.5 mg/dL; or *fulminant disease,* defined as hemodynamic shock or megacolon. Treatment begins with the initiation of antibiotics, either oral vancomycin or oral fidaxomicin. In the setting of a severe infection or in the case of an ileus, intravenous metronidazole or rectal vancomycin may be added. Antibiotic treatment is usually continued for 10 to 14 days. Recurrent episodes can be treated with the same antibiotics but may require a longer duration. Chronic colonizers with recurrent infections may require oral vancomycin prophylaxis while on other antibiotics. For recurrent disease, a fecal transplant can also be considered, which has proven to change the microbiome of the colon and may decrease the risk of recurrent infection.[114] Indications for surgery during an acute infection include peritonitis, worsening hemodynamic shock, perforation, or toxic megacolon. Delaying surgery in the setting of shock can increase mortality. Surgical options include a subtotal colectomy, current standard of care, and for select patients without perforation or peritonitis, a loop ileostomy with colonic lavage and antegrade vancomycin enemas.[115,116] The original procedure was described as initially performing a diagnostic laparoscopy to assess for colonic viability, then creating a loop ileostomy and infusing 8 L of warmed polyethylene glycol 3350/electrolyte solution into the colon, with postoperative antegrade vancomycin flushes (500 mg in 500 cc of lactated Ringer solution every 8 hours over 10 days) through a Malecot catheter into the distal limb of the ileostomy.[116] The original study and other small cohort studies have shown that this method reduces mortality and increases colonic preservation.[115,116]

PALLIATIVE CARE AND END OF LIFE

As the population ages and our abilities to extend life in the ICU improve, the incorporation of palliative care is a crucial skill set for the surgical intensivist. Palliative care is the patient- and family-centered approach focused on the alleviation of symptoms. This includes pain management and psychosocial support. Its integration into ICU care is critical.

It is imperative to understand that the term *palliative care,* although often inclusive of end-of-life care, is *not* synonymous with *withdrawal of care.* This is a common misconception, particularly among surgeons, and may lead to hesitation to involve a palliative care team early in a patient's course. Elderly, frail, and comorbid patients, in particular, may benefit from early engagement of a palliative care team.[117]

Recent literature suggests that surgeons often struggle to provide appropriate guidance to patients with severe surgical problems in the preoperative period.[118] Despite efforts to improve such preoperative deliberation,[119] insurmountable complications occur, and patients and their families may find themselves in the surgical ICU facing unexpected death. If this situation occurs, it is important for the surgeon and critical care physician to recognize impending death and address it in a frank and transparent manner with the patient and family.

Although these discussions are difficult and nuanced, if performed well, the patient's family and care team can often come to a resolution that has the patient's best interest in mind. Engaging local experts, including palliative care specialists and the hospital's ethics committee, can be quite beneficial and is recommended. Critical care physicians are an integral part of such processes.

SELECTED REFERENCES

Devlin JW, Skrobik Y, Gélinas C, et al. Clinical practice guidelines for the prevention and management of pain, agitation/sedation, delirium, immobility, and sleep disruption in adult patients in the ICU. *Crit Care Med.* 2018;46(9):e825-e873.

This most recent clinical practice guideline developed via the Society of Critical Care Medicine offers the most recent summary of supporting recommendations and associated literature gaps in the assessment, prevention, and treatment of pain, agitation/sedation, delirium, immobility (mobilization/rehabilitation), and sleep (disruption) in critically ill adults.

Girard TD, Exline MC, Carson SS, et al. Haloperidol and ziprasidone for treatment of delirium in critical illness. *N Engl J Med.* 2018;379(26):2506-2516.

In a multicenter randomized double-blind placebo-controlled trial of critically ill patients, haloperidol (typical antipsychotic) or ziprasidone (atypical antipsychotic), as compared with placebo, did not significantly alter the duration of delirium, survival, time to freedom from mechanical ventilation, or time to ICU and hospital discharge.

PEPTIC Investigators for the Australian and New Zealand Intensive Care Society Clinical Trials Group, Alberta Health Services Critical Care Strategic Clinical Network, Irish Critical Care Trials Group, et al. Effect of stress ulcer prophylaxis with proton pump inhibitors vs histamine-2 receptor blockers on in-hospital mortality among ICU patients receiving invasive mechanical ventilation: the PEPTIC randomized clinical trial. *JAMA.* 2020;323(7):616-626.

In this multicenter, five-country, cluster crossover randomized clinical trial, ICU stress ulcer prophylaxis with PPIs versus histamine-2 receptor blockers did not alter all-cause mortality (primary end point), upper GI bleeding, C. difficile infection, or ICU and hospital lengths of stay.

Singer M, Deutschman CS, Seymour CW, et al. The Third International Consensus definitions for sepsis and septic shock (Sepsis-3). *JAMA.* 2016;315(8):801-810.

This seminal work updates the definitions for sepsis and septic shock and facilitates earlier recognition and more timely management using these standardized metrics.

STARRT-AKI Investigators, Canadian Critical Care Trials Group, Australian and New Zealand Intensive Care Society Clinical Trials Group, et al. Timing of initiation of renal-replacement therapy in acute kidney injury. *N Engl J Med.* 2020;383(3): 240-251.

In this multinational randomized controlled trial of ICU patients with AKI, an accelerated strategy of RRT within 12 hours of meeting eligibility, compared with a standard strategy, was not associated with lower 90-day mortality and was possibly associated with more adverse events and dependence on RRT at 90 days.

In this multicenter randomized clinical trial, among patients with septic shock undergoing mechanical ventilation, a continuous infusion of hydrocortisone (200 mg/day) did not alter 90-day mortality more than placebo, but it shortened resolution of shock.

Venkatesh B, Finfer S, Cohen J, et al. Adjunctive glucocorticoid therapy in patients with septic shock. *N Engl J Med.* 2018; 378(9):797-808.

The full reference list appears on Elsevier eBooks+.

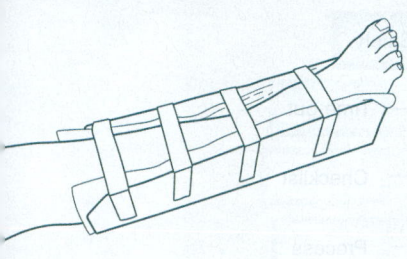

CHAPTER 47

Moving Operating Room Procedures to the Intensive Care Unit

Bradley M. Dennis, Rachel D. Appelbaum, and Jose J. Diaz

OUTLINE

Bedside surgical procedures have become a standard in many intensive care units (ICUs), replacing the operating room (OR) as the preferred location for select procedures in critically ill patients.[1] Performing appropriately selected procedures within the ICU limits the risk of transporting critically ill patients, facilitates flexibility in timing and scheduling, decompresses busy ORs, and reduces cost.[2-4] The ability to perform some operations at the bedside may be lifesaving in critically ill patients too unstable to transport safely to the OR. Advancements in monitoring and sedation, endoscopic and percutaneous techniques, and bedside imaging have enabled the transition of several procedures traditionally performed in the OR, endoscopy, and interventional radiology suites to the ICU. Procedures now regularly performed in the ICU include bedside laparotomy, tracheostomy, percutaneous endoscopic feeding access, percutaneous drainage procedures, placement of inferior vena cava filters, and initiation of extracorporeal circulatory life support (the latter covered in a separate chapter). In the unstable patient, other procedures may be performed at the bedside, including irrigation and debridement of wounds, orthopedic stabilization with external fixation, fasciotomies, amputations, and diagnostic laparoscopy.

Although bedside operative procedures can be performed safely, with complication rates equal to those in the OR, doing so mandates that cases are appropriately selected and that appropriate safety practices are consistently implemented. The ICU represents a complex environment in which to perform complex processes and procedures. Recognition of the numerous potentials for error and adverse events in such settings is important. Based on the experience of industry and other high-reliability organizations, prevention of error and adverse events requires standardization of processes and elimination of variability.[5] Protocols and safety practices specifically for bedside operative procedures should be in place to ensure the ability to perform these procedures safely, with low infection rates, and with the assurance of comfort and amnesia. In this chapter, we discuss the following topics: (1) the rationale for bedside surgical procedures; (2) the process of bringing the OR to the bedside; (3) systematic safety methodologies and practices to ensure safe performance of

bedside procedures; (4) selection of patients for bedside surgical procedures; and (5) specific considerations for common bedside procedures, such as bedside laparotomy, tracheostomy, percutaneous endoscopic feeding tubes, and bronchoscopy.

RATIONALE FOR BEDSIDE SURGICAL PROCEDURES

For good reasons, most surgical procedures are performed in the OR. The centralization of resources—including anesthesia personnel and equipment, surgical equipment, radiology, and specialized nursing and procedural support staff—and safety policies and principles make the modern surgical suite an ideal venue for most operations (Fig. 47.1). However, OR demand may exceed available resources, complicating timely access to the OR and scheduling of unplanned, urgent, or emergent cases. Competition for OR space may delay or prevent timely operative procedures for critically ill patients. Additionally, performance of procedures in the OR requires transportation of critically ill patients from the ICU and back, resulting in substantial resource use and costs. As the complexity and severity of illness of critical care patients have increased, so, too, have the risks related to their transport. The transport of critically ill patients frequently requires multiple personnel, including nursing staff, transport staff, respiratory care, and anesthesia staff. Furthermore, the change of venue and personnel caring for the patient necessitates detailed communication for handoff and transitions of care, representing a potential source of medical error. Consideration of transport to the OR should be evaluated in the same manner as other treatments by assessing risk versus benefit for the individual patient.[6] Each hospital should have guidelines for the inter- and intrahospital transport of critically ill patients to various parts of the hospital for imaging, tests, or procedures and to the OR to decrease this inherent risk.[7]

TAKING THE OPERATING ROOM TO THE BEDSIDE

Although the vast majority of surgical procedures should be performed in the OR, the ICU is a logical alternative location for some surgical procedures. The two locations are similar in many

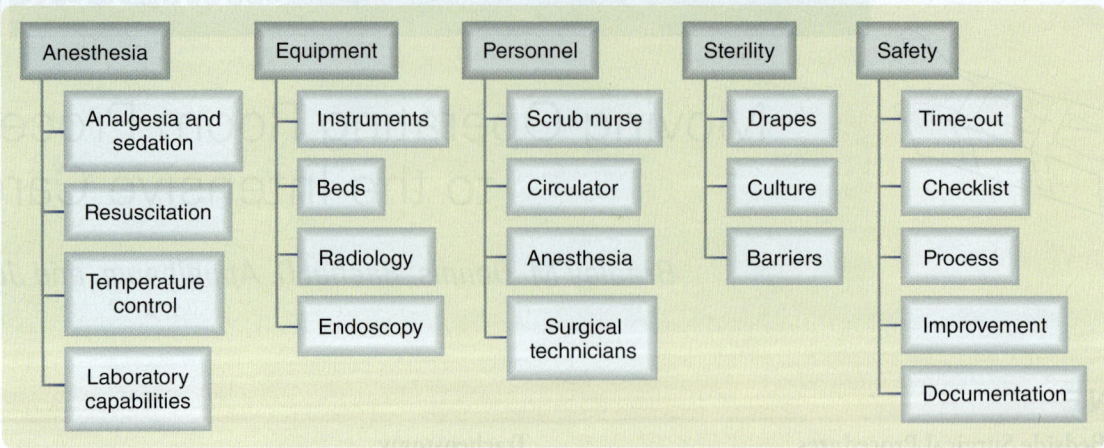

FIGURE 47.1 Resources available in the operating room.

ways. Both locations have equipment capable of real-time monitoring of cardiovascular, respiratory, and neurologic systems. The ICU and OR both have mechanical ventilation capability. In fact, many ICUs have ventilators with more advanced functionalities than their corresponding ORs. Although ICUs lack inhalational anesthetic administration capabilities, intravenous sedation and analgesia can be administered in the ICU to allow for the performance of bedside procedures. Lastly, and most importantly, there are analogous staff in the ICU. The roles of circulating OR nurses and anesthesia providers can be filled by the ICU team, which consists of a critical care nurse, respiratory therapist, and intensivist. The one crucial OR role not easily translated to the ICU setting is the scrub nurse or technician. Dedicated procedure support personnel have been described in the ICU setting to bridge this gap.[2] In this role, the procedure support nurse is responsible for many of the same functions as the scrub nurse. Dedicated procedure support personnel not only decrease the variability in how an individual procedure is performed, but they also play important roles in compliance with guidelines, both of which are significant factors in reducing error.

Multiple factors are required to create and maintain a successful system for performing bedside procedures (Fig. 47.2). Management guidelines may include standard operating procedures; preprocedure checklists, including time-out procedures; and sedation protocols. Appropriate access to supplies may require temporary storage of core equipment in an individual ICU with standardized restocking mechanisms, streamlining the supply

chain. Finally, a facilitative mindset among staff is vital to the success of such a system.

SAFETY PRACTICES FOR BEDSIDE SURGICAL PROCEDURES

To ensure the safety of operative procedures performed at the bedside in the ICU, systematic measures should be in place for appropriate patient selection; adequate expertise of supporting personnel; limited procedural variability; adequate monitoring and anesthesia; and facilitation of concise, accurate, and specific intrateam communication. Measures shown to increase safety in the OR are also appropriate for procedures performed at bedside in the ICU. Implementation of the Safe Surgery Saves Lives program developed by the World Health Organization (WHO) has been associated with a significant global reduction in perioperative morbidity and mortality.[8] The 10 safety objectives outlined in the WHO Guidelines for Safe Surgery 2009 are as follows[9]:

1. The team will operate on the correct patient at the correct site.
2. The team will use methods known to prevent harm from administration of anesthetics while protecting the patient from pain.
3. The team will recognize and effectively prepare for life-threatening loss of airway or respiratory function.
4. The team will recognize and effectively prepare for the risk of high blood loss.
5. The team will avoid inducing an allergic or adverse drug reaction for which the patient is known to be at significant risk.
6. The team will consistently use methods known to minimize the risk for surgical site infection.
7. The team will prevent inadvertent retention of instruments and sponges in surgical wounds.
8. The team will secure and accurately identify all surgical specimens.
9. The team will effectively communicate and exchange critical information for the safe conduct of the operation.
10. Hospitals and public health systems will establish routine surveillance of surgical capacity, volume, and results.

The use of specifically trained procedure support personnel to support bedside operative procedures within the ICU greatly facilitates reduction in variability, compliance with standard operative procedures, reduction of communication errors, and maintenance of appropriate skill sets. Depending on the volume of procedures to

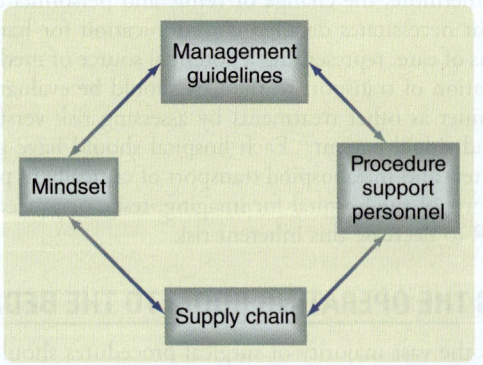

FIGURE 47.2 Fundamentals vital to the success of bedside surgical procedures.

be supported, these personnel can be dedicated to a specific unit or service or used to support bedside procedures on numerous services in multiple ICUs. Limiting this procedure support role to a small number of personnel allows a greater degree of expertise to be developed and is extremely valuable in maintaining procedural safety; this is particularly true with managing the airway and endotracheal tube during percutaneous tracheostomies. Additionally, these individuals are charged with the development and monitoring of safety practices and ensuring their application during all procedures.

Management guidelines, protocols, and standard operating procedures should be in place before the routine performance of bedside operative procedures. They should be in line with procedures developed for the OR and be easily accessible, and compliance should be monitored. Because of variations in specific personnel and practice patterns in various ICUs, documents may be customized to each location to ensure their appropriate application during bedside operative procedures. These documents should address the selection of appropriate cases, mandatory personnel, equipment, medications, and monitoring. An example of a bedside operative guideline is provided in Box 47.1.[3] All patients should have blood pressure, electrocardiography, pulse oximetry, end-tidal carbon dioxide, and ventilation routinely monitored throughout the procedures. Adequate personnel must be present to allow performance of the procedure, monitoring of sedation and anesthesia, medication administration, manipulation of ventilation if required, and documentation. The actual number of personnel required varies depending on the procedure and expertise of particular personnel. Analgesia and sedation must be ensured with appropriate medications under the direction of adequately credentialed personnel. Additionally, guidelines and protocols should include standards for adequate preparation, equipment, and instrument accounting.

The use of preprocedure time-outs and procedural checklists aid in ensuring appropriate safety practices. The use of these tools helps limit communication errors, facilitates compliance with standard operating procedures, and can aid in documentation and compliance monitoring. These tools should be consistent with practices employed in the OR to reduce variability where appropriate. Fig. 47.3 provides an example of such a procedural checklist. Ideally, these tools can be combined with forms required for documentation, and information can be captured for quality and performance analysis.

Ensuring a high degree of safety of bedside operative procedures and providing documentation of such when required mandate that mechanisms for tracking procedure performance, compliance monitoring, and adverse event review and reporting are developed. These mechanisms must be applicable locally to facilitate consistent, nonvariable performance and interface with global hospital safety mechanisms and initiatives. Development of process-mapping flow charts and diagrams facilitates the integration of unit-specific, departmental, and hospital-wide processes and helps delineate lines of communication and authority.

SELECTION OF PATIENTS FOR BEDSIDE SURGICAL PROCEDURES

As noted previously, if selected appropriately, bedside operative procedures can be performed with a similar risk of complications as when performed in the OR, at lower cost, and without transportation risks.[3,4] However, there are no randomized studies and few retrospective reviews that evaluate the safety of bedside operative procedures or help delineate what the appropriate patient populations and operative procedures are. The safety and efficacy of bedside procedures vary depending on the local experience and application of safety practices. As experience is gained, indications may broaden, and frequency may increase. The decision to perform an operative procedure at the bedside requires a careful risk-benefit analysis. This decision considers the difficulty and risk of transport; the complexity of the operation; the ability to achieve timely OR space; and the safety, ease, and cost savings of performing the procedure at the bedside. Most major operative procedures should be performed in the OR. In general, the indications for bedside operative procedures fall into two categories: (1) the patient requires a lifesaving intervention but is too unstable for transport to the OR and (2) low-complexity procedures in which the risk of transport, difficulties of OR scheduling, and cost and resource use of the OR favor a bedside procedure. Factors that generally favor performance of procedures in the OR include

---

BOX 47.1 Bedside Surgery Protocol

Indications
- Decompressive celiotomy for abdominal compartment syndrome
- Exploratory celiotomy for intraabdominal hemorrhage after damage control and packing
- Reexploration of a previously open abdomen for washout or closure
- Exploratory celiotomy to rule out intraabdominal sepsis in a patient with ventilatory requirements that prohibit safe transport to the operating room (OR)

Protocol
a. Intensive care unit (ICU) attending physician and operating surgeon will be present for the entire surgical procedure.
b. Informed consent will be obtained (if possible).
c. Preprocedure checklist will be reviewed by the bedside nurse.
d. Bedside nurse and a respiratory therapist will monitor patient and record procedure (conscious sedation sheet).
Indications to proceed to OR:
- Surgical bleeding
- Dead bowel

- Need to open another body cavity
- Surgeon preference
For laparotomies:
- A sterile perimeter will be set up in the patient's room. All individuals must wear a surgical head covering and mask.
- The ICU attending physician will oversee anesthetic management of the patient.
- General anesthesia will include narcotics, benzodiazepines, propofol, paralytics, and ventilator management.
- A sterile hand wash will be performed by the operating team.
- Preoperative antibiotics are indicated only if a new surgical wound is to be made (e.g., cefazolin [Ancef], 1–2 g intravenously).
- A povidone-iodine (Betadine)–chlorhexidine abdominal preparation will be used.
- A standard Bovie will be set up (when indicated).
- Wall suction canisters will be set up.
- A 4-L warm irrigation with normal saline will be used.
- A standard bedside celiotomy tray will be set up with suture on a sterile field.

SICU Procedure "TIME-OUT" Checklist

Complete this form (a) just prior to beginning the procedure and (b) at the location where the procedure is to be performed.

Patient's Name: _____   Medical record number: _____

Procedure Type: ☐ Planned nonemergent   ☐ Not planned nonemergent   ☐ Emergent

VERIFICATION

	Circle one	
1. Invasive procedure to be performed:		
2. H&P completed if patient admitted within past 24 hours	Yes	No
3. Informed consent obtained? (Verified by Bedside RN and Procedure RN)	Yes	No
4. Correct patient identity? ☐ Arm Band ☐ MRN ☐ Consent If procedure is emergent, Bedside RN, Procedure RN, and Physician performing procedure need to verify patient ID and initial this form.	Yes	No
5. Agreement on procedure (Agreement b/w Physician performing procedure and Procedure RN)	Yes	No
6. Correct side/site verified and marked? ☐ NA ☐ Right ☐ Left ☐ Site: (Verified and marked by Physician performing procedure and Procedure RN)	Yes	No
7. Correct equipment available? (Verified by Physician performing procedure and Procedure RN)	Yes	No
8. Required resources available? (Verified by Physician performing procedure and Procedure RN)	Yes	No
9. Ready to set up procedure? (Verified by Procedure RN)	Yes	No
9. Ready to proceed with procedure? (Verified by Procedure RN)	Yes	No

TIME-OUT: All individuals performing and assisting with the procedure are to review the checklist and sign below.

Physician performing procedure:			
Procedure RN name:			
Bedside RN name:			
Other:	Other:		Other:
Staff calling "TIME-OUT": (Title and signature)			

FIGURE 47.3 Surgical intensive care unit *(SICU)* procedure time-out checklist. *b/w*, Between; *H&P,* history and physical; *MRN*, medical record number; *NA*, not applicable; *RN*, registered nurse.

complex procedures, complex or extensive equipment needs, risk of encountering significant bleeding, need for insertion of prosthetic materials, significant lighting requirements, and lengthy procedures. Commonly performed bedside procedures in the ICU include percutaneous and open tracheostomy, percutaneous endoscopic gastrostomy (PEG) or percutaneous endoscopic transgastric

jejunostomy (PEGJ) tube placement, bronchoscopy, soft tissue debridement, decompressive laparotomy for abdominal hypertension, washout and packing removal after a damage control laparotomy, placement of inferior vena cava filters, and damage control orthopedic procedures (e.g., placement of external fixator). Occasionally, the condition of extremely critically ill patients can be temporized at the bedside by the performance of an operative procedure in the ICU with subsequent performance of the definitive operation in the OR.

LAPAROTOMY AND THE OPEN ABDOMEN

Laparotomy at the bedside in the ICU was initially a procedure of last resort in patients too sick to proceed to the OR—a heroic attempt to identify reversible intraabdominal pathology because the patient was near death.[3] However, the recognition of abdominal compartment syndrome (ACS) as a frequent complication of fluid resuscitation in acutely ill patients resulted in the acceptance of the "damage control" approach to the management of acutely ill patients with intraabdominal pathology. Historically, this led to an increase in the application of bedside laparotomy in the controlled settings of the ICU, although the incidence of this is decreasing in the United States with current-era resuscitation practices liberally using blood instead of fluid. Damage control and management of ACS use an open abdomen approach in which the fascia remains open, which necessitates the use of various temporary abdominal closure techniques. Indications for bedside laparotomy can be classified as emergent or semielective. Common emergent indications include (1) decompressive laparotomy for ACS, (2) control and packing for recurrent bleeding after a previous damage control laparotomy, and (3) suspicion of intraabdominal infection in patients too critically ill to be transported to the OR. Common semielective indications include (1) pack removal after damage control laparotomy, (2) irrigation and debridement of the open abdomen, (3) source control and surveillance for sepsis resulting from intraabdominal pathology, and (4) management of traumatic abdominal defects.

Historically, the most common emergent indication for ICU laparotomy was for decompression of abdominal hypertension. Recognition and understanding of the pathophysiology of increased intraabdominal pressure leading to organ system dysfunction—ACS—have increased significantly since first described as the measurement of intraabdominal pressure as an indication for abdominal reexploration. ACS can be classified as primary, resulting from intraabdominal processes, or secondary, resulting from bowel edema and intraabdominal fluid due to the treatment and resuscitation of extraabdominal pathology. Increasing intraabdominal pressure leads to alterations in abdominal perfusion pressure, restricted venous return, and reduction of pulmonary compliance. These alterations can lead to cardiac failure, pulmonary decompensation, and oliguria. Severe elevations in abdominal pressure can lead to organ hypoperfusion and ischemia, although the pressure at which this occurs may vary depending on mean arterial pressure. Grading systems for the degree of abdominal hypertension have been proposed, with grades III (21–25 mm Hg) and IV (>25 mm Hg) considered to be significantly elevated, and when coupled with new-onset organ dysfunction, this defines ACS.[10] Management of ACS involves measures to ensure adequate abdominal perfusion at lower pressures, but as intraabdominal pressure increases, abdominal decompression by laparotomy is indicated. Appropriate treatment requires recognition of the development of this syndrome.

The indirect measurement of bladder pressures via intravesicular catheter has become the gold standard because of its widespread availability and limited invasiveness. This technique is performed by clamping and attaching the drainage tubing of the Foley to a three-way stop, zeroing the system, and then injecting 25 mL of sterile saline into the bladder. Bladder pressures over 25 mm Hg are highly suspicious for ACS, but the intensivist must take the entire clinical picture into account. Bladder pressure measurements are contraindicated in bladder trauma, neurogenic bladder, and pelvic hematoma. It is important to note that bladder pressures will be potentially inaccurate if the patient is not completely sedated or lying flat.

The acceptance of damage control, an abbreviated laparotomy to salvage trauma patients with exsanguination, has led to an application of bedside laparotomy for control of recurrent bleeding within the abdomen before correction of the patient's systemic physiology and for removal of abdominal packs, irrigation, and debridement. Bedside laparotomy in the ICU is common in most major US academic and trauma centers where damage control and temporary abdominal closure for patients in extremis are frequently used. Numerous methods of temporary abdominal closure have been described and continue to evolve. In 2022, the Eastern Association for the Surgery of Trauma published a practice management guideline regarding techniques to manage the open abdomen. This systematic review and meta-analysis conditionally recommends the use of a fascial traction system over routine care when treating patients with an open abdomen after damage control laparotomy. This recommendation is based on the benefit of improved primary myofascial closure without worsening mortality or enterocutaneous fistula formation.[11]

The open abdominal approach is also applied to the general surgery population, most commonly for the management of abdominal sepsis with bowel edema and the inability to perform a fascial closure, hemodynamically unstable patients requiring damage control procedures, necrotizing soft tissue infection of the abdominal wall, diffuse peritonitis in patients at high risk of failure of source control, and mesenteric ischemia.[3] Damage control techniques with staged gastrointestinal reconstruction, serial abdominal washouts for source control, and delayed abdominal wall closure can be used in the management of these very complex patients. Controlled trials of these techniques are limited, and the indications and settings in which the open abdominal approach is most appropriate are not fully determined.

Surgical rescue of the critically ill patient has become an increasing area of awareness. In select critically ill patients with severe cardiopulmonary instability precluding transport to the OR, a resuscitative bedside laparotomy in the ICU may be indicated. Patients who require an emergent bedside laparotomy have an extremely high rate of death, with over 50% mortality. This information may be useful in the setting of preintervention counseling with patients' families.[12]

TRACHEOSTOMY

Tracheostomy is the most common surgical procedure in critically ill patients requiring prolonged mechanical ventilation.[13] Table 47.1 shows some of the common indications and contraindications for tracheostomy. Nearly all contraindications are relative ones, and most are temporary. Indications for tracheostomy in critically ill patients fall broadly into three categories: (1) upper airway obstruction, (2) prolonged mechanical ventilation, and (3) neurologic condition preventing safe extubation.

The ease and convenience of bedside tracheostomy in critically ill patients have made performance at the bedside the standard in many institutions. Open and percutaneous dilatational tracheostomy (PDT) can be performed safely at the bedside in the ICU.[2,14] Conversion from Jackson endotracheal tube size to tracheostomy size is shown in Table 47.2. Evidence-based guidelines

TABLE 47.1 Indications and Contraindications for Tracheostomy

INDICATIONS	CONTRAINDICATIONS
Upper airway obstruction	Recent anterior neck surgery (<7 days)
Difficult airway	High ventilator settings
Significant maxillofacial	Fraction of inspired oxygen >50%
trauma	Positive end-expiratory pressure
Angioedema	>10 cm H_2O
Upper airway tumors	Advanced ventilator modes
Neurologic condition preventing	Elevated intracranial pressure
safe extubation	Hemodynamic instability
Brain injury—acute or	Significant bleeding risk
progressive	Local infection or malignancy at
Spinal cord injury (including	proposed site
halo fixation)	Predicted early mortality
Severe agitation or delirium	
Prolonged altered mental	
status	
Prolonged mechanical ventilation	

do not recommend one specific technique over another with respect to reducing complications or mortality.[15] PDT has become widely used for elective tracheostomy in critically ill adult patients. Ciaglia and colleagues[16] first described elective PDT in 1985, and since that time, numerous modifications to the technique have been made. When comparing PDT with standard surgical tracheostomy performed in the OR via systematic review and meta-analysis, PDT suggested decreased wound infection and clinically relevant bleeding.[14] Percutaneous tracheostomy has also been demonstrated to be more cost-effective in critically ill ICU patients.[17] Periprocedural mortality related to PDT in randomized studies appears to be less than 0.2%.[2,14] The safety of bedside PDT was described in a single institutional retrospective analysis of more than 3000 consecutive procedures.[2] This case series revealed a periprocedural major complication rate of 0.15% and a periprocedural mortality rate of less than 0.1% within this population of critically ill patients. Additionally, this work demonstrated the safety of bedside PDT in patients of higher obesity classes. These data are useful for decisions regarding the indications for tracheostomy in critically ill patients; patients should be considered for tracheostomy when the risks of failure of extubation or airway loss resulting in death are estimated to be less than 1 in 1000.

Timing of tracheostomy is controversial in patients with predicted prolonged mechanical ventilation.[18] Most studies have shown no difference in relevant clinical outcomes such as mortality, pneumonia rates, and hospital length of stay.[17-19] Studies have

TABLE 47.2 Conversion from Jackson Endotracheal Tube Size to Tracheostomy Size

JACKSON SIZE	INNER DIAMETER WITH INNER CANNULA (MM)	INNER DIAMETER WITHOUT INNER CANNULA (MM)	OUTER DIAMETER (mm)
4	5.0	6.7	9.4
6	6.4	8.1	10.8
8	7.6	9.1	12.2
10	8.9	10.7	13.8

supported early tracheostomy (up to 7 days) versus delayed tracheostomy (after 7 days), with shorter ICU stays and less mechanical ventilation but with no difference in mortality in trauma and nontrauma populations.[19-23] However, a randomized study of medical ICU patients demonstrated a significant reduction in mortality (32% vs. 62%), pneumonia (5% vs. 25%), and accidental extubation (0 vs. 6) when early tracheostomy at 48 hours was compared with delayed tracheostomy at 14 to 16 days for patients predicted to require more than 2 weeks of mechanical ventilation.[24] The early group also had significantly decreased ICU length of stay and ventilator days. The largest randomized clinical trial studied >900 adult patients enrolled in 72 ICUs across 13 academic and 59 nonacademic UK hospitals, where early (within 4 days) was compared with late (after 10 days) tracheostomy. From a follow-up period of 30 days to 2 years, there was no mortality difference,[20] which is supported by a number of recent systematic reviews.[25,26] Notably, in this British trial, over 50% of those randomized to late tracheostomy did not require a tracheostomy due to liberation from mechanical ventilation and/or ICU discharge.[20]

The COVID pandemic presented new challenges to the bedside percutaneous tracheostomy. Because it is an aerosol-generating procedure, appropriate airborne and droplet precautions are required for proceduralist and procedural support personnel if the patient is still actively shedding virus. Appropriate timing of the procedure is a topic of some debate. Retrospective data and meta-analysis suggest that tracheostomy after 10 to 14 days of mechanical ventilation is associated with a lower duration of mechanical ventilation and ICU length of stay without increases in mortality.[27,28] In addition, the pandemic brought to the forefront the practice of tracheostomy in patients on extracorporeal membrane oxygenation (ECMO). Tracheostomy can be safely performed in this group at the bedside with appropriate hemostatic technique. Complications are higher overall, almost entirely related to bleeding, but percutaneous and open techniques showed no difference in complication rate.[29]

Reported perioperative complications of percutaneous tracheostomy include the following: peristomal bleeding from injury to the anterior jugular veins or thyroid isthmus, injury of the posterior trachea and/or esophagus by laceration through the back wall of the trachea, extraluminal placement by creating a false tract during placement of the tracheostomy tube, and loss of airway. Long-term complications have not been adequately studied in randomized trials to draw conclusions.

Major perioperative complications can be minimized by employing safety measures outlined in the previous sections. Using specifically trained support personnel to manage the airway is particularly helpful in limiting airway mishaps. Dedicated multidisciplinary tracheostomy teams have been shown to reduce time to decannulation, length of stay, and adverse events.[30] Additionally, one of two techniques should be used to ensure proper positioning of the tracheostomy tube and minimize risk of loss of airway by inadvertent extubation during the procedure: bronchoscopic guidance or a semiopen technique with blunt dissection to the anterior trachea. However, bronchoscopic guidance does not eliminate severe tracheal injuries, and involvement of experienced personnel is important to prevent these complications. Recently, the use of preprocedure ultrasound to identify the neck anatomy has been described as helpful in decreasing the potential risk of bleeding from crossing veins, identifying enlarged thyroid lobes, and decreasing the number of sticks.[31,32] This has been especially helpful with patients in the higher obesity classes. Long term, the incidence of serious tracheal stenosis after percutaneous tracheostomy is low, with reports of 6%,[33] and tracheal stenosis usually occurs early in the subglottic position. Subclinical tracheal stenosis is found in 40% of patients.[34] Follow-up of patients discharged from the ICU with tracheostomies is important to minimize and identify complications.

PERCUTANEOUS ENDOSCOPIC FEEDING TUBES

Gauderer and coworkers[35] first described PEG in 1980 for access into the stomach for enteral feedings using a "pull" technique. Various other techniques have since been described. The principle of a sutureless approximation of the stomach to the anterior abdominal wall has allowed the pull technique to become the most popular method used. The other two most commonly used techniques are the "push" and introducer techniques, both of which require the use of stay sutures to approximate the stomach to the anterior abdominal wall. Newer PEGJ tubes combine gastric and jejunal ports to allow distal feeding and proximal decompression.

Accepted primary indications for a PEG or PEGJ include inability to swallow, high risk of aspiration, severe facial trauma, and indications for mechanical ventilation for longer than 4 weeks.[36] Other indications include nutritional access for debilitated patients and patients with dementia with severe malnutrition. PEG tubes have been associated with reducing overall hospital costs.

Numerous gastrostomy and gastrojejunostomy tubes are commercially available. Most allow simple gastrostomy assessment with or without a valve. Some are flush with the skin and require a tube to be attached only during feeding. For critically ill patients with an increased risk of aspiration, multilumen PEGJ tubes are available. These tubes allow drainage of the stomach while feeding the proximal jejunum. A third lumen connects to a balloon that maintains apposition of the gastric and abdominal walls.

Enteral feeding through a newly placed percutaneous feeding tube can usually be initiated after 12 to 24 hours. Studies evaluating the efficacy of early initiation of enteral nutrition have demonstrated encouraging results; however, delayed feeding after percutaneous placement continues to be widely practiced. Dubagunta et al. performed a prospective study using a protocol standardizing enteral nutrition after 4 hours. They concluded that initiation of enteral feeding after PEG tube placement can be successfully completed with a systematic protocol and close observation. The protocol was safe and associated with significant cost savings by eliminating the need for inpatient hospitalization postprocedure.[37,38]

Contraindications for PEG placement include the following: no endoscopic access, significant ascites, severe coagulopathy, gastric outlet obstruction or previous gastric resection, gastric bypass surgery, survival of less than 4 weeks, inability to bring the gastric wall in approximation to the abdominal wall, and severe immunosuppression (white blood cell count <1). There are a few relative contraindications, such as an inability to transilluminate through the anterior abdominal wall, gastric varices, diffuse gastric cancer, and agitation requiring restraints. It may be nearly impossible to place a PEG in class III obese patients (body mass index >40 kg/m^2) because of the thickness of the abdominal wall. Anterior wall inflammation or infection should be treated before the procedure. If there are no other options, ascites may be drained before the procedure to facilitate PEG tube placement.[39] PEG tubes may be placed in the presence of a ventriculoperitoneal shunt or a dialysis catheter. However, placement should be separated by 1 to 2 weeks or more to minimize the risk of catheter infection.[40] History of a previous or recent laparotomy is not a contraindication for PEG. However, one may consider a preprocedure CT scan to confirm there is a clear window for PEG placement. A discrete indentation of the stomach when palpating the anterior abdominal wall and adequate transillumination should be ensured.[41]

PEG is thought to be a safe procedure whether it is performed in the gastrointestinal laboratory, the OR, or at bedside in the ICU. However, because PEG tube placement is frequently performed in debilitated or critically ill patients, complications are associated with a higher mortality than would be expected for most elective procedures.[42] Free intraperitoneal air after PEG is common and can persist for 4 weeks, although it should not be considered benign on initial evaluation.[43] Abdominal wall infection can occur as an early complication of PEG placement; an ample skin incision that prevents creation of a closed space around the feeding tube and administration of antibiotics before the procedure have been demonstrated to decrease PEG site infections.[44] Dislodgment of the PEG from the stomach can occur and may be life threatening. Dislodgment may occur acutely through the application of traction on the gastrostomy tube, pulling it partially or completely through the abdominal wall. Alternatively, the tube may necrose through the stomach wall if the internal PEG flange, disc, balloon, or bumper (i.e., buried bumper syndrome) applies too much pressure on the gastric wall. If this complication occurs before development of a fibrous tract during the initial 10 to 14 days, it should be considered a surgical emergency because gastric contents would spill into the abdominal cavity; operative closure of the gastrostomy is required. To minimize the risk of this complication, methods that prevent inadvertent movement of the gastrostomy tube should be used and meticulously followed. These methods include recording of the position of the gastrostomy tube at the skin surface immediately after the procedure with routine verification and application of binders or other devices that limit the inadvertent application of traction on the tube. Of note, the historical common practice of tube fixation to the external abdominal wall has been deemed a less critically important method, and it has even been abandoned at some major centers to limit external skin morbidities.

Patients requiring access for enteral nutrition are inherently at risk for healing issues due to malnutrition. Patients on high-dose steroids or chemotherapy present additional complexity to wound healing and are at increased risk for complications with feeding tube dislodgement. Hyperactive, delirious, or agitated patients are also at increased risk for tube complications; hence, they represent a relative contraindication for placement. As mentioned, the morbidity associated with early tube dislodgement is significant and often requires surgical exploration for gastric repair and tube replacement. Timratana et al. performed a small retrospective review of PEG placement when their group began to selectively place T-fasteners in high-risk agitated patients. They concluded the placement of T-fasteners may decrease overall morbidity if early tube dislodgement occurs and tubes can be nonemergently replaced.[45] Other institutions place nonremoval PEG tubes in these same populations, with a lower risk of dislodgement requiring laparotomy but higher rates of buried bumpers and soft tissue complications, along with the disadvantage of needing a second endoscopic procedure for PEG excision and removal when it is no longer required for enteral support.

BRONCHOSCOPY

Fiberoptic bronchoscopy of critical care patients is indicated for diagnostic and therapeutic purposes. Therapeutic indications include insertion of an endotracheal tube, removal of foreign bodies inadvertently aspirated, removal of mucous plugs, reversal of atelectasis in mechanically ventilated patients, suctioning of thick tenacious secretions, and diagnosis of obstructive pneumonia.[46]

Diagnostic bronchoscopy is most commonly used for obtaining pulmonary specimens for diagnosis and management of pneumonia.[47] Quantitative cultures obtained via fiberoptic bronchoscopy have been shown to eliminate the diagnosis of pneumonia in nearly 50% of patients with clinical signs of pneumonia, to decrease inappropriate antibiotic use, and to improve mortality compared with nonquantitative techniques. Standardization of culture techniques should be undertaken.

Currently, they exist as single-use flexible bronchoscopes (SFBs) or reusable flexible bronchoscopes (RFBs). Traditionally, RFBs have played a crucial role in the diagnosis and treatment of pulmonary diseases; however, they come with some limitations, including risk of cross-infection (2.8% risk), high maintenance cost, and long waiting times for decontamination.[48] In 2009, the Ambu company first invented an SFB. The greatest benefit of SFBs is the avoidance of cross-infection. Additionally, they are portable and easy to set up. They do not require endoscopy staff or a large bronchoscopy tower. Since its initial development, the SFB has been modified and improved, and it is used widely in clinical practice. The COVID-19 pandemic led to increased interest and use. Several studies have evaluated the efficacy of these bronchoscopes.[48] He et al. performed a prospective controlled study with 45 patients undergoing bronchoscopic biopsy. The authors concluded that SFBs are noninferior to RFBs in routine bronchoscopy, bronchoalveolar lavage, and biopsy.[49]

The risk associated with diagnostic bronchoscopy is related to the need for conscious sedation and the required medications if performed in a nonintubated patient. Medication use can possibly result in depressed mental status progressing to hypoventilation, airway vulnerability, and the risk of aspiration. The risks of the procedure itself are pneumothorax, hypoxia, airway hyperreactivity, pulmonary hemorrhage, loss of pulmonary reserve in patients on high ventilator settings, and systemic hypotension or hypertension.

SUMMARY

This chapter covered the rationale for bedside surgical procedures in the ICU, resources required, and safety practices and considerations for transitioning procedures from the OR to the ICU. Given the rising demand for OR resources in many healthcare systems, using the nimbler ICU environment with properly supported personnel and clear protocols can enhance throughput of patient care. With attention to patient selection, laparotomy for acute abdominal pathologies, tracheostomy, percutaneous endoscopic feeding access, and bronchoscopy have evolved into reliable, safe, and common bedside practices in many ICU environments around the world.

SELECTED REFERENCES

Delaney A, Bagshaw SM, Nalos M. Percutaneous dilatational tracheostomy versus surgical tracheostomy in critically ill patients: a systematic review and meta-analysis. *Crit Care.* 2006;10:R55.

This meta-analysis of percutaneous dilatational tracheostomy (PDT) versus standard open surgical tracheostomy supports the benefits of PDT.

Dennis BM, Eckert MJ, Gunter OL, et al. Safety of bedside percutaneous tracheostomy in the critically ill: evaluation of more than 3,000 procedures. *J Am Coll Surg.* 2013;216:858-865.

This article, which is the largest review of the safety of bedside percutaneous dilatational tracheostomy, documents safety across body mass index distribution.

Diaz Jr JJ, Mejia V, Subhawong AP, et al. Protocol for bedside laparotomy in trauma and emergency general surgery: a low return to the operating room. *Am Surg.* 2005;71:986-991.

This primary article examines outcomes of bedside laparotomy, with a protocol for indications and support.

Fagon JY. Diagnosis and treatment of ventilator-associated pneumonia: fiberoptic bronchoscopy with bronchoalveolar lavage is essential. *Semin Respir Crit Care Med.* 2006;27:34-44.

The indications, benefits, and performance of bronchoscopy for the diagnosis of pneumonia are reviewed.

Kirkpatrick AW, Roberts DJ, De Waele J, et al. Intra-abdominal hypertension and the abdominal compartment syndrome: updated consensus definitions and clinical practice guidelines from the World Society of the Abdominal Compartment Syndrome. *Intensive Care Med.* 2013;39(7):1190-1206.

This article provides a current-era review of the definitions and guidelines associated with the treatment of abdominal compartment syndrome.

Raimondi N, Vial MR, Calleja J, et al. Evidence-based guidelines for the use of tracheostomy in critically ill patients. *J Crit Care.* 2017;38:304-318.

This article provides a systematic review and evidence-based recommendations for the use of tracheostomy in critically ill patients, including technique, timing, cost, and special populations.

Van Natta TL, Morris Jr JA, Eddy VA, et al. Elective bedside surgery in critically injured patients is safe and cost-effective. *Ann Surg.* 1998;227:618-624.

This article is the first report on the safety and effectiveness of bedside surgical procedures.

Young D, Harrison D, Cuthbertson B, et al. Effect of early vs late tracheostomy placement on survival in patients receiving mechanical ventilation: the TracMan randomized trial. *JAMA.* 2013;309:2121-2129.

This is the largest randomized trial of early versus late tracheostomy in critically ill patients.

The full reference list appears on Elsevier eBooks+.

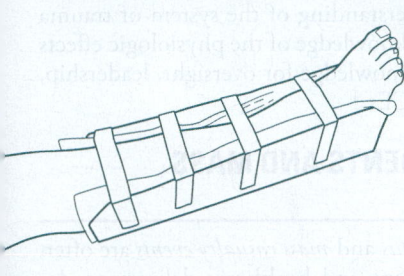

CHAPTER 48

The Surgeon's Role in Disaster Management

David Zonies, Michael Cheatham, and Joseph Johnson

INTRODUCTION

Mass casualty incidents (MCIs) or mass casualty events (MCEs) are characterized by a large number of people becoming injured or ill in a specific event or series of related events. These events can include anthropogenic (human-derived) intentional events (e.g., mass shootings, bombings), anthropogenic nonintentional events (e.g., industrial accidents, structure fires), and natural disasters (hurricanes, earthquakes). Although often unpredictable, such disaster events are increasing such that every medical provider and medical system must be prepared to respond. The most recent example of a long-duration disaster has been the response to the COVID-19 pandemic, in which systems were rapidly overwhelmed in terms of both physical capacity and capability.[1] Since the September 11, 2001, attacks, there has been a particular focus on education and preparation for such events, partly as a result of the increased number of events related to terrorist groups, civilian bombings, and large-scale shootings. This was amplified in 2013 at the Boston Marathon bombing, along with numerous mass shootings at schools and other public venues.[2-4]

One hallmark of most disasters is the presence of major traumatic injuries that require rapid triage, evaluation, and surgical treatment.[5,6] The surgeon plays a critical role in nearly every aspect of disaster management, from preparation and training to the execution and recovery phases. It is critical that surgeons be actively involved in all of the key nonclinical aspects of disaster care, particularly in the local and regional planning and preparatory activities. In many systems, these tasks have been assigned to nonsurgeons and even to nonclinicians, which can result in an unrealistic disaster plan and suboptimal clinical response to the actual event.

Another frequently underappreciated and misunderstood concept in disaster care is the critical role and importance of triage. Among the earliest changes in the way that patients are managed during an MCE is the "sifting and sorting" into categories and their priorities for receiving emergent/urgent care.[7] Although the injury severity and urgency of injured patients will vary somewhat between events, the majority of patients presenting for care will not have major or life-threatening injuries (Fig. 48.1). Further, these minimally injured patients tend to arrive before the more severely injured cohorts, rather than the most severely injured arriving first. This is because less severely injured patients are easier to transport by emergency medical services (EMS) or self-present to the closest emergency department (ED).

Because of the complex nature of disaster responses, high-quality triage may be the most critical physician-driven aspect of initial disaster management. All surgeons should be familiar with the principles and practices of triage in such situations. Appropriate and effective

Disaster injury severity on hospital arrival

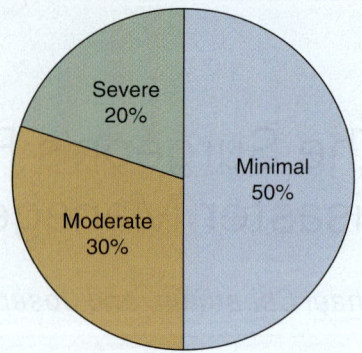

FIGURE 48.1 Most patients who present after a disaster are minimally injured. Approximately 20% of patients are severely injured and should be the focus of immediate interventions.

triage will set the stage for the success or failure of any disaster response by optimizing the match between the injuries and injury severity of the presenting patients and the available critical resources of the facility or system that will be providing care.[8-10]

Ultimately, the goal of any disaster response should be to (1) save the lives of those injured in the event, (2) restore the trauma center or hospital to normal operations as quickly as possible, and (3) learn from the MCI and revise the hospital disaster plan so as to improve future responses. An MCI has a far-reaching impact on a hospital and community, and the lasting effects extend well beyond the hours of the initial response.

HISTORY OF DISASTER

The term *triage* was coined by Napoleon Bonaparte's surgeon, Dr. Baron Larrey. Dr. Larrey poignantly described the importance of addressing the most seriously injured patients first. The military's earliest documented systems of triage date back to the 18th century, and triage is a principal component of disaster care. MCEs are becoming increasingly common, and there are many lessons that can be learned from both the military and civilian systems in terms of triage and trauma systems to optimize care and outcomes for as many casualties as possible.

Triage is a term with its roots in military medicine, and the practice of triage arose from the demands of large amounts of battlefield casualties during war; the original triage concepts were primarily focused on maximal salvage during battlefield injury. Dr. Larrey was known for his surgical leadership and skill and is credited with the development of the concept of "sorting" patients to salvage the greatest number of casualties in a resource-scarce battlefield environment. Dr. Larrey's principals of sorting also included evacuating patients according to the severity of wounding and prioritizing their care based on both the severity of the injury and the likelihood of survival.[11-13]

With each subsequent war since Napoleon's time, military and civilian medical communities have continued to advance the concepts of triage and mass casualty management. As the world becomes increasingly turbulent, with a higher frequency of MCEs, the potential and need for surgeons to be involved in such events are increasing. Surgeon leadership, hospital planning, and community preparation are the first steps to the successful management of these challenging events. Surgeon involvement in every tier of disaster management should be a professional expectation. Although the modern-day surgeon is rarely a prehospital provider,

surgeons' comprehensive understanding of the system of trauma care, combined with intricate knowledge of the physiologic effects of injury, gives them unique knowledge for oversight, leadership, and training in relation to MCEs.[4]

MASS CASUALTY INCIDENTS AND MASS CASUALTY EVENTS

The terms *mass casualty incidents* and *mass casualty events* are often used in emergency management and healthcare delivery to describe situations involving a large number of casualties. The term *mass casualty incident* typically refers to an event in which the number of injured or deceased individuals overwhelms the available resources and capabilities of the emergency response system in a specific location. This could include incidents such as natural disasters, industrial accidents, or large-scale transportation accidents. On the other hand, *a mass casualty event* is a broader term that encompasses a wide range of incidents, both intentional and unintentional, resulting in a significant number of casualties. MCEs may include acts of terrorism, pandemics, and other incidents that lead to a substantial impact on public health and safety. Although the terms are sometimes used interchangeably, MCIs are often more localized and immediate, whereas MCIs have a broader scope and may have long-lasting implications on a larger scale.

THE SPECTRUM OF CARE STANDARDS DURING A DISASTER RESPONSE

Disaster response in the hospital setting is a dynamic process that evolves through distinct phases—standard care, contingency care, and crisis care—when confronted with an MCI. Initially, healthcare systems operate under standard care protocols, assuming routine conditions where resources and infrastructure are adequate. However, when faced with an event that overwhelms the system's capacity, a transition to contingency care becomes imperative. During this phase, all healthcare providers adapt and modify practices to optimize the use of available resources without compromising the quality of care. This is an important distinction: During contingency operations, care quality is not significantly affected. Contingency care involves innovative approaches to maintain essential services while responding to the surge in demand.[1]

In the unfortunate event of a catastrophic escalation, hospitals may need to enter the crisis care phase. Here, the emphasis shifts from delivering optimal care to delivering the best possible care under extreme resource constraints. This stage often involves difficult decision-making, such as re-triaging patients based on the severity of their conditions and the likelihood of survival. Ethical considerations become paramount because resources, including medical supplies and personnel, may be insufficient to meet the overwhelming demand.

Effectively navigating these phases requires meticulous planning, coordination, and flexibility. This process will be described in detail later in this chapter. From a surgeon's perspective, preparedness includes not only physical resources like surgical supplies and infrastructure but also training to swiftly adapt to evolving circumstances. A seamless transition between standard care, contingency care, and crisis care is essential to ensure a resilient healthcare response capable of mitigating the impact of MCIs and safeguarding the well-being of those affected.

An important aspect of such a response is appreciating the differences between a surgical team's capability to deal with injury response and a hospital's capacity to manage a large number of patients. In the context of disaster response in hospitals, capacity and capability are distinct but interconnected concepts. *Capacity* refers to the ability of a hospital to accommodate and manage a certain volume of patients, considering factors such as available beds, staff, and resources. It quantifies the physical and logistical limits of the healthcare facility. On the other hand, *capability* refers to the hospital's proficiency in providing specific services and interventions, irrespective of its physical capacity. It encompasses the skills, expertise, and resources necessary to deliver effective medical care. Whereas capacity focuses on the quantity of care a hospital can provide, capability delves into the qualitative aspects of that care, emphasizing the expertise and resources needed for various medical scenarios. During a disaster response, understanding and balancing both capacity and capability are crucial for hospitals to efficiently and effectively manage a surge in patients while maintaining a high standard of care.

During an MCE, the goal of medical personnel is to provide the best possible care to the greatest number of people. In such situations, the standard of care may be compromised because of the sheer volume of patients.[14] Sufficient care is defined as the minimum level of care that is necessary to stabilize a patient's condition and prevent further deterioration. Standard care, on the other hand, is the level of care that would be provided under normal circumstances. During an MCE, medical personnel may have to prioritize patients based on the severity of their injuries and the likelihood of survival. This may mean that some patients receive only sufficient care while others receive standard care.

KEY DEFINITIONS

Under normal circumstances, the term *triage* most frequently applies to the sorting of trauma or critically ill patients in order to direct them to the medical treatment facility with the most appropriate level of capability. Accurate triage results in distributing patients to appropriate hospitals that can expertly manage their condition, whether it is traumatic injury, myocardial infarction, stroke, or sepsis. In terms of trauma, the standard civilian use of the term *trauma triage* refers to the day-to-day function of sending patients to the appropriate hospital/trauma center in order to avoid over- and undertriage. Basic triage optimizes and balances care delivery and resource allocation. Optimizing triage in the face of multiple casualties and potentially limited resources requires leadership, planning, and an established trauma system. Surgeon leadership in the triage process and the trauma system helps establish a well-organized response to disaster. Surgeon involvement in the triage planning and process should occur at every level in a healthcare system: individual, local, regional, and national.

Triage is the process of sorting patients to provide the greatest amount of good for the greatest (highest) number of patients. Success or failure is measured in lives saved or lives lost and resources wasted or appropriately used; success or failure depends on accurate and effective triage.[4]

- Field triage
  Accomplished at or near the scene of the event. The process by which EMS providers decide which hospital to send patients injured by a disaster or traumatic event. Involves collaboration within the field incident command system (ICS).

- Undertriage
  Occurs when seriously injured patients are transported to nontrauma centers or centers that do not have the expertise or capability to manage the severity of the injury.
- Overtriage
  Occurs when patients with minor or nonurgent injuries are transported to major trauma centers or triaged to an immediate care bed. In a disaster situation, this bogs down the system, results in significant bottlenecking, and can result in increased rates of adverse outcomes (Fig. 48.2).

> - The goal of field triage is to efficiently concentrate injured patients to major trauma centers without overwhelming these centers with patients who have minor injuries.
> - The national benchmarks for field trauma triage are set by the American College of Surgeons Committee on Trauma and are based on system-level rates of undertriage and overtriage.

- Hospital triage
  Sorting patients into predefined categories in order to determine their relative priority of treatment. Patients are separated into groups based on the local triage system that is used. Patients are sorted into categories: those not expected to survive even with treatment; those who will recover with minimal treatment; and the highest-priority group, those who will not survive without treatment.
- Mass casualty incident (MCI)
  Multiple injured patients present simultaneously, but adequate resources are present, and the system is not significantly stressed. An MCI for a large trauma center could be routine, but an MCI may result in a disaster scenario for a small hospital.
- Mass casualty event (MCE)
  Large-scale event that often results in overwhelming numbers of injured or ill patients, as well as frequent destruction or degradation of local infrastructure, which may include the healthcare facilities.

There is a critical distinction between an MCI and MCE that must be understood and appreciated by the treating surgeon.[15]

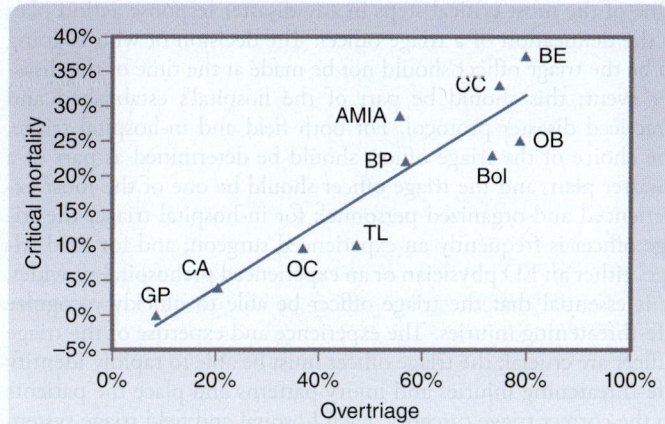

FIGURE 48.2 Relationship between overtriage and critical mortality. One must balance acceptable overtriage with risk of mortality because as it increases, resources are consumed, with resultant increased mortality, as seen in this series of disasters. *AMIA,* Buenos Aires; *BE,* Beirut; *BP,* Birmingham pubs; *Bol,* Bologna; *CA,* Craigavon; *CC,* Cu Chi; *OB,* Old Bailey; *OC,* Oklahoma City; *TL,* Tower of London.

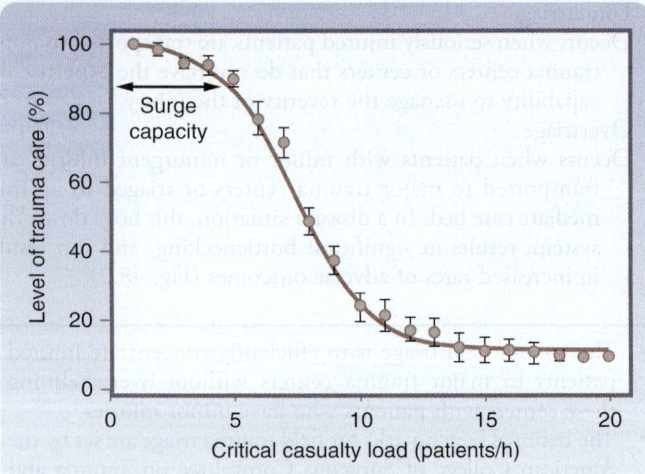

FIGURE 48.3 As patient volume rapidly increases, there is a logarithmic drop in capacity. The goal is to push capacity to the right and thereby increase the total volume of patients a system can manage.

Whereas an MCI requires little to no change in the usual practices and the standard of care, a larger disaster or MCE may result in alternative care pathways with a focus on optimizing group outcomes versus individual patient outcomes. The primary factor that distinguishes these two categories is the relationship between the presenting injuries and the available resources and expertise to care for them. This is commonly referred to as the *surge capacity* for a given facility or system. As shown in Fig. 48.3, the standard level of care can be maintained for a finite number of patients, but once this number is exceeded, there is a precipitous decline in the level of care and associated outcomes. A well-resourced major trauma center may be easily able to handle 20 severely injured patients from one incident, whereas a smaller rural nontrauma center may be overwhelmed with more than 2 or 3 severely injured patients.

HAVE A PLAN

Given the increased requirements placed on a system by an MCE, having a clear plan of action in the event of an MCE is critical to ensure maximal efficiency in the face of unusual circumstances. One of the most critical steps in any disaster response action plan is the delineation of a triage officer. The decision of who is going to be the triage officer should not be made at the time of the disaster event; this should be part of the hospital's established and practiced disaster protocol. For both field and in-hospital triage, the choice of the triage officer should be determined as part of a disaster plan, and the triage officer should be one of the most experienced and organized personnel; for in-hospital triage, the triage officer is frequently an experienced surgeon; and for field triage, either an ED physician or an experienced prehospital provider. It is essential that the triage officer be able to quickly recognize life-threatening injuries. The experience and expertise of the triage officer are crucial; the triage officer must be able to rapidly identify life-threatening injuries and injury patterns and place the patients in the correct triage category. Each hospital and field triage system should have redundancy in the personnel who can serve as the triage officer. Although most triage officers are surgeons, experienced providers in emergency medicine can be excellent triage officers. Disaster plans in the hospital should be rehearsed, and training should be provided. More than one potential triage officer should be identified and train for that role to provide redundancy in the

available expertise and also to prepare for scenarios in which the primary triage officer is injured, ill, or otherwise engaged or in which multiple triage points need to be established.

The location for the triage point(s) should be predetermined and clearly spelled out in the written disaster plan and any rehearsal drills. One of the most common errors that we have observed in hospital disaster planning is the development of only one triage plan and location, which fails to appreciate the highly variable nature of these events.[16,17] We recommend the development of at least two flexible triage schemas that allow for the different triage requirements that will be seen in smaller-scale MCIs versus larger-scale or disaster-type events. In general, smaller-scale incidents where all patients can be immediately brought inside the facility require only one primary triage point that is usually optimally located near the ED entrance. Larger-scale MCEs that exceed the available bed space or providers necessitate the establishment of an external primary triage site where patients are categorized, prioritized, and held until they can be moved into the facility (Fig. 48.4).[18,19] Secondary triage would then occur as patients are filtered into the facility and then directed to the appropriate location based on their needed level of care. The external triage location should have climate control, be well lit, and have prestocked supplies for immediate patient needs, including hemorrhage control and airway/breathing interventions. All patients who arrive at the facility must be triaged and ideally enter the hospital through one tightly controlled entry point, with all other facility entrances protected by assigned security personnel.

Field triage protocols benefit trauma systems, but for optimal effect, they must be tailored to local needs and tested in each system for sensitivity and specificity. Training should be provided, and protocols should have a built-in performance improvement mechanism and be monitored by experienced physicians and surgeons who can adjust the protocols when necessary (Figs. 48.5 and 48.6). The American College of Surgeons (ACS) Committee

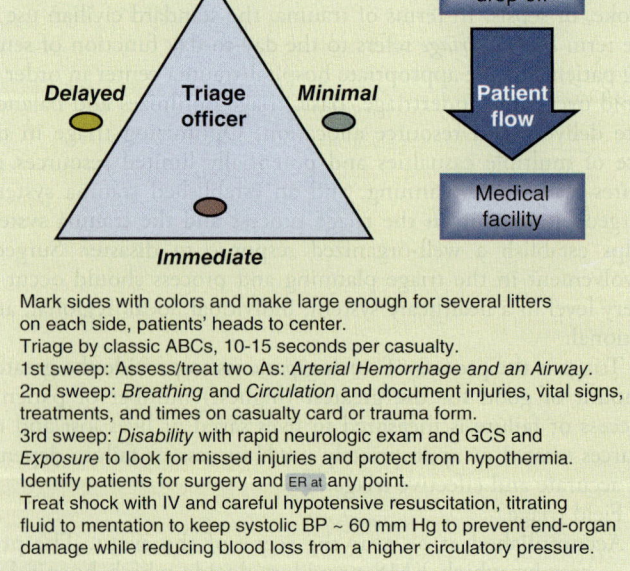

FIGURE 48.4 Prehospital allocation of patients through triage before hospital transport. *ABCs,* Airway, breathing, and circulation; *BP,* blood pressure; *GCS,* Glasgow Coma Scale.

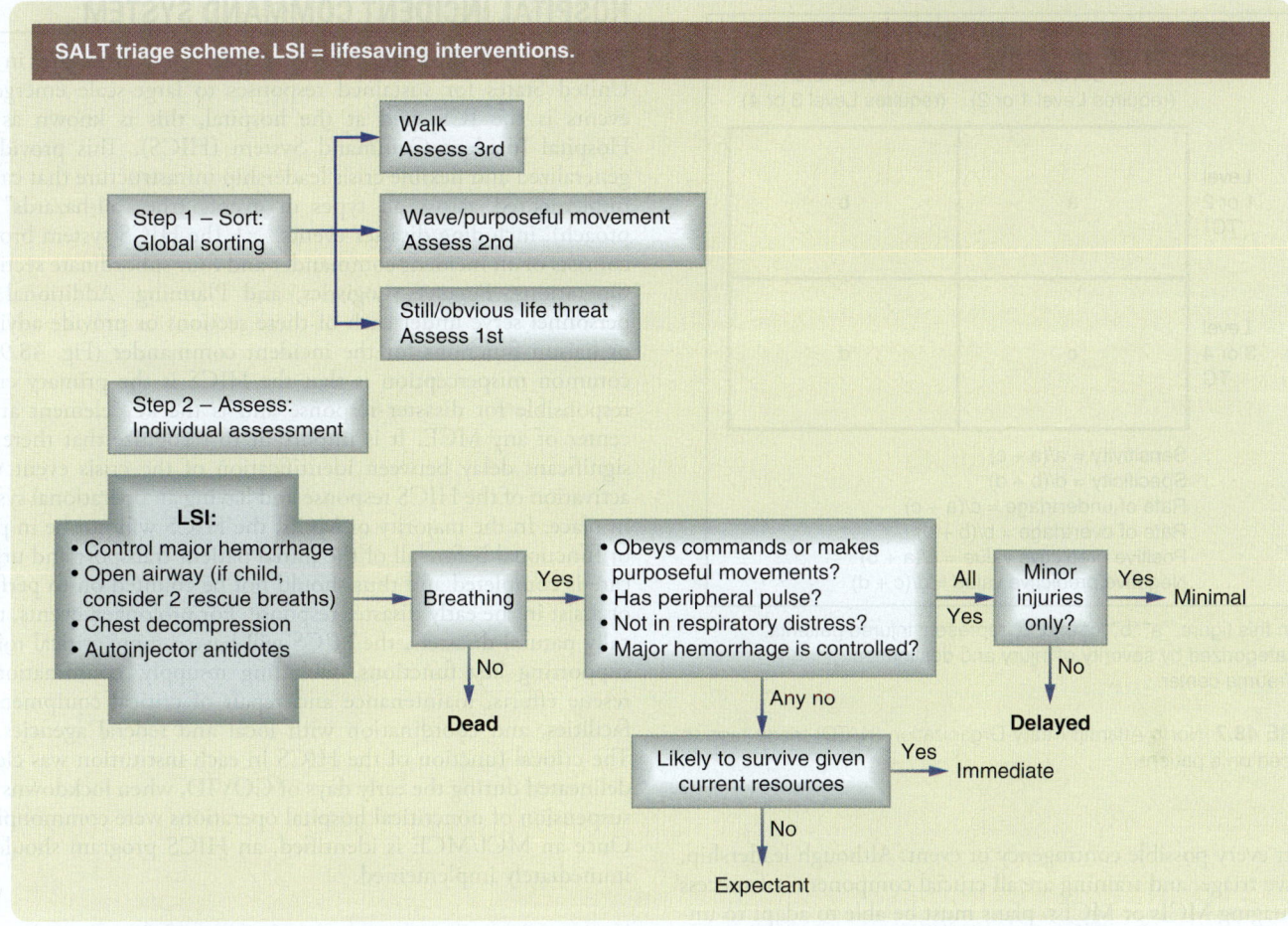

SALT triage scheme. LSI = lifesaving interventions.

Step 1 – Sort: Global sorting
- Walk — Assess 3rd
- Wave/purposeful movement — Assess 2nd
- Still/obvious life threat — Assess 1st

Step 2 – Assess: Individual assessment

LSI:
- Control major hemorrhage
- Open airway (if child, consider 2 rescue breaths)
- Chest decompression
- Autoinjector antidotes

Breathing — No → **Dead**

Breathing — Yes →
- Obeys commands or makes purposeful movements?
- Has peripheral pulse?
- Not in respiratory distress?
- Major hemorrhage is controlled?

All Yes → Minor injuries only?
- Yes → Minimal
- No → **Delayed**

Any no → Likely to survive given current resources
- Yes → Immediate
- No → Expectant

FIGURE 48.5 SALT (Sort, Assess, Lifesaving interventions, Treatment/transport) triage is one example of a triage schema to determine proper patient placement.

Triage and evacuation categories

- Standard NATO nomenclature is recommended, often called "DIME"
- **Delayed** (yellow tag) – may be life threatening, but intervention may be delayed for several hours with frequent reassessment – (fractures, tourniquet-controlled bleeding, head or maxillofacial injuries, burns)
- **Immediate** (red tag) – immediate attention required to prevent death; usually "AABC" issue – airway, arterial bleed, ventilation, circulatory
- **Minimal** (green tag) – ambulatory, minor injuries such as lacerations, minor burns, or musculoskeletal injuries; can wait for definitive attention
- **Expectant** (black tag) – survival unlikely, such as extensive burns, severe head injuries

FIGURE 48.6 Example matrix of allocation to trauma center levels based on injury severity.

on Trauma (COT) sets national benchmarks for the measurement of field triage accuracy.[20] System-level rates of overtriage and undertriage are established based on objective criteria. Overtriage significantly encumbers the system during MCIs and can result in preventable deaths and system failure. Mathematically, it is defined as 1 − specificity (Fig. 48.7). On the other hand, undertriage could

result in transport to nontrauma centers or triage to an inappropriate category at the hospital. This is mathematically defined as 1 − sensitivity (see Fig. 48.7). In usual trauma practice, there is a focus on avoiding undertriage at all costs while accepting the resultant high levels of overtriage. During disasters, this relationship changes to one in which there must be an equal or greater focus on avoiding overtriage as there is on minimizing undertriage in order to optimize outcomes and preserve scarce or critical resources (see Fig. 48.2).

Casualty identification and tracking can be a serious challenge in any disaster.[4] A large number of different triage cards are widely used and can be beneficial if their use is standardized and practiced within a given system. The most common triage cards used are standardized Field Triage Cards.[21,22] As shown in the example in Fig. 48.8, these cards can rapidly display critical information, including vital signs and major injuries, and then easily identify what category or priority has been assigned to that patient. Although these cards have the advantage of simplicity and ease of use, there are downsides and logistic challenges, such as the cards getting lost or not staying with the patient as they move through the system. Writing can also be obscured by blood or be illegible. Like everything else in a disaster response, practice must be provided, and the cards' use must be rehearsed.

The success or failure of a disaster response pivots on many different factors. The best plans may not be able to be implemented secondary to unforeseen events. Disaster planning cannot

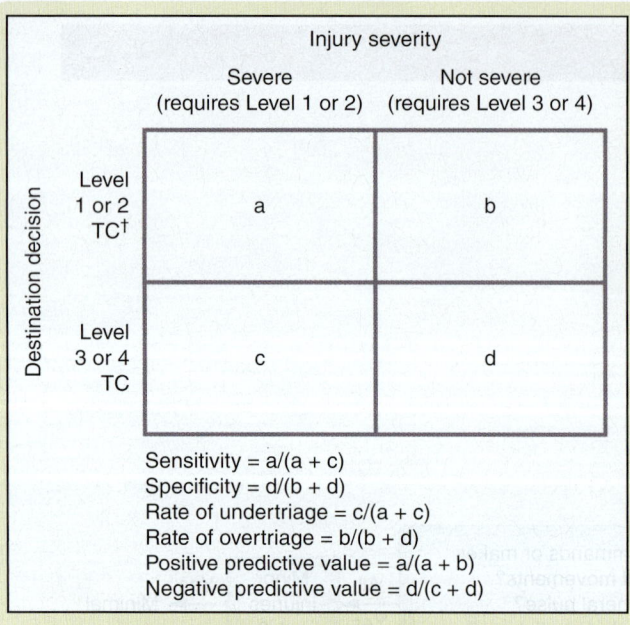

Sensitivity = a/(a + c)
Specificity = d/(b + d)
Rate of undertriage = c/(a + c)
Rate of overtriage = b/(b + d)
Positive predictive value = a/(a + b)
Negative predictive value = d/(c + d)

* In this figure, "a", "b", "c", and "d" represent injured patients, categorized by severity of injury and destination.
† Trauma center.

FIGURE 48.7 North Atlantic Treaty Organization (NATO) triage tags to be placed on a patient.

predict every possible contingency or event. Although leadership, effective triage, and training are all crucial components of success in managing MCIs or MCEs, plans must be able to adapt to unforeseen circumstances. No disaster is the same; however, triage principles and patient management concepts remain the same, but they must be adaptable to the situation.

When plans need to be quickly adapted because of the situation, leadership is crucial. If leaders are unable to adapt, the system will be unable to adapt. Triage, regional and in-hospital response, and overall disaster management are dynamic processes that unfold as the casualty-producing event progresses. Management of triage patients as they move through the system must be performed within the constraints of the scenario and environment and the considerations of the tactical situation.

THREAT ANALYSIS

The triage officer should be informed by the incident commander and prehospital providers to understand the tactical situation in order to appropriately manage resources and meet the goal of doing the best for the most. Awareness of the event, the situation, the estimated number of casualties, the risk for a secondary event, the effectiveness of field triage, and so forth gives the hospital triage officer the proper perspective to facilitate optimization of resources. The triage officer must have good situational awareness and ensure that casualties get treated in a timely and appropriate manner while using resources appropriately to maintain capability for the additional influx of casualties. Coordination and communication are key factors in being able to adapt; there must be redundancy and fail-safes in the communication systems so that as the system adapts to overcome situations not accounted for in disaster planning, all elements of the local and regional teams are kept aware.

HOSPITAL INCIDENT COMMAND SYSTEM

The currently used organizational plan and structure in the United States for sustained responses to large-scale emergency events is the ICS, and at the hospital, this is known as the Hospital Incident Command System (HICS). This provides a generalized and flexible crisis leadership infrastructure that can be implemented across all types of events (the "all-hazards" approach), including disaster events.[23,24] The HICS system broadly consists of an incident commander and four subordinate sections: Operations, Finance, Logistics, and Planning. Additional key personnel serve under each of these sections or provide advisory or liaison functions for the incident commander (Fig. 48.9). A common misperception is that the HICS is the primary entity responsible for disaster response and is the key element at the center of any MCE. It is important to recognize that there is a significant delay between identification of the crisis event with activation of the HICS response and having an operational system in place. In the majority of MCIs, the HICS will not be in place or functional before all of the initial patient transport and urgent care is completed and thus should not be counted on to perform or assist in the early disaster response. For prolonged events, typically natural disasters, the HICS will have a more critical role in supporting key functions, including resupply, coordination of rescue efforts, maintenance and repair of critical equipment or facilities, and coordination with local and federal agencies.[24,25] The critical function of the HICS in each institution was clearly delineated during the early days of COVID, when lockdowns and suspension of noncritical hospital operations were commonplace. Once an MCI/MCE is identified, an HICS program should be immediately implemented.

DRILLS AND TRAINING

Training for disaster events requires surgeon involvement at the local and regional levels. Effective leadership and training are foundational for a successful response to an MCI or MCE; although surgeons are not involved with point-of-injury care and only rarely with field triage, surgeon involvement with planning and training is extremely important. Any trauma system, even the most established, can be burdened by large volumes of patients. Successful triage requires significant training and sorting and prioritizing of casualties according to their injuries while considering the tactical situation and resources available; it is a skill that, in addition to training, requires education and leadership. Additionally, this skill is rarely practiced in clinical settings on this scale and requires frequent reeducation because it is outside of most clinicians' daily practice.

Although there are many triage categorization schemes, each hospital and trauma system should choose one, keep it simple, and train with it regularly (see Fig. 48.9).[9,17,26] Training requires a significant investment of time, energy, and resources; perfunctory training without stressing the weak areas in the process or involving the entire system will only lead to potential failures should the system be stressed with a disaster event. Surgeon leadership is necessary for disaster training; there is a tendency for triage and disaster training to involve prehospital providers and the initial hospital response, but the training does not get brought into the hospital beyond the ED phase of care. Not involving the operating rooms (ORs) and intensive care units (ICUs) in the disaster training makes the scenarios less realistic and can portend a false sense of success when patients get rapidly moved out of the ED to

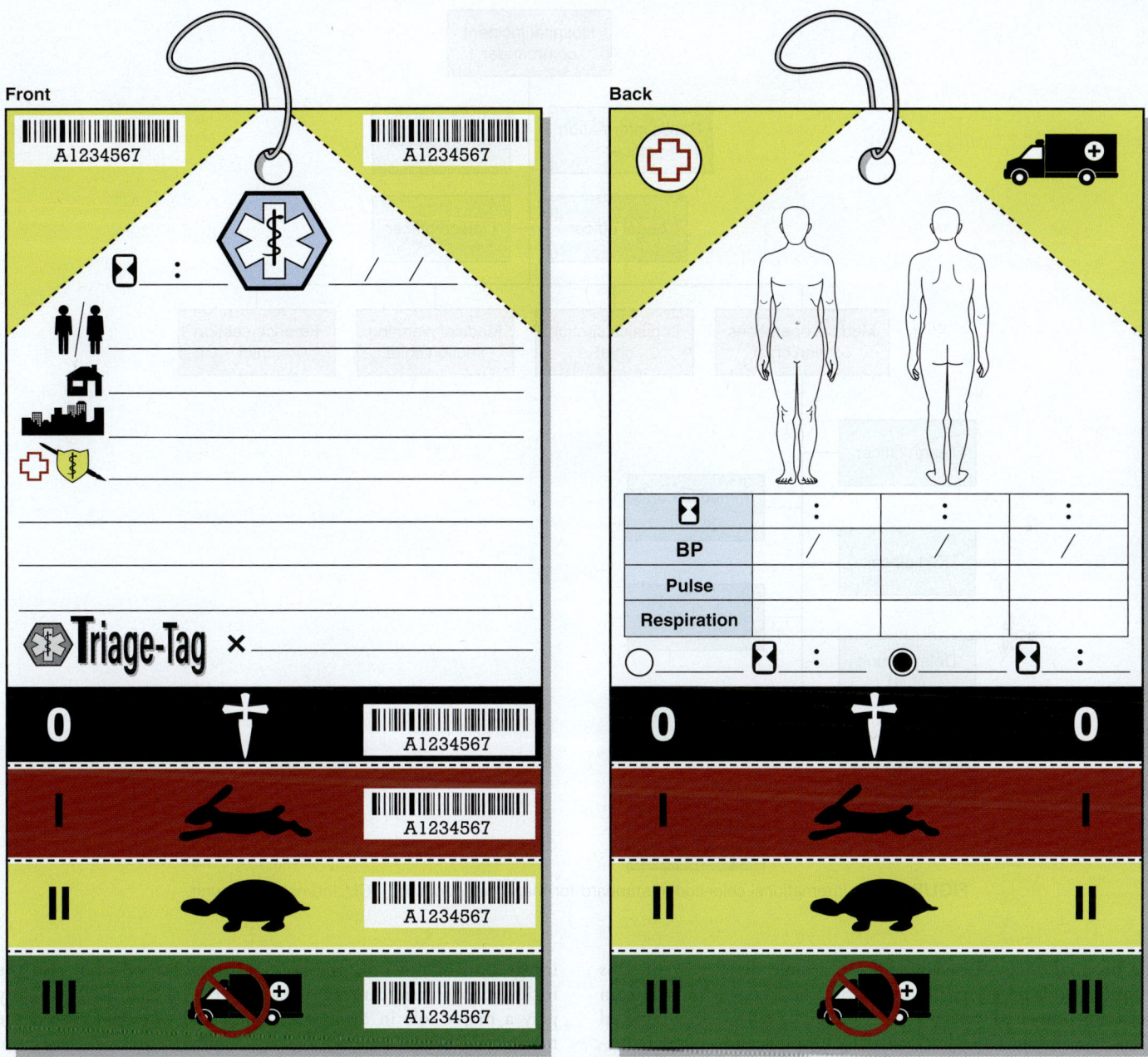

FIGURE 48.8 Example Hospital Incident Command System structure.

go to the ORs without planning for and understanding the time that it takes for multiple operations to occur.[16,27] Although the details and nuances may be second nature to the triage officer, weak areas in the system will be amplified in the event of a disaster scenario. Optimal real-world training is typically resource intensive, and surgeon involvement at all levels will improve the triage and initial response.

Regional readiness for disasters takes coordination, communication, and leadership.[16,18,28,29] The readiness of a hospital and of a community (local and regional readiness) for disaster events is a significant investment that will pay dividends if tragedy strikes. A community being caught off-guard without a rehearsed regional trauma plan will likely pay the price in terms of lives lost. Regional readiness involves coordination with all prehospital elements and first responders. In some communities, there are multiple Level 1 trauma centers, whereas others may have none.

Coordination with EMS is essential and can be challenging, given regional EMS organization and communication lines.[30,31] Surgeon involvement at the regional planning levels through regular trauma regional advisory councils will help with coordination and provide a systematic approach.

SURGE COMPONENTS

Although there should be a redundancy of capability, there should not be a redundancy of action; inefficiency must be avoided. As patients are being triaged to different hospitals in the system, both the capability and capacity must be considered, and this should be part of the triage training. *Capability* refers to the current clinical services that would be immediately available at the hospital (neurosurgery, vascular, interventional radiology). *Capacity*, on the other hand, refers to bed status, hospital status, blood available at

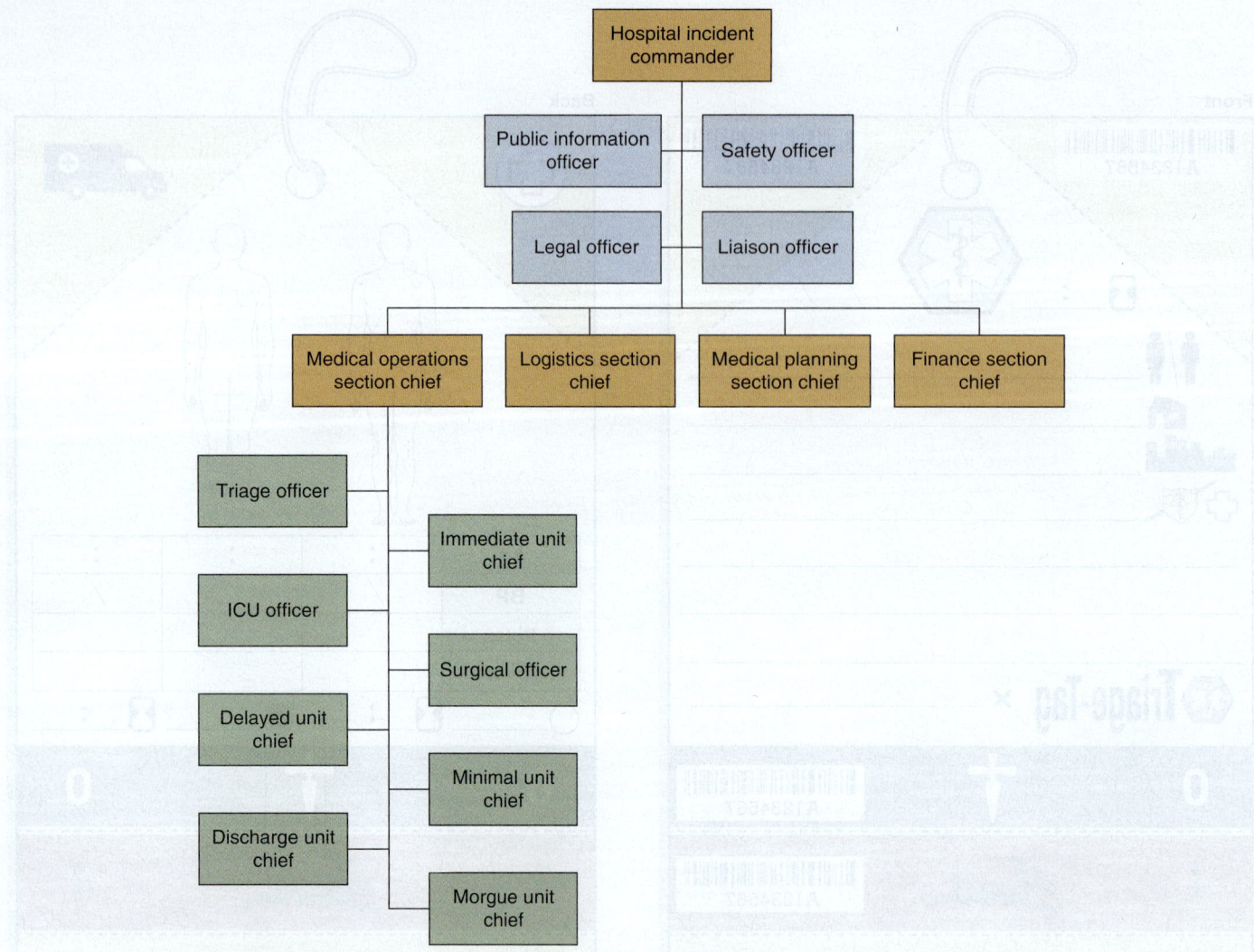

FIGURE 48.9 International color-coded standard for triage categorization. *ICU*, Intensive care unit.

the hospital, and OR availability. In a large disaster event, this information is necessary for appropriate field triage. Variations in both capability and capacity status should be rehearsed in regional disaster training. Coordination with hospital and regional incident command centers is necessary for this to occur successfully. Newer web-based tools are now widely available that can greatly aid this process by monitoring and continually updating the status and capabilities of all available hospitals in a given health system or region.[18,32]

SYSTEM INTEGRATION (LOCAL, STATE, FEDERAL)

Multiple systems come into play when considering a prepared community response for a disaster. Both local (in-hospital) and regional (field) triage coordination, planning, training, and process leadership will help minimize loss of life during an MCE, where casualties may be overwhelming. This is why systematic coordination and integration among the multiple hospitals, incident command, prehospital providers, and in-hospital elements are essential. Trauma system coordination occurs through the function of the ACS COT among Level 1 trauma centers; however, as more regional Level 2 trauma centers enter communities, it is imperative that surgeon leadership be involved in the integration of not only the regional triage process but also the incident command centers. These lower-level facilities frequently play a major role in disaster response and can even exceed the role played by the regional Level 1 trauma center. In the Route 91 shooting in Las Vegas that occurred in October 2017, most of the victims were brought to the Level 2 trauma centers around the shooting site.[33] Maintaining good lines of clinician communication and surgeon leadership among the regional trauma centers will continue to integrate and build the system to function well during large casualty events. This requires frequent contact between community sites and a process for delineating patient transport and disbursement from the incident scene that does not overwhelm one trauma center.

From an in-hospital perspective, the function of hospital departments, such as the blood bank, patient transport, radiology, postanesthesia care unit (PACU), ORs, and so forth, relies on integration and coordination within the hospital in order for there to be good patient flow and no bottlenecks. Without reliable integration of the functional areas of the hospital, there is more likely to be increased disorganization, chaos, and delays in patient care. Good system integration does not come without a significant training investment. Surgeon leaders, trauma directors, ED leadership, and nursing leadership must all participate in system integration with the incident command center and the hospital department. These plans cannot just be on paper; they have to be invested in with rehearsals and mock events that stress the system in order to determine the weak areas of system integration. When these weak points and bottlenecks are found, the disaster response plan can be modified and adapted to specific institutional necessities. Events that create large numbers of patients are naturally chaotic and stressful, and a systems integration plan (including backup mechanisms for communication between hospital departments) helps mitigate the chaos inherent to most disasters.

RESPONSE

The surgical management of multiple victims presenting in a mass casualty response should be simultaneously familiar and unfamiliar to a surgeon. The surgical principles and guidelines that govern the care of any traumatically injured patient remain the same. The initial emergent care of any MCI victim should follow standard Advanced Trauma Life Support principles (see Chapter 36). Biologic, chemical, and nuclear terrorism events will require additional specialized response training. Surgeons should consider this training so that they are prepared to provide surgical management for these less common MCEs. The rapidity of patient care during a mass casualty response is commonly heightened, with greater emphasis on damage control surgery and less emphasis on definitive surgical management to allow lifesaving care to be provided to the greatest number of victims in the shortest time possible. The following key lessons from previous MCEs highlight the impact and aftermath of caring for large numbers of victims as well as the importance of promptly returning the hospital to normal function.

HOSPITAL TRIAGE

As discussed previously, triage is an essential tool for ensuring that all patients receive the most appropriate care. Although triage is ideally performed at the scene to identify transport priorities, a recent survey of clinicians responding to worldwide disaster events identified that many victims self-transport, bypassing prehospital triage.[34] These clinicians identified the importance of hospital triage/re-triage as being essential to the success of a disaster response. Triage/re-triage upon arrival to the hospital ensures that all victims receive the necessary care balanced against the available resources.

Various paper and electronic tools have been advocated to facilitate communication and track victims during the triage process. To be effective, these tools must be used routinely on all victims and at all stages of the disaster response continuum. They should also be used during disaster drills so that all providers are familiar with their use in advance of an actual event. Electronic systems that integrate with the hospital's computerized health record may seem attractive, but experience in several large-scale MCEs has found such systems to be lacking.[34] Paper-based systems are easier to use initially but require subsequent manual entry of information into the computerized health record.

The focus during the initial assessment of the mass casualty victim is on immediate lifesaving interventions. Patient history, physical examination, radiographic imaging, and the documentation of these findings are frequently lacking because of the turmoil of the initial response. Previous MCEs have identified that every victim should be thoroughly reexamined and reimaged

as appropriate "once the dust has settled" to ensure that no injuries have been missed during the initial response.[34,35]

SURGE CAPACITY

Surge capacity is defined as the ability to increase staff, supplies, equipment, and patient care areas in response to a sudden rise in demand.[34] Advance planning that ensures operative and hospital surge capacity is vital to any mass casualty response. Although each event is different, preparing to accommodate a 20% increase in patient capacity is a reasonable approach during hospital disaster planning. Effective surge capacity is defined by several key principles[35,36]:

- Increase operative capacity:
  - Operative capacity can be rapidly augmented by canceling elective surgical procedures and redeploying available surgical and anesthesia staff. In the Pulse Nightclub mass shooting event in Orlando, 82% of admitted patients required surgery in the first 24 hours, highlighting the importance of operative surge capacity.[36] "Tiered staffing," in which specialized OR or ICU staff are paired with clinical staff from other hospital areas, may also be employed to augment patient care capacity. Another effective strategy involves using an experienced surgeon in the triage area to decide which victims need operative intervention next. This person could be the triage officer or another provider in addition to the triage officer, depending on patient load and operational planning for disaster events. This allows surgeons to remain in the OR rather than moving from triage area to OR and back. Preparing the OR and opening instruments/supplies while the next patient is being transported and anesthesia is induced is also an effective method for reducing turnover time in an MCE. Essential surgical specialties in the first 24 hours after a mass shooting include trauma surgeons, orthopedic and hand surgeons, and vascular surgeons, supported by emergency physicians, intensivists, anesthesia providers, and interventional radiologists.[36] Damage control procedures and multisystem injuries will require frequent trips to the OR in the days after an MCI. Dedicated ORs in the days after an MCE will accommodate those patients who require staged surgery.[36]
- Promptly discharge/downgrade eligible patients:
  - Nonsurgeons, resident physicians, advanced practice providers, and nurses can all function as "discharge teams," increasing hospital bed capacity for incoming victims by downgrading inpatients to lower-acuity beds or discharging appropriate patients to public areas while they await transport out of the hospital.[36]
- Repurpose existing patient care areas:
  - Surge capacity can be achieved by using existing areas of the hospital, such as ambulance bays, procedural areas, PACUs, and even classrooms to perform triage, emergent assessment, and intensive care activities. To be effective, this requires advance planning and practice during disaster drills rather than choosing surge areas in the "heat of the moment." Dedicated disaster supply carts can be created to equip these "surge unit" areas with the resources needed to achieve their intended purpose. These surge units can be created virtually in most computerized health records in advance and activated quickly to facilitate documentation and patient care when the need arises.

- Delegate tasks:
  - Appropriate use of available personnel and delegation of tasks is essential to a successful surge response and a prompt return to normal function. An effective surge response may require clinicians and hospital staff to assume nontraditional duties and perform necessary tasks that are outside of their usual duties.[35] Flexibility in assignments and willingness to perform whatever tasks are needed is an essential component of mass casualty response.[34]

VICTIM TRANSPORTATION

Recent large-scale disasters have demonstrated that many MCI victims present to hospitals via nonconventional means, including private and law enforcement vehicles, bypassing prehospital triage.[34] As such, MCI victims may arrive with little to no warning and with minimal prehospital care. Depending on the nature of the event, a relatively small percentage of victims may present for care via traditional ambulance transport. As those who are most mobile, the initial victims presenting from an MCI may be "walking wounded" patients who require minimal care. Careful triage of the initial wave of victims is essential to ensure that resources remain available for the more critically injured patients to follow.

VICTIM IDENTIFICATION

Disaster victims may be unable to provide information regarding their identity, necessitating the use of alias naming systems until the patient's true identity can be confirmed. In some events, underage victims have been found to have fake identification cards, further contributing to the confusion of the disaster response.[36] In other events, multiple nationalities and/or languages have been involved, requiring the availability of translators and subsequent embassy or consulate support.[35] Sufficient victim aliases should be registered in the hospital's computerized health record well in advance to reduce the burden on the hospital's business office when large numbers of victims present acutely. The advantage of such aliases is that trauma care can be immediately implemented without having to wait for patient registration. Such aliases should remain in use for the first 24 hours of patient care until the chaos of the MCE has abated to avoid the confusion inherent in changing aliases to actual patient names amid active resuscitation and mass transfusion protocols.

COMMUNICATION

Communication (or lack thereof) is a common opportunity for improvement in postdisaster after-action reports.[34] Effective mass casualty communication should consider five "audiences": (1) direct patient care team; (2) local, state, and federal government/law enforcement; (3) hospital staff; (4) victims' families and friends; and (5) community.

- Direct patient care team:
  - Those providing direct patient care need an effective method for communicating patient and resource needs. All mass casualty disaster plans should designate at least a primary and secondary communication system (such as cellular phones and very high-frequency radios). Some cellular phone carriers have systems in place that give priority in a disaster event to first responders and healthcare providers. Registration with such systems must occur in advance of an MCE. In the event of a mass power outage, "runners" may become necessary to

disseminate information between HICS and various areas of the hospital. Disaster drills should regularly test the communication tools chosen to ensure that they function properly in all areas of the hospital.

- Local, state, and federal government/law enforcement:
  - Effective communication channels and relationships with key leaders in government and law enforcement should be established well in advance of an MCE. Such relationships are extremely valuable during a disaster response. Disaster drills are an excellent opportunity to develop these relationships by inviting local officials and law enforcement to participate.
- Hospital staff:
  - Every hospital needs an effective system for notifying providers when an MCE has occurred.[34] Such systems should continue to attempt contact with providers until they respond and document when they do. Throughout the event, routine updates should be provided to hospital staff to inform them of the status of the disaster response and important security updates. This can occur via email or a secure hospital website.
- Victims' families and friends:
  - Hospital switchboards are commonly inundated with calls during an MCE by family and friends seeking information regarding loved ones. Messaging for hospital operators should be prepared in advance. A dedicated hotline telephone number to handle victim inquiries should be considered.
- Community:
  - During an MCE, normal hospital operations are frequently limited. The event may also place the local population at risk of injury. Communication with the community regarding the disaster response, alternatives for patient care, and any pertinent public health issues is essential.

BLOOD BANK AND MASSIVE TRANSFUSION

Massive transfusion protocols are now commonplace among trauma and nontrauma hospitals alike. MCEs, however, escalate the burden on hospital blood banks exponentially. Additional blood bank staff will be necessary to prepare the volume of blood products required. The large volume of blood products consumed will also rapidly exhaust even a busy trauma center's blood reserves. A close working relationship and advanced disaster planning with the hospital's blood supplier are essential to ensuring timely availability of blood products. Recent domestic mass shooting events, such as the Pulse Nightclub shooting, have highlighted the ability of the community to respond through blood donation, with over 26,000 units of blood being donated in 72 hours. Although lack of blood products is a common concern, recent MCEs have not identified blood product availability to be a limiting factor in disaster response.[34]

BLOOD-BORNE PATHOGENS

During an MCE, it is common for victims to be exposed to other victims' blood and body fluids.[36] Patients should be offered baseline testing for hepatitis B, hepatitis C, and human immunodeficiency virus (HIV).[37] Patients without previous hepatitis B vaccination should be started on a vaccination program, but postexposure prophylaxis against hepatitis C and HIV is not currently recommended. Because not all victims of disaster events may present to hospitals for medical care, these recommendations should be made known to the community through local television and newspapers.

PRESERVING EVIDENCE

Most MCEs will be considered crime scenes and require investigation by local, state, or federal law enforcement. As such, all victim clothing and belongings should be considered evidence, labeled, preserved with appropriate chain of custody, and held for law enforcement to examine. Appropriate documentation of all injuries sustained, as with any traumatically injured patient, is vital to subsequent investigation. Law enforcement will typically request to interview disaster victims, sometimes before they are reunited with family. Such requests must be balanced against each victim's ongoing care, resuscitation, and need for family notification.

SECURITY

In an MCE, hospital security is paramount. The hospital should be "locked down," with limited, monitored entrances and exits, until all potential threats to the facility have been identified. Hospitals should be considered as possible "secondary targets." Hospital security should plan to be self-sufficient because local law enforcement may be occupied with the disaster response and unable to provide security resources for the hospital.

FINANCE

Disaster response is costly. The finance chief within the HICS structure is tasked with keeping track of all disaster response–associated expenses and labor costs. This should include direct patient care costs and hospital staff compensation (including overtime) as well as the costs of disaster preparation. Government reimbursement for the financial costs incurred may (or may not) be available after the event, but appropriate documentation of expenses will be required.

THE MEDIA

Newspaper, radio, and especially television news crews will arrive soon after any MCI. This can be a distraction to patient care and can violate patient confidentiality if not handled appropriately.[35] Unified hospital messages, distributed through the HICS public information officer, are essential. Regular press conferences with hospital leadership should be scheduled. Surgeons are commonly asked to participate in such press conferences to describe the nature of the disaster, the number of victims, and the medical response required. Media training for surgeon leaders, such as trauma medical directors, should be part of any hospital's disaster planning. Hospital staff should be informed on how to respond to the media's request for comment as well as educated on appropriate social media posts surrounding the disaster response to protect patient confidentiality.[35]

ROLE OF THE HEALTH INSURANCE PORTABILITY AND ACCOUNTABILITY ACT

In a mass casualty situation, the usual rules regarding patient confidentiality, privacy, and disclosure function slightly differently. During Hurricane Katrina in 2005, the Department of Health and Human Services stated, "Health care providers can share patient information as necessary to identify, locate and notify family members, guardians, or anyone else responsible for the individual's care of the individual's location, general condition, or death." This statement allows hospitals and surgeons to disclose limited protected patient health information as needed to identify victims and notify family members of their condition.

FAMILIES AND FRIENDS

In an MCE, the hospital will quickly be inundated with family and friends requesting information about their loved ones. Hospital mass casualty plans must consider not only the family and friends of victims in the hospital but also those of victims who may be deceased at the scene. It frequently falls on hospital physicians and staff to notify families of deceased victims. While awaiting victim identification and notification of outcome, be prepared to provide family and friends with food, water, a place to rest, telephone chargers, translators, and medical care as needed.

COMMUNITY GIVING AND DONATIONS

MCEs commonly result in an outpouring of support from the community. Individuals and businesses will offer to donate their time and services to aid in the response. Donations of food items must be carefully evaluated. A "second-hit" attack on hospital staff through tainted food must always be considered. Donations of material goods also require hospital resources to accept and process them. Monetary donations to legitimate victims' resource funds are an alternative that allows the community to respond while minimizing the impact on hospital personnel and resources. Offers of assistance from healthcare providers outside the credentialed hospital staff must be carefully considered and should follow routine medical staff processes. Disaster responses tend to attract individuals claiming to be healthcare providers when, in fact, they are not.

VISITS FROM VERY IMPORTANT PERSONS

After a disaster response, it is common for elected officials to visit the trauma center/hospital and participate in press conferences.[35] Such visits can be helpful in gaining governmental support for the response efforts. These visits can also place a burden on the hospital, however, because the security required and diversion of hospital staff from patient care responsibilities. Well-intentioned visits from politicians, celebrities, and other prominent individuals immediately after the event can detract from patient care and require hospital resources that are best focused initially on the victims and their families. Such visits are more appropriately arranged for a later time when they can help encourage patients and staff.

STAFF COUNSELING

The impact of an MCE on hospital staff cannot be underestimated. A plan for staff counseling should be part of any hospital disaster plan.[35] Counselors should be made immediately available so that staff who wish to participate in critical incident stress debriefing may have that opportunity before they leave the hospital. Staff schedules should be adjusted to allow those who responded sufficient time to decompress before their next shift. It is important to recognize that individuals cope with the stress of an MCE in different ways. Some team members will wish to speak with a trained counselor, whereas others will simply want to spend time with individuals from their unit or department. Some will seek counseling immediately, whereas others may recognize the need for counseling days to weeks later. Some staff will require counseling for weeks to months after an MCE. Havron et al. studied surgical residents who responded to the 2016 Pulse Nightclub shooting; 30% met the criteria for posttraumatic stress disorder, and 30% met the criteria for major depression, as assessed at 3 and 7 months after the incident.[38]

RETURNING TO NORMAL OPERATIONS

During an MCE, normal clinical operations, including nonemergent surgery and usual trauma patient arrivals, are commonly placed on hold to focus on the victims of the event. The care of preexisting inpatients, as well as critical hospital services such as trauma care, stroke alerts, and myocardial infarction care, must continue, however. The hospital surge plan must include strategies for caring for both disaster victims and current inpatients. The goal of any hospital disaster plan must include the actions required to restore the trauma center/hospital to normal clinical operations as quickly as possible.

ROLE OF REGIONAL MEDICAL OPERATIONS CENTERS IN TRAUMA RESPONSE TO DISASTER

Role of Regional Medical Operations Coordination Centers in Trauma Response to Disaster (RMOCCs) can serve as a critical component in disaster response, providing a centralized hub for coordination, communication, and resource management across various healthcare entities within a specific geographic region. RMOCCs are relatively uncommon in most of the United States, with a few notable exceptions.[39] They serve to enhance the overall efficiency and effectiveness of the healthcare response during crises. The RMOCC acts as a bridge between individual hospitals, public health agencies, EMS, and other healthcare organizations, fostering collaboration and ensuring a unified approach to managing resources and responding to incidents. The overarching goal is to get the right patient to the right place at the right time.[40,41]

Use of an RMOCC involves real-time information exchange, resource allocation, and strategic decision-making. It facilitates the coordination of medical assets, personnel, and supplies to address the evolving needs of a disaster or public health emergency. The RMOCC enables a more cohesive and synchronized response, helping hospitals optimize their capacity and capability during challenging circumstances.

For example, during a large-scale natural disaster, such as a hurricane or a widespread infectious disease outbreak, an RMOCC would play a pivotal role. It could coordinate the distribution of medical supplies, manage patient transportation, and provide a centralized communication platform for healthcare providers to share critical information. By consolidating information and resources, the RMOCC ensures that healthcare facilities are adequately supported, reducing duplication of efforts and enhancing the collective ability to respond effectively to the demands of the emergency. The RMOCC concept exemplifies the importance of regional collaboration in safeguarding public health during crises.

A NATIONAL MODEL FOR DISASTER PREPAREDNESS

A national injury disaster plan does not currently exist in the United States.[42] A future national trauma and emergency preparedness system (NTEPS) would be the next level of coordination beyond RMOCCs to a larger geographic care coordination system.[43,44] Conceptually, a national system would ensure access to high-quality, lifesaving trauma care for anyone, regardless of their location.[1]

An NTEPS would support public health readiness and coordination of care during MCIs, ultimately saving more lives during larger MCEs. Such an established system would facilitate equitable access to high-quality emergency care across the United States.[39] Lessons learned in several states during the COVID-19 pandemic support such a novel approach. The strengths of highly functional state/regional care systems and RMOCCs would facilitate the work of individual surgeons who would be end users of such a care system.

POSTEVENT PROCESSING AND IMPROVEMENT

Among the most important and frequently overlooked aspects of improving disaster care at every level is the need to capture, process, and then act on the feedback and lessons learned from past events. This is critical for both actual disasters and training exercises. Although success or failure during an MCI or MCE may be based on accurate and effective triage, the success or failure of the next event depends on a structured after-action report (AAR) of each event in order to improve individuals, groups, and systems. Although there are many different formats and techniques for performing an effective AAR, they all have several characteristics in common that should be highlighted.

The AAR should be completed as soon after the event as possible to capture events while they are fresh in people's minds and ensure maximal participation. AARs should be completed at every level, from an individual department or area (ED, OR, ICU) up to the facility level and even the system level. The AAR should focus on gathering input in two categories: things that went well or worked and things that did not work or need to be improved. In particular, any obvious areas that resulted in suboptimal outcomes, patient/provider harm, or near misses should be identified. This should be done in an entirely nonjudgmental and nonpunitive manner, and input from all levels should be encouraged. A formal report of the AAR should be created and submitted up the chain of command to be integrated into the hospital- or system-level AAR. Finally, and most importantly, an action plan based on the AAR feedback and review should be created that identifies and prioritizes changes to be implemented to better prepare for future disaster events. Institutionalization of processes like this, with the aim of continual improvement of the delivery of care and focused on the patient at the center, characterize the "Learning Health System." This concept was emphasized and codified in a recent National Academies of Science, Engineering, and Medicine report, "Zero Preventable Deaths," calling for an overhaul of the national trauma systems in the United States.[29,45]

Several large-scale events in the relatively recent past are illustrative of postevent processing improvements throughout health systems, both those that responded to the events and those preparing for such disasters in other communities. One of the most cited successful examples was that of the citywide response to the Boston Marathon bombing in 2013. The scene triage and distribution of patients during this disaster allowed for rapid transport and care for a large population of critically injured patients.[3,46] Although this is a great example of how to distribute patients to trauma centers, the area of the attack was uniquely situated almost equidistant to five Level 1 trauma centers, allowing for access to the highest level of care in a time frame that is difficult to replicate in almost any other area of the country. Another aspect that was thoroughly studied during this attack was scene safety because the detonation of the second bomb raised concerns about the possibility of further attacks, specifically targeting first responders.

The Pulse Nightclub shooting in Orlando and the Route 91 shooting in Las Vegas both provided unique lessons relating to large-scale ballistic MCEs. Both of these demonstrated that large numbers of patients can appear at trauma centers via nonconventional means (civilian transport, police transport, etc.), which can make accurate assessment and on-scene triage exceedingly difficult. This emphasizes the need for accurate on-scene data and communication between centers regarding surge capacity because accurate patient flow from the scene to patient centers may be difficult to impossible to assess in real time at the scene of the incident. The Pulse Nightclub mass shooting clearly highlights the need for understanding of a center's true surge capacity; in this incident, 82% of patients required urgent surgery within the first 24 hours of arrival at the trauma center, placing a strain on resources.[36] In the Las Vegas shooting in 2017, most of the victims were brought to Level 2 centers around the site of the shooting. This highlights the need for involvement of Level 2 centers in regional training for MCIs and the critical nature of communication between all centers, regardless of designation level.[33]

In July of 2013, an Asiana Airline crash occurred in San Francisco, sending 187 patients to hospitals in the Bay Area. Most of these patients were non–English speaking, placing an unusual strain on the hospital systems based on both provider resources and translation ability. Given that San Francisco is a hub for travel to Asia from the United States, this is a somewhat unique aspect of mass casualty response for that city and provides a great example of how postevent processing can allow for improvement in a previously unthought-of area of mass casualty response.

In all of these specific examples, postevent processing allowed for identification of what portions of the systems performed admirably and what portions required improvement. Documentation and dissemination of this information within the involved systems allow for improvement in mass casualty response for possible future encounters, and publication of some of this information has allowed other health systems to refine their processes based on shared information.

SELECTED REFERENCES

Berwick DM, Downey AS, Cornett EA. A national trauma care system to achieve zero preventable deaths after injury: recommendations from a National Academies of Sciences, Engineering, and Medicine report. *JAMA*. 2016;316(9):927-928.

This commentary highlights the important release of the mission zero concept in military-civilian care, inclusive of MCI preparedness. Recommendations in the report include better digital capture of patient care experiences, coordination of performance improvement initiatives, timely knowledge dissemination, and patient-centered injury care. This report resulted in the development of enhanced military-civilian partnerships with the goal of deployment-ready preparedness.

Brunner J, Rocha TC, Chudgar AA, et al. The Boston Marathon bombing: after-action review of the Brigham and Women's Hospital emergency radiology response. *Radiology*. 2014; 273(1):78-87.

This study was an analysis of emergency resources and process turnaround times in response to the April 15, 2013, Boston Marathon bombing. The outcomes of interest were to identify opportunities for improvement for a receiving trauma center and ways to enhance an emergency operations plan. The importance of this study was to highlight the value of a postevent evaluation.

Dichter JR, Kanter RK, Dries D, et al. System-level planning, coordination, and communication: care of the critically ill and injured during pandemics and disasters: CHEST consensus statement. *Chest*. 2014;146(suppl 4):e87S-e102S.

This study evaluated system-level planning for disaster preparedness and response. This involves the collaboration of hospitals, health systems, and regional and national response. This reference provides guidance for system planning, coordination, communication, and response. A Delphi process was used, given the lack of evidence in the literature.

Khajehaminian MR, Ardalan A, Keshtkar A, et al. A systematic literature review of criteria and models for casualty distribution in trauma related mass casualty incidents. *Injury*. 2018; 49(11):1959-1968.

This study reviewed models and detailed approaches to criteria affecting the distribution of casualties during mass causality incidents. This is a systematic review of close to 500 criteria affecting patient distribution across more than 30 manuscripts. It is one of the first comprehensive reviews on this subject.

National Academies of Sciences Engineering and Medicine. Toward a Post-Pandemic World: Lessons from COVID-19 for Now and the Future: Proceedings of a Workshop. Washington, DC: National Academies Press; 2022.

This proceedings workshop was a retrospective evaluation of the COVID-19 response. As a component of the National Academies review, discussion of preparedness coordination was undertaken. The workshop focused broadly on key lessons and emerging data from ongoing pandemic response efforts that can be incorporated into current health systems to improve resilience and preparedness for future outbreaks.

Sauer LM, Romig M, Andonian J, et al. Application of the incident command system to the hospital biocontainment unit setting. *Health Secur*. 2019;17(1):27-34.

This article addresses the utility of the ICS, a standard tool for command, control, and coordination in disaster response. The manuscript describes lessons learned from after-action reviews of exercises.

The full reference list appears on Elsevier eBooks+.

Transplantation and Immunology

The following chapters appear only on Elsevier eBooks+:

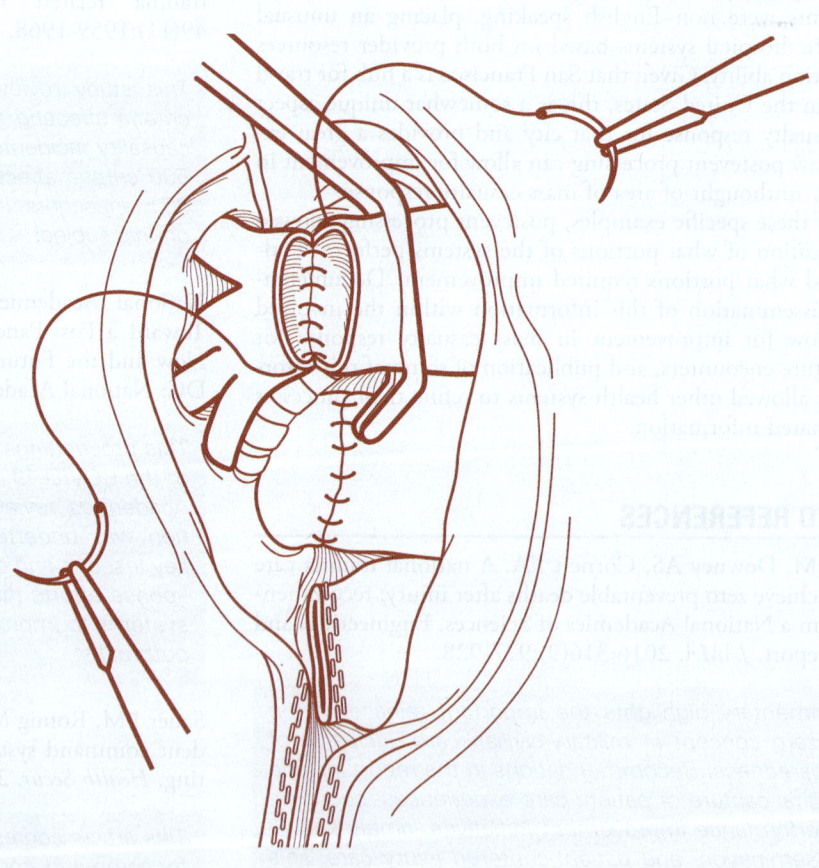

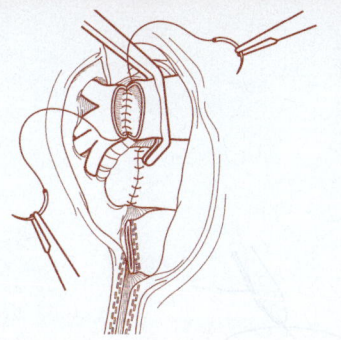

CHAPTER 49

Transplantation Immunobiology and Immunosuppression

William H. Kitchens, Idelberto Raul Badell, and Andrew B. Adams

OUTLINE

Please access Elsevier eBooks+ to view the video for this chapter.

Only a few short decades ago, there were no options for patients dying of end-stage organ failure. The concept of transplanting an organ from one individual to another was thought to be impossible. The evolution of clinical transplantation and transplant immunology is one of the bright success stories of modern medicine. It was through understanding of the immune response to the transplanted tissue that pioneers in the field were able to develop therapies to manipulate the immune response and to prevent rejection of the transplanted organ. Today, more than 25,000 transplants are performed annually, and over 100,000 patients are currently listed and awaiting an organ.

The concept of transplantation is certainly not new. History is replete with legends and myths recounting the replacement of limbs and organs. An oft-repeated myth of early transplantation is derived from the miracle of Saints Cosmas and Damian (brothers and subsequently patron saints of physicians and surgeons) in which they successfully replaced the gangrenous leg of the Roman deacon Justinian with a leg from a recently deceased Ethiopian (Fig. 49.1). It was not, however, until the French surgeon Alexis Carrel developed a method for joining blood vessels in the late 19th century that the transplantation of organs became technically feasible and verifiable accounts of transplantation began (Fig. 49.2). He was awarded the Nobel Prize in Medicine in 1912 "in recognition of his work on vascular suture and the transplantation of blood vessels and organs." Having established the technical component, Carrel himself noted that there were two issues to be resolved regarding "the transplantation of tissues and organs . . . the surgical and the biological." He had solved one aspect, the surgical, but he also understood that "it will only be through a more fundamental study of the biological relationships existing between living tissues" that the more difficult problem of the biology would come to be solved.

Forty years would pass before another set of eventual Nobel Prize winners, Peter Medawar and Frank Macfarlane Burnet, would begin to define the process by which one individual rejects another's tissue (Fig. 49.3).[1] Medawar and Burnet had developed an overall theory on the immunologic nature of self and the concept of immunologic tolerance. Burnet hypothesized that the definition of "self" was not preprogrammed, but rather actively defined during embryonic development through the interaction of the host's immune cells with its own tissue. This hypothesis implied that tolerance could be induced if donor cells were introduced to the embryo within this developmental period. Burnet was proven correct when Medawar showed that mouse embryos receiving cells from a different mouse strain accepted grafts from the strain later in life while rejecting grafts from other strains. These seminal studies were the first reports to demonstrate that it was possible to manipulate the immune system to accept allografts.[1]

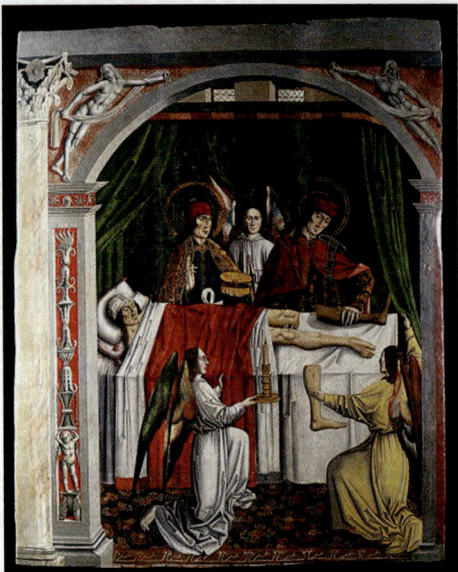

FIGURE 49.1 A 15th-century painting of Cosmas and Damian, patron saints of physicians and surgeons. The legend of the Miracle of the Black Leg depicts the removal of the diseased leg of Roman Justinian and replacement with the leg of a recently deceased Ethiopian man.

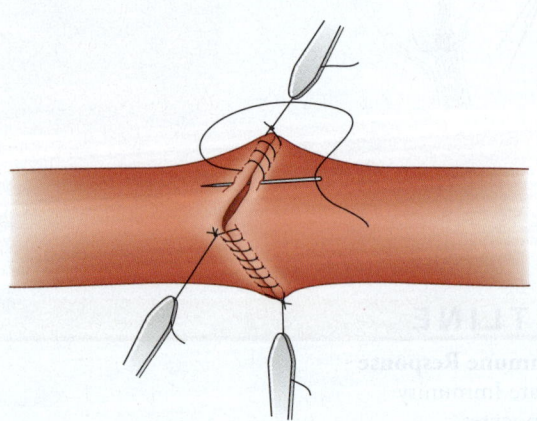

FIGURE 49.2 Triangulation technique of vascular anastomosis by Alexis Carrel. (Reprinted from Edwards WS, Edwards PD. *Alexis Carrel: Visionary Surgeon.* Springfield, IL: Charles C. Thomas; 1974.)

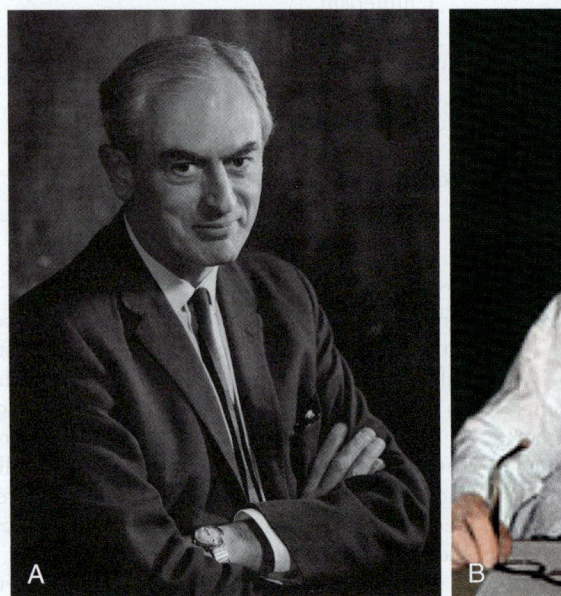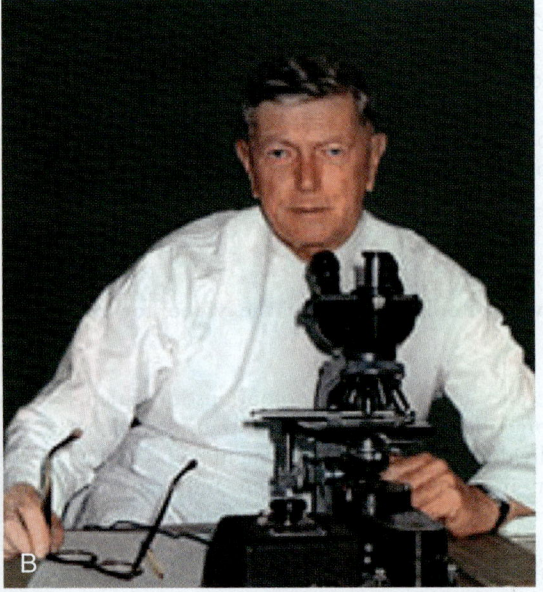

FIGURE 49.3 (A) Sir Peter Medawar. (B) Sir Frank Macfarlane Burnet. (A, Courtesy Bern Schwartz Collection, National Portrait Gallery, London. B, Courtesy Walter and Eliza Hall Institute of Medical Research.)

Shortly thereafter, Joseph Murray, Nobel Laureate 1990, performed the first successful renal transplant between identical twins in 1954.[2] At the same time, Gertrude Elion, who worked as an assistant to George Hitchings at Wellcome Research Laboratories, developed several new immunosuppressive compounds, including 6-mercaptopurine and azathioprine. Roy Calne, a budding surgeon-scientist who came from the United Kingdom to study with Murray, subsequently tested these reagents in animals and then introduced them into clinical practice, permitting nonidentical transplantation to be successful. Elion and Hitchings later shared the Nobel Prize in 1988 for their work on "the important principles of drug development." Subsequent discovery of increasingly effective agents to suppress the rejection response has led to

the success in allograft survival that we enjoy today. It is this collaboration between scientists and surgeons that has driven our understanding of the immune system as it relates to transplantation. In this chapter, we provide an overview of the immune response with specific attention to transplant immunity and the rejection process, review the specific immunosuppressive agents that are employed to prevent rejection, and provide a glimpse into the future of the field.

THE IMMUNE RESPONSE

The immune system, of course, did not evolve to prevent the transplantation of another individual's tissue or organs; rejection, rather, is a consequence of a system that has developed over thousands of years to protect against invasion by pathogens and to prevent subsequent disease. To understand the rejection process and in particular to appreciate the consequences of pharmacologic suppression of rejection, a general understanding of the immune response as it functions in a physiologic setting is required.

The immune system has evolved to include two complementary divisions to respond to disease: the innate and acquired immune systems. Broadly speaking, the innate immune system recognizes general characteristics that have, through selective pressure, come to represent universal pathologic challenges to our species (ischemia, necrosis, trauma, and certain conserved nonhuman molecules such as unmethylated CpG oligodeoxynucleotide DNA). The acquired arm, on the other hand, recognizes specific structural aspects of foreign substances, usually peptide or carbohydrate moieties, recognized by receptors generated randomly and selected to avoid self-recognition. Although the two systems differ in their specific responsibilities, they act in concert to influence each other to achieve an optimal overall response.

Innate Immunity

The innate immune system is thought to be a holdover from an evolutionarily distant response to foreign pathogens. In contrast to the acquired immune system, which employs an innumerable host of specificities to identify any possible antigen, the innate system uses a select number of protein receptors to identify specific motifs consistent with foreign or altered and damaged tissues. These receptors can exist on cells, such as macrophages, neutrophils, and natural killer (NK) cells, or free in the circulation, as is the case for complement. Whereas they fail to exhibit the specificity of the T-cell receptor (TCR) or antibody, they are broadly reactive against common components of pathogenic organisms, for example, lipopolysaccharides on gram-negative organisms or other glycoconjugates. Thus, the receptors of innate immunity are the same from one individual to another within a species and, in general, do not play a role in the direct recognition of a transplanted organ. They do, however, exert their effects indirectly through the identification of "injured tissue" (e.g., as is the case when an ischemic, damaged organ is moved from one individual to another).

Once activated, the innate system performs two vital functions. It initiates cytolytic pathways for the destruction of the offending organism, primarily through the complement cascade and NK cells. In addition, the innate system can shape the development of a concomitant acquired immune system response both through production of an immunomodulatory cytokine milieu and through enabling the activation and maturation of antigen-presenting cells (APCs). Macrophages and dendritic cells not only engulf foreign organisms that have been bound by complement but also distinguish pathogens, as they can be identified through receptors for foreign carbohydrates (e.g., mannose receptors). A highly evolutionarily conserved family of proteins known as *toll-like receptors (TLRs)* has been described to play an important role as activation molecules for innate APCs. They bind to pathogen-associated molecular patterns, motifs common to pathogenic organisms. Some examples of TLR ligands include lipopolysaccharide, flagellin (from bacterial flagella), double-stranded viral RNA, unmethylated CpG islands of bacterial and viral DNA, zymosan (β-glucan found in fungi), and numerous heat shock proteins. In contrast to pathogen-associated molecular patterns, which initiate a response to an infectious challenge, damage-associated molecular pattern molecules (DAMPs), also called *alarmins,* trigger the

innate inflammatory response to noninfectious cell death and injury. Many DAMPs are nuclear or cytosolic proteins or even DNA that is released or exposed in the setting of cell injury. These signals alert the innate immune system that injury has occurred and a response is required. DAMP receptors include some of the TLRs, including TLR2 and TLR4, but also a variety of other proteins, such as receptor for advanced glycosylation end-products (RAGE) and triggering receptor expressed on myeloid cells 1 (TREM-1). In the setting of a transplant surgery where an organ is cut out of one individual with a period of obligatory ischemia, cooled to near freezing, and then replaced in another individual, DAMPs play an active role in stimulating the innate inflammatory response. Once an injury or infectious insult has been identified, the cellular components of the innate system begin to initiate a response.

Monocytes

Mononuclear phagocytes are bone marrow–derived cells that initially emerge as monocytes within peripheral blood. In the setting of certain inflammatory signals, they home to sites of injury or inflammation, where they mature and become macrophages. Their function is to acquire, process, and present antigen as well as to serve as effector cells in certain situations. Once activated, they elaborate various cytokines that regulate the local immune response. They play a significant role in facilitating the acquired T-cell response through antigen presentation, and their cytokines induce substantial tissue dysfunction in sites of inflammation. Thus, their recruitment to sites of injury and cell death can subsequently provoke T-cell activation and rejection.

Dendritic Cells

Dendritic cells are some of the most potent APCs, and they are distributed throughout the lymphoid and nonlymphoid tissues of the body. Immature dendritic cells can be found along the gut mucosa, within the skin, and in other sites of antigen entry. Once they have encountered antigen in sites of injury, they undergo a process of maturation, including the upregulation of both major histocompatibility complex (MHC) molecules, class I and class II, as well as various costimulatory molecules. They also begin to migrate toward peripheral lymphoid tissue (i.e., lymph nodes), where they can interact with antigen-specific T cells and potentiate their activation. The dendritic cell is involved in the licensing of CD8+ T cells for cytotoxic function, stimulates T-cell clonal expansion, and provides signals for helper T cell (Th) differentiation. There are also subsets of dendritic cells that serve distinct functions in inducing and regulating the cellular response. For example, myeloid dendritic cells are more immunogenic, whereas plasmacytoid dendritic cells are more tolerogenic and may work to suppress the immune response. Follicular dendritic cells are another subset of dendritic cells largely restricted to lymph nodes, and they play a critical role in shaping B-cell responses to antigens and in promoting the development of long-lived memory B-cell and antibody-secreting cell responses.

Natural Killer Cells

NK cells are large granular lymphocytes with potent cytolytic function that constitute a critical component of innate immunity. They were initially discovered during studies focused on tumor immunology. A small subset of lymphocytes exhibited the ability to lyse tumor cells in the absence of prior sensitization, described as "naturally" reactive. These "natural killer" cells exhibited rapid cytolytic activity and existed in a relatively mature state (i.e., morphology characteristic of activated cytotoxic lymphocytes—large size, high protein synthesis activity with abundant endoplasmic reticulum, and rapid killing activity). Further studies have indicated that NK cells lyse cell targets that lack expression of self class I MHC, termed the *missing self hypothesis,* a situation that could arise as a result of viral infection with suppression of self class I molecules or in tumors under strong selection pressure of killer T cells. Since those initial studies, NK cells have been found to express cell surface inhibitory receptors, which include killer inhibitory receptors. These molecules function to deliver inhibitory signals when they bind self class I MHC molecules, thus preventing NK-mediated cytolysis on otherwise healthy host cells. NK cells produce various cytokines, including interferon-γ (IFN-γ), which may function to activate macrophages, which can in turn eliminate host cells infected by intracellular microbes. Similar to macrophages, NK cells express cell surface Fc receptors, which bind antibody and participate in antibody-dependent cellular cytotoxicity. NK cells also play an important role in the immune response after bone marrow transplantation and xenotransplantation. Their role in solid organ transplantation is less well defined, although there is some evidence that they may participate in acute and chronic allograft rejection.

Acquired Immunity

The distinguishing feature of the acquired immune system is specific recognition and disposition of foreign elements as well as the ability to recall prior challenges and to respond appropriately. Highly specific receptors, discussed later, have evolved to distinguish foreign from normal tissue through antigen binding. The term *antigen* is used to describe a molecule that can be recognized by the acquired immune system. An epitope is the portion of the antigen, generally a carbohydrate or peptide moiety, that actually serves as the binding site for the immune system receptor and is the base unit of antigen recognition. Thus, there may be one or many epitopes on any given antigen. The acquired response is divided into two distinct arms: cellular and humoral. The predominant effector cell in each arm is the T cell and B cell, respectively. Accordingly, the two main types of receptors that the immune system employs to recognize any given epitope are the TCR and B-cell receptor (BCR, or antibody). In general, individual T or B lymphocytes express identical receptors, each of which binds only to a single epitope. This mechanism establishes the specificity of the acquired immune response. The antigenic encounter alters the immune system such that future challenges with the same antigen provoke a more rapid and vigorous response, a phenomenon known as *immunologic memory.* There are vast differences in the way each division of the acquired immune response identifies an antigen. The BCR or antibody can identify its epitope directly without preparation of the antigen, either on an invading pathogen itself or as a free-floating molecule in the extracellular fluid. T cells, however, recognize only their specific epitope after it has been processed and bound to a set of proteins unique to the individual, which are responsible for presentation of the antigen. This set of proteins, crucial to antigen presentation, are termed *histocompatibility proteins* and, as their name suggests, were defined through studies examining tissue transplantation. The case of the immune response in tissue transplantation is unique and is discussed in its own section.

Major Histocompatibility Locus: Transplant Antigens

The MHC refers to a cluster of highly conserved polymorphic genes on the sixth human chromosome. Much of what we know about the details of the immune response grew from initial studies defining the immunogenetics of the MHC. Studies began in mice in which the MHC gene complex, termed *H-2,* was described by Gorer and Snell as a genetic locus that segregated with transplanted tumor survival. Subsequent serologic studies identified a similar genetic locus in humans called the *human leukocyte antigen (HLA) locus.* The products of these genes are expressed on a wide variety of cell types and play a pivotal role in the immune response. They are also the antigens primarily responsible for human transplant rejection, and their clinical implications are discussed later.

MHC molecules play a role in both the innate and acquired immune systems. Their predominant role, however, lies in antigen presentation within the acquired response. As mentioned earlier, the TCR does not recognize its specific antigen directly; rather, it binds to the processed antigen that is bound to cell surface proteins. It is the MHC molecule that binds the peptide antigen and interacts with the TCR, a process called *antigen presentation.* Thus, all T cells are restricted to an MHC for their response. There are two classes of MHC molecules: class I and class II. In general, CD8+ T cells bind to antigen within class I MHC, and CD4+ T cells bind to antigen within class II MHC.

Human Histocompatibility Complex

The antigens primarily responsible for human allograft rejection are those encoded by the HLA region of chromosome 6 (Fig. 49.4). The polymorphic proteins encoded by this locus include class I molecules (HLA-A, B, and C) and class II molecules (HLA-DP, DQ, and DR). There are additional class I genes with limited polymorphism (E, F, G, H, and J), but they are not currently used in tissue typing for transplantation and are not considered here. There are class III genes as well, but they are not cell surface proteins involved in antigen presentation directly, but instead include molecules that are pertinent to the immune response by various mechanisms: tumor necrosis factor-α (TNF-α), lymphotoxin β, components of the complement cascade, nuclear transcription factor-β, and heat shock protein 70. Other conserved genes within the HLA include genes necessary for class I and class II presentation of peptides, such as the peptide transporter proteins TAP1 and TAP2 and proteasome proteases LMP2 and LMP7.[3] Although other polymorphic genes, referred to as *minor histocompatibility antigens,* exist in the genome outside of the HLA locus, they play a less significant role in transplant rejection and are not covered here. It is, however, important to point out that even HLA-identical individuals are subject to rejection on the basis of these minor differences. The blood group antigens of the ABO system must also be considered transplant antigens, and their biology is critical to humoral rejection.

Although initially identified as transplant antigens, class I and class II MHC molecules actually play vital roles in all immune responses, not just those to transplanted tissue. HLA class I molecules are present on all nucleated cells. In contrast, class II molecules are found almost exclusively on cells associated with the immune system (macrophages, dendritic cells, B cells, and activated T cells) but can be upregulated and appear on other parenchymal cells in the setting of cytokine release caused by immune response or injury.

The importance to transplantation of MHC gene products stems from their polymorphism. Unlike most genes, which are identical within a given species, polymorphic gene products differ in detail while still conforming to the same basic structure. Thus, polymorphic MHC proteins from one individual are foreign

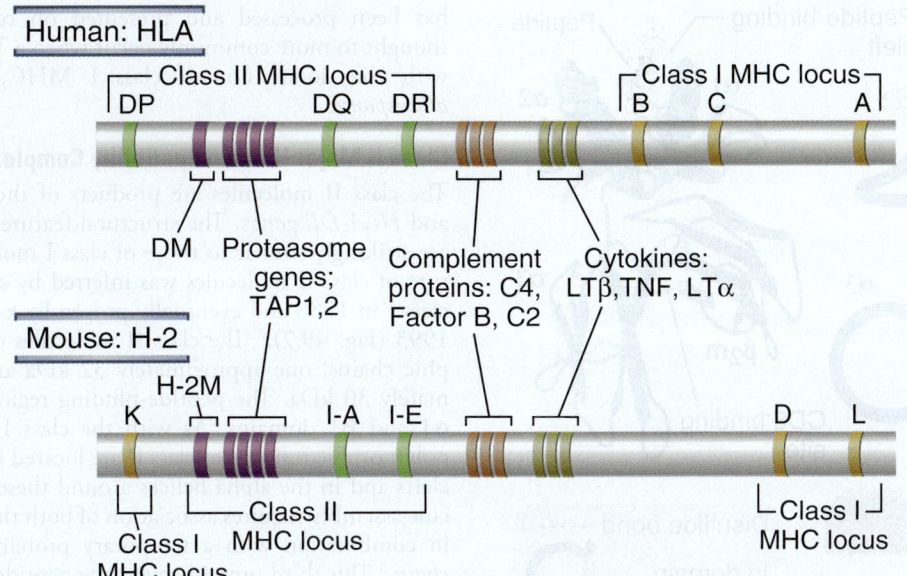

FIGURE 49.4 Schematic maps of human and mouse major histocompatibility complex *(MHC)* loci. The basic organization of the genes in the MHC locus is similar in humans and mice. *HLA,* Human leukocyte antigen; *LT,* lymphotoxin; *TAP,* transporter associated with antigen processing; *TNFα,* tumor necrosis factor-α. (Adapted from Abbas AK, Lichtman AH, Pillai S. *Cellular and Molecular Immunology.* 10th ed. Philadelphia: Saunders Elsevier; 2021.)

alloantigens to another individual. Recombination within the HLA locus is uncommon, occurring in approximately 1% of molecules. Consequently, the HLA type of the offspring is predictable. The unit of inheritance is the haplotype, which consists of one chromosome 6 and, therefore, one copy of each class I and class II locus (HLA-A, B, C, DP, DQ, and DR). Thus, donor-recipient pairings that are matched at these HLA loci are referred to as *HLA-identical allografts,* and those matched at half of the HLA loci are termed *haploidentical.* Note that HLA-identical allografts still differ genetically at other genetic loci and are distinct from isografts. Isografts are organs transplanted between identical twins and are immunologically indistinguishable and thus are not naturally rejected. The genetics of HLA is particularly important in understanding clinical living related donor transplantation. Each child inherits one haplotype from each parent; therefore, the chance of siblings being HLA identical is 25%. Haploidentical siblings occur 50% of the time, and completely nonidentical or HLA-distinct siblings occur 25% of the time. Biologic parents are haploidentical with their children unless there has been a rare recombination event. The degree of HLA match can also improve if the parents are homozygous for a given allele, thus giving the same allele to all children. Likewise, if the parents share the same allele, the likelihood of that allele being inherited improves to 50%. This is even more important in the field of bone marrow transplantation in which the risks of donor-mediated cytotoxicity and resultant graft-versus-host disease become a more relevant issue.

Each class I molecule is encoded by a single polymorphic gene that is combined with the nonpolymorphic protein β_2 microglobulin (chromosome 15) for expression. The polymorphism of each class I molecule is extreme, with 40 to 130 alleles per locus. Class II molecules are made up of two chains, α and β, and individuals differ not only in the alleles represented at each locus but also in the number of loci present in the HLA class II region. The polymorphism of class II is thus increased by combinations of α and β chains as well as by hybrid assembly of chains from one

class II locus to another. As the HLA sequence varies, the ability of various peptides to bind to the molecule and to be presented for T-cell recognition changes. Teleologically, this extreme diversity is thought to improve the likelihood that a given pathogenic peptide will fit into the binding site of these antigen-presenting molecules, thus preventing a single viral agent from evading detection by T cells of an entire population.[4]

Class I Major Histocompatibility Complex

The three-dimensional (3D) structure of class I molecules (HLA-A, B, and C) was first elucidated in 1987.[5] The critical structural feature of class I molecules is the presence of a groove formed by two α helices mounted on a β pleated sheet (Fig. 49.5). Within this groove, a 9–amino acid peptide, formed from fragments of proteins being synthesized in the cell's endoplasmic reticulum, is mounted for presentation to T cells (Fig. 49.6). Almost all the significant sequence polymorphism of class I is located in the region of the peptide-binding groove and in areas of direct T-cell contact. In general, all peptides made by a cell are candidates for presentation, although sequence alterations in this region favor certain sequences over others.

Human class I presentation occurs on all nucleated cells, and expression can be increased by certain cytokines, thus allowing the immune system to inspect and to approve of ongoing protein synthesis. IFNs (IFN-α, IFN-β, and IFN-γ) induce an increase in the expression of class I molecules on a given cell by increasing levels of gene expression. T-cell activation occurs when a given T cell encounters a class I MHC molecule carrying a peptide from a nonself protein presented in the proper context (e.g., viral protein is processed in an infected cell and the peptide fragments are presented on class I molecules for T-cell recognition). So-called *cross-presentation* may also occur in which certain APCs, namely, a subset of dendritic cells, have the ability to take up and process exogenous antigen and present it on class I molecules to CD8+ T cells.[6] In the case of transplantation, this activation is not only possible when foreign peptide is identified after the donor MHC

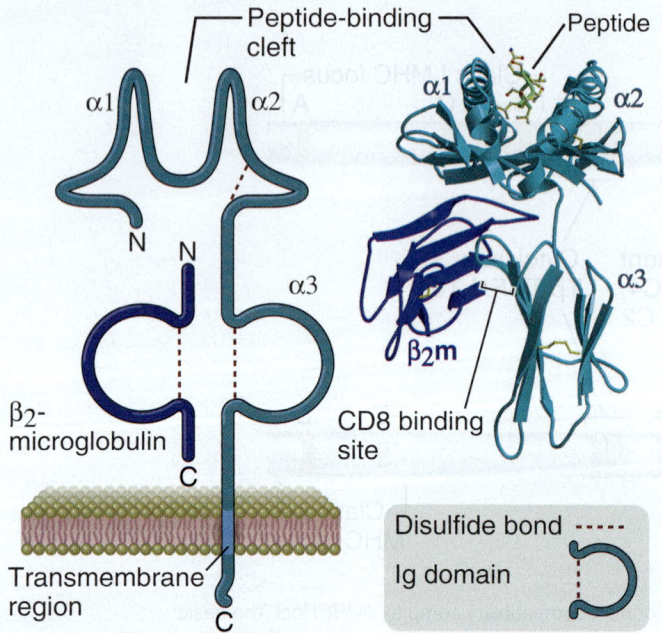

FIGURE 49.5 Structure of the major histocompatibility complex class I molecule. Class I molecules are composed of polymorphic (α) chain noncovalently attached to the nonpolymorphic β2-microglobulin (β2m), as shown in this schematic diagram and ribbon diagram of the extracellular structure of a class I molecule with a bound peptide. (Adapted from Abbas AK, Lichtman AH, Pillai S. *Cellular and Molecular Immunology*. 10th ed. Philadelphia: Saunders Elsevier; 2021.)

has been processed and presented on recipient APCs but is thought to more commonly occur when a T cell interacts directly with the donor nonself class I MHC, the so-called *direct alloresponse*.

Class II Major Histocompatibility Complex

The class II molecules are products of the *HLA-DP, HLA-DQ,* and *HLA-DR* genes. The structural features of class II molecules are strikingly similar to those of class I molecules. The 3D structure of class II molecules was inferred by sequence homology to class I in 1988 and eventually proven by x-ray crystallography in 1993 (Fig. 49.7).[7] The class II molecules contain two polymorphic chains, one approximately 32 kDa and the other approximately 30 kDa. The peptide-binding region is composed of the α1 and β1 domains. As with the class I molecule, significant polymorphic residues of class II are located in the peptide-binding clefts and in the alpha helices around these clefts. Class II molecule assembly requires association of both the α chain and β chain in combination with a temporary protein called the *invariant chain*.[8] This third protein covers the peptide-binding groove until the class II molecule is out of the endoplasmic reticulum and is sequestered in an endosome. Proteins that are engulfed by a phagocytic cell are degraded at the same time as the invariant chain is removed, allowing peptides of external sources 11 to 30 amino acids long to be associated with and presented by class II (see Fig. 49.6). In this way, the acquired immune system can inspect and approve of proteins that are present in circulation or that have been liberated from foreign cells or pathogens through

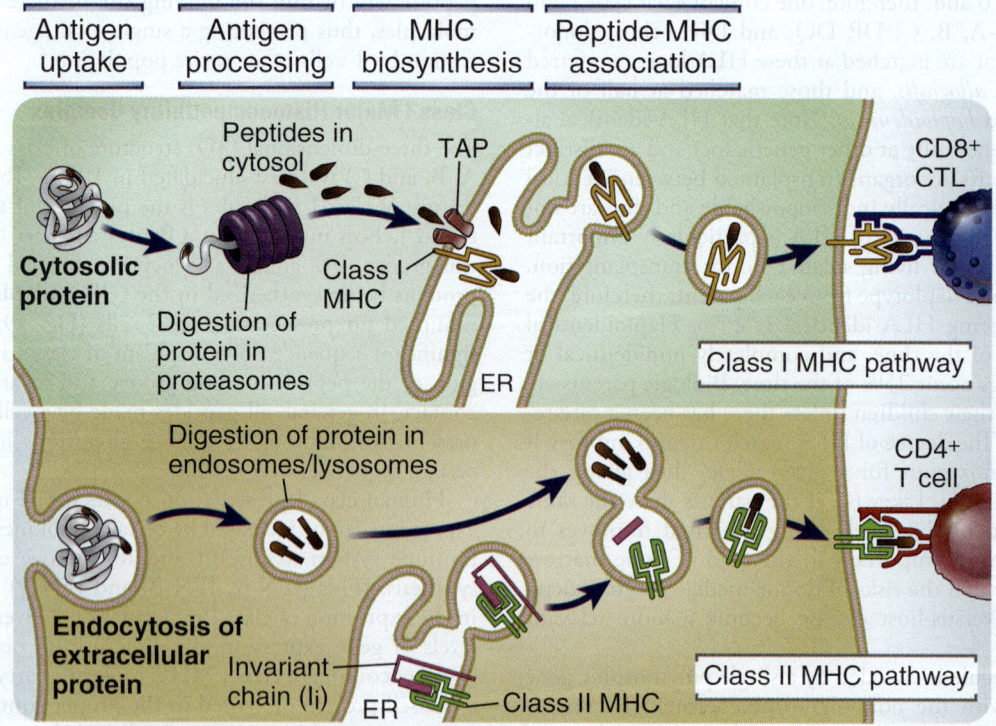

FIGURE 49.6 Pathways of antigen processing and presentation. In the class I major histocompatibility complex *(MHC)* pathway *(top panel)*, protein antigens in the cytosol are processed by proteasomes, and peptides are transported into the ER, where they bind to class I MHC molecules. In the class II MHC pathway *(bottom panel)*, extracellular proteins that are endocytosed are then degraded in lysosomes and bound to class II MHC molecules. *CTL,* Cytotoxic T lymphocytes; *ER,* endoplasmic reticulum; *TAP,* transporter associated with antigen processing. (Adapted from Abbas AK, Lichtman AH, Pillai S. *Cellular and Molecular Immunology*. 10th ed. Philadelphia: Saunders Elsevier; 2021.)

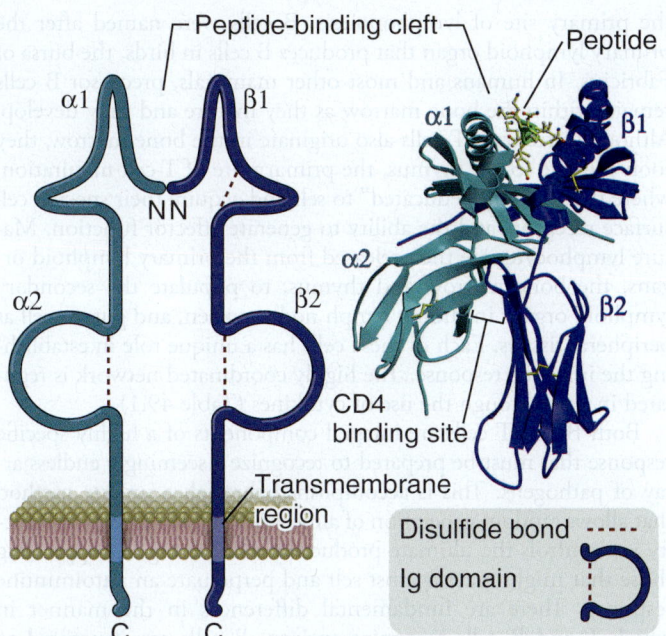

FIGURE 49.7 Structure of the major histocompatibility complex class II molecule. Class II molecules are composed of a polymorphic α chain noncovalently attached to a polymorphic β chain. Shown is a schematic diagram and ribbon diagram showing the extracellular structure of a class II molecule (HLA-DR1) with a bound peptide, resolved by x-ray crystallography. (Adapted from Abbas AK, Lichtman AH, Pillai S. *Cellular and Molecular Immunology*. 10th ed. Philadelphia: Saunders Elsevier; 2021.)

the phagocytic process. Accordingly, class II molecules, in contrast to class I molecules, are confined to cells related to the immune response, particularly APCs (macrophages, dendritic cells, B cells, and monocytes). Class II expression can also be induced on other cells, including endothelial cells, under the appropriate conditions. After binding class II molecules, CD4+ T cells participate in APC-mediated activation of CD8+ T cells and antibody-producing B cells. In the case of transplanted organs, ischemic injury at the time of transplantation accentuates the potential for T-cell activation by upregulation of both class I and class II molecules locally on the recipient. The trauma of surgery and ischemia also upregulates class II on all cells of the allograft, making nonself MHC more abundant. Host CD4+ T cells may then recognize donor MHC directly (direct alloresponse) or after antigen processing on the recipient's own MHC (indirect alloresponse) and then proceed to participate in rejection.

Human Leukocyte Antigen Typing: Implications for Transplantation

For the reasons already discussed, closely matched or less mismatched transplants are less likely to be recognized and rejected than are similar grafts differing by multiple alleles at the MHC. The degree of HLA matching has historically had clear influence on the prolongation of graft survival. Humans potentially have two different HLA-A, B, and DR alleles (one from each parent, six in total), and although now recognized as biologically important, the HLA-C, DP, and DQ loci have historically been administratively dismissed in general organ allocation. Reporting requirements on the genetic typing of donors have now been expanded to include HLA-C, DP, and DQ so that these HLA molecules can also be considered for the purpose of organ allocation. Whereas improvements in kidney transplantation and immunosuppressive

regimens have minimized some of the impact of matching, studies have demonstrated better renal allograft survival when the six primary alleles (A, B, and DR) are matched between donor and recipient, a so-called *six-antigen match* or *zero-antigen mismatch* (Fig. 49.8), and studies continue to show smaller but significant correlations between HLA mismatches and graft survival. HLA typing is not only important for the determination of MHC disparities between donors and recipients but is also critical for the avoidance of preformed HLA donor-specific antibodies that can exist in transplant recipients. Historically, MHC typing had been defined using serologic assays like the complement-dependent cytotoxicity (CDC) and microlymphocytotoxicity techniques that rely on antibodies to detect HLA antigens. These assays identify MHC antigens but suffer from low sensitivity and specificity, subjectivity in interpretation of results, and an inability to distinguish between closely related MHC molecules. Because of these logistical and performance limitations, they have been replaced by faster and more precise molecular techniques that define the actual nucleotide sequence of an individual's MHC.

Serologic typing via the CDC technique involved mixing patient lymphocytes with sera containing anti-HLA antibodies of known specificity, exogenous complement, and a vital dye (which is not taken up by intact cells). If a patient expressed an MHC matching the known anti-HLA antibody, the antibody would bind to patient lymphocytes, and added complement would lead to cell membrane disruption and visible uptake of vital dye under the microscope, confirming the MHC identity. However, as noted earlier, important antigen differences were not always identified this way, and the source of antibodies became more limiting as more relevant antigens were discovered. Thus, it has been supplanted by DNA-based molecular methods using polymerase chain reaction (PCR), including sequence-specific oligonucleotide (SSO), sequence-specific primers (SSPs), and sequence-based typing (SBT).

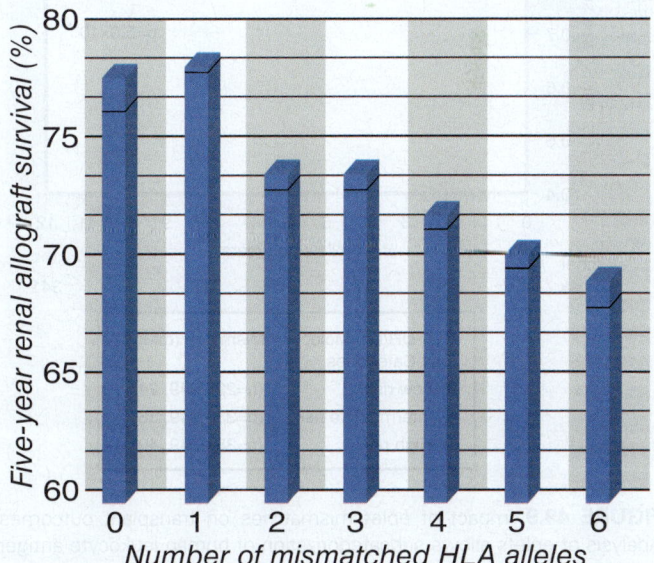

FIGURE 49.8 Influence of human leukocyte antigen *(HLA)* matching on renal allograft survival. Matching of HLA alleles between donor and recipient significantly improves renal allograft survival. The data are shown for deceased donor renal allografts stratified by number of matched HLA alleles. (Adapted from Abbas AK, Lichtman AH, Pillai S. *Cellular and Molecular Immunology*. 10th ed. Philadelphia: Saunders Elsevier; 2021.)

These advances in HLA typing have enhanced understanding of tissue compatibility between individuals, thus improving organ allocation—especially for recipients with preexisting HLA antibodies. Although the advent of PCR-based techniques transitioned tissue compatibility to more precise whole HLA antigen matching, rapidly advancing high-resolution molecular HLA typing techniques and next-generation sequencing have made it possible to view compatibility at the molecular and amino acid level. Molecular HLA typing data along with potent bioinformatics tools have combined to identify polymorphic amino acid clusters within whole HLA molecules that comprise the epitope specifically targeted by HLA-specific antibodies. These amino acid clusters, or "eplets," on or near the surface of the 3D HLA molecule can then be compared between donors and recipients as more precise determinants of compatibility compared with the whole HLA molecule or antigen. As such, HLA typing has evolved from crude measures of whole HLA antigen disparities between individuals to very high-resolution identification of the amino acids that form the epitopes on these large polymorphic HLA molecules that are specifically responsible for HLA compatibility and alloimmune outcomes (Fig. 49.9).

Cellular Components of the Acquired Immune System

The key cellular components of the immune system, T cells, B cells, and APCs, are hematopoietically derived and arise from a common progenitor stem cell. The development of the lymphoid system begins with pluripotent stem cells in the liver and bone marrow of the fetus. As the fetus matures, the bone marrow becomes

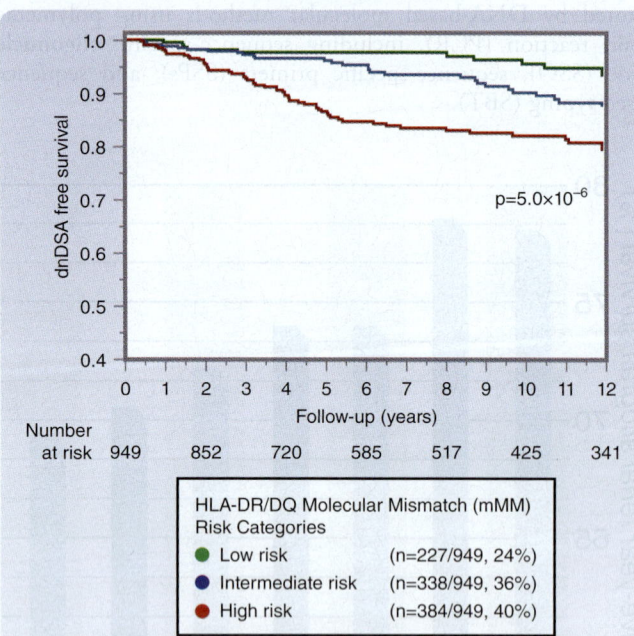

FIGURE 49.9 Impact of eplet mismatches on transplant outcomes. Analysis of eplets allows subcategorization of human leukocyte antigen (*HLA*)-DR and HLA-DQ mismatches between donor and recipient into those mismatches at low, intermediate, or high risk of allorejection. Use of these HLA-DR/DQ molecular mismatch risk categories accurately predicts the development of de novo donor-specific antibodies in renal transplant recipients. *dnDSA,* De novo donor-specific antibodies. (From Wiebe C, Balshaw R, Gibson IW, et al. A rational approach to guide cost-effective de novo donor-specific antibody surveillance with tacrolimus immunosuppression. *Am J Transplant.* 2023;23[12]:1882-1892.)

the primary site of lymphopoiesis. B cells were named after the primary lymphoid organ that produces B cells in birds, the bursa of Fabricius. In humans and most other mammals, precursor B cells remain within the bone marrow as they mature and fully develop. Although precursor T cells also originate in the bone marrow, they soon migrate to the thymus, the primary site of T-cell maturation, where they become "educated" to self and acquire their specific cell surface receptors and the ability to generate effector function. Mature lymphocytes are then released from the primary lymphoid organs, the bone marrow and thymus, to populate the secondary lymphoid organs including lymph nodes, spleen, and gut as well as peripheral tissues. Each of these cells has a unique role in establishing the immune response. The highly coordinated network is regulated in part through the use of cytokines (Table 49.1).

Both B and T cells are integral components of a highly specific response that must be prepared to recognize a seemingly endless array of pathogens. This is accomplished through a unique method that allows random generation of almost unlimited receptor specificity yet controls the ultimate product by eliminating or suppressing those that might react against self and perpetuate an autoimmune response. There are fundamental differences in the manner in which T and B cells recognize antigen. B cells are structured to respond to whole antigen and in response synthesize and secrete antibody that can interact with antigen at distant sites. T cells, on the other hand, are responsible for cell-mediated immunity and of necessity must interact with cells in the periphery to neutralize and eliminate foreign antigens. From the peripheral blood, T cells enter the lymph nodes or spleen through highly specialized regions in the postcapillary venules. Within the secondary lymphoid organ, T cells interact with specific APCs, where they receive the appropriate signals that in effect license them for effector function. They then exit the lymphoid tissues through the efferent lymph, eventually percolating through the thoracic duct and returning to the bloodstream. From there, they can return to the site of the immune response, where they encounter their specific antigen and carry out their predefined functions.

T-Cell Receptor

Considerable progress has been made in defining the mechanisms of T-cell maturation and the development of a functional TCR. The formation of the TCR is fundamental to the understanding of its function.[9] A central paradox of immunology for many years was how the immune system can encode millions of different antibodies and TCRs, given the fixed size of the human genome. This mystery was solved by Susumu Tonegawa, who was awarded the Nobel Prize in 1987 for his discovery of V(D)J recombination, the genetic mechanism that produces antibody and TCR diversity. The genetic locus encoding the α and β chains that comprise the TCR contains both a constant region (C) and a variable region that is assembled from a V genetic segment (with 52 options for the human β chain and ~70 for the α chain), a D genetic segment (2 options for the β chain and absent in the α chain), and a J segment (13 and 61 options, respectively). These V, D, and J segments are randomly assembled together by the RAG1 and RAG2 recombinases through a process of double-strand DNA breaks and nonhomologous DNA end joining, generating a "mixed-and-matched" recombined V(D)J segment that encodes the actual variable region of the TCR. Through this process of V(D)J recombination, a limited number of gene segments can generate millions of different TCR specificities (Fig. 49.10).

Regardless of the genes used, individual cells recombine to express a TCR with only a single specificity. These rearrangements

TABLE 49.1 **Summary of Cytokines**

CYTOKINE	SOURCE	PRINCIPAL CELLULAR TARGETS AND BIOLOGIC EFFECTS
Interleukin-1	Macrophages, endothelial cells, some epithelial cells	Endothelial cell: activation (inflammation, coagulation) Hypothalamus: fever Liver: synthesis of acute-phase proteins
Interleukin-2	T cells	T cells: proliferation, ↑ cytokine synthesis, survival, potentiates Fas-mediated apoptosis, promotes regulatory T-cell development NK cells: proliferation, activation B cells: proliferation, antibody synthesis (in vitro)
Interleukin-3	T cells	Immature hematopoietic progenitor cells: stimulates differentiation into myeloid lineage, proliferation of myeloid lineage cells
Interleukin-4	CD4+ T cells (Th2), mast cells	B cells: isotype switching to IgE T cells: Th2 differentiation, proliferation Macrophages: inhibition of IFN-γ–mediated activation Mast cells: stimulates proliferation
Interleukin-5	CD4+ T cells (Th2)	Eosinophils: activation, ↑ production B cells: proliferation, IgA production
Interleukin-6	Macrophages, endothelial cells, T cells	Liver: ↑ synthesis of acute-phase proteins B cells: proliferation of antibody-producing cells
Interleukin-7	Fibroblasts, bone marrow stromal cells	Immature hematopoietic progenitor cells: stimulates differentiation into lymphoid lineage T and B cells: important for survival during development as well as for T-cell memory
Tumor necrosis factor	Macrophages, T cells	Endothelial cells: activation (inflammation, coagulation) Neutrophils: activation Hypothalamus: fever Liver: ↑ synthesis of acute-phase proteins Muscle, fat: catabolism (cachexia) Many cell types: apoptosis
Interferon-γ	T cells (Th1, CD8+ T cells), NK cells	Macrophages: activation (increased microbicidal functions) B cells: isotype switching to IgG subclasses that facilitate complement fixation and opsonization T cells: Th1 differentiation Various cells: ↑ expression of class I and class II MHC, ↑ antigen processing and presentation to T cells
Type I interferons (IFN-α, IFN-β)	Macrophages: IFN-α Fibroblasts: IFN-β	All cells: stimulates antiviral activity including ↑ class I MHC expression NK cells: activation
Transforming growth factor-β	T cells, macrophages, other cell types	T cells: inhibition of proliferation and effector functions B cells: inhibition of proliferation, ↑ IgA production Macrophages: inhibits activation, stimulates angiogenic factors Fibroblasts: increased collagen synthesis
Lymphotoxin	T cells	Lymphoid organogenesis Neutrophils: increased recruitment and activation
BAFF (CD257)	Follicular dendritic cells, monocytes, B cells	B cells: survival and proliferation
APRIL (CD256)	T cells, follicular dendritic cells, monocytes	B cells: survival and proliferation
Interleukin-8	Lymphocytes, monocytes	Stimulates granulocyte activity Chemotactic activity
Interleukin-9	Activated Th2 lymphocytes	Enhances proliferation of T cells, mast cells
Interleukin-10	Macrophages, T cells (mainly regulatory T cells)	Macrophages and dendritic cells: inhibition of IL-12 production, stimulates expression of costimulatory molecules and class II MHC
Interleukin-11	Bone marrow stromal cells	Megakaryocytes: thrombopoiesis Liver: induces acute-phase proteins B cells: stimulates T-dependent antibody production
Interleukin-12	Macrophages, dendritic cells	T cells: Th1 differentiation NK and T cells: IFN-γ synthesis, increased cytotoxic activity
Interleukin-13	CD4+ T cells (Th2), NKT cells, mast cells	B cells: isotype switching to IgE Epithelial cells: increased mucus production Fibroblasts and macrophages: increased collagen synthesis
Interleukin-14	T cells, some B-cell tumors	B cells: enhances proliferation of activated B cells, stimulates Ig production
Interleukin-15	Macrophages, others	NK cells: proliferation T cells: proliferation (memory CD8+ T cells)

TABLE 49.1	Summary of Cytokines—cont'd	
CYTOKINE	**SOURCE**	**PRINCIPAL CELLULAR TARGETS AND BIOLOGIC EFFECTS**
Interleukin-17	T cells	Endothelial cells: increased chemokine production
		Macrophages: increased chemokine/cytokine production
		Epithelial cells: GM-CSF and G-CSF production
Interleukin-18	Macrophages	NK and T cells: IFN-γ synthesis
Interleukin-21	Th2, Th17, Tfh	Drives development of Th17 and Tfh
		B cells: activation, proliferation, differentiation
		NK cells: functional maturation
Interleukin-22	Th17	Epithelial cells: production of defensins, increased barrier functions
		Promotes hepatocyte survival
Interleukin-23	Macrophages, dendritic cells	T cells: maintenance of IL-17–producing T cells
Interleukin-27	Macrophages, dendritic cells	T cells: inhibits production of IL-17/Th17 cells, promotes Th1 differentiation
		NK cells: IFN-γ synthesis
Interleukin-33	Endothelial cells, smooth muscle cells, keratinocytes, fibroblasts	Th2 development and cytokine production

APRIL, A proliferation-inducing ligand; *BAFF*, B cell–activating factor; *G-CSF*, granulocyte-colony stimulating factor; *GM-CSF*, granulocyte-macrophage colony-stimulating factor; *IFN*, interferon; *Ig*, immunoglobulin; *IL*, interleukin; *MHC*, major histocompatibility complex; *NK*, natural killer; *NKT*, natural killer T cell; *Tfh*, T follicular helper.
Adapted from Abbas AK, Lichtman AH, Pillai S. *Cellular and Molecular Immunology*. 10th ed. Philadelphia: Saunders Elsevier; 2021.

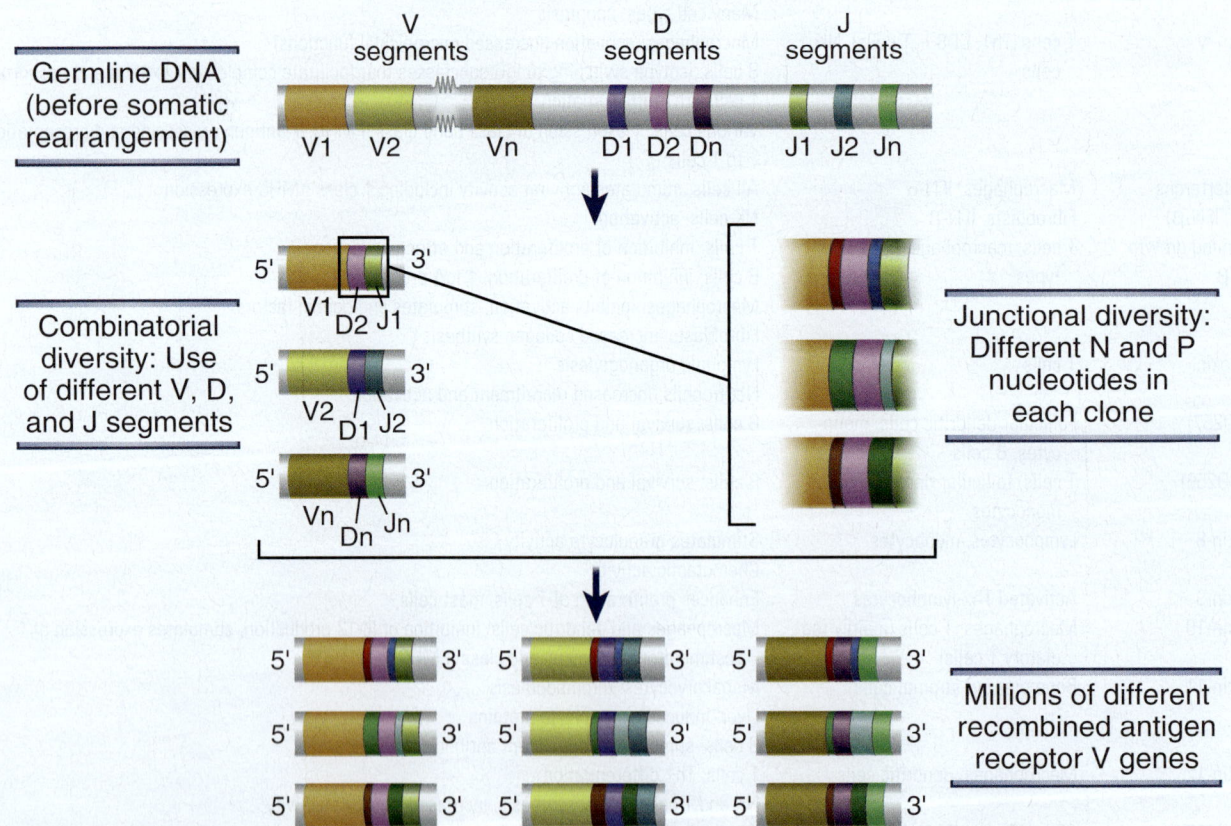

FIGURE 49.10 Diversity of antigen receptor genes. The variable regions of T-cell receptors and immuno-globulins are both produced by the genetic mechanism of V(D)J recombination. Several enzymes found only in lymphocytes (such as the RAG recombinases) mediate this special kind of nonhomologous DNA recombination event. Combinations of different V, D, and J gene segments from the germline DNA are derived, with the addition or removal of nucleotides at the joints. This process generates the mRNA of millions of different recombined antigen receptors. (Adapted from Abbas AK, Lichtman AH, Pillai S. *Cellular and Molecular Immunology*. 10th ed. Philadelphia: Saunders Elsevier; 2021.)

occur randomly and can theoretically produce 10^{10} different TCRs; however, 10^{10} T cells would weigh 500 kg and cannot all be contained in the human body. Based on computational models of homeostasis of multiclonal populations of T cells, it is estimated that approximately 10^9 naïve T-cell clonotypes (i.e., T cells with the same TCR specificity) are present at any point in time.[10] As a result, the frequency of naïve T cells available to respond to any given pathogen is relatively small, estimated to be between 1 in 200,000 and 1 in 500,000. These developing T cells also express both CD4 and CD8, accessory molecules that strengthen TCR binding to MHC. These accessory molecules further increase the binding repertoire of the population to include either class I or class II MHC molecules. If the process of T-cell maturation ended at this stage, there would be a host of T cells that could recognize self MHC–peptide complexes, resulting in an uncontrolled, global autoimmune response. To avoid the release of autoreactive T cells, developing cells undergo a process after recombination known as *positive and negative thymic selection* (Fig. 49.11).[11] Cells initially interact with the MHC-expressing cortical thymic epithelium, which produces hormones (thymopoietin and thymosin) as well as cytokines (e.g., interleukin [IL]-7) that are critical to T-cell development. If binding does not occur to self MHC, those cells are useless to the individual (e.g., they cannot bind self cells to assess for infection), and they are permitted to die by neglect through apoptosis, a process called *positive selection*. Thus, positive selection ensures that T cells are restricted to self MHC. Cells surviving positive selection then move to the thymic medulla and normally eventually lose either CD4 or CD8. If binding to self MHC in the medulla occurs with an unacceptably high affinity, there is an active process whereby death-promoting signals are delivered and programmed cell death is initiated, a process termed *negative selection*. Negative selection stands in contrast to the death that occurs by neglect when immature lymphocytes are not positively selected. Negative selection of T cells in the thymus is a form of central tolerance in the immune system, resulting in the deletion of a pathogenic autoreactive T-cell repertoire. Another possible, although less common, outcome of a high-affinity interaction with self peptide–MHC is the development of a regulatory T-cell (Treg) phenotype. The precise nature of this affinity threshold remains a matter of intense investigation and involves interaction with hematopoietic cells that reside in the thymus as well as medullary thymic epithelial cells. These thymically derived "natural" Tregs emerge from the thymus and are involved in the suppression of autoreactive T cells in the periphery, which is discussed later.

The only cells released into the periphery are those that can both bind self MHC and avoid activation by self-antigens.

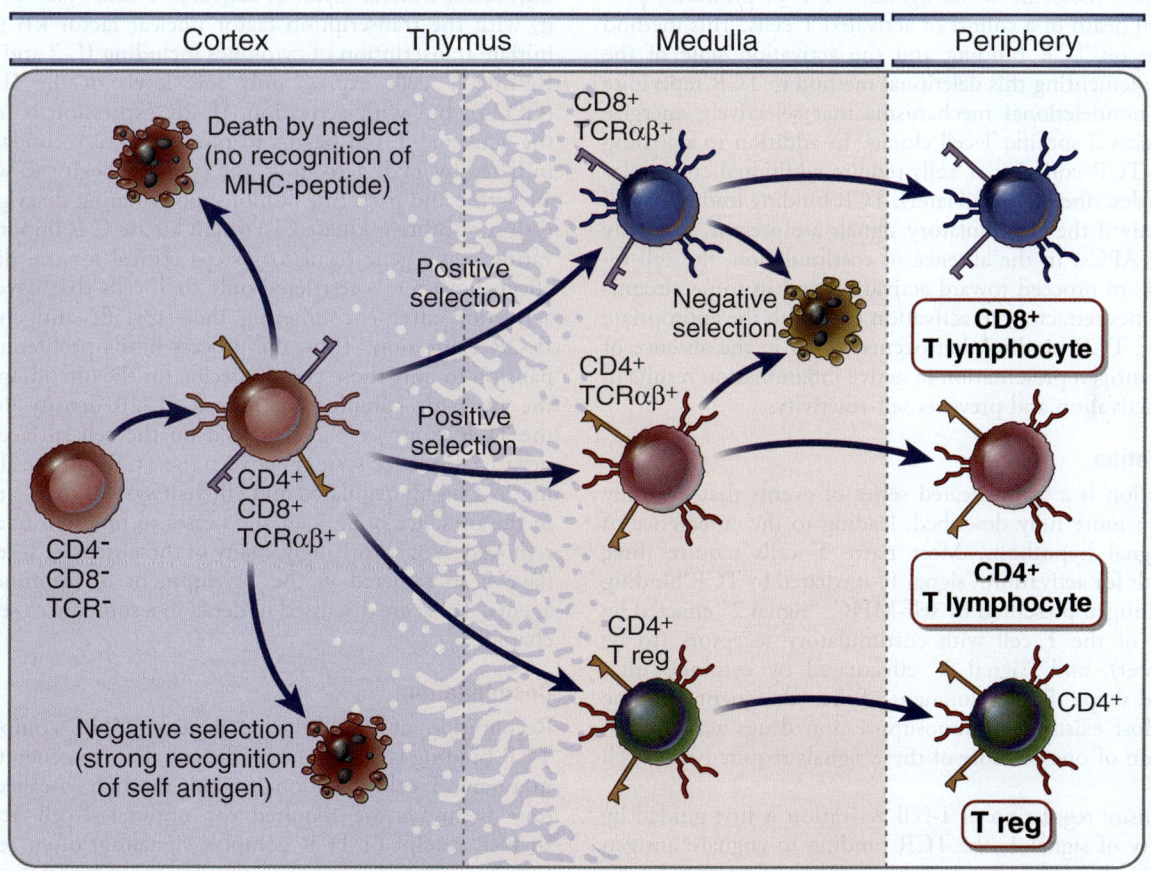

FIGURE 49.11 T-cell maturation in the thymus. Initially, bone marrow–derived T-cell precursors arrive in the thymic cortex lacking CD4, CD8, or a T-cell receptor *(TCR)* and are referred to as *double negative*. In the thymic cortex, these cells begin to express TCRs and the CD4 and CD8 coreceptors. Positive selection promotes the survival of T cells bearing TCR that can bind to self-major histocompatibility complex *(MHC)*, whereas negative selection promotes the deletion of T cells bearing autoreactive TCR. The T cells progress through a double-positive (expressing both CD4 and CD8) and eventually a single-positive stage, where they ultimately express only CD4 or CD8, depending on which class of MHC they restrict to. (Adapted from Abbas AK, Lichtman AH, Pillai S. *Cellular and Molecular Immunology.* 10th ed. Philadelphia: Saunders Elsevier; 2021.)

Whereas T cells are restricted to bind self MHC–peptide complexes without activation, the selection process does not consider foreign MHC. Thus, by random chance, some cells with appropriate affinity for self MHC survive and have inappropriately high affinity for the MHC molecules of other individuals. In the setting of transplantation, these recipient T cells are able to recognize donor MHC–peptide complexes because sufficient conserved motifs are shared between donor and self MHC molecules. However, because donor MHC was not present during the thymic education process, the binding of donor MHC by an "alloreactive" T cell leads to activation, and rejection ensues. The precursor frequency, or the number of alloreactive T cells, is much higher than the 1 in 200,000 or 1 in 500,000 T cells available to react toward any given antigen. Because T cells are selected to bind self MHC, the frequency specific for a similar, nonself MHC (i.e., alloreactive) is estimated to be between 1% and 10% of all T cells.[12]

In addition to thymic selection, it is now clear that mechanisms exist for peripheral modification of the T-cell repertoire, so-called *peripheral mechanisms of tolerance*. Many of these mechanisms are in place for removal of T cells after an immune response and downregulation of activated clones. CD95, a molecule known as *Fas,* is a member of the TNF receptor superfamily and is expressed on activated T cells. Under appropriate conditions, binding of this molecule to its ligand, CD178, promotes programmed cell death of a cohort of activated T cells. This method is dependent on TCR binding and the activation state of the T cell. Complementing this deletional method to TCR repertoire control are nondeletional mechanisms that selectively anergize (make unreactive) specific T-cell clones. In addition to signaling through the TCR complex, T cells require additional costimulatory signals (described in detail later). TCR binding leads to T-cell activation only if the costimulatory signals are present, generally delivered by APCs. In the absence of costimulation, the cell remains unable to proceed toward activation and in some circumstances becomes refractory to activation even with the appropriate signals. Thus, TCR binding that occurs to self in the absence of appropriate antigen presentation or active inflammation results in an aborted activation and prevents self-reactivity.

T-Cell Activation

T-cell activation is a sophisticated series of events that has only recently been more fully described, leading to the emergence of the three-signal hypothesis. Most naïve T cells require three unique signals for activation: "signal 1" mediated by TCR binding to cognate antigen presented by self-MHC, "signal 2" enacted by engagement of the T cell with costimulatory receptors (to be described later), and "signal 3" effectuated by cytokines that promote and shape the development of the subsequent immune response. Most existing immunosuppression drugs act through the disruption of one or more of these signals required for T-cell activation.

The exquisite regulation of T-cell activation is first guided by the specificity of signal 1, the TCR binding to cognate antigen presented by self-MHC. Because the number of potential antigens is high and the likelihood is that self-antigens vary minimally from foreign antigens, the nature of the TCR-binding event has evolved such that a single interaction with an MHC molecule is not sufficient to cause activation. In fact, a T cell must register a signal from approximately 8000 TCR-ligand interactions with the same antigen before a threshold of activation is reached. Each event results in the internalization of the TCR. Because resting T cells have low TCR density, sequential binding and internalization during several hours are required. Transient encounters are not sufficient. This threshold is reduced considerably by appropriate costimulation signals (detailed later).

Most TCRs are heterodimers composed of two transmembrane polypeptide chains, α and β. The $\alpha\beta$-TCR is noncovalently associated with several other transmembrane signaling proteins, including CD3 (composed of three separate chains, γ, δ, and ϵ) and ζ chain molecules as well as the appropriate accessory molecule from the T cell, either CD4 or CD8, which associates with its respective MHC molecule. Together, these proteins are known as the *TCR complex*. When the TCR is bound to an MHC molecule and the proper configuration of accessory molecules stabilizes its binding, a signal is initiated by intracytoplasmic protein tyrosine kinases (Fig. 49.12). These protein tyrosine kinases include p56lck (on CD4 or CD8), p59Fyn, and ZAP-70, the last two of which are associated with CD3. Repetitive binding signals combined with the appropriate secondary costimulation eventually activate phospholipase-γ1, which in turn hydrolyzes the membrane lipid phosphatidylinositol bisphosphate, thereby releasing inositol trisphosphate and diacylglycerol. Inositol trisphosphate binds to the endoplasmic reticulum, causing a release of calcium that induces calmodulin to bind to and activate calcineurin. Calcineurin dephosphorylates the critical cytokine transcription factor nuclear factor of activated T cells (NFAT), prompting it, with the transcription factor nuclear factor κB (NF-κB), to initiate transcription of cytokines including IL-2 and its receptor. Resting T cells express only low levels of the IL-2 receptor (CD25), but with activation, IL-2R expression is increased. As the activated T cell begins to produce IL-2 secondary to events initiated by TCR activation, the cytokine begins to work in both autocrine and paracrine fashions, potentiating diacylglycerol activation of protein kinase C. Protein kinase C is important in activating many gene regulatory steps critical for cell division. This effect, however, is restricted only to T cells that have undergone activation after encountering their specific antigen leading to IL-2R expression. Thus, the process limits proliferation and expansion to only those clones specific for the offending antigen. As the antigenic stimulus is removed, IL-2R density decreases and the TCR complex is reexpressed on the cell surface. There is a negative feedback system between the TCR and the IL-2R, resulting in a highly regulated and efficient system that is reactive only in the presence of antigen and ceases to function once antigen is removed. Not surprisingly, many of these steps in T-cell activation have been targeted in the development of immunosuppressive agents. These are discussed in detail in a subsequent section of this chapter.

Costimulation

Recognition of the antigenic peptide–MHC complex through TCR binding is usually not sufficient alone to generate a response in a naïve T cell. Additional signals through so-called costimulatory pathways are required for optimal T-cell activation.[13,14] In fact, receipt of TCR complex signaling, often referred to as signal 1, in the absence of costimulation, or signal 2, not only fails to achieve activation but also can lead to a state of inaction or anergy (Fig. 49.13). An anergic T cell is rendered unable to respond even if given both of the appropriate stimuli.[15] This characteristic of the immune system is thought to be one of the major mechanisms in tolerance to self-antigens in the periphery, crucial in the prevention of autoimmunity. Researchers have exploited this discovery using antibodies or receptor fusion proteins

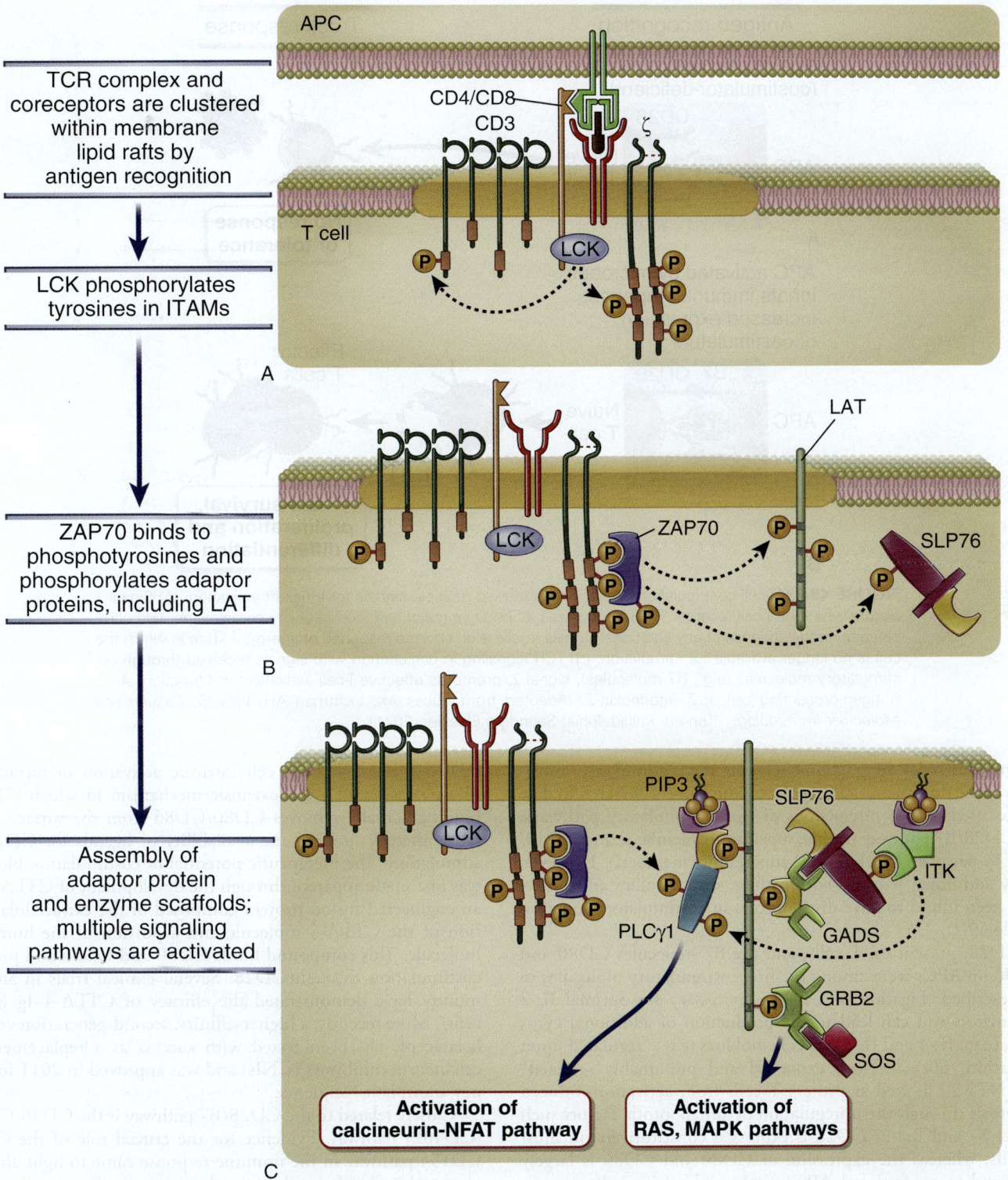

FIGURE 49.12 T-cell activation. On antigen recognition, there is a clustering of T-cell receptor *(TCR)* complexes and coreceptors that initiates a cascade of signaling events within the T cell. Tyrosine kinases associated with the coreceptors (e.g., Lck) phosphorylate CD3 and the ζ chain (A). The ζ chain association protein kinase (ZAP-70) subsequently associates with these regions and becomes activated. ZAP-70 phosphorylates various adaptor molecules, such as LAT (B). These adaptors become docking sites for other enzymes such as PLCγ1 and GDP-GTP exchange factors that ultimately activate downstream MAP kinase pathways (C). PLCγ1 activation specifically produces a rapid increase in cytosolic free calcium, which in turn activates the calcium-calmodulin–dependent phosphatase calcineurin. Calcineurin dephosphorylates cytoplasmic NFAT, which then translocates into the nucleus and serves as a critical transcription factor promoting the expression of various genes involved in proliferation and T-cell responses. (Adapted from Abbas AK, Lichtman AH, Pillai S. *Cellular and Molecular Immunology.* 10th ed. Philadelphia: Saunders Elsevier; 2021.)

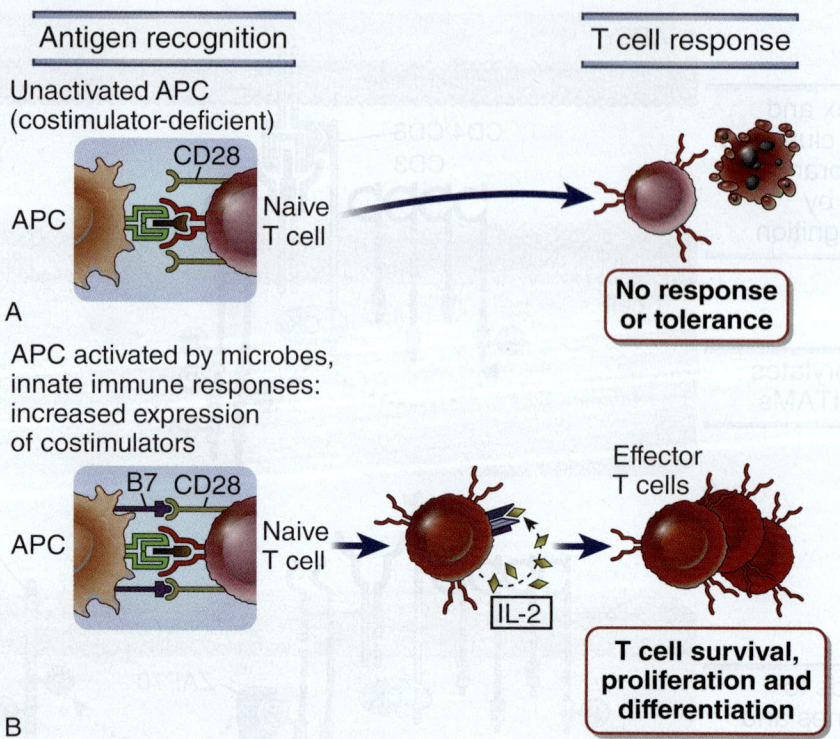

FIGURE 49.13 T-cell costimulation. Naïve T cells require multiple signals for efficient activation. (A) Signal 1 occurs when the T-cell receptor (TCR) recognizes its putative major histocompatibility complex–peptide combination. In the absence of any additional signals, there is an aborted response or anergy, a state in which the cell is no longer available for stimulation. (B) TCR signaling in conjunction with signals received through costimulatory molecules (e.g., B7 molecules), signal 2, promotes effective T-cell activation and function. *APC,* Antigen-presenting cell; *IL-2,* interleukin-2. (Adapted from Abbas AK, Lichtman AH, Pillai S. *Cellular and Molecular Immunology.* 10th ed. Philadelphia: Saunders Elsevier; 2021.)

designed to block interactions between key costimulatory molecules at the time of antigen exposure. Much of the research to date has focused on the interactions of two costimulatory pathways: the CD28/B7 pathway (Ig-like superfamily members) and CD40/CD154 pathway (TNF/TNFR superfamily members). However, many additional pairings within these same families and others have been found to have distinct roles in costimulatory function (Table 49.2).

CD28, present on T cells, and the B7 molecules CD80 and CD86 on APCs were among the first costimulatory molecules to be described. Ligation of CD28 is necessary for optimal IL-2 production and can lead to the production of additional cytokines (e.g., IL-4 and IL-8) and chemokines (e.g., "regulated upon activation, normal T-cell expressed and presumably secreted" ([RANTES]) as well as protect T cells from activation-induced apoptosis through the upregulation of antiapoptotic factors such as Bcl-X$_L$ and Bcl-2. CD28 is expressed constitutively on most T cells, whereas the expression of CD80 and CD86 is largely restricted to professional APCs, such as dendritic cells, monocytes, and macrophages. The kinetics of CD80/CD86 expression is complex, but they are typically increased with the induction of the immune response. Another ligand for CD80 and CD86 is CTLA-4 (CD152). This molecule is upregulated and expressed on the surface of T cells after activation, and it binds CD80/CD86 with 10 to 20 times greater affinity than CD28. CTLA-4 has been shown to have a negative regulatory effect on T-cell activation and proliferation, an observation supported by the fact that CTLA-4–deficient mice develop a lethal lymphoproliferative disorder. The negative regulatory effect of CTLA-4 is mediated through both cell intrinsic activation of intracellular phosphatases and a cell extrinsic mechanism in which CTLA-4 binding actually removes CD80/CD86 from the surface of the APC, thereby limiting the availability of ligands for CD28 costimulation. The therapeutic potential of costimulation blockade was first made apparent through the development of CTLA-4–Ig, an engineered fusion protein composed of the extracellular portion of the CTLA-4 molecule and a portion of the human Ig molecule. This compound binds CD80 and CD86 and prevents costimulation through CD28. Several clinical trials in autoimmunity have demonstrated the efficacy of CTLA-4–Ig (abatacept). More recently, a higher-affinity, second-generation version, belatacept, has been tested with success as a replacement for calcineurin inhibitors (CNIs) and was approved in 2011 for kidney transplant recipients.[16,17]

Closely related to the CD28/B7 pathway is the CD40/CD154 (CD40L) pathway. Evidence for the crucial role of the CD40/CD154 pathway in the immune response came to light after the observation that hyper-IgM syndrome results from a mutational defect in the gene encoding CD154. In addition to defects in the generation of T-cell–dependent antibody responses, patients with hyper-IgM syndrome also have defects in T-cell–mediated immune responses. CD40 is a cell surface molecule expressed on endothelium, B cells, dendritic cells, and other APCs. Its ligand, CD154, is primarily found on activated T cells. Upregulation of CD154 after TCR signaling allows signals to be sent to the APC through CD40; in particular, it is a critical signal for B-cell activation and proliferation. CD40 binding is required for APCs to stimulate a cytotoxic T-cell response. It leads to the release of

TABLE 49.2 Costimulatory Molecules

RECEPTOR	DISTRIBUTION	LIGAND	DISTRIBUTION	PRINCIPAL EFFECTS AND FUNCTIONS
CD28	T cells	CD80/CD86	Activated APCs	Lowers the threshold for T-cell activation Promotes survival, ↑ antiapoptotic factors Promotes Th1 phenotype
CD40	Dendritic cells, B cells, macrophages, endothelial cells	CD154	T cells, soluble platelets	Induces CD80/CD86 expression on APCs
CD27	T cells, NK cells, B cells	CD70	Thymic epithelium, activated T cells, activated B cells, mature dendritic cells	Enhances T-cell proliferation and survival Acts after CD28 to sustain effector T-cell survival Influences secondary responses more than primary Promotes B-cell differentiation and memory formation
CD30	Activated T cells, activated B cells	CD153	B cells, activated T cells	Maintains survival of primed and memory T cells Promotes Th2 > Th1
CD95 (Fas)	T cells, B cells, APCs, stromal cells	CD178 (FasL)	T cells, APCs, stromal cells	Involved in peripheral T-cell homeostasis through "fratricide," may deliver costimulatory signal
CD134 (OX40)	Activated T cells CD4+ > CD8+	CD252 (OX40L)	Activated T cells, mature dendritic cells, activated B cells	Important for CD4+ T-cell expansion and survival ↑ Antiapoptotic factors Functions after CD28 to sustain CD4+ T-cell survival Enhances cytokine production Augments effector and memory CD4+ T-cell function Promotes Th2 > Th1
CD137 (4-1BB)	Activated T cells CD8+ > CD4+ Monocytes, follicular dendritic cells, NK cells	4-1BBL	Mature dendritic cells, activated B cells, activated macrophages	Sustains rather than initiates CD8+ T-cell responses Functions after CD28 to sustain T-cell survival Important in antiviral immunity Promotes CD8+ effector function and cell survival
CD152 (CTLA-4)	Activated T cells	CD80/CD86	Activated APCs	Higher affinity for CD80/CD86 than CD28, inhibits T-cell response
HVEM	T cells, monocytes, immature dendritic cells	CD258 (LIGHT)	Activated lymphocytes, immature dendritic cells, NK cells	Augments T-cell responses, CD8+ > CD4+ Promotes dendritic cell maturation
		CD272 (BTLA)	Activated T cells, B cells, dendritic cells	Negative costimulator, inhibits IL-2 production BTLA remains expressed on Th1 but not Th2
		CD160	NK cells, cytolytic CD8+ T cells, γδ T cells	Negative regulator of CD4+ T-cell activation Inhibits proliferation and cytokine production
CD265 (RANK)	Dendritic cells	CD254 (TRANCE)	Activated T cells CD4+ > CD8+	Enhances dendritic cell survival, upregulates Bcl-xl, possibly enhances IFN-γ production
CD279 (PD-1)	T cells	CD274 (PD-L1)	T cells, B cells, APCs, some parenchymal cells	Inhibits activation, proliferation, and acquisition of effector cell function Th1 > Th2
		CD273 (PD-L2)	Dendritic cells, macrophages	Inhibits activation, proliferation, and acquisition of effector cell function Th2 . Th1
CD278 (ICOS)	Activated T cells, memory T cells	CD275 (ICOSL)	Dendritic cells, B cells, macrophages	Promotes survival and expansion of effector T cells, possibly promotes Th2 responses
GITR	Tregs, CD8+ T cells, B cells, macrophages	GITRL	B cells, dendritic cells, macrophages, endothelial cells	Marker for Tregs, allows proliferation of Tregs Promotes T-cell proliferation and cytokine production Negative regulator for NK function

APC, Antigen-presenting cell; *BTLA,* B and T lymphocyte–associated; *CTLA,* cytotoxic T lymphocyte–associated; *GITR,* glucocorticoid-induced tumor necrosis factor receptor; *GITRL,* glucocorticoid-inducted tumor necrosis factor receptor ligand; *HVEM,* herpes virus entry mediator; *ICOS,* inducible costimulator; *ICOSL,* inducible costimulator ligand; *NK,* natural killer; *PD,* programmed death; *RANK,* receptor activator of NFκB; *Treg,* regulatory T cell.

activating cytokines, particularly IL-12, and the upregulation of B7 molecules. It also initiates innate functions of APCs, including nitric oxide synthesis and phagocytosis. Interestingly, CD154 is also released in soluble form by activated platelets. Thus, sites of trauma that attract activated platelets simultaneously recruit the ligand required to activate tissue-based APCs, providing a link between innate and acquired immunity. Antibody preparations against CD154 have shown great promise in experimental models, but initial clinical trials were halted because of concern for unexpected thrombotic complications. There continues to be hope that anti-CD154 antibodies that bind distinct epitopes, Fc-silent domain antibodies devoid of cross-linking abilities, or antibodies directed toward CD40 may circumvent this issue (see "Immunosuppression" section).

Since earlier investigations, multiple other pairings of molecules have been characterized and shown to demonstrate costimulatory or coinhibitory activity. It is the sum of these positive costimulatory and negative coinhibitory signals that shapes the character and magnitude of the T-cell response.[18] CD278 (inducible costimulator, or ICOS) is a CD28 superfamily expressed on activated T cells, and its ligand, CD275 (ICOSL or B7-H2), is expressed on APCs. Unlike CD28, ICOS is not present on naïve T cells, but instead expression is upregulated after T-cell activation and persists on memory T cells. ICOS can function to boost activation of effector T cells in general but in particular plays a critical role in the function of T follicular helper (Tfh) cells, a specialized CD4+ T-cell subset involved in the germinal center reaction and generation of class-switched antibody. Another member of the CD28 superfamily, programmed cell death 1 (PD-1) (CD279), and its ligands PD-L1 (CD274) and PD-L2 (CD273), both B7 family members, have been shown to be involved in negative regulation of cellular immunity. More recently, coinhibitory molecules PD-1H (also known as *VISTA* for V domain Ig suppressor of T-cell activation) and B- and T-lymphocyte–associated (BTLA) have joined this list. Several members of the TNF/TNFR superfamily have been shown to play important roles in T-cell costimulation. These include CD134/CD252 (OX40/OX40L), CD137/CD137L (4-1BB/4-1BBL), CD27/CD70, CD95/CD178 (Fas/FasL), CD30/CD153, receptor activator of NF-κB/TNF-related activation-induced cytokines (RANK/TRANCE), and others. Furthermore, members of the CD2 family function in both costimulatory (i.e., CD2) and coinhibitory (i.e., 2B4) roles during the execution of an alloimmune response. Finally, the T cell–Ig mucin-like family of molecules has been shown to play important coinhibitory roles during alloimmunity, both on effector cells and on Tregs.

In addition to the multitude of costimulatory molecules, many other adhesion molecules expressed on the cell surface (intercellular adhesion molecules, selectins, integrins) control the movement of immune cells through the body, regulate their trafficking to specific areas of inflammation, and nonspecifically strengthen the TCR-MHC binding interaction. They differ from costimulation molecules in that they enhance the interaction of the T cell with other cell types and antigen without directly influencing the quality of the TCR response. There are two main families of cellular adhesion molecules within the immune system: the selectins and the integrins. The selectin family of adhesion molecules is responsible for "rolling"—the initial attachment of leukocytes to vascular endothelial cells at sites of tissue injury and inflammation before their firm adhesion (mediated by integrin binding). The selectin family of proteins is composed of three closely related molecules, each having differential expression on immune cells: L-selectin is expressed on leukocytes, P-selectin is expressed on platelets, and E-selectin is expressed on endothelium. Structurally, all selectins share an amino-terminal lectin domain that interacts with a carbohydrate ligand, an epidermal growth factor–like domain, and two to nine short repeating units that share homology with sequences found in some complement-binding proteins. In contrast to most other adhesion molecules that also possess some signaling or costimulatory functionality, selectins function solely to facilitate leukocyte binding to vascular endothelium. This selectin-mediated loose binding is converted into tight adhesion after activation of leukocyte integrins. Integrins are transmembrane receptors that serve as bridges for cell-cell as well as for cell–extracellular matrix interactions. Many are expressed constitutively on cells of the immune system (i.e., leukocyte function antigen 1) but on sensing inflammatory cytokine or chemokine signals, such as IL-8, are induced to change conformation that results in higher avidity interaction with integrin ligands, resulting

in leukocyte extravasation into inflamed tissue. Both selectins and integrins are potential therapeutic targets to inhibit access of donor-reactive T cells into the allograft and weaken proimmune interactions.

T-Cell Effector Functions

During thymic education, most T cells initially express both CD4 and CD8 molecules, but subsequently, T cells become either CD4+ or CD8+, depending on which MHC class they restrict to. Thus, these accessory molecules govern which type of MHC and, by extension, which types of cells a given T cell can interact with and evaluate. Because there is nearly ubiquitous expression of class I MHC, all cell types are surveyed. These class I molecules display peptides that are generated within the cell (e.g., peptides from normal cellular processes or from internal viral replication). T cells responsible for inspecting all cells express the accessory molecule CD8, which in turn binds to class I and specifically stabilizes a TCR interaction with a class I–presented antigen. Thus, CD8+ T cells evaluate most cell types and mediate destruction of altered cells. Appropriately, they have been termed *cytotoxic T cells.*

APCs are the predominant cell type that expresses class II MHC molecules in addition to class I. Class II molecules display peptides that have been sampled from surrounding extracellular spaces through phagocytosis and thus usually represent the presentation of newly acquired antigen. Cells initiating an immune response need to have access to this newly processed antigen. CD4 binds class II MHC and stabilizes the interaction of the TCR with the class II–peptide complex. Thus, under physiologic conditions, CD4+ T cells are first alerted to an invasion of the body by hematopoietically derived APCs that present their newly acquired antigen in the form of processed peptide in a class II molecule. As a consequence of their MHC restriction, these subpopulations of T cells have several different functions. CD4+ T cells typically contribute to the response in a helper or regulatory role, whereas CD8+ T cells are much more likely to play a part in cell elimination through cytotoxic functions.

After activation, CD4+ T cells initially play a critical role in the expansion of the immune response. After encountering an APC that expresses the specific antigenic peptide–MHC class II pairing, the CD4+ T cell can then signal back to the APC to promote factors that allow CD8+ T-cell activation. This process is accomplished by expression of specific costimulatory molecules and the release of certain cytokines. This licensing of CD8+ T cells for cytotoxic function is a key step within the immune response. This describes in part how CD4+ T cells become helper cells. More recently, there has been further elucidation of their cellular differentiation into several well-defined Th subsets, including Th1, Th2, Th17, and Tfh cells, which are largely defined on the basis of the distinct transcription factors they express and the cytokines they elaborate (Fig. 49.14). The main cytokine driving the differentiation of Th1 cells is IL-12, and mature Th1 cells mediate effector function through the release of IFN-γ and TNF. The predominant role of IFN-γ is to enhance macrophage function and activity as well as to promote cell-mediated immunity. Activated macrophages then proceed to ingest and to kill invading microbes, and at the same time, the acquired immune system is directed to produce antibodies that promote opsonization, thereby enhancing the overall process. Th2 cell differentiation, in contrast, is driven by the presence of IL-4 and results in release of IL-4, IL-5, IL-10, and IL-13, which ultimately inhibit macrophage activation and promote IgE production and eosinophil activation.

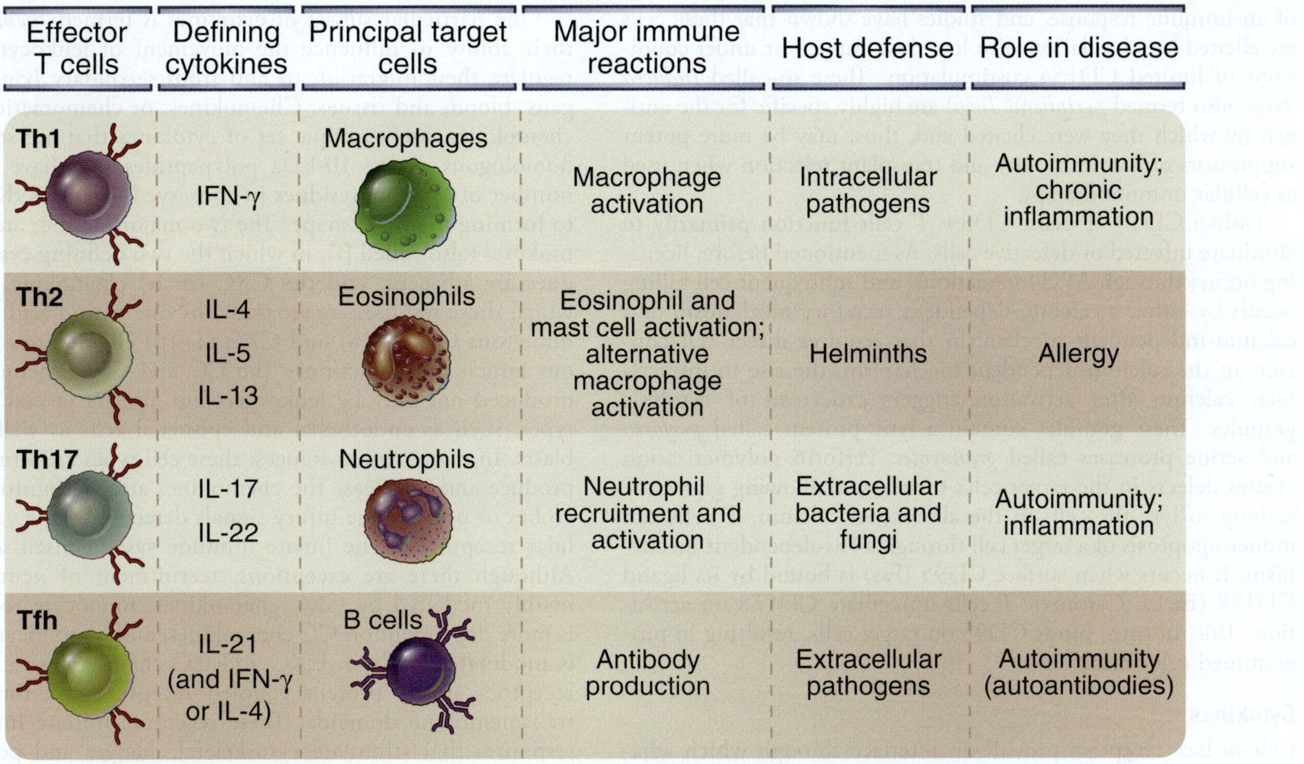

Effector T cells	Defining cytokines	Principal target cells	Major immune reactions	Host defense	Role in disease
Th1	IFN-γ	Macrophages	Macrophage activation	Intracellular pathogens	Autoimmunity; chronic inflammation
Th2	IL-4 IL-5 IL-13	Eosinophils	Eosinophil and mast cell activation; alternative macrophage activation	Helminths	Allergy
Th17	IL-17 IL-22	Neutrophils	Neutrophil recruitment and activation	Extracellular bacteria and fungi	Autoimmunity; inflammation
Tfh	IL-21 (and IFN-γ or IL-4)	B cells	Antibody production	Extracellular pathogens	Autoimmunity (autoantibodies)

FIGURE 49.14 T-cell subsets. Naïve CD4+ T cells may differentiate into distinct subsets of effector cells in response to antigen, costimulatory, or coinhibitory signals and cytokines. Th1 cells produce interferon-γ (IFN-γ), which activates macrophages to kill intracellular microbes. Th2 cells produce cytokines (interleukin [IL]-4, IL-5, and others) that stimulate immunoglobulin E production and activate eosinophils in response to parasitic infection. Th17 cells secrete IL-17 and IL-22; they play an important role in responses to fungi and contribute to several autoimmune inflammatory diseases. Tfh cells produce IL-21 and provide help to B cells for antibody production. (Adapted from Abbas AK, Lichtman AH, Pillai S. *Cellular and Molecular Immunology*. 10th ed. Philadelphia: Saunders Elsevier; 2021.)

Th17 cells are an inflammatory CD4+ subset that plays a major role in the protective immune response against fungal pathogens and extracellular bacteria. Th17 cells are generated in the presence of transforming growth factor-β (TGF-β) and IL-6 and are potent secretors of the inflammatory cytokines IL-17 and IL-23. Interestingly, in addition to their role in protective immunity, Th17 cells have been associated with several autoimmune diseases, including multiple sclerosis, rheumatoid arthritis, and psoriasis, and several immunomodulatory therapies are being developed to impair their activity in these patients. Finally, Tfh cells are ICOS+ PD-1+ cells that home to lymphoid germinal centers by virtue of their expression of the chemokine receptor CXCR5, where they provide help for the generation of class-switched, high-affinity IgG responses. Tfh cells provide this help in the form of CD154 expression and the secretion of IL-21.

An important feature of these CD4+ Th cells is the ability of one subset to regulate the activity of the other. For example, IL-10 produced by Th2 cells and Tregs negatively regulates transcription of IFN-γ mRNA. Thus, the initial steps in differentiation depend greatly on the surrounding immunologic milieu, which ultimately influences the character of the immune response. This unique cytokine environment that shapes developing immune responses constitutes "signal 3" of the three-signal hypothesis of T-cell activation. Furthermore, more recent fate mapping studies have revealed a high degree of plasticity between Th subsets, demonstrating that cells of one Th subset can, under certain conditions, transdifferentiate into another Th subset.

Another subset of CD4+ T cells that has been described to play a critical role in the ability of the immune system to temper its response is the Treg population. Tregs suppress immune responses either through direct cell-cell contact with effector cells or indirectly through their interaction with APCs. These cells not only have the ability to suppress cytokines, adhesion molecules, and costimulatory signals but are also able to focus this response by expression of integrins, which allows Tregs to home to the location of immune engagement. The most extensively studied population of Tregs are those CD4+ T cells that express the transcription factor FoxP3, the majority of which also express CD25 (the high-affinity α chain of the IL-2 receptor).[19] CD4+/CD25+/Foxp3+ Tregs play a critical role in maintaining peripheral self-tolerance and in preventing pathologic inflammation; indeed, both mice and humans that lack a functional Foxp3 molecule develop severe systemic autoimmunity. Thus, CD4+/CD25+/Foxp3+ T cells have been the target of numerous attempts to alter immune function and are being tested in clinical trials of cellular immunotherapy to control graft rejection after transplantation and to mitigate autoimmunity. Foxp3+ Tregs develop during T-cell thymic development after recognition of self-antigen in the thymus (with signal strength that is not sufficient to induce negative selection). These so-called *natural Tregs* (also termed *thymic Tregs*) express a TCR repertoire distinct from that of conventional T cells and are important for maintaining immune homeostasis and preventing autoimmunity. However, Foxp3+ Tregs can also develop extrathymically during the course of an immune response, and studies have shown that these cells are elicited by stimulation with low-dose antigen or under conditions of limited CD154 costimulation. These so-called *induced Tregs* (also termed *peripheral Tregs*) are highly specific for the antigen by which they were elicited and, thus, may be more potent suppressors of autoimmunity and transplant rejection when used as cellular immunotherapy.

Unlike CD4+ T cells, CD8+ T cells function primarily to eliminate infected or defective cells. As mentioned before, licensing occurs through APC interactions, and subsequent cell killing occurs by either a calcium-dependent secretory mechanism or a calcium-independent mechanism that requires direct cell contact. In the calcium-dependent mechanism, the rise in intracellular calcium after activation triggers exocytosis of cytolytic granules. These granules contain a lytic protein called *perforin* and serine proteases called *granzymes*. Perforin polymerization creates defects in the target cell's membrane, allowing granzyme activity to lyse the cell. In the absence of calcium, T cells can induce apoptosis of a target cell through a Fas-dependent mechanism. It occurs when surface CD95 (Fas) is bound by its ligand CD178 (FasL). Cytotoxic T cells upregulate CD178 on activation. This, in turn, binds CD95 on target cells, resulting in programmed cell death.

Cytokines

Cell surface receptors provide an interface through which adjacent cells can transfer signals vital to the immune response. Whereas this cell-to-cell contact is a critical component of cellular communication, soluble mediators are also used extensively to accomplish similar tasks. These polypeptides, termed *cytokines,* are critical to the development and function of both the innate and acquired immune processes. The action of cytokines, also known as *interleukins* (see Table 49.1), may be autocrine (on the same cell) or paracrine (on adjacent cells), but is usually not endocrine. They are released by multiple cell types and may function to activate, suppress, or even amplify the response of adjacent cells. The prototypical cytokine of T-cell activation is IL-2. Once a given T cell encounters its specific antigen in the setting of appropriate costimulation, it will subsequently produce and release IL-2 as well as other cytokines that will influence any cell within its vicinity. As mentioned before, Th cellular subsets are differentiated on the basis of the pattern of cytokine expression. Th1 cells, which mediate cytotoxic responses such as delayed-type hypersensitivity, express IL-2, IL-12, IL-15, and IFN-γ. Th2 cells support the development of humoral or eosinophilic responses and consequently express IL-4, IL-5, IL-10, and IL-13. Th17 cells, a more recently described subset, are distinguished by their production of IL-17, IL-21, and IL-22.

Cytokine receptors are now known to function through Janus kinase (JAK) signal transduction proteins. They convey signals to signal transducers and activators of transcriptions (STATs), DNA-binding proteins that translocate to the nucleus to influence gene transcription. As is the case with most of the immune response, this pathway is tightly regulated. For example, suppressors of cytokine signaling proteins act in a negative feedback loop to inhibit STAT phosphorylation by binding and inhibiting JAKs or competing with STATs for phosphotyrosine-binding sites on cytokine receptors. Evidence is emerging for the involvement of suppressors of cytokine signaling proteins in human disease, which raises the possibility that therapeutic strategies based on the manipulation of suppressors of cytokine signaling activity might be of clinical benefit.

One particular subset of cytokines is termed *chemokines* for their ability to influence the movement of leukocytes and to regulate their migration to and from secondary lymphoid organs, blood, and tissues. Chemokines, or chemotactic cytokine chemokines, are a unique set of cytokines that are structurally homologous, 8- to 10-kDa polypeptides that have a varying number of cysteine residues in conserved locations that are key to forming their 3D shape. The two major families are CC chemokines (also called β), in which the two defining cysteine residues are adjacent, and the CXC (or α) chemokine family, in which these residues are separated by one amino acid. There are numerous CC (1–28) and CXC (1–16) chemokines with various targets and functions. The CC and CXC chemokines are produced not only by leukocytes but also by several other cell types, such as endothelial and epithelial cells as well as fibroblasts. In many circumstances, these cell types are stimulated to produce and to release the chemokines after recognition of microbes or other tissue injury signals detected by the various cellular receptors of the innate immune system discussed earlier. Although there are exceptions, recruitment of neutrophils is mainly mediated by CXC chemokines, monocyte recruitment is more dependent on CC chemokines, and lymphocyte homing is modulated by both CXC and CC chemokines. Chemokine receptors are G protein–coupled receptors containing seven transmembrane domains. These receptors initiate intracellular responses that stimulate cytoskeletal changes and polymerization of actin and myosin filaments, resulting in increased cell motility. These signals may also change the conformation of cell surface integrins, increasing their affinity for their ligands, thus affecting migration, rolling, and diapedesis. Thus, chemokines work in concert with adhesion molecules, such as integrins and selectins, and their ligands to regulate the migration of leukocytes into tissues. Distinct combinations of chemokine receptors are expressed on various types of leukocytes, resulting in the differential patterns of migrations of those leukocytes. In addition to cytokines, a host of other soluble, small-molecule mediators are released during an immune response or with other types of inflammation. These function to increase blood flow to the area and to improve the exposure of the area to lymphocytes and the innate immune system.

B Cells and Antibody Production

The primary lymphoid organ responsible for B-cell differentiation is the bone marrow. Similar to all other cells in the immune system, B cells are derived from pluripotent bone marrow stem cells. IL-7, produced by bone marrow stromal cells, is a growth factor for pre-B cells. IL-4, IL-5, and IL-6 are cytokines that stimulate the maturation and proliferation of mature primed B cells. The principal function of B cells is to produce antibodies against foreign antigens (i.e., the humoral immune response) as well as to be involved in antigen presentation. B-cell development occurs through several stages, each stage representing a change in the genomic content at the antibody loci. During the differentiation process, a similar process of V(D)J recombination as described for TCR diversity occurs, resulting in a nearly unlimited array of antibody specificities (see Fig. 49.10).

Similar to the T cell and its receptor, each B cell has a unique membrane-bound receptor through which it recognizes specific antigen. In the case of the B cell, this Ig molecule may also be produced in a secreted form that can interact with the extracellular environment far from its cellular origin. Each mature B cell produces antibody of a single specificity.

Each antibody is composed of two heavy chains and two light chains. Five different heavy chain loci (μ, γ, α, ε, and δ) are found on chromosome 14, and two light chain loci (κ and λ) are located on chromosome 2. Ig has a basic structure of four chains, two of which are identical heavy chains and two of which are identical light chains (Fig. 49.15). Both heavy and light chains have a constant region as well as a variable antigen-binding region. The antigen-binding site is composed of both the heavy and light chain variable regions. The ability of antibody to neutralize microbes is entirely a function of this antigen-binding region.

In humans, there are nine different Ig subclasses or isotypes: IgM, IgD, IgG1, IgG2, IgG3, IgG4, IgA1, IgA2, and IgE. Heavy chain use defines the subtype of any given antibody. Whereas the variable regions are involved in antigen binding, the constant regions have functionality as well. The fragment crystallizable region, or Fc region, is in the tail portion composed of the two heavy chain constant regions. It interacts with Fc receptors on phagocytic cells of the innate immune system to facilitate opsonization and subsequent destruction of the antigen to which the antibody is bound as well as facilitating antigenic peptide

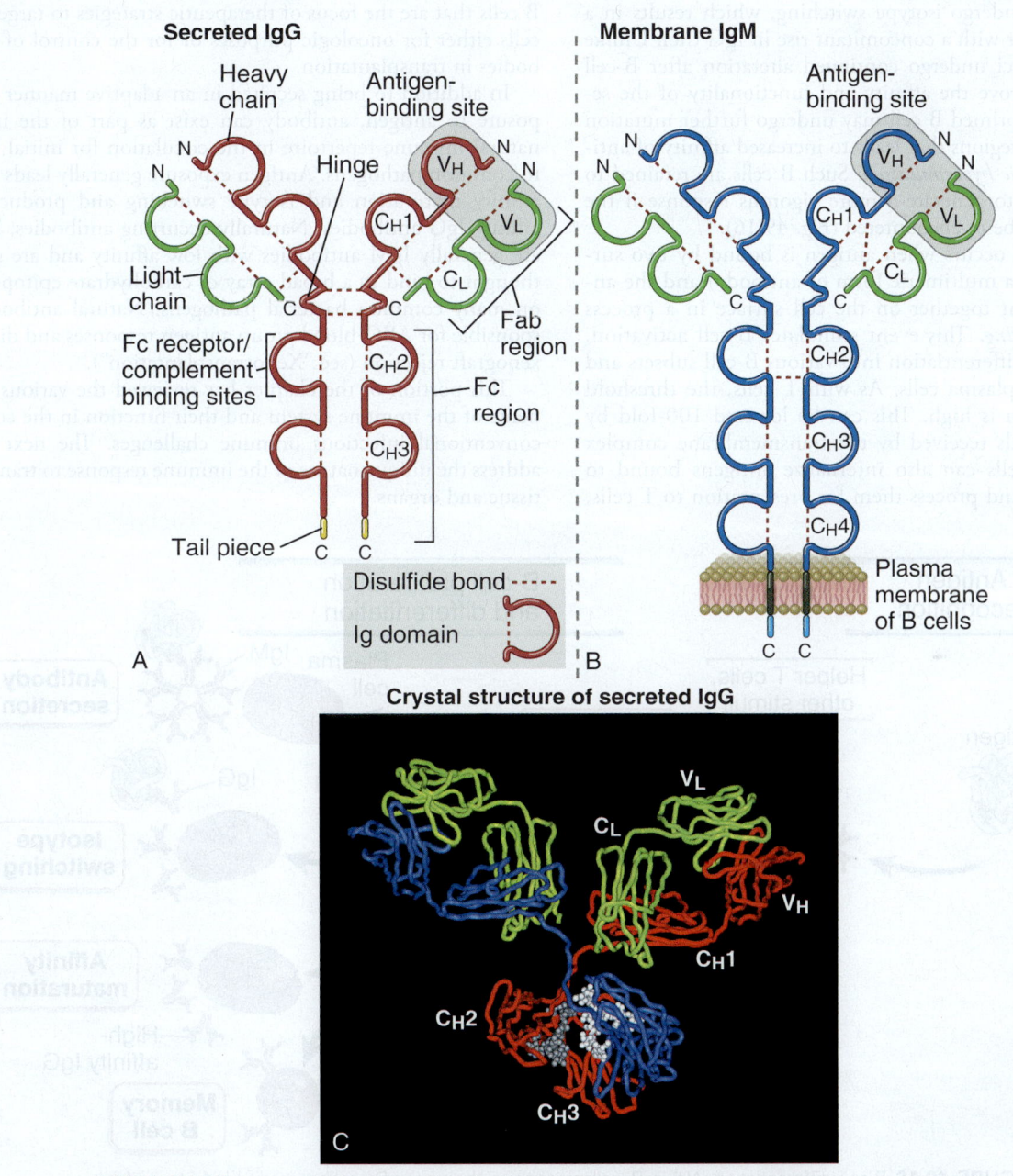

FIGURE 49.15 Structure of immunoglobulin (Ig). (A) Representation of secreted immunoglobulin G (IgG) molecule. The antigen-binding regions are formed by the variable regions of both light (V_L) and heavy (V_H) chains. The constant region of the heavy chain (C_H) is responsible for the Fc receptor and complement-binding sites. (B) Schematic diagram of membrane-bound immunoglobulin G (IgM). The membrane form of the antibody has C-terminal transmembrane and cytoplasmic portions that anchor the molecule in the plasma membrane. (C) X-ray crystallography representation of IgG molecule. Heavy chains are colored *blue* and *red*, light chains are colored *green*, and carbohydrates are shown in *gray*. (Adapted from Abbas AK, Lichtman AH, Pillai S. *Cellular and Molecular Immunology.* 10th ed. Philadelphia: Saunders Elsevier; 2021.)

processing. The Fc portion of IgM and some classes of IgG also serve to activate complement. Distinct immune effector functions are assigned to each isotype. IgM and IgG antibodies provide a pivotal role in the endogenous or intravascular immune response. IgA is primarily responsible for mucosal immunity and is largely confined to the gastrointestinal and respiratory tracts. Resting B cells that have not yet been exposed to antigen express IgD and IgM on their cell surface. After interaction with antigen, the first isotype produced is IgM, which is efficient at binding complement to facilitate phagocytosis or cell lysis. Further activation and differentiation of the B cell occur after interactions with CD4+ Tfh cells. B cells undergo isotype switching, which results in a decrease in IgM titer with a concomitant rise in IgG titer. Unlike the TCR, the Ig loci undergo continued alteration after B-cell stimulation to improve the affinity and functionality of the secreted antibody. A primed B cell may undergo further mutation within the variable regions that leads to increased affinity of antibody, termed *somatic hypermutation*. Such B cells are retained to provide the ability to generate a more vigorous response if the antigen happens to be re-encountered (Fig. 49.16).

B-cell activation occurs when antigen is bound by two surface antibodies (or a multimeric form of antibody) and the antibodies are brought together on the cell surface in a process known as *cross-linking*. This event stimulates B-cell activation, proliferation, and differentiation into various B-cell subsets and antibody-secreting plasma cells. As with T cells, the threshold for B-cell activation is high. This can be lowered 100-fold by costimulatory signals received by the transmembrane complex CD19-CD21. B cells can also internalize antigens bound to surface antibodies and process them for presentation to T cells,

thus participating in antigen presentation. As discussed earlier, B cells may provide and receive certain costimulatory signals. For example, B cells express CD40, and when bound by CD154 expressed on activated T cells, the result is upregulation of B7 molecules on the B cell and delivery of important costimulatory signals to T cells as well.

Plasma cells reside in the bone marrow and are distinguished histologically by their hypertrophied Golgi apparatus resulting from their high degree of protein synthesis. They secrete large amounts of monoclonal (single specificity) antibody and exhibit phenotypic and functional characteristics distinct from other B cells that are the focus of therapeutic strategies to target plasma cells either for oncologic purposes or for the control of alloantibodies in transplantation.

In addition to being secreted in an adaptive manner after exposure to antigen, antibody can exist as part of the innate or natural immune repertoire in the circulation for initial response to common pathogens. Antigen exposure generally leads to B-cell affinity maturation and isotype switching and produces high-affinity IgG antibodies. Naturally occurring antibodies, however, are generally IgM antibodies with low affinity and are generally thought to bind to a broad array of carbohydrate epitopes found on many common bacterial pathogens. Natural antibody is responsible for ABO blood group antigen responses and discordant xenograft rejection (see "Xenotransplantation").

This portion of the chapter has reviewed the various components of the immune system and their function in the context of conventional infectious immune challenges. The next sections address the unique nature of the immune response to transplanted tissue and organs.

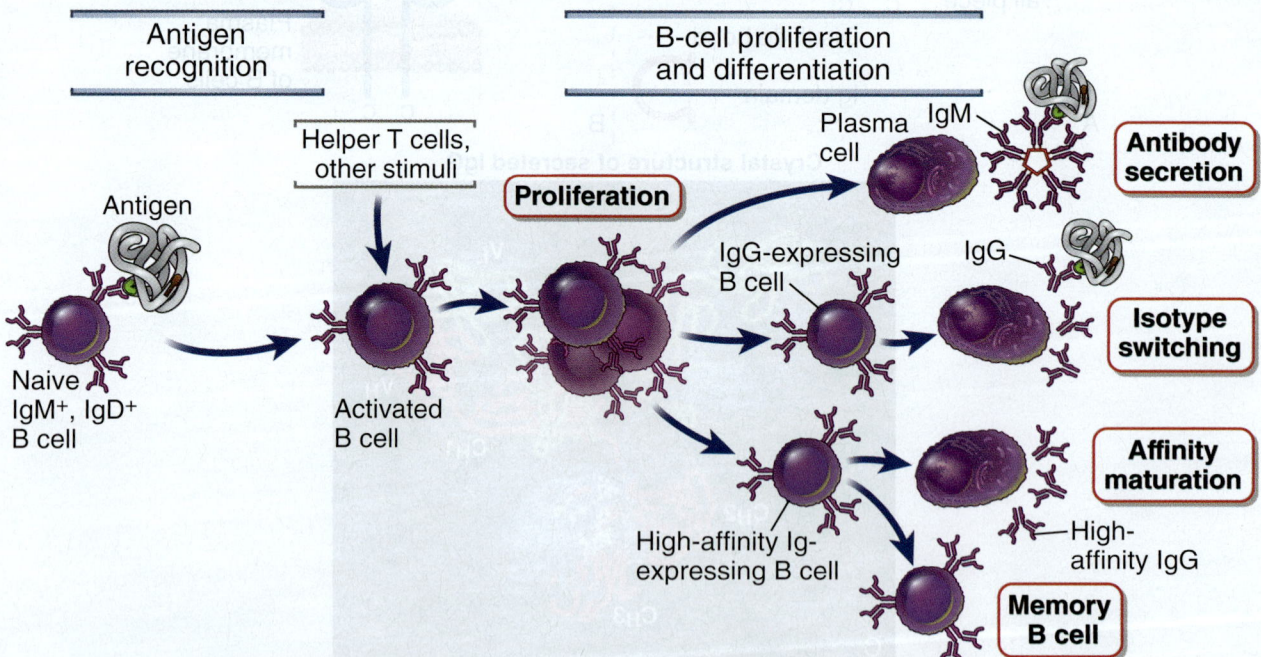

FIGURE 49.16 B-cell differentiation. Naïve B cells recognize their specific antigen as it binds to surface-bound antibody. Under the influence of helper T cells, costimulatory signals, and other stimuli, B cells become activated and clonally expand, producing many B cells of the same specificity. They also differentiate into antibody-secreting cells, plasma cells. Some of the activated B cells undergo heavy chain class switching and affinity maturation. Ultimately, a small subset become long-lived memory cells, primed for future responses. *Ig*, Immunoglobulin; *IgD*, immunoglobulin D; *IgG*, immunoglobulin G; *IgM*, immunoglobulin M. (Adapted from Abbas AK, Lichtman AH, Pillai S. *Cellular and Molecular Immunology*. 10th ed. Philadelphia: Saunders Elsevier; 2021.)

TRANSPLANT IMMUNITY

The study of modern transplant immunology is traditionally attributed to the experiments of Sir Peter Medawar, fueled by attempts to use skin transplantation as a treatment for burned aviators during World War II. While monitoring the victims with autologous (syngeneic) and homologous (allogeneic) skin grafts, he noted that not only did all allogeneic grafts universally fail promptly but also secondary grafts from the same donor were rejected even more vigorously, suggesting immune involvement. He pursued this hypothesis with extensive experiments in rabbits, wherein he confirmed his previous observation and noted the presence of a heavy lymphocyte infiltrate in the rejecting graft. It was N.A. Mitchison, working in the early 1950s, who definitively identified a role for lymphocytes in the rejection of foreign tissue. Subsequent studies in tumor immunology as well as work by Snell using strains of genetically identical mice identified the genetic basis for graft rejection as the MHC, known in humans as HLA and in mice as the H-2 locus. These series of experiments during a short period of several years demonstrated that rejection of transplanted tissue was an immunologic process, implicated lymphocytes as the principal effector cells, and identified the MHC as the primary source of antigen in the rejection response. These pivotal studies laid the groundwork for the transition of transplantation from the experimental to the clinical realm.

Whereas the technical skill for the transplantation of skin and other organs had been available for some time, the vigorous rejection of allografts had prevented its widespread use for many years. It was not until 1954, after Medawar's critical studies had been published, that the first successful organ transplantation was performed. Despite Medawar's claim that the "biologic force" responsible for rejection would "forever inhibit transplantation from one individual to another," Joseph Murray, a surgeon-scientist, persevered in his pursuit of making clinical transplantation a reality. At the time, there was evidence to suggest that the overall immunologic barrier was lacking between identical twins, and coincidentally, Murray was busily perfecting a surgical technique for kidney transplantation in dogs. In 1954, the opportunity presented itself to test the hypothesis. Richard Herrick, who had end-stage renal disease, was the first candidate, and his identical sibling, Ronald, was willing to donate a kidney for transplantation to his brother. Murray confirmed the lack of immunologic reactivity between the two brothers by first placing skin grafts from each twin onto the other. Once he confirmed the lack of a response, he used the technique that he had perfected in the canine model, performing the first successful kidney transplant between identical twins in December 1954.[2] The operation proceeded without complication, and the kidney functioned well without the need for immunosuppression. Despite this landmark advance in transplantation, the majority of individuals in need of a transplant did not have an identical twin to donate an organ. Thereafter, the focus of the field was appropriately directed toward the development of methods to control the rejection response.

During the 1950s and 1960s, several discoveries were made that were of the utmost importance for future successes in transplantation. After Gorer and Snell's description of the murine MHC system, Jean Dausset described the equivalent in humans using antibodies developed against HLA. This led to the first serologically based typing system for human transplant antigens. Snell and Dausset shared the Nobel Prize in 1980 for their observations.

In the late 1960s, Paul Terasaki reported on the significance of preformed antibody directed against donor MHC molecules and its impact on kidney graft survival.[20] He developed the microlymphocyte cytotoxicity test, allowing pretransplantation detection of recipient-derived antidonor antibody. This formed the basis for the physical crossmatch assay that is used today to screen potential donor-recipient pairings. These techniques, along with the development of new immunosuppressive compounds, including 6-mercaptopurine and azathioprine, led to the first successful kidney transplantation between relatives who were not identical twins and also to the first successful transplant using a kidney from a deceased donor.

Although early attempts at immunosuppression permitted extended allograft survival in selected patients, both the reproducibility and durability of results were far from adequate. In the 1970s, investigators sought novel treatments to improve the success rate for transplantation; these modalities included thoracic duct drainage and the use of antilymphocyte serum. Despite these efforts, the results for kidney transplantation remained poor, with the best centers achieving 1-year survival rates of 70% for living related kidney grafts and 50% for deceased donor kidney transplants. Then a chance discovery of a promising agent from a fungal isolate dramatically changed the outlook for kidney and other types of transplantation. Jean-François Borel identified an active metabolite, cyclosporine A (CsA), that showed selective in vitro inhibition of lymphocyte cultures but no significant myelotoxic effects. Promising results in dogs eventually led to clinical trials in humans, and the modern era of transplantation had begun.

The introduction of CsA ushered in the most dramatic improvement in the field of transplantation (Fig. 49.17). Liver and heart transplant survival rates doubled, and the improved immunosuppression encouraged transplant teams around the world to begin broader investigational use, transplanting lung, small bowel, and pancreas. Now, with the use of CsA and newer agents such as tacrolimus, 1-year graft survival has exceeded 90% for virtually all organs

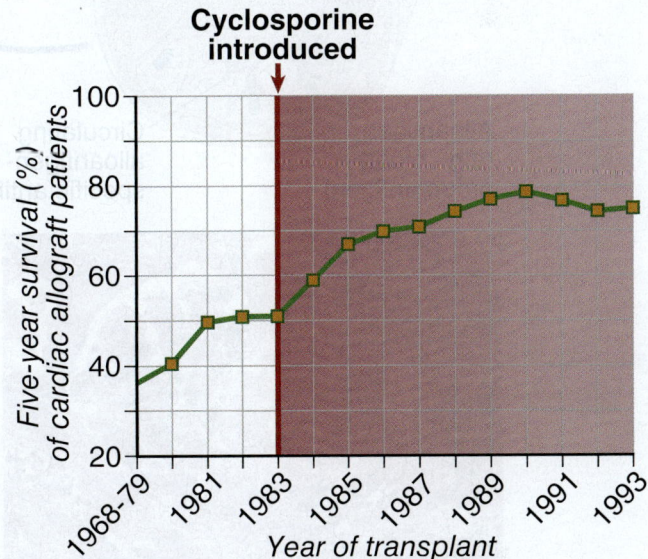

FIGURE 49.17 Influence of cyclosporine on transplant survival. Five-year survival rates for cardiac transplant recipients significantly increased with the introduction of cyclosporine in 1983. (Adapted from Abbas AK, Lichtman AH, Pillai S. *Cellular and Molecular Immunology.* 10th ed. Philadelphia: Saunders Elsevier; 2021.)

except the small intestine. Despite the discovery and clinical introduction of ever increasingly potent immunosuppressants, the field of transplantation has many areas in need of improvement. Drug-related side effects and the intractable problem of chronic rejection still plague practitioners. One area of focus of current research is the development of a clinically applicable strategy to promote "transplantation tolerance," thereby eliminating the pitfalls and shortcomings of current immunosuppressive therapy.

Rejection

There are three classic histopathologic definitions of allograft rejection that are based on not only the predominant mediator but also the timing of the process.

1. Hyperacute rejection occurs within minutes to days after transplantation and is primarily mediated by preformed donor-specific antibody (DSA) in the recipient.
2. Acute rejection is a process mediated most commonly by T cells but is often accompanied by an acquired antibody response and generally occurs within the first few weeks to months of transplantation (but can occur at any time).
3. Chronic rejection is a common contributing cause of long-term allograft loss and is an indolent fibrotic process that occurs over months to years. It is thought to be secondary to chronic immunologic injury from both T- and B-cell–mediated processes (including antidonor antibodies) but is difficult to completely separate from nonimmune mechanisms of chronic organ damage (e.g., drug toxicity and cardiovascular comorbid diseases).

Hyperacute Rejection

Although essentially untreatable, hyperacute rejection is nearly universally avoidable with the proper use of the lymphocytotoxic crossmatch or other means of detecting antidonor antibodies before transplantation. This form of rejection occurs when preformed antibodies against the donor, commonly referred to as *donor-specific antibodies,* are present in the recipient's system before transplantation (Fig. 49.18). These antibodies may be the result of "natural processes," such as the formation of antibody to blood group antigens, or the product of prior exposure to antigens with similar enough specificities as those expressed by the donor that cross-reactivity can occur. In the latter, sensitization is usually the result of prior transplantation, transfusion, or pregnancy but may also result from prior environmental antigen exposure. As expected, hyperacute rejection can occur within the first minutes to hours after graft reperfusion. Antibodies bind to the donor tissue or endothelium and initiate complement-mediated lysis and endothelial cell activation, resulting in a procoagulant state and immediate graft thrombosis. On histologic evaluation, there may be platelet and fibrin thrombi, early neutrophil infiltration, and positive staining for the complement product C4d on the endothelial lining of small blood vessels. Thankfully, this type of rejection is avoidable with pretransplantation testing by current crossmatch assays.

A physical crossmatch test is often employed to minimize the risk of hyperacute rejection. Similar to the lymphocytotoxicity assay described previously that is used for MHC class I typing, the physical crossmatch is performed by mixing cells from the donor

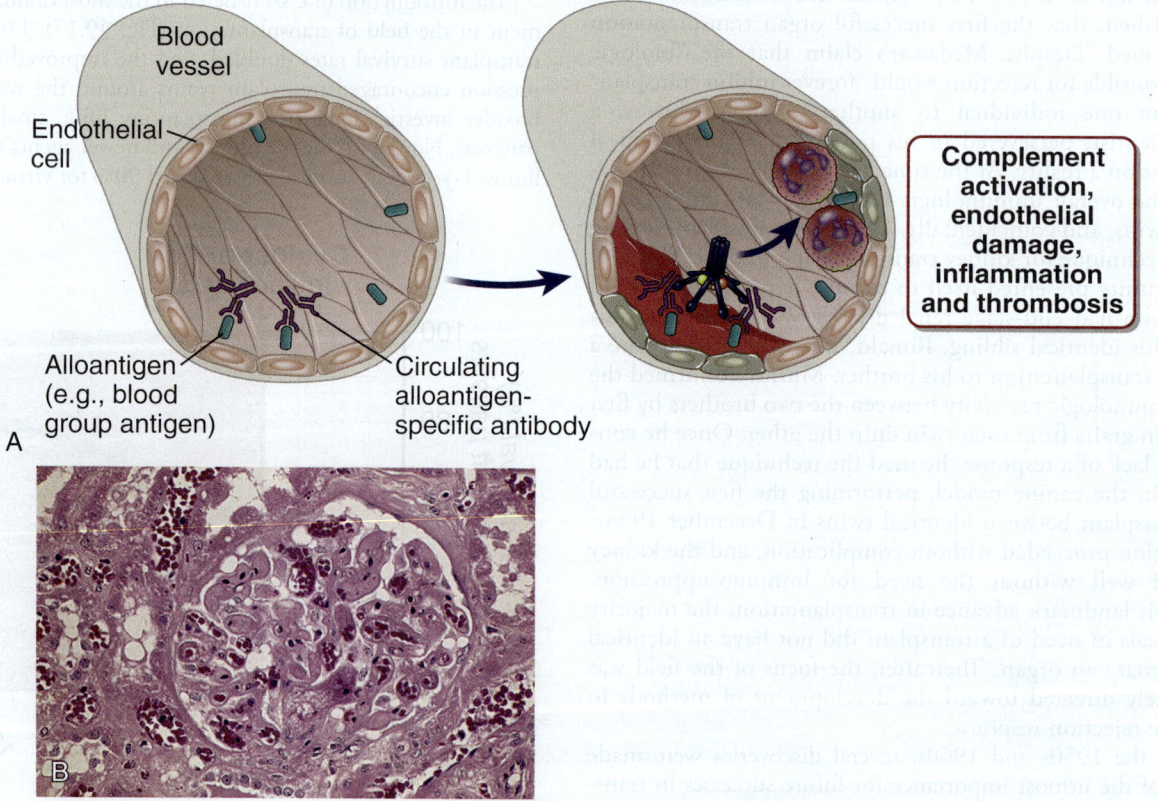

FIGURE 49.18 Hyperacute rejection. (A) In hyperacute rejection, preformed antibodies reactive with vascular endothelium activate complement and trigger rapid intravascular thrombosis and necrosis of the vessel wall. (B) Hyperacute rejection involving a glomerulus in a kidney allograft. Typical features include endothelial damage, thrombi, and leukocytic infiltration. (Adapted from Abbas AK, Lichtman AH, Pillai S. *Cellular and Molecular Immunology.* 10th ed. Philadelphia: Saunders Elsevier; 2021.)

with serum from the recipient and the addition of complement if needed. Lysis of the donor cells indicates that antibodies directed against the donor are present in the recipient's serum; this is called a *positive crossmatch*. Thus, a negative crossmatch assay coupled with proper ABO matching will effectively prevent hyperacute rejection in 99.5% of transplants. Newer crossmatch techniques have become increasingly sophisticated, including those directed at both class I and class II antibodies, flow cytometric techniques, and bead-based screening assays to exclude non-HLA antibodies. As a given patient's sensitivity status may change over time, a more common technique for screening a patient's sensitization status is to screen a potential recipient's serum against a panel of random donor cells representing the anticipated regional donor pool. Known as the *panel reactive antibody (PRA) assay*, the results are expressed as a percentage of the panel within the randomly selected cell set that lyses when recipient serum is added. Thus, a nonsensitized patient would be given a score of 0%, and a highly sensitized patient might have a PRA score up to 100%. These screens can now be performed without the need for cells by using polystyrene beads coated with HLA antigens (Fig. 49.19). In this situation, the laboratory detects all anti-HLA antibodies and determines a calculated PRA (cPRA) score on the basis of the expected frequency of the HLA types in the donor pool. In the event a compatible donor is not available for a highly sensitized recipient, clinical protocols exist to attempt desensitization that uses plasmapheresis or intravenous immunoglobulin (IVIG) to reduce circulating antibody and prevent hyperacute rejection.[21] However, the need for desensitization is decreasing with advancements in deceased donor allocation algorithms and living donor paired donor exchange programs aimed at avoiding crossmatch-positive donor-recipient pairs.

Acute Rejection

Of the three types of rejection, only acute rejection can be successfully reversed once it is established. T cells constitute the core element responsible for acute rejection, often termed *T-cell–mediated rejection*. There is also a form of acute rejection that is particularly aggressive and involves vascular invasion by T cells known as *acute vascular rejection*. Finally, a more recently recognized form of acute rejection mediated by the humoral immune system, known as *antibody-mediated rejection (AMR)*, is discussed briefly later. With the advent of increasingly effective immunosuppression, allograft loss from acute cellular rejection has become increasingly rare. Acute rejection can occur at any time after the first few postoperative days—the time needed to mount an acquired immune response; it most commonly occurs within the first 6 months after transplantation. Without adequate immunosuppression, the cellular response will progress during the course of days to a few weeks, ultimately destroying the allograft. As described earlier, there are two main pathways through which rejection can proceed: the direct and indirect alloresponses (Fig. 49.20). In either case, alloreactive T cells encounter their specific antigen (either processed donor MHC peptides indirectly presented on self MHC or directly recognized donor MHC), undergo activation, and promote similar rejection responses. The precursor frequency

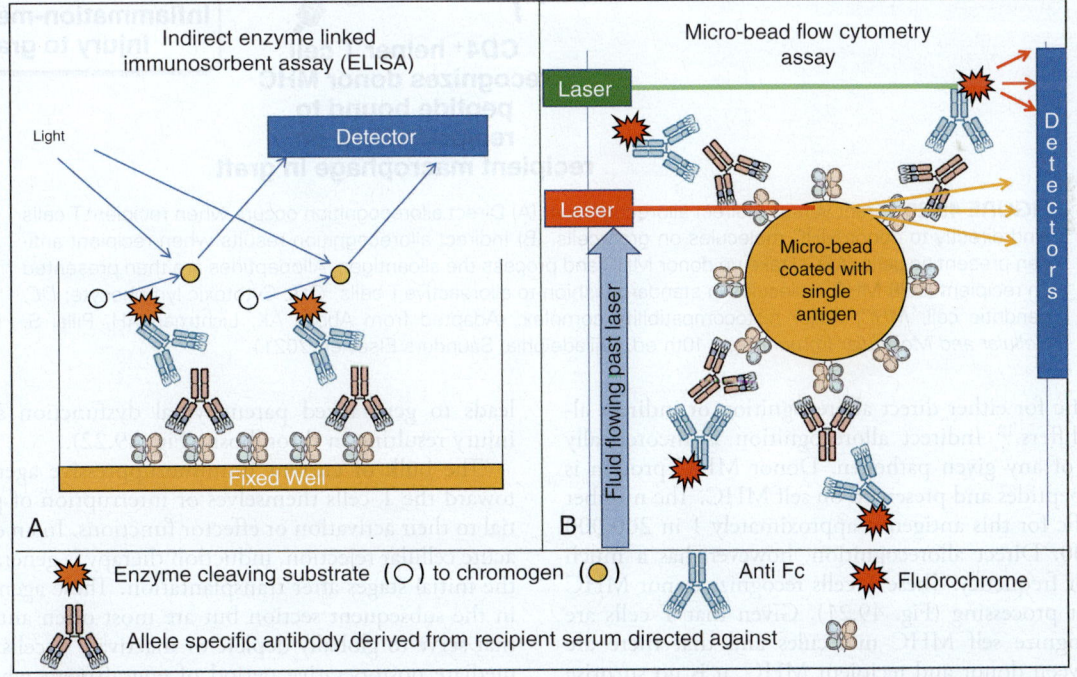

FIGURE 49.19 Solid-phase assays for detection of anti-HLA antibodies. (A) An indirect enzyme-linked immunosorbent assay *(ELISA)*. HLA molecules are immobilized in a well, test serum is added, and the plate is washed to remove all non–HLA-specific antibody. A reporter enzyme-tagged anti-immunoglobulin is added. After washing, a substrate is added that can be cleaved by the reporter enzyme to yield a chromogen detectable by a plate reader. (B) A microbead flow cytometry assay. Polystyrene microspheres embedded with fluorochromes for detection are coated in purified HLA molecules. Test serum is added to the beads and a secondary antibody labelled with a fluorophore is then added. The beads are then passed through a flow cytometer in which both bead identification and the presence of bound secondary antibody are detected. (Adapted from Sypek M, Kausman J, Holt S, et al. HLA epitope matching in kidney transplantation: an overview for the general nephrologist. *Am J Kidney Dis*. 2018;71[5]:720-731.)

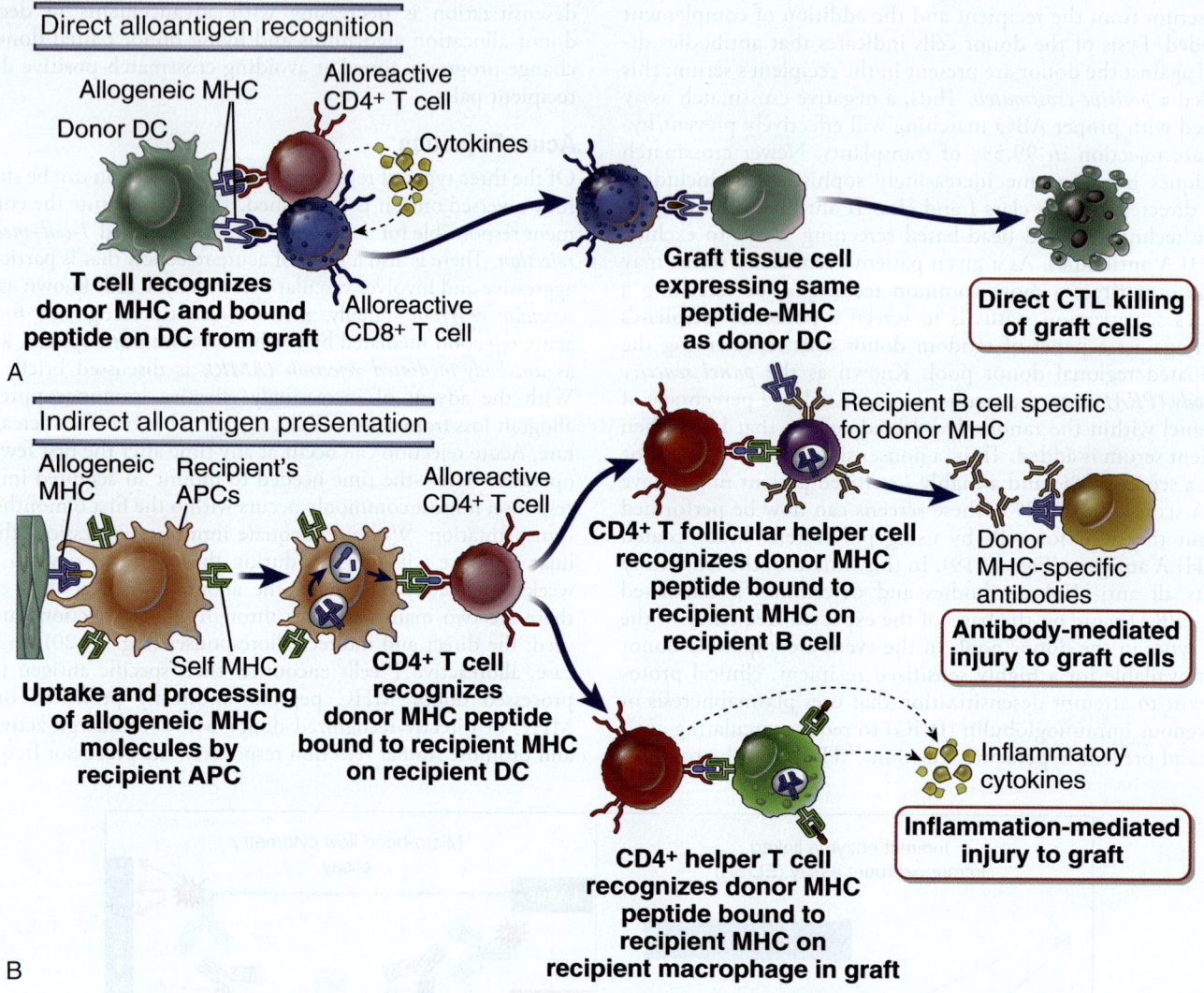

Direct alloantigen recognition

Donor DC
Allogeneic MHC
Alloreactive CD4+ T cell
Cytokines

T cell recognizes donor MHC and bound peptide on DC from graft

Alloreactive CD8+ T cell

A

Graft tissue cell expressing same peptide-MHC as donor DC

Direct CTL killing of graft cells

Indirect alloantigen presentation

Allogeneic MHC
Recipient's APCs
Alloreactive CD4+ T cell
Recipient B cell specific for donor MHC

Self MHC

Uptake and processing of allogeneic MHC molecules by recipient APC

CD4+ T cell recognizes donor MHC peptide bound to recipient MHC on recipient DC

CD4+ T follicular helper cell recognizes donor MHC peptide bound to recipient MHC on recipient B cell

Donor MHC-specific antibodies

Antibody-mediated injury to graft cells

Inflammatory cytokines

Inflammation-mediated injury to graft

CD4+ helper T cell recognizes donor MHC peptide bound to recipient MHC on recipient macrophage in graft

B

FIGURE 49.20 Direct versus indirect allorecognition. (A) Direct allorecognition occurs when recipient T cells bind directly to donor MHC molecules on graft cells. (B) Indirect allorecognition results when recipient antigen-presenting cells *(APCs)* take up donor MHC and process the alloantigen. Allopeptides are then presented on recipient (self) MHC molecules in standard fashion to alloreactive T cells. *CTL,* Cytotoxic lymphocyte; *DC,* dendritic cell; *MHC,* major histocompatibility complex. (Adapted from Abbas AK, Lichtman AH, Pillai S. *Cellular and Molecular Immunology.* 10th ed. Philadelphia: Saunders Elsevier; 2021.)

of T cells specific for either direct allorecognition or indirect allorecognition differs.[12] Indirect allorecognition is theoretically similar to that of any given pathogen. Donor MHC protein is processed into peptides and presented on self MHC. The number of T cells specific for this antigen is approximately 1 in 200,000 to 1 in 500,000. Direct allorecognition, however, has a much higher precursor frequency. These T cells recognize donor MHC directly without processing (Fig. 49.21). Given that T cells are selected to recognize self MHC molecules and that there are similarities between donor and recipient MHC, it is no surprise that a substantial number of T cells are alloreactive. Some estimates suggest that somewhere between 1% and 10% of all T cells are directly alloreactive.[12] This high precursor frequency likely overwhelms many of the regulatory processes in place to control the much lower cell frequencies involved in physiologic immune responses. These alloreactive T cells, once activated, move to attack the graft. Subsequently, there is massive infiltration of T cells and monocytes into the allograft, resulting in organ injury through direct cytolysis and a general inflammatory milieu that

leads to generalized parenchymal dysfunction and endothelial injury resulting in thrombosis (Fig. 49.22).

The bulk of current immunosuppressive agents are directed toward the T cells themselves or interruption of pathways essential to their activation or effector functions. In an effort to prevent acute cellular rejection, induction therapy is generally used during the initial stages after transplantation. These agents are discussed in the subsequent section but are most often antibody therapies that serve to globally deplete or inactivate T cells during the immediate postoperative period of engraftment when ischemia-reperfusion injury is most likely to promote immune recognition. Immunosuppressive regimens are frequently designed to favor more intensive initial immunosuppression in the immediate postoperative period and are then tapered to lower, less toxic levels over time.

T-cell–specific treatments lead to the prevention of acute rejection in approximately 70% of transplants, and when it does occur, it can be reversed in most cases. Similar to hyperacute rejection resulting from preformed antibody responses, T-cell presensitization

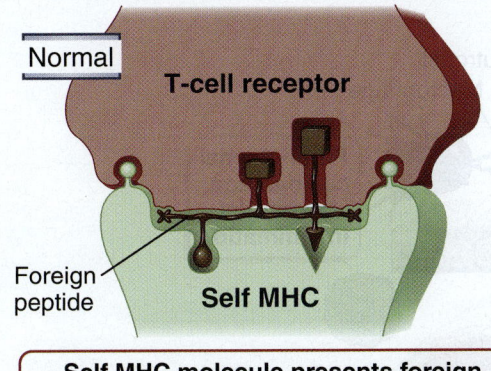

Normal

Self MHC molecule presents foreign peptide to T cell selected to recognize self MHC weakly, but may recognize self MHC–foreign peptide complexes well

A

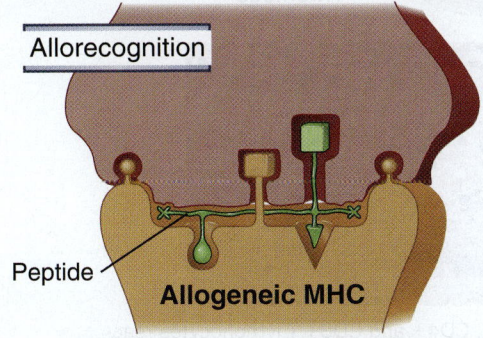

Allorecognition

The self MHC–restricted T cell recognizes a structure formed by both the allogeneic MHC molecule and the bound peptide

B

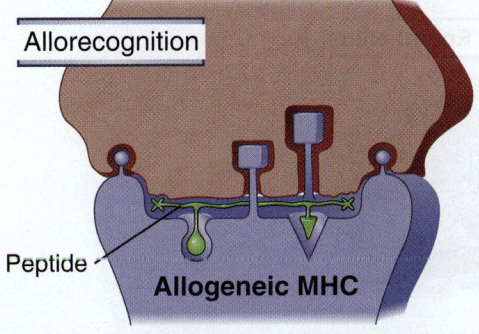

Allorecognition

The self MHC–restricted T cell recognizes the allogeneic MHC molecule whose structure resembles a self MHC–foreign peptide complex

C

FIGURE 49.21 Molecular basis for direct allorecognition. Recipient T cells may recognize donor major histocompatibility complex *(MHC)* molecules directly because of the similarities between MHC alleles but become activated because only T cells strongly reactive to self MHC were deleted in the thymus through negative selection. (A) Normally, T cells encounter self MHC complexed with foreign peptide and become activated in the appropriate context. (B) T cells may encounter allogeneic MHC complexed with endogenous peptide that together resemble self MHC bound with foreign peptide. (C) Alternatively, allogeneic MHC alone may contribute to allorecognition and T-cell activation independent of self peptide. (Adapted from Abbas AK, Lichtman AH, Pillai S. *Cellular and Molecular Immunology*. 10th ed. Philadelphia: Saunders Elsevier; 2021.)

will result in an accelerated form of cellular rejection mediated by memory T cells. It generally occurs within the first 2 or 3 days after transplantation and can be accompanied by a significant humoral response.

The humoral equivalent to acute cellular rejection is AMR. This occurs when offending antibodies specific for alloantigen exist in the circulation at levels undetectable by crossmatch assays or, alternatively, B-cell clones capable of producing DSA are activated and stimulated to produce de novo alloantibodies. These antibodies are thought to bind HLA antigens within the graft, recruit innate and adaptive immune mechanisms, and acutely injure the transplanted organ (Fig. 49.23). The former scenario is often seen in patients with a high PRA score that has decreased over time. Transplantation presumably leads to restimulation of memory B cells responsible for the donor-specific antibodies. The result is initial graft function, followed by rapid deterioration within the first few postoperative days. Implementation of a more aggressive immunosuppressive regimen, including higher doses of steroids combined with nonspecific antibody reduction by plasmapheresis or IVIG (nonspecific Ig), is occasionally successful in acutely reversing AMR.

Prompt recognition of acute rejection is essential to ensure optimal graft survival. Untreated rejection leads to expansion of the immune response to involve multiple pathways, some of which are less sensitive to T-cell–specific therapies. In addition, damage to the allograft, particularly for kidney, pancreas, and heart, is generally accompanied by a permanent loss of function that is proportional to the magnitude of involvement. Most acute rejection episodes are initially asymptomatic until the secondary effects of organ dysfunction occur. By this point, the rejection process has proceeded to a point that is often more difficult to reverse. Accordingly, monitoring for acute rejection is usually intense initially, particularly during the first year after transplantation. In general, any unexplained graft dysfunction should prompt biopsy and evaluation for the lymphocytic infiltration, antibody deposition, and parenchymal necrosis characteristic of acute rejection.

Novel Diagnostic Strategies for Acute Rejection

Since the dawn of transplantation, allograft biopsy has been the gold standard for the diagnosis of acute cellular rejection. Recently, several promising techniques have emerged to attempt diagnosis of acute rejection without biopsy, obviating the complications that occasionally arise with invasive interventions such as needle biopsy. One of the most promising of these new techniques for assessing the presence of acute rejection is the characterization of donor-derived cell free DNA (dd-cfDNA) in the serum. During processes of graft injury like acute rejection, dd-cfDNA is liberated into the circulation as donor allograft cells die or become inflamed, and sensitive PCR techniques can amplify and quantify this transplant-specific cfDNA. For example, one specific test analyzes single nucleotide polymorphisms (SNPs) across all 22 somatic chromosomes to optimize dd-cfDNA detection. The dd-cfDNA assays have found numerous clinical applications, such as capturing incipient rejection responses while switching or adjusting immunosuppression regimens, monitoring rejection treatment response, identifying rejection in patients with delayed or slow graft function, and substituting for invasive tissue biopsies in high-risk recipients (such as anticoagulated patients, for whom biopsy would be at increased risk of complication).[22] The Circulating Donor-Derived Cell-Free DNA in blood for diagnosing Acute Rejections

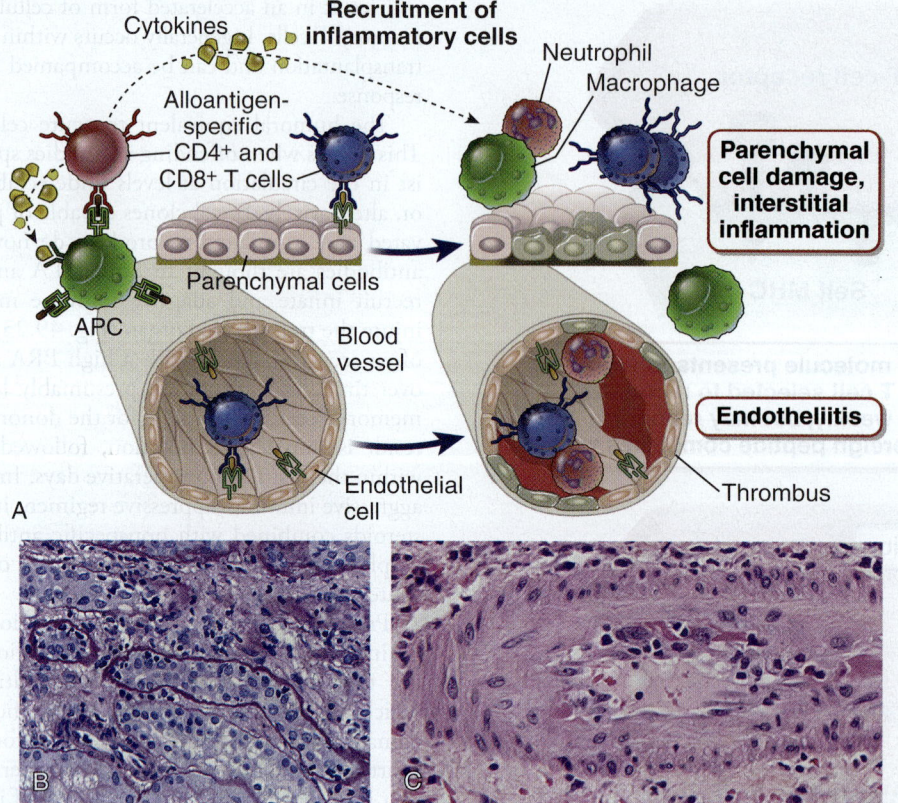

FIGURE 49.22 Acute cellular rejection. (A) In acute cellular rejection, CD4+ and CD8+ T lymphocytes reactive with alloantigens on endothelial cells in blood vessels, and parenchymal cells mediate damage to these cell types. (B) Acute cellular rejection of a kidney with inflammatory cells in the connective tissue around the tubules and between epithelial cells of the tubules (tubulitis). (C) Inflammation of the endothelial layer of a blood vessel (endotheliitis) in acute cellular rejection, with inflammatory cells damaging endothelium. *APC,* Antigen-presenting cells. (Adapted from Abbas AK, Lichtman AH, Pillai S. *Cellular and Molecular Immunology.* 10th ed. Philadelphia: Saunders Elsevier; 2021.)

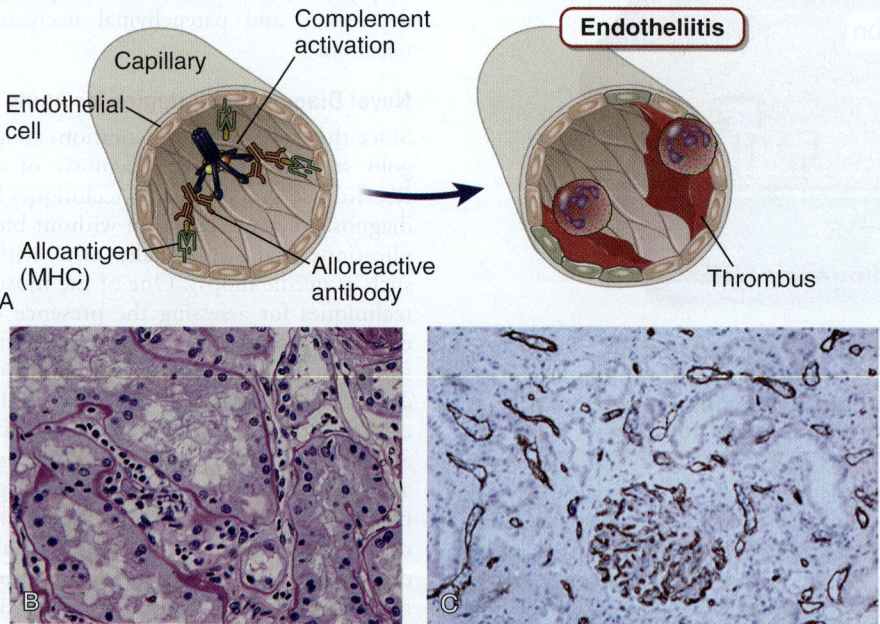

FIGURE 49.23 Acute antibody-mediated (humoral) rejection. (A) Alloreactive antibodies formed after engraftment may contribute to parenchymal and vascular injury. (B) Acute antibody-mediated rejection of a kidney allograft with inflammatory cells in peritubular capillaries. (C) Complement C4d deposition in capillaries in acute antibody-mediated rejection, revealed by immunohistochemistry as brown staining. *MHC,* Major histocompatibility complex. (Adapted from Abbas AK, Lichtman AH, Pillai S. *Cellular and Molecular Immunology.* 10th ed. Philadelphia: Saunders Elsevier; 2021.)

in Kidney Transplant Recipients (DART) study found that dd-cfDNA significantly outperformed serum creatinine in detecting active rejection in renal allograft recipients, especially for discriminating AMR. Similarly, the Resolution by AlloSure Differentiates Ambiguous Rejection (RADAR) study found that a dd-cfDNA level >0.5% can help risk-stratify patients with grade 1A or borderline rejection with respect to poor clinical outcomes such as estimated glomerular filtration rate (eGFR) decline, formation of de novo DSA, or future recurrent rejection episodes. The use of dd-cfDNA has also been validated for heart and lung transplant recipients.

Another US Food and Drug Administration (FDA)–approved assay measures adenosine triphosphate production by peripheral blood CD4+ T cells as a marker of global immune competence. This assay enables clinicians to determine which transplant recipients may be functionally over-immunosuppressed (and thus at increased risk of opportunistic infection) and which patients may be functionally under-immunosuppressed (and thus at increased risk of allograft rejection). Finally, some researchers are also exploring other noninvasive diagnostic tests for acute allograft rejection, such as use of urinary biomarkers in kidney transplant recipients. A variety of different urinary biomarkers such as IL-18, CXCL9, and CXCL10 have been validated for the diagnosis of renal allograft rejection. In total, although these assays promise to unlock future standards of noninvasive diagnostic testing, limitations on their sensitivity and specificity do not currently allow them to substitute for gold standard allograft biopsy. In particular, these assays may be too sensitive and not specific enough, having demonstrated difficulty distinguishing allograft rejection from other causes of allograft dysfunction such as urinary tract infection or BK nephropathy.

Chronic Rejection

Whereas the mechanisms of acute and hyperacute rejection are now well-described, chronic rejection remains less understood. True chronic rejection is an immune-based process derived from repeated or indolent T-cell–mediated rejection or AMR, but the clinical phenotype of chronic graft fibrosis and deterioration is often secondary to a combination of both immune and nonimmune effects. Appropriately, the term *chronic rejection* has been substituted with more descriptive terms: interstitial fibrosis and tubular atrophy (previously chronic allograft nephropathy) for kidneys, chronic coronary vasculopathy for hearts, vanishing bile duct syndrome for livers, and bronchiolitis obliterans for lungs.[23] The process is insidious, usually occurring during a period of years, but it can be accelerated and occur within the first year. Regardless of the organ involved, it is characterized by parenchymal replacement by fibrous tissue with a relatively sparse lymphocytic infiltrate but may contain macrophages or dendritic cells. Organs with epithelium show a disappearance of the epithelial cells as well as endothelial destruction. The events that ultimately trigger this response are certainly related to the transplantation, including but not limited to the response to alloantigen as well as myriad nonimmune factors such as ischemia-reperfusion injury, cytomegalovirus (CMV) infection, CNI toxicity, and posttransplant metabolic disease. These events set the stage for expression of various soluble factors, including TGF-β, leading to a remodeling of the parenchyma and ensuing fibrous replacement (Fig. 49.24). Chronic inflammatory insults can also evoke a process of epithelial-to-mesenchymal dedifferentiation, leading to epithelial cells that regress into fibrocytes. Although to date these processes remain essentially untreatable once

identified, several factors have been identified that predispose toward the development of chronic rejection. The most important of these is prior acute rejection episodes. Another important factor is the presence of DSA, which often portends premature allograft loss. Thus, the more effectively immune control is exerted to limit acute rejection episodes and the development of donor-specific antibodies in the early stages after transplantation, the less likely chronic rejection related to immune injury is to occur.

IMMUNOSUPPRESSION

Current immunosuppressive therapies in transplantation achieve excellent results, especially in terms of relatively short-term patient and allograft survival rates. Despite tremendous progress during the past 60 years, all agents designed to prevent rejection remain nonspecific to the alloimmune response. Given the redundancy of the immune system, recipients almost always need multiple agents to adequately control the normal immune response. In addition, none of these therapies specifically inhibit the response to the allograft; instead, most immunosuppressants target the immune response globally. In other words, all drugs that prevent rejection do so at the cost of suppressing the normal host response to bacterial and viral pathogens as well as tumor surveillance. Whereas some of the newer therapies are more precise in their mechanisms and selective for immune cells, many target not only the mediators of the immune response but also any cells undergoing maturation or division. Consequently, many nonimmune side effects are associated with immunosuppressive therapy that can directly or indirectly contribute to graft dysfunction and loss. In addition, the societal costs are not trivial, considering that transplant recipients may take dozens of pills a day at an annual cost of $10,000 to $15,000.

The most critical time for immune protection is the first few days to months after transplantation. The graft is fresh, and there is a heightened state of inflammation secondary to inevitable graft injury from ischemia-reperfusion as well as the physical transfer of the organ itself. In addition, this is the time of initial antigen exposure, which plays a large role in determining the long-term status of immune responsiveness. For this reason, immunosuppression is extremely intense in the early postoperative period and normally tapered thereafter. This initial conditioning of the recipient's immune system is known as *induction immunosuppression*. It most commonly involves depletion, or at least aggressive reduction, of T cells and consequently is tolerated only for a short time without lethal consequences. After this initial period, the agents used to prevent acute rejection for the remainder of the life of the transplanted organ are called *maintenance immunosuppressants*. These medications still carry with them a host of immune and nonimmune side effects that may also ultimately contribute to long-term graft failure. Immunosuppressants used to reverse an acute rejection episode are called *rescue agents*. They are generally the same as those agents used for induction therapy. The mechanisms of the various immunosuppressants are described here and detailed in Table 49.3.

Induction Therapy

Most of the current induction regimens involve the use of some depleting antilymphocyte antibody preparation. Their mechanism of action is probably not fully understood but involves some combination of either selective or nonselective depletion and inactivation. They cause profound immunosuppression,

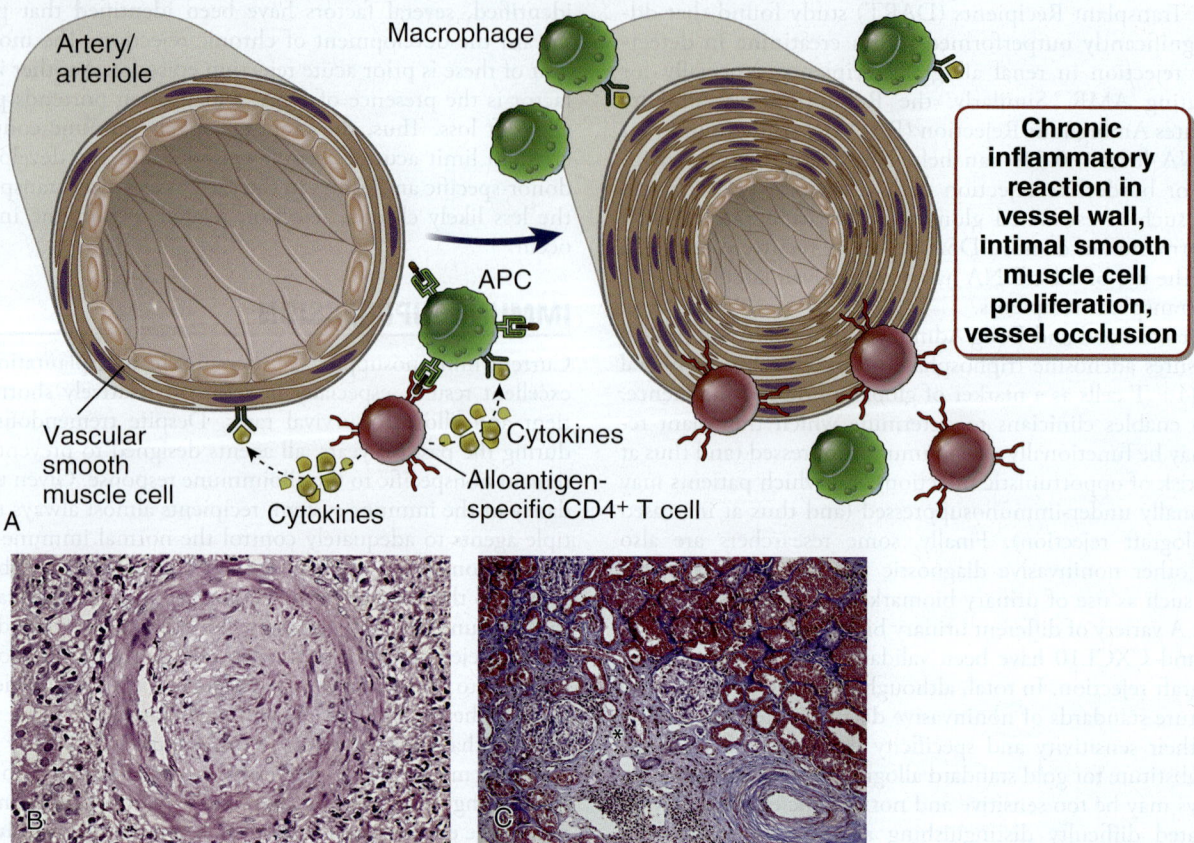

FIGURE 49.24 Chronic rejection. (A) In chronic rejection with graft arteriosclerosis, injury to the vessel wall leads to intimal smooth muscle cell proliferation and luminal occlusion. This lesion may be caused by a chronic inflammatory reaction to alloantigens in the vessel wall. (B) Chronic rejection in a kidney allograft with graft arteriosclerosis. The vascular lumen is replaced by an accumulation of smooth muscle cells and connective tissue in the vessel intima. (C). Fibrosis and loss of tubules in a kidney with chronic rejection *(lower left)* adjacent to relatively normal kidney *(upper right)*. The blue area shows fibrosis, and an artery with graft arteriosclerosis is present *(bottom right)*. (Adapted from Abbas AK, Lichtman AH, Pillai S. *Cellular and Molecular Immunology.* 10th ed. Philadelphia: Saunders Elsevier; 2021.)

placing the recipient at increased risk for opportunistic infections or malignancies such as lymphoma, and are consequently generally limited to short-term use on the order of days to weeks.

Antithymocyte Globulin

Antithymocyte globulin preparations are produced by immunizing another species with an inoculum of human thymocytes consisting primarily of lymphocytes, followed by collection of the sera and purification of the gamma globulin fraction. The result is a polyclonal antibody preparation that contains antibodies directed against a multitude of antigens on lymphocytes. The two most commonly used preparations are rabbit antithymocyte globulin (RATG) and horse antithymocyte globulin (ATGAM). RATG seems to be more effective than ATGAM at reducing the incidence of acute rejection episodes and consequently is the preferred preparation at most US transplantation centers.[24] The polyclonal preparation consists of hundreds of polyclonal antibodies that coat dozens of epitopes over the surface of the T cell. The result is T-cell clearance through complement-mediated lysis and opsonization. In addition to simple depletion mechanisms, the antisera also interfere with effective TCR signaling and can promote inappropriate cross-linking of key cell surface molecules, including adhesion and costimulatory receptors, resulting in unresponsiveness or anergy.

These preparations are used as induction agents as well as rescue treatment for acute rejection episodes. Most commonly, RATG is used as part of a multidrug induction protocol that includes a CNI, an antiproliferative agent such as mycophenolate mofetil (MMF), and prednisone. One strategy in renal transplantation is the sequential use of RATG followed by a CNI to avoid the nephrotoxic effects of the CNI in the early posttransplantation period as well as to maximize the effects of RATG by depleting or inactivating the majority of T cells at the critical time of graft introduction. More recently, RATG has been used as a key component of newer steroid-minimization or CNI-free regimens.[25,26]

Many of the side effects associated with RATG administration are related to its polyclonal composition. Surprisingly, only a small fraction of the known specificities are actually directed at defined T-cell epitopes. One major side effect is profound thrombocytopenia secondary to platelet-specific antibodies within the polyclonal preparation. In addition to T-cell depletion, leukopenia and anemia may also result. Overimmunosuppression is also a concern; given that these preparations are extremely effective at T-cell depletion, there is an increase in viral reactivation and primary viral infections, including CMV, Epstein-Barr virus (EBV), herpes simplex virus, and varicella-zoster virus. The effect on EBV-specific T cells also predisposes treated patients to a higher incidence of EBV-associated lymphoid malignant neoplasms. Overall, however,

TABLE 49.3 Summary of Immunosuppressive Drugs

DRUG	DESCRIPTION	MECHANISM	NONIMMUNE TOXICITY AND COMMENTS
Prednisone	Corticosteroid	Binds nuclear receptor and enhances transcription of IκB, which inhibits NF-κB and T-cell activation	Diabetes, weight gain, psychological disturbances, osteoporosis, ulcers, wound healing, adrenal suppression
Cyclosporine	11–Amino acid cyclic peptide from *Tolypocladium inflatum*	Binds to cyclophilin; complex inhibits calcineurin phosphatase and T-cell activation	Nephrotoxicity, hemolytic uremic syndrome, hypertension, neurotoxicity, gingival hyperplasia, skin changes, hirsutism, posttransplantation diabetes, hyperlipidemia
Tacrolimus (Prograf)	Macrolide antibiotic from *Streptomyces tsukubaensis*	Binds to FK-BP12; complex inhibits calcineurin phosphatase and T-cell activation	Effects similar to CsA but with lower incidence of hypertension, hyperlipidemia, skin changes, hirsutism, and gingival hyperplasia but higher incidence of posttransplantation diabetes and neurotoxicity
Sirolimus (Rapamycin)	Triene macrolide antibiotic from *Streptomyces hygroscopicus* from Easter Island (Rapa Nui)	Binds to FK-BP12; complex inhibits target of rapamycin and IL-2–dependent T-cell proliferation	Hyperlipidemia, increased toxicity of calcineurin inhibitors, thrombocytopenia, delayed wound healing, delayed graft function, mouth ulcers, pneumonitis, interstitial lung disease
Everolimus (Zortress)	Derivative of sirolimus, similar mechanism and toxicities		
Mycophenolate mofetil (CellCept)	Mycophenolic acid from *Penicillium stoloniferum*	Inhibits synthesis of guanosine monophosphate nucleotides; blocks purine synthesis, preventing proliferation of T and B cells	Gastrointestinal symptoms (mainly diarrhea), neutropenia, mild anemia
Azathioprine (Imuran)	Prodrug that undergoes hepatic metabolism to form 6-mercaptopurine	Converts 6-mercaptopurine to 6-thioinosine-5′-monophosphate, which is converted to thioguanine nucleotides that interfere with DNA and purine synthesis	Leukopenia, bone marrow depression, liver toxicity (uncommon)
Antithymocyte globulin	Polyclonal IgG from rabbits or horses immunized with human thymocytes	Blocks T-cell membrane proteins (CD2, CD3, CD45), causing altered function, lysis, and prolonged T-cell depletion	Cytokine release syndrome, thrombocytopenia, leukopenia, serum sickness
OKT3 (muromonab-CD3)	Anti-CD3 murine monoclonal antibody	Binds CD3 associated with the TCR, leading to initial activation and cytokine release, followed by blockade of function, lysis, and T-cell depletion	Severe cytokine release syndrome, pulmonary edema, acute renal failure, central nervous system changes
Basiliximab	Anti-CD25 chimeric monoclonal antibody	Binds to high-affinity chain of IL-2R (CD25) on activated T cells, causing depletion and preventing IL-2–mediated activation	Hypersensitivity reaction, uncommon
Daclizumab	Anti-CD25 humanized monoclonal antibody	Similar to that of basiliximab	Hypersensitivity reaction, uncommon
Rituximab	Anti-CD20 chimeric monoclonal antibody	Binds to CD20 on B cells and causes depletion	Infusion and hypersensitivity reactions, uncommon
Alemtuzumab	Anti-CD52 humanized monoclonal antibody	Binds to CD52 expressed on most T and B cells, monocytes, macrophages, and NK cells, causing lysis and prolonged depletion	Mild cytokine release syndrome, neutropenia, anemia, autoimmune thrombocytopenia, thyroid disease
Belatacept (LEA29Y)	High-affinity homologue of CTLA-4–Ig	Binds to CD80/CD86 and prevents costimulation through CD28	In clinical trials, results show improved glomerular filtration rate and improved outcomes to CsA

CsA, Cyclosporine A; *CTLA,* cytotoxic T lymphocyte–associated; *IgG,* immunoglobulin G; *IL,* interleukin; *NF-κB,* nuclear factor κB; *NK,* natural killer; *TCR,* T-cell receptor.
Adapted from Halloran PF. Immunosuppressive drugs for kidney transplantation. *N Engl J Med.* 2004;351:2715-2729.

the drug is well tolerated by most transplant recipients and is the most common form of induction treatment used in kidney transplantation. The most common symptoms are the result of transient cytokine release after antibody binding and cell lysis. Chills and fevers occur in up to 20% of patients, but this cytokine release syndrome is usually self-limited and treatable with antipyretics and antihistamines. In addition, this response is often tempered in patients receiving corticosteroids as part of the induction regimen.

Anti–IL-2 Receptor Antibodies

The cytokine IL-2 plays a critical role in T-cell activation and function. After antigen recognition and signal transduction through the TCR complex, expression of IL-2 and its receptor is markedly upregulated. The receptor consists of three chains: α (CD25), β (CD122), and the common cytokine receptor γ chain (CD132). These chains associate in a noncovalent manner to form the IL-2 receptor complex. The α chain, CD25, is a type I transmembrane protein that is responsible for the high-affinity binding of IL-2 on activated T cells and is critical for T-cell clonal expansion (Fig. 49.25). Given its importance in the cellular response, two nondepleting monoclonal antibodies (mAbs) specific for CD25 were developed and approved for use in transplantation: daclizumab and basiliximab.[27,28] The two antibodies differ in their composition in that daclizumab is humanized and

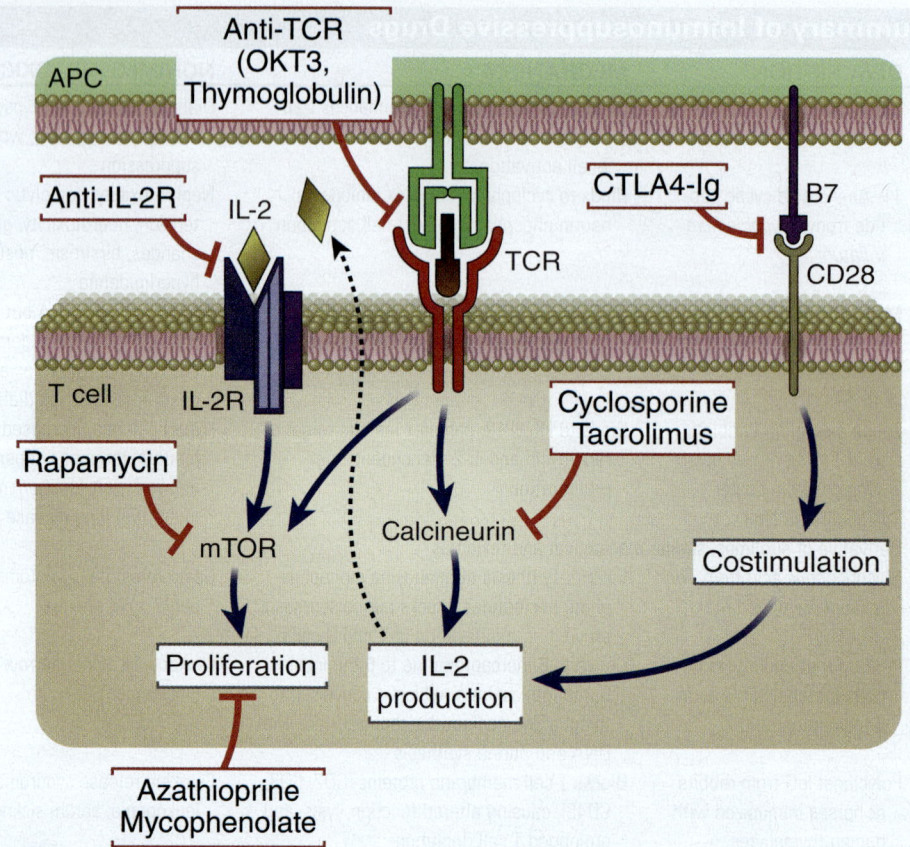

FIGURE 49.25 Molecular mechanisms of immunosuppression. Immunosuppressants may be small molecules, antibodies, or fusion proteins that block various pathways critical for T-cell activation. TCR activation is blocked by anti-TCR monoclonal and polyclonal antibodies such as OKT3 and thymoglobulin. Downstream signaling from TCR activation is blocked by calcineurin inhibitors such as cyclosporine and tacrolimus, which prevent the calcineurin-mediated dephosphorylation of NFAT necessary for the nuclear translocation of this critical transcription factor. Costimulation signals necessary for T-cell activation (such as CD28-B7 interaction) are interrupted by costimulatory blockade fusion proteins such as CTLA4-Ig and belatacept. IL-2 is a necessary cytokine permitting leukocyte proliferation, and this pathway is disrupted by both IL-2 receptor antagonists (such as basiliximab) and mTOR inhibitors such as rapamycin and everolimus. Antimetabolites such as azathioprine and mycophenolate interfere with nucleic acid metabolism and therefore disrupt cellular proliferation. Finally, prednisone (not shown) binds to cytoplasmic steroid receptors, which then translocate into the nucleus and function as transcription factors for multiple immunosuppressive genes. *CTLA,* Cytotoxic T lymphocyte–associated; *Ig,* immunoglobulin; *IKK,* IkB kinase; *IL,* interleukin; *mAb,* monoclonal antibody; *MMF,* mycophenolate mofetil; *MPA,* mycophenolic acid; *mTOR,* mammalian target of rapamycin; *NFAT,* nuclear factor of activated T cell; *TCR,* T-cell receptor. (Adapted from Abbas AK, Lichtman AH, Pillai S. *Cellular and Molecular Immunology.* 10th ed. Philadelphia: Saunders Elsevier; 2021.)

basiliximab is a mouse-human chimeric antibody. Both are directed against CD25 and function to block IL-2 binding. Because CD25 is preferentially expressed on recently activated T cells, the antibodies are semiselective in their effects, presumably affecting only T cells specific for the allograft that have been activated at the time of graft implantation. Once the T-cell response is well under way, effector T cells are much less dependent on CD25 expression, and these antibodies are much less effective. For this reason, both anti-CD25 antibodies are used during the induction phase only. Much like antithymocyte globulin, they have been shown to prevent or to reduce the frequency of acute rejection when they are used in combination with standard three-drug regimens.[27,28] However, in contradistinction to lymphocyte-depleting agents, daclizumab and basiliximab, although generally less potent, confer less risk of infection and malignancy posttransplant. More recently, they have been employed as part of regimens to reduce or eliminate

CNIs or within steroid-minimization protocols. These anti–IL-2R antibodies are well tolerated clinically, as they do not precipitate the same side effects seen with antithymocyte globulin, such as the cytokine release syndrome. Unlike the murine antibody OKT3 (see "OKT3" next), both daclizumab and basiliximab are the products of genetic engineering, with some or all of the structural components of the mouse antibody having been replaced with human IgG, and thus, they are much less likely to invoke neutralizing antibody responses themselves. Daclizumab has since been discontinued as a result of diminished demand, leaving basiliximab as the sole anti–IL-2 receptor option.

OKT3

Muromonab-CD3 (OKT3), a murine mAb directed against the human CD3 ε chain (a component of the TCR signaling complex), was approved by the FDA for use in patients in 1986 and is now of purely historical interest. It was the first commercially available mAb preparation for use in organ transplantation with T-cell specificity devoid of the unintended bystander effects observed with polyclonal preparations. OKT3 was shown to be superior to conventional steroid therapy in reversing rejection and consequently improved allograft survival.[29] Because OKT3 is a mouse antibody, it can elicit an immune response to itself, and the recipient will generate antimurine antibodies directed against the structural regions of the antibody or the actual binding site, thereby limiting its therapeutic effect. In addition, the cytokine release syndrome associated with OKT3 administration can be vigorous, resulting in hypotension, pulmonary edema, and myocardial depression. Because of this vigorous response, its immunogenicity, and the availability of alternative therapeutic options, OKT3 has been withdrawn from production.

Alemtuzumab

Alemtuzumab was originally developed in the oncology field for the treatment of lymphoma. It is a humanized antibody against human CD52, a cell surface protein expressed on most mature lymphocytes and monocytes but not on their stem cell precursors. It has been used not only in patients with lymphoma but also in autoimmune processes, such as multiple sclerosis and rheumatoid arthritis. Administration of alemtuzumab is extremely effective at reducing the number of T cells both in the peripheral blood and in secondary lymphoid organs. In addition, it depletes, to a lesser extent, both B cells and monocytes. Unlike other strategies, this depletion may last for weeks to months after dosing. Investigational studies in transplantation employing alemtuzumab as an induction agent have allowed minimization of immunosuppression, particularly when it is combined with a CNI.[30,31] Its optimal use in transplantation remains to be established.

Maintenance Immunosuppression

After the immediate posttransplant period of induction, transplant recipients continue on long-term maintenance immunosuppression. Practice has evolved to maintain patients on standard multidrug regimens that have facilitated lower doses of individual agents to minimize toxicity and enhanced the quality of net immunosuppression through the use of various mechanisms of action. With outstanding short-term transplant outcomes, chronic use of maintenance agents and their attendant off-target toxicities have driven dose-reduction protocols over time and efforts to develop more selective and less toxic novel therapies.

Corticosteroids

Steroids, in particular glucocorticoids, remain one of the most commonly employed medications to prevent rejection. They are almost exclusively used in combination with other agents with which they seem to act synergistically to improve graft survival. They may also be used in higher doses as induction or rescue therapy for acute rejection episodes. Although steroids possess potent immunosuppressive properties, they can contribute significantly to the morbidity of transplantation by their effects on wound healing and propensity to cause diabetes, hypertension, and osteoporosis. With the advent of more effective and alternative immunosuppressive options over time, there has been an emphasis on developing steroid-minimization or steroid-sparing protocols to avoid these well-known side effects. Nonetheless, low-dose steroids remain a common component of current standard immunosuppressive regimens.

Although the Nobel Prize was awarded more than 50 years ago for work on the hormones of the adrenal cortex, the mechanism of the immunosuppressive effect of glucocorticoids was only recently better understood.[32] Similar to other steroid hormones, glucocorticoids bind to an intracellular receptor after passing into the cytoplasm through nonspecific mechanisms. The receptor-steroid complex then enters the nucleus, where it acts as a transcription factor. One of the most important genes upregulated is the gene encoding IκB. This protein binds to and inhibits the function of NF-κB, a key activator of proinflammatory cytokines and an important transcription factor involved in T-cell activation. Through this mechanism, steroids also act to diminish transcription of IL-1 and TNF-α by APCs as well as to prevent upregulation of MHC expression. Phospholipase A2, and consequently the entire arachidonic acid cascade, is also inhibited. They decrease the leukocyte response to various chemokines and chemotactins and by inhibiting vasodilators, such as histamine and prostacyclin, thus dampen the inflammatory response globally. This broad antiinflammatory response quickly mollifies the intragraft environment and thus substantially improves graft function long before the offending cells have actually left the graft. The most commonly used oral glucocorticoid formulation is prednisone; its intravenous equivalent is methylprednisolone.

Antiproliferative Agents

Azathioprine. The purine analogue azathioprine was first described in the 1960s and remained a mainstay of immunosuppression for the next 30 years.[33] It is still used today in organ transplantation and in the treatment of some autoimmune diseases, such as autoimmune hepatitis. Similar to other antiproliferative agents, it is a nucleotide analogue that targets cells undergoing rapid division; in the case of an immune response, its goal is to limit the clonal expansion of T and B cells. Azathioprine undergoes hepatic conversion to several active metabolites, including 6-mercaptopurine and 6-thioinosine monophosphate. These derivatives inhibit DNA synthesis by alkylating DNA precursors and interfering with DNA repair mechanisms. In addition, they inhibit the enzymatic conversion of thioinosine monophosphate to adenosine monophosphate and guanosine monophosphate, effectively depleting the cell of adenosine. The effects of azathioprine are relatively nonspecific, and like other antiproliferative agents, it acts on all rapidly dividing cells requiring nucleotide synthesis. Consequently, its predominant toxicities are seen in the bone marrow, gut mucosa, and liver. Azathioprine has been used as a maintenance agent in combination with other medications, such as a corticosteroid and CNI. Although it has largely been replaced by MMF as the first-line antiproliferative agent, azathioprine remains the agent of choice during pregnancy.

Mycophenolate mofetil. MMF is an immunosuppressive agent with a similar mechanism of action to azathioprine. It is derived from the fungus *Penicillium stoloniferum*. Once ingested, it is metabolized in the liver to the active moiety mycophenolic acid. The active compound inhibits inosine monophosphate dehydrogenase, the enzyme that controls the rate of synthesis of guanosine monophosphate in the de novo pathway of purine synthesis, a critical step in RNA and DNA synthesis. Importantly, however, is the presence of a "salvage pathway" for guanosine monophosphate production in most cells except lymphocytes (hypoxanthine-guanine phosphoribosyltransferase–catalyzed guanosine monophosphate production directly from guanosine). Thus, MMF exploits a critical difference between lymphocytes and other body tissues, resulting in relatively lymphocyte-specific immunosuppressive effects. MMF blocks the proliferative response of both T and B cells, inhibits antibody formation, and prevents the clonal expansion of cytotoxic T cells.

Numerous clinical trials have evaluated MMF. Specifically, MMF has been shown to decrease the rate of biopsy-proven rejection and the need for rescue therapy compared with azathioprine.[34] Accordingly, MMF has replaced azathioprine in most standard three-drug immunosuppressive regimens, although recent evidence suggests that its therapeutic difference is less pronounced when it is used with more modern immunosuppressive therapies. It has also been used in combination with either a CNI or sirolimus by many centers in steroid-sparing protocols. However, MMF is not effective enough to be used alone without either steroids or CNIs. The major clinical side effects include leukopenia and diarrhea. An advanced, enteric-coated formulation of mycophenolate sodium (Myfortic) that only releases in the high pH environment of the small intestine has been developed to mitigate some of the gastrointestinal side effects of MMF.

Calcineurin Inhibitors

Cyclosporine A. Jean-François Borel is credited with the discovery of CsA in 1972 while working as a microbiologist for Sandoz Laboratories (now Novartis). He apparently was vacationing in Norway and while there had collected soil samples for analysis in search of new antibiotics. Although the samples failed to show any significant antimicrobial activity, they did show potent immunosuppressive characteristics. Further studies demonstrated that the active component is a cyclic, nonribosomal peptide of 11 amino acids produced by the fungus *Tolypocladium inflatum*.[35] The mechanism of action of CsA is mediated primarily through its ability to bind the cytoplasmic protein cyclophilin. The CsA-cyclophilin complex binds to the calcineurin-calmodulin complex within the cytoplasm and blocks the phosphatase activity of calcineurin, preventing the dephosphorylation and resulting activation of NFAT, a critical transcription factor involved in T-cell activation, including upregulation of the IL-2 transcript (see Fig. 49.25). The result is blockade of IL-2 production. Thus, CsA is used as a maintenance agent, blocking the initiation of an immune response, but it is ineffective as a rescue agent once IL-2 has already been produced. In addition, CsA acts to increase transcription of TGF-β, a cytokine involved in the normal processes that limit the immune response by inhibiting T-cell activation, reducing regional blood flow, and stimulating tissue remodeling and wound repair. As discussed later, the toxicity and side effects of CsA may be in large part related to the effects of TGF-β.

CsA has poor water solubility and consequently must be given in a suspension or emulsion. This becomes a particular concern in liver transplantation because the oral absorption of CsA is dependent on bile flow; fortunately, this was addressed through the development of a microemulsion form that is less bile dependent. CsA is metabolized by the hepatic cytochrome P450 enzymes, and blood levels are therefore influenced by agents that affect the P450 system. P450 inhibitors, which include ketoconazole, erythromycin, calcium channel blockers, and grapefruit juice, result in higher CsA levels; inducers of P450, including rifampin, phenobarbital, and phenytoin, result in lower CsA levels.

The discovery of CsA and its subsequent development as an immunosuppressant contributed enormously to the advancement of organ transplantation (see Fig. 49.17). It was first approved for clinical use in 1983 and led to substantial improvement in the outcome of deceased donor renal transplantation and permitted the widespread practice of heart and liver transplantation.[36]

Whereas its potent immunosuppressive activity was welcomed, its attendant toxicities were less than ideal. CsA induces the expression of TGF-β, and much of CsA's toxicity can be linked to increased TGF-β activity. One of the most important side effects of CsA is renal toxicity. CsA has a significant vasoconstrictor effect on proximal renal arterioles, resulting in a 30% decrease in renal blood flow. This action is most likely mediated through increased TGF-β levels that act to increase the transcription of endothelin, a potent vasoconstrictor, resulting in activation of the renin-angiotensin pathway and resultant hypertension. The remodeling effects of TGF-β also induce fibrin deposition, which is thought to play a role in the fibrosis typically seen during chronic allograft nephropathy. CsA frequently causes neurologic side effects consisting of tremors, paresthesias, headache, depression, confusion, somnolence, and, rarely, seizures. Hypertrichosis (increased hair growth) is another frequent side effect, predominantly occurring on the face, arms, and back in up to 50% of patients. Gingival hyperplasia may also occur. The use of CsA in combination with other immunosuppressive agents permitted lower doses of CsA to limit toxicity, but current mainstay immunosuppression now favors the CNI tacrolimus.

Tacrolimus. Tacrolimus was isolated from Japanese soil samples in 1984 as part of an effort to discover novel immunosuppressants. A macrolide produced by the fungus *Streptomyces tsukubaensis*, tacrolimus was found to possess potent immunosuppressive properties.[37] Similar to CsA, it blocks the effects of NFAT, prevents cytokine transcription, and arrests T-cell activation. The intracellular target is an immunophilin protein distinct from cyclophilin known as *FK-binding protein (FK-BP)*. In vitro, tacrolimus was found to be 100 times more potent in blocking IL-2 and IFN-γ production than CsA and is clinically more effective at preventing acute rejection.[38] Tacrolimus, like CsA, also increases TGF-β transcription, leading to both the beneficial and toxic effects of this cytokine. The side effect profile for tacrolimus is similar to that of CsA with regard to renal toxicity, but the cosmetic side effects, such as abnormal hair growth and gingival hyperplasia, are substantially reduced. Neurotoxicity, including tremors and mental status changes, is more pronounced with tacrolimus, as is its diabetogenic effect. Tacrolimus has been shown to be extremely effective for solid organ transplantation and has become the cornerstone drug of choice for most centers.

Mammalian Target of Rapamycin Inhibitors

Sirolimus and everolimus. Sirolimus (rapamycin) was isolated from a soil sample taken from Easter Island, a Polynesian island in the southeastern Pacific Ocean also known as Rapa Nui, hence the name rapamycin. It is a macrolide derived from the bacterium *Streptomyces hygroscopicus* with potent immunosuppressive properties. Everolimus is a derivative of rapamycin that possesses similar properties. Both are similar in structure to tacrolimus and bind to the same intracellular target, FK-BP, but neither agent affects calcineurin activity and consequently does not inhibit expression of NFAT or IL-2. Instead, the sirolimus–FK-BP complex inhibits the mammalian target of rapamycin (mTOR), specifically the mTOR complex 1 (see Fig. 49.25). mTOR is also called FRAP (FK-BP–rapamycin-associated protein) or RAFT (rapamycin and FK-BP target). RAFT-1 is a critical kinase involved in the IL-2 receptor signaling pathway. The result is inhibition of p70 S6 kinase activity, an enzyme essential for ribosomal phosphorylation, and arrest of cell cycle progression. Other receptors are also affected, including those for IL-4, IL-6, and platelet-derived growth factor.

Both sirolimus and everolimus are potent inhibitors of rejection in experimental models. Sirolimus and tacrolimus can act synergistically to impair rejection, but the combination can result in intolerable clinical toxicity. For example, the TRANSFORM trial found that the combination of everolimus and low-dose CNI was noninferior to standard immunosuppression with CNI and MMF in renal transplant recipients, although the rate of study discontinuation for adverse medicine effects was twice as high in the everolimus group than in the MMF group.[39] More often, sirolimus is used as an alternative to CNIs in a multidrug regimen or combined with other agents, allowing a reduction in the dose and minimization of side effects, including CNI-related nephrotoxicity or steroid-specific side effects. In addition to immunosuppressive properties, mTOR inhibitors have been shown to have promising antitumor effects as well. For example, sirolimus has been shown to promote programmed cell death in B-cell lymphomas, and everolimus has demonstrated activity against EBV. Thus, both agents may play an important role in the prevention of posttransplantation lymphoproliferative disorder (PTLD). Sirolimus and everolimus have also been used in the development of drug-eluting coronary stents to limit the rate of in-stent restenosis because of their antiproliferative properties. There is an increased incidence of hypercholesterolemia and hypertriglyceridemia with both agents that often requires treatment with cholesterol-lowering agents or discontinuation of the drug. Oral ulcers, wound healing complications (in particular an increased incidence of lymphoceles), elevated levels of proteinuria, pneumonitis, and thrombocytopenia remain frequent problems and limit universal application.

Costimulation Blockade

Belatacept. Costimulation is a critical component of naïve T-cell activation and has been extensively studied as a potential target for immune modulation in organ transplantation. One of the most important costimulation pathways is the interaction between CD28 and CD80/CD86. Signaling through CD28 allows effective IL-2 production and promotes cell survival through upregulation of antiapoptotic molecules. CD152 (CTLA-4) is another cell surface molecule expressed on activated T cells that is more effective in binding CD80 and CD86 than CD28. Once activated, T cells begin to express CD152, which interacts with CD80 and CD86 with a higher affinity and effectively interferes with CD28 binding and may deliver inhibitory signals to the T cell as part of a downregulatory mechanism for the immune response. CTLA-4–Ig is a fusion protein consisting of the extracellular component of CTLA-4 and the heavy chain of human IgG1 that was developed to block CD28-CD80/CD86 interactions and consequently to impair costimulation and T-cell activation (see Fig. 49.25). CTLA-4–Ig (abatacept) is used clinically for several autoimmune indications, including rheumatoid arthritis and psoriasis. However, the observed immunosuppressive strength of abatacept in preclinical transplant studies was suboptimal; thus, efforts to improve the efficacy of CTLA-4–Ig resulted in a novel mutant form, LEA29Y (belatacept). LEA29Y is a second-generation CTLA-4–Ig molecule that differs by two amino acid residues within the ligand binding domain, resulting in increased affinity for CD80 and CD86. The resultant improvement in binding affinity led to more potent immunosuppressive properties in vitro and in vivo.[17] Belatacept has since been tested in both preclinical nonhuman primate studies and phase III clinical trials in human renal transplantation and was FDA approved for use in kidney transplantation in 2011. Seven-year clinical trial data demonstrated improved long-term outcomes with better renal function and a significant reduction in the risk of patient death and allograft loss with belatacept in a CNI-free regimen compared with CsA-based immunosuppression.[16] Higher-than-expected acute rejection rates and logistic challenges related to intravenous infusion administration requirements have slowed large-scale uptake of belatacept. A few centers have employed belatacept with low-dose tacrolimus that is tapered off within the first year of transplant or thymoglobulin induction, achieving similar acute cellular rejection rates as conventional CNI-based immunosuppression regimens while achieving the long-term improvements in allograft eGFR that is associated with belatacept therapy. Belatacept cannot be used in recipients who are naïve to EBV infection because of higher associated rates of PTLD in these patients. With proven improvement in long-term transplant outcomes and a favorable toxicity profile, along with new-generation blockers and alternative delivery methods poised for clinical testing in transplantation, the future for costimulation-based immunosuppression strategies is bright.

B-Cell– and Antibody-Directed Therapies

Intravenous immune globulin. IVIG is composed of pooled plasma fractions from thousands of donors and essentially contains a representative sample of all antibodies found within that population. It is used frequently in the treatment of several autoimmune diseases, such as idiopathic thrombocytopenic purpura, Guillain-Barré syndrome, and myasthenia gravis as well as in patients with severe immune deficiencies featuring low or absent antibody levels. IVIG is also used in organ transplantation, specifically in the treatment of humoral rejection or before transplantation in highly sensitized recipients as a desensitization method in an attempt to reduce the PRA score and risk for hyperacute or early rejection. More recently, it has also been used as part of ABO-incompatible protocols. Although the immunosuppressive mechanism of IVIG is not known, it probably works through several mechanisms to alter the immune response, including neutralization of circulating autoantibodies and alloantibodies through antiidiotypic antibodies and selective downregulation of antibody production through Fc-mediated mechanisms.[40]

Rituximab. Rituximab is a murine antihuman CD20 chimeric antibody that was initially developed for the treatment of B-cell lymphoma and has since been used in the treatment of PTLD. CD20 is a cell surface protein expressed on all mature B cells but not on plasma cells. Rituximab binds to CD20 and facilitates antibody-dependent cellular cytotoxicity and CDC of B cells and promotes programmed cell death. More recently, rituximab has been used in a wide variety of autoimmune disorders and as a component in some investigational strategies designed as induction therapy in highly sensitized transplant recipients undergoing kidney transplantation or even in ABO-incompatible pairings. Some studies have indicated a reduction in the risk of AMR and antibody rebound posttransplant with rituximab, whereas others have shown no benefit. Therefore, additional clinical studies are needed to better define its optimal role in solid organ transplantation. Interestingly, the fact that CD20 is not expressed on antibody-producing plasma cells may explain the mixed clinical results with rituximab, and its beneficial effects may relate to the role of B cells in antigen presentation and memory B cells in antibody recall responses.

Antiplasma Cell Therapies

In an effort to specifically target antibody-secreting plasma cells, the anti-CD38 mAb daratumumab and two proteasome inhibitors have emerged. In contrast to CD20, CD38 is expressed on the surface of short- and long-lived plasma cells and may be a better target for the control of AMR resulting from plasma cell–derived alloantibodies. However, daratumumab mediates potent depletion of not only plasma cells but also potentially beneficial immunoregulatory T- and B-cell subsets. Therefore, the net effect of this anti-CD38 mAb remains to be carefully investigated in human transplantation. The proteasome inhibitors bortezomib and carfilzomib also selectively target antibody-producing plasma cells because of their high rate of Ig synthesis and reliance on their proteasomes to break down damaged proteins. The use of these agents to treat AMR in transplantation has also led to mixed results, and although proteasome inhibition may be effective at controlling acute antibody production, combination with other agents may be needed to achieve sustained control of alloantibodies and improve long-term outcomes in transplantation.

Eculizumab. The complement system is one of the main components of the innate immune response but also plays a significant role in regulating the adaptive immune system. Complement activation with formation of the membrane attack complex is the end point of a number of inflammatory processes that can cause damage to the transplanted organ. In particular, the role of complement in AMR or other processes that lead to immune complex deposition within the allograft or xenograft has recently been recognized as a potential target of therapeutic intervention. Eculizumab is a humanized mAb targeting the complement component C5. Its binding to C5 inhibits the formation of complement components downstream, including the split product C5a and membrane attack complex. It is approved to treat patients with paroxysmal nocturnal hemoglobinuria and atypical hemolytic uremic syndrome. More recently, there have been several reports employing eculizumab in solid organ transplantation as a means to treat or even to prevent AMR and other complement-mediated causes of renal allograft dysfunction and injury (e.g., atypical hemolytic uremic syndrome). Some efficacy has been observed when given prophylactically in combination with plasma exchange and IVIG in highly sensitized recipients at high risk for development of AMR. Unfortunately, it has not been universally effective, as a significant number of highly sensitized patients proceed to experience AMR despite treatment. This likely reflects the complexity of the processes leading to AMR, suggesting that additional mechanisms may be at play. Additional ongoing studies have shown promising early results with other complement-specific reagents, such as an inhibitor of C1 esterase (Berinert), but further trials are needed.

Novel Immunosuppressive Agents

The vast improvements in immunosuppression and transplant outcomes have led to a very high standard for new agents to overcome. Although agents in the clinical development pipeline have had rational mechanisms of action and strong preclinical efficacy, many have not met expectations and have failed to show efficacy and improved outcomes.

Selective CD28 antagonists. Costimulatory blockade has emerged as a promising immunosuppressive strategy in transplant patients. However, belatacept (the only costimulatory blockade drug currently clinically approved for transplant immunosuppression) blocks not only the T-cell activation signals mediated through CD28 but also the immunosuppressive signals mediated by CTLA-4. Several selective CD28 antagonists were developed to target the costimulatory pathways required for T-cell activation while leaving the suppressive signals

mediated by CTLA-4 intact. FR104 is an anti-CD28 monovalent Fab′ antibody. This monovalent Fab′ antibody was designed to prevent the CD28 cross-linking and resulting T-cell costimulation that would occur with divalent anti-CD28 mAb.[41] In nonhuman primate renal transplant models, FR104 was more efficacious in preventing acute cellular rejection than belatacept, with a trend toward higher frequencies of Tregs in FR104-treated animals.[42] FR104 is currently being studied in early phase kidney transplant clinical studies. Similarly, lulizumab, a pegylated anti-CD28 monovalent domain antibody (dAb), has been shown to prolong nonhuman primate renal allograft survival in sensitized recipients treated with a desensitization regimen of preoperative carfilzomib and lulizumab

CD40/CD154 pathway blockade. Beyond the CD28/B7 pathway, blockade of the CD40/CD154 costimulation pathway remains of significant interest in transplantation. Although the clinical development of CD154-specific therapies has been circuitous and challenged by an association with thromboembolic events in preclinical and clinical studies, experimentally targeting this pathway continues to show profound effects on alloimmunity. The recognition that anti-CD154 mAbs may cause thromboembolism by binding and cross-linking CD154 on platelets has spurred the pursuit of therapeutic agents that can disrupt CD40/CD154 signaling without cross-linking platelet-bound CD154. Initially efforts focused on the development of therapeutics targeting CD40, the receptor for CD154, thereby avoiding the previously seen thromboembolic complications. A few humanized anti-CD40 antibodies such as iscalimab (CFZ533) and bleselumab (ASKP1240) were developed and tested in clinical trials of patients undergoing kidney or liver transplantation. Unfortunately, development has not progressed after trials were halted because of concerns with increased rejection and/or infections. More recently, therapeutics designed to target CD154 have reemerged after alterations have rendered them Fc-silent, eliminating the potential for cross-linking of platelets and resultant thromboembolism. These Fc-silent anti-CD154 drugs include tegoprubart (AT-1501), dazodalibep (HZN-4920), and frexalimab (SAR441344). Tegoprubart is a humanized, Fc-silent anti-CD154 that is now being evaluated in a clinical trial of kidney transplant recipients. Results from this and other trials will be an important next step in realizing the potential of next-generation costimulation blockade reagents.

IL-6–directed therapies. Recently, several trials have explored the role of therapeutics targeting the IL-6 pathway to treat chronic active AMR, a common cause of late allograft loss after renal transplantation. IL-6 is a proinflammatory cytokine that has wide-ranging effects on B-cell and T-cell alloresponses. IL-6 promotes B-cell maturation into plasma cells and plays an important role in stimulating and maintaining germinal center formation and high-affinity antibody production, partly through its role as a potent stimulator of Tfh. Furthermore, IL-6 stimulates the development of proinflammatory Th17 cells while inhibiting the development and differentiation of suppressive Tregs. Interestingly, higher levels of IL-6 have been observed in rejecting human kidney, liver, and heart allografts.[43] Several groups have explored targeting the IL-6 pathway as either part of a desensitization strategy in highly sensitized transplant candidates or to treat chronic active AMR in transplant recipients. Tocilizumab, an anti–IL-6 receptor mAb, was effective in several desensitization regimens in highly sensitized transplant candidates. Several case studies have also demonstrated efficacy of tocilizumab in treating chronic active AMR, with significant reductions in DSA and stabilization of eGFR. A recent case-control series found that in lung transplant patients with chronic AMR, treatment regimens with tocilizumab had more clearance of DSA and lower rates of graft failure compared with treatment regimens without tocilizumab.[44] One phase II open-label study of clazakizumab (anti–IL-6) found that in 20 highly HLA-sensitized patients with end-stage renal disease awaiting kidney transplantation, clazakizumab along with plasma exchange and IVIG resulted in significant reduction in both class I and class II antibodies, enabling 18 of 20 patients to be successfully transplanted.[45] A recent randomized controlled clinical trial of clazakizumab in renal allograft recipients with chronic active AMR found that clazakizumab stabilized the eGFR after initiation of therapy and resulted in a significant reduction in DSA levels and C4d staining in the allografts.[46]

NOVEL THERAPIES TARGETING B CELLS AND ANTIBODIES

In addition to IL-6–directed therapies, some efforts to reduce alloantibody in highly sensitized transplant candidates have used the new drug imlifidase, a recombinant cystine protease derived from *Streptococcus pyogenes* that can rapidly cleave all four IgG subclasses. Imlifidase binds and cleaves just below the hinge region of IgG, and the resulting fragments can no longer mediate their antibody-dependent cytotoxic effects and are rapidly cleared from circulation. Some pilot studies have demonstrated that imlifidase can successfully allow transplantation of highly sensitized recipients, although the drug is limited by a "rebound effect" of DSA that could constrain long-term transplant success. Another novel B-cell–directed therapy with investigational use in transplantation is belimumab, an mAb directed against B-cell–activating factor (BAFF). BAFF is a soluble mediator secreted by a variety of cells (including monocytes and macrophages) that interacts with BCRs such as BAFF receptor (BAFF-R), B-cell maturation antigen (BCMA), and transmembrane activator and calcium modulator and cyclophilin ligand interactor (TACI). By disrupting BAFF signaling, belimumab suppresses B-cell survival and leads to reduced numbers of circulating B cells. One small trial of belimumab in renal transplant patients has been published, and it found belimumab was a safe adjunct therapy to conventional immunosuppression, although surprisingly no expected reduction in B cells in belimumab-treated patients was noted.[47]

Complications of Immunosuppression

The development of immunosuppressive agents was the key step in the advancement of the field of transplantation. Unfortunately, these same agents are responsible for much of the morbidity associated with organ transplantation as well. All current immunosuppressants function to a greater or lesser degree in a nonspecific fashion (i.e., global immunosuppression instead of donor-specific or allospecific immunosuppression). The consequence is occasional overzealous suppression of the immune system, resulting in infectious complications, primarily viral infections, as well as an increased risk of malignant disease. In addition, many of these agents modify the function of proteins and pathways required for normal cell function, and consequently, their inhibition results in undesired, nonimmune side effects, including direct organ injury.

Risk of Infection

There is a fine balance between sufficient immunosuppression to prevent rejection and preservation of the host response to nontransplant antigens and pathogens. Introduction of tissue from one individual to another always introduces the potential for transfer of new organisms. Currently, an extensive battery of testing is performed on both the donor and recipient before transplantation. These examinations have greatly decreased the potential exposure to the recipient, but no test is perfect, and testing can be limited by available technology and the time interval between procurement and implantation. Some infections may still be transferred unknowingly for various reasons, including early infection and lack of seropositivity. Infections may be donor derived, such as a CMV-positive organ placed into a CMV-negative recipient, or may arise from less commonly transferred viruses, resulting in primary infections of HIV, hepatitis C virus, hepatitis B virus, tuberculosis, *Trypanosoma cruzi*, West Nile virus, lymphocytic choriomeningitis virus, or rabies.[48]

The threat comes not only from new pathogens but, more importantly, from those to which the recipient has likely already been exposed and harbors in a state of dormancy or latency. Normally, these pathogens are controlled after the initial infection and remain quiescent. After the immune system is rendered impotent by pharmacologic suppression, these pathogens can spring to life and quickly become uncontrollable. Recipient-derived infections are much more common after transplantation than donor-derived infections. One common example is CMV reactivation. The majority of the population has been exposed to CMV at some point in their lives. In the setting of induction and maintenance immunosuppressive therapy in transplantation, CMV reactivation can occur, resulting in pneumonitis, hepatitis, pancreatitis, or colitis. CMV has also been implicated in the lesions of heart transplant recipients with chronic rejection, highlighting the interplay between the immune response and chronic viral infections or the inflammation they may induce. Other recipient-derived infections include tuberculosis, certain parasites (*Strongyloides stercoralis*, *T. cruzi*), viruses (e.g., CMV, EBV, herpes simplex, varicella-zoster, hepatitis B, hepatitis C, and HIV), and endemic fungi (e.g., *Pneumocystis jiroveci*, *Histoplasma capsulatum*, *Coccidioides immitis*, and *Paracoccidioides brasiliensis*).

Fortunately, patterns of opportunistic infections after transplantation have been altered by the use of routine antimicrobial prophylaxis. The risk for reactivation is highest approximately 6 to 12 weeks after transplantation and again after periods of increased immunosuppression for acute rejection episodes. Transplant programs use various prophylactic regimens, depending on the organs transplanted. Many regimens include pneumococcal vaccine, hepatitis B vaccine, and trimethoprim-sulfamethoxazole for *Pneumocystis* pneumonia and urinary tract infections; ganciclovir or valganciclovir for CMV infections; and clotrimazole troche or nystatin for oral and esophageal fungal infections. As immunosuppressive strategies have evolved, resulting in increases in both allograft and patient survival, the specific pathogens as well as the pattern of infection have also evolved. For example, the polyomaviruses BK and JC have been recognized to play a more important role in transplantation than previously understood. Infection with the polyomavirus BK has been found in association with a progressive nephropathy and ureteral obstruction, and the JC virus has been associated with progressive multifocal leukoencephalopathy. Detection of BK viral DNA in blood and urine has been useful for monitoring response to therapy, which includes minimizing immunosuppression and treatment with antiviral therapies.

Risk for Malignant Disease

The immune system not only plays a critical role in defending the host against attack from pathogens, it also plays an important role in the surveillance and detection of cancer, particularly those cancers driven by viral infection. The consequence is a nearly tenfold increase in rates of malignant disease. Skin cancers, particularly squamous cell cancers, are the most common malignant conditions in transplant recipients and account for substantial morbidity and mortality.[49] As expected, virally mediated tumors tend to occur much more frequently in transplant recipients. For example, human papillomavirus is associated with cancer of the cervix, hepatitis B and C viruses with hepatocellular carcinoma, and human herpesvirus 8 with Kaposi sarcoma. EBV, in particular, can be associated with the development of PTLD, a broad term used to describe EBV-associated lymphomas that occur in transplant recipients. PTLD varies from asymptomatic to life threatening, and, accordingly, treatment varies from simple reduction or withdrawal of immunosuppression to vigorous chemotherapeutic regimens. More recently, patients have been treated with antiviral agents targeting EBV or even chemotherapy including antibody therapy against the tumor cells, such as rituximab.

Nonimmune Side Effects

Although current immunosuppressants have become increasingly more specific, in general, they are still directed at pathways that play an important role in multiple systems other than immunity. Thus, inhibition of a pathway for the sake of immunosuppression can also lead to unintended consequences if the target is critical to other processes. For example, CNIs are potent suppressors of T-cell activation, but their activity not only decreases IL-2 transcription but also increases TGF-β expression. Elevated levels of TGF-β result in an increase in endothelin expression and eventually lead to hypertension. In addition, TGF-β is thought to play a critical role in the development of chronic allograft nephropathy, previously thought to be immune mediated but now likely to be, at least partly, secondary to nonimmune side effects secondary to CNI use.

Histologic evidence of CNI-associated nephrotoxicity is essentially universal in renal transplants by 10 years. Furthermore, these deleterious effects are not limited to only renal transplant recipients. The incidence of chronic renal failure in nonrenal transplant recipients is an astonishing 16.5%.[50] New-onset diabetes after transplantation is also an important problem, particularly in individuals receiving tacrolimus or steroids. The incidence of new-onset immunosuppressive-related diabetes mellitus approaches 30% in the first 2 years after renal transplantation, conferring a significantly higher risk of death. In addition to renal failure, hypertension, and diabetes, immunosuppressive therapy can lead to hyperlipidemia, anemia, and accelerated cardiovascular disease, which is a leading cause of death in long-term transplant survivors. Thus, it appears that the very reagents that ushered in a new era of short-term success in organ transplantation have proven to be major contributors to the demise of the transplanted organ or recipient over the long term. Clearly, there is a pressing clinical need to develop novel immunosuppressive agents that are effective and more specific yet less toxic, or to devise strategies to induce immune tolerance so that long-term immunosuppression may eventually be eliminated altogether.

TOLERANCE

Immunologic tolerance, or the maintenance of allograft function without immune suppression, has been fittingly thought of as the "holy grail" of transplantation biology, as it has been the subject of noble scientific pursuit that remains a mystery and has yet to be discovered. Self-tolerance, as discussed before, involves regulation of the immune response to prevent undesired effects toward host tissues or proteins. This is established and maintained through both central (i.e., thymic selection and deletion) and peripheral mechanisms. The ability to selectively inactivate the host response toward only the transplanted donor antigens while maintaining immunocompetence would be highly desirable. This would avoid the need for lifelong immunosuppression with its associated toxicities as well as eliminate chronic rejection, a major cause of late graft failure.

It has been more than 50 years since the first reports of acquired tolerance. The discovery of neonatal transplantation tolerance has been credited to Ray Owen, a geneticist who studied the inheritance of red blood cell antigens in cattle. He reported in 1945 that dizygotic twins had mixtures of their own cells and their twin partner's cells. Earlier observations had demonstrated that bovine dizygotic twins develop a fusion of their placentas during embryonic life. This results in a common intrauterine circulation and the unabated passage of sex hormones, explaining the phenomenon of freemartin cattle. Owen also recognized that this common circulation allows the exchange of hematopoietic cells during embryonic life and the establishment of a chimeric state. Interestingly, these calves did not develop isoantibodies to their twin, suggesting a state of immunologic tolerance.

Peter Medawar acknowledged the importance of Owen's observation and predicted that an exchange of skin grafts between dizygotic calves could verify the tolerance hypothesis, and together with his postdoctoral fellow, Rupert Billingham, he performed a series of grafting experiments that provided direct support for the concept of neonatally acquired transplantation tolerance. Subsequent experiments by Billingham, Leslie Brent, and Medawar demonstrated that neonatally acquired transplantation tolerance could be achieved in mice by inoculation of embryos or intravenous injection of newborn mice with allogeneic cells. Medawar shared the Nobel Prize in 1960 for the discovery of acquired immunologic tolerance.

Just as there are multiple methods to provide for self-tolerance in any given individual, there have been many proposed strategies to induce transplantation tolerance exploiting these pathways. Some of these include clonal deletion or elimination of donor-reactive cells, clonal anergy or functional inactivation of donor-reactive cells, and regulation or suppression of donor-reactive cells. There are rare reports of patients who have discontinued immunosuppression for various reasons and have not experienced rejection. Ongoing studies within this small population of operationally tolerant patients seek to determine what mechanisms are responsible for graft maintenance in the absence of immunosuppression. One such study suggests that those kidney transplant patients who discontinue their immunosuppressive treatments for whatever reason and continue to enjoy stable allograft function also have elevated numbers of naïve and transitional B cells in their peripheral blood compared with those patients who remain on immunosuppression, suggesting a role for this cell population in the tolerant state.[51] Interestingly, several populations of regulatory B cells (Bregs) have been described by different investigators, although these are not nearly as well described as the corresponding Treg population. These Bregs often express the immunosuppressive cytokine IL-10, and many described subsets are also positive for the surface marker T-cell immunoglobulin and mucin domain 1 (TIM-1).

There are numerous reports of intentionally induced tolerance in experimental models, but most of these are not effective when translated to higher animal models such as nonhuman primates. Although there are several exciting avenues of research and even clinical trials in humans, currently there is no proven regimen to reliably induce transplantation tolerance that would be widely applicable. Here are a few strategies of particular interest that are currently under investigation.

Lymphocyte Depletion

Most currently employed immunosuppressive regimens involve the use of induction therapy. Many rely on some form of antilymphocyte preparation, most commonly RATG, to eliminate or inactivate recipient cells at the time of transplantation. They are used in the very early posttransplantation period, which corresponds to the time when ischemia and reperfusion of the graft accompanied by the surgical trauma significantly increase immune recognition. These preparations successfully remove T cells from the circulation for several days, and those that are present remain anergic for some period. Use of these agents has significantly reduced the rate of acute rejection and allowed minimization of immunosuppression in several different protocols. A number of groups have undertaken clinical trials using early recipient T-cell depletion in combination with various other immunosuppressive strategies in an attempt to induce tolerance. The prevailing concept is one of T-cell clone reduction in an effort to allow existing tolerance mechanisms to be effective. Several studies have used alemtuzumab to induce profound T-cell depletion for this purpose. Despite achieving depletion that was similar to promising preclinical studies with respect to kinetics, magnitude, and effectiveness within the secondary lymphoid tissues, treatment with alemtuzumab alone or in combination with deoxyspergualin was not sufficient to induce tolerance in adult humans.[31] Newer studies have combined alemtuzumab with belatacept and rapamycin with promising results, although tolerance was not achieved.[52] The failure of these T-cell–centric approaches suggests that other components of the immune system, such as B cells, NK cells, or monocytes, may also need to be specifically targeted to achieve tolerance. Whereas depletion alone has not been able to establish tolerance, it has allowed minimization of immunosuppression to a single agent in some cases and likely facilitates other protolerant approaches.

Costimulation Blockade

T-cell activation requires not only interaction between the TCR complex and MHC-bound peptide but also sufficient costimulatory signals to promote a successful response. TCR ligation in the absence of appropriate costimulation results in T-cell inactivation or anergy. This mechanism is used presumably as a mechanism of peripheral tolerance to control any aberrant, self-reactive T cell that may have escaped the thymic selection process. Researchers have tried to exploit this through the development of antibodies or fusion proteins designed to block these costimulatory interactions. Interruption of costimulatory pathways at the time of transplantation should thus selectively inactivate or anergize only those cells specific for donor antigen, leaving nonreactive cells unaffected. Preexisting immunity and innate responses should be unaffected by this approach. There are multiple animal models of transplantation in which this has proven to be the case, particularly with simultaneous blockade of the CD28 and CD40 pathways.[53] This approach in both rodents and primates has resulted in prolonged survival of cardiac and renal allografts without the

need for any subsequent immunosuppression and without significant infectious or malignant side effects. However, the extrapolation of these results to clinical practice has been disappointing thus far. In the only human tolerance trial of costimulation blockade, hu5C8, a humanized anti-CD154 mAb, demonstrated limited efficacy and was associated with potential thromboembolic toxicity. Newly developed agents that block the CD28 pathway are now being tested as maintenance agents, which may pave the way for use in future tolerance trials. In addition, numerous other therapeutic reagents have been or are in development (such as antibodies to CD40, CD134 [OX40L], ICOS, and many other costimulatory pathways). It remains to be seen which of these will make it through the gauntlet of drug development, but there are exciting possibilities for future tolerance regimens.

Chimerism

Hematopoietic chimerism is associated with a particularly robust form of donor-specific tolerance. This approach involves both central and peripheral mechanisms for induction and maintenance of tolerance. Complete chimerism classically occurs in bone marrow transplantation where all bone marrow–derived cells in a recipient are eliminated and replaced by donor cells. However, the morbidity associated with the myeloablative conditioning required to achieve complete chimerism precludes it as a viable method of tolerance induction in solid organ transplantation. Hence, mixed chimerism refers to a recipient who possesses both self- and donor-derived hematopoietic cells after bone marrow transplantation and requires less morbid and milder forms of preconditioning to achieve. In chimeric states, similar to the normal physiologic process, donor marrow elements migrate to the thymus and participate in thymic selection, resulting in central deletion of potentially donor-reactive T cells. Presumably similar events occur within the bone marrow for B-cell selection. The peripheral compartment can be pharmacologically deleted in a nonspecific fashion at the time of transplantation, or alternatively, donor antigen delivered at the time of bone marrow infusion engages donor-reactive cells in the absence of appropriate costimulation as a result of concomitantly administered immunosuppression, causing peripheral deletion, anergy, or regulation and resulting in donor-specific nonresponsiveness.

In humans, successful bone marrow transplantation and complete chimerism allow the acceptance of subsequent organ allografts from the same donor in the absence of immunosuppression. Conventional bone marrow transplantation regimens, however, are typically myeloablative in nature, and the associated toxicities are too great for them to be employed as part of a solid organ tolerance trial. Newer advances in nonmyeloablative techniques with less toxicity have since paved the way for the clinical application and testing of mixed chimerism–based strategies. An initial trial to test the efficacy of a mixed chimerism strategy to induce tolerance was performed in highly selected patients suffering from both end-stage renal failure and multiple myeloma. These patients simultaneously received bone marrow and a kidney from an HLA-identical sibling. The regimen led to chimerism in all six patients; four had transient chimerism, and the remaining two progressed into full chimeras. Three patients remain operationally tolerant without any immunosuppression after a reported follow-up of up to 7 years. The same group of investigators reported on a similar protocol in haploidentical living related donor-recipient pairs that resulted in the successful induction of transient chimerism and tolerance. None of these patients possessed concomitant indications for bone marrow transplantation, such as multiple myeloma, as was the case in the first trial. One allograft was lost to irreversible humoral rejection, but remarkably, the other four recipients have sustained stable renal allograft function for up to 5 years after complete withdrawal of immunosuppressive drugs.[54] The conditioning regimen required resulted in profound T-, B-, and NK-cell depletion and substantial myelosuppression, leading to severe leukopenia and capillary leak syndrome. Interestingly, the biologic phenomenon that inspired the protocol, mixed chimerism, was not achieved in any patient, suggesting that the predominant effect is one of intensive induction.

Newer approaches have involved nonmyeloablative techniques combined with cell-based therapies to facilitate chimerism and tolerance induction. Cell-based therapies have consisted of a variety of different cell types, including modified hematopoietic stem cell preparations, Tregs, tolerogenic dendritic cells, and regulatory macrophages, among others. One notable phase II trial combined reduced-intensity conditioning with facilitator cell-enriched hematopoietic stem cell transplantation in HLA-mismatched living donor kidney transplant recipients. Of 31 subjects with more than 12 months of follow-up, 22 patients achieved stable donor chimerism and were weaned off immunosuppression. However, not all subjects achieved chimerism and discontinuation of immunosuppression, and several experienced recurrent autoimmunity and infectious complications resulting in graft loss.[55] Two patients developed graft-versus-host disease, resulting in one death. Therefore, although these approaches show promise for immunosuppression withdrawal in a portion of transplant recipients, the incidence and durability of tolerance, the rate and severity of graft-versus-host disease, and the long-term effects of intensive conditioning remain to be determined before these regimens find a role in clinical practice.

Adoptive Cell Transfer Therapy

Several groups have recently tried to achieve allograft tolerance through stimulation of peripheral tolerance via adoptive transfer of immunomodulatory cells. Several groups have sought to expand autologous polyclonal CD4+/CD25+/FoxP3+ Tregs and then adoptively transfer into an allograft recipient to generate durable peripheral tolerance against an allograft. This strategy has shown success in both nonhuman primate and some pilot human clinical trials, but it is generally limited by the difficulties of enriching and expanding Tregs ex vivo as well as by the less potent immunosuppressive effects of polyclonal rather than donor-specific Tregs. An alternative strategy to mitigate these difficulties is to rely on chimeric antigen receptor Tregs (CAR-Tregs). This strategy transduces autologous Tregs with the gene encoding a CAR, which recognizes donor-specific HLA molecules through a single-chain variable fragment (scFv) domain, which is a fusion protein of the variable's regions of the heavy and light chains of a donor-specific immunoglobulin. This scFv domain is usually coupled to the intracellular signaling domain of CD3ζ as well as additional intracellular costimulatory domains (such as CD28), allowing activation of the CAR-Treg after binding to donor-HLA molecules. CAR-Tregs allow the generation of a large quantity of allograft-specific Tregs, thus maximizing potential immunosuppression of alloimmunity. The STEADFAST trial is a phase I/II, first-in-human clinical trial of CAR-Tregs in recipients of living donor renal transplants, and it is currently enrolling. Finally, some investigators have also explored whether adoptive transfer of bone marrow–derived mesenchymal stem cells can confer allograft tolerance, given the well-described immunosuppressive effects of this cell population. One small pilot trial (the TRITON study) found that adoptive transfer of allogeneic mesenchymal stromal cells enabled early withdrawal of tacrolimus in many renal transplant patients without an increase in allorejection and with preserved renal function compared with a control group on conventional tacrolimus-based immunosuppression.[56]

NEW AREAS OF TRANSPLANTATION

Xenotransplantation

The most pressing problem in clinical transplantation is the shortage of available organs. More than 100,000 individuals are currently listed and awaiting organ transplantation. Several strategies have emerged to expand the available organ pool for patients with end-stage organ failure, including the dramatically increased use of matched-pairs kidney exchanges to increase the number of living donor transplants, the use of hepatitis B– or hepatitis C–infected donor organs in noninfected recipients, the use of HIV-infected donor organs in HIV-positive transplant candidates, and a significantly expanded use of organs from donors after cardiac death (abetted by improved donor organ procurement technologies such as normothermic machine perfusion and normothermic regional perfusion). Even with these developments, however, constraints of the organ supply significantly limit access to transplantation to many patients who could potentially benefit. Xenotransplantation, the use of organs from another species, has long been offered as a potential source of a nearly unlimited organ supply for transplant patients, although a host of significant immunologic, technical, and ethical barriers remain unresolved. Norman Shumway, the pioneering heart transplant surgeon at Stanford, once famously declared that "xenotransplantation is the future, and always will be." Although his pessimism has long seemed well-grounded, recent advents have poured renewed energy into the field of xenotransplantation.

Many of the earliest examples of vascularized xenotransplants were so-called *concordant xenotransplants,* using organs from closely related species, such as transplants of nonhuman primate organs into humans. In the 1960s, Keith Reemtsma of Tulane University performed a series of 13 chimpanzee kidney transplants into patients; although most patients died within 1 to 2 months, one of the patients lived for 9 months and even returned to work as a schoolteacher. Several other early pioneers in transplant, such as Tom Starzl (who performed the first successful human liver *allo*transplant) and James Hardy (who performed the first successful human lung *allo*transplant), also experimented with xenotransplants using primate organs, but with abysmal results. Perhaps the most famous early example of concordant xenotransplant was the "Baby Fae" case, where Dr. Leonard Bailey transplanted a baboon heart into a female infant with left hypoplastic heart syndrome in 1983.[57] This transplant attracted significant coverage in the lay media, and although technically successful, the patient died of acute rejection on postoperative day 20. Besides the lack of long-term survival in these early case series, the use of concordant xenotransplants is significantly limited by the fact that the need for donor organs far outstrips the available supply of nonhuman primates, potent ethical concerns about using primates as organ donors (given the close evolutionary link between humans and primates), and concerns that zoonotic viral transmission between primates and humans poses a threat that would outweigh the benefits of transplantation on a societal level. Given these factors, it is unlikely that concordant xenotransplantation will ever gain widespread application.

Most of the recent investigations of xenotransplantation have pursued discordant xenografts—transplantation between dissimilar species—most often using porcine donors. Pigs offer many advantages for xenotransplantation compared with nonhuman primates: they are better size matched for most adult humans compared with primates, there is an abundant worldwide supply of pigs, and there are far fewer ethical concerns regarding use of porcine organs (given that pigs have been raised for human consumption for millennia). However, discordant xenografts do pose more significant immunologic barriers, mainly because of the differential carbohydrate expression on the cell surfaces of pig cells compared with humans. Specifically, pigs possess an $\alpha(1$-$3)$-galactosyltransferase enzyme (GGTA1) and therefore express galactose-α-1,3-galactose (also known as α-Gal) sugar moieties on most cell surfaces. As humans lack this enzyme, they have a high degree of preformed IgM antibodies against cell surface carbohydrate moieties, particularly α-Gal. These so-called *natural antibodies* are similar to those antibodies that define the blood group antigens. In transplantation, they bind to the endothelial cells on the donor organ and induce a hyperacute rejection in concert with complement, precipitating an irreversible reaction of cell damage, thrombosis, and immediate graft failure. As with concordant xenografts, the remainder of the acquired and innate immune responses may also play an important role in the rejection process.

A major advance in the field of xenotransplantation was the development of genetic knockout pigs that lack the GGTA1 gene encoding $\alpha(1$-$3)$-galactosyltransferase in 2002, which significantly extended the function of xenograft hearts in a pig-to-primate preclinical transplant model (Fig. 49.26).[58] The advent of CRISPR/Cas9 transgenic techniques and refinement of somatic cell nuclear transfer enabled the generation of pigs possessing multiple genetic manipulations intended to prolong xenograft survival. Some of these manipulations delete other genes (such as *β4GalNT2* and *CMAH*) that produce non-Gal cell-surface glycans that are targets for human natural antibodies, thereby reducing the risks of hyperacute rejection. Other genetic manipulations added transgenic human complement-regulatory proteins such as human decay-accelerating factor (hDAF; CD55) and membrane cofactor protein (MCP, CD46), transgenes intended to quell xenorejection such as inhibitory HLA-E or HLA-G, and transgenes for human coagulation regulatory proteins such as thrombomodulin and endothelial protein C receptor (as many groups had observed a posttransplant thrombotic microangiopathy in xenograft organs, which was attributed to the inability of porcine regulatory proteins to interact with human thrombin and protein C). Finally, some groups used CRISPR/Cas9 to knock out the loci of porcine endogenous retroviruses (PERVs), which were the most concerning zoonotic infections that could theoretically infect recipients of porcine xenotransplants. Recently, a commercial company published their work generating a pig for use as a xenotransplant donor with 69 distinct genetic manipulations and demonstrated up to 2 years of renal xenograft survival using these donor pigs in a nonhuman primate model and clinically relevant immunosuppression.[59] Bolstered by recent rapid advances in the field and demonstrated long-term survival in pig-to-primate preclinical transplant models, investigators at the University of Alabama-Birmingham and NYU Langone Health have used a human decedent model to approach a step

closer to human clinical trials of xenotransplantation.[60] In these human decedent models, the families of brain-dead patients who are otherwise deemed not acceptable organ donors consent to have porcine xenograft kidneys or hearts transplanted into their loved ones, who continue to receive mechanical life support therapy for the duration of the experiment. Although the initial experiences with this decedent model were only for 54 to 72 hours, recently these institutions have extended the experiment for up to 2 months to better study the xenogeneic rejection responses. Investigators at the University of Maryland have now performed two life-sustaining porcine xenograft heart transplants in human patients who were otherwise not candidates for an allogeneic heart transplant. The first patient lived almost 2 months before succumbing, potentially because of an unrecognized porcine CMV in the donor heart (Fig. 49.27). The second patient died after almost 6 weeks from rejection, highlighting that significant challenges remain. Most recently, researchers at Massachusetts General Hospital transplanted a genetically modified porcine kidney into a patient whose dialysis access was failing. These early attempts of xenotransplantation into living patients have been approved by the FDA through their compassionate use exemption, but the field awaits the results of clinical trials before deciding whether the promise of widespread xenotransplantation to solve the organ shortage crisis can be realized.

Machine Perfusion

The shortage of available organs for transplant and the resulting burgeoning transplant waitlist is certainly one of the central challenges in transplantation today. One strategy to expand the supply of organs is to use normothermic machine perfusion of "marginal" organs that would otherwise be discarded, providing diagnostic or prognostic data and/or rehabilitating them and rendering them suitable for transplantation. These "marginal" organs might come from donors after circulatory death (DCDs), older donors, or steatotic donors (in the case of liver allografts). Both hypothermic and normothermic machine perfusion systems have been described, and there are conflicting data in the literature about which approach is superior. Use of machine perfusion helps minimize the ischemia-reperfusion injury that often accompanies prolonged cold static storage of organs in ice, greatly expanding the window of time in which the organs can be safely transplanted. Furthermore, machine perfusion systems also provide dynamic assessment of organ function by measurement of pH and lactate in the perfusion fluid of the machine, providing assurance that a marginal organ will not be a primary nonfunction (which would have particularly devastating consequences for organs such as the heart, lungs, and liver). Finally, there is some evidence that machine perfusion can remediate compromised allografts, allowing their posttransplant function to improve. Whereas DCDs were previously rarely employed in thoracic transplant, widespread use of machine perfusion has significantly expanded the supply and use of DCD heart and lung allografts in recent years. The advent of machine perfusion has also led to a recent dramatic expansion in the number of liver transplants performed using donors after cardiac death, as data from the International Randomized Trial to Evaluate the Effectiveness of the Portable Organ Care System (OCS) Liver for Preserving and Assessing Donor Livers for Transplantation (PROTECT trial) suggest that pumped livers have a lower incidence of early allograft dysfunction and lower

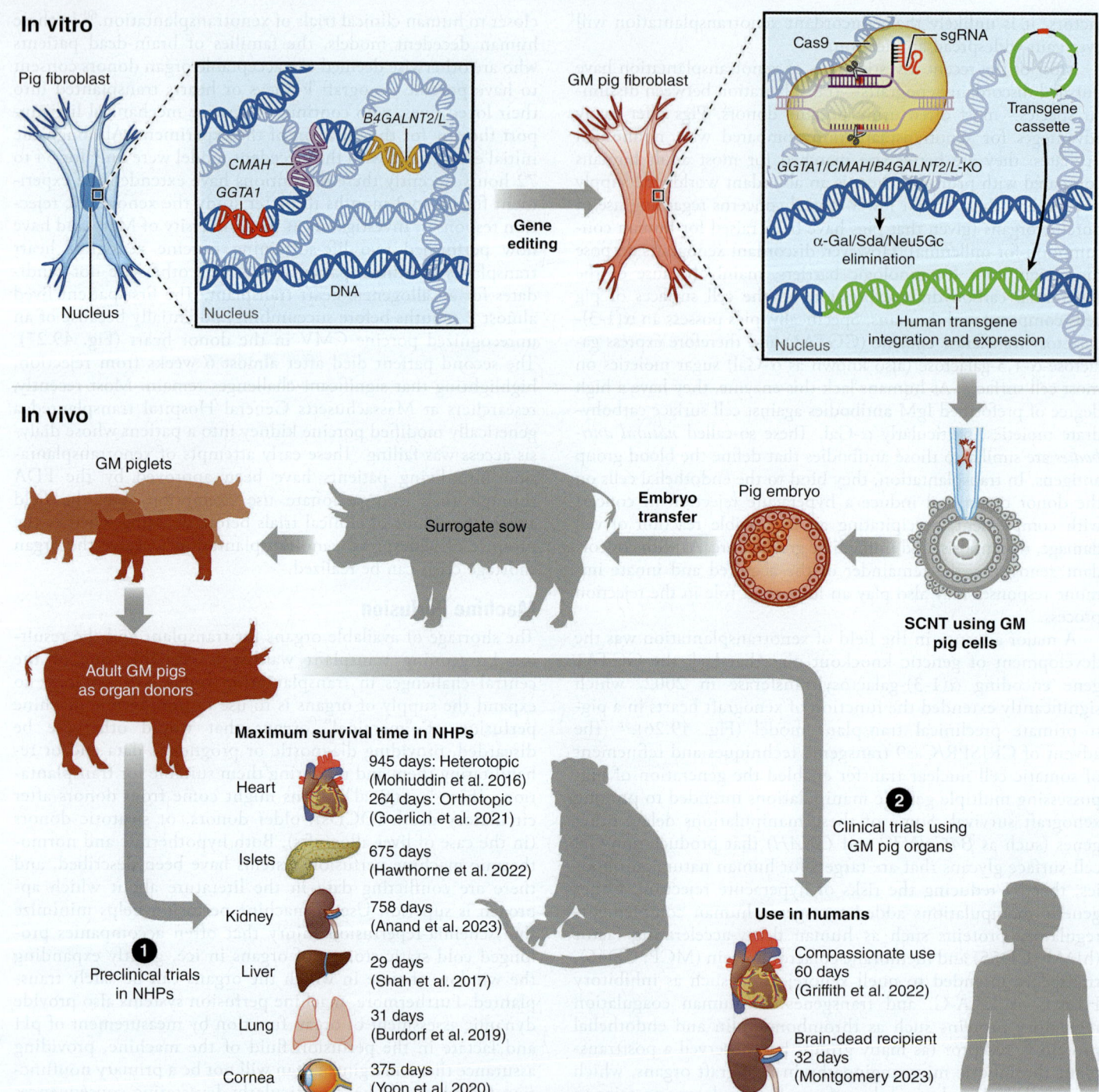

FIGURE 49.26 Advances in xenotransplantation. Using modern gene editing techniques such as CRISPR-Cas9, cloned pigs can be developed bearing multiple genetic modulations intended to render them better donors for xenotransplantation. Many of these genetic modifications target enzymes involved in creating cell surface carbohydrate moieties not present on human tissues, such as α-1,3-galactosyltransferase *(GGTA1)*, beta-1,4-*N*-acetyl-galactosaminyl transferase *(B4GALNT)*, and cytidine monophosphate-*N*-acetylneuraminic acid hydroxylase *(CMAH)*. These carbohydrates are prominent targets for natural antibodies that can provoke hyperacute rejection of xenografts. These genetically modified pigs have been used in preclinical transplant studies with nonhuman primate recipients, demonstrating substantially longer xenograft survival than historical experiments using nonmodified porcine donors. This success has led to several recent trials of xenografts in both human decedent models (where xenografts are transplanted into brain-dead human recipients who are kept alive with life support for the duration of experiment) and even some recent compassionate-use cases where porcine hearts were transplanted into human patients. *GM,* Genetically modified; *NHP,* nonhuman primate. (Adapted from Ali A, Kemter E, Wolf E. Advances in organ and tissue xenotransplantation. *Annu Rev Anim Biosci.* 2024;12:369-390.)

incidence of ischemic biliary strictures compared with allografts kept in cold static storage (Fig. 49.28).

Bioartificial Organs

The shortfall in organ availability has also led some investigators to explore the possibility that bioartificial organs might offer a new organ supply. Various bioengineering techniques have been employed to generate these bioartificial organs. Driven by the 3D printing revolution that has transformed many industries, some are exploring whether 3D bioprinting is a possibility, using microfluidics to "print" specific cells on a scaffold substrate in a bioreactor, thereby recapitulating tissues of interest. Currently, this technology is in its infancy. Another more developed strategy to develop bioartificial organs relies on decellularization of existing organs (such as organs recovered from donors but found to be unsuitable for transplant) by perfusing them with a detergent solution (usually sodium dodecyl sulfate). This decellularization leaves behind an extracellular matrix protein "scaffold" that can then be recellularized by perfusing it with a slurry of stem cells that help reconstitute a functioning organ. This strategy has been employed in porcine transplant models, showing transient function of bioartificial hearts, lungs, and renal allografts. The long-term survival of these bioartificial organs has not been observed, so it remains to be determined whether xenotransplantation or bioartificial organs might be the best ultimate strategy to expand our current organ supply.

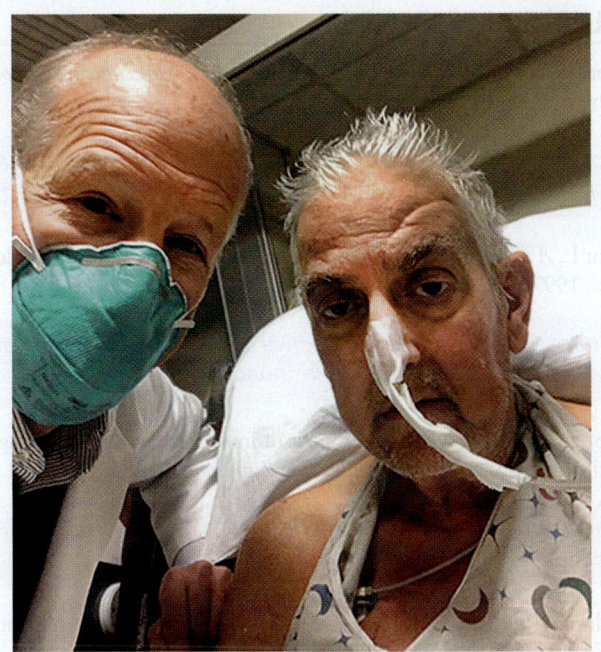

FIGURE 49.27 Progress in xenotransplantation. David Bennett (right) is shown with his cardiothoracic surgeon, Dr. Bartley Griffith, after receiving a cardiac xenograft from a genetically modified pig. Mr. Bennett survived almost 2 months posttransplant. (Courtesy the University of Maryland School of Medicine.)

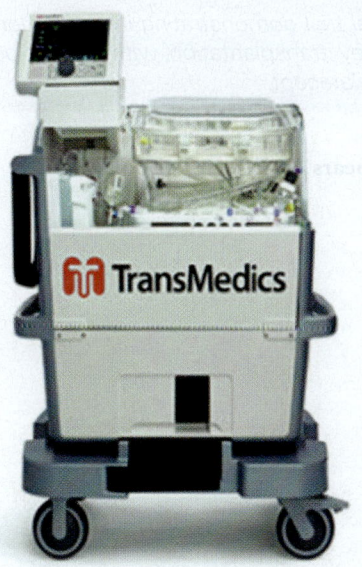

OCS Liver console

A

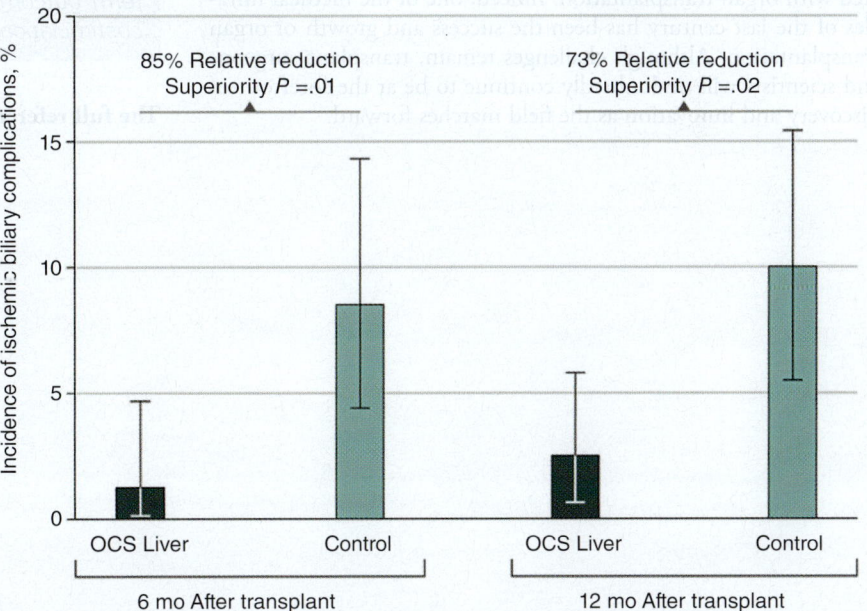

B

FIGURE 49.28 Normothermic machine perfusion. (A) The Transmedics Organ Care System, an FDA-approved normothermic machine perfusion system for use in liver transplantation. Similar pumps have also been used for heart and lung transplantation. (B) In the PROTECT trial, the incidence of both early allograft dysfunction and ischemic biliary strictures (shown) was far lower in liver allografts placed on the normothermic machine perfusion circuit after procurement compared with control allografts kept in cold static storage. OCS, Organ Care System. (Adapted from Markmann JF, Abouljoud MS, Ghobrial RM, et al. Impact of portable normothermic blood-based machine perfusion on outcomes of liver transplant: the OCS Liver PROTECT Randomized Clinical Trial. JAMA Surg. 2022;157[3]:189-198.)

CONCLUSION

More than a half-century has passed since the first successful solid organ transplantation. Today, thousands of patients with end-stage diseases undergo lifesaving transplantation each year. That which was once considered impossible is now an everyday occurrence, and most transplant recipients are leading healthy, productive lives with an organ from another individual functioning inside of them. The idea of replacing a diseased organ with a healthy one is simple in concept, yet the details of managing the rejection response is complex. The immune system typically generates a highly organized yet regulated response when challenged. Many of the principal details of the normal immune response were described by researchers examining the mechanisms of allograft rejection. In fact, surgeons garnered multiple Noble Prizes in Medicine for their significant contributions to the field. Whereas short-term allograft survival rates have steadily improved, long-term outcomes remain an area in need of significant improvement. The availability of adequate donor organs remains the most pressing issue restricting the majority of potential recipients from receiving a life-sustaining transplant. There continues to be progress in xenotransplantation and tissue engineering, and they may yet provide for an unlimited supply of safe, transplantable organs. There are significant drawbacks to current nonselective immunosuppressive therapies, such as increased risks of infections and malignant disease, economic constraints, and long-term metabolic toxicities, including renal insufficiency, diabetes, hyperlipidemia, and cardiovascular disease. Increasingly targeted immunosuppressive agents continue to be developed and tested. Ultimately, the goal is to achieve low-risk, donor-specific immunosuppression. The development of a safe, widely applicable regimen that reliably produces transplantation tolerance would eliminate many of the problems currently associated with organ transplantation. Indeed, one of the medical miracles of the last century has been the success and growth of organ transplantation. Although challenges remain, transplant surgeons and scientists will undoubtedly continue to be at the forefront of discovery and innovation as the field marches forward.

SELECTED REFERENCES

Abbas AK, Lichtman AH, Pillai S. *Cellular and Molecular Immunology*. 10th ed. Philadelphia: Saunders Elsevier; 2021.

Concise and well-established textbook of immunology that comprehensively surveys fundamental immunology.

Brent L. *A History of Transplantation Immunology*. San Diego: Academic Press; 1997.

Interesting historical perspective on the development and evolution of transplantation immunology.

Chong AS, Alegre ML. The impact of infection and tissue damage in solid-organ transplantation. *Nat Rev Immunol*. 2012;12:459-471.

Excellent review on the importance of the innate immune response in the rejection process.

Halloran PF. Immunosuppressive drugs for kidney transplantation. *N Engl J Med*. 2004;351:2715-2729.

Excellent overview of immunosuppression in the context of clinical transplantation.

Vincenti F, Rostaing L, Grinyo J, et al. Belatacept and long-term outcomes in kidney transplantation. *N Engl J Med*. 2016;374: 333-343.

Seminal report of clinical trial demonstrating improved long-term outcomes in kidney transplantation with the biologic costimulation blocker belatacept.

The full reference list appears on Elsevier eBooks+.

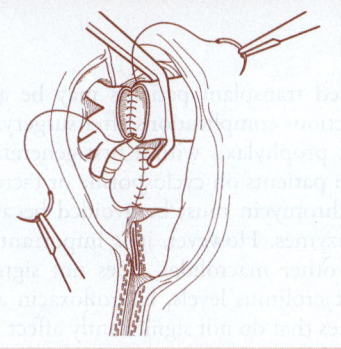

CHAPTER 51

Surgical Considerations in Transplant Patients Undergoing Nontransplant-Related Procedures and Operating in Patients With Portal Hypertension

Hassan Aziz, Jenna N. Whitrock, and Shimul A. Shah

OUTLINE

INTRODUCTION

With both short- and long-term survival rates improving after solid organ transplantation, a growing number of recipients need nontransplantation-related medical care, including elective or emergency surgery. Perioperative and intraoperative management principles are similar for transplant and nontransplant patients; however, there are a few key differences. This chapter discusses potential preoperative, intraoperative, and postoperative issues related to nontransplant surgery in transplant patients. It also highlights the principles of surgery in patients with portal hypertension.

OPERATING ON TRANSPLANT PATIENTS

Preoperative Risk Stratification

To develop an initial estimate of perioperative risk, clinicians must integrate information from patient history, physical examination, and laboratory tests. Significant coronary artery disease in transplant recipients undergoing noncardiac surgery is a common finding and therefore should be a preoperative consideration. Several clinical and surgical determinants can be used to stratify the cardiac risk. Patients with cardiac disease undergoing noncardiac surgery must be assessed for their clinical risk profile in relation to the surgery to be performed and its associated risks.[1]

Although successful kidney transplantation decreases the overall cardiovascular risk in patients with end-stage renal disease

(ESRD), cardiovascular disease is more prevalent in kidney transplant recipients than in the general population and remains the most common cause of death in kidney transplant patients. In addition, preexisting coronary artery disease progression can occur in posttransplant patients, largely because of immunosuppression contributing to de novo hyperlipidemia, hypertension, and diabetes. Because long-term studies on cardiac outcomes after nontransplant surgery in kidney transplant recipients are lacking, there are no specific recommendations for cardiovascular evaluation in transplant recipients. For previous kidney transplant patients undergoing nontransplant surgery, the American College of Cardiology/American Heart Association (ACC/AHA) guidelines for perioperative cardiovascular evaluation should be used to guide preoperative cardiovascular testing.[2]

Glucocorticoids

In the past, patients receiving azathioprine-based immunosuppression regimens frequently received chronic glucocorticoids, which caused characteristic side effects in many recipients. High perioperative doses of glucocorticoids are required in these patients because of adrenal suppression caused by high maintenance doses of steroids. In the era of more potent maintenance immunosuppressive agents such as tacrolimus, mycophenolate mofetil, and sirolimus, maintenance glucocorticoids are either reduced or avoided. As a result, adrenal suppression has become less problematic. It is generally unnecessary to administer high doses of glucocorticoids, and it may be contraindicated in some cases.[3]

The administration of high doses of glucocorticoids is not entirely benign and has occasionally been associated with gastritis, bleeding, induction of diabetes, and worsening of glycemic control. Although the cosyntropin test is often considered cumbersome, impractical, and somewhat unreliable, it can be used to help determine adrenal reserve in at-risk patients.

In those with adrenal insufficiency, glucocorticoids may be administered to patients starting at the time of anesthesia induction. Perioperative dosing of glucocorticoids depends on the surgical stress predicted to be caused by the procedure occurring. For example, in minor and moderately stressful procedures such as inguinal hernia repairs, colonoscopies, joint replacements, and colon resections, the patient's usual daily dose can be continued with 50 mg IV hydrocortisone given before incision followed by 25 mg IV every 8 hours for 24 hours before returning to the baseline dose. In major surgeries such as esophagectomy, hepaticojejunostomy, trauma, or major cardiac or vascular surgery, 100 mg IV hydrocortisone before incision followed by continuous IV infusion of hydrocortisone 200 mg for at least 24 hours or 50 mg every 8 hours for 24 hours followed by a taper can be given.[4] Perioperative infusion of glucocorticoids in this population may decrease the possibility of glucocorticoid deficiency as a cause of an adverse event such as hypotension, allowing the actual cause, like hemorrhage or volume depletion, to be identified and resolved.[5]

Another approach in managing patients on chronic glucocorticoids is to give half the baseline dose the day after surgery and resume the maintenance dose on the second postoperative day. Use of typical maintenance doses of glucocorticoids for this amount of time is unlikely to cause adverse effects. However, prolonged use of steroids can mask the signs and symptoms of infection and cause undesirable side effects, depicted in Fig. 51.1.

Mammalian Target of Rapamycin Inhibitors

The introduction of mammalian target of rapamycin (mTOR) inhibitors to the polydrug posttransplantation regimen led to an apparent increase in wound-related complications. This constitutes a serious clinical problem in the immediate posttransplantation period and in patients requiring further surgery while still receiving immunosuppressive drugs. In addition, studies have demonstrated that everolimus, administered as a single drug from the day of surgery onward, strongly interferes with restoring tissue strength in the intestinal tract and abdominal wall wounds.[6]

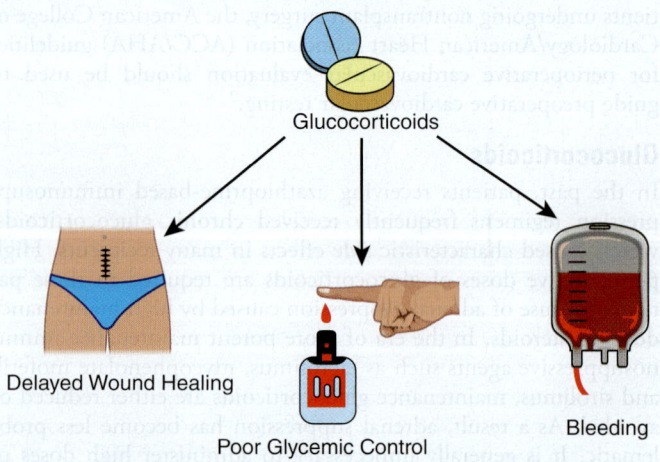

FIGURE 51.1 Potential complications from steroids.

Antibiotic Prophylaxis

Chronically immunosuppressed transplant patients may be at a higher risk of developing infectious complications after surgery. In most cases, routine antibiotic prophylaxis with a first-generation cephalosporin is sufficient.[7] In patients on cyclosporine or tacrolimus, erythromycin and clarithromycin must be avoided because they antagonize CYP 3A4 enzymes. However, it is important to note that azithromycin, like other macrolides, does not significantly affect cyclosporine or tacrolimus levels. Ciprofloxacin and clindamycin are safe alternatives that do not significantly affect the cyclosporine or tacrolimus levels.[8]

Surgical Outcomes

A recent study found that the incidence of emergency general surgery is significantly higher in transplant patients even after stratification by comorbidity burden.[7] In general, the published data suggest more complications in transplant patients undergoing nontransplant surgery than in nontransplant patients. For example, in patients undergoing cholecystectomy, mortality, morbidity, and length of stay were longer for kidney transplant recipients compared with nontransplant patients.[9] Similarly, in patients undergoing colorectal resections, in-hospital mortality was higher for kidney transplant recipients than nontransplant patients, as were overall complications. In addition, the length of stay was significantly longer and the cost was significantly greater in kidney transplant recipients than in nontransplant patients.[10–12] Similarly, studies have found that immunosuppressed patients experienced significantly higher rates of postoperative mortality after emergency surgery than immunocompetent patients undergoing surgery for diverticular disease.[13]

Wound Healing

Patients with chronic immunosuppression, even those receiving low doses of glucocorticoids, may have delayed wound healing after surgery.[14] Some immunosuppressive agents may exacerbate wound-healing complications during the immediate postoperative period.[14] Sirolimus is one example of an immunosuppressant that can lead to a higher incidence of adverse outcomes, such as wound complications. In one study, the incidence of allograft wound complications in the sirolimus group was significantly higher (47% vs. 8%) than the transplant recipients receiving tacrolimus.[15] There have also been reports of perigraft fluid collections, superficial wound infections, and incisional hernias associated with the use of sirolimus.[15,16]

Specific Surgical Problems

Transplant recipients have been shown to more commonly experience acute conditions requiring general emergency surgery, demonstrating a 3.6-fold higher incidence than their age-matched counterparts.[17] Surgical complications in transplant patients may be masked by chronic immunosuppressive therapy, which can lead to significant morbidity and mortality. A review of operative reports and common surgical incisions made for liver and kidney transplants is essential for operative planning (Fig. 51.2).

Acute appendicitis can be particularly difficult to diagnose in kidney or pancreatic transplant patients with transplanted organs in the right lower quadrant. The symptoms and signs are often uncharacteristic because the transplanted organ displaces the appendix superiorly (Fig. 51.3). The appendix is often perforated by the time a diagnosis is made, as these patients may either be asymptomatic or show no signs of a perforated viscus in terms of physical examination or laboratory data because of being

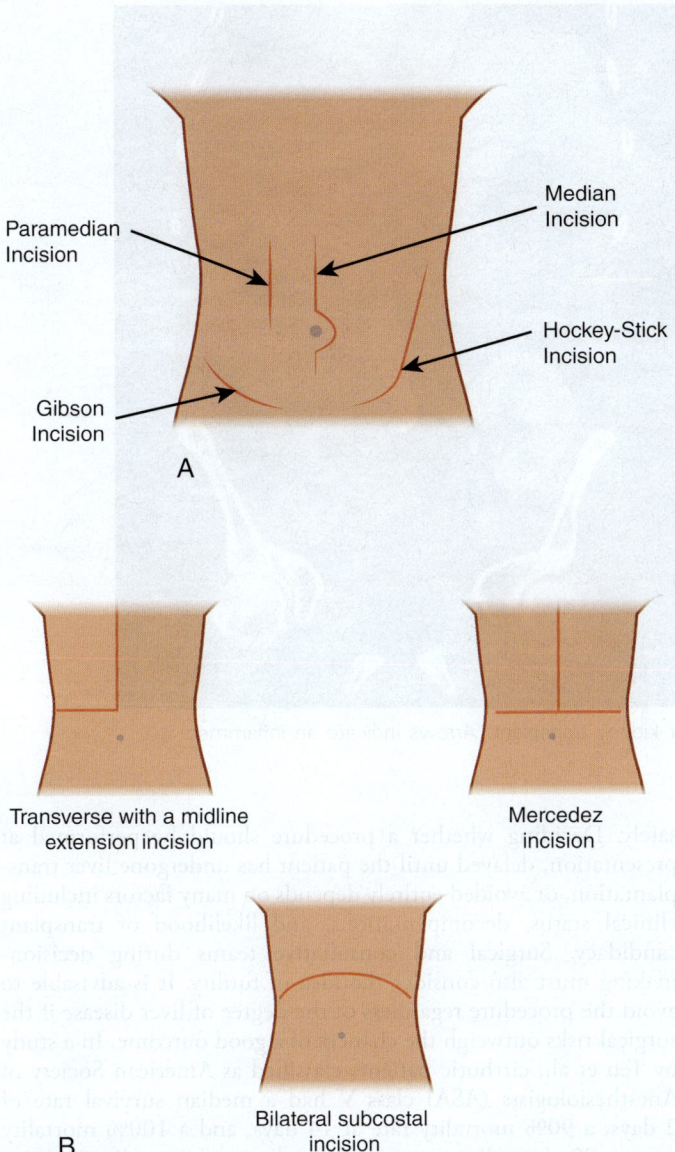

FIGURE 51.2 (A) Common incisions for kidney transplant. (B) Common incisions for liver transplant.

immunocompromised. Additionally, laparoscopic port placement may be challenging because of transplanted organ placement. For minimally invasive surgeries of the pelvis, such as colorectal or gynecologic procedures (e.g., colectomy or hysterectomy), attention should be paid to port placement. The transplanted kidney is placed retroperitoneally and should not be of concern to the operative surgeon. Upper gastrointestinal or hepatobiliary surgery, such as cholecystectomy, after a kidney transplant should be performed in the usual fashion, and port placement should not be affected.

Prior liver transplant and the formation of adhesions in the upper abdomen frequently lead to increased complexity in upper gastrointestinal surgery, such as sleeve gastrectomy. However, adhesions in transplant patients are typically less dense because of chronic steroid use and immunosuppression. Biliary anatomy after a liver transplant must also be considered, and operative reports from the transplant should be obtained preoperatively for any surgery involving the gastrointestinal tract, such as Roux-en-Y gastric bypass or total abdominal colectomy.

For example, if a Roux-en-Y hepaticojejunostomy was performed during the liver transplant, the surgeon should be aware before entry into the abdomen, if possible, so appropriate surgical planning can occur.

Other common surgical procedures performed after liver transplant are hernia repairs, especially umbilical and inguinal hernia repairs. Patients with ascites may develop incarceration of their umbilical or inguinal hernia as the ascites resolves after liver transplantation. Emergency repair of strangulated hernias should be performed. In cases of symptomatic or incarcerated hernias that do not require emergent intervention, it is ideal to wait 6 months to 1 year before interventions to allow patients to be weaned off steroids and most prophylactic medications. The use of mTOR inhibitors in transplantation surgery has been associated with increased wound complications and hernias. Animal studies have previously reported a negative effect of everolimus on anastomotic strength in rat intestines 7 days postoperatively.[18] This loss of strength was also accompanied by a decrease in the hydroxyproline content after 7 days, and the negative effect of everolimus on wound repair persisted for at least 4 weeks after the operation in this rodent model. Therefore, having the patient off mTOR inhibitors weeks before a planned surgery is ideal to help avoid unnecessary healing complications. Though no clinical studies describing differences in outcomes between open and laparoscopic hernia repair exist, the benefits of laparoscopic surgery seen in the general patient population, such as reduced postoperative pain, faster recovery, and fewer wound complications, remain true in transplant patients.

Dialysis access creation is occasionally needed after liver transplantation. The incidence of ESRD after nonrenal solid organ transplantation is increasing and is associated with a poor prognosis. The etiology of ESRD is multifactorial but is most commonly the result of calcineurin inhibitor nephrotoxicity. The impact of the dialysis modality on the survival of these patients remains unclear. An arteriovenous (AV) fistula is a better option than a peritoneal dialysis catheter, which is usually avoided in patients with recent liver transplants, ascites, or a current abdominal hernia.[19] Other factors to consider include adhesions after surgery, synthetic vascular grafts used during liver transplant, and concern for secondary peritonitis.[20] Peritoneal dialysis catheter placement should be avoided in patients being evaluated for liver transplantation because of several factors, including coagulopathy and thrombocytopenia, presence of abdominal wall varices, ascites, and inability to use it effectively after liver transplantation.

Repairing an abdominal aortic aneurysm (AAA) requires cross-clamping of the abdominal aorta to allow anastomosis between the distal and proximal aortas. In addition, a temporary bypass from the ipsilateral axillary artery to the femoral artery may be needed to ensure continuous arterial blood supply to the transplanted kidney. In this way, the aneurysm can be repaired precisely while reducing the risk of allograft thrombosis.

Tertiary hyperparathyroidism occurs in up to 40% of patients undergoing kidney transplants. Persistent elevation of serum parathyroid hormone can increase the risk for long-term bone loss and decrease allograft and patient survival after transplant. Parathyroidectomy has high cure rates and reduced graft failure rates.[21] However, recent data suggest that surgery may be underused compared with medical management in these patients. Therefore, these patients should be referred to endocrinology for hypercalcemia workup.

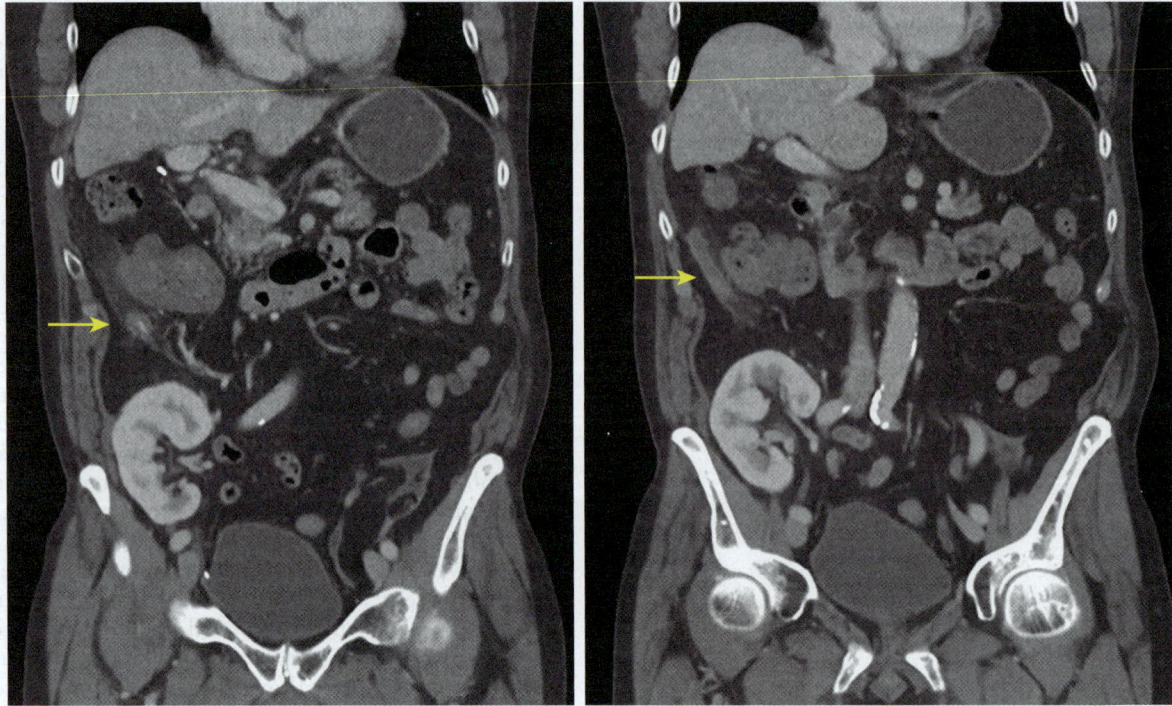

FIGURE 51.3 Acute appendicitis in a patient with prior kidney transplant. *Arrows* indicate an inflamed appendix.

OPERATING ON PATIENTS WITH PORTAL HYPERTENSION

Predicting Surgical Risk in a Patient With Cirrhosis

Surgical procedures that may be required in patients with cirrhosis can be categorized as procedures that improve a patient's quality of life, such as symptomatic hernia repairs, or as lifesaving procedures, such as cardiovascular surgery, cancer surgery, or emergency interventions. From simple procedures like umbilical hernia repairs (Fig. 51.4) to more complex liver resections for malignancy (Fig. 51.5), any surgery in a patient with cirrhosis poses unique challenges.

The first challenge for the care team is to assess the surgical risks before deciding whether the procedure can be carried out safely. Deciding whether a procedure should be performed at presentation, delayed until the patient has undergone liver transplantation, or avoided entirely depends on many factors including clinical status, decompensations, and likelihood of transplant candidacy. Surgical and consultative teams during decision-making must also consider the idea of futility. It is advisable to avoid the procedure regardless of the degree of liver disease if the surgical risks outweigh the chances of a good outcome. In a study by Teh et al., cirrhotic patients classified as American Society of Anesthesiologists (ASA) class V had a median survival rate of 2 days, a 90% mortality rate at 14 days, and a 100% mortality rate at 90 days. Postoperative mortality and complications increase with hepatic dysfunction, increased comorbidities, type of surgery, and decreased expertise of the management team.[22] The severity of liver disease appears to have the greatest impact on mortality risk. Another study found that cirrhotic patients undergoing coronary artery bypass graft had an eightfold increased risk of death compared with those without cirrhosis.[23] They also

FIGURE 51.4 Umbilical hernia in a patient with portal hypertension and large varices *(arrow)* seen.

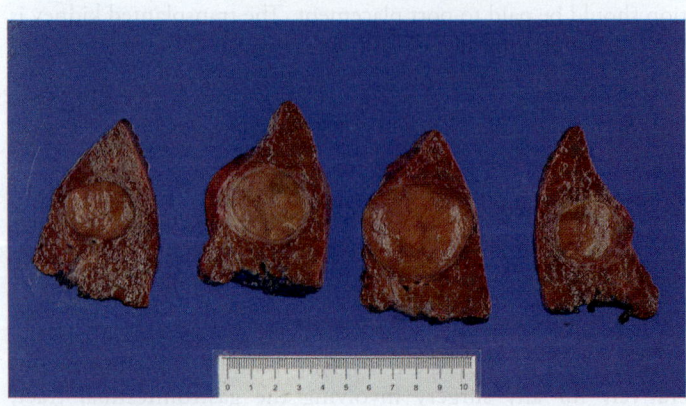

FIGURE 51.5 Malignancy in patients with cirrhosis.

found higher mortality rates in patients undergoing cholecystectomy, colectomy, or AAA repair.[23] Liver disease severity has traditionally been measured using the Child-Turcotte-Pugh (CTP) score (Child-Pugh class) and Model for End-Stage Liver Disease (MELD) score.

Child-Turcotte-Pugh Score

In patients with cirrhosis, the CTP score has been traditionally used to assess the severity of liver dysfunction and portal hypertension. Table 51.1 highlights the classification of CTP and its scoring system. Before the use of MELD scores, studies noted a good correlation between surgical mortality and Child-Pugh class when evaluated in combination with other variables.

Generally, patients with class A cirrhosis may be treated with surgery when there is no thrombocytopenia or clinically significant portal hypertension. Elective surgery is generally not considered for patients with class B or C cirrhosis.

However, recent analyses show less correlation between the Child-Pugh class and surgical outcomes, likely because of the low number of patients with Child-Pugh class C cirrhosis included in the modern series. In addition, patients with decompensated cirrhosis are more likely to avoid or not be offered surgery. Ascites, however, often correlates more reliably with poor surgical outcomes.

CTP scores have largely been supplanted by the MELD score for surgical risk stratification because of the subjective nature of assessing the severity of ascites and encephalopathy, which encapsulates the objective liver function–dependent components of the CTP score that are predictive of outcomes. In patients with severe portal hypertension but preserved hepatic synthetic function, the MELD score may be less effective, and the CTP score may be more useful.

Model for End-Stage Liver Disease Score

The MELD score was originally developed to predict mortality after transjugular intrahepatic portosystemic shunt (TIPS) placement. The MELD score can be calculated using the international normalized ratio (INR), serum creatinine level, and serum bilirubin level, with sodium also being considered in the more recent MELD-Na score. It has been shown that patients with preoperative MELD scores <16 have lower postoperative mortality rates than those with higher scores. Table 51.2 compares and contrasts the components of MELD and CTP scores.

An increase in the MELD score has been found to be positively correlated with postoperative mortality. Studies have shown that the most important predictors of mortality after surgery in patients with cirrhosis include the severity of cirrhosis as reflected by the MELD score, ASA classification and patient comorbidities, and age.[22] Others have shown that mortality is increased after surgery in the cirrhotic population for up to 90 days postoperatively after

TABLE 51.2 Components of MELD and CTP Scores

MELD SCORE COMPONENTS	CTP SCORE COMPONENTS
Bilirubin	Bilirubin
INR	INR
Creatinine	Serum albumin
Sodium (only included in MELD-Na)	Ascites
	Hepatic encephalopathy

CTP, Child-Turcotte-Pugh; *INR,* international normalized ratio; *MELD,* Model for End-Stage Liver Disease.

major surgery, independent of the type of surgery performed.[23] Not only has mortality been shown to increase in patients with cirrhosis after surgery, but studies have also demonstrated an increase in hospital cost and length of stay, even for those without portal hypertension.[24]

American Society of Anesthesiologists Classification

Since the early 1940s, the ASA physical classification system has been used as a measure of surgical anesthesia risk. ASA classification ranges from I to VI, with increasing classes representing increasing levels of comorbidities and illness, represented by Table 51.3. Although ASA score is correlated with surgical outcomes in some circumstances, it is generally regarded as a measure of disease severity or comorbidity rather than a direct predictor of outcomes, particularly in patients with cirrhosis. In addition, the classification system suffers from poor interobserver variability and is somewhat subjective. Moreover, there is no category for moderate diseases, only mild ones. Despite these weaknesses, ASA classification is still widely used for risk stratification before invasive procedures in the general surgical population and has been shown to correlate with increased mortality risk in patients with cirrhosis.[22–25]

Preoperative and Perioperative Evaluation and Management of the Patient With Cirrhosis

Patients with decompensated cirrhosis may be at high risk of complications from surgical procedures that are generally considered safe in the noncirrhotic population. A multidisciplinary medical and surgical team with extensive experience is essential for success. In this population, an informed decision about surgical procedures requires earnest, data-driven discussions with the patient and surgical teams.[23] The discussion should begin as early

TABLE 51.1 Child-Pugh Score

COMPONENT	1	2	3
Bilirubin	≤2 mg/mL	2–3 mg/mL	≥3 mg/mL
INR	≤1.6	1.7–2.2	≥2.3
Serum albumin	≥3.5 mg/mL	2.8–3.5 mg/mL	≤2.7 mg/mL
Ascites	None	Slight	Moderate
Hepatic encephalopathy	None	Grade 1 or 2	Grade 3 or 4
Class	**A = 5–6**	**B = 7–9**	**C = 10–15**

INR, International normalized ratio.

TABLE 51.3 ASA Classification

ASA CLASS	PATIENT DESCRIPTION
Class I	Normal healthy patient
Class II	Patient with mild systemic disease
Class III	Patient with severe systemic disease
Class IV	Patient with severe systemic disease that is a constant threat to life
Class V	Moribund patient who is unlikely to survive without intervention
Class VI	Patient who has been declared brain-dead

ASA, American Society of Anesthesiologists.
Excerpted from the ASA Physical Status Classification System, American Society of Anesthesiologists, 2020. asahq.org/standards-and-practice-parameters/statement-on-asa-physical-status-classification-system.

as possible in the process. For example, in patients undergoing elective or semielective procedures, ascites should be controlled, variceal bleeding should be reduced, acute hepatic encephalopathy should be treated preoperatively, and medical treatment should be continued to prevent recurrence. In addition, patients with cirrhosis are likely to have nonhepatic risk factors for surgical complications because of aging and the increasing prevalence of obesity, nonalcoholic steatohepatitis (NASH), and diabetes mellitus.[24]

There is evidence that class III obesity and cardiopulmonary disease are risk factors for morbidity and mortality regardless of liver disease severity. Most risk stratification scores do not include age; however, age is known to be an independent risk factor for medical and surgical complications. CTP and MELD scores predict surgical outcomes only in patients who are otherwise satisfactory candidates for surgery and have no significant comorbidities.[26] These complex patients often require cardiology and pulmonology consultations.

It is generally recommended that patients with cirrhosis avoid elective operations until liver disease can be optimally controlled. It is well-documented that patients with postoperative compensated cirrhosis may still be at risk for progression to decompensated cirrhosis. For chronic viral and autoimmune hepatitis, antiviral and immunosuppressive therapy must be adhered to strictly to prevent viral resistance and relapses.[27] To avoid treatment interruption, elective or semielective surgery may be delayed until therapy is completed. Patients with autoimmune hepatitis who cannot take oral medications such as corticosteroids may require alternative routes of drug administration.

For patients undergoing liver surgery, portal hypertension should be assessed. A measure such as the hepatic venous pressure gradient or the presence of gastroesophageal varices should be used instead of surrogate markers such as splenomegaly or thrombocytopenia.[28] Compared with patients without portal hypertension, patients with clinically significant portal hypertension have a double mortality rate and a threefold complication rate.[29]

Ascites

Practice guidelines recommend aggressive management of ascites before surgical procedures if possible. Ascites can restrict pulmonary function and delay recovery of lung function after surgery. A patient with ascites may also experience pulmonary aspiration during induction. Preoperatively, large-volume abdominal paracenteses should be performed in patients with symptomatic ascites, followed by intravenous administration of albumin 6 to 8 g/L of ascitic fluid removed.[30] According to practice guidelines, oral antibiotic prophylaxis can be started in patients with concern for development of spontaneous bacterial peritonitis or with low ascitic total protein concentrations once oral medications are tolerated. If a patient cannot take oral medications, third-generation cephalosporins such as ceftriaxone can be administered intravenously at 1 g every 24 hours until oral antimicrobials are tolerated. Patients with moderate to large pleural effusions that compromise respiratory function should be evaluated for preoperative thoracentesis. Blood products and intravenous fluids should be limited perioperatively to minimize the development of extracellular volume and ascites.[31] Surgical drains are usually avoided in the postoperative period because of infection concerns. These patients, however, may require serial paracentesis in the postoperative period.

TIPS placement before surgery has only been investigated in a few case reports and uncontrolled case series to reduce the risk of collateral vessels and intraabdominal variceal bleeding during surgery.[32] Although TIPS placement has been shown to reduce intraoperative blood transfusions, the available studies have been uncontrolled, and the frequency of complications such as hepatic encephalopathy was not reported.[33] Alternatively, studies comparing patients who underwent TIPS placement before liver transplantation with those who had not undergone TIPS placement revealed no differences in the need for red blood cell or plasma transfusions.[34] Furthermore, TIPS placed in the right atrium, inferior vena cava, or mesenteric veins of a patient undergoing nontransplant surgery may adversely affect future liver transplantation. Thus, preemptive TIPS placement before surgery is not recommended as a routine practice because of its unproven efficacy, lack of published evidence, high complication rates, and significant additional costs.

Hemostasis and Coagulation

Based on preoperative platelet counts and INRs, protocolized transfusion strategies do not reduce intraoperative or postoperative bleeding.[35] Patients with cirrhosis do not always have an increased risk of severe bleeding based on laboratory values alone. Procoagulant factor deficits are offset by anticoagulant protein deficits synthesized by the liver, resulting in a state of "rebalancing." As liver disease progresses, protein C deficiency may progress to thrombophilia in some patients. Therefore, preoperative blood transfusions are not always required. INR does not predict bleeding complications in patients with cirrhosis, and "prophylactic" preoperative fresh frozen plasma transfusion is not recommended. Although thrombocytopenia is common in patients with cirrhosis, in vitro and retrospective cross-sectional studies have shown that platelet counts above 50,000/μL are adequate to allow clot formation in most patients with cirrhosis.[36] Therefore, increasing platelet count with prophylactic transfusions may not be beneficial and can cause problems such as volume overload, thrombosis, and transfusion-related complications. It has recently been discovered that thrombocytopenia caused by idiopathic thrombocytopenic purpura can be treated with thrombopoietin analogs (romiplostim) and receptor agonists (eltrombopag, avatrombopag, and lusutrombopag).[35] During interferon-based antiviral therapy, eltrombopag is also approved for use in patients with cirrhosis caused by chronic hepatitis C to increase platelet counts. Only avatrombopag and lusutrombopag have been approved for general thrombocytopenia related to liver disease. In patients with cirrhosis, avatrombopag and lusutrombopag were effective in raising platelet counts above 50,000/μL in phase III clinical trials when administered before invasive procedures compared with placebo.[37]

Although there is no clear guidance in the literature for using these agents preoperatively in patients with cirrhosis, it seems reasonable to use them when the platelet count is less than 50,000/μL when undergoing an elective procedure associated with high bleeding risk. It is important to pay special attention to the possibility of thrombotic events such as portal vein thrombosis and other deep vein thromboses. These agents are currently being studied in clinical settings.

Patients with cirrhosis may have quantitative or qualitative abnormalities in their coagulation profile.[38] Low fibrinogen levels are associated with a higher risk of bleeding, whereas levels above 100 mg/dL inhibit clot formation in patients with cirrhosis.[36] Cryoprecipitate transfusions are a low-volume replacement for fibrinogen that do not significantly increase plasma volume. Despite the lack of controlled trials examining the efficacy of fibrinogen transfusion in patients with cirrhosis, it seems physiologically reasonable to resupply fibrinogen levels with cryoprecipitate before high-risk surgery to ensure adequate clot formation.

Viscoelastic testing (thromboelastography and rotational thromboelastometry) during intraoperative transfusions in large centers has been shown to reduce the need for red blood cell and plasma transfusions in surgical patients with cirrhosis. Therefore, viscoelastic testing should be considered before and during surgical procedures in patients with cirrhosis as a guide for a rational transfusion strategy.[39]

Assessing preoperative imaging to locate varices is an important aspect of preparing for these cases. Fig. 51.6 shows the common locations of these varices.

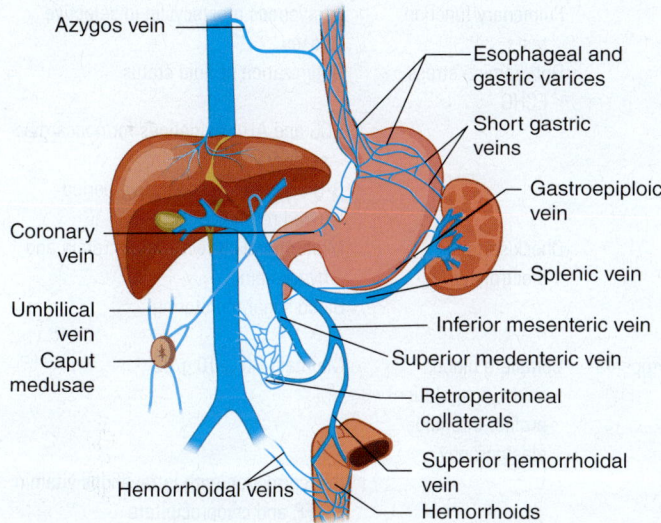

FIGURE 51.6 Sites of varices to be aware of anatomically when operating on patients with cirrhosis. (From Rikkers LF. Portal hypertension. In: Miller TA, ed. *Physiologic Basis of Modern Surgical Care.* St Louis: Mosby; 1988:417-428.)

Pain Control

Drug-related toxicity is particularly high in patients with cirrhosis because of altered drug metabolism and elimination. Therefore, opioid dosages and dosing intervals should generally be lower than the standard. Although randomized controlled trials have not been conducted in patients with cirrhosis, hydromorphone and transdermal fentanyl may be the preferred agents.[40] Tramadol, which has favorable hepatic metabolism, is also commonly used in this population.

As benzodiazepines are eliminated primarily through protein binding and hepatic metabolism, it is best to use short-acting benzodiazepines, such as midazolam. Although there is a misconception that acetaminophen, even in small doses, is contraindicated in patients with cirrhosis, a daily maximum of 2 g/day is generally acceptable. Patients with cirrhosis should avoid the routine administration of nonsteroidal antiinflammatory drugs (NSAIDs) because they can impair renal blood flow. Additionally, oral combination products containing acetaminophen or NSAIDs, especially when combined with opioids, should not be administered because they can cause accidental toxicity or overdose if the patient is unaware that acetaminophen is a component of the product.[41]

For patients with cirrhosis, polyethylene glycol solution may be used daily to maintain bowel regularity and minimize hepatic encephalopathy flare-ups. In the absence of comparative trials, rifaximin may be preferred in patients with hepatic encephalopathy who undergo primary bowel surgery because it generally causes less bowel distention than lactulose.

Table 51.4 shows the optimization strategies for patients with cirrhosis.

Rescue Liver Transplantation

It is important to determine if a patient is likely to be a candidate for liver transplantation before undergoing a surgical procedure. Before proceeding with surgery, it is essential to clarify the

---

TABLE 51.4 Optimization Strategies in Patients With Cirrhosis

PREOPERATIVE CONCERNS	PATHOPHYSIOLOGIC CHANGES	POTENTIAL COMPLICATIONS	ASSESSMENT	PERIOPERATIVE OPTIMIZATION
Nutrition and metabolism	Protein calorie malnutrition	Muscle wasting, impaired mobility, increased need for postoperative ventilation, impaired wound healing, sepsis, and delay in recovery	Serum albumin	Diet with high carbohydrate, high lipid content, and low in amino acid
	Depletion of glycogen storage		Anthropometric measurement	Protein intake of 1.0–1.5 g/kg daily
				Monitoring for hypoglycemia and hyperglycemia
				Vitamin B_1 in alcoholics
Portal hypertension and ascites	Portal hypertension	Decreased quality of life, spontaneous bacterial peritonitis, increased risk of abdominal wound dehiscence, recurrence of abdominal wall hernia, and respiratory compromise	Clinical evaluation Ultrasonography	Salt and water restriction, diuretics
				Ascitic fluid analysis
				SBP treatment and prophylaxis
				Large-volume paracentesis for uncontrolled ascites with albumin
				TIPS for refractory ascites
Renal	Low renal blood flow and low glomerular filtration rate	Acute kidney injury	Serum creatinine, GFR, and urine analysis	Fluid and electrolyte balance
	Raised aldosterone	Hepatorenal syndrome		Avoid nephrotoxic drugs, including contrast agents
				Combination of albumin and terlipressin or octreotide with midodrine in HRS

Continued

TABLE 51.4	Optimization Strategies in Patients With Cirrhosis—cont'd			
PREOPERATIVE CONCERNS	**PATHOPHYSIOLOGIC CHANGES**	**POTENTIAL COMPLICATIONS**	**ASSESSMENT**	**PERIOPERATIVE OPTIMIZATION**
Cerebral	Glial edema	Hepatic encephalopathy	Clinical assessment	Use of lactulose, metronidazole, and neomycin
	Increased permeability of blood-brain barrier		Serum ammonia level	Rifaximin and branched-chain amino acids
	Increased sensitivity to opioids			Treat infections, avoid diuretics, and constipation
				Correct electrolyte abnormalities
Pulmonary	Pleural effusion	Hypoxemia	Chest imaging	Optimize pulmonary functions
	Hepatopulmonary syndrome	Respiratory compromise	Bubble ECHO for HPS	Incentive spirometry
	portopulmonary hypertension		Pulmonary function tests	Intravenous prostacyclin in selective cases
Cardiac	Increased cardiac output, Systemic vasodilation	Cardiomyopathy	Dobutamine stress ECHO	Optimization of fluid status
				ACC and AHA guidelines for noncardiac surgery
				β-Blockers in perioperative period (need reference)
Electrolytes and metabolism	Hyponatremia (fluid overload)	Electrolyte disorders	Check serum electrolytes	Monitor and correct hyponatremia and hypokalemia
	Hypoglycemia (depletion of glycogen stores)			Blood sugar monitoring
Hematology	Thrombocytopenia, hypocoagulability, and hypercoagulability	Anemia, bleeding, thrombocytopenia	Complete blood count, coagulation profile, thrombo-elastography	Maintain Hb >10 g/dL
	Bone marrow suppression			INR correction with intravenous vitamin K, FFP, and cryoprecipitate
				May need DDAVP, recombinant factor VIIa, aprotinin, and tranexamic acid
				Prophylactic platelets transfusion for platelets <50,000

ACC/AHA, The American College of Cardiology/American Heart Association; *ECHO,* echocardiogram; *FFP,* fresh frozen plasma; *GFR,* glomerular filteration rate; *HPS,* hepatopulmonary syndrome; *HRS,* hepatorenal syndrome; *INR,* international normalized ratio; *TIPS,* transjugular intrahepatic portosystemic shunt.
From Newman KL, Johnson KM, Cornia PB, Wu P, Itani K, Ioannou GN. Perioperative evaluation and management of patients with cirrhosis: risk assessment, surgical outcomes, and future directions. *Clin Gastroenterol Hepatol.* 2020;18(11):2398-2414.e3.

position of patients who are not potential candidates for liver transplantation to prevent the patient's family and medical team from revisiting this issue if the patient's condition deteriorates postoperatively. In addition, it is important to determine whether the patient is a candidate for liver transplantation and if the planned surgery can be postponed until the patient has undergone transplantation. Despite uncertainty about how long the patient will be on the liver transplant waiting list, elective procedures such as orthopedic procedures may be best deferred. When a procedure cannot be delayed because of its adverse impact on the patient's quality of life, it is best to complete the liver transplant evaluation before the anticipated surgery. Choosing whether to undergo a liver transplant is not easy and depends, in part, on how quickly a liver transplant evaluation can be completed if the patient deteriorates after surgery and how likely the patient is to undergo a liver transplant. A preoperative evaluation for liver transplantation is recommended if the postoperative mortality risk is >15% at 3 months using an appropriate risk calculator or if the MELD score is >15 (a score that predicts an increased mortality rate).[42,43]

SELECTED REFERENCES

Coccolini F, Improta M, Sartelli M, et al. Acute abdomen in the immunocompromised patient: WSES, SIS-E, WSIS, AAST, and GAIS guidelines. *World J Emerg Surg.* 2021;16(1):40.

This paper presents the World Society of Emergency Surgery (WSES), Surgical Infection Society Europe (SIS-E), World Surgical Infection Society (WSIS), American Association for the Surgery of Trauma (AAST), and Global Alliance for Infection in Surgery (GAIS) joint guidelines on the management of acute abdomen in immunocompromised patients.

Fairfield CJ, Harrison EM, Wigmore SJ, VanWagner LB. Steroid-free versus steroid-containing immunosuppression for liver transplant recipients. *Clin Liver Dis (Hoboken).* 2020;16(5):191-195.

This study assessed the effects of steroid minimization or avoidance among liver transplant recipients compared with *steroid-containing immunosuppression protocols on mortality, graft loss, rejection, and infection in addition to a variety of secondary cardiometabolic outcomes.*

Gomez D, Acuna SA, Joseph Kim S, et al. Incidence and mortality of emergency general surgery conditions among solid organ transplant recipients in Ontario, Canada: a population-based analysis. *Transplantation.* 2023;107(3):753-761.

The study found that the incidence of emergency general surgery (EGS) conditions is significantly higher in recipients of organ transplantation, even after stratification by comorbidity burden. They also found a higher likelihood of death after EGS in transplant patients than in nontransplant patients.

Newman KL, Johnson KM, Cornia PB, Wu P, Itani K, Ioannou GN. Perioperative evaluation and management of patients with cirrhosis: risk assessment, surgical outcomes, and

future directions. *Clin Gastroenterol Hepatol.* 2020;18(11): 2398-2414.e3.

The authors conducted a comprehensive review of the literature from 1998 to 2018 and identified studies reporting perioperative outcomes in patients with cirrhosis.

Northup PG, Garcia-Pagan JC, Garcia-Tsao G, et al. Vascular liver disorders, portal vein thrombosis, and procedural bleeding in patients with liver disease: 2020 practice guidance by the American Association for the Study of Liver Diseases. *Hepatology.* 2021;73:366-413.

This article provides an overview of the current understanding of bleeding and thrombosis in patients with cirrhosis.

The full reference list appears on Elsevier eBooks+.

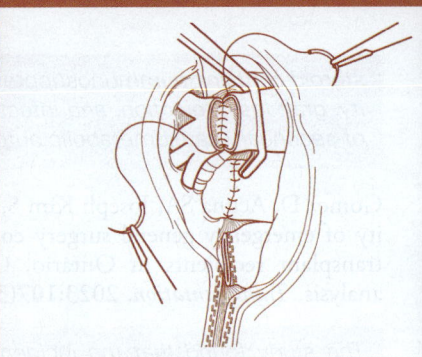

Kidney Transplantation

Muhammad Umaid Rabbani and Jayme E. Locke

OUTLINE

INDICATIONS FOR KIDNEY TRANSPLANTATION

The United States has a heavy chronic kidney disease (CKD) burden, with one in seven adults, or 37 million Americans, carrying the diagnosis. CKD is more common in people aged 65 years or older (34%) than in people aged 45 to 64 years (12%) or 18 to 44 years (6%).[1] Numerous studies have shown that patients who progress to end-stage kidney disease (ESKD) have a survival advantage and improved quality of life if they undergo kidney transplantation compared with remaining on dialysis, establishing kidney transplantation as the gold standard for the treatment of ESKD.[1] Long-term survival for patients after kidney transplant is significantly better in comparison to patients who remain on the transplant waiting list, with a 50% lower 5-year mortality risk among transplant recipients compared with waiting-list candidates.[2] Importantly, the aging US population is projected to increase the CKD prevalence and risk for progression to ESKD and thus drive increased demand for kidney transplantation.

CKD can be caused by numerous disease processes, some of which are more common than others. Hypertension and diabetes are the most common etiologies, with a unique pathophysiologic basis for causing chronic kidney damage. Hyaline arteriosclerosis, seen in hypertensive kidney disease, results from recurring injury to endothelium. This leads to leaking of plasma proteins and platelets, causing a cascade of events resulting in medial and intimal thickening.[3] Diffuse thickening of basement membranes and mesangial sclerosis are the prominent morphologic features seen in kidneys of patients with diabetes, which leads to nephrotic syndrome.[3] At the macrovascular level, diabetes leads to atherosclerosis of renal arteries, leading to progressive ischemia, which leads to scarring and loss of kidney function. Autosomal dominant polycystic kidney disease (ADPKD) is another common etiology causing progressive CKD, accounting for about 10% of CKD burden in the United States. The underlying defect lies in *PKD1* or *PKD2* gene expression, which leads to development of cysts from nephrons and progressive loss of renal parenchyma.[4]

Less common causes include systemic lupus erythematous, membranous nephropathy, minimal change disease, and membroproliferative glomerulonephritis (MPGN) type 1.

The most common indications for transplantation in the pediatric population are different as compared with adults because CKD is rare in children. For children below the age of 5, ESKD most commonly results from congenital anomalies of the kidney and urinary tract, such as renal aplasia, obstructive urologic malformations, and focal sclerosing glomerulosclerosis (FSGS). Reflux nephropathy, chronic glomerulonephritis, and polycystic and medullary cystic disease are even rarer causes of ESKD in children. An in-depth overview of indications seen in the pediatric population is beyond the scope of this chapter.

Patient Selection for Kidney Transplantation[5]

Across the United States, there are more than 250 transplant centers that perform kidney transplants. Every center has internal processes through which they evaluate patients to be considered for kidney transplantation. Existing guidelines encourage consideration of local factors when evaluating patients for kidney transplantation and emphasize the need to select patients for whom kidney transplantation will increase quality and/or quantity of life compared with dialysis. For example, it may not be suitable to have an 80-year-old undergo kidney transplantation and experience the potential diminished quality of life associated with immunosuppressive side effects if their life expectancy remains unchanged compared with remaining on dialysis.

Consideration for transplantation begins with referral from a general nephrologist. Ideally, candidates are referred for evaluation 6 to 12 months before anticipated dialysis initiation. This allows for possible preemptive transplantation, particularly when suitable living kidney donors are identified. Therefore, estimated glomerular filtration rate (eGFR) ≤ 30 mL/min/1.73 m^2 is the typical trigger most nephrologists use to initiate discussions with patients regarding referral for kidney transplantation. It is important to note, however, that disparities in access to preemptive referral and transplantation exist, particularly for ethnic minorities and those with poor social determinants of health.[6]

There are numerous medical conditions that may make a patient high risk or unsuitable for kidney transplantation. We can subdivide patient assessment for transplantation based on system:

- **Neurologic diseases:** Recovery from cerebrovascular accidents is variable. Some patients may never be candidates for transplantation after a stroke, depending on severity of residual neurologic deficits. Generally, a wait of 6 months is recommended after a stroke and 3 months after a transient ischemic attack (TIA). Those patients who have progressive central neurodegenerative disorder do not have improved quality of life or increased survival benefit after transplantation; hence, they are generally not considered for transplantation. Patients who have stable cognitive impairment but do not have an underlying neurodegenerative disorder are considered for transplantation if they have an appropriate social support structure or are able to demonstrate acceptable activities of daily living (ADLs). Candidates with ADPKD are at risk for intracerebral aneurysms. If there is a family history of subarachnoid hemorrhages or a personal history of unexplained headaches, they are usually screened with MRI of the head to rule out aneurysms before transplantation. Peripheral neuropathies are frequently encountered in ESKD patients, mostly as a result of a history of uncontrolled diabetes mellitus. Peripheral neuropathies do not exclude patients from kidney transplantation unless they are severely debilitated and are not expected to recover after a major operation because of the high risk of complications associated with immobilization in perioperative period.

- **Cardiovascular diseases:** Patients with ESKD need to be thoroughly investigated for possible underlying cardiovascular disease (CVD). Baseline workup includes an electrocardiogram (ECG) and echocardiogram (ECHO). Those who have good functional status and minimal risk factors for coronary artery disease (CAD) are initially screened with a nuclear medicine stress test. Some centers are more conservative with regard to using noninvasive cardiac stress tests, but based on local population characteristics, many centers routinely use stress tests as part of preoperative workup. If nuclear stress test is suggestive of underlying CAD, patients are referred to a cardiologist for further workup. High-risk patients with long-standing diabetes or a history of heavy smoking should be considered for left heart catheterization as part of initial workup. Those who have advanced triple-vessel disease or critical lesions are referred to cardiologists for further treatment before being considered. After cardiac stent placement, it is advisable to wait until the patient is off dual-antiplatelet therapy, typically a delay of 6 to 12 months, before wait-listing and/or transplanting the patient. If ECHO is suggestive of heart failure, patients are referred to a cardiologist for further evaluation. Having an ejection fraction of <30% is usually a contraindication for being considered for kidney transplant alone. Patients with severe uncorrectable pulmonary hypertension are also not candidates. Those patients with pulmonary artery pressures above 45 mm Hg are first evaluated by cardiology, but those with pressures above 60 mm Hg are not considered candidates for kidney transplantation alone. One needs to be aware of the reversible depressed ejection fraction that may be encountered in patients who have advanced CKD but have not initiated dialysis. Specifically, the reduced ejection fraction may simply reflect underlying volume overload, which can be corrected with dialysis initiation. Moreover, patients already on dialysis may also have reduced ejection fractions from volume overload secondary to inaccuracies in their dry weight, resulting in underdialysis of the patients. In both instances, optimization of volume control/status is initiated (e.g., dialysis initiation or more aggressive fluid removal), followed by repeat ECHO once euvolemia is achieved. Finally, patients with active symptoms concerning for CAD or valvular disease should be referred to a cardiologist for detailed workup and management before referral for kidney transplant evaluation.

- **Pulmonary diseases:** All patients should undergo x-ray of the chest as a minimum when undergoing evaluation for kidney transplant. Patients who are active smokers or have a heavy smoking history (≥30 pack-years) should undergo computed tomography (CT) scanning of the chest as well. Patients are encouraged and counseled regarding smoking cessation. Patients with irreversible severe obstructive or restrictive lung disease are not considered in isolation for kidney transplant and may be considered if they are candidates for lung transplantation.

- **Gastrointestinal diseases:** Patients should be evaluated with esophagoduodenoscopy (EGD) if they have long-standing history concerning for peptic ulcer disease. Any active inflammation/infection needs to be resolved before considering transplantation. Among labs done at the time of transplant evaluation are liver function tests, which necessitate further workup if abnormal. Patients with underlying cirrhosis need to be referred for simultaneous liver-kidney transplantation. In some rare cases, patients with early compensated cirrhosis may be able to undergo isolated kidney transplantation. Patients with underlying ulcerative colitis and Crohn's disease must have the disease under control before being considered. Colonoscopy is completed in all patients over the age of 45 for colorectal screening, and this is done earlier in patients with inflammatory bowel disease per disease-specific guidelines.

- **Hematologic diseases:** As the average age of the US population increases, a greater number of patients undergoing kidney transplant evaluation are found to have primary hematologic malignancies/disorders. Generally, patients with monoclonal gammopathy of undermined significance (MGUS) and smoldering multiple myeloma remain candidates for transplantation. Patients should, however, be counseled about the risk of disease progression before proceeding with transplantation. Cytopenia encountered in a routine laboratory workup should be carefully evaluated, and if the etiology is unclear, a referral to a hematologist should be made. If there is a history of unexplained blood clots, patients should be evaluated for thrombophilias, such as antiphospholipid antibodies. Anticoagulation preoperatively for hypercoagulable disorders is not contraindicated, but it is usual practice to discontinue novel anticoagulants (e.g., apixaban) and switch to warfarin while waiting for transplant. As previously discussed, patients on dual-antiplatelet therapy for cardiac stenting should complete the recommended treatment period before being considered. Aspirin can be continued through the perioperative period.

- **Peripheral arterial disease (PAD):** Pelvic CT scans can be leveraged to assess for arterial calcifications and ensure kidney transplantation remains technically feasible. For patients who have a history suggestive of underlying PAD, such as claudication or rest pain, noninvasive studies such as ankle-brachial index calculations and early referral to vascular surgery are recommended. If patients have a history of aorto-iliac occlusive disease that has been treated, they can still be transplanted if vessels (pelvic or intraabdominal) on preoperative imaging remain suitable for implantation of the graft.

- **Malignancy and preoperative cancer screening:** As the age of the patients requiring kidney transplantation continues to increase, we are encountering more patients who have previously been treated for malignancies. Here, we will focus on the most common malignancies encountered during kidney transplantation evaluation.
  - **Breast cancer:** Low-risk breast cancer patients, such as those being treated for ductal carcinoma in situ (DCIS) or stage I breast cancer, can be transplanted after completion of their recommended treatment without any waiting period. Length of endocrine therapy should not influence the decision to transplant. For high-risk breast cancer patients (stage III and above), a waiting period of 3 to 5 years after completion of standard therapy is recommended. Patients with inflammatory and metastatic breast cancer should not be transplanted.[7] Females who are 50 years of age and older should have a screening mammogram every 2 years while waiting for transplant.
  - **Colorectal cancer:** Patients with low-risk colorectal cancer (stage I and II) can be considered for transplantation after completion of treatment and remaining disease-free for 2 years. Those with high-risk cancers (stage III or IV) should be considered after completing treatment and being cancer-free for 5 years.[7] High-risk features include lymphovascular invasion, perineural invasion, signet net histology, poor differentiation, tumor perforation, inadequate lymph node assessment, and node-positive disease, all of which increase the risk of cancer recurrence even in nonmetastatic disease.[8] Screening colonoscopy is required for all standard-risk patients aged 45 years and older.
  - **Renal cell carcinoma (RCC):** ESKD patients are at increased risk of RCC. Most renal masses are incidentally discovered and are less than 4 cm in size. Those that are less than 4 cm can be safely monitored, but current standard practice is treatment of all masses suspicious for RCC, either through ablation or nephrectomy. If the rate of growth is more than 0.5 cm/year, or when the mass becomes 4 cm or greater, definitive treatment is indicated before proceeding with transplantation.[7,9] Incidentally discovered renal tumors less than 1 cm in size can be monitored.
  - **Prostate cancer:** Prostate cancer is the leading cause of cancer in males. All male patients 50 years and older are screened with a prostate-specific antigen (PSA) test. A repeat PSA screening every 1 to 2 years is recommended.[10]
  - **Gynecologic cancers:** Females 21 years and older are screened for cervical cancer with a Pap smear before being placed on a waiting list. Pap smears should be repeated every 3 years if normal. Low-risk gynecologic cancers that have risk of recurrence of less than 5% do not require any waiting period after completion of therapy. These include early stage (stage I, grade 1–2) endometrial; stage IA/B/C, grade 1 to 2, epithelial ovarian; and stage IA squamous/adenocarcinoma of cervix. With intermediate-risk cancers that have a 5% to 15% risk of recurrence, a 3-year wait time after completion of primary therapy is usually recommended. These include stage I and II endometrial cancers with high-risk features and stage IB cervical cancers. With high-risk disease with a recurrence chance of greater than 30%, a wait time of 5 years is recommended. These include high-stage endometrial,

ovarian, and cervical cancers, except stage IV disease, in which case patients are not considered candidates for transplant.

- **Infectious workup:** Patients undergoing transplantation will be initiated on immunosuppression; hence, part of the evaluation process involves comprehensive assessment for any underlying infectious disease process. Generally, any active viral, bacterial, or fungal infections will need to be adequately treated before transplantation. Active tuberculosis needs to be treated, and screening should be done on all potential recipients with chest x-ray and either purified protein derivative (PPD) skin test or interferon-gamma release assay. Urinary tract infections will be frequently encountered and should be treated before transplant. Patients with a history of renal cyst infections (e.g., polycystic kidney disease patients) should be managed on a case-by-case basis. Although the Kidney Disease Improving Global Outcomes (KDIGO) guidelines do not recommend routine preoperative prophylactic nephrectomy in these patients, a case may be made for those patients with other symptoms in conjunction with recurrent infections, such as considerable pain, recurrent cyst infections, or history of sepsis from cyst infections.[5] Human immunodeficiency virus (HIV) infection, if adequately treated and controlled, is not a contraindication to transplantation. HIV-positive recipients should be selected based on institutional criteria, just as with other standard recipients. HIV-positive recipients can receive kidneys from HIV-positive donors, which has decreased wait times for these patients in some parts of the United States from 8 years to less than 1 year.[11] HIV nephropathy may recur, and therefore, these patients should be closely monitored. Hepatitis C (HCV)-positive recipients should be assessed for possible underlying cirrhosis and the presence of an active infection. If decompensated, they need to be referred for simultaneous liver-kidney transplant evaluation. If there is active infection, it should ideally be treated before transplant unless patient consents to an HCV-positive organ and there is probability of being transplanted soon after being listed. Patients with mild stages of fibrosis or early cirrhosis can be transplanted in cases where they do not have portal hypertension. If there is evidence of invasive fungal infection, that needs to be appropriately treated before transplant, whereas mere colonization by fungi is not a contraindication for transplantation. Screening for *Coccidioides* species in endemic areas is important because a history of pretransplant active disease or seropositivity might require azole prophylaxis for life. With regard to parasitic infection, *Toxoplasma* screening should be done in all patients undergoing organ transplantation. *Strongyloides* and *Trypanosoma cruzi* screening should be done in highly endemic areas (Table 52.1).[12]

KIDNEY ALLOCATION SYSTEM

Presently, the US transplant system faces multiple challenges in kidney allocation, particularly with regard to equity. As a result of the increasing ability of centers to list more complicated patients as well as an ever-growing CKD/ESKD population, the wait list has progressively increased. The supply of organs has remained relatively constant, and as such, waiting times for a deceased donor kidney in some areas of the United States approach 10 years. Given the large gap between supply and demand, allocation rules exist and are founded on the basic premise of allocating organs to

TABLE 52.1 Recommendations for Initial and Follow-up Screening of Viral and Nonviral Pathogens in Kidney Transplant Candidates

PATHOGEN	TEST	REPEAT TESTING
Viral Infections		
HIV	IgG	If negative, repeat annually and at time of transplant
HCV	IgG	If negative, repeat annually and at time of transplant
HBV	Anti-HBs, anti-HBc, HBsAg	If negative, repeat annually and at time of transplant
CMV	IgG	If negative, repeat at time of transplant
EBV	VGA IgG or EBNA IgG	If negative, repeat at time of transplant
HSV	IgG	If negative, repeat at time of transplant
VZV	IgG	If negative, repeat at time of transplant and 4 weeks after vaccination
Measles, mumps, rubella	IgG	If negative, repeat at time of transplant and 4 weeks after vaccination
HTLV	IgG	None unless ongoing risk of exposure
Nonviral Infections		
Syphilis	IgG with confirmatory testing if IgG positive	None
Strongyloides	IgG	None
Chagas disease	IgG	None
Tuberculosis (in low prevalence areas)	Tuberculin skin test or Interferon-gamma release assay (IGRA)	Annually if ongoing risk of exposure
Malaria	Blood smear if clinically indicated	None

CMV, Cytomegalovirus; *EBNA,* Epstein-Barr virus nuclear antigen; *EBV,* Epstein-Barr virus; *HBc,* hepatitis B core antibody; *HBs,* hepatitis B surface antibody; *HBsAg,* hepatitis B surface antigen; *HBV,* hepatitis B virus; *HCV,* hepatitis C virus; *HSV,* herpes simplex virus; *HTLV,* human T-lymphotropic virus 1; *VGA,* viral capsid antigen; *VZV,* varicella-zoster virus.
Adapted from Chadban SJ, Ahn C, Axelrod DA. KDIGO clinical practice guidelines on the evaluation and management and management of candidates for kidney transplantation. *Transplantation.* 2020 Apr;104(4S1 suppl 1):S11-S103.

the sickest first and doing so without introducing or exacerbating disparities based on race/ethnicity, sex, or geography. Allocation processes aim to match higher-quality kidneys with those individuals with highest expected posttransplant survival within a certain geographic parameter around the donor hospital. Pediatric patients therefore take priority for objectively better organs, with kidneys with a kidney donor profile index (KDPI) <35% matched to them first. There are also efforts to prioritize disadvantaged population subgroups, such as individuals with a high panel reactive antibody (PRA; e.g., difficult to find a compatible match) or previous living kidney donors. It is a constantly evolving process, and at the time of writing this chapter, allocation policies remain in flux as the transplant community moves toward continuous distribution policies. Intricate details regarding existing and proposed allocation policies are beyond the scope of this chapter.

DECEASED DONOR KIDNEY EVALUATION

Selecting an appropriate kidney for a recipient is a complex decision-making process that takes into consideration multiple variables. Donor history, serum creatinine trend, urine output, kidney biopsy results, kidney anatomy, and KDPI are just some of the factors initially assessed. KDPI aims to score donor kidneys (scale: 0%–100%), with kidneys with the highest KDPIs projected to have the worst graft survival. KDPI uses several variables, including donor age, height, weight, ethnicity, history of hypertension, history of diabetes, cause of death, serum creatinine, HCV status, and whether the donation occurred after brain death or circulatory death. However, KDPI alone may not always be helpful in discerning appropriate kidneys from marginal ones. For example, KDPI can be falsely elevated in the setting of acute kidney injury, which may improve over time. Comorbid conditions

such as diabetes and hypertension may not always be known from history. Hemoglobin A1c (HbA1c) can give an indication about the level of diabetic control in a donor or raise suspicion of undiagnosed diabetes. Long-standing uncontrolled diabetes should be an indication for considering kidney biopsy even in the setting of normal serum creatinine or low KDPI. If hypertension is not diagnosed, one should be suspicious if the patient died of a hemorrhagic stroke, especially if a young donor.

Moreover, if the donor required renal replacement therapy during the organ-allocation process, it does not necessarily mean that the kidneys are not useable. Here, it becomes crucial to carefully assess kidneys once they have been procured to ensure they have not infarcted, and kidney biopsy is helpful in these scenarios to help rule out thrombotic microangiopathy, fibrin thrombi, or necrosis.

Generally, donor-recipient size mismatch has not been considered in adult kidney transplantation, but there is an increasing breadth of data suggesting that size difference does have an impact on the outcomes of the kidney transplant recipient. It is still unclear which anthropometric measurement is most dependable when matching donor-recipient size. Height differences between donor and recipient have been shown to have a correlation with outcome; for example, the use of kidneys from shorter donors in tall recipients leads to worse transplant outcomes.[13] On the other side of the spectrum, using larger kidneys in smaller recipients should also be carefully considered. Although unusual, having a large kidney implanted in a smaller recipient may lead to an inability to close fascia primarily or lead to vessel compression.

Frozen-section biopsy of kidneys has always been a contentious topic. Numerous studies now suggest minimizing use of kidney biopsy when choosing deceased donor kidneys. One of the commonly listed reasons for organ decline is kidney biopsy results. Most recently, published Organ Procurement and

Transplantation Network (OPTN) data demonstrated that nationally, the kidney discard rate has reached 25%. Performance of a kidney biopsy increases the odds of discard by three times, even when adjusted for donor characteristics. This association is strongest for low-risk (KDPI <20) kidneys.[14] There is a marked difference in histologic findings in sequential biopsies of the same kidney, with first biopsy findings having no association with posttransplant outcomes.[15] Therefore, across the United States, there is a movement to limit kidney biopsy on standard-criterion donors. OPTN has attempted to standardize the reporting of kidney biopsy results. In general, kidney biopsy reporting includes percentage of globally sclerotic glomeruli, presence or absence of nodular mesangial glomerulosclerosis, percentage of interstitial fibrosis and tubular atrophy, percentage of vascular disease/arteriosclerosis, and presence or absence of cortical necrosis and fibrin thrombi. Most centers across the United States use a threshold of 10% to 20% of glomerulosclerosis as a threshold for acceptance[16] because glomerulosclerosis >20% has been shown to positively predict graft loss.[17] However, in otherwise healthy patients who are 50 years of age and older, about 20% glomerulosclerosis may be observed; hence, certain kidneys with high glomerulosclerosis (up to 20%) may be considered after weighing donor history and recipient characteristics. Kidneys with a higher percentage of glomerulosclerosis may be appropriate in recipients with lower body mass index (BMI). Another option when considering kidneys with high glomerulosclerosis is to use both kidneys in the same recipient.

Historically, most centers decline kidney allografts that have fibrin thrombi on biopsies. Studies have shown that kidneys with fibrin thrombi can be safely used, with good outcomes, after ruling out any significant cortical necrosis. Diffuse glomerular fibrin thrombi are often observed in the setting of a donor cause of death from severe head trauma. Kidneys with diffuse glomerular fibrin thrombi seen on biopsy have a higher incidence of DGF, but overall, >90% are associated with good clinical outcomes.[20]

Donor cross-sectional imaging can be very useful in assessing blood vessels and give an indication of the degree of atherosclerosis. At the time of procurement when assessing kidney anatomy, the surgeon comments on their subjective assessment of the degree of atherosclerosis of the aortic patch and renal artery orifice. Hypothetically, having significant atherosclerosis of the renal artery should correlate with microscopic arteriosclerosis of smaller renal vessels, and this rationale has been used by centers to decline those kidneys with marked gross atherosclerosis. However, it has been shown that there is no correlation between the two.[18] The most obvious reason for this is the subjective differences in evaluation of gross macroscopic disease by different surgeons. Main renal artery arteriosclerosis is not associated with delayed graft function (DGF), eGFR at 1 year, or long-term graft survival.[18] Microscopic arteriosclerosis, on the other hand, is associated with posttransplant allograft outcomes. Allografts with arteriosclerosis have a higher incidence of calcineurin inhibitor nephrotoxicity and posttransplant anemia, as well as poorer long-term function.[19] Kidneys with mild to moderate arteriosclerosis can still be used in select recipients. When using such kidneys, one needs to be aware of their physiologic demand for higher blood pressure to maintain perfusion, especially in the initial postoperative period. Because of the high degree of discordance observed when reporting arteriosclerosis on frozen section versus permanent, it is prudent to rely more on other parameters when considering kidneys with high percentage of arteriosclerosis. Donor history and hypo-

thermic perfusion pump numbers offer additional data points to correlate with the degree of arteriosclerosis observed on frozen section. Allografts with abnormally reported histology are expected to have higher resistance and lower flow rates.

Recent severe acute respiratory syndrome coronavirus 2 (SARS-CoV-2, COVID-19) pandemic affected the field of transplantation as centers became rightfully wary of use of any donors that were COVID-19 positive. This was to protect not just the transplant recipients but also the healthcare teams involved in the process. At the outset of the COVID-19 pandemic, when there were limited therapies for treatment, no available vaccination, and a lack of understanding of modes of transmission, kidneys from donors infected with COVID-19 were universally declined because angiotensin receptors, which are expressed in kidneys, were identified as potential receptors for COVID-19 and could promote transmission.[21] With changing strains of the virus potentially leading to less severe disease, transplant center practices have evolved, and kidneys from low-risk COVID-positive donors are being accepted and transplanted. Low-risk features include a longer time since initial positive test, mild disease severity or no systemic signs, cycle threshold >35, no acute respiratory distress syndrome (ARDS), and no thrombosis. Kidney transplantation from carefully selected COVID-positive donors does not negatively affect early patient and graft survival.[22] There is a paucity of data on long-term outcomes.

LIVING KIDNEY DONOR SELECTION

Living kidney donors are crucial to close the organ-shortage gap. In the United States, living donor kidney transplants represent 30% of all kidney transplants performed annually. Every center in the United States has an established workflow around the evaluation of potential living kidney donors. The United Network for Organ Sharing (UNOS) and KDIGO are the two organizations that provide guidelines around the testing and workup of potential living kidney donors. An essential part of the approval process is to ensure that there is minimal risk to the donor in immediate term and minimal risk of developing ESKD in the long term after donation. These individuals are otherwise healthy people who are undergoing an operation they individually do not need. Therefore, any morbidity and mortality associated with the process of kidney donation is taken very seriously.

Historically, it was assumed that donating a kidney was not associated with increased risk for future development of ESKD, but more recent studies have demonstrated increased risk compared with healthy nondonor controls.[23] Particularly among vulnerable subpopulations, such as African American persons and obese persons.[24-26] Moreover, metabolic changes associated with kidney donation may, over time, increase risk of CVD. Recent reviews have shown that if the follow-up is extended beyond 15 years, there is an association of kidney donation with increased cardiovascular and all-cause mortality.[27] Kasiske et al. followed living donors for 9 years after donation and demonstrated that the donors had higher parathyroid hormone, homocysteine, and uric acid levels, and their mean small artery elasticity was significantly lower. However, at 9 years, donor and control urine protein, urine albumin, glucose, HbA1c, lipoprotein levels, and blood pressure were not much different.[27] Although it is important to note that most risks are reported as relative and the absolute postdonation risks remain very low, it is critical that all potential risks, no matter how small the magnitude, be communicated to persons considering living kidney donation, particularly for vulnerable subpopulations, to ensure the fidelity of the informed consent process:

- **Females:** Davis et al. reported that females who get pregnant after kidney donation do not have a statistically significant increased risk of preeclampsia/eclampsia, but there was a trend toward preeclampsia in the kidney donor group compared with controls.[28] Although there is a dearth of comprehensive data to suggest a proven increased risk of hypertension-related complications during pregnancy, females should be counseled adequately about these potential concerns.

- **Obese persons:** Increasing numbers of obese individuals are being evaluated as potential donors because the prevalence of obesity in the United States is on the rise. Various studies over the years have tried to establish a BMI cutoff, above which the risks of harm to the donor postdonation are substantial enough to warrant an absolute contraindication to living donation. Even donors who are overweight (BMI >27 kg/m^2), however, have been shown to have an increased risk of developing ESKD, although the strongest association remains among donors with a BMI above 30 kg/m^2.[24,25] Obese donors have an almost twofold higher risk for ESKD in comparison to nonobese donors. Apart from increased risk of developing ESKD, obese donors are at an increased risk of all-cause mortality, which has been reported as 30% higher compared with nonobese donors, regardless of development of ESKD.[24,25] With increasing average BMI of potential living donors, centers need to ensure it is communicated to the donors that with a BMI beyond 27 kg/m^2, there is an increased risk of end-stage renal disease (ESRD). Ideally, donors who are otherwise approved for donation but have a BMI above 30 should be counseled about weight loss before proceeding with kidney donation.

- **African American persons:** African American persons have a higher incidence of hypertension and ESKD compared with other ethnicities, and they have a statistically significant risk of developing hypertension and ESKD after kidney donation.[27,29] Therefore, when counseling African American donors, they should be informed of their increased risk for developing hypertension and ESKD after kidney donation.

When evaluating the potential living donor, it is the responsibility of the transplant center to perform a detailed consultation in which all the risks are explained in detail. Risk assessment is individualized for each patient. Although there are calculators available that can estimate an individual's lifetime risk of acquiring ESKD before donation, there are multiple variables that are not included in these calculators. One of the tools that is available online (http://www.transplantmodels.com) attempts to give a quantitative value to the risk of developing ESKD before kidney donation.[30] This is one tool that can allow physicians to appropriately counsel donors based on their individual risk (Fig. 52.1).

The standard evaluation appointment for the donor involves obtaining detailed history of the patient, including medication history and family history. Psychosocial assessment should ideally be done by a provider not involved in the care of the potential recipient. Assessment should be done in the absence of other family members who may influence the decision of the donor. Coercion needs to be ruled out during the interview. Social history is very important because once someone is found to be suitable as a donor, it is necessary to ensure adequate social support is in place

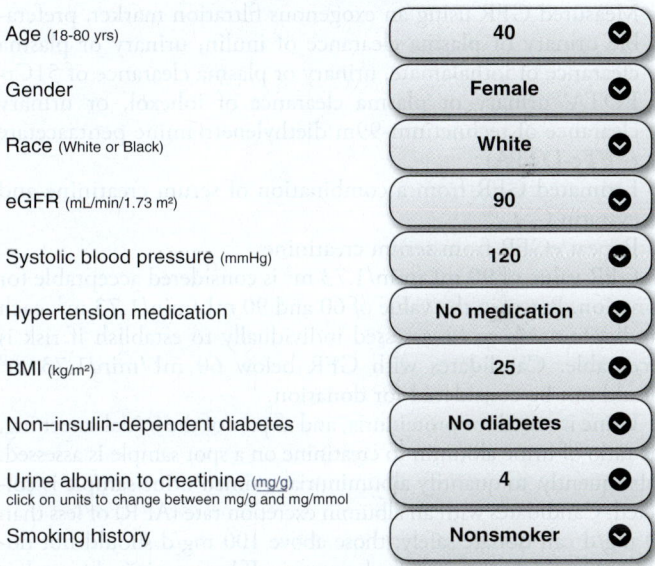

Projected incidence of end-stage renal disease:	
0.04% Predonation 15-year*	**0.30%** Predonation lifetime*
? Postdonation 15-year**	**?** Postdonation lifetime**

blue: <1%, green: 1-2%, yellow: 2-3%, orange: 3-5%, red: >5%

The predonation risks represent projections if a person does not donate a kidney. Details about estimating postdonation risk are provided below.

reset **print summary**

Patient characteristics:

Age (18-80 yrs)	40
Gender	Female
Race (White or Black)	White
eGFR (mL/min/1.73 m^2)	90
Systolic blood pressure (mmHg)	120
Hypertension medication	No medication
BMI (kg/m^2)	25
Non–insulin-dependent diabetes	No diabetes
Urine albumin to creatinine (mg/g) click on units to change between mg/g and mg/mmol	4
Smoking history	Nonsmoker

FIGURE 52.1 End-stage renal disease (ESRD) risk tool for kidney donor candidates. Example illustrates a hypothetical patient and their estimated lifetime risk of ESRD before donation. *BMI,* Body mass index; *eGFR,* estimated glomerular filtration rate. (From http://www.transplantmodels.com.)

to assist with postdonation recovery. Things to consider in these situations include work-related needs (e.g., time off) and any childcare obligations that may need to be covered.

On physical exam, attention needs to be paid to blood pressure, any previous abdominal surgical scars, and any hernias. Two blood pressure readings should be taken in the office to assess for white-coat hypertension. Ambulatory blood pressure monitoring is not required but is a common practice among centers to assess multiple blood pressure readings over multiple days.[31] For donors with borderline blood pressure, a blood pressure log helps in having a better understanding of their mean blood pressure. Individuals with uncontrolled hypertension are not candidates for donation. Individuals with controlled hypertension on a maximum of two agents may be considered with caution.[32] They need to be counseled in depth about their increased risk of developing ESKD and worsening hypertension with one kidney.[30,33]

These are rare circumstances. Most centers turn down individuals who have hypertension as potential donors.

Evaluation workup is extensive. Blood group needs to be tested and confirmed with a second test. Subtyping of blood group A donors is needed if the intended recipient has anti-A antibodies. Human leukocyte antigen (HLA) typing for major histocompatibility complex (MHC) class I and class II antigens, which are known to be most immunogenic, needs to be performed. Subsequently, the recipients are tested for donor-specific antibodies against these antigens.

As highlighted earlier, the most important part of the evaluation is establishing baseline kidney health of the donor. Per the 2019 commentary on the KDIGO 2017 guidelines, predonation kidney function evaluation involves measuring glomerular filtration rate (GFR) and not relying on serum creatinine concentration. The donor GFR needs to be expressed in mL/min/1.73 m². The first GFR can be the eGFR, most commonly calculated from serum creatinine concentration. The eGFR needs to be confirmed using one or more of the following calculations:

1. Measured creatinine clearance using 24-hour urine collection[34]
2. Measured GFR using an exogenous filtration marker, preferable urinary or plasma clearance of inulin, urinary or plasma clearance of iothalamate, urinary or plasma clearance of 51Cr-EDTA, urinary or plasma clearance of iohexol, or urinary clearance of technetium-99m diethylenetriamine pentaacetate (^{99m}Tc-DTPA)
3. Estimated GFR from a combination of serum creatinine and cystatin C
4. Repeat eGFR from serum creatinine

GFR value of 90 mL/min/1.73 m² is considered acceptable for donation. Between the value of 60 and 90 mL/min/1.73 m², each candidate needs to be assessed individually to establish if risk is acceptable. Candidates with GFR below 60 mL/min/1.73 m² should not be considered for donation.

Urine is tested for proteinuria, and as part of the initial screening, the ratio of urine albumin to creatinine on a spot sample is assessed. Subsequently, to quantify albuminuria, a timed urine sample is collected. Candidates with an albumin excretion rate (AER) of less than 30 mg/d can donate safely; those above 100 mg/d should not donate. Urine is also assessed for hematuria. If hematuria is detected, it can be confirmed with another sample. Cause of hematuria may be simple, such as a bladder infection or kidney stones. Some cases may warrant a cystoscopy to rule out bladder cancer or other urothelial malignancies. Eventually, patients with unexplained hematuria with no other identified cause will need a kidney biopsy to rule out pathologies such as Alport syndrome, IgA nephropathy, and thin basement membrane nephropathy disease. If nephrolithiasis is discovered, previous stone history needs to be obtained and recurrence risk assessed. Biochemical analysis can be done, which provides details of stone composition and may highlight underlying metabolic issues as a cause of recurrent stones, in which case it becomes unsafe to proceed with donation. It is important to consider that donors with one kidney will have much less tolerance for maintaining adequate renal function if they develop large stones in the remaining kidney. If an isolated kidney stone is discovered on imaging and the rest of the workup is not suggestive of risk of recurrent stones, the kidney with the stone should be donated.

Kidney donors undergo computed tomography angiography (CTA) of abdomen, and it is recommended that 3D reconstruction is done on those images to carefully assess anatomy before proceeding to the operating room. Cross-sectional imaging can be used to estimate the kidney volume. If there is a significant size difference between the kidneys, radionuclide scans can be used to assess individual kidney GFR. Radionuclide studies should also be conducted in situations where vascular anomalies or pelvic collecting system anomalies are encountered incidentally on preoperative imaging.

Donors with a history of type 1 diabetes should not donate. Those with type 2 diabetes are usually discouraged from donating because they have risk of progressive end-organ damage over the years. HbA1c and fasting blood glucose levels are checked as part of routine workup. History of active smoking is not an absolute contraindication for donating, but potential donors should be counseled about increased risk of developing ESKD with continued smoking after donation. Smokers may have poor-quality vessels, which may pose technical challenges when those kidneys are transplanted. Cross-sectional imaging can alert to any significant calcifications in the main artery, in which case the potential donor should not be approved.

Infectious workup includes testing for human immunodeficiency virus (HIV), hepatitis B (HBV), hepatitis C (HCV), Epstein-Barr virus (EBV), cytomegalovirus (CMV), and *Treponema pallidum*. These labs should be drawn within 28 days of donation as per regulations—ideally, as close as possible to the donation date. Donors need to be up to date with their cancer screening per their age group and recommended health screening protocols.

LIVING DONOR NEPHRECTOMY

Donor nephrectomy should ideally be performed with a minimally invasive technique using laparoscopic or robotic assistance. In those donors who have extensive surgical history, open technique may be justified. There is an increasing prevalence of robotic utilization in donor nephrectomies, although this method is not officially endorsed by KDIGO.[32]

Debriefing with anesthesia before incision is a critical step. This ensures both teams have rapport and continue communication throughout the case. Donors will be under general anesthesia for about 2.5 to 3 hours. After induction, a nasal or oral gastric tube is placed to keep the stomach decompressed. Urine output needs to be strictly monitored. Preoperative antibiotic prophylaxis to lower the risk of surgical site infection is recommended. Commonly, mannitol and/or furosemide are administered before cross-clamping. IV heparin between 2500 and 5000 units may also be requested before cross-clamping of renal vessels. Heparization needs to be reversed with protamine after removal of the kidney.

The surgeon should be present at the time of patient positioning. Before the patient is positioned, it is important to carefully mark planned surgical incision sites. In the approach described here, we describe a total laparoscopic technique without a hand assistance port specific to a left-sided nephrectomy. A suprapubic transverse 6-cm mark is made in location of a typical cesarean delivery site. This location is used for extraction of the kidney. A 12-mm supraumbilical incision site is marked, a 12-mm left flank incision site is marked, and a 5-mm subxiphoid site is marked. After the incision sites have been marked, the patient is positioned in right modified lateral decubitus position, with the left arm out and secured on an armrest. The bed is flexed to allow more working space by increasing the distance between the inferior rib margin and the anterior superior iliac spine. All bony prominences and pressure points are carefully padded. Entry is made at the supraumbilical port, which can be done with either Hasson technique or with a Veress needle. After pneumoperitoneum is established, appropriately sized trocars are placed in previously marked surgical sites. An additional trocar is placed at the suprapubic incision site through the planned incision mark to aid in retraction.

The key steps of the operation include the following:
1. Begin with mobilization of the descending colon medially, along the white line of Toldt, ensuring mesentery stays intact.

Release splenic flexure if needed to expose superior pole of the kidney. Medial extent of the mobilization ends with exposure of the ureter.

2. Identify the left ureter as it crosses over the common iliac artery.
3. Identify the gonadal vein and dissect cranially until it drains into renal vein.
4. Dissect renal vein along its superior and inferior border; identify adrenal vein superiorly and draining lumbar branches inferior or posterior to the renal vein. Ligate lumbar branches with a sealing device or stapler.
5. Identify renal artery, commonly along the inferior-posterior border of the renal vein; dissect circumferentially at the takeoff from aorta.
6. Once superior edge of renal artery is identified, it is safe to encircle the left adrenal vein and ligate.
7. Dissect adrenal gland off the superior aspect of the kidney.
8. Dissect the kidney off retroperitoneal fat with a vessel-sealing device.
9. Transect the gonadal with a stapler, and transect the ureter after doubly clipping distal ureter.
10. Position an EndoCatch bag in the midline after inserting it through the suprapubic port site.
11. Ensure diuretic per institutional protocol has been administered, and use a stapler to transect renal artery at the takeoff from aorta, followed by renal vein in a similar manner; maneuver kidney into the EndoCatch bag.
12. Swiftly extend the Pfannenstiel incision and open fascia superiorly and inferiorly, remove kidney, and pass it to the back table for flushing.
13. Bring peritoneum and fascia of extraction site together with clamps and reestablish pneumoperitoneum.
14. Ensure hemostasis at the stump sites.
15. Ensure descending colon mesentery is intact and position colon in anatomic location.
16. Close fascia at 12-mm port sites; close fascia at extraction site.

POSTOPERATIVE COURSE AND COMPLICATIONS

Most living donors are discharged home within 24 to 48 hours after the operation. Urine output is closely monitored postoperatively; hence, a Foley catheter is left in until postoperative day 1. Postoperatively, a low urine output should raise suspicion of possible bleeding or urine leakage from the ureter stump. Both need to be addressed expeditiously, with return to the operating room if confirmed. On postoperative day 1, it is safe to remove Foley catheter. If patient is unable to void, its cause should be evaluated. In the case of a full bladder with inability to urinate, a Foley catheter may need to be replaced and another void trial attempted the day after. An empty bladder can be a result of numerous causes. If underresuscitation is suspected, a fluid bolus may be needed. It is important to decompress the bladder because there is a higher risk of failure of Weck clips on the ureter if bladder is under pressure from distal obstruction, which will lead to intraperitoneal urine leakage, necessitating an exploration.

The most common postdonation complaint living donors experience is that of pain at incision sites and in shoulders. Shoulder pain is a result of diaphragm irritation postinsufflation. A multimodal regimen that includes narcotics and muscle relaxants is initiated to control pain. Early mobilization is necessary to prevent respiratory complications and decrease risk of deep venous thrombosis (DVT). By postoperative day 2, after ensuring

appropriate pain control and bladder emptying, patients can be discharged home.

Rates of postoperative complications are low. Most studies report an incidence between 7% and 9.9 %.[35] Obesity is associated with higher risk of perioperative complications, with donors with a BMI >30 kg/m^2 at a higher risk. Most common complication in the postoperative period is ileus.

No donor nephrectomy technique has been proven to be superior to the other. There are differences in warm ischemia time, risk of bleeding, and operative time in between techniques, but all techniques are equally safe, and optimal approach depends on surgeon preference and training. Laparoscopic donor nephrectomy and robotic-assisted donor nephrectomies are reported to have the highest warm ischemia time, but this is not significant enough to have an impact on graft survival. Retroperitoneoscopic donor nephrectomy has the highest amount of blood loss.[35] After fatal incidents, the US Food and Drug Administration (FDA) issued a black box warning for use of Hem-o-lok clips on renal artery at the time of nephrectomy; hence, nearly all centers now use staplers to transect renal artery.

DECEASED DONOR KIDNEY PROCUREMENT

As previously mentioned, deceased donors can either be donation after brain death (DBD) donors or donation after circulatory death (DCD) donors. It is primarily the responsibility of the organ procurement organization, not the transplant center, to ensure that all required brain death testing has been completed before allocation begins. Brain death testing protocols differ between states. As an organ procurement surgeon, it is crucial to confirm that the donor's chart has brain death testing and confirmatory notes completed and that brain death declaration has been done by a physician not involved in the organ transplant process.

For DBDs, the procurement operation has a few critical steps with regard to kidney procurement:

1. Begin xiphoid process–pubic symphysis incision in midline.
2. Carefully examine all intraperitoneal surfaces and organs to ensure no occult malignancy.
3. Release right colon by dissecting along white line of Toldt until duodenum is visualized, followed by Kocherization of duodenum.
4. Identify left renal vein crossing over the aorta to drain into inferior vena cava, which usually signifies extent of this dissection. Cephalad, the superior mesenteric artery is palpable in the small bowel mesentery.
5. Similarly, medialize the left colon by lifting the mesentery off the left kidney and releasing the colon by working along the white line of Toldt.
6. Identify ureters on both sides crossing over the common iliac arteries on either side; isolate location of transection as distally as possible.
7. Expose aorta before iliac bifurcation and place two umbilical tapes for control—this will be the site of cannulation.
8. Expose supraceliac aorta if chest is not open; otherwise, an aortic clamp can be placed on descending aorta in the chest at the time of cross-clamping.
9. Heparinize with 50 to 80 units/kg of body weight of donor; while waiting for heparin to circulate, ligate distal aorta with umbilical tape.
10. Transect aorta with digital control of proximal aorta, and cannulate with an appropriate cannula (usually between 18 and 20 Fr).

11. Use the junction of the atrium and inferior vena cava (IVC) as the site of outflow and transect while at the same time clamping descending aorta to ensure all flush flows into abdominal organs. Open preservation solution flush. Place ice on all organs.

12. While flush flows, use a bowel stapler to transect small bowel past the duodenum, and similarly staple across the small bowel and right colon mesentery to release bowel out of the abdomen for better exposure.

13. Once flush is completed, remove the cannula, dissect all lymphatic tissue anterior to the aorta until left renal vein is reached, and transect at the exact insertion into the IVC to allow adequate length on the left renal vein.

14. Transect the IVC above the insertion of right renal vein, which may be higher than expected (Fig. 52.2).

15. Staying anterior on the aorta, transect the anterior wall open until the takeoff of superior mesenteric artery; visualize the orifices of right and left renal artery; and completely transect aortic wall above these orifices, leaving an adequate patch with the orifices intact. Transect the aorta in the midline.

16. Transect ureter on the right and release it out of pelvis, leaving adequate tissue (mesoureter) around the ureter to preserve microvasculature for its blood supply.

17. Transect inferior vena cave above bifurcation, release the IVC along with aortic patch off the spine, and dissect the kidney from retroperitoneal fat to bring it out of the body.

18. Release left kidney in a similar manner.

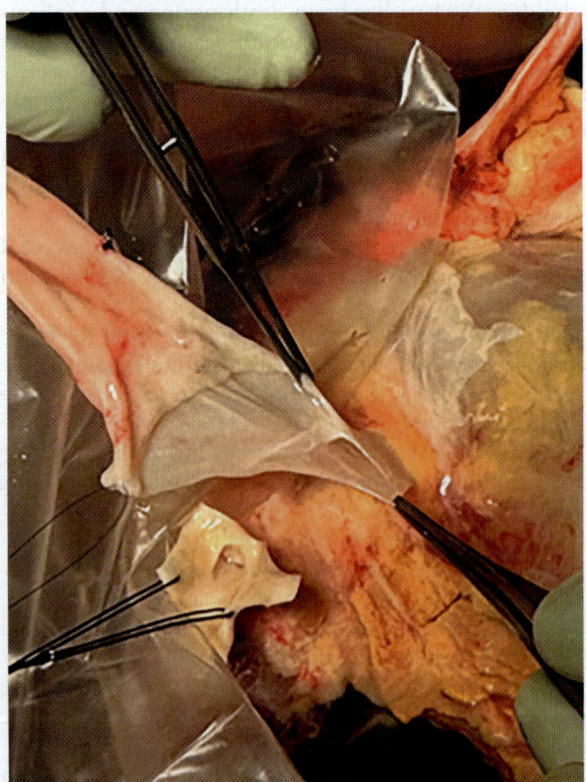

FIGURE 52.2 Procurement injury in a deceased donor in which the inferior vena cava (IVC) was transected below the right renal vein takeoff. This kidney was able to be used by reconstructing an extension graft. Donor IVC was completely transected and sewn end to end to the right renal vein.

For a DCD operation, the goal is to cannulate aorta as quickly as possible after donor has progressed. After getting into the abdomen from a midline incision, bowels are retracted superiorly, and blunt and sharp dissection is used to get down to aorta at the bifurcation. Once cannulated, a supra celiac aortic clamp is placed. This is followed by draining the venous system either in the abdomen at lower vena cava or in the chest. After flush is initiated, the remainder of the dissection occurs as described previously.

With recent advances in organ preservation techniques, it is becoming increasingly common that procured kidneys will be placed on a perfusion pump for storage. Hypothermic machine perfusion (HMP) continuously pumps cold preservation solution, in contrast to static cold storage, whereby after being flushed with preservation solution, the kidney is stored submerged in preservation solution with ice around it. There is a lower rate of DGF, along with improved long- and short-term graft survival in those kidneys that are placed on HMP pumps.[36] This is true for both DBD and DCD donors. It is therefore recommended to use HMP pumps where available. Parameters that can be assessed on HMP include renal resistance and flow rates. These parameters are only meant to assist in decision-making when using marginal kidneys and should not be the sole factor determining use versus discard of a kidney. Commonly agreed-on poor perfusion parameters include a renal resistance (RR) of >0.40 mm Hg/mL/min and flow rate less than 80 mL/min/100 g. However, these should only be used in conjunction with donor medical history and biopsy findings to assess concordance before considering discard.

BACK-TABLE PREPARATION OF KIDNEY GRAFT

Careful back-table preparation is crucial for a successful kidney transplant. There are no statistics or studies available at present to accurately predict how many kidney discards are a result of inadvertent procurement and/or back-table injuries.

The goal of the back table of a kidney graft is to have adequately exposed artery and vein with hemostatic control of all side branches. Removal of all extra adipose tissue around the kidney is recommended. Preparation of the ureter should focus on preserving the mesentery of the ureter. Closing of biopsy site if present and assessing for leaks at the completion of back table is strongly encouraged.

The kidney graft should be examined for any gross abnormalities or injuries that might make it not transplantable; for example, assess for any capsular tears, check that main artery is intact and orifice is patent, and similarly check that the vein is intact. Ureter entering the pelvic collecting system should be traced. At this point, it is usually acceptable to allow the recipient to be brought back to the room for induction and line placement while back-table preparation of the kidney is completed.

Kidney should be positioned in its anatomic position in the basin. Gentle traction on artery and vein can be accomplished through silk sutures at the corners of arterial patch and edge of vein. For left kidney, vein is prepared first. Dissection stops before the vein enters the renal hilum. This is followed by clearing the artery, ensuring no early branches to the kidney are inadvertently tied off. Vessel probes can be used to assess the trajectory of arterial branches. Methylene blue injection can be used to assess amount of parenchyma supplied by arterial branches. This can be useful when deciding to potentially ligate superior pole branches in situations where preservation of those branches will make the anastomosis challenging. Branches that supply less than 10% of the parenchyma can be safely ligated.[37] Some studies have assessed lower pole arterial branches to delineate ureteral blood supply. In our experience, lower pole branches need to always be preserved and separately prepared on back table if they are far apart on the aortic patch. It is crucial to visualize the whole artery because there may be areas close to hilum that have been injured during procurement (Figs. 52.3 and 52.4). Once vessels have been prepared, perinephric fat is cleared from the kidney. On the posterior aspect of the kidney, the surgeon should ensure that clearing of fat does not extend onto the pelvic collecting system, particularly when there is an extrarenal pelvis.

Biopsy site, if present, should be closed. It can be closed with a chromic suture in an interrupted U-stitch manner, or the site can be closed with running Prolene suture. One needs to ensure biopsy site is not too deep because that increases the risk of inadvertent injury to collecting system, which can lead to urine leak. Biopsy should not be done on inferior pole. If that is encountered, retrograde injection of diluted methylene blue can be used to assess if there is any brisk leakage. If that is encountered, reassessment can be done after repair to decide whether the kidney can be used. Preservation solution can then be injected into the artery and vein to assess for any major leaks.

Right kidney from a deceased donor comes with the IVC. Back-table preparation is similar except for preparation of this conduit. The vena cava is cleared off all tissues, and branches are ligated. Right renal vein is very thin, and generally, no sharp dissection is done to clear the tissue off the right renal vein. Small branches can be ligated carefully if they leak at the time conduit is tested. This vena cava conduit can be useful in scenarios where extra length is needed for a deep pelvis. This conduit can be prepared in different ways. For example, the superior caval orifice and orifice of takeoff of left renal vein can be joined

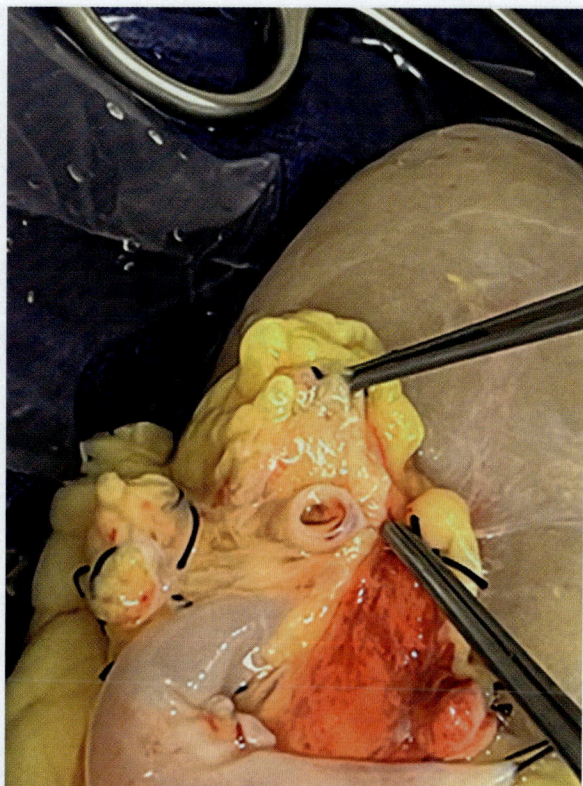

FIGURE 52.4 Artery was cut above the dissection to assess for possible reconstruction. Dissection extended past the first-order branches. This kidney was not used.

and then closed with a running Prolene in two layers (Figs. 52.5 and 52.6).

For right kidneys from living donors, venous conduit construction may be needed to have adequate vein length for anastomosis. Before a living right kidney donor is scheduled, it is important to ensure cadaveric vessels are available in case venous extension is required. If a venous extension is required, cadaveric iliac veins can be used. The cadaveric iliac vein, after being prepared, can then be anastomosed to right renal vein in an end-to-end manner. It is important to keep in mind that iliac vein may have valves; hence, with regard to orientation of conduit, anatomic caudal end of the iliac vein should be the end anastomosed to the renal vein.

KIDNEY TRANSPLANT OPERATION

A standard kidney transplant operation involves retroperitoneal placement of the kidney in right or left iliac fossa. During preoperative planning for kidney transplant, cross-sectional imaging is assessed to look for suitability of vessels for implantation. Because patients with long-standing ESKD will have calcifications of intimal and medial layers of the vessel wall, CT scans of the pelvis can guide placement of vascular clamps for arterial occlusion, avoiding calcified plaque areas. Similarly, it can help pick up the area most suitable for arterial anastomosis.

The preferred site of arterial anastomosis is the external iliac artery. If both external iliac arteries are severely calcified, the common iliac can be used for anastomosis. Previous surgical history of inguinal hernia repair will make retroperitoneal exposure challenging; hence, the opposite side to hernia repair

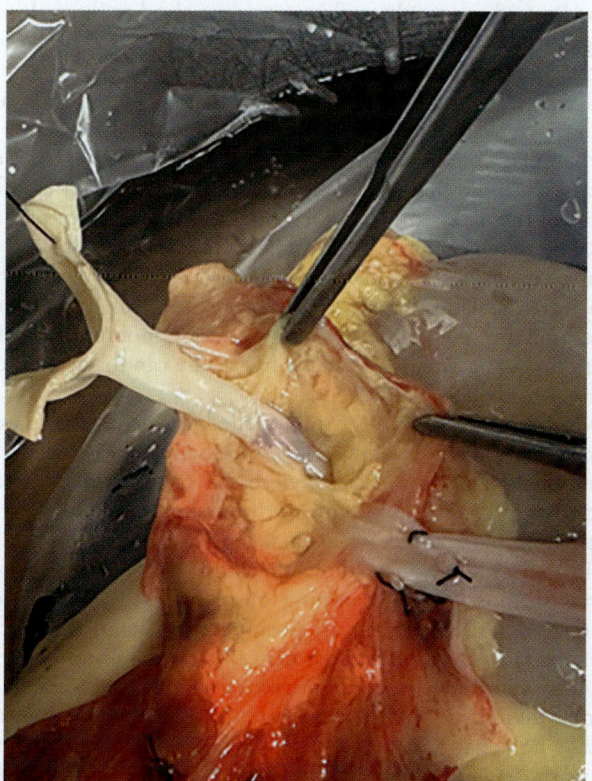

FIGURE 52.3 Renal artery dissection encountered at the hilum during back table preparation of kidney.

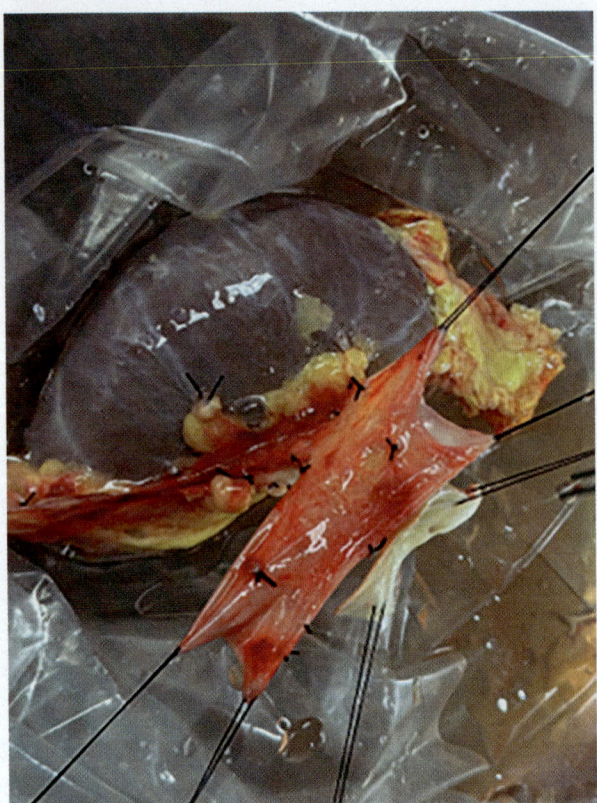

FIGURE 52.5 Right kidney on the back table with a cuff of inferior vena cava above the right renal vein.

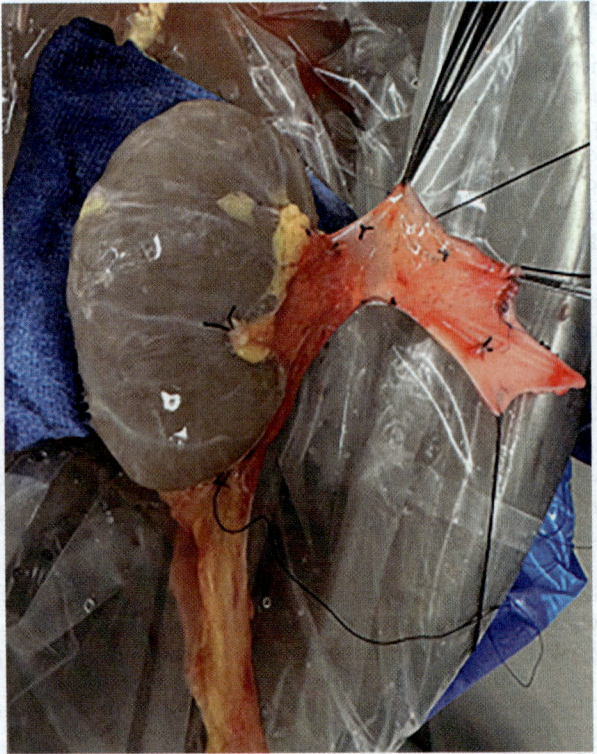

FIGURE 52.6 Reconstructed conduit for right renal vein with running Prolene across the top of vena cava extending onto left renal vein takeoff orifice.

may be better suited for implantation. With most inguinal hernia repairs now being done with laparoscopic techniques, patients may not remember the correct side during their history taking. CT scan will show signs of previous hernia repair, such as poor demarcation of planes on the side of hernia repair, and mesh can sometimes be visible as well on cross-sectional imaging. If there is hernia repair on the side with better blood vessels, it is generally recommended to still implant on that side even though vascular exposure on that side may be more challenging. Mesh can be traversed with heat cautery if encountered during dissection.

Anatomic landmarks that are helpful if marked on the abdominal wall include anterior superior iliac spine and pubic symphysis. A hockey-stick incision is made on the side where the kidney is going to be implanted. Incision should be roughly 2 to 4 cm medial to the anterior superior iliac spine (ASIS). The goal is to have minimal transection of musculature of lateral abdominal wall. Retroperitoneal space can be entered by transecting the linea semilunaris and gently moving the peritoneum medially. As the incision is extended cephalad, it may have to come through muscle layers of lateral abdominal wall as incision is extended laterally to have better exposure of right retroperitoneum. Caudally, incision is ideally extended to the pubic symphysis because this allows easier exposure of the bladder, especially in ESKD patients who have been anuric for multiple years and have atrophied and contracted muscular layers of the bladder.

When dissecting in the retroperitoneum, the round ligament in females can be ligated. In males, the spermatic cord is looped with a Penrose drain and retracted medially. Inferior epigastric vessels may be encountered in caudal aspect of the incision as they cross through the created space toward their course underneath the rectus abdominus muscle. These can be ligated if retraction is being limited as a result or if retractors may lead to them sheering. If ligated, leaving a longer stump at the proximal end allows for inflow options in situations of a known inferior pole artery or a missed artery, which may become evident after reperfusion of the kidney. After placement of retractors, external iliac artery and external iliac vein are exposed. All lymphatic channels anterior to the artery should be carefully ligated or coagulated. At the inferior aspect of the external iliac artery, one needs to be wary of a large crossing venous branch as it drains into the external iliac vein. Goal of exposure is to have an appropriate length of artery and vein for easy clamping and space for anastomosis. In atherosclerotic arteries, one needs to limit posterior mobilization of the artery because a circumferentially free artery can dissect and crack at sites of calcified plaque.

Minimize the amount of time needed for the kidney to be out of ice. Position the kidney in iliac fossa, and pull vessels to proposed site of anastomosis. In deceased donor kidney arteries, aortic patch can be used, and the vein should be cut to an appropriate length based on arterial length. Leaving an ice pack behind the kidney may allow the kidney to stay cold longer. Heparinization before clamping of vessels is a debated topic. There is no increased risk of postoperative hemorrhage if systemic heparin is administered; hence, it can be done in selected patients who may be at a high risk of vascular thrombosis. But overall, there is no difference in rates of thrombosis between patients who are administered systemic heparin before anastomosis versus those who are not.[38] Data are lacking to determine if systemic heparinization prevents venous thrombus formation of distal branches of clamped vein.

Venous anastomosis of the renal vein to the external iliac vein is performed first in an end-to-side manner with running 5-0 Prolene suture. This is followed by arterial anastomosis in an end-to-side manner between renal artery and external iliac artery with running 6-0 Prolene suture. For reperfusion, vein clamp is taken off first, followed by arterial clamp. The kidney is then warmed with irrigation. Hemostasis is secured.

Ureter is prepared by intentionally keeping it as short as possible for a tension-free anastomosis. Ureter is trimmed back to appropriate length, and if there is bleeding from the edges, this is a reassuring sign. Vascular bundles are ligated at the edge of the spatulated ureter. For ureteroneocystostomy, the bladder is back-filled with methylene blue–stained irrigation. Peritoneal reflection on superior and medial aspect of bladder is identified and swiped upward. Dissection on bladder wall is carried down through detrusor muscle to the mucosa. Mucosal entry should be made sharply, with anastomosis completed in two layers over a double-J stent. There is evidence that routine stenting of ureteroneocystostomy prevents major complications such as ureteral strictures and urine leakage.[39,40] The ureter is anastomosed to bladder mucosa with running polydioxanone (PDS) suture. Minimal handling of ureteral edges is recommended to prevent iatrogenic injury because ureteral wall is very fragile and can easily get crushed between tips of forceps. Second layer is of detrusor muscle on top of the ureter with a PDS suture. Once anastomosis is completed, Foley catheter can be unclamped to allow urine to start draining.

The length of time it takes to sew the kidney affects outcomes. The goal is to be swift but precise. Once out of ice, kidney should be reperfused, ideally in less than 45 minutes. An implantation time of more than 45 minutes increases risk of poor early graft function.[41] It is unclear if there is a difference in long-term outcomes. Some of the predictors of prolonged sew time include obese patients and use of right kidneys (because they are more likely to have multiple and longer arteries and more complex venous anastomosis).

SURGICAL COMPLICATIONS AND THEIR MANAGEMENT

1. **Transplant renal artery stenosis (RAS):** RAS is one the most common complications after renal transplant. Reported incidence is wide, ranging from 1% to 12%.[42] Early diagnosis is crucial for adequate treatment to prevent cortical necrosis and graft loss. Patients may present with worsening allograft function not explained by any other cause; refractory hypertension; and other signs of graft failure, such as fluid retention leading to volume overload. Patients with concern of RAS, based on ultrasound, should have confirmatory testing with a different modality, such as a magnetic resonance angiography (MRA). This limits administration of potentially nephrotoxic contrast to only at the time of therapeutic intervention such as angiogram and angioplasty. Ultrasound findings that suggest RAS include (1) an absolute peak systolic velocity (PSV) of 340 to 400 cm/sec at the anastomosis with normal waveforms, (2) a tardus parvus waveform, and (3) relatively reduced resistive indexes (RIs) from prior or RIs less than 0.5.[43] On an angiogram, a luminal narrowing of more than 50% with other concordant clinical findings suggestive of RAS should be treated. Most cases are resolved by percutaneous transluminal angioplasty with stent placement (Figs. 52.7 and 52.8). Not all renal artery stenoses will require intervention because routine postoperative surveillance imaging, such as Doppler ultrasound,

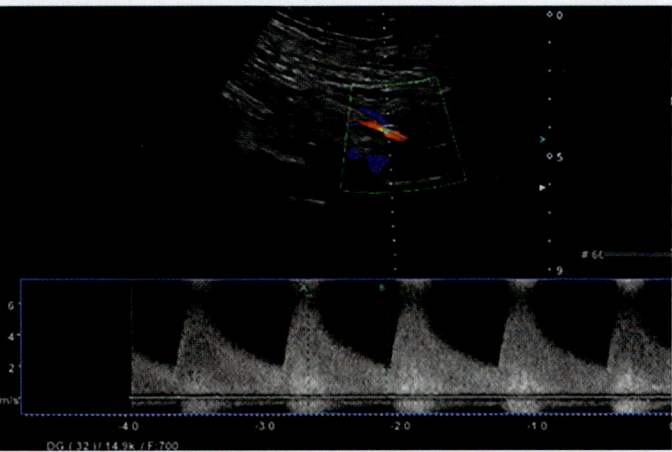

FIGURE 52.7 Ultrasound Doppler at 3 months after deceased donor renal transplantation of a 64-year-old male with increasing serum creatinine. Peak systolic velocity at the anastomosis is >600 cm/s.

can have findings that are consistent with RAS per radiologic criterion but have no clinical effect on the kidney.

2. **Renal artery thrombosis:** This is usually encountered in immediate postoperative settings, mostly within the first month after transplant. It is a surgical emergency and needs to be addressed promptly for any chances of graft salvage. Incidence is low at about less than 1%. Most of the cases are a result of technical issues. Intimal flap in the artery, external compression from a hematoma, dissection of the external iliac artery from clamp placement, and kinking of the artery at the time of fascial closure can all lead to renal artery thrombosis. Hyperacute rejection can also lead to renal artery thrombosis, but this is extremely rare, given advancements in immunologic matching between donors and recipients. Ultrasound will show an absence of arterial flow to renal parenchyma, and it can be confirmed by contrast-enhanced ultrasound. If patient was previously making urine, there may be an abrupt cessation of urine production, and there may be pain as a result of peritoneal irritation from an infarcting kidney. When encountered in the immediate postoperative setting, patient needs to be emergently taken back for exploration. The operating room team should be aware of the possibility of graft explant and reimplantation. If absence of flow is confirmed upon entry with visual inspection, inspection of vasculature, and Doppler examination, graft should be explanted by reclamping the vessels. Graft needs to be assessed on the back table and flushed with cold preservation solution. Artery needs to be assessed. If a dissection is present, it may not be salvageable if it extends into hilar branches; otherwise, an attempt should be made to cut back to healthy artery wall. If parenchyma flushes out well, this kidney may be able to be retransplanted. If there is a concern about timeline between renal artery thrombosis and reexploration, a kidney biopsy should be sent for frozen section. A finding of significant cortical necrosis will render the kidney not transplantable.

3. **Renal vein thrombosis:** This is a rare complication; the reported incidence in the literature ranges from 0.3% to 4.2%.[43] If it occurs in the immediate postoperative period, patients will have an abrupt drop in urine output, urine will appear sanguineous, and there may be pain from graft swelling. This can be life threatening because graft rupture can occur as a result

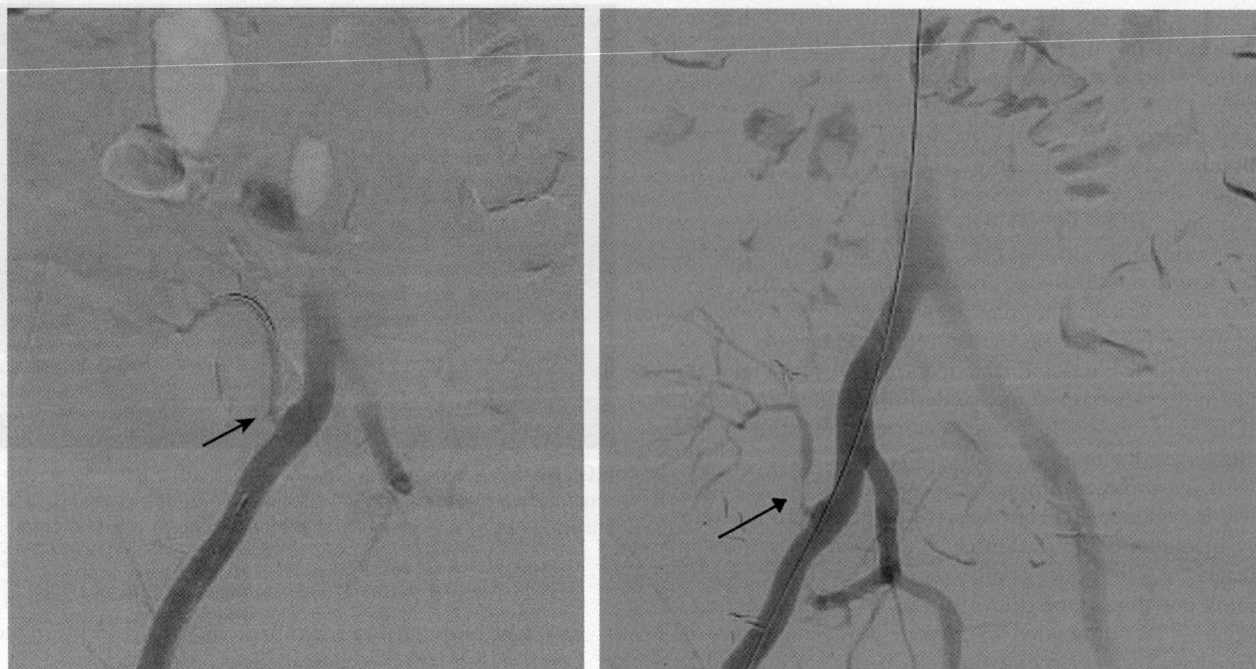

FIGURE 52.8 Angiogram of the same 64-year-old male before and after deployment of balloon expandable stent across the stenotic segment.

of patent inflow and occluded outflow. Ultrasound is the modality of choice and will show either a hypoechoic or anechoic clot; another characteristic finding is reversal of diastolic flow in renal artery on Doppler assessment. At the time of reexploration, direct thrombectomy can be attempted, and if unable to retrieve clot from renal vein, the team may need to explant the graft. Upon explant, graft needs to be flushed with cold preservation solution and assessed for viability before reimplantation.

4. **Peritransplant collections:** Depending on the time posttransplant, the differential for the etiology of fluid collection varies. Hematomas usually present within the first few days posttransplant. Patients may complain of pain in flank region because a hematoma can dissect into retroperitoneal fat on that side of the transplant. A drop in hemoglobin, along with an ultrasound showing peritransplant collection, will usually be sufficient to confirm the diagnosis. A noncontrast CT scan can better evaluate the extent of the hematoma as well. Reexploration and washout are recommended. The source of bleeding may not be found in most cases, but hematoma evacuation is necessary because it can compress vasculature and become infected, leading to future abscess formation. Small incidental hematomas that are found on surveillance ultrasound can be left alone. Peritransplant abscesses need to be dealt with aggressively and can often be managed percutaneously, but operative debridement should be strongly considered. Lymphoceles are another common collection that will be encountered in postoperative period. They are usually encountered between 2 weeks to 6 months after transplantation, with a peak incidence at 6 weeks.[44] There is a wide range of incidence reported from 1% to 50%.[45] Patients may present with symptoms of pain and pressure at site of transplant. On examination, surgical site swelling may be noticeable as well; there may be associated lower extremity swelling on the same side as a result of

compression of iliac vein. Labs can demonstrate worsening renal function. Surgical technique matters when clearing iliac artery because multiple lymphatic channels cross anterior to the vessel. The large ones should be ligated, and smaller ones should be coagulated. Lymphatic channels from the transplanted kidney hilum can leak as well; hence, careful ligation of excess tissue is important. Management involves percutaneous drainage, which has a high failure rate. After simple drainage fails, it can be followed by povidone-iodine sclerotherapy, which is a safe modality for management of primary symptomatic lymphoceles.[46] Surgical management involves creating a peritoneal window, which can be done both laparoscopically and open. When making this peritoneal window, careful attention needs to be paid to preoperative imaging to stay clear of ureter and hilar vascular structures. Once this fluid is drained, it should be sent off for Gram stain and culture. Fluid creatinine should also be assessed to rule out a urine leak.

5. **Urologic complications:** Most ureteral complications stem from a failure to preserve its blood supply during either procurement or back-table preparation. Transplanted kidney ureter is dependent on blood supply through the mesoureter. Any tissue on the inferior pole of the kidney surrounding the ureter needs to be preserved. Preservation of the inferior pole artery, if present, is critical because in those kidneys, the ureter will be dependent on it for the blood supply. Ureteral stenosis presents a few weeks to months after transplant; it is reported in the literature to have an incidence of 2.6% to 15%.[47] Patients will present with worsening renal function with hydronephrosis on ultrasound. Acute hydronephrosis can be managed by placement of a nephrostomy tube. A retrograde placement of a double-J stent can also be attempted, but in some cases, severity of stenosis may prevent a wire from passing. An antegrade nephrostogram can help assess the length of the

stenosis. Minimally invasive techniques that can be attempted before open surgery, such as balloon stenting and self-expanding metal stent placement, have been described in the literature. Open surgical technique depends on size and location of the stricture. If it is a short-segment stenosis at the anastomosis, it can be fixed by reimplantation of the healthy ureteral edge into the bladder. If stenosis is a long segment or too proximal, a ureteropyelostomy is needed, using the native ureter. In delayed presentations of ureteral stricture, it is important to rule out BK viremia. Urine leak in immediate postoperative period is either a result of surgical error or distal ureter necrosis caused by ischemia. Reported incidence is between 1.5% and 8.9%.[48] An attempt should be made to manage it conservatively with bladder catheterization, double-J stent placement if not previously stented, and drainage of urine in perinephric space with a percutaneous drain. Unless there is complete disruption of the ureteroneocystostomy, these maneuvers may work to seal the leak. If they do not work, open surgical techniques, as mentioned earlier for ureteral stenosis, will be needed.

SUMMARY

Kidney transplantation is an evolving field with many advances being made to diminish organ-shortage constraints and decrease waiting times for accessing lifesaving transplants. The current landscape of kidney transplantation aims to equitably increase access to organs by broadening the donor pool, improving allocation algorithms, and decreasing organ discard from deceased donors. Careful selection of transplant recipients is important to ensure maximal benefit from this limited resource. Success of a kidney transplant depends on careful selection of a donor organ and suitable recipient, as well as meticulous surgical technique to prevent postoperative surgical complications.

SELECTED REFERENCES

Bock MJ, Vaughn GR, Chau P, Berumen JA, Nigro JJ, Ingulli EG. Organ transplantation using COVID-19-positive deceased donors. *Am J Transplant.* 2022;22(9):2203-2216.

In the postpandemic world, this article explains the safety of use of organs from COVID-19–positive donors in certain settings.

Chadban SJ, Ahn C, Axelrod DA, et al. KDIGO clinical practice guideline on the evaluation and management of candidates for kidney transplantation. *Transplantation.* 2020;104(4S1 suppl 1):S11-S103.

This is a comprehensive review of the selection of a suitable kidney transplant recipient.

Lentine KL, Kasiske BL, Levey AS, et al. KDIGO clinical practice guideline on the evaluation and care of living kidney donors. *Transplantation.* 2017;101(8S suppl 1):S1-S109.

Most recent overview of the selection of living kidney donors.

Lentine KL, Naik AS, Schnitzler MA, et al. Variation in use of procurement biopsies and its implications for discard of deceased donor kidneys recovered for transplantation. *Am J Transplant.* 2019;19(8):2241-2251.

This article highlights the necessity of limiting kidney biopsies to only high-risk kidneys to decrease the organ discard rate.

Locke JE, Reed RD, Massie AB, et al. Obesity and long-term mortality risk among living kidney donors. *Surgery.* 2019;166(2):205-208.

Obese donors need additional counseling at time of donation, and this article brings forward objective data to be discussed at the time of informed consent.

The full reference list appears on Elsevier eBooks+.

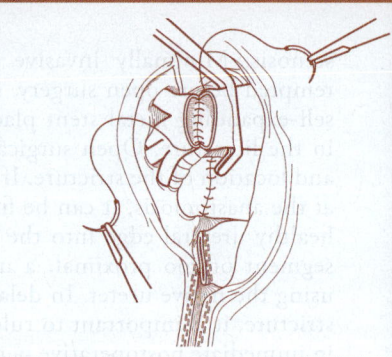

53 | CHAPTER

Liver Transplantation

Franklin Olumba, William C. Chapman Sr., and Majella Doyle

HISTORY

More than 90% of patients receiving a liver transplant in the United States will be alive 1 year after the surgery, and almost 88% will be alive after 3 years.[1] This extraordinary achievement arose as a result of the synthesis of a myriad of discoveries in disparate fields. Liver transplantation represents a triumph of scientific achievement, collaboration, and teamwork.

Seminal discoveries instrumental in developing transplantation trace back more than 100 years. These include the technical achievements of Alexis Carrel in creating vascular anastomoses in the first decade of the 20th century. While performing research on skin grafting for soldiers in World War II in the early 1940s, Sir Peter Medawar discovered graft loss was due to immunologic factors, specifically cell-mediated immunity.[2] His subsequent studies established the efficacy of steroids to protect against graft injury.[3] In 1952, the chemists Gertrude Eillion and George Hitchings at Burroughs-Wellcome synthesized azathioprine and 6-mercaptopurine, which would become cornerstones of early immunosuppressive therapy. In 1954, Joseph Murray proved transplantation could be successful by performing a renal transplant using an identical twin as a donor.[4] In 1959, Dr. Murray went on to demonstrate the feasibility of transplantation across immunologic barriers using total body irradiation to suppress the immune system.[5] All of these investigators earned a Nobel Prize in recognition of their accomplishments.

Despite these advancements allowing limited success for kidney transplantation, early attempts at human liver transplantation were marked by failure (expertly chronicled in the book *The Puzzle People* by Thomas Starzl).[6] Technical complexities of the operation, coagulopathy, metabolic derangements, and poor understanding of the immunologic basis of graft loss conspired to produce poor outcomes. The first attempt at human liver transplantation in 1963 by Dr. Starzl failed, as did subsequent attempts in Berlin, Boston, and Paris. Things looked so grim that Starzl himself placed a 3-year moratorium on liver transplantation, returning exclusively to the lab to determine how to best move forward.[6]

With advances in technique and immunosuppression, limited success was achieved. In the 1970s, Starzl reported 1-year survival rates around 30%.[7] Nearly two decades after the first liver transplant was attempted, Jean Borel discovered that cyclosporine, initially investigated as an antifungal agent, had immunosuppressive properties.[8] This discovery ushered in the modern era of liver transplantation as cyclosporine became the mainstay of antirejection therapy.

As outcomes improved, attention turned toward maximizing the number of available donors. In 1989, Mies and colleagues[9] in Brazil described two cases of liver transplantation from live adult donors into children, although neither achieved long-term survival. The first generally accepted successful living donor liver transplantation (LDLT) in a pediatric recipient was performed by Strong and colleagues.[10] A Japanese group led by Koichi Tanaka produced excellent outcomes using these techniques and established the reliability of this approach.[11] Approximately 10 years later, the first adult-to-adult LDLT using the left lobe was performed by Hashikura and colleagues.[12]

Other efforts to expand the donor pool include the use of grafts produced after circulatory determination of death and grafts with higher than previously accepted fibrosis or fat content for selected recipients. To this end, the past 10 years have seen a rapid increase in techniques that allow transplantation of more marginal grafts. These include ex vivo normothermic and hypothermic machine perfusion of any marginal grafts as well as normothermic regional perfusion of circulatory death grafts.

INDICATIONS

Indications for adult liver transplantation fall into two main categories: (1) symptomatic liver failure and (2) select liver tumors with tumor location or accompanying liver disease preventing proper oncologic resection. Disease states causing liver failure that may be successfully treated with transplant include noncholestatic and cholestatic cirrhosis (Box 53.1), cancer, fulminant hepatic failure, metabolic diseases, and biliary atresia as well as a relatively rare mix of other causes, including Budd-Chiari syndrome, hyperalimentation-induced liver disease, large adenomas, and polycystic liver disease. With the advent of effective antiviral therapy for hepatitis C, the most common reason patients are listed for liver transplantation is alcoholic liver disease, followed by metabolicassociated steatohepatitis (MASH), which rose dramatically in the late 2010s, followed by hepatitis C.

Noncholestatic Cirrhosis

The common theme in these diseases is hepatocyte injury. Although the liver has a unique potential to regenerate, over time, chronic hepatocyte injury results in stellate cell activation, leading to widespread collagen deposition. This process disrupts the unique liver microstructure that allows low-pressure portal blood flow, nutrient exchange, and bile secretion. This in turn leads to portal hypertension and associated varices and ascites. As hepatocyte synthetic and excretory function fails, coagulopathy, jaundice, hypoalbuminemia, fatigue, pruritus, and encephalopathy may occur. Additional complications, the development of which is poorly understood, include hepatorenal syndrome, hepatopulmonary syndrome, and portopulmonary hypertension. The term *noncholestatic* reflects that the primary injury is to the hepatocytes and not the bile ducts, even though patients can and often do present with jaundice.

Alcoholic

Alcoholic liver disease encompasses steatohepatitis, alcoholic cirrhosis, and alcoholic hepatitis.[13] The absolute number of patients listed with this diagnosis is growing, and chronic alcohol ingestion

---

BOX 53.1   Disease States Causing Liver Failure That May Be Successfully Treated With Transplant

Noncholestatic Cirrhosis
Alcoholic
Metabolic-associated fatty liver disease
Hepatitis C
Cryptogenic cirrhosis
Autoimmune cirrhosis
Hepatitis B
Drug or exposure induced

Cholestatic Cirrhosis
Primary biliary cirrhosis (PBC)
Primary sclerosing cholangitis (PSC)
Caroli disease
Choledochal cyst

---

remains the most common indication for liver transplantation, responsible for approximately 39% of all listings.[1] Ingestion of 30 g of alcohol per day seems to be a relevant threshold and will cause chronic liver damage in approximately 6% of people; risk increases with increasing use.[14] Screening for alcoholic liver disease (ALD) is recommended with biochemical testing and liver ultrasonography in any patients meeting harmful use criteria. These include greater than 3 drinks per day in males and greater than 2 drinks per day in females for a duration greater than 1 year. Not all patients meeting these criteria will have acute or chronic liver disease, but screening evaluation should still take place if history is elicited.

Toxicity of ethanol is incompletely understood but likely depends on conversion to acetaldehyde via alcohol dehydrogenase, catalase, or cytochrome P450. Over time, pericentral fibrosis progresses to panlobar fibrosis with associated manifestations of cirrhosis. The ratio of aspartate aminotransferase (AST) to alanine aminotransferase (ALT) is typically greater than 2, and transaminase elevation tends to be relatively mild (<500).

Alcoholic hepatitis is a subset of alcohol-associated liver disease that occurs in patients with a long history of alcohol use who present with an acute inflammatory syndrome with a bilirubin of greater than 3.0 mg/dL. Episodes can be self-limited or lead to complete liver failure. This diagnosis is increasingly common as an indication for liver transplantation.

Historically, decisions regarding whether to list a patient with ALD for transplantation depended on a period of sobriety before transplant, typically 6 months, because of concern for recidivism and injury to the transplanted liver. Policies vary by center, but in general, these guidelines have been relaxed over time because there is evidence from European studies to suggest good outcomes in patients transplanted for alcoholic hepatitis with shorter-duration abstinence of periods as long as 2 weeks.[15] Current practice guidance from the American Association for the Study of Liver Diseases on alcohol-associated liver disease recommends referral for transplant if the model for end-stage liver disease (MELD) is greater than 20.[16] Such patients with no improvement in liver disease after a 6-month period of abstinence are recommended to undergo liver transplantation evaluation if the MELD score in greater than 17.

Metabolic-Associated Fatty Liver Disease

Metabolic-associated fatty liver disease (MAFLD) is a recently coined term to describe a complex and heterogeneous disease phenotype with several causes. This shift represents our increasing understanding of the disease as one influenced by a panoply of factors, such as age, sex, ethnicity, environmental factors, diet, genetic predisposition, an individual's microbiota, and even their alcohol intake (Fig. 53.1).[17] The change in terminology also reflects the patient perspective because the term *nonalcoholic* can make light of the disease process and even assign blame for the patient's condition as well as its treatment.

The drivers of MAFLD for an individual will vary greatly based on factors present, and thus, the ways to address and study the disease also vary. This is among several reasons for the nomenclature change. MAFLD reflects a spectrum of disease, ranging from mild to moderate hepatic steatosis to the inflammatory condition known as *metabolic-associated steatohepatitis* (MASH; formerly known as *nonalcoholic steatohepatitis* [NASH]) and end-stage liver cirrhosis. It is important to recognize the full spectrum of disease because pathology such as hepatocellular carcinoma has been observed even in patients with moderate steatosis without MASH or cirrhosis.

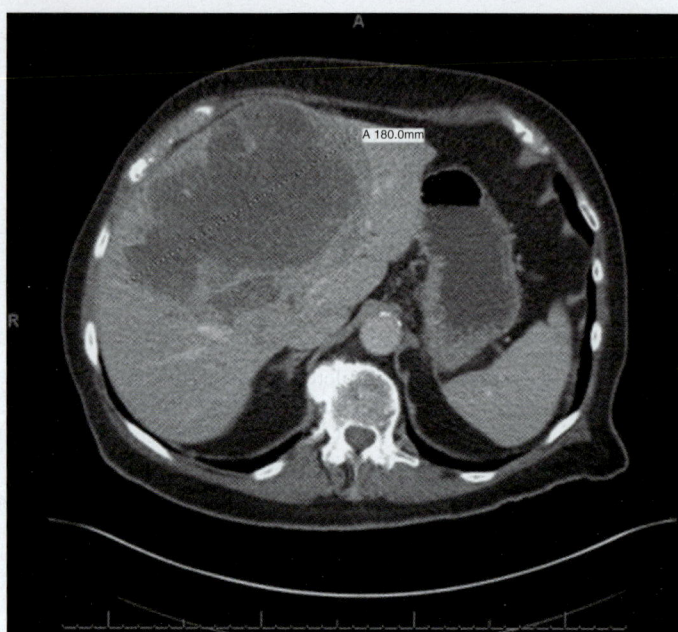

FIGURE 53.1 Heterogeneity of metabolic-associated fatty liver disease.

This spectrum of disease is more common in Western nations, affecting over 1 billion people worldwide. The prevalence of MAFLD worldwide is about 25%, with MASH prevalence worldwide being around 4% to 6%. In America, approximately 20% to 30% of adults meet criteria for some form of MAFLD, although only about 4% of patients with steatosis progress to cirrhosis. Still, MAFLD must be taken seriously because roughly 20% of patients progressing from hepatic steatosis to MASH will go on to develop liver cirrhosis over their lifetime.[18] MASH is now the second most common indication for liver transplantation in the United States. Biopsy in MASH demonstrates hepatocyte steatosis, ballooning degeneration, and lobular inflammation, most commonly in zone 3. Over time, the inflammation can progress to fibrosis, cirrhosis, and liver failure, leading to the need for liver transplantation. Before end-stage cirrhosis and liver failure, lower levels of hepatic steatosis can be reversible in some patients with diet and lifestyle modification as well as control of metabolic syndrome–associated comorbidities (diabetes, hyperlipidemia, and hypertension). MASH, however, has been historically difficult to treat. Very recent advances in the understanding of MASH pathophysiology have led to the development of Resmetirom, a thyroid hormone receptor β-selective agonist. This first-in-class treatment demonstrated biopsy improvement of MASH and MAFLD activity as well as low-density lipoprotein cholesterol levels in the treatment group compared with placebo in a phase III study and was FDA approved in March 2024.[19]

The growing incidence of MAFLD in the Western world has also begun to affect liver donation, with an increasing number of potential donors being unsuitable because of higher levels of steatosis and early MASH development on recovery biopsy.

Hepatitis C

In 2016, Bartenschlager, Rice, and Sofia were awarded the Lasker-DeBakey Clinical Medical Research Award for efforts instrumental in developing effective therapies for hepatitis C.[20] Their work, and that of many others, revolutionized the care and treatment of patients with advanced liver disease in two fundamental ways. First, it greatly reduced the burden of hepatitis C and the number of patients being listed with this diagnosis, and second, it allowed the use of organs from donors with hepatitis C, significantly increasing the organ supply. As a result, hepatitis C has gone from the most common to the third most common indication for liver transplantation in the United States, a truly remarkable achievement.

Patients who present with advanced cirrhosis should be considered for liver transplantation consistent with usual clinical indications. Patients with mild disease should be treated with the end goal of sustained virologic response (SVR), defined as undetectable hepatitis C virus (HCV) RNA in the serum or plasma either 12 weeks or 24 weeks after the end of therapy. Those achieving SVR may delay or arrest further disease progression and, in some cases, reverse fibrosis.[21] In patients with advanced disease, the decision to treat is individualized to the patient. Depending on the level of fibrosis, all patients, including those achieving SVR, must have regular posttreatment hepatocellular carcinoma (HCC) surveillance (as frequent as every 6 months) because the risk of cancer development remains.

Cryptogenic

Cryptogenic cirrhosis remains an ambiguous cause of liver disease and is a diagnosis of exclusion. Up to 30% of liver cirrhosis is due to cryptogenic cirrhosis as well as up to 10% of liver transplants. Ongoing scholarship suggests that many patients with cryptogenic cirrhosis share a lot of comorbidities with those diagnosed with MASH-related cirrhosis. Histopathologic evidence also demonstrates that during the natural progression of MASH, steatosis can disappear, leaving extensive fibrosis seen in cirrhosis without clear evidence of the preceding steatohepatitis. This has led many to believe most of what we consider cryptogenic cirrhosis is actually "burnout-stage" advanced MASH cirrhosis. Still, there are some groups finding distinct differences between cohorts of patients with cryptogenic cirrhosis and MASH cirrhosis, and debate continues on whether it should be its own pathologic entity.[22,23] The diagnosis, treatment, and decision-making remain similar to patients with MASH.

Autoimmune

Autoimmune hepatitis is an inflammatory disease of the liver with poorly understood etiology. Some accepted hypotheses include loss of immunologic tolerance against hepatocytes by the environment in some genetically predisposed individuals (possessing human leukocyte antigen [HLA]-DR3 and HLA-DR4 alleles) as well as possible molecular mimicry. It occurs mostly in females (75%), with a bimodal age distribution of patients in their 20s and in their 50s to 60s, although it is reported in both sexes and all age groups, including pediatric populations.[24] The course can be self-limited or recurrent, leading to chronic liver disease and cirrhosis requiring transplantation. Diagnosis is typically one of exclusion. Characteristic findings on laboratory evaluation include high elevations in AST and ALT, lesser elevations in alkaline phosphatase, and elevated gamma globulins. Antinuclear and anti–smooth muscle antibodies as well as IgG are often elevated. Histologic findings include a mononuclear cell infiltrate primarily in the portal regions, and piecemeal necrosis may be present at the periportal region. Most patients will have ductal injury, and plasma cell infiltrates are common. In the initial stages of the disease, fibrosis may be absent. As the disease progresses, fibrosis occurs and may develop into cirrhosis. Transplantation should be considered for patients who develop cirrhosis.

Hepatitis B

Approximately 3.8% of the world population has been exposed to hepatitis B, and nearly 296 million are chronic carriers,[25] making hepatitis B a major public health problem. Acute infection with hepatitis B is subclinical in 70% of patients. Approximately 30% will develop jaundice. Less than 1% will develop fulminant hepatic failure. These patients should be considered for emergent liver transplantation. In patients who develop chronic infection, progression to cirrhosis is influenced by the age of onset. For perinatal acquired infection, 90% will progress to chronic infection, with rates decreasing as the age of transmission increases.[25]

Up through the late 1990s, transplantation for patients with hepatitis B produced poor outcomes as a result of disease recurrence. This changed with the discovery of lamivudine, which, in combination with hepatitis B immunoglobulin, allowed successful transplantation of these patients. In current practice, patients with hepatitis B routinely receive liver transplants, and donors with hepatitis B can be used with appropriate antiviral therapy.

Cholestatic Liver Disease

The common thread in this group of diseases is chronic biliary damage. As ducts become injured, bile stasis occurs, leading to infection and a vicious cycle of damage, inflammation, and recurrent infection. Pruritis can be debilitating. Recurrent cholangitis may produce the classic Charcot triad of jaundice, fever, and right upper quadrant pain. Ongoing biliary damage predisposes the patient to the development of cholangiocarcinoma, especially in patients with primary sclerosing cholangitis (PSC).

Primary Biliary Cholangitis

Primary biliary cholangitis is an autoimmune disease in which inflammatory injury to the bile ducts results in cholestatic liver disease. Granulomatous destruction of the intralobar ducts resulting from loss of immune tolerance to biliary epithelial cells causes obstruction and jaundice.[26] Patients often suffer from jaundice and pruritis. Laboratory evaluation typically reveals elevated alkaline phosphatase, and positive antimitochondrial antibodies are often present. History often reveals fatigue and pruritis, with physical exam showing jaundice and xanthomata. Osteoporosis commonly develops. Positive antimitochondrial antibodies are the hallmark of the disease. The mainstay first-line treatment is the use of ursodeoxycholic acid, with several mechanisms of action suggested. Roughly 40% of patients do not respond to this therapy and will eventually require transplantation at higher rates than responders to initial therapy.

Primary Sclerosing Cholangitis

Patients with PSC develop fibrosis of the intrahepatic and/or extrahepatic biliary tree, leading to inflammation. The disease is more common in males. Diffuse structuring leads to jaundice, pruritis, fibrosis, recurrent biliary sepsis, and liver failure. Many patients with PSC also have a history of inflammatory bowel disease. These patients are at high risk for cholangiocarcinoma and require careful screening. Laboratory evaluation most commonly shows elevated alkaline phosphatase. In addition, gamma-globulin, serum immunoglobulin M levels, atypical perinuclear antineutrophil cytoplasmic antibodies, HLA DRw52a, antinuclear, anti–smooth muscle, anticardiolipin, thyroperoxidase, and rheumatoid factor may be elevated and can provide clues to the diagnosis. Antimitochondrial antibodies are generally negative in contrast to primary biliary cholangitis.

Patients with PSC carry a significant risk of cholangiocarcinoma of 13%. With the onset of cholangiocarcinoma, carbohydrate antigen 19-9 (CA 19-9) levels typically rise and should be followed serially.

Caroli Disease

Caroli disease is a poorly understood congenital disorder of the large intrahepatic bile ducts. Most commonly, the disease is transmitted in an autosomal recessive fashion associated with polycystic renal disease. When associated with congenital hepatic fibrosis, the term *Caroli syndrome* is used. Like PSC, stasis, recurrent infection, and ongoing fibrosis lead to liver failure in some patients, although the severity of disease is variable. Patients are at risk for the development of cholangiocarcinoma.

Acute Liver Failure

Acute liver failure (ALF) is a clinical syndrome of liver injury (elevated transaminases), hepatic encephalopathy, and coagulopathy (elevated prothrombin time [PT]/international normalized ratio [INR]) in patients without preexisting liver disease. Terminology can be confusing. In general, *fulminant liver failure, acute hepatic necrosis, fulminant hepatic necrosis,* or *fulminant hepatitis* can refer to the same clinical syndrome. Importantly, the presence of encephalopathy is required for the diagnosis and for listing in the most urgent category for liver transplant, a status 1A designation.

ALF can be further divided based on the duration between onset of symptoms and encephalopathy. Hyperacute liver failure occurs within 7 days of symptom onset; acute, from 7 to 21 days; and subacute, between 21 days and 26 weeks. The shorter the duration of symptoms, the more common it is for patients to develop cerebral edema. In contrast, patients with disease of longer duration more commonly present with portal hypertension.

The most common causes of ALF are given in Box 53.2, with acetaminophen overdose being the most common cause.

Patients with ALF present with challenging management decisions, centered around determining who needs a transplant and who will improve with supportive management. Although successful transplantation is associated with excellent survival (84% 1-year survival in the United States), it is still inferior to the survival rates of patients who spontaneously recover.[27] Contrarily, failure to list and perform a transplant in a patient who needs one will result in death. This is made more challenging by the need for an expeditious workup and, if needed, listing for transplantation. The challenge is typified by patients with acetaminophen overdose, who tend to be young but may have a history of multiple suicide attempts or poor social support, leading to challenges in treatment decision-making. Hospital mortality for patients with ALF can be predicted by the MELD system or the King's College Criteria, with evidence suggesting more

---

BOX 53.2 Common Causes of Acute Liver Failure

- Acetaminophen overdose
- Drug ingestion
- Indeterminate
- Hepatitis B
- Hepatitis A
- Autoimmune
- Ischemia
- Wilson disease

accurate mortality prediction among acetaminophen-associated ALF with the King's College Criteria.

Progression of hepatic encephalopathy to stage II can be used as a guideline to move forward with transplant, although this differs among transplant centers. More precise determination in these patients again uses the King's College Criteria.[28] In a patient with acetaminophen overdose, arterial pH less than 7.3 after resuscitation or high PT, creatinine, and grade III or IV encephalopathy suggest need for transplant. Use of serial computed tomography (CT) scans or an intracranial pressure monitor (bolt) can help guide therapy and, importantly, the decision to proceed with transplantation.

Malignant Neoplasms

Hepatocellular Cancer

In 2022 approximately 16% of transplants performed in the United States were performed for HCC as the primary indication.[1]

Initial efforts in performing liver transplantation for HCC produced dismal results, with very high recurrence rates. Over time, it became apparent that early-stage lesions did quite well; clinical evidence began to demonstrate the correlation between initial tumor size and number, risk of micrometastasis, and recurrence. The best set of clinical criteria based on this relationship was published by a group in Milan, eponymously defined as the *Milan Criteria*.[29] These early-stage lesions have equivalent survival to nonmalignant indications for transplantation. To prioritize these patients for transplant to receive a graft before the development of metastatic disease, exception points can be granted for patients with up to three lesions, each between 1 and 3 cm in diameter, or one lesion 2 to 5 cm in diameter. It is recommended that patients with HCC be managed in a multidisciplinary setting with the use of locoregional therapies, including transarterial chemoembolization, radiofrequency ablation, and radioembolization using Y90, to "downstage" patients into "within" Milan Criteria, with excellent results. Many guidelines are available for surgical management of HCC patients, including liver transplantation, with one of the more widely used and modified being the Barcelona Clinic Liver Cancer staging system (BCLC). This system factors tumor size and number, patient performance status, and liver function to classify patients into stages that correlate with treatment algorithms depending on group.[30] Recent modifications recognize the poor prognosis carried by high α-fetoprotein levels and require special exception point applications for these patients.

Many patients with hepatocellular cancer have significant underlying fibrosis or cirrhosis. The primary treatment modality for HCC is surgical resection. The determination must be made as to whether the underlying liver disease will allow successful resection. In general, 30% of the liver must be preserved to ensure adequate synthetic function; however, in the setting of significant liver disease, this proportion may be as high as 40% to 50% and can be prohibitive of resection depending, again, on tumor size and location. Severe portal hypertension with varices, significant ascites, debilitation, malnutrition, and encephalopathy are all contraindications to resection. In addition, the location of the lesion may also make resection impossible. Lesions adjacent to the confluence of major vascular or biliary structures may not allow surgical options. In this case, transplantation is the preferred treatment.

Chemotherapy and other locoregional therapies may be employed to halt the progression of disease while patients remain on the wait list.

Cholangiocarcinoma

Cholangiocarcinoma is a highly lethal primary liver lesion with poor long-term survival. In patients with perihilar lesions who are not surgical candidates, 3-year survival is nearly 0%. This is due to the aggressive nature of cholangiocarcinoma, with micrometastasis being present in most patients with visible lesions on imaging. Early reports from the Mayo Clinic demonstrated that chemoradiation protocols followed by liver transplantation provided good long-term survival for patients with early-stage hilar lesions.[31] Still today, few centers have adopted any criteria for transplanting patients with cholangiocarcinoma because all but the most carefully selected patients experience a survival benefit. Despite this benefit, 1- and 3-year disease recurrence rates are very high, leading some countries, such as Japan and Germany, to not offer transplantation as a therapeutic option. Centers listing and transplanting these patients report that these patients have been carefully selected and show equivalent survival to patients who undergo liver resection. There is still wide practice variation, with not all centers including radiation therapy and some choosing up-front transplantation for the smallest perihilar tumors. A key principle is the need to obtain a negative margin either with transplantation or resection.

Other

Budd-Chiari Syndrome

Budd-Chiari syndrome is a rare condition that occurs when hepatic venous outflow is occluded, typically due to thrombosis of the hepatic veins or vena cava at the level of the hepatic veins. It can also occur as a result of extrinsic compression. Presentation is variable and can be divided into acute, subacute, and chronic. Approximately 5% of patients will present with ALF. In these patients, ascites and pain are more common, whereas patients with chronic obstruction more frequently present with portal hypertension. An underlying hypercoagulable or other reason is identified in about 75% of patients[32] and should be actively sought with a hypercoagulable workup and imaging to look for masses (Fig. 53.2).[33]

In early stages, side-to-side portacaval shunt decompresses the liver and can provide excellent long-term survival. In patients with established fibrosis or cirrhosis, liver transplantation should

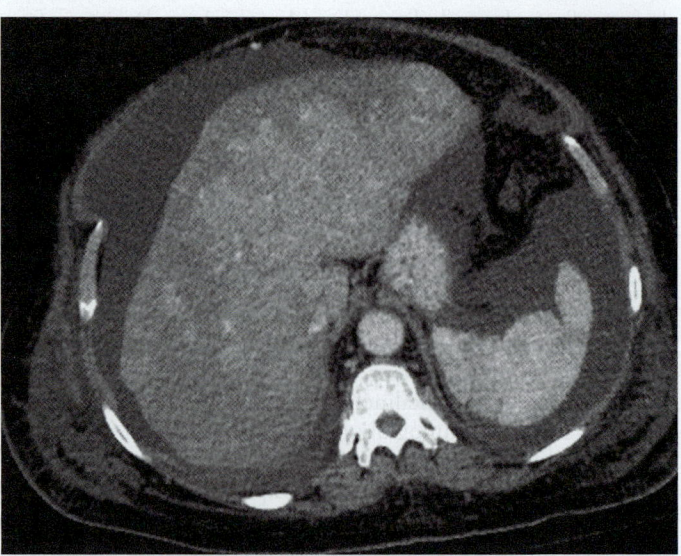

FIGURE 53.2 Budd-Chiari syndrome.

be considered. Operative planning must consider suitable outflow options, particularly side-to-side cavocavostomy.

Rare Causes of Liver Failure That Can Be Addressed With Liver Transplantation

Total Parenteral Nutrition/Hyperalimentation-Induced Liver Disease

In patients with short bowel syndrome or intestinal failure, liver failure can follow for reasons that are not well understood. In these patients, combined liver/intestinal transplant can be lifesaving.

Polycystic Liver Disease

In rare cases, patients with polycystic liver disease can present with debilitating pain, intestinal obstruction, malnutrition, hemorrhage, or liver failure. For these patients, liver transplantation may be indicated.

Hepatic Adenoma

Patients with large, unresectable hepatic adenomas may present with pain or bleeding and carry increased risk of malignancy. Transplant is indicated for symptomatic, large, unresectable lesions.

Metastatic Cancer

Certain types of metastatic disease can be treated with transplantation, including neuroendocrine tumors and unresectable colorectal liver metastases. Liver transplantation for metastatic cancers, including colorectal cancer, had been tried before, with demonstrated abysmal outcomes in the 1980s. The practice is slowly returning with better selection criteria for recipients. There has been growing literature on transplantation for unresectable colorectal liver metastases, with the initial study of 21 patients with unresectable colorectal liver metastases from Oslo, Norway (SECA-I), showing a 60% 5-year survival rate after liver transplantation. This trial was recently followed up in a 2020 report from the same group (SECA-II) demonstrating a 5-year survival of 83% and a 5-year disease-free survival of 35% in a highly selected cohort.[34] Although still not as common, more centers have begun to develop selection criteria based on these reports for the transplantation of unresectable colorectal liver metastases. This remains a controversial indication, but as will be discussed in a subsequent section, a new field of "transplant oncology" is emerging to revisit the idea of expanding liver transplant indication to many cancer types.

Hemangioendothelioma

Hemangioendothelioma is a slow-growing and rare malignancy. In the case of unresectable disease, transplant can provide excellent outcomes.

Wilson Disease

Occurring at a frequency of 1 in 30,000, Wilson disease is an autosomal recessive disease of copper transport. Over time, copper accumulation leads to cirrhosis. A small subgroup of patients will present with liver failure, which is generally an acute presentation on the background of undiagnosed cirrhosis. These patients benefit from transplant and have good long-term survival.

CONTRAINDICATIONS

As techniques and technologies for liver transplantation improved, the number of patients who could benefit increased at a rate that outpaced organ availability. To be good stewards of the limited resource, the decision-making around listing patients for liver transplant is more complex than in other areas of surgery. Contraindications are based on whether the patient can survive the operation and whether they can achieve long-term survival, including whether they can properly care for the organ.

Patients with advanced cardiac disease are usually excluded from consideration for transplant. Severe valvular disease can make intraoperative management prohibitively difficult. Hypotension may occur as a result of rapidly shifting intravascular volume with significant hemorrhage or clamping of major vasculature. This can also lead to life-threatening arrhythmias. A particularly difficult problem is pulmonary hypertension, which may result in unrecoverable right heart failure on reperfusion of the new liver. Patients with coronary heart disease are at risk for intraoperative myocardial infarction and may have accelerated progression of atherosclerosis as a result of immunosuppression after transplant.

Similarly, patients with severe respiratory conditions are generally not candidates for liver transplantation. Intraoperative hypoxia may be uncorrectable, and long-term outcomes are poor. Portopulmonary hypertension uncorrectable to less than 50 mm Hg is generally considered a contraindication, as is hepatopulmonary syndrome if the PaO_2 cannot be corrected on 100% oxygen.

Other contraindications include irreversible neurologic impairment. In the setting of encephalopathy, this can be difficult to determine. A careful history is needed to exclude chronic, progressive causes. Infection must be carefully considered but, in many cases, is not an absolute contraindication. For example, in patients with PSC and liver abscesses, liver excision may be the only way to eradicate the infection. Uncontrolled sepsis or other infection that will not be cured by the transplant is a relative contraindication. In most cases, extrahepatic cancer is a contraindication for transplant. Recent cancer may require a waiting period. The Israel Penn International Transplant Tumor Registry maintains a database that can provide guidance around waiting times needed for different types of cancer. Patients with human immunodeficiency virus (HIV), previously thought to be an absolute contraindication to transplant, can undergo successful transplantation. A 2013 congressional act, the HIV Organ Policy Equity (HOPE) Act, enabled transplantation from HIV-positive donor to HIV-positive recipient to take place under research protocols reviewable by the US Department of Health and Human Services. A recent multicenter prospective report in 2022 demonstrated the best outcomes to date, with 45 HIV-positive recipients (R+) without AIDS or evidence of opportunistic infection receiving either HIV-positive or HIV-negative donor livers (D− or D+). Compared with HIV-positive recipients who received livers from HIV-negative donors (D−/R+), HIV-positive recipients receiving livers from HIV-positive donors (D+/R+) had excellent 1-year survival (83.3% vs. 100%; $p = 0.04$), with no difference in rejection rates (10.8% vs. 18.2%; $p > 0.05$).[35] Such results merit further investigation but are promising for a future where HIV status will no longer be a relative contraindication, similar to HCV.

The transplant community generally feels that the ability to take care of the graft depends on adequate social and financial support and resources, so lack of this resource is an absolute contraindication to transplantation, although recent work suggests this may be a disadvantage to certain groups of patients.[36]

Active alcohol use is considered a contraindication for transplant, although selected centers will perform transplants in these patients, and in fact, the number of these transplants is increasing rapidly.[15] Liver transplant programs generally include social, psychiatric, and finance specialists to help sort out relevant issues.

Advances in surgical technique have made exclusion of patients for anatomic reasons very rare in experienced centers. Methods for dealing with difficult anatomy are discussed in the section on surgical considerations.

MELD AND ALLOCATION

Originally developed to predict 3-month mortality in patients after transjugular portosystemic shunt placement, the MELD was also found to accurately predict mortality in patients waitlisted for transplant. Currently, the MELD score (now on its third iteration) determines priority for liver transplantation. A great success of the system was in creating objective criteria (laboratory results) that were not subject to interpretation by individual centers, as was the case for grading of hepatic encephalopathy under the Child-Turcotte-Pugh system. In its original formulation in 2003, it was based on serum creatinine, INR, and bilirubin. Serum sodium was subsequently added to improve the predictive value of the score for those with a regular MELD score greater than 11. The latest iteration of the model (3.0) includes the variables of female sex and serum albumin as well as interaction terms between variables to correct previous disparities among females as well as create a more predictive model based on contemporary data.[37] The current calculation is included in Box 53.3. When a donor liver becomes available, a list of patients eligible to receive the transplant is generated, ranked by MELD score. The liver is offered sequentially to each person on the list until it is accepted.

Status 1 patients suffer from fulminant liver failure, with expected death on the order of days. These patients are prioritized above patients with MELD scores.

Although MELD is recognized as a good predictor of mortality, there are certain conditions thought to carry higher mortality than the MELD score would suggest. In particular, patients with hepatocellular cancer can be cured with liver transplantation, but many have low MELD scores because of preserved liver function and would likely not come to transplant before disease progression. For these patients, additional points are given, termed *exception points,* to reflect the desire of the community to prioritize them. Prioritization algorithms are reviewed and adjusted regularly to ensure equity among all waitlisted patients. Additional diagnoses generally accepted for additional points are listed in Boxes 53.4 and 53.5. If patients do not fit into these categories, a review board exists to consider special cases.

How organs are distributed across the country is a distinct question regarding which patients in a group receive priority for the transplant offer. This complex question is one of the most hotly debated in the transplant community. Within this decision resides the intersection of ethical principles of justice, utility, and fairness, as well as public preferences, resource utilization, and disparities in access and outcomes of care resulting from socioeconomic factors.[38] In February 2020, liver allocation policy radically

BOX 53.4   Common Indications for Exception Points for Liver Transplant

- Hepatocellular carcinoma
- Hepatopulmonary syndrome
- Portopulmonary hypertension (provided the mean arterial pressure can be maintained at <35 mm Hg with treatment)
- Familial amyloid polyneuropathy
- Primary hyperoxaluria
- Cystic fibrosis
- Hilar cholangiocarcinoma
- Hepatic artery thrombosis (occurring within 14 days of liver transplantation but not meeting criteria for status 1A)

BOX 53.5   Diagnoses That May Be Appropriate for Exception Points

- Recurrent cholangitis in patients with primary sclerosing cholangitis who are on antibiotic suppressive therapy or require repeated biliary interventions
- Refractory ascites
- Refractory hepatic encephalopathy
- Refractory variceal hemorrhage
- Portal hypertensive gastropathy leading to chronic blood loss
- Intractable pruritus in a patient with primary biliary cirrhosis

changed from donation service areas to "acuity circles" in an effort to reduce disparities based on geography that resulted in widely different median MELD scores at time of transplant depending on geographic location.[39] In practice, this created concentric donation circles around liver donor hospitals rather than offering livers based on where the recipient lived, ranging from 150 to 500 nautical miles. For example, when a donor offer becomes available at a hospital, that offer will be made first to any recipients considered status 1A (imminent risk of death within less than 1 week) within a 500-nautical-mile radius of the donor hospital. If no such recipient is found, it is first offered to any high-MELD recipients within 150 nautical miles, then any similar MELD recipients within 250 nautical miles, followed by 500 nautical miles until a high-MELD recipient is found. If no high-MELD recipient is found, the process repeats, with progressively lower-MELD recipients within 150, 250, and then 500 nautical miles being offered until a recipient match is found. This change to allocation policy was met with skepticism, with some believing it would lead to the net exportation of liver grafts from more resource-poor geographic areas. Many studies have been published since implementation, but more time is needed to determine the ultimate impact of the policy change as well as brainstorm improved policies.

In March 2023 the US Department of Health and Human Services announced plans to overhaul and reform the United Network for Organ Sharing (UNOS) in response to growing criticism of declining transplant outcomes and inefficient organ utilization rates. This led to the signing of the Securing the US Organ Procurement and Transplantation Network Act in September 2023, which promises to break up UNOS and award multiple contracts for organ administration networks. This will allow broader eligibility and more transparency in transplant allocations, including better performance-based metrics. Finally, whether and how to incorporate performance of local organ procurement organizations will be included for potential change as the landscape of American transplantation rapidly changes. Allocation

BOX 53.3   Current Calculation for the Model for End-Stage Liver Disease (MELD 3.0) Score

MELD = 1.33*(Female) + 4.56*ln(Serum bilirubin) + 0.82*(137 − Sodium) − 0.24*(137 − Sodium)*ln(Serum bilirubin) + 9.09*ln(INR) + 11.14*ln(Serum creatinine) + 1.85*(3.5 − Serum albumin) − 1.83*(3.5 − Serum albumin)*ln(Serum creatinine) + 6, Rounded to the nearest integer

INR, International normalized ratio.

thus remains a complex and hotly contested topic, with change anticipated in the coming years.

DONOR SELECTION

The ideal liver donor is young, healthy, and thin, with normal liver function tests and no history of liver disease or risk factors for infectious disease. The patient is pronounced brain dead and, with normal hemodynamics, is taken semielectively for the donation procedure. This "perfect" scenario is quite rare, however, and each deviation from these characteristics carries quantifiable risks. It is critical to consider that the risk of accepting any individual donor must be balanced with the risk of the potential recipient declining the liver and dying before receiving the next offer. From a public health standpoint, use of livers with high risk is, in general, preferable to not using the liver, given the number of waiting-list deaths.

Older donors carry additional risk of short- and long-term graft loss, and older age is an independent risk factor for mortality. Still, outcomes with older donors are very good.[40]

Donors with significant health problems need to be considered on a case-by-case basis. In general, disease in other organs should not be a contraindication to use of the liver. A notable exception is cancer, but this still must be considered on a case-by-case basis. Severe atherosclerosis can affect the hepatic artery, and this must be assessed at the time of donation.

Livers from patients who are obese may have MAFLD with or without MASH. In general, livers with more than 60% steatosis or with significant fibrosis for any reason should be used with caution, if at all, for only the most robust recipients. Bridging portal fibrosis and cirrhosis are typically contraindications for using any donor liver.

Interestingly, ongoing infection in the donor is not an absolute contraindication for use of the organ. Suspicion of viral etiology for the donor death, however, is typically an absolute contraindication for the use of any organs. Spread of the virus to immunosuppressed recipients can cause multiple deaths. Patients with risk factors for infection, such as intravenous drug abuse, carry a small risk of transmission of disease even though nucleic acid testing is routinely performed and is very sensitive for hepatitis C and HIV. The use of hepatitis C–infected donors is becoming routine given the success of specific antiviral therapy, and there is already some early evidence to suggest acceptable outcomes of HIV-positive donors only for HIV-positive recipients.

The standard liver donation comes from a deceased patient declared dead by brain death criteria. Brain death is declared by the patient's treatment team, independent of and before any family members being approached by a transplant services team for donation consent. Recipients of these grafts tend to have the best outcomes, although not as good as those of living donation, which is covered later in this chapter.[1] A class of organs can also be procured from donors declared dead based on circulatory criteria. These are termed *donation after circulatory death (DCD) organs*. In this case, after determination that the patient experienced a devastating, nonsurvivable injury and that the patient wishes to donate, support measures are withdrawn, and the patient is allowed to progress to death. Once the patient is declared dead by cessation of heartbeat, a "hands-off" period ranging from 5 minutes (in the United States) to as long as 15 to 20 minutes in some European countries is observed in case of autoresuscitation. A physician, typically the intensivist team, must confirm lack of pulse and heartbeat before the surgical team can proceed. A rapid perfusion technique with organ removal is performed by quickly opening the abdomen and cannulating the donor aorta to initiate a cold flush of preservation solution. DCD donors are a significant source of organs for transplant, with excellent outcomes in selected hands, and their use has increased over several years.[41] These organs are not without risk, however, because of both warm and cold ischemia. Each hour of cold ischemia increases risk of graft failure for DCD organs, and many donor comorbidities, such as macrosteatosis, have higher rates of graft loss in DCD organs than donation after brain death (DBD) donors. Ischemic cholangiopathy, a diffuse structuring disease, also occurs with more frequency in these donors compared with DBD livers, and this complication can, in some cases, require retransplantation.

PREOPERATIVE EVALUATION

Evaluation of a patient for liver transplantation is complex and seeks to determine whether a candidate would benefit from a transplant, whether there are alternative therapies available, and whether the predicted outcome is good enough to justify use of this scarce resource in this individual.

Workup therefore includes a detailed history and physical exam. Full laboratory evaluation is appropriate for patients, considering the magnitude of the operation. Cardiac and pulmonary workup is similarly essential, including stress testing and pulmonary function tests in patients with appropriate risk factors. All screening testing should be up to date, including mammography, colonoscopy, prostate cancer screening, and so forth.

Liver transplantation requires long-term follow-up and medications to prevent rejection and other complications. For this reason, adequate financial and social support must be available to the recipient. Patients in the United States meet with financial coordinators as well as social workers to ensure that they can adequately care for the organ postoperatively. This also assesses risk of recidivism in patients with a history of alcohol or other substance abuse.

SURGICAL CONSIDERATIONS

The major steps of the liver transplant operation are pictured in Fig. 53.3. Many techniques are used; here, we will outline a relatively common general approach. Access to the abdomen is generally obtained using a right subcostal incision and either a midline extension or a left subcostal extension, and sometimes both. Often, portal hypertension is severe, occurring in combination with severe coagulopathy. Care must be taken to prevent exsanguinating hemorrhage. Portal dissection involves ligating the right and left branches of the hepatic artery and transecting the bile duct high in the hilum. Ligation of lymphatics leaves only the intact portal vein for later transection before excision of the liver. The triangular and coronary ligaments are lysed. In an orthotopic placement, the inferior vena cava is encircled above the renal veins and the suprahepatic cava above the hepatic veins in preparation to remove the entire cava. The recipient liver is removed with the retrohepatic cava, and the donor liver is then placed with the donor cava anastomosed to the recipient cava both above the renal veins and below the diaphragm. In the piggyback technique, the caudate is dissected off the retrohepatic cava, leaving the recipient cava intact. The donor cava is anastomosed to the cloaca fashioned using the confluence of the three hepatic veins. Once this is done, the liver is perfused with saline to remove the potassium contained in the preservation solution. The portal vein anastomosis is performed, followed by the hepatic artery and then bile duct, usually in a duct-to-duct fashion (see Fig. 53.3).

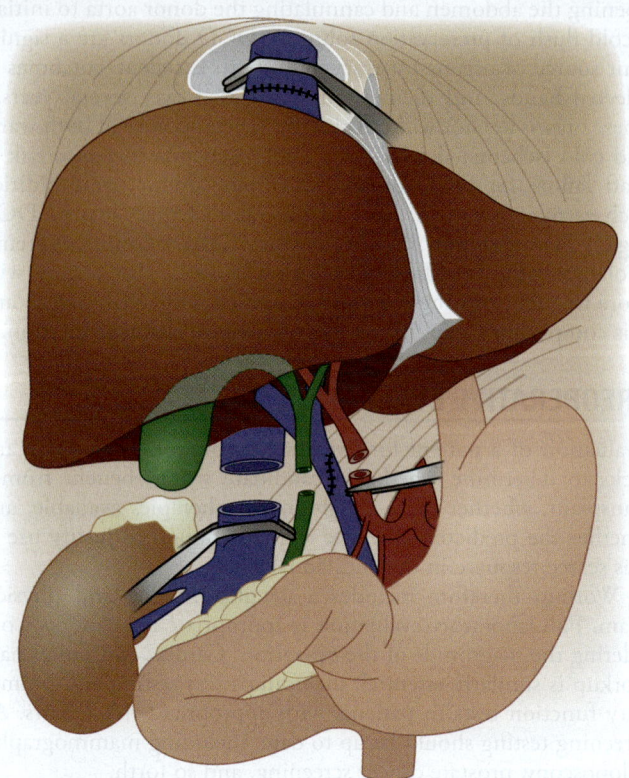

FIGURE 53.3 Steps of the liver transplant operation.

Major hemodynamic shifts occur during the operation. Patients with cirrhosis typically have very low systemic vascular resistance and can quickly become hypotensive with blood loss. Either total caval occlusion using the orthotopic technique or hepatic vein occlusion using the piggyback technique diminishes blood flow to the heart, causing hypotension and increased renal vein pressure, leading to kidney injury. After the liver is implanted, reperfusion leads to a massive bolus of volume to the right heart on opening the cava, which can lead to right heart strain or even failure, which can be life threatening.

In recipients with portal vein thrombosis, first attempts should be to open the vein with thrombectomy catheters and thromboendovenectomy if needed. If this fails, inflow can be obtained from the superior mesenteric vein, nearby varices, and even the left renal vein in patients in whom there is significant splenorenal shunting. For arterial inflow, much of the splanchnic circulation can be used, as can grafts from the suprarenal or infrarenal aorta. Difficult biliary anastomoses can be managed with a Roux-en-Y technique or even direct choledochoduodenostomy. A particularly difficult problem is trying to place a large liver into a small recipient. If the right lobe is very large, it can be difficult to perform the portal anastomosis. Similarly, if the liver is too large in the dorsal-ventral direction, the donor portal vein can lie on top of the recipient portal vein in a fashion where it cannot be cut back far enough to permit anastomosis. In this case, alternative inflow must be sought.

POSTOPERATIVE MANAGEMENT

After a complex surgery with significant hemodynamic derangements, good postoperative management is essential to ensure optimal outcomes. Liver transplantation creates some specific challenges.

Given the hemodynamic changes, patients often come out of the operating room after receiving a significant amount of fluid and blood products. It is critical to have a good sense of the patient's total body volume and intravascular volume. Most patients will be total volume overloaded, but intravascular volume can be low, normal, or high. The best way to determine total body volume status is an accurate patient weight, taking into account preoperative ascites. If the patient is massively volume overloaded but hypotensive, a vasopressor may mitigate the need for massive ongoing fluid resuscitation. Pulmonary artery catheters or noninvasive echocardiographic assessment may help determine intravascular volume to guide decision-making around fluids. Once the blood pressure is normalized, restoring whole body euvolemia is an important goal to prevent soft tissue and pulmonary edema. Volume management is complicated by potential ongoing bleeding and acute renal injury, which is common. Very careful attention must be paid to these possibilities.

Respiratory management consists of extubation as soon as feasible, with the understanding that many patients will be severely debilitated and may not be able to perform the work of breathing. In these cases, early tracheostomy is indicated.

Feeding should begin as early as is safe, and there should be a low threshold for placing a feeding tube should the patient demonstrate an inability to consume adequate calories after normal gastrointestinal (GI) function returns. Early ambulation and incentive spirometry are critical, and early discharge should be a goal to prevent nosocomial infection.

Most programs will use drains for additional fluid and to diagnose bile leaks. These should be inspected multiple times a day for output and color.

COMPLICATIONS AND THEIR TREATMENT

Regarding early complications, careful attention to the patient in the immediate postoperative setting is essential to ensure optimal outcomes. Frequent assessment of graft function is essential, and quick action must be taken when indicated. Postoperative hypotension can be caused by many factors, but bleeding must always be considered. Abdominal drains will usually, but not always, help establish this diagnosis. Drains can become clotted or sequestered from areas of massive hemorrhage. Frequent hematocrit checks should be obtained. Ongoing hemorrhage requiring continuous blood replacement is generally an indication to return to the operating room. The exception may be a patient with severe coagulopathy and or hypothermia, who may benefit from a longer observation period with factor replacement and warming to determine if the bleeding is surgical in nature. A good practice is to set a threshold transfusion limit, after which abdominal exploration is considered. In addition, patients who develop compartment syndrome must return to the operating room.

Primary nonfunction is a serious complication requiring retransplantation. The most common causes are an unrecognized procurement error; use of certain types of higher-risk grafts (fatty, fibrotic, DCD); or arterial complications after the transplant, such as hepatic arterial thrombosis. Typically, the patient will not wake up, the lactate will remain very high, bilirubin will continue to rise, and the AST and ALT will rise into the range of 5000 to 10,000 IU/L. In these cases, an ultrasound should be obtained to interrogate the artery, and plans should be made for urgent retransplantation.

Arterial complications not producing primary nonfunction occur in approximately 2% to 4% of patients.[42] This usually manifests as increased AST and ALT, elevated bilirubin, and poor synthetic function with elevated INR. Arterial stenosis or thrombosis can be diagnosed on ultrasound or contrast CT and must be

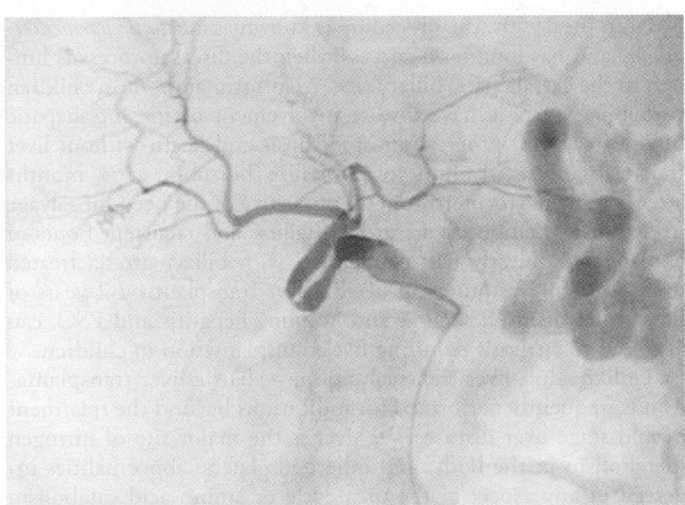

FIGURE 53.4 Hepatic artery stenosis demonstrated by arteriogram.

addressed as soon as possible if discovered. Early arterial thrombosis, even if not associated with primary nonfunction, should lead to relisting for transplantation (Fig. 53.4).

Portal vein stenosis or thrombosis may present with normal liver function tests and synthetic function. Over time, however, these patients develop signs and symptoms of portal hypertension and require intervention. Portal stents are often successful in these situations.

Biliary issues are the most common complication in the postoperative period and occur in approximately 20% of patients. This can present as bile in the drain in the case of a leak or in a patient who returns with a biloma. Stricture leads to increased bilirubin and alkaline phosphatase. Modern management of bile duct issues employs endoscopic management for stent placement and dilations. Early major biliary issues should prompt an ultrasound to ensure vessel patency and reoperation to check for bile duct ischemia and to consider reanastomosis, possibly as a Roux-en-Y reconstruction.

Rejection typically presents with elevated liver function tests and is diagnosed on biopsy, characterized by portal inflammatory infiltrate, bile duct injury, and endotheliitis. In many cases, mild rejection can be treated by raising the immunosuppression level and bolus steroids. More severe rejection may require antibody therapy.

Recurrent hepatitis C is becoming much less common with the advent of direct-acting antiviral therapy.

Late complications include arterial or portal venous structuring, bile duct strictures, and opportunistic infections. Chronic rejection is poorly understood and often leads to the need for retransplantation. Chronic immunosuppression often leads to renal dysfunction and increased risk of certain types of cancer, especially skin cancer associated with sun exposure.

IMMUNOSUPPRESSION

Liver grafts are recognized by the recipient as foreign based on major histocompatibility complex antigens. Hepatocytes express low levels of class I antigen and no class II antigen. During ongoing immune surveillance, T cells recognize the graft as foreign and initiate an immune response. Distinct from renal transplantation, liver transplantation does not require matching between donor and recipient HLA, although there is some concern that the effect of HLA mismatch may be greater than previously appreciated.

Modern immunosuppression offers a variety of classes of agents. Induction agents, if used, are administered at implantation. Choices include anti-thymocyte globulin, an anti–T-cell antibody that binds to and depletes T cells, delivering potent and relatively nonspecific immunosuppression. These are very potent agents that can increase the rate of infection. Basiliximab is an antibody to the interleukin-2 (IL-2) receptor, which blocks IL-2 signaling and is not as immunosuppressive as anti-thymocyte globulin.

Maintenance immunosuppression generally involves agents of three different classes. Steroids inhibit transcription of cytokines, the most important of which is IL-2, which downregulates the immunologic response to antigen. They also inhibit T-cell migration. Side effects are multiple and varied and include hypertension, fluid retention, cataracts, osteoporosis, diabetes, and increased risk of infection. Mycophenolate mofetil inhibits purine synthase, which decreases proliferation of T and B cells. The major side effect is GI upset. Calcineurin inhibitors block signal 2, which is required for T-cell activation. Calcineurin itself is a calcium-dependent phosphatase in T cells. Side effects include hypertension, renal toxicity (which can lead to renal failure), and lipid abnormalities.

The mainstay of immunosuppression for liver transplantation is tacrolimus, with over 90% of liver transplant recipients receiving this drug with mycophenolate and/or steroids. The practice of using induction agents, which have been shown to decrease acute rejection, has increased over time, and they are currently given to approximately 30% of patients.[1] The incidence of acute rejection by 1-year posttransplant is around 10% to 15% among patients using a T-cell–depleting agent and/or IL-2 receptor antibodies for induction.

LIVING DONOR LIVER TRANSPLANTATION, INCLUDING DONOR SELECTION

LDLT arose from the intersection of an improved understanding of segmental liver anatomy, technical advances in hepatic parenchymal transection, and urgency resulting from the inadequate supply of deceased donor liver allografts. LDLT draws on the ability of the liver to regenerate. A portion of liver with sufficient quality and mass, when provided with adequate arterial and venous inflow, as well as venous drainage, will re-create adequate mass to meet the metabolic demands of both donor and recipient. The first LDLT consisted of an adult segment II/III graft that included the left hepatic vein, left hepatic artery, left portal vein, and left hepatic duct that was transplanted into a small child. The field quickly developed to allow for adult-to-adult liver transplantation with right lobe grafts consisting of segments V/VI/VII/VIII, along with the right hepatic veins, right hepatic arteries, right portal veins, and right hepatic ducts and left lobe grafts consisting of segments II/III/IV along with the left hepatic vein, left hepatic arteries, left portal vein, and left hepatic ducts. The increase in the number of LDLTs has led to a better understanding of both recipient selection and donor risk, with significant improvements in patient and graft survival.

Donor

The safety of the donor is of paramount importance. Increased experience with LDLT in several high-volume centers helped define general criteria to maximize donor safety. Specifically, the donor should be left with an adequate amount of hepatic mass to ensure full recovery postoperatively. Donors with acute or chronic liver diseases or extrahepatic diseases that may subsequently impair regeneration are excluded from becoming living liver donors. Donors should undergo a thorough medical and psychosocial evaluation to ensure that they are able to donate and recover from surgery safely. A donor should be left with a residual liver volume of no less than 30%.[43] This may be increased if the donor is older or has hepatic steatosis. Although laparoscopic live liver donation has been reported, most centers perform an open hepatectomy.[44] Donation is associated with a mortality rate of 0.2%.[43] Forty percent of donors will experience at least one complication within the first year after donation. The most frequent complications include infection (13%–15%), bile leak/biloma (7%–9%), reoperation (2%–3%), and hernia (11%–16%).[43] Despite both short- and long-term complications, most donors would choose to donate again.

Recipient

Successful living donor transplantation requires a liver allograft of adequate parenchymal mass to support the recipient's metabolic needs, as determined by the donor graft-recipient weight ratio (GRWR). Although successful liver transplantation has been performed with living donor grafts resulting in GRWR as low as 0.5%, the risk of morbidity and mortality due to small-for-size syndrome significantly increases with decreasing GRWR. Small-for-size syndrome develops when the amount of functioning transplanted liver parenchyma is inadequate to support the recipient; it manifests with jaundice, coagulopathy, ascites, encephalopathy, and renal impairment that may progress to death. Retransplantation with a larger allograft may be necessary.

A GRWR of 0.8% to 1% is generally accepted as safe; however, donor liver quality and recipient degree of illness both affect the minimum safe GRWR. Donor steatosis, donor age older than 50 years old, and high recipient MELD score frequently necessitate higher GRWR up to or more than 1%.[43] Ensuring adequate hepatic arterial and portal venous inflow to the live donor allograft is of critical importance for immediate graft function and subsequent graft hypertrophy. Hepatic parenchymal mass is regulated based on portal vein flow, and inadequate portal flow resulting from portosystemic shunting can be deleterious to allograft regeneration and perpetuate graft failure. Alternatively, exposure of a healthy liver allograft to sudden and persistent portal hypertension can lead to centrilobular injury and small-for-size syndrome.

LDLT is technically challenging because of the microvascular and biliary reconstructions necessary between the donor graft and recipient. The biliary reconstructions are especially prone to complications, with biliary stricture occurring in nearly 30% of recipients. Despite the challenges, LDLT is currently associated with a 1-year patient survival of almost 93% and is an important and lifesaving option.[43]

PEDIATRIC LIVER TRANSPLANTATION

The indications for pediatric liver transplantation are generally grouped into diseases leading to cirrhosis, inborn errors of metabolism, primary hepatic malignancies, and ALF. Biliary atresia is the most common cause of end-stage liver disease in children and accounts for one-third of all pediatric liver transplants. It is a congenital disease of unknown etiology that leads to progressive fibroinflammatory obliteration of the biliary tree and the rapid development of cirrhosis. A diagnosis of biliary atresia should be suspected in all infants with persistent neonatal jaundice. Early intervention within the first several months of life is associated with superior outcome.[45] Reestablishing adequate biliary-enteric drainage before the development of end-stage liver disease is critical. This is typically accomplished by surgical anastomosis of the intestine to the biliary tree at the hepatic hilum. Pioneered by Kasai in the 1950s, the procedure is known as a *hepatic portoenterostomy* and has long-term success when the disease process is limited to the extrahepatic biliary tree.[46] Unfortunately, most children with biliary atresia have disease involvement of the intrahepatic biliary tree, with progression of cirrhosis and death without liver transplantation.[47] Failure to normalize bilirubin at 3 months after hepatic portoenterostomy is predictive of the need for salvage liver transplantation, as are growth failure and recurrent bouts of cholangitis.[48] Nearly half of children with biliary atresia treated with portoenterostomy will need a liver transplant by 2 years of life. Other diseases, such as autoimmune hepatitis and PSC, can also lead to cirrhosis requiring liver transplantation in children.

Unlike adult liver transplantation, pediatric liver transplantation is frequently performed for indications beyond the treatment of end-stage liver disease. The liver is the major site of nitrogen metabolism in the body, and inherited genetic abnormalities involved in any aspect of the urea cycle or amino acid catabolism can lead to the accumulation of toxic metabolites and neurologic injury. Significant enzymatic dysfunction within the urea cycle of either N-acetylglutamate, carbamoyl phosphate synthase I, ornithine transcarbamylase, or argininosuccinate lyase deficiency impairs the body's ability to dispose of nitrogenous waste through the conversion of ammonia to urea. The neurotoxic hyperammonemia that ensues, particularly in the interval shortly after birth, causes the rapid development of lethargy, cerebral edema, seizures, and death. Other enzyme deficiencies within the urea cycle, including those of argininosuccinate synthase or citrin with resultant citrullinemia, arginase with resultant hyperargininemia, and ornithine translocase deficiency with resultant hyperornithinemia and homocitrullinuria, result in more insidious hyperammonemia and progressive neurologic injury. Similarly, enzymatic dysfunction in amino acid catabolism, as seen in maple syrup urine disease, methylmalonic acidemia, propionic acidemia, and tyrosinemia, results in the accumulation of certain amino acids and their metabolites, with resultant cellular toxicity and neurologic injury. Children with inborn errors of nitrogen metabolism are particularly vulnerable to neurologic injury resulting from the metabolic stress associated with growth, injury, or infections. Routine viral infections of childhood, including common colds or influenza, can be life-threatening events. The synthetic function of the liver in patients with inborn errors of metabolism is normal, and liver transplantation is performed to provide normal enzymatic function and minimize or arrest further neurologic injury. Early liver transplantation minimizes or arrests neurologic injury.[49]

Liver transplantation treats primary malignancies of the liver, including hepatoblastoma and HCC. Hepatoblastoma arises from fetal or embryonal hepatocyte progenitor cells and is the most common primary pediatric liver malignancy. It is often diagnosed in children less than 3 years of age when they present with abdominal distention, feeding intolerance, or abdominal pain. The goal of treatment of hepatoblastoma is complete surgical resection. The PRETEXT (pretreatment extent of disease) classification is used to stage the extent of hepatic involvement and the likelihood of successful treatment with partial hepatectomy.[50] Although most hepatoblastomas can be successfully treated with partial hepatic resection, approximately 10% are surgically unresectable and benefit from liver transplantation, which provides for a 3-year survival of 75%, with most mortality secondary to disease recurrence.[51] HCC is very rare in the pediatric population and has a different pathology than that in adults. Excellent long-term survival approaching 80% at 5 years is reported with liver transplantation for HCC even when patients exceed the Milan Criteria.[52]

Most pediatric recipients who undergo orthotopic liver transplantation are younger than 5 years of age, and many receive a deceased donor whole liver allograft. However, the number of children needing a liver transplant greatly exceeds the number of pediatric whole liver deceased donors. This imbalance between the supply of size-appropriate pediatric deceased donors and demand of pediatric recipients necessitated the development of techniques for liver transplantation using reduced-size adult allografts. The introduction of deceased donor split liver allografts in 1998 allowed the transplantation of infants and small children using the left lateral section of an adult liver based on the vasculobiliary anatomy of the left lobe. LDLT further increased liver allograft availability for all pediatric patients with end-stage liver disease. The transplantation of left lateral segment and live donor grafts necessitates the use of a cava-preserving technique. The vascular anastomoses in infants and small children have an increased complication rate, and microvascular techniques and anticoagulation are routinely used to minimize thrombotic events. Long-term results for pediatric liver transplantation are excellent, with a 5-year graft survival of 85% for biliary atresia and by a 5-year graft survival slightly above 75% for hepatoblastoma and ALF (Fig. 53.5).[1]

New Technologies, Treatment Paradigms, and Advances

Machine Perfusion

Machine perfusion is an old technology made new again. It was pioneered by many surgical teams, such as Folkert Belzer's at the University of California, San Francisco (UCSF), in the late 1960s for short-term kidney preservation and transportation and was even described by Thomas Starzl for short-term liver preservation during the recipient operation. However, cost, safety, and contemporaneous advances in static preservation solutions that yielded some of the first reliable preservation solutions, such as Euro-Collins, prevented any serious adoption of the technology. After moving to the University of Wisconsin, Dr. Belzer and his colleague Dr. Southard would also help create a benchmark preservation solution in the late 1980s, solidifying cold storage as the standard of care.

Over 30 years later, clinical investigation of machine perfusion devices gained renewed interest, with groups in the United States and Europe publishing clinical series of liver transplants after hypothermic oxygenated machine perfusion. Groups in the UK and Netherlands began to publish trial series using normothermic machine perfusion devices before liver transplantation. Worldwide interest in machine perfusion has exploded in the last 10 years; many recognize its potential to recover, test, and possibly rehabilitate marginal livers before transplantation, helping reduce the organ shortage. Mechanisms of how machine perfusion benefits grafts are still debated, but many believe machine flow maintains sinusoidal endothelial cell integrity; oxygenation repletes mitochondrial adenosine triphosphate (ATP) stores; and in the case of normothermic machine perfusion (NMP), body temperature enables metabolic function and nutrient supplementation during preservation.[53] Hypothermic oxygenated perfusion (HOPE) has recently been shown in a randomized trial to have

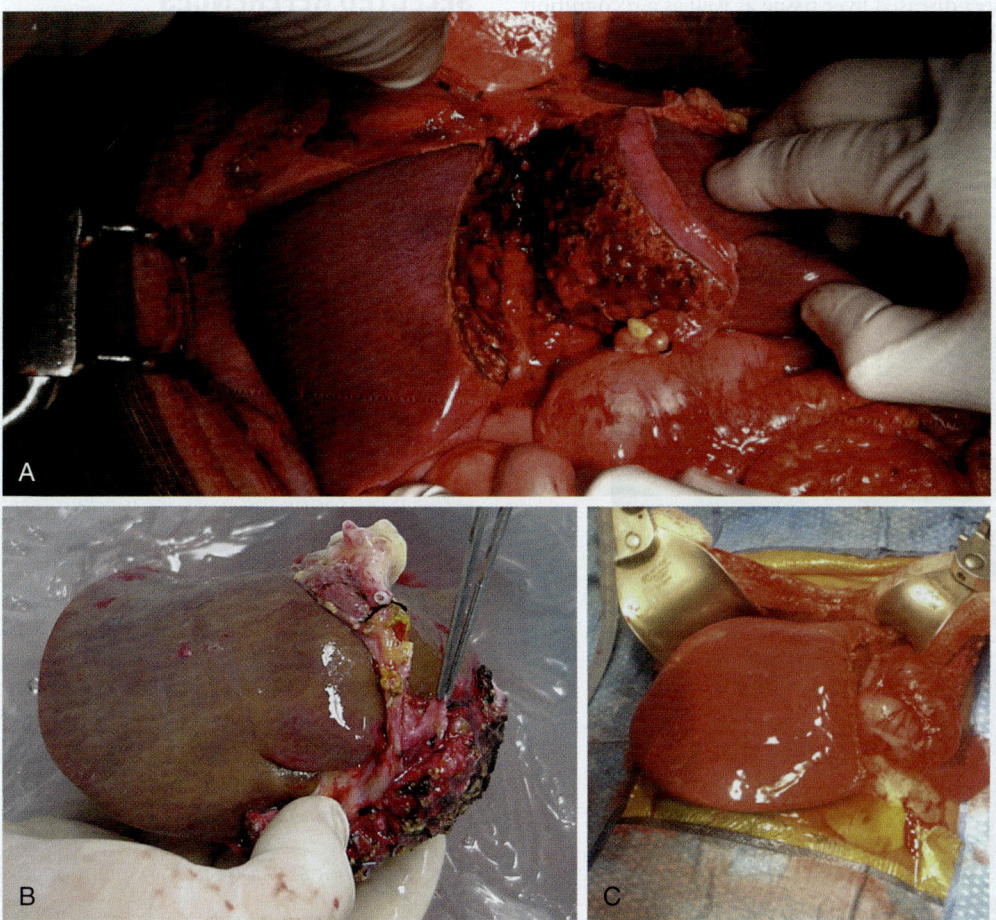

FIGURE 53.5 Split liver transplant for a child. (A) In situ resection of live donor graft. (B) Segment prepared for transplant. (C) Graft reperfused in recipient.

superior outcomes to static cold storage, with lower rates of early allograft dysfunction and a lower incidence of nonanastomotic biliary strictures, especially in DCD donors.[54] Randomized trials in NMP have also shown excellent outcomes and promising improvement in recovery of marginal donor organs.[53] There is ongoing investigation of the use of NMP for these marginal donors because the body temperature conditions enable metabolic assessment of liver grafts and enable improved logistics for transplant centers because perfusions can occur overnight, allowing surgeons to rest before cases (Fig. 53.6).[55] In addition to machine perfusion devices, there is growing literature on the use of extracorporeal membrane oxygenation (ECMO) devices on DCD donors before organ procurement in a technique called *normothermic regional perfusion* (NRP). The donor is cannulated for ECMO after withdrawal of support, and either the abdomen or the chest and abdomen are perfused for a period of 2 to 4 hours before procurement of abdominal and/or thoracic organs. This technique has gained popularity in many European countries, but there is still ethical debate on whether its use should be expanded in the United States, where not all regions of the country currently allow it.

Transplant Oncology

The indications for liver transplantation covered previously are numerous. As surgical techniques for both donor and recipient operations improve and knowledge of optimal preservation methods increases, so will the indications for an allograft. The concept of transplant oncology is an expansion of the multidisciplinary team for hepato-biliary tumors. It was born of our increased abilities to safely resect diseased liver tissue as well as a recognition that patients with liver tumors require a more coordinated and thoughtful approach to management that may also include transplantation. Over the past 30 years since the Milan Criteria, it has been feasible to safely transplant highly selected patients with unresectable colorectal liver metastases, intrahepatic and perihilar cholangiocarcinomas, neuroendocrine liver metastases, and hepatic hemangioendothelioma. Care for these complex hepato-biliary

tumors continues to progress, and multidisciplinary teams must include transplant surgery and medicine to extend the margins of traditional surgical oncology and determine how transplant immunology can be leveraged against tumor biologies that enable liver transplantation as cure.[56]

Xenotransplantation

As with many ideas in transplantation, xenotransplantation is not entirely new. Starzl undertook the first xenotransplant of nonhuman primate to human liver in 1966, which was unsuccessful. It was tried again in the 1990s by a few surgeons (including Starzl once more), with short-term success on the order of days. Since that time, decades of preclinical work in immunology and genomics have allowed for exponential growth in xenotransplantation. Specifically, the use of CRISPR-Cas9 to create the genetically engineered α1,3-galactosyltransferase KO (GalT-KO) pigs has successfully taken the field from small animal studies to clinical research protocols in humans, with promising results for kidneys.[57] With this same technique, the first gene-edited pig liver was transplanted in China in March of 2024. Despite this progress, our scientific understanding of xenotransplantation has outpaced our moral and ethical understanding. Much work must be done to understand all the true costs and risks for both nonhuman donors and human recipients if this breakthrough is to become future clinical practice.

SELECTED REFERENCES

Kim WR, Mannalithara A, Heimbach JK, et al. MELD 3.0: the model for end-stage liver disease updated for the modern era. *Gastroenterology*. 2021;161(6):1887-1895.e4.

Latest MELD scoring.

Kwong AJ, Kim WR, Lake JR, et al. OPTN/SRTR 2022 annual data report: liver. *Am J Transplant*. 2024;24(2S1):S176-S265.

Current liver transplantation by the numbers.

Mazzaferro V, Regalia E, Doci R, et al. Liver transplantation for the treatment of small hepatocellular carcinomas in patients with cirrhosis. *N Engl J Med*. 1996;334:693-699.

This work forms the basis for modern treatment of unresectable hepatocellular cancer.

Starzl TE. *The Puzzle People. Memoirs of a Transplant Surgeon*. Pittsburgh: University of Pittsburgh Press; 1992.

An engaging history of liver transplantation by its pioneer.

Sapisochin G, Hibi T, Toso C, et al. Transplant oncology in primary and metastatic liver tumors: principles, evidence, and opportunities. *Ann Surg*. 2021;273(3):483-493.

A comprehensive look at transplant oncology principles.

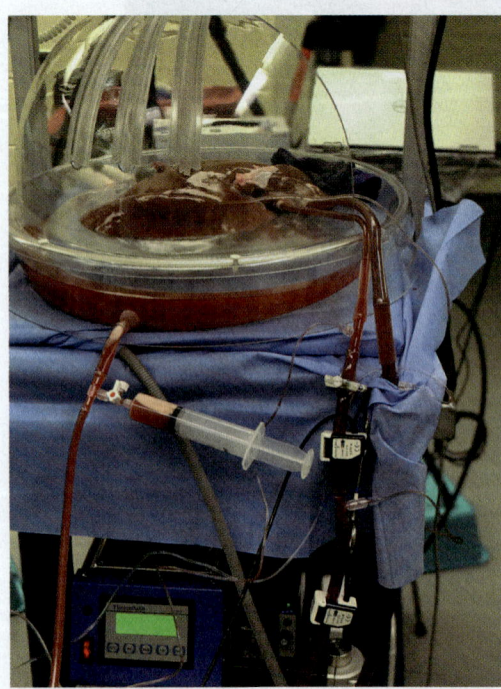

FIGURE 53.6 Machine perfusion of a liver.

The full reference list appears on Elsevier eBooks+.

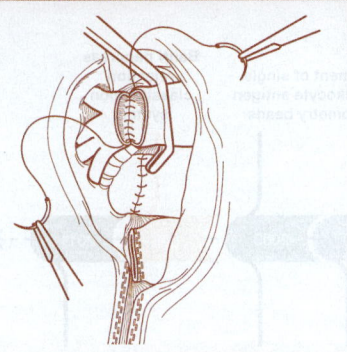

CHAPTER 54

Pancreas Transplantation

Tsukasa Nakamura, Jon S. Odorico, James F. Markmann, and Paul M. Schroder

OUTLINE

INTRODUCTION

Pancreas transplantation was the first treatment to successfully restore euglycemia with endogenous insulin production in patients with type 1 diabetes mellitus (T1DM). The early outcomes of whole organ pancreas transplantation were dismal. However, advances in surgical techniques, organ preservation, and immunosuppression over time have led to improved outcomes for pancreas transplant recipients, who now experience 85% to 90% 1-year graft survival and greater than 95% 1-year patient survival.[1] The remainder of this section will focus on providing a brief history of pancreas transplantation and related landmark events, which are summarized in Fig. 54.1.

The treatment of diabetes was revolutionized by the discovery of insulin by the Canadian research team led by Frederick Banting and Charles Best in 1921.[2] The discovery of this essential pancreatic hormone combined with performance of the first successful kidney transplant in 1954 led to the conceptualization of pancreas transplantation as a way to restore endogenous insulin production in T1DM. In 1966, the first human pancreas transplant was performed in combination with a kidney transplant for a patient with T1DM and end-stage renal disease (ESRD) by a team led by Richard Lillehei and William Kelly at the University of Minnesota in Minneapolis.[3] The procedure was performed using a duct-ligated segmental pancreas with cobalt-60 irradiation to limit pancreatic exocrine secretions. At that time, effective immunosuppressive agents were still not available, so a combination of azathioprine and prednisolone was employed. The pancreas graft was eventually explanted as a result of graft pancreatitis, thought

to be secondary to duct ligation and rejection, and ultimately, the patient succumbed 13 days after transplant. This first case highlighted difficulties in exocrine management and the need for improved immunosuppression and organ preservation in pancreas transplantation. Soon after the first, a second pancreas transplant was performed. This time, the recipient received a whole pancreas graft, including the duodenum, with construction of a cutaneous duodenostomy to manage exocrine secretion. However, the transplanted pancreas failed after 2 months as a result of rejection involving the duodenum, and the patient succumbed to sepsis 4 months posttransplant.[4] After several failed attempts relying on enteric exocrine drainage, segmental pancreas transplantation gained popularity up until the mid-1980s in order to avert implanting the highly antigenic duodenum. During this period, procedures such as pancreatic ductal ureterostomy[5] and neoprene polymer injection to permanently occlude the pancreatic duct[6] were employed. These techniques achieved up to 50 and 29 months of graft survival, respectively. Ultimately, bladder drainage with a duodenocystostomy replaced these other experimental techniques and became the standard method for managing exocrine secretions in the late 1980s.[7,8] However, as experience accumulated over the ensuing decades and urologic complications mounted, surgeons began to revisit enteric drainage approaches to managing exocrine secretions with duodeno-intestinal anastomoses in the mid-1990s.[9]

It is also noteworthy that the first living donor pancreas transplantation was performed in 1979, primarily to offer a preemptive opportunity for pancreas transplantation and minimize rejection rates by using related donors.[10] Another surgical consideration for pancreas transplant surgeons at this time was whether venous

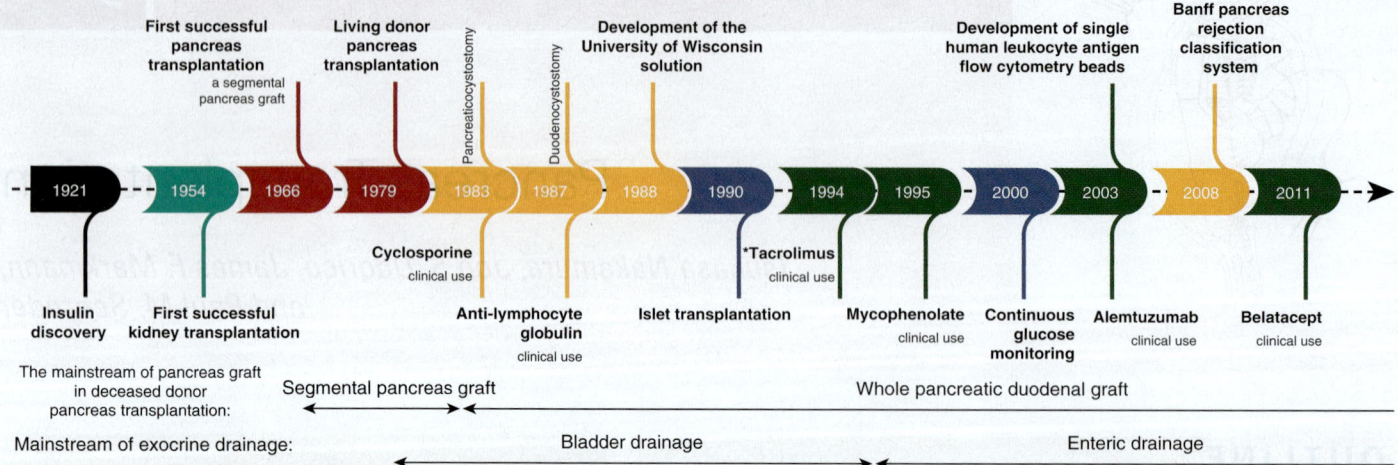

FIGURE 54.1 Landmarks in pancreas transplantation. * The first administration to humans was in 1989.[21]

drainage should occur through the portal or systemic venous system. For this reason, a portal venous drainage technique was employed, particularly in the 1980s, to create a more physiologic flow of insulin and prevent pseudohyperinsulinemia, although the causal relationship and clinical implications for posttransplant outcomes of this phenomenon were not completely understood.[11] Ultimately, portal venous drainage demonstrated no clear benefit in pancreas transplant outcomes; thus, systemic venous drainage of the pancreas graft remains the preferred method of venous drainage, particularly for its surgical simplicity.

Increasing volumes of organ transplantation led to the need for better preservation of organs for transport over longer distances. The first commercially available cold storage preservation solution was Collins solution, developed in 1969. Modifications to this formulation were made to prolong organ storage time, leading to the production of Euro-Collins solution by 1980. Soon afterward in the late-1980s, the University of Wisconsin (UW) solution was developed, and this solution and its competitor, histidine-tryptophan-ketoglutarate (HTK) solution, became the dominant cold storage solutions for abdominal organ preservation.[12] These advances in organ preservation allowed for an expansion in use of pancreases for transplant because they could be stored and transported over long distances and for longer periods of time.

As was the case for the entire field of organ transplantation, a major step forward in pancreas transplant outcomes came after the approval and routine use of cyclosporine A (CsA) in 1983.[13] The introduction of this agent into maintenance immunosuppression regimens dramatically reduced rates of allograft rejection. After this revolutionary advance in immunosuppression, a pancreas transplant without the duodenum employing pancreaticocystostomy[7] and a whole pancreas grafting with graft duodenocystostomy[8] were developed in 1983 and 1987, respectively. These successes led to bladder drainage becoming the main means of exocrine drainage until the mid-1990s. The ability to measure amylase level in urine as a biomarker of rejection conferred an important advantage in an era when acute pancreas graft rejection rates were still 50% to 70% or greater in the first year posttransplant. Nevertheless, bladder drainage is not a physiologic pathway for exocrine pancreas drainage, and the technique thus caused both acute and chronic complications, such as urinary tract infection, chemical cystitis and urethritis, and refractory acidosis, which often required surgical conversion to enteric drainage. For this reason, the mode of exocrine drainage of the pancreas was reevaluated, leading to a paradigm shift to enteric drainage for pancreas transplants in the mid- to late-1990s. At about the same time, other major immunosuppressants, tacrolimus and mycophenolate mofetil in particular, were introduced to the field of organ transplantation for more effective maintenance immunosuppression.[14,15] Finally, the recognition that early lymphocyte depletion improved transplant outcomes stimulated the development and clinical implementation of induction immunotherapy agents such as antithymocyte globulin and alemtuzumab, further reducing rates of early pancreas allograft loss from rejection.[16,17]

As another major step forward in organ transplantation in general, the single human leukocyte antigen (HLA) beads assay was developed by Paul Terasaki and his colleagues, which eventually enabled the prediction of physical cross-match results by a virtual cross-match, helping streamline organ allocation.[18]

The evolution of pancreas transplantation into the practice we know today is closely aligned with advances in surgical technique, organ preservation, and immunologic management. Although other major therapeutic options, such as islet transplantation and continuous glucose monitoring technology, were developed and clinically applied in 1990 and 2000, respectively,[19,20] pancreas transplantation is still recognized as the most durable and effective therapeutic option for restoring endogenous insulin production. The remainder of this chapter will focus on the current practice of pancreas transplantation, its outcomes, and what directions this field might take in the future to further improve outcomes (see Fig. 54.1).

PATIENT SELECTION

Historically, pancreas transplantation had been reserved for patients with T1DM because these patients had their islet mass destroyed by autoimmunity and were expected to benefit from restoration of islet mass by the pancreas graft while also reducing the threat of recurrent autoimmune destruction of islets by using immunosuppression and HLA mismatching. Patients with type 2 diabetes mellitus (T2DM) were traditionally not expected to benefit from pancreas transplantation because of a concern for reduced rates of achieving insulin independence as a result of peripheral insulin resistance and metabolic syndrome. However, pancreas transplantation for lean T2DM patients is on the rise, with favorable outcomes in terms of patient survival, graft survival, and glycemic control.[22] Despite these successes, there remains a paucity of data to understand the limits to successful outcomes in this population with regard to pretransplant insulin requirements, body mass index, and fasting C-peptide levels.

The majority of pancreas transplants are performed in combination with a kidney transplant as a simultaneous pancreas-kidney (SPK) transplant for patients with insulin-dependent diabetes mellitus and ESRD. In addition to meeting the requirements for kidney transplantation, patients should be requiring treatment with insulin. Decisions about moving forward with SPK transplantation versus kidney transplant alone or pancreas transplant after kidney transplant (PAK) are based on factors such as availability of a compatible, high-quality living donor kidney (LDK) or, in the absence of an LDK, the estimated wait time on dialysis as well as comorbidities and surgical risk associated with SPK transplant. Which option is best should be individualized and determined through multidisciplinary discussions with patients. Patients with insulin-dependent diabetes seeking pancreas transplant alone (PTA) should have documented significant complications of insulin therapy, such as impaired awareness of hypoglycemic events, including severe hypoglycemic events, or consistent failure of exogenous insulin therapy as well as normal stable renal function without evidence of significant proteinuria or diabetic nephropathy.[23] Another less frequent indication for pancreas transplant is endocrine and exocrine insufficiency associated with cystic fibrosis[24] or pancreatectomy. Other less common indications for pancreas transplantation include those who have undergone total pancreatectomy for chronic pancreatitis, with or without autoislet transplantation; those who have lost endogenous insulin production; and those who are on exogenous insulin therapy.[25] In these cases, the pancreatic allograft can treat both endocrine and exocrine insufficiencies.

All potential pancreas transplant recipients should undergo a full evaluation, including a thorough history and physical examination, to identify any existing medical conditions that may require optimization and prior surgery that would influence their candidacy for transplant. Contraindications to pancreas transplant include active malignant disease, active infection, severe peripheral vascular disease, severe cardiac or pulmonary disease, active IV drug abuse, and significant psychosocial barriers to compliance with posttransplant medical management. Laboratory evaluation should include serum chemistries, liver function testing, complete blood count, coagulation profile, urinalysis, fasting C-peptide, hemoglobin A1c (HbA1c), and autoantibody serologies as well as serology testing for hepatitis B and C, cytomegalovirus (CMV), Epstein-Barr virus (EBV), varicella-zoster virus (VZV), syphilis, human immunodeficiency virus (HIV), and tuberculosis. Imaging should include a chest x-ray and abdominal and pelvic CT imaging to evaluate the candidate's iliac vasculature and anatomy for surgical planning purposes. Cardiac risk stratification is an essential component of the evaluation because there is a high rate of silent atherosclerotic disease in the diabetic-uremic individual. All patients should undergo an electrocardiogram of the heart and cardiac stress testing at a minimum. In addition, all patients over age 50 or those with risk factors such as angina symptoms, smoking history, and iliac vascular disease should be considered for a resting echocardiogram and coronary angiography to evaluate for any intervenable ischemic cardiac disease before transplant. Physical examination should include pulse examination, particularly of the femoral, posterior tibial, and dorsalis pedis pulses, to gauge the degree of peripheral vascular disease that requires further workup. A psychosocial evaluation should also be performed to determine a candidate's social support and mental status before transplant to ensure appropriate resources are available to maintain compliance with medications and clinical follow-up posttransplant. Open wounds and amputations should be noted and ideally healed before transplantation. A frailty assessment is valuable as well.[26]

DONOR SELECTION

Donor selection for pancreas transplantation begins with a screening of donor characteristics. The pancreas can be procured and used successfully from both donation after brain death (DBD) and donation after circulatory death (DCD) donors, with similar outcomes, particularly with the use of newer technologies such as normothermic regional perfusion in the case of DCD.[27,28] However, successful donation of pancreas from DCD is generally limited to donor functional warm ischemia times of less than 30 minutes. The pancreas donor risk index (PDRI) is a useful tool for predicting pancreas graft outcomes, particularly with regard to early technical and ischemia-reperfusion injury–related outcomes, taking into account donor age, sex, terminal creatinine, body mass index, race, height, cause of death, type of donor (DBD or DCD), cold ischemia time, and whether or not is the organ will be used as a pancreas after kidney transplant.[29] Other high-risk factors to consider in the donor are HbA1c and past medical history of diabetes or prediabetes; obesity; traumatic injury to the pancreas, duodenum, or spleen; evidence or history of pancreatitis; chronic alcohol use; and any abnormal lesions in the pancreas, duodenum, or spleen. Evaluation of the pancreas during and after procurement on the back table is integral for a successful outcome and requires significant surgical experience. The ideal pancreas organ should be free of significant adipose tissue within the parenchyma. When palpated, the parenchyma should be soft and free of nodularity and able to be folded over on itself (i.e., supple). The parenchyma should be free of saponification or hemorrhage, and the duodenum should be free of injury. The superior mesenteric artery (SMA) and splenic artery should be of adequate size for reconstruction with donor iliac Y graft, usually at least 3 mm in size. It is important to note during procurement the presence of any aberrant arterial anatomy, such as inferior pancreaticoduodenal arteries arising from a replaced right hepatic artery. In this situation, the pancreas may be used; however, it is important to evaluate flow by flushing the SMA and observing the flush returning out of the gastroduodenal artery (GDA) stump to ensure there is enough collateral blood supply to perfuse the head of the pancreas.

Evaluation of the quality of the donor kidney should also be considered carefully using metrics such as the kidney donor profile index (KDPI) and anatomy of the right and left kidneys in order to choose an appropriate kidney for recipients of SPK transplant. It should also be noted that for higher-risk recipients, it may be wise to choose lower-risk organs so that higher recipient risks and higher donor risks are not stacked together.

PANCREAS PROCUREMENT

Donation After Brain Death

There are several methods to procure deceased donor grafts during multiorgan recovery, with a priority being avoidance of compromising the recovery and use of other organs. Two common approaches include procuring the pancreas separately or en bloc with the liver, emphasizing that an extensive in situ (in the warm) dissection should occur using a no-touch to light-touch technique on the pancreas for the purpose of facilitating a rapid post–cross-clamp extraction and minimizing surgical trauma to the pancreas. First, to decontaminate the duodenum, amphotericin B, nystatin, or povidone-iodine solutions are typically injected through an indwelling nasogastric tube, but this practice has not been determined to be essential. In general, a midline incision from the sternal notch to the pubic bone is made with or without a cruciate extension for internal visualization of abdominal organs. A transverse incision enables better exposure of the tail of the pancreas and spleen. Alternatively, division of the diaphragm bilaterally can facilitate upper abdominal exposure. The infrarenal abdominal aorta just above the bifurcation is accessed and encircled for vascular control early in the operation in case of DBD donor instability and for rapid recovery in the case of DCD donors. The supraceliac aorta is prepared in the thoracic or abdominal cavity for a cross-clamp. Initial visualization of the pancreas is facilitated by entry into the lesser sac and ligation of the gastrocolic omentum and short gastric vessels. Then, via Cattell-Braasch and Kocher maneuvers, the duodenum, head of the pancreas, ascending colon, and small intestine are mobilized. To maximize exposure, the stomach can be divided just proximal to the pylorus by using a gastrointestinal anastomosis (GIA) linear stapler. The pancreas should be palpated and photographed at this stage, and information is shared with the recipient surgical team. If the appearance is not ideal, the organ may be declined at this point. Of note, as the gastrohepatic ligament is divided to approach the supraceliac aorta, care should be taken to avoid injury to an accessory or replaced left hepatic artery. If present, the left gastric artery is preserved, and peripheral branches are divided close to the lesser curvature of the stomach. Furthermore, during the inspection of the hepatoduodenal ligament, if there is a replaced right hepatic artery or the proper hepatic artery arises from the SMA, the procurement method should be discussed with the liver team to determine how to allow for simultaneous safe recovery and preserve perfusion to both organs.

Next, the distal common bile duct is ligated and divided just above the head of the pancreas, and the gallbladder is incised to flush both the gallbladder and the common bile duct with saline. The GDA is also identified and looped. The left renal vein is dissected out and looped. Then the location of the root of the SMA is identified and separated from the surrounding ganglion tissues and encircled with a vessel loop. Ideally, additional time for in situ warm dissection is carried out before cross-clamping and in situ flush. The inferior border of the pancreas is mobilized from the pancreaticocolic ligament with ligatures of the mesentery structures, and the spleen is detached from the retroperitoneum. Then the pancreas is mobilized away from the retroperitoneum, with the spleen being used as a handle and using a no-touch technique. Identification and dissection of the inferior mesenteric vein (IMV) should be carried out to facilitate cannulation for in situ portal venous flushing. Careful dissection of the celiac bifurcation to expose the common hepatic artery and splenic artery, as well as exposure of the portal vein, are valuable to identify points of separation of the pancreas and liver in order to speed organ extraction. It is also important to avoid direct trauma to the pancreas surface or capsular injury during this dissection.

Heparin 300 to 500 units/kg (~30,000 units) is administered intravenously. After waiting for 3 to 5 minutes, the aortic cannula is inserted and secured by an umbilical tape. A cannula is also inserted into the IMV in the same fashion. The aorta is cross-clamped; UW preservation solution is flushed by gravity into the aorta and IMV; the supradiaphragmatic inferior vena cava (IVC)

is incised for venting to the thoracic cavity; and organs are cooled with slushed ice, including anterior and posterior to the pancreatic parenchyma. UW solution seems to be superior to HTK solutions and Celsior.[30] However, HTK and Celsior can be employed where preservation times are kept to less than 10 and 12 hours, respectively, and if low perfusion volumes are used.[31] According to the procurement team's plan, the pancreas is recovered separately in situ or en bloc with the liver. Regardless, the pancreas vessels (SMA and splenic artery) should be flushed again immediately on the back table with an additional 100 to 200 mL volume of cold UW solution.

The initiation of extraction of the pancreas after in situ flush begins with dividing the proximal jejunum with a GIA linear stapler, and the root of the mesentery is divided with a vascular stapler. The aorta is cut at the root of the SMA (minimal cuff) but retaining an aortic cuff with the celiac artery and the renal arteries. The right gastric artery is divided, and the GDA is also divided, taking care to avoid injury or stenosis of the common hepatic artery. Small branches to the pancreas from the common hepatic artery are ligated. The splenic artery is divided at the root and typically marked by a small monofilament suture. The portal vein is carefully inspected and divided at the point where an adequate length is secured both for the pancreas and the liver. This is usually about 1 cm above the head of the pancreas, which is generally near the origin of the coronary vein branch. Once the pancreas is extracted and separated from the liver and arteries flushed with additional UW solution, goodquality photos or video should be obtained, along with a surgical quality assessment, and shared with the recipient surgeon.

Donation After Circulatory Death

Pancreas transplants generally rely on controlled DCD. Currently, super-rapid recovery (SRR) or normothermic regional perfusion are two commonly applied approaches. Heparin is administered at a dose of 300 to 500 units/kg (30,000 units) 3 to 5 minutes before withdrawal of the life-support system. After the declaration of death, a midline incision and a median sternotomy with or without a transverse abdominal incision are made. The infrarenal aorta is approached and clamped just above the bifurcation, and an aortic cannula is inserted above the clamp and secured in place. In the case of SRR, in situ perfusion of the abdominal viscera with cold organ preservation solution is initiated. The IVC is divided in the abdominal cavity or in the right chest cavity or pericardium for exsanguination. The thoracic or abdominal aorta is cross-clamped, and slush ice is placed over all the organs. The rest of the recovery procedures generally follow those used for DBD procurement, with emphasis on rapid extrication, keeping the pancreas cold, and minimizing surgical trauma to the gland. In the case of abdominal normothermic regional perfusion, the abdominal aorta and IVC are cannulated with catheters that are then connected to an extracorporeal membrane oxygenation perfusion circuit for a period of time for viability assessment before proceeding with the procurement. As for DBD donors, once the pancreas is removed in DCD donors, it should again be flushed with cold preservation solution on the back table, and photos/videos, along with a quality assessment, should be provided to the recipient surgeon. It is generally recommended that pancreatic grafts be preserved for less than 12 hours. However, this period has been extended to up to 24 hours, with some compromise in outcomes, depending on the quality of the organ.[31]

Donation From Living Donor

The body and tail of the pancreas, along with the spleen, are procured for living donor pancreas transplantation akin to a distal pancreatectomy procedure. Extra caution should be taken to minimize trauma to both the pancreas remnant and the pancreas graft. After mobilization of the tail of the pancreas with the spleen, the celiac artery, the splenic artery, the common hepatic artery, and the left gastric artery are visualized. Then the pancreas is dissected from the portal vein and subsequently transected at the level of the left border of the portal vein. The open proximal pancreatic duct is typically oversewn with a fine Prolene suture, and bleeding from the pancreatic parenchyma is controlled by ligatures and fine sutures. After systemic heparinization, the proximal splenic artery and vein are clamped, then divided. The stumps are closed with nonabsorbable sutures. After the recovery, the pancreas is flushed from the splenic artery with UW organ preservation solution.

BACK TABLE

On the back table, a meticulous inspection should be performed to confirm the quality of the pancreatic graft, with particular focus on possible presence of prerecovery trauma, fibrosis, woodiness, mass, or pancreatitis and to assess whether any significant surgical recovery damage to the pancreatic capsule, duodenum serosa, or vessels (including inspection for the iliac Y graft), has occurred. Fig. 54.2 shows high- and low-quality grafts on the back table.

The SMA, splenic artery, and portal vein are identified. If the mesentery was divided using vascular staples, it is prudent to oversew the cut edge with nonabsorbable monofilament sutures to minimize risk of a hematoma. Additional tissues along the border of the pancreas are cleared with ligatures, taking care not to injure the pancreatic capsule or parenchyma. The spleen can be removed from the tail of the pancreas by suture ligation of the splenic artery and vein beyond the tail of the pancreas, although some surgeons prefer to defer this step until after reperfusion to use the spleen as a handle to manipulate the graft. The location of the ampulla of Vater may be confirmed by inserting a probe through the stump of the common bile duct, which should be re-tied thereafter. Then, after dissecting the first portion of the duodenum from the head of the pancreas, the proximal end of the duodenum is stapled and oversewn with seromuscular sutures. The distal end of the duodenum is generally dissected from the mesentery, shortened by stapling, and oversewn with seromuscular sutures as

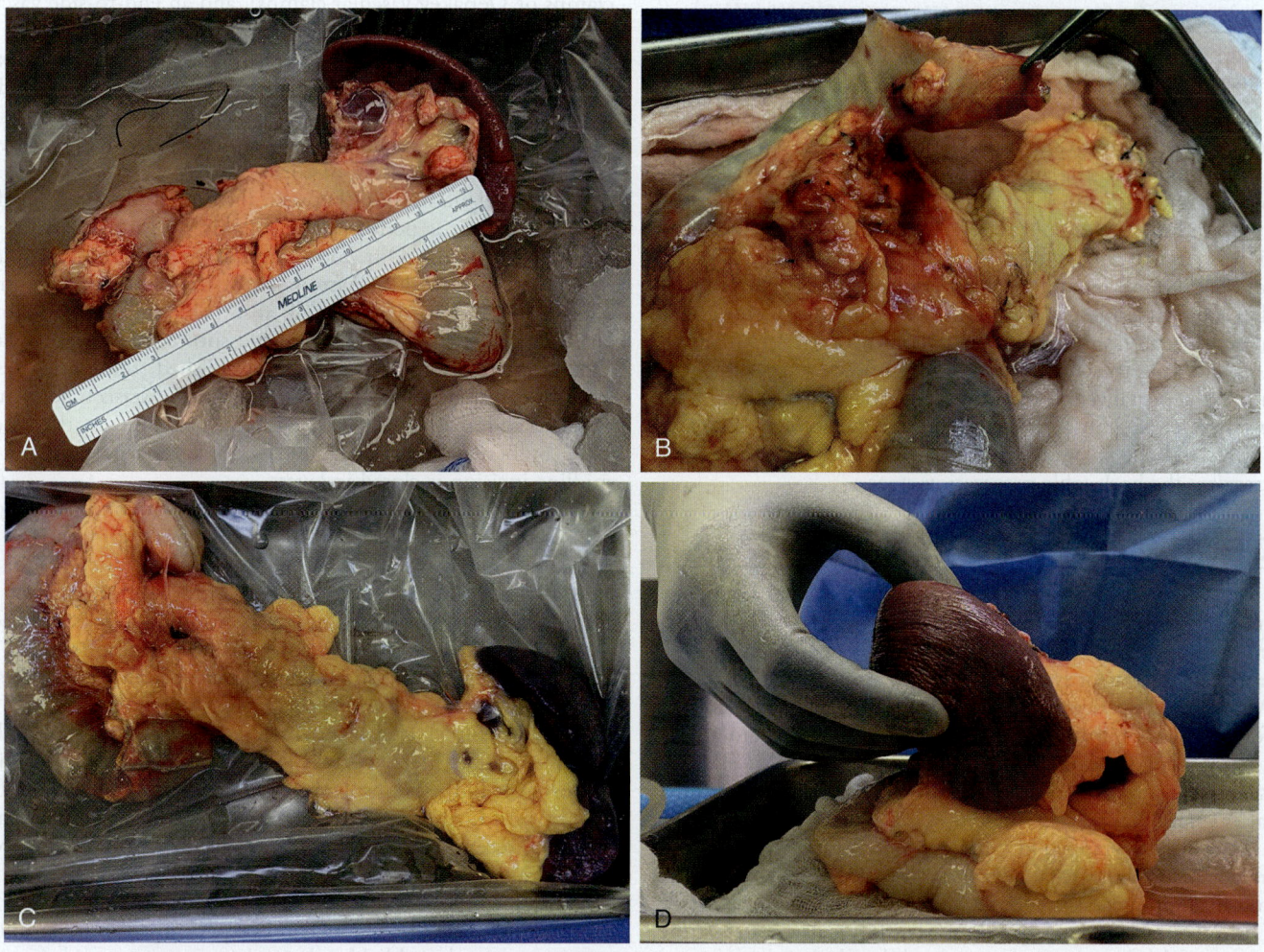

FIGURE 54.2 Back-table inspection of pancreas graft quality. (A) A high-quality pancreas after procurement. (B) Poor-quality pancreas as a result of procurement injury to head and duodenum. (C) Poor-quality pancreas with fatty infiltration of the parenchyma. (D) Poor-quality pancreas demonstrating firm, nonpliable parenchyma upon folding.

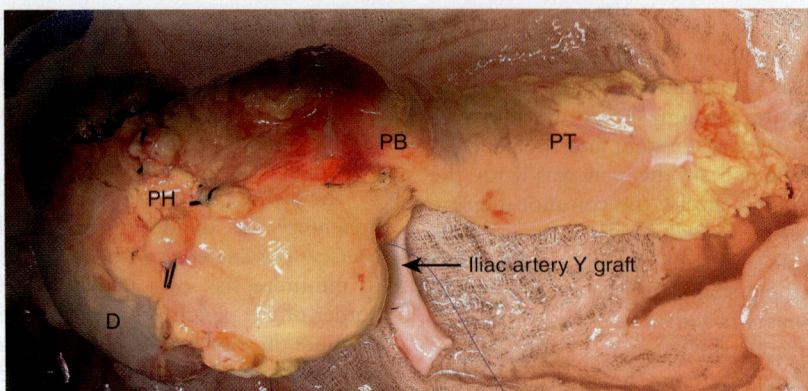

FIGURE 54.3 Pancreas allograft after back-table preparation. *D,* Duodenum; *PH,* pancreatic head; *PB,* pancreatic body; *PT,* pancreatic tail, respectively.

Back-table preparation of the pancreas for transplantation

➢ Careful inspection of quality of pancreas for transplant
➢ Removal of the spleen from the tail of pancreas
➢ Preparation of duodenum C-loop and oversewing staple lines
➢ Oversew the mesenteric staple line
➢ Preparation of the donor iliac Y graft
➢ Anastomosis of donor iliac Y graft to graft splenic artery and SMA

FIGURE 54.4 Back-table preparation of the pancreas graft for transplantation. *SMA,* Superior mesenteric artery.

---

performed for the proximal duodenum; however, some centers choose to complete the distal duodenal closure after exocrine drainage is established in the recipient. Additional tissue is cleared from around the SMA, splenic artery, and portal vein. Next, attention is paid to the reconstruction of the arteries. Usually, the donor iliac artery, including the internal and external arteries, used as a Y graft is anastomosed to the SMA and the splenic artery in an end-to-end fashion using 6-0 nonabsorbable monofilament sutures, allowing the creation of a single inflow orifice. Finally, if required, the portal vein is extended using the iliac vein. Fig. 54.3 shows a pancreas graft after completion of the reconstruction of the SMA and the splenic artery using a Y graft, and Fig. 54.4 summarizes the back-table preparation steps.

RECIPIENT TRANSPLANT OPERATION

The pancreas transplant operation begins with the patient positioned supine, arms abducted to 90 degrees, often with the kidney rest raised to help with retroperitoneal exposure. A long midline incision is made, and a retractor system is set up for exposure (Fig. 54.5).

A right medial visceral rotation (Cattell-Braasch maneuver) is performed by mobilizing the right colon, from the cecum all the way to the hepatic flexure, along the white line of Toldt. This allows for exposure of the retroperitoneal structures, namely, the distal IVC and iliac vessels. The bowel is then retracted superiorly and medially and wrapped in a moist towel. The ureter is retracted laterally to expose the distal IVC and right common iliac artery to permit maximum exposure for implantation of the pancreas graft.

Once the vessels are adequately exposed, it is useful to test the geometry of the pancreas graft and vessels by placing the pancreas in the desired orientation (our convention is to place head superior and tail inferior with plans for portal vein anastomosis to distal IVC and donor Y-graft anastomosis to the right common

iliac artery) to plan the clamp placements for anastomotic sites. A side-biting venous clamp is used to clamp the distal IVC, and an end-to-side anastomosis is performed between the donor portal vein (or donor iliac vein extension graft if patient is deep or portal vein is short) and recipient distal IVC using running nonabsorbable monofilament suture. Clamps are then placed on proximal and distal right common iliac arteries (padded Fogarty arterial clamps or DeBakey vascular clamps), and an end-to-side vascular anastomosis is performed between donor iliac artery Y graft and recipient right common iliac artery using running nonabsorbable monofilament suture. The pancreas graft is then reperfused by removing the venous clamp first, then the distal artery clamp, and finally the proximal artery clamp. Hemostasis is obtained by electrocautery, suture ligation, or clips.

The bowel anastomosis between the donor duodenum and recipient jejunum is performed at roughly 30 to 50 cm from the ligament of Treitz. Our convention is to perform a two-layer hand-sewn side-to-side anastomosis of the donor duodenum to recipient jejunum using running absorbable suture for the inner layer and interrupted nonabsorbable suture for the outer layer. Once exocrine drainage has been established, the kidney rest is lowered, another round of inspection for hemostasis is performed, and the abdomen is irrigated with warm saline. In the case of PTA, bulb suction surgical drains are placed if needed, and the midline incision is closed in layers.

Fig. 54.5 shows a diagram of SPK transplant and an image of the pancreas after reperfusion. In general, our approach is to implant the pancreas graft on the right and the kidney on the left side of the abdomen. Although implanting both organs on the same side or swapping the implant positioning may be needed in certain recipients based on vascular anatomy or prior surgical history, this alternative positioning may make percutaneous access to the organs for biopsy more challenging posttransplant. During SPK transplant, it is also our preference to perform the kidney transplant after the pancreas is implanted. Another strategy is to perform the kidney transplant portion of the SPK operation first, often while a pancreas graft is being prepared on the back table, although recent data show no advantage and possibly a disadvantage in outcomes with this approach.[32]

Variations to this procedure do exist. Up until the mid-1990s, exocrine drainage of the pancreas was performed through duodenocystostomy, but bladder-drained pancreas transplants were associated with higher rates of complications, as mentioned previously, including reflux pancreatitis, hematuria, urethral stricture, and urinary tract infections, compared with the current standard

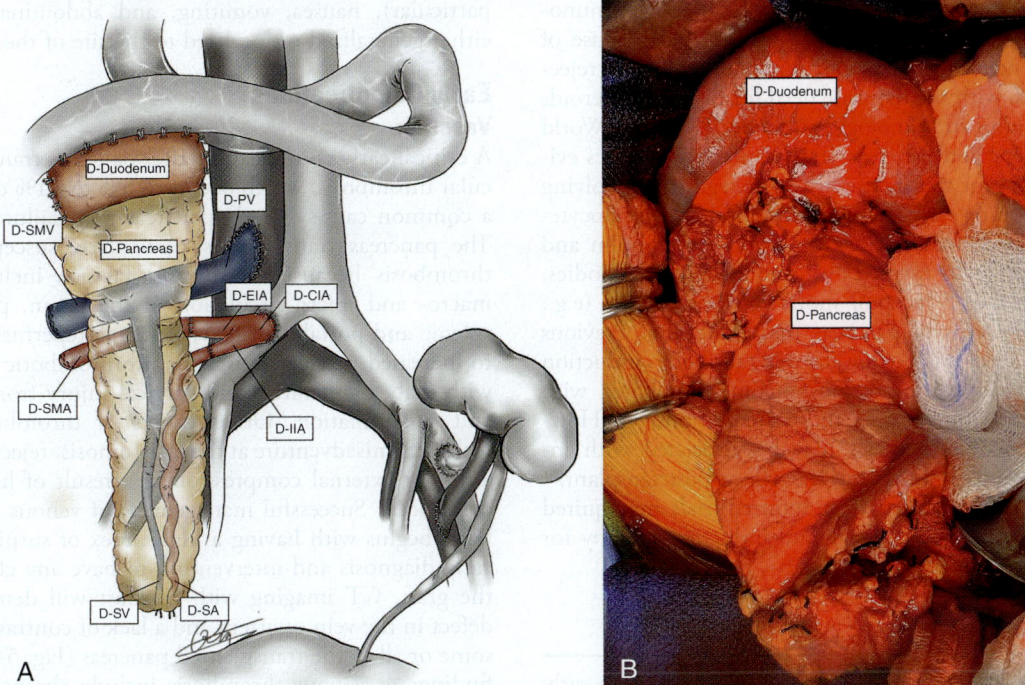

FIGURE 54.5 (A) Diagram of simultaneous pancreas and kidney transplantation with enteric exocrine and systemic portal vein drainage. The SMA and the splenic artery are reconstructed in an end-to-end fashion, using a donor iliac artery as a Y graft. A Y graft is anastomosed to the recipient common right iliac artery and the graft portal vein to the recipient inferior vena cava. A two-layer hand-sewn side-to-side duodenojejunostomy is created at around 30 to 50 cm distal to the ligament of Treitz. A renal graft is transplanted in the left iliac fossa. (B) Pancreas allograft after reperfusion in the recipient. *CIA,* Common iliac artery; *D,* donor; *EIA,* external iliac artery; *IIA,* internal iliac artery; *PV,* portal vein; *SA,* splenic artery; *SMA,* superior mesenteric artery; *SMV,* superior mesenteric vein; *SV,* splenic vein.

of enteric exocrine drainage.[33] Retroperitoneal placement of the pancreas graft is also described, particularly for PTA procedures with exocrine drainage via a duodenoduodenostomy.[34] Stapled enteric anastomosis may also be performed, although it can be challenging in cases where the donor duodenal segment has significant edema resulting from ischemia-reperfusion injury compared with the recipient intestine. Finally, portal venous drainage of the pancreas graft through anastomosis of the donor portal vein to the superior mesenteric vein (SMV) has been described but is not associated with significant benefit compared with systemic venous drainage.[35] This approach can be available when other outflow options, such as iliac veins, are thrombosed. Other creative solutions, such as the gonadal vein, can be employed under these circumstances. A brief outline of the steps for pancreas transplantation is shown in Fig. 54.6.

IMMUNOSUPPRESSION

The current standard immunosuppression regimen for pancreas transplantation consists of calcineurin inhibitors (CNIs; tacrolimus is favored over CsA); antimetabolite agents (mycophenolate mofetil/mycophenolic acid is favored over azathioprine or rapamycin); and steroids with T-cell–depleting induction therapies, such as antithymocyte globulin or alemtuzumab. The main concept is the same as in other solid organ transplants: to obtain sufficiently suppressed T- and B-cell immune responses while minimizing side effects, which is why solid organ transplantation has evolved to use multiple agents with different mechanisms

Surgical steps for pancreas transplantation
➤ Midline incision
➤ Exposure of the distal IVC and iliac vessels
➤ Placement of vascular clamps
➤ Anastomosis of graft portal vein to venous outflow
➤ Anastomosis of arterial Y graft to arterial inflow
➤ Removal of vascular clamps and graft reperfusion
➤ First round of hemostasis
➤ Anastomosis of graft duodenum to recipient bowel
➤ Second round of hemostasis and placement of drains
➤ Closure of abdomen in layers

FIGURE 54.6 Surgical steps for pancreas transplantation. *IVC,* Inferior vena cava.

of action. In terms of CNI options, tacrolimus is believed to achieve superior immunologic outcomes compared with CsA. Although there are several reported non–CNI-based approaches with the incorporation of the mammalian target of rapamycin (mTOR) inhibitors or costimulation blockade, such as cytotoxic T-lymphocyte–associated protein 4 (CTLA-4)-immunoglobulin, CNI-free immunosuppression is currently not supported by high-level evidence in the setting of pancreas transplantation.[36,37] Regarding antimetabolites, mycophenolate mofetil seems to be superior to azathioprine. However, in a setting in which mycophenolate is contraindicated, such as pregnancy, azathioprine is used as an alternative. It has been debated whether steroid avoidance (i.e., early steroid withdrawal) is associated with inferior immunologic and superior metabolic outcomes. Minimizing the use of steroids is likely beneficial to metabolic outcomes as long as rejection is not incurred, with the requisite need for high-dose steroids and the risk of inferior immunologic outcomes. The First World Consensus Conference on Pancreas Transplantation provides evidence-based support for the increased use of regimens involving steroid minimization or early steroid withdrawal.[31] Lymphocyte-depleting induction agents such as antithymocyte globulin and alemtuzumab are generally favored over nondepleting antibodies, such as interleukin (IL)-2 receptor monoclonal antibodies (e.g., basiliximab), in all forms of pancreas transplantation. Previous randomized controlled trials showed that antibody induction therapies offer superior immunologic outcomes compared with immunosuppression without using those medications.[38,39] However, antibody induction therapies may be associated with increased rates and severity of infectious side effects posttransplant.[31] Additional multicenter prospective randomized trials are required to establish a consensus about a standard induction therapy for pancreas transplant recipients.

SURGICAL COMPLICATIONS

Complications after pancreas transplant can be divided into early and late (>90 days posttransplant) complications. Nearly all complications after pancreas transplantation can be diagnosed through a history and physical, CT angiography, and pancreas biopsy. Alternative imaging modalities may be needed for patients with significant renal dysfunction where there is concern for contrast-induced nephropathy. In these instances, pancreas transplant ultrasonography with Doppler blood flow assessment (limited by operator dependence and limited windows because of overlying intestinal gas) or magnetic resonance imaging may be needed. Common signs and symptoms of complications include hyperglycemia, hyperamylasemia or hyperlipasemia, increased insulin requirements, electrolyte abnormalities (hyperkalemia in

particular), nausea, vomiting, and abdominal distention/pain, either generalized or localized to the site of the graft.

Early Complications
Vascular

A critical early complication after pancreas transplantation is vascular thrombosis, which occurs in 5% to 14% of recipients and is a common cause of early pancreas graft failure after rejection.[40] The pancreas transplant is particularly susceptible to vascular thrombosis because of multiple factors, including changes in macro- and micro-circulation of the organ, particularly in the splenic and portal vein flow; ischemia-reperfusion injury leading to increased vascular resistance; prothrombotic state of recipients with diabetes mellitus; and surgical injury from vessel clamping and inflammation. Other causes of thrombosis may include technical misadventure at the anastomosis, rejection, graft pancreatitis, or external compression as a result of hematoma or fluid collections. Successful management of venous or arterial thrombosis begins with having a high index of suspicion and requires early diagnosis and intervention to have any chance at salvaging the graft. CT imaging with contrast will demonstrate a filling defect in the vein or artery and a lack of contrast enhancement of some or all of the transplanted pancreas (Fig. 54.7A). Ultrasound findings of venous thrombosis include absence of venous flow, high resistive indices, and reversal of diastolic flow in the arteries (see Fig. 54.7B), whereas arterial thrombosis will be evidenced by lack of pulsatile flow in the arteries of the pancreas. Early venous thrombosis is managed with initiation of systemic anticoagulation therapy and immediate thrombectomy, either surgically or by percutaneous thrombolysis. Surgical thrombectomy may be performed via the ligated ends of the SMV or splenic vein of the graft. Endovascular techniques may also be applied in later presentations or when operative intervention carries higher risk. Percutaneous endovenous thrombolysis with aspiration thrombectomy is a technique that has been reported to have some success.[41] Arterial thrombosis is commonly associated with technical

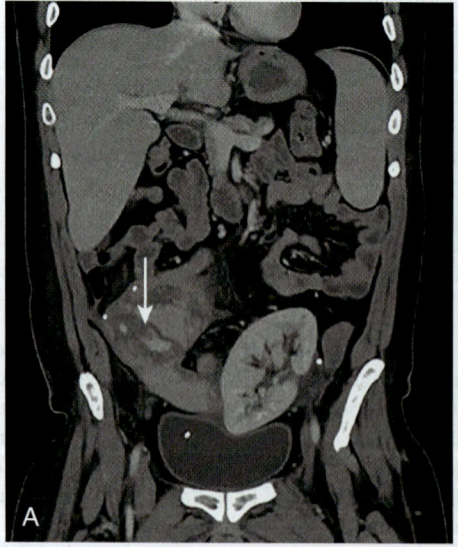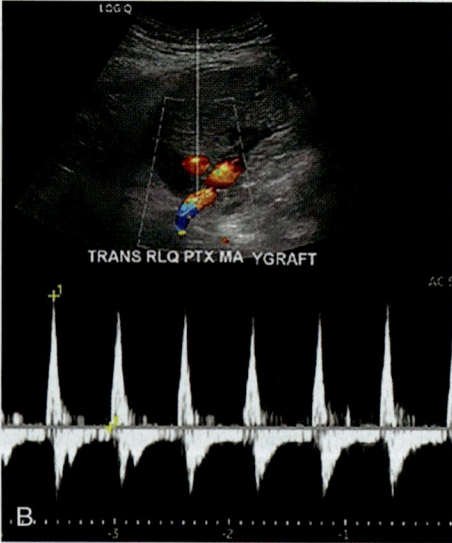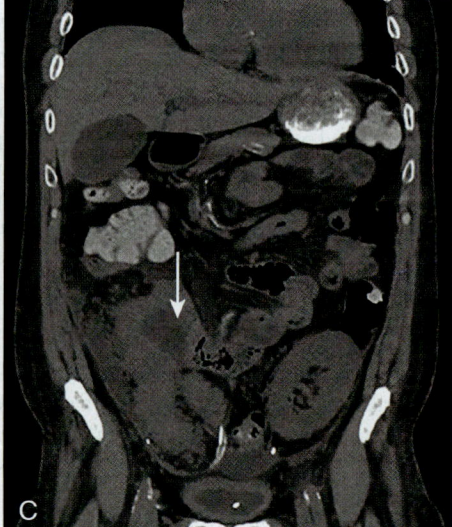

FIGURE 54.7 Early complications after pancreas transplantation. (A) CT imaging showing thrombus present in the peripheral portal vein system of the pancreas allograft, notated by the *arrow*. (B) Ultrasound of a pancreas transplant with acute proximal portal vein thrombus showing elevated velocities in the artery Y graft, reversal of diastolic flow in the artery, and lack of flow in the portal vein. (C) CT imaging showing peripancreatic fluid from an acute parenchymal leak, notated by *arrow*, after pancreas transplant.

problems at the anastomosis, and unless it is diagnosed immediately with emergent surgical intervention, the chances of graft salvage are poor, and early transplant pancreatectomy may be required. Endovascular intervention with transarterial catheter-directed thrombolysis has been described but with very limited success.[42] It should be noted that the dual arterial and SMA–splenic artery cross-circulation of the pancreas graft may allow preservation of parenchymal perfusion in the absence of splenic artery patency.

Incidental arterial and venous partial thromboses with preserved perfusion are relatively common after pancreas transplantation. These clots, if they occur, commonly involve the stumps of the SMA, SMV, splenic artery, or splenic vein and reflect vascular stasis in these segments. It is not clear at this time whether these clots merit anticoagulation or intervention. Many are incidentally detected on imaging studies and are inconsequential to long-term functional outcomes, even if not treated with anticoagulation.[43]

Bleeding

Bleeding is a relatively common complication after pancreas transplantation and is divided into intraabdominal/surgical site bleeding and gastrointestinal bleeding, and the expected frequency will vary depending on the type of pancreas transplant (SPK > solitary pancreas) and whether heparin is used during and after the operation. Intraabdominal bleeding can be from the vascular anastomoses, the parenchyma, or the retroperitoneum. Gastrointestinal bleeding in an enterically drained graft is almost universally from the intestinal anastomosis between the graft duodenum and the recipient intestine. Gastrointestinal bleeding may present as hematochezia or melanotic stools and is usually self-limited, although infusion of octreotide may help to stop persistent gastrointestinal bleeding by virtue of its visceral vasoconstricting effect. Patients experiencing refractory gastrointestinal bleeding may be suspected of having another source and should undergo nasogastric tube placement or upper endoscopy in an attempt to identify the bleeding source. Vascular bleeding is more often associated with vital sign changes, including hypotension, tachycardia, and a fall in hemoglobin levels. Imaging with ultrasound and CT may demonstrate evidence of evolving hematoma around the transplant site, and CT angiography may demonstrate extravasation of contrast to better localize bleeding. Early vascular bleeding complications are best treated with early reoperation to evacuate the hematoma and achieve hemostasis, whereas gastrointestinal bleeding rarely requires reoperation.

Infection

Early infections after pancreas transplantation (those occurring within the first 1–2 months) are generally bacterial infections related to the surgical procedure. The most common infection after pancreas transplantation is urinary tract infection. The most commonly isolated pathogens are *Enterobacteriaceae*, *Enterococci*, and *Candida*. Risk factors for urinary tract infection after pancreas transplantation include a prior history of urinary tract infections, prolonged urinary catheter use after transplant, urinary tract infection in the donor in patients receiving both kidney and pancreas grafts, use of ureteral stent in patients receiving pancreas and kidney transplant, and use of the bladder as the exocrine drainage modality.[44] Surgical site infections are also relatively common after pancreas transplantation because recipients are more susceptible, given the clean-contaminated nature of the procedure, the opening of the intestinal tract, the

presence of diabetes, and the more intense immunosuppressive regimens used to prevent rejection. The most common pathogens associated with superficial surgical site infections include *Staphylococcus aureus*, coagulase-negative *Staphylococci*, and gram-negative organisms (*Escherichia coli* and *Klebsiella* species). Deep surgical site infections are more commonly associated with *Enterococci*, *Streptococci*, anaerobes, other gram-negative bacteria, and *Candida* species.[45] Although diagnosis and treatment of superficial surgical site infections is generally straightforward, deep space infections can be more challenging. Diagnosis of deep space infections is often aided by contrast-enhanced CT imaging of the abdomen and pelvis.

Management of these early infections starts with prevention. Although there are no proven guidelines regarding perioperative antibiotics in solid organ transplant recipients, following the recommendations from the First World Consensus Conference and/or the clinical practice guidelines for antimicrobial prophylaxis in surgery from the Infectious Diseases Society of America is generally good practice; recommendations can be modified based on institutional experience and individual patient risk factors.[45] Optimal management of comorbidities (blood glucose control, temperature regulation during surgery), minimizing operative duration, using antibiotic irrigation solutions, and using fine surgical technique are all important factors in reducing the risk of surgical site infections in pancreas transplant recipients. Once diagnosed, an antibiotic regimen tailored to the offending organisms and source control are the mainstays of treatment for infections. Further management strategies may include removal of foreign bodies (ureteral stents, central lines, urinary catheters, etc.); percutaneous drain placement; and appropriate wound care, including debridement of devitalized tissue in the wound. For intraperitoneal infections, source control and debridement of devitalized tissue may require reoperation, depending on the source and location of the infection.

Leaks (parenchymal/enzyme or Enteric)

Deep surgical site infections often occur in the context of leaks after pancreas transplant, thus providing an ongoing source of bacterial contamination and/or nutrient-rich secretions. Leaks can be assertively categorized as either from the gastrointestinal tract (termed *enteric leaks*), most commonly the intestinal anastomosis or oversewn ends of the duodenum, or from the parenchyma of the pancreas itself (parenchymal or enzyme leaks). The physician should have a high index of suspicion for the development of an enteric leak from the enterically drained pancreaticoduodenal graft because signs and symptoms such as hypotension, tachycardia, leukocytosis, abdominal distention, or discomfort may be subtle in the context of immunosuppression. Placing surgical drains and monitoring the volume and character of the output in patients that are at high risk for leak is one strategy that can aid in early diagnosis. Similarly, an aggressive stance for inserting postoperative drains in developing fluid collections and evaluating the character of the output may provide an expeditious diagnosis. Abdominal imaging with a CT scan with per os (PO) and intravenous contrast is the best diagnostic test for leaks and will show fluid collections around the pancreas (see Fig. 54.7C) and may show extravasation of PO contrast at the site of the enteric anastomosis. Drains, either operative or postoperative, should be sampled frequently and tested for amylase and quantitative bilirubin. If both are present, these generally represent enteric leaks, but if only amylase is present, then this most likely represents a parenchymal/enzyme leak.[46] Gastrointestinal leaks are generally best treated with early reoperation. Small leaks can be treated with reinforcement of the anastomosis with additional sutures. However, larger leaks may require a redo of the anastomosis if an adequate amount of donor duodenum is left or a diversion of the intestinal stream away from the graft using a Roux-en-Y limb; in severe circumstances, transplant pancreatectomy may be necessary.[47] Risk factors for enteric leaks include older donor age, higher KDPI, higher PDRI, longer cold ischemic time (CIT), and SPK versus PTA.[47]

Leaks from the parenchyma of the pancreas may also occur and are generally either a result of surgical injury at the time of procurement or a consequence of significant ischemia-reperfusion injury. Parenchymal/enzyme leaks are diagnosed similarly by fluid sampling, but they are often self-limited. Checking surgical drains for amylase levels can help to determine the extent and improvement of pancreatic leaks over time. Persistent leaks may benefit from an octreotide infusion to slow the production of secretions by the pancreas. If the leak persists, then reoperation with evacuation, debridement, and additional drain placement may be necessary.

Late Complications

Late complications after pancreas transplantation also have a significant impact on graft function and survival. The most common cause of late death-censored graft failure is chronic rejection, which occurs in up to 15% of pancreas transplant recipients.[48] On the other hand, the most common cause of late *overall* graft failure is patient death, most commonly as a result of cardiovascular disease.[49] Immunologic complications such as acute and chronic rejection will be discussed separately. Here, we will discuss the late complications after pancreas transplant, including vascular complications, infections, and graft pancreatitis.

Vascular

Late complications of the vasculature after pancreas transplant are rare but can be a cause of graft loss and patient death. Mycotic pseudoaneurysm formation may develop in the setting of continued infection in the vicinity of vascular structures or chronic rejection. A dilated vascular segment, as the name may imply, is almost never appreciated; instead, this entity is an abnormal vascular-enteric connection that results in massive, life-threatening gastrointestinal bleeding. These may occur at the site of anastomoses as a result of disruption of the integrity of the vessel wall, usually in the setting of peripancreatic fluid collections, infection, or rejection episodes due to surrounding inflammation. The initial presentation of this entity may be subtle but usually includes a sentinel, self-limited bleeding event manifesting as hematemesis or hematochezia. Imaging with systemic CT angiography of the abdomen/pelvis (not visceral angiography) may demonstrate the bleeding point if it is active. Prompt endovascular intervention using either a covered stent or microparticle embolization, depending on the location and features of the bleeding point, if identified, is preferred to prevent evolution to catastrophic intestinal hemorrhage.[42] Stenting and embolization are generally considered temporizing procedures, with transplant pancreatectomy ultimately being required in many of these cases.

Infection

Although early infections are often related to the surgical procedure, late infections after pancreas transplantation are more frequently associated with opportunistic infections and reactivation of latent viruses. At 3 to 6 months after pancreas transplantation,

de novo opportunistic infections such as *Pneumocystis jiroveci* pneumonia, *Nocardia* spp., *Listeria monocytogenes*, *Toxoplasma gondii*, and fungal infections may present. In addition, reactivation of latent viruses may occur. The most common late infection after pancreas transplantation is reactivation of CMV, but others may also occur, such as herpes simplex virus (HSV) type 6, EBV, and VZV.[50] After 6 months, community-acquired infections become more common, such as community-acquired pneumonia or urinary tract infection. Opportunistic infections may still arise, and reactivation of latent viruses, particularly CMV and, in SPK patients specifically, BK polyomavirus, leading to nephropathy, is not uncommon.[43,51] Late infectious complications may also lead to tumor formation, such as anogenital condyloma associated with human papillomavirus and posttransplant lymphoproliferative disease associated with EBV.[50] Prevention is a key aspect of management of late infections. All pancreas transplant candidates are evaluated with a thorough history and physical exam as well as laboratory serology testing to evaluate for preexisting infection and determine exposure to prior infections, most notably CMV, EBV, HIV, hepatitis, toxoplasmosis, HSV, syphilis, VZV, and tuberculosis. This will help to determine appropriate antibacterial, antiviral, and antifungal prophylactic medication regimens as well as intervals for surveillance posttransplant. Reduction in immunosuppression in combination with antimicrobial agents is also important to facilitate clearance of late opportunistic infections.[44]

Graft Pancreatitis

Graft pancreatitis, defined as increased pancreatic enzymes, has been reported in roughly 20% of pancreas transplant recipients, may occur early or late after transplantation, and has many underlying causes.[52] The most important aspect of a diagnosis of graft pancreatitis is identifying the etiology, which thereby provides the opportunity for targeted therapy.[53] Graft pancreatitis that occurs immediately (postoperative day [POD] 1–3) after transplantation is usually a result of ischemia-reperfusion injury and is self-limited, although it may portend near-term future postsurgical complications.[54] Increased serum enzymes appearing somewhat later in the first week to 10 days after normalization is usually related to refeeding and, if the patient is without symptoms, may be related to ileus. Such mild increases in enzymes under these conditions are usually benign and self-limited and do not require specific treatment. However, if the patient develops signs and symptoms such as abdominal discomfort (particularly near the site of the transplant), fever, nausea, vomiting, and increased white blood cell count or creatinine, in conjunction with increased serum amylase and lipase levels, then contrast-enhanced CT imaging of the abdomen and pelvis is useful in helping to identify a source of the symptoms and distinguish a significant issue requiring intervention. Even if there is no intraoperative source of the increased enzymes or postsurgical complication, a CT scan in the first several weeks postoperatively commonly shows nonspecific stranding and edema around the transplanted pancreas. Graft pancreatitis, in the absence of intraabdominal findings that explain the increased enzymes, whether early (beyond the first several weeks) or late (>90 days), is graft rejection until proven otherwise and merits consideration for graft biopsy.

The causes for late graft pancreatitis are myriad and include acute or chronic rejection, CMV pancreatitis, intestinal obstruction, constipation, ventral or internal hernia with or without strangulation, ductal stricture, cystic lesions such as intraductal papillary mucinous neoplasm (IPMN), pseudocyst, and pancreatic graft cancer. Increased enzymes may also be a result of inflammation of the native pancreas or bowel perforation. The diagnosis can usually be confirmed after both cross-sectional imaging and pancreatic graft biopsy. In addition, because tissue-invasive CMV may cause graft pancreatitis, testing for CMV viremia by polymerase chain reaction can aid in focusing the differential diagnosis of pancreatitis. Rarer causes of graft pancreatitis may include duct obstruction, either with pancreatic duct stones or masses such as IPMN.[55] Mechanical intestinal obstruction distal to the pancreas in enteric-drained pancreas grafts may also lead to graft pancreatitis and increased serum enzymes. This can be related to adhesive disease, internal hernias, or incarcerated ventral hernias. In bladder-drained pancreas grafts, bladder outlet obstruction or atony resulting from diabetes-related neurogenic bladder may result in reflux pancreatitis.

Management of late graft pancreatitis begins with supportive care with IV fluid hydration, bowel rest, and possible nutritional supplementation with total parenteral nutrition if prolonged bowel rest is required. Additional treatments are targeted at the specific etiology of pancreatitis, once identified. For instance, treatment of rejection with increased immunosuppression; treatment of invasive CMV or CMV viremia with ganciclovir; or surgical intervention for mechanical bowel obstructions, particularly those associated with internal or ventral hernias, will most likely lead to improvement in the pancreatic enzyme levels in the blood if the diagnosis is correct. Bladder outlet obstruction leading to reflux pancreatitis in the bladder-drained pancreas graft may be treated initially with urinary catheter decompression of the bladder, but recurrent episodes may require conversion to enteric drainage. Complications of late graft pancreatitis, if ongoing inflammation is present, may include peripancreatic abscess, pancreatic necrosis, pancreatic fistula, or pseudocyst formation, the severity of which may dictate additional therapies such as drain placement, antibiotics, and in severe cases, transplant pancreatectomy.[56]

IMMUNOLOGIC COMPLICATIONS

Rejection

It is recognized that the mechanisms and types of rejection that occur after pancreas transplant are similar to those of other solid organ transplants. The main targets of acute T-cell–mediated rejection (TCMR) are the pancreatic ductal epithelium, pancreatic acinar cells, and vascular endothelium, reflecting the expression levels of the major histocompatibility complex (MHC). On the other hand, the endocrine cells of the islets of Langerhans are not considered an immediate and direct target of acute TCMR, given the low level of MHC expression.[57] Therefore, it is generally accepted that clinical hyperglycemia is not an early sign of TCMR; conversely, a finding of asymptomatic increased serum pancreatic enzymes is the earliest clinical manifestation of TCMR. In addition to TCMR, antibody-mediated rejection (ABMR) has been recognized recently to occur in the pancreas graft. ABMR is associated with donor-specific antibodies (DSAs) and/or C4d staining of the capillary endothelium. This condition typically causes disturbed microcirculation[58] and is associated with neutrophilic interacinar capillaritis on hematoxylin and eosin staining.[59] DSA can be divided into preformed (pretransplant) DSA and de novo (posttransplant) DSA, depending on the timing of when DSA is present. The role of preformed DSA is closely related to preoperative positive cross-match results and worse clinical outcomes in the early posttransplant course, whereas de novo DSA is associated with chronic allograft dysfunction, which is well recognized, especially in the fields of kidney and heart transplantation.[60] It has

also been reported that the presence of DSA, coupled with biopsy-proven signs of rejection, has a negative impact on allograft survival in the context of pancreas transplantation.[61] If not treated adequately, both TCMR and ABMR will eventually result in fibrosis and sclerosis of acinar lobules and deterioration of endocrine function, causing hyperglycemia and, ultimately, failure of the pancreas graft.

The diagnosis of pancreatic allograft rejection in the setting of SPK transplantation may also be assessed by monitoring and biopsy of the kidney allograft. Theoretically, rejection of both organs should occur concordantly; however, it has been reported that 20% to 40% of biopsies are discordant for rejection, with only the kidney or the pancreas involved.[62,63] Pancreas graft rejection in the setting of PAK and PTA transplants relies solely on monitoring the pancreas graft. Rejection of the pancreas is typically asymptomatic, especially in the early phases of the process. Therefore, in addition to monitoring regular laboratory data, especially amylase, lipase, and white blood cell counts, it is recommended to perform pancreas allograft biopsies. Pancreas allograft biopsies allow the determination of the precise grade of rejection; distinguish the presence or absence of ABMR; and distinguish other causes of enzyme elevations, such as CMV pancreatitis. Nonetheless, many centers will treat patients empirically for rejection if there is no other explanation found on imaging or blood tests for other causes of increased pancreatic enzymes. If the exocrine drainage route is through the bladder, urine amylase can be a useful marker of rejection. Whereas hyperamylasemia and/or hyperlipasemia are the most common signs of rejection, hyperglycemia is relatively rare and often a late finding. If hyperglycemia is present and rejection is diagnosed, this is generally considered a negative prognostic sign and is associated with a higher rate of short-term allograft failure, defined as a permanent return to insulin therapy. On the other hand, hyperglycemia in the early phases of pancreas transplantation without hyperamylasemia and hyperlipasemia may suggest thrombosis, infection, or tacrolimus toxicity rather than rejection. In addition, the recurrence of T1DM could also be a reason for hyperglycemia, as discussed later, but it is generally rare and experienced beyond the first year posttransplant.

A core-needle biopsy of the pancreas can be performed percutaneously with real-time ultrasound guidance with a ~6% complication rate[64] or laparoscopically when intestines are interposed between the graft and the abdominal wall. After biopsy, attention should be directed to monitoring for significant complications, such as pancreatic fistula, pancreatitis, and bleeding. An endoscopic duodenal cuff biopsy may be useful when a percutaneous pancreas biopsy is not possible. However, clinicians should be aware of possible pathologic discordance in the results between pancreas and duodenal biopsies in up to one-third of cases.[65] The Banff criteria advocated an allograft rejection grading schema, first in 2008[66]; it was then refined in 2011[67] and 2022.[59] The criteria include seven diagnostic categories for pancreas graft pathology, including rejection, T1DM recurrence, islet amyloid deposition, and other histologic diagnoses: (1) *Normal* indicates the absence or minimal inflammation without fibrosis. (2) *Indeterminate* indicates that septal inflammation exists but is overall not significant and does not meet the criteria for cell-mediated rejection. (3) TCMR is divided into three grades, I to III (mild, moderate, severe), and chronic active TCMR. (4) ABMR is diagnosed with evidence of DSA positivity, C4d deposition in interacinar capillaries, and morphologic changes. ABMR is also categorized into three grades, I to III (mild, moderate, severe). In addition, chronic active ABMR is defined if chronic lesions, such as parenchymal fibrosis, vascular remodeling, or chronic transplant arteriopathy, are identified. (5) Mild to severe graft fibrosis is staged according to the severity: stage I, <30% of the core surface; stage II, 30% to 60% of the core surface; stage III, >60% of the core surface. (6) Islet pathologies include ischemia, CNI toxicity, recurrence of T1DM, T2DM, and nonspecific reactive or regenerative changes. (7) The final category is other pancreatic lesions not related to rejection or any of the other pathologies.

Although control of TCMR has improved with advances in immunosuppressants, resulting in better short-term outcomes,[68] two major remaining challenges in pancreas transplantation are control of ABMR and securing better long-term graft survival. The first World Consensus Conference on Pancreas Transplantation published guidelines for therapeutic strategies based on three distinct patterns: first rejection, second rejection, and ABMR.[31] It is recommended to treat first or mild episodes of rejection or biopsy-proven grade I TCMR with steroid pulses, sparing T-cell–depleting antibodies. A general increase in maintenance immunosuppression is also recommended if the patient is able to tolerate it. The statement recommends that second-rejection episodes should be individualized and that T-cell–depleting antibodies should be used in most cases. Because of the lack of definitive evidence, treatment strategies for ABMR are largely based on those of renal transplantation. The main target is to control the humoral immune response. Therefore, IV immunoglobulins and plasma exchange with or without B-cell–depleting antibodies are reasonable considerations. In all cases, close posttreatment surveillance is paramount because relapses and rebounding enzyme elevations are not uncommon.

Recurrence

Diabetes may recur after pancreas transplantation, and it can negatively affect graft survival. Because T1DM has an autoimmune etiology, autoimmune destruction of pancreatic β cells of the graft may occur, but this is fortunately quite rare in mismatched deceased donor pancreatic allografts being treated with immunosuppression. The overall rate of developing T1DM after pancreas transplantation is thought to be relatively low,[49] partially owing to the impact of immunosuppressive agents used to prevent rejection. Conversely, recurrence cases have been reported in twins or HLA-identical siblings who underwent living-related partial pancreas transplantation with no or minimal immunosuppression, suggesting the importance of genetic factors and immunosuppression.[69] If a pancreas transplant is performed for T2DM or if there is significant weight gain, then significant insulin resistance may result in suboptimal glycemic control, which is more common, occurring 5% to 25% of the time, depending on the definition and time posttransplant.[70]

As an etiology, pancreatic islet–related autoantibodies have been identified and debated for their role in T1DM. Among them, insulin autoantibody (IAA), glutamic acid decarboxylase 65 (GAD65) antibody, insulinoma-associated protein-2 (IA-2) antibody, and zinc transporter 8 (ZnT8) autoantibody have been considered clinically relevant.[71] Several studies emphasized the importance of HLA sharing[69,72] and autoimmunity.[73] HLA-DR allele sharing, or the existence of HLA-DR3 and HLA-DR4 in the recipient's allele, and the appearance of multiple autoantibodies postoperatively are considered risk factors for recurrence.[72] On the other hand, T1DM recurrence was observed in recipients who underwent HLA-mismatched pancreas transplantation in which conventional immunosuppression was reduced. Therefore, the possibility of delaying the progression of T1DM recurrence has

been reported.[72] However, it is still unclear which specific populations have heightened vulnerability to T1DM recurrence.

OUTCOMES

There were 963 pancreas transplants performed in 2021, according to the most recent Organ Procurement and Transplantation Network (OPTN)/Scientific Registry of Transplant Recipients (SRTR) Annual Data Report. The vast majority, 68%, of pancreas transplants are performed in recipients with T1DM. An increasing proportion of pancreas transplants, 26%, are being performed for recipients with insulin-dependent T2DM. The 5-year survival for patients receiving a pancreas transplant is 92.2% for recipients with T1DM and 89.1% for recipients with T2DM. The 1-year and 10-year mortality rates for pancreas transplant recipients are as follows: PAK transplant, 2.8% and 20.1%; PTA transplant, 0% and 18.5%; and SPK transplant, 3.6% and 23.2%, respectively.[1]

Pancreas graft survival (or failure) rates have been difficult to track and report in the past because of inconsistencies in the definition of pancreas graft failure. However, in 2018 a consensus statement was published and has been implemented in OPTN policy that defines pancreas graft failure if a recipient experiences any one of the following: (1) undergoes transplant pancreatectomy, (2) is relisted for pancreas transplant, (3) is listed for islet transplant after undergoing pancreas transplant, (4) dies, or (5) has total daily insulin use of greater than or equal to 0.5 units/kg for 90 consecutive days.[74] Overall, pancreas graft failure rates at 1 year, 5 years, and 10 years after transplant are 6%, 15%, and 31%, respectively, but these outcomes are very much dependent on the type of transplant, center volume, sensitization to a particular donor, and retransplant status.

Most patients who receive a pancreas transplantation are also the recipients of a kidney transplantation as part of SPK or PAK. Notably, the kidney allograft survival in patients who receive a pancreas transplant is, on average, better than that in recipients with diabetes who receive a kidney transplant alone. The 10-year LDK graft survival rate of 69.8% in patients who received a PAK was significantly improved compared with 61% in similar insulin-dependent diabetic recipients of an LDK transplant alone. Similarly, the 10-year deceased donor kidney graft survival rates of 66% in the PAK group and 61% in the SPK group were superior to the kidney graft survival of 50.4% in diabetic recipients of deceased donor kidney alone.[75] The most recent 1-, 5-, and 10-year kidney graft failure rates for PAK were 6.3%, 14.7%, and 31%, respectively, and for SPK, they were 5.7%, 16.4%, and 32.3%, respectively.[1]

SUMMARY AND FUTURE PERSPECTIVES

Pancreas transplantation was initiated clinically in 1966. Difficulties in the procedure and a lack of effective immunosuppression and organ preservation led to a poor prognosis for a relatively long time. However, with improvements in surgical procedures, organ preservation, and immunosuppressive management, pancreas transplantation has become a fundamental therapeutic option not only for T1DM but also for selected recipients with insulin-dependent, low-risk T2DM as well as for patients after total pancreatectomy.

At present, there are several therapeutic options for T1DM: pancreas transplantation, islet transplantation, and insulin pump therapies in conjunction with continuous glucose monitoring. For patients with T2DM and/or severe obesity, medications, in addition to nutrition and exercise therapy, and bariatric surgery are options with specific indications. The sum of existing data indicates that pancreas transplantation seems to be superior in its effectiveness to islet transplantation and sensor-augmented insulin pump therapy, but it is inferior in terms of safety and invasiveness.[76] It is critically important to provide objective risk/benefit information on the multiple therapeutic options to patients during the consultation and evaluation phase for those considering pancreas transplantation.

There are several areas for future investigation in the field of pancreas transplantation and β-cell replacement therapy. Surgical techniques are evolving to more minimally invasive options, and the field of robotic surgery is growing, particularly in the field of transplantation, and may eventually provide a less invasive method of implanting pancreas grafts that could reduce postoperative pain and/or length of stay after transplant. Novel machine learning and artificial intelligence technologies are constantly being developed and refined, and if applied intelligently to transplantation practice, these may represent the future of enhanced diagnostics and complex donor–recipient matchings to maximize organ utilization and equity for pancreas transplant recipients. The possibility of ex vivo machine perfusion similar to the current revolution occurring in liver, lung, and heart transplantation may lead to the ability to store pancreas grafts for longer and possibly offer an opportunity to evaluate quality before transplant. More widespread use of normothermic regional perfusion for DCD donors in the United States has the potential to enhance use of pancreas grafts as it has for most of Europe. Novel immunosuppressive agents, such as biologic agents targeting other aspects of the immune response, such as costimulation blockade, or cellular therapies such as Treg therapies, may lead to more possibilities for pancreas transplant recipients to undergo immunosuppression withdrawal or at least get to CNI- and/or steroid-free maintenance regimens. Advances in genetic manipulation of other species have led to the clinical execution of xenotransplant more recently, which, with further improvements in technique and immunosuppression, may diminish the organ-shortage crisis. Other β-cell replacement technologies, such as stem cell–derived islets, islet encapsulation, and immunomodulation technologies, may provide additional β-cell replacement options for patients with diabetes or, if combined with three-dimensional printing or organoid ex vivo culture techniques, may lead to the development of a manufactured pancreas for transplant in the more distant future.

SELECTED REFERENCES

Amara D, Hansen KS, Kupiec-Weglinski SA, et al. Pancreas transplantation for type 2 diabetes: a systematic review, critical gaps in the literature, and a path forward. *Transplantation.* 2022;106(10):1916-1934.

Recent supportive evidence in pancreas transplantation for type 2 diabetes is discussed and also describes the requirement for further characterization regarding better candidacy of this population.

Boggi U, Vistoli F, Andres A, et al. First World Consensus Conference on pancreas transplantation: Part II—recommendations. *Am J Transplant.* 2021;21(suppl 3):17-59.

Practically important queries and useful deliberations/recommendations according to the first World Consensus Conference on Pancreas Transplantation are listed with clear arrangements.

Drachenberg CB, Buettner-Herold M, Aguiar PV, et al. Banff 2022 pancreas transplantation multidisciplinary report: refinement of guidelines for T cell-mediated rejection, antibody-mediated rejection and islet pathology. Assessment of duodenal cuff biopsies and noninvasive diagnostic methods. *Am J Transplant.* 2024;24(3):362-379.

This reference shows updated practical guidelines regarding the diagnosis and grading of both acute and chronic T cell-mediated or antibody-mediated rejection, including novel diagnostic approaches.

Kandaswamy R, Stock PG, Miller JM, et al. OPTN/SRTR 2021 annual data report: pancreas. *Am J Transplant.* 2023;23(2 suppl 1):S121-S177.

Objective statistical data of pancreas transplants in the United States is discussed in this report. This shows that the number of pancreas transplantation is slightly below 1,000/year. The mainstay (85%) of pancreas transplantation is performed as simultaneous pancreas-kidney transplantation. There is a trend of increasing proportions of pancreas transplants in type 2 diabetes population.

Kelly WD, Lillehei RC, Merkel FK, Idezuki Y, Goetz FC. Allotransplantation of the pancreas and duodenum along with the kidney in diabetic nephropathy. *Surgery.* 1967;61(6):827-837.

This report describes the beginning and challenges of pancreas transplantation in the transplant field.

The full reference list appears on Elsevier eBooks+.

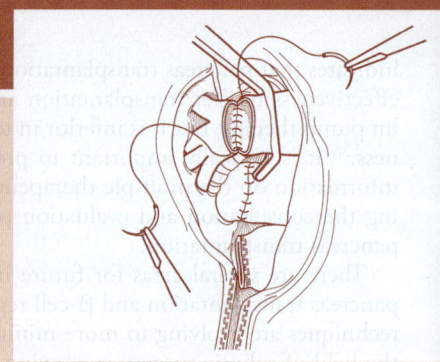

Islet Transplantation

Divyansh Agarwal, Tina Bharani, Chengyang Liu, Vijay Bhoj, and Ali Naji

INTRODUCTION

Type 1 diabetes mellitus (T1DM) is an autoimmune disease resulting from the selective destruction of insulin-producing islet β cells by autoreactive T lymphocytes.[1] Exogenous insulin therapy is the primary treatment approach for individuals with T1DM. However, attaining the desired glycemic targets with insulin usage can heighten the risk of severe hypoglycemic episodes (SHEs).[2] Although contemporary technologies for insulin administration and glucose monitoring offer promise, some patients remain resistant to even the most advanced strategies,[3] continuing to experience persistent SHEs. This situation can lead to the development of hypoglycemic unawareness,[4] greatly affecting their quality of life and, in some cases, resulting in mortality, affecting up to 10% of patients.[5] Both whole pancreas and pancreatic islet transplantation are well-established therapies to restore glucose homeostasis.[6]

The modern era of experimental islet transplantation took its first steps in the early 1970s. Pioneering research led primarily by Paul Lacy at Washington University[6] and Clyde Barker at the University of Pennsylvania[7] demonstrated the effectiveness of islet transplantation in normalizing blood sugar levels in rodent models of diabetes. This research also pinpointed the liver as the optimal engraftment site, following portal vein infusion of the isolated islets.[8] As a significant milestone, the first transplantation of deceased donor human islets was successfully carried out in the 1970s.[9]

Efforts to improve the quality and viability of isolated islets for transplantation[10,11] culminated in the development of an automated method for isolating human pancreatic islets, a breakthrough credited to Camillo Ricordi.[12] This innovative technique was subsequently applied in the first instance of allogeneic islet transplantation for T1DM, resulting in a brief period of insulin independence.[13] The real turning point, however, came in the year 2000 when the Edmonton group, led by James Shapiro and Ray Rajotte, achieved consistent success in attaining insulin independence in all seven consecutive patients with T1DM who received islets isolated from an average of two donor pancreases.[14] This pivotal achievement underscored the necessity of transplanting a sufficient mass of islet β cells to achieve insulin independence and emphasized the importance of avoiding the use of glucocorticoids in the immunosuppressive regimen to prevent islet toxicity and insulin resistance.

The success of the Edmonton protocol was confirmed in an international trial in 36 patients with T1DM.[15] Meanwhile, efforts in the United States have focused on improving the efficiency of both islet isolation and posttransplant islet engraftment to minimize the number of donor pancreases required to stabilize metabolic control and, when possible, eliminate the requirement for insulin therapy.[16,17] In 2005 the Minnesota group led by Bernard Hering introduced several modifications to peritransplantation management and reported consistent achievement of insulin independence in eight consecutive patients with T1DM who received islets isolated from a single donor pancreas.[18] This enhanced efficiency for allogeneic islet transplantation prompted a phase III multicenter licensure trial conducted by the Clinical Islet Transplantation (CIT) Consortium under the auspices of the US National Institutes of Health,[19] which confirmed its efficacy (primary end point met by 87% subjects at 1 year and by 71% at 2 years). This chapter presents our current knowledge about human islet transplantation, including long-term outcomes as well as future research directions of β-cell replacement therapy in the treatment of diabetes.

PRODUCTION, QUALITY ASSESSMENT, AND INFUSION OF ALLOGENEIC HUMAN ISLETS

The selection of hemodynamically stable deceased pancreas donors plays a pivotal role in determining the quantity and quality of procured islets for transplantation. A retrospective multicenter study identified donor factors associated with yields exceeding

400,000 islet equivalents (IEQs) and found that age, body habitus, hemodynamic status, HbA1c, peak glucose, aspartate aminotransferase (AST), alanine aminotransferase (ALT), amylase, and sodium levels were among the most predictive factors.[20]

In the United States, allogeneic islets have been considered a biologic drug and thus subject to the same regulatory rules applied to other cell therapies (e.g., genetically modified cells).[21] Based on this premise, a license-enabling phase III trial was initiated incorporating eight manufacturing facilities participating in the CIT Consortium. These sites implemented a harmonized process for the manufacture of allogeneic purified human pancreatic islet (PHPI) products. Selection of deceased donor pancreases and manufacturing, including the use of critical reagents for tissue dissociation, were standardized. Furthermore, the processing was conducted in compliance with Current Good Manufacturing Practices and Current Good Tissue Practices (Video 55.1). The quality systems and regulatory and operational strategies developed by the CIT Consortium yielded product lots that met the prespecified characteristics of safety, purity, potency, and identity. The CIT clinical protocol, master production batch record, and standard operating protocols are publicly available.[22]

After satisfactory release of the PHPIs, the islets are infused in the portal vein via percutaneous transhepatic catheterization, typically in collaboration with interventional radiology, or through a mini laparotomy to access a branch of the mesenteric vein (Figs. 55.1–55.2).

SELECTION OF RECIPIENTS FOR ISLET ALLOTRANSPLANTATION

Allogeneic islet transplantation has been conducted for individuals with T1DM in various modalities, including islet transplant alone (ITA) for nonuremic recipients,[19] simultaneous islet-kidney (SIK) transplantation for uremic recipients, and islet after previous kidney (IAK) transplantation for posturemic recipients.[23] ITA recipients are subjected to generalized immunosuppression to prevent islet allograft rejection. The decision to pursue ITA hinges on the severity of diabetes complications, particularly life-threatening hypoglycemic events. Recurrent hypoglycemia can profoundly affect individuals' confidence, professional lives, personal relationships, and daily activities, including driving, work performance, leisure activities, and sleep, while contributing to social exclusion and discrimination.[5] Evidence-based clinical practice recommendations identify individuals with T1DM complicated by IAH and recurrent SHEs as suitable candidates for islet or pancreas transplantation under specific conditions: if SHEs persist after following a structured stepped-care approach or undergoing a formalized medical optimization period that provides access to hypoglycemia-specific education, including behavioral therapies, insulin analogues, and diabetes technologies, all closely supervised by a specialist hypoglycemia service.[24]

Similarly, an optimal candidate for IAK should meet specific criteria: they should have been diagnosed with T1DM for at least 5 years, possess a stable kidney transplant, exhibit a lack of stimulated C-peptide, be identified as having impaired awareness of hypoglycemia, and have a history of SHEs within the past year, despite receiving medical care from an endocrinologist or diabetologist. Additionally, individuals who are unable to attain and sustain glycemic control without experiencing hypoglycemic episodes while aiming for a HbA1c ≥7.5% are also considered suitable candidates. On the contrary, individuals with a high body mass index (BMI) exceeding 30, a glomerular filtration rate (GFR) ≤40, a history of panel-reactive antibodies surpassing 50%, or the presence of anti–human leukocyte antigen (HLA)

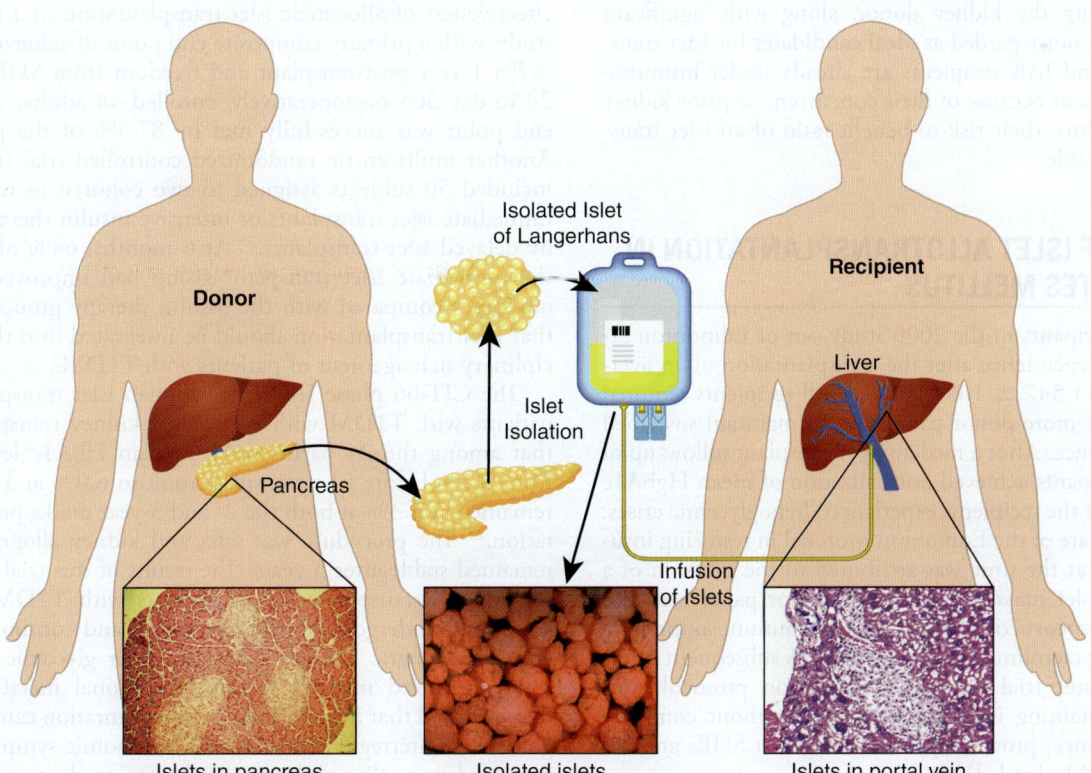

FIGURE 55.1 Islet transplantation as a β-cell replacement therapy involves infusion of insulin-secreting islet cells into the liver via the portal vein.

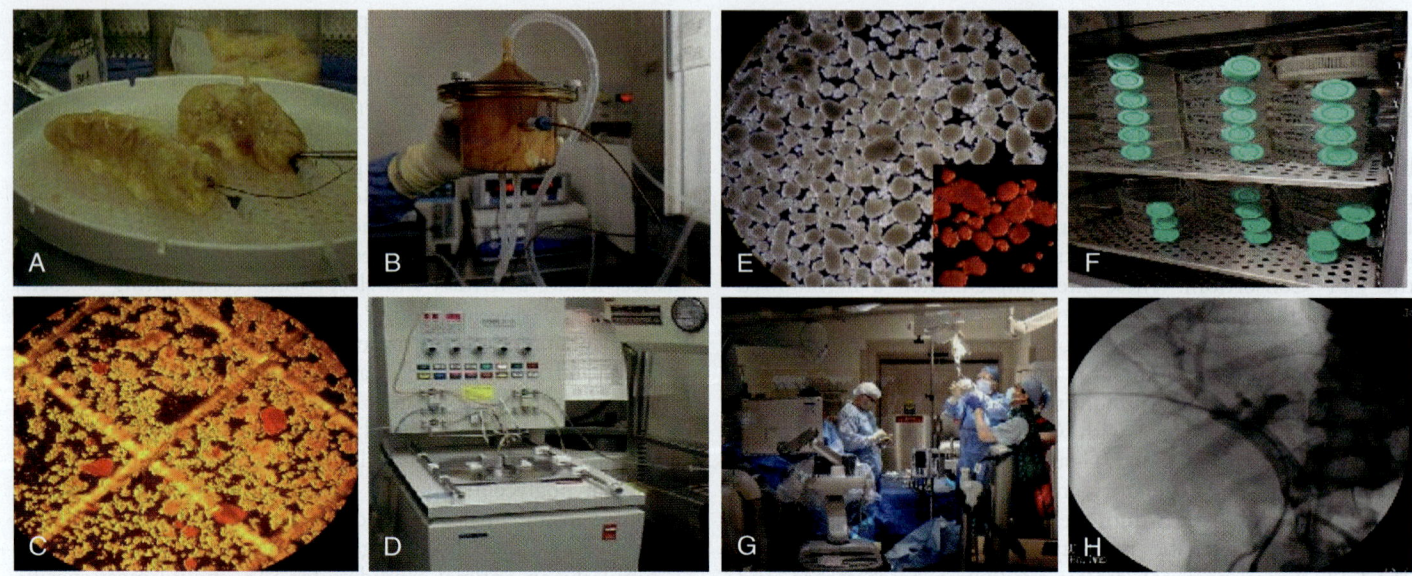

FIGURE 55.2 Steps involved in the isolation and infusion of purified human islets. Whole pancreas from deceased donor is brought to the Good Manufacturing Practices (GMP) facility. (A) The duodenal loop is dissected from the head of the pancreas with careful attention not to enter the bowel lumen. Next, the peripancreatic tissue is dissected from the head, body, and tail of the pancreas while avoiding damage to the pancreatic capsule. At this stage, the pancreas is sharply transected in the midbody, visualizing the lumen of the major pancreatic duct, which is then cannulated and infused with enzyme blend to disrupt the acinar tissue. (B) The tissue is then minced and transferred to an automated closed chamber (Ricordi) to continue further digestion. (C) Samples of the digest are intermittently stained with dithizone, a zinc-binding dye that specifically stains Zn-rich β cells, to assess for satisfactory separation of islets from exocrine cells. (D) Separation of the islets from exocrine tissue is achieved by a continuous density gradient centrifugation using a cell separator. (E) Isolated islets after COBE purification; *inset* shows staining with dithizone. (F) Pretransplant culture of islets in T-flasks for 48 to 72 hours at 22°C to 24°C. (G–H) Intraportal infusion of purified human islets under fluoroscopy via percutaneous transhepatic route after obtaining a portal angiogram.

antibodies targeting the kidney donor, along with significant comorbidities, are not regarded as ideal candidates for islet transplantation. SIK and IAK recipients are already under immunosuppressive treatment because of their concurrent or prior kidney transplantation; thus, their risk-to-benefit ratio of an islet transplant can be favorable.

OUTCOMES OF ISLET ALLOTRANSPLANTATION IN TYPE 1 DIABETES MELLITUS

The T1DM participants in the 2000 study out of Edmonton attained insulin independence after the transplantation of an average islet mass of 11,547 ± 1604 IEQ/kg. All recipients required islets from two or more donor pancreases to maintain sustained insulin independence. After a median posttransplant follow-up of 1 year, the participants achieved normalization of mean HgbA1c levels, and none of the recipients experienced hypoglycemic crises. The high success rate of the Edmonton protocol in restoring insulin independence at the time was attributed to the infusion of a required critical islet mass from multiple donor pancreases and the use of a glucocorticoid-free, low-dose immunosuppressive regimen involving tacrolimus and sirolimus.[14] A subsequent international multicenter trial using the Edmonton protocol confirmed that maintaining islet function, even without complete insulin independence, provided protection against SHEs and led to improved HgbA1c levels.[15]

Building on this work, the CIT-07 phase III trial, conducted at eight centers in North America, established the safety and effectiveness of allogeneic islet transplantation in T1DM.[19] The study, with a primary composite end point of achieving HgbA1c <7% 1-year posttransplant and freedom from SHEs from day 28 to day 365 postoperatively, enrolled 48 adults. The primary end point was successfully met by 87.5% of the participants. Another multicentric randomized controlled trial from Europe included 50 subjects assigned to two cohorts: to receive either immediate islet transplants or intensive insulin therapy followed by delayed islet transplants.[25] At 6 months, 64% of patients in the immediate islet transplant group had improved metabolic outcomes compared with the insulin therapy group, suggesting that islet transplantation should be integrated into the multidisciplinary management of patients with T1DM.

The CIT-06 phase III trial of human islet transplantation in patients with T1DM with established kidney transplants found that among the 24 participants, median HbA1c level dropped from 8.1% before islet transplantation to 6.0% at 1 year, and it remained at 6.3% at both the 2- and 3-year marks posttransplantation.[23] The procedure was safe, and kidney allograft function remained stable after 3 years. The results of this trial endorse the use of islet transplantation in patients with T1DM who have previously undergone kidney transplants and continue to experience problematic hypoglycemia and poor glycemic control despite optimized medical therapy. Additional metabolic studies have revealed that intraportal islet transplantation can help restore glucose counterregulation, reinstate autonomic symptom perception, and normalize endogenous glucose production in response to insulin-induced hypoglycemia in patients with long-standing T1DM.[26]

In further long-term follow-up studies of IAT and IAK recipients, the CIT-08 study demonstrated durable islet graft survival permitting achievement of glycemic targets in the absence of severe hypoglycemia for most appropriately indicated recipients having impaired awareness of hypoglycemia, with acceptable safety profile. Of the 48 IAT and 24 IAK recipients, insulin independence was achieved by 74% of the recipients, with more than one-half maintaining insulin independence during long-term 8-year follow-up.[27] In a remarkable 12-year follow-up of seven recipients who underwent the Edmonton protocol, sustained islet function was demonstrated. The median HbA1c level was 6.3%, and no patient encountered SHEs, opportunistic infections, or malignancy.[28]

IMPACT OF ISLET TRANSPLANTATION ON CHRONIC DIABETES COMPLICATIONS AND QUALITY OF LIFE

Studies over the past decade have highlighted the potential of islet transplantation to improve chronic diabetes complications, quality of life, and overall survival for patients with diabetes. In a prospective cohort study that explored the effects of ITA versus intensive medical therapy on the progression of microvascular diabetes complications, ITA recipients experienced a slower rate of decline in GFR and a reduced rate of retinopathy progression compared with those on medical therapy.[29] Furthermore, islet transplants have been associated with improvements in diabetes-specific patient-reported quality of life, including a diminished fear of hypoglycemia, a decrease in behaviors aimed at avoiding hypoglycemia, and reduced concerns regarding SHEs.[30] Participants in the CIT-06 and CIT-07 trials have also consistently reported significant and clinically meaningful enhancements in condition-specific health-related quality of life, along with more favorable self-assessments of their overall health.[31]

ADVERSE EFFECTS OF ISLET TRANSPLANTATION AND IMMUNOSUPPRESSION

Complications related to the islet transplantation surgical procedure itself, particularly intraportal islet infusion, encompass issues such as portal venous thrombosis, a temporary rise in liver enzyme levels, gallbladder perforation, and instances of bleeding. Portal thrombosis is a preventable complication if therapeutic anticoagulation is consistently maintained and the volume of infused packed cells is restricted to less than 5.0 mL.[32] Effective prevention of postprocedural bleeding can be achieved by ensuring the complete closure of the intraparenchymal catheter tract in the liver[33] or by employing a mini laparotomy approach to access a mesenteric vein for intraportal islet infusion.

Immunosuppression-related complications encompass calcineurin inhibitor (CNI)–induced nephrotoxicity, the potential development of islet donor–specific alloantibodies, and possible malignancy. Although GFR decline is common, it is primarily attributed to the acute effects of CNIs and partly to the correction of hyperfiltration after the restoration of near normoglycemia. Importantly, this decline in GFR appears to be stable in islet recipients over time. In the 2022 report of the international Collaborative Islet Transplant Registry, a total of 189 instances of neoplasms were reported in 101 out of 1373 islet recipients.[34] The most commonly diagnosed neoplasms included basal or squamous cell carcinoma ($N = 61$), thyroid cancer ($N = 5$), posttransplant lymphoproliferative disorder ($N = 5$), breast cancer ($N = 4$), and lung cancer ($N = 2$).

REGULATORY STATUS OF ALLOGENEIC HUMAN ISLET TRANSPLANTATION

Several countries, including Canada, the United Kingdom, Australia, and Japan, have either adopted islet transplantation as a standard of care or have granted regulatory approval for its use. In the United States, allogeneic pancreatic islets are considered a form of somatic cell therapy, therefore falling under the classification of biologic products and drugs. Consequently, they must receive approval through the submission of a Biologics License Application (BLA). There is currently a single BLA, petitioned by a nonacademic entity, for allogeneic islets issued by the US Food and Drug Administration to CellTrans.[35] At present, in the United States, islet allotransplantation remains investigational, and future approval would be crucial in expanding patient access to β-cell replacement therapies and fostering new advances in islet biology research.

RESEARCH PRIORITIES IN ISLET TRANSPLANTATION

Despite the efficacy of islet transplantation, major limitations hamper its widespread clinical application. These critical areas include a shortage of adequate supply of islets and the requirement for chronic immunosuppression. Significant progress has been made to address islet supply, and three key future research priorities stand out:

1. **Meeting islet supply and demand:** Given the limited availability of suitable deceased donor pancreases, stem cell–derived β cells have garnered recent attention,[36] especially given encouraging early clinical data that demonstrate the use of stem cell–derived islets in achieving insulin independence,[37] based on the immunosuppressive regimen used for transplantation of native pancreatic islets across the CIT-06 and CIT-07 studies. In view of the variability of islet yield from donor pancreas and to facilitate broader use of β-cell replacement strategies, modern cryopreservation techniques can be harnessed to help establish high-quality islet banks.[38]

2. **Establishing optimal microenvironment for islet engraftment:** Current clinical islet transplantation is based on intraportal infusion of pancreatic islets, associated with potential complications, including hemorrhage, portal vein thrombosis, inflammatory response, and amyloidosis, ultimately resulting in graft loss. The milieu in which islets are engrafted is also critically important for their survival. Making sites such as the subcutaneous space safe and easily accessible for islet engraftment and survival would be crucial to facilitate graft monitoring in the clinical setting.[39]

3. **Developing hypoimmunogenic islets to evade immune response:** Reducing or eliminating the need for long-term maintenance immunosuppression is a priority for long-term success of islet transplantation. Strategies based on short-term immunosuppression (using native islets) as well as encapsulation techniques (for stem cell–derived islets) without immunosuppression have provided a unique opportunity to minimize host immunosuppression.[40,41] Furthermore, innovations in gene editing have been employed for successful immune evasion to islet allografts.[42,43]

In summary, multiple phase III trials of islet allotransplantation have established its efficacy as a therapeutic option for individuals with T1DM with impaired hypoglycemic awareness.[44] Despite its clear advantages, the use of allogeneic human islet transplantation has been limited, largely because of inadequate islet supply and the risks associated with chronic immunosuppression. With significant progress in generating a sustainable supply of islets for transplantation, refining the procedures for their delivery and successful integration, and exploring strategies to eliminate the need for ongoing immunosuppression, we anticipate that islet transplantation will assume an important role in the comprehensive care of individuals with T1DM.

SELECTED REFERENCES

Shapiro AM, Lakey JR, Ryan EA, et al. Islet transplantation in seven patients with type 1 diabetes mellitus using a glucocorticoid-free immunosuppressive regimen. *N Engl J Med.* 2000;343(4):230-238. https://doi.org/10.1056/NEJM200007273430401

First report of islet transplantation based on the Edmonton protocol.

Hering BJ, Clarke WR, Bridges ND, et al. Phase 3 trial of transplantation of human islets in type 1 diabetes complicated by severe hypoglycemia. *Diabetes Care.* 2016;39(7):1230-1240. https://doi.org/10.2337/dc15-1988

Multicenter Phase 3 trial of the efficacy of human islet transplantation in Type 1 Diabetes.

Markmann JF, Rickels MR, Eggerman TL, et al. Phase 3 trial of human islet-after-kidney transplantation in type 1 diabetes. *Am J Transplant.* 2021;21(4):1477-1492. https://doi.org/10.1111/ajt.16174

Report of Feasibility and Impact and of Human Islet-after-Kidney Transplantation in Type 1 Diabetes.

Melton D. The promise of stem cell-derived islet replacement therapy. *Diabetologia.* 2021;64(5):1030-1036. https://doi.org/10.1007/s00125-020-05367-2

Review of the potential of stem-cell derived beta cell replacement therapy.

Yu M, Agarwal D, Korutla L, et al. Islet transplantation in the subcutaneous space achieves long-term euglycaemia in preclinical models of type 1 diabetes. *Nat Metabol.* 2020;2(10):1013-1020. https://doi.org/10.1038/s42255-020-0269-7

First report of successful long-term glycemic control after subcutaneous islet transplantation.

The full reference list appears on Elsevier eBooks+.

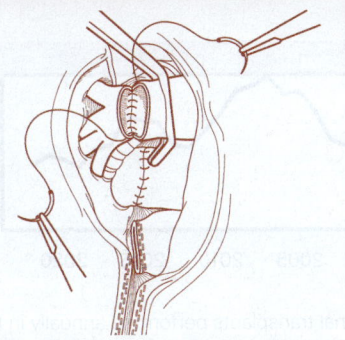

Small Bowel Transplantation

Imran J. Anwar and Debra L. Sudan

HISTORY

Intestine transplantation has become a lifesaving treatment option for patients with intestinal failure. The term *intestinal failure* encompasses multiple disorders of inadequate intestinal length or function that prevent adequate nutrient absorption. In contrast, *enteral autonomy* is a term describing the ability of an individual to absorb all nutrient needs from the gastrointestinal tract. For the subset of patients who have intestinal failure because of loss of bowel length, the terms *short gut syndrome* (SGS) and *short bowel syndrome* are used interchangeably. The causes of short bowel syndrome include congenital malformations, traumatic injury, infection, and ischemia. The absolute length of remnant bowel required to sustain nutrient absorption varies among individuals and on the basis of age. As a rule of thumb, however, short bowel syndrome and lack of enteral autonomy are expected after resection of more than 70% of the native intestine.

Intestinal failure may also describe a subset of patients with normal or nearly normal intestinal length but with abnormal function as a result of Crohn disease, motility disorders (such as intestinal pseudoobstruction and long-segment Hirschsprung disease), or diseases of the enterocytes (such as intestinal epithelial dysplasia). Disorders of intestinal function are less common than short bowel syndrome but share the same devastating consequences, leaving patients unable to absorb nutrients from the gut. In fact, before the 1960s, any cause of intestinal failure was nearly always fatal. Today, however, numerous treatment strategies have been developed, and the management of intestinal failure continues to vary greatly by treatment center. To better understand the natural history and clinical outcomes in these patients, several intestinal failure registries were established in the last years, both nationally and internationally. The International Intestinal Failure Registry (IIFR) is a global collaborative effort to track and report current trends in intestinal failure and began collecting data in 2021. There are currently 12 centers participating. In a pilot

phase study, The IIFR found that minimizing bowel resection at initial surgery and establishing bowel continuity were predictors of early enteral autonomy at 1 year, showing the feasibility and utility of an international registry.[1] Furthermore, several other national registries have been established over the past years.[2,3] These registries will allow us to better define the role of intestinal transplantation as a lifesaving therapy and which patients would most benefit from it.

The first investigation of intestine transplantation as therapy for intestinal failure is attributed to Alexis Carrel in 1905.[4] Given the lack of understanding of transplant immunology at that time, it was not surprising that these early efforts were unsuccessful. Approximately 50 years later, in 1959 (after the first reports of successful kidney transplantation), Walton Lillehei and colleagues[5] at the University of Minnesota published their successful experimental work transplanting intestines in a canine model. In 1962, Thomas Starzl (also working in a dog model) described transplantation of multiple abdominal organs, including the liver and entire gastrointestinal tract (from stomach through colon), termed *homotransplantation of multiple visceral organs.*[6] Human intestinal transplantation was subsequently attempted by Walton Lillehei and coworkers in 1967.[7] Like Anthony Carrel's work, this effort and several additional attempts during the next two decades were unsuccessful in achieving complete enteral autonomy, although several intestine recipients survived for several months after transplantation.[8] The primary reasons for failure were early technical complications and the inability to control rejection, leading to development of overwhelming infections or posttransplantation lymphoma.

The clinical course of intestinal failure was dramatically altered when Stanley Dudrick and associates[9] described hyperalimentation, which is arguably one of the most significant medical breakthroughs of the century. Their work demonstrated that puppies could achieve nearly normal growth patterns while exclusively sustained by hyperalimentation, more commonly referred to currently as *total parenteral nutrition (TPN)*. The clinical introduction of long-term TPN led to increased survival in individuals with intestinal failure, and contemporary studies have now reported overall survival in parenteral nutrition–dependent patients at 84% and 73% in pediatric populations[10] and 88% and 64% in adults[11] at 1 and 5 years, respectively. Given the success of parenteral nutritional support in the early 1970s and the abysmal results after early attempts at intestine transplantation, there was diminished enthusiasm for further clinical trials of intestine transplantation during this era.

Potentially fatal complications associated with TPN administration were identified as experience increased over time, including severe catheter-associated bloodstream infections; technical difficulties in maintaining venous access because of catheter-associated venous thrombosis; and cholestasis leading to liver failure, also referred to as *parenteral nutrition–associated liver disease (PNALD)* or *intestinal failure–associated liver disease (IFALD)*. Although a formal consensus definition for IFALD is lacking, it is often biochemically characterized as a conjugated bilirubin level greater than 2 mg/dL in patients who have been on TPN for longer than 2 weeks. IFALD develops in approximately 50% of pediatric patients and is closely related to the duration of TPN (>3 months).[12] Risk of IFALD-induced steatosis in adults receiving home parenteral nutrition is lower, with reported rates of 15% to 40%. Once IFALD develops, however, it is associated with a 43% 5-year mortality in patients with remnant jejunum and ileum length of less than 50 cm.[10]

Concurrent with reports of severe TPN-associated complications, cyclosporine immunosuppression was introduced, resulting in marked improvements in kidney and liver allograft survival. With advances in immunosuppression, there was renewed interest in the field of intestine transplantation. The first successful human isolated intestine allograft (with the achievement of enteral autonomy) was reportedly performed by Eberhard Deltz and colleagues[13] in 1988 with a living donor allograft procured from the sister of the 42-year-old recipient. Although rejection episodes recurred, these episodes were controlled with the use of cyclosporine, bolus steroids, and antilymphocyte treatments, eventually achieving enteral autonomy. A few months later, Grant and coworkers[14] performed the first cadaveric combined liver-intestine transplant to achieve complete enteral autonomy and more than 1-year patient and graft survival using cyclosporine. Despite these individual successes, 1-year expected patient survival after intestine transplantation using cyclosporine immunosuppression was approximately 25%, and failure to achieve enteral autonomy and risk for early death persisted.[8] In the early 1990s, the introduction of tacrolimus immunosuppression improved control of intestine allograft rejection, resulting in improved patient and graft survival after intestine transplantation.[15] Although this led to a mild increase in volume that peaked in 2007, the overall volume and experience with intestine transplantation have been dramatically less than with transplantation of other solid organ allografts, and intestinal transplant remains the least common form of solid organ transplantation. In the United States, the United Network for Organ Sharing (UNOS) has reported that only 3400 intestine transplants have been performed as of October 2023, with 82 performed in 2022 (Fig. 56.1). Since 2010, there has been a steady increase in adults waiting for intestinal transplant; in 2021, there were more adults compared with individuals <18 years old on the abdominal transplant waitlist. This is in part because of advances made in pediatric intestinal rehabilitation over the past several years.[16–18] A multicenter multinational study following a large

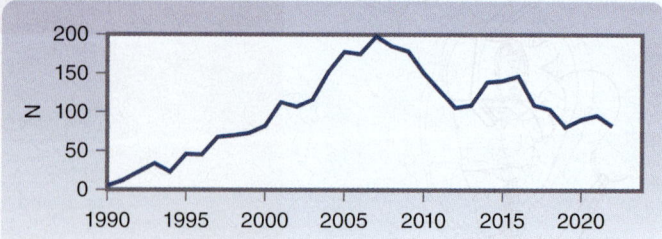

FIGURE 56.1 Number of intestinal transplants performed annually in the United States 1990–2023. (From https://insights.unos.org/OPTN-metrics/; accessed on October 10, 2023.)

cohort of pediatric patients with intestinal failure from 2010–15 found a survival rate of 90% at 6-year follow-up with a cumulative incidence of 53% of enteral autonomy and 16% transplant rates.[19] Favorable bowel anatomy (≥50% small bowel length, presence of ileocecal valve), small bowel syndrome as etiology, absence of portal hypertension, and treatment at high-volume transplantation center were associated with enteral autonomy.

INDICATIONS FOR INTESTINE TRANSPLANTATION

Dependence on parenteral nutrition alone is not considered an indication for intestine transplantation in light of the excellent survival of most patients receiving parenteral nutrition. Indications for transplantation of the intestine were initially proposed by experts in the field at the Sixth International Small Bowel Transplant Symposium in 2001 and further discussed at the XIV International Small Bowel Transplant Symposium in 2015.[20] These include irreversible intestinal failure *and* one of the following: (1) evidence of advanced or progressive intestinal failure–associated liver disease; (2) limited central venous access because of multiple thromboses of central veins; (3) life-threatening morbidity in the setting of indefinite TPN therapy, such as two intensive care unit (ICU) admissions; (4) invasive intraabdominal desmoids; (5) acute diffuse intestinal infarction with hepatic failure; and (6) failure of first intestinal transplant. Other potential indications include patients with high morbidity, poor quality of life, and severe fluid or electrolyte abnormalities that require frequent hospitalization, although these are not uniformly accepted.

Additionally, multivisceral transplant has been proposed as a treatment for diffuse portomesenteric thrombosis (Yerdel grade 4), as it is the only treatment that produces a definitive solution by completely replacing the portal system.[21–23] However, transplanting those patients carries increased hemorrhagic risk given extensive collateralization. Pre/perioperative embolization has been proposed as a means to decrease bleeding in those patients in certain centers.[23,24]

The international Intestinal Transplant Registry (ITR) has collected demographic and outcome data on intestine transplants worldwide since 1985. The most common primary underlying disease states prompting intestinal transplantation reported by the ITR are shown in Table 56.1. In both pediatric and adult patients, SGS accounts for about two-thirds of patients, although the SGS is secondary to different underlying pathologies, in part depending on the age of the patient; in pediatric patients, these include gastroschisis (38%), volvulus (25%), and necrotizing enterocolitis (23%), whereas in adults, ischemia (24%), Crohn disease (11%), volvulus (8%), and trauma (7%) are more common.[25,26]

TABLE 56.1 Underlying Conditions Necessitating Intestinal Transplantation

PEDIATRIC	INCIDENCE (%)	ADULT	INCIDENCE (%)
Short bowel syndrome	63	Short bowel syndrome	64
• Gastroschisis	22		24
• Volvulus	16	• Ischemia	11
• Necrotizing enterocolitis	14	• Crohn disease	10
	4		8
• Atresia	1	• Other	7
• Ischemia	1	• Volvulus	
• Trauma	3	• Trauma	
• Unspecified			
Motility disorders	18	Tumor	13
Malabsorption syndromes	8	Motility disorders	11
Retransplantation	8	Other	9
Other	5	Retransplantation	7

Adapted from Grant D, Abu-Elmagd K, Mazariegos G, et al. Intestinal Transplant Registry report: global activity and trends. *Am J Transplant*. 2015;15:210-219.

TABLE 56.2 Diagnostic Studies for Evaluation of the Intestine Transplant Candidate

DIAGNOSTIC STUDIES	TESTS AND PROCEDURES
Laboratory evaluation	Serum chemistries, liver function tests, complete blood count, prothrombin time–international normalized ratio, partial thromboplastin time, platelet count, albumin
Immunologic evaluation	HLA typing, HLA antibody, panel reactive antibody (PRA)
Serologic tests for infectious diseases	CMV immunoglobulin G/immunoglobulin M, EBV antibodies, hepatitis B virus, hepatitis C virus, HIV
Endoscopy	Upper gastrointestinal endoscopy, colonoscopy with biopsy
Pathology	Percutaneous liver biopsy
Radiographic evaluation	Upper gastrointestinal series with small bowel follow-through, barium enema
	Computed tomography of abdomen and pelvis, liver ultrasound
	Doppler ultrasonography of jugular and subclavian veins (or magnetic resonance venography) to assess patency
	Gastric emptying study, motility testing
	Two-dimensional echocardiography
Other	Nutrition, psychosocial, cardiopulmonary, and anesthesia assessment

CMV, Cytomegalovirus; *EBV*, Epstein-Barr virus; *HIV*, human immunodeficiency virus; *HLA*, human leukocyte antigen.

EVALUATION

Recipient Evaluation

Timely referral to an intestine transplantation center (before or soon after the development of complications of parenteral nutrition administration) is the first step for the potential intestine transplant candidate. Evaluation for transplantation includes determination of residual intestine length, anatomy and function, extent of complications of intestinal failure, and presence and extent of comorbid conditions. Although each center develops its own protocols, diagnostic studies frequently performed during the evaluation are listed in Table 56.2. After the evaluation, a multidisciplinary team (including transplant surgery, gastroenterology, anesthesia, social work, finance, nutrition, pharmacy, and medical psychology) determines whether a patient is an appropriate candidate on the basis of center-specific inclusion and exclusion criteria. If the patient is deemed a candidate, the center places the patient on a national waiting list. The allocation system then prioritizes recipients that are closest to a donor hospital. If no local candidate is identified, the distance progressively expands according to UNOS allocation guidelines. UNOS has developed allocation strategies for available cadaveric donor organs, which are publicly available (http://www.unos.org).

Donor Evaluation

An appropriate cadaveric donor is selected on the basis of compatible blood type and size of the donor compared with the recipient. Size is a significant consideration for the intestine donor because substantial loss of abdominal domain is common in the recipients who have typically undergone extensive resection. To address the problem of loss of domain, some centers have advocated that an ideal donor should have a body weight 50% to 75% that of the recipient.[27] Additionally, an extensive abdominal surgical history in the donor may preclude procurement.

Another important aspect of donor selection is cold ischemia time. Compared with other abdominal organs, intestinal allografts are particularly sensitive to cold ischemia owing to the highly vascularized and metabolically active mucosa. Prolonged cold storage of the graft may lead to loss of mucosal integrity and

thus bacterial translocation, intestinal inflammation leading to rejection, or, if severe, intestine perforation early after implantation; therefore, many protocols advise a maximum cold ischemia time of 6 to 8 hours. As a result, optimal small bowel donors are hemodynamically stable, require minimal vasopressor support, and are geographically close to the recipient transplant center.[28]

Similar to trends in other solid organ transplants, machine perfusion has been trialed by several groups in preclinical models, both as a means to minimize cold ischemia time and to decrease reperfusion injury. In a porcine model, Abraham et al.[29] devised a normothermic machine perfusion and reported successful transplantation of the machine-perfused small bowel. Hou et al.[30] showed overall improved recipient survival and decreased severity of ischemia-reperfusion injury after intestinal allograft preservation by a hypothermic machine perfusion compared with static cold storage in a porcine model. Although preliminary, these studies suggest that application of machine perfusion to intestine transplantation will in the long term allow improved intestine allograft preservation by decreasing ischemia-reperfusion injury and ischemia-reperfusion injury–related complications and allow for organ procurement in a geographically distant manner.

Lastly, viral serologic testing of the cadaveric donor for Epstein-Barr virus (EBV) and cytomegalovirus (CMV) is important because of the associated risk for primary viral transmission, leading to posttransplantation lymphoproliferative disorder (PTLD) and severe enteritis, respectively.[31]

Donor and Recipient Surgical and Technical Considerations
Isolated Intestine Transplantation

Isolated intestine (or small bowel) allografts typically include the entire jejunum and ileum with the associated vasculature, that is, the superior mesenteric artery (SMA) and vein (SMV) (Fig. 56.2). The most common variable in this type of allograft is the site of vascular transection (above or below the pancreas), which primarily depends on whether the pancreas from the intestine donor is allocated independent of the intestine allograft. In the neonatal donor or in any donor for whom the isolated pancreas has not been allocated separately for transplantation, the SMA is divided at the level of the aorta and the portal vein is divided at the superior border of the pancreas to provide maximum lengths of vessels to the intestine allograft. The donor jejunum is divided with a surgical stapler just distal to the ligament of Treitz, and the transverse colon is transected at the hepatic flexure. In contrast, in adult and older pediatric donors without significant aberrations in anatomy, isolated intestine can be safely procured while still allowing use of the liver and pancreas from the same donor for other recipients. In these circumstances, the donor operation requires additional careful dissection of the mesentery from the retroperitoneal organs, and the SMA and SMV are divided at the mesenteric root at the inferior border of the pancreas. Carotid or iliac arteries and iliac or jugular veins are also procured from the cadaveric donor to allow vascular reconstruction in the recipient.

During the recipient operation, arterial inflow is established by direct anastomosis of the donor SMA to the recipient infrarenal aorta or by interposition of a donor arterial conduit. Venous outflow from the allograft is provided by anastomosis of the donor SMV to the recipient portal vein or inferior vena cava, with or without an interposition of donor venous conduit. The continuity of the bowel is established proximally and distally by standard techniques for enteric anastomoses. Finally, a distal ileostomy/colostomy is created to allow routine monitoring of the graft (see Fig. 56.2).

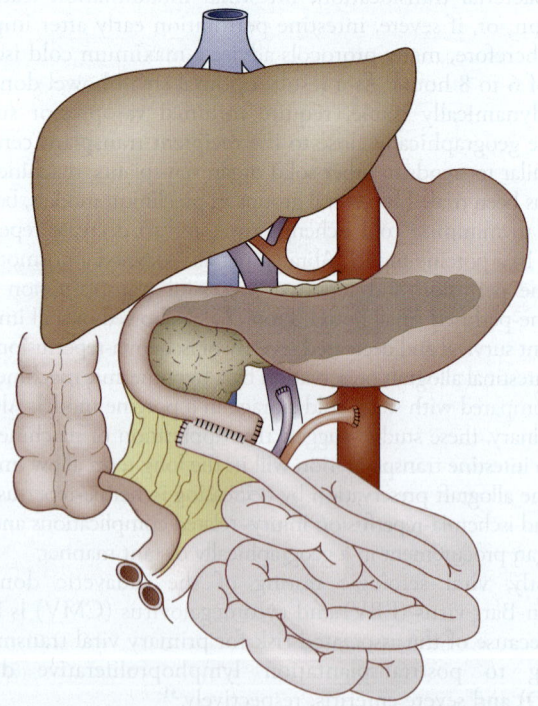

FIGURE 56.2 Isolated intestine transplant. Arterial inflow is established through anastomosis of the donor superior mesenteric artery with the recipient infrarenal aorta. Venous drainage is achieved by anastomosis of the donor superior mesenteric vein to the native portal vein or inferior vena cava. Bowel continuity is established through anastomosis of the proximal graft jejunum to the recipient duodenum, and the distal ileum is brought out as an ileostomy.

Intestine Allograft in Combination With Other Abdominal Organs

The nomenclature of grafts that include additional abdominal organs along with the intestine is less consistent than the isolated intestine graft and has varied over time and among various centers. A liver–small bowel graft as described by Grant and colleagues[14] refers to the individual liver and intestine grafts procured from the same cadaveric donor, but each implanted separately. The technical aspects of donor procurement for grafts planned to be implanted separately are the same as those described for isolated intestine transplantation and in standard liver procurement. This composite graft requires a loop of defunctionalized (Roux-en-Y) allograft small bowel for biliary drainage. In this situation, the pancreas allograft could potentially be allocated to a different recipient. The second variant of the liver and intestine allograft is the en bloc version, in which the liver and intestine, along with the duodenum and pancreas (or head of the pancreas), are procured and transplanted in continuity, thus preserving the extrahepatic biliary system (Fig. 56.3).[32] However, when the liver–small bowel graft is planned to be implanted en bloc, after complete mobilization of the abdominal organs along the avascular planes, the cadaveric donor procurement differs from that described before in that (1) no hilar dissection is performed (leaving the hepatic hilum, donor duodenum, and donor pancreas undisturbed, (2) the donor thoracic aorta is excised in continuity with the abdominal aorta (including the orifices of both the celiac axis and SMA), and (3) the donor spleen is typically removed from the tail of the pancreas on the back table. The sites for division of the bowel (just distal to the pylorus and proximal to the ileocecal valve) are similar to isolated intestine transplantation unless the stomach is included, which then makes the site of transection at the proximal stomach. The division of the inferior vena cava (above and below the liver) is the same as in isolated liver.

During the recipient operation, the native liver is excised along with most (or all) of the remnant small bowel to make room for the composite liver and intestine allograft. In some patients where the portal and splenic veins are patent and adequate room is present for the new allograft, the native foregut may be preserved. The extent of further native visceral resection (which may include the distal native stomach, native duodenum, pancreas, and spleen) is dependent on the extent or location of hilar or mesenteric root tumors; presence of enterocutaneous fistulas or anatomic abnormalities in any of these structures; presence of portal, splenic, and mesenteric thrombus; and/or loss of abdominal domain that precludes placement of the graft because of size discrepancy. The suprahepatic inferior vena cava anastomosis is performed first as in a liver-only transplantation procedure. Reconstruction of the vena cava can be performed in either caval replacement or piggyback fashion (largely dependent on the presence or absence of size discrepancy between the donor and recipient or preference of the center or surgeon). The caval anastomosis allows venous drainage of the composite organs because the donor portal system remains intact. Next, the arterial inflow is reestablished. Fig. 56.3A demonstrates use of the donor thoracic aorta as a conduit for arterial inflow to the donor celiac trunk and SMA. This donor aortic conduit may be anastomosed to the recipient's infrarenal aorta or supraceliac aorta, as shown in Fig. 56.3B. Once the graft is revascularized, bowel continuity is restored proximally and distally; however, the site of anastomosis depends on the recipient's anatomy and the extent to which native viscera have been removed. In Fig. 56.3A, the proximal bowel reconstruction is shown at the

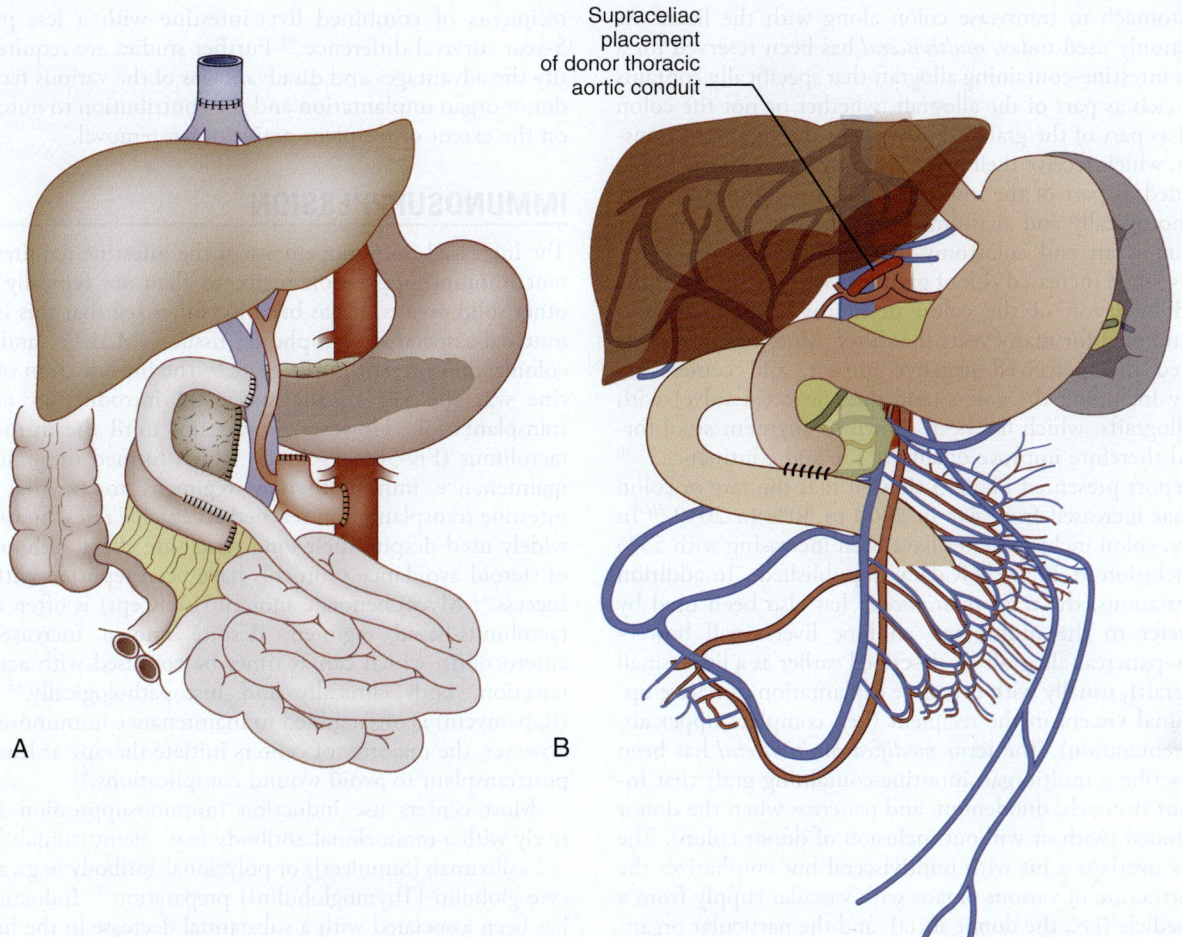

Supraceliac placement of donor thoracic aortic conduit

FIGURE 56.3 Liver-intestine-pancreas transplant. (A) The donor celiac axis and superior mesenteric arteries are left on an aortic conduit, which is anastomosed to the recipient aorta infrarenally. Venous outflow is through the anastomosis between the donor hepatic veins and the recipient suprahepatic inferior vena cava. The donor duodenum and the head of the pancreas (shown) or the entire donor pancreas are left intact to preserve the donor common bile duct. The donor jejunum is anastomosed to the native stomach, duodenum (shown), or proximal jejunum, depending on the native remnant anatomy. (B) Supraceliac placement of donor thoracic aortic conduit.

level of the native duodenum and allograft proximal jejunum, and the distal reconstruction is at the level of the allograft distal ileum and remnant native transverse colon. Alternatives include a proximal gastrogastrostomy and distal colocolostomy when the donor stomach and/or colon are included in the graft.

When the recipient foregut is retained, a portacaval (or splenorenal) shunt must be performed to allow venous drainage of the native foregut (stomach, pancreas, spleen, and duodenum) to prevent formation of esophagogastric varices or refractory ascites from venous outflow obstruction. In this instance, the proximal bowel reconstruction is performed between the proximal native remnant jejunum and the donor allograft proximal jejunum.

The strategic advantage of individual implantation is the potential to explant a failed intestine allograft without disrupting the liver allograft if discordant injury occurs after transplantation, which was clearly a concern in the early experience in light of the high incidence and recurrent nature of intestine allograft rejection. The advantages of the en bloc strategy are the simplified recipient operation and the decreased potential for technical complications, given that reconstruction of the biliary drainage and portal vein is not necessary. In addition, the en bloc strategy requires a single vascular anastomosis to either a cuff or conduit of

donor aorta, in contrast to individual reconstruction of the celiac artery and SMA, in which the grafts are implanted separately.[32] The major criticism of the nomenclature of the liver–small bowel for both of these techniques is that it does not distinguish when the donor duodenum and pancreas are included as part of the graft, nor does it distinguish what native viscera are retained or removed.

Other Technical Variations

Technical variations in the donor and recipient operations are common for multiorgan intestine-containing allografts; however, the nuances of these variations are difficult to assess in terms of contribution to patient outcomes because of the nonspecific nature of the nomenclature used to describe these techniques and inconsistency in use of the various terms. In addition to the liver–small bowel allograft described earlier, three additional terms are presently (or have been) used in reference to multiorgan intestine-containing allografts: cluster, multivisceral, and modified multivisceral grafts. In the initial papers using the term *multivisceral* in the description of multiorgan intestine-containing allografts in dogs, the graft included the entire gastrointestinal tract from proximal stomach to transverse colon along with the liver.[6] As more commonly used today, *multivisceral* has been reserved for a multiorgan intestine-containing allograft that specifically contains donor stomach as part of the allograft, whether or not the colon is included as part of the graft.[33] Historically, the right and transverse colon, which receive their arterial supply based on the SMA, were included as part of the intestine transplant. The colon was placed orthotopically and anastomosed to the recipient colon or brought out as an end colostomy. An early series from Pittsburgh[34] described increased risk of graft loss with inclusion of the colon, and inclusion of the colon in multivisceral grafts was largely abandoned for many years thereafter. More recent reports have refuted this perceived negative impact, and centers are increasingly including the colon (and thus ileocecal valve) with intestine allografts, which has been shown to augment stool formation and therefore improve quality of life and continence.[35,36] The ITR report presented in 2013 showed that the rate of colon inclusion has increased from 4% in 2000 to 30% in 2012.[26] In recent years, colon inclusion rates have been increasing with 55% of colon inclusion in 2021 (ITR data, unpublished). In addition to these variations, the term *multivisceral* has also been used by some to refer to the multiorgan en bloc liver–small bowel–duodenum–pancreas allograft (as described earlier as a liver–small bowel allograft), usually with extensive explantation of native upper abdominal viscera in the recipient (i.e., complete upper abdominal exenteration). The term *modified multivisceral* has been used to describe a multiorgan intestine-containing graft that includes donor stomach, duodenum, and pancreas when the donor liver is excluded (with or without inclusion of donor colon). The term *cluster* overlaps a bit with multivisceral but emphasizes the anatomic structure of various organs with vascular supply from a common pedicle (i.e., the donor aorta), and the particular organs included or excluded could be altered on the basis of the needs for the particular recipient. As originally described, the cluster graft was used primarily for the transplantations performed for tumor, and the organs included were selected on the basis of the extent of native organ involvement.[37]

For a number of years, there has been suspicion that the liver was protective immunologically for the intestine allograft[38]; however, data from the 2021 Organ Procurement and Transplantation Network/Scientific Registry of Transplant Recipients (OPTN/SRTR) have demonstrated equivalent long-term graft survival between isolated intestinal and combined intestine-liver grafts (Fig. 56.4).[39] Interestingly, the same report showed better 1-year survival for recipients of intestine-only allografts compared with

recipients of combined liver-intestine with a less pronounced 5-year survival difference.[40] Further studies are required to identify the advantages and disadvantages of the various techniques of donor organ implantation and the contribution to outcome based on the extent of recipient native organ removal.

IMMUNOSUPPRESSION

The increased immunogenicity of the intestine requires more potent immunosuppression regimens than are typically used with other solid organs. It has been hypothesized that this is related to mucosal-associated lymphoid tissue (MALT) and bacterial colonization present in the graft.[41] The introduction of cyclosporine was the key to the successful introduction of intestine transplantation. However, it was not until the introduction of tacrolimus (FK-506, Prograf), which formed the basis for most maintenance immunotherapy regimens today, that successful intestine transplantation reached acceptable rates. Steroids are still widely used despite their long-term side effect, although the use of steroid avoidance protocols have been reported with apparent success.[42] Mycophenolate mofetil (CellCept) is often added to a tacrolimus-based regimen, despite known increased risk of enterocolitis, which can at times be confused with acute cellular rejection, both clinically and histopathologically.[43] Sirolimus (Rapamycin) is often added to maintenance immunosuppression; however, the majority of centers initiate therapy at least 1 month posttransplant to avoid wound complications.[44]

Most centers use induction immunosuppression intraoperatively with a monoclonal antibody (e.g., alemtuzumab [Campath] or basiliximab [Simulect]) or polyclonal antibody (e.g., antithymocyte globulin [Thymoglobulin]) preparation.[44] Induction therapy has been associated with a substantial decrease in the incidence of early rejection, and the most recent review by the ITR suggests a survival advantage for depletional induction therapy.[26] As such, induction therapy is currently used in around 80% of all the intestine transplants performed.

Despite improved outcomes after the introduction of tacrolimus as well as induction therapy, long-term outcomes continue to remain inferior to other solid organ transplants, partly because of the immunogenicity of the allograft, leading to either rejection or complications related to over-immunosuppression. Although possible short-term outcomes have improved slightly in the past 2 to 3 years, there has not been any substantial improvement in graft survival outcomes from 2010–21. Several centers are now trialing novel strategies primarily targeting antibody-mediated injury and inflammatory responses (most commonly rituximab, vedolizumab, and infliximab) that aim to optimize immunosuppression and transplant conditions that would lead to long-term outcomes.

The Leuven immunomodulatory protocol (LIP), a multifactorial strategy, is perhaps the most promising strategy. It was designed to promote pro-tolerogenic T regulatory cells while avoiding calcineurin inhibitors and steroids and minimizing ischemia reperfusion injuries and consists of donor-specific blood transfusion, induction therapy, tacrolimus at lower-than-usual trough levels, steroid taper, and low-dose azathioprine as well as minimizing cold ischemia time and decontaminating the bowel.[45] The 5-year graft and patient survival rates in recipients on this protocol were 92%, and only 4/13 patients developed rejection, which were all controlled with steroids or thymoglobulin. No patient developed donor-specific antibodies (DSAs). Importantly, no patients developed graft-versus-host disease (GVHD) or PTLD, and infection rates have been low. Given that LIP is a

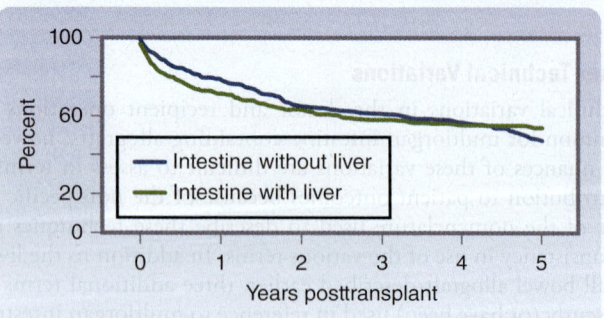

FIGURE 56.4 Graft survival within the first 60 months after transplantation among adult deceased donor intestine transplant recipients. (From Horslen SP, Wood NL, Cafarella M, Schnellinger EM. OPTN/SRTR 2021 annual data report: intestine. *Am J Transplant.* 2023;23:S264-S299.)

multifactorial strategy, it is impossible to tease out the contribution of each component to outcomes.

Belatacept (Nulojix), a modified version of CTLA4-Ig that interferes with the CD80/86-CD28 costimulatory pathway, remains seldom used in intestinal transplant recipients, with the only report in patients experiencing nephrotoxicity secondary to tacrolimus, which was associated with a high rate of rejection.[46] In a similar vein, sirolimus (Rapamycin) has been used in a pediatric intestinal transplantation cohort when recipients developed tacrolimus-related side effects and immunologic complications, which occurred in more than one-third of their cohort.[47] Graft survival, patient survival, and rejection rates were similar between patients maintained on tacrolimus and patients transitioned to sirolimus.

Similar to the anatomic considerations in surgical techniques and choice of induction agent, no specific maintenance regimen has proved to be superior to another, and centers continue to use regimens based on preference of the physician, experience, and needs of the individual patient.

COMPLICATIONS

Surgical and Perioperative Complications

Despite the advances in intestine transplantation, it remains a surgical procedure with high morbidity, and reported complication rates approach 50%. The most common types of technical complications are bowel anastomotic leaks, intestine perforations, and wound complications. These can be catastrophic and require a high index of suspicion because of the extensive immunosuppression and at times lack of typical signs and symptoms. The management of these surgical complications in the intestine allograft recipient uses standard surgical principles to provide coverage to the bowel loops, to drain or to debride infectious material or tissue, and to close enteric defects. Vascular complications are rare but include both bleeding and thrombosis. Postoperative hemorrhage may result from recipient coagulopathy (especially in the case of native or allograft hepatic dysfunction) and be amplified by the extensive dissection usually required as a result of multiple adhesions from previous surgeries. Thrombosis of arterial inflow or venous outflow conduits is typically associated with devastating sudden graft necrosis and results in patient or graft loss. Biliary complications can be largely avoided in liver-intestine transplantations by including the duodenum and pancreas, thus avoiding any hilar dissection, as noted before. Rare instances of intrahepatic biliary strictures caused by preservation injury, prolonged cold ischemia, or late immunologic injury have been observed.

Monitoring and Rejection

Unlike in hepatic or renal transplantation, no convenient serochemical marker exists to monitor intestinal function. Stool calprotectin and serum citrulline levels have been examined as potential markers, but because of limited access and prolonged testing time, neither of these tests is widely used at this time.[48,49] Pleximmune is a cell-based test that was approved by the FDA in 2014 to predict occurrence of acute cellular rejection in pediatric intestinal transplant recipients.[50] It is based on a mixed lymphocyte reaction (MLR) that quantifies allo-specific CD154[+] T-cytotoxic memory cells, a specific cell type that has been shown to correlate with rejection after intestinal transplant.[51] One of the major drawbacks of this assay is that it is only run by a single laboratory, requiring

centers to ship samples and at times leading to several days to get results back.

One advantage unique to intestinal transplants is that tissue for biopsy can be readily obtained endoscopically. Ileoscopy through the ostomy provides a method of visualizing the mucosa and directly obtaining tissue for pathologic examination. Routine ileoscopy and biopsy typically begin between postoperative days 5 and 7, and most centers will obtain biopsy specimens once or twice weekly for the first 1 to 3 months and as needed for symptoms thereafter.

Historically, rejection was frequent and often severe in intestine transplant recipients, with incidence as high as 70% to 80%.[14] More recently, with the evolution of various immunosuppressive strategies, a decrease in the incidence of rejection has been observed that correlates with improved patient survival.[38] Despite this, recipients of intestinal transplant continue to experience higher rates of rejection and graft loss than other solid organ transplants, and minimal improvement has been made over the past 10 years, emphasizing the need to improve immunosuppression and long-term management of these patients. Acute cellular rejection usually occurs in the early postoperative period (most commonly within 3 months) but can occur at any time. The most frequent clinical signs and symptoms of rejection may mimic those of viral gastroenteritis, including unexplained fever, abdominal pain or cramping, and increased stoma or stool output. Because of the insidious onset, lack of distinctive features, and absence of specific biomarkers, diagnosis may be delayed. For this reason, rejection remains closely associated with rates of graft failure and mortality.

Acute cellular rejection is characterized histologically in mild forms by an inflammatory response that is localized to the lamina propria and the crypts, with increased numbers of apoptotic bodies seen in the crypts but with maintenance of an intact mucosal lining and normal or nearly normal villous height. Moderate acute cellular rejection is defined by markedly increased inflammation within the lamina propria, increased apoptotic bodies within the crypts, and blunting or distortion of the villous architecture. In severe acute cellular rejection, the damage to crypts is so marked that the intestinal architecture may be lost and severe mucosal ulceration or exfoliation is identified.[52]

Recent investigation has also highlighted the contribution of antibody-mediated rejection (ABMR) in the setting of both acute and chronic events.[41] DSAs bind donor human leukocyte antigen (HLA) and are present in 11% to 31% of patients before transplant and develop de novo in up to 18% to 25% of patients posttransplant; their presence indicates up to 30% risk of graft loss within 2 years. Although the mechanisms are presently unclear, liver-containing allografts, compared with visceral allografts without liver, appear to afford protection with higher rates of preformed DSA clearance and lower rates of de novo DSA formation, leading to improved allograft survival.[41] Monitoring DSA is accomplished via enzyme-linked immunosorbent assay or HLA-bound microbead assay (Luminex); however, currently there is no consensus protocol in using these assays or for the treatment of DSA. In clinical investigation, however, DSA has been measured at 1-, 3-, 6-, and 12-month intervals after transplant (in addition to anytime rejection is clinically suspected) and is treated on a case-by-case basis.[53]

Once rejection has been established, treatment usually consists of large steroid doses and an increase in the target levels of maintenance immunosuppression. Resistant cases may be treated with more potent immunosuppression, such as rabbit antithymocyte globulin with or without additional immunosuppressive medications (e.g., sirolimus, mycophenolate mofetil).[54]

Several novel strategies have been trialed in the case of refractory rejection. Kroemer et al.[55] described 100% response rate (14/14 patients) after infliximab (Remicade), an anti–tumor necrosis factor (TNF)-α monoclonal antibody, in patients with refractory rejection. Mechanistically, the authors found that intragraft memory T-helper type 17 cells were a leading feature of refractory rejection and could be targeted by infliximab. Vedolizumab (Entyvio) is a monoclonal antibody against the α4β7 integrin, an integrin required for gut homing of inflammatory cells, and successfully treated refractory rejection after intestinal transplantation[56] and combined intestinal and abdominal wall transplant.[57] Clearly, those novel strategies ought to be evaluated in large, prospective clinical trials.

During treatment for rejection, the combination of increased immunosuppression and potential compromise of the gut mucosal barrier can lead to secondary infections, requiring close follow-up and a high index of suspicion for infections.

Infection

After intestinal transplantation, infection is a leading cause of morbidity and mortality and is the most common cause of graft loss.[26] Bacterial infections are prevalent, with incidence as high as 70% to 90% after intestine transplantation.[58] Initial infectious risk stems from ischemia-reperfusion injury, which may lead to loss of the gut mucosal barrier and bacterial translocation, intestinal anastomotic leak in the immediate postoperative period, and/or trigger immune activation leading to rejection. Rejection may lead to a similar impairment of the gut mucosal barrier. In addition, a number of preoperative and intraoperative factors contribute to a high rate of bacterial infection, including prolonged operative time, multiple blood transfusions, potential contamination from enteric spillage, preexisting liver disease, preexisting infections, and frequent need for prolonged central venous access. Bacterial infections can be manifested as translocation-related bacteremia, intraabdominal infection, catheter-related infections, pneumonia, or wound infections, with central line infections being the most common.[59] Organisms include typical gut flora such as *Escherichia coli, Klebsiella, Enterobacter,* and enterococci. Special consideration is also given to fungal infections (most commonly invasive candidiasis),[60] and most centers now incorporate antifungal prophylaxis as part of their perioperative regimen.

Viral infections (particularly with members of the herpesvirus family) are common in patients receiving intestine transplants, affecting approximately two-thirds of patients. CMV is a common pathogen with infection rates from 18% to 25% and a 7% incidence of invasive disease.[61] Donor and recipient CMV serologic status is an important predictor of posttransplantation CMV infection. Transplanting bowel from the CMV-positive donor to a CMV-negative recipient facilitates transmission and may increase the risk for tissue-invasive CMV, recurrent CMV, and ganciclovir-resistant CMV infection.[62]

Similar to rejection, the presentation of CMV infection may be insidious and ranges from mild symptoms (fever, increased stoma or stool output, cramping, and abdominal pain) to severe symptoms (intestinal ulceration, bleeding, perforation, or frank ischemia). The potential severity of primary CMV infections has led some to propose the restriction of transplantation from a CMV-positive donor intestine into a CMV-negative recipient. Because the symptoms of CMV infection may mimic those of intestine allograft rejection, biopsy of the allograft may be needed

to differentiate the two causes of graft injury. The presence of CMV inclusion bodies on hematoxylin and eosin stain or identification of CMV by immunohistochemistry or stool electron microscopy confirms the diagnosis of CMV enteritis. Fortunately, with appropriate antimicrobial treatment, typically IV ganciclovir (Cytovene) alone or in combination with CMV immune globulin (CytoGam), and reduction in immunosuppression, graft loss can be avoided in most cases.[63]

EBV, another member of the herpesvirus family, presents a unique challenge to intestine transplant recipients because of the association with development of PTLD. In intestine transplant recipients, the reported incidence of PTLD is 5% to 10%, which is considerably higher compared with kidney recipients (1%–2%), liver recipients (2%–5%), and lung-heart recipients (5%–10%).[64] In addition, EBV-associated PTLD is more common after primary infection and therefore more common in children than in adults. The incidence of PTLD has declined with modern immunosuppression and management, with an overall incidence of 19.2% in patients transplanted in 1985–95, 10% for patients transplanted in 1995–2001, and 6.2% for those transplanted in 2001–11.[26]

PTLD usually is manifested within the first year after intestine transplantation and has a variable presentation, ranging from mild to moderate symptoms of infection (fever, malaise, lymphadenopathy) to life-threatening malignant disease (solid masses at extranodal sites, such as the transplanted intestine, lung, liver, or central nervous system). Routine screening for seroconversion by a serum quantitative EBV polymerase chain reaction assay is common to try to identify primary infections before severe symptoms occur. Other risk factors for the development of PTLD include transplantation of organs from an EBV-positive donor to an EBV-negative recipient, use of more potent immunosuppression, history of rejection, and history of retransplantation.[65] Reduction of immunotherapy (with or without antiviral medication) is the first line of treatment with more severe cases (patients who develop Burkitt or T-cell lymphoma) requiring chemotherapy. Anti-CD20 monoclonal antibodies (e.g., rituximab) may also be useful in the treatment of PTLD when the EBV infection appears to be leading to B-cell tumors or proliferation. Surgical excision of localized disease, if possible (e.g., tonsillectomy, splenectomy, lobectomy, or enterectomy), is also highly effective. Despite these treatments, EBV-associated PTLD has a mortality rate exceeding 25%.[65]

Graft-Versus-Host Disease

GVHD occurs when donor lymphoid cells begin to target recipient tissues, most notably the epithelial cells in the skin and intestine. Because of the large amount of lymphoid tissue present in the intestine, before successful intestine transplantation, it was predicted that GVHD would be a prohibitive barrier. The reported incidence of GVHD is approximately 10% and, although not prohibitive to successful intestine transplantation, remains considerably higher than the incidence associated with other solid organ allografts.[66] In adults, increasing graft volume (e.g., colon and liver inclusion) is associated with higher rates of GVHD.[67,68] Increasing immunosuppression (commonly steroids and antithymocyte globulin) remains the mainstay treatment for GVHD, and outcomes remain poor, with survival rates below 50%.[67] Several centers use antilymphocyte treatments (anti-thymocyte globulin, anti-thymocyte globulin [equine]) in the donor to decrease the amount of passenger leukocytes with the transplanted intestine. The overall clinical benefit of this approach is currently unclear, with the largest case series of GVHD in intestinal transplant showing no benefit.[67]

OUTCOMES

Patient and Graft Survival

Patient and graft survival rates have improved with time. The 2015 ITR report analyzed 2699 patients from 82 transplant centers, finding overall patient survival of 77%, 58%, and 47% at 1, 5, and 10 years, respectively, for patients transplanted after 2000.[26] Data from the most recent OPTN/SRTR annual report have also shown that patient survival is influenced by patient age, with superior survival in recipients under age 18 compared with those above age 18 (5-year survival 62% vs. 43%, respectively; Fig. 56.5).[40] One-year patient survival was better in patients receiving intestine-alone allografts compared with liver-containing allografts (86.4% vs. 75.2%, respectively), but the difference narrowed at 5 years. The ITR report demonstrated overall graft survival rates of 71%, 58%, and 47% at 1, 5, and 10 years, respectively.[26] In the past 5 years, 1-year and 5-year conditional graft survival have dramatically improved, with both survival rates approaching 90% (unpublished data, ITR 2022). Sepsis is the leading cause of graft loss (50%), followed by rejection (13%), cardiovascular events (8%), PTLD (6.8%–9.9%), and technical complications (6.1%).[26] Age appears to influence the cause of graft loss, as children younger than 18 years are more likely than adults to lose grafts as a result of rejection (62.4% vs. 47.8%) and lymphoma (2.2% vs. 0%).[26] In general, graft function after transplantation is good in survivors; at 6 months posttransplant, 67% are free from TPN. In patients receiving a colon segment with their intestine graft, there is a 5% higher rate of freedom from parenteral nutrition or IV fluid support.

Cost

Given the substantial cost to manage intestinal failure, many patients rely on government payers (state Medicaid or Medicare) before transplantation. As a result of these financial constraints, access to experienced centers can be a challenge, as there are only 23 US centers performing intestinal transplant, which has led to differential access to multidisciplinary intestinal failure programs.[69] Estimates of the annual cost for home TPN range from $100,000 to $250,000, including costs of supplies and infusion solutions (ranging from $75,000 to $122,000) and costs of hospitalizations for parenteral nutrition–related complications (ranging from $10,000 to $196,000).[70] Comparatively, the cost of intestinal transplantation has been estimated between $130,000 and $250,000.[71] Despite the high cost of the initial transplant procedure, immunosuppressive medications, and subsequent hospitalizations, transplantation typically becomes cost-effective within 1 to 3 years.[71]

Quality of Life

Although intestinal transplantation may be the only lifesaving treatment for select patients with intestinal failure, many will suffer challenges related to healthcare-related quality of life following transplantation. A series published by the University of Pittsburgh Medical Center evaluated quality of life in patients who survived longer than 5 years after transplant, finding that 75% were able to maintain an occupation (including those who identified as either a student or homemaker). Postoperatively, 24% met diagnostic criteria for neuropsychiatric impairment (including hearing loss, developmental delay, depression, anxiety, and substance abuse), and self-reported surveys demonstrated improvement in domains of anxiety, cognitive ability, sleep, social support, and recreation after transplant (although depression and financial obligations were worsened).[72] In studies that specifically evaluate pediatric patients, 29% have developmental delay (often recognized before transplant) and 60% require specialized educational programming.[73] Parents of intestine recipients tend to perceive a slightly worse quality of life; however, pediatric patients rate their quality of life similar to that of normal age-matched children.[74]

CONCLUSION

The field of intestine transplantation has expanded slowly, in part because of successful widespread use of home TPN for the treatment of intestinal failure. PNALD and catheter-related complications (infections or venous thrombosis) remain the most frequent indications for intestine transplantation, although the incidence of PNALD is decreasing or delayed with the introduction of improved parenteral nutrition management strategies, particularly alternative lipid strategies. Intestine transplantation is no longer considered experimental and is offered to patients with life-threatening complications of parenteral nutrition administration or complete portomesenteric thrombosis. The transplant operation is frequently challenging because of patients' complex surgical history, altered anatomy, and presence of portal hypertension. Furthermore, the postoperative course is frequently complicated. However, after initial recovery, independence from TPN is achieved in most patients. Patient survival has been increasing, similar to survival on long-term TPN. These improvements in morbidity and mortality have led to acceptance of intestine transplantation as a standard treatment for intestinal failure in appropriately selected patients.

Future directions in the field of intestinal transplantation include conducting multi-institutional studies to aid in standardizing immunosuppression protocols, development of universal postoperative monitoring guidelines (including use of ileoscopy, biomarkers, and DSA testing), and elucidating the mechanisms underlying DSA-mediated rejection.

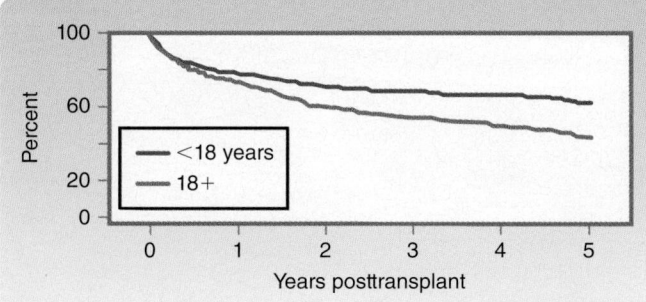

FIGURE 56.5 Patient survival among intestinal transplant recipients, 2014–16. (From Horslen SP, Wood NL, Cafarella M, Schnellinger EM. OPTN/SRTR 2021 annual data report: intestine. *Am J Transplant.* 2023; 23:S264-S299.)

SELECTED REFERENCES

Abu-Elmagd KM, Costa G, Bond GJ, et al. Five hundred intestinal and multivisceral transplantations at a single center: major advances with new challenges. *Ann Surg.* 2009;250:567-581.

A landmark single-center series that highlights outcomes between different transplant eras.

Ceulemans LJ, Braza F, Monbaliu D, et al. The Leuven immuno-modulatory protocol promotes T-regulatory cells and substantially prolongs survival after first intestinal transplantation. *Am J Transplant.* 2016;16(10):2973-2985.

A report on a novel multifactorial strategy to achieve improved outcomes after intestinal transplantation.

Cheng EY, Everly MJ, Kaneku H, et al. Prevalence and clinical impact of donor-specific alloantibody among intestinal transplant recipients. *Transplantation.* 2017;101:873-882.

A recent study characterizing the prevalence of donor-specific antibody and its association with accelerated intestinal graft rejection.

Deltz E, Schroeder P, Gebhardt H, et al. Successful clinical small bowel transplantation—report of a case. *Clin Transplant.* 1988;3:89-91.

A case report of what is considered the first successful living donor small intestine transplant.

Dudrick SJ, Vars HM, Rhoads JE. Growth of puppies receiving all nutritional requirements by vein. *Fortschr Parenteral Ernahrung.* 1967;2:16-18.

This is the landmark paper in which prolonged survival was demonstrated to be feasible in puppies using only hyperalimentation (intravenous nutrition, more commonly referred to today as parenteral nutrition).

Fryer JP. Intestinal transplantation: current status. *Gastroenterol Clin North Am.* 2007;36:145-159, vii.

A review of intestinal transplantation and its current practices.

Grant D, Abu-Elmagd K, Mazariegos G, et al. Intestinal Transplant Registry report: global activity and trends. *Am J Transplant.* 2015;15:210-219.

This is a summary of data from the Intestinal Transplant Registry database that includes statistics compiled from intestinal transplant recipients at transplant centers from 21 countries.

Horslen SP, Wood NL, Cafarella M, Schnellinger EM. OPTN/SRTR 2021 annual data report: intestine. *Am J Transplant.* 2023;23(2 Suppl 1):S264-S299.

The most recent report from the Organ Procurement and Transplantation Network that summarizes trends in intestinal transplantation over the past decade.

The full reference list appears on Elsevier eBooks+.

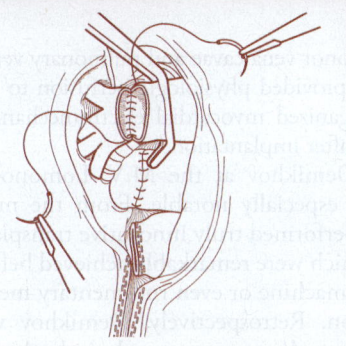

CHAPTER 57

Heart Transplantation

Jeffrey E. Keenan, Chetan Pasrija,
Ashish S. Shah, and Carmelo A. Milano

INTRODUCTION

Heart transplantation has evolved from an investigational procedure to a well-established treatment for end-stage heart failure.
Each era of heart transplantation has resulted in unique progress
toward the goal of a durable allograft and recipient survival. The
technical aspects of the procedure and rudimentary processes for
allograft preservation by hypothermia and flushing with preservative fluid were established in the 1960s, most notably in the

laboratories of Drs. Norman Shumway and Richard Lower of
Stanford University in Palo Alto, California. These advances set
the stage for the first clinical heart transplantation, performed by
Dr. Christian Barnard at the Groote Schuur Hospital in Cape
Town, South Africa, on December 3, 1967. In these early times,
survival was largely limited by poor understanding of immune-
mediated allograft rejection and a lack of effective immunosuppressive regimens. The advent of calcineurin inhibitors (CNIs) in
the early 1980s and ability to limit long-term high-dose steroids

enabled incremental improvement in survival, and heart transplantation became a well-established and highly effective therapy for end-stage heart failure.

Over the past two decades, there has been additional advancement in peritransplant recipient care, donor selection, and allograft preservation, which have collectively led to the continued growth of the field with improved outcomes. The rise of effective temporary and durable circulatory support devices has complemented the growth of heart transplantation and provided new means to bridge patients with advanced heart failure to heart transplantation. Additionally, current durable left ventricular assist device (LVAD) therapy achieves an average survival of greater than 6 years, enabling long-term, out-of-hospital bridging and, in some cases, an alternative therapy for patients with advanced heart failure when transplantation cannot be offered. Over the past 5 years, there have been marked advancements in allograft preservation technology and strategies. These advances include using hearts from donation after circulatory death (DCD) donors, which represents a new frontier in heart transplantation. Novel preservation techniques, including modification of donor storage temperature, perfusion-based devices, and strategies to evaluate the allograft during storage, also represent significant recent advances that appear to limit the incidence of primary graft dysfunction (PGD).

In this chapter, the current state of heart transplantation is presented, but the limitations are also described; future goals include being able to safely prolong ischemic time, immunologic tolerance off immunosuppression medication, elimination of long-term complications such as cardiac allograft vasculopathy (CAV), more effective use of the potential donor pool, and optimally integrating heart transplantation within the ever-improving landscape of mechanical circulatory support (MCS) technology.

HISTORY OF HEART TRANSPLANTATION

Early Investigations and the First Heart Transplants

It was not long after some of the earliest technical work in kidney transplantation that early pioneers in cardiothoracic surgery began to develop techniques for heart transplantation. It is worth noting the contributions of Alexis Carrel, often cited as the person who successfully established the technique for vascular anastomosis, and Charles Guthrie at the University of Chicago, who in collaboration may be credited with the first animal heterotopic heart transplantation in 1905.[1] In these experiments, the donor heart was implanted into the necks of the recipient animal with anastomotic connections made between the donor heart and the internal jugular vein and carotid artery of the recipient animal. The anastomotic configuration in these experiments was such that physiologic perfusion of the implanted heart was not achieved. However, there was sufficient coronary reperfusion for the implanted hearts to regain a brief period of myocardial activity. Perhaps most notable in these experiments, Carrel and Guthrie demonstrated that the transplanted heart could regain activity after a sustained period of ischemia and that anastomotic connection of the heart was technically feasible. In part for this work, Carrel was awarded the Nobel Prize in Medicine and Physiology in 1912.

Roughly three decades later, in the early 1930s Mann and colleagues built on the pioneering work of Carrell and Guthrie; in a dog model, they transplanted a heart into the neck of a recipient animal, connecting the internal carotid artery to the donor aorta and the donor pulmonary artery (PA) to the internal jugular vein of the

recipient while tying off the donor vena cavae and pulmonary veins. Hence, in this model, Mann provided physiologic perfusion to the donor heart and reported organized myocardial electromechanical activity for as many as 8 days after implantation.[1]

The work of Vladimir Demikhov at the M.V. Lomonosov Moscow State University is especially notable. From the mid-1940s to 1950s, Demikhov performed truly innovative transplantation procedures in dogs, which were remarkably achieved before the advent of the heart-lung machine or even rudimentary methods in myocardial protection. Retrospectively, Demikhov was likely the first in the world to make numerous technical achievements in heart transplantation, including (1) the first experiment in which a heterotopically transplanted intrathoracic heart supported the recipient circulation, (2) orthotopic heart-lung transplantation, and (3) isolated orthotopic heart transplantation inclusive of the development of the left atrial cuff anastomotic connection (as opposed to isolated pulmonary vein anastomosis). However, given Demikhov's isolation in post–World War II Russia, his work was unknown to the Western world until the early 1960s, and he was likely similarly unaware of the progress in the field in the Western world.[1]

Not long after Demikhov's experiments in Russia, pioneers in the Western world made gains to carry the field of heart transplantation forward.[1,2] The work of Marcus and colleagues at the University of Chicago in the early 1950s is notable for the use of cross-circulation support of a third dog for different heterotopic heart-lung and heterotopic heart transplantation models. In 1953, Neptune and colleagues used hypothermia preservation techniques to perform orthotopic heart-lung transplantation in dogs, in which the animals survived for up to several hours after transplantation, demonstrating to the world for the first time that a transplanted heart could fully support the recipient circulation. Webb and colleagues at the University of Mississippi described the use of a pump oxygenator (nascent heart-lung machine) to support the recipient animal in the process of orthotopic heart-lung transplantation (1957) and later in isolated orthotopic heart transplantation (1959). Also in 1959, Goldberg and colleagues at the University of Maryland reported successful orthotopic heart transplantation in a dog model. In their implantation, a left atrial cuff anastomosis was used as opposed to individual pulmonary venous anastomosis, vastly simplifying the technique. Later that year, Cass and colleagues at the Guy's Hospital in London, England, also reported an orthotopic heart transplantation model using a left atrial cuff anastomosis as Goldberg had, along with a right atrial cuff anastomosis. The so-called *biatrial anastomosis technique* reported by Cass was the foundational technique used clinically for several decades, although now it has largely been superseded by the bicaval technique.

Therefore, by the early 1960s, the groundwork underlying the technical aspects of orthotopic heart transplant had largely been established. However, refinement in allograft preservation techniques, the ability to control the immune system, and establishment of a process for identifying and managing potential donors and recipients was still needed before heart transplantation might become a clinical reality. In 1960, Dr. Norman Shumway, newly appointed chief of cardiac surgery at Stanford Hospital, and Dr. Richard Lower, a surgical resident, would perform the pivotal work that would catapult heart transplantation from an experimental procedure into a viable therapy (Fig. 57.1). Through the early 1960s Shumway and Lower refined the surgical techniques of orthotopic heart transplantation as well as early methods in allograft preservation with infusion of hypothermic saline and

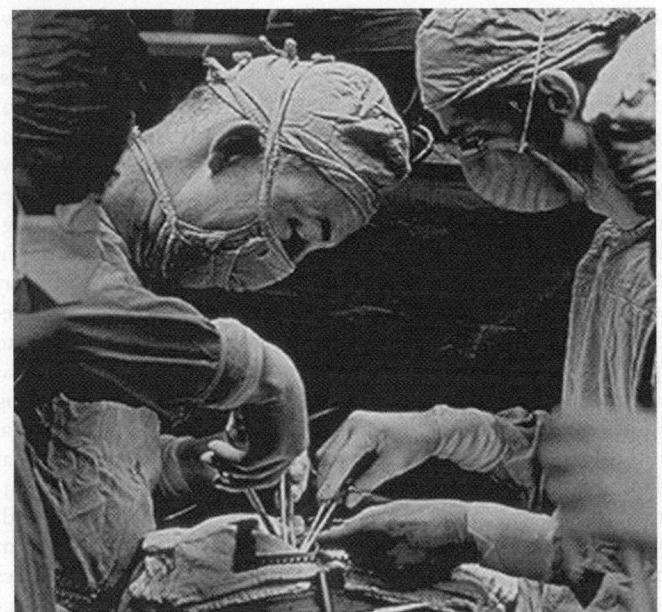

FIGURE 57.1 Dr. Norman Shumway performing Stanford's first clinical heart transplant on January 8, 1968, assisted by Dr. Edward Stinson. (From Baumgartner WA, Reitz BA, Gott VL, et al. Norman E. Shumway, MD, PhD: visionary, innovator, humorist. *J Thorac Cardiovasc Surg.* 2009;137[2]:269-277.)

storage at 4°C before implantation. They offered the first report of "longer-term" recipient canine survival for a period of up to 8 days in 1961.[1,3]

Indeed, through the early and mid-1960s, with growing experience in the Shumway and competitor laboratories, there was increasing confidence that human heart transplantation might be feasible and was nearing readiness for clinical application. One of the major challenges facing the field related to the ethical considerations around organ donation. The concept of neurologic death had not been defined, and unlike the kidney where one kidney could be removed from the donor without necessitating the donor's death, heart donation before the donor's death might be considered tantamount to murder. These concerns coupled with the technical capability to perform orthotopic heart transplantation contributed to the decision of Dr. James Hardy and his team at the University of Mississippi to move forward with what can be considered the first attempt at clinical transplantation in humans using a chimpanzee xenograft in 1964.[1,4] Along with Dr. Webb, Hardy and the Mississippi group had obtained considerable expertise in the laboratory using animal transplantation models and were contemporary leaders in the field along with the Shumway Stanford group. In his fascinating 1964 manuscript published in *Journal of the American Medical Association,* Hardy describes the management of a patient in cardiogenic shock after a myocardial infarction who faced imminent death, in whom the decision had been made to go forward with the first-ever attempt at human heart transplantation.[4] Hardy had hoped to use a human donor who had what was believed to be an unrecoverable neurologic injury. However, there had not been established agreement on the ethical basis to withdrawal life support for the purpose of organ donation. The putative donor did not expire in time for the decompensating recipient. As a backup option, Hardy and the Mississippi group instead used a xenograft procured from a chimpanzee and implanted this into the recipient. After implantation, the recipient was weaned from cardiopulmonary bypass (CPB) and

survived for approximately 1 hour supported by the chimpanzee allograft before the graft failed.

Although ill-fated and likely premature, Hardy's first attempt at clinical transplantation was emblematic of the fact that the field had progressed to the point where technical feasibility was no longer a barrier. As Hardy alluded in his manuscript, ethical considerations relating to human organ donation and how the process of organ donation was to be carried out were major challenges to confront. Recognizing the benefits of organ preservation that would come with heart donation from a "beating heart" donor led Shumway to become an advocate for establishment of death by neurologic criteria. At the time, no such neurologic criteria for death had been established, and it was certainly not codified into American law.[3] Although the field of transplantation along with advancement of mechanical ventilatory and other life support forced the medical and ethics community to grapple with the concept of a neurologic basis for death, the lack of accepted criteria for neurologic death in the medical community likely factored into some delay in Shumway moving forward with clinical transplantation.

The world changed on December 3, 1967, when Dr. Christian Barnard performed the first human-to-human heart transplantation at the Groote Schuur Hospital in Cape Town, South Africa (Fig. 57.2).[5] The recipient was Louis Washkansky, a 53-year-old male suffering from advanced ischemic cardiomyopathy. The donor was a 25-year-old female, Denise Darvall, who had suffered a severe neurologic injury after being struck by a motor vehicle. In this case, mechanical ventilatory support was withdrawn from the donor, and she was allowed to progress to cardiac arrest, with death being confirmed by the state's medical examiner, before Barnard rapidly placed the donor on CPB and resuscitated and cooled the donor heart before explanation. Washkansky was prepared for implantation in the adjacent operating room. The procedure was a technical success. The patient successfully was

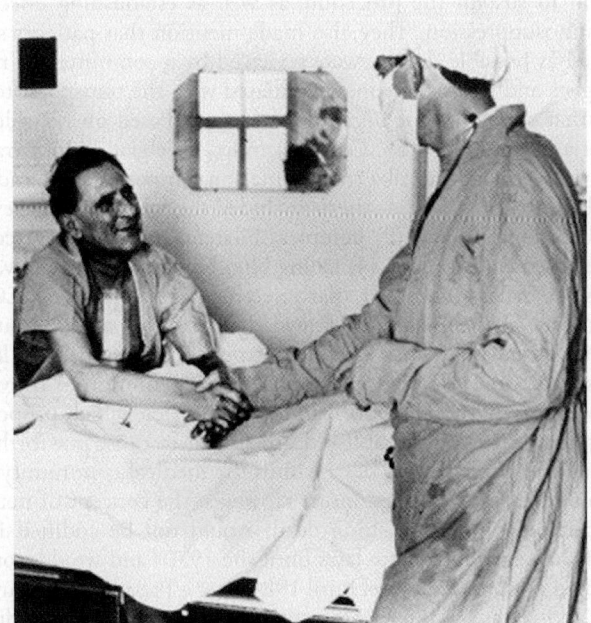

FIGURE 57.2 Dr. Christian Barnard and recipient Louis Washkansky a few days after the world's first human-to-human heart transplant, which was performed on December 3, 1967. (From Cooper DK. Christiaan Barnard and his contributions to heart transplantation. *J Heart Lung Transplant.* 2001;20[6]:599-610.)

weaned from CPB, extubated, and survived for 18 days before developing and succumbing to pneumonia.

Three days after the Barnard transplant, Dr. Adrian Kantrowitz and his team at Maimonides Medical Center in Brooklyn, New York, performed the world's second heart transplant. They performed transplantation on a 3-week-old neonate with tricuspid atresia using an anencephalic infant donor.[1] Kantrowitz and the Maimonides team had performed extensive work in the transplantation of juvenile dogs, positing the advantages of transplantation in organisms with immature immune systems. In this case, the implantation was performed under hypothermic circulatory arrest. Although technically successfully, the infant succumbed 6 hours after the procedure from severe metabolic and respiratory acidosis.

The world's third heart transplant was also performed by Barnard in Cape Town on January 2, 1968. Remarkably, the recipient, Philip Blaiberg, would go on to live for 19 months in what can be considered the first heart transplant with longer-term success. As with his first transplant, Barnard had used an immunosuppression cocktail of azathioprine and corticosteroids as developed by Calne and Starzl.[6] Additionally, he had administered an antilymphocyte serum after implantation in what may be considered the first use of an induction immunosuppression strategy in heart transplantation.[5] On autopsy, Blaiberg's transplanted heart demonstrated widespread coronary atherosclerosis, which would later be appreciated to be the consequence of chronic rejection known as *cardiac allograft vasculopathy*.

Shumway and the Stanford group performed the fourth heart transplantation on January 8, 1968. The patient lived for 15 days before succumbing to sepsis resulting from multiple abdominal complications. Shortly after this, Shumway published a manuscript describing the Stanford experience with their first two clinical transplantations.[7] In the report, Shumway and colleagues espoused the technical feasibility of heart transplantation but also highlighted the challenges facing them at the time, including identifying appropriate recipients for transplantation that are not too ill to sustain the procedure as well as establishing effective immunosuppression. They also made mention that patients submitted as possible donors were reviewed by a committee of neurologists and neurosurgeons unaffiliated with the transplant team and that suitability for organ donation was based on neurologic criteria elaborated by Dr. Guy Alexandre, a Belgian kidney transplant surgeon, at the Ciba transplantation symposium in London, England in 1966. These criteria included the following: (1) severe cerebrocranial injury, (2) complete bilateral mydriasis, (3) complete absence of reflexes, (4) failing blood pressure requiring vasopressive drugs, and (5) flat electroencephalogram (EEG).[8] Shumway himself would acknowledge that the use of beating heart donors in the early clinical experience was without legal basis.[3] Late in 1967, the publication of "A Definition of Irreversible Coma" by the Harvard Ad Hoc committee, which proposed neurologic criteria to establish death similar to those put forth by Alexandre, offered some basis within the medical community for the use of beating heart donors. However, the concept of neurologic criteria for establishing death would not be codified into California and other state laws until the 1970s and would not be codified at the federal level until 1981 after a President's Commission and release of the report entitled "Defining Death: Medical, Legal, and Ethical Issues in the Determination of Death."[9]

From the First Heart Transplants to Modern Practice

The earliest clinical heart transplants stirred a great deal of fervor around the world. Roughly 100 heart transplants were performed around the world in the year after Barnard's first transplant. However, early results were dismal. By the early 1970s, 1-year survival after transplant was no greater than 20%, and this caused most centers to discontinue their efforts in heart transplantation altogether. In fact, given these poor results with early clinical transplantation, through the 1970s and into the early 1980s only a few centers around the world, including Shumway at Stanford; Lower in Richmond, Virginia; Barnard in South Africa; Dr. Terence English at Papworth Hospital in Cambridge; and Dr. Chris Cabrol in Paris, continued clinical programs.[3] During this period, Shumway and the group at Stanford recognized that episodes of immune rejection were a major hindrance to longer-term survival and came to appreciate that rejection may occur at some level without obvious acute clinical manifestation. In 1973, Dr. Philip Caves, a visiting cardiac surgery fellow in the Shumway laboratory, was instrumental in the development and use of transvenous bioptome, a device that allowed for sampling of small portions of tissue from the right ventricle (RV) using a percutaneous approach. In collaboration with pathologist Dr. Margaret Billingham, analysis of such samples from experimental animal transplant models as well as clinical samples established the pathologic findings associated with immune rejection in heart transplantation and, importantly, provided means of grading the severity of rejection as well as the ability to detect subclinical rejection.[10] Integration of surveillance biopsies into the heart transplantation protocols helped elucidate the onset of rejection, enabling the titration of immunosuppression medications in response to subclinical rejection. Surveillance biopsies remain a crucial component of routine posttransplant care to this day.

Even with established expertise in surgical technique and improved understanding and recognition of rejection, longer-term outcomes for heart transplantation did not really take off until the advent of cyclosporin. Recognizing the importance of the work of Calne and Starzl, in 1980, Shumway and the Stanford group added cyclosporine to their immunosuppression regimen. Five years later, they reported dramatically improved outcomes, demonstrating 1-, 2-, and 3-year survivals of 83%, 75%, and 70%, respectively.[1] With this, there was rebirth in enthusiasm for heart transplantation in the United States and the world over, setting the stage for heart transplantation to emerge as a mainstream therapy for end-stage heart failure.

In the early 1980s as solid organ transplantation emerged as a viable and more widely used treatment strategy for organ failure, there was a need for consolidation and regulation of the practices surrounding organ transplantation. In the United States, Congress passed the National Transplant Act in 1984, which culminated in the formation of the Organ Procurement and Transplantation Network (OPTN), a national entity to ensure fair and equitable organ allocation. In 1986 the OPTN subsequently contracted with the nonprofit organization United Network of Organ Sharing (UNOS), which remains to this day the organization that oversees organ allocation and monitors performance of transplant centers. Other countries have formed their own processes and organizations for regulation of organ transplantation. Although practices in organ allocation are imperfect and subject to revision with the evolving field, consolidation has allowed more widespread and ideally more equitable opportunity for organ transplantation. In the United States, since the 1980s the number of heart transplantations performed annually has increased steadily to approximately 3500 at present. Over that same period survival outcomes have also steadily improved, and currently 1-year survival for transplantation recipients is approximately 90% and median survival is greater than 12 years.

HEART TRANSPLANT RECIPIENT SELECTION AND MANAGEMENT

Etiology, Pathophysiology, and Medical Management of Heart Failure

Worldwide, cardiovascular disease remains the leading cause of death, and its incidence continues to rise. Approximately 500,000 new cases of heart failure are diagnosed each year in the United States, with nearly 2 million new cases worldwide. Currently, over 22 million people in the world suffer from some degree of heart failure.

Heart failure is a complex clinical syndrome including a variety of symptoms, resulting from the heart being unable to maintain a normal circulation either at rest or with exertion. There are many different underlying etiologies for heart failure; for adult patients in developed countries, ischemic cardiomyopathy is most common, followed by idiopathic dilated cardiomyopathy, which typically afflicts a younger population. Other etiologies include valvular heart disease, viral myocarditis, congenital heart disease (CHD), restrictive myopathies including hypertrophic cardiomyopathy, and infiltrative conditions such as amyloidosis and sarcoidosis. Heart failure has been characterized by the American College of Cardiology (ACC) and American Heart Association (AHA) on a continuum of progressive stages (Fig. 57.3).[11] Those patients in the most advanced state of heart failure, or ACC/AHA stage D heart failure, represent patients whose heart failure is refractory to optimal guideline-directed medical therapy (GDMT) and whose condition is characterized by a high burden of symptoms that markedly limit daily life and recurrent hospitalizations. Such patients merit consideration for heart transplantation or MCS interventions.

For patients with advanced heart failure with systolic dysfunction, the heart and circulation initially attempt to compensate. The Frank-Starling mechanism provides an early compensation. Preload increases, resulting in increased ventricular end-diastolic pressure and volume; resting stroke volume and cardiac output are then temporarily maintained despite a decrease in ejection fraction (EF). However, increased diastolic pressures in the heart result in increased pulmonary or peripheral venous pressures and edema. Another component of the compensation is increased sympathetic nervous system stimulation and the release of the catecholamines (epinephrine and norepinephrine). This results in increased heart rate, contractility, and vasoconstriction. Other neurohormones are also activated, including the renin-angiotensin-aldosterone system and the release of vasopressin, which will cause further vasoconstriction, increased mean arterial pressure (MAP), and fluid retention. The release of these neurohormones can ultimately lead to changes in the structure and function of the heart, known as *ventricular remodeling*. Although helpful initially, remodeling eventually becomes detrimental as it leads to increased left ventricular (LV) wall tension, fibrosis, and further reduction of contractility. Oral heart failure medications attempt to modulate these compensatory mechanisms, which become deleterious but are more effective in patients with earlier stages (e.g., stage C) of heart failure.

Before patients with chronic heart failure are referred for heart transplantation or MCS therapies, they are treated medically with a combination of lifestyle modification and GDMT. In terms of lifestyle modification, patients should be encouraged to lose excess weight, remain active, and abstain from alcohol, tobacco, and illegal drugs. Their comorbid conditions, such as diabetes mellitus and hypertension, should also be treated and optimized. GDMT includes many medications that have been shown to help counteract the deleterious effects of the compensatory mechanisms that are activated during heart failure. Currently, four evidence-based

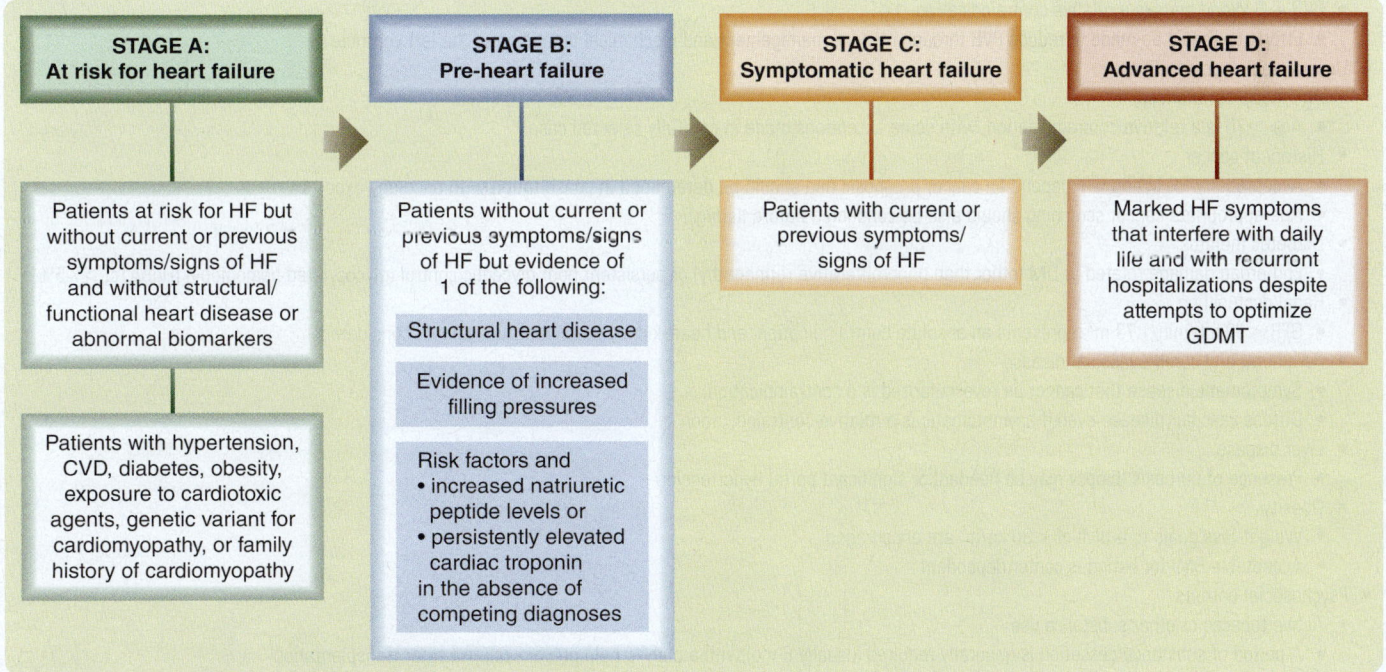

FIGURE 57.3 American College of Cardiology/American Heart Association stages of heart failure. *CVD,* Cardiovascular disease; *GDMT,* guideline-directed medical therapy; *HF,* heart failure. (From Heidenreich PA, Bozkurt B, Aguilar D, et al. 2022 AHA/ACC/HFSA guideline for the management of heart failure: a report of the American College of Cardiology/American Heart Association Joint Committee on Clinical Practice Guidelines. *J Am Coll Cardiol.* 2022;79[17]:e263-e421.)

therapies have been shown to improve outcomes in patients with reduced EF heart failure: renin-angiotensin-aldosterone inhibitors with or without a neprilysin inhibitor, β-adrenergic receptor blockers, mineralocorticoid-receptor antagonists (MRAs), and a sodium-glucose cotransporter-2 (SGLT2) inhibitor.[11]

Other medications, including hydralazine, nitrates, ivabradine, and vericiguat, have been shown to improve outcomes in certain subsets of patients with advanced heart failure. In addition, device therapies for heart failure include internal cardiac defibrillators and biventricular pacing systems, which have achieved reduced mortality and improved functionality, respectively, in select groups.[11] Percutaneous/transcatheter edge-to-edge repair (TEER) of secondary mitral insufficiency has also achieved clinical benefits in a randomized trial of patients with advanced heart failure.[11] However, these additional procedures should only be considered after patients have been optimized on GDMT. Notably, heart failure is generally a progressive disease, and patients may initially respond to GDMT or device therapy but later relapse with worse symptoms. When patients have failed GDMT and device therapy,

they should be evaluated for advanced therapies, which include durable LVADs and heart transplantation.[11]

Evaluation of the Potential Transplant Recipient: Indications and Contraindications

Potential candidates for heart transplantation should be evaluated by a multidisciplinary committee that includes cardiologists, cardiac transplant surgeons, social workers, care managers, psychiatrists, and advanced practice providers. Consideration for heart transplantation is reserved for patients who have ACC/AHA stage D heart failure or those whose condition is refractory to GDMT and other conventional forms of heart failure management. Even so, many patients with ACC/AHA stage D heart failure will have characteristics and comorbidities that may contraindicate transplantation in accordance with guidelines set out by the International Society for Heart and Lung Transplantation (ISHLT) (Table 57.1).[12] Ultimately, the decision of whether to proceed with heart transplantation should be individualized to the patient, with all the patient-specific factors carefully considered by the

---

TABLE 57.1   Indications and Contraindications to Heart Transplant Listing

Indications
- ACC/AHA Stage D HF
  - MCS dependence
  - Inotrope dependence
  - CPET with peak oxygen consumption ≤14 mL/kg/min if not on a β-blocker and ≤12 mL/kg/min if on a β-blocker (criteria may need to be altered in younger patients, obese patients, and those in whom maximal CPET could not be achieved)
  - Selective use of heart failure prognosis scores for ambulatory HF patients with ambiguous CPET results

Contraindications
- Elevated PVR
  - PVR >6 Wood units is an absolute contraindication (heart-lung transplantation should be considered)
  - PVR 4–6 Wood units is a relative contraindication
    - Efforts to should be made to reduce PVR through medical management and mechanical unloading of the left ventricle
- Unacceptable comorbidities
  - Age inappropriateness
    - Age >70 is a relative contraindication, with some exceptions made in carefully selected cases
  - History of cancer
    - Acceptability for listing will depend on cancer prognosis and should be determined in consultation with oncology experts
    - Age-appropriate cancer screening should also be conducted before listing
  - Diabetes mellitus
    - End-organ damage related to DM (other than nonproliferative retinopathy) or persistent poor glycemic control (glycosylated hemoglobin [HgbA1c] >7.5%)
  - Renal dysfunction
    - GFR <30 mL/min/1.73 m² represents an absolute contraindication, and heart-kidney transplantation should considered
  - Peripheral and cerebrovascular disease
    - Symptomatic disease that cannot be revascularized is a contraindication
    - Diffuse vascular disease even if asymptomatic is a relative contraindication
  - Liver disease
    - Presence of cirrhosis (biopsy may be needed) or significant portal hypertension
  - Obesity
    - Weight-loss goals to a BMI of <30 kg/m² are encouraged
    - Acceptable BMI for listing is center dependent
- Psychosocial barriers
  - Active tobacco or other substance use
    - A period of substance cessation is generally required (usually 6 mo) with a plan to help prevent relapse after transplantation
  - Inability or unwillingness to comply with medical therapy because of psychological/cognitive, social, or behavioral reasons

ACC, American College of Cardiology; *AHA,* American Heart Association; *BMI,* body mass index; *CPET,* cardiopulmonary exercise testing; *DM,* diabetes mellitus; *GFR,* glomerular filtration rate; *HF,* heart failure; *MCS,* mechanical circulatory support; *PVR,* pulmonary vascular resistance.
Adapted from Mehra MR, Canter CE, Hannan MM, et al. The 2016 International Society for Heart Lung Transplantation listing criteria for heart transplantation: a 10-year update. *J Heart Lung Transplant.* 2016;35(1):1-23.

multidisciplinary committee. Additionally, consideration for durable LVAD therapy often should be considered in parallel because many patients with stage D heart failure may also benefit from this therapy, and in some instances durable LVAD may be a preferable option to heart transplantation or be an appropriate modality to bridge a patient to heart transplantation.

Evaluating a patient with advanced heart failure includes history and physical examination, laboratory studies, and imaging. Relevant symptoms should be noted, including chest pain, edema, and dyspnea; symptom duration, prior treatments, severity, and disease progression should also be assessed. Medical history should also exclude any reversible causes for heart failure such as thyroid hormone disorders or alcohol abuse. The medical history should capture whether the patient has failed conventional oral heart failure medications and whether other, less invasive treatment options have been addressed such as chronic resynchronization therapy or treatment of functional mitral insufficiency. A physical examination, including evaluation of peripheral edema, jugular venous distention, detection of hepatomegaly, and ascites, along with heart auscultation for valvular abnormalities, is important. Auscultation of the lungs for wheezing or crackles can help provide information regarding a patient's fluid status.

In terms of laboratory studies, patients should undergo complete blood count, electrolyte measurement, renal and liver function, coagulation parameters, and brain natriuretic peptide. Significant electrolyte disturbances should be corrected. Significant renal or hepatic dysfunction should be assessed for reversibility, as severe irreversible kidney or liver disease is a contraindication for isolated heart transplantation. Patients may already have a left heart catheterization documenting coronary disease and heart function. However, a right heart catheterization is often necessary to measure pulmonary vascular resistance (PVR), which affects candidacy for heart transplantation. A PVR less than 4 Wood units is acceptable, 4 to 6 is borderline, and greater than 6 and irreversible is considered prohibitive. However, although initial PVR measurements are often elevated, they may respond to medical therapy or LV unloading with forms of MCS.

In some cases, cardiopulmonary exercise testing may be performed to further risk stratify a patient for risk of death and inform appropriate timing of transplant listing. For example, a VO$_2$ (oxygen uptake) max of <12 mL/kg/min while on a β-blocker, or <14 mL/kg/min while not, with a respiratory quotient >1.05, predicts poor transplant-free survival and supports need for listing. Patients who are more decompensated and require intravenous inotropes or MCS support do not require VO$_2$ max assessment.

Psychosocial screening and assessment of medical compliance is also typically part of the transplant evaluation process. This is important because long-term success in heart transplantation requires active participation of the recipient and their caregivers with frequent follow-up and high compliance with immunosuppression and other medication regimens. The inability or unwillingness to meet these requirements because of psychosocial factors, therefore, contraindicates heart transplantation because there can be no expectation for long-term benefit.

Age- and sex-appropriate cancer screening should be performed (e.g., colonoscopy, mammography, gynecologic/prostatic evaluation). Particularly for patients with ischemic cardiomyopathy, assessment for other atherosclerotic disease is important (e.g., carotid ultrasound and lower extremity noninvasive vascular studies). Potential recipients are also screened for anti–human leukocyte antigen (HLA) antibodies, which are more prevalent in females who have been pregnant and those with other allogenic exposures,

such as transfusions administered at the time of previous cardiac surgery, or prior transplant. Finally, computed tomography (CT) imaging of the chest is important, especially for those who have had prior intrathoracic surgery. Lastly, vaccination history and completion of routine vaccinations should proceed listing.

Recipient Bridging Strategies

There are several modalities to support recipients awaiting transplantation. As noted, the cornerstone of compensated heart failure optimization for patients with reduced EF is GDMT.[11] However, in patients with decompensated heart failure, additional circulatory support is needed to reverse the spiraling heart failure process.[13] The nature of the support required needs careful clinical and hemodynamic assessment and is dictated by the severity of the heart failure along with the relative contribution of right and left heart dysfunction. Most commonly, the first support strategy initiated is intravenous inotropic support. This can be safely done as an outpatient in appropriate cases and can progress from a single inotrope such as a β-adrenergic receptor agonist (dobutamine) or a cyclic adenosine monophosphate phosphodiesterase inhibitor (milrinone) to dual inotropic support. However, patients who remain in decompensated heart failure despite inotropic therapy may require MCS.

MCS can be classified as univentricular or biventricular and temporary or durable. Forms of left-sided temporary univentricular support include an intraaortic balloon pump (IABP) and an axial flow LVAD (Impella CP or 5.5).[13] Some physicians argue that these devices are, in effect, biventricular support, as decreasing the LV end-diastolic pressure results in less RV afterload and, thus, supports the RV as well. Forms of right-sided univentricular support include an axial flow RV assist device (Impella RP) and right-sided extracorporeal pump support with right atrial drainage and pulmonary arterial return. Right-sided extracorporeal support can be done percutaneously through the internal jugular or subclavian vein using specialized dual-lumen cannulas (e.g., Protek Duo or Spectrum). The ability to provide high level univentricular or biventricular support through peripherally inserted devices has been a major advance in the ability to bridge patients with end-stage heart failure to heart transplantation or durable MCS, which has occurred over the past 5 to 10 years. Historically, high-level temporary ventricular support required central implantation of cannulas connected to an extracorporeal circuit. Although this strategy is infrequently used in the current era, there are still selected situations where centrally cannulated extracorporeal ventricular assist devices (VADs) are rightfully employed to support a patient to transplant.

Temporary biventricular support can be accomplished with venoarterial extracorporeal membrane oxygenation (VA-ECMO) with drainage from the venous system and return to the arterial system. This is most commonly accomplished by peripheral cannulation through the common femoral vein and common femoral artery.[14] When cannulated in this fashion, placement of an antegrade perfusion catheter in the common femoral artery or superficial femoral artery distal to the arterial cannula is advisable to reduce the likelihood of lower limb ischemia. VA-ECMO in heart failure can also be complicated by ventricular distention caused by increased LV afterload accompanied with VA-ECMO coupled with poor native ventricular function. When LV distention with VA-ECMO occurs, it must be addressed to limit secondary myocardial injury and pulmonary edema. LV decompression in these circumstances is most commonly achieved with a peripherally inserted axial flow catheter-based LVAD (Impella CP or Impella 5.5). Other techniques, including atrial septostomy or direct LV venting, have also been described, but are not frequently used in adults in the contemporary era, given the effectiveness and relative ease of placement of the Impella devices. An alternative to VA-ECMO for temporary biventricular support is use of a univentricular device in the right and left ventricle separately, such as placement of an Impella RP or peripherally inserted dual-lumen cannula and Impella 5.5. Proponents of this strategy have advocated for ease of ambulating with this approach. Additionally, relative to VA-ECMO support, the temporary extracorporeal biventricular assist device (BiVAD) strategy also enables assessment of pulmonary function, which is essentially replaced with VA-ECMO. Outcomes for patients bridged from temporary MCS to transplant vary broadly based on patient acuity and amount of support required. The timing of MCS is also critical; failure to initiate support before after advanced end-organ dysfunction has occurred is associated with very poor outcomes.[15]

In patients who are not candidates for heart transplantation at the time of advanced heart failure, a bridge to transplant strategy can be accomplished with a durable VAD. Although most patients with heart failure have a component of biventricular heart failure, an isolated durable LVAD, with consideration for temporary RV support, is a commonly employed strategy. However, patients with severe biventricular failure may require durable biventricular support. This can be accomplished with placement of two durable VADs, such as the HeartMate 6 configuration, with two Heart-Mate 3 VADs placed in the right and left ventricle.[16] Other options for durable biventricular support include the SynCardia total artificial heart and devices under investigation such as the Bivacor total artificial heart.

Outcomes for patients with a durable LVAD undergoing transplant remain excellent with a 90% 1-year survival and 77% 5-year survival after transplant.[17] On the other hand, patients receiving a total artificial heart represent a particularly high-risk cohort with a waitlist mortality of nearly 10% and 1-year survival after transplant of 80%.[18,19]

DONOR SELECTION AND MANAGEMENT

Donation After Brain Death Versus Donation After Circulatory Death

Successful heart transplantation requires not only proper assessment and management of the recipient before and through the process of transplantation but also the proper selection and management of the organ donor as well as cardiac allograft preservation during the period from when the donor organ is explanted to when it is implanted in the recipient. As discussed, the dawn of the field of organ transplantation helped to catalyze the definition of death by neurologic criteria, which was codified into law in the United States in the 1970s and 1980s.[9] The criteria for neurologic death are met when there is an absence of brainstem reflexes, motor responses, or respiratory drive in a normothermic patient. There must also be a lack of potential interfering effects from metabolic derangements or neuroactive drugs. Although the field of heart transplantation has historically been based almost exclusively in the use of cardiac allograft donation after brain death (DBD), that has changed considerably over the past 5 years as advances in preservation strategies and techniques have made cardiac allograft DCD possible.[20] There is increasing use of DCD organs in heart transplantation in the United States and other countries, which has helped to expand the donor pool significantly.

The fundamental difference between DBD and DCD donors is that at the time of organ donation, DBD donors have been declared legally dead by neurologic criteria but still have a working cardiopulmonary system that provides gas exchange and circulation for end-organ perfusion. This allows for the organ procurement process to be carried out in a controlled fashion without any significant period of warm ischemia before the point where cold preservative solution is administered to the organs before explanation from the donor. This is in stark contrast to DCD, in which the potential organ donor does not meet criteria for neurologic death. In the DCD situation, life support is withdrawn, and there must be cessation of spontaneous circulation and other signs of life before the donor is then declared clinically dead. Generally, an additional interval of time (5 minutes most commonly) is required to ensure there is no recovery of circulation or other signs of life before the organ procurement process can begin. DCD, therefore, mandates a variable period of injurious warm ischemia to the donor organ. Accordingly, management of DBD versus DCD donors differs in important ways, as does the process of allograft preservation from these different types of donors.

Regardless of donor type, in the United States, the Federal Conditions of Participation of the Centers for Medicare and Medicaid Services mandates that hospitals notify their local organ-procurement organization (OPO) in a timely manner of an impending death. OPOs are regional nonprofit third-party organizations that operate under the supervision of OPTN/UNOS whose responsibilities include evaluating potential organ donors for organ donation suitability, approaching families regarding organ donation, participating in the care of the organ donor, and coordinating the process of organ allocation and procurement. Before declaration of brain death or in situations where the potential donor is not brain dead, the patient remains primarily under the care of the treating center and, with the family's consent, the OPO may assist and advise the treating center in obtaining certain bloodwork and other diagnostic studies, but decisions in care ultimately lie with the treating center. When the potential donor is declared brain dead, the OPO will assume the care of the donor and primarily direct additional evaluation.

General Principles in Heart Donor Assessment

Ultimately, the selection of an appropriate heart donor for a given recipient is highly individualized and requires detailed assessment of both donor and recipient factors. With respect to the donor, transthoracic echocardiography (TTE) is the cornerstone of heart assessment. TTE provides a detailed functional and morphologic assessment of the heart. Generally, hearts accepted should demonstrate normal RV and LV function as well as normal or near-normal valvular function. Mild reduction in LV function (EF >45%) may be acceptable in some circumstances. Importantly, it is not uncommon for the potential donor heart to have a period of depressed function after the inciting episode of cardiac arrest, brain death, or thoracic trauma. Often, this will improve within a period of days. So, it is prudent to serially repeat TTE assessments to monitor for improvement in ventricular function. In some instances, if visualization of the heart by TTE is inadequate, transesophageal echocardiography (TEE) can provide a clearer assessment. Echocardiographic assessment should be made with the potential donor off any inotropic infusions so that a sense of the true cardiac function can be obtained. Aside from ventricular function, other important information obtained by echocardiography should also be carefully considered. Any significant valvular pathology precludes organ use. The echocardiogram also measures ventricular hypertrophy; most centers will consider an LV wall thickness of up to 1.3 cm, although thresholds of what is acceptable vary by center as well as case-specific factors, most notably size of the donor. In general, it is appreciated that increasing ventricular hypertrophy is associated with increased difficulty in the process of allograft preservation as well as higher risk of early allograft dysfunction.[21]

Coronary angiography is another important diagnostic modality to consider in the evaluation of a potential donor. The presence of coronary artery disease in the donor can put the organ at risk of greater ischemic injury during allograft procurement and preservation and likely portends poorer long-term outcomes with respect to allograft vasculopathy. Given the increasing incidence of coronary disease with age, it is standard practice to obtain a coronary angiogram on any potential donor greater than 40 years of age. It is also routine practice to perform coronary angiography on potential donors greater than 30 years of age who have risk factors for coronary disease, such as diabetes mellitus, hypertension, smoking history, or history of methamphetamine or cocaine use.

Although perhaps not a standard part of the donor heart evaluation, most donors will have cross-sectional thoracic imaging by CT as part of their clinical care or transplant evaluation. This is important to review to assess for any anatomic variation or abnormalities and can be a useful tool to assist with donor-recipient size matching. Furthermore, in situations where there was significant chest trauma, it is important to review for the presence of sternal or rib fracture, presence of a pericardial effusion, or major thoracic vascular injury. Such findings portend a higher likelihood of myocardial contusion. This may influence the decision about whether to go forward with organ acceptance or at least heighten the concern to carefully assess for myocardial contusion at the time of organ procurement.

Apart from the diagnostic assessment of the donor heart, a detailed understanding of the potential donor's acute illness, cause of death, and past medical history should be obtained.[21] Important factors for consideration include the donor's age, size, cardiovascular-relevant comorbidities, infectivity profile, and substance use history. Many donors will have suffered a primary neurologic injury from either trauma or stroke, but increasingly, resulting in large part from the opioid overdose epidemic, donors may have suffered hypoxic brain injury after cardiac arrest. In situations where the putative donor experiences cardiac arrest and was later revived, it is important to understand the period of downtime and to gain confidence that the arrest was not of primary cardiac etiology (e.g., arrhythmia).

It is well appreciated that there is an inverse relationship between donor age and posttransplantation outcomes. Transplantation performed using relatively younger donor hearts is associated with improved early survival, presumably because of reduced rates of early allograft dysfunction. The reasons for this are complex and not fully delineated but likely relate to better resilience against ischemia as well as reduced levels of preexisting fibrosis, atherosclerosis, and valvular thickening in younger hearts. Although the optimal donor heart is a young heart, acceptable outcomes can be achieved across a wide spectrum of donor heart ages. Furthermore, the donor heart supply shortage along with the acute risk of a death that a patient with end-stage heart failure faces while on the waiting list necessitate that older donor hearts sometimes be considered. Most heart centers will consider hearts from donors up to 55 or 60 years old, but the majority of hearts transplanted are 40 years old or younger.

Relevant cardiovascular comorbidities include hypertension, diabetes mellitus, smoking, and substance use history. Patients with these comorbidities have higher rates of atherosclerosis and should undergo coronary angiography to rule out significant coronary disease. Selective use of donors with these comorbidities is appropriate provided that the echocardiogram and coronary angiography are reassuring. However, even in the absence of significant coronary disease, longstanding diabetes, hypertension, or smoking in the donor will often deter acceptance of the organ because of concern for the microvascular disease that accompanies these conditions, which may predispose to poorer posttransplant outcomes. Similarly, long-term substance use, particularly alcohol, cocaine, and methamphetamine, have well-established negative cardiovascular effects, and similar caution should be used before proceeding.

Infectious Considerations for Donor Heart Assessment

Given the critically ill state of potential donors, it is not uncommon for there to be some bacterial infection present at the time of donation. So long as this infection is localized and controlled with appropriate antimicrobial therapy, heart donation is usually not precluded. If there is bacteremia, there should be assurance of culture clearance after administration of pathogen-specific antimicrobial therapy as well as detailed valvular assessment by TEE to rule out endocarditis. Blood culture positivity for certain pathogens, including fungus and atypical or multidrug-resistant bacteria, generally preclude organ use. Other infectious conditions that preclude organ donation include meningitis and encephalitis as well as donors who test positive for syphilis, *Mycobacterium tuberculosis,* nontuberculosis mycobacteria, and some types of fungal infection including *Aspergillus* or *Cryptococcus*. In situations where there is a potentially concerning infection in the donor, it is appropriate to engage an infectious disease expert to provide guidance over the safety of donor organ use as well as posttransplant infectious management in the recipient if the organ is transplanted.

With regard to viral infectivity, OPTN/UNOS policy mandates screening of donors for hepatitis B/C, human immunodeficiency virus (HIV), cytomegalovirus (CMV), and Epstein-Barr virus (EBV) in addition to syphilis. Infection with human T-cell leukemia-lymphoma virus as well as systemic viral infections and prior related disease are contraindications to organ donation. HIV has historically been a contraindication to heart donation, but now with special designation some centers can perform transplantation of HIV-positive donors to HIV-positive recipients. Hepatitis C was also historically a contraindication to heart donation, but since the advent of effective antiviral therapies to eradicate hepatitis C, hearts from hepatitis C–positive donors are now routinely used. Recipients of these organs are treated with antiviral therapy after recovery from transplant, and there has been no apparent detriment in short- or long-term outcomes associated with these organs. Less commonly, hearts from hepatitis B–infected donors can be used, provided appropriate vaccination status and antiviral treatments are in place for the recipient. Use of hepatitis B and C hearts requires special consent from the recipient and engagement with infectious disease colleagues to ensure appropriate antiviral therapy. The emergence of COVID-19 over the past 5 years presented numerous challenges with the process of donor organ evaluation and transplantation. All potential donors are screened for COVID-19 infection. Early on, there was reluctance to consider heart donation from donors with COVID-19 infection, and there is possibility of myocardial involvement with this infection. However, there is growing experience with transplantation from donors with symptomatic and asymptomatic COVID-19 infection. Generally, reports on this matter have indicated that if the heart is otherwise a suitable organ for transplantation, it can be safely used without additional risk to the recipient.[22]

Immunologic Assessment: ABO Compatibility and Human Leukocyte Antigen Matching

In adult heart transplantation, ABO blood type matching is standard because of the well-described risk of hyperacute antibody-mediated rejection from preformed anti-ABO antibodies. Although ABO blood type–incompatible adult heart transplantation has occasionally been performed, sometimes intentionally, with specialized immunomodulatory regimens including the addition of rituximab and/or plasmapheresis, observed short-term outcomes in ABO-incompatible heart transplantation are markedly inferior compared with ABO-compatible heart transplantation.[23,24] Consequently, in current practice, ABO-compatible heart transplantation is the standard of care, and any intentional ABO-incompatible heart transplantation would be considered investigational and should be undertaken with a high level of caution.

Outside of blood type matching, the most significant cause of rejection is mismatch of HLA antibodies. In particular, a recipient with a high level of preformed or memory HLA antibodies to donor HLA antigens would be at high risk of acute and/or chronic rejection. However, even without significant preformed HLA antibodies, mismatch of donor-recipient HLA, in particular HLA-DR and HLA-DQ sub-types, has been associated with decreased long-term graft survival.

Mechanisms to manage preformed or memory HLA antibodies have been and continue to be developed and are termed *desensitization*. Desensitization techniques are based on the principle of eliminating preformed and memory HLA antibodies and preventing the development of new HLA antibodies. Drug-based approaches include monoclonal antibodies, such as rituximab, to eliminate memory B cells and chemotherapeutic agents, such as bortezomib, to eliminate plasma and antibody-producing cells. Plasmapheresis can also be used to remove circulating antibodies and replace recipient plasma with fresh plasma or albumin.

Size and Sex Matching

Size considerations between donor and recipient have a critical impact of survival after transplantation. Although many size-matching methods exist, including height, weight, and body surface area matching, determination of predicted heart mass (PHM) ratio has emerged as a validated and widely used method for donor-recipient sizing.[25,26] PHM is determined from a few simple variables including age, height, weight, and sex, which have been correlated to heart mass–based cardiac magnetic resonance imaging. Comparing donor to recipient PHM allows for a size ratio, with a PHM ratio of 1 considered optimal. It has been established that PHM ratio less than 0.85, suggesting a donor heart smaller than recipient, is associated with an increase in 1-year mortality.[26] PHM analyses have also suggested that significant oversizing is also associated with an increased 1-year mortality. Although the exact mechanisms of this are unknown, it may be that oversized donor hearts are anatomically restricted within the recipient's pericardial space.

Historically, used of hearts with a sex mismatch, in particular female donor to male recipient, was considered high risk. This is largely because of size considerations, with female hearts considered generally small for male recipients. However, in the setting of PHM ratio, the impact of sex mismatch remains unclear.[27] Still, sex-mismatch heart transplantation should be performed carefully, with consideration of donor transplant recipient risk factors including age, pulmonary hypertension, and other comorbidities.

Clinical Management of the Donor

For both potential DBD and DCD donors, the period leading up to organ donation is almost always associated with critical illness and commonly can be associated with hemodynamic instability, end-organ injury/dysfunction, and metabolic derangements. Therefore, to maximize the organ donation potential of a putative organ donor, fastidious critical care is required to optimize hemodynamics and volume resuscitation and to reverse any acute organ injury. In many ways, the principles of care for the potential donor are not different from those that guide the care of any critically ill patient. However, there are some special considerations for potential organ donors.

The neurologic injury associated with brain death, as well as severe neurologic injury short of brain death, adversely affects the cardiopulmonary system in a variety of ways. Early on, there can be a sympathetic surge as the body attempts to maintain cerebral perfusion. This is associated with systemic hypertension and increased myocardial strain, which can damage the heart.[28] Later, there is loss of sympathetic activation, which leads to vasodilation, low levels of circulating catecholamines, and reduced cardiac stimulation. These events can lead to depressed myocardial function, which can further be exacerbated by poor end-organ perfusion from hypotension related to intravascular volume depletion and vasoplegia. The care team must, therefore, actively work to achieve goal hemodynamic parameters geared toward supporting adequate end-organ perfusion. These include intravascular volume resuscitation to a goal central venous pressure (CVP) of 8 to 12 mm Hg and maintenance of systemic arterial pressure of >65 mm Hg, with the use of vasopressors as needed to counteract vasoplegia. Anemia should be corrected to a goal hemoglobin of 10 g/dL to help ensure adequate oxygen delivery. Maintenance of urine output of 1 mL/Kg/hour is a good marker of adequate end-organ perfusion, and frequent assessment of blood acid-base status and lactate levels is also helpful. In cases where there is associated renal injury, continuous renal replacement therapy may be required to help manage intravascular volume as well as serum electrolyte and acid-base balance. In instances where hemodynamic and resuscitation goals are not being met, it is appropriate to place a PA catheter to guide management.[28] Although the use of inotropes may be appropriate to support potential donors with a component of cardiogenic shock, the requirement for inotropes generally precludes consideration for heart use.

Aside from the importance of adequate volume resuscitation and hemodynamic optimization, hormone and electrolyte derangements are common among potential donors. There may frequently be dysfunction of the hypothalamic-pituitary-adrenal axis, and although there is not definitive evidence, it is probable that hormone replacement with thyroid hormone and vasopressin is appropriate in some donors for this reason. Additionally, when there are significant electrolyte abnormalities, particularly with sodium and potassium, these should be aggressively corrected.

CARDIAC ALLOGRAFT PRESERVATION

Donor Heart Procurement: Donation After Brain Death

Before the procurement procedure, the donor surgeon should review the echocardiogram, cardiac catheterization data (if obtained), inotropic or vasopressor drug dosages, blood typing, and brain death certification (or consent for withdrawal of care in DCD donors). It is also important to note if the lungs are being harvested, as this will affect the way the left atrium is divided. The subsequent steps include inspection, appropriate venting of the right and left heart, appropriate protective perfusate administration, and avoidance of heart distention.

Median sternotomy is performed in continuity with the midline laparotomy if there is simultaneous abdominal organ procurement. A pericardial cradle is created. LV and RV function are inspected. The aorta and left and right coronaries and branches are palpated to evaluate for presence of calcifications. These findings are conveyed to the recipient team. After the heart is accepted, the aorta and PA are dissected and isolated. The superior vena cava (SVC) and inferior vena cava (IVC) are circumferentially dissected. The Sondergaard groove may be dissected as well.

Once all teams are ready, IV heparin (400 U/kg) is administered, and a cardioplegia cannula is inserted through a purse string suture in the ascending aorta. The cold preservation flush lines are primed and connected to the cannula. The SVC may be ligated or clamped at the level of the innominate vein. The IVC is then divided above the diaphragm, venting the right heart. A cross-clamp is then applied to the ascending aorta, and the preservative is delivered into the aortic root. The left heart can then be vented through the left atrial appendage, the left atrial wall anterior to the left inferior pulmonary vein, or through Sondergaard groove. If the lungs are not being harvested, the pulmonary veins can be divided. Opening the pericardium into the pleural space helps drain blood and improve visualization. Cold slush is then placed on the heart. Care is taken to monitor aortic root pressure and avoid LV distention. If the LV distends, the infusion is stopped, and the heart can be manually compressed to alleviate distention. After completion of the preservation solution (1–2 L), the donor cardiectomy is performed. The remaining IVC is divided. The SVC is then divided high near the innominate vein, and the aorta is divided at the level of the aortic arch. The PA is divided either proximal or distal to its bifurcation depending on whether the lungs are being used. The heart is then elevated, providing appropriate visualization of the coronary sinus and the pulmonary veins at the pericardial reflection. In cases where the lungs are being procured, the left atrium is incised at the midpoint between the coronary sinus and pulmonary veins. Metzenbaum scissors are used to cut the left atrium, providing a minimum left atrial cuff on the heart of 1.5 cm while also allowing a left atrial cuff on the left and right pulmonary veins. When the lungs are not being procured, each pulmonary vein can be divided, and the entire left atrium is taken with the donor heart. Once donor cardiectomy is complete, a timely but complete inspection is performed. The heart should be inspected for patent foramen ovale (PFO), atrial or ventricular septal defects, valvular abnormalities, and appropriate cuff lengths. If there are any major concerns, these are immediately communicated to the implanting surgeon. Final preparation includes placement of the heart in an external ice packing box, the SherpaPak (Paragonix, Cambridge, MA), or ex vivo perfusion devices (Transmedics, Andover, MA) depending on storage and preservation strategy. The donor team will then transport the heart back to the recipient institution.

Communication between the donor and recipient teams is critical. The donor team should update the recipient team at each step of travel to and from the donor operating room. They should also keep the recipient team updated regarding anticipated cross-clamp and heparinization and when donor cardiectomy is complete and when the team is returning. Ideally, the recipient cardiectomy is completed as the donor heart team arrives at the recipient operating room.

Methods of Cardiac Allograft Preservation/Storage

Donor organ preservation is an area of active research, innovation, and discussion. The current standard of care for cardiac allograft storage for brain death donors remains storage in ice with a traditional cooler. Current ISHLT guidelines recommend storage in perfusate solution such that the ice does not directly touch the heart, with a temperature goal of 4°C. Although conventional ice storage has yielded what might be considered acceptable outcomes, significant shortcomings remain. For example, the rate of severe PGD requiring the use of MCS early posttransplant (to be reviewed in more depth later) consistently lies between 10% and 15% with ice storage. Moreover, most centers prefer not to extend the cold ischemic storage period beyond 4 hours, because of the associated increased risk of PGD beyond this point. This limits the geographic distance that a center may travel for a donor organ. Over the past decade, at least two novel strategies have emerged to enhance preservation and address some of these limitations.

First, studies have shown that severe hypothermia can lead to myocardial injury associated with the freeze-thaw process. Therefore, a device is commercially available that controls temperature at 4°C to 8°C during hypothermic static storage (SherpaPak, Paragonix Technology, Waltham, MA). Recent data from the Guardian registry have suggested less severe PGD when using the SherpaPak temperature-controlled system as compared with traditional ice storage.[29,30] Some case reports have also suggested that the period of cold ischemia using the SherpaPak may be extended beyond 4 hours with good results, although larger-scale studies are needed before this can be stated with certainty.

Second, a mobile ex vivo normothermic blood-based perfusion system (Organ Care System [OCS], Transmedics, Andover, MA) has recently been approved by the FDA for cardiac allograft preservation and storage for extended criteria brain death donors. For the Transmedics OCS, approximately 1 to 1.5 L of donor blood is obtained at the time of procurement. The blood is mixed with several additives, including thyroid hormone and epinephrine; this perfusate is circulated in a closed system with a pump oxygenator and is delivered into the aortic root and returned via the coronary sinus through a pulmonary arterial cannula. The left atrium is left open and vented. Coronary sinus flow is measured and is generally maintained between 600 and 900 cc/min, and MAP is maintained at 65 to 80 mm Hg, balancing myocardial oxygen consumption with myocardial edema. While the heart remains unloaded throughout the perfusion, it can be visually assessed for contractility. Moreover, arterial and venous lactate can be measured as an assessment of myocardial metabolism. A venous lactate lower than arterial lactate suggests metabolic activity and viability, whereas a venous lactate higher than arterial lactate suggests lactate production and potentially nonviability. Once the organ has been transported on the Transmedics OCS to the recipient site and the recipient team is ready for implantation of the donor heart, the donor heart is cooled and preservation solution is delivered down the aortic root to induce a diastolic arrest for implant. Although short-term clinical outcomes are not decidedly improved using the Transmedics OCS compared with cold static storage after brain-dead donation under standard risk conditions, it has proven utility for extended-criteria donors and particularly for cardiac allograft preservation in cases in which prolonged preservation is anticipated and has, therefore, helped expand the geographic distance that a center may travel for a donor organ.[31]

There is also a blood-based hypothermic (8°C) perfusion system now being evaluated in a clinical trial in the United States (XVIVO, Gothenburg, Sweden). Early data using this device in Australia have suggested it may reduce PGD in extended criteria brain-dead donors. Furthermore, the concept of ex vivo perfusion for more prolonged cardiac allograft preservation and interventions (e.g., small molecule administration and gene transfection) for organ conditioning remain an area of high research interest.

Considerations for Donation After Circulatory Death

As noted, the first clinical human heart transplantation performed by Dr. Christian Barnard in 1967 was technically done with a DCD allograft. However, with a few exceptions, DCD heart transplantation was largely abandoned because of concerns about ischemic injury in the withdrawal process and ethical concerns about reanimation of a donor heart. This has changed in the past decade as two strategies have emerged to allow resuscitation and evaluation of DCD hearts before using them for heart transplantation.

The first of these strategies is known as *direct preservation and perfusion (DPP)*. With DPP, after declaration of death and the specified waiting period, there is rapid entry into the mediastinum followed by administration of cold preservative down the aortic root and donor heart explantation. The heart is then placed on the Transmedics OCS for a period of normothermic ex vivo perfusion with reanimation. Evaluation of donor hearts using this system includes the ability to maintain lactate consumption as well as visual inspection of contractility, albeit limited to an unloaded heart. The first modern report of DCD heart transplantation was described by the St. Vincent's group in Australia in 2015. Using the Transmedics OCS, the St. Vincent's group reported three DCD heart transplants. Although two of the three had PGD requiring MCS, all were alive at follow-up ranging from 77 to 176 days.[32] Subsequently, a relatively large clinical trial conducted in the United States demonstrated comparable 6-month posttransplant survival between DCD hearts procured using DPP with the Transmedics OCS versus traditional DBD hearts.[20] The results from this study helped gain the Transmedics OCS FDA approval for the indication of DCD heart transplantation in 2022. This was a landmark development, as it established DCD heart transplantation using the Transmedics OCS as a standard-of-care option.

The second strategy that has emerged in recent years for DCD heart transplantation employs a resuscitation and assessment technique known as *normothermic regional perfusion (NRP)*. NRP involves rapid sternal entry with cannulation of the venous and arterial system and establishment of extracorporeal circulatory support after declaration of death and the specific waiting period. Abdominal NRP, via the femoral vein and artery, was initially adopted by abdominal transplant surgeons as a method to reestablish flow for optimization of abdominal organs on DCD procurement. However, thoracoabdominal (TA) NRP, involving cannulation of the right atrium and ascending aorta, was later established as a method to allow for thoracic and abdominal organ optimization, evaluation, and recovery. In all practices of NRP, cerebral blood flow is mechanically prevented before reestablishing in situ blood flow. With TA-NRP, this is performed with clamps to the head vessels. Although practices vary by institution, a PA vent or left atrial vent is often used to maintain ventricular decompression. Extracorporeal flow is maintained to achieve an indexed cardiac output above 2 L/min/m² and a MAP above 60 mm Hg. Theoretical benefits to NRP include a more physiologic reanimation, with hepatic and renal clearance of lactate, cytokines, and other potentially injurious chemokines. After a period of NRP support (usually 30–60 minutes), evaluation of donor hearts includes fully loading the heart and conducting visual, echocardiographic, and hemodynamic assessment. After assessment, and if accepted for transplantation, the heart is commonly preserved via standard cold preservation solution followed

by cold storage. Alternatively, the UK groups have reported used of NRP followed by normothermic machine perfusion for travel.

Outcomes associated with DCD heart transplantation when using the Transmedics OCS system have been evaluated prospectively, comparing outcomes associated with DCD hearts with standard brain death donors. Although there was more moderate or severe PGD (22% vs. 10%) in the DCD cohort, 6-month survival was similar: 94% in the DCD cohort and 90% in the DBD cohort, establishing noninferiority. Outcomes associated with NRP have been evaluated retrospectively. Of 100 TA-NRP cases performed at Vanderbilt University (unpublished data), the incidence of severe PGD was 10% with a 1-year survival of 93%. In total, early experience over the past decade has demonstrated both DPP and NRP to be viable strategies for DCD heart transplantation, with short-term outcomes comparable to traditional DBD heart transplantation achieved with both strategies. Consistent with this, over 500 DCD heart transplants have been performed over the past 5 years with volumes steadily increasing over that time frame.[33] Continued study into the longer-term outcomes for DCD heart recipients is warranted, as are continued refinement and organization of DCD organ procurement practices in order to optimize DCD organ use and outcomes.

SURGICAL TECHNIQUE

Recipient Operative Preparation

Before taking the recipient to the operating room, the patient's medical history should be thoroughly reviewed. Close attention should be paid to prior imaging, current MCS, and peripheral vascular access sites. Review of a prior chest CT is especially important in the setting of a redo sternotomy to minimize chance of injury to the heart and other vascular structures. Many transplant recipients will have had prior heart surgeries such as coronary artery bypass, surgery for congenital heart defects, or valvular surgery. Furthermore, there is an increasing population of patients who have had prior heart transplantation and require redo transplantation, usually for CAV. Finally, many recipients have had prior sternotomy or thoracotomy for placement of durable LVAD. For these redo situations, preoperative chest CT scans are paramount in planning reentry; reviewing not only axial views but also sagittal and coronal imaging and reconstructions may be helpful. From the history and the CT imaging, the surgeon decides whether institution of peripheral CPB should be done before the redo sternotomy. Multiple prior sternotomies and juxtaposition of vascular structures to the posterior sternal table would support a strategy for peripheral cannulation and CPB before redo sternotomy.

In the operating room, invasive monitoring is performed and includes radial arterial lines and central venous access. A Swan-Ganz catheter is also placed for evaluation of cardiac output, PA pressures, and mixed venous saturation. Some patients may also have an implanted automated internal defibrillator or permanent pacemaker. These devices should be reprogrammed, or a magnet is placed over the generator to convert to an asynchronous mode, compatible with electrocautery. The patient should be positioned supine with the arms tucked and with a shoulder roll.

The recipient is also treated with immunosuppression. Typically, 1 g of solumedrol is administered IV. Additionally, anti–lymphocyte antibody preparations may be given IV as induction immunosuppression (typically these are given intraoperatively but after CPB). After the transplant procedure, CNIs and antimetabolite agents such mycophenolate mofetil (MMF) and a steroid taper are administered orally as maintenance immunosuppression.

Orthotopic Heart Transplantation

Although heterotopic heart transplant has been described for patients with severely elevated PVR, this type of implant is infrequently performed. Modern strategies to address increased PVR include chronic mechanical LV unloading or combined heart-lung transplant for cases in which reversibility cannot be achieved. Orthotopic implants may use either a biatrial approach or a bicaval technique. As noted, Norman Shumway was instrumental in pioneering and refining the biatrial approach in which two pairs of atrial cuffs were sewn together: a left atrial cuff, which contains the confluence of the four pulmonary veins, and a right atrial cuff, which contains the confluence of the SVC and IVC. For the biatrial procedure, the donor heart is explanted by transecting the SVC and IVC, then the SVC is tied off and an incision is constructed from the IVC orifice superiorly to the right atrial appendage area. This opening is then sutured to the cuff of the recipient right atrium. The biatrial approach is less frequently applied and has given way to almost universal application of the bicaval technique. Relative to the biatrial approach, studies have concluded that the bicaval technique results in less sinus node dysfunction and need for permanent pacemaker and less atrial distortion manifesting as tricuspid insufficiency. Therefore, the remainder of the discussion regarding the implant procedure will focus on the orthotopic bicaval technique.

Considerations for the Recipient With Durable Left Ventricular Assist Device

Prior durable LVAD implantation poses unique challenges given the robust scarring induced by the LVAD. In addition, the outflow graft of the LVAD is an anterior mediastinal structure, which can be injured. Attention to a more lateral positioning of the outflow graft during the LVAD implant procedure may facilitate reentry for the transplant procedure. In addition, the use of thin Gore-Tex membrane (WL Gore and Associates, Newark, DEL) over the LVAD structures may reduce adhesions and facilitate the transplant procedure. Notably, the diaphragmatic pericardium, which is a common starting location for other types of redo dissection, is typically highly scarred with the outflow graft and, therefore, not the best starting point. The left lateral pericardium over the main PA and RV outflow tract is a better starting point for the dissection; from this point, the dissection can be conducted superiorly to the ascending aorta and inferiorly toward the apex and the LVAD pump. Some of this dissection usually can be done before CPB and is facilitated by using a Rultract retractor (Rultract, Cleveland, OH) for the left lateral exposure. Furthermore, a large portion of the outflow graft can be dissected free of adhesions before CPB. After CPB is initiated, the LVAD speed should be decreased, but the device should not be immediately turned off, as regurgitant volume with flow through the device can result in LV distention and lung injury. Once the entire LVAD is mobilized, the device is turned off and the outflow graft is clamped. The device is then removed from the LV apical attachment. In other situations, the LV apical area and the body of the LVAD pump can be densely adherent to various structures, including lung, pericardium, diaphragm, or chest wall. This dissection can be made easier by first removing the native heart, allowing for better exposure of the LVAD and LV apical area.

When peripheral cannulation is not required, CPB is typically initiated via aortic cannulation, and venous drainage is achieved via individual SVC and IVC cannulas. Circumferential dissection of the SVC and IVC with placement of umbilical tapes is necessary before the aorta is cross-clamped.

Recipient Heart Explantation

After aortic cross-clamp placement, the native heart explantation begins with a longitudinal incision along the right atrioventricular (AV) groove; this is carried superiorly onto the dome of the left atrium and inferiorly into the coronary sinus. This incision should remain very close to the AV groove, away from the IVC and, thus, avoid cutting into tissue that will serve as part of the IVC cuff. Once the right atrium has been opened, the left atrium is entered by an incision through the fossa ovalis. Next, the aorta and main PA are transected; care is used to retain most of the main PA (incising at the pulmonic valve) and a generous part of the ascending aorta (dividing at the sinotubular junction). Next, the left atrial incision is extended over the dome of the left atrium toward the base of the left atrial appendage. The left atrial incision is completed by continuing to divide along the course of the coronary sinus around the posterior leaflet of the mitral valve. After the native heart is removed, individual cuffs of the SVC and IVC are fashioned by extending the dissection of the intraatrial groove under the SVC and IVC, separating these structures from the underlying wall of the left atrium. Complete mobilization of the SVC and IVC cuffs back to the level of the umbilical tape is helpful. The SVC commonly contains old transvenous defibrillator or pacing leads, and these should be removed by careful dissection into the SVC; scar tissue around the leads should be mobilized up to the innominate vein; this should enable removal of residual lead material at the end, from the site of lead insertion (usually the subclavicular fossa where the leads have been inserted into the subclavian vein). The cuff of the left atrium can be further modified by excising the residual coronary sinus and removing the left atrial appendage. Previous use of clip devices in the recipient at the left atrial appendage can result in dense scarring, and it may be best to leave the old clip device as well as the obliterated left atrial appendage of the recipient. For the great vessels, initially maintaining additional length is advised, and excess vessel can be resected after sizing as the implant is performed. Placement of an LV vent through the right superior pulmonary vein into the left atrial cuff is recommended to remove blood volume that returns from the pulmonary veins (Fig. 57.4).[34]

Donor Heart Preparation

The donor heart is removed from storage and placed on ice. In the case of ex vivo warm perfusion storage, the heart is typically arrested on the perfusion device with Del Nido cardioplegia and removed from the device and placed on ice. If there are individual pulmonary veins, these are opened into a confluent left atrial cuff. The mitral valve is inspected. The interatrial septum is inspected from both the left and the right side; if there is a PFO, this can be closed primarily with a running Prolene suture. Next, the coronary sinus and tricuspid valve are inspected. The ascending aorta and main PA are separated with care to avoid coronary artery injury. The aortic and pulmonic valves should be inspected. Any material on any of the valves should be removed and sent for culture.

Heart Implantation

The first anastomosis is the left atrial cuff. This is started at the site of the left atrial appendage or left superior pulmonary vein. The donor heart is held or retracted toward the left side of the pericardium. Typically, a running 3-0 Prolene is used, and the initial

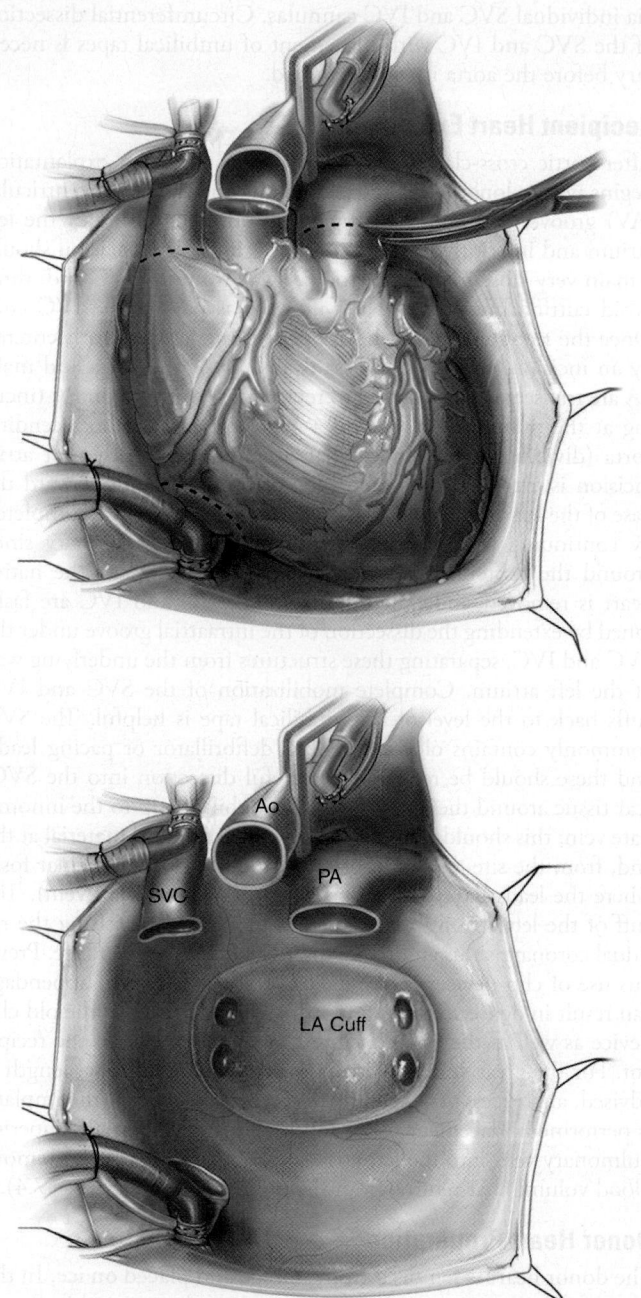

FIGURE 57.4 Recipient cardiectomy. Recipient cardiectomy is usually performed such that it is completed at the same time that the donor heart arrives in the operating room. The patient is placed on cardiopulmonary bypass; the aorta is cross-clamped, and the caval snares are tightened. The aorta and the pulmonary artery are separated, and the interatrial groove is developed. The great vessels are divided just distal to their respective valves. The superior vena cava is transected at the cavoatrial junction. A large cuff of inferior vena cava (IVC) is prepared by transecting the right atrium adjacent to the IVC (this incision is ideally made by carrying it medially through the ostium of the coronary sinus and laterally through the floor of the fossa ovalis). The left atrial cuff is prepared by entering the roof of the left atrium (this is facilitated by the development of the interatrial groove); this incision is extended to leave behind a generous cuff of posterior left atrial tissue, while observing the orifices of the four pulmonary veins. The left atrial appendage is also usually excised. *Ao,* Aorta; *LA,* left atrial; *PA,* pulmonary artery; *SVC,* superior vena cava. (From John R, Liao K. Orthotopic heart transplantation. *Oper Tech Thorac Cardiovasc Surg.* 2010;15[2]:138-146.)

direction of the anastomosis is from the left superior toward the left inferior pulmonary vein. The anastomosis is then continued toward the IVC or right inferior vein. Then, using the other limb of the running suture, the left atrial anastomosis is completed over the roof of the left atrium toward the right superior pulmonary vein.

After the left atrial anastomosis, there is variability in the order of the subsequent anastomoses. Some surgeons complete the aortic anastomosis next, enabling the remaining anastomoses to be completed after removal of the cross-clamp while the heart is reperfused. In certain cases, however, the posterior aspect of the PA and IVC anastomoses are poorly exposed after the aortic cross-clamp is removed. After completing the left atrial anastomosis, we typically perform the posterior wall of the IVC and PA anastomoses and then complete these after the aortic anastomosis and removal of the cross-clamp. Care must be taken to avoid redundancy in these anastomoses; in particular, the PA can kink leading to increased RV afterload. The SVC anastomosis is generally completed last; in some instances, the recipient SVC may be scarred from prior implantable cardiac defibrillator leads, and care must be used to prevent stenosis of the anastomosis; a locking running or interrupted technique may help prevent stenosis at the SVC anastomosis (Fig. 57.5).[34]

Considerations for Congenital Heart Defects

Transplantation of patients with congenital heart defects poses special challenges. In the case of a prior Fontan, the main PA is essentially absent. Furthermore, the SVC and IVC conduits need to be removed from the PAs. Once these are detached, the defects in the PAs need to be patched, typically with bovine pericardium or Gore-Tex membrane. Care must be taken to ensure each PA has adequate diameter. It is beneficial to have extra donor PA length, as the anastomosis to the neo–main PA may be more rightward than usual, or the donor PA may be used to augment either the right or left PA.

In the condition of transposition, the positions of the recipient aorta and PA are inversed. Additional length of the donor PA enables the anastomosis to be more rightward than usual. For these cases, a longer segment of donor aorta should also be acquired, enabling a more distal aortic anastomosis. With these measures, the positioning of the recipient great vessels can be accommodated.

Heart transplantation for individuals with situs inversus is challenging. A key requirement is that the IVC and SVC need to be extended from their native position, which is typically left of the midline to a position that is to the right of the midline. Prosthetic augmentation of the IVC and SVC can be accomplished with a Gore-Tex tube graft or vessels from the donor. Care is required to avoid kinking of these conduits. Furthermore, for these cases, the left pericardium should be removed down to the level of the phrenic nerve to generate space for the new heart.

ORGAN PROCUREMENT AND TRANSPORTATION NETWORK/UNITED NETWORK FOR ORGAN SHARING HEART ALLOCATION SYSTEM

Since its inception in 1984, OPTN has contracted with UNOS to oversee organ allocation and monitor transplant center performance. To date there have been three major iterations of OPTN/UNOS adult donor heart policy.[35] The most recent revision took effect in October 2018.[36] Before the adoption of the current

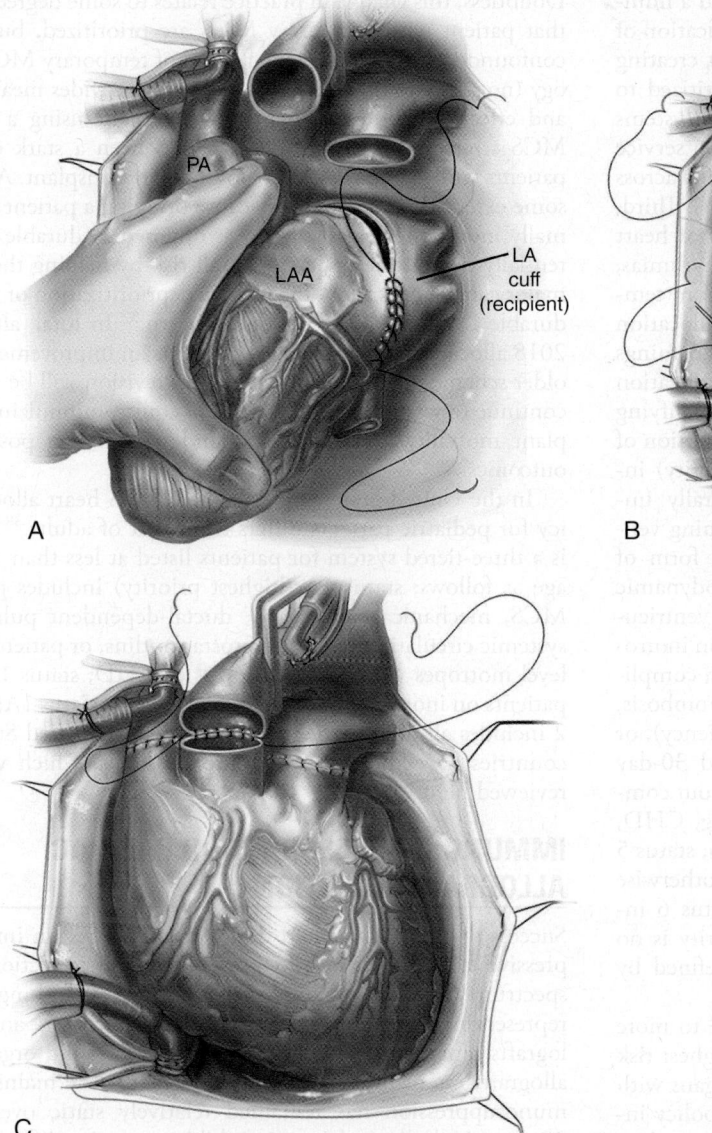
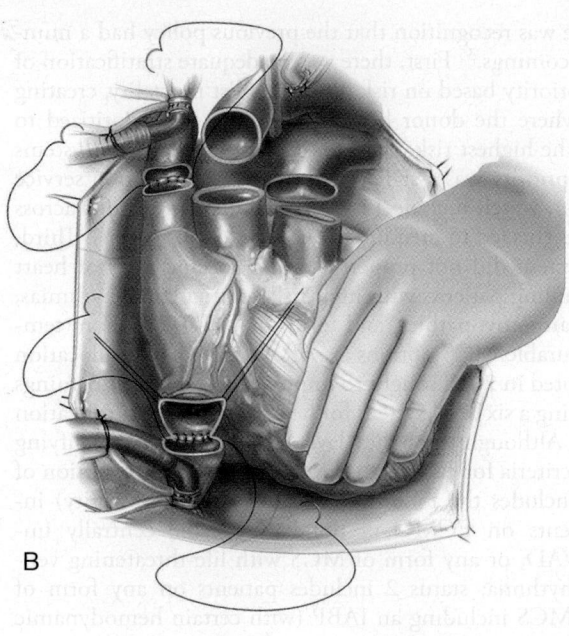

FIGURE 57.5 Orthotopic heart transplantation: Bicaval anastomosis technique. (A) Left atrial anastomosis. The left atrial anastomosis is always performed first by using a long 3-0 Prolene suture starting at the left atrial cuff adjacent to the left superior pulmonary vein and passing it through the donor left atrial cuff adjacent to the left atrial appendage. The initial few sutures are completed with the donor heart positioned at the level of the sternal edge, and the heart is subsequently lowered into the pericardial space. The posterior left atrial suture line is first completed and then subsequently the anterior suture line (as shown in the figure, this is facilitated by the assistant retracting the donor aorta and PA to provide adequate exposure of the left atrium). To minimize the risk of left atrial thrombus formation, an everting suture technique should be done to facilitate approximation of the smooth endocardial surfaces of donor and recipient left atrial tissue. A left ventricular vent can be passed through an opening between the two untied left atrial sutures that can help with deairing. During all the anastomosis, a cold saline-soaked laparotomy pad can be placed on the heart. In addition, continuous carbon dioxide is also run into the pericardial well. (B) Superior and inferior vena caval anastomosis. Next, the inferior and superior vena caval anastomoses are usually performed with 3-0 and 4-0 Prolene sutures, respectively. During performance of the inferior vena cava (IVC) anastomosis, care is taken to avoid deep sutures being placed in the region of the donor coronary sinus ostium to avoid potential injury. The donor right atrial appendage is medially oriented to facilitate proper orientation of the superior vena cava (SVC) anastomosis. This is important to avoid the SVC from being kinked or improperly aligned. Further, attention should be closely paid to avoid "purse-stringing" the SVC anastomosis to prevent inadvertent narrowing at the anastomotic level. (C) Pulmonary artery and aortic anastomosis. It is important to avoid excess length of the PA to avoid kinking at the level of the anastomosis. The median raphe on the PA may help orient the anastomosis, which is performed with 4-0 Prolene suture. Next, the aortic anastomosis is completed with 4-0 Prolene suture. If the recipient aortic tissue quality is suboptimal, a two-layer technique, with an inner layer of horizontal mattress suture and outer layer of running suture, can be performed to ensure adequate hemostasis. *LA*, left atrium; *LAA*, left atrial appendage; *PA*, pulmonary artery. (From John R, Liao K. Orthotopic heart transplantation. *Oper Tech Thorac Cardiovasc Surg.* 2010;15[2]:138-146.)

policy, there was recognition that the previous policy had a number of shortcomings.[35] First, there was inadequate stratification of allocation priority based on risk of waiting list mortality, creating situations where the donor hearts were often not prioritized to patients at the highest risk of death. Second, in the prior systems geographic priority was assigned with respect to donation service areas (DSAs), which include 11 arbitrarily defined regions across the country. This led to inequity in access to donor organs. Third, the prior system did not properly stratify specific sorts of heart failure, including patients with high-risk ventricular arrhythmias, restrictive cardiomyopathies, and forms of CHD, in whom temporary or durable MCS options are often limited. The allocation system adopted in 2018 sought to improve on these shortcomings by introducing a six-level system for heart allocation prioritization (Fig. 57.6). Although the policy lays out a number of qualifying details and criteria for each status level, a simplified description of each level includes the following: status 1 (highest priority) includes patients on ECMO, a nondischargeable centrally implanted BiVAD, or any form of MCS with life-threatening ventricular arrhythmia; status 2 includes patients on any form of temporary MCS including an IABP (with certain hemodynamic parameters met), total artificial heart, or life-threatening ventricular arrhythmias not on MCS; status 3 includes patients on inotropes with hemodynamic monitoring, durable LVAD with complications (e.g., device infection, hemolysis, pump thrombosis, severe right heart failure, bleeding, severe aortic insufficiency), or durable LVAD without complications for a designated 30-day period; status 4 includes patients on durable LVAD without complications, inotropes without hemodynamic monitoring, CHD, restrictive cardiomyopathy, or awaiting retransplantation; status 5 includes patients awaiting dual organ transplant not otherwise meeting criteria for higher allocation priority; and status 6 includes all other patients. Additionally, geographic priority is no longer based on DSA, but rather a series of zones defined by nautical distance from the donor organ.[36]

The primary goals of the new allocation policy were to more precisely prioritize organ allocation to the patients at highest risk of mortality and to provide more equitable access to organs with respect to geography. Criticisms of the new allocation policy included the fact that (1) status level designation is often dependent on treatment modality and this may not directly correlate to degree of heart failure or illness (e.g., discretionary decisions on how to support a patient with heart failure may influence a patient's status level, creating opportunity to "game" the system) and (2) expanding geographic access of donor organs would lead to increased distance traveled for donor organs, thereby increasing organ ischemic times, which may potentially affect outcomes.

Since the advent of the 2018 policy, there have been myriad publications examining its effects on transplant center activities and outcomes. Collectively, these studies have indicated that mortality on the waiting list has decreased, as have waiting times for organ transplant. Conversely, the average organ ischemic time has increased significantly (as much as 30 minutes) since the policy took effect, consistent with greater distance traveled for donor organs. Overall, posttransplant survival outcomes have remained stable in the pre- and post-2018 allocation policy eras. Therefore, it may be stated that the allocation policy change achieved the stated goals and has improved upon the prior policy.[37] Not surprisingly, since the adoption of the policy, there have been corresponding changes in transplant center behavior and perhaps the nature of management of advanced heart failure altogether. Centers are increasingly bridging patients to transplant with temporary MCS.

Doubtless, this change in practice relates to some degree to the fact that patient with temporary MCS are prioritized, but it is also confounded by the improving arsenal of temporary MCS technology (notably the Impella 5.5 device) that provides means to safely and effectively bridge patients to transplant using a temporary MCS strategy. Concurrently, there has been a stark decrease in patients with durable LVAD who undergo transplant. Although to some extent this is desirable because bridging a patient with minimally invasive temporary MCS as opposed to durable LVAD potentially decreases a patient's overall risk by helping them avoid a major cardiac operation, the relative deprioritization of patients on durable LVAD has caused some concern.[37] In total, although the 2018 allocation policy change represents an improvement over the older scheme, ongoing assessment and revision will be required to continue to work toward the ideals of equity, minimizing pretransplant mortality and morbidity, and maximizing posttransplant outcomes.

In the United States, the OPTN/UNOS heart allocation policy for pediatric patients differs from that of adults.[38] In brief, it is a three-tiered system for patients listed at less than 18 years of age as follows: status 1A (highest priority) includes patients on MCS, mechanical ventilation, ductal-dependent pulmonary or systemic circulation requiring prostaglandins, or patients on high-level inotropes with specified forms of CHD; status 1B includes patients on inotropes not meeting criteria for status 1A; and status 2 includes all other patients. Outside of the United States, other countries have their own allocation systems, which will not be reviewed here.

IMMUNOSUPPRESSION AND CARDIAC ALLOGRAFT REJECTION

Success of the transplanted donor heart hinges on immunosuppressive strategies aimed to prevent allograft rejection. On the spectrum of solid organ transplantation, with lung allografts representing the most immunogenic solid organ and liver allografts representing the least immunogenic solid organ, cardiac allografts are of moderate immunogenicity. The mainstay of immunosuppression has remained relatively static over the past 30 years, including calcineurin inhibition, antiproliferative agents, and corticosteroids.

Calcineurin Inhibitors

Tacrolimus and cyclosporine exert their effect on calcineurin through binding FK-binding protein and cyclophilin, respectively. This ultimately inhibits calcineurin, preventing transcriptional factor NFAT from producing interleukin (IL)-2 and other cytokines that lead to T-cell activation, proliferation, and differentiation.

Antiproliferative Agents

MMF, a cornerstone antiproliferative agent and cell-cycle inhibitor, operates through selective inhibition of inosine monophosphate dehydrogenase, a key enzyme in de novo purine synthesis.[39] MMF depletes guanosine nucleotides preferentially in T and B lymphocytes and inhibits their proliferation, thereby suppressing cell-mediated immune responses and antibody formation. MMF also has the secondary effects of preventing antigen-presenting cells, such as dendritic cells, from acting on T cells. Azathioprine, an older agent in this category, is a prodrug that is metabolized to 6-mercaptopurine, interfering with DNA synthesis and, thus, impeding lymphocyte proliferation.

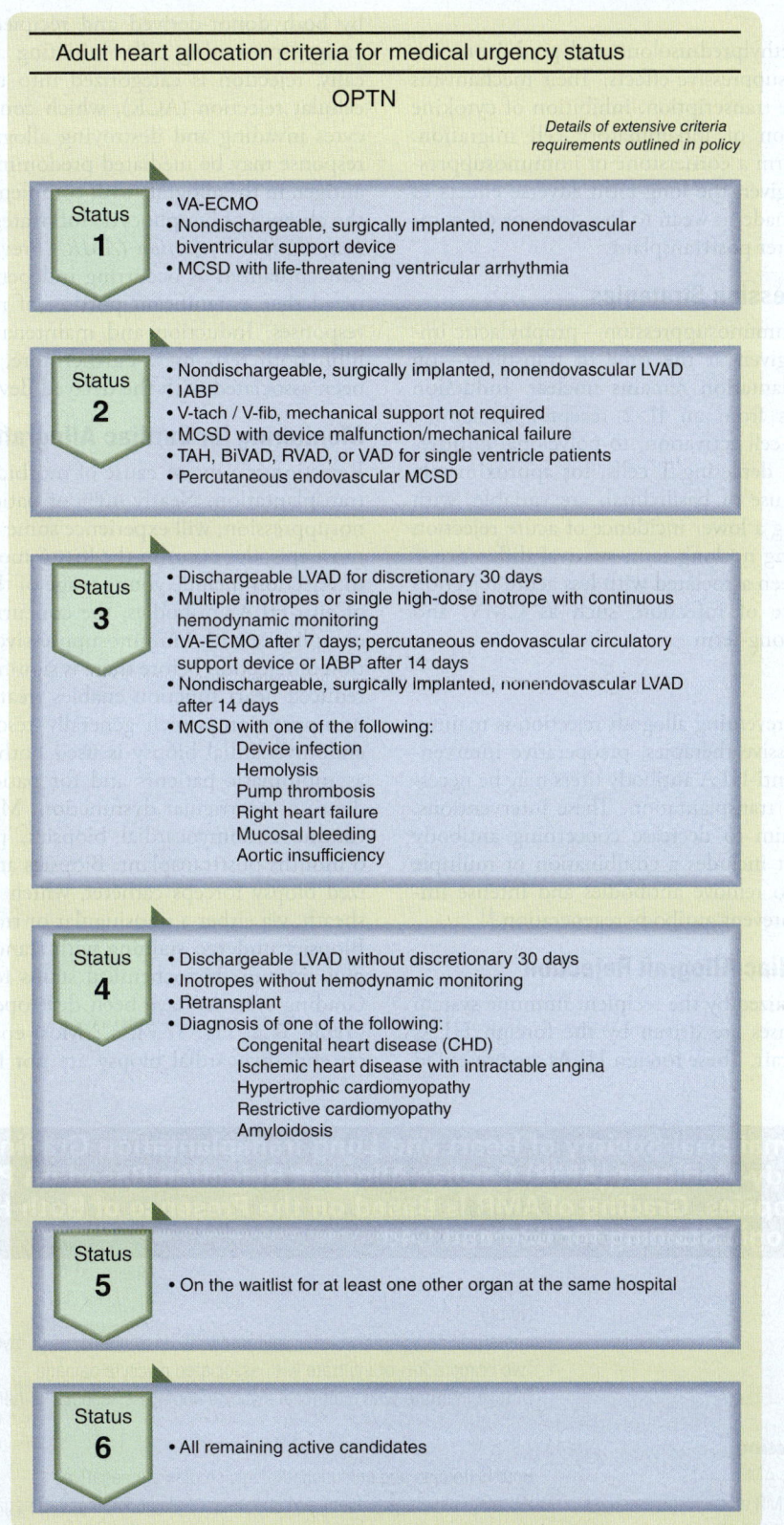

Adult heart allocation criteria for medical urgency status

OPTN

Details of extensive criteria requirements outlined in policy

Status 1
- VA-ECMO
- Nondischargeable, surgically implanted, nonendovascular biventricular support device
- MCSD with life-threatening ventricular arrhythmia

Status 2
- Nondischargeable, surgically implanted, nonendovascular LVAD
- IABP
- V-tach / V-fib, mechanical support not required
- MCSD with device malfunction/mechanical failure
- TAH, BiVAD, RVAD, or VAD for single ventricle patients
- Percutaneous endovascular MCSD

Status 3
- Dischargeable LVAD for discretionary 30 days
- Multiple inotropes or single high-dose inotrope with continuous hemodynamic monitoring
- VA-ECMO after 7 days; percutaneous endovascular circulatory support device or IABP after 14 days
- Nondischargeable, surgically implanted, nonendovascular LVAD after 14 days
- MCSD with one of the following:
  - Device infection
  - Hemolysis
  - Pump thrombosis
  - Right heart failure
  - Mucosal bleeding
  - Aortic insufficiency

Status 4
- Dischargeable LVAD without discretionary 30 days
- Inotropes without hemodynamic monitoring
- Retransplant
- Diagnosis of one of the following:
  - Congenital heart disease (CHD)
  - Ischemic heart disease with intractable angina
  - Hypertrophic cardiomyopathy
  - Restrictive cardiomyopathy
  - Amyloidosis

Status 5
- On the waitlist for at least one other organ at the same hospital

Status 6
- All remaining active candidates

FIGURE 57.6 Organ Procurement and Transplantation Network/United Network of Organ Sharing (OPTN/UNOS) criteria for medical urgency status infographic. This infographic provides an overview of the listing status for heart allocation priority for patients awaiting heart transplantation. Full details of this policy can be found on the OPTN website https://optn.transplant.hrsa.gov/professionals/by-organ/heart-lung/adult-heart-allocation/. *BiVAD,* Biventricular assist device; *IABP,* intraaortic balloon pump; *LVAD,* left ventricular assist device; *MCSD,* mechanical circulatory support device; *RVAD,* right ventricular assist device; *TAH,* total artificial heart; *V fib,* ventricular fibrillation; *V tach,* ventricular tachycardia; *VAD,* ventricular assist device; *VA-ECMO,* venoarterial extracorporeal membrane oxygenation.

Corticosteroids

Corticosteroids such as methylprednisolone and prednisone exhibit broad-based immunosuppressive effects. Their mechanisms include modulation of gene transcription, inhibition of cytokine production, and suppression of inflammatory cell migration. Although corticosteroids form a cornerstone of immunosuppression after transplantation, given the long-term adverse effects of corticosteroids, efforts are made to wean to low doses or off completely after the first year after posttransplant.

Induction Immunosuppression Strategies

The impact of induction immunosuppression—prophylactic immunosuppressive therapy given at the time of transplant—on survival after heart transplantation remains unclear. Induction immunosuppression ranges from an IL-2 receptor antagonist (basiliximab), mitigating T-cell activation, to polyclonal antithymocyte antibodies (ATGs), depleting T cells, for approximately 6 months. Results on the use of basiliximab are variable, with some authors demonstrating a lower incidence of acute rejection but multiple studies showing no long-term survival difference.[40] Induction with ATG has been associated with less acute rejection but an increased incidence of infection, such as CMV, and malignancy-related deaths long-term.

Desensitization

Although the mainstay of preventing allograft rejection is maintenance with immunosuppressive therapies, preoperative interventions in patients with high anti-HLA antibody titers may be necessary to safely proceed with transplantation. These interventions, known as *desensitization,* aim to decrease concerning antibody levels to a safe threshold. It includes a combination of multiple rounds of plasmapheresis to remove antibodies and intense immunosuppressive drugs to prevent antibody regeneration.[41]

Pathophysiology of Cardiac Allograft Rejection

Cardiac allografts are recognized by the recipient immune system as foreign. Immune responses are driven by the foreign HLAs present on cells of the allograft. These foreign HLAs are presented by both donor-derived and recipient dendritic cells and other antigen-presenting cells, initiating an immune response. Clinically, rejection is categorized into two types. The first is acute cellular rejection (ACR), which consists of activated T lymphocytes invading and destroying allograft tissue. Second, immune response may be mediated predominantly by antibody to foreign antigen in the allograft with complement activation, but largely in the absence of lymphocytic infiltrates; this process is termed *antibody-mediated rejection (AMR).* Previously, ACR and AMR were conceptualized as occurring independently, but it is now recognized that a significant portion of rejection cases involve mixed responses. Induction and maintenance immunosuppression inhibit both responses. Furthermore, both ACR and AMR have been associated with the delayed development of CAV.

Monitoring for Cardiac Allograft Rejection

Rejection is a major cause of morbidity and mortality after heart transplantation. Nearly 40% of patients, despite optimal immunosuppression, will experience some degree of ACR or AMR, and most episodes occur in the first 6 months. Factors that predispose to rejection include younger age of the recipient, the preexistence of anti-HLA antibodies, the concurrence of infection, and noncompliance with immunosuppressive medications. Early recognition of rejection before there is significant myocardial damage and reduced heart function enables treatment with increased immunosuppression, which generally resolves the process. Therefore, endomyocardial biopsy is used both on a protocolized basis for asymptomatic patients and for patients with symptoms or evidence of ventricular dysfunction. Most centers use protocols for routine endomyocardial biopsies, particularly during the first 6 months posttransplant. Biopsies are performed using a specialized biopsy forceps catheter, which is delivered through a small sheath, via either a transjugular or transfemoral venous approach. Biopsies undergo staining with standard hematoxylin and eosin, plus immune-histochemical stains for C3d and C4d for AMR. Grading systems have been developed for both ACR and AMR (Table 57.2, Fig. 57.7).[42,43] Most episodes of rejection identified on endomyocardial biopsy are not hemodynamically significant

---

TABLE 57.2   International Society of Heart and Lung Transplantation Grading System for Cellular and Antibody-Mediated (AMR) Cardiac Allograft Rejection Based on Pathology From Endomyocardial Biopsies. Grading of AMR Is Based on the Presence of Both Histologic Findings and Immunopathologic Staining for C3d and C4d

Cellular Rejection

Grade 0R	No rejection
Grade 1R, mild	Interstitial and/or perivascular infiltrate with up to one focus of myocyte damage
Grade 2R, moderate	Two or more foci of infiltrate with associated myocyte damage
Grade 3R, severe	Diffuse infiltrate with multifocal myocyte damage ± edema, ± hemorrhage, ± vasculitis

Antibody-Mediated Rejection

pAMR 0: negative for pathologic AMR	Both histologic and immunopathologic studies are negative
pAMR1 (H+): Histopathologic AMR alone	Histologic findings present and immunopathologic findings are negative
pAMR1 (I+): Immunopathologic AMR along	Histologic findings are negative and immunopathologic findings are present
pAMR2: Pathologic AMR	Both histologic and immunopathologic findings are present
pAMR3: Severe pathologic AMR	Severe AMR with histopathologic findings of interstitial hemorrhage, capillary fragmentation, mixed inflammatory infiltrates, endothelial cell pyknosis and/or karyorrhexis, and marked edema

Adapted from Colvin MM, Cook JL, Chang P, et al. Antibody-mediated rejection in cardiac transplantation: emerging knowledge in diagnosis and management: a scientific statement from the American Heart Association. *Circulation.* 2015;131(18):1608-1639; Stewart S, Winters GL, Fishbein MC, et al. Revision of the 1990 working formulation for the standardization of nomenclature in the diagnosis of heart rejection. *J Heart Lung Transplant.* 2005;24(11):1710-1720.

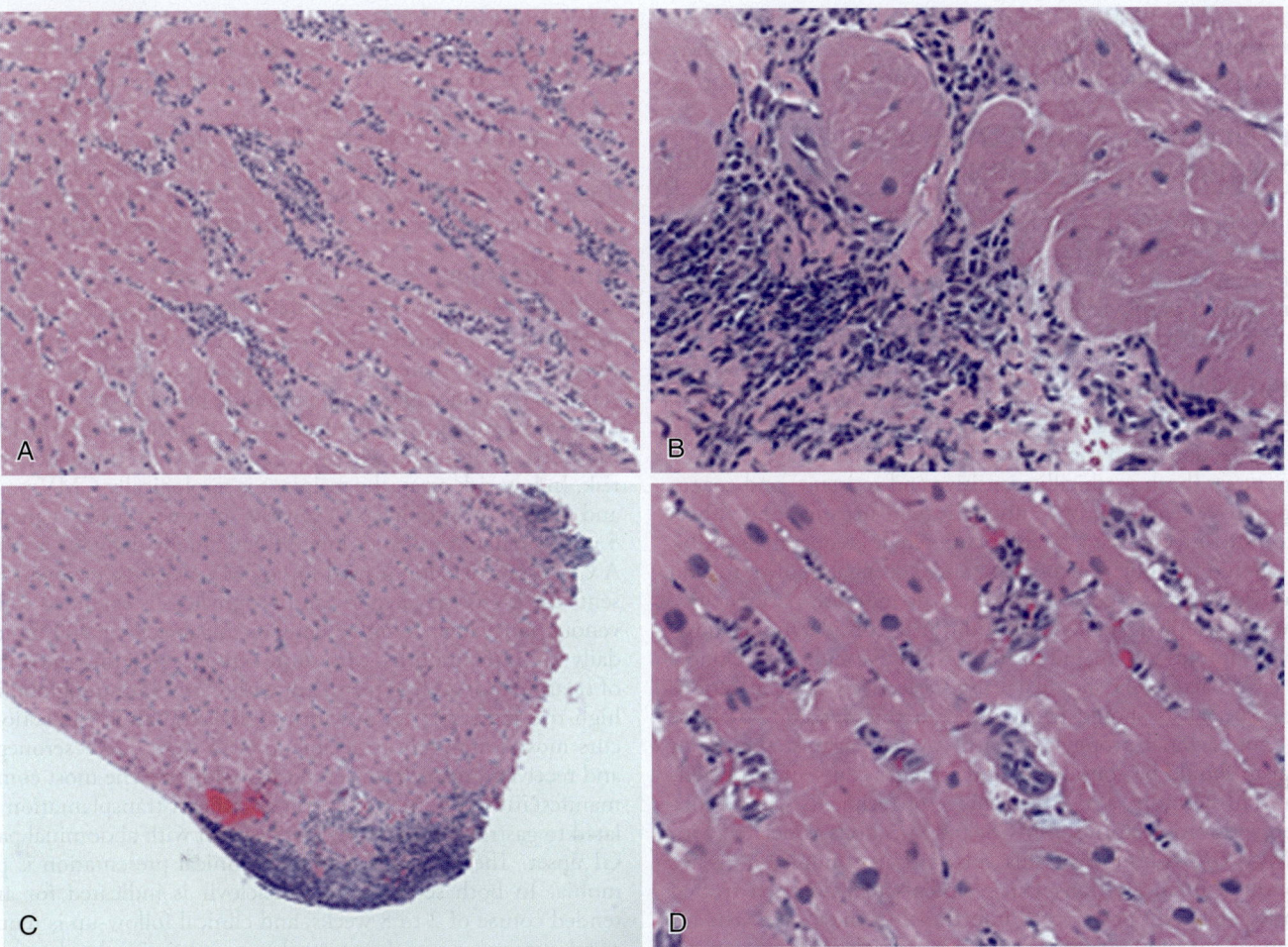

FIGURE 57.7 Histology of allograft immune rejection. (A) Hematoxylin and eosin (H&E)–stained slide at 20× demonstrating ISHLT grade 2R (high grade) acute cellular rejection (ACR). Based on the International Society of Heart and Lung Transplant (ISHLT) criteria, grade 2R is defined by the presence of at least two separate foci of dense perivascular and interstitial T-cell–dominant lymphocytic infiltrates associated with myocyte damage. (B) H&E-stained slide at 40× demonstrating a focus of myocyte damage in ACR with dense perivascular and interstitial T-cell–dominant lymphocytic infiltrate. (C) H&E-stained slide at 20× demonstrating a Quilty lesion, an endocardial-based lesion composed of mixed B- and T-cell lymphocytes and macrophages but without myocardial necrosis. In contrast to ACR, Quilty lesions are not treated with increased immuno-suppressive therapy. (D) H&E-stained slide at 40× demonstrating histologic features of antibody-mediated rejection. Macrophages and/or mononuclear cells distend and fill the capillary and venular lumens. Swollen or activated endothelial cells are usually seen more diffusely. Immunofluorescent studies (not pictured) show endothelial complement, commonly C4d, deposition.

and are treated with increasing levels of CNI or steroid boluses. More severe ACR warrants anti–lymphocyte antibody preparations, and AMR may be treated with plasmapheresis, intravenous immunoglobulin, and monoclonal anti–B-cell agents.

In an effort to reduce invasiveness, many centers are decreasing the frequency of routine endomyocardial biopsy (EMB) and trialing other tests for detection of rejection. This is particularly important for pediatric heart transplant recipients for whom EMB requires sedation or general anesthesia. Recent studies have investigated the use of gene expression profiling (GEP) of peripheral blood to detect rejection after heart transplant. E-IMAGE was a randomized trial of GEP versus EMB that enrolled 60 patients between 2 and 6 months after heart transplant. Patients were managed with GEP or EMB, and a GEP score ≥30 between 2 and 6 months or ≥34 after 6 months posttransplant prompted a follow-up EMB. There were no

significant differences in the composite primary end point of death, retransplantation, rejection with hemodynamic compromise, or graft dysfunction at 18 months. Also, there was no difference in CAV.[44] CARGO II was an observational study that also suggested that a GEP score of less than 34 early after transplant defined patients who were at low risk for rejection.[45]

Aside from GEP, donor-derived circulating cell-free DNA is increasingly used within solid organ transplantation to monitor for rejection. Donor-derived DNA can be found in recipient serum, and levels are increased during rejection.[46] These levels may identify and quantitate severity of rejection, and clinical trials are examining this. High-sensitivity troponin in serum may also correlate with rejection and indicate severity; these levels are being investigated as a noninvasive method to detect rejection. Finally, cardiac magnetic resonance imaging demonstrates changes during rejection, including increased volume, reduced function, perfusion alterations, altered T1 and T2 mapping, and late gadolinium enhancement. Clinical trials are seeking to define a set of these changes, which would accurately predict rejection.

ANTIMICROBIAL PROPHYLAXIS AND OPPORTUNISTIC INFECTION

Immunosuppressive therapy associated with cardiac transplantation increases the incidence of infection in general, and antimicrobial prophylaxis has become a standard for certain infections. Antimicrobial prophylaxis can be divided into strategies to prevent possible bacterial, viral, or fungal infections.

Bacterial Infections

Bacterial infections after heart transplant are most typically surgical site infections, and the most common organisms are *Staphylococcus aureus* (both methicillin sensitive and resistant) and coagulase-negative *Staphylococcus*, although gram-negative and fungal surgical site infections are rarely encountered. Preoperative antibiotics should include vancomycin and a cephalosporin to add gram-negative coverage. Most centers do not use perioperative antifungal prophylaxis. Several additional considerations, however, are important, including donor-positive cultures. Donors who have bacteremia should be used selectively, and infectious disease specialists should be involved in this decision. In these cases, antibacterial prophylaxis with coverage against the donor organism should be considered, and a longer course may be beneficial. Furthermore, a high percentage of recipients will be supported with various forms of MCS, and infections associated with the MCS are common in this subset. For example, it is not uncommon for heart transplant recipients to have been treated recently for LVAD power cord infections. In these cases, the involvement of an infectious disease specialist is warranted; furthermore, use of perioperative antibacterial prophylaxis with coverage against the organism that caused the previous infection is warranted. In addition, tissue from the surgical field can be cultured to rule out any colonization or lingering infection. If these tissue cultures become positive, a 6-week course of focused antimicrobial therapy is indicated. A final situation is when the median sternotomy incision is not fully closed at the end of the transplant; commonly for concerns related to coagulopathy and compression of the RV of the new heart, the incision may be incompletely closed, with plans for a delayed complete closure. In these situations, a more prolonged course of antibiotics is warranted, and our center typically continues therapy for 1 week after the final closure.

Mediastinitis after heart transplantation has been reported in 1% to 2% of cases. Early aggressive management is important, and failure to recognize and drain such infection can rapidly lead to bacteremia and death. In some cases, an enlarged pericardial space from previous cardiomegaly poses additional challenges; multiple soft tissue flaps may be required to fully obliterate the dead space that occurs with reopening of the sternal incision. Poor wound healing associated with immunosuppression makes management of mediastinitis after heart transplant particularly challenging, and outcomes are inferior to those seen with similar infections after other types of heart surgery.

Heart transplant recipients can also develop nosocomial bacterial pneumonia and urinary tract infections, which represent more serious events given the immunosuppressed status. There is probably increased risk for these types of infections among recipients who have remained hospitalized with intravascular catheters for extended periods before their transplant. This subgroup is increasing, given an allocation system that favors temporary MCS as a mechanism to bridge patients. Nosocomial bacterial pneumonia and urinary tract infections are treated in a standard manner, with antibiotic therapy guided by culture results. Bacteremia and sepsis can ensue at a higher frequency relative to nontransplant patients. These events emphasize the importance of early extubation and removal of intravascular catheters and urinary bladder catheters.

Viral Infections

Viral infections are also the focus for additional perioperative prophylactic regimens. CMV can cause a variety of serious infections in solid organ transplant recipients. The CMV serologic status of the donor and recipient should be used to stratify the risk of posttransplant CMV infection, and antiviral prophylaxis is modified according to whether there is low, intermediate, or high risk. In low-risk cases, the recipient is serologically CMV positive, and common prophylaxis consists of intravenous ganciclovir 5 mg/kg daily or valganciclovir 900 mg orally daily for 3 months. A CMV-positive donor used for a CMV-negative recipient represents the high-risk category, and prophylaxis is extended to intravenous ganciclovir 5 mg/kg daily or valganciclovir 900 mg orally daily for 3 to 6 months, with some centers extending the duration of treatment or adding treatment with CMV immunoglobulin for high-risk patients.[47] Even with prophylaxis, clinical infection occurs most commonly in recipients who were CMV seronegative and received organs from seropositive donors. The most common manifestation of CMV infection after heart transplantation is related to gastrointestinal (GI) involvement with abdominal pain or GI upset. The next most common clinical presentation is pneumonia. In both settings, IV ganciclovir is indicated for an extended course of 2 to 8 weeks, and clinical follow-up is required, as relapses can occur. Importantly, an association has been established between CMV infection and the development of CAV, emphasizing the importance of both prophylaxis and early identification of any infection and treatment.

Heart transplant recipients are also at increased risk for EBV infection. However, there are conflicting data regarding the use of antiviral prophylaxis for EBV. Preemptive monitoring of donor-positive and recipient-negative high-risk situations is warranted. Symptoms of EBV infection may be nonspecific and include fever, cough, and sore throat. The diagnosis can be confirmed serologically and with nucleic acid testing (NAT). Treatment should include consideration for reduction of immunosuppression. There is an association between EBV infection and lymphoproliferative disorders and lymphoma; approximately half of patients with lymphoproliferative disorders post–heart transplant will have had associated EBV infection.

Fungal Infections

Invasive pulmonary aspergillosis has been reported in heart transplant recipients with rates between 1.6% and 14%. The higher rates are associated with outbreaks linked to construction or areas of contamination.[48] These infections occur most commonly during the first year after the transplant. Risk factors for the development of this infection include pretransplant airway colonization, reoperation, postoperative need for dialysis or MCS, and culture evidence of intensive care unit (ICU) contamination. The role of antifungal prophylaxis for *Aspergillus* is unclear; high-risk centers have employed either prophylactic systemic agents or inhaled amphotericin. Furthermore, in high-risk settings, some centers have described the use of screening chest CT scans for early identification of lesions. Treatment of active infection in an immunosuppressed patient is challenging; agents that have shown effectiveness include voriconazole and amphotericin B. Mortality from invasive *Aspergillus* infection exceeds 50%; earlier recognition and combined medical treatment and surgical resection may improve outcomes.

Coccidioides is another fungus that can cause invasive infection after heart transplant. There is insufficient evidence to support routine prophylaxis, but recipients in endemic regions and transplants performed using donors who have a history of infection should receive prophylaxis with 6 to 12 months with fluconazole.

Another fungus that can become important after heart transplant is *Pneumocystis jiroveci*, which causes *Pneumocystis carini* pneumonia (PCP), a diffuse lung infection, leading to acute respiratory failure. The preferred prophylaxis for *Pneumocystis jiroveci* infection is trimethoprim-sulfamethoxazole for 6 to 12 months, with dapsone or atovaquone serving as alternative agents if there is an allergy to the primary agent. This same prophylaxis may be effective for *Toxoplasma gondii,* which can cause a parasitic protozoan infection. This parasite may be most important when transplants occur between a recipient who has not been exposed and a donor who harbors the organism. Infection with this agent can involve the brain with neurologic and psychiatric symptoms.

Considerations for Hepatitis C

Historically, use of donors, who were seropositive or NAT positive for hepatitis C was limited because of reduced outcomes among recipients receiving these hearts, both in terms of increased mortality and morbidity. It was observed that the majority of these recipients would develop hepatitis C infection, with a significant percentage progressing to advanced liver disease. Furthermore, studies concluded that use of hepatitis C donors may result in higher rates of CAV. However, with the advent of direct-acting antiviral drugs such as Harvoni (ledipasvir/sofosbuvir), hepatitis C infection after transplant can be irradicated in the vast majority of recipients, and subsequent survival outcomes appear to be equivalent to recipients who receive hepatitis C–negative donor organs.[49] In parallel with increased application of direct-acting antiviral therapy, a recent report described that the use of hepatitis C–positive donors for heart transplantation in the United States increased from 0.12% in 2015 to 12.9% in 2021. Furthermore, in more than 1000 heart transplant recipients for whom hepatitis C donors were used, equivalent 1- and 3-year survival outcomes relative to transplants from negative donors were shown; furthermore, there was no difference in rates of acute rejection.[50] Over 90% of recipients who receive hearts from NAT-positive donors will develop hepatitis C viremia within the first year after the transplant, thus justifying prophylactic application of direct-acting antiviral therapy. In practice, however, most centers monitor these recipients with serial serologic testing or NAT and initiate therapy when there is evidence for viremia. Given the recent increased use of hepatitis C donors, the long-term impact of this practice remains to be studied; long-term survival as well as rates of CAV and malignancy should be followed.

Considerations for Hepatitis B

Donors with active hepatitis B infection, defined by the presence of serum hepatitis B surface antigen, have also been used for heart transplantation, and there is increased risk for viral transmission in these cases. This risk may be mitigated for recipients who have been successfully immunized and show hepatitis B surface antibody positivity. This emphasizes the utility of vaccination for patients with heart failure who may become potential heart transplant recipients. Recipients of hepatitis B surface antigen–positive hearts require prophylaxis with a potent antiviral such as lamivudine, tenofovir, or entecavir, and hepatitis B immunoglobulin is administered regardless of the immune status of the recipient (hepatitis B surface antibody positive or negative). The duration of antiviral prophylaxis is not well defined. All of these recipients should undergo posttransplant monitoring for hepatitis B infection.

SURVIVAL AND QUALITY-OF-LIFE OUTCOMES

Survival Outcomes

Survival rates after heart transplantation have progressively improved over time. The ISHLT registry data demonstrate that the contemporary survival rates at 1, 5, and 1- years posttransplant stand at approximately 90%, 75%, and 60%, respectively.[51,52] Additionally, median survival for heart transplant recipients is now greater than 12 years, and median survival conditional on 1-year survival is greater than 14 years (Fig. 57.8). These encouraging figures are attributed to advancements in immunosuppressive therapies, surgical techniques, and the adoption of advanced organ preservation methods.

Quality-of-Life Outcomes

In addition to improved survival rates, heart transplantation has been associated with a marked improvement in recipients' quality of life. Patients often report enhanced energy levels, improved exercise tolerance, and a reduction in symptoms such as shortness of breath and fatigue, significantly contributing to an overall improvement in their quality of life. Many individuals are able to return to work, resume daily activities, and partake in physical exercises, underscoring the transformative impact of heart transplantation on their well-being.

Studies have used various measures, including quality-of-life scores, to evaluate physical, emotional, and social aspects of recipient well-being and have consistently shown a meaningful and positive impact on recipients' quality of life after heart transplantation. Furthermore, psychological assessments often reveal significant improvements in mental health, including a reduction in depression and anxiety levels and an increased sense of overall well-being.[53]

COMPLICATIONS AND ADVERSE EVENTS

Bleeding

Bleeding is always possible after heart transplantation but is of greater concern in specific scenarios. First, many heart transplant cases constitute reoperative surgery; for example, patients with ischemic cardiomyopathy may have had remote coronary bypass surgery, and such cases have mediastinal scarring and pericardial adhesions, the dissection of which results in greater postoperative bleeding. Other patients who come for heart transplant surgery may have been on anticoagulants such as warfarin that are not completely reversed at the time of the surgery. Furthermore, many patients are on different forms of MCS at the time of surgery, which may cause thrombocytopenia, platelet dysfunction, and acquired von Willebrand condition. Other recipients have liver congestion and dysfunction secondary to right heart failure, resulting in reduced levels of clotting factors. In the operating

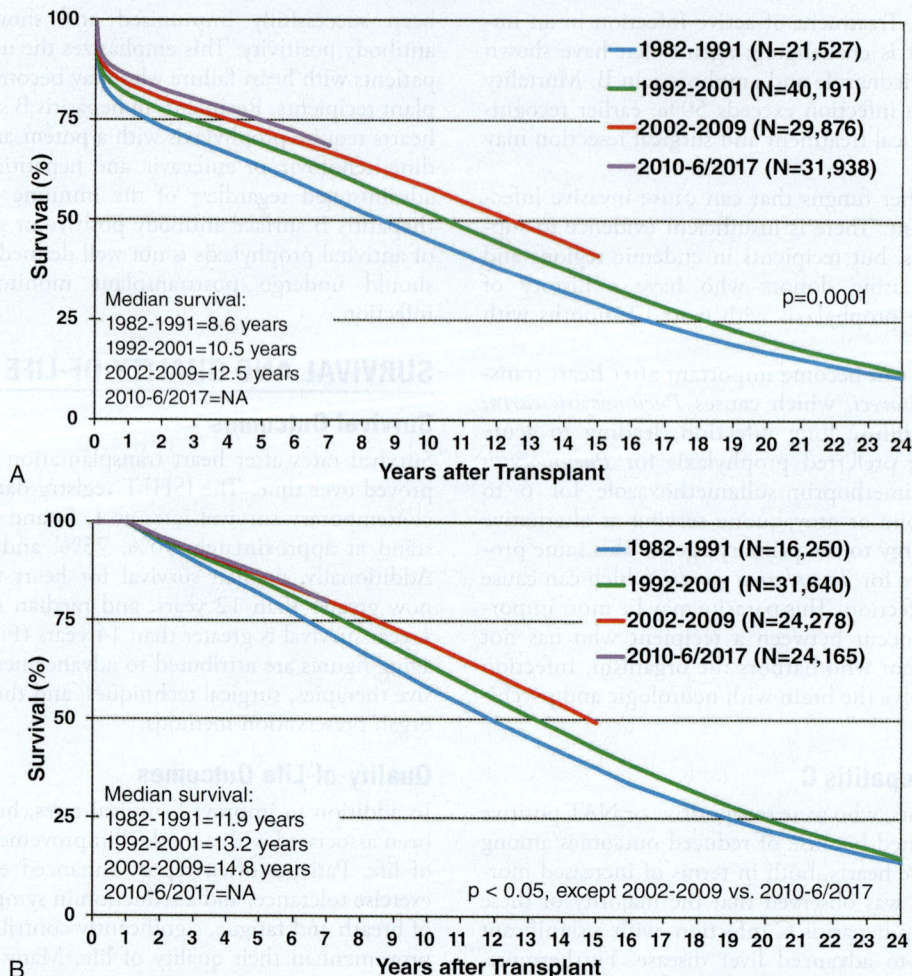

FIGURE 57.8 (A) Survival after heart transplantation. Above shows Kaplan-Meier survival after heart transplantation in adults, stratified by era. (B) Kaplan-Meier survival after heart transplantation in adults conditional on 1-year survival, stratified by era. (From Khush KK, Cherikh WS, Chambers DC, et al. The International Thoracic Organ Transplant Registry of the International Society for Heart and Lung Transplantation: thirty-sixth adult heart transplantation report – 2019; focus theme: donor and recipient size match. *J Heart Lung Transplant*. 2019;38[10]:1056-1066.)

room, after administration of protamine and ensuring surgical hemostasis, correction of coagulopathy should be guided by platelet count, fibrinogen level, and rotational thromboelastometry. In addition to platelets and cryoprecipitate, additional agents such as prothrombin complex concentrate or synthetic activated factor VII can be administered to correct for factor deficiencies. Additionally, hypothermia and hypocalcemia may predispose to bleeding and should be corrected. Major bleeding can result in periods of hypotension and hypoperfusion to the allograft, and this has been identified as a cause for early graft dysfunction. Ongoing bleeding in the ICU, after coagulation abnormalities and thrombocytopenia have been corrected, mandates expeditious return to the operating room. Patients with severe coagulopathy will have greater postoperative mediastinal blood loss, and delayed sternal closure may be practiced to ensure removal of any retained blood or clot before final closure.

Primary Graft Dysfunction

PGD is defined as immediate dysfunction of the allograft without an obvious cause such as severe antibody-mediated rejection. The

ISHLT has published a consensus statement on this adverse event and has created a grading system that divides events into right versus left heart and categorizes degree of dysfunction: mild, moderate, and severe (Table 57.3).[54] The etiology of PGD is often unclear and likely multifactorial. Donor characteristics, the preservation strategy, and recipient factors may all contribute to PGD. Associations with higher rates of PGD have been made with older donor age, DCD donors, longer cold static storage times, and posttransplant bleeding. PGD is commonly attributed to some deficiency in preservation.

Severe PGD carries a mortality of up to 40%. In the operating room, treatment consists of maximizing graft performance and mechanically supporting the circulation. A preliminary step is to establish an AV synchronous rhythm and maintain a heart rate of 80 to 100 beats/minute. After optimizing heart rate and rhythm, preload should be optimized. Frequently, MAP and coronary perfusion pressure are low and must be supported with vasopressors. An extended period of unloaded reperfusion with CPB is commonly employed to allow recovery from ischemic insult. Inotropic infusions such as epinephrine, dopamine, dobutamine, and milrinone are used to

TABLE 57.3 International Society of Heart and Lung Transplantation Definition of Severity Scale for Primary Graft Dysfunction (PGD)

PGD-Left Ventricle (PGD-LV)

Mild PGD-LV: One of the following criteria must be met	• LVEF ≤40% by echocardiography • Hemodynamics with RAP >15 mm Hg, PCWP >20 mm Hg, CI <2.0 L/min/m² (lasting more than 1 hour) requiring low-dose inotropes

Moderate PGD-LV: Must meet one criterion from I and another criterion from II	I. One criteria from the following:
	  • LVEF ≤40% by echocardiography
	  • Hemodynamics with RAP >15 mm Hg, PCWP >20 mm Hg, CI <2.0 L/min/m² (lasting more than 1 hour) requiring low-dose inotropes
	II. One criteria from the following:
	  • High-dose inotrope—inotrope score >10[a]
	  • Newly placed IABP (regardless of inotropes)

Severe PGD-LV	• Dependence on left or biventricular mechanical support including ECMO, LVAD, BiVAD, or percutaneous LVAD (excludes the requirement for IABP)

PGD-Right Ventricle (PGD-RV)

PGD-RV: Requires either I and II or III alone	I. Hemodynamics with RAP >15 mm Hg, PCWP >20 mm Hg, CI <2.0 L/min/m² (lasting more than 1 hour) requiring low-dose inotropes II. TPG <15 mm Hg and/or pulmonary artery systolic pressure <50 mm Hg III. Need for RVAD

[a]Inotrope score = dopamine (×1) + dobutamine (×1) + amrinone (×1) + milrinone (×15) + epinephrine (×100) + norepinephrine (×100) with each drug dosed in µg/kg/min.

BiVAD, Biventricular assist device; *CI*, cardiac index; *ECMO*, extracorporeal membrane oxygenation; *IABP*, intraaortic balloon pump; *LVAD*, left ventricular assist device; *PCWP*, pulmonary capillary wedge pressure; *RAP*, right atrial pressure; *RVAD*, right ventricular assist device; *TPG*, transpulmonary pressure gradient.

Adapted from Kobashigawa J, Patel J, Azarbal B, et al. Report from a consensus conference on primary graft dysfunction after cardiac transplantation. *J Heart Lung Transplant.* 2014;33(4):327-340.

stimulate improved contractility. If an adequate circulation cannot be achieved, MCS must be used. Intraaortic balloon counter pulsation can be initially tried and may provide improvement in the circulation. At our institution, severe PGD is commonly supported with venoarterial ECMO using either central or peripheral cannulation. Fortunately, for patients with severe PGD after heart transplant, ventricular function often recovers significantly with a period of mechanical support, enabling the ECMO to be weaned off within several days of transplant. Retransplant is infrequently used for severe PGD but may be considered in cases where other organ system function recovers but allograft failure persists.

Although typically it is an immediate finding in the operating room, PGD can also manifest during the first 24 hours after the transplant surgery, in the ICU setting. When there is delayed hemodynamic decline, cardiac tamponade must be ruled out, and in general these patients should be surgically reexplored.

Reports have suggested higher rates of severe PDG after transplant using DCD donors. This may be related to the ischemic insult associated with cardiac death. Fortunately, this PGD appears to be short lived and readily reversible with short periods of mechanical support. In a randomized controlled trial, despite higher rates of PGD, overall survival after heart transplant using DCD donors was equivalent to that achieved with brain-dead donors.[20] Furthermore, some centers are reporting improving rates of PDG after cardiac transplant with DCD, perhaps attributed to increasing experience with these types of donors.

Right Ventricular Failure

Isolated RV failure can occur as a form of PGD. Right heart failure can also occur in the setting of increased PVR, which is a common sequela of chronic left heart failure. PVR is often dynamic and highly sensitive to common perturbations such as hypoxia and hypercarbia; therefore, it is important to maintain appropriate oxygenation and ventilation during recovery from heart transplantation to avoid triggering further increase in PVR. If there is evidence or concern for RV failure, echocardiography will demonstrate decreased RV contractility, RV dilation, and an underfilled LV. On invasive monitoring, cardiac output will be low along with an elevated CVP. Early aggressive hemodynamic support is crucial, as often RV function can improve over time. When treating RV dysfunction, a rhythm that has AV synchrony and a rate of 80 to 100 beats/minute is desirable. Pharmacologic treatments should include intravenous dobutamine and milrinone. MAP should be supported to ensure adequate coronary perfusion, and inhaled agents, such as nitric oxide or epoprostenol, should be used to selectively lower PVR. Many centers use inhaled pulmonary vasodilators routinely after heart transplantation. Minimizing fluid resuscitation and prioritizing diuresis can also help if the CVP is high. If RV dysfunction is severe, temporary right ventricular assist device placement may be required.

Heart Rhythm Disturbances After Heart Transplantation

Sinus and AV node dysfunction are common immediately after reperfusion. The mechanism for this dysfunction probably relates to ischemia, but hypothermic injury and surgical trauma are also possible. Temporary epicardial pacing wires are placed to achieve AV synchronous activation and adequate rate. This electrical dysfunction typically resolves within 24 hours. Less than 5% of heart transplants display significant impairment of sinus or AV node function beyond 5 days, and this is addressed with a permanent pacemaker system. Atrial fibrillation may occur during the perioperative period and is typically temporary and should be treated with conventional agents to chemically cardiovert, such as amiodarone, and control rate, such as calcium channel blocking agents or β-adrenergic receptor blocking agents. Late atrial fibrillation or ventricular dysrhythmias may occur with acute rejection or CAV, and further diagnostic testing for these conditions is warranted.

Cardiac Allograft Vasculopathy

CAV is a vascular condition that affects both the arteries and veins of the allograft; the classic histology is progressive smooth muscle cell proliferation within the intima leading to luminal compromise (Fig. 57.9). The condition differs from typical atherosclerosis in that it affects both the arterial and venous sides and affects the vessels in a more diffuse manner with less focal lipid or calcium deposits. CAV occurs in varying levels of severity in approximately 50% of transplant recipients by 10 years. Risk factors include both ACR and AMR. An association has been described between viral infection (such as CMV and hepatitis C) and more aggressive CAV. As it progresses, patients experience coronary insufficiency but may only have atypical symptoms such as dyspnea or syncope, because the hearts are denervated. The late stages of CAV result in fibrotic replacement of the myocardium and LV dysfunction.

Monitoring for CAV most commonly involves routine coronary angiography, which is scheduled every 1 or 2 years. The frequency of these studies is center specific but may be more frequent when disease is identified and treatment started, or less frequent for low-risk patients. Multiple other modalities have been described to diagnose or quantitate CAV. Concurrent intravascular imaging using intravascular ultrasound (IVUS) or optical coherence tomography permits examination of the vessel wall for neointimal hyperplasia and is more sensitive than angiography alone to detect early CAV. Reports have also described the use of noninvasive imaging modalities to detect ischemia and as adjunctive strategies to diagnose CAV and determine the severity of the vascular lesions. Dobutamine or exercise stress echocardiography, nuclear myocardial perfusion imaging, positron emission tomography, and cardiac magnetic resonance imaging have all been shown to demonstrate ischemic changes associated with CAV after heart transplant.

Treatment options for CAV include prophylactic medication and interventions for established disease. Statin therapy has been shown to reduce CAV and improve long-term outcomes regardless of lipid levels and should be considered for all heart transplant recipients. Another class of medications that has been shown to be effective for CAV is the mammalian target of rapamycin (mTOR) inhibitors; the two agents that are clinically available are sirolimus (rapamycin) and everolimus. These agents have been shown to prevent or delay progression of CAV, especially when used within 2 years of the transplant; these agents are immunosuppressive, and when added to a patient's drug regimen, typically they are substituted for the CNI or MMF. A meta-analysis of 14 studies of patients receiving mTOR inhibitors (sample sizes of 23–644) showed 61% relative reduction in CAV for the treated group.[55] A large single-center nonrandomized analysis of 402 patients compared a calcineurin-based regimen with sirolimus with complete calcineurin withdrawal. The sirolimus group experienced reduced CAV, quantitated by IVUS, as well as reduced CAV-related events and all-cause mortality.[56] Notably, use of mTOR inhibitors is frequently limited by adverse side effects, including increased ACR when calcineurin inhibition is stopped.

Interventions for CAV include percutaneous coronary interventions (stenting) and even coronary artery bypass surgery. These interventions should be reserved for cases that include significant disease of the proximal coronary arterial tree, as these interventions cannot address the more distal disease. For percutaneous coronary interventions, newer-generation, drug-eluting stents are favored, as in-stent restenosis rates are high. Coronary artery bypass surgery for this condition is associated with increased morbidity and mortality with uncertain long-term outcomes. For younger patients with severe CAV, particularly when it is symptomatic and with declining LV function, retransplant should be considered. CAV remains the most common reason for retransplantation

Malignancy

Heart transplant recipients are at an increased risk to develop a malignancy compared with the general population caused in part by chronic systemic immunosuppression. The risk of new malignancy in 10-year heart transplant survivors is roughly 20%. In a recent study reviewing the ISHLT database, there was increasing frequency of new malignancies for 5-year survivors of 12.4%.[57] The most common malignancy is skin cancer, including squamous cell and basal cell carcinoma, followed by prostate, lung, and posttransplant lymphoproliferative disorder (PTLD) including lymphoma. The presence of each type of malignancy significantly reduces overall survival. Risk factors for the development of malignancy after heart transplant include older age of the recipient, history of smoking, and use of specific immunosuppressive agents such as IL-2 receptor antibody preparations. PTLD is found in around 1% of patients at 5 years and can be associated with EBV infection of B lymphocytes. This can lead to lymphoid proliferation in any body system. Given the increased incidence for malignancies, enhanced screening is recommended posttransplant and, most importantly, annual dermatologic examination. In addition, more tailored immunosuppression may enable reductions, which in turn could reduce malignancy rates.[57]

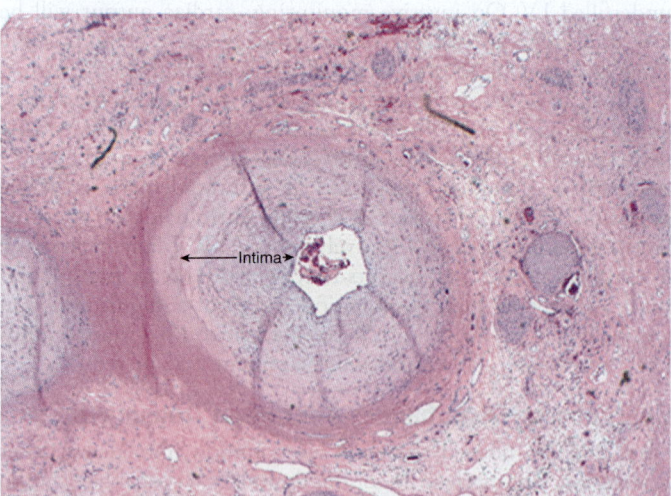

FIGURE 57.9 Histopathology of cardiac allograft vasculopathy. Photomicrograph of H&E-stained slide at 20× demonstrating chronic allograft vasculopathy involving an epicardial coronary artery. Concentric fibromuscular intimal *(arrow)* and medial thickening with luminal stenosis is a hallmark feature resulting from host allorecognition of donor human leukocyte antigen on coronary endothelium, T-cell and endothelial activation, vascular smooth muscle proliferation, and intimal or medial thickening.

PEDIATRIC HEART TRANSPLANTATION

Indications

Heart transplantation in pediatric patients remains an important option for children with end-stage heart failure. Heart transplantation in this patient population poses a particularly difficult decision, as it must be balanced against other possible therapies that can be offered to the child. The most common indication for heart transplant in the pediatric population within North America is CHD, with New York Heart Association stage III or IV symptoms.[58] However, as outcomes of surgical interventions for CHD have improved, indications for transplant must be individual and dynamic. This indication is closely followed by dilated cardiomyopathy, with an increasing prevalence of heart transplant for this indication in older pediatric patients. Other indications for surgery include severe myocarditis, intractable arrythmias, and retransplantation.

Outcomes

Outcome after pediatric heart transplantation varies significantly by recipient age at the time of transplant. For children <1 year old, median survival is 22.3 years. This is compared with 18.4 years for those 1 to 5 years, 14.4 years for those 6 to 10 years, and 13.1 years for those 11 to 17 years. Interestingly, 10-year survival, conditional on survival to 1 year, is 83%.[59] Patients with a diagnosis of CHD have the highest perioperative and early postoperative mortality compared with other diagnoses of heart failure. This difference persists out of 3 years but is no longer present by 10 years posttransplant. Survival for CHD is 79% at 3 years and 68% at 10 years. Comparatively, survival for dilated cardiomyopathy is 88% at 3 years and 70% at 10 years. Among patients with CHD, single ventricle patients with prior staged surgical palliation have a significantly lower 10-year survival at 53%. Other factors associated with early postoperative mortality include need for preoperative or postoperative extracorporeal MCS, preoperative dialysis, preoperative prolonged intubation, and other markers of preoperative organ failure. Causes of death are similar to the adult population and include allograft rejection, infection, and CAV.

CARDIAC RETRANSPLANTATION

Given a median posttransplant survival of approximately 12 years, most patients who receive heart transplantation are not returned to normal life expectancy. Therefore, some patients are vetted for retransplantation, and the registry of the ISHLT shows that approximately 2.5% of all heart transplants are retransplants. Furthermore, this rate appears to be similar between the United States and other countries and has been relatively stable for the past decade.

There are a range of different scenarios and indications in which cardiac retransplant may be considered. The most common indication is CAV. Frequently, this condition is asymptomatic and first identified on surveillance angiography, with a characteristic appearance of diffuse pruning of the coronary tree. With progression of the condition, patients begin to experience dyspnea, syncope, dysthymias, and sudden death. CAV is the leading cause of late death after cardiac transplantation.

In contrast to CAV, where patients may be considered for retransplant late after the initial procedure, other indications include early graft failure. Retransplant has been used as a treatment for severe PGD in which the transplanted heart never recovers function. Typically, such a patient might be supported on temporary MCS devices such as VADs or VA-ECMO as a bridge to a second transplant.

Other indications for retransplant include severe acute rejection with failure of functional recovery. Again, such scenarios are rare, as most rejections will demonstrate recovery with treatment. A final group of patients have nonspecific loss of graft function in which the exact etiology for the graft failure is not understood.

Retransplant poses a variety of challenges. First, given that donor organs are in limited supply, the concept of providing a single individual with multiple allografts has been challenged from an ethical standpoint. This argument is strengthened by the observation that outcomes after retransplant are generally inferior to those after primary transplants. On the other hand, pediatric transplant, which has been strongly supported, generally is part of a larger strategy that must include a plan for retransplant if normal longevity is held as a goal.

Another common challenge to retransplantation is extracardiac organ dysfunction, in particular, renal function. Patients who have been maintained on immunosuppressive regimens, including CNIs, frequently over time will develop significant irreversible renal insufficiency, which may preclude retransplant. Furthermore, many heart transplant recipients may develop donor-specific anti-HLA antibodies, which subsequently interfere with donor organ matching, increase wait time, and contribute to reduced outcomes. The presence of HLA antibodies is greater among patients who have received a transplant versus those who are naïve to alloantigen exposure. Finally, care must be taken to evaluate candidates for retransplant for malignancy, acknowledging that there is an increased risk which accrues over time.

From a technical perspective, additional challenges exist. First, significant adhesions can develop around previous suture lines. The authors' approach has been to resect all of the previous anastomoses, essentially removing the entire previous allograft. Furthermore, redundancy of the aortic anastomosis can lead the ascending aorta to project anteriorly and, thus, increases the risk of sternal reentry. This feature emphasizes the importance of preoperative CT imaging in planning the procedure. Lastly, chronic immunosuppression in the recipient of the retransplant probably retards wound healing and may contribute to an increased risk of wound healing complications.

Given these challenges, the inclusion and exclusion criteria for retransplant are generally more stringent than those of primary transplant. Retransplantation is most often considered in a younger cohort relative to primary heart transplant, with avoidance of recipients who experienced early primary graft failure or early failure because of severe rejection.[60] Even so, short- and long-term survival is lower in heart retransplant recipients compared with first-time heart transplantation. Not only is 1-year survival significantly lower, but survival conditional on 1-year survival is also lower with retransplantation. When examining ISHLT data for all heart transplantations performed between 1982 and 2016, 1-year survival for retransplantation is 68.9% with a median survival of 6.6 years, median survival conditional on 1-year survival of 11.6 years, and 10-year survival of 38%. Survival with retransplantation has improved in the most recent era between 2009 and 2016, with 1-year survival for retransplantation of 80% compared with 85.4% for primary adult heart transplants and 5-year survival of 68.6% versus 74.6%, respectively. Similar outcomes have been found when analyzing the UNOS database between 1995 and 2012, with estimated survival at 1, 3, 5, 10, and 15 years after retransplantation of 80%, 70%, 64%, 47%, and 30%, respectively.[60]

COMBINED HEART AND OTHER ORGAN TRANSPLANTS

The presence of heart failure with other concomitant end-organ dysfunction poses a barrier to isolated heart transplantation. Consideration of dual organ transplantation requires collaboration between several disciplines and clear guidelines for assessment and listing of the dual organ transplant candidate.

Heart-Kidney Transplantation

Chronic kidney disease (CKD) is defined as a glomerular filtration rate (GFR) <60 mL/min/1.73 m^2 or at least one marker of kidney damage for a minimum of 3 months. CKD is present in 40% to 60% of patients with heart failure. However, consensus guidelines recommend consideration of heart-kidney transplant in patients with a GFR <30 mL/min/1.73 m^2.[61] Patients with a GFR ranging between 30 and 44 represent a "gray" zone, where dual organ transplant should be considered on an individual basis. Evidence of small kidney size, proteinuria, or other irreversible factors may also push toward dual organ transplantation.

Patients who undergo simultaneous heart-kidney transplant have improved survival and less rejection than patients who undergo isolated heart transplantation. However, a high incidence of posttransplant dialysis remains—between 26% and 37%. Immunosuppression will vary by center, but often includes an induction immunosuppression agent.

Newer UNOS guidelines have also brought forward consideration of kidney after heart transplant. With the "safety net" guidelines, patients who receive an isolated heart transplant but are on dialysis or have a GFR <20 mL/min/1.73 m^2 are eligible to receive high-sequence (sequence B-D) donor kidneys. Data regarding these newer guidelines are forthcoming.[62]

Heart-Liver Transplantation

Liver disease in the setting of heart failure is common, representing between 15% and 50% of patients with chronic heart failure. Heart failure can lead to hepatic congestion and ischemia and, over time, to chronic liver disease. Moreover, patients with heart failure may have metabolic disorders such as familial hypercholesterolemia or transthyretin amyloidosis that can also affect the liver. Isolated heart transplantation in the setting of cirrhosis is associated with a mortality rate of nearly 50%. As such, pathologically confirmed cirrhosis is now an established contraindication to isolated heart transplant.[61]

Evaluation of liver disease in the setting of heart failure includes assessment of liver enzymes, liver function, and calculation of a Model for End-stage Liver Disease (MELD) score. Imaging remains a critical modality for assessment, including hepatic ultrasound, CT, and magnetic resonance imaging. Hepatic elastography is a newer imaging technique to further assess for fibrosis. If there is concern for possible cirrhosis or portal hypertension after these clinical assessments, liver biopsy with measurement of portal pressures should be conducted to provide histologic assessment of the presence of cirrhosis and hemodynamic determination of the presence of portal hypertension. If either cirrhosis or portal hypertension is confirmed, dual heart-liver transplantation should be considered as opposed to isolated heart transplantation.

The most common approach for heart-liver transplant is sequential, where the heart transplant is performed first on CPB, followed by the liver transplant after the patient has been weaned off bypass. Venovenous or venoarterial extracorporeal support is often used while clamping the IVC during the liver transplant to prevent rapid shifts in hemodynamics with a new cardiac allograft. Another approach is simultaneous heart-liver transplant, where the IVC remains connected. The simultaneous approach has the benefits of decreased hepatic ischemic time and potentially better hepatic function from the new allograft when weaning off CPB.

Heart-Lung Transplantation

Cardiac and pulmonary disease are intrinsically related, and end-stage heart or lung disease can lead to chronic disease of the other organ. Historically, heart-lung transplantation was performed for isolated pulmonary disease because of the poor outcomes with isolated lung transplantation. However, with the marked improvement in isolated lung transplant survival, indications for combined heart-lung transplant have since changed. The most common indication for combined transplant is CHD resulting in end-stage cardiac disease as well as end-stage pulmonary disease or pulmonary vascular disease. Other common indications include acquired heart disease leading to fixed, severe pulmonary hypertension (PVR above 4 Woods units despite vasodilator challenge) and primary lung disease with severe pulmonary hypertension leading to irrecoverable RV failure. Unfortunately, it can be difficult to determine whether RV recovery is expected after isolated lung transplant in the setting of severe pulmonary hypertension.[63]

Technically, combined heart-lung transplantation can be performed through a sternotomy or transverse thoracosternotomy (clamshell) incision. Airway anastomosis is most commonly performed via a tracheal anastomosis, whereas historically it was performed as a bibronchial anastomosis because of concern about airway ischemia. On the other hand, the cardiac anastomoses are limited to the aortic and right atrial or bicaval anastomosis(es), given the heart-lung bloc.

Posttransplant survival after heart-lung transplant has steadily improved over time. Recent registry data suggest a 1-year survival after heart-lung transplant of 84% from 2012 to 2021.[63] This is compared with a 1-year survival of 63% in the previous decade. Median graft survival appears to be nearly 6 years, mimicking the graft survival associated with isolated lung transplantation. Graft and patient survival after heart-lung transplantation is predominantly dictated by the pulmonary allograft, and monitoring for infection and rejection is focused on this as well.

CARDIAC XENOTRANSPLANTATION

Modern xenotransplantation dates back to the 1960s, when Keith Reemtsma performed a series of chimpanzee-to-human kidney transplants, with one patient surviving for 9 months.[64] As discussed, the first cardiac xenotransplant was attempted in 1964, when James Hardy performed a cardiac xenotransplant using a chimpanzee donor.[4] Finally, Leonard Bailey at Loma Linda University performed a baboon-to-human heart transplant into an infant with hypoplastic left heart syndrome. The patient survived for 21 days.[65]

Since these early efforts, research over the past 40 years has focused on use of swine as the donor species for xenotransplantation. Central to the success of swine xenotransplantation was development of gene modifications to knock out the α-galactose

1,3-galactose (Gal) carbohydrate. Additional gene modifications to form the critical three-gene knockout swine were done with the β1,4-N-acetylgalactosyltransferase gene, which results in Sda carbohydrate and CMP-N-acetylneuraminic acid hydroxylase, responsible for Neu5Gc synthesis. With these three-gene knockouts as a backbone and additional gene modification additions over time, swine-to-baboon animal studies were quite promising with greater than 9-month survival.[66] This led to the first two swine-to-human cardiac xenotransplants, performed by a team led by Dr. Bartley P. Griffith at University of Maryland. The first swine-to-human cardiac xenotransplant was performed in a 57-year-old patient who was bridged from long-term extracorporeal support and was not felt to be a candidate for conventional human-to-human heart transplantation or durable MCS. The procedure was a technical success, and the xenograft demonstrated excellent early function. Remarkably, the patient survived for 60 days after the implant before succumbing to xenograft failure related to rejection and possibly reactivation of latent porcine CMV and porcine roseolovirus.[67] Nevertheless, the path forward for cardiac xenotransplantation remains exciting. Greater understanding of rejection pathways, infection-rejection interactions, and requisite immunosuppression is needed, but, after this landmark achievement, it seems highly possible that clinical cardiac xenotransplantation will become a part of the advanced heart failure management landscape in the years to come.

CONCLUSION

Norman Shumway's development of the surgical technique for cardiac transplantation led many centers both in the United States and around the world to perform clinical cases. Unfortunately, these first pioneering heart transplants in the late 1960s and early 1970s did not achieve successful long-term survival, with many of the recipients expiring in less than 1 year. Important changes in the immunosuppressive regimen to include the CNI cyclosporine A and routine endomyocardial biopsies for early identification of rejection resulted in substantial improvement in long-term survival. As a result of these improvements, more centers started heart transplantation programs. Annual heart transplant procedures in the United States rose to roughly 3500 cases per year. Within the past decade, several additional developments have further expanded the therapy, mainly by expanding the donor pool and enabling more potential recipients to receive the therapy. Use of donors with active hepatitis C became safe with the development of direct-acting antiviral medications, which could be administrated after the transplant to prevent serious hepatitis C infection. Further expansion occurred as the result of increased donors related to death from drug overdose, in particular, narcotic overdose. Finally, groups in the United Kingdom and Australia demonstrated that use of specific reperfusion strategies enabled use of hearts from donors who were declared dead on the basis of circulatory cessation. Previously, these DCD donors were not felt to be suitable for cardiac donation because of concerns that the associated ischemia would result in significant irreversible injury and reduced graft function. A randomized study in the United States using reperfusion with ex vivo warm blood perfusion demonstrated that recipients randomized to a DCD donor were transplanted more quickly and had equivalent short-term survival. Some centers have now substantially increased use of DCD, with up to 30% of total cases being from DCD. Together these changes have resulted in a near doubling of total heart transplants performed in the United States—currently around 4000 cases per year.

The future looks bright for heart transplantation. Still over 50% of consented donors are not used for heart allograft donation in the United States. Ongoing clinical trials with novel organ preservation strategies may enable successful use of these higher-risk donors. Furthermore, current immunosuppressive medications remain nonspecific, and clinical trials are ongoing with agents that may focus inhibition on pathways more specific to the alloimmune response. One such agent is belatacept, which inhibits costimulatory pathways necessary to amplify T-lymphocyte alloimmune responses. Finally, two recent xenotransplants using genetically modified pigs have demonstrated the feasibility of xenotransplantation at least in the short term, enabling consideration of larger-scale clinical trials.

SELECTED REFERENCES

Geller BJ, Sinha SS, Kapur NK, et al. Escalating and de-escalating temporary mechanical circulatory support in cardiogenic shock: a scientific statement from the American Heart Association. *Circulation.* 2022;146(6):e50-e68.

Supporting the circulation, either medically with inotropes or with temporary mechanical support, is critical for successfully managing patients with advanced heart failure and cardiogenic shock in the modern era. This statement from the AHA provides a framework for circulatory support strategies in patients with advanced heart failure/cardiogenic shock in order to bridge them to native recovery or long-term therapies, including durable mechanical circulatory support or heart transplantation.

Heidenreich PA, Bozkurt B, Aguilar D, et al. 2022 AHA/ACC/HFSA guideline for the management of heart failure: a report of the American College of Cardiology/American Heart Association Joint Committee on Clinical Practice Guidelines. *J Am Coll Cardiol.* 2022;79(17):e263-e421.

Heart failure arises from a variety of etiologies and exists on a spectrum of severity. These current ACC/AHA guidelines provide a comprehensive description of contemporary heart failure management, from guideline-directed medical therapy for stable heart failure, to corrective interventions, to escalation of therapy including mechanical circulatory support or heart transplantation in the most advanced cases of heart failure.

Khush KK, Cherikh WS, Chambers DC, et al. The International Thoracic Organ Transplant Registry of the International Society for Heart and Lung Transplantation: thirty-sixth adult heart transplantation report – 2019; focus theme: donor and recipient size match. *J Heart Lung Transplant.* 2019;38(10):1056-1066.

This statement from the ISHLT provides contemporary data relating to long-term survival after heart transplantation. Survival has continued to improve with time, and median survival after heart transplantation is currently greater than 12 years.

Mehra MR, Canter CE, Hannan MM, et al. The 2016 International Society for Heart Lung Transplantation listing criteria for heart transplantation: a 10-year update. *J Heart Lung Transplant.* 2016;35(1):1-23.

> Many factors affect whether a patient should or should not be considered for heart transplantation. These 2016 guidelines from the ISHLT outline indications as well as contraindications for proceeding with heart transplant listing.

Stinson EB, Dong E Jr, Schroeder JS, et al. Initial clinical experience with heart transplantation. *Am J Cardiol.* 1968;22(6):791-803.

> This 1968 publication from Dr. Norman Shumway and the Stanford group describes some of the earliest human-to-human transplants ever performed. Technical details behind the biatrial transplant are described, and insights related to early methods for allograft preservation as well as some of the ethical and practical challenges facing the field of heart transplantation at the time are gained.

The full reference list appears on Elsevier eBooks+.

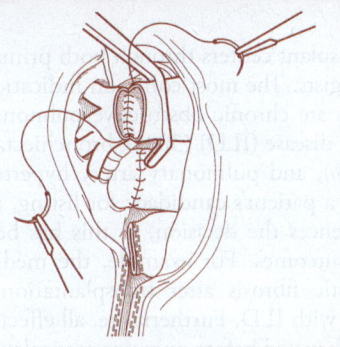

CHAPTER 58

Lung Transplantation

Jason M. Gauthier, Douglas Tran, Christine L. Lau, Alexander S. Krupnick, and Daniel Kreisel

INTRODUCTION

Lung transplantation is the only cure for a multitude of end-stage lung diseases. Among patients in the United States, 74% are predicted to achieve a ≥2-year survival benefit. Recent 1- and 5-year survival rates are 85% and 54%, respectively, figures that have substantially improved since lung transplantation was made a clinical reality in the early 1980s.[1] These achievements are a result of advances on several fronts, most notably of which is donor-recipient selection, perioperative management, immunosuppression strategies, and reducing risk factors for rejection. Many of these insights have arisen from investigations over the past two decades, built upon the substantial progress that was made in the 1980s and 1990s.

The first lung transplant was done in 1963 by James Hardy at the University of Mississippi (Fig. 58.1). After years of experimentation on animals, Dr. Hardy and colleagues performed a single lung transplant at the University of Mississippi on a recipient with a left mainstem bronchial tumor and postobstructive pneumonia. The donor died of a massive myocardial infarction, and, as such, this also represented the first donation after circulatory death (DCD) donor. Unfortunately, the recipient succumbed to renal failure on postoperative day 18. The lung graft functioned immediately after the surgery, and despite the early mortality, the surgery was a monumental achievement.[2] Dr. Hardy's operation quickly spurred interest at other institutions that similarly had poor early outcomes because of infection, bleeding, and rejection. Early pioneers in the field, including Denton Cooley, Walton Lillehei, and Christian Barnard, performed lung transplantations over the next decade, but there were no long-term successes. In the 20 years after the first lung transplant in humans, advances in surgical technique and immunosuppression substantially aided the understanding of why early attempts were unsuccessful long term.

In 1983, Joel Cooper, G. Alec Patterson, and colleagues at the University of Toronto performed the first single lung transplant for interstitial pulmonary fibrosis in a patient who lived for 7 years, dying of renal failure. This procedure represented the first lung transplant with long-term success.[2,3] In the ensuing years the technique for en bloc double lung transplantation was perfected in a canine model. In 1986 the Toronto group performed double lung transplantation for the first time in a human for a patient with emphysema.[4] The advent of the double lung transplantation substantially increased enthusiasm for the procedure, with the number of lung transplants performed worldwide increasing from 45 in 1987 to over 400 by 1990. Since this time there has been a nearly year-over-year increase in the number of lung transplants performed annually, with 2569 transplants done in 2021.[1]

Although outcomes have substantially improved since the early years of the specialty, the procedure still carries substantial short-term risks, and long-term outcomes are inferior to other solid organs. The Achilles heel of lung transplantation is no longer early mortality, as was the case in the first two decades after its inception. In the modern era, chronic rejection is the main cause of mortality in recipients, affecting about 50%. Chronic rejection is the principal reason for the 10-year survival rates falling to 33%.[5]

The following chapter will focus on topics most relevant to lung transplantation in the perioperative setting because these are most relevant to surgeons. We will also discuss the current knowledge surrounding chronic rejection and the risk factors that can be targeted to minimize it.

RECIPIENT SELECTION

The demand for suitable donor lungs has surpassed the supply for decades. As such, it is paramount that recipients are chosen carefully such that those undergoing transplantation have the highest odds of success. The ideal lung transplant candidate is one with an end-stage respiratory illness who has failed available nontransplant interventions and does not have medical comorbidities that may limit their survival. As such, the absolute contraindications to lung transplantation include conditions that significantly increase the risk of adverse postoperative outcomes, such as nonadherence to therapy, substance abuse, or end-organ dysfunction. Relative contraindications include recipient characteristics that have been associated with increased risk for an adverse

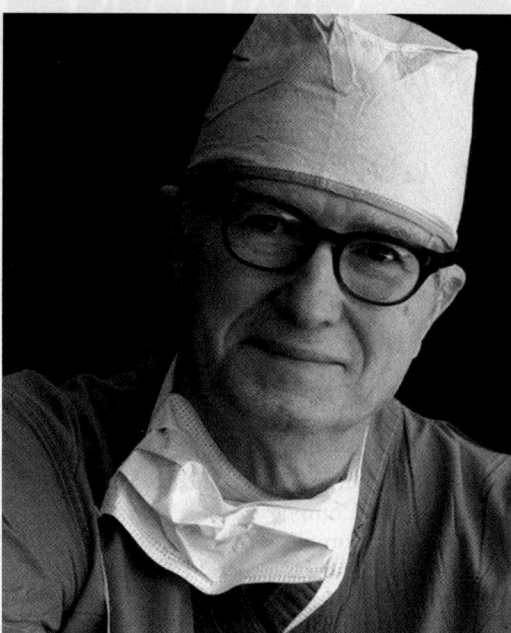

FIGURE 58.1 Dr. James Hardy at the University of Mississippi. (From Aru GM, Call KD, Creswell LL, et al. James D. Hardy: a pioneer in surgery [1918 to 2003]. *J Heart Lung Transplant.* 2004;23[11]:1307-1310, Figure 1.)

Patients are referred to transplant centers through both primary care providers and pulmonologists. The most common indications among transplanted recipients are chronic obstructive pulmonary disease (37%), interstitial lung disease (ILD) (30%), bronchiectasis (including cystic fibrosis; 19%), and pulmonary artery hypertension (4%). When considering a patient's candidacy for listing, the primary lung pathology influences the decision, as this has been shown to significantly alter outcomes. For example, the median survival of patients with cystic fibrosis after transplantation is 10 years, but 5 years for those with ILD. Furthermore, all effective medical therapies should be exhausted before pursuing transplantation. For instance, the number of cystic fibrosis–related lung transplants has significantly decreased in some countries after the availability of highly effective cystic fibrosis transmembrane conductance regulators. Lung retransplantation accounts for about 4% of transplants in the modern era, a figure that has increased in the past two decades. Retransplantation survival is inferior to that of primary recipients, but careful selection of these patients, including consideration of why the graft failed initially, results in acceptable outcomes.

The workup is focused on ascertaining surgical risk and estimating the probability of long-term survival assuming adequate graft function. Preoperative studies generally included high-resolution chest CT, echocardiogram, quantitative lung perfusion scan, bronchoscopy, pulmonary function tests, age-appropriate health screening, and right and left heart catheterization. All patients are discussed in a multidisciplinary manner through the transplant center before a listing decision is made.

The modern-day lung allocation system prioritizes patients with an urgent need for transplant, such as those mechanically ventilated or on extracorporeal membrane oxygenation (ECMO); such treatments are known as a *bridge to transplantation* and at times are initiated before a patient has been listed. ECMO and mechanical ventilation before transplantation have been associated with inferior

outcome to a lesser degree. Some centers, particularly those high in volume, will list patients with relative contraindications. The presence of multiple relative contraindications in a potential recipient must be closely considered because the detriment is thought to be multiplicative in terms of increasing risk. The absolute and relative contraindications to lung transplantation are summarized in Table 58.1.

TABLE 58.1   Absolute and Relative Contraindications to Lung Transplantation

Risk factors can change over time and may not be a contraindication for referral but when present at the time of listing or while listed for lung transplantation may increase risk for poor transplant outcomes. There was 100% consensus (24 committee members) for the content of the entirety of this table.

Absolute Contraindications:

- Candidates with these conditions are considered too high risk to achieve successful outcomes post lung transplantation.
- Factor or condition that significantly increases the risk of an adverse outcome posttransplant and/or would make transplant most likely harmful for a recipient.
- Most lung transplant programs should not transplant patients with these risk factors except under very exceptional or extenuating circumstances.

1. Lack of patient willingness or acceptance of transplant
2. Malignancy with high risk of recurrence or death related to cancer
3. Glomerular filtration rate <40 mL/min/1.73 m² unless being considered for multiorgan transplant
4. Acute coronary syndrome or myocardial infarction within 30 days (excluding demand ischemia)
5. Stroke within 30 days
6. Liver cirrhosis with portal hypertension or synthetic dysfunction unless being considered for multiorgan transplant
7. Acute liver failure
8. Acute renal failure with rising creatinine or on dialysis and low likelihood of recovery
9. Septic shock
10. Active extrapulmonary or disseminated infection
11. Active tuberculosis infection
12. HIV infection with detectable viral load
13. Limited functional status (e.g., nonambulatory) with poor potential for posttransplant rehabilitation
14. Progressive cognitive impairment
15. Repeated episodes of nonadherence without evidence of improvement (Note: For pediatric patients, this is not an absolute contraindication, and ongoing assessment of nonadherence should occur as they progress through different developmental stages.)
16. Active substance use or dependence including current tobacco use, vaping, marijuana smoking, or IV drug use
17. Other severe uncontrolled medical condition expected to limit survival after transplant

TABLE 58.1 Absolute and Relative Contraindications to Lung Transplantation—cont'd

Risk Factors With High or Substantially Increased Risk:

- Candidates with these conditions may be considered in centers with expertise specific to the condition.
- We may not have data to support transplanting patients with these risk factors, or there is substantially increased risk based on the currently available data, and further research is needed to better inform future recommendations.
- When more than one of these risk factors are present, they are thought to be possibly multiplicative in terms of increasing risk of adverse outcomes.
- Modifiable conditions should be optimized when possible.

1. Age >70 years
2. Severe coronary artery disease that requires coronary artery bypass grafting at transplant
3. Reduced left ventricular ejection fraction <40%
4. Significant cerebrovascular disease
5. Severe esophageal dysmotility
6. Untreatable hematologic disorders, including bleeding diathesis, thrombophilia, or severe bone marrow dysfunction
7. BMI >35 kg/m^2
8. BMI <16 kg/m^2
9. Limited functional status with potential for posttransplant rehabilitation
10. Psychiatric, psychological, or cognitive conditions with potential to interfere with medical adherence without sufficient support systems
11. Unreliable support system or caregiving plan
12. Lack of understanding of disease and/or transplant despite teaching
13. *Mycobacterium abscessus* infection
14. *Lomentospora prolificans* infection
15. *Burkholderia cenocepacia* or *gladioli* infection
16. Hepatitis B or C infection with detectable viral load and liver fibrosis
17. Chest wall or spinal deformity expected to cause restriction after transplant
18. Extracorporeal life support
19. Retransplant <1 year after initial lung transplant
20. Retransplant for restrictive CLAD
21. Retransplant for AMR as etiology for CLAD

Risk Factors:

- Risk factors with unfavorable implications for short- and/or long-term outcomes after lung transplant.
- Although acceptable for lung transplant programs to consider patients with these risk factors, multiple risk factors together may increase risk for adverse post–lung transplant outcomes.

1. Age 65–70 years
2. Glomerular filtration rate 40–60 mL/min/1.73 m^2
3. Mild to moderate coronary artery disease
4. Severe coronary artery disease that can be revascularized via percutaneous coronary intervention before transplant
5. Patients with prior coronary artery bypass grafting
6. Reduced left ventricular ejection fraction 40–50%
7. Peripheral vascular disease
8. Connective tissue diseases (scleroderma, lupus, inflammatory myopathies)
9. Severe gastroesophageal reflux disease
10. Esophageal dysmotility
11. Thrombocytopenia, leukopenia, or anemia with high likelihood of persistence after transplant
12. Osteoporosis
13. BMI 30–34.9 kg/m^2
14. BMI 16–17 kg/m^2
15. Frailty
16. Hypoalbuminemia
17. Diabetes that is poorly controlled
18. Edible marijuana use
19. *Scedosporium apiospermum* infection
20. HIV infection with undetectable viral load
21. Previous thoracic surgery
22. Prior pleurodesis
23. Mechanical ventilation
24. Retransplant >1 year for obstructive CLAD

AMR, Antibody-mediated rejection; *BMI,* body mass index; *CLAD,* chronic lung allograft dysfunction; *HIV,* human immunodeficiency virus; *IV,* intravenous.
From Leard LE, Holm AM, Valapour M, et al. Consensus document for the selection of lung transplant candidates: an update from the International Society for Heart and Lung Transplantation. *J Heart Lung Transplant.* 2021;40(11):1349-1379, Table 2.

outcomes, presumably because of debilitation. Therefore, every effort should be made to have patients being bridged to transplantation awake and able to participate in rehabilitation programs before transplantation. To this end, many centers have developed ambulatory ECMO programs, and ECMO as a bridge to transplant in the modern era has been shown to have similar survival to those non-bridged patients.[6] It has been shown that such "awake ECMO" before transplantation improves survival.

Another preoperative consideration that must be given to potential lung transplant recipients is whether to plan a single or double lung transplant. Satisfactory outcomes have been reported for each approach, and the decision is influenced by institutional practice patterns. Although no guidelines exist to govern this clinical dilemma, available evidence collectively suggests that double lung transplantation results in improved pulmonary function tests, freedom from chronic rejection, and better long-term survival after surgery. Single lung transplantation has the theoretical advantage of increasing the benefit to society given that one donor can provide lungs for two recipients. Among donors who contributed to a single lung transplant, however, it has been shown that only 43% donated both lungs, making this theoretical benefit less clear. Furthermore, the decision to perform a single or double lung transplantation is often made intraoperatively and discussed more later.

Recipient sensitization to donor antigens must also be carefully considered. Donor-specific antibodies, which most commonly occur after a prior organ transplantation, pregnancy, or blood transfusion, have been associated with antibody-mediated rejection and chronic lung allograft dysfunction (CLAD). Before adding a recipient to the waitlist, a common approach is to screen the person for compatibility with the general population; this is usually done via a panel reactive antibody (PRA) assay that tests a candidate's serum for reaction with lymphocytes from a large proportion of blood donors. The PRA estimates the probability of a positive crossmatch with the general population. Around 80% of potential recipients are not sensitized. Highly sensitized candidates, often defined as a PRA $\geq$80%, are considered high risk for the development of donor reactive antibodies and several complications after transplantation. Highly sensitized candidates have a longer waitlist time and increase in waitlist mortality. As a result, many centers consider high sensitization a contraindication to lung transplantation. Multiple strategies have been developed to successfully transplant highly sensitized candidates. One such strategy is a "virtual crossmatch" of donor antigens and recipient antibodies; this approach has been shown to be predictive of a negative actual crossmatch with high accuracy. Recipient "desensitization" is another strategy whereby highly sensitized recipients are treated with pre- or peritransplant multimodal therapies such as plasmapheresis, solumedrol, and/or rituximab. Although promising results have been seen with some desensitization protocols, such protocols vary considerably among institutions, and a standard of care has not been established.

LUNG ALLOCATION

Historically waitlist candidates were matched with donors based on their time on the waitlist, such that patients who had been on the waitlist the longest were prioritized for a transplant. This "first come, first serve" basis was suboptimal for several reasons. First, the most critically ill patients who would benefit most from a time-sensitive transplant could be behind less sick patients because of the time spent on the waitlist. Second, institutional practices govern when a patient should be placed on the waitlist, with some patients being waitlisted early in the disease course, before their need for a transplant. Additionally, prioritization based on waitlist time presented an opportunity for "gaming" of the system. In 2005 a more equitable system of lung allocation was established through the United Network for Organ Sharing (UNOS), whereby recipients are matched with a donor based on a lung allocation score (LAS) that is calculated based on their acuity and estimated length of survival postoperatively. With the LAS system, an algorithm is used to match donors with recipients in a

stepwise fashion based on the LAS, blood type, age, and distance between the two hospitals, with initial matches being made within a 250-mile radius. The advent of the LAS had several major implications, translating into a lower waitlist mortality and nearly double the amount of lung transplants being done.

In March 2023 a new method of lung allocation was implemented by the Organ Procurement and Transplantation Network based on a lung composite allocation score (CAS), replacing the LAS. In contrast to the LAS system, the lung CAS system integrates all variables in a continuous fashion and results in a single weighted score that is unique for each donor-recipient match. The major recipient variables and their respective maximum weights are summarized as follows:

- Medical urgency (25 points)
- Likelihood of survival >5 years posttransplant (25 points)
- Biologic challenges in matching (blood type, height, or sensitivity) (15 points)
- <18 years of age when listed for a transplant (20 points)
- Prior living organ donor (5 points)

The geographical variable in the LAS system was initially included to reduce ischemic time for the organ; this variable's weight is reduced in the lung CAS. Lung allocation under the new policy is expected to decrease deaths on the waitlist by 36% to 47% and increase the number of transplants among high-acuity recipients.[7]

DONOR SELECTION

There has been a record increase in US organ donation rates for the past 11 years in a row, presumably in part because of society's awareness of organ shortages and policies at the state level. Despite this increase, a persistent shortage of suitable donor lungs has remained, with lungs being used from only 23% of potential lung donors in the United States. Increasing the donor pool is one way to expand access for waitlist candidates, but these efforts must be carefully balanced with the potential for transplanting allografts with poor quality.

The historically used "ideal" lung donor criteria was established based on clinical experience and expert consensus rather than data-driven evidence. The main tenets of an ideal lung donor include the following:

- Age <55 years
- <20 pack-year smoking history
- Lack of chest trauma or prior cardiopulmonary surgery
- Negative sputum cultures and/or Gram stain
- Bronchoscopy without purulent secretions
- ABO compatibility
- PaO_2/FiO_2 (P/F) ratio >300
- Clear chest radiograph (CXR)
- Appropriate size match with recipient

Strict adherence to these guidelines is apt to result in inappropriately low utilization rates. Given the shortage of donor lungs that meet the ideal criteria, some centers have transplanted lungs outside of these guidelines for quite some time now, which are referred to as *marginal* or *extended* criteria donors. UNOS data have demonstrated that 80% of transplants in the recent era use extended criteria lungs, and 42% of transplants performed use lungs with two or more variables outside of the ideal donor criteria.[8] Studies on these variables show that extended criteria donors do not always result in inferior outcomes, and when they do, the risk-benefit ratio may still be acceptable for a recipient. For example, it has been shown in both adult and pediatric recipients that use of lungs previously

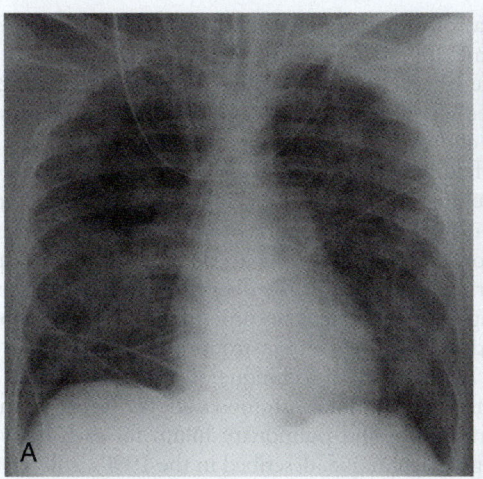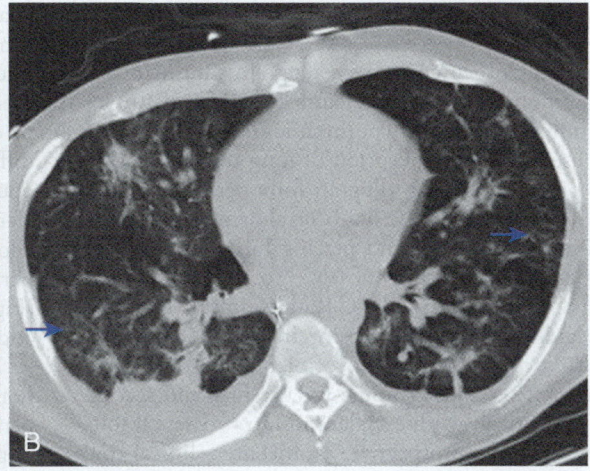

FIGURE 58.2 (A) CXR and (B) CT scan from a potential lung donor with findings of interstitial lung disease on chest CT scan. (From Gauthier JM, Bierhals AJ, Liu J, et al. Chest computed tomography imaging improves potential lung donor assessment. *J Thorac Cardiovasc Surg*. 2019;157[4]:1711-1718.e1, Figure 2.)

declined by at least three centers does not lead to inferior outcomes.[9] A recipient risk-adjusted model has suggested that donor P/F ratio, abnormal CXR, age, purulent secretions on bronchoscopy, and bacteremia/fungemia do not significantly influence recipient survival. Importantly, in this model donor smoking history did result in decreased survival. Although randomized, multi-institutional trials examining extended versus ideal lung donors are lacking, the available literature supports acceptance of extended criteria donor lungs on a case-by-case basis, and use of lungs with one or two variables outside of the ideal criteria is unlikely to adversely affect outcomes.

CT imaging was traditionally not a component of lung donor criteria because of cost and inconsistent availability of this technology at donor hospitals. In the modern era, however, around 60% of potential lung donors receive a CT scan. CT scans have created a valuable opportunity for donor assessment, as some lung pathology may be missed through evaluation with traditional means (i.e., CXR), such as structural lung disease (Fig. 58.2). A recent study found that CT findings of structural lung disease (emphysema and ILD) significantly decreased odds of lung utilization from potential donors.[10] Importantly, donor-recipient size match based on total lung capacity improves recipient survival, and methods have been established to accurately size match donors with recipients using donor CT scans.[11] As such, donor CT scans appear to be an important tool for remote evaluation of potential donors before the resource intensive "fly-out" for procurement.

Another area of interest in recent years to increase the donor pool is use of organs from drug overdose donors. Sadly, the US opioid epidemic has resulted in a drastic increase in "unintentional deaths," with this category being the main cause of death in those less than 45 years of age. Traditionally, organs from drug overdose donors were not used because of concerns of transplanting organs harboring a blood-borne illnesses. Improvements in screening and mainstream treatments for diseases such as HIV and hepatitis C have brought into question whether a lack of utilization is appropriate. UNOS data have revealed that heart donation from drug overdose donors does not result in adverse recipient survival. Although data on drug overdose donors in the setting of lung transplantation are limited, it stands to reason that recipient outcomes will similarly be unaffected, and if a blood-borne illness is contracted, modern medical therapy can suppress or cure it.

Four percent of all lung transplants performed in the United States from 2015–20 employed lungs from DCD donors, a figure that has risen from 1% in 2005–10.[12] Increased use of DCD lungs would surely expand the donor pool, but several concerns exist that limit their use. Inherent to DCD procurement is some degree of increased warm ischemia, which may lead to allograft injury. To this end, some have reported increased rates of airway complications and inferior survival among recipients receiving lungs from DCD donors. These concerns explain why only half of US transplant centers use DCD lungs, with higher-volume centers using more DCD lungs than lower-volume centers.[12,13] However, most studies now suggest that there is no difference in outcomes using DCD and donation after brain death (DBD) donor lungs. Another barrier to increasing the use of DCD organs is the consent process, which varies considerably worldwide. For example, several European countries have an "opt-out" (presumed consent) system for organ donation, whereas the United States operates in an "opt-in" (explicit consent) system. Single-center studies from Europe have shown that DCD lung donations account for 15% to 45% of all lung transplants (compared with 4% in the United States).[14] Finally, a significant amount of potential DCD donors do not progress to death, and "negative" fly-out rates of up to 40% have been reported.[15] These obstacles can be overcome with national policies and institutional investment that facilitate the use of DCD organs.

The advent of specialized donor care facilities (SDCFs) has also presented a unique opportunity to improve donor utilization. In the SDCF model DBD donors are transported to a free-standing medical facility in geographic proximity to a major transplant center. Donor management, organ allocation, and the procurement procedure are all performed at the SDCF, and use of the SDCF model has been associated with decreased surgeon travel time, increased organ yield, and use of extended criteria donors for multiorgan transplantation. The SDCF model also appears to be cost-effective, particularly with regard to management of heart and lung donors.[16] SDCFs may also facilitate lung focus resuscitation protocols that have been shown to increase lung utilization rates. Importantly, the recent changes to the lung allocation process may have an impact on the efficacy of SDCFs, and studies are warranted in the new era of this allocation system.

LUNG PRESERVATION

During traditional lung procurement, the allograft is flushed with a preservation solution, fully inflated, and then placed on ice (4°C). This traditional method of hypothermic static cold storage has been widely used since the inception of lung transplantation and is known to preserve the lung allograft for a period of 6 to 8 hours. However, lung storage at 4°C has been shown to be deleterious to mitochondrial function, and placing lung grafts on ice can result in allograft temperatures of 0°C. To this end, it was recently shown that lung storage at 10°C leads to improved mitochondrial health and lung function in a porcine model; this strategy was applied to a cohort of human recipients with a median preservation time of 12.5 and 14 hours for the first and second implanted lung, respectively, with excellent results.[17] These results were recently extended to a prospective, multicenter clinical trial whereby 70 transplants using donor lungs with an overnight procurement were not allowed to start until 6 a.m. and matched with controls using a traditional 24/7 schedule. Importantly, there were no differences in outcomes, demonstrating that prolonged cold storage at 10°C is safe.[18]

Ex vivo lung perfusion (EVLP) is a relatively new method of lung preservation whereby donor lungs are ventilated and perfused outside of the body before implantation in the recipient (Fig. 58.3). The technology allows for assessment of donor lungs through a variety of biochemical and physiologic measurements for up to 24 hours at normothermic temperatures. EVLP has been used principally to assess extended criteria and DCD lungs before acceptance by a transplant center. The Toronto group has demonstrated that EVLP can be used to increase the donor pool using "high-risk" extended criteria donor lungs (i.e., DCD status, P/F ratio <300 mm Hg, poor compliance) with equivalent short- and long-term recipient outcomes. Several EVLP protocols have been published, with the most widely adopted pathway being transportation of donor lungs to an EVLP center for initiation of EVLP before acceptance. Commercially available portable EVLP devices are also being used that allow for onsite initiation of EVLP at the donor hospital, which is maintained during transport to the transplant center (Fig. 58.4).[19] EVLP has presented a window of opportunity for treatment and/or reconditioning of donor lungs before implantation. Multiple interventions via EVLP have been demonstrated with good results over the past decade, including fibrinolysis of pulmonary embolisms, recruitment of atelectasis, delivery of high-dose antibiotics, and bioengineering with cellular and gene therapies. For example, the Toronto group recently demonstrated with a porcine model that intermittent 4-hour cycles of EVLP could be used to store porcine lungs for 3 days with satisfactory early outcomes, highlighting the tremendous potential that this technology has to increase the donor pool and organ sharing possibilities.[20]

TECHNICAL ASPECTS OF LUNG TRANSPLANTATION

The first reported lung transplants, performed by both Jim Hardy at the University of Mississippi in 1963 and the Toronto lung transplant team in 1983, involved single lung implants with the bronchial, arterial, and venous anastomosis performed through a posterolateral thoracotomy.[2,3] As the development of the field led to the exploration of the advantage of double lung transplantation, attempts to implant both lungs were initially performed en bloc, with airway continuity restored through a single tracheal anastomosis through a median sternotomy. However, it soon became apparent that this technique was likely to result in a high rate of tracheal dehiscence and technical failure.[3] Although the median sternotomy was the original and often still the exposure of choice in select centers, limitations of this approach include difficulty in dissection of the posterior chest wall, control of intraoperative bleeding, and tracheal anastomotic complications. The clamshell anterior thoracotomy provides excellent exposure and allows for simultaneous access to both pleural spaces and to the pericardial space for the dissection and anastomosis of the grafts[21] (Fig. 58.5). This has become the exposure of choice at our center and many other centers around the world.

As the modern technique of sequential double lung transplantation emerged, the anastomoses are performed at the junction of the pericardium and pulmonary hilum for each individual organ. The original technique, described in the 1990s, still serves as the basis for the technical aspects of lung transplantation implantation in the majority of centers.[21] Technical aspects involve the dissection of the superior and inferior pulmonary veins, which sit in the most ventral portion of the hilum, followed by the pulmonary artery and bronchus. The vascular structures are divided using stapling devices while the bronchus is transected sharply. Limited dissection is performed in and around the bronchus to preserve its blood supply and allow for optimization of healing. As the bronchial anastomosis relies on systemic arterial circulation for its vascular supply—the portion of the dual pulmonary circulation that is not surgically restored at the time of implantation—this aspect of the implant remains the most precarious. Airway complications can range from ischemic injury to stenosis.[22] Early in the development of lung transplantation, the recognition that high-dose corticosteroids resulted in excessive bronchial dehiscence[23,24] led to multiple ancillary techniques to augment healing. These efforts went as far as wrapping omentum around the bronchial structures.[25] After both clinical and experimental investigation, however, the current successful techniques for the bronchial anastomosis depend on very short bronchial stumps[26] and running monofilament suture anastomoses.[27]

With the advent of robotically assisted thoracic surgery, clinical efforts have also been directed for using this technique for lung transplantation as a possible method of decreasing pain and improving quality of life in recipients. This approach involves the use of specialized robotic instruments and a high-definition camera system that allow for small incisions to minimize trauma to the chest. The group from Cedars-Sinai Medical Center in Los Angeles reported the first series with minimal rates of ischemic injury and reasonable operating times in eight patients.[28]

Although the majority of lung transplants are performed in adults for acquired disease, a total of 25 out of 2569 lung transplants reported to the Scientific Registry of Transplant Recipients were younger than 17 years of age.[1] This number, however, has substantially decreased over the past couple of years because of improved care for conditions such as pulmonary hypertension and cystic fibrosis. Pediatric lung transplantation presents unique challenges because of the smaller size of both donor and recipient organs. Donor lungs must be carefully matched to the recipient's chest size to ensure a proper fit. Surgeons must also adapt their surgical techniques to the smaller anatomy, often requiring finer suturing and meticulous dissection to achieve successful outcomes. In addition to the technical difficulties, pediatric patients do not have ease of access to a dedicated children's program and often suffer long wait times and increased mortality.[29] To address some of these issues, select centers have advocated for living donor lobar lung transplantation, a procedure where a healthy living donor donates a portion of their lung to the recipient.

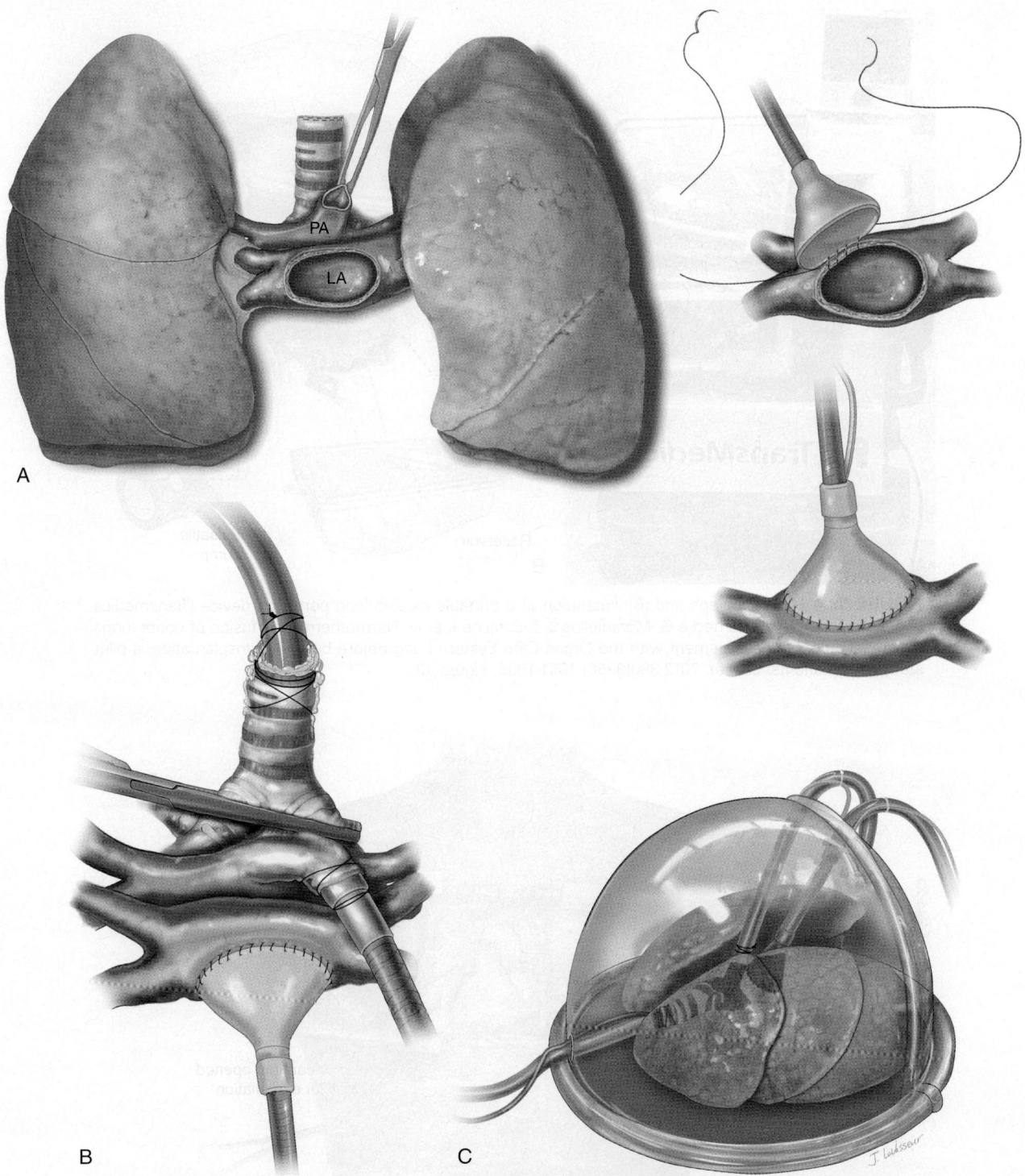

FIGURE 58.3 (A) Donor lung bloc prior to cannulation for ex vivo lung perfusion (EVLP). (B) Airway and vascular anastomoses for the EVLP circuit. (C) Donor lungs on EVLP. *LA,* Left atrium; *PA,* pulmonary artery. (From Cypel M, Keshavjee S. Ex vivo lung perfusion. *Oper Tech Thorac Cardiovasc Surg.* 2014;19:433-442, Figure 1A, 3C, and 4.)

Although originally described in 1990 in Los Angeles,[30] this technique has been popularized in Japan, where cadaveric DBD can be hindered by systemic and societal issues. This procedure involves the recovery of a right lower and left lower from two living donors, who are usually the parents, with implantation into the orthotopic position.[31]

INTRAOPERATIVE MECHANICAL SUPPORT

The options for lung transplantation include no extracorporeal mechanical support, the use of full cardiopulmonary bypass, or the use of ECMO. A full cardiopulmonary bypass circuit includes inflow and outflow cannulas as well as a blood reservoir and pump

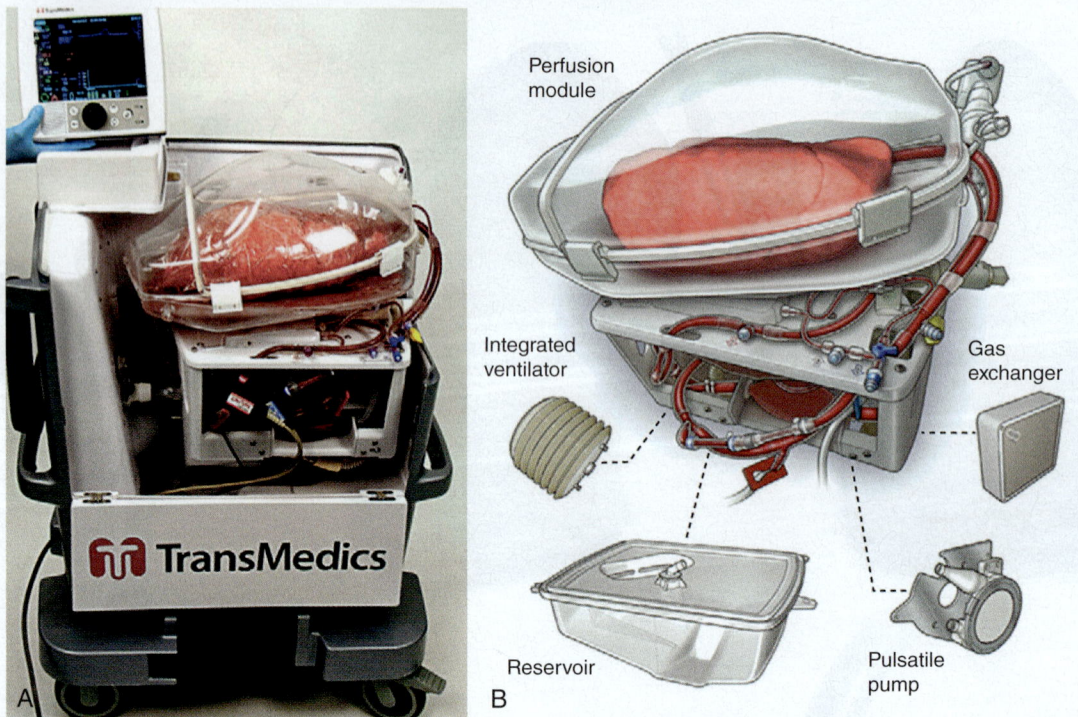

FIGURE 58.4 (A) Photograph and (B) illustration of a portable ex vivo lung perfusion device (Transmedics Organ Care System). (Warnecke G, Moradiellos J, Tudorache I, et al. Normothermic perfusion of donor lungs for preservation and assessment with the Organ Care System Lung before bilateral transplantation: a pilot study of 12 patients. *Lancet.* 2012;380[9856]:1851-1858, Figure 19.)

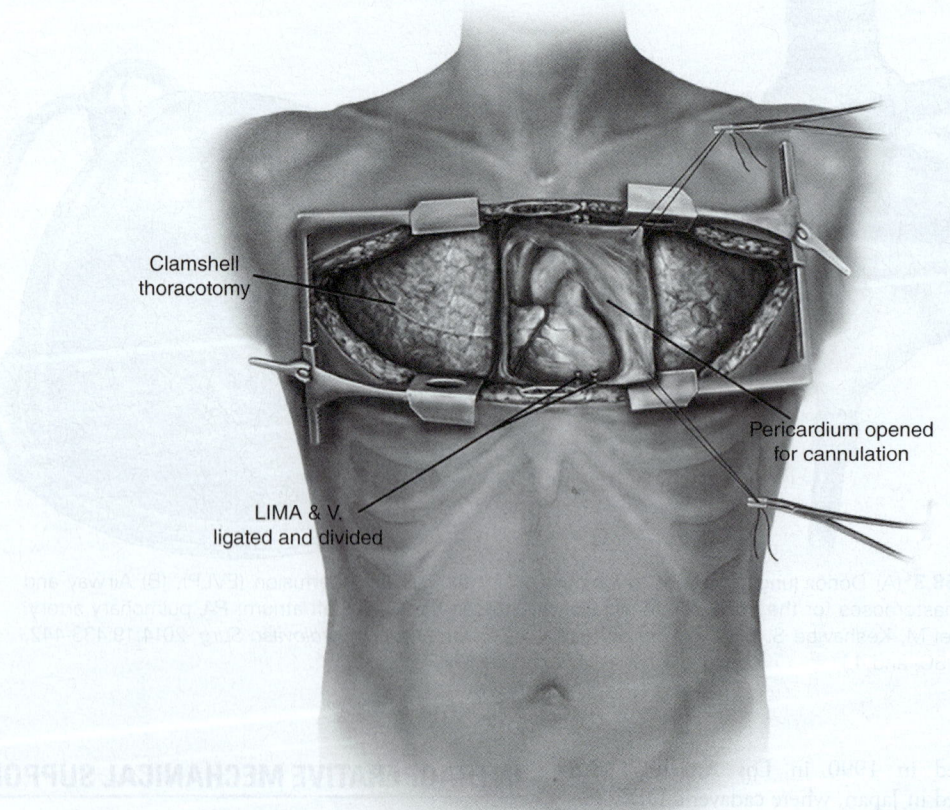

FIGURE 58.5 Surgical approaches for lung transplantation (clamshell incision). *LIMA,* Left internal mammary artery; *LIMV,* left internal mammary vein. (Hayanga JW, D'Cunha J. The surgical technique of bilateral sequential lung transplantation. *J Thorac Dis.* 2014;6[8]:1063-1069, Figure 2.)

suckers that allow for the direct return of blood from the operating field to the circuit. Although such a setup has many advantages, such as easy control of the circulation and intravascular status because of the ability to rapidly return any lost blood to the patient, there are multiple disadvantages as well. The large blood surface interface requires a high level of anticoagulation and results in the elaboration of many proinflammatory cytokines.[32] Based on this, many centers have advocated for the use of ECMO as a means of intraoperative circulatory support during lung transplantation. Unlike full cardiopulmonary bypass, the ECMO circuit is a closed system with no direct air/blood interface and less surface area for exposure to plastic components of the circuit. Thus, less, or even no, anticoagulation is required, and lower levels of proinflammatory cytokines are elaborated intraoperatively. In 2022 the American Association for Thoracic Surgery rendered an expert consensus document on the use of mechanical circulatory support in lung transplantation.[33] Recommendations of this 16-person panel included the use of ECMO support intraoperatively through central canulation of the aorta and right atrium as the preferred method for circulatory support during lung transplantation. The examined data concluded that the use of such a system does not hinder chest closure, may be safely used with minimal or no anticoagulation, can decrease the chance of ischemia/reperfusion injury, and may still allow for sternal-sparing lung implantation. The only clear indication for the use of full cardiopulmonary is when concomitant intracardiac repair is required along with lung transplantation.

POSTOPERATIVE CONSIDERATIONS AND IMMUNOSUPPRESSION

Postoperative care in lung transplant recipients requires a multidisciplinary approach to be effective for long-term success. Several tenets of postoperative care are specifically unique to lung transplant recipients. Immunosuppression can be divided into (1) induction in the immediate perioperative period, (2) maintenance agents designed to prevent acute rejection, and (3) agents used to reverse the course of diagnosed acute rejection. In recent years, the evolution of immunosuppressive strategies has led to more tailored and precise approaches, aiming to strike a balance between protecting the graft and minimizing side effects.

Induction agents are medications administered at the time of transplant surgery or shortly thereafter to provide powerful initial suppression of the recipient's immune system. These induction agents help prevent acute rejection of the transplanted organ at the time of implantation and during the direct postoperative period. There is no standardized regimen that is outlined for lung transplantation recipients, and each regimen is center specific. Furthermore, the rationale for such therapy in lung transplantation is based on results in other organs because studies of induction immunosuppression for the lung are small and retrospective in nature with conflicting results. Nevertheless, there is a trend suggesting that induction agents decrease the incidence of acute rejection and provide improvements in long-term outcomes without a significant increase in infectious complications or adverse side effects.[34-36] Some common immunosuppressive induction agents used in lung transplantation include:

1. Antithymocyte globulin (ATG), which is a polyclonal antibody preparation derived from the serum of rabbits or horses immunized with human thymocytes. ATG works by targeting and depleting T lymphocytes through a process known as *antibody-dependent cellular cytotoxicity*. Because the initial recognition of alloantigen depends on recognition of foreign major histocompatibility complex on donor graft by T cells, such depletion helps prevent acute rejection of the transplanted organ. When using ATG, it is important to monitor the patient's white blood cell and platelet count, as severe thrombocytopenia and leukopenia can occur on initiation. ATG has also been associated with significant pulmonary infiltrates and acute respiratory distress syndrome, which significantly increase mortality.

2. Monoclonal antibodies as induction agents have been proven to significantly reduce rates of both acute and chronic rejections. Basiliximab is a monoclonal antibody that specifically inhibits interleukin (IL)-2 receptors on the surface of activated T cells. By blocking these receptors, basiliximab reduces T-cell activation and proliferation, which are critical processes in the immune response. Daclizumab, a similar agent to basiliximab, is a monoclonal antibody that targets IL-2 receptors on T cells. Alemtuzumab is another monoclonal antibody that targets CD52, a protein found on the surface of B and T cells. In addition to these agents, high-dose corticosteroids are often administered.

Unlike induction immunosuppression, which is often omitted at the time of implantation, maintenance immunosuppressive agents are an essential component of the long-term care of lung transplant recipients. These medications are administered after the initial transplantation procedure to prevent the recipient's immune system from rejecting the transplanted lungs. The goal is to strike a balance between suppressing the immune response to prevent rejection and minimizing the risk of infections and medication-related side effects. The core immunosuppression for lung transplantation consists of calcineurin inhibitors such as tacrolimus (Prograf) and cyclosporine (Neoral). Calcineurin is a serine/threonine protein phosphatase that participates in a number of cellular processes and calcium-dependent signal transduction pathways. Calcineurin inhibitors bind to specific proteins called *cyclophilins* (for cyclosporine) and *FK-binding proteins* (for tacrolimus). These drug-protein complexes then bind to calcineurin, preventing its activation by blocking calcineurin's function as a transcription factor. This is such a powerful pathway of immunoactivation that the modern era of successful organ transplantation only began after the discovery of this class of drugs.[37]

Medications like mycophenolate mofetil (CellCept) and azathioprine (Imuran) inhibit the proliferation of immune cells through disruption of DNA synthesis and are known as *antiproliferative agents*. For cells with high proliferation rates such as T cells and B cells, these inhibitors act as a significant barrier to immunoactivation and the generation of a productive immune response. In addition to these two classes of agents, corticosteroids, such as prednisone or other agents in this class, are often used initially after transplantation to control inflammation and prevent acute rejection. The dosing of corticosteroids is quickly tapered postoperatively because of the high side effect profile, but it is rare to discontinue this class of drugs after lung transplantation.

Individualized immunosuppressive regimens: The specific combination and dosages of maintenance immunosuppressive agents vary from patient to patient and are determined by the transplant team based on factors such as the recipient's medical history, previous response to medications, and risk of rejection. For patients who receive lung transplantation, they are often discharged on triple-drug maintenance therapy consisting of a calcineurin inhibitor, an antiproliferative agent, and a corticosteroid. The agents of choice vary from center to center, and patients are closely followed in the outpatient setting to progressively taper these medications as they progress in order to balance immunosuppression and infection risk.

Perioperative and prophylactic medications for infection: Perioperative antibiotics are administered to prevent infections that can occur immediately after transplantation. The selection of antibiotics is guided by donor culture results to ensure the most effective coverage against potential pathogens. The duration of antibiotic therapy typically ranges from 5 to 14 days, depending on the patient's risk factors and the absence of signs of infection.

Inhaled antibiotics are medications that are administered directly into the lungs through inhalation and are commonly used in postoperative lung transplants with positive donor cultures and to prevent both acute and chronic rejection. They are used to treat respiratory infections, particularly those involving the lower respiratory tract. Many studies have shown that the usage of inhaled antibiotics has been associated with better long-term outcomes, as lung transplant recipients are at higher risk of multidrug-resistant respiratory infections throughout their course as an organ recipient. Examples of inhaled antibiotics include but are not limited to:

Tobramycin: Tobramycin is commonly used in lung transplant recipients to prevent and treat respiratory infections, particularly those caused by gram-negative bacteria like *Pseudomonas aeruginosa.* Inhaled tobramycin is frequently used as a prophylactic antibiotic to reduce the risk of posttransplant infections and as a treatment for lung infections. It helps maintain lung function and reduces the risk of CLAD, a condition that can lead to graft failure.

Colistimethate sodium: Colistimethate sodium is used in lung transplant recipients to treat infections caused by multidrug-resistant gram-negative bacteria, including *P. aeruginosa.* It is reserved for serious infections when other antibiotics have failed or when there is a high likelihood of multidrug-resistant pathogens.

Aztreonam: Aztreonam is used to treat respiratory infections caused by *P. aeruginosa,* particularly in patients with cystic fibrosis. Like inhaled tobramycin, aztreonam is employed to manage bacterial infections and prevent complications posttransplant. It can be part of a comprehensive treatment plan to prevent graft rejection.

Itraconazole: Itraconazole is primarily an antifungal medication used to treat fungal infections, including those affecting the lungs.

Amikacin: Amikacin is another aminoglycoside antibiotic used to treat respiratory infections, especially those caused by gram-negative bacteria. It may be considered in lung transplant recipients with specific bacterial infections that are resistant to other antibiotics or as part of a multidrug regimen.

Levofloxacin: Levofloxacin is a fluoroquinolone antibiotic used in the treatment of chronic lung infections, particularly in non–cystic fibrosis bronchiectasis. Levofloxacin can be beneficial in preventing or managing respiratory infections in lung transplant recipients, especially in those with bronchiectasis or other underlying lung conditions.

Inhaled antibiotics are preferred in some cases because they can deliver the medication directly to the site of infection in the lungs, resulting in higher drug concentrations and fewer systemic side effects compared with oral or intravenous antibiotics. They are typically administered using nebulizer devices, inhalers, or specialized inhalation systems designed for these medications.

In patients who are culture negative with no signs of infection, there are multiple prophylactic medications that patients will remain on indefinitely to mitigate the risk of a significant infection. The specific medications and regimens may vary depending on the recipient's medical history, immunosuppression protocol, and local guidelines. It can be notably difficult to balance these medications, the immunosuppressive regimens, and the overlapping adverse side effects. The use of these medications is often closely monitored by the transplant team, as each is associated with their own unique side effect profile. Some common prophylactic infection medications for lung transplant recipients include:

- Trimethoprim-sulfamethoxazole to prevent *Pneumocystis jirovecii* pneumonia.
- Azithromycin to prevent *Mycobacterium avium* complex infections.
- Ciprofloxacin or levofloxacin for bacterial coverage.
- Antivirals: Lung transplant recipients are at risk of viral infections, particularly from cytomegalovirus (CMV) and herpes simplex virus (HSV). Agents include:
  - Valganciclovir or ganciclovir for CMV prophylaxis.
  - Acyclovir or valacyclovir for HSV prophylaxis.
- Antifungals: Fungal infections, such as invasive aspergillosis and candidiasis. Agents include:
  - Fluconazole for *Candida* prophylaxis.
  - Itraconazole, voriconazole, or posaconazole for *Aspergillus* prophylaxis.

Lung transplant recipients should also receive vaccinations according to a specific schedule to prevent infections such as influenza, pneumonia, and hepatitis. These vaccinations are typically administered once the patient's immune system is stable posttransplant.

OUTCOMES AND POSTOPERATIVE COMPLICATIONS

Early Postoperative Complications

Primary graft dysfunction (PGD), as defined by the International Society of Heart and Lung Transplantation (ISHLT), is a syndrome of acute lung injury that can be seen in the early postoperative period after lung transplantation. PGD is thought to be the result of ischemic-reperfusion injury, with an incidence rate ranging from 11% to 25%. Mortality rates for those who develop PGD can be as high as 30% within the first 30 days, and many studies have shown that the presence of PGD leads to higher rates of rejection and worse long-term survival. PGD is typically graded on a standardized scale per ISHLT guidelines, ranging from PGD grade 0 to 3. These grades are assigned at specific time points, beginning with single lung reperfusion or second lung reperfusion, and continue for 72 hours after transplant, with assessments at 24-hour intervals. The severity of PGD is determined based on the presence of pulmonary edema observed on CXR and the P/F ratio regardless of the presence of mechanical ventilation (Fig. 58.6 and Table 58.2). It is important to note that the use of ECMO support postoperatively, regardless of the time of cannulation, is categorized as PGD grade 3 if pulmonary infiltrates are present and if the primary reason for ECMO is hypoxia. However, individuals on ECMO support postoperatively without pulmonary infiltrates and with indications other than hypoxia should be classified as "ungradable."

Atrial fibrillation (AF) and other atrial arrhythmias are relatively common after lung transplantation, with an occurrence rate of as high as 50% of patients. Some preoperative risk factors for AF include prior history of atrial arrhythmias, advanced age,

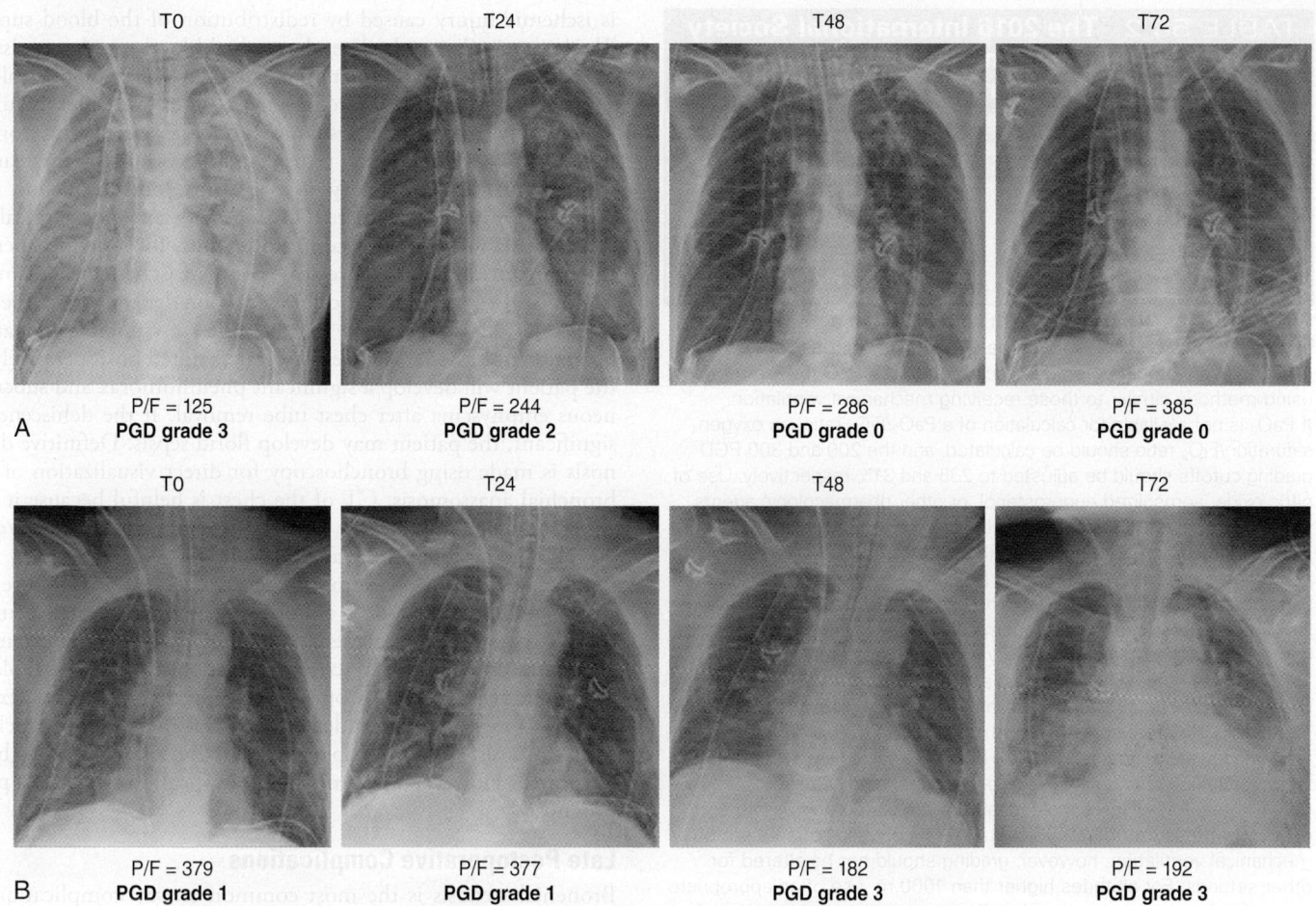

FIGURE 58.6 CXRs from two lung transplant recipients demonstrating (A) early, transient and (B) late, increasing PGD. *P/F ratio*, PaO_2/FiO_2; *PGD*, primary graft dysfunction. (Van Slambrouck J, Van Raemdonck D, Vos R, et al. A focused review on primary graft dysfunction after clinical lung transplantation: a multilevel syndrome. *Cells.* 2022;11[4]:745, Figure 1.)

pulmonary fibrosis, enlarged atria, and a history of coronary artery disease. In lung transplantation, the manipulation and implantation of the pulmonary veins as a single venous cuff to left atrial tissue are thought to play a role in arrhythmia because the pulmonary veins are a common origin for atrial arrhythmias. Atrial arrhythmias may require medication or, in severe cases, electrical cardioversion.

Excess fluid accumulation in the pleural space is a common complication after lung transplantation. These effusions develop ipsilaterally to the transplanted lung with a combination of blood and lymphatic drainage. In the days directly after transplantation, it is known that there is an increase in alveolar permeability because of ischemic-reperfusion–related inflammation, denervation, and disruption of the native lymphatics. It is important to point out that lymphatic drainage after lung transplantation does not reestablish itself for at least 2 weeks after implantation[38]; thus, pulmonary edema remains a major issue after lung transplantation. This can result in prolonged chest tube requirements and strict fluid management. It is generally accepted that chest tubes can be removed when the output reaches 150 to 200 mL/24 hours.

Pneumothorax is the presence of air in the pleural space, which can cause lung collapse. For patients who undergo any thoracic intervention, there is always a risk of developing a pneumothorax even with a chest tube in place. Factors such as donor-recipient size mismatch can contribute to the development of a pneumothorax

if the transplanted lung cannot fill the entire space. Any pleural injury at the time of transplant can also result in air leaks leading to a pneumothorax. It is important to note that if a new pneumothorax develops 7 to 10 days after transplant, a patient should undergo a bronchoscopy to evaluate the bronchial anastomosis for possible dehiscence.

Complications related to vascular anastomotic complications carry a large morbidity and mortality but are overall rare, with a rate of 1% to 3%. These complications include kinking of the vessel, vessel misalignment, vessel stenosis, vessel thrombosis, and vessel dissection. The usage of intraoperative transesophageal echocardiography intraoperatively to evaluate pulmonary artery and pulmonary vein flow can provide a means of early detection for any vascular complications. Pulmonary venous complications are generally noted within a few hours after surgery and present with unilateral or focal areas of pulmonary infiltrates because of pulmonary congestion. These patients can suffer from hypoxia and subsequent hemodynamic instability. Pulmonary artery complications are often diagnosed later because the patient will often develop pulmonary artery hypertension with associated hypoxia. As the transplanted lungs have their bronchial blood supply, they are at elevated risk for infarction if pulmonary artery blood flow is compromised.

Management of vascular complications can vary depending on the degree and etiology. For those with mild obstruction, conservative

TABLE 58.2 The 2016 International Society for Heart and Lung Transplantation Primary Graft Dysfunction Definition

GRADE	PULMONARY EDEMA ON CHEST X-RAY	PAO₂/FIO₂ RATIO
PGD grade 0	No	Any
PGD grade 1	Yes	>300
PGD grade 2	Yes	200–300
PGD grade 3	Yes	<200

Grade severity notes: Patients with no evidence of pulmonary edema on chest x-ray are considered grade 0. Absence of invasive mechanical ventilation should be graded according to the PaO_2/FiO_2 ratio, using methods similar to those receiving mechanical ventilation.
If PaO_2 is not available for calculation of a PaO_2/FiO_2 ratio, an oxygen saturation/FiO_2 ratio should be calculated, and the 200 and 300 PGD grading cutoffs should be adjusted to 235 and 315, respectively. Use of nitric oxide, aerosolized epoprostenol, or other pharmacologic agents that may improve oxygenation should not change grading methods.
Use of extracorporeal lung support (ECLS) with bilateral pulmonary edema on chest x-ray image should be graded as grade 3, and ECLS use should be explicitly recorded. The use of ECLS for nonhypoxic indications without pulmonary edema on chest x-ray imaging should be considered ungradable and explicitly recorded separately.
Time window notes: PGD is graded at four points: every 24 hours and over the first 72 hours after transplantation (T0, T24, T48, and T72 hours). Time starts at reperfusion of second lung. T0, T24, T48, and T72 have time windows ± 6 hours. If multiple blood gas values are available, the worst PaO_2/FiO_2 ratio on a given calendar day should be used.
Other notes: PaO_2/FiO_2 should ideally be measured on positive end-expiratory pressure of 5 cm H_2O at FiO_2 of 1.0 while patients are on mechanical ventilation; however, grading should not be altered for other settings. For altitudes higher than 1000 m, use of an appropriate correction factor is recommended. For comparative purposes, single lung transplantation is recommended to be reported separately from bilateral lung transplant without change in grading methodology.
Fio₂, Fraction of inspired oxygen; *Pao₂*, partial pressure of arterial oxygen; *PGD*, primary graft dysfunction.
Snell GI, Yusen RD, Weill D, et al. Report of the ISHLT Working Group on Primary Lung Graft Dysfunction, part I: definition and grading – a 2016 Consensus Group statement of the International Society for Heart and Lung Transplantation. *J Heart Lung Transplant.* 2017; 36(10):1097-1103, Table 4.

management with outpatient intervention is a viable option. Balloon angioplasty dilation for stenosis or systemic anticoagulation for mild thrombosis is often enough to manage these mild pathologies. If the stenosis or thrombosis is significant enough to cause an acute infarction of the lung, this is an indication for emergent reoperation and surgical intervention; however, the mortality is generally very high. The timing of when the stenosis is noted plays a key role in determining what interventions can be offered. For patients in the early postoperative period, significant stenosis causing hypoxia and hemodynamic compromise will need surgical intervention. If these issues are noted in the outpatient setting, endovascular interventions such as angioplasty or balloon dilation, with or without stenting, can be used. Overall prognosis of these complications varies significantly and depends on the severity and time of diagnosis as well as the intervention used.

Bronchial dehiscence and complications are decreasing in frequency after lung transplantation but still carry a significant morbidity if they do occur. One reason for bronchial complications

is ischemic injury caused by redistribution of the blood supply. The lung, similar to the liver, has a dual blood supply consisting of deoxygenated pulmonary and oxygen-rich systemic blood supply. Under normal circumstances, the bronchial cartilage relies primarily on the systemic bronchial circulation for its blood supply. Because lung transplantation occurs by the reanastomosis of the pulmonary artery, veins, and bronchus, the systemic bronchial vessels rely on ingrowth and not surgical reanastomosis to reestablish continuity. Thus, for a defined period the bronchus undergoes a relative phase of ischemia that can result in dehiscence. The clinical presentation depends on the severity of the dehiscence, as it can be either a complete or partial breakdown. Either a persistent air leak is noted postoperatively or the patient will develop a significant pneumothorax and subcutaneous emphysema after chest tube removal. If the dehiscence is significant, the patient may develop florid sepsis. Definitive diagnosis is made using bronchoscopy for direct visualization of the bronchial anastomosis. CT of the chest is helpful because it can show bronchial wall defects, narrowing of the airway, wall irregularities, and air around the anastomosis.

Management of anastomotic defects depends on the severity. For small defects that are 4 cm or less, conservative management such as chest tube placement, aspiration monitoring, extended antibiotic and antifungal coverage, endobronchial stent placement, and serial bronchoscopies to track healing has shown excellent outcomes. For larger defects, surgical interventions such as reanastomosis, flap bronchoplasty, or retransplantation has been advocated. However, any bronchial complication portends a poor prognosis.

Late Postoperative Complications

Bronchial stenosis is the most common airway complication in lung transplant and usually occurs 2 to 3 months later. This stenosis can occur either at the site of the anastomosis or at a nonanastomotic segmental branch; however, the latter is rare. Vanishing bronchus syndrome is a severe form of nonanastomotic stenosis of the bronchus intermedius that is associated with a high morbidity and mortality. Bronchial stenosis is thought to be the result of chronic inflammation and immunologic cytolytic airway damage over a prolonged period, leading to scar tissue and overall narrowing of the airway. However, as described earlier, it can also be the result of an initial ischemic injury leading to scarring. Bronchial stenosis can lead to symptoms like cough, wheezing, and decreased airflow with notable declines in forced expiratory volume in 1 second (FEV_1) and peak expiratory flow. Diagnosis is done though bronchoscopy, but CT of the chest with 3D reconstruction is often helpful with interventional planning.

Standard forms of management include endoscopic intervention such as balloon dilation and stent placement. If granulation tissue is present contributing to the stenosis, removal of the tissue using cryotherapy, electrocautery, or argon laser before balloon dilation has been successful. Some data suggest that topical application of mitomycin C after debridement may reduce the incidence of granulation tissue, but these data are controversial.[39] For mild obstructions, serial dilation and close follow-up for recurrence are sufficient for management. For patients who are unable to maintain airway patency, the usage of removable airway stents for 2 to 3 months has been found effective because it allows the airway to heal and remodel.

Bronchomalacia is a potential postoperative complication that can occur after lung transplantation, although it is relatively rare. It is defined as narrowing of the bronchial airway by 50% or more during exhalation and is mostly seen 3 to 4 months after transplant as a dynamic stenosis. Patients present with dyspnea, cough, possible stridor, and recurrent airway infection. On spirometry, they will show an obstructive airway disease pattern with a drop in FEV_1, peak expiratory rate, and forced expiratory flow. Diagnosis is done using bronchoscopy and CT of the chest with 3D reconstruction. Asymptomatic patients do not require intervention; however, if patients do become symptomatic, it can be managed using nocturnal noninvasive positive pressure and airway stenting.

Chronic Lung Allograft Dysfunction

CLAD refers to a progressive and irreversible decline in the function of the transplanted lungs over time. CLAD is a broad term that encompasses various clinical and pathologic entities that are hard to reverse once they occur. The common denominator for this form of rejection is scar tissue accumulation and fibrosis. The

prevalence of CLAD has been persistent, with an occurrence rate of 50% at 5 years and contributes to significant overall mortality of lung transplant recipients at 5 years.

Subtypes of CLAD are defined based on spirometry, clinical parameters, and imaging, with the two recognized subtypes being defined as bronchiolitis obliterans syndrome (BOS) and restrictive allograft syndrome (RAS). BOS was the first subtype of CLAD identified and is characterized by progressive airflow limitation caused by small airway inflammation and fibrosis (Fig. 58.7A). It is defined as a ≥20% decline in FEV_1 for the best postoperative baseline over 2 measurements with a ≥3-week interval between measurements. BOS severity is graded on a scale from 0 to 3 based on spirometry. RAS is characterized by reduced lung compliance and can be challenging to diagnose because of its subtle presentation. It is accepted that RAS, or restrictive CLAD, is another form of chronic rejection, but with a distinct phenotype when compared with BOS (see Fig. 58.7B). RAS is characterized by restrictive lung

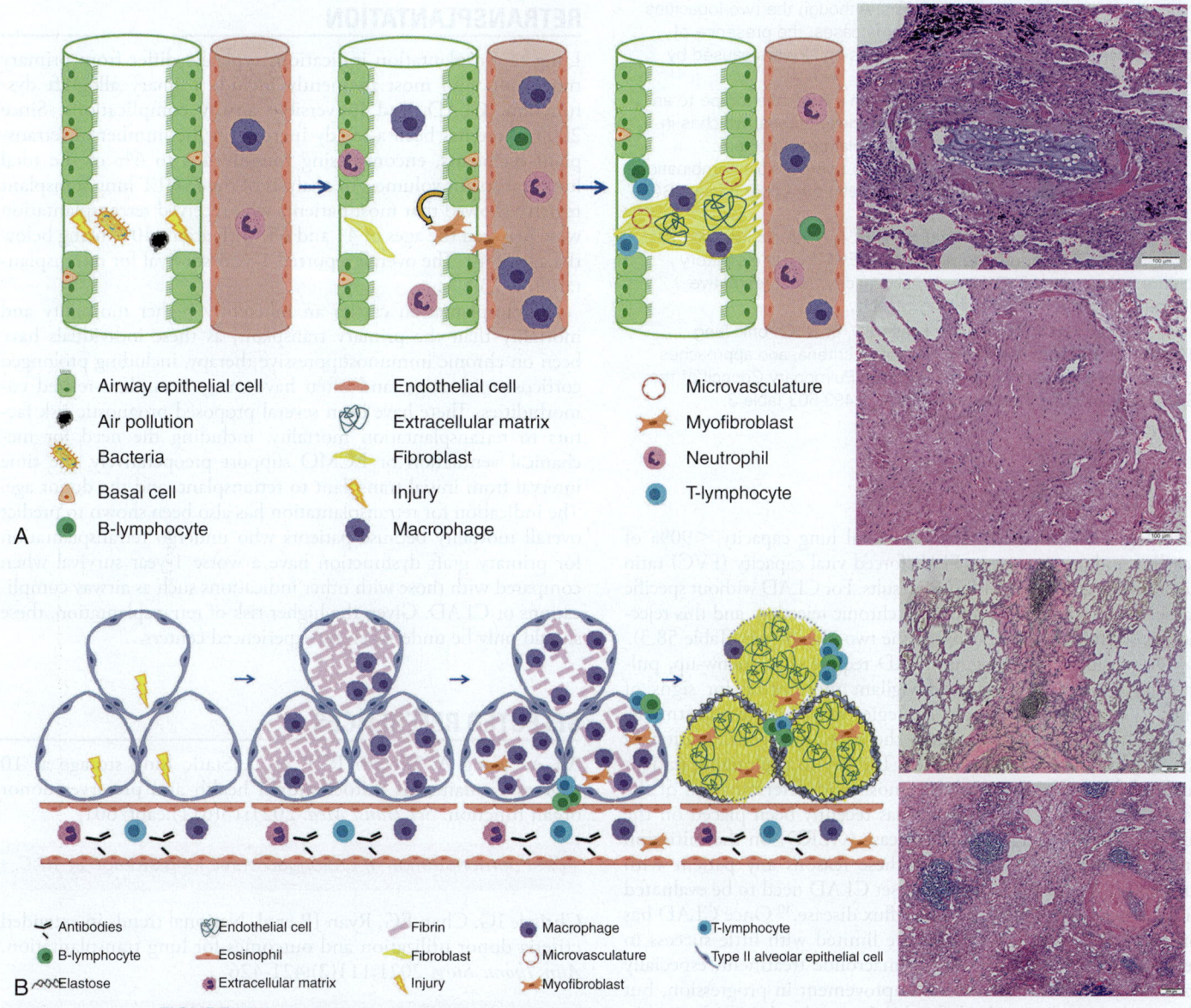

FIGURE 58.7 Histologic representation of (A) bronchiolitis obliterans syndrome and (B) restrictive allograft syndrome. (Verleden SE, Von der Thüsen J, Roux A, et al. When tissue is the issue: a histological review of chronic lung allograft dysfunction. *Am J Transplant.* 2020;20[10]:2644-2651, Figures 1 and 2.)

Legend for A:
- Airway epithelial cell
- Air pollution
- Bacteria
- Basal cell
- B-lymphocyte
- Endothelial cell
- Extracellular matrix
- Fibroblast
- Injury
- Macrophage
- Microvasculature
- Myofibroblast
- Neutrophil
- T-lymphocyte

Legend for B:
- Antibodies
- B-lymphocyte
- Elastose
- Endothelial cell
- Eosinophil
- Extracellular matrix
- Fibrin
- Fibroblast
- Injury
- Macrophage
- Microvasculature
- Myofibroblast
- T-lymphocyte
- Type II alveolar epithelial cell

TABLE 58.3 Basic Phenotypes of Chronic Lung Allograft Dysfunction

EMPTY CELL	OBSTRUCTION[a] (FEV$_1$/FVC <0.7)	RESTRICTION[b] (TLC DECLINE ≥10% FROM BASELINE)	CT OPACITIES[c]
BOS	Yes	No	No
RAS	No	Yes	Yes
Mixed[d]	Yes	Yes	Yes
Undefined[e]	Yes	No	Yes
Empty Cell	Yes	Yes	No

[a]Obstruction is defined by a fall in FEV$_1$ (as described in the text) and associated with other indices of airflow limitation (FEV$_1$/FVC ratio <0.70).

[b]Restriction is properly defined as a ≥10% reduction in baseline TLC.

[c]Refers to parenchymal opacities and/or increasing pleural thickening consistent with a diagnosis of pulmonary and/or pleural fibrosis and likely to cause a restrictive physiology, rather than the airway-based changes consistent with bronchiectasis. Although the two (opacities and bronchiectasis) may coexist, in some cases, the presence of bronchiectasis may reflect traction changes on airways caused by fibrotic parenchymal opacities.

[d]By definition, all cases that transition from a BOS phenotype to an RAS phenotype and vice versa will meet these criteria, which is in accord with histopathologic findings at explant/postmortem.

[e]Undefined means definite CLAD, but with two possible combinations of variables, making it difficult to categorize in the upper panels (BOS, RAS, or mixed phenotype).

BOS, Bronchiolitis obliterans syndrome; CLAD, chronic lung allograft dysfunction; CT, computed tomography; FEV1, forced expiratory volume in 1 second; FVC, forced vital capacity; RAS, restrictive allograft syndrome; TLC, total lung capacity.

From Verleden GM, Glanville AR, Lease ED, et al. Chronic lung allograft dysfunction: definition, diagnostic criteria, and approaches to treatment-a consensus report from the Pulmonary Council of the ISHLT. *J Heart Lung Transplant.* 2019;38(5):493-503 Table 3.

pathology with a noted decline in total lung capacity <90% of baseline and an increase in FEV$_1$/forced vital capacity (FVC) ratio higher when compared with prior results. For CLAD without specific cause, it is assumed to be a form of chronic rejection, and this rejection exists on a spectrum between the two phenotypes (Table 58.3).

Diagnosing and managing CLAD require close follow-up, pulmonary function testing, and vigilant monitoring for signs of graft dysfunction. Treatment strategies may involve adjustments to immunosuppression, targeted therapies, and consideration of retransplantation in certain cases. The key to prolonging patient survival from CLAD is early diagnosis and determination of the initiating cause. A big emphasis has recently been placed on the role of gastroesophageal reflux disease (GERD) on the initiation and progression of CLAD. For these reasons any patient with known GERD or signs of early onset CLAD need to be evaluated and surgically treated to prevent reflux disease.[40] Once CLAD has progressed, therapeutic options are limited with little success in reversing the disease. The use of macrolide treatment, especially azithromycin, has shown some improvement in progression, but the mechanism is poorly defined.[41] It may be that azithromycin is able to reduce airway inflammation and the associated neutrophilia causing direct damage to the airways, allowing for stabilization of FEV$_1$ in these select patients. Other approaches that have been tried, including the administration of montelukast, a cysteinyl leukotriene receptor antagonist, has been shown to decrease the rate of FEV$_1$ decline compared with control groups.[42] Another promising therapy is the use of a technique called *extracorporeal photopheresis*. This cell-based therapy relies on leukapheresis to isolate leukocytes from the lung graft recipient followed by treatment with methoxsalen and ultraviolet light to induce apoptosis, after which the cells are returned to the patient. Although the exact mechanism is still being deciphered, it is suspected that the introduction of apoptotic cells downregulates multiple aspects of the immune response to the allograft. Clinical trials have demonstrated an improvement in CLAD after such therapy, and ongoing work focuses on expanding and better understanding this form of therapy.[43] Nevertheless, despite such efforts, CLAD remains the leading cause of long-term graft loss in lung transplant recipients because most patients will succumb to this form of rejection.

RETRANSPLANTATION

Lung retransplantation indications typically differ from primary transplants and most frequently include primary allograft dysfunction, CLAD, and irreversible airway complications. Since 2005, there has been a steady increase in the number of retransplant recipients, encompassing roughly 4% to 6% of the total lung transplant volume. An analysis of the ISHLT lung transplant registry showed that most patients who received retransplantation were between the ages of 41 and 65, with about 40% being below the age of 40. The overall reported 1-year survival for retransplantation is 73.8%.

Retransplantation carries an inherently higher morbidity and mortality than the primary transplant, as these individuals have been on chronic immunosuppressive therapy, including prolonged corticosteroid usage, and often have many transplant-related comorbidities. There have been several proposed prognostic risk factors to retransplantation mortality, including the need for mechanical ventilation or ECMO support preoperatively, the time interval from initial transplant to retransplant, and the donor age. The indication for retransplantation has also been shown to predict overall mortality because patients who undergo retransplantation for primary graft dysfunction have a worse 1-year survival when compared with those with other indications such as airway complications or CLAD. Given the higher risk of retransplantation, these should only be undertaken by experienced centers.

SELECTED REFERENCES

Ali A, Wang A, Ribeiro RVP, et al. Static lung storage at 10 degrees C maintains mitochondrial health and preserves donor organ function. *Sci Transl Med.* 2021;13(611):eabf7601.

First demonstration of prolonged static lung storage at 10°C.

Christie IG, Chan EG, Ryan JP, et al. National trends in extended criteria donor utilization and outcomes for lung transplantation. *Ann Thorac Surg.* 2021;111(2):421-426.

Trends in extended criteria donor use and recipient outcomes in the modern era.

Expert Consensus Panel, Hartwig M, van Berkel V, et al. The American Association for Thoracic Surgery (AATS) 2022 Expert Consensus Document: the use of mechanical circulatory support in lung transplantation. *J Thorac Cardiovasc Surg.* 2023;165(1):301-326.

Consensus recommendations on mechanical circulatory support in the peritransplantation period.

Leard LE, Holm AM, Valapour M, et al. Consensus document for the selection of lung transplant candidates: an update from the International Society for Heart and Lung Transplantation. *J Heart Lung Transplant.* 2021;40(11):1349-1379.

Consensus recommendations on evaluation and selection of lung transplant candidates.

Pasque MK, Cooper JD, Kaiser LR, et al. Improved technique for bilateral lung transplantation: rationale and initial clinical experience. *Ann Thorac Surg.* 1990;49(5):785-791.

Common technique of bilateral lung transplantation via a clamshell thoracotomy.

The full reference list appears on Elsevier eBooks+.

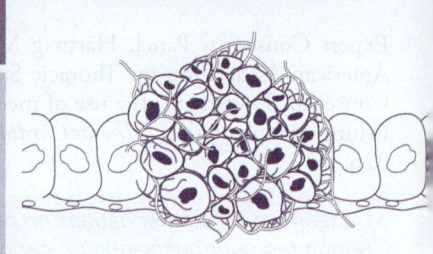

Melanoma and Cutaneous Malignancies

Michael E. Egger, Georgia M. Beasley, Douglas S. Tyler, and Kelly M. McMasters

MELANOMA

Historical descriptions of what was likely melanoma can be found in the writings of Hippocrates. John Hunter provided the first modern published account of the surgical treatment of melanoma in 1787. René Laennec, who identified metastatic melanoma deposits in distant viscera, described it as "cancer noire" and subsequently named the disease *melanosis*. Our understanding of melanoma, its clinical behavior, molecular mechanisms, and targetable pathways, has steadily improved over decades of research.

Epidemiology

Even though melanoma accounts for less than 2% of skin cancer cases, it is currently the fifth most common cancer in males and females in the United States when the other forms of less serious skin cancers (squamous cell carcinoma [SCC] and basal cell carcinoma [BCC]) are not counted.[1] Melanoma also causes the majority of skin-cancer–related deaths. The American Cancer Society estimated that there would be 97,610 new cases of melanoma diagnosed in the United States in 2023, with 7990 deaths.[1] In terms of absolute numbers, the greatest numbers of new cases and deaths related to melanoma are found in North America and Europe; however, the highest incidence rates of melanoma are in Australia and New Zealand.[2] The age-standardized incidence rate of melanoma in Australia and New Zealand is 41.6 per 100,000

person-years; the next highest is in Western Europe (19.4 per 100,000 person-years). The estimated cumulative risk of developing melanoma by age 74 in Australia and New Zealand approaches 1 out of 20 (4.7%).[2] The incidence of melanoma has steadily increased in the United States over the past 45 years, with the exception of a decrease in incidence in 2020 related to a decrease in incidences of all cancers in the Surveillance, Epidemiology, and End Results (SEER) registry as a result of the COVID-19 pandemic (Fig. 63.1). The root causes of this overall increase are not well understood but are likely related to both increased sun exposure and improved detection.

The degree of pigmentation in the skin is a relative protective factor against cutaneous melanoma; those with lighter skin tones are at increased risk. As a result, cutaneous melanoma is predominantly a disease of non-Hispanic White populations. In particular, patients with a fair complexion, blonde or red hair, and blue eyes are at increased risk, as are those who sunburn easily, have a tendency to develop freckles, or have an inability to tan. According to SEER data, in the United States from 2000–20, the average annual age-adjusted melanoma incidence per 100,000 persons is 34.7 for non-Hispanic White males and 22.5 for non-Hispanic White females, compared with 4.6 for Hispanic males and 4.2 for Hispanic females, 8.0 for Native American Indian males (including Alaska Natives) and 6.3 for females, 1.5 for Asian/Pacific Islander males and 1.2 for females, and 1.1 for Black

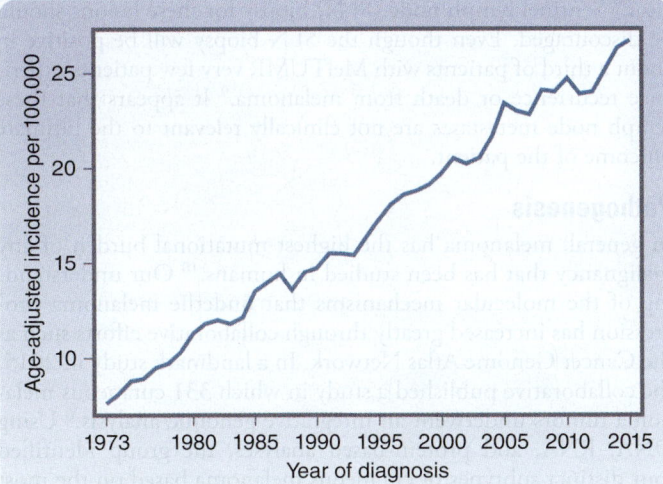

FIGURE 63.1 Age-adjusted incidence of cutaneous melanoma in the United States, 1973–2015. (From Surveillance, Epidemiology, and End Results [SEER] database.)

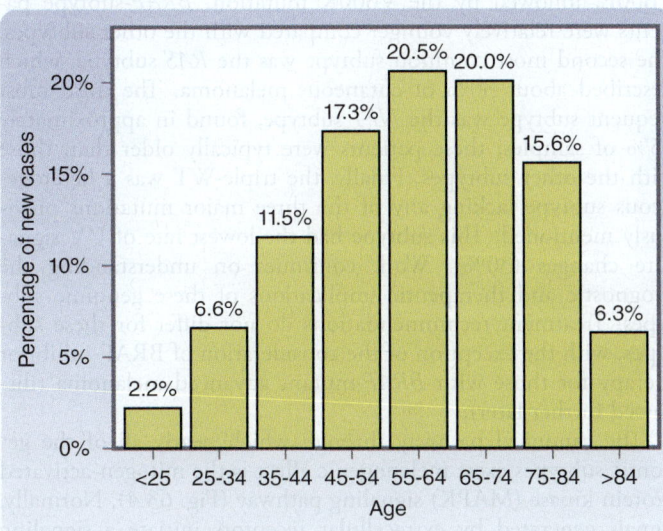

FIGURE 63.2 New cases by age group: cutaneous melanoma in the United States, 1973–2015. (From Surveillance, Epidemiology, and End Results [SEER] database.)

males and 1.0 for Black females. Melanoma incidence is slightly higher in males compared with females across race/ethnicities.

Melanoma is predominantly seen in middle-aged adults, although it occurs across all ages (Fig. 63.2). Importantly, approximately one in six new cases of melanoma occur in patients <45 years old. Genetic risk factors for melanoma include high-risk skin types (Fitzpatrick types I and II), family history of melanoma, and xeroderma pigmentosum. Patients with a prior history of melanoma or other skin cancers, as well as those with a large number of melanocytic nevi, dysplastic nevi, or giant congenital nevi, are also at increased risk. The estimated incidence of developing a second cutaneous melanoma 5 and 10 years after a first cutaneous melanoma is 3.9% and 6.7%, respectively.[3] Environmental risk factors include episodes of intense intermittent sun exposure associated with severe blistering sunburns, immunosuppression, and upper socioeconomic status. Childhood sun

exposure is believed to contribute to an increase in melanoma risk, although adult sun exposure continues to be a contributing factor to melanoma risk as well.

There is a clear association between ultraviolet (UV) radiation exposure and the development of melanoma. Intermittent, intense UV radiation exposure appears to be a strong causative factor for melanoma, as opposed to chronic sun exposure and the associated risk of nonmelanoma skin cancers (NMSCs). UV light can be classified as either UVA or UVB; UVA has a longer wavelength and penetrates more deeply into the skin than UVB. Although UVA radiation has long been known to play a major role in skin aging and wrinkling, growing evidence has implicated UVA radiation as a cause of melanoma. UVA is the predominant wavelength in tanning beds. Emerging evidence has demonstrated an epidemiologic link between tanning bed use (even without sunburn) and melanoma.[4,5] Another major risk factor for melanoma is UVB exposure from natural sunlight, especially among those with fair skin. UVB damages the skin's more superficial epidermal layers and is the chief cause of sunburns. A UV signature consistent with mutations caused by UV damage was found in over 90% of three of the four melanoma subtypes identified in the Cancer Genome Atlas project.[6]

From a public health perspective, melanoma is a cancer for which there are clear primary prevention strategies that can prevent its development and reduce preventable deaths. Recommendations for reducing the risk of melanoma include avoidance of sunbathing and tanning beds, use of sun-protective clothing, and use of sunscreens. From a policy standpoint, one strategy that has been used on a state-by-state basis in the United States is the ban on indoor tanning bed use by minors (age <18). Some countries, including Brazil and Australia, have banned commercial indoor tanning salons outright.

Precursor Lesions

Melanomas frequently arise de novo in otherwise normal skin; however, up to 40% may arise within preexisting lesions, including dysplastic nevi, congenital nevi, and Spitz nevi. Upward of 5% to 10% of melanoma patients will have a family history of the disease. Variously termed *dysplastic nevus syndrome, familial atypical multiple mole–melanoma syndrome,* and *B-K mole syndrome,* these syndromes include patients with melanoma in one or more first- or second-degree relatives and large numbers of melanocytic nevi (often >100). These nevi will often be classified as atypical or dysplastic on close clinical and histologic examination. Other cancers may also be present in the family history, particularly pancreatic cancer. These patients require detailed dermatologic evaluation several times annually, with periodic biopsies of the most suspicious lesions. The most common pathogenic variant found in hereditary melanomas is the *CDKN2A* gene.[7]

In general, a dysplastic nevus is a 6- to 15-mm macular (flat) pigmented skin lesion with indistinct margins and variable color. The clinical distinction between a nevus with dysplasia and a nevus without dysplasia is often difficult; therefore, these lesions require careful monitoring over time to evaluate for progression. Most nevi are benign, but some may reflect early atypia associated with increased intracellular growth signaling and can progress to invasive disease with the accumulation of additional mutations. Although most dysplastic nevi do not progress to melanoma, suspicious lesions require biopsy. Dysplastic nevi are typically described as having mild, moderate, or severe dysplasia on histologic examination. Nevi with mild dysplasia usually do not require excision with negative margins but should be closely observed over time. It has been common practice to excise moderately or severely dysplastic nevi with negative margins, although wide local excision (WLE) is unnecessary. However, there is controversy about whether moderately dysplastic nevi require negative-margin excision. Moderately dysplastic nevi have a very low risk of "recurring" or developing an invasive melanoma at the biopsy site if they are not excised to negative margins; however, these patients have an increased risk of developing melanoma at other sites.[8] Thus, the presence of dysplastic nevi can be considered a marker of increased risk of developing cutaneous melanoma. The risk of melanoma in those patients with congenital nevi is proportional to the size and number of nevi. Small- or medium-sized congenital nevi represent a low risk and therefore are observed unless they change in appearance. Giant congenital nevi (>20 cm in diameter) are rare and are estimated to occur in anywhere from 1 in 20,000 to 1 in 500,000 newborns, but they carry an increased lifetime risk for the development of melanoma (Fig. 63.3). These patients are also at increased risk for other tumors, particularly sarcomas. Complete excision should be considered when possible. At a minimum, these patients should undergo regular dermatologic evaluation.

A Spitz nevus is a rapidly growing, pink or brown, benign skin lesion with little or no risk for further progression to melanoma. Whereas benign Spitz nevi are most common in children, lesions in adults are more likely to have atypical features or represent melanoma with spitzoid features. A class of melanocytic tumors is now characterized by its existence on the spectrum between benign nevi and invasive melanoma. These tumors are now commonly referred to as *melanocytic tumors of uncertain malignant potential* (MelTUMP). This term will generally include lesions categorized as melanocytic tumors, melanocytomas, or atypical Spitz tumors. Based on the available evidence, management of these tumors should include WLE. Most studies report a 10-mm margin, but the exact margin necessary for optimal clinical outcomes is not

clear.[9] Sentinel lymph node (SLN) biopsy for these lesions should be discouraged. Even though the SLN biopsy will be positive in about a third of patients with MelTUMP, very few patients experience recurrence or death from melanoma.[9] It appears that these lymph node metastases are not clinically relevant to the ultimate outcome of the patient.

Pathogenesis

In general, melanoma has the highest mutational burden of any malignancy that has been studied in humans.[10] Our understanding of the molecular mechanisms that underlie melanoma progression has increased greatly through collaborative efforts such as the Cancer Genome Atlas Network. In a landmark study in 2015, the collaborative published a study in which 331 cutaneous melanoma tumors underwent an integrative genomic analysis.[6] Using DNA, RNA, and protein-based analyses, the group identified four distinct subtypes of cutaneous melanoma based on the most prevalent significantly altered genes: mutant *BRAF,* mutant *RAS,* mutant *NF1,* and triple-wild-type (WT).

The *BRAF* subtype was the most common genomic subtype in cutaneous melanoma, comprising approximately one-half of all cutaneous melanoma cases. The most common mutation was V600E, followed by the V600K mutation. *BRAF*-subtype patients were relatively younger compared with the other subtypes. The second most common subtype was the *RAS* subtype, which described about 30% of cutaneous melanoma. The third most frequent subtype was the *NF1* subtype, found in approximately 15% of samples; these patients were typically older than those with the other subtypes. Finally, the triple-WT was a heterogeneous subtype lacking any of the three major mutations previously mentioned. This subtype had the lowest rate of UV signature changes (30%). Work continues on understanding the prognostic and therapeutic implications of these genomic subtypes. Treatment recommendations do not differ for these subtypes, with the exception of the consideration of BRAF-inhibitor therapy for those with *BRAF*-mutant advanced melanoma (discussed further later).

The canonical pathway through which nearly all of the genomic subtypes exert melanogenic effect is the mitogen-activated protein kinase (MAPK) signaling pathway (Fig. 63.4). Normally, signals generated by extracellular receptors initiate a signaling cascade that passes down the MAPK pathway to modulate gene expression in the nucleus. Gain-of-function mutations affecting any of the constituent steps along this cascade (*BRAF* and *RAS* subtypes) or loss of inhibitory steps *(NF1)* can result in unchecked cellular growth.

Gain-of-function mutations alone are likely not enough to generate melanoma; *BRAF* mutations are observed in high frequencies in other benign or preinvasive melanocytic lesions.[11] Additional loss of key tumor suppressor genes is necessary for further neoplastic development. For instance, an inactivating mutation in the gene *CDKN2A* occurs in many familial melanomas. A well-characterized gene with key roles in cell cycle control, *CDKN2A* codes for two separate tumor suppressor proteins, INK4A (p16INK4A) and ARF (p14ARF). In the event of DNA damage or activated oncogenes, INK4A prevents the cyclin-dependent kinase 4 from stimulating the cell to progress through the cell cycle. Through the regulation of p53 levels, ARF also acts as a tumor suppressor in the face of DNA damage or amplified growth signals. ARF prevents degradation of p53, allowing this key regulatory protein to accumulate and either arrest the cell cycle or initiate apoptosis. Loss of either ARF or INK4A, therefore,

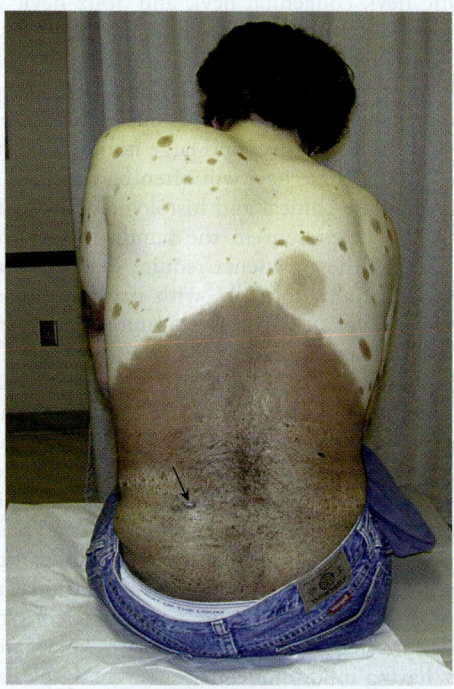

FIGURE 63.3 Giant congenital nevus of the trunk with an associated melanoma *(arrow).*

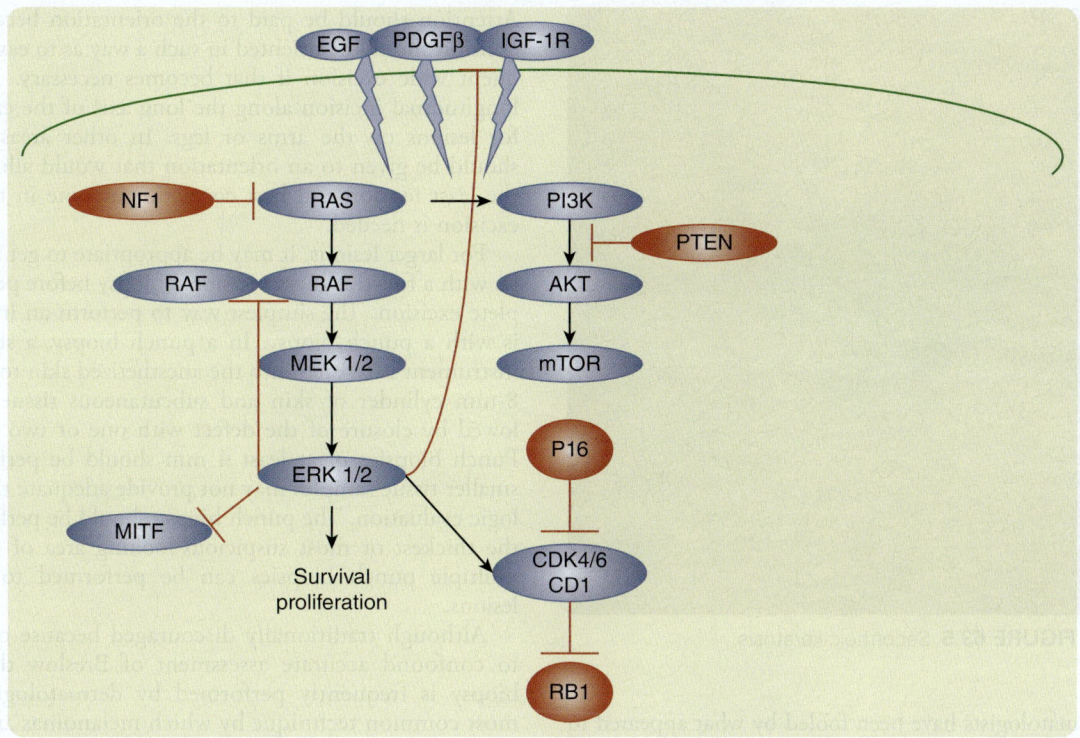

FIGURE 63.4 The mitogen-activated protein kinase (RAS-RAF-MEK-ERK) and PI3/AKT pathways, two canonical pathways in melanoma pathogenesis. (From Amaral T, Sinnberg T, Meier F, et al. The mitogen-activated protein kinase pathway in melanoma part I—activation and primary resistance mechanisms to BRAF inhibition. *Eur J Cancer.* 2017;73:85-92.)

removes a checkpoint in the cell cycle, increasing the risk of uncontrolled replication.

The second major canonical pathway in melanoma pathogenesis is the PI3/AKT pathway (see Fig. 63.4). The PI3/AKT pathway is potentially altered in all four genomic subtypes. Phosphatidylinositol 3,4,5-trisphosphate (PIP_3) stimulates AKT to increase cellular proliferation through the mammalian target of rapamycin (mTOR) signaling molecule. Phosphatase and tensin homologue (PTEN), whose gene is located on chromosome 10, inhibits PI3/AKT signaling. Loss of PTEN occurs in approximately 25% to 50% of nonfamilial melanomas and is a common culprit pathway for the development of resistance to therapies targeting BRAK/MEK inhibition.

Initial Evaluation

Melanoma commonly presents as an irregular pigmented skin lesion that has grown or changed over time (Box 63.1). The ABCDE criteria are used to guide diagnosis and the decision to perform a biopsy of suspicious cutaneous lesions (see Box 63.1). The first and most important step in the evaluation of a patient diagnosed with melanoma is a thorough history and physical

examination. The history should elicit factors related to the primary melanoma, including duration, change over time, and symptoms such as itching or bleeding. Other risk factors, such as sun exposure, tanning bed use, immunosuppression, prior history of cancer, and family history, should be queried. A detailed physical examination should specifically include a complete skin examination, with inspection and palpation of the skin to detect any other suspicious skin lesions, including in-transit disease. Palpation of the cervical, axillary, and inguinal lymph nodes should always be performed, with palpation of the epitrochlear or popliteal nodes as appropriate for distal upper or lower extremity melanomas. Although it is widely recognized that a skin examination should be part of the routine physical examination by primary care physicians and others, it is rarely adequately performed. A full skin examination requires only that the patient undress, and it may take only 1 minute to perform a complete survey. Many lives have been saved by early detection of melanomas by physicians who took the time to carefully and fully evaluate the skin.

Most melanomas occur de novo, but some can arise within a congenital or acquired nevus. Even for experienced clinicians, distinguishing between a benign nevus and an early melanoma can be difficult. Benign pigmented lesions are so prevalent that it is challenging to detect an early melanoma among many benign lesions. The most common benign pigmented skin lesions are seborrheic keratoses (Fig. 63.5). Known for their propensity to accumulate over time in elderly patients, typically these are scaly, waxy, raised lesions with a stuck-on look that makes them appear as if they could easily be scraped off with a fingernail. The characteristic appearance is usually completely diagnostic, and these lesions do not need to be removed. However, even the most

BOX 63.1	**ABCDE Criteria of Suspicious Skin Lesions**
A	**A**symmetry
B	Irregular **B**orders
C	**C**olor variegation
D	**D**iameter >6 mm
E	**E**volution or changes over time

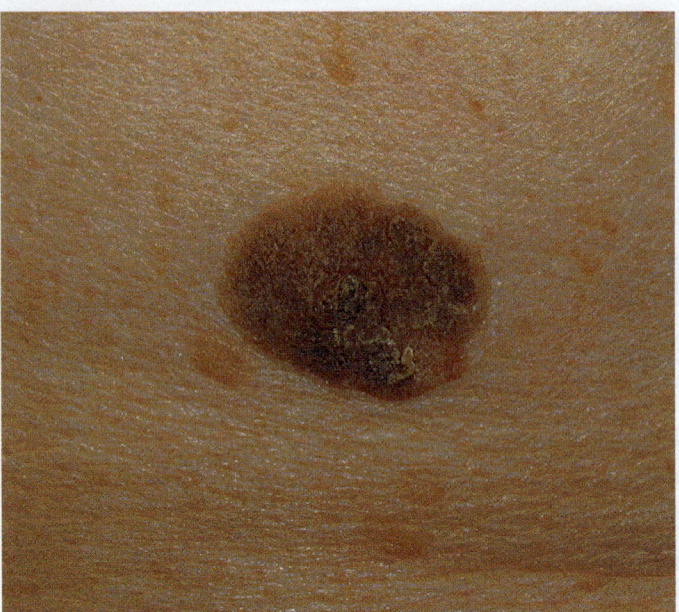

FIGURE 63.5 Seborrheic keratosis.

experienced dermatologists have been fooled by what appeared to be an irritated seborrheic keratosis that turned out to be melanoma.

Additional atypical presentations include amelanotic melanoma; these lesions are not pigmented and present as a raised pink or flesh-colored skin lesion. A high index of clinical suspicion is needed, and particular attention should be paid to any history of change in a lesion. If a patient presents with a skin lesion that has changed in size, color, or shape and/or is itching or bleeding, there should be a low threshold for biopsy. Telling a patient that "we should keep an eye on it" usually means that it will be ignored.

Given the increased awareness of this disease, in the present time, it is uncommon for patients to have advanced regional or distant metastatic disease at the time of initial melanoma diagnosis. Nonetheless, roughly 10% of patients will present with regional disease, and up to 5% may present with metastases. *Regional disease* refers to the lymphatic spread of tumor to the regional nodal basin, which are the lymph nodes that receive the first drainage from the site of the primary tumor. In-transit melanoma is a form of regional lymphatic metastasis in which the tumor spreads within the draining lymphatic channels and becomes evident as cutaneous or subcutaneous nodules between the site of the primary tumor and regional lymph nodes. *Distant metastasis* refers to the hematogenous spread of melanoma to distant organs. Although uncommon at the time of initial diagnosis, it is important to elicit symptoms of metastatic disease, such as any masses, neurologic symptoms or headaches, anorexia, weight loss, bone pain, or respiratory symptoms.

Biopsy

Primary care physicians, in addition to dermatologists and surgeons, should be trained to perform a skin biopsy. There are three basic types of skin biopsy—excisional, incisional (including punch biopsy), and shave biopsy. An excisional biopsy completely removes a pigmented skin lesion and is particularly well suited to diagnose and completely remove small lesions. Using local anesthesia, a narrow-margin excision is performed, with the subsequent defect closed by suture repair. The depth of excision should extend to the subcutaneous fat to ensure a full-thickness biopsy.

Attention should be paid to the orientation because a fusiform excision should be oriented in such a way as to easily allow subsequent wide excision if that becomes necessary. In particular, a longitudinal incision along the long axis of the extremity is best for lesions on the arms or legs. In other areas, consideration should be given to an orientation that would allow closure with the least tension and best cosmetic outcome in the event wider excision is needed.

For larger lesions, it may be appropriate to get a tissue diagnosis with a full-thickness incisional biopsy before performing complete excision. The simplest way to perform an incisional biopsy is with a punch biopsy. In a punch biopsy, a sharp disposable instrument is twisted into the anesthetized skin to remove a 2- to 8-mm cylinder of skin and subcutaneous tissue, generally followed by closure of the defect with one or two simple sutures. Punch biopsies of at least 4 mm should be performed because smaller tissue samples may not provide adequate tissue for pathologic evaluation. The punch biopsy should be performed through the thickest or most suspicious-looking area of the lesion, and multiple punch biopsies can be performed to sample larger lesions.

Although traditionally discouraged because of the potential to confound accurate assessment of Breslow thickness, shave biopsy is frequently performed by dermatologists and is the most common technique by which melanomas are biopsied and diagnosed. Shave biopsy is performed by elevating the skin lesion with forceps or inserting a small needle beneath the lesion, followed by shaving the lesion with a razor blade or scalpel. Hemostasis is achieved using topical agents or by electrocautery. The patient then treats the area with topical ointment, and the wound heals by secondary intention. Because a shave biopsy is easy to perform and does not require sutures, it is a popular method of biopsy. However, a potential drawback to the use of a shave biopsy to diagnose melanoma is that the lesion may be transected, compromising the ability to accurately assess tumor thickness. To circumvent this problem, dermatologists often perform deep shave or saucerization biopsies, which completely remove the lesion down to subcutaneous fat. In the hands of experienced clinicians, this can be an effective biopsy technique. In reviewing the pathology report of a newly diagnosed melanoma, surgeons should take care to note whether the deep margin is free of tumor.

All pigmented lesions should be sent for pathologic evaluation using fixation and permanent section. Ablation of pigmented skin lesions using cryotherapy, cautery, or lasers should be specifically discouraged; there are many examples of prolonged delays in diagnosis as a result of these practices.

Pathology

The biopsy report is the most important piece of information needed by the surgeon to evaluate a new skin lesion and develop a treatment plan. Given the consequences of a missed diagnosis of melanoma, pathologists often have a low threshold to classify equivocal lesions as melanoma. When the diagnosis is not clear and there is equivocation as to whether the lesion is an invasive melanoma or a premalignant lesion, the prudent decision is to treat such lesions as an early invasive melanoma with a 1-cm-margin WLE. Although melanoma in situ does not invade beyond the basement membrane into blood vessels and lymphatics, it may be considered a premalignant lesion given that there remains a significant likelihood of progression to invasive melanoma. For this reason, margins of at least

5-mm are recommended for these lesions (see the "Wide Local Excision" section).

Histology. Histologically, invasive cutaneous melanoma is divided into four major types based on growth pattern and location: lentigo maligna melanoma, superficial spreading melanoma, acral lentiginous melanoma (ALM), and nodular melanoma. All melanomas initially proliferate in the basal layer of the skin. As they multiply, these cells expand radially in the epidermis and superficial dermal layer, termed the *radial growth phase.* With time, growth begins in a vertical direction, and the skin lesion may become raised and palpable, known as the *vertical growth phase.* The vertical growth phase allows invasion into the deeper layers of the skin, where the tumor may ultimately achieve metastatic potential by invasion of blood vessels and lymphatic channels. Although the histologic subtype is not a major factor in prognosis, some histologic subtypes progress to the vertical growth phase earlier in tumor development and are therefore more likely to present at an advanced stage.

The most common histologic type is superficial spreading melanoma (Fig. 63.6). It is not necessarily associated with sun-exposed skin and most commonly appears on the trunk and proximal extremities. As the name suggests, superficial spreading melanoma initially appears as a flat pigmented lesion growing radially. These lesions are often asymmetric with irregular borders and can display a wide variety of pigments. Untreated, these melanomas will subsequently develop a vertical growth phase, invade more deeply into the skin, and possibly ulcerate.

Lentigo maligna melanoma occurs most commonly on the sun-exposed areas of older individuals and presents as a flat, dark, variably pigmented lesion with irregular borders and a history of slow development (Fig. 63.7). Lentigo maligna melanomas may become relatively large before diagnosis because the slow progression can escape the patient's notice. The prognosis of lentigo maligna melanoma is better than that for the other subtypes because of the superficial nature of these tumors. Nonetheless, these lesions can pose challenging management problems because of their propensity to develop in cosmetically challenging areas, such as the face. The histologic extent of the lesion may extend well beyond the clinically apparent borders of the pigmented lesion, hampering efforts to achieve negative margins. Before proceeding with complex tissue flaps for closure, it is prudent to ensure

negative margins. This may necessitate delaying the closure until the final pathology report indicates negative margins of excision.

ALM is classified by its anatomic site of origin. These tumors develop in the subungual areas beneath fingernails and toenails and on the palms of the hands and soles of the feet (Fig. 63.8). This is the most common type of melanoma in non-White patients. The histologic appearance of ALMs is similar to melanomas arising on the mucous membranes. The diagnosis is often made at an advanced stage, which accounts for the generally poor prognosis of these tumors. Subungual ALMs are often mistaken for subungual hematomas, leading to a delay in diagnosis. The distinguishing feature of subungual melanomas is that they do not change in position underneath the nail, whereas a hematoma should migrate distally with growth of the nail. Biopsy of subungual melanomas can be accomplished by performing a digital block with local anesthesia and removing the nail or by performing a punch biopsy through the nail itself.

Nodular melanomas are raised papular lesions that can occur anywhere on the body and tend to develop a vertical growth pattern early in their course (Fig. 63.9). These melanomas can have atypical presentations that do not always conform to ABCDE criteria, including a higher rate of amelanotic lesions compared with the other subtypes. Nodular melanomas often have a poor prognosis because of greater average tumor thickness and frequent ulceration at initial presentation.

A fifth type of melanoma that has a distinct histologic character is desmoplastic melanoma. These lesions are characterized by a combination of melanoma cells with a prominent stromal fibrosis. The diagnosis can be challenging, and the presentation may be delayed because these lesions are often amelanotic. Desmoplastic melanomas are classified as either pure or mixed, depending on the degree of desmoplasia present. Desmoplastic melanomas have a greater propensity for local recurrence and often exhibit neurotropism. Pure desmoplastic melanomas have a low risk of lymph node metastases, and some have advocated forgoing an SLN biopsy in these lesions. Mixed desmoplastic melanomas have lymph node metastatic rates that are similar to those of other histologic subtypes; therefore, SLN biopsy should be considered for the usual indications in these lesions.[12]

Depth assessment. Dr. Wallace Clark first described a classification system for melanoma that correlated with survival in 1969.

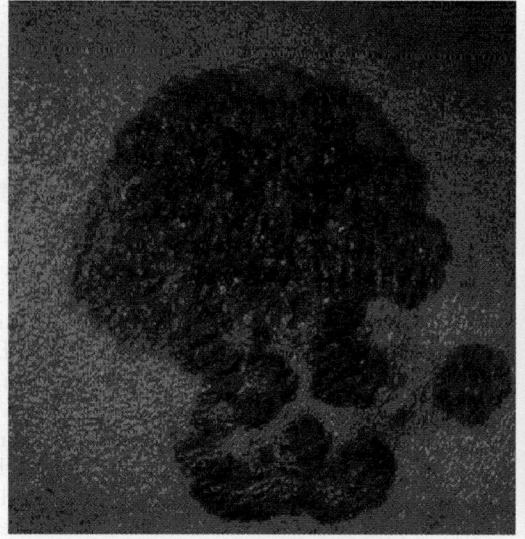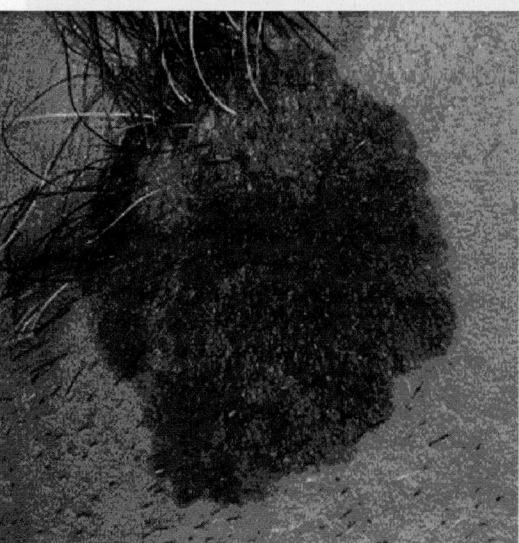

FIGURE 63.6 Superficial spreading melanoma.

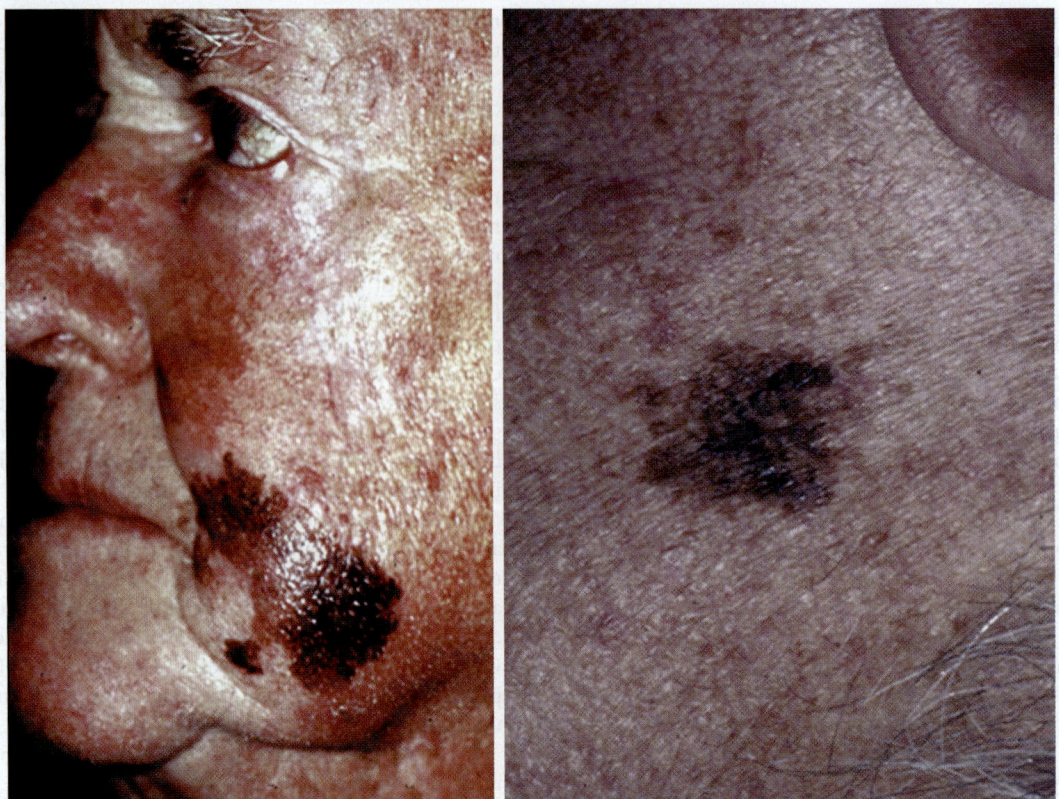

FIGURE 63.7 Lentigo maligna melanoma.

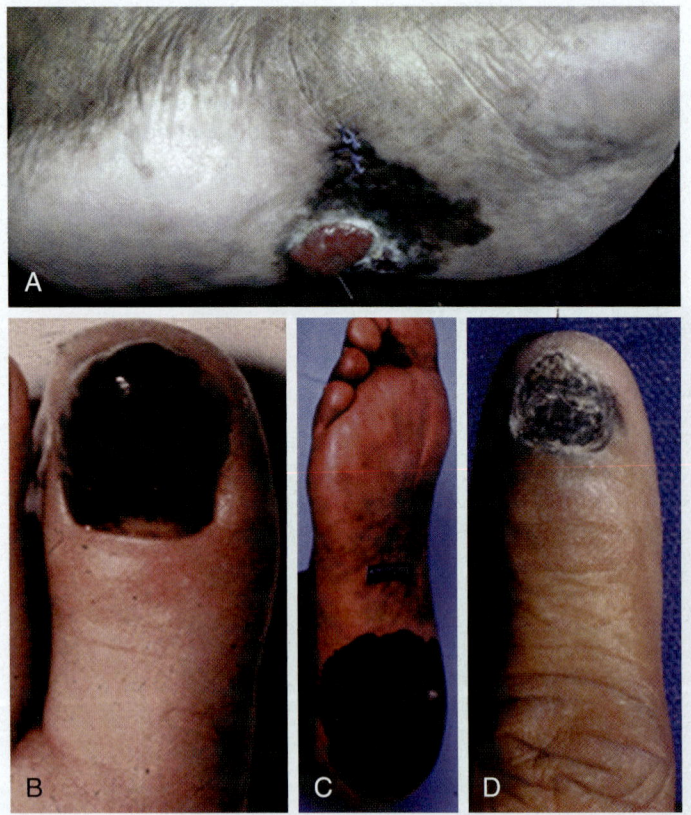

FIGURE 63.8 Acral lentiginous melanoma of the plantar foot (A), toenail (B), heel (C), and fingernail (D).

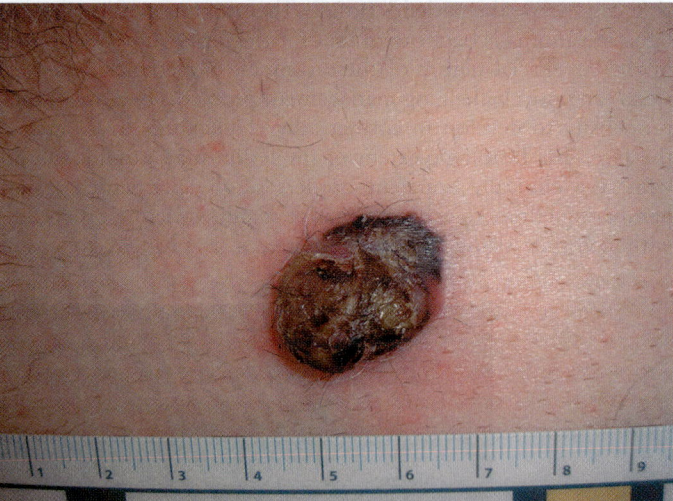

FIGURE 63.9 Nodular melanoma.

Known as *Clark's level of invasion,* this classification was based on the extent of invasion into the anatomic layers of the skin. Shortly after Clark introduced his levels of invasion, Dr. Alexander Breslow described a simpler system based on a measurement of the vertical thickness of the melanoma. Now known as *Breslow's thickness,* this is the distance from the top of the granular layer down to the lowest tumor cell. Over time, Breslow thickness has largely supplanted Clark level because it has been shown to have less variability between pathologist interpretations and, as such, is a more accurate method of predicting prognosis. Melanomas are commonly referred to as *thin* (<1 mm Breslow thickness), *intermediate* (1–4 mm), and *thick* (>4 mm). As the thickness of the melanoma increases, the prognosis worsens.

STAGING

American Joint Committee on Cancer Staging

The American Joint Committee on Cancer (AJCC) Melanoma Staging Committee uses a tumor-node-metastasis (TNM) classification for cutaneous melanoma based on an analysis of data gathered from centers across North America, Europe, and Australia. Important prognostic factors in the staging system include Breslow thickness, ulceration, nodal status, and other manifestations of lymphatic spread (e.g., satellite lesions, in-transit disease) as well as the presence of distant metastatic disease. Taking all these factors into consideration, the system provides good discrimination of survival among different patient groups. There are two types of staging classifications provided by the AJCC: Clinical staging is what can be determined by biopsy of the primary lesion and physical examination, whereas pathologic staging is only complete once a full assessment of the regional lymph nodes, when indicated, is performed—usually by SLN biopsy.

T Stage

The 8th edition of the AJCC staging guidelines designates T classification based on Breslow thickness measured to the nearest one-tenth of a millimeter while further subclassifying T1 to T4 based on ulceration. The cutoff points for designating T1 to T4 melanoma are 1.0, 2.0, and 4.0 mm. Ulceration is a critically important prognostic factor. It is defined histologically by the absence of an intact epithelium over the melanoma. Across all T classifications, ulceration portends a worse prognosis. The 8th edition of the AJCC staging system made an important change to the subclassification of T1 melanomas. T1b melanomas are now defined as the presence of either (1) ulceration at any thickness or (2) thickness of 0.8 to 1.0 mm without ulceration. Mitotic rate, which was adopted in the AJCC 7th edition, is not used to designate T1b melanomas in the 8th edition.

N Stage

For patients with regional lymph node disease, independent prognostic factors include the number of involved nodes and nodal tumor burden at the time of staging, in addition to the thickness and ulceration status of the primary tumor. Tumor burden is characterized as either clinically occult disease detected by SLN biopsy or clinically apparent disease that is subsequently confirmed pathologically. Clinically apparent nodal disease includes palpable, enlarged lymph nodes or those lymph nodes identified on imaging as abnormal and confirmed by needle biopsy to contain metastatic melanoma. In a change from the 7th edition, the current 8th edition of the AJCC staging guidelines stratifies nonnodal regional disease, which includes in-transit cutaneous and/or subcutaneous metastases, microsatellite, or satellite metastases, by N category according to the number of regional lymph nodes (N1c, N2c, or N3c).

M Stage

The 8th edition AJCC staging guidelines stratify M categories by both anatomic site of distant disease and serum lactate dehydrogenase (LDH) levels. Four subgroups are defined by distant skin, soft tissue, and nonregional lymph nodes (M1a); lung (M1b); non–central nervous system viscera (M1c); and central nervous

system (M1d). Elevated serum LDH levels further subclassify M1a to M1d groups with a (0) or (1) designation. An elevated serum LDH level indicates a worse prognosis across all types of metastatic disease.

Additional Factors

Several factors that have consistently been shown to affect survival are not incorporated into the current AJCC staging system. Older patients have a greater risk of melanoma mortality than younger patients despite the fact that younger patients are more likely to have nodal metastasis. Patients with axial (trunk, head, and neck) melanomas have a worse prognosis than those with extremity tumors. Females have a better prognosis than males for reasons that are unclear.

Surgeons involved in the care of melanoma patients should also be familiar with several additional features that are commonly mentioned in pathology reports. Tumor-infiltrating lymphocytes (TILs) can indicate the presence of a host immune response and are associated with a more favorable prognosis. TILs are classified as brisk, nonbrisk, or absent. Brisk indicates that TILs infiltrate diffusely throughout the lesion or along the base, whereas nonbrisk indicates only a focal presence of lymphocytes. *Regression,* defined as partial or complete loss of tumor cells, has not clearly been shown to be an important factor affecting metastasis or survival. There is no compelling evidence that the presence of regression should be used as an indication for SLN biopsy. Although nodular melanoma and ALM often present at a more advanced stage, once controlling for tumor thickness and other factors, there is no survival difference based on histologic subtype.

Even though mitotic rate is no longer used to subclassify T1 melanoma, the AJCC does suggest that it should continue to be reported in pathology reports and in prospective research datasets. The number of mitoses per square millimeter is an important predictor of survival across all thickness categories, and the presence of mitoses in thin (<1.0 mm) melanoma may still be used to select patients for SLN biopsy (especially in the 0.8- to 1.0-mm thickness category).

Beyond American Joint Committee on Cancer tumor-nodemetastasis staging. Staging systems must perform dual functions that are at odds with one another. On one hand, a staging system should try to identify as many groups as possible that have distinct survival differences. On the other hand, a good staging system should not be overly complex. Thus, the AJCC staging system provides a parsimonious classification of patients into relatively large categories, within which there still remains a fair amount of heterogeneity with regard to prognosis. For these reasons, clinical prediction tools are becoming more popular to provide precise, patient-specific assessments of risks using multiple clinical and pathologic risk factors. Two examples of these prediction tools are the AJCC electronic prediction tool (http://www.melanomaprognosis.org) and the Melanoma Calculator (http://www.melanoma-calculator.com), which is based on data from the Sunbelt Melanoma Trial. Ultimately, tools like these will allow for more accurate risk assessments that can be used to formulate patient-specific treatment and surveillance plans.

Gene expression profile testing. The next logical extension to using clinical and pathologic factors to predict outcomes in melanoma is to add genomic profiling information. Multiple studies of gene expression profiling of formalin-fixed, paraffin-embedded primary melanoma tissue have shown promising results. In terms of risk of recurrence, at least two commercially available tests using primary melanoma tissue, a 31-gene expression profile, and a clinicopathologic gene expression profile have demonstrated a convincing ability to identify early-stage patients at high risk of recurrence.[13,14] The tests may also provide risk stratification in terms of the risk of having a positive SLN biopsy.[15] However, no studies have demonstrated improvement in outcomes from treatment decisions based on the results of these tests.

How these tests should be used and integrated into decision-making for patients with melanoma is not entirely clear. The extent to which these tests offer improvement in our risk stratification for either recurrence or SLN positivity over our existing clinical calculators and nomograms that use more readily available clinical and pathologic features is not readily apparent from the literature. That is, the *marginal* additional prognostic information from these tests has not been clearly demonstrated. Although these tests may provide prognostic information, there are no data to support their use for clinical decision-making in place of or in conjunction with existing clinical and pathologic features.

Additional workup and imaging. Most melanoma patients who seek surgical consultation already have the diagnosis confirmed. Patients clinically staged with localized stage I or II disease do not require any further tests unless symptoms or physical examination prompts further evaluation. Liver function tests or serum LDH levels were commonly ordered in the past; however, there is no evidence that blood tests are helpful for detecting metastatic disease in patients with localized melanoma. Similarly, additional imaging studies are unnecessary for most patients with localized disease, although patients with thick primary tumors can be considered for imaging to detect metastatic disease. Patients who can be considered for presurgical imaging include those with T4 tumors because a minority of these patients will have metastatic disease not appreciated on clinical examination. Identification of this metastatic disease before resection and SLN biopsy can eliminate the need for SLN staging and expedite treatment for metastatic disease. From a practical standpoint, many of these patients with thicker tumors who are SLN negative (IIB/IIC) will be considered for adjuvant therapy (see later discussion) and will accordingly undergo imaging before initiation of adjuvant therapy. Thus, imaging before surgery can streamline their postsurgical workup and adjuvant therapy initiation.

In patients with stage III disease detected by SLN biopsy, additional imaging workup is controversial. The probability of detecting actual disease in patients with microscopic nodal metastasis using radiographic studies such as positron emission tomography (PET) and computed tomography (CT) scanning is low. Patients with advanced stage III disease who have clinically detectable nodal metastasis or patients in earlier disease stages that present with symptoms suggestive of metastasis should undergo further imaging studies. The distinction between stage III and IV melanoma is important in deciding the appropriate treatment options, and imaging can determine the extent and resectability of any metastatic lesions in stage IV disease. For these advanced presentations, PET/CT or CT scans of the chest, abdomen, and pelvis and magnetic resonance imaging (MRI) of the brain are generally recommended. The National Comprehensive Cancer Network (NCCN) routinely updates guidelines, including the appropriate workup, surgical treatment, and adjuvant therapy, for patients with melanoma. These are available for reference online at http://www.nccn.org.

TREATMENT

Wide Local Excision

Historically, aggressive surgical resection was recommended for cutaneous melanoma. Excision margins of 5 cm were surgical

TABLE 63.1 **Recommended Margins of Wide Local Excision (WLE)**

THICKNESS	WLE MARGIN[a]
in situ	0.5 cm
<1 mm	1 cm
1–2 mm	1–2 cm[b]
>2–4 mm	2 cm
>4 mm	2 cm[c]

[a]Lesser margins may be justified in specific cases in order to achieve better functional or cosmetic outcome.

[b]A 1-cm margin may be associated with a slightly greater risk of local recurrence in this Breslow thickness category.

[c]There is no evidence that margins >2 cm are beneficial; however, greater margins may be considered for advanced melanomas when local recurrence risk is high.

dogma for much of the previous century. Beginning in the 1970s, studies began to report no adverse outcomes in patients who underwent excision with narrower margins. Since that time, multiple randomized controlled trials evaluating excision margins have established the current guidelines, which are summarized in Table 63.1. The principal determinant for appropriate excision margins is the thickness of the primary tumor.

Based largely on clinical experience and consensus guidelines, 5-mm excision margins are generally recommended for melanoma in situ. There are two potential issues with 5-mm margins for melanoma in situ. One is that negative pathologic margins may not be routinely achieved with gross 5-mm margins; a near 100% margin-negative rate can be achieved with gross margins closer to 10 mm versus 5 mm. The second issue is that there may be some diagnostic uncertainty with melanoma in situ. In those situations in which an invasive component is found once the entire tumor is excised (as opposed to the biopsy specimen), a 5-mm gross margin would be inadequate, and reexcision would be needed for an oncologically sound operation. With this in mind, it may be prudent to attempt 1-cm margins for some melanoma in situ lesions in anatomic areas that will allow for easy primary closure.

In general, the randomized trials that have focused on margins of excision have focused on intermediate-thickness melanoma. The general consensus and practice for thin (<1.0 mm) melanomas is that 1-cm margins are sufficient. Several randomized controlled trials have evaluated the margins needed for intermediate-thickness melanoma. As in most solid organ malignancies, no benefit in overall survival (OS) has been shown with wider excision margins for melanoma, although locoregional recurrence may be influenced by the margin of excision.

The British Collaborative Trial randomized 900 patients with melanomas ≥2 mm in thickness to a 1-cm versus 3-cm margin excision. Locoregional recurrences (defined as recurrence within 2 cm of excision or in-transit recurrence) were higher in the group with 1-cm margins compared with the group with 3 cm margins (hazard ratio [HR] 1.26, $p = 0.05$), with no difference in OS.[16] Based on this study, 1-cm margins are generally considered inadequate for intermediate or thick melanomas. The Swedish Melanoma Study group trial randomized 936 patients in nine European centers with cutaneous melanoma ≥2 mm in thickness to 2-cm versus 4-cm margins of excision. No statistically significant difference in OS was found, and the local recurrence rates were not statistically different.[17] Based on these trials and others, the general consensus is that 2-cm margins should be attempted for all melanoma ≥2.0 mm in thickness. For 1- to 2-mm-thick lesions, 2-cm margins are recommended, although narrower (1 cm) margins are acceptable in areas in which wider margins are not anatomically feasible. These narrower margins come with the understanding that local recurrence may be higher with 1-cm margins.

There is continued interest in determining whether 2-cm margins are necessary for all intermediate-thickness melanomas or whether 1-cm margins could be adequate. In a pilot study to assess the feasibility of such a randomized clinical trial, the use of a 2-cm margin in patients with a thickness >1 mm was associated with an increased need for complex reconstruction, increased wound necrosis rate, and no difference in patient-reported outcomes compared with the use of a 1-cm margin.[18] These findings have set the stage for the larger, multicenter international Melanoma Margins Trial (MelMarT-II) randomized clinical trial powered to answer the question of whether there is a difference in local recurrence between a narrower or wider margin.

Technique

WLE can be performed under local anesthesia in most cases, although general anesthesia is preferred for patients who will also undergo SLN biopsy or lymphadenectomy. The appropriate margins of excision are measured from the edge of the lesion or previous biopsy scar. This is usually achieved with a fusiform incision that encompasses the margins of excision to allow primary closure (Fig. 63.10). The incision is carried down to the muscular fascia so that all of the skin and underlying subcutaneous tissue are in the margin of excision. Excision of the fascia is not necessary in most cases but may be performed for patients with thick primary tumors and limited subcutaneous tissue in whom the deep margin is of concern. The specimen is submitted for permanent section pathology; frozen section analysis of margins is not performed. In most cases, the incision is closed by mobilizing the skin without the

need for complex tissue rearrangement or skin grafting. Rotational tissue flaps or skin grafts maybe necessary, especially for those requiring 2-cm margins in the head/neck region or distal extremities. In these anatomic areas, grafting or tissue rearrangements are useful techniques to achieve skin closure. Tumors arising in proximity to structures such as the nose, eye, and ear may require a compromise of conventionally oncologically sound margins to avoid deformities or disabilities. Subungual melanomas are treated with amputation of the distal digit. For fingers, ray amputations are unnecessary because the melanoma commonly involves only the distal phalanx, and amputation at the distal interphalangeal joint is sufficient. In all cases, resection should achieve histologically negative margins. Pathologic margins that are negative but correspond to a gross margin <1 cm may have a slightly higher risk of local recurrence, but limited evidence exists to support additional resection for these close margins.[19]

Mohs micrographic surgery (MMS) involves the sequential tangential excision of skin cancers with immediate pathologic margin assessment. It is used most often for NMSCs, such as squamous cell and BCCs, with good results. In melanoma, MMS is used primarily for in situ lesions, although some centers have begun to use MMS for invasive melanoma. MMS is preferred for cosmetically sensitive areas, such as the face, where it may minimize the skin defect while still achieving negative margins of excision. Success can be highly operator dependent and requires full pathologic examination of the excised margins. Although there have been several single-institution reports indicating that MMS results in low local recurrence rates for melanoma, it remains controversial.[20,21] In general, MMS is not considered oncologically acceptable for melanoma, except in the hands of experienced centers in highly selected cases.

Evaluation and Management of Regional Lymph Nodes

The evaluation and management of regional lymph nodes in melanoma have changed rapidly in the past three decades. Elective lymph node dissection to stage clinically node-negative patients is a relic of the past. SLN biopsy has been widely adopted and is the foundation of the assessment of intermediate and thick cutaneous melanoma. Indications have changed for a completion lymph node dissection (CLND) after a tumor-positive SLN biopsy based on two landmark studies. Altogether, the evaluation and management of the regional lymph nodes in melanoma has evolved over time based on clinical research and the willingness of surgical investigators to question the status quo.

Sentinel Lymph Node Biopsy

Since it was introduced by Dr. Donald Morton in 1992, the SLN biopsy has become an indispensable tool in staging patients with cutaneous melanoma.[22] The accuracy of the technique has been well validated, and it is now a required part of staging for melanoma >1.0 mm in thickness, according to the AJCC. The status of the SLNs is the single most important prognostic factor in melanoma patients without clinical evidence of nodal metastases. The results from the SLN biopsy directly affect treatment and surveillance decisions. A thorough understanding of the indications for SLN across the spectrum of melanoma thickness and the technical execution of the operation is critical for any surgeon who treats melanoma.

Indications. SLN biopsy is relatively simple and straightforward to perform; however, it is not without morbidity and costs. Like other staging tests, it should not be overused in patients at

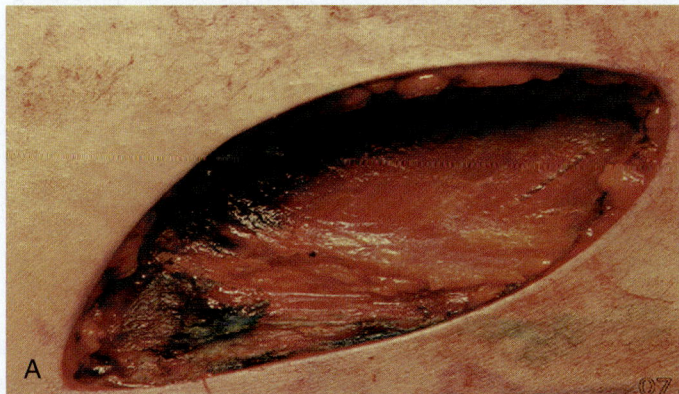

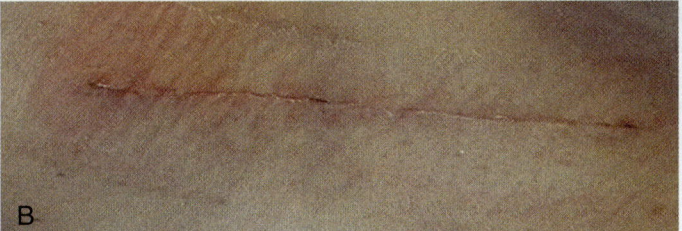

FIGURE 63.10 Fusiform incision (A) allowing primary closure (B) for wide local excision of melanoma.

low risk for lymph node metastases or with comorbidities that make general anesthesia prohibitively risky. The NCCN guidelines recommend consideration of SLN biopsy in all patients with T2 or greater (>1.0 mm) melanomas and in those with thinner lesions with a 5% or greater risk of a positive SLN. Some controversy exists regarding the circumstances under which SLN biopsy should be offered to patients with thin (T1) melanomas.

In the United States, approximately 70% of melanomas present as thin melanomas (defined as ≤1.0 mm in thickness). Although the overall risk of nodal metastasis in these patients is estimated at 5% or less, certain subsets of this population have rates of nodal disease that approach those seen with thicker lesions. Routine use of SLN biopsy is not recommended for thin melanomas, but if these lesions have any features that are associated with an increased risk for nodal spread, then SLN biopsy may be indicated. Features of the primary lesion that have been linked to an increased risk of nodal metastasis include ulceration and mitotic rate (≥1 mitosis/mm²).

The changes to the AJCC staging classification of T1 melanomas have complicated the assessment and risk stratification of thin melanomas for SLN biopsy. Previously, a T1b melanoma was defined by the presence of either ulceration and/or ≥1 mitosis/mm². Because these two factors are the strongest risk factors for SLN metastases in thin melanoma, it made for a fairly straightforward recommendation that SLN biopsy be considered for T1b melanomas. However, now T1b is defined by either ulceration or thickness of 0.8 to 1.0 mm, with no consideration for mitotic rate. T1b is a group defined by a slightly worse survival than T1a, but it is not necessarily a group with a higher risk of SLN metastases. Mitotic rate, although not formally considered in the AJCC staging criteria, should still be used to identify thin melanomas with an increased risk of SLN metastases. Other factors that can be used to identify higher-than-average-risk thin melanomas include age and thickness ranging from 0.8 to 1.0 mm.[23] Younger patients with thin melanomas have an increased risk of SLN metastases. Our general practice is to offer SLN biopsies to any patient with an acceptable risk of general anesthesia who has a T1 melanoma with ulceration or those between 0.8 and 1.0 mm thick with a mitotic rate ≥1 mitosis/mm². We selectively offer

SLN biopsy to younger patients without these adverse features, especially with thickness approaching 1.0 mm.

Technical details. The technical details of a proper SLN biopsy are worthy of attention. All patients should undergo preoperative lymphoscintigraphy, typically performed on the day before or the same day as the WLE and SLN biopsy operation (Fig. 63.11).[24] Technetium-99 sulfur colloid (0.5 mCi) should be injected into the dermis, raising a wheal, in four aliquots around the melanoma or biopsy site. It is important to inject the tracer into the normal skin approximately 0.5 cm away from the melanoma or scar from the biopsy and not into the melanoma itself or biopsy scar. A common mistake is to inject the radioactive tracer too deeply, into the subcutaneous tissue, which will result in failure to detect a sentinel node. If no sentinel nodes are identified after the initial injection, a repeat injection should be performed with the proper technique by an experienced clinician. In almost all cases, this will result in identification of sentinel nodes. Imaging is performed with a gamma camera, with dynamic and static images that allow identification of lymphatic channels and sentinel nodes. Although patterns of lymphatic drainage can be predictable at times, lymphoscintigraphy often identifies lymph nodes in locations that are not anticipated. This is especially true for melanomas in ambiguous lymphatic drainage areas, such as the trunk, head, or neck, where anatomic predictions of nodal spread are unreliable. In such cases, lymphoscintigraphy may identify sentinel nodes in more than one nodal basin. Furthermore, it is not uncommon to identify sentinel nodes outside the traditional cervical, axillary, and inguinal nodal basins. So-called *interval, intercalated,* or *in-transit nodes* may be found in subcutaneous locations or between muscle groups. For distal upper or lower extremity melanomas, it is important to assess the presence of epitrochlear or popliteal sentinel nodes, respectively. These interval nodes have the same risk of harboring melanoma cells as sentinel nodes in traditional nodal basins; therefore, it is recommended that they be removed at the time of sentinel node biopsy. In addition, 85% of the time, the interval lymph node is the only positive node, even for those patients with other SLNs identified in traditional basins. Therefore, all sentinel nodes identified by preoperative lymphoscintigraphy should be removed (Fig. 63.12).

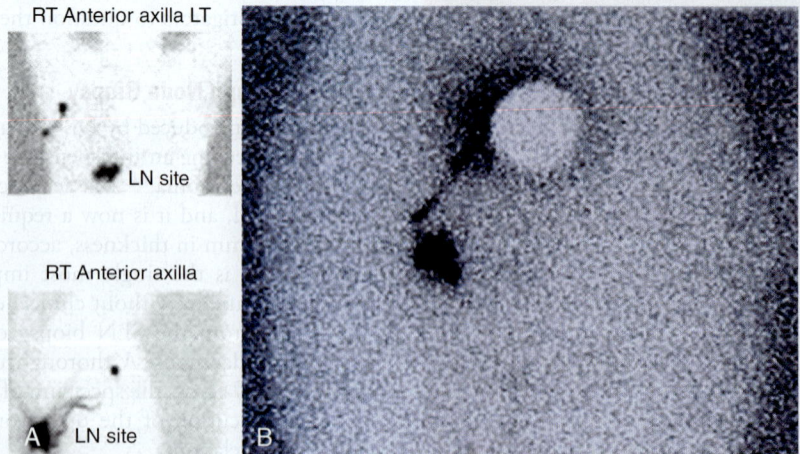

FIGURE 63.11 Preoperative lymphoscintigraphy can aid in identification of sentinel lymph nodes. (A) Melanoma of the back with drainage to the axilla. (B) Periumbilical melanoma with drainage to the left inguinal lymph nodes. *LN,* Lymph node; *LT,* left; *RT,* right.

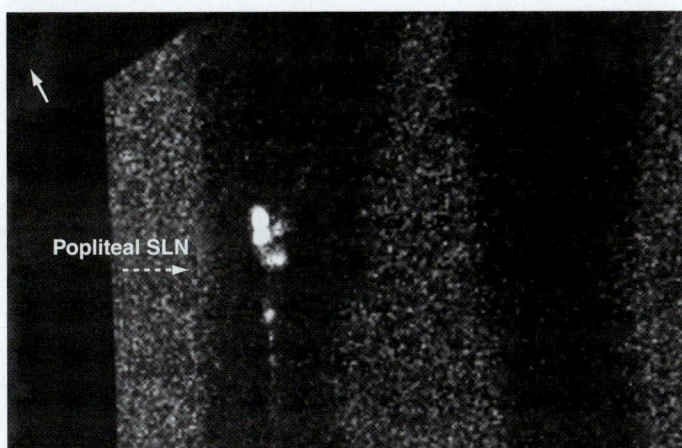

FIGURE 63.12 Popliteal sentinel lymph node *(SLN)* on lymphoscintigraphy.

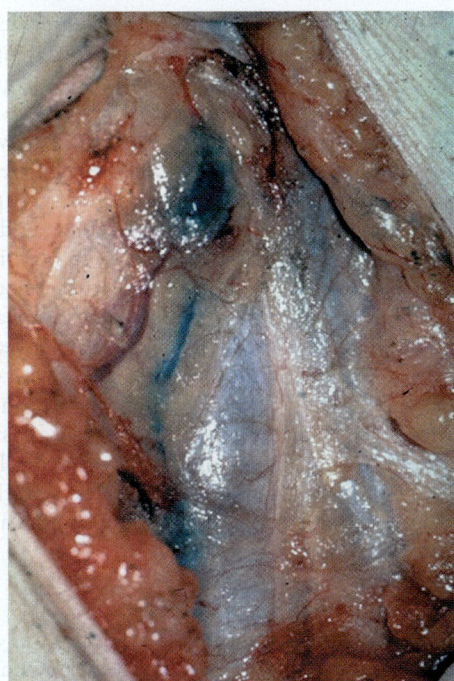

FIGURE 63.14 Blue lymphatic channels leading to a blue sentinel lymph node.

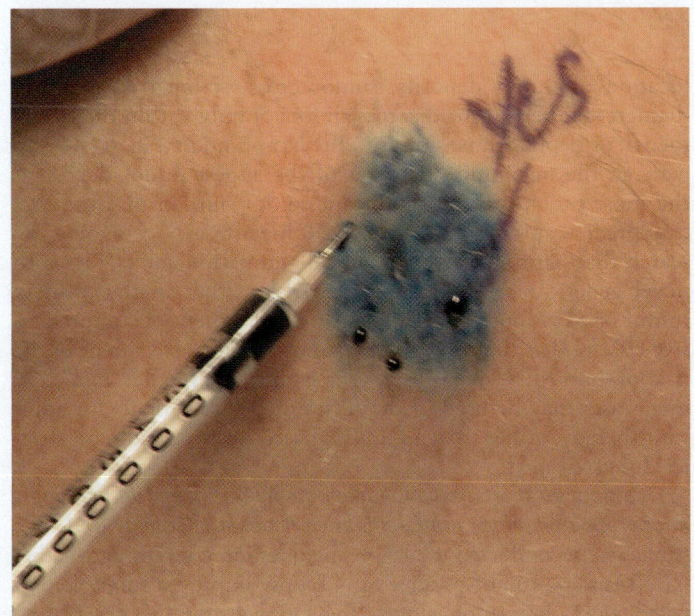

FIGURE 63.13 Intradermal injection of isosulfan blue dye for intraoperative lymphatic mapping and sentinel lymph node biopsy.

At operation, which is generally performed under general anesthesia, a vital blue dye (e.g., isosulfan blue or methylene blue) is injected into the dermis around the melanoma site in a manner similar to that for injection of the radioactive tracer (Fig. 63.13). This combined lymphatic mapping technique allows for the identification of the sentinel nodes in 99% of patients. Because the blue dye will not persist in the sentinel nodes for prolonged periods, it is injected just before the operation. Because blue dye will persist in the skin for many months after injection, it is best to inject it within the margins of the planned WLE. A handheld gamma probe is used to identify the location of the sentinel node(s), and dissection is performed to identify blue lymphatic channels entering into any blue lymph nodes (Fig. 63.14). A sentinel node is defined as any lymph node that is the most radioactive node in the nodal basin, any node that is blue, any node that has a radioactive count of 10% or higher of the most radioactive node in that basin, or any node that is palpably abnormal or

visually suspicious for tumor. All such nodes require resection. By following these guidelines, the risk of a false-negative SLN biopsy is minimized. Although multiple radioactive lymph nodes may be evident within a nodal basin on lymphoscintigraphy, many of these represent mildly radioactive second-echelon nodes and not true sentinel nodes. There is often a poor correlation between the number of nodes visualized on the lymphoscintigram and the number of SLNs identified. In general, the average number of sentinel nodes identified is two per nodal basin.[25] Sentinel nodes should be sent for permanent section histopathology with immunohistochemical stains for melanoma markers (e.g., S-100, HMB-45, and Melan-1). Immediate frozen section histology should be avoided because even expert pathologists have difficulty diagnosing micrometastatic melanoma in the SLN on frozen sections.

SLN biopsy is more challenging in the head and neck than for other regions because of the rich lymphatic drainage network in this location. Correspondingly, the false negative rate for SLN biopsy is generally higher for melanomas in these locations. Cross-sectional imaging, such as with a single-photon emission computed tomography (SPECT), can allow the surgeon to identify the exact anatomic location of the SLNs more accurately than with the planar lymphoscintigrams. Precise knowledge of the anatomy in this region is essential to avoid inadvertent neurologic injury. Parotid SLNs can be identified and removed, usually without the need for superficial parotidectomy. However, if there is any concern for facial nerve injury, superficial parotidectomy may be a safer option. A common site for cervical SLN is directly adjacent to the spinal accessory nerve, which should be visualized and preserved.

Multicenter selective lymphadenectomy Trial-I. The only randomized control trial to compare outcomes between SLN biopsy and nodal observation is the first Multicenter Selective Lymphadenectomy Trial (MSLT-I).[26] The trial randomized 1347 patients with intermediate-thickness melanoma (1.2–3.5 mm thick) and 314 patients with thick melanoma (>3.5 mm thick) to either

SLN biopsy or observation. Patients with disease identified by SLN biopsy underwent immediate completion lymphadenectomy. The frequency of nodal metastasis across all groups was 20.8% and was similar within each treatment arm. No difference in 10-year melanoma-specific survival was found between SLN biopsy and observation group in either the intermediate-thickness (81.4% vs. 78.3%, $p = 0.18$) or thick melanoma groups (58.9% vs. 64.4%, $p = 0.56$). However, improved 10-year disease-free survival (DFS) was observed with SLN biopsy in both intermediate and thick melanomas. The status of the sentinel node was the strongest predictor of recurrence or death from melanoma: in patients with intermediate-thickness melanoma, 10-year survival was 85.1% with a negative SLN biopsy, compared with 62.1% for positive nodes (HR 3.09, $p < 0.001$). Interestingly, on subgroup analysis limited only to patients with nodal metastasis (disease identified either on SLN biopsy or that developed while under observation), improved melanoma-specific survival, DFS, and distant DFS were observed in the SLN biopsy arm among patients with intermediate-thickness lesions.

Lymph Node Dissection

Historical. Lymph node dissection historically was an important component of the surgical treatment of melanoma, but with the development of the SLN biopsy technique and an improved understanding of the biology of melanoma, it has become less important. Before the use of SLN biopsy, an elective lymph node dissection of the draining regional nodal basin was often performed for high-risk melanomas in order to identify early, clinically occult lymph node metastases and provide accurate staging. The SLN technique accomplishes the same objectives with decreased morbidity; therefore, elective lymph node dissection is of historical interest only. Lymph node dissection does still play an important role in the treatment of melanoma; therefore, the surgeon treating melanoma should be familiar with the technical details of the operation and its indications.

Completion lymphadenectomy. Completion lymphadenectomy or CLND is used to remove the remaining lymph nodes in a regional nodal basin that is found to have metastatic melanoma by SLN biopsy. A wide range of prognoses exists in stage III, SLN-positive melanoma. CLND allows one to identify nonsentinel node metastases. This is an important prognostic factor because multiple studies have demonstrated that metastases to the nonsentinel nodes represent an additional echelon of metastatic disease with more aggressive biology and worse prognosis compared with disease limited to the SLNs. CLND may have a potential therapeutic benefit by removing additional lymph nodes with micrometastatic disease, improving DFS, as seen in MSLT-I. CLND does, however, greatly increase the short- and long-term morbidity to the patients. Complications include wound complications, paresthesias, and permanent lymphedema. Only 15% to 20% of patients with SLN-positive micrometastatic lymph node disease have additional micrometastatic nonsentinel nodes after CLND; thus, five out of six patients undergoing CLND for SLN-positive disease derive no therapeutic benefit from the procedure and experience all the morbidity associated with the CLND.

Efforts to predict non-SLN metastases have focused on clinical and pathologic factors that identify high- and low-risk patients in whom a CLND could either be selectively omitted (in patients at low risk for non-SLN disease) or in whom a CLND would be particularly beneficial. Multiple different scoring systems evaluating the burden of micrometastatic disease within the lymph node have been developed, with criteria including the

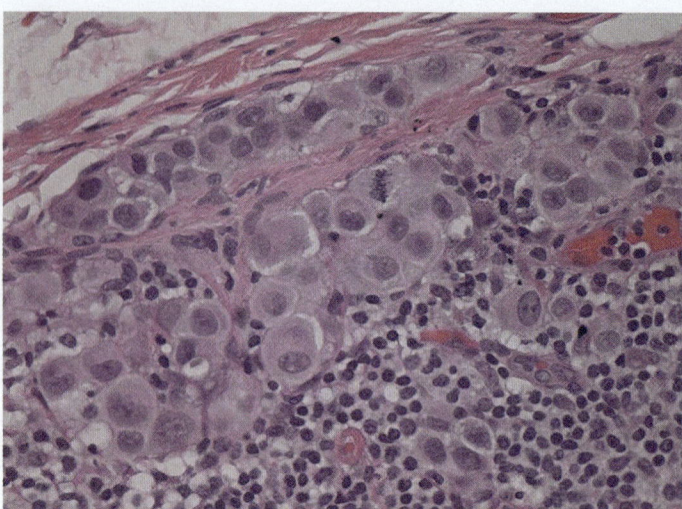

FIGURE 63.15 Subcapsular micrometastatic melanoma deposits within the lymph node.

location of tumor deposits, tumor cross-sectional area, tumor diameter (either summed across all foci or only within the largest focus), or depth of invasion into the lymph node (Fig. 63.15). In general, the maximum diameter of the largest tumor deposit is the most prognostically significant tumor burden measure that can predict survival and non-SLN metastases.[27] Ongoing research that harmonizes these clinical and pathologic factors with novel genetic markers of increased risk, either in the primary tumor or SLN biopsy, will allow the development of comprehensive risk models that can give a patient-specific assessment of the risk of non-SLN metastases. The ability to predict non-SLN metastases may be used in the future to select patients for adjuvant therapy, rather than a CLND, based on two landmark studies discussed next.

Multicenter selective lymphadenectomy Trial-II and dermatologic cooperative oncology group-selective lymphadenectomy trial. Two studies were conducted to answer the question concerning whether CLND after a tumor-positive SLN biopsy improved survival compared with observation alone. The rationale for the observation approach is that, as discussed earlier, upward of 85% of patients do not have any additional micrometastatic disease after a positive SLN biopsy; therefore, no survival benefit is achieved from routine CLND.

The Dermatologic Cooperative Oncology Group-Selective Lymphadenectomy Trial (DeCOG-SLT) study was a multicenter, randomized clinical trial conducted in Germany, the results of which were published in 2016.[28] In the study, 483 patients with a positive SLN biopsy were randomized to either a CLND of the positive lymph node basin or observation. The trial was closed early because of difficulties in accrual and low event rates; the planned enrollment was 550. With a median follow-up of 35 months, there was no difference in the primary end point, distant metastasis–free survival (DMFS), between the two groups (77% vs. 75%). There were no differences in recurrence-free survival (RFS) or OS. Subgroup analysis of the primary end point based on micrometastatic tumor burden (≤1 mm or >1 mm) showed no differences in DMFS. The study has been criticized as being underpowered and failing to meet accrual, but it is an important study that establishes the safety of an observation strategy with SLN-positive melanoma.

The Multicenter Selective Lymphadenectomy Trial-II (MSLT-II) was a larger, multicenter randomized clinical trial that confirmed the findings of the DeCOG study. In MSLT-II, 1939 patients with a tumor-positive SLN biopsy were randomized to a CLND or observation, which consisted of ultrasound-based surveillance of the involved nodal basin.[29] There was no difference in the primary end point, melanoma-specific survival, between the two groups. The 3-year melanoma-specific survival rate was 86% in both groups, whereas the 3-year DFS rate was numerically (but not statistically) greater in the CLND group compared with the observation group (68% vs. 63%, $p = 0.05$). There was an increase in the cumulative incidence of non-SLN metastases in the observation group versus the CLND group (26% vs. 20% at 5 years, $p = 0.005$).

Taken together, the findings of DeCOG-SLT and MSLT-II have been practice changing. Only in very selective circumstances, in which there is a high degree of concern for non-SLN metastases and failure of regional nodal control or inability to follow the observation surveillance strategy, is CLND considered after a positive SLN. The DeCOG and MSLT-II studies firmly establish that it is safe and reasonable to avoid CLND for the vast majority of patients with a positive SLN. The issues of this approach and the selection of patients for adjuvant therapy will be discussed later.

Therapeutic lymph node dissection. The routine use of therapeutic lymph node dissection (TLND), which is a lymphadenectomy of a regional nodal basin with clinically apparent nodal metastases, in conjunction with adjuvant immunotherapy for patients with clinically apparent stage III disease was commonplace but is increasingly being supplanted by a neoadjuvant approach with a more limited targeted lymph node dissection (discussed further later). For patients with suspected nodal metastases based on palpable lymph nodes or radiographic abnormalities, a fine-needle aspiration biopsy should be obtained to confirm the diagnosis. On occasion, benign lymphadenopathy may be found, but in a patient with cutaneous melanoma, palpable lymph nodes should be concerning for metastatic disease until proven otherwise. Palliative resection of bulky, painful regional lymphadenopathy can be considered, recognizing that there will be a high risk of regional and distant metastatic recurrence in the absence of

effective adjuvant therapy (Fig. 63.16). However, more commonly today, these patients would start treatment with systemic therapies, reserving the TLND for individuals with advanced locoregional disease that is unresponsive to systemic therapies.

A TLND should remove all the fibrofatty and lymphatic tissue in the involved regional nodal basin according to standard anatomic boundaries. For the axilla, a thorough level I, II, and III axillary dissection is performed. This includes complete removal of all fibrofatty tissue around the axillary vein, thoracodorsal and medial pectoral neurovascular bundles, and long thoracic nerve. The pectoralis minor muscle may need to be divided near its insertion on the coracoid process in order to clear bulky level II and III nodes. On rare occasions, the pectoralis major muscle may need to be divided as well. The axillary vein may be ligated and divided if it becomes involved with tumor, often with less consequence in terms of edema than one might anticipate.

Inguinal lymph node dissection includes the superficial inguinal (femoral) lymph nodes and may also include dissection of deep or pelvic (internal iliac, external iliac, and obturator) nodes. There is no consensus as to when pelvic nodal dissection should be performed for patients with macroscopic disease confined to the superficial inguinal nodal basin. For patients with palpable nodal disease or with imaging suggestive of involved pelvic lymph nodes, the deep nodes should be dissected in most cases. Metastasis to Cloquet's node, which links the femoral and iliac nodal chains underneath the inguinal ligament, has traditionally been a common indication for pelvic nodal dissection. Similarly, gross involvement of multiple femoral nodes is another traditional indication for pelvic dissection.

For cervical lymphadenectomy, a functional neck dissection with sparing of the internal jugular vein and spinal accessory nerve is usually sufficient. The need for superficial parotidectomy may be guided by the lymphoscintigraphy and SLN results. Epitrochlear or popliteal lymphadenectomy is frequently unnecessary but requires careful attention to the particular anatomy in these regions (Fig. 63.17).

Adjuvant Therapy

As with most solid organ malignancies, the dismal prognosis historically associated with advanced melanoma was the result

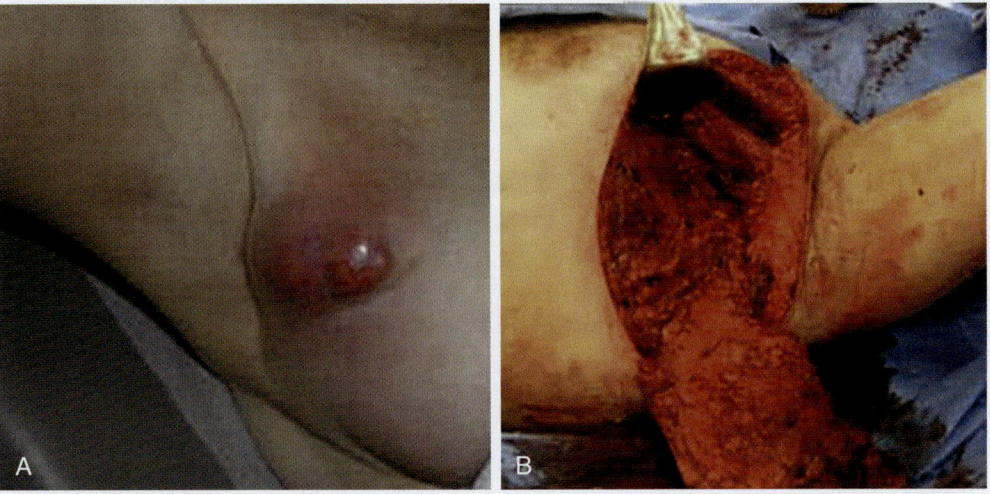

FIGURE 63.16 (A) Advanced axillary lymph node metastases. (B) Levels I, II, and III axillary lymph node dissection.

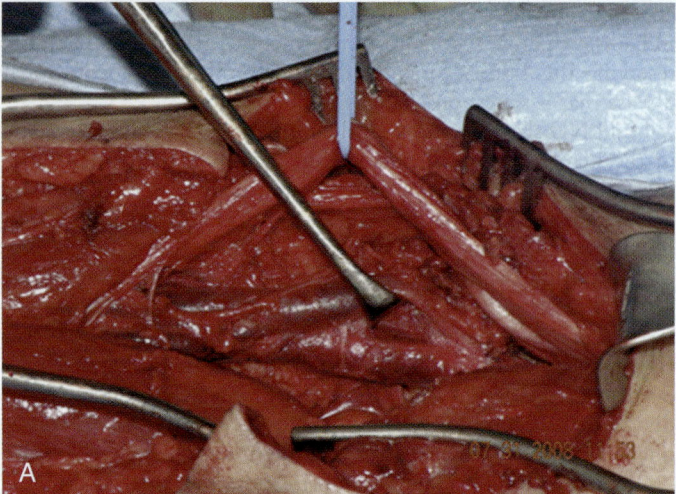

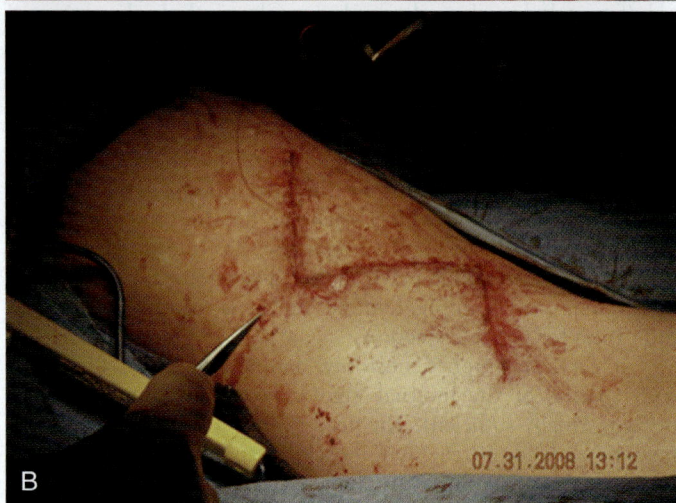

FIGURE 63.17 (A) Popliteal lymph node dissection with exposed popliteal artery and vein. (B) Closure.

of a lack of effective systemic therapies. Melanoma biology has historically trumped the locoregional disease control strategies of the surgeon. With the exception of some increase in the sophistication of our understanding of the evaluation and management of the regional lymph nodes, vis-á-vis SLN biopsy and indication for completion lymphadenectomy, the operative treatment of melanoma has not changed much in the past few decades. The same cannot be said for systemic treatment options. It is an exciting time to be treating melanoma; advances in targeted therapy and immunotherapy have been occurring at breakneck speed. We now have multiple adjuvant therapy options that are safe and effective and offer melanoma patients the hope for durable disease remission after operative therapy (Table 63.2).

Historical

Before 2015, the only adjuvant systemic therapy approved for melanoma by the US Food and Drug Administration (FDA) was high-dose interferon-α2b. This drug was quite toxic, with a prolonged treatment course and numerous serious adverse events. Therapy was typically delivered for 1 month via IV therapy, followed by 11 months of thrice weekly subcutaneous injections. Common side effects included influenza-like symptoms, fatigue, malaise, anorexia, neuropsychiatric side effects, and hepatic toxicity.

The therapy was marginally effective at best and quite toxic at worst. The FDA approval was based largely on the Eastern Cooperative Oncology Group E1684 trial, in which high-risk patients with palpable nodal disease experienced short-term disease-free and OS benefit with adjuvant interferon; longer follow-up demonstrated a modest difference in DFS only. Alternative dosing strategies, including intermittent dosing and the use of pegylated interferon-α2b, were tried. The Sunbelt Melanoma Trial demonstrated that in lower-risk patients with a single positive SLN, there was no benefit to adjuvant interferon in terms of disease-free or OS.

TABLE 63.2 Summary of Adjuvant Therapy Trials for BRAF/MEK Inhibition and Immunotherapy in Cutaneous Stage III Melanoma

TRIAL NAME	STUDY POPULATION	INTERVENTION TREATMENT	CONTROL TREATMENT	PRIMARY OUTCOME	NOTES
EORTC 18071[31]	IIIA (with >1-mm micro-metastasis), IIIB, IIIC (with no in-transit metastases)	Ipilimumab 10 mg/kg every 3 weeks × 4, then every 3 months × 3 years	Placebo	Improved recurrence-free survival (HR 0.76, 95% CI 0.64–0.89)	Improved overall survival at 5 years (65.4% vs. 54.4%, HR 0.72, 95% CI 0.58–0.88)
COMBI-AD (Long et al., Dummer et al.)[30]	IIIA (with >1-mm micro-metastasis), IIIB, IIIC BRAF V600 mutation	Daily dabrafenib/trametinib × 12 months	Placebo	Improved relapse-free survival (RFS; 5-yr RFS 52% vs. 36%, HR 0.51, 95% CI 32–41)	—
CheckMate 238 (Larkin et al.)[32,33]	Completely resected IIIB, IIIC, or IV	Nivolumab every 2 weeks × 12 months	Ipilimumab 10 mg/kg every 3 weeks × 4, then every 12 weeks × 12 months	Improved 5-yr RFS with nivolumab (50% vs. 39%, HR 0.72, 95% CI 0.60–0.86)	5-yr overall 76% with Nivolumab and 72% ipilimumab
EORTC 1325 (Eggermont, et al.)[34]	IIIA (with >1-mm micrometastasis), IIIB, IIIC (with no in-transit metastases)	Pembrolizumab every 3 weeks × 12 months	Placebo	5-yr recurrence-free survival 55.4% vs. 38.3% (HR 0.61, 95% CI 0.51–0.72)	—

CI, Confidence interval; EORTC, European Organisation for Research and Treatment of Cancer; HR, hazard ratio.

The summary assessment of adjuvant interferon for melanoma is that it reproducibly improved DFS and had minimal effect on OS at the cost of serious toxicity. Better adjuvant therapy options were needed; these options came in the form of targeted therapy and immunotherapy.

Targeted Therapy

The first successful targeted therapy developed for melanoma was vemurafenib, a small molecule tyrosine kinase inhibitor targeted against the V600E *BRAF* mutation. *BRAF* is one of the recognized driver mutations in melanoma that is present in about half of all cutaneous melanoma cases. Building on the initial successful trials in metastatic melanoma, BRAF inhibition as a treatment concept evolved into dual BRAF-MEK inhibition in order to overcome some of the resistance issues seen with single-agent BRAF inhibition (Fig. 63.18). The promising experience with BRAF-MEK inhibition in metastatic melanoma led to the development of an adjuvant trial for patients with resected stage III BRAF-mutant melanoma.

The landmark 2017 COMBI-AD trial published 5-year data in 2020.[30] In this multicenter, international study, 870 patients with completely resected stage III melanoma with either the *BRAF* V600E or V600K mutation were randomly assigned to dual BRAF (dabrafenib) and MEK (trametinib) inhibition therapy or placebo for 12 months after resection. The initial findings were as follows: 3-year relapse-free survival was improved from 39% to 58% in the treatment group (HR 0.47), and 3-year OS was improved from 77% to 86% (HR 0.57), although the level of improvement in survival did not cross the prespecified interim analysis boundary. At 5 years, the percentage of patients who were alive without relapse was 52% (95% confidence interval [CI] 48–58) with dabrafenib plus trametinib and 36% (95% CI 32–41) with placebo (HR for relapse or death, 0.51; 95% CI 0.42–0.61); OS at 5 years was not analyzed because the number of events for final survival analysis had not been reached. The therapy was well tolerated, with a reasonable adverse-event profile. Importantly, the trial enrolled patients with stage III disease who had undergone a completion lymphadenectomy for SLN-positive disease. High-risk micrometastatic disease was selected by only enrolling patients with a lymph node metastasis of >1 mm.

Immunotherapy

Adjuvant immunotherapy developed in a similar manner to BRAF-targeted therapy, in which early experience with the treatment of metastatic disease developed into an adjuvant therapy concept. The first immunotherapy agent to gain approval for adjuvant therapy was the monoclonal anti–cytotoxic T-lymphocyte–associated protein 4 (CTLA-4) antibody ipilimumab in 2015. In activated T cells, the CTLA-4 receptor traffics to the extracellular membrane, where it inhibits costimulatory ligands on antigen-presenting cells (APCs) and thereby prevents continued stimulation of the T cells by APCs. By blocking CTLA-4, ipilimumab effectively prolongs the T-cell response. The FDA approved ipilimumab based on the initial findings of the European Organisation for Research and Treatment of Cancer (EORTC) 18071 study published in 2015.[31] In this trial, 951 patients with resected stage III melanoma were randomized to treatment with ipilimumab at a dose of 10 mg/kg for up to 3 years or placebo. Five-year RFS was 40.8% in the ipilimumab group compared with 30.3% (HR 0.76), and the 5-year OS rate was improved from 54.4% to 65.4% (HR 0.72). These benefits did not come without increased risk of serious adverse events and even death from adjuvant ipilimumab. Serious adverse events occurred in 54% of the patients treated with ipilimumab compared with 26% of the placebo group. Five patients (1.1%) died as a result of complications from adjuvant ipilimumab. The promising results from this trial led to the first new drug approved by the FDA for adjuvant therapy of melanoma in nearly 20 years. However, the side effects and risk of death were of significant concern.

The newer programmed cell death 1 (PD-1) inhibitors nivolumab and pembrolizumab offered the promise of safer, better-tolerated immunotherapy with a response that was just as effective and durable as ipilimumab. The interaction of a PD-1 receptor with its ligands PD-L1 and PD-L2 promotes T-cell anergy and apoptosis. The CheckMate 238 trial demonstrated that adjuvant nivolumab was more effective than ipilimumab at preventing recurrence in resected stage III and stage IV melanoma.[32] In this trial, 906 patients with complete resection of stage IIIB, IIIC, or IV (as defined by AJCC 7th edition) melanomas were randomly assigned to 1 year of adjuvant nivolumab or ipilimumab. At a minimum follow-up of 62 months, RFS with nivolumab remained superior to ipilimumab (HR 0.72; 95% CI 0.60–0.86; 5-year rates of 50% vs. 39%). Five-year DMFS rates were 58% with nivolumab versus 51% with ipilimumab. Five-year OS rates were 76% with nivolumab and 72% with ipilimumab (75% data maturity: 228 of 302 planned events).[33] The relative benefit of nivolumab compared with ipilimumab was consistent across multiple subgroups, including age, sex, stage (IIIB,

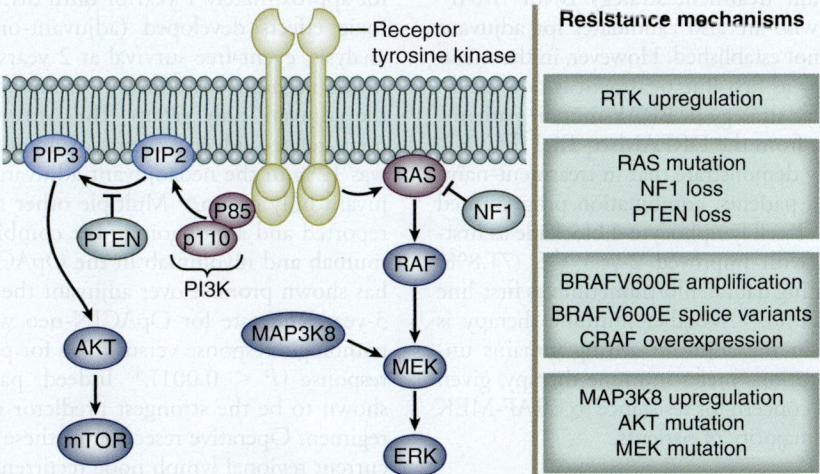

FIGURE 63.18 BRAF/MEK signaling pathway and potential mechanisms of resistance. (From Welsh SJ, Rizos H, Scolyer RA, Long GV. Resistance to combination BRAF and MEK inhibition in metastatic melanoma: where to next? *Eur J Cancer.* 2016;62:76-85.)

IIIC, and IV), ulceration, and micro- versus macro-metastatic lymph node disease. Adjuvant pembrolizumab has also been reported to improve RFS in resected stage III melanoma. In the EORTC 1325 (KEYNOTE-054) trial, 1019 patients with resected stage III melanoma (by 7th edition AJCC) were randomized to 1 year of adjuvant pembrolizumab or placebo.[34] The 5-year rate of RFS was 55.4% versus 38.3% for placebo (HR 0.61, 95% CI 0.51–0.72).[34] The low rate of serious adverse events reported in the pembrolizumab group (14.7%) was similar to that of nivolumab in the CheckMate 238 trial. Like nivolumab, pembrolizumab was effective across multiple subgroups, including PD-L1 expression, sex, stage (IIIA, IIIB, IIIC), number of positive lymph nodes, micro- versus macro-metastatic lymph node disease, ulceration, and BRAF-mutation status.

Based on these landmark trials, the PD-1 inhibitors nivolumab and pembrolizumab have become the preferred adjuvant immunotherapy option for patients with resected stage III and IV melanoma. Ipilimumab has fallen out of favor because of its toxicity profile compared with the PD-1 inhibitors, but it may still play a role in salvage therapy or in combination with PD-1 inhibitors (discussed in more detail later). A trial combining both adjuvant nivolumab and ipilimumab versus nivolumab (CheckMate 915) in resected stage III/IV melanoma did not show improvement in RFS, and grade 3 or 4 adverse events were reported in 32.6% of patients receiving the combination.[35] The preference for nivolumab or pembrolizumab is usually institution specific because there are no data to suggest that one is more effective than the other. All patients in these adjuvant studies underwent completion lymphadenectomy for SLN-positive disease; however, the current treatment strategy for SLN-positive disease in light of the MSLT-II and DeCOG studies is to forgo completion lymphadenectomy in favor of nodal surveillance. A large multicenter retrospective analysis showed that the 24-month RFS in patients not receiving CLND after a positive SLN biopsy was 64%, similar to the 24-month RFS rate of patients in the trials.[36] However, those without CLND had a higher rate of relapse in the regional nodal basin.

Future adjuvant studies that include nivolumab plus relatlimab (anti–LAG-3 antibody) are underway. The combination of relatlimab (also an immune checkpoint inhibitor) and nivolumab provided greater progression-free survival (PFS) compared with nivolumab alone in metastatic melanoma, and the strategy is now being applied to the adjuvant setting.[37]

What the optimal adjuvant treatment strategy is for BRAF-mutant melanoma patients who are also candidates for adjuvant immunotherapy is currently not established. However, in the metastatic setting, immune therapy as first-line treatment is now established as the optimal treatment strategy in BRAF-mutant patients. Randomized prospective data from the DREAMseq Trial (ECOG-ACRIN EA6134) now clearly demonstrate that in treatment-naïve BRAF600-mutant melanoma patients, combination programmed cell death protein 1/cytotoxic T-cell lymphocyte-4 blockade as first-line treatment is associated with improved 2-year OS (71.8%) compared with patients initiating dabrafenib/trametinib as first-line treatment (2-year OS of 52.1%).[38] Whether immune therapy is also a more durable choice in the adjuvant setting remains unknown; however, many institutions prefer immune therapy, given data in metastatic disease and concern for resistance to BRAF-MEK inhibition that develops in a majority of patients.

Adjuvant Therapy For Stage IIB/IIC

Given that the prognosis for stage IIB and IIC melanoma (with a negative SLN biopsy) remains poor and is actually worse than that

for IIIA patients, two trials were initiated to examine adjuvant therapy after excision and a negative SLN in this population. KEYNOTE 716 randomized IIB or IIC patients with a negative SLN biopsy to pembrolizumab or placebo. At a median follow-up of 20.9 months (16.7–25.3) in the pembrolizumab group and 20.9 months (16.6–25.3) in the placebo group, 72 (15%) patients in the pembrolizumab group and 115 (24%) in the placebo group had a first recurrence or died (HR 0.61, 95% CI 0.45–0.82); grade 3 or 4 adverse events occurred in 16% of pembrolizumab patients and 4% in the placebo group.[39] This trial led to the FDA approval of adjuvant pembrolizumab in these patients in the spring of 2022. Similarly, CheckMate 76K randomized stage IIB/C patients to adjuvant nivolumab versus placebo; nivolumab significantly prolonged RFS compared with placebo; FDA approval is pending.[40]

Finally, another adjuvant therapy is the mRNA-based personalized cancer vaccine (PCV). In brief, KEYNOTE-942 is a randomized study of adjuvant pembrolizumab plus mRNA-4157 versus pembrolizumab alone. The resected tumor undergoes genetic sequencing to identify 20 neoantigen epitopes; the sequences encoding up to 34 patient-specific epitopes are transcribed and loaded onto a single mRNA molecule. On administration, the mRNA-based PCV mRNA-4157 is thought to be taken up and translated by APCs. Then, the expressed epitopes are presented via major histocompatibility complex (MHC) molecules on the surface of the APCs, leading to an induction T-cell–dependent immune responses that specifically target and destroy the patient's cancer cells that express these neoantigens. Updated results in the first 157 patients show that the 18-month RFS rates were 78.6% (95% CI 69%–85.6%) for combination therapy versus 62.2% (95% CI 46.9%–74.2%), and DMFS was also significantly improved in the combination group.[41]

Neoadjuvant Therapy

For clinically detectable (e.g., palpable lymph node) stage III or IV disease amenable to surgical resection, neoadjuvant therapy is now a standard-of-care approach after the results of SWOG1801. In this phase II randomized trial, patients with clinically detectable, measurable stage IIIB to IVC melanoma that was amenable to surgical resection were randomized to three doses of neoadjuvant pembrolizumab, surgery, and 15 doses of adjuvant pembrolizumab (neoadjuvant-adjuvant group) or to surgery followed by pembrolizumab (200 mg intravenously every 3 weeks for a total of 18 doses) for approximately 1 year or until disease recurred or unacceptable toxic effects developed (adjuvant-only group). In a landmark analysis, event-free survival at 2 years was 72% (95% CI 64–80) in the neoadjuvant-adjuvant group and 49% (95% CI 41–59) in the adjuvant-only group. The percentage of patients with treatment-related adverse events of grade 3 or higher during therapy was 12% in the neoadjuvant-adjuvant group and 14% in the adjuvant-only group.[42] Multiple other neoadjuvant trials have been reported and are ongoing. The combination of neoadjuvant ipilimumab and nivolumab in the OpACIN and OpACIN-neo trials has shown promise over adjuvant therapy; the reported estimated 3-year RFS rate for OpACIN-neo was 95% for patients with a pathologic response versus 37% for patients without a pathologic response (P < 0.001).[43] Indeed, pathologic response has been shown to be the strongest predictor of RFS for any neoadjuvant regimen. Operative resection of these patients for persistent or recurrent regional lymph node recurrence still plays a role; however, we predict that these operations will become less common or deescalate in the future as our immunotherapy treatments improve. Efforts such as the Personalized Response-Directed Surgery and

Adjuvant Therapy (PRADO) study, in which patients achieving a major pathology response after neoadjuvant ipilimumab and nivolumab in a single index lymph node had TLND omitted, are an important step.[44] Patients with no TLND had lower surgical morbidity. However, 4 of the 60 patients developed regional recurrence, and 3 of 4 then underwent TLND. Neoadjuvant trials are ongoing to consider the appropriate regimen, duration, timing, and need for adjuvant therapy after pathologic assessment. Much like metastatic disease, choice of therapy will likely be dependent on patient factors and ability to tolerate treatment; ipilimumab + nivolumab, relatlimab + nivolumab, and anti–PD-1 monotherapy may all be reasonable choices in the appropriate patient. Given SWOG1801 data, any patient with clinically detectable stage III or higher melanoma should be given full consideration for neoadjuvant therapy. There will, of course, be subsets of patients who are not candidates for whom risk may outweigh benefit (e.g., autoimmune disease), but SWOG1801 results should be considered practice changing.

Radiation Therapy

Although melanoma has been historically felt to be relatively resistant to radiation, several newer studies suggest that there may be roles for radiation treatment in the adjuvant and palliative settings as well as a potential adjunct to systemic immunotherapy. Adjuvant radiation therapy may have a role in select patients at high risk for lymph node basin recurrence after lymphadenectomy. In long-term follow-up of the Australia and New Zealand Melanoma Trials Group (ANZMTG) 01.02/Trans-Tasman Radiation Oncology Group (TROG) 02.01 trial, adjuvant radiation therapy after regional lymphadenectomy reduced the cumulative incidence of lymph node field relapse from 36% to 21% (adjusted HR 0.52).[45] The trial randomized 250 patients considered to be at high risk for nodal recurrence to either adjuvant radiotherapy (48 Gy in 20 fractions) or observation after lymphadenectomy. High risk was defined as one or more involved parotid nodes, two or more cervical or axillary nodes, three or more involved inguinal nodes, presence of extra nodal extension, or maximum diameter of the largest lymph node greater than 4 cm (3 cm for cervical nodes). After long-term follow-up, there remained no difference in OS or RFS. Adjuvant radiation therapy does appear to offer some improvement in control of regional lymph node disease in high-risk patients after lymphadenectomy; however, the importance of this regional control with disease that is clearly at high risk for systemic metastases is not clear. It is likely that patients with high-risk regional nodal disease would derive more benefit from better adjuvant systemic therapy (immunotherapy) to reduce the risk of metastatic recurrence rather than adjuvant radiation therapy to improve nodal basin disease control. For select patients with contraindications to adjuvant therapy and/or a large burden of disease in the SLN, adjuvant radiation to the nodal basin may be considered to decrease local recurrence.

Treatment of Locoregional Recurrent Disease

Local Recurrence

Recurrence within 5 cm of the WLE scar or skin graft is considered a local recurrence and represents aggressive tumor biology associated with poor OS (Fig. 63.19). Recurrence risk increases with tumor thickness and has been estimated as 0.2%, 2%, 6%, and 13% for melanomas less than 0.75 mm, 0.75 to 1.5 mm, 1.5 to 4 mm, and larger than 4 mm, respectively. Treatment for local recurrence can be operative resection to histologically negative margins. However, patients with local recurrences that are dermal

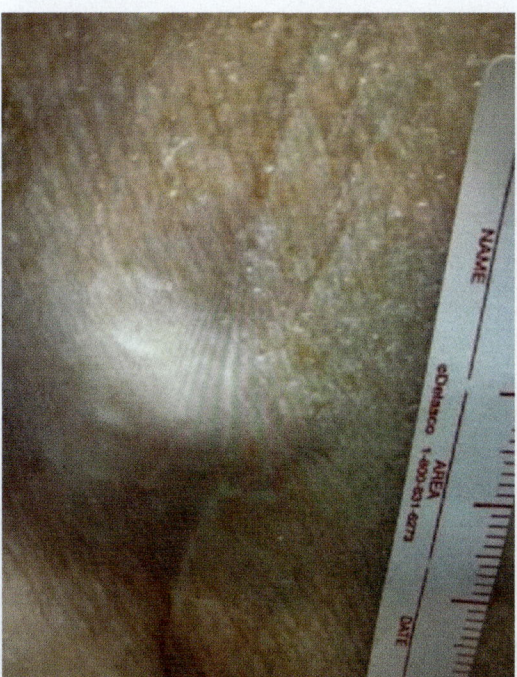

FIGURE 63.19 Local recurrence of melanoma within the scar of the primary melanoma excision.

(lack epidermal component) are also considered recurrent stage III melanoma. In the appropriate patient, adjuvant or neoadjuvant therapy can also be an option. Factors such as burden of disease, disease-free interval, number of recurrences, age, and ability to tolerate therapy should be considered.

In-Transit Disease

In-transit tumors, either at presentation or as a recurrence after initial local therapy, are subcutaneous or cutaneous tumor nodules between the primary tumor site and draining nodal basin formed by tumor deposits within the lymphatic channels (Fig. 63.20). They are often subtle in appearance, lack pigmentation, and may only be appreciated as a palpable nodule. Fine-needle aspiration or core biopsy can confirm the diagnosis. Once diagnosed, whole body imaging should be performed because there is a high risk of distant metastatic disease (around 75% of patients will eventually develop nodal and distant disease). Limited in-transit disease may be adequately treated with simple excision to negative margins, but similar to local recurrence, these patients are candidates for neoadjuvant and adjuvant therapies, and a high suspicion for a more aggressive disease biology must be in the mind of the surgeon.

Historically, extensive or recurrent in-transit disease confined to the extremity was treated with regional chemotherapy. Methods of delivering high-dose chemotherapy into the limb that was otherwise isolated from the rest of the body included hyperthermic isolated limb perfusion or isolated limb infusion. Melphalan was the most common chemotherapy agent delivered into the circuit. Isolated limb infusion was developed as a less invasive, less resource-intensive technique with comparable oncologic outcomes and less limb toxicity. These treatments are used less often now because intralesional and systemic immunotherapies are now preferred as an effective way to achieve locoregional disease control of in-transit disease with less morbidity for patients.

Talimogene laherparepvec (T-VEC) is a herpes simplex virus type 1–derived oncolytic immunotherapy that is serially injected

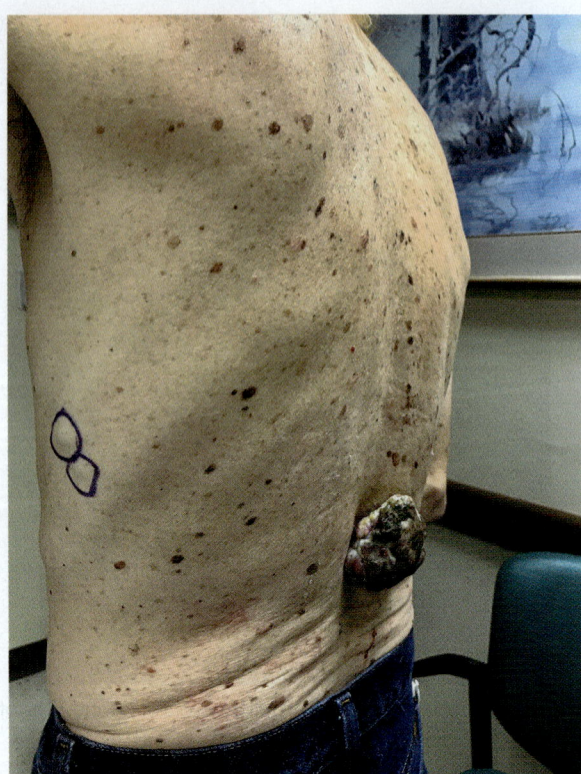

FIGURE 63.20 In-transit metastases *(circled on left flank)* between the large primary tumor of the mid–lower back and the draining nodal basin.

into palpable target lesions to induce both a direct local effect and potentially a systemic response. In the Oncovex (GM-CSF) Pivotal Trial in Melanoma (OPTiM) trial, 436 patients with unresected stage IIIB to IV melanoma by 7th edition AJCC staging were randomized to either serial intralesional T-VEC injection or granulocyte-macrophage colony-stimulating factor as a control.[46] A durable response rate of 16% was seen in the T-VEC group compared with 2% in the control group (odds ratio 8.9). The overall response rate was also greater in the T-VEC group (26% vs. 6%), and median OS was marginally improved (23 months vs. 19 months). The best responses were seen in IIIB, IIIC, and M1a disease. Based on this trial, T-VEC received FDA approval for intralesional therapy of stage III or IV cutaneous melanoma. There was enthusiasm for adding T-VEC to immune therapy with the concept of increasing response to immune therapy while creating an inflamed tumor microenvironment with T-VEC. However, a randomized trial comparing T-VEC to T-VEC plus pembrolizumab did not show an improvement in PFS or OS for the combination in anti–PD-1 naïve patients.[47] Use of T-VEC in a patient not appearing to respond to initial anti–PD-1 therapy is still being investigated.

Given the success of T-VEC, multiple intralesional agents are being developed for treatment-naïve or anti–PD-1–refractory patients, including other oncolytic viruses and immune agonists. Regional infusion of chemotherapy continues to have a role, mostly in salvage situations in which immunotherapy has been ineffective and the disease remains isolated to an extremity. These situations are increasingly uncommon as our experience with intralesional and systemic immunotherapy continues to grow.

Current Approaches
Current Approach to Patient with Final Stage IIB/C and Microscopic Stage III Disease

Patients with final pathologic diagnosis IIB/IIC (with negative SLN biopsy), in addition to patients with microscopically detected stage III disease (IIIA with 1 mm in lymph node or more, IIIB, IIIC, or microsatellites in final excision), are now all eligible for adjuvant anti–PD-1 therapy in addition to targeted BRAF-MEK for stage III. As many as 50% of patients within this group may never develop recurrence, and we urgently need improved risk stratification to understand which patients in this group can safely forego adjuvant therapy and avoid exposure to side effects.

Current Approach to Patient with Clinically Detected Stage III and Higher Disease

For patients presenting with palpable or clinically evident stage III or IV disease potentially amenable to surgical resection (local recurrences, in-transit disease, dermal metastases, lymph node recurrence, isolated stage IV disease), there are now numerous approved options that can be individualized based on patient factors. First and foremost, all patients should have restaging scans to determine extent of disease and, if not done yet, testing for a BRAF mutation. Factors such as disease-free interval, associated illnesses (e.g., autoimmune diseases are a relative contraindication to immune therapy), and morbidity of surgery should be considered. For frail patients with small, isolated recurrences, surgical excision alone may be adequate. For patients with rapid, multiple synchronous cutaneous recurrences or continued isolated cutaneous recurrence, consideration of T-VEC is warranted, but most patients should be strongly considered for either neoadjuvant or adjuvant immune therapy as first-line treatment because immune therapy has demonstrated improvements in OS. Other therapies can then be considered for immune therapy failures. Indeed, single-agent anti–PD-1 continues to be effective in achieving a complete response in only about 30% of patients, so it is likely that many patients will need additional therapies, which can include addition of ipilimumab, relatlimab, T-VEC, surgery when feasible, or clinical trials.

For patients presenting with lymph node recurrences or significant dermal metastases, neoadjuvant therapy should be considered standard if the patient is otherwise an appropriate candidate for immune therapy. At select centers, consideration of the adjuvant mRNA vaccine after resection is an option. The choice between neoadjuvant therapy or resection to facilitate generation of the vaccine will be one that needs to be addressed. The numerous effective options ultimately mean that therapy can be tailored to individual patients to achieve optimal disease control and balance side effects.

TREATMENT OF METASTATIC DISEASE

Treatment options for metastatic melanoma have expanded greatly in the past decade (Table 63.3). Metastatic melanoma, which once carried a dismal prognosis measured in months, can now be treated effectively with multiple agents that prolong survival and improve quality of life. It is indeed an exciting time to be treating melanoma as our therapies expand and our ability to treat patients with metastatic disease continues to improve.

Historical

Historically, the only two agents approved for metastatic melanoma were dacarbazine and high-dose interleukin-2. These agents

TABLE 63.3 Summary of Important Targeted Therapy and Immunotherapy Trials for Metastatic Melanoma

TRIAL NAME	STUDY POPULATION	INTERVENTION TREATMENT	CONTROL TREATMENT	PRIMARY OUTCOME	NOTES
Robert et al.[48]	Previously untreated, unresectable IIIB or IV	Ipilimumab 10 mg/kg + dacarbazine	Dacarbazine	Improved overall survival (OS) with ipilimumab + dacarbazine (median OS 11.2 vs. 9.1 months, HR 0.72)	
COMBI-v (Robert et al.)[52]	Unresectable stage III or IV melanoma with *BRAF* V600E or V600K mutations	Dabrafenib + trametinib	Vemurafenib	Improved OS at 12 months (72% vs. 65%, HR 0.69, 95% CI 0.53–0.89)	Stopped early for efficacy, improved objective response rate (64% vs. 51%)
CheckMate 067 (Wolchok et al.)[49]	Previously untreated, unresectable III or IV	Nivolumab + ipilimumab Nivolumab alone	Ipilimumab	Improved OS in nivolumab/ipilimumab (HR 0.55) and nivolumab alone (HR 0.65) versus ipilimumab alone	6.5-year follow-up Median OS in months: 72.1 (ipilimumab + nivolumab), 36.9 (nivolumab), 19.9 (ipilimumab), Median MSS: not reached (ipilimumab + nivolumab), 58.7 (nivolumab), 21.9 (ipilimumab)
KEYNOTE-006 (Schacter et al.)[67]	Unresectable stage III or IV	Pembrolizumab every 2 or 3 weeks	Ipilimumab	OS better in both pembrolizumab groups compared with ipilimumab (HR 0.68 compared with ipilimumab for both treatment regimens)	No differences in q2 week or q3 week pembrolizumab
RELATIVITY-047 (Tawbi et al.)[37]	Treatment-naïve, unresectable melanoma	Relatlimab + nivolumab q4 weeks	Nivolumab q4 weeks	Median PFS 10.1 months for relatlimab + nivolumab versus 4.6 months for nivolumab (HR for progression or death 0.75)	Grade 3/4 toxicity 18.9% for relatlimab + nivolumab, 9.7% for nivolumab

CI, Confidence interval; *HR,* hazard ratio; *MSS NR,* melanoma-specific survival not reached; *PFS,* progression-free survival.

were found to induce moderate response rates without any benefit in OS. Biochemotherapy, which was a highly toxic combination of cytotoxic chemotherapy with interleukin-2 and interferon, would sometimes result in limited successes. This approach was never able to demonstrate a consistent improvement in OS. Some individuals would respond well and achieve a durable response; however, these events were too infrequent to demonstrate a benefit to a large population of patients. These therapies were associated with significant toxicity and potentially fatal complications. Better therapies for metastatic melanoma were desperately needed.

Immunotherapy

Melanoma was always considered a cancer that was susceptible to immunotherapy treatment strategies. Before the development of immune checkpoint blockade, interleukin-2, interferon, granulocyte-macrophage colony-stimulating factor, and multiple vaccines were tried in an attempt to boost the inherent immune response to melanoma. Through a better understanding of the regulation of the immune response, newer strategies focusing on blocking the negative-feedback systems that suppress T-cell activity were developed, specifically the CTLA-4 and PD-1 pathways (Fig. 63.21).

Ipilimumab is a monoclonal anti–CTLA-4 antibody that was the first systemic agent to demonstrate improved OS in patients with metastatic melanoma. In one of the early randomized trials to show that ipilimumab could improve survival, 502 patients with metastatic melanoma were randomized to standard-of-care dacarbazine or dacarbazine plus ipilimumab.[48] The group treated with ipilimumab had improved OS at 1 and 3 years (HR 0.72). Based on this study and other subsequent studies, ipilimumab was

approved by the FDA for metastatic melanoma. Significant autoimmune toxicities, including potentially fatal bowel perforations, prompted additional studies to find less toxic but equally effective immunotherapy options.

Multiple randomized clinical trials have demonstrated that PD-1 inhibitors can improve survival in patients with metastatic melanoma. Patients treated with pembrolizumab alone or nivolumab alone have improved OS compared with those treated with ipilimumab alone.[49] The PD-1 inhibitors have an improved safety profile compared with ipilimumab and are more effective; thus, they have become the preferred first-line agents for metastatic melanoma. Combining PD-1 inhibitors (nivolumab) with CTLA-4 inhibition improves response rates, survival, and also toxicity. Long-term data with a minimum 7.5-year follow-up for patients treated with nivolumab plus ipilimumab demonstrated a median OS of 72.1 months (nivolumab + ipilimumab), 36.9 months (nivolumab), and 19.9 months (ipilimumab), whereas melanoma-specific survival was not reached for nivolumab + ipilimumab; it was 49.4 months for nivolumab and 21.9 months for ipilimumab.[50] When nivolumab or ipilimumab alone were used, the rates of serious adverse treatment-related events were 21% and 28%, whereas when these were used in combination, the rates of serious adverse treatment-related events doubled to 59%.[49]

In March 2022, the FDA approved nivolumab and relatlimab for patients with unresectable melanoma based on a randomized trial showing greater benefit with regard to PFS than anti–PD-1 therapy alone.[37] Relatlimab is a first-in-class human IgG4 LAG-3–blocking antibody that binds to LAG-3 and restores the effector function of exhausted T cells; it is a distinct inhibitory immune

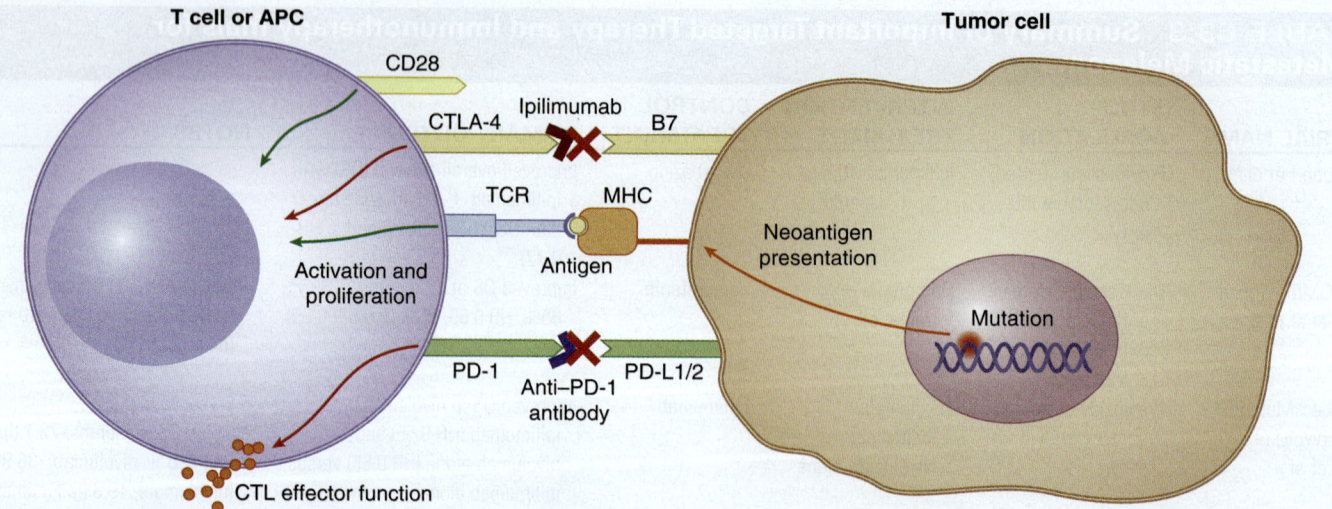

FIGURE 63.21 The cytotoxic T-lymphocyte–associated protein 4 *(CTLA-4)* and programmed cell death 1 *(PD-1)* pathways that are integral to immunotherapy for melanoma. *APC,* Antigen-presenting cell; *CTL,* cytotoxic T lymphocyte; *MHC,* major histocompatibility complex; *TCR,* T-cell receptor. (From Herzberg B, Fisher DE. Metastatic melanoma and immunotherapy. *Clinical Immunol.* 2016;172:105-110.)

checkpoint. The toxicity of this regimen is double that of nivolumab alone (18.9% in combination vs. 9.7% nivolumab only).

The next generation of immunotherapy for melanoma will likely include the use of TILs. The TIL technique involves the isolation and expansion of tumor-specific T cells collected from the peritumor stroma and was initially described in the 1980s. With this technique, these melanoma-specific TIL cells are clonally expanded, then reinfused into the patient after lymphodepletion with high-dose, nonmyeloablative chemotherapy. TIL infusion is also followed by high-dose interleukin-2. The TIL cells then enhance the patient's own adaptive immunity in order to evoke a heightened immune response to the tumors. In a recent phase II trial in 153 patients treated with lifileucel, 81.7% of whom had received prior immune checkpoint therapy, the objective response rate was 31.4%, with grade 3 or 4 toxicities in greater than 30% of patients.[51] This therapy is not yet FDA approved.

Targeted Therapy

The first agent used to target metastatic melanoma with the V600E *BRAF* mutation was vemurafenib. For BRAF-mutant patients, vemurafenib demonstrated significant improvement in overall and PFS and was approved by the FDA for treatment of BRAF-mutant metastatic melanoma. The major issue with single-agent BRAF inhibition, including vemurafenib and dabrafenib, is the development of treatment resistance. This is not the result of a change in the target *BRAF* gene; rather, it is felt to be the result of upregulation of alternative signaling pathways, including the MAPK pathway. Dual BRAF-MEK inhibition with trametinib and dabrafenib has been shown to improve overall response rates and survival compared with single-agent trametinib or dabrafenib in BRAF-mutant metastatic melanoma.[52] There are currently three approved BRAF and MEK inhibitor combinations, including dabrafenib plus trametinib, vemurafenib plus cobimetinib, and encorafenib plus binimetinib, all of which possess a comparable 18-month PFS range of 30% to 40% with their own unique side-effect profiles. However, concerns over durability and resistance remain. Randomized prospective data from the Doublet, Randomized Evaluation in Advanced Melanoma Sequencing

(DREAMseq) Trial (ECOG-ACRIN EA6134) now clearly demonstrate that in treatment-naïve BRAF600-mutant melanoma patients, combination programmed cell death protein 1/cytotoxic T-cell lymphocyte-4–blockade as first-line treatment is associated with improved 2-year OS (71.8%) compared with patients initiating dabrafenib/trametinib as first-line treatment (2-year OS of 5.1%).[38] Dual BRAF-MEK inhibition is a good treatment option for patients with BRAF-mutant metastatic melanoma who cannot tolerate immunotherapy, usually because of existing autoimmune comorbidities. Additionally, for patients with symptomatic and high-burden disease where a fast response is preferable, targeted therapy may also be preferred as a first choice. Patients not eligible for immunotherapy with BRAF-wild-type melanoma continue to have limited effective treatment options.

Current Approach

Options for a patient presenting with metastatic melanoma not amenable to surgical resection now include anti–PD-1 monotherapy, nivolumab + relatlimab, nivolumab + ipilimumab, T-VEC, and BRAF-MEK therapy (for 50% of patients with activating BRAF mutations). Disease burden, patient fitness and comorbidities, symptoms, and other factors allow for tailoring of therapy. As discussed, immune therapy should be considered the first-line option. Among immune therapy options, nivolumab + ipilimumab has the highest response rates and durability and yet the highest toxicity. For patients with brain metastases, nivolumab + ipilimumab, in addition to stereotactic radiosurgery, may be needed. For healthy patients and large disease burden, nivolumab + ipilimumab is strongly considered. Unless frail, most patients with moderate to low disease burden are initiated on nivolumab + relatlimab. For patients who fail initial anti–PD-1 monotherapy, the addition of ipilimumab (changing to nivolumab + ipilimumab regimen) is associated with a 30% response rate. Treatment with nivolumab + relatlimab after failure of nivolumab or nivolumab + ipilimumab appears to be less effective. Finally, it is important to remember that a large portion will initially fail current immune therapy regimens or develop recurrence after initial response and will need alternative treatment strategies. Targeted therapy plays a role in those patients. Additionally, ongoing efforts to target pathways of immune therapy resistance are in clinical trials. Many patients will also still need surgeries for treatment failures and symptomatic disease.

Surveillance

There are no definitive guidelines on appropriate follow-up for patients with resected melanoma who are disease-free, although the NCCN does offer some suggested surveillance approaches. The general principle that should be considered is that the intensity of the surveillance strategy and incorporation of imaging studies should be individualized according to the patient's risk and likely site of recurrence. Most recurrences are detected within the first 5 years after treatment, although melanoma is notorious for delayed recurrences, sometimes decades after treatment, in seemingly low-risk lesions.

Patients with early-stage, localized disease (0–II) are at low risk of recurrence and should be observed by history and physical examination at least every 6 months for the first 3 years and at least annually thereafter. A careful history is necessary to elicit symptoms such as new skin lesions, nodal masses, pain, headaches, neurologic changes, weight loss, and gastrointestinal and pulmonary symptoms. Patients should be educated about common symptoms and signs of recurrence so that they can report any important changes that arise between scheduled visits. Physical examination should include a complete skin inspection, including palpation to detect regional nodal or in-transit recurrence. Most recurrences in these patients will be reported by the patients themselves.

For stage III melanoma and those with high-risk stage II disease (thick and/or ulcerated primaries), a reasonable follow-up schedule is a history and physical examination every 3 or 4 months for the first 3 years, every 6 months for the next 2 years, and annually thereafter. The use of laboratory tests and imaging tests such as CT, MRI, or PET/CT is controversial but not unreasonable for these patients. Even though there has never been any proven benefit to early detection of recurrent melanoma with radiographic or laboratory studies, it stands to reason that in this age of effective immunotherapy for metastatic melanoma, there may be some utility in early detection of low-volume disease. Patients with stage IV melanoma will have regular clinical, laboratory, and radiologic evaluations to monitor the response to treatment.

The survivorship team, which will likely include the surgeon, dermatologist, and potentially the medical oncologist, should consider both recurrence of the primary melanoma and development of a second primary melanoma. Melanoma survivors have a tenfold increased risk of a subsequent melanoma compared with the general population and a cumulative risk of the development of a second primary melanoma of approximately 5%.[53] Melanoma survivors should have regular skin examinations for the rest of their lives.

Metastasectomy

Although most patients with stage IV melanoma will present with disseminated lesions that are not amenable to resection, patients with limited metastatic disease should be considered for resection if the disease is stable or responds to systemic therapy. Operative resection may not only offer symptom palliation, but also, in some highly selected patients, it may provide a survival advantage similar to that seen after lymphadenectomy for advanced stage III patients. Resection of oligometastatic disease in well-selected patients can lead to 5-year survival rates ranging from 15% to 40%.

Even patients with brain metastases may benefit from complete resection, further emphasizing that complete extirpation of all disease may be the best treatment, even for advanced disease. Careful selection of patients is paramount. Important things to consider in evaluating a patient for resection of metastatic disease include the patient's underlying functional status and comorbidities, the location and number of metastatic lesions, and the features reflective of the underlying tumor behavior, such as the disease-free interval from the time of primary resection. Failure to respond to systemic immunotherapy is usually a poor prognostic sign that signifies aggressive disease biology. However, medical and surgical oncologists are more often encountering the phenomenon of mixed response to immunotherapy or a single site of persistent disease (oligoprogression). Oftentimes in patients with multiple sites of metastatic disease, there will be a good radiologic response to immunotherapy in most, but not all, of the distant metastases. In these situations, if these nonresponding sites are amenable to resection, it may benefit patients to perform metastasectomy to remove the nonresponding lesions.

SPECIAL SITUATIONS AND NONCUTANEOUS MELANOMA

Unknown Primary Melanoma

Unknown primary melanoma occurs in up to 15% of patients presenting with clinically detected stage III or stage IV melanoma and no preceding diagnosis of a primary cutaneous melanoma. A diagnosis of unknown primary melanoma should prompt a thorough skin examination, including the perianal area, external genitalia, nail beds, scalp, and external auditory canal. Endoscopic evaluation of the oral cavity and nasopharynx as well as of the anus and rectum can identify mucosal melanoma. Females should undergo a thorough pelvic examination, and an ophthalmology examination may be required to rule out ocular melanomas. PET/CT and MRI of the brain are warranted to assess the extent of disease.

Some hypothesize that unknown primary melanomas arise from benign nevus cells already trapped within lymph nodes. Alternatively, cutaneous melanoma is known to undergo spontaneous regression in rare cases, presumably as a result of an immune response to the primary tumor. Therefore, a history of a prior pigmented skin lesion that has disappeared or clinical evidence of vitiligo should not be dismissed. Patients may provide a history of pigmented skin lesions that have been excised, cauterized, or treated with lasers. Pathology review of any previously excised skin lesions should be performed. Although pathology review of all prior lesions is ideal, this can be challenging in practice.

In the setting of lymph node metastasis without a primary lesion, the patient should be treated as a patient with stage III melanoma, as discussed earlier. Interestingly, patients with unknown primary melanomas who present with lymph node involvement have equivalent or possibly better OS compared with patients with a known primary lesion. This may suggest a stronger immune response in these patients that resulted in regression of the primary melanoma.

Melanoma and Pregnancy

As many as one-third of females diagnosed with melanoma are of childbearing age; treatment of melanoma in pregnant females involves some difficult decision-making. Whether there is a link between pregnancy and the overall risk for development of melanoma is not well understood. Early studies suggested that hormonal changes during pregnancy led to increasing pigmentation and an environment conducive to melanoma development; however, current evidence does not support this theory. Any nevus or pigmented lesion with suspicious changes during pregnancy should not be attributed to hormones or the expected physiology of pregnancy; appropriate workup is required. Some evidence has suggested worse outcomes for melanoma in pregnancy; however, after controlling for other relevant risk factors, it appears that the prognosis of patients with melanoma treated during pregnancy is no different from that of nonpregnant patients.[54]

The evaluation and treatment of a pregnant patient with melanoma should follow guidelines similar to those for the nonpregnant patient. There is no therapeutic benefit to early termination of the pregnancy. WLE can be safely performed under local anesthesia. Based on experience with pregnant patients with breast cancer, SLN biopsy may be performed if indicated by the pathologic factors of the primary tumor, although vital blue dye should not be used. Not only is there an unknown risk to the fetus, but there is also an estimated 1 in 10,000 risk of an anaphylactic reaction if isosulfan blue dye is used. Lymphoscintigraphy is considered safe because the dose used is well below the teratogenic threshold.[55] Nevertheless, some physicians and patients are uncomfortable with the use of radioactive materials during pregnancy. In such situations, WLE under local anesthesia with a 1-cm margin can be performed, with wider margin excision and SLN biopsy reserved until after the baby is delivered. The placenta should be examined pathologically for evidence of melanoma in females who develop melanoma during pregnancy as a marker for metastasis as well as possible transmission to the child. For patients who have tumors with poor prognostic factors, it may be advisable to wait 2 to 3 years before the next pregnancy because this represents the time during which recurrence is most likely.

Noncutaneous Melanoma

The neural crest cells from which melanocytes develop migrate predominantly to the skin during fetal development; however, they will also localize to several other organs and tissues. As a result, melanoma may arise in other locations, including the mucosal surfaces, within the eye, or in the leptomeninges.

Ocular Melanoma

Within the eye, melanocytes are found in the retina and uveal tract (iris, ciliary body, and choroids). In the United States, ocular melanoma is the most common intraocular malignant neoplasm in adults. Primary treatment consists of enucleation or iodine-125 brachytherapy, although other options include photocoagulation and partial resection. Unlike cutaneous melanoma, given the lack of lymphatic vessels in the uveal tract, metastatic spread of ocular melanoma occurs hematogenously. Metastases develop almost exclusively in the liver. Resection is rarely possible because the pattern of metastases is often a diffuse, miliary one. Dedicated liver imaging is needed to detect these lesions. Ocular melanoma is less responsive to immunotherapy compared with cutaneous melanoma. In January 2022, the FDA approved tebentafusp, a bispecific gp100 peptide–HLA-directed CD3 T-cell engager, for patients with unresectable metastatic uveal melanoma (only patients who are HLA-A*02:01) based on a randomized phase III trial showing OS at 1 year of 73% in the tebentafusp group versus 59% in the control arm.[56] For liver-only metastatic uveal melanoma,

percutaneous liver perfusion that delivers high-dose melphalan with use of a specialized catheter and perfusion circuit to isolate the liver from systemic circulation is currently in clinical trials.

Mucosal Melanoma

The most common sites for mucosal melanoma are the head and neck (oral cavity, oropharynx, nasopharynx, and paranasal sinuses), anal canal, rectum, and female genitalia. Because of the occult location of many of these lesions, patients tend to present with more advanced disease and have a poor prognosis. These tumors should be excised to negative margins when possible. Given the high risk of metastatic disease, extensive local resections, such as abdominoperineal resection or pelvic exenteration, do not improve OS. These procedures may still be necessary for local disease control. Radiation therapy may be used to improve locoregional disease control. In general, the role of SLN biopsy has not been well established. For anal melanoma, a negative SLN biopsy in the superficial inguinal region would omit that region from the radiation fields. The response rate to immunotherapy for mucosal melanoma is lower than that of cutaneous melanoma, but it is still improved over cytotoxic chemotherapy regimens.

NONMELANOMA SKIN CANCERS

NMSC represents the most common type of malignant neoplasm in the world. In the United States, it is estimated that almost one in five Americans will develop NMSC during their lifetime. Approximately 80% are BCC, with SCC representing nearly 20%. Much rarer types of NMSC make up the remainder of cases. Sun exposure is the predominant risk factor. Similar to cutaneous melanoma, the overall incidence of NMSC is increasing. Accurate estimates of NMSC incidence are difficult to ascertain because many are treated without obtaining a histologic diagnosis, and most cases are not reported in cancer registries. The American Cancer Society estimated there are more than 5 million cases of BCC and SCC diagnosed in over 3 million people per year in the United States. Patients diagnosed with a BCC or SCC have an increased risk of additional cancers, including a second NMSC, melanoma, and nonskin cancers. For this reason, patients with a prior diagnosis of skin cancer require long-term surveillance.

Squamous Cell Carcinoma
Presentation and Risk Factors

Risk factors for development of SCC include exposure to sunlight, susceptible skin types, compromised immunity, environmental exposures, and underlying genetic disorders. Most SCCs occur on sun-exposed surfaces, particularly the head and neck. In susceptible individuals (those with fair skin, blond hair, and blue eyes), prolonged sun exposure correlates directly to an increased risk for SCC. In contrast to melanoma or BCC, the cumulative effect of chronic UV radiation likely plays a larger role in SCC than intermittent, intense exposures. As with melanoma, individuals with dark complexions have a lower risk of SCC, even with prolonged sun exposure. The risk for SCC increases with occupational or recreational sun exposure, advancing age, and proximity to the equator. The amount of sun exposure is also proportional to the incidence of known precursor lesions for SCC, including actinic keratosis.

UV radiation, and UVB in particular, increases the risk of SCC through several mechanisms. One mechanism is the direct carcinogenic effect of UV light on the frequently dividing keratinocytes within the basal layer of the epidermis. Unrepaired mutations from UV-light damage can drive tumor proliferation and growth. UVB-induced silencing of the *p53* tumor suppressor gene occurs in more than 90% of SCCs. With loss of p53, keratinocytes are unable to arrest the cell cycle or initiate apoptosis in the face of cellular damage from UV radiation. With subsequent mutations, cells can then progress from dysplasia to in situ or invasive disease.

Occupational and environmental carcinogens, including arsenic, organic hydrocarbons, ionizing radiation, and cigarette smoke, are associated with an increased risk for SCC. Genetic disorders, including xeroderma pigmentosum and albinism, are associated with increased risk for many types of skin cancer, including SCC. A history of chronic inflammation from burn scars (Marjolin ulcer), draining sinuses, infections (including osteomyelitis), and nonhealing ulcers can precede the development of SCCs. In the setting of chronic nonhealing wounds or even with previously healed wounds that subsequently break down, biopsy may be prudent to rule out SCC.

Immunosuppression is a well-established risk factor for SCCs of the skin, particularly with the suppression of cell-mediated immunity after solid organ transplantation. Skin cancer is the most frequent malignant neoplasm in organ transplant recipients, with SCC and BCC representing 95% of these cancers. Whereas the risk of BCC increases tenfold after transplantation, the incidence of SCC in posttransplant patients is 65 times that of the normal population (Fig. 63.22). SCCs that develop in immunosuppressed patients are more aggressive and have an increased risk of systemic metastases. The intensity of immunosuppression and the duration of therapy both correlate with the risk of malignancy. Whereas malignant neoplasms develop in 10% to 27% of patients after 10 years of immunosuppression, this number increases to 40% to 60% after 20 years. Other

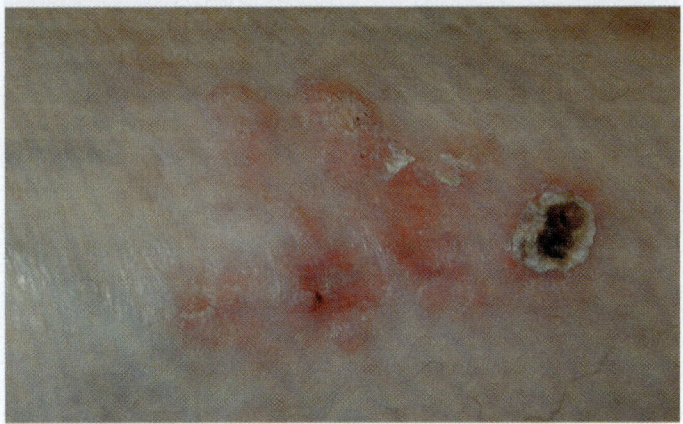

FIGURE 63.23 Squamous cell carcinoma with red, scaling skin.

conditions associated with impairments of cell-mediated immunity (lymphoma, leukemia, autoimmune disease, etc.) are associated with an increased risk of SCC. Human papillomavirus, an infection associated with immunosuppression, is a proposed risk factor for the development of SCCs. BRAF inhibition used to treat melanoma is also associated with the development of SCC.

Most SCCs begin with a proliferation of keratin cells in the basal layer of the epidermis that appear as red or pink areas, clinically termed *actinic keratoses* (solar keratoses). Local symptoms may wax and wane for a period of many months. Lesions are scaling, with an uneven surface and an erythematous base (Fig. 63.23). Individual lesions are usually smaller than 1 cm in diameter and appear in chronically sun-damaged skin. The diagnosis is both clinical and histologic because actinic keratoses share many microscopic features with SCC in situ. The risk of malignant transformation of actinic keratosis to SCC is approximately 0.01% to 0.6% over 1 year and up to 2.5% over 4 years. Bowen disease, which appears histologically as SCC in situ, initially manifests as a reddened area that progresses to thickened plaques of variable size. When it is confined to the glans penis or vulva, Bowen disease is sometimes referred to as *erythroplasia of Queyrat*.

Invasive SCCs are palpable scaling lesions that become ulcerated centrally and have elevated, firm edges. In addition to spreading horizontally, these lesions may grow vertically and become fixed to underlying tissue. They may be confused with keratoacanthoma, a benign lesion that can also thicken and ulcerate. Biopsy may be required to differentiate between these two conditions.

Treatment

Unlike melanoma, SCC T category is based on the diameter of the lesion. Other high-risk features for SCC of the skin have been defined by the NCCN (Table 63.4). These high-risk features include assessment of size, location, histology, and individual patient factors. Most SCCs can be treated with local excision with excellent results. The typical margin of excision is a gross 5-mm resection, although MMS can be used when a cosmetically sensitive area demands skin conservation. MMS may also be preferred for recurrent or high-risk tumors. For higher-risk lesions, 10-mm margins are recommended.

Field therapies, which treat a generalized area but do not define the status of the margin, can also be used. Examples of field

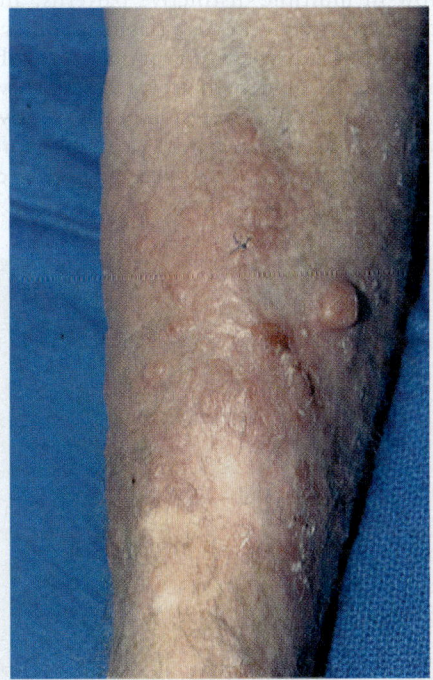

FIGURE 63.22 Multiple squamous cell carcinomas on the forearm of a patient on immunosuppression after kidney transplant.

TABLE 63.4 Risk Factors for Local Recurrence or Metastases in Squamous Cell Carcinoma of the Skin

	LOW RISK	HIGH RISK
Location/Size	Area L <20 mm	Area L ≥20 mm
	Area M <10 mm	Area M ≥10 mm
		Area H
Borders	Well defined	Poorly defined
Primary versus recurrent	Primary	Recurrent
Immunosuppression	No	Yes
Site of prior radiation therapy or chronic inflammatory process	No	Yes
Rapidly growing tumor	No	Yes
Neurologic symptoms	No	Yes
Degree of differentiation	Well or moderately differentiated	Poorly differentiated
Acantholytic (adenoid), adeno-squamous (showing mucin production), desmoplastic, or metaplastic (carcinosarcoma-tous) subtypes	No	Yes
Depth, thickness, or Clark level	<2 mm, or I, II, III	≥2 mm, or IV, V
Perineural, lymphatic, or vascular involvement	No	Yes

Area H = "mask areas" of face (central face, eyelids, eyebrows, periorbital nose, lips [cutaneous and vermillion], chin, mandible, preauricular and postauricular skin/sulci, temple, ear) genitalia, hands, and feet
Area M = cheeks, forehead, scalp, neck, and pretibial
Area L = trunk and extremities (excluding pretibial, hands, feet, nail units, and ankles)

therapies include radiation therapy, cryosurgery, photodynamic therapy, electrodessication and curettage, and topical agents like imiquimod. Cryotherapy is best suited for small superficial lesions and can be expected to achieve local control rates greater than 90%. Treated areas are allowed to heal slowly by secondary intention, often resulting in pale scars. Curettage may be used for patients with superficial lesions less than 2 cm in size. In precursor lesions of SCC, such as actinic keratosis, cryotherapy is a commonly performed therapy. Alternative treatments include topical 5-fluorouracil, electrodessication and curettage, carbon dioxide laser, dermabrasion, and chemical peel. Tissue biopsy is indicated when the actinic keratosis is raised or recurrent after topical therapy.

SLN biopsy may have a role in high-risk lesions because clinically occult lymph node metastases may be identified in 7% to 20% of patients. The indications for SLN biopsy and subsequent nodal management strategy (completion lymphadenectomy with or without radiation therapy) are not as well defined as they are for cutaneous melanoma. Adjuvant radiation to the primary tumor is recommended by the NCCN for any SCC with extensive perineural or large nerve involvement.

Locally advanced or metastatic SCC of the skin is fortunately rare. Systemic cytotoxic chemotherapies are usually platinum based, with variable response rates. Targeted epidermal growth factor receptor agents have been used with moderate success as primary and salvage systemic therapy for metastatic SCC.[57] However, immune therapies have also made an impact on advanced SCC. Cemiplimab and pembrolizumab (anti–PD-1 therapies) are both FDA approved for locally advanced SCC, with overall response rates ranging from 30% to 50%.[58] In a neoadjuvant trial of cemiplimab in patients with resectable stage II and higher SCC, pathologic complete response was observed in 51% (95% CI 39%–62%) of patients.[59] Therefore, strong consideration for neoadjuvant therapy should be given for advanced SCC in patients who can be given anti–PD-1 therapies.

Basal Cell Carcinoma

Presentation and Risk Factors

BCC is the most common NMSC, and lesions are most commonly found on the sun-exposed areas of the head and neck. Risk factors for development of BCC are similar to those for SCC, although basal cell lesions are more often associated with intense, intermittent exposure to UV radiation. The hedgehog (Hh) signaling pathway is a key signaling pathway in embryonic development but is largely inactive in mature adult tissue. The pathway is mutated in up to 90% of BCCs. In the presence of Hh signaling peptides, the Patched (PTCH) receptor releases the transmembrane Smoothened (SMO) protein, allowing SMO to initiate a signaling cascade that activates the expression of several target genes. Normally, PTCH will inhibit SMO in the absence of Hh signals. Both activating mutations in SMO and inactivating mutations in PTCH have been linked to BCC, ultimately leading to unrestricted growth signaling.

In contrast to SCCs and actinic keratoses, there is no precursor skin lesion for BCCs. These lesions may have an appearance that varies from nodules in the skin to a large nonhealing sore with drainage and crusting. In comparison to SCCs, they have a slow growth rate, often leading to a delay in diagnosis. BCCs commonly infiltrate locally but rarely metastasize. Metastases are associated with advanced age and large, neglected lesions. The primary site will often undergo resection multiple times before metastases appear. Once metastatic disease develops, the median survival decreases to less than 1 year.

BCCs grow in multiple distinctive patterns, and although there is not a universally accepted classification system, there are several common subtypes. The nodular growth pattern is characterized by a well-defined, elevated lesion with a waxy appearance (Fig. 63.24). As the lesion grows, pearly opalescent nodules develop along the margins. A central depression with umbilication or ulceration and rolled edges is a classic sign.

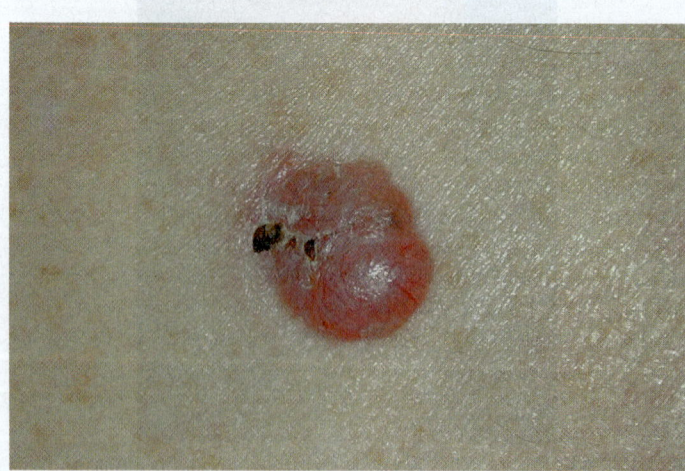

FIGURE 63.24 Nodular basal cell carcinoma.

Distinct blood vessels (telangiectasia) may be seen across the surface or along the edges of the lesion. Although most BCCs are pink or skin-colored, they may also have shades of brown or black pigmentation, thereby mimicking a benign mole or melanoma. Cystic BCCs are less common but have a distinctive translucent appearance. Their blue or gray appearance may lead to misdiagnosis as a blue nevus. Superficial BCCs have more macular growth patterns and may extend over the surface of the skin in a multicentric pattern. The center can ulcerate, and the margins are often irregular and ill defined. These lesions may appear similar to those of psoriasis, tinea, or eczema. In micronodular lesions, there may be several mildly elevated pink or red lesions that pepper the skin. Associated with a more aggressive growth pattern, these lesions often have extension well beyond visible changes in the skin surface. The white-scarring varieties of this growth pattern are termed *morpheaform BCC;* these lesions are among the most locally invasive subtypes and can penetrate deep into the underlying subdermis (Fig. 63.25).

Treatment

Because the vast majority of BCCs are locally confined, treatment is directed at a margin-negative resection. Similar to SCC, a gross 5-mm margin is usually adequate for local disease control. For higher-risk lesions, wider margins may help reduce local recurrence, but the exact width of the margins has not been defined. MMS can be used for the same indications as SCC. High-risk features of BCC have been defined by the NCCN (Table 63.5).

Similar to local SCCs, field therapies can be used for BCC, including radiation therapy, cryosurgery, photodynamic therapy, electrodessication and curettage, and topical agents like imiquimod. Adjuvant radiation therapy for high-risk lesions can reduce the risk of local recurrence. Evaluation of the lymph nodes by SLN biopsy is not necessary for BCC because lymph node metastases are exceedingly rare.

TABLE 63.5 Risk Factors for Recurrence in Basal Cell Carcinoma of the Skin

	LOW RISK	HIGH RISK
Location/size	Area L <20 mm Area M <10 mm	Area L ≥20 mm Area M ≥10 mm Area H
Borders	Well defined	Poorly defined
Primary versus recurrent	Primary	Recurrent
Immunosuppression	No	Yes
Site of prior radiation therapy	No	Yes
Pathologic subtype	Nodular, superficial	Aggressive growth pattern
Perineural invasion	No	Yes

Area H = "mask areas" of face (central face, eyelids, eyebrows, periorbital nose, lips [cutaneous and vermillion], chin, mandible, preauricular and postauricular skin/sulci, temple, ear) genitalia, hands, and feet
Area M = cheeks, forehead, scalp, neck, and pretibial
Area L = trunk and extremities (excluding pretibial, hands, feet, nail units, and ankles)
Aggressive growth pattern: having (mixed) infiltrative, micronodular, morpheaform, basosquamous, sclerosing, or carcinosarcomatous differentiation features in any portion of the tumor.

In the very rare circumstances in which locally advanced or metastatic BCC develops and cannot be resected, there have been major advances in systemic therapy based on the Hh signaling pathway. The small molecule inhibitor of the Hh pathway vismodegib demonstrated a 30% response rate in locally advanced BCC and a 43% response rate in metastatic BCC; the complete response rate was 21%.[60] Long-term follow-up confirmed the durability of response in both the metastatic and locally advanced patients, with a median duration of response of nearly 15 months in the metastatic patients and 26 months in the locally advanced patients.[61] A second Hh pathway inhibitor, sonidegib, has shown similar efficacy, with objective response rates on the order of 30% to 40% in metastatic or locally advanced BCC.[62] Immune checkpoint therapies also have activity for metastatic BCC, with response rates of around 30% in patients with advanced BCC who failed Hh inhibitor treatment.[63]

Merkel Cell Carcinoma

Merkel cell carcinoma (MCC) is a rare but aggressive malignant neoplasm of the skin. It is locally aggressive, with high local recurrence rates, and has the potential for regional and distant metastases. There is debate as to whether Merkel cells arise from epidermal or neural crest progenitors, but on histologic evaluation, MCC may be indistinguishable from small cell carcinoma and other small round blue cell tumors. The incidence of MCC appears to be rising at a faster rate than that of cutaneous melanoma; the reasons for this are unclear. Up to 80% of MCCs are associated with the Merkel cell polyomavirus (MCPyV).[64] Up to 50% of patients with new MCC will have evidence of MCPyV antibodies, and serologic levels of MCPyV in patient blood correlate with overall tumor burden. Many sites are obtaining MCPyV serologies within 2 to 3 months of initial diagnosis, and if detectable, serologic testing can be used to detect recurrence.

MCC usually appears as a painless, raised nodule, often red or purplish, but it can be of the same color as the surrounding skin (Fig. 63.26). It is more commonly found in sun-exposed areas. Workup is similar to melanoma, in that a tangential shave biopsy

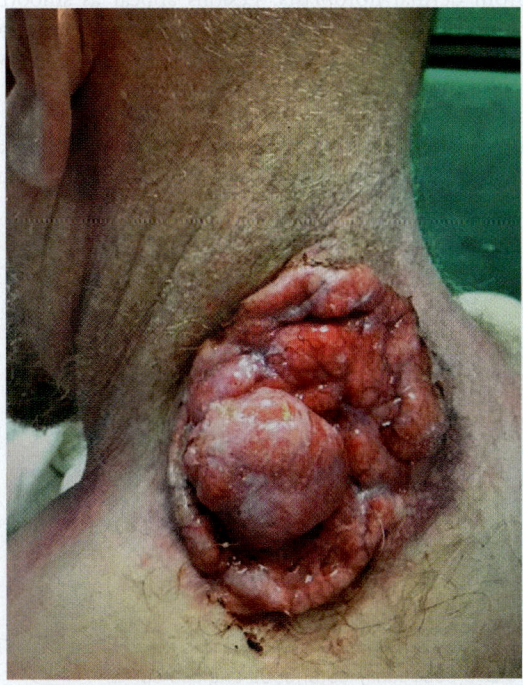

FIGURE 63.25 Locally advanced basal cell carcinoma.

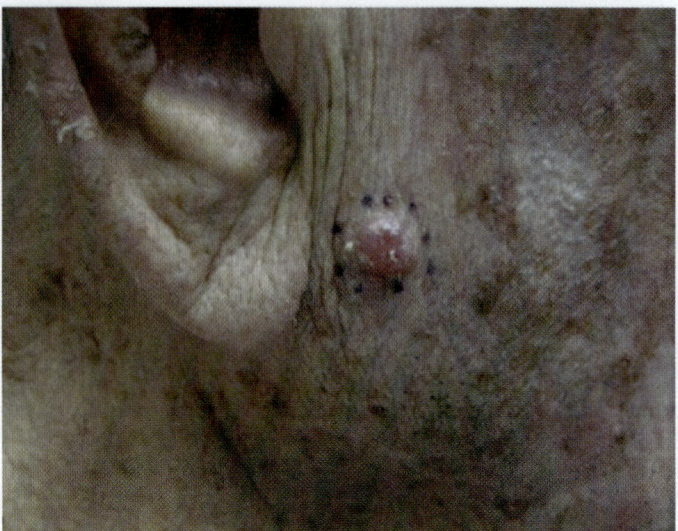

FIGURE 63.26 Merkel cell carcinoma.

or punch biopsy makes the diagnosis. An experienced dermatopathologist may be needed to confirm the diagnosis. A careful clinical examination of the draining lymph node basis is required because MCC will often present with clinically apparent lymph nodes. Clinically staging with radiographic imaging, such as cross-sectional CT scan, is reasonable.

The AJCC has a separate staging system for MCC, based on maximum tumor diameter rather than depth of invasion. The primary treatment is WLE (1- to 2-cm margins), although MMS has been used for some lesions where tissue conservation is necessary. SLN biopsy is generally recommended for all T stages of MCC to identify patients with occult regional lymphatic metastases, which may occur in up to one-third of cases. Nodal status affects prognosis, and patients with nodal disease have a significantly decreased OS. MCC is a relatively radiosensitive tumor, and adjuvant radiation has been shown to reduce the local recurrence rate at the primary tumor site. If the SLN is positive, adjuvant radiation to the nodal basin or consideration of CLND may decrease the rate of regional recurrence and improve OS. Further smaller trials have supported adjuvant anti–PD-1 after resection of high-risk MCC (including SLN positive). The Surgically Treated Adjuvant Merkel cell carcinoma with pembrolizumab (STAMP)/EA6174 study randomized 280 patients to observation or adjuvant pembrolizumab after surgery for MCC (stage I–IIIB), and results are pending.

For metastatic MCC, a response rate of approximately 50% has been reported with the PD-1 inhibitor pembrolizumab; these responses, like those with melanoma, appear durable.[65] The PD-L1 inhibitor avelumab has also shown good responses in advanced MCC.[66] Combination checkpoint therapy has also been shown to be effective.

Other Cutaneous Malignancies

Cutaneous Angiosarcoma

Cutaneous angiosarcoma is a rare, aggressive soft tissue sarcoma derived from blood or lymphatic vessel endothelium. Cutaneous angiosarcoma predominantly occurs in elderly Whites and most commonly arises on the head and neck. In addition, angiosarcoma has been observed in the setting of chronic lymphedema after axillary dissection for breast cancer (Stewart-Treves syndrome) and may arise in irradiated tissues after prolonged intervals. The typical finding is a smooth, firm or spongy subcutaneous growth that develops a violaceous erythema similar to a bruise (Fig. 63.27). Advanced tumors may grow in excess of 10 cm in size and become ulcerated. On histologic evaluation, angiosarcomas are high grade and often multifocal, with skip areas of normal-appearing skin. Abnormal, pleomorphic, malignant-appearing endothelial cells are pathognomonic. Like most sarcomas, the principal route of metastatic spread is hematogenous, although it falls into the small category of sarcomas with an increased propensity for lymph node metastases. Treatment consists of complete resection with histologically negative margins and radiotherapy of the involved field. Like most sarcomas, a gross margin of approximately 2 cm is attempted at the time of operation to achieve the desired negative pathologic margin. SLN biopsy is not usually performed. Lymph node dissection is indicated for regional lymph node metastases in the absence of metastatic disease. There is no consensus about the role of adjuvant chemotherapy.

Dermatofibrosarcoma Protuberans

Dermatofibrosarcoma protuberans (DFSP) is a low-grade sarcoma arising from dermal fibroblasts. Lesions appear as smooth, flesh-colored nodules in or immediately beneath the skin and generally occur in relatively young patients between 20 and 50 years of age. Most appear on the trunk (50%), with the remainder on the proximal extremities (20%–35%) or in the head/neck region (10%–15%). DFSP grows slowly, so the lesions are usually not grossly very large at the time of diagnosis unless they have been

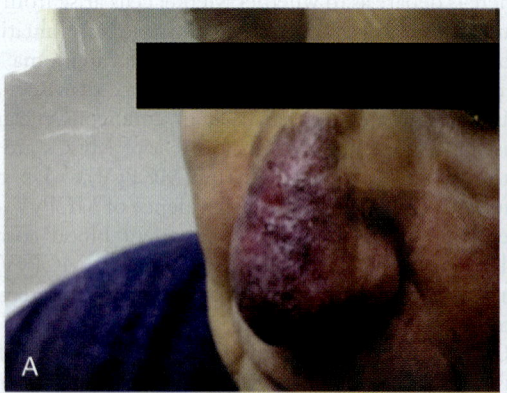
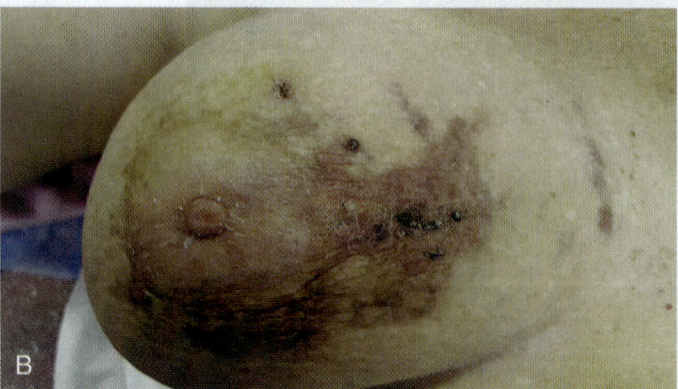

FIGURE 63.27 Primary cutaneous angiosarcoma of the nose (A) and secondary cutaneous angiosarcoma of the breast in the setting of radiation therapy for breast cancer (B).

neglected for a long period of time. Their external appearance belies their true character because tumor cells will frequently invade the underlying soft tissues and contribute to incomplete excision and local recurrence. A margin-positive resection is an all-too-common occurrence when managing DFSP. Treatment consists of WLE with a gross 2- to 4-cm margin. Specimen orientation and pathologic analysis of margins are required. Because the margins are often microscopically positive and the wide margin of excision often requires flap reconstruction, a temporary wound coverage strategy, such as with a negative-pressure dressing, may be employed to confirm histologically negative margins before flap reconstruction. Another strategy is to "map out" the planned margin of excision with punch biopsies in the office to confirm that the planned excision will be adequate before surgery. Distant metastases are uncommon and are often preceded by multiple local recurrences. A variant of DFSP is associated with fibrosarcomatous change on pathologic examination; these lesions have a more aggressive character with a higher risk for distant metastases. Adjuvant radiation therapy may be considered for margin-positive resection or for recurrences. Imatinib has been used with reasonable results in patients with locally advanced or metastatic disease and sometimes as neoadjuvant therapy in an attempt to improve the odds of negative-margin resection for advanced tumors or in anatomically constrained areas.

Kaposi Sarcoma

Kaposi sarcoma is a low-grade soft tissue malignant neoplasm that arises from lymphatic vascular endothelial cells in the skin. The incidence of Kaposi sarcoma has been increasing over the past several decades because it is most often seen in patients with acquired immunodeficiency syndrome (AIDS) and other immunosuppressed states. Human herpesvirus 8 has been identified as the causative agent of Kaposi sarcoma in patients infected with human immunodeficiency virus (HIV). There is also a classic variant not associated with an immunosuppressed state seen on the lower extremities of older males of eastern European and Mediterranean descent. The clinical picture is variable; asymptomatic purple to brown bruises develop and progress to spots, plaques, or nodules on both lower extremities. In AIDS patients, the most effective treatment is aggressive antiretroviral therapy. Symptomatic skin lesions can be treated with radiation therapy, intralesional injection of chemotherapeutic agents, cryotherapy, or excision.

Extramammary Paget Disease

Extramammary Paget disease (EMPD) is a rare form of adenocarcinoma that arises from apocrine glands of the skin, most commonly in the perianal area, vulva, and scrotum. The clinical appearance is that of an erythematous plaque, but white or depigmented areas with crusts and scaling may also be present. The size is variable, from smaller than 1 cm to an entire area in the anogenital region. Because EMPD can have many clinical characteristics in common with eczema, bacterial and fungal infections, and nonspecific dermatitis, the diagnosis is often made by biopsy of lesions not responding to standard therapies. In most cases, EMPD is confined to the epidermis and is well controlled with excision. When invasion of the deeper structures occurs, the disease becomes increasingly difficult to control, and the mortality rate approaches 50%. Because EMPD is also associated with an increased risk for simultaneous internal malignant neoplasms in the genitourinary and gastrointestinal tracts, a complete

workup includes a survey of these locations via endoscopy. Standard treatment is surgical resection extending to histologically negative margins, which may require a number of procedures to achieve because the histologic changes are best seen on permanent section. Patients require close clinical follow-up because local recurrences are common. Radiation therapy may reduce the incidence of local recurrence after excision.

SELECTED REFERENCES

Amaria RN, Prieto PA, Tetzlaff MT, et al. Neoadjuvant plus adjuvant dabrafenib and trametinib versus standard of care in patients with high-risk, surgically resectable melanoma: a single-centre, open-label, randomised, phase 2 trial. *Lancet Oncol.* 2018;19:181-193.

This randomized phase II study established the safety and efficacy of a neoadjuvant therapy approach to BRAF-mutant, resectable stage III melanoma. Expect more trials in the future to build off of this study design, in which on-treatment biopsies and pathologic response to t'herapy are end points to neoadjuvant immunotherapy studies.

Cancer Genome Atlas Network. Genomic classification of cutaneous melanoma. *Cell.* 2015;161:1681-1696.

An important publication from the Cancer Genome Atlas Network that defines four genomic subtypes of cutaneous melanoma. Potential markers of responsiveness to immunotherapies are reported as well.

Faries MB, Thompson JF, Cochran AJ, et al. Completion dissection or observation for sentinel-node metastasis in melanoma. *N Engl J Med.* 2017;376:2211-2222.

The published results of MSLT-II, which establish level I evidence that a completion lymphadenectomy after a positive SLN biopsy does not improve survival. This is a practice-changing study that has altered the way micrometastatic stage III melanoma is treated.

Long GV, Hauschild A, Santinami M, et al. Adjuvant dabrafenib plus trametinib in stage III BRAF-mutated melanoma. *N Engl J Med.* 2017;377:1813-1823.

This randomized trial demonstrated a survival benefit with adjuvant dual BRAF/MEK inhibition in resected stage III BRAF-mutant melanoma.

Weber J, Mandala M, Del Vecchio M, et al. Adjuvant nivolumab versus ipilimumab in resected stage III or IV melanoma. *N Engl J Med.* 2017;377:1824-1835.

A randomized, multicenter clinical trial that has established the efficacy of adjuvant nivolumab for resected stage III and IV melanoma.

The full reference list appears on Elsevier eBooks+.

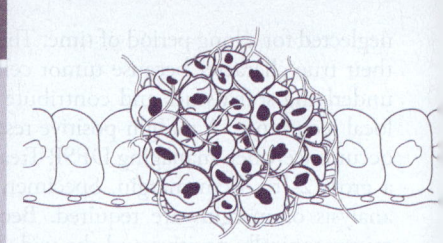

Sarcomas of the Soft Tissues, Retroperitoneum, and Bone

*Heather G. Lyu, Elizabeth J. Lilley, Shalin S. Patel,
Chandrajit P. Raut, and Christina L. Roland*

OUTLINE

SOFT TISSUE AND RETROPERITONEAL SARCOMA

Epidemiology

Soft tissue sarcomas (STSs) are a diverse group of approximately 70 distinct neoplasms that can arise from virtually any anatomic site and can affect the very young as well as the elderly. STSs originate from a variety of tissue types, including skeletal muscle, adipose cells, blood and lymphatic vessels, and other connective tissue derived from a common mesodermal origin (Fig. 64.1 and Table 64.1). Also included are peripheral nerves derived from the neuroectoderm. Clinical behaviors of mesodermal tumors occupy a wide spectrum, from indolent low-grade neoplasms, such as benign lipomas, to tumors with aggressive tumor biology, such as angiosarcoma or desmoplastic small round cell tumors. STSs are relatively rare, with 13,400 estimated new cases and an estimated 5140 deaths for the year 2023.[1] This accounts for 1% of cancer incidence and 2% of cancer-related deaths in the United States. The diagnosis of patients with STS is challenging because they are rare in the general population, and a number of common, non-neoplastic conditions can mimic STS (Box 64.1).

Although there is a great deal of overlap between the various STS subtypes, the most traditional categorization separates trunk and extremity STSs from abdominal and retroperitoneal sarcomas. Before these varieties are discussed in detail, this chapter first reviews core concepts that are relevant to all STSs. These core concepts include STS etiology, staging, and clinical evaluation. This is followed by a more detailed discussion of trunk and extremity STS and retroperitoneal sarcoma and the common histologic subtypes relevant to each anatomic section.

Large published series demonstrate that extremity and trunk STSs are more common than intraperitoneal and retroperitoneal STSs.[2] Among extremity STSs, the proximal limb is more commonly affected than the distal portion, with the thigh being the most common location, accounting for 44% of patients. The age at diagnosis and the histologic STS subtype are often closely linked. Rhabdomyosarcoma, hemangioma, neurofibroma, and alveolar soft parts sarcoma tend to disproportionately affect children and young adults. Most STS occurs sporadically, but other well-documented causes include germline mutations, radiation exposure, and environmental exposure, which are discussed later.

RISK FACTORS

Germline Mutations

Although most STSs arise sporadically, there are some known germline mutations and genetic syndromes that have been

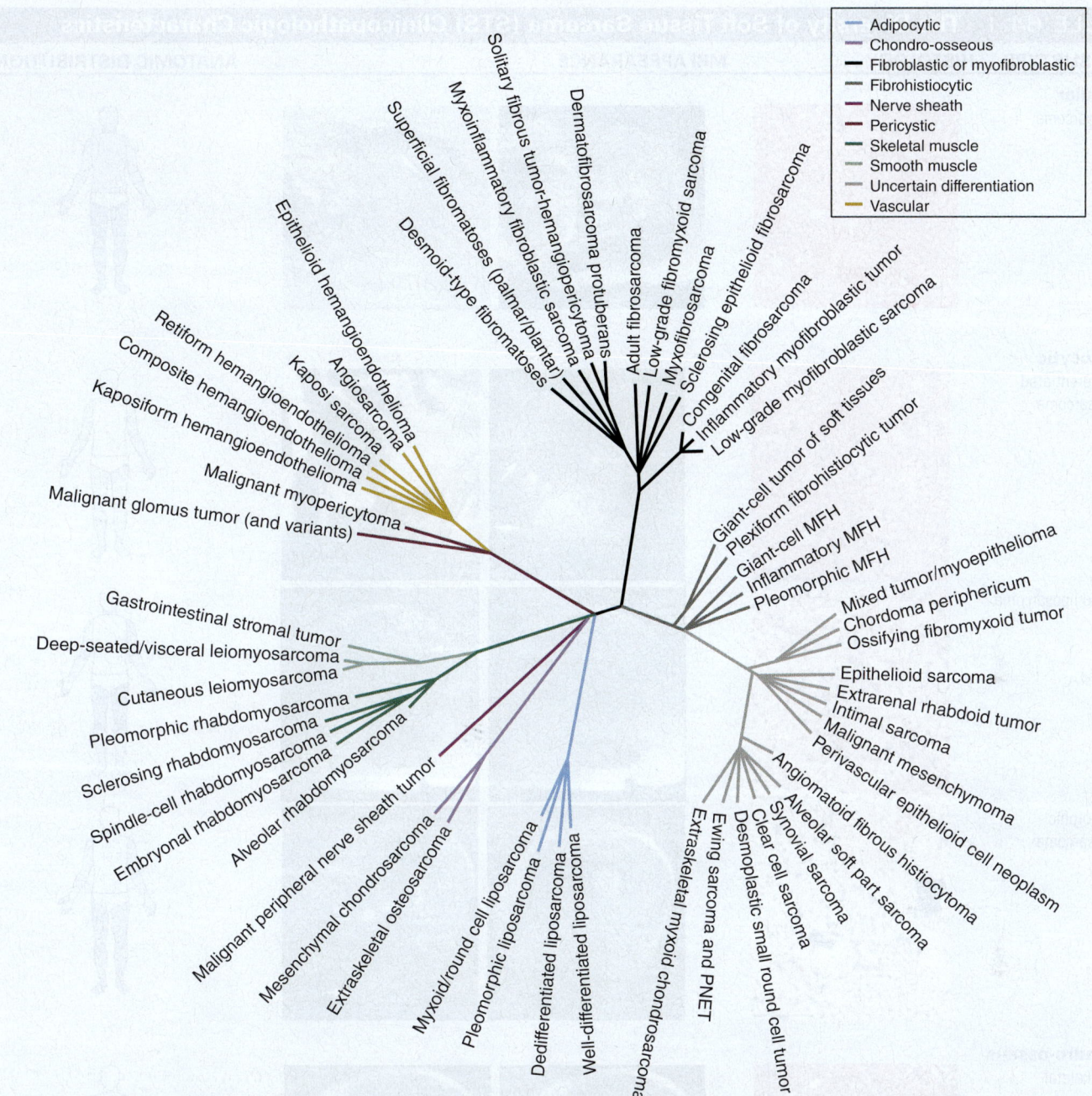

FIGURE 64.1 Taxonomy of soft tissue sarcoma. This unrooted phylogeny shows about 60 sarcoma subtypes, as originally defined by the World Health Organization International Agency for Research on Cancer, amended and updated on the basis of current knowledge. The classification reflects relationships among lineage, prognosis (malignant, intermediate or locally aggressive, intermediate or rarely metastasizing), driver alterations, and additional parameters. Branch lengths are determined by nearest-neighbor joining of a discretized distance matrix based on the aforementioned variables. Initial branching reflects differences in lineage, with associated lineages appearing closer in distance (such as skeletal and smooth muscle). Subsequent branching denotes similarity in prognosis, whether they are translocation associated, and, if so, the genes shared among distinct fusions (in this order). Although this taxonomy is incomplete because many subtypes lack sufficient global molecular profiling data on which to base a phylogeny, this initial formulation minimally reflects the relationships among lineage and major molecular lesions in the subtypes. The illustration excludes 52 benign types of tumor. *MFH,* Undifferentiated pleomorphic sarcoma; *PNET,* primitive neuroectodermal tumor. (From Taylor BS, Barretina J, Maki RG, et al. Advances in sarcoma genomics and new therapeutic targets. *Nat Rev Cancer.* 2011;11:541-557.)

TABLE 64.1   The Diversity of Soft Tissue Sarcoma (STS) Clinicopathologic Characteristics

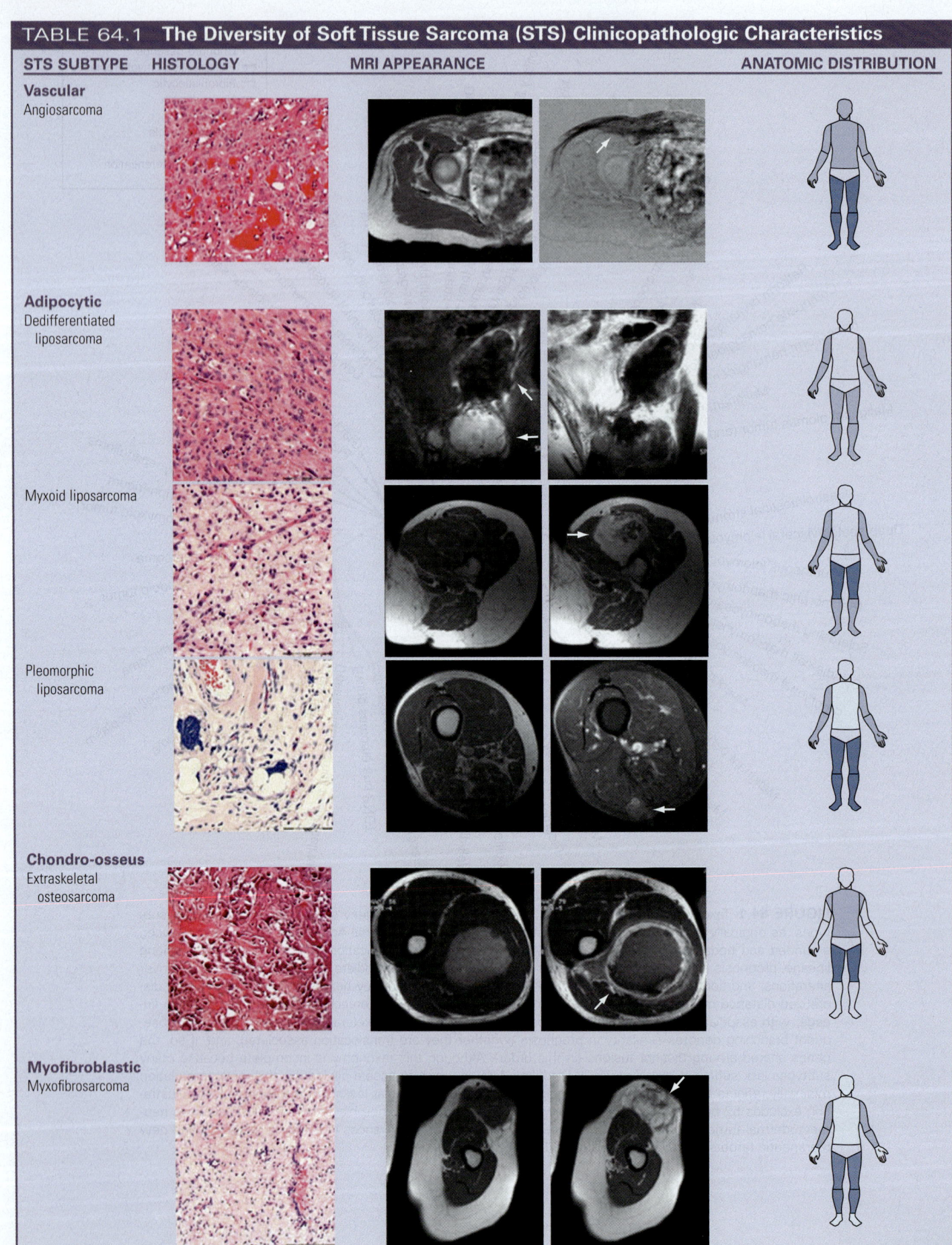

STS SUBTYPE	HISTOLOGY	MRI APPEARANCE		ANATOMIC DISTRIBUTION
Vascular Angiosarcoma				
Adipocytic Dedifferentiated liposarcoma				
Myxoid liposarcoma				
Pleomorphic liposarcoma				
Chondro-osseus Extraskeletal osteosarcoma				
Myofibroblastic Myxofibrosarcoma				

TABLE 64.1   The Diversity of Soft Tissue Sarcoma (STS) Clinicopathologic Characteristics—cont'd

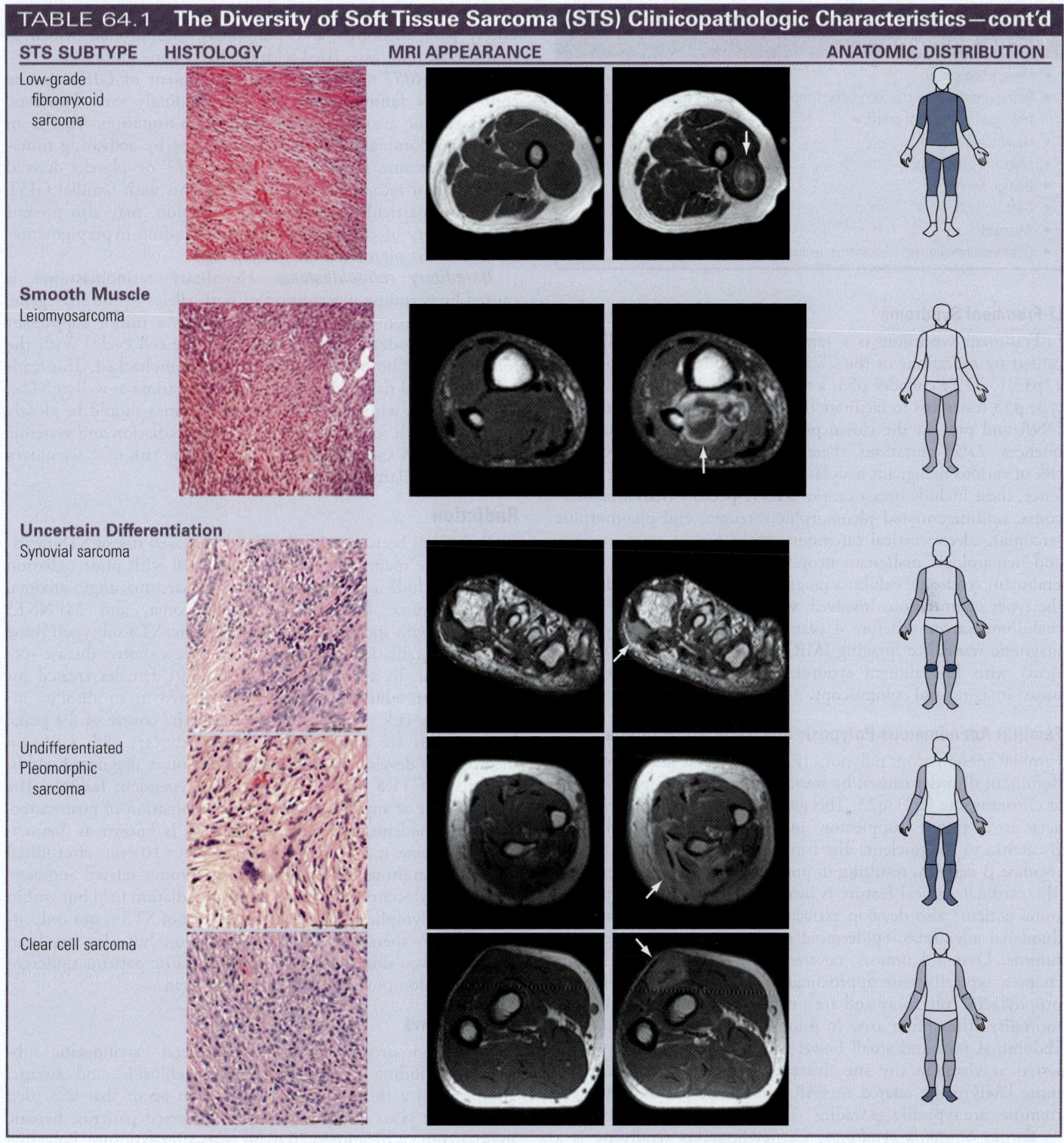

STS SUBTYPE	HISTOLOGY	MRI APPEARANCE	ANATOMIC DISTRIBUTION
Low-grade fibromyxoid sarcoma			
Smooth Muscle Leiomyosarcoma			
Uncertain Differentiation Synovial sarcoma			
Undifferentiated Pleomorphic sarcoma			
Clear cell sarcoma			

Adapted from van Vliet M, Kliffen M, Krestin G, et al. Soft tissue sarcomas at a glance: clinical, histological, and MR imaging features of malignant extremity soft tissue tumors. *Eur Radiol.* 2009;19:1499-1511.
MRI, Magnetic resonance imaging.

associated with an increased risk of developing sarcomas. In patients with a significant family history of STSs or various cancers that meet the pattern of the following syndromes, genetic counseling and testing may be warranted.

Neurofibromatosis Type 1

Neurofibromatosis type 1 (NF1) is an autosomal dominant condition caused by mutations of the *NF1* gene, which is located at

chromosome 17q11.2. *NF1* encodes the protein neurofibromin, a tumor suppressor of the *ras* oncogene signaling pathway. In addition to the ubiquitous development of multiple cutaneous neurofibromas, these patients have a 10% risk for development of a malignant peripheral nerve sheath tumor (MPNST), which is covered in more detail later in this chapter. NF1 is also related to a variety of other tumors, including gastrointestinal stromal tumors (GISTs), schwannomas, and gliomas.

BOX 64.1 Entities That May Mimic Soft Tissue Sarcoma

- Hypertrophic scar
- Retroperitoneal lymphadenopathy: lymphoma, germ cell tumor, or metastasis from gastrointestinal primary
- Hematoma
- Myositis ossificans
- Benign lipoma
- Cyst
- Abscess
- Cutaneous malignant neoplasms, including melanoma

Li-Fraumeni Syndrome

Li-Fraumeni syndrome is a rare autosomal dominant disorder caused by mutations of the *TP53* gene, located at chromosome 17p13.1. *TP53* encodes p53, a tumor suppressor protein. Wild-type p53 functions to facilitate the clearance of damaged cellular DNA and prevent the clonal propagation of these mutated sequences. *TP53* mutations, therefore, contribute to an increased risk of various malignant neoplasms. In order of decreasing prevalence, these include breast cancer, STS (especially rhabdomyosarcoma, undifferentiated pleomorphic sarcoma, and pleomorphic sarcoma), adrenocortical carcinoma, brain cancer, osteosarcoma, and hematologic malignant neoplasms. Patients affected by Li-Fraumeni syndrome exhibit a range of phenotypes, depending on the types of mutations involved, with some patients developing rhabdomyosarcoma before 4 years of age. Annual whole body magnetic resonance imaging (MRI) has been advocated for patients with Li-Fraumeni syndrome, in addition to dedicated breast imaging and colonoscopy.[3]

Familial Adenomatous Polyposis and Gardner Syndrome

Familial adenomatous polyposis (FAP) syndrome is an autosomal dominant disorder caused by mutation of the *APC* gene located at chromosome 5q21-q22. This gene also encodes a protein that acts as a tumor suppressor, inhibiting the localization of β-catenin to the nucleus. The truncated mutant protein fails to regulate β-catenin, resulting in unchecked cellular proliferation. The cardinal clinical feature is innumerable colonic polyps, but some patients also develop extracolonic manifestations, such as duodenal adenomas, epidermoid cysts, osteomas, and desmoid tumors. Desmoid tumors, covered in more detail later in this chapter, typically arise approximately 5 years after FAP-related prophylactic colectomy and are a major source of morbidity and mortality. They often arise in prior surgical sites, including the abdominal wall and small bowel mesentery, but can be manifested at virtually any site. Intraabdominal tumors are much more likely to be related to FAP, whereas desmoids of the extremities are typically sporadic.

Carney-Stratakis syndrome. Carney-Stratakis syndrome is a rare dyad of familial paraganglioma and GIST that is associated with germline mutations in the succinate dehydrogenase (SDH) genes *SDHB, SDHC,* and *SDHD.* It is characterized by allelic losses around the chromosomal loci of the SDH subunit, leading to an SDH deficiency.[4] It is an autosomal dominant disorder with incomplete penetrance. The tumors often manifest in the first three decades of life. As with other SDH-deficient GISTs, they are more frequently associated with female sex and younger age. They are almost always more likely to be multifocal and are more likely to have lymph node metastases as opposed to non–SDH-deficient GISTs.[5] First-line treatment is usually surgery. It is important to note that this is distinct from the Carney triad (the association of GIST, paraganglioma, and pulmonary chondroma, which is sporadic and not associated with the SDH gene mutation).

Familial GIST syndrome. The development of GISTs in the context of a familial syndrome is exceedingly rare. However, GISTs can be associated with a germline mutation. This is an autosomal dominant disorder characterized by activating mutations in tyrosine kinase genes, either *KIT* or platelet-derived growth factor receptor *(PDGFR)*-α. Patients with familial GIST syndrome, particularly with a *KIT* mutation, may also present with a variety of clinical phenotypes, including hyperpigmentation, urticaria pigmentosa, and dysphagia.

Hereditary retinoblastoma. Hereditary retinoblastoma is caused by germline inactivation of both alleles of the *RB1* gene, located at chromosome 13 q14.2. *RB1* is a tumor suppressor gene that encodes a protein regulating the cell cycle. With the inactivation of both alleles, cells can grow unchecked. This leads to an increased risk of developing retinoblastoma as well as STSs.

Individuals with hereditary retinoblastomas should be closely monitored with surveillance imaging after radiation and systemic therapy, which can significantly increase the risk of a secondary cancer, particularly bone and STSs.

Radiation

Radiation has been associated with an increased risk of STS development. The main STS subtypes associated with prior radiation exposure include unclassified pleomorphic sarcoma, angiosarcoma, leiomyosarcoma, fibrosarcoma, osteosarcoma, and MPNST.[6] Compared with sporadic forms of these same STS subtypes, those arising after radiation exposure tend to have a shorter disease-specific survival. In a large cohort of 122,991 females treated for breast cancer, adjuvant radiation contributed to an absolute increase in the risk of STS of 0.13% over the course of 10 years. Patients who are treated for childhood cancers with radiation therapy who develop a secondary STS are often diagnosed within a median of 11.8 years, also in a dose-dependent fashion. The development of angiosarcoma after a combination of postmastectomy lymphedema and radiation therapy is known as *Stewart-Treves syndrome;* it also has a latency of about 10 years after initial therapy. Interestingly, Stewart-Treves syndrome–related angiosarcoma usually occurs outside the previous radiation field but within the zone of lymphedema. An increased risk of STS is not only attributable to therapeutic doses of radiation but also has been linked to lower doses encountered by pediatric patients undergoing routine computed tomography (CT) scan.

Carcinogens

Hepatic angiosarcoma is related to several carcinogenic substances, including Thorotrast, polyvinyl chloride, and arsenic. Thorotrast is a thorium-based IV contrast agent that was used between the years 1930 and 1955. In affected patients, hepatic angiosarcoma is diagnosed 20 to 30 years after exposure. Polyvinyl chloride is an extremely common form of plastic, but prolonged and unprotected exposures have been linked to the development of hepatic angiosarcoma.

STAGING

The American Joint Committee on Cancer/Union for International Cancer Control (AJCC/UICC) tumor-node-metastasis (TNM) staging systems are the most widely used tool for prognostic prediction in many cancer types. Previous versions of AJCC/UICC did not differentiate among disease sites; however, the most recent 8th edition includes four different site-specific staging systems: trunk and extremities, retroperitoneum, head and neck, and abdomen and thoracic visceral organs. The separate schemas for GIST, bone sarcoma, uterine sarcoma, Kaposi sarcoma, and dermatofibrosarcoma protuberans (DFSP) are maintained. The importance of the size of the primary STS to prognosis is well described (Fig. 64.2), but the size thresholds specified by previous AJCC editions have been challenged. The 8th edition subsequently incorporated more granular variables for tumor dimension. Now T1 tumors are defined as 5 cm or less, T2 tumors are >5 to ≤10 cm, T3 tumors are >10 to ≤15 cm, and T4 tumors are >15 cm.[7] Overall, regional lymph node involvement for STS is uncommon (2%–10%). The most common STS subtypes with an increased risk of lymph node metastases are angiosarcoma, rhabdomyosarcoma, undifferentiated pleomorphic sarcoma, epithelioid sarcoma, and clear cell sarcoma. Although regional nodal involvement is an important prognosticator of survival, patients with a single lymph node, multiple positive nodes, and distant metastatic disease all have similar survival.[2] Some groups have proposed the use of sentinel lymph node dissection for epithelioid sarcoma, clear cell sarcoma, and rhabdomyosarcoma in the pediatric population, but the utility of the technique has never been successfully established in STS in a well-designed clinical trial. Nevertheless, the 8th edition incorporates N1 status for stage IV patients. Overall, the schema for the 8th edition AJCC staging system is a significant update over the 7th edition (Tables 64.2 and 64.3).

Many have cited the ongoing limitations of the AJCC/UICC staging system for sarcomas, particularly because it does not currently include histologic subtypes, one of the most important prognostic factors in sarcoma. Anaya and colleagues[8] demonstrated that a more descriptive and clinically relevant method of estimating prognosis involves segregating patients into three histologic groups: well-differentiated liposarcoma, dedifferentiated or pleomorphic liposarcoma, and all other retroperitoneal sarcoma histologic types. Studies validating the recent AJCC/UICC staging system for sarcomas using the Surveillance, Epidemiology, and End Results (SEER) database and the National Cancer Database (NCDB) have both demonstrated its suboptimal performance.[9,10]

TABLE 64.2	American Joint Committee on Cancer Staging for Soft Tissue Sarcomas
Primary Tumor (T)	
Primary tumor cannot be assessed	TX
No evidence of primary tumor	T0
Tumor 5 cm or less in greatest dimension	T1
Tumor more than 5 cm and less than or equal to 10 cm in greatest dimension	T2
Tumor more than 10 cm and less than or equal to 15 cm in greatest dimension	T3
Tumor more than 15 cm in greatest dimension	T4
Regional Lymph Nodes (N)	
Regional lymph nodes cannot be assessed	NX
No regional lymph node metastasis	N0
Regional lymph node metastasis	N1
Distant Metastasis (M)	
No distant metastasis	M0
Distant metastasis	M1

TABLE 64.3	Anatomic Stage and Prognostic Groups for Soft Tissue Sarcomas			
GROUP	**T**	**N**	**M**	**GRADE**
Stage IA	T1	N0	M0	G1, GX
Stage IB	T2–4	N0	M0	G1, GX
Stage II	T1	N0	M0	G2, G3
Stage IIIA	T2	N0	M0	G2, G3
Stage IIIB	T3, T4	N0	M0	G2, G3
Stage IV	Any T	N1[a]	M0	Any grade
	Any T	Any N	M1	Any grade

[a]For retroperitoneal sarcoma, N1 disease is designated as stage IIIB, not stage IV.

AJCC stage for STS is largely driven by tumor grade. The two most commonly applied grading systems are the French Fédération Nationale des Centres de Lutte Contre le Cancer (FN-CLCC) system and the National Institutes of Health (NIH) system. The FNCLCC is a score based on the sum of three categories: tumor differentiation, mitotic rate, and amount of tumor necrosis. The NIH system is similar, but for certain STS subtypes, it requires that the pathologist state the degree of tumor cellularity and pleomorphism, which can limit its reproducibility. When the FNCLCC and the NIH systems were compared, the FNCLCC system was found to be superior in estimating the risk of distant metastasis and survival. The AJCC staging system states that the FNCLCC system is preferred over the NIH system.[11]

Nomograms have been developed in response to the fact that standard staging systems, such as the AJCC, do not adequately consider the relevant parameters (such as histology) and therefore may not accurately estimate the prognosis of patients with STS. No fewer than 13 different nomograms have been published for STS alone. The nomograms were developed to address a number of oncologic outcomes but most typically predict local recurrence or overall survival (Fig. 64.3). Some of them also addressed a prior shortcoming of the AJCC staging system by being specific to site of origin. In general, the nomograms are reported to more accurately prognosticate outcome than traditional staging systems, but

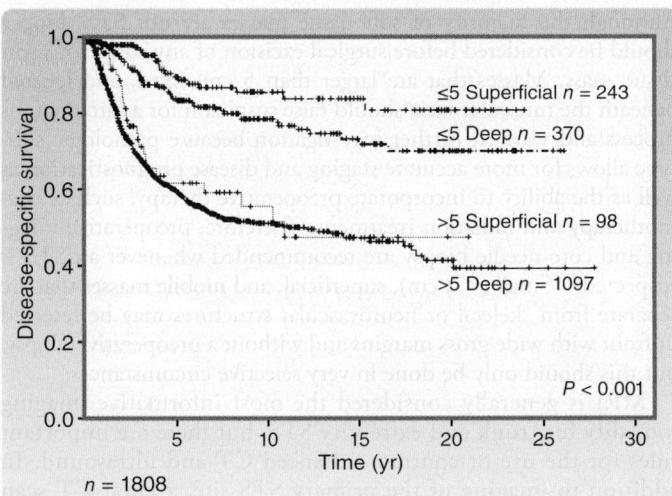

FIGURE 64.2 Importance of size and depth among primary high-grade soft tissue sarcoma tumors. (From Brennan MF, Antonescu CR, Moraco N, et al. Lessons learned from the study of 10,000 patients with soft tissue sarcoma. *Ann Surg.* 2014;260:416-422.)

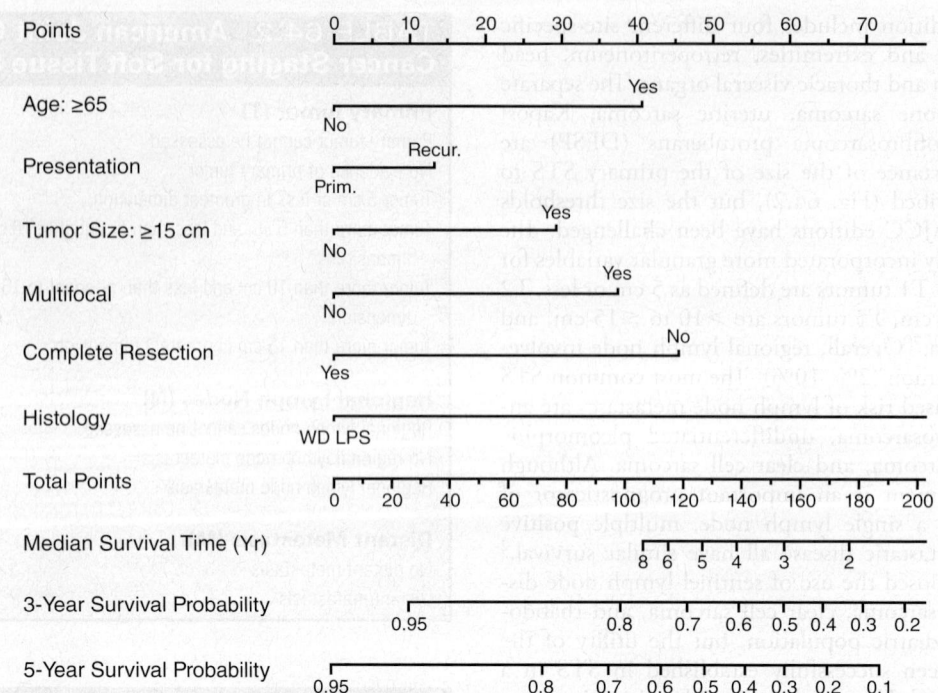

FIGURE 64.3 Postoperative nomogram for median 3- and 5-year overall survival prediction in patients with nonmetastatic, resectable, retroperitoneal sarcoma. *WD LPS,* Well-differentiated liposarcoma. (From Anaya DA, Lahat G, Wang X, et al. Postoperative nomogram for survival of patients with retroperitoneal sarcoma treated with curative intent. *Ann Oncol.* 2010;21:397-402.)

few have been validated in a dataset beyond that which was used to generate the nomogram. Nonetheless, they can provide meaningful information that, when used appropriately, can have an impact on the care of patients with STS.

Gene Fusions and Molecular Testing

Gene fusions have been identified as important driver mutations in a number of tissue types, including various STS subtypes. Although approximately one-third of STSs have been found to harbor gene fusions, not all fusion products are pathogenetically relevant (i.e., "driver mutations"). Thus, the utility of gene fusions lies in their use as diagnostic tools and also as potential therapeutic targets. Gene fusions are but one example of how mutations manifest in STS. An ever-expanding array of platforms is available in the molecular analysis of these patients, including fluorescence in situ hybridization (FISH), reverse transcription–polymerase chain reaction (RT-PCR), and next-generation sequencing (NGS). In one study, molecular analysis changed the clinical diagnosis in 13% of patients, often sparing the patient the toxicity of a nontherapeutic chemotherapy regimen. In particular, the diagnosis was changed in 23% of patients initially suspected to have dedifferentiated liposarcoma.[12] The routine use of molecular analysis is likely to grow in this field as additional gene mutations and fusion events predictive of response to specific systemic agents are discovered. For example, a platform called Complex INdex in SARComas (CINSARC) consists of a group of 67 genes that have been demonstrated to predict metastasis-free survival. These genes, which are associated with mitosis and chromosome management, show promise in being able to predict prognosis more effectively than histologic grade, even in patients with grade 1 tumors. Although these early data have not been prospectively validated, they demonstrate the potential role of routine molecular analysis for STS patients in the future.

TRUNK AND EXTREMITY SARCOMA

Presentation

For patients presenting with a trunk or extremity sarcoma, the most common clinical presentation is a patient with a painless mass without prior evaluation. When STS is included in the differential diagnosis, appropriate oncologic staging should be undertaken. A detailed history and physical examination are important in determining the likelihood of STS versus other more common mimicking diagnoses, such as hypertrophic scar, myositis ossificans, hematoma, or cyst (see Box 64.1).

Diagnosis

Although the majority of soft tissue masses are not STS, biopsy should be considered before surgical excision of any suspicious soft tissue mass. Masses that are larger than 5 cm, fixed, and located beneath the muscular facia should raise suspicion for a sarcomatous process and warrant further investigation because pathologic subtype allows for more accurate staging and disease prognostication as well as the ability to incorporate preoperative therapy, such as chemotherapy and radiation treatment. Therefore, preoperative imaging and core-needle biopsy are recommended whenever an STS is suspected.[13] Small (<2 cm), superficial, and mobile masses that are separate from skeletal or neurovascular structures may be resected upfront with wide gross margins and without a preoperative biopsy, but this should only be done in very selective circumstances.

MRI is generally considered the most informative imaging modality for trunk and extremity STS, but there are important roles for the use of contrast-enhanced CT and ultrasound. In addition to imaging of the primary STS site, a chest CT scan should generally be obtained because this is the most frequent site of metastasis. When available, the biopsy results may prompt consideration of additional imaging. For example, a

CT scan of the abdomen and pelvis should be considered for patients with more aggressive histologic types, such as myxoid or round cell liposarcoma, epithelioid sarcoma, angiosarcoma, and leiomyosarcoma. Paraspinal MRI may also be considered for myxoid liposarcoma. Brain imaging may be considered to exclude metastasis from alveolar soft part sarcoma, clear cell sarcoma, and angiosarcoma.

Biopsy of the suspected sarcoma should generally be performed via percutaneous core-needle biopsy. Given the scant amount of tissue procured, a fine-needle aspirate is generally unsatisfactory. An image-guided core-needle biopsy is more likely to provide a reliable diagnosis, providing more information about tissue architecture to help distinguish individual histologic types of sarcoma. To decrease the risk of local recurrence, the core biopsy approach should be planned so that the entire needle trajectory can be easily incorporated into the forthcoming surgical resection volume. If the first core-needle biopsy attempts are nondiagnostic, repeat biopsy is recommended, but an incisional biopsy may be considered. Here, again, it is critical to plan the incision so that the entire bi-

opsy trajectory is ultimately included within the resection volume and along the planned course of the incision for future resection.

Armed with radiographic and pathologic information, an ideal treatment plan should be constructed by a multidisciplinary team, preferably at a high-volume STS center. Multidisciplinary teams include representatives from surgical oncology, medical oncology, diagnostic radiology, pathology, and radiation oncology. The goal of a multidisciplinary discussion is to assess which treatment modalities are most appropriate for each patient and in what sequence each modality should be implemented (Fig. 64.4). Up to 74% of patients who undergo an unplanned trunk or extremity sarcoma resection have residual disease at the time of re-resection; a multidisciplinary approach may preclude a nononcologic resection. Thirty-day mortality, rates of limb preservation, and overall survival have been linked to care delivered at high-volume STS centers.[14]

Treatment

Treatment of extremity STS poses a particular challenge with respect to balancing the goal of maintaining limb function against

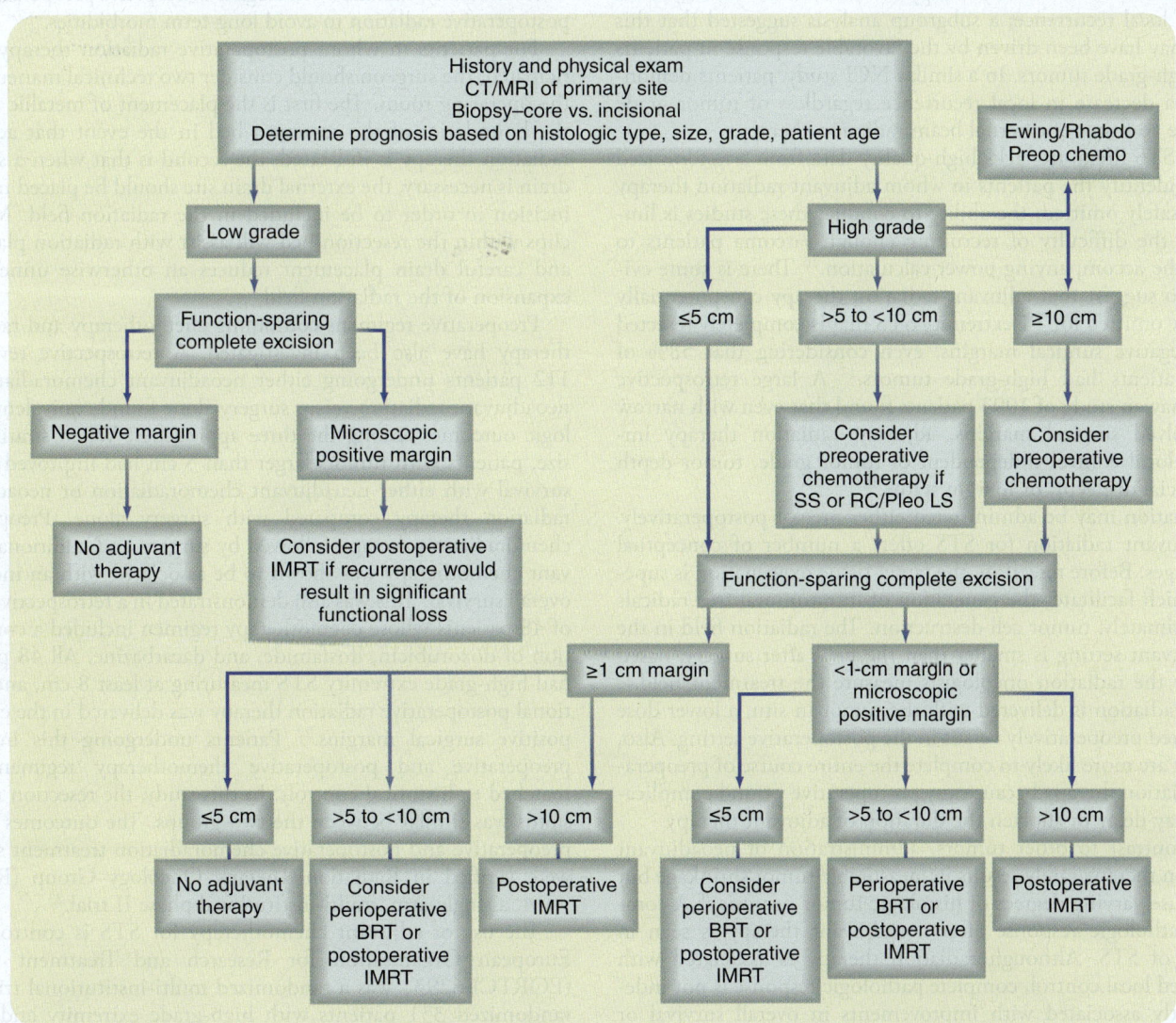

FIGURE 64.4 Algorithm for the management of primary (with no metastases) extremity or trunk soft tissue sarcoma using a biologic rationale (i.e., size and grade of tumor). *BRT*, Brachytherapy; *CT*, computed tomography; *EBRT*, external beam radiation therapy; *IMRT*, intensity-modulated radiation therapy; *MRI*, magnetic resonance imaging; *RC/Pleo LS*, round cell–pleomorphic liposarcoma; *SS*, synovial sarcoma.

the extent of resection for local tumor control. Historically, extremity amputation was routinely performed for STS. However, data from clinical trials have prompted a shift toward limb preservation in these patients, which is the standard of care. The ability to offer limb preservation is a result of improvements in the multidisciplinary care of these patients, particularly local control with perioperative radiation therapy. A seminal trial conducted at the National Cancer Institute (NCI) proposed that extremity STS resection might be addressed by a limb-sparing approach instead of amputation.[15] In this study, 43 patients with high-grade extremity STS were randomized to undergo a limb-sparing operation followed by adjuvant radiation therapy and chemotherapy versus amputation and adjuvant chemotherapy. There were four local recurrences in the limb-sparing group compared with none in the amputation group, but this difference was not statistically significant. Importantly, disease-free and overall survival rates were equivalent between the two groups. To address the role of radiation therapy in STS, a trial from Memorial Sloan Kettering Cancer Center evaluated 126 patients who were randomized to limb-sparing STS resection with or without adjuvant brachytherapy. In this trial, brachytherapy was associated with improved rates of local recurrence; a subgroup analysis suggested that this result may have been driven by the favorable response in patients with high-grade tumors. In a similar NCI study, patients demonstrated a decrease in local recurrence regardless of tumor grade with the addition of external beam radiation therapy.

The STS literature lacks high-quality data from a randomized trial to identify the patients in whom adjuvant radiation therapy can be safely omitted; the ability to conduct these studies is limited by the difficulty of recruiting enough sarcoma patients to satisfy the accompanying power calculation.[16] There is some evidence to suggest that adjuvant radiation therapy can potentially be safely omitted for T1 extremity STS that is completely resected with negative surgical margins, even considering that 58% of these patients had high-grade tumors.[17] A large retrospective Scandinavian study of 1093 patients found that even with narrow or involved surgical margins, adjuvant radiation therapy improved local control independent of tumor grade, tumor depth (superficial or deep), or margin status.[18]

Radiation may be administered either pre- or postoperatively. Neoadjuvant radiation for STS offers a number of conceptual advantages. Before resection, the target tissue oxygenation is superior, which facilitates the generation of intratumoral free radicals and, ultimately, tumor cell destruction. The radiation field in the neoadjuvant setting is smaller than the field after surgery, based on how the radiation oncologists measure the treatment field.[19] When radiation is delivered with the tumor in situ, a lower dose is required preoperatively versus in the postoperative setting. Also, patients are more likely to complete the entire course of preoperative radiation therapy because any postoperative wound complications may delay or shorten the duration of adjuvant therapy.

In contrast to other tumors, administration of neoadjuvant radiation therapy rarely results in measurable tumor shrinkage but may cause varying degrees of histologic tumor necrosis.[20] A complete pathologic response after neoadjuvant therapy is seen in <10% of STS. Although radiation therapy is associated with improved local control, complete pathologic response is not independently associated with improvements in overall survival or local recurrence rates in STS patients.[21] Also, patients with a positive surgical margin after undergoing preoperative radiation therapy do not appear to derive a significant reduction in local recurrence by administration of a postoperative radiation boost.

The optimal timing of perioperative radiation treatment is still debated. A landmark clinical trial randomized patients with extremity STS to receive either neoadjuvant or postoperative radiation therapy, with a primary end point of 120-day wound complications. In this trial, neoadjuvant external beam radiation therapy was associated with an increased risk of postoperative wound complications (35% vs. 17%; $p = 0.001$).[19] However, long-term toxicity in terms of fibrosis and joint stiffness was significantly higher in patients treated with postoperative radiation therapy. Although the authors reported a statistically significant difference in overall survival favoring the neoadjuvant arm, survival was a secondary end point, and the trial was not properly powered to evaluate this parameter. One would expect that another conceptual advantage of choosing a neoadjuvant approach would be to decrease the incidence and consequences of positive surgical margins by delivering tumoricidal doses preoperatively to the areas most at risk. However, the existing randomized trial showed equivalent rates of negative surgical margins in patients receiving preoperative versus postoperative radiation therapy (83% and 85%, respectively).[19] Given the absence of a significant survival advantage of either modality, radiation oncologists often prefer preoperative over postoperative radiation to avoid long-term morbidities.

For patients in whom postoperative radiation therapy is anticipated, the surgeon should consider two technical maneuvers in the operating room. The first is the placement of metallic clips at the boundaries of the resection bed in the event that adjuvant radiation therapy is indicated; the second is that when a surgical drain is necessary, the external drain site should be placed near the incision in order to be included in the radiation field. Metallic clips within the resection bed will assist with radiation planning, and careful drain placement reduces an otherwise unnecessary expansion of the radiation field.

Preoperative regimens combining chemotherapy and radiation therapy have also been investigated. A retrospective review of 112 patients undergoing either neoadjuvant chemoradiation or neoadjuvant radiation versus surgery alone found equivalent oncologic outcomes among the three approaches. When stratified by size, patients with tumors larger than 5 cm had improved overall survival with either neoadjuvant chemoradiation or neoadjuvant radiation therapy compared with surgery alone. Preoperative chemoradiation therapy followed by surgery and additional adjuvant chemotherapy was shown to be associated with an increased overall survival. This was also demonstrated in a retrospective study of 48 patients whose chemotherapy regimen included a combination of doxorubicin, ifosfamide, and dacarbazine. All 48 patients had high-grade extremity STS measuring at least 8 cm, and additional postoperative radiation therapy was delivered in the event of positive surgical margins.[22] Patients undergoing this intensive preoperative and postoperative chemotherapy regimen were matched to historical controls. In this study, the resection margin status was similar between the two groups. The outcomes of this preoperative and postoperative chemoradiation treatment schema were verified in Radiation Therapy Oncology Group (RTOG) 9514, a single-arm, multi-institutional phase II trial.[23]

The use of adjuvant chemotherapy for STS is controversial. European Organisation for Research and Treatment Center (EORTC) 62931 was a randomized multi-institutional trial that randomized 351 patients with high-grade extremity and trunk wall STS to receive adjuvant chemotherapy (doxorubicin, ifosfamide, and the hematopoietic growth factor lenograstim) versus no chemotherapy.[24] The overall and relapse-free survivals were equivalent in both groups. However, a meta-analysis of 1953 patients who had participated in 18 trials showed that those patients who received adjuvant doxorubicin-based chemotherapy had significant improvements in local, distant, and overall recurrence. The addition of ifosfamide is associated with a statistically significant improvement in survival.[25]

A phase III randomized controlled trial performed in 32 centers across Europe compared the use of three cycles of standard chemotherapy with histology-tailored regimens based on sarcoma subtype.[26] Patients in the control group received epirubicin/ifosfamide, and those randomized to receive tailored treatment were given trabectedin for myxoid liposarcoma, gemcitabine/docetaxel for undifferentiated pleomorphic sarcoma, gemcitabine/dacarbazine for leiomyosarcoma, high-dose ifosfamide for synovial sarcoma, or etoposide/ifosfamide for MPNSTs. After enrolling 287 patients, the study was closed at the third futility analysis when it was found that patients receiving histology-tailored regimens had worse disease-free and overall survival compared with the standard arm.

Based on the existing data, adjuvant doxorubicin and ifosfamide should be considered the standard of care. However, it is worth noting that the reported survival benefits are modest. Consequently, it is important to weigh the toxicities of chemotherapy against the potential benefit in patient selection for adjuvant systemic treatment. Because of the abundance of conflicting data, consensus guidelines, such as those of the National Comprehensive Cancer Network and the European Society for Medical Oncology, remain guarded in their recommendation for adjuvant chemotherapy as the standard of care.

A recent development in the sarcoma treatment paradigm has been the introduction of immunotherapy. Some initial studies have demonstrated some benefit of immune checkpoint inhibition for specific histologies, most notably undifferentiated pleomorphic sarcoma and alveolar soft parts sarcoma. However, the role of immunotherapy in the treatment of STS is still not well studied, and further studies on potential targets for tailored treatments are needed.

Another treatment strategy that has been employed in patients with locally advanced extremity STS is regional chemotherapy, namely, limb perfusion. More commonly used in the treatment of locally advanced melanoma, this involves placement of both IV and intraarterial catheters that are positioned within the affected limb proximal to the tumor. The combination of the limb vasculature and the intravascular catheters completes a circuit through which hyperthermic chemotherapy is circulated. A tourniquet proximal to the tips of the catheters separates the limb circulation from the systemic circulation to minimize systemic chemotherapy toxicity. The most common perfusion agents used are melphalan, tumor necrosis factor-α, and interferon-γ. Isolated limb perfusion is often combined with other modalities, namely, surgery. The technical demands and potential for local toxicities limit the application of this therapy. Currently, only one randomized trial has compared regional chemotherapy with other standard STS therapies. Overall, the published data are insufficient to conclusively establish the role of regional chemotherapy in the care of extremity STS. Furthermore, tumor necrosis factor-α, which is felt to be a key component of the infusion, is not regularly available in all countries, including in the United States.

The question as to what constitutes an adequate STS resection margin is complex, but the following is clear: the volume of tissue that is resected has clear implications for the postoperative function of the limb, and a quantitative definition of an adequate surgical margin has never been defined in a randomized, prospective format. Whereas advances in rehabilitation medicine and

prosthetic construction have significantly improved the functional capacity of patients who undergo extremity STS resection, the aforementioned data demonstrate that the goal of effective tumor extirpation with the smallest functional deficit is possible. Unlike in the melanoma literature, patients with extremity STS have never been randomized to compare surgical margin widths. Retrospectively, the local recurrence rate after resection of extremity STS with a microscopic margin of 1 cm or more is superior to when the margin is less than 1 cm.[27] However, in a different retrospective study, the only factor associated with an increased risk of local recurrence was tumor at the margin of resection.[28]

Patients presenting after surgery with positive margins on final pathology should be offered re-resection; re-resection in this setting has been shown to be associated with a decreased risk of local recurrence.[29] As with primary resections, the pursuit of clear surgical margins should be weighed against the natural history of extremity STS and the risk of a permanent functional deficit. Even in the setting of multimodality therapy, the risk of distant metastasis consistently outweighs the risk of local recurrence in high-grade tumors.

The gross morphology of STS is such that during resection, the plane of least resistance is usually along a tumor pseudocapsule. The pseudocapsule is a characteristic plane of thickened tissue that radiographically and during intraoperative assessment gives the impression of representing the interface between tumor and normal tissue. However, resections along the pseudocapsule plane often result in involved margins and should be avoided when possible. Traditionally, a 1- to 2-cm grossly negative margin beyond the pseudocapsule is recommended, but this may be difficult to achieve in certain anatomic sites and may be unnecessary in dealing with low-grade tumors.[13] Neoadjuvant therapy may be associated with formation of a more robust tumor pseudocapsule populated by fewer tumor cells.[30] Ultimately, the final resection margin is only as good as the closest margin in any region of the tumor; extending resections to increase morbidity in one region is not necessary if a closer margin exists in another region.

STS tumors tend to metastasize hematogenously to the lungs, liver, and bone. Tumor grade is the most important predictor of distant metastasis, with only a 43% rate of metastasis-free survival in patients with high-grade tumors.[31] Other important predictors of metastasis include tumor size, bone or neurovascular involvement, tumor depth (superficial vs. deep), and histology. The prevalence of pulmonary metastases among patients previously treated for extremity STS is approximately 19%. Isolated pulmonary metastases could be resected whenever feasible.[32] A prolonged disease-free interval between initial STS treatment and development of lung metastasis is generally a favorable prognostic factor. Repeated pulmonary metastasectomy for patients with stable disease is also a consideration. Patients who are not candidates for metastasectomy because of disease burden or biology of the disease should be evaluated for ablative or systemic therapies. Typical systemic agents for metastatic STS include doxorubicin, dacarbazine, ifosfamide, gemcitabine, docetaxel, eribulin, pazopanib, regorafenib, and olaratumab.

Surveillance

Because of the considerable risk for recurrence, close postoperative surveillance is essential for STS patients. In general, these patients should undergo a physical examination every 3 to 6 months for 2 or 3 years, then every 6 months for the next 2 years, and then annually. For patients with extremity STS, radiographic surveillance of the chest (chest CT) and the primary site should also be undertaken in patients with high-grade disease or histologies that are more likely to metastasize. The modality (CT vs. MRI) for imaging the primary site and the frequency should be individualized to the patient and the tumor characteristics. The most informative preoperative imaging modality is favored, but consideration should also be given to avoiding unnecessary radiation exposure by ultrasound or MRI. The imaging frequency for STS patients has not been rigorously studied, but a shorter imaging frequency may be appropriate for a patient with close surgical margins or a patient with a particularly aggressive histologic subtype.

RETROPERITONEAL AND VISCERAL SARCOMA

Retroperitoneal sarcoma represents approximately 15% of all STS. The sequestered location of the retroperitoneum probably accounts for the fact that the average tumor size at presentation is 15 cm.[33] The most frequent retroperitoneal sarcoma subtypes are liposarcoma, leiomyosarcoma, and undifferentiated pleomorphic sarcoma. The predominant intraperitoneal STS subtypes are GIST and leiomyosarcoma. The average age at presentation is 54 years, and there is an equal male-to-female distribution. In most series, the overall 5-year survival of patients presenting with retroperitoneal sarcoma is 33% to 39%. Even after optimal resection, at least 70% of patients will relapse. In one large retrospective series, approximately 12% of patients presented with metastatic disease, predominantly pulmonary or hepatic.

The presentation of retroperitoneal sarcomas is variable, depending on the size and location of the tumor. Some are asymptomatic and incidentally discovered. Symptomatic tumors may manifest with abdominal pain, weight loss, early satiety, nausea, emesis, back or flank pain, paresthesias, and weakness. CT and MRI are widely used for the evaluation of retroperitoneal sarcoma because of their excellent spatial resolution and reproducible axial image acquisition. The advantages of CT scan include rapid image acquisition, nearly universal availability, and a concise image set that can be more intuitive for the nonradiologist to interpret. The advantages of MRI include a wider range of soft tissue differentiation, but the disadvantages include patient discomfort, more limited availability, and a greater number of implant-related contraindications compared with CT scan. These imaging modalities can be complementary, and at times, both provide useful information. The patient must be carefully evaluated along with the imaging studies to verify that the retroperitoneal mass does not represent an unappreciated lymphoma, germ cell tumor, or metastasis from another primary tumor.

Management of retroperitoneal sarcomas can vary based on histologic subtypes. Preoperative biopsies are recommended in order to help guide perioperative treatment decisions, especially with respect to neoadjuvant treatment strategies and surgical planning. A retrospective review of retroperitoneal sarcoma patients who underwent surgery showed that those who underwent a preoperative biopsy were more likely to receive neoadjuvant therapy and undergo a complete tumor resection.[34] With the increasing use of targeted therapies, preoperative tissue sampling may become more important. Limitations of a biopsy include the possibility of seeding and sampling error. Studies have shown that the rate of needle tract seeding from a percutaneous approach is low.[35,36] Sampling errors leading to possible preoperative downstaging of disease can be mitigated by obtaining tissue samples from the most concerning regions under image guidance. When possible, treatment should proceed with a complete gross resection. In the retroperitoneal sarcoma literature, the concept of

margin status is different from that for extremity STS. Because extremity STS tumors are usually smaller than retroperitoneal sarcoma tumors, microscopic evaluation of the entire surgical specimen margin is often feasible. Given the much larger tumor dimensions of most retroperitoneal sarcomas and proximity to the entire abdominal contents, it is not practical and often impossible to microscopically evaluate 100% of the surgical specimen margin surface area. Consequently, most of the retroperitoneal sarcoma literature refers to complete gross resection (R0/R1). In one large series, complete gross resection was achieved in 80% of initial sarcoma resections, 57% of operations for first recurrence, 33% of operations at second recurrence, and 14% of operations at third recurrence. In 75% of patients, achieving complete gross resection may mean resecting contiguous or inseparable adjacent organs, such as the kidney, bowel, adrenal, pancreas, and vascular structures. Resection requiring pancreaticoduodenectomy, major vascular resection, or splenectomy was more likely to result in a major postoperative complication, but a major postoperative complication does not appear to adversely affect long-term survival or recurrence.[37]

Predicting histologic invasion on the basis of gross intraoperative findings can be inaccurate. Before the era of modern CT technology, patients who underwent nephrectomy as a result of intraoperative evidence of suspected involvement during retroperitoneal sarcoma resection were further evaluated for histologic evidence of sarcoma invasion. In 73% of cases, the nephrectomy specimen did not contain STS. Predictors of poor prognosis include gross residual disease after resection, unresectable disease (either metastatic or locally advanced), and high tumor grade. Patients with an R0/R1 resection have a median survival of 103 months compared with 18 months for patients with incomplete resections. Even with optimal chemotherapy and radiation therapy, the median survival of patients with unresectable disease is 10 months.[38] Patients who undergo complete resection should have active surveillance because the risk of local recurrence and distant metastasis after 5 years is 23% and 21%, respectively. Timing of resection of recurrent retroperitoneal sarcoma is complex and individualized and should be considered after multidisciplinary evaluation, ideally at a high-volume center.

In contrast to extremity sarcoma, the role of multimodality therapy is more controversial in retroperitoneal sarcoma. Given the success of adjuvant radiation in extremity STS, this approach has been applied to retroperitoneal sarcoma. However, the 60- to 70-Gy dose that is typically used for extremity STS is not feasible in the adjuvant setting for retroperitoneal sarcoma because of the adverse effects on surrounding bowel and visceral organs. Even dose reduction to 50 to 55 Gy can result in significant enteritis. These tolerability issues prompted consideration of neoadjuvant radiation for retroperitoneal sarcoma. An advantage of neoadjuvant radiation is that the in situ tumor displaces the bowel anteriorly, thus facilitating the delivery of a higher radiation dose posteriorly (Fig. 64.5). Two retrospective studies demonstrated that the neoadjuvant approach is well tolerated and that long- and short-term oncologic outcomes are favorable compared with historical cohorts treated with resection alone.[39,40] A recent randomized, phase III trial (EORTC-62090: STRASS) comparing patients with retroperitoneal sarcoma who underwent preoperative radiation and surgery versus surgery alone demonstrated no differences in recurrence-free survival and overall survival between the groups.[41] A post hoc subgroup analysis by subtype and grade suggested that preoperative radiation may improve outcomes for patients with liposarcoma and low-grade retroperitoneal sarcomas;

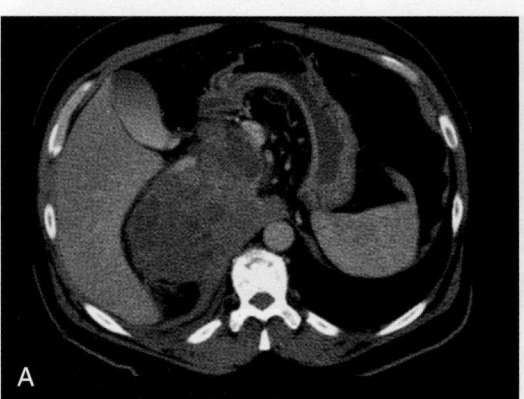 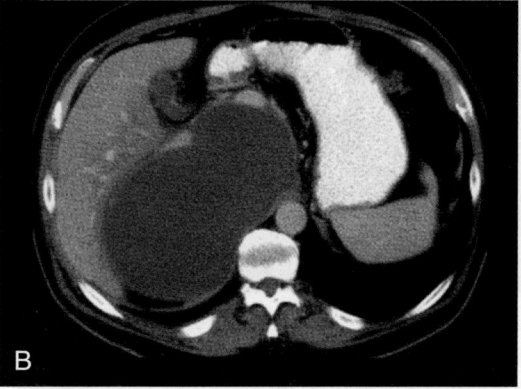

FIGURE 64.5 Liquefaction of a high-grade retroperitoneal sarcoma before (A) and after (B) administration of 60-Gy preoperative radiation therapy. The tumor was subsequently resected with negative surgical margins, and no viable tumor was histologically identifiable.

however, this was not a preplanned study, and the cohorts were relatively small.

For patients with metastatic retroperitoneal sarcoma, single or combination therapy with anthracyclines can be used as first-line therapy. A second-line regimen is gemcitabine and docetaxel. Thus far, the experience with immunotherapy agents in STS patients has been limited. One encouraging finding is that patients with undifferentiated pleomorphic sarcoma or dedifferentiated liposarcoma have a somewhat more promising objective response rate than those with other STS subtypes when treated with pembrolizumab, a programmed death-1 inhibitor.[42] In an open-label phase II trial, combined programmed death-1 inhibitor and cytotoxic T-lymphocyte–associated protein 4 (CTLA-4) inhibition showed very poor response rates in patients with metastatic sarcoma.[43] Novel agents undergoing further study include trabectedin, tyrosine kinase inhibitors, MDM2 antagonists, peroxisome proliferator-activated receptor gamma agonists, and CDK4 antagonists.

COMMON SUBTYPES

Lipomatous Tumors

Lipomas are adipocytic tumors that can arise from any part of the body. By definition, they are benign neoplasms, but they can cause symptoms as a consequence of the adjacent structures that the lipoma displaces. Lipomas are encapsulated and devoid of nodularity or thick internal septations. They are generally homogeneous but may contain calcifications or hemorrhage secondary to trauma. There can be a great deal of clinical overlap between a lipoma and liposarcoma. The CT and MRI features that have been demonstrated to be associated with liposarcoma include tumor size larger than 10 cm, presence of thick (more than 2 mm) septa, presence of nonadipose areas, and lesions that are less than 75% adipose tissue. Lipomas are effectively treated by a simple excision beyond the capsule of the tumor, whereas the treatment of liposarcoma involves a more complex resection with attention to adequate negative margins and the input of a multidisciplinary care team specializing in STS.

Overall, liposarcoma is the most frequent STS subtype and represents 45% of all retroperitoneal sarcomas. There are three histologic varieties: well-differentiated and dedifferentiated liposarcoma, pleomorphic liposarcoma, and myxoid/round cell liposarcoma, listed in order of decreasing frequency. Well-differentiated and

dedifferentiated liposarcomas typically arise from the retroperitoneum versus the extremities, whereas the inverse is true for pleomorphic and myxoid/round cell liposarcoma. Compared with well-differentiated liposarcoma, the dedifferentiated variety has a worse prognosis because there is a higher risk of distant metastasis compared with well-differentiated liposarcoma. Local recurrence is common in both types. The malignant behavior of well-differentiated and dedifferentiated liposarcomas is attributable to the amplification of chromosome 12q13-15, which accounts for the upregulation of *MDM2* and *CDK4*. Both well-differentiated and dedifferentiated retroperitoneal liposarcomas are often multifocal. *Myxoid* and *round cells* are descriptive terms based on their histologic appearance. These liposarcoma varieties are characterized by distinct translocations such as *FUS-DDIT3* located at t(12;16)(q13;p11) and more rarely *EWSR1-DDIT3* located at t(12;22)(q13;q12). Multiple tumor-promoting pathways, including MET, RET, and PI3K/Akt, are activated as a result of these translocations. Myxoid liposarcomas are radio- and chemosensitive and are associated with a 10-year disease-specific survival of 87%. The round cell variety, which is considered a poorly differentiated type of myxoid liposarcoma, has worse outcomes, with distant metastasis rates of up to 21%. Pleomorphic liposarcomas are also poorly differentiated and have a poor prognosis. The are no known targetable mutations because the genetic underpinnings of the disease are widely variable.

It is ideal to distinguish well-differentiated from dedifferentiated retroperitoneal liposarcomas because of differences in natural history and management. MRI and CT scans are useful in making this distinction but can be difficult when the tumors are large and heterogeneous in appearance. The imaging characteristics that raise suspicion of a dedifferentiated histology were described in a study with a cohort of 78 patients with retroperitoneal liposarcoma. These included tumor hypervascularity, areas of necrosis or cystic change, adjacent organ invasion, and areas of focal nodular or water density.[44] These authors proposed a clinical algorithm in which patients with evidence of focal nodularity or water density underwent biopsy of suspicious areas in order to clarify the specific histology (Fig. 64.6). Both well-differentiated and dedifferentiated liposarcomas can be distinguished from lipomas and other poorly differentiated STS subtypes on the basis of MDM2 and CDK4 immunohistochemistry.

For extremity liposarcomas, the goal is a limb-sparing resection with negative surgical margins. Extremity well-differentiated liposarcomas (commonly called *atypical lipomatous tumors*) have a low

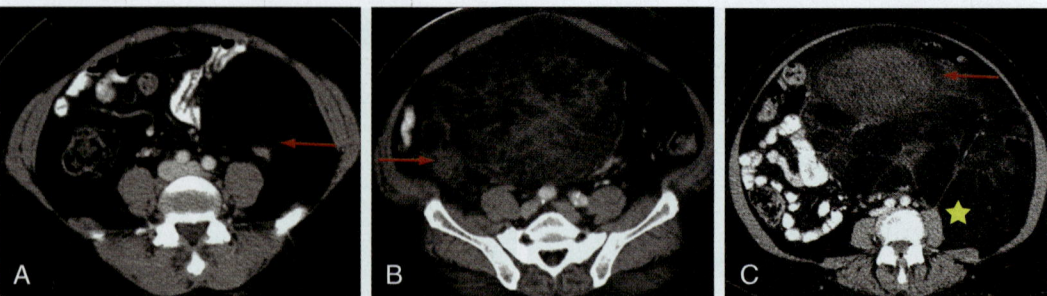

FIGURE 64.6 Variability in computed tomography appearance of retroperitoneal liposarcoma. (A) Simple, predominantly fatty, well-differentiated tumor; the *arrow* marks the inferior mesenteric vein. Thin septa are appreciable within the tumor. (B) A hypercellular well-differentiated tumor with a focal nodular or water density area *(arrow)*. (C) This tumor contains well-differentiated areas *(star)* as well as dedifferentiated elements *(arrow)*.

risk of distant metastasis and a favorable overall survival, and a more limited resection is warranted. The risk of local recurrence can be reduced with perioperative, preferably neoadjuvant, radiation therapy.

The treatment of patients presenting with retroperitoneal liposarcomas is more complex. The principal goal is a gross complete resection; incomplete resections with residual disease are associated with an increased risk of mortality.[45] Traditionally, retroperitoneal sarcomas are resected with a generous gross margin and the resection of organs and structures that are contiguous with or invading the tumor when feasible. More recently, some have advocated for a complete compartmental resection, which is defined as the resection of any and all adjacent organs, even if they are not directly involved with the tumor.[46] The complete compartmental resection approach results in frequent multivisceral resections, with the following organs resected in more than 50% of cases: spleen, pancreas, diaphragm, adrenal gland, and kidney.[46] However, when there is an unavoidably close margin on one side of the tumor, the resection of contiguous but uninvolved organs in another area to get negative margins may not be necessary. Proponents of a more conservative approach in which only tumor-contiguous organs are removed point out that 15% of patients who have recurrence after undergoing standard resection do so beyond the compartmental bounds of their initial tumor.[47] These out-of-field recurrences are unlikely to have been prevented with an aggressive complete compartmental resection strategy, and patients who may eventually benefit from nephrotoxic systemic chemotherapy are adversely affected by a potentially unnecessary complete compartmental resection–related nephrectomy. Understanding the patterns of recurrence is essential in surgical planning and determining the extent of resection. Although grossly incomplete resections should be avoided, a margin-negative resection is not possible in many situations.

The decision to resect recurrent retroperitoneal liposarcoma is based on the rate of recurrent tumor growth. Patients whose recurrence demonstrates growth of less than 0.9 cm/mo benefit from complete resection of the recurrence, whereas recurrent tumor growth of more than 0.9 cm/mo is associated with poor outcome.[48] Palliative chemotherapy is also an option for patients presenting with unresectable recurrence. A subgroup analysis of a randomized phase III trial comparing eribulin versus dacarbazine for either extremity or retroperitoneal liposarcoma showed that eribulin was associated with an improvement in overall survival (15.6 vs. 8.4 months). Based on these data, single-agent eribulin is now approved in the palliative setting for patients with liposarcoma.

Malignant Peripheral Nerve Sheath Tumors

MPNSTs are malignant tumors of neural origin. These tumors occur in roughly equal frequency sporadically or as a manifestation of neurofibromatosis, which results from an inherited mutation in *NF1*. There is no consensus in the literature as to whether MPNST in the setting of NF1 carries a worse prognosis than spontaneous cases. Although MPNSTs arise from a peripheral nerve or the nerve sheath, they are often painless on presentation. The most common age at presentation is 20 to 50 years. Historically, other names have been applied to MPNST, such as *malignant schwannoma, neurogenic sarcoma,* and *neurofibrosarcoma.* The term *malignant schwannoma* is avoided because not all MPNSTs actually arise from Schwann cells. Atypical neurofibromas are a rare precursor to MPNST and should be excised. MPNSTs are generally aggressive tumors, with a local recurrence rate of about 20% and a 10-year disease-specific survival of more than 40%. Tumor size is a key prognostic factor. Treatment of these tumors is similar to that of other STS subtypes, with a focus on margin-negative resection. Although it has not been studied prospectively in the MPNST population, most retrospective reports agree that (neo)adjuvant radiation therapy is indicated to decrease the rate of local recurrence, but it does not improve survival. Similarly, studies have reported mixed results from neoadjuvant and adjuvant chemotherapy with ifosfamide and an anthracycline. Several recent clinical trials of targeted therapies have failed to show a benefit, and complete surgical resection remains the only effective therapy.

Desmoid Tumor

Desmoid tumors, also known as *desmoid fibromatosis* or *aggressive fibromatosis,* are an uncommon group of fibroblastic tumors. Approximately 75% to 85% of cases arise sporadically; the remainder are related to Gardner syndrome, a variant of FAP. Among the sporadic cases, recent pregnancy and antecedent trauma (including surgery) are recognized risk factors. These tumors are two to three times more common in females than in males, and peak incidence occurs between the ages of 30 and 40 years. Approximately 20% of FAP patients develop desmoid tumors, and a common presentation involves a desmoid in the surgical incision/abdominal wall or the small bowel mesentery. Desmoid tumors are usually preceded by colonic polyposis in FAP patients and represent the second leading cause of death in FAP patients. A detailed family history should be obtained from patients presenting with desmoid tumors to rule out unappreciated FAP, and screening colonoscopy should be considered.

The molecular underpinnings of desmoids are related to the Wingless and Int-1 (WNT) signaling pathway. In sporadic cases, *CTNNB1* mutations result in the expression of a stabilized form of β-catenin, which ultimately accumulates and is transported to the nucleus, where it exerts its proliferative effects through activation of transcription factors. In the setting of FAP, β-catenin stabilization is caused by *APC* mutations. Specific *APC* codon mutations appear to confer a higher desmoid risk than other codon mutations. Desmoid tumors have also been found to highly express NOTCH1 and HES1.

Clinically, the most common areas of origin include the extremity, peritoneal cavity, abdominal wall, and chest wall. Presentation is varied based on the tumor location: Patients may present with a painful or asymptomatic firm mass, bowel obstruction, or bowel ischemia. Desmoid tumors are usually slow-growing but, on occasion, do grow aggressively. Distant metastases are extremely rare. On radiographic evaluation, these tumors are generally homogeneous and solid in appearance and may have a distinct or an infiltrating boundary. Cross-sectional imaging with CT scan or MRI is useful but not diagnostic, and tissue sampling with core-needle biopsy is indicated to rule out other STS subtypes.

Treatment of these tumors can be challenging and has evolved in recent years. Resection with widely negative margins was once the standard of care but is no longer the primary treatment modality. Local recurrence after surgery is common and is associated with larger tumor size, extraabdominal location, and older age. In addition, spontaneous regression is known to occur in 20% to 30% of cases. Consequently, treatment has shifted away from surgery to an initial active surveillance approach, preferably at a center experienced in management of desmoid tumors, with treatment (medical, preferably) reserved for progressive or symptomatic disease. Sorafenib, pazopanib, and cytotoxic chemotherapy are effective for patients with desmoid tumors that have failed active surveillance or require upfront treatment because of size or symptoms.[49]

Other local treatment options for desmoid tumors include radiation and cryotherapy. In retrospective studies, radiation therapy alone or in combination with surgical resection improves local control compared with surgery alone. Cryoablation has been shown to be effective in retrospective series for small or moderate-sized extraabdominal desmoid tumors. Systemic treatment options include hormonal therapy (e.g., tamoxifen), NSAIDs, tyrosine kinase inhibitors, and conventional cytotoxic chemotherapy regimens. Recent studies on targeted therapy have also shown promise. Nirogacestat is an oral medication that blocks the activity of gamma-secretase, which activates the NOTCH pathway. In an international phase III randomized trial, nirogacestat was associated with improvement in progression-free survival, symptom burden, function, and quality of life compared with placebo.

Angiosarcoma

Angiosarcoma is a malignant tumor that arises from the endothelial lining of blood vessels and therefore can arise from almost any site. Angiosarcomas are rare, accounting for 2% of all STS. Approximately 40% are radiation associated.[50] In decreasing order of frequency, the most common sites are the skin, breast, liver, and spleen. Angiosarcoma is typically diagnosed in the seventh and eighth decades. Although most angiosarcoma is sporadic, risk factors for secondary angiosarcoma include previous therapeutic radiation exposure and lymphedema (see previous section). Compared with primary angiosarcoma, secondary angiosarcoma has a higher frequency of cutaneous and regional lymph node involvement. Approximately 20% of patients present with metastasis, most frequently to the lung.[50] On histologic evaluation, these tumors range from well differentiated, mimicking hemangioma, to poorly differentiated. Consistent with this, there is a wide variety of cytogenetic changes. On immunohistochemical examination, CD31 and FLI-1 are the most consistent markers.

Resection with negative margins is the mainstay of treatment for both primary and secondary angiosarcomas. On microscopic examination, these tumors often infiltrate well beyond the area of gross involvement, and therefore, a wide margin is needed with at least 2 cm of normal tissue surrounding the tumor. For patients with head and neck angiosarcoma, this can present a reconstructive challenge. For those arising within the hair-bearing region of the scalp, locoregional recurrence rates are high, and systemic therapy with adjuvant radiation therapy may be a reasonable alternative. Radiation-associated angiosarcoma that arises within the breast after breast-conserving therapy is managed with mastectomy. Even after resection, the outcome is poor, with a 5-year disease-specific survival of 53%.[50] A more radical resection involving mastectomy with, importantly, all of the irradiated breast skin, compared with a more conservative simple mastectomy with only a wide excision of the involved skin, has been associated with a better 5-year crude cumulative incidence of local recurrence (23% vs. 76%) and distant metastasis (18% vs. 47%), respectively.[51] In that series, the 5-year disease-specific survival was 86% with more radical surgery compared with 46% with more conservative surgery. In the cohort with resectable disease, tumor size larger than 5 cm and histologic evidence of an epithelioid component are indicators of poor prognosis. These tumors are often locally advanced and unresectable at presentation. Fortunately, these tumors are responsive to chemotherapy and radiation therapy, and neoadjuvant treatment may facilitate complete surgical resection. Although local recurrence is common after surgery, the most common site of recurrent disease is new distant metastasis. Angiosarcoma metastasizes hematogenously. The lungs are the most common site of metastasis, which may manifest with hemopneumothorax. Breast angiosarcoma may metastasize to the liver. The median survival for stage IV angiosarcoma is 8 to 12 months. In the unresectable or metastatic setting, paclitaxel and doxorubicin are the most typical agents. Radiation therapy is also used for angiosarcomas that are not thought to be incited by prior radiation exposure. In recent trials, pazopanib was found to control disease progression in some patients, particularly for cutaneous angiosarcoma.[52]

Dermatofibrosarcoma Protuberans

DFSP is an uncommon STS that affects approximately 1 in 4.2 million patients in the United States. This tumor affects males and females equally and appears to be more common in Black patients than in Whites. The typical range of presentation is between the fourth and seventh decades. The trunk, upper extremity, and lower extremity are equally frequent sites of DFSP, followed by the head and neck. On physical examination, DFSP appears as a firm, indurated nodule with red or brown pigmentation. On histologic evaluation, DFSP is within the dermal or subdermal tissue layers and does not penetration into the epidermis.

Cytogenetically, the majority of DFSP cases will display the t(17;22)(q22;q13) translocation, which fuses the *COL1A1* and platelet-derived growth factor B genes and accounts for its overexpression of platelet-derived growth factor B. In difficult cases, this gene fusion can be detected by FISH hybridization. Because of its somewhat bland visual appearance and the lack of associated pain, DFSP can initially be mistaken for a hypertrophic scar or keloid. Large DFSPs can undergo fibrosarcomatous transformation and are treated similar to other STSs with wide resection with or without radiation therapy.

DFSPs recur almost exclusively locally. Consequently, the treatment is resection with wide margins. As is true with most STSs, there are no well-designed clinical trials to define an adequate margin, but 2- to 3-cm margins are generally accepted as sufficient. Local recurrence can be successfully treated with wide resection, but radiation can be considered for recurrent disease. DFSP rarely metastasizes, and the 5-year survival is >99%. In cases where metastasis occurs, it often implies degeneration to fibrosarcoma. Because of the upregulation of platelet-derived growth factor B, patients with unresectable disease may be treated with neoadjuvant imatinib.[53]

Undifferentiated Pleomorphic Sarcoma

Since 2013, tumors that once were classified as malignant fibrous histiocytoma are now referred to as *unclassified* or *undifferentiated pleomorphic sarcoma* (UPS). UPS accounts for 10% to 20% of STSs. White race, male sex, older age, and prior radiation exposure are associated with increased incidence. UPS is a diagnosis of exclusion, and therefore, careful histologic, immunohistochemical, and molecular analysis by a pathologist with STS expertise is crucial. The most common disease sites are the extremities and trunk. Treatment consists of surgical resection with 2-cm margins, and radiation improves local control. Unresectable disease is treated with anthracycline plus ifosfamide chemotherapy. Neoadjuvant anthracycline plus ifosfamide may also be considered for high-risk cases. Recent studies have shown that neoadjuvant treatment with immune checkpoint inhibitors may improve survival.[35,54,55]

Gastrointestinal Stromal Tumor

GIST is the most common variety of visceral STS. These tumors are believed to originate from the interstitial cells of Cajal within the gastrointestinal myenteric plexus, which are thought to function as pacemaker cells in the viscera, mediating contractions. They can emanate from any part of the alimentary tract but are most common in the stomach (40%–60%), jejunum or ileum bowel (24%–30%), and colon or rectum (5%–15%). Cajal cells and GISTs share common markers for CD117 and a calcium-activated chloride channel called *DOG1*. In morphologic appearance, GIST is classically a spindle cell neoplasm of smooth muscle origin and is distinguished from other smooth muscle STSs based on expression of CD34, CD117, and DOG1 and lack of smooth muscle staining. CD117, also known as the *KIT* gene, encodes a tyrosine kinase transmembrane receptor called *c-kit*. The c-kit receptor is a proto-oncogene that belongs to the PDGFR superfamily. The natural c-kit ligand is a stem cell factor, and its binding causes tyrosine kinase receptor homodimerization; autophosphorylation; and activation of multiple pathways, including RAS, RAF, MAPK, AKT, and STAT3. Certain mutations of the c-kit receptor confer constitutive activation of the receptor, which ultimately results in cellular proliferation. The *PDGFRα* gene, also found on chromosome 4, bears striking similarity to c-kit. Overall, approximately 70% of GISTs have *KIT* gene mutations, and 7% have *PDGFRα* mutations. GISTs with wild-type *KIT* and *PDGFRα* genotypes are characterized by a number of other mutations affecting *SDH, BRAF, KRAS,* and *NF1. SDH* mutations are related to GIST in patients affected by the Carney-Stratakis syndrome, and *NF1* mutations drive GIST formation in patients with NF1.

The clinical presentation of these tumors is variable, with some asymptomatic tumors being identified incidentally and others found for workup of symptoms, including pain, nausea, vomiting, or gastrointestinal bleeding resulting from tumor ulceration through the mucosa. On endoscopic examination, GIST usually appears as a smooth submucosal tumor that extrinsically impinges on the visceral lumen as opposed to an ulcerated mucosal mass. Some GISTs are pedunculated on the serosal layer and do not contribute to intestinal obstruction. CT imaging demonstrates that these tumors are well encapsulated and generally have heterogeneous contrast enhancement because of regions of necrosis within the tumor. Metastasis is most commonly to the liver, omentum, and peritoneal surface. Because these are submucosal tumors, endoscopic forceps biopsies are often nondiagnostic. Tumors situated between the ligament of Treitz and the ileocecal valve can be localized by double-balloon enteroscopy or capsule endoscopy. An endoscopic ultrasound-guided needle biopsy generally shows a spindle cell neoplasm; if sufficient tissue is available, this can be submitted for CD117 evaluation. Preoperative biopsy for suspected GIST is not mandatory if a surgery-first approach is taken but should be considered for larger tumors with multivisceral involvement where neoadjuvant imatinib is indicated. Appropriate preoperative staging for GIST includes a contrast-enhanced CT scan of the chest, abdomen, and pelvis. Small gastric GIST (<2 cm) with low mitotic count have low risk of progression and can be managed with active surveillance with serial endoscopy or imaging until they grow or become symptomatic. Localized lesions are treated with resection with grossly negative surgical margins. Obtaining wide surgical margins has not been demonstrated to improve local recurrence rates or overall survival. Given the rarity of lymph node involvement, lymphadenectomy is not mandatory for GIST. Care should be taken not to compromise the capsule of the tumor because rupture can lead to tumor seeding. As long as the risk of tumor rupture is not elevated, consideration of minimally invasive surgical resection techniques is appropriate.

The AJCC 8th edition staging system has a schema that separates GISTs based on anatomic site of origin: gastric and omental tumors versus nongastric tumors (Tables 64.4–64.6). The anatomic site of origin is important from both a surgical planning and a prognostic standpoint, with gastric GISTs having a better prognosis than jejunal/ileal tumors and colorectal GISTs having a worse prognosis. Several tools exist to predict prognosis after resection. The Memorial Sloan Kettering Cancer Center (MSKCC) group nomogram is validated to predict the probabilities of 2- and 5-year recurrence-free survival without adjuvant treatment after complete resection based on the size of the resected GIST, the mitotic rate, and the anatomic site of origin.[35] Another prognostic tool is the Armed Forces Institute of Pathology criteria, designed to predict the risk of progressive disease after resection without adjuvant therapy based on mitotic rate, size, and anatomic site of origin. The modified NIH criteria were established using several datasets, including the Armed Forces Institute of Pathology criteria, and have subsequently been validated (Table 64.7).[56,57]

These prognostic scores can be used to assess the need for adjuvant therapy; however, they do not account for the GIST molecular phenotype, which affects both long-term prognosis and response to therapy. In general, the presence of a *KIT* mutation is

TABLE 64.4 American Joint Committee on Cancer Staging for Gastrointestinal Stromal Tumor

Primary Tumor (T)

TX	Primary tumor cannot be assessed
T0	No evidence of primary tumor
T1	Tumor 2 cm or less
T2	Tumor >2 cm, ≤5 cm
T3	Tumor >5 cm, ≤10 cm
T4	Tumor >10 cm

Regional Lymph Nodes (N)

N0	No regional lymph node metastasis
N1	Regional lymph node metastasis

Distant Metastasis (M)

M0	No distant metastasis
M1	Distant metastasis

Histologic Grade (G)

GX	Grade cannot be assessed
G1	Low grade; mitotic rate ≤5 per 5 mm^2
G2	High grade; mitotic rate >5 per 5 mm^2

From Amin MB, Edge SB, Greene FL, et al. *AJCC Cancer Staging Manual.* 8th ed. New York: Springer; 2017.

TABLE 64.5 Anatomic Stage and Prognostic Groups for Gastric and Omental Gastrointestinal Stromal Tumor

GROUP	T	N	M	GRADE
Stage IA	T1 or T2	N0	M0	Low
Stage IB	T3	N0	M0	Low
Stage II	T1	N0	M0	High
	T2	N0	M0	High
	T4	N0	M0	Low
Stage IIIA	T3	N0	M0	High
Stage IIIB	T4	N0	M0	High
Stage IV	Any T	N1	M0	Any rate
	Any T	Any N	M1	Any rate

From Amin MB, Edge SB, Greene FL, et al. *AJCC Cancer Staging Manual.* 8th ed. New York: Springer; 2017.

TABLE 64.6 Anatomic Stage and Prognostic Groups for Nongastric[a] Gastrointestinal Stromal Tumor

GROUP	T	N	M	GRADE
Stage IA	T1 or T2	N0	M0	Low
Stage II	T3	N0	M0	Low
Stage IIIA	T1	N0	M0	High
	T4	N0	M0	Low
Stage IIIB	T2	N0	M0	High
	T3	N0	M0	High
	T4	N0	M0	High
Stage IV	Any T	N1	M0	Any rate
	Any T	Any N	M1	Any rate

[a]Nongastric includes small bowel, colorectal, esophageal, mesentery, and peritoneal.
From Amin MB, Edge SB, Greene FL, et al. *AJCC Cancer Staging Manual.* 8th ed. New York: Springer; 2017.

TABLE 64.7 Assessing the Prognosis of Resected Gastrointestinal Stromal Tumor

		RISK OF TUMOR PROGRESSION WITHOUT ADJUVANT THERAPY	
TUMOR SIZE	MITOTIC RATE (mitoses/mm^2)	GASTRIC ORIGIN	SMALL BOWEL ORIGIN
≤2 cm	≤5	0%	0%
	>5	0%[a]	50%[a]
>2 cm, ≤5 cm	≤5	1.9%	4.3%
	>5	16%	73%
>5 cm, ≤10 cm	≤5	3.6%	24%
	>5	55%	85%
>10 cm	≤5	12%	52%
	>5	86%	90%

[a]These values are based on small sample sizes, which limits their clinical applicability.
Adapted from Miettinen M, Lasota J. Gastrointestinal stromal tumors: review on morphology, molecular pathology, prognosis, and differential diagnosis. *Arch Pathol Lab Med.* 2006;130:1466-1478.

highly associated with response to tyrosine kinase inhibitors. Again, because of the similarities to the c-kit and *PDGFRα*, some patients with wild-type *KIT* are sensitive to tyrosine kinase inhibition. Systemic therapy is indicated in the neoadjuvant setting for locally advanced or unresectable tumors, in the adjuvant setting for high-risk GIST, and for treatment of metastatic GIST. Imatinib, the best studied of these systemic agents, is an oral tyrosine kinase inhibitor of c-kit. Imatinib was demonstrated to be associated with a dramatic improvement in the median overall survival of metastatic GIST from 20 months to 57 months.[58] In the adjuvant setting after complete surgical resection, two randomized studies have demonstrated improved disease-free recurrence.[59,60] The ACOSOG Z9001 was a double-blind trial that randomized patients with a grossly negative GIST resection to receive imatinib versus placebo for 1 year. All tumors were larger than 3 cm and

were c-kit positive by immunohistochemistry. One year of adjuvant imatinib was associated with a statistically significant improvement in recurrence-free survival versus placebo (98% vs. 83%, respectively).[59] A subsequent Z9001 follow-up study demonstrated a persistent improvement in recurrence-free survival but did not demonstrate any improvement in overall survival.[61] In a separate trial, patients were randomized to 1 versus 3 years of adjuvant imatinib after resection of c-kit–positive GIST. This trial stipulated that patients must have high-risk disease per the NIH consensus criteria. The 3-year duration of therapy was associated with improvements in both recurrence-free and overall survival.

Joensuu and colleagues[62] published the first data describing the parameters associated with tumor recurrence after resection in patients already treated with adjuvant imatinib. Datasets from two of the aforementioned three randomized trials were used to construct and validate a risk stratification score. Two such scores were developed. The five-parameter score includes mitotic count, organ of origin, size, tumor rupture, and duration of imatinib therapy. The two-parameter score includes mitotic count and organ of origin. These data support a 3-year duration of imatinib therapy and indicate that nongastric site of disease and high mitotic count adversely affect recurrence-free survival. Because the previous risk assessment schemas were developed using patients who had never been treated with adjuvant imatinib, this stratification score may prove to be clinically relevant. The Postresection Evaluation of Recurrence-Free Survival for Gastrointestinal Stromal Tumors With 5 Years of Adjuvant Imatinib (PERSIST-5) phase II clinical trial showed that of the 46 patients who completed 5 years of adjuvant imatinib, no patient with sensitive mutations experienced tumor recurrence.[63]

The specific *KIT* exon in which the GIST mutation resides affects the molecular and clinical phenotype. For example, a *KIT* mutation in exon 13 resides within the tyrosine kinase domain and confers susceptibility to imatinib therapy. Conversely, exon 9 mutations, which are observed principally in small bowel or colon GIST, correspond to the extracellular domain of the c-kit receptor and are less sensitive to imatinib. Genetic analysis should be performed at the time of diagnosis to determine the precise mutation because this may alter treatment recommendations.[64] Avapritinib was associated with progression-free survival in patients with imatinib-resistant GIST, including the *PDGFRα* D842V mutation.[65] Other available tyrosine kinase inhibitors include sunitinib, regorafenib, and ripretinib. Patients with *SDH*-deficient GISTs are generally younger, have multiple gastric GISTs, and are resistant to tyrosine kinase inhibitors.

Leiomyosarcoma

Leiomyosarcoma is a malignant smooth muscle tumor that can originate from virtually any part of the body. The most common sites are the retroperitoneum and peritoneal cavity, namely, the uterus. About 25% arise from the trunk and extremities. Overall, after liposarcoma, leiomyosarcoma is the second most frequent STS subtype.[2] Peak incidence of leiomyosarcoma is in the sixth and seventh decades. Retroperitoneal and uterine leiomyosarcomas are more common in females, but there is a male predominance in other leiomyosarcoma sites. Predisposing risk factors include prior radiation exposure and immunosuppression with Epstein-Barr virus–related tumor promotion. Leiomyoma, a common benign soft tissue tumor, is not a precursor to leiomyosarcoma.

Histologically, leiomyosarcomas are generally heterogeneous, well-circumscribed tumors with a cystic or necrotic central area. These tumors stain positive for desmin and smooth muscle actin. There are a wide variety of cytogenetic aberrations seen in these tumors, but no reliable or pathognomonic markers.

A macroscopically complete resection is the mainstay of treatment for leiomyosarcoma. Depending on the size and location of the tumor (especially retroperitoneal), neoadjuvant chemotherapy may be a consideration. For uterine leiomyosarcoma, a total abdominal hysterectomy with bilateral oophorectomy is indicated. Retroperitoneal tumors that invade or are intimately associated with the inferior vena cava (IVC) require special planning. The intraoperative options include tumor resection with ligation of the IVC or reconstruction with a patch or interposition graft. Tumors involving the IVC typically have a great deal of collateralization already in place. For tumors requiring segmental resection of the infrahepatic IVC, if the collaterals can be preserved, ligation without reconstruction may be an acceptable maneuver because postoperative lower extremity edema is well tolerated.

Regardless of the organ of origin, adjuvant therapy is not currently recommended, although this is the subject of ongoing trials, including the EORTC STRASS-2 study. Metastasis occurs via hematogenous spread, mainly to the lung and liver. Despite promising findings from a phase II trial, olaratumab, a recombinant human monoclonal antibody that binds PDGFRα, in combination with doxorubicin was not found to improve overall survival for patients with unresectable or metastatic STS over doxorubicin alone, resulting in its withdrawal from the market.[66] Systemic treatment for advanced leiomyosarcoma includes regimens with doxorubicin, ifosfamide, docetaxel, and gemcitabine.

BONE SARCOMA: EPIDEMIOLOGY CORE CONCEPTS

Bone Microenvironment

An understanding of the bone microenvironment affects the macroscopic management of skeletal tumors. In the absence of tumor, bone is a dynamic and symbiotic organ, actively maintained by cells that respond to stimuli such as injury, stress, or metabolic need. Osteoblasts represent a terminal differentiation of a mesenchymal stem cell. They generate a collagen matrix, which is then mineralized. When osteoblasts become surrounded by the matrix they create, they are deemed *osteocytes*, and they serve to maintain the bony environment. Osteoclasts are multinucleated cells derived from a hematopoietic lineage (macrophages), which resorb bone. The constant interplay of those cells (osteoblast, osteocyte, osteoclast) is necessary to maintain bone health. The marrow space is also home to other significant cell populations, such as mesenchymal stem cells. The active and ongoing homeostasis of bone and its intramedullary inhabitants generate a microenvironment rich in growth factors and signaling molecules, making it an ideal soil for osteophilic tumors.

In the setting of bone metastases, intravascular tumor cells are attracted to the microenvironment of bone because it is both preconditioned for tumor cell arrival by circulating factors and because it is inherently attractive as a result of the proteins, signaling molecules, and cells that it contains (Fig. 64.7). That concept was first coined the "seed and soil" theory by Dr. Stephen Paget in 1889.[67] For example, mesenchymal stem cells return (in part) to the bone marrow as a result of a signaling pathway involving the CXCL12 chemokine and the CXCR4 receptor. Intramedullary mesenchymal stem cells secrete CXCL12, and circulating stem cells that express the correlating CXCR4 receptor are recruited to the marrow space. Similarly, in the setting of metastatic breast cancer as an example, tumor cells express CXCR4 receptor and therefore can also be recruited to the marrow space via the chemokine CXCL12.[68] In general, cell-signaling molecules produced in the marrow space are recognized by tumor-based receptors and represent one example of how the bone microenvironment influences tumor deposition. Other players involved in homing of tumor cells to bone include, but are not limited to, exosomes/oncosomes, adhesion molecules, platelets, and circulating stem cells.[69]

Once in the bone microenvironment, in what is deemed the "vicious cycle," tumor cells hijack the endogenous cells of bone to create an environment that fosters their own growth. Normally, the balance of lysis and bone formation in bone is maintained through the strategic production of signaling proteins. For example, receptor activator of nuclear factor-κB ligand (RANKL) is generated by osteoblasts and recognized by its osteoclast receptor (RANK). When bound, RANKL stimulates osteoclastogenesis.[70] Osteoprotegerin is a decoy receptor secreted by osteoblasts, which inhibits RANKL binding and therefore inhibits osteoclastogenesis.[71] Tumor cells can disturb

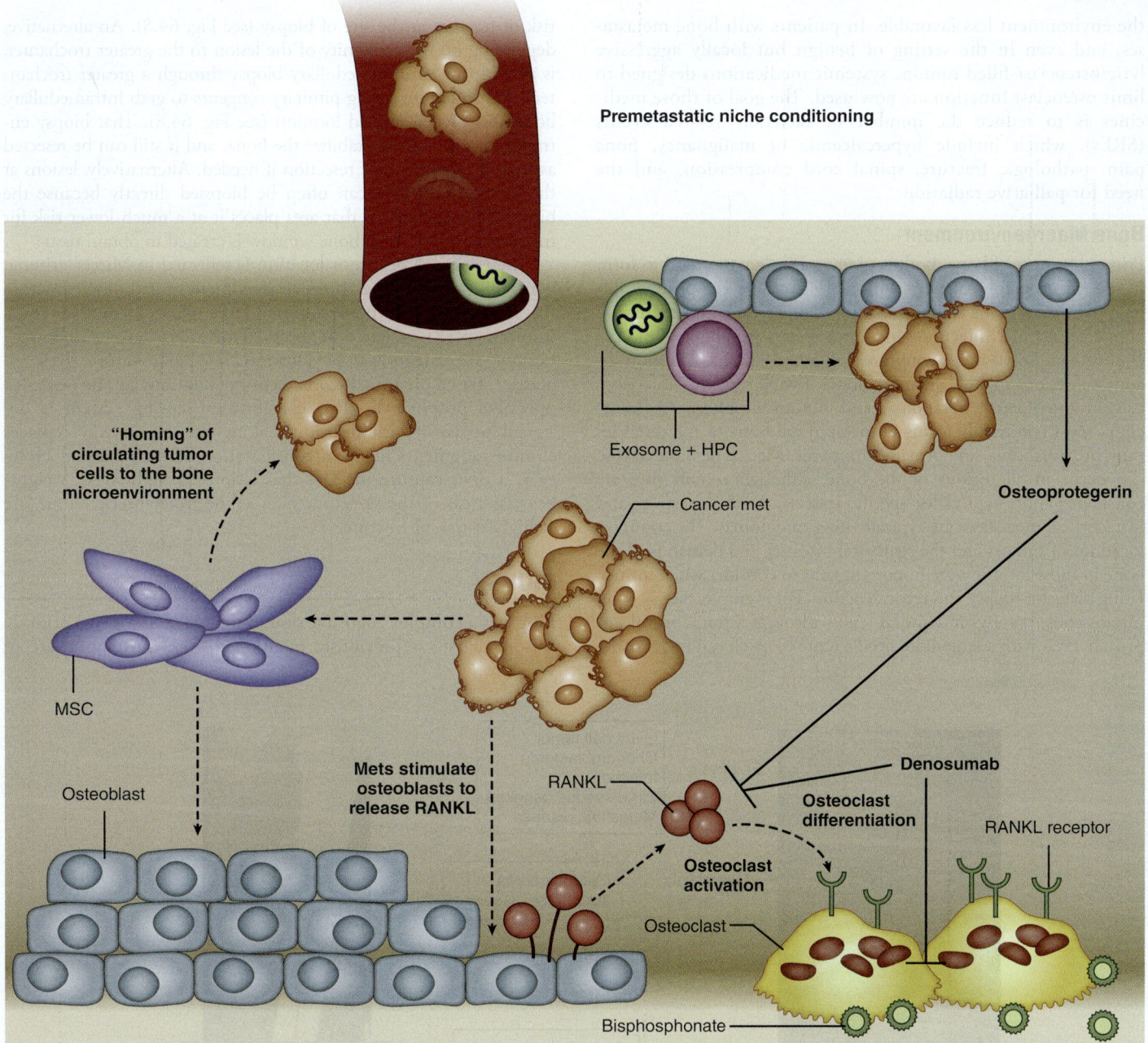

FIGURE 64.7 Circulating metastatic cancer cells find the bone microenvironment through a complex series of steps. Before their arrival, circulating factors optimize the bone (premetastatic niche conditioning). Cells are then recruited to the bone by signaling molecules called *chemokines* (homing). Once in the bone, tumor cells hijack normal bone metabolism (the vicious cycle). Medical therapies used in the treatment of metastatic bone cancers exploit the understanding of the vicious cycle. Denosumab is a human monoclonal antibody that binds the receptor activator of nuclear factor-κB ligand *(RANKL)* and directly inhibits osteoclastogenesis. Zoledronic acid is a bisphosphonate that is taken up by and then inhibits activated osteoclasts. *HPC,* Hematopoietic progenitor cell; *MSC,* mesenchymal stem cell. (Adapted from Cook LM, Shay G, Araujo A, et al. Integrating new discoveries into the "vicious cycle" paradigm of prostate to bone metastases. *Cancer Metastasis Rev.* 2014;33:511-525.)

bone homeostasis in a variety of ways. Tumor cells can directly stimulate osteoblasts to generate RANKL, which is the most prominent cytokine inducer of osteoclastogenesis.[72,73] Alternatively, tumor-secreted matrix metalloproteinase-7 can cleave extracellular matrix where bound and inactive RANKL resides, thereby releasing the active form of RANKL.[74] Once overactive osteoclastogenesis is initiated, tumor growth is fueled by this aggressive bone degradation, which frees an abundance of growth factors that can drive tumor proliferation.

This chapter is not intended to cover all aspects of the microenvironment tumor–native bone interplay. However, an appreciation of those complex relationships is important. Medical therapies can target not only tumor cells (the seed) but also the soil—essentially preventing tumor growth by making the environment less favorable. In patients with bone metastases, and even in the setting of benign but locally aggressive lytic/osteoclast-filled tumors, systemic medications designed to limit osteoclast function are now used. The goal of those medicines is to reduce the number of skeletally related events (SREs), which include hypercalcemia of malignancy, bone pain, pathologic fracture, spinal cord compression, and the need for palliative radiation.

Bone Macroenvironment

Primary tumors of bone, both benign and malignant, tend to form in specific geographic regions of bone (Fig. 64.8). The primary differential diagnosis of epiphyseal tumors includes giant cell tumor, chondroblastoma, infection, and intraosseous ganglion. Clear cell chondrosarcoma is a less common epiphyseal lesion. Common diaphyseal lesions include adamantinoma, Ewing sarcoma, infection, osteoid osteoma/osteoblastoma, and fibrous dysplasia. Osteosarcoma most commonly forms in metaphyseal bone of the distal femur, proximal tibia, and proximal humerus. Metastatic bone disease can occur in all regions of the bone, although certain sites are considered more typical for specific cancers. Acral metastases and intracortical metastases are typically lung carcinomas. The common locations of tumors and the structural integrity and demands of the bone in those locations are important facts to consider when formulating plans for biopsy and reconstruction. For example, biopsy of an intraosseous, diaphyseal femoral lesion through a transcortical approach, even with a large-bore needle (core biopsy), can increase the

risk of fracture at the site of biopsy (see Fig. 64.8). An alternative, depending on the proximity of the lesion to the greater trochanter, is to perform an intramedullary biopsy through a greater trochanteric starting point, using pituitary rongeurs to grab intramedullary bone at a predetermined location (see Fig. 64.8). That biopsy entrance site does not destabilize the bone, and it still can be resected as part of a wide tumor resection if needed. Alternatively, lesions at the metaphyseal flare can often be biopsied directly because the biomechanical stress in that area places it at a much lower risk for fracture, even if a small bone window is created to obtain tissue.

The relevance of tumor location is reflected in Mirels' criteria, which allow for a more objective assessment of pathologic fracture risk in patients with bone tumors (Table 64.8). In that system, a numeric score is assigned to observed metastatic lesions in bone.[75] Lesions are categorized by location, size, and nature (lytic vs. blastic). Based on a total score, recommendations can be made for operative prophylaxis. This classification/scoring system is designed to assist with decision-making but in no way replaces clinical judgments made in consideration of each patient. However, it does capture the fact that lesions in high-stress, weight-bearing areas of the skeleton, such as the trochanteric femur, are at highest risk of fracture.

BIOPSY

Biopsy is a complex cognitive skill in the skeleton for two primary reasons. First, as previously mentioned, one must be aware of

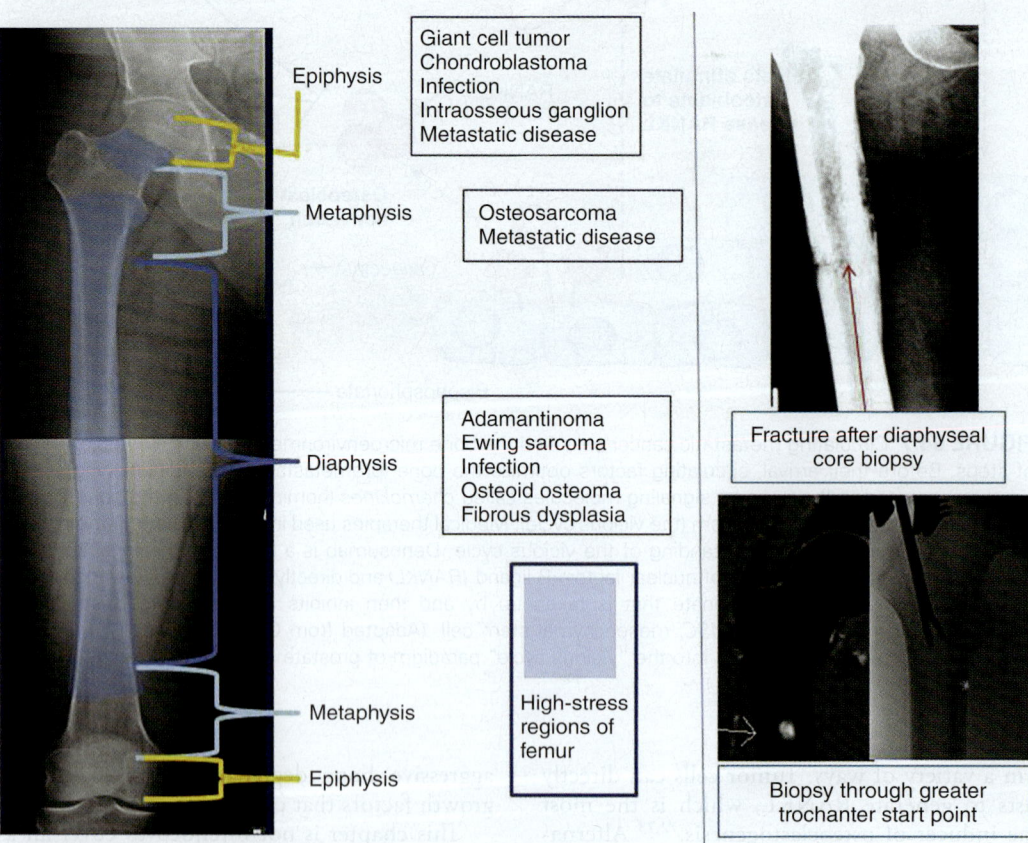

FIGURE 64.8 The location of tumors helps to narrow the differential diagnosis. Biopsy in certain locations can increase the risk of fracture in long bones. Pictured is an example of a fracture created in the diaphyseal femur after a core-needle biopsy. Biopsy through the greater trochanter, an intramedullary nail starting point, is a biomechanically safer option.

TABLE 64.8 Mirels Scoring System

SCORE	SITE OF LESION	SIZE OF LESION	LESION TYPE	PAIN
1	Upper limb	$> \frac{1}{3}$ cortex	Blastic	Mild
2	Lower limb	$\frac{1}{3} - \frac{2}{3}$ cortex	Mixed	Moderate
3	Trochanteric	$> \frac{2}{3}$ cortex	Lytic	Functional

The Mirels scoring system allows assessment of fracture risk. There are four factors (site, size, lesion type, pain) that are assigned a numeric score of 1 to 3. The four scores are added together. If the overall score is more than 9, prophylactic fixation is indicated. A score of less than 7 can often be treated with radiation and medical therapies. Despite the utility of the scoring system, clinical judgment must always be taken into consideration regarding a specific patient.[75]

what approaches might further destabilize the bone in question. Second, one must place the biopsy tract in a location that accommodates future wide resection. Specifically, if a diagnosis of primary malignancy is rendered, a wide resection must include the biopsy tract, which harbors malignant cells. If a significant hematoma forms after bone biopsy, then larger resection may be needed to obtain adequate margins (Fig. 64.9).

There are different modalities of bone biopsy. Fine-needle aspirate is rarely used unless there is a significant extraosseous soft tissue component that is accessible or significant bony lysis. Core biopsy, often performed with CT scan guidance, can be performed through intact cortices (with adjunct use of a combined biopsy/drill system) or through areas of soft tissue extension. Incisional biopsy is a surgical procedure during which a carefully planned small incision is made in line with the tumor, with respect to neurovascular structures and bone biomechanics. Open biopsy allows for acquisition of the most tissue as compared with other techniques. If the cortex is intact, a high-speed burr is often used to create a less-than-dime-sized window into the bone. Meticulous hemostasis must be obtained to prevent contamination of surrounding tissues. Often, Surgicel and Gelfoam are packed into defects created in the soft tissue extraosseous component of the tumor, and then the tumor capsule and superficial layers are closed meticulously. If the cortex has been violated, bone wax or a small plug of bone cement is often used to prevent intramedullary extravasation of blood and tumor into the biopsy tract.

Inappropriately placed biopsy tracts can change the nature of the surgery required—even changing a potential limb-salvage candidate into a patient requiring an amputation. Biopsy placement and execution are critical. It has been conclusively shown in several studies that surgeons inexperienced in musculoskeletal oncology principles have a three to four times increased rate of complication from a poorly placed biopsy site.[76-78]

The biopsy result is the most important factor driving a patient's care. The tissue obtained allows one to render a diagnosis and build a treatment pathway. As such, when a biopsy is performed, it is critical that the surgeon has a basic understanding of how to make a correct diagnosis. Surgical pathology tissue review includes histologic evaluation and immunohistochemistry. The challenge in sarcoma care has previously been interobserver reliability with regard to diagnosis. The molecular pathology of bone tumors—identification of genetic signatures that correlate to skeletal neoplasia—allows for consistency in diagnoses and is

emerging as a powerful tool in the care of bone tumor patients. Table 64.9 documents the pathognomonic mutations associated with various bone tumors.[79]

STAGING

A critical part of biopsy planning includes a global understanding of the nature of a tumor—whether it is localized or part of a more systemic process. Patient history and physical examination are vital parts of evaluation. Physical examination must include chaperoned breast examination or prostate examination in patients who potentially may have a process that is metastatic to bone. A series of radiologic studies is then performed to characterize the scope of the disease process. When a patient presents with an isolated bone lesion that may represent a malignancy, especially without antecedent history of cancer, the following studies or labs are typically obtained:

- MRI of the entire affected bone with contrast—identifies a soft tissue component of the tumor that, if present, may be easier to sample and also helps to identify skip metastases.
- CT scan of the chest, abdomen, and pelvis with and without IV and oral contrast—screens for common osteophilic carcinomas, including breast, lung, renal, thyroid, and prostate, and also helps to establish whether solid organ metastases are present.
- CT with two-dimensional reconstructions of the affected bone—allows a better three-dimensional understanding of how the tumor has affected the bone.
- Whole body bone scan—identifies other possible osseous sites/metastases.
- Plain radiographs of the affected bone—show where in the bone the tumor is located (epiphyseal, metaphyseal, diaphyseal), show what the tumor is doing to the bone (lytic, blastic), show what the bone is doing to the tumor (containment vs. failure to contain), and show the matrix of the lesion (bone, cartilage, fibrous, etc.).
- Laboratory evaluation to include prostate-specific antigen, serum electrophoresis, calcium to rule out hypercalcemia of malignancy, lactate dehydrogenase, alkaline phosphatase, complete blood count with differential, comprehensive metabolic panel, sedimentation rate, and C-reactive protein.

There are two primary staging systems used to describe skeletal sarcoma. In the Musculoskeletal Tumor Society Staging System, or Enneking system,[80] stage I refers to a low-grade skeletal sarcoma, stage II refers to a high-grade skeletal sarcoma, and stage III represents metastatic disease, either regional or distant. The letter A refers to intracompartmental tumor localization, whereas the letter B refers to extracompartmental extension. An example of extracompartmental extension would include an osteosarcoma with extraosseous soft tissue mass or a pathologic fracture through an osteosarcoma, resulting in hematoma contamination. The AJCC staging system has been updated.[81] Tumors are described by grade (I, low; II, high; III, tumor of any grade with skip metastasis; IV, tumor of any grade with distant metastasis) and size (<8 cm, A; >8 cm, B). Staging systems, in general, are designed to reflect prognosis and therefore guide treatment algorithms.

Enneking also developed a staging system for benign bone tumors.[82] In the Enneking system, tumors are characterized as latent (1), active (2), or aggressive (3). Aggressive benign tumors often have a higher risk of local recurrence. Although aggressive benign tumors still can be technically resected in an intralesional fashion, resection must be meticulous, often using high-speed

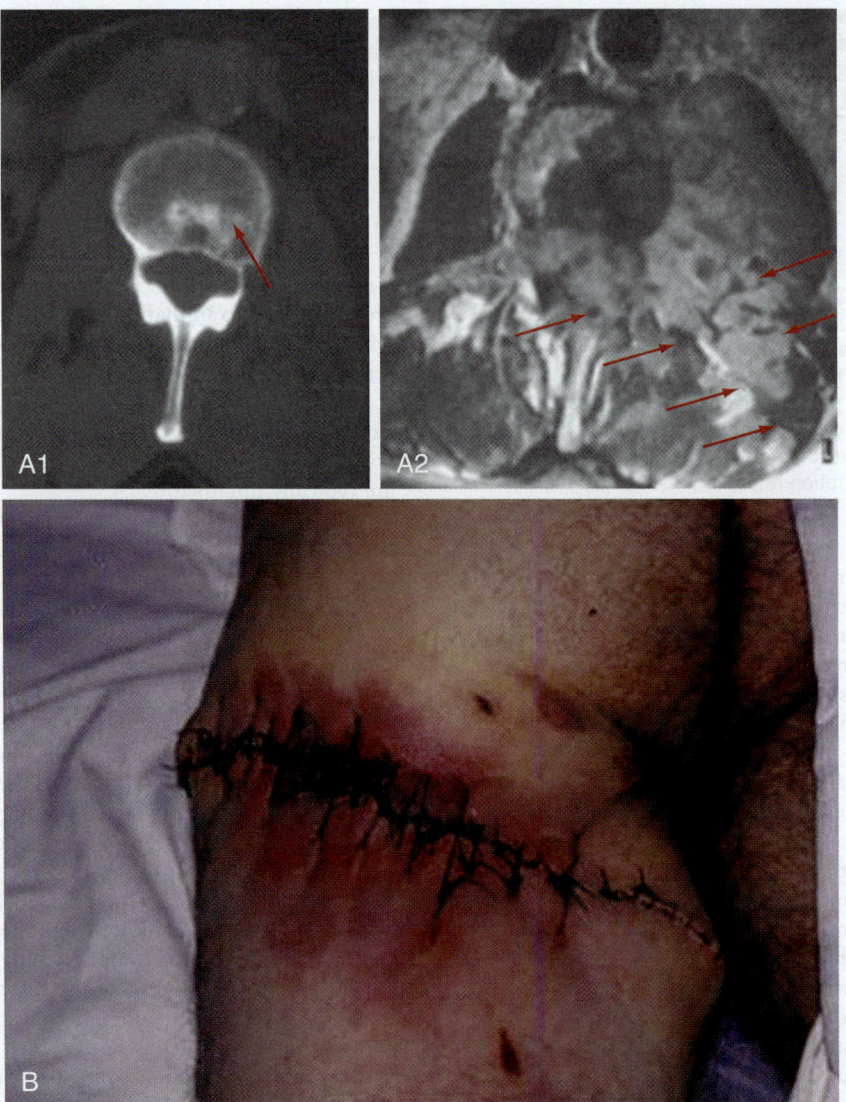

FIGURE 64.9 When planning a biopsy location, one must consider that the biopsy tract will be contaminated and, in the case of malignant tumors, will require resection. (A1) A computed tomography–guided biopsy tract into the vertebral body is demonstrated by the *arrow.* (A2) *Arrows* indicate the extent of biopsy tract recurrence. (B) An excellent example of an inappropriate biopsy, which mandated an otherwise unnecessary amputation in the patient. Biopsies must be performed in line with the incision that will eventually be required to resect a tumor. The entire biopsy tract must be resected. Therefore, a biopsy incision is typically small and strategically placed.

burrs and other adjuvants. The most important factor in preventing recurrence is likely to be adequacy of resection.[83]

ONCOLOGIC RESECTION

There are four types of resection: (1) intralesional, (2) marginal, (3) wide, and (4) radical. The type of margin reflects the surgical dissection plane relative to the tumor or capsule of the tumor. Intralesional resections involve an incision made into the substance of tumor. Intralesional resections in bone are typically exemplified by curettage or debulking. They are used in the setting of benign bone tumors and tumors that are metastatic to bone. Marginal resections theoretically involve resection of the tumor around its capsule and, by definition, leave microscopic disease behind. Wide resections involve resection of the tumor with a surrounding rim of normal tissue, designed to remove the entirety

of a tumor with a margin of normal tissue. Radical resections include not only the tumor and a rim of normal tissue but also the entirety of the compartment in which the tumor resides. Wide resections are more commonly used in the treatment of skeletal sarcomas, as opposed to radical resections.

SKELETAL RECONSTRUCTION

The type of reconstruction needed often depends on the type of resection that is indicated. It also depends greatly on the reparative potential of the bone. For example, children can regenerate bone at a higher rate than adults, and therefore, in the setting of benign tumors such as aneurysmal bone cyst, bone graft might be used in a child, whereas in an adult bone, cement might be used. Another important factor is the posttreatment impact of a tumor on bone. For example, a lytic lesion caused by multiple myeloma

TABLE 64.9 Skeletal Neoplasia DNA Alterations

TUMOR	SUPPRESSOR GENE	ONCOGENE	TRANSLOCATIONS	CHROMOSOME LOSS	CHROMOSOME GAIN	PROTEIN CHANGE
Osteosarcoma	RB, p53 INK4A, INK2A	CDK4, FOS, cMYC MDM2, MET		6q, 13q, 15q, 17p, 18q	1q, 5p, 6p, 7q, 8q, 12q, 17p, 19q	
Ewing sarcoma	KCMF1	CD99	t(11;22)(q24;q12) EWS-FLI1 t(21;22)(q22;q12) EWS-ERG			
Chondrosarcoma		IDH1, IDH2		1p, 5q, 6p, 9p, 14q, 22q	7p, 12q, 21q	
Osteochondroma	EXT1, EXT2					
Enchondroma					12q	IHH-PTHrP
Aneurysmal bone cyst			t(16;17)(q22;p13) CDH11-USP6			
Fibrous dysplasia		GNAS1		20q		G$_S$
Giant cell tumor		TPX2 H3F3	Telomeric fusions	1q	20q	RANKL Histone

G_s, Mutation in alpha-subunit of the G_S stimulatory protein leading to activation and inappropriate cyclic adenosine monophosphate production (cAMP); *IHH-PTHrP*, Indian hedgehog-PTH-related protein; *RANKL*, receptor activator of nuclear factor-κB ligand.

has a better chance of healing after medical therapies than a lytic lesion caused by lung cancer. The potential for bone regeneration at the site of tumor relates in many ways to the stromal content of the tumor. Lymphoma of bone is predominantly cellular, whereas lung carcinoma in bone has a significant stromal component. The footprint of the tumor cannot be erased in stromal-heavy tumors.

Skeletal Stabilization Used in Intralesional Resections

Skeletal stabilization/reconstruction comes in many forms. Plates and screws that span defects can be used after curettage of lesions. Bone strength can be augmented through the insertion of polymethylmethacrylate (bone cement) into skeletal defects, along with plates and screws (rebar) (Fig. 64.10). Intramedullary nail fixation is a common strategy for prophylaxis of diaphyseal

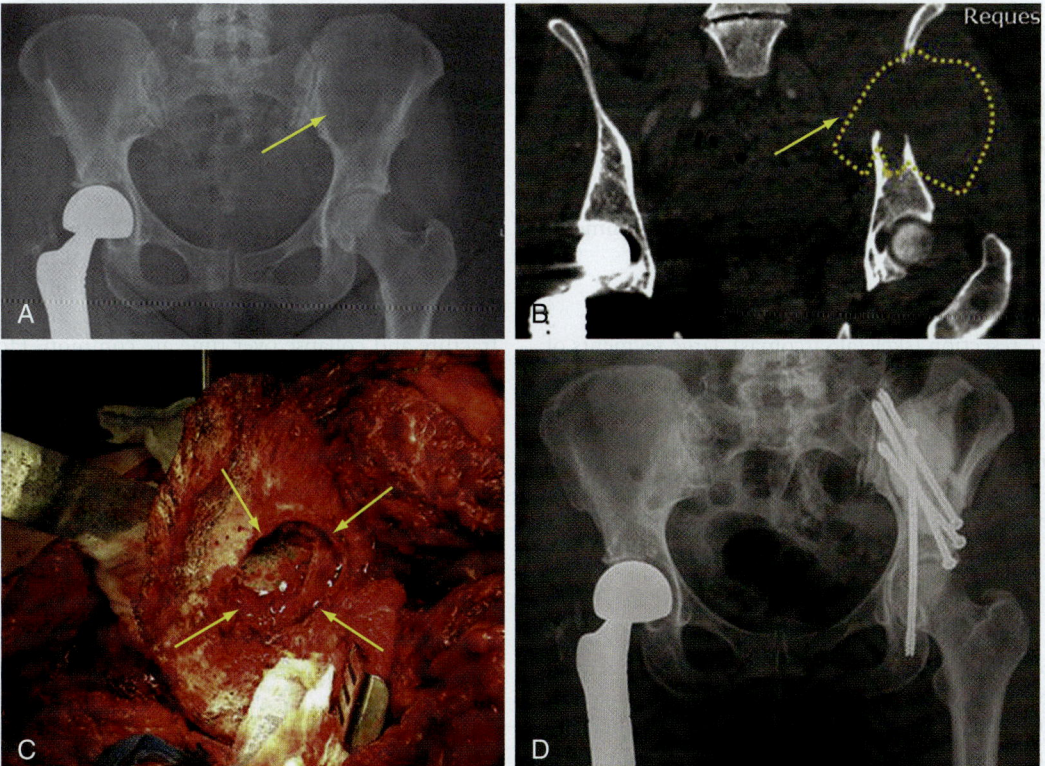

FIGURE 64.10 The patient had a prior right proximal femur metastatic lesion treated with proximal femur resection and megaprosthesis. She then developed a large, lytic, painful left iliac wing lesion, which required intralesional resection and reconstruction using cement and 7.3-mm cannulated screws. (A) Anteroposterior pelvis x-ray shows the lytic defect *(arrow)*. (B) Computed tomography scan two-dimensional coronal reconstruction view shows not only the bony defect but also the associated soft tissue mass *(arrow and dotted line)*. (C) Intraoperative view of the bony defect *(arrows)*. (D) Postoperative anteroposterior pelvis.

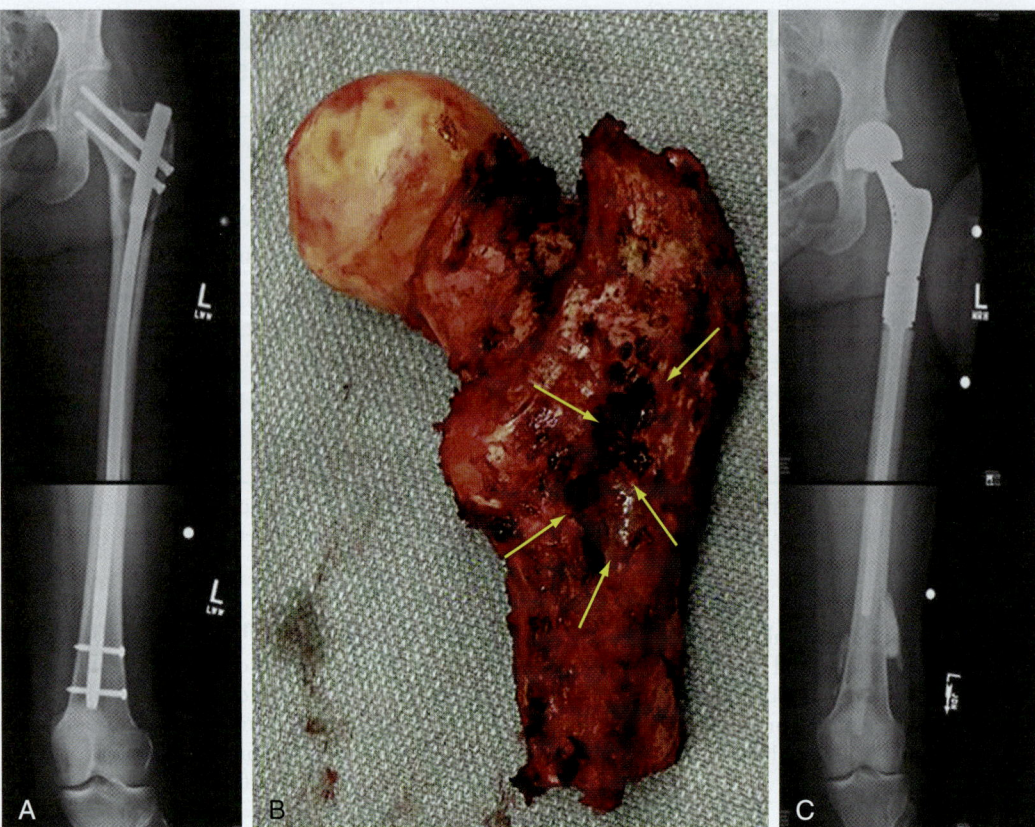

FIGURE 64.11 This patient had intramedullary nail stabilization and palliative radiation of the left femur for treatment of a peritrochanteric metastatic renal cell carcinoma lesion. (A) Despite appropriate attempt at stabilization and adjuvant therapies, she had persistent pain. A left proximal femoral resection and proximal femur megaprosthesis was performed. (B) Gross specimen revealed persistent lysis of the bone *(arrows)*. (C) A long-cemented stem proximal femur endoprosthesis was used for reconstruction.

lesions, especially in the femur (Fig. 64.11). In the setting of metastatic disease with palliation as a goal, the reconstruction strategy selected should impart immediate stability and immediate full weight-bearing potential whenever possible.

Skeletal Reconstruction Used in Wide Resections

In the case of wide resection (skeletal sarcomas), large segments of bone are resected (see Fig. 64.11B–C). In those cases, reconstruction often involves the use of intercalary allografts or metal components, osteoarticular allografts, allograft-prosthetic composites, arthroplasty using megaprosthesis, or arthrodesis. Autologous vascularized free tissue transfer, such as vascularized free fibulas, can also be an option. Amputation is also always an alternative in select cases.

Allograft

When a patient is identified who will require a large bulk allograft, templated x-rays of the bone needed (or the contralateral bone if there is too much deformity) are obtained. Approved tissue banks harvest materials with meticulous sterility and then can assess whether any in-stock cadaveric allografts match the bone being requested.[84] Allografts can be harvested with soft tissue attachments, and in that case, the host tendons can be sewn into the allograft attachment sites. Allografts can be fortified with cement augmentation, if possible, and then secured to the native bone using plates and screws (Fig. 64.12). Allografts are obviously non-viable scaffolds, and therefore, ultimate healing at the native

bone–allograft interface depends on the native bone use of the allograft as a scaffold through which new bridging bone is formed. Intercalary allografts are essentially bony placeholders and can often be secured in situ through the use of intramedullary stabilization. Osteoarticular allografts include implantation of a new joint surface. In weight-bearing joints, osteoarticular allograft fracture and collapse over time are common. However, especially in the growing child, they allow for delay of arthroplasty and generation of additional bone stock.

The means of reconstruction is often dictated by the weight-bearing demands of the bone in question. For example, an osteoarticular allograft is a good option for the proximal humerus—a technically non–weight-bearing limb. An allograft with soft tissue attachments allows the rotator cuff tendons to be sewn to the implant, thereby potentiating some overhead mobility. An osteoarticular allograft in the distal femur may be more problematic because of weight-bearing demands. Therefore, arthroplasty may be preferred.

Arthroplasty

Arthroplasty is a common reconstruction strategy used after tumor resections that include portions of a joint (Fig. 64.13). The so-called megaprosthesis is named such because large modular metal implants are combined to restore length to the limb and replace large bone defects. Those metal replacements are either potted into the bone using bone cement or press fit into the long bone canal. Bone cement offers immediate stability but an

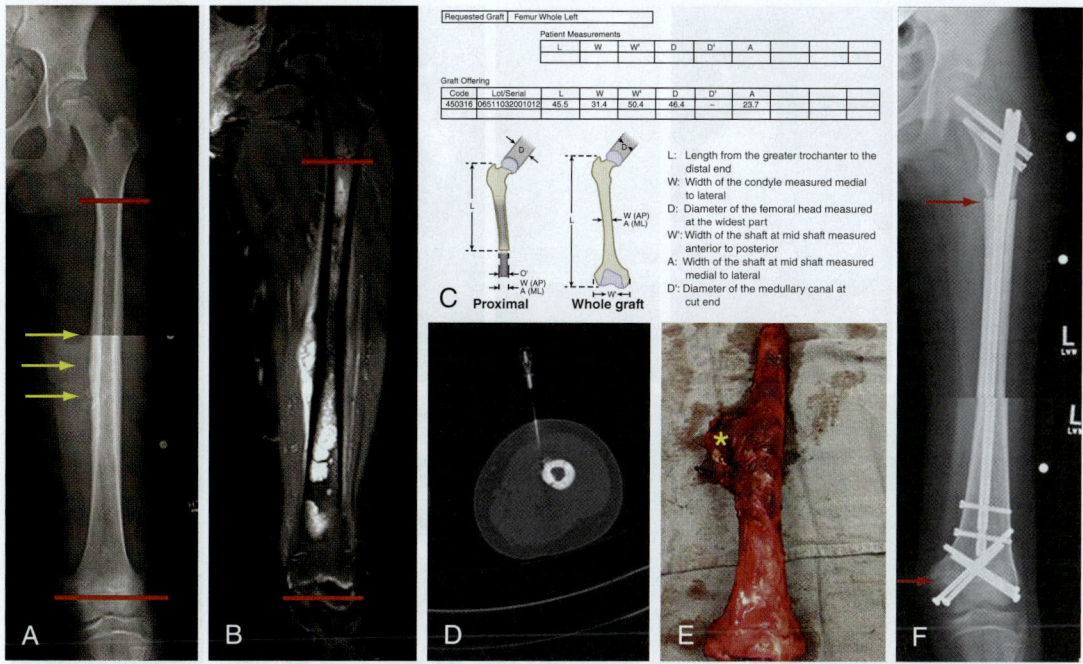

FIGURE 64.12 Allograft reconstruction can be used in osteoarticular, intercalary, or allograft-prosthetic composite reconstructions. An 11-year-old with an extensive left femoral diaphyseal osteosarcoma with multiple skip metastases. (A) Anteroposterior femur x-ray demonstrates periosteal reaction *(yellow arrows)*. Anticipated resection is denoted with *red lines*. (B) Magnetic resonance imaging (MRI) shows the extent of tumor, which does not extend distal to the physis. Proximal extent of tumor extends to the inferior aspect of the lesser trochanter. MRI allows planning of intercalary femoral resection. (C) Allograft matched. (D) Biopsy tract. (E) Resection performed with negative margins, and it includes the medial biopsy tract *(*)*. (F) Anteroposterior femur x-ray postresection. *Red arrows* indicate allograft–native bone interfaces.

increased chance of aseptic loosening over time.[85] Press-fit stems require ingrowth or ongrowth of host bone over time around the stem periphery. In the case of the proximal humerus and proximal femur, no additional resurfacing of the acetabulum or glenoid is typically done. For distal femur or proximal tibia tumors, the tumor-unaffected side of the joint requires resurfacing to accommodate a hinge mechanism.

Amputation

Amputation is indicated in the setting of primary tumors when an adequate margin cannot be obtained through the use of limb salvage or when the functional result achieved through limb salvage is worse than that achieved by amputation. Amputation may be indicated in the setting of metastatic or advanced cancers for the purposes of palliation.

SKELETAL SARCOMAS

The American Cancer Society estimates that 3970 new cases of primary bone cancers would be diagnosed in 2023.[86] In adults, 40% of primary bone cancers are chondrosarcomas, 28% are osteosarcomas, 10% are chordomas, 8% are Ewing sarcomas, and 4% are skeletal sarcomas of bone not otherwise specified. In children, osteosarcoma is the most common primary bone tumor (56%), followed by Ewing sarcoma (28%) and chondrosarcoma (6%). The incidence of skeletal sarcomas is approximately equal in the pediatric and adult populations.

The modern-day algorithm for treatment of bone sarcomas, which includes neoadjuvant chemotherapy, wide resection, and adjuvant chemotherapy, was a serendipitous discovery in

the 1970s.[87] During that time, intensive chemotherapy was administered to many teenagers with nonmetastatic osteosarcoma of the extremities after biopsy while they awaited fabrication of a custom endoprosthesis. After several months, the tumor was surgically removed, and the implant was inserted to preserve the limb. The resected bone was then examined histopathologically for evidence of chemotherapy effect. A survival benefit was noted in children who had received chemotherapy. That observation evolved into the modern-day treatment algorithm for skeletal sarcoma, which includes neoadjuvant chemotherapy, wide surgical resection, and subsequent adjuvant chemotherapy.

Wide margins of resection are mandated for skeletal sarcomas. The surgical goal is a local recurrence rate of less than 7%. Early studies by Simon et al.[88] and Link et al.[89] documented equivalent local recurrence and survival rates between limb salvage and amputation for distal femoral osteosarcoma. Cure rates are approximately 67% for extremity sarcomas, whereas axial tumors in the pelvis or spine have a worse prognosis (33%) for a similar tissue type.[90,91]

It has been demonstrated that limb salvage is more cost-effective over a period of decades than immediate amputation in the teenage population.[92] Implant survival is complicated in the short term by infection (allografts) and in the long term by aseptic loosening (metal).[93] Ten-year implant survival rates for metallic prostheses range from 50% to 80% in the proximal tibia, distal femur, and proximal femur, respectively.[94] Wound healing, especially while administering chemotherapy, is enhanced with healthy local flaps. Rotational flaps are often used around the knee to improve prosthetic coverage. For example, in proximal tibia resections, a medial gastrocnemius flap is

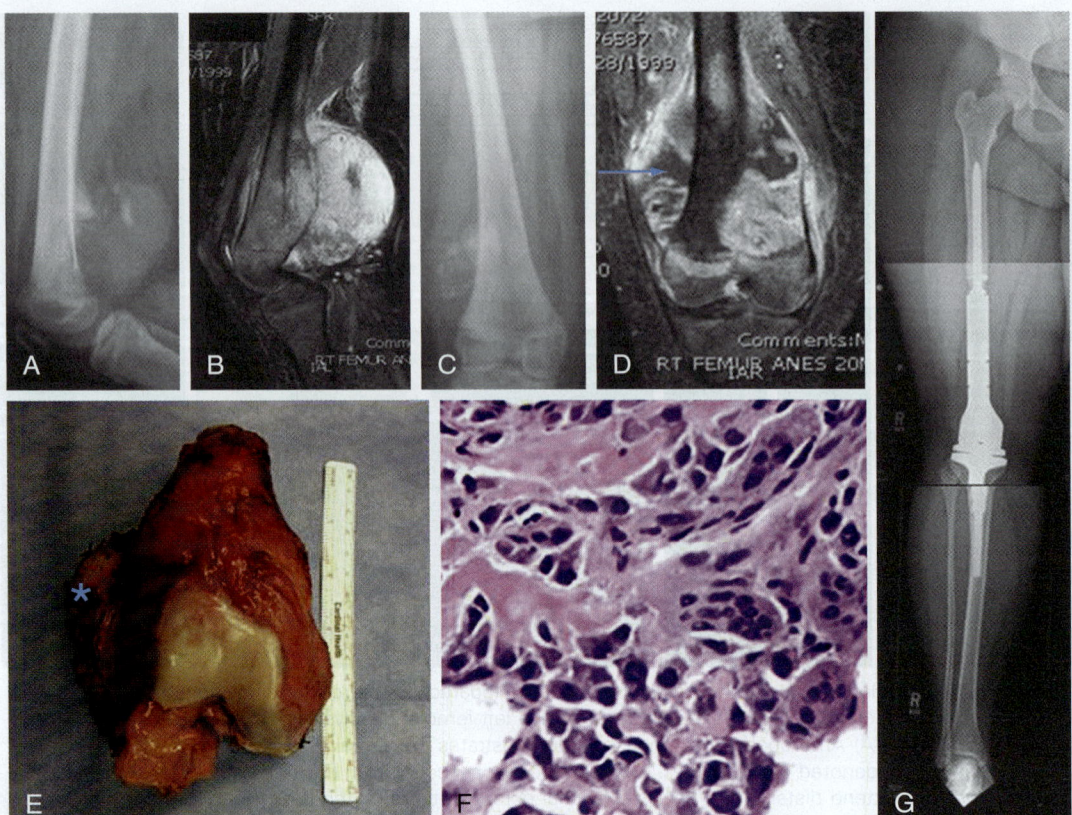

FIGURE 64.13 Endoprostheses are used to reconstruct periarticular malignant tumors. (A) Lateral x-ray of distal femur shows aggressive bone tumor with large soft tissue extension. (B) Magnetic resonance imaging (MRI) T2 sagittal shows true extent of bone involvement and soft tissue mass. (C) Anteroposterior distal femur x-ray demonstrates osteoblastic matrix. (D) MRI T2 coronal shows planned biopsy trajectory—lateral to access soft tissue mass *(arrow)*. (E) Resection specimen with biopsy tract *(*)*. (F) Histology analysis shows malignant cells with lacelike osteoid matrix. (G) Right distal femur endoprosthesis using press-fit fixation into the femoral canal.

needed to cover the prosthesis and reconstruct the extensor mechanism.

Osteosarcoma

Osteosarcoma, or osteogenic sarcoma, is defined as a malignant tumor that produces neoplastic osteoid. Neoplastic cartilage or fibrous tissue may be present. There are many types of osteosarcoma, and they vary by location (intraosseous, surface, or extraskeletal), grade, and etiology. Spontaneous osteosarcomas are most common, but some osteosarcomas occur in the genetic syndromes of Li-Fraumeni and hereditary retinoblastoma as well as in postradiation scenarios. There is a bimodal age of tumor occurrence. Conventional osteosarcomas occur in the first two decades of life, whereas posttreatment or secondary (malignant transformation) osteosarcomas occur much later. Survival is best predicted by the degree of chemotherapy-induced necrosis.[95] Nonmetastatic extremity osteosarcoma with greater than 90% chemotherapy-induced necrosis has survival rates of 80% at 5 years. Pelvic osteosarcoma with less than 90% chemotherapy-induced necrosis has a survival rate of approximately 30%.[90,91]

Ewing Sarcoma

Ewing sarcoma and primitive neuroectodermal tumors are small blue cell (microscopic appearance) malignancies of bone that cytogenetically represent the same entity. They share a common translocation, t(11;22)(q24;q12), in 85% of cases. Molecular cloning of the translocation reveals fusion between the 5′ end of the *EWS* gene from the 22q12 chromosome and the 3′ end of the 11q24 *FLI1* gene.[96] This tumor is sensitive to chemotherapy and radiation treatment. Because Ewing is considered a systemic disease, primary treatment centers around systemic chemotherapy, usually six cycles before and after local treatment, either surgery, radiation therapy, or a combination, depending on tumor and anatomic factors.

Chondrosarcoma

Chondrosarcoma is a malignant skeletal neoplasm that produces hyaline cartilage (Fig. 64.14D1–D2). Several pathologic subtypes exist in which the neoplastic cells produce unusual matrices. Histopathology alone does not predict biologic behavior. Rather, a combination of histopathology, age, location, and radiographic appearance yields the best predictor of tumor aggressiveness. A low-grade cartilage tumor of the phalanx may have the same microscopic appearance as a pelvic chondrosarcoma. It would be exceedingly rare to die of a phalanx cartilage tumor. However, local control is notoriously difficult to achieve in pelvic chondrosarcomas, and long-term cure rates require massive resection. Secondary chondrosarcomas occur after malignant transformation of benign cartilage tumors such as enchondroma or osteochondroma.

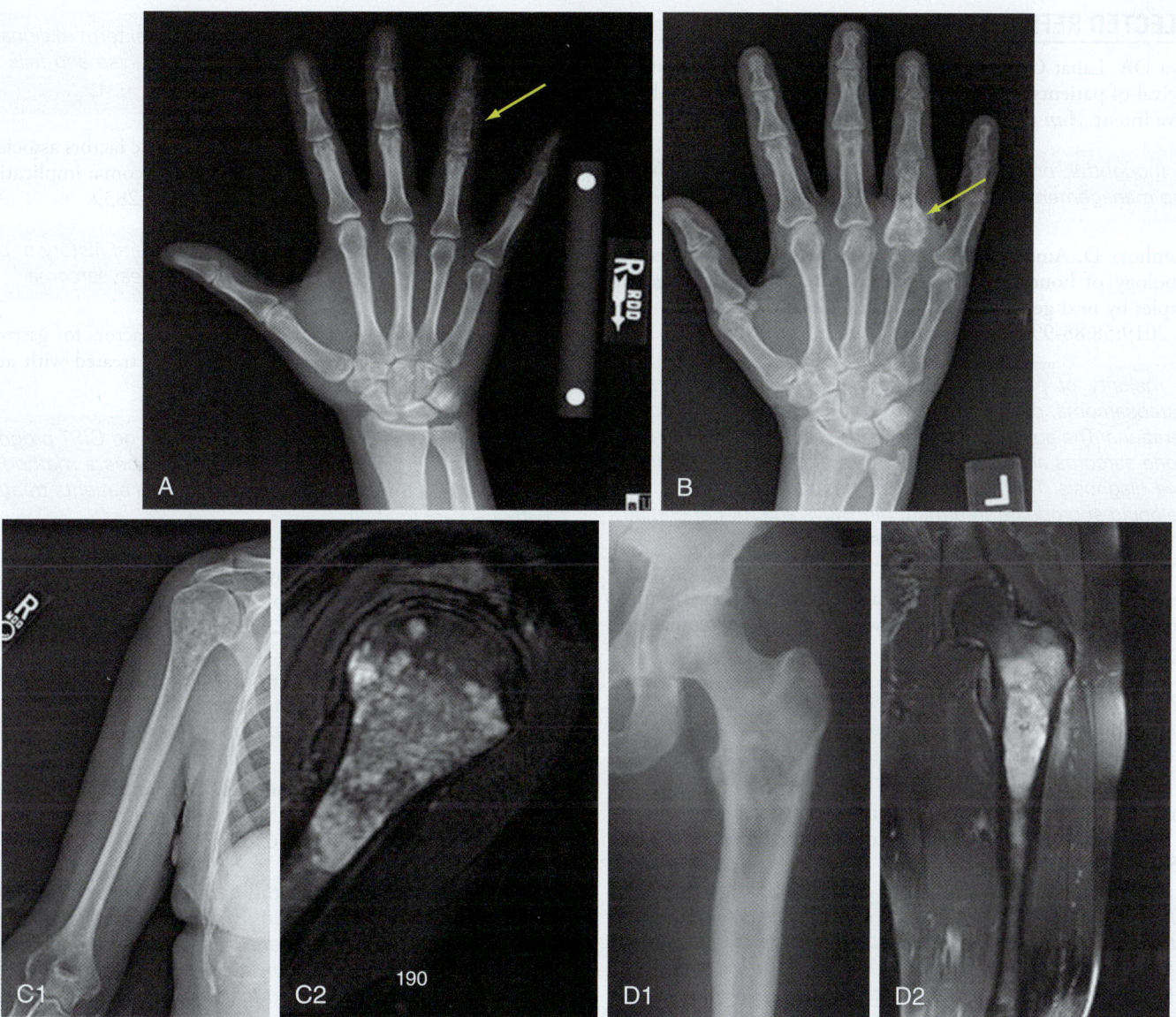

FIGURE 64.14 The differential diagnosis of cartilage lesions depends on clinical and radiographic information. (A) Middle phalanx expansile lesion with internal calcification presenting as pathologic fracture is a typical presentation for enchondroma. (B) Although the more distal a cartilage lesion is, the less likely it is malignant, another patient presented with an aggressive proximal phalanx lesion, marked by pain, periosteal reaction, and internal calcification, and she was diagnosed with chondrosarcoma. (C) Patient has a proximal humerus cartilage lesion with expected calcification on anteroposterior proximal humerus x-ray without destruction of surrounding cortex (C1). The lesion is lobular in nature, as is apparent on MRI (C2). The patient is being followed radiographically. (D) In comparison, another patient had an aggressive-appearing lesion in the left proximal femur, causing bony distortion (D1), which on MRI was associated with surrounding bone edema (D2). The patient was diagnosed with a high-grade chondrosarcoma and treated with proximal femoral resection, megaprosthesis.

SUMMARY

Sarcomas represent a diverse group of rare tumor types that all require a nuanced and robust understanding of connective tissue tumor biology, anatomy, and multimodal treatment regimens. The heterogeneity of this group of diseases poses significant diagnostic and treatment challenges, and successful management requires the ability to effectively work within the context of a multidisciplinary oncology team. Recent discoveries relating to the molecular and genetic underpinnings and the tumor microenvironment demonstrate that although they are rare, these tumors may offer opportunities in the development of novel targeted therapies.

SELECTED REFERENCES

Anya DA, Lahat G, Wang X, et al. Postoperative nomogram for survival of patients with retroperitoneal sarcoma treated with curative intent. *Ann Oncol.* 2010;21:397-402.

A thoughtful, pragmatic, and easily applicable approach to the management of retroperitoneal sarcomas.

Baumhoer D, Amary F, Flanagan AM. An update of molecular pathology of bone tumors. Lessons learned from investigating samples by next generation sequencing. *Genes Chromosomes Cancer.* 2019;58:88-99.

A majority of primary bone tumors, excluding high-grade osteosarcoma, can now be defined by molecular genetic alterations. The ability to identify distinct molecular markers in bone sarcoma allows one to more reliably determine definitive diagnosis. The right diagnosis has ramifications for developing appropriate treatment pathways and for generating meaningful research study groups.

Brennan MF, Antonescu CR, Moraco N, et al. Lessons learned from the study of 10,000 patients with soft tissue sarcoma. *Ann Surg.* 2014;260:416-422.

The largest surgical series of STSs demonstrates a number of key concepts that relate to natural history and management of patients with this disease.

Enneking WF, Spanier SS, Goodman MA. A system for the surgical staging of musculoskeletal sarcoma. *Clin Orthop Relat Res.* 1980;153:106-120.

This surgical staging system for musculoskeletal sarcomas stratifies bone tumors and STSs by the grade of biologic aggressiveness, by the anatomic setting, and by the presence of metastasis. It consists of three stages: I—low grade; II—high grade; and III—presence of metastases. These stages are subdivided by whether the lesion is anatomically confined (a) within a compartment or (b) beyond a compartment in ill-defined fascial planes and spaces. It has proven to be the most correlative system for predicting sarcoma outcomes.

Fizazi K, Carducci M, Smith M, et al. Denosumab versus zoledronic acid for treatment of bone metastases in men with castration-resistant prostate cancer: a randomised, double-blind study. *Lancet.* 2011;377:813-822.

In this phase III randomized controlled trial, denosumab was shown to be better than zoledronic acid in the prevention of SREs. The results reflect the importance of understanding the bone microenvironment in which tumors proliferate. Denosumab is a human monoclonal antibody targeted against receptor activator of nuclear factor κB ligand. Zoledronic acid is a bisphosphonate that inhibits the activated osteoclasts.

Fletcher CD, Gustafson P, Rydholm A, et al. Clinicopathologic re-evaluation of 100 malignant fibrous histiocytomas: prognostic relevance of subclassification. *J Clin Oncol.* 2001;19:3045-3050.

This illustrates the concept that the historical term malignant fibrous histiocytoma is pathologically imprecise and fails to accurately predict outcome.

Heslin MJ, Lewis JJ, Nadler E, et al. Prognostic factors associated with long-term survival for retroperitoneal sarcoma: implications for management. *J Clin Oncol.* 1997;15:2832-2839.

An important article demonstrating the natural history of patients undergoing resection for retroperitoneal sarcoma.

Joensuu H, Eriksson M, Hall KS, et al. Risk factors for gastrointestinal stromal tumor recurrence in patients treated with adjuvant imatinib. *Cancer.* 2014;120:2325-2333.

Whereas most retrospective reviews focus on GIST prognosis after resection alone, this article describes a methodology to stratify the risk of GIST recurrence in patients treated with adjuvant imatinib.

Joensuu H, Eriksson M, Sundby Hall K, et al. One vs three years of adjuvant imatinib for operable gastrointestinal stromal tumor: a randomized trial. *JAMA.* 2012;307:1265-1272.

In demonstrating superior recurrence-free and overall survival, this trial established the duration of adjuvant imatinib for patients with a high risk for GIST after resection.

Mankin HJ, Mankin CJ, Simon MA. The hazards of the biopsy, revisited. Members of the Musculoskeletal Tumor Society. *J Bone Joint Surg Am.* 1996;78:656-663.

This investigation reviewed the hazards associated with biopsies of primary malignant musculoskeletal sarcomas and demonstrated that there were troubling rates in errors in diagnosis and technique, which adversely affected patient care. In addition, it was noted that patients had a decreased incidence of biopsy-related complications or adverse change in outcome when biopsy was performed in a sarcoma care center. On the basis of those observations, whenever possible, musculoskeletal tumor biopsies should be done in a tertiary-type sarcoma center by an orthopedic oncologist or collaborating musculoskeletal radiologist.

O'Sullivan B, Davis AM, Turcotte R, et al. Preoperative versus postoperative radiotherapy in soft-tissue sarcoma of the limbs: a randomised trial. *Lancet.* 2002;359:2235-2241.

The National Cancer Institute of Canada/Canadian Sarcoma Group SR2 clinical trial represents the only prospective randomized comparison of preoperative versus postoperative radiation therapy for extremity sarcoma.

Pisters PW, Pollock RE, Lewis VO, et al. Long-term results of prospective trial of surgery alone with selective use of radiation for patients with T1 extremity and trunk soft tissue sarcomas. *Ann Surg.* 2007;246:675-681.

Compelling data supporting the selective use of adjuvant radiation for early-stage soft tissue sarcoma.

Rosenberg SA, Tepper J, Glatstein E, et al. The treatment of soft-tissue sarcomas of the extremities: prospective randomized evaluations of (1) limb-sparing surgery plus radiation therapy compared with amputation and (2) the role of adjuvant chemotherapy. *Ann Surg.* 1982;196:305-315.

> *This phase III National Cancer Institute (NCI) study paved the way for a generation of studies examining the role of limb-sparing surgery in the setting of multimodal therapy.*

Rougraff BT, Kneisl JS, Simon MA. Skeletal metastases of unknown origin. A prospective study of a diagnostic strategy. *J Bone Joint Surg Am.* 1993;75:1276-1281.

> *In 85% of patients, the primary site of metastatic origin was identified with the use of a CT scan of the chest, abdomen, and pelvis. This diagnostic strategy was simple and highly successful for the identification of the site of an occult malignant tumor before biopsy in patients who had skeletal metastases of unknown origin. In a patient presenting with a skeletal lesion suspicious for a metastatic lesion with an unknown primary, CT scan is the test of choice to identify the primary lesion. In an era when insurance approval of such tests is increasingly more difficult, it is important to advocate for patients to receive this standard of care examination.*

Simon MA, Aschliman MA, Thomas N, et al. Limb-salvage treatment versus amputation for osteosarcoma of the distal end of the femur. *J Bone Joint Surg Am.* 1986;68:1331-1337.

> *This study compared three groups of patients who had a limb-sparing procedure, an above-the-knee amputation, or disarticulation of the hip for osteosarcoma of the distal femur. The use of a limb-salvage procedure for osteosarcoma of the distal end of the femur did not shorten the disease-free interval or compromise long-term survival.*

Taylor BS, Barretina J, Maki RG, et al. Advances in sarcoma genomics and new therapeutic targets. *Nat Rev Cancer.* 2011; 11:541-557.

> *A unique perspective on the taxonomy and classification of soft tissue sarcoma, driven by the molecular genetics of this diverse tumor family.*

van Vliet M, Kliffen M, Krestin GP, et al. Soft tissue sarcomas at a glance: clinical, histological, and MR imaging features of malignant extremity soft tissue tumors. *Eur Radiol.* 2009;19:1499-1511.

> *This article is a concise atlas of STS that correlates the natural history of the disease with the imaging and histologic characteristics.*

The full reference list appears on Elsevier eBooks+.

65 CHAPTER

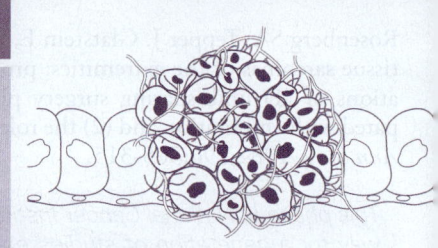

Gastrointestinal Stromal Tumors

Mark Antkowiak, Ronald P. DeMatteo, and Jason K. Sicklick

OVERVIEW

Gastrointestinal stromal tumors (GISTs) are the most common soft tissue sarcoma and the most common mesenchymal tumor of the gastrointestinal (GI) tract. GISTs are thought to originate from interstitial cells of Cajal (ICCs) and can appear anywhere throughout the GI tract. They are most often located in the stomach and small bowel. Understanding of GIST biology has changed dramatically over the past 25 years. The discovery of KIT (CD117) overexpression in these tumors prompted investigation into the molecular underpinnings of GISTs, and it is now known that mutations in the *KIT* proto-oncogene cause constitutive activation of the KIT protein in a majority of GISTs. However, GISTs that do not harbor primary *KIT* mutations often exhibit a very different biology and natural history. Now, with the advent of next-generation sequencing (NGS), other driver mutations have been discovered in genes, including *PDGFRA, SDHx* subunits, and *NF1*. Understanding of the molecular basis of GISTs has led to significant advances in treatment, including the development of systemic therapies targeting the KIT and PDGFRA receptor tyrosine kinases (RTKs). These agents have shown dramatic clinical responses in patients with *KIT*-mutant and *PDGFRA*-mutant GISTs. Although significant advances have been made in understanding the biology of GISTs, there remains much to be discovered. This chapter will present current knowledge of the major

aspects of GISTs, including molecular drivers, clinical evaluation, pathology, surgical management, and medical treatment.

EPIDEMIOLOGY

GISTs comprise approximately 1% to 2% of all primary GI tract tumors and are the most common mesenchymal neoplasm of the gut.[1] GISTs can occur anywhere in the GI tract, including the esophagus, stomach, small bowel, colon, and rectum. The majority of GISTs occur in the stomach or small bowel, representing 40% to 60% or 25% to 30% of all GISTs, respectively.[1] There have been rare reports of extraintestinal GISTs, typically occurring in the mesentery, omentum, pelvis, liver, or pancreas.[2] It is unclear whether these are primary extraintestinal tumors or represent metastatic disease secondary to undetected primary GIST.

The incidence of GISTs in the United States is approximately seven to eight new cases per million annually.[3] Worldwide, the incidence is more variable, ranging from 2.1 to 19.7 cases per million annually.[4,5] But the true incidence of GISTs is difficult to determine accurately because the methods for diagnosing and documenting GISTs have changed over time, and GISTs can be clinically silent during a patient's lifetime, only to later be discovered incidentally on autopsy,[6] where up to one in four individuals have occult, microscopic gastric GISTs.

GISTs are most often diagnosed in adults, with the median age at diagnosis of 65 to 69 years.[3,4] GISTs rarely occur in patients under the age of 40. Although somatic mutations are most common for all patients presenting with GISTs, younger patient populations are more likely to harbor germline mutations in *SDHx* subunit genes or *NF1*.[7,8]

The incidence of GISTs is similar in male and female patients, with very slight male predominance.[4] However, in patients with SDH-deficient tumors, SDH-deficient GISTs occur twice as commonly in females. Racial differences in the incidence of GISTs have also been found in multiple studies, including a recent epidemiologic study of the Surveillance, Epidemiology, and End Results (SEER) database, which found that the incidence of GISTs in Black patients was 1.37 cases per 100,000 compared with 0.65 cases per 100,000 in White patients, with a rate ratio of 2.12 between these two populations.[3,9] Moreover, GIST is slightly more common in Asian Pacific Islanders, with an incidence of 1.1 cases per 100,000. This may partially explain the higher incidences seen in Asian countries, beyond screening bias, for gastric adenocarcinoma.

ETIOLOGY

Cell of Origin

GIST likely arises from ICCs, colloquially referred to as *intestinal pacemaker cells*. Originally discovered in the late 19th century by the pathologist Santiago Ramon y Cajal, these cells are thought to play an important role in slow-wave gut peristalsis.[10] The ICCs reside between nerve endings and smooth muscle cells in the submucosal and muscularis propria layers of the bowel wall (Fig. 65.1), consistent with the typical presentation of GISTs as submucosal tumors. But our knowledge of how GISTs arose was once considerably less clear. Historically, stromal tumors of the GI tract were presumed to be leiomyomas or leiomyosarcomas because of their histologic similarities to smooth muscle cells. However, with advances in immunohistochemistry in the late 20th century, several studies pointed out that GISTs have a unique histologic signature compared with other intestinal stromal tumors, namely, the nearly ubiquitous overexpression of KIT and CD34.[11,12] Interestingly, almost no true leiomyomas or leiomyosarcomas demonstrate expression of these markers.[13] With this discovery, a key question remained: If the signature of these tumors is different from that of other stromal tumors, which cells give rise to GISTs? A key insight into this question came by examining the expression pattern of KIT and CD34 in stromal cells of the gut, where the ICCs also express both markers.[14] This insight led directly to the hypothesis that ICCs (or a common precursor) give rise to GIST. More recently, the origins of different GIST subtypes have been questioned. Telocytes, or fibroblast-like cells expressing PDGFRA and CD34, were postulated as the ICC equivalent in a patient with germline *PDGFRA*-mutant GIST.[15] Moreover, smooth muscle cells of the small intestine have been shown to give rise to *BRAF*

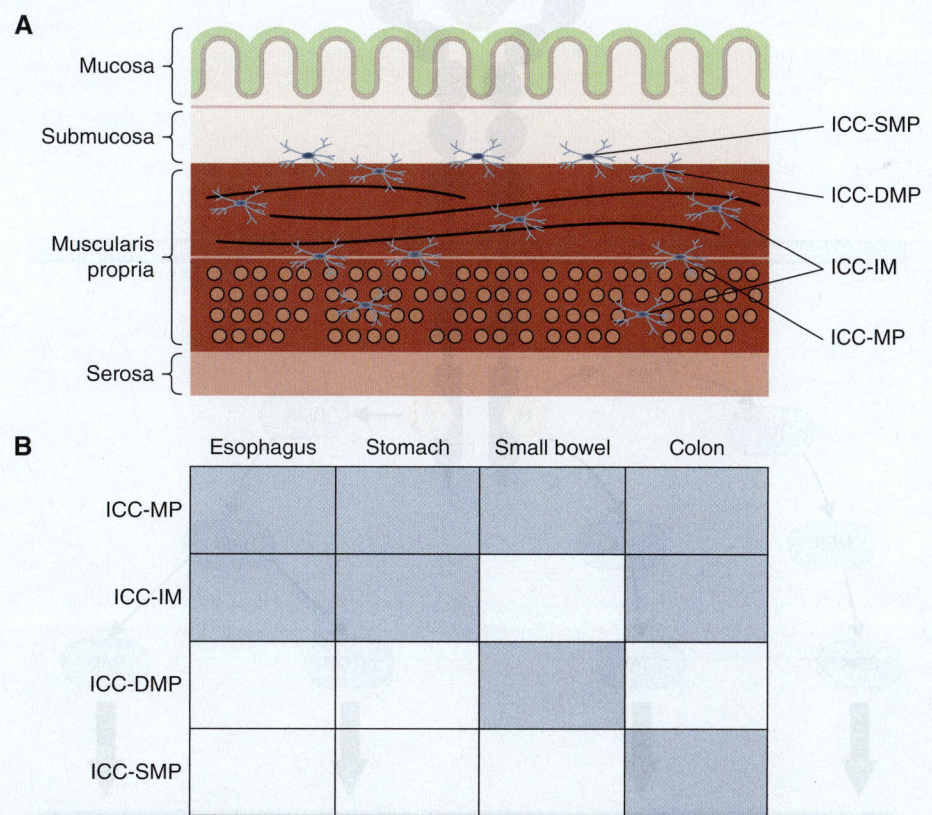

FIGURE 65.1 Interstitial cells of Cajal *(ICCs)* in the bowel wall. (A) Schematic representation of the location of ICCs in the submucosal and muscularis layers of the bowel wall. There are four subtypes of ICCs depending on the location within the bowel wall: (1) ICC-SMP in the submucosal plexus, (2) ICC-DMP in the deep myenteric plexus, (3) ICC-IM in the longitudinal or circular muscularis, and (4) ICC-MP in the myenteric plexus. In the bowel wall, these cells are typically located between enteric neurons and play a key role as the pacemaker cells of the gastrointestinal tract. (B) Predominant ICC subtype found in different areas of the gastrointestinal tract.

V600E–mutant GIST in a mouse model.[16] Thus, there may be several cell types that give rise to different GIST subtypes based on tumor location and driver mutations.

Molecular Drivers

One of the key discoveries that led to a better understanding of GIST biology was the finding that KIT overexpression almost always occurs in GIST. This clue led to investigations into the potential role of *KIT* mutations in driving tumor biology, and this was discovered to be the case.[17] The majority of newly diagnosed GISTs harbor *KIT* mutations.[17,18] KIT is an RTK that belongs to the platelet-derived growth factor receptor (PDGFR) superfamily. In normal physiology, monomeric KIT receptors on the cell membrane interact with the KIT ligand (KITLG), which is also known as *stem cell factor* (SCF). Upon ligand binding, the receptor dimerizes, causing autophosphorylation, activation of downstream signaling pathways, and cellular responses (Fig. 65.2). Canonically, the downstream signaling pathways regulated by KIT signaling include the MAPK (RAS/RAF/MEK/ERK), PAM (PI3KCA/AKT/mTOR), and JAK/STAT pathways.[17] In the majority of GISTs that are driven by oncogenic *KIT* mutations, there is ligand-independent dimerization, and therefore, the downstream signaling

pathways become constitutively active and cause uncontrolled cellular proliferation and oncogenesis.

But just because GIST expresses KIT does not imply that the tumor cells have a KIT mutation. In fact, as our understanding of GIST has grown, clinicians have found that not all GISTs exhibit *KIT* mutations or even overexpress KIT.[18] Even though the drivers of *KIT* wild-type tumors are different from those in *KIT*-mutant GIST, these tumors were often treated with therapies targeting *KIT* mutations. Unsurprisingly, these tumors did not respond well. The advent of NGS represented a leap forward in our understanding of GISTs, and multiple other driver mutations have since been discovered, including *PDGFRA, SDHx, NF1,* and *BRAF* mutations.[17,18] These differing mutational profiles are tightly associated with differences in tumor biology and treatment responses.

Mutations in *PDGFRA*,[18,19] which also encodes an RTK belonging to the same superfamily (i.e., PDGFR), can also activate downstream signaling pathways that result in uncontrolled cellular proliferation and oncogenesis.[17] GISTs that do not harbor a mutation in *KIT* or *PDGFRA* are sometimes referred to as *KIT/PDGFRA wild-type GISTs*. In this group, the most common driver mutations affect *SDHx* genes, and thus, these GISTs are known as *succinate dehydrogenase (SDH)-deficient GISTs*.[20] SDH is

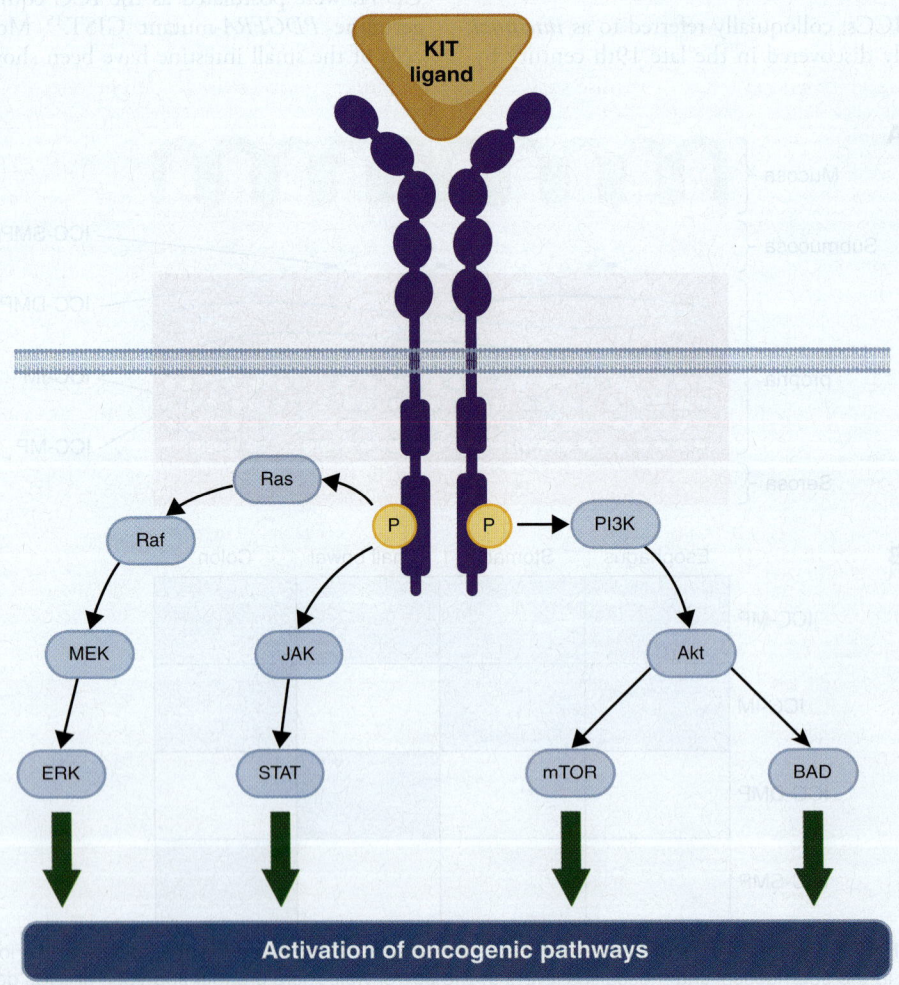

FIGURE 65.2 Major KIT signaling pathways. Binding of KIT ligand, otherwise known as *stem cell factor* (SCF), leads to dimerization of the KIT receptor and autophosphorylation. Once active, the KIT receptor activates multiple downstream signaling pathways, including the MAPK (i.e., RAS/RAF/MEK/ERK), JAK/STAT signaling pathway, and PI3KCA/AKT/mTOR signaling pathways. Together, these pathways lead to increased cell proliferation, increased cell survival, and decreased apoptosis.

an enzyme complex that functions in the citric acid cycle, where it catalyzes the oxidation of succinate to fumarate. Inherited (i.e., germline) loss-of-function mutations in any of the four SDH subunits *(SDHA, SDHB, SDHC, SDHD)* can cause formation of gastric GISTs when there is loss of heterozygosity in the second allele, leading to loss of SDH expression. In turn, these are called *SDH-deficient GISTs* because they lack SDHB expression when expression of any subunit is lost. In other words, negative SDHB staining is a positive biomarker for this GIST subtype. Most recently, it was discovered that epigenetic changes in the DNA promoter of the *SDHC* gene can also lead to *SDHC* silencing and SDH-deficient GIST without germline mutations. These nonhereditary gastric GISTs that generally only occur in young females are now often referred to as *SDH-epimutant GISTs.*[17,21] After SDH-deficient GISTs, other driver mutations include *NF1* (germline and somatic), *BRAF, ETV6-NTRK3, FGFR1* gene fusions, and unknown/unclassified mutations, in descending order of prevalence.[20,22-24]

Hereditary Syndromes

GISTs are typically caused by somatic gene mutations that are sporadic in nature. But a subset of GISTs is caused by germline mutations known to cause hereditary syndromes. These syndromes include neurofibromatosis type 1 (NF1), familial GIST syndrome, and Carney-Stratakis syndrome.[24-26] When assessing patients with GISTs, it is important to take a thorough family history to rule in or out any of these syndromes. Those suspected to have an underlying familial syndrome should be referred for further genetic counseling and possibly additional germline testing to confirm the diagnosis because these may be treated differently and have different prognoses.

NF1 is a multisystemic autosomal-dominant genetic disorder caused by mutations in the *NF1* gene. Manifestations include development of skin lesions, neurofibromas, and increased risk for various malignancies. Patients with NF1 have an increased risk for development of GISTs, most frequently occurring in the small bowel, and patients often have recurrent and multifocal disease. NF1-related GISTs often have spindle cell morphology. In contrast to sporadic disease, these patients rarely have mutations in *KIT* or *PDGFRA* but nevertheless overexpress KIT in most cases.[24]

Familial GIST syndrome is caused by mutations in *KIT* or *PDGFRA* and is characterized by a predisposition to GIST development. Patients with familial GIST syndrome can develop GISTs from a young age and can have multifocal disease. In addition, patients with germline *KIT* mutations may also present with skin hyperpigmentation, dysphagia, and urticaria pigmentosa, and when the syndrome is caused by germline *PDGFRA* mutations, they may present with inflammatory fibroid polyps.[25,26]

Carney-Stratakis syndrome is caused by germline *SDHx* mutations and features a dyad of increased risk for GIST and development of paragangliomas (previously called *extraadrenal pheochromocytoma*). These patients also may develop GISTs at a young age, and they typically have germline mutations in *SDHA, SDHB, SDHC,* or *SDHD.* They all can cause SDH deficiency. Much remains unclear about how deficiency of the SDH enzyme drives oncogenic transformation in GISTs and paragangliomas.[27]

Nonhereditary Syndrome

Like Carney-Stratakis syndrome, **Carney triad** is characterized by an increased risk for GIST and paraganglioma development. But patients with Carney triad also have a predisposition for development of pulmonary chondromas. Patients with Carney triad often have SDH-deficient tumor expression as a result of epigenetic silencing of *SDHC.* Because of this, Carney triad is not considered a hereditary syndrome.[21]

CLINICAL EVALUATION

Presentation

Most GISTs are asymptomatic and are discovered incidentally on cross-sectional imaging or endoscopy. GISTs will often appear as well-encapsulated, homogeneous masses on cross-sectional imaging and/or as smooth submucosal masses arising from layer 4 of the stomach on endoscopic examination. However, presentation will vary depending on the size and location of the tumor.[28]

Small GISTs are typically asymptomatic or minimally symptomatic. When located in the upper GI tract, patients may experience unspecified abdominal pain, early satiety, bloating, or dyspepsia; in the lower GI tract, tumors are likely to present as abdominal pain or bloating.[7,28] Larger tumors may present with similar symptoms that are magnified in intensity and may additionally present with nausea, vomiting, constipation, evidence of acute or chronic GI bleeding, or palpable mass. Symptoms rarely relate to compression of adjacent organs, such as obstructive symptoms for intestinal compression or blockage and obstructive jaundice resulting from compression of the biliary tree.[7,28]

Although GISTs are typically submucosal, they may occasionally ulcerate through the mucosa. When this occurs, GISTs may present with bleeding and may cause anemia, melena, or hematemesis. In addition, a sinus tract into the tumor may result in infection and fever. Rarely, GISTs may also rupture into the intraperitoneal space, resulting in tumor dissemination, intraperitoneal bleeding, and/or peritonitis.[7,28]

Patients may also present with multifocal or metastatic disease, often without symptoms or less commonly with symptoms similar to patients with solitary tumors. Multifocal GI primary disease is more common for patients with hereditary causes of GIST. For patients with metastatic disease, the most common sites of metastases are the liver, omentum, and peritoneal surfaces.[7] GISTs rarely metastasize to lymph nodes, with the exception of the SDH-deficient GISTs and those caused by gene fusions (e.g., *ETV6-NTRK3* or *FGFR1*).

Pediatric, adolescent, and young adult patients are more likely to present with familial syndromes. For those with Carney-Stratakis syndrome or Carney triad, patients may exhibit symptoms related to excess catecholamine/metanephrine secretion, including hypertension, headaches, and tachycardia.

Differential Diagnosis

The differential diagnosis for submucosal tumors includes both benign and malignant tumors. Many submucosal tumors present with similar symptoms to GISTs, and the diagnosis of these tumors relies on biopsy and histopathologic assessment. Benign tumors that may present similarly to GISTs include leiomyoma, schwannoma, hemangioma, desmoid tumors, plexiform fibromyxoma, glomus tumors, and pancreatic rests, whereas malignant tumors include leiomyosarcoma, lymphoma, neuroendocrine tumors, and metastatic tumors. All of these tumor types may masquerade as GISTs. Because of the similarity in presentation and often indistinguishable features on cross-sectional imaging, histopathologic assessment provides the greatest degree of diagnostic clarity and should ultimately guide management, although definitive preoperative histologic confirmation is not always possible.

Imaging

When suspected, GISTs should be evaluated with cross-sectional imaging. Typically, contrast-enhanced computed tomography (CT) imaging of the abdomen and pelvis is sufficient. However, in cases where a patient is unable to undergo CT imaging, magnetic resonance imaging (MRI) is another option. This may be particularly useful in rectal GIST, where MRI provides better visualization of the tumor.[28] On cross-sectional imaging, GISTs will often appear as smooth and highly enhancing masses (Fig. 65.3).[29] Small GISTs will typically appear homogeneous, whereas large GISTs are more likely to appear heterogeneous because of tumor necrosis, intratumoral hemorrhage, and/or cystic degeneration.[29] Chest imaging is generally only indicated in advanced disease because GIST rarely metastasizes to the lungs. In cases of diagnostic uncertainty, positron emission tomography (PET)/CT can be considered, but it is typically not necessary when the tumor is adequately visualized on CT or MRI.

Diagnostic Procedures

In addition to cross-sectional imaging, suspected GISTs should be evaluated with endoscopy and endoscopic ultrasound (EUS). Tumor location and accessibility are important factors in determining whether a tumor can be assessed via esophagogastroduodenoscopy, double-balloon enteroscopy, or colonoscopy. In addition to better characterizing the tumor, endoscopy can be used to aid in biopsy and histopathologic assessment.

Endoscopically, GISTs typically appear as a submucosal mass with smooth margins and normal overlying mucosa. Bulging of the tumor into the stomach or bowel and, rarely, ulceration may be observed (Fig. 65.4). EUS can confirm the layer of origin of the tumor and whether the tumor is intramural or extramural.[30,31]

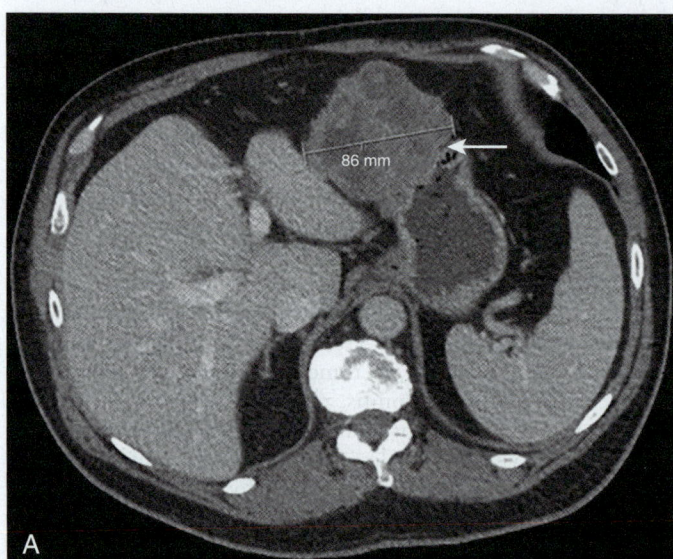

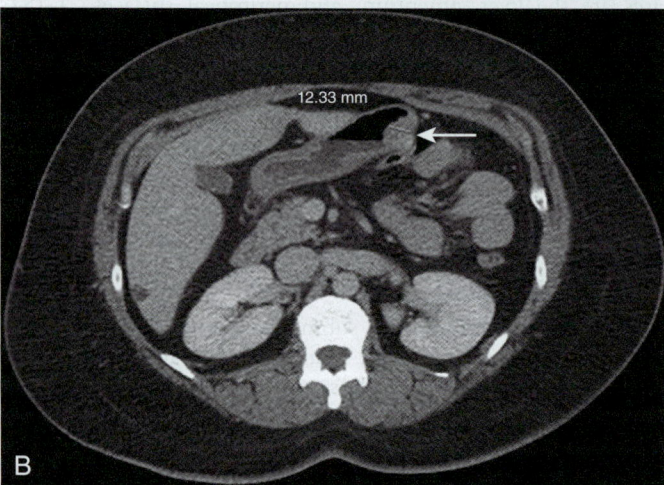

FIGURE 65.3 Representative computed tomography (CT) images of gastrointestinal stromal tumors (GISTs). On CT imaging, GISTs will often appear as enhancing masses. (A) CT findings of a patient with an approximately 8.6-cm GIST on the lesser curvature of the stomach *(arrow)*. (B) CT findings of a patient with a small GIST along the greater curvature of the stomach *(arrow)*.

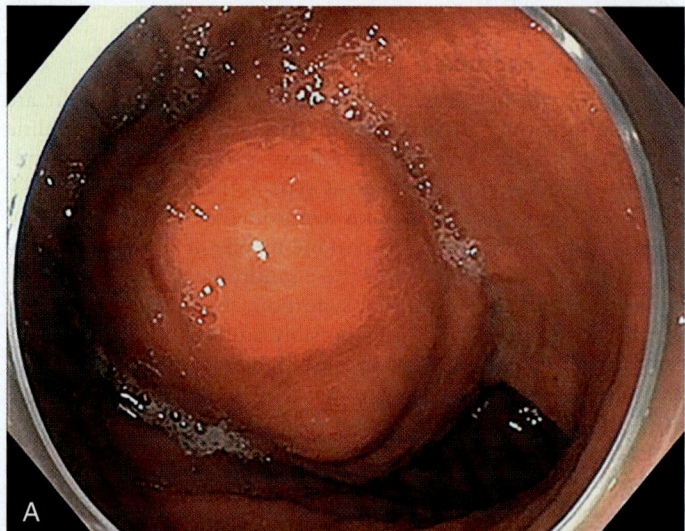

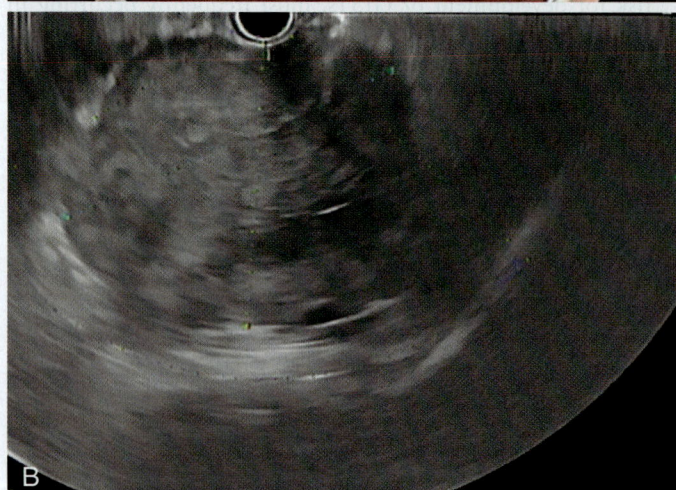

FIGURE 65.4 Representative endoscopic images of gastrointestinal stromal tumors (GISTs). Endoscopically, GISTs typically appear as smooth, well-defined submucosal masses that may bulge into the gut lumen. Typically, the overlying mucosa is normal. Ulceration is a higher-risk feature and can be associated with bleeding at presentation. Endoscopic ultrasound (EUS) typically shows hypoechoic, homogeneous lesions with well-defined borders, but EUS should be used to evaluate for high-risk features, including irregular borders, cystic cavities, echogenic foci, and heterogeneity. (A) Endoscopic findings of a gastric GIST. (B) Accompanying EUS findings.

GISTs are typically visualized as hypoechoic, homogeneous masses with well-defined margins in the muscularis mucosa or muscularis propria. Additionally, certain high-risk features, including irregular borders, cystic cavities, ulceration, echogenic foci, and heterogeneity, can be seen.[30,31]

As previously mentioned, while the patient is undergoing endoscopic evaluation, biopsy of the suspected lesion should be performed, although it is not always diagnostic. A mucosal biopsy alone is insufficient to make the diagnosis. EUS with core-needle biopsy (CNB) or fine-needle aspiration (FNA) should be performed. Histopathologic examination of a suspected GIST is critical to confirm the diagnosis. Additionally, obtaining adequate tissue in patients with suspected multifocal disease, borderline resectable disease, or unresectable disease provides additional material for mutational profiling to guide treatment, including eligibility for neoadjuvant therapy.[30]

As alluded to earlier, several options exist for biopsy of the lesion, including EUS-guided FNA, EUS-guided CNB, and percutaneous biopsy. EUS-guided sampling is preferred to endoscopic sampling alone because of inadequate sampling for submucosal tumors.[32] Although EUS-guided FNA is sufficient for diagnosis, evidence suggests that EUS-guided CNB may allow for superior diagnostic yield.[32] Percutaneous biopsy may be performed for patients with inaccessible tumors or metastatic tumors or for patients in whom EUS-guided biopsy was unsuccessful. Historically, percutaneous biopsy was believed to carry at least a theoretical risk of peritoneal seeding of the tumor as a result of disruption of the tumor capsule. There is now evidence that rates of this are less than 1%, leaving percutaneous biopsy as a valid alternative approach.

PATHOLOGY

Once obtained, tissue should be comprehensively assessed via histopathologic, immunohistochemical, and molecular analyses.[30] The pathologist should note several key parameters, including the tumor site of origin; tumor size; tumor focality; mitotic rate; margin status (for resected tumors); immunohistochemical results, including KIT (CD117), DOG-1, and SDHB expression; and sequencing results (if available).

Histology

Histologically, GISTs can be grouped into three morphologic subtypes—spindeloid, epithelioid, and mixed. Approximately 70% of tumors have spindle cell morphology, followed by 20% epithelioid and 10% mixed.[13] GISTs with spindle cell morphology are typically composed of relatively uniform eosinophilic cells arranged in fascicles or whorls and nuclei that are uniform and ovoid in appearance, often with nuclear palisading.[13] Epithelioid GISTs typically have rounded cells with eosinophilic or clear cytoplasm with relatively uniform nuclei that are round to ovoid in appearance.[13] Epithelioid GISTs are more likely to harbor PDGFRA or SDH subunit mutations.[33] Mixed type GISTs often have both spindle cell–like and epithelioid morphology that may show intermingling or distinct separation between the cell types.[13] Other rare features that can be identified histologically include myxoid stroma, neuroendocrine features, signet ring variants, and lymphocytic infiltrates.[13] Mitotic rate should be assessed for all tumors and represented as total mitoses per 5 mm² in the most proliferative area of the tumor.[30]

Immunohistochemistry

In addition to histologic assessment, suspected GISTs should undergo immunohistochemistry staining for key markers, including KIT (CD117) and DOG-1 (ANO1). KIT overexpression is now widely used as a criterion for pathologic diagnosis of GISTs, with a reported sensitivity of 95%.[11–14,17,18] Although most GISTs demonstrate KIT overexpression, this is not always caused by mutations in the KIT gene itself. Indeed, some tumors with KIT overexpression lack mutations in KIT and might instead exhibit mutations in other genes, such as NF1 or SDHx.[24,33]

Approximately 5% of GISTs do not demonstrate KIT overexpression on immunohistochemistry.[18] This group is genetically diverse and can include PDGFRA- and SDHx-mutant GISTs. This group also includes a subset of KIT-mutant tumors where KIT is expressed at normal levels, and these are presumably a result of epigenetic silencing. This subset of tumors appears to be enriched in patients after treatment with tyrosine kinase inhibitors (TKIs),[34] probably by clonal selection.

Other markers have been studied for the evaluation of GISTs, including ANO-1, PKC-theta, Nestin, CD34, ASMA, Desmin, and S100. Of these, ANO1 (also known as DOG-1, for Discovered on GIST-1) has shown high sensitivity in the diagnosis of GISTs and is now commonly used for histologic diagnosis.[34,35] In general, tumors with immunohistochemistry positive for both KIT and ANO1 are confirmed to be GISTs. Additionally, immunohistochemistry for SDHB can provide useful diagnostic information and help identify SDH-deficient tumors (i.e., lacking SDHB expression) that may be related to hereditary syndromes.

Molecular Analysis

The advent of NGS has revolutionized understanding of the mutational profiles of GISTs. It is now standard practice to perform sequencing or mutational analysis on GISTs to guide treatment.[30,36] Both the National Comprehensive Cancer Network (NCCN) and European Society for Medical Oncology (ESMO) guidelines recommend molecular testing for suspected GISTs, particularly in patients who are being considered for systemic targeted therapy because it may have variable clinical efficacy depending on the tumor mutational profile.[30,36] If broader panel sequencing is not available, assessment of individual mutations (beginning with KIT) can be performed. For some patients who are candidates for up-front resection, mutational analysis may not alter management and hence need not be performed.

As mentioned, approximately 95% of all GISTs demonstrate KIT overexpression, and of these, about 80% demonstrate KIT mutations that result in constitutive activation (most common mutations in GIST; Table 65.1).[17,18] These pathologic KIT mutations most often occur in exons 11 and 9, representing approximately 70% and 15% of GISTs that harbor KIT mutations, respectively.[18] Other less common mutations can occur in exons 13/14 (adenosine triphosphate [ATP]-binding pocket [AP]) and/or 17/18 (activation loop [AL]). Mutations in KIT exon 11 have been found to cause dysfunction of an autoinhibitory intracellular domain of the receptor, which in turn causes constitutive activation.[17] Other KIT mutations can affect different protein domains that can result in abnormal activation of the receptor. KIT exon 9 mutations alter the KIT ligand-binding site. Mutations in exons 13, 14, 17, and 18, although rare, have been observed in patients who have developed resistance to certain TKIs.[17]

PDGFRA is the second most commonly mutated gene in GISTs, representing approximately 10% to 15% of all tumors.[17,19] Mutation most often occurs in exon 18 and 12, comprising approximately 90% and 9% of cases, respectively.[19] The missense mutation D842V in exon 18 is particularly significant because it confers primary resistance to imatinib, the most commonly used

TABLE 65.1	**Most Common GIST Mutations**	
DRIVER MUTATION	**SPECIFIC MUTATION**	**OVERALL FREQUENCY**
KIT	All mutations	60%–70%
	Exon 11	50%–60%
	Exon 9	6%–9%
	Exon 13, 14, 17, 18	1%–4%
PDGFRA	All mutations	10%–15%
	Exon 18 D842V	8%–9%
	Exon 18 non-D842V	4%–5%
	Exon 12	1%–2%
	Exon 10, 14	<1%
Other genes	All mutations	10%–15%
	SDHA, SDHB, SDHC, SDHD	5%–8%
	NF1	2%–3%
	BRAF V600E	<1%
	ETV6-NTRK3 fusions	<1%
	FGFR fusions	<1%

GIST, Gastrointestinal stromal tumor.
Adapted from Blay, JY et al. Gastrointestinal stromal tumours. *Nat Rev Dis Primers.* 2021;7(1):22.

TKI in GISTs.[19] *PDGFRA* mutations can also rarely occur in exons 10 and 14.[19]

GISTs that do *not* carry *KIT* or *PDGFRA* mutations comprise approximately 10% to 15% of all GISTs.[17] Of these, *SDHx* mutations are the most common.[20] SDH-deficient GISTs often have a poor response to therapy with TKIs. Other mutations include those in *NF1, BRAF* V600E, and *NTRK* or *FGFR1* gene fusions.[17,20,22,23] GISTs that do not harbor *KIT* or *PDGFRA* mutations are more likely to be found in the pediatric, adolescent, and young adult populations.

Interestingly, the location of the GIST tumor often relates to the underlying mutation (Fig. 65.5). For example, SDH-deficient GISTs predominate in the stomach and are rarely found as intestinal tumors, whereas *NF1*-mutant GISTs typically occur in the small bowel.[20,24] Also, a recent study found that nearly all proximal gastric GISTs harbor *KIT* mutations, but distal gastric GISTs have a much higher likelihood of harboring *PDGFRA* or *SDHx* mutations.[37]

TREATMENT

The treatment of GISTs has undergone a significant evolution over the past several decades. In the past, GISTs were typically managed operatively, with few treatment options available for unresectable or metastatic tumors. Radiation therapy and chemotherapy often demonstrated low to no efficacy. With the discovery of oncogenic *KIT* mutations and the realization that these genomic alterations drive GIST biology, targeted therapy with TKIs (especially imatinib) quickly became a viable option for previously untreatable tumors. However, surgical therapy continues to play a central role in the management of GISTs, and there are now various TKIs that can be used. Our understanding of GIST biology has become much more complex, and managing patients diagnosed with GISTs should be discussed by a multidisciplinary tumor board that includes surgical oncologists, medical oncologists, radiologists, and pathologists, among others. New guidelines published by the NCCN establish an algorithmic approach to the management of GISTs (Fig. 65.6).[30]

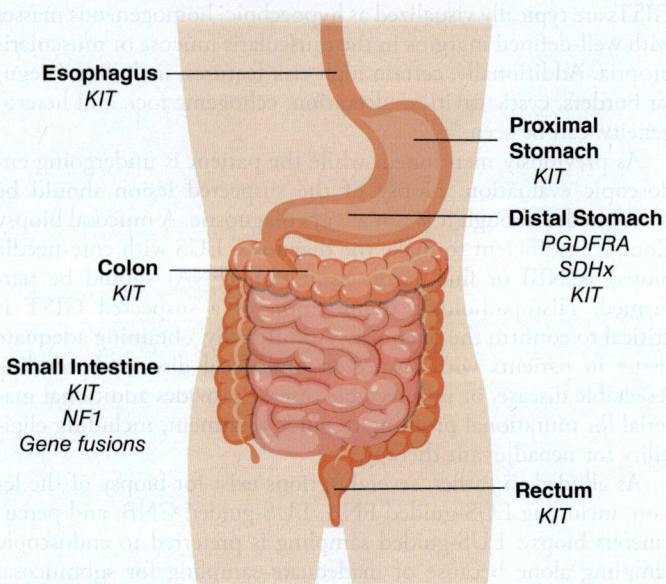

FIGURE 65.5 Most common mutations by location in the gastrointestinal tract. The driver mutations of gastrointestinal stromal tumors (GISTs) vary according to location in the gut. Overall, *KIT* mutations predominate throughout the gastrointestinal tract. Interestingly, *SDHx*- and *PDGFRA*-mutant GISTs most commonly occur in the distal stomach, whereas *NF1*-mutant GISTs almost exclusively occur in the small bowel.

Surgical Treatment

Surgical management remains a cornerstone in the management of GIST. Surgical resection may be offered to patients with localized, locally advanced, or metastatic disease. Candidacy for surgery depends on the evaluation of the patient's surgical risk, extent of disease, tumor size, and tumor location. Because GISTs can occur throughout the GI tract, surgical therapy should be individualized for each patient. Where feasible, resection is typically pursued, either immediately or after neoadjuvant therapy. The role of neoadjuvant therapy depends both on the extent of disease and the location of the tumor. Operative therapy should follow general oncologic principles, including full macroscopic and microscopic resection when feasible, avoidance of disruption of the tumor capsule to prevent peritoneal seeding of the tumor, and exploration of the abdomen to assess for peritoneal or hepatic metastases.

Small Gastrointestinal Stromal Tumors (<2 Centimeters in Size)

The management of small GISTs that are up to 2 cm in size is generally conservative based on the general consensus guidelines of the NCCN and ESMO.[30,36] The natural history of these tumors is unclear, as are the rate of growth and the metastatic potential. Most tumors are indolent, but a subset can have more aggressive biology.[38] In appropriate surgical candidates, all esophageal, small bowel, and colorectal tumors should be resected, regardless of size, because tumors in these locations tend to have more aggressive biology.[30] Gastric tumors that express high-risk features on EUS (e.g., irregular borders, cystic spaces, ulceration, echogenic foci, or heterogeneity) or have high-risk features when biopsied (including high mitotic index) should also be resected.[30] For patients with gastric tumors less than 2 cm in size

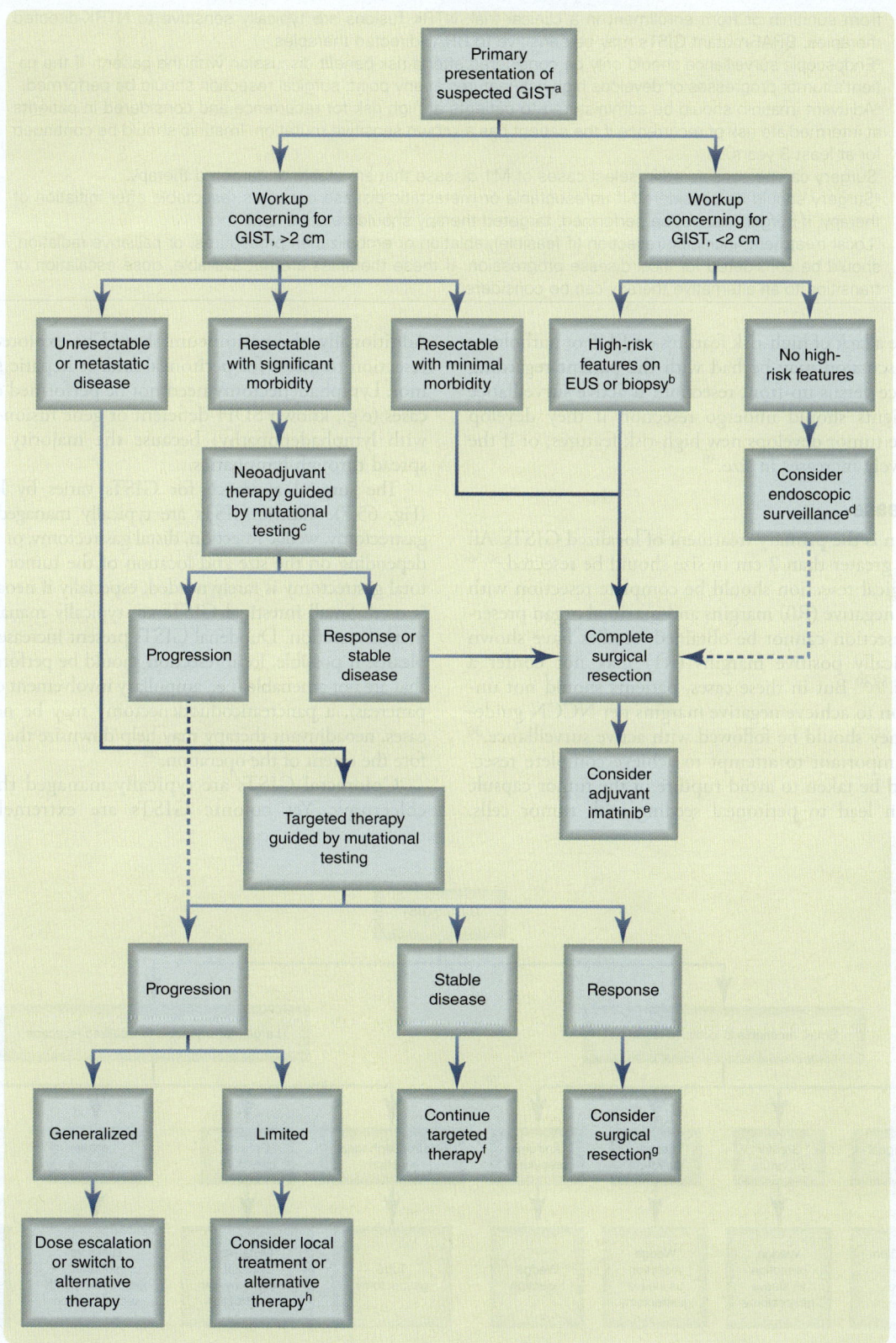

FIGURE 65.6 National Comprehensive Cancer Network (NCCN) algorithm for gastrointestinal stromal tumors *(GIST)* management. *EUS,* Endoscopic ultrasound.

[a]On primary presentation of GISTs, patients should undergo workup, including imaging, endoscopy, and tumor molecular testing, if medical therapy is being considered.

[b]High-risk endoscopic ultrasound features include irregular borders, cystic spaces, ulceration, echogenic foci, and heterogeneity. High-risk pathologic features include number of mitoses and/or tumor necrosis.

[c]Neoadjuvant therapy should be guided by mutation. Imatinib is effective for most KIT- and PDGFRA-mutant GISTs, except for PDGFRA D842V, for which avapritinib may be effective. SDH-deficient tumors may benefit

Continued

from sunitinib or from enrollment in a clinical trial. NTRK fusions are typically sensitive to NTRK-directed therapies. BRAF-mutant GISTs may be sensitive to BRAF-directed therapies.

dEndoscopic surveillance should only be considered after a risk-benefit discussion with the patient. If the patient's tumor progresses or develops high-risk features at any point, surgical resection should be performed.

eAdjuvant imatinib should be administered to patients at high risk for recurrence and considered in patients at intermediate risk of recurrence if the patient has a known sensitive mutation. Imatinib should be continued for at least 3 years.

fSurgery can be considered in select cases of M1 disease that are stable on targeted therapy.

gSurgery should be considered if unresectable or metastatic disease becomes resectable after initiation of therapy. If surgery cannot be performed, targeted therapy should be continued.

hLocal treatment, including resection (if feasible), ablation or embolization procedures, or palliative radiation, should be considered for local disease progression. If these therapies are not available, dose escalation or transition to an alternative therapy can be considered.

that demonstrate a lack of high-risk features on EUS or pathology, a risk-benefit discussion may be had with the patient regarding active surveillance versus up-front resection. If active surveillance is pursued, patients should undergo resection if they develop symptoms, if the tumor develops new high-risk features, or if the tumor progressively increases in size.[30]

Localized Disease

Surgical resection is the primary treatment of localized GISTs. All localized GISTs greater than 2 cm in size should be resected.[30,36] The goal of surgical resection should be complete resection with microscopically negative (R0) margins and maximal organ preservation. If R0 resection cannot be obtained, studies have shown that microscopically positive margins (R1) may not confer a worse prognosis.[39,40] But in these cases, patients should not undergo re-resection to achieve negative margins per NCCN guidelines. Instead, they should be followed with active surveillance.[30] Although it is important to attempt to achieve complete resection, care should be taken to avoid rupture of the tumor capsule because this can lead to peritoneal seeding with tumor cells.

Additionally, the peritoneum should be explored at the time of resection to assess for peritoneal and/or hepatic spread of the tumor. Lymphadenectomy need not be performed except in specific cases (e.g., known SDH-deficient or gene fusion–positive tumors with lymphadenopathy) because the majority of GISTs rarely spread through lymphatics.

The surgical approach for GISTs varies by location and size (Fig. 65.7). Gastric GISTs are typically managed through partial gastrectomy, wedge resection, distal gastrectomy, or total gastrectomy, depending on the size and location of the tumor. Overall, though, total gastrectomy is rarely needed, especially if neoadjuvant imatinib is used. Small intestinal GISTs are typically managed through segmental resection. Duodenal GISTs present increased operative complexity. If possible, local resection should be performed, but in cases that are not amenable (i.e., ampullary involvement or adhesion to the pancreas), a pancreaticoduodenectomy may be necessary. In these cases, neoadjuvant therapy may help downsize the tumor and therefore the extent of the operation.[30]

Colorectal GISTs are typically managed through standard colectomy. Yet colonic GISTs are extremely rare. Unlike

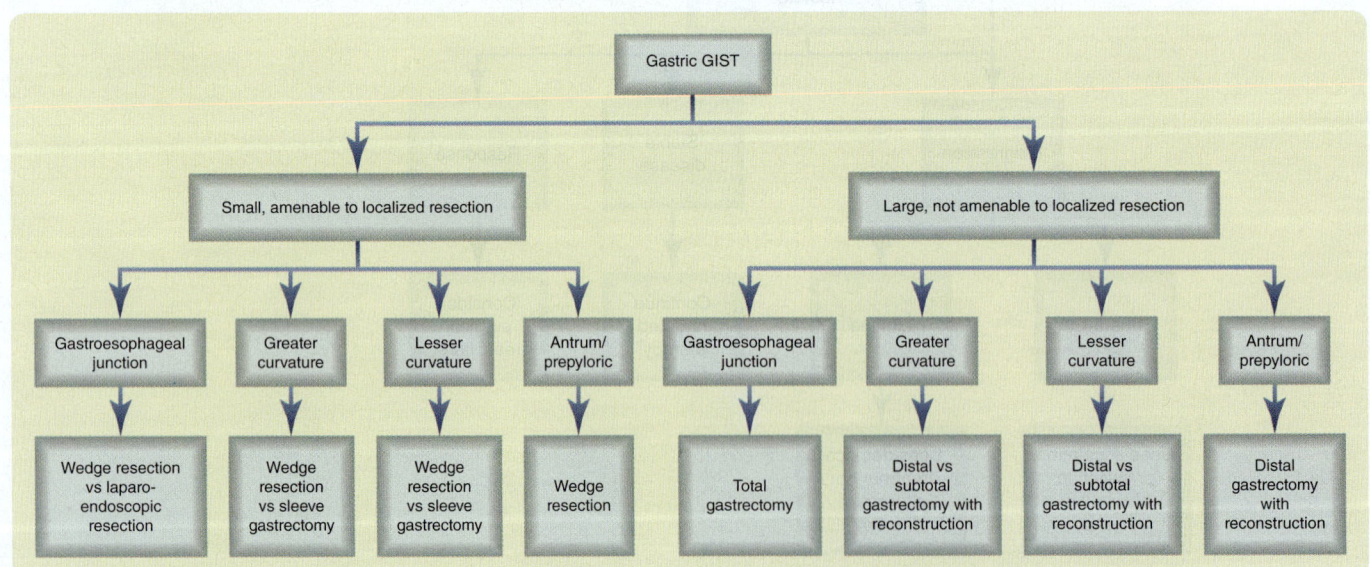

FIGURE 65.7 Surgical treatment of gastric gastrointestinal stromal tumors *(GISTs)*. The procedure chosen for resection of gastric GISTs depends on the size and location of the tumor. Smaller tumors are usually amenable to localized resection, whereas larger tumors may require more extensive procedures. Small tumors are most often managed by wedge resection or sleeve gastrectomy, depending on the location of the tumor. Tumors in the gastroesophageal junction may benefit from laparo-endoscopic resection. Larger tumors may need to be managed with distal or subtotal gastrectomy with subsequent reconstruction (e.g., Billroth I, Billroth II, or Roux-en-Y reconstruction). Large gastroesophageal junction or cardia tumors may require a total gastrectomy.

colorectal adenocarcinoma, mesenteric excision is not necessary because, as previously mentioned, GIST rarely spread through the lymphatic system. Rectal GISTs can be challenging to manage depending on the size and location of the tumor relative to the anal verge. Larger and more distal tumors may require more extensive surgery, including low anterior resection or even abdominoperineal resection. As with duodenal GISTs, neoadjuvant therapy should be considered, with the goal of shrinking the tumor to allow for location resection, including via a transanal approach.[30]

Esophageal GISTs and gastric GISTs near the gastroesophageal junction can also be difficult to manage because of the anatomy of the esophagus. Local resection can be attempted if the tumor is small and confined to the distal esophagus. However, for larger tumors, an esophagectomy may be necessary. Again, as with other GISTs in challenging locations, neoadjuvant therapy should be considered before surgical intervention.[30]

Resection of a GIST requires following the aforementioned oncologic principles. When technically feasible and safe, minimally invasive techniques (including laparoscopic and robotic) have equivalent outcomes to open surgical resection, but they typically result in lower morbidity and shorter hospital stays.[41] Depending on surgeon experience, minimally invasive techniques should be used for resection of localized GISTs.

Locally Advanced Disease

Traditionally, there was a long-held belief that GISTs only push against adjacent organs or structures but do not invade them. With increased experience, however, it was found that this is not always true. As with localized tumors, the goal in treatment of locally advanced GIST is R0 resection. But this is more difficult to achieve with larger tumors and/or those invading adjacent organs/structures. Therefore, to maximize the potential benefit of resection, neoadjuvant therapy with TKIs (e.g., imatinib) can be administered.[30] Neoadjuvant therapy will often shrink the tumor and allow downsizing of the tumor and often the scope of the operation. This is particularly important for tumors in difficult-to-access locations.

Patient-specific treatment that is known to be effective for the mutational status of the tumor should be used. It is critical to assess the mutational profile of the tumor when possible before initiating neoadjuvant therapy because not all GISTs are sensitive to imatinib treatment.[17,19] For example, *PDGFRA* D842V–mutant tumors have primary imatinib resistance and may instead benefit from treatment with avapritinib,[17,19,30] whereas other *PDGFRA* mutations are often sensitive to imatinib. The duration of neoadjuvant therapy before resection needs to be individualized. Most data support 6 months or more before resection because this can allow R0 resection in up to 80% of cases.[42,43] Patients should be serially monitored while undergoing neoadjuvant therapy. Resection can be considered when there is no further tumor shrinkage (i.e., serial scans show no substantial change in size) or when further tumor shrinkage will not affect the approach or morbidity of the operation.

Patients with non-*KIT/PDGFRA* mutations should undergo individualized assessment for neoadjuvant therapy. Neoadjuvant avapritinib can be considered for *PDGFRA* D842V mutations, NTRK-directed therapies can be considered for *NTRK* fusions, sunitinib or enrollment in clinical trials can be considered for SDH-deficient tumors, and BRAF-directed therapies (e.g., BRAF plus MEK inhibitors) can be considered for *BRAF* V600E mutations.[30]

Metastatic Disease

The role of surgery in metastatic and recurrent GIST is less clear. Before resection, patients should undergo treatment with TKI therapy that is targeted to the tumor's mutational profile.[30] Depending on response to neoadjuvant therapy, selected patients may be considered for cytoreductive surgery. These include patients with potentially resectable disease with treatment-responsive disease or stable disease. Those with unifocal progression may be considered for operation in select circumstances, whereas resection is generally not recommended in the setting of multifocal progression.[44,45] Nevertheless, there are no level 1 data proving that resection of metastatic GIST improves progression-free or overall survival (OS). Furthermore, patients offered surgical management for metastatic disease tend to have better outcomes when they are earlier in their disease course and on first- or second-line therapies rather than third-line or later treatments.

The goals of operative management are resection of the primary tumor and all known/visible metastatic disease. Cytoreduction provides the theoretical benefit of lowering the risk of tumor resistance to therapy and decreasing clonal heterogeneity. Conceptually, by decreasing the tumor burden and hence the number of cells exposed to therapy, there are fewer chances for a cell to develop resistance to the therapy and thus fewer chances for a tumor resistant to therapy to arise. Targeted therapy controls tumor growth in approximately 80% of patients, but complete response is uncommon. Moreover, most tumors eventually develop resistance.[46,47] As such, cytoreductive surgery theoretically may prolong long-term disease control.

Several studies have attempted to assess the efficacy of cytoreductive surgery in patients with metastatic disease. Because of poor accrual of patients, no randomized controlled trials have been completed. Nevertheless, the results of multiple retrospective studies showed promise that cytoreductive surgery may portend better disease control and longer OS in highly selected patients.[44,45] On the other hand, for patients who show poor response to targeted therapy, cytoreductive surgery does not appear to improve outcomes.[44,45] Therefore, surgery should be avoided in patients who demonstrate generalized tumor progression while receiving treatment with targeted therapy. For patients who do undergo cytoreductive surgery, systemic therapy should be continued indefinitely because interruption of therapy leads to rapid progression in most patients with advanced GIST.[48]

Medical Treatment

Systemic therapy for GISTs has evolved significantly over the past two decades. Since the discovery of oncogenic *KIT* mutations as a key driver of GIST, advances have been made in therapies targeting these mutations. Imatinib, the oldest and most studied of these agents, is an oral TKI that inhibits both the KIT and PDGFR RTKs. This small molecular inhibitor was originally developed to inhibit the BCR-ABL fusion protein found in chronic myelogenous leukemia (CML). Imatinib is thought to work as a competitive inhibitor of the ATP-binding domain of RTKs, ultimately inhibiting activation and downstream signaling (Fig. 65.8). Initially, this drug was approved to treat CML, and shortly thereafter, it was approved for treatment of GIST. Treatment with imatinib has shown remarkable responses in patients with GIST and is now used as the first-line agent for neoadjuvant therapy, adjuvant therapy, and metastatic disease. Since the discovery of imatinib, many other TKIs have been developed, including sunitinib, regorafenib, and ripretinib, among others.

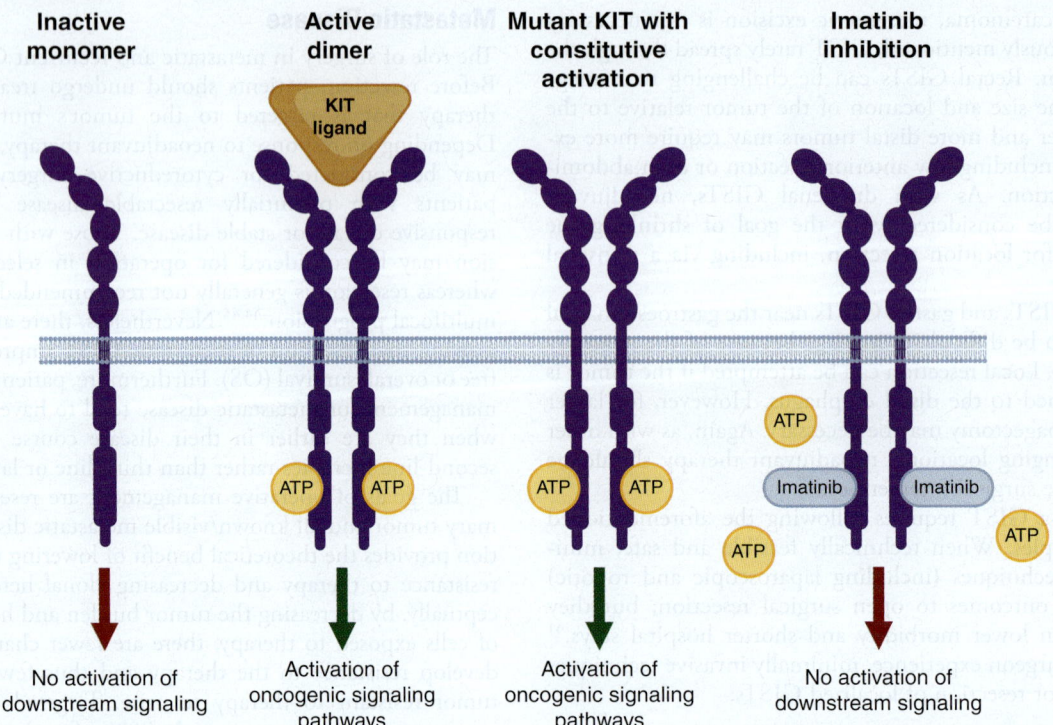

Inactive monomer	Active dimer	Mutant KIT with constitutive activation	Imatinib inhibition

FIGURE 65.8 Imatinib mechanism of action. Imatinib is an oral tyrosine kinase inhibitor that acts on both KIT and PDGFRA receptor tyrosine kinases (RTKs). Imatinib acts as a competitive inhibitor of the adenosine triphosphate *(ATP)*-binding domain, preventing ATP binding and autophosphorylation. The receptor is consequently rendered inactive and cannot activate oncogenic downstream signaling pathways.

Neoadjuvant Imatinib

For patients who present with locally advanced GIST, neoadjuvant therapy may allow a patient to avoid a complex multivisceral resection, decrease blood loss, decrease the scope or morbidity of an operation, or facilitate the resection of a previously unresectable tumor.[30] Additionally, neoadjuvant therapy may decrease the size of tumors in difficult-to-access locations, including the esophagus, duodenum, and rectum. However, before initiating neoadjuvant imatinib, the tumor mutational status should be assessed when feasible to tailor therapy as appropriate.

After starting neoadjuvant therapy, tumor response should be assessed with serial imaging every 8 to 12 weeks, although the first scan is often performed in approximately 3 weeks to assess for tumor response, such as changes in tumor perfusion or size. If the tumor responds to therapy, imatinib should be continued until tumor shrinkage is no longer observed or until further tumor shrinkage would no longer affect the scope or morbidity of the operation.[30] Typically, this period is 6 months or longer, depending on the individual patient's tumor response.[42,43] For patients with larger tumors, neoadjuvant therapy can continue for up to 10 to 12 months. Beyond 12 months, neoadjuvant therapy is controversial, and some data suggest that continuing neoadjuvant therapy for longer periods may increase the likelihood of recurrence.[49]

If feasible after completion of neoadjuvant therapy, the tumor should be resected. After resection, the patient should continue adjuvant imatinib therapy depending on the pretreatment risk of recurrence, as will be discussed later.[30,50,51] If the tumor is unresectable after neoadjuvant therapy, imatinib therapy should be continued.[30,48]

In the absence of molecular testing, which is not recommended, patients who show no response to imatinib therapy should be considered for second- or third-line therapy.[30] For patients with GIST who harbor *PDGFRA* D842V mutations, imatinib should be avoided.[17,19] These patients may proceed immediately to resection if the tumor is resectable. If not, neoadjuvant avapritinib can be considered.[30] Little evidence exists for the use of avapritinib in this clinical scenario. GISTs with other mutations should have treatment tailored to the specific mutational profile of the tumor.

Adjuvant Imatinib

After resection, patients with GIST are at risk for tumor recurrence. Multiple factors affect the risk of recurrence, including tumor size, tumor location, presence of tumor rupture, and mitotic index. In patients believed to be at high risk for tumor recurrence, adjuvant imatinib has been shown to improve recurrence-free survival (RFS) and OS.

ESTIMATING RISK OF RECURRENCE

Much work has been done in attempting to create a model that accurately estimates the risk of recurrence and identifies patients likely to benefit from adjuvant imatinib. Some of the most well-established models include the modified National Institutes of Health (NIH) consensus criteria, the Armed Forces Institute of Pathology (AFIP) prognostic model, the Memorial Sloan Kettering (or Gold) nomogram, and the Joensuu heatmaps (Table 65.2).[13,52–55]

The earliest model attempting to estimate the risk of recurrence in patients with GISTs was the NIH consensus criteria.

TABLE 65.2 Modified NIH Consensus Criteria

RISK CATEGORY	TUMOR SIZE (CM)	MITOTIC INDEX (PER 5 MM²)	PRIMARY TUMOR SITE
Very low	<2.0	≤5	Any
Low	2.1–5.0	≤5	Any
Intermediate	2.1–5.0	>5	Gastric
	<5.0	6–10	Any
	5.1–10.0	≤5	Gastric
High	Any	Any	Tumor rupture
	>10 cm	Any	Any
	Any	>10	Any
	>5.0	>5	Any
	2.1–5.0	>5	Nongastric
	5.1–10.0	≤5	Nongastric

NIH, National Institutes of Health.
Adapted from Joensuu H. Risk stratification of patients diagnosed with gastrointestinal stromal tumor. *Hum Pathol*. 2008;39(10):1411-1419.

Created in 2002, this model categorized tumors into four broad categories: very low risk, low risk, medium risk, and high risk. Categorization of tumors was determined solely by tumor size and mitotic rate.[13] This model was later revised in 2008 with the inclusion of the presence of tumor rupture during resection, and it is now known as the *modified NIH consensus criteria*.[53]

After the NIH model, the AFIP prognostic model was developed. This model was created using data from a cohort of 1900 patients and estimates the risk of recurrence through a combination of tumor size, mitotic rate, and tumor location. This model categorizes tumors into five broad categories: no risk, very low risk, low risk, intermediate risk, and high risk.[52]

Although these models categorize tumors into broad categories of risk, Gold et al. attempted to quantitatively estimate the risk of recurrence. The Gold nomogram uses tumor size, tumor location, and mitotic index to quantitatively estimate the risk of recurrence. This model was created to predict the probabilities of 2- and 5-year RFS using two independent GIST cohorts.[55]

To better estimate recurrence risk, the Joensuu heatmap recognizes that the relationship between mitotic count, tumor size, and risk of recurrence is nonlinear. Therefore, they developed heatmaps to estimate recurrence risk based on this nonlinear relationship. These heatmaps also integrate data regarding tumor location and presence of tumor rupture during resection to more accurately reflect each clinical scenario.[54]

Although multiple methods for estimating risk of recurrence have been developed over time, ultimately, these prognostication tools show relatively similar performance.[54] Because many of these tools are built on similar data (i.e., tumor size and mitotic rate), little additional information about the underlying tumor biology can be inferred by the model. With the advent of NGS, additional information pertaining to each patient's tumor biology is now available and may provide future insights to estimate the risk of tumor recurrence more accurately.

Nevertheless, although the specific criteria for determining which patients will benefit most from adjuvant imatinib therapy have not been fully established, patients at high risk for recurrence often benefit from adjuvant imatinib therapy. Clinicians should carefully weigh the risks and benefits of initiating adjuvant therapy, and decisions should be individualized for each patient.

TREATMENT EFFICACY

The benefit of adjuvant imatinib therapy has been assessed in multiple phase III trials, most notably in the American College of Surgeons Oncology Group (ACOSOG) Z9001 and Scandinavian Sarcoma Group (SSG) XVIII trials.[50,51]

The ACOSOG Z9001 trial was a multicenter, double-blind trial that assessed the efficacy of imatinib in 713 patients with immunohistochemically KIT-positive GISTs of 3 cm or larger. Patients were randomized to receive either adjuvant imatinib for 1 year or placebo after grossly negative resection. The primary end point of the trial was RFS. The trial was stopped early after patients in the imatinib arm were found to have significantly longer RFS. At a median follow-up of 20 months, 1-year RFS was 98% in the imatinib group versus 83% in the control group. There was no difference in OS. Subgroup analysis showed improved outcomes in all risk categories of the imatinib group but greatest benefit in high-risk groups.[51]

The SSG XVIII trial was a prospective, open-label trial that enrolled 397 patients with high-risk GIST defined by modified consensus criteria (i.e., tumor size >10 cm; mitotic index >10 mitoses per 5 mm²; tumor size >5 cm and mitotic index >5 mitoses per 5 mm²; or tumor rupture). Patients were randomized to receive adjuvant imatinib for either 1 or 3 years after resection. The primary end point compared was RFS. At a median follow-up of 54 months, the 3-year imatinib arm demonstrated a 5-year RFS of 66%, compared with 48% for the 1-year arm. Five-year OS was improved in the 3-year imatinib arm, with an OS of 92% versus 82%.[50]

After the SSG XVIII trial, the Postresection Evaluation of Recurrence-Free Survival for Gastrointestinal Stromal Tumors With 5 Years of Adjuvant Imatinib (PERSIST-5) trial attempted to evaluate whether 5 years of adjuvant imatinib provided additional improvement of outcomes in patients. Although this study lacked a control arm, it showed that of the 46 patients who completed 5 years of adjuvant imatinib, no patient with imatinib-sensitive mutations experienced tumor recurrence.[56]

Together, these trials not only definitively establish the efficacy of adjuvant imatinib therapy after GIST resection but also demonstrate that adjuvant treatment for at least 3 years postoperatively is beneficial in patients with GISTs at high risk for recurrence. It is now standard practice to administer adjuvant imatinib for 3 years postoperatively to patients at high risk for recurrence, and current guidelines additionally recommend consideration of adjuvant imatinib for patients at intermediate risk for recurrence with known sensitive mutations.[30] In clinical practice, physicians will often recommend lifelong adjuvant therapy in high-risk patients to minimize the risk of recurrence, but this has not been studied in clinical trials.

Targeted Therapy for Metastatic Disease

The introduction of targeted therapies has revolutionized management of metastatic GIST. Imatinib is now considered standard first-line therapy and has shown astounding efficacy. Before initiating therapy with imatinib, the mutational profile of the tumor should be assessed, and the choice of therapy should be individualized depending on the mutational status. Patients with mutations known to be resistant to imatinib should receive mutation-specific therapy or be referred to a specialized care center for consideration of enrollment into clinical trials.

TREATMENT WITH TYROSINE KINASE INHIBITORS

For patients with metastatic *KIT-* or *PDGFRA*-mutant GISTs, treatment with imatinib can induce rapid, profound, and sustained clinical responses. In one of the first trials assessing the effect of imatinib on patients with advanced GISTs, over 80% of patients had either a partial response or stable disease when treated with imatinib.[57] In a long-term follow-up analysis of this study, patients treated with imatinib had a median OS of 57 months at a median follow-up time of 63 months.[58] This represents a dramatic difference from the standard of care at the time, for which patients with advanced GISTs had an estimated median OS of 20 months.

Although responses can be dramatic, complete responses are rare.[57,58] Many patients who demonstrate initial response to therapy subsequently develop resistance to imatinib and progress. After initiation of imatinib therapy, median time to progression is estimated at 2 to 3 years.[59,60] If patients do not experience progression, treatment should continue indefinitely because interrupting treatment leads to disease progression.[48]

Response should be monitored using serial cross-sectional imaging (i.e., CT or MRI) every 8 to 12 weeks. Several criteria exist for evaluating tumor response, including the Response Evaluation Criteria in Solid Tumors (RECIST) criteria, which are based on tumor measurements, and the Choi criteria, which measure tumor density in addition to tumor dimensions.[61,62] The Choi criteria have been found to better correlate with disease-specific survival and tumor progression.[61,62]

Effect of Dose

The standard dose of imatinib is 400 mg. Two randomized controlled trials have assessed the efficacy of higher imatinib doses.[59,60] One trial found no difference in OS or progression-free survival (PFS) for higher doses of imatinib, whereas the second trial found a significantly higher PFS rate with higher imatinib doses at a 25-month median follow-up. However, this difference disappeared with longer median follow-up times.[59,60] No difference in OS was observed in either trial. A subsequent meta-analysis of these two trials demonstrated that the subgroup of patients with *KIT* exon 9 mutations had significantly longer PFS and response rates on higher doses of imatinib.[63] Given these data, patients with *KIT* exon 9 mutations should receive 800 mg imatinib.

Treatment for *PDGFRA* D842V Mutations

Certain mutations confer primary resistance to imatinib. Most notably, tumors with a *PDGFRA* D842V mutation are often resistant to imatinib therapy.[17,19] For these patients, avapritinib is effective as an initial therapy.[64] Avapritinib is a selective TKI that targets both KIT and PDGFRA. The best current evidence for avapritinib is an open-label, phase I clinical trial that examined 56 patients with *PDGFRA* D842V mutations.[64] At a median follow-up of 28 months, 1-year PFS was 83%. Moreover, 88% of patients demonstrated either complete or partial response to therapy during the initial trial, which rose to 91% on long-term follow-up analysis.[64] Although avapritinib tends to cause more significant medication-related side effects compared with imatinib (e.g., anemia, edema, and hyperbilirubinemia; CNS toxicity, including cognitive dysfunction, memory impairment, confusional state, amnesia, and encephalopathy), this drug nevertheless represents a promising medication for patients with *PDGFRA* D842V mutations.

Treatment of Refractory Disease

Some patients either do not respond to imatinib therapy or develop secondary resistance after initially responding to the therapy. Resistance to imatinib in *KIT*-mutant GIST is most commonly a result of acquired mutations affecting the ATP-binding pocket (exon 13/14) or AL (exon 17/18) of KIT.[17] Therapeutic options for these patients include dose escalation or transition to sunitinib, the standard second-line agent for patients with tumors refractory to imatinib. Sunitinib is a TKI that shows activity against both KIT and PDGFR as well as VEGF receptors. The efficacy of sunitinib was demonstrated in an international phase III clinical trial.[65] This study found that at a median follow-up of 42 months, patients in the sunitinib group had a median PFS of 27 weeks compared with 6 weeks in the placebo group. A total of 7% of patients demonstrated a partial response, and 58% of patients had stable disease.[65] Unfortunately, disease progression occurred at a median of approximately 6 months.

For patients with disease refractory to sunitinib, the standard third-line treatment is regorafenib. Regorafenib also targets KIT, PDGFR, and VEGF receptors. The efficacy of regorafenib was evaluated in a double-blind placebo-controlled phase III trial in 199 patients with GIST refractory to sunitinib.[66] Compared with placebo, patients receiving regorafenib had a PFS of approximately 19 weeks versus 4 weeks. Patients receiving regorafenib showed a partial response rate of 4.5% and stable disease in 71.4%.[66] Median time to progression was approximately 5 months.

In cases where imatinib, sunitinib, and regorafenib all prove ineffective, therapy with other TKIs may be attempted. Ripretinib is now approved as fourth-line therapy.[30] It is a promising new TKI that acts as a switch-control inhibitor to stabilize target kinases in an inactive form. Ripretinib efficacy was evaluated in a phase III trial in 129 patients with GIST refractory to or intolerant of imatinib, sunitinib, and regorafenib.[67] At a median follow-up of 6 months, patients receiving ripretinib had a median PFS of 6.3 months and a median OS of 15 months, compared with 1 month and 6 months with placebo, respectively.[67] In the ripretinib-treated group, 9% of patients demonstrated partial response, and 47% of patients demonstrated stable disease. Ripretinib was later assessed in a phase III trial for superiority versus sunitinib as a second-line therapy for GISTs refractory to imatinib.[68] This trial found that ripretinib is not superior to sunitinib in PFS, but ripretinib showed improved patient tolerability. Based on these results, sunitinib continues to be regarded as the standard-of-care second-line therapy for patients with GISTs resistant to imatinib.[30]

Even with the plethora of available TKIs, treatment of refractory disease represents a difficult clinical problem. As the disease progresses, fewer medications are available for treatment, and PFS typically decreases with each new medication.

TREATMENT FOR TUMORS POORLY RESPONSIVE TO TRADITIONAL TYROSINE KINASE INHIBITORS

SDH-deficient tumors represent an important subset of tumors that do not harbor *KIT* or *PDGFRA* mutations. Because of their unique biology, SDH-deficient tumors often respond poorly to imatinib. Optimal treatment for patients with SDH-deficient tumors has not been established, although some patients may respond to sunitinib or regorafenib.[20] There is an ongoing need for investigation into therapeutic options for these patients. Thus, patients should be referred to a specialized care center.

Like SDH-deficient tumors, tumors that harbor other mutations have distinct clinical management. Treatment should be individualized and guided by mutational status. For example, treatment with larotrectinib or entrectinib may be effective for patients with *ETV6-NTRK* mutations, and treatment with dabrafenib and trametinib may be effective for patients with *BRAF* V600E–mutant GIST.

Surveillance

There are no evidence-based guidelines for GIST surveillance after resection. GISTs most often spread hematogenously or directly into the abdominal cavity, and relapses most frequently occur in the liver and/or peritoneum. The most recent NCCN guidelines recommend serial imaging every 3 to 6 months for 3 to 5 years after resection, followed by annual evaluation indefinitely.[30] ESMO guidelines recommend a similar pattern of surveillance for patients at high risk for recurrence but advocate for individualized surveillance plans for patients at lower risk of recurrence.[36] For patients with low-risk or very low-risk tumors, the utility of routine surveillance is not as clear, but follow-up surveillance imaging should be considered.[36]

CONCLUSION

GIST represents an important disease for which key insights into tumor biology have led to remarkable advances in treatment. After the early discovery that most GISTs demonstrate KIT overexpression, genomic studies have revealed a complex and varied mutational landscape. *KIT*-mutant GISTs predominate, but many other subtypes exist, including GISTs with *PDGFRA*, *SDH*, and *NF1* mutations, among others. Surgery remains a cornerstone in the treatment of GISTs and has now become possible in previously unresectable tumors through the administration of neoadjuvant therapy. Additionally, PFS in patients after surgery has been revolutionized through the administration of adjuvant imatinib therapy. Amazingly, patients with metastatic disease have shown profound and sometimes durable responses to targeted therapy, raising questions about the optimal role of surgical management in these individuals. Nevertheless, much remains to be discovered with regard to both the biology and clinical management of GIST.

SELECTED REFERENCES

Corless CL, Barnett CM, Heinrich MC. Gastrointestinal stromal tumours: origin and molecular oncology. *Nat Rev Cancer.* 2011;11(12):865-878.

> In this review, Corless et al. highlight the most common mutations underlying GIST and elucidate the molecular mechanisms driving tumor biology.

Dematteo RP, Ballman KV, Antonescu CR, et al. Adjuvant imatinib mesylate after resection of localised, primary gastrointestinal stromal tumour: a randomised, double-blind, placebo-controlled trial. *Lancet.* 2009;373:1097-1104.

> In the ACOSOG Z9001 landmark trial, DeMatteo et al. demonstrate that patients with GISTs of 3 cm or larger have improved RFS with adjuvant imatinib therapy and that patients at high risk for recurrence derive the greatest benefit from therapy.

Demetri GD, von Mehren M, Blanke CD, et al. Efficacy and safety of imatinib mesylate in advanced gastrointestinal stromal tumors. *N Engl J Med.* 2002;347(7):472-480.

> In this landmark phase II trial, Demetri et al. demonstrate for the first time the remarkable efficacy of imatinib in treating patients with GIST.

Joensuu H, Eriksson M, Sundby Hall K, et al. One vs three years of adjuvant imatinib for operable gastrointestinal stromal tumor: a randomized trial. *JAMA.* 2012;307(12):1265-1272.

> In the SSG XVIII landmark trial, Joensuu et al. show that patients at high risk for recurrence have improved OS and RFS when treated with adjuvant imatinib for 3 years versus 1 year postoperatively.

Joensuu H, Vehtari A, Riihimäki J, et al. Risk of recurrence of gastrointestinal stromal tumour after surgery: an analysis of pooled population-based cohorts. *Lancet Oncol.* 2012;13(3):265-274.

> In this article, Joensuu et al. discuss the different methodologies for estimating risk of recurrence in patients with operable GIST, compare predictions from each method, and develop the Joensuu heatmap method.

The full reference list appears on Elsevier eBooks+.

Benign Diseases of Head and Neck

Sepehr Shabani and Orly M. Coblens

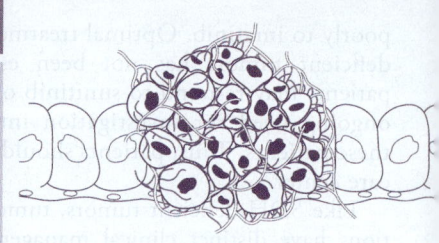

▶ **Please access Elsevier eBooks+ to view the videos for this chapter.**

NORMAL ANATOMY AND HISTOLOGY

The normal histology of the upper aerodigestive tract varies based on the cells, tissues, and function required of each site. The upper aerodigestive tract can be conceptualized to start with the openings to the nose, mouth, and throat. The nose consists of the nasal vestibule, nasal cavity, and nasopharynx. The mouth is anatomically characterized by the red lip and the oral cavity up to the oropharynx. The throat is also called the pharynx, which consists of oropharynx, hypopharynx, and larynx.

The shape of the nasal vestibule is maintained by underlying septal, upper lateral, and lower lateral cartilages, and externally, it is a cutaneous structure lined by keratinizing squamous epithelium that has sebaceous and sweat glands as well as hair follicles. The limen nasi, or mucocutaneous junction, is where the epithelium changes to a ciliated pseudostratified columnar (respiratory) epithelium that lines the sinus and nasal cavities except for the olfactory epithelium at the roof of the nasal cavity. The olfactory epithelium is a specialized tissue composed of supporting cells and bipolar olfactory neural cells with odorant receptors on cilia that face the nasal cavity and axons that coalesce to form the olfactory nerve (cranial nerve [CN] I). It passes through the cribriform plate on the deep surface within the cranium. As with the nasal cavity, the paranasal sinuses are also lined by respiratory epithelium; however, it tends to be thinner and less vascular than that of the nasal cavity.

The nasal cavity begins at the anterior nasal vestibules and contains the bony and cartilaginous nasal septum, structures of the lateral nasal wall, and the olfactory cleft. The paranasal sinuses are divided into paired maxillary and ethmoid sinuses and the central sphenoid and frontal sinuses, which are usually completely separated by septae into right and left halves. Structures of the lateral nasal wall include the inferior, middle, and superior turbinates and the superior, middle, and inferior meatus, named for the turbinate

superior to them. The maxillary, anterior ethmoid, and frontal sinuses drain via the infundibulum into the middle meatus, whereas the nasolacrimal duct drains into the inferior meatus.

The four paired paranasal sinuses lie lateral and superior to the nasal cavity. The frontal sinuses are the most anterior and superior air cavities that lie within the frontal bone and drain into the nasal cavity via the frontal recesses into the middle meatus. The ethmoid sinuses are a honeycomb-like bony labyrinth located medial to the orbits and inferior to the anterior cranial fossa. The lamina papyracea is the thin lateral wall of the ethmoid sinus that constitutes the medial wall of the orbit. The anterior and posterior ethmoid cavities are separated by the basal lamella of the middle turbinate, with the anterior ethmoids draining into the middle meatus and the posterior ethmoids draining via the sphenoethmoidal recess into the posterior nasal cavity. The sphenoid sinus lies in the middle of the sphenoid bone and is the most posterior and central of the sinuses. The vital structures of the optic nerves, carotid arteries, and cavernous sinuses are immediately adjacent to the lateral walls of the sphenoid sinus, whereas the sella turcica and optic chiasm are immediately superior to the central and posterior superior sinus roof. Additionally, the very lateral boundaries of the sphenoid sinus are adjacent to the second division of the trigeminal nerves (V2) and the vidian nerves. The maxillary sinuses drain into the middle meatus and are bound posteriorly by the pterygopalatine fossa, laterally by the zygomatic process of the maxilla, superiorly by the orbital floor, and inferiorly by the palate.

The nasopharyngeal lining varies from squamous to respiratory epithelium in an inconsistent manner. The adenoidal pad, which lies in the nasopharynx, is lymphoid tissue containing germinal centers without capsules or sinusoids and, like the palatine and lingual tonsils, contains a specialized lymphoepithelium with a discontinuous basement membrane and an intermixing of stromal, immune, and epithelial cells. The oral cavity is lined by nonkeratinized, stratified squamous epithelium with minor salivary glands throughout the submucosa and within the muscular tissue of the tongue. The oral cavity transitions to the oropharynx at the junction between the hard and soft palates and at the anterior tonsillar pillar. Waldeyer's ring is formed by lymphoid tissues of the bilateral palatine tonsils, adenoids, lingual tonsils, and adjacent submucosal lymphatics. Like the adenoids, the palatine tonsils contain germinal centers without capsules or sinusoids, but, in contrast to the adenoids, the tonsils have crypts lined by stratified squamous epithelium with the lymphoepithelial cells residing at the base of the crypts. The junction between the oropharynx and hypopharynx is a horizontal line at the top of the hyoid bone. The hypopharynx is lined by nonkeratinizing, stratified squamous epithelium. Seromucous glands are found throughout the submucosa of the hypopharynx, in the lower two-thirds of the epiglottis, and in the potential space between the true and false vocal folds known as the *ventricle.* The larynx consists of the supraglottis, glottis, and immediate subglottis. The lining of the larynx transitions from nonkeratinizing, stratified squamous epithelium of the epiglottis and true vocal folds to pseudostratified, ciliated respiratory epithelium of the false vocal fold, ventricle, and subglottis. The thyroid, cricoid, and arytenoid cartilages are composed of hyaline cartilage, whereas the epiglottis, cuneiform, and corniculate cartilages are composed of elastic-type cartilage.

The external ear is a cutaneous structure supported by cartilage that is lined with keratinizing squamous epithelium and associated adnexal structures. The external third of the external auditory canal is unique in that it contains modified apocrine glands that produce cerumen. The middle ear is lined with respiratory epithelium and houses three ossicles, which are important for conducting sound.

Numerous noncancerous changes in squamous epithelium can be seen in the upper aerodigestive tract. *Leukoplakia* describes any white mucosal lesion, and *erythroplakia* describes any red mucosal lesion. Both are clinical descriptions and should not be used as diagnostic terms. Erythroplakia is more concerning than leukoplakia because it is more often associated with an underlying malignant lesion and has increased malignant potential. *Hyperplasia* refers to thickening of the epithelium, whereas *parakeratosis* is an abnormal presence of nuclei in the keratin layers, and *dyskeratosis* refers to any abnormal keratinization of epithelial cells and is found in dysplastic lesions.

Oral Cavity

There are seven subsites to the oral cavity (Fig. 66.1), and each should be understood separately because the pathologic as well as surgical and reconstructive considerations can be quite distinct.

Lip

The lip starts at the junction of the facial skin and vermillion border and ends at the point where the upper and lower lips meet when the mouth is closed. The oral commissures are the lateral most aspects of the lip and are important anatomic considerations because size and position are important for oral competence and mouth opening.

Oral Tongue

The oral tongue extends from the floor of mouth to the circumvallate papillae posteriorly. The base of tongue (and lingual tonsils) is not anatomically part of the oral tongue or the oral cavity. The tongue is a muscular organ made of four intrinsic muscles and four extrinsic muscles, which are anchored to bone and/or aponeurosis. Lesions in the tongue can be described by location, including lateral border, dorsal tongue, or ventral tongue. The oral tongue plays a critical function in speech articulation and the oral phase of swallowing. If bilateral lingual arteries and/or hypoglossal nerves are sacrificed as part of tumor extirpation, vascularity and function will be compromised; therefore, if the tumor extent allows, effort should

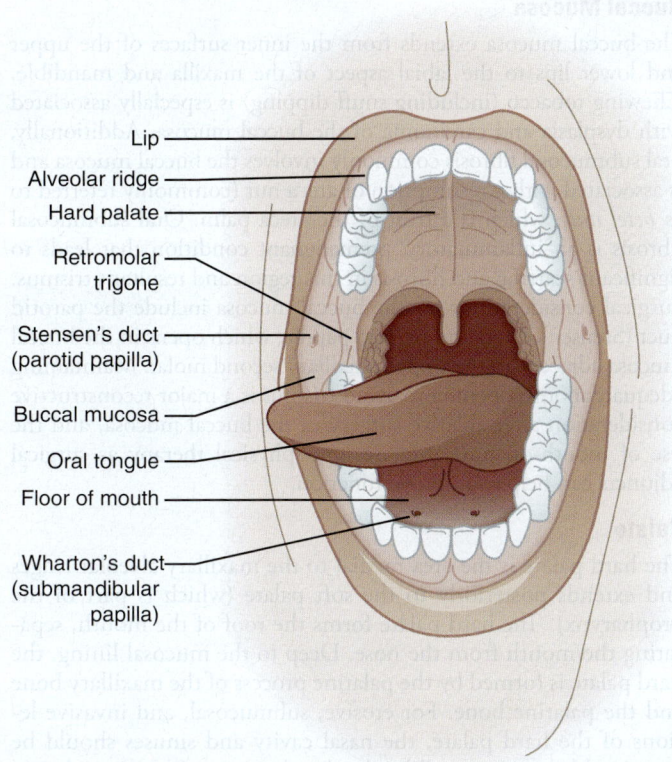

FIGURE 66.1 Anatomy of oral cavity and its subsites.

Labels: Lip; Alveolar ridge; Hard palate; Retromolar trigone; Stensen's duct (parotid papilla); Buccal mucosa; Oral tongue; Floor of mouth; Wharton's duct (submandibular papilla)

be made to maintain the neurovascular bundle to one side of the tongue. If total glossectomy is required for adequate tumor extirpation, the risk of aspiration is greatly increased, and patients may require a total laryngectomy to avoid recurrent aspiration pneumonia. Reconstruction after glossectomy considers optimizing tongue mobility for speech and swallowing, maintenance of adequate oral bulk for propulsion of food boluses, and minimizing the risk of aspiration. In cases where the extrinsic tongue muscles are separated from the hyoid bone, a hyoid and/or laryngeal suspension procedure should be considered to decrease risk of aspiration.

Floor of the Mouth

The floor of the mouth extends from the lingual surface of the mandible to the ventral tongue anteriorly and to the glossotonsillar sulcus (or anterior tonsillar pillars) posteriorly. The left and right sides are separated by the lingual frenulum, and just lateral to the frenulum on each side is the papilla of the submandibular duct (Wharton's duct). The submandibular duct papilla should be cannulated and protected in surgeries involving the floor of mouth whenever possible, and redirection with sialodochoplasty can be performed to maintain submandibular gland salivary flow. The submandibular duct in the floor of mouth is also the most common site of salivary stones, which can oftentimes be successfully removed endoscopically. In addition, the lingual nerve (a branch of trigeminal V3 cranial nerve) travels in the floor of mouth quite superficially and is crossed by the submandibular duct. Finally, the sublingual gland lies in the floor of mouth and can be the source of a ranula (a fluid-containing cyst that forms in the mouth under the tongue and can protrude into the neck) or malignancy. The floor of the mouth plays an important role in separating the tongue from the mandible, which is necessary for tongue mobility and a major consideration in oral cavity reconstruction.

Buccal Mucosa

The buccal mucosa extends from the inner surfaces of the upper and lower lips to the labial aspect of the maxilla and mandible. Chewing tobacco (including snuff dipping) is especially associated with dysplasia and carcinoma of the buccal mucosa. Additionally, oral submucosal fibrosis commonly involves the buccal mucosa and is associated with consumption of areca nut (commonly referred to as *betel nut*), which is a fruit of the areca palm. Oral submucosal fibrosis is an inflammatory, premalignant condition that leads to significant scarring and fibrosis in this region and resultant trismus. Surgical considerations for the buccal mucosa include the parotid duct (Stensen's duct) and parotid papilla, which opens in the buccal mucosa adjacent to the upper/maxillary second molar. Maintaining adequate mouth opening to avoid trismus is a major reconstructive consideration after ablative surgery of the buccal mucosa, and the use of mouth-opening exercises and physical therapy as surgical adjuncts can help to improve function.

Palate

The hard palate is the area medial to the maxillary alveolar ridges and extends posteriorly to the soft palate (which is part of the oropharynx). The hard palate forms the roof of the mouth, separating the mouth from the nose. Deep to the mucosal lining, the hard palate is formed by the palatine process of the maxillary bone and the palatine bone. For erosive, submucosal, and invasive lesions of the hard palate, the nasal cavity and sinuses should be examined because a small hard palate lesion could be just the tip of more substantial minor salivary gland, nasal, or paranasal sinus pathology. For example, in immunocompromised patients, invasive fungal sinusitis can present as a palatal erosion, and although not a cancer, it carries a high mortality and must be diagnosed and treated expeditiously. There are several benign conditions of the palate, with some that mimic a mass or cancer. Torus palatini is a common and benign bone growth in the center hard palate, which only requires surgical removal if it interferes with function, such as adequate fitting of upper dentures. Necrotizing sialometaplasia is a self-limited ulcerative inflammatory lesion of minor salivary glands that can mimic carcinoma on physical examination and requires clinical suspicion for appropriate diagnosis and avoidance of inappropriate treatment.

Tumors of the hard palate can arise from the stratified squamous mucosa, with the most frequent malignancy being squamous cell carcinoma (SCC), or from minor salivary glands. Because of the thick mucoperichondrium that is fixed to the bone, hard palate malignancies typically require removal of bone for adequate margin, and surgical approaches include infrastructure maxillectomy or total maxillectomy, depending on extent of tumor.

Alveolus

The alveolus (or alveolar ridge) and the accompanying gingiva extend from the gingivobuccal sulcus laterally to the floor of mouth and hard palate and make up the dental surfaces of the maxilla and mandible. SCC is the most common malignancy of the alveolus and is much more common at the lower gingiva. Upper gingival primaries often extend onto the hard palate, and many surgical considerations are the same for both. Adequate tumor resection requires resection of the alveolar ridge mucosa and underlying periosteum. The periosteum of the mandible is a strong tumor barrier, and tumors that abut the bone may be resected along with the adjacent periosteum only. Tumors adherent to the periosteum should undergo excision with at least a marginal mandibulectomy, which involves resection of the superior or

inner cortical portions of the mandible, with preservation of a continuous rim. If there is more than superficial cortical erosion of the mandible, the marrow space is at risk of harboring malignancy, and thus, a segmental mandibulectomy is required for adequate margin control. In many cases of alveolar primary tumors, dental extraction is required for both exposure and osteotomies. Reconstructive considerations of the alveolus include maintaining tongue mobility if adjacent floor of the mouth is also resected, vestibule height if adjacent buccal mucosa/inner lip is resected, and dental restoration with prosthesis or implants if possible.

Retromolar Trigone

The retromolar trigone is the region defined by the ascending ramus of the mandible, starting on each side just posterior to the last molar tooth and ending adjacent to the tuberosity of the maxilla. Numerous adjacent subsites of the oral cavity (buccal mucosa, upper and lower alveolar ridge) and oropharynx (anterior tonsil pillar and soft palate) are immediately adjacent to the retromolar trigone, making exact identification of the primary site difficult. In addition, the attached gingiva in this region is extremely thin, and the inferior alveolar nerve enters the mandible through the mandibular foramen near this region of the mandible. For these reasons, tumors in the retromolar trigone have a higher propensity for bone invasion, and the inferior alveolar nerve is at greater risk when performing marginal mandibulectomy in this region.

Oropharynx

Anatomic borders of the oropharynx include the circumvallate papillae anteriorly, plane of the superior surface of the soft palate superiorly, plane of the hyoid bone inferiorly, pharyngeal constrictors laterally and posteriorly, and medial aspect of the mandible laterally. Subsites within the oropharynx include the base of the tongue, inferior surface of the soft palate and uvula, anterior and posterior tonsillar pillars, glossotonsillar sulci, pharyngeal tonsils, and lateral and posterior pharyngeal walls. There are very few benign pathologies within this tissue site—most pathologies consist of malignancies that require treatment.

Hypopharynx

The hypopharynx is posterior and lateral to the larynx and extends inferiorly from the horizontal plane of the top of the hyoid bone to a horizontal plane extending posteriorly from the inferior border of the cricoid cartilage. The hypopharynx is composed of three distinct subsites and includes the bilateral pyriform sinuses, posterior hypopharyngeal wall, and postcricoid space. The postcricoid area extends inferiorly from the two arytenoid cartilages of the larynx to the inferior border of the cricoid cartilage, connecting the pyriform sinuses and forming the anterior hypopharyngeal wall. The pyriform sinuses are inverted, pyramid-shaped potential spaces medial to the thyroid lamina; they begin at the pharyngoepiglottic folds and extend to the cervical esophagus at the inferior border of the cricoid cartilage. Again, very few benign pathologies exist in this region.

Larynx

The larynx serves critical functions for breathing, airway protection during swallowing, and voice. The normal functions of the larynx are to provide airway patency, protect the tracheobronchial tree from aspiration, provide resistance for Valsalva maneuvers and coughing, and facilitate phonation. To understand the pathology and surgical approaches to the larynx, thorough knowledge of the 3D anatomy of the larynx and its subsites is needed (Fig. 66.2). Using the cartilage framework of

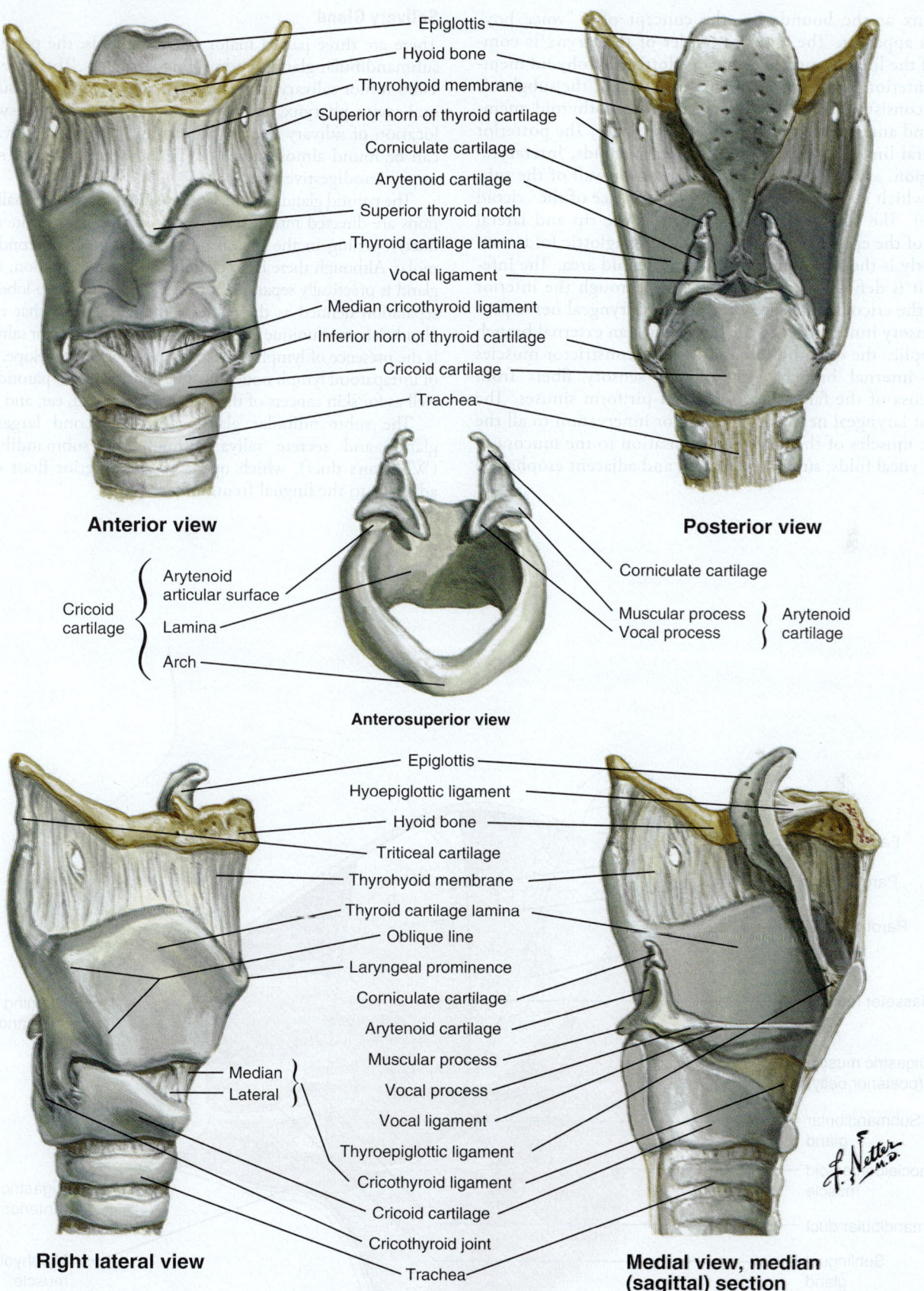

Anterior view

- Epiglottis
- Hyoid bone
- Thyrohyoid membrane
- Superior horn of thyroid cartilage
- Corniculate cartilage
- Arytenoid cartilage
- Superior thyroid notch
- Thyroid cartilage lamina
- Vocal ligament
- Median cricothyroid ligament
- Inferior horn of thyroid cartilage
- Cricoid cartilage
- Trachea

Posterior view

- Corniculate cartilage
- Muscular process } Arytenoid
- Vocal process } cartilage

Cricoid cartilage {
- Arytenoid articular surface
- Lamina
- Arch

Anterosuperior view

Right lateral view

- Epiglottis
- Hyoepiglottic ligament
- Hyoid bone
- Triticeal cartilage
- Thyrohyoid membrane
- Thyroid cartilage lamina
- Oblique line
- Laryngeal prominence
- Corniculate cartilage
- Arytenoid cartilage
- Muscular process
- Vocal process
- Vocal ligament
- Thyroepiglottic ligament
- Cricothyroid ligament
- Cricoid cartilage
- Cricothyroid joint
- Trachea

Median }
Lateral }

Medial view, median (sagittal) section

FIGURE 66.2 Framework anatomy of larynx.

the larynx as the boundaries, the concept of a "voice box" becomes apparent. The anterior border of the larynx is composed of the lingual surface of the epiglottis, thyrohyoid membrane, anterior commissure, and anterior wall of the subglottis (which consists of the thyroid cartilage, cricothyroid membrane, and anterior arch of the cricoid cartilage). The posterior and lateral limits of the larynx are the arytenoids, interarytenoid region, aryepiglottic folds, and posterior wall of the subglottis (which is the mucosa covering the surface of the cricoid cartilage). The superior limit anteriorly is the tip and lateral borders of the epiglottis, laterally is the aryepiglottic folds, and posteriorly is the arytenoids and interarytenoid area. The inferior limit is defined as the plane passing through the inferior edge of the cricoid cartilage. The superior laryngeal nerve provides sensory innervation to the larynx with an external branch that supplies the cricothyroid and inferior constrictor muscles and an internal branch with afferent sensory fibers from the mucosa of the false vocal folds and piriform sinuses. The recurrent laryngeal nerve supplies motor innervation to all the intrinsic muscles of the larynx and sensation to the mucosa of the true vocal folds, subglottic region, and adjacent esophageal mucosa.

Salivary Gland

There are three paired major salivary glands: the parotid glands, submandibular glands, and sublingual glands. There are also up to 1000 minor salivary glands located submucosally throughout the oral cavity, pharynx, and larynx (Fig. 66.3). Given the widespread location of salivary glands, tumors and lesions of salivary glands can be found almost anywhere in the head and neck region and upper aerodigestive tract.

The parotid glands are the largest salivary glands, and salivary secretions are directed into the oral cavity via the parotid duct (Stensen's duct) opening in the buccal mucosa next to the second maxillary molar. Although there is no capsular or fascial separation, the parotid gland is practically separated into superficial and deep lobes, with the separation defined as the plane of the facial nerve that runs in the gland. A feature unique to the parotid among the major salivary glands is the presence of lymph nodes within the fascial envelope. Treatment of intraparotid lymph nodes must be considered for parotid cancers as well as for skin cancers of the face, temple, eyelid, ear, and scalp.

The submandibular glands are the second largest salivary glands and secrete saliva through the submandibular duct (Wharton's duct), which opens in the anterior floor of mouth, adjacent to the lingual frenulum.

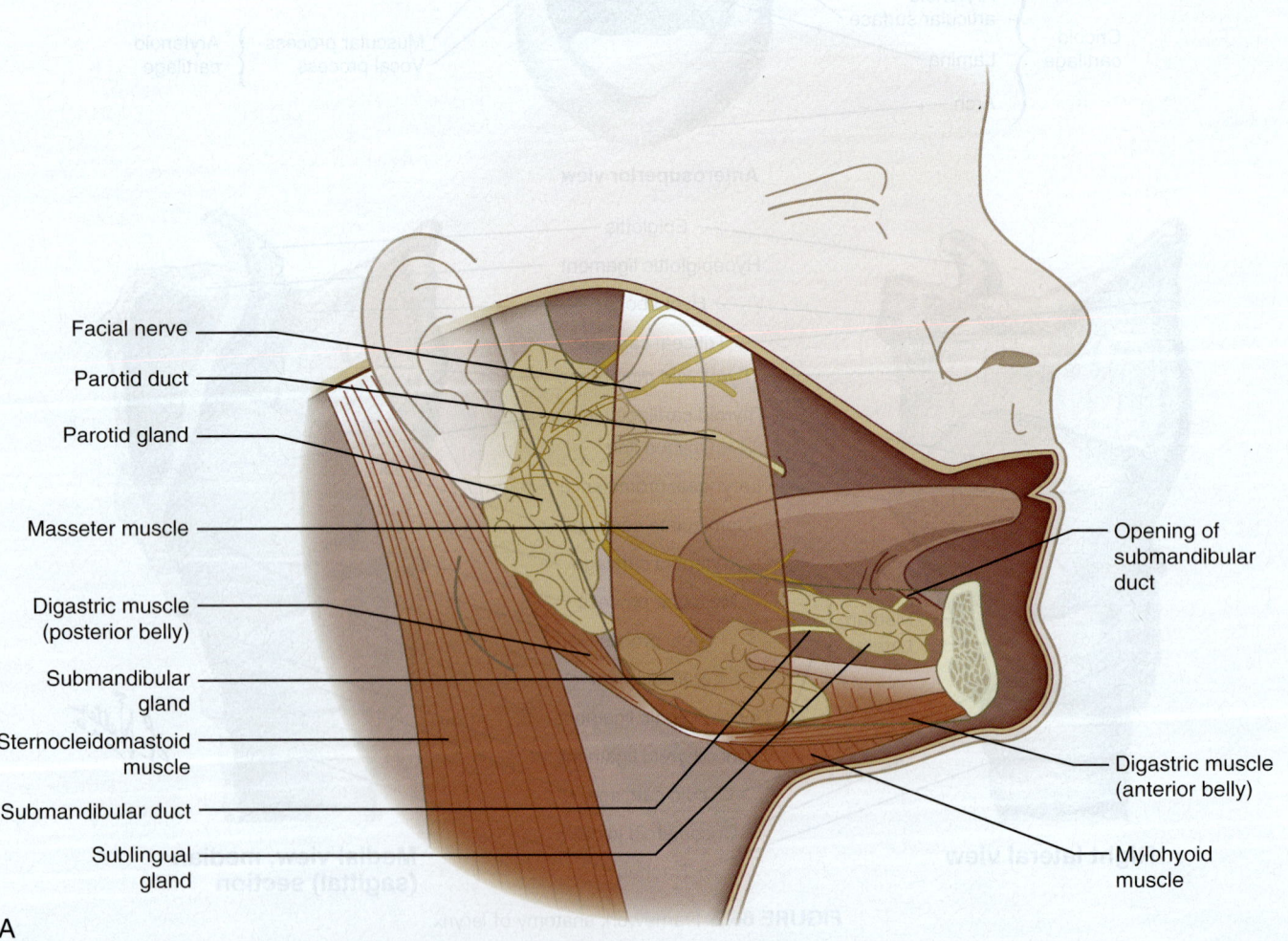

Facial nerve
Parotid duct
Parotid gland
Masseter muscle
Digastric muscle (posterior belly)
Submandibular gland
Sternocleidomastoid muscle
Submandibular duct
Sublingual gland

Opening of submandibular duct
Digastric muscle (anterior belly)
Mylohyoid muscle

A

FIGURE 66.3 Anatomic distribution of the major salivary glands (A)

Continued

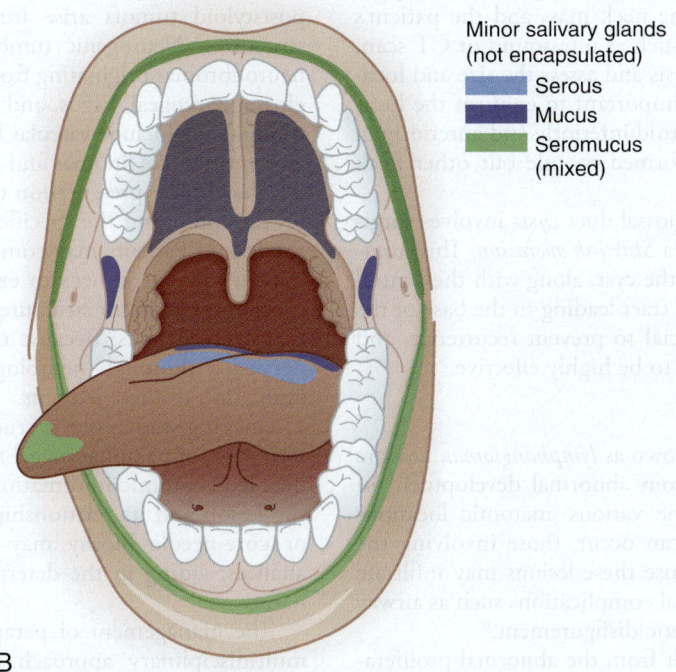

Minor salivary glands
(not encapsulated)
- Serous
- Mucus
- Seromucus (mixed)

FIGURE 66.3, cont'd and minor salivary glands (B).

The final pair of major salivary glands, the sublingual glands, are found in the floor of the mouth, superficial to the lingual nerve and mylohyoid muscle, and drain into the floor of the mouth via the ducts of Rivinus, some of which also drain into the Wharton's duct. There are numerous minor salivary glands, and they drain individually through the mucosa without named ducts.

CONGENITAL

Congenital masses of the neck present a complex and varied set of anomalies originating from aberrations in embryonic development. Understanding these anomalies is crucial for accurate diagnosis and appropriate management. This overview explores common types of congenital neck masses, their clinical features, diagnostic modalities, and treatment approaches.

Branchial Cleft Cysts

One prevalent category of congenital neck masses is branchial cleft cysts. During embryonic development, the branchial arches and clefts play a crucial role in the formation of the head and neck structures. The branchial clefts, also known as *pharyngeal clefts,* are paired structures that form between the branchial arches.[1] Normally, these clefts fuse and disappear by the end of the fetal period. However, if remnants persist, they can give rise to branchial cleft cysts. They are typically found along the anterior border of the sternocleidomastoid muscle. It is important to recognize and manage branchial cleft cysts promptly because they have the potential for recurrent infections.[2]

Branchial cleft cysts typically present as painless, fluctuant masses in the lateral neck. These cysts are often discovered in early childhood or adolescence but can become symptomatic later in life. Infections may occur, causing pain, swelling, and redness. Additionally, the cysts may cause discomfort or difficulty swallowing if they compress nearby structures.[1]

Branchial cleft cysts are classified into four types based on their anatomic location and embryonic origin. Each type corresponds to a specific branchial arch and cleft, and the classification helps guide surgical management. Type II cysts, arising from the second branchial cleft, are the most common, comprising approximately 95% of cases.[2]

Diagnosing branchial cleft cysts involves a combination of clinical evaluation and imaging studies. Fine-needle aspiration (FNA) may be performed to rule out other neck masses or infections. Imaging modalities such as ultrasound, computed tomography (CT), or magnetic resonance imaging (MRI), can provide valuable information about the size, location, and relationship of the cyst to surrounding structures.[2]

Surgical excision is the primary treatment for branchial cleft cysts, and the approach may vary depending on the cyst type and location. Complete removal of the cyst and its tract is essential to prevent recurrence. Surgical intervention is generally well tolerated, and the prognosis after successful excision is excellent.[1,2]

Thyroglossal Duct Cyst

The thyroglossal duct cyst is a congenital anomaly that arises from the persistence of the thyroglossal duct during embryonic development. The thyroid gland originates as a diverticulum from the floor of the pharynx and descends through the neck to its final location via the thyroglossal duct. Although the duct normally disappears as the thyroid gland descends to its final position in the neck, anomalies can occur along the tract, leading to the formation of cysts.[3]

Thyroglossal duct cysts typically present as painless, midline neck masses. Mostly seen in pediatric patients, these masses are often located just below the hyoid bone and may move in a craniocaudal fashion during swallowing or tongue protrusion. Although cysts are usually asymptomatic, they can become infected, causing pain, redness, and swelling. Rarely, they can cause difficulty swallowing or breathing and can have malignant potential.

The diagnosis of thyroglossal duct cysts is primarily clinical, based on the characteristic midline neck mass and the patient's medical history. Imaging studies, such as ultrasound or CT scan, can be used to confirm the diagnosis and assess the size and location of the cyst.[4] Imaging is also important to confirm the location and existence of a normal thyroid inferiorly and anteriorly in the neck. FNA may also be performed to rule out other neck masses or malignancies.

Definitive treatment for thyroglossal duct cysts involves surgical excision, a procedure known as a *Sistrunk operation.* This surgical technique includes removal of the cyst, along with the central portion of the hyoid bone and the tract leading to the base of the tongue. Complete excision is crucial to prevent recurrence, and the Sistrunk operation has proven to be highly effective.[5]

Lymphatic Malformations

Lymphatic malformations, also known as *lymphangiomas,* are rare congenital anomalies that arise from abnormal development of the lymphatic system. Among the various anatomic locations where lymphatic malformations can occur, those involving the neck pose unique challenges because these lesions may infiltrate adjacent tissues, leading to potential complications such as airway obstruction, dysphagia, and cosmetic disfigurement.[6]

Lymphatic malformations result from the abnormal proliferation or dilation of lymphatic vessels during embryonic development. The exact etiology remains elusive, with some cases associated with genetic factors, whereas others appear sporadic. Recent research has highlighted the involvement of vascular endothelial growth factor receptor 3 (VEGFR-3) mutations in the pathogenesis of lymphatic malformations, providing valuable insights into potential targeted therapeutic approaches.[7]

In the neck, they may manifest as painless, soft masses, often discovered at birth or in early childhood. They often enlarge during periods of illness, which assists in their initial diagnosis.

Accurate diagnosis relies on a combination of clinical evaluation and imaging studies. Ultrasonography, MRI, and CT scans can provide valuable information about the extent and nature of the malformation.[8] FNA or biopsy is generally avoided because of the risk of complications and potential for inaccurate representation of the lesion's full extent.

The management of lymphatic malformations requires a multidisciplinary approach. Treatment options include observation, sclerotherapy, surgical excision, and in select cases, systemic therapies. Sclerotherapy, involving the injection of sclerosing agents such as OK-432 or bleomycin, has emerged as a less invasive alternative to surgery, particularly for extensive lesions.[9]

NEOPLASM

Parapharyngeal Space

Parapharyngeal space tumors are a rare and diverse group of neoplasms that arise within the potential space located between the deep fascial layers of the neck. This anatomic region is bounded by the skull base superiorly, the hyoid bone inferiorly, and the lateral pharyngeal wall medially.[10] Parapharyngeal space tumors can present with various clinical manifestations, posing diagnostic challenges because of their proximity to vital neurovascular structures and the intricate nature of the anatomy in this region.

These tumors can be broadly classified into two categories based on their location within the parapharyngeal space: prestyloid and poststyloid. Prestyloid tumors originate from the salivary glands, most commonly the deep lobe of the parotid gland, whereas poststyloid tumors arise from neurogenic and nonneurogenic structures. Neurogenic tumors are frequently schwannomas or neurofibromas originating from the cranial nerves, particularly the glossopharyngeal, vagus, and sympathetic nerves. Nonneurogenic tumors may include vascular lesions, lymphatic malformations, or rare entities like lipomas and minor salivary gland tumors.[10,11]

The clinical presentation of parapharyngeal space tumors varies depending on the specific structures involved and the size of the lesion. Patients may complain of a painless, slowly enlarging mass in the lateral neck or experience symptoms related to compression of adjacent structures, such as dysphagia, otalgia, or cranial nerve deficits. Because the potential involvement of cranial nerves, a thorough neurologic examination is essential in the evaluation of these patients.

Imaging studies play a crucial role in the diagnosis and characterization of parapharyngeal space tumors. CT and MRI provide detailed anatomic information, helping to delineate the extent of the lesion and its relationship to surrounding structures.[11] FNA or core-needle biopsy may be performed for histopathologic analysis, aiding in the determination of the tumor's origin and nature.

The management of parapharyngeal space tumors requires a multidisciplinary approach. Treatment strategies may include surgical excision, radiation therapy, or a combination of both, depending on the histologic type, size, and location of the tumor. The surgical approach can be transoral, transcervical, or a combination of both, with the goal of achieving complete resection while preserving neurovascular structures and minimizing postoperative morbidity.[12]

Salivary Gland Diseases
Nonneoplastic Salivary Disease

Nonneoplastic diseases of salivary glands are most commonly obstructive, infectious, or inflammatory and typically manifest as enlargement and tenderness of the affected gland(s). Viruses and or aerobic/anaerobic bacteria are the most common infectious causes and are associated with acute onset and rapid resolution after appropriate therapy. More persistent and indolent granulomatous infections can be caused by typical or atypical tuberculosis, toxoplasmosis, actinomycosis, and *Bartonella henselae* (cat-scratch disease). Bacterial sialadenitis is typically unilateral and painful, purulence can often be expressed from the ductal opening with deep palpation, and sometimes skin changes are evident (Fig. 66.4). Bacterial salivary gland infections are associated with dehydration (or ductal obstruction) and are more common in elderly or infirm patients who may be on dehydrating medication. Sudden and acute swelling of a single major salivary gland typically indicates ductal obstruction and can be caused by salivary stones, strictures, thick saliva, or bacterial infection. Viral sialadenitis is typically bilateral and can be caused by the mumps virus as well as several other more common viral infections that affect the upper aerodigestive tract. Multiple, large, bilateral cysts of the parotid glands (lymphoepithelial cysts) can be seen in patients with poorly controlled HIV infection.

A major cause of salivary obstruction is salivary stones (sialolithiasis) that cause gland swelling, which is often worsened upon eating. Small stones in the parotid or submandibular duct can be managed with salivary endoscopy, by which the stones can be removed. However, in the case of large stones, removal of the gland is often necessary to prevent recurrent infections. Obstructive or

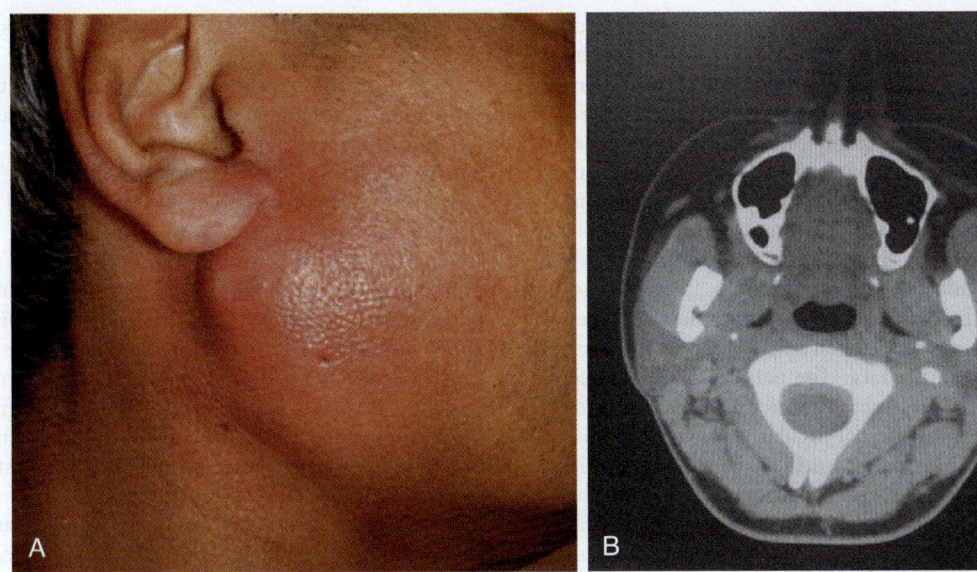

FIGURE 66.4 (A) Acute right parotitis with infection caused by obstruction of Stensen's duct by a salivary stone. (B) Computed tomography scan showing parotid stone within the left duct (not during active infection).

inflammatory sialadenitis can also be a manifestation of systemic diseases, such as Sjogren syndrome, sarcoidosis, or immunoglobulin G4 (IgG4)-related disease. In addition, patients treated with radioactive iodine for thyroid cancer are much more prone to developing obstructive sialadenitis, which can be immediately associated with treatment or occur up to 1 year after completion of therapy.

Benign Neoplasms of the Salivary Glands

Salivary neoplasms manifest as masses either within one of the major salivary glands or submucosally when arising from a minor salivary gland. Deep lobe parotid tumors can present as what appears to be unilateral tonsil hypertrophy or soft palate bulge, which is caused by mass effect within the parapharyngeal space pushing the palatine tonsil medially within the oropharynx. Deep lobe parotid tumors may have no outward signs or symptoms and are frequently found incidentally on imaging. Warthin's tumors are the second most common benign salivary neoplasm and are fluorodeoxyglucose 18F (^{18}F-FDG) avid by positron emission tomography (PET) imaging because of the high mitochondrial content of oncocytes within the tumor. When Warthin's tumors are found by staging or restaging PET imaging of cancer patients, they raise concern for metastasis or second primary malignancy. These can be assessed with FNA. They also have a malignant potential, and surgical excision is recommended.

Pretreatment evaluation of salivary gland masses may include cross-sectional imaging (CT or MRI) and/or FNA. FNA, either with direct palpation or under image guidance (ultrasound or CT), can help identify benign versus malignant salivary tumors. The benefit of FNA in the workup of salivary gland tumors is controversial because cytologic accuracy varies based on the experience of the cytologist and is not definitive, with the sensitivity of distinguishing benign from malignant tumors being approximately 80%.[13] In addition, most parotid tumors are benign (80%), and surgical removal is recommended for almost all, regardless of pathology, because of their malignant potential. Advocates of FNA tout the value of identifying a malignancy before surgery for improved patient counseling, patient expectations, and surgical planning (i.e., the likelihood of facial nerve sacrifice, the extent of parotidectomy, and the need for concomitant neck

dissection). In addition, intraoperative frozen section pathologic analysis of the tumor can help guide the extent of surgery and avoid the need for reoperation after pathologic diagnosis.

Most salivary neoplasms (~75%) are found in the parotid gland, and most parotid salivary tumors are benign. As a rule, the larger the salivary gland, the more likely a tumor within that gland is benign; for example, the probability of a tumor being malignant in the parotid, submandibular, and sublingual/minor salivary glands is approximately 25%, 50%, and 75%, respectively. The most common benign neoplasm is pleomorphic adenoma, followed by Warthin's tumor (also known as *papillary cystadenoma lymphomatosum*).

Treatment for benign salivary tumors is surgical removal, either parotidectomy, submandibular gland excision, or wide local excision of the minor salivary gland with margin control. Removal of benign salivary gland tumors upon detection improves the accuracy of histopathologic diagnosis, avoids more difficult dissection, and lowers the risk of patient morbidity (e.g., facial nerve injury, aesthetic concerns) by removal of the tumor before it enlarges. Removal of benign tumors also prevents malignant transformation that can occur with some histologies, particularly transformation of pleomorphic adenoma to an aggressive cancer, carcinoma ex pleomorphic adenoma. On the other hand, some benign tumors may be observed based on patient preference, patient suitability for surgery, patient life expectancy, and histopathology. Patients with Warthin tumors that are not enlarging or that were incidentally found or that occur in patients with metastatic cancer or in patients with contraindications to surgery may be appropriate for observation because this tumor has very low malignant potential. Additionally, these tumors are very commonly bilaterally in patients with a strong smoking history.

Surgical Technique

Submandibular gland excision is classically performed by creating a transcervical incision, raising subplatysmal flaps, and protecting the marginal mandibular branch of the facial nerve. The Hayes-Martin maneuver of dividing the facial vein at the inferior aspect of the gland and raising it with the gland fascia can protect the facial nerve branch because it travels superficially to this vein. The superior aspect of the gland is then dissected free (with division of the facial artery); the inferior aspect of the gland is dissected off the anterior belly of the digastric muscle; and the gland is freed from the posterior border of the mylohyoid muscle, which is retracted medially-superiorly, revealing the lingual nerve, submandibular ganglion, and the submandibular duct. The hypoglossal nerve can be identified with medial-inferior retraction of the mylohyoid muscle. Finally, the gland is dissected free posteriorly, and the facial artery is once again divided along the posterior aspect of the gland.

For parotidectomy, the most common incision is a cervicomastoid incision, as described by Blair in 1912 and modified by Bailey in 1941. Skin flaps are raised in a subplatysmal plane in the neck and over the parotid fascia in the face. The parotid gland is freed from the sternocleidomastoid muscle, often requiring division of the greater auricular nerve and external jugular vein, and the posterior belly of the digastric muscle is identified. Next, the parotid gland is dissected from the tragal cartilage, proceeding deep to the tympanic and mastoid bones and the lateral aspect of the tympanomastoid suture line. The tissue between the digastric dissection and mastoid dissection is carefully divided, and the parotid gland is retracted medially. The main trunk of the facial nerve is identified at the tympanomastoid suture line, at the level of the digastric muscle approximately 1 cm anterior, inferior, deep to the tragal pointer. The nerve and its branches are followed distally, dividing the overlying parotid tissue to expose the nerve. The tumor is removed en bloc with visualization and dissection of the nerve branches. Mobilization of nerve branches is required for large or deep lobe tumors (Fig. 66.5). Facial nerve electromyographic monitoring can be used if available per surgeon preference.

Sinonasal Benign Neoplasm

Sinonasal benign neoplasms arise within the sinonasal cavity, with most arising from the epithelial lining. Schneiderian papilloma (also called *sinonasal papilloma*) is the most common benign tumor of the nasal cavity,[14] and patients present with unilateral nasal

congestion and/or epistaxis. This benign tumor is associated with local destruction and has potential for malignant transformation. Schneiderian papilloma should be on the differential diagnosis for any unilateral sinonasal mass (Fig. 66.6). Sinonasal papilloma is classified into three groups:

1. Septal papilloma. These tumors usually begin growing on the septum; they are exophytic and not associated with malignant degeneration.
2. Inverted papilloma (most common). These tumors usually arise along the lateral nasal wall and have an inverted growing pattern with local destruction. Inverted papillomas have an approximately 10% to 15% malignant degeneration rate.
3. Cylindrical cell papilloma (very rare). An oncocytic variant, and like inverted papilloma, these tumors most commonly originate from the lateral nasal wall. These tumors have equal or slightly higher potential for malignant transformation compared with inverted papilloma.

The treatment of choice for sinonasal papillomas is complete resection with negative margins. In the case of inverted papilloma and cylindrical papilloma, removal of bone at the base of the tumor is important to prevent recurrence. With complete removal of sinonasal papilloma, recurrence rates are low. Open and endoscopic approaches are safe and effective for resection of these tumors; however, endonasal endoscopic approaches are preferred when possible because they avoid a lateral rhinotomy and associated facial scar.

Other benign nasal lesions include hemangioma, benign fibrous histiocytoma, fibromatosis, leiomyoma, ameloblastoma, myxoma, and fibromyxoma as well as fibro-osseous and osseous lesions, such as fibrous dysplasia, ossifying fibroma, and osteoma. Growth of tumors, weakness of the skull base, or the combination can allow intracranial tumors or normal tissues to extend into the nasal cavity, presenting as encephaloceles, meningoceles, dermoids, or pituitary tumors.

CT and MRI are important imaging studies to obtain for evaluation of sinonasal and skull base tumors because they provide complementary information. Together, these imaging studies help

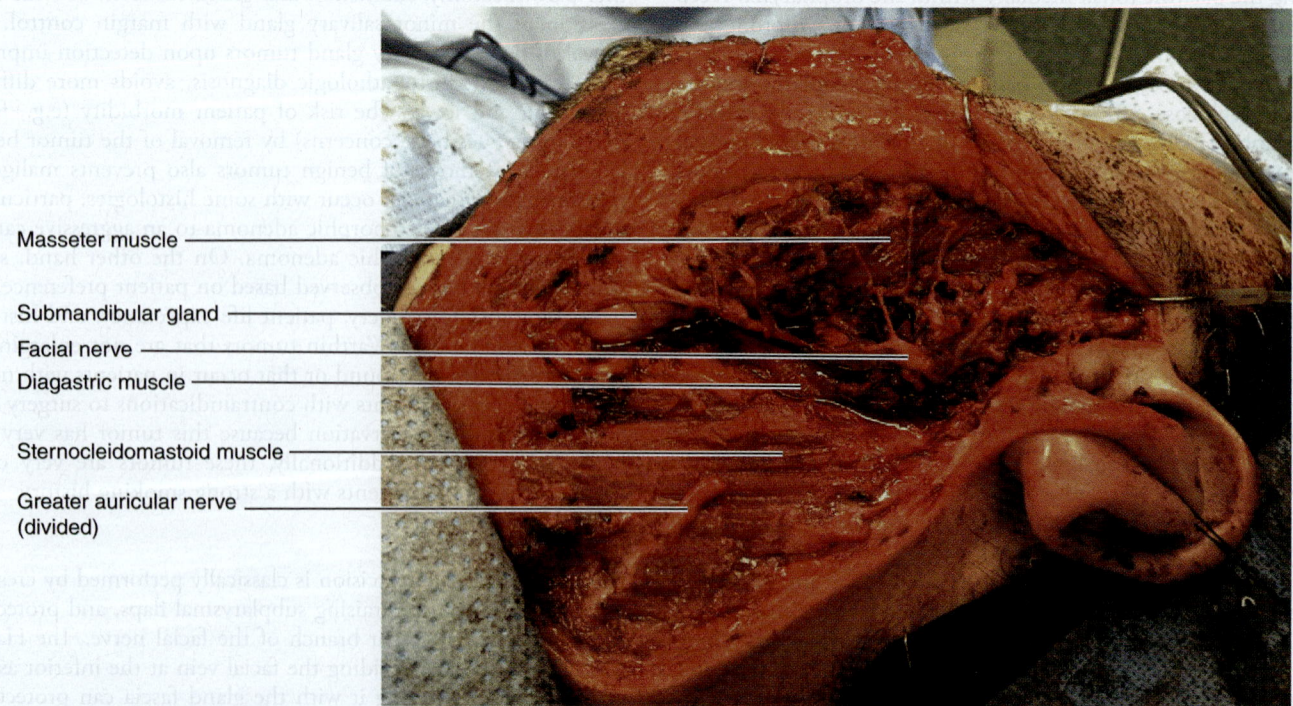

Masseter muscle

Submandibular gland

Facial nerve

Diagastric muscle

Sternocleidomastoid muscle

Greater auricular nerve (divided)

FIGURE 66.5 Total parotidectomy with identification and preservation of all facial nerve branches.

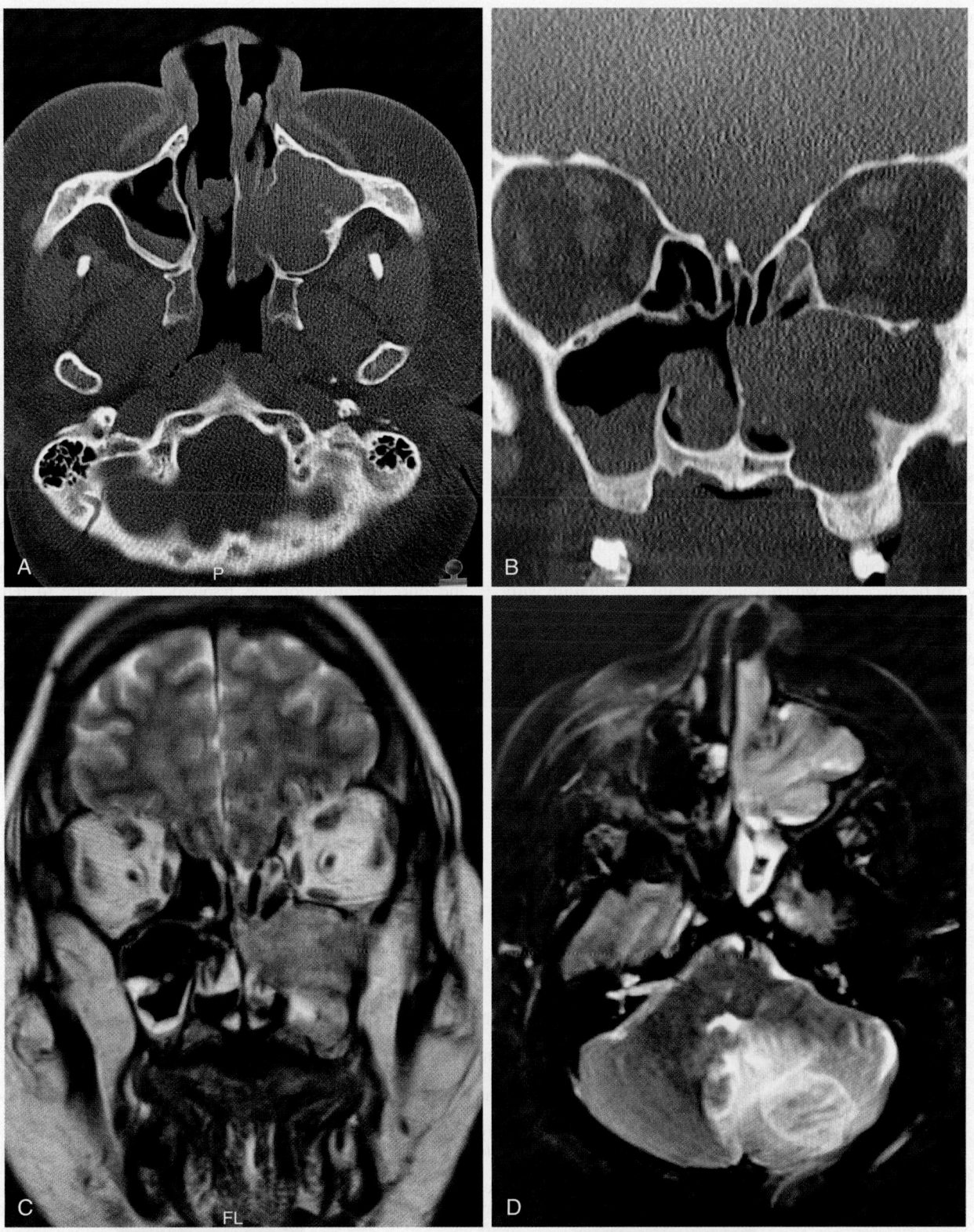

FIGURE 66.6 (A) Axial computed tomography (CT) of an inverted papilloma showing base of the tumor in the lateral maxillary wall with hyperostosis noted. (B) Coronal CT of an inverted papilloma showing base of the tumor in the lateral maxillary wall with hyperostosis noted. (C) Coronal T1 magnetic resonance imaging (MRI) showing soft tissue boundaries of the tumor filling the maxillary sinus, abutting the orbital wall but without orbital soft tissue invasion. (D) Axial T2 MRI showing the soft tissue tumor filling the maxillary sinus but with T2 hyperintense signal in the sphenoid sinus showing mucus instead of tumor in the sphenoid.

clinicians narrow the potential differential diagnoses because they also assist in the identification of intracranial connections, involvement or impingement on critical structures (e.g., orbit, cranial nerves), and tumor vascularity. T2-weighted MRI images are more sensitive to differentiate tumors from obstructed secretions within the nasal or sinus cavities, whereas CT images help identify bony destruction. Identification of structures involved by or adjacent to the tumor assists with diagnostic, treatment, and surgical planning. It is particularly important to determine if the tumor breaches the skull base because intracranial involvement can increase the risk of cerebrospinal fluid (CSF) leak, even with diagnostic biopsy.

POSTOPERATIVE OTORHINOLARYNGOLOGIC CONSIDERATIONS

Epistaxis

Routine epistaxis is generally controlled with constant pressure of the nostrils. This puts compression on the anterior septal plexus, called *Kiesselbach's plexus,* which is the most common site of bleeding. Pressure should be held continuously for at least 10 to 20 minutes without checking for resolution. Patient should sit forward and breathe gently through their mouth. If this is not sufficient, spray both nostrils with oxymetazoline spray and hold pressure again. In patients with facial trauma, these techniques should be attempted but may not be successful, which would warrant consultation with an otorhinolaryngologist. Altered anatomy may warrant different management techniques, including nasal packing, and operative versus interventional radiologic control of the sphenopalatine artery may be necessary. Another important aspect to consider is blood pressure because hypertension can either cause epistaxis or increase the bleeding. And finally, determine reversible causes of anticoagulation. After resolution of bleeding, patient should use nasal saline spray multiple times a day. Avoid nose blowing, and if supplemental oxygen is required, ensure that it is humidified air.

Cuts to Lips/Tongue

Most injuries to the lip or tongue heal on their own. Oral tongue injuries can bleed significantly. Applying pressure with an oxymetazoline-soaked gauze at the site of the injury can help to decrease bleeding and allow for better evaluation. If the injury is significant and causing deformity, consider primary closure with absorbable sutures in two layers—deep muscle and the superficial mucosa. One can also consider consultation with otorhinolaryngology. After these injuries, a liquid diet is recommended for a few days until healing takes place. Lip lacerations can be iatrogenic, such as through intubation, or via trauma. Again, pressure with oxymetazoline-soaked gauze can be applied to achieve hemostasis to better assess the injury. At times, a suture is required; however, most heal by secondary intention. If the laceration is deep and/or involves the vermillion border, suturing will provide the best cosmetic and functional outcome. It is crucial to line up the vermillion edges to achieve optimal cosmetic results. Occasionally, a deep suture with an absorbable stitch is necessary as well.

Sialolithiasis and Sialadenitis

These conditions of the salivary glands present with swelling and pain. They are common in patients with fluid or dietary restrictions. It is believed that the dehydration leads to thickened saliva and stasis of secretions. The overwhelming majority of patients are managed conservatively: increase hydration, apply warm compresses, and provide gentle massage along the gland and sialogogues (lemon wedges or sour candies). Occasionally, if there is no resolution, gram-negative coverage with antibiotics may be necessary. Most salivary stones (sialolithiasis) cases require treatment with antibiotics, and once the infection has resolved, a procedure to remove the stones might be needed to prevent recurrent infection.

Oropharyngeal/Laryngeal Edema

Patients can experience swelling within the upper aerodigestive tract from manipulation during surgery and intubation. Although the swelling is often self-resolving, it can cause difficulty breathing, speaking, and swallowing. Usual treatment involves 24 to 72 hours of high-dose IV steroids—dexamethasone 8 mg every 8 hours.

Dysphonia After Intubation

Often, dysphonia is discovered in patients after prolonged intubation or cardiothoracic surgery. If this is a sudden change after surgery that is not improving within 48 hours, it is recommended to evaluate vocal fold function via flexible laryngoscopy (Fig. 66.7).

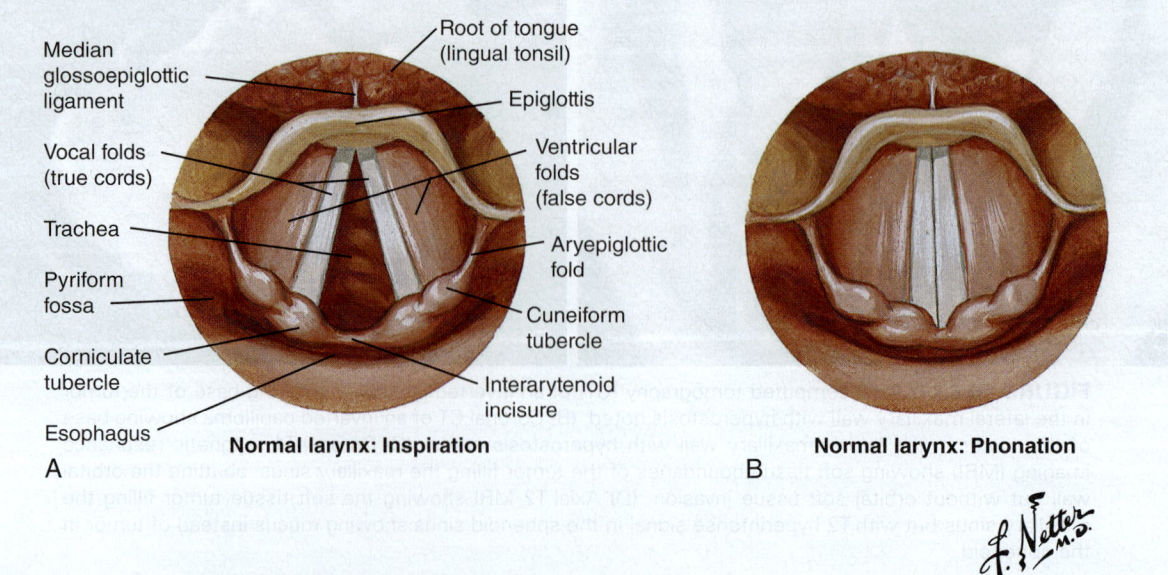

Median glossoepiglottic ligament
Root of tongue (lingual tonsil)
Epiglottis
Vocal folds (true cords)
Ventricular folds (false cords)
Trachea
Aryepiglottic fold
Pyriform fossa
Cuneiform tubercle
Corniculate tubercle
Interarytenoid incisure
Esophagus
Normal larynx: Inspiration
A

Normal larynx: Phonation
B

f. Netter
m.d.

FIGURE 66.7 Endoscopic view of larynx during inspiration (A) and phonation (B).

At times, dysphonia can be a result of vocal fold immobility. This can be managed as an outpatient; however, in a select patient population at high risk of aspiration, early intervention with vocal cord injection and/or speech therapy should be considered.

SELECTED REFERENCES

Colbert SD, Seager L, Haider F, Evans BT, Anand R, Brennan PA. Lymphatic malformations of the head and neck-current concepts in management. *Br J Oral Maxillofac Surg.* 2013;51(2):98-102.

This reference provides an overview of parapharyngeal space (PPS) tumors, which are rare and often challenging to diagnose due to their deep location. It discusses the anatomical considerations, clinical presentations, and imaging techniques like CT and MRI used for diagnosis. Treatment options, including surgical approaches and potential complications, are reviewed, highlighting the importance of careful preoperative planning.

Khandawala PS. Parapharyngeal space tumors. *Int J Head Neck Surg.* 2011;2(2):95-99.

This article provides an overview of parapharyngeal space tumors. It discusses the anatomical considerations, clinical presentations, and imaging techniques like CT and MRI used for diagnosis. Treatment options, including surgical approaches and potential complications, are reviewed, emphasizing the importance of careful preoperative planning to assure safe surgical planning due to deep location.

Lisan Q, Laccourreye O, Bonfils P. Sinonasal inverted papilloma: from diagnosis to treatment. *Eur Ann Otorhinolaryngol Head Neck Dis.* 2016;133:337-341.

This reference reviews the diagnosis and treatment of sinonasal inverted papilloma, a benign but locally aggressive tumor of the nasal cavity and paranasal sinuses. It discusses the clinical presentation, imaging techniques like CT and MRI for diagnosis, and the importance of histopathological confirmation. Various treatment options, primarily surgical resection using endoscopic techniques, are evaluated for effectiveness and recurrence rates.

The full reference list appears on Elsevier eBooks+.

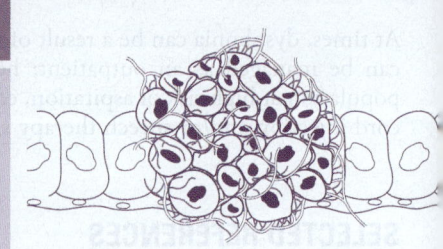

67 CHAPTER

Head and Neck Cancer

Alice Yu, Ehab Hanna, and Maie St. John

OUTLINE

INTRODUCTION

Cancers of the head and neck span a vast array of etiologies, subsites, and morbidities. Accordingly, the treatment modalities and surgical options for these diseases are similarly broad; management can involve specialists from head and neck surgery, plastics and reconstructive surgery, radiation oncology, medical oncology, oral maxillofacial surgery, maxillofacial prosthetics, oculoplastic surgery, and dentistry. Because of critical nature of the anatomy involved in these malignancies, patient outcomes are related not only to the characteristics of tumor biology but also the location of the lesions.

Collectively, head and neck cancers (HNCs) represent the sixth most common cancer subtype globally. These cancers are classically of epithelial origin—squamous cell carcinoma (SCCA) comprises 90% of etiologies—and are associated with tobacco use

and alcohol consumption.[1] Locations of HNCs are grossly divided into eight subsites: oral cavity, oropharynx, larynx, hypopharynx, trachea, nasopharynx, nasal cavity and paranasal sinuses, and salivary glands (Fig. 67.1).

Surgical excision, lymph node dissection, radiation therapy, and systemic therapy are all commonly used in the treatment of HNC. Because most patients present without distant metastasis (90%), surgical excision is often considered the mainstay of therapy unless tumors are deemed unresectable.[2] For patients with unresectable cancers, debulking is generally not a viable management strategy. Instead, such patients will often undergo radiation with or without systemic therapy or pursue palliative treatment.

Surgical resection of these tumors often creates defects that would confer significant morbidity if left untreated. Expert reconstruction of such defects can improve functional and cosmetic outcomes and prevent complications for patients after therapy.

Head and Neck Cancer Regions

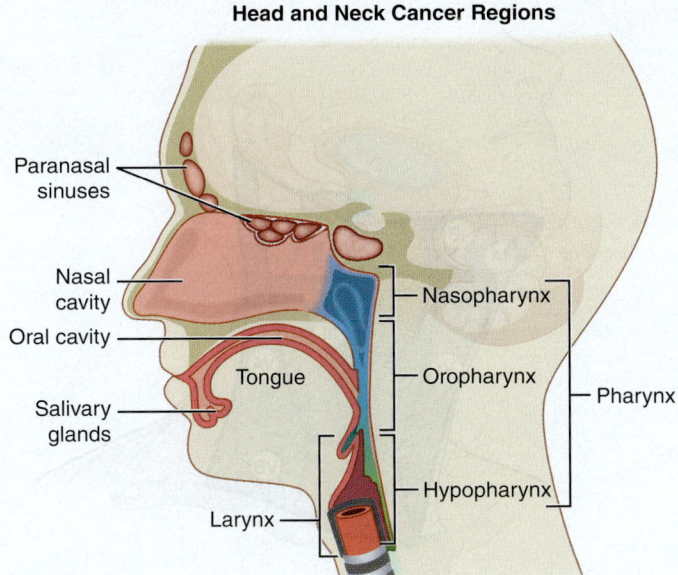

FIGURE 67.1 Subsites of head and neck cancer. Pharynx anatomy.[73] (National Cancer Institute. Copyright 2012 Terese Winslow LLC, US government has certain rights.)

As such, reconstruction is an ever-present consideration during surgical planning to confer both form and function. Choice of surgical reconstructive options include free tissue transfers, rotational or translational tissue flaps, or partial- and full-thickness skin grafts, which can be used to reconstruct a range of defects, from cutaneous to osseous. In selected patients, prosthetic reconstruction is the simplest and most effective method of restoring form and function.

Treatment of HNCs requires a nuanced understanding of tumor biology; options for surgical, adjuvant, and neoadjuvant therapies; and methods to improve patient quality of life. In this chapter, we will discuss each of these aspects of HNC in turn to elucidate the important considerations involved in management of these patients.

PATHOLOGY

As is common across all cancers, HNCs occur as the result of accumulation of mutations in genes involved in cell signaling pathways, such as *TP53, CDKN2A, PI3K, EGFR,* and *HRAS.*[3] In the classic understanding of this disease, HNC patients were usually male, in their sixth or seventh decade of life, with prior exposure to tobacco or alcohol. The use of both alcohol and tobacco leads to a synergistic increase in risk, with the combination of the two having a multiplicative effect compared with either alone.[4] Although these effects are seen in most HNCs, they are particularly important for laryngeal cancers, where the population attributable risk for disease was reported to be 89%.[4]

However, despite the traditional understanding of the association of HNC with tobacco and alcohol, within the past decade, there has been increasing awareness of the role of human papillomavirus (HPV) in the development of HNCs—most commonly within the oropharynx. HPV-positive cancers occur in a younger cohort of patients and are associated with improved survival outcomes and differing patterns of disease metastasis. Accordingly, the mutational profile varies between HPV-positive and HPV-negative

HNCs, with HPV-positive tumors displaying fewer mutations in canonical tumor suppressor genes, such as *TP53* and *CDKN2A,* in favor of activating mutations, such as those in the oncogene *PIK3CA,* or loss of the tumor suppressor genes *TRAF3* and *ATM.*[5,6] Other viruses, such as Epstein-Barr virus (EBV), have been implicated in the formation of nasopharyngeal carcinomas.

HPV-associated HNCs occur primarily in the oropharynx, most commonly causing tonsillar and base-of-tongue tumors. The prevailing explanation for the association between HPV and the oropharynx is that high-risk strains of HPV preferentially infect mucosal surfaces, such as tonsillar and base-of-tongue tissue. These areas are uniquely susceptible to HPV infection and promote evasion of immune surveillance because of the deep crypts present in the tissue. Moreover, the discontinuous basement membrane in the oropharyngeal epithelium predisposes to spread of HPV infections.[7] Although the carcinogenesis of HPV-infected cells usually involves the deactivation of p53 and retinoblastoma protein (pRb) by HPV-synthesized proteins E6 and E7, these cancers have a significant degree of expressional heterogeneity, with differential expression of immunologic response genes, viral integration of HPV, *PIK3CA* mutations, and chromosome 16q losses.[5]

EPIDEMIOLOGY

The incidence of HNC is approximately 600,000 new cases globally, making HNCs cumulatively the sixth most common cause of cancer.[2] HNCs also represent the ninth most common cause of death from cancer, with 325,000 deaths annually. The overall incidence of these diseases is increasing, with a predicted 30% rise by the year 2030.[8] Given the association of HNCs with tobacco and alcohol, the uptrend in cancer rates appears to be at odds with global trends of diminishing tobacco use. These rates are driven in large part by the growing role of HPV in HNC as well as the delay in vaccinating males against high-risk strains of HPV. In fact, HNCs have recently overtaken cervical cancers as the most common malignancy caused by HPV infection. Moreover, oral cancer is expected to rise in regions where chewing of betel quid, with or without tobacco, is common, such as Southeast Asia.

The median age of diagnosis is 66 years for HPV-negative HNC and 53 years for HPV-positive HNC. Males are two to four times more likely than females to develop HNC. The average 5-year survival for patients with HNCs is roughly 66%, although this figure varies widely depending on subsite and disease stage on presentation.[2] Particularly in the case of HPV-negative cancers, patients present with advanced stages of disease, which can limit options for curative treatment. However, mortality has broadly improved over the past few decades as a result of improved detection, surgical techniques, and adjuvant therapeutic options. Notably, morbidity and mortality in oropharyngeal cancer have improved dramatically in the past few decades, both because HPV-positive cancers carry more favorable outcomes than HPV-negative malignancies and because the advent of robotic-assisted surgeries has reduced the morbidity experienced by patients undergoing surgical resection of oropharyngeal squamous cell carcinoma. As such, prognosis is most favorable for HPV-positive oropharyngeal carcinoma, with a 5-year survival rate of 87%. Other subsites carry 5-year survival rates ranging from 69% in the oral cavity to 51% in the hypopharynx.[6]

The main risk factors for HNCs include tobacco use, betel nut use, and alcohol consumption. High-intensity, chronic tobacco use markedly increases the risk of all head and neck squamous cell carcinomas, although particularly in the case of laryngeal carcinoma—some reports have stated that the odds ratio (OR) of cancer in patients with heavy tobacco use was 10 in oral and oropharyngeal cancers and reached up to 40 in laryngeal cancers compared with nonsmokers. Smoking cessation was associated with 33% to 80% reduced risk.[9] Betel quid, or a mixture of areca nut, with or without tobacco, is a risk factor for HNC that is more common in Asian countries. Use of betel quid carries an OR of roughly 8 for developing HNC compared with nonusers and is particularly associated with oral cancers (OR 18.5).[4] When used alone, alcohol appears to have a moderate effect on increasing risk of HNC, particularly in oropharyngeal and hypopharyngeal cancers, although abstinence of more than 20 years was associated with reversion of risk to that of nonusers.[10]

Risk factors for HPV-associated HNC differ from those for HPV-negative HNC. The defining risk factor for HPV-positive oropharyngeal cancer is sexual behavior, such as early age of first sexual exposure, multiple sexual partners, and number of lifetime oral sexual partners. Cigarette smoking can further increase this risk by causing dysplastic changes; immunosuppression is also linked to a higher risk of HPV-positive HNC due to chronic infection or reactivation. Vaccination appears to reduce the risk of oropharyngeal cancer, with multiple meta-analyses indicating a 50% risk reduction in patients who had received HPV vaccines.[11] This observed protective effect has prompted a recent revision in CDC guidelines to include males in the target demographic for receiving the HPV vaccination.

WORKUP AND TREATMENT: OVERVIEW

Presenting Symptoms

Patients with HNC may present with a variety of symptoms, depending on location. However, the most common presenting complaints across all different subsites are pain, neck mass, dysphagia, dysphonia, and weight loss. Unfortunately, because of the general nature of these symptoms, patients often experience a delay in treatment while infectious etiologies are ruled out. Often, patients will undergo several rounds of antibiotics before receiving imaging studies or biopsies ultimately confirming their diagnosis.

Physical Examination

The physical examination of HNC patients is crucial in providing clinical staging and diagnostic information. Where possible, direct visualization and palpation to assess the size, appearance, and invasion is advised to inform the clinician of the extent of tumor spread and possibility of surgical resection. For oral cavity and oropharyngeal cancers, a thorough oral cavity examination can readily provide information about the characteristics of the tumor, whether exophytic, endophytic, or ulcerative. In nasopharyngeal or laryngeal cancers, endoscopic evaluation, either through rigid or flexible endoscopy, may also provide visual information regarding tumor characteristics. Endoscopic evaluation allows closer inspection of the base of the tongue, vallecula, and laryngeal inlet; moreover, assessment of vocal fold movement can often determine whether tumor spread has involved the recurrent laryngeal nerve in patients with and without dysphonia (Fig. 67.2).

Assessment of the head and neck for regional metastases is advised to aid in clinical staging in HNC patients. Facial lymph node stations include occipital, mastoid, superficial parotid, deep parotid, preauricular, infraauricular, intraglandular parotid, buccinator, nasolabial, and mandibular. Neck lymph nodes are broadly classified into six lymph node levels based on location.

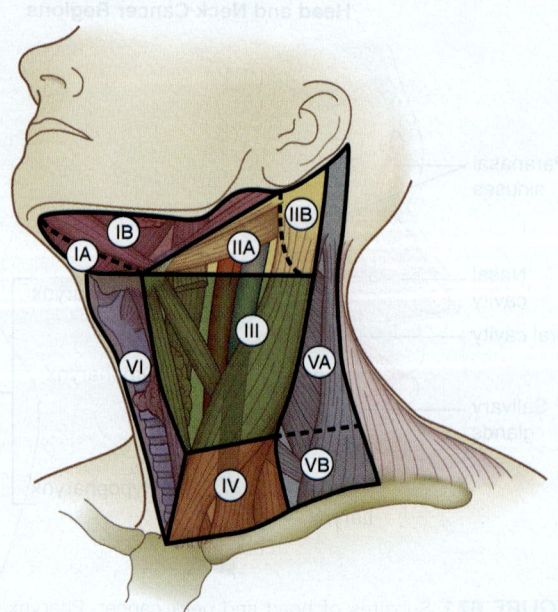

FIGURE 67.2 Lymph node stations of the neck.[74] (National Cancer Institute. Copyright 2016 Terese Winslow LLC, US government has certain rights.)

Level I is described as submental and submandibular lymph nodes; levels II–IV denote the superior, middle, and inferior internal jugular chain lymph nodes, respectively; level V demarcates the posterior triangle; and level VI refers to the anterior or central compartment of the neck. Common patterns of metastasis can be described via lymph node levels; oral cavity cancers commonly metastasize to levels I–III, whereas oropharyngeal cancers travel to levels II–IV. Lymphadenopathy seen in distant levels, such as level V, may suggest a more advanced degree of spread and thus a poorer prognosis.[12]

The cranial nerve examination is an additional critical component of the physical examination of HNC patients. Because of the density of critical vessels and nerves in the head and neck region, cranial nerve deficits may often lend important diagnostic information regarding local tumor spread before imaging has been performed. Deficits in the trigeminal or facial nerves can occur in oral, oropharyngeal, and certain salivary gland cancers, whereas extraocular movements may be compromised in nasopharyngeal or paranasal sinus tumors that invade the orbit or cavernous sinus.

Imaging

Diagnostic imaging for HNCs can be accomplished with the use of computed tomography (CT) scans with concurrent use of intravenous contrast. However, when possible, magnetic resonance imaging (MRI) provides clearer soft tissue discrimination, allowing for the differentiation of the mass from surrounding edema to determine the boundaries of tumor extension. However, because CT scans are more widely available and provide a high-quality examination with rapid acquisition time, they are often relied on in the diagnosis of HNC because of their accessibility. Additionally, CT scans also provide valuable information regarding invasion of surrounding bony structures.

Specifically, MRI imaging is preferred for assessment of local spread in nasopharyngeal, paranasal sinus, salivary, oral cavity, and oropharyngeal cancer because of its greater soft tissue discrimination. T2-weighted short-tau inversion recovery (STIR) images often provide the most value in differentiating tumor from fibrosis because fluid, inflammation, and subacute blood products appear hyperintense on T2 images, whereas fibrous tissue, calcification, protein-rich fluid, and flow voids appear hypointense. Moreover, STIR sequences often display some degree of fat suppression, which can allow more sensitivity in detection of smaller lesions. Diffusion-weighted imaging can also help with discrimination of tumors from surrounding edema. In this case, hypercellular tumors would demonstrate diffusion restriction and low apparent diffusion coefficient (ADC) values compared with edema, whose relative acellularity would correspond to high ADC values.[13]

Ultrasound is commonly used as a rapid method for assessment of the undiagnosed neck mass to distinguish malignant from nonmalignant etiologies such as cysts or abscesses. Cysts or abscesses often appear as a simple collection of hypoechoic fluid on ultrasound, whereas malignant metastases may appear more solid, with scattered calcifications or a lack of other physiologic morphologic characteristics. Given the lack of exposure to radiation, ultrasound can prove a useful diagnostic tool in children. Moreover, to obtain pathologic diagnosis, ultrasound-guided fine-needle aspiration or biopsy is standard for masses whose locations are amenable to in-office sampling.

Positron emission tomography–computed tomography (PET/CT) imaging is used to determine staging in HNC by using radiolabeled glucose (fluorodeoxyglucose [FDG, 18F]) to detect areas of increased metabolic activity. Of note, several areas in the head and neck can appear with falsely increased FDG uptake due to inflammation or physiologic activity. Particularly, tonsillar tissue, such as lymphoid tissue, often appears with high standardized uptake values (SUVs) without corresponding malignancy.[14] One method for determining whether this detected uptake is physiologic or concerning for malignancy is the degree of symmetry in uptake; because it is unlikely to present with bilateral tonsillar cancer, symmetric uptake is more likely to suggest noncancerous etiologies. Vocal folds present another area at risk for false positives on PET/CT—whereas edema or muscular activity may result in bilateral increased FDG uptake, patients with unilateral vocal cord paralysis or unilateral granuloma may also present with asymmetric SUVs in the vocal folds. In these cases, fiberoptic laryngoscopy or even biopsy may be necessary to rule these sites out as locations for possible malignancy.[15]

Staging Overview

HNCs are staged by subsite per the American Joint Committee on Cancer (AJCC)/International Union Against Cancer (UICC) tumor-node-metastasis (TNM) staging guidelines. Importantly, this staging system underwent a revision in 2017 to the 8th edition of the staging system.[16] The most significant modifications in the 8th edition of AJCC guidelines concerned the inclusion of depth of invasion in the grading of oral cavity cancers; the inclusion of extranodal extension in N staging as an indication for upstaging in certain subsites of HNC; the subdivision of nasopharynx, oropharynx, and hypopharynx; and finally, the separate staging system for HPV-positive and HPV-negative oropharyngeal cancers.[17] Staging for individual subsites will be covered in their respective subsections.

Treatment Overview

Broadly, treatment of HNC generally involves ablative surgery with possible adjuvant radiotherapy with or without chemotherapy, primary radiotherapy alone, or concurrent chemoradiotherapy.

For patients who present at too late of a stage for curative treatment, palliative chemoradiotherapy or systemic therapy are viable options.

Neck Dissection

Surgical techniques for resection vary by site; however, common among various types of HNC is the need for neck dissection. HNCs often present with regional spread to cervical lymph nodes without evidence of metastasis to more distant sites. Neck dissection has been used for more than a century for the removal of nodal metastasis. The traditional approach for evacuation of nodal metastasis—the radical neck dissection—involved en bloc removal of lymph node tissues superiorly, from the inferior border of the mandible to the clavicle inferiorly, as well as the lateral border of the strap muscles medially to the anterior border of the trapezius laterally. Along with the lymph node packet, the spinal accessory nerve, internal jugular vein (IJV), and sternocleidomastoid muscle (SCM) were resected. Although a radical neck dissection may be required for patients with widely disseminated neck disease, it entails significant morbidity for the patient and may not always prove necessary for clearance of cervical disease. The modified radical neck dissection was developed to resect the lymph node packet while preserving the spinal accessory nerve, the IJV, and/or the SCM. In both radical and modified radical neck dissections, levels I–V are completely excised.

However, for many patients with HNC, cervical disease is limited to few lymph nodes in predictable lymph node levels; for instance, oral cavity cancers commonly metastasize to levels I–III, whereas oropharyngeal cancers may spread to levels II–IV. As such, selective neck dissections with use of adjuvant radiotherapy present an attractive option for surgeons to preserve maximal function while clearing regional spread. Selective neck dissections fall into four main categories based on the levels removed: supraomohyoid (levels I–III), often used in treatment of SCCA of the oral cavity; lateral neck (levels II–IV), used in treatment of SCCA of the larynx, oropharynx, and hypopharynx; anterior neck (level VI), used for cancers of the midline structures of the neck, such as the thyroid, larynx, pyriform sinus, or trachea; and regional node dissection, used in cutaneous malignancies to excise lymph node packets closest to the tumor. For most patients with HNC, site-specific selective neck dissection is preferred.

For patients who clinically appear to have no cervical metastases (cN0), either on examination or imaging, elective neck dissections have proven controversial. Although these procedures involve the morbidity of an additional neck incision, particularly for early-stage oral or oropharyngeal cancers for which resection would not require operation within the neck, for certain patients with increased risk of regional spread or difficulty in presenting for follow-up, this additional step may be beneficial. Several randomized controlled studies have been done determining the utility of elective neck dissection in prolonging disease-free survival, with varying results; multiple studies concluded that elective neck dissection showed a statistically significant improved regional control rate compared with patients managed with observation. Retrospective studies have concurred that both regional control rates and overall survival are improved with elective neck dissection.[18]

Less invasive procedures, such as sentinel lymph node biopsy, in cN0 patients have been investigated; however, several challenges have arisen. In traditional applications of sentinel lymph node biopsy, in which radiotracer is injected peritumorally, injection can prove difficult for nuclear medicine specialists because of HNC present in areas close to critical structures, such as the oropharynx or the larynx. More recent studies have evaluated intravenous delivery of biomarkers attached to fluorescent dyes targeted against tumor-specific antigens, such as endothelial growth factor receptor (EGFR).[19] These antibodies are infused before resection; after binding to tumor tissue, the fluorescent component of the antibodies is then able to be traced intraoperatively to locate and excise the sentinel node for pathologic analysis. Although these methods may gain popularity in the future, they are not yet widely applied in most institutions.

Importance of Pathologic Findings

Treatment recommendations for surgery and adjuvant therapy versus medical management are described in the National Comprehensive Cancer Network (NCCN) guidelines. Generally, clinical management depends on TNM staging, subsite, and presence of adverse pathologic features, such as margin status, perineural invasion, lymphovascular invasion, extranodal extension, and depth of invasion (in oral cavity cancer).

Margin status is of key importance when determining the course of treatment. Positive margin status can serve as an indication for re-resection if a clear margin is believed to be obtainable; otherwise, the addition of radiotherapy with systemic therapy may be considered depending on disease stage and invasion. To determine whether complete surgical resection has been achieved, intraoperative frozen section analysis of margins is both sensitive and specific; however, errors still exist. One study of 1796 frozen/fixed margin specimen pairs noted discordance in 3.1% of pairs within HNC, with 1.9% false negatives and 1.1% false positives.[20]

Extranodal extension is defined as extension of nodal metastases beyond the lymph node capsule and can be diagnosed either pathologically or clinically through clear extension on radiographic imaging or palpation. Upon physical examination, these nodes feel fixed and immobile. This finding reflects the aggressiveness of tumor biology and is a criterion for nodal upstaging in both clinical and pathologic staging. Presence of extranodal extension similarly serves as a strong indication for adjuvant radiotherapy with chemotherapy. Pathologic findings that also predict poorer outcomes are lymphovascular invasion or perineural invasion, where cancer is seen to invade either lymphatic, vascular, or neural structures intratumorally. The evidence for the advantage of adjuvant therapies with these histopathologic features is less clear than that for extranodal extension or margin positivity; nevertheless, addition of radiotherapy or chemotherapy can be considered depending on clinician judgment or clinical gestalt.

Neck Dissection Complications

Although they are generally well tolerated, neck dissections are not without risks, including the following:

Infection: Many resections in HNC do not meet standards of sterility because they involve clean-contaminated spaces such as the oral cavity and the airway. However, neck dissections that are kept separate from these dissections without violation of contaminated spaces are considered "clean." As such, neck dissections alone do not benefit from prophylactic antibiotics. However, clean-contaminated head and neck surgeries have an infection rate of up to 80%, warranting perioperative antibiotics for at least 24 hours postoperatively. Additional antibiotics for 3 to 5 days have not shown appreciable benefit over 24 hours. Thus, suspicion of contamination during cases combining neck dissection with clean-contaminated tumor resections warrants use of prophylactic antibiotics. Generally, cefazolin is used in these cases, although amoxicillin-clavulanate and clindamycin with gentamicin have demonstrated similar efficacy.[21,22]

Bleeding: As with any other surgery, a risk of bleeding and hematoma exists in the postsurgical period, often in the first few days after surgery. Of note in neck dissections, brisk bleeding and large hematoma can cause a risk of airway compromise, necessitating immediate evacuation and control of hemorrhage to regain airway patency. In cases of slower bleeding in free flap patients, evacuation of hematoma may be preferable to placement of a pressure dressing because pressure can occlude blood supply to the tissue graft.

Nerve injury: Several nerves are in danger of damage or even transection during a neck dissection. These nerves are particularly imperiled in cases with prior irradiation, surgery, or extensive disease distorting the normal architecture of structures within the neck. Nerves at highest risk of injury include the marginal mandibular branch of the facial nerve and the greater auricular nerve. Paresis of the marginal mandibular nerve results in facial droop at the corner of the mouth. This nerve travels above the submandibular gland and is often encountered in dissections involving levels I and II. The greater auricular nerve originates from the cervical plexus from vertebral levels C2–C3 and innervates cutaneous sensation to the parotid gland and posterior auricular region. The greater auricular nerve exits the posterior aspect of the SCM at Erb's point and is frequently encountered in lateral neck dissections. Studies from various institutions have reported temporary injury rates to these nerves to be as high as 32.5% (to marginal mandibular nerve) and 36.1% (to greater auricular nerve).[23] The spinal accessory nerve is also encountered in lateral neck dissections, and injury to this cranial nerve can result in weakness in shoulder movement. Injury to this nerve occurs less frequently, perhaps because of its more robust nature. Phrenic injury can also occur, although its course is usually deep enough to avoid serious injury.

Chyle leak: Chyle leaks can occur in patients with level IV neck dissections; the incidence rate is reported to be approximately 3%.[24] Although they most commonly occur on the left side, chyle leaks may also present on the right after bilateral or, rarely, right neck dissections.[25] One retrospective study suggested that use of suture ligation or monopolar electrocautery during dissection was associated with lower rates of chyle leak compared with use of the harmonic scalpel.[24] Treatment involves testing fluid output for triglycerides; medical management includes medium-chain triglyceride diets, fluid and electrolyte repletion, octreotide therapy, or pressure dressings. In refractory or high-volume (defined as chylous leak of greater than 300 mL/day) cases, more definitive treatment may be necessary, including surgical ligation or percutaneous lymphangiography.

Carotid artery blowout: A rare but devastating complication of neck dissection is carotid artery blowout syndrome (CBS), which entails the often-sudden rupture of the carotid artery. Risk factors for CBS include radiation therapy, salivary fistulas, neck dissection, and advanced tumor stage. Generally, the area of rupture occurs proximal to the carotid bifurcation and co-presents with soft tissue necrosis or mucocutaneous fistulas.[26] CBS can be discovered incidentally on clinical examination or imaging, after self-limiting episodes of sentinel bleeding, or with high-volume hemorrhage. In the case of the latter, immediate management involves control of hemorrhage with manual and focused pressure until emergent definitive management. One meta-analysis reported that half of patients presented with some form of sentinel bleed before a life-threatening hemorrhage; 90% of these events were managed with endovascular embolization, stenting, or vessel sacrifice.[27]

In the case of more complicated ruptures, surgical intervention may be indicated. Mortality occurs in approximately half of patients with CBS.[27] However, even in the case of survival, the damage to the common carotid artery entails significant neurologic morbidity in up to 60% of patients. As such, care must be taken to prevent CBS by ensuring proper coverage of the carotid artery during closure, particularly in patients with risk factors for poor wound healing, such as malnutrition, uncontrolled diabetes, or prior radiation.[28]

Reconstruction

Given the critical nature of the anatomy involved in HNCs, reconstruction must consider safety, functionality, and aesthetics. Although the classic method of closing defects created in the resection of HNC involves use of free tissue transfer, pivotal flaps and skin grafts are often used as well. Next, we review several options for reconstruction of HNC defects.

Skin Graft

Skin grafts are commonly used to cover superficial or extensive defects. They are classified as split- or full-thickness grafts depending on the depth of tissue harvested; split-thickness grafts consist of epidermis and part of the dermis, whereas full-thickness grafts take both epidermis and the full thickness of dermis. For both split- and full-thickness skin grafts, close contact between the transposed tissue and recipient site is important to ensure appropriate vascularization and graft viability—oftentimes, this is achieved with a wound bolster or a negative-pressure dressing. These restrictions limit the applicability of skin grafts to different wound beds; specifically, exposed bone, irradiated tissue, cartilage, and tendon have poor rates of graft survival because of their limited vascularity.

Split-Thickness Skin Grafts

Skin grafts are used for various purposes in HNC reconstruction. Often, split-thickness skin grafts are used to repair graft harvest sites such as the radial forearm or fibula. For primary cancer defects, they may be used in situations where the soft tissue defect is not large enough to warrant a free tissue transfer but is too large to close primarily. They may also be employed in certain cases to close large primary defects over which an obturator or prosthesis may be placed. Some examples of this include maxillectomy patients who require palatal obturators or patients requiring an orbital exenteration who are reconstructed with orbital prostheses after surgery. Split-thickness skin grafts can be considered for patients who are too medically ill to undergo the prolonged anesthesia required for a free flap. Moreover, they can be used in delayed reconstruction of large defects wherein the primary site is allowed to granulate in or heal with a collagen tissue matrix. After the first layer of tissue develops, split-thickness skin grafts may be placed over the wound bed to complete the closure at a later stage. However, despite their various uses, for the majority of HNC resection defects, split-thickness skin grafts are not preferred because they experience contracture and are often associated with poor matching in terms of skin color and thickness.

Full-Thickness Skin Grafts

Full-thickness skin grafts consist of epidermis and full-thickness dermis; because of the inclusion of dermis, these grafts resist contracture and appear more akin to native skin compared with split-thickness skin grafts. Facial defects in regions such as the temple or nose are amenable to full-thickness skin grafts; however, because of the size of the graft defect for larger reconstructions, full-thickness grafts are predominantly used for smaller defects in cosmetically important areas.

Regional flap. In the 1980s, before the refinement of microvascular surgical techniques, rotational pedicled flaps, such as pectoralis myocutaneous or latissimus dorsi flaps, were commonly used to reconstruct large HNC defects. However, although these regional flaps have the advantages of shorter operative time and accessibility for surgeons of various training backgrounds, they have fallen out of favor as the standard of care for closing HNC defects because they have higher rates of flap failure than free tissue transfer. Moreover, because they remain tethered to the original site of the vascular pedicle, usage of these flaps is necessarily limited by distance of the defect from the harvest site. Nevertheless, these regional pedicled flaps are still commonly applied because of their versatility and relative ease of harvest.

First, patients who are not ideal candidates for free tissue transfer may be more appropriate for regional flap. Older patients with peripheral arterial disease, abnormal vasculature, or cardiopulmonary medical comorbidities who may not tolerate the length of general anesthesia needed for free tissue transfer are included in this population. Additionally, patients who have experienced flap failure after prior resection or require salvage surgery after disease recurrence may require use of a regional flap because there may be limited options for recipient vessels in the head and neck region.

Free flap. Free tissue transfers are considered to be the gold standard for reconstruction of most HNC defects. Because of their flexibility in shape, size, recipient location, and tissue composition, free flaps provide reconstructive options that allow HNC surgeons to resect tumors from both primary and recurrent disease that previously would have been deemed untreatable as a result of the extent of defect created. These flaps may be taken from a variety of different locations, including the radial forearm, lateral arm, lateral thigh, rectus, latissimus dorsi, and gracilis muscle. When considering which donor site to harvest from, the length of the vascular pedicle, area of harvestable tissue, tissue composition, and diameter of both harvested and recipient vessels must all be considered. Although the range of options for harvest sites available for free tissue transfer is wide, the mainstays of reconstruction are radial forearm and anterolateral thigh free flaps for soft tissue defects that require fascio-cutaneous tissue and fibular free flaps for defects that require osteocutaneous reconstruction.

Radial forearm free flap. The radial forearm free flap is the quintessential flap used for reconstruction of HNCs, particularly for oral cavity and oropharyngeal defects. This site may donate cutaneous, fascial, and/or osseous tissue to recipient sites. The tissues used for these transfers include the skin from antecubital fossa to wrist, brachioradialis muscle, and radial bone. This flap is often preferred over other sites given the thin and pliable nature of the tissue harvested, which allows for reconstruction in areas, such as the oral cavity, where excess bulk would be undesirable. Although osteocutaneous transfer is possible from this site, given the small size of the radial bone, these flaps often provide insufficient bony tissue for adequate reconstruction.

The vascular supply of radial forearm flaps is primarily the radial artery, its two venae comitantes, and the cephalic vein. Because harvest of this flap involves sacrifice of the radial artery, care must be taken to ensure that the ulnar artery provides adequate blood supply to the hand to avoid distal necrosis. The Allen test, wherein both the radial and ulnar artery are occluded before the pressure on the ulnar artery is released, is a rapid test to determine the adequacy of the ulnar artery. If release of the ulnar artery is sufficient to restore capillary refill while the radial artery is still occluded, the patient is determined to be able to undergo radial forearm free flap harvest. However, if any doubt exists, Doppler checks of ulnar arterial flow can be used as a more definitive assessment. Provided the Allen test is reassuring, selection of the nondominant hand is preferred when selecting laterality. Given the lack of laxity in the donor site, split-thickness skin grafts are often taken to close these defects. Postoperative care involves immobilization of the forearm with the wrist held in extension for approximately 1 week to ensure adequate contact between the skin grafts and the harvest site.

Anterolateral thigh flaps. Anterolateral thigh flaps are septocutaneous or musculocutaneous flaps that are commonly used in cases where the defect is too large for radial forearm flaps. These flaps also have thin, pliable skin with a long vascular pedicle, contributing to their versatility. As such, they can be used for defects of the oral cavity, tongue, oropharynx, and skull base. However, variability exists depending on patient anatomy. First, the width of the pedicle depends on the level of fat deposition for patients, which can make anterolateral thigh free tissue transfers too bulky for functional reconstruction. Moreover, the vascular supply to the skin varies in that arterial perforators enter the skin between the anterior superior iliac spine to the lateral edge of the patella. As such, anterolateral thigh flaps are designed around the perforator to ensure proper vascular supply by identifying the perforators using a Doppler probe before surgical planning.

The anterolateral thigh flap is supplied by the lateral circumflex femoral artery and its venae comitantes; because the anatomy of the perforators varies, it can be either septocutaneous or musculocutaneous depending on the path of the perforators before reaching the deep fascia of the cutaneous portion of the flap. The donor site can often be closed primarily, which contributes to improved recovery times.

Fibular free flaps. Bony defects in the head and neck are primarily closed with three main types of free tissue harvest: fibular, iliac crest, and scapular free flaps. Because iliac crest and scapular grafts entail increased morbidity and difficulties with harvesting due to positioning, fibular free flaps are often preferred by head and neck reconstructive surgeons. These flaps are commonly used to reconstruct maxillary or mandibular defects and can provide a long segment of vascularized bone with a thin skin paddle. When harvesting this graft, to preserve ankle stability inferiorly and protect the common peroneal nerve superiorly, 6 to 8 cm of fibula are left on either side of the fibula while the remainder is taken. To ensure reliable blood supply to the skin paddle, cutaneous perforators must be identified before designing the cutaneous portion of the graft. The peroneal artery and vein provide blood supply for this free tissue graft; as such, preoperative angiography with CT angiogram is recommended to ensure adequate distal arterial supply to the foot. Donor sites are imbricated then covered with a split-thickness skin graft. Patients wear a splint for the week after surgery, with ambulation initiated as early as the patient can tolerate.

Flap failure factors: rates, risks, irradiation. With the advancements in microvascular free flap surgeries achieved in the past few decades, free flap success rates have been reported by many sources to be over 95%. However, given the potentially devastating consequences of flap failure, flap loss remains highly feared. Most flap failures occur within 48 hours of surgery; commonly, these failures occur as a result of thrombosis of the venous and, less frequently, the arterial anastomosis. Other risk factors for flap failure include peripheral arterial disease, which can compromise

the integrity of donor vessels; smoking, which can result in vasoconstriction; and diabetes, which can impair wound healing. Although radiotherapy exposure can limit the regenerative ability of tissues, it has been extensively shown not to be correlated with rates of flap failure. Improper head positioning, which can lead to redundancy and "kinking" of vascular anastomoses, can result in thrombosis, as can extrinsic compression such as tracheostomy ties or oxygen masks. Rarely, flaps may fail after postoperative day 7—causes for these failures include vascular pedicle compromise but also entail infection causing wound breakdown and poor graft survival.

Flap success is monitored via several means depending on institutional preferences. Some common methods include Doppler, capillary refill, temperature, and scratch-test checks. In the first few days, flaps are monitored by physician or nursing staff every 1 to 2 hours. In the event of flap failure detection, further intervention is indicated. Depending on the degree of flap failure and the timeline and etiology for failure, reconstructive surgeons may choose to immediately bring the patient back to the operating room for revascularization, perform an additional rotational or free tissue transfer, or observe to allow the failed tissue to fully declare its extent before considering further reconstruction. Emergency surgery is the first-line therapy for patients with clear evidence of flap failure. Salvage surgery after flap failure has a success rate of approximately 50% in the literature and entails inspection of the arterial and venous connections for thrombosis. Heparinized saline can be used to irrigate the vessels, and thrombectomy may be performed if a thrombus is visualized. Because the duration of ischemia is important to the rates of flap survival, flap takebacks are emergent surgeries. For patients without overt signs of flap failure but evidence of venous congestion, leech therapy can be used with moderate rates of success; however, use of this therapy for intraoral flaps can be difficult because patients must be monitored for possible aspiration risk. Second free flaps may be indicated, with a success rate of 85% to 94%; however, patients who experience failure of two free tissue transfers usually should not undergo a third.

Inoperable tumors. Although surgery is the mainstay of most advanced HNCs, a subset of patients with advanced disease are considered unresectable. These inoperable tumors have two categories: locoregionally unresectable disease and patients who present with distant metastases. *Unresectable tumors* are defined as lesions whose complete removal is either not feasible or would cause unacceptably high morbidity. Specifically, involvement of the cervical vertebrae, deep muscles or fascial planes of the neck, skull base, or carotid artery precludes patients from surgery as a means to achieve a total resection. Patients with metastatic disease are also considered nonsurgical candidates because evidence of spread to distant sites indicates an inability to clear most of the disease burden with surgery. In these cases, chemoradiotherapy or palliation is preferred.

Radiation: options, deescalation trials. The most frequently used form of adjuvant therapy in HNCs is radiotherapy; moreover, it may also be used as the primary treatment modality for either unresectable tumors or for patients who prefer not to undergo surgery. For patients who choose primary treatment with radiation therapy, doses are 70 to 74 grays (Gy), whereas adjuvant therapy doses are 60 to 66 Gy. It is not uncommon for patients to undergo targeted radiotherapy in various locations with a variety of dosage strengths depending on the relative risk of involvement—for example, a patient undergoing primary treatment of an oropharyngeal cancer may receive 70 Gy in the primary tumor site but 50 Gy in an uninvolved lymph node basin.[29]

Radiation therapy carries its own toxicity profile, particularly in the head and neck. The effect of radiation on skin, salivary glands, and the tissues of the neck can result in side effects such as xerostomia, skin breakdown, thickened secretions, taste changes, hypothyroidism, dysphagia, carotid artery stenosis, and osteoradionecrosis. Traditional three-dimensional conformal radiotherapy was used to deliver uniform doses to areas within a designated field, thus incurring significant morbidity. Now, modern radiation therapies use intensity modulation of photon therapy based on the likelihood of disease in various areas, administering lower doses of therapy to tissue that is not grossly involved in tumor extension. Examples of these techniques are intensity-modulated radiation therapy (IMRT) and volumetric-modulated arc therapy (VMAT). In VMAT, further dose distribution differences can be achieved compared with IMRT, given the treatment gantry can move at varying speeds and rates of dose delivery, thus allowing faster delivery of therapy.[30] Proton therapy is also often used in HNCs in critical areas, such as those originating from the nasopharynx, skull base, or oropharynx, because of its steep distal fall-off.[31]

Nevertheless, radiotherapy still entails morbidity for patients. Because of the toxicities involved with high doses of radiotherapy, several trials have looked at deescalating the doses of radiation needed in the treatment of HPV-associated oropharyngeal cancer. The rationale for these trials includes the fact that many HPV-associated oropharyngeal tumors are highly radiosensitive, and patients experience good rates of survival when presenting with less advanced stages. These trials have looked toward either reducing the role of chemotherapy, reducing the dosage of radiotherapy after induction chemotherapy, or reducing the dosage of radiotherapy as an adjuvant therapy. Although most of these trials remain in various phases of clinical development and have not been incorporated into broader practice, they carry implications that aim to improve patients' quality of life after treatment for these diseases.[32]

Systemic therapy: chemotherapy, immunotherapy.
Chemotherapy for HNC is less commonly used as a primary modality of treatment compared with surgery or radiotherapy, and although it is sometimes used in the neoadjuvant (induction) setting, it is more commonly used in conjunction with radiotherapy. The most frequently used chemotherapeutic agents are platinum-based agents, which include cisplatin and carboplatin. Their mechanism of action is through formation of covalent bonds within DNA that inhibit replication and transcription. Taxanes, including docetaxel and paclitaxel, are frequently used to induce mitotic arrest because they cause microtubule dysfunction, which inhibits protein transport and cell division. 5-fluorouracil, a fluorinated pyrimidine, is another agent that is used in combination with other agents because it inhibits DNA synthesis for cells in the S-phase of the cell cycle. Although biologic agents such as programmed cell death 1 (PD-1)/programmed cell death ligand 1 (PD-L1) inhibitors (pembrolizumab, nivolumab) and EGFR inhibitors (cetuximab) have proven revolutionary in other fields, their application in HNC is rapidly evolving.

Organ-preserving trials/primary chemoradiotherapy.
Although traditionally, treatment of HNC involves surgery, removal of head and neck organs entails significant morbidity, particularly for speech and swallowing functions. In the 1990s, there was a push toward using chemoradiotherapy to avoid the negative consequences of tumor resection. Organ-preserving trials using primary chemoradiotherapy have been attempted, with varying levels of success among the subsites of HNC. Most notably, trials aimed at organ preservation in patients with laryngeal cancer who would otherwise require a total laryngectomy experimented with first treating patients with induction chemotherapy, followed by definitive radiotherapy. Salvage total laryngectomy was reserved as a definitive treatment for patients who did not respond to primary chemoradiotherapy. These studies found that select patients experienced similar survival outcomes as patients who underwent total laryngectomy but experienced less morbidity. These trials identified a group of patients for whom primary chemoradiotherapy could avoid the possibility of losing vital organs and began a wave of the use of primary chemoradiotherapy for treating HNCs. Currently, patients with HPV-positive oropharyngeal cancer, nasopharyngeal cancer, advanced laryngeal cancer, and certain hypopharyngeal cancers may undergo chemoradiotherapy with treatment success. However, for oral cavity cancers, surgical ablation and reconstruction are still preferred.

Common procedures during surgical resection of head and neck cancer.
Resection and reconstruction are not the only surgical considerations when treating HNC patients. Because the extent of surgical resection, postsurgical edema, and HNCs themselves closely abut or even frankly involve the airway, evaluation for tracheostomy must be performed on any patient undergoing HNC therapy. Furthermore, the anatomy involved in the swallowing mechanism is commonly affected in treatment of oropharyngeal, oral, hypopharyngeal, and laryngeal cancers, which can necessitate placement of a gastrostomy tube.

Tracheostomy tube placement.
For patients with patent airways undergoing HNC resection, tracheostomy tube placement is often chosen for prophylactic airway protection in anticipation of postoperative edema and swelling. For example, patients with large base-of-tongue defects after reconstruction may experience upper airway obstruction necessitating a tracheostomy tube. Another instance includes patients who undergo separation of the floor-of-mouth muscles from the mandible, which can cause collapse of soft tissue structures into the oropharyngeal airway. Moreover, bilateral neck dissections may cause significant enough swelling to result in airway compression and serve as an indication for tracheostomy tube placement.[33]

Careful consideration of whether patients may experience a compromised airway in the postoperative period is necessary because patients with HNC and free tissue flap reconstruction often present challenging intubations for healthcare providers as a result of airway swelling, intraoral flap volume, and altered anatomy. It is often advisable to err on the side of tracheostomy tube placement to avoid emergent intubation or tracheostomy on a postoperative HNC patient in respiratory distress. Additionally, because patients undergo restructuring of their oral cavity and pharynx, the tracheostomy tube allows for easy suctioning and airway clearance for patients who are unable to clear secretions as a result of upper airway swelling. Many patients who undergo complete surgical resection can be decannulated once postoperative swelling diminishes, although some patients with subglottic stenosis secondary to cancer treatment or tracheostomy tube placement may experience persistent tracheostomy tube dependence after the period of active treatment.

Tracheostomy tubes may also be placed on patients who do not undergo primary surgical resection. For patients with large oral, oropharyngeal, hypopharyngeal, or laryngeal masses with risk of airway compromise, a clear surgical airway may be necessary both for airway protection and secretion clearance. Additionally, patients with friable masses and the risk of bleeding in the airway without a clear embolization target may require the additional airway protection afforded by a cuffed tracheostomy tube. Many of these patients will remain dependent on the tracheostomy tube throughout the course of treatment and potentially afterward. Voice outcomes are variable depending on the ability to tolerate a Passy-Muir valve and tumor involvement of the glottis. Speech outcomes are highly dependent on the extent of oral cavity resection, reconstruction, and rehabilitation.

Gastrostomy tube dependence. For lesions that affect the swallowing function, gastrostomy tube insertion may be necessary. Patients with oral, oropharyngeal, hypopharyngeal, or laryngeal lesions may experience dysphagia related to surgical resection or radiotherapy, presenting an aspiration risk. Often, these patients will require gastrostomy tube placement in the peritreatment period, which may be removed, depending on the location and extent of the tumor as well as the posttreatment recovery of swallowing function. Patients with persistent dysphagia after therapy may see benefit through working with specialists in swallowing function, such as speech and language pathologists; however, a certain percentage of HNC patients—estimated to be approximately 17% of those who undergo free tissue flap reconstruction—may remain dependent on the gastrostomy tube for life.[34]

Surveillance. After remission of HNC, patients should regularly follow up with an HNC surgeon for surveillance for recurrence. This may take the form of physical examinations conducted at regular intervals, fiberoptic laryngoscopy to assess for locoregional recurrence, MRI/CT or PET/CT scans, or molecular testing. In general, NCCN guidelines suggest follow-up every 1 to 3 months for the first year, every 2 to 6 months for the second year, and every 4 to 8 months for years 3 through 5. The majority (80%–90%) of recurrences occur within 2 years of conclusion of treatment.[35] NCCN guidelines also recommend imaging within the first 6 months after treatment, although no formal guidelines exist for imaging beyond the immediate posttreatment period. In general, further imaging can be guided by clinician judgment and suspicion of recurrence. Circulatory biomarkers have been of particular interest, especially for HPV-positive oropharyngeal carcinoma. Numerous studies have investigated the effectiveness of measuring levels of circulating tumor DNA as a rapid way of detecting the presence or recurrence of HNC. The negative and positive predictive values of these assays have yet to be fully determined, with studies reporting positive predictive values ranging from 63% to 98%.[36,37] Nevertheless, further investigation into these rapid methods of tumor detection has important implications for the ease of tumor surveillance for patients in the future.

Oral cavity cancer

Introduction. Oral cavity cancer is the most common type of HNC, with more than 377,000 cases reported worldwide in 2020.[38] The oral cavity comprises seven clear subsites: lips, buccal mucosa, alveolar ridge, retromolar trigone, floor of mouth, oral tongue, and hard palate. Importantly, these various sublocations have different areas of common lymph node metastasis. Lesions of the upper lip will commonly spread to levels IB and II as well as perifacial nodes. Cancers of the lower lip tend to metastasize first to levels IA and IB, with some spread into level II. The upper alveolar ridge drains to levels IB and II, whereas the lower alveolar ridge and floor-of-mouth tumors descend to levels IA, IB, and II. Retromolar trigone tumors travel farther to levels IIA, IIB, and III, whereas metastases of hard palate and buccal mucosa tumors can be found in levels IB and II. Understanding patterns of metastases is important during the preliminary evaluation of these patients because assessing lymph node levels can provide information as to whether the degree of regional metastasis has progressed further than the expected station for the primary location.

PATHOPHYSIOLOGY AND EPIDEMIOLOGY

The vast majority (>95%) of oral cavity cancers are squamous cell carcinomas, although salivary gland tumors, sarcomas, lymphomas, and melanomas may also occur. Risk factors for development of oral squamous cell carcinoma include tobacco or betel quid usage as well as alcohol consumption. The combined use of alcohol with tobacco synergistically increases the risk of HNC by 45 times, more than can be explained by either alone. Poor oral hygiene and repetitive trauma can also contribute to development of oral cavity malignancies.[39] Overall, 5-year survival rates of oral cavity squamous cell carcinoma (OCSCC) have improved dramatically over the past few decades, improving from 59% in 1990 to 70% in 2011. These rates vary by subsite, with one study reporting that of all OCSCCs from 1975 to 2004, oral tongue cancers displayed the highest rates of cause-specific mortality.[40] However, when examined at stages II, III, and IV, this study found that patients with hard palate and retromolar trigone cancers fare more poorly compared with their counterparts with oral tongue cancer. Locoregional disease-free survival rates among T2–T4 OCSCC patients have been reported to be approximately 60%, whereas overall disease-free survival (including distant metastases) is approximately 50%.[41] The most common locations of distant metastasis include lung, liver, and bone, with pulmonary metastases being by far the most likely.

PRESENTATION

Patients with OCSCC present with oral lesions of varying appearances and textures. Often, these patients will have been sent for biopsy and further workup after routine dental examinations with areas of leukoplakia or erythroplasia. Leukoplakia is frequently caused by chronic irritation second to repetitive trauma or poor dentition; although its malignant potential is limited, transformation to squamous cell carcinoma (Marjolin ulcer) can occur and is a reason for these lesions to be monitored. Erythroplasia has five to seven times the likelihood of transformation to malignancy and warrants biopsy and further workup. Bleeding, halitosis, and pain can also occur as presenting symptoms.

DIAGNOSIS AND WORKUP

During the initial examination of a patient presenting with concern for oral malignancy, adequate visualization and palpation are key. These lesions are often located in areas of the oral cavity that are readily overlooked; as such, it is important to systematically examine all subsites of the oral cavity to determine the full extent of the primary lesion and to assess whether secondary areas of concern exist. Moreover, palpation of the depth of the lesion is important; depth of invasion of oral cavity cancers is an important indicator of prognosis, and physical manipulation can provide an expedient way of assessing the invasion of the mass. Imaging with MRI or CT of the face and neck can provide information regarding disease spread, and PET/CT lends information regarding distant metastases.

STAGING

Current AJCC guidelines regarding the staging of oral cancer rely on the correlation of a standard TNM staging system to a stage from I to IV. Recent 8th edition AJCC guidelines published in 2017 incorporated additional clinical characteristics into determination of staging, most notably extranodal extension and depth of invasion.[17] Tumors can be staged clinically, through radiographic imaging and clinical examination, or pathologically, with specimens obtained through surgical resection. Although the primary tumor (T) staging remains constant across clinical and pathologic staging, grading of nodal metastasis (N) more strongly weights clinically detectable extranodal extension by upgrading patients with any amount of extranodal extension to N3b. These new revisions aim to prognosticate patients with greater granularity, and reports suggest that the system is more accurate in stratifying survival of OCSCC patients according to stage. These reports describe 5-year disease-specific survival rates of close to 90% for patients with stages I, II, and III, 75% for stage IVa, and around 50% for stage IVb.[16]

TREATMENT

Historically, the mainstay of treatment of oral cavity cancer has been surgery with adjuvant therapy. Surgical resection of early-stage tumors can usually be managed transorally without need for lip split or mandibulotomy; however, in cases where tumor expansion precludes adequate visualization with a transoral approach, greater exposure is often necessary, with greater functional and cosmetic morbidity. Often, these cases will necessitate reconstruction of the oral cavity with a free tissue transfer, not only to close the resection bed but also to preserve speech and swallowing outcomes. Invasion of tumor into mandible must also be assessed both pre- and intraoperatively for oral cavity cancers. For cases where the tumor invasion is limited to the superficial aspects of the cortex, marginal resection may suffice; however, if the tumor extension has significant involvement of the bony cortex or medullary cavity, more drastic measures, such as segmental mandibulectomy or partial maxillectomy, must also be performed to achieve adequate resection margins. In cases of mandibular resection, bony reconstruction with an osteocutaneous free tissue transfer is commonly performed. For maxillary defects, free flap may be considered, although prostheses are often used, with or without free tissue grafts, to reconstruct oroantral defects.

Primary chemoradiotherapy can be administered for patients who choose not to undergo surgery, because of either medical comorbidities prohibiting surgery, advanced extension of the tumor such as to be unresectable, or patient preference. Radiation can, in certain cases, be administered as a single agent, but chemotherapy is never used as a single agent in the treatment of oral cavity cancer. Delivery of radiation is often limited by side effects of high doses of radiation to the oral cavity; these include xerostomia, dysgeusia, dysphagia, and osteoradionecrosis. Techniques such as IMRT, where maximal radiation dosages are applied to tumor tissue to minimize side effects, have had some, although not complete, success in mitigating adverse effects of radiation. Organ-preservation trials are currently still under development, but preliminary results suggest that patients who receive surgery with adjuvant therapy have similar overall and disease-free survival rates as those who receive primary chemoradiotherapy. However, those who eschew surgical treatment may experience greater toxicity from chemoradiotherapy as a result of definitive rather than adjuvant-level doses.

OROPHARYNGEAL CANCER

Introduction

The oropharynx is composed of the base of the tongue, tonsillar complex, soft palate, and pharyngeal wall. Treatment of oropharyngeal cancers has changed dramatically over the past decade. Beginning with the advent of robotic-assisted oral surgery, patients who previously required mandibulotomies to adequately expose the oropharynx for tumor resection were able to achieve similar results without significant morbidity. Moreover, the discovery of the role of HPV in development of oropharyngeal cancer has led to a stratification in the staging system according to HPV status because HPV-driven disease is associated with markedly different outcomes and treatment. Moreover, the rising incidence of HPV-associated oropharyngeal cancer is projected to continue increasing, with oropharyngeal squamous cell cancer (OPSCC) being the most common cancer caused by HPV in the United States.

Pathophysiology and Epidemiology

The oropharynx houses structures that are key in speech and swallowing. These structures are composed of mucosal surfaces and lymphoid tissue, which serve as the basis of current understanding of disease etiology in OPSCC. Most notably, it is believed that the crypts in tonsillar and base-of-tongue tissue are particularly amenable to HPV virus infection and replication, accounting for the association between HPV and OPSCC.[42] The posited theory of disease formation includes viral infection of basal stem cells, followed by gradual progression from abnormal cell proliferation to frank malignancy through the acquisition of oncogenic mutations. Moreover, tobacco and alcohol are readily exposed to these areas and increase the risk of development of non–HPV-associated tumors. Although squamous cell carcinoma is by far the most prevalent cause of oropharyngeal cancer, salivary glands and lymphoid tissue present in the oropharynx can also be sources of malignancy, with salivary gland cancers and lymphoma being far more rare tumors in this anatomic region.

Although oropharyngeal cancers are relatively uncommon, they tripled in incidence from 1988 to 2004 in the United States as a result of the rising incidence of HPV-associated cancers.[42] CDC guidelines now recommend that males aged 9 to 45 should receive the HPV vaccine; however, the high prevalence of unvaccinated males in the United States suggests that the incidence of OPSCC will continue to increase in upcoming years. Patients with HPV-positive oropharyngeal cancer display markedly improved outcomes compared with those with HPV-negative disease; 5-year overall survival rates have been reported to be over 90% for HPV-associated tumors and 40% to 60% in HPV-negative cancers.[43] Locoregional or distant recurrence occurs within 5 years for 10% of HPV-positive patients and 26% of HPV-negative patients.[35] Although it is rare for oropharyngeal cancer to be metastatic upon presentation, oropharyngeal cancer spreads primarily to lungs, liver, and bone.

Presentation, Diagnosis, and Workup

Frequently, patients may present because of a neck mass; however, persistent pharyngeal swelling is not uncommon. As in most HNCs, patients may commonly be referred after failing several rounds of antibiotics for a presumed abscess or infection. Nonspecific symptoms such as sore throat may further obfuscate the clinical picture. Clinical history that includes weight loss, hemoptysis, dysphagia, dysphonia, or unilateral ear pain is more suggestive of head and neck malignancy.

As with all forms of HNC, a thorough physical examination, with particular attention paid to lymph node levels and isolating the primary lesion, is recommended. For all patients, flexible laryngoscopy is useful in determining the extent of the lesion; however, in patients who present with a neck mass of unknown origin, this examination is particularly crucial for determining where the initial lesion occurred. Some patients may present without a clearly identified primary lesion and cervical lymph nodes positive for disease; in this case, direct laryngoscopy under general anesthesia in the operating room is advised to more assiduously identify a primary site.

CT scans and MRI of the face and neck are also useful for radiographically determining extent of the lesion; PET/CT should be used to rule out malignancy during evaluation for surgery. Because oropharyngeal lesions affect the complex of muscles essential for swallowing, patients may present with dysphagia or aspiration symptoms. As such, a modified barium swallow study and fiberoptic endoscopic evaluation of swallowing can prove useful for presurgical management of patients to determine whether patients may warrant gastrostomy tube placement.

Staging

Staging for oropharyngeal carcinoma is dependent on HPV status, a modification that was added in the 8th edition of the AJCC tumor-staging guidelines. T staging remains largely the same for both groups, with size demarcating T1 to T3 and extension into local structures differentiating T4a from 4b in HPV-negative tumors. HPV-positive tumors also include a T0 designation for tumors with proven disease without a clear primary source; HPV-positive tumors also combine all locally advanced cancers into one T4 staging group. Whereas HPV-negative oropharyngeal tumors are graded on the same clinical and pathologic N-staging system as oral cancers, oropharyngeal cancers simply use the number of lymph nodes involved to designate cancers as N1 or N2. Similarly, the cumulative staging system based on TNM score is the same as in oral cancer for HPV-negative oropharyngeal disease; however, HPV-positive staging reflects the more treatment-sensitive tumor biology of these cancers by downstaging HPV-positive tumors relative to HPV-negative tumors with the same TNM staging.

Treatment

Treatment strategies for oropharyngeal cancer have shifted dramatically over the years. Before the advent of transoral robotic surgery, mandibulotomies were often required to obtain the exposure needed for complete resection. As such, some patients were diverted to primary chemoradiotherapy to avoid such surgical morbidity. However, as minimally invasive strategies have become available, surgical therapy has regained its place in the overall treatment strategy, particularly for lower-stage disease. Finally, the advent of highly radiosensitive HPV-positive tumors has heralded an era of radiation therapy alone for these cancers; moreover, several trials have investigated the success of deescalating the dose of radiation therapy to avoid deleterious effects of radiation on patients' quality of life. Because of the high percentage of oropharyngeal cancers that present with cervical metastases, neck dissection or radiation is almost always indicated for these cancers.

Popularized in the 2010s, transoral robotic surgery revolutionized treatment for patients with oropharyngeal cancer by significantly reducing operative time, surgical morbidity, and the need for free tissue transfer and improving swallowing function. Although OPSCCs can be surgically managed with transoral robotic surgery, locally invasive disease may still require more extensive procedures to fully expose the extent of the tumor. These include lingual release, lateral and suprahyoid pharyngotomies, and approaches that require mandibulotomy. In these cases, sufficient tissue is often removed to necessitate use of a free tissue transfer, most commonly a radial forearm free flap.

As a result of the noted radiosensitivity of HPV-positive oropharyngeal cancers, radiation with or without chemotherapy has increasingly been used as a primary treatment strategy. Several randomized control trials have shown no difference between radiation

and surgery for survival or swallowing outcomes in early-stage tumors.[44,45] However, a recent study showed that patients who received primary surgery showed improved survival and swallowing outcomes compared with those who underwent primary chemoradiotherapy, although this study noted that patients were incompletely matched by cancer stage.[46] Nevertheless, given the success of radiation therapy in treating HPV-positive oropharyngeal cancer, several other trials have investigated the effectiveness of deescalating the radiation dose from the standard therapy of 66 Gy to 60 Gy, thus reducing the risk of deleterious effects such as xerostomia or dysphagia.[47] Finally, further trials have investigated the use of chemotherapy induction to stratify patients who are strong responders to systemic therapy to determine whether patients would be appropriate for deescalation therapy.[48] However, these trials remain in progress and are not common practice for treatment of HPV-positive OPSCC.

LARYNGEAL CANCERS

Introduction

The larynx comprises three unpaired cartilages (epiglottis, thyroid, and cricoid) and three paired cartilages (arytenoid, corniculate, and cuneiform) as well as a series of ligaments and intrinsic and extrinsic muscles. Together, these structures function to facilitate the highly orchestrated processes of speech and swallowing. Nevertheless, despite the intricacy of laryngeal anatomy, laryngeal cancers are generally categorized as supraglottic, glottic, or subglottic. The supraglottic region spans from the epiglottis to the apices of the vestibular folds, whereas the glottis includes the region 1 cm below (Fig. 67.3). The subglottis begins 1 cm below the vestibular apices and extends to the cricoid cartilage. The larynx contains several spaces that are important

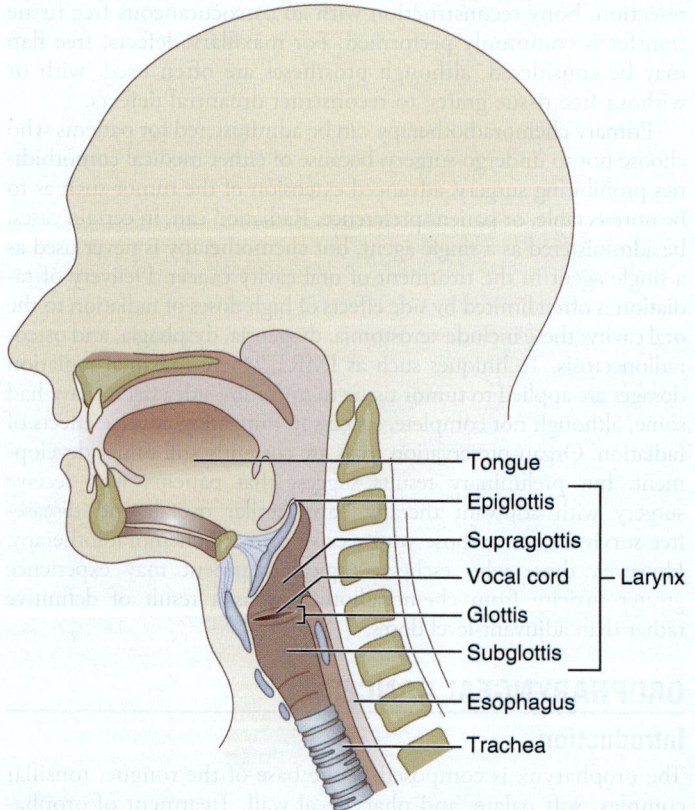

FIGURE 67.3 Anatomy of the larynx.[75] (National Cancer Institute. Copyright 2012 Terese Winslow LLC, US government has certain rights.)

Labels in figure: Tongue, Epiglottis, Supraglottis, Vocal cord, Glottis, Subglottis, Esophagus, Trachea, Larynx

to understanding locoregional spread of disease. Specifically, the pre-epiglottic space lies anterior to the epiglottis and contains significant lymphatic drainage pathways. This space is contiguous laterally with the paraglottic space, which surrounds the laryngeal ventricle and serves as a common pathway to extralaryngeal spread of laryngeal cancers.

Pathophysiology and Epidemiology

Within the three subsites of the larynx, supraglottic cancer is the second most common subcategory of laryngeal cancer, with 30% to 40% of laryngeal cancers occurring in this region (Fig. 67.3). Glottic cancer is the most common, comprising 50% to 60% of laryngeal lesions; subglottic tumors are the least common, constituting 1% to 5% of laryngeal lesions. Squamous cell carcinomas constitute the vast majority of laryngeal cancers. Although lower-risk strains of HPV have been known to affect the larynx with disease such as recurrent respiratory papillomatosis, there is no proven association between HPV and laryngeal squamous cell carcinoma development. As with other HNCs, smoking and alcohol usage predispose patients to laryngeal cancer. Some studies have reported that smoking cessation reduces the risk of laryngeal cancer by 60% after 10 to 15 years of cessation; however, the risk remains elevated relative to the general population. Nevertheless, the benefits of smoking cessation continue to accrue over time.[49]

Survival outcomes vary significantly based on tumor stage at presentation. Early glottic cancers have 5-year overall survival rates of over 90%, regardless of treatment modality. A randomized controlled trial of surgery compared with radiotherapy in 234 patients showed that the 5-year survival was 92% after radiotherapy and 100% after surgery for T1 tumors.[50] Patients with T2 tumors performed similarly well after treatment, with overall survival rates of 90% to 97% after 5 years.[51] However, late-stage tumors have a more guarded prognosis, with 5-year survival rates reported from 50% to 60%.[52]

Presentation

Because of the proximity of these tumors to the vocal cords, patients may often present with vocal changes ranging from hoarseness to a muffled-sounding voice. Obstruction of the airway can result in dyspnea, and encroachment on pharyngeal nerves can impair swallowing. Referred otalgia may also occur as a result of a sensory network between cranial nerves V, VII, IX, and X and cervical nerves C2 and C3. Patients may also be asymptomatic and present only with an isolated cervical metastasis. As with other cancers, patients may also present with "B-symptoms" of chills, weight loss, and night sweats. Patients with glottic cancers may present earlier than those with tumors of the supra- or infraglottis as a result of vocal changes.

Diagnosis, Workup, and Staging

A detailed physical examination, including flexible laryngoscopy and videostroboscopy, can lend information regarding cervical metastasis, tumor extension, and vocal cord involvement, all of which are critical to staging. CT and MRI scans help with radiographic description of disease extent; although MRI is often preferred for detection of locoregional spread in HNCs, CT scans are more sensitive for detecting cartilaginous invasion in laryngeal squamous cell cancers. At most centers, biopsies are done through direct laryngoscopy under general anesthesia, affording clinicians a form of direct visualization superior to fiberoptic laryngoscopy.

Treatment

Treatment of laryngeal carcinoma varies dramatically based on stage and location. Early supraglottic cancers can be managed with endoscopic transoral laser microsurgery (TLM) without significant deleterious effects on speech. Similarly, glottic cancers can frequently be treated surgically with TLM cordectomy or radiation therapy with equally positive outcomes. Subglottic cancers, compared with glottic or supraglottic cancer, always require some form of surgery, often with adjuvant therapies postoperatively. TLM can also be used for subglottic cancers, but often, more extensive surgeries, such as horizontal partial laryngectomy, may be indicated for tumors with deeper invasion into surrounding structures. Partial or total laryngectomy may be indicated for early laryngeal cancers that fail initial treatment.

Treatment for advanced laryngeal cancers incurs significantly greater morbidity. Paradigms in laryngeal cancer management have shifted in recent decades from the goal of immediate cure to organ preservation with salvage therapy after publication of the Radiation Therapy Oncology Group (RTOG) 91-11 trial. This trial addressed whether the use of induction chemotherapy to stratify patients who could be treated with radiation versus surgery was successful in ensuring laryngectomy-free survival in patients with late-stage disease. The results found that chemoradiation was more effective than induction chemotherapy or radiation alone.[53] The Veterans Affairs Study Group also investigated the role of induction chemotherapy followed by radiotherapy and found that patients who underwent this strategy had similar outcomes to those who underwent total laryngectomy.[54] Generally, these results suggest that nonsurgical treatment can safely be pursued in many patients with up to T3 tumors.

However, for very advanced, progressive, or recurrent disease, surgical resection is the best option. Endoscopic TLM surgery can be used up to the stage of select T3 and T4 tumors; however, the more common procedures to address more advanced tumors include both voice-sparing and voice-sacrificing laryngectomies. There are limitations to the clinical scenarios in which these procedures may be performed; it depends on extension of the tumor to the contralateral side or the vocal cords. In patients with tumors that cannot be safely resected with these organ-sparing surgeries, total laryngectomy is the gold standard for complete resection. Some studies have indicated that patients with T4 tumors should directly undergo total laryngectomy rather than organ conservation because the advanced stage of disease necessitates surgical resection. The 5-year survival rate for T3 disease ranges from 50% to 80%, whereas the 5-year survival for T4 tumors after total laryngectomy ranges from 30% to 60%.[55] For patients who receive total laryngectomy as salvage for failed organ-preservation therapy, 5-year overall survival is estimated to be roughly 60%.[56]

HYPOPHARYNGEAL CANCERS

Pathophysiology and Epidemiology

Hypopharyngeal cancers are a rare malignancy of the head and neck, constituting 3% to 4% of all cases of HNC.[57] Anatomically, the hypopharynx demarcates the region inferior to the hyoid bone to the inlet of the cervical esophagus. The hypopharynx comprises three regions: the pyriform sinus, the postcricoid area, and the posterior pharyngeal wall. Hypopharyngeal cancer presents most commonly in the piriform sinus, constituting 70% of cases.[58] Patients with hypopharyngeal cancer often present with late-stage disease and experience poor survival outcomes. Advanced disease may spread into more anterior structures of the neck, involving larynx and vocal function. Like most HNCs, the most common etiology of hypopharyngeal cancer is SCCA; risk factors of the disease include tobacco and alcohol use. Patients with hypopharyngeal cancer experience 5-year survival rates of 65% to 80% for early-stage cancers and 20% to 50% for late-stage disease.[59]

Presentation, Diagnosis, and Workup

Many patients present with either neck mass or associated symptoms, such as weight loss, dysphagia, or dysphonia. Because of the rarity of the disease and hidden nature of the anatomy, patients often will not present until the tumor has advanced to affect their speech or swallowing function. Many patients will present with significant weight loss or even malnutrition. As such, nutritional optimization and a gastrostomy tube may be required before initiation of therapy. Patients will require imaging with CT/MRI and PET/CT for appropriate disease staging before deciding on management. Fiberoptic and direct laryngoscopy are also recommended for evaluation of tumor extension.

Treatment

Although early-stage tumors may be managed with surgery or radiation alone, the majority of hypopharyngeal cancers will require more extensive resection and multimodal therapy. Surgical options include partial laryngo-pharyngectomy or supracricoid hemilaryngectomy. In more advanced cases, total laryngectomy and possible total pharyngectomy may be required. In these cases, free tissue flaps or rotational flaps must be used to close the defect made. Although tumor bulk affects critical functions such as swallowing and speech, debulking is usually not recommended, given the rapid rate of recurrence. However, if patients present with grossly extensive disease, it would be wise to discuss the possibility of palliative chemoradiation.

When considering nonsurgical options, chemoradiation has been used both in therapy (in organ-preserving trials) and palliation. Although other HNCs show poor utility of chemotherapy, several studies have demonstrated a survival benefit to the concurrent use of chemotherapy with radiotherapy.

NASOPHARYNGEAL CARCINOMA

Introduction

The nasopharynx begins at the posterior choanae and extends to the superior portion of the hard palate. Nasopharyngeal carcinoma is an SCCA that arises from this area, most commonly from the fossa of Rosenmüller, which is a recess that lies posterior to the eustachian tube and its distal cartilaginous extension, or the torus tubarius. Histologically, these tumors are classified into three categories: keratinizing squamous, nonkeratinizing squamous, and undifferentiated. Undifferentiated cancers hold the worst prognosis.

Pathophysiology and Epidemiology

Nasopharyngeal carcinoma is a rare variant of HNC, accounting for 0.7% of all cancers in 2018.[60] Interestingly, this disease has a strong geographic preference, with more than 70% of new cases occurring in East and Southeast Asia. In particular, Chinese patients from Guangdong and Inuits from Alaska have relatively high rates of nasopharyngeal carcinoma squamous cell carcinoma (NPSCC). The main risk factor associated with development of these tumors is consumption of salted fish, which contains the carcinogenic compound nitrosamine. EBV has also been linked to development of NPSCC because patients with these cancers have a higher rate of elevated EBV titers compared with controls. EBV

infection is more closely linked to the undifferentiated nonkeratinizing subtype of NPSCC.[61]

Presentation

Nasopharyngeal carcinoma affects a younger population compared with HNC patients, with peak incidence occurring between 40 and 59 years of age.[61] Common symptoms on presentation include nasal obstruction or epistaxis. Local extension can be associated with eustachian tube dysfunction, which may result in otitis media with effusion, otalgia, and tinnitus. Because of the proximity to the skull base, extension of nasopharyngeal carcinoma superiorly can affect the contents of the cavernous sinus, resulting in cranial nerve III, IV, and VI palsies. As with most HNCs, metastasis will often travel first to cervical lymph nodes; thus, painless neck mass is a common presenting symptom.

Diagnosis, Workup, and Staging

The workup for nasopharyngeal carcinoma requires a thorough physical examination with assessment for cervical lymphadenopathy, fiberoptic scope examination, and ear examination. Imaging studies include MRI, CT, and PET/CT, with a preference for MRI over CT scan, given better visualization of tumor extension. Of note, measurement of plasma EBV DNA before treatment is recommended for appropriate staging and prognostication.

The updated 8th edition AJCC guidelines incorporate both tumor extension into surrounding structures and EBV status. T1 staging involves nasopharyngeal, oropharyngeal, and nasal cavity involvement. Parapharyngeal extension or extension into the medial or lateral pterygoids or prevertebral muscles qualifies tumors as T2. T3 involves invasion into bony structures and paranasal sinuses, and T4 denotes tumors with intracranial extension or cranial nerve, orbit, parotid, or hypopharyngeal involvement. Nodal and distant metastatic staging remains like other HNCs. EBV DNA presence in a patient with an isolated lymph node without a clear primary source is assumed to be nasopharyngeal carcinoma and thus treated accordingly.

Treatment

Unlike other HNCs, the treatment of nasopharyngeal carcinoma is largely nonsurgical, with surgery reserved for situations required for recurrent tumors too bulky for radiotherapy or brachytherapy. For primary tumors, NPSCC is usually radiosensitive and responds well to IMRT, with good local control rates of greater than 90% at 3 years.[62] Chemotherapy may be added to radiotherapy, particularly in the cases of advanced locoregional disease, either as neoadjuvant, concurrent, or adjuvant therapy. In cases of locoregional failure after primary chemoradiotherapy or persistent disease in cervical lymph nodes, brachytherapy and radical neck dissection may be considered. Another indication for surgical management for patients with nasopharyngeal carcinoma includes patients who may not be able to tolerate a second course of radiation. Additionally, nasopharyngectomy may be considered for resection of localized disease in patients in whom clear margins may be achieved. Five-year disease-free survival after surgical salvage therapy is approximately 50%.[63]

NASAL/PARANASAL SINUS CANCERS

Introduction, Pathophysiology, and Epidemiology

Cancers of the paranasal sinuses and nasal cavity are rare, constituting approximately 3% of all HNCs. These tumors include the nasal cavity, which spans from the nasal vestibule to the posterior choanae, as well as the paranasal sinuses, or the ethmoid, maxillary, sphenoid, and frontal sinuses. Approximately half of these tumors originate in the nasal cavity, whereas the rest predominantly originate from the maxillary or ethmoid sinuses. Although tumors of this region are usually benign—the most common of which being inverted papilloma or fungiform papilloma—these benign papillomas may sometimes evolve into SCCA. Adenocarcinomas, adenoid cystic carcinomas, melanomas, and olfactory neuroblastomas may also occur in this anatomic region. Nonepithelial tumors that can also present in the sinonasal cavity include sarcomas and rhabdomyosarcomas, although these are far less common. Sinonasal undifferentiated carcinoma is a rare and malignant tumor that occurs in the nasal cavity and paranasal sinuses. Primary cancers of the kidneys, breasts, and lungs may also rarely metastasize to the paranasal sinuses. Exposures to wood dust, leather tanning, paint, chromium compounds, and industrial fumes have all been linked to sinonasal cancers.

Presentation, Diagnosis, and Workup

Similar to nasopharyngeal carcinomas, patients may present with symptoms of nasal obstruction and epistaxis. Patients may also present with symptoms like those of chronic sinusitis, including congestion, facial pressure or pain, and anosmia. Numbness in the distribution of the supraorbital or maxillary nerves can present in cases of tumor extension. In the workup of sinonasal or nasal cavity cancer, nasal endoscopy is important for visualization of the tumor and can be used to aid in-office biopsy. MRI scans can be used to assess soft tissue extension, whereas CT scans are most appropriate for evaluation of bony extension. Contrast is indicated in these cases to gain visualization of tumor vascularity. PET/CT can be used to detect malignancies. In cases of suspicion for intracranial extension, lumbar puncture may be necessary to diagnose leptomeningeal spread.

Staging

T staging for sinonasal cancers is dependent on extension into surrounding structures. T1 tumors remain limited to the primary site of origin, such as the nasal cavity or maxillary sinus. T2 tumors have extended into another location, such as an adjacent sinus. T3 tumors involve extension into the inferior or lateral orbital wall, palate, or cribriform plate, whereas T4a tumors have anterior orbital extension, cutaneous involvement, extension into sphenoid or frontal sinuses, or involvement of the pterygoid plates. T4b tumors are highly advanced, with intracranial involvement. Nodal and metastatic staging for sinonasal cancers follows the same staging system described for other HNCs.

Treatment

Surgical resection is considered first line for sinonasal cancers. For tumors without extensive bony extension or advancement into soft tissue structures, endoscopic techniques for ablation are often sufficient for curative therapy. However, for patients with more advanced disease, maxillectomy may be required to achieve clear margins. Unlike oral or oropharyngeal defects, maxillectomies may not be reconstructed or obturated at the time of the initial operation to allow postoperative debridement and monitoring. These defects may be reconstructed with a temporalis flap, a free tissue transfer, or obturation with a prosthesis. Certain locations of tumors may prove more challenging for total surgical resection, such as the sphenoid sinus, because both its deep location and proximity to critical neurovascular structures can make ablation challenging. As such, outcomes for sinonasal cancers depend on location within the

sinonasal cavity. Radiation therapy can be used as an adjuvant or neoadjuvant, although tumors are variably responsive, depending on their tumor biology. Chemotherapy has also been demonstrated to play an important role in induction therapy before primary treatment with surgery or definitive radiotherapy or chemoradiotherapy.[64] Studies have reported a 2-year survival rate of 77% when induction chemotherapy was performed.[64] Similarly, induction chemotherapy may improve outcomes in sinonasal undifferentiated carcinoma, with patients with a strong response to induction chemotherapy also showing robust responses to chemoradiotherapy regimens, thereby avoiding the morbidity of surgical resection.[65]

SALIVARY GLAND CANCERS

Introduction

Although HNCs at most subsites are of squamous origin, salivary gland cancers are the notable exception. The major salivary glands are the parotid, submandibular, and sublingual glands, whereas the minor glands are scattered throughout the upper aerodigestive tract. Because of its larger size, the parotid gland is the source of the majority of salivary gland tumors. Most of these tumors are benign, with salivary gland malignancies making up only 5% of HNCs. Although the parotid gland is the site of the greatest number of malignant salivary gland cancers, tumors in the sublingual or submandibular glands are more likely to be cancerous, with 40% to 45% of submandibular gland tumors and 70% to 90% of sublingual tumors being malignant.[66]

Pathophysiology and Epidemiology

As previously mentioned, most salivary gland tumors are benign, such as pleomorphic adenoma, papillary cystadenoma lymphomatosum (Warthin tumor), oncocytoma, and basal cell adenoma. When malignant tumors occur in the salivary glands, they are most commonly metastases from nonmelanoma and melanoma cutaneous cancers. However, the most common primary cancers of the salivary glands are mucoepidermoid carcinoma and adenoid cystic carcinoma. Other malignancies that can occur include acinic cell carcinoma, adenocarcinoma, polymorphous low-grade adenocarcinoma, carcinoma ex pleomorphic adenoma, primary SCCA, and salivary duct carcinoma. Mesenchymal tumors, such as rhabdomyosarcoma or fibrosarcoma, may also occur but are rare. Lymphoma may also occur infrequently as a primary lesion in the salivary glands.

The most common cancer of the parotid gland is mucoepidermoid carcinoma, which comprises 30% to 35% of all salivary gland cancers. This cancer is graded according to the relative proportion of mucoid and epidermoid cells, with a higher percentage of epidermoid cells being correlated with more aggressive behavior. Nodal metastasis is uncommon in mucoepidermoid carcinoma; as such, a neck dissection is not usually indicated without evidence of cervical metastasis. The 5-year survival rate for low-grade tumors is 97%, with only a 10% chance of locoregional recurrence. However, for high-grade cancers with more epidermoid behavior, locoregional recurrence occurs 40% of the time, with 5-year overall survival reported as 26%.[67]

Adenoid cystic carcinoma is the second most common parotid malignancy but the most common cancer of the submandibular and minor salivary glands. Its histologic features determine prognosis, with the most common pattern being a cribriform pattern, wherein collections of nests of cells are organized with pseudocystic spaces. In tubular adenoid cystic carcinomas, glands of tumor cells with single central lumens occur; in solid tumors, tumors grow in sheets without any visible organization. Degree of presence of solid components within adenoid cystic tumors is correlated with negative survival outcomes.[68] Although these tumors are slow growing, local—not regional—recurrences are common. Characteristically, this tumor has a high degree of perineural invasion, contributing to local recurrences even after complete resection. Because of its indolent spread, prognosis is measured after 10 years, which has been reported to be around 60%. Interestingly, 42% of patients will experience only distant metastasis without any locoregional recurrence.[69]

Acinic cell carcinoma is the third most common type of salivary gland malignancy, constituting about 20% of all cancers from this region. These cancers tend to be indolent, with possibility for recurrence long after surgical resection. Like mucoepidermoid carcinoma, histologic grading greatly determines prognosis, with 10-year survival rates for low-grade carcinoma of approximately 90% and rates for high-grade acinic cell carcinoma of around 33%.[70]

Salivary duct carcinoma is a rare but aggressive salivary malignancy that pathologically resembles ductal carcinoma of the breast. It occurs most commonly in submandibular or minor salivary glands, with a high rate of regional and distant metastasis and locoregional recurrence. Many salivary ductal carcinomas can be found within pleomorphic adenomas, with prior pleomorphic adenomas occurring in 20% to 70% of patients with salivary ductal carcinoma.[71] Interestingly, as in many breast cancers, HER2 expression can be seen in salivary duct carcinomas, with higher expression correlated with poorer survival.[72]

Presentation, Workup, and Staging

Salivary gland cancers usually present as asymptomatic masses, although they may be associated with pain. Ulceration is uncommon in salivary gland malignancies. Careful physical examination and neck examination for cervical lymphadenopathy are recommended. Fine-needle aspiration is recommended but may be insufficient to provide a definitive tissue diagnosis. MRI is recommended for visualization of extension into soft tissues, whereas CT is used to assess bony invasion in cases with a high index of suspicion for malignant spread. PET/CT may be used to assess spread. Staging of these tumors is determined after surgical excision, with T staging determined by size until stage IV, after which tumor extension into local structures drives T stage. Regional lymph node staging is determined similarly to other HNCs.

Treatment

Most salivary gland cancers are treated by complete surgical excision; depending on the histologic grade and risk for metastasis, radiation therapy may be included. Neck dissection for the clinically negative neck is controversial, with one sect arguing that because exact tumor pathology is not always known before surgery, neck dissection should always be performed. The opposing opinion posits that patients can instead be stratified for neck dissection by clinical characteristics such as patient age, tumor size, and local extension. Adjuvant radiation is used for high-grade tumors, evidence of perinodal metastasis, high tumor stage, or positive surgical margins. Extensive resection may also require surgical reconstruction with free tissue transfer, particularly for advanced-stage tumors.

CONCLUSION

HNCs are varied but rely on similar principles of diagnosis, staging, and treatment. The vast majority of cancers are squamous in origin and can be managed primarily with surgery with the possibility of adjuvant therapy. Because of the critical nature of structures in the region, free tissue transfer, tracheostomy, and gastrostomy tube must always be considered when planning surgical resection. Close multidisciplinary collaboration with colleagues in radiation oncology, hematology oncology, dentistry, and plastic and reconstructive surgery is critical to ensuring optimal patient care.

SELECTED REFERENCES

Argiris A, Karamouzis MV, Raben D, Ferris RL. Head and neck cancer. *Lancet*. 2008;371(9625):1695-1709.

A broad overview of basic treatment options in HNC. Largely focused on squamous cell carcinoma, this article addresses various aspects of epidemiology and treatment in the management of HNC. However, it does not include current efforts to deescalate therapy in oropharyngeal cancer.

Berman TA, Schiller JT. Human papillomavirus in cervical cancer and oropharyngeal cancer: one cause, two diseases. *Cancer*. 2017;123(12):2219-2229.

A review of the epidemiology and rising significance of HPV-positive oropharyngeal cancers. Importantly, these numbers may be affected by the advent of patients who have received the HPV vaccine; however, the wave of people who did not receive vaccination will surely significantly affect patient populations for decades to come.

Chamoli A, Gosavi AS, Shirwadkar UP, et al. Overview of oral cavity squamous cell carcinoma: Risk factors, mechanisms, and diagnostics. *Oral Oncol*. 2021;121:105451.

An in-depth analysis of genetic mechanisms implicated in the development of oral cancer.

Hoffman HT, Porter K, Karnell LH, et al. Laryngeal cancer in the United States: changes in demographics, patterns of care, and survival. *Laryngoscope*. 2006;116(suppl 111):1-13.

An in-depth analysis of the care and outcomes of laryngeal cancer patients.

Rosenberg AJ, Vokes EE. Optimizing treatment de-escalation in head and neck cancer: current and future perspectives. *Oncologist*. 2021;26(1):40-48.

A broad overview of various new efforts to deescalate treatment therapy to improve quality of life in HNC patients. In particular, efforts to deescalate therapy for patients with HPV-associated cancers have been investigated in recent years.

Zanoni DK, Patel SG, Shah JP. Changes in the 8th edition of the American Joint Committee on Cancer (AJCC) Staging of Head and Neck Cancer: rationale and implications. *Curr Oncol Rep*. 2019;21(6):52.

A good review of the recent changes made to the AJCC staging guidelines for HNC. Most relevantly for the general practitioner, oral cancer staging now includes depth of invasion as a negative prognostic indicator for oropharyngeal cancers and p16 positivity as a positive prognostic indicator.

The full reference list appears on Elsevier eBooks+.

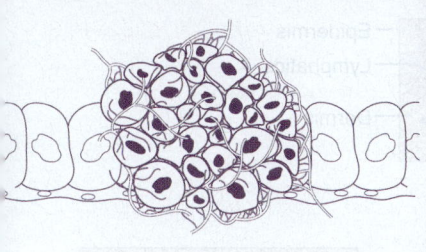

CHAPTER 68

Diseases of the Breast

Roi Weiser, V. Suzanne Klimberg, and Kelly K. Hunt

OUTLINE

BREAST ANATOMY, DEVELOPMENT, AND PHYSIOLOGY

Breast Anatomy

The anatomic structures relevant to the understanding of breast diseases and their management include the breast; the underlying chest wall and musculature; and the axillary, internal mammary, and supraclavicular areas. The breast is located between the skin and the subdermal layer of adipose tissue and the superficial pectoral fascia, overlying the pectoralis major muscle (Fig. 68.1).

Located deep to the pectoralis major muscle, the pectoralis minor muscle is enclosed in the clavipectoral fascia, which extends laterally to fuse with the axillary fascia. Multiple fibrous bands termed the *suspensory ligaments of Cooper* run between the chest wall and the dermis, providing shape and structure to the breast. Because these ligaments are anchored into the skin, edema of the breast or infiltration of Cooper ligaments by cancer can produce dimpling of the otherwise smooth surface of the breast, producing an "orange skin" appearance known as *peau d'orange*.

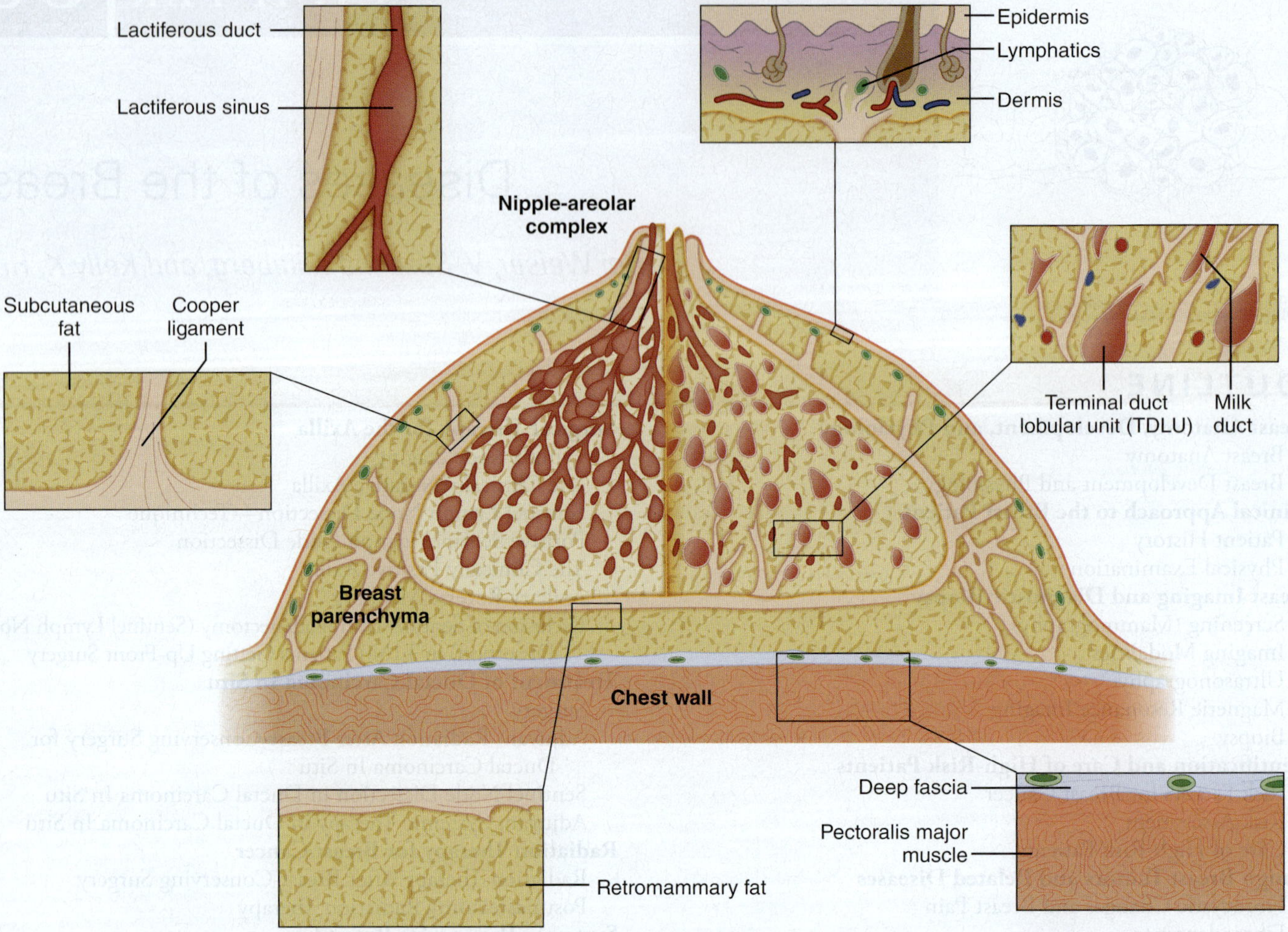

Lactiferous duct

Lactiferous sinus

Epidermis

Lymphatics

Dermis

Nipple-areolar complex

Subcutaneous fat   Cooper ligament

Terminal duct lobular unit (TDLU)   Milk duct

Breast parenchyma

Chest wall

Deep fascia

Pectoralis major muscle

Retromammary fat

FIGURE 68.1 Cutaway diagram of a mature resting breast. The breast lies cushioned in fat between the overlying skin and the pectoralis major muscle. The skin and the retromammary space under the breast are rich with lymphatic channels. Cooper ligaments, the suspensory ligaments of the breast, fuse with the overlying superficial fascia just under the dermis, coalesce as the interlobular fascia in the breast parenchyma, and then join with the deep fascia of the breast over the pectoralis muscle. The system of ducts in the breast is configured like an inverted tree, with the largest ducts just under the nipple and successively smaller ducts in the periphery. After several branching generations, small ducts at the periphery enter the breast lobule, which is the milk-forming glandular unit of the breast.

The mature breast is composed of three principal tissue types: (1) glandular epithelium, (2) fibrous stroma, and (3) adipose tissue. The breast also contains lymphocytes and macrophages. In adolescents, the predominant tissues are epithelium and stroma. In postmenopausal females, the glandular structures involute and are largely replaced by adipose tissue. The glandular apparatus of the breast is composed of a branching system of ducts, organized in a radial pattern spreading outward from the nipple-areolar complex (NAC; see Fig. 68.1). There are 15 to 20 lobes, each ending with a lactiferous duct, opening at the nipple. Each of these major ducts has a dilated portion (lactiferous sinus) below the NAC and progressively branches and ultimately ends in the terminal ductules or acini (Figs. 68.2 and 68.3). The acini are the milk-forming glands of the lactating breast and, together with their small efferent ducts or ductules, are known as *terminal duct lobular units* (TDLUs) or *lobules*. The TDLUs are invested in a specialized loose connective tissue that contains capillaries, lymphocytes, and other migratory mononuclear cells. This intralobular stroma is clearly distinguished from the denser and less cellular interlobular stroma and the adipose tissue within the breast.

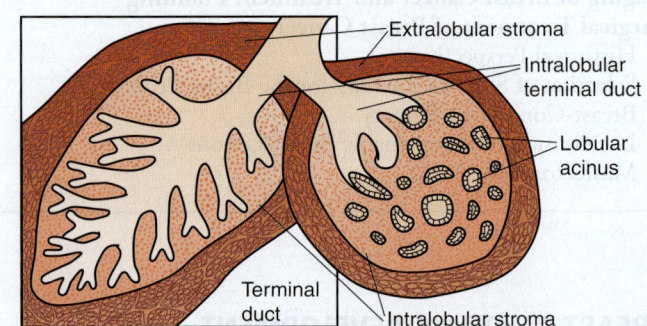

Extralobular stroma

Intralobular terminal duct

Lobular acinus

Terminal duct

Intralobular stroma

FIGURE 68.2 Mature resting terminal duct lobular unit. At the distal end of the ductal system is the lobule, which is formed by multiple branching events at the end of terminal ducts, each ending in a blind sac or acinus, and is invested with specialized stroma. The lobule is a three-dimensional structure but is seen in two dimensions in a histologic thin section, as demonstrated in the right lobule in this figure. The intralobular terminal ductule and acini are invested in loose connective tissue containing a modest number of infiltrating lymphocytes and plasma cells. The lobule is distinct from the denser interlobular stroma, which contains larger breast ducts, blood vessels, and fat.

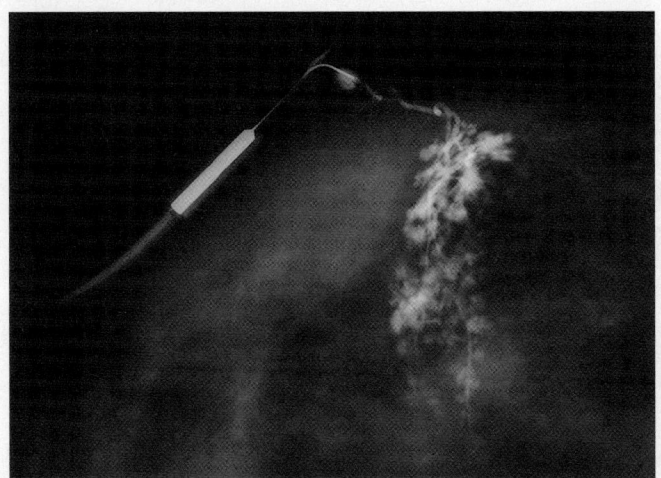

FIGURE 68.3 Injection of contrast material into a single ductal system (ductogram). Occasionally used to evaluate surgically significant nipple discharge, ductography is performed by cannulation of an individual duct orifice and injection of contrast material. This ductogram opacifies the entire ductal tree, from the retroareolar duct to the lobules at the end of the tree. It also demonstrates the functional independence of each duct system; there is no cross-communication between independent systems.

The entire ductal system is lined by epithelial cells, which are surrounded by specialized myoepithelial cells that have contractile properties and serve to propel milk formed in the lobules toward the nipple. Outside the epithelial and myoepithelial layers, the ducts of the breast are surrounded by a continuous basement membrane containing laminin, type IV collagen, and proteoglycans. The basement membrane layer is an important boundary, differentiating noninvasive breast cancer, ductal carcinoma in situ (DCIS), from invasive breast cancer (see "Pathology of Breast Cancer" later). Invasion or infiltration of the wall of the duct gives tumor cells access to the lymphatics and blood vessels that twine around the outside of the ducts, giving it metastatic potential.

A major route of breast cancer metastasis is through the lymphatic system; therefore, an understanding of the patterns of regional spread is important for optimal locoregional control. Lymphatic channels are abundant in the breast parenchyma and dermis. Specialized lymphatic channels collect under the nipple and areola and form the Sappey plexus, named for the anatomist who described them in 1885. Lymph flows from the skin to the subareolar plexus and then into the interlobular lymphatics of the breast parenchyma. Appreciation of lymphatic flow is important for performing successful sentinel lymph node (SLN) surgery (see "Lymph Node Staging" later). Of the lymphatic flow from the breast, 70% to 80% is directed into the axillary lymph nodes. A minor amount of the lymphatic flow from the breast goes through the pectoralis muscle and into more medial lymph node groups (Fig. 68.4). Lymphatic drainage also occurs through the internal mammary lymph nodes as the predominant drainage in 2% to 3% of patients and as a secondary route in combination with axillary drainage in approximately 20% of patients.

The axillary lymph nodes, grouped by location, are typically described as three anatomic levels defined by their relationship to the pectoralis minor muscle (see Fig. 68.4). Level I nodes are located lateral to the lateral border of the pectoralis minor muscle. Level II nodes are located posterior to the pectoralis minor muscle as well as anterior to the pectoralis minor and posterior to the

pectoralis major (*Rotter's* or interpectoral nodes). Level III nodes are located medial to the pectoralis minor muscle and include the infraclavicular nodes. The apex of the axilla is defined by the costoclavicular ligament *(Halsted ligament),* at which point the axillary vein passes into the thorax and becomes the subclavian vein. Lymphatic drainage continues after level III nodes to supraclavicular nodes, which are considered outside the anatomic boundaries of the axilla. Functionally, the lymph nodes in the axilla drain lymphatics from the upper extremity, chest wall, upper abdomen, and back, in addition to the breast. Boneti and colleagues[1] described the anatomic drainage of the lymphatics from the arm within the axilla (Fig. 68.5). Although traditional teaching described the arm's lymphatic drainage as following the axillary vein, either above it or closely below it, Boneti showed arm lymphatics to have various patterns of crossing the axilla (sling, apron, twine, etc.), some of which reach several centimeters inferior to the axillary vein, well within the boundaries of an axillary lymph node dissection (ALND). This functional anatomy of axillary lymphatics helps us understand the role of axillary surgery as a cause of breast cancer–related lymphedema and also the possible surgical strategies for its prevention (see "Surgical Therapy for the Axilla" later).

The axillary anatomy, beyond the lymphatic structures, consists of several important structures. Its surgical boundaries are made up of the serratus anterior muscle and chest wall at the medial aspect; the latissimus dorsi, teres major, and subscapularis at the posterior aspect; the pectoralis major and minor muscles at the anterior aspect; and the axillary vein at the superior aspect. There are several neurovascular structures important for the execution of axillary surgery. The first, coursing deep and close to the chest wall on the medial side of the axilla, is the long thoracic nerve (see Fig. 68.4), also known as the *external respiratory nerve of Bell,* which innervates the serratus anterior muscle. This muscle helps fix the scapula to the chest wall during shoulder adduction and arm extension, and its division during surgery can cause a winged scapula deformity; it should therefore be preserved. The second major nerve encountered during axillary dissection is the thoracodorsal nerve, which innervates the latissimus dorsi muscle. This nerve arises from the posterior cord of the brachial plexus and enters the axillary space under the axillary vein, close to the entrance of the long thoracic nerve. The thoracodorsal nerve, as a neurovascular bundle, crosses the axilla to the medial surface of the latissimus dorsi muscle. The thoracodorsal nerve and vessels are also preserved during axillary surgery. The third, the medial pectoral nerve, named for its derivation from the medial cord of the brachial plexus, innervates the pectoralis major muscle and lies within a neurovascular bundle that wraps around the lateral border of the pectoralis minor muscle. The pectoral neurovascular bundle is a useful landmark because it can help identify the position of the axillary vein, which is just cephalad and deep to the bundle. This neurovascular bundle should be preserved, if possible, during any lymphadenectomy. There are also three to five sensory intercostal brachial or brachial cutaneous nerves that cross the axilla horizontally and supply sensation to the upper inner surface of the arm and the skin of the chest wall along the posterior margin of the axilla. Lymphatics run along these nerves as well. Dividing these nerves results in cutaneous anesthesia in these areas and potentially a chronic and uncomfortable pain syndrome in a small percentage of patients. The possibility of this outcome should be explained to patients before axillary surgery. Preservation of the most superior nerve maintains sensation to the posterior aspect of the upper part of the arm without compromising the axillary dissection in most patients. Taking these nerves with their associated lymphatics may lead to lymphedema of the chest wall.

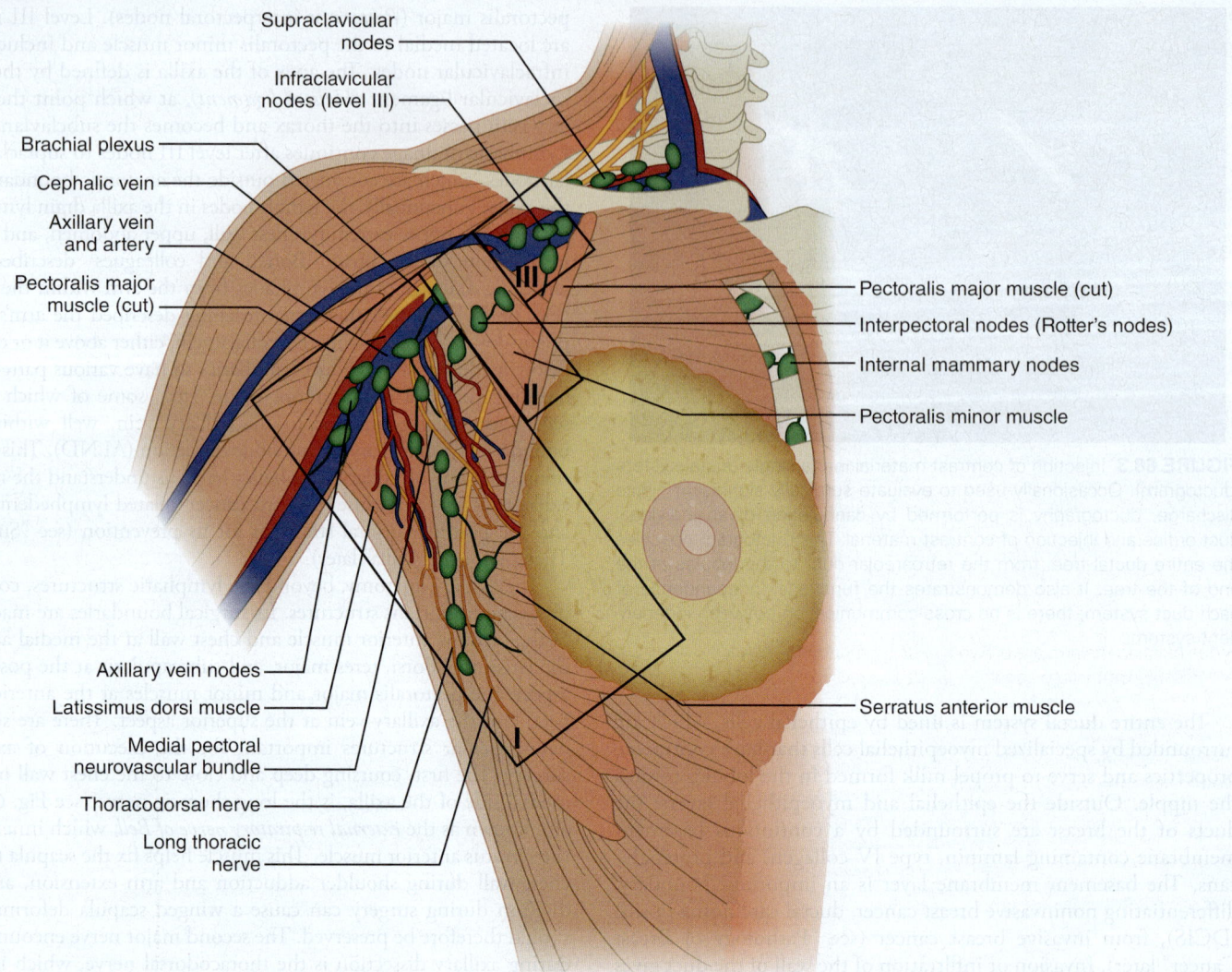

Supraclavicular
nodes

Infraclavicular
nodes (level III)

Brachial plexus

Cephalic vein

Axillary vein
and artery

Pectoralis major
muscle (cut)

III

II

I

Axillary vein nodes

Latissimus dorsi muscle

Medial pectoral
neurovascular bundle

Thoracodorsal nerve

Long thoracic
nerve

Pectoralis major muscle (cut)

Interpectoral nodes (Rotter's nodes)

Internal mammary nodes

Pectoralis minor muscle

Serratus anterior muscle

FIGURE 68.4 Lymphatic drainage of the breast. The lymph nodes in the axilla are grouped by location depending on their relationship to the pectoralis minor muscle: group I, lateral to the muscle; group II, at the level of the muscle; group III, medial to the muscle. The infraclavicular nodes in the axilla (level III) are continuous with the supraclavicular nodes in the neck. Nodes between the pectoralis major and minor muscles, called the *interpectoral nodes* (also known as *Rotter's lymph nodes*), are part of level II. The sentinel lymph node is functionally the first node or nodes in the axillary chain and, anatomically, is usually found in the external mammary group (level I). The relative positions of the long thoracic, thoracodorsal, and medial pectoral nerves are shown. These major nerves should be preserved during surgery.

Breast Development and Physiology

In utero, the milk bud develops from the ectodermal thickening in the pectoral area and extends as the milk streak (mammary ridge) from the axilla to the inguinal area. At 9 weeks of gestation, the milk streak begins to atrophy to normally form a single pair of bilateral glands. When less than the normal atrophy of the milk streak occurs, then polymastia (accessory breast[s]) and/or polythelia (accessory nipple[s]) occur, located along the milk line from the axilla to the pubis. True polythelia refers to more than one nipple serving a single breast, which is rare. Accessory breast tissue is commonly located above the breast in the axilla and can present as an enlarging mass during pregnancy that can persist after the termination of lactation. Rarely, congenital amastia or athelia (absence of breast tissue or nipple) occurs as a result of failure of the milk bud. Unilateral rudimentary breast development is more

common, as is adolescent hypertrophy of one breast compared with the other. *Poland syndrome* is a disorder that presents as a unilateral variable loss of the breast tissue, pectoralis major and minor, and serratus anterior muscles as well as several ribs.

Ninety percent of newborns will have a breast secretion that is commonly referred to as *witches' milk* that is the result of elevated maternal hormones and prolactin levels. If the secretion sequesters within the nipple, it can cause a mass or lactocele that will resolve on its own in 3 to 4 weeks, as will the discharge.

Before puberty, the breast is composed primarily of dense fibrous stroma and scattered ducts lined with epithelium. In the United States, puberty, as measured by breast development and the growth of pubic hair, begins between the ages of 9 and 12 years, and menarche (onset of menstrual cycles) begins at approximately 11 to 14 years of age. These events are initiated by

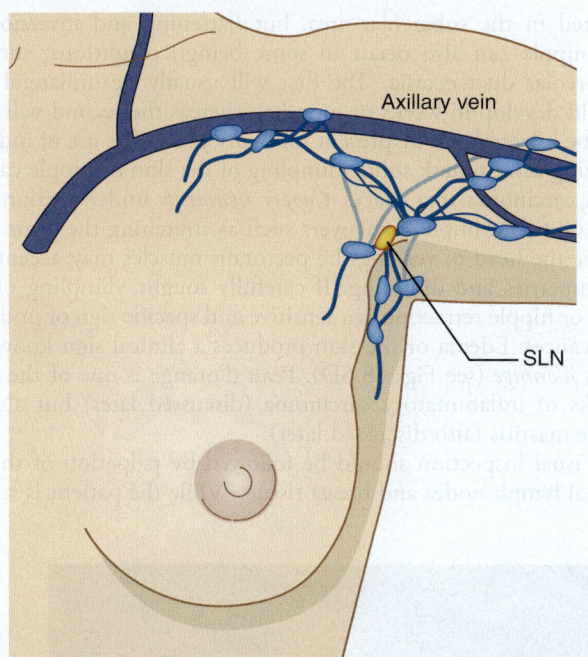

FIGURE 68.5 Axillary anatomy of lymphatics draining the arm. Lymph nodes draining the arm are drawn in *blue* (one potential pattern of drainage is illustrated, but many additional patterns have been described). Lymph nodes draining the breast and chest wall are drawn in *green*. A sentinel node is drawn in *yellow*. The axillary reverse mapping procedure (described later) allows for the differentiation between these nodes and preservation of nodes draining the arm. *SLN,* Sentinel lymph node. (Adapted from Boneti C, Korourian S, Diaz Z, et al. Scientific Impact Award: axillary reverse mapping [ARM] to identify and protect lymphatics draining the arm during axillary lymphadenectomy. *Am J Surg.* 2009;198:482-487.)

low-amplitude pulses of pituitary gonadotropins, which increase serum estradiol concentrations. In the breast, this hormone-dependent maturation (thelarche) entails increased deposition of fat, the formation of new ducts by branching and elongation, and the first appearance of lobular units. This process of growth and cell division is under the control of estrogen, progesterone, adrenal hormones, pituitary hormones, and the trophic effects of insulin and thyroid hormones. There is evidence that local growth factor networks are also important. The exact timing of these events and the coordinated development of both breast buds may vary from the average in individual patients. The term *prepubertal gynecomastia* refers to symmetric enlargement and projection of the breast bud in a female before the average age of 12 years, unaccompanied by the other changes of puberty. This process, which may be unilateral, should not be confused with neoplastic growth and is not an indication for biopsy.

The postpubertal mature or resting breast contains fat, stroma, lactiferous ducts, and lobular units. During phases of the menstrual cycle or in response to exogenous hormones, the breast epithelium and lobular stroma undergo cyclic stimulation. The dominant process appears to be hypertrophy and alteration of morphology rather than hyperplasia. In the late luteal (premenstrual) phase, there is an accumulation of fluid and intralobular edema. This edema can produce pain and breast engorgement.

These physiologic changes can lead to increased nodularity and may be mistaken for a malignant tumor. Ill-defined masses in premenopausal females are generally observed throughout the course of the menstrual cycle before any intervention is undertaken. With

pregnancy, there is a diminution of the fibrous stroma and the formation of new acini or lobules, termed *adenosis of pregnancy*. After birth, there is a sudden loss of placental hormones, which, combined with continued high levels of prolactin, is the principal trigger for lactation. The actual expulsion of milk is under hormonal control and is caused by the contraction of the myoepithelial cells that surround the breast ducts and terminal ductules. There is no evidence for innervation of these myoepithelial cells; their contraction appears to occur in response to the pituitary-derived peptide oxytocin. Stimulation of the nipple appears to be the physiologic signal for continued pituitary secretion of prolactin and acute release of oxytocin. When breastfeeding ceases, the prolactin level decreases, and there is no stimulus for the release of oxytocin. The breast returns to a resting state and to the cyclic changes induced when menstruation resumes.

Menopause is defined as cessation in menstrual flow for at least 1 year; in the United States, it usually occurs between the ages of 40 and 55 years, with a median age of 51 years. Menopause may be accompanied by symptoms such as vasomotor disturbances (hot flashes), vaginal dryness, urinary tract infections, and cognitive impairment (possibly secondary to interruption of sleep by hot flashes). Menopause results in involution and a general decrease in the epithelial elements of the resting breast. These changes include increased fat deposition, diminished connective tissue, and the disappearance of lobular units. The persistence of lobules, hyperplasia of the ductal epithelium, and cyst formation, as well as an increase in breast density, can occur under the influence of exogenous ovarian hormones, usually in the form of postmenopausal hormone replacement therapy (HRT).

CLINICAL APPROACH TO THE BREAST PATIENT

Patient History

When taking care of a patient with a suspected breast disease, several elements in the patient's history are pertinent. These include information that would convey the patient's risk for breast cancer as well as the symptoms she or he is experiencing that would help the clinician develop a differential diagnosis.

Some patients may be asymptomatic, arriving for routine assessment or as a result of findings on screening imaging. The patient should be asked about the history of a mass, breast pain, nipple discharge, swelling of the breast, and any skin changes. If a mass is present, and regarding any other complaint, the patient should be asked how long it has been present and whether it has grown or if its size fluctuates with the menstrual cycle. If a cancer diagnosis is suspected, inquiries about constitutional symptoms, bone pain, headaches, weight loss, and respiratory changes should be made to direct investigations that could reveal evidence of metastatic disease. The patient should also be asked about any prior breast conditions, including prior breast imaging and biopsies performed and their pathologic findings and, of course, any history of prior breast cancer.

Regarding the patient's risk for breast cancer, inquiries should include the patient's demographics, such as age and ethnicity. They should include elements regarding the patient's lifelong exposure to estrogen as well as the patient's reproductive history, including age at menarche; age at menopause; history of pregnancies, including age at first full-term pregnancy; lactation; and exposure to exogenous estrogen in the form of HRT or contraception. If the patient has had a hysterectomy, it is important to determine whether the ovaries were removed. In premenopausal females, a recent history of pregnancy and lactation should be noted. The family history should detail any known genetic abnormalities as well as any cancer, but especially of the breast and ovaries, and the menopausal status or age of any affected relatives at diagnosis. Radiation to the chest at a young age should also be noted because it, too, confers a higher risk of developing breast cancer.

Physical Examination

The physical examination of the breast begins with the patient in the upright sitting position. The breasts are visually inspected for obvious masses, asymmetries, and skin changes, such as dimpling or frank invasion and ulceration. The nipples are examined and compared for the presence of retraction, nipple inversion, or excoriation of the superficial epidermis, such as that seen with Paget disease (Fig. 68.6B). Paget disease (discussed later) produces a dermatitis-like appearance that begins in the nipple, whereas benign skin conditions, such as eczema, usually originate in the areola. Retraction of the nipple can be seen with carcinomas located in the subareolar area, but flattening and inversion of the nipple can also occur in some benign conditions, such as subareolar duct ectasia. The first will usually be unilateral and would develop in weeks or months, whereas the second will usually be bilateral and be present for many years. The use of indirect lighting can unmask subtle dimpling of the skin or nipple caused by a carcinoma that places *Cooper ligaments* under tension (see Fig. 68.6C). Simple maneuvers such as stretching the arms high above the head or tensing the pectoralis muscles may accentuate asymmetries and dimpling. If carefully sought, dimpling of the skin or nipple retraction is a sensitive and specific sign of underlying cancer. Edema of the skin produces a clinical sign known as *peau d'orange* (see Fig. 68.6D). Peau d'orange is one of the hallmarks of inflammatory carcinoma (discussed later) but also of acute mastitis (also discussed later).

Visual inspection should be followed by palpation of the regional lymph nodes and breast tissue. While the patient is still in

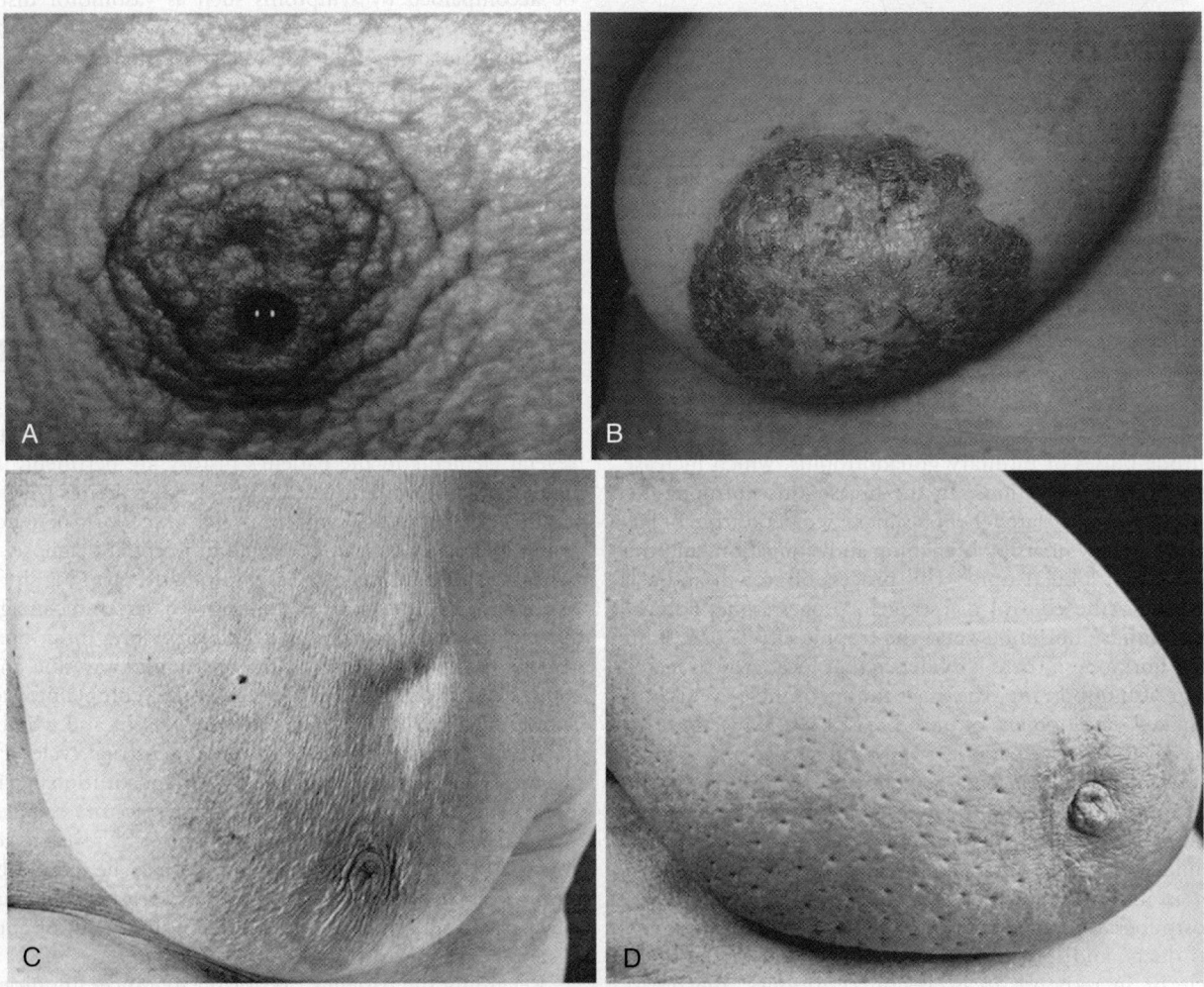

FIGURE 68.6 Common physical findings during breast examination. (A) Nipple discharge. Discharge from multiple ducts or bilateral discharge is a common finding in healthy breasts. In the case shown, the discharge is from a single duct orifice and may signify underlying disease in the discharging duct. In this patient, a papilloma was the source of her symptoms. (B) Paget disease of the nipple. Malignant ductal cells invade the epidermis without traversing the basement membrane of the subareolar duct or epidermis. The disease appears as a psoriatic rash that begins on the nipple and spreads off onto the areola and into the skin of the breast. (C) Skin dimpling. Traction on Cooper ligaments by a scirrhous tumor distorts the surface of the breast and produces a dimple best seen with angled indirect lighting during abduction of the arms upward. (D) Peau d'orange ("skin of the orange") or edema of the skin of the breast. This finding may be caused by dependency on the breast, lymphatic blockage (from surgery or radiation), or mastitis. The most feared cause is inflammatory carcinoma, in which malignant cells plug the dermal lymphatics—the pathologic hallmark of the disease.

the sitting position, the examiner supports the patient's arm and palpates each axilla from a posterior and/or anterior approach to detect the presence of enlarged axillary lymph nodes. The supraclavicular and infraclavicular spaces are similarly palpated for enlarged nodes. Then the patient lies down, and the breast is palpated. Palpation of the breast is always done with the patient lying supine on a solid examining surface, with the arm stretched above the head. The breast is best examined with compression of the tissue toward the chest wall, with systematic palpation of each quadrant and the tissue under the NAC. Palpable masses are characterized according to their size, shape, consistency, and location (hour and distance from the nipple) and whether they are fixed to the skin or underlying musculature. Benign tumors, such as fibroadenomas and cysts, can be as firm as carcinomas; usually, these benign entities are distinct, well circumscribed, and movable. Carcinoma is typically firm but less circumscribed, and moving a carcinoma produces a drag of adjacent tissue. Cysts and fibrocystic changes can be tender with palpation of the breast; however, tenderness is rarely a helpful diagnostic sign. Ultrasonography can be used as an extension of your physical exam, delineating normal ridges from worrisome masses and cystic from solid masses (see "Ultrasonography" section).

BREAST IMAGING AND DIAGNOSTIC BIOPSY

Screening (Mammography)

Screening mammography is performed in asymptomatic females to detect occult breast cancer. This approach assumes that breast cancers identified through screening will be smaller, have a better prognosis, and require less aggressive treatment than cancers identified by palpation. The potential benefits of screening are weighed against the cost of screening and the number of false-positive studies that would prompt additional workup, biopsies, potential complications, and patient anxiety.

Guidelines for screening are based on the female's lifetime risk of having breast cancer. For screening purposes, a female is considered to be at average risk if she does not have a personal history of breast cancer, a strong family history of breast cancer, or a genetic mutation known to increase the risk of breast cancer (e.g., the *BRCA* gene) and has not had chest radiation therapy (RT) before the age of 30. In addition, several calculators offer an estimation of a female's lifetime risk for breast cancer, which can further assist in guiding screening (see "Care of High-Risk Patients" later).

Eight heterogeneously designed prospective randomized trials of screening mammography have been performed, with almost 650,000 females participating. In these trials, among females 39 to 49 years old, screening mammography reduced the risk of breast cancer death by 15% (relative risk [RR] 0.85; credible interval [CrI] 0.75–0.96). In the six trials that included females 50 to 59 years old, screening mammography reduced the risk of breast cancer death in this age group by 14% (RR 0.86; CrI 0.75–0.99). Two trials included females 60 to 69 years old, and screening mammography reduced the risk of breast cancer death in this age group by 32% (RR 0.68; CrI 0.54–0.87). Only one trial included females older than 70 years, and data were insufficient to recommend routine screening in this age group. Although the randomized trials of screening mammography did not enroll females older than 74 years, breast cancer risk increases with age, and the sensitivity and specificity of mammography are highest in older females, whose breast tissue has usually been replaced by fat. It is therefore reasonable to continue mammographic screening in older females who are in good general health and who would be considered appropriate candidates for surgery.[2]

Table 68.1 summarizes the current recommendations for screening by the leading medical societies for average-risk females.[3-6] Recommendations are based on the current data available as to the risk reduction, the number of females needed to be

TABLE 68.1 Screening Mammogram Guidelines of the Leading Medical Societies for Average-Risk Patients

	STARTING AGE	FREQUENCY	STOPPING AGE	IS CLINICAL BREAST EXAM RECOMMENDED?	SUPPLEMENTAL IMAGING
American Cancer Society (ACS)[a]	40–44: optional 45: recommended	40–54: annually ≥55: every other year or annually	As long as in good health and life expectancy ≥10 years	No	
United States Preventive Services Task Force (USPSTF)[b]	40	Biennially	≥75: no sufficient data		Dense breasts: no sufficient data to recommend supplemental ultrasound or MRI
American Society of Breast Surgeons (ASBrS)[c]	40	Annually	As long as life expectancy ≥10 years		Dense breasts: consider supplemental imaging
National Comprehensive Cancer Network (NCCN)[d]	40	Annually		Breast encounter (including exam): annually from 40 Every 1–3 years from 25	Dense breasts: consider supplemental imaging

[a]Oeffinger KC, Fontham ETH, Etzioni R, et al. Breast cancer screening for women at average risk: 2015 guideline update from the American Cancer Society. *JAMA.* 2015;314(15):1599.
[b]U.S. Preventive Services Task Force Final Recommendation Statement. *Breast cancer: Screening.* https://www.uspreventiveservicestaskforce.org/uspstf/recommendation/breast-cancer-screening. Accessed January 18, 2025.
[c]American Society of Breast Surgeons. Position Statement on Screening Mammography. Accessed November 19, 2023. https://www.breastsurgeons.org/docs/statements/Position-Statement-on-Screening-Mammography.pdf.
[d]Bevers TB, Niell BL, Baker JL, et al. NCCN Guidelines® insights: breast cancer screening and diagnosis, version 1.2023. *J Natl Compr Canc Netw.* 2023;21(9):900-909.

invited for screening to prevent one breast cancer death, and the potential for harm from additional testing and biopsies. These recommendations are updated periodically by the different societies and are made public through their publications and on their websites (see Table 68.1). We recommend discussing breast cancer risk with females in their 20s, including an assessment of their risk for breast cancer. For those with an average risk, screening mammography should be recommended from the age of 40 and continued annually as long as the patient is a candidate for surgery. This should, of course, be part of shared decision-making between patient and physician, taking into account the particular patient's preference as far as onset, termination, and frequency of screening.

The imaging modality recommended for screening is 2D mammography or tomosynthesis (3D mammography). Yearly MRI is recommended for high-risk patients, including younger females with previous breast cancer, females with a known pathologic germline mutation, those with a significant family history of breast cancer, those with additional risk factors that convey a >20% lifetime risk of breast cancer, and potentially for patients with dense breasts. Some recommend using ultrasound (US) for screening, either as a sole modality or in conjunction with a mammogram, in younger patients or those with dense breasts. The addition of these supplemental modalities to screening mammography increases the breast cancer detection rate, with about 5 additional cancers detected per 1000 exams. This increased detection rate comes with the price of an over 10% recall and increased biopsy rate as well as financial toxicity.[7]

Imaging Modalities

Mammography

The primary imaging modality for screening asymptomatic females is mammography. During mammography, the breast is compressed between plates to reduce the thickness of the x-rayed tissue, separate adjacent structures, and improve resolution. On screening mammography, two views of each breast are obtained, mediolateral-oblique (MLO) and craniocaudal (CC), and read at a later time, usually in batches. For further evaluation of abnormalities identified on the two views of screening mammogram or of clinical findings or symptoms, diagnostic mammography is indicated. Diagnostic mammography includes additional views of the breast to allow better evaluation of suspicious findings, such as the mediolateral view, axillary view, implant displaced view, magnification views, compression views, and many others. These are read at the time of performance, so additional views may be performed as needed.

Mammographic abnormalities include clustered microcalcifications and areas of abnormal density (e.g., masses, architectural distortions, asymmetries). These can be correlated to areas of palpable findings if those exist (Fig. 68.7). The Breast Imaging Reporting and Data System (BI-RADS) is a widely used score developed by the American College of Radiology (ACR) to standardize and categorize the degree of suspicion of malignancy for detected abnormalities on mammography, US, or MRI (Table 68.2) (the ACR supplies a useful "Quick Reference" for the BI-RADS scoring on its website: https://www.acr.org/-/media/ACR/Files/RADS/BI-RADS/BIRADS-Reference-Card.pdf).[8] This grading system also aids in choosing patients for image-guided biopsy and avoiding unnecessary biopsies. Of patients with nonpalpable mammographic findings for whom diagnostic biopsy is recommended, 75% to 80% have benign findings. Therefore, a less invasive and less costly approach is preferred whenever feasible.

The sensitivity of mammography is limited by breast density, and 10% to 15% of clinically evident breast cancers have no visible abnormality on mammography. Higher breast density reduces mammographic accuracy and is an independent risk factor for breast cancer. A mammographic report therefore starts with an assessment of the density of the imaged breast, using the BI-RADS classification: A—fatty; B—scattered fibroglandular density; C—heterogeneously dense; and D—extremely dense. Some would advocate for supplemental imaging, with either US or MRI, for females with BI-RADS C and D dense breasts.

Since its advent in the mid-20th century, there have been numerous technical advancements in mammography. *Digital mammography* acquires digital images and stores them electronically, allowing manipulation and enhancement of images to facilitate interpretation. Digital mammography appears to be superior to traditional film-screen mammography for detecting cancer in younger females and those with dense breasts. *Computer-assisted diagnosis* (CAD) consists of software analysis of the digital images to detect abnormalities and prompt further investigation. There have been conflicting reports as to the potential of CAD to increase the sensitivity and specificity of mammography and US over review by the radiologist alone. Machine learning and artificial intelligence are used in the newest versions of this software. *Tomosynthesis* (digital 3D mammography) acquires multiple sectional images of the compressed breast from different angles and, similarly to a CT scan, translates them into a 3D image, which is presented in section form. This aids in separating overlapping breast tissues seen on 2D mammography and better delineates small masses, microcalcifications, and distortions from ducts and vessels. The Screening with Tomosynthesis or Standard Mammography-2 (STORM-2) prospective trial compared 2D and 3D mammography. This trial, in which 9672 patients were randomized between the two modalities, showed a significantly higher detection rate of breast cancer in the tomosynthesis group, with a slightly higher false-positive and recall rate and a modest increase in radiation dose to the patient. Another emerging innovation is *contrast-enhanced mammography*. Iodine-based contrast is delivered by intravenous injection before mammography, taking advantage of the cancer's abnormal neoangiogenesis to enhance suspicious lesions. It has been shown in retrospective trials to increase cancer detection and reduce false-positive rates compared with standard mammography. Furthermore, it has been shown to approach the accuracy of MRI, providing a potential alternative modality for screening high-risk patients.[9] Contrast-Enhanced Mammography for the Improvement of Surveillance in Women With a Personal History of Breast Cancer is a phase III trial currently investigating whether a contrast-enhanced mammogram can improve screening for females previously diagnosed with breast cancer. According to retrospective studies, new or recurrent breast cancer may be discovered earlier and treated less invasively when such patients are screened with contrast-enhanced mammography compared to standard mammographic surveillance.

Ultrasonography

US is useful in determining whether a lesion detected by mammography is solid or cystic. In addition, it is useful to further characterize suspicious lesions because malignant lesions tend to appear as irregular, spiculated, hypoechoic, more "tall" than "wide," and with acoustic shadowing. US can also be useful for discriminating lesions in patients with dense breasts and in characterizing the lymphatic basins. Moreover, US is most useful for image-guided aspirations, biopsies, and marker placement. Nevertheless, US is not useful as a breast cancer screening tool because of its high dependence on the operator performing the freehand

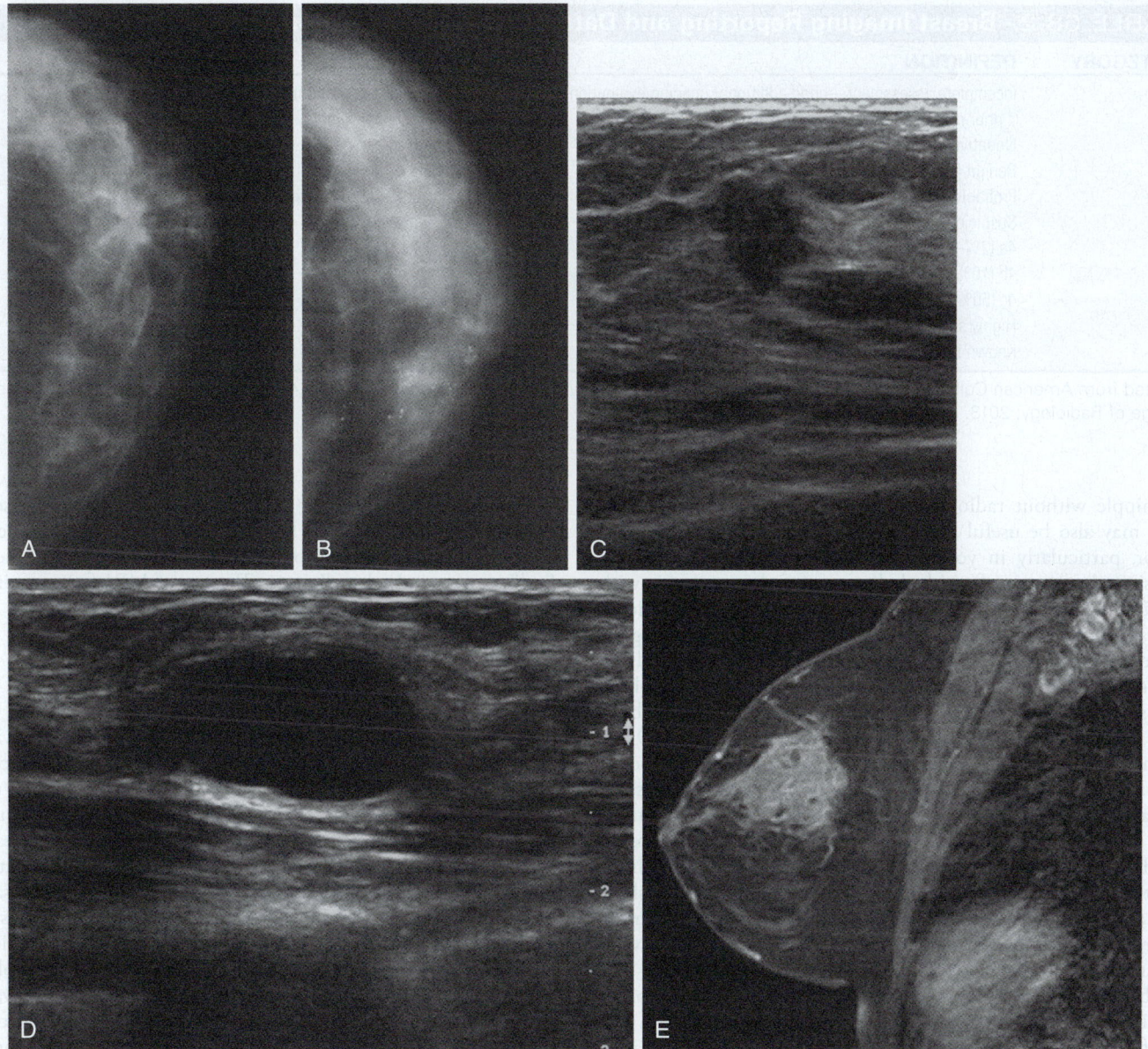

FIGURE 68.7 Mammography, ultrasound, and magnetic resonance imaging (MRI) findings in breast disease. (A) Stellate mass in the breast. The combination of density with spiculated borders and distortion of surrounding breast architecture suggests a malignancy. (B) Clustered microcalcifications. Fine, pleomorphic, and linear calcifications that cluster together suggest the diagnosis of ductal carcinoma in situ. (C) Ultrasound image of breast cancer. The mass is solid, contains internal echoes, and displays an irregular border. Most malignant lesions are taller than they are wide. (D) Ultrasound image of a simple cyst. On ultrasound, the cyst is round with smooth borders, there is a paucity of internal sound echoes, and there is increased through-transmission of sound with enhanced posterior echoes. (E) Breast MRI showing gadolinium enhancement of a breast cancer. Rapid and intense gadolinium enhancement reflects increased tumor vascularity. Lesion contour and size may also be assessed by MRI.

exam and the lack of standardized screening protocols. The American College of Radiology Imaging Network (ACRIN) 6666 trial randomized high-risk females to screening mammography plus US versus mammography alone and showed that the combination of mammography plus US resulted in the detection of an additional 4.2 cancers per 1000 females. However, the use of US resulted in more false-positive events and required more callbacks and biopsies.[10] Furthermore, there are no data available showing that the use of screening US can reduce mortality caused by breast

cancer. Automated breast US overcomes some of the issues of freehand US but is not widely used.

Magnetic Resonance Imaging

MRI is increasingly being used for the evaluation of breast abnormalities. It is useful for identifying the primary tumor in the breast in patients who present with axillary lymph node metastases without mammographic evidence of a primary breast tumor (the unknown primary tumor) or in patients with Paget disease of

TABLE 68.2   Breast Imaging Reporting and Data System Final Assessment Category

CATEGORY	DEFINITION	MANAGEMENT
0	Incomplete assessment—need additional imaging evaluation or prior mammograms for comparison	Obtain additional mammogram views or additional modality (ultrasound or magnetic resonance imaging)
1	Negative (0% chance of malignancy)	Annual screening
2	Benign finding (0% chance of malignancy)	Annual screening
3	Probably benign finding (<2% malignant)	Short-interval follow-up (6 months)
4	Suspicious abnormality	Perform biopsy
	4a (2%—10% malignant)	
	4b (10%–50% malignant)	
	4c (50%–95% malignant)	
5	Highly suggestive of malignancy (>95% malignant)	Perform biopsy
6	Known biopsy-proven malignancy	As indicated

Adapted from American College of Radiology. *Breast Imaging Reporting and Data System Atlas (BI-RADS Atlas)*. 5th ed. Reston, VA: American College of Radiology; 2013.

the nipple without radiographic evidence of a primary tumor. MRI may also be useful for assessing the extent of the primary tumor, particularly in young females with dense breast tissue; assessing the extent of residual disease after lumpectomy with positive margins; evaluating the presence of multifocal or multicentric cancer; screening of the contralateral breast; and evaluating invasive lobular cancers. Some surgeons use MRI preoperatively to determine eligibility for breast conservation; however, no high-level data show that the use of MRI to guide decision-making about local therapy improves local recurrence rates or survival. Other diagnostic indications include assessment of treatment response after neoadjuvant chemotherapy. It can also be used for assessing implant rupture or assessing the breast when silicone injections have been used. Clinical trials are examining modifications to healthy breast tissue identified with breast MRI, which may indicate the onset of cancer development. These will potentially show that a female's risk of developing breast cancer may be more accurately determined by combining breast tissue indicators with breast imaging, such as MRI.

The sensitivity of MRI is greater than 90% for the detection of invasive cancer but only 60% or less for the detection of DCIS. The specificity of MRI is only moderate compared with mammography or US because there is significant overlap in the appearance on MRI of benign and malignant lesions. A meta-analysis of 22 studies reporting the detection of contralateral breast cancer by MRI revealed a mean incremental cancer detection rate of 4.1% and a positive predictive value of 47.9%. This high rate of detection may result partly from selection bias; however, it is of significant concern that more than 50% of the abnormalities detected on MRI represented false-positive findings, resulting in the need for additional imaging studies and biopsies.

The Comparative Effectiveness of MRI in Breast Cancer (COM-ICE) trial was a multicenter trial that recruited 1623 females aged 18 years or older with newly diagnosed breast cancer to assess the clinical efficacy of contrast-enhanced MRI.[11] Patients had standard clinical and radiologic examinations and were randomly assigned to undergo MRI or no further imaging. The primary end point was the proportion of patients undergoing another surgical procedure (reexcision or mastectomy) within 6 months. There was no statistically significant difference in reoperation rates between patients who did or did not undergo MRI. The contralateral breast cancer detection rate in the COMICE trial was 1.6%, significantly lower than that reported in other trials. This trial was criticized because

MRI-guided biopsy was not available at all centers to assess suspicious findings identified on MRI. This situation led to numerous mastectomies without pathologic verification that the suspicious findings were indeed malignant. The use of MRI for screening is discussed later.

Biopsy
Fine-Needle Aspiration
Historically, fine-needle aspiration (FNA) was a common tool used in the diagnosis of breast masses. FNA can be done with a 22-gauge needle, an appropriately sized syringe, and an alcohol preparation pad. The needle is repeatedly inserted into the mass while constant negative pressure is applied to the syringe. In this way, multiple areas of a mass can be sampled. Suction is released, and the needle is withdrawn. The fluid and cellular material within the needle are submitted in physiologically buffered saline or fixed immediately on slides in 95% ethyl alcohol, and the slides are submitted for cytologic evaluation of the aspirated material. A limitation of FNA in evaluating solid masses is that cytologic evaluation does not differentiate noninvasive lesions from invasive lesions if malignant cells are identified. If FNA demonstrates malignancy, a core-needle biopsy (CNB) is still required for definitive histologic diagnosis before surgical intervention.

One clinical scenario in which FNA still has utility is in the evaluation of a second suspicious lesion in the ipsilateral breast of a patient with a known malignancy. In this case, FNA can be used to determine whether the second lesion is malignant and confirm a diagnosis of multifocal breast cancer. This information can aid in determining the appropriate surgical plan. A second clinical scenario in which FNA is commonly used is in the evaluation of lymph nodes that are suspicious on either physical examination or imaging, such as high-resolution ultrasonography of the regional nodal basins. Suspicious lymph nodes can be evaluated by FNA to determine whether metastatic disease is present. In this situation, FNA has a reported sensitivity of approximately 90% and a specificity of up to 100%. Determining whether the tumor has spread to the lymph nodes is an important step in the initial staging of breast cancer that provides prognostic information and helps determine appropriate management strategies. In the setting where neoadjuvant therapy is to be used and targeted axillary dissection (TAD; discussed later) might be considered, a clip can be placed in the positive node for future localization.

Core-Needle Biopsy

CNB is the method of choice for sampling breast lesions. Biopsies can be performed with trigger devices requiring multiple entries or with vacuum-assisted devices that require only a single insertion. The size of a CNB ranges from 8 to 14 gauge. CNB can be performed under mammographic (stereotactic), US, or MRI guidance. Mass lesions that are visualized by US can be sampled under US guidance; calcifications and densities that are best seen on mammography are sampled under stereotactic guidance. During stereotactic CNB, the breast is compressed, most often with the patient lying prone on the stereotactic CNB table or sitting upright. A robotic arm and biopsy device are positioned based on computed analysis of mammographic images to triangulate the location of the lesion. After a local anesthetic is injected, a small skin incision is made, and a core biopsy needle is inserted into the lesion to obtain the tissue sample with vacuum assistance. There are standards for the appropriate number of core samples to be obtained for each type of abnormality being sampled. A clip should be placed to mark the site of the lesion to allow for future localization and excision, particularly for small lesions that may be difficult to find after extensive sampling or when neoadjuvant therapy is to be considered. The specimens biopsied should be imaged to confirm that the targeted lesion has been adequately sampled and to guide pathologic assessment of the tissue. A mammogram of the breast should also be obtained to confirm adequate sampling of the target lesion and to ensure the location of the marking clip is appropriate. A similar approach is used for US-guided and MRI-guided biopsies.

Excisional Biopsy

The use of a minimally invasive procedure, such as CNB, is the preferred approach for the diagnosis of breast lesions. The use of a surgical excisional biopsy as a diagnostic procedure increases costs and results in delays of definitive surgery for patients with cancer.[12] Less than 10% of patients who undergo CNB have inconclusive or discordant results and require surgical biopsy for definitive diagnosis. Biopsy results that are not concordant with the targeted lesion (e.g., a highly suspicious spiculated mass on imaging and normal breast tissue on CNB) necessitate surgical excision.

IDENTIFICATION AND CARE OF HIGH-RISK PATIENTS

Risk Factors for Breast Cancer

Identification of factors associated with an increased incidence of breast cancer development is important in general health screening for females (Box 68.1). Risk factors for breast cancer can be divided into several broad categories: patient demographics and lifestyle, chest wall radiation, lifetime exposure to estrogen, family and genetic risk factors, personal history of breast cancer, and histologic risk factors. It is important to note that 30% of postmenopausal breast cancer cases are attributed to potentially modifiable risk factors.

Patient Demographics and Lifestyle

Age is probably the most important risk factor for breast cancer development. The age-adjusted incidence of breast cancer continues to increase with the advancing age of the female population. Breast cancer is rare in females younger than 20 years and constitutes less than 2% of total cases. Thereafter, the incidence

---

> **BOX 68.1** Risk Factors for Breast Cancer
>
> **Demographic and Lifestyle Risk Factors**
> Increased age
> Female sex
> Shift work (nighttime)
> Obesity
> Smoking
> Alcohol consumption
> Physical inactivity
> High-fat and low-fiber diet
>
> **Personal History of Chest Radiation Before the Age of 30**
> *Hormone Exposure*
> Early age at menarche (onset of menses before age 11)
> Older age of menopause (onset of menopause after the age of 55)
> Nulliparity and fewer live births
> Age at first live birth (first full-term pregnancy after age 30)
> Lack of breastfeeding
> Use hormone replacement therapy, contraception, and other forms of exogenous hormones
>
> **Genetic Predisposition**
> Family history of breast cancer
> Carrying a known germline mutation predisposing to breast cancer
>
> **Personal History of Breast Cancer**
> *Breast Histology*
> Dense breasts
> Proliferative breast disease without atypia (fibrocystic changes with severe hyperplasia, papillomas, papillomatosis, sclerosing adenosis, radial scar)—relative risk (RR) 1.3 to 1.9
> Proliferative disease with atypia (atypical ductal hyperplasia and atypical lobular hyperplasia)—RR 3.7 to 4.2
> Lobular carcinoma in situ (LCIS)—RR >7

Data from Hartmann LC, Sellers TA, Frost MH, et al. Benign breast disease and the risk of breast cancer. *N Engl J Med.* 2005;353:229; London SJ, Connolly JL, Schnitt SJ, et al. A prospective study of benign breast disease and the risk of breast cancer. *JAMA.* 1992;267:1780; Dupont WD, Parl FF, Hartmann WH, et al. Breast cancer risk associated with proliferative breast disease and atypical hyperplasia. *Cancer.* 1993;71:1258.

---

increases and peaks at the eighth decade of a female's life, with a cumulative lifetime incidence of 12.9%.[13]

Sex is also an important risk factor because most breast cancers occur in females. Breast cancer does occur in males; however, male breast cancer constitutes less than 1% of breast cancer cases in the United States. Nevertheless, males are usually diagnosed at a more advanced stage than females. Variation in the incidence of breast cancer worldwide, with higher incidences in North America and Europe compared with Africa and East Asia, attests to the association between economic development as well as social and lifestyle factors and breast cancer. Shift work (nighttime), obesity, smoking, alcohol consumption, physical inactivity, and a high-fat and low-fiber diet have all been shown to be risk factors for breast cancer.

Chest Wall Radiation

In patients with cancers requiring mantle irradiation (e.g., Hodgkin lymphoma), especially before the age of 30, the risk of future breast cancer is estimated at twofold to fourfold. The risk of breast cancer starts to increase about 8 years after radiation. These patients are considered to be at high risk and are recommended to start breast cancer screening at 25 to 30 years of age.

Hormone Exposure

Reproductive milestones that increase a female's lifetime estrogen exposure are thought to increase the risk for breast cancer. These include early onset of menarche before the age of 11, late onset of menopause after the age of 55, nulliparity or fewer pregnancies, and a first live childbirth after age 30 years. There is a 10% reduction in breast cancer risk for each 2-year delay in menarche and a 12% risk with menopause after age 55 compared with before; a first full-term pregnancy before age 18 years compared with after 30 is associated with half the risk for development of breast cancer. Breastfeeding has been reported to reduce breast cancer risk, with a 4% reduction in risk for every 12 months of breastfeeding. This effect may be secondary to a decrease in the number of lifetime menstrual cycles. Compared with sex, age, histologic risk factors, and genetics, reproductive risk factors are relatively mild in terms of their contribution to risk (RR 1.1–2.0). However, in contrast to family history or histologic factors, reproductive risk factors have a large influence on breast cancer prevalence in populations.

Exogenous hormone use is also associated with a higher risk of breast cancer. Therapeutic or supplemental estrogen and progesterone are taken for various conditions, with the two most common scenarios being contraception in premenopausal females and HRT in postmenopausal females. Other indications for the use of exogenous hormones include menstrual irregularities, polycystic ovaries, fertility treatment, hormone insufficiency states, and gender-affirming therapy. Studies have suggested that breast cancer risk is increased by up to 20% in current or past users of oral contraceptives but that the risk decreases as the interval after cessation of use increases.

The use of HRT was studied in the Women's Health Initiative, a prospective, randomized controlled trial in which healthy postmenopausal females 50 to 79 years old received various dietary and vitamin supplements and postmenopausal HRT. The study assessed the benefits and risks associated with HRT, a low-fat diet, and calcium and vitamin D supplementation and their effects on rates of cancer, cardiovascular disease, and osteoporosis-related fractures. During the period from 1993–98, at 40 centers in the United States, 16,608 females were randomly assigned to receive combined conjugated equine estrogens (e.g., Premarin, 0.625 mg/day) plus medroxyprogesterone acetate (2.5 mg/day) or placebo. Screening mammography and clinical breast examinations were performed at baseline and yearly thereafter. The study reached a stopping rule at 5.2 years of follow-up, at which time there were 245 cases of breast cancer (invasive and noninvasive) in the combined HRT group versus 185 cases in the placebo group. Of greater concern was that breast cancer was more likely to be diagnosed at a more advanced stage in females receiving combination HRT. An additional subgroup, who had undergone a hysterectomy, received estrogens only as their HRT. After 7 years of follow-up, they had similar rates of breast cancer as those receiving placebo (RR for the estrogen group 0.80; 95% CI 0.62–1.04). Females in the treatment arm did have a higher need for short-interval mammographic follow-up examinations compared with the placebo group (36.2% vs. 28.1%).

These findings were corroborated in a meta-analysis of prospective studies investigating HRT use and its effect on breast cancer incidence. It included 108,647 postmenopausal females who developed breast cancer, 51% of whom received HRT. It showed that nearly all HRT types, except vaginal estrogens, were associated with a higher breast cancer risk, with increased risk with longer use of HRT and a more pronounced risk in patients treated with combination estrogen and progesterone formulations compared with those treated with estrogen-only formulations. Risk persisted after ceasing to use HRTs, and the longer the treatment duration, the longer it persisted.[14]

Family History of Breast Cancer and Genetic Risk Factors

Many studies have examined the relationship between family history of breast cancer and the risk for breast cancer. First-degree relatives (mothers, sisters, and daughters) of patients with breast cancer have a 1.5-fold increased risk of breast cancer when one family member is affected and a twofold to fourfold excess risk if more than one relative is affected. The risk is much higher if the affected first-degree relative has premenopausal-onset and bilateral breast cancer. In families with multiple affected members, particularly with bilateral and early-onset cancer, the absolute risk in first-degree relatives can approach 50%, consistent with an autosomal dominant mode of inheritance.

Genetic and familial factors are estimated to be responsible for about 10% of all breast cancer cases, accounting for 25% of cases in females younger than 30 years. The first described germline mutations were in the *BRCA* (BReast CAncer) gene. Germline mutations inactivate a single inherited allele in every cell, with a somatic event occurring in the remaining allele, causing cancer. In 1990, King and colleagues identified a region on the long arm of chromosome 17 (17q21) that contained a cancer susceptibility gene, and the *BRCA1* gene was described in 1994 as a tumor suppressor gene with disease susceptibility inherited in an autosomal dominant fashion. A second susceptibility gene, *BRCA2*, located on chromosome 13, was discovered in 1995. Females with *BRCA1 or BRCA2* mutations have a lifetime breast cancer risk of over 60%. In addition to being at increased risk for breast cancer, females with mutations in *BRCA1* or *BRCA2* are at increased risk for ovarian cancer (39%–58% lifetime risk for *BRCA1* carriers and 13%–29% risk in *BRCA2* carriers). *BRCA1/2* mutation carriers also have a higher risk for pancreatic cancer, prostate cancer (more with *BRCA2*), and male breast cancer (more with *BRCA2*).

Deleterious mutations in *BRCA1* or *BRCA2* are rare in the general population. The frequency of mutations is approximately 1 in 1000 (0.1%) in the population of the United States. Certain relatively closed populations may have higher prevalence rates and show a preference for certain mutations, termed *founder mutations*. Examples of such mutations in *BRCA1* include the 185delAG and 5382insC mutations, found in 1.0% of Ashkenazi Jews (Jews of Eastern European descent), and the C4446T mutation, found in French-Canadian families. Examples of founder *BRCA2* mutations include the 617delT mutation, present in 1.4% of the Ashkenazi population; the 8765delAG mutation, present in the French-Canadian population; and the 999del15 mutation, found in 0.6% of the Icelandic population. The penetrance of a gene refers to the chance that carriers of mutations in the gene will develop breast cancer. The initial estimates of the penetrance of *BRCA1* and *BRCA2* mutations were high, but the penetrance of *BRCA1* and *BRCA2* mutations more recently has been estimated to be 56% (95% CI 40%–73%).

The histopathology of *BRCA1*-associated breast cancer is generally unfavorable compared with *BRCA2*-associated cancer, with a higher prevalence of tumors that are high-grade and triple receptor negative (triple negative). In comparison, *BRCA2*-associated cancers are more commonly hormone receptor positive. Overall mortality rates in patients with *BRCA1*- or *BRCA2*-associated breast cancer are similar to mortality rates in females with sporadic breast cancer of similar histology and stage.

TABLE 68.3 Germline Genetic Mutations Conferring a Higher Risk for Breast Cancer

MUTATION	RISK OF BREAST CANCER	RISK FOR OTHER CANCERS/ SYNDROMES
BRCA1	>60% Male: 0.2%–1.2%	Ovarian: 39%–58% Pancreatic: <5% Prostate: 7%–26%
BRCA2	>60% Male: 1.8%–7.1%	Ovarian: 13%–29% Pancreatic: 5%–10% Prostate: 19%–61% Melanoma
ATM	20%–40%	Ovarian: 2%–3% Pancreatic: 5%–10% Prostate
BARD1	20%–40%	
CDH1	41%–60% (more ILC)	Gastric (hereditary diffuse gastric cancer)
CHEK2	20%–40%	Colorectal
MLH1, MSH2, MSH6, PMS2, EPCAM	<15%	Ovarian Pancreatic Colorectal, uterine, and others
NF1	20%–40%	Neurofibromatosis syndrome
PALB2	41%–60% Male: 0.9%	Ovarian: 3%–5% Pancreatic: 5%–10%
PTEN	40%–60%	Cowden syndrome
RAD51C/D	20%–40%	Ovarian: 10%–15%
STK11	32%–54%	Peutz-Jeghers syndrome
TP53	>60%	Li-Fraumeni syndrome

ILC, Invasive lobular carcinoma.
Adapted from the NCCN guidelines version 3.2023.

In recent years, several additional germline mutations that confer a higher risk for breast cancer have been described, and these are now included in current commercial gene panels. Several of these mutations are related to known genetic syndromes, such as the *TP53* gene and Li-Fraumeni syndrome, *PTEN* and Cowden syndrome, and *STK11* and Peutz-Jeghers syndrome, with each syndrome having its associated manifestations. Additional genes include *PALB2*, a gene related to *BRCA2*, along with *ATM*, *CHEK2*, and *CDH1* (associated with diffuse gastric cancer syndrome as well as with lobular breast cancer). Each of these mutations confers a breast cancer risk of 20% to over 60% lifetime risk, and, in addition, each is associated with an elevated lifetime risk of nonbreast cancers. Screening recommendations for these patients are derived from their respective risk of developing breast or other cancers. See NCCN Clinical Practice Guidelines in Oncology for a list of genetic mutations and their risk for breast cancer and other cancers as well as management recommendations (Genetic/Familial High-Risk Assessment: Breast, Ovarian, Pancreatic, and Prostate at nccn. org/professionals/physician_gls/pdf/genetics/bopp.pdf).

Personal History of Breast Cancer and Other Histologic Risk Factors

A history of cancer, invasive or DCIS, in one breast increases the likelihood of a second primary cancer, usually in the contralateral breast (70%), with about 5% of breast cancer survivors developing a new breast cancer. The magnitude of risk depends on the age at diagnosis of the first primary cancer, estrogen receptor (ER) status of the first primary cancer, and use of adjuvant systemic chemotherapy and endocrine therapy. The incidence of contralateral breast cancer and recurrences has decreased in recent years thanks to improvements in adjuvant systemic treatments, with the actual 5-year risk for contralateral cancer varying from 1% to 2%.[15] This risk increases with a family history of breast cancer.

Histologic abnormalities other than cancer, as diagnosed by breast biopsy, are also associated with an increased risk of breast cancer and constitute an important category of breast cancer risk factors. These abnormalities include lobular carcinoma in situ (LCIS) and proliferative changes with or without atypia. Classic LCIS is not considered a precursor for cancer but rather a risk factor for breast cancer. Pleomorphic and florid LCIS, on the other hand, are more aggressive and are considered and treated as cancer precursors, much like DCIS. Classic LCIS is typically an incidental finding at biopsy for another condition and does not manifest as a palpable mass or suspicious microcalcifications on mammography. In a report on more than 5000 biopsies performed for benign disease, LCIS was found in 3.6% of cases. Classic LCIS confers a sevenfold risk ratio for developing breast cancer, based on data from the Connecticut Tumor Registry. In that report, 40% of cancers that developed were DCIS, the invasive carcinomas were predominantly of ductal and not lobular histology, and 50% of cancers occurred in the contralateral breast of the LCIS. LCIS is therefore considered only a histologic marker for increased breast cancer risk and not a cancer precursor, with an estimated added risk of 1% per year, longitudinally. For most patients with a diagnosis of LCIS, a conservative approach is favored, with close observation, high-risk screening, and consideration for chemoprevention. Some patients will opt for prophylactic mastectomies for risk reduction.

Dense breasts on mammography, with BI-RADS C or D, and no histologic abnormalities are associated with a 1.5- to 2-fold risk of breast cancer compared with those with BI-RADS A and B dense breasts. Higher breast density can also hinder the identification of other underlying breast pathologies. Regardless, additional breast histologies that might confer a higher risk for malignancy can be broadly divided into nonproliferative and proliferative epithelial changes. Nonproliferative changes include fibrocystic changes with no, usual, or mild to moderate hyperplasia of luminal cells within breast ducts; these do not significantly increase a female's lifetime risk for development of breast cancer. Proliferative changes within the breast ductal system have been divided by Dupont and Page into lesions with or without atypia; both are associated with an increased risk of breast cancer. Proliferative changes without atypia, including fibrocystic changes with severe hyperplasia, papillomas, sclerosing adenosis, and radial scars, are associated with a 1.3- to 1.9-fold increased risk of breast cancer. Radial scars are complex sclerosing lesions, appearing as spiculations on imaging and containing microcysts, epithelial hyperplasia, and adenosis with central sclerosis. Radial scars generally require excision to rule out an underlying carcinoma.

Proliferative changes with atypia include atypical ductal hyperplasia (ADH) and atypical lobular hyperplasia (ALH). The risk of developing breast cancer in females with ADH or ALH is approximately four to five times the risk in the general population. The estimated risk is further influenced by age at diagnosis, menopausal status, and family history (e.g., family history of breast cancer and atypical hyperplasia increases the risk to almost nine times that of the general population). The annual risk for the development of breast cancer in a female with ADH or ALH is 0.5% to 1% per year. ADH has a >20% rate of upgrade upon excision, and excision is generally recommended, but observation could be considered based on patient risk factors as well as the volume of disease and whether the lesion was completely excised or adequately sampled during biopsy. The upgrade risk for ALH might be lower than that for ADH, so excision recommendations could be tailored to patient and lesion characteristics (e.g., whether ALH was an incidental finding and how many TDLUs were involved). See the American Society of Breast Surgeons (ASBrS) guidelines on the management of high-risk lesions at https://www.breastsurgeons.org/docs/statements/asbrs-ccs-concordance.pdf.

Risk Assessment

Several risk assessment models have been developed to help estimate a patient's risk for developing breast cancer. Each tool incorporates different known risk factors and does not incorporate others and therefore could over- or underestimate certain populations. When estimating an individual's risk, clinicians should acquaint themselves with these different models and choose the appropriate one for the clinical scenario.

A model for assessing breast cancer risk, known as the *Gail model,* was developed from case-control data in the Breast Cancer Detection Demonstration Project. (This model is available for clinical use at http://www.cancer.gov/bcrisktool.) In developing the model, factors influencing the risk for breast cancer were identified as age, race, age at menarche, age at first live birth, number of previous breast biopsies, presence of proliferative disease with atypia, and number of first-degree female relatives with breast cancer. The model does not include detailed information about genetic factors and may underestimate the risk for *BRCA1* or *BRCA2* mutation carriers and overestimate the risk for noncarriers. The model should not be used in females with a diagnosis of LCIS or DCIS. Other limitations include incorporation of only first-degree relatives and only those with breast cancer, without taking the age of diagnosis into account, therefore underestimating risk in patients with a strong family history of breast and other cancers and those with known genetic mutations. In addition, it is not accurate for non-European (non-White) patients. A specific model, the CARE model, was developed to more accurately assess the risk for breast cancer in the Black population. The Gail model for breast cancer risk was used in the design of the Breast Cancer Prevention Trial, which randomly assigned females at high risk (defined as >1.66% risk in 5 years) to receive tamoxifen or a placebo, and in the design of the Study of Tamoxifen and Raloxifene (STAR), which randomly assigned females at high risk to receive tamoxifen or raloxifene.

The Tyrer-Cuzick model was developed with data from the International Breast Cancer Intervention Study (IBIS). It estimates the risk of breast cancer and of carrying a mutation in the *BRCA1/2* gene (online calculator available at https://ibis.ikonopedia.com/). It incorporates, apart from a female's age, weight, and height, hormonal and reproductive history (age of menarche, age at first live birth, age at menopause, and use of HRT), *BRCA1/2* status, whether she has undergone a breast biopsy in the past, and whether that biopsy showed atypical findings or LCIS as well as detailed family history of breast and ovarian cancer and *BRCA1/2* status. It includes the largest number of breast cancer risk factors and so requires more time to complete. It is estimated to be more accurate than the Gail model in predicting breast cancer risk in patients with considerable family history or hormonal and reproductive risk factors. Several other models have been designed to assess the risk of harboring a mutation in *BRCA1* or *BRCA2*: The Couch model predicts the risk for a mutation in the *BRCA1* gene, and the BRCAPro model, developed by Myriad Genetics Laboratories,

estimates the risk of *BRCA1* and *BRCA2* mutations. Such models have estimated that the incidence of clinically significant *BRCA1* or *BRCA2* mutations in the general population is approximately 1 in 300 to 500.

The Claus model is based on assumptions about the prevalence of high-penetrance breast cancer susceptibility genes. The Claus model provides individual estimates of breast cancer risk according to decade of life based on knowledge of first-degree and second-degree relatives with breast cancer and their age at diagnosis. Many other models have been developed for specific populations, all with similar discriminatory power as compared with the nonspecific traditional models. Increased mammographic density is associated with a high risk for breast cancer. However, models including breast density have only minimal discriminatory power. Other well-known risk factors not included in most, if not all, risk assessment tools are alcohol consumption, body weight, and physical activity.

The National Comprehensive Cancer Network (NCCN) guidelines recommend genetic testing in specific patients with breast cancer: patients diagnosed with breast cancer before the age of 50; or patients diagnosed at any age with triple-negative breast cancer, multiple primary breast cancers, invasive lobular carcinoma (ILC) with a family history of diffuse gastric cancer, those with male breast cancer, patients with Ashkenazi Jewish heritage, and those with a family history of breast cancer at an age younger than 50 years, male breast, ovarian, pancreatic, or high-risk prostate cancer. Testing is also recommended if genetic testing would aid in systemic treatment decisions with polyadenosine diphosphate-ribose polymerase (PARP) inhibitors or olaparib (discussed later under "Systemic Therapy for Breast Cancer"). These guidelines indicate testing for a majority of breast cancer patients. The ASBrS has taken a more permissive approach and recommends making genetic testing available to any patient with a personal history of breast cancer, advocating its potential to affect treatment recommendations as well as the screening recommendations for family members (ASBrS guidelines are available at https://www.breastsurgeons.org/docs/statements/Consensus-Guideline-on-Genetic-Testing-for-Hereditary-Breast-Cancer.pdf).

Commercial genetic testing has become more accessible as a result of reduced cost and offers multigene panel testing. These include, in addition to the *BRCA1* and *BRCA2* genes, additional genes that have been recognized to increase the risk for breast cancer, as mentioned earlier. These include *ATM, BARD1, CDH1, CHEK2, NF1, PALB2, PTEN* (Cowden syndrome), *RAD51C, STK11,* and *TP53* (Li-Fraumeni syndrome). In addition, different companies provide additional preliminary-evidence genes for testing, such as *ABRAXAS1, AKT1, BRIP1, DICER1, EPCAM, FANCC, FANCM, MRE11, MUTYH, PIK3CA, RECQL, RINT1, SDHB, SDHD,* and *XRCC2*. Genetic testing results should be interpreted in conjunction with a patient's history and clinical scenario to determine both the relevance and potential penetrance of the pathogenic mutations. Recommendations for screening and potential risk reduction treatments are outlined by the different associations, including the NCCN and the ASBrS. Of note, individuals identified with a variant of uncertain significance (VUS) should not be acted upon because there is still not enough information to determine whether these specific mutations are indeed pathogenic.

Care of High-Risk Patients

In practice, clinicians assess risk factors, employ risk models, and consider the factors that are important to individual patients in making recommendations about breast cancer screening and prevention. The clinician should take into account the limitation of each risk model, and risk should be calculated within the context of an individual's personal and family history, with the risk models functioning as a starting point. Increased risk for breast cancer is defined as a 5-year calculated risk of 1.66% or higher by the Gail model; a 20% or higher lifetime risk based on histologic, family, and genetic factors; or history of thoracic radiation between the ages of 10 and 30 years. This risk assessment can provide a context for recommendations for supplemental screening as well as primary prevention strategies appropriate to the individual's risk level. For patients found to be at high risk for the development of breast cancer, options include close surveillance with clinical breast examination, mammography, and breast MRI, along with interventions to reduce risk, such as chemoprevention or a bilateral prophylactic mastectomy and/or salpingo-oophorectomy. Patients carrying known pathogenic mutations should be managed according to the recommendations for the specific gene mutation, regarding their risk for both breast cancer and other types of cancer.

Close Surveillance

Surveillance guidelines for individuals at high risk for breast cancer were established in 2002 by the NCCN and the Cancer Genetics Studies Consortium and have been updated since. These guidelines are based primarily on expert opinion; screening guidelines for high-risk individuals are not established by prospective trials. Recommendations start with breast awareness from the establishment of the high-risk state, with clinical encounters that include risk assessment, consideration for genetic counseling and testing, and a clinical breast exam between twice a year and annually, beginning in the early 20s. In addition, imaging with annual tomosynthesis is recommended starting from the diagnosis of the histologic risk factor (ADH/ALH/LCIS), 10 years earlier than the youngest family member affected by breast cancer, or 8 years after receiving thoracic RT, but not before the age of 30 years old (25 years for RT). Nonetheless, studies of females with known BRCA1 or BRCA2 mutations found that 50% of the detected breast cancers were diagnosed as interval cancers; that is, they were diagnosed between screening episodes and were not identified during the course of routine screening. This observation prompted many groups to add annual screening MRI to screening mammography, with some groups recommending doing the two examinations simultaneously and others recommending staggering the two examinations.

The American Cancer Society has recommended a risk-adjusted model. Annual MRI screening, as an adjunct to annual screening mammography, is recommended beginning at age 30 years for females at high lifetime risk for breast cancer development, defined as those with a history of radiation to the chest at age 10 to 30, a known genetic mutation with increased risk for breast cancer, or a lifetime risk of approximately 20% to 25% or greater based on risk assessment models. Females at moderately increased lifetime risk (15%–20%) are advised to discuss the benefits and limitations of adding MRI screening with their physicians. MRI is not recommended for females with a lifetime risk of less than 15%.[3]

Chemoprevention of Breast Cancer

Drugs currently approved for reducing breast cancer risk are the selective ER modulators (SERMs) tamoxifen and raloxifene and aromatase inhibitors (AIs). Tamoxifen has been proven beneficial for the adjuvant treatment of patients with ER-positive breast cancer (see "Endocrine Therapy" later on) and has been used as adjuvant treatment for breast cancer for several decades. In this scenario, it is known to reduce the incidence of a second primary breast cancer in the contralateral breast by 47%, as demonstrated by the Early Breast Cancer Trialists' Collaborative Group (EBCTCG) overview analysis. This observation prompted several prospective randomized trials that evaluated tamoxifen for chemoprevention in healthy females at increased risk for breast cancer.

The FDA approved the use of tamoxifen for risk reduction in patients at high risk for breast cancer based on the National Surgical Adjuvant Breast and Bowel Project (NSABP) P-1 trial.[16] In this trial, 13,388 females who were 35 to 59 years old (both pre- and postmenopausal) with a cumulative 5-year breast cancer risk of 1.7% or higher based on the Gail model, healthy females aged 60 or older, and females with a history of LCIS were randomly assigned to 20 mg daily tamoxifen or placebo for 5 years. In this study, tamoxifen reduced the risk for invasive breast cancer by 43% through a 7-year follow-up, with a more pronounced risk reduction of 59% in females with LCIS and 75% in females with ADH or ALH. Nevertheless, it showed no change in all-cause mortality, and the risk reduction was noted only for ER-positive cancers. In addition, noted side effects included menopausal symptoms, an over twofold increase in the incidence of endometrial cancer, and a threefold increase in the incidence of pulmonary embolism in patients 50 years and older. Data as to the efficacy of tamoxifen for the reduction of breast cancer risk in BRCA1 and BRCA2 mutation carriers were limited as a result of small numbers, because mutation testing was not routinely performed on P-1 study participants. That being said, a trend toward reducing the risk of breast cancer was seen in BRCA2 mutation carriers but not in BRCA1 mutation carriers, probably because of the difference in development of ER-positive tumors in each of these subgroups.

Three other tamoxifen prevention trials were conducted at approximately the same time as the NSABP P-1 trial, including the Italian Tamoxifen Prevention Study, the Royal Marsden Hospital Pilot Tamoxifen Chemoprevention Trial, and the International Breast Cancer Intervention Study-I (IBIS-I). The Italian and Royal Marsden studies did not show any benefit of tamoxifen over placebo in terms of reduced incidence of breast cancer. There were some differences in the study populations and trial designs, which may explain the negative results compared with the P-1 trial. The IBIS-I trial showed a 32% reduction in the incidence of breast cancer with tamoxifen, slightly lower than the risk reduction in P-1 but confirming the risk reduction benefit of tamoxifen. Subsequently, a meta-analysis of all the tamoxifen prevention trials found that tamoxifen reduced the risk of breast cancer by 38% in study participants. This analysis also confirmed the increased risks of endometrial cancer and venous thromboembolic events seen with tamoxifen use.

The NSABP P-2 trial (STAR trial) compared tamoxifen with raloxifene (a second-generation SERM) in postmenopausal females. This comparison was based on the findings from the Multiple Outcomes of Raloxifene Evaluation (MORE) trial, which included 7700 females who received a placebo versus raloxifene for the prevention and treatment of osteoporosis. In the MORE trial, at an average of 3 years of follow-up, there was a 54% reduction in the incidence of breast cancer and no increase in uterine cancer in females taking raloxifene. The STAR trial enrolled 19,747 females at increased risk for breast cancer, based on the Gail model or personal history of LCIS, and randomized them to tamoxifen or raloxifene. It demonstrated that there was no difference in breast cancer incidence between tamoxifen and ral-oxifene at 4 years, each estimated to reduce the risk for invasive breast cancer by approximately 50%. At a median follow-up of 8 years, raloxifene was 24% less effective in reducing the risk for breast cancer than tamoxifen, although it had a more favorable toxicity profile, with a 45% reduction in the risk for endometrial cancer and a 25% reduction in thromboembolic events.

Use of AIs in the adjuvant setting has been shown to prevent more contralateral breast cancers than tamoxifen in postmeno-pausal females with early-stage breast cancer. This led to their evaluation for chemoprevention. The National Cancer Institute of Canada Clinical Trials Group completed the Mammary Prevention 3 (MAP.3) trial investigating the AI exemestane. In this study, 4560 postmenopausal females who had at least one of several breast cancer risk factors (≥60 years old; Gail model 5-year risk score >1.66%; personal history of ADH, ALH, or LCIS; or prior DCIS with mastectomy) were randomly assigned to exemestane or pla-cebo. After a median follow-up of 35 months, exemestane was associated with a 65% relative reduction in the annual incidence of invasive breast cancer. Adverse events occurred in 88% of subjects in the exemestane group and 85% of subjects in the placebo group ($P = 0.003$), with significant differences noted in the development of endocrine, gastrointestinal, and musculoskeletal symptoms. Exemestane has not been approved by the FDA as a chemopreven-tive agent; however, it has a category 1 recommendation for breast cancer prevention in the NCCN clinical practice guidelines. The IBIS-II trial similarly evaluated anastrozole versus placebo in a population of 3864 high-risk individuals, defined as those with a family history of breast cancer or a personal history of DCIS, LCIS, or ADH. It showed that anastrozole resulted in a 53% reduction in the incidence of breast cancer.

Based on these trials, patients at a higher risk for breast cancer, defined as a 5-year risk of 1.7% or more based on the Gail model, a 10-year risk of 5% or more based on the Tyrer-Cuzick model, or a personal history of LCIS or ADH/ALH, should be individu-ally counseled. Depending on age, menopausal status, BRCA1/2 status, prior hysterectomy, thromboembolic event risk, and so forth, the most appropriate chemopreventive drug should be sug-gested. An option for reduced-dose tamoxifen, with 5 mg daily for 3 years instead of 20 mg for 5 years, is available for those who are symptomatic or unable to take the higher dose.

Prophylactic Mastectomy

Bilateral prophylactic mastectomy (BPM) has been shown to re-duce the risk of breast cancer development in high-risk females by 90%. This was first reported in 1999 by Hartmann and col-leagues, who retrospectively reviewed a group of 639 females with a family history of breast cancer who underwent prophylactic mastectomy. These females were divided into high-risk ($n = 214$) and moderate-risk ($n = 425$) groups based on their family history. Both groups were shown to have a 90% and 89% reduction in breast cancer incidence compared with a control group based on the Gail model (for moderate-risk females) and the sisters of high-risk probands (for high-risk females).[17]

Several groups reported on prospective studies in BRCA1 and BRCA2 mutation carriers treated with prophylactic mastectomy versus surveillance and showed that mastectomy is highly effective in preventing breast cancers. More recently, a meta-analysis includ-ing 2555 patients showed a risk reduction of 89% in BRCA1/2 mutation carriers undergoing BPM. It further showed that prophy-lactic bilateral salpingo-oophorectomy (PBSO) in 7323 BRCA1/BRCA2 mutation carriers reduces the risk of breast cancer by 45%.

Nevertheless, this meta-analysis showed no statistically significant improvement in all-cause mortality in BRCA1/BRCA2 mutation carriers undergoing BPM, whereas an improved all-cause and breast cancer–specific mortality was seen with PBSO.[18] The available data suggest that BRCA mutation carriers should be counseled to con-sider risk-reducing surgeries as a strategy to reduce cancer incidence and potentially improve survival.

The use of risk-reducing surgery in females who are not known to have pathogenic mutations in BRCA1 or BRCA2 is controver-sial. Risk-reducing surgery can be considered in females who are carriers of mutations other than BRCA1/BRCA2, such as PALB2, PTEN, ATM, and CHEK2, although data are insufficient to determine its advantage, and the decision should be tailored based on the individual's family history. Similar recommendations would be made to females who are mutation carriers with primary breast cancer regarding a contralateral prophylactic mastectomy (CPM) as part of their cancer treatment. Regarding females who are not mutation carriers, trends have suggested that more females with newly diagnosed breast cancer are choosing to undergo CPM as a strategy for reducing the risk of contralateral breast cancer. Studies have shown that the risk of contralateral breast cancer is 0.1% to 0.6% a year in the average-risk population, and although CPM would reduce this risk, it does not have a survival benefit and is associated with both a twofold increase in postop-erative complications and potential negative effects on long-term quality of life. The ASBrS and the Society of Surgical Oncology have published consensus statements regarding the use of CPM; these statements do not recommend the routine use of contralat-eral mastectomy in sporadic cancer patients, but because many females request such procedures, the statements favor a shared-decision model.[19] Nevertheless, these statements discourage CPM in average-risk females with unilateral breast cancer, those with advanced primary cancer (T4, N3, or stage IV), females with high risk for postoperative complications, BRCA-negative patients in BRCA-positive families, and males with breast cancer.

BENIGN BREAST TUMORS AND RELATED DISEASES

This section serves as an overview of several of the more common benign conditions of the breast.

Fibrocystic Changes and Breast Pain

The condition previously referred to as *fibrocystic disease* represents a spectrum of clinical, mammographic, and histologic findings and is common during the fourth and fifth decades of life, generally lasting until menopause. An exaggerated response of breast stroma and epithelium to various circulating and locally produced hor-mones and growth factors is frequently characterized by the constel-lation of breast pain, tenderness, and nodularity. Symptomatically, the condition manifests as premenstrual cyclic mastalgia, with pain and tenderness to touch. Treatment with Danocrine, Lupron, or tamoxifen is effective but has significant side effects. Noncyclic mastalgia is likely idiopathic and is more difficult to treat. Females 30 years and older with noncyclic mastalgia should undergo breast imaging with mammography and ultrasonography in addition to a physical examination. If examination reveals a mass, this should become the focus of subsequent evaluation. Occasionally, a simple cyst may cause cyclical or noncyclic breast pain, and aspiration of the cyst usually resolves the pain. In the case of large cysts, which will quickly recur after aspiration, percutaneous excision with a vacuum-assisted device will be definitive.

Referred pain can be a significant cause of breast pain as well, the most common source of which is scapulothoracic bursitis. It can be cyclical but is most often noncyclical. The confluence of afferent signals from the shoulder and the dorsal horn of the spinal cord can cause referred pain from the shoulder in the distribution of the intercostal nerves along the axilla, the breast, and the arm. Trigger point injections, with short- and long-acting analgesics as well as steroids along the medial scapular border, to access the scapulothoracic bursa, are both diagnostic and therapeutic for this malady. Subsequent heat and nonsteroidal and antiinflammatory drugs are recommended to help alleviate the inflammation after injection.[20] Of note, mastalgia can be worrisome to many females. However, breast pain is not usually a symptom of breast cancer; pain without other signs or symptoms of breast cancer is uncommon, occurring in only approximately 7% of breast cancer patients.

Patients with fibrocystic changes have clinical breast findings that range from mild alterations in texture to dense, firm breast tissue with palpable masses. Fibrocystic changes are usually seen on mammography as diffuse or focal radiologically dense tissue. Palpable or multiple small cysts can be seen on US and are typical of fibrocystic disease. Histologically, in addition to macrocysts and microcysts, females with fibrocystic changes may have identified solid elements, including adenosis, sclerosis, apocrine metaplasia, stromal fibrosis, and epithelial metaplasia and hyperplasia.

Cysts within the breast parenchyma are fluid-filled, epithelial-lined cavities that vary in size from microscopic to large palpable masses. A palpable cyst develops in at least 1 in every 14 females, and 50% of cysts are multiple or recurrent. The pathogenesis of cyst formation is not well understood; however, cysts appear to arise from the destruction and dilatation of lobules and terminal ductules. Microscopic studies showed that fibrosis at or near the lobule, combined with continued secretion, results in the unfolding of the lobule and expansion of an epithelial-lined cavity containing fluid. Cysts are influenced by ovarian hormones, a fact that explains their variation with the menstrual cycle. Most cysts occur in females older than 35 years, and the incidence steadily increases until menopause and sharply declines thereafter. Cysts with or without fibrocystic disease are uncommon in postmenopausal females. New cyst formation in older females is generally associated with exogenous HRT.

Most patients with simple cysts, confirmed by US, do not require further evaluation and do not require cyst aspiration if not symptomatic. If aspirated, cyst fluid can be straw-colored, opaque, or dark green and may contain debris. If the cyst resolves after aspiration and the cyst contents are not grossly bloody, the fluid does not need to be sent for cytologic analysis. If the cyst recurs multiple times (more than twice is a reasonable rule), CNB should be performed to evaluate any solid elements. Patients with complex cysts with solid intracystic components also require additional evaluation with a biopsy of the solid components. The entire cystic structure can be percutaneously removed with a vacuum-assisted core-needle device if recurrent and symptomatic.[21] Surgical removal of a cyst is usually not indicated but may be required if the cyst recurs multiple times, if needle biopsy reveals findings of atypia, if there is incomplete removal of the mass, or if the cyst is large and painful for the patient. Of note, intracystic carcinoma is exceedingly rare. Rosemond reported that only three cancers were identified in more than 3000 cyst aspirations (0.1%).

Fibroadenomas

Fibroadenomas are benign solid tumors composed of stromal and epithelial elements. They are the second most common tumor in the breast (after carcinoma) and the most common tumor in females younger than 30 years. They most often arise during the late teens and early reproductive years and are rarely seen as new masses in females after age 40 or 45 years. Clinically, fibroadenomas manifest as firm masses that slide easily under the examining fingers and may be lobulated or smooth. They may increase in size over several months or wax and wane with the menstrual cycle. Mammography is of little help in discriminating between cysts and fibroadenomas; however, ultrasonography can readily distinguish between them. On excision, fibroadenomas are well-encapsulated masses that may detach easily from surrounding breast tissue.

Fibroadenomas are benign tumors, although neoplasia may develop in the epithelial elements within them. Cancer in a newly discovered fibroadenoma is exceedingly rare (0.2%). When a tissue diagnosis confirms that the breast mass is a fibroadenoma, the patient can be reassured that surgical excision is not needed. An excisional biopsy is warranted when there is suspicion of a phyllodes tumor (discussed later in "Rare Tumors"), either clinically with a tumor >3 cm in size or rapidly growing or if it is histologically difficult to distinguish. If the mass is symptomatic or the patient prefers removal, surgical excision could also be considered. The mass can be removed with open excisional biopsy or via a percutaneous approach for smaller masses.[21]

Two subtypes of fibroadenoma are recognized. *Giant fibroadenoma* is a descriptive term applied to a fibroadenoma that attains an unusually large size (typically >5 cm). Excision is usually recommended. The term *juvenile fibroadenoma* refers to a large fibroadenoma that occasionally occurs in adolescents and young adults and histologically is more cellular than the usual fibroadenoma. They can be observed if smaller than 5 cm in size and with no concerning features. If larger than 5 cm, growth is observed, or they persist to adulthood, excisional biopsy is warranted and is usually curative.

Breast Infections and Abscess

There are two general categories of infections of the breast: lactational infections and chronic subareolar infections associated with duct ectasia. Lactational infections are thought to arise from the entry of bacteria through the nipple into the duct system and are characterized by fever, leukocytosis, erythema, and tenderness. Infections of the breast are most often caused by *Staphylococcus aureus* or streptococci species and may manifest as cellulitis with breast parenchymal inflammation and swelling, termed *mastitis,* with or without an underlying abscess. US evaluation can assist in characterizing a breast abscess and help to guide needle aspiration. Treatment requires antibiotics (depending on the risk for methicillin-resistant *S. aureus* [MRSA] colonization) and regular emptying of the breast. True abscesses require drainage. Initial attempts at drainage should include needle aspiration; surgical incision and drainage should be reserved for abscesses that do not resolve after aspiration and treatment with antibiotics. In such cases, abscesses are generally multiloculated.

In females who are not lactating, a chronic relapsing form of infection may develop in the subareolar ducts of the breast, which is variously known as *periductal mastitis* or *duct ectasia*. This condition appears to be associated with smoking and diabetes. The infections are most often mixed infections that include aerobic and anaerobic skin flora. A series of infections with resulting inflammatory changes and scarring may lead to retraction or inversion of the nipple, masses in the subareolar area, and occasionally a chronic fistula from the subareolar ducts to the periareolar skin. Palpable masses and mammographic changes may result from the infection and scarring; these can make surveillance for breast cancer more challenging.

Subareolar infections may initially manifest as subareolar pain and mild erythema. Warm soaks and oral antibiotics may be effective treatments at this stage. Antibiotic treatment generally requires coverage for aerobic and anaerobic organisms. If an abscess has developed, needle aspiration is required in addition to antibiotics. Surgical incision and drainage are reserved for abscesses that do not resolve with these more conservative measures. Repeated infections are treated by excision of the entire subareolar duct complex after the acute infection has resolved completely, together with intravenous antibiotic coverage. Rarely, patients have recurrent infections requiring excision of the nipple and areola.

Idiopathic Granulomatous Mastitis

Idiopathic granulomatous mastitis (IGM) is a benign inflammatory process in the breast, presenting as a unilateral single mass or as multiple tender breast masses, with possible underlying abscesses as well as skin inflammation and ulceration. It is more common in the Hispanic, Middle Eastern, and Southeast Asian populations. IGM can easily be mistaken for either an infectious process or an aggressive carcinoma. Biopsy shows nonnecrotizing granulomatous lesions and should also be sent for culture and possibly analyzed to exclude fungal or mycobacterial infection and sarcoidosis, although cultures rarely grow anything.

Some small IGM processes could resolve spontaneously over months. Other more extensive and persistent processes are more difficult to treat. Surgical management is not recommended because it might result in an open, poorly healing wound. Antibiotic treatment directed against *Corynebacterium* species (shown to have an association with IGM)—with doxycycline, clindamycin, azithromycin, or levofloxacin, or culture driven—is a possible first-line treatment. Some advocate alternating antibiotics every month. Systemic treatment with steroids is an additional avenue for treatment, with methotrexate for those unable to tolerate steroids or who experience exacerbation on taper. Recently, intralesional injections of steroids have shown promising results.[22]

Nipple Discharge

The appearance of discharge from the nipple (see Fig. 68.6A) of a nonlactating female is a common condition and is rarely associated with an underlying carcinoma. In one review of 270 subareolar biopsies for discharge from one identifiable duct and without an associated breast mass, carcinoma was found in only 16 patients (5.9%). In these cases, the fluid was bloody or tested strongly positive for occult hemoglobin. In another series of 249 patients with discharge from a single identifiable duct, breast carcinoma was found in 10 patients (4%). In eight of these patients, a mass lesion was identified in addition to the discharge. Therefore, in the absence of a palpable mass or suspicious findings on mammography, discharge is rarely associated with cancer.

It is important to establish whether the discharge comes from one breast or both breasts; determine whether it comes from multiple duct orifices or just one; and characterize the discharge, specifically whether it contains blood. Nipple discharge that is bilateral and comes from multiple ducts is not usually a cause for surgery. A milky discharge from both breasts is termed *galactorrhea*. In the absence of lactation or a history of recent lactation, galactorrhea may be associated with increased production of prolactin, which should be tested in the serum. However, true galactorrhea is rare and is diagnosed only when the discharge is milky (contains lactose, fat, and milk-specific proteins). Bilateral bloody

spontaneous discharge is likely endocrine in nature and is associated with pregnancy and hypothyroidism.

The most common cause of spontaneous nipple discharge from a single duct is a solitary intraductal papilloma (60%–80%) in one of the large subareolar ducts under the nipple. Another cause (20%) is subareolar duct ectasia producing inflammation and dilatation of large collecting ducts under the nipple, yielding discharge from multiple ducts. Cancer is a very unusual cause of discharge in the absence of other signs. However, papillomas that are located away from the NAC are at higher risk of malignancy (20%). Physical exam and imaging should be performed to identify any underlying pathology that can be sampled and acted upon. Without a diagnosis, bloody discharge from a single duct often requires surgical excision of the involved duct to establish a diagnosis and control the discharge.

Papillomas and Papillomatosis

Solitary intraductal papillomas are true polyps of epithelial-lined breast ducts. Solitary papillomas are most often located close to the areola but may be present in peripheral locations. Most papillomas are smaller than 1 cm but can grow to 4 or 5 cm. Papillomas located close to the nipple are often accompanied by bloody nipple discharge. Less frequently, they are discovered as a palpable mass under the areola or as a density seen on mammogram. Papillomas with atypia on histology have an upgrade rate to DCIS or invasive cancer in about 50% of cases and should therefore undergo excision. Excision is also recommended when papillomas are accompanied by bloody discharge or a palpable mass. Excision can be performed through a circumareolar incision, identification of the involved duct using a lacrimal probe or dye, and excision of that duct. Small incidental papillomas with no atypia have an upgrade rate of less than 10% and can therefore be closely followed. The presence of papillomatosis or multiple papillomas in a patient's breast has been shown to increase the risk of developing breast cancer, even without the presence of atypia upon biopsy.

Hamartomas and Adenomas

Hamartomas and adenomas are benign proliferations of variable amounts of epithelium and stromal supporting tissue. A hamartoma is a discrete nodule that contains closely packed lobules and prominent, ectatic extralobular ducts, with varying amounts of stroma. On physical examination, mammography, and gross inspection, a hamartoma is indistinguishable from a fibroadenoma. Adenomas are benign cellular neoplasms of ductules packed closely together so that they form a sheet of tiny glands without supporting stroma. Tubular adenomas form in premenopausal females, and lactating adenomas form during pregnancy and lactation. Biopsy and sometimes an excisional biopsy is required to establish the diagnosis.

Fat Necrosis

Fat necrosis may follow an episode of trauma to the breast or be related to a prior surgical procedure (tissue mobilization or fat grafting) or RT. It can mimic cancer on mammography by producing a palpable mass or density that may contain calcifications. Calcifications are characteristic of fat necrosis and can often be visualized on US as well. Histologically, fat necrosis is composed of lipid-laden macrophages, scar tissue, and chronic inflammatory cells. These lesions have no malignant potential.

Galactocele

A galactocele is a milk retention cyst that is round, well circumscribed, and easily movable within the breast. A galactocele generally occurs after the cessation of lactation or when feeding frequency has declined significantly, although galactoceles may occur 6 to 10 months after breastfeeding has ceased. The pathogenesis of galactocele is unknown, but inspissated milk clogging a duct is thought to be responsible. The cyst is usually located in the central portion of the breast or under the nipple. Needle aspiration is both diagnostic and therapeutic and produces thick, creamy material that may be tinged dark green or brown. Although it appears purulent, the fluid is sterile. Repeated aspiration or surgery is reserved for symptomatic patients or infected galactoceles. Additional pathologies that can affect the breastfeeding patient include nipple blebs (obstruction of the nipple pore ducts as a result of inflammation), nipple injury or dermatitis, and breast engorgement, among others.

Gynecomastia

Hypertrophy of breast tissue in males is a clinical entity for which there is frequently no identifiable cause. It should be differentiated from pseudogynecomastia, which is simply an increase in breast fat. Pubertal hypertrophy occurs in males between the age of 13 years and early adulthood and can be unilateral or bilateral. Unless it is unilateral or painful, it may pass unnoticed and regress into adulthood. Surgical intervention is usually not warranted but could be considered if gynecomastia fails to regress with observation, is unilateral, or is cosmetically unacceptable. Gynecomastia in males over 50 years old, or senescent gynecomastia, is also common. It can be caused by commonly used drugs, such as digoxin, thiazides, estrogens, phenothiazines, theophylline, cannabis, and many more. In addition, gynecomastia may be a systemic manifestation of hepatic cirrhosis, renal failure, malnutrition, hypogonadism, testicular tumors, and hyperthyroidism, and therefore, an underlying condition should be sought.

Upon exam, it presents as a smooth, firm, saucer-shaped, and symmetrically distributed mass beneath the areola, which is frequently tender. Underlying carcinomas are usually not tender, are asymmetrically located beneath or beside the areola, and may be fixed to the overlying dermis or the deep fascia. Mammography and ultrasonography can be used to discriminate between gynecomastia and a suspected malignancy. A nipple-sparing mastectomy can be performed to remove the enlarged breast. A donut of deepithelized skin around the nipple is then enfolded to remove the excess skin, as one would do for a Benelli reduction mammoplasty.[23]

EPIDEMIOLOGY OF BREAST CANCER

It has been estimated that 297,790 cases of invasive breast cancer and 55,720 cases of in situ breast cancer were diagnosed in 2023 in the United States. Breast cancer is the second leading cause of cancer-related deaths in females, second to lung cancer, with approximately 43,700 estimated deaths caused by breast cancer in 2023 in the United States.[24] Breast cancer is also a global health problem, being the world's most prevalent cancer, with more than 2 million cases diagnosed and 685,000 deaths from breast cancer worldwide each year. The overall incidence of breast cancer was increasing until approximately 1999 because of increases in the average life span, lifestyle changes that increase the risk for breast cancer, and improved survival rates for other diseases. Breast cancer incidence decreased from 1999 to 2006 by approximately 2% per year. This decrease may be attributed to a reduction in the use of HRT after the initial results of the Women's Health Initiative were published but may also be the result of a reduction in the use of screening mammography (70.1% of females ≥40 years old

were screened in 2000 vs. 66.4% in 2005). Since the mid-2000s, breast cancer incidence has increased by 0.5% a year. This has been attributed in part to an increase in the population's body weight and a decrease in the fertility rate.

Survival rates in females with breast cancer have steadily improved over the past several decades, with 5-year survival rates of 63% in the early 1960s, 75% during the years 1975 to 1977, 87% during 1995 to 1997, and 91% during 2012 to 2018. The largest decreases in death rates from breast cancer have been in females younger than 50 years (decrease of 3.2% per year), although breast cancer death rates have also decreased in females older than 50 years (by 2% per year). The decreased mortality from breast cancer is thought to be the result of earlier detection via mammographic screening (with an understandable lead-time bias), a decreased incidence of breast cancer, and improvements in therapy.

Worldwide, higher incidence rates of breast cancer (>80 per 100,000) are seen in Australia and New Zealand, Western Europe, North America, and Northern Europe, whereas lower rates (<40 per 100,000) are seen in Central America, Eastern and Middle Africa, and South-Central Asia. These differences reflect differences in the prevalence of reproductive, hormonal, and behavioral risk factors as well as the availability of screening programs in high- versus low-income regions. Worldwide mortality, on the other hand, is highest (>20 per 100,000) in Melanesia, Western Africa, and Micronesia/Polynesia. This is mainly due to late-stage presentation and inadequate access to high-quality care.[25] In the United States, there are differences in breast cancer incidence by race and ethnicity, with the highest incidence in White females (133.7 per 100,000), followed by Black females (127.8), American Indian/Alaska Natives (111.3), Asian/Pacific Islanders (101.3), and Hispanics (99.2). Mortality, conversely, is highest in Black females, 40% higher than in White females. This disparity is partly a result of a higher incidence of triple-negative breast cancer (TNBC) and later-stage diagnosis in the Black population, although mortality is higher across all stages and subtypes.[13]

PATHOLOGY OF BREAST CANCER

Noninvasive (In Situ) Breast Cancer

Noninvasive neoplasms of the breast were previously broadly divided into two major types, LCIS and DCIS (Box 68.2). LCIS is no longer regarded as a neoplasm of the breast in the 8th edition of the American Joint Committee on Cancer (AJCC) staging system but is regarded as a risk factor for the development of breast cancer. LCIS is recognized by its conformity to the outline of the normal lobule, with expanded and filled acini (Fig. 68.8A). One variant of LCIS, pleomorphic LCIS, is a distinct, more aggressive histopathologic subtype. Pleomorphic LCIS shows marked nuclear pleomorphism compared with classic LCIS, with one or more lobules being distended by discohesive cells with irregularly shaped, high-grade nuclei. Pleomorphic LCIS may or may not be associated with comedonecrosis and calcifications. If pleomorphic LCIS is associated with calcifications, it may be detected mammographically. The natural history of pleomorphic LCIS is unknown, and there is debate regarding treatment, with most recommending pleomorphic LCIS be treated with surgical excision similar to DCIS.

DCIS is more morphologically heterogeneous than LCIS, and pathologists recognize five main types of DCIS: micropapillary, papillary, cribriform, solid, and comedo types. The latter three types are shown in Fig. 68.8. DCIS is recognized as discrete spaces filled with malignant cells, usually with a recognizable basal cell layer composed of presumably normal myoepithelial cells. The four morphologic types of DCIS are rarely seen as pure lesions;

BOX 68.2 Classification of Primary Breast Cancer

Noninvasive Epithelial Cancers (15%–20%)

Ductal carcinoma in situ or intraductal carcinoma

- Papillary, cribriform, solid, and comedo types

Invasive Epithelial Cancers (Percentage of Total)

Invasive lobular carcinoma (5%–15%)

Invasive ductal carcinoma (70%–80%)

- Invasive ductal carcinoma, not otherwise specified (50%–70%)
- Tubular carcinoma (2%–3%)
- Mucinous or colloid carcinoma (2%–3%)
- Medullary carcinoma (5%)
- Invasive cribriform carcinoma (1%–3%)
- Invasive papillary carcinoma (1%–2%)
- Adenoid cystic carcinoma (1%)
- Metaplastic carcinoma (1%)

Mixed Connective and Epithelial Tumors (<5%)

Phyllodes tumors, benign and malignant (<1%)

Carcinosarcoma (<1%)

Angiosarcoma (<1%)

DCIS lesions are usually of mixed morphology. The papillary and cribriform types of DCIS are generally lower-grade lesions and may take longer to transform into invasive cancer. The solid and comedo types of DCIS are generally higher-grade lesions. The grade and ER status of DCIS are eventually much more important than its architectural pattern in terms of prognosis and treatment.

As the cells inside the ductal membrane grow, they tend to undergo central necrosis. The necrotic debris in the center of the duct undergoes coagulation and finally calcifies, leading to the tiny, pleomorphic, and frequently linear forms of microcalcifications that can be seen on mammography. In some patients, an entire ductal tree may be involved in the malignancy, and the mammogram shows typical calcifications that can span from the nipple extending posteriorly into the breast (termed *segmental calcifications*). If not treated, DCIS can transform into an invasive cancer, usually recapitulating the morphology of the cells inside the duct. In other words, low-grade cribriform DCIS tends to be associated with low-grade invasive lesions that retain some cribriform features. DCIS frequently coexists with invasive cancers, and when this is the case, the two phases of the malignancy are usually morphologically similar.

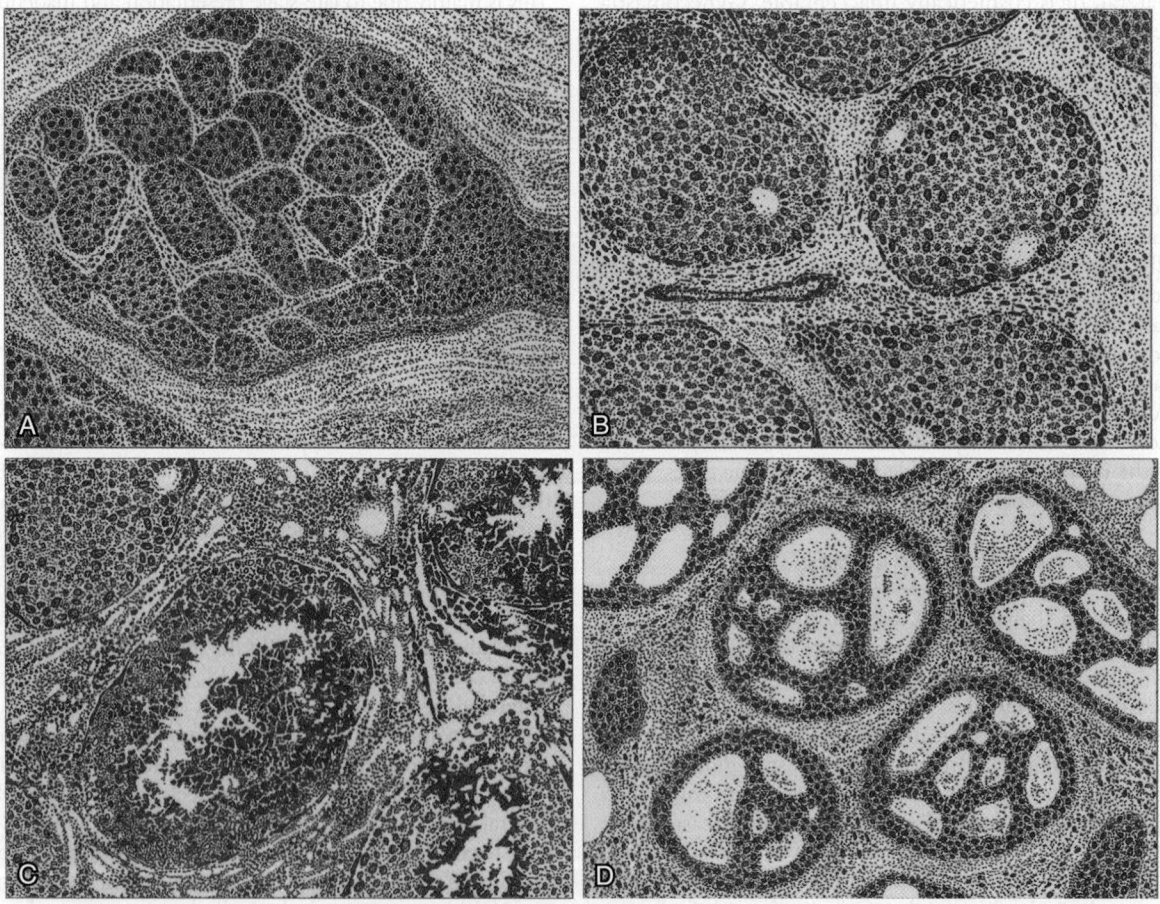

FIGURE 68.8 Noninvasive breast cancer. (A) Lobular carcinoma in situ (LCIS). The neoplastic cells are small with compact, bland nuclei and are distending the acini but preserving the cross-sectional architecture of the lobular unit. (B) Ductal carcinoma in situ (DCIS), solid type. The cells are larger than in LCIS and are filling the ductal rather than the lobular spaces. However, the cells are contained within the basement membrane of the duct and do not invade the breast stroma. (C) DCIS, comedo type. In comedo DCIS, the malignant cells in the center undergo necrosis, coagulation, and calcification. (D) DCIS, cribriform type. In this type, bridges of tumor cells span the ductal space and leave round punched-out spaces.

Invasive Breast Cancer

Invasive breast cancers are recognized by their lack of overall organized architecture with infiltration of cells haphazardly into a variable amount of stroma or formation of sheets of continuous and monotonous cells without respect for the form and function of a glandular organ. Pathologists broadly divide invasive breast cancer into ductal and lobular histologic types, which probably do not reflect histogenesis and imperfectly predict clinical behavior. Invasive ductal cancer (IDC) tends to grow as a cohesive mass; it appears as discrete abnormalities on mammograms and is often palpable as a discrete lump in the breast. ILC tends to permeate the breast in a single-file nature, which explains why it remains clinically occult and often escapes detection on mammography or physical examination until the disease is extensive. Most ILCs are characterized by a mutation in the *CDH1* gene, causing loss of E-cadherin. The growth patterns of invasive ductal and lobular carcinomas are shown in Fig. 68.9.

IDC, also known as *infiltrating ductal carcinoma,* is the most common form of breast cancer; it accounts for 50% to 70% of invasive breast cancers. ILC accounts for 5% to 15% of breast cancers, and mixed ductal and lobular cancers have been increasingly recognized and described in pathology reports. When invasive ductal carcinomas take on differentiated features, they are named according to the features that they display. If the infiltrating cells form small glands lined by a single row of bland epithelium, they are called *infiltrating tubular carcinoma* (see Fig. 68.9C). The infiltrating cells may secrete copious amounts of mucin and appear to float in this material. These lesions are called *mucinous* or *colloid tumors* (see Fig. 68.9D). Tubular and mucinous tumors are usually low-grade (grade 1) lesions; these tumors each account for approximately 2% to 3% of invasive breast carcinomas.

Medullary cancer is characterized by bizarre invasive cells with high-grade nuclear features, many mitoses, and a lack of an in situ component (see Fig. 68.9E). The malignancy forms sheets of cells in an almost syncytial fashion, surrounded by an infiltrate of small mononuclear lymphocytes. The borders of the tumor push into the surrounding breast rather than infiltrating or permeating the stroma. In its pure form, medullary cancer accounts for only approximately 5% of breast cancers; however, some pathologists have described a so-called *medullary variant* that has only some features of the pure form. These tumors are uniformly high grade, ER and progesterone receptor (PR) negative, and negative for the human epidermal growth factor receptor 2 (HER2/neu; HER2) cell surface receptor.

Another rare subtype of breast cancer that is typically high grade and negative for ER, PR, and HER2 is metaplastic carcinoma. Most metaplastic carcinomas are node negative, but they have a high potential for metastatic spread, and 10% of patients present with de novo metastatic disease. Even patients presenting with localized metaplastic carcinoma have a poor prognosis: approximately 50% experience local or distant relapse.

Although tumor histologic subtype has a bearing on a patient's prognosis, tumor staging, histologic grade, and molecular markers have a more crucial influence, driving both prognosis and treatment. Tumor grade reporting is based on the Nottingham Histologic Score. It is made up of three categories, each receiving 1 to 3 points: (1) the percentage of tumor area forming glandular/tubular structures (>75% = 1, 10%–75% = 2, <10% = 3), (2) nuclear pleomorphism, and (3) mitotic rate. The sum of the three categories defines the grade of the tumor: 3 to 5 is grade 1 (well differentiated), 6 to 7 is grade 2 (moderately differentiated), and 8 to 9 is grade 3 (poorly differentiated).

Molecular Markers

Numerous molecular markers have been reported to affect breast cancer outcomes, including molecules in the steroid hormone receptor pathway (ER and PR), molecules in the HER pathway (HER family), angiogenesis-related molecules, cell cycle–related molecules (e.g., cyclin-dependent kinases), apoptosis modulators, proteasomes, cyclooxygenase-2, peroxisome-proliferator-activated receptor γ, insulin-like growth factors (insulin-like growth factor family), transforming growth factor-γ, platelet-derived growth factor, and *p53.* Most of these markers are not routinely tested on breast cancer specimens at the time of diagnosis. Those routinely reported are ER, PR, and HER2. Classification based on these markers reflects tumor biology and prognosis and defines targets for available systemic treatment; for example, before the discovery of ER, all breast cancers were considered potentially sensitive to endocrine therapy, whereas currently, ER and PR status predict which patients may benefit from and should receive adjuvant endocrine therapy, and patients whose tumors are ER negative can be spared endocrine therapy. ER and PR are identified based on immunohistochemical testing and are reported based on the percentage of tumor cells expressing these receptors. Over 1% expression would be defined as an ER/PR-positive tumor. Nevertheless, 1% to 10% expression of ER, would be defined as low ER expression, with limited data as to the benefit of endocrine therapy in these patients.

A second important predictive factor in breast cancer, discovered in 1985, is HER2. This protein is the product of the *erb-B2* gene and is amplified in approximately 20% of human breast cancers. HER2 is a member of the epidermal growth factor receptor family of receptor tyrosine kinases. HER2 protein overexpression is measured clinically by immunohistochemistry and scored on a scale from 0 to 3+, defined by the percentage of stained cells and the intensity of that staining. Scoring of 0 or 1+ is defined as HER2 negative, a score of 3+ is HER2 positive, and 2+ is considered equivocal. In cases of equivocal results, in situ hybridization (ISH) is performed with a single HER2 probe. If the average number of HER2 copies is <4 per cell, the tumor is defined as HER2 negative, and if it is 6 or higher, the tumor is HER2 positive. For those with 4 to 6 copies, ISH with dual tracer is performed, and if the HER2/CEP17 ratio is equal to or over 2, the tumor is defined as HER2 positive. HER2 positivity predicts the response of tumors to treatment with antibodies directed against the extracellular domain of HER2, such as trastuzumab and pertuzumab (discussed later under "Human Epidermal Growth Factor Receptor 2 Based Targeted Therapy").

An additional immunohistochemical marker reported for breast cancer specimens is Ki-67. The expression of Ki-67 in breast cancer cell nuclei is associated with tumor cell proliferation and growth and is considered a proliferation marker. It is reported as the percentage of positive nuclei to the staining.

ER/PR, HER2, and Ki-67 status are used to classify and stage breast cancer as well as guide treatment. However, breast cancer is a heterogeneous disease, and different breast cancers behave in different ways. For example, some ER-positive tumors are indolent and not life threatening, whereas other ER-positive tumors are very aggressive. In 2000, Perou et al. described the heterogeneity of breast cancer on a molecular level through gene expression profiling. They showed that the variation in gene expression correlated with variation in growth rate and signaling pathways. It further correlated with the known tumor markers, ER/PR, HER2, and Ki-67. Microarray experiments use thousands of gene transcripts (messenger RNAs) to provide a snapshot of the

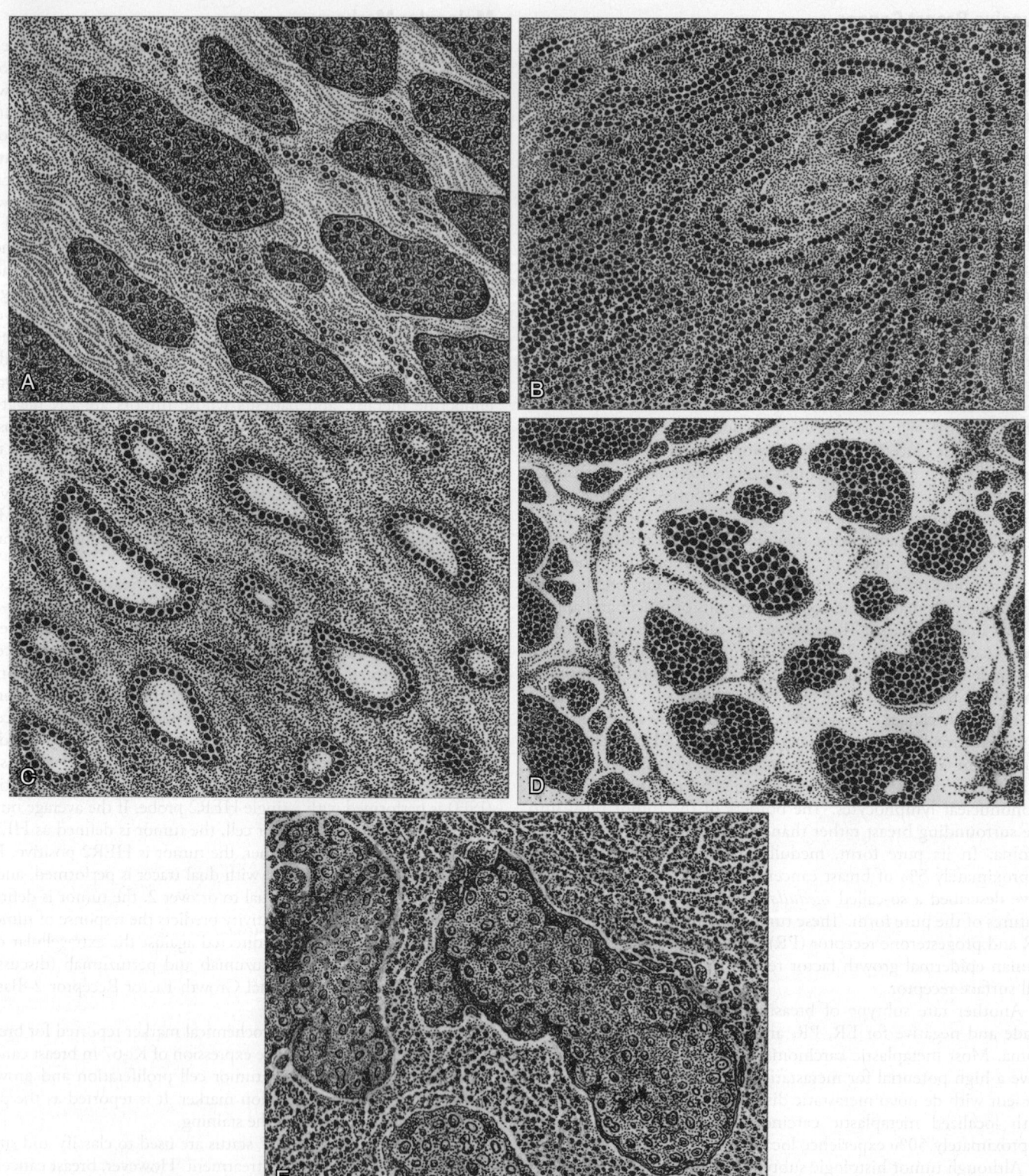

FIGURE 68.9 Invasive breast cancer. (A) Invasive ductal carcinoma, not otherwise specified. The malignant cells invade in haphazard groups and singly into the stroma. (B) Invasive lobular carcinoma. The malignant cells invade the stroma in a characteristic single-file pattern and may form concentric circles of single-file cells around normal ducts (targetoid pattern). (C) Invasive tubular carcinoma. The cancer invades as small tubules, lined by a single layer of well-differentiated cells. (D) Mucinous or colloid carcinoma. The bland tumor cells float like islands in lakes of mucin. (E) Medullary carcinoma. The tumor cells are large and very undifferentiated, with pleomorphic nuclei. The distinctive features of this tumor are the infiltration of lymphocytes and the syncytium-appearing sheets of tumor cells.

with higher grade and higher Ki67 expression. Basal-like tumors express proteins in common with myoepithelial cells at the base of mammary ducts (in contrast to the milk-producing luminal cells). Females who have a pathogenic mutation in *BRCA1* (but not *BRCA2*) are much more likely to develop a basal-like cancer (triple negative) than other subtypes. It is important to note that because these categories were developed using differing technologies than immunohistochemistry, categorization based on gene expression correlates, but does not exactly overlap with categorization based on immunohistochemical staining.

To adapt this technology for clinical application, investigators have created different genomic assays in which only selected critical genes are tested. The expression of these limited numbers of genes tested provides a similar predictive ability as a genome-wide analysis. The most used genomic assay in the United States is the 21-gene Recurrence Score (RS) assay (Oncotype DX, Exact Sciences, Madison, WI), composed of 16 cancer-related genes and 5 reference genes, analyzed using a paraffin-embedded breast tumor specimen with reverse transcription polymerase chain reaction (RT-PCR). It provides a score between 1 and 100, with a higher score signifying a higher risk of distant recurrence with endocrine therapy alone. It has also been shown to predict the benefit of adding chemotherapy to systemic endocrine therapy in early-stage ER-positive, HER2-negative breast cancer with zero to three positive lymph nodes (see 'Systemic Therapy for Breast Cancer" later). Another multigene assay for determining prognosis is the MammaPrint 70-gene breast cancer recurrence assay (Agendia, Amsterdam, Netherlands). The MammaPrint assay analyzes data from 70 genes to develop a risk profile. The test provides a simple readout of low-risk or high-risk diseases. This tool can be used for risk assessment in patients with ER-positive or ER-negative tumors. Additional genomic assays include PAM50 (Prosigna; Veracyte, San Francisco, CA), EndoPredict (Myriad Genetics, Salt Lake City, UT), and Breast Cancer Index (Biotheranostics, San Diego, CA). Tests based on critical combinations of genes will likely increasingly be used to guide clinical decision-making regarding breast cancer treatment.

Other Tumors of the Breast

Phyllodes Tumors

Tumors of mixed connective tissue and epithelium constitute an important group of unusual primary breast tumors. On one end of the spectrum are benign fibroadenomas, which are characterized by a proliferation of connective tissue and a variable component of compressed ductal elements. Clinically more challenging are phyllodes tumors (<1% of breast neoplasms), which contain a biphasic proliferation of stroma and mammary epithelium. First called *cystosarcoma phyllodes,* these tumors are now called *phyllodes tumors* in recognition of their usually benign course. These tumors range from benign phyllodes, which behave similarly to fibroadenomas, to malignant phyllodes, which are locally aggressive, can degenerate into sarcomatous lesions, and have metastatic potential. Histologically, benign phyllodes tumors, although similar to fibroadenomas, show whorled stroma forming larger clefts lined by epithelium that resemble clusters of leaflike (phyllodes) structures.

Phyllodes tumors usually occur in females in their 40s. Clinically, they present as firm lobulated masses that can range in size, with an average size of approximately 5 cm, and are slowly or rapidly growing. It is exceedingly rare for phyllodes to metastasize to axillary lymph nodes. When trying to differentiate from a fibroadenoma, the diagnosis is suggested by the larger size (>3 cm), history of rapid growth, and occurrence in older patients. CNB is

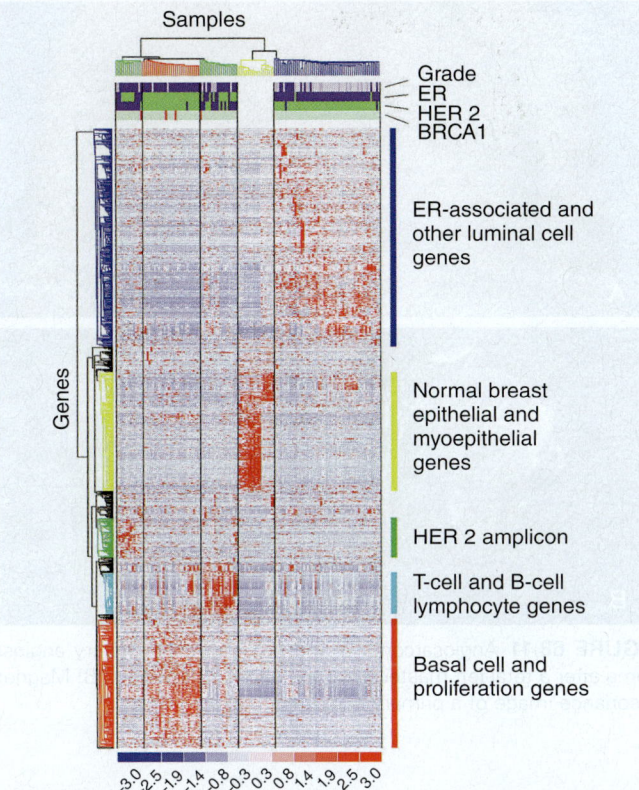

FIGURE 68.10 Microarray representation of human breast cancer. This portrayal of global gene expression is called a *heat map,* with shades of *red* indicating high gene expression and shades of *blue* indicating low gene expression relative to a mean across tissue samples. Tissue samples are present across the top in columns, and individual genes are in rows down the side; the intersection is an individual gene in a particular sample. A computer-clustering algorithm aligns samples with similar gene expression and genes with similar expression patterns in the samples (two-way clustering). This illustration provides an unbiased look at breast cancer according to gene expression. The dendrogram at the top depicts the degree of similarity of the tissue samples: *yellow,* normal breast epithelium; *blue,* predominantly ER-positive cancers; *red,* basal-like or triple-negative cancers; and *green,* HER2-positive cancers (in two clusters defined by the degree of lymphocytic infiltrate). The *stripes* at the top indicate grade (shades of *darker purple* are higher grades), ER expression (*purple* is positive; *green* is negative), and HER2 (*purple* is positive; *green* is negative). *BRCA1* mutation was determined for other reasons in this experiment. *ER,* Estrogen receptor; *HER2,* human epidermal growth factor receptor 2. (Courtesy Dr. Andrea Richardson, Department of Pathology, Brigham and Women's Hospital, Boston, MA.)

molecular phenotype of an individual cancer. A typical microarray experiment, commonly known as a *heat map,* is shown in Fig. 68.10, with colors indicating levels of gene expression. It shows the clustering of breast cancer into four subtypes: luminal A tumors (40% to 60% of cases) correlate with strongly ER-positive expression, possible PR expression, negative HER2 expression, low to intermediate grade, and low levels of Ki-67; luminal B tumors (20% to 30% of cases) correlate with positive but lower ER/PR expression, negative HER2 expression, higher grade, and higher Ki-67 expression; HER2-enriched (10% to 20% of cases) tumors express HER2 and can have positive or negative expression or ER/PR; and basal-like tumors (10% to 20%) are usually triple receptor negative (negative for ER, PR, and HER2 expression),

preferred over cytology for diagnosis, although it is difficult to classify phyllodes tumors based on limited sampling. If CNB is equivocal, a final diagnosis is best made by excisional biopsy followed by careful pathologic review. After a phyllodes tumor is diagnosed, it is classified into benign, borderline, or malignant based on stromal cellular atypia, mitotic activity, infiltrative margins, and the presence of pure stroma without an epithelial component.

Local excision or an excisional biopsy of a benign phyllodes tumor, similar to a fibroadenoma, is curative. Intermediate or borderline phyllodes and malignant phyllodes should be treated by a wide excision of 1 cm or more to achieve negative margins to reduce the risk of local recurrence. When the tumor is large compared with the size of the breast, a total mastectomy may be required. No axillary staging is indicated. Adjuvant radiation can be considered for patients with borderline or malignant phyllodes undergoing breast-conserving surgery (BCS). Affected patients are at some risk for local recurrence, most often within the first 2 years after excision. Close follow-up with examination and imaging allows early detection of recurrence. Metastases from malignant phyllodes tumors occur via hematogenous spread, most commonly to the lungs. They are usually treated with chemotherapy similar to sarcomas, with limited benefit.

Angiosarcoma

Angiosarcoma, a rare vascular tumor (1% of all breast tumors), may occur de novo in the breast parenchyma (primary) or within the dermis of the breast after irradiation, usually for previous breast cancer (secondary). Stewart-Treves syndrome is a secondary angiosarcoma that has developed in the upper extremity of patients with lymphedema, historically 10 to 15 years after radical mastectomy and irradiation. Clinically, primary angiosarcomas generally form an ill-defined mass within the parenchyma of the breast, whereas secondary angiosarcomas arise in the area of irradiated skin as reddish, brown to purplish raised vascular proliferations that may go unrecognized for some time because they may be difficult to distinguish from atypical vascular proliferations in irradiated skin (Fig. 68.11). Mammography is unrevealing in most cases of angiosarcoma. Histologically, angiosarcoma is composed of an anastomosing tangle of invasive blood vessels in the dermis and superficial subcutaneous fat. These tumors are graded based on pleomorphic nuclei, frequency of mitoses, and stacking of the endothelial cells lining neoplastic tissue.

In the absence of metastatic disease at initial evaluation, surgery is the only modality with curative potential. Patients should be managed by a multidisciplinary team experienced in the care of these rare patients. Surgery is performed to secure negative skin margins, which is the single most important determinant of long-term outcomes. The extent of resection depends on the size of the tumor compared with the breast, with some proposing a 3-cm margin and usually requiring a total mastectomy. A split-thickness skin graft or myocutaneous flap may be needed to replace a large skin defect created by the resection. Metastasis to regional nodes is extraordinarily rare, and axillary dissection or staging is not required. Because of the high risk of local recurrence, for patients who present with primary angiosarcoma, adjuvant irradiation is considered for high-risk tumors. Neoadjuvant or adjuvant chemotherapy should be considered in high-risk patients based on differentiation, size (over 3–5 cm), and spread. Metastatic spread occurs hematogenously, most commonly to the lungs and bone and less frequently to the abdominal viscera, brain, and contralateral breast. Outcomes are based on grade and size and range from 28% to 82% 10-year survival.

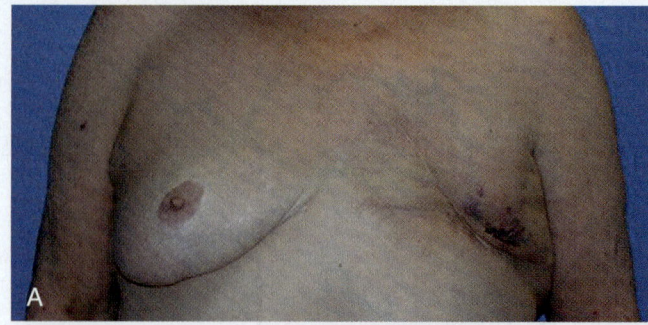
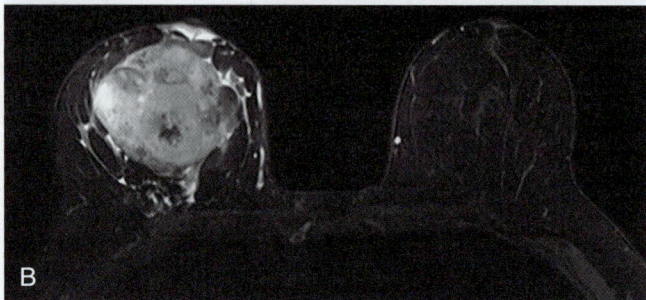

FIGURE 68.11 Angiosarcoma of the breast. (A) Secondary angiosarcoma after a total left mastectomy and adjuvant radiation. (B) Magnetic resonance image of a primary angiosarcoma.

STAGING OF BREAST CANCER AND TREATMENT PLANNING

Breast cancer staging is based on the tumor-node-metastasis (TNM) classification system, and the most widely used system is produced and updated periodically by the AJCC. Staging is performed to group patients into risk categories that define prognosis and guide treatment recommendations for patients with a similar prognosis. With advances in diagnosis and treatment, the most recent 8th edition has become more complex. To the original variables of T classification (primary tumor size and involvement of adjacent organs), N classification (status of regional lymph node involvement), and M classification (presence or absence of distant metastases), several other variables have been added. These include subcategories added within each classification (e.g., microscopic involvement of primary tumor, lymph nodes, or distant sites; the presence of circulating tumor cells; or evidence of tumor in bone marrow), but also tumor histologic grade, biologic markers (ER, PR, and HER2 status), genomic assays (the Oncotype DX score, where applicable), and tumor response to neoadjuvant systemic treatment.[26] A staging website or calculator is best used to determine the stage (e.g., https://www.komen.org/breast-cancer/diagnosis/stages-staging/).

Some prefixes and suffixes are used with the "clinical TNM" (cTNM; determined before treatment by physical exam and imaging) and "pathologic TNM" (pTNM; based on pathologic evaluation of primary tumor and lymph nodes after definitive surgical treatment) staging systems to designate special cases. These do not affect the stage group but indicate specific considerations. These prefixes and suffixes include the "m" suffix, which signifies multiple primary tumors, pT(m)NM; the "y" prefix, which denotes patients who have received systemic therapy before surgery, ypTNM; and the "r" prefix, which indicates a recurrent tumor, rTNM. For example, a patient with a 3-cm, grade 3, ER–, PR–, HER2+ tumor in her left breast, with clinically positive and mobile lymph nodes in her left axilla and no distant metastasis on imaging, who was treated with neoadjuvant systemic therapy and underwent BCS and axillary dissection, with complete response in the breast but only partial response in the nodes, with 2 positive nodes out of 15 in the axillary dissection would be staged as clinical stage IIB (cT2, cN1, cM0) and pathologic stage IIA (ypT0, ypN1, M0).

In clinical practice, physicians use the anatomic stage grouping in addition to important clinical and biologic factors to determine risks and guide treatment recommendations. Treatment modalities include surgery, both therapeutic and reconstructive; RT; and systemic therapy. Each discipline has multiple treatment options, taking into consideration patient and tumor characteristics as well as additional factors, such as patient genetic status and family history, the patient's family planning expectations, and the patient's personal preferences. Each discipline's choice of treatment as well as the sequencing of treatments could affect treatment considerations of other disciplines. This is especially important in the era of neoadjuvant systemic therapy, affecting the ability to deescalate breast and axillary surgery, which could influence the choice for adjuvant radiation and additional systemic treatment. For these reasons, the management of patients with breast cancer should be done in a multidisciplinary context, with open and continuous communication between disciplines, to develop and implement the optimal patient-centered treatment plan. In the upcoming sections, we delineate the different surgical considerations and options alongside the medical and radiation treatments. The multidisciplinary team takes all these into account when discussing the specific patient and devising a course of action.

A history and physical examination, in addition to appropriate imaging studies, are important to establish the extent of the disease and assign a clinical stage. The NCCN provides guidelines regarding the use of laboratory and radiologic testing in patients at initial diagnosis based on the clinical stage. CT scans, bone scans, and other imaging studies are generally reserved for patients with clinically positive nodes, abnormalities on blood chemistry tests or chest radiographs, and symptoms based on history and physical examination and for patients with locally advanced or inflammatory breast cancer. Thorough imaging of the ipsilateral and contralateral breast is performed to look for areas of concern other than the index lesion. Breast MRI may be used in selected cases to define the extent of the tumor and look for additional breast lesions or to document response to neoadjuvant chemotherapy; however, there is no high-level evidence demonstrating that the use of MRI to guide decisions regarding local therapy improves local recurrence rates or survival.

In the absence of distant metastatic disease, surgery is a central part of treatment. In patients with very early breast cancer, surgery would be the first intervention, with resection of the tumor and surgical staging of the regional lymph nodes. Pathologic assessment of the primary tumor size and regional lymph node status, defining the pathologic stage, provides an estimate of prognosis and helps inform decisions about adjuvant systemic treatment and RT. Patients with locally advanced disease and inflammatory breast cancers should receive neoadjuvant systemic therapy before surgery. This is dependent on a multitude of factors and is further discussed in the "Neoadjuvant Systemic Therapy for Operable Breast Cancer" section later.

SURGICAL TREATMENT OF BREAST CANCER

Surgery is a central pillar in the care of locoregional breast cancer and is an essential component in any treatment plan with a curative intent. Surgery is key to establishing a diagnosis when an excisional biopsy is necessary to remove and characterize high-risk lesions. It is indispensable in treating breast cancer through resection as well as staging and assessing response to treatment. The selection of surgical procedures is based on patient characteristics and other clinical and pathologic variables. Patient characteristics, including age, family history, menopausal status, and overall health, are assessed. Some patients may undergo genetic testing for *BRCA* or other gene mutations at the time of diagnosis. Patients with a known *BRCA* mutation or other high-risk features can consider bilateral mastectomy for treatment of the index breast and reduction of the risk of contralateral breast cancer. The location of the tumor within the breast and tumor size relative to breast size are evaluated. Patient preferences for breast preservation versus mastectomy are determined. For patients considering mastectomy, options for immediate versus delayed reconstruction are discussed. All are considered in the context of multimodal therapy, taking into consideration the timing of systemic therapy and indications for adjuvant radiation. The importance of multidisciplinary consideration cannot be stressed enough because each modality affects the other.

Historical Perspective

Through the mid-20th century, breast cancer was thought to arise in the breast and progress to other sites largely via centrifugal spread. In this model, more extensive surgical procedures were expected to reduce mortality by resecting locoregional disease before it could spread to distant sites. This model was supported, in part, by the results of the Halsted radical mastectomy, which was the first procedure that demonstrated improvements in breast cancer survival relative to the local excision of tumors. Introduced in the 1880s, the radical mastectomy included the removal of the breast, overlying skin, and underlying pectoralis muscles in continuity with the regional lymph nodes along the axillary vein up to the costoclavicular ligament. The procedure often required a skin graft to cover the large skin defect that was created. This approach was well suited to breast cancer biology of the time, when most tumors were locally advanced, frequently with chest wall or skin involvement and extensive axillary nodal disease. Radical mastectomy provided improved local control and led to an increasing population of long-term survivors. Radical mastectomy continued to be the mainstay of surgical therapy into the 1970s, when investigations into the deescalation of surgery ensued. The accepted terminology and what is included in each type of mastectomy are shown in Box 68.3.

The NSABP B-04 trial was one of the first large trials to investigate alternatives to radical mastectomy. Breast cancer patients with clinically negative nodes were randomly assigned to radical mastectomy, total mastectomy with irradiation of the chest wall and regional nodes, or total mastectomy alone, with delayed axillary dissection if nodes became clinically enlarged. Patients did not receive systemic therapy. Patients with clinically positive nodes were randomly assigned to radical mastectomy or total mastectomy with irradiation of the chest wall and regional lymphatics. At 25 years of follow-up, overall survival (OS) and disease-free survival (DFS) were equivalent in all treatment arms within the node-positive and node-negative groups. The results of NSABP B-04 showed radical mastectomy to have no advantage over total mastectomy, demonstrating the safety of less aggressive surgery, ending the era of radical mastectomy as the hallmark of breast surgery. Of note, of the patients with clinically node-negative disease who underwent radical mastectomy, 38% were found to have nodal metastases at surgery, yet only 18% of patients

BOX 68.3   Types of Mastectomies and the Tissue Included in Each Resection

	BREAST TISSUE (BETWEEN PECTORALIS AND SKIN FLAP)	NIPPLE-AREOLAR COMPLEX (NAC)	SKIN OVER BREAST BEYOND NAC	AXILLARY CONTENT— LEVELS I AND II	PECTORALIS MAJOR AND MINOR
Radical mastectomy	+	+	+	+[a]	+
Modified radical mastectomy	+	+	+	+	
Total mastectomy	+	+	+		
Skin-sparing mastectomy	+	+			
Nipple skin-sparing mastectomy	+				

[a]Radical mastectomy traditionally includes removal of the axillary content in levels I, II, and III.

TABLE 68.4   Randomized Trials Comparing Breast Conservation Versus Mastectomy

TRIAL	NO. PATIENTS	MAXIMUM TUMOR SIZE (CM)	SYSTEMIC THERAPY	FOLLOW-UP (YEARS)	% SURVIVAL LUMPECTOMY + XRT	% SURVIVAL MASTECTOMY	LOCAL RECURRENCE (BCT) (%)
NSABP B-06[b]	1851	4	Yes	20	47	46	14[a]
Milan Cancer Institute[c]	701	2	Yes	20	44	43	8.8[a]
Institute Gustave-Roussy[d]	179	2	No	14	73	65	13
National Cancer Institute[e]	237	5	Yes	10	77	75	16
EORTC 10801[f]	868	5	Yes	10	65	66	17.6
Danish Breast Cancer Group[g]	905	None	Yes	6	79	82	3

[a]Includes only females whose excision margins were negative.
[b]Fisher B, Anderson S, Bryant J, et al. Twenty-year follow-up of a randomized trial comparing total mastectomy, lumpectomy, and lumpectomy plus irradiation for the treatment of invasive breast cancer. N Engl J Med. 2002;347:1233.
[c]Veronesi U, Cascinelli N, Mariani L, et al. Twenty-year follow-up of a randomized study comparing breast-conserving surgery with radical mastectomy for early breast cancer. N Engl J Med. 2002;347:1227.
[d]Arriagada R, Le M, Rochard F, et al. Conservative treatment versus mastectomy in early breast cancer: Patterns of failure with 15 years of follow-up data. J Clin Oncol. 1996;14:1558.
[e]Jacobson J, Danforth D, Cowan K, et al. Ten-year results of a comparison of conservation with mastectomy in the treatment of stage I and II breast cancer. N Engl J Med. 1995;332:907.
[f]van Dongen J, Voogd A, Fentiman I, et al. Long-term results of a randomized trial comparing breast-conserving therapy with mastectomy: European Organization for Research and Treatment of Cancer 10801 Trial. J Natl Cancer Inst. 2000;92:1143.
[g]Blichert-Toft M, Rose C, Andersen J, et al. Danish randomized trial comparing breast conservation therapy with mastectomy: six years of life-table analysis. Danish Breast Cancer Cooperative Group. J Natl Cancer Inst Monogr. 1992;11:19.
BCT, Breast-conserving therapy; EORTC, European Organization for Research and Treatment of Cancer; NSABP, National Surgical Adjuvant Breast and Bowel Project; XRT, radiation therapy.

undergoing total mastectomy without axillary dissection or RT developed axillary recurrence requiring delayed dissection.

Next, investigations into alternatives to total mastectomy, in the form of BCS, took place. Six prospective clinical trials that included more than 4500 patients compared mastectomy versus breast-conserving therapy (BCT; Table 68.4). In all these trials, there was no survival advantage for the use of mastectomy over breast preservation. The largest of these trials, NSABP B-06, enrolled 1851 patients with tumors up to 4 cm in diameter and clinically negative or positive lymph nodes. Patients were randomly assigned to undergo modified radical mastectomy, lumpectomy and axillary dissection, or lumpectomy and axillary dissection with postoperative irradiation of the breast without an extra boost to the lumpectomy site. All patients with histologically positive axillary nodes received chemotherapy. At 20 years of follow-up, OS and DFS were the same in all three treatment groups.

NSABP B-06 provided valuable information about rates of ipsilateral breast cancer recurrence after lumpectomy, with or without breast irradiation. At 20 years of follow-up, local recurrence rates were 14.3% in females treated with lumpectomy and RT and 39.2% in females treated with lumpectomy alone ($P < 0.001$). For patients with positive nodes who received chemotherapy, the local recurrence rate was 44.2% for lumpectomy alone and 8.8% for lumpectomy plus RT.

Another important trial that evaluated BCT was the Milan I trial. This trial enrolled patients with smaller tumors and used more extensive surgery and RT than the NSABP B-06 trial. There were 701 females with tumors up to 2 cm and clinically negative nodes randomly assigned to undergo radical mastectomy or quadrantectomy with axillary dissection and postoperative irradiation. Patients with pathologically positive nodes received chemotherapy. OS at 20 years did not differ between the two groups. Locoregional failure rates differed between the groups: Chest wall recurrence occurred in 2.3% of females who underwent radical mastectomy, and ipsilateral breast tumor recurrence occurred in 8.8% of females who underwent quadrantectomy and RT (20-year follow-up). After quadrantectomy, local failure rates were higher in younger females, with rates of

1% per year in females younger than 45 years and 0.5% per year in older females.

Three other randomized trials in patients with operable breast cancer found no survival benefit to mastectomy over BCT. In the European Organization for Research and Treatment of Cancer (EORTC) Trial 10801, in which 868 females were randomly assigned to modified radical mastectomy or lumpectomy and irradiation, there was no difference in survival at 10 years. This trial included patients with tumors up to 5 cm, and 80% of females enrolled had tumors larger than 2 cm. Positive margins were allowed, and the results showed lower rates of local recurrence with clear versus involved margins. In the Institut Gustave-Roussy trial, 179 females with tumors smaller than 2 cm were randomly assigned to modified radical mastectomy or lumpectomy with a 2-cm margin of normal tissue around the cancer. No differences were observed between the two surgical groups in risk for death, metastases, contralateral breast cancer, or locoregional recurrence at 15 years of follow-up. In the United States National Cancer Institute trial, 237 females with tumors 5 cm or smaller were randomly assigned to lumpectomy with axillary dissection and RT or modified radical mastectomy. No differences were seen in OS or DFS rates at 10 years. With this evidence, BCT has become a standard alternative to mastectomy.

In parallel to the deescalation of surgery, there were considerable advances in systemic therapy for breast cancer. Up to the 1970s, despite the use of radical mastectomy and even after more extensive surgical procedures, such as radical mastectomy with en bloc resection of the internal mammary and supraclavicular nodes, many females continued to die of metastatic disease. This eventually led to a shift in the theory of primary centrifugal spread to the more modern theory that breast cancer spreads centrifugally to adjacent structures and via lymphatics and blood vessels to distant sites.

In the modern era, breast cancer treatment includes local and regional approaches (surgery and RT) in addition to medical therapies designed to treat systemic disease. Multimodality treatment approaches were the first to show significant improvements in locoregional control and survival. Because breast cancer was being recognized at earlier stages, radical mastectomy was abandoned in favor of more conservative surgical approaches in combination with RT. The result was dramatic reductions in the extent of surgery required for local control of breast cancer and decreases in treatment-related morbidity. With the understanding that breast cancer is a heterogeneous disease, current treatment is tailored for each patient and guided by molecular properties of the individual patient's tumor, the size and location of the tumor, lymphatic spread, the patient's genetic and family history, and other risk factors as well as their age and comorbidities. Because radical mastectomy conceptually and practically included surgery for the breast and the axillary nodal basins en bloc, the modern surgical approach can be seen as conceptually separating surgical planning for the primary tumor in the breast from lymph node surgery in the axilla. The upcoming segments will follow the same understanding.

Selection of Surgical Therapy for the Breast Primary

The results of the aforementioned trials established BCT, defined as BCS and adjuvant RT, as equivalent to mastectomy in terms of patient survival. The choice of surgical treatment is therefore individualized. With these criteria and current surgical and RT approaches, local recurrence rates after lumpectomy and RT are less than 5% at 10 years at many large centers. Each patient

---

BOX 68.4 Contraindications to Radiation

Absolute
- Pregnancy
- Homozygous for *ATM* mutation

Relative
- Connective tissue diseases, especially systemic scleroderma and systemic lupus erythematosus[a]
- Prior radiation to breast or chest wall
- Severe pulmonary disease
- Severe cardiac disease (if tumor is left-sided)
- Inability to lie supine
- Inability to abduct arm on affected side
- *p53* mutation[b]

[a]Other collagen vascular diseases are not contraindications to radiation, although patients should not be taking immunosuppressants, such as methotrexate, because they are radiosensitizers.
[b]Patients with *p53* mutations are highly susceptible to radiation-induced cancers.

---

desiring BCS should be evaluated as to the appropriateness of this approach based on their individual circumstances. There are several considerations for surgical planning:

1. *Willingness and ability to receive radiation*: Patients who desire BCS should be willing to attend postoperative RT sessions and undergo postoperative surveillance of the treated breast. To better understand the implications, consultation with a radiation oncologist may be arranged before the planned surgery. Patients with contraindications to RT, as outlined in Box 68.4, should not be considered for BCT. Of note, although pregnancy is an absolute contraindication to RT, many patients pregnant at diagnosis can complete their pregnancy and receive RT after delivery.

2. *Tumor size*: The trials examining the safety of BCT included tumors smaller than 5 cm. Nevertheless, in current practice, lumpectomy is considered when the tumor, regardless of size, can be excised with clear margins and an acceptable cosmetic result. Therefore, a significant factor in determining whether BCT is feasible is the relationship between tumor size and breast size. In patients with larger tumors, several approaches could allow BCT in a patient who otherwise would not qualify. Neoadjuvant systemic therapy (discussed later) is considered for patients for whom adjuvant systemic chemotherapy would likely be recommended. Neoadjuvant trials have shown that rates of BCT are higher in patients treated with neoadjuvant therapy, with good response in the tumor. Another strategy is to consider oncoplastic breast surgery (discussed later) with local tissue rearrangement or pedicled myocutaneous flaps (e.g., latissimus dorsi) for better cosmetic results.[27]

3. *Tumor characteristics*: Although high nuclear grade, presence of lymphovascular invasion (LVI), and negative ER and PR status have all been linked to increased local recurrence rates, none of these factors is considered a contraindication to breast conservation. Invasive lobular cancers, included in the mastectomy-versus-BCT trials, and cancers with an extensive in situ component can also be treated with lumpectomy if clear margins can be achieved. Atypical hyperplasia (ductal and lobular) and LCIS at resection margins do not increase local recurrence rates. Patients with multicentric tumors are usually treated with mastectomy because it is difficult to perform more than one BCS in the same breast with acceptable cosmesis. The

recently published American College of Surgeons Oncology Group (ACOSOG)/Alliance recently published the results of the Z11102 trial, a prospective single arm phase II study in females with multiple ipsilateral breast cancers (MIBCs), demonstrated the safety of BCT with adjuvant radiation inpatients with two to three ipsilateral tumors, showing a 3.1% 5-year local recurrence rate with a median follow-up of 66.4 months. The majority of patients in the trial had T1 tumors that were ER+ and pathologically node negative, most patients had two foci of disease, and almost all had preoperative MRI. Local recurrence rates were higher in patients with ER+ disease who did not receive endocrine therapy and patients who did not have a preoperative MRI. [28]

4. *Patient characteristics and preference:* Local recurrence rates after BCS are higher for younger females than for older females, but there are no age limitations on BCT. Local recurrence rates are reduced in patients of all ages with the use of RT. A radiation boost to the tumor bed has been shown to reduce local failures after lumpectomy with negative margins, particularly in younger females. Recent studies have identified subgroups of patients who can undergo BCS with the omission of adjuvant radiation (discussed later). Ultimately, after considering all other factors, patient preference between BCT and mastectomy is central to the decision process.

Breast-Conserving Surgery
Technical Aspects

Resection of the primary tumor, either invasive or in situ, with preservation of the breast, has been referred to by many terms, including *lumpectomy, partial mastectomy, segmental mastectomy, segmentectomy, tylectomy,* and *wide local excision.* BCS removes the malignancy with a surrounding rim of grossly normal breast parenchyma while conserving the remainder of the breast tissue. In the operating room (OR), the surgeon determines the location of the tumor with palpation in cases of palpable tumors, or with the aid of a localization device in cases where the tumor is not palpable (the different techniques are discussed shortly). An incision is performed over the tumor or at a distant location, allowing for a less apparent scar. Dissections are performed toward and around the tumor, and it is excised in its entirety (Fig. 68.12). The breast specimen is oriented, and its edges are inked before sectioning. Specimen radiography should be performed for all nonpalpable lesions or if there are microcalcifications associated with the palpable tumor. If a margin appears to be close or is positive histologically on intraoperative assessment, reexcision to remove more tissue from that margin frequently achieves a clear margin and allows conservation of the breast. Orientation of the surgical specimen allows for directed reexcision of involved margins rather than reexcision of the entire lumpectomy cavity and improves the cosmetic result by reducing the amount of normal breast parenchyma that is excised.

There is level I evidence that cavity shave margins at the time of the lumpectomy reduce positive margins and the need for reexcision. The larger the volume of excision, the better the margin clearance, but the poorer the cosmetic result. [29] The surgical defect created after lumpectomy is inspected for hemostasis, and clips are left in the cavity for future orientation (i.e., planning for adjuvant radiation). The cavity and incision are then closed cosmetically. There is increasing interest in the use of advancement flap closure and other oncoplastic surgical techniques to maximize the cosmetic result. Axillary surgery is performed on the same occasion and will be discussed shortly.

Margins

The appropriate margin width for lumpectomy specimens has been debated. Although the NSABP B-06 trial defined a negative margin as "no ink on tumor," other trials evaluating BCT did not specify a required margin width or did not evaluate microscopic margins. The optimal margin width has been open to interpretation, resulting in substantial variability in treatment and recommendations regarding the need for reexcision for "positive" margins. The Society of Surgical Oncology (SSO) and the American Society for Radiation Oncology (ASTRO) convened a multidisciplinary panel to address the question of what margin width is required to minimize the risk of ipsilateral breast tumor recurrence. [30] The panel used a meta-analysis of margin width and ipsilateral breast tumor recurrence from a systematic review of 33 studies including 28,162 patients. Positive margins, defined as ink on invasive carcinoma or DCIS in the context of invasive cancer, were associated with a twofold increase in ipsilateral breast tumor recurrence risk compared with negative margins, defined as "no ink on tumor." The risk was not affected by any specific clinicopathologic features, including favorable biology, use of endocrine therapy, or administration of a radiation boost. In addition, more widely clear margins than "no ink on tumor" did not significantly decrease the ipsilateral breast tumor recurrence risk, including in patients with unfavorable biology, lobular cancers, or cancers with an extensive intraductal component. The panel concluded that "no ink on tumor" should be used as the standard for an adequate margin in invasive breast cancer.

SSO, ASTRO, and the American Society of Clinical Oncology (ASCO) convened a similar consensus conference on margin width in DCIS and identified a margin of 2 mm as an appropriate negative margin for DCIS. [31] Based on a meta-analysis of 20 studies and 7883 patients, a 2-mm margin was found to confer improved ipsilateral breast cancer recurrence compared with a 0- or 1-mm margin. Margins wider than 2 mm were not found to significantly decrease ipsilateral breast tumor recurrence compared with 2-mm margins. [32] The use of adjuvant whole breast RT has been demonstrated in prospective trials to decrease the risk of local recurrence. The use of endocrine therapy in patients with ER-positive DCIS can further decrease the risk for local recurrence and reduce the risk for development of new contralateral and ipsilateral breast cancers.

Localization of Nonpalpable Breast Lesions

Nonpalpable malignancies, usually detected during screening, require localization before BCS. As mentioned earlier, during the biopsy of suspected breast lesions, a clip is placed at the biopsy site to allow for future localization. This clip and associated lesions can be localized for excision in a number of techniques. The traditional method for localization is wire localization: Before surgery, either under US or mammographic guidance, a wire is placed into the breast, with its hook-shaped tip slightly beyond the target lesion. This second procedure (the initial biopsy and clip placement is the first procedure) has several disadvantages, including a painful procedure for patients, commonly accompanied by vaso vagal events, the risk of wire displacement and failure in clip retrieval, and scheduling issues because this second procedure usually occurs on the day of surgery. To overcome these disadvantages, several alternative techniques have been developed.

Several markers have been developed to be placed at the biopsy site, usually placed in a second procedure next to the biopsy marking clip. These markers include radioactive ^{125}I seeds, radar reflectors (e.g., Savi Scout; Penn Medicine, Philadelphia, PA), radiofrequency identification tags, and magnetic seeds (e.g., Magseed;

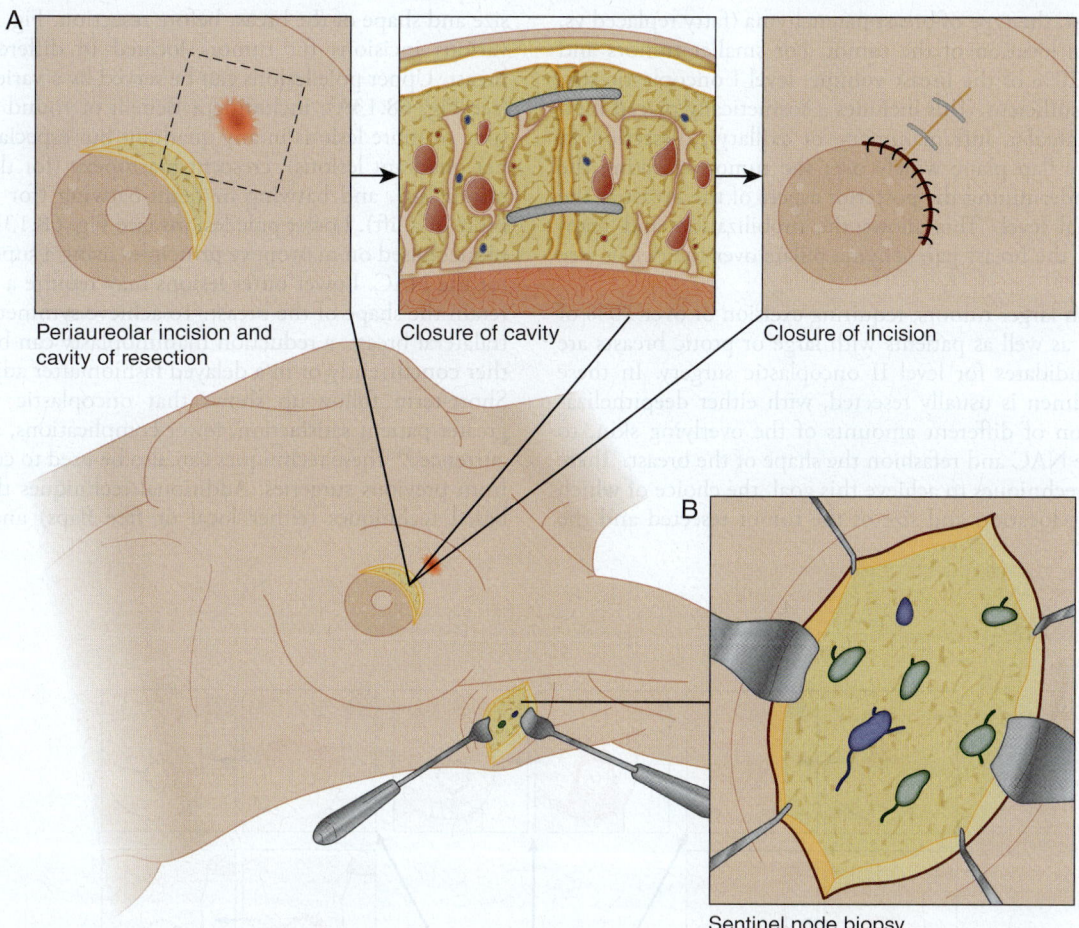

FIGURE 68.12 Breast-conserving surgery and sentinel lymph node dissection. (A) Incisions to remove malignant tumors are placed directly over the tumor or around the areola. After the partial mastectomy has been completed, the parenchymal defect is closed after raising the necessary skin flaps *(inset)* to prevent a cosmetic deformity. (B) A transverse incision below the axillary hairline is used for sentinel node dissection, which may be located by percutaneous mapping with the gamma probe to detect a hot spot from the radiolabeled colloid. It is extended through the clavipectoral fascia, and the true axilla is entered. The sentinel node is located by staining with blue dye *(inset)*, radioactivity, or both and is dissected free as a single specimen.

A label in the figure reads "Periaureolar incision and cavity of resection", "Closure of cavity", "Closure of incision", and "Sentinel node biopsy".

Edomag, Cambridge, UK). Each is localized using a probe in the OR. Alternative, less costly techniques adequate for rural and lower-resource communities and countries are available. If the lesion is visible with US, then intraoperative US can be used for localization. A newer technique, fluoroscopic intraoperative neoplasm or node detection (FIND), uses fluoroscopy to find the radiopaque clip placed at the time of the original CNB. It avoids any other procedures before surgery and provides a dynamic localization technique most surgeons are acquainted with.[33] With all localization techniques, after excision, a specimen radiograph should be performed to confirm that the targeted lesion and localization device have been excised.

Oncoplastic Techniques

When the primary tumor is resected using an incision directly over the tumor and then the skin is closed, several deformities can occur. These include retraction of the skin into the cavity once the seroma reabsorbs, displacement of the NAC (i.e., bird-beak deformity with a downward turning nipple after resection of a lower

pole lesion), and asymmetry of the breast. These deformities can make it difficult for patients to wear tight-fitting clothing, because significant asymmetry may be evident, having a detrimental effect on their body image and quality of life. These deformities can be further accentuated by adjuvant radiation, also complicating future corrective surgery.

The term *oncoplastic surgery* has been popularized to stress the importance of achieving the best possible esthetic result in the context of resecting the tumor with adequate oncologic margins. The goal is to provide optimal cosmesis and symmetry with the opposite breast while retaining as much of the natural breast size and contour as possible. The surgeon should consider oncoplastic techniques in any breast surgery, but especially whenever resection of over 20% of breast tissue is planned, the resection is from an area associated with poor cosmetic outcome, or when resection may lead to nipple malposition.

When choosing the appropriate oncoplastic technique, the surgeon must take into account the patient's breast size and level of ptosis, the size of the tumor to be resected in comparison to the size of the breast, the type of breast parenchyma (fatty replaced vs. dense), and the location of the tumor. For smaller tumors and resection of <20% of the breast volume, level I oncoplastic surgery is usually sufficient. This includes a cosmetically placed incision (e.g., periareolar, inframammary, or axillary), dissection in the mastectomy flap plane widely over the tumor, resecting the tumor, then undermining the posterior aspect of the breast at the pectoralis fascial level. This allows the mobilization and reapproximation of the breast parenchyma pillars over the defect (see Fig. 68.12).

Patients with larger tumors, requiring excision of over 20% of breast volume, as well as patients with large or ptotic breasts are often good candidates for level II oncoplastic surgery. In these cases, the specimen is usually resected, with either deepithelization or resection of different amounts of the overlying skin, to recentralize the NAC and refashion the shape of the breast. There is a myriad of techniques to achieve this goal, the choice of which depends on the location and size of the tumor resected and the

size and shape of the breast before resection. Fig. 68.13 shows the various incisions for tumors located in different parts of the breast. Upper pole lesions can be served by a variety of techniques (see Fig. 68.13A), including a Benelli or round block technique (one or more lesions in any quadrant but especially for upper inner quadrant lesions), crescent mastopexy (for those who need a minor lift), and batwing or hemi-batwing (for those who need more of a lift). Lower pole lesions (see Fig. 68.13B) may use techniques based on mastopexy principles using a superior pedicle flap for the NAC. Lower outer lesions may require a J- or V-plasty to retain the shape of the breast. To achieve symmetry with the contralateral breast, a reduction mammoplasty can be performed, either concurrently or in a delayed fashion after adjuvant radiation. Short-term follow-up shows that oncoplastic techniques have greater patient satisfaction, fewer complications, and less local recurrence.[34] These techniques can also be used to correct defects left from previous surgeries. Additional techniques that include flap-based techniques (either local or free flaps) and implant-based

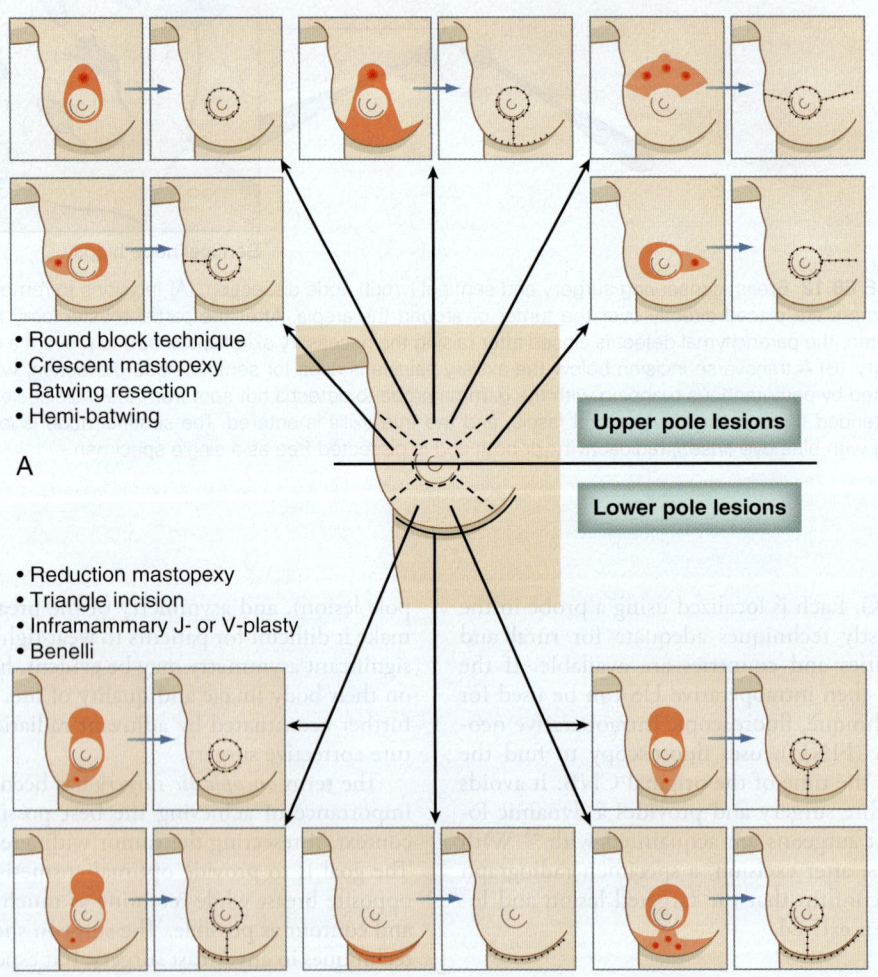

FIGURE 68.13 The various incisions for tumors located in different parts of the breast. (A) Upper pole lesions can be served by a variety of techniques, including round block, crescent mastopexy, and batwing or hemi-batwing. (B) Lower pole lesions may use techniques that require a mastopexy based on a superior pedicle flap, including reduction mastopexy, triangle incision, J- or V-plasty, and Benelli. (Adapted from Fitoussi A, Berry MG, Couturaud B, et al. *Oncoplastic and Reconstructive Surgery for Breast Cancer: The Institut Curie Experience*. Paris: Springer; 2008.)

techniques are beyond the scope of this chapter and are discussed elsewhere.

Immediate repair of a BCS defect with oncoplastic surgery, involving tissue advancement and local tissue rearrangement, is almost always preferred to a delayed repair and provides an optimal solution. Furthermore, performing oncoplastic reconstruction at the time of tumor resection has not been associated with delay in delivery of adjuvant systemic therapy or radiation. If a cosmetic defect occurs after BCS and RT, reconstruction of the treated breast is generally not recommended for 1 to 2 years after RT has been completed. In fatty replaced and irradiated tissue, there is a higher rate of tissue necrosis, seroma formation, and infection. The use of vascularized tissue from outside the radiation field is the favored approach for correcting defects after radiation. If the main deformity is caused by asymmetry with the contralateral breast, a contralateral mastopexy can be considered. In general, surgical procedures on the irradiated breast should be minimized because healing and recovery are impaired even when the skin appears healthy.

Mastectomy

Indications

Certain patients still require mastectomy, including those with tumors that are large relative to breast size, tumors with extensive calcifications on mammography, tumors for which clear margins cannot be obtained on wide local excision, and patients with contraindications to breast irradiation (see Box 68.4). Patient preference for mastectomy or a desire to avoid radiation is also a valid indication for mastectomy. Some patients with high-risk genetic mutations and a diagnosis of breast cancer will opt for an ipsilateral therapeutic mastectomy and a CPM.

Technical Details

Simple or *total mastectomy* refers to the complete removal of the mammary gland, including the nipple and areola. *Modified radical mastectomy* refers to the removal of the mammary gland, nipple, and areola, with the addition of a complete ALND (Fig. 68.14; see Box 68.3). For either a total mastectomy or a modified radical mastectomy, an elliptical skin incision is planned to include the

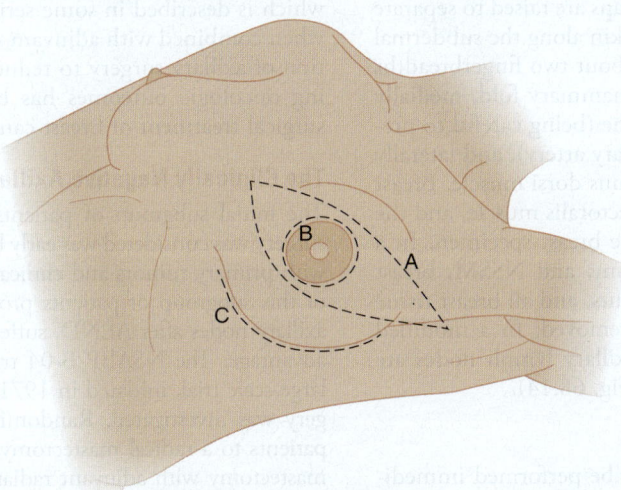

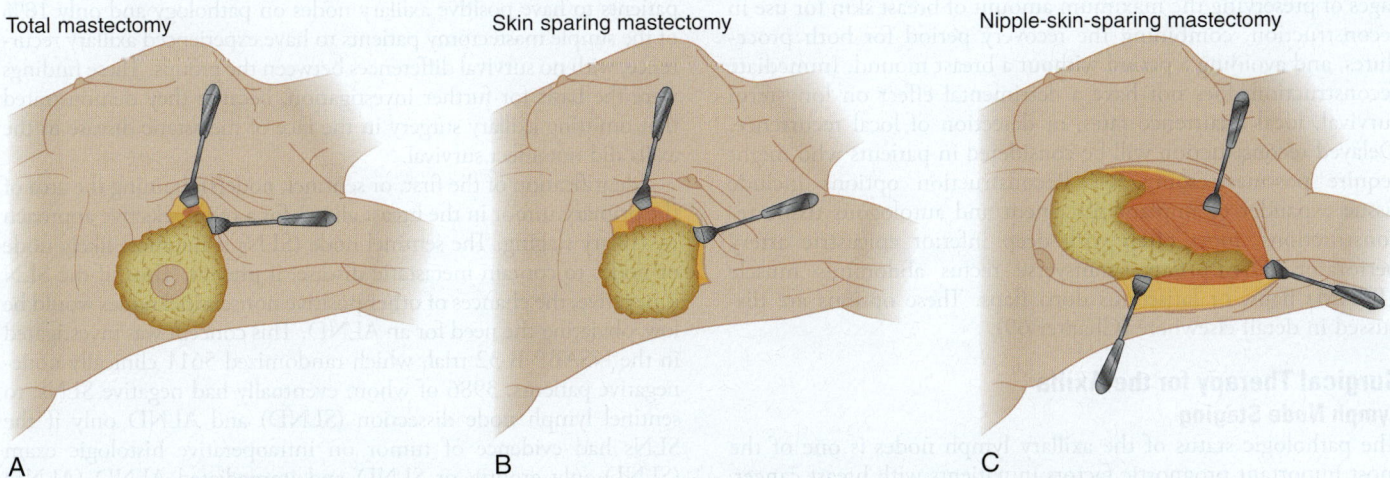

Total mastectomy   Skin sparing mastectomy   Nipple-skin-sparing mastectomy

A   B   C

FIGURE 68.14 Total, skin-sparing and nipple-skin-sparing mastectomies. For patients undergoing mastectomy without reconstruction, skin incisions are generally transverse and include the skin over the central breast and nipple-areolar complex (A). Circumareolar incisions are most common for patients undergoing skin-sparing mastectomy with immediate reconstruction (B). An inframammary incision is shown for nipple–skin–sparing mastectomy, although additional incisions have been described for this procedure (C). Skin flaps are raised to separate the gland is dissected off the overlying skin and then the gland is dissected off the underlying muscle. A mastectomy divides the breast from the axillary contents and stops at the clavipectoral fascia. If axillary staging or axillary lymph node dissection is planned, this is performed through the same incision or a separate transverse axillary incision.

nipple and areola and usually any previous excisional biopsy scars. It is important to know whether immediate or delayed reconstruction is planned or if the patient has chosen an aesthetic flat closure ("to go flat"). For an aesthetic flat closure, sufficient skin should be taken to allow smooth closure of skin flaps without redundant skin folds. The aim is to create a smooth chest wall, which will also facilitate the comfortable use of a breast prosthesis if desired.

If immediate reconstruction is planned, a skin-sparing mastectomy may be performed in which only the NAC is removed, and the maximum amount of skin is left for use in the reconstruction. Nipple-skin-sparing mastectomy (NSSM) has been used with increasing frequency for selected patients with breast cancer. Multiple studies have shown the safety and feasibility of this approach, with many series showing low recurrence rates in patients undergoing NSSM. NSSM has also been demonstrated to be safe in patients undergoing prophylactic mastectomy for risk reduction, including *BRCA1* and *BRCA2* gene mutation carriers.[35] If NSSM is chosen, there are several potential locations for incisions, including the inframammary fold, periareolar, a radial incision, and a lateral/axillary incision.[36]

After incisions have been made, skin flaps are raised to separate the underlying gland from the overlying skin along the subdermal plexus. This continues superiorly up to about two fingerbreadths from the clavicle, inferiorly to the inframammary fold, medially to a fingerbreadth or two from the midline (being careful to preserve the branches of the internal mammary artery), and laterally toward the axilla and down to the latissimus dorsi muscle. Breast tissue is separated from the underlying pectoralis muscle, and the pectoral fascia is generally taken with the breast specimen. In a total mastectomy, skin-sparing mastectomy, and NSSM, breast tissue is separated from the axillary contents, and all breast tissue superficial to the fascia of the axilla is removed. In a modified radical mastectomy, the level I and II axillary lymph nodes are taken en bloc with the breast tissue (see Fig. 68.14).

Postmastectomy Breast Reconstruction

If breast reconstruction is chosen, it may be performed immediately, on the same day as mastectomy, or as delayed reconstruction months or years later. Immediate reconstruction has the advantages of preserving the maximum amount of breast skin for use in reconstruction, combining the recovery period for both procedures, and avoiding a period without a breast mound. Immediate reconstruction does not have a detrimental effect on long-term survival, local recurrence rates, or detection of local recurrence. Delayed reconstruction will be considered in patients who might require postmastectomy RT. Reconstruction options include tissue expander or implant placement and autologous tissue reconstructions, most often with deep inferior epigastric artery perforator (DIEP) flaps, transverse rectus abdominis muscle (TRAM) flaps, or latissimus dorsi flaps. These options are discussed in detail elsewhere (Chapter 69).

Surgical Therapy for the Axilla
Lymph Node Staging

The pathologic status of the axillary lymph nodes is one of the most important prognostic factors in patients with breast cancer. Identification of metastatic tumor deposits in the axillary nodes indicates a poorer prognosis and often prompts a recommendation for more aggressive systemic and locoregional therapies. Patients can present with clinically involved nodes (cN1–3 in the TNM staging system), evident on physical exam or imaging and proven by biopsy, or clinically uninvolved nodes (cN0), who after axillary surgery will either still have a negative axilla (pN0) or will prove to have microscopically occult nodal involvement diagnosed histologically after surgical excision (cN0, but pN1–3). Currently, management of the clinically positive versus the clinically negative axilla differs substantially.

Since the introduction of Halsted's radical mastectomy, axillary surgery has been a routine component of the surgical management of breast cancer. It provides prognostic information about axillary nodal status and plays a therapeutic role in regional control by removing axillary disease in patients with positive nodes. ALND, either as part of a modified radical mastectomy or separate from the surgical approach in the breast, includes clearance of node-bearing tissue within the axilla, defined as the space between the pectoralis major muscle anteriorly, the latissimus dorsi muscle posteriorly, the chest wall medially, and the axillary vein superiorly. Axillary dissection is the main source of morbidity in patients with early-stage breast cancer, both in the postoperative period and long term. Morbidity includes acute and chronic pain and paresthesias; reduced range of motion to the shoulder joint; and most dreaded, lymphedema of the ipsilateral arm, which is described in some series to affect up to 80% of patients when combined with adjuvant radiation. As a result, the deescalation of axillary surgery to reduce morbidity without compromising oncologic outcomes has become an ongoing effort in the surgical treatment of breast cancer.

The Clinically Negative Axilla

The initial subgroup of patients in which deescalation of axillary surgery was considered was early breast cancer patients who presented with primary tumors and clinically uninvolved nodes. Sixty percent of this subgroup of patients proves to have pathologically negative axillary nodes after ALND, suffering morbidity with no therapeutic advantage. The NSABP B-04 trial, mentioned earlier, was the first large-scale trial, initiated in 1971, in which omission of axillary surgery was investigated. Randomizing 1079 clinically node-negative patients to a radical mastectomy, a simple mastectomy, or a simple mastectomy with adjuvant radiation demonstrated no difference in OS, distant metastasis-free survival, or DFS, whether ALND was performed or not. It nevertheless found 38% of radical mastectomy patients to have positive axillary nodes on pathology and only 18% of the simple mastectomy patients to have experienced axillary recurrence, with no survival differences between the groups. These findings were the basis for further investigation, because they demonstrated that omitting axillary surgery in the face of metastatic disease in the axilla did not affect survival.

Identification of the first, or sentinel, node(s) draining the area of the primary tumor in the breast allows for a more selective approach to axillary staging. The sentinel node (SLN) is the most likely node or nodes to contain metastatic disease, if present. Thus, if the SLN is negative, the chances of other positive nonsentinel nodes would be low, obviating the need for an ALND. This concept was investigated in the NSABP B-32 trial, which randomized 5611 clinically node-negative patients, 3986 of whom eventually had negative SLNs, to sentinel lymph node dissection (SLND) and ALND only if the SLNs had evidence of tumor on intraoperative histologic exam (SLND-only group), or SLND and immediated ALND (ALND group). It showed a lower rate of morbidity, including lower limited range of motion, pain, and lymphedema rates, in the SLND-only group compared with the ALND group; no difference in OS, DFS, or regional recurrence between the two groups was found, demonstrating that when the sentinel node is negative, SLND alone without further ALND is appropriate for patients with clinically negative lymph nodes.[37] Furthermore, the detection rate was 97% in this trial, and the false-negative rate (FNR) was 9.8%. A randomized trial conducted at the European Institute of Oncology and numerous single-institution reports confirmed the findings from the NSABP B-32 trial showing that the SLND technique is accurate, with FNRs of 0% to 11%, establishing SLND, from the 1990s on, as an essential standard component in the surgical care of patients with early breast cancer and clinically negative nodes.

Sentinel Lymph Node Dissection—Technique

In an SLND, often called *sentinel lymph node biopsy* (SLNB)—a misnomer—a tracer, injected into the breast, passes through the lymphatics to the first draining node(s), where it accumulates. In the B-32 trial, both technetium-99m (^{99m}Tc)-labeled sulfur colloid and a vital blue dye, isosulfan blue (Lymphazurin), were used. Nowadays there are additional tracers, such as indocyanine green and magnetic particles, which can be used. Lymphatic mapping can be performed with a combination of these agents or with a single agent. Studies indicate that using the combination technique may result in a lower FNR. Preoperative lymphoscintigraphy can provide information on the specific nodal basins draining the primary tumor. Using a peritumoral injection technique, approximately 70% to 80% of patients have drainage to the axilla, <20% have drainage to the axilla and the internal mammary nodal basin, 2% to 3% have drainage to the internal mammary nodal basin alone, and up to 8% do not show any drainage to the regional nodal basins. If a subareolar or subdermal injection technique is used, drainage is seen almost exclusively in the axillary nodal basin. A dose of 2.5 mCi of ^{99m}Tc-labeled sulfur colloid can be injected on the day before surgery, for preoperative lymphoscintigraphy; this allows for adequate activity to remain in the sentinel nodes for the intraoperative lymphatic mapping procedure the following day without the need for reinjection. Alternatively, for surgeons not using preoperative lymphoscintigraphy, 0.5 to 1.0 mCi of ^{99m}Tc-labeled sulfur colloid can be injected in the operating suite at the begining of surgery to avoid preoperative pain and vasovagal events.

In the operating suite, 3 to 5 mL of blue dye can also be injected, and the injection site is massaged to facilitate the passage of the dye through the lymphatics. A handheld gamma probe is used to transcutaneously localize the area of increased radioactivity; this helps guide the placement of the incision for the sentinel node procedure (see Fig. 68.12). After the incision is made, an area of increased radioactivity is localized with the handheld gamma probe, and the surgeon visualizes blue lymphatic channels leading to the sentinel node. Careful dissection is performed to avoid prematurely disrupting the afferent lymphatics. If a blue-stained lymphatic channel or a specific area of radioactivity ("hot spot") cannot be identified, the primary tumor can be resected to remove the site of injection, decreasing the background shine-through radioactivity. The sentinel node is identified and removed, after which the nodal basin is checked again to confirm that the level of radioactivity has decreased. If the level of radioactivity remains high, additional sentinel nodes may remain in the nodal basin, and additional dissection should be completed to remove all sentinel nodes. Published studies have demonstrated an average of two or three sentinel nodes per patient. This is a procedure that can be performed as an outpatient procedure and does not require a drain. Patients have a more rapid return to full mobility and can return to work and other activities weeks sooner than after an ALND. Long-term morbidity, including lymphedema, numbness, and chronic pain, is greatly reduced.

It is important to note that the identification of the sentinel node allows for a more detailed analysis of a limited number of nodes compared with the larger number of nodes in an ALND. In general, pathologists will section the sentinel node along its short axis and submit all the sections for paraffin embedding of the tissues. The paraffin blocks are sectioned and examined with hematoxylin-eosin staining of sections from each block. For SLNs, pathologists perform a more detailed analysis with step-sectioning of the paraffin blocks and immunohistochemical staining for cytokeratin, which enhances sensitivity by allowing the detection of micrometastases. The NSABP B-32 trial provided an opportunity to investigate the clinical significance of occult metastatic disease. For patients with negative sentinel nodes by hematoxylin-eosin staining, additional sections were evaluated by cytokeratin immunohistochemistry to identify occult metastases. The 5-year DFS rate was 86.4% for patients with occult metastases compared with 89.2% for patients without occult metastases (absolute difference = 2.8%), and the 5-year OS rate was 94.6% for patients with occult metastases compared with 95.8% for patients without occult metastases (absolute difference = 1.2%).[38] These differences were statistically significant given the large number of patients enrolled in the study; however, because the absolute differences were small, the NSABP investigators concluded that the presence of occult metastases was not clinically significant. This conclusion was confirmed by the ACOSOG Z0010 trial, which was designed to evaluate the significance of sentinel node and bone marrow micrometastases in patients with early-stage breast cancer undergoing BCT.[39] In that study, the 5-year DFS rates for patients with immunohistochemistry-positive and immunohistochemistry-negative sentinel nodes were 90% and 92%, respectively ($P = 0.82$), and the 5-year OS rates were 95% and 96%, respectively ($P = 0.64$). These findings suggested that micrometastases in SLNs (defined as metastases 0.2–2.0 mm in size) were likely not clinically significant, a finding that was further confirmed in the International Breast Cancer Study Group (IBCSG) 23-01 and Spanish Sentinel Node (AATRM) trials, which randomized patients with micrometastases on SLND to completion ALND versus observation.[40,41]

Positive Sentinel Lymph Node Dissection

When the sentinel node contains metastatic disease, the likelihood of additional involved nodes is directly proportional to the size of the primary breast tumor, the presence of lymphatic vascular invasion, and the size of the lymph node metastasis. Although ALND has been standard practice for patients with positive sentinel nodes, the need for ALND in all patients with a positive sentinel node has been called into question because many patients have small-volume metastases, and the sentinel node is often the only positive node. A meta-analysis of studies evaluating patients with positive sentinel nodes showed that 53% of patients have additional positive nodes at ALND. In the case of micrometastatic disease in the sentinel nodes, the rate of nonsentinel node involvement is 20%, and for patients with isolated tumor cells, it is less than 12%. In addition, as the NSABP B-06 trial has taught us, not excising all lymphatic involvement does not necessarily affect survival. These findings led the ACOSOG to initiate a prospective randomized trial in 1999 designed specifically to evaluate the impact of omitting ALND on survival and locoregional recurrence in clinically node-negative SLN-positive patients with early-stage breast cancer.[42,43] ACOSOG Z0011 enrolled patients with clinical T1 or T2 breast cancer with one or two positive sentinel nodes who were planning to undergo BCS and whole breast irradiation (WBI). Patients were randomly assigned to undergo completion ALND or no further surgery (SLND alone). The primary end point of the Z0011 study was OS; secondary end points were locoregional recurrence and lymphedema. Patients enrolled in the Z0011 study had relatively favorable disease characteristics: the median age was 55 years, 70% of patients had T1 tumors, 82% had ER-positive tumors, 71% had only one positive sentinel node, and 44% had micrometastases. At a median follow-up of 9.3 years, the 10-year OS was 86.3% in the SLND-alone group and 83.6% in the ALND group ($P = 0.02$). The 10-year DFS was 80.2% in the SLND-alone group and 78.2% in the ALND group ($P = 0.32$). Ten-year regional recurrence did not differ significantly between the two groups. The Z0011 study investigators concluded that ALND may be safely omitted in patients with early-stage breast cancer with one or two positive sentinel nodes who are undergoing BCS and receive whole breast radiation and systemic therapy. It should be noted, however, that there was no significant difference in lymphedema seen between the groups. This may be because this trial included WBI, which included the level I axilla or higher in most patients. This study did not include mastectomy patients.

The After Mapping of the Axilla: Radiotherapy or Surgery? (AMAROS) trial randomized patients with T1 or T2 disease and clinically node-negative disease but positive SLNs to completion ALND or axillary radiation.[44,45] Most tumors were T1 (80%), and most had only one positive sentinel node (76%). There were 248 mastectomy patients included out of 1166 patients randomized (18%). Despite this limited number, axillary recurrence rates for mastectomy and BCS patients were similar, whether they underwent completion ALND or adjuvant radiation. As a result of these trials, the ASBrS endorses omission of an ALND in a patient found to have micrometastases to their SLNs (applicable to those with one or two positive SLNs undergoing BCS and WBI and those undergoing mastectomy with one or two, possibly three, positive SLNs) if they will be receiving adjuvant axillary radiation. The Liberty trial is currently examining the omission of ALND in patients undergoing mastectomy with positive SLNs, with the hope of shedding more light on this subgroup of patients. That being said, population-based studies are showing that clinicians are omitting ALND in patients with positive SLNs who would not qualify for the aforementioned randomized controlled trials and would fall outside of their criteria, such as patients with T3 tumors, those with more than two or three positive SLNs, those with clinically positive nodes, or those who choose not to have indicated adjuvant radiation or systemic treatment.

The Clinically Positive Axilla

Patients who present with clinically palpable lymph nodes should be evaluated with axillary ultrasonography and fine-needle aspiration biopsy (FNAB) of the nodes. If axillary metastasis is confirmed, patients can proceed directly to standard axillary node dissection or be considered for preoperative chemotherapy. Historically, all patients undergoing neoadjuvant systemic treatment underwent an ALND thereafter, regardless of their response to treatment. Current systemic neoadjuvant regimens achieve an over 50% pathologic complete response (pCR) rate in the axilla, most prominently in patients with triple-negative and HER2-positive tumors. In these patients, an ALND could theoretically be avoided.

ACOSOG Z1071 was a phase II trial investigating the accuracy of SLND in detecting a pCR in patients with initial clinically positive axilla treated with neoadjuvant chemotherapy. It included females with N1–N2 disease, SLND was performed with dual tracer, and patients had to have at least two SLNs retrieved. All 756 patients in the trial underwent an SLND as well as a completion ALND. The primary end point was the FNR, which exceeded the prespecified threshold of 10% because 39 of the 310 patients (12.6%) with residual axillary disease had negative SLNs. Similar results were found in the European Sentinel Neoadjuvant (SENTINA) and Canadian Sentinel Node Biopsy Following Neoadjuvant Chemotherapy (SN FNAC) trials. The results of these studies suggest that surgical technique is critical in reducing the FNR for SLND in patients with initially clinically node-positive disease receiving neoadjuvant chemotherapy. Upon reanalysis of the Z1071 results, the presence of a clip that was placed before neoadjuvant treatment in the biopsy-proven node, within the SLND specimen, was found to lower the FNR to 6.2%.[46,47] Targeted axillary dissection (TAD), a combination of SLND and retrieval of the clipped node, has been shown to result in an FNR as low as 1.4%.[48] Trials are ongoing to determine if, in the neoadjuvant setting, it is safe to omit ALND if the SLN or TAD is negative.

As for patients with a clinically negative axilla receiving neoadjuvant systemic treatment, SLND after systemic treatment was historically reported to be less accurate. A meta-analysis of the published studies on sentinel node surgery after chemotherapy suggested that this technique is accurate; a more recent comparison showed that FNRs after chemotherapy compared favorably with FNRs observed in patients who undergo surgery first.[49] Current recommendations for patients with a clinically negative axilla who receive neoadjuvant systemic treatment with persistently negative axilla before surgery are to undergo axillary staging with SLND. If they have a positive SLN or an SLN cannot be identified upon surgery, completion ALND is currently indicated. The Alliance A011202 trial is evaluating patients with an initially clinically node-positive axilla who have a good response to neoadjuvant therapy but still have positive SLNs at surgery. Patients are randomized to completion ALND versus axillary radiation with no further surgery.

Currently, ALND remains the standard of care for patients with locally advanced breast cancer or inflammatory breast cancer; patients with a positive sentinel node who have more than three positive nodes, those who are scheduled for mastectomy, and those who will not receive WBI; and patients with clinically positive or negative nodes who have a positive SLND or TAD after neoadjuvant chemotherapy.

Axillary Reverse Mapping

Alternative or complementary procedures to the standard ALND, aiming at reducing the rate of lymphedema, have been suggested. The most well studied of these is axillary reverse mapping (ARM). This technique, developed by Klimberg and colleagues, allows for the intraoperative identification of the lymphatic drainage of the upper extremity and its preservation. During this procedure, split mapping is performed, with the surgeon injecting blue dye in the arm and isotope in the breast. This allows the surgeon to identify and preserve the blue lymphatics draining the arm, unless they carry radioactivity, signifying they also function as primary drainage of the breast, practically an SLN. In these cases, these blue nodes are resected with the ALND specimen, and their lymphatic bunch is ligated. In a 26-month median follow-up of a phase II trial of 654 patients receiving SLND or ALND with ARM, the rate of lymphedema was less than 1% and 6%, respectively.[50] When any cut lymphatics were reapproximated, the rate of lymphedema was nil for either group. Alliance 221702 is a randomized trial that will further determine the efficacy of ARM. Additional intraoperative techniques have been developed to lower the rate of lymphedema, including the lymphatic microsurgical preventive healing approach (LYMPHA), in which a microsurgical lympho-venous bypass is performed with the blue lymphatics draining the arm, or simplified-LYMPHA (S-LYMPHA), a similar nonmicrosurgical procedure.

Exclusion of Sentinel Lymphadenectomy (Sentinel Lymph Node Dissection) in T1N0 Patients Getting Up-Front Surgery

The Sentinel Node Versus Observation After Axillary Ultrasound (SOUND) study, a prospective, randomized trial, was supported by the European Institute of Oncology of Milan. It is a step forward in the conservative approach to axillary surgery.[51] The theory was that distant DFS for patients with axilla observation would not be worse than for axillary surgical staging if there were no discernible axillary lymph node metastases at the time of diagnosis. In order to rule out suspicious lymph node involvement, patients with cT1N0 breast cancer who were candidates for BCS had an axillary US. Patients underwent US-guided FNA cytology when they had a single "doubtful" (ambiguous but not suspicious) lymph node. Randomization was used to assign patients to either SLND ± ALND or no axillary surgical staging (observation) if they had either negative cytology of the solitary questionable lymph node or negative axilla ultrasonography results. Of the 1463 patients who were randomized, 697 patients in the experimental arm did not receive SLND, and 708 patients in the control arm did. Age, menopausal status, molecular subtype, tumor size and grade, biomarkers, adjuvant systemic medication, and RT were all well matched among the patients in both experimental arms. In both arms, the average tumor size was 1.2 cm. In both arms, 98% of patients received RT. Distant DFS with a median follow-up of 5.8 years was 98.0% in the observation arm and 97.7% in the SLND arm (hazard ratio [HR] 0.84, 90% CI 0.45–1.54, P = 0.024). The survival after omitting axillary surgery was not inferior to that after surgical staging in patients with cT1N0 tumors and a negative pretreatment axillary US.

TREATMENT OF DUCTAL CARCINOMA IN SITU

DCIS, or intraductal cancer, accounts for approximately 20% of all newly diagnosed breast cancers. It was anticipated that more than 51,400 new cases of DCIS would be diagnosed in 2022. Most cases of DCIS are detected during screening mammograms as an area of clustered calcifications without an associated palpable abnormality. Rarely, DCIS manifests as a palpable mass or as unilateral, single-duct nipple discharge.

Findings on mammography in patients with DCIS include clustered calcifications without an associated density in 75% of patients, calcifications coexisting with an associated density in 15%, and a density alone in 10%. The calcifications seen on a mammogram generally correspond to areas within the involved duct in which there is often necrosis and debris. DCIS calcifications tend to cluster closely together, are pleomorphic, and may be linear or branching, suggesting their ductal origin.

DCIS is viewed as a precursor to IDC, with long-term follow-up studies and modeling studies reporting progression to invasive cancer in 10% to 64% of patients. This wide range is probably due to the variability in DCIS pathology and presentation. Larger lesions, those presenting with a palpable mass, high-grade DCIS, and DCIS presenting in premenopausal patients have a higher rate of upgrading to an invasive carcinoma upon excision.

Surgery

Treatment recommendations for a patient with DCIS are based on the extent of disease within the breast, histologic grade, ER status, and presence of microinvasion as well as the patient's age and preference. Surgical options and considerations are similar to those for invasive cancer and include mastectomy, BCS with irradiation, and BCS alone, the purpose of which is to remove the lesion with negative margins. Negative margins are considered as no tumor within 2 mm of the inked resection margin.[31] Local recurrence of DCIS is approximately 1% to 2% per year when treated with BCT versus 1% to 2% lifetime when treated with mastectomy, whereas the survival rates with either treatment are the same, 98% to 99%. Reasons to choose a mastectomy versus BCS would be the same as for invasive cancer and have been discussed earlier.

Adjuvant Radiation After Breast-Conserving Surgery for Ductal Carcinoma In Situ

The use of RT after lumpectomy was investigated in four prospective randomized trials (Table 68.5), the results of which are remarkably consistent, showing a reduction of in-breast recurrence of both DCIS and invasive cancer of about 50%. In the NSABP B-17 trial, 818 females with DCIS were randomly assigned to lumpectomy alone versus lumpectomy plus 50 Gy of postoperative WBI. The addition of radiation to surgery decreased the ipsilateral recurrence rate from 35% to 19.8% (P < 0.001), as shown by 17-year actuarial recurrence data. The addition of radiation also decreased the incidence of invasive breast cancer, from 19.6% to 10.7% (P < 0.00001), and produced a smaller decrease in the incidence of in situ recurrence, from 15.4% to 9% (P < 0.001).[52] In the EORTC 10853 trial, 1010 females with DCIS were randomly assigned to lumpectomy alone versus lumpectomy plus 50 Gy of RT. Radiation reduced the 10-year breast recurrence rate from 26% to 15% (P < 0.0001) and reduced the rate of invasive recurrences from 13% to 8% (P = 0.0011).[53] The UK ANZ (United Kingdom, Australia, and New Zealand) trial, which included 1701 patients, was a large, randomized trial that simultaneously evaluated the benefits of RT and tamoxifen after BCS for patients with DCIS. This trial also demonstrated that RT reduced the risk of breast cancer recurrence (HR 0.41; P < 0.0001) and ipsilateral DCIS and invasive breast cancer recurrence (HR 0.38 and 0.32; P < 0.0001)[54] Finally, the Swedish Ductal Carcinoma in Situ (SweDCIS) trial included 1046 patients with DCIS. After a median follow-up of 20 years, the cumulative incidence of breast recurrence was 32% in the group that underwent surgery only versus 20% in the group that underwent surgery plus RT (P < 0.0001).[55] Similar findings were seen in the NRG Oncology/Radiation Therapy Oncology Group (RTOG) 9804 trial, which randomized patients with low- to intermediate-grade DCIS, 2.5 cm or smaller, with 3-mm or larger margins of excision. It showed 7.1% versus 15.1% in-breast recurrence with and without adjuvant radiation, respectively (HR 0.38; P = 0.0007) and 5.4% versus 9.5% invasive recurrence, respectively. On multivariate analysis, it showed radiation and tamoxifen to be the only variables associated with a reduced in-breast recurrence.[56]

Attempts have been made to identify subsets of DCIS for which wide excision without irradiation would provide sufficient local control. Silverstein[57] derived the Van Nuys criteria for classifying DCIS from a series of patients with DCIS treated by wide excision with and without RT. A system was proposed to identify patients who do not need RT because they have a low DCIS nuclear grade, a small lesion (<1.4 cm), older age (>60), and

TABLE 68.5 Randomized Trials of Lumpectomy for Ductal Carcinoma In Situ: Impact of Radiation Therapy and Tamoxifen

| TRIAL | NO. PATIENTS | FOLLOW-UP (YEAR) | LOCAL RECURRENCE RATES (%) | | | |
			LUMPECTOMY	LUMPECTOMY + XRT	LUMPECTOMY + XRT + TAMOXIFEN	PVALUE
NSABP B-17[a]	818	17.25	35	19.8		<0.001
EORTC 10853[b]	1010	10	26	15		<0.00001
UK ANZ[c]	1701	12.7	26	10	6	<0.0001
SweDCIS[d]	1046	20	32	20		<0.0001
NSABP B-24[a]	1804	13.6		16.6	13.2	0.025
NRG Oncology/ RTOG 9804[e,f]	636	13.9	15.1	7.1		0.0007
ECOG-ACRIN E5194[g]	665	12	14.4%—low risk 24.6%—high risk			

[a]Wapnir IL, Dignam JJ, Fisher B, et al. Long-term outcomes of invasive ipsilateral breast tumor recurrences after lumpectomy in NSABP B-17 and B-24 randomized clinical trials for DCIS. *J Natl Cancer Inst.* 2011;103(6):478-488.

[b]EORTC Breast Cancer Cooperative Group, EORTC Radiotherapy Group, Bijker N, et al. Breast-conserving treatment with or without radiotherapy in ductal carcinoma-in-situ: ten-year results of European Organisation for Research and Treatment of Cancer randomized phase III trial 10853—a study by the EORTC Breast Cancer Cooperative Group and EORTC Radiotherapy Group. *J Clin Oncol.* 2006;24(21):3381-3387.

[c]Cuzick J, Sestak I, Pinder SE, et al. Effect of tamoxifen and radiotherapy in women with locally excised ductal carcinoma in situ: long-term results from the UK/ANZ DCIS trial. *Lancet Oncol.* 2011;12(1):21-29.

[d]Wärnberg F, Garmo H, Emdin S, et al. Effect of radiotherapy after breast-conserving surgery for ductal carcinoma in situ: 20 years follow-up in the randomized SweDCIS Trial. *J Clin Oncol.* 2014;32(32):3613-3618.

[e]Inclusion criteria were tumors 2.5 cm or smaller, final margins 3 mm or more, and low-intermediate grade.

[f]McCormick B, Winter KA, Woodward W, et al. Randomized phase III trial evaluating radiation following surgical excision for good-risk ductal carcinoma in situ: long-term report from NRG Oncology/RTOG 9804. *J Clin Oncol.* 2021;39(32):3574-3582.

[g]Solin LJ, Gray R, Hughes LL, et al. Surgical excision without radiation for ductal carcinoma in situ of the breast: 12-year results from the ECOG-ACRIN E5194 Study. *J Clin Oncol.* 2015;33(33):3938-3944.

EORTC, European Organization for Research and Treatment of Cancer; *NSABP,* National Surgical Adjuvant Breast and Bowel Project; *SweDCIS,* Swedish Ductal Carcinoma In Situ trial; *UK ANZ,* United Kingdom, Australia, and New Zealand; *XRT,* radiation therapy.

wide surgical margins (>1 cm). Silverstein reported low breast recurrence rates with surgery alone for patients with favorable Van Nuys scores. However, in a prospective trial testing this approach, investigators from Harvard enrolled 158 patients from the most favorable Van Nuys subset (low-grade or intermediate-grade DCIS <2.5 cm, with a minimum 1-cm margin on excision) and were unable to reproduce the results; the Harvard investigators stopped the trial early because the rates of recurrence exceeded the predefined stopping rules. More recently, Eastern Cooperative Oncology Group (ECOG) investigators reported the result of a relatively large prospective single-arm study, ECOG-ACRIN (American College of Radiology Imaging Network) E5194, of surgery with negative margins of at least 3 mm without RT for patients with favorable subsets of DCIS. Patients with low-grade or intermediate-grade DCIS measuring 2.5 cm or smaller had 5- and 12-year rates of ipsilateral breast recurrence of 6.1% and 14.4%, respectively. In contrast, patients with high-grade disease measuring 1 cm or smaller had much higher 5- and 12-year ipsilateral breast recurrence rates of 15.3% and 24.6%, respectively.[58]

Taken together, the data from these trials of treatment for DCIS suggest that adjuvant radiation should be recommended for most patients with DCIS undergoing BCS to lower the chances for ipsilateral in-breast recurrence. The one subgroup that appears to have favorable outcomes without radiation is patients with small, low-grade, or intermediate-grade lesions. The Alliance for Clinical Trials in Oncology initiated the Comparison of Operative Versus Monitoring and Endocrine Therapy (COMET) trial in 2018 to evaluate the safety of omission of surgery in patients with low-risk DCIS. COMET is a phase III randomized trial comparing active surveillance to guideline-concordant care

(surgery, radiation, and endocrine therapy). The primary end point is to assess the ipsilateral invasive breast cancer rate at 2, 5, and 7 years. The study has completed accrual and will report on clinical outcomes and patient-reported outcomes in the near future.

Sentinel Node Dissection in Ductal Carcinoma In Situ

DCIS, by definition, represents breast cancer contained within an intact basement membrane and without access to lymphatic or vascular channels. However, when ALND was performed during mastectomy for DCIS, positive nodes were found in 3.6% of cases, as indicated by a review of more than 10,000 patients in the National Cancer Database. These positive nodes probably result from microinvasive disease in the primary tumor that was not detected on routine pathologic analysis.

Sentinel node surgery is currently recommended in patients undergoing mastectomy for DCIS because 20% to 30% of patients with DCIS on a diagnostic CNB are found to have invasive cancer on detailed evaluation of the excised specimen. The addition of sentinel node surgery to mastectomy adds minimal morbidity and avoids the need for ALND if invasive cancer is identified (sentinel node mapping has lower success rates after mastectomy). For patients undergoing BCS for DCIS, SLND may be considered for patients with a higher risk of upgrading to invasive cancer upon excision: patients with larger areas of DCIS, a palpable mass, and those with high-grade histology or with high suspicion of microinvasion.

The recent publication of the SentiNot trial offers an alternative to SLND during breast surgery in DCIS patients. In this study, patients with DCIS undergoing mastectomy or those with high-risk DCIS (mass forming, grade 3, or grade 2 and >2 cm) undergoing BCS underwent an injection of superparamagnetic iron oxide (SPIO) during breast surgery, without an SLND. The SPIO accumulated in the sentinel nodes and allowed for delayed SLND in patients whose final pathology revealed invasive disease. Of the 254 patients participating, 78.7% were able to avoid up-front SLND.[59]

Adjuvant Systemic Therapy in Ductal Carcinoma In Situ

Because the prevalence of lymphatic spread or metastatic disease in patients with DCIS without demonstrable invasion is low (<1%), systemic chemotherapy is not required. Hormonal therapy may be used for the prevention of new primary tumors and to improve local control after BCT but is generally recommended only when the DCIS is positive for ER on immunohistochemistry.

The use of tamoxifen has been shown to reduce the risk of development of new breast cancers in high-risk females, including females with a previous breast cancer (see "Chemoprevention for Breast Cancer" earlier). The NSABP B-24 protocol evaluated the benefit of tamoxifen for patients with DCIS. In this trial, 1804 females who had undergone lumpectomy and RT for DCIS were randomly assigned to 5 years of tamoxifen or placebo. Study criteria allowed enrollment of patients with positive margins, and ER was not measured. At 13 years of follow-up, the addition of tamoxifen to lumpectomy and RT decreased the incidence of ipsilateral breast cancer recurrence from 16.6% to 13.2% and reduced the risk for contralateral breast cancer by 40% (from 8.1% to 4.9%) (see Table 68.5).[52] Subsequent analyses demonstrated that the benefit from tamoxifen is seen only in females with ER-positive DCIS. Patients at highest risk for local recurrence, and most likely to benefit from tamoxifen, were patients with positive margins, comedonecrosis, a mass on physical examination, and age younger than 50 years. For individual patients, the benefits of tamoxifen are weighed against its side effects, including risk for endometrial carcinoma, thromboembolic events, hot flashes, and cataracts.

The International Breast Cancer Intervention Study II (IBIS-II) DCIS trial examined the use of anastrozole as an adjuvant treatment in patients with DCIS. It enrolled 2980 postmenopausal females who underwent an excision of a hormone receptor–positive DCIS and randomized them to 5 years of daily anastrozole or tamoxifen. After a median follow-up of 7.2 years, there were no differences between the groups in recurrence rates, mortality, or side effects.[60] The NSABP B-35 trial enrolled a similar cohort of 3083 patients and also randomized them to anastrozole or tamoxifen for 5 years. With a median follow-up of 9 years, the researchers were able to show the superiority, in terms of breast cancer–free survival, of adjuvant anastrozole over tamoxifen in postmenopausal patients younger than 60.[61] Generally speaking, adjuvant endocrine therapy can reduce the risk of breast cancer recurrence in patients with DCIS by about 50%. Nevertheless, the decision to use endocrine therapy as adjuvant treatment should take into account the type of surgery the patient received, BCS versus mastectomy, and the objective of treatment (reducing local recurrence vs. contralateral breast cancer); the patient's age and comorbidities (recurrence incidence rises with time from surgery); the characteristics and risk factors of the DCIS resected; and the specific side-effect profile and patient tolerance.

RADIATION THERAPY FOR BREAST CANCER

Adjuvant RT is offered to many breast cancer patients after surgery. This includes radiation to the breast when BCS has been performed, radiation to the nodal basins (axillary, supraclavicular, and internal mammary) in high-risk patients and those with nodal involvement, and postmastectomy radiation to the chest wall in high-risk patients undergoing mastectomy. By eradicating residual occult disease after surgery, adjuvant radiation has been shown to improve locoregional control as well as breast cancer–related mortality. To reduce morbidity associated with radiation, efforts have been made to find alternatives to the standard radiation regimens, such as hypofractionation of treatment and partial breast irradiation in place of standard whole breast radiation after BCS, and to identify subgroups of patients who can forgo adjuvant radiation.

Radiation Therapy After Breast-Conserving Surgery

For patients with invasive breast cancer treated with BCS, adjuvant irradiation of the breast has been conclusively demonstrated to reduce the probability of a breast recurrence and improve outcome. The EBCTCG published a meta-analysis of the data from 10,801 females who participated in randomized trials of BCS with or without RT. Adjuvant radiation was shown to reduce 10-year local and distant recurrence rates by 15.4% in node-negative patients (from 31% to 15.6%, $P = 0.00005$) and by 21.2% in node-positive patients (from 63.7% to 42.5%, $P < 0.00001$). The 15-year breast cancer deaths were reduced by 3.3% (from 20.5% to 17.2%, $P = 0.005$) and 8.5% (from 51.3% to 42.8%, $P = 0.01$), respectively. These recurrence and mortality benefits were found to vary depending on the patient's age, the grade and hormonal status of the primary tumor, the extent of surgery, and endocrine therapy use, with minimal reduction in breast cancer–related deaths in patients with low- to intermediate-risk characteristics.[62] Based on these data, RT after BCS is considered as a standard. Adding nodal radiation to breast radiation in node-positive and high-risk node-negative patients has also been shown to reduce the risk of local recurrence as well as breast cancer–related and overall mortality and has increased in popularity with the deescalation in axillary surgery.[63]

Most trials attempting to define subgroups of patients who could potentially avoid radiation after lumpectomy have been unsuccessful. The only group identified that might be able to avoid irradiation safely is patients older than 70 years who undergo lumpectomy and adjuvant hormonal therapy for stage I ER-positive breast cancer. In Cancer and Leukemia Group B (CALGB) 9343, OS rates at 10 years were similar with or without radiation (67% and 66%, respectively). Nevertheless, 98% of patients receiving tamoxifen and WBI, compared with 90% of those receiving tamoxifen alone, were free from local and regional recurrences.[64] The Post-Operative Radiotherapy in Minimum-Risk Elderly (PRIME-II) trial similarly found improved local control but no benefit as far as OS, distant recurrence, regional recurrence, or breast cancer–specific survival in a similar cohort of 1326 females 65 years or older with 3-cm or smaller hormone receptor–positive tumors undergoing BCS and randomized to WBI or no radiation.[65]

Historically, RT after lumpectomy has consisted of a 5- to 8-week treatment course, which can be a hardship for patients. An important Canadian trial successfully compared this historical schedule (of 50.0 Gy in 25 fractions over 35 days) with a more abbreviated WBI schedule (42.5 Gy in 16 fractions over 22 days).[66] Based on long-term outcome results from this and similar studies showing equivalent local recurrence rates as well as cosmetic outcomes, the 3-week hypofractionated scheme became the preferred adjuvant radiation regimen after BCS in patients with negative margins and negative nodes. There has also been significant interest in shortening the treatment course to 1 week, with the Faster Radiotherapy for Breast Cancer (FAST)-Forward trial demonstrating noninferiority of a 1-week regimen of 26 Gy in five sessions compared with the 3-week regimen regarding local recurrence and effect on normal tissue in 5 years.[67] Long-term follow-up of this ultrafast hypofractionation schedule is still pending.

An additional approach to deescalate and decrease the burden of adjuvant radiation is limiting the radiation field by focusing the radiation exclusively on the area around the tumor bed. This approach, called *partial breast irradiation* (PBI), may be performed with brachytherapy catheters, balloon catheters, intraoperative radiation, or external-beam radiation. The NRG (NSABP B-39/RTOG 0413) trial randomly assigned 4216 females who had recently undergone lumpectomy to receive either WBI or accelerated PBI. Females enrolled in the study could have up to three positive axillary nodes. Twenty-five percent of the group had DCIS, 65% had stage I breast cancer, and 10% had stage II disease. The majority of females also had hormone receptor–positive tumors. Females who were assigned to the WBI arm after adjuvant chemotherapy received daily treatment with 2.0 Gy/fraction of radiation totaling 50 Gy with a sequential boost to the surgical site. Those assigned to accelerated PBI before adjuvant chemotherapy received a total of 10 treatments given twice daily, with 3.4 to 3.85 Gy given as either brachytherapy or 3D external-beam radiation. The 10-year cumulative incidence of ipsilateral breast tumor recurrence was very low in both groups, at 4.6% for patients in the accelerated PBI arm versus 3.9% for those in the

WBI arm, but did not meet equivalence. There were no differences in distant DFS, OS, or DFS.[68] ASTRO published a consensus statement highlighting appropriate selection criteria that should be considered if patients are to be treated with PBI outside the context of a clinical trial (Table 68.6).[69] Most would suggest that accelerated PBI would be suitable for older patients with low-risk DCIS or those with T1 invasive cancer excised with clear margins, hormone-positive tumors, and node-negative disease.

Postmastectomy Radiation Therapy

For patients with T1N0 or T2N0 breast cancer, mastectomy and SLND provide effective local control, and RT is not required. In contrast, patients with stage III breast cancer have high rates of locoregional recurrence after treatment with a modified radical mastectomy and adjuvant or neoadjuvant chemotherapy. Clinical trial data indicate that postmastectomy RT (PMRT), including radiation to the chest wall and the axillary, infraclavicular, supraclavicular, and internal mammary nodal basins, can significantly improve the outcome of patients who would be expected to have a 20% to 40% risk of locoregional recurrence without RT.

Three prospective randomized trials addressed the role of PMRT. In the Danish Breast Cancer Cooperative Group Trials, premenopausal females with stage II or III breast cancer were randomly assigned to chemotherapy alone or chemotherapy plus chest wall and nodal irradiation (protocol 82b); postmenopausal females were randomly assigned to tamoxifen alone or tamoxifen plus RT (protocol 82c).[70] Most patients had node-positive

TABLE 68.6   **American Society for Radiation Oncology Guidelines for Accelerated Partial Breast Irradiation**

FACTOR	"SUITABLE" GROUP	"CAUTIONARY" GROUP	"UNSUITABLE" GROUP
Patient Factors			
Age (years)	≥50	40–49	<40
Tumor Factors			
Tumor size (cm)	≤2	2.1–3.0	>3
T stage	Tis or T1	T0 or T2	T3 or T4
Margins	Negative by at least 2 mm	Close (<2 mm)	Positive
Histology	Invasive ductal carcinoma or other favorable subtypes	Invasive lobular carcinoma	NA
Pure DCIS	When: screen-detected grade 1–2 2.5 cm or smaller Resected with 3-mm or larger margins	≤3 cm and does not meet suitability criteria	>3 cm
Grade	Any	NA	NA
LVI	None	Limited/focal	Extensive
ER status	Positive	Negative	NA
Multicentricity	Unicentric	NA	If present
Multifocality	Clinically unifocal with total size ≤2 cm	Clinically unifocal with total size 2.1–3 cm, microscopic multifocality allowed	Clinically multifocal or microscopically multifocal >3 cm
Nodal factors			
N stage	pN0	NA	pN1–3
Treatment factors			
Neoadjuvant chemotherapy	Not allowed	NA	If used

DCIS, Ductal carcinoma in situ; *ER*, estrogen receptor; *LVI*, lymphovascular invasion; *NA*, not available.
Adapted from Correa C, Harris EE, Leonardi MC, et al. Accelerated partial breast irradiation: executive summary for the update of an ASTRO evidence-based consensus statement. *Pract Radiat Oncol.* 2017;7(2):73-79; Smith BD, Arthur DW, Buchholz TA, et al. Accelerated partial breast irradiation consensus statement from the American Society for Radiation Oncology (ASTRO). *J Am Coll Surg.* 2009;209:269.

disease, but some high-risk node-negative patients with T3 or T4 tumors were included. In the British Columbia study, premenopausal females with node-positive breast cancer were randomly assigned to chemotherapy alone or chemotherapy plus chest wall and nodal irradiation.[71] In addition to reducing locoregional recurrences, as expected, PMRT significantly improved distant recurrence rates and OS in all three trials.

In 2005, the EBCTCG published the results of a meta-analysis of trials of PMRT, which included data from 9933 patients treated with mastectomy and axillary clearance with or without PMRT. PMRT decreased the 5-year isolated locoregional recurrence rate for patients with lymph node–positive disease from 23% to 6% and reduced the 15-year breast cancer mortality rate from 60.1% to 54.7% ($P = 0.0002$). The most recent analysis from this group, which included 8135 females, suggested that benefits of PMRT were not seen in patients with node-negative disease but were significant in patients with one to three positive lymph nodes and patients with four or more positive lymph nodes regarding local control and breast cancer–specific mortality.[72]

There is consensus that patients with four or more positive lymph nodes or other features characteristic of stage III disease should be counseled to undergo RT. However, the use of PMRT for patients with stage II disease is controversial because many US series have reported that locoregional recurrence rates after standard modified radical mastectomy and adjuvant chemotherapy are only 12% to 15%, much lower than rates reported in the clinical trials of PMRT and the EBCTCG meta-analysis. Based on this disparity, it is reasonable to consider PMRT only for selected patients with stage II disease, such as patients with nodal metastasis with extracapsular extension, LVI, age 40 years or younger, close/positive surgical margins, or a nodal positivity ratio (ratio of positive nodes to total nodes examined) of 20% or greater and patients who have undergone less than a standard level I or II axillary dissection.

With improved systemic treatments and high pCR rates to neoadjuvant therapy, investigations into the deescalation of treatment based on response to neoadjuvant treatment are ongoing. The NRG Oncology/NSABP B-51/RTOG 1304 trial is questioning the need for regional nodal irradiation in cases of complete response in the nodal basin to neoadjuvant systemic therapy. The Alliance A011202 trial is questioning the need for both axillary surgery and radiation in patients with residual disease in the nodal basin based on sentinel node dissection after neoadjuvant systemic treatment, randomizing patients to ALND with nodal basin (infra/supraclavicular and internal mammary) irradiation or to radiation to the axilla and regional nodal basins without an ALND.

SYSTEMIC THERAPY FOR BREAST CANCER

Despite advances in locoregional therapy, a significant proportion of females with breast cancer develop metastatic disease within 5 to 10 years after diagnosis. Most patients who develop metastatic breast cancer die of their disease. Metastatic disease is the principal cause of death from breast cancer.

Systemic therapy in patients with resectable disease is used to treat and prevent the recurrence of microscopic metastatic breast cancer. For females with stage IV breast cancer, systemic therapy is given to palliate symptoms from cancer and potentially prolong survival. Current thinking is that metastasis occurs early in the progression of breast cancer, probably before initial clinical evaluation in most patients. This concept argues for the administration of systemic therapy in concert with local treatment. What is missing

at present is the ability to detect occult metastatic disease accurately in order to select appropriate patients to receive systemic treatment.

The first prospective trials of systemic therapy for breast cancer combined oophorectomy, to deprive patients of estrogen, with radical mastectomy. Since these early trials, hundreds of prospective studies of systemic therapy have been conducted involving thousands of females. Medications used to treat early breast cancer have their foundation in the treatment of advanced disease. In general, treatments that are used effectively to improve outcomes for patients with incurable breast cancer are estimated to have an increased impact on outcomes for patients with earlier stages of breast cancer, who have smaller volumes of disease and potentially less resistance to therapy. When medications are identified that improve outcomes for patients with stage IV breast cancer, they are often brought forward into clinical studies for earlier stages of the disease.

Goals of Therapy and Assessment of Potential Benefits and Risks From Therapy

For patients with stage I to III invasive breast cancer, the goal of treatment is cure. In selecting treatment, the potential benefits of therapy (reduction in the risk of recurrence) are considered together with the potential harms of treatment. Patient preferences, particularly preferences regarding adjuvant therapy, are carefully considered. Some patients believe that the reduction in risk of recurrence with adjuvant therapy is not worth the adverse effects of the therapy, particularly in the case of chemotherapy. Often, several long discussions with the patient are essential to determine the treatment that best suits that patient.

The risk of systemic recurrence increases with increasing stages of the disease. The biologic characteristics of an individual tumor also influence the risk of systemic recurrence. The most commonly used breast cancer biomarkers—ER, PR, and HER2—not only affect prognosis but also predict response to different systemic therapies. In general terms, tumors that have no ER or PR expression and tumors with high levels of HER2 are associated with worse cancer outcomes than tumors that are strongly positive for ER and PR and have negative or normal levels of HER2. For most patients, the risk of recurrence is estimated using population-based statistics. Current federal and international guidelines use stage and biologic characteristics in the development of treatment recommendations to guide decisions regarding systemic therapy for breast cancer (Fig. 68.15).

Multigene assays, such as the 21-gene RS assay, have been developed in an attempt to identify a specific molecular phenotype of a tumor in an individual patient and use the phenotype to predict the response to therapy or provide information regarding prognosis. The Oncotype DX assay was developed from a candidate pool of 250 genes and narrowed to a specific 21-gene panel based on three independent studies of the candidate genes. This assay was validated first in patients with ER-positive, lymph node–negative breast cancer (NSABP B-14). The Oncotype DX assay was found to be prognostic for OS and predictive of the benefits of systemic therapy, with higher recurrence scores predicting increased benefit from chemotherapy and lower scores predicting lesser benefit from chemotherapy and increased benefit from endocrine therapy. This assay has also been validated in subsequent studies. The Oncotype DX assay can help clinicians estimate the benefits of therapy for patients with ER-positive breast cancer and zero to three positive lymph nodes. For patients with low recurrence scores, chemotherapy appears to have

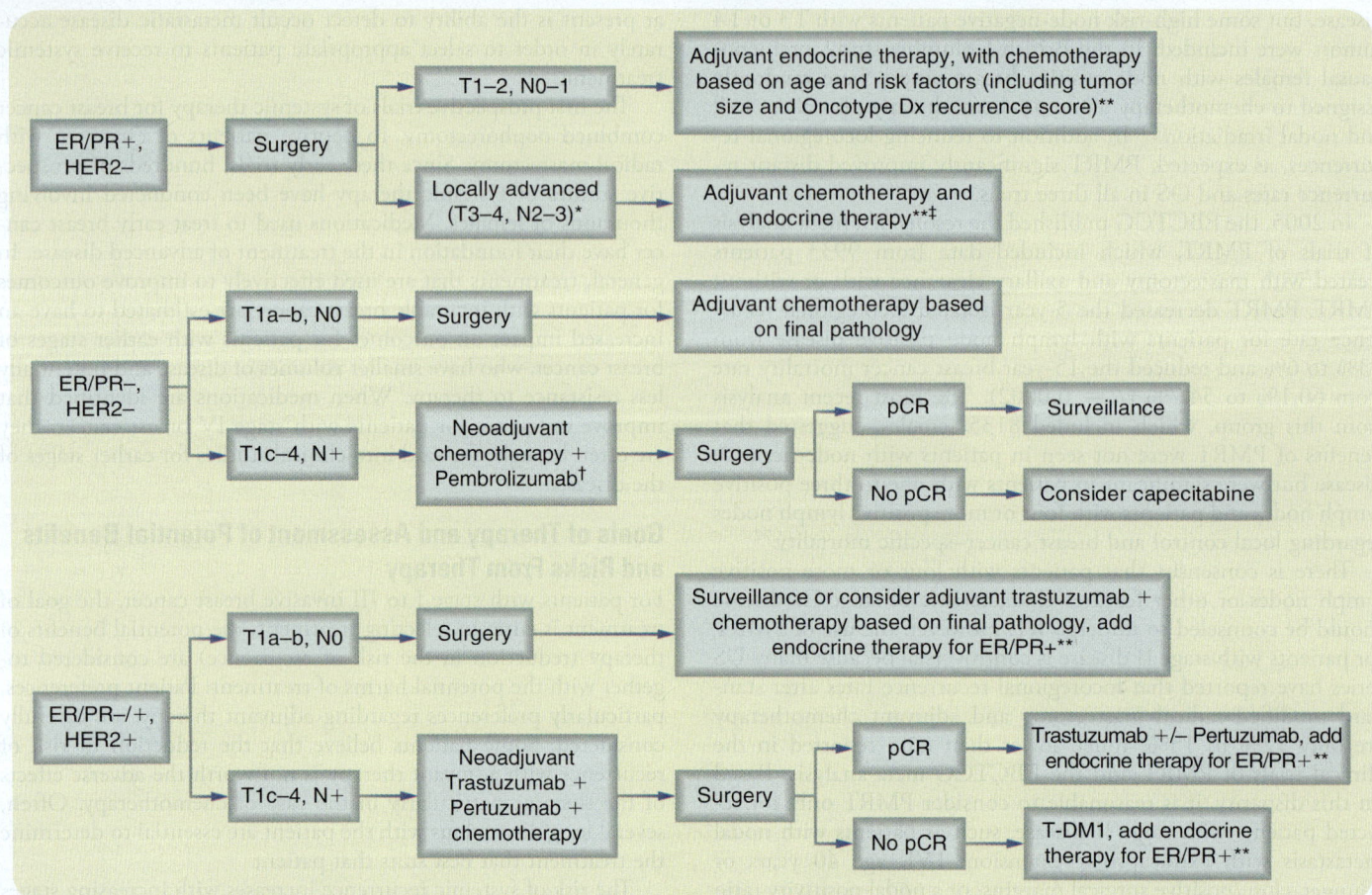

FIGURE 68.15 Systemic treatment schema for locoregional operable breast cancer. This is a general schema for systemic treatment choices divided by hormonal status of tumors. There are many nuances in deciding on systemic treatment for patients with breast cancer, which are beyond the scope of this chapter. This schema provides general principles, and each patient should be discussed in a multidisciplinary setting to decide on the recommended systemic treatment as well as the sequence of treatment modalities (surgery, radiation, reconstruction, and systemic treatment). *A neoadjuvant systemic approach can be considered for high-risk or locally advanced patients. **GnRH/LHRH analogues can be considered for premenopausal patients. †Pembrolizumab is continued in the adjuvant setting. ‡Consider CDK4/6 inhibitors in high-risk patients.

marginal benefit in terms of reducing the risk of distant recurrence, but for patients with high recurrence scores, chemotherapy offers significant benefit. A cooperative group trial, the Trial Assigning Individualized Options for Treatment (Rx) (TAILORx), was conducted to determine the benefit of chemotherapy in patients with intermediate recurrence scores. This trial included 9719 females with hormone receptor–positive, HER2-negative, axillary node–negative breast cancer.[73] Patients with recurrence scores less than 11 received endocrine therapy alone. Patients with recurrence scores greater than 25 received chemotherapy followed by endocrine therapy. There were 6711 patients who had intermediate recurrence scores of 11 to 25 and were randomly assigned to receive either chemotherapy followed by endocrine therapy or endocrine therapy alone. Endocrine therapy alone was noninferior to chemotherapy followed by endocrine therapy in the analysis of invasive DFS, invasive disease recurrence, second primary cancer, and OS at 9 years of follow-up. Some benefit of chemotherapy was found in females 50 years of age or younger with a recurrence score of 16 to 25. Therefore, chemotherapy is not recommended for patients with hormone receptor–positive, HER2-negative, and node-negative disease and recurrence scores

of less than 25 for females over 50 years of age or recurrence scores of less than 16 for those under 50 years of age. The Rx for Positive Node, Endocrine Responsive Breast Cancer (RxPONDER) trial was conducted to determine the benefit of chemotherapy in patients with one to three positive nodes and a low-intermediate recurrence score. In this trial, 5018 patients with hormone receptor–positive and HER2-negative breast cancer, one to three positive axillary nodes, and a recurrence score of 25 or lower were randomized to chemotherapy followed by endocrine therapy or endocrine therapy alone. Postmenopausal patients were not found to benefit from the addition of chemotherapy to endocrine therapy, with similar 5-year invasive DFS, new primary cancer rates, and OS, whereas premenopausal females showed a 5-year invasive DFS benefit from chemotherapy followed by endocrine therapy (93.9%) compared with endocrine therapy alone (89%; HR 0.6; $P = 0.002$), with a similar benefit in distant relapse-free survival.[74]

Chemotherapy

The main classes of chemotherapeutics used to treat early-stage breast cancer include anthracyclines (e.g., doxorubicin, epirubicin) and taxanes (e.g., paclitaxel, docetaxel). The anthracyclines, which act as topoisomerase II inhibitors and antimetabolites, have high levels of activity in the treatment of breast cancer. When anthracyclines are delivered as single agents for the treatment of metastatic breast cancer, responses to therapy are generally seen in 45% to 80% of patients. The 2005 EBCTCG analysis noted that compared with nonanthracycline, cyclophosphamide, methotrexate, 5-fluorouracil (CMF)-type therapies, anthracyclines are associated with a 16% reduction in the risk of death and an 11% reduction in the risk of recurrence.[75] Anthracyclines are associated with the potential long-term toxic effect of cardiomyopathy, which may lead to congestive heart failure, often many years after treatment. The risk of cardiac dysfunction resulting from anthracyclines is dose dependent, and current anthracycline-containing chemotherapy regimens are associated with a risk of cardiac dysfunction of 1.5% to 3%. An additional risk of anthracycline-based chemotherapy is the risk of developing leukemia (<1%).

Taxanes (microtubule inhibitors) have significant activity in the treatment of metastatic breast cancer and are active not only in tumors without exposure to chemotherapy but also in anthracycline-resistant tumors. Numerous clinical trials have evaluated the use of taxanes for the treatment of early-stage breast cancer. A meta-analysis of the use of taxanes in 13 different studies from the Intergroup Trial C9741/Cancer and Leukemia Group B (CALGB) trial 9741 found improvement in DFS (HR 0.83; 95% CI 0.79–0.87; $P <$ 0.0001) and OS (HR 0.85; 95% CI 0.79–0.91; $P <$ 0.0001). The antitumor activity of paclitaxel depends on the timing of treatment: more frequent administration of paclitaxel (weekly compared with every 3 weeks) improves outcomes. The activity of docetaxel depends less on the timing of treatment, and docetaxel is generally administered on an every-3-week schedule. The two taxanes, when given at their optimal dose and schedule, produce equivalent outcomes. The taxanes are associated with the potential permanent toxic effect of peripheral neuropathy but do not cause a long-term increased risk of cardiac dysfunction or second cancers.

Chemotherapy is generally administered with combinations of medications to take advantage of nonoverlapping toxic effects and to maximize different mechanisms of action in targeting tumor cells. The largest comprehensive analysis to date of the benefits of polychemotherapy for breast cancer is the EBCTCG analysis published in 2012. This analysis summarized data from randomized trials that were initiated between 1973 and 2003. The authors presented individual patient data from trials comparing a taxane-plus-anthracycline–based regimen versus a non–taxane-containing regimen with the same or higher cumulative doses of each non taxane component ($n = 44,000$), trials comparing one anthracycline-based regimen versus another ($n = 7000$) or versus CMF ($n = 18,000$), and trials comparing polychemotherapy versus no chemotherapy ($n = 32,000$).[76] Based on the drug dosages and the anthracycline used (either doxorubicin [Adriamycin; A] or epirubicin [E]), regimens were defined as including standard CMF, standard Adriamycin/Cytoxan (AC), Cytoxan/Adriamycin/fluorouracil (CAF), or Cytoxan/epirubicin/fluorouracil (CEF). The meta-analysis showed that compared with no chemotherapy, the use of CMF or standard AC reduced the recurrence rate by one-third at 8 years and produced a 20% to 25% reduction in breast cancer mortality. The addition of more chemotherapy (i.e., CAF or CEF compared with CMF or AC) resulted in an additional proportional reduction of 15% to 20% in breast cancer mortality. On average, the taxane-plus-anthracycline–based control regimens were superior to standard AC but were not superior to anthracycline regimens with extra cycles (i.e., CAF or CEF). In analyses comparing taxane-based and anthracycline-based

regimens, the proportional risk reductions were not significantly affected by age, tumor size, nodal status, tumor grade, or ER status. Taken together, these data suggest that independent of age or tumor characteristics, a chemotherapy regimen that includes a taxane or anthracycline regimens with higher cumulative dosages reduced breast cancer mortality by approximately one-third. Recent evidence, including pooled analyses from the PlanB and Simultaneous Study of Docetaxel Based Anthracycline Free Adjuvant Treatment Evaluation (SUCCESS) C phase III trials, demonstrates that docetaxel/cyclophosphamide (TC)-based adjuvant therapy can safely replace anthracycline-containing regimens in many early HER2-negative breast cancer patients.[77]

Human Epidermal Growth Factor Receptor 2–Based Targeted Therapy

HER2 gene amplification or protein overexpression occurs in approximately 20% to 25% of breast cancers. Amplification leads to protein overexpression, measured clinically by immunohistochemistry and scored on a scale from 0 to 3+. Alternatively, fluorescence ISH directly detects the quantity of HER2 gene copies; the normal copy number is 2 (see "Molecular Markers" earlier).

Trastuzumab is a humanized monoclonal antibody developed to target the extracellular domain of the HER2 receptor. When trastuzumab is used as a single agent for the treatment of metastatic breast cancer, response is seen in approximately 30% of patients. Trastuzumab combined with chemotherapy is even more effective, with synergy seen with multiple agents. Trastuzumab-based chemotherapy regimens improve PFS and OS for patients with metastatic disease. Given the promising activity of trastuzumab against metastatic disease, numerous trials of trastuzumab for adjuvant and neoadjuvant therapy have been conducted; these trials demonstrated improved outcomes for patients with stage I to III breast cancer. The Herceptin Adjuvant (HERA) trial ($N = 5090$) enrolled patients with HER2-positive breast cancer and randomly assigned them to trastuzumab treatment (for 1 or 2 years) versus observation after completion of chemotherapy. In a comparison of 1-year of trastuzumab treatment versus observation, trastuzumab reduced the risk of a breast cancer–related event by 46% (HR 0.54; 95% CI 0.43–0.67; $P <$ 0.001) and improved OS by 34% (HR 0.66; 95% CI 0.47–0.91; $P <$ 0.0115). Treatment with trastuzumab for 2 years was not more effective than 1 year of treatment, and 6 months was inferior, which established 1 year of treatment as the standard of care.

Long-term follow-up of the NSABP B-31 and NCCTG-N9831 adjuvant trials, which were similar in study design, demonstrated that the initial benefit seen with adjuvant trastuzumab persisted, with an improvement in 10-year OS from 75.2% to 84%.[78] Patients receiving trastuzumab-based therapy in NSABP B-31 (AC followed by paclitaxel-trastuzumab) had an increased risk of cardiac dysfunction, with a 3-year event rate of 4.1% versus 0.8% in the control arm. Patients with lower ejection fraction at the initiation of therapy, older age, or hypertension were at the highest risk of cardiac dysfunction.

The Breast Cancer International Research Group (BCIRG) 006 trial used a non–anthracycline-containing regimen as one of its treatment groups and showed equivalence in outcome between AC followed by docetaxel-trastuzumab (AC-TH) and docetaxel combined with carboplatin and trastuzumab (TCH).[79] Both trastuzumab-containing treatments were superior in terms of DFS to the control treatment of AC followed by docetaxel, with an HR of 0.61 (95% CI 0.48–0.76; $P <$ 0.001) for the AC-TH group and an HR of 0.67 for the TCH group (95% CI

0.54–0.83). Rates of cardiac toxicity were markedly lower in the TCH group (0.37%) compared with the AC-TH group (1.87%).

Pertuzumab is another humanized monoclonal antibody designed to target the extracellular HER2 dimerization domain, binding to a different epitope than trastuzumab. The addition of pertuzumab to adjuvant chemotherapy with trastuzumab in node-positive or high-risk node-negative patients has been shown in the Adjuvant Perjeta and Herceptin in Initial Therapy in Breast Cancer (APHINITY) trial to improve 3-year DFS. The NeoSphere trial randomized patients to neoadjuvant trastuzumab and pertuzumab with or without single-agent docetaxel, trastuzumab with docetaxel, and pertuzumab with docetaxel, with postoperative anthracycline-based adjuvant chemotherapy for all arms and docetaxel added to those randomized to the trastuzumab and pertuzumab-only arm. Patients receiving docetaxel with pertuzumab and trastuzumab (THP) had the highest pCR rate (46%) compared with the other three arms (17%–29%), with equivalent rates of adverse events, apart from higher rates of diarrhea. The TRYPHAENA trial randomized 225 patients with HER2-positive tumors 2 cm or larger with or positive nodes with a 1:1:1 ratio to docetaxel, carboplatin, trastuzumab, and pertuzumab (TCHP); 5-fluorouracil, epirubicin, cyclophosphamide (FEC), trastuzumab and pertuzumab followed by docetaxel, trastuzumab and pertuzumab (THP); or FEC followed by THP. pCR rates were highest in the TCHP group (64%), with 55% and 56% pCR in the FEC-THP–containing groups.[80] The findings of these trials have established the use of trastuzumab and pertuzumab with chemotherapy in the neoadjuvant setting for patients with HER2-positive tumors that are 2 cm or larger or with positive nodal disease as the standard of care. For patients with smaller tumors, treatment would usually start with surgery, with chemotherapy and trastuzumab, with or without pertuzumab, in the adjuvant setting based on final pathology.[81]

Patients with a pCR after neoadjuvant systemic treatment have been shown to have improved prognosis compared with those who do not experience a pCR. The response to treatment also allows identification of higher-risk patients based on residual disease after neoadjuvant therapy, and their adjuvant treatment can thus be tailored accordingly. Patients who experience a pCR would generally continue adjuvant trastuzumab with or without pertuzumab for a year. Those who do not experience a pCR have an indication for adjuvant ado-trastuzumab emtansine (T-DM1) for 14 cycles. T-DM1 is an antibody-drug conjugate of trastuzumab and the cytotoxic agent emtansine, a microtubule inhibitor. The KATHERINE trial randomized 1486 patients with residual HER2-positive tumors (either primary or nodal) after neoadjuvant treatment containing taxanes and trastuzumab to receive adjuvant trastuzumab or T-DM1. Adjuvant T-DM1 was shown to reduce the risk of breast cancer recurrence or death by 50%, with a 3-year RFS of 88.3% in the T-DM1 group and 77.0% in the trastuzumab group.

Additional drugs targeting HER2 in combination with trastuzumab are being evaluated, including the tyrosine kinase inhibitors (TKIs) lapatinib, neratinib, pyrotinib, and tucatinib. Neratinib after adjuvant treatment with trastuzumab has been shown in the ExteNET trial to improve RFS rates, especially in patients with HER2-positive and hormone receptor–positive tumors and patients with high-risk larger tumors, although at the cost of a higher rate of adverse events. Adding lapatinib to trastuzumab in the neoadjuvant setting has been shown to improve pCR and possibly improve RFS and OS, but this comes at a price of increased grade 3 or higher adverse events. To date, the TKIs are used more frequently in the metastatic setting.

Endocrine Therapy

One of the original targeted therapy approaches in breast cancer was the use of oophorectomy to reduce systemic estrogen production. Most breast cancers (>70%) express ER or PR or both; interruption of the production of estrogen or the ability of estrogen to interact with the ER has been associated with improved DFS and OS for females with metastatic breast cancer. This therapeutic approach is associated with a generally favorable adverse-effect profile compared with the adverse effects of chemotherapy.

Tamoxifen

Tamoxifen is a selective ER modulator that has antagonistic and weak agonistic effects. It is generally well tolerated; the most common side effect is hot flashes or vasomotor symptoms, which occur in less than 50% of patients. Potentially serious but rare effects include an increased risk of thromboembolic events and uterine cancer, in addition to increased cataract formation in older patients.

Clinical trials of tamoxifen as treatment for early-stage breast cancer began in the 1970s. In 2005, the EBCTCG meta-analysis reported data on more than 80,000 females treated in clinical trials. Tamoxifen administered for 5 years was found to reduce the risk of recurrence of breast cancer for patients with hormone receptor–positive disease by 41% (recurrence rate ratio 0.59; standard error [SE] 0.03). The risk of death from breast cancer was reduced by approximately one-third (death rate ratio 0.66; SE 0.04). Tamoxifen was shown to be beneficial for premenopausal and postmenopausal females and had a similar magnitude of benefit for patients with lymph node–positive and lymph node–negative disease. The duration of therapy with tamoxifen was also evaluated; 5 years of therapy was found to be superior to only 1 to 2 years of therapy in terms of breast cancer recurrence (15.2% proportionate reduction; $P < 0.001$) and death from breast cancer (7.9% proportionate reduction; $P = 0.01$).

Tamoxifen therapy for more than 5 years has been investigated, and results from the two largest studies with the longest follow-up were recently reported. The Adjuvant Tamoxifen: Longer Against Shorter (ATLAS) trial showed an approximately 25% reduction in the rate of recurrence and approximately 3% reduction in mortality risk in females taking 10 years of tamoxifen versus 5 years, with the benefit being most pronounced after year 10.[82] These findings were confirmed in the Adjuvant Tamoxifen-to Offer More (aT-Tom) trial, in which patients were also randomly assigned to 5 years versus 10 years of tamoxifen. There was a decrease in breast cancer recurrence rates and breast cancer mortality rates in patients treated for a longer duration. In light of these findings, ASCO recently updated its guidelines regarding adjuvant endocrine therapy. For premenopausal or perimenopausal females, tamoxifen for 5 years is recommended. After 5 years, if the patient is still premenopausal, she should be offered an additional 5 years of tamoxifen therapy, and if proven to be postmenopausal, she should be offered an additional 5 years of tamoxifen or an AI.[83]

Aromatase Inhibitors

AIs block the conversion of the hormone androstenedione into estrone by inhibition of the aromatase enzyme. This enzyme is present in adipose tissue, breast tissue, breast tumor cells, and other sites. Multiple generations of medications that block the aromatase enzyme have been evaluated; less specific agents, such as aminoglutethimide, also suppress the production of other hormones, and this is associated with unacceptable side effects. Selective or third-generation AIs purely block the final step of conversion of hormones into estrogen and are not associated with the broad hormone suppression seen with earlier AIs. Selective AIs, which include the nonsteroidal AIs anastrozole and letrozole and the steroidal AI exemestane, are unable to suppress ovarian function completely in a premenopausal or perimenopausal female and are used only in postmenopausal females. Selective AIs as a group have similar adverse effects, including hot flashes, vasomotor symptoms, joint symptoms, myalgias, bone loss, and vaginal dryness.

Several different trial designs have been used to evaluate AIs as adjuvant therapy. Direct comparisons of 5 years of a selective AI versus 5 years of tamoxifen demonstrated improvement in cancer outcomes for anastrozole and letrozole. The Arimidex, Tamoxifen, Alone or in Combination (ATAC) trial demonstrated that 5 years of anastrozole significantly improved DFS by 17% compared with 5 years of tamoxifen (HR 0.83; 95% CI 0.73–94; $P = 0.05$). In addition to reducing the risk of distant recurrence (distant DFS HR 0.86; 95% CI 0.74–0.99; $P = 0.04$), anastrozole reduced the risk of development of contralateral breast cancers by 42%.[84] The EBCTCG meta-analysis showed similar findings, with 5 years of AI reducing breast cancer–related mortality rates by about 15% compared with 5 years of tamoxifen.[85]

Administration of selective AIs for 2 to 3 years after tamoxifen for 2 to 3 years has been compared with 5 years of tamoxifen treatment. The use of all three modern AIs after 2 to 3 years of tamoxifen was associated with better cancer outcomes than the use of tamoxifen alone, with equivalent results to 5 years of AIs.[86,87] In addition, trials examining extended adjuvant therapy with AIs up to 10 years, after 5 years of tamoxifen or AIs, show either no DFS benefit or only a modest benefit and suggest more pronounced benefit for patients with high-risk disease.[88] As a result, the recent ASCO guidelines recommend extended AI therapy for up to 10 years for postmenopausal patients with node-positive, hormone receptor–positive breast cancer. For those with node-negative disease, extended AI therapy can be considered based on risk factors and is not recommended for patients with low-risk node-negative disease.[83]

Ovarian Ablation

The EBCTCG meta-analysis evaluated premenopausal females who were treated with ovarian ablation or suppression and found that this treatment reduced the risk of relapse and death from breast cancer.[75] Compared with the use of CMF chemotherapy, the use of ovarian ablation with goserelin as a treatment for lymph node–positive, stage II breast cancer in premenopausal females resulted in equivalent outcomes in terms of DFS (HR 1.01; $P = 0.94$) and OS (HR 0.99; $P = 0.94$). Even with this high level of activity, the optimal role for the addition of ovarian ablation is unknown.

Results were reported from two phase III trials that evaluated the use of an AI with ovarian suppression in premenopausal patients with hormone receptor–positive early breast cancer. These trials were the Tamoxifen and Exemestane Trial (TEXT) and the Suppression of Ovarian Function Trial (SOFT).[89] TEXT was designed to evaluate 5 years of the AI exemestane plus ovarian suppression with a gonadotropin-releasing hormone agonist versus tamoxifen plus a gonadotropin-releasing hormone agonist. SOFT was designed to evaluate 5 years of exemestane plus ovarian suppression versus tamoxifen plus ovarian suppression versus tamoxifen alone. The addition of ovarian suppression to either tamoxifen or exemestane showed a benefit in 8-year DFS and OS rates, with improved recurrence rates in patients treated with exemestane and ovarian suppression. As a result, females with

hormone receptor–positive high-risk breast cancer with an indication for systemic chemotherapy are recommended to receive ovarian suppression together with their adjuvant endocrine therapy.[90] Starting ovarian suppression 2 weeks before the first chemotherapy dose can help preserve ovarian function in younger females, regardless of the tumor's hormonal status.

Additional Systemic Therapy Options

Cyclin-dependent kinase (CDK) inhibitors, selective to CDK4 and 6, block the retinoblastoma tumor suppressor protein phosphorylation and prevent progression through the cell cycle. Palbociclib, abemaciclib, and ribociclib have been shown to improve progression-free survival (PFS) and OS in the metastatic setting. In the adjuvant setting, several studies (Palbociclib Collaborative Adjuvant Study [PALLAS] and PENELOPE-B) have failed to show a benefit for palbociclib. In contrast, adding abemaciclib to endocrine therapy in the adjuvant setting in the MonarchE trial has been shown to improve DFS and distant recurrence-free survival (RFS) in patients with high-risk hormone receptor–positive, HER2-negative breast cancer and was subsequently approved in this patient population by the FDA. High-risk was defined as four or more positive nodes or one to three positive nodes with one of the following risk factors: grade 3 tumors, tumor size 5 cm or larger, or Ki-67 of 20% or higher.[91] Similar preliminary results were seen in the New Adjuvant Trial With Ribociclib (NATALEE) trial, which randomized patients to adjuvant endocrine therapy with or without ribociclib.

A recent addition to chemotherapy regimens for patients with TNBC includes the anti–programmed cell death 1 (PD-1) antibody pembrolizumab. The addition of pembrolizumab to paclitaxel and carboplatin followed by doxorubicin or epirubicin and cyclophosphamide in the neoadjuvant setting has been shown in the KEYNOTE-522 trial to increase pCR rates from 51% to 65%, independent of programmed cell death ligand 1 (PD-L1) status.[92] Pembrolizumab since has been approved in the neoadjuvant setting for high-risk (stage II and III) TNBC, with continuation of treatment in the adjuvant setting. The addition of atezolizumab to nab-paclitaxel followed by AC in the Impassion031 trial showed similar results, with increased pCR from 41% to 58%.[93] Its use has not yet been incorporated into the care of breast cancer patients.

The PARP inhibitor olaparib is indicated in the adjuvant setting for patients with HER2-negative disease and a *BRCA1/2* mutation. It was shown in the OlympiA trial, when given for 1 year after standard neoadjuvant/adjuvant chemotherapy, to improve 4-year invasive DFS (82.7% with olaparib vs. 75.4% with placebo) as well as OS and distant DFS.[94] Trials are ongoing with further combinations, such as phosphoinositide 3 kinase (PI3K)/protein kinase B (Akt)/mammalian target of rapamycin (mTOR) inhibitors, cyclin-dependent kinase 4 and 6 (CDK4/6) inhibitors, anti–PD-(L)1 antibodies, endocrine therapy, and newer anti–HER2 agents.[95]

Neoadjuvant Systemic Therapy for Operable Breast Cancer

Chemotherapy has traditionally been administered as adjuvant therapy after completion of surgery. Neoadjuvant therapy, the administration of systemic chemotherapy or endocrine therapy before surgery, has several theoretical advantages, including the potential to lower the volume of microscopic metastatic disease; decrease drug resistance by treating tumors before resistance has developed; increase the efficacy of treatment because the vascular system has not been disrupted by surgery; reduce the size of the tumor before surgery, allowing the deescalation of surgery; and permit evaluation of the response to treatment in vivo, allowing adjustment in adjuvant therapies. In addition, it has been shown that response to neoadjuvant chemotherapy correlates with survival outcomes. In the NSABP B-18 trial, after 9 years of follow-up, the DFS rate in patients achieving a pCR in the neoadjuvant therapy arm was 75% compared with 58% in patients who had any residual invasive disease after chemotherapy. A meta-analysis of 12 randomized trials evaluating neoadjuvant chemotherapy found that a pCR, defined as either no invasive disease in the breast or axilla or no invasive or in situ residual disease, was associated with improved event-free survival and OS.[96] The association between pCR and long-term outcomes was strongest in patients with aggressive tumor subtypes, including patients with TNBC and patients with HER2-positive, hormone receptor–negative breast cancer.

The use of neoadjuvant systemic therapy in breast cancer patients has increased in recent years for two practical reasons affecting patient care: the potential for deescalation of surgery thanks to the downstaging of the tumor in the breast and regional nodes and the ability to tailor adjuvant therapy, with escalation or deescalation, based on tumor response. Neoadjuvant treatment can allow for deescalation of surgery in the breast through a reduction in tumor size, converting inoperable tumors to operable ones, making tumors that would require mastectomy amenable to lumpectomy, and shrinking larger tumors to allow an improved cosmetic outcome with BCS. Several prospective randomized trials evaluating the efficacy of chemotherapy and endocrine therapy administered as neoadjuvant versus adjuvant therapy have all demonstrated increased rates of breast conservation with the use of neoadjuvant systemic therapy. The NSABP B-18 trial included 1523 patients and found no survival advantage (or detriment) in patients who received preoperative doxorubicin and cyclophosphamide chemotherapy versus the same regimen delivered postoperatively. The breast conservation rate was higher in females completing neoadjuvant chemotherapy, and the rate of in-breast recurrence in females who underwent neoadjuvant therapy followed by BCS was not significantly different from the rate of in-breast recurrence in females who underwent BCS before adjuvant chemotherapy.

One must take into consideration that by the end of neoadjuvant systemic therapy, a percentage of patients will have complete resolution of the tumors by clinical examination and imaging. This percentage ranges from 10% to 15% in patients with hormone receptor–positive tumors to approximately 65% to 70% in patients with HER2-positive tumors receiving trastuzumab and pertuzumab in combination with chemotherapy. To enable resection of the primary tumor or biopsy-proven axillary nodes, the clinician should be sure to have a metallic clip placed under image guidance in the primary tumor site or biopsy-proven positive node before neoadjuvant chemotherapy is initiated. This clip can facilitate identification of the original tumor site for excision after therapy. There are also ongoing efforts to identify patients who have experienced a pCR before surgery, with the possibility of omitting surgery in selected patients.[97]

Management of the axilla in patients undergoing neoadjuvant therapy has also evolved. The timing of SLND has been debated, with a few centers performing SLND before neoadjuvant therapy in patients with clinically negative nodes to inform decisions about systemic and RT and out of concern that lymphatic mapping after neoadjuvant treatment would be less accurate. Several meta-analyses of single-institution and multicenter studies concluded that SLND is feasible and accurate after neoadjuvant chemotherapy, resulting in sentinel node identification rates of approximately 91% to 96% and FNRs of 6.0% to 10.5%.[98,99] In light of increasing

pCR rates in node-positive patients after neoadjuvant treatment, the necessity of an ALND has been questioned. As mentioned earlier, it has been shown that in patients with limited axillary involvement, TAD, in which the clipped node is removed in addition to SLNs, provides an adequate sampling of the axilla, with FNRs as low as 1.4%. This approach has gained much support and is advocated by NCCN guidelines in patients with good clinical responses in the axillary nodes after neoadjuvant systemic treatment. Some advocate for SLND without the need to clip nodes as long as a dual mapping technique is used and at least three sentinel nodes are retrieved at the time of surgery.

The second practical reason for the neoadjuvant approach is the ability to learn about the biology of the tumor and its response to treatment in vivo. This can serve as a research platform and help in the identification of patient and tumor characteristics that can predict response to therapy. However, it can also provide prognostic information and help direct adjuvant treatment choices in individual patients. As outlined earlier, there are several clinical scenarios in which adjuvant treatment decisions are based on the response to neoadjuvant therapy. These include HER2-positive patients who would receive a T-DM1 as adjuvant treatment and TNBC patients who would be considered for adjuvant capecitabine if they did not achieve a pCR after neoadjuvant treatment.

Finally, because new and more targeted regimens have been and will continue to be introduced, accurate assessment of the residual tumor burden in the breast and regional nodes will become increasingly important in terms of defining prognosis and determining what personalized adjuvant therapy is needed. Nevertheless, neoadjuvant chemotherapy has potential disadvantages in terms of loss of prechemotherapy prognostic information (e.g., axillary lymph node status, actual invasive tumor size), which may have an impact on decision-making concerning postmastectomy RT.

TREATMENT OF SPECIAL CONDITIONS

Locally Advanced and Inflammatory Breast Cancer

Patients with locally advanced breast cancer include patients with large primary tumors (>5 cm), tumors involving the chest wall, those with skin involvement, ulceration or satellite skin nodules, inflammatory carcinoma, bulky or fixed axillary nodes, and clinically apparent internal mammary or supraclavicular nodal involvement (stages IIB, IIIA, IIIB, and IIIC disease). Central to treatment is the concept that the disease is advanced on the chest wall, in regional lymph nodes, or both, with no evidence of metastasis to distant sites. These patients are recognized to be at significant risk for the development of metastases, and treatment must address the risk of local and systemic relapse. Experience before the 1970s demonstrated that surgery alone provided poor local control, with local relapse rates of 30% to 50% and mortality rates of 70%. Similar results were reported when RT was the sole modality of treatment. Current management includes surgery, RT, and systemic therapy, with the sequence and extent of treatment determined by specifics of the patient's tumor subtype, staging, and comorbid conditions.

Although inflammatory breast cancer is rare, accounting for approximately 1% to 5% of all breast tumors, it is the most aggressive subtype of breast cancer. The hallmark of inflammatory breast cancer is diffuse tumor involvement of the dermal lymphatic channels within the breast and overlying skin, often without a discrete underlying tumor mass. Inflammatory breast cancer manifests clinically as erythema, edema, and warmth of the breast as a result of lymphatic obstruction. There may be no abnormality on mammography beyond skin thickening, and a palpable mass is not required for the diagnosis. The term *peau d'orange* is used to describe the orange-peel appearance of the skin resulting from edema and dimpling at sites of hair follicles (see Fig. 68.6D). The history should reveal a rapid onset of the disease, with progression over weeks to 3 months. Neglected primary breast tumors that lead to secondary inflammatory changes within the breast should not be categorized as inflammatory breast cancer. Inflammatory cancer is a purely clinical diagnosis and can occur with tumors of ductal or lobular histology and any receptor status. The pathologic hallmark of inflammatory cancer is the presence of tumor cells within dermal lymphatics, but this is often missed because of sampling error and is not a prerequisite for diagnosis. Axillary nodal metastases are common, and there is a significant risk for distant metastases. SLNB is not performed for inflammatory breast cancer as it has been shown to have a high FNR in these patients, and therefore, ALND should always be performed.

Current treatment approaches emphasize the use of combined-modality treatment, including neoadjuvant chemotherapy, modified radical mastectomy without immediate reconstruction, and postmastectomy RT, with appropriate adjuvant systemic therapy. With trimodal treatment, locoregional recurrence rates were as low as 6.9% in a large single-institution experience, with a distant recurrence rate of 35.1% during a 5-year median follow-up period.[100]

Breast Cancer in Older Adults

Several studies have explored options that reduce the extent of surgery and RT for older females with breast cancer. In the CALGB 9343 trial and the PRIME-II trials described earlier, older females were randomly assigned to lumpectomy with or without irradiation. As mentioned earlier, both trials reported inferior local control but no difference in 10-year survival in patients either 65 or 70 years of age or older with hormone receptor–positive, HER2-negative tumors, 2 to 3 cm or smaller, with or without whole breast radiation.[64,65] The low rates of local recurrence and the significant rates of death from other comorbid conditions led to the acceptance of wide excision and endocrine therapy without adjuvant breast irradiation for selected older patients with small ER-positive tumors and clinically negative axillary nodes. Several studies have also questioned the need for SLNB in older patients with early hormone receptor–positive breast cancer. They have shown no difference between patients who underwent axillary staging and those who did not regarding DFS and OS.[101,102] This led the SSO to issue a recommendation, as part of its Choosing Wisely campaign, to avoid routine SLND in clinically node-negative females 70 years or older with early-stage hormone receptor–positive, HER2-negative breast cancer, as long as they are treated with adjuvant endocrine therapy.

Paget Disease

First described by Paget in 1874, Paget disease accounts for 1% or less of breast malignancies. It is characterized clinically by nipple erythema and irritation with associated pruritus and may progress to crusting and ulceration. The condition may spread outward from the nipple and onto the areola and surrounding skin of the breast (see Fig. 68.6). The differential diagnosis of scaling skin and erythema of the NAC includes eczema, contact dermatitis, postradiation dermatitis, and Paget disease. Many benign skin conditions affecting the breast, such as eczema, frequently begin on the areola, whereas Paget disease originates on the nipple and secondarily involves the areola. A biopsy of the skin of the nipple should be performed; a specimen containing Paget cells confirms the diagnosis.

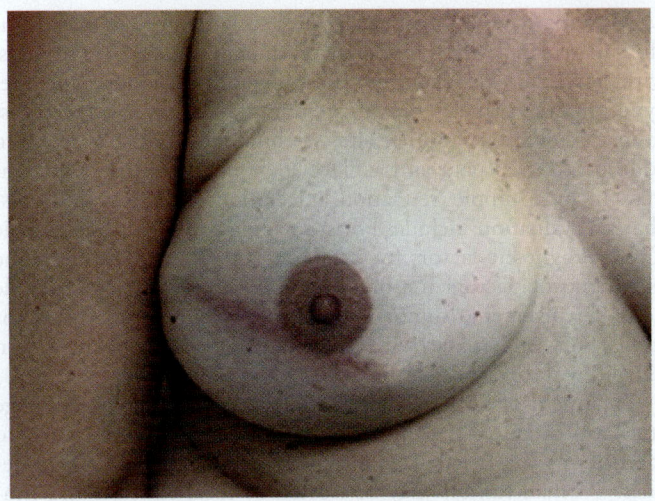

FIGURE 68.16 Three-dimensional tattoo of the nipple-areolar complex.

Pathologically, a Paget cell is a large, pale-staining cell with round or oval nuclei and large nucleoli located between the normal keratinocytes of the nipple epidermis. Carcinoma cells spread into the lactiferous sinuses, invade across the junction of epidermal and ductal epithelial cells, and enter the epidermal layer of the skin of the nipple. Paget cells do not invade through the dermal basement membrane and are categorized as carcinoma in situ. More than 95% of patients with Paget disease have an underlying breast carcinoma. Paget disease may be accompanied by a palpable mass in slightly more than 50% of patients. A palpable mass or mammographic findings raise the chances of an underlying invasive breast cancer, which is identified in more than 90% of such patients. Those without these findings will more often have an underlying DCIS.

Treatment of Paget disease includes mastectomy with axillary staging or wide local excision of the nipple and areola to achieve clear margins, axillary staging, and adjuvant RT. For many patients, lumpectomy with a Grisotti flap or other oncoplastic reconstruction, with adjuvant irradiation, provides an acceptable cosmetic appearance and obviates the need for mastectomy and breast reconstruction. Nipple-areolar reconstruction can be performed 4 to 6 months after RT or via 3D tattooing (Fig. 68.16). For patients considering lumpectomy, thorough preoperative evaluation is required to rule out occult multicentric disease.

Breast Cancer in Males

Less than 1% of new breast cancer cases (2800 estimated in 2023 in the United States) and deaths (530) occur in males. The median age at diagnosis is 68 years, 5 years older than in females, and it is usually diagnosed at a more advanced stage than in females because of a lack of awareness.[103] Risk factors include increasing age; radiation exposure; and factors related to abnormalities in estrogen and androgen balance, including testicular disease, infertility, obesity, and cirrhosis. Risk factors related to a genetic predisposition include Klinefelter syndrome (47,XXY karyotype), family history, and *BRCA* gene mutations (particularly *BRCA2* mutations). Gynecomastia is not a risk factor.

Histologically, 90% of breast cancers in males are invasive ductal carcinomas. Of these, approximately 80% to 90% are hormone receptor positive, 10% to 15% overexpress HER2, and less than 5% are TNBC. DCIS represents 10% of cases. Given the absence of terminal lobules in the normal breast in males, ILC and LCIS are rarely seen.

Most males with breast cancer present with a breast mass, usually subareolar. There is nipple involvement in up to 50% of cases, with potential skin changes. The differential diagnosis includes gynecomastia, primary breast carcinoma, metastasis to the breast from carcinoma at another site, sarcoma, and breast abscess. In addition to local pain and axillary adenopathy, initial symptoms may include nipple retraction, ulceration, bleeding, and discharge. Evaluation includes breast imaging studies and diagnostic CNB. Prognostic factors for breast in males are the same as prognostic factors for breast cancer in females and include nodal involvement, tumor size, histologic grade, and receptor status. Survival in males with breast cancer is similar to survival in females with breast cancer matched for age and stage.

Treatment of breast carcinoma in males depends on the stage and local extent of the tumor, with treatment options similar to the options for females, as outlined in 2020 by ASCO guidelines.[104] Small tumors may be treated by local excision and irradiation or by mastectomy. Sentinel node biopsy is effective for staging breast cancer in males. Breast tumors in males more commonly involve the pectoralis major muscle, probably because breast tissue in males is scant. If the underlying pectoral muscle is involved, a modified radical mastectomy with excision of the involved portion of the muscle is an adequate treatment, but it may be combined with postoperative RT. Adjuvant systemic therapy for breast cancer in males is the same as adjuvant therapy for breast cancer in females, including chemotherapy and targeted therapy. Most breast cancers in males are hormone receptor positive. Adjuvant endocrine therapy with tamoxifen is indicated for patients with node-positive disease and high-risk patients with node-negative disease. Those with contraindications to tamoxifen can be treated with gonadotropin-releasing hormone (GnRH) agonists/antagonists with an AI. Males diagnosed with breast cancer treated with BCT should be followed with ipsilateral mammogram, with a contralateral mammogram recommended for those with a germline genetic mutation.[104]

Breast Cancer During Pregnancy

The diagnosis of breast cancer during pregnancy occurs in 1 out of 3000 to 10,000 pregnancies. The diagnostic and treatment options are similar to those for nonpregnant patients, apart from several considerations. Mammography is not contraindicated, and US is useful in characterizing the breast lesion. MRI with gadolinium should be avoided during pregnancy. The considerations relevant for treatment recommendations are the desire to avoid irradiation as well as endocrine and HER2-directed therapy during the entire pregnancy and to avoid chemotherapeutic agents during the organogenesis phase of the first trimester. Surgery, including SLND, can be safely performed during pregnancy. BCS is as safe as mastectomy, and adjuvant radiation can be postponed until after delivery with the administration of neoadjuvant/adjuvant systemic therapy in the interim.

Recently, the results of the Positive trial have been published, demonstrating that temporary interruption of adjuvant endocrine therapy in order to attempt pregnancy in patients with prior hormone receptor–positive breast cancer is safe. It enrolled 516 females, 42 years old or younger, 93.4% of whom had stage I or II breast cancer, who received 18 to 30 months of adjuvant endocrine therapy and desired pregnancy, into this single-arm trial. The 3-year incidence of breast events was 8.9% in the study group compared with 9.2% in an external control cohort, and 74% of patients were able to have at least one pregnancy, and 64% had a live birth.[105]

SELECTED REFERENCES

Brabender DE, Klimberg VS, Sener SF. What's new in surgical oncology breast. *J Surg Oncol.* 2024;129:10-17.

This article reviews some of the most important clinical trials in the past 5 years.

Clarke M, Collins R, Darby S, et al. Early Breast Cancer Trialists' Collaborative Group (EBCTCG): effects of radiotherapy and differences in the extent of surgery for early breast cancer on local recurrence and 15-year survival: an overview of the randomized trials. *Lancet.* 2005;366:2087-2106.

This overview analysis by the Early Breast Cancer Trialists' Collaborative Group showed the benefit of radiotherapy on survival in patients with breast cancer.

Domchek S, Friebel TM, Singer CF, et al. Association of risk-reducing surgery in BRCA1 or BRCA2 mutation carriers with cancer risk and mortality. *JAMA.* 2010;304:967-975.

This was the first trial to demonstrate the survival benefit of risk-reducing surgery in BRCA1- and BRCA2-mutation carriers.

Early Breast Cancer Trialists' Collaborative Group (EBCTCG). Effects of chemotherapy and hormonal therapy for early breast cancer on recurrence and 15-year survival: an overview of the randomized trials. *Lancet.* 2005;365:1687-1717.

This overview analysis by the Early Breast Cancer Trialists' Collaborative Group showed the benefit of chemotherapy and hormonal therapy on survival based on the stage of disease and hormone receptor status.

Fisher B, Anderson S, Bryant J, et al. Twenty-year follow-up of a randomized trial comparing total mastectomy, lumpectomy, and lumpectomy plus irradiation for the treatment of invasive breast cancer. *N Engl J Med.* 2002;347:1233-1241.

This randomized trial showed no difference in survival between total mastectomy and breast-conserving surgery with or without radiation.

Fisher B, Costantino JP, Wickerham DL, et al. Tamoxifen for prevention of breast cancer: Report of the National Surgical Adjuvant Breast and Bowel Project P-1 Study. *J Natl Cancer Inst.* 1998;90:1371-1388.

In this first randomized trial for breast cancer prevention in a high-risk population, patients were assessed for risk based on the Gail model and randomly assigned to receive 5 years of tamoxifen or placebo. The use of tamoxifen reduced breast cancer incidence by approximately 50%.

Fisher B, Jeong JH, Anderson S, et al. Twenty-five-year follow-up of a randomized trial comparing radical mastectomy, total mastectomy, and total mastectomy followed by irradiation. *N Engl J Med.* 2002;347:567-575.

This report showed no difference in survival between radical mastectomy and total mastectomy with or without radiation.

Giuliano AE, Ballman KV, McCall L, et al. Effect of axillary dissection vs no axillary dissection on 10-year overall survival among women with invasive breast cancer and sentinel node metastasis: the ACOSOG Z0011 (Alliance) Randomized Clinical Trial. *JAMA.* 2017;318:918-926.

This randomized trial showed no benefit to completion of axillary lymph node dissection in selected patients with early-stage breast cancer and positive sentinel lymph nodes.

Krag DN, Anderson SJ, Julian TB, et al. Sentinel-lymph-node resection compared with conventional axillary-lymph-node dissection in clinically node negative patients with breast cancer: overall survival findings from the NSABP B-32 randomised phase 3 trial. *Lancet Oncol.* 2010;11:927-933.

In this randomized trial of sentinel lymph node dissection versus axillary dissection in early-stage breast cancer, there was no difference in overall survival or locoregional recurrence among patients undergoing sentinel node surgery versus standard axillary surgery.

Perou CM, Sorlie T, Eisen MB, et al. Molecular portraits of human breast tumours. *Nature.* 2000;406:747–752.

This article provided the first description of molecular subtypes of breast cancer using microarray analysis.

Rossouw JE, Anderson GL, Prentice RL, et al. Risks and benefits of estrogen plus progestin in healthy postmenopausal women: principal results from the Women's Health Initiative randomized controlled trial. *JAMA.* 2002;288:321-333.

In this long-term follow-up study of participants in the Women's Health Initiative, the risks and benefits of hormone replacement therapy in postmenopausal females were demonstrated.

The full reference list appears on Elsevier eBooks+.

69 | CHAPTER

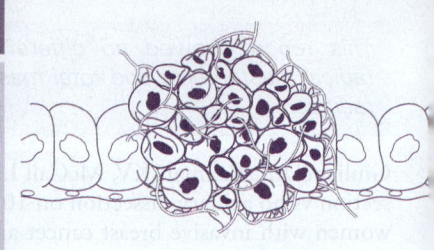

Plastic Surgical Considerations in Cancer Surgery

Margaret Roubaud, Eva Roy, Erin Taylor, Colby Hyland, Z-Hye Lee, Sahil Kapur, and Andrea Pusic

---

GOALS OF RECONSTRUCTION

Large defects in the body can occur after tumor resection and radiation treatment. The restoration of the body as close as possible to its premorbid form is the main goal of reconstruction after ablative surgery. The availability of reconstructive techniques allows for large tumors that would otherwise be unresectable, and in this sense, reconstructive surgeons are key enablers for all surgical oncologists. Especially in areas like the head and neck and the extremities, the availability of tissue is limited, and many tumors cannot be resected without the use of free tissue transfer to cover the defects.

Choosing the correct modality of reconstruction requires keeping in mind the two main goals: to restore function and to optimize aesthetics. Meticulous planning between the oncologic and reconstructive surgeons is necessary to plan incisional access to avoid compromise of potential reconstructive options. In general, replacing "like with like" is the most important reconstructive principle. A thorough defect analysis is performed to identify which critical structures are missing such as skin, fat, muscle, and nerves, and the reconstructive plan should ideally have components to replace the corresponding tissue. Simply "closing the hole" is no longer an acceptable goal in reconstruction. Successful social reintegration of patients after they have survived their cancer is paramount, and the aesthetic outcomes must be prioritized as much as functional outcomes. In general, the aesthetic unit should be treated as a whole, and incisions should ideally be hidden as much as possible within relaxed tension lines and natural creases of the body. This is particularly true in cosmetically sensitive areas, such as the face. Tissues can change over time, and the ideal reconstruction should anticipate these changes so that the patient has the optimal aesthetic and functional result not only right after surgery but also as they age. Furthermore, reconstruction must consider changes that will occur with adjuvant treatment. For example, radiation in particular causes significant tissue atrophy of both muscle and fasciocutaneous tissue; therefore, extra bulk is often incorporated into the reconstruction.

Finally, secondary procedures are not uncommon after oncologic reconstruction. Liposuction or defatting of a reconstructive flap is sometimes necessary to improve the contour of the newly placed tissue and improve the overall aesthetic result. These revision procedures are typically performed 3 to 6 months after reconstruction or after all adjuvant therapy is complete.

Preoperative Considerations in Reconstruction of the Oncologic Patient

When evaluating a patient for any surgery, the provider must consider all aspects of a patient's health. In elective cases, patients should be physically, emotionally, and oncologically appropriate candidates for reconstruction. Issues such as diabetes, smoking, and disease remission should be resolved. However, in urgent cases, when disease burden requires resection and reconstruction is necessary for function, little time may be available for comorbidity optimization. The acknowledgment of "high-risk" patients requiring surgery necessitates early active management.

Patients who are considered at increased risk for reconstructive surgical complications include those who present with medical diagnoses or physical conditions that predispose them to infection, tissue necrosis or dehiscence, perioperative morbidity, or reconstructive failure. The consequences of these complications include pain, long-term disability, scarring, and, most important, possible delay in adjuvant treatments that could affect oncologic outcome or even survival. Although a single high-risk factor alone may not preclude a reconstruction, patients with multiple risk factors should be judiciously evaluated and advised.

Advanced Age

Cancer disproportionately affects elderly individuals. For example, nearly 75% of breast cancer is diagnosed in patients over 65 years. With the rapidly increasing elderly population, cancer treatment providers must consider this select group. For example, historically, some surgeons did not offer breast reconstruction in elderly patients, with one study finding the biggest single predictor for offering reconstruction being a patient under age 50 years.[1] Although age is always a consideration regarding the overall health and tolerance of a surgical candidate, increasing data across multiple disciplines have demonstrated that the global health of the patient is more predictive of successful outcomes than chronology alone.

In a recent review from the United Kingdom, the authors found that breast reconstructive surgery is well tolerated in the elderly population, with complication rates comparable to a younger group.[2] Importantly, in areas such as social functioning and emotional well-being, patients with reconstructive surgery displayed better outcomes than those without. These data are reinforced by multiple other studies with similar findings, demonstrating both comparable safety and patient satisfaction in the elderly population undergoing reconstructive surgery.

When determining relevant risk factors in older populations, many studies have demonstrated that patient frailty may be more predictive of surgical complications than age. The Canada Study of Health and Aging (CSHA) developed a 70-item frailty index (CSHA-FI) that was based on this concept and assessed cognitive function, nutritional status, gait, grip strength, and comorbidities. The CHSA-FI has been shown to be strongly associated with adverse outcomes.[3] The American College of Surgeons NSQIP database initially developed an 11-factor modified frailty index (mFI-11), and, more recently, Subramaniam et al. have demonstrated a simplified 5-factor modified frailty index (mFI-5) that is an equally effective predictor of mortality and postoperative complications in all subspecialties.[4] The factors comprising the mFI-5 include functional status, diabetes, history of chronic obstructive pulmonary disease, history of congestive heart failure, and hypertension requiring medication. Cuccolo et al. examined patient frailty versus age on outcomes after pedicled flap reconstruction. Although increased age was associated with increased risk of complications, the mFI-5 held much stronger predictive capacity.[5]

In summary, age should be considered a single factor in overall patient capacity for reconstruction but should not be used as a method of exclusion. Perioperative risk stratification, such as using the mFI-5, is a better predictor of complications than age alone.

Smoking

For decades, smoking has been linked to cancer-related deaths and nicotine-induced vascular insufficiency. In the patient with cancer, smoking is not only associated with higher risk of perioperative infection but also tissue necrosis, poor wound healing, and thrombosis.

In the breast cancer literature, in both alloplastic and autologous reconstruction, smoking has been found to increase the risk of developing postoperative complications. A study of independent risk factors for postoperative complications of autologous or implant-based reconstruction showed smoking was associated with the highest number of early overall complications. When smoking was combined with other potential risk factors such as obesity or preoperative radiation, the risk for complications rose exponentially.[6]

Although former smokers remain with an elevated lifetime risk of cancer, the reduced risk of perioperative complications has been replicated in multiple randomized controlled trials. A meta-analysis by Mills et al. pooled data from six randomized controlled trials regarding smoking cessation. Compared with controls, cessation programs were found to reduce overall risk of complications by 41%, postoperative wound-healing complications by 52%, and surgical site infections (SSIs) by 60%.[7] Furthermore, a significantly lower complication rate was observed in the trials that used a duration of smoking cessation 4 weeks or greater, with each week of smoking cessation progressively reducing postoperative risk out to 6 weeks.

The diagnosis of cancer can often induce anxiety and maladaptive coping mechanisms, including cigarette use. However, during initial consultation the oncologic treatment team may have a counseling opportunity at a time when concerned patients are most receptive to the idea of smoking cessation. In a meta-analysis regarding the effectiveness of smoking cessation interventions, the authors found that a smoker had approximately one in eight chances of quitting without aid.[8] However, this rate was doubled with the use of nicotine replacement therapy (NRT) and more than doubled when smoking cessation medications were used appropriately. Interestingly, in a randomized controlled trial, smoking cessation with NRT was shown to reduce postoperative complications as much as smoking cessation alone.[9] Therefore, although absolute nicotine cessation for at least 4 weeks is the optimal recommendation for patients, NRT and adjunct medications may provide the highest chance of adherence to a cessation regimen with minimal wound-healing complications.

Obesity

For a multitude of socioeconomic reasons, many industrialized nations are facing an increasing obesity epidemic. If current trends continue, 30% of the US population will be obese (BMI $>30 \text{ kg/m}^2$) by 2050. Obesity contributes to chronic medical comorbidities such as hypertension, diabetes, and cardiovascular disease. It has also been linked to increased rates of cancer, especially in hormone-sensitive tumors such as endometrial cancer. In the reconstruction population, obesity is associated with increased risk of seroma, wound-healing complications, infection, and reconstructive failure.

Every reconstructive surgeon must decide their particular limit for different types of reconstruction in the obese patient. Importantly, different classes of obesity may do better than others. In a large breast reconstruction study by Fischer et al., the authors demonstrated that progressive obesity, defined by the World Health Organization class I to III obesity guidelines, was associated with higher rates of overall perioperative morbidity, length of stay, operative time, and anesthesia risk.[10] In particular, class III obese patients experienced a 5.3% higher risk of return to the operating room and a 1.7% higher rate of flap or implant loss within 30 days. However, BMI alone should not be considered an exclusion to reconstruction. A large study of outcomes after prepectoral breast implant reconstruction found that despite a tendency for class II and III obese patients to experience increased perioperative morbidity and reconstruction loss, on multivariate analysis, the presence of diabetes and smoking was more predictive of any complication than obesity.[11] These results suggest that although obesity should be considered, the global health of the patient and control of obesity-associated morbidities should be considered before excluding from reconstruction. Ultimately, success is dependent on the correct selection of the appropriate reconstructive technique for the patient body habitus and health. For example, the thickness of soft tissue flap may vary greatly between patients with class I versus class III obesity. This becomes extremely important when reconstruction requires an exact fit in a limited field, such as pharyngeal repair or distal extremity coverage.

Nutrition

Proper wound healing is dependent on a patient's reserve of nutritional building blocks. Unfortunately, the cancer patient faces many obstacles in this area. Neoadjuvant chemotherapy, tumor-induced soft tissue wasting, and general fatigue may limit patient oral intake. In particular, cancers of the head and neck region or gastrointestinal tract may severely affect the ability to consume nutrients despite a desire to do so. Furthermore, tolerance of chemotherapy may depend on steroid tapers, which in turn exacerbate preexisting diabetes and tissue fragility. In the presence of open wounds or fistulas, protein deficiency is exaggerated.

Although the basics of nutrition are outside of the scope of this text, several factors warrant consideration in the patient with cancer. Preoperative hemoglobin A1c (120-day cycle), prealbumin (half-life 3 days), and albumin (half-life 20 days) may provide preoperative insight into patient condition. Hemoglobin A1c may require temporary correction with insulin and endocrine specialty intervention. Prealbumin below 10 mg/dL and albumin below 2.7 g/dL indicate moderate to severe malnutrition. These patients benefit from preoperative nutritional supplement, either in oral drinks or tube feeding.

Timing of Reconstruction

The timing of reconstruction is most often dictated by the status of the tumor and oncologic treatment. Reconstruction can be performed in an immediate or delayed fashion. Immediate reconstruction is considered when a patient needs restoration of a vital structure, such as the pharynx or abdominal wall, or when their physiologic reserve allows extended time under anesthesia. When immediate reconstruction is performed, tissue planes are readily accessible, and the wound bed has little or no fibrotic tissue. In contrast, when the reconstruction is delayed, scar tissue, fibrosis, and wound contracture can inhibit optimal aesthetic and functional outcomes. However, delayed reconstruction may be necessary when margins are not clear, as in permanent section evaluation for melanoma, or when the patient requires significant postoperative radiation that will damage the reconstruction, such as in breast reconstruction.

Chemotherapy

Chemotherapy refers to drugs or medicines that treat cancer. They may be given alone or in combination therapy. Traditional or standard chemotherapy uses drugs that are cytotoxic and target different phases of the cell cycle. These drugs may cause damage to normal cells as well as cancer cells and can cause side effects such as neutropenia and nausea. They are generally divided by

their mechanism of action, such as alkylating agents (that keep the cell from reproducing by damaging its DNA), antimetabolites (interfere with DNA or RNA building blocks by substitution), antitumor antibiotics such as anthracyclines (interfere with enzymes involved in copying DNA), topoisomerase inhibitors/plant alkaloids (interfere with topoisomerase enzyme to prevent DNA separation and copying), and mitotic inhibitors/plant alkaloids such as taxanes and vinca alkaloids (which keep enzymes from making proteins for mitosis).

Other drugs designed to treat cancer may include those labeled as targeted therapies, hormone therapy, or immunotherapy. These targeted therapies work by finding specific proteins or receptors that certain cancer cells possess. An example is trastuzumab, which targets the cancer cell signaling protein HER2, which is overactive in about 25% of breast cancers. Hormone therapy drugs work to suppress different actions of hormones that make some cancers grow. An example of this is androgen suppression therapy and the drug leuprolide to reduce the level of testosterone in the treatment of prostate cancer. Immunotherapy uses a patient's immune system to recognize and attack cancer cells. Pembrolizumab (Keytruda) is an example of an immunotherapy drug. It works by blocking the T-cell protein programmed cell death 1 (PD-1), a normal immune inhibitor, to help the T cells find and attack cancer cells.

In reconstruction, knowledge of a patient's recent chemotherapy or drug regimen can help predict certain responses after surgery. Chemotherapeutic agents that inhibit normal cell metabolism may interfere with pathways required for effective wound healing. These include disruption of inflammation-induced responses such as cell migration, extracellular matrix production, and angiogenesis. Patients on extensive neoadjuvant therapy regimens may require monitoring of their absolute neutrophil count (ANC) and demonstration of count "recovery" before open or surgical procedures are attempted. A patient who is on an adjuvant regimen that causes profound neutropenia may not be a great candidate for elective hardware or implant placement. If a foreign device, such as tissue expander, is required, then limiting access of the port or chances for bacterial contamination is paramount during the neutropenic phase.

Because of the explosion in chemotherapeutic drug development and varied effects on wound healing, multidisciplinary discussion is encouraged. Many agents can be safely timed with surgery and radiation to provide the best outcome to cancer patients. Reconstruction must work with cancer-curing modalities to optimize the chance of survival. The medical oncologist, resecting surgeon, and reconstructive surgeon should have an open line of communication when planning operative interventions.

Radiation

Radiation oncology uses high-energy electromagnetic radiation to treat oncologic diseases. It can be delivered in a variety of forms, dependent on the particular characteristics of radiation that benefit the patient and tumor biology. The total radiation dose and fractionation vary, depending on clinical goals of the patient treatment plan. It is given in multiple settings, including the neoadjuvant, adjuvant, and palliative circumstance. Radiation kills tumor cells by irreversibly damaging their DNA. As such, tissues and organs have known dose and volume levels that must be respected to avoid late permanent injury.

In the reconstructive field, it is important to not only understand the dose of radiation a patient will have or has received but also the fractionation. Fractionation is the process of dividing the total dose into smaller equal doses that are delivered over a set time. This process exploits the inherit biologic differences between tumor and normal cells to maximize tumor cell death while minimizing normal cell damage. Standard dose fractions range from 1.8 to 2 gray (Gy). Hypofractionation refers to the delivery of larger doses per fraction (>2 Gy) over a shorter period. Accelerated fractionation refers to standard fraction sizes given in a shorter period (i.e., twice daily). Cell radiobiologic response dictates the optimization of fractionation. These cell responses include repair, repopulation, redistribution, and reoxygenation.

Radiation can be delivered externally via high- or low-energy beams or internally via implanted radiation sources. External beam radiation therapy (EBRT) is most common and delivered from an external source. Patients are immobilized on a treatment table while multiple radiation beams are stereotaxically targeted from various angles, converging on the desired target. In contrast, brachytherapy is the practice of directly delivering radiation by placing radioactive sources in the tumor or tumor bed. The advantage is delivery of high doses of radiation directly to the tumor while sparing normal tissues. It is commonly used for locally contained, small-volume disease, which can be accessed by an applicator device, such as prostate or cervical cancer. Intraoperative radiation therapy (IORT) is radiation that is delivered to a tumor bed during surgery. It allows the delivery of radiation to a tumor bed of interest after resection and is most commonly seen in locally advanced or recurrent colorectal cancers.

Radiation side effects are classified as either acute or late reactions. Acute reactions are related to the depletion of rapidly dividing cells. These reactions include desquamation and associated erythema, nausea, diarrhea, and reduced blood cell counts. These effects are temporary as the cell lines recover. In contrast, late reactions, such as tissue or pulmonary fibrosis, are caused by microvascular damage or the depletion of terminally differentiated cells. As such, these reactions are less likely to resolve.

In general, a patient who has received neoadjuvant radiation is given 4 to 6 weeks before surgery for this acute reaction to pass. However, surgery is time dependent because it is important to resect the tumor before the tumor cell biology is unfavorable. Similarly, adjuvant radiation is likely to occur 4 to 6 weeks after surgery, when the early phase of wound healing has been completed. As the reconstructive surgeon, is important to consider these timelines when planning reconstructive technique. In a patient destined for adjuvant radiation, although one reconstructive technique may seem "less involved" to reconstruct a defect, such as a skin graft, its time to complete healing and poor resistance to radiation may make it less favorable than a "more complicated" technique such as a free flap. When considering a patient who has received neoadjuvant radiation, a defect that has had recent radiation may be highly irritated and prone to friability, vasospasm, and dehiscence. In these instances, vascularized tissue from another region may promote better wound healing. An example of this is the transfer of vascularized tissue of the abdomen, such as a pedicled vertical rectus abdominis myocutaneous (VRAM) flap, to the perineum after neoadjuvant radiation and colorectal resection. Lastly, radiation often changes the volume and contour of transferred tissues. As such, patients may undergo delayed reconstruction in breast cancer to prevent damage to an aesthetically favorable reconstruction, or the surgeon may "overcorrect" volume in a situation where delay is not possible, such as head and neck reconstruction.

Resection Margins

Perhaps the most difficult reconstructive challenge is predicting the size of the anticipated defect. Whereas cancers on the skin surface may be amenable to predictable margins, such as those delineated for melanoma, deep tissue cancers are often prone to intraoperative margin evaluation and possible further resection. Reconstructive plans should always have a first-, second-, and third-line option to account for growing defect size and/or the resection of favorable donor sites. For example, a first-line pedicled flap, such a latissimus dorsi flap for trunk reconstruction, may be rendered obsolete if its vascular pedicle is resected with tumor. A mandible reconstruction in oral cancer may require both a bone flap and a soft tissue flap if the tumor extends onto the buccal surface or deep into the floor of mouth. Successful oncologic reconstructive plans are flexible to account for surprise pathology or difficult anatomy.

UNIQUE RECONSTRUCTIVE CONSIDERATIONS BY ANATOMIC AREA

Head and Neck

Head and neck cancer can dramatically affect a patient's function and quality of life. Surgical resection is the mainstay of treatment, and defects in the head and neck region can significantly affect speech, respiration, alimentation, and cosmesis. Radiation therapy is an important adjuvant therapy but can further negatively affect function by causing xerostomia, scar contracture, impaired wound healing, and osteoradionecrosis.

Tumors involving the upper aerodigestive tract pose significant challenges because of the functional importance of this area as a conduit for alimentation, articulation and speech, and airflow for oxygen exchange. Areas that can potentially be affected include the tongue, floor of the mouth, buccal mucosa, oropharynx, nasopharynx, hypopharynx, and cervical esophagus. Each area requires variable tissue characteristics for reconstruction, but the overall focus is to provide reliable wound coverage while maximizing function.[12]

The entirety of head and neck reconstruction is outside the scope of this chapter. However, certain principles dominate the field. Bony defects that compromise three-dimensional (3D) structure usually require bone replacement for optimal function. Free tissue transfer of bone is generally performed using a fibula, scapula, or iliac crest. Soft tissue defects that compromise the airway or mucosal structures require resilient tissue replacement to resist the detrimental effects of bacteria and saliva. Small defects may be amenable to local tissue flaps; however, many require free tissue transfer as well. The most common flaps are the anterolateral thigh and radial forearm. See Fig. 69.1 for an example of a partial glossectomy defect reconstructed with free lateral arm flap. Lastly, resections of the external structure of the scalp, face, or neck will lead to highly visible defects. Plastic surgery colleagues possess an armamentarium of reconstructive techniques that can restore functional defects in these areas while minimizing aesthetic devastation. This is important to patient quality of life after cancer, specifically, social interaction with families and loved ones. Resecting a cancer is not sufficient if the resultant defect creates patient isolation and resultant psychosocial depression.

When planning head and neck reconstruction, the reconstructive surgeon must constantly consider the most important goals and potential complications. Three important areas deserve special consideration, discussed next.

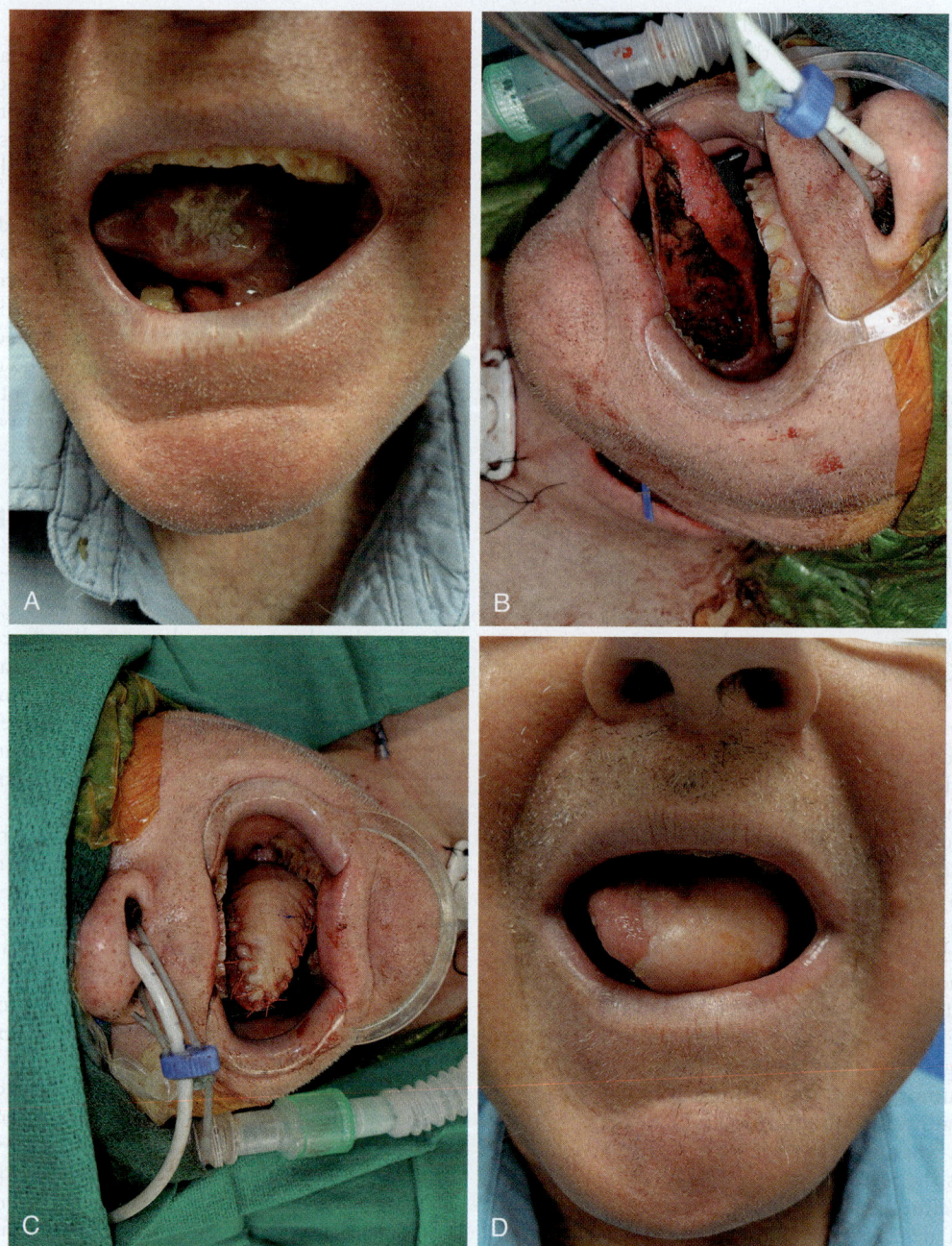

FIGURE 69.1 (A) Patient presented to the clinic with ulcerative squamous cell carcinoma of left lateral tongue. (B) The patient underwent left partial glossectomy and neck dissection by the head and neck surgery team. (C) The plastic surgery team harvested a lateral arm free flap, which was used to reconstruct the volume and surface of the tongue. The anastomosis was performed to ipsilateral facial vessels in the neck. (D) The patient had excellent postoperative contour and speech after radiation.

Airway

Airway management after head and neck reconstruction is a fundamental aspect of the perioperative care of patients.[13] This is especially true with reconstruction of defects involving the oral cavity. Airway edema and the presence of a bulky flap often compromise the upper airway in the immediate days after surgery. Elective tracheostomy has been classically advocated as the safest option, although some centers advocate for delayed extubation, typically the day after surgery while the patient stabilizes. Tracheostomy has several advantages including a secure airway, early discontinuation of mechanical ventilation, decreased sedation

requirements, and improved pulmonary mechanics. Furthermore, tracheostomy provides expedient access to the airway in cases of emergent return to the operating room for flap compromise or other complications. Attempting reintubation in these scenarios can be extremely stressful and unsafe, especially if there is increased flap or neck swelling, which is not uncommon in this setting. However, tracheostomies are not without potential risks including obstructed or displaced tracheostomy tubes, tracheoesophageal fistula, pneumonia, and tracheal stenosis. Therefore, in select patients, delayed extubation in the intensive care unit can be a reasonable option. This strategy maintains a safe airway while airway edema subsides and prevents airway compromise in case of an immediate postoperative surgical complication. Patients with delayed extubation have a faster return to speech and possibly reduced hospital stay. Ultimately, choosing the optimal method for airway management requires a multidisciplinary discussion between the ablative surgeon, the reconstructive surgeon, and the anesthesia team to reduce morbidity.

Fistula

Fistulas of the head and neck region are a common and well-known complication after reconstruction.[14] A fistula is an abnormal connection between two spaces, and in the head and neck region, it typically forms between the pharynx and the skin. It can occur after neck dissection, glossectomy, laryngectomy, or any other ablative surgery, resulting in an opening between the aerodigestive tract and the surrounding neck tissues. Fistulas can be devastating, as they can lead to prolonged open wounds, severe infections, and carotid blowouts.

Several factors have been correlated with an increased risk of fistula formation. In particular, total laryngectomy patients are at higher risk of having a pharyngocutaneous fistula when they have a previous history of radiation and malnutrition. In addition, postoperative hypothyroidism has also been correlated with fistula formation risk. Therefore, optimization with nutritional supplementations is critical for these patients. Many recent studies have shown that the use of vascularized tissue to close or reinforce the pharyngeal defect significantly reduces the risk of pharyngocutaneous fistula.[15] Both pedicled and free flaps can be used to patch the pharyngeal defect after total laryngectomy or to onlay over a primary pharyngeal closure as an additional layer of protection. The most common flaps used in this scenario include the pedicled myocutaneous pectoralis flap, the radial forearm free flap, and the anterolateral thigh free flap.

The management of a fistula can be variable depending on its severity. Conservative management with appropriate local wound care can be effective in some scenarios. The surrounding tissues should be kept free from excessive secretions, and the wound bed should be debrided regularly. Dry packing and the classic wet-to-dry dressing are the most effective ways to prevent saliva from pooling in cavities. Minimizing contamination is essential to healing; therefore, patients should be maintained on strict nothing by mouth with enteral feedings via nasogastric or gastrostomy tube. A barium swallow study should be performed before starting an oral diet to confirm fistula closure.

Fistulas that result in an uncontrolled infection with destruction of tissues or systemic symptoms require urgent operative intervention. Collection of spit and bacteria in the neck near the great vessels can lead to carotid blowout, which is the most devastating sequelae of fistulas. Any patient who presents with signs of infection in the neck should be evaluated with a computed tomography scan to determine the proximity of the infection to the carotid artery. The threshold for a washout in the operating room remains low in this setting. During the operative debridement, cultures should be taken to guide antibiotic therapy, and the size of the fistula should be assessed to determine the chances for closure with conservative measures. The pectoralis major muscle flap is the gold standard for the closure of large fistulas, as the robust muscle can be used to seal areas with tenuous tissue quality and obliterate dead space. In general, fistulae can delay adjuvant treatments such as radiation; therefore, timely intervention is often key to avoid delays in care.

Facial Paralysis

Loss of facial nerve function can be devastating with partial or complete inability to use the muscles of facial movement. The functional consequences are profound, leading to brow ptosis obstructing the visual field, incomplete eye closure, paralytic ectropion of the eyelids, inability to smile, and loss of oral competence. In addition, this condition significantly affects social interactions because of an inability to adequately convey emotion, leading to significant psychological distress. Although there are numerous etiologies for facial paralysis, including idiopathic, congenital, and traumatic causes, oncologic procedures that result in facial paralysis pose unique reconstructive challenges, which include older age, concurrent soft tissue defects, need for postoperative radiation therapy, and limited life expectancy. Immediate nerve grafting and nerve transfers yield the best functional results because these methods allow for functional restoration of the native facial musculature. Radiation therapy may delay but does not ultimately prevent nerve recovery and should not be a contraindication for nerve reconstruction. In patients who present with long-standing facial paralysis in a delayed fashion, static procedures such as fascial sling for the lower face and periocular procedures such as browlift, upper eyelid gold weight placement, and canthoplasty procedures can be used to improve overall function. Dynamic reconstruction in this population requires the transfer and neurotization of a functional muscle such as the gracilis to replace the entire neuromuscular unit and is currently mostly used to restore patients' smiles.[16]

Breast

With the passage of the Women's Health and Cancer Rights Act (WHCRA) in 1998, patients have the right to breast reconstruction covered by insurance.[17] Breast reconstruction coverage includes symmetry procedures of the contralateral breast without restrictions on time frame of surgery. This federal law has reduced financial barriers and increased access to breast reconstruction, increasing breast reconstruction rates steadily.

Breast reconstruction can be performed in the immediate or delayed setting with mastectomy. Immediate reconstruction refers to reconstruction at the time of mastectomy. A very individualized approach should be taken when deciding timing of reconstruction, such as the patient's goals, stage, and type of breast cancer. Immediate breast reconstruction is typically indicated for breast cancers that do not require immediate postmastectomy radiation therapy.[18] The benefits of immediate breast reconstruction include reduction in overall number of surgical procedures, preservation of the breast soft tissue envelope, and improved aesthetic outcomes. Additionally, some patients benefit psychologically with maintenance of body image. However, immediate breast reconstruction can lead to a longer surgical and anesthesia duration with associated risks.

Delayed breast reconstruction occurs after mastectomy on a separate procedure date. There are a variety of reasons to perform delayed breast reconstruction, including need for postmastectomy radiation therapy, adjuvant chemotherapy, or hormone therapy. Delayed reconstruction may be indicated for more advanced carcinomas to monitor treatment response before definitive reconstruction. Immediate breast reconstruction is contraindicated in breast cancers with aggressive pathology, such as inflammatory breast cancer, because reconstruction may delay postmastectomy radiation treatment. Patient comorbidities may also necessitate staging reconstruction until they are optimized, such as a high BMI, uncontrolled diabetes, and active tobacco smoking, in order to allow for a safe and successful reconstruction. Obesity significantly increases the risk of wound dehiscence in both implant-based and autologous breast reconstruction.[19] Active smoking can lead to significant mastectomy-skin necrosis leading to implant failure or flap loss. Overall, immediate breast reconstruction has become more prevalent than delayed reconstruction, and implant-based reconstruction has become more prevalent than autologous reconstruction.[20] However, oncologic treatment plans, patient comorbidities, patient preferences, and surgeon judgment affect reconstruction timing and type of reconstruction.

Types of reconstruction should be thoroughly discussed with patients. With mastectomy, patients should be aware of the options of mastectomy without reconstruction, implant-based reconstruction, or autologous reconstruction. Mastectomy without reconstruction with aesthetic chest wall closure may be preferred by patients who do not want to undergo additional procedures for breast mound reconstruction. Both implant-based reconstruction and autologous reconstruction may be performed in one or two stages. Two-stage reconstruction has a first-stage tissue expander, which can be partially filled, placed at the time of mastectomy. Tissue expanders have the benefit of allowing the mastectomy skin and nipple, if present, to recover from mastectomy given the significant reduction in blood flow to the tissue after mastectomy. Over the following weeks, the tissue expanders undergo fills in clinic with injection of sterile saline through the built-in port, identified through a magnet, until the patient reaches their desired size. As long as patients do not require postmastectomy radiation therapy or chemotherapy, they can then undergo tissue expander–to–permanent implant exchange once they reach their desired size. For patients who require radiation therapy, tissue expander–to–implant exchange or definitive autologous reconstruction is delayed to allow for healing of tissues, which can range from 6 to 12 months after radiation therapy.

Direct-to-implant breast reconstruction is implant placement at the time of mastectomy. Candidates for direct-to-implant surgery include patients with preference for approximately the same breast size or smaller, an adequately perfused skin flap after mastectomy, and no signs of nipple blood flow compromise if nipple-sparing mastectomy. Because nipple-sparing mastectomy allows for preservation of the full breast soft tissue envelope, direct-to-implant is often performed in the setting of nipple-sparing mastectomy. With a nipple-sparing mastectomy, an inferolateral inframammary fold incision is often used because of the improved aesthetic appearance of the incision hidden within the shadow of the breast and improved nipple blood flow.[21] Other incisions performed with nipple-sparing mastectomy include a periareolar incision with lateral extension, horizontal radial incision, or a vertical incision inferior to the nipple. The benefits of the direct-to-implant approach include one operation; however, patients may opt for revision procedures with direct-to-implant reconstruction.

Implant-based reconstruction can be performed in a total submuscular plane, a subpectoral plane, or a prepectoral plane. To prevent high rates of capsular contracture, or contraction around the implant, muscle or acellular dermal matrix is typically used to cover the implant. Total submuscular coverage of the implant is performed with the pectoralis major muscle, anterior serratus muscle, and superior edge of the rectus abdominus fascia. Subpectoral reconstruction is performed with elevation of the inferior edge of the pectoralis major muscle and inferior attachment to the sternum with inferior coverage with acellular dermal matrix. Prepectoral reconstruction is performed with complete coverage with acellular dermal matrix on the anterior surface of the implant, sparing chest wall muscles from elevation. Total submuscular and subpectoral reconstruction have the disadvantage of animation deformity, or visible activation of muscles with movement, increased postoperative pain, and longer recovery times. The advantages of subpectoral breast reconstruction include reduction of rippling of the implant. Prepectoral breast reconstruction has the advantage of no animation deformity and reduced postoperative pain. The disadvantages to prepectoral reconstruction are increased implant visibility with sharper transition from the chest wall to the implant and increased implant rippling; however, second-stage fat grafting can ameliorate these challenges.

When counseling patients on implant-based breast reconstruction, the type of implant used should be discussed. Implant choices include saline versus silicone, smooth versus textured, and round versus anatomic-shaped implants. Textured implants have been associated with breast implant–associated anaplastic large cell lymphoma (BIA-ALCL), which is a rare type of T-cell lymphoma. BIA-ALCL most commonly presents with a late-onset seroma around the breast implant.[22] Workup and treatment involve a multidisciplinary team approach with implant removal, en bloc versus total capsulectomy, and possible chemotherapy. Because of the association with BIA-ALCL with textured implants, most implants and tissue expanders used now are smooth. Anatomic implants are textured to prevent rotation, so most implants are not only smooth but also round. Most patients opt for silicone implants over saline because of a more natural feel and appearance of silicone implants over saline implants. The FDA recommends silicone implants be monitored with ultrasound or MRI 5 years after placement and every 2 to 3 years thereafter to ensure no silicone implant leak. Benefits of implant-based reconstruction include no additional donor site morbidity, shorter duration of procedure, and faster recovery compared with autologous reconstruction. Complications associated with implant-based reconstruction include infection, capsular contracture, BIA-ALCL, and breast implant–associated illness.

Autologous breast reconstruction involves transferring tissue from one area of the body to the breast for reconstruction. There are a variety of autologous breast reconstruction donor sites, including the abdomen, back, thighs, and buttock. See Fig. 69.2 for an example of deep inferior epigastric perforator (DIEP) reconstruction in a patient undergoing bilateral nipple-sparing mastectomy. The optimal donor site and candidacy for autologous breast reconstruction depend on the BMI, body habitus, prior surgeries, comorbidities, breast size, and goals of a patient. Abdominal-based flaps include the DIEP flap, superficial inferior epigastric artery flap, and transverse rectus abdominis myocutaneous (TRAM) flap. Nonabdominal-based flaps include the superior gluteal artery perforator flap, inferior gluteal artery perforator flap, diagonal upper gracilis flap, and profunda artery perforator (PAP) flap. Free flap reconstruction often uses a co-surgeon model, with one microsurgeon performing flap elevation and the other microsurgeon performing chest vessel recipient exposure, which reduces operative times. Currently, the most commonly used flap is a DIEP free flap. Preoperative imaging such as CTA or MRI angiography can help identify perforators. The benefit of a DIEP flap is that it is muscle sparing over the pedicled or free TRAM flap. TRAM flaps have increased donor site morbidity with higher risk of hernia, bulge, and abdominal wall laxity; therefore, abdominal wall mesh is often used to repair the abdominal wall. Thus, the TRAM flap has become less favorable because of its donor site morbidity and availability of DIEP flap.[23]

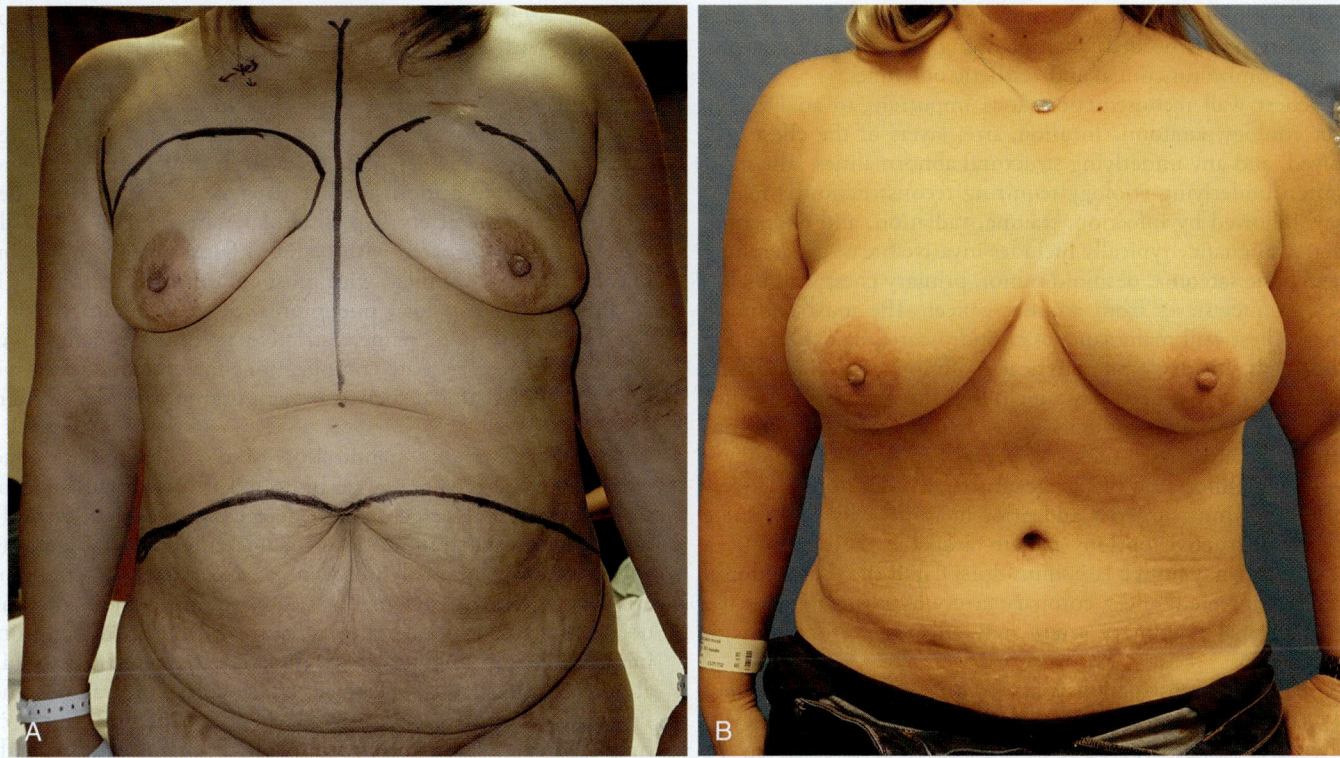

FIGURE 69.2 (A) The patient presented with ductal carcinoma in situ and known genetic mutation. She requested bilateral prophylactic mastectomies. (B) The patient underwent immediate reconstruction with bilateral deep inferior epigastric perforator flaps, which achieved her desired volume and shape.

Rates of autologous flap donor site morbidity are significantly higher in patients with BMI >35. Free flap procedures are contraindicated in patients who are active smokers and have blood clotting disorders. Donor site availability is based on tissue available for reconstruction, patient goals for reconstruction size, and prior surgeries, such as abdominoplasty or liposuction, which may limit available options. Advantages of autologous breast reconstruction include a more natural appearance and feel of the breast reconstruction, better match to the contralateral breast in unilateral reconstruction, and higher rates of breast satisfaction in patients. Disadvantages of autologous breast reconstruction include donor site morbidity and longer operative and recovery time.

Hybrid breast reconstruction occurs when an autologous reconstruction is combined with implant-based reconstruction. The pedicled latissimus dorsi flap in combination with an implant is used as a salvage option in patients who require soft tissue resurfacing of the breast but are not candidates for DIEP flap reconstruction. A less common option for breast reconstruction is autologous fat grafting alone, but often only smaller breast sizes can be achieved and multiple fat-grafting procedures are required.

Lymphatic Surgery

Lymphatic surgery is an emerging field within reconstructive surgery with the goal to prevent and treat lymphedema. Patients with breast cancer undergoing axillary lymph node dissection, postmastectomy radiation therapy, and chemotherapy have increased risk of lymphedema, with rates ranging from 25% to 40%. Patients with inflammatory breast cancer have the highest rates of lymphedema at 50.6%.[24] Lymphatic surgery provides both preventive and treatment options for lymphedema through microsurgery and supermicrosurgery techniques.[25] Regarding lymphedema prevention in high-risk patients, prophylactic lymphovenous bypass (LVB), also known as *LYMPHA,* can be performed after axillary lymph node dissection with microanastomosis of open draining lymphatic channels to nearby veins in the axilla. Prophylactic LVB has been shown to decrease rates of lymphedema from 30% to 40% to 4% to 13%.[26]

Established lymphedema is treated first with conservative decongestive therapy (CDT) managed through lymphedema-certified physical therapists. CDT includes manual massage, wearing arm sleeve garments, and pneumatic compression. In the setting of established lymphedema, LVB and vascularized lymph node transplant (VLNT) can be performed to treat lymphedema physiologically. LVB creates a new pathway to avoid obstructed lymphatic vessels that leads to dermal backflow in lymphedema. VLNT transfers lymph nodes from elsewhere in the body to the axilla or area affected greatest by lymphedema symptoms. Common donor sites for lymph nodes include superficial groin lymph nodes, omentum, and supraclavicular lymph nodes. A prospective study examining DIEP with VLNT and LVB versus DIEP with VLNT alone demonstrated both groups to have subjective improvement in symptoms.[27] Lymphatic surgery at the time of breast reconstruction to treat established lymphedema has been shown to be safe and efficacious for patients.

Trunk and Chest Wall

Chest wall reconstruction is designed to restore the integrity and function of the chest wall. Three main goals of chest wall reconstruction are completion of necessary resection, restoration of the rigid chest wall to prevent physiologic flair, and soft tissue coverage.[28] Soft tissue coverage seals the pleural space, protects viscera of vital organs and the great vessels, and prevents infection.

A multidisciplinary approach with the oncologic, thoracic, and plastic surgeons is needed when planning chest wall reconstruction to optimize functional and aesthetic outcomes.

In chest wall reconstruction, it is important to analyze the defect etiology, anatomic location, size, layers of the chest wall involved, and any underlying structural abnormalities. The most common underlying etiology requiring reconstruction is malignancy, followed by infection, trauma, radiation, and congenital defect. Malignancy typically includes invasive breast cancer, lung cancer, bone sarcoma, desmoid tumor, primary chest wall malignancy, or metastases from another cancer. The most common primary chest wall malignancy is chondroscarcoma.[29] Obtaining a thorough history and physical is imperative; identifying previous thoracic procedures—including thoracotomies; cardiac procedures, including coronary artery bypass graft; and previous abdominal surgeries, such as open cholecystectomies or ileostomies—affects available reconstructive options. Understanding previous surgeries and prior incisions will help dictate what reconstructive options remain available. For example, a thoracotomy may limit a latissimus dorsi flap if the thoracodorsal artery is transected, and a coronary artery bypass graft with use of the internal mammary artery may affect a pectoralis major turnover flap.

Soft tissue reconstruction is an essential component in chest wall reconstruction. This may be required to reconstruct the layers of the chest wall, whether preventing bronchial leak, sealing the pleural space, or providing coverage of vital structures or hardware. Local and regional flaps include the pectoralis major turnover, pectoralis major advancement, latissimus dorsi, rectus abdominis, serratus anterior, serratus posterior, deltoid, and omental flaps.

Anteriorly, pectoralis major flaps are quite versatile, as they can be used as advancement flaps based on the thoracoacromial artery, turnover flaps based on the internal mammary artery, or myocutaneous flaps. Pectoralis advancement flaps are useful for defects of the upper sternum and manubrium, and turnover flaps are beneficial for defects of the lower sternum. Other flaps that can be used anteriorly include the rectus abdominis flap, which can be turned upward on the superior epigastric artery and vein. This robust flap is based on the muscle but can include large cutaneous components. Similarly, the omental flap can be used alone or in conjunction with a muscle flap. It is helpful in providing soft tissue coverage over vital structures such as the heart, lung, and thoracic esophagus. However, the omentum requires obligate harvest from the intraperitoneal space; therefore, it can lead to increased risk of abdominal hernias, adhesions, and bowel obstruction.

The latissimus dorsi musculocutaneous flap has also been a workhorse flap because of its large size and mobility.[30] It particular, it can be used for both posterior and anterior defects, because of its primary blood supply originating from the thoracodorsal vessels near the axilla. Releasing the latissimus dorsi from all its insertions gives it a very large arc of rotation for coverage. It can be moved superiorly toward the neck and shoulder or anteriorly over the chest wall. Conversely, the latissimus dorsi may be folded over in the posteromedial direction, based on its second blood supply from intercostal perforators.

Posteriorly, other local rotational flaps provide important coverage in addition to the latissimus. The trapezius muscle is used for small defects near the superior spine, and the lumbar artery perforator flaps are good for inferior spine coverage. Medialization of the paraspinous muscles provides durable coverage over hardware frequently placed for spinal tumors.

See Fig. 69.3 for an example of posterior chest wall reconstruction with a combination of trapezius and latissimus dorsi flaps.

As there is an abundance of local flaps, free flaps are not always needed. However, for larger defect sizes or when local options are not available, microvascular free flaps may be indicated.[31] Preferred options for free flaps to this area include deep inferior epigastric artery flap, anterolateral thigh flap, and radial forearm flap. Compared with pedicled flaps, postoperative complication rates are similar, with most common complications including partial flap loss, pneumonia, acute respiratory distress syndrome, infection, pain, restrictive pulmonary deficits, and local recurrence.[32,33] Late complications may include issues with the prosthetic material such as broken titanium barrier or hernia development.

In regard to bony stabilization of the chest wall, thoracic wound skeletal repair may be indicated if more than four consecutive ribs are resected or if the defect is greater than 5 cm. For skeletal reconstruction, options include autograft, allograft, and prosthetic implants. Polypropylene or expanded polytetrafluoroethylene mesh, methyl methacrylate, titanium mesh, acellular dermal matrix, or bone grafts or flaps can be used. When thinking about the optimal prosthetic material, characteristics to think about include rigidity, inertness, malleability, and radiolucency. Polypropylene mesh is semirigid, which is beneficial, but it can fragment, cause seroma formation, or become infected. Expanded polytetrafluoroethylene mesh is also semirigid, malleable, and flexible, but it is higher cost and also is associated with seroma formation. Methyl methacrylate, which becomes rigid through exothermic reaction, is often placed between two pieces of Prolene or other mesh, creating a methyl methacrylate sandwich. Benefits of methyl methacrylate include quick fixation, cost-effectiveness, easy customization per patient, and no additional donor site (i.e., rib graft) is required. Negatives with methyl methacrylate include poor anchorage and fixation, risk of fracture, and infection. Acellular dermal matrix, which is semirigid, becomes vascularized and incorporated into the chest wall, with benefits of reduced risk of infection. Titanium plates provide rigid fixation but have the risk of fracture, extrusion, and infection. Overall, a variety of synthetic materials are available to reconstruct the chest wall with different preferences of the surgeon and different benefits for each individual patient. As new technology develops, virtual 3D models have assisted in helping plan reconstruction. One technique is shaded surface displace volume rendering (SS-VRT) that creates a 3D depiction from a CT scan to help determine the volume and space of the area to be resected and reconstructed.[34]

In particular, chest wall reconstruction in the setting of sternotomy defects and osteoradionecrosis must first focus on obtaining a healthy wound bed. Initial management includes antibiotics, drainage and debridement of all devitalized tissue, cultures, and imaging.[35,36] Surgical debridement in collaboration with the cardiothoracic surgery team is necessary, followed by local wound care and negative pressure wound therapy if actively infected. Local wound care involves wet-to-dry dressing changes with normal saline or sodium hypochlorite solutions. If sternal wires or infected hardware is within the wound bed, then removal may be required. Negative pressure wound therapy promotes healthy granulation tissue and contraction in the wound bed size. In addition, incisional vacuums have been shown to be helpful once the incision has been closed to help prevent infection and dehiscence.

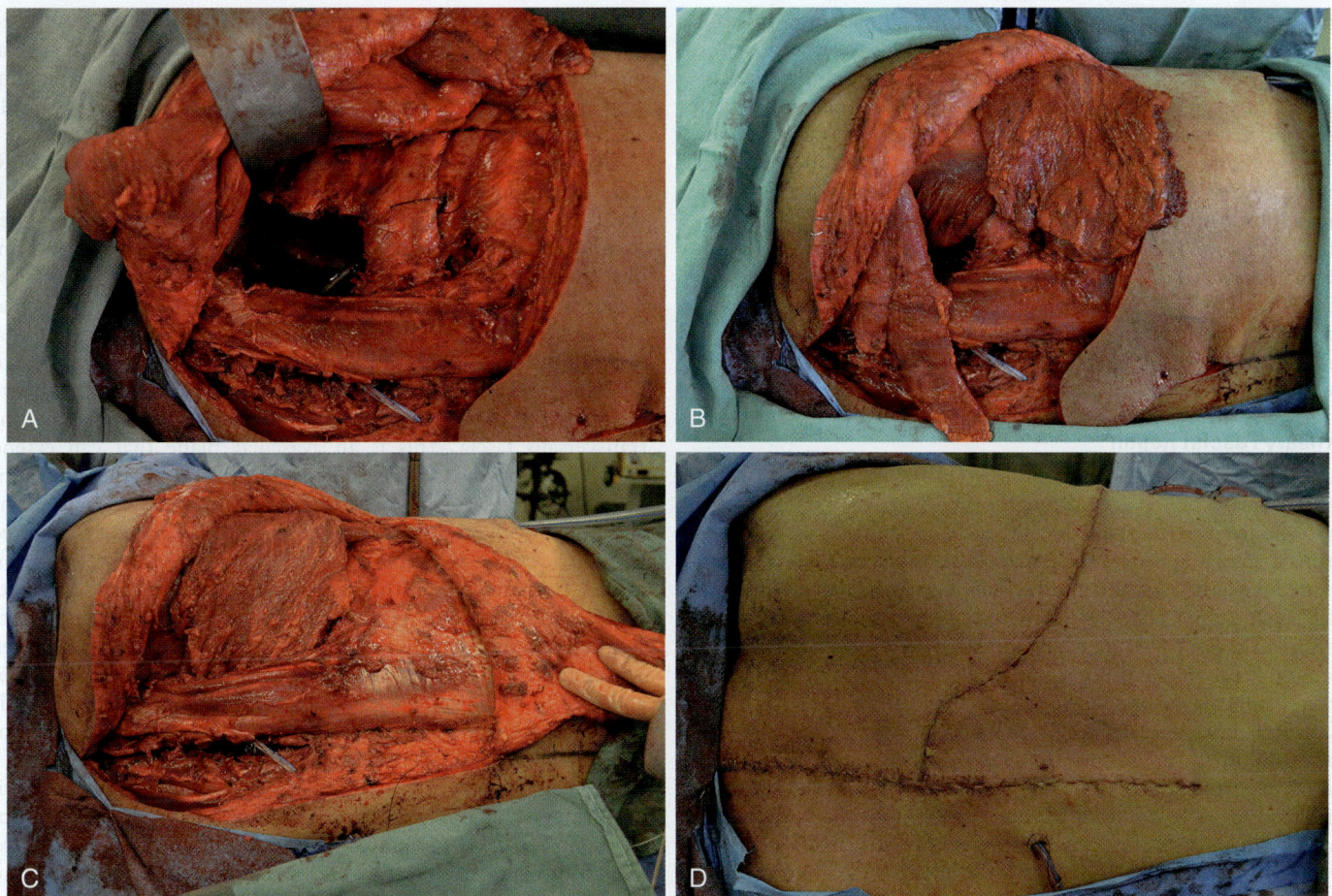

FIGURE 69.3 (A) Plastic surgery was consulted for reconstruction of a large posterior thoracic defect including lung, pleura, rib, and muscle. (B) Two rotational flaps were harvested from the back for obliteration of the thoracic opening and full coverage of the radiated field. (C) The trapezius flap was placed intrathoracically for dead space control and pleural fistula prevention, while the latissimus dorsi was used for bony chest wall coverage. (D) The patient was closed primarily over the flaps with no need for additional soft tissue.

Some reconstructive surgeons advocate for rigid fixation of the sternum and ribs, whereas other reconstructive surgeons do not advocate for rigid fixation given the sternal-rib joints are not rigid in a natural physiologic state. Hardware prevents friction between sternal segments, which may prevent infection; however, in the setting of established infection, hardware may become contaminated, thus presenting additional problems. In patients with a history of significant radiation, chest wall mobility may be stabilized by long-standing fibrosis. Most treatment involves aggressive debridement and vascularized flap coverage. In the setting of previous radiation, liberal excision of rib and sternum must be performed to remove all elements potentially suffering from osteoradionecrosis, or recurrent sinus tracts may occur.

Abdominal Wall

The structural composition of the abdominal wall can be thought of as a musculoaponeurotic girdle composed of muscle layers bound by fascia that coalesce into static supports. The ventral abdominal wall consists of longitudinally oriented rectus abdominis muscles enclosed between the anterior and posterior rectus sheaths, which receive contributions from the external oblique, internal oblique, and transversus abdominis muscles and the transversalis fascia. It extends from the xyphoid to the pubis and is bound laterally by the linea semilunaris.

A laparotomy is generally performed by dividing the midline linea alba. Poor healing and weakened scar formation along this area, amplified by increased intrabdominal pressure and lateral pull of the abdominal musculature, can lead to the development of hernia defects. The incidence of ventral hernia after laparotomy ranges from 1% to 20%, and hernia recurrence rates range from 20% to 48%.[37] The main objective of hernia repair is to attain primary fascial closure, reduce tension along the closure, and provide reinforcement to the abdominal wall fascia. With long oncologic abdominal surgeries, tissue edema and swelling are significant. The oncologic reconstructive surgeon uses hernia repair techniques that provide robust repairs while allowing for bowel edema and necessary ostomies or ileal conduits.

Preoperative Optimization

Although the need for expedient surgery in tumor removal may not allow enough time for preoperative optimization, when possible modifiable risk factors such as glucose control, tobacco use, and obesity should be optimized to improve outcomes.

Elevated blood glucose greater than 200 mg/dL and hemoglobin A1c greater than 6.5 are associated with threefold higher wound dehiscence rates.[38] Multiple trials and observational studies have demonstrated that smoking tobacco reduces tissue perfusion and leads to necrosis and abscess formation. Smoking is a known risk for hernia repair failure. Although patients with cancer may not have sufficient time for smoking cessation before surgery, they must be counseled extensively that postoperative use significantly affects their chance of hernia recurrence. Obesity is yet another potentially modifiable risk factor that can materially affect outcomes. A study out of MD Anderson Cancer Center that reviewed 511 abdominal wall reconstruction patients with a mean follow-up of 32 months demonstrated that obesity contributed to higher rates of surgical site occurrence (SSO) but not hernia recurrence. Most patients in the study had a BMI of less than 40. BMI of 32 was to be an inflection point for increased complications.[39] Studies from other institutions have consistently demonstrated threefold higher rates of hernia recurrence in patients with BMI greater than 40.[40]

Primary Fascial Repair

After reduction of a hernia or resection of tumor, the defect should ideally be repaired through primary approximation of the myofascial edges reinforced with deep mesh placement. When primary fascial approximation cannot be achieved because of increased tension along the midline, mesh is used to bridge myofascial layers at the edges of the defect. Primary reinforced fascial repair is a major determinant of improved postoperative outcomes because it provides a more robust multilayered closure compared with a single-layer bridged repair. A study out of MD Anderson Cancer Center that reviewed 535 consecutive patients with a mean follow-up of 30 months showed a fivefold higher rate of hernia recurrence and twice the rate of overall complications in bridged repairs compared with cases in which primary reinforced fascial closure was performed. The interval to hernia recurrence was also found to be ninefold shorter in the bridged group.[41] In light of the benefits of primary fascial repair, tension reduction techniques such as anterior component separation (ACS) and transversus abdominis release (TAR) have become popular. These techniques leverage the layered anatomy of the abdominal wall to reduce tension across the closure and increase chances of primary fascial repair.

ACS is a surgical technique in which the external oblique fascia is incised near the linea semilunaris to reduce the lateral force exerted by the external oblique muscle on the rectus complex and midline closure. ACS initially described in the 1960s was popularized by Ramirez in 1990.[42] The traditional description of this technique involves elevation of overlying abdominal skin and soft tissue from the midline to 2 cm lateral to the linea semilunaris. The external oblique fascia is then divided 2 cm lateral to the linea semilunaris, and the muscle is elevated off the internal oblique, allowing the internal oblique, transversus muscle, and posterior rectus sheath to move medially. These maneuvers allow additional medial migration of the rectus complex at the epigastrium (3 cm), midline (5 cm), and inferiorly (2 cm). Five centimeters of medial migration bilaterally along the midline can enable surgeons to close defects of up to 10 cm and reduce the need for bridged repair. The dissection also maintains complete neurotization of the muscle complex, as it spares the plane between the internal oblique and transversus muscles, which contain the neurovascular bundles.

One of the major drawbacks of traditional open ACS is the need to elevate an extensive amount of overlying soft tissue, which leads to higher seroma and abscess rates. Division of periumbilical perforators leads to hypoperfusion of the midline skin and increased rates of soft tissue necrosis. Perforator-sparing techniques such as endoscopic and nonendoscopic minimally invasive

approaches consequently gained popularity. When compared with traditional open ACS, perforator-sparing approaches such as minimally-invasive component separation (MICS) have demonstrated lower rates of skin dehiscence (11% vs. 28%; $p < 0.011$) and wound-healing complications (14% vs. 32%; $p < 0.026$).[43]

Posterior component separation, generally referred to as TAR, is an extension of the Rives-Stoppa repair.[44] The posterior rectus sheath is dissected off the rectus muscle laterally up to the linea semilunaris. The thoracolumbar-intercostal neurovascular bundles entering the rectus complex are visualized, and the posterior leaflet of the internal oblique fascia medial to the neurovascular bundles is incised. This opens the interval between internal oblique and transversus abdominis that contains the neurovascular bundles. The transversus abdominis muscle is then divided to open up the plane between the transversus abdominis and the transversalis fascia. This is an avascular plane that can extend laterally to the psoas muscles. A large piece of synthetic mesh is generally placed in this protected plane to widely reinforce the abdominal wall. Transversus abdominis release has been reported to allow for almost 10 cm of medial migration of the rectus complexes. Proponents hail this technique because it avoids transection of medial rectus perforators and allows for placement of synthetic mesh in a protected plane that prevents contact between bowel and mesh. TAR has been reported to have low SSI (9.1%) and SSO (18%) rates along with very low rates of hernia recurrence (3.7%) at 31.5 months.[45] Head-to-head comparisons between anterior and posterior component separations have a significant amount of heterogeneity with respect to how ACS is performed. The TAR approach has been shown to have superior SSO and SSI rates compared with open ACS, which is not unexpected given that all medial skin perforators are transected and large areas of dead space are created with the traditional open technique. When compared with the perforator-sparing or MICS approach, the difference between outcomes is less significant.[46] Large prospective, less heterogenous studies are needed to provide a better comparison between the techniques.

Mesh Types

Mesh reinforcement of hernia repairs has been clearly demonstrated to reduce hernia recurrence by almost 50%. However, there is an ongoing discussion about what mesh type is most appropriate. Meshes can be broadly categorized as synthetic, bioprosthetic, or biosynthetic.[47]

Synthetic meshes are generally made from polymers such as polypropylene, polyester, and polytetrafluoroethylene (PTFE) and can differ with respect to density of material and pore size. Lightweight, macroporous materials have the advantage of inducing more type I collagen production, better long-term incorporation, and less scarring or fibrosis but have a higher mesh fracture rate. Heavyweight, microporous material, on the other hand, can develop bridging fibrosis and significant patient discomfort because of their poor compliance. Microporous material such as PTFE encapsulates rather than integrates, which reduces their ability to clear infection and may require explantation.

Bioprosthetic materials include acellular dermal matrices, intestinal submucosa, or ovine rumen that has been processed, decellularized, and sometimes cross-linked. These materials have a superior ability to integrate and clear infection and hence can be used in contaminated settings. This is especially important in the oncologic setting, where bowel and bladder resections are common. However, biologic meshes do have some drawbacks. Some studies comparing the results of synthetic and bioprosthetic mesh materials have generally demonstrated higher rates of hernia recurrence with bioprosthetic meshes. However, this may be dependent on technique. Long-term studies using bioprosthetic mesh reported from MD Anderson Cancer Center have demonstrated superior outcomes. In a recent study of 725 patients, 44% of repairs were completed in clean-contaminated and 14% in contaminated/infected settings, with a median follow-up of 34 months. SSO rate was 27% and hernia recurrence rate was only 13%. Long-term durability of bioprosthetic mesh repair was further demonstrated in a subset of these patients, with a median follow-up of 82 months, who were noted to have a hernia recurrence rate of 16%.[48] Obesity, bridged repair, and stoma presence were noted to be independent predictors of hernia recurrence.

A third group of more recently introduced mesh materials known as biosynthetic mesh are gaining popularity because they can resorb over time to avoid long-term complications of permanent mesh materials. The quick resorption rate could potentially contribute to a higher hernia recurrence. These meshes are created from resorbable materials such as polyglycolic acid (PGA), polylactic acid, trimethyl carbonate (TMC), and poly-4-hydroxybutyrate and tend to resorb between 6 and 18 months. The COBRA study prospectively evaluated 104 patients who underwent abdominal wall reconstruction with Gore BIO-A (PGA/TMC) mesh that resorbs in 6 months. Hernia recurrence was noted to be 14% at 2 years with an SSO rate of 28%.[49] Another biosynthetic mesh (Phasix) that is resorbed at 12 to 18 months was noted to have a hernia recurrence rate of 22% at 5 years.[50] More in-depth studies and longer follow-up are needed to better understand the indication of these mesh types.

Soft Tissue Management

In addition to myofascial repair and reinforcement, management of the overlying soft tissue can affect the outcome of hernia repair as it affects rates of contamination, infection, and mesh incorporation. Soft tissue defects in the cancer population are generally sustained in the tumor excision or flap harvest for pelvic reconstruction. Depending on the size and location, these defects can be managed using local tissue rearrangement, pedicled flaps, or free flaps. The tissue flap option that is used to repair the soft tissue defect should not be simultaneously used to reconstruct the myofascial defect. Using a single flap to restore musculofascial integrity and reconstruct the overlying soft tissue compromises both the durability of the hernia repair and the vascularity of the soft tissue component. To provide a framework to guide soft tissue choice, the ventral abdominal wall can be subdivided into the epigastric, paraumbilical, and hypogastric regions.[51]

Epigastric defects can extend from the xyphoid process to an imaginary transverse line connecting the caudal tips of the costal margins. Local flap options include adjacent tissue transfer or pedicled perforator flaps. Adjacent tissue transfer options such as rotation advancement, VY advancement, or keystone flaps are chosen based on the laxity of tissue and its vascularity. Scarring because of prior surgery or radiation may limit these options. Perforator-based flaps can be designed around the internal mammary or intercostal perforators and rotated into the defect. For larger defects, regional pedicled flap options such a rectus abdominis muscle or rectus abdominis myocutaneous flap can be used. The omentum flap can potentially be used but requires an obligate hernia to transfer the flap from its intrabdominal location. The thigh and back provide the mainstay for free tissue transfer choices if defect size precludes local options.

The paraumbilical region of the abdominal wall affords the highest degree of both myofascial and soft tissue laxity. The increased soft tissue laxity in this region allows local options such as wide undermining, VY advancement, rotation advancement, or keystone flaps to resurface larger areas than is possible in other locations of the abdominal wall. Moderate- to large-sized defects in this location are also amenable to reconstruction using bipedicled fasciocutaneous flaps. These flaps are oriented longitudinally and designed to maintain a 3:1 length-to-width ratio to maintain blood supply from the superior and inferior poles. They are elevated off the rectus or oblique fascia, leaving the superior and inferior poles connected at the level of the groin and costal margin. The flaps are then advanced medially, and the exposed donor site fascia is skin grafted. To reduce the probability of hypoperfusion at the midline, a wider portion of the flap is left connected at the poles, which may limit the extent of medial migration. Although the paraumbilical location affords the highest soft tissue laxity of adjacent soft tissue, it is also the farthest from any of the nutrient vessel options needed to vascularize free flaps. To reconstruct large defects, free flaps are harvested from the thigh and anastomosed to the deep inferior epigastric or internal mammary vessels with the use of interposition vein grafts.

The hypogastric region is bordered by the arcuate line superiorly, the pubic symphysis inferiorly, and the coalescence of the linea semilunaris and inguinal ligament laterally. Although the lack of soft tissue laxity precludes many local options, proximity to the lateral circumflex femoral vessels allows for multiple thigh-based pedicled flap options. The anterolateral thigh flap can be elevated on the descending branch of the lateral circumflex vessels and transposed to this region by routing the pedicle deep to the rectus femoris muscle and superficial to the inguinal ligament via a subcutaneous tunnel. Care must be taken to avoid compression of the pedicle. Depending on the vascular anatomy, if the pedicle reach is limited and if extrinsic compression cannot be avoided, the flaps are harvested as free flaps.

In certain cases, soft tissue excess associated with increased dead space, increased tension on the incision, or poor tissue quality needs to be addressed. A vertical, horizontal, or combination (fleur de leis) panniculectomy is performed at the time of the hernia repair.

Pelvis and Perineal Reconstruction

The deep pelvis, genitourinary tract, and perineum provide a unique challenge to the reconstructive surgeon. Complex 3D anatomy and functional requirements demand thoughtful and durable reconstruction. Aesthetic considerations, in particular with regard to sexuality, are of great concern to many patients. Recent studies document the increasing trend of plastic surgery flap reconstruction of pelvic oncologic defects in the last 20 years, with decreasing risk of wound breakdown and secondary procedures for dehiscence.[51–53] Reconstructive plastic surgery is of paramount importance to patients undergoing challenging resections, for both physiologic and emotional healing.

Preoperative Considerations

Before operation, preoperative consult with a reconstructive surgeon is critical to establish a physiologic baseline and discuss postoperative expectations. Open discussion regarding postoperative functional and aesthetic changes ahead of time dramatically reduces anxiety for the patient and sets realistic goals for both patient and surgeon. This conversation gives the patient a sense of ownership in their postoperative outcome and restores a sense of control.

Neoadjuvant radiation is extremely common in cancers affecting the pelvis and genital tracts. Although absolutely beneficial and required, it unequivocally makes tissue healing slower and delayed. Radiation therapy induces a cascade of cellular events that begins with the influx of inflammatory cells causing erythema, desquamation, and ulceration and results in chronic changes from fibroblast proliferation including inelastic and thickened skin. At the time of preoperative consult, many patients present with ongoing stigmata of radiation treatment, including poor skin laxity, alopecia, decreased vascularity of soft tissue, and labial or introital strictures. Jakowatz et al. found that patients receiving pelvic radiation before exenteration had a significantly higher complication rate (67%) compared with those who did not receive radiation (26%).[54] When discussing reconstructive surgery, the patient should be advised early that their surgical sites will require careful attention to hygiene and positioning to prevent undue burden on physiologically stressed tissue.

Previous surgical history must be discussed in depth. Prior caesarian sections or pelvic surgeries may have damaged important vascular pedicles to reconstructive flaps. The reconstructive workhorse flap, the omental flap, is often scarred and frozen because of previous exploratory laparotomies or prior debulking procedures. Diverting ostomies affect one half of the abdominal wall and may alter the use of important flaps such as the VRAM. Liposuction, which is frequently considered "nonoperative" by patients, can disrupt superficial vascular perforators. In the thigh or abdomen, this may render a local flap unusable and must be a point of discussion.

Regardless of age or orientation, sexual function and activity must be discussed. Frequently, patients have ceased intimate relations because of pain, tumor-related discharge, or radiation changes and strictures. However, many patients, when carefully asked, will say that they wish to resume activity in the future if possible. Patients may have strongly charged and emotional reactions to the changes that have occurred to their genital and pelvic structures as a result of cancer. Most worry that their partner, or future partner, may find them undesirable based on surgical changes. Many are frightened when considering penetrating intercourse because of postradiation burning and pain. It is extremely important to tease out the patient's desire for sexual intercourse as they are now versus how they may feel when fully healed. Maintenance of sexual function and prevention of the psychological sequelae of surgery are fundamental issues.

For patients who have interest in penetrating intercourse in the future, surgery affecting the vagina or perineum should be reconstructed with adequate soft tissue to prevent scarring or stricture. See Fig. 69.4 for an example of insufficient soft tissue reconstruction causing stricture after radiation. Furthermore, the patients should be advised that postoperative maintenance, such as daily dilation or penetration, will be required to keep a reconstructed vault open. Patients must be told genital sensation changes are the rule, rather than the exception. In male patients, surgery near the prostate or deep pelvis may significantly impair erectile function and should be counseled by their urologist. Lastly, if the partner is present, it is important to consider their feelings regarding sexuality.

Intraoperative Considerations

Reconstruction is highly dependent on the size of resection and the components removed. Small, narrow male pelvises may

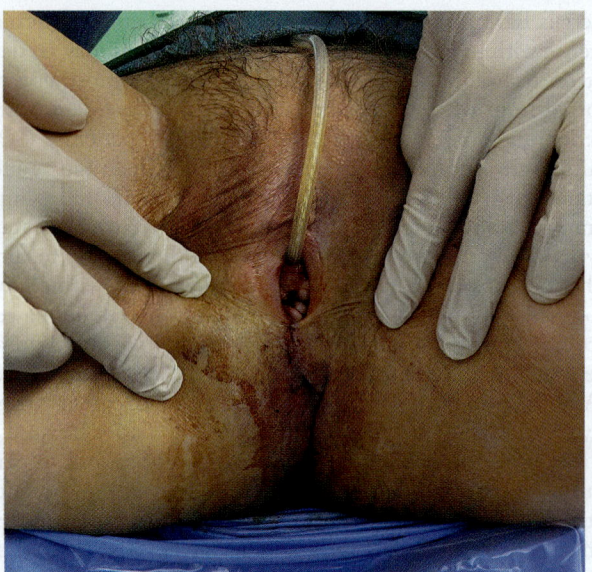

FIGURE 69.4 This is an example of a patient with resultant stricture after closure without sufficient soft tissue replacement. The patient presented after previous vaginal introitus resection with primary closure and adjuvant radiation. She complained of severe webbing and stricture that prevented intercourse and caused excoriation when sitting.

require less tissue to reconstruct an abdominoperineal resection (APR); however, a broad female pelvis with vaginal resection will likely require a large-volume flap. The reconstruction of the pelvis and perineum is affected by the size of the pelvic outlet and components removed.

In many instances of pelvic reconstruction, the rectum, uterus, prostate, or bladder may be taken. This creates a large pelvic dead space. If the pelvic floor is left bereft of sufficient soft tissue, fluid collections and potential abscess may occur. Small bowel may migrate to the pelvic floor. In radiated patients, bowel adhesions near the pelvic floor may result in eventual fistula. If substantial pelvic floor musculature is removed, herniation of intraabdominal contents is possible. For these reasons, sufficient vascularized soft tissue should be brought to the pelvis when more than one structure is removed.

The omental flap is a workhorse flap for obliteration of pelvic dead space. It is large and fan-shaped with a reliable arterial arcade fed by three vascular branches: the right, middle, and left omental vessels. These vessels originate from the right and left gastroepiploic vessels. The flap may be isolated on one of its vascular pedicles, usually the right gastroepiploic, as it is larger, and will retain sufficient vasculature inflow to supply the entire flap. Ligation of the additional pedicles allows the flap to be advanced deeper into the pelvis. As a free flap, it can be up to 40 × 60 centimeters in size, although as a pedicled flap it more commonly provides 20 × 30 cm at the target location. Studies have documented the favorable use of the omentum for pelvic dead space obliteration.[55] It is an excellent choice for a narrow pelvis when the external defect is minimal, such as a male APR. However, its size may limit its use in larger defects and provides no cutaneous paddle. When a large or external defect is present, an abdominal-based flap may be preferred.

In cases where the omental flap is prohibitively scarred and small, alternative sources of tissue may come from the abdominal wall. The rectus muscle may be harvested alone or in combination with its fascia and overlying cutaneous tissue, also known as a

VRAM flap. Both the rectus flap alone and the VRAM require isolation of the flap on the deep inferior epigastric artery and vein system. These vessels are readily isolated as they branch from the external iliac artery and vein before the inguinal canal. The rectus flap is helpful for small defects but may prove to be insufficient in a broad gynecoid pelvis. Furthermore, the muscle will undergo atrophy over time from ligation of the motor nerves. Alternatively, the VRAM flap can be designed with variable sizes of skin and subcutaneous tissue. Modifications such as the extended VRAM, which incorporates tissue near the costal cartilages, allows the flap to reach nearly 30 to 40 centimeters from its vascular pedicle and may be up to 10 cm wide. For the reconstructive surgeon, the VRAM provides extreme flexibility to reconstruct a variety of defects.

Importantly, it must be discussed that the traditional VRAM does create an incisional hernia of the abdominal wall that requires repair. Fascial and muscle-sparing techniques have been popularized to avoid this comorbidity, but patients must be counseled regarding the potential for bulge, hernia, or weakness in the future. When a traditional VRAM is taken, or even a fascial-sparing VRAM, some surgeons advocate mesh placement in comorbid patients. This mesh is used to reinforce the abdominal wall repair prophylactically, especially if an ostomy is present. Frequently, a biologic mesh is chosen for its resistance to bacterial contamination. Techniques to minimize wound-healing issues, such as perforator and fascial-sparing harvest, can improve outcomes. When two ostomies are required, such as when there is a complete pelvic exenteration, the necessary ileal conduit will be on the patient's right side and the colostomy on the left. In this scenario, it is best to harvest the VRAM before ostomy positioning and then reinforce both after both ostomies are seated. Two ostomies on the abdominal wall create a high-risk situation for hernia formation. Prophylactic reinforcement is helpful because reentering the pelvic exenteration abdomen for hernia repair is fraught with peril. Valuable insight regarding abdominal wall repair is discussed previously in the chapter. See an example of VRAM harvest and abdominal closure with component separation and mesh in Fig. 69.5.

Of note, it is important to know that as robotic and laparoscopic extirpative surgery advances, so does flap harvest. Several studies now demonstrate excellent results with the use of robotically harvested rectus abdominis muscle flap for pelvic dead space obliteration.[56] Alternatively, if the abdominal wall is inaccessible or unavailable, local tissue flaps from the thigh may be considered for pelvic dead space fill. However, these flaps remain second choice unless an external defect is present. Even with certain external defects, the reach of such flaps at the gracilis or profunda artery perforator may be limited. See Fig. 69.5 for a male pelvis after robotic total pelvic exenteration reconstructed bilateral gracilis flaps.

Vaginal Reconstruction

Because of its proximity to the rectum and anus, vaginal defects are common after extensive colorectal resection. Vaginal defects after oncologic resection vary from mucosal excision to full circumferential loss. Pusic describes an algorithmic approach to vaginal reconstruction based on defect classification.[57] In these classifications, defects are described as partial (type I) or total (type II) and further subclassified based on location. The authors describe the use of three workhorse flaps for reconstruction of these defects, including the rectus abdominis, gracilis, and Singapore flaps. This algorithm demonstrates the choice of flap based

on location as well as body habitus and is highly valuable as a reference.

With small defects of the vagina (less than one-third the circumference), primary repair of the vaginal wall may be possible. However, if a patient has previously undergone radiation or surgery, constriction and atrophy of the tissue may prevent sufficient laxity for repair. It is especially important to have asked a patient about their sexual activity preoperatively for this reason. If a patient desires a vagina sufficient for penetration, the vault must be reconstructed with enough depth and laxity for this purpose. Additionally, if the vaginal mucosa is intact but heavily thinned by the resection, reinforcement with a rotational flap such as the omentum or rectus may prevent ulceration or breakdown in high-risk patients.

In regard to vaginal repair of over one-third of the circumference, such as a type IA or IB, several options exist. As previously discussed, the VRAM is an extremely reliable source of tissue with multiple design permutations available. For resections that are near or involve the cervix, such as posterior vaginectomy, the cutaneous paddle of the VRAM provides exceptional lining of the vault, and the subcutaneous tissue provides posterior dead space obliteration or perineal reconstruction. Multiple authors cite the VRAM as the best choice for posterior vaginal defects (Fig. 69.6).[57-59] In more involved vaginectomies or total vaginectomies, the VRAM may be tubularized and inset as a neovagina. For total vaginectomy, it is recommended to provide a cutaneous paddle at least 9×9 cm so as to allow a 3-cm circumference and 8- to 9-cm depth. In females who are obese or have significant central adiposity, the cutaneous paddle may be prohibitively thick for inset. In these instances, the rectus flap may be harvested with the anterior fascia or posterior peritoneum alone. This surface is then skin grafted or allowed to mucosalize secondarily. Skin grafting may slightly decrease secondary contraction but is prone to poor take given the difficulty of graft stabilization.

Alternatives to abdominal-based vaginal reconstruction include local rotational flaps from the thigh. The gracilis muscle and/or its overlying cutaneous tissue may be dissected as a rotational flap on the medial femoral circumflex artery and venae comitantes. The skin paddle may be designed vertically (for increased intrapelvic length) or transversely. The gracilis is located just posterior to the adductor longus muscle and anterior to the adductor magnus. In thin patients, the gracilis flap is exceptionally pliable and valued for ease of inset. It is very useful for treating vaginal fistulas when no laparotomy is performed. However, it may also be insufficient in size for larger defects. In these cases, bilateral gracilis flaps may be harvested and used in conjunction. This is especially useful for low or total vaginectomy defects, such a Pusic type IIB. In high-volume centers, surgeons may need to reconstruct defects after recurrent cancer resection, which removes a previous flap. The gracilis can also serve as an important second-line flap for this purpose.

An alternative to the gracilis flap is the PAP flap. This flap is based on perforators traveling through the adductor magnus muscle or between the adductor muscle septums. In the right patient, it has exceptional use for low vaginal or introital defects. It may also be designed vertically or horizontally. As with all flaps, body habitus will largely determine the bulk and reach of any of these local flaps.

An additional flap that is highly useful for anterior (Pusic type IA) or low vaginal defects is the Singapore flap. This flap incorporates thin, pliable fasciocutaneous groin tissue (lateral to labia) based on the posterior labial artery perforators, which is a

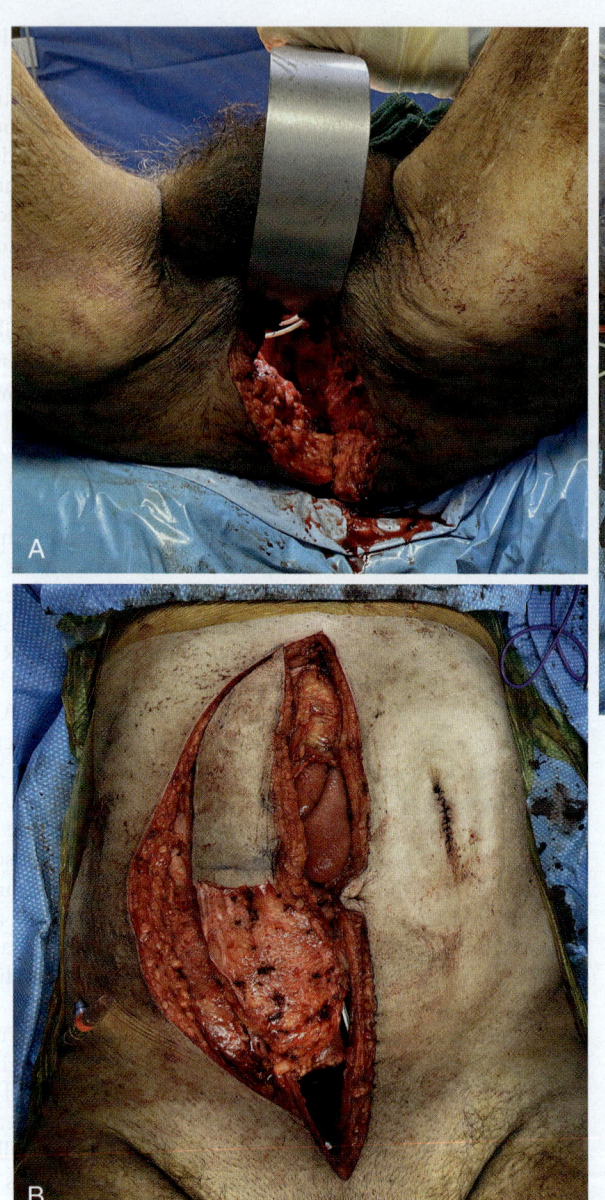

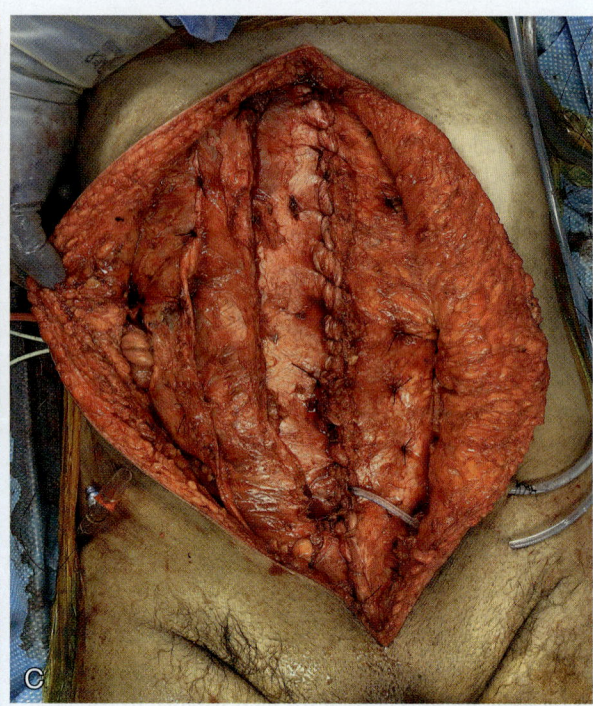

FIGURE 69.5 (A) This image demonstrates a large pelvic defect in a male pelvis after robotic total pelvic exenteration. (B) Because of the extent of dead space in the deep pelvis, the patient required a rotational vertical rectus abdominis myocutaneous (VRAM) flap for closure of the pelvis and perineum. The flap is partially deepithelialized to allow this portion to remain intrapelvic and the epithelialized portion to be externalized and line the perineum. (C) The patient's abdomen is closed with unilateral right anterior component separation and underlay biologic mesh around the ileal conduit and colostomy.

continuation of the perineal artery. These flaps may be designed up to 6 × 15 centimeters. The Singapore flap is raised unilaterally or bilaterally and rotated medially for repair of defects near the introitus. See Fig. 69.7. It is exceptionally useful in patients with vaginal fistulas that require healthy vascularized tissue for closure. Because of its proximity to the vagina, it may be less reliable in patients who have been radiated or undergone multiple previous local excisions. Ultrasound-guided (Doppler) investigation of available perforators is highly valuable in such instances.

In vaginal reconstruction, if the vaginal introitus is involved, it cannot be overstated that sufficient soft tissue surface area must be restored. Without sufficient tissue, the perineal and introital tissues are prone to stricture, webbing, and excoriation. Painful tears

and scar banding may occur and prohibit not only sexual activity but routine sitting and stair climbing.

Vulvar Repair

Similar to the vagina, the vulva is frequently implicated in tumors that affect the perineal region. The vulva is a collective term for the female external genitalia that includes the mons pubis, labia majora, labia minora, clitoris, and vestibule. The vestibule is the triangular space between the labia minora where the urethra and vagina open. All structures are important considerations in peripelvic female reconstruction.

The labia majora and labia minora serve both functional and aesthetic purposes to the female genitourinary tract. As protection for sensitive structures, their loss may cause exquisite sensitivity or

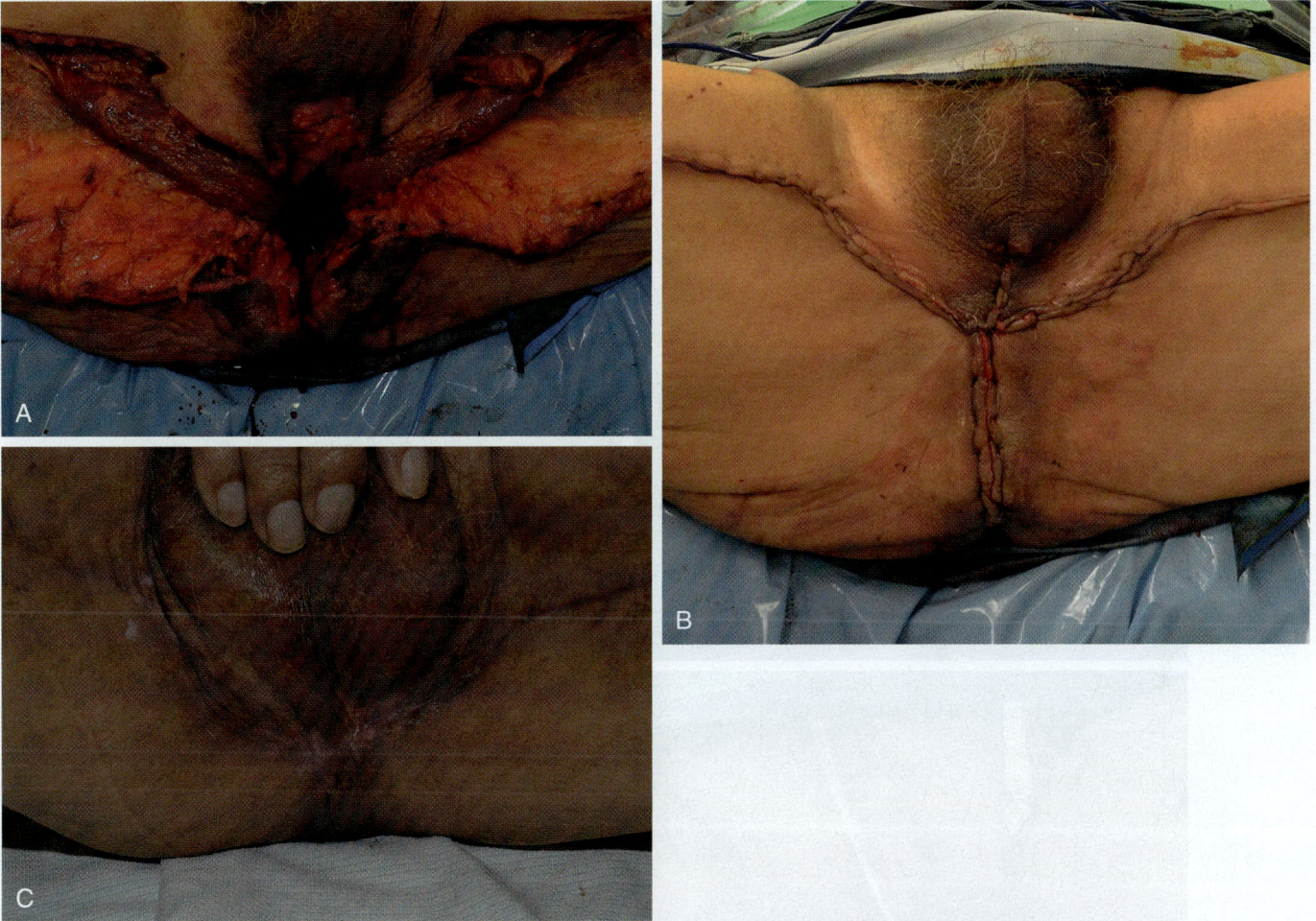

FIGURE 69.6 (A) This male patient underwent robotic-assisted abdominoperineal resection. Because of the narrow outlet of the male pelvis, rotational bilateral gracilis flaps were sufficient to line the outlet with vascularized muscle and prevent bowel prolapse. (B) The patient was closed primarily over the muscle. (C) The patient healed without issue.

dyspareunia. In particular, the labia major make up prominent folds of cutaneous tissue that protect the orifices of the urogenital triangle. The labia minora unite superiorly to protect the clitoris. Aesthetically, many patients feel disfigured or unattractive if these structures are removed.

Isolated vulvar cancer, including cancers of the labia, is rare, accounting for less than 5% of female genital cancers. However, resection of labial and vulvar structures is common in combination with other peripelvic cancers. Vulvar reconstruction attempts to restore genitalia, body image, sexual function, micturition, and defecation. Several algorithms have been proposed based on location and size of the defect.[60–61a] The vulva is generally divided into the upper third (mons pubis to labia), the middle third (labia proper), and the lower third (vaginal orifice and perineum).

In general, upper-third defects less than 20 cm² can be closed primarily or with adjacent tissue transfer. In multiparous females, the upper abdomen may be recruited in "abdominoplasty fashion" to cover defects of the mons. In larger defects, local rotational flaps, such as the anterolateral thigh flap, may be needed to restore adequate soft tissue. The anterolateral thigh flap is based on the descending branch of the lateral femoral circumflex artery and its associated venae comitantes. The pedicle travels in the septum between the vastus lateralis and rectus femoris muscles and gives

several musculocutaneous or septocutaneous perforators to the overlying thigh skin. The flap can be designed with skin paddles up to 8 × 20 cm and still undergo primary closure of the donor site. It may be rotated above or below the rectus femoris muscle based on necessary pedicle length.

Middle-third defect reconstruction, including those of the labia major and labia minora, is highly dependent on defect size. Small resections of the labia major (up to 2 cm) and labia minora (up to 1 cm) may be amenable to primary closure alone. Larger resections require local tissue flap coverage, including the previously mentioned Singapore, gracilis, and profunda artery perforator flaps. Several unique designs have been described in case series, including Sawada's lotus flap for vulvoperineal reconstruction.[62] In elderly patients or those with significant gluteal laxity, random pattern gluteal fold flaps may be designed that advance buttock tissue from the lateral buttock and thigh toward the perineum. This flap was initially described by Yii and Niranjan and later modified by Hashimoto.[63,64] The flap is located in the triangle formed by the ischial tuberosity, anus, and vaginal orifice. The fascia is lifted over the gluteus maximus to preserve fasciocutaneous blood supply from the internal pudendal perforators.

The lower third of the vulva includes the vaginal orifice and perineum. This area is surrounded by a rich supply of vascular

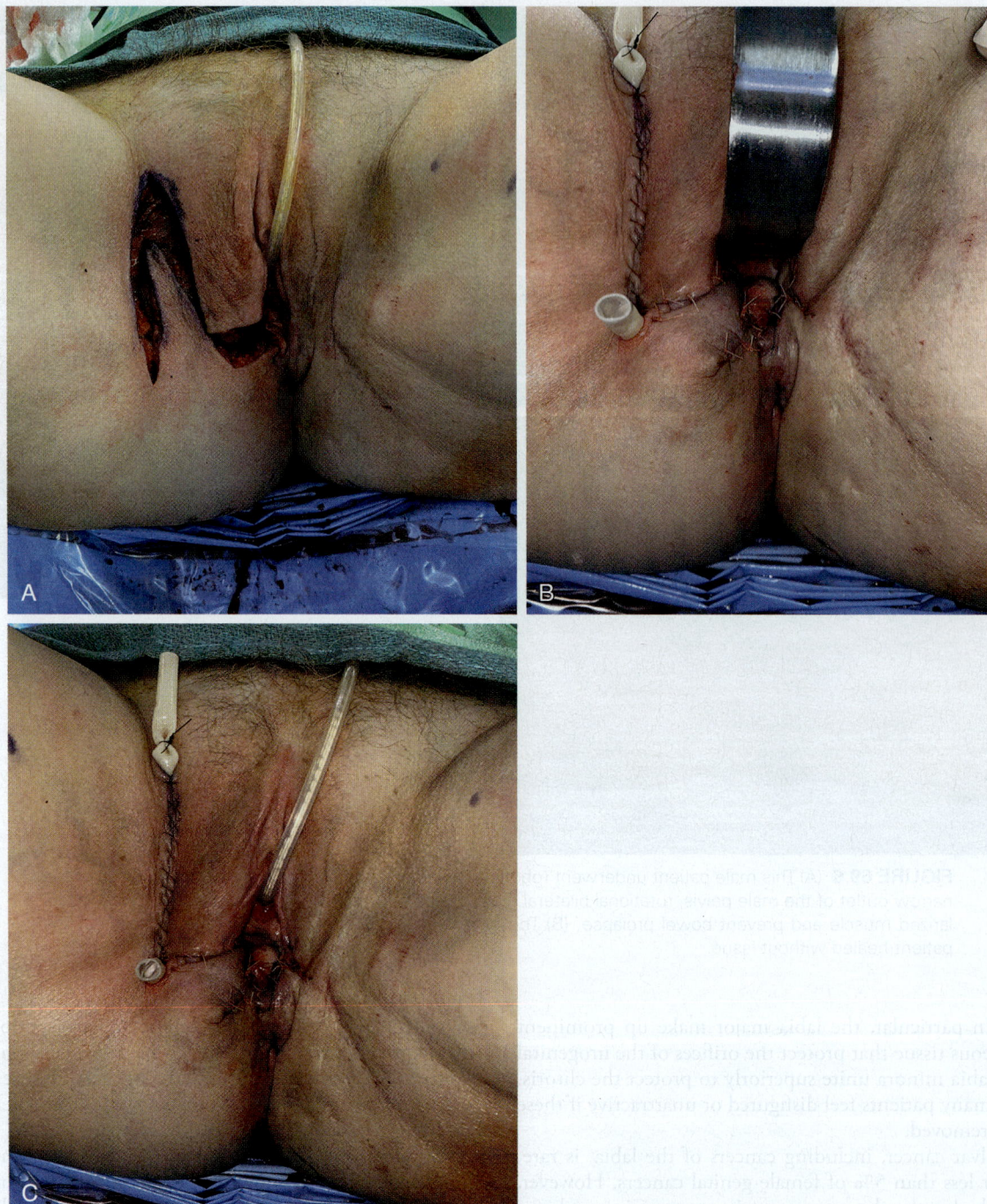

FIGURE 69.7 (A) A 50-year-old female patient presented with painful introital contracture after previous vaginal resection and radiation. After surgical release of the contracture, a unilateral Singapore flap was designed to replace the missing soft tissue. (B) The Singapore flap is rotated medially and sewn into the vaginal release and introitus. (C) After complete scar release and soft tissue replacement, the patient healed and resumed normal sitting and sexual activity at 3 months.

perforators. This region may be reconstructed using random pattern local flaps, such as the previously described gluteal fold flap, or by axial pattern flaps such as the Singapore flap. Again, it cannot be overstated that sufficient soft tissue is required in this area to prevent painful contraction or excoriation. Bilateral local flaps may be required in large defects. In defects that result from pelvic exenteration, the VRAM flap is still the gold standard because of the ability to obliterate pelvic dead space while relining the external surface area. A combination of flaps may be used in unique

defects when different subunits of the pelvis and perineum are resected (Fig. 69.8).

Postoperative Considerations

Although the reconstruction of the genitourinary and pelvic area is largely a surgical maneuver, postoperative care determines outcome. Without careful protection of surgical sites and graduated physical activity, reconstructive sites are prone to dehiscence and infection. Even with flap reconstruction, the risk of infection and

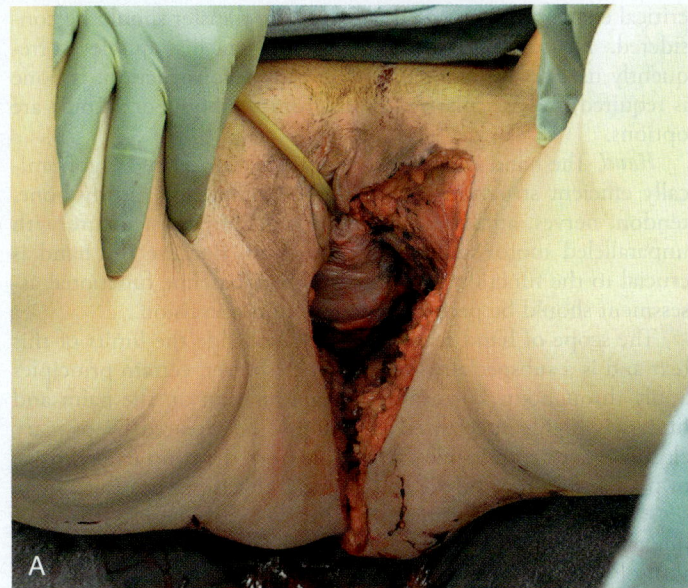

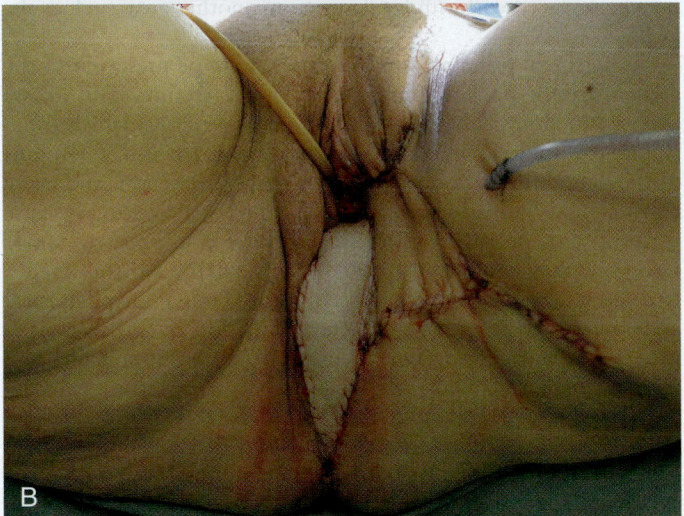

FIGURE 69.8 (A) This patient underwent a resection including a posterior vaginectomy, abdominoperineal resection (APR), and left vulvar resection. (B) A vertical rectus abdominis myocutaneous flap was used to reconstruct the vaginectomy and APR defects, while a V to Y local flap was designed from the thigh to reconstruct the vulvar defect.

pelvic abscess approaches 10%, and delayed wound healing may occur in 10% to 66% of patients.[54,65,66]

Sitting protocols are especially important to protect a new perineal reconstruction. After any rotational flap to the pelvis or perineum, it is recommended that sitting is limited significantly for a minimum of 5 days. Dependent pressure from body weight or positioning can cause ischemia and reconstructive flap loss. Furthermore, ischemia and bacterial contamination create a perfect environment for wound infection and dehiscence. Physical therapy is consulted and present postoperative day 1 so that the patient is taught to "log roll" out of bed and avoid shearing on the surgical site. Patients are allowed to ambulate short distances, such as 100 feet, up to four times a day, but are not allowed to sit at any time. This includes no sitting for transfers or toileting. As such, a Foley catheter is recommended for 5 days to limit urination on the surgical sites and to avoid sitting to urinate. A bedpan may be used for bowel movements if an ostomy is not present.

After 5 days, the patient begins a sitting protocol, which includes sitting 5 minutes four times daily (QID) the first day, 10 minutes QID the second day, 15 minutes QID the third day, and advancing as such every day until 1 hour is reached. If a patient demonstrates signs of early dehiscence or surgical site strain, this is delayed.

Surgical drains are left in all surgical sites until less than 20 cc for 2 days in a row. In particular, drains are not removed while the patient is in the early postoperative period when physical activity and sitting have yet to be fully resumed. The perineal region, secondary to the urogenital and anorectal systems, has been shown to have the highest counts of bacterial contamination in the body. In the pelvic and perineal regions, simple fluid collections will break down suture lines and form abscesses. In areas of dependency, especially those that are previously radiated, seromas will persist up to 3 weeks after surgery. Avoiding wound contamination and/or subsequent infection by urine or stool creates an environment highly susceptible to complication. The use of abundant and reliable drainage is critical.

Limitation of lifting and strenuous activity is also very important. If any abdominal surgery has taken place, patients are advised to avoid lifting anything over 10 pounds for 6 weeks. This prevents undue pressure on the abdominal repair or early ostomy. Some surgeons prefer patients to wear an abdominal binder during this period, although this is not required. Light walking or gentle stretching is recommended, but vigorous athletic activity is held until 6 weeks. This helps prevent shear and breakdown in difficult areas such as the perineum.

After reconstruction of the vaginal cavity or perineum, the area is highly prone to stricture. This is exacerbated in patients who have undergone radiation therapy. There is a careful balance between allowing sutures lines to strengthen and heal and starting scar massage and dilation to prevent contracture. In general, if a patient has healed without complication, a speculum examination is performed at 4 weeks postoperatively. If the speculum examination reveals all sutures lines intact and all tissues viable, then the patient is advised to begin dilation. Medical-grade dilators are available from a variety of companies. In general, they are sized from smallest to largest with increasing length and width. If the speculum passes easily on an adult female, it is usually recommended to start with a mid-range size and advise dilation twice daily with water-based lubricant. The patient is advised to pass the dilator into the cavity three times, gently holding and removing at each pass. At the end of 2 weeks, if there is no tightness and no pain, they then advance to the next size. Once they are able to pass the maximal size dilator, they may resume intercourse. If the patient is not resuming penetrating intercourse at least once a week, then they need to maintain dilation at least three times a week.

Extremity

Multimodality therapy has expanded the indications for limb salvage in patients with cancers of the extremities. Limb salvage, however, must not be performed at the expense of an oncologically adequate resection. In addition, preserving a limb that is nonfunctional, insensate, or painful provides no benefit over amputation. In fact, some patients may do better with a prosthesis if rehabilitation is faster. Indications for amputation after extirpative surgery include major neurovascular compromise, significant loss of muscle bulk causing a nonfunctional limb, infection or fractures that compromise reconstruction and delay adjuvant therapy, poor nutrition, serious medical conditions, and a lack of patient motivation or compliance with rehabilitation.

Defects from surgery for soft tissue and bony neoplasms, such as sarcomas, generally require larger margins than many other tumors and therefore reconstruction with pedicled or free flaps. Neoadjuvant therapy often decreases tumor size and facilitates limb salvage, but radiation therapy may also hinder wound healing and necessitate a nonirradiated tissue flap closure to provide coverage of neurovascular structures, tendons, bone, and endoprostheses.

In limb reconstruction, bony defects can be repaired with prosthetics, allografts, bone grafts, or vascularized bone flaps. Bones may also be temporarily shortened and plated, with later bone lengthening procedures such as bone transport. Free and pedicled muscle flaps not only provide well-vascularized wound coverage but can also be neurotized to provide functional muscle. Tendon transfers may be performed to allow functioning muscle bellies to take over the function of resected ones. Microsurgical techniques can be used to repair or graft damaged nerves, thereby restoring motor and sensory functions. However, because nerve regeneration occurs at a rate no faster than 1 mm/day, some muscle end plates may die before reinnervation occurs. If reinnervation is expected to take more than 12 to 18 months, some patients may be better served with tendon transfers or amputation.

At a minimum, functional upper limb reconstruction should provide a stable shoulder joint and restore elbow flexion, median nerve sensibility, and prehensile grip.[67,68] Functional lower limb reconstruction should provide at least stable hip and knee joints, moderate knee flexion and extension, and tibial nerve sensation on the plantar foot.[69] This allows the patient to feed and clothe themselves and ambulate with assistive devices. Ultimately, if a limb is amputated, fillet of digit or fillet of arm or leg flaps can be used as tissue transfers to cover open wounds.[70] In this operation, the uninvolved soft tissue portions of the distal limb are isolated on the neurovascular structures and transferred as a pedicle or free flap.

Upper Extremity

Proximal arm, elbow, and forearm. Proximal arm wounds, such as those around the humerus, can be covered with local flaps from the trunk and cervical region. Common flaps include the pectoralis major flap or pedicled latissimus dorsi flap. These flaps can be used to repair defects in the shoulder, axilla, and upper arm. The pedicled latissimus dorsi muscle flap can also be used as a functional muscle transfer to restore elbow flexion or extension in many patients.

Very high tumors of the proximal arm and shoulder joint, including the scapular region, may require amputation. If the brachial plexus or vascular supply to the arm is involved in tumor, it renders the distal arm unsalvageable. In these instances, a shoulder disarticulation (amputation at the glenohumeral joint) or forequarter amputation (amputation of the humerus, scapula, acromion, clavicle) may be required. If the periscapular tissue is involved, it may not be possible to close a defect with the local tissue. A common indication for a fillet-of-arm flap is the forequarter amputation. In this surgery, the distal, healthy forearm soft tissues and/or bone is salvaged as a free flap to reconstruct the chest wall. For oncologic purposes, this process requires that all tumor is above the elbow and one joint space away.

Soft tissue defects in the elbow and forearm are commonly reconstructed with local flaps, such as a pedicled reverse radial forearm or an ulnar forearm flap. Because of the paucity of muscle bellies in the distal forearm, other local options are scarce. If

critical elements are exposed, a free tissue transfer should be considered. Neurotized latissimus dorsi or gracilis muscle is frequently used for functional muscle belly reconstruction. If bone is required, free vascularized grafts from the fibula or scapula are options.

Hand. The hand is one of the most specialized and ergonomically efficient structures in the body. Comprising mostly bone, tendon, nerves, and skin, the hand is a compact structure with unparalleled motor and sensory function. Because the hand is crucial to the functions of everyday life, a baseline functional assessment should be performed before tumor excision.

The scope of hand reconstruction is outside the limits of this text and is a subspeciality of its own. However, certain principles apply throughout. For example, glabrous skin on the palm and fingers is highly specialized and should be repaired by primary closure whenever possible. Skin grafts from the contralateral palm or plantar foot may be the best match if this is not possible. Some sensation, especially at the fingertips, is better preserved by secondary healing than replacement with an alternate tissue. The skin of the dorsum of the hand is thin with moderate laxity and may be replaced with similar tissue from another area, such as the groin.

As a general principle, digit length should be preserved to the greatest extent possible during oncologic resection. This allows proper function of the extensor and flexor tendons, which function like a pulley system and require a fine balance. The tendons of the hand are surrounded in vascularized paratenon, and every effort should be made not to strip them of this covering because it can lead to necrosis or rupture. If they are stripped by tumor resection, they should be covered by vascularized tissue, even a free flap if necessary. Bone grafts can be used to replace phalangeal and metacarpal resections. When amputation is necessary, it is generally performed through the most distant joint possible.

When neural structures are involved, primary nerve repair or a nerve graft may be used to preserve adequate function. Epineurial or interfascicular repairs are typically performed depending on the nerve and location. Small sensory branches can be spared from the extremities and make useful grafts. A commonly harvested nerve is the sural nerve from the lower leg.

When large resections of the hand disrupt the soft tissue envelope, bone, and/or tendons but the hand is otherwise salvageable, many reconstructive surgeons will stage the reconstruction. The hand cannot tolerate a large amount of scar tissue without affecting joint function or the fine tendon pulley system. In some instances, Hunter rods may be placed in the locale of previous tendons. Hunter rods are soft silicone rods that can be placed to maintain the tendon gliding mechanism and covered with a free flap. Once the soft tissue is stabilized, tendon grafting or transfers may be performed.

Lower Extremity

Oncologic extirpation in the lower extremity can result in defects of the groin, thigh, knee, lower leg, and foot. The most common tumor in the lower extremity is sarcoma.

Thigh. When defects occur in the groin or thigh, many times they can be closed by adjacent tissue transfer of redundant thigh subcutaneous tissue or pedicled flaps. After groin dissection, the proximal femoral vessels are often exposed, and the neighboring sartorius muscle can be transposed for coverage. For larger defects, the most common flaps in this region are a pedicled rectus abdominis myocutaneous flap or an anterolateral thigh/vastus lateralis flap. With massive defects of the thigh, free tissue transfers can be performed, and the femoral and deep femoral vessels are usually good recipients. End-to-side anastomoses are commonly performed in the lower extremity to preserve blood flow to the distal limb. Innervated muscle transfers, such as free latissimus dorsi innervated flap, can help restore knee extension when the anterior compartment is resected. These innervated flaps capitalize on the motor nerve of the donor muscle, such as the thoracodorsal nerve to the latissimus, and coapt the nerve to the resected proximal nerve, such as the femoral. Over time, usually 6 to 9 months, the muscle will reinnervate and will help power the knee. Although it cannot be guaranteed to achieve full strength, most patients will attain baseline stability and function for everyday activities of living.

Knee and Lower Leg

In the knee and leg, many defects are associated with osteotomies related to tumor resection. Bony defects in the distal femur and proximal tibia are usually reconstructed with an allograft or endoprosthesis. For large defects, microsurgical bone transfers may be used to augment an allograft or endoprosthesis. An example of this is the Capanna technique, which combines the use of a large cadaveric allograft with an intermedullary vascularized fibular flap to allow for immediate rigid fixation of the allograft but potential accelerated bony union through the vascularized fibula bone. Hardware failure, nonunion, and infection are always potential complications of bony reconstruction, and vascularized tissue may help prevent these issues.

Soft tissue coverage of defects in the knee and proximal one-third of the lower leg can be achieved with pedicled gastrocnemius muscle flaps. The medial or lateral heads of the gastrocnemius can be separated and used as individual pedicled muscle flaps, or both heads can be used to provide more coverage. If both heads of the gastrocnemius muscle are to be used for reconstruction, the soleus muscle must be preserved to provide plantar flexion of the foot. Alternatively, when soft tissue coverage is required in the middle third of the leg, the soleus muscle is used, as it has better reach in this area. See Fig. 69.9 for an example of a rotational gastrocnemius muscle for coverage of lower extremity hardware.

In comparison to the more proximal thigh and leg, reconstructing the distal third of the leg with local or regional muscle flaps is not usually possible because of sparse amount of local tissues available. In the distal third of the leg, most muscle bellies have become tendinous and tightly fixed to the bone. Small local flaps may cover defects up to 5 cm, but larger defects or radiated areas mandate free tissue transfer. Generally, wounds in this region are repaired with free fasciocutaneous or myocutaneous flaps. Three sets of vessels are present in the lower leg: the anterior tibial, posterior tibial, and peroneal vessels. Any of these can be suitable for free flap anastomosis. The lower leg and foot can survive off a single vessel, if necessary, although it is preferable to leave at least two systems intact. See Fig. 69.10 for an example of free anterolateral thigh flap for coverage of radiated distal lower extremity wound.

For this reason, microsurgical reconstruction of the lower extremity is an integral part of limb salvage. The successful salvage of a limb depends on proper application of orthopedic and plastic surgery principles, including debridement of nonviable tissue, bony stabilization, and vascularized soft tissue coverage. Initial outcome studies by Gustilo, Byrd, and Godina in the 1970s and 1980s demonstrated that early (within 1 week) microsurgical reconstruction of the lower limb has superior outcomes. However, as adjuvant wound modalities have developed, such as the wound

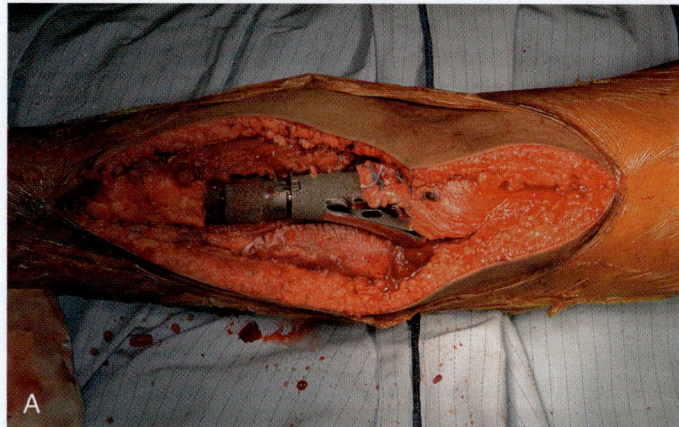

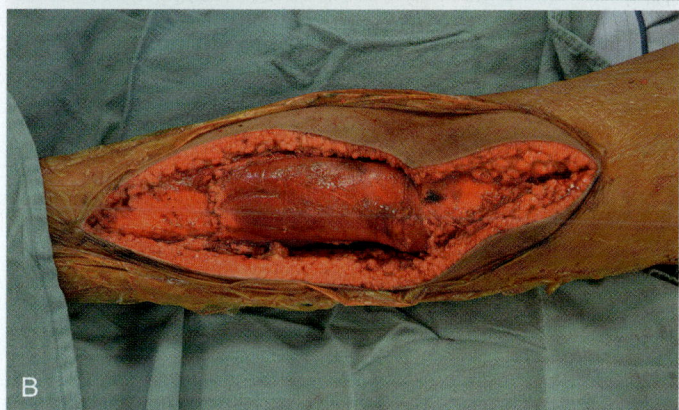

FIGURE 69.9 (A) This image demonstrates the defect of a 20-year-old female patient with proximal tibia tumor resection requiring endoprosthetic reconstruction. (B) A medial gastrocnemius flap was harvested from the posterior calf and rotated anteriorly for complete hardware coverage.

vacuum, new data suggest that in situations where a wound cannot be immediately covered, such as if oncologic margins are pending, then these wounds can be temporized and closed as soon as possible.

Of note, microsurgical reconstruction of the distal extremity is one of the most challenging extremity procedures for a reconstructive surgeon. Distal venous pooling, lymphedema, and radiation all make blood egress challenging. Successful reconstruction requires strict adherence to gradual dangling of the extremity with gravity, delayed ambulation, and careful management of swelling. Most patients who will require a microsurgical flap will need at least a 7- to 10-day hospital stay with additional outpatient physical therapy.

Foot

Like the hand, the foot is extremely specialized. It bears the entire weight of the body and, therefore, must have extremely durable coverage. Additionally, it must have fine sensation to protect against frequent trauma and infection. Because of this, sacrifice of the tibial nerve during tumor extirpation and subsequent rendering of the plantar foot insensate is a strong indication for amputation with few exceptions.

Similar to the hand, very small oncologic resections are best repaired with primary closure or secondary healing. Small defects are repaired with skin grafts and local flaps. Because of the paucity of muscle and soft tissue in the lower leg, few local flaps are available for foot reconstruction. The reverse sural artery rotation flap

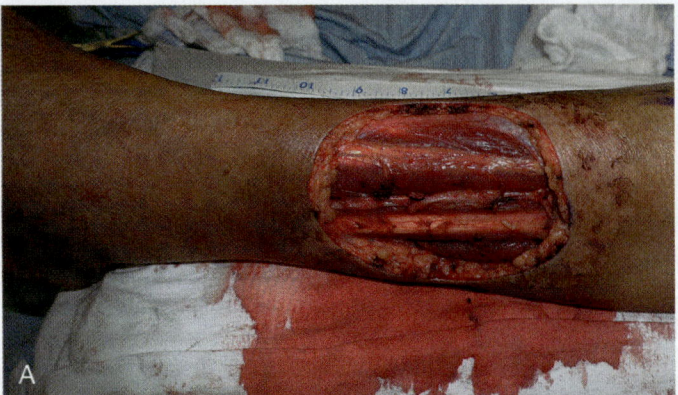

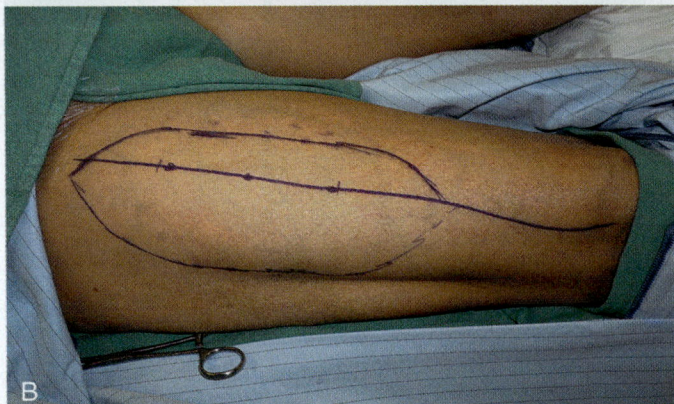

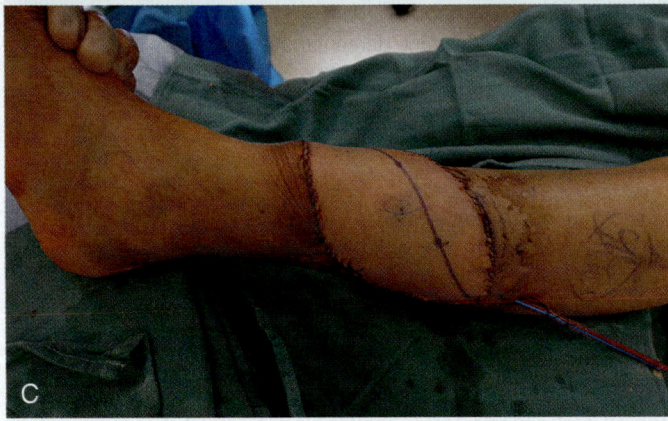

FIGURE 69.10 (A) This elderly patient required resection of a sarcoma over the distal third of the lower extremity. She also required preoperative radiation, which made the tissues fibrotic and the wound unstable. (B) A right fasciocutaneous anterolateral thigh flap was harvested and the donor site closed primarily. (C) The anterolateral thigh flap was anastomosed to the posterior tibial vessels on the medial side of the leg, with the flap providing excellent coverage over the defect. The patient was able to resume ambulation within 1 week.

can repair small defects at the heel or malleolus. The medial plantar artery flap includes the glabrous skin of the instep and can be moved short distances from the non–weight-bearing area of the foot to the weight-bearing surface. However, both these flaps are limited in their reach.

When defects reach over 5 cm, they must be reconstructed with a free flap. However, flap selection is critical because large bulky flaps will prevent shoe donning. Smaller but durable muscles such as the gracilis or serratus anterior can be used and then covered with a skin graft. Fasciocutaneous flaps such as the lateral forearm

flap are also used for foot reconstruction and can be designed to include sensory innervation. Insensate muscle and fasciocutaneous flaps are susceptible to pressure ulceration and so must be vigilantly monitored for the breakdown of skin and soft tissue. If a flap remains bulky after healing, then additional revision or debulking procedures may be required and staged about 6 to 12 months later.

Lastly, similar to the forequarter amputation of the upper extremity, large tumors involving the pelvis and hip joint may compromise the neurovascular structures of the lower extremity. In these instances, an internal (sparing the limb) or external (removing the limb) hemipelvectomy may be required. In instances where an internal hemipelvectomy is performed, the goal is to restore the pelvic domain and obligate hernia with mesh and soft tissue. If the iliac bone is resected from the sacrum, stabilizing vascularized bone grafts may be required. If the limb requires removal, a free fillet of leg flap may be required to restore the soft tissue of the pelvis for sitting and prosthetic donning.

New Advancements

As with most areas of surgery, the field of plastic and reconstructive surgery is constantly evolving to improve patient outcomes. For the oncologic patient, posttreatment quality of life is paramount to a "successful" paradigm.

Surgical Management of Chronic Pain and the Amputee

Chronic residual limb pain and phantom limb pain are debilitating outcomes of traumatic and oncologic amputation. In general amputees, 10% to 76% report residual limb pain and up to 85% report phantom limb pain.[71,72] Because of this, many amputees suffer not only from the initial insult of amputation but also the chronic consequences.

Neuromas are masses of disorganized axons that form after a nerve is ligated and send painful and distressing signals to the brain. Phantom pain develops with neuromas as the neural efferent-afferent loop is disrupted from the amputated limb to the brain. Fortunately, in the past decade, there have been emerging and promising microsurgical treatments for the treatment of postamputation pain. Kuiken and Dumanian pioneered work in the surgical technique of targeted muscle reinnervation (TMR), which coapts mixed major nerves (those that contain motor and sensory fibers) to available motor nerves in the surrounding tissue using microsurgical sutures in the epineurium.[73,74] The recipient motor nerves are available because their respective muscles have lost their distal insertion with the amputation and are rendered nonfunctional. Trophic stimulus from the denervated muscle transmitted through the recipient nerve encourages regenerative and physiologic healing of the amputated major mixed nerves. Similarly, Cederna and colleagues have published their novel work with regenerative peripheral nerve interfaces (RPNIs), which use free autologous muscle wrapped around the proximal amputated nerve to provide trophic regenerative stimulus from denervated muscle.[75] Both techniques give the amputated proximal nerve a target for regeneration and encourages the nerve to "heal," as opposed to the surgical standard of care, which consists of burying or crushing the amputated nerve fascicles.

Both strategies have recognized the need to provide a physiologic end organ for nerve regeneration to prevent and reduce symptomatic neuroma formation. Additionally, by reestablishing a neural efferent-afferent closed loop, this may reduce aberrant pain perception in the sensorimotor cortex and decrease phantom pain. Although developed in parallel, both TMR and RPNI techniques have been shown to capitalize on directed trophic motor nerve stimulus and have excellent early results in the treatment, and prevention, of amputation-associated limb pain.[76] TMR and RPNI are now being trialed in other forms of surgical resection, such as mastectomy-associated nerve pain. It is important to know that in studies to date, neither technique has been shown to make a patient's pain worse or result in inferior outcomes. TMR and/or RPNI can be performed in an immediate or delayed fashion, although performing the nerve management immediately appears to have the greatest benefit for pain prevention.

Lastly, it is important to understand that the TMR and RPNI were initially developed for the control of myoelectric prosthetics. Myoelectric prosthetics function by detecting electromyographic signals on remaining muscle on the amputee and translating these signals into multiple coordinated movements on a highly specialized prosthetic. TMR and RPNI surgical nerve transfers were designed to create specific muscle sites in the amputee that these prosthetics could detect. Fortuitously, treated patients were found to have less pain after their neuromas were resected, and the nerves coapted to healthy remaining motor nerves. Although TMR and RPNI remain highly important for developing myoelectric prosthetics, these techniques are most broadly applicable for pain control. Myoelectric prosthetics remain cost-prohibitive for most patients and require a heavy battery; therefore, they require further technologic advancement for broader application.

OUTCOME ASSESSMENTS IN PLASTIC SURGERY

Measuring, interpreting, and acting upon outcomes is critical across healthcare disciplines. Outcomes enable understanding the impact of interventions, quality improvement, innovation, research, and reimbursement benchmarking. Although the general utility and need for outcomes in healthcare delivery can be recognized, which types of outcomes and when to collect them may vary significantly by patient population, clinical indication, and specialty.

Originating primarily within the "outcomes movement" of the 1980s, healthcare outcomes were initially designed to mitigate geographic practice variation, insurer competition, and healthcare costs. Although these early outcomes centered mainly on easily measurable, physician-driven metrics like mortality and readmission rates, healthcare outcomes have since evolved to be more inclusive of the patient experience, such as the physical, emotional, and social tolls of healthcare from the patient's perspective, or patient-reported outcomes (PROs). Advances in measurement theory and psychometrics have since enabled rigorous and scientific measurement of PROs, known as patient-reported outcome measures (PROMs).[77,78]

In plastic surgery, improving the quality of life of patients from their own unique perspective is commonly the indication for performing surgery. For example, whereas an oncologic surgeon may prioritize evidence-based outcomes for mortality and recurrence rates in their surgical planning for a patient with breast cancer, a plastic surgeon may prioritize unique patient-centered outcomes in their surgical planning for breast reconstruction, such as sensation and satisfaction with breast shape. In the field of plastic surgery, both clinical outcomes (e.g., infection rates, readmission rates) and patient-centered outcomes play important roles.

Clinical Outcomes

Clinical outcomes pertinent to other surgical fields also are applicable to plastic surgery (e.g., rates of infection, hematoma, readmission, and mortality). Plastic surgeons have created dedicated registries and databases to systematically record clinical outcomes. One such example is the Tracking Operations and Outcomes for Plastic Surgeons (TOPS) database, akin to the National Surgical Quality Improvement Program (NSQIP) database used across general surgery specialties. There are also device- and procedure-specific outcomes databases, such as the National Breast Implant Registry (NBIR), which specifically records outcomes related to implants used in breast reconstruction and augmentation. Owing to specific concerns regarding known outcomes of implants, such as BIA-LCL, as well as outcomes under active investigation, such as breast implant illness, plastic surgery–specific outcomes databases are key for research, quality, and safety surveillance.

Importantly, reconstructive outcomes are often directly dependent on both antecedent and subsequent oncologic care and their respective outcomes. Thus, plastic surgeons must be mindful of the pre- and postoperative oncologic plan for patients undergoing reconstruction. For example, the extent and depth of oncologic resection may affect the complexity of reconstructive care, which can range from local wound care to microsurgical free flap coverage. Chemoradiation affects healing, especially when using devices or implants, which may influence either the timing or choice of reconstruction (e.g., breast implants vs. autologous reconstruction). High recurrence rates and low survival outcomes may hinder reconstruction efforts, as demonstrated in inflammatory breast cancer, where immediate reconstruction is typically contraindicated. Finally, common functional deficits from oncologic care, such as lymphedema or sensation loss, may inform innovative and novel approaches for lymphatic and nerve reconstruction, respectively. As such, close collaboration and communication of known and foreseeable outcomes is essential between oncologic and reconstructive surgeons. Table 69.1 lists examples of oncologic care that may affect reconstruction.

TABLE 69.1	Components of Oncologic Care and Impact on Plastic Surgery Outcomes
ONCOLOGIC CARE COMPONENT	**POTENTIAL IMPACT ON PLASTIC SURGERY**
Need for chemotherapy or radiation therapy	Higher risk of poor wound healing; consider delayed reconstruction, use of autologous tissue flaps over implants; optimize nutrition
High recurrence rates/low survival	Consider delaying reconstruction or less complex reconstruction
Lymphatic dissection and/or lymph node removal	Consider prophylactic lymphatic reconstruction techniques at the time of dissection
Nerve transection/excision during cancer resection	Consider microsurgical neurotization techniques at time of resection or reconstruction
Hardware placement/exposed bone	Consider more complex soft tissue reconstruction for hardware and bone coverage
Required resection depth, size, involved structures	Reconstructive plan affected by type and size of tissue required to re-create form and function
Psychosocial needs and coping	Consider social support structure and psychotherapy, especially for patients with history of mental illness or high degree of reconstruction complexity

BREAST-Q™
Reconstruction module (Post operative) 2.0

This question is about NIPPLE reconstruction. If you did <u>not</u> have nipple reconstruction, please skip to question 11. If you did have nipple reconstruction, please answer question 10 below.

10. In the past 2 weeks, how <u>satisfied or dissatisfied</u> are you with:

	Very dissatisfied	Somewhat dissatisfied	Somewhat satisfied	Very satisfied
a. The shape of your reconstructed nipple(s)?	1	2	3	4
b. How your reconstructed nipple(s) and areola(s) look?	1	2	3	4
c. How natural your reconstructed nipple(s) look?	1	2	3	4
d. The color of your reconstructed nipple/areolar complex?	1	2	3	4
e. The height (projection) of your reconstructed nipple(s)?	1	2	3	4

FIGURE 69.11 Representative image of the BREAST-Q PROM questionnaire.

Patient-Reported Outcomes

PROs are key outcome metrics for plastic surgeons, as reconstructive surgery often aims to achieve the goals known to and reported by patients themselves. PROMs are typically survey tools that translate qualitative reports about health and well-being into rigorously quantifiable data, such as survey response about pain or satisfaction after chest wall reconstruction. PROMs then can be used to track outcomes over time in individual patients as well as across different patients and patient populations.

The BREAST-Q is one example of a PROM that has been used in both research and routine clinical care. The BREAST-Q contains different modules, or scales (i.e., measurements), that can be used by physicians, researchers, and patients according to the clinical indication of interest, for example, with satisfaction with breasts, physical well-being, psychosocial well-being, and sexual well-being. A representative survey question from the BREAST-Q is shown in Fig. 69.11.[79]

PROMs serve many functions and exist across medical specialties. Here, we outline three key ways in which PROMs have and can be used in plastic surgery. First, they can be used in research. In plastic surgery, there are often many reasonable reconstructive options for a given indication. PROMs are therefore useful to provide head-to-head comparison of outcomes that matter most to patients. For example, after mastectomy for breast cancer, patients may opt for implant-based reconstruction or autologous reconstruction using their own tissue, such as with DIEP reconstruction. In one study, patients undergoing autologous reconstruction were found to have greater satisfaction and health-related quality of life 3 to 4 years postoperatively.[80]

Second, PROMs can be used in routine clinical care. Research has shown that PROMs can enhance patient-provider communication, reduce healthcare utilization, and increase patient satisfaction with care.[81,82] As such, many efforts are currently underway at various institutions to incorporate PROMs into clinical care, akin to vital signs measurement at clinic visits. Given that many oncologic patients receive multidisciplinary care, including from surgical and medical oncologists, radiation

oncologists, and plastic surgeons, PROMs may provide a relevant timeline of outcomes across the cancer care continuum relevant to multiple specialties.

Third, PROMs may be used in quality and reimbursement.[83] Given that PROMs enable rigorous and quantifiable measurement of outcomes important to patients, PROMs are well poised to serve as key metrics for quality improvement initiatives, as well as innovation, in the field of plastic surgery. Additionally, although not widespread, quality metrics informed by PROMs may be used to benchmark reimbursements in insurer negotiations.

SELECTED REFERENCES

Colwell AS, Taylor EM. Recent advances in implant-based breast reconstruction. *Plast Reconstr Surg.* 2020;145(2):421e-432e.

Breast reconstruction with implants has advanced as a result of emerging techniques. These new techniques include nipple- and skin-reducing incision patterns, biologic mesh, prepectoral placement, and direct-to-implant techniques.

Cuccolo NG, Sparenberg S, Ibrahim MS, et al. Does age or frailty have more predictive effect on outcomes following pedicled flap reconstruction? An analysis of 44, 986 cases. *J Plast Surg Hand Surg.* 2020;54(2):67-76.

The 2005–2016 ACS-NSQIP databases were queried to identify 44,986 cases involving pedicled flaps based on CPT codes. Although increased age does contribute to risk of postoperative complications, the 5-factor modified frailty index (mFI-5) appears to hold much stronger predictive capacity. These findings stress the importance of optimizing preoperative comorbidities to reduce the risk of poor postoperative outcomes.

Dumanian GA, Potter BK, Mioton LM, et al. Targeted muscle reinnervation treats neuroma and phantom pain in major limb amputees: a randomized clinical trial. *Ann Surg.* 2019;270:238.

> Targeted muscle reinnervation (TMR) is a novel method of nerve coaptation at amputation. The amputated nerve is co-apted to local motor nerves to restore nerve continuity. This randomized trial of the technique demonstrates reduced residual limb neuroma pain as well as phantom limb pain.

Isaac KV, Elzinga K, Buchel EW. The best of chest wall reconstruction: principles and clinical application for complex oncologic and sternal defects. *Plast Reconstr Surg.* 2022;149(3):547e-562e.

> Advances in reconstructive techniques have expanded the resectability of large complex oncologic tumors by safely and reliably restoring chest wall integrity in an immediate fashion with minimal or no secondary deficits. This article discusses the evaluation and management of oncologic chest wall defects, reviews controversial considerations in chest wall reconstruction, and provides an algorithm for the reconstruction of complex chest wall defects. Respiratory preservation, semirigid stabilization, and longevity are key when reconstructing chest wall defects.

Roubaud MS, Hassan AM, Shin A, et al. Outcomes of targeted muscle reinnervation and regenerative peripheral nerve interfaces for chronic pain control in the oncologic amputee population. *J Am Coll Surg.* 2023;237(4):644-654.

> TMR and regenerative peripheral nerve interfaces (RPNIs) are novel surgical techniques to manage ligated nerves during amputation. In this retrospective review of oncologic amputees, TMR and RPNI were shown to reduce expected residual limb and phantom limb pain, despite preexisting chemoradiation and preamputation limb pain.

Santosa KB, Qi J, Kim HM, Hamill JB, Wilkins EG, Pusic AL. Long-term patient-reported outcomes in postmastectomy breast reconstruction. *JAMA Surg.* 2018;153(10):891-899.

> Patients were recruited from 11 centers (57 plastic surgeons) across North America for the Mastectomy Reconstruction Outcomes Consortium study, a prospective, multicenter trial, from 2012 to 2015. The patients were assessed with the BREAST-Q patient-reported outcome instrument before surgery and at 2 years after surgery. At 2 years, patients who underwent autologous reconstruction were more satisfied with their breasts and had greater psychosocial well-being and sexual well-being than did those who underwent implant reconstruction. These findings can inform patients and their clinicians about expected satisfaction and quality-of-life outcomes of autologous versus implant-based procedures and further support the adoption of shared decision-making in clinical practice.

Soltanian H, Garcia RM, Hollenbeck ST. Current concepts in lower extremity reconstruction. *Plast Reconstr Surg.* 2015;136(6):815e-829e.

> The principles of lower extremity reconstruction are discussed for both traumatic and oncologic defects. A review of the Gustilo-Anderson open fracture classification and local and free flap reconstructive options is presented.

Squitieri L, Bozic KJ, Pusic AL. The role of patient-reported outcome measures in value-based payment reform. *Value Health.* 2017;20(6):834-836.

> Pressure to improve the quality of patient care and control costs has caused a rapid shift from traditional volume-driven fee-for-service reimbursement to value-based payment models. Under the 2015 Medicare Access and Children's Health Insurance Program Reauthorization Act, providers will be evaluated on the basis of quality and cost efficiency and ultimately receive adjusted reimbursement as per their performance. Although current performance metrics do not incorporate patient-reported outcome measures (PROMs), many wonder whether and how PROMs will eventually fit into value-based payment reform. This article summarizes the findings of the second annual Patient-Reported Outcomes in Healthcare Conference, in the context of recent literature and guidelines, to inform implementation of PROs in value-based payment models. Recommendations for evaluating key perspectives and measurement goals are made to facilitate appropriate use of PROMs to best benefit and amplify the voice of our patients.

Thorarinsson A, Frojd V, Kolby L, et al. Patient determinants as independent risk factors for postoperative complications of breast reconstruction. *Gland Surg.* 2017;6:355-367.

> High BMI, history of radiotherapy, and smoking are independent risk factors for many types of both early and late postoperative complications in breast reconstructive surgery. Combining these risk factors multiplies the risk of postoperative complications.

Weichman KE, Matros E, Disa JJ. Reconstruction of peripelvic oncologic defects. *Plast Reconstr Surg.* 2017;140:601e.

> Peripelvic reconstruction most commonly occurs in the setting of oncologic ablative surgery. The peripelvic area contains several distinct reconstructive regions, including vagina, vulva, penis, and scrotum. Each area provides unique reconstructive considerations. Local, pedicled, and free flap reconstructive options are elucidated based on region.

The full reference list appears on Elsevier eBooks+.

70 CHAPTER

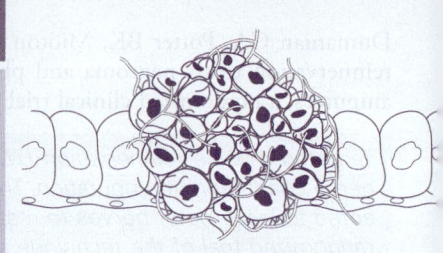

Peritoneal Malignancy and HIPEC

Konstantinos Chouliaras, Konstantinos I. Votanopoulos,
and Edward A. Levine

OUTLINE

History
    Peritoneum
    Peritoneal Fluid Circulation
Preoperative Considerations
Technical Aspects
Hyperthermic Intraperitoneal Chemotherapy

Appendiceal Tumors
Mesothelioma
Colorectal Cancer
Ovarian Cancer
Gastric Cancer
Future Directions

HISTORY

The majority of peritoneal malignancies arise from gastrointestinal (GI) and gynecologic cancers, with peritoneal mesothelioma being less common. Other rare sources of peritoneal surface malignancy (PSM), such as urachal, sarcoma, and GI stromal tumors, are occasionally encountered. Although the term *PSM* is often used interchangeably with *carcinomatosis,* it seems more precise to reserve the term *PSM* for cases in which the disease is predominantly confined to peritoneal surface locations and without deep parenchymal or systemic components (most commonly, low-grade appendiceal or ovarian cancer and peritoneal mesothelioma). This distinction ensures a better understanding of the pathophysiology of metastasis and facilitates clearer communication in clinical contexts. PSM represents a formidable challenge to surgeons and oncologists, given the difficulties in both diagnosis and treatment. These cases present at an advanced stage with significant burden of disease. Symptoms can have either an insidious or abrupt presentation. Obtaining a diagnosis before the tumor burden becomes overwhelming is often challenging as a result of difficulties in identifying small-volume peritoneal implants, even with state-of-the-art imaging.

Historically, the field of PSM has been criticized for the paucity of level 1 evidence demonstrating its efficacy. However, there now is a growing body of evidence that includes several randomized clinical trials and better delineates the role of cytoreductive surgery (CRS) and intraperitoneal (IP) therapies. Tumor-debulking surgery was first reported for ovarian cancer by Joe Meigs in New York in 1934.[1] Yet it was not until the 1970s that systematic study of IP chemotherapy agents was undertaken. The synergistic effect of hyperthermia and IP chemotherapy was first reported by Spratt et al. in 1980.[2] In the 1990s, there was ongoing interest in expanding its use for GI cancers. During that time, the

fundamental principles of CRS were established. Several publications detailed peritonectomy techniques in an attempt to standardize both the operative approach[3] and the calculation of peritoneal tumor burden.

In the past three decades, several centers have published their experience with CRS, with a goal of extirpating all gross disease, combined with hyperthermic intraperitoneal chemotherapy (HIPEC) to address microscopic residual disease.[4,5] Notably, there is variation in techniques, duration, and chemotherapeutic agents between leading centers. Recognizing the need for standardization of the technique, several consensus statements have been published to promote a more consistent approach.[6] IP chemotherapy has advantages over systemic chemotherapy, including the ability to achieve substantially higher tissue concentration with lower levels of systemic absorption and attendant adverse effects. Its one-time administration allows for better tolerance and reduces issues with accumulated toxicity. As targeted approaches based on molecular markers such as MSI, HER2, RAS, and BRAF advance, there is renewed interest in exploring novel agents for chemoperfusion or combination approaches before and after radical surgical resection.

PERITONEUM

The peritoneum is the largest and most complex serous membrane in the human body. Understanding of peritoneal anatomy is essential for diagnosis, surgical treatment, and drug administration. The peritoneal cavity contains the stomach, small bowel (with the exception of the second and third portions of the duodenum), and most of the colon, with the greater and lesser omentum dividing the peritoneal cavity into the greater and lesser sacs (Fig. 70.1). The lesser sac is contained behind the lesser and greater omentum, stomach, and transverse colon and communicates

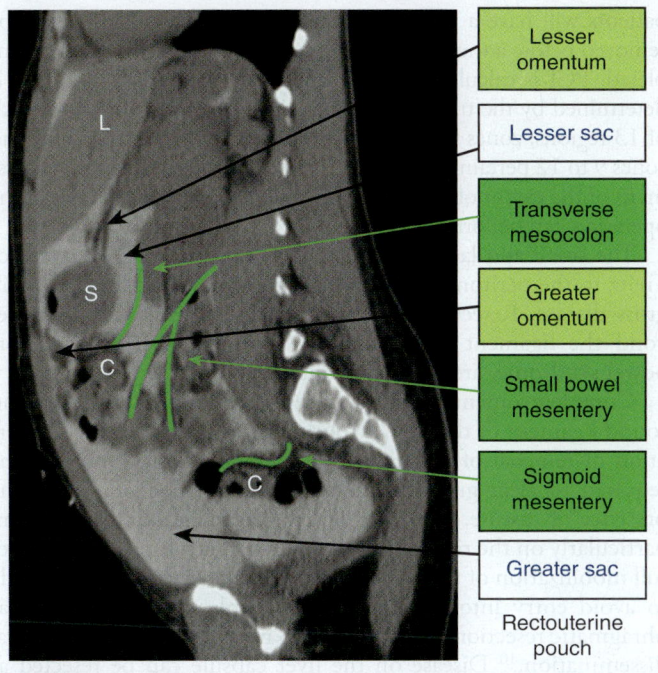

FIGURE 70.1 Sagittal image from a CT peritoneogram illustrating the mesenteries, greater and lesser sac, and omenta. *L*, Liver; *S*, stomach; *C*, colon. (From Ceelan WP, Levine E. *Intraperitoneal Cancer Therapy. Principles and Practice.* CRC Press; 2015.)

Labels: Lesser omentum; Lesser sac; Transverse mesocolon; Greater omentum; Small bowel mesentery; Sigmoid mesentery; Greater sac; Rectouterine pouch

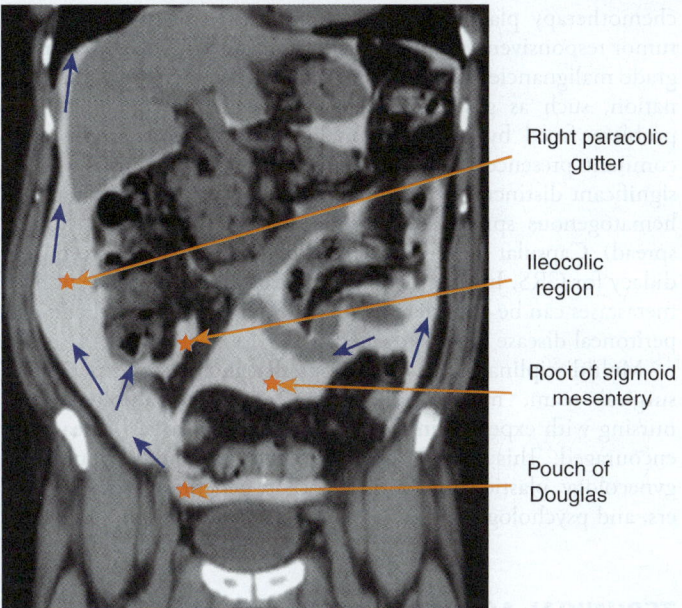

FIGURE 70.2 Coronal image from a CT peritoneogram with associated diagram showing the direction of flow of peritoneal fluid *(blue arrows)* and sites of maximum fluid stasis *(orange stars)*. (From Ceelan WP, Levine E. *Intraperitoneal Cancer Therapy. Principles and Practice.* CRC Press; 2015.)

Labels: Right paracolic gutter; Ileocolic region; Root of sigmoid mesentery; Pouch of Douglas

with the greater sac through the foramen of Winslow. The omentum is a duplication of the visceral peritoneum and plays a key role in the pathophysiology of peritoneal metastases. Histologically, the peritoneum contains mesenchymal cells as well as an epithelial lining, called the *mesothelium,* made up of a single layer of simple cuboidal epithelium. It serves a protective function for all the viscera and facilitates smooth movement of all the visceral organs, with minimal lubrication. Besides its protective role, it has immunologic properties and plays an important part in tissue repair and scar formation.

Peritoneal Fluid Circulation

The pattern of fluid flow and dynamics creates areas of possible stasis that represent common locations where peritoneal disease is encountered. In general, peritoneal fluid circulates in a clockwise orientation (Fig. 70.2). The surgeon should seek disease in the rectovesical/rectouterine pouch (pouch of Douglas), right paracolic gutter, right subhepatic space, and the hepatorenal fossa (pouch of Morrison), which represent the most common areas to identify peritoneal implants. These locations, along with a thorough, systematic search of the entire peritoneal cavity, need to be examined upon review of preoperative imaging and at exploration to accurately measure the extent of disease.

PREOPERATIVE CONSIDERATIONS

CRS, with or without HIPEC, is a substantial operative undertaking, and thorough preoperative evaluation and discussions are mandatory. Pathologic confirmation of peritoneal dissemination should be obtained. The extent of disease in the peritoneal cavity and the lack of extraabdominal metastatic sites must be determined with computed tomography (CT) and/or magnetic resonance imaging (MRI) scans. Tumor marker levels should be obtained before surgery (carcinoembryonic antigen [CEA], carbohydrate antigen [CA] 19-9, and CA125) for GI and gynecologic disease.

Patient selection is critical to achieving optimal outcomes after CRS and HIPEC. Preoperative assessment must suggest that resection of the primary tumor and the metastatic disease is feasible. Patient and technical factors, as well as assessment of tumor biology, are critical components in the decision-making process. Functional status plays a very important role, and we routinely use Eastern Cooperative Oncology Group (ECOG) functional status to standardize reporting for documentation and research purposes. Resection is offered to patients with an ECOG of 0 or 1; however, highly selected patients with ECOG 2 status may be considered. Thorough and multidisciplinary evaluation of patient comorbidities is essential and is focused primarily on cardiac, pulmonary, and psychosocial issues, with liberal use of subspecialty consultant input. Preoperative evaluation should ensure likely patient tolerance of these frequently lengthy operations and their attendant significant fluid shifts and operative stresses.

A preoperative systematic assessment of the extent of disease is mandatory. We routinely employ high-quality cross-sectional imaging such as multiphase CT scans with intravenous (IV) and oral contrast. In challenging cases with concerns of extraabdominal metastases, we consider positron emission tomography–CT (PET/CT) scans. MRI offers further advantages, particularly in the assessment of the liver, when there are concerns about parenchymal lesions that might affect resectability, and also in the assessment of pelvic disease that might necessitate radical approaches, such as exenteration.[7]

An understanding of tumor biology is essential before embarking on extensive potentially morbid operations. These cases are better served in established centers with teams experienced in the management of peritoneal surface disease cases with a multidisciplinary team. Thorough review of prior imaging, operative records, and pathology slides cannot be emphasized enough. This becomes even more critical in rare cancers. Preoperative chemotherapy plays an important role in better understanding tumor responsiveness and pattern of spread, particularly for high-grade malignancies with a propensity for hematogenous dissemination, such as gastric and colon cancer. A frequent clinical problem faced by peritoneal malignancy surgeons is the concomitant presence of liver masses and peritoneal metastases. A significant distinction has to be made between parenchymal (via hematogenous spread) or capsular liver lesions (via peritoneal spread). Capsular metastases do not preclude a patient from candidacy for CRS. In cases of colorectal cancer, the presence of liver metastases can be considered with CRS only if all the hepatic *and* peritoneal disease can be resected.[8]

Multidisciplinary case discussions that include an experienced surgical team, medical oncology, radiology, pathology, and nursing with expertise in the evaluation of peritoneal disease are encouraged. This team is optimally complemented by urology, gynecology, plastic surgery, pharmacists, geneticists, social workers, and psychologists.

TECHNICAL ASPECTS

The goal of cytoreduction is removal of all gross disease while minimizing impact on long-term organ function. Select patients with very low peritoneal disease burden may be treated with minimally invasive approaches; however, most cases are best explored with a generous midline incision. In the authors' experience, ureteral stenting is used liberally to facilitate identification and reduce the probability of unrecognized ureteral injury; this is particularly true in cases when extensive pelvic dissection is expected in a reoperative field. After making the incision, a self-retaining retractor is placed. The abdomen must be thoroughly and completely explored at this point, which requires lysis of any preexisting adhesions[9]

The peritoneal tumor burden is then evaluated and quantified with the Peritoneal Carcinomatosis Index (PCI) score. Occasionally,

patients will have a significant omental cake that may need to be removed before a thorough assessment of the abdomen can be completed. PCI is calculated at the time of the operation. The PCI is determined by the tumor size, which is scored from 0 to 3 for each of 13 regions; zones 0 to 8 cover the abdomen topographically, and zones 9 to 12 pertain to the small bowel (Fig. 70.3). After this assessment of the extent of visceral involvement, a plan for conduct of the operation can be formulated.

The small and large bowel are then run from the ligament of Treitz to the peritoneal reflection, with removal or ablation of all gross disease. Resections leaving the patient with <100 cm beyond the ligament of Treitz, with attendant permanent short bowel syndrome, are rarely warranted.

Complete omentectomy and resection of the falciform and round ligament of the liver is routinely performed, as is consideration of removal of the lesser omentum. Peritonectomy may be required to clear gross disease and is performed only with the presence of disease. Stripping of the diaphragmatic peritoneum, particularly on the right side, is frequently performed and requires full mobilization of the right lobe of the liver. Every effort is made to avoid entry into the pleural space unless full-thickness diaphragmatic resections are necessary to minimize the risk of pleural dissemination.[10] Disease on the liver capsule can be resected as individual metastases when limited in number. The liver capsule can be stripped off via hepatic capsulectomy if larger areas of disease are present.

Standardized reporting of the completeness of tumor cytoreduction achieved is essential to determine patient prognosis and facilitate comparisons and research efforts. R resection status is determined upon completion of the cytoreduction and divided into R0, complete removal of all visible tumor and negative cytologic findings or microscopic margins; R1, complete removal of all visible tumor and positive postperfusion cytologic findings or microscopic margins; R2a, minimal residual tumor, nodule(s) measuring 0.5 cm or less; R2b, gross residual tumor, nodule greater than 0.5 cm but less than or equal to 2 cm; and R2c,

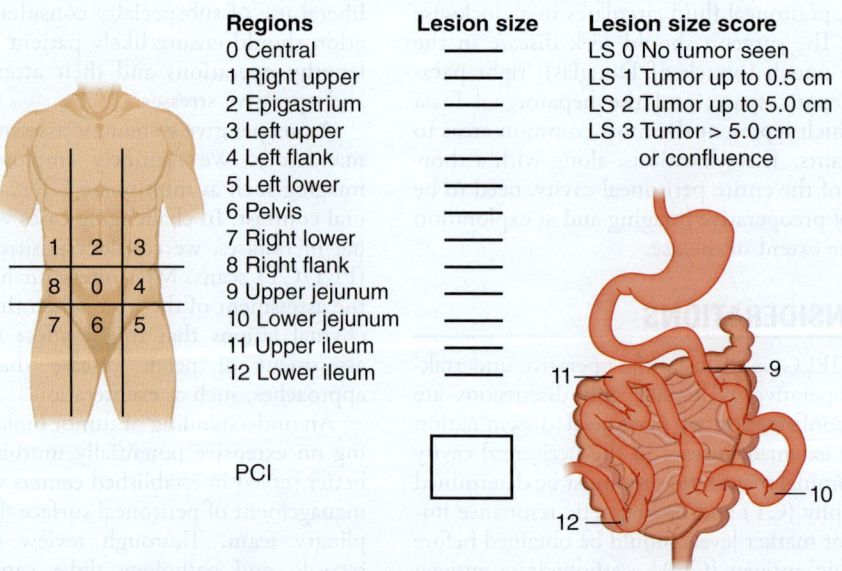

Regions	Lesion size	Lesion size score
0 Central	——	LS 0 No tumor seen
1 Right upper	——	LS 1 Tumor up to 0.5 cm
2 Epigastrium	——	LS 2 Tumor up to 5.0 cm
3 Left upper	——	LS 3 Tumor > 5.0 cm
4 Left flank	——	or confluence
5 Left lower	——	
6 Pelvis	——	
7 Right lower	——	
8 Right flank	——	
9 Upper jejunum	——	
10 Lower jejunum	——	
11 Upper ileum	——	
12 Lower ileum	——	

PCI

FIGURE 70.3 Peritoneal Carcinomatosis Index *(PCI)* scoring system based on lesion size *(LS)* for 13 regions.

extensive disease remaining, nodules greater than 2 cm. The completeness of cytoreduction (CC) score ranges from 0 to 3. CC 0 or 1 is indicative of a complete cytoreduction, leaving residual tumors smaller than 2.5 mm, whereas a score of 2 or 3 shows an incomplete cytoreduction.[11]

HYPERTHERMIC INTRAPERITONEAL CHEMOTHERAPY

After a complete cytoreduction, we establish a circuit for hyperthermic IP chemotherapy, with a closed technique, for 120 minutes of perfusion (variability exists among centers, with some using shorter perfusion times). Two inflow and two outflow cannulas with Y connectors are used to complete the circuit.[12] The patient's core temperature and inflow and outflow temperature are monitored throughout the perfusion and in close coordination with the anesthesiologists. We target an outflow temperature of 40°C and manipulate inflow up to 44°C to maintain this target. The patient is typically actively cooled during the hyperthermic perfusion with a cooling blanket and an air blower on ambient or cool setting. Mitomycin C is the most commonly used chemotherapeutic agent for GI primaries, whereas cisplatin or carboplatin is the chemotherapy of choice for ovarian cancer and peritoneal mesothelioma. Our group has extensive experience with iterative HIPEC, and oxaliplatin is sometimes used for repeat perfusion in appendiceal and colorectal cases.[13,14] Nephroprotection with sodium thiosulfate, given intravenously, is considered when cisplatin is used. More frail patients and patients with prior hematologic compromise can have the HIPEC dose reduced or the perfusion time shortened.

After completion of the perfusion, all cannulas are removed, and the abdomen is reexplored. Hemostasis is then ensured, and anastomoses are inspected or, if not performed before perfusion, are then completed. Should a colostomy or ileostomy be required, it is created at this point. The patient is then definitively closed and taken to the recovery unit.

Appendiceal Tumors

Despite the rarity of appendiceal tumors, their incidence is rising, estimated to approach 1 per 100,000.[15] Commonly, these are initially diagnosed via an appendectomy for appendicitis or found incidentally on imaging. Carcinoid tumors represent nearly half of the malignant lesions of the appendix but are less commonly encountered with peritoneal metastases. The Peritoneal Surface Oncology Group International (PSOGI) supports World Health Organization (WHO) nomenclature that has been widely accepted for primary appendiceal neoplasms: low-grade appendiceal mucinous neoplasm (LAMN), high-grade appendiceal mucinous neoplasm (HAMN), and mucinous adenocarcinoma with or without signet ring cells.[16]

Pseudomyxoma peritonei is a clinical syndrome of mucinous ascites that describes accumulation of mucin. Pseudomyxoma can be associated with or without epithelial cells in the mucin and is nearly always a result of peritoneal dissemination after appendiceal tumor rupture (Fig. 70.4). Carr et al. described diagnostic criteria for intraabdominal mucin to assist in the characterization of pseudomyxoma peritonei that range from acellular mucin, low-grade mucinous carcinoma peritonei or disseminated peritoneal adenomucinosis (DPAM) to high-grade mucinous carcinoma peritonei or peritoneal mucinous carcinomatosis (PMCA) with or without signet ring cells.

The systemic treatment of appendiceal cancer has been historically extrapolated from the treatment of colorectal cancer

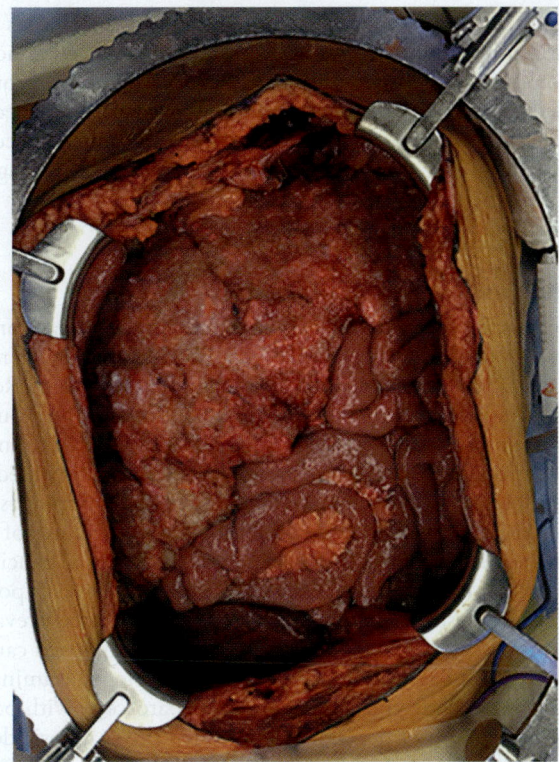

FIGURE 70.4 Omental "cake" obscuring complete Peritoneal Carcinomatosis Index evaluation from low-grade appendiceal neoplasm with relative small bowel sparing. (Visualized through a midline laparotomy incision.)

despite strong evidence that these represent genetically different entities.[17,18] In the past four decades, there has been a significant accumulation of experience in the treatment of these tumors. CRS and HIPEC have been established as an effective modality in the treatment of these tumors with a track record for safety and efficacy.[19,20] In the only completed randomized clinical trial for treatment of appendiceal tumors to date, Levine et al. studied the difference in hematologic toxicities with mitomycin C versus oxaliplatin and found similar overall and progression-free survival (PFS); however, there was more leukopenia and a slightly worse short-term quality-of-life score in the mitomycin arm.[21]

Modern systemic chemotherapy has been used primarily for patients who are not surgical candidates and is most efficacious for high-grade carcinoma.[22] The role of perioperative chemotherapy is still unclear in appendiceal neoplasms, with some studies even reporting a detrimental impact on survival after preoperative chemotherapy.[23,24] For low-grade disease, a recent randomized crossover trial showed no benefit of 6 months of fluoropyrimidine-based systemic chemotherapy compared with observation.[25] This builds on a body of literature, primarily retrospective studies, that has established CRS and HIPEC as the primary modality of treatment, with little role for systemic chemotherapy.[26,27]

Appendiceal Tumors Ex Goblet Cell

Ex goblet cell appendiceal tumors, also called *goblet cell carcinoid* or *adenocarcinoid,* demonstrate mixed pathologic features of a neuroendocrine tumor and adenocarcinoma at the same time. These tumors demonstrate significant heterogeneity, and the Tang classification has been used to differentiate them pathologically as well as predict outcomes.[28] Typical goblet cell carcinoids were categorized in group A, whereas group B was classified as adenocarcinoma ex goblet cell with signet ring features, and group C included poorly differentiated adenocarcinomas. Localized tumors are typically treated with right hemicolectomy, particularly in the setting of goblet cell adenocarcinoma, whereas stage IV patients with peritoneal dissemination are considered for CRS with HIPEC.[29,30]

Mesothelioma

Peritoneal mesothelioma is a very rare subtype of intraabdominal cancer that occurs from the malignant transformation of mesothelial cells. A recent Surveillance, Epidemiology, and End Results (SEER) database analysis estimated the incidence to be around 1 case per million person-years,[31] or only 300 to 400 cases annually in the United States. Despite its rarity, it is further subdivided into histopathologic subtypes: epithelioid (the most common), sarcomatoid (the rarest), and a mixed subtype sharing features of both called *biphasic*. Given the low incidence, there is a paucity of dedicated clinical trials, and systemic treatment is extrapolated from pleural mesothelioma, which is nearly 10 times as prevalent. Diagnosis can be challenging, and percutaneous biopsies can frequently be nondiagnostic or nonspecific. Cytologic examination of ascites is rarely diagnostic. Diagnostic laparoscopy with peritoneal biopsies is often necessary to establish the diagnosis definitively and obtain adequate tissue sample. The treatment of the epithelioid and highly select biphasic cases is primarily CRS and HIPEC in centers experienced with this disease.[32–34]

Various chemotherapeutic agents have been used for IP perfusion, with the backbone being a platinum agent such as cisplatin or carboplatin. Sarcomatoid peritoneal mesothelioma cases are best treated nonoperatively, with systemic chemotherapy alone. The first-line systemic treatment is nivolumab and ipilimumab, extrapolated from the CheckMate 743 trial, which demonstrated improved overall survival (OS) compared with platinum-based chemotherapy and pemetrexed (former standard of care).[35] Cisplatin and pemetrexed with or without bevacizumab are still used for unresectable disease. A recent phase II trial showed a 40% objective response rate with atezolizumab and bevacizumab after progression on platinum-pemetrexed chemotherapy in a prospective cohort of 20 patients.[36]

Well-differentiated Papillary/benign Cystic Peritoneal Mesothelioma

Benign and preinvasive mesothelial tumors are very rare and pose a challenge in management because of very limited data, mainly from small case series or case reports (Fig. 70.5). Benign cystic peritoneal mesotheliomas, previously called *peritoneal inclusions cysts,* are primarily diagnosed in females of childbearing age and tend to cluster in the pelvis. The moniker *benign* can be misleading because these lesions can be progressive. The primary treatment is surgical resection and CRS with hyperthermic IP chemotherapy, which has been reported to decrease recurrences.[37] However, we reserve surgery for patients with proven progressive disease for these subtypes. After surgery, recurrences are common, and surgical resection is typically recommended for worsening symptomatic disease.

Colorectal Cancer

Colorectal cancer remains the third most common cancer in the United States in both males and females. Peritoneal dissemination

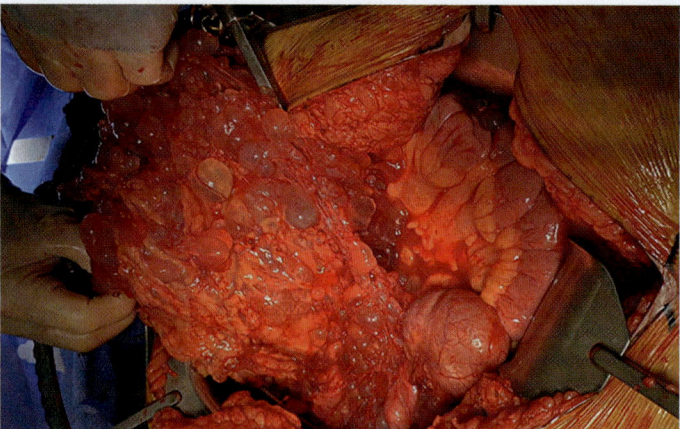

FIGURE 70.5 Cystic mesothelioma, greater omentum, with substantial tumor burden displayed via midline laparotomy.

is found in approximately 10% of cases and is the second most common cause of death attributable to colorectal cancer, after liver metastases. Because of significant challenges in the diagnosis and treatment, patients with peritoneal carcinomatosis have a poorer prognosis compared with liver or lung metastases.[38] The development of CRS and HIPEC has opened new possibilities in a disease that was previously viewed with nihilism. Laparoscopic evaluation before CRS is a useful tool for selecting patients for CRS. We use a laparoscopic PCI score >20 as a contraindication for CRS and HIPEC.

Several large retrospective studies have been published documenting the role of CRS + HIPEC in carefully selected patients who can achieve complete cytoreduction.[39] The first randomized clinical trial was from the Netherlands, and despite criticisms regarding the design, type of chemotherapy used, and inclusion of patients with appendiceal cancer, it paved the way for additional trials. Remarkably, it found a near doubling of survival in patients undergoing CRS and HIPEC compared with systemic therapy. It included patients with peritoneal carcinomatosis and reported improved survival after CRS and HIPEC with mitomycin C compared with systemic therapy with or without palliative surgery.[40] More recently, the French randomized controlled trial PRODIGE 7 compared CRS and HIPEC versus CRS alone with modern systemic chemotherapy. Even though there was no OS benefit associated with HIPEC, the results published represent significant improvement compared with historical results, with a median OS of 41 months in both arms and 5-year survival of 39.4% versus 36.7% in the HIPEC versus CRS-alone arm.[41] This study has been strongly criticized for using a brief 30-minute oxaliplatin perfusion as the HIPEC agent. Nevertheless, it clearly demonstrated that CRS should be the standard of care in resectable cases of peritoneal dissemination because it reported the best outcomes ever for patients in this setting.

Earlier diagnosis has been a challenge for peritoneal carcinomatosis. Therefore, several groups have assessed the role of second-look operations or adjuvant HIPEC in preventing peritoneal recurrence in high-risk patients. The results to date have been mixed. A Spanish phase III trial reported significantly improved locoregional recurrence rates after cytoreduction and HIPEC (1 hour of mitomycin C at 30 mg/M^2) versus cytoreduction alone in a group of patients with T4 tumors and no carcinomatosis.[42]

A similar Dutch trial (COLOPEC) did not show improvement in peritoneal metastasis-free survival with prophylactic HIPEC for perforated or T4 colorectal cancers, albeit using an attenuated chemoperfusion of oxaliplatin for 30 minutes.[43] A French phase III trial assessed the role of systematic second-look surgery and HIPEC in patients with high-risk tumors or completely resected peritoneal or ovarian metastases, concluding that there was no disease-free survival benefit with the addition of HIPEC (oxaliplatin for 30 minutes).[44] In light of the current evidence, adjuvant or "prophylactic" HIPEC is considered investigational and should be performed in the setting of a trial, although the Spanish T4 trial is suggestive of a modest benefit. Clearly, there is a pressing need for more sensitive modalities to achieve early diagnosis of peritoneal recurrences.

A significant proportion of patients with peritoneal carcinomatosis are also diagnosed with liver or lung metastases. In an analysis of phase III trial data, only 2% of patients were found to have isolated peritoneal metastases, whereas 11% were found to have other metastatic sites besides peritoneal.[38] The optimal timing and chemotherapy regimen for the management of peritoneal metastases remains under investigation. A recent phase II trial showed radiologic responses in 28%, and pathologic responses in 38%, of patients who underwent CRS and HIPEC after 3 months of chemotherapy (FOLFOX/CapeOx/FOLFIRI).[45] Even though liver metastases do not represent an absolute contraindication for cytoreduction and HIPEC, the timing and selection of patients need to be done in a multidisciplinary setting and by experienced teams. In a multi-institutional analysis, excellent outcomes were reported from CRS/HIPEC and liver resection, whether simultaneous or in a two-stage approach. Median OS was 47.6 months, severe morbidity was 32.3%, and perioperative mortality was 4%.[46]

Ovarian Cancer

Epithelial ovarian cancer is the leading cause of death from gynecologic cancer in the United States. Peritoneal dissemination is very common, and optimal cytoreduction followed by adjuvant chemotherapy has been the standard of care for many years. Several phase III randomized clinical trials and pooled analyses have demonstrated the efficacy of IP chemotherapy and demonstrated improved PFS and even OS compared with IV chemotherapy alone.[47-49] However, these results have been criticized because of increased rates of hematologic toxicities, renal toxicity, and difficulty in tolerating all intended treatment cycles. A trial that compared IV carboplatin/paclitaxel versus IP carboplatin/IV paclitaxel and IP cisplatin/IP paclitaxel (all arms included bevacizumab) showed no difference in PFS between IV and IP chemotherapy arms.[50]

The management of these patients with neoadjuvant chemotherapy followed by interval debulking is being more commonly used. This approach is particularly helpful in patients with a high volume of disease upon presentation and other significant comorbidities precluding them from upfront debulking. In a recent analysis of long-term survival data from the Ovarian Cancer Hyperthermic Intraperitoneal Chemotherapy-1 (OVHIPEC-1) trial, the addition of HIPEC to interval debulking led to improved survival outcomes compared with interval debulking alone, with median OS of 44.9 versus 33.3 months.[51] The management of these patients is complex and individualized; even though IP chemotherapy is an acceptable addition to optimal debulking, its role in ovarian cancer is not typically as a first-line therapy for all patients with advanced disease.

Gastric Cancer

Even though gastric cancer is less common in Western Europe and the United States, it remains a significant global health problem, particularly in Asia. Gastric cancer has a clear propensity for metastases to the peritoneal cavity. All patients with suspected locoregional disease should be considered for diagnostic laparoscopy with biopsy of suspicious lesions and peritoneal washings.[52] Positive peritoneal cytology is considered M1 disease, and systemic therapy remains the first-line standard of care. However, survival outcomes have been dismal, with median OS of less than 12 months for patients with peritoneal disease resulting from gastric cancer. Several studies, primarily from Asia, have investigated the role of CRS and IP chemotherapy in gastric cancer. The PHOENIX-GC trial was a phase III randomized clinical trial that compared IP paclitaxel and IV paclitaxel versus IV S-1 plus cisplatin on a two-to-one ratio. Even though the trial did not meet its primary end point of median survival, there was a trend toward improved survival with the IP paclitaxel of 17.7 versus 15.2 months and improvement in baseline ascites.[53] In a Chinese phase III trial, patients with gastric cancer and synchronous peritoneal metastases were randomized to CRS versus CRS and HIPEC with cisplatin and mitomycin C. Median survival was improved in the HIPEC arm at 11 months versus 6.5 months in the CRS-alone arm.

Primarily retrospective studies and small randomized trials have been conducted in the Western Hemisphere to assess the role of CRS + HIPEC. The Gastrectomy With Metastasectomy Plus Systemic Chemotherapy (GYMSSA) trial randomized patients to CRS, HIPEC, and systemic therapy versus systemic therapy alone. All patients in the experimental arm had a complete cytoreduction, and median survival was 11.3 months versus 4.3 months in the systemic therapy arm.[54] More recently, the German GASTRIPEC trial compared CRS alone with CRS + HIPEC using mitomycin C and cisplatin with standard perioperative chemotherapy in both arms. The study was closed because of slow accrual, and median survival was the same in both arms at 13.9 months. However, PFS doubled in the CRS + HIPEC arm to 7.1 months from 3.5 months, and distant metastases–free survival increased as well.[55] In summary, CRS and HIPEC should be considered for patients with limited peritoneal disease (we suggest a PCI <6) after a good response to systemic therapy, particularly in the setting of a trial.

The role of palliative gastrectomy in patients with limited metastatic disease was investigated in the REGATTA trial. Patients were randomized to gastrectomy followed by systemic therapy versus systemic therapy alone, and at 2 years, OS was 25.1% versus 31.7%, respectively. The study was closed early as a result of futility and because patients who had total gastrectomy could not tolerate oral S-1.[56] The group from MD Anderson has published encouraging results from using repeated laparoscopic HIPEC with and without cytoreduction in a group of patients with gastric cancer and peritoneal metastases after maximal treatment with systemic therapy.[57,58]

An area of active research is the use of adjuvant or "prophylactic" HIPEC in patients with high-risk gastric cancer. The interim safety results of the European Gastric Cancer Hyperthermic Intraperitoneal Chemotherapy (GASTRICHIP) trial showed no difference in morbidity after perfusion with oxaliplatin over 30 minutes in combination with IV 5-fluorouracil (5-FU) leucovorin.[59] A Japanese trial is investigating the role of prophylactic HIPEC using IP paclitaxel and the role of the same regimen to clear cytology-positive disease without gross peritoneal metastases.[60] Several questions remain in the treatment of peritoneal carcinomatosis resulting from gastric cancer, and despite the scarcity of level 1 data, there is a growing body of evidence demonstrating efficacy of IP chemotherapy for select patients with limited disease and after response to systemic therapy.

FUTURE DIRECTIONS

Four decades into the development of CRS and HIPEC in the treatment of peritoneal malignancies, there are still unanswered questions. It must be kept in mind that CRS with compete resection of apparent disease is the cornerstone of therapy for patients with peritoneal metastasis. Further, it must be emphasized that HIPEC is a treatment platform for drug delivery. As such, it will be modified in regard to agents, pressurized delivery, duration, and temperature with ongoing research. For many types of peritoneal metastasis, CRS and HIPEC should be applied with systemic therapies, not in lieu of them.

Incremental progress has been made with improvement of survival from peritoneal metastases associated with several primary cancers. There is a need for more multi-institutional collaboration and cooperative trials to move the field forward. New technologies, such as circulating tumor cells and circulating tumor DNA, offer new ways to evaluate and monitor for recurrence.[34,61] Further, the development of patient-derived organoids provides a new high-throughput platform to investigate tumor susceptibility to different chemotherapeutic agents and represents a new frontier in personalized medicine.[62,63] Treatment of peritoneal metastasis has moved from therapeutic nihilism to mainstream therapy, offering selected patients the real possibility of long-term survival with excellent quality of life.

SELECTED REFERENCES

Forsythe SD, Sasikumar S, Moaven O, et al. Personalized identification of optimal HIPEC perfusion protocol in patient-derived tumor organoid platform. *Ann Surg Oncol.* 2020;27(13):4950-4960.

This study demonstrated feasibility of organoid platforms in the preclinical personalized evaluation of HIPEC regimens in appendiceal and colon cancer carcinomatosis patients. Furthermore, it showed lack of efficacy of the high-dose, short-duration oxaliplatin HIPEC regimen in colon cancer, with more than 50% of treated colon cancer organoid patients alive postperfusion.

Franko J, Shi Q, Meyers JP, et al. Prognosis of patients with peritoneal metastatic colorectal cancer given systemic therapy: an analysis of individual patient data from prospective randomised trials from the Analysis and Research in Cancers of the Digestive System (ARCAD) database. *Lancet Oncol.* 2016;17(12):1709-1719.

In this analysis, the presence of peritoneal metastases was shown to have a prognostic impact on survival of patients having peritoneal metastases, demonstrating worse outcomes among stage IV colon cancer patients.

Levine EA, Stewart JH 4th, Shen P, Russell GB, Loggie BL, Votanopoulos KI. Intraperitoneal chemotherapy for peritoneal surface malignancy: experience with 1,000 patients. *J Am Coll Surg.* 2014;218(4):573-585.

Single-center experience establishing performance status and completeness of cytoreduction as key prognostic factors of survival outcomes after cytoreduction and HIPEC. A statistically significant difference in survival was noted based on institutional experience as well as type of primary tumor.

Levine EA, Votanopoulos KI, Shen P, et al. A multicenter randomized trial to evaluate hematologic toxicities after hyperthermic intraperitoneal chemotherapy with oxaliplatin or mitomycin in patients with appendiceal tumors. *J Am Coll Surg.* 2018; 226(4):434-443.

First completed prospective randomized clinical trial on appendiceal tumors; showed similar survival rates after perfusion with mitomycin C versus oxaliplatin. Leukopenia was statistically more common after perfusion with mitomycin, whereas oxaliplatin led to more thrombocytopenia after HIPEC.

Quenet F, Elias D, Roca L, et al. Cytoreductive surgery plus hyperthermic intraperitoneal chemotherapy versus cytoreductive surgery alone for colorectal peritoneal metastases (PRODIGE 7): a multicentre, randomised, open-label, phase 3 trial. *Lancet Oncol.* 2021;22(2):256-266.

Phase III randomized clinical trial that showed no difference in survival outcomes between cytoreduction versus cytoreduction and HIPEC after 30-min perfusion with high-dose oxaliplatin in patients with colorectal peritoneal metastases. Median overall survival was upwards of 41 months in both arms, solidifying cytoreductive surgery as the most effective modality in the treatment of colorectal peritoneal metastases.

The full reference list appears on Elsevier eBooks+.

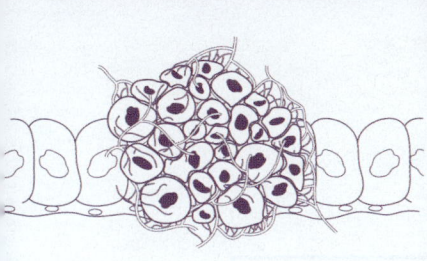

CHAPTER 71

Surgeon's Approach to Lymphadenopathy

Jennifer Zhang, Giorgos Karakousis, and John Miura

INTRODUCTION

Lymphadenopathy remains a common clinical condition that affects patients of all age groups. It refers to the swelling of lymph nodes, which can occur in isolation or could be more generalized on presentation. When initially discovered, lymphadenopathy can pose a diagnostic dilemma because the underlying etiology is broad and includes malignancies, infection, autoimmune disorders, medications, and iatrogenic causes. For surgeons, patients with new lymphadenopathy remain a common clinical scenario. The critical task in approaching these patients is determining whether their presentation is associated with a benign self-limited process versus a malignancy or other serious condition requiring immediate attention. As a result, establishing a systematic approach for surgeons remains paramount when evaluating lymphadenopathy cases to ensure the workup remains safe and effective and avoids the potential for unnecessary procedures. This chapter reviews the evaluation of patients with lymphadenopathy, with particular emphasis on differential diagnoses, diagnostic imaging, biopsy techniques, pathology, and clinical management.

DIAGNOSTIC CONSIDERATIONS

Given the numerous causes that can lead to lymphadenopathy, the initial diagnostic considerations should include the patient's age, lymph node location (isolated vs. generalized), duration of lymphadenopathy, antecedent events (recent infections, new medications/immunizations), extranodal signs and symptoms, and physical examination findings. A thorough initial assessment will often assist in refining the diagnostic evaluation (Fig. 71.1).

Among the pediatric population, lymphadenopathy is common, with up to 50% of children developing a palpable lymph node at any one time.[1] For the vast majority of children, lymphadenopathy reflects a benign reactive process secondary to a self-limiting infection. Lymphadenopathy due to a neoplastic process is extremely rare among younger patients, with only 0.4% of unexplained lymphadenopathy cases being attributable to cancer among individuals less than 40 years of age.[2] Conversely, in older adults, new lymphadenopathy can be a more worrisome finding, with a greater percentage of cases (4%) due to malignancy.

The ascertainment of recent exposures and past medical history is also a critical component in the evaluation of patients with lymphadenopathy. Obtaining a thorough history that includes prior cancers, recent infections, travel, medications, recent immunizations, and sexual history can aid in the diagnostic workup. Additionally, certain symptoms may help narrow the diagnosis. Fevers, although nonspecific, could suggest either an infectious or malignant cause. However, the presence of constitutional "type B" symptoms that include fever, night sweats, and unintentional weight loss may suggest an underlying lymphoproliferative disorder. As for an autoimmune process, extranodal signs and symptoms such as arthralgias, muscle weakness, and skin rash could also accompany the lymphadenopathy.

The duration of the lymphadenopathy can also assist in the diagnostic assessment. For lymphadenopathy that lasts less than 2 weeks or lasts longer than 12 months without a change in size, or if the patient reports a fluctuation in lymph node size, the likelihood of it being caused by a malignant process is extremely low.[3]

PHYSICAL EXAMINATION

Patients evaluated for new lymphadenopathy should undergo a thorough lymphatic examination (cervical, axillary, inguinal, epitrochlear, popliteal) that takes into consideration common lymphatic drainage patterns (Table 71.1). Determining whether the lymphadenopathy is isolated or generalized will further refine the examination and help assist in determining whether additional ancillary diagnostic tests (blood work, imaging) are necessary. The

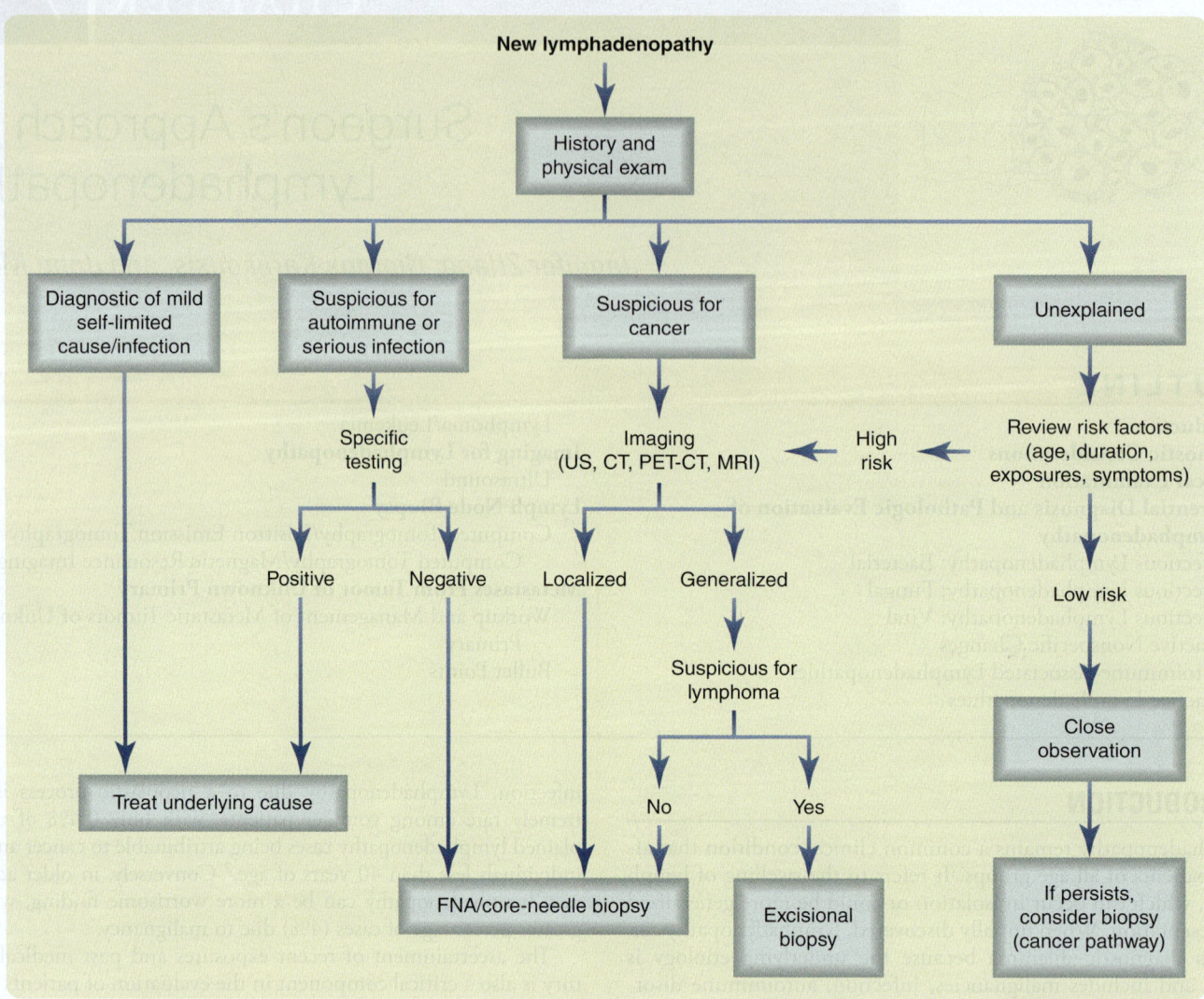

FIGURE 71.1 Algorithm for evaluating new lymphadenopathy of uncertain etiology. *CT,* Computed tomography; *FNA,* fine-needle aspiration; *MRI,* magnetic resonance imaging; *PET,* positron emission tomography; *US,* ultrasound.

TABLE 71.1 Peripheral Lymph Node Basins: Location, Drainage Pattern, Differential Diagnosis

LOCATION	DRAINAGE PATTERN	DIFFERENTIAL DIAGNOSIS
Submandibular/ Submental	Lower face, mouth, lips, tongue, salivary glands	Infection, mononucleosis, lymphoma, head and neck cancer, melanoma or other cutaneous skin cancers
Cervical	Scalp, neck, upper back, thorax	Infection, mononucleosis, lymphoma, head and neck cancer, melanoma or other cutaneous skin cancers
Supraclavicular	Mediastinum, lungs, esophagus, thorax, abdomen/ retroperitoneum (via thoracic duct)	Infection (bacterial/fungal); lung/thoracic, esophageal, retroperitoneal, or GI cancer; lymphoma; melanoma or other cutaneous skin cancers
Axillary	Upper extremity, thoracic wall, breast	Infection, lymphoma, breast cancer, skin cancer (melanoma, cutaneous squamous cell carcinoma)
Epitrochlear	Forearm, hand	Infection, lymphoma, sarcoidosis, melanoma or other cutaneous skin cancers
Inguinal	Lower extremities, penis, scrotum, vulva, vagina, perineum, gluteal region, lower abdominal wall, anus	Infections of the lower extremities or abdominal wall, sexually transmitted infections, lymphoma, melanoma or other cutaneous skin cancers, GU/GI/GYN malignancy
Popliteal	Lower leg, sole of foot	Infections of the lower extremity, melanoma or other cutaneous skin cancers

GI, Gastrointestinal; *GU,* genitourinary; *GYN,* gynecologic.

quality of the enlarged lymph nodes should also be assessed. Lymph node qualities can include size, tenderness, warmth, consistency (firm vs. fluctuant), and fixed versus mobile. Tender lymph nodes often reflect an inflammatory or reactive process caused by an infection but can also be seen with aggressive malignancies that result in rapid enlargement of the lymph node, resulting in hemorrhage or necrosis.[4] As a result, the qualitative characteristics of lymphadenopathy are usually inadequate in differentiating benign versus malignant causes. Additional examination findings, although infrequent, could include concomitant splenomegaly, which occurs with infectious mononucleosis and lymphoproliferative processes (lymphoma, leukemia) (Table 71.1).

DIFFERENTIAL DIAGNOSIS AND PATHOLOGIC EVALUATION OF LYMPHADENOPATHY

The differential diagnosis for lymphadenopathy can be broadly categorized into infectious, noninfectious benign, and malignant etiologies (Table 71.2).[4,5] Pathologic evaluation is critical in arriving at a diagnosis for otherwise unexplained lymphadenopathy.

Infectious Lymphadenopathy: Bacterial

Bacterial infections can cause regional lymphadenopathy and lead to acute lymphadenitis.[6] These are often due to soft tissue infections caused by *Staphylococcus aureus* or group A streptococcus. In the early acute phase, there is an increase in eosinophilic proteinaceous material and neutrophils and macrophages. Sometimes bacteria can be seen on histology, and a tissue Gram stain may be a useful tool.[5] Definitive diagnosis requires culture of infected tissue.

TABLE 71.2 Differential Diagnosis of Lymphadenopathy

INFECTIOUS	NONINFECTIOUS BENIGN	MALIGNANT
Bacterial:	Reactive nonspecific changes:	Hodgkin lymphoma:
• Soft tissue infections	• Reactive follicular hyperplasia	• Nodular lymphocyte-predominant
• Tuberculosis	• Reactive paracortical hyperplasia	• Classic type
• Cat-scratch disease		
• Syphilis		
Fungal:	Autoimmune-associated lymphadenopathies:	Non-Hodgkin lymphoma:
• Coccidioidomycosis	• Rheumatoid arthritis	• Lymphoblastic leukemia/lymphoma
• Histoplasmosis	• Systemic lupus erythematosus	• Mature B-cell lymphoma
• Cryptococcosis		• Mature T-cell lymphoma
Viral:	Reactive lymphadenopathies:	Tumor metastases:
• Epstein-Barr virus	• Rosai-Dorfman	• Breast
• Human immunodeficiency virus	• Kimura disease	• Melanoma
• Cytomegalovirus	• Castleman disease	• Head and neck
• Herpes simplex virus	• Sarcoidosis	• Other

Adapted from Gaddey HL, Riegel AM. Unexplained lymphadenopathy: evaluation and differential diagnosis. *Am Fam Physician.* 2016;94: 896-903; Miranda RN, Khoury JD, Medeiros LJ. *Atlas of Lymph Node Pathology.* New York: Springer; 2013.

Mycobacterium tuberculosis lymphadenitis is the most common extrapulmonary manifestation of tuberculosis. This usually presents as painless lymphadenopathy involving the cervical lymph nodes.[5,7] Necrotizing granulomatous inflammation and caseous necrosis can be seen histologically. *M. tuberculosis* can be identified by acid-fast stains and appears as bright-red bacilli. Atypical mycobacteria, such as *M. marinum, M. kansaii,* and *M. avium-intracellulare,* can cause lymphadenitis in immunocompromised patients, such as those with human immunodeficiency virus or hairy cell leukemia. A histologic hallmark of atypical mycobacterial lymphadenitis is the concomitant existence of suppurative and nonnecrotizing granulomatous inflammation. Acid-fast bacilli can also be identified on histology.[8]

Bartonella henselae is the pathogenic organism responsible for cat-scratch lymphadenitis. The associated lymphadenopathy is usually unilateral and appears 1 to 3 weeks after a cat-inflicted injury, with accompanying fever and fatigue in some cases. *B. henselae* can be visualized within the lymph node using the Warthin-Starry silver stain[9] and is associated with an increase in macrophages and small areas of necrosis.[5]

Treponema pallidum infection can lead to syphilitic lymphadenitis during any of the three stages of disease.[5] During the primary syphilis stage, inguinal lymph nodes are most commonly affected in the regional area of primary infection. Cervical lymphadenopathy is the second most common site. Generalized lymphadenopathy can occur in the secondary syphilis stage 6 to 8 weeks after initial onset of infection and can involve the femoral, cervical, and axillary lymph node basins. Laboratory screening tests can be used as a first step, but confirmatory tests specific for *T. pallidum* must be performed in light of a positive screening test.

Infectious Lymphadenopathy: Fungal

Fungal lymphadenitis can present in patients who are immunosuppressed and includes histoplasmosis, cryptococcosis, and coccidioidomycosis. Patients often have additional affected organ systems, such as pulmonary and central nervous system. Diagnosis can be made based on fungal antigens, serologic studies, and/or fungal cultures. Enlarged lymph nodes can be seen demonstrating granulomas and yeast on histopathology.[5] Necrotizing granulomas or calcifications can be seen in histoplasmosis. Periodic acid–Schiff (PAS) stains can identify *Histoplasma capsulatum, Cryptococcus neoformans,* and *Coccidioides* organisms.

Infectious Lymphadenopathy: Viral

Epstein-Barr virus (EBV) is the causative agent of infectious mononucleosis. Symptoms can include pharyngitis, fever, and lymphadenopathy.[10] A monospot serologic test can identify heterophile antibodies that agglutinate horse red blood cells and is a sensitive screening test. Polymerase chain reaction (PCR) can be performed if a diagnosis cannot be reached.[11] Caution is advised against lymph node biopsy, especially in young people, given that the characteristic histopathologic features may produce a false-positive diagnosis of lymphoma. On histopathology, there is interfollicular or paracortical expansion of lymphocytes, plasma cells, and dendritic cells. In situ hybridization of EBV RNA or immunostaining for latent membrane protein-1 (LMP-1) can help identify the virus.

Human immunodeficiency virus (HIV) primarily targets CD4 T cells and leads to immunodeficiency. Lymph nodes may or may not be enlarged. Cervical, axillary, and head and neck nodal basins are the most common locations of lymphadenopathy.[12] In acute-stage disease, follicular hyperplasia with numerous lymphoid follicles can be seen in the cortex and medulla. End-stage or late-stage disease is characterized by lymphocyte depletion and lymphoid follicles with few lymphocytes and an increase in dendritic cells and histiocytes.[5,13] Serologic testing for HIV antigens should be done to establish a diagnosis.

Cytomegalovirus lymphadenitis is associated with a mixed reactive pattern on histology, with lymph nodes demonstrating follicular, paracortical, and interfollicular hyperplasia. Herpes simplex virus (HSV) lymphadenitis can show multinucleation of immune and epithelial cells as well as areas of focal necrosis and follicular hyperplasia within the lymph node. Of note, HSV lymphadenitis can occur in tandem with lymphoma.[5,13]

Reactive Hyperplasia

Reactive follicular hyperplasia is most commonly seen in children and may account for 75% of lymphadenopathies seen in children. It is seen in 20% to 30% of adult lymphadenopathies because lymphadenopathies due to malignancy increase with age, but it is nonetheless the most common manifestation of reactive lymphadenopathy.[14,15] An increase in number and size of B-cell–containing lymphoid follicles is evident in reactive follicular hyperplasia. This can happen in response to infection and autoimmune diseases, although in some instances, the specific cause cannot be definitively determined. Follicular hyperplasia can often be associated with hyperplasia of other lymph node compartments.[5] It is critical to distinguish reactive follicular hyperplasia from a neoplastic lymphoid proliferation such as follicular lymphoma (see later discussion), which can be differentiated based on morphologic differences, immunohistochemistry, and possibly flow cytometry. For example, the immunohistochemical marker B-cell lymphoma 2 (BCL-2) is usually not expressed by B cells found in reactive follicular hyperplasia but is often expressed in follicular lymphoma.[5,6]

Reactive paracortical hyperplasia is associated with the paracortical zone of the lymph node, which is enriched in T cells, dendritic cells, and histiocytes. Inflammatory stimuli that cause a T-cell response can lead to paracortical zone expansion, including infection, vaccination, and drugs.[5] The viruses that most commonly cause reactive paracortical hyperplasia are herpes simplex virus, EBV, and cytomegalovirus, although, similar to reactive follicular hyperplasia, sometimes no definitive cause can be identified. The proliferation marker Ki-67 may be increased on immunostaining, and viral immunostains may be helpful as a diagnostic adjunct. T-cell lymphoma should be ruled out with additional molecular studies as necessary.

Autoimmune-Associated Lymphadenopathies

A variety of autoimmune diseases can be associated with lymphadenopathy, including rheumatoid arthritis and systemic lupus erythematosus (SLE). Up to 75% of patients with rheumatoid arthritis can have either generalized or localized lymphadenopathy, with cervical, supraclavicular, and axillary lymph node basins being most commonly affected. Lymph node changes can include reactive follicular hyperplasia with varying follicle sizes and a starry-sky pattern in large germinal centers. Eosinophilic deposits are often present in germinal centers and will demonstrate positive PAS staining. B-lymphocyte immunohistochemistry will demonstrate positivity for CD10 and BCL-6 while being negative for BCL-2.[5,13]

SLE can be commonly associated with lymphadenopathy,[16] either localized or generalized, often involving cervical, mesenteric,

axillary, inguinal, and retroperitoneal lymph nodes. During the active untreated phase of the disease, lymph nodes can be necrotic and hemorrhagic, with paracortical hyperplasia and necrosis on histology. Over time, granulation tissue and PAS+ hematoxylin bodies can be seen.[5]

Reactive Lymphadenopathies

Rosai-Dorfman disease is a benign proliferation of histiocytes with massive lymphadenopathy.[17,18] The etiology is unknown. On histopathology, the lymph node demonstrates dilated sinuses filled with a proliferation of histiocytes with abundant eosinophilic cytoplasm and a prominent nucleolus. On immunohistochemistry, it is associated with S100 positivity and negative for CD1a.[5,13]

Kimura lymphadenopathy is a chronic inflammatory disorder affecting subcutaneous tissue and regional lymph nodes of the head and neck, mainly seen in young Asian males.[19] Lymph nodes demonstrate reactive follicular hyperplasia and extensive eosinophilia with microabscesses. IgE deposits can be seen in germinal centers. Cytopathology is of limited importance in the diagnosis of Kimura disease.[5,13]

Castleman disease usually presents as a localized and benign lymphoproliferative lesion in young adults. Histopathology demonstrates large follicles with involuted germinal centers, with follicular dendritic cells positive for CD21, CD23, CD35, and epidermal growth factor receptor (EGFR).[5,13] Excision alone is often curative.

Sarcoidosis is a systemic granulomatous disease that is often a diagnosis of exclusion. Most patients with sarcoidosis present with intrathoracic lymphadenopathy and pulmonary disease,[20] with imaging showing bilateral hilar lymphadenopathy and possibly lung nodules. Sarcoidosis can involve any organ and is histologically characterized by nonnecrotizing granulomatous inflammation. Lymph nodes are often involved with granulomas without signs of acute inflammation or necrosis. Erythrocyte sedimentation rate and serum angiotensin-converting enzyme levels are often elevated. It is important to rule out lymphoma and leukemia because these malignant diseases can coexist in the same lymph node biopsy specimen as sarcoidosis.[5,13]

Lymphoma/Leukemia

Hodgkin lymphoma (HL) is organized into two major categories, nodular lymphocyte predominant and classic.[21] Classic type makes up approximately 90% to 95% of all HL and includes nodular sclerosis, lymphocyte-rich, mixed cellularity, and lymphocyte-depleted subtypes. These neoplasms arise from germinal center B-cell precursor cells and transform into the malignant Reed-Sternberg and Hodgkin cells. Over 90% of the cells within the neoplasm are reactive immune cells, including lymphocytes, histiocytes, plasma cells, and neutrophils. Nodular lymphocyte-predominant HL stains positively for CD20 on immunohistochemistry and negatively for CD30 and CD15, which stain classic HL.[22] Staging is based on degree and location of lymph node or organ involvement.

In general, fine-needle aspiration (FNA) is a safe and accurate tissue-sampling technique in the evaluation of lymphadenopathy, particularly in the evaluation of suspected nonlymphoproliferative malignancies. Lymph node FNA has approximately 90% accuracy with rare false-positive results.[23,24] False-negative diagnoses are more commonly seen, possibly due to partial lymph node involvement or insufficient sampling. It is important to note, however, that FNA is less sensitive for the diagnosis of lymphomas compared with metastatic carcinoma or melanoma. Core-needle biopsy has demonstrated reasonable accuracy for lymphoma in the setting of cervical lymphadenopathy.[25] Although FNA or core-needle biopsy may be very reasonable first starting points for otherwise unspecified lymphadenopathy, if there is high suspicion for lymphoproliferative disorder (or if the results of needle biopsy are nondiagnostic), consideration for excisional lymph node biopsy would be indicated. For HL specifically, identification of Reed-Sternberg cells can be greatly facilitated with excisional biopsy. In circumstances where a lymph node is not readily accessible for excisional biopsy, a combination of core-needle biopsies and FNA in conjunction with appropriate ancillary testing may be sufficient for a diagnosis.

Lymphoblastic leukemia/lymphoma comprises B-lymphoblastic leukemia/lymphoma (B-ALL/LBL) and T-lymphoblastic leukemia/lymphoma (T-ALL/LBL).[26] B-cell lymphomas are more common than T-cell lymphomas and are most commonly seen in children. They display a high degree of molecular heterogeneity, with multiple classifications, including *ETV6-RUNX1* positive, *BCR-ABL1* positive, and hyperdiploidy.[22] Lymph node histopathologic findings in B-LBL and T-LBL are very similar and difficult to distinguish from one another. In general, the lymph node architecture becomes completely replaced with the neoplasm, which appears as monomorphous lymphoblasts infiltrating the lymph node capsule and extending into perinodal soft tissue. Immunostains can help distinguish between T- and B-cell neoplasms. Almost all B-ALL/LBL neoplasms will express CD19, CD79a, and TdT, and most will express CD10, CD22, and CD20. T-ALL/LBL neoplasms often express CD7, CD52, and CD3.[22]

Mature B-cell lymphomas involving lymph nodes include a wide range of neoplasms, such as chronic lymphocytic leukemia, mantle cell lymphoma, diffuse large B-cell lymphoma, and follicular lymphoma.[27] Lymph nodes are often diffusely replaced by lymphoma. Immunophenotyping and molecular analyses are important in identifying the underlying diagnosis. Chronic lymphocytic leukemia is often positive for CD5 and negative for CD10. Mantle cell lymphomas are positive for CD23, cyclin D1, and SOX11. Diffuse large B-cell lymphomas are generally positive for B-cell markers such as CD19, CD20, CD22, and CD79a.[22]

Follicular lymphoma is one of the most common lymphomas in Western society.[28] It is a malignancy that involves germinal center B cells. The lymph node architecture is often completely effaced by neoplastic follicles that extend through the capsule and into perinodal soft tissue. Follicular lymphomas are usually positive for CD19, CD20, CD22, CD79a, and BCL-6 and negative for CD5. The molecular hallmark of follicular lymphoma is the t(14;18)(q32;q21) rearrangement, which results in overexpression of BCL-2. Fluorescence in situ hybridization or PCR can be used to identify this rearrangement. About 30% of patients with follicular lymphoma will transform to diffuse large B-cell lymphoma, which is high grade and associated with resistance to therapy and short median overall survival.[5,13,29] Positron emission tomography (PET)/CT is preferred over CT for staging because PET/CT has been found to alter therapy and is associated with a decreased rate of histologic transformation.[30] In addition, PET/CT can help identify lymph nodes with the highest fluorodeoxyglucose (FDG) uptake, which can then be targeted for excisional biopsy.

Mature T-cell lymphomas involving lymph nodes include peripheral T-cell lymphoma, adult T-cell lymphoma, and anaplastic large-cell lymphoma. T-cell lymphomas are less common than B-cell lymphomas. They generally are seen to replace the lymph node architecture and can be distinguished from B-cell lymphomas by showing positivity for T-cell markers such as CD2 and CD3.[22]

IMAGING FOR LYMPHADENOPATHY

In most cases of unexplained lymphadenopathy, imaging is an important adjunct during the diagnostic evaluation. Imaging allows for more accurate characterization of the abnormal lymph nodes and overall distribution of the lymphadenopathy as well as assisting in guiding the biopsy approach, which is of particular importance in oncology to ensure a definitive diagnosis can be rendered. Common imaging techniques include ultrasound (US), computed tomography (CT), PET/CT, or magnetic resonance imaging (MRI).

Ultrasound

US, which may be a combination of gray scale and/or Doppler sonography, is well established and commonly used for evaluating lymphadenopathy. Multiple nodal characteristics can be assessed, such as nodal site, size, shape, internal architecture, and vascular pattern (Fig. 71.2). Although no single sonographic criterion can accurately differentiate a reactive from a malignant lymph node, when combined with the clinical history, it can frequently help to further differentiate the two processes, with reported sensitivity and specificity of 97% and 93%, respectively.[31]

Size: The size of normal lymph nodes varies and depends on their location. Cervical lymph nodes tend to be the smallest, whereas axillary and inguinal lymph nodes can be much larger. Given the inconsistency in nodal size throughout the body, size alone is insufficient for differentiating a reactive versus malignant process.[32] However, assessment of nodal size can be beneficial during surveillance imaging; fluctuations in size may be more suggestive of a reactive process, whereas interval enlargement would increase the suspicion for an underlying cancer and the need for biopsy.[33]

Shape: Normal lymph nodes have a classic oval or reniform shape. Reactive processes, which can lead to nodal enlargement, tend to preserve the classic lymph node architecture. In contrast, when lymph nodes develop a rounded shape, this finding is more concerning for a malignant process. The "shape index," which is defined as the ratio between the short and long axis of the node, has been proposed as a criterion to differentiate benign and malignant nodes.[34] Normal lymph nodes commonly have a long-axis diameter two times the short-axis diameter. As a result, lymph nodes that have a shape index greater than 0.5 correspond to a rounded shape, which is more concerning for a malignant node.

Hilum: Normal lymph nodes possess an echogenic hilum as a result of the blood vessels and fatty tissue that reside within this space. When tumor infiltrates the normal nodal tissue, this can result in the loss of an echogenic hilum, or "fatty hilum."[35] Up to 92% of benign lymph nodes will have a preserved echogenic hilum as compared with only 4% of malignant nodes.

Additional sonographic characteristics: Normal, reactive, and malignant lymph nodes tend to have a hypoechoic cortex. However, if necrosis or calcifications are noted on US, despite the presence of a hypoechoic cortex, these specific sonographic features are often suggestive of a malignant node.[36] Lastly, Doppler US can be a useful adjunct in assessing vascular distribution.[37] Hilar flow, which describes blood flow branching radially from the hilum, is commonly seen in normal nodes. Conversely, peripheral flow is more frequently observed in malignant

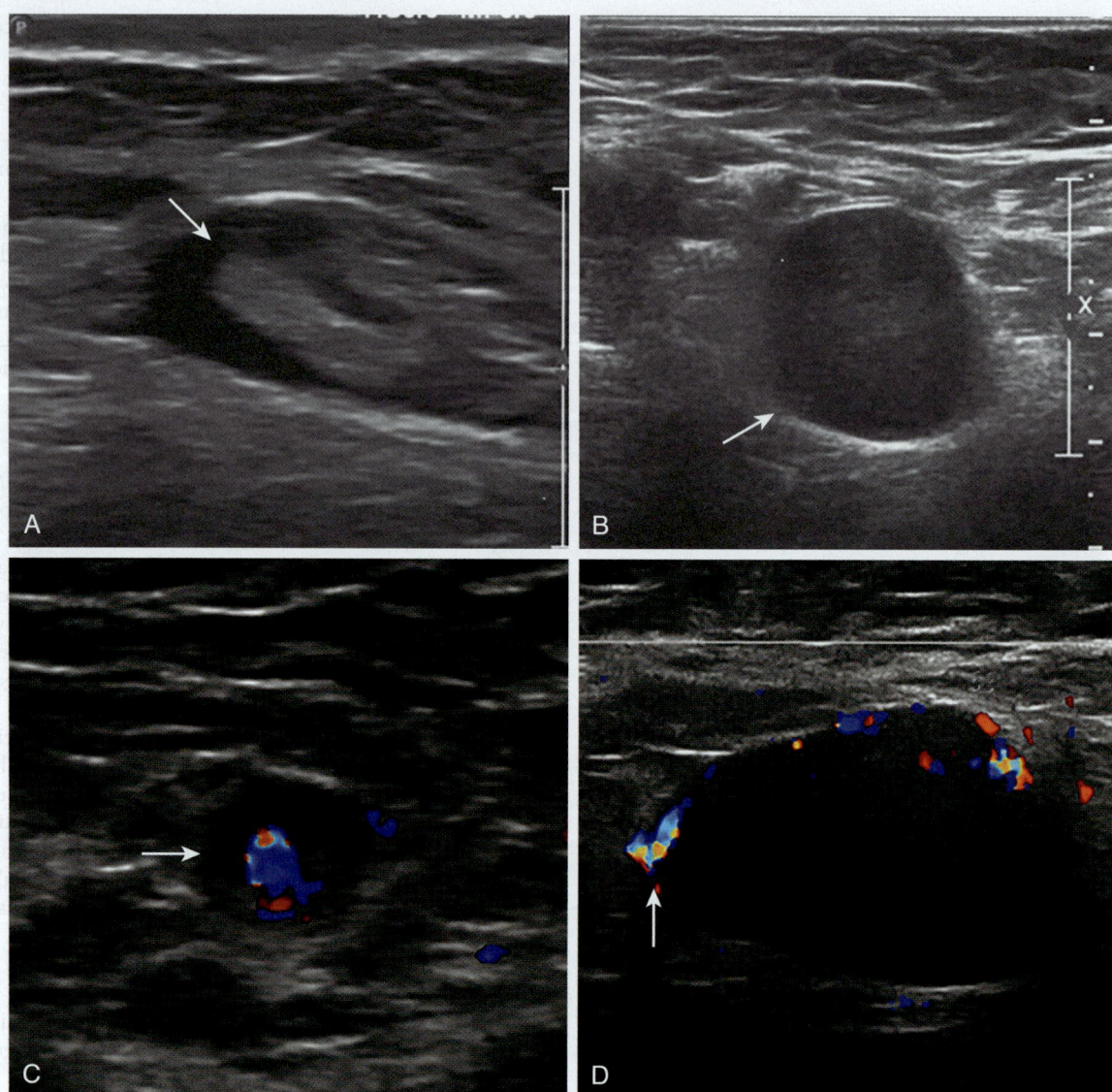

FIGURE 71.2 Ultrasound characteristics of benign versus malignant lymph nodes. (A) Normal oval-shaped axillary lymph node with preserved fatty hilum *(arrow)*. (B) Malignant lymph node with rounded shape *(arrow)* and loss of fatty hilum. (C) Normal lymph node with hilar blood flow. (D) Abnormal lymph node with peripheral blood flow *(arrow)*.

nodes. As tumor infiltrates the nodal cortex, this can lead to the displacement of hilar vessels to the periphery of the node, resulting in blood flow occurring around the edges.

Computed Tomography/Positron Emission Tomography–Computed Tomography/Magnetic Resonance Imaging

CT, PET/CT, and MRI are effective imaging modalities for evaluating lymph node size, character (necrotic/cystic), and distribution. If there is concern for generalized lymphadenopathy, these imaging techniques can quickly determine the extent of the lymphadenopathy and the lymph node basins involved and evaluate the relationship of the lymphadenopathy to surrounding anatomic structures. Additionally, cross-sectional imaging allows for assessment of mediastinal, mesenteric, and retroperitoneal lymphadenopathy, lymph node basins not easily evaluated by ultrasound or physical examination.[38] Radiographic size thresholds for determining abnormal lymphadenopathy have been proposed, but

depending on the location and size cutoff, this will ultimately affect the sensitivity and specificity of the study. Unlike CT and MRI, where the primary metric captured is size, PET/CT has the additional advantage of assessing lymph node function/metabolism, whereby standardized uptake values (SUVs) are measured, leading to an increase in study accuracy. Of the three imaging techniques, PET/CT maintains the highest sensitivity (94%) and specificity (96%) in identifying malignant lymph nodes.[38] With CT or MRI, the reported sensitivity and specificity in the evaluation of abnormal lymphadenopathy are 90% and 94% and 86% and 94%, respectively.[39]

LYMPH NODE BIOPSY

If there is any concern for malignancy, or the lymphadenopathy is unexplained or persistent despite appropriate targeted laboratory studies, lymph node biopsy should be considered. Determining which lymph node to biopsy is extremely important because it increases the likelihood of making a diagnosis and avoids additional unnecessary procedures.

Traditionally, the most abnormal node or, in the setting of isolated lymphadenopathy, a single node is targeted for biopsy. If the adenopathy is diffuse and no single node predominates, clinicians have several options that could help guide the biopsy approach and technique. When involving the superficial lymph node basins, all other diagnostics being comparable, one can consider the order of anatomic biopsy preference to be guided by efforts to reduce surgical morbidity. Occasionally, the lymphadenopathy may be confined to deeper compartments. For mediastinal lymphadenopathy, depending on the location, sampling may require a bronchoscopy or mediastinoscopy. Early engagement of thoracic surgery and/or interventional pulmonology may be beneficial in these scenarios. There are several approaches to addressing isolated mesenteric/retroperitoneal lymphadenopathy. Depending on the location, biopsy approaches can be by image guidance, endoscopic, or surgical (laparoscopic/robotic/open). Lastly, if lymphoma is suspected, PET/CT can be extremely helpful for identifying the lymph node with the greatest SUV.[40] This will ensure that the highest-grade lymphoma is being captured, which is important for treatment planning (Fig. 71.3). This may be particularly relevant in the setting of follicular lymphoma when there may be concern for transformation to large B-cell lymphoma.

There are several biopsy options available, but the approach will depend on the location of the lymphadenopathy and suspected diagnosis.

Fine-needle aspiration (FNA): FNA is a widely used biopsy technique that is effective, is low risk, and consumes low resources.[41] The biopsy can be done in clinic and may occasionally require image guidance. When the cytologic analysis is combined with immunohistochemistry studies, its accuracy is high, with a low false-positive rate (0.9%).[42] Solid organ malignancies (head and neck, lung, breast, gastrointestinal) and cutaneous malignancies (melanoma, cutaneous squamous cell carcinoma) can frequently be diagnosed by FNA. Given the lack of tissue obtained, limitations of FNA include inability to run ancillary diagnostic tests (next-generation sequencing) and a high false-negative rate (3.4%).[42] Additionally, assessment of nodal architecture is not possible. As a result, if lymphoma is suspected, FNA will often be ineffective at rendering a definitive diagnosis.[43]

Core-needle biopsy: If more tissue is required to establish a diagnosis or special studies such as immunophenotypic, genetic, or molecular analyses are anticipated, then core-needle biopsy is an effective approach. Additionally, nodal architecture can occasionally be captured, allowing for appropriate lymphoma evaluation.[44] For lymph nodes that are not easily accessible and for which a surgical approach would yield significant morbidity, core-needle biopsy should be considered over an open surgical biopsy.

Excisional/open biopsy: In cases where needle biopsy is inconclusive or lymphoma is suspected, excisional biopsy can be considered.[40,45] Although the most invasive of the three biopsy techniques, it allows for complete histologic and architectural lymph node assessment. Most excisional lymph node biopsies are performed under general anesthesia, but for superficially located nodes, the procedure can be selectively performed with monitored anesthesia care (MAC) or local anesthesia. Morbidity, albeit low, is most common after excisional biopsy compared with the other approaches. Complications include bleeding, infection, seroma/lymphocele development, nerve injury, and lymphedema, with most cases being self-limiting and mild in severity.

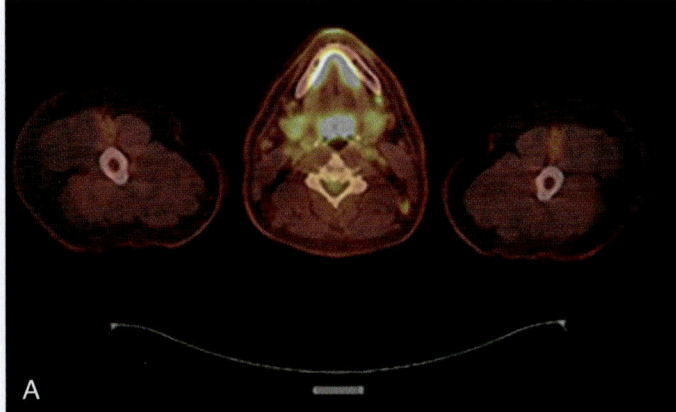
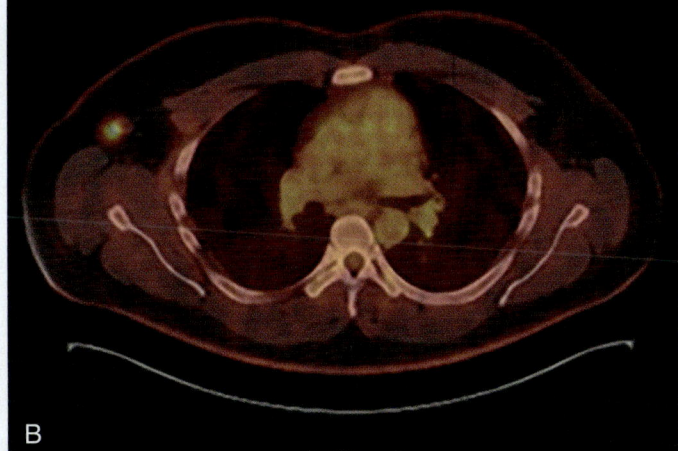
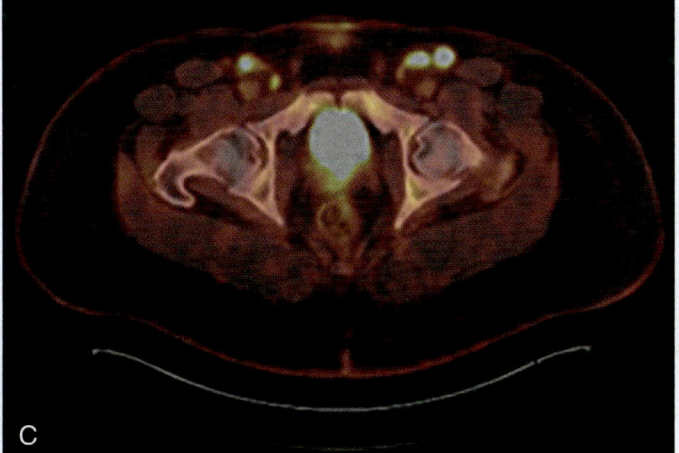

FIGURE 71.3 Seventy-year-old male with a history of new lymphadenopathy. Positron emission tomography scan revealed hypermetabolic lymph nodes in the (A) cervical, (B) axillary, and (C) inguinal lymph node basins. The inguinal lymph nodes had the highest standardized uptake value (14). Excisional biopsy of the inguinal lymph node revealed a grade 3A follicular lymphoma.

METASTASES FROM TUMOR OF UNKNOWN PRIMARY

Lymphadenopathy can sometimes be due to metastases from a nonhematologic malignancy to the regional nodal basin. The histologic pattern of lymph node metastases is often similar to that of the primary tumor, except in cases of very poorly differentiated tumors. Determination can be made between adenocarcinoma, squamous cell carcinoma, melanoma, and neuroendocrine tumors. There are also associated histologic features, such as mucus secretion, signet ring cells, papillary architecture, keratin pearls, clear cell features, and melanin pigmentation, which may help give clues as to the tumor of origin. Immunohistochemistry can be particularly helpful. Cytokeratin staining can help identify a malignancy of epithelial origin. Synaptophysin can be used to identify neuroendocrine tumors, and S100 can help identify tumors of melanocyte origin. Breast metastases to lymph nodes often express estrogen and progesterone receptors, whereas thyroid transcription factor-1 (TTF-1) can help identify the thyroid as a source of cervical lymphadenopathy and the lung as a source of mediastinal lymphadenopathy.

Workup and Management of Metastatic Tumors of Unknown Primary

The site of lymphadenopathy may provide important clues to the origin and site of the primary tumor (Table 71.3).

In cases of axillary lymphadenopathy with pathologic findings from FNA suggestive of a breast primary, a core-needle biopsy of the lymph node is typically required to allow staining for estrogen receptor (ER), progesterone receptor (PR), and human epidermal growth factor receptor 2 (HER2). Every effort should be made to identify the presence and location of the breast primary using a combination of mammogram, ultrasound, and MRI. Treatment will likely involve neoadjuvant chemotherapy followed by definitive surgery and radiation in those without metastatic disease.[46] Postmenopausal patients with ER-positive and HER2-negative disease who have a low nodal burden can sometimes proceed straight to surgery followed by adjuvant chemotherapy, as determined by number of lymph nodes involved on final pathology or Oncotype DX of the primary tumor.[47] In fewer than 1% of cases, the tumor is occult, and a breast primary cannot be identified on imaging. In these cases, the breast can be treated with either mastectomy or radiation. Patients going to up-front surgery will require axillary dissection with removal of levels I and II axillary

lymph nodes. Patients undergoing neoadjuvant chemotherapy can have the most suspicious lymph node clipped, followed by a sentinel lymph node biopsy with retrieval of the clipped node in cases where lymphadenopathy clinically resolves with chemotherapy.[48] Should the sentinel lymph node biopsy be positive for residual nodal disease, a completion axillary dissection would be warranted. Strong consideration should be given to avoidance of excisional biopsy to obtain a diagnosis in cases of suspected breast cancer because the success of a second sentinel lymph node biopsy performed after an initial sentinel lymph node biopsy before neoadjuvant chemotherapy may be significantly lower.[49]

In cases of suspected primary melanoma, a thorough history and physical examination will be critical in identifying any potential lesions. Ideally, a core-needle biopsy or FNA would be performed for diagnosis rather than excisional biopsy, particularly for a single enlarged pathologic node, to allow for the possibility of neoadjuvant therapy. Complete staging imaging (ideally with PET/CT and brain imaging) and *BRAF* mutation testing should be obtained. In cases of resectable nodal disease, either up-front surgery with wide local excision of the primary tumor (if identified) and a therapeutic lymph node dissection or neoadjuvant therapy can be pursued. Major pathologic response (<10% viable tumor) to neoadjuvant immune checkpoint blockade (with the programmed cell death 1 [PD-1] inhibitor pembrolizumab) has been shown to correlate with durable disease-free survival after surgery, and there are data to support that such an approach combined with adjuvant therapy may yield more favorable outcomes with respect to event-free survival compared with adjuvant therapy alone.[50] Moreover, a neoadjuvant approach may obviate the need for more extensive lymphadenectomies with associated morbidity if an index node removal demonstrates a major pathologic response. A therapeutic lymph node dissection, which remains the standard approach for disease localized to a nodal basin, requires an anatomically complete dissection of the involved nodal basin. In the axilla, a level I–III dissection should be performed. In the groin, an inguinofemoral dissection is sufficient for clinically evident nodal disease, although therapeutic iliac and obturator lymph node dissection may be considered if imaging shows resectable lymphadenopathy at these locations. Systemic adjuvant therapy options consist of immunotherapy with nivolumab or pembrolizumab, or a BRAF/MEK inhibitor for patients with *BRAF V600* activation mutations. In high-risk patients, adjuvant radiation may be selectively considered to the nodal basin based on location, number of involved lymph nodes, and presence of extracapsular extension.

For cervical lymphadenopathy concerning for a head and neck primary, a history and complete head and neck examination, including examination of the skin, nasopharynx, oropharynx, hypopharynx, and larynx and palpation of the oropharynx, should be performed with mirror and fiberoptic examination. Image-guided FNA of the lymph node should be performed to help differentiate between a likely head and neck malignancy and other pathologies, such as thyroid cancer, lymphoma, or melanoma. Workup entails a CT or MRI with contrast of the skull base through the thoracic inlet. If targeted imaging fails to identify a primary, PET/CT should be performed before additional interventions, such as examination under anesthesia and more invasive workup studies. Human papillomavirus (HPV) and EBV testing can be performed for squamous cell or undifferentiated histology. For cervical node levels I, II, III, and upper V, an examination under anesthesia, biopsy of areas of

LOCATION OF LYMPHADENOPATHY	ORIGIN OF PRIMARY TUMOR[a]
High cervical	Nasopharynx, tonsils, tongue, thyroid, larynx, face and scalp
Low cervical	Pulmonary, intraabdominal
Virchow's lymph node (left supraclavicular)	Intraabdominal and pelvic (gastric)
Axillary	Breast, upper extremities, trunk
Inguinal	Lower extremities, cervix, vulva, endometrium, ovary, rectum, anus, penis, prostate
Pelvic	Prostate, testes, gynecologic organs, lower extremities

TABLE 71.3 Regional Lymph Node Metastases and Common Origins of Primary Tumors

[a]Melanoma can present at any of these nodal basin sites.

Adapted from Miranda RN, Khoury JD, Medeiros LJ. *Atlas of Lymph Node Pathology.* New York: Springer; 2013; Medeiros LJ. *Loachim's Lymph Node Pathology.* Philadelphia: Wolters Kluwer Health; 2022.

concern, tonsillectomy, and direct laryngoscopy and nasopharyngeal assessment should be performed. For cervical node levels IV and lower V, an examination under anesthesia, direct laryngoscopy, esophagoscopy, and bronchoscopy should be performed. Subsequent treatment will be based on standard regimens for the primary tumor. For thyroglobulin-negative and calcitonin-negative adenocarcinoma occult primaries, a neck dissection, and if high in the neck, parotidectomy, should be performed. For squamous cell occult primaries, appropriate neck dissection or possibly radiation should be performed.

Bullet Points

1. Differential for lymphadenopathy is broad and includes benign and malignant etiologies.
2. If suspicion is high for malignancy or for benign etiology, either symptomatic or for which diagnostic tissue could influence medical management, a lymph node biopsy may be warranted.
3. Methods of lymph node biopsy include FNA, core-needle biopsy, and surgical excisional lymph node biopsy. The decision for biopsy type should take into account potential morbidity of biopsy methods and amount of tissue needed for accurate histologic diagnosis. FNA is usually effective at diagnosis for tumors metastatic to lymph node, whereas core-needle biopsy may provide additional tissue if molecular diagnostics are needed to guide therapy. Surgical biopsy is often indicated in cases where lymphoproliferative disorder is suspected to obtain lymph node architecture and adequate tissue for flow cytometry and other ancillary studies.
4. Ultrasound is a particularly sensitive, specific, and cost-effective diagnostic imaging modality for assessing potentially pathologic lymphadenopathy and for nodal ultrasound surveillance; PET/CT (using SUV avidity) may be particularly helpful in helping to target a specific node or nodal basin in cases of lymphoma where there may be a mixed pattern of disease (with higher- and lower-grade components)
5. In cases of isolated node lymphadenopathy with the potential for nodal metastasis from an unknown primary, special attention should be given to avoiding excisional biopsy of the isolated node and considering the possibility of a potential role for neoadjuvant therapy.
6. Management of localized lymphadenopathy of unknown primary will vary by tumor histology; regional therapeutic lymphadenectomy with appropriate anatomic level of dissection and neoadjuvant therapy may be appropriate considerations.

SELECTED REFERENCES

Cheson BD, Fisher RI, Barrington SF, et al. Recommendations for initial evaluation, staging, and response assessment of Hodgkin and non-Hodgkin lymphoma: the Lugano classification. *J Clin Oncol.* 2014;32:3059-3068.

> *Consensus guidelines for the initial diagnosis and evaluation of suspected lymphoma patients.*

Gordon MJ, Smith MR, Nastoupil LJ. Follicular lymphoma: the long and winding road leading to your cure? *Blood Rev.* 2023;57:100992.

> *Follicular lymphoma is the second most common non-Hodgkin lymphoma and is characterized by the t(14;18) translocation with increased expression of BCL-2.*

Kuehn T, Bauerfeind I, Fehm T, et al. Sentinel-lymph-node biopsy in patients with breast cancer before and after neoadjuvant chemotherapy (SENTINA): a prospective, multicentre cohort study. *Lancet Oncol.* 2013;14:609-618.

> *The SENTINA trial demonstrated a decrease in detection rate of a second sentinel lymph node biopsy performed after an initial sentinel lymph node biopsy for staging and subsequent neoadjuvant chemotherapy.*

Patel SP, Othus M, Chen Y, et al. Neoadjuvant-adjuvant or adjuvant-only pembrolizumab in advanced melanoma. *N Engl J Med.* 2023;388:813-823.

> *The addition of neoadjuvant pembrolizumab increased event-free survival compared with the adjuvant-only group in resectable stage III or IV melanoma.*

Torabi M, Aquino SL, Harisinghani MG. Current concepts in lymph node imaging. *J Nucl Med.* 2004;45:1509-1518.

> *Comprehensive review of the different imaging modalities commonly used for the identification and characterization of lymphadenopathy*

The full reference list appears on Elsevier eBooks+.

The Spleen

Meredith Christina Mason, Joshua Winer, and Seth Concors

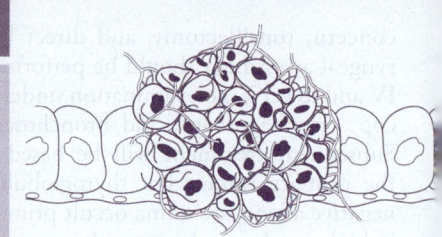

SPLENIC ANATOMY

The spleen is the largest lymphatic organ in the body; it measures 7 to 13 cm in length and weighs up to 250 g. It develops as a discernible organ from mesenchymal cells in the dorsal mesogastrium during week 5 of embryogenesis. The spleen is initially adherent to dorsal pancreatic bud and ultimately separates from the pancreatic bud and settles into the left uppermost aspect of the abdomen in the intraperitoneal cavity. Anatomically, it is located in the upper abdomen protected by ribs 9, 10, and 11. In healthy adults, it is not palpated below the costal margin. In infants, however, it is palpable below the costal margin at the midaxillary line. The spleen has both a diaphragmatic surface and visceral surface, which abuts the greater curvature of the stomach, splenic flexure of the colon, apex of the left kidney, and tail of the pancreas (Fig. 72.1). Peritoneal reflections along these surfaces suspend the spleen in the peritoneal cavity (Fig. 72.2). The splenophrenic ligament is along the diaphragmatic surface, whereas the gastrosplenic, splenorenal, and splenocolic ligaments are related to the visceral surface. In patients without portal hypertension, the splenophrenic and splenocolic ligaments are relatively avascular. The gastrosplenic ligament carries the short gastric vessels in its superior aspect and the left gastroepiploic in its inferior aspect. The splenorenal ligament houses the splenic artery and vein as well as the tail of the pancreas. The tail of the pancreas abuts the splenic hilum in 30% of individuals and is within 1 cm of the hilum in 70% of cases.

Vascular Anatomy

The splenic artery, a branch of the celiac trunk, together with its branches of the short gastric arteries provide the arterial blood supply to the spleen. The splenic artery is a tortuous vessel that gives off multiple branches (up to 16–18) to the pancreas as it travels along its posterior aspect (Fig. 72.3). There are two common variations of the splenic artery with regard to the relation between the splenic artery branches and the hilum of the spleen: the magistral type, which branches into terminal and polar arteries near the hilum of the spleen, and the distributed type, which arborizes much more proximally and distantly from the hilum. A distributed anatomy of the artery is found in 70% of the population.

The splenic artery commonly branches into four to six polar arteries, which go to lobes of the spleen dividing into terminal arteries within the organ, and six short gastric arteries, which often are connected, or come off of, the superior polar artery.

The large splenic vein, which travels posteriorly to the pancreas, is created by the union of several splenic veins and the left gastroepiploic vein, joining with pancreatic branches, and often the inferior mesenteric vein, to form the portal vein with the superior mesenteric vein.

The spleen is encased within a fibroelastic capsule. From the capsule, trabeculae extend and compartmentalize the spleen into lobules. The spleen is also segmented by the divisions of the splenic vessels as they branch within the organ and merge with these trabeculae (Figs. 72.4 and 72.5). The arterioles branch into even smaller vessels and leave these trabeculae to merge with the splenic pulp, where their adventitia is replaced by a covering of lymphatic tissue that continues until the vessels thin to capillaries. There are two general types of tissue within the spleen known as white and red pulp. The majority of the spleen is red pulp, and the vasculature, connective tissue, and venous sinuses are the key aspects of this portion. The lymphatic sheaths make up the white pulp of the spleen and are interspersed among the arteriolar branches as lymphatic follicles. The white pulp interfaces with the red pulp at the marginal zone of the spleen. It is in this marginal zone that the arterioles lose their lymphatic tissue, and the vessels evolve into thin-walled splenic sinuses and sinusoids. The sinusoids then merge into venules, draining into veins that travel along the trabeculae to form larger splenic veins that mirror their arterial counterparts.

SPLENIC FUNCTION

The spleen has four main functions in humans.

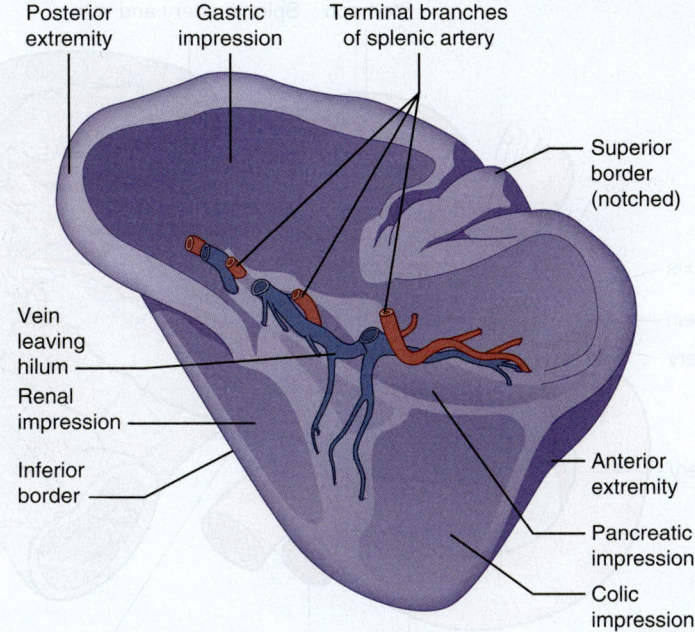

FIGURE 72.1 The spleen and its visceral surface relationships. (From Ellis H. Anatomy of splenectomy for ruptured spleen. *Surgery [Oxford].* 2010;28:226-228.)

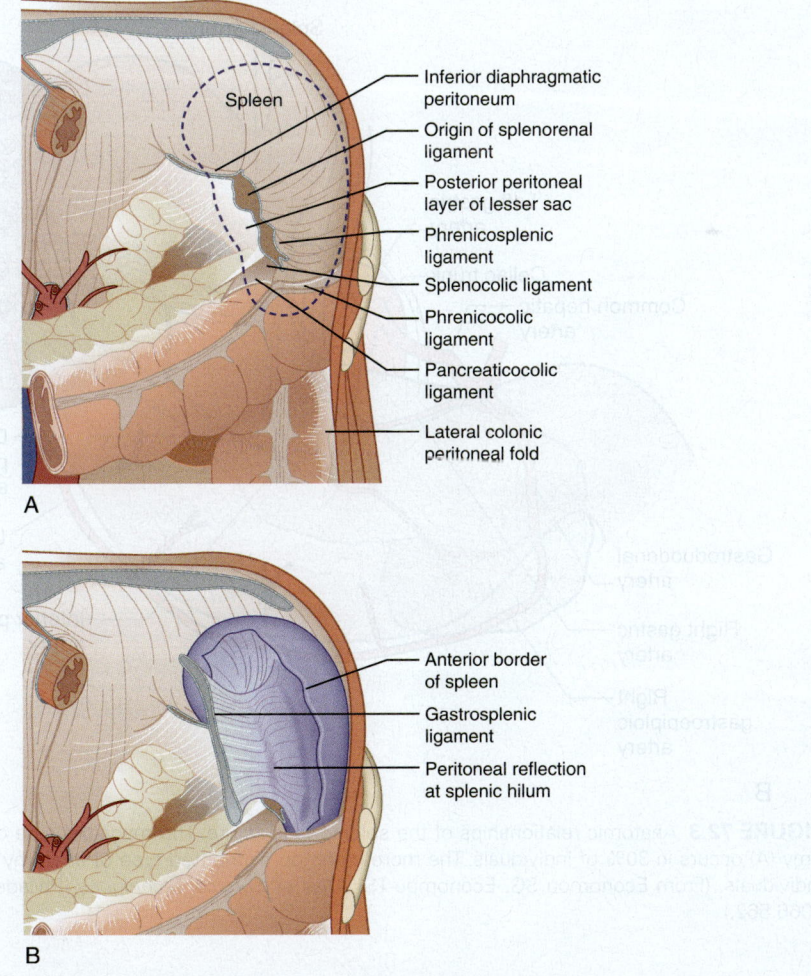

FIGURE 72.2 (A) Posterior peritoneal attachments. (B) Anterior peritoneal attachments. (From Ellis H. Anatomy of splenectomy for ruptured spleen. *Surgery [Oxford].* 2010;28:226-228.)

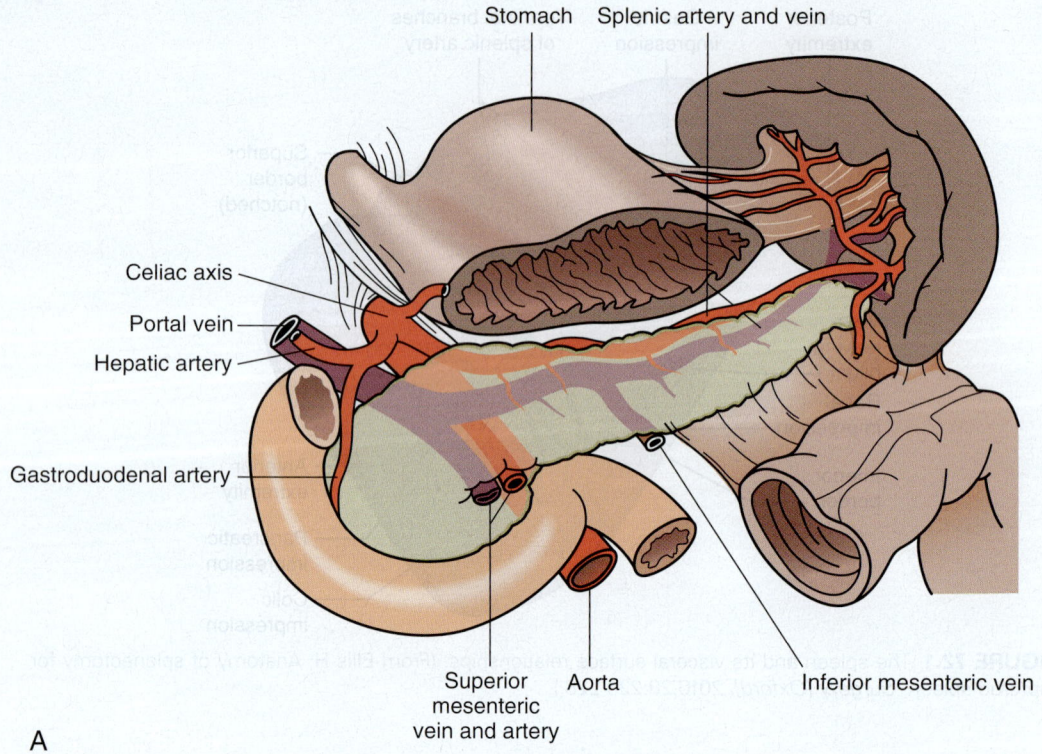

A

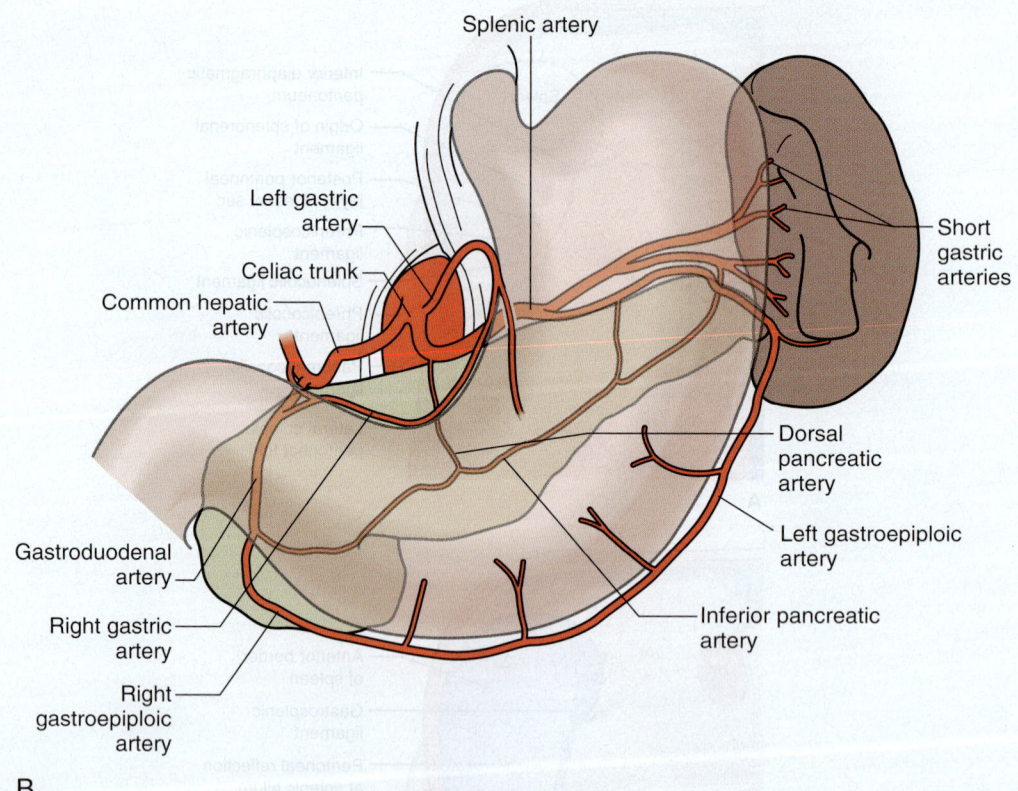

B

FIGURE 72.3 Anatomic relationships of the splenic vasculature. The magistral type of splenic artery anatomy (A) occurs in 30% of individuals. The more common distributed type of anatomy (B) occurs in 70% of individuals. (From Economou SG, Economou TS. *Atlas of Surgical Techniques*. Philadelphia: WB Saunders; 1966:562.)

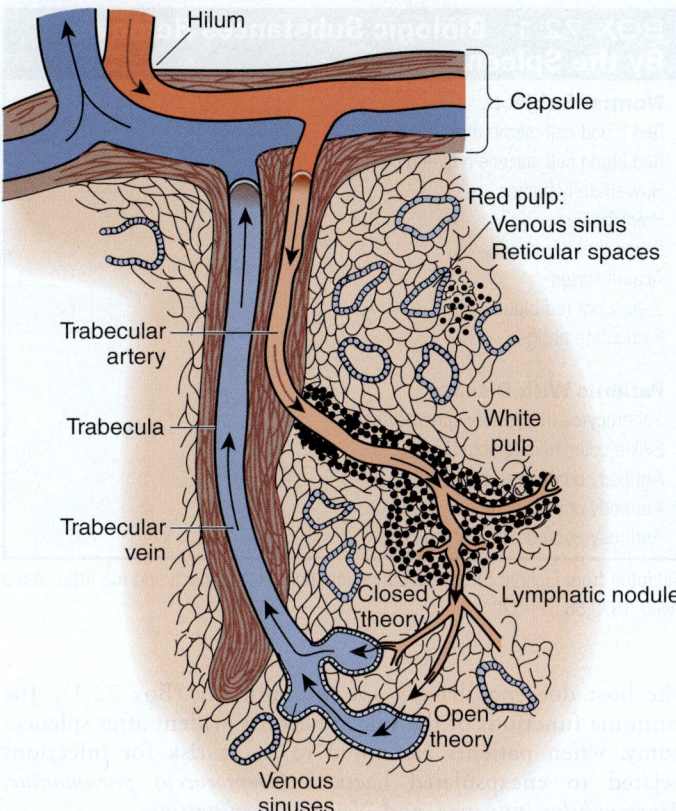

FIGURE 72.4 Structure of the sinusoidal spleen showing the open and closed blood flow routes. (From Bellanti JA. *Immunology: Basic Processes.* Philadelphia: WB Saunders; 1979.)

Hematopoietic

Between 3 and 5 weeks of fetal life, the spleen is a key producer of white and red blood cells and continues along with the liver as gestation progresses. The bone marrow begins to ramp up production during the fifth month of gestation, and under normal conditions, the spleen has no significant hematopoietic function beyond this point. However, in certain pathologic conditions such as myelodysplastic syndrome, the spleen is one of the main organs involved in extramedullary erythropoiesis.

Reservoir

The spleen functions as a reservoir specifically for platelets. Normally one-third of the platelets are pooled within the spleen. Thus, patients with splenomegaly are able to sequestrate a large volume of platelets (up to 80%) with resultant thrombocytopenia.

Filtration

The splenic filtration process consists of two methods of blood flow: the closed and open systems. In the closed system, blood flows directly from arteries to veins. In the open system, the blood flows through the arterioles and then trickles through a sievelike parenchyma made up of reticuloendothelial cells into the splenic sinuses before draining into the venous system (see Figs. 72.4 and 72.5). The cellular elements of blood are directed toward these reticuloendothelial cells, in which cellular cleansing processes take place. These include removal of senescent

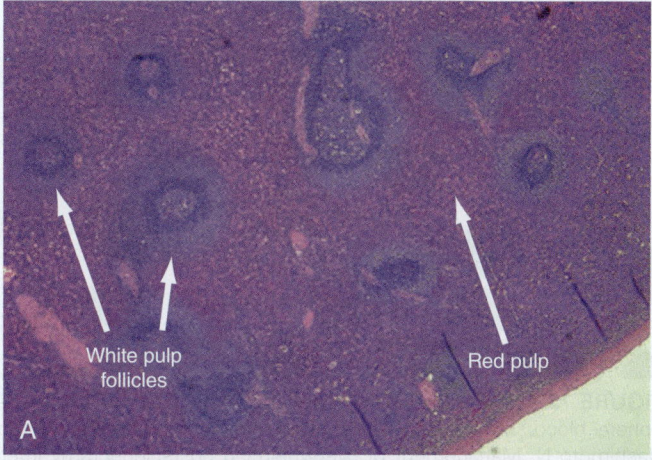

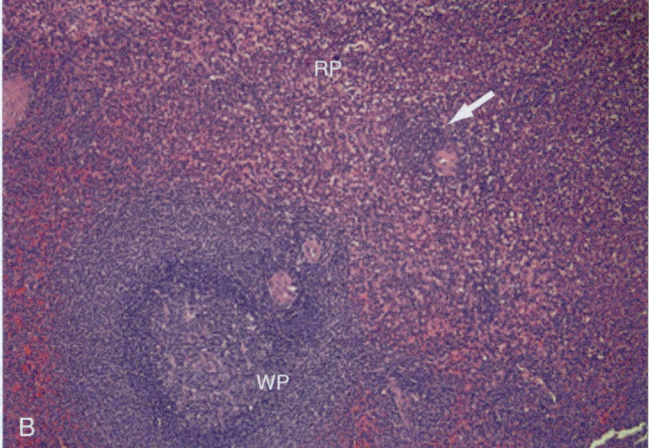

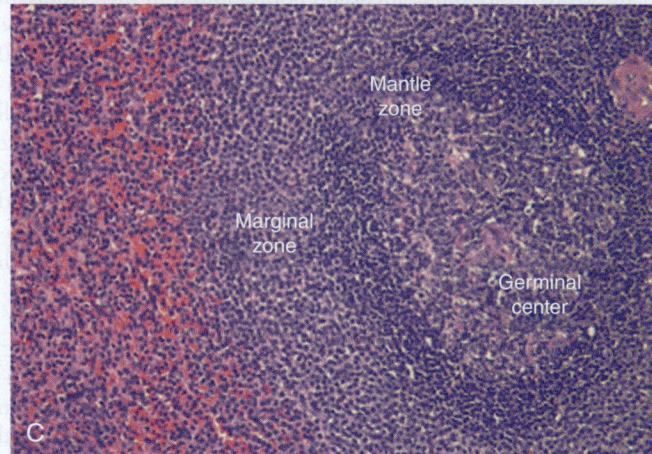

FIGURE 72.5 Normal human spleen on hematoxylin-eosin staining. (A) Low-power photomicrograph showing relationship and relative proportions of red and white pulp. (B) Medium-power photomicrograph (*arrow* indicates periarterial lymphoid sheath). (C) High-power photomicrograph showing detailed secondary follicle architecture. *RP,* Red pulp; *WP,* white pulp (secondary follicle). (From Pernar LIM, Tavakkoli A. Anatomy and physiology of the spleen. In: Yeo CJ, ed. *Shackelford's Surgery of the Alimentary Tract.* 8th ed. Philadelphia: Elsevier; 2019:1595.)

cells, cellular inclusions (e.g., RBC nucleoli) and parasites, and the sequestration of red blood cells (RBCs) (for maturation) and platelets (reservoir). The plasma is directed to the lymphoid tissue, where soluble antigens stimulate the production of antibodies.

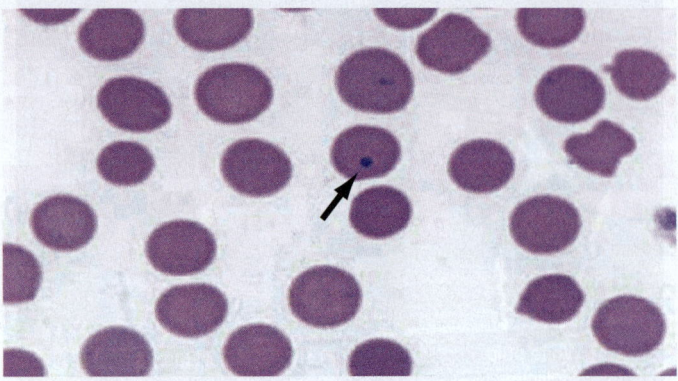

FIGURE 72.6 The presence of Howell-Jolly bodies *(arrow)* on the peripheral blood smear is suggestive of asplenia or hyposplenism. (From Hashimoto N. Management of overwhelming postsplenectomy infection syndrome. *Clin Surg.* 2016;1:1148.)

RBC morphology, and thus RBC function, is maintained by splenic filtration. Normal RBCs are biconcave and deform easily. This plasticity allows passage through the microvasculature and optimizes the exchange of oxygen and carbon dioxide. Imperfect RBCs with inclusions such as Howell-Jolly bodies (nuclear remnant), Heinz bodies (denatured hemoglobin), Pappenheimer bodies (iron granules), and abnormally structured cells such as acanthocytes (spur cells) and codocytes (target cells) cause these RBCs to undergo removal in the spleen.

The presence of Howell-Jolly bodies on a peripheral blood smear is one of the most characteristic findings in asplenia, whether surgical or medical (hemoglobinopathies) (Fig. 72.6). Howell-Jolly bodies are strongly basophilic inclusion bodies found in the cytoplasm of RBCs and represent nuclei remnants that were unable to be cleared by the spleen. Aged RBCs with decreased plasticity (>120 days) become trapped and destroyed in the spleen. Abnormal erythrocytes that result from hemoglobinopathies such as sickle cell anemia, hereditary spherocytosis (HS), thalassemia, or pyruvate kinase deficiency (PKD) are also trapped and destroyed by the spleen. The overall effect is worsening anemia, splenomegaly, and sometimes autoinfarction of the spleen. Similarly, the spleen is involved in platelet destruction in immune thrombocytopenia (ITP), formerly known as *idiopathic thrombocytopenia purpura.*

Immunity

The spleen assists in managing the immune response by antibody synthesis and phagocytosis. Asplenic patients have been found to express subnormal immunoglobulin M levels, and their peripheral blood mononuclear cells exhibit a suppressed immunoglobulin response. Other factors involved in the immune response are opsonins, such as properdin and tuftsin. Opsonins, produced in the spleen, exhibit reduced serum levels after splenectomy. Properdin, a globulin protein also known as *factor P,* initiates the alternate pathway of complement activation; this increases the destruction of bacteria and abnormal cells. Tuftsin, a tetrapeptide, enhances the phagocytic activity of mononuclear phagocytes and polymorphonuclear leukocytes. Absence of a circulating mediator appears to result in suppressed neutrophil function. The spleen also plays a key role in cleaving tuftsin from the heavy chain of immunoglobulin G; thus, circulating levels of tuftsin are subnormal in asplenic patients. Additionally, splenic filtration may be particularly important for removal of microorganisms for which the host does not have a specific antibody (Box 72.1). The immune functions of the spleen become evident after splenectomy, when patients are noted to be at risk for infections related to encapsulated bacteria *Streptococcus pneumoniae, Haemophilus influenza,* and *Neisseria meningitidis.*

SPLENECTOMY

Splenectomy may be indicated for conditions other than trauma. These indications encompass mainly hematologic disorders in addition to other mass lesions and splenic vascular lesions that are discussed elsewhere in this textbook.

Benign Hematologic Conditions
Immune Thrombocytopenia

ITP is the most common hematologic indication for splenectomy. Previously known as *idiopathic thrombocytopenic purpura,* the naming was adjusted to *immune thrombocytopenia* in 2009 to reflect a better understanding of the disease process and the absence of purpura in most cases.[1] ITP is characterized by a low platelet count below 100×10^9/L despite normal bone marrow and the absence of other causes of thrombocytopenia that could be responsible for the finding.[2] The pathogenesis is not fully understood; however, immunoglobulin G autoantibodies directed toward the platelet membranes are believed to be responsible for platelet destruction within the reticuloendothelial system by macrophages and cytotoxic T cells. In addition to the destruction, there is dysfunction of megakaryocytes with a low level of thrombopoietin.

ITP has a heterogenous clinical presentation and course and can be classified as either primary—without any underlying cause—or secondary—related to an autoimmune or infectious cause. Primary ITP is further classified into three subtypes based on disease chronicity: newly diagnosed (within 3 months), persistent (3–12 months), and chronic (greater than 12 months). Secondary ITP is the result of a known cause such as medication induced, infectious, or rheumatologic conditions (i.e., systemic lupus erythematosus). Presentation of ITP can vary, and bleeding episodes may be minor (including bruising and petechiae) or severe, including life-threatening gastrointestinal or intracerebral hemorrhage.[3] In general, patients with ITP have significantly impaired health-related quality of life and have a 1.3- to 2.2-fold higher mortality rate than the general population.[4,5]

The diagnosis of primary ITP involves the exclusion of other causes of thrombocytopenia—pregnancy, drug induced thrombocytopenia (e.g., heparin, quinidine, quinine, sulfonamides), viral infections, and hypersplenism (Box 72.2). Mild thrombocytopenia may be seen in approximately 6% to 8% of otherwise normal pregnancies and in up to 25% of females with preeclampsia. Drug-induced thrombocytopenia is thought to occur rarely, in approximately 20 to 40 cases/million users of common medications, such as trimethoprim-sulfonamide and quinine. Other medications, such as gold salts, have a higher incidence—almost 1% of users. Viral infection (e.g., hepatitis C, human immunodeficiency virus [HIV] infection, rarely Epstein-Barr virus infection) can be responsible for thrombocytopenia independent of splenic sequestration. Bacterial infection, specifically *Helicobacter pylori*, has also been linked to infection-related thrombocytopenia that improves with eradication.

ITP more commonly occurs in females, with bimodal age distribution peaking between 1 to 5 years old and >60 years of age.[6] The clinical manifestation of ITP in children is unique, with sudden-onset severe thrombocytopenia; complete spontaneous remissions are seen in approximately 80% of affected children.

Management of ITP depends primarily on the severity. Asymptomatic, low-risk patients with platelet counts higher than 30,000/mm^3 may be observed without further intervention. Platelet counts of 50,000/mm^3 and higher are rarely associated with clinical sequelae, even with invasive procedures. Initial medical treatment of patients with platelet counts below 30,000/mm^3 and symptoms such as mucous membrane bleeding, high-risk conditions (e.g., active lifestyle, hypertension, peptic ulcer disease), or platelet counts below 20,000 to 30,000/mm^3, even without symptoms, is glucocorticoid administration (prednisone 0.5–2 mg/kg/day or dexamethasone 50 mg/day for 4 days).[2] Clinical response with increases in platelet levels to higher than 50,000/mm^3 is seen in up to two-thirds of patients within 1 to 3 weeks of initiating treatment. Of patients treated with steroids, 25% will experience a complete response. Initial hospitalization for treatment may be required for patients with platelet counts <20,000/mm^3. Platelet transfusion is indicated only for those who experience severe hemorrhage. Intravenous immune globulin is important for the treatment of acute bleeding, in pregnancy, or for patients being prepared for operation, including splenectomy. This dose usually increases the platelet count within 3 days; it also increases the efficacy of platelet transfusions.

In adults with ITP who are corticosteroid dependent or corticosteroid unresponsive, second-line therapy may include rituximab (375 mg/m^2/week intravenously for 4 weeks), thrombopoietin receptor antagonists (TPO-RAs; eltrombopag, romiplostim), or splenectomy. There are no clear guidelines for which second-line therapy is preferred, and the American Society of Hematology suggests that treatment should be individualized based on duration of ITP, frequency of bleeding episodes, comorbidities, age, social support, cost, and availability.[2] In a 2019 meta-analysis, aggregate response rates at 1 month for splenectomy, TPO-RA, and rituximab were 86.7%, 65.7%, and 62.1%, respectively.[2]

For patients with ITP less than 1 year, spontaneous remission may be possible, and secondary treatment with either TPO-RA or rituximab is generally preferred. However, for those patients who are corticosteroid unresponsive or dependent beyond 1 year, splenectomy should be considered. In the pediatric population, splenic preservation is preferred, and high rates of spontaneous remission are seen; therefore, medical therapy is recommended over splenectomy when feasible.[7] Splenectomy is also the treatment of choice for patients with incomplete response to glucocorticoid treatment and for pregnant females in the second trimester who have also failed to respond to steroid treatment or intravenous immune globulin therapy with platelet counts below 10,000/mm^3 without symptoms or below 30,000/mm^3 with bleeding problems.[8]

Splenectomy represents a desirable second-line treatment option for patients who value a durable medication-free response. Most patients will exhibit improved platelet counts within 10 days postoperatively, and durable platelet responses are associated with patients who have platelet counts of 150,000/mm^3 by postoperative day 3 or more than 500,000/mm^3 by postoperative day 10. Two large systematic reviews have reported response rates after splenectomy of 66% and 72%.[9,10] Careful evaluation for splenules

---

BOX 72.2 Differential Diagnosis of Immune Thrombocytopenia (ITP)

Falsely Low Platelet Count

In vitro platelet clumping caused by EDTA-dependent or cold-dependent agglutinins, insufficiently anticoagulated specimen, glycoprotein IIb/IIIa inhibitors (e.g., abciximab)

Giant platelets that are miscounted as WBC rather than platelets by automated counters

Common Causes of Thrombocytopenia

Pregnancy (gestational thrombocytopenia, preeclampsia, HELLP syndrome)

Drug-induced thrombocytopenia (common drugs include heparin, quinidine, quinine, sulfonamides, acetaminophen, cimetidine, ibuprofen, naproxen, ampicillin, piperacillin, vancomycin, linezolid, glycoprotein IIb/IIIa inhibitors)

Viral infections such as HIV, HCV, EBV (infectious mononucleosis), rubella

Helicobacter pylori

Malaria

Hypersplenism caused by chronic liver disease

Alcohol

Nutrient deficiencies (e.g., vitamin B$_{12}$, folate, copper)

Rheumatologic/autoimmune disorders (e.g., systemic lupus erythematosus, rheumatoid arthritis)

Other Causes of Thrombocytopenia Mistaken for ITP

Myelodysplasia

Congenital thrombocytopenias

Thrombotic thrombocytopenic purpura and hemolytic-uremic syndrome

Chronic disseminated intravascular coagulation

Thrombocytopenia Associated With Other Disorders

Autoimmune diseases, such as systemic lupus erythematosus

Lymphoproliferative disorders (chronic lymphocytic leukemia, non-Hodgkin lymphoma)

EBV, Epstein-Barr virus; *EDTA*, ethylenediaminetetraacetic acid; *HCV*, hepatitis C virus; *HELLP*, hemolysis, elevated liver enzymes, and low platelet levels; *HIV*, human immunodeficiency virus; *WBC*, white blood cell.

Adapted from George JN, El-Harake MA, Raskob GE. Chronic idiopathic thrombocytopenic purpura. *N Engl J Med.* 1994;331:1207-1211.

should be undertaken, using both preoperative imaging and a systematic operative approach. In their evaluation of 394 patients treated with laparoscopic splenectomy, Katkhouda and colleagues noted 15% of patients with accessory spleens.[11] Retained accessory spleen should be considered in the differential diagnosis for refractory ITP after splenectomy. Workup may include radionucleotide scans, and resection should be considered for patients who are adequate surgical candidates.

Hereditary Anemias

Hereditary anemia is classified into (1) defects of the RBC membrane (e.g., HS); (2) defects in erythrocyte enzyme (e.g., glucose-6-phosphate dehydrogenase [G6PD] deficiency); and (3) defects in hemoglobin synthesis (e.g., thalassemia, sickle cell anemias [hemoglobin S]).

The decision to perform splenectomy, particularly among patients with hemolytic disorders, needs to be individualized. The benefits of surgery need to be balanced against risk of overwhelming postsplenectomy infection syndrome (OPSI), arterial/venous thromboembolism, and pulmonary arterial hypertension.[12]

Hereditary Spherocytosis

HS is the third most common inherited anemia, following sickle cell disease and thalassemia, and results from an autosomal dominant or recessively inherited defect in the erythrocyte cell membrane. Mutations affecting the production of cytoskeleton proteins such as spectrin, ankyrin, band 3 (anion exchanger AE1), and band 4.2 lead to the loss of the usual biconcave erythrocyte shape.[13] These erythrocytes lack deformability, are more rigid, and have increased osmotic fragility, leading to trapping and destruction in the spleen. Clinically, HS presents with moderate hemolytic anemia, jaundice, folate deficiency, and splenomegaly. Diagnosis is made by hematologic workup, including peripheral blood smear demonstrating spherocytes, elevated lactate dehydrogenase, increased indirect bilirubin, absence of decreased haptoglobin, increased osmotic fragility, and negative Coombs test result.

Splenectomy is indicated in severe HS, when hemoglobin is <8 g/dL, and moderate HS, with hemoglobin 8 to 12 g/dL based on individual metrics, including spleen size and quality-of-life parameters.[12] Splenectomy should be delayed until 6 years to preserve immunologic function of the spleen and to reduce the risk of OPSI. Challenging clinical scenarios in HS remain, including the role for partial splenectomy below 6 years of age and the role for concurrent splenectomy and cholecystectomy, and are outside the scope of this review.

Hereditary elliptocytosis, hereditary pyropoikilocytosis, hereditary xerocytosis, and hereditary hydrocytosis also result in anemia secondary to RBC membrane abnormalities. Splenectomy may be indicated in cases of severe anemia with these conditions, except hereditary xerocytosis, which results in only mild anemia of limited clinical significance.[14]

Hemolytic Anemia Caused by Erythrocyte Enzyme Deficiency

PKD and G6PD deficiency are the predominant hereditary conditions associated with hemolytic anemia. PKD is an autosomal recessive disease, resulting in insufficient pyruvate to maintain RBC membrane structure and spleen-mediated RBC destruction. G6PD deficiency is an X-linked disease, resulting in a deficiency of nicotinamide adenine dinucleotide phosphate (NAPDH), high RBC susceptibly to oxidative stress, and episodic stress-related hemolysis. Splenectomy is indicated

in patients with severe PKD, particularly among those with high transfusion requirements.[12] A recent international, multicenter registry suggested that splenectomy reduced transfusion in 91% of cases; however, transfusion dependency and moderate anemia persist in >50% of patients. These data suggest that the decision to perform splenectomy should be individualized based on burden of disease.[15] Similarly, splenectomy in G6PD deficiency should be considered in cases of symptomatic splenomegaly or transfusion dependence.

Hemoglobinopathies

Sickle cell disease and thalassemia are the two most clinically important inherited hemoglobinopathies and may necessitate splenectomy. Sickle cell disease is a point mutation in the β globin gene resulting in a single amino acid substitution (valine for glutamic acid) in the sixth position of the β chain of hemoglobin A. Sickle cell disease results from homozygous inheritance of the defective hemoglobin (hemoglobin S), although it can be seen when hemoglobin S is inherited along with other hemoglobin variants, such as hemoglobin C or sickle cell β-thalassemia. In African Americans, 8% are heterozygous for hemoglobin S (sickle cell trait) and approximately 0.5% are homozygous for hemoglobin S. The affected hemoglobin chains become rigid, sickle shaped, and unable to deform under reduced oxygen conditions. These misshapen cells are unable to pass through the microvasculature, resulting in capillary occlusion, thrombosis, and ultimately microinfarction, frequently in the spleen. These episodes of vasoocclusion and progressive infarction result in autosplenectomy. The thalassemias are a group of autosomal recessive disorders with a disproportional α-to-β chain ratio, resulting in precipitation of the unpaired chain and subsequent RBC destruction. Thalassemia is classified into two main types depending on which globin chain is defective: α-thalassemia and β-thalassemia. Splenomegaly, hypersplenism, and splenic infarction are commonly seen in patients with sickle cell disease and thalassemia.

Acute splenic sequestration crises are life-threatening disorders in children with sickle cell disease or sickle β-thalassemia. In this condition, there is a rapid drop in hemoglobin level because of vasoocclusion and splenic RBC sequestration, leading to life-threatening hypovolemic shock. Patients with acute splenic sequestration crisis present with severe anemia, abdominal pain, splenomegaly, and reticulocytosis. Treatment for acute splenic sequestration includes resuscitation, followed by consideration of splenectomy (in particular after two episodes), given high rates of recurrence and associated high mortality.[12,16]

Hypersplenism related to sickle cell disease is characterized by transfusion-dependent anemia, leukopenia, and thrombocytopenia. Splenectomy may be indicated in patients with sickle cell disease, with pressure effects caused by splenomegaly or failure to thrive. Despite being recommended in these scenarios, there is limited evidence demonstrating an improvement in hemoglobin levels or overall survival, which may be related to increases in thromboembolism.[12,16]

Splenic abscesses may also be seen in patients with sickle cell anemia. These patients present with fever; abdominal pain; and a tender, enlarged spleen. Most patients with splenic abscesses will present with leukocytosis, thrombocytosis, and Howell-Jolly bodies on peripheral smear, indicating a functional asplenia. *Salmonella* and *Enterobacter* spp. are common pathogens. These patients require resuscitation and antibiotics and may require urgent splenectomy after stabilization.

Malignant Disease
Hematopoietic Neoplasm

Lymphomas. Hodgkin lymphoma (HL) is a group of malignant conditions that are characterized by the presence of Reed-Sternberg cells. HL usually affects adults in their 20s and 30s with a second peak in adults over the age of 50. Rarely, patients present with constitutional symptoms such as night sweats, weight loss, and pruritus, but more typically, patients present with asymptomatic lymphadenopathy that usually involves the cervical nodes. Historically, splenectomy played a critical role in patients with HL and was part of a standard staging laparotomy. However, current staging is performed with cross-sectional imaging, and treatment includes radiation and chemotherapy, with splenectomy reserved for patients with symptomatic splenomegaly.

Non-Hodgkin lymphoma (NHL) is a group of malignant neoplasms derived from progenerates of B cells, T cells, mature B cells, and mature T cells. Splenomegaly is common in NHL and may present with cytopenia because of hypersplenism. Splenectomy is indicated for patients with symptomatic splenomegaly, which may present as abdominal pain, early satiety, and fullness. It may also be indicated for patients who develop refractory anemia, neutropenia, and thrombocytopenia associated with hypersplenism.

Splenectomy may also be indicated in the diagnosis and treatment of splenic marginal zone lymphoma, a subtype of NHL previously termed *splenic lymphoma*. This is a rare subtype of NHL, accounting for <1% of patients. Most present with splenomegaly, lymphocytosis, anemia, and thrombocytopenia.[17] Diagnosis of splenic marginal zone lymphoma is challenging and can definitively be made on splenic histology. If clinical suspicion is high for splenic marginal zone lymphoma, splenectomy may be indicated for diagnosis. Splenectomy is also indicated for symptomatic splenomegaly and with suspected large cell transformations on PET/CT scan. In patients with spleen-predominant disease, splenectomy may provide durable improvement in splenic sequestration and improve survival.[17]

Leukemia

Hairy cell leukemia. Hairy cell leukemia, accounting for approximately 2% of adult leukemias, is characterized by splenomegaly, pancytopenia, and neoplastic mononuclear cells in the peripheral blood and bone marrow with characteristic cytoplasmic projections. Typically indolent in course, hairy cell leukemia was historically treated with interferon and splenectomy. However, more recently purine analogues and targeted agents (rituximab and anti-BRAF therapy) represent the mainstay of medical therapy. Splenectomy may remain a valid treatment option for patients with splenomegaly and low bone marrow involvement, refractory/relapsed disease, splenic rupture, pregnancy, or transfusion-dependent splenic sequestration.[18]

Chronic lymphocytic leukemia. Chronic lymphocytic leukemia (CLL) is the most common leukemia in the Western world and is characterized by the progressive accumulation of relatively morphologically normal, mature, but functionally incompetent lymphocytes. Low-risk CLL (formerly stage 0) involves bone marrow and blood lymphocytosis only; intermediate-risk CLL (formerly stages I and II) involves lymphocytosis and lymphadenopathy in any site or splenomegaly, hepatomegaly, or hepatosplenomegaly; and high-risk CLL (formerly stages III and IV) involves lymphocytosis and anemia or thrombocytopenia. Medical treatment is reserved for fit patients with symptomatic disease and advanced stages. Splenectomy is rarely indicated in CLL, aside from symptomatic splenomegaly or rare cases of splenic rupture.

Chronic myelogenous leukemia. Chronic myelogenous leukemia (CML) is a myeloproliferative disorder that develops as a result of a neoplastic transformation of myeloid elements. CML is characterized by the progressive replacement of normal diploid elements of the bone marrow with mature-appearing neoplastic myeloid cells. Although CML can be asymptomatic at presentation, patients commonly present with fever, fatigue, malaise, effects of pancytopenia (e.g., infections, anemia, easy bruising), and occasionally splenomegaly. Peripheral blood smear analysis shows leukocytosis of white blood cell count up to 100,000/μL. The gold standard for the diagnosis of CML is expression of the BCR-ABL fusion oncogene.

CML usually presents with an asymptomatic chronic phase but may progress to an accelerated phase associated with fever, night sweats, and progressive splenomegaly and a blastic phase characterized by anemia, opportunistic infections, and bleeding.

Targeted therapy with kinase inhibitors, cytotoxic chemotherapy, and bone marrow transplant is used in treatment of CML. Symptomatic splenomegaly and hypersplenism in CML can be effectively treated with splenectomy, but there does not appear to be a survival benefit when it is performed during the early chronic phase. Surgery is ultimately reserved for patients with symptomatic splenomegaly or hypersplenism.

Nonhematologic Tumors of the Spleen

Although lymphoma is the most common primary tumor of the spleen, other splenic lesions are common and can typically be differentiated based on imaging characteristics and clinical presentation. Hemangiomas are frequently incidentally identified on cross-sectional imaging and have been identified in up to 14% of patients at autopsy.[19] The natural course of hemangiomas is indolent, and rupture, hypersplenism, and malignant degeneration are rare and occur late in the course. Hemangiosarcomas are typically <2 cm, round, and have immediate homogenous enhancement on CT. They are rare and may be related to environmental exposure; they are also aggressive and associated with poor prognosis.

Inflammatory myofibroblastic tumor (IMF), previously known as *inflammatory pseudotumor,* is uncommon and potentially linked to Epstein-Barr virus exposure. These lesions are typically large (>10 cm), with characteristic central stellate calcifications on imaging, and are composed of inflammatory and myofibroblastic spindle cells.[20] These tumors have intermediate malignant potential and should be resected.

Lymphangiomas, most commonly seen in children, are endothelium-lined cysts that can lead to splenomegaly secondary to cyst enlargement. These are usually benign tumors; however, malignant degeneration is rarely possible. Imaging typically identifies thin septa within a multiloculated cyst. Splenectomy is appropriate for symptomatic lesions.[21]

Additional rare benign and borderline malignant splenic lesions may be seen. Splenic sarcoidosis is present in up to 40% of patients with systemic disease and may portend poorer prognosis. Litoral cell angioma is a rare vascular tumor that results in splenomegaly and may be associated with autoimmune conditions. If suspected, splenectomy is indicated for diagnosis and treatment. Sclerosing angiomatoid nodular transformation is another rare vascular tumor, typically mistaken for IMF on imaging; splenectomy is effective, with no reported recurrences. Splenic hamartomas are also rare and challenging to identify on imaging and are usually identified after diagnostic splenectomy on pathology.

Secondary metastatic splenic neoplasms are rare and thought to be the result of a lack of afferent lymphatics and are seen in up to 7% of autopsies of patients with cancer. The most common primary tumors for splenic metastases are breast, lung, and melanoma. Splenectomy may be considered in appropriate surgical candidates, with symptomatic or solitary lesions.

Miscellaneous Benign Conditions

Splenic Cysts

Splenic cysts have been seen with increasing frequency since the advent of CT and ultrasound scanning. They are classified as parasitic and nonparasitic cysts. The nonparasitic cysts are further divided into true cysts and pseudocysts. True cysts are lined with epithelium and may be considered congenital and account for 10% of all splenic cysts.

Parasitic cysts occur in areas of endemic hydatid disease (*Echinococcus* spp.). Radiographic imaging, usually with ultrasound, reveals cyst wall calcifications or daughter cysts, and although hydatid disease is uncommon in North America, this diagnosis must be excluded before invasive procedures are undertaken that might result in spillage of the cyst contents. Rupture of the cyst and expulsion of contents into the abdomen may precipitate anaphylactic shock and intraperitoneal infection. Serologic testing is helpful for verifying the presence of these parasites. Splenectomy is the treatment of choice. As with hydatid cysts of the liver, the cysts may be sterilized by injection of a 3% sodium chloride solution, alcohol, or 0.5% silver nitrate.

Nonparasitic true cysts of the spleen account for approximately 10% of all splenic cysts. These epithelial cells are often positive for carbohydrate antigen 19-9 and carcinoembryonic antigen by immunohistochemistry. Patients with splenic epidermoid cysts may have elevated serum levels of one or both of these tumor markers. These cysts, however, are benign and are often asymptomatic and discovered incidentally. Patients may complain of abdominal fullness, early satiety, pleuritic chest pain, shortness of breath, and left shoulder or back pain. On physical examination, an abdominal mass may be palpable. Rarely, splenic cysts present with acute symptoms related to rupture, hemorrhage, or infection. Diagnosis is best made by CT, and operative intervention is indicated for those with symptomatic or large cysts. Total or partial splenectomy may provide appropriate treatment.

Nonparasitic pseudocysts represent the remaining 70% to 80% of splenic cysts. A history of prior trauma can typically be elicited. Pseudocysts of the spleen are not lined with epithelium. Radiologic imaging usually reveals a smooth, unilocular, thick-walled lesion, sometimes with focal calcifications. Asymptomatic, small (<4 cm) pseudocysts do not require treatment and may involute with time. Symptomatic pseudocysts are treated surgically with total or partial splenectomy. Percutaneous drainage has also been reported for splenic pseudocysts, although this has higher recurrence and should generally be reserved for poor surgical candidates.

Splenic Abscess

Splenic abscess is an unusual but potentially life-threatening illness if not promptly identified and treated, with mortality rates from 15% to 20% in immunocompetent patients and up to 80% in immunocompromised patients. Malignancy, polycythemia vera, endocarditis, prior trauma, hemoglobinopathies, urinary tract infections, intravenous drug use, and acquired immunodeficiency syndrome may preclude patients to develop abscesses.

Approximately 70% of splenic abscesses result from hematogenous spread of the infective organism, typically from endocarditis, osteomyelitis, and intravenous drug use. Spread may also occur in a contiguous fashion from local infections of the colon, kidney, or pancreas. Gram-positive cocci (commonly *Staphylococcus, Streptococcus,* or *Enterococcus* spp.) and gram-negative enteric organisms are common. *Mycobacterium tuberculosis, Mycobacterium avium, Actinomyces,* and fungal abscesses have also been described, typically in immunosuppressed patients.

Splenic abscesses present with nonspecific symptoms: vague abdominal pain, fever, peritonitis, and pleuritic chest pain. Splenomegaly is not typical. CT is the preferred method for diagnosis. Treatment of splenic abscesses depends on whether the abscess is unilocular or multilocular. Unilocular abscesses are often amenable to percutaneous drainage, along with antibiotics, with high success rates. Multilocular lesions, however, are usually treated with splenectomy, drainage of the left upper quadrant, and antibiotics.

Wandering Spleen

Wandering spleen is a rare finding, seen in children and in females between the ages of 20 and 40 years. Wandering spleen may be related to failure of normal embryologic attachments to form or hormonal changes leading to laxity in splenic ligaments. Without typical attachments, the splenic pedicle is unusually long and prone to torsion.

Intermittent abdominal pain, splenomegaly from venous congestion, and severe abdominal pain are suggestive of wandering spleen caused by intermittent torsion of the splenic pedicle. A mobile mass may be palpable on physical examination. CT provides confirmation of the diagnosis, with the spleen located outside its usual position. A noncontrasted spleen or whorled appearance of the vascular pedicle provides additional evidence for the condition and may be helpful in choosing splenopexy or splenectomy.

Other Considerations

Splenic Trauma

Vascular conditions. Splenectomy could be indicated for vascular conditions that will be discussed elsewhere in this textbook. These vascular disorders are portal hypertension (see Chapter 51), splenic artery aneurysm (see Chapter 105), and splenic vein thrombosis.

Preoperative Considerations

As part of preoperative planning, several factors should be considered before deciding on the optimal operative approach (Box 72.3). In general, in patients who have sustained blunt trauma who either fail nonoperative/embolization management or are hemodynamically unstable at presentation, open splenectomy is still the standard of care.[22] Most other indications, including malignancy and massive splenomegaly, are still recommended to be attempted minimally invasively, with a hand-assist option as an available modification.[23,24] Diagnostic adjuncts such as CT or MRI are useful in operative planning and counseling the patient, specifically in determining splenic size/volume, potential accessory spleens, and presence of varices, and it is important to be prepared to change approach when the situation requires.[25]

Apart from surgical approach, preoperative medical optimization must also be considered. Specifically, as discussed in the earlier sections, for patients with ITP or hemolytic anemias such as thalassemia or sickle cell, discussion with the patient's hematologist should address expected need for blood product transfusions, steroid administration and/or tapering, and other treatments such as immunoglobulins.[26]

Laparoscopic Splenectomy

As with a majority of organ resections, a minimally invasive approach to splenectomy is the preferred method for resecting the spleen. The laparoscopic technique was first described in 1991,[24] and many studies have supported its use, with favorable outcomes and patient safety. Compared with an open surgical approach, potential disadvantages of the laparoscopic technique may be longer relative operating times and increased difficulty removing large spleens; however, the well-described benefits of reduced length of hospital stay (and hospital costs by proxy) and decreased morbidity and mortality more than justify these relative limitations.[30]

Most splenectomies can be safely completed minimally invasively, though the reported conversion rate to open surgery is between 0% and 20%.[31] Risk factors associated with conversion to open surgery include intraoperative hemorrhage, lack of surgical experience, significant intraabdominal adhesions, massive splenomegaly, and obesity.[32] As with other minimally invasive procedures, there is a learning curve, and with increasing experience, conversion to open splenectomy declines.[31]

In previously published investigations, laparoscopic outcomes and safety are considered equivalent to those of open splenectomy. Although older literature suggests open splenectomy should be used in cases of malignancy, newer data report similar oncologic outcomes with shorter length of stay, lower morbidity, and lower 30-day mortality, similar to outcomes reported for benign disease.[27,33]

Minimally invasive splenectomy should still be carefully considered, even in special populations. Portal hypertension with associated risk of uncontrollable operative hemorrhage was previously considered to be a relative contraindication for minimally invasive splenectomy. However, with advancement in laparoscopic techniques and improvements in laparoscopic energy devices and staplers, laparoscopic splenectomy can be safely performed in patients with portal hypertension.

Patient positioning. The laparoscopic technique may be performed in the lateral or supine position, depending on surgeon's preference, concomitant surgery, and patient's body habitus. The lateral technique is the most commonly used position. For all positions, the patient is placed on the operating table so that the kidney rest can be raised to maximize the space between the iliac crest and costal margin. The patient is tilted in a reverse Trendelenburg position to facilitate retraction of the viscera caudally away from the left upper quadrant.

In the right lateral decubitus position (Fig. 72.7), the patient is placed in a 60-degree right-side-down position using a beanbag

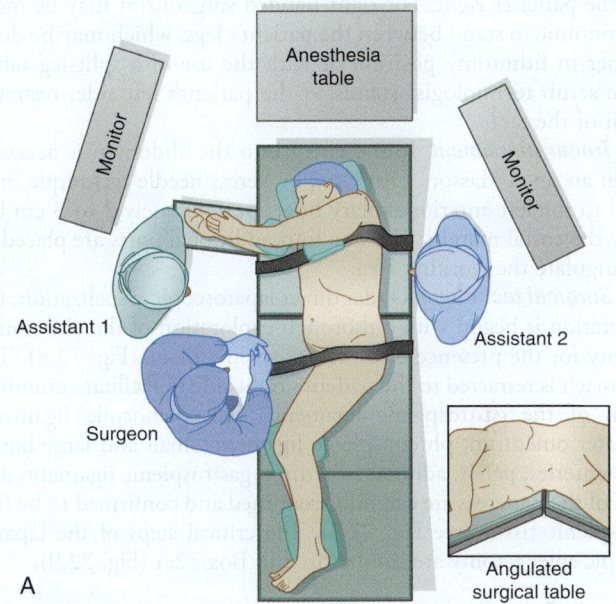

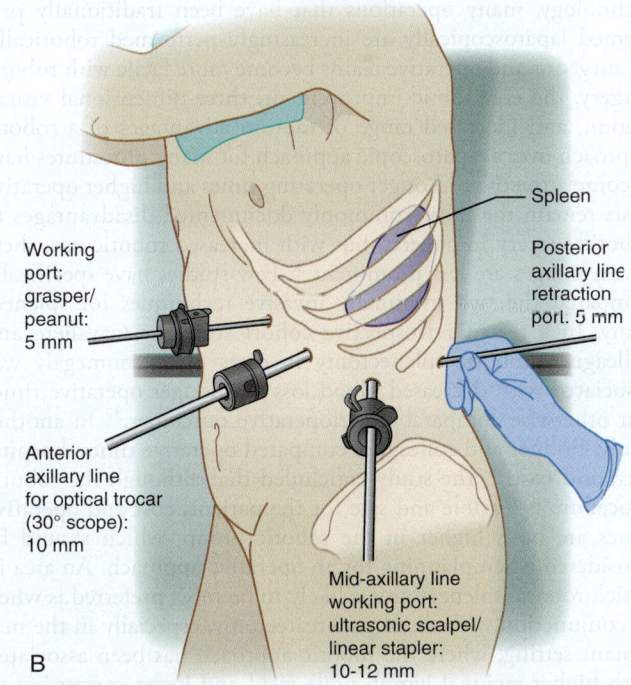

FIGURE 72.7 (A) Patient positioning and (B) trocar placement: lateral decubitus position. (Copyright Lianne Krueger Sullivan. From Jenkins M, Parikh M, Pachter HL. Technique of splenectomy. In: Yeo CJ, ed. *Shackelford's Surgery of the Alimentary Tract.* 8th ed. Philadelphia: Elsevier; 2019:1600.)

and axillary roll. In this case, the patient's left arm is placed on an arm board or supported by a splint with protection of all pressure points. With this approach, the surgeon and scrub technologist stand to the patient's right and the surgical assistants stand to the patient's left.[34] The spleen will then be allowed to suspend from its diaphragmatic attachments, and this allows gravity to retract the stomach, omentum, and colon. Additionally, the splenic hilum will be under some tension, which allows for ease of dissection. Alternatively, in the supine position, the surgeon stands to the patient's left, and the first assistant and camera assistant stand to the patient's right. For right-handed surgeons, it may be more ergonomic to stand between the patient's legs, which may be done either in lithotomy position or with the use of a split-leg table. The scrub technologist stands to the patient's left side, near the foot of the table.

Trocar placement. Initial entry into the abdomen is accessed with an open Hasson, Optiview, or Veress needle technique, medial to the left anterior axillary line, approximately 2 to 3 cm below the costal margin. Three to four additional ports are placed to triangulate the working area.

Surgical technique. Under direct laparoscopic visualization, the operation is begun with a thorough exploration of the abdominal cavity for the presence of accessory splenic tissue (Fig. 72.8). The stomach is retracted to the patient's right side to facilitate examination of the gastrosplenic ligament. The splenocolic ligament, greater omentum, phrenosplenic ligament, small and large bowel mesenteries, pelvis, adnexal structures, gastrosplenic ligament, and tail of the pancreas are carefully examined and confirmed to be free of splenic tissue (see Fig. 72.8). The critical steps of the laparoscopic splenectomy are summarized in Box 72.4 (Fig. 72.9).

Robotic Splenectomy

With increased access to and surgeon comfort with using robotic technology, many operations that have been traditionally performed laparoscopically are increasingly performed robotically. As surgeons and operative teams become more facile with robotic surgery, the ergonomic improvement, three-dimensional visualization, and increased range of motion advantages of a robotic approach over a laparoscopic approach for many procedures have become attractive.[35] Longer operating times and higher operative costs remain the most commonly documented disadvantages to robotic surgery in general, but with increased robotic use, these disadvantages are less prominent.[36] Few studies have specifically compared the two minimally invasive techniques for splenectomy. In a recent retrospective cohort study by Cavaliere and colleagues, robotic splenectomy in cases of splenomegaly was associated with decreased blood loss and longer operative times but otherwise comparable perioperative outcomes.[37] In another study, Bodner and colleagues compared operative times, hospital stay, and cost.[38] The study concluded that although the robotic procedure is feasible and safe for the patient, cost and operative times are both higher in the robotic group, which should be considered when planning for an operative approach. An area in which robotic splenectomy is likely to be most preferred is when in conjunction with distal pancreatectomy, especially in the malignant setting, where the robotic approach has been associated with higher regional lymph node yield and lower conversion to open rate.[39]

Short-Term Complications After Splenectomy

Splenectomy, like any other surgical procedure, is associated with risk of postoperative complications, regardless of the surgical

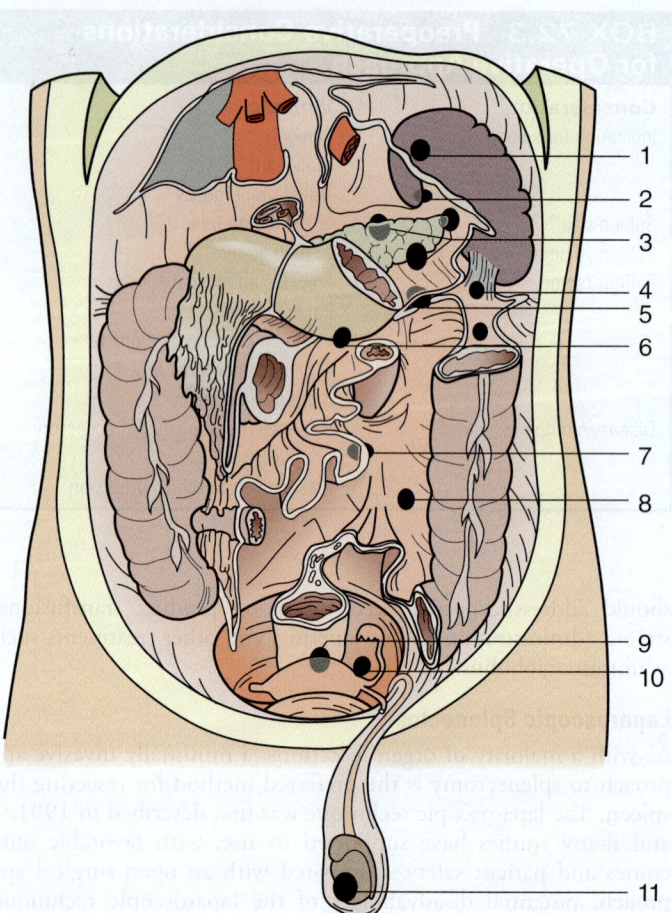

FIGURE 72.8 Usual location of accessory spleens: *(1)* gastrosplenic ligament, *(2)* splenic hilum, *(3)* tail of the pancreas, *(4)* splenocolic ligament, *(5)* left transverse mesocolon, *(6)* greater omentum along the greater curvature of the stomach, *(7)* mesentery, *(8)* left mesocolon, *(9)* left ovary, *(10)* Douglas pouch, and *(11)* left testis. (From Gigot JF, Lengele B, Gianello P, et al. Present status of laparoscopic splenectomy for hematologic diseases: certitudes and unresolved issues. *Semin Laparosc Surg.* 1998;5:147-167.)

BOX 72.4   Critical Steps of Laparoscopic Splenectomy

1. Position patient in right lateral decubitus with operating table flexed to 45 degrees
2. Mobilize splenic flexure of the colon
3. Incise lateral peritoneal attachments to the spleen (tip: leave ~1cm of peritoneal cuff along the lateral spleen to facilitate grasping and retracting; see Fig. 72.9)
4. Enter lesser sac along medial border of spleen
5. Visualize short gastric vessels, main splenic vascular pedicle, and tail of the pancreas
6. Ligate and divide short gastric vessels with laparoscopic energy device
7. Circumferentially dissect splenic vascular pedicle near the hilum and ligate and divide with laparoscopic stapler, avoiding injury to tail of the pancreas
8. Divide final splenophrenic attachments at the superior pole and place in laparoscopic retrieval bag
9. Remove spleen by morcellating (benign only) and remove through an enlarged port site (see Fig. 57.9; for malignant disease, spleen must be extracted intact through an appropriate incision)
10. Avoid spillage of any splenic tissue into the abdominal cavity

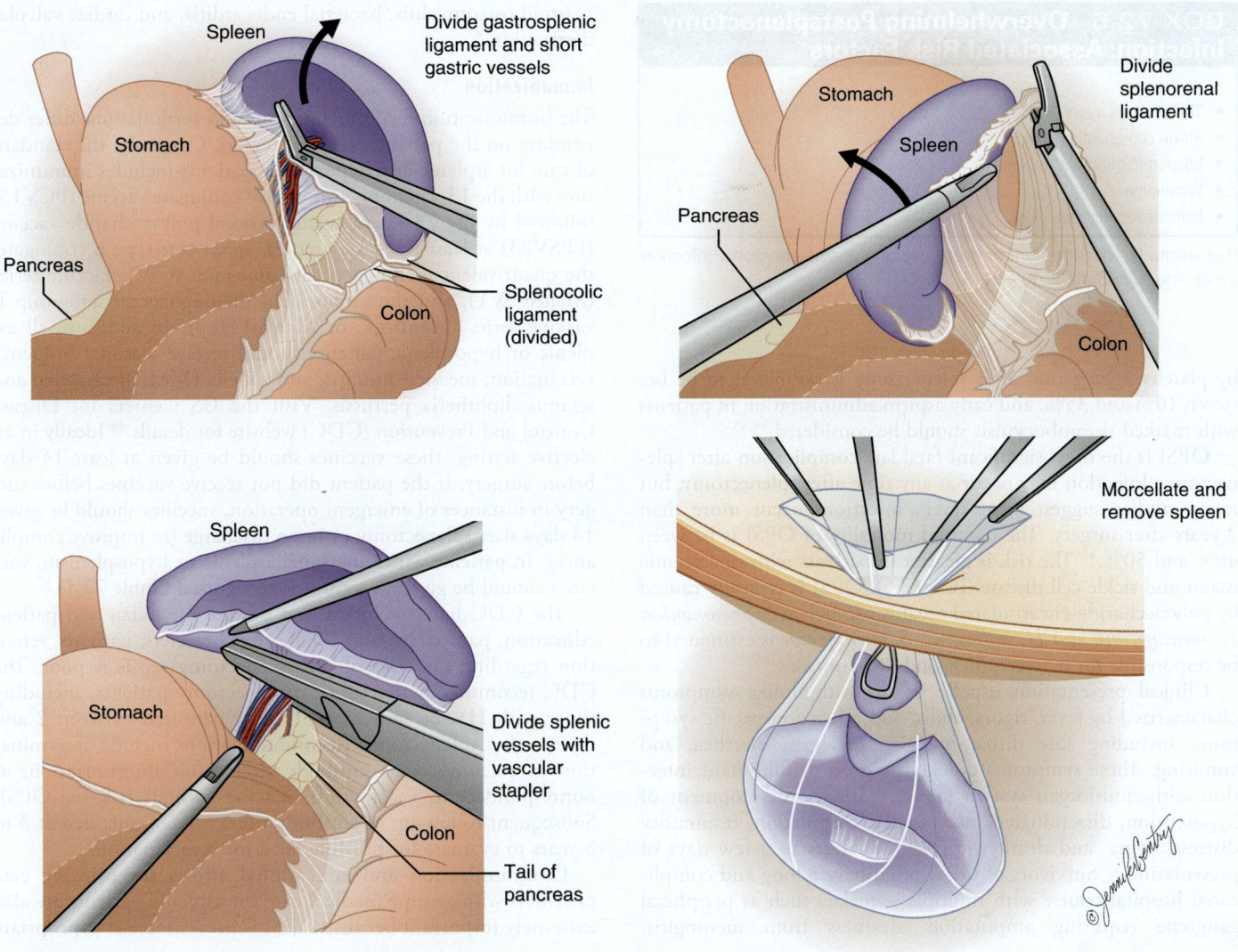

FIGURE 72.9 Surgical technique. (Copyright Jennifer N. Gentry. From: Jenkins M, Parikh M, Pachter HL. Technique of splenectomy. In: Yeo CJ, ed. *Shackelford's Surgery of the Alimentary Tract.* 8th ed. Philadelphia: Elsevior; 2019:1600.)

approach. In the immediate postoperative period, intraabdominal hemorrhage as a result of slipped ligature from the hilar vessels or other small vascular tributaries is one of the most common complications. Other well-described short-term complications include pneumonia, left-sided pleural effusion, colon injury, and pancreatic fistula from unrecognized pancreatic tail injury during splenic hilum dissection.[28,40] Pancreatic fistula, which may clinically manifest with abdominal pain, early satiety, fever, and leukocytosis with left shift is typically managed with percutaneous drainage. These must be managed appropriately in order to avoid infection and pseudoaneurysm with bleeding. Another important, yet rare, complication is gastric perforation at the greater curvature of the stomach, caused by iatrogenic injury to the greater curvature during dissection of the short gastric arteries. This commonly requires reoperation and may lead to chronic fistula if associated with concomitant pancreatic injury. Venous thromboembolism is another serious complication after splenectomy. It is thought to be related to reactive thrombocytosis after splenectomy; however, the

correlation is not entirely clear. Abdominal venous thrombosis, also known as *postsplenectomy thrombosis of the splenic, mesenteric, and portal veins*, has an incidence of 8% to 10%, with splenic size and myeloproliferative disorder reported to be the main risk factors.[41,42] Presentation is usually with nonspecific postoperative gastrointestinal symptoms of abdominal pain and ascites. Management is typically nonsurgical with administration of systemic anticoagulation. Currently there is an increasing role for interventional radiology with catheter-based thrombolysis, stents, and/or thrombectomy.[43]

Late Morbidity After Splenectomy

Postsplenectomy thrombocytosis occurs most commonly in patients with myeloproliferative disorders (e.g., CML, polycythemia vera, essential thrombocytosis), which can result in thrombosis of the mesenteric, portal, and renal veins and can be life-threatening, leading to both risk of hemorrhage and thromboembolism. The risk for deep venous thrombosis and pulmonary embolism caused

BOX 72.5   Overwhelming Postsplenectomy Infection: Associated Risk Factors

- Young age
- Thalassemia major (8.2%)
- Sickle cell anemia (7.3%)
- Idiopathic thrombocytopenia (2.1%)
- Lymphoma
- Immunosuppression

Hashimoto N. Management of overwhelming postsplenectomy infection syndrome. *Clin Surg.* 2016;1:1148.

by platelet aggregation after splenectomy is estimated to be between 10% and 35%, and early aspirin administration in patients with marked thrombocytosis should be considered.[44,45]

OPSI is the most significant fatal late complication after splenectomy. Infection may occur at any time after splenectomy, but many studies suggest most severe infections occur more than 2 years after surgery. The reported mortality of OPSI is between 40% and 50%.[46] The risk is greatest in patients with thalassemia major and sickle cell disease (Box 72.5). OPSI is typically caused by polysaccharide-encapsulated organisms, such as *S. pneumoniae*, *N. meningitidis*, and *H. influenzae*. *S. pneumoniae* is estimated to be responsible for between 50% and 90% of cases.

Clinical presentation usually begins with flulike symptoms characterized by fever, rigors, chills, and other nonspecific symptoms, including sore throat, malaise, myalgias, diarrhea, and vomiting. These symptoms quickly progress to fulminant infection with multiorgan system failure, with the development of hypotension, disseminated intravascular coagulation, respiratory distress, coma, and death within a few hours to a few days of presentation.[47] Survivors of OPSI often have a long and complicated hospital course with multiple sequelae, such as peripheral gangrene requiring amputation, deafness from meningitis,

mastoid osteomyelitis, bacterial endocarditis, and cardiac valvular destruction.[47]

Immunization

The immunization recommendations and formulations differ depending on the patient's age and region. Currently, the standard of care for asplenic and hyposplenic patients includes immunization with the 13-valent pneumococcal conjugate vaccine (PCV13) followed by the 23-valent pneumococcal polysaccharide vaccine (PPSV23) at least 8 weeks later, *H. influenzae* type b conjugate, the quadrivalent meningococcal conjugate ACWY vaccine series (MenACWY), and the monovalent meningococcal serogroup B vaccine series (MenB-4C or MenB-FHbp). In addition, all asplenic or hyposplenic patients should receive seasonal influenza vaccination; measles, mumps, and rubella (MMR); varicella; and tetanus diphtheria pertussis. Visit the US Centers for Disease Control and Prevention (CDC) website for details.[48] Ideally in an elective setting, these vaccines should be given at least 14 days before surgery. If the patient did not receive vaccines before surgery in instances of emergent operation, vaccines should be given 14 days after splenectomy or upon discharge (to improve compliance). In patients with functional asplenia or hyposplenism, vaccines should be given as soon it is recognized (Table 72.1).[47]

The CDC has concluded that despite physician and patient education, pamphlets, and MedicAlert bracelets, patients' retention regarding the risks of postsplenectomy sepsis is poor. The CDC recommends that all postsplenectomy patients, including those with HS, be revaccinated and reeducated between 2 and 6 years after splenectomy. Recommendations include determination of pneumococcal antibody titers after immunization, as nonresponders to vaccination may be at high risk for OPSI. Subsequent follow-up of antibody titers is recommended at 3 to 5 years to evaluate for possible need for revaccination.

Communication and educational efforts for primary care providers who assume medical care for asplenic patients are also extremely important because OPSI is preventable if appropriate

TABLE 72.1   Centers for Disease Control and Prevention Vaccine Recommendations for Asplenic Patients[a,b]

	PNEUMOCOCCAL VACCINATION	MENINGOCOCCAL VACCINATION	*HAEMOPHILUS INFLUENZAE* TYPE B VACCINATION
Children	Immunologically naïve 2–6 years[c]: PCV13 followed by PVC13 8 weeks later; PPSV23 8 weeks later; repeat PPSV23 at 5 years Immunologically naïve 6–18 years[c]: PCV13 followed by PPSV23 8 weeks later; repeat PPSV23 at 5 years	MenACWY series AND MenB series[d]	Hib once if 15 months or older and previously not vaccinated
Adults (age 19 and older)	Immunologically naïve[c]: PCV13 followed by PPSV23 8 weeks later; repeat PPSV23 every 5 years	MenACWY or MPSV4 2 months apart; repeat MenACWY every 5 years AND MenB series[d] once	Hib once

[a]First vaccination should be administered at least 2 weeks before splenectomy if elective.
[b]Even with vaccination, oral antibiotic prophylaxis with penicillin V or amoxicillin should be considered for children under 2 years of age or high-risk postsplenectomy patients.
[c]For patients who have previously received any PCV or PPSV23 or a combination of these vaccinations, the recommendations vary and are outlined in the CDC guidelines accessible online.
[d]MenB-4C 2 doses 1 month apart or MenB-FHbp 3 doses, 1 each at 0, 2, and 6 months.
Hib, H. influenzae type b; *MenACWY*, meningococcal 4-valent conjugate; *MPSV4*, meningococcal 4-valent polysaccharide; *PCV13*, 13-valent pneumococcal conjugate vaccine; *PPSV23*, pneumococcal 23-valent polysaccharide.
From Pernar LIM, Tavakkoli A. Anatomy and physiology of the spleen. In: Yeo CJ, ed. *Shackelford's Surgery of the Alimentary Tract.* 8th ed. Philadelphia: Elsevier; 2019:1595.

precautions are taken. CDC immunization guidelines for 2023 have recommended the following vaccines in addition to what has been discussed earlier for asplenic patients: tetanus (Tdap or Td), human papillomavirus (HPV), MMR, varicella, zoster, influenza, hepatitis A (hep A) and hepatitis B (hep B), and meningococcal.

Antibiotics

Significant controversy still exists about antibiotic prophylaxis in postsplenectomy patients. The primary goal of prophylaxis is to prevent OPSI, particularly secondary to pneumococcal infection, which is the most common cause of OPSI. However, OPSI secondary to penicillin-sensitive pneumococcal infection has been reported in children and adults receiving penicillin prophylaxis.

There are two general approaches for antibiotic prophylaxis in asplenic or hyposplenic patients. One is daily prophylactic dosing and the other is maintaining an emergency supply. There is variability of practice among different societies. For example, the Australian Spleen Society recommends daily antibiotic prophylaxis for children up to age 16 or a minimum up to age 5 or 3 years after splenectomy. In addition, they recommend lifelong prophylaxis for immunocompromised states and an emergency supply of oral antibiotics for postsplenectomy adults, with instructions to begin taking the medication at the onset of a febrile illness or rigors if there is no access to immediate medical evaluation.[49]

The oral antibiotic of choice is amoxycillin or oral penicillin. For patients with confirmed hypersensitivity or significant allergy, the second choice is a macrolide. For the emergency supply, we recommend the use of amoxycillin plus clavulanate, and for penicillin-allergic patients, macrolides or quinolones are acceptable alternatives.

There is evidence that the risk of OPSI is lowest in patients who exhibit the greatest understanding of the infectious risks of asplenia.[50] This highlights the importance of education of the patient, particularly at follow-up visits, to ensure compliance with antibiotic and vaccine prophylaxis. It is important to note

any asplenic or hyposplenic patient who presents with rigors or fever, who must be started immediately on aggressive broad-spectrum empiric antibiotic coverage, even without culture data.

SELECTED REFERENCES

Feldman LS. Laparoscopic splenectomy: standardized approach. *World J Surg.* 2011;35:1487-1495.

This article provides an overview of indications and technique for laparoscopic splenectomy.

Gigot JF, Jamar F, Ferrant A, et al. Inadequate detection of accessory spleens and splenosis with laparoscopic splenectomy. A shortcoming of the laparoscopic approach in hematologic diseases. *Surg Endosc.* 1998;12:101-106.

This article provides good technical tips for splenectomy

Kanhutu K, Jones P, Cheng AC, et al. Spleen Australia guidelines for the prevention of sepsis in patients with asplenia and hyposplenism in Australia and New Zealand. *Intern Med J.* 2017;47:848-855.

Comprehensive guidelines for the prevention of sepsis in asplenia and hyposplenism.

Lambert MP, Gernsheimer TB. Clinical updates in adult immune thrombocytopenia. *Blood.* 2017;129:2829-2835.

This study provides the latest clinical guidelines for the management of immune thrombocytopenia.

The full reference list appears on Elsevier eBooks+.

Endocrine Disorders

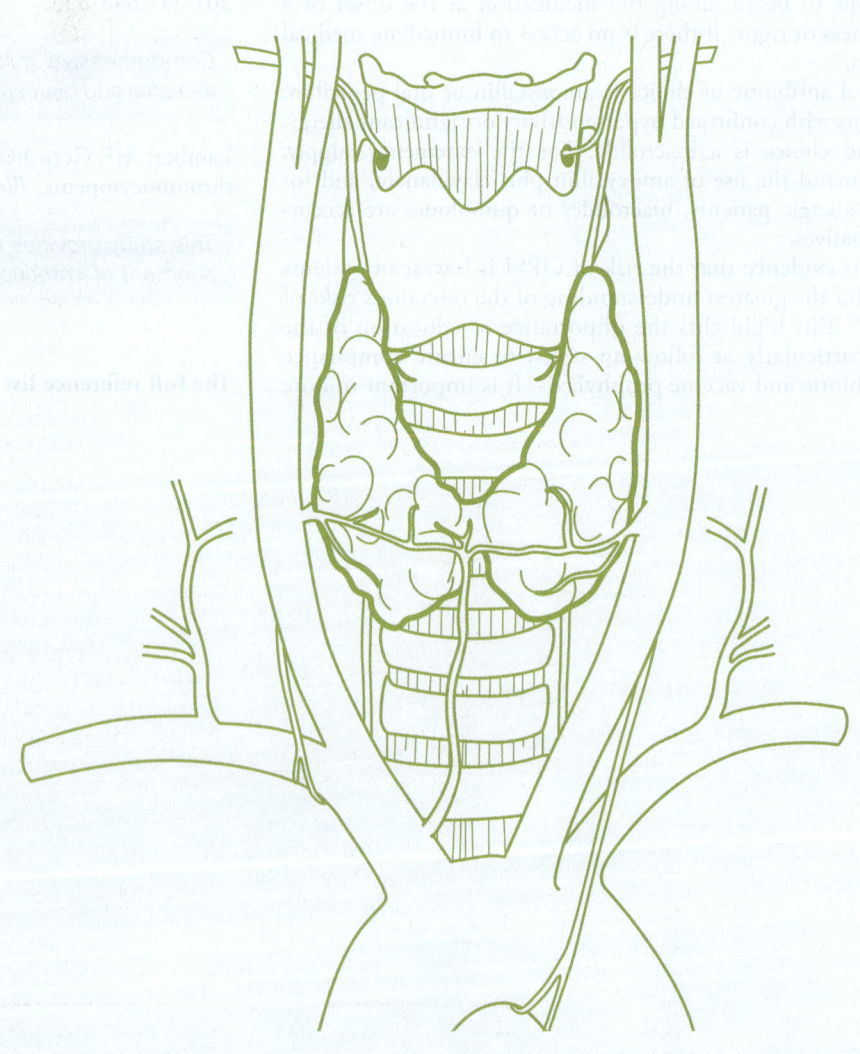

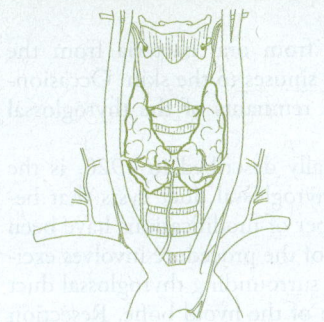

CHAPTER 73

The Thyroid

Timothy Ullmann, Jina Kim, Brenessa Lindeman, and Julie Ann Sosa*

OUTLINE

THYROID EMBRYOLOGY AND ANATOMY

Embryology

The thyroid gland originates from the median and lateral thyroid anlages—embryologic precursor tissues—which follow separate embryologic paths before fusing and forming a single gland.

*Disclosure: JAS is a member of the Data Monitoring Committee of the Medullary Thyroid Cancer Consortium Registry supported by Novo Nordisk, Astra Zeneca, and Eli Lilly. Institutional research funding is received from Exelixis and Eli Lilly. TU has participated in research funded by Blueprint Pharmaceuticals.

Median Thyroid Anlage

In utero, thyroid development begins with the median thyroid anlage, which is a thickening of the endodermal epithelium of the foregut in the floor of the pharynx. This thickening becomes an outpouching of the endoderm adjacent to the myocardial cells. As it descends caudally, along with the myocardial cells, the median thyroid anlage becomes a bilobed diverticulum with a median tubal structure called the *thyroglossal duct,* which keeps the structure connected to the tongue. The thyroglossal duct becomes a solid structure in the fifth week, after which it fragments and disappears. The obliteration of this structure leaves the foramen cecum at the base of the tongue superiorly and, when present, the pyramidal lobe inferiorly. The thyroid continues to descend to its final position anterior to the trachea by the seventh week. The cells derived from the median thyroid anlage arrange to form follicles and produce thyroid hormone by the tenth week of gestation.

Lateral Thyroid Anlage

The lateral thyroid anlage arises from the pharyngeal endoderm and fuses to the median anlage in the fifth week during its embryologic descent. The lateral thyroid anlage is comprised in part from cells of the ultimobranchial bodies, which originate from the fourth and fifth pharyngeal pouches. It is from these ultimobranchial bodies that the calcitonin-secreting parafollicular C cells arise. (The median anlage does not carry these cells.) The lateral thyroid anlage comprises approximately one-third of the total mass of the eventual thyroid gland.

Anomalies in the embryologic development of the thyroid gland can lead to a variety of conditions, some of which can be pathologic (Fig. 73.1).

Thyroglossal Duct Cyst

The normal development and subsequent obliteration of the thyroglossal duct are connected to that of the hyoid bone, which forms starting at the seventh week of gestation and functionally divides the thyroglossal tract into superior and inferior aspects. When the thyroglossal duct does not completely obliterate and the epithelial duct cells remain, a thyroglossal duct cyst may arise from a persistent connection between the thyroid gland and the foramen cecum. This scenario typically presents as a painless midline neck mass at or near the level of the hyoid, although it can be found near the base of the tongue or at the thyroid gland proper.

These cysts can become infected from oral bacteria from the tongue and can also form fistulous sinuses to the skin. Occasionally, thyroid tissue can develop in remnants of the thyroglossal duct along its tract.

The Sistrunk procedure, originally described in 1920, is the surgical treatment of choice for thyroglossal duct cysts that become chronically infected. A number of modifications have been described, but the key component of the procedure involves excision of the entirety of the cyst and surrounding thyroglossal duct tract, including the central portion of the hyoid bone. Resection of a small portion of the tongue is no longer thought to be necessary in the majority of cases.

Ectopic Thyroid Tissue

Aberrant thyroid tissue can be found anywhere along the normal path of development and descent of the thyroid gland, from the foramen cecum down to the anterior mediastinum. The development of an undescended thyroid can lead to the formation of a lingual thyroid gland near the base of the foramen cecum. This abnormal thyroid tissue often is associated with inadequate thyroid hormone production with subsequent goitrous enlargement, which in turn can lead to local compressive symptoms of the upper neck, such as airway obstruction and dysphagia. Surgical excision is occasionally necessary for these cases.

The other common locations for ectopic thyroid tissue are along the path of the thyrothymic tract, which originates from the third pharyngeal pouch and pulls along the inferior parathyroid glands and lower poles of the thyroid lobes via the descending path of the thymus gland. Foci of normal thyroid tissue along this tract are typically referred to as *thyroid rests*. These rests can occur

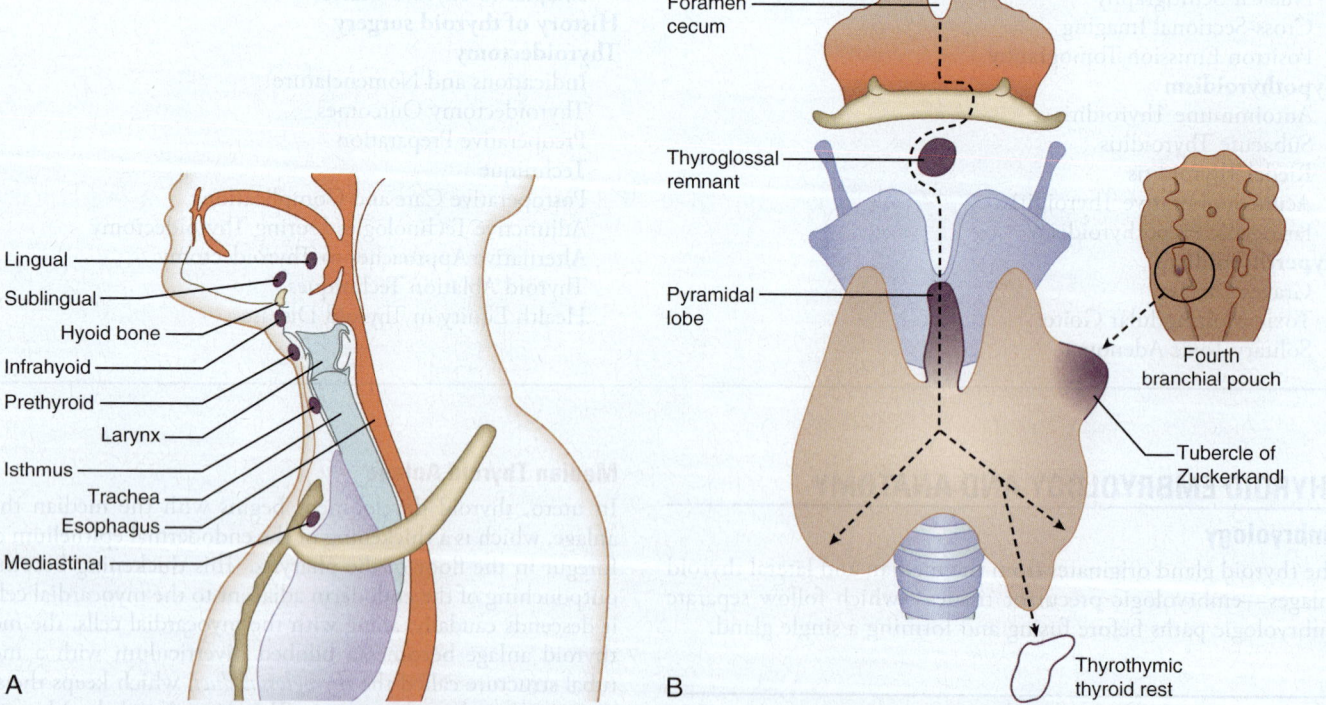

FIGURE 73.1 (A) Schema illustrating some common sites for midline ectopic thyroid masses. (B) A summary of the major medial and lateral embryologic elements of the thyroid gland and their potential adult anatomic consequences. (From Agarwal A, Mishra AK, Lomardi CP, et al. Applied embryology of the thyroid and parathyroid glands. In: Randolph GW, ed. *Surgery of the Thyroid and Parathyroid Glands*. 2nd ed. Philadelphia: Elsevier Saunders; 2013:18.)

in up to 50% of people and are typically not thought to be pathologic findings in and of themselves, although they occasionally may be mistaken for pathologic lymph nodes or parathyroid glands. Rests either can be connected to the thyroid gland proper by a thin stalk or can exist as completely separate structures. Primary intrathoracic goiters are thought to arise from enlargement of intrathoracic thyroid rests. Surgical treatment of thyroid rest tissue may occasionally be indicated if clinically relevant; examples of this include thyroid cancer requiring resection of a thyroid rest as a part of thyroidectomy or local compressive symptoms from an intrathoracic goiter. Another example of ectopic thyroid tissue is struma ovarii, which is a rare ovarian tumor with thyroid tissue comprising more than 50% of the overall mass. It is most commonly part of a teratoma and can be benign or malignant.

Anatomy

The normal thyroid gland is reddish-brown in color and rubbery in texture, with an adult gland typically weighing about 20 g. The thyroid gland typically is situated behind the sternohyoid and sternothyroid strap muscles and the superficial and middle layers of the deep cervical fascia.

When viewed in an anteroposterior plane, the shape of the thyroid resembles the silhouette of a butterfly, with two lateral lobes connected by an isthmus draped over the upper trachea just caudal to the cricoid cartilage. A normal-sized thyroid lobe is typically 4 to 6 cm in height and 1.3 to 1.8 cm in both transverse and anteroposterior dimensions. The isthmus typically has a thickness of 2 to 3 mm. In half to three-quarters of people, a pyramidal lobe extends superiorly from the isthmus and represents the caudal remnant of the thyroglossal duct. The right and left thyroid lobes make up the majority of the gland's volume. Each lobe's height extends from the level of the mid to upper aspect of the thyroid cartilage down to the fifth to sixth tracheal rings. Laterally, the lobe extends to the sternocleidomastoid muscle and carotid artery, with a small posterolateral projection or lump known as the *tubercle of Zuckerkandl*. The capsule enveloping the thyroid also forms separate "pseudolobules" within the parenchyma of the gland itself; these coalesce into a solid ligamentous structure at the posterolateral aspect of the upper trachea called the *suspensory ligament of Berry*. The tubercle of Zuckerkandl and Berry ligament are relatively constant anatomic landmarks for identification of the distal recurrent laryngeal nerve (RLN), which typically runs just posterior to these structures.

Blood and Lymphatic Supply

The thyroid is a highly vascular gland with abundant and redundant blood supply (Fig. 73.2). The arterial supply to the thyroid gland generally derives from two bilateral pairs of arteries. The superior thyroid arteries originate from the external carotid arteries and divide as they enter the superior poles of the thyroid lobes. The inferior thyroid arteries are branches from the thyrocervical trunks of the subclavian arteries. Because they branch fairly proximally from the thyrocervical trunk, their course runs cephalad and posterior to the carotid sheath before making a turn and entering the midthyroid lobes. In about 2% of people, a third artery called the thyroid ima artery arises directly from the aorta or innominate artery. This artery follows a midline path and enters the thyroid isthmus or the inferior poles of the thyroid lobes. The direction of the inferior thyroid artery as it enters the thyroid gland is another important landmark used for the identification of the RLN, which typically crosses the artery perpendicularly as it travels into the larynx (see later).

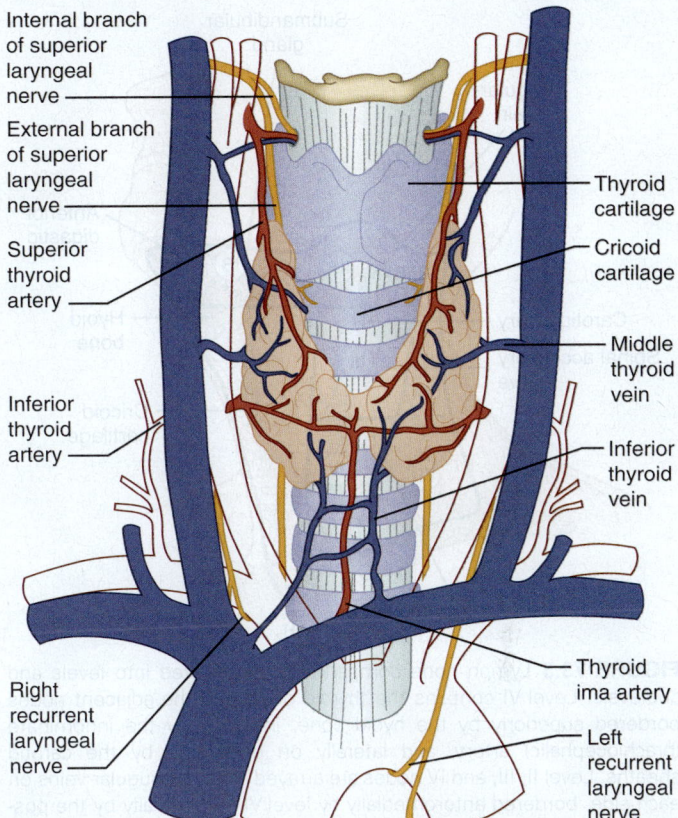

FIGURE 73.2 Anatomy of the thyroid gland and surrounding structures. (From McHenry CR. Thyroidectomy for nodules or small cancers. In: Duh QY, Clark OH, Kebebew E, eds. *Atlas of Endocrine Surgical Techniques*. Philadelphia: Elsevier Saunders; 2010:7.)

Branches of the inferior and superior arteries also supply the parathyroid glands. It is traditionally thought that the inferior thyroid arteries supply both superior and inferior parathyroid glands, but there can be significant anatomic variation around the arterial supply to the superior glands, which can be supplied by the inferior thyroid artery alone, the superior thyroid artery alone, or both.

There are three main venous drainage pathways from the thyroid gland. The superior thyroid veins typically run parallel to the superior thyroid arteries and drain into the internal jugular veins. The inferior thyroid veins run in a caudal direction from the inferior poles of the thyroid lobes and drain into the innominate veins. The middle thyroid veins are highly variable but typically arise from the lateral aspect of the midthyroid lobes; they drain into the internal jugular veins.

Much like the blood supply, the lymphatic network in and around the thyroid gland is rich and extensive. Lymphatic vessels course within the thyroid and drain into regional cervical lymph nodes. There is a standardized method and nomenclature for organizing the cervical lymph nodes into seven discrete "levels" (Fig. 73.3). An understanding of the pattern of lymphatic drainage from the thyroid is particularly important for understanding the surgical management of thyroid cancer (see "Thyroid Cancer" section later). The bulk of lymphatic drainage from the thyroid first goes to the perithyroidal lymph nodes in the central neck collectively grouped as level VI, which includes the lymph nodes

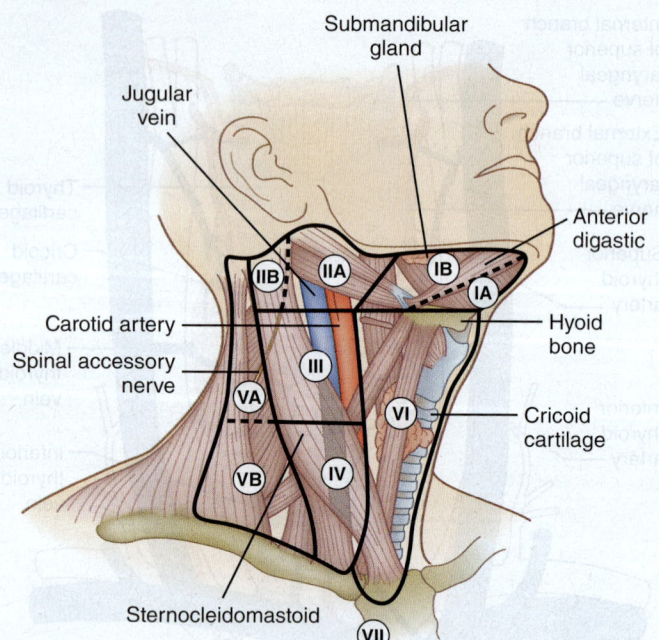

Jugular vein

Submandibular gland

Anterior digastic

Carotid artery

Spinal accessory nerve

Hyoid bone

Cricoid cartilage

Sternocleidomastoid

IIB IIA IB IA III VA VI VB IV VII

FIGURE 73.3 Lymph node compartments separated into levels and sublevels. Level VI contains the thyroid gland and the adjacent nodes bordered superiorly by the hyoid bone, inferiorly by the innominate (brachiocephalic) artery, and laterally on each side by the carotid sheaths. Level II, III, and IV nodes are arrayed along the jugular veins on each side, bordered anteromedially by level VI and laterally by the posterior border of the sternocleidomastoid muscle. Level III nodes are bounded superiorly by the level of the hyoid bone and inferiorly by the inferior aspect of the cricoid cartilage; levels II and IV are above and below level III, respectively. The level I node compartment includes the submental and submandibular nodes above the hyoid bone and anterior to the posterior edge of the submandibular gland. Level V nodes are in the posterior triangle, outside the lateral edge of the sternocleidomastoid muscle. Levels I, II, and V can be further subdivided as noted in the figure. The inferior extent of level VI is defined as the suprasternal notch. Many authors also include the pretracheal and paratracheal superior mediastinal lymph nodes above the level of the innominate artery (sometimes referred to as level VII) in central neck dissection.

between the two carotid arteries and bounded by the hyoid bone superiorly and the sternal notch inferiorly. This compartment extends inferiorly as level VII from the sternal notch to the brachiocephalic artery inferiorly. The lateral neck jugular lymph nodes (levels IIa, III, and IV) as well as those in the posterior triangle of the neck (particularly level Vb) also drain lymphatics from the thyroid, typically in transit from the central neck lymph nodes. Skip metastases that avoid level VI and extend directly from the primary tumor (typically in the superior pole of the thyroid) to the lateral neck are exceptional cases that occur in less than 15% of patients. Other levels of the neck are rarely associated with regional thyroid cancer metastases.

Nerves Associated With the Thyroid Gland

The thyroid is directly supplied by a network of tiny autonomic nerves arising from the superior and middle cervical sympathetic ganglia and parasympathetic fibers derived from the vagus nerve. The two most important nerves associated with the thyroid gland for the surgeon are the RLN and the external branch of the superior laryngeal nerve (EBSLN). It is critical that the thyroid

surgeon have a thorough understanding of the normal and anomalous paths of these nerves, such that these structures can be better preserved during thyroidectomy.

The RLN and EBSLN are the main nerves responsible for the function of the larynx. Each nerve is paired, with a right and left side. The RLN is by far the more important nerve and innervates the motor function of all of the intrinsic laryngeal muscles except for the cricothyroid. It carries sensory fibers from the lower larynx as well as minor motor and sensory fibers from the trachea and esophagus. Unilateral injury to the RLN leads to paralysis of the ipsilateral vocal fold, with typical symptoms ranging from voice complaints such as hoarseness and vocal fatigue to aspiration. Bilateral RLN injury with subsequent bilateral vocal fold paralysis may require tracheostomy for airway control if the paralyzed vocal folds rest in a median position preventing adequate air exchange; alternatively, the risk of persistent aspiration and respiratory tract infections is high if the resting vocal folds remain in an abducted position. The EBSLN innervates the cricothyroid muscles, and it contributes to vocal fold tone and tension. EBSLN injury leads to difficulties with achieving high pitch and vocal projection and volume. The nerve became a historical focus of attention after the famous opera singer Amelita Galla-Curci developed difficulty singing high notes after thyroidectomy; this was thought to be because of injury to it during surgery, although subsequent historical reports dispute this claim.

The anatomy of the left and right RLNs differs based on their embryologic development (Fig. 73.4). Both RLNs are derived from the sixth branchial arches below the sixth aortic arches. As the fifth and sixth aortic arches above the RLNs subsequently regress in embryogenesis, the two nerves then anchor to, and follow, the right and left fourth aortic arch structures, which develop into differing arteries—the right subclavian artery and the aortic arch, respectively. Both nerves loop back, or "recur," into the neck because of the heart and great vessels descending into the thorax, bringing the RLNs down with them. The left RLN loops under the ligamentum arteriosum at the aortic arch and travels in the tracheoesophageal groove until it reaches the thyroid. The right RLN loops under the right carotid-subclavian artery junction and migrates to the cricothyroid joint at the insertion into the larynx. Because of the lateral location of the right carotid-subclavian junction and the shorter length of the course of the right RLN, this nerve can be identified traveling in a slightly anterior plane and an oblique direction compared with the left RLN, which tends to stay relatively deep and straight in the tracheoesophageal groove.

There are a number of anatomic landmarks that can aid in identification and characterization of the RLN. The tubercle of Zuckerkandl typically lies just anterior and lateral to the nerve. There is an intimate relationship between the nerve, Berry ligament, and inferior thyroid artery at the level of the cricoid cartilage. Here, the nerve crosses the artery (usually posteriorly) and typically curves anteriorly toward the ligament before diving posteriorly again into the laryngeal insertion point at the cricothyroid joint. There are numerous anatomic variations of the course of the nerve and its relationship with the three structures, particularly with respect to how anteriorly the nerve can be positioned. In addition, the RLN may branch more proximally in up to 20% to 30% of cases, and preservation of all of the branches is important to preserve nerve function; this is particularly true for the anterior branches, which predominantly provide motor innervation.

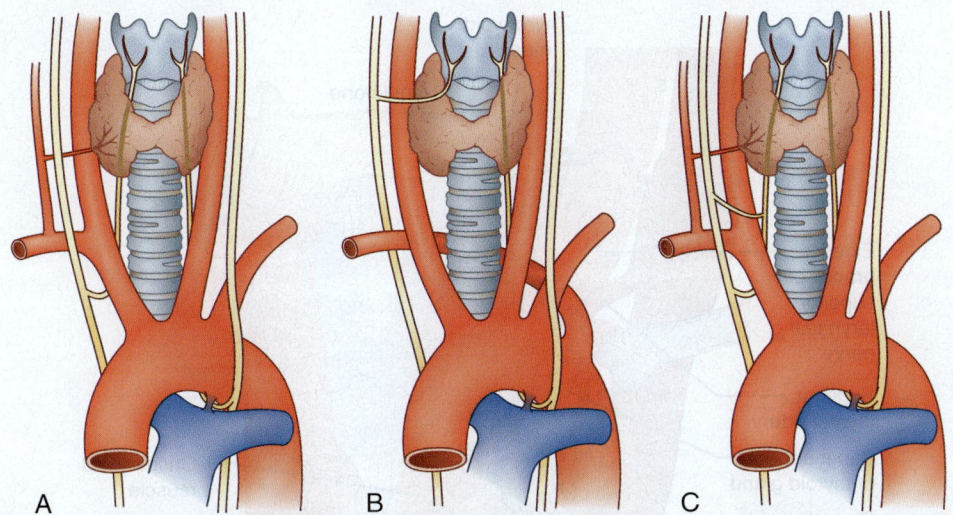

FIGURE 73.4 Anomalous variations in the course of the right recurrent laryngeal nerve. (A) The normal course of the recurrent laryngeal nerve arises from the vagus after it passes beneath the subclavian artery. A nonrecurrent laryngeal nerve arises from the vagus and courses medially into the larynx in the setting of an aberrant origin of the right subclavian artery. (B) A nonrecurrent laryngeal nerve arises from the vagus and courses medially into the larynx in the setting of an aberrant origin of the right subclavian artery. (C) The unusual coexistence of a nonrecurrent laryngeal nerve and the recurrent laryngeal nerve forms a common distal nerve.

The RLN also may course in a nonrecurrent fashion, instead branching in a direct path from the cervical vagus nerve (see Fig. 73.4). On the right side, this is associated with—and likely secondary to—an aberrant right subclavian artery arising directly from the aortic arch instead of the innominate artery (called the *lusoria artery*). This artery arises distal to the left subclavian artery and crosses the midline posterior to the esophagus. Because of the absence of a normal right subclavian-carotid junction to pull down the right RLN during embryologic development, the right RLN follows a straight path from the vagus nerve to the larynx. A right-sided non-RLN occurs in up to 1% of people. A left-sided nonrecurrent nerve can occur in the extremely rare scenarios of a patient with situs inversus and a right-sided aortic arch.

Like the RLN, the superior laryngeal nerve arises from the vagus nerve. The EBSLN branches off at the hyoid bone and runs along the inferior pharyngeal constrictor muscle before running parallel to the upper aspect of the superior pole thyroid vessels and then terminating in the cricothyroid muscle. Although the EBSLN is typically fairly high above the thyroid lobe, care must be taken when ligating and dividing the superior pole vessels during thyroidectomy because the anatomic variations in the EBSLN can run quite close to the vessels and the upper thyroid lobe and must be dissected away as the superior pole of the gland is taken down (Fig. 73.5).

THYROID HISTOLOGY AND PHYSIOLOGY

Histology

The thyroid is composed mainly of two epithelial cell types. The first and predominant type is the follicular cell, which is responsible for the production and secretion of thyroid hormone (Fig. 73.6). The second type is the parafollicular C cell, which secretes calcitonin. The histologic architecture of the thyroid is arranged into spherical follicles containing colloid. Colloid is made up of thyroglobulin

(Tg), which is the noniodinated precursor to active thyroid hormone and acts as a reservoir. The parafollicular C cells are located within the interfollicular stroma and are mainly found in the lateral aspect of the mid and upper thyroid lobes.

Normal Thyroid Physiology

Thyroid Hormone

The synthesis of thyroid hormones is a complex multistep process that occurs within the thyroid follicle unit. The process is dependent on the presence of iodine and is outlined as follows:

- Follicular cells actively transport iodide anions across the cell membrane from the bloodstream into the cytoplasm via the Na/I symporter transmembrane protein. The concentration of iodine within the follicular cells is normally manyfold higher than that of the systemic circulation because of this active transport.
- Iodide then moves toward the follicular cell border with the colloid stores, and the anions are oxidized to form the neutral I_2 molecule. This form of iodine can pass through the cell membrane into the colloid.
- Colloid stores Tg, which contains a multitude of tyrosine residues. Colloid also contains the enzyme thyroid peroxidase (TPO), which catalyzes the next major step in thyroid hormone synthesis, which is the iodination of tyrosine residues on Tg. A tyrosine residue iodinated by a single iodine molecule leads to the formation of the molecule monoiodotyrosine and that iodinated by two iodine molecules leads to diiodotyrosine (DIT).
- The DIT and monoiodotyrosine molecules form covalent bonds with one another to constitute the active forms of thyroid hormone tetraiodothyronine, or thyroxine (T_4), formed by two DITs and carrying four iodine molecules, and triiodothyronine (T_3), formed by a DIT and monoiodotyrosine and carrying three iodine molecules. When stimulated

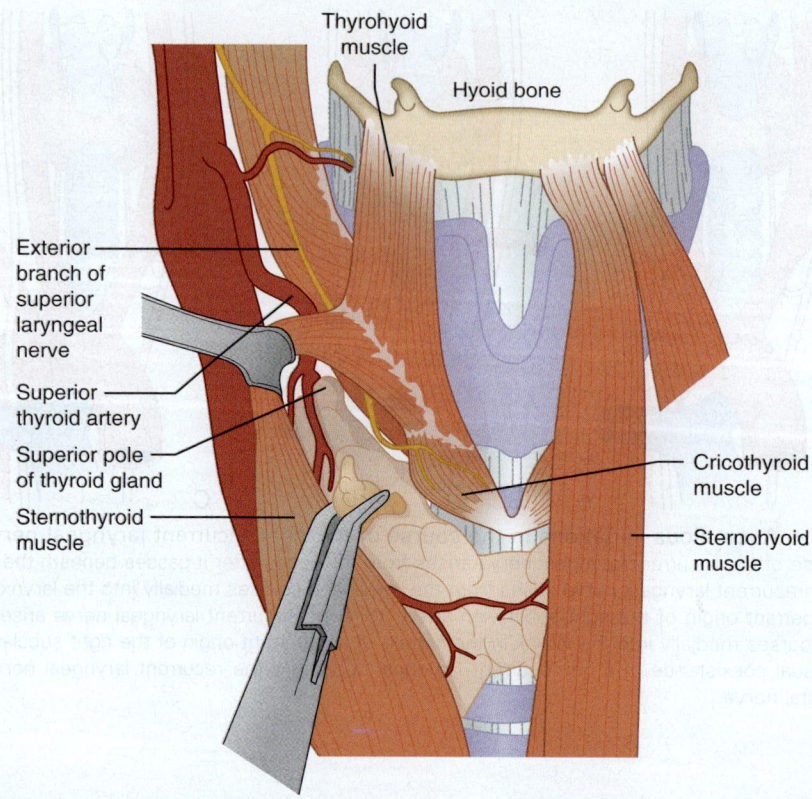

FIGURE 73.5 Dissection and ligation of the superior-pole thyroid vessels should be performed as far caudally on the thyroid gland as possible to avoid injury to the external branch of the superior laryngeal nerve. (From Randolph GW. Surgical anatomy, intraoperative neural monitoring, and operative management of the RLN and SLN. In: Duh QY, Clark OH, Kebebew E, eds. *Atlas of Endocrine Surgical Techniques.* Philadelphia: Elsevier Saunders; 2010:105.)

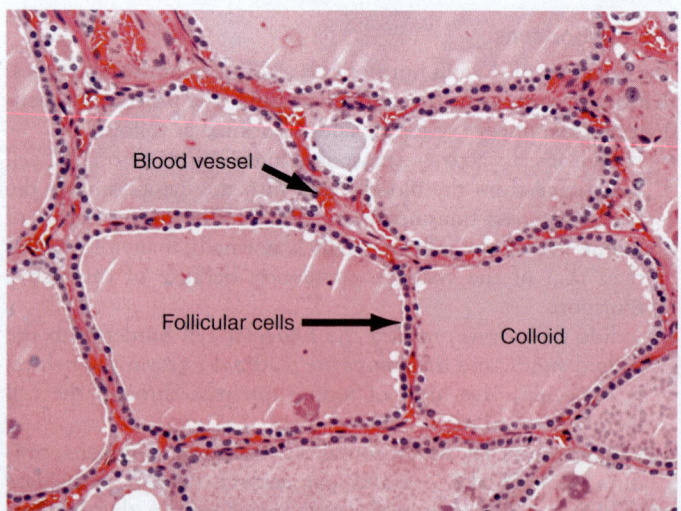

FIGURE 73.6 Photomicrograph of normal thyroid parenchyma with hematoxylin and eosin staining. The follicular unit contains colloid at the center, and each follicle is surrounded by a single layer of well-ordered, cytologically normal follicular cells. The parafollicular spaces contain blood vessels and parafollicular cells.

by thyroid-stimulating hormone (TSH), the follicular cells transport the activated thyroid hormones from the colloid center into the bloodstream (Fig. 73.7).

Once in the bloodstream, greater than 99% of circulating thyroid hormones are bound to transport proteins such as albumin and T_4-binding globulins; less than 1% exists in free form. This allows a relatively tight degree of control of thyroid hormone diffusion into target cells, in that the bound hormones will be released if circulating free levels decrease. Although there is normally a higher concentration of T_4 compared with T_3, T_3 is the more potent form, and in fact many target organs such as the brain, liver, gut, skeletal muscle, and thyroid are able to convert T_4 to T_3 through the deiodinase system that removes one of the iodine molecules.

Iodine plays a primary role in thyroid hormone physiology, and it is predicated on there being an adequate supply in the body. The average daily iodine requirement for adult humans is 0.1 mg, and this is entirely derived from dietary intake. The thyroid is the target for the overwhelming majority of the body's iodine stores. Seafood such as fish, shrimp, and seaweed are rich in iodine stores. Since 1924, the United States has iodized salt, which effectively has eliminated iodine deficiency in this country. Many regions of the world remain at risk for iodine deficiency despite worldwide efforts to improve access to iodized salt; the World Health Organization estimates that 54 countries remain iodine deficient.

Thyroid hormone is critical for normal bodily function. On a cellular level, T_4 and T_3 bind to mitochondrial receptors, leading to increased adenosine triphosphate (ATP) production, oxygen consumption, and glucose oxidation in a calorigenic process that releases heat. Therefore, thyroid hormone function is often referred to in shorthand as the primary driver of the basal metabolic rate. It is hypothesized that virtually all cells in the body are end-targets for thyroid hormone, mostly through their actions with

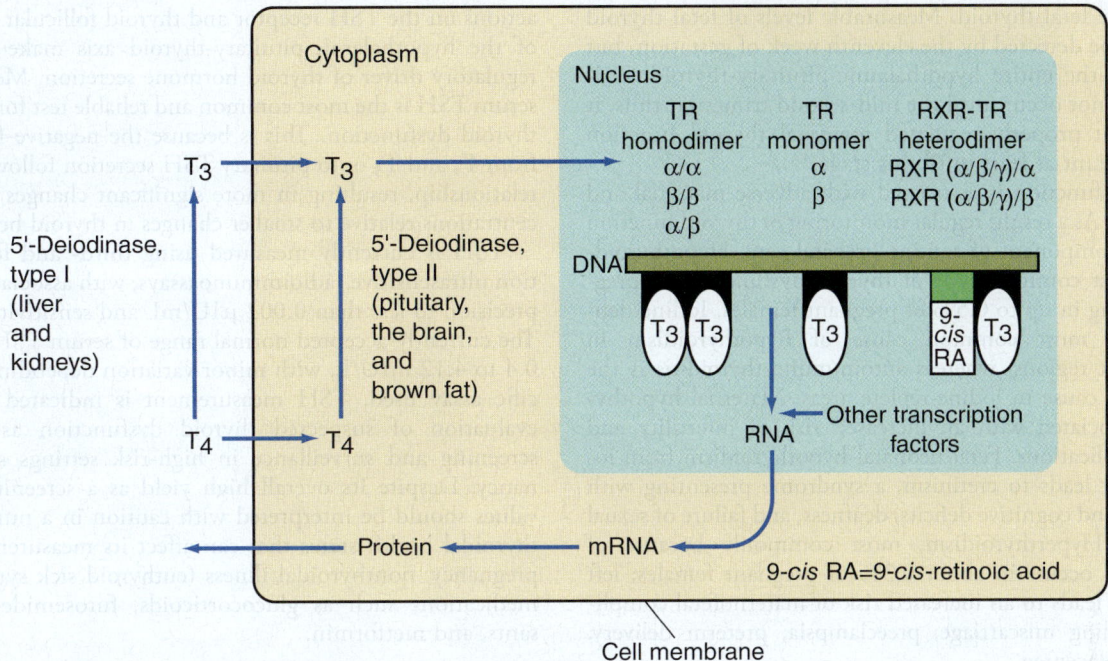

FIGURE 73.7 Cellular and molecular events involved in thyroid hormone function. Thyroxine (T_4) is converted in the periphery and in the cytoplasm of the cell into triiodothyronine (T_3). T_3 travels to the nucleus, where it binds to a thyroid hormone receptor (TR) (homodimer, monomer, or heterodimer). TR binding leads to RNA transcription in association with other transcription factors; messenger RNA is subsequently expressed and then translated into protein.

regard to stimulating lipid and carbohydrate metabolism. Thyroid hormone is critical for normal in utero and childhood growth and development, especially with respect to neurologic function. The cardiovascular system is an important target of thyroid hormone, which increases cardiac output and vasodilatation. Normal reproductive function is highly dependent on thyroid hormone (see later).

The regulation of thyroid hormone production is tightly controlled by interactions between the hypothalamus, pituitary, and thyroid glands. Low circulating levels of T_4 and T_3 stimulate the hypothalamus to release thyrotropin-releasing hormone, which in turn stimulates the release of TSH from the anterior pituitary. TSH stimulates the formation of thyroid hormones by binding to its receptor on the thyroid follicular cells, leading to both increased transport of iodine and transport and release of T_4 and T_3 from the colloid into the bloodstream. Conversely, elevated circulating thyroid hormone levels lead to a negative feedback loop, with downregulation of thyrotropin-releasing hormone and TSH from the hypothalamus and pituitary, respectively.

Calcitonin

The thyroid gland also produces calcitonin from the parafollicular C cells, but the production of calcitonin is not regulated by the same processes that govern that of thyroid hormone. The primary known function of calcitonin is to decrease the serum concentration of calcium through its end-effect actions on bone (increasing osteoblast and decreasing osteoclast activity), gut (decreasing calcium absorption), and kidney (increasing urinary calcium excretion), and its release is stimulated by elevated serum calcium levels. However, the absence of calcitonin does not lead to a noticeable change in calcium homeostasis—as it would for

parathyroid hormone (PTH)—and so its ultimate importance for normal physiologic function remains poorly understood.

Thyroid Physiology in Pregnancy

Normal pregnancy induces significant changes in thyroid hormone function because of its critical importance for early fetal development. Although multiple fetal processes depend on thyroid hormone, including overall growth, metabolic regulation, and bone maturation, neuronal and brain development are the most critical, as evidenced by the finding of severe neurocognitive deficits in babies born to mothers with untreated hypothyroidism.

During the first trimester, maternal thyroid hormone production rises significantly, with total T_4 concentrations increasing up to 1.5 times that of the nonpregnant state. Although the details are not completely elucidated, it is thought that this rise is at least in part because of the rapidly increasing levels of human chorionic gonadotropin, which shares a common alpha subunit with TSH and acts as a TSH agonist. This can occasionally lead to a phenomenon known as *transient gestational thyrotoxicosis* occurring only in the first trimester and resolving spontaneously.

The rise in T_4 concentration is also accompanied by a concomitant increase in T_4-binding globulin concentration in the bloodstream, which results in greater binding of the circulating T_4 and relative stability in free T_4 levels. Because of the increased demands for thyroid hormone production, the daily recommended iodine intake during pregnancy also rises. Maternal T_4 is transported to the fetal circulation via specialized thyroid hormone transporters in the placenta.

Maternal thyroid hormone production increases and peaks during the first trimester of pregnancy and declines steadily afterward; this likely coincides with the development and early function of the fetal thyroid. Measurable levels of fetal thyroid hormone can be detected by the eleventh week of gestation, but maturation of the entire hypothalamic-pituitary-thyroid feedback axis does not occur until the mid-second trimester; thus, it is thought that properly regulated maternal thyroid function remains important at least until this stage.

Thyroid dysfunction is associated with adverse maternal and fetal outcomes. As a result, regular monitoring of thyroid function is a standard component of routine prenatal care. Hypothyroidism is the most common type of thyroid dysfunction in pregnancy, occurring in up to 0.5% of pregnant females. Iodine deficiency is the most common cause of hypothyroidism in iodine-deficient regions, whereas autoimmune thyroiditis is the most common cause in iodine-replete areas. Maternal hypothyroidism is associated with an increased risk of infertility and perinatal complications. Fetal/neonatal hypothyroidism from iodine deficiency leads to cretinism, a syndrome presenting with severe growth and cognitive deficits, deafness, and failure of sexual development. Hyperthyroidism, most commonly because of Graves disease, occurs in about 0.3% of pregnant females; left untreated, this leads to an increased risk of maternofetal complications, including miscarriage, preeclampsia, preterm delivery, and abruptio placentae.

Thyroid Physiology in Nonthyroidal Illness (Euthyroid Sick Syndrome)

Many acute and chronic nonthyroidal disease states can affect thyroid function measurement. This phenomenon, commonly called *euthyroid sick syndrome* or *nonthyroidal illness syndrome,* leads to the finding of abnormal thyroid function tests in the setting of nonthyroidal illness in a patient without preexisting thyroid disease. The most common finding is low serum T_3 concentrations, with decreases in T_4 also seen in more severe disease states. TSH concentrations remain relatively normal to slightly elevated, but not to the degree of true hypothyroidism. Patients do not exhibit any signs of clinical thyroid dysfunction.

The pathophysiology behind euthyroid sick syndrome remains poorly understood, although several theories exist. Some believe that conversion of T_4 to T_3 in the target tissues is impaired during nonthyroidal illness because of decreased activity of peripheral deiodinase enzymes (in particular, deiodinase type 2). Others have investigated the role of cytokines such as tumor necrosis factor-α, interleukin-1, and interleukin-6 in decreasing thyroid hormone production at the level of the thyroid follicular cell. Others hypothesize that the inhibition of thyroid hormone binding to various thyroid-binding proteins may lead to inaccurate measurement of true free hormone levels. Regardless of theory, it is generally believed that patients with this phenomenon are in fact euthyroid and do not have intrinsic thyroid dysfunction.

Common states associated with euthyroid sick syndrome in surgical patients include sepsis, fasting/starvation, trauma, thermal injury, and myocardial infarction. Many medications such as corticosteroids and amiodarone also can affect thyroid function measurement. There is no treatment for euthyroid sick syndrome other than treating the underlying condition, which resolves the thyroid function test abnormalities.

THYROID BIOMARKERS

Thyroid-Stimulating Hormone

TSH is a 28-kDa glycoprotein secreted from the anterior pituitary gland in a pulsatile fashion; it follows a circadian rhythm. Its actions on the TSH receptor and thyroid follicular cells as a part of the hypothalamic-pituitary-thyroid axis make it a primary regulatory driver of thyroid hormone secretion. Measurement of serum TSH is the most common and reliable test for screening for thyroid dysfunction. This is because the negative feedback loop from T_4 and T_3 onto pituitary TSH secretion follows a log-linear relationship, resulting in more significant changes in TSH concentrations relative to smaller changes in thyroid hormone levels.

TSH is currently measured using third- and fourth-generation ultrasensitive radioimmunoassays, with associated degrees of precision to less than 0.002 μIU/mL and sensitivity up to 97%. The currently accepted normal range of serum TSH for adults is 0.4 to 4.12 mIU/L, with minor variation depending on the specific assay used. TSH measurement is indicated as a part of evaluation of suspected thyroid dysfunction as well as for screening and surveillance in high-risk settings such as pregnancy. Despite its overall high yield as a screening test, TSH values should be interpreted with caution in a number of nonthyroidal health states that can affect its measurement, such as pregnancy, nonthyroidal illness (euthyroid sick syndrome), and medications such as glucocorticoids, furosemide, anticonvulsants, and metformin.

Tetraiodothyronine and Triiodothyronine

Serum measurement of T_4 and T_3 is an important confirmatory component in the evaluation of thyroid dysfunction. The vast majority of both thyroid hormones in systemic circulation are bound to plasma proteins such as T_4-binding globulins, with less than 0.2% of the hormones available in the free, biologically active states. Because of this, measurement of free T_4 and free T_3 levels are more accurate in reflecting thyroid function compared with measuring total hormone levels, which can be falsely affected by the presence of various circulating transporter proteins.

The measurement of TSH and free T_4 are the most commonly paired thyroid function tests because of their accurate interpretability in the majority of scenarios, including the diagnosis and treatment monitoring of thyroid dysfunction. Free T_3 is not as useful for the diagnosis of hypothyroidism, but it can be useful for the confirmation of other conditions such as hyperthyroidism and euthyroid sick syndrome. All forms of thyroid hormones are measured using modern competitive immunoassays, with mild variations in normal ranges depending on the method and manufacturer. Normal reference ranges are also age dependent, with different standards for pediatric and adult populations.

Thyroid Autoantibodies

The measurement of serum thyroid autoantibodies is useful in the diagnosis of various autoimmune thyroid diseases, although their variable sensitivities and specificities require caution in test interpretation. The three most commonly measured autoantibodies today are anti-TPO (TPOAb), anti-Tg (TgAb), and anti-TSH receptor (TRAb).

Measurement of TPOAb is the most accurate and commonly used screening test for autoimmune thyroiditis. TPOAb is positive in over 90% of patients with autoimmune thyroiditis as well as 80% of patients with Graves disease. However, it also has a false-positive rate of 10% to 15%. Measurement of TgAb is commonly performed, with 80% sensitivity for autoimmune thyroiditis and 30% sensitivity for Graves disease and a similar false-positive rate as TPOAb. Importantly, the presence of TgAb interferes with the interpretation of Tg measurement for the surveillance of differentiated thyroid cancer (DTC; see later). TPOAb is usually measured by ultrasensitive immunoradiometric assays; TgAb also can be measured with this method, although other techniques such as radioimmunoassays or enzyme-linked immunosorbent assays are also acceptable. These two tests are often ordered together and are generally readily available in most clinical laboratories.

Measurement of TRAb is typically reserved for diagnostic confirmation of Graves disease because it is positive in over 90% of patients with the diagnosis. TRAb measurement is typically performed in one of two ways: (1) a TSH receptor-binding inhibitory immunoglobulin bioassay, which detects immunoglobulins inhibiting the binding of TSH to the recombinant TSH receptor, and (2) a thyroid-stimulating immunoglobulin (TSI) bioassay, which more specifically detects the stimulatory subtype of TRAb that activates the TSH receptor on thyroid follicular cells. TSI measurement has been hypothesized to more closely correlate with the severity of active Graves disease. According to the 2016 American Thyroid Association (ATA) guidelines for hyperthyroidism, initial evaluation of thyrotoxicosis can include measurement of TRAb, determination of radioactive iodine (RAI) uptake, or measurement of thyroidal blood flow on ultrasonography. Thyrotoxicosis related to Graves disease will demonstrate elevated TRAb, elevated iodine uptake in the thyroid gland, and/or elevated thyroidal blood flow. In a study employing a theoretical model of 100,000 patients in a US-managed care system, using TRAb to diagnose Graves disease reduced costs and provided faster diagnosis.[1]

Thyroglobulin

Tg is a large, 660-kDa glycosylated protein that acts as a precursor protein for the active iodinated forms of thyroid hormone. Although the majority of Tg is stored in colloid within the thyroid follicles, a small amount of Tg escapes into the systemic circulation during the conversion process to T_4 and T_3 and is thus detectable in peripheral blood. Tg can be particularly elevated in patients with DTC, although with low diagnostic utility for routine measurement or before total thyroidectomy. On the other hand, postoperative serum Tg measurement after total thyroidectomy with RAI for DTC remains among the most sensitive cancer biomarkers in existence today, with the caveat that its accuracy depends on the absence of TgAb.

Current widely used immunoassay methods for Tg measurement include enzyme-linked immunosorbent assay, enzyme-multiplied immunoassay, fluorescence polarization immunoassay, and immunochemiluminometric assay. All of these immunoassay methods have made Tg measurement highly sensitive and specific, such that it is possible to detect Tg down to the 0.1 ng/mL level. For postoperative surveillance of DTC, the sensitivity of Tg measurement can be augmented further with TSH stimulation, either after withdrawal of thyroid hormone or after injection of recombinant human TSH (rhTSH). A stimulated Tg of more than 1 to 2 ng/mL is considered higher risk for persistent or recurrent disease in the postthyroidectomy setting.[2]

The accuracy of serum Tg testing is highly dependent on the absence of TgAb, which must be obtained at the same time. TgAb is present in 10% to 15% of the general population and can limit the interpretability of postoperative Tg measurement. Even in these scenarios, TgAb often can be used as a crude surrogate biomarker because autoantibodies can disappear over time after the successful treatment of thyroid cancer; in addition, an increase in TgAb levels can signify disease recurrence.[3] Newer Tg assays that employ mass spectrometry offer reasonable detection capability even in the presence of TgAb, with sensitivities down to 0.5 ng/mL, approaching those of the immunoassays.

Calcitonin

Calcitonin is a 32–amino acid protein secreted by the parafollicular C cells. Normally, serum calcitonin levels are highest in infancy, decline rapidly in early childhood, then remain relatively stable through adulthood (although absolute levels can fluctuate minute to minute). Calcitonin does not appear to play a significant role in calcium homeostasis despite its known mechanisms of action at the level of the bone, gut, and kidney. Serum calcitonin is the most sensitive biomarker for the detection and surveillance of medullary thyroid cancer (MTC), which is a malignancy of the parafollicular C cells. This test is performed in patients with—or family members at risk for—MTC or multiple endocrine neoplasia type 2 (MEN2; see later). There is controversy around the utility of measuring serum calcitonin as a routine screening test in the evaluation of a thyroid nodule.[4] Calcitonin is currently measured using a variety of methods, including radioimmunoassays, enzyme-linked immunosorbent assay, and immunochemiluminometric assay, with differing sensitivities, specificities, and reference ranges.

THYROID IMAGING

Neck Ultrasound

Neck ultrasonography is the preferred modality for routine radiographic evaluation of the thyroid gland because it offers the most accurate visualization of thyroid nodular disease and allows for the concomitant ability to perform percutaneous fine-needle aspiration (FNA) biopsy of thyroid lesions (see later). Neck ultrasound provides information about overall thyroid size and vascularity, presence and risk stratification of thyroid nodules, and presence of suspicious cervical lymphadenopathy; in addition, it can be used to localize parathyroid disease. Advantages of ultrasound include the fact that it is noninvasive and portable for the clinic and it is not associated with radiation exposure.

One potential disadvantage of neck ultrasound is that the study quality is highly dependent on having a skilled operator; this issue is amplified by practice- and institution-specific variations on what specialties perform ultrasound because radiologists, surgeons, pathologists, and medical endocrinologists all may be trained in its performance. Efforts to standardize the quality of neck ultrasound have included common ultrasound training and credentialing pathways regardless of specialty as well as standardized templates for neck ultrasound reporting.

The normal sonographic appearance of the thyroid is homogeneously echogenic with a uniform echotexture (Fig. 73.8). Pathologic findings on thyroid ultrasound are described in the appropriate sections next.

Nuclear Scintigraphy

Thyroid scintigraphy is performed using either technetium-99m pertechnetate or a radiolabeled iodine nuclide (typically ^{123}I or ^{131}I). Depending on the specific study, the tracer can be administered intravenously, orally, or via inhalation, and images are obtained anywhere from 30 minutes (for intravenous [IV] injection) to 24 hours (for oral administration) afterward. The thyroid normally displays symmetric uptake bilaterally. Nodular disease can be classified into whether there is increased focal uptake (the so-called "hot" nodule, Fig. 73.9) or not (the "cold" nodule). Classically, "hot" nodules in the setting of hyperthyroidism are thought

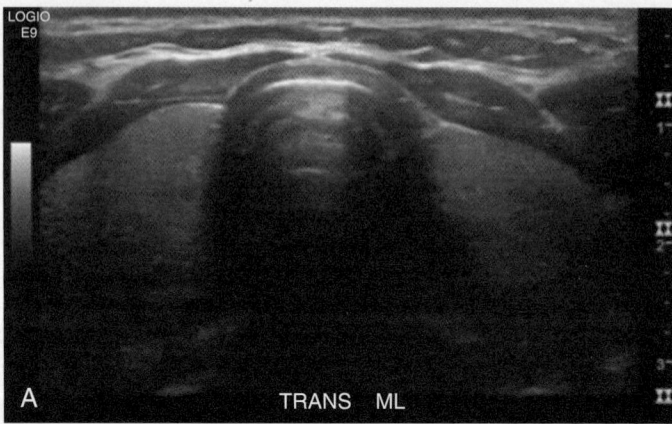

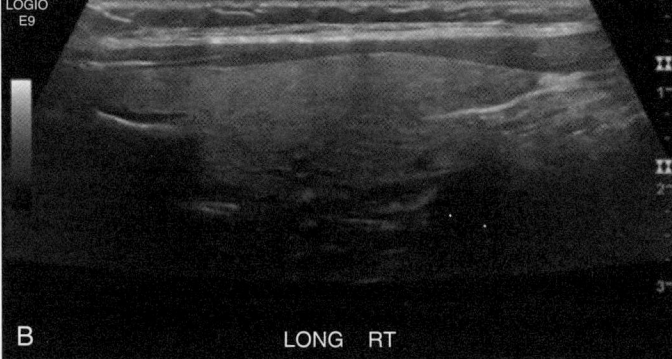

FIGURE 73.8 Normal appearance of the thyroid gland on neck ultrasound. Note the homogeneous echogenicity with uniform echotexture of the gland. (A) Transverse midline view with the two lobes on either side of the trachea. (B) Longitudinal view of the right thyroid lobe. *ML*, Midline; *RT*, right.

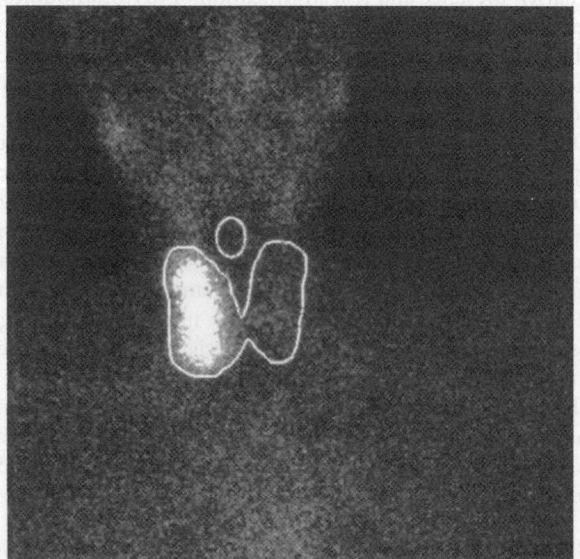

FIGURE 73.9 ^{131}I scan demonstrating an area of increased uptake in the right lobe of a 32-year-old patient with increased thyroid function test values and a palpable nodule. This scan is consistent with a toxic or hyperfunctioning nodule.

to be benign toxic nodules with extremely low risk of malignancy, whereas "cold" nodules carry a 15% risk of malignancy.

Improvements in ultrasonography and cross-sectional imaging over the past few decades have rendered thyroid scintigraphy obsolete in all but a few scenarios. A thyroid uptake scan is useful for the

differential diagnosis of hyperthyroidism by determining whether increased radiotracer uptake occurs diffusely throughout the gland as in the case of Graves disease or in more discrete "hot" nodules in cases of solitary toxic adenoma or toxic multinodular goiter (TMG). In addition, radiolabeled iodine scans (usually referred to as *RAI scans*) are commonly performed to assess for, and treat, persistent/recurrent or metastatic disease in the setting of DTC (see later).

Cross-Sectional Imaging

Computed tomography (CT) or magnetic resonance imaging (MRI) scans can be useful adjuncts to ultrasound for specific indications because they can provide precise cross-sectional anatomic assessment of the thyroid gland relative to the other structures in the neck, including the larynx and trachea, esophagus, muscles, and major vascular structures. These modalities are helpful particularly for two scenarios: substernal (intrathoracic) goiter and advanced thyroid cancer (Fig. 73.10). CT and MRI have improved ability over ultrasound in visualizing the infraclavicular

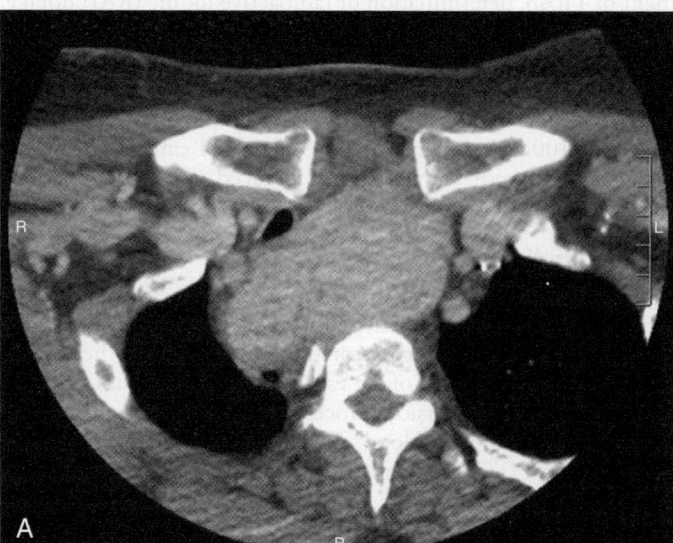

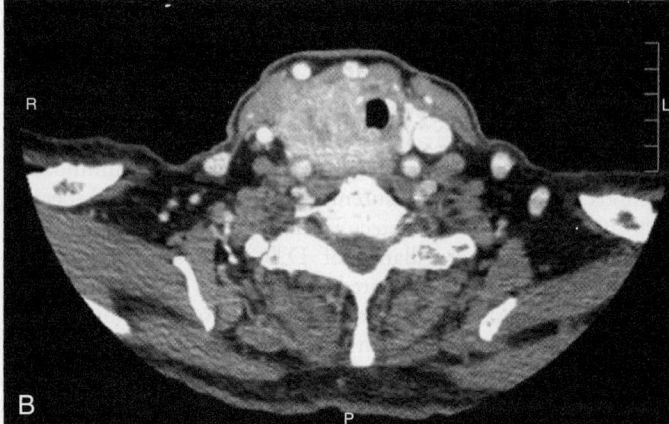

FIGURE 73.10 Computed tomography (CT) scans provide useful anatomic information about the thyroid in selected scenarios. (A) Contrast-enhanced CT scan demonstrating a left-sided substernal goiter extending into the posterior mediastinum and crossing over to the right side with tracheal compression and deviation of both the trachea and esophagus. (B) Contrast-enhanced CT scan of a bulky, locally advanced follicular thyroid cancer originating in the right lobe with invasion into the lateral tracheal wall and esophagus and obliteration of the right internal jugular vein.

mediastinum. In addition, cross-sectional imaging more readily detects vascular anomalies such as the lusoria artery that can alert the surgeon to complex anatomic situations (e.g., presence of non-RLN) and assist with perioperative planning. Many surgeons prefer CT over MRI because of its greater ease of interpretation as well as its superiority over MRI in the detection of cervical lymph node metastases.

If ordered, cross-sectional thyroid imaging should evaluate not just the neck but a wide craniocaudal dimension from the skull base to the tracheal bifurcation in order to accurately assess the extent of intrathoracic goiter or malignancy. Both CT and MRI can be performed with or without IV contrast, depending on the clinical scenario. For evaluation of substernal goiter, a noncontrast CT or MRI is sufficient. On the other hand, IV contrast is indicated for clinical suspicion of advanced thyroid cancer such as locally advanced tumors or those with multiple and/or bulky lymph node metastases in the preoperative setting. Contrast-enhanced images are best for assessing local invasion into neighboring structures, particularly the aerodigestive tract.

On noncontrast CT scan, the thyroid appears homogeneous and mildly hyperattenuating compared with the surrounding muscles, whereas iodinated contrast administration leads to fairly bright diffuse enhancement. On MRI, the thyroid can be mildly hyperintense on both T1- and T2-weighted images, with bright enhancement on gadolinium contrast administration. Incidental thyroid nodules can be found in up to 9% of neck CT or MRI scans. Iodine is generally cleared within 4 to 8 weeks after iodinated contrast administration, which generally does not cause a clinically significant delay in postoperative RAI administration for DTC.

Positron Emission Tomography

Positron emission tomography (PET, typically coupled with CT or MRI) is most frequently performed with the administration of [18F]-fluorodeoxyglucose (FDG) radiotracer, which is taken up in tissues with elevated metabolism of glucose. The normal thyroid takes up [18F]-FDG to a similar level as surrounding skeletal muscle. The role of [18F]-FDG PET is limited to selected cases of higher-risk thyroid cancers, such as for surveillance and staging for RAI-refractory DTC.

PET is not recommended for the routine evaluation of thyroid disease. However, with greater use of these scans, along with other cross-sectional modalities for cancer surveillance purposes, incidental thyroid nodular disease is being detected by PET scans with increasing frequency. Up to 3% of PET scans identify incidental thyroid nodules. PET-positive nodules are generally associated with an elevated risk of malignancy, particularly compared with thyroid nodules found incidentally on other imaging studies (20% on average),[5] but this fact does not supersede the need for standard evaluation with neck ultrasound and FNA biopsy before consideration of surgical management.

HYPOTHYROIDISM

Hypothyroidism is a disorder characterized by inadequate thyroid hormone production and/or availability in peripheral target tissues. Hypothyroidism is a common disorder in the world, although the specific causes differ depending on geography. The most common cause overall is iodine deficiency, which is primarily encountered in the developing world because of lack of sufficient dietary iodine; the same pathophysiology leads to an elevated risk of developing endemic goiter. In the developed world, the most

common causes include autoimmune thyroiditis and iatrogenic hypothyroidism as a result of thyroidectomy or RAI treatment with insufficient thyroid hormone supplementation or replacement.

With respect to the hypothalamic-pituitary-thyroid axis, the overwhelming majority of causes of hypothyroidism are primary—that is, the lack of thyroid hormone production is the result of causes at the level of the thyroid. A small percentage of cases may be the result of inadequate secretion of TSH from the pituitary or thyrotropin-releasing hormone from the hypothalamus, which are referred to as *secondary* or *tertiary hypothyroidism*, respectively.

The symptoms and signs of hypothyroidism can range from mild to no symptoms to the classic presentation of cold intolerance, fatigue, puffiness and weight gain, dry skin, and hair loss. Myxedema represents an extreme of symptomatic hypothyroidism in which patients develop a constellation of severe findings, such as altered mental status or coma, hypothermia, bradycardia, and electrolyte abnormalities, with an increased risk of cardiomegaly, pericardial effusion and ascites, and shock. Myxedema typically occurs as a decompensation of chronic hypothyroidism because of an acute physiologic stressor, such as trauma, infection, or an acute cardiovascular event.

Thyroid function tests, and particularly TSH, are highly sensitive for screening for hypothyroidism. In adults, primary hypothyroidism is generally suspected when serum TSH levels are above 4.12 mIU/L, although normal ranges differ depending on age as well as pregnancy.[6] Further testing typically includes measurement of thyroid hormones, including free T_4 and T_3 levels. Elevated TSH levels with decreased free T_4 and T_3 levels are diagnostic of primary hypothyroidism. Elevated TSH levels with relatively normal levels of thyroid hormones are considered to be subclinical or mild hypothyroidism.

Hypothyroidism is fortunately easily treatable with pharmacologic agents such as levothyroxine (LT_4) or liothyronine (LT_3), which are synthetic versions of T_4 and T_3, respectively. LT_4 is recommended as the first-line therapy in most patients for the treatment of hypothyroidism and is available in oral, intramuscular, and IV forms. The rationale for LT_4 lies in the body's ability to convert the exogenously administered T_4 into T_3 by deiodinases in the peripheral tissues. Other therapeutic strategies include a combination of LT_4 and LT_3, LT_3 alone, and desiccated thyroid extracts; all strategies were developed under the hypothesis that LT_4 administration alone may be insufficient to replicate the normal euthyroid state, whether the result of inadequate in vivo conversion to T_3 or the absence of some other heretofore undescribed molecule(s). None of these options is recommended currently as routine first-line therapy. Regarding combination LT_4 and LT_3 therapy, multiple randomized controlled trials have failed to demonstrate superiority over LT_4 monotherapy in various outcomes, including achievement of target TSH and thyroid-specific symptoms and thyroid-specific health outcomes. Further research is needed to study the possible benefit of combination therapy in selected patients with low serum T_3 levels or persistent symptoms on monotherapy. Both LT_3 monotherapy and thyroid extract regimens have some preliminary supporting evidence on short-term outcomes and preference, but high-quality, long-term data on safety and equivalent efficacy are lacking.

Autoimmune Thyroiditis

Autoimmune thyroiditis is the most frequent cause of hypothyroidism in iodine-replete populations. The most common type is chronic lymphocytic thyroiditis, otherwise known as *Hashimoto thyroiditis.* This disorder is found predominantly in females at up to a 10:1 female-to-male incidence ratio. In addition, there is a strong hereditary component, with first-degree relatives of patients with Hashimoto thyroiditis having a ninefold risk of also developing the disease. The etiology of Hashimoto thyroiditis is the presence of circulating autoantibodies to thyroid antigens, resulting in a chronic autoimmune destructive process involving the formation of immune complexes and complement in the basement membrane of follicular cells. This leads to the infiltration of lymphocytes into the thyroid follicles and eventually results in fibrosis, which decreases the effective number of follicles able to produce thyroid hormones.

The biochemical workup for Hashimoto thyroiditis includes measurement of thyroid function tests as well as circulating thyroid autoantibodies, including TPOAb and TgAb (see earlier), which are present in 95% and 60% of patients, respectively. Euthyroid and subclinically hypothyroid patients with elevated autoantibody titers are at greater risk of progressing to overt hypothyroidism. In addition, thyroid autoantibody measurement is recommended in patients at higher risk of developing hypothyroidism, including those with other autoimmune diseases or taking drugs such as lithium or amiodarone.[6]

There is typically no role for imaging studies in the workup and diagnosis of Hashimoto thyroiditis. However, patients with Hashimoto thyroiditis will frequently have symptoms of neck discomfort, pain, and globus sensation, necessitating neck ultrasound for diagnostic workup. Sonographic characteristics of Hashimoto thyroiditis include coarse, heterogeneous, and hypoechoic parenchymal echotexture with increased vascularity, often with the presence of fine echogenic septae producing a pseudonodular appearance that can sometimes be confused with discrete thyroid nodules (Fig. 73.11). The size of the thyroid may range from diffusely or focally enlarged to small and atrophic, and there may be mildly enlarged and more numerous perithyroidal lymph nodes from the autoimmune inflammatory process. Hashimoto thyroiditis has been associated with an increased risk of papillary thyroid cancer (PTC), but possibly with a slight

improvement in prognosis based on several single-institution surgical series. As a result, any suspicious thyroid nodules or lymph nodes in the setting of Hashimoto thyroiditis should be worked up with FNA biopsy.

Cytologic features of Hashimoto thyroiditis include a moderately cellular specimen with aggregates of follicular cells with oncocytic changes, minimal colloid, and infiltration of mature lymphocytes. Giant cells, plasma cells, macrophages, histiocytes, and eosinophils also may be seen. Primary thyroid lymphoma, a rare thyroid malignancy with an annual incidence of 2 per 1 million, is associated with Hashimoto thyroiditis and can often be difficult to distinguish based on cytology because of similarities around having large numbers of lymphoid cells and lymphoid follicles with decreased colloid.

The second most common type of autoimmune thyroiditis is postpartum thyroiditis, which can occur in up to 10% of females within the first 2 to 12 months of the postpartum period. The pathogenesis of postpartum thyroiditis appears to have similarities and parallels to that of Hashimoto thyroiditis in that (1) hypothyroidism may be preceded by a short thyrotoxic state, (2) it is often associated with the presence of circulating TPOAb, and (3) postpartum thyroiditis is associated with a tenfold risk of ultimately developing Hashimoto thyroiditis. Postpartum thyroiditis is typically short-lived, with resolution in 2 to 4 months. A short course of exogenous thyroid hormone supplementation/replacement may be necessary.

Subacute Thyroiditis

Subacute thyroiditis, also known as *de Quervain disease* or *subacute granulomatous thyroiditis,* is a relatively uncommon disease found primarily in the developed world. It has a female preponderance, with a 2:1 female-to-male ratio, and typically occurs in the fourth decade of life. The pathogenesis remains poorly understood, but the disease often occurs after a viral prodrome, such as an upper respiratory infection. The hallmark of the clinical presentation for de Quervain thyroiditis is pain and swelling in the thyroid region, along with low-grade fevers, dysphagia, and severe fatigue. Biochemical findings may include an elevated erythrocyte sedimentation rate, which is diagnostic. As with autoimmune thyroiditis, de Quervain thyroiditis can be associated with transient hyperthyroidism followed by hypothyroidism. Cytopathologic characteristics from FNA biopsy include the presence of multinucleated giant cell granulomas. Histopathology shows evidence of granulomatous changes in the thyroid follicles. The follicles are enlarged, with infiltration by mononuclear cells, neutrophils, and lymphocytes.

The time course of de Quervain thyroiditis is typically 2 to 5 months, and most patients return to a euthyroid state spontaneously. Because of its self-limited course, no specific treatments are indicated except for symptomatic relief of pain and/or temporary treatment of clinical hypothyroidism. The pain associated with de Quervain thyroiditis can be treated with nonsteroidal antiinflammatory drugs; more severe cases can be treated with a course of corticosteroids. Surgery is not typically indicated for treatment of de Quervain thyroiditis, and reassurance and emotional counseling are often necessary, particularly during the painful phase of the disease.

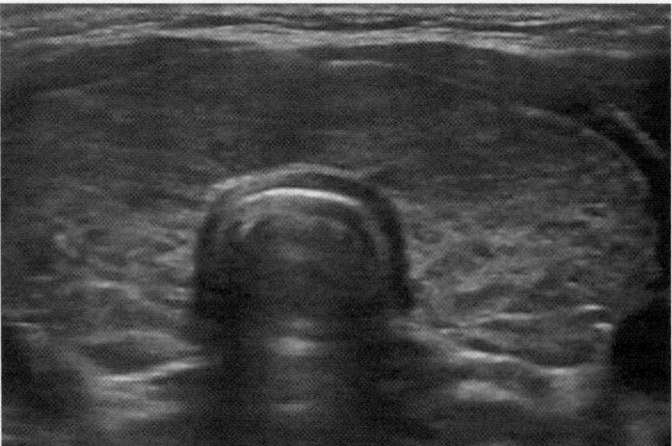

FIGURE 73.11 Sonographic features of Hashimoto thyroiditis. In this image, the thyroid gland is enlarged, predominantly hyperechoic, and diffusely heterogeneous, with irregular echotexture and poorly defined hyperechoic regions separated by fibrous strands. (From Andrioli M, Valcavi R. Sonography of normal and abnormal thyroid and parathyroid glands. *Front Horm Res.* 2016;45:1-15.)

Riedel Thyroiditis

Riedel thyroiditis, also known as *Riedel struma* or *chronic fibrous thyroiditis,* is an extremely rare and poorly understood inflammatory process causing diffuse destruction and fibrosis of the thyroid. The primary theories for the etiology of this disease are that it is either an autoimmune process or a specific fibrotic disorder related to multifocal fibrosclerosis. The most relevant finding in Riedel thyroiditis is the presence of an extremely firm and constricting gland that can be very uncomfortable for patients. The fibrotic process often extends into surrounding structures, including the aerodigestive tract and RLN, which may cause clinically significant airway obstruction, dysphagia, and dysphonia.

Patients with Riedel thyroiditis have the biochemical markers of hypothyroidism. Imaging is necessary to rule out other causes of the dramatic local symptoms. Ultrasound characteristics often demonstrate a diffusely hypoechoic gland with ill-defined borders. FNA cytology reveals dense fibrotic changes but cannot be reliably distinguished from fibrotic changes often associated with anaplastic thyroid cancer (ATC).

Medical treatment for the inflammatory component of Riedel thyroiditis traditionally consists of corticosteroids and tamoxifen. Other agents such as mycophenolate and rituximab also have been used. Thyroid hormone supplementation/replacement is used to treat the associated hypothyroidism. Surgical resection is often indicated to rule out malignancy such as ATC or primary thyroid lymphoma or to treat aerodigestive tract obstruction. Surgery is usually extremely challenging because of the firmness of the gland and obliteration of normal planes and landmarks. Partial resection of only the affected components is recommended, with simple wedge resection of the isthmus being the most common surgical therapy for relief of tracheal compression. There is no evidence to suggest that Riedel thyroiditis is associated with an increased risk of thyroid malignancy.

Acute Suppurative Thyroiditis

Acute suppurative thyroiditis is rare and defined as an acute pyogenic infection of the thyroid gland. The most common underlying cause is infection of a congenital pyriform sinus fistula that tracks and communicates with the thyroid. The clinical presentation of acute thyroiditis is that of a bacterial infection: fever, severe unilateral pain and swelling at the thyroid gland (typically left-sided), and cervical lymphadenopathy. The most common organisms include the *Staphylococcus* and *Streptococcus* species, but other aerobic or anaerobic species also may be involved. The thyroiditis also can lead to thyroid abscess formation; rarely, it can lead to even more serious sequelae, including retropharyngeal abscess, tracheal obstruction, mediastinitis, and jugular venous thrombosis.

Thyroid function tests are rarely useful in the diagnosis of acute suppurative thyroiditis; rather, other biochemical findings of acute systemic illness and sepsis are more useful, such as a complete blood count marked by a leukocytosis with a left shift. Ultrasound with FNA biopsy can be useful for bacterial culture and speciation of any abscess fluid. Treatment consists of targeted antibiotics as well as percutaneous drainage of any identified abscess. Acute thyroiditis does not generally lead to long-term hypothyroidism requiring thyroid hormone supplementation.

Iatrogenic Hypothyroidism

Aside from postthyroidectomy hypothyroidism caused by the absence of sufficient thyroid parenchyma, pharmacotherapy is the primary cause of iatrogenic hypothyroidism. The number and variety of medications and therapies that are associated with hypothyroidism are extensive (Box 73.1). The most common medications associated with hypothyroidism include RAI (^{131}I),

---

BOX 73.1 Medications That May Cause Iatrogenic Hypothyroidism

Inhibition of Thyroid Hormone Synthesis or Secretion
Aminoglutethimide
Lithium
Perchlorate
Thalidomide
Thionamides (methimazole, propylthiouracil)
Iodine-containing medications
  Amiodarone
  Iodinated IV contrast
  Guaifenesin
  Kelp
  Potassium iodide
  Topical antiseptics

Immune Dysregulation
Interferon alfa
Interleukin-2
Alemtuzumab
Ipilimumab
Nivolumab
Pembrolizumab

TSH Suppression
Dopamine

Destructive Thyroiditis
Sunitinib

Increased Type 3 Deiodinase Activity
Sorafenib

Increased T₄ Clearance and TSH Suppression
Bexarotene

T₄, Tetraiodothyronine or thyroxine; *TSH*, thyroid-stimulating hormone.

---

antithyroid thionamides (such as methimazole and propylthiouracil [PTU]), amiodarone, lithium, immune modulators, and kinase inhibitors.

The etiology of drug-induced hypothyroidism depends on the specific agent. In the case of RAI therapy, the often-expected hypothyroidism is caused by direct destruction of the thyroid follicular cells by the delivered radioactive agent. Thionamides such as methimazole and PTU directly inhibit T$_4$ and T$_3$ synthesis (as well as block peripheral conversion of T$_4$ to T$_3$ in the case of PTU). The antiarrhythmic agent amiodarone can lead to both hypothyroidism and hyperthyroidism caused by a number of mechanisms, including inability to escape from the Wolff-Chaikoff effect from the drug's high iodine content, inhibition of deiodinase activity, inhibition of thyroid hormone entry into the periphery, and direct cytotoxic thyroiditis (see later). Lithium may act by directly inhibiting the cyclic adenosine monophosphate (cAMP)–dependent pathway, leading to thyroid hormone formation in the thyroid follicle. Tyrosine kinase inhibitors (TKIs) such as sunitinib and vandetanib cause hypothyroidism in different ways, including direct destructive autoimmune thyroiditis, reduction in vascular endothelial growth factor (VEGF)–related thyroid vasculature, and reduction of thyroid iodine uptake.

Treatment of drug-related hypothyroidism usually consists of removal of the offending agent if possible as well as thyroid hormone supplementation/replacement as necessary.

HYPERTHYROIDISM

Hyperthyroidism is defined as a clinical state of elevated thyroid hormone action in tissues, usually because of inappropriately high constitutive secretion of thyroid hormone from the thyroid. The degree of severity of hyperthyroidism is typically divided into two groups: overt (suppressed TSH levels with concomitant elevations in free T_4 or T_3) and subclinical (suppressed TSH with normal free T_4 and T_3). Both overt and subclinical hyperthyroidism can lead to clinically significant symptoms or signs, although subclinical disease is more likely to be milder in presentation.

The clinical symptoms and signs of hyperthyroidism are broad, reflecting the fact that thyroid hormone exerts an effect on nearly every organ system. Overt hyperthyroidism can cause a litany of effects, including tremor, heat intolerance, tachycardia and atrial fibrillation, increased gastrointestinal motility, muscle weakness, anxiety, and embolic events. Uncontrolled hyperthyroidism can rarely cause severe cardiovascular complications, including cardiomyopathy and congestive heart failure that can even progress to cardiovascular collapse and death. Subclinical hyperthyroidism typically has milder manifestations along this same disease symptomatology.

The prevalence of hyperthyroidism worldwide is approximately 2.5%.[7] The most common causes of hyperthyroidism—Graves disease, TMG, and solitary toxic adenoma—are all those in which thyroidectomy plays an important, if not primary, role in management. These three disease states are discussed in further detail next. Other causes of hyperthyroidism are listed in Box 73.2, and amiodarone-induced thyrotoxicosis (AIT) is also discussed.

Graves Disease

Graves disease, named after Dr. Robert J. Graves who first described the condition in the 1830s, is an autoimmune disease characterized by the constitutive activation of the TSH receptor by TRAb, which results in increased synthesis and secretion of thyroid hormone. Graves disease is the most common cause of hyperthyroidism in the United States, with an estimated incidence of 30 cases per 100,000 persons per year. The disease has a female predominance, with an 8:1 female-to-male ratio, and typically presents during younger adult life, with a typical patient age range of between 20 and 40 years.

Because of its autoimmune etiology, Graves disease can have other manifestations in addition to the classic symptoms and signs of hyperthyroidism. The most common is Graves orbitopathy, which occurs in up to 25% to 30% of patients. In this process, autoimmune reactions at the orbital and periorbital soft tissues lead to proptosis, eyelid retraction, chemosis, periorbital edema, and diminished ocular muscle motility (Fig. 73.12); if left untreated, the orbitopathy can lead to vision loss from corneal lesions or optic nerve compression. Skin manifestations also can occur, including pretibial myxedema and acropachy (edema at the digits). Other autoimmune conditions that have been associated with Graves disease include Hashimoto thyroiditis, lupus, rheumatoid arthritis, pernicious anemia, and Addison disease, among others.

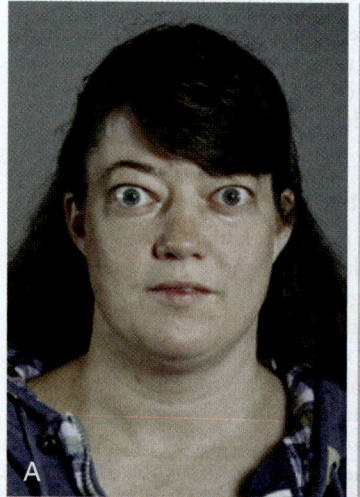
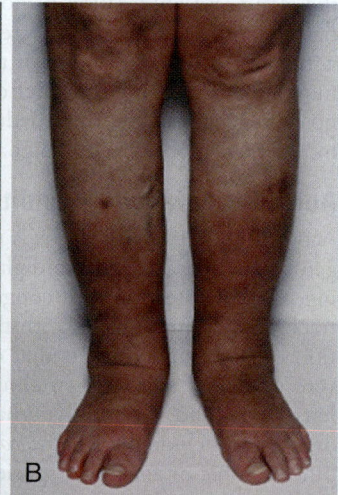
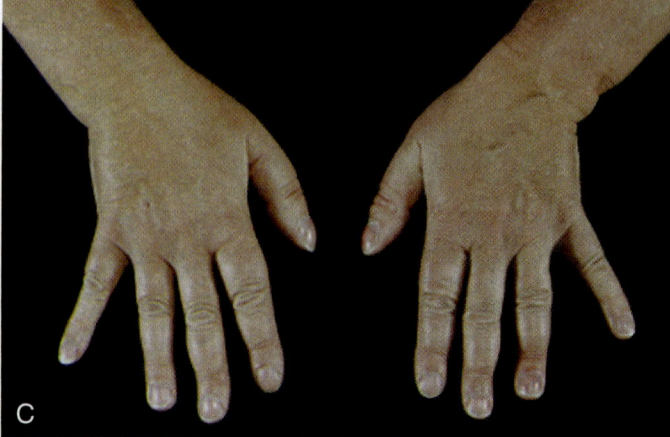

FIGURE 73.12 Extrathyroidal manifestations of Graves disease. (A) Orbitopathy. (B) Dermopathy (pretibial myxedema). (C) Acropachy. (From Al-Shoumer KAS, Gharib H. Hyperthyroidism: toxic nodular goiter and Graves' disease. In: Randolph GW, ed. *Surgery of the Thyroid and Parathyroid Glands 2.* Philadelphia: Elsevier Saunders; 2013:53.)

BOX 73.2   Causes of Hyperthyroidism

Associated With Normal/Elevated RAI Uptake

Graves disease
Toxic multinodular goiter
Toxic adenoma
Trophoblastic disease
TSH-producing pituitary adenoma
Thyroid hormone resistance

Associated With No/Minimal RAI Uptake

Painless thyroiditis
Amiodarone-induced thyroiditis
Subacute thyroiditis
Iatrogenic thyrotoxicosis
Struma ovarii
Acute thyroiditis
    Follicular thyroid cancer metastases
Palpation thyroiditis

RAI, Radioactive iodine; *TSH,* thyroid-stimulating hormone.

The biochemical workup for Graves disease typically includes thyroid function tests, including TSH, free T_4, and T_3 as well as measurement for TRAb (typically with TSI but also with TSH receptor-binding inhibitory immunoglobulin in selected scenarios). The presence of TRAb is diagnostic for Graves disease. Imaging may consist of neck ultrasound and/or nuclear medicine thyroid uptake scan, depending on the indications. Sonographic features may include a diffusely hypervascular gland, often with heterogeneous echogenicity; thyroid nodular disease may also be identified. Nuclear scintigraphy using either ^{99m}technetium pertechnetate or ^{123}I may help differentiate TSI-negative Graves disease from toxic nodular disease based on diffuse versus nodular uptake pattern. Cross-sectional imaging of the head may be useful for the evaluation of orbitopathy.

The three management options for Graves hyperthyroidism include antithyroid medications, RAI ablation, and thyroidectomy. In the United States, RAI is the most employed treatment option, although antithyroid medication is being used more frequently as a first option; nearly one-third of patients may be able to achieve long-term remission with medication alone. In truth, each of the three treatment options comes with its own unique set of advantages and disadvantages as well as indications and contraindications, which must be tailored according to individual patient values and preferences. The 2016 ATA guidelines on the management of hyperthyroidism provide a helpful evidence-based summary of the clinical scenarios that would most favor a particular option for treatment (Table 73.1).[8]

In general, thyroidectomy is the preferred modality in the following situations: presence of severe eye disease, failure or contraindications to other treatment options, need or desire for rapid reversal of hyperthyroidism, presence of concomitant suspicious thyroid nodules, large goiters with locally compressive symptoms, and pregnancy or postpartum/breastfeeding states. Although thyroidectomy is a first-line treatment option, in practice, it is often relegated to a secondary role because of perceived risks associated with general anesthesia and surgery. Although RAI ablation is often billed as extremely low-risk or no-risk, emerging evidence suggests a higher rate of secondary malignancy than previously reported.[9]

For patients choosing surgical management, the recommended extent of surgery is a total or near-total thyroidectomy, which is associated with a nearly 0% risk of recurrent hyperthyroidism. In contrast, subtotal thyroidectomy is associated with a 5% to 10% risk of recurrence from the presence of residual thyroid tissue. Although the risk of thyroidectomy-specific complications (including permanent hypoparathyroidism, RLN injury, and neck hematoma) is higher in Graves disease than for other indications, the absolute risks remain low, particularly in the hands of higher-volume surgeons, and there are no differences between total/near-total and subtotal thyroidectomy groups. The rate of permanent RLN injury is 0% to 2%, permanent hypoparathyroidism is 0.6% to 6%, and neck hematoma is 0.3% to 0.7% for total thyroidectomy performed in the setting of Graves disease.[10] The risk of complications from remedial thyroidectomy is up to tenfold higher than initial thyroidectomy, which further underscores why subtotal thyroidectomy (with its risk of recurrent disease) is no longer favored.

Patients ideally should be rendered euthyroid before thyroidectomy with antithyroid medications, but recent studies suggest that the risk of thyroid storm during thyroidectomy in actively thyrotoxic patients is minimal.[11] The most commonly used antithyroid drug is methimazole because PTU was found to be more often associated with liver failure resulting in the need for transplantation.[12] β-Blockers may be added for patients who remain hyperthyroid and/or tachycardic. High-concentration potassium iodide solutions, including Lugol solution or super saturated potassium iodide (SSKI), can be given for 7 to 10 days before surgery; they are thought to be beneficial for decreasing thyroid blood flow and vascularity of the gland and help to rapidly achieve a euthyroid state via the Wolff-Chaikoff effect. Their use

TABLE 73.1 Clinical Situations That Favor a Particular Modality as Treatment for Graves Hyperthyroidism

CLINICAL SITUATIONS	RADIOACTIVE IODINE	ANTITHYROID DRUG	SURGERY
Pregnancy	×	√√/!	√/!
Comorbidities with increased surgical risk and/or limited life expectancy	√√	√	×
Inactive Graves ophthalmopathy	√	√	√
Active Graves ophthalmopathy	!	√√	√√
Liver disease	√√	!	√
Major adverse reactions to antithyroid drugs	√√	×	√
Patients with previously operated or externally irradiated necks	√√	√	!
Lack of access to a high-volume thyroid surgeon	√√	√	!
Patients with high likelihood of remission (especially females and those with mild disease, small goiters, and negative or low-titer TRAb)	√	√√	√
Patients with periodic paralysis	√√	√	√√
Patients with right pulmonary hypertension or congestive heart failure	√√	√	!
Elderly with comorbidities	√	√	!
Thyroid malignancy confirmed or suspected	×	-	√√
One or more large thyroid nodules	-	√	√√
Coexisting primary hyperparathyroidism requiring surgery	-	-	√√

√√ = Preferred therapy; √ = acceptable therapy; ! = cautious use; - = not first-line therapy but may be acceptable depending on the clinical circumstances; × = contraindication.
From Ross DS, Burch HB, Cooper DS, et al. 2016 American Thyroid Association guidelines for diagnosis and management of hyperthyroidism and other causes of thyrotoxicosis. *Thyroid.* 2016;26:1343-1421.

may not be helpful or needed in selected situations. All other associated medical and surgical comorbidities should be optimized, including repurposing of cholestyramine or lithium to decrease circulating free thyroid hormone levels.[13] Preoperative optimization of calcium and vitamin D status, including preoperative supplementation with calcitriol, has been shown to decrease the postoperative risk of transient hypocalcemia.

Thyroid storm is a rare state of life-threatening physiologic decompensation in patients with severe, uncontrolled hyperthyroidism, which often occurs after an inciting stressor event. The symptoms can be dramatic and severe, including fever; cardiac effects including hypertension, tachycardia, arrhythmia, and congestive heart failure; mental status changes including agitation, stupor, and coma; and hepatic failure. Treatment is multimodal and consists of β-blockade, antithyroid medications, potassium iodide, corticosteroids, mechanical cooling therapies, and intensive supportive care. Plasmapheresis also has been reported to rapidly decrease circulating thyroid hormone levels and should be considered as another option in the armamentarium in severe cases, although its use is limited by cost and availability.[14]

Toxic Multinodular Goiter

TMG is an enlarged nodular thyroid containing one or more autonomously functioning nodules leading to a state of hyperthyroidism. This condition is also known as *Plummer disease,* so named after Henry Plummer of the Mayo Clinic in 1913. TMG is the second most common cause of hyperthyroidism in the United States after Graves disease. Among the elderly and those who live in iodine-deficient regions, TMG is the most common cause of hyperthyroidism. TMG has a female predominance, with an approximately 5:1 female-to-male ratio, and typically affects adults above the age of 50 years.

Autonomously functioning nodules in TMG often result from mutations in the TSH receptor gene leading to constitutive synthesis and secretion of thyroid hormones. These "warm" or "hot" nodules are rarely malignant and typically do not require biopsy. However, they can coexist with other nonfunctioning nodules in the same gland, which should be evaluated independently (see "Thyroid Nodule" section later).

The workup of TMG consists of both biochemical and radiographic testing. As with Graves disease, thyroid function tests are mandatory in order to diagnose hyperthyroidism. In addition, a survey of thyroid antibodies (including TRAb) is necessary to identify coexisting autoimmune thyroiditis and rule out Graves disease. Nuclear scintigraphy is a first-line imaging study and, in the case of TMG, can identify the location and distribution of autonomously functioning nodules and/or regions. In addition, ultrasound is highly recommended as a correlative study to assess overall thyroid size and characterize any nonfunctioning nodules that may require biopsy.

The three management options for TMG—antithyroid medication, RAI, and thyroidectomy—are the same as those for Graves disease, but with some differences. First, antithyroid medication is generally not advocated as a long-term management strategy except for patients in whom the other two options are absolutely contraindicated, such as in some elderly or otherwise ill or frail patients with limited life expectancy. Because this disease state is not autoimmune in nature, autonomous nodules do not undergo remission with medical therapy. Second, RAI with ^{131}I is the most common definitive treatment for TMG in the United States; however, the dose of radiation is typically higher (and, by extension, the risk of treatment failure and need

for retreatment) than in Graves disease because of lower uptake of iodine in TMG. Third, both RAI and surgery should be preceded by optimal preoperative treatment of the hyperthyroid state, which typically includes methimazole with or without β-blockade. SSKI and Lugol solutions are not indicated for TMG as they are for Graves disease because the high iodine concentration may not achieve a temporary euthyroid state from the Wolff-Chaikoff effect. They induce hyperthyroidism from the Jod-Basedow phenomenon.

Near-total or total thyroidectomy is the generally recommended surgical treatment of TMG. As in the case of Graves disease, complete extirpation can be performed with a similarly low rate of complications as subtotal thyroidectomy while at the same time virtually eliminating the risk of disease recurrence.

Solitary Toxic Adenoma

A toxic adenoma is a single autonomously functioning nodule existing within an otherwise normal or nontoxic nodular thyroid gland. The main theory around its pathogenesis focuses on constitutively activating mutations in the TSH receptor gene, although the prevalence of these mutations is not universal and varies widely by geography. Toxic adenoma affects females at a median age of 50 to 60 years, with a mild female predominance. Toxic adenoma shares many, if not most, of the diagnostic approach and workup with TMG; in fact, the ATA guidelines on the management of hyperthyroidism combine the two groups together in their treatment recommendations.

The treatment philosophy for toxic adenoma generally follows the same principles as those for TMG—namely, that antithyroid medications are not effective for long-term remission, and either RAI or thyroidectomy is the preferred method for definitive treatment. Thyroidectomy is typically limited to unilateral lobectomy addressing the side of the toxic adenoma; this strategy is associated with a near-universal cure for the hyperthyroidism. Near-total or total thyroidectomy is indicated only in the presence of other factors, such as bilateral nodules with suspicion for cancer or a large and/or symptomatic goiter. Thermal ablation techniques, discussed in further detail later in this chapter, have shown variable resolution of hyperthyroidism for toxic adenomas compared with surgery or RAI. Therefore, RFA is not recommended as first-line treatment for large toxic adenomas, but it can be considered in young patients with small toxic adenomas. Small nodules (<12 mL in volume) with volume reduction exceeding 80% are more likely to experience resolution of hyperthyroidism.[15]

Amiodarone-Induced Thyrotoxicosis

Amiodarone is an antiarrhythmic medication used frequently for atrial or ventricular tachyarrhythmias. Molecularly, amiodarone is an iodine-rich compound with structural similarities to T_4 that contains 37% iodine content by molecular weight; a normal dosing schedule can deliver over 100 times the daily dietary iodine requirement. AIT occurs in up to 6% of patients taking this medication.

Two distinct mechanisms are proposed in the development of AIT. Type 1 AIT is caused by the Jod-Basedow phenomenon, in which the high iodine load potentiates excess thyroid hormone synthesis and release. Type 1 AIT is more common in patients with preexisting hyperthyroid disease. Type 2 AIT usually occurs in patients with no preexisting thyroid disease and is caused by a destructive thyroiditis from direct drug toxicity on follicular cells, leading to release of preformed thyroid hormone. Mixed forms of AIT also can occur.

Medical treatment of AIT typically consists of methimazole, with corticosteroids added to address the thyroiditis in type 2 AIT. The decision to halt amiodarone treatment must be determined carefully on an individual basis in consultation with the treating cardiologist in order to ensure continuity of adequate antiarrhythmic therapy in these often high-risk patients. Total thyroidectomy is recommended for patients who are unresponsive to aggressive medical therapy. Although thyroidectomy is associated with more risks for AIT compared with most other indications (with perioperative mortality of 9%–10%), delay in surgery carries an even higher risk of mortality.[16]

NONTOXIC GOITER

A nontoxic goiter is defined as any benign, noninflammatory enlargement of the thyroid gland that is not associated with hyperthyroidism. The causes of nontoxic goiter can be broadly divided into diffuse and nodular enlargement, which roughly lead to the respective entities of endemic/diffuse and sporadic multinodular goiter, each with their own pathogenesis, risk factors, and management strategies.

Endemic (Diffuse) Goiter

Strictly defined, endemic goiter occurs in more than 10% of a given population; however, the only known cause of endemic goiter is dietary iodine deficiency, which predisposes people predominantly to diffuse goiter from persistent TSH stimulation, leading to diffuse follicular epithelial hyperplasia. In effect, the terms *endemic goiter* and *diffuse goiter* have functionally become synonymous.

It is estimated that more than 2 billion people worldwide are exposed to iodine-deficient diets.[17] In iodine-deficient populations, a palpable goiter can be detected in up to 40% to 90% of individuals, and hypothyroidism can be found in up to 50%. The risk of goiter and hypothyroidism increases proportionally with the severity of iodine deficiency. There is a female predominance in the prevalence of endemic goiter (approximately two to three times higher than in males), and its incidence increases by age group because of its environmental etiology.

The morbidity and mortality from endemic goiter are a result of its association with chronic untreated hypothyroidism and cretinism as much as—if not more than—the local effects on the neck because of its size. Instituting proper iodine supplementation in iodine-deficient populations has been shown to be an effective strategy for decreasing the incidence of these diseases.

Nontoxic Multinodular Goiter

Sporadic multinodular goiter is the most common cause of nontoxic goiter in the United States and other developed nations with iodine-rich diets, with an incidence of approximately 5%. Although there is a known stepwise pathophysiologic process in which iodine deficiency can first cause diffuse follicular hyperplasia and subsequently stimulate nodule formation, the causes of the majority of sporadic multinodular goiter remain unknown. The incidence of multinodular goiter increases with age, probably paralleling the age-related incidence of thyroid nodules in general.

Substernal Goiter

Substernal (or retrosternal) goiter is defined broadly as a goiter with a significant proportion of the gland extending inferiorly through the thoracic inlet and into the mediastinum. The incidence of substernal goiter is estimated at 0.02% in the general population, with 60% occurring among patients who are over the age of 60 years.[18] There are a number of subtypes of substernal goiter. The most common subtype extends into the anterior mediastinum. The second subtype extends posteriorly to the great vessels, trachea, and/or RLN, sometimes crossing over to the contralateral neck. The third and least common subtype is the isolated mediastinal goiter with no connection to the normal cervical orthotopic gland and with unique blood supply from the chest.

Substernal goiters are more likely than cervical goiters to be associated with local compressive symptoms, including shortness of breath/orthopnea and dysphagia. This is because the mediastinal extension of the goiter pushes against and compresses the normal thoracic inlet structures (trachea, esophagus, vascular structures) within a fixed bony space bound by the ribs and vertebrae. Tracheal compression is of particular concern because minor degrees of goiter enlargement and resultant narrowing of tracheal diameter can lead to dramatic reductions in ventilatory flow (Poiseuille's law) in a relatively short period. In contrast, primarily cervical goiters are often capable of dramatic growth without causing significant compressive symptoms because of the expandability of the surrounding cervical soft tissues. Vocal cord paralysis from RLN compression is extremely rare, and the presence of vocal cord dysfunction should raise the concern for malignancy harbored within the goiter.

Workup

The workup of nontoxic goiter consists of thyroid function testing to rule out hyperthyroidism and imaging studies to assess for goiter extent and presence of nodules. The mainstay for thyroid imaging is neck ultrasound, which offers the highest resolution description of thyroid size/volume, presence or absence of significant thyroiditis, and characterization of thyroid nodules. As stated in the ATA guidelines, every nodule at least >1 cm should be evaluated for suspicious sonographic features on an individual basis, and FNA should be performed preferentially based on suspicion for malignancy according to a number of criteria outlined by the ATA and the American College of Radiology (ACR).[19]

Cross-sectional imaging with either CT or MRI is essential for the assessment of—and preoperative planning for—substernal goiter and is indicated for any patient with significant compressive symptoms and/or sonographic evidence of inferior extension past the clavicle (see Fig. 73.10A and Fig. 73.13). Cross-sectional imaging is useful because it provides information about the degree of tracheoesophageal deviation/compression, laterality of dominant substernal lobe, inferior-most extent, anterior versus posterior pattern of extension, presence of cross-over to the contralateral chest, and presence of a separate intrathoracic "rest." Unless there is concern for malignancy, the need for contrast enhancement is typically unnecessary.

Management

The management options for nontoxic goiter generally consist of nonoperative surveillance, TSH suppression with thyroid hormone supplementation, RAI ablation, and thyroidectomy. Small nontoxic goiters generally can be followed expectantly with periodic thyroid function testing and neck imaging. TSH-suppressive therapy with LT$_4$ is often employed by endocrinologists as a first-line treatment option, particularly for smaller goiters. The results of several large-scale trials are somewhat mixed but do appear to show goiter size reductions in about 30% of patients; however, these results must be balanced against the drawbacks of therapy,

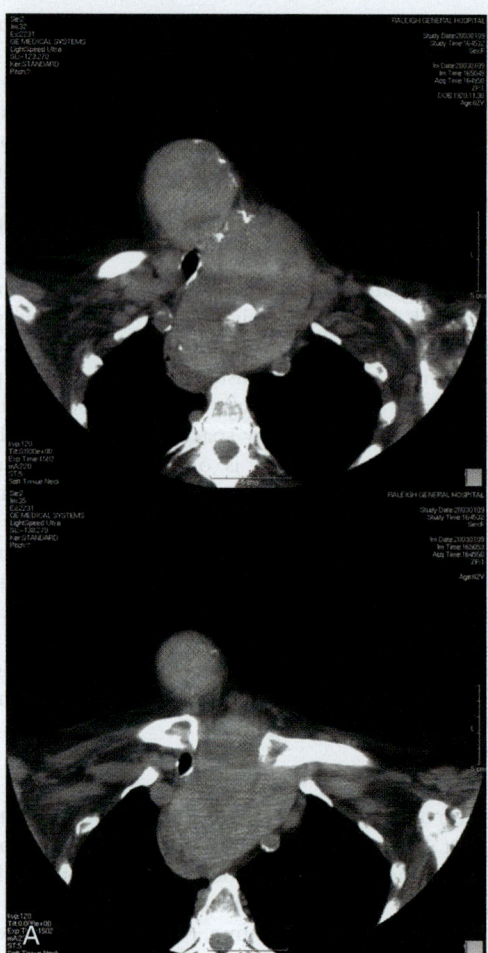

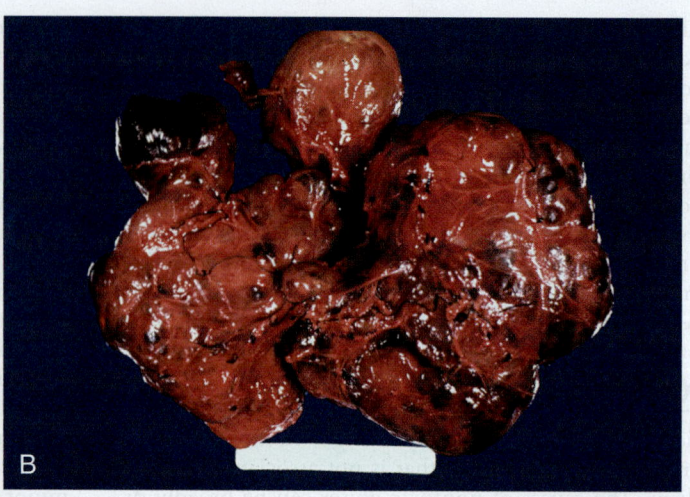

FIGURE 73.13 (A) Computed tomography scan at the level of the thoracic inlet demonstrating a heterogeneous, large thyroid mass that involves both lobes of the thyroid and displaces the trachea. It has extended into the anterior mediastinum. This patient ultimately proved to have a large multinodular goiter. (B) Gross picture of the resected multinodular goiter.

including the need for lifelong suppression and the long-term effects of subclinical hyperthyroidism on the heart and bone.[20] RAI ablation can reduce goiter size by up to 50% over a 1-year period, and it is an increasingly popular treatment option in many developing countries where access to thyroidectomy is limited. However, the effect of RAI is gradual; acute transient thyroiditis can occur, which may exacerbate local symptoms, and it is ineffective for larger goiters.

The absolute indications for thyroidectomy in nontoxic goiter include local compressive symptoms, substernal extension (which often presents with compressive symptoms), presence of nodules suspicious or diagnostic for malignancy in which prolonged ultrasound surveillance would be hampered, and patient preference (assuming that the patient is otherwise an acceptable surgical candidate). The extent of thyroidectomy, specifically unilateral lobectomy versus total thyroidectomy, can be tailored to the individual patient and goiter scenario. Total or near-total thyroidectomy is typically the procedure of choice; subtotal thyroidectomy is associated with an unacceptably high rate of recurrence in the long term (>50% in some studies). However, unilateral lobectomy may suffice in certain scenarios, such as a single-side dominant goiter with a relatively normal contralateral lobe and in patients predicted to have poor adherence to daily thyroid hormone replacement.

Thyroidectomy for substernal goiter presents a unique challenge depending on the amount and pattern of intrathoracic extension, specifically in relation to the probability of requiring partial or complete sternotomy. Most substernal goiters can be resected via standard cervical thyroidectomy incision because the majority of substernal goiters are anterior and extend inferiorly to a point no lower than the superior aspect of the aortic arch on cross-sectional imaging. These goiters can readily be retrieved via cervicotomy with proper neck extension and patient positioning. On the other hand, goiters extending farther inferiorly than the aortic arch, extending posteriorly, and/or crossing the midline from the dominant side are significantly more difficult and may require sternal split and partial or even total median sternotomy. Thoracic surgery assistance is useful, especially for the more difficult substernal goiters requiring sternotomy or other mediastinal access.

THYROID NODULE

A thyroid nodule is a commonly identified discrete lesion within the thyroid gland. Up to 5% of females and 1% of males in iodine-replete areas have palpable thyroid nodules, and with the advent of ever-improving high-resolution ultrasound, the frequency of thyroid nodules has been estimated to be as high as

19% to 68% because of imaging's ability to pick up nonpalpable, incidentally discovered thyroid nodules, or "incidentalomas." Although thyroid nodules are quite common, the majority do not require extensive (or any) workup, and the vast majority do not require surgical intervention. The primary reasons for surgical intervention for thyroid nodules include (1) concern for malignancy, (2) hyperfunction, and (3) locally compressive symptoms.

The management of thyroid nodules (and thyroid cancer) is the subject of much active research and controversy. Multiple organizations have published clinical practice guidelines over the past 25 years. The ATA guidelines were first published in 1996 and updated over the years, most recently in 2006, 2009, and 2015, and arguably remain the most comprehensive, current, and cited among thyroidologists.[19] Much of this section will reflect the evidence and recommendations contained in the most recent iteration of the ATA guidelines.

Clinical Presentation and Workup

The majority of thyroid nodules are benign and asymptomatic, and as mentioned earlier, many are now diagnosed as "incidentalomas." Several clinical findings on history or physical exam raise the suspicion for thyroid cancer. These include patient age <20 years or >70 years, male sex, locally compressive or infiltrative symptoms such as hoarseness or dysphagia, firm and/or immobile nodule, nodules >3 to 4 cm, cervical lymphadenopathy, history of neck irradiation, and history of thyroid cancer in first-degree family members. Although less common, the suspicion for a hyperfunctioning nodule or toxic adenoma is raised when there are symptoms or signs of thyrotoxicosis, including palpitations, atrial fibrillation, anxiety, insomnia, weight loss, heat intolerance, diaphoresis, and increased defecation.

The workup of thyroid nodules typically includes assessment of thyroid function with serum TSH as a screening test as well as neck ultrasound (Fig. 73.14). The finding of a suppressed TSH

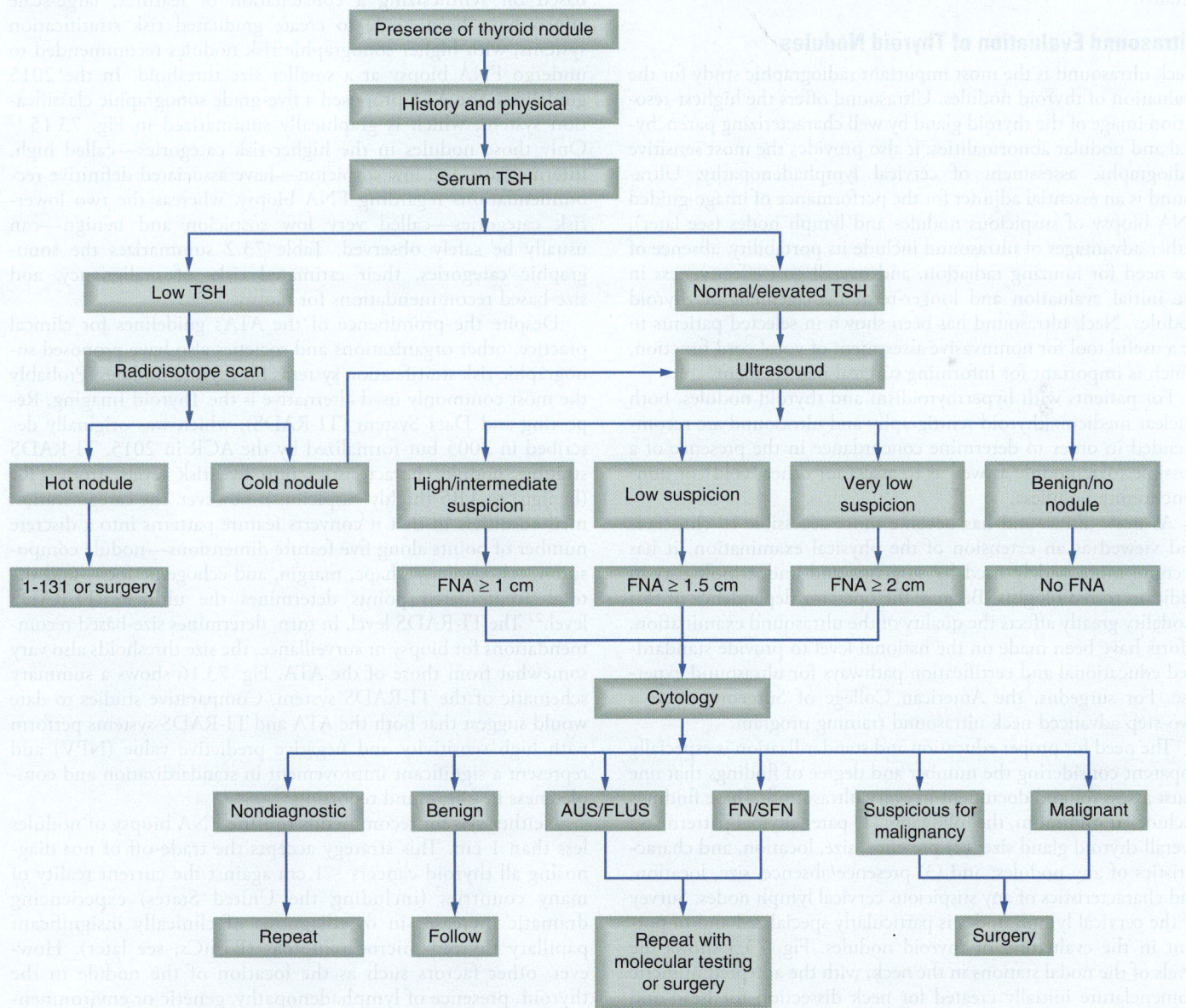

FIGURE 73.14 Workup of a thyroid nodule. *AUS,* Atypia of undetermined significance; *FLUS,* follicular lesion of undetermined significance; *FN,* follicular neoplasm; *FNA,* fine-needle aspiration biopsy; *SFN,* suspicious for follicular neoplasm; *TSH,* thyroid-stimulating hormone.

level also may trigger further workup of hyperthyroidism as detailed earlier, including thyroid antibody workup and thyroid nuclear medicine scintigraphy. Further workup for malignancy always includes FNA biopsy (see later) and, depending on the concern for locally advanced or metastatic behavior, may include cross-sectional imaging.

The majority of thyroid nodules are benign neoplasms and include colloid nodules, degenerative cysts, nodular hyperplasia, and follicular adenomas. Of note, the 2022 World Health Classification of Thyroid Neoplasms has designated oncocytic adenomas of the thyroid as a distinct classification; the term *Hürthle cell* is now discouraged because it is a historical misnomer.[21] The most common malignant diagnosis is PTC, and in decreasing order of frequency also includes follicular thyroid cancer (FTC), oncocytic carcinoma of the thyroid (OCA), MTC, poorly differentiated thyroid cancer (PDTC), and ATC; other rare malignancies, including primary thyroid lymphoma and metastasis to the thyroid gland, can occur (see the "Thyroid Cancer" section later for more details).

Ultrasound Evaluation of Thyroid Nodules

Neck ultrasound is the most important radiographic study for the evaluation of thyroid nodules. Ultrasound offers the highest-resolution image of the thyroid gland by well characterizing parenchymal and nodular abnormalities; it also provides the most sensitive radiographic assessment of cervical lymphadenopathy. Ultrasound is an essential adjunct for the performance of image-guided FNA biopsy of suspicious nodules and lymph nodes (see later). Other advantages of ultrasound include its portability, absence of the need for ionizing radiation, and overall cost-effectiveness in the initial evaluation and longer-term management of thyroid nodules. Neck ultrasound has been shown in selected patients to be a useful tool for noninvasive assessment of vocal cord function, which is important for informing surgical management.

For patients with hyperthyroidism and thyroid nodules, both nuclear medicine thyroid scintigraphy and ultrasound are recommended in order to determine concordance in the presence of a possible toxic nodule as well as to assess for other "cold" or nonfunctioning nodules.

As neck ultrasound has become more accessible to clinicians and viewed as an extension of the physical examination, it has become more widely used by surgeons and endocrinologists in addition to radiologists. Because the operator dependence of this modality greatly affects the quality of the ultrasound examination, efforts have been made on the national level to provide standardized educational and certification pathways for ultrasound expertise. For surgeons, the American College of Surgeons offers a two-step advanced neck ultrasound training program.

The need for proper education and standardization is especially apparent considering the number and degree of findings that one must assess for and document in every ultrasound. These findings include, at minimum, the following: (1) parenchymal pattern and overall thyroid gland size; (2) presence, size, location, and characteristics of any nodules; and (3) presence/absence, size, location, and characteristics of any suspicious cervical lymph nodes. Survey of the cervical lymph nodes is particularly specialized and important in the evaluation of thyroid nodules. Fig. 73.3 shows the levels of the nodal stations in the neck, with the accepted numeric nomenclature initially created for neck dissection for head and neck cancers. Thorough examination must be performed particularly of the pretracheal and paratracheal nodes of the central neck and mediastinum (levels VI and VII, respectively) as well as the

lateral jugular chain nodes (especially levels IIa/IIb, III, IV, and Vb).

Sonographic Risk Stratification of Thyroid Nodules

The sonographic characteristics in thyroid nodules that appear to confer the highest risk of malignancy—specifically PTC—include (1) the presence of microcalcifications, (2) hypoechogenicity, (3) irregular margins, and (4) a taller-than-wide nodule shape. Size is also thought to be a predictor and is clinically relevant, although whether size is an independent predictor is controversial. Intranodular vascularity has historically been thought to also be predictive of malignancy but is likely more correlated with FTC than PTC. Although each individual ultrasound characteristic is relatively unreliable in isolation for predicting malignancy, the combination provides improved specificity. On the opposite end of the spectrum, features such as spongiform pattern or a purely cystic appearance dramatically decrease the risk of malignancy.

Because the sonographic interpretation for malignancy is based on synthesizing a constellation of features, large-scale efforts have been made to create graduated risk stratification systems, with higher sonographic risk nodules recommended to undergo FNA biopsy at a smaller size threshold. In the 2015 guidelines, the ATA proposed a five-grade sonographic classification system, which is graphically summarized in Fig. 73.15.[19] Only those nodules in the higher-risk categories—called high, intermediate, and low suspicion—have associated definitive recommendations regarding FNA biopsy, whereas the two lower-risk categories—called very low suspicion and benign—can usually be safely observed. Table 73.2 summarizes the sonographic categories, their estimated risks of malignancy, and size-based recommendations for biopsy.

Despite the prominence of the ATA's guidelines for clinical practice, other organizations and societies also have proposed sonographic risk stratification systems for thyroid nodules. Probably the most commonly used alternative is the Thyroid Imaging, Reporting and Data System (TI-RADS), which was originally described in 2005 but formalized by the ACR in 2015. TI-RADS stratifies nodule characteristics into five risk levels, from TR1 (benign) to TR5 (highly suspicious); however, the categorization method differs in that it converts feature patterns into a discrete number of points along five feature dimensions—nodule composition, echogenicity, shape, margin, and echogenic foci—and the total accumulated points determines the ultimate TI-RADS level.[22] The TI-RADS level, in turn, determines size-based recommendations for biopsy or surveillance; the size thresholds also vary somewhat from those of the ATA. Fig. 73.16 shows a summary schematic of the TI-RADS system. Comparative studies to date would suggest that both the ATA and TI-RADS systems perform with high sensitivity and negative predictive value (NPV) and represent a significant improvement in standardization and completeness in ultrasound reporting.[23]

Neither system recommends routine FNA biopsy of nodules less than 1 cm. This strategy accepts the trade-off of not diagnosing all thyroid cancers <1 cm against the current reality of many countries (including the United States) experiencing dramatic increases in overdiagnosis of clinically insignificant papillary thyroid microcarcinomas (PTmCs; see later). However, other factors such as the location of the nodule in the thyroid, presence of lymphadenopathy, genetic or environmental risk factors, patient age, and patient preference may take precedence in influencing whether a subcentimeter thyroid nodule is biopsied.

ATA NODULE SONOGRAPHIC PATTERN RISK OF MALIGNANCY

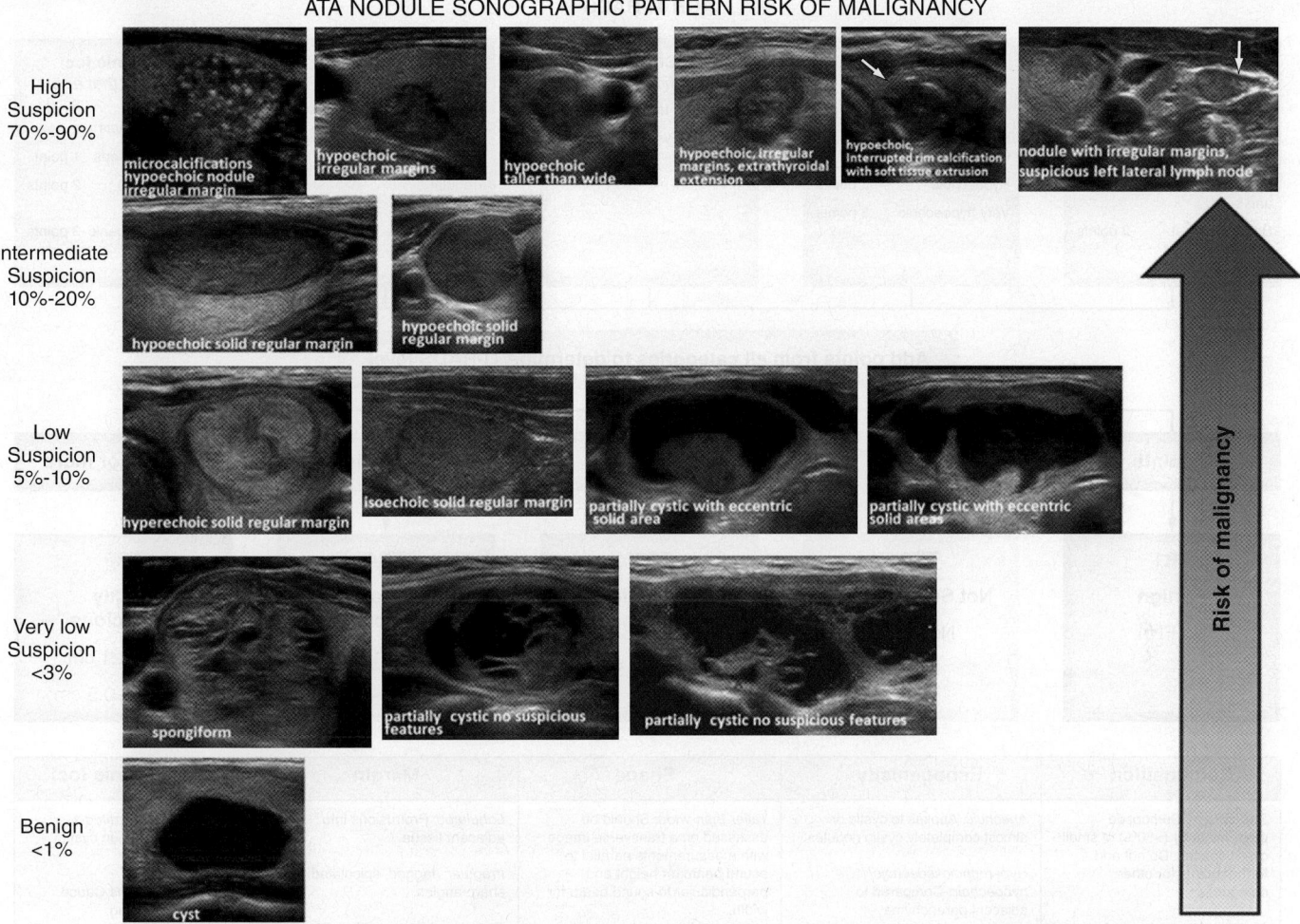

FIGURE 73.15 American Thyroid Association *(ATA)* nodule sonographic patterns and risk of malignancy. (From Haugen BR, Alexander EK, Bible KC, et al. 2015 American Thyroid Association management guidelines for patients with thyroid nodules and differentiated thyroid cancer. *Thyroid.* 2016;26:1-133.)

TABLE 73.2 Sonographic Patterns, Estimated Risk of Malignancy, and FNA Guidance for Thyroid Nodules

SONOGRAPHIC PATTERN	SONOGRAPHIC FEATURES	ESTIMATED RISK OF MALIGNANCY	FNA SIZE CUTOFF (LARGEST DIMENSION)
High suspicion	Solid hypoechoic nodule or solid hypoechoic component of a partially cystic nodule **with** one or more of the following features: irregular margins (infiltrative, microlobulated), microcalcifications, taller-than-wide shape, rim calcifications with small extrusive soft tissue component, evidence of ETE	>70%–90%	Recommend FNA at ≥1 cm
Intermediate suspicion	Hypoechoic solid nodule with smooth margins **without** microcalcifications, ETE, or taller-than-wide shape	10%–20%	Recommend FNA at ≥1 cm
Low suspicion	Isoechoic or hyperechoic solid nodule or partially cystic nodule with eccentric solid areas **without** microcalcification, irregular margin or ETE, or taller-than-wide shape	5%–10%	Recommend FNA at ≥1.5 cm
Very low suspicion	Spongiform or partially cystic nodules **without** any of the sonographic features described in low-, intermediate-, or high-suspicion patterns	<3%	Consider FNA at ≥2 cm; observation without FNA also reasonable
Benign	Purely cystic nodules (no solid component)	<1%	No biopsy; aspiration reasonable for symptomatic or cosmetic drainage

ETE, Extrathyroidal extension; *FNA,* fine-needle aspiration.
From Haugen BR, Alexander EK, Bible KC, et al. 2015 American Thyroid Association management guidelines for adult patients with thyroid nodules and differentiated thyroid cancer: the American Thyroid Association Guidelines Task Force on Thyroid Nodules and Differentiated Thyroid Cancer. *Thyroid.* 2016;26:1-133.

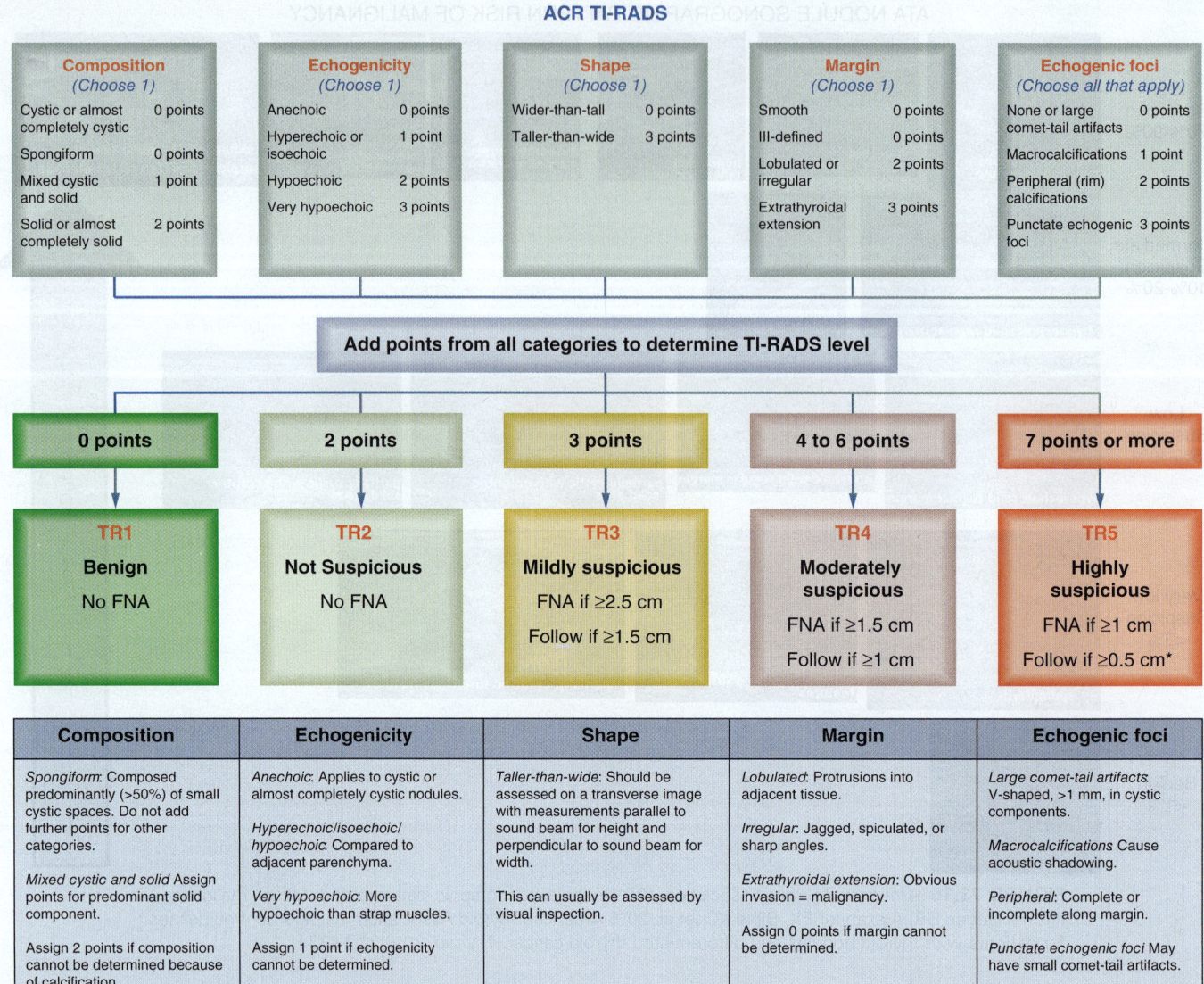

ACR TI-RADS

Composition *(Choose 1)*	Echogenicity *(Choose 1)*	Shape *(Choose 1)*	Margin *(Choose 1)*	Echogenic foci *(Choose all that apply)*
Cystic or almost completely cystic — 0 points	Anechoic — 0 points	Wider-than-tall — 0 points	Smooth — 0 points	None or large comet-tail artifacts — 0 points
Spongiform — 0 points	Hyperechoic or isoechoic — 1 point	Taller-than-wide — 3 points	Ill-defined — 0 points	Macrocalcifications — 1 point
Mixed cystic and solid — 1 point	Hypoechoic — 2 points		Lobulated or irregular — 2 points	Peripheral (rim) calcifications — 2 points
Solid or almost completely solid — 2 points	Very hypoechoic — 3 points		Extrathyroidal extension — 3 points	Punctate echogenic foci — 3 points

Add points from all categories to determine TI-RADS level

0 points	2 points	3 points	4 to 6 points	7 points or more
TR1 Benign No FNA	**TR2** Not Suspicious No FNA	**TR3** Mildly suspicious FNA if ≥2.5 cm Follow if ≥1.5 cm	**TR4** Moderately suspicious FNA if ≥1.5 cm Follow if ≥1 cm	**TR5** Highly suspicious FNA if ≥1 cm Follow if ≥0.5 cm*

Composition	Echogenicity	Shape	Margin	Echogenic foci
Spongiform: Composed predominantly (>50%) of small cystic spaces. Do not add further points for other categories. *Mixed cystic and solid* Assign points for predominant solid component. Assign 2 points if composition cannot be determined because of calcification.	*Anechoic*: Applies to cystic or almost completely cystic nodules. *Hyperechoic/isoechoic/hypoechoic*: Compared to adjacent parenchyma. *Very hypoechoic*: More hypoechoic than strap muscles. Assign 1 point if echogenicity cannot be determined.	*Taller-than-wide*: Should be assessed on a transverse image with measurements parallel to sound beam for height and perpendicular to sound beam for width. This can usually be assessed by visual inspection.	*Lobulated*: Protrusions into adjacent tissue. *Irregular*: Jagged, spiculated, or sharp angles. *Extrathyroidal extension*: Obvious invasion = malignancy. Assign 0 points if margin cannot be determined.	*Large comet-tail artifacts*: V-shaped, >1 mm, in cystic components. *Macrocalcifications* Cause acoustic shadowing. *Peripheral*: Complete or incomplete along margin. *Punctate echogenic foci* May have small comet-tail artifacts.

Refer to discussion of papillary microcarcinomas for 5–9 mm TR5 nodules.

FIGURE 73.16 The American College of Radiology *(ACR)* Thyroid Imaging, Reporting and Data System *(TI-RADS)* lexicon, TR levels, and criteria for fine-needle aspiration *(FNA)* biopsy, *TR* = TI-RADS classification (eg. TR1, TR2, etc.). (From Tessler FN, Middleton WD, Grant EG, et al. ACR Thyroid Imaging, Reporting and Data System [TI-RADS]: white paper of the ACR TI-RADS Committee. *J Am Coll Radiol.* 2017;14:587-595.)

Ultrasound elastography is a technique that measures the stiffness of a thyroid nodule. It was originally developed with the promise of incrementally improving ultrasound's noninvasive risk assessment of malignancy. Initial results were promising, although follow-up results have been mixed on validation studies.[24] Elastography is a highly specialized technique with unique equipment, and it is most effective for only a small subset of nodules. Currently, elastography is not recommended for routine use in the evaluation of thyroid nodules, but it may be useful for selected cases in specialized centers.

Fine-Needle Aspiration Cytology

FNA biopsy is the most accurate and cost-effective invasive procedure in the workup of thyroid nodules. For all thyroid nodules, FNA has a mean sensitivity of over 80% and a mean specificity of over 90%. Although FNA can technically be performed without ultrasound guidance for palpable nodules, the accuracy overall with ultrasound assistance is superior. FNA is performed with a small-gauge needle (typically 23–27 gauge), and it may be performed with capillary or suction techniques. Ideally, the adequacy of the specimen can be confirmed at the time of the procedure with on-site cytopathologic evaluation. The excellent discriminatory ability and extremely low complication rate of FNA have rendered biopsy methods with larger-bore needles such as core-needle biopsy obsolete.

The indications for FNA biopsy are described in greater detail earlier and are largely dependent on the risk profile of the thyroid nodule on ultrasound. For example, FNA would be recommended for higher-risk pattern nodules classified as ATA high-suspicion or TI-RADS TR5; in other words, solid hypoechoic nodules with microcalcifications that are at least 1 cm should be considered for biopsy, whereas very low-risk nodules that are spongiform have higher size cutoffs for biopsy or can be observed. Risk factors other than sonographic profile can reduce the threshold for performing FNA biopsy, including positive family history of thyroid cancer, history of significant radiation exposure, and PET-positivity. FNA should only be performed if the results would influence patient management. For instance, small- to moderate-sized thyroid nodules in the extreme elderly or those with prohibitive surgical risk, or in patients without other concerning features who are already proceeding with thyroidectomy, do not require FNA.

Historically, cytologic findings from FNA were broadly categorized into three categories: benign, malignant, and indeterminate. Although this system was generally helpful for the majority of thyroid nodules with highly predictive benign and malignant features, its drawbacks included (1) significant variability in pathology evaluation and reporting and (2) inability to more finely discriminate features within the broadly termed "indeterminate" category. To address these limitations, the National Cancer Institute convened a State of the Science conference in 2007 to develop a consensus for cytologic terminology known as the *Bethesda System for Reporting Thyroid Cytopathology;* an updated third version was published in 2023 and is described here.[25] This system formalized six diagnostic categories of FNA cytology, with an estimation of cancer risk associated with each category based on literature review and expert opinion. These categories, in increasing numerical order, are (1) nondiagnostic/unsatisfactory, (2) benign, (3) atypia of undetermined significance (AUS), (4) follicular neoplasm (FN), (5) suspicious for malignancy, and (6) malignant (Fig. 73.17). Table 73.3 provides a breakdown of these categories and their associated malignancy risk in addition to the possible changes in malignancy risk if the histopathologic diagnosis of noninvasive follicular thyroid neoplasm with papillary-like nuclear features (NIFTP; see later) were no longer to be included as a malignancy.

The broad institution of the Bethesda classification system across virtually all major centers has led to significant improvements in standardization of care, communication of cancer risk with other clinicians and patients, and research efforts. Validation studies in large numbers of patients have shown overall good concordance in the FNA reporting patterns and malignancy rates. However, there is significant variability in the risk of malignancy in each category, particularly in the AUS category.[26] This has led to the recommendation for each individual institution to define its own patient population's malignancy risks for each of the Bethesda categories by correlating cytology to surgical histopathology from surgical specimens.

Molecular Testing of Fine-Needle Aspiration Specimens

Although no FNA cytology can completely rule out or rule in malignancy in a thyroid nodule, the cytologic diagnoses of benign (Bethesda category II) and malignant (Bethesda VI) are highly accurate with an error rate of less than 3%. On the other hand, the remaining "indeterminate" categories—particularly AUS and follicular neoplasm (Bethesda III and IV, respectively)—are associated with a cancer risk anywhere from 6% to 40%, with Bethesda III nodules falling in the 6% to 30% range and the Bethesda IV nodules in the 10% to 40% range. Bethesda V lesions (suspicious for malignancy) are also technically indeterminate, but because these are associated with a 50% to 75% risk of malignancy, they are typically managed similarly to malignant (Bethesda VI) cytology.

Traditionally, the malignancy risk associated with Bethesda III or IV cytology in a thyroid nodule led to the recommendation of diagnostic thyroid lobectomy, but because the majority of these nodules are still ultimately benign on final pathology, efforts have been made in molecular genetics to improve prediction capability and reduce the number of unnecessary thyroidectomies. Advancements in molecular genetics have enabled the creation of relatively affordable high-throughput DNA- or RNA-based assays for creating molecular profiles or signatures of cytology samples that would provide more accurate assessment of malignancy risk in thyroid nodules. There are multiple commercial providers for these tests, but the two most prominent tests are the Afirma (Veracyte, San Francisco, CA) and ThyroSeq (CBLPath, Rye Brook, NY).

The Afirma product was the first molecular test commercially available in this space. Its first-generation assay, the Gene Expression Classifier, employed proprietary machine learning algorithms on a 167-gene mRNA microarray to separate nodules' gene expression signatures into "benign" and "suspicious" categories. The Gene Expression Classifier test's accuracy was first evaluated in 2012 in a study of surgically excised thyroid nodule specimens, and it was found to demonstrate excellent sensitivity and NPV (90% and ~95%, respectively), but with relatively poor specificity and positive predictive value (PPV; ~50% and 38%, respectively) for Bethesda III and IV nodules. Subsequent studies have largely validated the original study's findings, but many of them have been limited by the lack of a true negative (i.e., benign) reference standard.[27]

TABLE 73.3 The 2023 Bethesda System for Reporting Thyroid Cytopathology Implied Risk of Malignancy and Recommended Clinical Management

DIAGNOSTIC CATEGORY (BETHESDA NUMBER)	RISK OF MALIGNANCY IF NIFTP ≠ CANCER	RISK OF MALIGNANCY IF NIFTP = CANCER	USUAL MANAGEMENT
Nondiagnostic (I)	5%–18%	5%–20%	Repeat FNA with ultrasound guidance
Benign (II)	0%–4%	2%–7%	Clinical and sonographic follow-up
AUS (III)	6%–24%	~13%–30%	Repeat FNA, molecular testing, or lobectomy
FN (IV)	17%–28%	23%–34%	Molecular testing or lobectomy
Suspicious for malignancy (V)	58%–74%	67%–83%	Near-total thyroidectomy or lobectomy
Malignant (VI)	94%–96%	97%–100%	Near-total thyroidectomy or lobectomy

AUS, Atypia of undetermined significance; *FN,* follicular neoplasm; *FNA,* fine-needle aspiration; *NIFTP,* noninvasive follicular thyroid neoplasm with papillary-like nuclear features.
From Ali SZ, Balcoch ZW, Cochand-Priollet B, Schmitt FC, Viehl P, VanderLaan PA. The 2023 Bethesda system for reporting thyroid cytopathology. *Thyroid.* 2023;33:1039-1044.

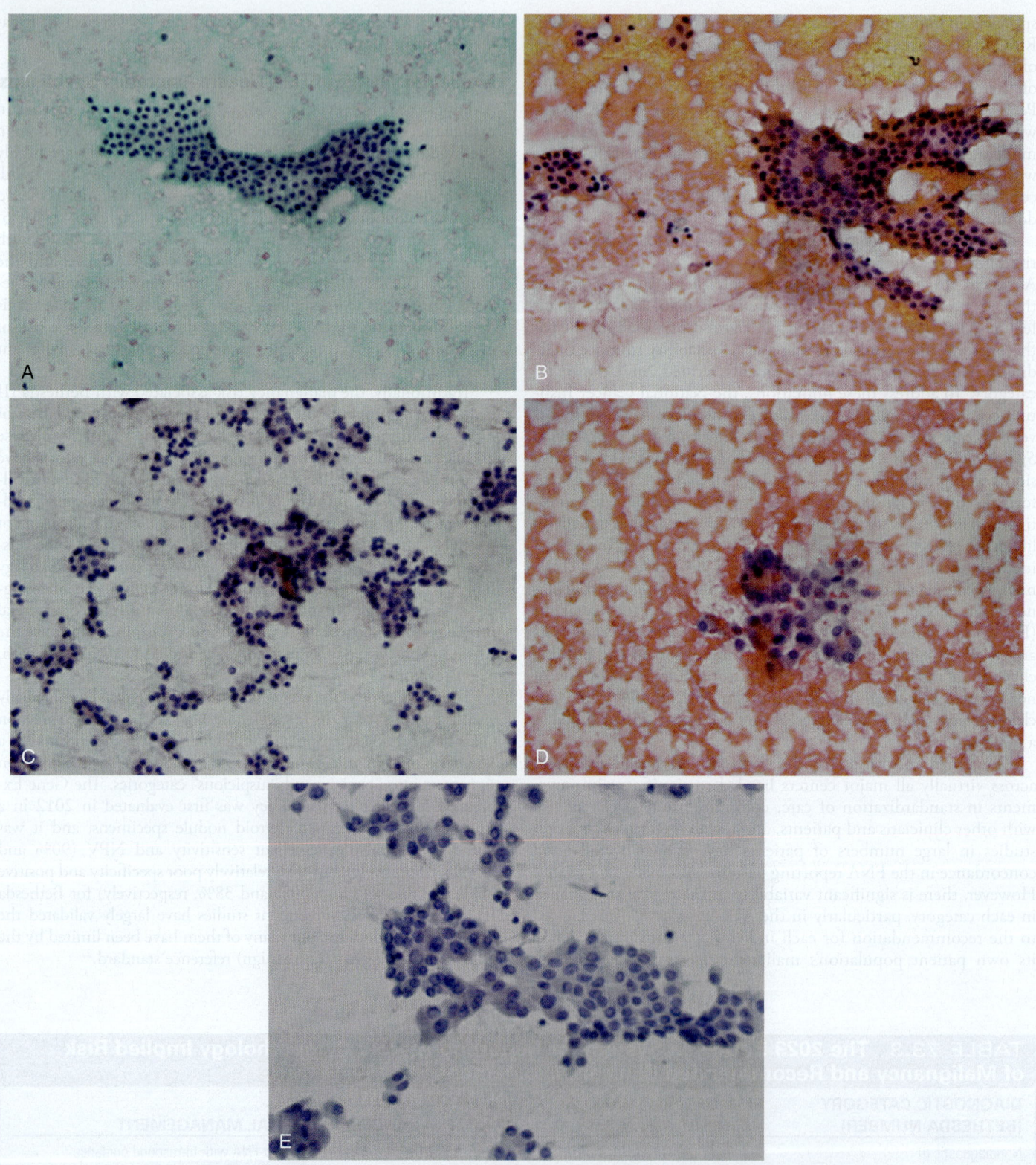

FIGURE 73.17 Representative cytologic features of thyroid fine-needle aspiration specimens arranged according to the Bethesda classification for prediction of malignancy. (A) Category II: benign colloid nodule with bland-appearing follicular cells arranged in a macrofollicular pattern and abundant colloid in the background. (B) Category III: atypia of undetermined significance; follicular cells show nuclear enlargement of most nuclei with occasional intranuclear grooves. (C) Category IV: follicular neoplasm with highly cellular aspirate composed of uniform follicular cells arranged in microfollicles. (D) Category V: suspicious for papillary thyroid cancer (PTC); these representative microfollicular groups show nuclear enlargement and pale chromatin and rare intranuclear grooves and pseudoinclusions. (E) Category VI: PTC demonstrating a large sheet of neoplastic cells with enlarged oval "Orphan Annie eye" nuclei; multiple intranuclear pseudoinclusions are also present. (Courtesy Elham Khanafshar, MD, MS, Department of Pathology and Laboratory Medicine, University of California, San Francisco.)

To address its limitations as a "rule-in" test because of its poor specificity and PPV, the newest Afirma product, the Genomic Sequence Classifier (GSC), improved the core machine learning algorithm for its larger gene expression array of 10,196 genes and included seven other upstream components, evaluating for a number of genetic mutations highly specific for malignancy. The performance of the GSC was recently evaluated in a multi-institutional blinded validation study on 191 cytology samples from 183 patients. For Bethesda III and IV lesions, the GSC demonstrated incremental improved performance compared with the Gene Expression Classifier, with sensitivity, specificity, NPV, and PPV of 91%, 68%, 96%, and 47%, respectively, based on a 24% cancer prevalence. Oncocytic neoplasms remained an area of weakness in the GSC; it accurately predicted oncocytic adenomas and carcinomas of the thyroid in only 10/17 and 1/9 specimens, respectively.[27]

The ThyroSeq product approaches molecular classification differently from Afirma, in that it employs next-generation DNA sequencing technology to detect the presence or absence of a discrete list of known gene mutations and gene fusions associated with thyroid cancer. This technology is based on work described by Nikiforov and colleagues[28] at the University of Pittsburgh, and the second version of the product (termed v2) evaluating 13 mutations and 42 fusions demonstrated promising results in their single-institution studies, with sensitivities and specificities in the low 90% range, PPV in the high 60% to 80% range, and NPV over 95%. These initial data originally generated excitement that perhaps the ThyroSeq v2 would offer ideal accuracy characteristics because the PPV appeared to approximate that of Bethesda V cytology while maintaining excellent NPV; however, subsequent validation studies showed less impressive results.[29]

The newest-generation ThyroSeq product (termed v3) improves the number of genes in its mutational panel and incorporates other genetic information, such as changes in gene copy number as well as some gene expression data. Steward and colleagues[29] conducted a prospective, blinded, multicenter study of the ThyroSeq v3 in 286 cytologically indeterminate FNA samples with known surgical pathology results. In Bethesda III and IV nodules, the test had a sensitivity and specificity of 94% and 82%, respectively, and an NPV and PPV of 97% and 66%, respectively, based on a cancer/NIFTP prevalence of 28%. Importantly, the test correctly predicted Hürthle cell (now oncocytic) adenomas and carcinomas in 62% and 100% of cases, respectively.[29]

The early data for both the Afirma GSC and ThyroSeq v3 suggest promising improvements over previous-generation products, and subsequent management guidelines for thyroid nodules will likely incorporate molecular testing to a greater degree. Ultimately, the decision whether or not to use molecular testing needs to be placed in the context of other variables that go into clinical decision-making. First, whether to proceed with thyroidectomy may rest on factors other than the results of an FNA biopsy, let alone molecular testing. Second, the price of these assays is not insignificant, and their institutional setting–specific incremental value and cost-effectiveness must be considered. Third, patients should be counseled about the inherent uncertainties in the therapeutic and long-term clinical implications of pursuing molecular testing.

THYROID CANCER

Thyroid cancers are generally classified into DTC, PDTC, MTC, and ATC. Other thyroid malignancies, including primary thyroid lymphoma, thyroid sarcoma, and metastases to the thyroid gland, are rare. DTCs consisting of PTC, FTC, and OCA are considered "differentiated" because they arise from the thyroid follicular epithelial cells and generally retain the ability to organify iodine. PDTC and ATC are also thought to arise from follicular cells but are more clinically aggressive compared with DTC because of their loss of differentiation. MTC, unlike the other tumors described, arise from the neuroendocrine parafollicular C cells.

DTC makes up the vast majority of thyroid cancers, with PTC and FTC representing 84% and 11%, respectively, of all thyroid cancer diagnoses. MTC represents 2%, and ATC occurs in 1% of all cases. Thyroid cancer overall carries an excellent prognosis, primarily because of the predominance of PTC, whereas ATC is among the most aggressive and lethal solid tumors of any organ system, with a nearly 100% mortality rate.

Incidence

Approximately 54,000 new cases of thyroid cancer are diagnosed each year in the United States, with over 2000 annual deaths. There is a more than threefold female predominance in incidence, and over the last several decades, thyroid cancer became the fastest-growing cancer among American females, with an incidence that tripled in the United States; similarly dramatic increases were seen in other developed and developing countries throughout the world.[30] Whereas many authors attributed the vast majority of the increase to overdiagnosis given overall stability of mortality rates at 0.5 deaths per 100,000, a more recent review of the same dataset revealed substantial increases in the incidence of larger and advanced-stage PTC concomitant with the increase in the smaller and likely more indolent tumors.[31] Specifically, Lim and colleagues found that the incidence-based mortality actually increased both overall in all PTCs and particularly in the advanced-stage tumors, suggesting that there was in fact a true increase in the occurrence of thyroid cancer.[31] Although incidence of distant metastatic disease in DTC has increased over the last several decades, survival for these patients remains static at only 50% 10 years after diagnosis.[32] As the 2009 and 2015 ATA Guidelines for DTC have generally recommended less aggressive management to avoid treatments with fewer benefits than risks, recent analysis has shown that the proportion of patients receiving thyroidectomy alone without postoperative RAI has increased from 2006 to 2018.[33] Performance of thyroid lobectomy increased only slightly from 2015 to 2018, potentially indicating that clinicians are exercising more caution about its utility. It is likely that the rate of lobectomy will increase in the coming years as more data and guidelines emerge supporting its use.

Differentiated Thyroid Cancer

The primary cancers arising from the thyroid follicular epithelial cells are PTC, FTC, and OCA. Despite some differences in biologic and clinical behavior, DTCs are generally approached and managed similarly.

PTC, as mentioned earlier, is the most common type of thyroid cancer overall, comprising 84% of all incident cases. There is a female predominance, with a 3:1 female-to-male ratio, and peak incidence is in the third to fifth decades of life. PTC disseminates primarily via the lymphatic route and affects the cervical lymph nodes in the central and lateral compartments (see later); however, distant metastases do occur in up to 3% to 5% of patients, typically to lung and bone. Histologically, PTC is characterized by complex branching papillae with pseudoinclusions, nuclear grooving, and psammoma bodies (Fig. 73.18A). The so-called

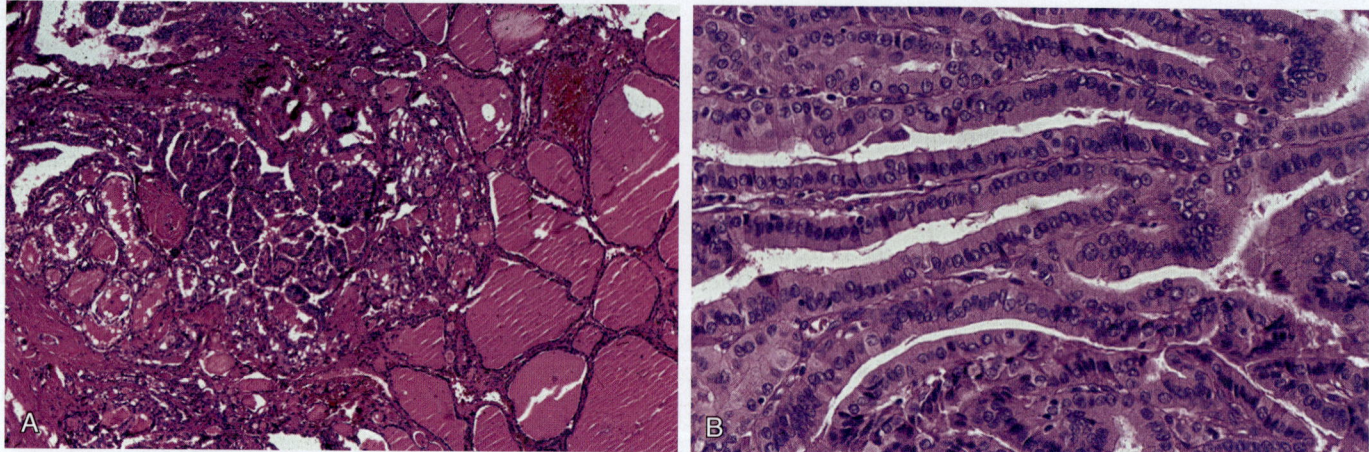

FIGURE 73.18 (A) Hematoxylin and eosin (H&E) staining of a thyroid mass reveals papillary projections consistent with papillary thyroid cancer (PTC). (B) H&E staining of PTC shows cells with an increased height-to-width ratio in a single row of cells. This is the so-called tall cell variant of PTC, which is associated with a poorer prognosis than well-differentiated PTC.

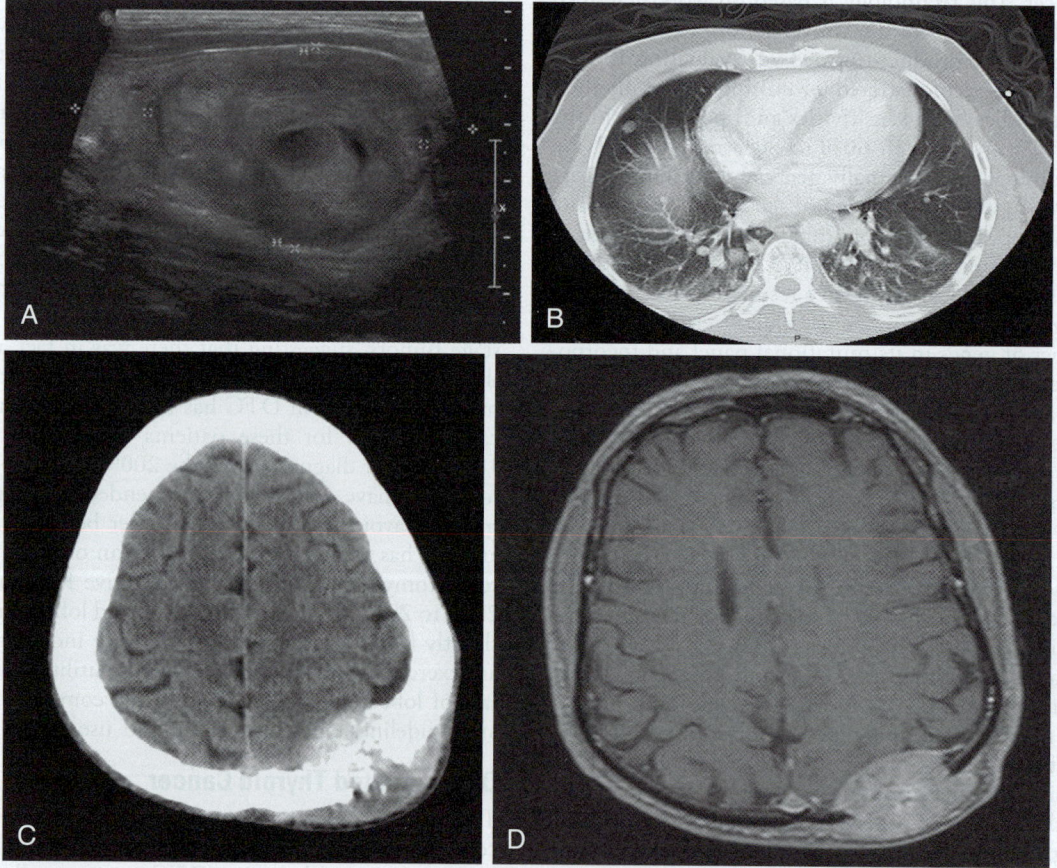

FIGURE 73.19 Metastatic follicular thyroid cancer (FTC); all images are from the same patient. (A) Preoperative ultrasound demonstrates a 6.7-cm mass in the left lobe of the thyroid; pathology demonstrated FTC. (B) Computed tomography (CT) image of the chest demonstrates multiple pulmonary metastases. (C) CT image of the head demonstrates left parietal bone metastasis. (D) Magnetic resonance imaging of the head demonstrates left parietal bone metastasis with an epidural component and mass effect on the brain.

follicular variant of PTC (fvPTC) has a similar prognosis to classical PTC and histologically has well-defined follicles with minimal papillary projections. Other less common but more aggressive histologic subtypes of PTC include tall cell (see Fig. 73.18B), hobnail, diffuse sclerosing, and columnar variants, which together comprise less than 1% of all PTCs.

FTC is the second most common type of DTC. FTC occurs in older adults, with peak incidence in the fourth and sixth decades. As in the case of PTC, the incidence of FTC is female-predominant, with a 3:1 female-to-male ratio. In contrast to that of PTC, the pattern of spread of FTC is hematogenous, typically to the lungs and bone (Fig. 73.19). Regional nodal metastases occur in less than 10% of cases. Cytologically, FTC can range from having virtually normal-appearing follicular cells to those with various abnormal features, including nuclear atypia, discohesion, hypercellularity, and microfollicles; thus, FTC cannot be reliably diagnosed by FNA. FTC can only be definitively diagnosed on histologic examination based on the presence of capsular and/or vascular invasion (Fig. 73.20A).

OCA is a new term in the 2022 World Health Organization classification of thyroid neoplasms, replacing the misnomer Hürthle cell carcinoma, to designate invasive, malignant follicular cell neoplasms with at least 75% oncocytic cells (see Fig. 73.20B).[21] It is less common, accounting for 5% of DTCs in the United States. OCA occurs in older adults, with peak incidence in the sixth and seventh decades. Metastases can occur via lymphatic and hematogenous routes, and distant metastases are present in up to 20% of patients at initial diagnosis. Five-year overall survival is about 85%, but only 24% for patients with distant metastases at

diagnosis. OCA is less RAI-avid compared with other DTCs, which makes OCA more difficult to treat if there is disease recurrence. RAI treatment is potentially associated with improved survival in patients with OCAs that are 2 to 4 cm.

Low-Risk Follicular Thyroid Neoplasms

The 2022 WHO classification of thyroid neoplasms has three distinct categories: benign, low-risk, and malignant.[21] Low-risk follicular thyroid neoplasms include noninvasive follicular thyroid neoplasm with papillary-like nuclear features (NIFTP), thyroid tumors of uncertain malignant potential (UMP), and hyalinizing trabecular tumor (HTT). Low-risk neoplasms have the potential to metastasize, but the incidence of metastasis is extremely low.

Historically, NIFTP was known as the noninvasive encapsulated follicular variant of papillary thyroid cancer (fvPTC). In 2016, a multidisciplinary group of thyroidologists performed a pivotal retrospective analysis of 109 patients with the encapsulated variant and 101 patients with invasive fvPTC; patients had a median follow-up period of 13 years (range, 10–26 years) for the encapsulated variant group and 3.5 years (range, 1–18 years) for the invasive fvPTC group. The authors found that none of the patients with encapsulated fvPTC died or had evidence of disease after treatment, compared with a 12% rate of adverse oncologic outcomes in the invasive fvPTC cohort. Based on these findings, the authors proposed a change in terminology from encapsulated fvPTC to "noninvasive follicular thyroid neoplasm with papillary-like nuclear features," or NIFTP (Fig. 73.21), with the goal being to more accurately reflect the indolent nature of this tumor as well as to deemphasize the connotations of malignancy from the name.[34] Thyroid lobectomy is considered adequate treatment for NIFTP, and further treatment such as TSH suppression or RAI is not required.[35]

HTTs are well-demarcated thyroid nodules with PTC-like nuclear changes, but they demonstrate a unique intratrabecular hyaline material that is not seen in other neoplasms. Also, HTT has a distinct molecular change: *GLIS* gene rearrangements define HTT and are not found in other thyroid neoplasms. HTT almost

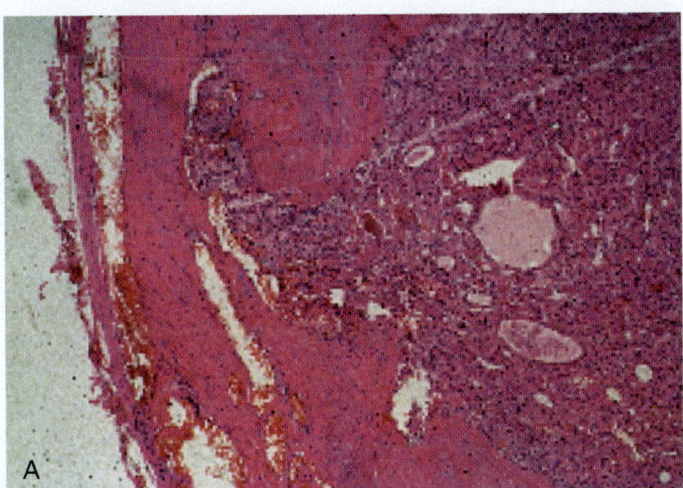

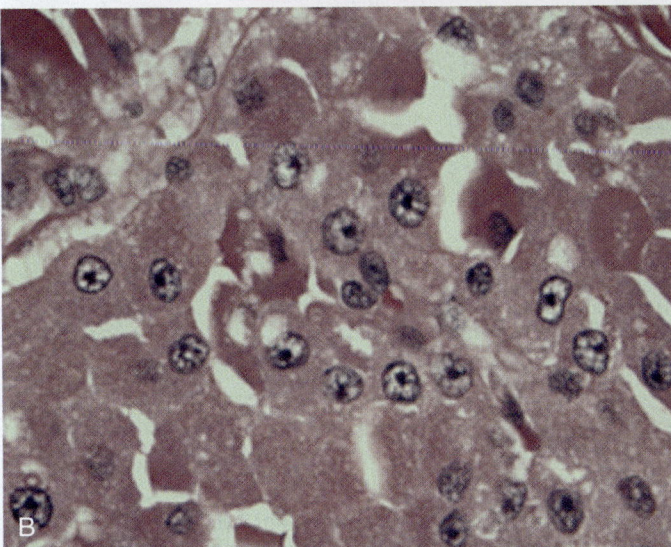

FIGURE 73.20 (A) Hematoxylin and eosin (H&E) staining of a follicular lesion. High-power examination reveals capsular invasion by follicular cells, which is consistent with a diagnosis of follicular thyroid cancer. (B) H&E staining of oncocytic carcinoma of the thyroid showing vesicular nuclei with irregular macronucleoli. (From Freeman JL, Kim DS. Hürthle cell tumors of the thyroid. In: Randolph GW, ed. *Surgery of the Thyroid and Parathyroid Glands 2*. Philadelphia: Elsevier Saunders; 2013:207.)

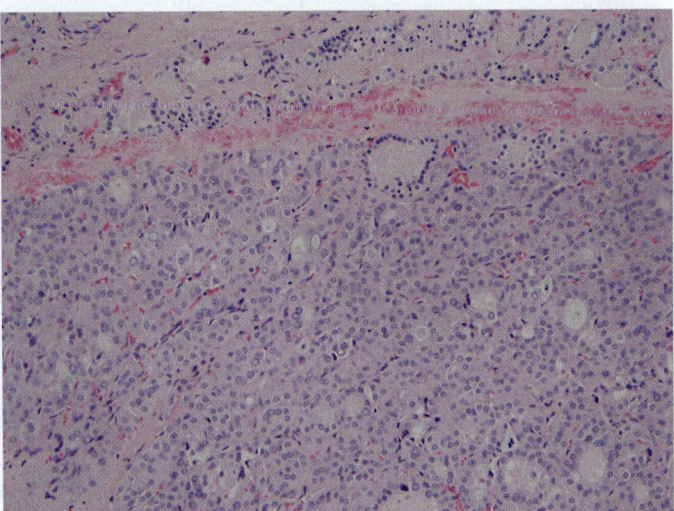

FIGURE 73.21 Noninvasive follicular thyroid neoplasm with papillary-like nuclear features is a well-circumscribed/encapsulated microfollicular-pattern neoplasm with no capsular or vascular invasion. The neoplastic cells show nuclear features similar to those of papillary thyroid cancer. (Courtesy Elham Khanafshar, MD, MS, Department of Pathology and Laboratory Medicine, University of California, San Francisco.)

always follows a benign course; therefore, thyroid lobectomy is considered adequate treatment. In general, thyroid lobectomy with clinical and imaging surveillance is favored for NIFTP and HTT because they almost always follow a benign course. However, UMP tumors require closer follow-up because their metastatic potential is uncertain.

Thyroid Follicular Cell Neoplasia and Oncogenesis

The two major molecular pathways governing thyroid follicular cell oncogenesis are the mitogen-activated protein kinase (MAPK) signaling and the phosphatidylinositol 3-kinase/protein kinase B (PI3K/AKT) pathways (Fig. 73.22). Together, these pathways govern normal thyroid cell survival and function; perturbations at multiple points in these pathways have been directly linked to the pathogenesis of thyroid cancer. In 2014, the Cancer Genome Atlas project consortium published its results from a comprehensive, multiplatform, next-generation genomic sequencing analysis of 496 PTCs.[36] This seminal study confirmed the dominant and typically mutually exclusive roles of driving somatic genetic

alterations in the MAPK and PI3K/AKT pathways in PTC. The results of the Cancer Genome Atlas are estimated to have increased the proportion of PTCs that can be identified based on molecular signature using current genome sequencing technology from 75% to over 96%. This has translated into improved molecular testing methods to facilitate the preoperative diagnosis of thyroid cancer (see earlier).

The MAPK signaling pathway is activated by growth factors binding to cell-surface transmembrane tyrosine kinase receptors. This triggers an intracellular signaling cascade that ultimately regulates the intranuclear transcription of genes responsible for cellular growth/proliferation, differentiation, migration, and survival. In the MAPK pathway, the proto-oncogene *BRAF* is most frequently mutated in PTC; it is typically a point mutation with a glutamate-for-valine substitution at residue 600 (p.V600E). The *BRAFV600E* mutation occurs early in oncogenesis, resulting in dedifferentiation and tumor growth. This mutation is found in up to 60% of all PTCs. The second most common type of mutations found in PTC involve the RAS family of genes. These mutations

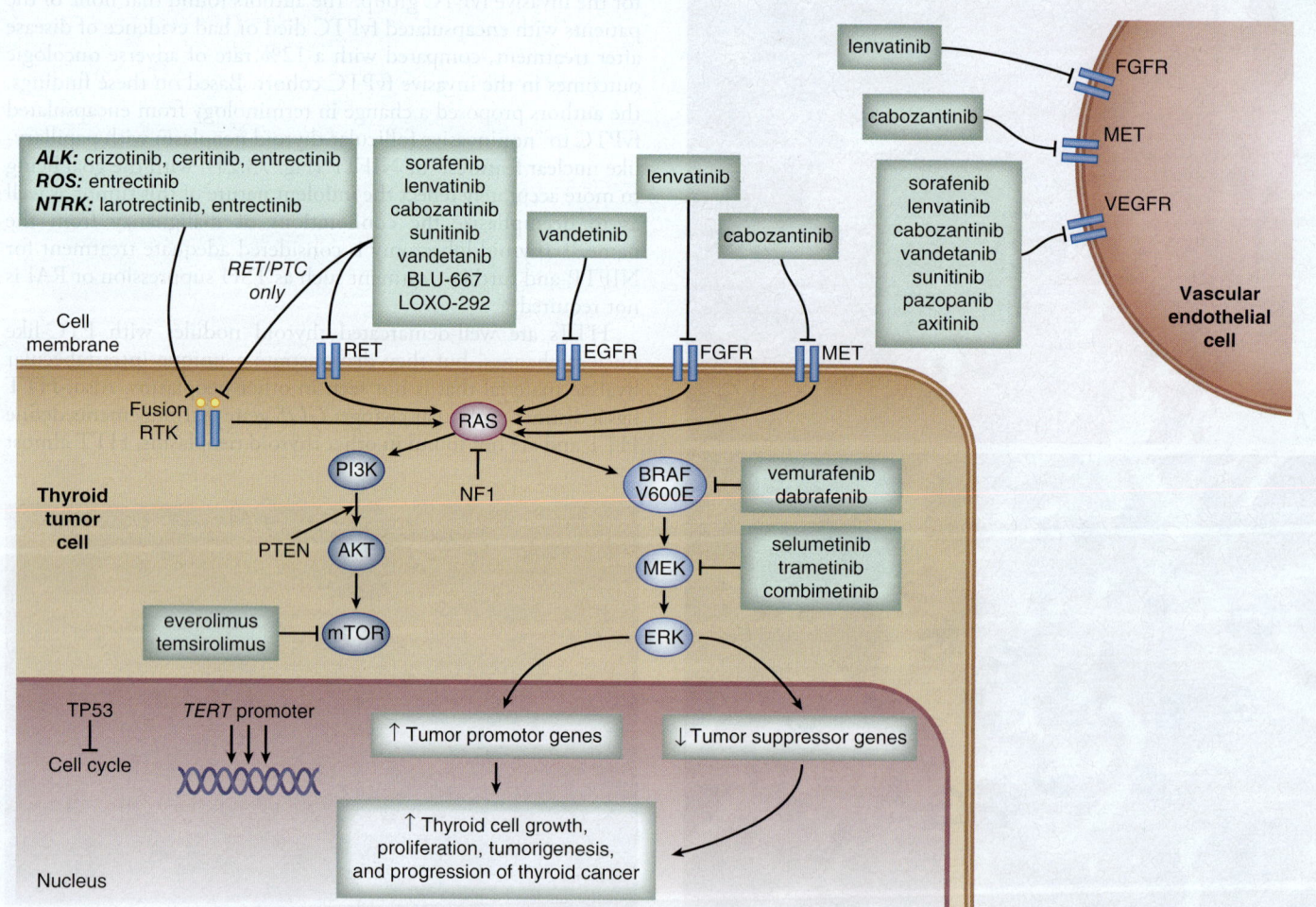

FIGURE 73.22 Schematic of the two most common pathways and genetic alterations associated with thyroid follicular cell oncogenesis: the MAPK and the PI3K-AKT pathways. Also shown are the current targeted therapies studied in thyroid cancer. *AKT,* Protein kinase B; *ALK,* anaplastic lymphoma kinase; *ERK,* extracellular signal–regulated kinase; *EGFR,* epidermal growth factor receptor; *FGFR,* fibroblast growth factor receptor; *MAPK,* mitogen-activated protein kinase; *mTOR,* mammalian target of rapamycin; *NTRK,* neurotrophic tropomyosin receptor kinase; *PI3K,* phosphatidylinositol 3-kinase; *PTC,* papillary thyroid cancer; *RTK,* receptor tyrosine kinase; *TERT,* telomerase reverse transcription; *VEGFR,* vascular endothelial growth factor receptor. (From Rao SN, Cabanillas ME. Navigating systemic therapy in advanced thyroid carcinoma: from standard of care to personalized therapy and beyond. *J Endocr Soc.* 2018;2:1109-1130.)

occur in 20% to 30% of PTCs and are more common in fvPTCs. Unlike BRAF, RAS can activate both the MAPK and PI3K-AKT pathways.

The PI3K/AKT pathway, like the MAPK pathway, involves a series of phosphorylation reactions, starting with a transmembrane protein kinase. This leads to the activation of AKT, which in turn phosphorylates proteins both in the cytosol and the nucleus. Downstream targets of AKT regulate apoptosis, proliferation, cell-cycle progression, cytoskeletal integrity, and energy metabolism. This pathway is thought to be particularly relevant to the development of FTC; further supporting this theory is the finding that mutations in *PTEN* (an inhibitor of AKT activation) are found in both sporadic FTC and FTC associated with Cowden syndrome (a hereditary disorder characterized by multiple hamartomas—particularly of the skin and mucous membranes—macrocephaly, and an increased risk of other solid organ cancers such as breast, endometrial, and colorectal cancer).

Rearrangements of the *RET* proto-oncogene, which are present in 5% to 10% of all PTCs, are characteristic of PTCs linked to radiation exposure. These translocations result in the kinase domain of RET being fused with another protein, most commonly CCDC6, resulting in a constitutively active kinase that triggers carcinogenesis through MAPK and PI3K/AKT activation. *RET*-rearranged PTCs are associated with more aggressive features, including multifocal tumors, extrathyroidal extension, and distant metastases, than *BRAFV600E* or *RAS* mutant tumors.[37]

Telomerase reverse transcriptase *(TERT)* promoter mutations are found in up to 27% of PTCs and especially in those that also have mutations affecting the MAPK pathway, such as *RAS* mutations and *BRAFV600E*. *TERT* promoter mutations upregulate expression of TERT, enabling unlimited cellular proliferation. *TERT* mutations are associated with aggressive clinical and histologic features as well as RAI resistance and high risk of cancer recurrence, especially when present with *BRAF* mutation.

Risk Factors

The two most studied and validated risk factors for PTC include a history of ionizing radiation exposure and a family history of DTC.

The association of ionizing radiation exposure in childhood and adolescence in particular is clear for PTC and perhaps ATC.[38] Acute environmental exposures from catastrophic occurrences, such as the Chernobyl nuclear accident and nuclear bombings in Hiroshima and Nagasaki, have dramatically demonstrated the impact of radiation on thyroid follicular cell oncogenesis. Atomic bomb survivors in Japan have been found to have an increased risk of thyroid nodules and PTC up to 50 years after the incident, with a linear radiation dose response. Medical sources of irradiation, such as external beam radiation therapy to the head and neck as well as historical practices such as radiation therapy in the 1950s and 1960s for acne and tonsillitis, also have been linked to the subsequent development of PTC. Children and adolescents are particularly vulnerable, with even low-dose radiation exposure (e.g., equivalent to a single chest x-ray) increasing PTC risk in a dose-dependent fashion.

A strong family history of DTC has also been shown to increase the risk of DTC. Known hereditary cancer syndromes with specific single-gene mutations are associated with higher incidence of DTC: familial adenomatous polyposis (which predisposes to PTC), Gardner syndrome (PTC), Cowden syndrome (FTC and occasionally PTC), Carney complex (PTC and FTC),

and Werner syndrome (PTC and FTC). In addition, a separate entity known as *familial non-MTC* was coined to describe families with two or more first-degree relatives diagnosed with DTC in the absence of other hereditary cancer syndromes. Familial non-MTC tumors are thought to be more aggressive and portend a worse prognosis than their sporadic counterparts.[39] However, the exact inheritance pattern and genetics underlying familial non-MTC remain poorly understood.

Obesity also has consistently been identified as a risk factor for DTC.[38] There has been a close parallel increase in the trends of obesity prevalence and the incidence of thyroid cancer. A pooled analysis of 22 prospective studies found that thyroid cancer risk was associated with multiple markers of obesity, including waist circumference, body mass index (BMI), and BMI gain between young adulthood and study baseline. Kitahara and colleagues analyzed the National Institutes of Health (NIH)–AARP Diet and Health Study data to show that overweight and obesity may have contributed to one out of every six new PTC cases in patients older than 60 by 2015.[40] In addition, PTCs in obese patients have been associated with more aggressive tumor characteristics.

Other environmental exposures have been hypothesized to increase the risk of DTC. Hoffman and colleagues[41] published a case-control study of patients with PTC and demonstrated a link between the levels at home of certain common flame-retardant chemicals to increased odds of PTC, particularly decabromodiphenyl ether and tris(2-chloroethyl) phosphate. An increased risk of DTC also has been reported in clusters of volcanic areas around the world, including Hawaii, Iceland, French Polynesia, New Caledonia, and Sicily; this may be the result, in part, of exposure to heavy metals and other toxic compounds from gas, ash, and lava emissions from volcanoes that contaminate ground water and food sources.[42] The underlying mechanisms for all of these potential environmental carcinogens remain unclear and require further study.

Clinical Presentation

The classic presentation of DTC is that of an asymptomatic, palpable thyroid nodule discovered by either patients or physicians during routine examination. Palpable thyroid nodules are present in approximately 5% of the population, the majority of which are benign. With the improvements in high-resolution ultrasonography and other imaging modalities, thyroid nodules—and by extension thyroid cancer—have become more commonly diagnosed in asymptomatic individuals, as described earlier.

DTCs are typically slow-growing, painless, and often asymptomatic. Acute pain is more typical of a benign process such as thyroiditis or an acute bleed into a benign cyst; however, pain can also be indicative of less common and more aggressive thyroid cancers such as MTC, primary thyroid lymphoma, and ATC. Concerning features include rapid growth of the nodule and symptoms such as hoarseness, coughing, or dysphagia, which could signal local invasion into surrounding structures such as the RLN and aerodigestive tract (Fig. 73.23).

On physical examination, palpable DTC can vary from soft to firm in texture on palpation. Firm and fixed masses may suggest locally advanced disease. Patients may have palpable or imaging-detected cervical lymphadenopathy.

Imaging Workup

To adequately inform initial surgical treatment, the quality of preoperative imaging is paramount. The most important imaging

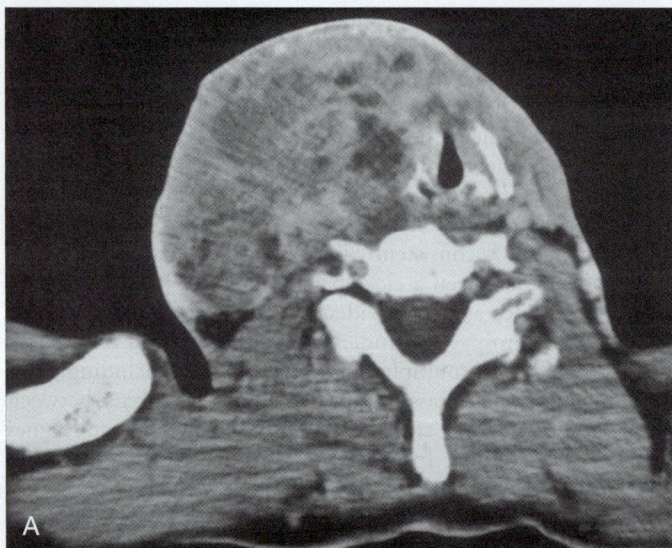

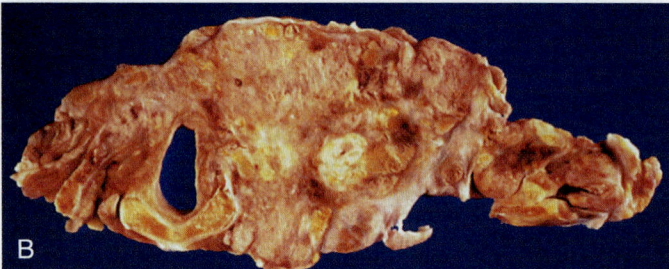

FIGURE 73.23 (A–B) Rapidly enlarging thyroid mass in a 70-year-old patient. Computed tomography image demonstrates displacement of the larynx and lateral involvement of both jugular veins. The patient died within 6 months of rapidly progressing follicular thyroid cancer.

modality for surgical planning is comprehensive thyroid ultrasound with lymph node mapping of the bilateral central and lateral neck compartment lymph nodes. Preoperative ultrasound is the most sensitive test for the characterization of thyroid nodules as well as identification of pathologic lymphadenopathy, with its results affecting the extent of initial surgical therapy in over 30% of patients.

Cross-sectional imaging (contrast-enhanced CT or MRI of the neck and chest) and intraluminal imaging (laryngoscopy, bronchoscopy, or esophagoscopy) may be required in patients with potentially more advanced local and regional disease. Clinical manifestations that may lead the clinician to obtain these additional studies include concerning symptoms such as voice changes and dysphagia; respiratory symptoms such as cough or hemoptysis; and palpable evidence of rapidly enlarging, bulky, and/or fixed disease on physical examination. Sonographic indications include evidence of bulky disease, disease extending into the chest or extending posteriorly, and extrathyroidal extension.

The routine use of PET scanning in preoperative planning is not recommended.

Staging

There have been many proposed staging systems over the years for estimating disease-specific mortality from DTC, but the American Joint Committee on Cancer (AJCC) and Union for International Cancer Control Tumor, Node, Metastasis (TNM) classification has emerged as the most widely accepted and easily understood. The current 8th edition of the TNM system, which took effect in

TABLE 73.4   Summary of the AJCC 8th Edition Staging System for DTC

TNM STAGE GROUPING PATIENTS AGED <55	TNM STAGE GROUPING PATIENTS AGED ≥55	AJCC STAGE
Any T, Any N, M0	T1/2, N0/NX, M0	I
Any T, Any N, M1	T1/2, N1, M0	II
	T3a/3b, Any N, M0	
-	T4a, Any N, M0	III
-	T4b, Any N, M0	IVA
-	Any T, Any N, M1	IVB

AJCC, American Joint Committee on Cancer; *DTC*, differentiated thyroid carcinoma; *TNM*, tumor-node-metastasis.
Data from Amin MB, Edge SB, Greene FI, et al. *AJCC Cancer Staging Manual*. 8th ed. New York: Springer; 2018.

early 2018, is summarized in Table 73.4. The 8th edition has made a number of major changes that better optimize prediction and stratification of patient survival.[43] These include the following:

1. The age cutoff for staging, which was originally established to reflect the survival benefit of younger age, was increased from 45 to 55 years at diagnosis.
2. Minimal extrathyroidal extension detected only on histologic examination—as opposed to gross extrathyroidal extension—was removed from the definition of T3 disease, effectively eliminating this factor from staging.
3. N1 (regional nodal) disease no longer upstages a patient ≥55 years to stage III.
4. T3a is a new category for tumors >4 cm confined to the thyroid gland.
5. T3b is a new category for tumors of any size demonstrating gross extrathyroidal extension into the strap muscles.
6. Level VII lymph nodes were reclassified as central neck lymph nodes (N1a) as opposed to lateral neck lymph nodes to be more anatomically consistent.
7. The presence of distant metastases in patients ≥55 years was reclassified from stage IVC to stage IVB.

The downstream effect of the changes made to the 8th edition is to downstage many patients; as a result, patients with higher-stage disease experience a worse prognosis in the new system, thus better discriminating prognosis between stages and more accurately reflecting the overall relatively low risk of thyroid cancer mortality. Under the 8th edition, the estimated disease-specific survival in younger patients is expected to be 98% to 100% for stage I and 85% to 95% for stage II, and in older patients >55 years 98% to 100%, 85% to 95%, 60% to 70%, and less than 50% for stage I, II, III, and IV disease, respectively.[44]

Although systems such as TNM are important for making initial estimates of disease-specific mortality, the fact remains that the vast majority of patients will have excellent long-term survival. Therefore, what is arguably more clinically relevant to patients with DTC is the risk of disease recurrence, which is an outcome that systems such as TNM are not designed to measure. In response, the ATA proposed in its 2009 guidelines a system for estimating the initial risk of recurrence based on a number of clinicopathologic features, with a three-tiered risk classification that stratified patients into low-risk (~3%), intermediate-risk (~21%), and high-risk (~68%) categories.[45] In the 2015 updated guidelines, it was acknowledged that even within these three tiers, the level of risk depends on many individual tumor

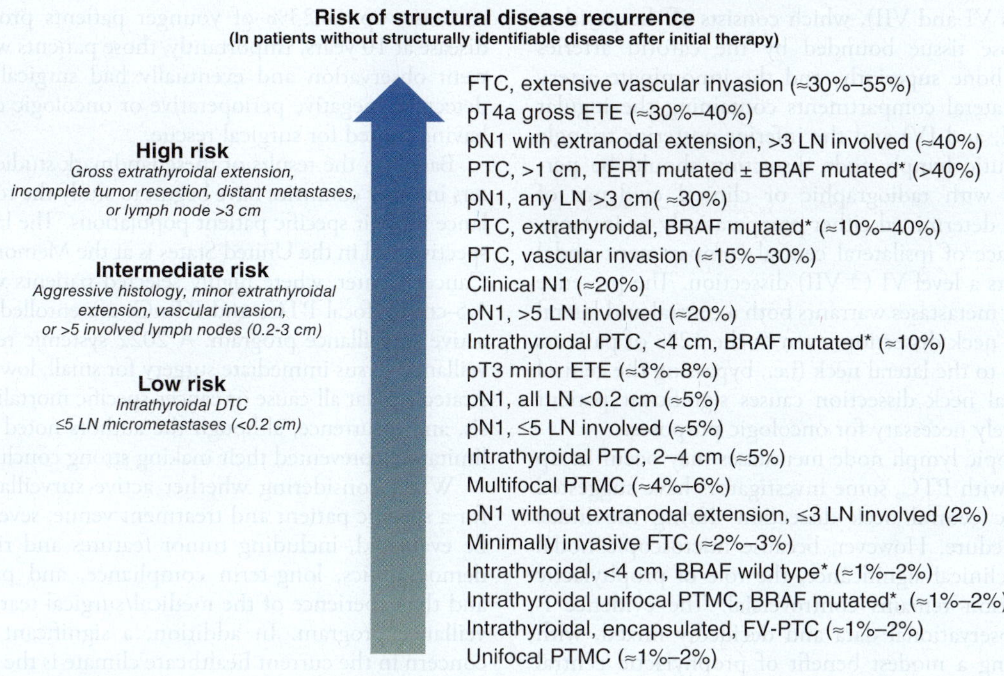

Risk of structural disease recurrence
(In patients without structurally identifiable disease after initial therapy)

High risk
*Gross extrathyroidal extension,
incomplete tumor resection, distant metastases,
or lymph node >3 cm*

Intermediate risk
*Aggressive histology, minor extrathyroidal
extension, vascular invasion,
or >5 involved lymph nodes (0.2-3 cm)*

Low risk
*Intrathyroidal DTC
≤5 LN micrometastases (<0.2 cm)*

FTC, extensive vascular invasion (≈30%–55%)
pT4a gross ETE (≈30%–40%)
pN1 with extranodal extension, >3 LN involved (≈40%)
PTC, >1 cm, TERT mutated ± BRAF mutated* (>40%)
pN1, any LN >3 cm(≈30%)
PTC, extrathyroidal, BRAF mutated* (≈10%–40%)
PTC, vascular invasion (≈15%–30%)
Clinical N1 (≈20%)
pN1, >5 LN involved (≈20%)
Intrathyroidal PTC, <4 cm, BRAF mutated* (≈10%)
pT3 minor ETE (≈3%–8%)
pN1, all LN <0.2 cm (≈5%)
pN1, ≤5 LN involved (≈5%)
Intrathyroidal PTC, 2–4 cm (≈5%)
Multifocal PTMC (≈4%–6%)
pN1 without extranodal extension, ≤3 LN involved (2%)
Minimally invasive FTC (≈2%–3%)
Intrathyroidal, <4 cm, BRAF wild type* (≈1%–2%)
Intrathyroidal unifocal PTMC, BRAF mutated*, (≈1%–2%)
Intrathyroidal, encapsulated, FV-PTC (≈1%–2%)
Unifocal PTMC (≈1%–2%)

FIGURE 73.24 The risk of structural disease recurrence for differentiated thyroid cancer after initial therapy exists on a continuum of risk estimates. The three-tiered American Thyroid Association modified initial risk stratification system is shown in the left-hand column. *ETE,* Extrathyroidal extension; *FTC,* follicular thyroid cancer; *FV-PTC,* follicular variant papillary thyroid cancer; *LN,* lymph node; *PTC,* papillary thyroid cancer; *PTMC,* papillary thyroid microcarcinoma. (From Haugen BR, Alexander EK, Bible KC, et al. 2015 American Thyroid Association management guidelines for adult patients with thyroid nodules and differentiated thyroid cancer: the American Thyroid Association Guidelines Task Force on Thyroid Nodules and Differentiated Thyroid Cancer. *Thyroid.* 2016;26:1-133.)

characteristics and actually exists on a continuum (Fig. 73.24). Molecular testing and profiling will likely enhance clinical staging systems.

The ATA guidelines have proposed a system that dynamically changes the initial risk estimates based on the clinical course of disease and response to therapy.[19] The four response-to-initial-therapy categories in this system include the following:

1. "Excellent response": no clinical, biochemical, or structural evidence of disease (translating to a 1%–4% risk of recurrence)
2. "Biochemical incomplete response": abnormal Tg or rising anti-Tg antibody levels in the absence of localizable disease (translating to 50% achieving no-evidence-of-disease status either spontaneously or with additional therapy and a 20% risk of developing structural disease)
3. "Structural incomplete response": persistent or newly identified locoregional or distant metastases (disease-specific mortality as high as 11% with locoregional disease and 50% with distant metastases)
4. "Indeterminate response": nonspecific biochemical or structural findings that cannot be confidently classified as either benign or malignant, including patients with stable or declining anti-Tg antibody levels without definitive structural evidence of disease (15%–20% will have structural disease identified during follow-up)

Surgical Management

Surgery is the mainstay of therapy for DTC. With the appropriate choice of operation and in the hands of a high-volume surgeon (see later), thyroidectomy is extremely safe and effective. The appropriate extent of thyroidectomy depends on multiple

factors, including the extent of disease and the patient's perioperative risk, with official recommendations evolving over the past several years.

In the past, total thyroidectomy was the traditionally recommended treatment for the majority of DTCs that measure at least 1 cm. However, ipsilateral thyroid lobectomy has become an acceptable alternative to total thyroidectomy for low-risk unilateral DTCs between 1 and 4 cm without extrathyroidal extension or evidence of metastatic disease, and it is the recommended surgical option for DTCs that are less than 1 cm. This shift in recommendations resulted from data in large observational database studies demonstrating equivalent survival between selected patients undergoing either total thyroidectomy or lobectomy for DTCs between 1 and 4 cm.[46] Thus, total thyroidectomy is now the preferred evidence-based approach only for those DTCs at higher risk for recurrence and/or disease-specific mortality. Such scenarios include the following:

- Tumor ≥4 cm
- Clinically evident nodal metastases
- Gross extrathyroidal extension
- Evidence of metastatic disease
- Radiation-induced DTC
- Familial nonmedullary thyroid cancer
- Multifocal bilateral DTC

In addition to total thyroidectomy for DTCs with clinical and/or radiographic evidence of cervical lymph node metastases, therapeutic compartment-based lymph node dissection is recommended. The lymph node compartments in the neck follow a standardized nomenclature, which is shown in Fig. 73.3. The most relevant nodal stations for thyroid cancer include the central compartment (levels VI and VII), which consists of the perithyroidal lymphoadipose tissue bounded by the carotid arteries laterally, the hyoid bone superiorly, and the innominate artery inferiorly, and the lateral compartments containing the jugular groups (levels II, III, and IV) and the inferior posterior triangle (level Vb). Therapeutic lymph node dissection should be performed in patients with radiographic or clinical evidence of metastatic disease as determined either preoperatively or intraoperatively. The presence of ipsilateral central compartment nodal involvement warrants a level VI (±VII) dissection. The presence of lateral neck nodal metastases warrants both a central and lateral compartment-based neck dissection, even in the 12% of patients with skip metastases to the lateral neck (i.e., bypassing the central neck nodes). Radical neck dissection causes significant patient morbidity and is rarely necessary for oncologic purposes.

Because microscopic lymph node metastases may occur in up to 80% of patients with PTC, some investigators have suggested routine prophylactic central neck dissection during the index thyroidectomy procedure. However, because microscopic nodal disease is rarely of clinical significance, the role of prophylactic central neck dissection remains controversial. The evidence is largely based on observational data and decidedly mixed, with some studies showing a modest benefit of prophylactic central neck dissection in reducing long-term locoregional recurrence. However, central neck dissection has been associated with a higher risk of temporary and permanent hypoparathyroidism, although this effect is blunted when the operation is performed by experienced surgeons.[47] Currently, the ATA guidelines suggest that prophylactic central neck dissection should be considered for certain higher-risk patients with cN0 papillary thyroid carcinomas with more advanced primary tumors (T3 or T4) and clinically involved lateral neck nodes and/or if the information would be helpful in guiding additional therapy.

For locally invasive primary tumors involving structures such as the strap muscles, trachea, esophagus, larynx, and RLN, careful preoperative planning with cross-sectional imaging and (rarely) endoscopic studies is critical (see earlier). Consultation and assistance from allied specialties, including thoracic surgery and otolaryngology, are recommended for complex tumors requiring segmental laryngotracheal or esophageal resection. The oncologically ideal goal of gross total resection of all visible tumor should be balanced against the potential life-changing morbidity of radical resections.

Active Nonoperative Surveillance of Papillary Thyroid Cancer

Despite advances in the management of higher-risk cancers as described earlier, arguably the most striking advance in the management of DTC in the past decade has been the dramatic deescalation of treatment for smaller thyroid cancers, which now includes nonoperative active surveillance for PTmCs, tumors smaller than 1 cm.

This treatment option has been best studied in the Japanese population. The initial report published in 2010 by Ito and colleagues[48] studied 340 patients with unilateral PTmCs who underwent once- or twice-yearly ultrasound and observation/surveillance over a mean period of 74 months. The proportion of patients in whom the tumors grew by 3 mm or more was 16% at 10 years and in whom new cervical nodal metastases were detected was 3.4% at 10 years.[48] A subsequent report by the same group of 1235 patients undergoing observation showed that patients >60 years had extremely slow progression to any form of clinical disease, with an overall rate of 2.5% at 10 years. In contrast, up to 23% of younger patients progressed to clinical disease at 10 years. Importantly, those patients who initially underwent observation and eventually had surgical resection had no detectable negative perioperative or oncologic consequences from having waited for surgical rescue.

Based on the results of these landmark studies from Japan, centers in other countries have begun to study the role of active surveillance in their specific patient populations. The largest ongoing prospective trial in the United States is at the Memorial Sloan-Kettering Cancer Center, where highly selected patients with no more than 1.5-cm unifocal PTCs and PTmCs are enrolled into a regimented active surveillance program. A 2022 systemic review of active surveillance versus immediate surgery for small, low-risk DTC demonstrated similar all-cause or cancer-specific mortality, distant metastasis, and recurrence, although the authors noted that methodologic limitations prevented their making strong conclusions.[49]

When considering whether active surveillance is appropriate for a specific patient and treatment venue, several attributes must be evaluated, including tumor features and risk profile; patient demographics, long-term compliance, and patient preferences; and the experience of the medical/surgical team running the surveillance program. In addition, a significant and controversial concern in the current healthcare climate is the geography-specific cost-effectiveness implications of long-term surveillance versus surgery.[50] Further research is needed to better identify those lowest-risk patients in whom active surveillance would benefit the most, possibly with the incorporation of molecular testing.

Postoperative Thyroid-Stimulating Hormone Suppression

In many patients after thyroidectomy for DTC, TSH suppressive doses of thyroid hormone medication are recommended to prevent hypothyroidism and to reduce the risk of TSH-stimulated tumor growth and recurrence. TSH suppression has been shown to improve overall survival in patients with stage II, III, and IV cancer; however, the degree of suppression required for survival benefit remains a point of controversy, and overall, there has been a trend toward less aggressive suppression over time.[51]

The TSH goals depend on both the risk of recurrence after initial treatment and the presence of comorbid conditions that may increase the risks of hyperthyroidism, such as older age, atrial fibrillation, and osteoporosis. For patients with low- to intermediate-risk tumors, serum TSH can initially be maintained between 0.1 and 0.5 mU/L, whereas patients with high-risk tumors should be kept initially at a TSH level of <0.1 mU/L if possible. The TSH level also may be allowed to increase closer to the normal range in patients who have an excellent response to therapy.

Radioactive Iodine

RAI therapy with ^{131}I for DTC relies on thyroid follicular cells' unique ability to take up iodine (see "Normal Thyroid Physiology," earlier). DTC is generally very iodine avid, at least initially, albeit at a lesser degree than normal thyroid follicular cells because of reduced expression of the sodium-iodide symporter. Thus, RAI is a useful adjunct in the treatment of PTC and FTC—as well as certain cases of OCA—despite its relative iodine nonavidity, whereas it plays no role in cancers that do not take up iodine, such as PDTC, MTC, and ATC.

In DTC, RAI is typically administered after thyroidectomy. There are generally two broad indications for RAI. The first indication is to ablate any residual normal thyroid tissue remaining after thyroidectomy. The rationale for this is threefold: (1) the elimination of normal thyroid tissue increases the specificity of both postoperative serum Tg and subsequent ^{131}I scanning for detection of recurrent disease, (2) remnant ablation prevents subsequent de novo thyroid cancer formation in the remnant tissue, and (3) it can be used at higher doses to treat microscopic disease as adjuvant therapy to prevent clinical recurrences. The second indication for RAI is to treat clinically detectable disease that cannot be addressed by surgery.

The role for postthyroidectomy RAI has become much more selective in the past decade, largely because of convincing evidence of the lack of benefit of RAI in patient with low-risk DTC. These patients include those with intrathyroidal tumors smaller than 4 cm without high-risk histologic features or small multifocal cancers. Multiple large database studies and systematic reviews have demonstrated no benefit of RAI in these patients with respect to either disease recurrence or mortality. In 2022, a randomized controlled trial found no benefit in terms of disease-free survival for patients with low-risk PTCs treated with total thyroidectomy and RAI versus total thyroidectomy alone.[52] However, the literature suggests some benefit of RAI for intermediate-risk patients. For example, a 21,870-patient study from the National Cancer Database demonstrated a 29% reduction in the risk of death in intermediate-risk thyroid cancer, with an even greater benefit in younger patients.[53] Further research is necessary to determine the specific subgroups in the intermediate-risk category that would benefit the most. RAI is routinely recommended for high-risk cancers to potentially decrease rates of recurrence and death. When considering ^{131}I therapy, postoperative serum Tg level and neck ultrasound can be considered: The risk of persistent or recurrent disease in cases with undetectable Tg levels (<0.2 ng/mL with thyroid hormone replacement or <1 ng/mL after TSH stimulation) in the absence of Tg antibodies with a normal neck ultrasound is very low.

RAI should be administered in patients in a low-iodine state and in a setting of high TSH levels to stimulate maximal iodine uptake by thyroid tissue. Two methods of TSH stimulation exist: administration of recombinant human TSH (rhTSH) and thyroid hormone withdrawal. The dose of RAI administered depends on the risk profile of the thyroid cancer and the indication(s) for RAI. Generally, remnant ablation doses of RAI fall in the 30 to 50 mCi range, whereas treatment-level doses are typically in the 100 to 150 mCi range. As long as there is evidence that thyroid cancer remains iodine-avid, repeated treatments with RAI are appropriate, assuming acceptable toxicity profiles. Dosimetry also can be used to help guide dosing regimens that optimize therapeutic activity while minimizing toxicity. The adverse effects of RAI include sialadenitis, nasolacrimal duct obstruction, transient tumor/thyroid swelling, infertility, and development of secondary malignancies (particularly leukemia); the risks of all of these occurrences are dose dependent. The maximal cumulative lifetime exposure to RAI is somewhat controversial but generally approximates 600 mCi. Pregnancy and breastfeeding are absolute contraindications to RAI.

Adjuvant Therapies

External beam radiotherapy (EBRT) plays a limited but important palliative role for selected situations in DTC. There are no randomized clinical trials, and EBRT practice patterns vary, so many of the recommendations rely on expert opinion and single-institution studies. The main indications for EBRT include local control of unresectable locally advanced macroscopic or microscopic residual disease after thyroidectomy (particularly in tumors thought to be RAI nonavid and affecting the aerodigestive tract)

as well as treatment of symptomatic distant metastatic foci that are RAI nonavid.

Other treatment options for local control of recurrent and/or metastatic disease exist in a limited number of centers. These include percutaneous ethanol or radiofrequency ablation for cervical nodal metastases, radiofrequency ablation of lung or bone metastases, and palliative embolization of bone metastases. In addition, there is much research activity around newer targeted systemic therapies for RAI-refractory disease (see later).

Targeted therapies. Most targeted therapies consist of TKIs. TKIs are typically reserved for patients with iodine-refractory disease because they are not curative therapy, and they can have significant side effects, including on the cardiac, renal, and hematologic systems, leading to a decrease in quality of life.[54] If available, use of genetic or molecular profiling of the tumor should be performed to identify potential therapeutic targets for a selective inhibitors against BRAF (e.g., dabrafenib), NTRK (e.g., larotrectinib, entrectinib), RET (e.g., selpercatinib, pralsetinib), or other kinases (e.g., RAS, MEK, FGFR). If no mutational targets are identified, patients are eligible for multikinase inhibitor therapy such as sorafenib, lenvatinib, cabozantinib, vandetanib, or sunitinib. These medications block several pathways responsible for tumor proliferation and survival but are considered "tumoristatic," as they eventually lose their responsiveness to tumor resistance. MKIs are typically considered for patients in whom the sum of tumor diameter is ≥2 cm and the lesions have progressed in the last 12 months or for patients suffering from DTC-related symptoms.[55] Recent interest has grown about what is known as redifferentiation therapy for RAI-refractory DTC. As more than 40% of PTCs harbor a *BRAFV600E* mutation, and this is associated with downregulated expression of the of the Na-I symporter (NIS), these tumors are often less sensitive to RAI. Some preclinical studies have shown redifferentiation of cells through inhibition of BRAF or MEK, thus promoting NIS restoration and RAI avidity. However, a recent phase III trial of the MEK1-2, RAS, and *BRAFV600E* inhibitor selumetinib did not improve the complete response rate in high-risk patients with DTC.[56]

Follow-up

After initial treatment of DTC, most patients are seen at 3- to 6-month intervals with biochemical testing and ultrasonography. ATA low-risk patients are expected to do well with low recurrence rates that would probably not be apparent for at least 3 to 5 years. Therefore, they return for follow-up in the first 6 to 12 months with serum lab testing (Tg antibody levels, thyroid function tests) and neck ultrasound. Follow-up then becomes less frequent if they demonstrate excellent response to therapy. ATA intermediate-risk patients also are followed at 6-month intervals with biochemical testing and more intensive ultrasound follow-up than ATA low-risk patients. ATA high-risk patients are evaluated every 2 to 3 months, using the same biochemical testing but with appropriate cross-sectional or functional imaging studies. Because of the more aggressive nature of their tumor, treatment response can be evaluated in the first 6 to 12 months for ATA high-risk patients, allowing timely, tailored changes to management.

The use of Tg as a marker in patients who have not undergone total thyroidectomy is an area of controversy. A recent systematic review and meta-analysis of Tg levels in patients who underwent thyroid lobectomy alone, total thyroidectomy alone, or total thyroidectomy followed by RAI revealed that the clinical utility of Tg measurement to identify recurrent or metastatic disease was low after partial thyroidectomy.[57] After total thyroidectomy, a cutoff of >1 to 2.5 ng/mL had high sensitivity for recurrent or metastatic disease.

Medullary Thyroid Cancer

MTC is an uncommon thyroid malignancy, comprising only 2% of all incident thyroid cancers in the United States.[31] Hazard and colleagues first coined the term *medullary* in 1959 to describe a unique thyroid tumor with nonfollicular characteristics and amyloid-containing stroma. Unlike DTC, MTC arises from the neuroendocrine parafollicular C cells, which secrete the polypeptide calcitonin (Fig. 73.25). MTC usually occurs as a sporadic tumor, but 25% of cases, on average, occur in the context of hereditary syndromes linked to germline mutations in the *RET* proto-oncogene, such as MEN types 2A and 2B (MEN2A and MEN2B, respectively) as well as familial MTC syndrome.

Clinical Presentation

The typical clinical presentation of MTC depends on whether the disease is sporadic or hereditary. Sporadic MTC usually presents

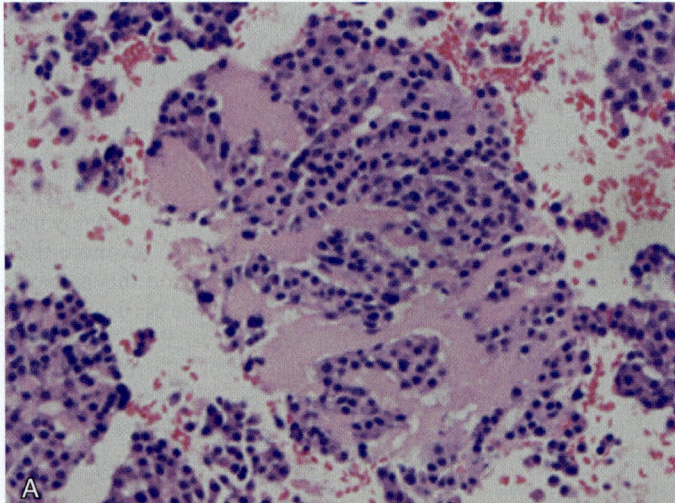

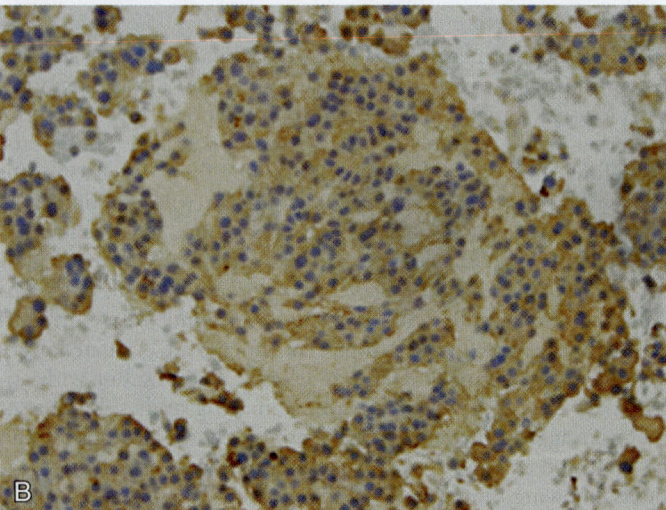

FIGURE 73.25 Medullary thyroid cancer (MTC). (A) Hematoxylin and eosin (H&E) staining of an MTC specimen showing plasmacytoid morphology with eccentric round nuclei, "salt-and-pepper" chromatin, small nucleoli, and amyloid infiltrate. (B) MTC exhibits cytoplasmic positivity on calcitonin staining. (Courtesy Elham Khanafshar, MD, MS, Department of Pathology and Laboratory Medicine, University of California, San Francisco.)

between the fourth and sixth decades of life; the most common presentation (occurring in up to 50% of cases) is a palpable neck mass from the primary tumor itself or from associated lymphadenopathy. These tumors are usually unifocal and, based on the distribution of C cells in the thyroid, often arise in the superior lateral thyroid lobes. In patients with sporadic MTC with a palpable thyroid nodule, cervical nodal metastases are present in up to over 70% of cases and distant metastases in 10% to 15% of cases. The most common locations of distant metastasis are the liver, mediastinum, lungs, and bone.

Hereditary MTC presents at a younger age compared with sporadic MTC; patients with familial MTC or MEN2A typically present in the third decade of life, and patients with MEN2B present before the second decade. Depending on the specific *RET* mutation, hereditary MTC can present very early in life within the first months to year (see later). Unlike in sporadic MTC, hereditary MTC often presents as multifocal disease. Fortunately, most patients with hereditary MTC are now identified at an earlier age by genetic screening of at-risk family members (see later). Hereditary MTC also can present during the diagnosis and workup of an associated disease, such as pheochromocytoma or primary hyperparathyroidism.

In both sporadic and hereditary MTC, elevated levels of circulating calcitonin can lead to diarrhea, flushing, and weight loss. Uncommonly, MTC also can produce a number of other hormones, such as carcinoembryonic antigen (CEA), adrenocorticotrophic hormone, chromogranin, and somatostatin, which can lead to paraneoplastic syndromes such as Cushing and carcinoid syndromes.

RET and Medullary Thyroid Cancer

The *RET* proto-oncogene is the most important gene associated with MTC. *RET* is located on chromosome 10q11.2 and encodes a transmembrane tyrosine kinase receptor with regulatory effects on cell growth and survival. Virtually all patients with a hereditary form of MTC have one of over 100 described germline mutations in *RET,* with each mutation portending a unique profile of MTC aggressiveness and frequency of other syndromic manifestations (e.g., pheochromocytoma, primary hyperparathyroidism, cutaneous lichen amyloidosis, and Hirschsprung disease). Mutations in codon C634 are the most common.

The 2015 revised ATA guidelines around the management of MTC proposed a modified risk classification system for hereditary MTC aggressiveness based mainly on the type of *RET* mutation identified in order to better inform the timing of prophylactic thyroidectomy in affected family members.[4] This classification has three risk categories: highest risk, high risk, and moderate risk. The highest-risk category includes patients with MEN2B and the codon M918T mutation in whom macroscopic MTC and nodal metastases can present within the first year of life; in these patients, total thyroidectomy is recommended as soon as possible in the first few months of life. The high-risk category comprises patients with the codon C634 and A883F mutations in whom thyroidectomy is recommended by the age of 5 years or sooner in the presence of elevated serum calcitonin levels. The moderate-risk category includes patients with all other mutations in whom either annual surveillance or thyroidectomy may be pursued. Fig. 73.26 shows the ATA management algorithm for patients with *RET* germline mutations.

RET testing in sporadic MTC is also important in two respects. First, apparently sporadic MTCs may in fact be the initial manifestation of a hereditary syndrome. Therefore, all patients

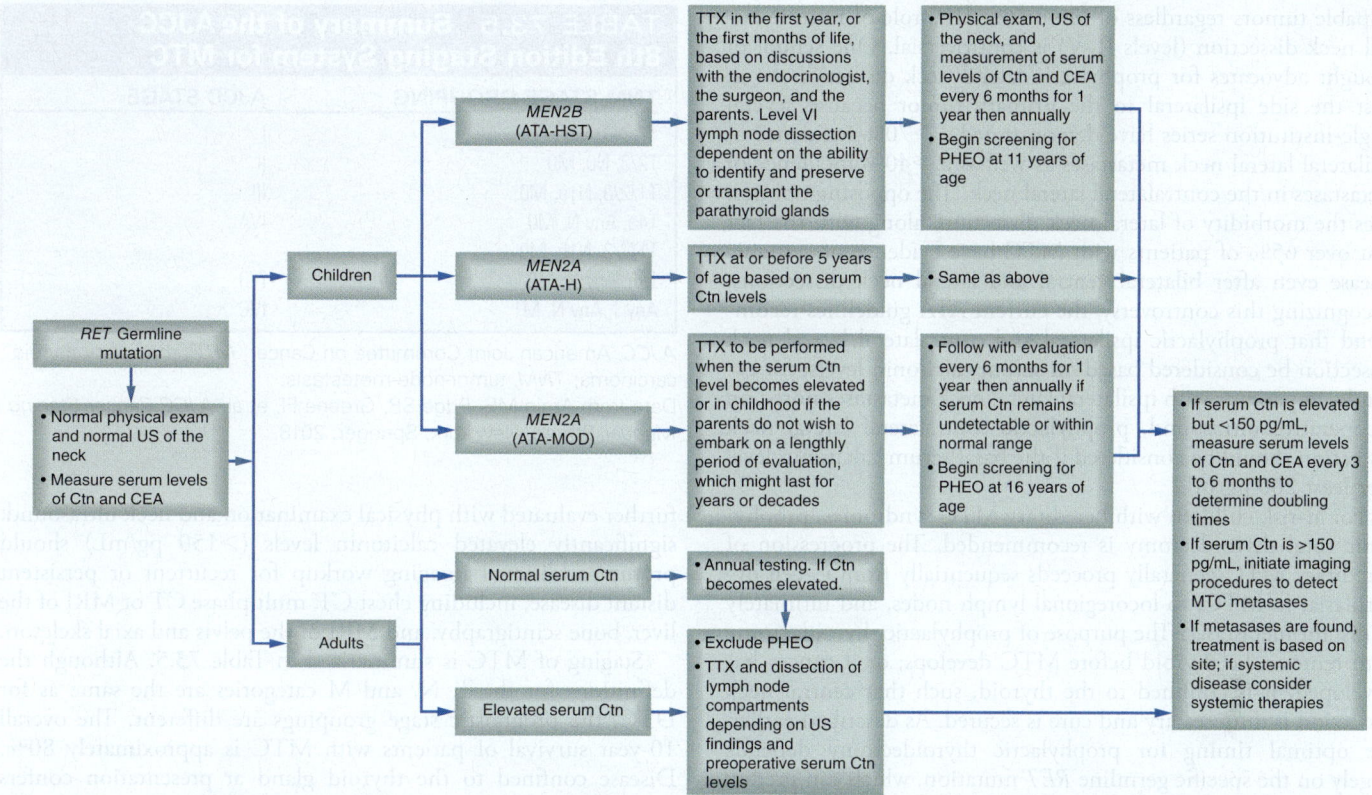

FIGURE 73.26 Recommended management of patients at risk for hereditary medullary thyroid cancer (MTC) based on positive *RET* germline mutation detected on genetic screening. *ATA-MOD*, American Thyroid Association Moderate Risk; *ATA-H*, American Thyroid Association High Risk; *ATA-HST*, American Thyroid Association Highest Risk; *CEA*, carcinoembryonic antigen; *Ctn*, calcitonin; *MEN2*, multiple endocrine neoplasia type 2; *PHEO*, pheochromocytoma; *TTX*, total thyroidectomy. (From Wells SA Jr, Asa SL, Dralle H, et al. Revised American Thyroid Association guidelines for the management of medullary thyroid carcinoma. *Thyroid.* 2015;25:567-610.)

with a diagnosis of MTC or C-cell hyperplasia should undergo genetic testing to rule out hereditary disease. Second, approximately 50% of sporadic MTCs have somatic *RET* mutations, which are associated with a higher incidence of nodal metastases, persistent disease, and disease-specific mortality. Therefore, they warrant more aggressive surveillance and treatment.

Workup

MTC can be definitively diagnosed by FNA biopsy, from which cytology can demonstrate the presence of stromal amyloid and absence of thyroid follicular cells. Measurement of elevated calcitonin levels in the FNA washout fluid increases the accuracy of FNA to 98%. Once MTC is diagnosed, measurement of serum calcitonin and CEA is recommended to establish a pretreatment baseline. Measurement of serum calcitonin and CEA as a screening test in the absence of cytologically confirmed MTC, on the other hand, is controversial. ATA guidelines recommend that a serum calcitonin of at least 100 pg/mL should be considered suspicious for MTC. In addition, a calcitonin value of at least 500 pg/mL before treatment should raise the suspicion for distant metastases. Notably, serum calcitonin can be elevated because of multiple states other than MTC, including autoimmune thyroiditis, hyperparathyroidism, lung cancer, and age <3 years. Serum CEA is not a specific biomarker for MTC and thus is more useful as an adjunctive test. CEA is often elevated in more aggressive MTCs that have lost calcitonin secretory function, thus acting as a marker for dedifferentiation. Measurement of

both serum calcitonin and CEA is recommended to establish a pretreatment baseline and to track disease progression.

Neck ultrasound is the most important preoperative imaging study in MTC in that it provides sensitive characterization of thyroid lesions and cervical lymph nodes. Cross-sectional imaging of the neck and chest (preferably CT with IV contrast) may be indicated depending on the suspicion for bulky or locally advanced disease. In higher-risk patients such as those with high-burden cervical disease, symptoms suspicious for distant metastases, or serum calcitonin levels ≥500 pg/mL, radiographic survey for distant metastases should be performed. The most common tests include multiphase CT or MRI of the liver, axial MRI, and bone scintigraphy.

All patients with hereditary MTC should be biochemically screened for pheochromocytoma and primary hyperparathyroidism. If a pheochromocytoma is identified, treatment for the pheochromocytoma should precede that of MTC in virtually all cases. Primary hyperparathyroidism can be surgically managed at the time of thyroidectomy for MTC if present concurrently.

Surgical Treatment

The surgical treatment for MTC is divided into that for clinically evident disease versus that performed as a prophylactic measure at an early age in hereditary MTC syndromes.

Clinically evident MTC is treated with, at a minimum, total thyroidectomy and bilateral central neck dissection, as central nodal metastases are present in more than 70% of cases with palpable tumors regardless of tumor size. The role of routine lateral neck dissection (levels II–V) is controversial. One school of thought advocates for prophylactic lateral neck dissection on at least the side ipsilateral to the primary tumor because several single-institution series have demonstrated a >70% incidence of ipsilateral lateral neck metastases as well as a >40% incidence of metastases in the contralateral lateral neck. The opposing opinion cites the morbidity of lateral neck dissection, along with the fact that over 65% of patients with MTC have evidence of systemic disease even after bilateral central and lateral neck dissections. Recognizing this controversy, the current ATA guidelines recommend that prophylactic ipsilateral and contralateral lateral neck dissection be considered based on serum calcitonin levels; for example, in patients with ipsilateral lateral neck metastases noted on preoperative ultrasound, prophylactic contralateral lateral neck dissection should be considered if the basal serum calcitonin level is at least 200 pg/mL.

For at-risk children with hereditary MTC syndromes, prophylactic total thyroidectomy is recommended. The progression of hereditary MTC generally proceeds sequentially from C-cell hyperplasia, to MTC, to locoregional lymph nodes, and ultimately to distant metastases. The purpose of prophylactic thyroidectomy is to remove the thyroid before MTC develops; or if cancer has developed, it is confined to the thyroid, such that central neck dissection is unnecessary and cure is secured. As described earlier, the optimal timing for prophylactic thyroidectomy depends largely on the specific germline *RET* mutation, which can predict typical age of MTC onset as well as aggressiveness of disease. This must be balanced with the risk of surgical complications in children and infants, which are elevated compared with adolescents and adults even in the hands of experienced surgeons.[58]

Management of the parathyroid glands during thyroidectomy in patients with MEN2A is unique because of the 20% penetrance of primary hyperparathyroidism. As mentioned earlier, screening for primary hyperparathyroidism should be done before thyroidectomy. For biochemically diagnosed primary hyperparathyroidism, a four-gland exploration should be performed at the time of thyroidectomy, with intentional resection performed only for enlarged glands. Most cases of primary hyperparathyroidism in MEN2 involve a single parathyroid adenoma. If a normal parathyroid gland is devascularized during surgery, it should be autotransplanted into a heterotopic site (e.g., the nondominant forearm) for ease of access because of the risk of primary hyperparathyroidism developing in the transplanted tissue later in life.

For patients with familial MTC, MEN2B, or sporadic MTC undergoing thyroidectomy, devascularized parathyroids may be autotransplanted into the sternocleidomastoid because these patients are not at increased risk for primary hyperparathyroidism.

Postoperative Surveillance and Prognosis

MTC is associated with an overall 50% rate of disease recurrence; therefore, close postoperative monitoring should begin as soon as 3 months after surgery with a check of serum calcitonin and CEA levels. If these values are negative or in the normal range, they should be repeated at 6-month intervals for the first year and then annually thereafter. The doubling time of calcitonin (and to a lesser extent CEA) is an accurate estimate of MTC growth as well as a prognostic indicator. A calcitonin doubling time of less than 6 months is associated with a 5-year survival rate of 25%, compared with 92% if the doubling time is ≥6 months.[59] Elevated calcitonin levels raise the suspicion of recurrence and should be

TABLE 73.5   Summary of the AJCC 8th Edition Staging System for MTC

TNM STAGE GROUPING	AJCC STAGE
T1, N0, M0	I
T2/3, N0, M0	II
T1/2/3, N1a, M0	III
T4a, Any N, M0	IVA
T1/2/3, N1b, M0	
T4b, Any N, M0	IVB
Any T, Any N, M1	IVC

AJCC, American Joint Committee on Cancer; *MTC,* medullary thyroid carcinoma; *TNM,* tumor-node-metastasis.
Data from Amin MB, Edge SB, Greene FI, et al. *AJCC Cancer Staging Manual.* 8th ed. New York: Springer; 2018.

further evaluated with physical examination and neck ultrasound; significantly elevated calcitonin levels (>150 pg/mL) should prompt additional imaging workup for recurrent or persistent distant disease, including chest CT, multiphase CT or MRI of the liver, bone scintigraphy, and MRI of the pelvis and axial skeleton.

Staging of MTC is summarized in Table 73.5. Although the definitions for the T, N, and M categories are the same as for DTC, the prognostic stage groupings are different. The overall 10-year survival of patients with MTC is approximately 80%. Disease confined to the thyroid gland at presentation confers an excellent long-term prognosis with 5-year overall survival approaching 95%. The presence of cervical nodal metastases is associated with a reduction in survival to approximately 75%, and distant metastases are associated with compromised survival further to 35%.

Despite its widespread use, the current AJCC TNM staging system has been modeled largely after that used for DTC. However, MTC is inherently distinct from DTC, so the generalizability of one staging system to another is likely not appropriate. Adam and colleagues proposed a revision in the staging groups based on a recursive partitioning analysis using the National Cancer Database and the Surveillance, Epidemiology, and End Results (SEER) databases to better divide MTC patients into four groups with more similar overall survival.[60] The proposed revision led to a more useful and stepwise downward progression of survival estimates compared with the existing TNM system, with 5-year overall survival of 92% to 94%, 86% to 87%, 69% to 81%, and 33% to 35% for stages I, II, III, and IV disease, respectively.

Targeted therapy. The *RET* mutations that underlie many cases of MTC have been found to be an effective therapeutic target. *RET*-targeting TKIs have emerged as an effective targeted therapy, although resistance can occur. Currently, optimal timing for initiation of TKI in MTC is unclear, and ATA guidelines recommend initiating TKI therapy for patients with radiographic evidence of disease progression or symptomatic disease.[4]

TKIs for MTC can be multitargeted or *RET*-specific. Vandetanib and cabozantinib are two multitarget TKIs that have been approved by the US Food and Drug Administration (FDA). Both drugs demonstrated significantly longer progression-free survival for patients with locally advanced or metastatic MTC who received the treatment drug compared with placebo. Other multitarget TKIs that have been investigated in the treatment of MTC include sunitinib, sorafenib, lenvatinib, and anlotinib. More recently, the US FDA approved selpercatinib and pralsetinib for

RET-altered MTC because these TKIs are more RET-specific and have an improved side effect profile. However, patients can develop resistance to these newer TKIs as well. Future strategies in the treatment of MTC will need to address optimal timing of TKI therapy and ways to overcome resistance mutations.

Anaplastic Thyroid Cancer

ATC is an extremely aggressive undifferentiated tumor of follicular cell origin. ATC is uncommon, comprising approximately 1% of all thyroid cancers.[31] The mean age at diagnosis is 65 years, with a 2:1 female-to-male incidence ratio; a history of multinodular goiter and/or previous thyroidectomy exists in up to 50% of patients. ATC is thought to arise from DTC of follicular cell origin (particularly PTC), based on the coexistence of PTC in at least 30% of cases as well as longitudinal case studies demonstrating dedifferentiation and transformation from DTC to ATC over time. On a molecular level, the dedifferentiation event in ATC may involve mutations in the TP53 and PIK3CA genes or genes in the catenin family.

Patients with ATC typically present with a rapidly enlarging neck mass. Unlike in other thyroid tumors, local cervical symptoms are frequent and severe and include neck pain, dyspnea, cough/hemoptysis, dysphagia, and hoarseness. Over half of patients have cervical lymphadenopathy, and 15% to 50% of patients have distant metastases at the time of presentation. The most common sites of distant metastases include the lungs, bone, and brain; other sites may include the skin, liver, kidneys, pancreas, heart, and adrenal glands.

Diagnosis and Staging

Because of its rapidity in growth and spread, timely diagnosis is of the essence when ATC is suspected. Diagnosis can be confirmed with FNA (~60% cases), but this can often be challenging because of the lack of cell differentiation. When FNA is not diagnostic, core biopsy is typically helpful, particularly with ultrasound guidance to identify particular solid areas or those of most concern; incisional biopsy is typically not required.[61] Cytologic features of ATC include mixed patterns of spindled, pleomorphic giant, and squamoid cells with mitotic figures, atypical mitoses, and extensive necrosis. ATCs typically do not secrete or stain for Tg, although differentiated components of tumors may retain the ability to make Tg (Fig. 73.27). Staging for ATC should proceed expeditiously because of the rapid progression of disease. Imaging includes neck ultrasound and cross-sectional imaging of the neck and mediastinum to assess the extent of locoregional disease. Unlike in DTCs or MTCs, PET scan is recommended for a metastatic survey in the initial evaluation of ATC because of its intense PET avidity. Management of ATC should follow the 2021 ATA guidelines, which highlight the increasing role of molecular targeted therapies for patients with ATC.[61]

According to the AJCC TNM system, all ATCs are considered stage IV disease because it is the most lethal type of thyroid cancer, with 1-year overall survival of 20%. Prompt staging and multidisciplinary management are essential because of the associated high mortality. [18F]-FDG PET/CT of the whole body is preferred for staging ATC because it can identify metastases that may not be detected on CT alone. However, if PET/CT is not available, IV contrast-enhanced CT of the neck, chest, abdomen, and pelvis can be obtained. Although brain metastases are uncommon at presentation, they are associated with worse prognosis. Therefore, the ATA has recommended brain MRI as part of the initial staging algorithm for ATC when clinically indicated.

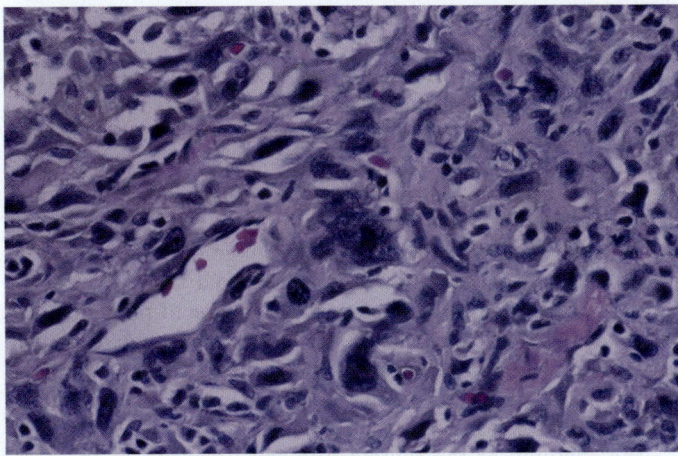

FIGURE 73.27 Anaplastic thyroid cancer. Hematoxylin and eosin staining showing marked nuclear pleomorphism, oval to spindle-shaped cells, and multinucleated tumor cell. (From Baloch ZW, Livolsi VA. Surgical pathology of the thyroid gland. In: Randolph GW, ed. *Surgery of the Thyroid and Parathyroid Glands 2.* Philadelphia: Elsevier Saunders; 2013:420.)

Surgical Management

Once diagnosis and staging of ATC are completed, resectability of the primary tumor should be evaluated. Patients with disease limited to the neck may be candidates for resection. Surgery should aim to achieve an R0 or R1 resection, which has been associated with longer survival. Extent of surgery typically involves total thyroidectomy with lymph node dissection. More radical resection to involve major vascular structures, esophagus, trachea, or larynx is generally not recommended because of the poor prognosis of ATC and should be discussed within a multidisciplinary team with consideration of molecular testing. Although a tracheostomy may be felt to be necessary as part of the initial surgery, especially depending on the extent of bilateral neck dissection, many patients with ATC do not require tracheostomy unless they endorse stridor or acute airway distress.

Adjuvant Therapy

Studies have demonstrated that survival and local disease control are optimized with R0/R1 resection, followed by radiotherapy and chemotherapy. Radiotherapy should aim to begin within 6 weeks after surgery. The 2021 ATA guidelines recommend cytotoxic chemotherapy involving a taxane, with or without anthracyclines or platin, in patients with ATC who receive definitive-intention radiation.

Targeted systemic therapies are increasingly being applied in ATC, especially for patients with advanced or initially unresectable disease. BRAF^V600E is the most common targetable mutation in ATC, and in 2018, dabrafenib/trametinib (BRAF/MEK inhibitor combination) was approved by the US FDA for use in BRAF^V600E-mutated ATC. BRAF-directed therapy can produce prompt tumor regression, and it is recommended for use in patients with distant metastases from BRAF^V600E-mutated ATC. Neoadjuvant use of BRAF/MEK inhibition has been explored to render an unresectable primary tumor resectable. Emerging data suggest that neoadjuvant BRAF inhibitory therapy followed by surgical resection can potentially lead to prolonged survival.

HISTORY OF THYROID SURGERY

The history of thyroid surgery began more than 1000 years ago.[62] Most records agree that the first thyroidectomy was performed for endemic goiter by the legendary surgeon Abu al-Qasim in 952 AD, although the patient was said to have barely survived because of torrential blood loss during the procedure. The majority of the ensuing millennium did not see encouraging advancements in either the understanding of the thyroid gland's function or its safe extirpation. In the 12th century, Roger Frugardii of the Italian Salerno school described a morbid method of thyroid removal involving the insertion of hot iron setons through the skin and into the gland, with gradual superficialization of the gland until the seton and thyroid tissue penetrated through the skin and were removed. This type of procedure exemplified what the early Catholic Church deemed to be the brutality and uncouthness of surgery, which led to a retreat of surgery from the mainstream of medicine and science during much of medieval European history.

The anatomy of the thyroid was first described in the early 16th century by Leonardo da Vinci; unfortunately, he did not understand the thyroid gland's function beyond its filling in an empty space in the neck between muscle layers in order to protect the trachea from the sternum. As the study of anatomy and surgery became more culturally acceptable during the Renaissance, additional incremental advancements in the understanding of thyroid anatomy occurred. The term *thyroid* was first coined by the anatomist Thomas Wharton in 1646; it was a derivation of the Greek word *thyreos,* or "shield."

Advancements in thyroid surgery were relatively few and far between until well into the 19th century. Wilhelm Fabricius described a case in the mid-1600s of a "rash" and "audacious doctor" who performed the first thyroidectomy using scalpels for a goiter in a 10-year-old female patient who died on the operating table; this surgeon was reported to have been imprisoned as a result. The first well-documented successful partial thyroidectomy was performed in 1791 by Pierre Joseph Desault during the French Revolution, and other surgeons reported small case series of successful thyroidectomies over the ensuing 50 years. Notable among them was the German surgeon Johann Hedenus, whose 0% mortality rate after the removal of six "suffocating" goiters was considered remarkable for the time. Despite this, thyroid surgery was still associated with (at a minimum) a 40% mortality rate in the early to mid-1800s, such that the leading surgical figures and professional associations of the time emphatically advised against performing thyroidectomy. Thyroid surgery was deemed by Liston "a proceeding by no means to be thought of," by Diffenbach as "most thankless, most perilous...foolhardy performances," and by Gross as "... horrid butchery. No honest and sensible surgeon would ever engage in it." The French Academy of Medicine frankly banned thyroid surgery during this time.

Starting in the mid-19th century and continuing on into the early 20th century, the course of thyroid surgery rapidly evolved from a dangerous and morbid endeavor into a safe, elegant, and modern practice. The practice of surgery as a whole advanced because of the triple developments of anesthesia, antisepsis/infection prophylaxis, and instrumentation for hemostasis. Thanks in large part to these innovations, the surgical giants of the day were able to more carefully study and refine surgical thyroidology. Theodor Billroth's foray into thyroid surgery was initially marked by 16 deaths among 36 thyroidectomies; however, he was able to dramatically reduce his mortality rate to 8% after introducing newer methods of hemostasis and antisepsis in his surgical practice. Theodor Kocher, Billroth's pupil, is widely regarded as the "father of modern thyroid surgery." He performed more than 5000 thyroidectomies during his career, with an associated mortality rate of 0.5%, which was widely attributed to his extreme meticulousness in antisepsis and hemostatic techniques. His remarkable surgical results as well as his seminal research contributions to the understanding of thyroid function led to his receiving the Nobel Prize in Medicine and Physiology in 1909, the first Nobel ever awarded to a surgeon. The Australian surgeon Thomas Dunhill is credited for his excellent results pioneering a safe bilateral operation of unilateral complete thyroid lobectomy with contralateral subtotal thyroid lobe resection for thyrotoxicosis, an operation that still bears his name today.

William Stewart Halsted's stature as the "father of modern surgery" and creator of the contemporary American surgical residency program makes it sometimes easy to overlook his many contributions to thyroid surgery. His research elucidated parathyroid blood supply as well as "ultraligation" of the distal thyroid artery branches to avoid parathyroid gland devascularization and avoid postoperative tetany. He also performed experiments that supported the mechanistic connection between hypoparathyroidism and tetany and its reversal with either calcium supplementation or parathyroid transplantation. Halsted further improved upon the techniques he learned from Billroth and Kocher by improving surgical instrumentation for hemostasis and introducing surgical gloves for sterile technique. Two of his trainees, George Crile and Frank Lahey, went on to become luminaries in thyroid surgery. Ultimately, Halsted wrote that thyroid surgery "typifies perhaps better than any other operation the supreme triumph of the surgeon's art."

Charles Mayo and his medical colleague Henry Plummer demonstrated the safe conduct of thyroidectomy for Graves disease with preoperative iodine preparation. Mayo's surgical volume and superlative outcomes far exceeded other contemporaries and led to his reputation for being the "father of American thyroid surgery."

Additional innovations over the past century have undoubtedly improved the conduct of modern thyroid surgery, but the influence around the turn of the 20th century of the previously mentioned luminaries, and particularly Kocher, remain unmatched.

THYROIDECTOMY

Indications and Nomenclature

Broadly speaking, the indications for thyroidectomy include the following:
1. Hyperthyroidism for which nonsurgical management has failed or is not preferred
2. Goiters with or without local compressive symptoms
3. Thyroid nodules and thyroid cancer

The extent of thyroid resection was a topic of much discussion historically, but in modern practice, the vast majority of thyroid resections fall under two categories: *total thyroidectomy,* in which all or nearly all of the visible thyroid gland is excised, and *thyroid lobectomy* (also referred to as *hemithyroidectomy*), in which all of the visible thyroid on one side is excised along with the isthmus and, if present, the pyramidal lobe. *Near-total thyroidectomy,* in which less than 1 g of remnant thyroid tissue is left at the ligament of Berry, is also commonly performed. *Subtotal thyroidectomy,* in which 3 to 5 g of thyroid tissue is left, is less commonly performed today. The rationale for these lesser-extent lobar resections has been to protect the RLN and blood supply to the parathyroids as well as to preserve thyroid function without the need for thyroid hormone replacement. Lastly, *isthmusectomy* is resection of only the thyroid isthmus and pyramidal lobe.

Thyroidectomy Outcomes

There are over 130,000 thyroidectomies performed annually in the United States, making thyroidectomy one of the most common surgical procedures. The rate of thyroidectomy was noted to increase in pace with the increased number of thyroid biopsies and diagnoses of thyroid cancer.[63] Deescalation of therapy for DTC has led to substantial reduction in the use of postthyroidectomy RAI and a slight increase in thyroid lobectomy compared with total thyroidectomy from 2000–18, although this is projected to continue to increase over time.[33] Thyroidectomy has evolved from a dangerous and morbid operation historically (see earlier) to a generally safe procedure, most of which likely can be performed safely in the outpatient setting.

Despite its safety, thyroidectomy is associated with a risk of complications such as RLN and EBSLN injury, hypoparathyroidism, and neck hematoma (see later), which, although rare, can nevertheless lead to significant patient morbidity and disability when they occur. Various efforts to minimize these complications and optimize thyroidectomy outcomes exist. One approach is to standardize the teaching and performance of thyroidectomy technique, such as that found in the *Operative Standards for Cancer Surgery* initiative by the American College of Surgeons, in an effort to minimize the potentially harmful effects of significant deviations of technique from evidence-based norms.[64]

Other efforts to study and improve thyroidectomy have focused on concentrating expertise and referral patterns into more experienced hands because surgeon experience measured by operative volume has been clearly established as an important and modifiable determinant of thyroidectomy outcomes. A large body of literature has demonstrated that higher-volume surgeons on average have fewer complications, shorter hospital stays, and lower costs. The threshold for what qualifies as a "high-volume" surgeon has been studied extensively; a recent study of 16,954 patients undergoing total thyroidectomy between 1998 and 2009 in the Nationwide Inpatient Sample database demonstrated on restricted cubic splines analysis that patient outcomes improved with increasing surgeon volume up to a threshold of 26 cases per year.[65] Data such as these will be important for setting minimum case volume thresholds for professional society credentialing and volume-based referral initiatives.

Preoperative Preparation

All patients undergoing thyroidectomy should have biochemical assessment of thyroid function as well as appropriate imaging studies, particularly neck ultrasound. As described in more detail earlier, thyroid nodular disease or malignancy should be assessed with FNA biopsy as indicated. For operations performed for hyperthyroidism, patients should ideally be rendered euthyroid by the time of operation with antithyroid medication with or without β-blockade, although the operation sometimes can be safely performed in a hyperthyroid state. For Graves disease, Lugol solution or SSKI also can be administered within 10 days of surgery per surgeon preference for rapid correction of thyroid function. Measurement of serum calcium levels should be performed in patients at risk for concurrent primary hyperparathyroidism, such as those with MEN2A.

Assessment of Voice and Laryngeal Function

Voice assessment is critical before thyroidectomy because vocal cord dysfunction is one of the most important complications of thyroid surgery. Vocal cord dysfunction can lead to significant decrement in quality of life, and it is one of the most frequent causes of medicolegal action. All preoperative voice assessments include a thorough patient history around voice changes and abnormalities, prior history of surgery that may have been associated with the risk of injury to the vagus verve or the RLN, and the surgeon's assessment of the voice.

Laryngoscopy is an indispensable tool in the objective preoperative assessment of vocal cord function and must be performed in patients at higher risk for vocal cord paralysis, including those with a history of voice changes or prior relevant surgical history or thyroid cancers with fixed masses, posteriorly extending extrathyroidal extension, or bulky metastases. The role of routine preoperative laryngoscopy for all patients regardless of risk assessment is controversial. Proponents of routine laryngoscopy in all patients cite (1) its ability to confirm preoperative vocal cord dysfunction in up to 3.5% of patients with benign thyroid disease and in up to 8% of patients with thyroid cancer; (2) its ability to definitively diagnose preoperative dysfunction is important for operative management in these cases, and (3) vocal cord paralysis can be associated with a normal voice in up to 20% of cases.[66] On the other hand, proponents of selective laryngoscopy state that the true incidence of preoperative vocal cord dysfunction in patients with a truly negative risk assessment by history and physical examination is closer to 0.5% and that subjecting all thyroid surgery patients to laryngoscopy is not cost-effective.[67]

Transcutaneous laryngeal ultrasound has emerged as a noninvasive alternative to laryngoscopy for assessment of vocal cord function in selected patients undergoing thyroidectomy. Studies in both Asian and Western patients have demonstrated high accuracy of laryngeal ultrasound for the detection of vocal cord paralysis (sensitivity and specificity 93%–100% and 97%–100%, respectively) as well as broad applicability in thyroid surgery practices, with over 74% of examinations able to adequately visualize the vocal cords for assessment.[68] In addition to its noninvasiveness, other advantages of this modality include its low cost, rapid learning curve, and increased efficiency if performed as part of another ultrasound examination. It is less reliable in older and male patients largely because of inability of the transducer to penetrate beyond thyroid cartilage calcification.

Current American Association for Endocrine Surgeons (AAES) guidelines for thyroid surgery recommend that all patients undergoing thyroid surgery have noninvasive preoperative voice assessment as a part of the physical examination, with the selective use of laryngoscopy for patients with preoperative voice abnormalities, history of cervical or upper chest surgery, or known thyroid cancer with posterior extrathyroidal extension or extensive nodal metastases.[69] Laryngeal ultrasound is mentioned as a potentially useful adjunct in the AAES guidelines.

Technique
Anesthesia and Positioning

Most thyroidectomies are performed under general endotracheal anesthesia. A neuromonitoring-specific endotracheal tube with contact electrodes for the vocal cords can be used if intraoperative neuromonitoring (IONM) is planned (see later). The patient is placed supine with both arms tucked. The back is raised 20 degrees, and the neck is extended by placing a soft roll behind the scapulae, with the head resting on a foam or gel ring; this brings the thyroid up to a more anterior and superior position in the neck, which is particularly helpful for glands that have substernal extension. The head is well supported to prevent neck hyperextension and postoperative posterior neck pain.

Intraoperative preincision neck ultrasound can be useful for confirming the findings of preoperative imaging and identifying any possible new findings as well as for assessing the overall anatomy of the thyroid to facilitate incision placement and operative planning.

Incision and Initial Exposure of the Thyroid

A centrally placed transverse incision is made between the sternal notch and the cricoid cartilage, with effort made to place the incision in a normal skin line of the neck for cosmetic purposes (Fig. 73.28). The length of the incision is typically 4 to 5 cm but should be sized based on the volume of the gland being excised as well as patient factors, such as body habitus and degree of neck extension. The incision is extended through the platysma muscle, and subplatysmal flaps are raised up to the thyroid cartilage superiorly and down to the sternal notch inferiorly. Care is taken to identify the anterior jugular veins draped between platysma and the strap muscles.

The strap muscles are separated in the midline via an incision through the superficial layer of the deep cervical fascia starting at the sternal notch and extending cephalad to the thyroid cartilage. For a cancer operation, dissection of the thyroid gland is generally begun on the side of the suspected tumor. The sternohyoid, which is the more superficial of the strap muscles, is separated from the

deeper sternothyroid muscle by blunt dissection. This dissection can be taken as far laterally until the ansa cervicalis is visible at the lateral border of the sternothyroid; this maneuver is useful for thyroid mobilization, particularly for larger goiters. The sternothyroid is then dissected off of the underlying thyroid capsule, and with the thyroid steadily retracted and rotated anteromedially, the carotid sheath is identified laterally (Fig. 73.29). For mobilization of larger glands, the sternothyroid may be partially or completely divided near its superior attachment to the thyroid cartilage, to be reapproximated during closure. The middle thyroid vein is identified laterally and ligated and divided.

Dissection and Release of the Superior Pole

The superior pole attachments are separated from the surrounding muscles and exposed mostly in a blunt fashion with a small peanut sponge or other dissector. These exposure maneuvers are carried out superolaterally and posteriorly, with downward and lateral countertraction of the thyroid using large Kelly or Allis

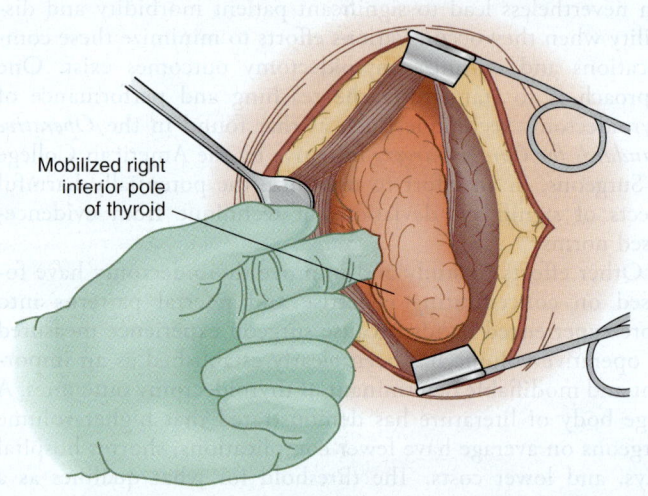

Mobilized right inferior pole of thyroid

A

Mobilization of thyroid near inferior thyroid artery and recurrent laryngeal nerve

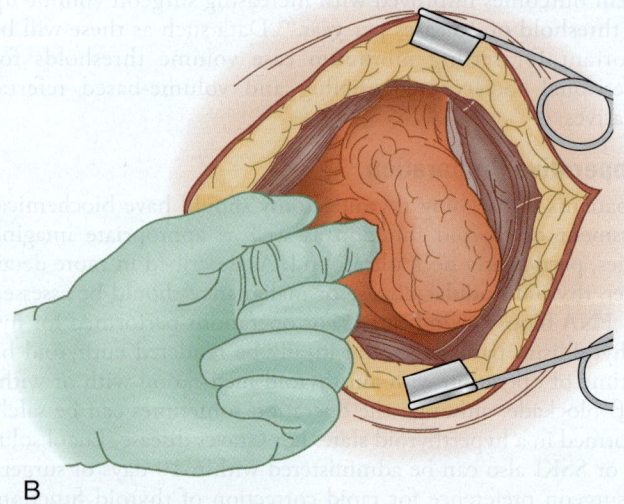

B

Mobilization of right lobe with ligation of middle thyroid vein

FIGURE 73.28 Image depicting a cervicotomy incision to facilitate exposure. After creation of a subplatysmal plane, the strap muscles (sternohyoid and sternothyroid) are separated by dividing the tissues in the avascular midline plane from the thyroid cartilage to the suprasternal notch. The thyroid lobe is exposed by mobilizing the strap muscles away from the lobe by means of lateral retraction on the muscles. The middle vein is exposed, divided, and ligated. (From Sabiston DC Jr, ed. *Atlas of General Surgery*. Philadelphia: Saunders; 1995.)

FIGURE 73.29 (A–B) The thyroid lobe is retracted medially to allow the posterolateral surface of the thyroid to be exposed. (From Sabiston DC Jr, ed. *Atlas of General Surgery*. Philadelphia: Saunders; 1995.)

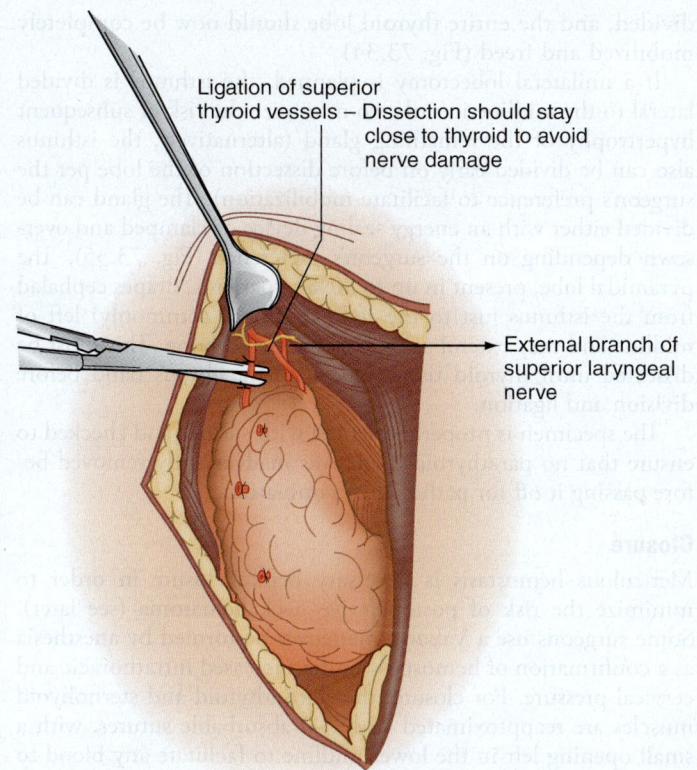

Ligation of superior
thyroid vessels – Dissection should stay
close to thyroid to avoid
nerve damage

External branch of
superior laryngeal
nerve

FIGURE 73.30 Downward and lateral traction exposes the superior-pole vessels, including branches of the superior thyroid artery. The external branch of the superior laryngeal nerve courses along the cricothyroid muscle just medial to the superior pole vessels. To avoid injury to this nerve, the superior-pole vessels are divided individually as close as possible to the point where they enter the thyroid gland. (From Sabiston DC Jr, ed. *Atlas of General Surgery*. Philadelphia: Saunders; 1995.)

clamps (Fig. 73.30). This exposes the superior-pole thyroid vessels as well as some connective tissue lateral to the superior pole. These lateral tissues are carefully mobilized to below the level of the cricothyroid muscle, as the RLN passes through the Berry ligament and dives deep into the laryngeal insertion point at the level of the cricoid cartilage.

The superior pole is similarly separated from the cricothyroid muscle medially with gentle blunt dissection. There is an avascular space between the medial superior pole and the cricothyroid muscle, often referred to as the *space of Reeves,* which is helpful for progressive dissection of the superior pole vessels. These vessels are individually isolated, ligated, and divided; the use of energy-sealing devices may replace or augment manual ligation. Care must be taken to divide these vessels close to the surface of the thyroid in order to prevent injury to the EBSLN; neuromonitoring can also assist in its identification and preservation (see later). Division and release of the superior pole vessels allow for easy sweeping of the remaining filmy tissues away from the posterior aspect of the superior pole via blunt dissection. At this point in the dissection, the superior parathyroid gland is often identified behind the mid-superior pole at the approximate level of the cricoid cartilage.

Mobilization of Inferior Pole and Medial Rotation of the Thyroid Lobe

The mobilization of the lateral and inferior aspects of the thyroid lobe includes identification of the inferior parathyroid gland.

With the inferior thyroid lobe grasped with an Allis or large Kelly clamp and retracted anteromedially, the inferior pole vessels entering anterolateral to the tracheal surface are ligated and divided. Retraction of the strap muscles exposes the carotid artery laterally, and the thyroid is progressively rotated and delivered from the wound in an anteromedial direction. The lymphoadipose tissues immediately adjacent to the lateral aspect of the thyroid are dissected off with a combination of sharp dissection with fine-tipped dissectors and ligation of small vessels as well as blunt sweeping with the peanut sponge.

The inferior parathyroid is usually encountered during these maneuvers as the posterolateral thyroid is exposed. The location of the inferior parathyroid gland is less constant than that of the superior gland, but it is invariably located on a plane anterior to the RLN and inferior to the inferior thyroid artery as this blood vessel crosses the RLN. In its typical location, the inferior gland is often adherent to the posterolateral surface of the inferior thyroid lobe. All normal parathyroid glands should be carefully dissected and swept away from the thyroid on as broad a vascular pedicle as possible in order to prevent devascularization.

Identification of the Recurrent Laryngeal Nerve and Completion of Lobectomy

Once the superior and inferior attachments of the thyroid lobe are freed, the majority of the gland aside from its tracheal attachments can be delivered from the incision with anteromedial rotation and retraction. Judicious retraction is performed with either a peanut sponge or with a finger wrapped with gauze. Care must be taken not to use excessive force when retracting the thyroid at this point because this may stretch the RLN at its tethering points at the Berry ligament and the larynx, which can increase the risk of neuropraxic injury.

The course of the right and left RLN varies considerably. The left RLN is typically situated deeper and more medially and runs in a straighter cephalocaudal direction along the tracheoesophageal groove, whereas the right RLN takes a more superficial and oblique course and may pass either anteriorly or posteriorly to the inferior thyroid artery (Fig. 73.31). Two commonly used rules of thumb for RLN identification are (1) it is located within 1 cm anteromedial to the superior parathyroid gland, at the level where the nerve crosses the inferior thyroid artery, and (2) its course through the ligament of Berry is also situated just underneath and medial to the tubercle of Zuckerkandl, the small posterior protuberance of the midthyroid lobe. Utmost care must be taken not to transect any substantial structures or tissues in this area until the RLN, inferior thyroid artery, and blood supply to the parathyroid glands are dissected and confidently identified (Fig. 73.32).

Once the parathyroids and RLN are identified and preserved, the remainder of the thyroid may be dissected in a more superficial plane off of the trachea, including the ligament of Berry. The course of the RLN here can vary such that it travels just under, within, or even anterior to the ligament of Berry; this requires careful mobilization of the nerve while the thyroid is peeled off this area (Fig. 73.33). Fine dissection of tissues with the judicious use of manual pressure, small clips, ties, and bipolar forceps is encouraged because this area contains tiny vessels that can nevertheless bleed and obscure the operative field. Occasionally, it may be appropriate to leave a tiny amount of thyroid tissue in the interest of protecting the nerve. The rest of the attachments to the anterior trachea are then

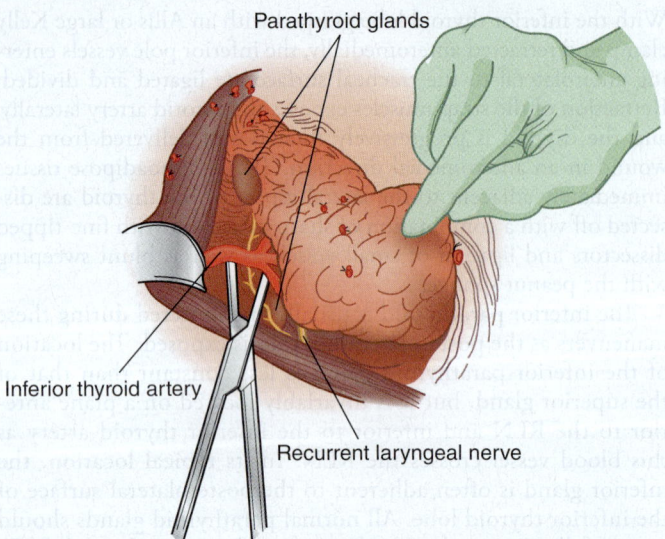

Parathyroid glands

Inferior thyroid artery

Recurrent laryngeal nerve

FIGURE 73.31 As the thyroid is retracted medially, gentle dissection is used to expose the parathyroid glands, inferior thyroid artery, and recurrent laryngeal nerve (RLN). The RLN usually passes deep to the inferior thyroid artery but may lie anterior to it. It is best found by careful dissection just inferior to the artery. The nerve can then be traced upward, and its position in relation to the thyroid can be determined. Parathyroid glands that lie on the thyroid surface can be mobilized with their vascular supply and preserved. (From Sabiston DC Jr, ed. *Atlas of General Surgery.* Philadelphia: Saunders; 1995.)

Ligation and division of distal branches
of inferior thyroid artery for total thyroidectomy

Ligament of Berry

Parathyroid

Inferior thyroid
artery

Recurrent laryngeal
nerve

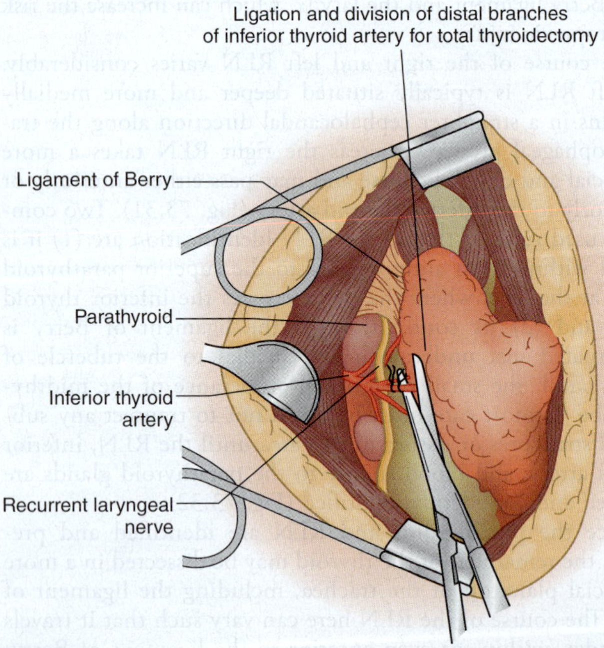

FIGURE 73.32 To complete the lobectomy, branches of the inferior thyroid artery are divided at the surface of the thyroid gland. The inferior thyroid veins can then be ligated and divided. Superiorly, the connective tissue (ligament of Berry), which binds the thyroid to the tracheal rings, is carefully divided. Several small accompanying vessels are usually present, and the RLN is closest to the thyroid and most vulnerable at this point. Division of the ligament allows the thyroid to be mobilized medially. (From Sabiston DC Jr, ed. *Atlas of General Surgery.* Philadelphia: Saunders; 1995.)

divided, and the entire thyroid lobe should now be completely mobilized and freed (Fig. 73.34).

If a unilateral lobectomy is planned, the isthmus is divided lateral to the midline in order to minimize the risk of subsequent hypertrophy of the remaining gland (alternatively, the isthmus also can be divided early on before dissection of the lobe per the surgeon's preference to facilitate mobilization). The gland can be divided either with an energy sealing device or clamped and oversewn depending on the surgeon's preference (Fig. 73.35). The pyramidal lobe, present in up to 80% of patients, drapes cephalad from the isthmus just to the right or (more commonly) left of midline and may extend as high as the hyoid bone. This must be dissected until thyroid tissue tapers into a fibrous band before division and ligation.

The specimen is properly oriented with sutures and checked to ensure that no parathyroid tissue was inadvertently removed before passing it off for pathologic examination.

Closure

Meticulous hemostasis is necessary before closure in order to minimize the risk of postoperative neck hematoma (see later). Some surgeons use a Valsalva maneuver performed by anesthesia as a confirmation of hemostasis under increased intrathoracic and cervical pressure. For closure, the sternothyroid and sternohyoid muscles are reapproximated with 3-0 absorbable sutures, with a small opening left in the lower midline to facilitate any blood to exit the deeper resection bed and into the superficial spaces. The platysma is reapproximated with similar sutures, and the skin is closed with a fine subcuticular suture. No drain is required in the majority of cases.

Postoperative Care and Complications

Postoperatively, patients are positioned in a low Fowler position, with the head and shoulders elevated at least 10 to 20 degrees in order to maintain low venous pressure in the neck. Diet is advanced quickly as the patient emerges from the effects of anesthesia. For patients who have undergone total thyroidectomy, serum calcium levels may be tracked periodically during the hospital stay. Prophylactic oral calcium supplementation can be administered, and additional supplementation may be given for symptomatic hypocalcemia. Prophylactic calcitriol also may be started preoperatively in patients at higher risk of postoperative hypocalcemia, such as those with Graves disease. Some surgeons measure preclosure intraoperative PTH or postoperative intact PTH levels within a few hours of the operation to help guide the dosing of calcium/calcitriol supplementation. There are several variations of these strategies with evidence-based literature, and any one of them would be helpful in the prevention and treatment of postoperative hypocalcemia. Patients who had undergone first-time unilateral lobectomy do not require any biochemical evaluation or calcium supplementation.

The vast majority of patients are discharged within 2 to 24 hours after surgery, with most procedures being performed in the outpatient setting. Patients having undergone total thyroidectomy are prescribed thyroid hormone replacement at a weight-based dose. Some surgeons prescribe a time-limited course of prophylactic calcium supplementation. Opioid analgesics are virtually never needed upon discharge. Most patients can return to work or full activity within 1 week and are typically seen for a postoperative check and pathology review within 2 weeks.

The length of hospital stay after thyroidectomy has evolved. Historically, patients undergoing thyroidectomy have been

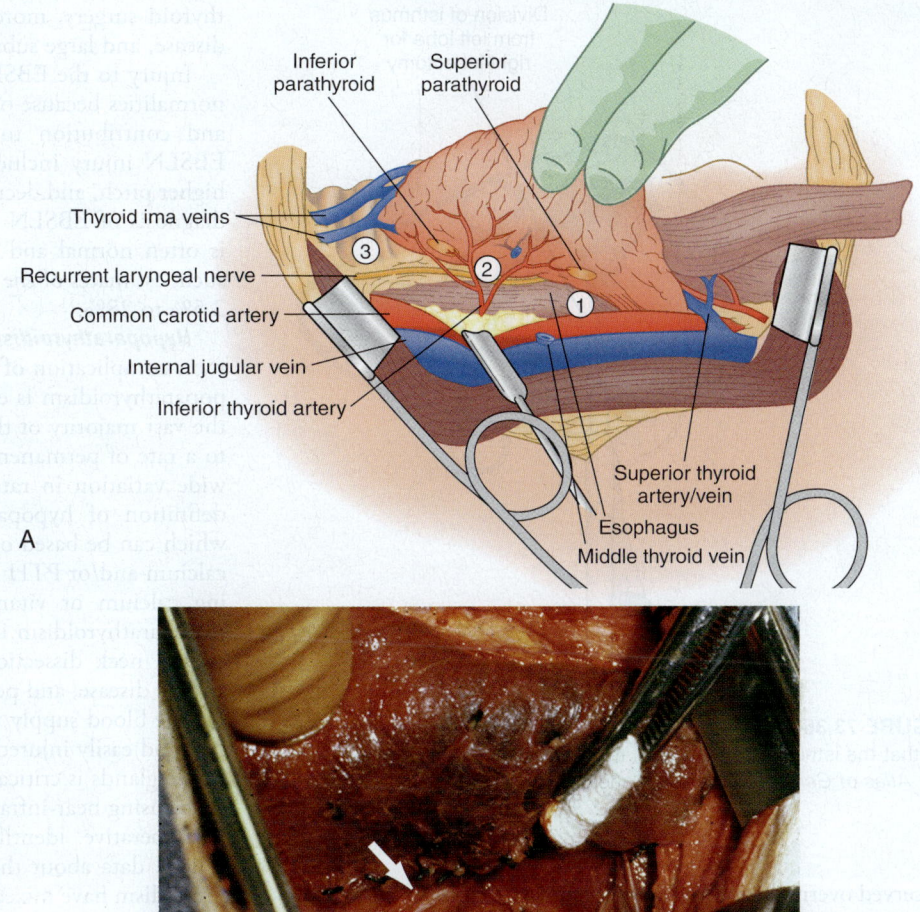

Inferior parathyroid
Superior parathyroid
Thyroid ima veins
Recurrent laryngeal nerve
Common carotid artery
Internal jugular vein
Inferior thyroid artery
Superior thyroid artery/vein
Esophagus
Middle thyroid vein

FIGURE 73.33 (A) During thyroidectomy, the recurrent laryngeal nerve *(RLN)* is at greatest risk for injury at the ligament of Berry *(1)* during ligation of branches of the inferior thyroid artery *(2)* and at the thoracic inlet *(3)*. (B) Intraoperative photo of the RLN in the tracheoesophageal groove *(arrow)*. (A, From Kahky MP, Weber RS. Complications of surgery of the thyroid and parathyroid glands. *Surg Clin North Am.* 1993;73:307-321.)

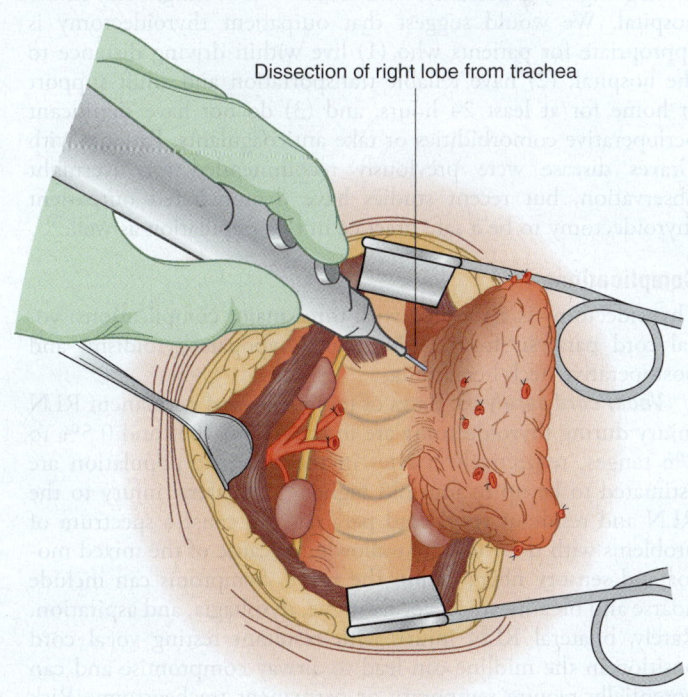

Dissection of right lobe from trachea

FIGURE 73.34 Dissection of the medial tracheal attachments is minimally vascular. Dissection is extended under the isthmus, and the specimen is divided so that the isthmus is included with the resected lobe. The pyramidal lobe also is included if present. (From Sabiston DC Jr, ed. *Atlas of General Surgery*. Philadelphia: Saunders; 1995.)

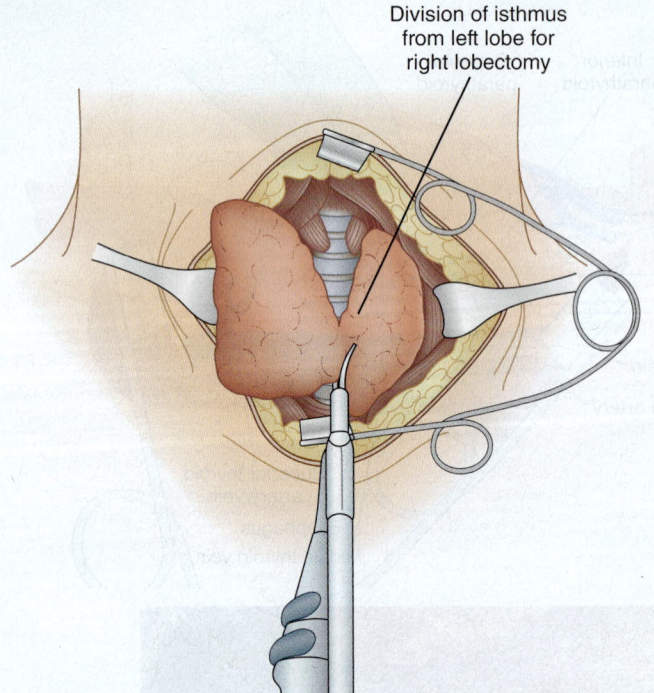

Division of isthmus
from left lobe for
right lobectomy

FIGURE 73.35 The thyroid can now be divided with an energy device so that the isthmus is included in the specimen. (From Sabiston DC Jr, ed. *Atlas of General Surgery.* Philadelphia: Saunders; 1995.)

observed overnight so that complications, particularly neck hematoma (see later), could be identified and managed expeditiously. Over the past decade, however, outpatient thyroidectomy has become a safe alternative for many selected patients undergoing routine thyroidectomy because the rate and sequelae of neck hematoma have been shown to be acceptable and, like those undergoing thyroidectomy, with at least one overnight stay in the hospital. We would suggest that outpatient thyroidectomy is appropriate for patients who (1) live within driving distance to the hospital, (2) have reliable transportation and adult support at home for at least 24 hours, and (3) do not have significant perioperative comorbidities or take anticoagulants. Patients with Graves disease were previously recommended for overnight observation, but recent studies have demonstrated outpatient thyroidectomy to be a safe practice in this population as well.[70]

Complications

Thyroidectomy is associated with three major complications: vocal cord paralysis from RLN injury, hypoparathyroidism, and postoperative neck hematoma.

Vocal cord paralysis. Rates of temporary and permanent RLN injury during thyroidectomy are in the 4% to 10% and 0.5% to 2% ranges, respectively[71]; rates in the pediatric population are estimated to be up to fourfold higher.[58] Unilateral injury to the RLN and resultant vocal cord paralysis can cause a spectrum of problems with the voice or swallowing because of the mixed motor and sensory fibers within the nerve. Symptoms can include hoarse and breathy voice, vocal fatigue, dysphagia, and aspiration. Rarely, bilateral RLN injury with resultant resting vocal cord position in the midline can lead to airway compromise and can potentially require temporary or permanent tracheostomy. Risk factors for RLN injury include low surgeon volume, reoperative

thyroid surgery, more extensive surgery for malignancy, Graves disease, and large substernal goiter.

Injury to the EBSLN also can lead to postoperative voice abnormalities because of its innervation of the cricothyroid muscle and contribution to vocal cord muscle tone. Symptoms of EBSLN injury include vocal fatigue, decreased ability to reach higher pitch, and decreased ability to project the voice. Definitive diagnosis of EBSLN injury is challenging because laryngoscopy is often normal and may require electromyographic studies; as such, estimates of the rate of injury are imperfect and range from 2.5% to 28%.[71]

Hypoparathyroidism. Hypoparathyroidism is the most common complication of thyroid surgery. The rate of temporary hypoparathyroidism is estimated to be as high as 5% to 15%, but the vast majority of these cases resolve within 6 months, leading to a rate of permanent hypoparathyroidism of 1% to 3%.[72] The wide variation in rates is in part because of differences in the definition of hypoparathyroidism in the published literature, which can be based on biochemical evidence of decreased serum calcium and/or PTH levels or symptomatic hypocalcemia requiring calcium or vitamin D supplementation. Risk factors for hypoparathyroidism include bilateral neck exploration, extensive central neck dissection, reoperative surgery, thyroidectomy for Graves disease, and pediatric patients.

The blood supply to the parathyroid glands is extremely delicate and easily injured, so meticulous dissection and preservation of the glands is critical. Although use of parathyroid autofluorescence using near-infrared (NIR) spectrum light holds promise for intraoperative identification and preservation of parathyroid glands, data about their use to prevent postoperative hypoparathyroidism have mixed results, showing no or a small difference.[73]

All thyroidectomy specimens should be checked for inadvertently resected parathyroid tissue; if parathyroid tissue is present and confirmed by either frozen section or intraoperative PTH aspiration, then the parathyroid tissue can be preserved on ice, minced, and autotransplanted into the sternocleidomastoid muscle before closure. Some high-volume endocrine surgical units administer prophylactic calcium with or without calcitriol supplementation in patients undergoing total thyroidectomy, with higher-risk populations (e.g., patients with Graves disease, pediatric patients) receiving preoperative administration as well.[72]

Postoperative neck hematoma. Postoperative neck hematoma occurs in 0.1% to 1.1% of patients undergoing thyroidectomy. Various studies have identified a number of different risk factors for hematoma, particularly male sex, advanced age, bilateral operation, Graves disease, and use of anticoagulants.[74] The danger lies not in the effect of blood loss on circulating blood volume, but rather on the local compressive effect on the trachea leading to rapid airway compromise. Neck hematoma typically presents with pain, oozing from the incision, ecchymosis, and firm swelling overlying the resection bed and incision. Patients can develop stridor with rapid airway collapse.

The vast majority of hematomas occur within the first 6 hours after the operation, 20% of cases occur between 6 and 24 hours, and very few cases occur afterward.[75] The key to management is early recognition and management. Depending on clinical status, the patient can be transported immediately back to the operating room for opening of the incision under a controlled setting with anesthesia availability; however, if the patient exhibits signs of impending airway collapse, the incision should be opened immediately wherever the patient may be. Because of this possibility, instruments for emergent opening of the incision should be present at the bedside at all times. When opening the incision, all three layers to the thyroidectomy bed—the skin, platysma, and strap muscles—must be opened to allow for maximal decompression.

Adjunctive Technologies During Thyroidectomy
Energy Sealing Devices and Hemostatic Agents

Technologies for minimizing the risk of bleeding after thyroidectomy generally fall under two categories: energy sealing devices, which are used as adjuncts or replacements for traditional clamp/tie or clipping methods for ligation of bleeding vessels, and hemostatic agents, which are typically placed on the thyroid resection bed as adjuvant methods mainly for controlling oozing-type bleeding. Energy sealing devices clamp down with force on blood vessels and apply one of two different types of energy—bipolar radiofrequency or ultrasonic vibration—to fuse the clamped tissues together. These devices are used for ligation of major structures such as the superior pole vessels, and some surgeons use them also for dissection of finer vessels around the RLN and the parathyroid glands; however, because their primary limitation is the radial spread of thermal energy and potential for damage to neighboring structures, care must be taken when using them around these critical structures. Multiple meta-analyses have demonstrated that energy sealing devices are associated with equivalent outcomes compared with traditional clamp-tie methods with respect to operative blood loss and rate of postoperative neck hematoma, along with improved operative times.[75]

Hemostatic agents also fall under multiple mechanistic groups: topical hemostats, which facilitate clotting at a bleeding surface; sealants, which prevent leakage from vessels; and adhesives, which bond tissues together. Different products can have overlapping mechanisms. A recent meta-analysis grouping studies of all hemostatic agents together showed improvements compared with conventional hemostatic methods in terms of drain output and length of postoperative hospital stay, but no significant differences were observed in the risk of hematoma formation.[76]

Intraoperative Neuromonitoring

IONM systems for the RLN involve the use of electrical stimulator probes to deliver electrical current to the vagus nerve or RLN, which leads to an electromyographic signal at the vocal cord detected by contact electrodes embedded on the surface of the endotracheal tube. All IONM systems use intermittent direct stimulation of the vagus and RLN with electrical current delivered via contact probe before, during, and after thyroid resection; some surgeons also add continuous stimulation of the vagus nerve via a flexible cuff electrode to monitor for fluctuations in the quality and integrity of the nerve signal in real time during the dissection. The IONM systems also can be used to stimulate and test integrity of the EBSLN.

The adoption of IONM has increased over the past 15 years, and in some countries, the routine use of IONM is mandatory. Despite the widespread adoption, the added benefit of IONM for reducing the risk of RLN injury remains controversial. Although multiple systematic reviews and meta-analyses have historically failed to demonstrate a significant benefit of routine IONM in reducing RLN injury rates during thyroidectomy, more recent data from multiple studies suggest that IONM was independently associated with reduced risk for short- and long-term vocal cord dysfunction.[77] Proponents of IONM cite its benefit in higher-risk operative scenarios, such as reoperative

surgery, surgery for malignancy, thyrotoxicosis, or substernal goiter,[78] and the reduction in the risk of bilateral RLN injury.

The 2018 guidelines from the International Neural Monitoring Study Group recommend standardized IONM practices during thyroidectomy, which include the following steps:

1. Initial vagal nerve stimulation to confirm intact RLN function and electrode position
2. Visual identification and direct stimulation of the RLN during the course of thyroid lobectomy
3. Final reconfirmation of intact RLN function with vagal nerve stimulation after completion of thyroid lobectomy

In addition, the International Neural Monitoring Study Group guidelines highlight the importance of surgeons' practicing and familiarizing themselves with IONM to be able to comprehensively troubleshoot equipment issues from true loss of RLN-signaling events.[79]

Fluorescent Imaging Aids for Parathyroid Identification

Because parathyroid identification during thyroidectomy is critical for the prevention of hypoparathyroidism, there has been renewed interest in newer technologies for intraoperative parathyroid imaging. The most prominent technologies under investigation currently are those that detect fluorescence from the parathyroid.

Parathyroid tissue autofluoresces in the NIR spectrum when exposed to a laser at a wavelength of 285 nm. Since this discovery in 2011, subsequent studies have demonstrated that parathyroid autofluorescence can be reliably detected both ex vivo and in vivo. Detection can either be done by spectroscopy using a contact probe or specialized NIR spectrum cameras, with parathyroid glands that can be located in 76% to 100% of cases.[80] The potential advantages of this technology are its noninvasiveness and avoidance of an exogenously administered fluorophore. Current disadvantages include its limited penetration to up to only a few millimeters' depth; subtle and subjective fluorescence images with current-generation cameras and image processing software, including false positives from brown fat and metastatic lymph nodes; and requirement for white (visible-spectrum) light to be turned off or minimized for the signal to be detected.

Exogenously administered fluorophores can aid in identification by more dramatically fluorescing the parathyroid glands. The fluorophore of greatest interest currently is indocyanine green, a water-soluble tricarbocyanine dye that rapidly binds to proteins in plasma after IV injection. Indocyanine green is a commonly used dye with low toxicity and a variety of clinical uses in other surgical procedures, and its use has been studied in both thyroidectomy and parathyroidectomy.

Alternative Approaches to Thyroidectomy

The techniques detailed earlier describe conventional thyroidectomy via an open, anterior cervicotomy approach that has become the standard of care worldwide. As techniques have been refined and technologies have improved, various efforts to minimize the cosmetic effect of a visible neck incision have been investigated. From a historical perspective, the most direct and straightforward means to this end was to decrease the length of the standard cervicotomy incision from 6 to 8 cm down to 3 to 4 cm using traditional instruments and 1.5 to 2.5 cm with the aid of endoscopic instruments. A number of variations have been described with differing terminology, including *minimally invasive, video-assisted, videoscopic/endoscopic,* and *mini-open,* all of which have demonstrated reasonable feasibility and safety in carefully selected patients.

In addition, various investigators have described nontraditional techniques that place incisions in hidden places away from the visible part of the neck, with subcutaneous and/or subplatysmal dissection using minimally invasive surgical instruments to the thyroidectomy area of interest. These so-called "remote access" approaches have largely been developed and widely adopted in Asia and have subsequently established a small but growing niche in the United States and Europe. All require the use of either laparoscopic or robotic instruments, and virtually all can be performed using insufflation of a closed space with CO_2 gas or with a gasless technique using custom long-tunneled retractors.

There are several different remote access approaches described in the literature differentiated by where the "hidden" incision is placed; the most common sites are the axilla, nipple-areolar complex or chest, retroauricular area at the hairline (the so-called "facelift" approach), and oral cavity. The most common approaches in the United States are the axillary and transoral approaches.

Transaxillary thyroidectomy using laparoscopic instruments via three small port incisions was first described in Japan in 2000 but first gained traction in the United States in 2007 based on excellent results from South Korea using a robotic, gasless technique with a single incision in the axilla. The initial American experience was marked by an upsurge of complications, including brachial plexus injury, tracheoesophageal injury, lymph leak, and hematoma, which was exacerbated by a combination of inadequate surgeon training and aggressive marketing by the medical device industry. After issuance of warnings by the US FDA in 2013, the manufacturers of the da Vinci surgical robotic system (Intuitive Surgical, Sunnyvale, CA) withdrew active support for robotic thyroidectomy, which led to an abrupt plateau in the adoption of robotic thyroidectomy cases. Since this initial turbulent experience, robotic transaxillary thyroidectomy has benefited from systematic study and steadier reintroduction in only a handful of more experienced centers. A recent experience of 301 cases in the United States revealed excellent technical feasibility (one conversion to open thyroidectomy) and safety (1.3% permanent RLN injury, 1.1% permanent hypoparathyroidism, 0.3% neck hematoma), with only one patient suffering from an approach-specific complication (arm lymphedema, which resolved with conservative management) and no recurrences among the 133 patients who had cancer identified histologically.[81]

Among all of the remote access approaches, only the transoral route offers the potential of avoiding an incision at the skin altogether. However, there were many theoretical concerns around removing the thyroid through the mouth, not least of which was introducing a new risk of infection from oral flora and injury to other structures in the oral cavity as well as at the chin. The most adopted technique was popularized in Thailand and uses laparoscopic instruments and gas insufflation via three small port incisions in the oral vestibule (Fig. 73.36). The largest published experience is a 425-patient case series from Thailand revealing zero cases of permanent RLN injury or permanent hypoparathyroidism, one case of neck hematoma requiring open thyroidectomy, and three intraoperative conversions to open thyroidectomy. With respect to approach-specific complications, three patients (0.7%) had transient mental nerve palsy, and no patients experienced a postoperative infection.[82] Other groups have replicated these results.

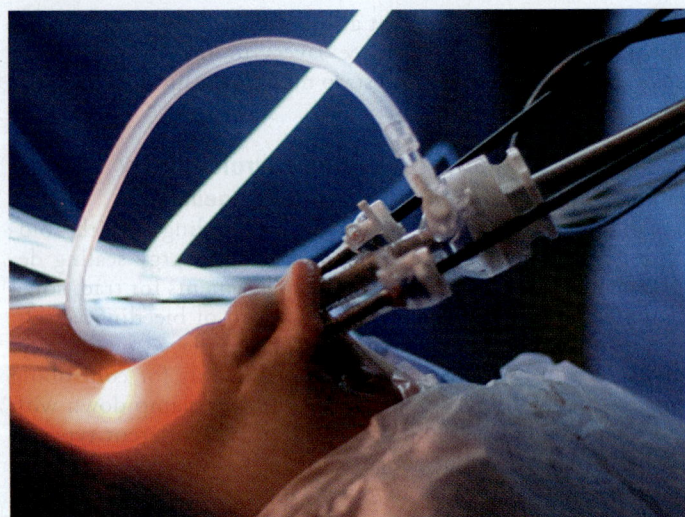

FIGURE 73.36 Transoral endoscopic thyroidectomy vestibular approach. Three laparoscopic ports are placed in the oral vestibule, and dissection is carried out down to the subplatysmal plane in the neck.

These excellent results have led to early adoption of the technique in the United States. However, with lessons learned from prior experiences around the rollout of transaxillary thyroidectomy, greater efforts are in place to introduce this technique in a more organized and responsible manner. Greater emphasis now exists on ensuring proper training, credentialing, and outcomes-tracking procedures for surgeons, and adoption is mainly occurring in larger, high-volume institutions at this time. Based on broad consensus, the selection criteria for transoral thyroidectomy have remained relatively constrained in the early phase of its adoption. It is with these quality control efforts that transoral thyroidectomy—and other future innovations—will be introduced in a manner that both fosters innovation and protects patient safety.

Thyroid Ablation Techniques

Ablation techniques have been recognized as an effective method for reducing thyroid nodule volume while preserving thyroid function, predominantly in benign disease states. Ablation techniques employ either chemical ablation or thermal ablation to achieve thyroid nodule volume reduction.

Chemical ablation is typically performed by injecting 95% to 99% dehydrated alcohol into a thyroid nodule under ultrasound guidance. Ethanol is left in situ or aspirated out after a period of time. Ethanol causes coagulative necrosis via cellular dehydration and ischemic necrosis via small vessel thrombosis, which in turn causes nodule volume reduction. Ethanol ablation is an effective technique for predominantly cystic nodules, which can recur if simply aspirated.

Thermal ablation uses different energy mechanisms to heat tissue and cause coagulative necrosis. It is best suited for patients with compressive symptoms or cosmetic complaints that can be attributed to a single or dominant thyroid nodule. Thermal ablation techniques include radiofrequency ablation, laser ablation, microwave ablation, and high-intensity focused ultrasound.

- Radiofrequency ablation uses a high-frequency alternating current (200–1200 kHz) to agitate tissue ions and cause heat production.

- Laser ablation uses single or multiple optical fibers to create a focused beam of light energy onto tissue, which causes heat.
- Microwave ablation generates an electromagnetic field (900–2500 MHz) to oscillate polar water molecules and generate heat.
- High-intensity focused ultrasound delivers ultrasound waves to generate heat at a target location, which then causes formation of microbubbles. Expansion and collapse of microbubbles induce hemorrhage through cavitation.

Radiofrequency Ablation

Symptomatic, nonfunctional, benign thyroid nodules are the most widely accepted indication for radiofrequency ablation. Thyroid nodules should appear with a very low to low suspicion for malignancy by the ATA classification for thyroid nodules (ACR TI-RADS 1, 2, or 3) or intermediate suspicion (ACR TI-RADS 4) with benign cytology. Two benign biopsies of the thyroid nodule are recommended before ablation. Functional nodules may be ablated, but resolution of hyperthyroidism is less predictable than after RAI or surgery. Therefore, RFA is considered best for patients with small toxic adenomas and contraindications to RAI or surgery.

RFA has been explored for treating indeterminate nodules and primary thyroid cancer, but it is not considered a first-line treatment currently for these indications. Because RFA does not allow for histologic analysis, nor does it prevent metastasis, it is not recommended for indeterminate nodules. Incomplete RFA treatment in other tumor types has led to tumor progression. Although RFA has been used to treat recurrent PTC and PTmC, further investigation is needed before considering RFA as a first-line treatment in malignant thyroid disease.

For benign thyroid nodules, RFA can effectively reduce nodule volume by 65% at 6 months and 77% at 12 months. Nodule volume reduction is also accompanied by improvement in local compressive symptoms and cosmesis. Compared with surgery, RFA is associated with improved preservation of thyroid function and better health-related quality of life.

Like any other procedure, RFA also introduces potential complications. There is risk of RLN injury, as in surgery, because of proximity of the RLN to the thyroid. Accurate RLN injury rates are currently lacking; one systematic review and meta-analysis identified a 1.4% rate of subjective voice change (temporary or permanent) after RFA.[83] Thyroid nodule rupture, thought to be caused by delayed bleeding resulting in thyroid capsule disruption, is the second most common complication after voice change. Hematoma can occur if an anterior jugular vein or a significant perithyroidal vein is crossed with the probe. Tracheal necrosis or airway compromise can occur from penetration or ablation near the trachea.

As thermal ablation techniques such as RFA have been introduced in North America, the ATA and international thyroid societies have recently released guidelines for safe adoption.[84] Clinicians interested in incorporating thermal ablation techniques into their practice are recommended to have comprehensive knowledge and experience in the management of thyroid nodules, neck anatomy, ultrasound imaging and FNA of the thyroid, and ultrasound risk stratification of thyroid nodules. Training should include extensive practice on phantom models, and initial thyroid nodule ablation should be performed with a proctor.

Health Equity in Thyroid Disease

The presence of disparities in care related to thyroid cancer has recently come to light. Given the indolent nature and favorable prognosis of most DTC, this disease process is somewhat unique, in that disparities in access to care may result in overdiagnosis and overtreatment of advantaged groups while simultaneously leading to underdiagnosis and undertreatment of disadvantaged groups.[85] Indeed, health insurance coverage has been shown to have a direct correlation with thyroid cancer incidence[86]; uninsured or otherwise socioeconomically disadvantaged patients have higher rates of negative prognostic indicators such as lymphovascular invasion, extrathyroidal extension, positive margins, and distant disease.[87] Socioeconomic status (SES), race, and ethnicity predict access to care and advanced presentation. Patients who are uninsured or underinsured are less likely to undergo total thyroidectomy, have formal lymphadenectomy, and adjuvant RAI than patients with private insurance, whereas Black patients, those >65 years of age, and with lower SES are less likely to be treated in accordance with ATA guidelines.[88] Sadly, this also translates into patient outcomes, with Black patients suffering higher 5-year mortality from DTC than White patients, even after adjustment for SES plus tumor- and treatment-related variables.[89] Davis and colleagues proposed strategies that can be used to combat health disparities in thyroid cancer diagnosis and treatment, including expanding Medicaid, providing insurance reimbursement for travel and other ancillary expenses, avoiding unnecessary in-person visits, and expansion of access to high-volume experts, including across states.[85]

SELECTED REFERENCES

Adam MA, Pura J, Gu L, et al. Extent of surgery for papillary thyroid cancer is not associated with survival: an analysis of 61,775 patients. *Ann Surg.* 2014;260:601-605.

This analysis from the National Cancer Database showing that lobectomy for selected papillary thyroid cancers was not associated with worse survival was an important paper that changed treatment guidelines.

Ali SZ, Baloch ZW, Cochland-Priollet B, et al. The 2023 Bethesda system for reporting thyroid cytopathology. *Thyroid.* 2023;33(9):1039-1044.

This paper on the current Bethesda classification system for reporting thyroid cytopathology provides updated data on risk of malignancy in light of the new WHO classification of thyroid neoplasms.

Haugen BR, Alexander EK, Bible KC, et al. American Thyroid Association management guidelines for adult patients with thyroid nodules and differentiated thyroid cancer: the American Thyroid Association Guidelines Task Force on Thyroid Nodules and Differentiated Thyroid Cancer. *Thyroid.* 2016;26:1-133.

The 2015 American Thyroid Association guidelines are arguably the most comprehensive and widely used evidence-based guidelines on the management of thyroid nodules and differentiated thyroid cancer.

Ito Y, Miyauchi A, Inoue H, et al. An observational trial for papillary thyroid microcarcinoma in Japanese patients. *World J Surg.* 2010;34:28-35.

> This landmark paper from Japan was the first to demonstrate the safety and feasibility of nonoperative surveillance of papillary thyroid microcarcinomas.

Lim H, Devesa SS, Sosa JA, et al. Trends in thyroid cancer incidence and mortality in the United States, 1974–2013. *JAMA.* 2017;317:1338-1348.

> This updated analysis from the Surveillance, Epidemiology, and End Results database demonstrated that mortality from advanced-stage papillary thyroid cancer rose in parallel with the increasing incidence of thyroid cancer overall, suggesting that the rise in cancer incidence could not be fully attributed to overdiagnosis.

The full reference list appears on Elsevier eBooks+.

SELECTED REFERENCES

Adam MA, Aral J, Goi L, et al. Is the extent of surgery for papillary thyroid cancer ... associated with survival: an analysis of 61,775 patients. *Ann Surg.* 2014;260:601-605.

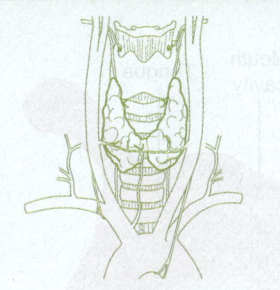

Parathyroid

Yinin Hu and John A. Olson, Jr.

HISTORY OF PARATHYROID SURGERY

In 1850, Sir Richard Owen, professor of the Royal College of Surgeons of England, presented the first record of what is now accepted as a parathyroid gland. He described, within an Indian rhinoceros, the dissection of a "small, compact yellow glandular body attached to the thyroid at the point where the vein emerged." Although others later described similar structures in other animals, it was ultimately Swedish medical student Ivar Victor Sandstrom who first described "glandulae parathyroideae" in a series of 50 human cadavers in 1880.

In 1879, Theodore Billroth performed a total thyroidectomy that was complicated by tetany. Anton Wolfer recognized the condition as the result of surgery but did not directly implicate the parathyroid. Eugene Gley, a physiologist at the College de France in Paris, reported fatal tetany after parathyroidectomy and thyroidectomy in animal models in 1891. Frederick von Recklinghausen first described osteitis fibrosa cystica that same year. The first decade of the 20th century saw a bevy of advancements in parathyroid physiology. Max Askanazy linked osteitis fibrosa cystica to parathyroid hormone (PTH), and Jacob Erdheim provided one of the earliest descriptions of parathyroid enlargement with a series of six autopsies of persons afflicted with osteomalacia. In 1909, Berkeley and Beebe used bovine parathyroid extract to alleviate parathyroidectomy-induced tetany.[1] In this era, a common hypothesis was that parathyroid hyperplasia was compensatory to bone disease and that parathyroid glands detoxified

plasma of excess calcium. Indeed, biochemist James Collip first patented parathyroid extract in 1925 as a treatment for osteitis fibrosa cystica. Contesting this theory was Viennese pathologist Friedrich Schlagenhaufer, who suggested in 1915 that parathyroid hyperplasia was not a sequela of bone disease but rather its instigator. Hyperparathyroidism became more readily diagnosed after the invention of the autoanalyzer by Leonard Skeggs in 1951.[2] Increased awareness of hypercalcemia led to recognition of parathyroid hyperactivity as its most common cause.

The history of parathyroidectomy is almost as long as that of PTH itself. William Halsted described autotransplantation of parathyroid tissue in a dog model in 1907, a practice that remains relevant today. Although incidental parathyroidectomy during thyroidectomy has been described since the late 1800s, the origin of *intentional* parathyroidectomy remains contested. Bland Sutton in London described resection of an infero-thyroidal mass causing airway obstruction sometime before 1918. This was reported to have been a parathyroid post hoc. However, the first parathyroidectomy performed for hypercalcemia is typically attributed to Viennese surgeon Felix Mandl. The patient, Albert Gahne, presented with osteitis fibrosa cystica in 1925. Mandl first acted on Collip's theory of detoxification and transplanted four cadaveric parathyroids into Gahne's rectus, to no avail. He then tested Schlagenhaufer's theory by performing a cervical exploration. This resulted in resection of a 2.5-cm mass caudal to the thyroid. Gahne improved dramatically but recurred 6 years later and died after a futile reexploration. Early surgical philosophy for the treatment of hyperparathyroidism strongly favored subtotal parathyroidectomy (SPTX) to minimize delayed recurrence despite a 10% rate of postoperative tetany.[2] This dogma was challenged by Oliver Cope, who in 1958 reported that nearly 80% of cases were due to single-gland hyperplasia. In subsequent years, SPTX became recategorized as the preferred treatment for secondary hyperparathyroidism (SHPT) due to vitamin D deficiency or renal insufficiency.

Parathyroid localization has been a unique surgical challenge for nearly a century. US merchant marine captain Charles Martell famously presented to Massachusetts General Hospital in 1926 as the first American patient diagnosed with hyperparathyroidism. He reportedly underwent five futile explorations before a 3-cm parathyroid adenoma (PA) was removed from his mediastinum.[3] The first successful parathyroidectomy for hyperparathyroidism in the United States is credited to Isaac Olch, who removed a 3-cm parathyroid tumor from an Illinois farmer, Elva Dawkins, at Barnes Hospital in St. Louis in 1926. As selective parathyroidectomy slowly became the preferred treatment for primary hyperparathyroidism (PHPT) in the 1950s, preoperative parathyroid localization gained subsequent appeal. Parathyroid localization in its modern form evolved from parathyroid ultrasonography in the 1960s to include molecular imaging in the 1970s and, ultimately, four-dimensional computed tomography (4D CT) in 2006. Complementing these technologies was the advent of intraoperative PTH measurement as a surgical adjunct in 1988—the final piece to shape today's widespread practice of targeted parathyroidectomy.

EMBRYOLOGY

Understanding parathyroid embryology provides insight into the parathyroid's surgical anatomy and its operative approach. Pharyngeal pouches are bilateral endodermal protrusions lateral to the pharynx derived from epithelium surrounded by neural crest–type mesenchymal cells. Human parathyroids develop from the third and fourth pharyngeal pouches, with differentiation driven by drosophila glial cell missing gene *(GCM2)*, which is also a requisite for PTH production (Fig. 74.1). Mutations in *GCM2* in humans can result in hypo- or hyperparathyroidism and are one genetic contributor to familial isolated hyperparathyroidism.

The third pharyngeal pouch gives rise to the thymus and inferior parathyroids, whereas the superior parathyroids and lateral thyroid originate from the fourth pharyngeal pouch. Separation and caudal migration of the thymic-parathyroid primordium away from the pharynx occurs in the fifth and sixth weeks of gestation.[4] Once parathyroid and thymus separate, the thymic lobes continue their migration into the mediastinum, leaving the inferior parathyroids behind in the lower neck. The variable timing of this separation is believed to contribute to the well-reported anatomic distribution of ectopic inferior parathyroids, the most common location of which is intrathymic. The migration may also leave a "trail" of *GCM2*-positive cell clusters along the path of descent, providing one theoretical explanation for cases of supernumerary parathyroids. In a similar pattern, the paired superior parathyroids separate from the fourth pharyngeal pouch in conjunction with the lateral thyroid and travel caudally in unison. Because of the shorter distance of travel and less variable timing of separation, the superior parathyroids are less frequently ectopic and more likely to be found within the capsule of the upper poles of the thyroid.

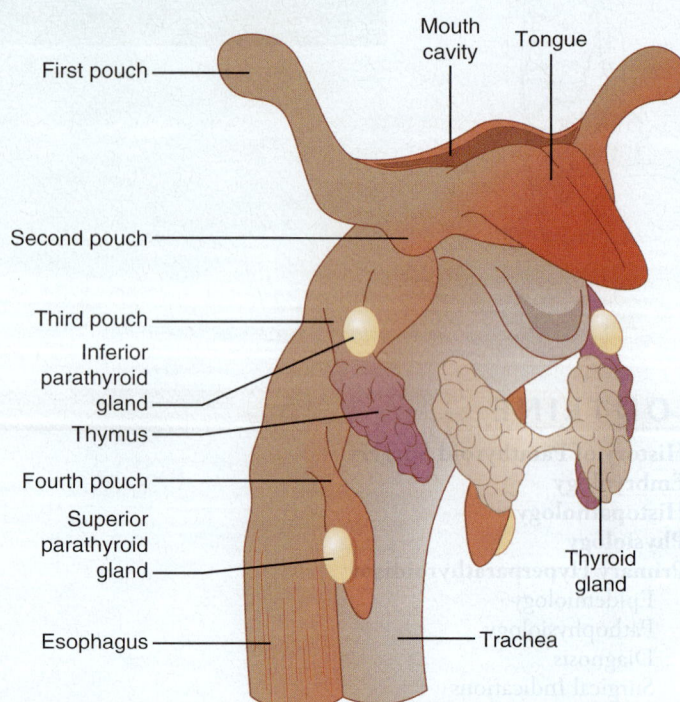

FIGURE 74.1 The pharynx and adjacent structures are depicted between the sixth and seventh weeks of embryologic development. The thyroid gland has descended to its normal location in the neck. The inferior parathyroid glands and thymus are seen arising from the third pharyngeal pouches. The superior parathyroid glands are seen arising from the fourth pharyngeal pouches.

HISTOPATHOLOGY

Grossly, normal parathyroids are typically smooth, soft, ovoid or lenticular structures measuring roughly $5 \times 3 \times 2$ mm in dimension with a yellow-tan appearance (Fig. 74.2). Fat content increases with age; thus, older patients tend to have glands with a paler-yellow appearance compared with younger counterparts, in whom the glands are typically reddish brown. Typical weight is 30 to 40 mg but highly variable. Frozen section is occasionally used intraoperatively to differentiate parathyroid from a thyroid rest, lymph node, or perithyroidal fat. In this context, parathyroid typically lacks the calcium oxalate crystals detectable with polarized light microscopy in thyroid tissue and has more structure and cellular clustering than the scattered lymphocytes and histocytes found in lymph nodes.

On microscopy, the parathyroid is encapsulated, with septa that divide the parenchyma into ill-defined lobules. The dominant cell types are chief cells and oxyphil cells. Chief cells are round with centrally located nuclei and small nucleoli. Cytoplasm is typically clear or faintly eosinophilic and often contains lipids that give it a slightly vacuolated appearance. They are the primary functional cell type in the gland and are responsible for PTH synthesis and secretion. Oxyphils are larger than chief cells and are arranged in clusters or sheets. As their name indicates, these cells contain a granular eosinophilic cytoplasm with abundant mitochondria.

In contrast to normal parathyroids, PAs typically weigh 200 mg to several grams and vary greatly in dimension. Grossly, PAs are well circumscribed, smooth, and may contain hemorrhagic or cystic components. Stromal fat content is lower than normal

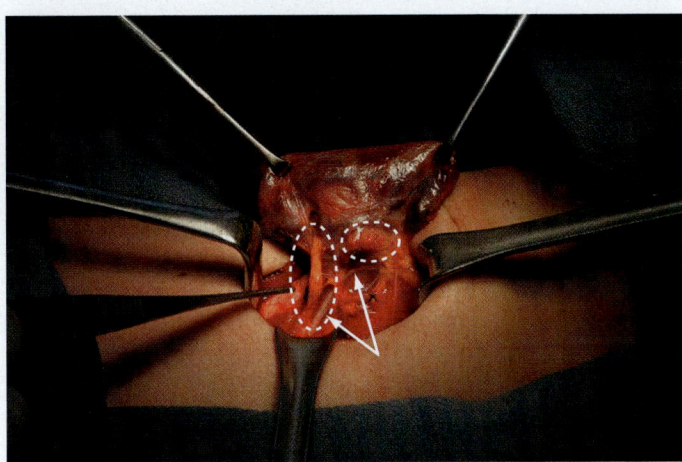

FIGURE 74.2 Intraoperative photograph demonstrating normal left superior and inferior parathyroid glands surrounded by adipose tissue and their relationship to the thyroid and the recurrent laryngeal nerve (*right side* of image is rostral, and *left side* is caudal; *dashed lines* encircle the parathyroid glands, and the *arrows* point to the left recurrent laryngeal nerve).

glands, lending the PA its red-brown coloration even in older patients. A rim of normal parathyroid tissue is often noted on pathology reports. Cellular atypia—usually indicated by enlarged, irregular, or multiple nuclei—does not imply a malignant or premalignant lesion. However, PA cells usually show low mitotic activity (<1 per 10 hpf), and findings of increased mitotic activity or necrosis should raise suspicion of carcinoma or atypical tumor.[5]

Parathyroid hyperplasia is a diffuse increase in parenchymal cell content, which can include proliferation of chief cells, oxyphils, or both in several or all parathyroid glands. When hyperplasia is unequal across all four glands, gross differentiation from adenoma can be challenging. This is particularly true if a clear secondary etiology for hyperplasia is unable to be established. Although the prevailing view is that most PAs are monoclonal cellular proliferations, recent data suggest that a substantial number of parathyroid tumors are polyclonal and that polyclonal tumor status is associated with multiple-gland disease.[6]

Parathyroid carcinoma (PCA) is among the rarest malignancies in humans and accounts for less than 1% of cases of PHPT. Grossly, PCA is characterized by obliteration of capsule and tissue planes and infiltration into surrounding structures such as the thyroid, fat, trachea, recurrent laryngeal nerve, or esophagus. According to the World Health Organization (WHO), histology diagnosis of PCA requires at least one of the following conditions: (1) angioinvasion, (2) lymphatic invasion, (3) perineural invasion, (4) invasion into adjacent structures, or (5) metastatic disease. In intermediate cases of clear cellular atypia in the absence of one of the aforementioned criteria—that is, increased mitotic activity (>5 per 10 hpf) and/or Ki67 index (>5%)—the WHO applies the term *atypical parathyroid tumor*.[7] Additional features include sheetlike growth pattern, consistent nuclear atypia, and the presence of intratumoral fibrous bands. The change from the prior nomenclature of *atypical parathyroid adenoma* to *atypical parathyroid tumor* reflects the recognition that the boundary between these diagnoses is most likely a continuum, and metastatic recurrence in atypical adenoma has been reported. In recent years, advanced immunohistochemical markers have further assisted in differentiating between benign and malignant cases. Adenomas typically retain expression of parafibromin, retinoblastoma protein

(RB), and adenomatous polyposis coli protein (APC). Loss of expression of these markers, overexpression of p53, and Ki-67 index >5% combine to favor a diagnosis of atypical parathyroid tumor or PCA.

PHYSIOLOGY

Within parathyroid chief cells, PTH is created through cleavage from pre-pro-PTH and stored in its biologically active form, intact PTH. This ready supply facilitates secretion within seconds and, together with the hormone's rapid extracellular degradation, allows for exquisite regulation of serum calcium. Renal and hepatic metabolism cleaves intact PTH into carboxyl- and amino-terminal fragments. Intact PTH has a plasma half-life of 3 to 4 minutes, a feature that greatly facilitates intraoperative decision-making through venous sampling of PTH level.

PTH is regulated predominantly by serum calcium via the calcium-sensing receptor (CaSR), which is a dimerized G protein–coupled receptor that acts on downstream kinases, including protein kinase C, ERK$_{1/2}$, p38, and JNK.[8] The net result is inhibition of both PTH synthesis and secretion and activation of intraglandular PTH degradation. The relationship between serum calcium and PTH levels is often described as an inverse sigmoidal curve (Fig. 74.3). The steep midportion of the curve alludes to a physiologic calcium set point around which the PTH response to calcium concentration is greatly magnified. In normal conditions, calcium fluctuation by 0.1 mg/dL can induce a noticeable change in PTH concentration within minutes. For example, when serum calcium is below the physiologic set point, CaSR-mediated responses include increased intact PTH secretion from parathyroid chief cells, inhibition of PTH cleavage into inert carboxy-terminal fragments, stabilization of PTH mRNA, and chief cell proliferation.[9]

Additional PTH regulators include phosphate and calcitriol. Phosphate stimulates PTH secretion and chief cell proliferation both directly and indirectly through induction of hypocalcemia. The mechanism of direct stimulation is thought to be due to noncompetitive inhibition of CaSR.[10] This phenomenon is important because persistent hyperphosphatemia is thought to be

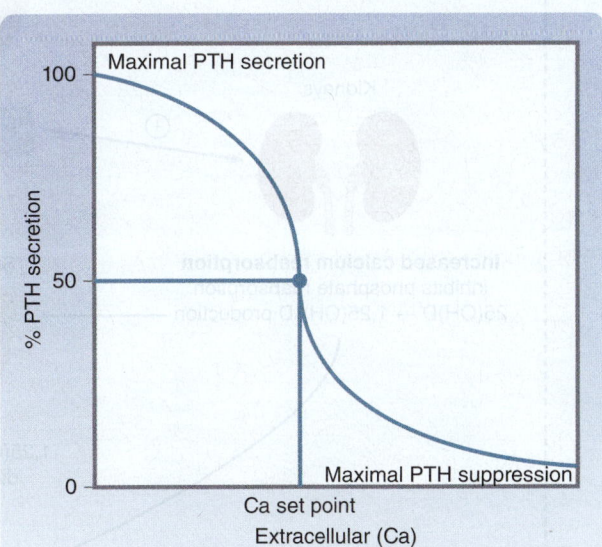

FIGURE 74.3 Inverse sigmoidal relationship of parathyroid hormone *(PTH)* to changes in extracellular calcium concentration and the calcium set point. *Ca,* Calcium.

one of the principal drivers of SHPT in the setting of chronic kidney disease (CKD). Calcitriol (1,25(OH)2D3) reduces PTH production and secretion by binding vitamin D receptors on chief cells to suppress PTH gene expression and by upregulating expression of CaSR. In the setting of CKD, there is a reduction in both renal conversion of 25(OH)D3 into calcitriol and chief cell vitamin D receptor expression, considerably stunting calcitriol's inhibitory effect.[11] Finally, fibroblast growth factor-23 (FGF23) promotes renal phosphate wasting, which results in decreased PTH secretion. Although parathyroid does express the FGF23 receptor αKlotho, whether FGF23 has a direct inhibitory effect on parathyroid secretion remains unclear.

PTH-mediated calcium regulation is enacted primarily through activation of receptor PTH1R, which binds both PTH and PTH-related protein (PTHrP). PTH1R binds to the amino-terminal section of PTH, which is structurally similar in PTHrP. Although the carboxy-terminus of PTH is classically thought of as inactive, there is mounting evidence that this fragment antagonizes PTH-mediated effects and induces hypocalcemia by inhibiting bone resorption.

In skeletal bone, stimulation of PTH1R results in maturation of osteocytes into mature osteoblasts that function to increase bone formation. However, PTH also indirectly mediates bone resorption through osteoclast-activating regulators produced by osteoblasts and progenitors. These include receptor activator of nuclear factor-kappa B (RANK), its corresponding ligand RANKL, and osteoprotegerin. The anabolic effect dominates in the setting of transient or intermittent PTH elevation, justifying

the use of recombinant PTH in treatment of osteoporotic post-menopausal females. Conversely, the catabolic effect dominates when PTH is chronically elevated, as is the case in osteoporosis as a result of PHPT or SHPT.

In the nephron, most filtered ionized calcium is reabsorbed by the proximal tubule via sodium-dependent passive transport. Although PTH does not directly modulate calcium transport in this segment, there is clear evidence that it inhibits sodium reabsorption. This may indirectly lead to reduced calcium reabsorption; however, in vivo studies have yielded variable results to date.[12] Phosphate is also predominantly reabsorbed in the proximal tubule, and there is strong evidence that PTH inhibits this process and induces phosphate wasting. This occurs through a reduction in apical membrane expression of sodium phosphate cotransporters NaPi-2a, NaPi-2c, and PiT2. Lastly, the proximal tubule is the principal site of conversion of inactive 25(OH)D3 into active calcitriol via 1-α hydroxylase. PTH stimulates synthesis of 1-α hydroxylase and inhibits the activity of 24-hydroxylase, the cumulative effect of which is an increase in serum concentration of biologically active calcitriol (Fig. 74.4).

The distal convoluted tubule is responsible for reabsorbing roughly 5% of filtered calcium via active transport. The primary apical channel that drives calcium uptake from the lumen is transient receptor potential vanilloid 5 (TRPV5). Once intracellular, calcium is shuttled to the basolateral membrane and secreted via a sodium-calcium exchanger (NCX1) and calcium-ATPases (PMCA4). Within the distal convoluted tubule, PTH binding to PTH1R enhances TRPV5 expression and regulates TRPV5

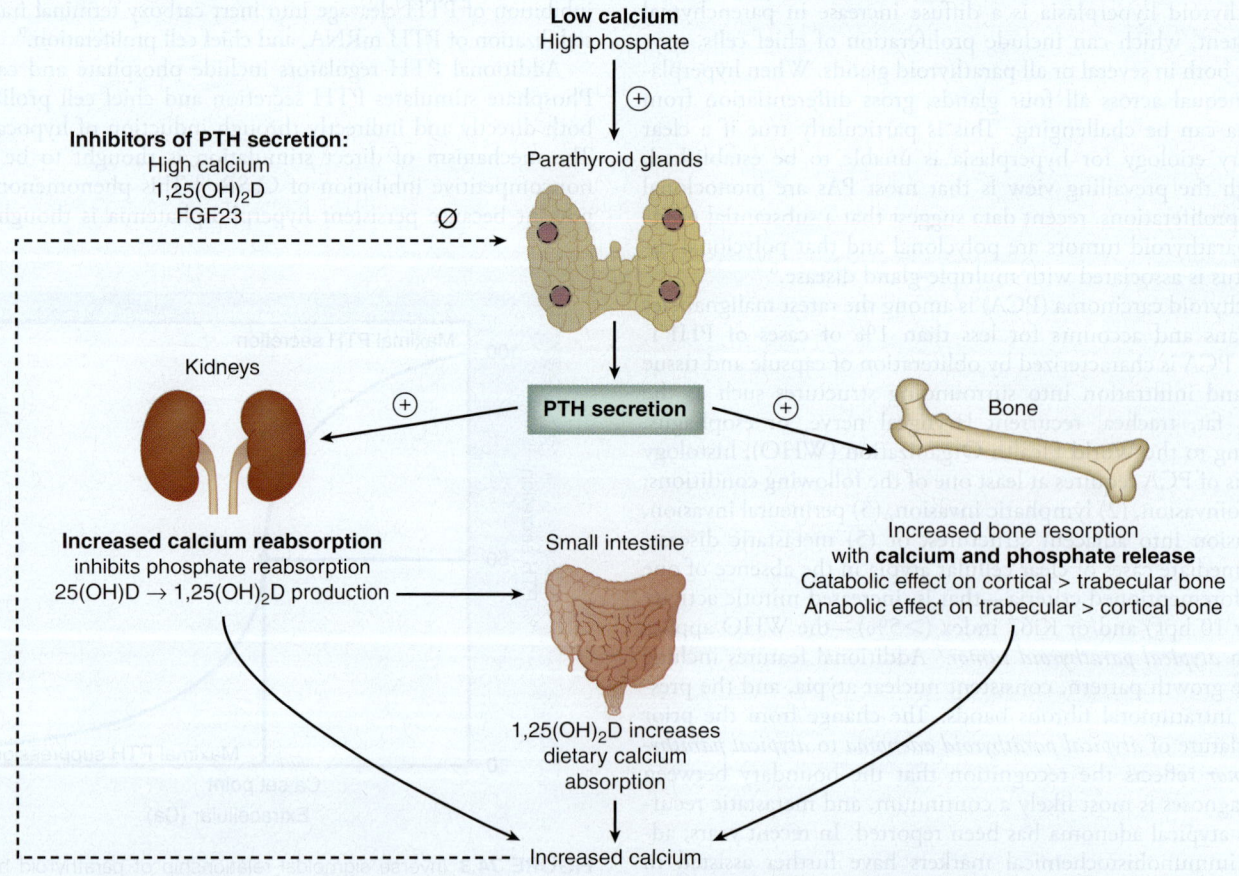

FIGURE 74.4 Regulators of parathyroid hormone *(PTH)* secretion and PTH effects on calcium homeostasis. *FGF23*, Fibroblast growth factor 23; *25(OH)D*, 25-hydroxyvitamin D; *1,25(OH)₂D*, 1,25-dihydroxyvitamin D.

function through hormone-dependent phosphorylation via protein kinase A. Finally, PTH stimulates conversion of 25(OH)D3 into calcitriol, which itself also amplifies TRPV5 expression. The net effect is dramatically increased apical membrane uptake and transcellular shuttling of calcium from the lumen to the basolateral membrane.[12]

PRIMARY HYPERPARATHYROIDISM

Epidemiology

Before the introduction of the chemistry autoanalyzer in 1974, PHPT typically presented with symptomatic hypercalcemia. After this breakthrough, and with increasing attention to osteoporosis screening in recent decades, detection of PHPT gradually rose. Recent estimates among the US population indicate a prevalence of 233 per 100,000 in females and 85 per 100,000 in males. Overall incidence is roughly 50 cases per 100,000 person-years. Incidence increases with age across both sexes and is highest among African American females.[13] Childhood exposure to ionizing radiation increases the risk of PHPT in later years. Lithium decreases CaSR sensitivity to calcium, thereby dampening negative feedback and promoting PHPT. Familial syndromes that involve PHPT with variable penetrance include multiple endocrine neoplasia (MEN) type 1, hyperparathyroidism–jaw tumor syndrome (HPT-JT), MEN2A, MEN4, and familial isolated primary hyperparathyroidism (FIHP). Corresponding germline mutations are *MEN1* (MEN1), *RET* (MEN2A), *CDKN1B* (MEN4), *CDC73* (hyperparathyroidism–jaw tumor), and *GCM2* or *CASR* (FIHP).

Pathophysiology

At its core, PHPT entails a disconnect in the physiologic feedback relationship between calcium and PTH secretion, resulting in an increase in the concentration of calcium necessary to suppress PTH. This may be due to chief cell proliferation or a decrease in the concentration of CaSR within the parathyroid, ultimately resulting in one of three biochemical patterns. In most cases, PHPT manifests with hypercalcemia and elevated PTH. However, PTH may be inappropriately normal (>20 pg/mL) in a patient with hypercalcemia (normohormonal PHPT) or inappropriately elevated in a patient with high-normal calcium (normocalcemic PHPT).

Before the modern era of biochemical screening and testing, PHPT often manifested with recurrent nephrolithiasis or osteitis fibrosa cystica. Additional symptoms include polyuria, polydipsia, constipation, pancreatitis, and renal deficiency. Osteitis fibrosa cystica is characterized by chronic bone pain, pathologic fractures (usually vertebral), bone cysts, and brown tumors. It is now rarely observed in developed nations because most cases of PHPT are diagnosed well before this terminal manifestation. Patients presenting with this symptom profile have usually undergone exhaustive testing for PHPT and should raise suspicion of alternative causes, such as mutations in *FGF23*.

Pathologically elevated PTH chronically activates PTH1R, resulting in bone resorption, increased calcium resorption from the distal convoluted tubule, phosphaturia, and elevated synthesis of 1,25(OH)2D3. There is preferential loss of bone density at cortical sites, most prominently in the distal radius. However, there is evidence that PHPT induces trabecular deterioration in the vertebrae as well, and there is an increased risk of vertebral fracture despite relative preservation in vertebral bone density on dual-energy x-ray absorptiometry (DXA).[14]

About 10% of patients with PHPT present with, or have a history of, nephrolithiasis. Rate of asymptomatic nephrolithiasis is likely significantly higher, and there are proponents of screening renal ultrasound for patients newly diagnosed with PHPT. Of note, nephrolithiasis in the setting of PHPT is not itself associated with reduced estimated glomerular filtration rate (eGFR); however, renal insufficiency is more common among patients with PHPT (15%) than among the general population. Mechanisms for PTH-mediated renal insufficiency are under investigation; current theories include impaired filtration secondary to nephrocalcinosis and hypercalcemia-induced sodium excretion that leads to a reduction in total body water.[14] This effect appears to be quite gradual, and two small, randomized trials comparing surgery versus observation for asymptomatic PHPT failed to show improvement in eGFR after parathyroidectomy at 1- and 2-year follow-up.

Manifestations of PHPT outside of the skeletal and renal systems have been extensively reported but are difficult to prove. These "soft" signs include neuropsychologic findings such as anxiety, cognitive dysfunction, and fatigue thought to be mediated by dysregulation of neurotransmitter synapses because of hypercalcemia. Although observational studies have suggested that these symptoms improve after parathyroidectomy, prospective data have been inconclusive. Similarly, large observational studies have suggested an increased risk of cardiovascular mortality in patients with severe PHPT, possibly mediated by increased vascular stiffness or valve calcification. Whether these risks are meaningful in mild PHPT—which constitutes most modern diagnoses—and whether they are reversible with surgical therapy is unknown. Finally, variable associations have been made between PHPT and gastrointestinal symptoms such as chronic constipation, pancreatitis, and peptic ulcer disease. Ultimately, however, consensus criteria for surgical referral focus on skeletal and renal sequelae (discussed later) because these are supported by more consistent scientific evidence and are more conducive to measurement and follow-up.

Given the unclear cause-and-effect relationship between the biochemical abnormality of PHPT and signs and symptoms of the disease as well as the increased appreciation of multiple-gland disease in series of bilateral exploration compared with unilateral exploration, it is debated whether all cases of apparent PHPT are in fact primary as opposed to polyclonal expansion of chronically stimulated parathyroid glands from a yet-unrecognized metabolic process involving bone and/or kidney.

Diagnosis

Diagnostic and treatment evaluation for PHPT should always incorporate three essential and independent components. The first is to confidently establish a diagnosis of PHPT via a thorough history, physical exam, and biochemical evaluation. Imaging of any form does not contribute to this first step. Upon establishing the diagnosis, the second step is to determine whether a patient possesses a meaningful indication for parathyroidectomy. Only after affirming both the diagnosis and surgical indication does parathyroid localization commence as the third and final step in workup.

Diagnosis of PHPT typically starts with either the recognition of classical PHPT symptoms (osteoporosis, pathologic fractures, recurrent nephrolithiasis, bone pain) or a biochemical profile showing hypercalcemia. Hyperparathyroidism and malignancy are the two most common causes of persistently elevated serum calcium. Other causes, which are readily excluded by a thorough history, include vitamin D intoxication, chronic granulomatous disease, and calcium-boosting medications such as lithium and thiazide diuretics.

A typical initial biochemical panel for evaluation of hypercalcemia includes a comprehensive metabolic panel, total serum calcium, intact PTH, and 25(OH)D3. Non–parathyroid-mediated hypercalcemia is usually associated with suppressed PTH (<20 pg/mL). Elevated PTH or inappropriately normal PTH (>20 pg/mL) in the setting of hypercalcemia is usually indicative of PHPT. Marked PTH elevation (>150 pg/mL) should raise consideration for either PCA or renal insufficiency, although benign PHPT remains the most likely diagnosis. Differential diagnoses also include vitamin D deficiency and familial hypocalciuric hypercalcemia (FHH). Normal or elevated 25(OH)D3 excludes SHPT caused by vitamin D deficiency. If 25(OH)D3 is low, intact PTH should be repeated once vitamin D is repleted. There is little role for ionized calcium in the workup for PHPT; however, one may consider this as an adjunct in the diagnostic evaluation of normocalcemic hyperparathyroidism.

For patients with hypercalcemia and normal or mildly elevated PTH, 24-hour urinary calcium is recommended to rule out FHH. Elevated or normal 24-hour urinary calcium is consistent with PHPT, whereas calcium excretion <100 mg over 24 hours is suggestive of FHH. Calcium-creatinine clearance ratio (CCCR) can further aid in FHH diagnosis and is calculated as CCCR = (24-hour urine Ca × serum Cr) ÷ (serum Ca × 24-hour urine Cr). CCCR <0.01 is the most frequently quoted threshold for diagnosis of FHH; however, there is considerable overlap with PHPT. Vitamin D repletion must be ensured when interpreting CCCR, and confirmatory genetic testing for CaSR mutations is recommended to definitively establish FHH.[15] This workup is ultimately meaningful, however, because FHH is a benign hypercalcemic condition that has no deleterious repercussions and is not improved by parathyroidectomy. Along with serum 25(OH)D3, 24-hour urine calcium can also help differentiate between PHPT and SHPT due to renal insufficiency, particularly for cases of normohormonal hypercalcemia. In the latter condition, both 25(OH)D3 and urinary excretion are typically low.

Surgical Indications

There is general consensus that patently symptomatic PHPT—kidney stones, pathologic fractures—should undergo definitive surgical treatment with parathyroidectomy. However, in the modern era of pervasive biochemical testing, most patients present with asymptomatic PHPT detected via workup for incidentally discovered hypercalcemia. For these patients, both the American Association for Endocrine Surgery (AAES) and the American Society for Bone and Mineral Research (ASBMR) recommend definitive surgical treatment for any patient who satisfies one or more of the following criteria[16]:

1. Serum calcium exceeding upper limit of normal by ≥1.0 mg/dL (0.25 mmol/L)
2. DXA scan with T-score ≤–2.5 at lumbar spine, total hip, femoral neck, or distal radius
3. Vertebral fracture
4. eGFR <60 mL/min
5. Nephrolithiasis or nephrocalcinosis
6. Age <50 years

The ASBMR recommends parathyroidectomy for patients with 24-hour urine calcium excretion >250 mg/day for females and >300 mg/day for males, whereas the threshold delineated by the AAES is >400 mg/dL without sex stratification. The ASBMR does not recommend surgical referral for PHPT associated with impaired cognition, cardiovascular conditions, or impaired quality of life because of insufficient evidence.[16] Conversely, the AAES

expands indications to include patients with neurocognitive/neuropsychiatric symptoms, cardiovascular disease, and those unwilling to comply with medical management. Our practice tracks with the ASBMR's narrower criteria, but we have noted many cases of improved quality of life with alleviation of vague symptoms after successful parathyroidectomy, and patient preference is strongly considered.

Localization

Once a firm diagnosis and a clear indication for surgery are established, the evaluation of PHPT shifts to preoperative localization. Broadly, the objective of preoperative localization is to help minimize the extent of surgical exploration and identify ectopic parathyroid(s). Localization studies have little utility in establishing a diagnosis, and rarely do they contribute to a recommendation for parathyroidectomy. Although localizing technology is constantly evolving—particularly in the realm of molecular imaging—the core modalities that are available to most surgical practices are ultrasonography, sestamibi scintigraphy, and 4D CT.

Ultrasonography is perhaps the most pervasive form of parathyroid localization and is often performed by surgeons themselves. Sonographically, a PA is typically homogeneous and hypoechoic, with well-defined borders and peripheral vascularity (Fig. 74.5). A grossly enlarged gland in a standard anatomic location is readily identified even by novice sonographers. However, small, intrathyroidal, or ectopic adenomas can be difficult to identify with confidence. Ultrasonography has the added advantage of identifying concurrent thyroid pathology, which may facilitate the treatment of multiple conditions through one surgical exploration. In experienced hands, a surgeon-performed ultrasound (SUS) can correctly localize a PA in nearly 90% of cases, and some studies have shown accuracy that exceeds sestamibi. These findings may encourage some to forego sestamibi entirely, particularly because availability of nuclear imaging could be rate limiting for surgical workup. However, it is important to recognize that ultrasonography is notoriously operator dependent, and accuracy as low as 74% has been reported.

^{99m}-Technetium sestamibi (MIBI) is absorbed by both thyroid and parathyroid via mitochondria. Within the parathyroid, oxyphil cells preferentially retain the MIBI radiotracer for a longer period than does thyroid tissue because of their greater concentration of mitochondria. In a typical MIBI protocol, images are captured immediately after tracer injection and at a 2-hour delay phase. Persistent tracer retention at the delayed phase is representative of parathyroid tissue (Fig. 74.6). Of note, thyroid nodules often retain MIBI tracer as well and can mislead interpretation. In these cases, a dual tracer protocol (i.e., 123-iodine) can facilitate a subtraction scan to better delineate between thyroid and parathyroid tissue. A standard planar MIBI scan provides very little anatomic detail, particularly along the anterior-posterior axis. Augmentation with single-photon emission computed tomography (SPECT) provides a three-dimensional correlate to the MIBI tracer. SPECT has been shown to improve sensitivity relative to MIBI, typically in the 90% to 97% range. In many facilities, SPECT can be fused with traditional computed tomography (CT) to provide further cross-sectional detail.

In 4D CT, the "fourth dimension" reflects differential enhancement over time after contrast administration. A typical 4D CT protocol includes a precontrast phase, an arterial phase, and a delay phase (60–80 s after injection). Parathyroid tissue has rapid arterial-phase uptake with rapid washout on delay phase. This allows differentiation from thyroid tissue, which has arterial

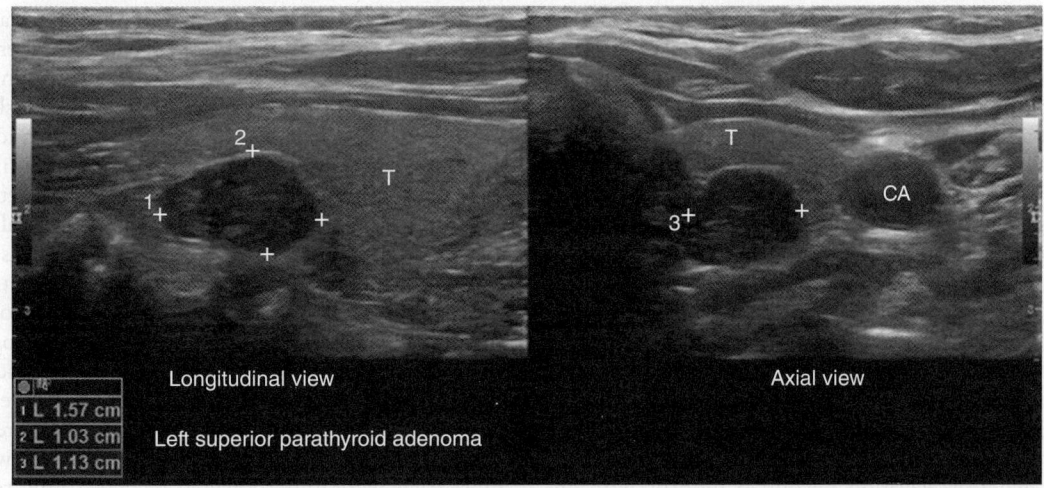

FIGURE 74.5 High-resolution ultrasound images demonstrating a 1.57- × 1.03- × 1.13-cm hypoechoic mass posterior to the superior pole of the left lobe of the thyroid gland in longitudinal and axial views, which corresponded to a left superior parathyroid adenoma. Parathyroid gland marked by measuring points. *CA,* Carotid artery; *T,* thyroid.

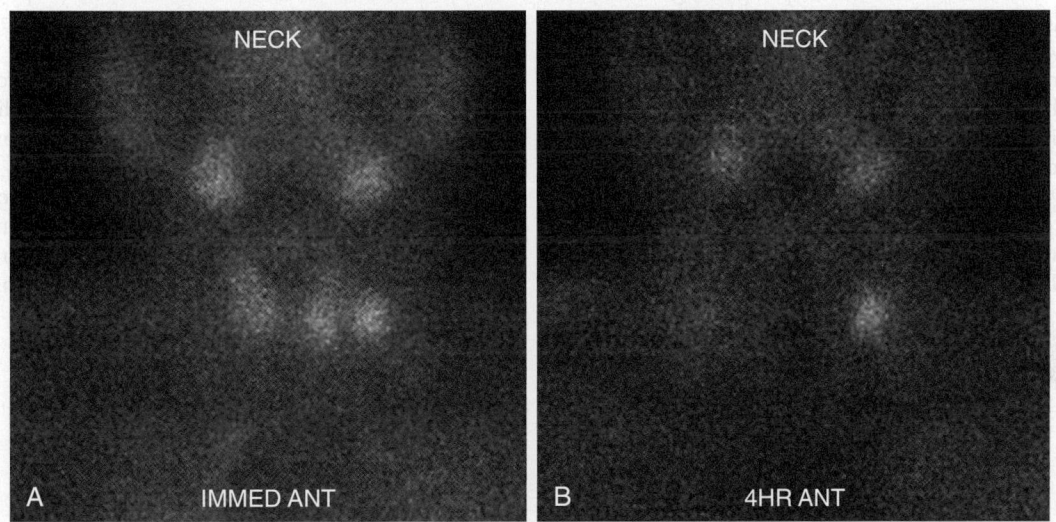

FIGURE 74.6 (A) A focal area of abnormal radiotracer accumulation lateral to the thyroid gland on an immediate technetium 99m sestamibi image. (B) A 4-hour delayed image.

enhancement and more prolonged retention, and from cervical lymph nodes, which have minimal arterial enhancement. Pooled accuracy in a meta-analysis composed of 34 studies was 73%.[17] Compared with MIBI, 4D CT has superior anatomic detail and may facilitate localization of smaller or ectopic parathyroids. Although the overall radiation dose is similar between 4D CT and MIBI, preferential radiation to the thyroid is roughly fiftyfold higher with 4D CT than with MIBI. The clinical significance of this is debatable, however, because it translates to a lifetime absolute increase in thyroid cancer risk of 0.1% for a 20-year-old female.

In recent years, positron emission tomography with CT (PET/CT) has been adopted at some centers as another localization option for challenging cases. In a retrospective single-institution study of 84 cases, PET/CT with ^{11}C-methionine outperformed MIBI, subtraction scintigraphy, and ultrasound in sensitivity.[18] Magnetic resonance imaging (MRI) has also seen some utility for parathyroid localization. On MRI, parathyroid tissue has low- to moderate-signal on T1 and tends to have high intensity on

T2. Compared with CT, MRI has advantages of avoiding ionizing radiation and intravenous contrast, but detection rates are mediocre. In general, both PET/CT and MRI are relegated to reoperative cases in which standard imaging modalities are unrevealing, all noninvasive imaging has been exhausted, and a suspected adenoma remains elusive. Selective venous sampling and selective arteriography do not provide anatomic detail but may help direct reexploration by providing general information on laterality and cervical versus mediastinal origin of PTH secretion.

Although institutional practices vary, our approach to localization begins with SUS. For patients with PTH ≥100 pg/mL and a clear single-gland adenoma on SUS, we proceed with targeted parathyroidectomy. For patients with equivocal SUS findings or PTH <100 pg/mL (for whom multigland disease or small adenomas are more likely), 4D CT is recommended. MIBI with SPECT-CT is reserved for cases in which there are discordant or negative findings on SUS and 4D CT or for suspected ectopic anatomy. If localization is unsuccessful after these three modalities have been employed, we proceed with planned four-gland exploration. PET/CT is considered for cases of reoperative disease with negative results on other imaging modalities, and selective venous sampling is used if all noninvasive modalities have been exhausted (Fig. 74.7).

Outcomes After Surgery

Because most patients with PHPT present with biochemical and DXA abnormalities rather than overt clinical symptoms, assessment of surgical outcomes requires long-term follow-up and persistent surveillance. Surgical efficacy may be measured via rate of cure and improvement or stabilization in end-organ performance. Cure from PHPT is defined as normalization of calcium and PTH at 6 months or greater after parathyroidectomy. Elevation of either marker within 6 months after surgery is considered persistent disease, whereas elevation beyond 6 months with an initial interval of normalization is considered recurrent disease. Variable rates of cure after parathyroidectomy have been reported, typically ranging from 90% to 99%. However, selection and publication bias must be considered, and it is generally accepted that there exists a volume-outcome relationship regarding efficacy of the index operation.

Surgical approach varies by institution. Minimally invasive parathyroidectomy (MIP) entails targeted removal of only the parathyroid(s) identified as abnormal on preoperative imaging, with intraoperative PTH (ioPTH) measurement to help determine adequacy of resection. Bilateral neck exploration (BNE), also called *four-gland exploration,* entails visual inspection of all four parathyroid glands with resection of those that appear grossly pathologic. Hybrid approaches involving BNE with ioPTH are a third option. In a meta-analysis of observational studies and

randomized trials, no difference in cure rate was noted between BNE and MIP. BNE was associated with higher rates of postoperative hemorrhage, hypocalcemia, and recurrent laryngeal nerve injury; however, the absolute differences in risks were low. On the other hand, it is speculated that multigland disease may be an underrecognized phenomenon, and routine BNE might yield more durable normocalcemia. Further details on operative approach are included in the section on Surgical Technique.

Although achievement of normocalcemia is easy to capture via routine screening laboratory panels, definitive proof of improvement or stabilization in end-organ function is challenging. In a systematic review of randomized trials comparing surgery versus nonoperative management, parathyroidectomy provided little to no effect on bone marrow density at the lumbar spine or femoral neck, left ventricular ejection fraction, renal impairment, or all-cause mortality at 12 to 24 months follow-up.[19] However, most trials were underpowered to detect long-term sequelae because the meta-analysis included a total of only 447 participants. The review also highlighted the importance of length of follow-up. Ten-year outcomes from the Scandinavian Investigation of Primary Hyperparathyroidism randomized trial (SIPH) provided clear evidence of treatment effect from parathyroidectomy. Patients in the observation arm experienced decreases in average T-score (ΔT) at all compartments over time. Compared with these controls, the 10-year ΔT of parathyroidectomy patients was 0.41 higher at the radius and 0.58 higher at the lumbar spine. However, an absolute increase in average T-score from baseline was only noted at the lumbar spine (+0.36).[20] To summarize, there are randomized prospective data to support that parathyroidectomy provides better *preservation* of bone density compared with observation and that it *improves* bone density at the lumbar spine. Across large, population-level longitudinal cohort

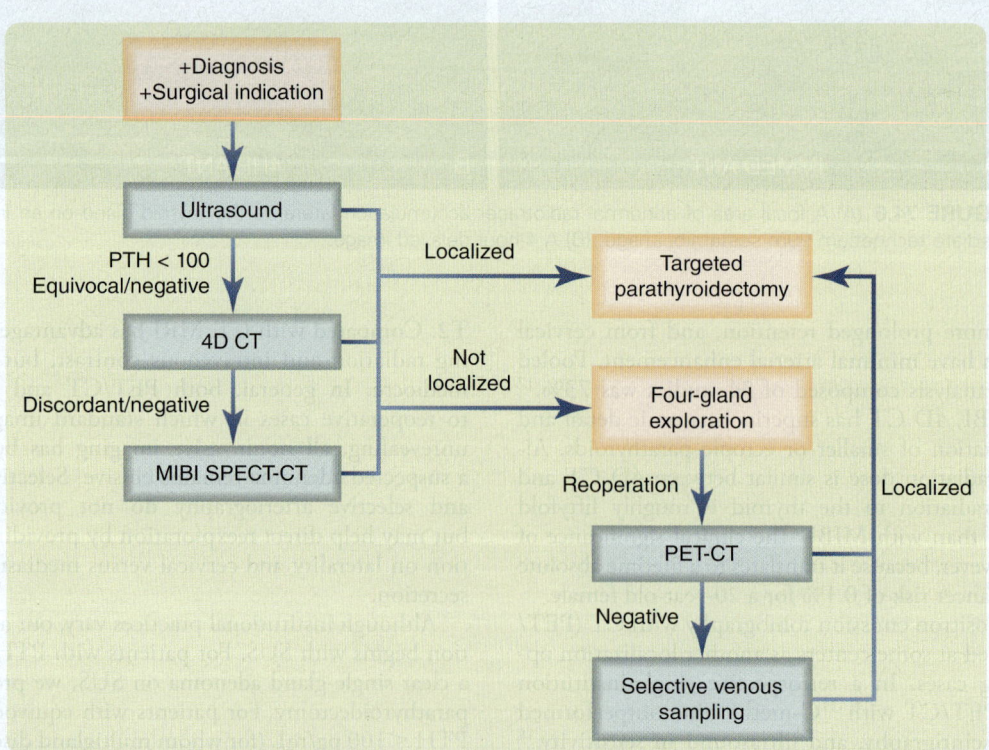

FIGURE 74.7 Approach to localization in primary hyperparathyroidism. *4D CT,* Four-dimensional computed tomography; *MIBI,* sestamibi; *PET,* positron emission tomography; *PTH,* parathyroid hormone; *SPECT,* single-photon emission computed tomography.

studies, this benefit translates to a significant reduction in long-term probability of fracture.

The effects of parathyroidectomy on extraskeletal end-organ function are less definitive. In the Medicare population, parathyroidectomy is associated with a lower incidence of major cardiovascular events and cardiovascular mortality compared with nonoperative counterparts, with an absolute risk reduction of roughly 1.5%.[21] However, randomized trials have shown no effect of parathyroidectomy on left ventricular ejection fraction at 24 months.[19] There are also scarce data to indicate that parathyroidectomy improves renal function among patients with impaired eGFR. In a retrospective study of the Danish National Patient Registry, parathyroidectomy was not associated with any change in eGFR among patients with impaired kidney function at baseline.[22] In a large target trial emulation study of a US veteran population, parathyroidectomy was associated with a reduced probability of eGFR decline compared with nonoperative management, but only in a subgroup of patients younger than 60 years of age.[23] Among patients who present with PHPT and a history of nephrolithiasis, parathyroidectomy is not associated with a reduction in future kidney stone events; however, follow-up beyond 5 years is lacking. Across three randomized trials that reported quality-of-life outcomes, two identified significant benefits over observation. However, the benefited domains differed, and a third trial found no difference between arms at 2-year follow-up.[19]

Taken together, these data may be summarized as follows: (1) There is tier 1 evidence that parathyroidectomy improves bone mineral density (BMD) compared with observation. (2) Population-level data suggest that parathyroidectomy is associated with reductions in long-term fracture risk and cardiovascular events. (3) Parathyroidectomy may be associated with a lower probability of significant eGFR decline among patients <60 years of age. For all other purported benefits of parathyroidectomy, we maintain a conservative stance during patient counseling but have observed that many patients seem to feel better after parathyroidectomy. Predicting such improvement has not been reliable, though.

Nonoperative Management

Calcium supplementation is frequently discouraged among patients with PHPT and hypercalcemia, and some physicians even recommend active restriction of dietary calcium intake. However, because of the inverse sigmoidal relationship between PTH and serum calcium, restriction of calcium intake results in minimal change in serum calcium level and may exacerbate PTH elevation. The Endocrine Society recommends *against* dietary calcium restriction and supports calcium supplementation consistent with general population guidelines (1000–1200 mg daily from all sources). Similarly, vitamin D supplementation does not worsen hypercalcemia in the setting of PHPT. Vitamin D deficiency is detrimental because the physiology of PTH regulation responds with further elevation in PTH. In a meta-analysis of retrospective studies, vitamin D supplementation was associated with lower PTH levels without worsening hypercalcemia. As such, the ASBMR recommends vitamin D supplementation on an individual basis to attain recommended normal levels of 25(OH)D3 (typically > 30 ng/mL).

The ASBMR recommends pharmacologic management of PHPT among patients who meet surgical indications but who are not appropriate surgical candidates or who are unable to achieve a surgical cure.[16] Medical management has two main objectives: preservation or improvement of BMD and reduction in hypercalcemia.

There is tier 1 evidence that bisphosphonates—most commonly alendronate—significantly improve BMD in the setting of PHPT. In one randomized, placebo-controlled crossover trial, alendronate increased BMD at the total hip, femoral neck, and lumbar spine and significantly reduced bone turnover markers. Risedronate has also been shown to increase lumbar spine BMD; however, its effects at other sites are less consistent. In a prospective observational study of postmenopausal females, parathyroidectomy outperformed a 2-year course of risedronate in tibial BMD improvement. As an antiresorptive drug class, bisphosphonates have no effect on serum calcium level, and unlike parathyroidectomy, there are no compelling data to suggest that bisphosphonates reduce long-term fracture risk.

Denosumab is another antiresorptive monoclonal antibody that acts through binding of RANKL, which in turn blocks osteoclast maturation and function. Like bisphosphonates, denosumab improves BMD and reduces bone turnover without affecting serum calcium. Although there is no randomized trial comparing denosumab to placebo in the setting of PHPT, observational data suggest that denosumab treatment is associated with reduced levels of alkaline phosphatase and an increase in BMD at the femoral neck and total hip. In one small retrospective study, patients treated with denosumab experienced comparable improvement in BMD at the lumbar spine, total hip, and femoral neck as those who underwent parathyroidectomy.

Among patients for whom correction of hypercalcemia is the primary goal of treatment, cinacalcet is the pharmacologic treatment of choice. As a calcimimetic, cinacalcet reduces serum calcium and PTH with minimal impact on BMD. In a meta-analysis of four randomized clinical trials, cinacalcet was found to significantly increase the likelihood of normocalcemia and reduce serum PTH levels compared with placebo.[24] However, there was no effect on BMD or urinary calcium. The DENOCINA trial randomized osteopenic or osteoporotic patients with PHPT to placebo, denosumab alone, or combination cinacalcet plus denosumab. BMD improved in patients who received denosumab, whereas calcium normalized in most patients who received cinacalcet.[25] Taken together, these studies suggest that bisphosphonates should be considered first-line therapy in osteoporotic patients with PHPT who cannot undergo surgery, whereas denosumab may be a second-line option. Cinacalcet may be added to correct significant hypercalcemia. Notably, no pharmacologic treatment has been shown to reduce fracture risk or cardiovascular events. Thus, patients who meet consensus indications for parathyroidectomy should be counseled that surgery is the most durable and comprehensive treatment.[16]

Hypercalcemic Crisis

Hyperparathyroidism-induced hypercalcemic crisis (HIHC) is a rare, potentially life-threatening condition that is variably reported as hyperparathyroid crisis, parathyroid storm, or parathyroid crisis. Incidence is reported as between 2% and 7% of PHPT cases and is confounded by inconsistent diagnostic criteria. A common definition is albumin-corrected serum calcium >14 mg/dL in the setting of elevated PTH and clinical symptoms. Unlike PHPT, HIHC has a female-to-male incidence ratio closer to 1:1 and mortality as high as 7%.

Among patients with PHPT, HIHC is usually precipitated by a second physiologic insult. Examples include dehydration, steroid use, surgery, thiazide diuretics, and infection. Presenting symptoms are typically neurologic and/or gastrointestinal: altered mental status, severe fatigue, anorexia, vomiting, and pain. Pancreatitis has been reported in up to 10% of cases. Cardiac signs typical of severe hypercalcemia include shortened QT interval and arrhythmia. Degree of hormonal elevation is generally more severe in HIHC than in noncrisis, and PTH in the range of 300 to 960 pg/mL is typical. Severe hypercalcemia with normal or minimally elevated PTH should prompt assessment for a second contributing etiology in addition to PHPT, such as advanced malignancy, sarcoidosis, and thyrotoxicosis.

Initial treatment of HIHC is pharmacologic correction of hypercalcemia. Most patients are hypovolemic, so intravenous normal saline is a critical first step and may be expected to drop serum calcium by roughly 2 mg/dL. After establishing euvolemia and consistent urine output, loop diuretics are introduced to reduce renal calcium resorption. Bisphosphonates inhibit bone resorption and are frequently used, but they typically do not take effect until 48 hours after initiation. Intravenous zoledronic acid is superior to pamidronate in restoring normocalcemia in malignancy and may have a faster time to onset; however, it is contraindicated in acute kidney injury. Calcitonin has rapid onset and is a useful bridge until bisphosphonates take effect. Calcitonin promotes calciuresis and can lower calcium by 1 mg/dL within 2 to 6 hours. Tachyphylaxis tends to develop within 48 hours; thus, combination therapy with bisphosphonates is recommended over calcitonin alone. For refractory cases and in patients with renal insufficiency, dialysis with a low-calcium dialysate is effective. In more recent years, other temporizing agents, such as denosumab and cinacalcet, have been described. Because of limited experience, these are generally reserved for patients for whom there is an anticipated delay in surgery.

Parathyroidectomy is recommended once the patient is medically optimized. There does not appear to be a clear advantage to expediting resection. As is the case with PHPT, most cases of HIHC are due to a single abnormal parathyroid gland, although the incidence of ectopic location and PCA are higher. As such, diagnostic workup and localization processes are largely the same for HIHC as for noncrisis cases, with ultrasound and sestamibi SPECT-CT commonly used. In surgical series, parathyroids resected for HIHC are significantly larger, and carcinoma is present in up to 10% of cases. Although the incidence of multigland disease has been reported to be as high as 24%, single-gland adenoma remains the most common culprit. Targeted parathyroidectomy guided by intraoperative PTH monitoring is reasonable (see "Surgical Technique"); however, in our practice, routine contralateral exploration is also performed because the repercussions of persistent or recurrent HIHC can be dire. In experienced hands, rates of operative success and normocalcemia at 6 months are similar between HIHC and noncrisis PHPT.

SECONDARY AND TERTIARY HYPERPARATHYROIDISM

Epidemiology

SHPT is a broad term that describes parathyroid hyperplasia and elevated PTH as an adaptive response to another physiologic insult. The two most common etiologies are vitamin D deficiency and CKD. Because isolated vitamin D deficiency is readily recognized and easily corrected, this section will focus on hyperparathyroidism because of CKD. Compensatory PTH elevation typically begins once eGFR drops to 45 mL/min. On initiation of dialysis, hyperparathyroidism is nearly ubiquitous. Persistent hyperparathyroidism with hypercalcemia—that is, tertiary hyperparathyroidism—is reported in roughly one-fifth of patients who undergo kidney transplantation.

Pathophysiology

Hyperparathyroidism develops in the setting of CKD primarily as a result of 1,25(OH)2D3 deficiency resulting from 1α-hydroxylase downregulation. Concurrent hyperphosphatemia also plays a role in upregulating PTH secretion (see Physiology). Persistently elevated PTH exacerbates renal osteodystrophy and is associated with a greater risk of osteoporosis and fracture. Histologically, parathyroids are initially characterized by polyclonal proliferation and diffuse hyperplasia. During this early phase, vitamin D and calcimimetics are effective at reducing PTH levels. Over time, there is gradual reduction in expression of vitamin D and calcium receptors on parathyroid cells, and super-physiologic secretion of PTH becomes autonomous. These changes are accompanied by evolution to nodular hyperplasia, and monoclonal adenomatous glands have also been described. This latter entity can be difficult to discern from normocalcemic PHPT.

After transplantation, early phases of SHPT are often reversible; however, advanced SHPT typically persists. In this setting, elevation of PTH with normocalcemia is generally referred to as *persistent SHPT*, whereas concurrent elevation of both PTH and serum calcium is referred to as *tertiary hyperparathyroidism* (THPT). For most patients with SHPT, serum PTH drops between 3 to 12 months after kidney transplant, with a greater likelihood of remission among patients with restored eGFR. However, roughly one in five patients evolve to long-term THPT with concurrent hypercalcemia.[26] Across retrospective datasets, THPT has been associated with delayed allograft function, higher rate of allograft failure, and higher all-cause mortality.[27] Vascular calcification and nephrocalcinosis have been proposed as potential mechanisms for this relationship; however, it remains unproven whether THPT is the instigator or the consequence of poor allograft function.

Nonoperative Management

Unlike PHPT, medical management is first line for early SHPT. The mainstays of pharmacologic treatment are vitamin D supplementation and cinacalcet. In observational studies, vitamin D supplementation in dialysis patients has been consistently associated with reduced PTH levels and improved survival. However, there is considerable risk of hypercalcemia, and consensus guidelines from the Kidney Disease Improving Global Outcomes (KDIGO) group recommend against routine supplementation in predialysis patients. Excess vitamin D may be detrimental because induced hypercalcemia and hyperphosphatemia have been linked to vascular calcification and myocardial fibrosis in animal models. With progression toward end-stage renal disease, parathyroid resistance to vitamin D develops. Although dose escalation may temporize SHPT and delay transition to nodular hyperplasia, this approach is ultimately limited by hypercalcemia and hyperphosphatemia.

Calcimimetics—most commonly cinacalcet—increase the sensitivity of parathyroid calcium receptors and increase vitamin D receptor expression. Both effects result in reduced PTH secretion and are accompanied by lower serum calcium and phosphorous. These ancillary effects on serum electrolytes make combination therapy with vitamin D appealing. Monotherapy cinacalcet has been shown to be as effective as vitamin D in lowering PTH via the PARADIGM trial.[28] The EVOLVE trial showed that cinacalcet lowered the rate of composite cardiovascular events, heart failure, and all-cause mortality compared with placebo in dialysis patients ≥65 years with severe SHPT.[29] The main drawbacks of cinacalcet are cost and incidence of nausea and vomiting in up to one-third of patients. After withdrawal of cinacalcet, calcium and

PTH tend to rebound significantly within 12 months. Currently, whether vitamin D monotherapy or combination therapy with cinacalcet is first line for SHPT remains controversial.

Surgical Indications and Outcomes

Early SHPT is typically asymptomatic, but prolonged disease may manifest with bone pain, weakness, and poor quality of life. Persistent hypercalcemia, hypophosphatemia, and anemia are common. Unlike PHPT, there is no consensus set of criteria for surgical referral. Most centers recommend surgery for SHPT or THPT that is symptomatic or has persistent electrolyte derangements despite maximal medical management. Degree of PTH elevation is a consideration: KDIGO recommends maintaining PTH at two to nine times the normal range (upper limit $\leq$585 pg/mL), but target thresholds of $\leq$500 or $\leq$800 have also been cited. In large retrospective series, patients with SHPT or THPT who undergo parathyroidectomy experience a significant increase in BMD and a lower risk of hip fracture.[30] Patients who undergo parathyroidectomy for SHPT while on dialysis tend to have durable treatment effect after subsequent transplant, with lower rates of developing THPT and need for posttransplant cinacalcet.[31] However, less than 5% of transplanted patients undergo parathyroidectomy for SHPT in the pretransplant setting.[32]

There is persistent debate regarding the indications for and timing of parathyroidectomy for THPT. Iatrogenic hypercalcemia due to vitamin D and/or cinacalcet in the SHPT setting typically improves within a month after transplantation once these drugs are stopped. However, a delayed phase of recurrent hypercalcemia is commonly noted roughly 6 months thereafter. In part because of these fluctuations over the first year, consideration of parathyroidectomy is typically deferred until 9 to 12 months after transplantation. Because persistent use of vitamin D supplementation or its analogs after kidney transplantation is limited by hypercalcemia, treatment options for THPT are predominantly cinacalcet or parathyroidectomy. In one retrospective series, early referral to parathyroidectomy (<278 days) was associated with improved preservation of posttransplant kidney function.[33] Despite the deleterious relationship between THPT and allograft function, there is no consistent evidence that parathyroidectomy improves long-term allograft survival. In a small randomized trial comparing parathyroidectomy versus cinacalcet, there was no difference between groups in rate of normocalcemia, PTH level, BMD, or creatinine.[34] Nevertheless, acknowledging low-quality evidence, the AAES supports parathyroidectomy as the treatment of choice for THPT and recommends surgical referral within 12 months posttransplant should patients experience persistent hypercalcemia.[35] Retrospective series have shown that parathyroidectomy for THPT may result in a transient reduction in eGFR by approximately 25%.[26] However, in most studies, allograft function recuperates to at least preparathyroidectomy levels by approximately 1 year, suggesting that this detriment is secondary to hemodynamic shifts during surgery rather than a durable pathophysiologic effect.

Choice of Surgery

The most common operations performed for SHPT and THPT are SPTX and total parathyroidectomy with autotransplantation (PTX-AT). In a small, randomized trial, PTX-AT outperformed SPTX in calcium normalization and clinical symptoms. PTX-AT has the added advantage that delayed reoperation to excise additional parathyroid tissue, if necessary, is less complex in the forearm than in a reoperative cervical field. However, data from the National Surgical Quality Improvement Program show that PTX-AT is associated with longer operating time and length of stay. In a meta-analysis of 18 studies and over 3500 patients, there was no difference between techniques in symptomatic improvement, persistent disease, recurrence rate, or reoperation. Persistent disease was present in 6% of SPTX patients and 2% of PTX-AT, and rates of reoperation were 5.3% and 5.8%, respectively. PTX-AT was associated with longer operating time and length of stay and a higher rate of long-term vitamin D supplementation.[36] Taken together, these data suggest that SPTX and PTX-AT are both highly effective at treating THPT, with PTX-AT trading more prolonged recovery for slightly increased short-term efficacy. The AAES recommends SPTX as the preferred option for patients with enlargement of all four parathyroids but acknowledges surgeon preference remains a key contributor.[35] Further details on surgical principles are available in the Surgical Technique section.

Postoperative Management

Regardless of surgical approach, recovery after parathyroidectomy for SHPT and THPT is more complex than for PHPT. This translates to longer length of stay and higher complication and readmission rates. Hungry bone syndrome (HBS) is a common phenomenon after SPTX and PTX-AT. It is reported in roughly 13% of patients undergoing parathyroidectomy for PHPT and up to 50% of patients undergoing surgery for SHPT or THPT.[37,38] Risk of HBS is lower for THPT than for SHPT and lower for SPTX than for PTX-AT.[35] Nearly all patients experience transient hypocalcemia after TPX-AT. HBS is defined as hypocalcemia for >4 days after surgery and is secondary to unchecked osteoblastic calcium uptake accompanying the dramatic decrease in serum PTH that follows parathyroidectomy. If uncorrected, symptoms include paresthesia, perioral numbness, and muscle locking, whereas severe disease can result in arrhythmia, tetany, and seizures.

Anticipation and prompt management of HBS are key to efficient postoperative recovery. Most centers employ immediate postoperative oral calcium carbonate and calcitriol, and some implement these medications preemptively before surgery for up to 1 week. Hypocalcemia refractory to oral supplementation is treated with intravenous calcium gluconate. Typically, native calcium levels nadir at between 2 and 3 days after surgery, after which intravenous calcium may be transitioned gradually to an oral regimen. Hypomagnesemia and hypophosphatemia are common accompaniments as a result of bone deposition, and these require vigilant supplementation. Rates of persistent hypocalcemia and hypoparathyroidism are not often reported but may be in the 5% to 20% range, depending on choice of operation and duration of vitamin D supplementation.[39,40]

Calciphylaxis

Calciphylaxis, also referred to *as calcific uremic arteriolopathy*, is a highly morbid condition usually reported among dialysis patients, although it can also afflict those in earlier stages of CKD. Nonuremic calciphylaxis is also described but is rare. First described by Hans Selye via a series of animal experiments, the condition became recognized in human subjects in 1969. Clinically, the disease presents with ischemic, painful, persistent skin wounds that progress to ulceration and infection (Fig. 74.8). Ischemia of muscle, viscera, and eyes have also been described. Pathogenesis is thought to be via small vessel calcification, and histologic inspection of skin biopsies often shows microthrombosis and fibrointimal hyperplasia. However, because of its rarity, most human data take the form of case series and case-control studies, and its mechanism remains under investigation.

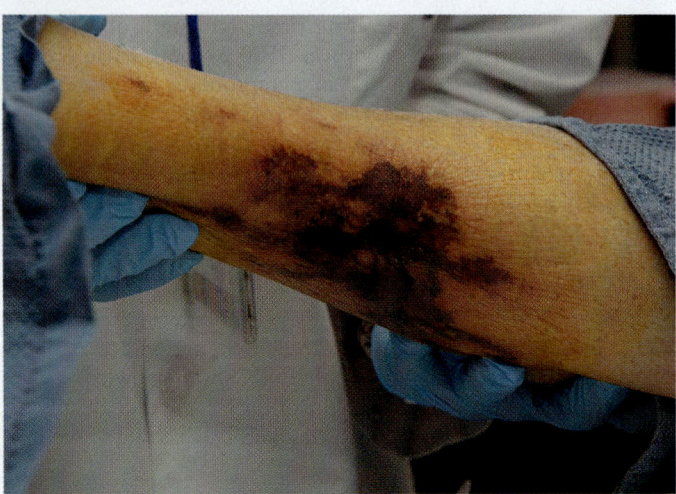

FIGURE 74.8 A violaceous skin lesion with ischemia and eschar formation resulting from calciphylaxis.

Risk factors for calciphylaxis vary across reports. Dysregulation of calcium and phosphorous due to abnormal mineral bone metabolism is thought to contribute to small vessel deposition and is compounded by iatrogenic effects from vitamin D or its analogs. However, calciphylaxis is not exclusive to patients with severe hypercalcemia or those with very elevated PTH. Other proposed risk factors include female sex, autoimmune disease, hypercoagulability, obesity, and medications that increase serum calcium. The relationship between warfarin and calciphylaxis is particularly notable. Although its intended therapeutic action is repression of vitamin K–dependent coagulation factors, it also affects vitamin K–dependent factors that inhibit vascular calcification, such as matrix Gla protein, thereby inducing vascular calcification in animal models. The relationship in humans is not fully understood, however, and tissue ischemia in patients who recently started warfarin must also raise consideration of warfarin-induced necrosis.

Because risk factors are inconsistent and clinical presentation varies widely, confirming a diagnosis of calciphylaxis can be challenging. There is no laboratory marker that establishes calciphylaxis, but a thorough workup for comorbid and contributing conditions should include a liver panel, bone turnover markers, hypercoagulation panel, and evaluation for autoimmune disease. Sequelae of calciphylaxis, such as local infection and sepsis, must be assessed continuously because these are the most common pathways to mortality. A punch or incisional biopsy that includes the edge of a suspected calciphylactic lesion and adjacent normal skin establishes the diagnosis. Histologic signs include calcification, thrombosis, and fibrointimal hyperplasia of arterioles, along with septal panniculitis.

Treatment of calciphylaxis is supportive and multidisciplinary. Wound care is paramount, with chemical debridement of small, noninfected ischemic ulcerations and surgical debridement of larger or infected areas of necrotic tissue. Surgical strategies include serial debridement with negative-pressure appliances, skin grafts, and hyperbaric oxygen, although no one protocol is supported by high-level evidence. Pain control is multimodal and adjusted for renal clearance. Cinacalcet, sodium thiosulfate, and phosphate binders are used to control serum PTH, and vitamin D and its analogs should be discontinued or used very judiciously. The Evaluation of Cinacalcet Hydrochloride Therapy to Lower Cardiovascular Events (EVOLVE) trial comparing cinacalcet to placebo noted a threefold lower rate of calciphylaxis in the cinacalcet arm.[41] The role of parathyroidectomy in calciphylaxis is controversial. Although some recommend early resection, an alternative approach is to restrict surgery for refractory cases with PTH > 300 ng/mL despite cinacalcet. If parathyroidectomy is indicated, SPTX or PTX-AT is preferred over more limited resections to avoid persistent or recurrent disease.

PARATHYROID CARCINOMA

Epidemiology

PCA is among the rarest solid organ malignancies in humans, accounting for less than 1% of PHPT. Because of its rarity, robust data on risk factors and even diagnostic criteria are lacking. A history of neck irradiation, younger age at diagnosis, and advanced kidney disease have been linked to PCA, but the condition remains rare in all patient strata. Most cases are sporadic, but both germline and somatic mutations have been characterized as pathogenic in a subset of cases. These included inherited mutations in *CDC73* (HPT-JT), *MEN1* (MEN1), *RET* (MEN2A), *TP53,* and *PRUNE2* as well as down- and upregulation via abnormal DNA methylation.

Diagnosis and Imaging

Preoperative diagnosis of PCA is rarely conclusive, and most cases of PCA are established after index resection, either on pathologic assessment or delayed recurrence at locoregional or distant sites. In fact, the criteria to establish a pathologic diagnosis of PCA have been debated over recent years. Current histologic features that confirm PCA, according to the WHO, are any of the following: (1) angioinvasion, (2) lymphatic invasion, (3) perineural invasion, (4) invasion into surrounding structures, or (5) confirmed metastatic disease.[42] It has been proposed that classic PA and PCA fall on a histologic spectrum, without a clear delineation. As such, borderline cases that feature nuclear pleomorphism, increased mitotic activity, necrosis, fibrotic bands, Ki-67 >5%, or pseudocapsular invasion without clear malignant criteria are collectively classified as "atypical parathyroid tumors."[43] The nomenclature has changed from prior WHO renditions, in which it was called *atypical parathyroid adenoma.* This reflects the acknowledgment that metachronous recurrence (local or distant) has been reported in roughly 3% of atypical cases.

Preoperative evaluation for PCA requires a high index of suspicion. Unlike PHPT, PCA tends to present with severely elevated serum calcium, often >3 mg/dL above the upper limit of normal. PTH levels are similarly elevated to greater than threefold the normal range, and values 10 times the normal range have been reported. Alkaline phosphatase elevation >300 IU/L may be indicative of high bone turnover associated with PCA, but this is not a sensitive threshold. Although most cases of PHPT are recognized incidentally on laboratory testing, PCA has a higher rate of end-organ complications. Presenting symptoms include nephrolithiasis, renal insufficiency, pathologic fracture, osteitis fibrosa cystica, and hypercalcemic crisis. Symptoms from mass effect and local invasion may be present, including dysphagia, compression, palpable mass, and vocal cord palsy. These latter findings are more commonly noted in nonfunctioning PCA—which constitutes roughly 10% of cases—and portend a worse prognosis as a result of delay in diagnosis.

Noninvasive imaging plays an important role in diagnosis, staging, and surgical planning. Sonographic features that may differentiate PCA from benign adenoma include size >3 cm, ill-defined margins, heterogeneity, invasion of surrounding structures, adenopathy, calcification, and greater depth-to-width ratio. However, no one feature is pathognomonic, and with the exception of regional invasion, all may be found in benign or atypical cases. Sestamibi, with or without SPECT-CT, serves not only to localize the primary tumor but also can demonstrate metastatic lesions as well. Cross-sectional anatomy is best evaluated via 4D CT or MRI and should be performed preoperatively for patients who have a biochemical and clinical presentation that places them at high risk for PCA. When performed, CT is extended to include the chest and abdomen to assess for metastatic disease. Routine positron emission tomography is not indicated for staging but may be effective for suspected recurrence or in cases of nonfunctioning PCA that are not sestamibi avid.

Needle biopsy or aspiration is not recommended because tract site tumor implants have been reported. Moreover, aspirated specimens are frequently ineffective at differentiating between benign adenoma and atypical tumors, and they do not address any of the criteria for confirming PCA. However, needle aspiration may have a role in establishing a diagnosis of metachronous metastatic recurrence, particularly among patients with a suspicious distant lesion that is not sestamibi avid. In such cases, fine-needle aspiration with PTH washout may be diagnostic.

Treatment

Initial treatment of suspected PCA focuses on managing signs and symptoms of hypercalcemia. Patients presenting in hypercalcemic crisis should be temporized pharmacologically (see "Hyperparathyroid-Induced Hypercalcemic Crisis"). Once the patient is stabilized, imaging is obtained to localize the offending parathyroid and assess for locoregional and distant extent of disease.

The only curative treatment for PCA is resection based on oncologic principles. Margin positivity is associated with significantly worse overall survival; thus, en bloc resection of the ipsilateral thyroid lobe is recommended because the parathyroid is often adherent to the adjacent thyroid. Most cases of PCA are not recognized preoperatively and are instead diagnosed on pathology after resection for presumed benign PHPT. In fact, less than 15% of cases undergo en bloc resection, and incomplete resection is reported in up to two-thirds of cases. After index surgery, if calcium and PTH remain elevated and pathologic inspection reveals positive margin(s), reoperation after interval imaging is advised. On the other hand, for patients with normalization of calcium and PTH in the setting of an R1 resection, the incremental benefit of reexploration may not justify the accompanying elevated risk of nerve injury.

There are no robust data on adjuvant therapy. PCA is resistant to radiation, and its role in locoregional control should be restricted to margin-positive or recurrent cases that are not amenable to reoperation. There is no role for adjuvant chemotherapy in PCA. Systemic therapy for recurrent disease is relegated to cases for which metastatic lesions are not amenable to surgery and hypercalcemia progresses despite maximal treatment with appropriate agents. In these very rare instances, case reports have documented efficacy of temozolomide, mammalian target of rapamycin (mTOR) inhibitors, and antiangiogenic tyrosine kinase inhibitors. In most cases, response is assessed not via traditional radiographic criteria but by improvement in severity of hypercalcemia.

Outcomes After Surgery

PCA is currently staged via the American Joint Committee on Cancer (AJCC) 8th edition classification scheme. T1 is localized to the parathyroid, T2 entails invasion into adjacent thyroid, T3 indicates invasion into other surrounding structures, and T4 describes invasion into major blood vessels (i.e., carotid, subclavian) or spine. N1a describes nodal metastases in levels VI or VII of the central neck, whereas N1b indicates involvement of stations I through V or retropharyngeal nodes. Distant metastases are classified as M1.[44] Because of disease rarity, prognostic stratification by risk factors is challenging. Larger tumor diameter and incomplete resection are associated with worse survival, but there is no consistent relationship between N1 disease and mortality. As such, routine central neck dissection does not serve a clear therapeutic or prognostic role.

Overall, PCA is a relatively indolent cancer. Five-year survival is estimated at 85% to 91%, whereas 10-year survival ranges from 50% to 85%.[45] However, recurrence is common, estimated in some series to be over 50%, with locoregional recurrence outnumbering metachronous metastases. Electrolyte derangements and recurrent hyperparathyroidism are indicative of recurrence, and long-term morbidity is driven by persistent PHPT rather than local effects. Re-resection of local recurrence and/or metastasectomy are aimed at attaining disease control and palliation of endocrinopathy. Multiple palliative operations may be performed for a single patient. Normalization of PTH and calcium via noncurative resection can have a durable impact on both survival and quality of life.

HEREDITARY HYPERPARATHYROIDISM

Most cases of PHPT are sporadic, whereas less than 5% of cases harbor a heritable mutation. Among these, most are attributable to genes well known to confer PHPT—sometimes in isolation, more commonly as one entity within a syndrome of other disorders. Understanding associated diseases directly affects management and surveillance, whereas identifying the genetic culprits holds implications for prognosis and screening of family members. There is no single consensus guideline for genetic testing in PHPT. It is commonly recommended to consider germline testing for patients with two affected primary relatives, anyone with PCA, those with recurrent PHPT, and patients <40 years of age.[46] A summary of genetic abnormalities found in sporadic and heritable hyperparathyroidism is provided in Table 74.1.

Multiple Endocrine Neoplasia Type 1

The *MEN1* gene was first identified in 1997, but cases that likely reflect MEN1 have been documented as early as 1927 by Harvey Cushing, who recorded a patient with a pancreatic islet cell tumor, PHPT, and acromegaly. The syndrome's autosomal dominant pattern of inheritance was described by Paul Wermer in the 1950s, hence its initial eponym *Wermer syndrome*. MEN1's corresponding protein, menin, has diverse roles in transcription modulation, DNA repair, cell signaling, and mitosis. MEN1 is characterized by multigland parathyroid hyperplasia, pancreatic neuroendocrine tumors (NETs), and pituitary adenomas. There is close to 100% penetrance of PHPT by the fifth decade. Disease onset is earlier than in sporadic cases, with biochemical derangements noted in childhood or adolescence and symptomatic presentation typically in the third decade. PHPT due to MEN1 tends to have more end-organ effects than sporadic cases, with lower BMD and higher rates of nephrolithiasis and CKD.[47]

Associated conditions include anterior pituitary adenomas, which most frequently secrete prolactin or somatotropin but may also be nonfunctional. Gastropancreatic NETs are often the most

TABLE 74.1   Genetic Abnormalities Associated With Sporadic and Inherited Forms of Primary HPT: Disorder, Genes, Inheritance, Phenotype, and Recommended Surgical Approach

DISORDER	GENES	INHERITANCE	PHENOTYPE	AGE[a]	SURGICAL APPROACH[b]
Sporadic					
Parathyroid adenoma and hyperplasia	PRAD1, CCND1 (20%–40%), MEN1 (12%–35%), CDC73, CDKN1B, AIP	Sporadic	Isolated pHPT with single adenoma, double adenoma, or four-gland hyperplasia	>45	Minimally invasive parathyroidectomy with ioPTH or bilateral exploration
Parathyroid carcinoma	RB1, CDC73, MEN1, microRNA-296	Sporadic	pHPT secondary to parathyroid carcinoma	>45	En bloc resection
Inherited					
MEN1	MEN1	AD	pHPT (95%) in third decade, pNETs (40%), pituitary adenomas (30%), adrenocortical and thyroid tumors, meningioma, facial angiofibromas, lipomas	25–45	Subtotal parathyroidectomy and transcervical thymectomy
MEN2A	RET	AD	pHPT (15%–35%), MTC (99%), pheochromocytoma (50%), lichen planus, amyloidosis, Hirschsprung disease	38	Resection of only visibly enlarged parathyroid glands. Address or rule out pheochromocytoma first
MEN4	CDKN1B	AD	pHPT (80%), pituitary adenoma (40%), pNETs, adrenal, thyroid, gonadal and renal tumors	50	Same as MEN1
Familial isolated HPT	MEN1, CDC73, CASR, GCM2, CDKN1B	AD	Isolated pHPT, parathyroid carcinoma (GCM2 mutation)	39	Bilateral neck exploration with resection of enlarged glands only versus subtotal parathyroidectomy. En bloc resection for parathyroid cancer
HPT-JT	CDC73	AD	pHPT in second or third decade, parathyroid carcinoma (35%), ossifying fibromas of mandible and maxilla, renal cysts, hamartomas and Wilms tumor, uterine tumors	32	Minimally invasive parathyroidectomy with ioPTH or bilateral exploration. En bloc resection for parathyroid cancer

[a]Age = mean age at presentation of primary HPT in years.
[b]Surgical approach to HPT associated with the disorder.
AD, Autosomal dominant; HPT, hyperparathyroidism; HPT-JT, hyperparathyroidism–jaw tumor syndrome; ioPTH, intraoperative parathyroid hormone; MEN, multiple endocrine neoplasia; MTC, medullary thyroid cancer; pHPT, primary hyperparathyroidism; PTH, parathyroid hormone; pNET, pancreatic neuroendocrine tumors.
Adapted from Silva BC, Cusano NE, Bilezikian JP. Primary hyperparathyroidism. Best Pract Res Clin Endocrinol Metab. 2018;32:593-607; Bilezikian JP, Cusano NE, Khan AA, et al. Primary hyperparathyroidism. Nat Rev Dis Primers. 2016;2:16033; Wilhelm SM, Wang TS, Ruan DT, et al. The American Association of Endocrine Surgeons guidelines for definitive management of primary hyperparathyroidism. JAMA Surg. 2016;151:959-968; El Lakis M, Nockel P, Gaitanidis A, et al. Probability of positive genetic testing results in patients with family history of primary hyperparathyroidism. J Am Coll Surg. 2018;226:933-938.

life-limiting component of MEN1 and affect up to 80% of patients. Gastrinomas of the pancreatic head or second portion of the duodenum—the so-called "gastrinoma triangle"—are most common. Gastrin excess leads to hypersecretion of gastric acid and multiple recurrent ulcers of the stomach and duodenum, that is, Zollinger-Ellison syndrome. Other hormone products include insulin, vasoactive intestinal peptide, and glucagon, each with its own pathognomonic clinical signs. Other conditions linked to MEN1 include lung NETs, breast cancer, and thymic NETs. Most NETs within the MEN1 spectrum are either indolent (lung, breast, pituitary) or have variable malignant behavior (pancreatic NETs) and are manageable via resection and pharmacologic control of systemic effects. However, thymic NETs are increasingly recognized for their unusually aggressive natural history. Despite being prevalent in 2% to 8% of MEN1 patients, they are responsible for 20% of deaths, and most cases present with metastatic disease.[47]

The traditional surgical management of MEN1 PHPT is SPTX with cervical thymectomy. The philosophy is similar to

management of SHPT, focusing on establishing durable control without inducing long-term hypocalcemia. However, it is increasingly recognized that hyperplasia in the setting of MEN1 is often asynchronous, and subtotal parathyroidectomy (or PTX-AT) in children or adolescents may induce prolonged hypoparathyroidism during an important phase of bone deposition. In recent years, reports of less-than-subtotal parathyroidectomy have gained traction. This approach is usually guided by 4D CT or parathyroid venous sampling to direct resection to the side of the neck with more dominant hyperplasia. Single-institution cohorts have shown that unilateral parathyroidectomy and thymectomy may produce durable control of PHPT with negligible risk of prolonged hypoparathyroidism.[48]

Multiple Endocrine Neoplasia Type 2a

The first patient with the grouping of medullary thyroid cancer, pheochromocytoma, and parathyroid enlargement was described by John Sipple in 1961, hence the name Sipple syndrome. Other associated features include cutaneous lichen amyloidosis. Pattern of inheritance is autosomal dominant, via activating mutations in the *RET* receptor tyrosine kinase proto-oncogene. The most common affected codons are 634 (85%), 609, and 618.[49] *RET* mutations are also associated with MEN2B and familial medullary thyroid cancer, but these are not affiliated with PHPT.

PHPT is a feature of 20% to 30% of cases of MEN2A and is most frequent among cases with a codon 634 mutation. Conversely, medullary thyroid cancer is nearly 100% penetrant. Thus, surgical treatment of PHPT is technically challenging because most patients have previously undergone total thyroidectomy by the time PHPT manifests. Unlike MEN1 and most other heritable PHPTs, MEN2A is typically characterized by one or more benign PA(s) rather than diffuse hyperplasia of all four glands. The surgical approach, therefore, leans more toward the philosophy of sporadic PHPT rather than that of MEN1 or SHPT/THPT. Although practice patterns vary, one common approach is preoperative localization followed by four-gland exploration with resection of any parathyroid(s) that appear hyperplastic. Similarly, if one or more enlarged parathyroids are encountered at the time of total thyroidectomy in the setting of known MEN2A, empiric parathyroidectomy should be performed.

Multiple Endocrine Neoplasia Type 4

Germline mutation in *CDKN1B,* which encodes the cyclin-dependent kinase inhibitor p27, is associated with acromegaly and PHPT. This disorder was first described in 2006 in both humans and rat models and has phenotypic overlaps with MEN1. In 2019, a multigenerational Danish family was reported that included members with PHPT who segregated with mutations in *CDKN1B.* Like MEN1, MEN4 presents with diffuse parathyroid hyperplasia and pituitary adenomas. Uniquely, however, MEN4 is also linked to testicular and cervical cancer and adrenal Cushing disease.[50] The surgical treatment of choice is SPTX or PTX-AT.

Hyperparathyroidism–Jaw Tumor Syndrome

Although advanced PHPT can result in giant cell bone lesions as a component of osteitis fibrosa cystica in <5% of cases (i.e., "brown tumors"), ossifying fibromas isolated to the maxilla and/or mandible are indicative of HPT-JT. These lesions lack the multinucleated giant cells characteristic of brown tumors. HPT-JT was first described in 1990 and is inherited in an autosomal dominant fashion. The genetic culprit is inactivation of *CDC73,* which encodes the parafibromin tumor suppressor protein.

Associated features include mixed epithelial and stromal tumors of the kidney, renal cysts, and Wilms tumor. Uterine soft tissue tumors, including leiomyomas and adenosarcomas, have also been linked to HPT-JT. Unlike MEN1 and MEN2A, HPT-JT is associated with an elevated risk of PCA, affecting one in five patients.[49] Risk of malignancy is even higher among patients with a frameshift or deletion mutation of *CDC73,* which is also commonly identified as a somatic mutation in isolated PCA. Like MEN2A, HPT-JT is typically characterized by single-gland parathyroid disease. Thus, focused parathyroidectomy guided by preoperative localization is appropriate. Because of the predisposition for PCA, a low threshold for en bloc ipsilateral thyroidectomy should be considered for cases in which the abnormal parathyroid is firm, adherent to the thyroid, or intracapsular.

Familial Isolated Hyperparathyroidism

For patients with a family history of PHPT suggestive of autosomal dominant inheritance who do not fit into one of the previously described syndromes based on genetic testing or phenotype, FIHP may be considered as a provisional diagnosis of exclusion. Over the last 20 years, as features of HPT-JT and MEN4 have become more thoroughly described, some patients originally classified as FIHP have been reassigned. Many cases of presumed FIHP lack germline mutation of any known PHPT pathway genes. Both *MEN1* and *CDC73* have been implicated, but these cases may represent MEN1 or HPT-JT with incomplete penetrance. Several studies have identified *GCM2* in a subset of FIHP. *GCM2* encodes a transcription factor expressed in chief cells, and activating mutations of the inhibitory domain are thought to result in FIHP. Because the parathyroid phenotype of FIHP varies greatly depending on genotype, routine bilateral exploration with either SPTX or resection only of grossly abnormal glands—guided by intraoperative PTH (ioPTH)—is reasonable.

SURGICAL TECHNIQUE

For most experienced surgeons, resecting a well-localized PA within a standard cervical location is a straightforward operation. However, challenges arise when multigland disease, supernumerary glands, and ectopic locations come into play. Intraoperative technologies have been directed at assisting in the identification of parathyroid tissue, but none supplants operative experience, anatomic familiarity, and meticulous dissection. Careful respect of embryologic tissue planes is critical because bleeding within the surgical field quickly obscures the delineation of parathyroid from surrounding tissues. Once the gland is identified, dissection is focused on avoidance of capsular disruption, which can lead to parathyromatosis and the need for additional, higher-risk operations. In the context of BNE, exposure of parathyroids that are anticipated to be normal requires close attention to native vasculature because compromise of the feeding pedicle can cause temporary or even permanent hypoparathyroidism. Although novel surgical approaches such as transaxillary and transoral endoscopic or robotic parathyroidectomy have given options to patients who wish to avoid a cervical incision, core surgical principles have not changed.

The superior parathyroid glands are classically located posterior to the superior thyroid poles, posterior and lateral to the trajectory of the recurrent laryngeal nerve bilaterally (Fig. 74.9). Their positions are relatively predictable compared with the more variable anatomy of the lower glands and are typically close to the intersection between the middle thyroid vein and the recurrent laryngeal nerve. The inferior parathyroid glands are usually located inferior and posterior to the lower poles, medial to the recurrent laryngeal nerves, along the tracheoesophageal groove. The four glands, in sequence of average proximity to the nerve, are right upper (closest), followed by left upper, left lower, and right lower.

Ectopic parathyroids are reported in up to 16% of cases. The most common scenario is of an ectopic lower parathyroid within the cervical or superior mediastinal thymus (Fig. 74.10). It is for this reason that a cervical thymectomy is commonly performed accompanying SPTX or PTX-AT or for cases in which ioPTH fails to respond appropriately despite BNE. Other common ectopic positions include the carotid sheath, superiorly along the superior thyroid pole vessels, retroesophageal, and retropharyngeal. Parathyroid glands uncommonly may be found under the thyroid capsule or even within the thyroid gland itself. This has led to the practice of ipsilateral thyroid lobectomy if a gland cannot be found. We uncommonly perform blind thyroid lobectomy and favor ultrasound or bivalving the thyroid lobe, especially if an internal jugular PTH gradient of 10% is demonstrated. Thorough

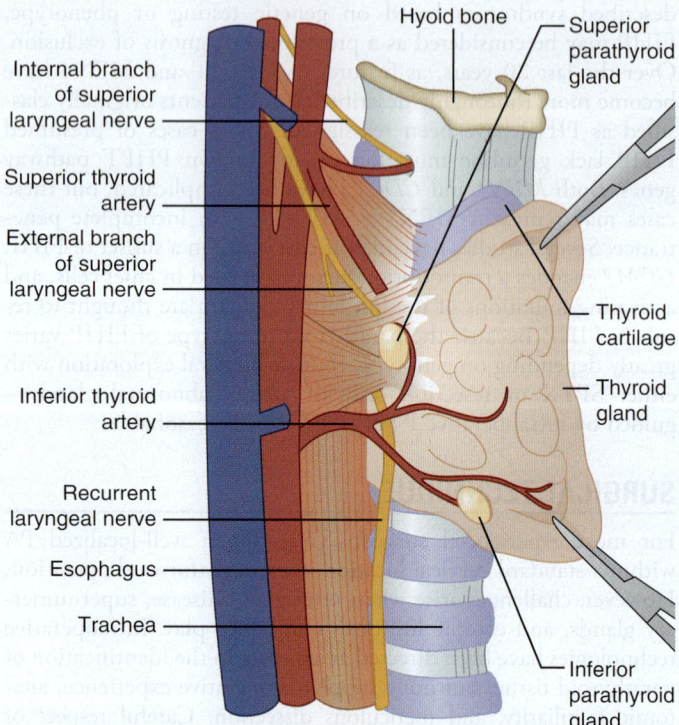

FIGURE 74.9 The superior and inferior parathyroid glands and their normal anatomic relationships are depicted with the right lobe of the thyroid gland retracted anteriorly and medially.

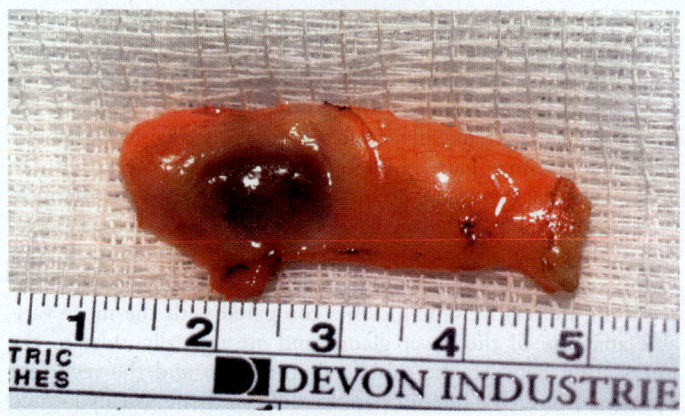

FIGURE 74.10 Ectopic intrathymic parathyroid adenoma.

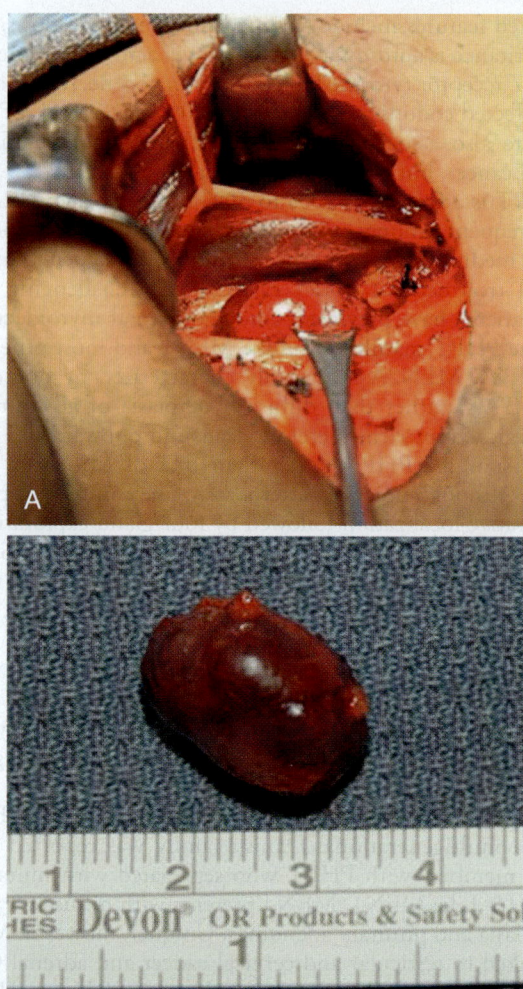

FIGURE 74.11 (A) An intraoperative photograph of an ectopic parathyroid gland in the left carotid sheath present between the internal jugular vein and common carotid artery. The vagus nerve is retracted with a vessel loop anteromedially, and the common carotid artery is retracted laterally. (B) Ex vivo ectopic parathyroid adenoma excised from the left carotid sheath.

exploration of each of these positions—within the constraints of the cervical incision—is indicated for inadequate ioPTH response (Fig. 74.11).

Intraoperative measurement of PTH level is a requisite component of MIP and is frequently used in BNE as well. Because the systemic half-life of PTH is between 3 and 5 minutes in most patients, ioPTH is typically measured before excision of the abnormal parathyroid gland and at 5- and 10-minutes after excision. Because manipulation of the hyperplastic or adenomatous gland may result in a brief spike in PTH secretion, preoperative levels are typically drawn at both induction of general anesthesia and immediately before ligation of the parathyroid vascular pedicle. When ioPTH is used, successful surgery is defined by the Vienna criteria (reduction in ioPTH by at least 50% within 10 minutes of excision compared with highest preexcision baseline) or the

Miami criteria (satisfaction of Vienna criteria plus normalization of ioPTH). Rigorous adherence to these criteria has reduced the rate of persistent PHPT after surgery to <5% in most large series.

SPTX describes planned resection of three parathyroid glands with partial resection of the fourth gland. Typical technique involves BNE with identification of all four glands and assigning the smallest gland for the planned remnant. A portion of that gland is excised, leaving a 40- to 80-mg remnant (roughly one to two times the size of a normal gland) with an intact vascular pedicle. Viability of the remnant can be assessed using visual inspection of color and bleeding at the cut edge. The remaining three glands are then excised after marking the location of the in situ remnant with permanent suture for future identification in the setting of recurrence. With PTX-AT, all four glands are excised, and a portion of one gland is morcellated sharply into <1-mm sections, then aspirated in 1 mL of normal saline. The mixture is then immediately injected into muscle—typically the brachioradialis or sternocleidomastoid—either percutaneously or via cut-down. If direct exposure is obtained, development of a pocket within well-vascularized muscle with meticulous hemostasis is encouraged because surrounding hematoma will compromise incorporation of the implant.

The challenge of accurately identifying and preserving parathyroids and their vasculature during operative exploration has led to advancements in intraoperative parathyroid imaging. The most common techniques harness intrinsic or extrinsic fluorophores to locate tissue using near-infrared fluorescence detectors. Parathyroid tissue emits autofluorescence at 820 nm when excited with a near-infrared laser. This forms the basis of probe-based detector systems, which house both a near-infrared laser and a photodiode detector. The system has been shown to detect parathyroid tissue with sensitivity and accuracy exceeding 90%.[51] However, successful localization of parathyroid tissue does not imply preserved blood flow. For this, intravenous injection of indocyanine green (ICG) may be used in conjunction with perfusion angiography to generate an intraoperative map of both the parathyroid gland and its contributing vascular pedicle. An important limitation of these technologies is the depth of near-infrared light penetration within tissue, which is limited to approximately 5 mm. Thus, both techniques are primarily used to confirm the presence of parathyroid after the presumed gland has already been fully exposed. As such, implementation is more relevant to avoidance of inadvertent parathyroid excision or devascularization in the context of thyroidectomy rather than initial localization during planned parathyroidectomy.

Complications after parathyroidectomy are rare when performed by experienced surgeons. Knowledge of these risks can guide safe postoperative management. Transient hypocalcemia occurs in 1.6% of MIP and up to 13.2% of BNE, and permanent hypocalcemia occurs in less than 0.2% of cases. Thus, single-gland excisions in the context of MIP do not require postoperative calcium assessment or supplementation, although some surgeons take an individualized approach to postoperative calcium supplementation after BNE. In the context of SHPT or THPT, subtotal or total parathyroidectomy is associated with a significantly elevated risk of temporary hypocalcemia. Temporary vocal cord palsy occurs in <1% of cases and is not consistently different by approach across studies. Although permanent vocal cord palsy is higher with BNE in several studies, the absolute risk is <0.2%. Although intraoperative neuromonitoring of the recurrent laryngeal nerve is widely used, there is no prospective evidence proving its efficacy in reducing the rate of nerve injury

in parathyroidectomy. Postoperative hemorrhage is reported in <1% of BNE and <0.5% of MIP; nevertheless, its occurrence may be life threatening. Therefore, although most parathyroidectomies may be performed on an outpatient basis, an observation period of 4 to 6 hours after surgery is recommended.

SELECTED REFERENCES

Bilezikian JP, Khan AA, Silverberg SJ, et al. Evaluation and management of primary hyperparathyroidism: summary statement and guidelines from the fifth international workshop. *J Bone Miner Res.* 2022;37(11):2293-2314.

A consensus guideline on the management of primary hyperparathyroidism.

Dream S, Kuo LE, Kuo JH, et al. The American Association of Endocrine Surgeons Guidelines for the definitive surgical management of secondary and tertiary renal hyperparathyroidism. *Ann Surg.* 2022;276(3):E141-E176.

Consensus guidelines for management of secondary and tertiary hyperparathyroidism.

Lundstam K, Pretorius M, Bollerslev J, et al. Positive effect of parathyroidectomy compared to observation on BMD in a randomized controlled trial of mild primary hyperparathyroidism. *J Bone Miner Res.* 2023;38(3):372-380.

Tier 1 evidence for consideration of parathyroidectomy over medical management in primary hyperparathyroidism.

Park HS, Lee YH, Hong N, Won D, Rhee Y. Germline mutations related to primary hyperparathyroidism identified by next-generation sequencing. *Front Endocrinol (Lausanne).* 2022;13:853171.

Summary of germline mutations relevant to heritable primary hyperparathyroidism.

The full reference list appears on Elsevier eBooks+.

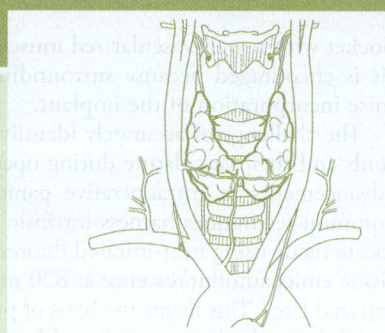

75 | CHAPTER

The Adrenal Glands

Heather Wachtel and Matthew A. Nehs

OUTLINE

HISTORY

The adrenal glands were first described by the Italian anatomist Bartolomeo Eustachi in 1564 as "glandulae quae renibus incumbent," or "glands lying on the kidney." The German comparative anatomist Albert von Kölliker (1817–1905), who noted the presence of the adrenals in a number of vertebrate species, is credited with first identifying two distinct portions of the adrenal gland: the cortex and the medulla. Although Thomas Addison described the clinical features of primary adrenal failure in 1855, it was not until nearly a century later that the adrenal hormones were fully isolated and characterized. Adrenaline (or epinephrine) was first isolated from adrenal extract at the turn of the century circa 1900. Steroid hormones were crystallized from cortical extract ("cortin") by Swiss and American investigators in the 1930s, but their highly similar chemical structures made isolation of the individual compounds challenging. Edward Kendall, Tadeus Reichstein, and Philip Hench jointly received the 1950 Nobel Prize in Physiology or Medicine for their groundbreaking work on the adrenocortical hormones. The Austrian-born endocrinologist Hans Selye first described the stress response in mammals in 1936 and made major contributions to the understanding of the hypothalamic-pituitary-adrenal (HPA) axis. Roger Guillemin, Andrew Schally, and Rosalyn Yalow were awarded the Nobel Prize in 1977 for characterizing the peptide hormones of the brain that underlie the HPA axis as we now understand it.[1,2]

ANATOMY AND EMBRYOLOGY

General and Developmental Aspects

The adrenal glands are paired, orange/yellow-colored structures that are positioned superior and slightly medial to the kidneys in the retroperitoneal space (Fig. 75.1). They are flattened and roughly pyramidal or crescent shaped, weighing approximately 4 g each. The adrenals are among the most highly perfused organs in the body, receiving 2000 mL/kg/min of blood, after only the kidney and thyroid. In most respects, the cortex and medulla can be considered two completely distinct organs that happen to co-localize during development. The two portions have disparate embryologic origins. The primordial cortex arises from the coelomic mesodermal tissue near the cephalic end of the mesonephros during the fourth to fifth week of gestation. Biosynthetic activity can be detected as early as the seventh week. Cortical cell mass dominates the fetal adrenal at 4 months of development, and steroidogenesis is maximum during the third trimester. The adrenal medulla arises from the ectodermal tissues of the embryonic neural crest. It develops in parallel with the sympathetic nervous system, beginning in the fifth to sixth week of gestation. From their original position adjacent to the neural tube, neural crest cells migrate ventrally to assume a paraaortic position near the developing adrenal cortex. There, they differentiate into chromaffin cells that make up the adrenal medulla.

This course of embryologic development yields certain surgically relevant sequelae. Both cortical and medullary tissue can be found at extraadrenal sites (Fig. 75.2). The range of potential sites is wider for chromaffin tissue than for cortical tissue. Pheochromocytomas may arise in extraadrenal sites more commonly than previously believed. When they are extraadrenal, pheochromocytomas are also termed *paragangliomas*.

Relationships

The right adrenal gland abuts the posterolateral surface of the retrohepatic vena cava. The right adrenal fossa is bounded by the right kidney inferolaterally, diaphragm posteriorly, and bare area of the liver anterosuperiorly. The left adrenal gland lies between the left kidney and aorta, with its inferior limb extending farther caudad toward the renal hilum than the right adrenal. The other relationships of the left adrenal gland are the diaphragm posteriorly and the tail of the pancreas and splenic hilum anteriorly. Each adrenal gland is enveloped by its proper capsule, in addition to sharing Gerota's fascia with the kidneys. The adrenal capsules are immediately associated with the perirenal fat.

Vasculature

Knowledge of the macroscopic vascular anatomy of the adrenal glands is essential to proper surgical management. It is important to conceptualize that although the arterial supply is *diffuse,* the

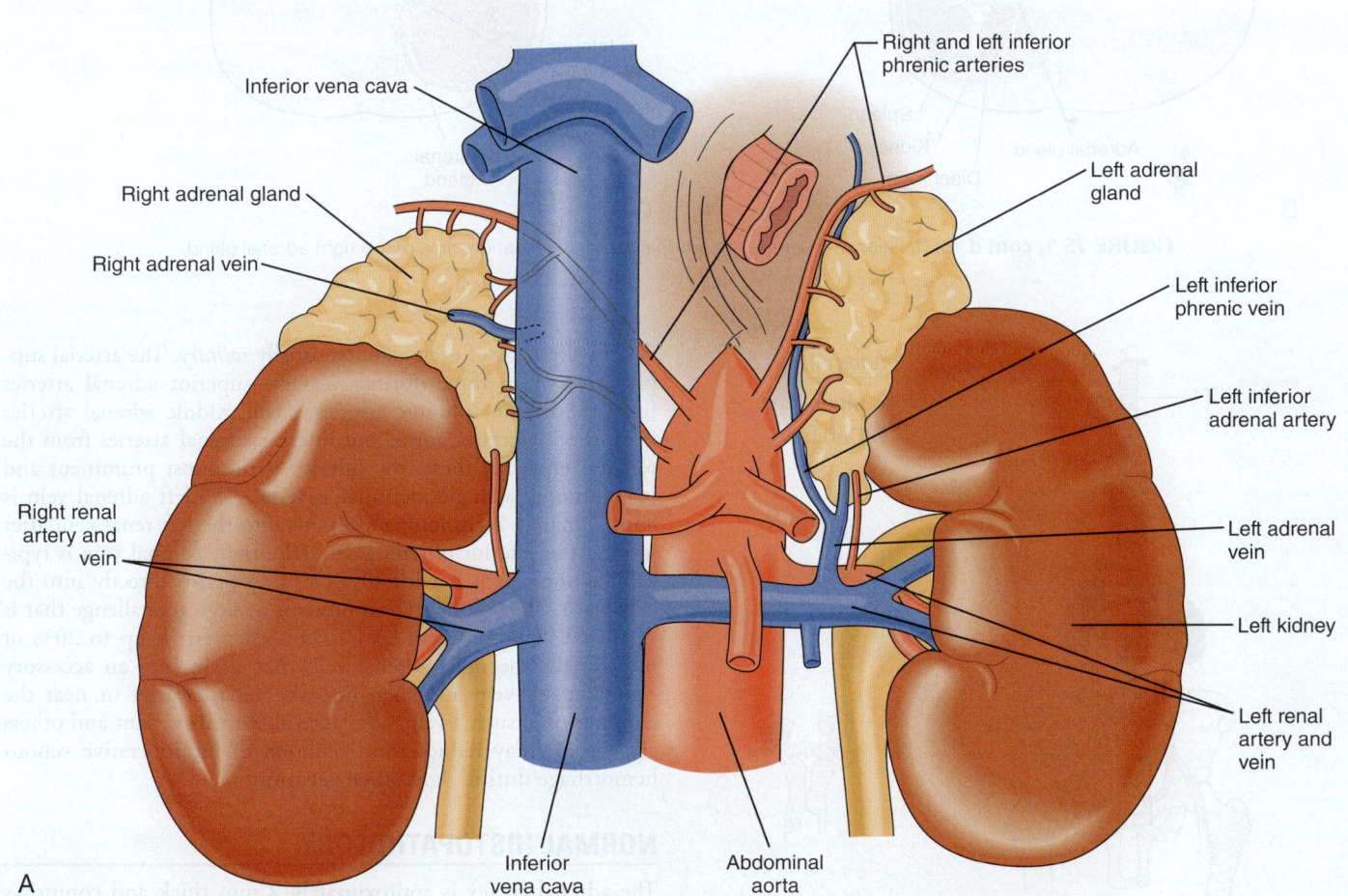

FIGURE 75.1 Anatomy of the adrenal glands. (A) Left and right adrenal glands in situ.

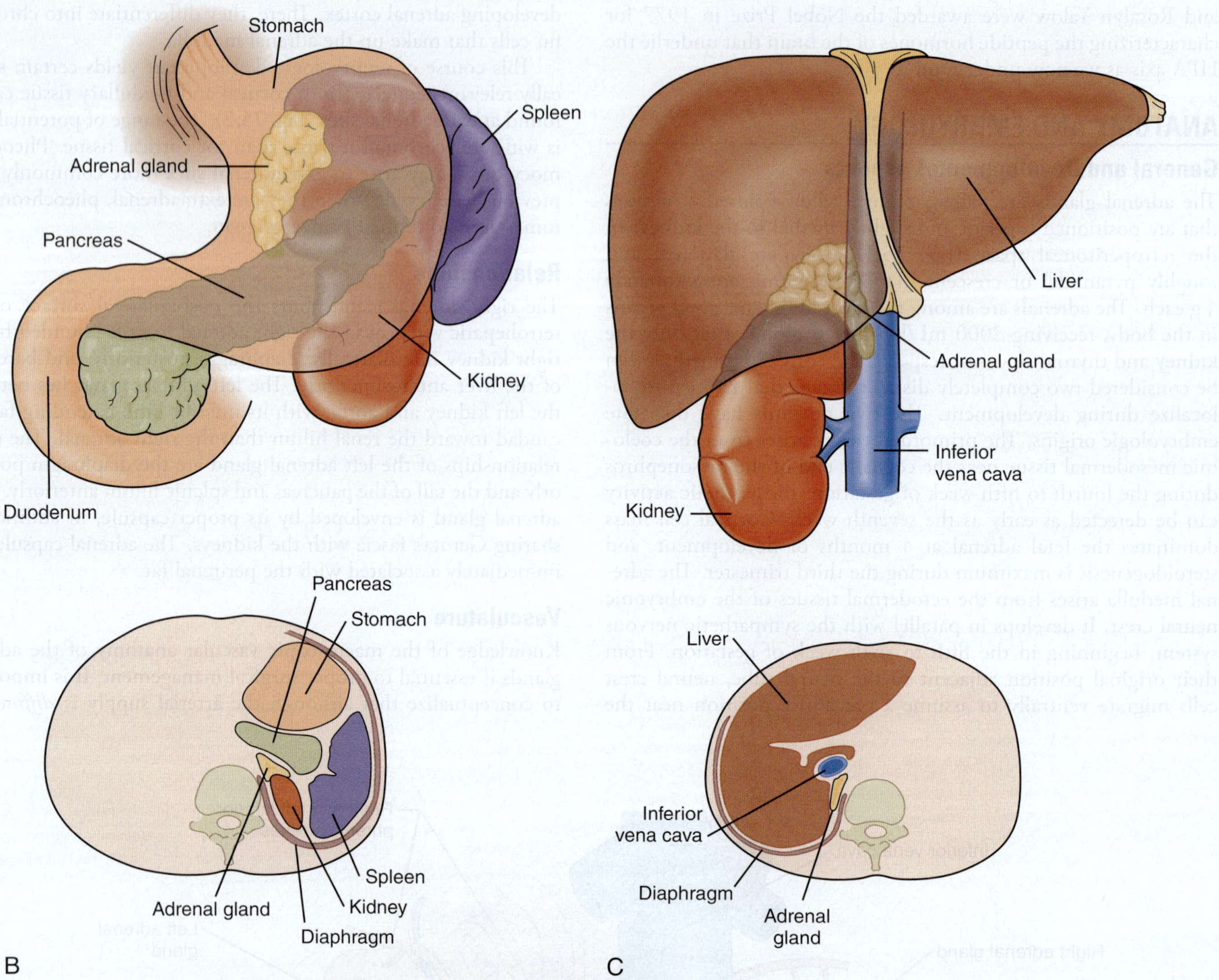

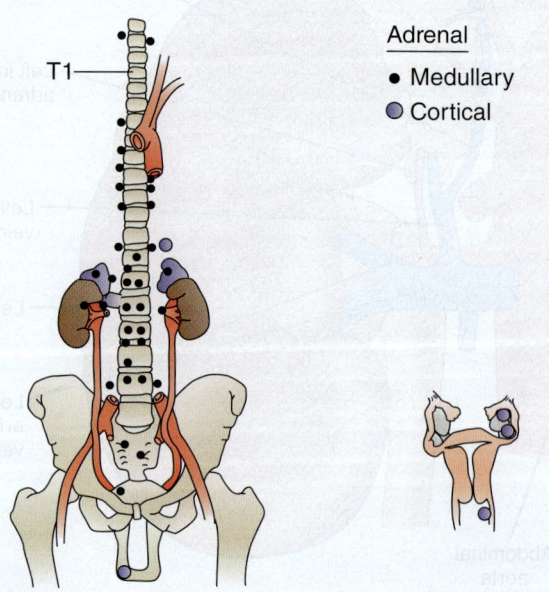

Stomach

Spleen

Adrenal gland

Pancreas

Kidney

Duodenum

Pancreas

Stomach

Liver

Adrenal gland

Inferior vena cava

Kidney

Liver

Spleen

Adrenal gland   Kidney

Diaphragm

Inferior vena cava

Diaphragm

Adrenal gland

B

C

FIGURE 75.1, cont'd (B) Relationships of the left adrenal gland. (C) Relationships of the right adrenal gland.

T1

Adrenal
- Medullary
- Cortical

FIGURE 75.2 Sites of extraadrenal cortical and medullary tissue.

venous drainage of each gland is usually *solitary*. The arterial supply arises from three distinct vessels—superior adrenal arteries from the inferior phrenic arteries, small middle adrenal arteries from the juxtaceliac aorta, and inferior adrenal arteries from the renal arteries. Of these, the inferior is the most prominent and is commonly a single identifiable vessel. The left adrenal vein is approximately 2 cm long and drains into the left renal vein after joining the inferior phrenic vein.[3] The right adrenal vein is typically as short as it is wide (0.5 cm) and drains directly into the vena cava. This configuration presents a surgical challenge that is discussed in more detail later in this chapter. In up to 20% of individuals, the right adrenal vein may drain into an accessory right hepatic vein and then into the vena cava, at or near the confluence of such a vein. Vigilance about this variant and others (Fig. 75.3) may reduce the likelihood of intraoperative venous hemorrhage during right adrenalectomy.

NORMAL HISTOPATHOLOGY

The adrenal cortex is approximately 2 mm thick and comprises more than 80% of the mass of the gland. It is made up of three

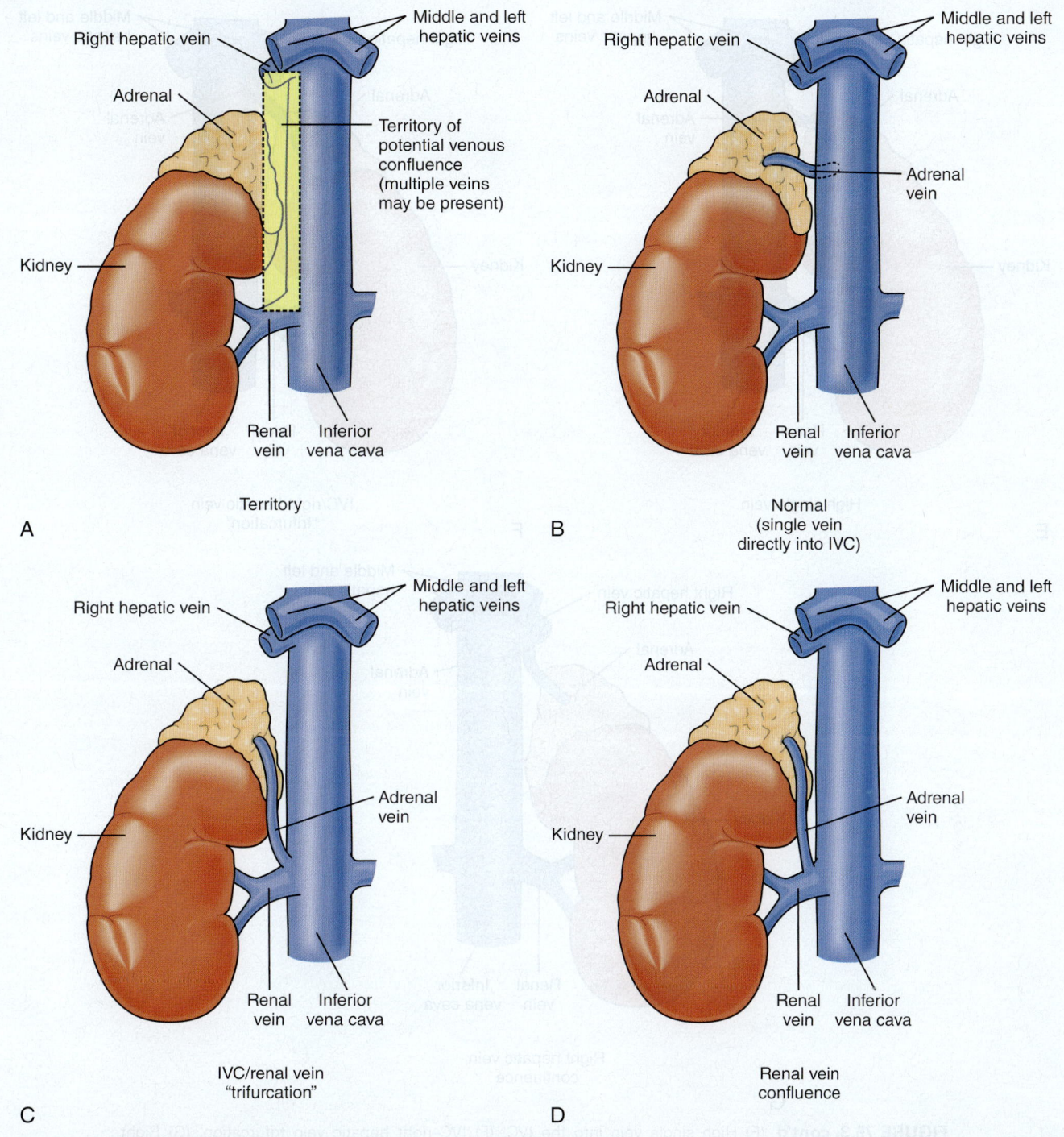

FIGURE 75.3 Variations in right adrenal vein anatomy. (A) Territory of potential right adrenal vein confluence. (B) Normal (>80%); single vein directly into the inferior vena cava *(IVC)*. (C) IVC–renal vein trifurcation. (D) Renal vein confluence.

Continued

the cells their name. In contrast to the cortex, the adrenal medulla is richly endowed with autonomic nerve fibers and ganglion cells. Sympathetic fibers synapse directly with the chromaffin cells, constituting an interface between the nervous and endocrine systems.

The microvasculature of the adrenal gland functionally unites the cortex and medulla in a portal system configuration that is designed to enhance the stress response. The adrenal arteries arborize extensively before entering the capsule to form a subcapsular plexus. Blood flows centripetally through capillaries in the zona glomerulosa and zona fasciculata before forming a deep plexus

layers (lipid-laden zona glomerulosa, zona reticularis) is a thin layer of relatively small cells with moderately eosinophilic lipid-poor cytoplasm; it has an undulating inner border and normally does not form a complete circumferential layer. Most of the adrenal cortex is formed by the zona fasciculata, a middle layer composed of long radial columns of large, clear, lipid-laden cells. The inner zona reticularis is made up of small nests of compact, eosinophilic cells. The adrenal medulla consist of clusters and short cords of chromaffin cells, which are large, polyhedral, and packed with basophilic secretory granules. Catecholamine within these granules yield a brown reaction when treated with chromium salts, giving

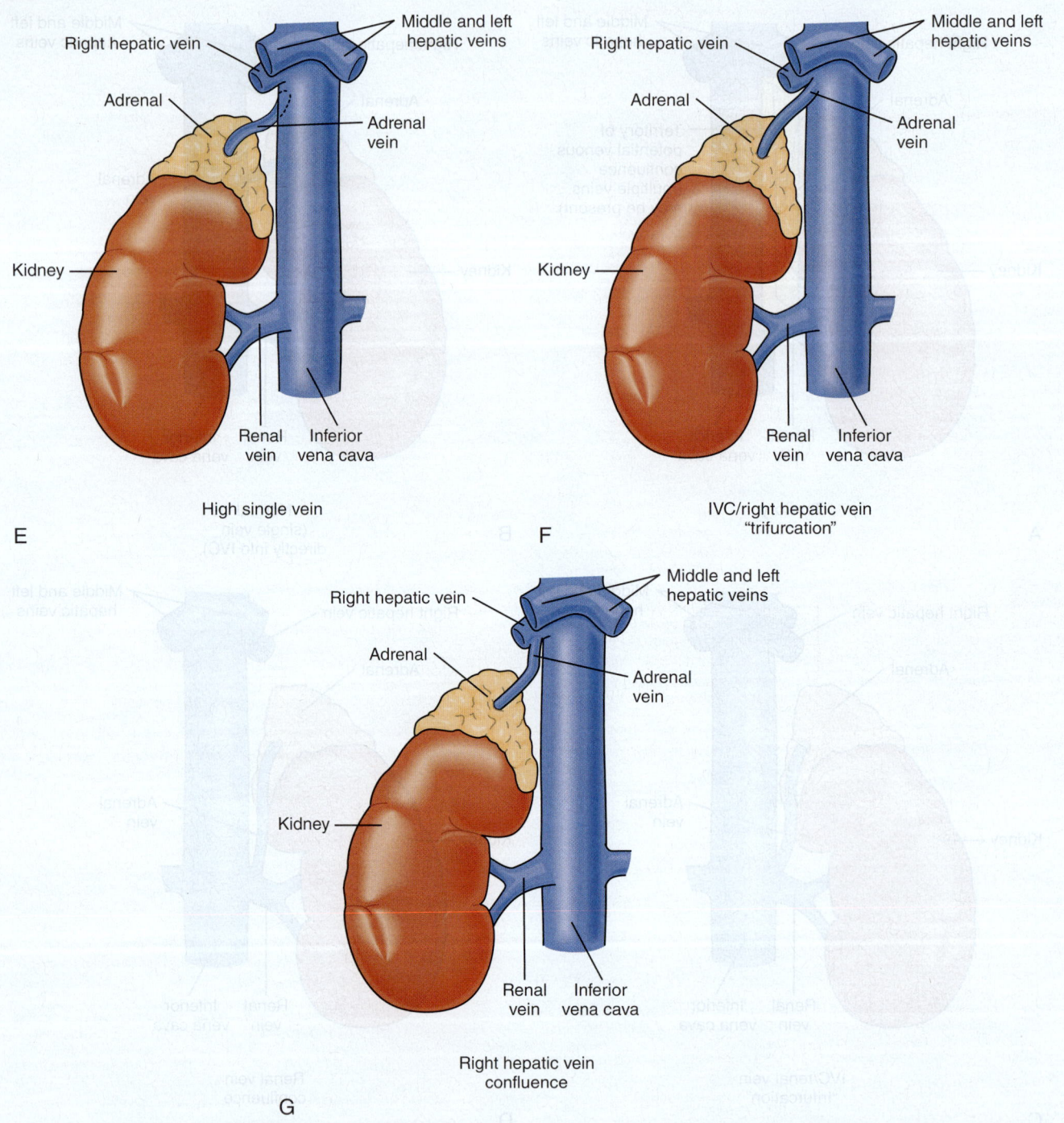

E   High single vein

F   IVC/right hepatic vein "trifurcation"

G   Right hepatic vein confluence

FIGURE 75.3, cont'd (E) High single vein into the IVC. (F) IVC–right hepatic vein trifurcation. (G) Right hepatic vein confluence.

layers (Fig. 75.4). The outer *zona glomerulosa* is a thin layer of relatively small cells with moderately eosinophilic, lipid-poor cytoplasm. It has an undulating inner border and normally does not form a complete circumferential layer. Most of the adrenal cortex is formed by the *zona fasciculata,* a middle layer composed of long radial columns of large, clear, lipid-laden cells. The inner *zona reticularis* is made up of small nests of compact, eosinophilic cells. The adrenal medulla consists of clusters and short cords of chromaffin cells, which are large, polyhedral, and packed with basophilic secretory granules. Catecholamines within these granules yield a brown reaction when treated with chromium salts, giving

the cells their name. In contrast to the cortex, the adrenal medulla is richly endowed with autonomic nerve fibers and ganglion cells. Sympathetic fibers synapse directly with the chromaffin cells, constituting an interface between the nervous and endocrine systems.

The microvasculature of the adrenal gland functionally unifies the cortex and medulla in a portal system configuration that is adapted to enhance the stress response. The adrenal arteries arborize extensively before entering the capsule to form a subcapsular plexus. Blood flows centripetally through capillaries in the zona glomerulosa and zona fasciculata before forming a deep plexus

generate testosterone, estrone, and estradiol from androstenedione. Oxidation of 17-hydroxypregnenolone by 3β-hydroxysteroid dehydrogenase followed by action of CYP21A2 and CYP11B1 yields cortisol, the active glucocorticoid hormone in humans. Aldosterone is generated by the oxidation of corticosterone by CYP11B2 within the zona glomerulosa. CYP17 expression is confined to the zona fasciculata and zona reticularis, accounting for the synthesis of glucocorticoids and adrenal sex steroids in these regions.

Steroid Hormone Physiology and Metabolism

Steroid hormones belong to a general class of low-molecular-weight, lipophilic signaling molecules that act by entering cells and binding to intracellular receptors. This group of hormones also includes thyroid hormone, retinoids, and vitamin D. Hormone binding results in alterations in gene expression that show a delayed and prolonged response compared with changes induced by peptide hormones, which act by binding to cell surface receptors. In the circulation, endogenous steroid hormones are largely bound to highly specific binding globulins. Serum levels of these proteins—and hence free hormone levels—can be altered by certain physiologic and disease states, such as pregnancy, nephrotic syndrome, and cirrhosis. Metabolism of both endogenous and pharmacologic steroids generally proceeds through hydroxylation, sulfonation, or conjugation to glucuronic acid in the liver, followed by urinary excretion. The regulation and physiologic actions of individual steroid hormones are discussed here.

Glucocorticoids

The release of corticotropin-releasing factor into the hypothalamic-pituitary portal system by hypothalamic neurons results in adrenocorticotropic hormone (ACTH) secretion by the anterior pituitary. ACTH binds to a G protein–coupled receptor on the adrenocortical cell surface and stimulates glucocorticoid secretion. Steroidogenesis is acutely upregulated by increased steroidogenic acute regulatory protein-mediated cholesterol transport and pregnenolone synthesis by CYP11A1. ACTH is released in a pulsatile fashion that normally displays a circadian rhythm. The highest level of ACTH, and therefore cortisol, is generally detected on waking, with levels gradually declining throughout the day to reach a nadir in the early evening. This pattern must be considered in evaluating patients for glucocorticoid deficiency or excess.

Glucocorticoid hormones have broad-ranging effects on almost all organ systems in the body. As a rule, they generate a catabolic state that characterizes the body's response to stress. The hormones are so named because they cause alterations in carbohydrate, protein, and lipid metabolism that have the net effect of increasing blood glucose concentrations. Hepatic glucose output is elevated by the upregulation of gluconeogenesis, and net glycogen deposition occurs. Glucose uptake by peripheral tissues is directly inhibited. Glucocorticoids stimulate lipolysis with release of free fatty acids into the circulation, and a general state of insulin resistance is induced, resulting in protein catabolism. Fatty acids and amino acids serve as energy sources and substrates for gluconeogenesis. In the cardiovascular system, glucocorticoids exert a permissive and enhancing effect on catecholamine signaling by sensitizing arterial smooth muscle cells to β-adrenergic stimulation and increasing catecholamine concentrations in neuromuscular junctions. Cardiac contractility and peripheral vascular tone are thus maintained, explaining why the hemodynamic collapse that accompanies acute adrenal insufficiency can be remedied by glucocorticoid administration.

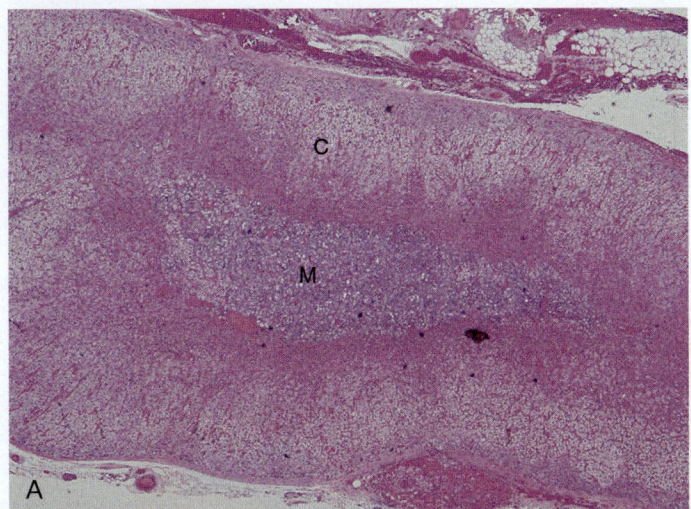

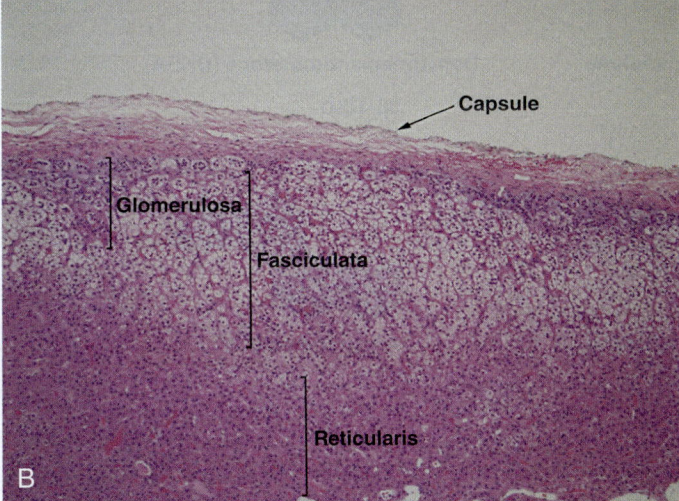

FIGURE 75.4 Normal adrenal histopathology. (A) Low-power view showing the adrenal cortex *(C)* and medulla *(M)*. (B) Medium-power view demonstrating individual layers of the adrenal cortex. The thickness of the zona glomerulosa varies along its length (hematoxylin and eosin stain). (Courtesy Dr. Anthony Gill.)

within the zona reticularis. From there, steroid-enriched postcapillary blood enters the medulla, where cortisol drives the expression of phenylethanolamine *N*-methyltransferase (PNMT). PNMT is responsible for the conversion of norepinephrine to epinephrine and is not expressed in extraadrenal paragangliomas.

BIOCHEMISTRY AND PHYSIOLOGY

Adrenal Steroid Biosynthesis

Adrenal steroid biosynthesis begins with the transport of cholesterol to the inner mitochondrial membrane by the steroidogenic acute regulatory protein (Fig. 75.5). Cholesterol then undergoes a series of oxidative reactions catalyzed predominantly by membrane-associated enzymes belonging to the cytochrome P450 (CYP) family. Cleavage of the cholesterol side chain yields the hormonally inactive compound pregnenolone, the immediate precursor to the adrenal steroid hormones. Serial oxidation by CYP17 converts pregnenolone and progesterone into the major adrenal sex steroids dehydroepiandrosterone (DHEA) and androstenedione. Additional enzymatic steps confined to the gonads

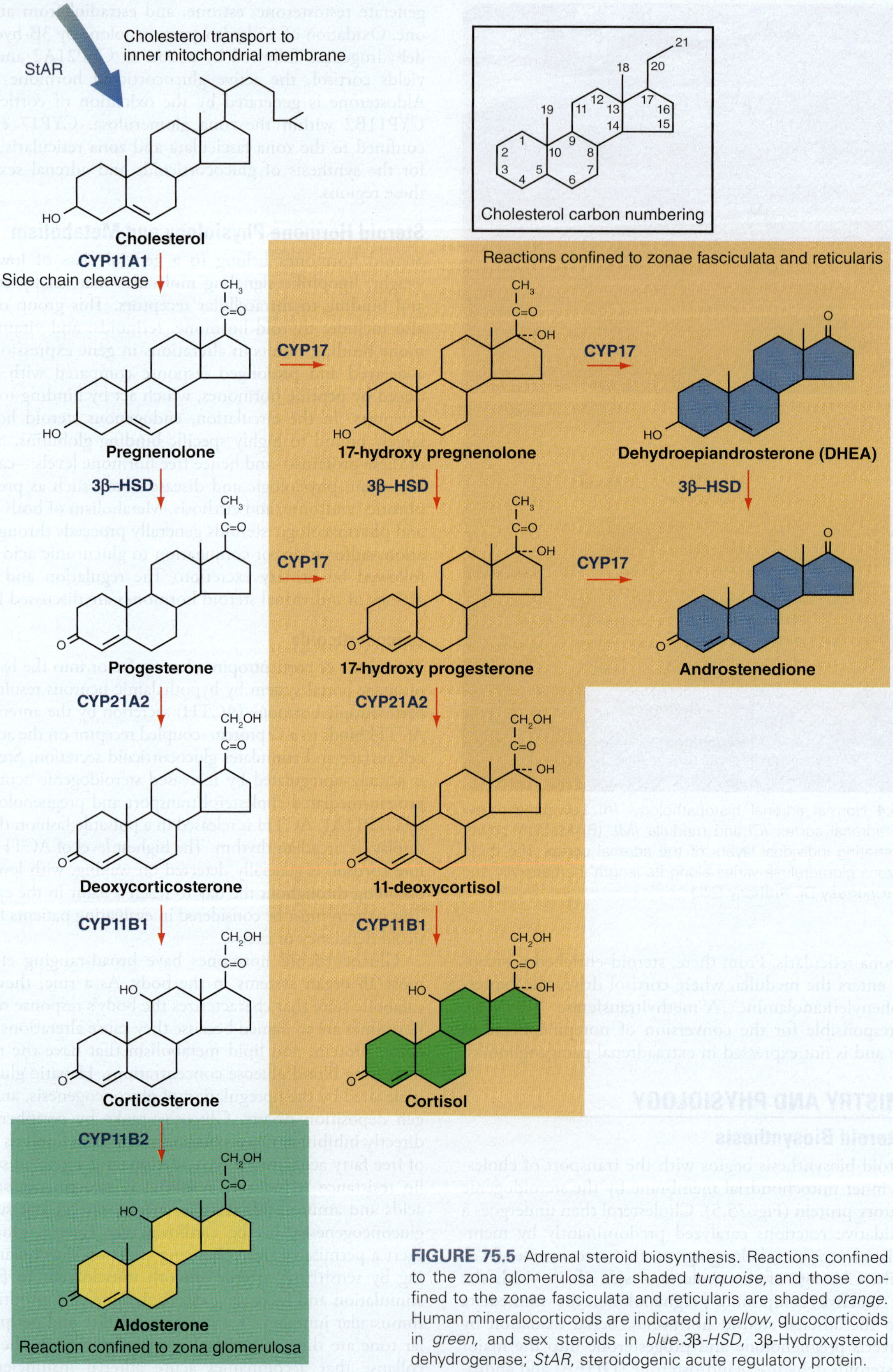

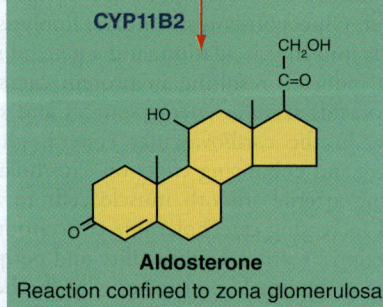

FIGURE 75.5 Adrenal steroid biosynthesis. Reactions confined to the zona glomerulosa are shaded *turquoise*, and those confined to the zonae fasciculata and reticularis are shaded *orange*. Human mineralocorticoids are indicated in *yellow*, glucocorticoids in *green*, and sex steroids in *blue*. *3β-HSD*, 3β-Hydroxysteroid dehydrogenase; *StAR*, steroidogenic acute regulatory protein.

Glucocorticoids are potent antiinflammatory and immuno-suppressive agents. Acutely, glucocorticoids reduce circulating lymphocyte and eosinophil counts while increasing neutrophil counts. Lymphocyte apoptosis is promoted, cytokine and immunoglobulin production is decreased, and histamine release is suppressed. Glucocorticoids also reduce prostaglandin synthesis through inhibition of phospholipase A2.

Mineralocorticoids

Aldosterone release from the zona glomerulosa is principally regulated by angiotensin II and the blood potassium level. The renin-angiotensin-aldosterone axis is responsive to sodium delivery to the distal convoluted tubule of the kidney. Low sodium delivery, which occurs in states such as hypovolemia, shock, renal artery vasoconstriction, and hyponatremia, stimulates the release of renin from the juxtaglomerular apparatus. The prohormone angiotensinogen is synthesized by the liver and is cleaved to inactive angiotensin I by renin. Further cleavage of angiotensin I by angiotensin-converting enzyme (ACE) in the lungs and elsewhere yields angiotensin II, a potent vasoconstrictor and stimulator of aldosterone release. Hypokalemia reduces aldosterone release by suppressing renin secretion and also by acting directly at the zona glomerulosa. Hyperkalemia has the opposite effect.

Aldosterone regulates circulating fluid volume and electrolyte balance by promoting sodium and chloride retention by the distal tubule. Potassium and hydrogen ions are secreted into the urine. Acutely, expansion of the extracellular fluid volume and a rise in blood pressure are observed after aldosterone infusion. Negative feedback occurs primarily through an increase in sodium delivery to the distal tubule, suppressing renin release.

Adrenal Sex Steroids

Secretion of the adrenal androgens androstenedione, DHEA, and DHEA-S (the sulfonated derivative of DHEA, synthesized in the adrenal and liver) is regulated by ACTH and other incompletely understood mechanisms. Of the three, androstenedione is produced in the smallest quantities. The physiologic effects of adrenal sex steroids are generally weak in comparison with the gonadal sex steroids, particularly in males. In females, peripheral conversion of DHEA and DHEA-S to more potent androgens, including androstenedione, testosterone, and dihydrotestosterone, supports normal pubic and axillary hair growth and may play a role in maintaining libido and a sense of well-being.

Catecholamine Biosynthesis and Physiology

Synthesis of catecholamines in the adrenal medulla begins with the hydroxylation of tyrosine, a rate-limiting step that generates dihydroxyphenylalanine (L-dopa) in the cytosol (Fig. 75.6). Decarboxylation of L-dopa generates dopamine, which is then β-hydroxylated to form norepinephrine. Epinephrine is created by the action of phenylethanolamine N-methyltransferase, which, unlike the other enzymes involved in catecholamine synthesis, is localized to the chromaffin cells of the adrenal medulla and organ of Zuckerkandl. Sympathetic stimulation of the adrenal medulla results in the release of stored catecholamines into the circulation. Basal levels of adrenal catecholamine secretion are normally low, although large (up to fiftyfold) increases in levels may be observed in response to major physiologic or psychological stressors. Target tissue responses are mediated by α- and β-adrenergic receptors. α-Adrenergic receptors display greater affinity for norepinephrine compared with epinephrine, and the opposite is true for β-adrenergic receptors. Stimulation of $β_1$-adrenergic receptors in the myocardium results in increased heart rate and contractility. Stimulation of $β_2$-adrenergic receptors results in smooth muscle relaxation in tissues such as the uterus, bronchi, and skeletal muscle arterioles. $α_1$-Adrenergic receptors mediate vasoconstriction in tissues such as the skin and gastrointestinal tract. $α_2$-Adrenergic receptors exist in presynaptic locations in the central nervous system, where they mediate attenuation of sympathetic outflow. The net effect of adrenal catecholamine release is to augment blood flow and oxygen delivery to the brain, heart, and skeletal muscle, which are essential to the fight-or-flight response, but at the expense of other organ systems.

Catecholamine Clearance

Catecholamines are potent and short-acting compounds, with a plasma half-life on the order of 1 minute. Their presence in synapses and the circulation exhibits tight negative regulation by both reuptake and degradation. Degradation pathways merit some discussion because they generate the metabolites commonly measured in the biochemical evaluation of pheochromocytoma (see later). Epinephrine and norepinephrine are inactivated by one or both of the enzymes monoamine oxidase and catechol-O-methyltransferase (see Fig. 75.6). Initial methylation by catechol-O-methyltransferase yields metanephrine and normetanephrine, which can be detected in plasma and urine. Their relatively stable plasma levels, which contrast with the high-amplitude fluctuations seen in plasma epinephrine and norepinephrine levels, make them attractive diagnostic markers.[4] The sequential action of monoamine oxidase and catechol-O-methyltransferase generates the major final product, vanillylmandelic acid. Catecholamine metabolites are excreted in the urine, sometimes after sulfonation or conjugation to glucuronic acid in the liver.

ADRENAL INSUFFICIENCY

Types of Adrenal Insufficiency

Primary Adrenal Insufficiency (Addison Disease)

Originally described in patients with tuberculous destruction of the adrenal glands, Addison disease is a rare condition that manifests with weakness and fatigue, anorexia, nausea or vomiting, weight loss, hyperpigmentation, hypotension, and electrolyte disturbances (hyponatremia and hyperkalemia). Hyperpigmentation, previously believed to be caused by elevated levels of pro-opiomelanocortin and its cleavage product, α-melanocyte-stimulating hormone, is now believed to result from ACTH-induced melanogenesis.[5] Hormonal insufficiency caused by intrinsic adrenal disease arises from three general mechanisms: congenital adrenal dysgenesis/hypoplasia, defective steroidogenesis, and adrenal destruction. Of these, adrenal destruction from autoimmune causes is the most common, followed by infectious adrenalitis (e.g., tuberculous, fungal, viral), adrenal replacement by metastatic tumor, and adrenal hemorrhage (Waterhouse-Friderichsen syndrome). The last occurs in the setting of septicemia caused by meningococcal or other organisms and is more common in pediatric and asplenic patients.

Secondary Adrenal Insufficiency

Secondary adrenal insufficiency is a relatively common disorder resulting from ACTH deficiency, often occurring in the setting of pharmacologic steroid withdrawal. Patients receiving high supraphysiologic doses of glucocorticoids (more than the equivalent of 20 mg of prednisone daily; Table 75.1) for more than 5 days and

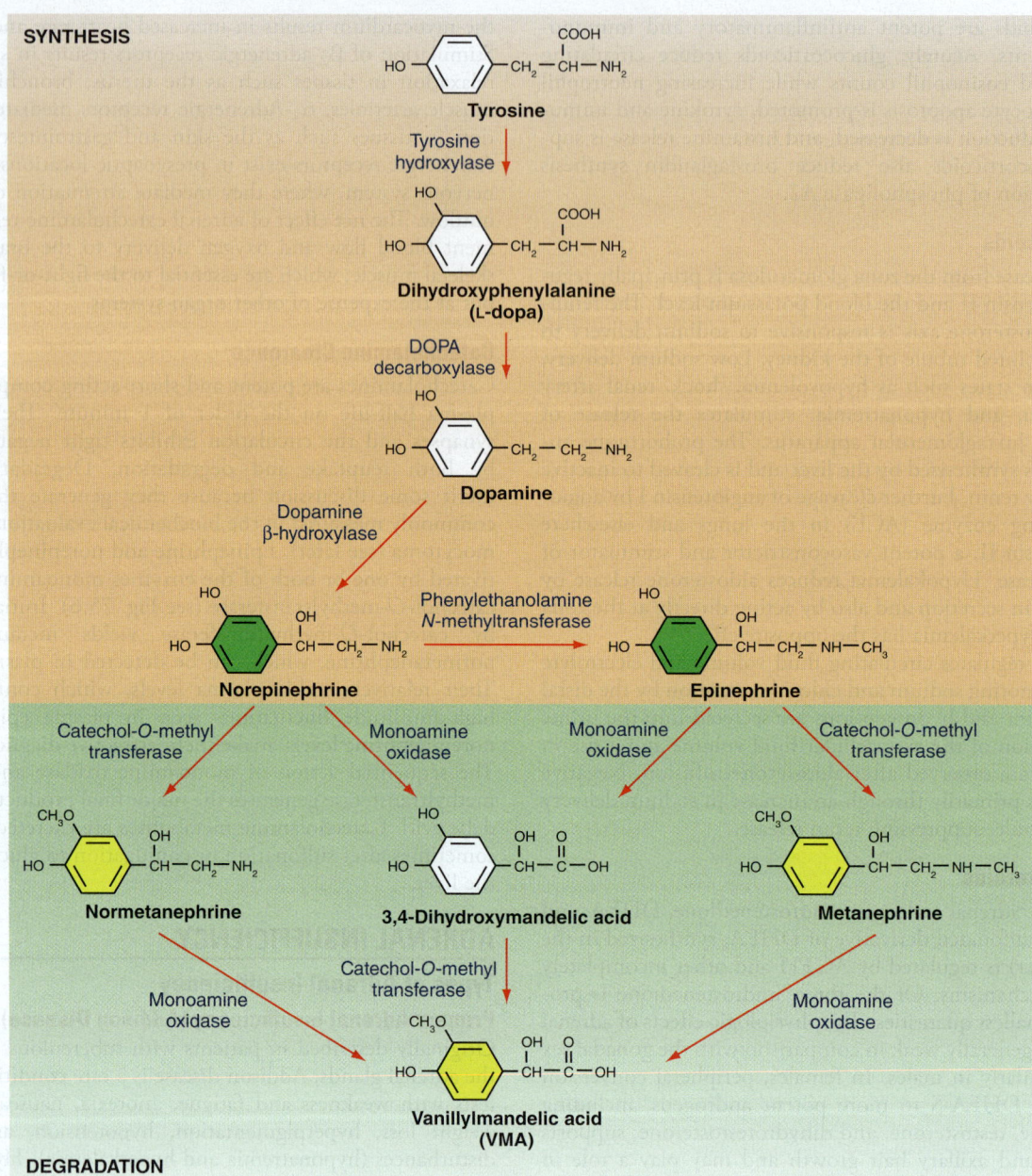

FIGURE 75.6 Catecholamine biosynthesis and metabolism. Synthetic steps are shaded *orange*, and degradative steps are shaded *turquoise*. Major catecholamines are indicated in *green*, and major metabolites are in *yellow*.

TABLE 75.1   Properties of Endogenous and Commonly Used Pharmacologic Glucocorticoids

COMPOUND	IV/PO[a]	COMMON TRADE NAME	RELATIVE POTENCY	DAILY PHYSIOLOGIC DOSE	DOSING INTERVAL
Cortisol = hydrocortisone	Both	Cortef (PO) Solu-Cortef (IV)	1×	20 mg	q8–12h
Cortisone	PO	—	0.8×	25 mg	q8–12h
Prednisone	PO	—	4×	5 mg	q24h
Prednisolone	PO	—	4×	5 mg	q24h
Methylprednisolone	Both	Medrol (PO) Solu-Medrol (IV)	5×	4 mg	q24h
Dexamethasone[b]	Both	Decadron	25×	1 mg	q24h

[a]Oral and intravenous dosages are similar.
[b]Does not cross-react with the cortisol assay.
IV, Intravenous; *PO,* orally.

those receiving low supraphysiologic doses for more than 3 weeks are at risk for HPA axis suppression. Surgical cure of Cushing syndrome likewise results in glucocorticoid withdrawal. The rate of recovery from HPA axis suppression varies in accordance with the duration and severity of previous glucocorticoid excess, and the need for glucocorticoid supplementation may last several years.[6] Other less common causes of secondary adrenal insufficiency include panhypopituitarism caused by neoplastic or infiltrative replacement, granulomatous disease, and pituitary hemorrhage or infarction. Pituitary infarction may occur in the setting of severe postpartum hemorrhage (Sheehan syndrome).

Adrenal Insufficiency in the Critically Ill

Studies have suggested that critically ill patients with sepsis or systemic inflammatory response syndrome may be affected by acute reversible dysfunction of the HPA axis. The incidence of the disorder is approximately 30% in critically ill patients, although this figure may be higher in those with septic shock. Whether these patients incur increased mortality because of adrenal insufficiency remains to be defined. Proposed mechanisms of reversible HPA axis dysfunction include adrenal ACTH resistance and decreased responsiveness of target tissues to glucocorticoids. Glucocorticoid supplementation in septic patients has been the topic of at least 42 randomized controlled trials. Among these studies, corticosteroid administration was associated with a small reduction in 30-day mortality (1.8% absolute risk reduction) and faster shock reversal. There appears to be an inverse relationship between survival benefit and glucocorticoid dose, with physiologic (i.e., replacement) doses yielding a possible benefit and high supraphysiologic doses demonstrating significant harm. Adverse effects of corticosteroid administration in this patient population include hypernatremia, hyperglycemia, and muscle weakness. Earlier trials suggested that patients with severe septic shock, particularly those requiring vasopressors, may benefit from 5- to 7-day courses of glucocorticoids up to 300 mg/day or less of hydrocortisone or equivalent. As more recent data have not confirmed a significant survival benefit, glucocorticoid use should be individualized in critically ill patients.[7]

Adrenal Crisis

Acute adrenal insufficiency, or adrenal crisis, is a life-threatening condition that typically occurs in individuals with already marginal adrenocortical function who are subjected to a significant acute physiologic stressor, such as infection or trauma. Sudden and complete loss of adrenal function, as occurs with Waterhouse-Friderichsen syndrome and certain hypercoagulable states, can also be manifested with adrenal crisis. Clinical findings include shock, abdominal pain, fever, nausea and vomiting, electrolyte disturbances, and occasionally hypoglycemia. Mineralocorticoid deficiency, resulting in an inability to maintain sodium and intravascular volume, is the primary pathogenic mechanism, although diminished cardiovascular responsiveness to catecholamines caused by glucocorticoid deficiency also plays a role. Treatment for suspected adrenal crisis should not be delayed while awaiting the results of diagnostic testing. The treatment of adrenal crisis centers around large-volume intravenous resuscitation with isotonic saline and glucocorticoid administration in the form of hydrocortisone (100 mg intravenous bolus followed by 75 mg every 8 hours) or dexamethasone (4 mg intravenously every 24 hours). Dexamethasone is long acting and carries the advantage of not interfering with biochemical assays of endogenous glucocorticoid production. Mineralocorticoid replacement is not an early priority

because the sodium- and fluid-retaining effects of mineralocorticoids are not manifested until several days after administration. Fluid and electrolyte balance can be rapidly achieved by saline infusion.

Diagnosis and Treatment

Diagnosis

As is true for most endocrine disorders, the diagnosis of adrenal insufficiency depends on maintaining sufficient clinical suspicion for the disease. The clinical manifestations have been discussed earlier. Surgeons are most likely to encounter patients with adrenal insufficiency in the intensive care unit, trauma suite, or operating room when treating patients with steroid-dependent chronic illnesses. Routine and provocative biochemical testing is necessary to confirm the diagnosis (Fig. 75.7). The first step is to document inadequate cortisol production, which can be done by measuring

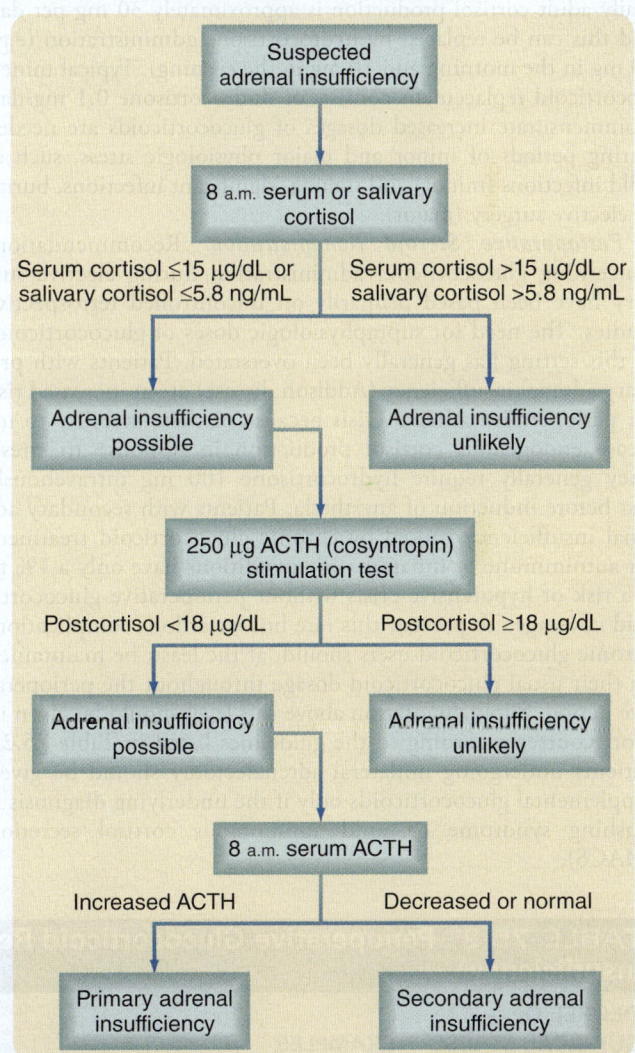

FIGURE 75.7 Algorithm for the diagnosis of adrenal insufficiency. The adequacy of cortisol production is initially assessed with morning cortisol level measurement. Patients with low or borderline values undergo provocative adrenocorticotropic hormone *(ACTH)* stimulation testing, with serum cortisol levels measured before and 30 to 60 minutes after the administration of ACTH. Failure to mount an adequate response to ACTH usually establishes the diagnosis of adrenal insufficiency. The cause of adrenal insufficiency is then investigated with a morning ACTH level measurement.

morning levels of cortisol in the serum or saliva. In most patients, morning serum cortisol concentration higher than 15 µg/dL or morning salivary cortisol concentration higher than 5.8 ng/mL effectively excludes adrenal insufficiency. Patients whose levels fall below these thresholds should undergo provocative testing. A high-dose cosyntropin stimulation test is performed by administering 250 µg cosyntropin and measuring serum cortisol levels 30 to 60 minutes later. A positive test result (i.e., a stimulated cortisol level less than 18 µg/dL) is strongly suggestive of adrenal insufficiency. After the diagnosis of adrenal insufficiency has been made, a morning ACTH level is determined to differentiate between primary and secondary adrenal insufficiency.

Treatment

The treatment of adrenal crisis has been discussed. The goal of maintenance therapy for chronic adrenal insufficiency is to replace physiologic glucocorticoid and mineralocorticoid levels. Daily adult cortisol production is approximately 30 mg per day, and this can be replaced by hydrocortisone administration (e.g., 20 mg in the morning and 10 mg in the evening). Typical mineralocorticoid replacement consists of fludrocortisone 0.1 mg/day. Commensurate increased dosages of glucocorticoids are needed during periods of minor and major physiologic stress, such as mild infections (minor) and trauma, significant infections, burns, or elective surgery (major).

Perioperative Steroid Administration. Recommendations concerning glucocorticoid administration during elective surgery have been based primarily on uncontrolled retrospective studies. The need for supraphysiologic doses of glucocorticoids in this setting has generally been overstated. Patients with primary adrenal insufficiency (Addison disease) are at increased risk for perioperative adrenal crisis because of their inability to increase endogenous cortisol production in response to stress. They generally require hydrocortisone 100 mg intravenously just before induction of anesthesia. Patients with secondary adrenal insufficiency caused by chronic glucocorticoid treatment for autoimmune or inflammatory conditions have only a 1% to 2% risk of hypotensive crisis without perioperative glucocorticoid coverage. To prevent this rare but hazardous complication, chronic glucocorticoid users should, at the least, be maintained on their usual glucocorticoid dosage throughout the perioperative period. Supplementation above this level should be given in short courses according to the guidelines listed in Table 75.2.[8] Patients undergoing unilateral adrenalectomy should be given supplemental glucocorticoids only if the underlying diagnosis is Cushing syndrome or mild autonomous cortisol secretion (MACS).

DISEASES OF THE ADRENAL CORTEX

Primary Aldosteronism

Epidemiology and Clinical Features

Primary aldosteronism, the unregulated release of excess aldosterone from one or both adrenal glands, was first described by Jerome Conn in 1954. Primary aldosteronism classically manifests with resistant hypertension and hypokalemia, although studies have revealed that most patients may be normokalemic, depending on the population screened. Hypokalemia is likely a manifestation of severe or late-stage disease. The prevalence of primary aldosteronism has been the topic of considerable debate. It was generally believed to affect approximately 1% of hypertensive patients. Widespread application of the aldosterone-to-renin ratio as a screening test in certain centers led to reports of a 10% to 40% prevalence of primary aldosteronism among hypertensive patients. There is some consensus that these higher figures reflect strong referral bias and that the actual prevalence in unselected hypertensive patients is likely to be 7% or less.[9] Nonselective use of the aldosterone-to-renin ratio to identify patients with primary aldosteronism is known to decrease the fraction of patients with surgically correctible disease (unilateral aldosteronoma) significantly, although the absolute number of surgically treatable cases has increased.

The mean age at diagnosis for primary aldosteronism is approximately 50 years, and the disease has a slight male predilection. Most patients are asymptomatic, although patients with significant hypokalemia may report muscle cramps, weakness, or paresthesias. Patients typically have moderate to severe hypertension that is refractory to medical therapy. It is common for patients with primary aldosteronism to require two to four antihypertensive medications. Responsiveness to mineralocorticoid antagonists such as spironolactone or eplerenone may be seen—a feature that is predictive of a good response to surgical treatment.

Primary aldosteronism is a potentially curable cause of significant cardiovascular disease. A study comparing 270 subjects with biochemically confirmed primary aldosteronism with case-matched hypertensive controls has revealed that primary aldosteronism is associated with a significantly increased risk of stroke, myocardial infarction, arrhythmias including atrial and ventricular fibrillation, and heart failure.[10] These results add to existing evidence indicating that the adverse cardiovascular sequelae of primary aldosteronism are more pronounced than those caused by blood pressure elevation alone. Surgical correction of primary aldosteronism leads to regression of many of these adverse physiologic changes.

TABLE 75.2	Perioperative Glucocorticoid Regimens for Patients With Secondary Adrenal Insufficiency[a]		
DEGREE OF SURGICAL STRESS	**EXAMPLES**	**INTRAOPERATIVE GLUCOCORTICOID DOSAGE**	**GLUCOCORTICOID TAPER**
Minor	Procedures under local anesthetic, most out-patient procedures, inguinal hernia repair	None (take usual morning steroid dosage)	None (continue to take usual dosage)
Moderate	Routine abdominal, peripheral vascular, or orthopedic surgery	Hydrocortisone 50 mg or equivalent before procedure	Hydrocortisone 25 mg every 8 hours for 24 hours, then resume usual dosage
Major	Resection of gastrointestinal cancer, cardio-pulmonary bypass	Hydrocortisone 100 mg or equivalent before procedure	Hydrocortisone 50 mg every 8 hours for 24 hours, then taper by half every day to usual dosage

[a]Caused by chronic pharmacologic steroid use.

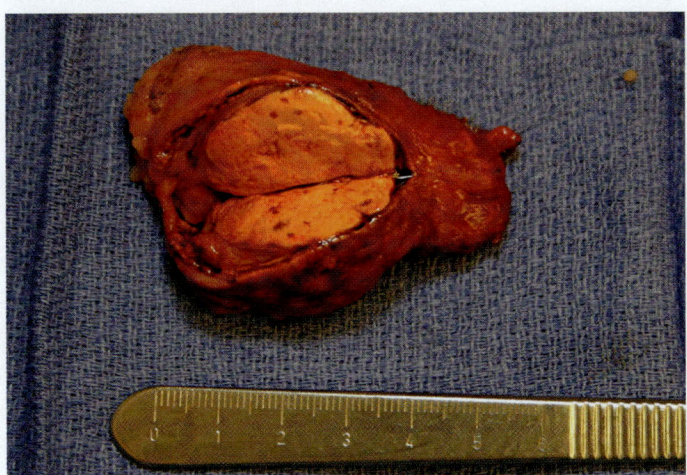

FIGURE 75.8 Classic canary-yellow aldosteronoma.

TABLE 75.3 Causes of Primary Aldosteronism

	SCREENING[a]	
CAUSE	SELECTIVE (%)	NONSELECTIVE (%)
Aldosterone-producing adenoma	60	30
Bilateral adrenal hyperplasia (idiopathic hyperaldosteronism)	35	65
Aldosterone-producing adrenocortical carcinoma	<1	<1
Familial hyperaldosteronism		
Type I (glucocorticoid-remediable aldosteronism)	<1	<1
Type II (non–glucocorticoid-remediable aldosteronism)	<1	<1

[a]Rates of specific pathologic processes are highly dependent on the pattern of screening (selective vs. nonselective).

The most common causes of primary aldosteronism are unilateral aldosterone-producing adenomas (aldosteronomas; Fig. 75.8) and bilateral adrenal hyperplasia (also termed *idiopathic hyperaldosteronism;* Table 75.3). In the past, aldosteronoma was present in more than 60% of cases, but this number has decreased substantially as nonselective screening with the aldosterone-to-renin ratio has been applied. This phenomenon may reflect increased detection of hyperplasia, which is characterized by milder biochemical abnormalities than aldosteronoma. Recent sequencing has revealed somatic mutations in genes coding for ion channels and ATPase in 94% of aldosterone-producing adenomas.[11]

Diagnosis and Localization

Biochemical diagnosis. The goal of diagnostic testing is to identify patients with primary aldosteronism and to perform subtype differentiation to optimize management. Biochemical screening should be performed in all patients with hypertension and unexplained hypokalemia, hypertension and an adrenal nodule, hypertension and sleep apnea, early-onset hypertension, and treatment-resistant hypertension. Establishing the diagnosis of primary aldosteronism begins with determining the ratio of plasma aldosterone concentration to plasma renin activity (expressed here as ng/dL divided by ng/[mL • hr]; Fig. 75.9). This

test is optimally performed after discontinuation of interfering medications. Variable cutoff values for the aldosterone-to-renin ratio have been used in the literature, with the most commonly cited value of 30 yielding a sensitivity of approximately 90%. Some centers have advocated a lower threshold of 20; this increases sensitivity at some cost to specificity and conceptually reflects appreciation of the clinical gravity of failing to diagnose surgically correctable hyperaldosteronism.[12] A subset of patients with essential hypertension will have suppressed renin levels, which may result in false elevations of the aldosterone-to-renin ratio. Thus, the inclusion of an absolute aldosterone concentration higher than 15 mg/dL increases the specificity of initial screening. Patients who test positive and are younger than 30 years should be genetically screened for glucocorticoid-remediable aldosteronism (familial hyperaldosteronism type I), especially if they have a family history of early-onset hypertension. This rare autosomal dominant condition results in abnormal regulation of aldosterone synthesis by ACTH and can be medically treated.

Confirmatory biochemical testing is aimed at demonstrating inappropriately high (nonsuppressible) aldosterone levels by creating a state of hypervolemia-sodium excess. This may be done with either intravenous saline loading (2–3 L of isotonic saline given during 4–6 hours, followed by measurement of plasma aldosterone) or oral salt loading (200 mEq = 5000 mg sodium daily for 3 days, followed by measurement of 24-hour urine aldosterone excretion). Some centers administer high-dose fludrocortisone (0.1 mg every 6 hours) during oral salt loading to increase the specificity of suppression testing, but this method has not been widely adopted.

Subtype differentiation. After the diagnosis has been confirmed, subtype differentiation to determine unilateral versus bilateral causes of hyperaldosteronism is performed. Studies may include adrenal venous sampling (AVS), anatomic imaging, and sometimes functional scanning. The fact that most aldosteronomas are smaller than 15 mm in maximum dimension poses some challenges to localization. Thin-cut (3 mm) adrenal computed tomography (CT) scanning may have utility in identifying small adrenal nodules (Fig. 75.10). Additionally, primary aldosteronism can be caused by microscopic islands of CPY11B2 overexpressing cells that are only detectable postoperatively on immunohistochemical staining. This fact highlights the importance of adrenal vein sampling before offering surgical management of primary aldosteronism.

The gold standard for subtype differentiation is AVS. This test relies on the simultaneous measurement of cortisol and aldosterone levels in the peripheral circulation (inferior vena cava) and left and right adrenal veins (Fig. 75.11). More than a threefold elevation of the cortisol concentration in a sample relative to peripheral blood indicates successful cannulation of an adrenal vein and is referred to as the *selectivity index.* Lateralization is indicated by an unbalanced ratio of aldosterone to cortisol in the left and right adrenal veins, with the ratio on one side being fourfold higher than the other to identify the culprit gland. Considerable controversy exists about which patients should undergo AVS, an invasive procedure with a 90% technical success rate in experienced hands. There is clear consensus that AVS should be applied in all cases in which the biochemical diagnosis of primary aldosteronism has been confirmed and thin-cut adrenal CT reveals no abnormalities or bilateral abnormalities. Of the remaining patients who have a unilateral mass on CT scan, a small but not insignificant fraction (2%–10%) will represent false-positive localization and have persistent hyperaldosteronism after unilateral

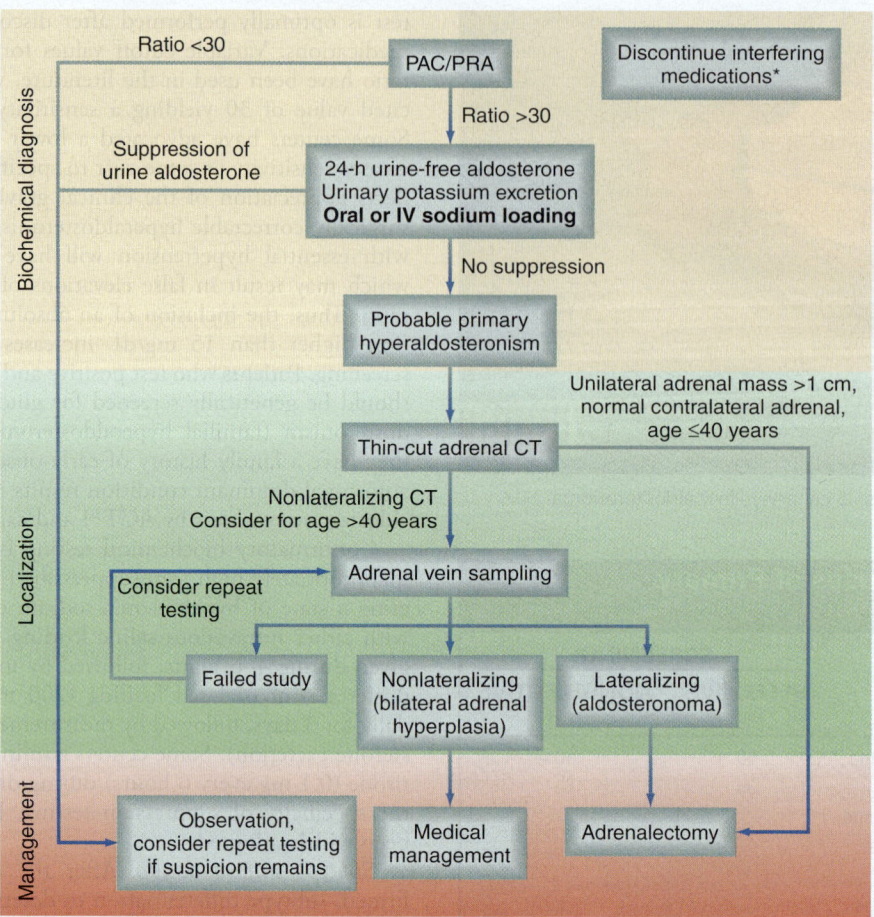

*Including spironolactone, ACE inhibitors, diuretics, β-blockers.

FIGURE 75.9 Algorithm for diagnosis, localization, and management of primary aldosteronism. Initial screening is done with determination of the PRA/PAC ratio, followed by confirmatory testing with sodium loading. After the biochemical diagnosis has been established, noninvasive localization is attempted with computed tomography *(CT)*. Patients with clear CT evidence of a unilateral abnormality can proceed to adrenalectomy with a more than 90% cure rate. Adrenal vein sampling is done in patients with equivocal CT findings and older patients, especially those older than 60 years, because nonfunctional cortical adenomas are found in 4% or more of this population and can cause false-positive CT localization. *ACE,* Angiotensin-converting enzyme; *PAC,* plasma aldosterone concentration, in ng/dL; *PRA,* plasma renin activity, in ng/(mL • hr).

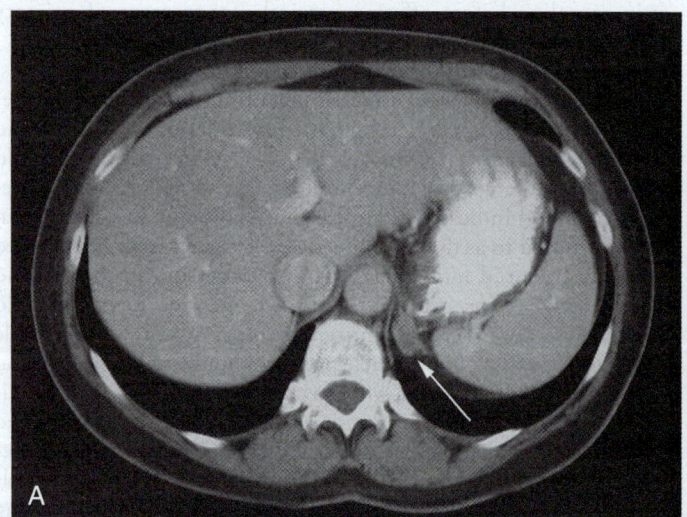

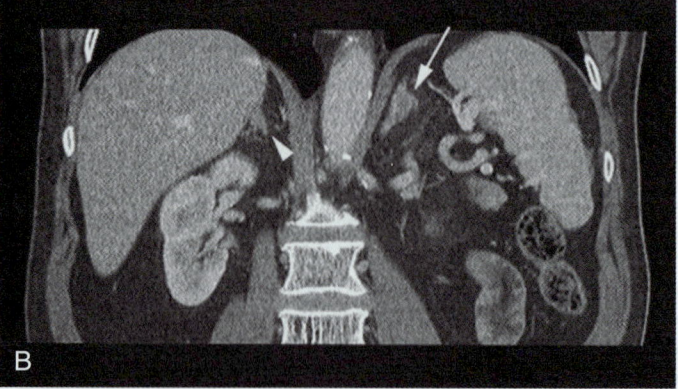

FIGURE 75.10 Appearance of aldosteronoma on anatomic imaging. (A) Venous phase, contrast-enhanced computed tomography (CT) scan demonstrating a 2-cm left aldosteronoma *(arrow)*. (B) Late arterial phase, coronal CT scan demonstrating a 1.7-cm left aldosteronoma *(arrow)* and a normal right adrenal gland *(arrowhead)*.

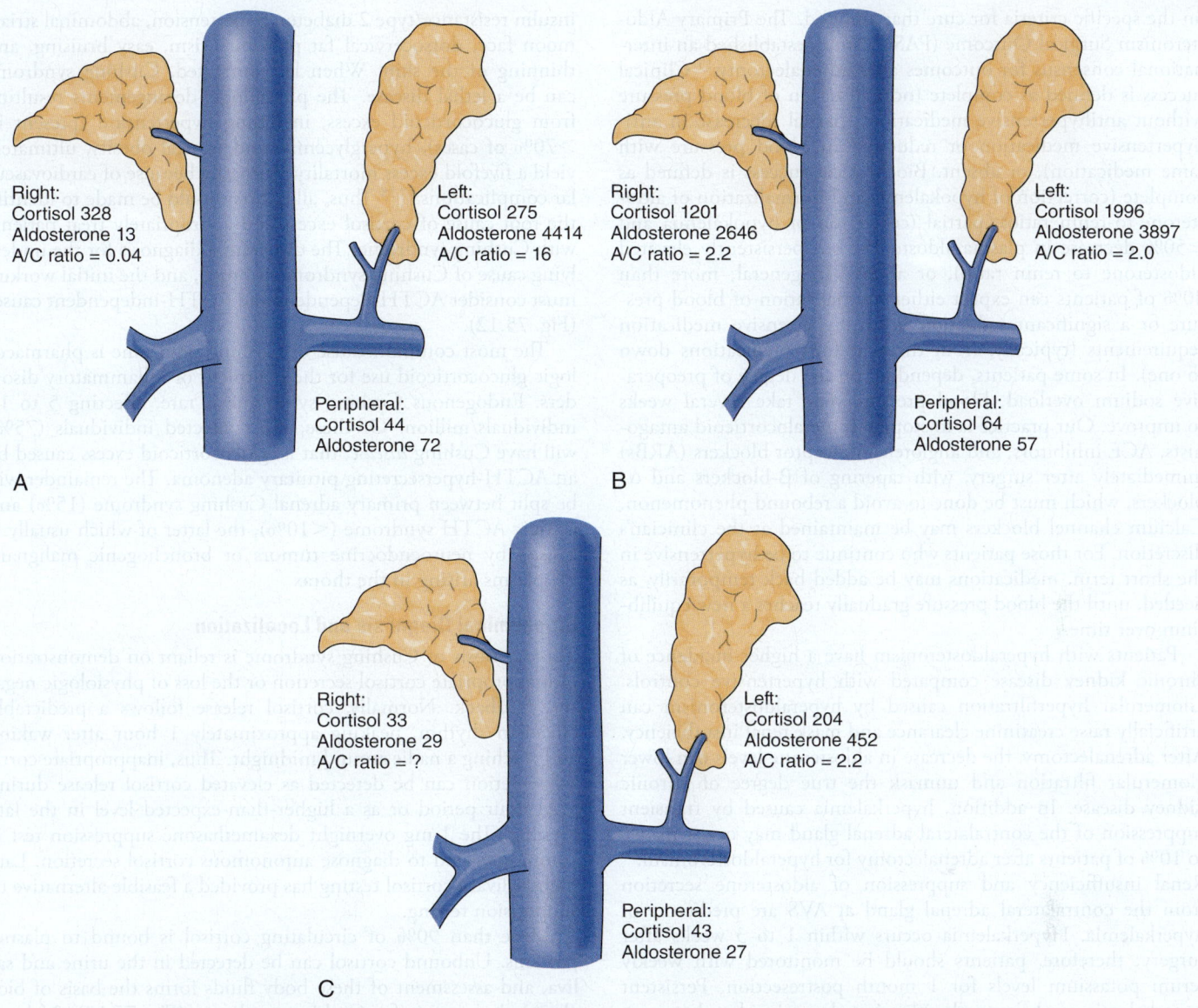

FIGURE 75.11 Possible outcomes of adrenal vein sampling for primary aldosteronism. Aldosterone is expressed in ng/dL, cortisol in μg/dL. (A) Successful study lateralizing strongly to the left adrenal. (B) Successful study, nonlateralizing. Stimulation with adrenocorticotropic hormone yielded high adrenal vein cortisol levels. (C) Failed study. The right adrenal vein was not cannulated. *A/C*, Aldosterone:cortisol ratio.

Right:
Cortisol 328
Aldosterone 13
A/C ratio = 0.04

Left:
Cortisol 275
Aldosterone 4414
A/C ratio = 16

Peripheral:
Cortisol 44
Aldosterone 72

A

Right:
Cortisol 1201
Aldosterone 2646
A/C ratio = 2.2

Left:
Cortisol 1996
Aldosterone 3897
A/C ratio = 2.0

Peripheral:
Cortisol 64
Aldosterone 57

B

Right:
Cortisol 33
Aldosterone 29
A/C ratio = ?

Left:
Cortisol 204
Aldosterone 452
A/C ratio = 2.2

Peripheral:
Cortisol 43
Aldosterone 27

C

adrenalectomy. In these patients, the adrenal mass represents a nonfunctioning cortical adenoma, and the true underlying diagnosis is a contralateral microaldosteronoma or bilateral adrenal hyperplasia, the latter of which is not surgically remediable.

Because patients 40 years and older are more likely to possess nonfunctioning adrenal cortical adenomas, some authors have advocated AVS in all patients 40 years of age and older, and others have recommended universal application of this test in the evaluation of primary aldosteronism.[12] Young patients with a unilateral cortical adrenal mass larger than 1 cm in diameter and a normal contralateral adrenal gland on CT can proceed directly to adrenalectomy, as their management is rarely changed by AVS results, whereas those without definitive CT localization undergo AVS.[13] In consideration of the body of literature, we advocate for more liberal application of AVS for patients 40 years and older.

Practically speaking, approximately 30% to 40% of patients being evaluated for primary aldosteronism undergo AVS when it is applied to select patients. The usefulness of the test is limited by its low success rate in some reports (40%–80%), with the most common reason for incomplete AVS being failure to cannulate the right adrenal vein. Frequently, however, sufficient lateralizing information is provided during AVS to guide surgical treatment, even when the study is not bilaterally selective.[14] AVS is also limited by access, as it may only be available at specialized centers.

Surgical Management and Outcomes

Minimally invasive adrenalectomy is the preferred procedure for the management of aldosteronoma and most other adrenal tumors.[15] Cure of primary aldosteronism is defined by clinical and biochemical end points. Reductions in blood pressure, antihypertensive medication requirements, and plasma and urine aldosterone levels and resolution of hypokalemia (if previously present) are observed as soon as 24 hours after successful surgery. Overall cure rates range from 75% to 95% at specialty centers, depending on the specific criteria for cure that are used. The Primary Aldosteronism Surgical Outcome (PASO) study established an international consensus for outcomes after adrenalectomy.[15] Clinical success is defined as complete (normalization of blood pressure without antihypertensive medication), partial (decrease in antihypertensive medication or reduction in blood pressure with same medication), or absent. Biochemical success is defined as complete (correction of hypokalemia and normalization of aldosterone-to-renin ratio), partial (correction of hypokalemia and ≥50% decrease in plasma aldosterone but persistently elevated aldosterone to renin ratio), or absent. In general, more than 80% of patients can expect either normalization of blood pressure or a significant reduction in antihypertensive medication requirements (typically, from three to four medications down to one). In some patients, depending on the degree of preoperative sodium overload, blood pressure may take several weeks to improve. Our practice is to stop all mineralocorticoid antagonists, ACE inhibitors, and angiotensin receptor blockers (ARBs) immediately after surgery, with tapering of β-blockers and α-blockers, which must be done to avoid a rebound phenomenon. Calcium channel blockers may be maintained at the clinician's discretion. For those patients who continue to be hypertensive in the short term, medications may be added back temporarily, as needed, until the blood pressure gradually reaches a new equilibrium over time.

Patients with hyperaldosteronism have a higher incidence of chronic kidney disease compared with hypertensive controls. Glomerular hyperfiltration caused by hyperaldosteronism can artificially raise creatinine clearance and mask renal insufficiency. After adrenalectomy, the decrease in aldosterone levels can lower glomerular filtration and unmask the true degree of chronic kidney disease. In addition, hyperkalemia caused by transient suppression of the contralateral adrenal gland may occur in 5% to 10% of patients after adrenalectomy for hyperaldosteronism.[16] Renal insufficiency and suppression of aldosterone secretion from the contralateral adrenal gland at AVS are predictors of hyperkalemia. Hyperkalemia occurs within 1 to 3 weeks after surgery; therefore, patients should be monitored with weekly serum potassium levels for 1 month postresection. Persistent hyperkalemia can be treated with mineralocorticoid replacement therapy (fludrocortisone).

A subset of patients with the following preoperative clinical characteristics experience reduced benefit from surgical treatment and continue to require antihypertensive medications after operation: males older than 45 years, family history of hypertension, long-standing hypertension, requirement of more than two antihypertensive medications, and nonresponse to spironolactone. These factors may indicate a component of essential hypertension or irreversible cardiovascular alterations caused by chronic disease, or both. On the basis of these clinical features, patients should be appropriately counseled as to what they should expect to gain from surgery.

Cushing Syndrome
Epidemiology and Clinical Features

The clinical features of glucocorticoid excess were first documented by Harvey Cushing in 1912 in his book, *The Pituitary Body*. He described a young female of "extraordinary appearance" who developed obesity, hirsutism, amenorrhea, easy bruising, and extreme muscle weakness. When evaluating a patient for Cushing syndrome, clinical signs and symptoms that can be present include visceral and truncal obesity, muscle weakness and atrophy,

insulin resistance/type 2 diabetes, hypertension, abdominal striae, moon face, dorsocervical fat pad, hirsutism, easy bruising, and thinning of the skin. When left untreated, Cushing syndrome can be a lethal disease. The physiologic derangements resulting from glucocorticoid excess, including hypertension (present in >70% of cases), hyperglycemia, and truncal obesity, ultimately yield a fivefold excess mortality, primarily because of cardiovascular complications.[17,18] Thus, all efforts should be made to identify the root cause of cortisol excess and appropriately treat patients with Cushing syndrome. The differential diagnosis for the underlying cause of Cushing syndrome is broad, and the initial workup must consider ACTH-dependent and ACTH-independent causes (Fig. 75.12).

The most common cause of Cushing syndrome is pharmacologic glucocorticoid use for the treatment of inflammatory disorders. Endogenous Cushing syndrome is rare, affecting 5 to 10 individuals/million. Of these, most affected individuals (75%) will have Cushing *disease,* that is, glucocorticoid excess caused by an ACTH-hypersecreting pituitary adenoma. The remainder will be split between primary adrenal Cushing syndrome (15%) and ectopic ACTH syndrome (<10%), the latter of which usually is caused by neuroendocrine tumors or bronchogenic malignant neoplasms arising in the thorax.

Biochemical Diagnosis and Localization

The diagnosis of Cushing syndrome is reliant on demonstration of inappropriate cortisol secretion or the loss of physiologic negative feedback. Normally, cortisol release follows a predictable circadian rhythm, peaking approximately 1 hour after waking and reaching a nadir around midnight. Thus, inappropriate cortisol secretion can be detected as elevated cortisol release during a 24-hour period or as a higher-than-expected level in the late evening. The 1-mg overnight dexamethasone suppression test is commonly used to diagnose autonomous cortisol secretion. Late night salivary cortisol testing has provided a feasible alternative to suppression testing.

More than 90% of circulating cortisol is bound to plasma proteins. Unbound cortisol can be detected in the urine and saliva, and assessment of these body fluids forms the basis of biochemical screening for Cushing syndrome (Fig. 75.13); 24-hour urine collection for urine-free cortisol should be performed at least twice for initial screening. Unequivocally elevated levels should prompt immediate further testing to determine the cause and subtype of Cushing syndrome (i.e., primary adrenal cause, pituitary cause, and ectopic ACTH syndrome). Patients with moderately elevated 24-hour urine cortisol levels should undergo confirmatory testing with two late night salivary cortisol measurements. A high cutoff value of 550 ng/mL has a sensitivity of 93% and specificity of 100%.[19]

ACTH-independent. Primary adrenal Cushing syndrome, also termed *ACTH-independent Cushing syndrome,* is caused by autonomous adrenal cortisol production and therefore is generally associated with an undetectable ACTH level (<5 pg/mL) because of feedback inhibition. The underlying pathologic process is variable, with solitary adrenal adenoma found in approximately 90% of cases, adrenocortical carcinoma (ACC) in less than 10%, and bilateral micronodular or macronodular hyperplasia in less than 1%. Almost all these lesions, except micronodular hyperplasia, are readily apparent on CT scans.

ACTH-dependent. Hypercortisolemia associated with normal or elevated ACTH levels is indicative of ACTH-dependent Cushing syndrome, most commonly caused by a pituitary corticotroph

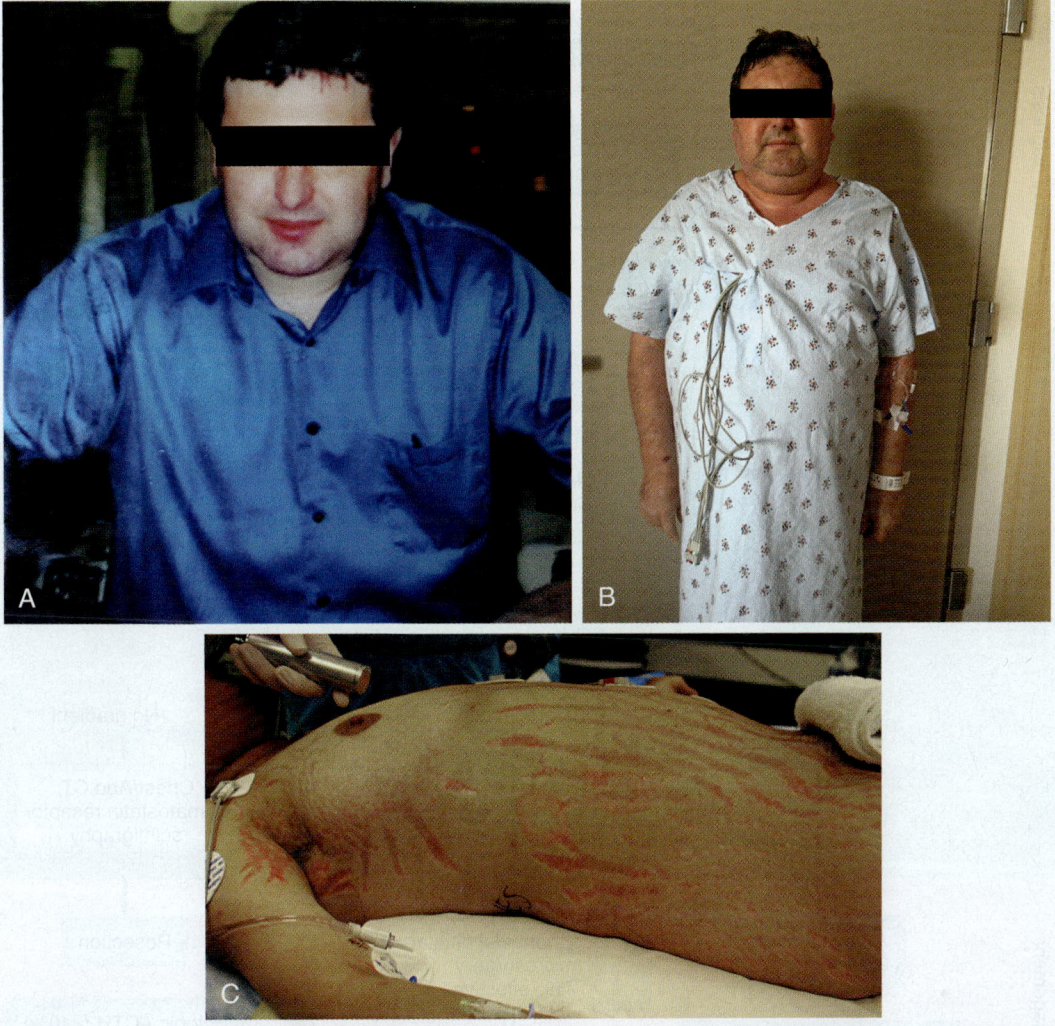

FIGURE 75.12 Clinical manifestations of Cushing syndrome. (A) Appearance of a male patient before development of Cushing syndrome. (B) Same patient 1 year after development of Cushing syndrome. (C) Purple abdominal and axillary striae in a male patient with Cushing syndrome.

microadenoma (Cushing disease). Suspicion for ACTH-dependent Cushing syndrome should prompt pituitary imaging and high dose dexamethasone suppression testing, that is, serum or urine cortisol measurement after administration of 2 mg of dexamethasone every 6 hours during 48 hours. Dexamethasone is chosen because it does not cross-react with biochemical assays for cortisol. Corticotroph adenomas are commonly suppressed in response to high-dose dexamethasone administration, whereas ectopic ACTH sources are completely lacking in feedback inhibition. Slightly more than 50% of corticotroph microadenomas are visible on pituitary magnetic resonance imaging (MRI). Detection of a pituitary mass larger than 6 mm in diameter in a patient with ACTH-dependent Cushing syndrome that is suppressed with high-dose dexamethasone justifies proceeding to pituitary surgery.[20] In the absence of a demonstrable mass, bilateral inferior petrosal sinus ACTH sampling with corticotropin-releasing factor stimulation should be pursued. Demonstration of a central-to-peripheral ACTH gradient in a study performed by a skilled physician is sufficient to diagnose Cushing disease. The absence of a clear gradient should prompt CT imaging of the chest and abdomen and, occasionally, somatostatin receptor scintigraphy to identify an ectopic ACTH source.

Surgical Management and Outcomes

Perioperative and postoperative glucocorticoid administration is obviously essential in the care of patients with Cushing syndrome. For patients undergoing adrenalectomy for Cushing syndrome, perioperative stress-dose steroids (e.g., hydrocortisone 100 mg intravenously every 8 hours for 24 hours) are recommended. In the most common scenario of resection of a solitary adrenal Cushing adenoma, steroids can usually be tapered to physiologic replacement levels during the course of several weeks. However, a subset of patients with Cushing syndrome of longer duration and severity will demonstrate lasting HPA axis suppression, requiring glucocorticoid supplementation for longer periods, sometimes longer than 1 year.

The management of patients who undergo pituitary surgery for Cushing disease is variable. In some centers, glucocorticoids are withheld during the immediate postoperative period to provide a window during which early remission may be assessed.[21] A subnormal morning cortisol level on postoperative day 1 or 2 is indicative of cure. Glucocorticoid supplementation is then resumed until the HPA axis recovers, usually for at least 6 months. Because of the significant risk of postoperative adrenal crisis in patients with Cushing syndrome of all subtypes, glucocorticoid

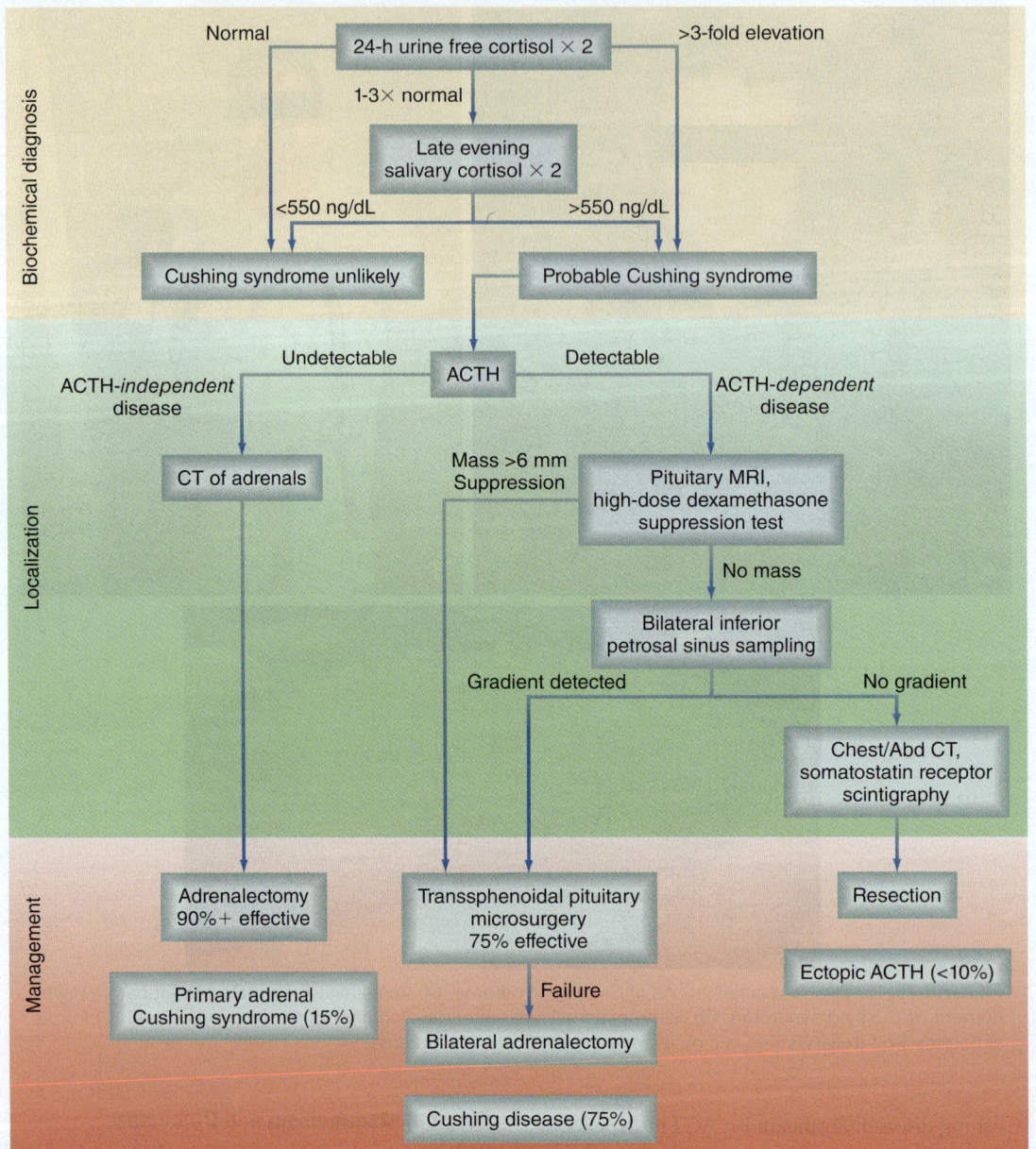

FIGURE 75.13 Algorithm for the diagnosis, localization, and management of endogenous Cushing syndrome. A biochemical diagnosis can be established with an unequivocally elevated 24-hour urine-free cortisol level (greater than a threefold elevation) or an elevated late evening salivary cortisol level. Most cases of Cushing syndrome are caused by Cushing disease (pituitary corticotroph microadenoma) in which the plasma adrenocorticotropic hormone *(ACTH)* level is elevated. An undetectable ACTH level establishes the diagnosis of ACTH-independent Cushing syndrome and prompts adrenal imaging. Bilateral adrenalectomy is considered for patients with Cushing disease not cured by transsphenoidal surgery. *Abd,* Abdomen; *CT,* computed tomography; *MRI,* magnetic resonance imaging.

management is ideally done in conjunction with an experienced endocrinologist.

Adrenalectomy is more than 90% effective in the treatment of primary adrenal Cushing syndrome. Resolution of symptoms typically takes months to years, and certain deleterious physiologic effects regarding bone density, body composition, and inflammation are extremely persistent.[22] Failures may result from local and occasionally distant tumor recurrence in the case of malignant disease. For Cushing disease, pituitary microsurgery, typically performed via a transnasal transsphenoidal approach, is approximately 90%

successful in expert hands. Remission rates may be improved by reoperation or pituitary irradiation for patients whose basal cortisol levels do not fall appropriately after initial surgery. Laparoscopic or retroperitoneoscopic bilateral adrenalectomy may be considered for patients with Cushing disease in whom pituitary surgery and medical management have failed. Patients with Cushing syndrome are hypercoagulable and carry a risk of venous thromboembolism of up to 5% after pituitary or adrenal surgery. Chemical thromboprophylaxis should be considered, although there are insufficient data to determine the optimal duration and dosage.[23,24]

Special Case: Mild Autonomous Cortisol Secretion

MACS has replaced the term *subclinical Cushing syndrome*. Patients with MACS typically have incidentally discovered adrenal masses and biochemical evidence of cortisol hypersecretion without overt signs or symptoms of Cushing syndrome. This disease entity has been incompletely characterized with respect to its physiologic consequences and natural history. A serum cortisol level of >50 nmol/L (>1.8 µg/dL) after a 1-mg dexamethasone suppression test is considered consistent with MACS in the absence of overt signs or symptoms of hypercortisolism.

Hypertension, dyslipidemia, and impaired glucose tolerance appear to be more prevalent among individuals with MACS compared with normal individuals. Retrospective studies suggest that this subset of patients experiences improvement in obesity, hypertension, glycemic control, and dyslipidemia when they are treated surgically.[25] Furthermore, a randomized controlled trial comparing surgery with observation in 45 patients with MACS noted more frequent resolution of hypertension and other metabolic conditions in the surgically treated group.[26] We observe a continuum of disease ranging from subclinical to overt Cushing syndrome, which arises as a function of both symptom severity and the perceptiveness of the treating physician. Patients along the entire spectrum appear to benefit from restoration of normal cortisol physiology. We therefore recommend surgery for patients with MACS and comorbid conditions associated with hypercortisolism who are appropriate surgical candidates, especially for patients with larger (3- to 4-cm) tumors and those whose tumors enlarge on serial imaging studies.

Sex Steroid Excess

Adrenal tumors causing clinical features of sex steroid excess are rare. Most of these tumors are virilizing (as opposed to feminizing) and may be manifested at a late stage in association with an ACC. Almost all feminizing tumors are malignant, whereas approximately one-third of virilizing tumors are malignant. Of ACCs, 20% cause virilization, with most of these cases occurring in children. An additional 24% of ACCs will display mixed features of Cushing syndrome and virilization.[27] Virilizing tumors may be biochemically detected by measurements of 24-hour urine testosterone, DHEA, and DHEA-S. Although minimally invasive adrenalectomy remains the preferred procedure for most adrenal tumors, the high probability of malignancy in sex steroid–producing tumors merits close radiographic and intraoperative inspection for evidence of invasion or metastasis. Open adrenalectomy should be considered for obviously malignant tumors.

Adrenocortical Carcinoma

ACC is a rare tumor with an annual incidence of approximately 1/million. It demonstrates no significant sex predilection. At the time of presentation, ACCs tend to be very large (mean tumor size, 9–13 cm) and have usually spread beyond the confines of the adrenal gland.[28] Historically, 5-year overall survival rates have been in the 15% to 20% range. Among patients who undergo surgical resection, 5-year survival is approximately 40%, a figure that has essentially remained unchanged during the past two decades.[29] A higher risk of death is associated with increasing age of the patient, poorly differentiated or high-grade tumors, positive surgical margins, and presence of distant metastases. More than 50% of ACCs are functional. Cushing syndrome is most commonly seen, followed by virilization. Radiographic evaluation is primarily performed with CT, which typically reveals a heterogeneous mass with irregular or indistinct borders, central necrosis, and invasion of adjacent structures (Fig. 75.14). Metastases to lymph nodes, liver, and lungs may be found; therefore, preoperative staging evaluation with a minimum of CT scan of the chest is indicated. Fluorodeoxyglucose (FDG) position emission tomography (PET)/CT may be of benefit in patients with a high suspicion for metastatic disease.

Surgery is the only potentially curative treatment for ACC. Therefore, aggressive surgery is typically indicated for isolated tumors or locoregional disease. Classic teachings recommend open surgery; however, for small stage 1 and stage 2 tumors, survival appears similar for open and minimally invasive techniques when performed by experienced surgeons.

Treatment of large ACCs requires radical resection, which is most commonly achieved by an open approach. Complete resection can be achieved in up to 70% of patients in experienced hands. This frequently involves en bloc resection of adjacent organs or regional lymphadenectomy. Particular care must be taken in dealing with right-sided ACCs because direct tumor thrombus extension into the inferior vena cava and sometimes the right side of the heart may be observed. Tumors demonstrating intravascular extension may need to be resected while the patient is on cardiopulmonary bypass to reduce the likelihood of lethal intraoperative tumor embolization.[30]

Patients who undergo incomplete resection of ACCs have extremely limited life expectancy (median survival <1 year). Even those who undergo successful surgery are prone to development of local recurrence and metastases, which typically occur within 2 years. The principal chemotherapeutic agent for the treatment of ACC is mitotane [*o,p*-DDD, or 1,1-dichloro-2-(*o*-chlorophenyl)-2-(*p*-chlorophenyl)ethane], a derivative of the insecticide DDT that is a direct adrenocortical toxin. Mitotane has been used clinically as an adjuvant to surgery and as primary therapy in individuals with unresectable or metastatic disease. A multinational retrospective study examining the efficacy of adjuvant mitotane after radical surgery has demonstrated a significant improvement in recurrence-free survival.[31] The use of mitotane is

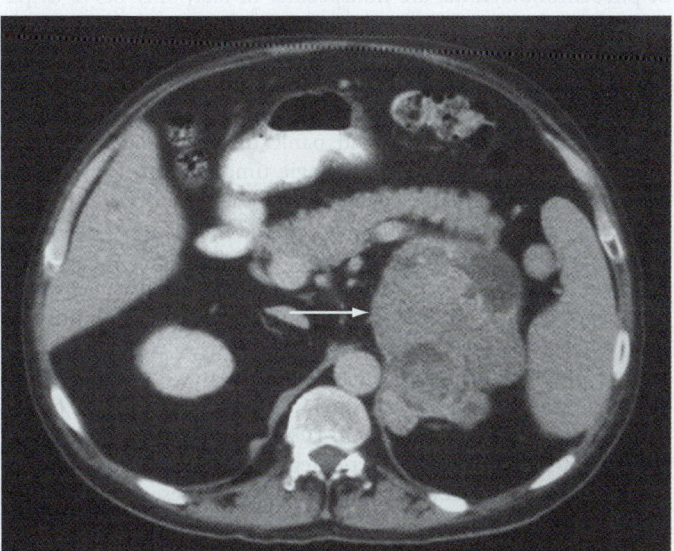

FIGURE 75.14 Computed tomography scan demonstrating a 10-cm left adrenocortical carcinoma. Note the area of central necrosis *(arrow)*.

limited by significant, dose-dependent gastrointestinal and neurologic toxicity. The multinational First International Randomized Trial in Locally Advanced and Metastatic Adrenocortical Carcinoma Treatment (FIRM-ACT) trial randomized 304 patients with locally advanced or metastatic ACC to receive etoposide, doxorubicin, cisplatin, and mitotane or streptozotocin and mitotane. There was a significantly improved response rate and progression-free survival in the former group, but median overall survival remained poor in both groups (14.8 vs. 12.0 months).[32] Several other trials are examining targeted agents such as epidermal growth factor inhibitors, insulin-like growth factor I inhibitors, antiangiogenic agents, and broad-spectrum tyrosine kinase inhibitors. There is also an emerging interest in individualized therapy based on genomic and expression profiling of tumors.

DISEASES OF THE ADRENAL MEDULLA

Pheochromocytoma

Epidemiology and Clinical Features

The first account of pheochromocytoma was published in 1886 by Felix Frankel, who described a young female suffering from intermittent attacks of palpitations, anxiety, vertigo, and headache. Autopsy revealed bilateral adrenal tumors that stained brown when treated with chromium salts. Because of the characteristic positive chromaffin reaction, these adrenomedullary tumors are termed *pheochromocytoma* (dusky-colored tumor, from the Greek *phaios*, dusky). Successful surgical management of pheochromocytoma was initially described in 1926 by César Roux followed by Charles Mayo in 1927.[33]

Pheochromocytoma affects approximately 0.2% of hypertensive individuals. Males and females are affected equally. The peak incidence in sporadic cases is between the ages of 40 and 50 years, whereas familial cases tend to manifest at earlier ages. A subset of patients present with the classic triad of headache, diaphoresis, and palpitations, although almost all patients will display at least one of these symptoms. Hypertension is present in 90% of cases and may be episodic or sustained. The principal challenge in making the diagnosis of pheochromocytoma arises from the fact that essential hypertension is common and the clinical features suggestive of pheochromocytoma are nonspecific. In fact, only 0.5% of patients with hypertension and suggestive features will ultimately prove to have the disease. The differential diagnosis of pheochromocytoma is broad, encompassing diverse processes such as hyperthyroidism, hypoglycemia, coronary artery disease, heart failure, stroke, drug-related effects, and panic disorder. Pheochromocytoma has been described as a biologic time bomb because of the potentially lethal cardiovascular effects of the bioactive compounds secreted by these tumors. Thus, despite the challenges in diagnosis, clinicians should screen for this disease aggressively and seek appropriate treatment for affected patients. Conversely, a growing number of pheochromocytomas identified incidentally on imaging may be minimally secreting; these so-called "silent pheos" may require a high clinical index of suspicion for diagnosis.

Previously, pheochromocytoma was termed the *10% tumor,* suggesting that 10% are bilateral, 10% malignant, 10% extraadrenal, and 10% familial. Discoveries regarding the genetic underpinnings of pheochromocytoma have challenged these old axioms, as discussed below.

Special Case: Pheochromocytoma in Pregnancy. Pheochromocytoma during pregnancy, although rare, is potentially fatal for the mother and child. When diagnosed in the antenatal period,

pheochromocytoma results in 12% fetal mortality. Unrecognized pheochromocytoma or paraganglioma during pregnancy is associated with a twenty-sevenfold increase in maternal and fetal complications[34] α-Adrenergic blockade is associated with better outcomes, whereas surgery during pregnancy is not associated with clear risk reduction. Therefore, all pregnant patients with a diagnosis of pheochromocytoma or paraganglioma should be treated with α-blockade. If the diagnosis is made within the first 24 weeks of pregnancy, adrenalectomy may be considered in the second trimester, whereas surgery should be postponed until after delivery if the diagnosis is made in the third trimester.

Biochemical Diagnosis and Localization

Establishing the biochemical diagnosis of pheochromocytoma is based on the detection of elevated levels of catecholamines and their metabolites in body fluids. Measurements of 24-hour urine levels of these compounds have long been the cornerstone of biochemical testing. In 2002, measurement of free (unconjugated) metanephrines in plasma was introduced as an alternative screening tool for pheochromocytoma. Plasma free metanephrine testing carries an extremely high sensitivity, approaching 99%, and is recommended as the initial screening test. However, the specificity of plasma free metanephrine testing is 89% at best, with specificities at most laboratories likely to be in the 85% range or below. Given that pheochromocytoma is a rare diagnosis that is sought within a large pool of hypertensive individuals, false-positive test results are a major problem. It has been estimated that false-positive test results outnumber true-positive test results by as much as 30:1 when plasma free metanephrine testing is used as a principal screening tool.[35]

Therefore, the primary usefulness of plasma free metanephrine testing is to exclude pheochromocytoma when the test result is negative (Fig. 75.15). When the test result is positive, confirmatory testing with 24-hour urine levels of catecholamines and their metabolites is recommended. Many drugs and conditions are capable of confounding catecholamine-based testing, contributing further to the problem of false-positive results. These include sympathomimetics (present in many cold remedies), phenoxybenzamine (frequently initiated when suspicion for pheochromocytoma is raised), acetaminophen (which interferes with the plasma free metanephrine assay), many psychotropic drugs (notably tricyclic antidepressants), and major physical or psychological stressors. Results of tests performed during episodes of acute pain, critical illness, or urgent hospitalization may be misleading. The presence of confounding factors is extremely common in the population being screened because they represent manifestations or treatments of competing diagnoses.

The operating characteristics of catecholamine-based plasma and urine tests are listed, along with corresponding cutoff values, in Table 75.4. Cutoff values for 24-hour urine tests are deliberately set high to maximize specificity; these values are approximately double the upper 95% reference range in most laboratories. A urine collection may be considered positive if total metanephrines or any single catecholamine fraction (e.g., epinephrine, norepinephrine, and dopamine) is elevated above its cutoff value. This approach maintains high specificity and yields an acceptable sensitivity of 88%.[36] Importantly, it takes into account the fact that pheochromocytomas synthesize and metabolize catecholamines and that tumors may possess heterogeneous secretory profiles, depending on their relative expression of synthetic and degradative enzymes (see Fig. 75.6).

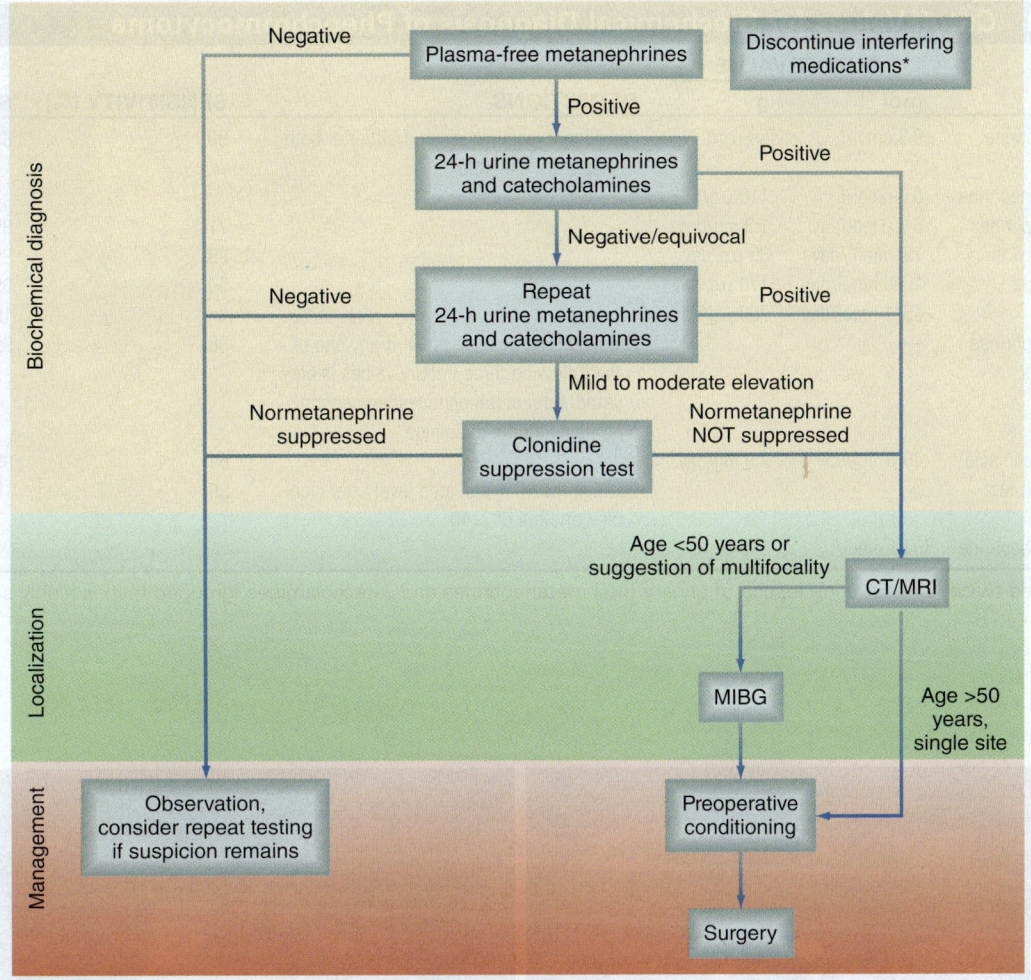

*Including sympathomimetics, phenoxybenzamine, acetaminophen, many psychotropic drugs.

FIGURE 75.15 Algorithm for the diagnosis, localization, and management of pheochromocytoma. Initial plasma free metanephrine testing can effectively exclude the diagnosis if the result is negative. A 24-hour urine collection for catecholamines and their metabolites is generally performed twice, with cutoffs approximately twice the upper limit of normal being criteria for positivity (see Table 75.4). Clonidine suppression testing can be used for the small fraction of patients in whom the diagnosis remains uncertain after urine testing. Localization with computed tomography (CT) or magnetic resonance imaging (MRI) follows biochemical confirmation of the diagnosis, with metaiodobenzylguanidine (MIBG) scanning performed for younger patients and those otherwise at risk for multifocal disease. Phenoxybenzamine is given in escalating doses for at least 2 weeks before surgery.

Two 24-hour urine collections for catecholamines and their metabolites are sufficient to make (or to exclude) the diagnosis of pheochromocytoma in almost all cases. Clonidine suppression testing, the measurement of plasma free normetanephrine levels after the oral administration of 0.3 mg clonidine, may help clarify equivocal test results but is very rarely used. Anatomic localization may be performed with MRI or CT. MRI is slightly more sensitive, but CT often yields better anatomic definition for operative planning (Fig. 75.16). The specificity of either modality is only 70% because of the high prevalence of incidental adrenal nodules. Scintigraphy with [131]I- or ^{123}I-labeled metaiodobenzylguanidine (MIBG; Fig. 75.17) can be performed in select patients in whom multifocal or malignant disease is suspected. MIBG scanning is highly specific for pheochromocytoma but carries a sensitivity of only 77% to 90%. PET and PET/CT using novel radionuclides such as ^{18}F-L-dihydroxyphenylalanine (^{18}F-DOPA; Fig. 75.18) and ^{18}F-dopamine are highly sensitive and superior to MIBG

scanning in the imaging of pheochromocytoma. Currently, the best PET/CT radiopharmaceutical for the localization of pheochromocytoma is ^{68}Ga-DOTATATE, which has a rate of lesion detection (97.6 %), which is higher than FDG PET/CT (49%) and ^{18}F-FDOPA PET/CT (75%).[37] However, the availability of these techniques remains confined to a small number of academic centers worldwide.

Perioperative Care

Throughout the first half of the 20th century, perioperative mortality rates in the treatment of pheochromocytoma ranged from 26% to 50%. Currently, the mortality rate in most specialty centers is approximately 1%. This dramatic improvement can largely be ascribed to advances in pharmacology, physiology, anesthesia, and perioperative medical care. The adverse perioperative hemodynamic changes most commonly observed with pheochromocytoma are intraoperative hypertension and postoperative

TABLE 75.4 Cutoff Values for Biochemical Diagnosis of Pheochromocytoma

TEST[a]	CUTOFF VALUE		DEFINITIONS	SENSITIVITY (%)	SPECIFICITY (%)
	mol	g			
Plasma free metanephrine	0.3 nmol/L	59 µg/L	Paired test, positive result if either or both values are elevated	99	85–89
Plasma free normetanephrine	0.6 nmol/L	110 µg/L			
Urinary total metanephrines	6.6 µmol/day	1.3 mg/day		71	99.6
Urinary epinephrine	191 nmol/day	35 µg/day		29	99.6
Urinary norepinephrine	1005 nmol/day	170 µg/day		50	99.6
Urinary dopamine	4571 nmol/day	700 µg/day		8	100
Urinary total metanephrines and catecholamines	—		Grouped test, positive result if any one of the following three urinary values is elevated: total metanephrines, epinephrine, norepinephrine, dopamine	88	99
Urinary vanillylmandelic acid	40 µmol/day	7.9 mg/day		64	95
Clonidine suppression test			Positive result = elevated level after clonidine and fall of <40	96	100
Plasma free normetanephrine	0.61 nmol/L	112 µg/L			

[a]When it is performed twice, 24-hour urine testing of urinary total metanephrines and catecholamines (grouped test) is highly sensitive and highly specific.

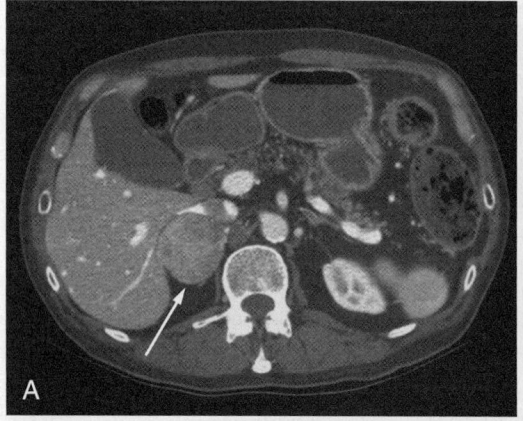

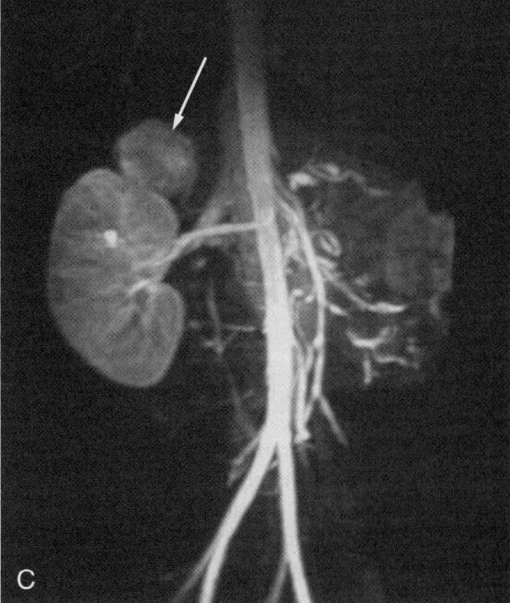

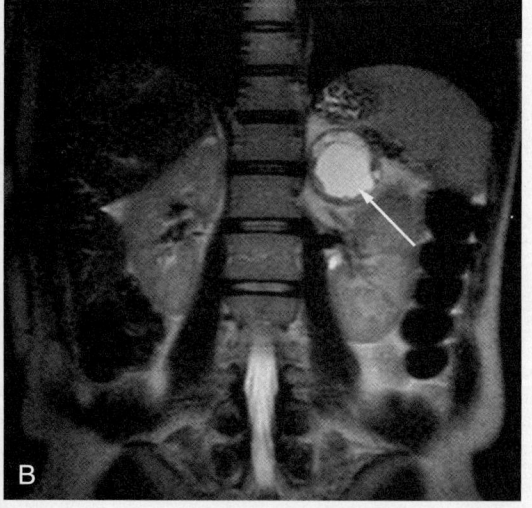

FIGURE 75.16 Appearance of pheochromocytoma on anatomic imaging. (A) Venous phase, contrast-enhanced computed tomography scan demonstrating a right adrenal pheochromocytoma *(arrow)*. The heterogeneity in the inferior vena cava represents swirling of contrast material, not tumor thrombus or invasion. (B) Coronal T2-weighted magnetic resonance imaging scan demonstrating a left adrenal pheochromocytoma with central cystic change *(arrow)*. (C) Left anterior oblique magnetic resonance angiographic reconstruction demonstrating a right adrenal pheochromocytoma *(arrow)*.

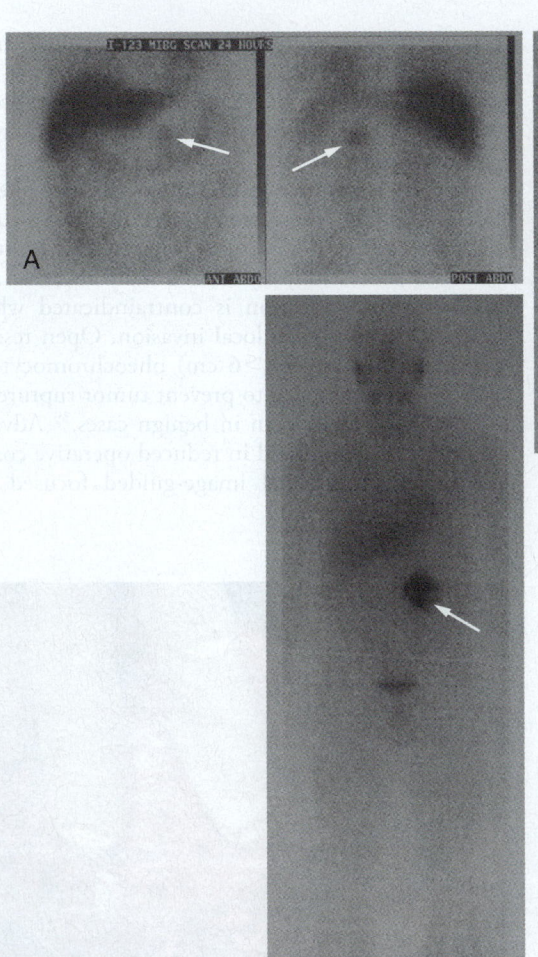
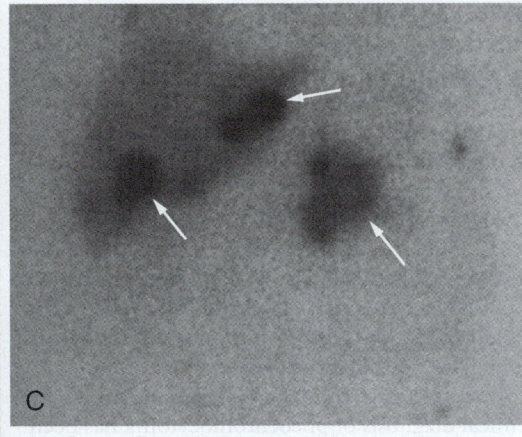

FIGURE 75.17 Appearance of pheochromocytoma on functional imaging (metaiodobenzylguanidine [MIBG] scanning). (A) ^{123}I-MIBG scan of the abdomen demonstrating an isolated left adrenal pheochromocytoma *(arrows)*. Physiologic radiotracer uptake is noted in the liver, right colon, and transverse colon. (B) Whole body ^{131}I-MIBG scan demonstrating a large, left, paraaortic extraadrenal pheochromocytoma *(arrow)*. Physiologic radiotracer uptake is noted in the liver, salivary glands, and bladder. (C) ^{131}I-MIBG scan of the abdomen demonstrating malignant pheochromocytoma, with local recurrence in the left adrenal bed and liver metastases *(arrows)*.

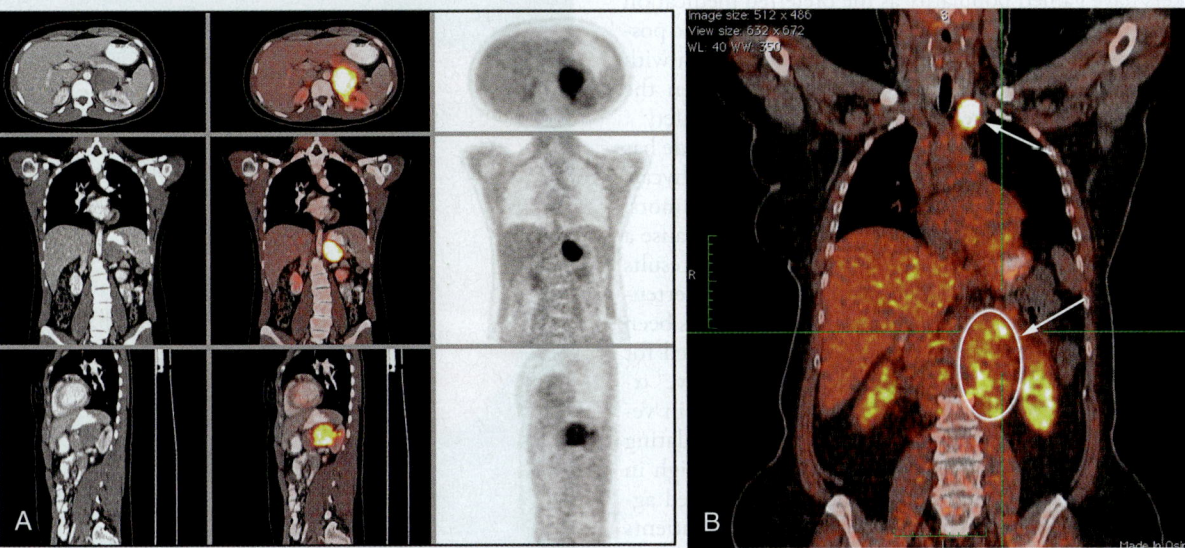

FIGURE 75.18 (A) Appearance of pheochromocytoma on functional imaging (^{18}F-L-dihydroxyphenylalanine [^{18}F-DOPA]). (B) ^{18}F-DOPA positron emission tomography/computed tomography scan in a patient with malignant multifocal pheochromocytoma. Diffuse uptake above background is seen in the region of the left adrenal gland and left periaortic region, where a locally invasive tumor was found at surgery *(arrow)*. A second area of intense tracer uptake is seen in the left paratracheal region, where a carotid sheath paraganglioma was found *(arrow)*. The patient is an *SDHB* mutation carrier.

hypotension. Intraoperative hypertension may be caused by stimulation of catecholamine release by anesthetic induction agents as well as by direct manipulation of the tumor. Postoperative hypotension may be profound. It results from a state of chronic hypovolemia created by the presence of excess circulating catecholamines. Sudden withdrawal of this stimulus after tumor removal leads to peripheral arteriolar vasodilatation and a dramatic increase in venous capacitance, which together may precipitate cardiovascular collapse. In their early report of a large successful case series, investigators at the Mayo Clinic described the use of intraoperative α-adrenergic blockade followed by aggressive volume repletion and the administration of α-adrenergic agonists in the immediate postoperative period.[38]

The principles of perioperative care remain the same today. As soon as the biochemical diagnosis of pheochromocytoma has been confirmed, α-adrenergic blockade should be initiated to protect against hemodynamic lability. Nonselective (phenoxybenzamine) and selective (prazosin, doxazosin) α-adrenergic antagonists demonstrate similar outcomes. Our practice is to start with phenoxybenzamine 10 mg twice daily. The dosage can be titrated upward every 2 to 3 days to a maximum of 40 mg three times daily to achieve normalization of heart rate and blood pressure. The period of preoperative conditioning should last at least 10 to 14 days to allow adequate reversal of α-adrenergic receptor downregulation. This restores sensitivity to vasopressor agents, which can then be used to treat the patient postoperatively. Phenoxybenzamine is a nonspecific, noncompetitive (irreversible), long-acting (half-life of 24 hours) α-adrenergic antagonist. It is associated with side effects including postural hypotension and significant nasal congestion but provides the most complete α-blockade among available agents, and its pharmacokinetics permit serum drug levels to decay in parallel with catecholamine levels postoperatively. Calcium channel blockers may be added for patients who have inadequate blood pressure control after titration of an α-blocker. The cost and availability of phenoxybenzamine in the United States have become highly variable in recent years, making it an impractical choice for a significant number of patients. For this reason, selective α-blockers have gained popularity as the preferred medication for preoperative conditioning in some centers. Because of the possibility of increased intraoperative hemodynamic fluctuation with this approach, the experience and communication between the anesthesia and surgical teams are critical to ensure patient safety.

β-Blockers may be administered after adequate α-blockade has been achieved for the subset of patients with persistent tachycardia, who often have predominantly epinephrine-secreting tumors. β-Blockers should never be the first agent administered because a decrease in peripheral vasodilatory β-receptor stimulation results in unopposed α-adrenergic tone, which may exacerbate hypertension. Preoperative volume expansion with isotonic fluids has been advocated in the past. However, in our experience, the need for this is significantly reduced when aggressive preoperative α-blockade has been achieved because the resultant increase in venous capacitance restores euvolemia gradually by stimulating thirst. Clinical suspicion for hypovolemia should remain high in the postoperative period, and patients should be resuscitated aggressively if they become hypotensive or oliguric. Some patients may require vasopressors after tumor removal, especially if preoperative α-blockade is incomplete.

Surgical Management and Outcomes

Successful operative treatment of pheochromocytoma is dependent on close communication between the surgeon and anesthesiologist.

Invasive hemodynamic monitoring is required, and fluid management must be meticulous. Manipulation of the tumor should be minimized, and the anesthetic team should be prepared to administer supplemental intravenous α- and β-blockers as well as vasopressors when necessary.

Surgery is curative in more than 90% of pheochromocytoma cases. Although these tumors are highly vascular and tend to adhere to adjacent structures (Fig. 75.19), most of them can be removed successfully by a minimally invasive approach. Minimally invasive resection is contraindicated when preoperative imaging demonstrates local invasion. Open resection should be considered for larger (>6 cm) pheochromocytomas depending on surgeon experience to prevent tumor rupture, which can lead to local recurrence even in benign cases.[39] Advances in surgical technique have resulted in reduced operative complication rates. Specifically, functional image-guided focused exploration has

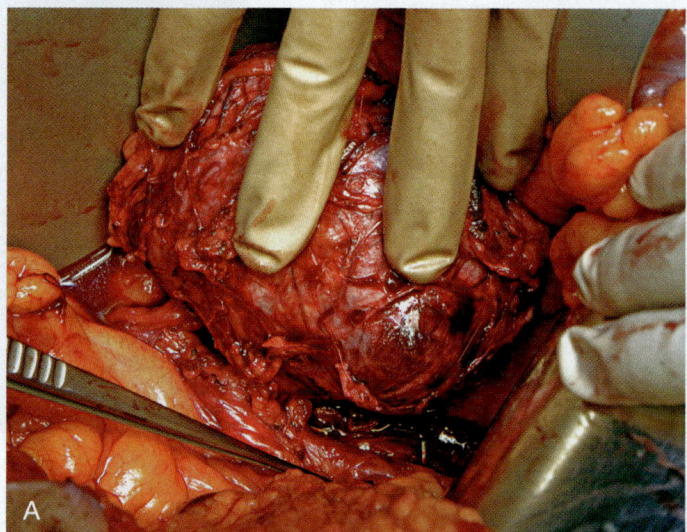

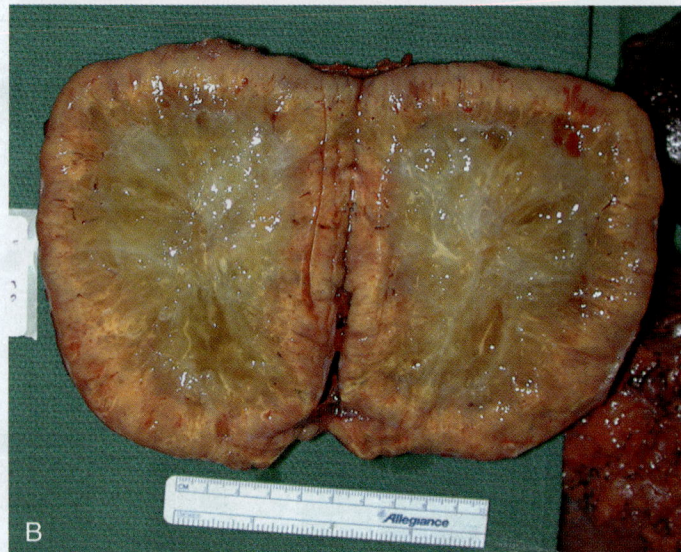

FIGURE 75.19 Gross appearance of pheochromocytoma. (A) Open resection of a left paraaortic extraadrenal pheochromocytoma (depicted in Fig. 75.17B) through an infracolic approach. The patient's head is to the right. The tumor is being rotated medially by the surgeon's hand to reveal the left ureter, indicated by forceps. (B) Left adrenal pheochromocytoma. (A, Courtesy Dr. Stan Sidhu.)

replaced bilateral adrenal and retroperitoneal exploration, leading to diminished rates of solid organ injury.

Molecular Genetics of Pheochromocytoma

Familial pheochromocytomas are much more common than previously believed. Before 2000, pheochromocytoma was known to be associated with multiple endocrine neoplasia type 2 (MEN2) syndromes (40%–50% penetrant), von Hippel-Lindau syndrome (10%–20% penetrant), and neurofibromatosis type 1 (1%–5% penetrant). Succinate dehydrogenase, which is made up of four subunits and two coassembly units, is a protein complex localized to the mitochondria and catalyzes essential steps in oxidative phosphorylation. Germline mutations in the genes encoding the succinate dehydrogenase subunits (SDHA, SDHB, SDHC, SDHD, SDHAF2) are causatively associated with hereditary pheochromocytoma and paraganglioma. More than 20 driver genes have been documented in pheochromocytoma and paraganglioma, and at least one-third of patients with pheochromocytoma have a germline mutation.[40] Germline genetic testing is therefore indicated for all patients with pheochromocytoma and paraganglioma. The discovery of a germline mutation may influence prognosis and surveillance, prompt additional investigations, and enable early identification of affected family members.

Familial cases are manifested at an earlier age and are more likely to be multifocal (Table 75.5). Succinate dehydrogenase B (SDHB) mutation carriers have high rates of extraadrenal (abdominal or thoracic) pheochromocytomas and malignant disease, whereas patients with pathogenic variants in succinate dehydrogenase D (SDHD) tend to present with multiple tumors and hormonally inactive paragangliomas of the head and neck. The lifetime penetrance of pheochromocytoma or paraganglioma in succinate dehydrogenase mutations is estimated at more than 75%. Cortical-sparing adrenalectomy should be considered in cases of familial pheochromocytoma where the risk of contralateral pheochromocytoma is high. Preservation of at least one-third of one adrenal gland is necessary to allow for adequate cortical function without the need for exogenous steroids.[39]

Metastatic Pheochromocytoma

Depending on the underlying genotype, 2.5% to 40% of pheochromocytomas will metastasize. Survival at 5 years ranges from 20% to 45% in the setting of metastatic disease.[41] No histopathologic criteria for determining metastasis have demonstrated the ability to predict the clinical course accurately. Metastasis is defined as the presence of pheochromocytoma in non-chromaffin-derived tissues to distinguish metastatic disease from multifocal primary tumors. The most common sites of metastasis are the axial skeleton, lymph nodes, liver, lung, and kidney. Treatment of primary and recurrent disease centers on surgical resection, which, even in the absence of cure, may have significant palliative benefits in terms of managing mass effect in critical anatomic locations and reducing the systemic impact of catecholamine excess.[42]

Metastatic pheochromocytomas are minimally responsive to radiotherapy and conventional chemotherapy. ^{131}I-MIBG radionuclide therapy achieves a complete or partial response rate of 22% in select patients with metastatic pheochromocytoma.[43] Peptide receptor radioligand therapy with ^{177}Lu-DOTA-SSA is widely used in Europe for metastatic disease but remains in clinical trial status in the United States. Chronic medical management of catecholamine excess should be performed with α_1-adrenergic selective blockers because of their favorable side effect profile. No targeted therapies exist yet for metastatic disease.

OTHER ADRENAL DISEASES

Incidentally Discovered Adrenal Mass (Incidentaloma)
Epidemiology and Differential Diagnosis

Incidentally discovered adrenal masses, also termed *incidentalomas,* are discovered through imaging performed for unrelated disease. Their existence as a clinical entity is a byproduct of advanced medical imaging. Incidentalomas were first described in the early 1980s, when CT scanners became more prevalent in developed nations, and they have become a common clinical problem as the use of CT and MRI has become widespread. Incidentalomas have been found in up to 8% of autopsies and approximately 4% of abdominal imaging studies. The prevalence increases to as high as 10% in patients older than 60 years.[44]

The differential diagnosis of adrenal incidentaloma is broad and includes secreting and nonsecreting neoplasms (Fig. 75.20). In patients with a history of malignant disease, metastatic disease is the most likely cause of adrenal masses (see later, "Metastases to the Adrenal Gland"). In patients without a clear history of malignant disease, at least 80% of incidentalomas are nonfunctioning cortical adenomas or other benign lesions that do not require surgical management. Thus, in most patients, the most important aspect of management is to identify the subset of adrenal masses that are likely to have a clinical impact.

TABLE 75.5	Hereditary Syndromes Associated With Pheochromocytoma	
SYNDROME	**GENE MUTATION**	**PHENOTYPE**
Hereditary leiomyomatosis and renal cell carcinoma syndrome (HLRCC)	FH	Leiomyomas, renal cell carcinomas
Hereditary pheochromocytoma	HIF2A/EPAS1	Familial polycythemia, somatostatinomas
Hereditary pheochromocytoma	MAX	Unknown
Neurofibromatosis type 1 (von Recklinghausen disease)	NF1	Neurofibromas, café au lait spots, Lisch nodules (benign iris hamartomas)
Multiple endocrine neoplasia type 2A	RET	Medullary thyroid cancer, primary hyperparathyroidism
Multiple endocrine neoplasia type 2B	RET	Medullary thyroid cancer, marfanoid habitus, mucosal neuromas
Familial paraganglioma syndrome	SDHA, SDHB, SDHC, SDHD, SDHAF2	Gastrointestinal stromal tumors, renal cell carcinomas
Hereditary pheochromocytoma	TMEM127	Renal cell carcinomas
von Hippel-Lindau	VHL	Retinal angioma, central nervous system hemangioblastoma, renal cell cancer, primitive neuroectodermal tumor, pancreatic and renal cysts

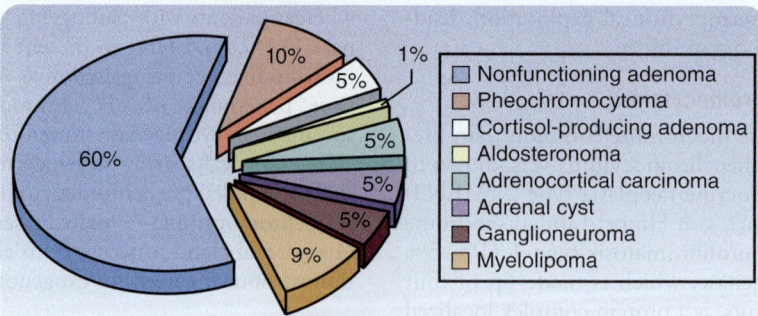

FIGURE 75.20 Differential diagnosis of adrenal incidentaloma in patients without a history of malignant disease. Approximate proportions of the various pathologic processes are shown.

Clinical Evaluation and Surgical Management

The evaluation of the adrenal incidentaloma integrates hormonal evaluation with size criteria. The principles and methods of hormonal evaluation have been discussed in the tumor-specific sections (see earlier) and are generally applicable to incidentalomas.

Evaluation begins with history taking, with a focus on prior malignant disease, hypertension, and symptoms of glucocorticoid or sex steroid excess. Biochemical investigations for hormonally active tumors are followed by consideration of size criteria (Fig. 75.21). In a general sense, surgery is recommended for hormonally active tumors and those that carry a significant risk of malignancy. ACCs represent less than 2% of adrenal tumors measuring 4 cm or smaller and roughly 6% of those measuring 4 to 6 cm. Tumors larger than 6 cm carry a more than 25% risk of malignancy. Because CT and MRI underestimate adrenal tumor size by approximately 20%, an effect that is exaggerated in smaller tumors, our practice is to remove all incidentalomas measuring 4 cm or larger in low-risk surgical patients. We strongly consider removal of those measuring 3 to 4 cm, particularly in younger patients who wish to avoid the burden of surveillance imaging.

Factors that should be considered in surgical decision-making for this latter group include suspicious imaging characteristics, the patient's age and surgical risk, growth on interval imaging, and the patient's preference. Characteristics suggestive of a benign lesion on CT scan include homogeneous appearance, well-defined borders, high lipid content, rapid washout of contrast material, and low degree of vascularity. Features that are concerning for malignancy include irregular or ill-defined borders, necrosis, internal calcifications or hemorrhage, and high vascularity. ^{18}F-FDG PET is usually reserved for suspicious cases and has high sensitivity and specificity for distinguishing between benign and malignant adrenal lesions, although it cannot differentiate between a metastasis and primary ACC. If observation is chosen, patients should undergo repeated imaging in 6 to 12 months and then on an annual basis for several years, given the fact that 5% to 25% of adrenal masses may increase in size.

It must be emphasized that CT-guided biopsy is rarely helpful in the evaluation of adrenal masses and may be hazardous. The diagnosis of primary adrenal malignancy cannot reliably be established based on cytologic criteria alone. Therefore, the use of adrenal biopsy is generally confined to patients with a history of extraadrenal malignancy in whom a tissue diagnosis would be anticipated to change management.[45] In all cases, pheochromocytoma must be excluded before attempting such a procedure to avoid precipitating a potentially fatal hypertensive crisis.

As with the other disease processes that have been discussed, most adrenal incidentalomas can be removed via a minimally invasive approach, except for those displaying obvious malignant features on imaging. No upper size limit to this approach has been established, and tumors measuring 15 cm have been successfully removed by experienced surgeons using a minimally invasive approach.

Metastases to the Adrenal Gland
Epidemiology and Clinical Features

The adrenal glands are common sites of metastasis because of their rich vascular supply. Autopsy studies have revealed that approximately 25% of patients with carcinomas eventually develop adrenal involvement. In 50% of these cases, metastatic disease is bilateral. The primary cancers that most often spread to the adrenals are those of the lung, gastrointestinal tract, breast, kidney, pancreas, and skin (melanoma). Patients with isolated adrenal metastases represent a very small subset of the total. However, these individuals are of particular interest to the surgeon and oncologist because resection of isolated adrenal metastases may improve survival, particularly in conjunction with systemic therapy.

Clinical Evaluation and Surgical Management

Evaluation of patients presenting with isolated adrenal metastases must involve careful exclusion of extraadrenal disease with CT or MRI (including the head in cases of breast cancer or melanoma and triphasic contrast-enhanced CT evaluation of the liver plus 3-mm slices through the lungs for gastrointestinal malignant neoplasms) as well as bone and PET scans, when appropriate. Patients presenting with isolated bilateral adrenal metastases (Fig. 75.22) must be evaluated for adrenal insufficiency because of replacement of all normal adrenal tissue with tumor, which may occur in up to 30% of these patients. This is best performed with measurement of morning cortisol and ACTH levels. Cortical insufficiency should be adequately treated before operation to avoid perioperative adrenal crisis.

Most adrenal metastases are well encapsulated and are thus amenable to minimally invasive resection; however, significant fibrosis may be observed in metastatic disease, particularly tumors that have previously been treated with local radiation therapy. Complete adrenal metastasectomy has yielded mean survival rates of up to 3 years compared with 12 months for patients undergoing incomplete resection and 6 months for patients not undergoing surgical therapy.[46]

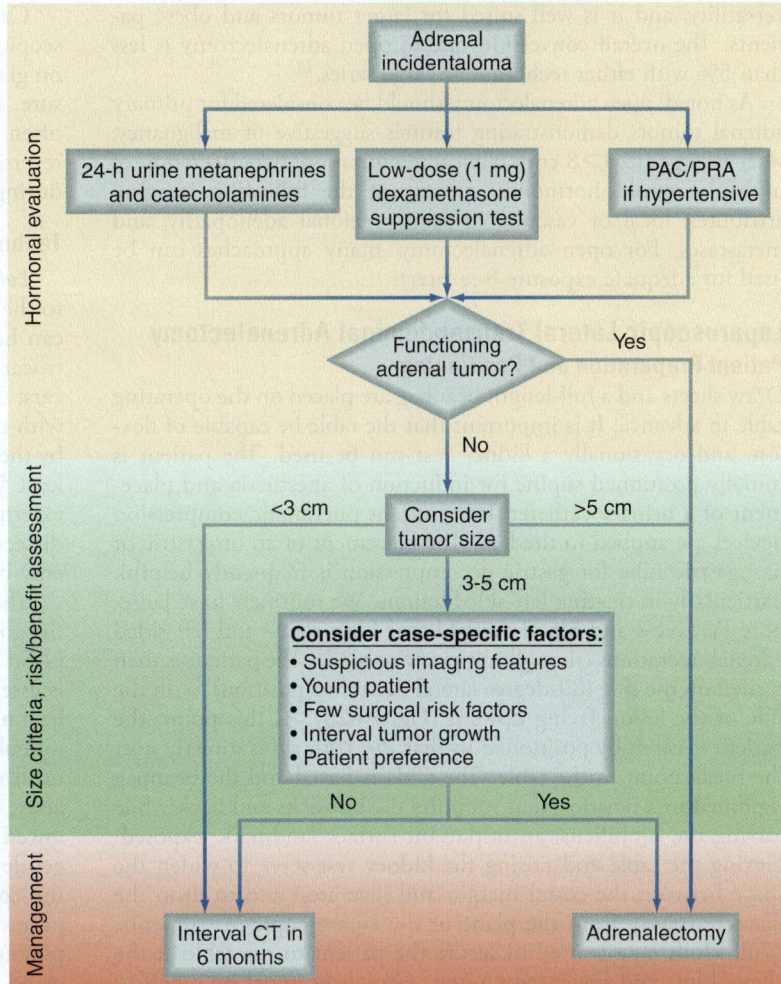

FIGURE 75.21 Algorithm for the management of an adrenal incidentaloma. Adrenalectomy is recommended for all patients with functional tumors. For nonfunctioning tumors, the risk for malignancy is assessed according to size. Tumors larger than 5 cm on computed tomography carry a more than 25% risk for malignancy and need to be removed. Those smaller than 3 cm can be safely observed. Case-specific factors must be considered for intermediate-sized tumors. *CT,* Computed tomography; *PAC,* plasma aldosterone concentration, in ng/dL; *PRA,* plasma renin activity, in ng/(mL • hr).

Within the algorithm figure:

- Adrenal incidentaloma
- Hormonal evaluation:
  - 24-h urine metanephrines and catecholamines
  - Low-dose (1 mg) dexamethasone suppression test
  - PAC/PRA if hypertensive
- Size criteria, risk/benefit assessment:
  - Functioning adrenal tumor? — Yes → Adrenalectomy; No →
  - Consider tumor size — <3 cm / 3-5 cm / >5 cm
  - Consider case-specific factors:
    - Suspicious imaging features
    - Young patient
    - Few surgical risk factors
    - Interval tumor growth
    - Patient preference
    - No / Yes
- Management:
  - Interval CT in 6 months
  - Adrenalectomy

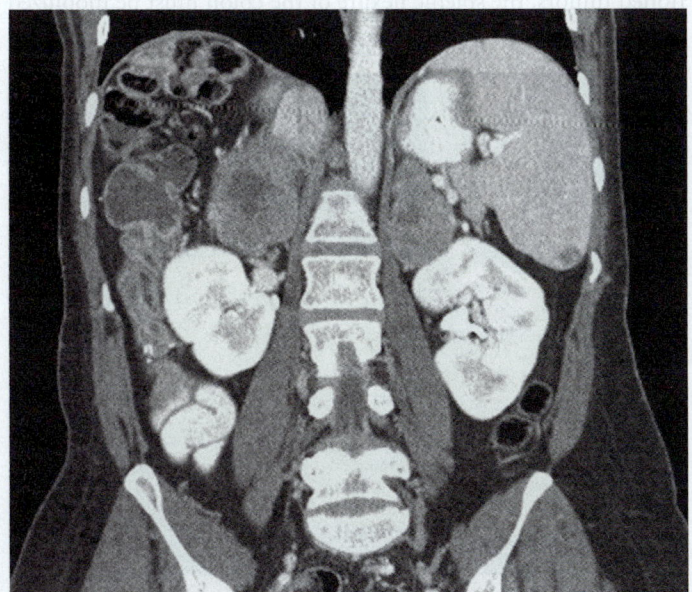

FIGURE 75.22 Isolated bilateral 7-cm adrenal metastases from colorectal cancer causing adrenal insufficiency. The patient had undergone previous right colectomy and right hepatectomy. Bilateral adrenal metastasectomy was performed laparoscopically.

TECHNICAL ASPECTS OF ADRENALECTOMY

Choice of Operative Approach

Because the adrenal glands are medial and posterior structures, conventional open surgery requires large incisions for adequate exposure. Minimally invasive approaches to adrenalectomy, however, greatly decrease length of hospitalization, pain, and operative blood loss and have a lower rate of postoperative complications such as hernia and wound infection. Similar degrees of benefit are observed with laparoscopic transabdominal and posterior retroperitoneoscopic approaches. One randomized controlled trial demonstrated reduced postoperative pain and faster recovery after the posterior retroperitoneoscopic approach.[47] We currently employ both techniques and favor the retroperitoneoscopic approach for tumors smaller than 6 cm, for bilateral tumors, and in patients with a history of extensive prior abdominal surgery. The retroperitoneoscopic approach is more challenging in older, obese male patients because of increased retroperitoneal fat, making initial entry and orientation more difficult. Severe obesity (body mass index >35) results in compression of the retroperitoneum by the abdominal viscera when the patient is in the prone position and is a relative contraindication to the retroperitoneoscopic approach, depending on the surgeon's experience. The lateral transabdominal technique offers a wider operative field and greater versatility, and it is well suited for larger tumors and obese patients. The overall conversion rate to open adrenalectomy is less than 5% with either technique in large series.[48]

As noted, open adrenalectomy should be considered for primary adrenal tumors demonstrating features suggestive of malignancy, such as large size (>8 cm), clinical feminization, hypersecretion of multiple steroid hormones, or any of the following imaging attributes: local or vascular invasion, regional adenopathy, and metastases. For open adrenalectomy, many approaches can be used for adequate exposure (see later).

Laparoscopic Lateral Transabdominal Adrenalectomy
Patient Preparation and Positioning

Draw sheets and a full-length beanbag are placed on the operating table in advance. It is important that the table be capable of flexion, and occasionally a kidney rest can be used. The patient is initially positioned supine for induction of anesthesia and placement of a urinary catheter. Intermittent pneumatic compression devices are applied to the legs. The placement of an orogastric or nasogastric tube for gastric decompression is frequently helpful, particularly in treating left-sided lesions. We routinely have large-bore IV access and blood available for both right- and left-sided adrenal operations (though it is rarely needed). The patient is then turned on the side (80-degree lateral decubitus position), with the side of the lesion facing upward (Fig. 75.23). At this point, the patient is carefully positioned so that the 10th rib is directly over the break point in the table. The table is flexed and the beanbag rigidified in a position that supports the buttocks and back while leaving the umbilicus, an important surface landmark, exposed. Flexing the table and raising the kidney rest serve to widen the space between the costal margin and iliac crest and to drop the iliac crest away from the plane of the laparoscopic instruments. Wide cloth tape is used to secure the patient to the table at the chest, hips, and lower extremities. Great care must be taken to protect bone prominences and points of potential peripheral nerve compression in the extremities (e.g., peroneal nerve). The surgical preparation is carried from the nipple line to the pubis and from the umbilicus to the midline of the back. It is essential to prep while considering the need for conversion to open surgery, if required.

Careful positioning is essential for technical success in laparoscopic adrenalectomy. As will be discussed, the surgeon is reliant on gravity to serve as a retractor for providing the necessary exposure. Having the patient securely fixed to the table permits the often extreme positioning with respect to pitch (Trendelenburg, reverse Trendelenburg) and roll (tilting left, right) that is necessary during the operation.

Technique

Left adrenal. Initial peritoneal access is achieved 2 cm inferior to the costal margin in the midclavicular line (Palmer point). This can be performed with the Veress technique or using an optical trocar in most cases. We generally use four radially dilating trocars. The ports are equally distributed along the costal margin, with the posterior port placed as far lateral-posterior as permitted by the position of the colon (Fig. 75.24). It is advisable to leave at least 5 cm (four fingerbreadths) between each port to minimize external interference of the laparoscopic instruments. For tissue dissection, we employ the hook monopolar cautery and an energy-based tissue sealing or dividing device.

The lateral attachments of the spleen are taken down first, with the goal of rotating the left upper quadrant viscera anteromedially. Great care must be taken to avoid a capsular tear of the spleen. It is essential to not rush this step, as a bleeding spleen capsule will be a nuisance throughout the operation and will distort the natural coloration of tissue planes. Splenic mobilization is continued until the greater curvature of the stomach becomes visible at its apex, at which point the spleen and tail of the pancreas are allowed to fall anteriorly with rightward tilting of the table and gentle use of the fan retractor, if necessary. It is critical to achieve the correct plane of dissection precisely during this part of the procedure because the tail of the pancreas and splenic vessels are potentially vulnerable to injury. At this point, the left adrenal gland and the left kidney are under/posterior to Gerota's fascia. The spleen and pancreas are both anterior to Gerota's fascia. Thus, it is *essential* to dissect underneath Gerota's fascia when looking for the adrenal gland. In patients with large or inferiorly positioned tumors, the splenic flexure of the colon must be mobilized

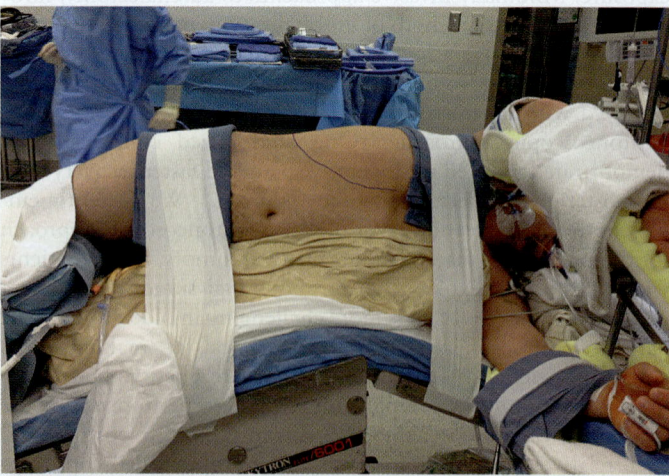

FIGURE 75.23 Positioning of the patient for left lateral transabdominal laparoscopic adrenalectomy.

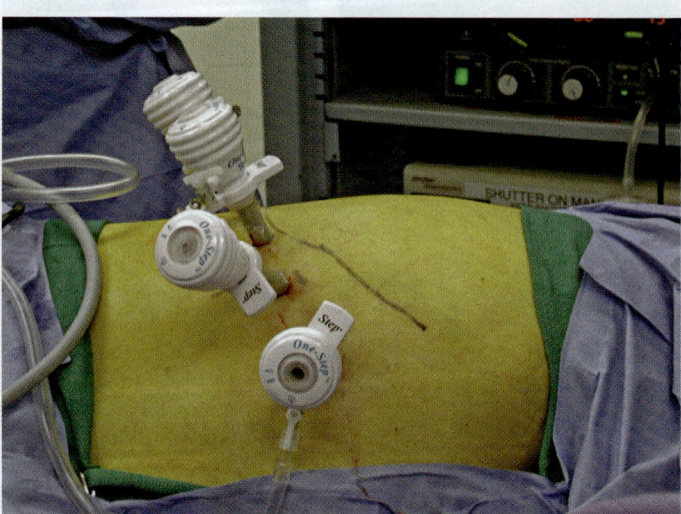

FIGURE 75.24 Port placement for right laparoscopic adrenalectomy. The patient is lying right-side up, with the head toward the right. The *marked line* denotes the costal margin. Ports are placed approximately 2 cm inferior to the costal margin, spaced about four fingerbreadths apart.

caudally by dividing the splenocolic ligament. We use an open book technique, which involves developing the cleftlike plane just medial to the adrenal gland and lateral to the aorta (Fig. 75.25). The left-hand page of the book is composed of the spleen, tail of the pancreas, and greater curvature of the stomach (everything anterior to Gerota's fascia). The right-hand page of the book is made up of the kidney and adrenal tumor. The left crus of the diaphragm is a useful landmark that leads the surgeon to the left inferior phrenic vein.

As mentioned in the anatomy section of this chapter, the left inferior phrenic vein courses along the medial aspect of the left adrenal gland before joining with the left adrenal vein. By developing the cleft of the open book, moving from superior to inferior, the adrenal vein is encountered at the inferomedial aspect of the adrenal gland. The small adrenal arteries that lie within this plane can be handled with energy-based coagulation. The left adrenal vein is carefully dissected out, coagulated or clipped, and divided. The inferior tip of the left adrenal gland may extend caudally, approaching the renal hilum within millimeters. However, because the left adrenal vein is rather long (2 cm), it is generally not necessary to expose the renal vasculature during left adrenalectomy. Many patients have a superior pole renal artery branch that approaches the inferior aspect of the left adrenal gland. Injury to this structure must be carefully avoided by keeping dissection close to the adrenal capsule while the specimen is elevated away from the medial aspect of the superior pole of the left kidney. Also, it is essential to study the CT or MRI preoperatively to look for supernumerary and accessory renal arteries.

The adrenal gland is liberated by completing dissection circumferentially and posteriorly, separating the specimen from the superior pole of the kidney and posterior abdominal wall. These attachments are deliberately divided last because they aid in suspending the adrenal gland on the lateral-superior wall of the operative field, providing exposure of the medial vascular plane during the critical initial portion of the procedure. The tumor is placed into a resilient catchment device and extracted. Tumor morcellation can be considered if it is known to be benign but should never be performed if the mass is potentially ACC. If noncutting trocars are used, only the skin will need to be closed.

Right adrenal. Laparoscopic right adrenalectomy is, in some respects, a mirror image of the procedure just described. During right adrenalectomy, the left-hand page of the open book is made up of the kidney and adrenal tumor and the right-hand page is composed of the bare area of the liver (Fig. 75.26). To gain access to the appropriate plane, the right triangular ligament of the liver must first be completely mobilized and the liver allowed to rotate anteromedially. On the right side, the colon usually lies well inferior to the operative field. When

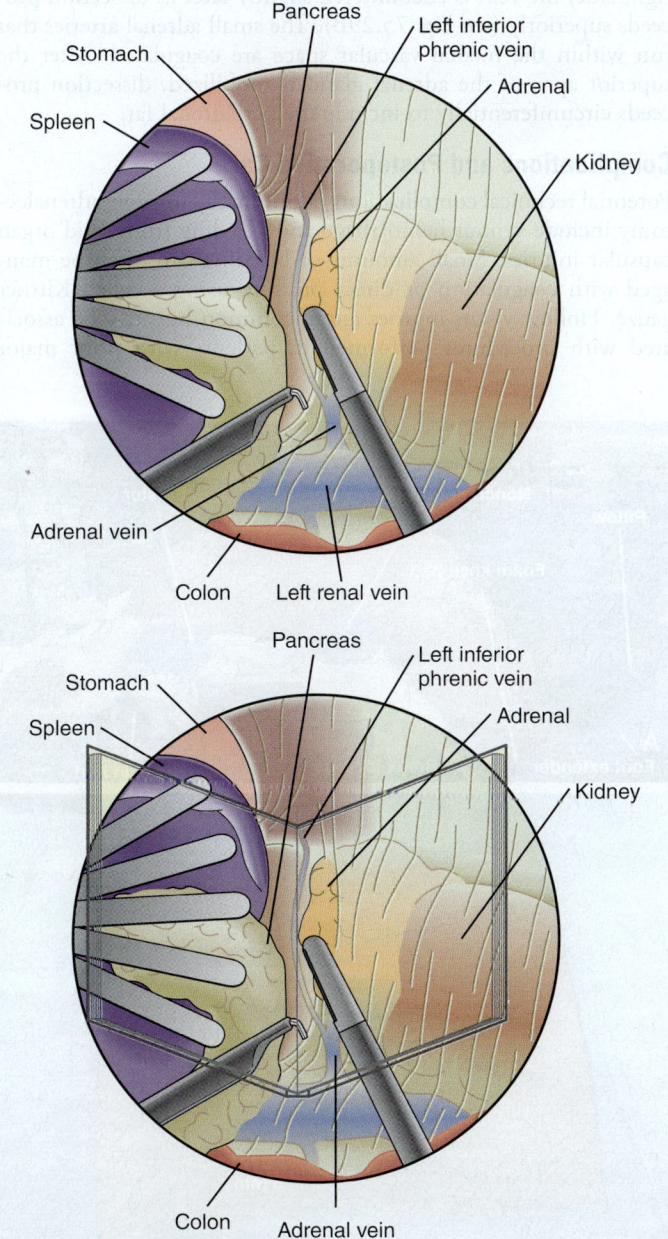

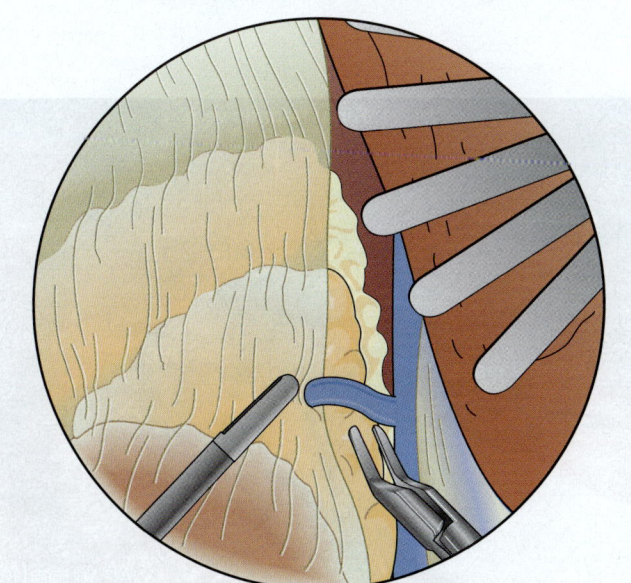

FIGURE 75.25 Technique of left laparoscopic adrenalectomy. The spleen and pancreatic tail have been mobilized and retracted anteromedially to expose the adrenal gland. The cleft of the open book is developed in a superior-to-inferior direction to identify the inferior phrenic vein and adrenal vein.

FIGURE 75.26 Technique of right laparoscopic adrenalectomy. The liver has been mobilized and retracted medially to expose the adrenal gland and inferior vena cava. The space just medial to the adrenal gland is developed to identify the adrenal vasculature.

developing the space between the adrenal gland and inferior vena cava from superior to inferior, the surgeon must be mindful of adrenal vein variants, as illustrated in the anatomy section of this chapter (see Fig. 75.3). The right adrenal vein is a potentially perilous structure to manage because it is short, wide, variable, and confluent, with thin-walled, large-capacitance vessels (the inferior vena cava in more than 80% of cases, followed by the renal vein, and, uncommonly, the right hepatic vein) that can bleed briskly if directly injured (e.g., by the cautery), lacerated from undue traction on adjacent structures, or sheared by clips. A significant second adrenal vein may be found in up to 10% of patients. By methodically dissecting one layer at a time and moving from superior to inferior, all potential adrenal vein variants can be encountered in a controlled fashion (Fig. 75.27). The adrenal vein must be dissected out delicately, definitively ligated, and then divided. Loss of control of the adrenal vein stump should be avoided; should this occur, conversion to an open procedure may be necessary.

Of note, the junction of the inferior vena cava and right renal vein is frequently difficult to identify. In vivo, the transition is a gradual curve rather than the 90-degree takeoff depicted in anatomy texts. Therefore, it cannot be used as a reliable anatomic landmark for identification of the adrenal vein. After control of the vein, the remaining mobilization of the right adrenal gland is straightforward because the inferomedial limb generally does not reach as far down toward the renal hilum as on the left side.

Posterior Retroperitoneoscopic Adrenalectomy

Posterior retroperitoneoscopic adrenalectomy was popularized in 1994 by Walz and associates.[49,50] The retroperitoneal approach has several advantages, including avoidance of mobilization of the solid organs that is necessary with transabdominal approaches, elimination of the need for repositioning during bilateral adrenalectomy, and avoidance of anterior adhesions in patients with extensive prior abdominal surgery. One disadvantage is the relatively small working space, which makes the retroperitoneal technique best suited for tumors smaller than 7 cm in diameter.

A prone position is used, with supports placed under the lower chest and pelvic girdle so that the abdomen is allowed to hang anteriorly (Fig. 75.28A). Three ports are placed inferior to the 12th rib (see Fig. 75.28B) using a direct cut-down technique for initial access. Relatively high insufflation pressures of 20 to 28 mm Hg are used and have caused no complications in regard to air emboli, hypercapnia, or clinically significant soft tissue emphysema. The working space is initially created by bluntly dissecting the retroperitoneal contents anteriorly away from the ports. The upper pole of the kidney is mobilized and reflected inferiorly to expose the adrenal gland. Mobilization of the adrenal gland begins near the crus of the diaphragm, at the inferomedial aspect of the gland. This is where the left adrenal vein is almost always encountered early in the procedure (Fig. 75.29A). On the right side, the vein is encountered slightly later as dissection proceeds superiorly (see Fig. 75.29B). The small adrenal arteries that run within the medial vascular space are coagulated. After the superior apex of the adrenal gland is mobilized, dissection proceeds circumferentially to include the periadrenal fat.

Complications and Postoperative Care

Potential technical complications of minimally invasive adrenalectomy include venous hemorrhage and bleeding from solid organ capsular injuries. Small amounts of bleeding can often be managed with coagulation or direct pressure using a rolled Kittner gauze. Hollow viscus injuries are uncommon but may be associated with procedures performed in patients with prior major

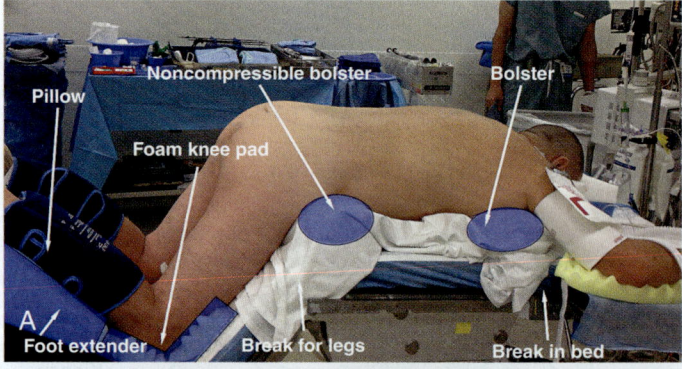

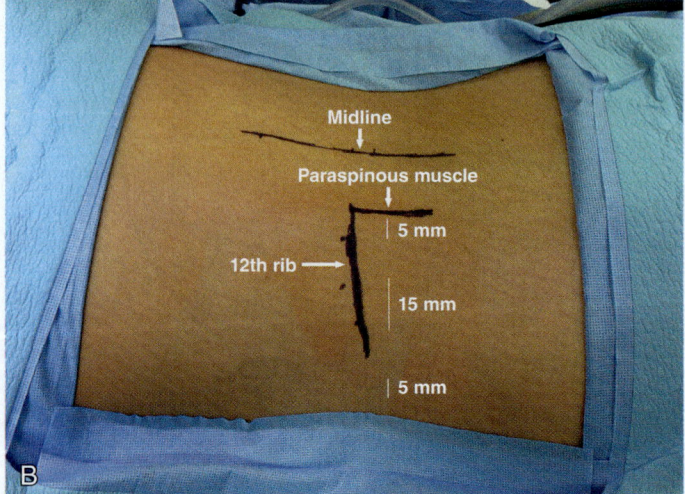

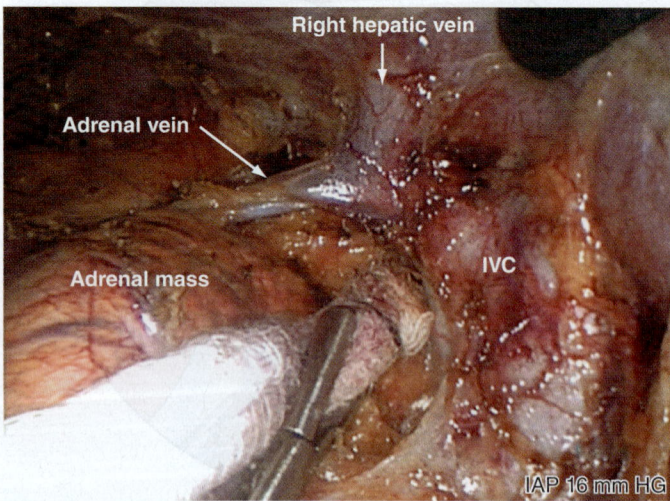

FIGURE 75.27 Right adrenal vein variant. This solitary adrenal vein arises from the superior apex of the gland and drains into the confluence of the inferior vena cava (*IVC*) and right hepatic vein, as shown in Fig. 75.3F.

FIGURE 75.28 (A) Positioning of the patient for posterior retroperitoneoscopic adrenalectomy. (B) Port placement for posterior retroperitoneoscopic adrenalectomy.

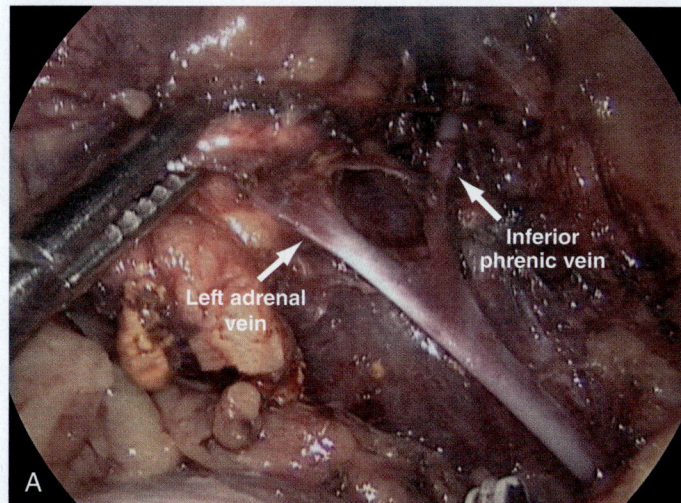

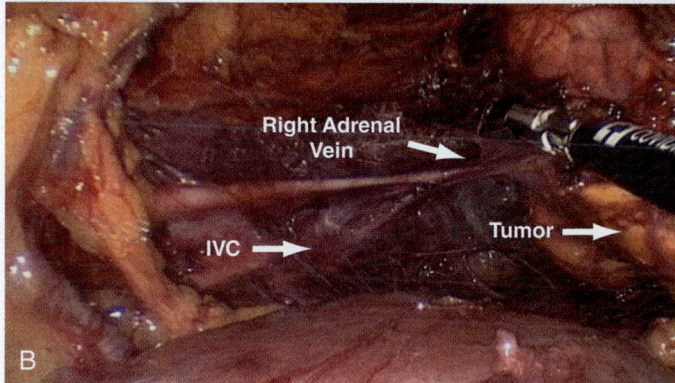

FIGURE 75.29 (A) Posterior view of the left adrenal vein. (B) Posterior view of the right adrenal vein. *IVC,* Inferior vena cava.

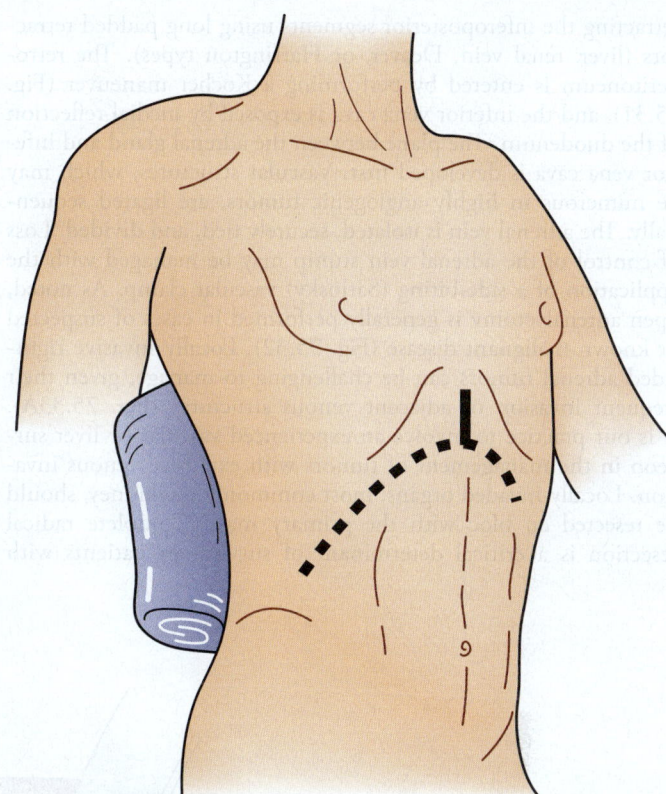

FIGURE 75.30 Positioning of the patient for open right adrenalectomy.

abdominal surgery. Pancreatic injuries and fistulas have been reported with left-sided procedures; these are rare complications, as are port site hernias and port site metastases in cases of malignant disease. Violation of the tumor capsule and tumor spillage can lead to tumor recurrence, especially in the case of pheochromocytoma. Patients undergoing minimally invasive adrenalectomy for Cushing syndrome are at risk for surgical site infections because of their catabolic and immunosuppressed state. These include port site infections in 5% of patients and, rarely, subphrenic abscesses requiring catheter drainage. One complication specific to the retroperitoneal approach is injury of the subcostal nerve causing relaxation or hypoesthesia of the abdominal wall, which occurs in 8% of cases and is usually temporary.

Patients who undergo minimally invasive adrenalectomy recover rapidly. Most patients, including those treated for pheochromocytoma and Cushing syndrome, can leave the hospital on the first postoperative day. In the treatment of adrenal tumors, successful outcomes hinge on excellent perioperative medical management as much as technical skill, particularly in cases of pheochromocytoma and Cushing syndrome, as discussed.

Open Anterior Transabdominal Adrenalectomy
Patient Preparation and Positioning
An epidural catheter or local injection with liposomal bupivacaine may be used for pain control for open adrenal surgery. The patient is positioned supine, with the ipsilateral side slightly elevated on a bolster (Fig. 75.30). A urinary catheter, orogastric or nasogastric

tube, and intermittent pneumatic compression devices are placed. The surgical preparation is carried from the nipple line to the pubis and down to the table on either side. Operative exposure involves trade-offs, and we prefer to customize the incision with several factors in mind. The most important of these relate to the size of the tumor and the size of the patient. For thin patients with large tumors, a midline approach from xiphoid to pubis is preferred. It provides outstanding exposure and preserves the rectus abdominus and oblique muscles. This approach is especially important for patients with professions that require physical labor (e.g., construction, plumbing). For patients with high visceral fat and more round abdomens, we prefer a large subcostal incision, which can extend bilaterally for better exposure. Other exposures such as thoracoabdominal or modified Makuuchi can be employed in specific circumstances.

Technique
Left adrenal. A left adrenal mass can be approached in the same way as was described in the laparoscopic approach. This method aims to preserve the spleen and tail of the pancreas. However, many large left-sided adrenal masses are tethered by the pancreas and the spleen is stuck posteriorly, which makes it vulnerable to capsular tears. In these cases, we begin with complete splenic flexure mobilization of the colon, entering the lesser sac, and then dividing the tail of the pancreas along with the splenic artery and vein in order to gain access to the medial portion of dissection along the left diaphragmatic crus.

Right adrenal. Open right adrenalectomy begins with complete mobilization of the right lobe of the liver, including the lateral attachments and the falciform ligament. The adrenal can be exposed by rotating the liver medially or, more commonly, retracting the inferoposterior segments using long padded retractors (liver, renal vein, Deaver, or Harrington types). The retroperitoneum is entered by performing a Kocher maneuver (Fig. 75.31), and the inferior vena cava is exposed by medial reflection of the duodenum. The plane between the adrenal gland and inferior vena cava is developed first. Vascular structures, which may be numerous in highly angiogenic tumors, are ligated sequentially. The adrenal vein is isolated, securely tied, and divided. Loss of control of the adrenal vein stump may be managed with the application of a side-biting (Satinsky) vascular clamp. As noted, open adrenalectomy is generally performed in cases of suspected or known malignant disease (Fig. 75.32). Locally invasive right-sided adrenal tumors can be challenging to manage, given their frequent invasion of adjacent venous structures (Fig. 75.33A). It is our practice to involve an experienced vascular or liver surgeon in the management of tumors with extensive venous invasion. Locally invaded organs, most commonly the kidney, should be resected en bloc with the primary mass. Complete radical resection is a critical determinant of survival in patients with malignant adrenal tumors; in some cases, this can be achieved only if immediate venous reconstruction is performed (see Fig. 75.33B).

Complications and Postoperative Care

Technical complications of open adrenalectomy include venous hemorrhage, tumor embolization in cases with intravascular tumor extension, and solid-organ injury. Postoperative complications are similar to those associated with other major abdominal procedures. Most patients experience return of bowel function within 3 to 4 days and are able to leave the hospital on postoperative day 5 to 7.

ACKNOWLEDGMENT

The current authors, Heather Wachtel and Matthew Nehs, have updated and edited this version of the chapter from a previous version that was edited by Michael Yeh, Masha Livits, and Quan Yang Duh.

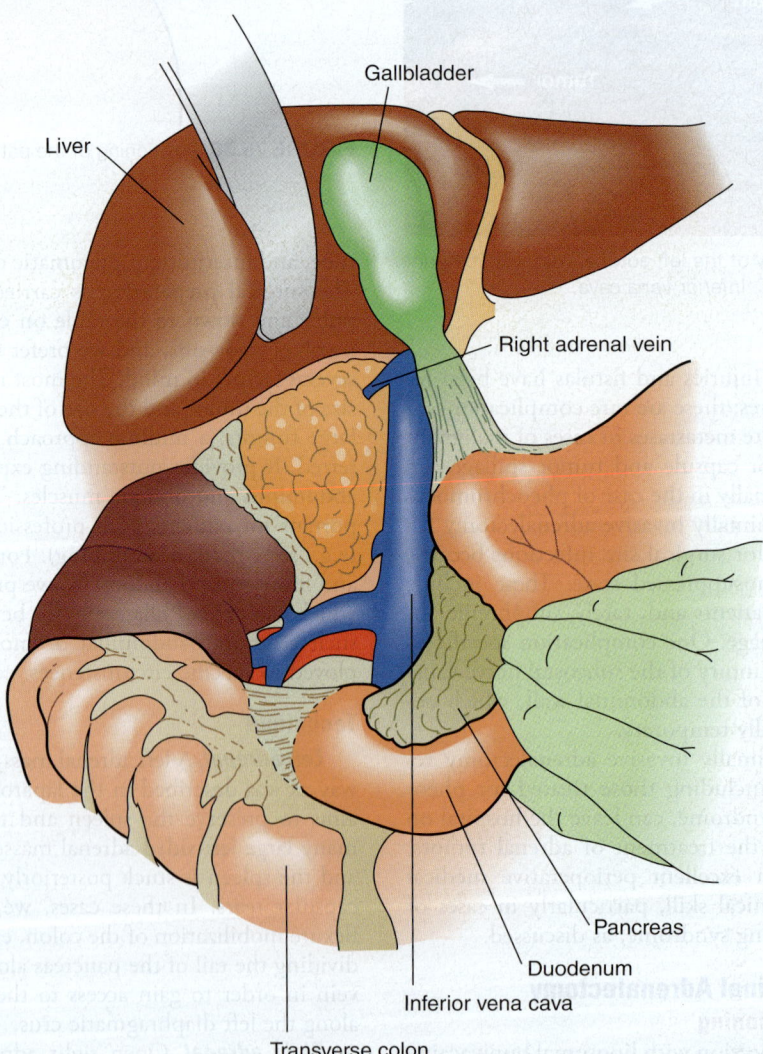

FIGURE 75.31 Open right adrenalectomy. The right lobe of the liver and the hepatic flexure of the colon have been completely mobilized. The retroperitoneum is entered, and the duodenum and head of the pancreas are reflected medially (Kocher maneuver) to expose the adrenal gland and inferior vena cava.

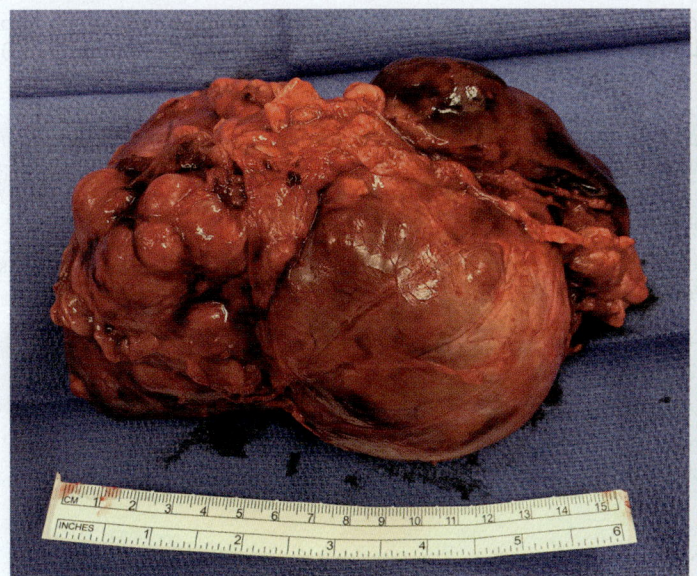
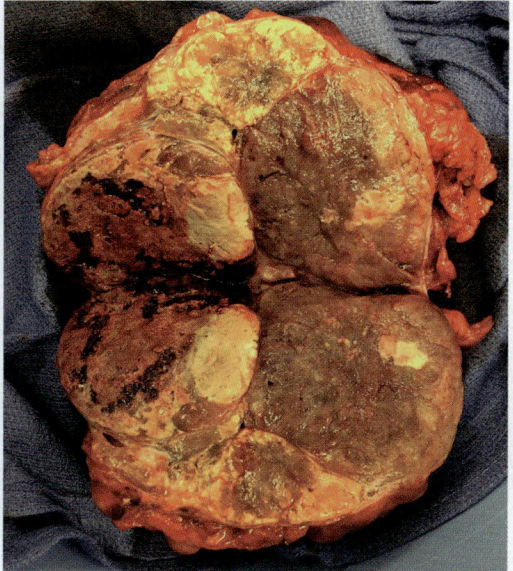

FIGURE 75.32 Gross appearance of adrenocortical carcinoma.

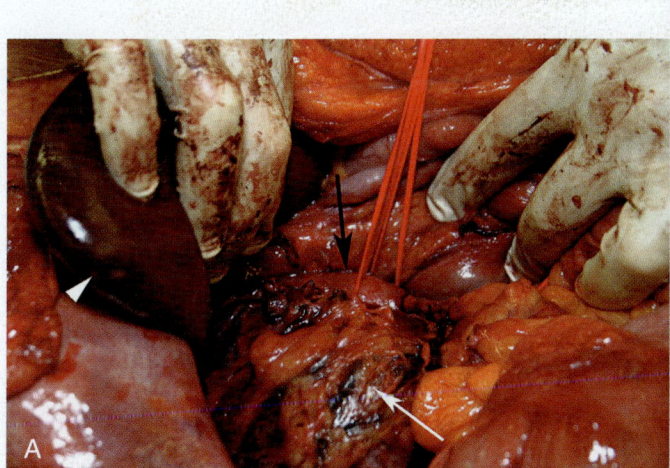
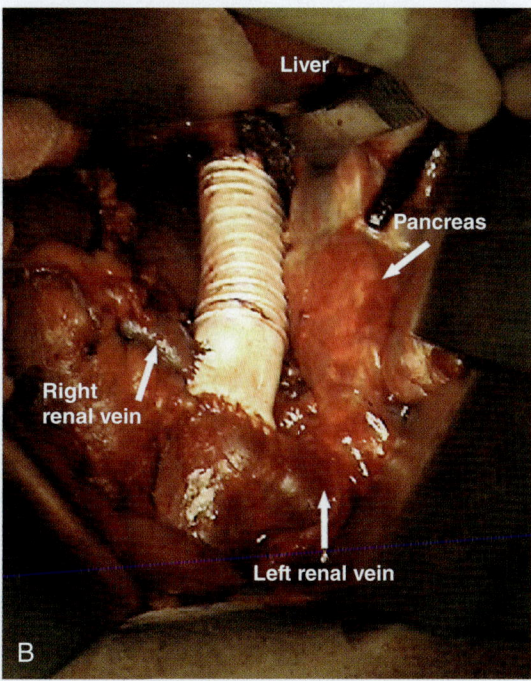

FIGURE 75.33 (A) Open resection of a right adrenocortical carcinoma invading the inferior vena cava. The patient's head is to the left. The liver *(arrowhead)* is retracted cephalad. The *white arrow* indicates the tumor; the *black arrow* indicates the inferior vena cava, which is encircled with vessel loops. (B) The infrahepatic inferior vena cava has been replaced with a polytetrafluoroethylene graft.

SELECTED REFERENCES

Chen Y, Scholten A, Chomsky-Higgins K, et al. Risk factors associated with perioperative complications and prolonged length of stay after laparoscopic adrenalectomy. *JAMA Surg.* 2018;153:1036–1041.

The largest single-institution series on laparoscopic transperitoneal adrenalectomy.

Fassnacht M, Terzolo M, Allolio B, et al. Combination chemotherapy in advanced adrenocortical carcinoma. *N Engl J Med.* 2012;366:2189-2197.

Until recently, mitotane has been the only accepted systemic therapy for patients with adrenocortical cancer. This randomized study of 304 patients in Europe showed improved progression-free survival in patients treated with multidrug chemotherapy in addition to mitotane.

Fishbein L, Leshchiner I, Walter V, et al. Comprehensive molecular characterization of pheochromocytoma and paraganglioma. *Cancer Cell*. 2017;31(2):181-193.

The first complete molecular characterization of pheochromocytoma and paraganglioma in the Cancer Genome Atlas identified both germline and somatic driver mutations.

Gifford RW Jr, Kvale WF, Maher FT, et al. Clinical features, diagnosis and treatment of pheochromocytoma: a review of 76 cases. *Mayo Clin Proc*. 1964;39:281-302.

A landmark account of the biochemical, pharmacologic, and physiologic advances that allowed collaborators at the Mayo Clinic to treat 76 patients with pheochromocytoma while experiencing only one death.

Walz MK, Alesina PF, Wenger FA, et al. Posterior retroperitoneoscopic adrenalectomy—results of 560 procedures in 520 patients. *Surgery*. 2006;140:943-948.

The largest single-institution series on this procedure, written by the developers of the technique.

Yip L, Duh Q, Wachtel H, et al. American Association of Endocrine Surgeons guidelines for adrenalectomy: executive summary. *JAMA Surg*. 2022;157(10):870-877.

Consensus guidelines from the American Association of Endocrine Surgeons on adrenalectomy.

The full reference list appears on Elsevier eBooks+.

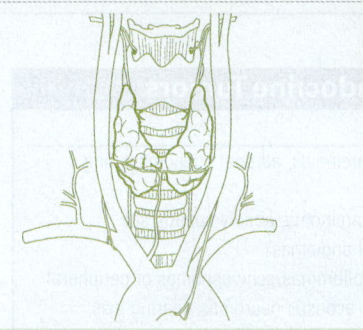

CHAPTER 76

Pancreatic Neuroendocrine Tumors

Scott K.Sherman and James R.Howe

INTRODUCTION

The German pathologist Paul Langerhans first described endocrine islet cells of the pancreas in 1869, and in 1902, Albert Nicholls reported a tumor of these islet cells.[1] Throughout the 20th century, clinical syndromes of hormonal excess from carcinoma-like "carcinoids" and different types of "islet cell tumors," including insulinomas, gastrinomas, VIPomas, and others, were identified and their associated hormones described.[2,3] Autosomal dominant genetic syndromes that include islet cell tumors as prominent features, such as multiple endocrine neoplasia type 1 (MEN1) and von Hippel-Lindau (VHL), were recognized and their responsible genes identified.[4,5] Although these tumors may be associated with clinical syndromes that include hormone production consistent with endocrine islet cell origin, contemporary research indicates that pancreatic neuroendocrine tumors (PNETs) likely arise from pluripotent stem cells in the pancreatic ductal or acinar system.[6] Unlike the more common and aggressive pancreatic ductal adenocarcinomas, PNETs usually show less aggressive behavior and exhibit distinct genetic alterations. Improved pancreatic imaging has led to increased diagnosis of nonfamilial neuroendocrine tumors that do not produce hormone excess. Indeed, it is now clear that these sporadic, nonfunctional PNETs represent the majority (90%) of neuroendocrine tumors of the pancreas.[7–9] The mainstay of PNET treatment remains surgical resection, which achieves excellent survival outcomes in localized disease. Increasingly, it is appreciated that low-grade, small tumors <2 cm may often be safely observed with minimal risk of growth or metastasis.[10,11] Localized functional tumors, those greater than 2 cm, and those with higher-risk features such as grade 2 tumors should generally be considered for resection. In metastatic tumors, resection of the primary tumor and cytoreduction of metastases can control symptoms in functional tumors and potentially increase survival in nonfunctional tumors. For advanced, unresectable, or metastatic high-grade disease, hormonal therapies like somatostatin analogues (SSAs), targeted kinase inhibitors, chemotherapy, and peptide receptor radionuclide therapy (PRRT) may delay progression and improve quality of life.

EPIDEMIOLOGY

Neuroendocrine tumor (NET) incidence of all sites steadily increased by 6.4-fold from the late 20th to early 21st century. Although still less common than lung, small bowel, and rectal NETs, PNETs now show an age-adjusted incidence in the United States of around 0.82 per 100,000 person-years. This remains much lower than the incidence of pancreatic adenocarcinoma (13.3 per 100,000), but it has increased from 0.2 per 100,000 in 1985 to 0.5 in 2000 and continues to rise.[7] Increased detection owing to higher sensitivity and use of cross-sectional imaging surely accounts for some of this, and early-stage disease shows the greatest increase in incidence.[12] Additional factors contributing to rising PNET diagnoses remain unknown. Similarly increased PNET incidence has been reported in Canada, Europe, Australia, and Asia.[13-18] In distinction from adenocarcinomas, PNETs tend to grow slowly and survival is relatively long (median nearly 100 months even with regional nodal metastases), contributing to a prevalence of 0.003% in the population, representing nearly 10% of all patients with pancreatic malignancy.[7,19]

As with other NETs, PNET incidence increases with age. Median age at diagnosis is in the late sixth decade of life,[17,20] and incidence is 0.5 per 100,000 among 40-year-olds compared with 2.5 per 100,000 among 70-year-olds.[21] Incidence may be higher among Black Americans, with rates reported to be 25% to 100% higher compared with Whites,[7,15,22] although others have reported no difference after adjustment for confounders.[21] Females are less likely to develop PNETs (45%/55% female/male distribution).[21]

Between 5% and 15% of PNETs arise in association with an autosomal dominant hereditary syndrome, depending on the population studied (Table 76.1). In a series of 383 resected PNETs, 6% of patients had a known hereditary syndrome, a number that rose to 16% among those diagnosed before age 50. Of the known hereditary syndromes, MEN1 was most common,

TABLE 76.1 Hereditary Syndromes Associated With Pancreatic Neuroendocrine Tumors

SYNDROME	RISK OF PNET	GENE	OTHER ASSOCIATIONS
MEN1	60%–80%	*MEN1* Ch11q13	Parathyroid hyperplasia; pituitary adenomas; thymic carcinoids; adrenal adenomas; lung carcinoid
VHL	5%–17%, up to 40% with some mutations	*VHL* Ch3p25-26	Cerebellar and spinal hemangioblastomas; renal cell carcinoma; endolymphatic sac tumors; pheochromocytoma; pancreatic cysts; retinal angiomas
NF1	0%–10%	*NF1* Ch17q11	Café au lait spots; freckles in skin folds; multiple neurofibromas/schwannomas of peripheral nerves; pheochromocytoma; scoliosis; meningiomas; acoustic neuromas/hearing loss; Lisch nodules in iris
TSC	1%	*TSC1* 9p34 *TSC2* 16p13	Hamartomas of multiple organs (heart, lungs, kidneys, lymphatics, eyes, brain); neurologic problems; skin lesions (fibromas, focal hypopigmentation)
Cowden syndrome	Case reports	*PTEN* 10q23	Hamartomas and cancers of the breast, thyroid, uterus, colorectum, kidney, and skin; trichilemmoma; macrocephaly

MEN1, Multiple endocrine neoplasia type 1; *NF1*, neurofibromatosis type 1; *PNET*, pancreatic neuroendocrine tumor; *TSC*, tuberous sclerosis; *VHL*, von Hippel-Lindau.

followed by VHL (65% and 26%, respectively).[20] Pancreatic microadenomas represent one of the "three Ps" of MEN1 (with four-gland parathyroid hyperplasia and pituitary tumors being the others). Patients with MEN1 tend to develop multiple tumors. Nearly 100% of patients develop pancreatic microadenomas (<0.5 cm) by age 50, and larger tumors develop in around 75% of patients, with penetrance increasing with age.[23] Many of these tumors are nonfunctional, but around half of patients with MEN1 develop gastrinomas (residing in either the pancreas or duodenum), and 20% may develop pancreatic insulinomas.[23] In addition to thymic neuroendocrine neoplasms, metastatic PNETs rank among the most common causes of disease-specific death in MEN1.[24,25]

VHL syndrome is autosomal dominant and results in failure of VHL protein to promote degradation of hypoxia-inducible factor (HIF), leading to constitutive HIF activation and development of multiple tumors.[26] Nonfunctional PNETs occur in around 20% of patients with VHL, at a median age in the mid-30s, and arise less commonly than cystic pancreatic lesions (~50%). Relative frequencies of PNETs versus other VHL manifestations such as central nervous system hemangioblastomas, renal cell carcinomas, retinal hemangiomas, pheochromocytomas, and cystic pancreatic lesions vary depending on the subtype of VHL disease and specific mutation present.[27] Type I VHL arises from truncation mutations or exon deletions and carries a lower risk of PNET (10%), whereas type II disease from missense mutations has a higher risk of developing PNETs of nearly 40%.[28]

Other hereditary syndromes associated with PNETs include tuberous sclerosis (TSC) and neurofibromatosis type 1 (NF1). In TSC, patients develop hamartomas of many organs, and PNETs are an uncommon manifestation, occurring in 1% of patients.[26] Most patients with TSC developing PNETs have mutations in *TSC2* as opposed to *TSC1*. In NF1, characterized by multiple benign neurofibromas, café au lait skin spots, and increased risk of gliomas, leukemia, and pheochromocytoma, around 10% of patients develop PNETs.[23,26] Mutations inactivating the TSC1/TSC2 protein complex or NF1 lead to loss of inhibition of mammalian target of rapamycin (mTOR) signaling and PNET development.[23] The gene responsible for Cowden syndrome, *PTEN*, also inhibits mTOR signaling. Although *PTEN* mutations sometimes exist in sporadic PNETs, and PNETs have been reported in Cowden syndrome, they remain an uncommon site of disease in these patients.[29,30]

Genetic testing for these syndromes should be performed in first-degree relatives of known patients. In MEN1 and VHL, disease features often develop in children, and testing should occur as early as possible.[11,27,31] Screening for PNETs in VHL should commence by age 15, as PNETs have developed in patients in their early teens.[31] For those without a known germline/familial diagnosis, testing for MEN1 and VHL should be considered in patients with other manifestations of these syndromes (especially hypercalcemia), those with a suggestive family history, those developing PNETs at a young age, or those with multifocal tumors. Genetic diagnoses facilitate screening for associated conditions, such as hyperparathyroidism in MEN1 and pheochromocytoma in VHL, before planning pancreatic intervention and adherence to syndrome-specific guidelines for screening for other disease manifestations.[32,33] Additionally, the unique behavior of PNETs in these syndromes affects surgical decision-making, as detailed later.

GRADE AND STAGE

Grade and stage are the most important prognostic features for PNETs. Historical series and current national databases tend to capture grade based on cellular differentiation alone. More recently, the Ki-67 index, or percentage of cells undergoing mitosis as determined by immunohistochemical (IHC) staining, has superseded differentiation as the key determinant of NET grade, and this is the single clinical parameter most indicative of a PNET's likely behavior and clinical course.[11,34] As set out in the 2004 World Health Organization (WHO) classification of endocrine tumors and updated most recently in 2022, the revised WHO grading of NETs separates them into grade 1 (<3% staining), grade 2 (3%–20% staining), and grade 3 (>20% staining), with grade strongly corresponding to differential survival.[3,34,35] Analyses of large European and American series found that grade 1 PNETs have a 5-year survival of 75% to 90%, compared with 62% to 63% in grade 2 and 7% to 12% in grade 3.[9,36] Around 90% of PNETs are grade 1 to 2, with 10% showing high-grade (grade 3) features at diagnosis.[9] An additional important distinction among grade 3 tumors is whether they have a well-differentiated histologic appearance (referred to as *G3 NETs*), as compared with

TABLE 76.2 AJCC Staging and WHO Grading of Pancreatic Neuroendocrine Tumors

AJCC 8TH EDITION STAGING FOR WELL-DIFFERENTIATED PNETS				WHO PNET GRADING		
DEPTH	NODES	METASTASES	STAGE	KI-67	DIFFERENTIATION	GRADE
T1 (<2 cm)	N0	M0	I	<3%	Well	G1 NET
T2 (2–4 cm)	N0	M0	II	3%–20%	Well	G2 NET
T3 (>4 cm or invading duodenum or distal bile duct)	N0	M0	II	>20%	Well	G3 NET
T4 (invasion of other adjacent organs or invasion of celiac or superior mesenteric arteries)	N0	M0	III	>20%	Poor	G3 NEC
T1–T4	N1	M0	III			
T1–T4	N0–1	M1	IV			

AJCC, American Joint Commission on Cancer; *NEC,* neuroendocrine carcinoma; *PNET,* pancreatic neuroendocrine tumor; *WHO,* World Health Organization.
From Rindi G, Mete O, Uccella S, et al. Overview of the 2022 WHO classification of neuroendocrine neoplasms. *Endocr Pathol.* 2022;33(1): 115-154; Lloyd RV, Osamura RY, Klöppel G, Rosai J. *Classification of Tumours of Endocrine Organs.* 4th ed. IARC Press; 2017; Amin MB, Edge SB, Greene FL, et al. *AJCC Cancer Staging Manual.* 8th ed. Springer International Publishing; 2017.

poorly differentiated, high-grade neuroendocrine carcinomas (NECs), typically with Ki-67 in excess of 50% to 70% (Table 76.2).[3] Well-differentiated G3 NETs tend to retain somatostatin receptor (SSTR) expression and grow more slowly with corresponding longer survival, whereas G3 NECs tend to show absent SSTR2 expression, unique genetic alterations, aggressive behavior, and poor survival.[3,37]

Staging in well-differentiated PNETs adheres to the American Joint Commission on Cancer (AJCC) 8th edition tumor-node-metastasis (TNM) system (see Table 76.2).[38] This staging system attempts to capture the extent of the primary tumor and, indirectly, resectability, as well as whether distant metastases exist. Distant metastases are present upon diagnosis in around 40% of patients in population-based studies, with some series reporting metastases in up to 60% of patients; at least 20% of patients have nodal metastases without distant metastases.[21,39] The 7th edition AJCC staging system followed the same definitions as exocrine pancreatic cancer. Although the exocrine pancreatic TNM designations still apply to poorly differentiated, high-grade NECs, they insufficiently discriminate outcomes in well-differentiated NETs, and the 8th edition modified the stage classifications in alignment with the system first proposed by the European Neuroendocrine Tumor Society (ENETS).[3,40,41] In the AJCC 8th edition, tumors <2 cm are T1, 2 to 4 cm are T2, T3 is >4 cm, and T4 tumors invade the celiac or superior mesenteric arteries or adjacent organs other than the duodenum or common bile duct. Nodal metastases indicate N1 disease. Stages I and II specify no nodal metastases and T1–T3 disease. Nodal metastases or T4 local extent define stage III, and distant metastases define stage IV. This system improves upon the 7th edition for survival discrimination by stage and has been validated in multiple populations.[42,43] A multicenter validation cohort of 1086 patients with PNET found median survival in stages I to IV of not reached, 115, 101, and 72 months, respectively.[43]

MOLECULAR FEATURES

Genetic alterations seen in sporadic PNETs differ from those present in adenocarcinoma. Mutations in *KRAS* and *TP53*, virtually ubiquitous in pancreatic adenocarcinoma, are absent in well-differentiated PNETs.[29,44] The much less common, high-grade, poorly differentiated pancreatic NECs typically show mutations in *TP53, RB1,* or both.[45] In well-differentiated tumors, mutations in *MEN1,* mTOR pathway genes (including *PTEN, TSC1, TSC2,* and *PIK3CA),* and *DAXX/ATRX* commonly occur and are seen in around 44%, 15%, and 43% of tumors, respectively.[29,39]

Increased mTOR pathway signaling results from mutations in mTOR inhibitory genes and correlates with worse prognosis and more aggressive behavior.[23] Presence of unrestricted mTOR signaling in some PNETs forms the molecular rationale for treatment with mTOR inhibitors, such as everolimus.[46] In addition to these changes, clinically sporadic PNETs demonstrate a high prevalence of germline mutations in DNA repair genes, including *MUTYH, CHEK2,* and *BRCA2,* which were found in 11% of patients.[47]

Menin, encoded by *MEN1,* is a histone methyltransferase and cell cycle regulator responsible for the autosomal dominant MEN1 syndrome in those with germline mutations.[19] In MEN1 syndrome, germline inactivation of one copy of *MEN1* combined with somatic mutation of the other copy leads to the development of multiple pancreatic neuroendocrine microtumors.[23] In sporadic tumors, biallelic mutation or inactivation of *MEN1* similarly leads to dysregulation of the G1/S cell cycle transition and malignant transformation.[19]

The death domain associated protein *(DAXX)* and α-thalassemia/mental retardation syndrome X-linked *(ATRX)* genes function together in a transcription/chromatin remodeling complex that localizes to telomeres.[29] Mutually exclusive alterations in either *DAXX* or *ATRX* produce chromatin instability and a loss of normal telomere maintenance. Alternative lengthening of telomeres (ALT) occurs in the presence of compromised DAXX/ATRX activity, which is a telomerase-independent mechanism of tumor immortalization that can be detected by IHC.[23,29,48] With their role as tumor suppressors important to maintaining chromosomal stability, loss of *DAXX/ATRX* and the presence of the ALT phenotype in PNET cells lead to malignant transformation and confer a worse prognosis.[49,50] In PNETs, the presence of ALT predicts increased recurrence risk.[51] In an international cohort of 1322 NETs, DAXX/ATRX-negative or ALT-positive nonfunctional PNETs had 5-year recurrence-free survival rates of 40% and 42%, respectively, compared with 85% and 86%, respectively, for DAXX/ATRX-intact or ALT-negative tumors.[52] Current recommendations suggest routine molecular assessment for either *DAXX/ATRX* mutation or presence of the ALT phenotype in PNETs.[3]

Perhaps the most distinctive molecular feature of most well-differentiated PNETs is high expression of SSTRs on the cell surface. Increased SSTR expression occurs in around 90% of well-differentiated PNETs, and clinicians exploit this phenomenon for imaging and treatment.[46,53] High-grade tumors and insulinomas more commonly have low SSTR expression, with SSTR2-negative staining by IHC present in around 85% of high-grade PNETs/ NECs and 40% of insulinomas.[45,46] In tumors with elevated SSTR expression, synthetic SSAs decrease hormone production and impair growth, improving progression-free survival (PFS).[54,55] SSAs conjugated to radioisotopes permit preferential accumulation of those isotopes in tumor cells, allowing for tumor-specific imaging (^{68}Ga or ^{64}Cu) or radiotherapy (^{90}Y or ^{177}Lu PRRT).[56,57]

CLINICAL FEATURES

The clinical features of functional PNETs differ from those of nonfunctional tumors. Functional tumors are defined by the presence of a clinical syndrome and elevated hormone levels. These present with symptoms related to the excess hormone being produced and may lead to their recognition at an earlier stage. Nonfunctional tumors are often silent until quite advanced, when large tumors or liver metastases give rise to symptoms that lead to workup. Increasingly, clinicians discover less advanced nonfunctional PNETs on imaging obtained for unrelated complaints. Functional NETs of the small bowel often produce large amounts of serotonin and, particularly when more advanced, give rise to classic "carcinoid syndrome" symptoms of serotonin excess, including flushing, diarrhea, carcinoid heart disease, and hemodynamic lability, in as many as one-third of patients.[58] In the pancreas, functional NETs much less commonly produce excess serotonin, and clinical carcinoid syndrome is exceedingly rare.[59] Instead, functional PNETs classically elaborate a single pancreatic hormone for which they are named. These pancreatic hormoneomas and the constellations of symptoms that define them are reviewed next. These clinical syndromes have captured great academic interest, but it should be noted that even the most common represent only a fraction of all PNETs, and most are vanishingly rare (Table 76.3).

Insulinoma

Insulinomas are the most common functional PNET, with an incidence of 1 to 4 per million per year, and were the first described.[60] Insulinomas can autonomously produce large quantities of insulin, leading to potentially life-threatening hypoglycemia.[61] In 1924, shortly after Frederick Banting and Charles Best identified insulin and demonstrated its use in correcting hyperglycemia in juvenile diabetes in 1921–22,[62] the American surgeon Seale Harris suggested that hypoglycemia in five patients might result from excessive endogenous insulin secretion. William Mayo reported a patient in 1926 with severe hypoglycemia found to have a widely metastatic pancreatic tumor on exploration. On autopsy, injection of a preparation of this patient's liver metastases lowered blood glucose in rabbits, marking the first report of metastatic insulinoma. The first cure after resection of a localized insulinoma by Canadian surgeon Roscoe Graham was reported in 1929, and soon after, Whipple and Frantz described the insulinoma triad of hypoglycemic symptoms, low blood glucose, and symptomatic relief with restoration of normoglycemia.[32]

Suspicion of insulinoma usually follows episodes of symptomatic hypoglycemia during exercise or fasting. Biochemical diagnosis requires laboratory evidence of hypoglycemia with inappropriately high insulin or proinsulin during a 72-hour period of fasting, with concurrent C-peptide testing to exclude surreptitious insulin administration.[63,64] Some patients with hypoglycemia have tumors that produce proinsulin rather than insulin, but these cases are rare.[65] Standard contrast-enhanced CT or MRI imaging localizes most insulinomas, which are hypervascular and may enhance on

TABLE 76.3   Functional Pancreatic Neuroendocrine Tumors

TUMOR	CELL OF ORIGIN	INCIDENCE (CASES PER MILLION PER YEAR)	CLINICAL FEATURES	COMMENTS	REFERENCES
Insulinoma	β cell	1–4	Whipple triad: Hypoglycemic symptoms (sweating, tremors, blurred vision, confusion, seizures) during fasting, hypoglycemia, correction with restoration of normoglycemia	Tend to present early, usually localized, low-grade, can be cured by resection. May be multiple in MEN1.	32,60,62,64
Gastrinoma	G cell	1–1.5	Severe reflux, diarrhea, recurrent ulceration of stomach, duodenum, upper jejunum	Most located in duodenum, 25% in pancreas. 20%–30% of gastrinomas associated with MEN1. More often metastatic to nodes or liver.	75,150
Glucagonoma	α cell	0.1	Necrolytic migratory erythema, glossitis, cheilitis, hyperglycemia, weight loss, thromboembolism	Symptomatic patients have severe protein wasting, may require TPN before intervention.	32,76–78,151
VIPoma		0.05–0.2	Profuse watery diarrhea, hypokalemia, achlorhydria, hypercalcemia, flushing	Neurotransmitter stimulating enteric smooth muscle contraction, pancreas secretion.	33,82
Somatostatinoma	D cell	0.01–0.05	Diabetes, diarrhea/steatorrhea, cholelithiasis		85,152
PPoma	Y cell	Case reports	No clinical syndrome	Tend to be large at diagnosis.	90

MEN1, Multiple endocrine neoplasia type 1 *PPoma*, pancreatic polypeptidoma; *TPN*, total parenteral nutrition; *VIPoma*, vasoactive intestinal peptidoma.

arterial and venous sequences.[63] Many lesions are isoenhancing on CT, and MRI has greater sensitivity at 70% to 90%, making high-field MRI with contrast and diffusion-weighted sequences a good option for localization.[66,67] Even highly symptomatic insulinomas may be small, making some tumors difficult to find. Endoscopic ultrasound (EUS) reports high success rates in finding small tumors and allows simultaneous biopsy.[63] For very small tumors failing less invasive methods, localization through selective arterial stimulation with venous sampling facilitates resection.[67] This method combines selective angiography to illuminate the tumor's hypervascular features with selective arterial calcium administration, which stimulates insulin release. Angiography and measurement of insulin in the hepatic veins after selective calcium injection can isolate the tumor location to the head, body, or tail of the pancreas with >94% accuracy.[63] Insulinomas frequently overexpress glucagon-like peptide-1 (GLP-1R), and radioisotope-labeled agents targeting this receptor show potential for imaging small tumors.[61]

Insulinomas remain localized to the pancreas, solitary, low grade, and <2 cm in more than 90% of cases, but some can show higher grade, larger size, and metastases. Patients with MEN1 often have multiple tumors. Small, localized insulinomas have excellent survival approaching 100% with resection, whereas those >2 cm or with metastases have 10-year survival below 30%.[64] For metastatic insulinomas, diazoxide improves hypoglycemia in around 50% of patients, but side effects are common. Diazoxide should be stopped at least a week before surgery because of risk of intraoperative hypotension.[68] For patients failing diazoxide, SSAs may help, but can show less benefit than in other hormonal excess syndromes due to lower rates of SSTR overexpression. In some cases, hypoglycemia may actually worsen with SSAs due to glucagon inhibition.[26] Other interventions used for PNETs, including everolimus, chemotherapy, liver-directed therapies, and PRRT, can also be employed.

Gastrinoma

In 1955 Zollinger and Ellison described two young females with recurrent perforated upper GI ulcers who were found to have very high acid secretion and non–β-cell pancreatic tumors. They suggested that these patients represented a syndrome where a new form of pancreatic tumor secreted an unidentified hormone (they wrongly suspected glucagon), causing excessive acid secretion.[69] Gastrin, which is synthesized by G cells located mainly in the gastric antrum, had been identified in 1905, but that gastrinoma was the cause of Zollinger-Ellison syndrome (ZES) only became clear in 1967 when gastrin was isolated from a PNET.[1] Gastrinomas tend to originate within the "gastrinoma triangle," defined by the base of the cystic duct, the junction of the second and third portion of the duodenum, and the neck of the pancreas.[70] Most arise in the duodenum, with around 25% located within the pancreas. As in Zollinger and Ellison's first patient, whose father died of a peptic ulcer and sister of an insulinoma, 20% to 30% of patients with a gastrinoma have MEN1.[32,69]

Gastrinomas remain difficult to diagnose. Symptoms such as reflux and diarrhea are widespread and nonspecific, and improvement with proton pump inhibitors (PPIs) can mask true hypergastrinemia. Even with documented hypergastrinemia, whether this results from pharmacologic acid suppression or gastrinoma may remain uncertain. Gastrin above 10 times the upper limit of normal confirms ZES. In other cases, the gold standard for biochemical diagnosis requires documenting elevated gastrin at a confirmed gastric pH of <2 and a dramatic increase during a secretin stimulation test. Such testing, however, is rarely performed

due in part to its complexity but also because of the danger of discontinuing PPIs and provoking gastrin secretion in a patient suspected of the disease, which can precipitate GI perforation. More commonly, a mass seen in the pancreas or duodenum on cross-sectional imaging and/or EUS in a suspicious clinical context produces the diagnosis. Gastrinomas within the pancreas are usually visualized by a combination of MRI and ^{68}Ga-DOTA-PET; however, sensitivity is lower for small duodenal tumors.[32] Some patients with negative localization studies other than nodal disease will have normal gastrin levels after resection and are thought to have their primary tumors originate within lymph nodes.[71]

Gastrinomas behave more aggressively than insulinomas, with liver metastases present in 30% of patients at diagnosis and nodal metastases in 60%.[32,72] Controlling acid secretion with high-dose PPIs decreases complications caused by ulceration and perforation. Surgical resection improves hypergastrinemia and may improve survival, but metastatic recurrences are common, with about half of patients whose gastrin levels initially normalize developing recurrent hypergastrinemia at 10 years.[73–75] Treatment for metastatic disease follows the multimodal strategies employed for nonfunctional PNETs.

Glucagonoma

Glucagon was first isolated in 1923, and in 1942 the dermatologist William Becker reported on the clinical features of malignant glucagonoma in a patient with hyperglycemia, necrolytic migratory erythema of the legs, which spread to the trunk, glossitis, and weight loss who was found to have a metastatic pancreatic tumor on autopsy.[32] In 1966, glucagon was first isolated from a metastatic pancreatic tumor in a patient with glucagonoma symptoms.[76] Glucagonomas are extremely rare, with an incidence of around 1 in 10 million.[77] Around half are metastatic at presentation, and only ~60% of confirmed glucagonomas produce both hyperglycemic symptoms and the characteristic dermatologic findings.[78] Biochemical diagnosis is by measurement of fasting glucagon greater than 500 pg/mL.[33] Persistently high glucagon leads to severe malnutrition and protein wasting. Amino acid infusion or parenteral nutrition improves dermatologic symptoms, and in very symptomatic patients may be necessary before surgical intervention.[79,80] Ten-year survival approaches 100% in resected patients without metastases and was reported at 52% in 87 resected metastatic glucagonomas.[78]

Vasoactive Intestinal Peptidoma

Vasoactive intestinal peptide (VIP) is a neurotransmitter found in the central nervous system and multiple organs throughout the body, including neuroendocrine pancreatic cells.[33] Verner and Morrison first reported the VIPoma syndrome of watery diarrhea, hypokalemia, and achlorhydria (WDHA syndrome) in two patients found to have PNETs in 1958.[81] After isolation of VIP and development of a blood assay, elevated VIP was documented in a patient with a PNET in 1973.[82] Patients with VIPoma syndrome may have 6 to 8 L of diarrhea per day, leading to severe electrolyte abnormalities and potentially fatal arrhythmias.[81,83] Facial flushing and hypercalcemia can be seen, and VIPomas may develop in the setting of MEN1.[82] Most VIPomas develop in the pancreas; however, as VIP-producing cells exist throughout the body, extrapancreatic VIPomas may also occur. Pancreatic VIPomas are found most commonly (70%) in the body and tail of the gland.[82] Markedly elevated fasting VIP (>200 pg/mL) in the setting of profuse diarrhea provides a biochemical diagnosis of VIPoma, whereas slightly elevated VIP can occur in heart failure or renal disease.[33] VIPomas may metastasize to the liver (21%), with 5-year survival of >90% for localized versus 60% for metastatic tumors.[84] Surgical and medical therapies follow those for other PNETs.

Somatostatinoma

Somatostatinomas arise in the pancreas, duodenum, or jejunum and produce high levels of somatostatin (SST), which inhibits multiple gut hormones, including insulin, glucagon, gastrin, secretin, cholecystokinin, and others.[85] First described in 1977, the somatostatinoma syndrome includes diabetes, cholelithiasis, and often diarrhea/steatorrhea caused by reduced pancreatic endocrine and exocrine function.[86-88] Only a few hundred reports exist in the literature, with an incidence estimated at 1 in 40 million.[85] Some PNETs without clinical features of somatostatinoma stain for SST on IHC. These should be considered nonfunctional, SST-positive PNETs, with somatostatinomas being defined by high serum SST and clinical symptoms of hypersomatostatinemia.[33]

In addition to these better-described, but still rare, functional PNETs, other extraordinarily rare PNETs have been reported to produce adrenocorticotropic hormone (ACTH) (and ectopic Cushing syndrome), parathyroid hormone–related peptide, calcitonin, and growth hormone–releasing hormones.[33] These should be resected when possible.

Pancreatic Polypeptidoma

Pancreatic polypeptide (PP) is a 36–amino acid hormone secreted by PP (also known as *upsilon*) cells mainly in the right side of the pancreas and was first isolated in 1968 as a contaminant during purification of chicken insulin.[89,90] Pancreatic polypeptidomas (PPomas) are extremely rare, with fewer than 100 reported in the literature, and they secrete high levels of PP, which normally functions in response to food to inhibit pancreatic secretion and stimulate gastric secretion.[91] PPomas do not produce a clinical syndrome; they are often recognized because of their large size, producing mass-effect symptoms in the head of the pancreas, or because of metastatic disease.[90]

Nonfunctional Pancreatic Neuroendocrine Tumors

Nonfunctional tumors do not cause syndromes associated with hormonal excess and account for up to 90% of PNETs.[8] As they produce no characteristic symptoms early in their course, nonfunctional tumors more often present with more advanced stage, and more than half have metastasized to nodes or liver at the time of diagnosis.[12] Some have detectable hormonal production on IHC or tumor marker investigations, but in the absence of clinical symptoms, these are termed nonfunctional.[26] Presenting symptoms include mass-effect symptoms of obstructive jaundice or duodenal obstruction for tumors in the head or uncinate or early satiety with larger tumors of the body and tail. The increasing incidence of PNETs is likely due in part to the frequency of abdominal imaging being performed for a variety of abdominal symptoms,[21] where these tumors may be picked up with or without corresponding liver metastases.

DIAGNOSIS

The diagnosis of a PNET may result from workup for a clinical syndrome in the case of functional tumors, but whether functional or not, confirmation will require the finding of a mass within the pancreas. This is commonly achieved by a CT scan, often done for another abdominal symptom. Characteristically

PNETs enhance on the arterial phase and will look whiter than the normal pancreas because of the higher density of blood vessels, especially in functional PNETs. Nonfunctional PNETs can less commonly appear as hypodense. It is important to have both arterial and venous phases,[92] as when only a standard venous phase CT is done, the lesion may or may not be seen, as the differential enhancement from the normal pancreas will have passed (Fig. 76.1). A biphasic CT can pick up lesions as small as 5 mm in size and should not miss many lesions >10 mm in size (Fig. 76.2). A CT scan gives excellent anatomic detail of the relationship of the tumor to the important vascular structures, such as the superior mesenteric and splenic veins, as well as the superior mesenteric artery, celiac axis, and splenic arteries. These are important determinants to resectability and can be viewed in axial, coronal, and sagittal planes to aid in operative planning. CT scans also can detect enlarged regional nodes, peritoneal disease, and liver metastases.

The other principal anatomic imaging modality is MRI. PNETs should look hypodense on T1 images and generally show enhancement on T2 sequences (Fig. 76.3).[93] Magnetic resonance cholangiopancreatography images can also be obtained, which nicely delineate the pancreatic and biliary ductal systems. An MRI scan with gadoxetic acid (Eovist) is the preferred scan for imaging the extent and distribution of liver metastases and will often demonstrate more and smaller lesions than revealed by CT. Another advantage to MRI over CT scans for diagnosis and surveillance is the lack of ionizing radiation and lower nephrotoxicity of contrast agents. Many surgeons may prefer CT because of fewer sequences, less susceptibility to respiratory artifact, greater coverage of the abdomen and pelvis, and better discrimination of nodal and peritoneal metastases. However, high-quality MRI offers the highest sensitivity for liver metastases and can show vascular and anatomic relationships in great detail.

Functional PET imaging represents another imaging category that can be extremely useful in working up patients with PNET. Whereas most NETs will not be detected by standard 18 F-fluorodeoxyglucose–positron emission tomography ([18]FDG/PET), NET functional studies, abbreviated as DOTA-PET, take advantage of the high expression of SSTRs on these tumors. Modified octreotide peptides are chelated to radioactive isotopes to bind to these receptors and can be imaged by PET, which has completely replaced the earlier generation of scans (^{111}In-pentetreotide scintigraphy).[56] DOTA-PET imaging agents in the United States, include ^{68}Ga-DOTATATE, ^{68}Ga-DOTATOC, and ^{64}Cu-DOTATATE. These PET scans can be fused with CT or MRI images captured at the same time, with or without IV contrast (Fig. 76.4). These scans can confirm that suspicious lesions are actually NETs, and uptake can be seen in primary tumors, nodes, and metastases. They are therefore helpful for determining the extent of disease and scan the whole body for potential metastases. They may reveal bone metastases not seen on CT scans, mediastinal nodes, supraclavicular nodes, and other areas of potentially resectable disease that the surgeon might not have otherwise recognized. In interpreting these images, high uptake is expected in the spleen, kidneys, bladder, ureters, adrenals, and pituitary as well as some background uptake within the liver and bowel. False-positive uptake is frequently seen in the uncinate process of the pancreas and sometimes in the tail of the pancreas, which can be further confused by the presence of accessory spleens. It is therefore important to not rely exclusively on a DOTA-PET scan for surgical decision-making for primary PNETs. Instead, other anatomic imaging can confirm that an abnormality exists in the

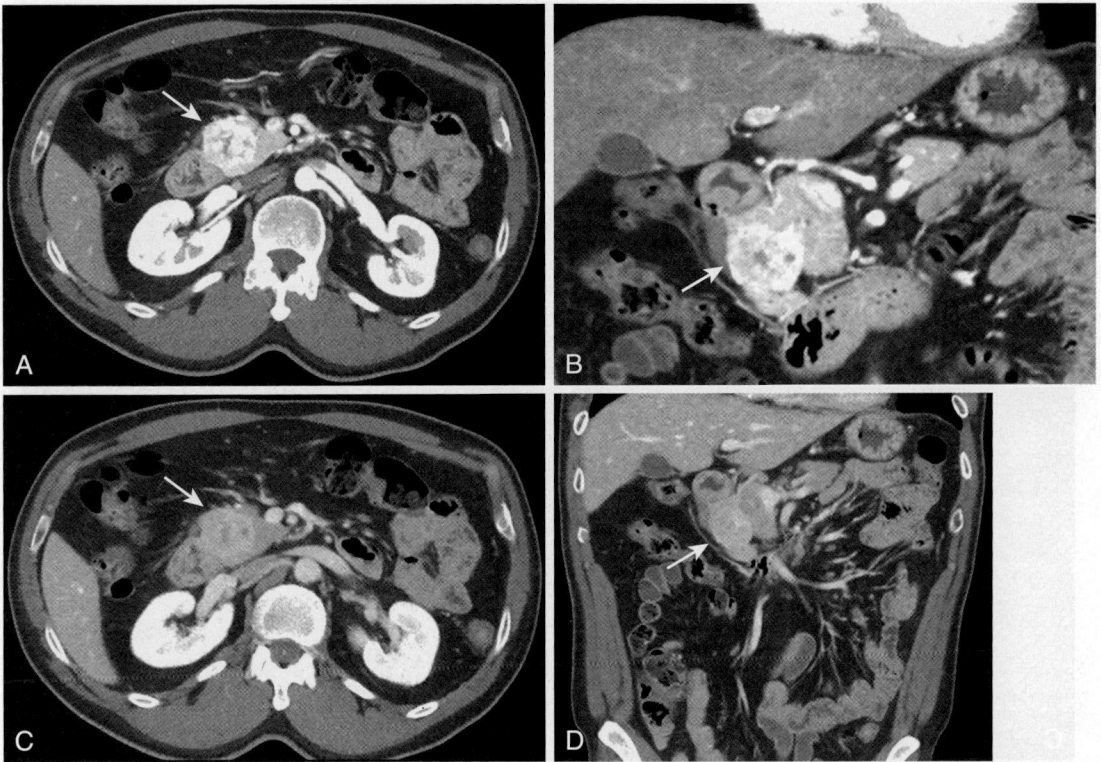

FIGURE 76.1 Comparison of arterial versus venous phase computed tomography for nonfunctional PNET. Transaxial (A) and coronal slices (B) in the arterial phase demonstrate a 4.1 × 3.5 cm enhancing mass in the pancreatic head *(white arrow)*. Transaxial (C) and coronal images (D) on the venous phase still show some enhancement, but significantly less than the arterial phase. *PNET,* Pancreatic neuroendocrine tumor.

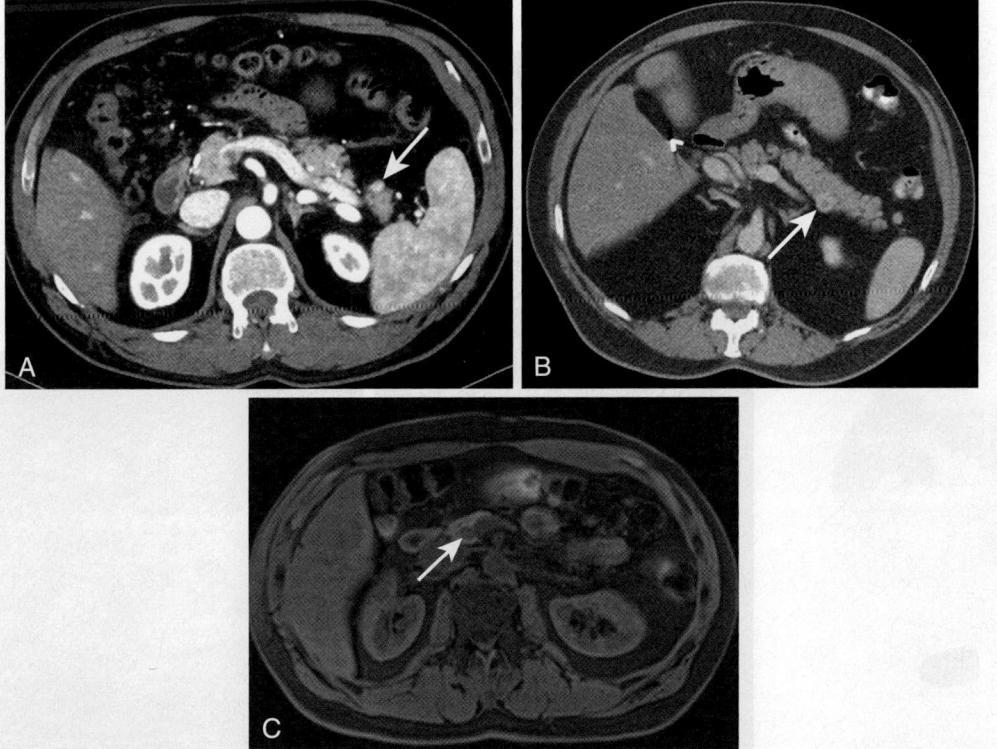

FIGURE 76.2 Transaxial arterial phase computed tomography (CT) showing an incidentally found, 8-mm, arterially enhancing lesion in the pancreatic tail (A), likely a PNET *(arrow)*. Enhancing 10-mm lesion incidentally found in the pancreatic body on transaxial CT (B), and 10-mm lesion of the pancreatic head on T1-weighted magnetic resonance image in a patient with symptomatic hypoglycemia (C). *PNET,* pancreatic neuroendocrine tumor.

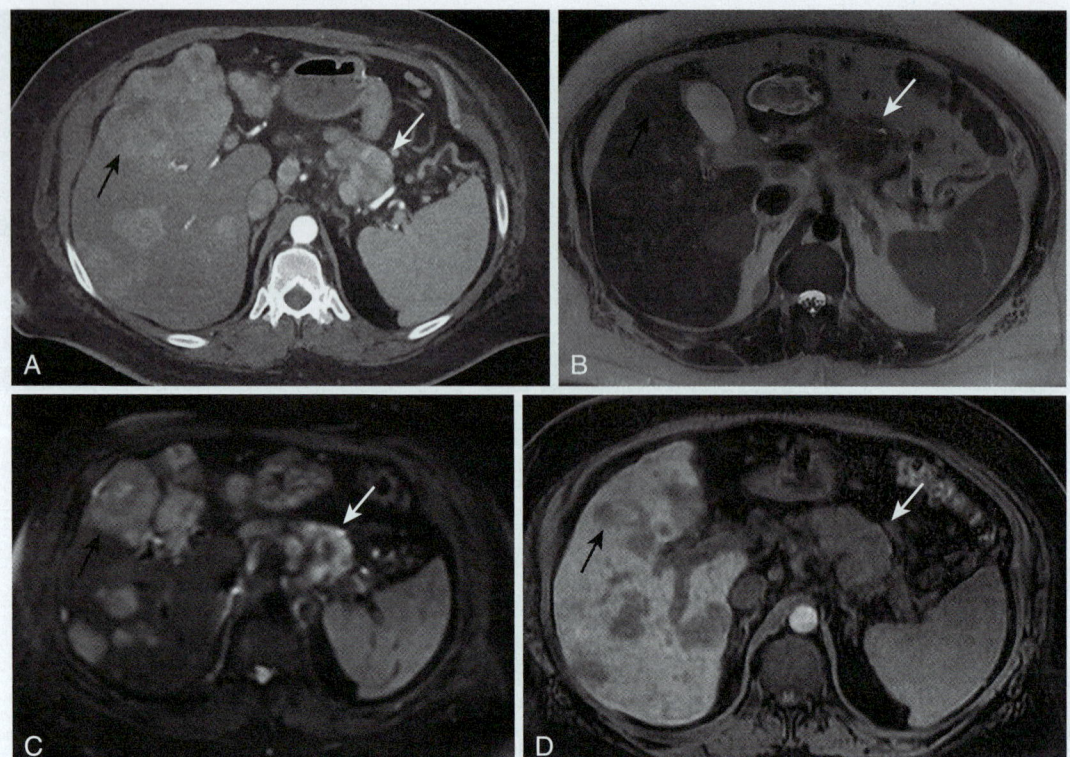

FIGURE 76.3 Transaxial arterial phase computed tomography (CT) (A) in a patient with a large pancreatic tail neuroendocrine tumor *(white arrows)* with nodal and liver metastases *(black arrow),* as compared with transaxial magnetic resonance imaging (MRI) with T2 (B), diffusion (C), and T1 sequences (D). Note the distinct information conveyed on different MRI sequences, with diffusion images showing the best delineation of liver lesions.

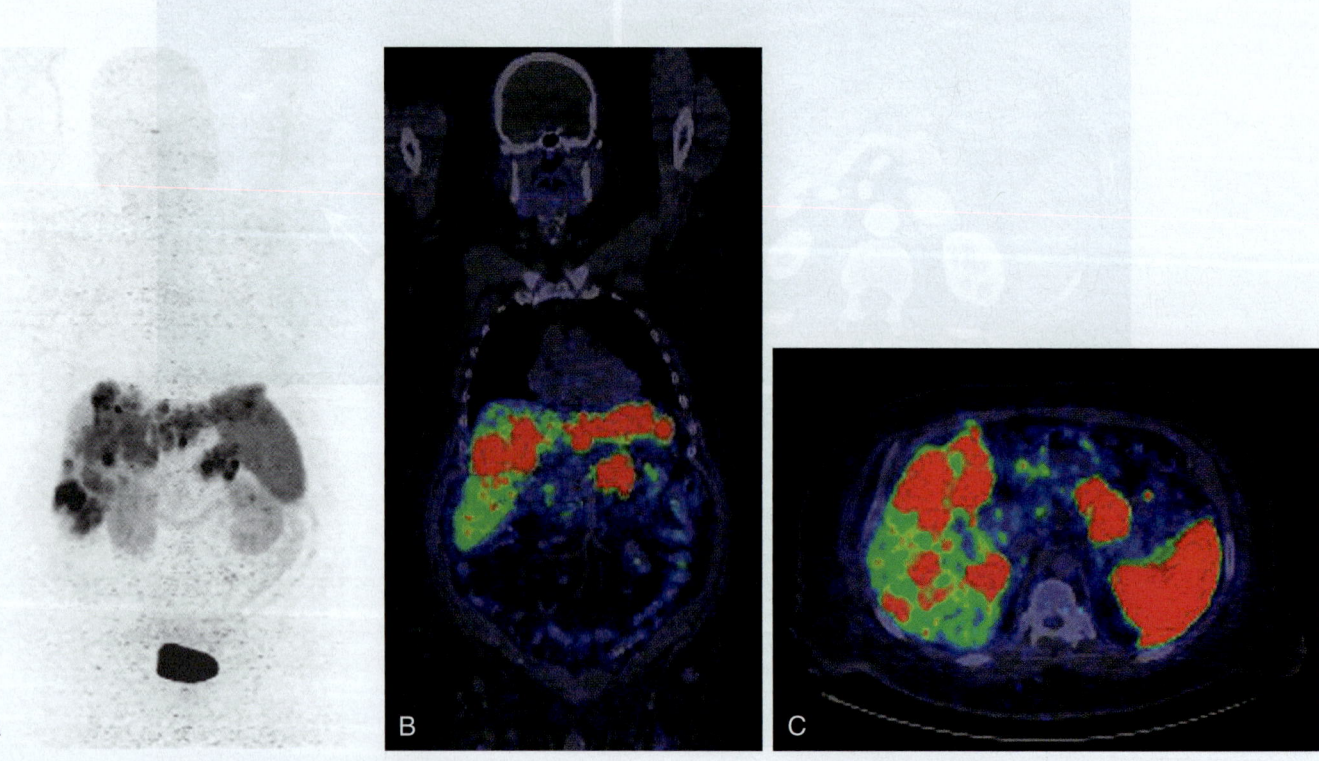

FIGURE 76.4 ^{64}Cu-DOTATATE scan of the same patient in Fig. 76.3. The maximum intensity projection image (A) gives an overview of the whole body, which shows many liver metastases, a large primary tumor, and enlarged nodes. The coronal fused computed tomography image (B) gives more anatomic information, as does the transaxial view (C). On this scan, areas of high somatostatin uptake are shown in *red.*

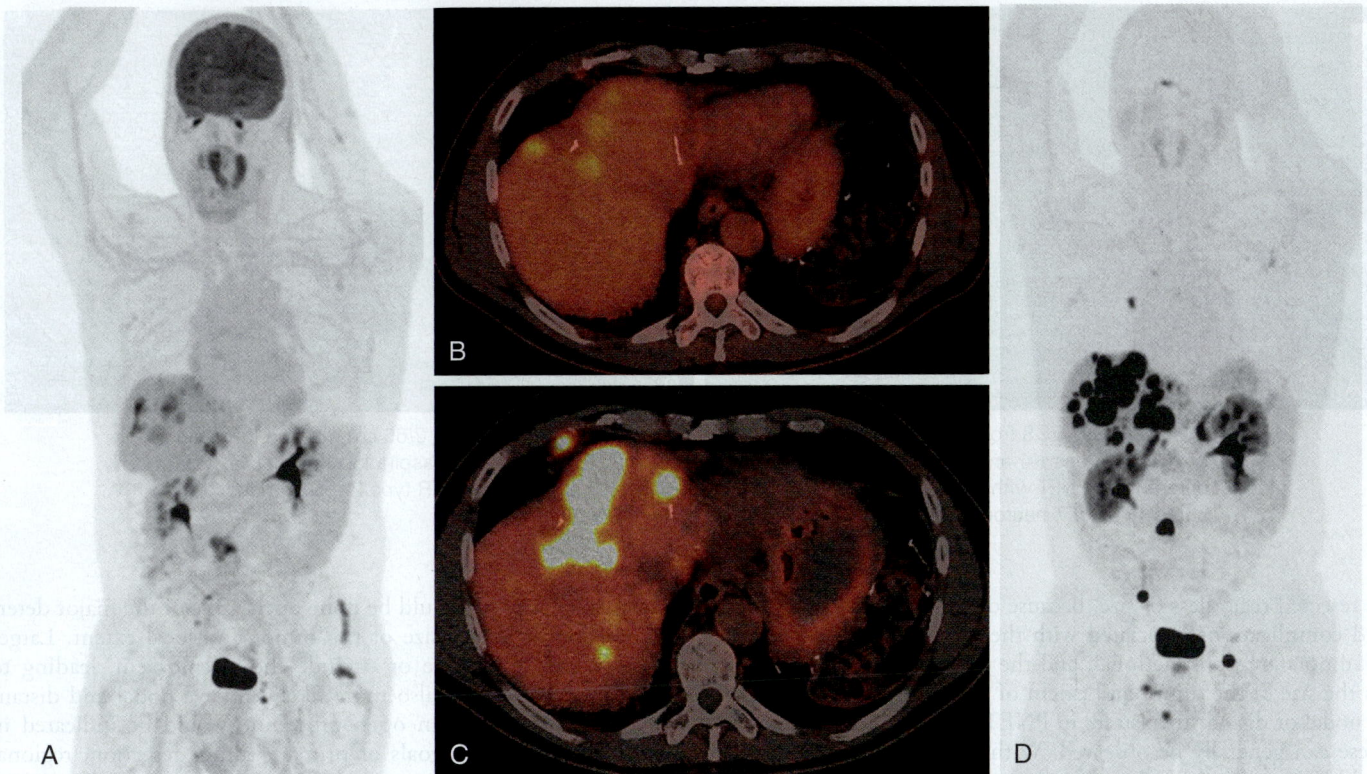

FIGURE 76.5 Comparison of ^{18}FDG/PET and ^{68}Ga-DOTATOC PET/CT scans taken 2 weeks apart in a patient with progressive PNET liver metastases. Surgical specimens from 7 months earlier revealed well-differentiated liver tumors with Ki-67 of 18%, 42%, and 67%. The ^{18}FDG/PET MIP image (A) reveals a few areas of uptake in the liver also seen on the transaxial fused image (B). The ^{68}Ga-DOTATOC transaxial fused CT image (C) and the MIP reveal higher levels of uptake in the liver as well as in L4, left ischium, and right iliac bone. ^{18}FDG/PET, 18 F-fluorodeoxyglucose–positron emission tomography; MIP, maximum intensity projection; PET/CT, positron emission tomography–computed tomography; PNET, pancreatic neuroendocrine tumor.

region suggested by the PET scan and to rule out that it might be a false positive. An important limitation of DOTA-PET scans is that higher-grade tumors often fail to express SSTRs and may not be detected. These less common higher-grade tumors represent a clinical situation where standard ^{18}FDG/PET scans may show disease, and some patients with high-grade tumors may require both types of PET scans for workup (Fig. 76.5).

When a mass is suspected, EUS provides another means for high-resolution imaging evaluation and allows for diagnostic biopsy (Fig. 76.6). This requires sedation and is more invasive, but it can confirm the presence of a pancreatic lesion and show its relationship to adjacent organs and structures. One can also perform fine-needle aspiration (FNA) or core biopsy to confirm the histology, and other pathologic features can be determined that might affect the decision to operate, like Ki-67,[94] the presence of DAXX/ATRX, and/or ALT status.[3,95]

Biochemical testing for PNETs includes testing for hormone elevation indicative of a functional tumor and for other, more generic NET markers.[96] For insulinoma, fasting glucose, c-peptide, a sulfonylurea screen, and insulin are useful. For gastrinoma, a serum gastrin is checked, but this may be falsely elevated by PPI use. VIP, glucagon, and, less commonly, SST round out the commonly evaluated functional hormones. Rare tumors may make ACTH or parathyroid hormone (PTH)–related protein, which would be suggested by Cushing syndrome or hypercalcemia. Patients with hyperparathyroidism should be screened for MEN1. PP has been used for monitoring patients with PNET, but can be

highly variable. Chromogranin A (CGA) is a general NET marker that can be useful in following patients with PNET, especially those with metastases. Pancreastatin, a subfragment of CGA, is also useful in many patients and is less affected by PPI use than CGA.[97] Serotonin is elevated in a fraction of patients with PNET. These hormone levels should be checked preoperatively, and levels that are found to be elevated may be helpful for determining tumor recurrence or progression in follow-up.

Analysis of pathology specimens should conform to the current WHO standards and includes differentiation status and Ki-67 and/or mitoses in order to be able to accurately assign grade.[98] Other useful pathologic determinants on tumor biopsies are the NET IHC markers CDX2, Islet1, PAX6, or PAX8. These transcription factors can help to confirm whether NET liver metastases or pancreatic tumors originate from the small bowel (CDX2 positive) or pancreas (Islet1, PAX6, or PAX8 positive).[99] Other important features in higher-grade tumors are the status of p53 and Rb, as these are lost more commonly in NECs. The status of the DAXX and ATRX proteins and ALT are also useful for helping to determine prognosis.[3,100] For patients where there is suspicion of MEN1, VHL, NF, or TSC, germline genetic testing should be performed to understand whether these patients are at risk for other tumors.[96]

SURGICAL MANAGEMENT

Surgical resection is the preferred treatment for PNETs, but decision-making can be complex. Most functional tumors should

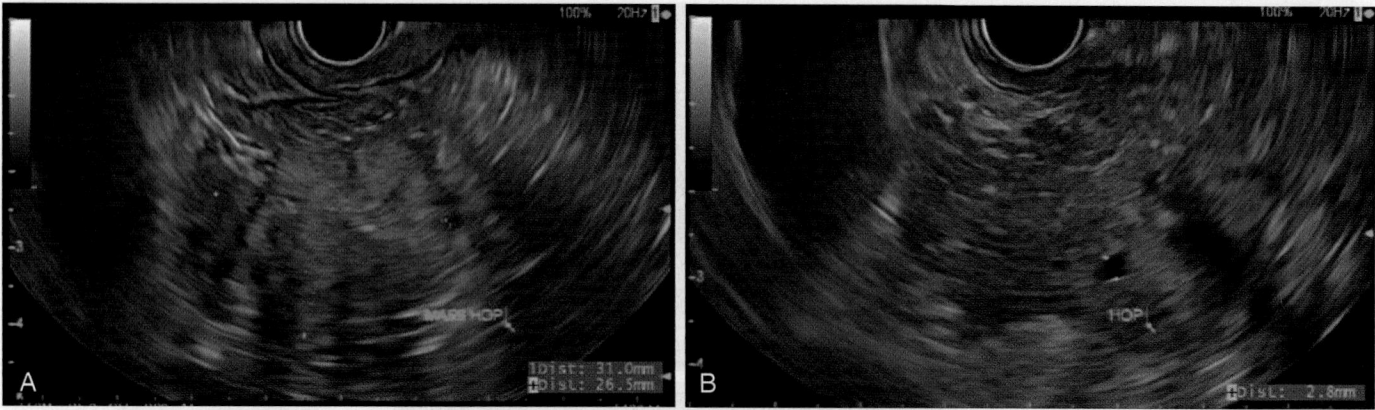

FIGURE 76.6 EUS from same patient shown in Fig. 76.1, demonstrating a 3.1 × 2.65 cm mass in the head of the pancreas (A) and a nondilated pancreatic duct 2.8 mm (B). Fine-needle aspiration revealed a well-differentiated NET with Ki-67 of 0.32%, with 70% of cells staining positive for SSTR type 2. *EUS,* Endoscopic ultrasound; *NET,* neuroendocrine tumor; *SSTR,* somatostatin receptor.

be resected regardless of size, because of the hormonal symptoms and complications associated with them. However, the majority of tumors are nonfunctional, and the decision to resect depends on the size of the tumor and extent of spread. In general, the risk of nodal or distant metastases in PNETs <1 cm is quite low, and these can generally be observed. With the increasing use of CT and MRI for a variety of conditions, small, incidentally discovered PNETs are common. Smaller, low-grade, nonfunctional tumors usually remain stable in size without metastases for long periods and can be observed. Tumors >2 cm, with higher Ki-67, or that show growth have an increased risk of nodal and distant metastases and should generally be resected in patients with reasonable performance status.[11] More controversial is the appropriate treatment of PNETs 1 to 2 cm in size, which again may remain small, but do have a low-intermediate risk of metastasis. The ASPEN trial in Europe is prospectively comparing results of resection versus observation of patients with these size tumors.[101] The decision to resect can be further influenced by the age of the patient (younger patients will need very long follow-up), their performance status, the location in the pancreas (tumors in the head requiring pancreaticoduodenectomy [PD] with higher risk of complications), and the grade of the tumor. Some have also suggested using FNA to identify tumors with DAXX/ATRX loss and ALT positivity, which suggest higher metastatic risk.[95]

If surgery is indicated, the choice of procedure depends primarily on the tumor's anatomic location. Perhaps the simplest procedure is enucleation, which is just an excision with narrow margins from within the pancreatic parenchyma (Fig. 76.7). This is best suited to benign lesions like insulinomas but can also be performed in lesions with malignant potential if the tumor is on the edge of the pancreas and at least 3 mm away from the main pancreatic duct. Enucleation can help to preserve pancreatic endocrine and exocrine function by removing minimal normal pancreatic tissue, but at the cost of increased risk of pancreatic fistula. When larger tumors are to be enucleated, regional nodal dissection should also be performed where possible.[11] Pancreatic parenchymal preservation takes on special importance in patients with genetic syndromes such as MEN1 or VHL, where multiple small, low-grade tumors will develop over the patient's lifetime.[31]

If the tumor is in the tail or distal body, then distal pancreatectomy (DP) is preferred. Important considerations here are whether to remove the spleen or not and whether it can be performed laparoscopically or should be done open. One of the major determinants again is the size of the tumor and local extent. Larger tumors tend to invade or occlude the splenic vein, leading to varices, and these are also more likely to have nodal and distant metastases. As such, an open procedure would be indicated in order to achieve the goals of primary tumor resection, regional nodal dissection, and liver cytoreduction, if necessary (Fig. 76.8). Some of these larger tumors will require partial gastrectomy or colectomy. For smaller tumors confined to the pancreas, laparoscopic DP has been shown to have similar complication rates as open procedures and with quicker recovery (Fig. 76.9).[102] Some prefer to use a 7- to 8-cm incision and a hand port for improved tactile feedback, to facilitate dissection, and for removal of the specimen with the spleen, if required. Splenectomy may not be necessary in all cases if the pancreas can be dissected off the splenic vessels. One may even transect the splenic artery and vein proximally and distally and keep the spleen if the short gastric vessels can be preserved, as popularized by Warshaw (see Fig. 76.9D).[103]

Smaller tumors in the body or neck of the pancreas can be treated by central pancreatectomy (CP), where the pancreas is divided proximal and distal to the primary tumor. This requires dissecting out the superior mesenteric vein (SMV) and splenic vein to keep these intact, then division of the pancreas over or to the left of the SMV, usually with a stapler, or, alternatively, it can be oversewn. The pancreas is then dissected off the splenic vein distally with preservation of the splenic artery to >1 cm beyond the tumor. The pancreas is divided sharply distally and bleeding vessels controlled. Regional nodal dissection to remove nodes along the splenic artery, celiac axis, and hepatic artery can also be carried out. A pancreaticojejunostomy to the distal pancreatic duct is next performed using a Roux-en-Y limb. For larger tumors in this location and in those with distal pancreatic atrophy, an extended DP may be preferable. Central resection will improve the potential for preserving endocrine and exocrine function, but with a higher risk of pancreatic leak.[104] Because these leaks are generally manageable with a surgical drain (with occasional need for an interventional radiology–placed drain), CP may be preferred for smaller lesions in this location.

If the tumor is in the head or uncinate process and not amenable to enucleation, then a PD (Whipple procedure) will be necessary (Fig. 76.10). This can be a classic Whipple procedure with associated gastric resection or pylorus-preserving. Laparoscopic and

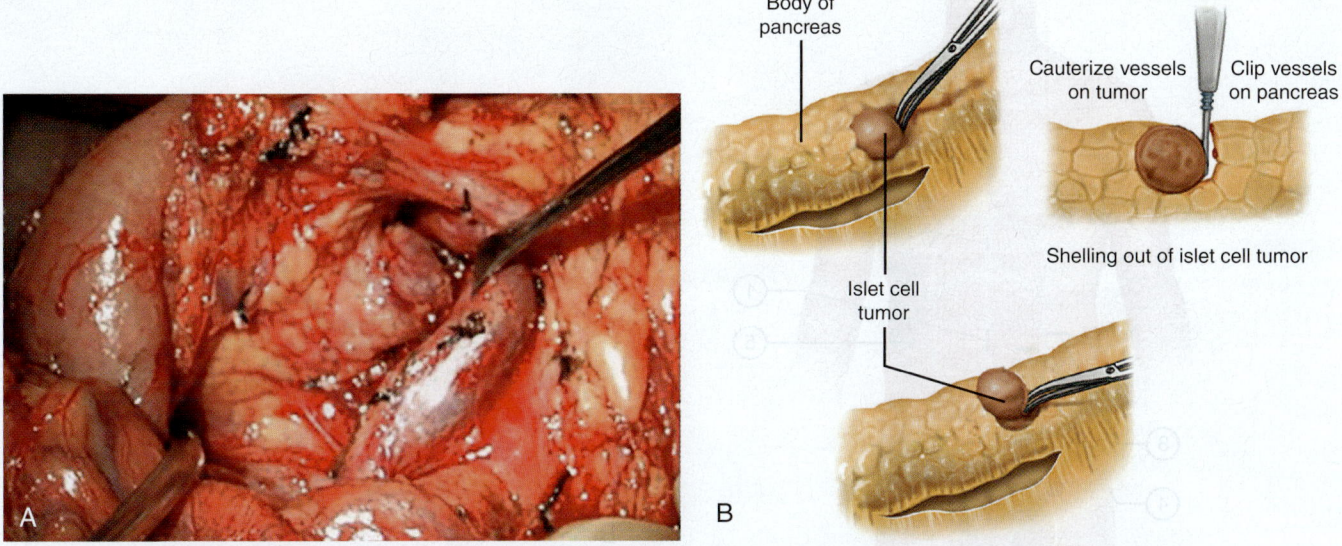

FIGURE 76.7 Enucleation of an insulinoma from the pancreatic uncinate region. The superior mesenteric vein is being pulled laterally *(right)* to expose the tumor, which is hard and white in color, standing out from the yellow pancreatic tissue. The duodenum is seen to the left of the pancreas (A). Steps of enucleation (B), which include dissection of the lesion from the normal pancreatic parenchyma and cauterization or ligation of pancreatic vessels. (A, Reproduced from Maxwell JE, Howe JR. Pancreatic neuroendocrine tumors: classification, clinical picture, diagnosis, and therapy. *Blumgart's Surgery of the Liver, Biliary Tract and Pancreas.* 6th ed. Elsevier; 2016:997-1006. B, Reproduced from Howe JR. *Atlas of Endocrine and Neuroendocrine Surgery.* Springer; 2017.)

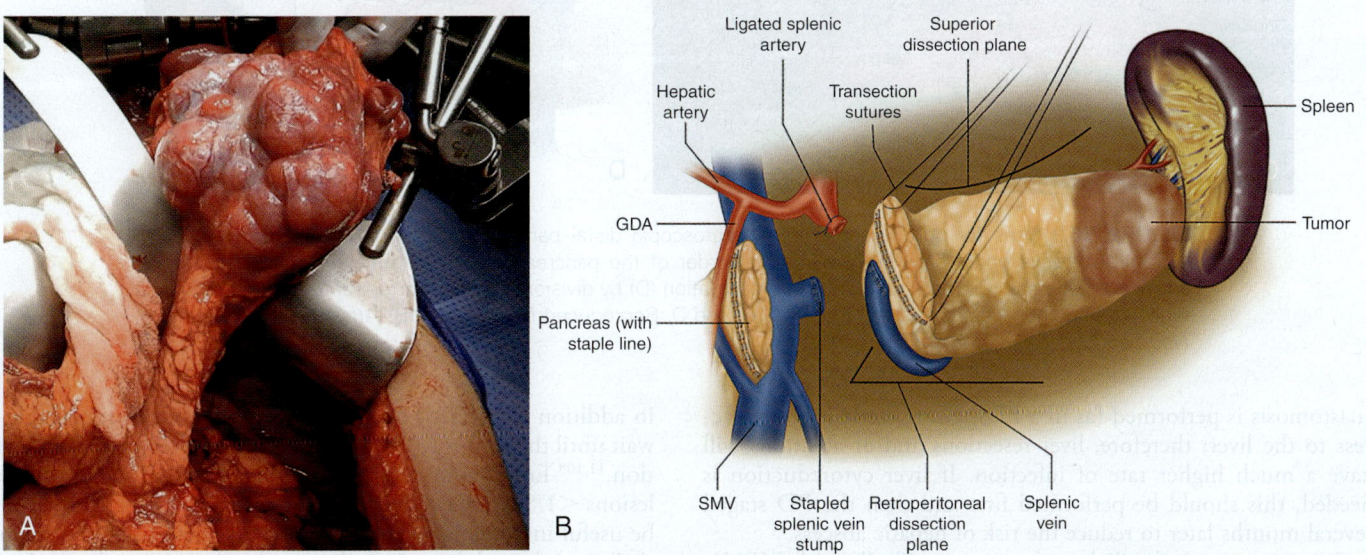

FIGURE 76.8 Lobulated PNET in tail of the pancreas (A). The normal pancreatic parenchyma is seen at left, and the tip of the spleen is visible just at the upper left of the tumor. Distal pancreatectomy specimen (B) after transection of the splenic artery and vein and pancreatic parenchyma. *GDA,* Gastroduodenal artery; *PNET,* pancreatic neuroendocrine tumor. (A, Reproduced from Scott AT, Howe JR. Evaluation and management of neuroendocrine tumors of the pancreas. *Surg Clin North Am.* 2019;99[4]:793-814; B, Reproduced from Howe JR. *Atlas of Endocrine and Neuroendocrine Surgery.* Springer; 2017.)

robotic PD are being performed with increasing frequency with good results in some centers, but require advanced skills, and there is a significant learning curve.[105,106] As with all of these procedures, careful consideration should be given to the tumor's relationship to vascular structures, and if there is involvement of the SMV, consideration should be given to neoadjuvant capecitabine/temozolomide chemotherapy or PRRT to shrink the tumor. In

general, PNETs are less likely to invade the SMV than pancreatic adenocarcinoma, and they can frequently be carefully dissected off the vein or hepatic artery. Occasionally, vein resection may be needed, which should not preclude resection if reconstruction is possible because of the good prognosis for resected PNETs. Another important consideration is whether there are liver metastases that need to be addressed or not. Once a biliary-enteric

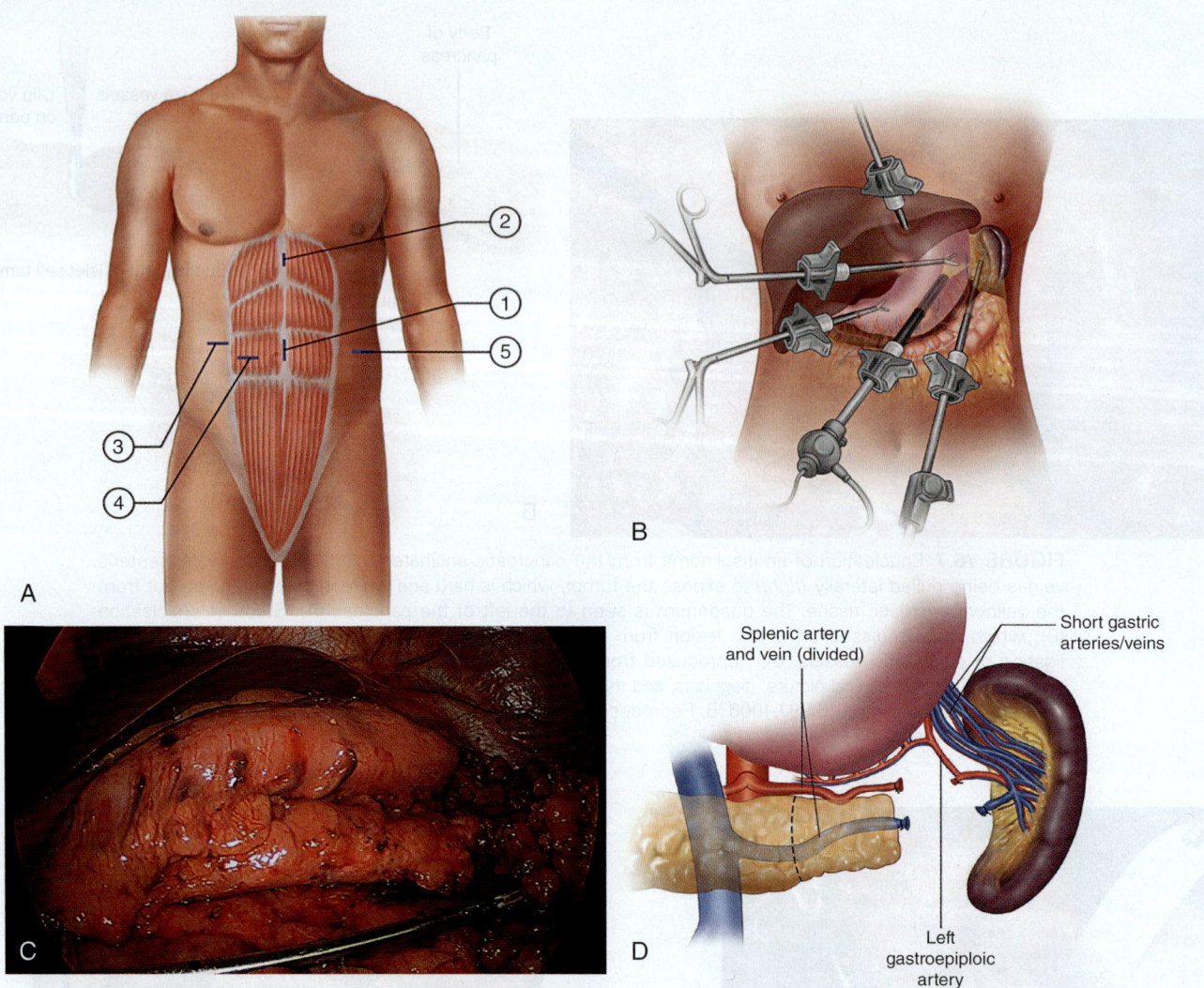

FIGURE 76.9 Sites for port placement for laparoscopic distal pancreatectomy (A), with ports in place (B). Intraoperative photo showing the inferior border of the pancreas dissected out with stomach sitting above the pancreas (C). Method of splenic preservation (D) by division of splenic artery and vein with tumor while leaving short gastric vessels intact. (A, B, and D, Reproduced from Howe JR. *Atlas of Endocrine and Neuroendocrine Surgery.* Springer; 2017.)

anastomosis is performed (as in a PD), gut bacteria have free access to the liver; therefore, liver resections and/or ablations will have a much higher rate of infection. If liver cytoreduction is needed, this should be performed first and then the PD staged several months later to reduce the risk of hepatic abscess.[11]

In patients with familial syndromes, specifically with MEN1, VHL, and, less frequently, TSC, there are additional considerations. These patients are born with germline mutations that affect every diploid cell in their body, and the potential for multifocal metachronous tumors is extremely high. Therefore, operative planning needs to take into account the likelihood of future tumors and later need for additional pancreatic operations. In MEN1, it is recommended to wait until the largest lesion is >2 cm in size before performing surgery, and the resection should incorporate all or most of the lesions present.[107] This can be very difficult, as there may be small tumors distributed throughout the gland. In such situations, leaving the smaller tumors (<5 mm) alone may be the best option, while enucleating and resecting the larger lesions. In VHL, the situation becomes even more complex because patients may also have extensive pancreatic cystic lesions

in addition to NETs. For patients with VHL, it is reasonable to wait until the tumor is >3 cm in size before recommending resection.[11,108] Enucleation is preferred when possible, and concurrent lesions <1.5 cm may be left alone.[31] A new drug (belzutifan) may be useful in patients with VHL to shrink these tumors or reduce their growth, and drugs including sunitinib, pazopanib, sorafenib, and others may be helpful for medical therapy of advanced disease.[109] Before any operation in a patient with known VHL, testing plasma metanephrines/normetanephrines to rule out pheochromocytoma is essential. A comparison of PNETs resected in patients with TSC versus sporadic PNETs found no recurrence or metastasis in the TSC group, suggesting potentially better tumor biology and a more conservative approach.[110]

National databases report that about two-thirds of patients with PNET have liver metastases.[111] Management recommendations for well-differentiated PNET liver metastases differ sharply from those for more aggressive histologies, such as colorectal adenocarcinoma. In functional PNETs, cytoreduction can improve symptoms even if all of the tumor cannot be eliminated, whereas in nonfunctional tumors, cytoreduction may help to improve

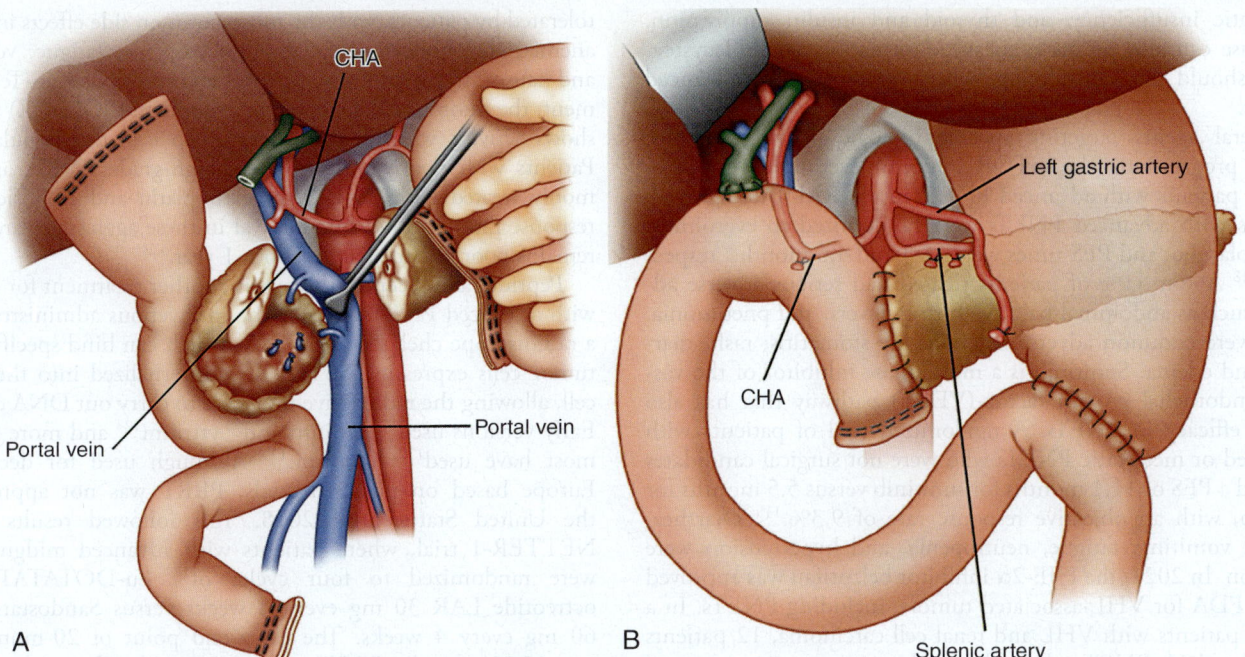

FIGURE 76.10 Division of pancreas, stomach, and jejunum for PNET in pancreatic head during pancreatico-duodenectomy (A). Reconstruction (B) with hepaticojejunal, pancreaticojejunal, and gastrojejunal anastomoses. *CHA*, Common hepatic artery; *PNET*, pancreatic neuroendocrine tumor. (Reproduced from Howe JR. *Atlas of Endocrine and Neuroendocrine Surgery.* Springer; 2017.)

survival. Although controversy exists as to the extent of cytoreduction necessary to warrant an operation, if >70% to 90% of the tumor can be debulked from the liver, it is probably worth attempting in well-selected candidates.[112] As mentioned, if a patient requires a PD, then a staged hepatic cytoreduction procedure followed by a Whipple procedure later on would be the preferred approach.[11] If the patient is to have a DP, CP, or enucleation, cytoreduction can be performed at the same procedure. These cytoreductive procedures are rarely curative because micrometastases are often present, and recurrence rates are as high as 94% by 5 years.[113] Because of this and the frequent presence of bilobar and numerous tumors, parenchymal-sparing approaches are preferable.[11] This means resecting superficial lesions by wedge resections or enucleations, which have very low rates of local recurrence despite minimal margins because these tumors tend to push rather than invade the adjacent liver parenchyma. Deeper lesions may be treated with concurrent ablative techniques, such as microwave ablation, which can allow for treatment of many lesions when facilitated by intraoperative ultrasound. These procedures are well tolerated and result in minimal bleeding. However, great caution must be used with lesions sitting along major portal structures, as the heat generated can impair inflow or lead to bile duct strictures. For these lesions, irreversible electroporation, which may spare normal tissues better, is a reasonable ablative alternative.[114]

MEDICAL THERAPY FOR PANCREATIC NEUROENDOCRINE TUMORS

A characteristic shared by most NETs that can be exploited for diagnosis and therapy is a high density of SSTRs. These G protein–coupled receptors activate antisecretory and antiproliferative pathways upon ligand binding. Their ligand is SST, a peptide of 14 or

28 amino acids made in the brain, hypothalamus, GI tract, and pancreas. SST is an inhibitory hormone that reduces secretion of insulin, glucagon, gastrin, other GI hormones, pancreatic enzymes, and neuropeptides. Native SST has a short half-life of 2 to 3 minutes, but the synthetic 8–amino acid analog octreotide also has excellent binding affinity and improved half-life of 90 to 120 minutes. Octreotide was initially used to treat patients with acromegaly, but soon found utility in managing the debilitating diarrhea and flushing in patients with carcinoid syndrome.[115] A depot form of octreotide (octreotide-LAR) was formulated in 1997 that allowed for sustained levels in the body for up to 28 days. This made treatment of a variety of conditions more practical with once-monthly rather than three-times-daily subcutaneous injections.[116]

SSAs can help patients with functional PNETs through their antisecretory effects. They have proven useful in managing hypoglycemia in patients with insulinoma, can reduce gastric acid levels in those with gastrinoma, reduce diarrhea in patients with glucagonoma, and decrease levels of VIP from VIPomas.[117] They also hold utility for those with nonfunctional tumors through their antiproliferative effects. The PROMID randomized trial showed improved PFS in patients with advanced midgut NETs treated with long-acting octreotide as compared with placebo (14.3 vs. 6 months).[54] This led to approval of SSAs for advanced midgut NETs and, by extrapolation, to PNETs as well. A similar randomized trial (CLARINET) using another long-acting SSA (lanreotide) in patients with GEP-NETs also showed improvements in PFS versus placebo (not reached vs. 18 months); the median PFS in the PNET patient subgroup was 29.7 months.[55] For patients with metastatic PNETs, treatment with SSAs after surgical management is often the preferred first line of therapy to halt progression. Side effects are usually mild with these agents and may include loose stools, abdominal cramping, flatulence, pancreatic insufficiency, and thyroid and insulin suppression. Their use can also promote gallstone formation, so cholecystectomy should be considering when operating on advanced PNETs.

Several agents targeting specific biologic pathways reduce PNET progression. The mTOR inhibitor everolimus improves PFS in patients with advanced PNET. In the RADIANT-3 trial, patients with advanced PNETs were randomized to everolimus versus placebo, and PFS times were 11.3 and 4.6 months, respectively.[118] About 41% of patients treated had serious adverse advents, such as abdominal pain, vomiting, fevers, and pneumonia. Less severe common adverse reactions are stomatitis, rash, diarrhea, and edema. Sunitinib is a multikinase inhibitor of the vascular endothelial growth factor (VEGF) pathway that has also shown efficacy in PNETs. A randomized trial of patients with advanced or metastatic PNETs who were not surgical candidates revealed a PFS of 11.1 months for sunitinib versus 5.5 months for placebo, with an objective response rate of 9.3%.[119] Diarrhea, nausea, vomiting, fatigue, neutropenia, and hypertension were common. In 2021, the HIF-2α inhibitor belzutifan was approved by the FDA for VHL-associated tumors, including PNETs. In a trial of patients with VHL and renal cell carcinoma, 12 patients who also had PNETs showed an objective response rate of 77%.[109] The drug commonly causes decreased hemoglobin/anemia, hypoxia, and fatigue, among other side effects. Whether these impressive response rates in PNETs will apply to patients without VHL remains to be seen, and phase II clinical trials that include advanced, sporadic PNETs and pheochromocytoma/paraganglioma are underway (NCT04924075).

For patients with advanced, well-differentiated PNETs, the oral chemotherapy combination of capecitabine and temozolomide (Cap/Tem) has shown response rates of 40% and improved PFS versus temozolomide alone (22.7 vs. 14.4 months).[120] Overall survival (OS) was similar in both groups (58.7 vs. 53.8 months). This combination can be extremely useful in the neoadjuvant setting for shrinking both primary and metastatic lesions before attempted resection and cytoreduction as well as for treating patients with progressive disease (Fig. 76.11). The combination is generally well

tolerated by patients, with the most common side effects including anemia, thrombocytopenia, granulocytopenia, fatigue, vomiting, and nausea. In patients who progress after previous Cap/Tem treatment, the fluorouracil, leucovorin, oxaliplatin (FOLFOX) regimen shows activity, with response rates of 45% in this population.[121] Patients with poorly differentiated, high-grade PNETs are commonly treated with cisplatin or carboplatin and etoposide, with response rates of 30%, but survival in these aggressive carcinomas remains poor at a median of about 1 year.[122]

Peptide radioreceptor therapy is another treatment for patients with advanced PNETs. This is the intravenous administration of a radioisotope chelated to an SSA, which can bind specifically to tumor cells expressing SSTRs. It is internalized into the tumor cell, allowing the radioactive molecule to carry out DNA damage. Early versions used[111] indium and[90] yttrium[123] and more recently most have used[177] lutetium.[124] Although used for decades in Europe based on phase II trials, PRRT was not approved in the United States until 2018. This followed results of the NETTER-1 trial, where patients with advanced midgut NETs were randomized to four cycles of[177] Lu-DOTATATE plus octreotide LAR 30 mg every 4 weeks versus Sandostatin LAR 60 mg every 4 weeks. The early end point of 20-month PFS was 65.2% for the PRRT versus 10.8% for the control group ($p < 0.001$).[125] Based on this study and several from Europe, the FDA approved PRRT for patients with advanced PNET and GI NET with SST-avid tumors. PRRT is generally used after surgical cytoreduction when there has been progression on SSAs, but can also be used in unresectable or borderline resectable PNETs in a neoadjuvant setting.[126] This therapy is well tolerated, but 2% may develop myelodysplastic syndrome or leukemia in long-term follow-up.[127]

There are a variety of options for the medical treatment of functional tumors. Excess gastric acid secretion can be managed by PPIs and further enhanced with SSAs.[128] For insulinoma, diazoxide can be very helpful in raising blood sugars, as well as frequent meals.[129] For unresectable VIPomas and glucagonomas, SSAs may be useful to help control the hypersecretory state.[130]

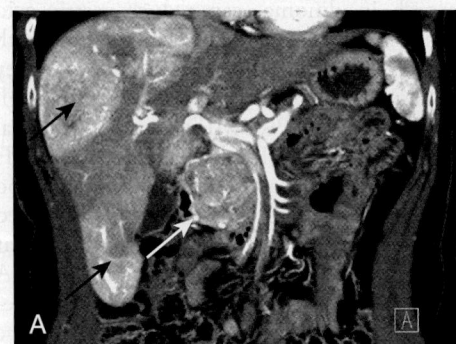
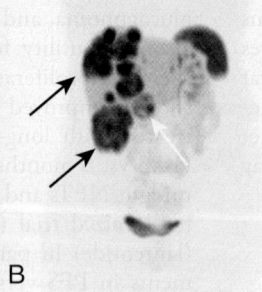
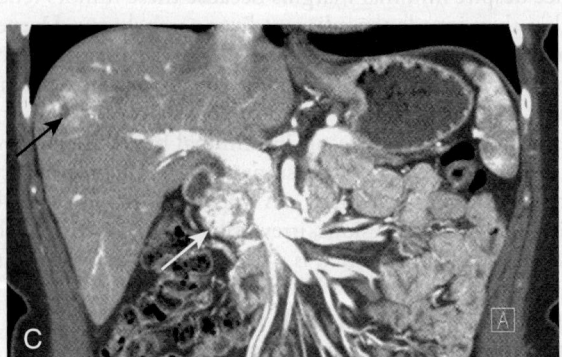

FIGURE 76.11 Coronal CT of patient with PNET in head of the pancreas (A). The *white arrow* shows the primary tumor, and *black arrows* show large liver metastases. ^{68}Ga-DOTATOC MIP image (B) showing liver metastases *(black arrows)* and primary tumor *(white arrow)*. Coronal CT (C) after 12 months of neoadjuvant capecitabine and temozolomide chemotherapy, showing substantial decrease in the size of liver *(black arrow)* and primary tumors *(white arrow)*. *MIP,* Maximum intensity projection; *PNET,* pancreatic neuroendocrine tumor.

OUTCOMES

Pancreatic surgery in general is well recognized for its relatively high morbidity and mortality rates.[131] Mortality for PD ranges from 2% to 16%, which correlates with hospital volume,[132] and should be <5% in high-volume centers.[133,134] Major complications such as pancreaticobiliary leaks, delayed gastric emptying, hemorrhage, abscess, aspiration, and pulmonary embolism are also common. Most pancreatic surgery outcome studies reflect primarily patients with adenocarcinoma, and complication rates may differ for operations performed for PNETs. The morbidity and morbidity also depend on whether PD, DP, CP, or enucleation is performed. A systematic review of pancreatectomies performed for PNETs revealed in-hospital mortality rates of 6%, 4%, 4%, and 3% for these respective procedures.[135]

The pancreas is often less fibrotic and more commonly has a nondilated duct in patients with PNETs, which increases the risk of pancreatic fistula.[136] One review found a pancreatic fistula rate was 45% for enucleation, 58% for CP, 14% for DP, and 14% for PD.[135] Delayed gastric emptying is more common after PD and CP (18% and 16%, respectively), as is postoperative hemorrhage (7% and 4%, respectively).[135] Rates of reintervention and readmission are higher with PD and enucleation of head lesions (46% and 49%) and lower for DP and enucleation of tail lesions (19% and 24%).[137]

The most common long-term complications related to pancreatic resections are exocrine and endocrine insufficiency. The risk of these sequelae generally correlate with how much pancreas is removed, favoring procedures such as enucleation and CP. In a Dutch study of patients with PNET, exocrine insufficiency was seen in 55% having PD, 8% with DP, and 5% after enucleation.[137] One US center found the incidence to be 36% in those having PD or DP.[138] Exocrine insufficiency is also influenced by whether gastric antrum and duodenum are present, receipt of chemotherapy and/or radiation, the patency of the pancreaticoenteric anastomosis, and whether the patient is receiving SSAs. Symptoms may include steatorrhea, flatulence, bloating, abdominal cramping, nausea, weight loss, and oily/yellow stools. Fecal elastase levels in a random stool sample may be helpful in making the diagnosis but are less reliable than in chronic pancreatitis. Pancreatic enzyme replacement therapy with 50 to 75,000 units of lipase per meal and 25 to 50,000 units for snacks are recommended starting doses in patients with exocrine insufficiency, and some would start these perioperatively.[139] Standard encapsulated porcine pancreatic enzymes can be expensive, and for some, chewable over-the-counter papaya extract can be a reasonable alternative.

Endocrine insufficiency is also common after pancreatic resections, and in a series of over 1700 patients having PD or DP, endocrine insufficiency (defined by the need for pharmacologic intervention) occurred in 20% of patients. Risk factors included higher BMI, smoking, family or personal history of diabetes, and DP over PD, possibly because of a higher density of islet cells in the tail of the pancreas. Patients should be followed by fasting glucose and hemoglobin A1c levels and educated on the symptoms (polyuria, polydipsia, blurred vision) and long-term complications of hyperglycemia (stroke, coronary artery, renal, and peripheral vascular disease).[138] Glycemic control must be monitored postoperatively and in follow-up, and patients may need to be on oral hypoglycemics or insulin if hemoglobin A1c remains elevated.

In patients with functional tumors, resection of the primary tumor may allow for the disappearance of symptoms. However, if residual nodal or metastatic disease is present, symptoms and elevated hormone levels may persist. The highest chance for cure would be in patients with insulinoma where the tumors are generally small but are detected early because of the pronounced symptoms of hypoglycemia. Other functional tumors are less likely to be localized, and cure will be more difficult. In a high-volume-center series of resected PNETs, one-quarter were functional tumors (17% insulinoma, 3% glucagonoma, 3% gastrinoma, 2% other), and the hazard ratio (HR) for PFS was significantly reduced as compared with nonfunctional tumors (HR 0.272, $p = 0.012$ by multivariate analysis).[140]

In the Surveillance, Epidemiology, and End Results program (SEER) database, 8944 PNETs were recorded between 2000 and 2016. The median OS of the entire group was 68 months, increasing from 46 months between 2000 and 2008 to 85 months between 2009 and 2016. Five-year OS was excellent for localized tumors, at 83.2%, diminishing to 67.4% in those with regional nodal disease and 28.1% with metastatic disease. In patients with metastatic grade 1 and 2 tumors who had surgery, median OS was 84 months versus 18 months in those not having surgery.[21] In the Verona database of 587 patients with resected PNET, where only 13% had stage IV disease and the median tumor size was 2.0 cm, the median disease-specific survival (DSS) was 269 months for all patients. Vascular invasion, higher tumor grade, and liver metastases were independent risk factors for decreased survival.[140]

Some controversy exists over the risks associated with smaller PNETs (<2 cm). In a study of the National Cancer Database (NCDB), Sugawara et al. compared survival of patients with localized, nonfunctional PNETs ≤1 cm and 1.1 to 2.0 cm. Over 80% of each group had resection, and resection was associated with improved survival for the 1.1- to 2.0-cm group (HR 0.58, $p < 0.001$) but not for the <1-cm group. The median OS was not reached in the <1-cm group, and incidence of nodal metastases was 6.1% versus a median OS of 186 months and 10% nodal metastases in the 1.1- to 2.0-cm group. They concluded that select patients with 1.1- to 2.0-cm tumors may benefit from resection (<65 years old, no comorbidities, and distal pancreas location).[141] A European study from 16 centers reviewed their experience with 210 resected PNETs <2 cm. Of these, 10.6% had positive nodes and 5.9% developed metastases (liver, nodes, lung), with 1 local recurrence. The 5-year OS was 96.2%, with 5-year DSS of 100% in the <10-mm group and 87.3% in the 11- to 20-mm group. Higher tumor grade (grade 2 to 3), biliary or pancreatic dilatation, and tumor size 11 to 20 mm were independent risk factors for recurrence.[142] The morbidity and mortality of pancreatic surgery need to be carefully factored versus the risk of decreased survival from the tumor. This risk in PNETs <10 mm appears negligible, and for tumors 11 to 20 mm, resection might be reserved for good-risk patients with grade 2 to 3 tumors and/or ductal dilatation.

In MEN1, the problem of multifocality can make the choice of operation challenging.[25] Furthermore, up to three-quarters of patients will develop new tumors in the remnant pancreas, sometimes requiring completion pancreatectomy.[143] In a study of 603 patients with MEN1 with duodenopancreatic tumors with median follow-up of 6.9 years, 67 patients died. Distant metastases developed in 36 patients; 46 of the deaths were considered NET related, 8 were non-NET cancer related, and 13 were the result of other medical conditions.[144] An older study following 57 patients with MEN1 with PNETs and ZES found that liver metastases occurred in 23% of patients and 14% had an aggressive growth pattern. Three deaths were attributed to ZES, and

8 patients died of other causes.[145] In a Dutch study of 69 patients with MEN1 with PNETs having surgery, 10 patients developed liver metastases, and all of these patients had primary tumors >3 cm; no liver metastases were seen in patients with tumors <2 cm.[146]

In patients with VHL, PNETs <3 cm also rarely metastasize; therefore, because of their multifocality and the complexity of coexistent cystic lesions, it has generally been recommended to delay resection until they reach >3 cm in size.[31,147] Recommendations from North American Tumor Society (NANETS) suggest that patients with PNETs >3 cm, a tumor doubling time of <500 days, or germline mutations in exon 3 of the *VHL* gene should be considered for surgical resection.[11]

SURVEILLANCE AND FOLLOW-UP

The European Society of Medical Oncology (ESMO) recommends that for follow-up of PNET patients that a CT or MRI be performed every 3 to 6 months for R0/R1 resected grade 1 or 2 GEP-NETs, decreasing to every 2 to 3 months for grade 3 NECs. In patients with advanced disease, the intervals should be the same, and surveillance should be lifelong, but intervals can be increased to 1 to 2 years as follow-up time increases.[148] Recent ENETS guidelines for nonfunctional PNETs resected with curative intent (including metastatic) suggest anatomic imaging (CT chest, abdomen, and pelvis or abdominal MRI) be performed at 3 to 6 months after surgery, then every 6 to 12 months for 5 years, then every 1 to 2 years until 10 years, and every 5 years thereafter. If liver metastases are being followed, this should be every 3 months, preferably by MRI. A DOTA-PET scan should be considered every 1 to 2 years to more fully evaluate for metastases, and chromogranin A levels may help assess tumor burden. If metastatic disease is not resected, then recommendations are similar, but the importance of using the same modality (preferably MRI with liver disease) is stressed so that response evaluation criteria for solid tumors (RECIST) criteria can accurately be used to determine whether changes in treatment are needed.[149]

SELECTED REFERENCES

de Herder WW, Rehfeld JF, Kidd M, Modlin IM. A short history of neuroendocrine tumours and their peptide hormones. *Best Pract Res Clin Endocrinol Metab*. 2016;30(1):3-17.

This is an excellent history of the discovery of neuroendocrine tumors and the hormones they produce.

Hofland J, Falconi M, Christ E, et al. European Neuroendocrine Tumor Society 2023 guidance paper for functioning pancreatic neuroendocrine tumour syndromes. *J Neuroendocrinol*. 2023;35(8):e13318.

This paper from the European Neuroendocrine Tumor Society (ENETS) reviews and provides guidance for the diagnosis, treatment, and follow-up of patients with functional PNETs.

Howe JR, Merchant NB, Conrad C, et al. The North American Neuroendocrine Tumor Society consensus paper on the surgical management of pancreatic neuroendocrine tumors. *Pancreas*. 2020;49(1):1-33.

This is a consensus paper from the North American Tumor Society (NANETS) on the management of a wide variety of clinical issues related to patients with PNETs.

Kos-Kudła B, Castaño JP, Denecke T, et al. European Neuroendocrine Tumor Society (ENETS) 2023 guidance paper for nonfunctioning pancreatic neuroendocrine tumours. *J Neuroendocrinol*. 2023;35:e13343.

This paper from ENETS reviews and provides guidance for the diagnosis, treatment, and follow-up of patients with nonfunctional PNETs.

Sonbol MB, Mazza GL, Mi L, et al. Survival and incidence patterns of pancreatic neuroendocrine tumors over the last 2 decades: a SEER database analysis. *Oncologist*. 2022;27(7):573-578.

This is a recent update on the epidemiology and outcomes of patients with PNETs in the United States.

The full reference list appears on Elsevier eBooks+.

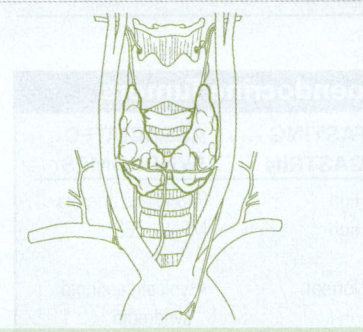

CHAPTER 77

Neuroendocrine Neoplasms (Carcinoid Tumors)

Andrea Gillis, Sophie Dream, and Herbert Chen

INTRODUCTION

Neuroendocrine neoplasms or tumors (NETs), classically called *carcinoid tumors,* encompass tumors that derive from neuroendocrine cell origin. The term *carcinoid* implies benignity and, given the propensity for these tumors to metastasize, is now generally considered a misnomer. The median age of incidence is 60.5 years. They are rare, but increasing in incidence, with an annual age-adjusted incidence of 6.98 per 100,000 persons in 2012.[1] The majority of NETs occur throughout the gastrointestinal (GI) tract and are commonly classified based on their embryologic site of origin: foregut, midgut, or hindgut. As these tumors arise from neuroendocrine cells, they can occur in other locations throughout the body, including the lungs, thymus, and bronchi, but less commonly.

NETs of the GI tract are generally not associated with hormone hyperproduction but can cause carcinoid syndrome, especially in cases with metastasis. In contrast to these GI tract NETs, bronchopulmonary and thymic NETs can cause both carcinoid syndrome and Cushing syndrome.

GASTROENTEROPANCREATIC NEUROENDOCRINE TUMORS

The majority of neuroendocrine/carcinoid tumors are found within the GI tract (55%). Neuroendocrine tumors of the intestinal tract are categorized by grade and/or differentiation.[2] Well-differentiated NETs are distinguished from poorly differentiated neuroendocrine carcinomas. Grading is divided into three groups from low (G1), to intermediate (G2), to high grade (G3) based on mitotic rates, cell appearance, Ki-67 proliferation rates (determined by immunohistochemical staining for nuclear Ki-67 protein expression), and clinical features such as local or angioinvasion. Low-grade, well-differentiated NETs carry a favorable prognosis, with 5-year survival ranging to >98% with appropriate treatment. The majority of NETs are "nonfunctioning," meaning not secreting metabolically active substances such as gastrin, serotonin, insulin, and vasoactive intestinal peptides

(VIPs). Additional classification relates to the tumor's cell of origin, which influences NET presentation, metastatic potential, and prognosis.

CT scans may be a useful diagnostic tool or may incidentally find these tumors. The use of multiphasic contrast-enhanced CT scan with a timed arterial and venous phase is crucial to identifying these lesions, which are hyperenhancing on arterial phase and isoenhancing on delayed phases. MRIs are particularly useful for identifying metastases such as within the liver. Because NETs tend to overexpress somatostatin receptors, functional imaging targeting somatostatin receptors are the most sensitive for diagnosing and staging neuroendocrine neoplasms. For example, somatostatin receptor–positron emission tomography (PET) scans (^{68}Ga-DOTATATE) are now the gold standard for reliably identifying these tumors. This test uses gadolinium, which binds to somatostatin receptors to allow for localization and staging.

Gastric

Gastric carcinoids or NETs comprise about 7% of all digestive NETS.[3–5] These tumors originate from the histamine-containing enterochromaffin-like (ECL) cells of the embryonic foregut. Of all gastric neoplasms, NETs are quite rare (about 1.8%), with an incidence of 0.5 per 100,000 persons.

Clinical and histologic features of gastric NETs can be divided into three subtypes (Table 77.1). Type I gastric NETs are the most common (70%–80%). These tend to present as multiple small, benign tumors. Their formation is associated with the loss of parietal cells and chronic atrophic gastritis leading to G-cell hyperplasia and hypergastrinemia from lack of inhibitory feedback.[6] ECL cells are then upregulated and become hyperplastic and then dysplastic tumors. When atrophic gastritis is associated with parietal cell or intrinsic factor antibodies, the patient is diagnosed with pernicious anemia.

Type II gastric NETs (5%) are associated with multiple endocrine neoplasia type 1 (MEN1) and Zollinger-Ellison syndrome (ZES). These tumors are driven by ectopic gastrin-producing

TABLE 77.1 Common Characteristics of the Three Types of Gastric Neuroendocrine Tumors

TYPE	PREVALENCE	MALIGNANT POTENTIAL	SIZE	LOCATION	GASTRIC PH	FASTING GASTRIN	ASSOCIATED SYNDROMES
Type I	70%–80%	Usually benign	Small (≤1 cm)	Fundus or body	High: pH >4–7	High	Pernicious anemia
Type II	5%	Malignant potential but usually indolent	Large (1–2 cm)	Fundus, body, antrum	Low: pH <2	High	MEN1, ZES
Type III	10%–15%	Highly malignant with metastatic potential	Large (>2 cm)	Fundus or antrum	Normal: pH <4	Normal	Atypical carcinoid syndrome

MEN1, Multiple endocrine neoplasia type 1; *ZES*, Zollinger-Ellison syndrome.

G cells (gastrinomas), usually in the duodenum or pancreas. Their development is thought to be induced by the presence of hypergastrinemia that is independent of normal inhibitory feedback. Clinically, these tumors tend to be larger than type I tumors with a higher risk of lymph node metastasis (5%–35%). The diagnosis of a type II gastric NET mandates screening for MEN1-associated tumors (pituitary and parathyroid; see later).

Type III gastric NETs (15%–25%) are also usually large (similar to type II) but are not associated with hypergastrinemia or any aberrant gastric physiology. Similar to gastric adenocarcinoma, these tumors are highly aggressive with a tendency to metastasize (usually to lymph nodes, followed by liver). Type III gastric NETs are associated with an impaired 5-year survival rate (25%–30%) compared with other gastric NETs (70%–99%). They are also associated with "atypical carcinoid syndrome" because of the possibility of overproduction of 5-hydroxytryptophan (5-HTP) (see "Carcinoid Syndrome" later) (see Table 77.1).

Diagnosis of gastric NETs is usually incidental given their indolent nature. They are likely to be discovered on routine endoscopy where a mass is found. Both mass and normal gastric tissue should be sampled in order to subtype these tumors by looking for the presence (or absence) of G-cell hyperplasia, atrophic gastritis, and/or ECL hyperplasia. Once diagnosed, as with all gastric tumors, endoscopic ultrasound (EUS) should be completed to assess for lymph node involvement and depth of invasion, as this will dictate treatment. CT or MRI may be used for evaluation of metastatic disease. Serum chromogranin A (CgA) is measured as a biomarker and prognostic factor for all neuroendocrine neoplasms.

The treatment for gastric NETs should consist of wide local excision.[7] Negative margins without any specified length cutoff ("no tumor on ink") is sufficient given the typical indolent nature of these tumors. The exact surgical approach depends on tumor size, level of invasion, and presence of high-risk features. Those type I and II gastric NETs without evidence of lymph node involvement and no greater than submucosal invasion can be treated endoscopically with snare polypectomy or endoscopic mucosal resection (EMR). All type III gastric NETs or large (>1 cm), high-risk type I and II gastric NETs should be managed aggressively with wedge or partial gastrectomy and lymph node dissection. Those patients with numerous gastric NETs not amenable to wedge resections may require a total gastrectomy. Those with type II gastric NETs must have the culprit gastrinoma resected as well, if possible.

Small Intestine

The small intestine and appendix are the most common sites for gastroenteropancreatic (GEP) NETs. Small intestinal NETs comprise about 30% of small intestinal neoplasms. The median age at presentation is in the seventh decade.

Duodenal NETs are extremely rare, usually small, and remain localized. Most are located in the first or second part of the duodenum, and about 20% are located in the periampullary region. All duodenal NETs should be removed if diagnosed before metastases given concern for obstruction. The approach to removal depends on size, location, and lymph node involvement. Endoscopic resection can be selected for submucosal, nonampullary tumors <10 mm.[8,9] Between 1 and 2 cm, endoscopic resection or surgical resection can be considered. Large (>2 cm) or ampullary duodenal NETs or those with lymph node involvement should be surgically removed, which may necessitate a pancreaticoduodenectomy based on proximity to the pancreatic duct.

Most small intestinal NETs are located in the last 2 feet of the terminal ileum. Ileal NETs may be aggressive, with 35% associated with metastases. Diagnosis of NETs, as with all small bowel tumors, is generally illusive. Video capsule endoscopy or balloon-assisted enteroscopy may be helpful in localizing small intestinal NETs. Unfortunately, small bowel NETs typically do not clinically manifest until they have reached a large, symptomatic size—on average 3.5 cm or once they have metastasized. The symptoms usually consist of a partial/intermittent small bowel obstruction caused by either intussusception or luminal obstruction. Additionally, a dense desmoplastic reaction as a result of the NET may occur, exacerbating a small bowel obstruction. In advanced stages, mesenteric and nodal involvement may obstruct venous drainage and lead to ischemia. Given the significant risk of multiple tumors (20%–30%) and metastasis, all small bowel NETs are recommended to undergo full staging before resection.

Surgical treatment is the standard of care. Minimally invasive (laparoscopic) or open surgical resection may be considered. Segmental resection along with locoregional lymphadenectomy is required to enhance disease-free survival. In widely metastatic disease, there are data that tumor debulking may increase long-term survival, but this is controversial.

Appendix

Appendiceal NETs are the most common neoplasm affecting the appendix (60%–80%).[10] Lymph node metastasis rates increase with tumor size, affecting 15% of appendix NETs <1 cm, 47% of those 1 to 2 cm, and 86% of those larger than 2 cm. The 10-year survival rate ranges from 91% to 100% based on these sizes, with larger sizes portending worse survival.

Appendix tumors tend to present earlier than intestinal NETs elsewhere because of obstruction of the appendiceal lumen causing appendicitis.[11,12] This leads to many appendix NETs being diagnosed incidentally on final pathology. Several series report the prevalence of incidental NETs in appendectomy specimens to be about 1% to 1.5%.

All symptomatic and asymptomatic appendiceal tumors are recommended to be resected if known preoperatively given their malignant potential. The size of the appendiceal tumor dictates the operative management via an algorithm based on National

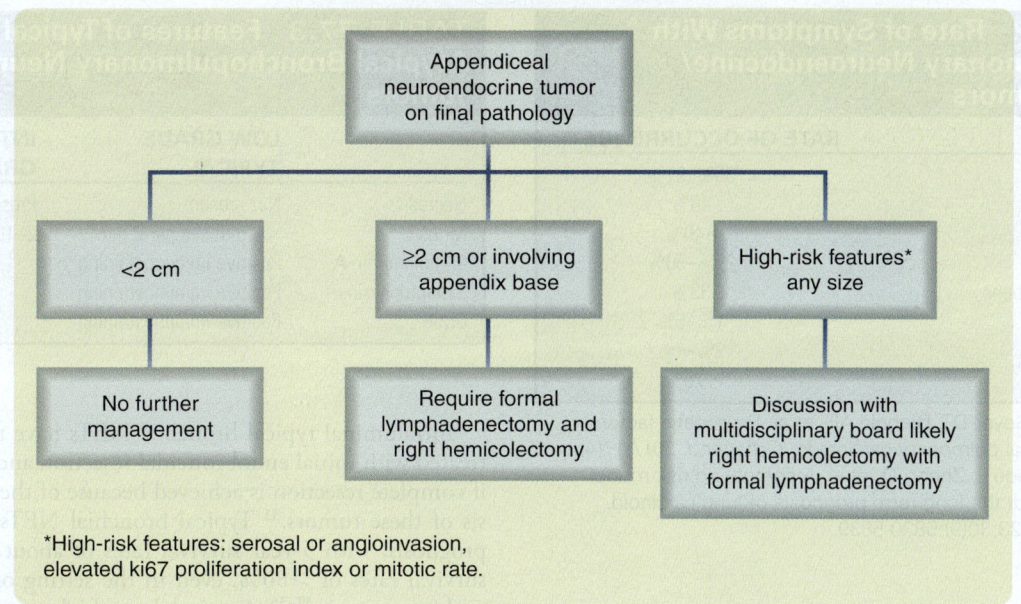

FIGURE 77.1 Management algorithm for appendiceal neuroendocrine tumors. (From Hoehn RS, Rieser CJ, Choudry MH, et al. Current management of appendiceal neoplasms. *Am Soc Clin Oncol Educ Book.* 2021;41:1-15.)

Comprehensive Cancer Network (NCCN) recommendations (Fig. 77.1).[13] Larger tumors and tumors with higher risk of recurrence (high Ki67, poorly differentiated) mandate more aggressive, wider resections than appendectomy alone, including right hemicolectomy. This allows for a tumor basin lymphadenectomy along the ileocolic vasculature for staging.

Colon and Rectal

Colorectal NETs comprise the "hindgut" NETs. Colon and rectal NETs are typically found on routine colonoscopy. On endoscopy, colorectal NETs appear as a small, yellowish, waxy-looking sessile or submucosal polyp. They rarely produce serotonin, limiting the usefulness of 24-hour urine 5′-hydroxyindoleacetic acid for diagnosis or monitoring but may secrete somatostatin. Less than half of colorectal NETs will manifest with symptoms, including bleeding or changes in bowel habits.

Colonic NETs make up 16% of all GI NETs.[14] They are rare, but tend to be aggressive, with 40% rated as high grade. The average tumor size is 5 cm, and over 65% have nodal or distal metastases. Colonic NETs carry the worst prognosis of all luminal GI NETs.[15] Across all stages, colonic NETs carry an average 5-year survival rate of 40% to 70%, with cecal tumors having the best prognosis.

Rectal NETs comprise 34% of all GI NETs and have an excellent prognosis, especially if <2 cm (5-year overall survival 76%–88%). If low grade and <2 cm in size, colorectal NETs can be resected endoscopically with polypectomy and do not require formal staging.[16] However, larger or high-risk colonic NETs require full staging and a formal segmental resection. Similarly, high-risk rectal NETs mandate a total mesorectal excision because of the need for lymph node staging.

Pancreatic

NETs of the pancreas (pNETs) are rare among NETs (9%); however, among all NETs, pNETs carry the worse overall 5-year survival (74%, all stages).[4,17] These tumors will be thoroughly discussed in a subsequent chapter of this volume.

BRONCHOPULMONARY NEUROENDOCRINE TUMORS

Bronchopulmonary NETs comprise a group of rare lung malignancies made up of carcinoid/NET, small cell lung carcinoma, large cell neuroendocrine carcinoma, and diffuse idiopathic pulmonary neuroendocrine cell hyperplasia.[18,29] The age-adjusted incidence of lung NETs was 1.49 per 100,000 persons.[1] This section of the chapter will focus on bronchopulmonary NETs that arise from the enteroendocrine (also known as *argentaffin* or *Kulchitsky*) cells of the lung.

The majority of bronchopulmonary NETs develop spontaneously and occur in the fifth and sixth decades of life. They account for a minority of lung cancers, with typical and atypical NETs of the lung representing less than 2% of lung tumors. Cigarette smoking has been associated with an increased odds ratio of developing pulmonary NETs, but the mechanism is unclear.[19]

Bronchial NETs usually present as centrally located endobronchial lesions, but also may present as peripheral lung nodules. They may secret serotonin, adrenocorticotropic hormone (ACTH), somatostatin, and bradykinin. Patients with bronchopulmonary NETs may be asymptomatic; however, the majority of patients will present with symptoms including cough, wheezing, chest pain, hemoptysis, and/or bronchial obstruction. Bronchial obstruction can result in lung hyperinflation, atelectasis, and recurring pneumonia distal to the site of tumor obstruction. Typical bronchial NETs may also be associated with lung hypoplasia, which may be the result of a reactive neuroendocrine hyperplasia.[20]

Although rare (Table 77.2), bronchopulmonary NETS may present with a secretory tumor that may cause carcinoid syndrome (see later) or produce ACTH resulting in Cushing syndrome (see Table 77.2). Classic features of Cushing syndrome include hypertension, hyperglycemia, weight gain, fatigue, easy bruising, thinning skin, striae, and mood disturbances.

When suspecting hypercortisolism, patients should be screened with a 1-mg overnight dexamethasone suppression test, two or

TABLE 77.2 Rate of Symptoms With Bronchopulmonary Neuroendocrine/Carcinoid Tumors

SYMPTOM	RATE OF OCCURRENCE
Cough	35%–91%
Dyspnea	46%
Chest pain	~40%
Hemoptysis	25%–50%
Recurrent lung infections	33%
Carcinoid syndrome	1%–5%
Cushing syndrome	2%–4%
Asymptomatic	~25%

From Ramirez RA, Beyer DT, Diebold AE, et al. Prognostic factors in typical and atypical pulmonary carcinoids. *Ochsner J.* 2017;17(4): 335-340; Wang T, Zhou J, Zheng Q, et al. A competing risk model nomogram to predict the long-term prognosis of lung carcinoid. *Ann Surg Oncol.* 2023;30(9):5830-5839.

TABLE 77.3 Features of Typical and Atypical Bronchopulmonary Neuroendocrine Tumors

	LOW-GRADE TYPICAL	INTERMEDIATE-GRADE ATYPICAL
Necrosis	Not present	Present
Mitosis	<2 mitoses per 2 mm^2	2–10 mitoses per 2 mm^2
Chromogranin A	Positive immunostaining	
Synaptophysin	Positive immunostaining	
CD56	Positive immunostaining	

more midnight salivary cortisol tests, or a 24-hour urine cortisol test.[23] Next, if patients do have hypercortisolism, an elevated morning ACTH and high-dose dexamethasone testing failing to suppress can elucidate the etiology as ACTH dependent from a nonpituitary source.

Bronchopulmonary NETs are often found incidentally on imaging. The majority of these tumors affect the mainstem or lobar bronchus. Initial evaluation is performed with CT chest with contrast and multiphasic axial abdominal imaging. Centrally located tumors can be further assessed with bronchoscopy, where these tumors appear as pink and rounded with a lobulated surface; irregular margins are more likely in atypical carcinoids. Biopsy can be safely done using bronchoscopy to confirm neuroendocrine cells.[24]

The 2022 WHO classification categorizes bronchopulmonary and thymic NETs/carcinoid tumors as low-grade typical and intermediate-grade atypical tumors based on the characteristics noted in Table 77.3.[25] Typical NETs are more likely to be well differentiated and less aggressive, whereas atypical NETs are more likely to be peripherally located, tend to be more aggressive, and are more likely to metastasize to local and regional lymph nodes and to distant sites, including the liver, bones, and brain. Atypical NETs may harbor *p53, BCL2,* or *BAX* gene mutations. Characteristics that confer worse prognosis include atypical carcinoid syndrome, increased age, male sex, larger tumor size, higher Ki-67 index (>10%), lymph node involvement, or metastatic disease.[21,22,26] Atypical tumors, centrally located tumors, and larger tumors are associated with more advanced lymph node metastasis.[27]

The overall prognosis of bronchopulmonary NETs is favorable when compared with other lung malignancies, with the majority of lung NETs being typical tumors. The goal of treatment for bronchial NETs is surgical resection, achieving an R0 or complete resection. Typical bronchial carcinoids can be treated with wedge resection in cases of peripheral tumors that are smaller than 2 cm in size, without lymph node involvement, or in patients with poor functional status when an anatomic resection is prohibitive. Anatomic lobectomy or segmentectomy is considered the standard of care for larger tumors, including lymph node dissection or sampling. In cases of atypical carcinoids, radical lymph node dissection is suggested because of the higher incidence of lymph node involvement in these patients.[28–30]

Intraluminal typical bronchial NETs have the potential to be treated with initial endobronchial resection and regular follow-up if complete resection is achieved because of the favorable prognosis of these tumors.[31] Typical bronchial NETs have an excellent prognosis, with 5-year survival rates of about 90% and 10-year survival rates of >80%, even in the setting of identified lymph node metastasis.[32–36] Atypical bronchial carcinoids have 5-year survival rates of 22% to 100% and 10-year survival rates of about 42% to 67%, with nodal metastasis having a significant impact on survival.[21,33,35,36] In cases where patient factors make surgical resection impractical, radiation therapy can be used. In advanced disease, patients are treated with adjuvant chemotherapy with cisplatin or carboplatin and etoposide and radiotherapy.[30]

THYMIC NEUROENDOCRINE TUMORS

Thymic neuroendocrine (or carcinoid) tumors are rare and make up about 5% of anterior mediastinal tumors.[31] They have a strong male predominance and are associated with MEN1 syndrome. Thymic NETs generally present as a large mass and often are locally invasive or have distant metastasis on initial presentation. Although the majority of these tumors are nonsecretory, they can produce ACTH. They are histologically classified by differentiation as well differentiated (low-grade typical), moderately differentiated (intermediate-grade atypical), or poorly differentiated/anaplastic (high-grade large cell neuroendocrine carcinoma or small cell neuroendocrine carcinoma), similarly to bronchopulmonary NETs (see Table 77.3). Patients with thymic carcinoids often present asymptomatically with a mass found on imaging, but may also present with chest pain, cough, and dysphagia related to mass effect in the mediastinum.

Thymic NETs are often discovered incidentally on screening chest x-ray or for mediastinal symptoms. Thymic NETs initially can be evaluated with contrast-enhanced chest CT scan, which can help delineate the presence of local invasion, regional metastasis, and features that may be indicative of multiple thymic tumors. On imaging, these tumors are lobulated and may demonstrate areas of necrosis or hemorrhage.

Tissue biopsy may be needed to rule out other tumors that have similar appearance on imaging that can be medically treated, including germ cell tumors or lymphoma. In cases where the tumor cannot be completely excised with thymectomy, tissue diagnosis with CT-guided fine-needle aspiration or endoscopic or bronchoscopy biopsy should be used to obtain tissue diagnosis. Cases where these less invasive approaches do not yield adequate tissue may necessitate surgical biopsy with mediastinoscopy, video-assisted thoracoscopy, or anterior mediastinotomy.

Once a thymic NET is diagnosed on tissue biopsy, additional abdominal cross-sectional imaging and baseline somatostatin receptor imaging (PET–DOTATATE) is performed for staging, tumor localization, and to confirm the presence of somatostatin overexpression. The overall mortality rate for thymic NETs is high, with the 5-year survival rate ranging from 25% to 56%. Patients who are treated with surgical resection, who have smaller tumors, and who have lower stage disease have improved survival.[37,38]

Thymic NETs are treated with resection, with complete surgical resection (R0) being the treatment of choice, as it confers the best overall survival.[31] In cases where complete resection is not possible, local radiation therapy can control residual disease. The addition of adjuvant chemotherapy with cisplatin or carboplatin and etoposide is suggested for poorly differentiated neuroendocrine carcinomas even in the setting of complete resection.

MULTIPLE ENDOCRINE NEOPLASIA TYPE 1 AND NEUROENDOCRINE TUMORS

Bronchial and thymic NETs occur in up to 25% of patients with MEN1.[39,40] These tumors are more likely to occur in males with MEN1, with some reports showing a 10:1 male-to-female predominance. Smoking has also been shown to be a risk factor for the development of thymic NETs in patients with MEN1. Although thymic NETs present late in MEN1, they are the second most common cause of death in patients with this condition, accounting for up to 20% of MEN1-associated mortality.[41] In this patient population, bronchial NETs have a more indolent course than thymic NETs.

Initial screening in patients diagnosed with MEN1 for bronchopulmonary and thymic NETs is important given the malignant potential. Screening with chest x-ray or chest CT with contrast is recommended for males over the age of 25 with MEN1 for thymic NETs, with repeat screening every 1 to 3 years. Imaging protocols for screening and surveillance are controversial because many MEN1-associated bronchopulmonary NETs have low rates of growth and high overall survival.[42] Biochemical evaluation is appropriate if patients exhibit clinical manifestations of carcinoid or Cushing syndrome related to serotonin or ACTH secretion, respectively.

Patients with type II gastric NETs should be evaluated for MEN1 given this syndromic association. An evaluation for the associated disorders of the pituitary and parathyroid should be ruled out.

METASTATIC NEUROENDOCRINE DISEASE

Metastatic disease because of NETs is fairly common, with rates ranging from 12% to 74% at presentation.[43] The liver and lymph nodes are the most frequent sites of metastatic disease, followed by bone, adrenal glands, and brain. Overall NET prognosis is heavily influenced by metastasis. In the United States, localized NET median overall survival is >30 years, those with regionally metastatic disease have a median overall survival of 10.2 years, and those with distant metastatic disease have a median overall survival of 12 months.[1] At times, NETs may be initially diagnosed from a biopsy of a metastasis. The primary tumor site should be delineated, if possible, to guide treatment.

Ideal treatment of metastatic neuroendocrine disease is surgical resection.[43] However, the level of tumor burden may not be safe or amenable to complete resection. Treatment of unresectable metastatic NET should consist of symptom management and tumor burden control, if able. Debulking of disease may improve

overall survival even if complete cure is not achievable, although this is controversial. Deciding on exact staging and sequencing of surgical resection is complex and should be made in conjunction with a multidisciplinary team.

Those with liver metastases may present with carcinoid syndrome (see later) or a variety of symptoms related to the hypersecretion of neuroendocrine hormones. These secretory syndromes should be managed for symptom relief. Specific hormonal hypersecretion can be targeted with, for example, proton pump inhibitors for gastrinomas, diet control and glucagon for insulinomas, and metyrapone/ketoconazole for ACTH hypersecretion.

Systemic therapy may be offered to shrink tumor burden and control all refractory hormonal hypersecretion.[44] This may include long-acting somatostatin analogues (SSAs) such as lanreotide or a serotonin inhibitor (telotristat). Kinase inhibitors (sunitinib), mammalian target of rapamycin (mTOR) inhibitors (everolimus), and radionuclide somatostatin therapy have also been used as second-line therapy. Cytotoxic agents are considered in patients with progressive disease who are not responsive to other treatments but have not been show to improve progression-free survival or disease-free survival.[30] CgA should be serially measured to monitor for response if downtrending.

At times, liver-directed therapies may be used in conjunction with or as a bridge to surgical resection. This may include ablative therapies such as radiofrequency or microwave ablation or regional therapies including transarterial chemoembolization, transarterial radioembolization, or peptide receptor radionuclide therapy (PRRT). These therapies may treat or shrink liver metastases, allowing a parenchymal-sparing liver resection that may be more tolerable to the patient. These therapies may also be used for palliative intent for symptom control.

Surgically, primary tumor resection and all metastatic disease caries the highest 5-year survival rates. In those with extensive metastatic disease that may be unresectable, debulking or cytoreduction may improve overall survival but is controversial.[45] Additional systemic treatment modalities may be offered in conjunction as well. For those patients with unresectable or medically unresponsive liver metastases, liver transplant may be considered an additional modality. Although rarely used in the United States, the 5-year survival rate for patients undergoing liver transplantation for unresectable NETs was 84% compared with 34% in those without surgical treatment.[46]

Overall survival in those with metastatic disease depends on the level of tumor burden, primary site tissue type, grade, and presence of high-risk features (Fig. 77.2).

CARCINOID SYNDROME

Carcinoid syndrome is uncommon and occurs in 10% to 30% of carcinoid cases.[47–49] It is driven by an overproduction of serotonin or tachykinin by neoplastic cells. In excess, this hormone can cause episodic skin flushing (reported in over 90%), edema (typically lower extremity), diarrhea (60%), and wheezing/dyspnea on exertion (15%). The typical flushing experienced by patients with carcinoid syndrome can range from violaceous, full body, episodic, or lasting multiple days. Diarrhea is extremely common and is often watery, postprandial, and explosive. Serotonin causes systemic vascular vasodilatation as well as fibrosis formation, which can increase risk of right-sided valvular dysfunction and heart failure.[49] The common cardiac manifestations are pulmonary stenosis (90%), tricuspid insufficiency (47%), and

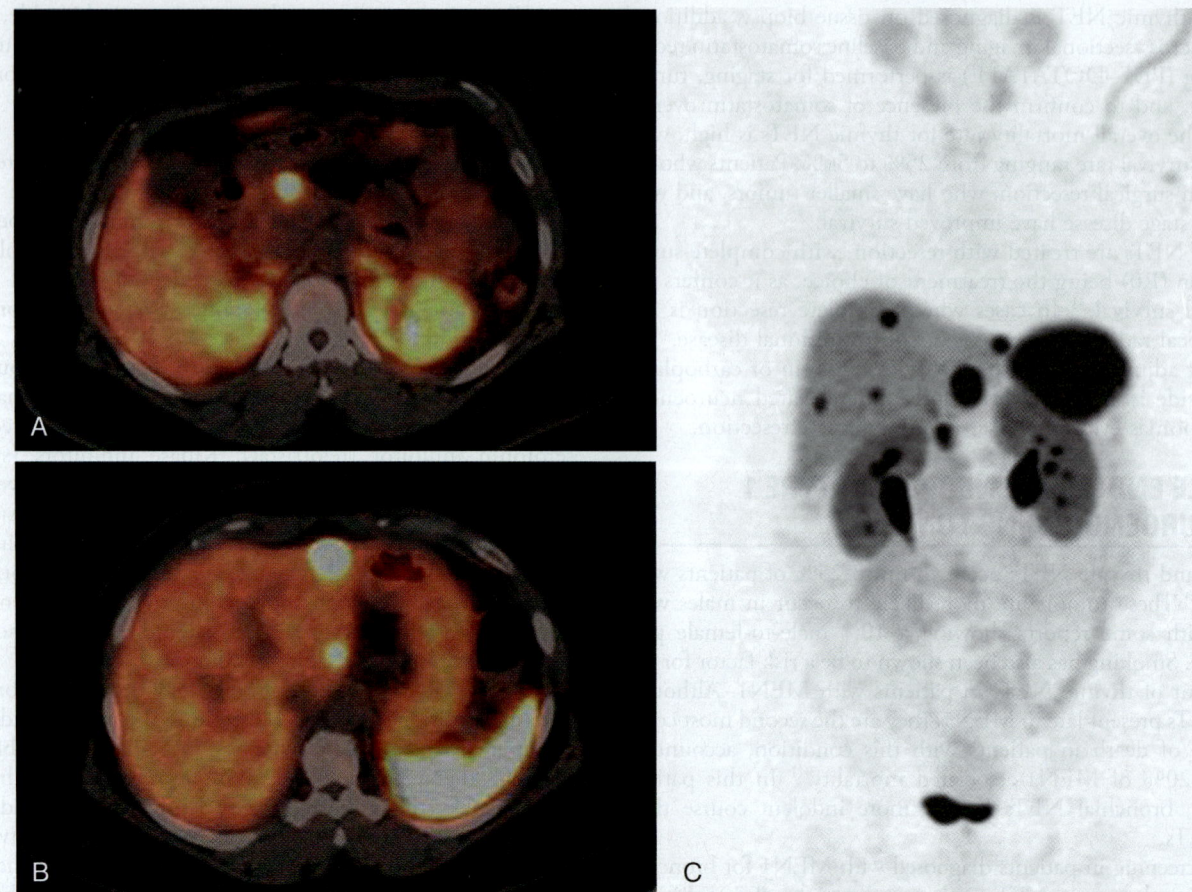

FIGURE 77.2 A 40s-year-old patient with a clinical diagnosis of hypergastrinemia. PET–DOTATATE scan was significant for head-of-pancreas pNET (initially occult on computed tomography scan) and numerous liver metastases (biopsy positive for well-differentiated pNET). (A) Axial cut demonstrating head-of-pancreas hyperintense region. (B) Axial cut demonstrating two of six hyperintense liver metastases. (C) Coronal cut demonstrating head-of-pancreas NET and six liver metastases. *NET,* Neuroendocrine tumors; *pNET,* neuroendocrine tumor of the pancreas;

tricuspid stenosis (42%). Atypical carcinoid syndrome is typically mediated by histamine production. Rarely, type III gastric NETs may cause this with a presentation of flushing that is extremely red, patchy, or pruritic.

Typically, serotonin, tachykinin, and metabolites are removed from systemic circulation by the liver. Therefore, excess secretion is usually clinically silent until liver metastases develop. Those patients with NETs that develop symptomatic carcinoid syndrome portend a worse prognosis than those without (median overall survival 4.7 years compared with 7.1 years). Several metabolites of serotonin may be measured, including 5-HTP, which can be measured in a 24-hour urine collection and may be used to monitor disease progression. 5-HTP can also be elevated in the urine in those without carcinoid syndrome after consuming certain foods. CgA is another well-established biomarker for carcinoid syndrome. It is elevated in more than 80% of patients with NETs.

Chronic carcinoid syndrome is treated by reducing the culprit hormone levels and tumor burden, if able. This includes surgical resection or debulking as well as medical management. Long-acting

SSAs such as octreotide are the standard of care, especially in those with unresectable disease, and have been shown to improve progression-free survival as well as quality of life. Those with refractory or progressive disease on SSAs may be trialed on PRRT. This therapy consists of dispensing a radiolabeled SSA therapy such as lutetium-177-DOTATATE (^{177}Lu).

Carcinoid crisis is a severe potential complication in those with uncontrolled carcinoid syndrome. It occurs upon a sudden release of serotonin or other vasoactive metabolites either spontaneously or from either tumor manipulation (biopsy or surgical resection), use of sympathomimetic drugs (amphetamines, albuterol), or upon receipt of cytolytic therapies (hepatic embolization). Patients may present with hemodynamic instability, severe flushing, profuse diarrhea, and ventilation difficulties from diffuse bronchospasm.

Treatment of carcinoid crisis consists of octreotide (both as an IV bolus and continuous infusion), IV fluid resuscitation, corticosteroids, and vasopressors as needed based on patient hemodynamics. Octreotide can also be used as a preventive measure before, during, and after maneuvers that may manipulate the tumor. Although potentially fatal, carcinoid crisis is rare.

SELECTED REFERENCES

Gluckman CR, Metz DC. Gastric neuroendocrine tumors (carcinoids). *Curr Gastroenterol Rep.* 2019; 21(4):13. doi:10.1007/s11894-019-0684-7.

> *Comprehensive update on the latest understanding of physiology and treatment of gastric neuroendocrine tumors.*

Grozinsky-Glasberg S, Davar J, Hofland J, et al. European Neuroendocrine Tumor Society (ENETS) 2022 guidance paper for carcinoid syndrome and carcinoid heart disease. *J Neuroendocrinol.* 2022;34(7):16.

> *Expert guidance and review of treatment of carcinoid syndrome and carcinoid heart disease.*

Harrelson A, Wang R, Stewart A, et al. Management of neuroendocrine tumor liver metastases. *Am J Surg.* 2023;226(5):623-630.

> *Comprehensive systematic review on the latest evidence for treating metastatic neuroendocrine tumors to the liver.*

Shah MH, Goldner WS, Benson AB, et al. Neuroendocrine and adrenal tumors, version 2.2021, NCCN Clinical Practice Guidelines in Oncology. *J Natl Compr Canc Netw.* 2021;19(7):839-868.

> *Extensive information and guidelines regarding staging and diagnosis of all-site neuroendocrine tumors.*

Singh S, Bergsland EK, Card CM, et al. Commonwealth Neuroendocrine Tumour Research Collaboration and the North American Neuroendocrine Tumor Society Guidelines for the diagnosis and management of patients with lung neuroendocrine tumors: an international collaborative endorsement and update of the 2015 European Neuroendocrine Tumor Society expert consensus guidelines. *J Thorac Oncol.* 2020;15(10):1577-1598.

> *The largest international organization of neuroendocrine tumor physicians' guidelines for evaluation and management of thoracic neuroendocrine tumors.*

The full reference list appears on Elsevier eBooks+.

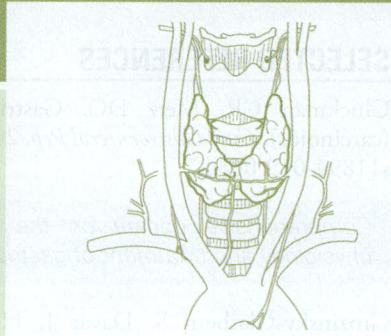

The Multiple Endocrine Neoplasia Syndromes

Samuel J. Enumah, Gerard M. Doherty, and Elizabeth G. Grubbs

The multiple endocrine neoplasia (MEN) syndromes are a consequence of genetic alterations that lead to the development of tumors in endocrine organs and tissues. MEN type 1 (MEN1) is caused by a genetic change in menin, a tumor suppressor gene. MEN type 2 (MEN2) is related to changes in the *RET* (REarranged during Transfection) proto-oncogene. MEN type 4 (MEN4) is a rare clinical entity with features similar to MEN1 but caused by a genetic mutation in the cyclin-dependent kinase CDKN1B, a tumor suppressor gene.

Each of the MEN syndromes manifests as a phenotypic expression of different tumors. MEN1 includes pituitary adenomas, parathyroid adenomas in multiple glands, and neuroendocrine tumors (NETs) of the pancreas and gastrointestinal system. MEN1 carriers may also develop thymic carcinoid tumors, lipomas, adrenal adenomas, ependymomas, and angiofibromas.[1] MEN2 is divided into MEN2A and MEN2B. Patients with MEN2A present with medullary thyroid cancer (MTC), pheochromocytomas, and parathyroid tumors. MEN2B is characterized by MTC, pheochromocytomas, mucosal neuromas, marfanoid features, and ganglioneuromatosis of the gastrointestinal tract. Management for these conditions involves screening, surveillance, and medical and surgical intervention.

MULTIPLE ENDOCRINE NEOPLASIA TYPE 1

Epidemiology and Genetics

MEN1 is rare in the general population, with a prevalence of 1 to 3 per 100,000.[2] MEN1 germline mutations are found in 1% to 18% of patients with reportedly sporadic primary hyperparathyroidism (PHPT).[3] Patients with pituitary tumors have MEN1 less than 3% of the time. For NETs, the presence of MEN1 mutations varies based on the type of tumor. The clinical manifestations of MEN1 vary across all ages. In general, clinical evidence of MEN1 develops by 50 years of age in 75% of individuals with MEN1

mutations. There does not appear to be any racial or ethnic predisposition, and autosomal dominance inheritance suggests that MEN1 affects male and female patients equally, though this may vary by subtype of clinically evident tumors.[4,5] Overall survival in MEN1 carriers is difficult to estimate and varies because many series combine patients with similar manifestations of a particular clinical entity. For example, in patients presenting with MEN1-related gastrinomas, survival after 5 and 10 years was 83% and 65%, respectively.[6]

MEN1 is a hereditary syndrome inherited in an autosomal dominant pattern. It develops after a germline mutation and loss of heterozygosity in the MEN1 (menin) gene, leading to the development of tumors. Menin, found on chromosome locus 11q13, functions as a tumor suppressor gene. Tumor suppressor genes regulate cell proliferation and growth. MEN1 mutations often result in a truncated menin protein, which leads to a loss of menin expression.[7]

Genetic cloning was used to identify menin, a 610–amino acid protein.[8] Endocrine and nonendocrine cells express varying levels of menin, which is located primarily in the cell nucleus. In addition to the functions noted earlier, menin has a role as a pro-on-cogenic factor in mixed lineage leukemia (MLL) by interacting with MLL-1 fusion proteins to cause leukemia. Also, it has been linked to an increased risk of developing breast cancer, possibly through estrogen receptor regulation.[9]

More than 1600 mutations in the menin gene have been described, and roughly 15% are somatic and 85% are germline.[10] Nearly 70% of MEN1 germline mutations are considered pathogenic, often because of frame-shift mutations (42%), nonsense mutations (14%), or splicing defects (11%).[3] The mutations are spread out over the coding region as opposed to existing in clusters. Around 5% of patients with MEN1 do not have any evident germline mutation within the known coding region, and these may be related to mutations in promoter regions that have not yet been described.

Current clinical practice guidelines recommend that patients suspected to have MEN1 and relatives of patients with known MEN1 receive genetic testing.[11] Asymptomatic relatives should receive MEN1 germline mutation testing because presence and timing of clinical manifestations of the disease vary. Appropriate genetic testing can often help individuals without a mutation avoid unnecessary tumor screening. Around 10% to 20% of individuals with MEN1 may not have a mutation identified. For this reason, the diagnosis of MEN1 is made clinically in patients with two or more MEN1-associated tumors or in a patient with one MEN1-associated tumor and a first-degree relative with MEN1.[3] Regardless of a genetic or clinical diagnosis, all patients with MEN1 should undergo routine screening for various associated tumors. Of note, germline mutations of the *CDKN1B* gene are associated with the development of parathyroid adenomas, pituitary adenomas, and PNETs, and this syndrome is known as *MEN4*. Given the clinical similarity to MEN1, this may account for persons who meet clinical criteria for MEN1 but lack a known mutation of the MEN1 gene. MEN4 is a relatively newer MEN categorization, and investigation is ongoing to better understand this entity.

Clinical Presentation and Management

MEN1 is classically described as an inheritable autosomal dominant disorder that manifests as tumors of the parathyroid, pancreas, and pituitary (3 Ps). The pancreatic tumors represent a subset of the broader category of gastropancreatic NETs that are found in these patients. Patients with MEN1 also have an increased risk of developing NETs, including meningiomas, angiofibromas, carcinoid tumors, and lipomas. The most common

presentation (nearly 100% penetrance) of MEN1 involves PHPT.[2] Often characterized as four-gland hyperplasia, these patients actually have multiple parathyroid adenomas in separate glands. In many cases, the PHPT is the initial clinical presentation of the syndrome.

MEN1 affects male and female patients equally and does not appear to have any specific association with race. If left untreated, patients with MEN1 have a 50% probability of death by 50 years of age.[11] Previously, peptic ulcer disease secondary to Zollinger-Ellison syndrome (ZES) led to significant morbidity (e.g., bleeding, perforation, fistula) and mortality in this patient population. Complications from hypersecretion were the main cause of death in patients with MEN1 and ZES. However, the introduction of medications to control gastric acid production (histamine H_2 receptor antagonists and proton pump inhibitors [PPIs]) has dramatically improved control of the disease, and acute and chronic control of acid hypersecretion is possible in most patients.[12]

Signs and symptoms of MEN1 are related to involvement of specific endocrine glands or tissues and are the result of either hormone overproduction or mechanical effects of benign and malignant tumors. Thus, diagnosis of MEN1 often occurs when evidence of hormone excess or tissue involvement produces identifiable clinical manifestations leading to diagnosis of the syndrome or when asymptomatic family members screen positive for a MEN1 mutation. An algorithm for diagnosis and surveillance is demonstrated in Fig. 78.1. Given the rare nature of the disease process, recent literature highlights the lack of high-quality evidence to guide treatment in this specific population. Much of the previous information relies on observational studies.[13] Certain recommendations (screening, surveillance) may expose patients to

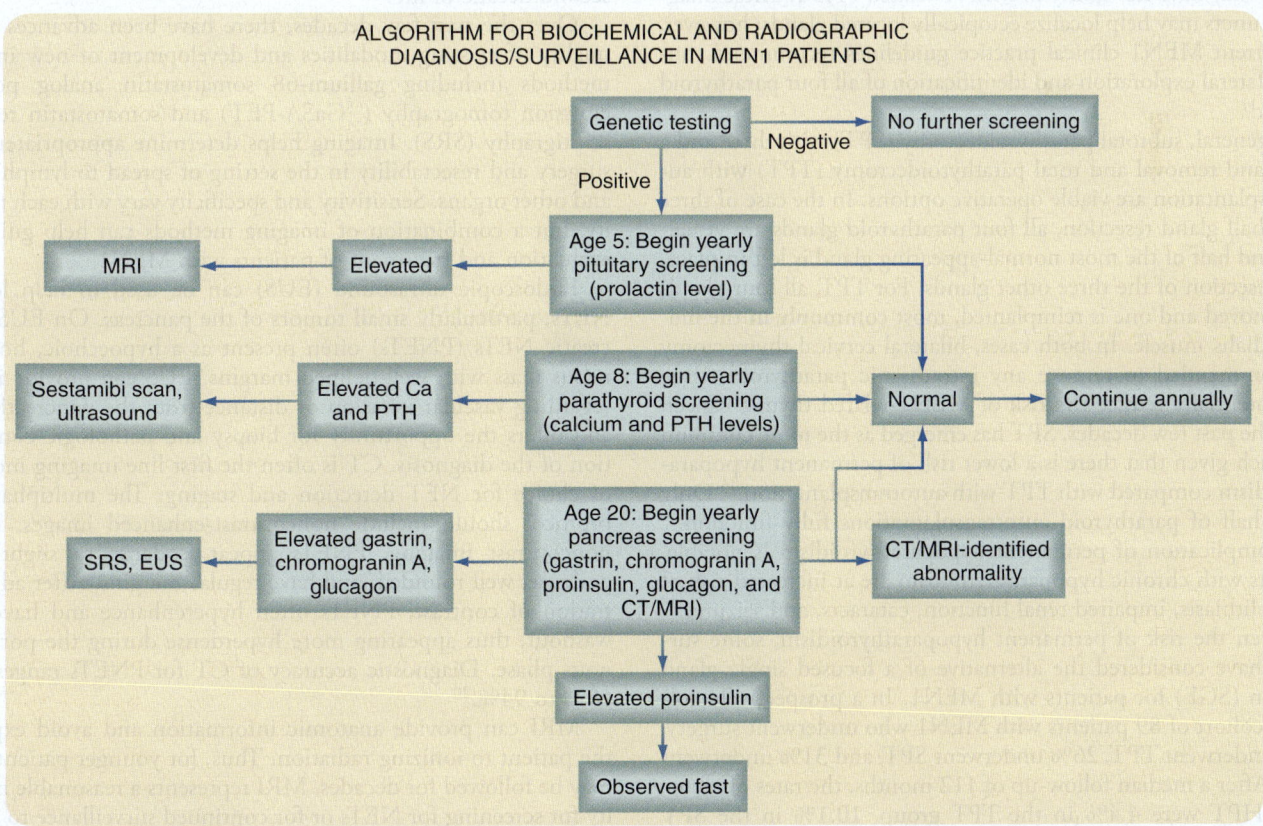

FIGURE 78.1 Algorithm for screening and management in multiple endocrine neoplasia type 1 *(MEN1)* syndromes. *CT,* Computed tomography; *EUS,* endoscopic ultrasound; *MRI,* magnetic resonance imaging; *PTH,* parathyroid hormone; *SRS,* somatostatin receptor scintigraphy.

ionizing radiation and false-positive results; each clinical decision should weigh associated benefits and risks for the individual patient. Overall, the goal of treatment rests on medical or surgical intervention to control hormonal hypersecretion or tumor spread. Although patients with MEN1 may have multiple types of tissues affected, parathyroid, enteropancreatic, and pituitary tissues are often described.

Parathyroid

PHPT is the most consistently observed feature of patients with MEN1. Similar to the sporadic form of PHPT, patients may present with evidence of diminished bone health (e.g., osteopenia, osteoporosis), kidney and ureteral stones, or general symptoms of fatigue, memory loss, depression, or anxiety. Additionally, many patients may be asymptomatic. The biochemical diagnosis of PHPT involves increased serum calcium levels and inappropriately nonsuppressed parathyroid hormone (PTH) levels. Generally, around 90% to 95% of patients with PHPT present with a sporadic form of the disorder, and 5% to 10% of PHPT is caused by germline mutations. In general, compared with the sporadic form, patients with MEN1-related PHPT present at an earlier age, with an equal male-to-female ratio, and with a greater severity of bone and renal involvement.[14]

Surgical intervention is the standard treatment for patients with symptomatic MEN1 with PHPT. The optimal timing for asymptomatic patients is not known, and surgeon experience and patient preference should be taken into account.[11] Although preoperative imaging (e.g., ultrasound, sestamibi scan, four-dimensional computed tomography [CT]) is often used in sporadic PHPT to identify potential targets for focused resection, these studies may have less utility in MEN1-related PHPT. These imaging adjuncts may help localize ectopically located glands; however, the current MEN1 clinical practice guidelines recommend routine bilateral exploration and identification of all four parathyroid glands.[11]

In general, subtotal parathyroidectomy (SPT) with three and a half gland removal and total parathyroidectomy (TPT) with autotransplantation are viable operative options. In the case of three and a half gland resection, all four parathyroid glands are visualized, and half of the most normal-appearing gland is left in place, with resection of the three other glands. For TPT, all four glands are removed and one is reimplanted, most commonly in the brachioradialis muscle. In both cases, bilateral cervical thymectomy is recommended to remove any intrathymic parathyroid tissue and potentially reduce the risk of MEN1-related thymic cancer. Over the past few decades, SPT has emerged as the more common approach given that there is a lower risk of permanent hypoparathyroidism compared with TPT with autotransplantation.[15] Only about half of parathyroid autotransplantations fully function.[16] The complication of permanent hypoparathyroidism is notable. Patients with chronic hypoparathyroidism are at increased risk of nephrolithiasis, impaired renal function, cataracts, and seizures.[17]

Given the risk of permanent hypoparathyroidism, some surgeons have considered the alternative of a focused single gland excision (SGE) for patients with MEN1. In a prospectively collected cohort of 89 patients with MEN1 who underwent surgery, 43% underwent TPT, 26% underwent SPT, and 31% underwent SGE. After a median follow-up of 112 months, the rates of recurrent PHPT were 4.4% in the TPT group, 10.1% in the SPT group, and 21.3% in the SGE group, and the rates of permanent hypoparathyroidism were 32%, 17%, and 0%, respectively.[18] A systematic review and meta-analysis involving 25 studies and 947 patients with MEN1 comparing less than subtotal parathyroidectomy (LSPT) to SPT identified that the risk of permanent hypoparathyroidism was 4% in the LSPT group and 20% in the SPT group, but the LSPT approach carried more than a fourfold increased odds of persistent hyperparathyroidism.[15] Weighing the risk of hypoparathyroidism against the likelihood of recurrence should be performed in the individual patient, but, in general, SPT is recommended as the first procedure.

Enteropancreatic Neuroendocrine Tumors

For patients with MEN1, the second most common tumors are enteropancreatic NETs. They occur in 55% to 70% of patients, and they may be functional or nonfunctional and benign or malignant.[2] Among various types, functional MEN1 tumors include gastrinomas (most common functional MEN1 tumor), insulinomas, and vasoactive intestinal peptidomas. Management aims to control hormone excess, prevent disease progression, and control symptoms. For functional tumors, hormone levels can be useful to follow over time to determine disease recurrence. For nonfunctional tumors, chromogranin A or pancreatic polypeptide may be useful. Unlike sporadic NETs, there are commonly multiple NETs in patients with MEN1. For functional NETs, screening for patients with MEN1 involves evaluation of gastrin, glucose, insulin, vasoactive intestinal peptide, glucagon, chromogranin A, and pancreatic polypeptide at 6- to 12-month intervals. Any abnormal elevation of these levels warrants further workup with imaging. For certain types of nonfunctional tumors (e.g., pancreatic), there remains debate about the optimal timing of initiating screening through use of imaging modalities (magnetic resonance imaging [MRI] or CT), but screening may start as early as the second decade of life.[19]

Over the past few decades, there have been advances in the quality of existing modalities and development of new imaging methods including gallium-68 somatostatin analog positron emission tomography (^{68}GaSA-PET) and somatostatin receptor scintigraphy (SRS). Imaging helps determine appropriateness of surgery and resectability in the setting of spread to lymph nodes and other organs. Sensitivity and specificity vary with each modality, but a combination of imaging methods can help guide the evaluation and treatment of patients with MEN1.

Endoscopic ultrasound (EUS) can be used to help localize NETs, particularly small tumors of the pancreas. On EUS, pancreatic NETs (PNETs) often present as a hypoechoic, homogeneous mass with well-defined margins. EUS can provide insight regarding vascular invasion or distance from the pancreatic duct and offers the opportunity for biopsy and pathologic confirmation of the diagnosis. CT is often the first-line imaging modality of choice for NET detection and staging. The multiphase CT protocol should include noncontrast-enhanced images. In the noncontrast imaging, PNETs appear isodense to slightly hypodense, well rounded, and have regular margins. After administration of contrast, PNETs often hyperenhance and have slow washout, thus appearing more hyperdense during the portal venous phase. Diagnostic accuracy of CT for PNETs ranges from 69% to 94%.[20]

MRI can provide anatomic information and avoid exposing the patient to ionizing radiation. Thus, for younger patients who may be followed for decades, MRI represents a reasonable modality for screening for NETs or for continued surveillance to follow known tumors longitudinally. MRI is performed in a multiphase fashion with noncontrast, arterial, and portal venous phases. Generally, the sensitivity ranges from 54% to 100% and the specificity ranges from 78% to 100% in detecting PNETs; the sensitivity and specificity increase for larger tumors.[21] On T1 imaging, PNETs appear hypoisointense amidst hyperintense pancreatic parenchyma. On T2 imaging, the lesions are hyperintense, and, similar to CT, these lesions hyperenhance during the arterial phase with slow washout.[20]

Functional imaging tests offer additional insight into enteropancreatic NETs. Various nuclear medicine tests can identify functional lesions that express somatostatin receptors (SSTRs). SSTRs are expressed in many different types of tissue including the pituitary, pancreas, gastrointestinal tract, thyroid, kidney, blood vessels, and peripheral nervous system, and different tumors (e.g., carcinoids, pheochromocytomas, paragangliomas, neuroblastomas) show a wide variety of SSTR expression. The radiotracers used are somatostatin analogues and have a high affinity for specific subtypes of SSTRs. SSTR scintigraphy has a sensitivity that ranges from 40% to 70% and a specificity that ranges from 92% to 100%. Alternatively, ^{68}GaSA-PET CT has a sensitivity ranging from 88% to 93% and specificity ranging from 88% to 95%.[20] This functional PET imaging technique has lower radiation dose and lower liver uptake compared with SRS. Additionally, PET/CT may play a vital role in detecting metastases when other cross-sectional imaging has failed to identify certain lesions. Dual tracer imaging with 68Ga-DOTATATE and 18F-fluorodeoxyglucose (18F-FDG) PET/CT may offer a promising opportunity to help identify local and metastatic NETs and may be able to predict response to treatment.[22]

For patients with MEN1, approximately 50% of functional enteropancreatic NETs that develop are gastrin-secreting tumors called *gastrinomas*. Conversely, 20% of patients with gastrinomas have MEN1. The typical appearance of a gastrinoma is seen in Fig. 78.2. Classically, these patients have ZES, which is characterized by recurrent multiple peptic ulcers, abdominal pain, chronic diarrhea, and gastroesophageal reflux. Providers should maintain a high index of suspicion in patients with recurrent ulcers, multiple ulcers that occur in atypical locations, that fail to respond to usual therapy, or that occur in the setting of PHPT. Diagnosis of ZES requires the presence of both acid in the stomach and elevated fasting serum gastrin levels after the patient has stopped taking acid-suppressive medication (generally 2 weeks off PPIs and 2 days off H$_2$ receptor antagonists). The diagnosis is definitive if the gastrin level is greater than 1000 pg/mL with gastric acid present (which may be determined by measuring a gastric pH level). Atrophic gastritis (pernicious anemia) can be a confounding diagnosis with elevated gastrin levels, but there is no acid in the stomach. In patients whose levels do not meet the diagnostic threshold, a secretin stimulation test can be performed. Serum gastrin levels are measured at 2 and 15 minutes after intravenous secretin administration, and levels greater than or equal to 200 pg/mL are considered diagnostic of ZES.

The role of surgical management for MEN1-associated gastrinoma remains controversial. Patients with MEN1 often have multiple tumors and nodal metastases, and so the cure rate is relatively low, though the disease is relatively indolent in terms of metastatic disease affecting survival. Medical management with PPIs and H$_2$ blockers is often deployed given that it is difficult, if not impossible, to cure patients with MEN1 or achieve long-term eugastrinemia. Providers can work with patients to determine their preferences and tailor the surgical approach individually based on malignant behavior and morbidity involved in resection. Of note, in patients with co-occurring PHPT and gastrinoma, parathyroidectomy is recommended because surgical resection has been shown to be associated with decreased basal acid output and lower gastrin levels.[23] Hypercalcemia is associated with an increase in circulating gastrin levels, and parathyroidectomy may help lower calcium and gastrin levels.

Insulinomas are characterized by hypersecretion of insulin causing hypoglycemia. The β-islet cell tumors secrete insulin even when plasma glucose concentrations are low. Hyperinsulinemia leads to decreased gluconeogenesis and increased glycogen synthesis, which contributes to hypoglycemia. Incidence is 1 to 4 per million per year. Around 7% of cases are associated with MEN1 syndrome.[24] Insulinomas represent up to 30% of functional PNETs in patients with MEN1. Patients often present with "Whipple triad," including (1) fasting glucose levels less than 50 mg/dL, (2) symptoms of hypoglycemia (headache, palpitations, confusion, hunger, fatigue), and (3) resolution of symptoms upon administration of glucose. The hypoglycemic episodes are divided into neuroglycopenic and adrenergic categories. Neuroglycopenic symptoms are caused by a reduction in central nervous system glucose supply and lead to impaired cognition, disorientation, memory deficits, and visual disturbances. Adrenergic symptoms are caused by sympathetic nervous system activation and include anxiety, tremor, diaphoresis, and palpitations. Patients often experience symptoms during fasting periods (e.g., upon awakening from overnight fast or during exercise).

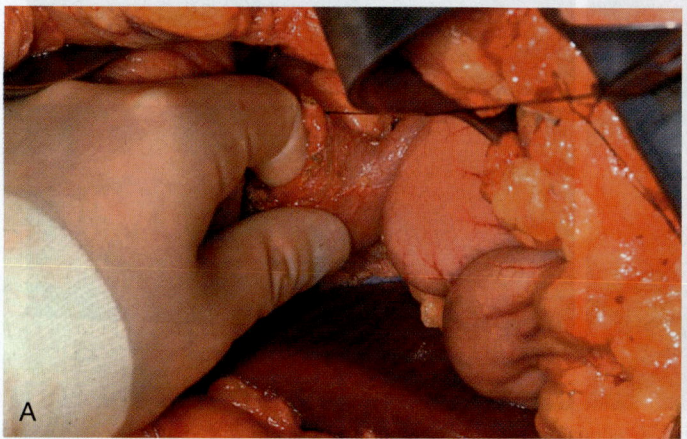
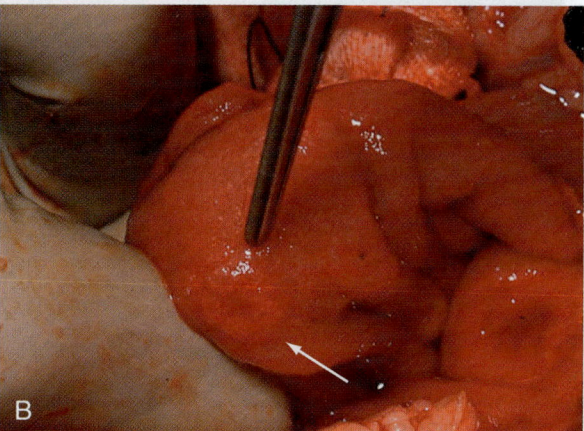

FIGURE 78.2 Gastrinoma, intraoperative findings. (A) Duodenotomy and palpation of the duodenal wall. (B) Typical appearance of a gastrinoma in the duodenal wall, indicated by *arrow*.

The differential diagnosis for patients with hypoglycemia is broad, and it is important to consider alternative explanations when patients present with low blood glucose. Exogenous insulin administration remains high on the differential, and a detailed history should be obtained from the patient to rule out this possible cause. Additionally, oral hypoglycemics, renal failure, liver dysfunction, autoimmune disease (e.g., systemic lupus erythematosus), and multiple myeloma can all contribute to states of insulin biochemical disturbances.[25]

The diagnosis of insulinoma is made during a monitored 72-hour supervised fast during which plasma glucose, insulin, and C-peptide levels are measured every 6 hours. An elevated insulin level with a low glucose level is diagnostic. However, a 48-hour fast may be adequate and as accurate and may replace the 72-hour fast. Oral hypoglycemic agents should be discontinued. To establish the diagnosis, these six criteria may be met: blood glucose ≤40 mg/dL, insulin >36 pmol/L, proinsulin ≥5 pmol/L, C-peptide ≥200 pmol/L, β-hydroxybutyrate ≤2.7 mmol/L, and absence of urine or plasma sulfonylurea metabolites.[25]

Insulinomas may be multifocal and occur throughout the pancreas and are best imaged by CT and EUS. They can be difficult to locate and may be identified at operative exploration with or without intraoperative ultrasound, whose sensitivity ranges from 70% to 95%. Fig. 78.3 demonstrates the use of intraoperative ultrasound to identify an insulinoma. Anatomic imaging, including CT, MRI, and EUS, has varying sensitivities—all less than 50%. Arterial calcium stimulation with selective hepatic vein sampling was historically used, but the invasive nature of this test has led to decreased use. Glucagon-like peptide-1 receptor (GLP-1R) imaging offers an alternative less invasive option given that GLP-1R is mainly expressed on pancreatic β cells. Intraoperative aspiration of the lesion and use of a rapid assay for insulin can confirm the diagnosis.

Surgery is the mainstay of treatment for insulinomas, but medical options exist. After confirmation of the diagnosis, many patients may receive diazoxide, which acts on potassium channels on β-pancreatic islet cells and contributes to decrease insulin secretion.[25] Diazoxide can be given in doses of 50 to 300 mg/day, and side effects include congestive heart failure, peripheral edema, renal dysfunction, and weight gain. Diazoxide should be stopped at least 1 week before surgery to avoid intraoperative hypotension. Potential additional medical therapies also include phenytoin, verapamil, streptozocin, and everolimus. Surgical intervention commonly involves enucleation, and this approach is generally used for benign, superficial tumors less than 2 cm. For larger tumors and those with suspicion for malignant features, a formal anatomic resection is often undertaken. Lesions of the distal body and tail undergo distal pancreatectomy, whereas patients with larger insulinomas localized to the head of the pancreas may undergo pancreaticoduodenectomy. In patients with MEN1 with multiple pancreatic tumors, it may be helpful to ensure that the functional tumor is included in the resection using a study such as selective arterial calcium infusion with hepatic vein insulin sampling. The remaining functional tumors (glucagonomas, VIPomas, and somatostatinomas) comprise less than 5% of functional PNETs in MEN1.

Most enteropancreatic NETs in patients with MEN1 are nonfunctional PNETs. These lesions do not have an associated clinical

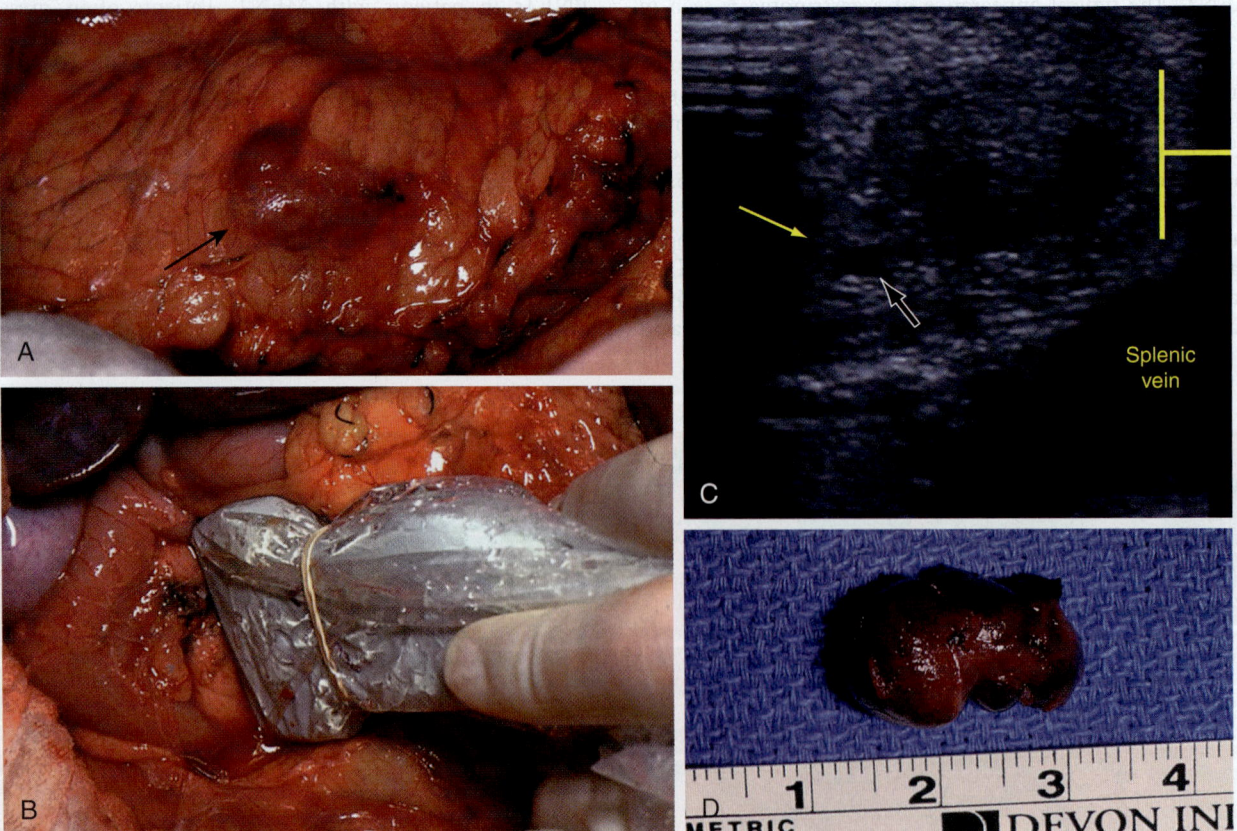

FIGURE 78.3 Insulinoma. (A) Insulinoma, reddish in appearance, posterior body of pancreas, indicated by *arrow.* (B) Intraoperative ultrasound used to identify insulinoma and define relationship to vessels and pancreatic duct. (C) Ultrasound image of insulinoma. (D) Resected insulinoma.

syndrome and are diagnosed on surveillance imaging or after the development of symptoms related to mass effects of tumor. For patients with MEN1, surveillance for nonfunctional PNETs should begin at age 13 years.[19] Surgical decision-making centers around the need for multiple operations and potential for the development of multiple tumors and metastases. In a systematic review of nonfunctioning PNETs encompassing 13 studies and 370 unique patients, tumor size and grade were the most important prognostic factors.[26] These findings suggest that tumors less than 2 cm can undergo watchful waiting and serial imaging. Higher-grade lesions may be considered for surgical resection regardless of size, though data are insufficient to provide a clear recommendation.[27] Surgical resection is recommended for nonfunctioning PNETs ≥2 cm.

Pituitary Gland

The prevalence of pituitary adenomas in patients with MEN1 ranges from 30% to 60% and often occurs in the fourth decade of life.[28] One percent of patients with pituitary adenomas have MEN1. Patients with MEN1 often present with PHPT before showing clinical evidence of a pituitary adenoma. Pituitary tumors can cause symptoms through hormone secretion or from local effects of the tumor. Most tumors are benign, unifocal, and secrete hormones including prolactin, growth hormone, or corticotropin. In a group of 268 patients with MEN1, 51.8% had pituitary adenomas and 57% of these were functional, most commonly prolactin-secreting adenomas.[28] Screening for pituitary adenomas should include annual prolactin and insulin-like growth factor-1 (IGF-1) measurements beginning at age 5 years and MRI evaluation every 3 years.[29] MEN1-related pituitary tumors are larger and more often secrete multiple hormones (e.g., prolactin and adrenocorticotropin-secreting hormone) compared with the sporadic form. Treatment for pituitary tumors in MEN1 includes both medical and surgical therapy. Medical therapy aims to control hormone excess. Unfortunately, a lower proportion of patients with MEN1 with functional pituitary adenomas achieve normalization of pituitary hormone concentrations compared with the sporadic tumor population. Surgical intervention is reserved for patients who fail to normalize hormone levels after initiation of the appropriate pharmacologic intervention or those who develop symptoms related to mass effect on the optic chiasm.

Other Tumors

Other MEN1-related tumors include carcinoids of the thymus, bronchi, and gastrointestinal tract; adrenocortical tumors; and cutaneous tumors (e.g., lipomas, facial angiofibromas, and collagenomas). Thymic carcinoid tumors are likely to be malignant, aggressive, and have a poor prognosis. Unfortunately, there is not an optimal screening method given the lack of data. Nevertheless, CT and MRI are recommended every 1 to 2 years for earlier detection. Surgery is the preferred treatment. Historically, transcervical thymectomy was thought to prevent thymic carcinoids. However, in a review of 122 patients with MEN1 who underwent cervical thymectomy at the time of parathyroidectomy, only one incidental thymic carcinoid was discovered.[30] Additionally, nine patients developed thymic carcinoid tumors during the follow-up period after a median of 36 months. Thus, preventive transcervical thymectomy is not recommended outside of planned parathyroidectomy, and specific follow-up and imaging protocols may allow for detection of thymic carcinoids. Adrenal tumors are common, and approximately 20% of patients have some adrenal hyperplasia. Compared with incidental adrenal tumors, patients

with MEN1 exhibit adrenocortical carcinoma and primary hyperaldosteronism more frequently and pheochromocytoma less frequently.[31] There are no established guidelines for management of adrenal tumors for the MEN1 population. Recommended management is similar to incidental adrenal masses, and surgical resection is indicated for size (≥4 cm), growth, suspicion for malignancy, and excess hormone production.

MULTIPLE ENDOCRINE NEOPLASIA TYPE 2

MEN2 is an autosomal dominant hereditary syndrome caused by germline mutations in the *RET* proto-oncogene. MEN2 is divided into MEN2A and MEN2B and includes various tumor types (Fig. 78.4). MEN2A classically presents with MTC, pheochromocytoma, and PHPT. MEN2A can be further subclassified into specific phenotypes including classical MEN2A, MEN2A with cutaneous lichen amyloidosis, MEN2A with Hirschsprung disease, and familial MTC. MEN2B is characterized by MTC, pheochromocytoma, ganglioneuromas, and marfanoid features. In the following sections, the genetics, clinical presentation, and management of MEN2 are detailed.

Epidemiology and Genetics

The prevalence of MEN 2A and MEN2B is approximately 20 and 2 per million, and the incidence for these two entities ranges from 8 to 28 and 1 to 3 per million live births, respectively.[32] The *RET* proto-oncogene is located on chromosome 10q11.2 and codes for a tyrosine kinase membrane receptor. Each of the MEN2 syndromes occurs as a result of a *RET* germline mutation. Mutations that result in the development of MTC are missense mutations that cause a gain-of-function mutation. The *RET* protein is formed by an extracellular ligand-binding domain, a transmembrane domain, and a cytoplasmic tyrosine kinase domain (Fig. 78.5). The intracellular tyrosine kinase subdomains are involved in intracellular signal transduction pathways. Unlike other receptor tyrosine kinases, *RET* activation occurs through a multiprotein ligand complex as opposed to direct receptor ligand interaction.[32] Activation of the *RET* complex results in *RET* dimerization and promotes cell signaling, differentiation, growth, and survival. Specific mutations in *RET* can result in unregulated gene activation and tumor development.

RET participates in a number of cell signaling pathways and is expressed in multiple neural crest tissues, including thyroid parafollicular cells (C cells), parathyroid glands, adrenal chromaffin cells, enteric ganglia, and peripheral and central neurons. Mice with mutated *RET* genes have renal agenesis and lack neurons throughout the digestive tract, suggesting that *RET* also plays a role in renal and neuronal development. Inactivating *RET* mutations are associated with Hirschsprung disease in humans, a defect in the development of enteric neurons resulting in megacolon and constipation in infancy. Unlike MEN1, strong genotype-phenotype correlations exist in MEN2, and specific *RET* mutations can predict the onset and aggressiveness of the disease. Prophylactic thyroidectomy is offered to improve survival. Patients with reportedly sporadic MTC may carry *RET* mutations, and they should be offered genetic testing.

For patients with MEN2 clinical presentation, the standard of care includes sequencing of the *RET* gene to identify germline mutations. Providers can anticipate and test for involved coding regions related to the MEN2 type known to the kindred or suspected based on clinical findings. All offspring of known kindreds should be offered genetic counseling and genetic testing early in

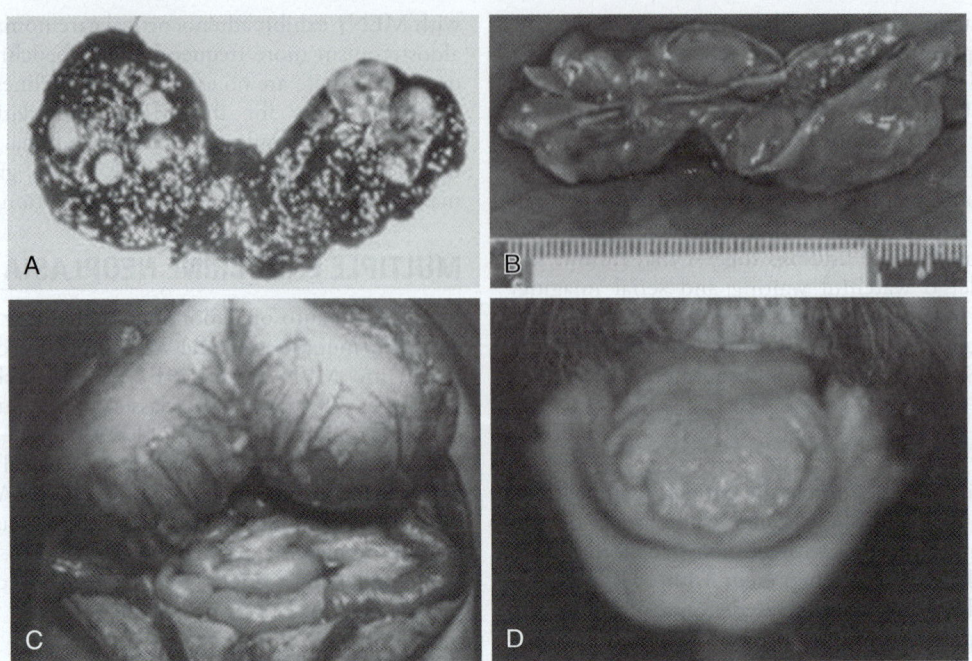

FIGURE 78.4 Clinical manifestations of multiple endocrine neoplasia type 2 (MEN2) syndromes. (A) Multifocal medullary thyroid cancer. (B) Adrenal medullary hyperplasia. (C) Megacolon in Hirschsprung disease. (D) Mucosal neuromas found in MEN2B.

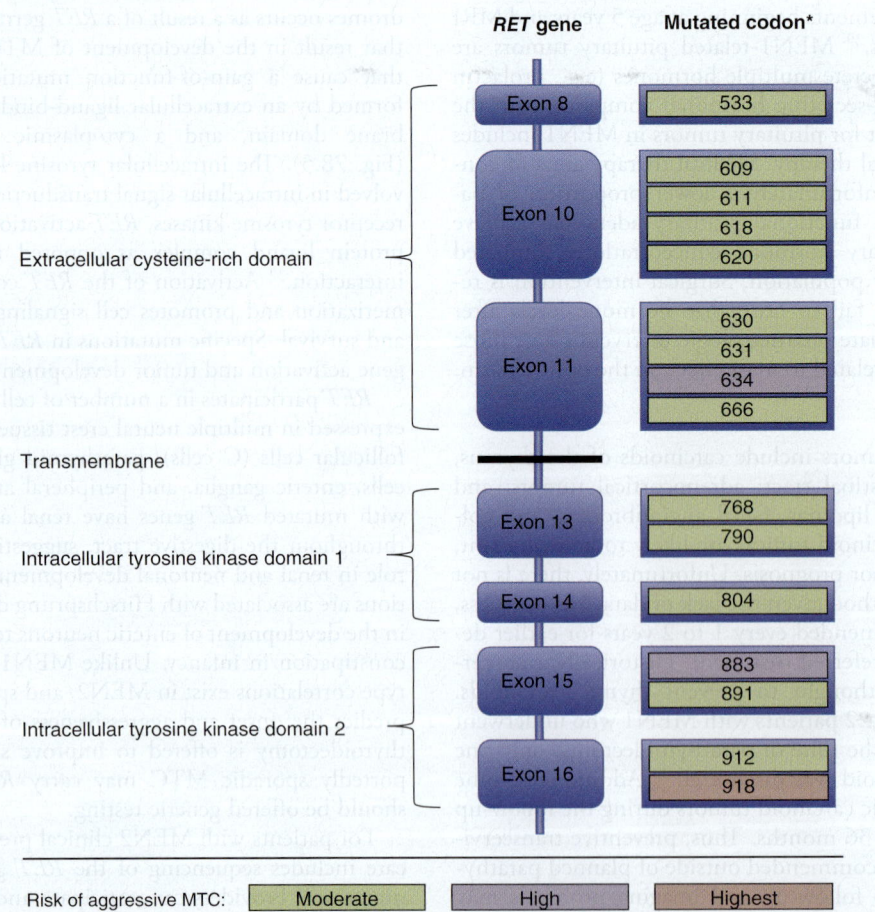

FIGURE 78.5 *RET* gene codons according to exon and medullary thyroid cancer (MTC) risk group. (Reprinted from Mathiesen JS, Effraimidis G, Rossing M, et al. Multiple endocrine neoplasia type 2: a review. *Semin Cancer Biol.* 2022;79:163-179.) * see Table 2 in the original source article for specific mutations.

life.[33] In certain cases, the presenting tumor known to occur within MEN2 may be the first evidence of the syndrome. Further, some presentations may occur as de novo mutations, and the absence of family history should not preclude testing. Additional recommendations for testing include infants or young children with Hirschsprung disease, parents whose infants or children have the physical phenotype of MEN2B, and patients with cutaneous lichen amyloidosis.[33]

CLINICAL PRESENTATION AND MANAGEMENT

Multiple Endocrine Neoplasia Type 2A

MEN2A is the most common subtype of the MEN2 syndromes, comprising the majority of cases (95%). The hallmark characteristic of MEN2A is the development of MTC in nearly 100% of patients, though there are mutations with lower or later in life penetrance patterns. In addition to MTC, pheochromocytoma develops in 30% to 50% of patients and PHPT in up to 5% to 15%.[32] The degree of penetrance of each tumor type is associated with specific codon mutations, and all patients are at risk for the development of multiple tumors.

MEN2A contains four subclassifications: classical MEN2A, MEN2A with cutaneous lichen amyloidosis, MEN2A with Hirschsprung disease, and familial MTC (FMTC). Cutaneous lichen amyloidosis is uncommon and typically occurs with codon 634 mutations. It is characterized by the symptom of pruritus, and it is thought that repeated scratching leads to amyloid deposition in the papillary dermis of the skin. As a result, patients develop cutaneous plaques, often located on the back. In this group, the prevalence of MTC, pheochromocytoma, and PHPT is 95%, 50%, and 5%, respectively.[32] Hirschsprung disease may also occur in patients with MEN2A. The disease is characterized by the congenital absence of ganglion cells within the myenteric and submucosal plexus of the distal colon. In newborns, the presentation often includes abdominal distention, constipation, and megacolon that occurs because of aganglionosis. In patients with MEN2A/Hirschsprung disease, there are mutations in codons 609, 618, or 620. In these kindreds, nearly 20% have Hirschsprung disease, and patients with MEN2A should be counseled regarding the possibility of the disease in offspring. Hirschsprung disease occurring outside of the setting of MEN2A is from inactivating, or loss-of-function, RET mutations. Hirschsprung disease affects approximately 7% of patients with MEN2A overall. In this group, the prevalence of MTC, pheochromocytoma, and PHPT is 77%, 17%, and 3%, respectively.[32]

Over time, multiple definitions of FMTC have emerged. FMTC is characterized by the identification of a RET mutation in families with MTC with no history of pheochromocytoma or PHPT. Although all patients ultimately develop MTC, on average, they are diagnosed in their mid-40s, approximately 20 years later than MTC associated with MEN2A. Multiple RET germline variants of different codons (e.g., 533, 768, and 804) are associated with FMTC. Many of the common variants are able to cause pheochromocytoma or PHPT, which makes it difficult to distinguish between classic MEN2A and FMTC.[32]

Multiple Endocrine Neoplasia Type 2B

Approximately 5% of MEN2 cases fall within the classification of MEN2B. As in MEN2A, the hallmark characteristic of MEN2B is the development of MTC. Approximately 50% of patients with MEN2B develop pheochromocytomas. Patients with MEN2B have a characteristic appearance with elongated facies, a marfanoid body habitus, ophthalmologic and skeletal abnormalities (e.g., pectus excavatum and scoliosis), and mucosal neuromas of the lips and tongue. Ganglioneuromatosis throughout the gastrointestinal tract contributes to esophageal dysmotility, abdominal bloating, intermittent constipation, and diarrhea. MEN2B often develops in infancy and tends to be aggressive with early metastasis. The majority of patients with MEN2B have germline mutations in exon 16, codon M918T, whereas less than 5% have mutations in codon A883F. MTC is the cause of death in approximately 65% of patients with the M918T variant.[34] Those with A883F mutations may have a milder, less aggressive form of MTC.

Medullary Thyroid Cancer

MTC represents less than 5% of all thyroid cancers.[32] Unlike papillary and follicular thyroid cancers, MTC arises from the parafollicular C cells, which produce calcitonin. Treatments such as suppression of thyroid-stimulating hormone and radioactive iodine (RAI) are not used, as C cells are not sensitive to these therapies. Approximately 25% of MTC is familial, and C-cell hyperplasia precedes the development of MTC. Although MTC may present as an indolent malignancy, there are distinct differences in outcomes among different codon mutations. In a German single-center database of 263 patients with MTC who underwent an operation, overall 10-year survival was 76.%, 94.3%, and 89.9% in the highest risk (codon 918), high (codons 634 and 883), and moderate risk (all other RET mutations) groups, respectively.[35] Independent predictors of worse disease-specific survival were increasing age, stage III/IV at diagnosis, and highest-risk group designation. Within MEN2A, the time of onset of MTC differs among genotypes, although the survival is the same once MTC is diagnosed.[36]

Once clinically apparent, MTC may present as a central neck mass. Symptoms from local effects such as compression or hoarseness may be present because of tumor invasion. MTC may be multifocal, and total thyroidectomy is recommended—certainly in those individuals harboring a germline mutation. Diagnosis can be made with fine-needle aspiration biopsy, and, in addition to the presence of parafollicular cells and staining for calcitonin, the tissue has amyloid staining properties in most cases. Importantly, amyloid goiter secondary to amyloid light chain amyloidosis can also present with amyloid deposits within the thyroid, but this is rare.[37] Nearly half of patients have lymph node metastases if the diagnosis is made clinically rather than based on calcitonin levels. Evaluation for lymph node disease should be done, including the central compartment (level VI) and the lateral compartment (levels II, III, IV, and V). MTC with distant metastases (outside of the neck) is considered incurable. Nearly 20% of patients with MTC with a palpable neck mass have metastases at diagnosis. In a single-center study, the most common sites of metastasis were lung (52%), bone (28%), and the mediastinum (20%).[38]

C cells secrete calcitonin, which is a useful surrogate marker for both diagnosis and recurrence as calcitonin is produced by nearly all MTC. Historically, provocative testing for calcitonin with pentagastrin was performed as a screening test; however, pentagastrin is no longer available in the United States. Most MTCs produce carcinoembryonic antigen (CEA), and CEA levels are often helpful for monitoring patients. However, CEA can be normal in advanced disease so it may play a limited role.[39]

Ultrasound is the most sensitive method of imaging the neck in patients with primary, persistent, or recurrent MTC and is useful for obtaining fine-needle aspiration biopsies of either thyroid nodules or suspicious-appearing lymph nodes in the neck. CT of the neck may be useful in planning surgery with apparently bulky disease. CT and MRI may be used to evaluate for metastatic disease for the chest and abdomen. In some cases of MTC, the tumor expresses SSTRs, and ^{68}Ga-DOTA-somatostatin analogue PET/CT may offer additional information regarding sites of disease. However, the prevalence of tumor avidity on these imaging scans may be low in the setting of metastatic disease.[40]

Surgery for Medullary Thyroid Cancer

Surgery for MTC in patients with MEN2 occurs in one of two settings: (1) to resect clinically apparent disease diagnosed by the finding of a biopsy-proven thyroid cancer or cervical malignant lymphadenopathy or (2) to prevent potential tumor development or spread in the prophylactic setting. For patients with clinically evident disease, preoperative workup includes a biochemical evaluation (calcitonin and CEA) as well as imaging to determine the extent of tumor involvement. Depending on preoperative calcitonin level, workup may also include cross-sectional imaging of the chest, abdomen, and pelvis to evaluate for distant metastases. Additionally, preoperative plasma or 24-hour urine metanephrines is necessary to exclude the possibility of a concomitant pheochromocytoma. If discovered, surgery for pheochromocytoma should precede thyroidectomy.

Total thyroidectomy should be performed in all patients with hereditary MTC because approximately 90% of patients with a familial form of MTC will have bilobar, multifocal disease. The initial operation should include a bilateral central (level VI) lymph node dissection given that the rate of lymph node metastases to level VI is high.[41] Additionally, reoperation carries higher risks of recurrent laryngeal nerve injury and hypoparathyroidism. Both the ipsilateral and contralateral lateral nodal compartments (levels II–V) are also frequently involved. The occurrence rates of lateral node metastases depend on primary tumor size as well as extent of involvement of the central compartment, and preoperative calcitonin and CEA levels can positively correlate with the presence of lateral node metastases.[33] Guidelines recommend a patient-tailored approach when considering lateral neck dissection at the time of the initial operation because the compartment is anatomically separate from the central neck. Careful attention should be paid to the identification of the parathyroid glands at operation. Ideally, they should be maintained in situ, but in situations where this is not possible, they may be autotransplanted into either the sternocleidomastoid muscle or to the brachioradialis muscle of the forearm depending on the likelihood of developing PHPT.

The goal of preventive surgery in patients with *RET* mutations is to limit the potential for metastatic spread of MTC and to improve overall survival. Improved survival is linked to performing thyroidectomy and central node dissection when calcitonin levels are either undetectable or very low and when there is no clinically apparent MTC. Therefore, preventive thyroidectomy is recommended in infants, children, and adolescents, and recommendations are stratified according to the mutation present.[33]

In the 2015 American Thyroid Association (ATA) guidelines, the management of MTC was updated.[33] Moderate-risk carriers (ATA-MOD) include all *RET* mutations other than M918T, C634, and A883F, and these individuals should begin annual screening with physical and ultrasound examination as well as calcitonin measurements done at 6- to 12-month intervals beginning at the age of 5 years. The timing of thyroidectomy can then

be determined using calcitonin levels. The follow-up period in this group may extend for several years, and there is potential for loss of continuity, and these factors should be considered when timing preventive surgery. Those in the ATA-H risk category (C634 or A883F mutations) should be considered for a preventive thyroidectomy performed at the age of 5 years, or earlier if serum calcitonin levels dictate otherwise. Inclusion of central lymph node dissection at the time of total thyroidectomy is based on preoperative calcitonin levels as well as intraoperative inspection of lymph nodes. For the ATA-HST risk category (M918T), patients should have a total thyroidectomy within the first year of life. Surgeons may perform central lymph node dissection at the initial operation based on the presence of clinically suspicious level VI lymph nodes and their ability to identify and preserve parathyroid glands.[31] Children operated on at an earlier age are more likely to have a biochemical cure and improved survival. In a cohort of 345 patients with MEN2B, early thyroidectomy (before 1 year) was compared with post–1 year thyroidectomy, and 83% of patients who underwent early thyroidectomy were in biochemical remission compared with 15% in the post–1 year group.[34]

Outcomes for patients with MTC are largely dependent on the age and stage at the time of surgical management. Ultimately, carriers of *RET* mutations require lifelong follow-up not only for detection of recurrent MTC but also to monitor and adjust thyroid hormone levels after total thyroidectomy. Calcitonin and CEA levels should be measured 3 to 6 months postoperatively, and future cadence of follow-up based on this result and subsequent doubling time of calcitonin and CEA.

Recurrent and Metastatic Disease

Approximately 50% of patients with MTC have either persistent or recurrent disease after initial operation. After surgery, these patients are identified by physical examination (e.g., palpable neck mass), rising calcitonin levels, or radiographic abnormalities. Depending on the degree to which calcitonin rises, distant metastatic disease should be considered and evaluated. Regional recurrences limited to the neck are best managed with repeat operation versus continued observation for small-volume stable disease. Reoperative neck surgery should be focused on treating compartments with imageable or biopsy-proven disease, with the operation done in a compartment-oriented fashion for previously nonoperated compartments.

Historically, limited options beyond surgery existed for management. Postoperative RAI is not indicated. External beam radiation therapy and traditional chemotherapy are of limited benefit for the management of recurrent disease in the neck. Recently, targeted therapies involving tyrosine kinase inhibitors have emerged as potential agents for metastatic MTC and *RET*-fusion thyroid carcinomas. Vandetanib and cabozantinib are oral agents that target *RET,* vascular endothelial growth factor (VEGF), and epidermal growth factor receptor (EGFR). In a trial of 331 patients, the median progression-free survival was 21.4 months in the vandetanib group compared with 8.4 months in the placebo group.[42] In this trial, nearly 36% of patients receiving vandetanib required dose reductions, often because of side effects. More recently, specific *RET* kinase inhibitors have emerged (e.g., selpercatinib, pralsetinib), and these agents appear to have fewer side effects and have demonstrated notable responses for MTC patients.[43,44] A clinical trial comparing the progression-free survival of selpercatinib versus vandetanib is ongoing and may soon offer evidence to support certain systemic treatments in *RET* mutant MTC.[45]

Pheochromocytoma

Pheochromocytomas are tumors arising from the chromaffin cells of the adrenal medulla (Fig. 78.6). These cells secrete catecholamines, which are produced in excess in the setting of a pheochromocytoma. The typical clinical presentation includes sweating, tremulousness, headache, flushing, palpitations, anxiety, and episodic hypertension. Typical age at diagnosis is in the fourth or fifth decade of life. Identification of a pheochromocytoma before surgical management of MTC is critical to avoid intraoperative hypertensive crisis and stroke or death. If a pheochromocytoma is identified, then in almost all situations, an adrenalectomy would be performed first to normalize catecholamine levels before thyroidectomy.

Compared with sporadic pheochromocytomas, MEN2-associated pheochromocytomas occur in younger patients, are often bilateral, and have higher baseline metanephrine levels. In a series of 345 patients with MEN2B, 50% presented with bilateral pheochromocytomas by age 30 years, and a similar penetrance was found for patients with MEN2A *RET* 634 codon by age 40 years.[46] Overall, penetrance is dependent on the specific *RET* mutation. MEN2 pheochromocytomas tend to be benign, but given the potential for recurrence and bilaterality, patients require lifelong monitoring. Pheochromocytomas can be malignant, but this is uncommon, occurring less than 5% of the time.[46]

Screening recommendations are stratified by the ATA risk categories, where highest-, high-, and moderate-risk patients begin screening at the ages of 11, 11, and 16 years, respectively.[33] Measurements of plasma free metanephrines and normetanephrines or 24-hour urinary metanephrines and normetanephrines should be done annually, at a minimum. If elevated levels are identified, imaging should be done with either CT or MRI of the abdomen to evaluate for the presence of an adrenal mass.

Patients confirmed to have a pheochromocytoma should undergo surgical resection. Patients should receive preoperative α-blockade to minimize the risk of intraoperative hypertensive crisis. The procedure of choice for operative management is either a laparoscopic or retroperitoneoscopic adrenalectomy, and the selection of the procedure depends on the expertise of the surgeon. The safety of either of these procedures is well established. Minimally invasive adrenalectomies are associated with a shorter hospital stay and less postoperative pain compared with open adrenalectomy. Laparoscopic transabdominal adrenalectomy may be better for larger lesions. If there is any radiologic concern for malignancy (e.g., invasion of adjacent organs or structures), an open adrenalectomy is preferred.

A major concern surrounding operation for MEN2 pheochromocytoma is that it is likely to either be bilateral or recur over time, and patients will potentially need multiple operations. When possible, a cortical-sparing or partial adrenalectomy should be performed to avoid permanent adrenal insufficiency. Situations where cortical-sparing adrenalectomy is preferred include patients who have had the contralateral adrenal gland removed and small tumors where there is a portion of normal-appearing adrenal gland that could potentially be left in situ. Treatment plans should be individualized, and the decision to perform a cortical-sparing adrenalectomy should be weighed against the risks of developing another pheochromocytoma over the patient's lifetime.

Primary Hyperparathyroidism

Debate exists about the prevalence of PHPT in the MEN2 population given different definitions of PHPT across studies. Approximately 8% to 35% of patients with MEN2A may develop PHPT, though the likelihood of development may be based on which mutation is present.[47] PHPT tends to occur earlier and is commonly seen in patients with codon 634 mutations. The recommended age at which screening and annual surveillance should begin follows the recommendations for pheochromocytoma. Moderate- and high-risk-category patients should begin annual testing of calcium and PTH levels at the ages of 11 and 16 years, respectively.[33]

Options for surgical management are similar for patients without MEN2 and include focused parathyroidectomy (removal of abnormal-appearing glands), SPT, and TPT with autotransplantation. Over time, the surgical management of PHPT in the setting of MEN2A has evolved to focus on only removing abnormal-appearing glands and monitoring intraoperative PTH levels.

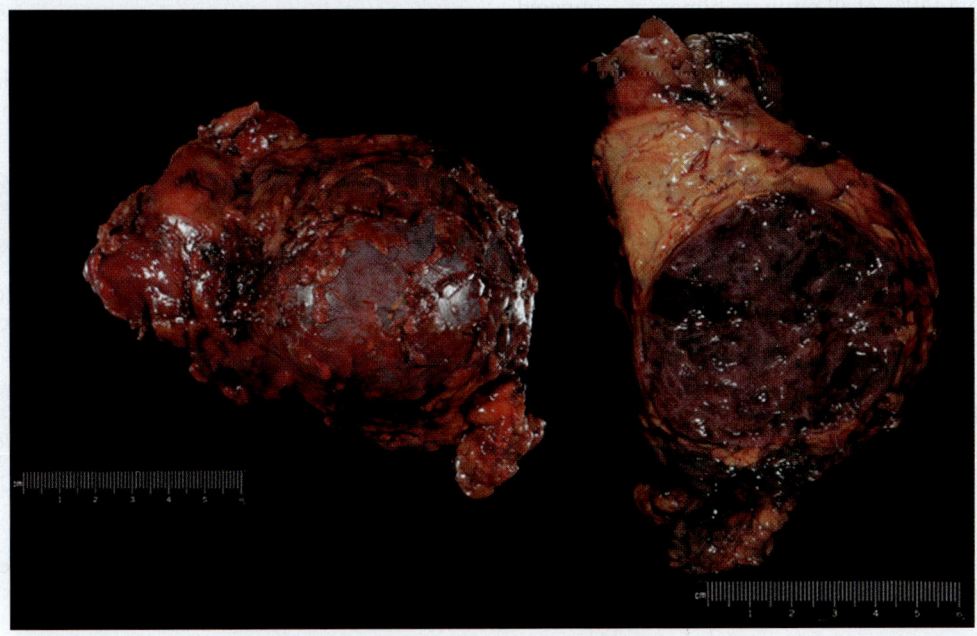

FIGURE 78.6 Resected pheochromocytoma specimen.

The rate of both persistent and recurrent disease is low even with focused or image-guided parathyroidectomy. In planning for a focused parathyroidectomy, preoperative imaging should be obtained. Patients who develop PHPT after a thyroidectomy for MTC should have imaging before undergoing reoperative neck surgery to localize the abnormal gland or glands.

MULTIPLE ENDOCRINE NEOPLASIA TYPE 4

MEN4 is a rare and more recently categorized group of the MEN syndromes. Classically, MEN4 shares clinical similarity with MEN1, and patients present with PHPT, pituitary adenomas, and NETs. However, MEN4 differs from MEN1 in that patients often present at an older age and with milder clinical features.[48] In 2002, a novel MEN syndrome was identified in rats and labeled as MENX. Subsequent studies in humans identified that the *CDKN1B* tumor suppressor gene encoded the cell cycle inhibitor p27, and analysis of patients with MEN1 who had tested negative for germline MEN1 mutations identified *CDKN1B* mutations in a subset of this group. Subsequently, MEN4 was recognized as its own clinical entity in 2007.[48]

Thus far, approximately 80 cases have been identified in the literature. The estimated prevalence is fewer than one per million. The *CDKN1B* gene codes for p27, which acts as a tumor suppressor. When p27 binds cyclin-dependent kinase subunit CDK4, the retinoblastoma protein cannot undergo phosphorylation and the cell cycle is arrested.[49] Studies suggest p27 may play a role in cell cycle progression, cellular migration, and mitotic spindle stability. Additionally, menin may epigenetically modulate *CDKN1B* expression, though further studies are needed to determine whether these associations are drivers or consequences of tumor development.[48]

Similar to MEN1, patients with MEN4 often present with PHPT (>90% of cases), and this is often the first manifestation. The mean age at diagnosis is in the fifth decade of life. Approximately 40% of patients with MEN4 have evidence of pituitary adenomas, with the mean age of onset in the fourth decade of life. Although prolactinomas are the most common subtype (65%) of pituitary tumors in patients with MEN1, adrenocorticotropin hormone (ACTH)–secreting pituitary tumors are more common in patients with MEN4 (40% of all pituitary tumors as compared with 5% in MEN1).[48] NETs are less frequent, occurring in 20% of patients with MEN4 compared with 50% of patients with MEN1.[50] Similar to MEN1, the most common type of functional NET for patients with MEN4 is a gastrinoma.

There is no consensus or widely recognized guidelines for screening, surveillance, or management of patients with MEN4. All patients with clinical evidence of MEN1 should be tested for MEN1. If these tests are negative, patients may have MEN4 and should undergo next-generation sequencing to investigate a germline mutation in *CDKN1B*. Given the paucity of cases and limited existing literature, it is difficult to determine optimal timing of screening or surveillance or to provide definitive recommendations on medical or surgical intervention. In general, guidelines for patients with MEN1 are adopted or modified to help guide treatment in this patient population.

CONCLUSION

Over time, management of MEN has evolved, and our understanding of the natural history and underlying genetic mutations has helped predict the course of the disease and tailor care to the individual patient. Patients with MEN1 can be offered treatment for hyperparathyroidism and appropriate surveillance to avoid sequelae of malignant progression of NETs. Patients with MEN2 may be offered preventive surgery and be cured of MTC. More recently, patients with MEN4 may benefit from identification of the underlying mechanism and placed within their own unique group as we work to better understand screening, surveillance, and treatment in this population. Exclusion of the presence of a mutation in known kindreds can avoid lifelong unnecessary testing. Over time, surveillance and treatment will be tailored to each patient as more is learned about the pathogenesis of these diseases.

SELECTED REFERENCES

Castinetti F, Waguespack SG, Machens A, et al. Natural history, treatment, and long-term follow up of patients with multiple endocrine neoplasia type 2B: an international, multicentre, retrospective study. *Lancet Diabetes Endocrinol.* 2019;7(3):213-220.

This international and multicenter retrospective study of M918T RET mutantations includes 345 patients from 48 centers. The study provides long-term follow-up data to demonstrate that early thyroidectomy (before age 1) led to long-term cure in 83% of patients.

Newey PJ, Newell-Price J. MEN1 surveillance guidelines: time to (re)think? *J Endocr Soc.* 2022;6(2):bvac001.

This is a review about surveillance guidelines for patients with MEN1.

Ruggeri RM, Benevento E, De Cicco F, et al. Multiple endocrine neoplasia type 4 (MEN4): a thorough update on the latest and least known MEN syndrome. *Endocrine.* 2023;82(3):480-490.

This review provides a recent update about multiple endocrine neoplasia type 4 (MEN4) and provides insights about the molecular genetics and clinical features of this syndrome.

Thakker RV, Newey PJ, Walls GV, et al. Clinical practice guidelines for multiple endocrine neoplasia type 1 (MEN1). *J Clin Endocrinol Metab.* 2012;97(9):2990-3011.

These are the most recently published guidelines for multiple endocrine neoplasia type 1.

Wells SA Jr, Asa SL, Dralle H, et al. Revised American Thyroid Association guidelines for the management of medullary thyroid carcinoma. *Thyroid.* 2015;25:567-610.

These are the most recently published management guidelines for medullary thyroid carcinoma written by a consensus group of experts in the field.

The full reference list appears on Elsevier eBooks+.

Abdominal Wall Hernias

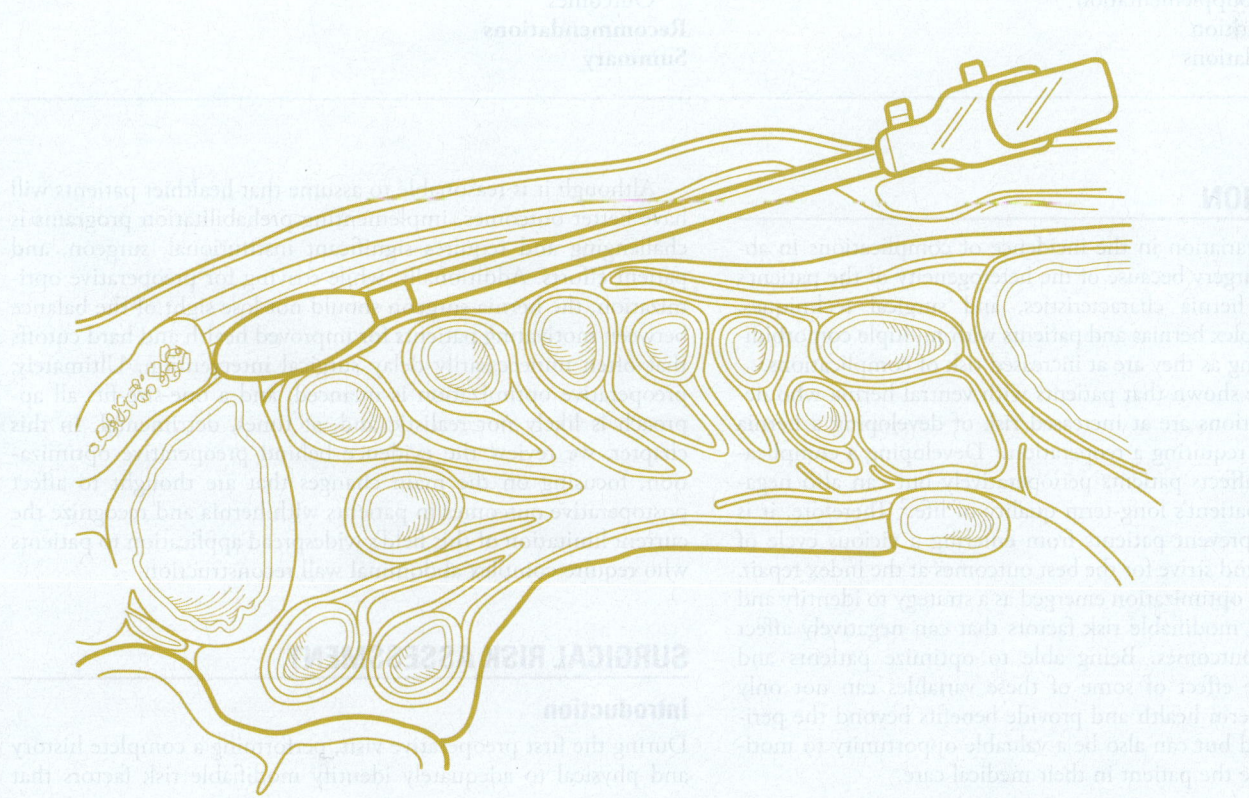

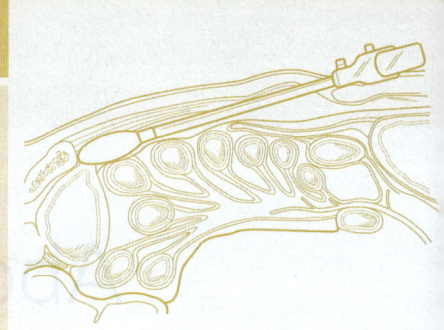

79 CHAPTER

Preoperative Management of the Hernia Patient

Sergio Mazzola Poli de Figueiredo, Aldo Fafaj, Benjamin Poulose, Alfredo Carbonell, and Michael J. Rosen

INTRODUCTION

There is wide variation in the incidence of complications in abdominal wall surgery because of the heterogeneity of the patient's comorbidities, hernia characteristics, and surgical techniques. Managing complex hernias and patients with multiple comorbidities is challenging as they are at increased risk of complications.

Studies have shown that patients with ventral hernia who develop complications are at increased risk of developing a hernia recurrence and requiring a reoperation.[1] Developing a complication not only affects patients perioperatively but can also negatively affect a patient's long-term quality of life.[2] Therefore, it is paramount to prevent patients from entering a vicious cycle of complications and strive for the best outcomes at the index repair.

Preoperative optimization emerged as a strategy to identify and intervene upon modifiable risk factors that can negatively affect hernia repair outcomes. Being able to optimize patients and minimizing the effect of some of these variables can not only promote long-term health and provide benefits beyond the perioperative period but can also be a valuable opportunity to motivate and involve the patient in their medical care.

Although it is reasonable to assume that healthier patients will have better outcomes, implementing prehabilitation programs is challenging and requires significant institutional, surgeon, and patient efforts. Additionally, while striving for preoperative optimization, the hernia surgeon should not lose sight of the balance between motivating patients for improved health and hard cutoffs that often unnecessarily delay surgical intervention. Ultimately, preoperative optimization is nuanced, and a one-size-fits-all approach is likely not realistic and, at times, detrimental. In this chapter, we review the evidence behind preoperative optimization, focusing on the main changes that are thought to affect postoperative outcomes in patients with hernia and recognize the current limitation of this field's widespread application to patients who require complex abdominal wall reconstruction.

SURGICAL RISK ASSESSMENT

Introduction

During the first preoperative visit, performing a complete history and physical to adequately identify modifiable risk factors that can be targeted with preoperative optimization is paramount. With the recent advancement in technology and artificial intelligence, surgical risk assessment is an area of exponential interest, and several tools have emerged to assist surgeons in assessing preoperative risk.

Outcomes

The American College of Surgeons (ACS) Universal Surgical Risk Calculator used data from a large database (National Surgical Quality Improvement Project [NSQIP]) and was one of the first tools developed to assess surgical risk using several patients and operative characteristics in a wide range of surgical procedures.[3] One of the main drawbacks of this tool is the lack of granular hernia information and operative techniques, limiting its applicability to patients with hernia.

Given these limitations, other surgical risk calculators were developed for patients with hernia, like the Carolinas Equation for Determining Associated Risks Application (CeDAR) and the Outcomes Reporting App for Clinician and Patient Engagement (ORACLE). The CeDAR app was developed using prospectively collected data from a hernia-specific registry from a single center and can be assessed on smartphones, allowing ease of patient participation during surgical risk discussions.[4] However, it is essential to highlight that the CeDAR app was developed for patients undergoing open ventral hernia repair (VHR) and when reporting complications can be misinterpreted. The CeDAR app reports complications as a composite score and, in essence, reports the overall complication rate, including minor and major morbidity events, which can overestimate actual surgical risk for an individual patient.

The ORACLE risk calculator was developed using a large, national, hernia-specific database (Abdominal Core Health Quality Collaborative [ACHQC]) with more than 10,000 patients undergoing elective VHR with mesh, regardless of operative approach (open, laparoscopic, or robotic). This software can also be downloaded on smartphones, allowing more effortless patient engagement and shared decision-making.[5] This app has the advantage of reporting more granular complications including specific wound events (surgical site occurrence [SSO], surgical site infection [SSI], and SSO requiring a procedural intervention), readmissions, and hernia recurrence. However, the data are reported with confidence intervals (CIs) for more accurate representation, which may be confusing for patients to interpret.

Recommendations

The use of risk assessment tools can assist surgeons and patients in assessing surgical risk and motivate patients to pursue preoperative optimization by allowing them to visualize the impact of preoperative strategies in minimizing surgical risks.

PHYSICAL ACTIVITIES AND PREHABILITATION PROGRAMS

Introduction

Functional activity is strongly correlated with favorable outcomes postoperatively, which is one of the main rationales for pursuing preoperative optimization. Prehabilitation is defined as preoperative methods focusing on improving a patient's functional capability to withstand any postoperative inactivity, functional decline, or eventual postoperative complication. Although some studies suggest a possible benefit with prehabilitation, most have heterogeneous design or lack statistical power, and even fewer include patients undergoing hernia repair.

Outcomes

The PREHAB study, an international, multicenter, randomized controlled trial (RCT), evaluated the effect of a 4-week supervised prehabilitation program in 269 patients undergoing colorectal cancer surgery and found fewer severe complications and medical complications in patients randomized to prehabilitation.[6] In this trial, patients underwent supervised physical training with 1-hour sessions three times a week incorporating aerobic and strength exercises, nutritional interventions supervised by a registered dietitian, anxiety-coping interventions provided by psychology-trained personnel, and a smoking cessation program if indicated.[6] Although the results of this trial are impressive, the amount of time, effort, and ancillary support can be overwhelming for many hernia practices.

In one of the few randomized trials evaluating prehabilitation in VHR, 118 patients were randomized to standard counseling or a prehabilitation program involving a nutritionist and physical therapist with weekly group meetings, daily checklist evaluating nutrition, and exercise program including a DVD with different physical activities.[7,8] In contrast to the PREHAB trial, this study provided access and training information rather than a formal supervised exercise program. Although the early results of the trial showed a lower rate of hernia-free and complication-free rates with prehabilitation, this was not observed in the 2-year follow-up study that showed no difference in hernia-free and complication-free patients between the groups (72.9% vs. 66.1%, $p = 0.42$).[7,8] Interestingly, patients who completed the prehabilitation program did not have sustained weight loss, and approximately half of patients in both groups gained weight from baseline. It is also important to highlight that five patients in the prehabilitation group (8.5%) and one patient in the standard counseling group (1.7%) underwent emergent hernia repair for acute incarceration during the study period.[8]

A large database study using the ACHQC found on multivariable analysis that higher patient-reported exercise level was associated with lower odds of postoperative complication and readmission.[9] However, even patients who reported only sporadic physical activity (once a month) had lower odds of complications and readmissions when compared with patients with no reported physical activity.[9] This highlights that any level of preoperative physical activity may affect postoperative recovery and benefit patients.

Recommendations

Growing evidence in general surgery literature supports prehabilitation programs that include physical activities, especially supervised exercise programs, which can provide better postoperative outcomes. However, few studies evaluate preoperative physical activity programs in patients undergoing abdominal wall surgery. Although there is great potential in implementing these programs, a lot of resources and effort are necessary to implement prehabilitation programs. It remains important to stress to patients in clinic that they can still perform exercise as tolerated because most patients are hesitant to undergo any level of exercise due to the fear of making their hernia larger. A significant amount of time is also necessary to achieve meaningful results through prehabilitation programs, which significantly delays surgical intervention and may increase the risk of a surgical emergency such as acute incarceration, obstruction, or strangulation. Given that the data are still limited, further studies are still required to justify the implementation of prehabilitation programs in patients undergoing hernia repair.

BODY MASS INDEX AND WEIGHT MANAGEMENT

Introduction

The prevalence of obesity is increasing yearly; nearly half of Americans will be obese by 2030, and 1 in 4 Americans are expected to have a BMI >35 kg/m^2.[10] Several studies have linked a higher BMI with an increased risk of hernia recurrence and wound complications in patients with abdominal wall hernias.[11-13] However, most studies identifying this trend include patients with mostly open repair and used large databases or systematic reviews and meta-analyses lacking substantial hernia-specific details.

Although BMI is the most common measurement of obesity, it can be quite inaccurate, particularly in patients with high muscle mass and extremes of height. A Belgian statistician (Lambert Adolphe Francois Quetelet) developed the BMI in the 19th century, and it has proven to have great value when evaluating large populations and public health trends.[14] However, given that patients can have different adipose tissue distribution and different phenotypes of obesity, BMI accuracy is limited when applied at an individual level. Recently, volumetric measurements on CT have emerged as a valuable tool to estimate the impact of obesity on postoperative outcomes. Schlosser et al. measured the abdominal subcutaneous fat volume in preoperative CT scans of patients undergoing open VHR and found that it was associated with the need for panniculectomy, readmissions, and wound complications.[15]

Kaoutzanis et al. used the NSQIP database including 25,172 patients undergoing VHR and found that BMI >30 kg/m^2 was a significant predictor of postoperative SSIs (odds ratio [OR] 1.49); however, open surgery was the strongest risk factor with OR 3.54.[11] It is essential to highlight that most of these studies lack important details, such as granular hernia and operative technique details, which can affect complication and recurrence rates.

The operative approach is an important consideration during operative risk assessment. Minimally invasive surgery (MIS) significantly reduces wound morbidity in obese patients undergoing hernia repairs.[11,16] Given that obese patients are at increased risk of wound complications, minimally invasive repairs can be particularly useful in obese patients, and the International Endohernia Society (IEHS) guidelines currently provide a grade A recommendation, suggesting that MIS techniques should be preferred in obese patients.[17] Obviously not all hernias can be repaired in an MIS approach, and these data are likely reserved for small- to medium-sized hernias.

Tsereteli et al. compared 134 patients with BMI >40 kg/m^2 with 767 patients with BMI <40 kg/m^2 undergoing laparoscopic intraperitoneal onlay mesh (IPOM) and found fewer hernia recurrences (8.3% in morbidly obese and 2.9% in nonmorbidly obese) but no difference in the rate of complications.[18] However, it is important to highlight that hernia defects were not closed in these patients, which can affect hernia recurrence, particularly in obese patients.

Laparoscopic and robotic retromuscular repairs, such as the extended totally extraperitoneal (eTEP) approach, has also been reported in obese patients. In one of the most extensive series of MIS retromuscular repairs, Addo et al. evaluated 461 patients with BMI >35 kg/m^2 and BMI <35 kg/m^2 and found no differences in hernia recurrence or complications.[19] This highlights that MIS can affect outcomes in obese patients and may play an important role when enrolling patients and balancing the risks and benefits of preoperative optimization programs.

Medical Nonpharmacologic Weight Loss Programs

In the previously discussed RCT, Bernardi et al. found no differences in the percentage of hernia-free and complication-free patients undergoing a prehabilitation program with access and training information versus standard counseling.[8] However, it is important to highlight that only 22% of patients in the prehabilitation group met the 7% total body weight loss goal,[7] highlighting the limitations of prehabilitation programs that do not offer supervised training activities or pharmacologic or surgical weight loss interventions. One observational study with 191 hernia patients reported a mean weight loss of 6 kg in patients who participated in a weight loss program compared with 1.8 kg in patients who did not enroll.[20] One of the most relevant findings of this study is that 55% of patients enrolled in a prehabilitation program were lost to follow-up and only 9 out of 80 patients (11%) enrolled in a program met the weight loss goal and underwent hernia repair.[20] These studies highlight how challenging it is to successfully implement such programs because patient engagement is poor and few patients meet their weight loss goals.

A small retrospective study by Rosen et al. evaluated the effect of a multidisciplinary approach with a low-calorie diet (<800 kcal/day) and protein-sparing fast (1.2–1.5 g/kg/day of protein according to ideal body weight) supervised by weight loss specialists in 25 patients with BMI greater than 35 kg/m^2.[21] The average duration of the preoperative program was 17 months, and patients lost approximately 18% of their initial weight and a mean BMI decrease of 9 points. Interestingly, 88% of patients could maintain their weight loss at 18-month follow-up postoperatively.[21] The protein-sparing fast supervised by a weight loss specialist appears to be a valuable strategy for medical weight loss.

Medical Pharmacologic Weight Loss

Several medications are approved for pharmacologic weight loss. However, the data on preoperative use of these medications are lacking, and no studies include patients undergoing abdominal wall surgery. A small nonrandomized study evaluated the use of phentermine-topiramate for 3 months preoperatively and postoperatively in patients with BMI >50 kg/m^2 undergoing laparoscopic sleeve gastrectomy (LSG).[22] Patients with adjunct weight loss medication lost two times more weight preoperatively than patients undergoing LSG only. The postoperative weight loss at 12- and 24-month follow-up was also greater in the phentermine-topiramate group.[22]

The current, most effective pharmacologic group for medical weight loss is the glucagon-like peptide-1 (GLP-1) agonists. Several RCTs with different GLP-1 agents have reported substantial and sustained reductions in body weight compared with placebo. In an RCT of patients including 338 patients, GLP-1 agonist use was associated with up to 24.2% mean weight reduction after 48 weeks.[23] Unfortunately, there is a lack of studies examining the preoperative use of GLP-1 agonists in the literature. Pharmacologic medical weight loss can be associated with significant side effects and requires a specialized follow-up program, which is better suited for primary care physicians and weight management specialists with experience with these medications. Further studies are needed to evaluate the role of these agents in the preoperative optimization of patients undergoing abdominal wall surgery.

Metabolic and Bariatric Surgery

Despite bariatric surgery being more effective than nonsurgical weight loss in multiple RCTs, there is still no consensus on the exact role of neoadjuvant bariatric surgery in preoperative optimization. Although surgical weight loss is highly effective, not all patients are appropriate candidates for metabolic surgery. These procedures can also result in unique complications and malnutrition that can potentially affect outcomes. At the same time, the weight loss provided by these interventions can increase abdominal wall compliance, reduce wound complications, reduce recurrence rates, and provide better control of comorbidities like diabetes.

Morrell et al. evaluated 20 patients who underwent LSG with complex ventral hernias, and 16 subsequentially underwent VHR on average 22.6 months after the first visit to the abdominal wall surgeon clinic.[24] Two patients required reoperation related to the LSG: one laparoscopic reexploration for bleeding and another required laparoscopic resleeving because of retained fundus and stalled weight loss. A 22.2% average decrease in BMI was noted, and two patients sustained hernia-related complications while waiting for an elective operation; both developed small bowel obstruction in which one required an emergent operation. No recurrences were seen on average follow-up of 20.9 months.[24]

In another case series of complex abdominal wall hernias that underwent neoadjuvant metabolic surgery, Schroeder et al. evaluated 12 patients (6 LSG, 6 laparoscopic Roux-en-Y gastric bypass [LRNYGB]) and reported no reoperations or complications.[25] The average excess BMI loss was 64.6%, and the mean BMI at hernia repair was 33 kg/m² versus 48 kg/m². The average time to undergo hernia repair was 22.3 months, and two patients were repaired emergently: one for strangulation and another for obstruction. Two patients developed superficial SSIs treated with antibiotics only, and no recurrences were noted on the mean follow-up of 21.9 months.[25]

Several studies have also described performing VHR simultaneously as laparoscopic bariatric surgery, especially for smaller defects. An analysis of 988 patients with concomitant VHR using the NSQIP database and propensity score matching found that patients with simultaneous VHR had higher 30-day morbidity, including reoperations and readmissions.[26] Chan et al. also reported synchronous VHR and bariatric surgery in 45 patients with placement of coated polypropylene or polytetrafluoroethylene mesh, with no recurrences noted at median follow-up of 13 months. However, two (4.4%) patients developed mesh infection that required drainage and antibiotics without mesh removal, and one patient required diagnostic laparoscopy for drainage of intraabdominal abscess.[27] We recommend caution with using intraperitoneal coated meshes in the setting of contamination because of higher rates of mesh infection and lower rates of mesh salvage with intraperitoneal meshes.[28]

Studies have also compared performing staged VHR with synchronous VHR before or during LSG. In a retrospective study with propensity score matching, 6.7% recurrence was noted in the staged group and 24% in the concurrent surgery group at a median 4.6-year follow-up.[29] BMI at hernia repair was 34.1 kg/m² after a mean of 21.5 months in the bariatric-first group and 42.4 kg/m² in the synchronous group. Most patients in both groups had hernias size >7 cm, and most patients underwent open retromuscular repair with mesh.[29] A retrospective study with propensity score matching evaluating patients with small (<4 cm) umbilical hernias compared patients with simultaneous LSG or VHR after weight loss after LSG and found similar rates of recurrence and complications in both groups.[30] Patients who underwent simultaneous VHR and LSG had a mean BMI of 42.7 kg/m², and patients with delayed repair achieved a mean BMI of 31 kg/m² approximately 13.7 months after LSG.[30]

The Society of American Gastrointestinal and Endoscopic Surgeons (SAGES) published detailed recommendations on the management of obese patients with hernias.[31] In their guidelines, a staged approach is recommended when possible. Still, some patients might require concomitant repair because of hernia anatomic location, history of recent small bowel obstruction, or need to reduce the bowel from the hernia sac for an anastomotic procedure in patients for whom LSG is not appropriate. In cases where concomitant hernia repair is reasonable, the authors recommend primary closure for smaller hernias and bridged repair with biologic or bioresorbable meshes as a temporizing measure for medium to large hernias. Empty hernia defects >10 cm may also be left alone, as the risk of incarceration is theoretically lower. Regarding the timing of hernia repair after bariatric surgery, SAGES recommends waiting until the nadir weight loss is achieved. However, it is reasonable to perform VHR in symptomatic patients who continue to lose weight despite BMI <35 kg/m² and in patients whose nadir weight continues to exceed the ideal BMI for hernia repair despite multiple weight loss interventions.[31]

Recommendations

We encourage preoperative weight loss in obese patients because it can promote overall health and potentially improve outcomes, particularly in complex hernias. It is essential to acknowledge that achieving meaningful weight loss can be extremely challenging and may require a significant number of resources to establish successful medical weight loss programs, require more invasive interventions such as neoadjuvant bariatric surgery, and take a substantial amount of time to achieve a weight loss goal before hernia repair, which can expose these patients to the risk of an emergent hernia operation.

We believe that strict BMI or weight loss cutoffs are not beneficial. The decision to proceed with surgery in obese patients should be individualized because some patients may never achieve significant weight loss or have significant symptoms that would benefit from earlier hernia repair. Additionally, we recommend MIS approaches when feasible, and if an open approach is required, we would avoid procedures that require undermining of large areas of skin and soft tissue. We use a medical weight loss program for 3 to 6 months in most obese patients and refer them to our metabolic institute, which includes medical and surgical weight loss. However, if significant symptoms are present or weight loss is not achieved despite multiple interventions within this period, VHR should be considered with appropriate risk-benefit discussions with the patients.

NUTRITIONAL SUPPLEMENTATION

Introduction

Poor nutritional status has been described as one of the leading risk factors for postoperative morbidity. Still, there is a lack of evidence supporting preoperative nutritional optimization, especially in patients undergoing abdominal wall surgery.

Nutritional Status Assessment

Several nutritional markers and nutritional scores can be valuable adjuncts in assessing nutritional risk preoperatively. In one study using the NSQIP database with 65,192 patients, serum albumin <3.5 g/dL was associated with an increased risk of major complications, mortality, and readmissions. Complications were decreased with each 0.1 g/dL increase in albumin levels.[32] Although albumin levels are one of the most used nutritional markers, hypoalbuminemia can occur in patients with chronic inflammation and has a relatively long half-life (approximately 3 weeks), limiting the applicability of using albumin alone for nutritional assessment in the preoperative setting. Prealbumin is another serum marker that can be more useful to assess short-term nutrition because it has a short half-life of approximately 3 days. However, prealbumin is also an acute phase reactant, and its level can be inaccurate in patients with ongoing inflammatory status. Adding C-reactive protein (CRP) levels can help assess inflammatory status and understand how it can interfere with nutritional serum markers. We believe that an increasing ratio of prealbumin and albumin associated with decreased levels of CRP can be a helpful sign of improved nutrition and a positive nitrogen balance.

In addition to laboratory and anthropometric values to assess nutrition, preoperative imaging can be a helpful adjunct. As patients undergoing abdominal wall surgery often have preoperative CT scans, this can add valuable information regarding nutritional status and provide accurate prognostic information. Although fat distribution in preoperative CT has been shown to correlate with postoperative outcomes, Schlosser et al. found that sarcopenia and psoas muscle size on CT was not associated with adverse outcomes in patients undergoing open VHRs.[15,33]

Obtaining volumetric data from CT scans may require computer skills, which can be highly user dependent, and specialized software that can perform such measurements. Using an image-based deep learning model, artificial intelligence can predict abdominal wall reconstruction complexity and postoperative infection, outperforming expert surgeons.[34] Further development of this technology will enhance preoperative planning and improve surgical risk discussion with patients.

Nutritional Supplementation

Although most patients undergoing abdominal wall surgery are not severely malnourished, patients with extensive comorbidities and complex hernias, such as enterocutaneous fistulas, can present in a catabolic state and potentially benefit from preoperative nutritional interventions. Patients should maintain at least a normocaloric diet with a protein intake of 1.2 g/kg, associated with dietary consultation and oral nutritional supplementation (ONS), if appropriate.[35]

The enteral route should always be preferred, but in some cases of patients who are malnourished or at severe nutritional risk and unable to meet energy requirements by the enteral route, parenteral nutrition (PN) should be considered.

Immunonutrition

In addition to addressing malnutrition, immunonutrition (IN) is another consideration preoperatively, as surgery can induce several metabolic alterations leading to increased catabolism and an inflammatory state. Immune-enhanced diets (IEDs) include arginine, glutamine, omega-3 fatty acids, and nucleotides. Several basic science studies have shown that these nutrients can reduce proinflammatory proteins and counteract stress-induced decreases in T-cell cytokine production and antigen-presenting cell

activity.[36,37] Supplementing these preoperatively theoretically can overcome the deficiency that can occur after the stress response from surgery.

A large meta-analysis containing 83 RCTs evaluating IN in patients undergoing abdominal surgery found that although a benefit was seen with IED, considering all trials, these effects disappeared when excluding trials at high or unclear risk of bias. The authors also noted that industry-founded trials were more likely to report positive effect in overall complications.[38] In another meta-analysis containing only RCTs comparing IEDs with regular ONS, no differences were seen in outcomes, suggesting that ONS is an acceptable alternative to IN, especially because ONS contains elements used in IN like arginine, omega-3, and other nutrients like proteins, minerals, and vitamins.[39]

In abdominal wall surgery, there is a lack of studies evaluating IN. In a small RCT of 40 patients undergoing enterocutaneous fistula takedown, patients in the intervention group were preoperatively administered arginine and glutamine supplementation for 7 days. Patients who underwent immune supplementation had lower interleukin-6 (IL-6) and CRP levels and also fewer infectious complications and fistula recurrence.[40] Although this trial provides positive results with IN in abdominal wall surgery, the number of patients was small, limiting the applicability of their findings.

Recommendations

A combination of anthropometric measurements, laboratory values, and CT volumetric analysis can be used to assess preoperative nutritional status. In malnourished patients, we recommend a normocaloric and high-protein diet with ONS if appropriate. PN is reserved for patients unable to tolerate EN. No high-quality evidence supports IN in patients undergoing abdominal surgeries; our approach is to selectively offer ONS or IEDs for 5 to 7 days to highly motivated patients.

MANAGEMENT OF DIABETES MELLITUS

A considerable body of evidence exists regarding the negative effect of uncontrolled diabetes mellitus (DM) in both basic science and clinical outcomes after cardiac, orthopedic, and general surgery.[41–43] However, despite being one of the most challenging concerns of public health, the management of diabetes remains poorly studied in the field of hernia repair.

Pathophysiology

The wound-healing process is complex and depends on numerous molecular pathways, which are modulated in the presence of DM. In vivo studies looking at impaired wound healing in the presence of DM have found a modulated local and systemic response to injury in the presence of DM because of impaired growth factor expression, severely impaired angiogenesis during the various stages of wound healing, increased production and release of proinflammatory cytokines, impaired function of macrophages and stem cells, and diminished apoptosis.

Outcomes

Glycemic control is typically assessed by measuring HbA1c. This value represents the percentage of glycosylated hemoglobin, which spans the lifetime of the erythrocyte. This is a test of choice because it reflects glycemic control over approximately 3 months.[44] A large systematic review and meta-analysis looked at the impact of glycemic control on outcomes in cardiac surgery by reviewing

30 studies including 30,000 patients.[41] In this study, low preoperative HbA1c (<7.5%) was associated with a lower risk of sternal wound infections when compared with patients with HbA1c >7.5% (risk ratio 0.50; 95% CI 0.32–0.80; $p = 0.003$). In addition, both early and late mortality improved with better glycemic control. Hernia-specific data are sparse. The European Hernia Society conducted a systematic review to evaluate patient prehabilitation before VHR. With regard to DM, only five publications were considered for analysis.[45] Four of these studies were retrospective reviews that reported increased risk for SSOs and hernia recurrence in diabetic patients. The other study was another expert consensus statement based on systematic reviews.[46] However, the data gathered were not from hernia-specific studies and showed increased odds of 1.69 to 5.8 for postoperative complications when HbA1c was >6.0% to 7.0%. A more recent retrospective review of prospectively collected data on the hernia-specific ACHQC database looked at the association of HbA1c and outcomes of VHRs in diabetic patients.[47] The patients were divided into two groups (HbA1c <8% and HbA1c ≥8%). After analyzing over 2000 patients, this study found no clinically significant differences in the rates of wound complications, reoperations, readmissions, length of stay, or mortality.

Recommendations

Poorly controlled diabetes has been shown to have a negative impact on wound morbidity in several types of surgeries. These results are often extrapolated into the field of hernia surgery, so the consensus has been to avoid elective hernia repair in patients with HbA1c >8%. However, as more hernia-specific studies are being presented, this notion is being challenged. At this time, we recommend that all diabetic patients should have their HbA1c checked before surgery. For those with HbA1c >8%, the surgeon must determine whether it is the result of poor compliance or lack of medical access. A referral to endocrinology is preferred for those with poorly controlled diabetes, and the surgeon should emphasize the importance of glycemic control on the patient's overall health. Currently, there is no evidence to recommend delaying hernia repair until the HbA1c is lowered to some arbitrary cutoff. Finally, DM, especially type 2, may be associated with morbid obesity. Referral to either medical or surgical weight loss before elective hernia repair may be beneficial in this select group of patients.

MANAGEMENT OF SMOKING

Worldwide, it is estimated that 33% of adult males and 7% of adult females are active smokers despite growing evidence that smoking is a leading cause of death.[48] Similar to the negative impact of poorly controlled diabetes, there is no shortage of studies highlighting the risk of smoking in patients undergoing surgical procedures in several surgical specialties such as gastrointestinal, orthopedic, and urology.[49–52] However, recent data have challenged this perceived increased risk in smokers undergoing hernia repair.

Pathophysiology

The detrimental effects of smoking on overall health are ubiquitous. These include reduced ability to heal wounds, immunosuppression, susceptibility to infections, increased risk of cardiovascular disease, and decreased respiratory function.[51] Regarding wound healing, smoking releases reactive oxygen species, producing a proinflammatory state and impairing wound proliferation and remodeling.[53]

More specifically, smoking increases the overall neutrophil cell count by as much as 20%, which in turn leads to the release of proinflammatory substrates such as tumor necrosis factor (TNF)-α, IL-1, IL-8, and granulocyte-macrophage colony-stimulation factor from alveolar macrophages.[54] In addition, smoking has been shown to inhibit fibroblast chemotaxis, migration, and proliferation as well as reduced collagen I and III production.

OUTCOMES

In the context of VHR, there have been several large-pool registry studies demonstrating that smoking increases the risk for wound infection. An NSQIP review by DeLancey et al. analyzing 220,000 ventral and inguinal hernias showed that smokers had increased risk for wound infection: superficial: OR 1.34 (95% CI 1.22–1.48); deep: OR 1.31 (95% CI 1.11–1.54); organ space: OR 1.45 (95% CI 1.17–1.79); and dehiscence: OR 1.41 (95% CI 1.11–1.80). However, the actual percentage differences of any wound complication were much smaller: 2.58% in current smokers and 1.69% in nonsmokers.[55] Analyzing patients in the ACHQC, Petro et al. compared current smokers with never-smokers and found similar rates of SSI (4.1% vs. 4.1%, $p = 0.98$), SSOs requiring procedural intervention (SSOPI) (6.2% vs. 5.0%, $p = 0.43$), reoperation (1.9% vs. 1.2%, $p = 0.39$), and all 30-day morbidity (7.5 vs. 6.6, $p = 0.60$). Smokers had higher rates of SSOs (12.0% vs. 7.4%, $p = 0.03$), which was driven by increased seromas.[56] In their retrospective propensity score matching analysis, Kudsi et al. reported comparable results when looking at clinical outcomes of robotic VHR between smokers and nonsmokers. SSOs and infections were similar when comparing smokers to nonsmokers (7.6% vs. 5.4%, $p = 0.472$; 5 vs. 0, $p = 0.060$, respectively).[53]

Recommendations

The large body of evidence implicating smoking in postoperative complications certainly outnumbers the results in hernia-specific populations. Importantly, the most cited large data pools lack the granularity of hernia-specific techniques and often produce statistically significant results that may not be clinically relevant. When considering the body of evidence against smoking and the negative effects on general health, all surgeons should encourage smoking cessation before any operative procedures. Preoperative counseling should be provided, and appropriate referrals should be made for those motivated to quit smoking. However, the surgeon should be truthful when presenting the data to smokers being evaluated for hernia repair. Historically, the authors viewed smoking as a contraindication to hernia repair. Currently, we continue to encourage patients to quit smoking. However, we will now proceed with surgery even if the patient has failed to quit, understating that for Centers for Disease Control and Prevention (CDC) class I hernia repairs there is an increased risk of SSOs, but the majority of these do not require further intervention. Importantly, a prerequisite for such a drastic change in practice is outcomes tracking. The surgeon must be aware of their current clinical outcomes and should be able to track any signals once a change in practice is implemented.

IMMUNOSUPPRESSION

Immunosuppression represents a unique set of challenges in the context of hernia repair, as a significant portion of this cohort are solid organ transplant patients who rely on these medications to prevent rejection. These challenging groups of patients are thought to be at increased risk for developing wound complications and hernia recurrence because of their immunosuppressed state.

Pathophysiology

The most common classes of immunosuppressive drugs encountered by the hernia surgeon include calcineurin inhibitors (cyclosporine and tacrolimus), antimetabolites (azathioprine and mycophenolate mofetil), mammalian target of rapamycin (mTOR) inhibitors (sirolimus or everolimus), TNF inhibitors, and steroids. Cyclosporine is a cyclical peptide that binds to intracellular cyclophilin, and together they act to inhibit calcineurin.[57] This results in the inhibition of T-cell proliferation and differentiation. Tacrolimus also blocks calcineurin by binding to the FK506-binding proteins (FKBPs) in a mechanism like cyclosporine. Azathioprine and mycophenolate mofetil inhibit purine synthesis, reducing B and T cells. Sirolimus and everolimus, like tacrolimus, bind to FKBP but affect the signal transduction pathway by blocking the activity of mTOR. This affects the phosphatidylinositol-3 kinase-Akt signaling pathway, which is an important checkpoint for cell growth and proliferation as well as proinflammatory factors IL-2, IL-15, and vascular endothelial growth factor, which are critical for wound healing. TNF is a central component of the inflammatory response. It is activated by macrophages, which, in turn, activate several signaling pathways including mitogen-activated protein (MAP) kinase, caspases, and nuclear factor-kB. These pathways lead to increase expression of other inflammatory cells (B and T cells), inflammatory cytokines (IL-1, IL-6), cell adhesion molecules, matrix metalloproteinase, and inducers of apoptosis.

Outcomes

A large registry-based study looked at the effect of immunosuppression, including corticosteroid treatment, on the outcomes of inguinal hernia repair in over 2000 patients.[58] When looking at immunosuppression (yes vs. no), there were no significant differences in SSIs (0.65% vs. 0.70%, $p = 1.000$) or seromas (1.22% vs. 1.57%, $p = 0.382$). Another study looked at the risk factors for hernia recurrence, SSO, and those requiring procedural intervention in 166 patients who underwent incisional hernia repair after abdominal transplantation.[59] Interestingly, immunosuppression had a lower risk of SSO and SSOPI (OR 0.33, 95% CI 0.11–1.00, $p = 0.05$; OR 0.14, 95% CI 0.02–0.88, $p = 0.036$). Finally, Kushner et al. looked at wound morbidity in immunosuppressed patients undergoing open or robotic bilateral transversus abdominis release.[60] Of the 321 patients included in the study, 20% were on chronic immunosuppression. When looking at chronic immunosuppression (yes vs. no), there were no significant differences in SSO (20.6% vs. 21.3%, $p = 0.92$), SSI (14.3% vs. 10.8%, $p = 0.50$), SSOPI (3.2% vs. 5.4%, $p = 0.48$), or readmission for wound-related compilations (1.6% vs. 4.3%, $p = 0.33$). Inhibitors of mTOR deserve special attention. Both animal and human studies have shown a significant decrease in wound strength and delayed healing.[57] As for the inhibitors of TNF, a large multicenter prospective cohort study of 947 patients studied the use of this class of medication and the risk for postoperative infectious complications in patients undergoing surgery for irritable bowel disease (IBD).[61] The rates of any infection (18.1% vs. 20.2%, $p = 0.469$) and SSI (12.0% vs. 12.6%, $p = 0.889$) were similar for patients currently exposed to TNF inhibitors when compared with the unexposed, respectively.

Recommendations

In general, calcineurin inhibitors and antimetabolites should be continued in the perioperative period. Trough levels of calcineurin inhibitors should be monitored daily to determine the appropriate dosage and ensure appropriate maintenance therapy levels. If elective surgery is planned, mTOR inhibitors should be stopped 4 to 6 weeks before surgery in consultation with the patient's transplant team. Currently, there is not enough evidence to suggest stopping TNF inhibitors before surgery. Patients on chronic steroids may require stress doses depending on the length of therapy and drug dosage at home. Finally, immunosuppressed patients, especially transplant patients, require a multidisciplinary team effort, including the transplant team and pharmacy.

PREOPERATIVE ADJUNCTS FOR VENTRAL HERNIA REPAIR

A critical component for the successful treatment of ventral hernias is closure of the midline. However, for complex hernias, this may not always be possible. Incomplete fascial closure, also referred to as a *bridged repair,* has been associated with increased SSI and recurrence rates. Component separation techniques were developed as effective means to close complex defects. However, even with advancements made with these techniques, loss-of-domain hernias often have chronic muscle retraction, reducing the compliance of the abdominal wall, which, in turn, hinders the reduction of hernia contents inside the abdomen and subsequently fascial closure. Three main preoperative adjuncts have been developed to facilitate fascial closure in complex hernias: botulinum toxin A (BTA), soft tissue expanders, and progressive preoperative pneumoperitoneum (PPP).

Pathophysiology

BTA is a neurotoxin that is produced by the bacterium *Clostridium botulinum.* This toxin, typically injected under ultrasound guidance, blocks the release of the neurotransmitter acetylcholine, resulting in temporary muscle paralysis. With regard to hernia repair, BTA is thought to cause relaxation and elongation of the lateral abdominal wall musculature (external oblique, internal oblique, and transversus abdominis muscles), which are thought to increase abdominal wall compliance and facilitate fascial closure.[62] PPP, first used in 1947, is a technique where the intraabdominal cavity is filled with, most commonly, ambient air via an intraperitoneal catheter. The volume of gas is gradually increased until a predetermined volume is reached or the patient can no longer tolerate it. The theorized effects of this technique, which acts as a pneumatic soft tissue expander, include elongation of soft tissues, improvement in respiratory capacity, and tension-free abdominal closure.[63] Soft tissue expanders are implants placed subcutaneously, between the internal and external obliques, posterior rectus sheath, or intramuscularly. After a period of 1 to 6 months, the expansion of the implants is started and continued until adequate soft tissue is recruited. This may result in the mobilization of abdominal wall fascia and soft tissue to allow for reconstruction.[64]

Outcomes

Although the use of these preoperative adjuncts is increasing, data that objectively justify clinical benefits are lacking and consist of mostly retrospective reviews. A retrospective propensity-scored matched study looked at patients who underwent abdominal wall reconstruction with (75 patients) and without BTA (145 patients).

Patients with BTA had higher fascial closure rates (92% vs. 81%, $p = 0.036$).[65] A subsequent study by the same group showed no difference in fascial closure rates when BTA and preperitoneal mesh placement were compared with component separation alone (100% vs. 90.5%, $p = 0.11$, respectively).[62] A different propensity-scored matched study looked at the ACHQC registry and compared the fascial closure rate with and without BTA use.[66] There was no difference in fascial closure rates between treatments with and without BTA (86% vs. 85.2%, $p = 0.934$, respectively). Regarding PPP, a systematic review and meta-analysis looked at 53 articles for a total of 1216 patients. In this study, the pooled data showed 86% fascial closure rates; however, there was no comparison arm. Of note, the authors found a 12% rate of complications associated with this procedure. Although the majority were minor (abdominal pain, subcutaneous emphysema, and dyspnea), there were two hollow viscus perforations and five deaths thought to be related to PPP.[67] Finally, tissue expansion data are even more lacking when compared with BTA and PPP. Tissue expansion is mainly used when there is inadequate soft tissue coverage, and a systematic review of 14 studies including 103 patients highlighted the feasibility of this technique.[68] However, the authors also highlighted the potential for complications during the expansion phase, which included wound infection ($n = 11$), hematoma ($n = 8$), and rupture of the implant ($n = 3$). After the reconstruction, the main complications included recurrence ($n = 12$), skin necrosis ($n = 6$), and mortality ($n = 2$).

Recommendations

It is important to highlight that the use of BTA is off-label when injected into the lateral abdominal wall musculature. The US Food and Drug Administration (FDA) requires the botulinum toxin manufacturers to include a black box warning about the possible risks associated with the systemic spread of the toxin, including death. To date, there is no high-quality objective evidence that BTA, which adds significant cost to the hernia repair, aids with fascial closure. At this time, the use of BTA in abdominal wall reconstruction should be limited to uses in a trial context. Tissue expanders and PPP can be valuable when there is inadequate soft tissue coverage, so these procedures should be in the surgeon's armamentarium. A multidisciplinary effort should be made when employing this technique, including providers who have experience with tissue expanders.

PREHOSPITAL SCRUB

Preoperative showering with an antiseptic agent such as chlorhexidine gluconate (CHG) has been a well-accepted practice among many surgical specialties to reduce the skin flora. However, it is not clear that this practice results in fewer SSIs.

Pathophysiology

Chlorhexidine has both bacteriostatic and bactericidal properties. It is a positively charged molecule that is attracted to the negatively charged bacterial cell wall, forming strong adsorption of phosphate-containing molecules.[69] This is followed by penetration through the bacterial cell wall, damaging its integrity and resulting in outflow of cytoplasmic components such as potassium, limiting the function of enzymes associated with the cytoplasmic membrane. Finally, CHG causes cytoplasmic coagulation and precipitation by forming complexes with phosphorylated molecules such as nucleic acids and adenosine triphosphate.

Outcomes

When looking to give recommendations for the use of CHG, the World Health Organization (WHO) conducted a systematic review to assess the effectiveness of CHG when compared with plain soap. Nine studies including more than 17,000 adult patients investigated preoperative bathing or showering with an antimicrobial soap compared with plain soap and found that bathing with CHG soap does not significantly reduce SSI rates compared with bathing with plain soap (OR 0.92; 95% CI: 0.80–1.04). Specific to hernia surgery, Prabhu et al. analyzed 3924 patients, and multivariate logistic regression modeling showed that the CHG scrub group had a higher incidence of SSOs (OR 1.34; 95% CI 1.11–1.61) and SSIs (OR 1.46; 95% CI 1.03–2.07) when compared with the no CHG group.[70] After these results, some of the study's authors stopped using prehospital CHG as part of the quality improvement initiative. They looked at the data 4 years after this change, and when 4276 patients were analyzed, the rates of SSO, SSIs, and SSOPIs at 30 days were similar before and after prehospital CHG discontinuation.[71]

RECOMMENDATIONS

In their global guidelines for preventing SSI, the WHO recommends that it is good clinical practice for patients to bathe or shower before surgery with a plain or antimicrobial soap. Currently, there is no evidence to recommend the use of prehospital CHG to reduce the rate of wound infections after hernia repair.

SUMMARY

In this chapter we described the current evidence on preoperative optimization of the patient with a hernia and provided several evidence-based recommendations as follows:

1. Preoperative optimization strategies can be a valuable opportunity to motivate patients to improve general health and minimize the impact of modifiable risk factors on postoperative outcomes.
2. The current evidence behind preoperative optimization in hernia repair is limited and likely overemphasized by current guidelines. Further high-quality studies are needed before making strong recommendations that have significantly affected patients undergoing abdominal wall surgery.
3. It is important to acknowledge that, most of the time, a significant amount of effort and time is required for patients to achieve meaningful weight loss. These patients are subject to the risk of undergoing an emergency operation that is associated with worse outcomes than in an elective setting.
4. We strongly discourage the use of cutoffs to select patients for operative interventions. We recommend the use of a patient-centered approach based on the patient's symptoms, baseline comorbidities, preoperative risk assessment, and surgical approach to determine the need and length of preoperative optimization in comorbid patients.
5. Patients with multiple modifiable risk factors likely benefit more from preoperative optimization strategies than patients with isolated risk factors.
6. A multidisciplinary effort is paramount to establishing optimal preoperative optimization strategies to promote a greater impact on postoperative outcomes.
7. There is no evidence to recommend delaying hernia repair until the HbA1c is lowered to an arbitrary cutoff.

8. Continue to encourage patients to quit smoking. However, the surgeon may proceed with surgery even if the patient has failed to quit depending on the complexity of the case and technique used.

9. For elective surgeries, mTOR inhibitors should be stopped 4 to 6 weeks before surgery in consultation with the patient's transplant team.

10. The use of BTA in abdominal wall reconstruction should be used in a trial context, and tissue expanders and PPP can be valuable adjuncts for achieving soft tissue coverage.

SELECTED REFERENCES

Al-Mansour MR, Vargas M, Olson MA, Gupta A, Read TE, Algarra NN. S-144 lack of association between glycated hemoglobin and adverse outcomes in diabetic patients undergoing ventral hernia repair: an ACHQC study. *Surg Endosc.* 2023;37:3180-3190.

> This study evaluated the impact of HbA1c in patient undergoing ventral hernia repair using the Abdominal Core Health Quality Collaborative database. The patients were divided into two groups HbA1c <8% and HbA1c >8%. There was no association between HbA1c and operative outcomes in diabetic patients undergoing elective ventral hernia repair.

Alzatari R, Hassanein R, Doble J, Huang LC, Poulose BK. Determining the impact of individual ventral hernia repair complications on patient-reported quality of life. *Hernia.* 2023;27:687-694.

> This study performed a propensity score matched analysis using the Abdominal Core Health Quality Collaborative comparing HerQLes scores at 1-year following ventral hernia repair in patients that had complications or no complications. The study found that developing wound complications had a significant negative impact in quality of life at 1 year in patients undergoing ventral hernia repair.

Bernardi K, Olavarria OA, Dhanani NH, et al. Two-year outcomes of prehabilitation among obese patients with ventral hernias. *Ann Surg.* 2022;275:288-294.

> This is a 2-year follow-up study of a blinded randomized control trial evaluating the impact of prehabilitation in obese patients seeking ventral hernia repair. There were no differences in 2-year outcomes in obese patients who underwent prehabilitation versus standard care.

Horne CM, Augenstein V, Malcher F, et al. Understanding the benefits of botulinum toxin A: retrospective analysis of the Abdominal Core Health Quality Collaborative. *Br J Surg.* 2021;108:112-114.

> This study evaluated the role of chemical component separation utilizing botulinum toxin A in patients with large ventral hernias using the Abdominal Core Health Quality Collaborative. This study did not demonstrate improved fascial closure rates, decreased need for component separation or improved patient reported outcomes with the use of botulinum toxin A.

Petro CC, Haskins IN, Tastaldi L, et al. Does active smoking really matter before ventral hernia repair? An AHSQC analysis. *Surgery.* 2019;165:406-411.

> This study evaluated patients undergoing elective clean open ventral hernia repair using the Abdominal Core Health Quality Collaborative. Current smokers were propensity matched to patients who never smoked. There was increased rates of surgical site occurrences, wound cellulitis and seromas with smoking, but no differences in surgical site infections, surgical site occurrences requiring procedural intervention, reoperations and overall 30-day morbidity.

The full reference list appears on Elsevier eBooks+.

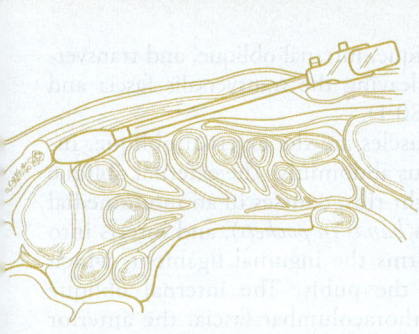

CHAPTER 80

Ventral Hernias

Richard Lu, Julie L. Holihan, Thomas Clements, Genevieve Chartrand, Luciano Tastaldi, Paul Taehoon Kim, and Igor Belyansky

OUTLINE

▶ Please access Elsevier eBooks+ to view the videos for this chapter.

INTRODUCTION AND ANATOMY

A ventral hernia (VH) is an anatomic defect of the anterior abdominal wall leading to herniation of preperitoneal or intraperitoneal contents and is seen as a bulge by the patient. VHs can be categorized as spontaneous or acquired. Examples of spontaneous VHs include umbilical hernias and epigastric hernias. The majority of acquired VHs are the result of surgical incisions, referred to as *incisional hernias*. It is estimated that 12% of major open abdominal surgical incisions and 3% of major minimally invasive operation incisions will develop an incisional hernia. The greatest risk of development occurs in the first 5 years. Traumatic hernias are also a type of acquired VH. Although not considered a true hernia (given the absence of a fascial defect and hernia sac), *diastasis recti* refers to progressive stretching of the linea alba leading to separation of the rectus abdominis muscles and manifests as a midline bulge that is frequently confused for a hernia.

Ventral hernia repair (VHR) of both spontaneous and acquired hernias remains one of the most common surgical procedures performed by general surgeons. A recent study demonstrated that in the United States, rates of VHR increased to over 600,000 between 2006 and 2016.[1] In recent decades, the landscape of VHR has evolved dramatically with the advent of many new materials to reinforce the abdominal wall and several new surgical techniques, including minimally invasive approaches. Despite these advances, hernia recurrence rates after VHR remain high, up to 40% in some studies.[2] This observation demonstrates that there is still significant room for improvement in hernia repair outcomes and that no single silver bullet exists against VH. Surgeons must maintain a broad armamentarium to provide tailored approaches to hernia patients. The goal of VHR should be to durably repair and restore abdominal wall anatomy with the lowest possible rate of complications.

A clear understanding of abdominal wall anatomy, including musculoaponeurotic structures, blood supply, and innervation, is imperative for the surgeon performing VHRs. The anterior abdominal wall is a hexagonal area defined superiorly by the costal margin and xiphoid process; laterally by the midaxillary line; and inferiorly by the symphysis pubis, pubic tubercle, inguinal ligament, anterior superior iliac spine (ASIS), and iliac crest. Layers of the anterior abdominal wall from anterior to posterior include skin, subcutaneous tissue, superficial fascia, deep fascia, muscle, transversalis fascia, preperitoneal fat and areolar tissue, and peritoneum. The superficial fascia of the abdominal wall is composed of both Camper's and Scarpa's fascia fused into a single layer above the umbilicus. Below the umbilicus, the division between a fatty outer anterior layer, Camper's fascia, and a membranous inner layer, Scarpa's fascia, becomes apparent. Camper's fascia is continuous with the superficial adipose tissue and may vary in thickness depending on patient body habitus. It extends inferiorly with the superficial thigh fascia and extends inferiorly to the scrotum in males and labia majora in females.

The anterior abdominal wall is formed mainly by rectus abdominis muscles and their associated fascia. The rectus abdominis muscles are covered by anterior and posterior fascia, the anterior and posterior rectus sheath. Fusion of bilateral rectus abdominis fascia in the midline forms the linea alba, which extends from the xiphoid process to the pubic symphysis. This critical structure is typically more well defined above the umbilicus. The lateral abdominal wall is formed by the external oblique, internal oblique, and transversus abdominis muscles, each with its own associated fascia. Their insertion to the lateral edge of the rectus abdominis forms the linea semilunaris.

The arcuate line is located midway between the umbilicus and symphysis pubis and is the anatomic point where the posterior rectus sheath transitions from being a fusion of the posterior fascial layer (or lamella) of the internal oblique and transversus abdominis aponeuroses cranially to being the transversalis fascia and parietal peritoneum only caudally. Above the arcuate line, the anterior rectus sheath is formed by contributions of the external oblique and the anterior lamella of the internal oblique aponeuroses. Below the arcuate line, the anterior rectus sheath is

composed of the external oblique, internal oblique, and transversus abdominis aponeuroses, leaving the transversalis fascia and peritoneum posteriorly (Fig. 80.1).

The lateral abdominal muscles are the external oblique, internal oblique, and transversus abdominis. The external oblique originates from the lower eight ribs, courses in an inferomedial orientation (often referred as *hands in pockets*), and inserts into the pubic crest. Its fascia forms the inguinal ligament, which extends from the ASIS to the pubis. The internal oblique muscles originate from the thoracolumbar fascia, the anterior two-thirds of the iliac crest, and the lateral portion of the inguinal ligament. The muscle fibers course in a superomedial direction (opposite to the external oblique) and insert into the inferoposterior borders of the 10th to 12th ribs superiorly and into the pubic crest inferiorly. The transversus abdominis muscles are the deepest of the lateral abdominal wall. They originate from the anterior three-fourths of the iliac crest, the lateral third of the inguinal ligament, and the inner surface of the lower six costal cartilages, where they interlock with fibers of the diaphragm. The origin is muscular but transitions into a broad flat aponeurosis medially and fuses with the posterior layer of the internal oblique fascia before inserting into linea alba. Below the arcuate line, the condensation of the transversus abdominis and internal oblique aponeuroses forms the

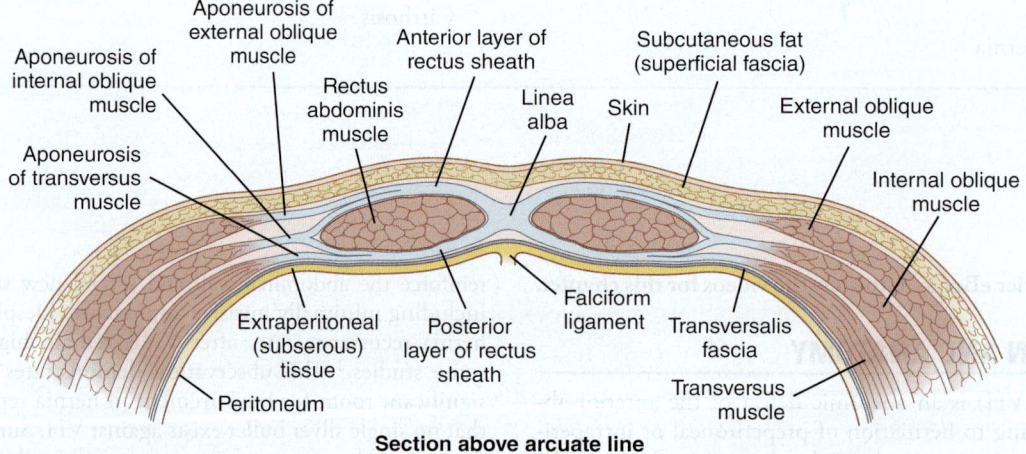

Section above arcuate line

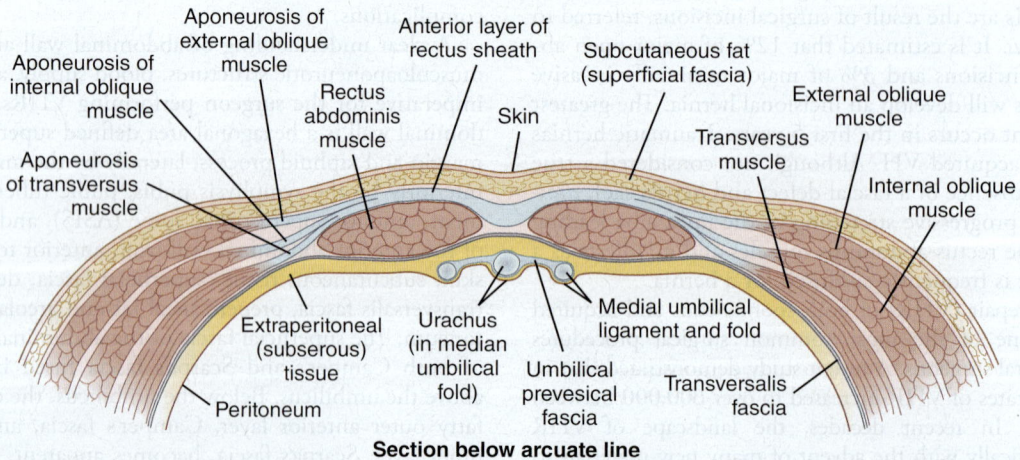

Section below arcuate line

FIGURE 80.1 Cross-sections of the rectus abdominis muscle and aponeurosis above and below the arcuate line.

conjoint tendon, which inserts into the pubic crest. Importantly, the transversus abdominis extends medially to the linea semilunaris and contributes to the posterior rectus sheath. The muscle fibers of the transversus abdominis muscle are more medial in the upper abdomen and become more lateral in the lower abdomen.

The blood supply to the abdominal wall is divided into three zones as described by Huger et al.[3] Zone I includes the upper- and mid central abdomen and is supplied by the superior epigastric artery (SEA) and the deep inferior epigastric artery (DIEA). Zone 2 includes the midline and lateral lower abdominal wall and is supplied by the epigastric arcade, superficial inferior epigastric, superficial external pudendal, and superficial circumflex iliac arteries. Zone 3 includes the lateral abdominal wall and is supplied by the musculophrenic, lower intercostal, and lumbar arteries (Fig. 80.2).

Both the SEA and DIEA lie on the posterior aspect of the rectus muscles and supply the rectus abdominis, subcutaneous tissue, and skin through musculocutaneous perforators. The two branching vascular systems converge within the rectus abdominis muscle at a point between the xiphoid process and the umbilicus.

The blood supply to the lateral abdominal wall includes the musculophrenic artery, deep circumflex iliac artery, and branches of the lower intercostal and lumbar arteries. These vessel arcades course within the plane between the transversus abdominis and internal oblique muscles (Fig. 80.3).

Motor and sensory innervation of the abdominal wall originates from branches of the intercostal nerves (T7–L1). Motor innervation is supplied by the nerve roots from T7–T12 intercostals and iliohypogastric and ilioinguinal nerves. These nerve roots travel perpendicularly in the lateral abdominal wall in between the transversus abdominis and the internal oblique muscle (the transversus abdominis plane) and pierce the posterior rectus sheath at the level of the linea semilunaris. After entering the posterior rectus sheath, the neurovascular bundles segmentally innervate the rectus abdominis muscle. Intraoperative identification and preservation of the neurovascular bundles are critical to maintain rectus abdominis trophism and avoid inadvertent injuries to the linea semilunaris.

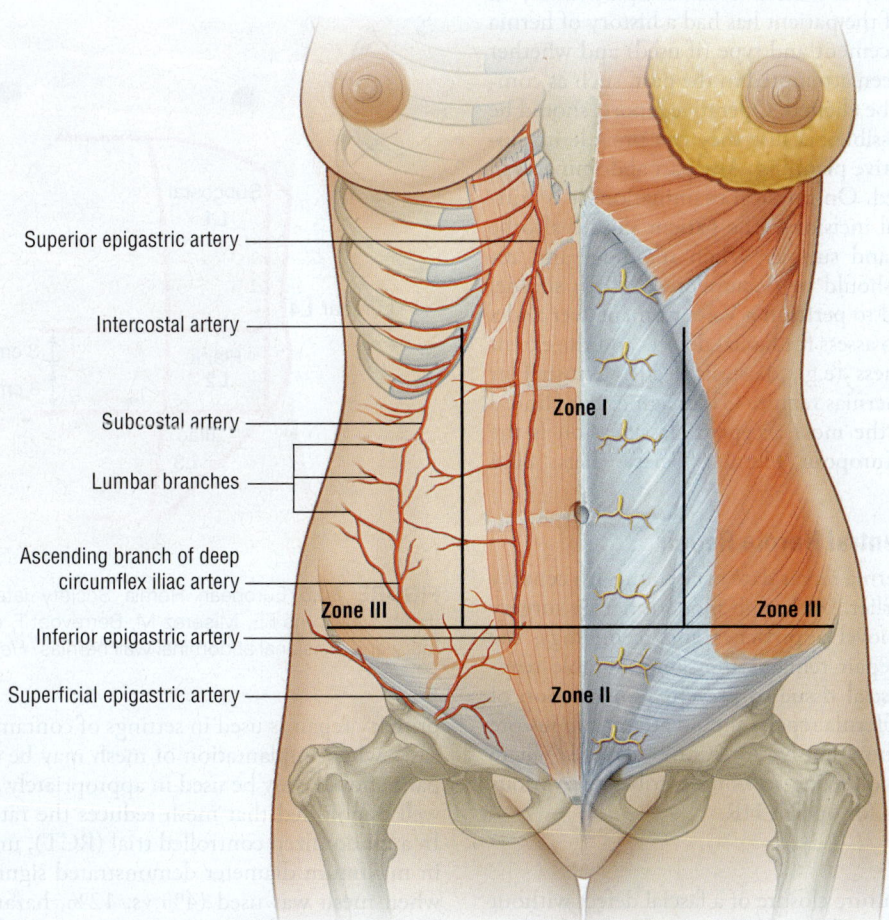

FIGURE 80.2 Zones of blood supply to the abdominal wall as described by Huger and colleagues. It is critical to consider the blood supply of not only the deeper abdominal wall layers but also the superficial layers to prevent wound complications. (From Neligan PC, Buck DW. Abdominoplasty and lipoabdominoplasty. In: Neligan PC, Buck DW, eds. *Core Procedures in Plastic Surgery*. 2nd ed. Elsevier; 2020:93-105.)

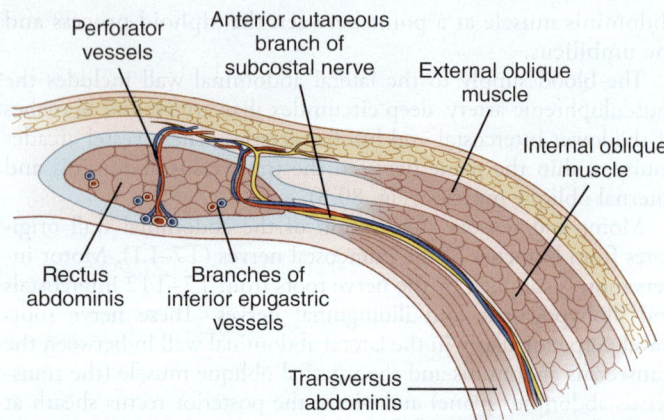

FIGURE 80.3 Cross-section of the lateral abdominal wall detailing location of intercostal neurovascular bundle traveling between the transversus abdominis and internal oblique muscles.

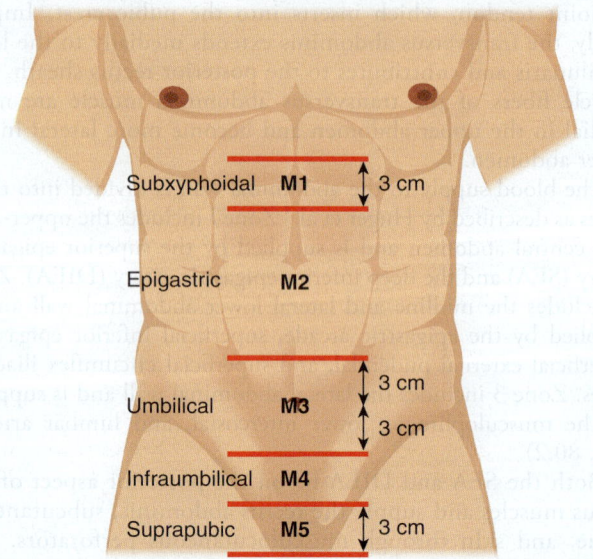

FIGURE 80.4 European Hernia Society midline hernia classification. (From Muysoms FE, Miserez M, Berrevoet F, et al. Classification of primary and incisional abdominal wall hernias. *Hernia.* 2009;13[4]: 407-414.)

MANAGEMENT OF VENTRAL HERNIAS

Diagnosis

A thorough history and physical examination should be performed. When interviewing the patient, risk factors for hernia development, symptoms, and effects on quality of life should be investigated. Surgical history is critical to obtain, particularly in the setting of recurrence. If the patient has had a history of hernia repair, details on mesh placement and type (if used) and whether a complex approach had been attempted in the past, such as component separation, should be elicited. Operative reports should be sought and obtained if possible because they can provide invaluable information for operative planning. Any past abdominal wall imaging should be reviewed. On physical examination, it is critical to note all past surgical incisions. The patient should also be examined both standing and supine. When standing, any abdominal wall asymmetry should be documented. When supine, the patient should be asked to perform a Valsalva maneuver and a straight bilateral leg raise to assess for fascial defects and the extent of abdominal wall weakness (e.g., diastasis recti). Unusual or complex presentations of hernias require CT imaging. For clinical documentation purposes, the most accepted classification is the one developed by the European Hernia Society (Figs. 80.4 and 80.5).[4]

Open Approaches to Ventral Hernia Repair

The first reports of open hernia repair date back to the 4th century BCE and possibly even earlier.[5] Although modern hernia surgery employs a multitude of novel approaches and technology, the basic tenant of a hernia repair remains the same: durable reapproximation of healthy fascial tissue to prevent re-herniation of intraabdominal contents. Hernia repairs should attempt to restore native anatomy and distribute tensive forces over the area where the hernia formed.[6,7] The following section describes the various approaches and techniques for open VHR.

Primary Repair

A *primary repair* refers to suture closure of a fascial defect without the use of a mesh prosthesis. This technique is often used in patients with small, primary fascial defects such as umbilical or epigastric hernias <2 cm.[8–10] In general, primary repair should be avoided for incisional hernias, given a significantly higher recurrence rate compared with repair using mesh. However, sometimes

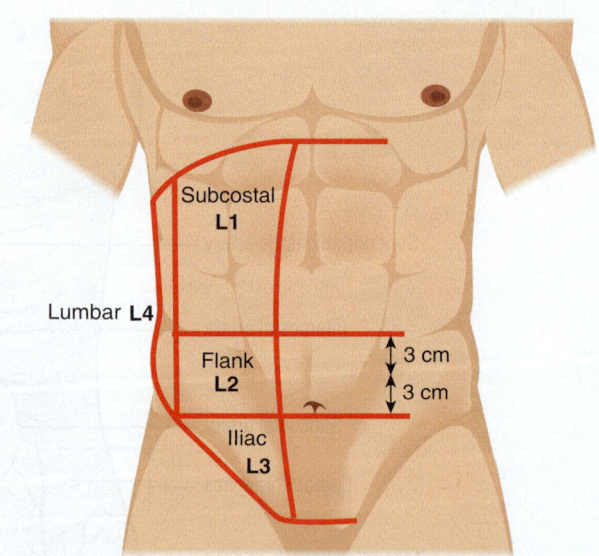

FIGURE 80.5 European Hernia Society lateral hernia classification. (From Muysoms FE, Miserez M, Berrevoet F, et al. Classification of primary and incisional abdominal wall hernias. *Hernia.* 2009;13[4]:407-414.)

primary repair is used in settings of contamination or in emergent cases when implantation of mesh may be ill-advised. Primary repairs should only be used in appropriately selected patients as it is well established that mesh reduces the rate of hernia recurrence. In a randomized controlled trial (RCT), umbilical hernias <4 cm in maximum diameter demonstrated significantly less recurrence when mesh was used (4% vs. 12%, hazard ratio [HR] = 0.31, 95% confidence interval [CI] 0.12–0.80).[11] With smaller hernias (1–2 cm), the absolute risk reduction from mesh use becomes more modest (2% vs. 8%, HR = 0.23, 95% CI 0.05–1.07) compared with larger (2- to 4-cm) defects (9% vs. 22%, HR = 0.39, 95% CI 0.12–1.30).[11]

Advocates of primary repair argue that avoidance of mesh implantation and its associated complications is worth the modest increase in recurrence of smaller defects. Guidelines differ in size cutoffs for recommending primary versus mesh repair, with some recommending the use of mesh in hernias >1 cm and others for hernias >2 cm.[6,7] Data extrapolated from the STITCH trial suggest that a small bites approach (0.5-cm × 0.5-cm bites) with a 4:1 ratio of suture to incision length using slowly absorbable suture minimizes the risk of hernia during laparotomy.[12] This approach is often applied to hernia repair. When deciding on an approach to small primary hernias, it is important to discuss the expected outcomes and absolute risk reduction with the use of mesh. Patients may desire to forego mesh placement and accept a higher risk of recurrence.

Fascial healing is a complex process that can take over a year to complete. Between the eighth postoperative day and second month, there is a rapid increase in fascial strength to about 50% of its original strength. This time frame corresponds to the beginning of the proliferative phase of wound healing to the end of collagen synthesis.[13] This time frame also suggests that at least a slowly absorbable suture material should be selected. A rapidly absorbing suture would otherwise risk failure before the expected significant regain in fascial strength. Although some select permanent suture for fascial closure in hernia repair, the authors typically do not choose this suture for fascial closure because it may lead to foreign body sensation and suture granulomas.

Before the introduction of mesh in the 1960s, multiple different techniques for the primary closure were described using both absorbable and nonabsorbable suture materials. The modified Mayo technique involves overlapping the edges of the fascia, creating fascial redundancy with two separate suture lines in an interrupted fashion, also colloquially referred to as *pants over vest*.[14] The "keel" repair used the dissected hernia sac to create redundancy posteriorly with anterior rectus sheath relaxing incisions to take tension off the midline repair. Steel wire repairs were used with reportedly good effect, but difficulty in replications of these results and application of the technique led to its disuse.[15] Currently, modern evidence for open primary repair is increasingly sparse, largely because of its abandonment in favor of mesh repair.

Mesh Repair

The introduction of mesh in the 1960s significantly reduced hernia recurrence rates, and mesh technology continues to evolve to this day.[11,16] Meshes can be classified as either permanent or absorbable. Permanent meshes are typically made from synthetic polymers, such as polypropylene, polyester, or polytetrafluoroethylene (PTFE), which will resist degradation by the patient's immune response. These synthetic meshes are typically used for definitive VHR and abdominal wall reconstruction. Each mesh varies in weight (g/cm^2), porosity, and hydrophilicity and may feature a composite design with an antiadhesive barrier. It is important to note that mesh weight should only be compared between meshes made from the same material. Ultra-lightweight polypropylene and lightweight polyester meshes have been shown to have increased central mesh failure.[16] Macroporous lightweight polypropylene mesh has demonstrated higher rates of bacterial clearance compared with other weights and porosities.[17] When synthetic mesh is placed in an intraperitoneal position, it must either be a composite mesh with an antiadhesive barrier or made of expanded polytetrafluoroethylene (ePTFE), which resists tissue incorporation. In the event of infection, composite meshes, especially PTFE, often require removal.

Absorbable meshes can be categorized into biologic and biosynthetic types. Biologic meshes are composed of acellular collagen matrices derived from either animal or human tissue and are gradually degraded by the host's biologic processes. Biologic meshes are classified based on their source material (including species and tissue type), postharvest processing techniques (e.g., cross-linked vs. non–cross-linked), and sterilization methods (e.g., gamma radiation, ethylene oxide gas sterilization, or nonsterilized). They are often preferred in contaminated cases, where permanent mesh is typically contraindicated due to the higher risk of infection. However, the use of biologic mesh has fallen out of favor recently because of high associated recurrence rates and costs.[18] Biosynthetic meshes are constructed from synthetic materials that absorb over time, such as polyglactin in Vicryl Mesh (Ethicon, Inc., Somerville, NJ). Polyglactin is rapidly absorbable and hydrolyzes completely in 2 to 3 months. These absorbable meshes are often used in contaminated fields where fascial closure is desired but the use of permanent synthetic mesh is prohibited. Other materials include poly-4-hydroxybutyrate (P4HB), which is found in Phasix Mesh (BD, Franklin Lakes, NJ) and is degraded over 12 and 18 months, and polyglycolide-trimethylene carbonate copolymer, which is found in GORE BIO-A Tissue Reinforcement (W.L. Gore & Associates, Inc., Newark, DE) and is degraded in about 6 months.[19,20] Further studies are necessary to better ascertain the optimal use for these materials. Mesh can be placed in several different locations, each with its own risks and benefits (Fig. 80.6).

Intraperitoneal underlay repair. *Intraperitoneal,* or "underlay," *mesh* refers to a mesh placed deep to the parietal peritoneum. Mesh placed in this position must be coated with an antiadhesion barrier or be absorbable to allow for direct contact with the bowel. Underlay mesh can be placed minimally invasively (most common) or via an open approach with the use of transfascial fixation sutures.

To perform this technique with an open approach, a midline incision is made. The hernia contents are completely reduced. Adhesions to the anterior abdominal wall are taken down circumferentially around the fascial defect to allow for adequate mesh overlap. The hernia defect is measured to determine mesh size. Correctly sizing the mesh is technically challenging in these cases because the mesh must be placed when the incision is open and lie flat when the fascia is closed. An oversized mesh will wrinkle with defect closure, whereas an undersized mesh will be prone to failure. Although wide overlap (>4–5 cm) is often advocated in laparoscopic underlay approaches, studies have not consistently shown that degree of mesh overlap is a significant predictor of recurrence in open procedures.[21] The authors still recommend aiming for a 5-cm mesh overlap in open procedures. Skin flaps are created by dissecting the subcutaneous tissue away from the anterior rectus fascia to facilitate the placement of transfascial sutures. The mesh is then secured circumferentially with these sutures, which are passed through the abdominal wall and along the mesh's edge. After all sutures are placed, the mesh is parachuted into position and tied down above the fascia. It is important to measure the location of the transfascial sutures to prevent wrinkling of the mesh when closing the hernia defect. The anterior rectus sheath is closed with a slowly absorbable suture. If large skin flaps are created, subcutaneous drain placement should be considered to prevent seroma formation.

Proponents of open underlay techniques argue that the mesh's placement provides a mechanical advantage against outward

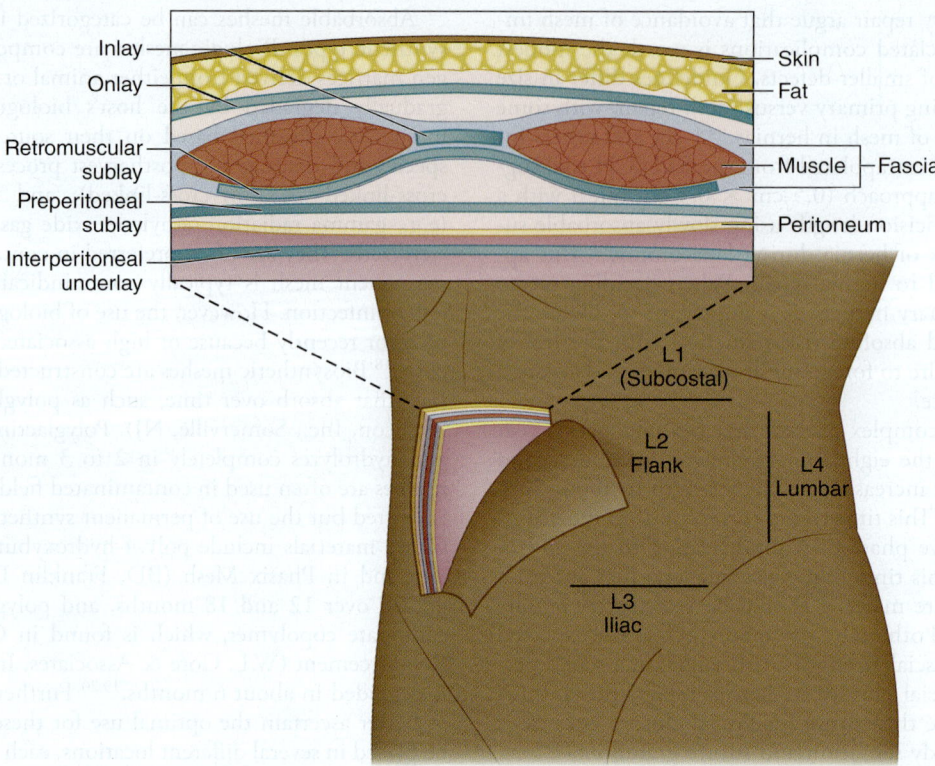

FIGURE 80.6 Mesh positions for ventral hernia repair. (Courtesy Board of Regents at the University of Texas System.)

intraabdominal pressure. Additionally, positioning the mesh away from the skin reduces the risk of contamination and lowers the likelihood of superficial surgical site infections (SSIs). Although underlay mesh placement is still commonly used in minimally invasive approaches, the rise of sublay techniques (see next section) has largely replaced open underlay approaches. Recent meta-analyses have shown sublay techniques to be superior in both recurrence and SSI rates compared with underlay techniques.[22]

Retromuscular sublay repair. Mesh placed in the retrorectus position is also known as a *retromuscular sublay,* or "Rives-Stoppa," repair. This technique of opening the posterior rectus sheath and placing mesh in the retrorectus space was described contemporarily by Rives in 1985[23] and later Stoppa in 1987.[24] This technique places the mesh deep to the rectus muscle and superficial to posterior sheath, parietal peritoneum, and sometimes hernia sac. This technique offers two key advantages: The mesh is placed outside the peritoneum, so a coated mesh is not needed, and it provides a highly vascularized area that supports better mesh integration.

This procedure is carried out by performing a laparotomy, reducing any herniated viscera, and lysing any anterior abdominal wall adhesions. The hernia sac should be carefully preserved because it can sometimes be needed later for closure of the posterior layer. On each side, the rectus muscle is identified, and the posterior sheath is opened at its medial attachment to the linea alba. It is critical not to cause an iatrogenic injury to the linea alba. The hernia sac should be left attached to the posterior sheath if possible. The posterior rectus sheath incisions are carried cranially and caudally. The retrorectus space is then developed laterally toward the semilunar line, where the neurovascular bundles of the rectus muscles are encountered (as shown in Fig. 80.3) and

protected. The extent of dissection depends on the size of the fascial defect and area necessary for mesh overlap, but it should be carried at least 5 cm superior and inferior to the defect. Superiorly, this dissection can extend past the costal margin and xiphoid process to the central tendon of the diaphragm. Inferiorly, the dissection can be carried below the pelvic brim into the space of Retzius. In most cases, surgeons will attempt to achieve at least 5 cm of mesh overlap from the hernia defect. However, the size of the cavity is largely determined by the anatomic constraints of the retrorectus space, and mesh is usually sized to occupy the entire extent of this space. A transversus abdominis release (TAR) allows for development of the retrorectus space beyond the linea semilunaris. The TAR technique will be described later in the chapter. Any holes in the posterior sheath are closed using absorbable suture. The posterior rectus sheath and hernia sac (if needed) are closed using a running, absorbable suture. The mesh is trimmed to the size of the retrorectus space and positioned flat against the posterior layer. Mesh fixation is not needed but can be performed based on surgeon preference.[25] Some options for mesh fixation include interrupted sutures, transfascial fixation, and fibrin sealant. In our practice, mesh fixation is typically not used. The anterior rectus fascia is then closed using slowly absorbable suture.

Sublay mesh placement has been shown to be superior to both onlay and underlay mesh in terms of SSI and recurrence rates.[22,26] In a meta-analysis of mesh location in open VHR, sublay mesh placement was associated with significantly lower recurrence rates and SSI rates compared with onlay, inlay (bridge), and underlay mesh placement. These results have led to a significant shift toward sublay mesh placement when doing open procedures. Open "Rives-Stoppa" repairs have improved over the years, with recent studies showing recurrence rates ranging from 7% to 11%.[25–28]

Preperitoneal sublay repair. In addition to the retrorectus plane, *sublay mesh* may also refer to mesh placed in the preperitoneal plane. The benefit of the preperitoneal plane is that it is not bound by the semilunar line like the retrorectus plane. In addition, a preperitoneal approach is less anatomically altering than a retrorectus repair because no fascial layers are incised. Preperitoneal repairs have gained popularity, with excellent results in expert hands. Heniford et al. have demonstrated excellent results even in large and complex hernias.[29] However, a preperitoneal dissection can be technically challenging to perform because the peritoneum can be extremely thin and difficult to dissect.

The procedure begins similarly to other open VHRs with a laparotomy, reduction of hernia contents, and lysis of adhesions. The preperitoneal space is entered and developed laterally, inferiorly, and superiorly to the fascial defect. The hernia sac should be protected and left in continuity with the preperitoneal flap because it can be used to facilitate closure of the flap later. The preperitoneal plane is dissected to allow for at least 5 cm of mesh overlap circumferentially. Once an adequate flap has been dissected, the space is measured, and a mesh is cut to size. Any holes in the peritoneal flap should be closed with absorbable suture. The hernia sac can be used to patch holes or facilitate closure of the flap if needed. The peritoneal flap is then closed with running absorbable suture. Mesh is placed in the preperitoneal space with optional fixation. The anterior rectus fascia is closed with running, slowly absorbable suture.

Bridging/Inlay repair. A bridging repair (inlay) is used when the fascial edges of a hernia defect cannot be closed primarily, and a mesh prosthesis must be used to bridge the gap between fascial edges. After a midline incision, the hernia contents are reduced, and adhesions to the anterior abdominal wall are lysed. The anterior rectus sheath should be cleared 1 cm circumferentially so that it can be clearly identified. The fascia is closed, starting from both the superior and inferior ends of the incision. The fascia is closed as much as possible from both ends. When it is no longer possible to close the fascia without undue tension, a mesh is sewn to the fascial edges using running suture.

This technique is often employed in the setting of extremely large defects where fascial approximation cannot be achieved. It is also used in some reoperative hernia surgeries where advanced techniques and tissue planes have already been used, in the emergency setting, after treatment of pathologies such as abdominal compartment syndrome (ACS), or with massive traumatic tissue loss.

Bridging mesh techniques are wrought with poor outcomes. Bridged repair has the highest recurrence rate among any of the mesh locations. It also leads to the poorest functional results because the linea alba (or fascial continuity in nonmidline hernias) is not restored. Although this technique is at times necessary in patients with massive hernias, every effort should be made to reoppose the fascia. Despite this, large retrospective studies have shown that although bridging repair is associated with a high degree of patient-perceived bulge, it does demonstrate quality-of-life benefits compared with preoperative patient-reported scores.[30] In addition, such a repair is sometimes the only option.

Onlay repair. Mesh that is placed anterior to the anterior rectus sheath is considered an onlay repair. After hernia sac reduction, the anterior rectus sheath edges are cleared so that they are clearly identifiable. The fascia is closed using running, slowly absorbable suture. Skin flaps are developed between the anterior rectus fascia and the subcutaneous tissue circumferentially to allow for wide mesh overlap (at least 5 cm). The mesh is secured in place using either interrupted or running suture directly between the mesh and the fascia. Care must be taken to sew the mesh to the fascia and not to the subcutaneous tissue to prevent migration, and dissecting skin flaps in the appropriate plane will ensure this. Subcutaneous tissue and skin are closed over the mesh per surgeon preference.

Onlay mesh has the advantage of keeping mesh out of the abdominal cavity and may be a valuable tool for patients at high risk for laparotomies as a result of dense adhesions or inability to tolerate prolonged operative times for a complex repair. However, it is associated with high rates of surgical site occurrences (SSOs), infections, and hernia recurrence.

Component Separation

Component separation refers to the creation of myofascial advancement flaps to assist with medialization of the rectus muscle and primary fascial closure. *Component separation* can refer to the division of either the external oblique muscles (anterior component separation) or transversus abduminus muscles (posterior component separation). These techniques are most often employed when the linea alba cannot be reapproximated because of the size of the hernia defect.

External oblique release (anterior component separation). Anterior component separation was initially described in 1990 by Ramirez and colleagues. It involves the division of the external oblique fascia and musculature. The amount of release it provides is debatable but is approximately 3 to 10 cm per side.[31]

The open anterior component separation begins with laparotomy, reduction of hernia contents, and lysis of adhesions to the anterior abdominal wall. Subcutaneous flaps are developed between the anterior rectus fascia and subcutaneous fat. The flaps are extended laterally to the linea semilunaris. The aponeurosis of the external oblique is incised 2 cm lateral to the semilunar line, and the external oblique muscle fibers are completely divided. This division is extended superiorly over the rib and inferiorly to the inguinal ligament. The space between the divided external and internal oblique muscle is developed. In addition, the posterior rectus sheath is incised and opened along the edge of the linea alba. This maneuver allows for medialization of the rectus muscles and closure of larger defects. The repair can then be performed with the surgeon's preferred mesh location. Finally, drains are placed in subcutaneous space.

The large skin flaps required for this procedure are associated with significant wound complications. As such, modifications to this procedure have been developed, including periumbilical perforator–sparing techniques, oblique release through separate incisions, and endoscopic release. A periumbilical perforator–sparing anterior component separation is performed similarly to a traditional open anterior component separation, but the periumbilical perforators, which lie in a 3-cm radius around the umbilicus, are preserved. Another approach is to use separate incisions to perform the release. Rather than creating skin flaps, small incisions are made along the semilunar line. The external oblique is divided as far cranially and caudally as possible through each incision, and a new incision is made once the limit is reached. Finally, with an endoscopic component separation, a small incision is made in the upper or lower quadrant at the semilunar line, and a balloon dissector is used to create a vertical tunnel in the subcutaneous space.[32] Two additional trocars are placed under direct vision. The external oblique is identified and divided using electrocautery from the costal margin to the inguinal ligament.

The initial use of the anterior component separation technique helped improve recurrence rates of large ventral incisional hernias from 50% down to 4.2% to 10% for large hernias.[33,34] The anterior component separation has been a mainstay in the armamentarium of abdominal reconstruction surgeons for many years and continues to be employed with good results. However, it has fallen out of favor with many hernia surgeons because of a high rate of wound complications and the development of the posterior component separation.

Transversus abdominis release (posterior component separation). Developed by Novitsky and colleagues in 2012, the TAR has quickly become a key instrument in abdominal wall reconstruction. The procedure allows for up to 8 cm of medialization depending on technique, avoids SSI complications from large skin flaps, allows for wide retromuscular sublay mesh placement, and can be performed via minimally invasive approaches.[35]

The anatomic considerations of the Rives-Stoppa and preperitoneal repair techniques, along with the mechanical theory of the anterior component separation, evolved into the development of the posterior component separation technique. The procedure is performed as a continuation of the Rives-Stoppa retrorectus dissection and can provide mesh overlap beyond the constraint of the linea semilunaris, and it offers increased fascial medialization. After development of the retrorectus space to the linea semilunaris as marked by the neurovascular bundles, the posterior lamellae of the internal oblique and underlying transverse abdominis muscle fibers are divided medially to the linea semilunaris. Once the muscle fibers are completely divided, the underlying transversalis fascia and/or peritoneum is visualized. This dissection is extended cranially and caudally, extending from under the diaphragm superiorly to the arcuate line inferiorly. The release can be started using either a "top-down" or "bottom-up" approach. The top-down approach involves beginning the TAR at the superior portion of the muscle and carrying it down toward the arcuate line. The muscle fibers of the transversus abdominis are more medial superiorly and thus more easily identifiable in this area. The transverse abdominis becomes more aponeurotic inferiorly. With the bottom-up approach, the arcuate line is identified. The posterior lamellae of the internal oblique aponeurosis and the underlying transverse abdominis (typically the aponeurotic portion) are divided medially to the linea semilunaris, beginning from the arcuate line up to the costal margin. Once the transverse abdominis is completely divided, the retromuscular space is developed laterally. Bare muscle can be seen superficial to the flap and confirms the true retromuscular or pretransversalis plane. If bare muscle fibers are not seen, the posterior layer is likely solely the peritoneum. Although it is safe to be in either the preperitoneal or pretransversalis plane, the surgeon must be able to identify which plane they are in throughout the operation. No muscle should be left of the posterior layer. Otherwise, the dissection has occurred in the incorrect plane. In addition, care should be taken to leave the muscular fibers of the diaphragm up when the superior dissection is performed because otherwise, an iatrogenic Morgagni hernia may occur. The retromuscular space is typically developed until the posterior layer lies flush with the intraabdominal viscera. The posterior layer is closed with running slowly absorbable suture. Mesh is placed in the retromuscular sublay plane with wide overlap to the full extent of the dissected retromuscular space. Mesh can be fixated with transfascial sutures to Cooper's ligament/pubis and to the costal margin if desired; however, fixation is optional. Although data are limited, drains are often placed in the transversus abdominus plane to control potential seroma or hematoma formation, which may impede mesh integration.

This technique has demonstrated excellent results, with recurrence rates under 5%.[34,36,37] The TAR is limited by the requirement for access to the retrorectus plane and may be complicated by previous repairs, transfascial sutures, previous stomas, transperitoneal tacks, or denervation of the rectus muscle resulting from previous surgery through chevron or Kocher incisions. Additionally, performing a TAR after an anterior component release is controversial due to the risk of abdominal wall destabilization, particularly along the linea semilunaris, when posterior component separation follows a previous anterior component separation.

Minimally Invasive Approaches to Ventral Hernia Repair

Minimally invasive approaches are permeating all aspects of surgery, including hernia repair and abdominal wall reconstruction. Although the general steps of each operation remain the same, the minimally invasive surgery (MIS) approach requires specific knowledge relating to positioning, instrumentation, and possible complications.

A key aspect of MIS is trocar placement and selection. The surgeon must place ports such that they are triangulating the area of interest. Increasing use of robotic surgery has made port placement more forgiving because there is less ergonomic strain with certain angles. Radially expanding blunt-tip trocars are often used because they are less traumatic and reduce port site bleeding. Upsizing of the trocar for mesh deployment may be necessary to prevent damage to the mesh. As with open cases, mesh contact with skin should be avoided to decrease contamination with skin flora.

Similar to open hernia repair, some cases may require extensive adhesiolysis. Accidental enterotomy or serotomy can occur. Based on the experience of the surgeon and whether contamination is limited, the injury may be addressed with MIS and the hernia repair performed immediately.[38] However, conversion to laparotomy should be considered if the extent of injury and contamination cannot be addressed in a minimally invasive fashion. After bowel injury repair, the surgeon may choose to delay hernia repair after a period of observation and parenteral antibiotics.

In addition to reducing the hernia, closure of the defect before placing mesh results in fewer instances of recurrence, bulging, and seroma (Fig. 80.7). The general benefits seen with MIS, such as decreased wound complications, are applicable to VHR and abdominal wall reconstruction.[39]

Intraperitoneal Underlay Repair

Minimally invasive intraperitoneal underlay mesh repair (IPUM) was the first minimally invasive VH technique described by LeBlanc et al. in 1992.[40] It is now a widespread technique because of its relatively technical simplicity and shorter learning curve while offering benefits of MIS, such as diminished SSI and length of stay.[41] Similar to the open approach, the MIS IPUM approach involves placing the mesh intraperitoneally. The location of the mesh is classically referred to as *underlay* because it is under the peritoneum and secured to the abdominal wall.

There are several options for port size and placement. MIS surgeons often opt for a triangulation approach and will place the ports along the side of the patient that increases surgeon mobility by decreasing the physical limitations of the patient's legs or chest. Of note, care should be taken not to place ports through the linea semilunaris because this may increase the risk of port site hernias. The herniated contents are then reduced, and the posterior fascia

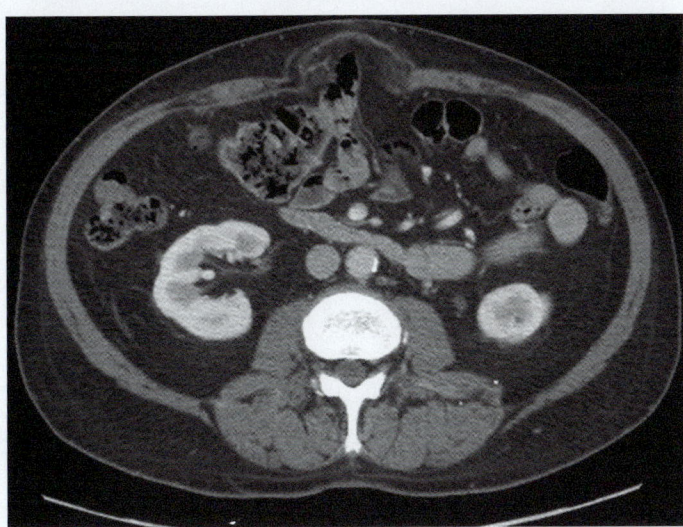

FIGURE 80.7 Abdominal CT scan after intraperitoneal underlay mesh repair without defect closure. The mesh has conformed to the defect, resulting in bulging and eventration of mesh.

should be cleared of any adipose tissue to encourage good apposition of mesh to fascia. Closure of the hernia defect is preferred because it decreases the rate of pseudorecurrence, which occurs when the mesh is secured at its periphery but bulges through the original defect like a trampoline. Wide defects that are unable to be approximated may not be the best suited for IPUM, and a more advanced technique may be necessary.

Two common options for mesh fixation in this approach are tacks or transfascial sutures, both of which have been associated with increased postoperative pain. The mesh is in direct contact with the underlying intraperitoneal viscera, and a composite mesh with an antiadhesive barrier should be selected. Intraperitoneal mesh can potentially lead to adhesions and bowel erosion with fistula development. Despite a wide array of composite meshes and other innovations, there has yet to be a proven barrier developed against these issues. Furthermore, when using 10-mm ports to insert the mesh, care must be taken to close the port site to decrease the risk of port site hernias. Refer to Video 80.1 for further details.

Transabdominal Preperitoneal Repair

More recently, the MIS transabdominal preperitoneal (TAPP) repair has gained popularity to address the limitations of the MIS IPUM approach, such as intraperitoneal mesh and the necessity of using a coated mesh. The port placement and importance of defect closure are analogous to the IPUM technique. This is a versatile technique because of the extent to which the preperitoneal space can be developed. However, preperitoneal dissection can be challenging due to the thin nature of the peritoneum and prior surgeries that may have violated the peritoneum.

A rule of thumb is to place the camera port about 15 cm away from the hernia. This allows 5 cm of mesh overlap, 5 cm for adequate peritoneal flap coverage of the mesh, and an additional 5 cm to visualize the initiation of the flap. After port placement, the herniated contents are reduced. An incision is made in the peritoneum, and the preperitoneal space is developed. As the surgeon begins the procedure, they must correctly identify the plane that lies between the peritoneum and the posterior rectus sheath, lateral to the hernia defect. Once the plane is dissected on either side of the hernia, the surgeon can then reduce any

preperitoneal adipose tissue. The dissection continues in that plane beyond the hernia to provide a sufficiently large peritoneal flap to cover the entire mesh. The hernia defect is then closed with absorbable barbed suture, such as V-Loc (Medtronic, Minneapolis, MN) or Stratafix (Ethicon, Raritan, NJ), and an uncoated synthetic mesh is secured to the abdominal wall with interrupted sutures. The peritoneal flap is then closed with absorbable barbed suture, with care to close any other fenestrations in the peritoneum that may have been made. If the peritoneal flap cannot be dissected or there is an excessive amount of peritoneal defects, the surgeon may convert to another approach, such as IPUM or retromuscular repair. Refer to Video 80.2 for further details.

Subcutaneous Onlay Repair

In 2018, Claus et al. reported the subcutaneous onlay laparoscopic approach (SCOLA).[42] This is an anterior minimally invasive approach that can simultaneously repair diastasis and midline hernias. Traditionally, diastasis was addressed by plastic surgeons through transverse lower abdominal incision, plication, and removal of excess skin. SCOLA offers a novel MIS approach, particularly useful for patients who do not require dermolipectomy.

The technique begins by placing the three ports along the Pfannenstiel incision line. If done laparoscopically, the midline suprapubic port will be 11 mm, and the lateral ports will be 5 mm.

When inserting the port, the dissection stops at the anterior aponeurosis of the rectus abdominis muscle. Pressure in this space can reach up to 10 mm Hg, and the surgeon can dissect the tissue from the aponeurosis toward the xiphoid cranially and the ribs laterally (Fig. 80.8).

The umbilical stalk is typically transected and re-created later during closure. Once this is accomplished, the hernia sac can be opened and the content reduced. With the use of a running barbed suture, the hernia defect can be closed and any diastasis recti plicated. As with other hernias, the use of a polypropylene mesh, here placed in an onlay position, reduces the risk of recurrence. Various methods can be used to keep this mesh in place, such as glue, sutures, or tacks. A drain is left in typically left in place.

Complications associated with this technique are mainly seroma formation but also include recurrences and wound infections. Of note, the patient population chosen for SCOLA repair had small hernias (<4 cm) and diastasis (<4 cm). The initial series has shown some positive results, and SCOLA may be appropriate in carefully selected patients. Refer to Video 80.3 for further details.

Retrorectus Sublay Repair

Larger (4- to 8-cm) midline hernias or hernias associated with a diastasis may benefit from the Rives-Stoppa repair.[43] The MIS Rives-Stoppa repair follows the same general steps as an open approach as described earlier in the chapter. Although the pertinent anatomy for an open retromuscular repair is the same for an MIS approach, there are stark differences in the operative approach and setup. Whereas open approaches typically begin with a midline incision to gain exposure, a minimally invasive approach has many incisional options. The location of the hernia and anatomic constraints, such as rectus abdominis width and bony prominences, will dictate the ideal location for initial port placement. Furthermore, a retromuscular repair may be performed using either a transabdominal or extraperitoneal approach, depending on patient factors. The patient is typically positioned supine in a flexed position with the arms tucked to increase mobility around

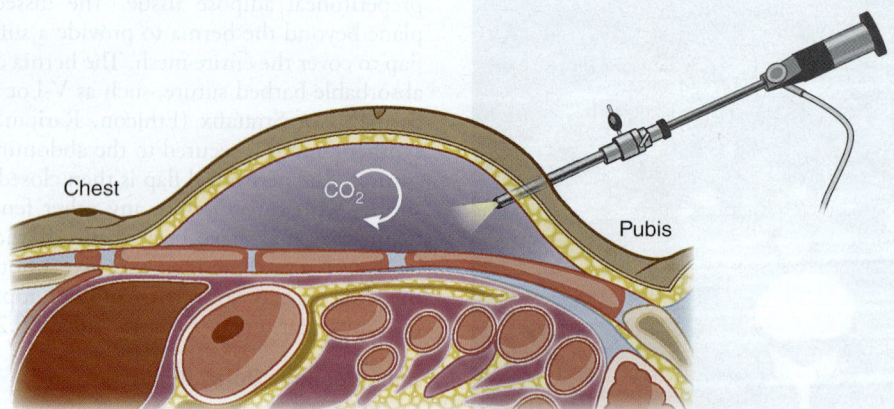

FIGURE 80.8 Insufflation of subcutaneous space during subcutaneous onlay laparoscopic approach. (From Claus CMP, Malcher F, Cavazzola LT, et al. Subcutaneous onlay laparoscopic approach [SCOLA] for ventral hernia and rectus abdominis diastasis repair: technical description and initial results. *Arquivos Brasileiros de Cirurgia Digestiva.* 2018;31[4].)

the patient. Flexion of the patient allows the chest and thighs to drop slightly away from the operative field to increase the operative working room of the surgeon and prevent robotic arm collision. Examples of robotic port placement are shown later; however, the same principles apply to traditional laparoscopy, such as triangulation of the working ports and the target. A retrorectus repair is limited laterally by the linea semilunaris. If further retromuscular space is required for hernia management, a TAR will be necessary.

A transabdominal retromuscular approach begins with establishment of pneumoperitoneum and placement of intraperitoneal ports. The retrorectus space is entered by incising the medial attachment of the posterior rectus sheath, and the retrorectus space is developed. Opposing ports are placed if necessary, and the contralateral retrorectus space is developed. The hernia defect is approximated with absorbable barbed suture, and plication of the linea alba is performed if necessary. An uncoated mesh is placed within the retromuscular space, and the posterior layer is closed. Although bridging peritoneum may suffice, it is our practice to approximate the posterior rectus sheaths if there is not excessive tension. It is critical to ensure any defects in the posterior layer are addressed to prevent intraparietal hernias.

The enhanced or extended totally extraperitoneal (eTEP) approach for retromuscular repair begins with direct access to the retrorectus space. The eTEP approach relies on the "crossover maneuver," which uses the midline preperitoneal space to bridge the bilateral retrorectus spaces.[44] Thus, a relative contraindication to this approach is a xiphopubic incision that may have significantly disrupted the midline preperitoneal space. In these cases, a transabdominal approach is preferred. Preoperative imaging is critical in determining if there is a safe plane for crossover. The authors prefer optical entry with advancement of the port through the rectus muscle and stopping just superficial to the posterior rectus sheath. The retrorectus space is then developed until other working ports can be placed.

Once the interface of the posterior rectus sheath and the linea alba is clearly visualized, an incision is made on the medial aspect of the posterior rectus sheath approximately 0.5 cm away from the linea alba to prevent iatrogenic injury to this critical structure.

Depending on location above or below the umbilicus, the adiposity from either the falciform or umbilical ligaments will be

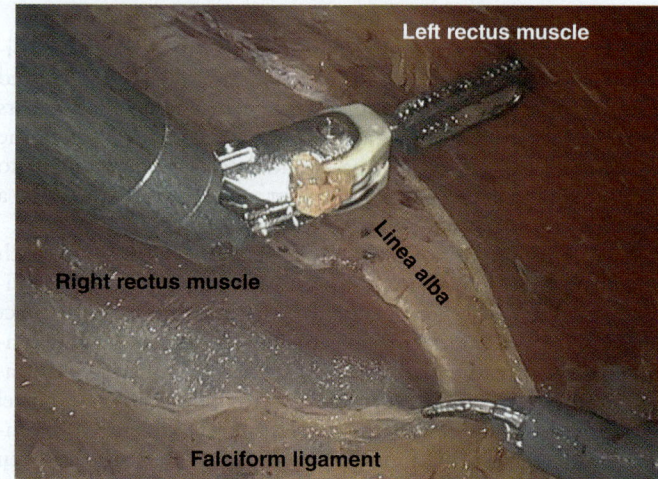

FIGURE 80.9 Completion of extended totally extraperitoneal crossover. Both rectus abdominis muscles and linea alba are clearly visualized. The posterior rectus sheaths and falciform ligament remain as the posterior layer.

encountered. The linea alba is then cleared of this adipose tissue until the contralateral posterior rectus sheath is visualized. This is then incised, exposing the contralateral rectus abdominis muscle. At this point, the "crossover" has been completed (Fig. 80.9).

As the dissection is continued, the hernia defect(s) are encountered and should be reduced. The retrorectus space is developed until adequate space for mesh overlap is achieved. The hernia defects are closed with absorbable barbed suture, and the linea alba is typically plicated to address any diastasis that is encountered. As mentioned, we routinely attempt to approximate the posterior rectus sheaths. If excessive tension is encountered, bridging peritoneum is sufficient. A medium-weight macroporous polypropylene mesh is placed, and the space is deflated under visualization. Refer to Video 80.4 for further details.

Transversus Abdominis Release

Patients who are candidates for MIS TAR are those patients with hernia defects 6 to 14 cm wide who have no more than 20% intraabdominal domain loss.[43] A TAR is useful for hernias that

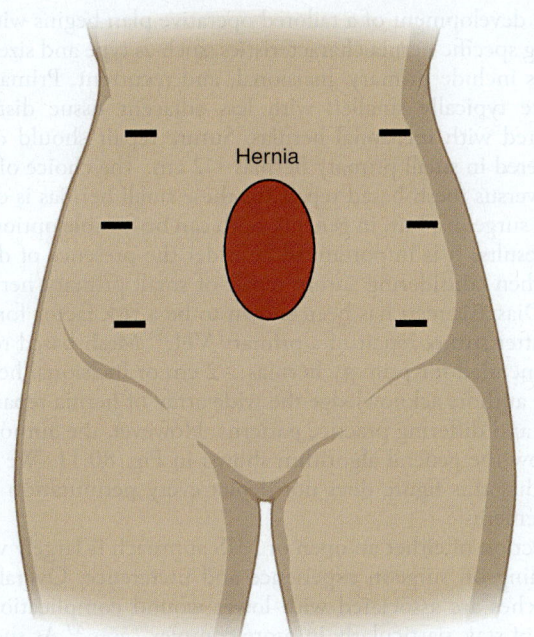

FIGURE 80.10 Port placement for minimally invasive surgery transversus abdominis release.

either would not have adequate mesh overlap from a retrorectus repair or hernias that are lateral to linea semilunaris. Any atrophic skin may be removed at the end of the case once the MIS portion is completed. Port placement is as illustrated in Fig. 80.10.

Initial access and the establishment of pneumoperitoneum can be performed with Veress needle, optical entry, or an open cutdown technique. After placing additional working ports, the first step often involves careful lysis of adhesions because these patients often have had multiple surgeries. The TAR dissection begins with a posterior rectus sheath release, stepping away laterally approximately 2 to 3 mm from the medial contributions of posterior rectus sheath to the linea alba and releasing this fascial structure from subxiphoid space to the arcuate line. Once in the retrorectus space, blunt dissection superficial to the posterior rectus sheath, in combination with judicious use of electrocautery, is used to dissect the retrorectus space. This dissection is limited laterally by the linea semilunaris. Neurovascular bundles that penetrate the posterior lamella of internal oblique are kept up with the underside of the rectus abdominis muscle, and care is used to identify and not injure these critical structures. Additional care is given to identify the deep inferior epigastric vessels on the dorsal portion of the rectus abdominis muscle. Some of the medial branches of this vessel may need to be ligated during the release of posterior rectus sheath. A TAR is then initiated by dividing two structures: first, the posterior lamella of internal oblique, followed by division of transversus abdominis muscle and/or aponeurosis and entering the space superficial to transversalis fascia and peritoneum.

This release is performed from the subxiphoid space, curving the release from subxiphoid fat pad, staying inferior to the insertion of the medial diaphragm fibers into the posterior rectus sheath, and staying medial and parallel to subcostal margin and, once below the level of costal margin, staying medial to neurovascular fibers and linea semilunaris. The release is extended past the arcuate line, which completely detaches the posterior rectus

sheath from its lateral attachments to the linea semilunaris. The actual transversus abdominis muscle is only divided at the upper aspect of the abdominal wall because the muscle fiber contributions of the transversus abdominis muscle in that region are quite prominent. The transversalis fascia and peritoneal layer are then dissected from the underside of transversus abdominis muscle. This dissection can be taken past the midaxillary line and above the costal margin, exposing the fibers of the diaphragm cranially and the myopectineal orifices caudally, offering the ability to address any additional subcostal, subxiphoid, and groin hernias that may be present.

Consequently, the posterior flap can be advanced up to 10 cm medially or more. The anterior myofascial flap also receives aggressive advancement due to two fascial releases of posterior components of abdominal wall—the posterior rectus sheath release followed by the release of the posterior lamella of internal oblique and transversus abdominis muscle complex.

The posterior flaps are reapproximated in the midline with a running suture, and the mesh is placed in the developed retromuscular space. The defect in the anterior layer is closed, which is facilitated by decreasing pneumoperitoneum to 5 to 7 mm Hg. An uncoated mesh is trimmed to size and placed in the retromuscular space. A retromuscular drain may be placed, and the abdomen is desufflated. Refer to Video 80.5 for further details.

Anterior Component Separation

Anterior component separation can also be performed with an MIS approach.[45] The surgeon typically begins by inserting ports on one side along the linea semilunaris and performing the dissection on the same (ipsilateral) side. Once the ipsilateral release is completed, the surgeon can place additional ports on the contralateral side. As with open technique, the MIS technique involves visualization of the entire anterior rectus sheath and identification of the linea semilunaris.

A fascial incision on the external oblique fascia, 1 to 2 cm lateral to the semilunar line, is then made in a cranial-to-caudal direction. The external oblique muscle itself can then be bluntly dissected off the underlying internal oblique muscle laterally to allow for medialization of the midline myofasciocutaneous flap. The superficial fascia and the linea alba are closed with a running suture technique. The mesh is inserted and deployed such that it lies flush on the anterior fascia. Onlay repairs mandate mesh fixation with suture, given its propensity to migrate in that position. A subcutaneous drainage is typically warranted. This relatively simple technique permits midline reapproximation and mesh placement outside the abdominal cavity. Complications such as flap ischemia and wound infections, although reduced with MIS approaches, are still seen.

Selection of Operative Technique

Hernia disease is a prevalent problem yet incredibly diverse. It is difficult to convey the complexity of hernia disease, which is determined by many factors, such as location, size, patient comorbidities, clinical acuity, and history of prior repairs. No VH classification system has been universally adopted, thus adding to the complexity of selecting management strategies. It is critical to approach each hernia patient with a tailored approach incorporating strong consideration for preoperative optimization, careful and individualized procedural selection, and comprehensive postoperative management. A surgeon requires a comprehensive understanding of abdominal wall anatomy and function as well as the various operative techniques and their potential pitfalls, as described earlier in this chapter, because complications can be devastating.

Patient selection is critical, and individual characteristics must be considered for a tailored approach. Factors including sex, BMI, social history, smoking status, functional status, and medical comorbidities (e.g., diabetes) can affect clinical outcomes. Refer to Chapter 79 for more details on preoperative management of the hernia patient. In terms of sex, studies have demonstrated female sex as independent risk factor for worse outcomes after hernia repairs, ventral or incisional, with increased adverse outcomes and chronic pain.[46] It is uncertain why such a disparity exists. Nevertheless, this is important to keep in mind because there may be less room for error in this patient population. It may also highlight the importance of a thorough preoperative conversation to set realistic goals and expectations. For female patients of childbearing age, it is important to consider their pregnancy and family plans. For those with asymptomatic or mildly symptomatic hernias, it is best to reserve definitive treatment until they have no plans for additional pregnancies because pregnancy may pose an increased risk for hernia recurrence. For patients with symptomatic hernias who are planning for future pregnancies, primary closure should be offered if possible. Although there certainly is a higher chance of recurrence, this approach does not disrupt any planes within the abdominal wall and preserves the more definitive tissue reinforcement-based repair options for the future if there is a recurrence. Complex abdominal wall reconstruction should be avoided in these patients, given the risk of postoperative abdominal wall compliance reduction.

Patient presentation and hernia symptomatology should be considered. Small asymptomatic hernias that contain preperitoneal fat or omentum can be monitored with a low risk of incarceration or bowel strangulation. Hernias that cause discomfort, pain, or intermittent obstructive symptoms should undergo repair. Hernias that present with acute incarceration should undergo urgent surgical intervention if reduction cannot be achieved promptly. Strangulated hernias certainly need surgical exploration. If there is bowel compromise that requires resection, primary repair is typically recommended because of the potential risk of mesh infection. If there is no bowel compromise, depending on the hernia characteristics and patient factors, definitive repair may be considered. However, it is typically not recommended to pursue complex repair with component separation in the acute setting. If it is a large or complex hernia that would require component separation, the primary or bridging repair and even skin closure alone may be considered, with plans for future abdominal wall reconstruction when the patient is better optimized.

Management of diastasis recti is a trending topic without consensus on its management. Diastasis can be a common incidental finding on examination or CT scan without evidence of abdominal wall dysfunction, and there is a lack of agreement on when diastasis is pathologic. Patients with diastasis recti may present with abdominal wall dysfunction with ongoing abdominal and back pain, in addition to having difficulty engaging their core. These patients typically benefit from physical therapy but can also benefit from surgical correction of their diastasis. Patients undergoing more extensive abdominal wall reconstruction for a complex hernia should have their diastasis addressed because it can serve as a weak point of the repair. For small VHs, diastasis should be considered a risk factor for recurrence after primary repair, and mesh placement should be considered.[47,48]

The development of a tailored operative plan begins with considering specific hernia characteristics, such as type and size. Types of VHs include primary, incisional, and recurrent. Primary hernias are typically smaller, with less adjacent tissue disruption compared with incisional hernias. Suture repair should only be considered in small primary hernias <2 cm. The choice of suture repair versus mesh-based repair for these small hernias is debated among surgeons, but, in general, both can be feasible options with good results. It is important to consider the presence of diastasis recti when considering suture repair of small primary hernia defects. Diastasis recti has been shown to be a risk factor for recurrence after suture repair of a primary VH.[48] Mesh-based repair is recommended for primary hernias >2 cm or incisional hernias.

The authors acknowledge the wide array of hernia repair techniques and differing practice patterns. However, the authors tend to follow the general algorithm shown in Fig. 80.11. We understand that this figure does not depict every permutation of VH management.

Selection of either an open or MIS approach is largely variable depending on surgeon experience and preference. Overall, MIS approaches are associated with lower wound complications and length of stay, particularly in more complex cases.[49] As such, our group generally prefers an MIS approach over an open approach for this reason if it is safe and feasible. An open approach is typically favored for small suture repairs or in cases where extensive tissue manipulation is necessary. These may include cases such as those with very large fascial defects (>15 cm), dense intraabdominal adhesions, necessity to excise large pieces of mesh or foreign bodies, bowel resection or fistula takedown, or need for extensive soft tissue rearrangement (e.g., panniculectomy). A hybrid approach in which a portion of the case is performed both MIS and open can also be considered and may reap the benefits of both approaches.[50] Long-term follow-up of outcomes, especially recurrence rates, will be important as the algorithmic approach to these complex hernia repairs continues to evolve.[51]

Regarding size, it is important to have a general concept of small, moderate, and large hernias; however, size is only one factor when deciding on the optimal operative approach. The hernia defect sizes discussed here are suggestions only and not concrete rules. Other considerations include anatomic details such as the width of the rectus abdominis muscles, hernia location, hernia-to-neck ratio, and abdominal wall compliance. For hernias 2 to 5 cm in size, preperitoneal, intraperitoneal, or retromuscular mesh repairs can be considered. For 6- to 8-cm defects, component separation will likely be needed with a Rives-Stoppa or retrorectus repair. Preperitoneal or intraperitoneal approaches can be considered for patients with good abdominal wall compliance, although it will be difficult to bring the fascial edges back together without too much tension. For 8- to 12-cm defects, Rives-Stoppa and potentially a TAR would likely be warranted, depending on the patient's abdominal wall compliance and rectus abdominis muscle width. Studies have shown that a ratio of the total rectus width to defect width greater than 2 can predict successful fascial closure with retrorectus dissection alone.[52] Anterior component separation can also be considered. For 12- to 15-cm hernias, it is likely that a component separation will be needed. For much larger, complex hernias, additional adjuncts such as Botox injections or progressive pneumoperitoneum may be necessary, but these are beyond the scope of this chapter.

Operative management of recurrent hernias is highly dependent on the patient's surgical history. It is critical to obtain all prior operative reports if possible. Imaging may add invaluable

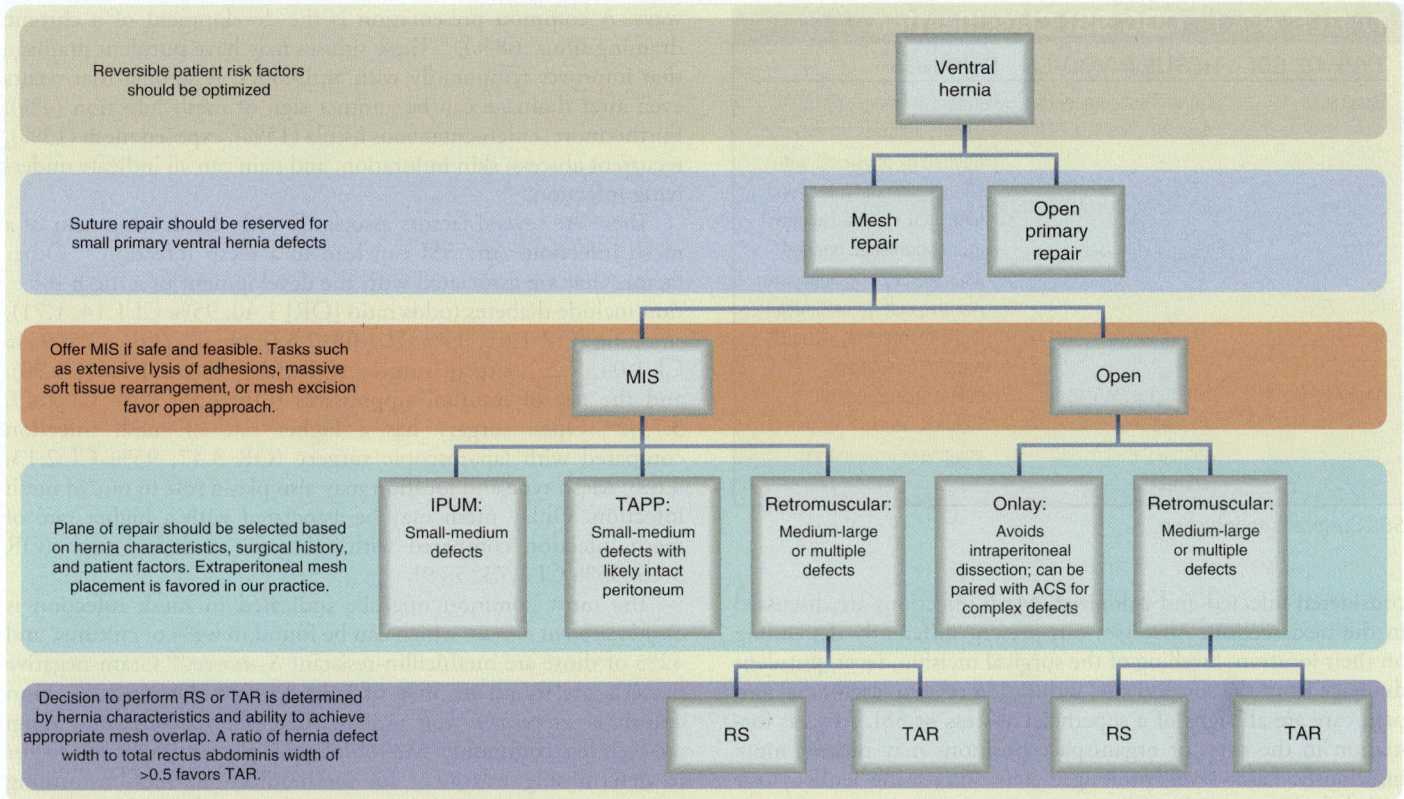

FIGURE 80.11 Management of ventral hernias. *ACS,* Anterior component separation; *IPUM,* intraperitoneal underlay mesh repair; *MIS,* minimally invasive surgery; *RS,* Rives-Stoppa; *TAPP,* transabdominal preperitoneal; *TAR,* transversus abdominis release.

information, including location of prior implants, fixation devices, and their relationship to the hernia defect. A recurrence after simple primary repair should be treated as an incisional hernia with an appropriate mesh-based repair for the hernia's characteristics. Recurrences after mesh-based repairs are tackled differently based on location of the prior mesh. The general concept is to perform a repair in a different plane compared with the last repair. For recurrences after an onlay repair, underlay or sublay repairs should be considered. Open or hybrid approaches may be needed if planning for mesh explantation or soft tissue resection. Recurrences after preperitoneal sublay or underlay repairs should be managed with either an onlay or retromuscular approach. Recurrences after retromuscular repairs can be challenging because most were likely performed for larger and more complicated hernias initially. If the recurrent hernia is small, an onlay or underlay repair may be considered. Large or more complex recurrence may necessitate a redo retromuscular repair, although it may be technically challenging.

Recurrent hernias can sometimes present with infectious complications, such as chronic abscesses or fistulas from mesh erosion. Staged approaches should be considered in the presence of active infection. The goal of the first stage is to achieve source control, which typically calls for the excision and removal of all foreign body material, including sutures and/or mesh. If a fistula has formed due to prior mesh placement, the mesh and involved viscera should be resected. Definitive hernia repair can be considered at least 6 months after clearance of active infection.

COMPLICATIONS

Complications are common after VHR. Complications can occur in the early postoperative period, similar to most wound complications, or in the long term, such as chronic pain or hernia recurrence. The clinical significance of each complication varies greatly. In this section, complications after VHR are discussed.

Infection

SSIs, as defined by the CDC, are complications caused by infection at the surgical incision site or from an intraabdominal process that leads to a collection of fluid, pus, or a culturable organism.[53] This includes abscess, necrotizing soft tissue infection, anastomotic failure, and mesh infection, among others. The infections are further classified by their location and what interventions are needed for resolution (Table 80.1).

The rate of SSI after VHR is highly variable in the literature, ranging from 4% to 21%.[54,55] Even a superficial SSI can be problematic. It is well established that patients who develop an infection are at higher risk of developing a hernia recurrence.[56] Furthermore, mesh infection can be a challenging problem, leading to chronic wounds and requiring reoperation.

An abscess is an infection involving a space-occupying collection of pus surrounded by inflammatory tissue. These collections can be in the superficial surgical site (skin and subcutaneous adipose), deep surgical site (fascial and muscle layers), and organ space (intraabdominal cavity). In hernia surgery, a mesh that is contained in the same space where an abscess has formed is

TABLE 80.1	CDC SSI Classification	
TYPE OF SSI	TISSUE INVOLVED	FINDINGS
Superficial	Skin and subcutaneous tissue	Purulent drainage, positive wound cultures, or incision opened by physician with clinical signs of infection (does not include cellulitis)
Deep	Fascia and muscle	Purulent drainage, opened/aspirated by physician with positive culture or clinical signs of infection, abscess present on imaging
Organ/space	Deep to fascia/muscle in area that was manipulated during surgery	Purulent drainage, positive cultures, abscess present on imaging or examination

SSI, Surgical site infection.

considered infected and colonized. Mesh infections are discussed in the next section. Abscesses can present differently depending on their location. Swelling of the surgical incision, fever, purulent drainage from the surgical site, induration of skin, erythema, and pain care are all signs of a superficial abscess or SSI. Abscess formation in the deep or organ/space positions may present more insidiously. Pain, fever, prolonged ileus, increasing leukocytosis with left shift, and thrombocytosis can often indicate a deep or organ/space infection. Abscesses must be dealt with promptly. Systemic infection, necrotizing soft tissue infection, wound dehiscence, and mesh colonization are all possible complications of untreated wound infection.

The most effective treatment for abscess is drainage (in the absence of a prosthetic, such as mesh). Small abscesses (<3 cm) that are not amenable to drainage can be treated with antibiotics. RCT evidence has shown that for intraabdominal infections, antibiotic therapy can be stopped 4 days after adequate source control has been achieved.[57] In superficial wound infections, drainage can be performed at the bedside through the wound or through percutaneous drainage. Subcutaneous collections that can be adequately drained and have no signs of spreading or systemic infection do not require antibiotic therapy. Resolution of symptoms, leukocytosis, fever, and restoration of normal gastrointestinal function are all signs of resolving abscess. In cases of small (<3-cm) or undrainable collections, the optimal duration for antibiotics in these cases is not clear, with some practitioners advocating that many of these collections do not need treatment at all. Equally unclear is the indication for repeated imaging examination. Deterioration in symptoms or biochemical metrics are indications for intervention or repeat investigation, usually with cross-sectional imaging. Routine follow-up imaging is used by some surgeons, but the optimal indication for this has yet to be elucidated.

The incidence of mesh infection ranges from 1% to 8% in the literature.[58] Unlike superficial or deep SSIs, which must be diagnosed within 90 days according to CDC definition, a mesh infection can be diagnosed for up to 1 year after surgery.[53] In some cases, it can take even longer for a mesh infection to be diagnosed. It has been reported that the mean time from hernia repair to presentation of mesh infection is 19.9 months.[59] This delay likely leads to an underreporting of the true incidence of mesh infection in the literature. Mesh infection can present in a variety of different

ways. A common presentation is the development of a chronic draining sinus (68%).[60] These sinuses may have purulent drainage that improves temporarily with antibiotics. A seroma that recurs even after drainage can be another sign of mesh infection (4%). Furthermore, enterocutaneous fistula (15%), exposed mesh (13%), recurrent abscess, skin induration, and pain can all indicate underlying infection.

There are several factors associated with the development of a mesh infection. Any SSI can lead to a mesh infection.[61] Other factors that are associated with the development of a mesh infection include diabetes (odds ratio [OR] 1.40; 95% CI 1.14, 1.71), smoking (OR 1.65; 95% CI 1.08, 2.52), obesity (OR 2.75; 95% CI 1.04, 7.27), urgent surgery (OR 3.10; 95% CI 1.61, 5.98), and the use of immunosuppressives (OR 2.35; 95% CI 1.49, 3.73).[62] Open surgery has a higher rate of mesh infection compared with laparoscopic surgery (OR 3.47; 95% CI 2.13, 5.62). Mesh type and location may also play a role in rate of mesh infection. Onlay mesh may be associated with a higher rate of mesh infection compared with sublay or underlay mesh (OR 3.16; 95% CI 1.73, 5.79).

The most common microbe indicated in mesh infection is *Staphylococcus aureus,* which can be found in 64% of cultures, and 42% of those are methicillin-resistant *S. aureus.*[60] Gram-negative bacteria are found in 35% of cultures, and the most common culprit is *Escherichia coli* (13%). Anaerobic bacteria and fungi are seen less commonly. Microbiology is also an important factor in determining treatment for mesh infection. Biofilm-forming organisms, such as *Staphylococcus,* are much more difficult to clear from mesh surfaces.

The type of mesh is important in determining if a mesh can be salvaged. Macroporous polypropylene mesh in an extraperitoneal position has the highest rate of mesh salvage at 72.2% of cases. Microporous polypropylene and polyester mesh have not been shown to be as infection resistant, with salvage rates of 3.1% and 3.2%, respectively. PTFE and composite meshes are unlikely to be salvaged.[59] Biosynthetic and biologic meshes were developed with the intention of being resistant to bacterial infection and therefore avoiding permanent mesh colonization. However, RCTs have shown comparable rates of SSI and increased recurrence rates when using biologic mesh versus synthetic mesh.[63] However, mesh explantation may be less likely with biologic mesh.[64] As such, with microporous polypropylene, biologic, or biosynthetic mesh, it is reasonable to attempt antibiotic therapy and drainage of any fluid collections as a first-line treatment for mesh infection. In the case of microporous polypropylene, polyester, PTFE, or composite mesh, antibiotic therapy can be attempted, but mesh explantation is likely to be required to adequately treat the infection.

There are several strategies for the treatment of a mesh infection. Conservative management with antibiotics alone can be attempted, but mesh salvage rates are low (21%).[59] Drainage, local debridement, and negative-pressure wound therapy (NPWT) can be used, with mesh salvage rates of 18% to 35%. Mesh explantation is often required. Mesh can be either partially or completely explanted. Infection recurrence is more likely with partial mesh excision compared with complete excision (58% vs. 25%; OR 4.15; 95% CI 2.30, 7.47). However, the rate of hernia recurrence is likely lower with partial compared with complete excision (10% vs. 40%; OR 0.25; 95% CI 0.04, 1.62).[65]

Seroma

A seroma is a sterile collection of inflammatory fluid. Seromas are common after many different types of surgery. The extent of intraparietal and/or subcutaneous dissection and the presence of a prosthesis make hernia surgery especially susceptible to seroma formation. The rate of seromas after VHR ranges from 3% to 52.4%, depending on the technique used.[34,66,67] The risk of seromas increases in emergency surgeries, patients with high BMI, large skin flaps, component separation, onlay mesh placement, and biologic mesh usage.[66] Seromas are often harmless. However, they can lead to secondary infection or compromise mesh integration.

The treatment of seromas depends on their size, location, and chronicity. Many seromas will resolve spontaneously. For seromas that are minimally symptomatic with no signs of infection, observation is the most appropriate treatment. Prophylactic antibiotics are not indicated. If the seroma is large or prolonged or if there are significant symptoms (e.g., pain or drainage from wound), seromas can be aspirated in an outpatient setting. Multiple aspirations or even drain placement may be required for complete resolution. Seromas refractory to percutaneous intervention may require surgical excision.

Drains are sometimes left in the surgical field to prevent seromas, but this is controversial and surgeon dependent. There is concern that drains may leave a patient more susceptible to infection. However, a recent meta-analysis suggests that drains reduce seroma rate (OR 0.34; 95% CI 0.12–0.96) with no increase in infection.[68] Drains should be considered if large subcutaneous flaps are developed, with retrorectus repair, or when component separation is performed. Drains are removed when output is minimal (30 mL/day) over 2 to 3 consecutive days or when a certain time point is met.[66]

Hematoma

Hematomas are collections of blood in a surgical space. The rate of hematoma after VHR has been reported as high as 7%.[5] Hematomas can present with hemodynamic compromise, pain, swelling, or orthostatic symptoms or can be clinically silent. Although many hematomas are self-limited, some require repeat intervention. Risk factors for postoperative hematoma include subcutaneous or intraparietal dissection, perioperative therapeutic anticoagulation, and component separation.[66,69,70] Patients who undergo posterior component separation are more likely to develop a hematoma than those with anterior component separation (OR 1.81; 95% CI 1.26–2.61).[34]

Management of postoperative hematomas is dependent on clinical presentation. Patients presenting with hemodynamic compromise should be adequately resuscitated, and individuals nonresponsive to resuscitation should return to the operating room for hematoma evacuation and source control. Those who are stable but who have had a clinically detectable bleeding episode often undergo cross-sectional imaging to identify its location. Consideration can be given to returning to the operating room if there is concern that the hematoma will interfere with mesh incorporation or is at high risk of infection. Stable, minimally symptomatic hematomas may be observed.

Chronic Pain

The definition of chronic pain can vary among studies, but it is generally accepted that pain still present at 1 year postoperative is considered chronic pain.[71,72] Approximately one-quarter of patients undergoing VHR will report some form of chronic discomfort or pain. Risk factors for postoperative pain include younger age, female sex, preoperative narcotic use, Carolinas Comfort Scale (CCS) preoperative pain score ≥2, and early

postoperative pain.[71,73] Different techniques for mesh fixation have been implicated in causing more acute and chronic postoperative pain, but the data do not support this.[74] It is thought that minimizing penetrating fixation may decrease chronic pain.

Chronic pain can be debilitating, and patients should be counseled about the risk of postoperative pain while discussing the risks and benefits of the procedure. Patients should be counseled that postoperative pain after VHR can last for several months, and it is generally unwise to return to the operating room before 6 to 8 months. Patients presenting with postoperative pain after hernia repair should be thoroughly interviewed and examined to determine the exact quality and location of the pain. Nonsteroidal antiinflammatory drugs (NSAIDs) are helpful during these initial few months. If neuropathic pain is suspected, the addition of gabapentin or pregabalin can be considered. For pain that persists for more than 1 year, physical examination findings should be correlated with the surgery performed and imaging findings to see if a surgical cause for the pain could exist. Transfascial sutures and tacks have been implicated in certain patients with chronic pain, and removal of these can be considered if the pain correlates to their location. Anterior cutaneous nerve entrapment syndrome (ACNES) generally presents as pain along the lateral edge of the rectus muscle and is frequently misdiagnosed.[75] Mesh can sometimes be the etiology of chronic pain. Although mesh explantation may be offered, it is difficult to know preoperatively if removing a mesh will improve pain. Patients who undergo mesh explantation are likely to develop a recurrent hernia. Mesh removal should be considered as a last resort if there is no obvious problem with the mesh. If no surgical cause for chronic pain can be identified, patients should be referred to a pain specialist. Other modalities, such as regional anesthetic techniques, cryoablation, physiotherapy, and cognitive therapy, may be employed to treat chronic pain.

Intraparietal Hernia

An *intraparietal hernia* refers to herniation within the layers of the abdominal wall, such as the peritoneum or posterior rectus sheath. The traditional example of a primary intraparietal hernia is a Spigelian hernia. With the advent of retrorectus and component separation procedures, iatrogenic intraparietal hernias are becoming increasingly common. With a sublay mesh placement, a preperitoneal or retromuscular plane is developed. If there is breakdown of the posterior layer, intraperitoneal viscera may herniate within the layers of the abdominal wall. Intraparietal hernias can occur with underlay mesh placement as well. Abdominal contents can herniate between the mesh and anterior abdominal wall. Intraparietal hernias often present insidiously, much like internal hernias. Patients may complain of vague or intermittent crampy abdominal pain and obstruction. Often, cross-sectional imaging will be reported as normal postoperative anatomy because there is no defect in the anterior abdominal wall where one traditionally looks for a hernia. Surgeons should review the images in an attempt to identify the location of the mesh in relation to the bowel. Although rare, early postoperative bowel obstructions may be caused by an intraparietal hernia secondary to posterior layer dehiscence in retromuscular hernia repair. Interparietal hernias require operative intervention. Depending on the nature of the original operation, minimally invasive techniques may be used to reduce the intraparietal hernia and address the defect primarily with underlay mesh reinforcement if necessary and feasible (Fig. 80.12).

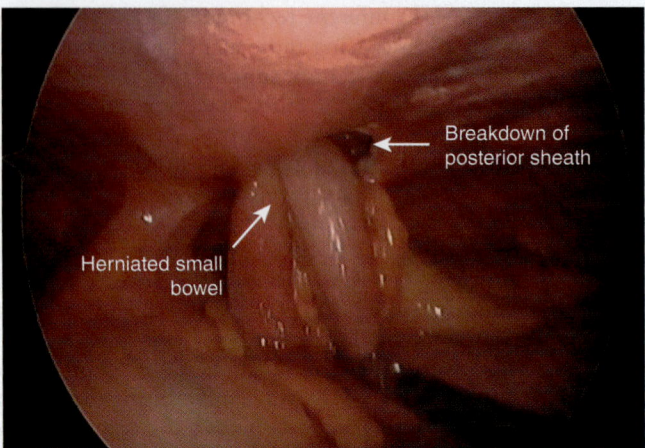

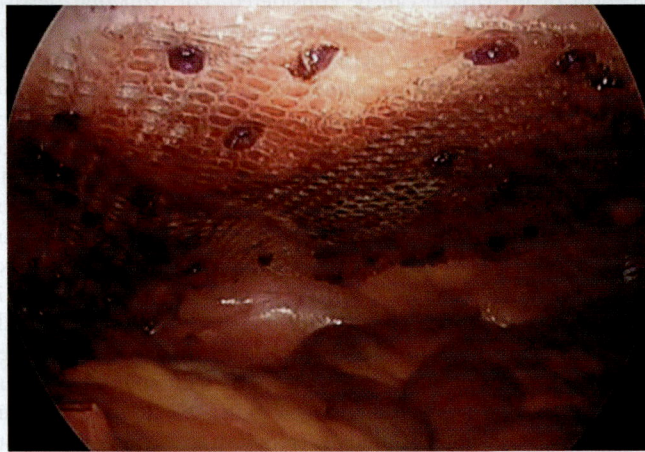

FIGURE 80.12 Before and after laparoscopic reduction of intraparietal hernia from posterior layer dehiscence with intraperitoneal underlay mesh repair.

Abdominal Compartment Syndrome

The repair of large and complex hernias can lead to intraabdominal hypertension. As a hernia gets larger, the amount of tension needed to close the abdominal cavity increases. Intraabdominal pressure increases proportionately. Intraoperatively, this can be noted by increases in airway pressure. Intraabdominal pressure can be estimated from bladder pressure, which is normally 5 to 7 mm Hg. It is considered intraabdominal hypertension when the pressure exceeds 12 mm Hg. In general, intraabdominal hypertension is not clinically impactful at lower pressures (12–20 mm Hg). However, at high pressure, intraabdominal hypertension can lead to ACS, which is characterized by respiratory, cardiac, renal, and gastrointestinal dysfunction. ACS is diagnosed by an intraabdominal pressure ≥20 mm Hg coinciding with acute-onset organ dysfunction. Prevention and early diagnosis of ACS are critical because the mortality rate of ACS is up to 60%.[76] The World Society of the Abdominal Compartment Syndrome (WSACS) recognizes ACS as a distinct class of compartment syndrome termed *quaternary compartment syndrome*. Risk factors for the development of ACS include positive fluid balance, hypoproteinemia, ratio of hernia sac to abdominal cavity volume (ACV) greater than 25%, and elevated BMI.[76,77]

The traditional treatment of ACS is decompressive laparotomy. However, the treatment of quaternary compartment syndrome can sometimes be nonoperative. Intraoperatively, mean airway pressures are monitored. Upon closure, if the mean airway pressure rises significantly (7–10 mm Hg), consideration should be given to keeping the patient intubated and paralyzed to allow for accommodation and muscle relaxation. In most cases, the intraabdominal pressure will decrease to appropriate levels in the next 24 to 48 hours, allowing for extubation. Patients who are extubated postoperatively who subsequently develop ACS should be intubated, sedated, and paralyzed, and abdominal pressure should be closely monitored. If unsuccessful, decompressive laparotomy may be needed. A high index of suspicion must be maintained to allow for the prompt diagnosis and treatment of ACS in the postoperative setting. Because of the risk of ACS, large, hernias involving domain loss should only be performed in an appropriate setting with access to intensive care unit (ICU) care.

Venous Thromboembolism

Patients undergoing VHR are at high risk of thromboembolic complications. Rates of venous thromboembolism in incisional hernia have been reported from anywhere between 0.2% and 7.9%.[78,79] Patients should begin postoperative chemical deep vein thrombosis (DVT) prophylaxis as soon as possible. Concerns of postoperative bleeding with early administration of DVT prophylaxis have not been demonstrated in the literature. Signs and symptoms of DVT or pulmonary embolism (PE), such as shortness of breath, calf swelling, unexplained tachycardia, and hypoxia, should be expeditiously investigated, and a high index of suspicion should be maintained in this patient population.

SPECIAL CONSIDERATIONS

Recurrence

The rate of hernia recurrence varies in the literature, ranging from 15% to 40%. It is therefore important for the surgeon to identify risk factors of recurrence to optimize the surgical outcomes.[80] Preoperative risk factors include smoking, diabetes, chronic obstructive pulmonary disease, American Society of Anesthesiologists (ASA) grade III to IV, and steroid use. Patients with higher BMIs also have higher odds of recurrence. In patients with VHs, 60% have BMIs greater than or equal to 30 kg/m^2.[81] Surgeons may encourage patients to lose weight before surgery. However, weight loss is challenging in these patients because the symptoms associated with the hernia can limit physical activities. Furthermore, delaying elective procedures increases the risk of hernia incarceration or strangulation.

Postoperative SSOs are associated with an increased risk of hernia recurrence. These include infections, seromas, hematomas, and wound dehiscence. The risk of SSI increases with higher BMIs, with the highest risk of SSI in patients with a BMI greater than 42 kg/m^2.[81] Minimally invasive approaches are thought to be protective against complications such as SSOs, given the decrease in wound and dead space area. A study demonstrated no significant differences in clinical outcomes with MIS retromuscular repairs in patients with a BMI either above or below 35 kg/m^2.[82] Smoking is associated with impaired wound healing because it affects oxygen delivery to the tissues. Smoking cessation for 4 weeks before elective surgery can decrease the risk of SSI in open cases.[83] Other systemic postoperative complications, such as pneumonia or urinary tract infection, increase the odds of recurrence. It is well known that hernia recurrence can lead to a vicious cycle of diminishing returns.[84] Increasingly, patients who develop hernia recurrences are being sent to multidisciplinary hernia centers to provide comprehensive care for these challenging cases.

Skin, Soft Tissue, and Dead Space Management in Abdominal Wall Reconstruction

Hernia repair should be done in a holistic fashion, with care to address the skin and subcutaneous tissue in conjunction with the underlying hernia defect. Over time, large hernias stretch the overlying skin. Leaving excess skin can increase the risk of SSOs and SSIs because of the large potential space for seroma formation that can lead to breakdown of skin closure. Thin skin may also necrose and ulcerate. To avoid wound breakdown and its associated complications, consideration should be given to excising the excess overlying skin.[85] Depending on the amount of redundant tissue, some patients may additionally benefit from a panniculectomy. During panniculectomy, excessive undermining of the remaining lipocutaneous flaps can disrupt blood flow from the perforators and compromise tissue vascularity. It is critical to consider other prior abdominal surgeries that may further compromise blood supply to the lipocutaneous flaps.

When dealing with SSO or SSI, healing by secondary intention with daily dressing changes is an option for small, superficial wounds. Large, clean, granulated wounds can benefit from skin grafts or flaps. Very rarely, regional muscular or fasciocutaneous flaps may be considered for larger wounds. Lastly, wounds may benefit from NPWT, which has been shown to improve blood flow and granulation tissue formation and decrease contamination.[86,87]

Physiologic fluid will accumulate in dead space. In the short term, this can cause issues with mesh incorporation and increase the risk of mesh infection and seroma formation. There are different ways to manage fluid buildup. When dealing with subcutaneous space, the surgeon can choose to place layered progressive sutures to approximate the defect. Closed suction drains can also direct fluid out of the surgical site. Surgeons may choose a combination of those techniques. More recently, NPWT over closed incisions, such as the PREVENA (3M, St. Paul, MN), have been used because it has been shown to reduce wound-healing complications, dehiscence, and seroma formation.

Acute Presentation

VHs that are reducible or chronically incarcerated with minimal symptoms can be repaired electively. Acutely incarcerated hernias or strangulated hernias require urgent surgical intervention. VH width-to-neck ratios greater than 2.5 are associated with an increased risk of emergency surgeries.[88] Emergent cases can present with acute pain, obstructive symptoms such as nausea or vomiting, overlying skin changes, and fever. Additional laboratory and radiologic studies, such as white blood cell count and lactate levels and CT imaging, can help with the diagnosis; however, strangulated hernias can be diagnosed on history and physical examination alone. Adequate volume resuscitation and broad-spectrum antibiotics should be initiated in the emergency department.

The goals of surgery are to relieve bowel obstruction and resect any necrotic bowel and/or tissue. Historically, VHs repaired in the emergent setting were closed primarily to avoid the risk of mesh infection. Recent evidence has shown more subtlety in decision-making.[89] Intraoperatively, the surgical field can be classified and help determine treatment options (Table 80.2).

For patients with intestinal obstruction but no signs of strangulation or need for bowel resection (class I wound), synthetic mesh is recommended. In cases with strangulated bowel needing resection without gross enteric contamination (class II wounds), using mesh does not increase the 30-day wound-related morbidity and decreases the risk of hernia recurrence. For patients with

TABLE 80.2	Surgical Wound Classification
Class I	Clean
Class II	Clean-contaminated
Class III	Contaminated
Class IV	Dirty-infected

TABLE 80.3 Traumatic Abdominal Wall Hernia Grading Scale

GRADE	REGION	DESCRIPTION
I	Abdominal wall	Contusion of subcutaneous tissue
II	Abdominal wall	Abdominal wall muscle hematoma
III	Abdominal wall	Disruption of a single abdominal wall muscle layer
IV	Rectus	Complete anterior abdominal wall muscle disruption
	Flank	
	Lumbar	Complete lateral abdominal wall muscle disruption
		Complete posterior abdominal wall muscle disruption
V	Rectus	Anterior disruption with herniation
	Flank	Flank lateral disruption with herniation
	Lumbar	Lumbar posterior disruption with herniation
VI	Rectus	Anterior herniation with evisceration
	Flank	Flank lateral herniation with evisceration
	Lumbar	Lumbar posterior herniation with evisceration

bowel necrosis and/or bowel perforation (class III–IV wounds), primary repair is indicated. In class III to IV wounds where the hernia is too large for primary repair, skin closure may be the only option. The surgeon should not attempt any component separation technique because these should be reserved for elective situations. The use of biologic mesh had been advocated in contaminated cases; however, this has fallen out of favor with time, given its high cost and unacceptable recurrence rates.[18]

Traumatic Abdominal Wall Hernias and the Open Abdomen

In 2021, the Western Trauma Association (WTA) published its guidelines regarding the management of a rare traumatic entity: the blunt abdominal wall hernia.[90] The traumatic abdominal wall hernia (TAWH) occurs when blunt traumatic forces induce a disruption in the abdominal wall. These can occur in the lumbar, flank, and ventral locations. Annually, there are approximately 15,000 TAWHs, which represents an incidence of <1% in blunt trauma. As with other traumas, TAWH has a grading scale (Table 80.3).

The WTA retrospectively reviewed the registry in 20 trauma centers. In over a third of TAWH cases, there was concomitant bowel injury, indicating a significant need for immediate laparotomy. The decision on timing of TAWH repair is difficult because the patient may have concomitant injuries precluding surgery. Physiologic status and overall injury burden were both higher in the nonoperative group. Definitions of early versus late repair vary in the literature; however, this study defined early repair as during the index hospitalization, with late being sometime after discharge. Early repairs were typically performed within

48 hours. Less than a third of patients had mesh repairs, which may be a result of either small injury size or concerns over contamination. Also, 90% of the repairs were performed open. Late repairs are done after discharge, and the average timing was 1 year after injury. In this late-repair group, more than three-fourths of the patients required mesh placement. However, 68.4% of the late group was performed open, whereas the rest were performed with laparoscopy (15.8%) or robotics (15.8%). The rate of hernia recurrence was 11.5% in the early-repair group compared with 15.8% in the late-repair group, but this was not statistically significant.

The term *open abdomen* represents conditions when the fascia of the abdominal wall is not reapproximated after a laparotomy.[91] This can occur after a damage control laparotomy, in the treatment of ACS, or when a second-look intervention is planned as management for an intraabdominal disease (e.g., bowel ischemia). The open-abdomen patient is at risk for multiple complications, such as fluid and protein loss, fistulas, VHs, and challenging abdominal wall closure.

To prevent contamination and protect the viscera, various temporary closure methods can be used. Some surgeons opt for simple skin closure or the use of nonpermeable, inert membranes. Most surgeons will use negative-pressure dressings, which, in addition to intraabdominal fluid management, can prevent fascial edge retraction. Indeed, with negative-pressure dressings, fascial closure can be achieved 89% of the time, as compared with 59% with non–negative-pressure approaches. Patients are then often managed in the ICU setting with multidisciplinary teams involving critical care physicians, surgeons, and nutritionists.

Before closing an abdomen, the surgeon must be certain that intraabdominal infections are controlled and that the patient's physiology will be able to sustain the closure. Timing of closure is partly determined by the etiology of the open abdomen as well as the clinical state of the patient. In trauma, abdominal closure is preferred within 48 hours. In situations where primary closure is unfeasible, options include negative-pressure dressings, mesh bridging, and abdominal reapproximation anchors (ABRA system). Once the acute condition is resolved, many patients will develop incisional hernias.

Parastomal Hernias

With approximately 100,000 to 120,000 new ostomies being created in the United States annually and an incidence of parastomal hernia development in nearly half of these patients, parastomal hernias pose a significant clinical burden. Management of parastomal hernias is challenging, with high recurrence rates of nearly 70%, in addition to higher SSOs and morbidity of stomal-related complications. One of the key aspects of a sound hernia repair is to obliterate the hernia defect. However, this cannot be completely done in the setting of a parastomal hernia because a fascial aperture must exist for the conduit. Most parastomal hernias may be managed nonoperatively; however, a third of these patients will require operative intervention. Ascertaining whether the ostomy can be reversed is imperative because ostomy reversal is the best treatment for parastomal hernia repair. However, if the ostomy cannot be reversed, various surgical options exist. Re-siting of the ostomy has fallen out of favor recently because of the chance for a de novo incisional hernia at the prior ostomy site and a parastomal hernia at the new ostomy site. Given its unacceptably high rates of recurrence, primary repair of a parastomal hernia should only be performed in an acute setting where the main clinical goal is management of threatened bowel or other hernia complications.

Regarding mesh repair, the two most common parastomal hernia repair techniques are the keyhole and Sugarbaker repairs.

The keyhole repair technique uses a mesh in which a slit and aperture are made so that the ostomy conduit can pass through (Fig. 80.13). A Sugarbaker technique is performed by lateralizing the ostomy conduit and then placing a mesh over the conduit and hernia (Fig. 80.14).[92]

The Sugarbaker repair has been found to have lower hernia recurrence rates compared with a keyhole repair; however, there were similar overall rates of complications, reoperations, stoma outlet obstruction, mesh infection, and postoperative bleeding.[93] Recently, a modified Sugarbaker technique has been described that uses a TAR and retromuscular mesh placement, but long-term data are still lacking regarding this technique.[94,95] It is important to consider that a synthetic mesh is in apposition to the bowel and may result in erosion, obstruction, or other severe complications.

Loss of Domain

The term *loss of domain* (LOD) is used to describe large VHs in which a significant amount of the abdominal contents are in the hernia sac outside of the confines of the abdomen walk. Quantitatively, the Sabbagh formula can be used to calculate the index of LOD. This volumetric method is the ratio of the incisional hernia volume (IHV) over the sum of the ACV and IHV. These volumes can be calculated from CT scans. A value of 20% or greater is generally considered a hernia with LOD.[96] In addition to affecting the patient's quality of life both aesthetically and functionally, hernias with LOD present a significant surgical challenge.[97] The etiology of these large hernias is usually secondary to midline laparotomies, although primary VHs with LOD can be seen. The incidence is on the rise as the population ages and with obesity becoming more prevalent. The giant hernias develop from a chronic process of linea alba disruption and lateral retraction of the abdominal muscles, followed by muscle atrophy and fibrosis. The abdominal viscera protrude into the hernia sac, the intraabdominal pressure will decrease, and there will ultimately be diaphragmatic muscle flattening. The dorsal muscle groups are no longer counterbalanced by the abdominal wall, and spine strain will ensue. In some cases, portal and mesenteric venous stasis may develop, resulting in bowel wall edema and digestive issues.

Most LOD hernias are not emergency cases; therefore, patients can be optimized for surgery.[96] Smoking cessation, nutritional optimization, blood glucose control, and improved cardiovascular function via prehabilitation are avenues to increase surgical success. Weight loss, although challenging, can decrease the volume of content that must be reduced in the abdominal cavity. Although there is a paucity of large studies to support this, omentectomy, right colectomy, and segmental small bowel resections can also reduce the visceral content that will be reduced in extreme cases. Adjuncts to complex VHR, such as progressive pneumoperitoneum, with or without botulinum toxin injection, can increase the ACV while allowing a functional abdominal wall reconstruction. The surgeon must be aware of possible negative sequelae caused by the reduction of hernia contents, such as respiratory compromise and intraabdominal hypertension, which may lead to ACS.

Cirrhosis

The incidence of abdominal wall hernias in patients with cirrhosis is 20% to 40%, and the increased morbidity and mortality in the setting of chronic liver disease pose challenges in management of these patients. A high-volume single-institution study found that

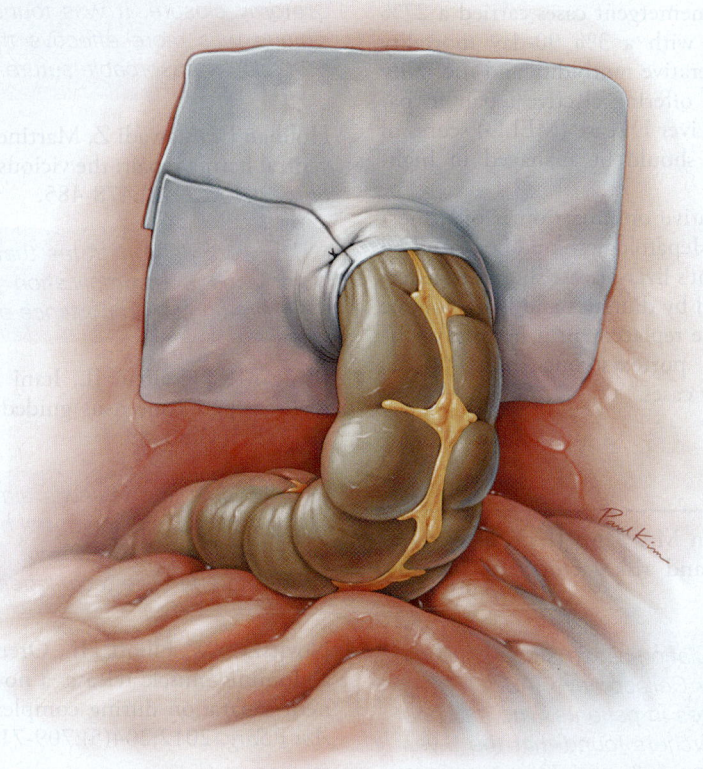

FIGURE 80.13 Keyhole repair of a parastomal hernia. (From Novitsky YW. Atlas of Robotic General Surgery. Elsevier; 2022, Figure 16.12.)

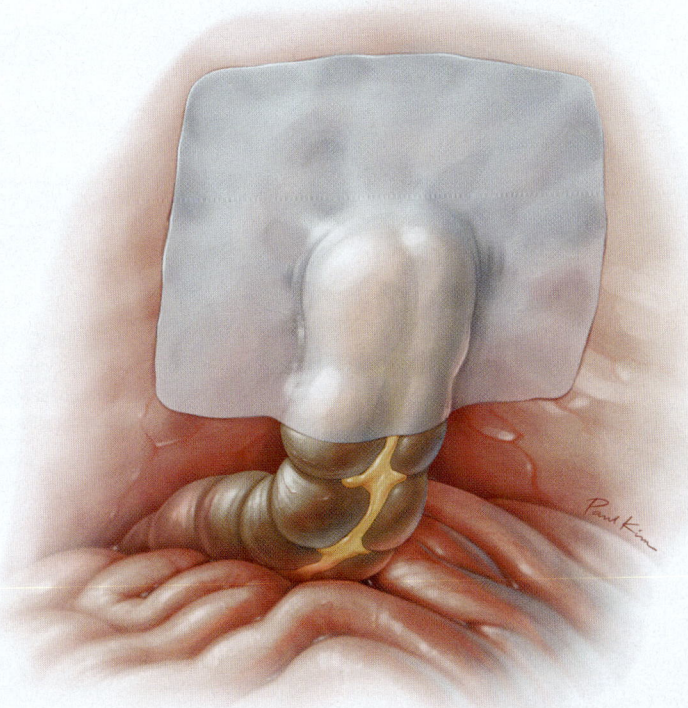

FIGURE 80.14 Sugarbaker repair of a parastomal hernia. (Atlas of Robotic General Surgery. 2022.)

emergent cases carried a 60% morbidity and mortality rate, with a 10% 90-day mortality rate. Nonemergent cases carried a 27% overall morbidity and mortality with a 3% 90-day mortality rate.[98] The high degree of postoperative morbidity and mortality in the emergent setting supports offering elective repair in patients with Model for End-Stage Liver Disease (MELD) scores of <20 if possible. These patients should be managed in high-volume hepatobiliary centers.

In elective situations, preoperative optimization is of utmost importance in cirrhotic patients. Hepatology should be consulted early, and the severity of the patient's liver disease should be ascertained. Ascites should be managed by diuretics and large-volume paracentesis with adequate volume replacement if necessary. The use of transjugular intrahepatic portosystemic shunt (TIPS) should be considered in refractory cases.

SELECTED REFERENCES

Bhardwaj P, Huayllani MT, Olson MA, Janis JE. Year-over-year ventral hernia recurrence rates and risk factors. *JAMA Surg.* 2024;159(6):651-658.

This recent retrospective, population-based study used the Abdominal Core Health Quality Collaborative (ACHQC) registry to evaluate recurrence rates in patients who had prior ventral hernia repair. The researchers found that the 5-year recurrence rate was greater than 40% and 70% in patients with and without mesh, respectively.

Deerenberg EB, Harlaar JJ, Steyerberg EW, et al. Small bites versus large bites for closure of abdominal midline incisions (STITCH): a double-blind, multicentre, randomised controlled trial. 2015;386(10000):1254-1260.

This RCT sought to find the ideal technique for midline laparotomy closure. It was found that small bites suture technique was more effective than traditional large bites with 2-0 slowly absorbable suture.

Holihan JL, Alawadi Z, Martindale RG, et al. Adverse events after ventral hernia repair: the vicious cycle of complications. *J Am Coll Surg.* 2015;221(2):478-485.

This work demonstrates that previous ventral hernia repair increases the complication profile of subsequent repairs, highlighting the importance of initial hernia prevention.

Liang MK, Holihan JL, Itani K, et al. Ventral hernia management: expert consensus guided by systematic review. *Ann Surg.* 2017;265(1):80–89.

This systematic review's aim was to achieve a consensus on best practices in ventral hernia management. Aspects of ventral hernia management, including preoperative optimization and operative techniques, are discussed.

Novitsky YW, Elliott HL, Orenstein SB, Rosen MJ. Transversus abdominis muscle release: a novel approach to posterior component separation during complex abdominal wall reconstruction. *Am J Surg.* 2012;204(5):709-716.

This publication describes the posterior component separation technique by Novitsky et al., which has now been widely adopted.

The full reference list appears on Elsevier eBooks+.

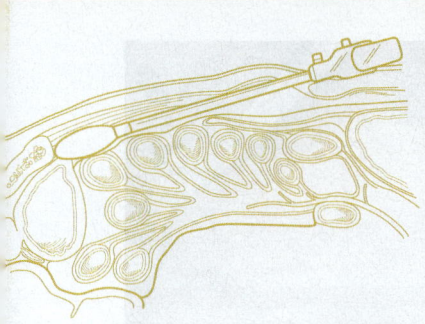

CHAPTER 81

Hernias of the Abdominal Wall: Atypical Locations

Dina Podolsky, Philip George, David John Morrell, Michael Turturro, and Yuri Novitsky

OUTLINE

INTRODUCTION

Atypical hernias present a particular challenge to the surgeon. A robust knowledge of abdominal wall anatomy is required to diagnose and repair these defects. Although many types of atypical hernias are reported in the literature, this chapter will focus on flank, lumbar, spigelian, obturator, intraperitoneal, sciatic, paramedian, and perineal hernias. Atypical hernias exist in different areas of the abdomen and have different physiologic causes, but the principles of hernia repair remain consistent: reduce the hernia contents, reapproximate the fascial defect, and reinforce the repair using mesh with wide overlap while preserving adjacent anatomic structures. Coupled with these objectives in mind, the surgeon should factor in the patient's medical and surgical history, risk factors for wound healing, resources available to the surgeon, and the surgeon's skill set to select the optimal repair that can be offered. This chapter will review the atypical hernias, their location, diagnostic methods, and the approaches to repair in an open and minimally invasive fashion.

MODERN TECHNICAL ADVANCES

Over the past few years, with the increased use of robotic surgery, minimally invasive options for repair are becoming more prevalent. Similarly, there has been renewed interest in placing mesh in extraperitoneal spaces, such as the preperitoneal and retromuscular planes. This allows for better ingrowth to the abdominal wall and reduced interface with bowel compared with intraabdominal mesh placement. Extraperitoneal mesh

can also be offered in an open fashion with similar results for recurrence; however, this approach is associated with greater wound morbidity and prolonged recovery. There may be more of a benefit with open approaches in those hernias with associated loss of domain, patients who cannot tolerate pneumoperitoneum, concurrent infection, severe intraabdominal adhesions, or previous mesh. A hybrid approach is also possible with a majority of the dissection and creation of the extraperitoneal space done minimally invasively with conversion to open to reapproximate the fascial defect and perform soft tissue reconstruction if needed.

SPIGELIAN HERNIAS

Relevant Anatomy

The Spigelian aponeurosis is formed from the membranous portions of the internal oblique and the transversus abdominis located laterally to the rectus and just medial to the semilunar line.[1] Defects in this Spigelian aponeurosis result in Spigelian hernias; however, because the external oblique does not contribute to the Spigelian aponeurosis, the hernia contents are typically covered by an intact external oblique (Fig. 81.1). Spigelian hernias almost always occur at or below the arcuate line, due to the absence of posterior rectus fascia in the area. The interparietal nature of these hernias can result in significant angulation of their contents; thus, they have a higher risk of strangulation and obstruction.[2] For that reason, it is recommended to repair these hernias even if they are asymptomatic.

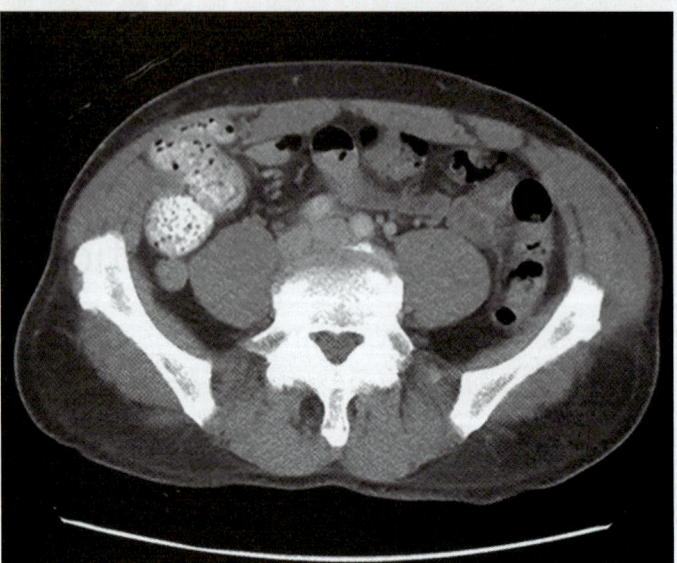

FIGURE 81.1 Right-sided spigelian hernia. Note the intact overlying external oblique muscle.

Etiology

Spigelian hernias are commonly small, present later in life, and can be difficult to detect on physical examination. These hernias can occur spontaneously or in the setting of previous surgical incisions because the naturally weak area is prone to forming hernias even from smaller incisions, including trocar sites.

Presentation

Due to the intact external oblique, a defect may not be appreciated on examination; however, a bulge or asymmetry may be present. Patients typically report pain or swelling on their lateral, lower abdominal wall. A dynamic ultrasound can be used for diagnosis; however, a noncontrast CT scan of the abdomen and pelvis is a more accurate test to allow for better delineation of the anatomy as well as assist in choosing the best operative approach.

In rare cases, a patient can present with diastasis of the semilunar line instead of a true hernia. Instead of an isolated bulge, it presents as an elongated ovoid ridge along the semilunar line (Fig. 81.2). Diastasis is more commonly seen in older and thin females. A CT scan is helpful to distinguish between a diastasis or a true defect as it is difficult to discern on physical examination (Fig. 81.3). Diastasis rarely causes symptoms and more often presents as a cosmetic complaint.

Surgical Repair

Our preference for repair of Spigelian hernias is a robotic transabdominal preperitoneal approach (TAPP). A total of three ports are placed across the abdomen at or slightly above the level of the umbilicus and triangulated toward the defect. The contents of the hernia are reduced, and a peritoneal flap is then created to ensure at least a 5-cm overlap around the defect. It is easiest to start medially at the medial umbilical ligament and work toward the anterior superior iliac spine (ASIS). The medial dissection is completed first, bluntly dissecting toward the space of Retzius until the pubic symphysis and Cooper's ligaments are identified. Laterally, the preperitoneal dissection is taken to the psoas muscle, and transitioning into a pretransversalis plane is frequently necessary to ensure adequate mesh overlap (Fig. 81.4). Once the peritoneal flap has been created, the defect is closed and an appropriately

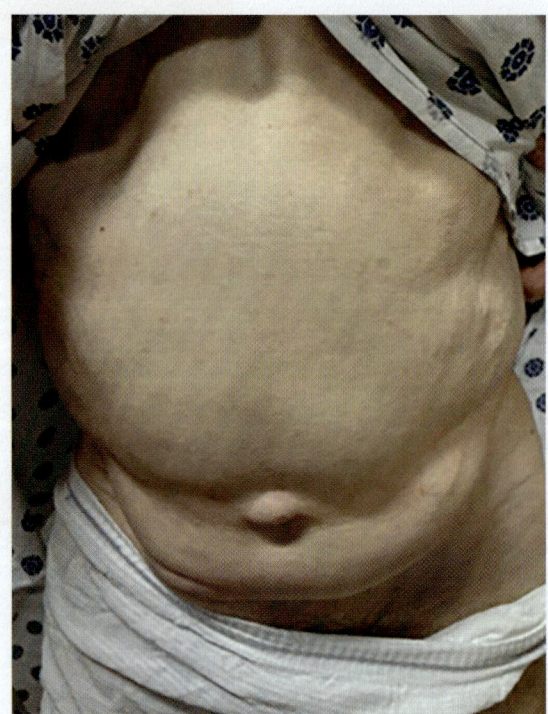

FIGURE 81.2 Patient with bilateral Spigelian aponeurosis diastasis.

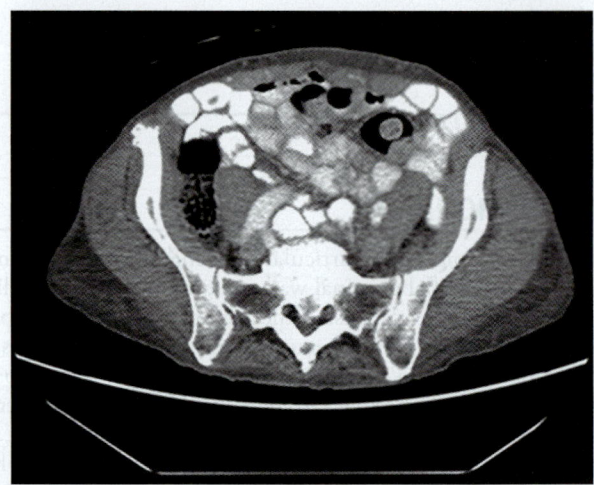

FIGURE 81.3 Axial CT scan of semilunar line diastasis showing no discernable defect in the transversus abdominis or internal oblique muscles.

sized mesh is placed in the preperitoneal pocket and is secured to the abdominal wall. The peritoneum is then closed over the mesh with a running suture. These are considered ambulatory procedures and patients routinely go home the same day in our practice.

For patients who might not be able to tolerate pneumoperitoneum, in recurrences after posterior repair or in larger defects, an open repair might be warranted. A transverse or oblique incision is made over the defect, which should be marked beforehand as the defect and associated contents may be difficult to palpate while the patient is supine. The external oblique is frequently intact over the hernia and will need to be incised in the direction of its fibers. Once the external oblique is opened, the hernia contents are identified and reduced into the abdomen. The fascial edges of the internal oblique and transversus abdominis anteriorly are

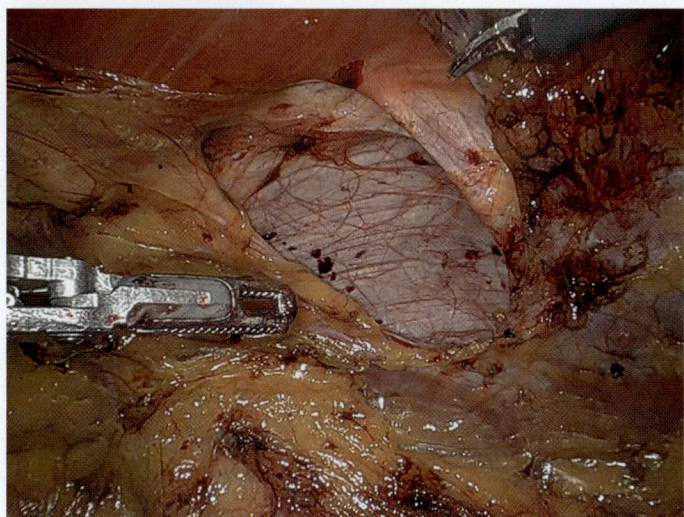

FIGURE 81.4 Intraoperative visualization of a right-sided Spigelian hernia occurring below the arcuate line.

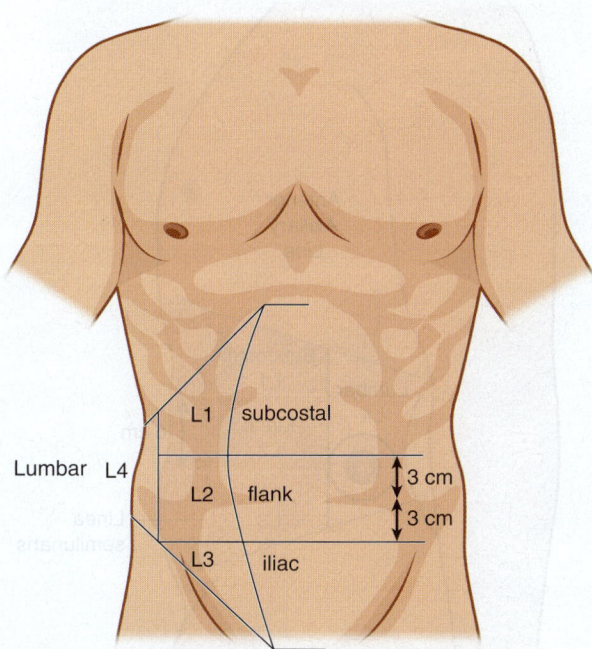

FIGURE 81.5 European Hernia Society classification of lateral hernias divided into four compartments: *L1*, the subcostal compartment; *L2*, the flank compartment; *L3*, the iliac compartment; and *L4*, the lumbar compartment.

cleared from the external oblique, and posteriorly any intraabdominal adhesions should be taken down. The defect is closed in layers, with the internal oblique and transversalis fascia reapproximated first, followed by the external oblique. Our preference is to use a slowly absorbable suture for fascial closure. For defects that are 2 cm or less, mesh augmentation may not confer a benefit; however, for larger defects, a mesh can be placed either preperitoneally or as an onlay. Our preference is to use an uncoated macroporous synthetic mesh in these situations. If mesh is placed in an onlay position, it must be well secured to prevent migration or bunching to maximize tissue ingrowth. Fibrin glue can also be used as an adjunct to suture fixation of the mesh; however, our practice is to use fixation with absorbable sutures. For onlay repairs we typically place a drain that is removed on follow-up visit around 2 weeks postoperatively. Spigelian hernia repairs are typically performed as outpatient surgeries.

Outcomes

The most common adverse outcomes after Spigelian hernia repair are hernia recurrence, seroma, hematoma, and infection; however, the risk profile is low. Minimally invasive repairs have a low rate of recurrence (0%–5%), a decreased length of stay, and earlier return of physical activity.[3–5]

Lateral Hernias

The European hernia society classifies lateral hernias as any fascial defect lateral to the rectus muscle.[6] The area can be broken up into four compartments: lumbar, subcostal, flank, and iliac (Fig. 81.5). These compartments are bordered by the subcostal margin superiorly, the iliac crest inferiorly, the lateral border of the rectus sheath medially, and the lumbar region laterally. Lateral hernias can be a challenge to repair due to their distortion of the abdominal wall and proximity to retroperitoneal nerves (Fig. 81.6). There can also exist a great challenge for closure of mesh overlap if the defect extends to costal margin or pelvic brim.

Relevant Anatomy

For the purposes of this section, we will group lumbar and flank hernias together because they are frequently diagnosed and treated the same. Although referred to interchangeably with flank

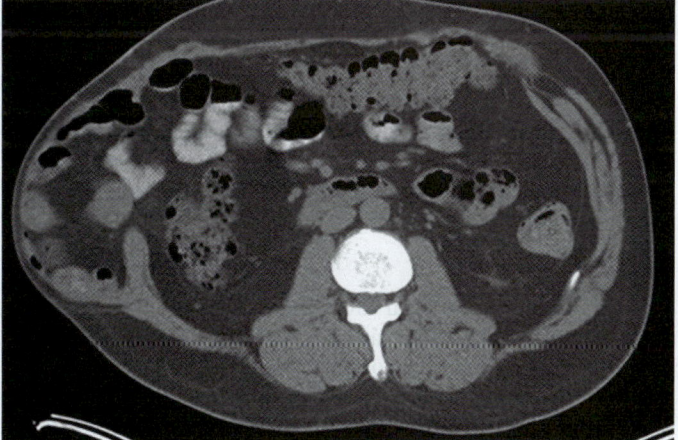

FIGURE 81.6 Iatrogenic flank hernia with incarcerated bowel contents.

hernias, lumbar hernias are located laterodorsal to the anterior axillary line between the costal margin and the inguinal region (Fig. 81.7). Although flank hernias are almost always incisional in nature, lumbar hernias can sometimes be found as primary hernias. Primary lumbar hernias are further classified anatomically based on the superior (Grynfeltt-Lesshaft) and inferior (Petit) lumbar triangles (Fig. 81.8). The superior lumbar triangle is bounded superiorly by the 12th rib and the inferior border of the serratus posterior, medially by the quadratus lumborum and sacrospinalis muscles, and laterally by the posterior border of the internal oblique.[7] The floor is formed by the aponeurosis of the transversus abdominis muscle, and the roof consists of the external oblique and latissimus dorsi muscles. The inferior lumbar triangle boundaries are the iliac crest inferiorly, the posterior

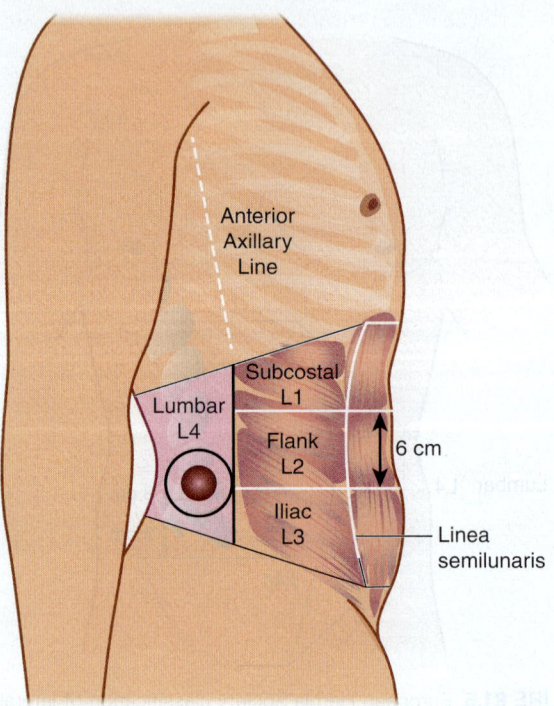

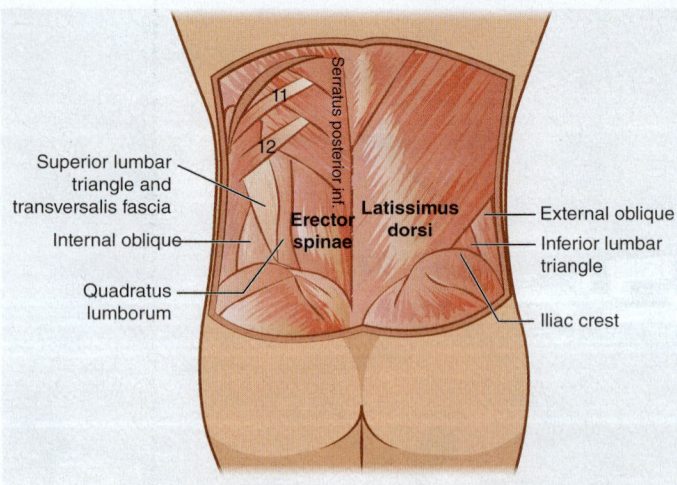

FIGURE 81.8 Anatomic boundaries of the superior and inferior lumbar triangles. (From Behrang Amini, based on Fig. 1 from Orcutt TW. Hernia of the superior lumbar triangle. *Ann Surg.* 1971;173[2]:294-297.)

FIGURE 81.7 Boundaries of flank and lumbar hernias as defined by the European Hernia Society. Flank hernias are located lateral to the rectus sheath, whereas lumbar hernias are lateral to the anterior axillary line. (From Khetan M, Kalhan S, John S, Sethi D, Kannaujiya P, Ramana B. MIS retromuscular repair of lateral incisional hernia: technological deliberations and short-term outcome. *Hernia.* 2022;26[5]:1325-1336.)

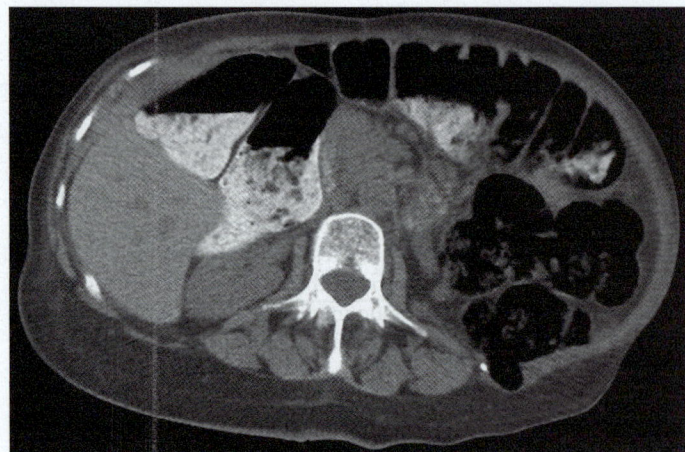

FIGURE 81.9 Patient with history of left nephrectomy with a resultant multiply recurrent left flank incisional hernia.

border of the internal oblique laterally, and lateral border of the latissimus dorsi medially. The floor consists of the internal oblique muscle, transversus abdominis muscle, and posterior lamina of the thoracolumbar fascia.

Etiology

Primary hernias occur near areas that weaken the posterior abdominal wall such as perforating neurovascular pedicles through both the inferior and superior lumbar triangles. Acquired hernias result from traumatic injuries or from prior surgical incisions. Procedures that involve a lumbar incision (e.g., nephrectomy; Fig. 81.9) have a high incidence of lumbar incisional hernia with one series estimating the incidence of postoperative herniation to be as high as 30%.[8]

Presentation

These hernias require high clinical suspicion to accurately diagnose because they are uncommon and can be asymptomatic. Primary lumbar hernias are even more rarely encountered in routine general surgical practice, previously estimated to be encountered only once during a general surgeon's career.[9] CT is a critical component of diagnosis and subsequent operative planning. Given the anatomic location of these hernias, the herniated contents frequently consist of extraperitoneal fat and can result in asymptomatic presentations. Despite this, incarceration appears to occur frequently especially in primary lumbar hernias with one systematic review noting an incidence of 31%.[10] Another systematic review estimated that 9% of these patients will present acutely

and require emergent surgical intervention.[11] Given the high rate of incarceration, repair of lateral hernias should be considered once diagnosed. Ultimately these hernias present rarely in surgical practice with incisional lumbar and flank hernias comprising less than 20% of all incisional hernia repairs and only 420 primary lumbar hernias reported in the literature.[12]

Surgical Repair

Current society guidelines recommend referral to specialized hernia centers for repair of the previously mentioned hernias.[13] Repair necessitates a solid understanding of the anatomy of the posterior abdominal wall with use of best hernia repair practices. In patients that are good candidates for a minimally invasive approach, we typically employ a robotic TAPP repair (Fig. 81.10). This repair takes advantage of the thicker layer of preperitoneal fat lateral to the semilunar line and has the benefit of excluding the mesh from the intraabdominal viscera. Depending on how lateral the hernia is, we either place the patients in a supine tilted fashion or place patients in a lateral decubitus position with the bed flexed to increase the space between the ASIS and the costal margin. The lateral extent of the preperitoneal dissection continues into the

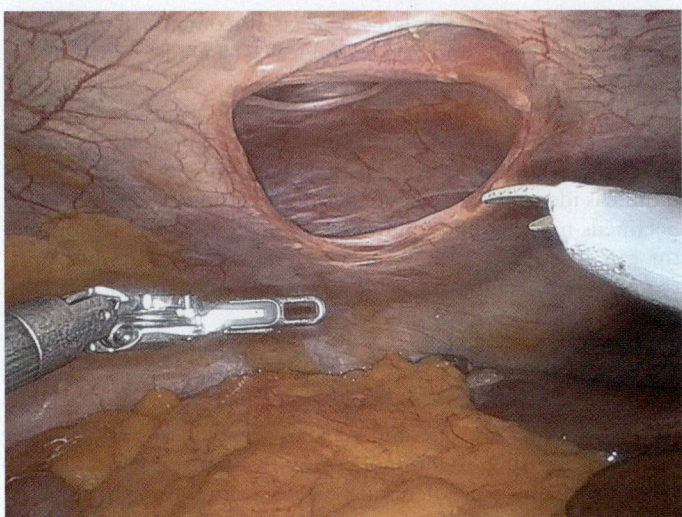

FIGURE 81.10 Visualization of right-sided incisional flank hernia.

pararenal space to the quadratus lumborum. The investing fascia of the quadratus lumborum and psoas muscles should be left intact to protect the ilioinguinal, iliohypogastric, genitofemoral, and lateral femoral cutaneous nerves. The ureter and gonadal vessels should be identified and preserved in this space as well. The dissection is sometimes carried below the costal margin or into the spaces of Retzius and Bogros if more overlap is needed. The goal of the repair is to reapproximate the obliques to the semilunar line (Fig. 81.11), and preperitoneal dissection is done to create a sufficient space for wide mesh overlap of the hernia.

In patients that are poor candidates for minimally invasive repair, an open approach can be done with the patient positioned similar to that for the preferred robotic approach. In patients with an incisional lateral hernia, the prior incision is used; otherwise, the incision is made directly over top of the hernia bulge or 2 to 3 cm superior to the ASIS. In the case of partial-thickness defects, frequently the external oblique muscle is intact and the dissection is carried down to the muscle, which is divided in the direction of the fibers to split the muscle and expose the hernia. After reducing the hernia contents, the preperitoneal plane is entered and a

preperitoneal dissection similar to that described in our robotic approach is undertaken to perform a preperitoneal underlay mesh-based repair. We do not use transfascial suture fixation in these patients, opting instead for fibrin sealant fixation to avoid possible entrapment of surrounding neurovascular structures.

OBTURATOR HERNIAS

Relevant Anatomy

The obturator canal starts in the pelvis and exits in the medial portion of the upper thigh. This part of the thigh is referred to as the obturator or adductor region and is bound by the pubic arch, perineum, and gracilis muscle medially; the femur laterally; the pubic bone superiorly; and the insertion of the adductor inferiorly.[14] The obturator canal contains the obturator nerve, artery, and vein. The function of the nerve is to adduct the leg, and injury to this nerve may cause a noticeable decrease in function. Large, intact vascular connections between the obturator and the external iliac systems are called the corona mortis and can be visualized during minimally invasive repair. Not all patients have robust communications present. Most obturator hernias are located medially to the vessels and most commonly the sac can be found in front of the external obturator muscle. Typically, there is a small "fat plug" associated with the canal, which in a routine inguinal hernia surgery should be left in situ (Fig. 81.12).

Etiology

Obturator hernias are protrusions through the obturator canal and are remarkably rare, making up less than 1% of all hernias, with a majority of the literature published in the form of case reports.[15] Typically, obturator hernias affect elderly, thin females due to their triangular pelvis coupled with the atrophy of preperitoneal fat surrounding the obturator vessels. Other risk factors include chronic obstructive pulmonary disease (COPD), chronic constipation, or ascites, all of which cause increased intraabdominal pressure. Due to their location, they can be confused with either a femoral or inguinal hernia; however, when incarcerated they carry a high risk of strangulation with morbidity as high as 14%. This could be due to the difficulty in diagnosing this hernia

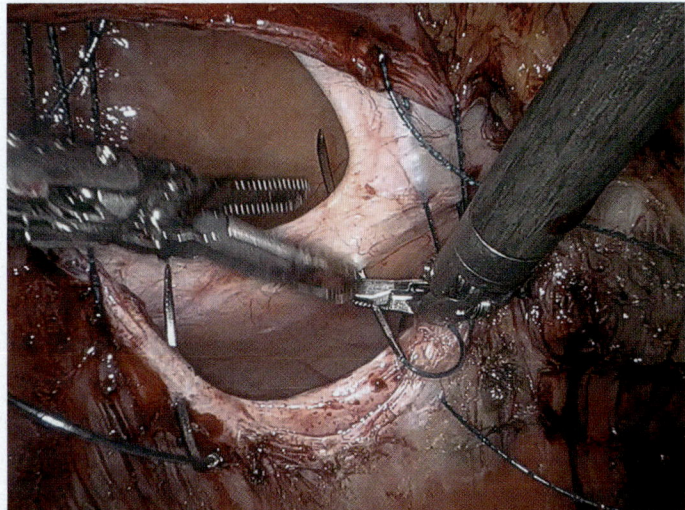

FIGURE 81.11 Reconstruction of components of the semilunar line during flank hernia repair.

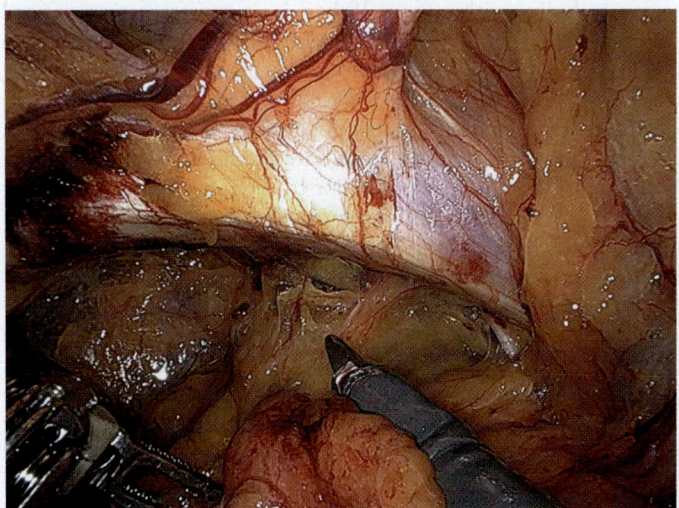

FIGURE 81.12 Visualization of obturator "fat plug" and associated nerve and vein underneath the pelvic brim.

leading to a delay in treatment, and a high clinical suspicion should be practiced in these scenarios.

Clinical Presentation and Evaluation

Because of the anatomic location of the obturator canal, diagnosing an obturator hernia on physical examination alone is incredibly challenging without adjunct imaging. One unique physical examination finding is pain in the anteromedial aspect of the thigh (Howship-Romberg sign), which is relieved with thigh flexion. This is caused by direct compression of the obturator nerve by the hernia contents. Unlike other hernias, one more common presenting symptom is bowel obstruction (up to 50%). Due to the bony pelvis and its associated interference, an ultrasound also may not be as useful as a CT scan in identifying an obturator hernia. Laparoscopy should be considered a diagnostic option as well.

Surgical Repair

A minimally invasive approach is preferred for obturator hernias because the visualization is much better compared with open repair. The setup for an obturator hernia repair is similar to the approach taken to repair an inguinal or femoral hernia. Three trocars are placed in a line at the umbilicus and triangulated toward the hernia. The patient is placed in steep Trendelenburg position, and the pelvis is inspected to identify the obturator hernia and a possible concurrent femoral or inguinal hernia. A peritoneal flap is started in a similar place to an inguinal hernia repair, near arcuate line, and is extending laterally to the abdominal side wall. Preperitoneal dissection is then performed down toward the pubic bone. Medially the space of Retzius is entered with identification of Cooper's ligament and pubic symphysis. Laterally the parietal plane is entered to protect the genital branch of the genitofemoral nerve and the lateral femoral cutaneous nerve. These nerves and the associated retroperitoneal fat should remain on the abdominal wall laterally and not taken down with the peritoneal flap. The dissection is then continued medially, parietalizing the spermatic vessels and vas deferens in males, whereas the round ligament is commonly ligated in females to assist with mesh overlap and exposure. Dissection proceeds until the obturator space is seen. At this point, inguinal and femoral hernias should be reduced. The obturator hernia contents should be reduced, and great care must be taken to avoid injuring the obturator vessels or nerve including with cautery. If there is no contamination or need for bowel resection, we recommend mesh reinforcement. The mesh should be placed medially in the space of Retzius covering the defect roughly 4 cm medially to the defect and 4 cm inferior to the defect. We typically fixate the mesh to Cooper's ligament. While closing the peritoneal flap, care should be taken so that the peritoneum does not slide anterior to the mesh because this may result in a recurrence. If done in an elective setting, patients are typically discharged on the day of surgery.

An open repair can also be undertaken in patients who do not qualify for minimally invasive surgery. A transabdominal approach with preperitoneal dissection through a lower midline incision is preferred. The patient should be positioned in Trendelenburg position to help facilitate exposure. If there is difficulty in reducing the contents, an inferomedial incision in the membrane can be made to enlarge the defect, taking care to avoid damage to the neurovascular bundle. The mesh should be placed in a preperitoneal pocket with generous overlap. In the scenario where a bowel resection is indicated, most of these defects are closed with permanent suture either in an interrupted or

purse-string fashion. For larger defects in contaminated fields, a flap of peritoneum and retroperitoneal fat may be used to close the defect.

An alternative to the transabdominal approach is the obturator approach, which consists of making an incision just lateral to and along the border of the adductor longus muscle. The obturator bundle is identified at the interface of the adductor longus and the pectineus muscles, and followed proximally it reveals the obturator canal. A plug can be used to obliterate the obturator canal space. When fixating the plug, care must be taken to avoid the obturator neurovascular bundle.

PERINEAL HERNIAS

Perineal hernias are rare and repair is challenging. Most occur iatrogenically after abdominoperineal resection or perineal prostatectomy. This type of hernia results from a weakness in the pelvic musculature allowing pelvic viscera or other organs to protrude. Symptoms may include bowel obstruction or urinary dysfunction. Primary perineal hernias most commonly affect older, multiparous females and are frequently identified during a rectovaginal examination. MRI or CT scan imaging can confirm the diagnosis and help delineate anatomy to decide which approach for repair is possible.

Perineal hernias can be repaired either by perineal or abdominal approach or a hybrid of the two. The goal of repair is to reduce the pelvic contents and close the defect if possible. If primary closure is not possible because of the bony pelvic anatomy, a coated mesh with bony or ligamentous fixation can be used to prevent the protrusion of intraabdominal viscera. Augmented tissue or flap reconstruction may also be an option and varies regarding surgeon preference and available vascularized anatomy. Unfortunately, because of the rarity of these hernia defects, there are no randomized trials available that discuss which surgical approach is optimal. A meta-analysis of repairs shows no advantage of perineal over abdominal approach.[16] There was also no difference in recurrence between primary versus mesh versus flap repair with perineal repairs overall resulting in around a 22% recurrence rate.

INTERPARIETAL HERNIAS

Interparietal hernias result from herniation between the layers of the abdominal wall. Apart from the previously discussed Spigelian hernia, these hernias are almost always incisional. Given the partial-thickness herniation of these defects, they are frequently challenging to diagnose, and patients will frequently present with intestinal obstruction. CT is an important diagnostic tool in operative planning for these patients with hernias in atypical locations.

Given the increasing frequency of posterior component separation techniques being used in ventral hernia repair, two types of interparietal hernias bear mentioning: posterior rectus sheath herniation and semilunar line herniation. Both typically result from technical errors during the index hernia repair. As with other interparietal hernias, CT is a necessary step in the diagnosis and management of these patients and a high level of suspicion needs to be maintained.

Interparietal herniation can occur via a posterior rectus sheath defect after posterior component separation ventral hernia repair (Rives-Stoppa and transversus abdominis release techniques). During re-creation of the visceral sac via closure of the posterior rectus sheath, missed fenestrations or excessive tension on the closure can result in a herniation through the posterior rectus sheath (Fig. 81.13). Any patient presenting with signs and symptoms of bowel obstruction in the postoperative period after a retrorectus or retromuscular repair should be promptly evaluated for this complication.

Interparietal herniation can occur via semilunar line injury during transversus abdominis release procedures (Fig. 81.14). Herniation at this site results from improper intraoperative identification of the semilunar line with inadvertent division of the anterior lamella of the internal oblique during attempted division of the fibers of the transversus abdominis muscle. When this rare

complication is identified, referral to a center specializing in complex abdominal wall surgery is recommended given the technical challenges associated with recurrent hernia repair after a transversus abdominis release procedure.

Discussion of operative approaches to manage these hernias is difficult given the variability in presentation as well as the anatomic structures involved. Furthermore, these are rare hernias with the literature describing repairs consisting of limited case reports.[17,17a] A straightforward repair of these hernias can involve laparoscopic-assisted intraperitoneal mesh placement, acting as a buttress to the posterior layer breakdown; however, larger defects need more extensive repair at a specialized center (Figs. 81.15 and 81.16). As with all hernias, management is based on the surgeon's clear understanding of abdominal wall anatomy coupled with wide mesh overlap of the hernia defect to limit recurrence.

SCIATIC HERNIAS

These hernias are extremely rare and occur at the site of the greater sciatic foramen (Fig. 81.17). Although there are no large series of cases, many case reports have been published.[18] A review of these

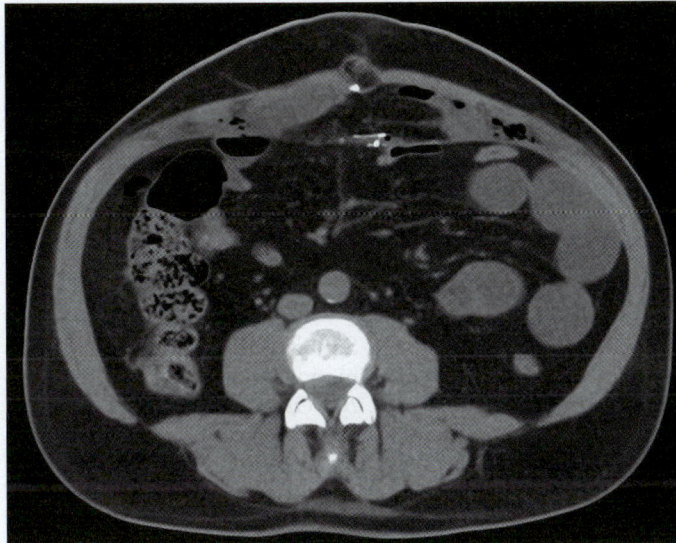

FIGURE 81.13 Interparietal hernia occurring after a retrorectus hernia repair because of posterior rectus sheath breakdown with small bowel herniating into the retrorectus space.

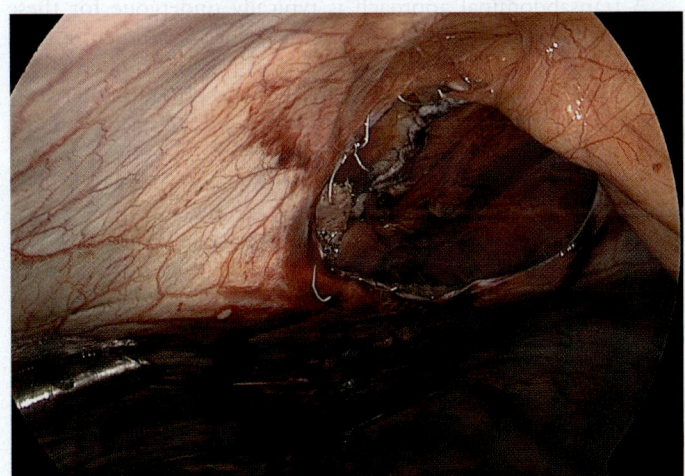

FIGURE 81.15 Posterior sheath breakdown after stapled Rives-Stoppa hernia repair.

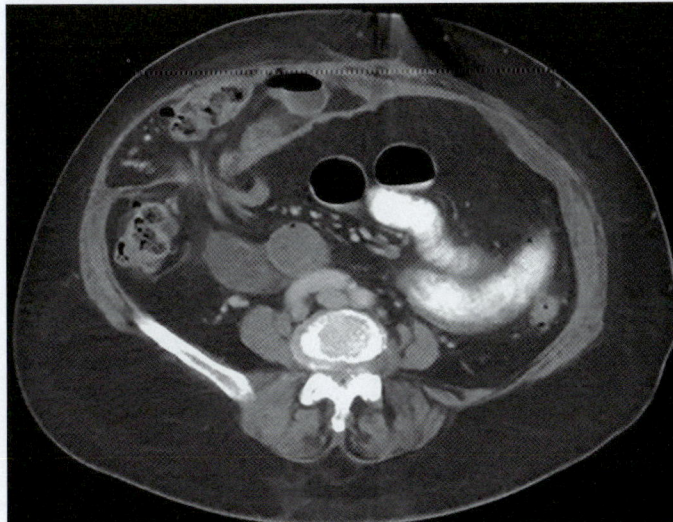

FIGURE 81.14 Interparietal hernia occurring in a patient presenting with small bowel obstruction from herniation at the right semilunar line secondary to a semilunar line injury from prior transversus abdominis release ventral hernia repair.

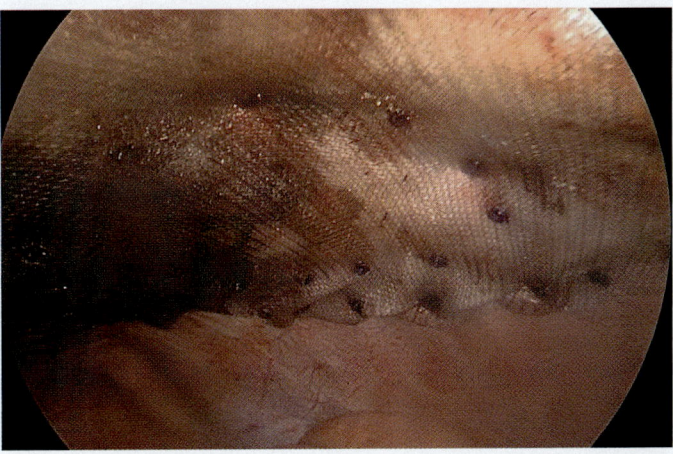

FIGURE 81.16 Intraperitoneal mesh repair of posterior sheath breakdown.

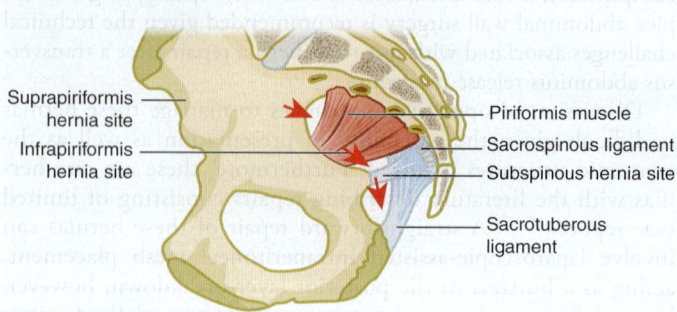

FIGURE 81.17 Anatomy and potential sites of hernia formation. (Adapted from Kavic, MS, et al. Hernias of the pelvic wall. In: LeBlanc, K, Kingsnorth, A, Snadersf, D, ed. *Management of Abdominal Wall Hernias*: Switzerland: Springer Cham; 2013:15-23.)

case reports from 1900–2008 yielded only 78 reports involving 99 patients.[19] Patients are typically asymptomatic until bowel obstruction occurs. Presentation of these hernias can manifest as a slowly enlarging mass or swelling near the gluteal area, or sciatic neuralgia. Repair of these hernias is recommended, and a minimally invasive approach should be undertaken when possible.[20]

A transabdominal approach is typically undergone for these hernias, and any incarcerated bowel is reduced with gentle traction. Steep Trendelenburg positioning can assist with visualization. Care is taken to not injure either the obturator nerve or vessels or the sciatic nerve or vessels, which are inferolateral to the obturator vessels. The ureter also courses inferior to this dissection plane and should be identified and protected. A flat synthetic mesh is used to cover the defect and is secured to Cooper's ligament. Plug mesh can be used; however, this may increase the risk of nerve damage. Alternatively, an open, transgluteal approach may be used with an incision over the hernia at the posterior edge of the greater trochanter. The hernia defect may be visualized after opening the gluteus maximus muscle, and the muscle and defect edges are closed in layers.

PARAMEDIAN HERNIAS

Off-midline incisions are encouraged by the European Hernia Society (EHS) to decrease risk of hernia formation.[21] Most paramedian incisions are made to perform operations in the retroperitoneal space, particularly anterior approaches to lumbar fusions, or repair of abdominal aortic aneurysm. A paramedian incision versus a midline incision has been shown to decrease incidence of hernia formation.[22] In the event a paramedian hernia occurs, principles of repair remain the same: reapproximating the mid rectus fascia with adequate mesh coverage. The particular challenge from a paramedian hernia repair is due to the close proximity to the midline and the semilunar line. If opting for a retromuscular repair and mesh placement, care must be taken to not disrupt these lines of anatomy. An open onlay approach or minimally invasive TAPP or intraperitoneal onlay mesh approach is reasonable and allows for wide mesh coverage, without the risk of injuring intact linea alba or semilunar line.

CONCLUSION

Atypical hernias are rare forms of hernias that may be encountered in a general surgery practice. Although their anatomy and presentation may be unique, their repair still follows traditional teaching of defect closure and mesh augmentation. A high level of clinical suspicion should be maintained for patients with symptoms and a history of off-midline or lateral incisions.

SELECTED REFERENCES

Henriksen NA, Kaufmann R, Simons MP, et al. EHS and AHS guidelines for treatment of primary ventral hernias in rare locations or special circumstances. *BJS Open.* 2020;4(2):342-353.

Important conglomeration of recommendations of atypical hernias or typical hernias in less common circumstances.

Moreno-Egea A, Baena EG, Calle MC, et al. Controversies in the current management of lumbar hernias. *Arch Surg.* 2007; 142(1):82-88.

Detailed systematic review regarding lumbar hernia diagnosis and management.

The full reference list appears on Elsevier eBooks+.

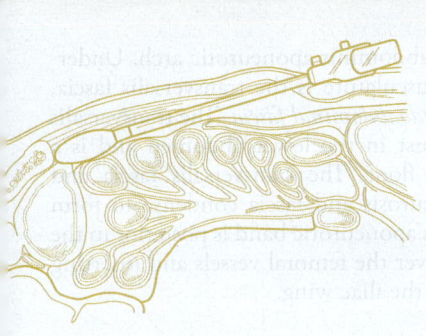

Inguinal Hernias

Richard Lu, Jorge Daes, David Lourie, Alexandra Z. Agathis, Luciano Tastaldi, Leandro Totti Cavazzola, Brian P. Jacob, and Flavio Malcher

OUTLINE

 Please access Elsevier eBooks+ to view the videos for this chapter.

INTRODUCTION

Inguinal hernia repair (IHR) is one of the most common surgical procedures performed worldwide, with over 20 million performed annually. It is among the top-five most common major ambulatory operations performed in males over 18 years of age in the United States.[1] The landscape of hernia surgery has evolved significantly over the past decade, driven by the increasing adoption of minimally invasive (MI) techniques and the integration of advanced technologies such as robotic assistance. The vast array of repair techniques suggests that there is not a perfect solution.[2] Despite these advances, inguinal hernias continue to cause significant morbidity and healthcare costs. Although many patients are treated successfully, research suggests that recurrence rates range from 1.7% to 10%. Approximately 10% to 15% of groin hernia recurrences will need reoperative intervention. The negative consequences of groin hernia surgery can be devastating. About 10% to 12% of patients who have groin hernia surgery develop ongoing pain that can lead to long-term disability, and 1% to 3% of patients experience severe, lasting pain.

The lifetime occurrence of developing a groin hernia is 27% to 43% in males and 3% to 6% in females.[2] Inguinal hernias are classified as direct or indirect. A direct hernia defect is within Hesselbach's triangle, which is bordered by the inguinal ligament inferiorly, the inferior epigastric vessels laterally, and the lateral border of the rectus abdominis muscle medially. Indirect inguinal hernias pass through the deep inguinal ring, which is lateral to the inferior epigastric vessels. Two-thirds of inguinal hernias are indirect, and the remainder are direct. Femoral hernias comprise only 3% of groin hernias, but their true incidence may be higher given that they are often misdiagnosed. The female-to-male ratio for femoral hernias is about 10:1. Although femoral hernias occur more frequently in females than in males, inguinal hernias remain the most common hernia in females. Indirect inguinal hernias are the most common inguinal hernia type for both males and females. Femoral and indirect inguinal hernias occur more frequently on the right side as a result of a delay in atrophy of the processus vaginalis after the normal slower descent of the right testis to the scrotum during fetal development. The higher incidence of right femoral hernias is thought to be attributed to the sigmoid colon blocking the left femoral canal.

PERTINENT ANATOMY

Open techniques are typically associated with anterior approaches, whereas MI methods often involve posterior approaches to groin hernia repair. A thorough understanding of inguinal anatomy from both anterior and posterior perspectives is essential.

Anterior Anatomy

Internal Oblique Muscle and Aponeurosis

Deep to the skin and subcutaneous tissues are the superficial circumflex iliac, superficial epigastric, and external pudendal vessels, which arise from and drain to the proximal femoral vessels. These can be ligated for operative exposure if necessary. The external oblique (EO) is the most superficial of the lateral abdominal wall muscles, and its aponeurosis is the most superficial boundary of the inguinal canal. The muscle fibers of the EO run inferiorly and medially, and the aponeurosis is formed by a superficial and deep layer. The inferior edge of the EO aponeurosis forms the inguinal (Poupart) ligament and extends from the anterior superior iliac spine (ASIS) to the pubic tubercle. This structure turns posteriorly to form the shelving edge of the inguinal ligament. The inguinal ligament has a medial extension (the lacunar ligament) that inserts onto the pubis. The external or superficial inguinal ring is an ovoid aperture that is superolateral to the pubic tubercle and conveys the spermatic cord as it exits from the inguinal canal toward the scrotum.

Internal Oblique Muscle and Aponeurosis

The internal oblique (IO) muscle is the middle layer of the lateral abdominal musculoaponeurotic complex. In the upper abdomen, its fibers course superiorly and laterally and are directed more inferiorly in the inguinal region. In 5% of patients, the aponeuroses of the medial aspect of the IO and transversus abdominis join to form the conjoint tendon. The conjoint tendon is most evident at the pubic tubercle, where these muscles insert. The IO muscle fibers continue inferiorly to become the cremaster muscle fibers as they encircle the spermatic cord and attach to the tunica vaginalis of the testis. Preserving these fibers during open IHR is crucial to minimize the risk of chronic groin pain, which can result from injury to the genital branch of the genitofemoral (GF) nerve.

Transversus Abdominis Muscle and Aponeurosis and Transversalis Fascia

Much of the transversus abdominis muscle runs transversely throughout the abdomen; however, it courses in a slightly oblique and downward direction in the inguinal region. The aponeurosis of the transversus abdominis covers both anterior and posterior surfaces of the abdominal wall, with its lower margin arching with the IO muscle over the internal inguinal ring to form the transversus abdominis aponeurotic arch. Underlying the abdominal wall musculature is the transversalis fascia, which is also known as the *endoabdominal fascia*. The transversalis fascia tends to be more robust in the lower abdomen and is a component of the inguinal floor. The transversalis fascia and transversus abdominis aponeurosis and fascia condense to form the iliopubic tract (IPT). This aponeurotic band is posterior to the inguinal ligament, crossing over the femoral vessels and inserting on the ASIS and inner lip of the iliac wing.

Inguinal Canal

The inguinal canal extends between the internal and external inguinal rings and is located cephalad to the inguinal ligament. The inguinal canal is bound by the EO aponeurosis superficially, with its floor composed of the transversus abdominis muscle and transversalis fascia. The IO and transversus abdominis musculoaponeuroses form the cephalad wall, whereas the inguinal and lacunar ligaments form the inferior wall. *Hesselbach's triangle* refers to the margins of the floor of the inguinal canal. These are the inferior epigastric vessels as the superolateral border, the rectus sheath as the medial border, and the inguinal and pectineal ligaments as the inferior border. In males, the inguinal canal contains the spermatic cord, and in females, it contains the round ligament. The spermatic cord is composed of cremaster muscle fibers, the vas deferens, the testicular vessels, the genital branch of the GF nerve, lymphatics, and the processus vaginalis (Fig. 82.1).

The iliohypogastric nerve, ilioinguinal nerve, and genital branch of the GF nerve are commonly exposed in anterior operative approaches to inguinal hernias. The iliohypogastric and ilioinguinal nerves provide sensation to the skin of the groin, base of the penis, and ipsilateral upper medial thigh. Proximally, the iliohypogastric and ilioinguinal nerves travel beneath the IO muscle

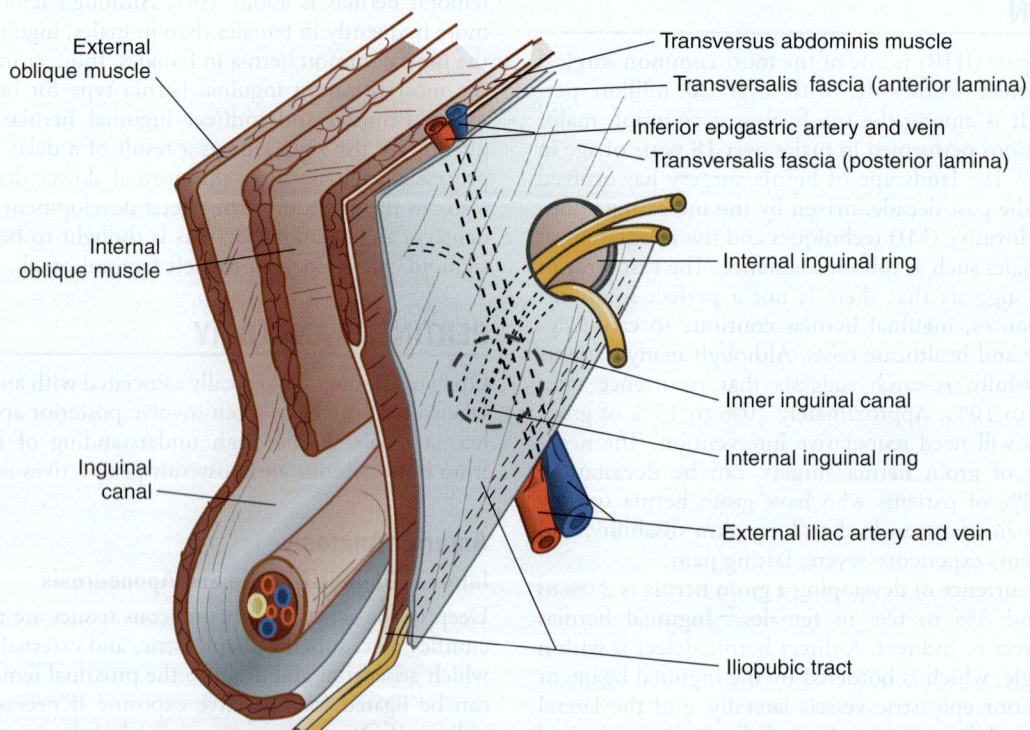

External oblique muscle
Internal oblique muscle
Inguinal canal

Transversus abdominis muscle
Transversalis fascia (anterior lamina)
Inferior epigastric artery and vein
Transversalis fascia (posterior lamina)
Internal inguinal ring
Inner inguinal canal
Internal inguinal ring
External iliac artery and vein
Iliopubic tract

FIGURE 82.1 Nyhus's classic parasagittal diagram of the right midinguinal region illustrating the muscular aponeurotic layers separated into anterior and posterior walls. (From Nyhus LM, Condon RE, eds. *Hernia*. 4th ed. Philadelphia: JB Lippincott; 1995:57-63.)

to a point just superomedial to the ASIS. These two nerves then penetrate the IO muscle, traveling under the EO aponeurosis. The main trunk of the iliohypogastric nerve courses on the anterior surface of the IO muscle and aponeurosis medial and superior to the internal ring before piercing the EO aponeurosis to innervate the skin. Occasionally, the iliohypogastric nerve gives off an inguinal branch that joins the ilioinguinal nerve. The ilioinguinal nerve runs anterior to the spermatic cord and branches at the external ring. The genital branch of the GF nerve innervates the cremaster muscle and provides sensory innervation to the lateral scrotum and labia. This nerve accompanies the cremaster vessels as a neurovascular bundle in males but follows the round ligament in females.

Posterior Anatomy

The Myopectineal Orifice

The medial aspect of the superior gap between the pelvis and the thigh is the myopectineal orifice. In 1956, the French anatomist and surgeon Henri René Fruchaud first described the term and the concept of a weakened myopectineal orifice as the cause of hernias in the inguinal region.[3] Wide reinforcement of the myopectineal orifice has become the foundation for our modern hernia repair of the adult groin. A posterior view of the right hemipelvis and associated musculature is shown in Fig. 82.2.

Femoral and Iliopectineal Area

Starting with the isolated right bony hemipelvis, the inguinal ligament, or Poupart's ligament, can be seen in Fig. 82.3. The inguinal ligament is the inferior border of the EO muscle and extends from the medial bony projection of the pubic tubercle to the ASIS.

The gap below the inguinal ligament is divided into two spaces by another condensation of the iliopsoas fascia, known as the *iliopectineal arch*. The medial aspect is vascular, and the lateral is muscular (Fig. 82.4).

The lateral muscles include the iliacus and major psoas muscles (iliopsoas complex). They share a common tendon as they exit the pelvis inferiorly, which inserts on the medial aspect of the femur. The femoral nerve (FN) runs deep within the psoas muscle and emerges laterally as it passes beneath the inguinal ligament. The FN is rarely encountered during routine MI IHR. The tendinous

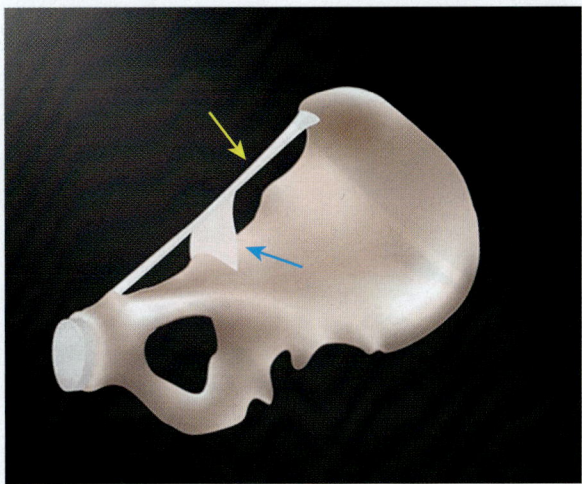

FIGURE 82.3 Poupart's or inguinal ligament *(yellow arrow)* spanning from the anterior superior iliac spine to the pubis. The iliopectineal arch *(blue arrow)* provides a septum between two spaces.

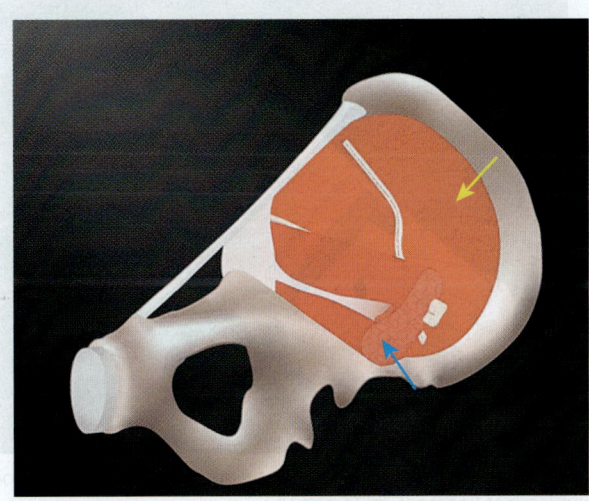

FIGURE 82.4 Muscular compartment lateral to the iliopectineal arch containing the iliacus muscle *(yellow arrow)* and psoas major *(blue arrow)*.

structure anterior to the psoas major is not its tendon, which can only be seen from the anterior view of the pelvis, but rather the tendon of the psoas minor muscle. The lateral femoral cutaneous nerve exits from the lateral border of the psoas and travels over the iliacus muscle. The nerve can be singular, but many branches are often found. Injury to the lateral femoral cutaneous nerve can lead to pain, numbness, or tingling in the lateral thigh, a condition known as *meralgia paresthetica*.

The lateral muscular aspect of the iliopectineal arch is covered by the iliopsoas fascia, which protects the surrounding nerves and should be preserved during hernia repair to prevent nerve injury. The pectineus muscle covers the floor of the vascular gap and inserts into the pectineal line, a ridge of bone, via the pectineal or Cooper's ligament (Fig. 82.5).

Posterior to the pubic arch and between it and the ischium is an opening known as the *obturator foramen*. The obturator muscle narrows inferiorly to exit the pelvis via the obturator foramen and then inserts on the femur. Anteriorly, it leaves a small gap for the passage of the neurovascular structures. This

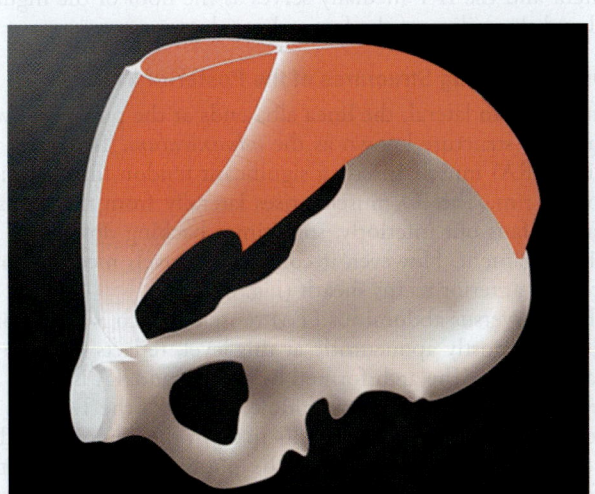

FIGURE 82.2 Posterior view of the right hemipelvis and associated abdominal musculature.

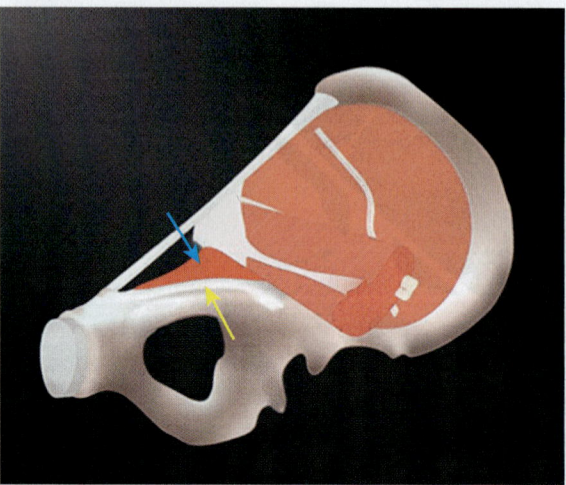

FIGURE 82.5 Cooper's ligament *(yellow arrow)* formed by the tendon of the pectineus muscle *(blue arrow)*.

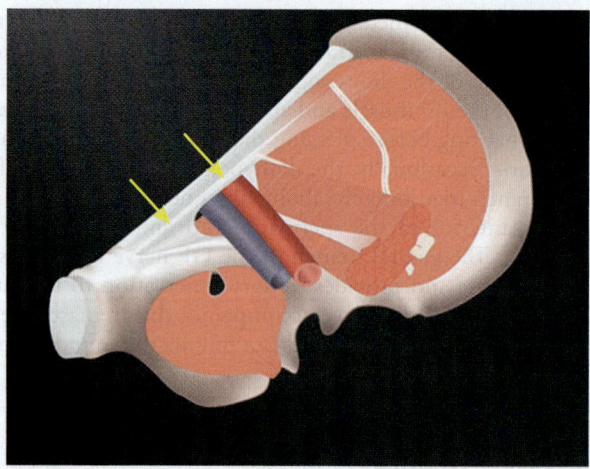

FIGURE 82.7 Femoral canal with the iliopubic tract (marked by *yellow arrows*), which is more lateral than the lacunar ligament.

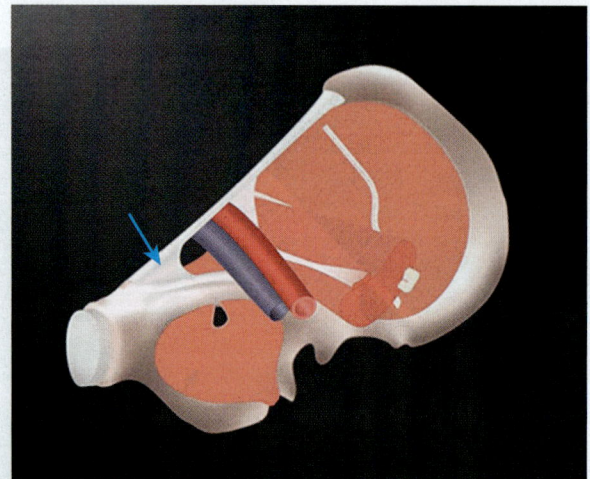

FIGURE 82.6 Femoral canal without iliopubic tract. Note the location of the lacunar ligament *(blue arrow)*.

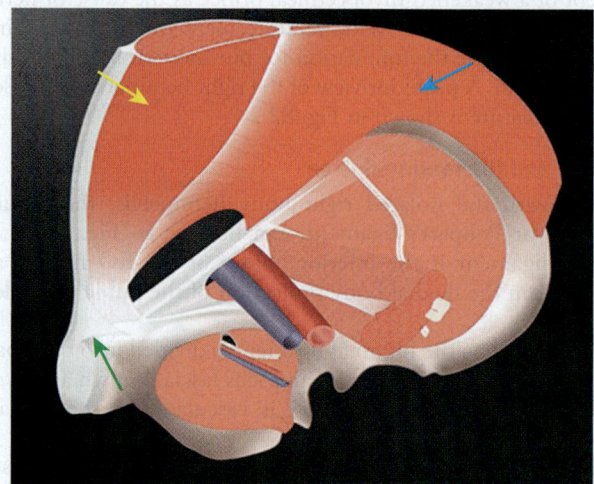

FIGURE 82.8 Relationship of the adminiculum *(green arrow)*, rectus abdominis muscle *(yellow arrow)*, and internal oblique muscle *(blue arrow)* with the posterior wall.

gap conveys the iliac artery and vein, which then continue as the femoral artery and vein once they pass the inguinal ligament. Medial to the vein is a recess of the transversalis fascia, the femoral canal, which is visible anteriorly. A portion of the most medial aspect of the inguinal ligament fans out and inserts into the pectineal rim to form the lacunar ligament. There are two major misconceptions commonly propagated. First is that the medial border of the femoral canal is the lacunar ligament (Fig. 82.6). This is typically not the case unless there is a sizeable femoral hernia significantly extending medially. Second is that the inguinal and lacunar ligaments are visible from the posterior wall. The correct anatomy becomes apparent when details of the IPT are considered. The IPT is formed as a condensation of the transversalis fascia, running parallel but posterior to the inguinal ligament (Fig. 82.7).

The IPT extends from the iliopectineal fascia (not the ASIS as commonly described) to the pubic tubercle, where it provides a triangular fascial extension that inserts into Cooper's ligament. The medial border of this extension is the medial limit of the femoral canal, which now appears smaller in Fig. 82.7. The medial border of the femoral canal is sometimes divided to reduce an

incarcerated femoral hernia safely. The space between the inguinal ligament and the IPT medially serves as the floor of the inguinal canal and the ceiling of the femoral canal.

Medial Supporting Structures of the Posterior Wall

From medial to lateral, the linea alba ends at the pubic area with a triangular structure known as the *adminiculum*. The rectus abdominus (RA) muscle inserts a significant tendon inferiorly into the pubic rim. The IO muscle arises laterally from the iliopsoas fascia and fans out inferiorly, sometimes backing down into the inguinal ligament. However, it commonly travels medially to reinforce the anterior rectus sheath (Fig. 82.8).

The transversus abdominus (TA) muscle, which is posterior to the IO and mostly aponeurotic at this level, reflects into the inguinal ligament. The arch formed by the IO and TA is called the *falx inguinalis* or *TA arch*. The middle tendon of the TA joins the IO tendon in about 5% of patients to form the conjoint tendon. The conjoint tendon inserts into the pubis, which adds further reinforcement to the posterior wall (Fig. 82.9).

The EO muscle, which is aponeurotic in the medial inguinal area, covers the anterior inguinal canal and leaves an inferolateral

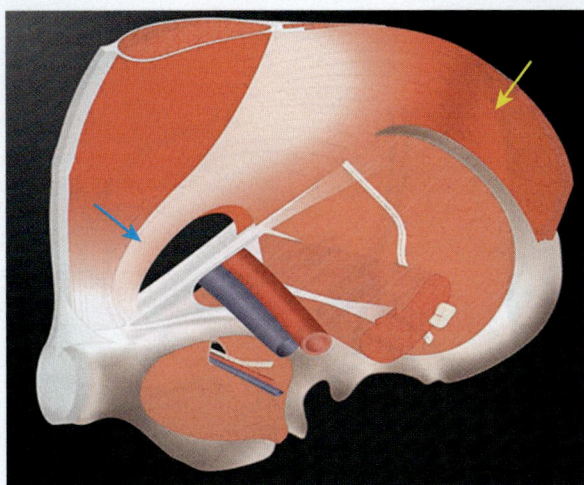

FIGURE 82.9 Relationship of the transversus abdominis muscle and the posterior wall *(yellow arrow)* and conjoint tendon *(blue arrow)*.

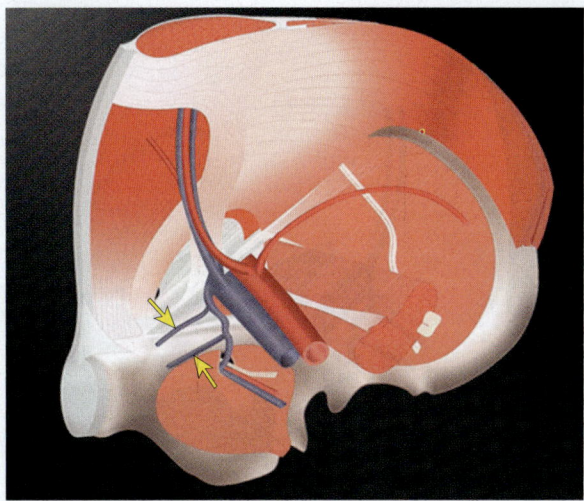

FIGURE 82.10 Origin of corona mortis vessels *(yellow arrows)*, which connect the inferior epigastric and obturator vessels.

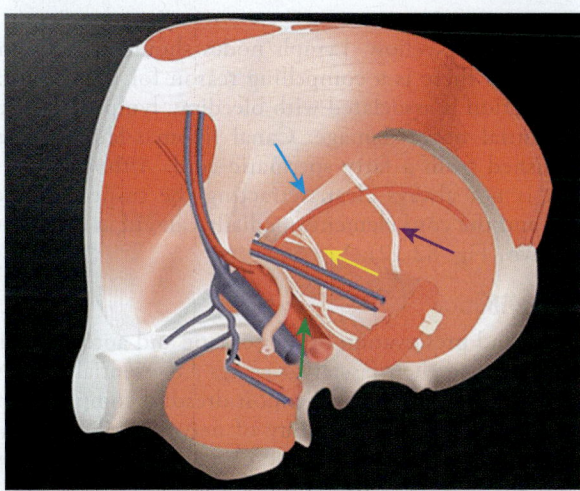

FIGURE 82.11 Transversalis sling *(blue arrow)* and its relationship to the genitofemoral nerve. Both the genital branch *(green arrow)* and femoral branch *(yellow arrow)* travel posterior to the horizontal limb of the transversalis sling, with the femoral branch coursing more lateral than the genital branch. The lateral femoral cutaneous *(purple arrow)* runs lateral to both branches of the genitofemoral nerve.

gap known as the *external* or *superficial inguinal ring*. The inferior border of the EO muscle is the inguinal ligament.

The posterior sheath of the RA muscle classically ends a third of a distance between the umbilicus and the pubis at the arcuate line, also known as the *semicircular line of Douglas*. However, it can extend lower, sometimes reaching the pubis. A fascial condensation of the transversalis fascia and the TA muscle extends medial to the arcuate line to reach the IPT. This is known as the *interfoveolar* or *Hesselbach's* ligament and is another reinforcement structure of the posterior wall. Hesselbach's ligament splits the inguinal canal into a medial and a lateral portion and usually supports the epigastric vessels. The accessory obturator vein (and sometimes also the artery) crosses the pubic rim to connect the obturator with the epigastric vessels and often gives off medial parallel branches called the *superior and inferior ramus branches*. This arrangement of vessels constitutes a circular connection known as the "crown of death" or *corona mortis*. Careful dissection in this area is of utmost importance to avoid inadvertent bleeding (Fig. 82.10).

Hesselbach's ligament, the conjoint tendon, and Henle's ligament buttress the transversalis fascia, which covers the entire area and prevents the development of hernias. Weakness of the transversalis fascia and absence or displacement of the supporting structures of the posterior wall cause direct hernias. Direct hernias typically occur medial to the epigastric vessels within Hesselbach's triangle. However, they can also appear lateral to the epigastric vessels if the supporting structures are absent or displaced.

The Internal Ring and the Cord Elements

The lateral border of Hesselbach's ligament forms the internal edge of the deep or internal ring. In the male embryo, the gubernaculum testis pulls the vas deferens and the internal spermatic vessels into the internal ring. In the female, the round ligament is the analog of the gubernaculum and enters the internal ring to insert into the labia majora. The first structure that the cord elements pass through on their way to the inguinal canal is not the opening of the transversus abdominis at the internal ring but a lesser-known microfascia called the *transversalis sling* (TS), which partially surrounds these elements. The TS is a condensation of the TA aponeurosis and the transversalis fascia and has horizontal and vertical limbs. As such, the TS serves as an important anatomic landmark during MI IHR. The GF nerve runs on the anterior surface of the psoas major, which has variable branches, although still predictable in location. Its fibers run below the TS to provide sensory innervation to the anteromedial thigh. Nerve distribution is variable, but the genital branch typically runs parallel to the iliac artery and passes under the horizontal limb of the TS, after which it angles anteriorly to enter the inguinal canal. The femoral branch of the GF nerve runs more laterally and courses under the horizontal limb of the TS (Fig. 82.11).

The cord elements are bound together by a fascial envelope derived from the urogenital fascia. Herniated preperitoneal fat, often referred to as *lipoma of the inguinal canal* because of its pseudocapsule, can be found anterolateral to the cord elements and above the horizontal limb of the TS. This arrangement helps differentiate canal lipomas from lymph nodes. Lipomas of the canal also tend to be lighter in color, whereas lymph

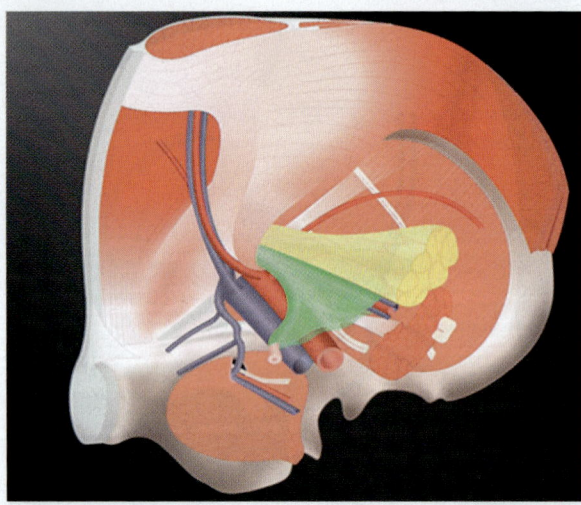

FIGURE 82.12 The urogenital fascia *(green)* envelops the cord elements. Canal or cord lipomas are located anterolateral to the cord elements *(yellow)*.

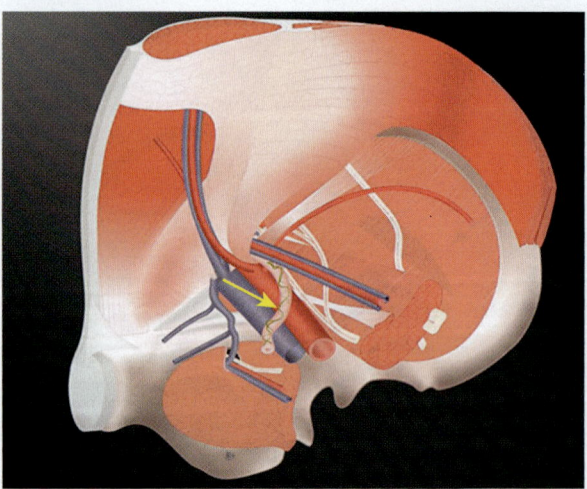

FIGURE 82.13 Autonomic innervation of the testicle is provided by the paravasal nerves *(yellow arrow)*, which travel along the vas deferens. Preserving these nerves is important during dissection of the hernia sac.

nodes are darker yellow. Lymph nodes should be left undisturbed unless there is a compelling reason for biopsy because their dissection is associated with bleeding, lymphatic leakage, and potential nerve damage. Canal lipomas should also be distinguished from a fatty spermatic cord. Although the distinction is not always clear, retracting the suspected lipoma laterally and the cord elements medially can aid in differentiating the two (Fig. 82.12).

Nerve Distribution

Awareness and preservation of the somatic and autonomic neural structures and their fascial coverings are essential to prevent neuropathy, which is one of the most dreadful complications of IHR. Despite the wide variability of nerve distribution in the posterior wall, there are anatomic clues that can help prevent nerve injury.

Nerves in the posterior inguinal wall are in a trapezoidal or triangular region, medial and inferior to the IPT and lateral to the spermatic vessels. This area has been dubbed the "triangle of pain." No mechanical fixation or careless dissection should take place in this area. However, studies have shown in cadaver dissections that nerves can enter the thigh above the IPT, with a few entering 1 cm above the IPT.[4] Based on this, it has been recommended to expand the triangle of pain by shifting the superolateral border 2 cm above an imaginary line drawn between the ASIS and the internal inguinal ring. Injury to the genital branch of the GF nerve tends to occur with aggressive dissection within the triangle of pain, which should be avoided. This is also typically the cause of injury to lateral nerves, such as the iliohypogastric and ilioinguinal nerves that course between the TA and IO muscles, which are not routinely visible during MI IHR.

The paravasal nerves are responsible for the autonomic innervation of the testicle. These nerves travel from the pelvic and hypogastric plexi and run along the vas deferens to innervate the testicle. Injury to the paravasal nerves can result in deep testicular visceral pain, as opposed to the scrotal pain of somatic dermatomal distribution. Dissection of the hernia sac with minimal manipulation of the cord elements is a fundamental strategy to avoid this complication (Fig. 82.13).

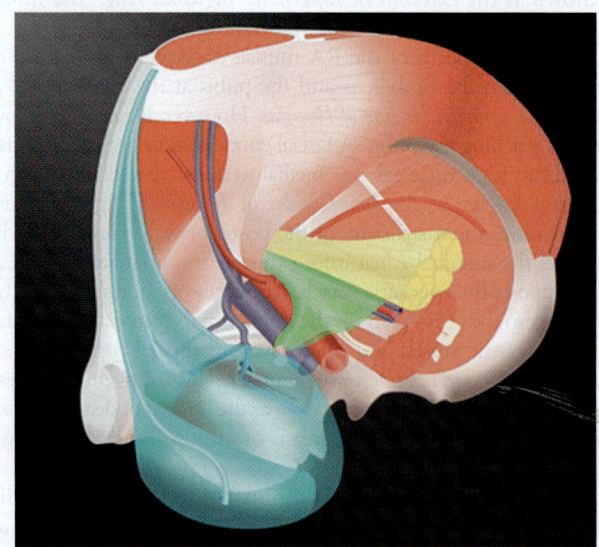

FIGURE 82.14 The umbilical-vesical fascia *(blue)* surrounds the bladder. Anterior to this fascia is the prevesical space of Retzius.

The Umbilical-Vesical Fascia and Associated Microfascia

The umbilical-vesical fascia is derived from embryonic structures. The median ligament, a remnant of the urachus, is at the midline. On each side are the medial ligaments, which correspond to the remnants of the umbilical arteries. These remnants may occasionally still contain patent vessels and bleed if divided. This fascia surrounds the bladder, and under it is the blood supply and autonomic innervation of the bladder. Anterior to this fascia is the prevesical space, or space of Retzius (Fig. 82.14).

The posterior transversalis fascia, or intermediate fascia, is an extension of the posterior rectus sheath and has a different level of development. The intermediate fascia divides the medial or parietal compartment from the lateral or visceral compartment. The careful division of the intermediate fascia is an essential aspect of the MI IHR to achieve a critical view of the myopectineal orifice.

MANAGEMENT OF INGUINAL HERNIAS

Diagnosis

A detailed history and clinical exam should be conducted to gather information about risk factors for hernia development, symptoms, and their impact on quality of life. A thorough surgical history should be obtained because this may have a significant impact on operative management. A history of extensive abdominal or pelvic surgery may preclude a MI preperitoneal approach. In the setting of recurrence after an open anterior approach, a posterior MI approach may be warranted. In contrast, a failed MI approach may warrant an open anterior approach. A surgeon must attempt to obtain all prior operative reports, particularly those of prior hernia repairs. This can provide invaluable information about distorted anatomy and previously placed implants, such as mesh or fixation devices.

Clinical examination alone is recommended for confirming the diagnosis of an evident groin hernia. Examinations should be performed in both the standing and supine positions. If no obvious groin bulge is visualized, a Valsalva maneuver may aid in the diagnosis. Small hernias may require direct palpation of the external inguinal ring for a bulge. One should be suspicious of a femoral hernia if a bulge is discovered below the inguinal ligament.

Ultrasound (US) is a useful adjunct in the setting of vague groin swelling or occult groin hernias. CT or dynamic MRI is useful when US is negative or nondiagnostic. Imaging may also be useful for cases of recurrence or extreme presentations, such as massive scrotal hernias.

Treatment

Nonoperative Management

Given the natural tendency for groin hernias to progress with time, the discovery of a symptomatic hernia typically warrants operative repair. However, patients with minimal or no symptoms present a challenge to clinicians because they must balance the risk of hernia-related complications and those associated with operative repair. Fitzgibbons and colleagues performed a prospective randomized trial of watchful waiting for males with asymptomatic or minimally symptomatic inguinal hernias. The study randomized over 700 males to either watchful waiting or open tension-free hernia repair. No deaths were attributed to the study at 2-year follow-up, and the risk of hernia incarceration in the watchful waiting group was extremely low at 0.3% of study participants. Nearly a quarter of those in the watchful waiting arm crossed over to the operative group as a result of pain interfering with activity.[5] A later report demonstrated that the crossover rate to the surgical group increased to 68% at 10 years, with almost 80% of males older than 65 years of age receiving surgical repair. Patients who had surgery later did not experience increased surgical site infections or recurrence rates compared with those assigned to early repair.[6] These studies demonstrate that watchful waiting is a safe option for patients with asymptomatic or minimally symptomatic inguinal hernias and that operative outcomes are no different from those undergoing immediate repair. It is important to note that these results should not be applied to females because they were not included in this study. In addition, femoral hernias were not included in these studies and typically warrant timely surgical repair, given their greater risk of strangulation than inguinal hernias. Patients opting for nonoperative management may have some symptomatic improvement with the use of a hernia truss.

Operative Management—Open Techniques

Anterior approaches. Anterior hernia repairs are the most common technique for inguinal hernias worldwide. Current best practices recommend tension-free repairs, which can be done in various ways. Older tissue-based repair methods are rarely used today, except in cases of contamination or concurrent bowel resection, where using a mesh prosthesis may not be advisable.

Certain technical aspects of the procedure are consistent across all anterior repairs. The open hernia repair procedure begins with a transverse or slightly curved incision made just above the inguinal ligament and approximately a fingerbreadth below the internal inguinal ring. Topographically, the internal inguinal ring is situated midway between the ASIS and the pubic tubercle on the same side. Dissection then proceeds through the subcutaneous tissues and Scarpa's fascia. The EO fascia and the external inguinal ring are first identified, after which the EO fascia is incised through the superficial inguinal ring to expose the inguinal canal. It is crucial to identify and carefully handle the ilioinguinal nerve, iliohypogastric nerve, and genital branch of the GF nerve to prevent inadvertent transection or entrapment. Awareness of nerve location is important to prevent damage because this is the main cause of postoperative chronic pain after inguinal hernia surgery. The spermatic cord is mobilized at the pubic tubercle using a combination of blunt and sharp dissection techniques. Improper mobilization, particularly laterally, can lead to confusion in identifying tissue planes and essential structures, potentially resulting in harm to the spermatic cord structures or disruption of the inguinal canal floor.

The cremaster muscle, a part of the mobilized spermatic cord, is separated parallel to its fibers from the underlying cord structures. The cremaster artery and vein, which join the cremaster muscle near the deep inguinal ring, can often be avoided but may need to be sacrificed. In the past, some surgeons advocated skeletonizing the spermatic cord. However, it is advisable to minimize disruption to the cremasteric fibers and vasculature to reduce the risk of injury to the genital branch of the GF nerve. With an indirect hernia, the hernia sac is situated deep to the cremaster muscle and anteromedial to the spermatic cord structures. Usually, spreading the cremaster muscle longitudinally is sufficient to expose an indirect sac. The hernia sac should be carefully separated from adjacent cord structures and dissected to the level of the internal inguinal ring. If the sac is large, it is opened and examined for visceral contents, although this step is unnecessary for small hernias. The sac can either be mobilized and placed within the preperitoneal space or ligated at the level of the internal ring, with any excess sac being excised. If dealing with a large hernia sac, electrocautery may be used for division to facilitate ligation. There is no need to remove the distal portion of the sac. For broad-based sacs, it may be more practical to reduce them into the peritoneal cavity rather than ligate them. Direct hernia sacs protrude through the floor of the inguinal canal medial to the epigastric vessels and can be reduced below the transversalis fascia before repair. This requires incising the weakened floor (transversalis fascia) to reveal the underlying preperitoneal fat, which can then be mobilized from the neck of the direct defect, and any other component of the direct hernia is reduced. Once the floor of the inguinal canal is opened, one should look for a femoral hernia, which, if present, will be found in the preperitoneal space medial to the femoral vein. After this exploration, the redundant transversalis fascia is excised, and the floor can often be reapproximated using a continuous absorbable suture. A cord lipoma, which is retroperitoneal fat that has herniated through the deep inguinal ring, should be suture-ligated and excised. Cord lipomas can serve as a mechanism for recurrence and can also be a persistent postoperative bulge felt by patients.

During the dissection of the hernia sac, one should take care to recognize the components of the hernia sac. A sliding hernia presents a unique challenge in managing the hernia sac. A *sliding hernia* is defined as a hernia in which part of the hernia sac comprises visceral peritoneum covering a retroperitoneal organ, typically the colon or bladder. In such cases, the grossly redundant portion of the sac should be excised, with care not to injure any viscera involved with the sac, and the peritoneal defect is then closed. The viscera and sac can then be reduced.

Tissue Repairs

Although the use of tissue repairs has significantly diminished because of their high recurrence rates, they still find relevance in specific clinical scenarios. Tissue repairs are indispensable when dealing with strangulated hernias necessitating bowel resection because the use of synthetic mesh prostheses is contraindicated. Several options are available for tissue repairs, including the IPT, Shouldice, Bassini, and McVay repairs.

The IPT repair is performed by approximating the transversus abdominis aponeurotic arch to the IPT using interrupted sutures (Fig. 82.15).

The repair begins at the pubic tubercle and extends laterally beyond the internal inguinal ring. It is worth noting that although this repair was initially described with a relaxing incision (as elaborated on later), many surgeons who employ this technique do not perform a relaxing incision as part of the procedure.

The Shouldice repair emphasizes a multilayer imbricated reconstruction of the posterior wall of the inguinal canal. It is considered the best tissue-based approach according to recent guidelines and expert consensus.[2] Although no studies exist comparing the learning curves of different nonmesh techniques, the Shouldice is not an easy technique to learn. At the Shouldice Hospital, surgeons are only considered qualified after 300 cases.[2] The repair is done using a continuous running suture technique. After completion of the dissection, the posterior wall of the inguinal canal is meticulously reconstructed by superimposing running suture lines, progressing from the deeper to more superficial layers. The initial suture line secures the transversus abdominis aponeurotic arch to the IPT. Subsequently, the IO and transversus abdominis muscles and

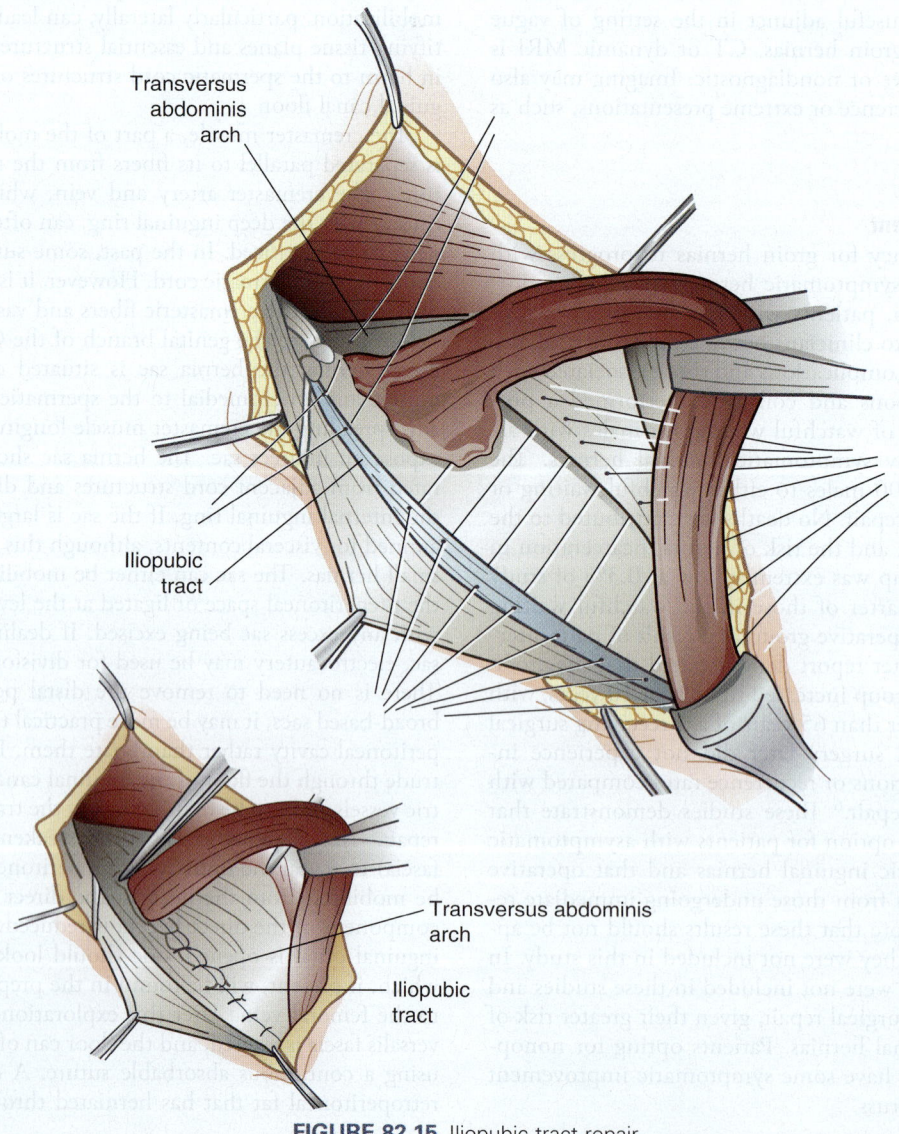

FIGURE 82.15 Iliopubic tract repair.

aponeuroses are sutured to the inguinal ligament. The Shouldice repair is known for its remarkably low recurrence rate and a high degree of patient satisfaction, particularly in highly selected patients.

The Bassini repair is performed by suturing the transversus abdominis and IO musculoaponeurotic arches, or the conjoint tendon when present, to the inguinal ligament. This once-popular technique represents the fundamental approach to nonanatomic hernia repairs and was the prevailing method employed before the emergence of tension-free repair methods.

The Cooper's ligament repair, often referred to as the *McVay repair,* has been a popular choice for addressing various types of groin hernias, including direct hernias, large indirect hernias, recurrent hernias, and femoral hernias. In this procedure, interrupted nonabsorbable sutures are used to approximate the edge of the transversus abdominis aponeurosis and Cooper's ligament. When the medial aspect of the femoral canal is reached, a transition suture is placed to incorporate Cooper's ligament and the IPT, making it effective for the repair of femoral hernias when present. Lateral to this transition stitch, the transversus abdominis aponeurosis is secured to the IPT. A key principle of this repair involves the use of a relaxing incision. This is performed by reflecting the EO aponeurosis cephalad and medial, which exposes the anterior rectus sheath. A curvilinear incision is then made, starting 1 cm above the pubic tubercle and extending along the anterior sheath toward its lateral border. This technique reduces tension on the suture line, resulting in decreased postoperative pain and a lower risk of hernia recurrence. The fascial defect created by this incision

is covered by the body of the rectus muscle, preventing herniation at the site of the relaxing incision. The McVay repair is particularly well suited for addressing strangulated femoral hernias because it obliterates the femoral space without the need for mesh.

Other novel tissue-based approaches have been described in the literature. For example, the Desarda hernia repair technique focuses on reinforcing the inguinal canal while preserving the patient's native tissues. In this procedure, a strip of the patient's EO aponeurosis is used to reconstruct the weakened inguinal floor. These tissue-based hernia repair techniques serve as valuable options in specific clinical scenarios where mesh prostheses are not suitable. Each technique has its own set of indications and is chosen based on the unique characteristics of the patient and the hernia being treated.

Tension-Free Anterior Inguinal Hernia Repair

Tension-free repair has become the most common approach to IHR. Recognizing that tension is a primary contributor to hernia recurrence, modern hernia practices typically use a synthetic mesh prosthesis to bridge the hernia defect, a concept popularized by Lichtenstein. There are several options for mesh placement in anterior inguinal herniorrhaphy, including the Lichtenstein approach, plug and patch technique, and sandwich technique involving both anterior and preperitoneal mesh pieces. However, recent guidelines suggest that a flat piece of mesh is preferred over three-dimensional meshes.[7]

In the Lichtenstein repair (Fig. 82.16), a piece of prosthetic nonabsorbable mesh is customized to fit the inguinal canal, with a

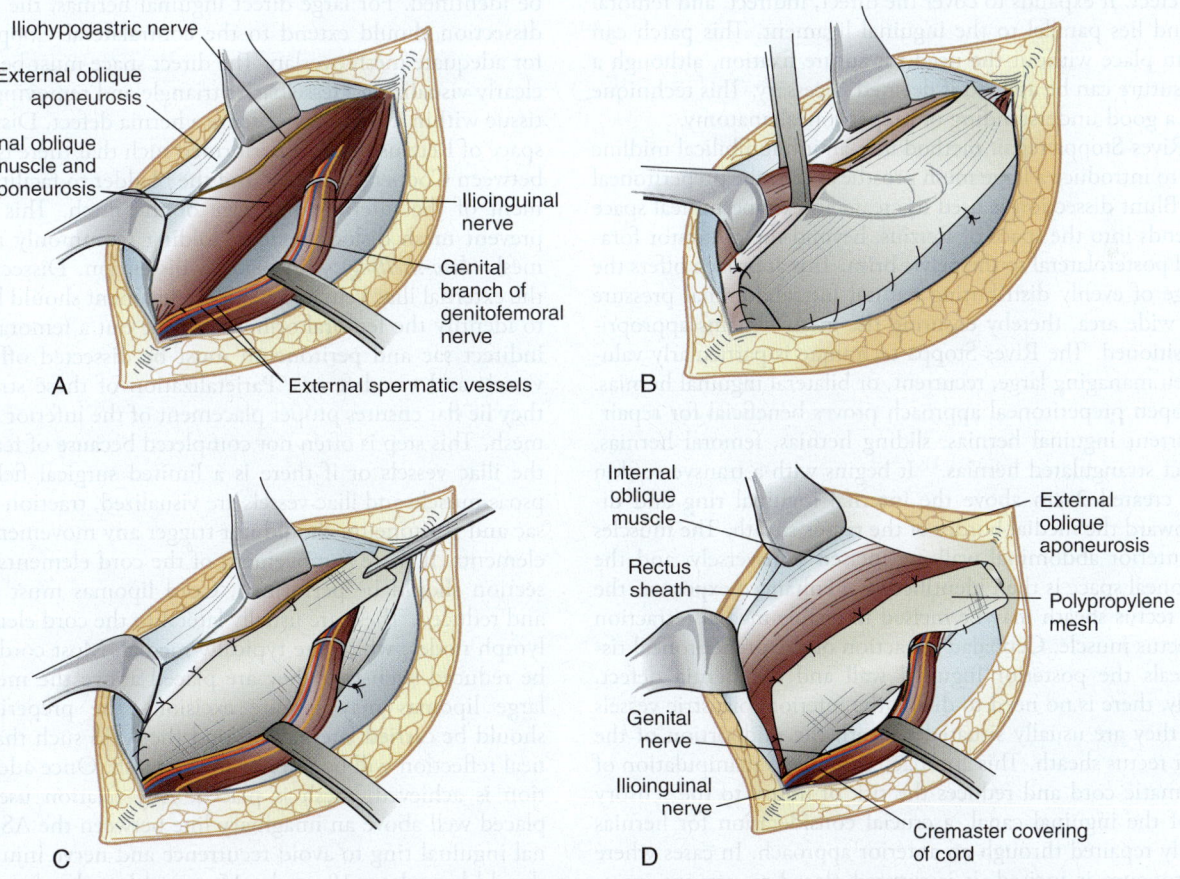

FIGURE 82.16 Lichtenstein repair. A polypropylene mesh is placed in an onlay position to provide a tension-free repair. (A) The relationship of the spermatic cord, myofascial layers, and neurovascular structures before mesh placement. (B) The inferolateral edge of the mesh is secured to the shelving edge of the inguinal ligament. (C) The superomedial aspect of the mesh is secured to the conjoint tendon. The superior portion of the mesh is split in preparation of forming a new internal inguinal ring. (D) The tails of the mesh are crossed to create a new internal inguinal ring.

slit cut into the distal lateral edge to accommodate the spermatic cord. Various preformed, commercially available prostheses are suitable for this purpose, or a surgeon can trim their own mesh construct. The periosteum overlying the pubic tubercle is exposed and dissected medially toward the midline of the pubis for at least 2 cm. Mesh fixation directly to the pubic tubercle is avoided to minimize the risk of chronic groin pain and osteitis. The inferolateral edge of the mesh is sutured to the shelving edge of the inguinal ligament, starting adjacent to the pubic tubercle but not into it, using a nonabsorbable suture. The medial aspect of the mesh generously overlaps the pubic tubercle by at least 2 cm. This suture is taken to a point lateral and superior to the internal inguinal ring and tied. Interrupted sutures are then placed to secure the superomedial aspect of the mesh to the conjoint tendon, with care to prevent injury or entrapment of the ilioinguinal and iliohypogastric nerves. The tails created by the slit are sutured together around the spermatic cord, forming a new internal inguinal ring. Special care is taken to safeguard the ilioinguinal nerve and genital branch of the GF nerve from entrapment, either by placing them with the cord structures as they pass through the newly fashioned internal inguinal ring or avoiding their enclosure in the repair.[8]

Posterior Approaches

An alternative tension-free mesh repair approach involves the preperitoneal placement of a self-expanding polypropylene patch.[9] A pocket is crafted within the preperitoneal space through gentle dissection, and a preformed mesh patch is introduced into the hernia defect. It expands to cover the direct, indirect, and femoral spaces and lies parallel to the inguinal ligament. This patch can remain in place without the need for suture fixation, although a tacking suture can be applied if deemed necessary. This technique requires a good understanding of preperitoneal anatomy.

The Rives-Stoppa repair method uses an infraumbilical midline incision to introduce a large mesh prosthesis into the preperitoneal space.[10] Blunt dissection is used to create an extraperitoneal space that extends into the space of Retzius, beyond the obturator foramen and posterolateral to the pelvic brim. This approach offers the advantage of evenly distributing natural intraabdominal pressure across a wide area, thereby ensuring the mesh remains appropriately positioned. The Rives-Stoppa technique is particularly valuable when managing large, recurrent, or bilateral inguinal hernias.

The open preperitoneal approach proves beneficial for repairing recurrent inguinal hernias, sliding hernias, femoral hernias, and select strangulated hernias.[11] It begins with a transverse skin incision created 2 cm above the internal inguinal ring and directed toward the medial border of the rectus sheath. The muscles of the anterior abdominal wall are incised transversely, and the preperitoneal space is then identified. For enhanced exposure, the anterior rectus sheath may be incised to enable medial retraction of the rectus muscle. Cephalad retraction of the preperitoneal tissues reveals the posterior inguinal wall and the hernia defect. Generally, there is no need to divide the inferior epigastric vessels because they are usually situated beneath the midportion of the posterior rectus sheath. This approach minimizes manipulation of the spermatic cord and reduces the risk of injury to the sensory nerves of the inguinal canal, a crucial consideration for hernias previously repaired through an anterior approach. In cases where the peritoneum is incised, it is sutured closed to prevent intraperitoneal contents from protruding into the operative field. Identification and suturing of the transversalis fascia and transversus abdominis aponeurosis to the IPT using permanent sutures is a key component of this approach. For femoral hernias addressed

via this technique, closure of the femoral canal is accomplished by securing the repair to Cooper's ligament. The use of a mesh prosthesis is a common choice to obliterate the defect in the femoral canal, particularly for large hernias.

Operative Management—Minimally Invasive Techniques

The most used MI techniques for IHR are the transabdominal preperitoneal (TAPP), totally extraperitoneal (TEP), and enhanced-view totally extraperitoneal (eTEP) approaches. These are all approaches to preperitoneal IHR and may all be performed with traditional or robotic-assisted laparoscopic surgery. Regardless of the technique chosen, the critical view of the myopectineal orifice (CV of the MPO) should always be obtained to reduce complications and recurrence.[12]

The Critical View of the Myopectineal Orifice

The CV of the MPO was described to standardize the dissection performed during an MI IHR. The protocol to achieve this was developed based on the best available evidence that demonstrated fewer hernia recurrence and complications.[12] Obtaining the CV of the MPO is important to ensure a safe dissection with adequate mesh overlap of the MPO. It is important to note that all of the following steps must be performed to achieve the CV of the MPO, but not necessarily in the order described. The pubic tubercle must be identified and dissected past the midline, and the ipsilateral Cooper's ligament in relation to the hernia defect must be identified. For large direct inguinal hernias, the preperitoneal dissection should extend to the contralateral Cooper's ligament for adequate mesh overlap. The direct space must be identified by clearly visualizing Hesselbach's triangle and removing any adipose tissue within it that may obscure a hernia defect. Dissection in the space of Retzius must be performed such that there is at least 2 cm between Cooper's ligament and the bladder to facilitate flat placement of the inferomedial edge of the mesh. This is critical to prevent mesh dislodgment or folding (commonly referred to as mesh *clam-shelling*) with bladder distention. Dissection between the external iliac vein and Cooper's ligament should be performed to identify the femoral orifice and rule out a femoral hernia. The indirect sac and peritoneum must be dissected off the gonadal vessels and vas deferens. Parietalization of these structures until they lie flat ensures proper placement of the inferior border of the mesh. This step is often not completed because of fear of injuring the iliac vessels or if there is a limited surgical field. Once the psoas muscle and iliac vessels are visualized, traction of the hernia sac and peritoneum should not trigger any movement of the cord elements. If there is movement of the cord elements, further dissection should be performed. Cord lipomas must be identified and reduced. These are usually lateral to the cord elements, unlike lymph nodes, which are typically medial. Most cord lipomas can be reduced such that they are placed above the mesh; however, large lipomas may require excision. The preperitoneal space should be carried laterally beyond the ASIS such that the peritoneal reflection will be inferior to the mesh. Once adequate dissection is achieved, mesh is placed. Any fixation used should be placed well above an imaginary line between the ASIS and internal inguinal ring to avoid recurrence and nerve injury. The mesh should be at least 10 cm by 15 cm, although a larger mesh may be needed for adequate MPO coverage. The mesh should adapt to the contour of the space and cord elements without significant memory and should lie flat, without creases or folds. It is not recommended to split the mesh for pass-through of the cord elements. Deflation of the space should be performed with visualization to ensure the mesh does not fold. If this occurs, the mesh may need to be repositioned, or further preperitoneal dissection may need to be performed to prevent mesh migration during deflation. Please refer to Video 82.1 for further details.

Transabdominal Preperitoneal Inguinal Hernia Repair

The most common MI inguinal hernia approach is a TAPP. The technique of abdominal access and establishment of pneumoperitoneum is performed at the discretion of the surgeon. A camera port is typically placed in the midline at least 15 cm from the pubis to allow ample working room. Two additional working ports are placed lateral to the camera port on each side of the abdomen. A peritoneal flap is initiated by incising the peritoneum medially at a distance 4 to 6 cm superior to the hernia defect and carrying this incision laterally to the ASIS. Dissection then continues to achieve a critical view of the myopectineal orifice, as described earlier. Once the mesh is placed, the peritoneal flap should be closed to exclude the mesh from the peritoneal cavity, avoid dislodgement of the mesh, and prevent visceral adhesions. Please refer to Video 82.2 for further details.

Total Extraperitoneal Inguinal Hernia Repair

The total extraperitoneal repair (TEP) is an MI inguinal hernia mesh repair technique that allows access to the preperitoneal

space by an anterior approach without entering the peritoneal cavity. It was first introduced in 1993 by McKernan and colleagues.[13] Patients are typically positioned supine with their arms tucked. The TEP procedure begins with retrorectus access. A 1- to 2-cm infraumbilical incision is made, and the anterior rectus sheath is identified. Stay sutures are placed, and the anterior rectus sheath is incised, revealing the underlying rectus abdominis muscle. The muscle fibers are then spread to reveal the posterior rectus sheath. This retromuscular/preperitoneal space can then be established from the incision down to the level of the pubic tubercle. The space is widened with assistance of different techniques, such as balloon-mediated separation or manual endoscopic-assisted dissection (Fig. 82.17).

Once the space is developed, insufflation is established via a Hasson cannula. Two additional 5-mm ports are inserted along the midline inferiorly or laterally based on surgeon preference.

Dissection to achieve the critical view of the myopectineal orifice is performed. Once the mesh is placed, the preperitoneal space is deflated under direct visualization to ensure stable positioning of the mesh.

Enhanced-View Totally Extraperitoneal Inguinal Hernia Repair

The enhanced-view totally extraperitoneal (eTEP) approach to IHR was described in 2009 as an evolution of the TEP approach. The goal of eTEP was to improve the operative field to facilitate an

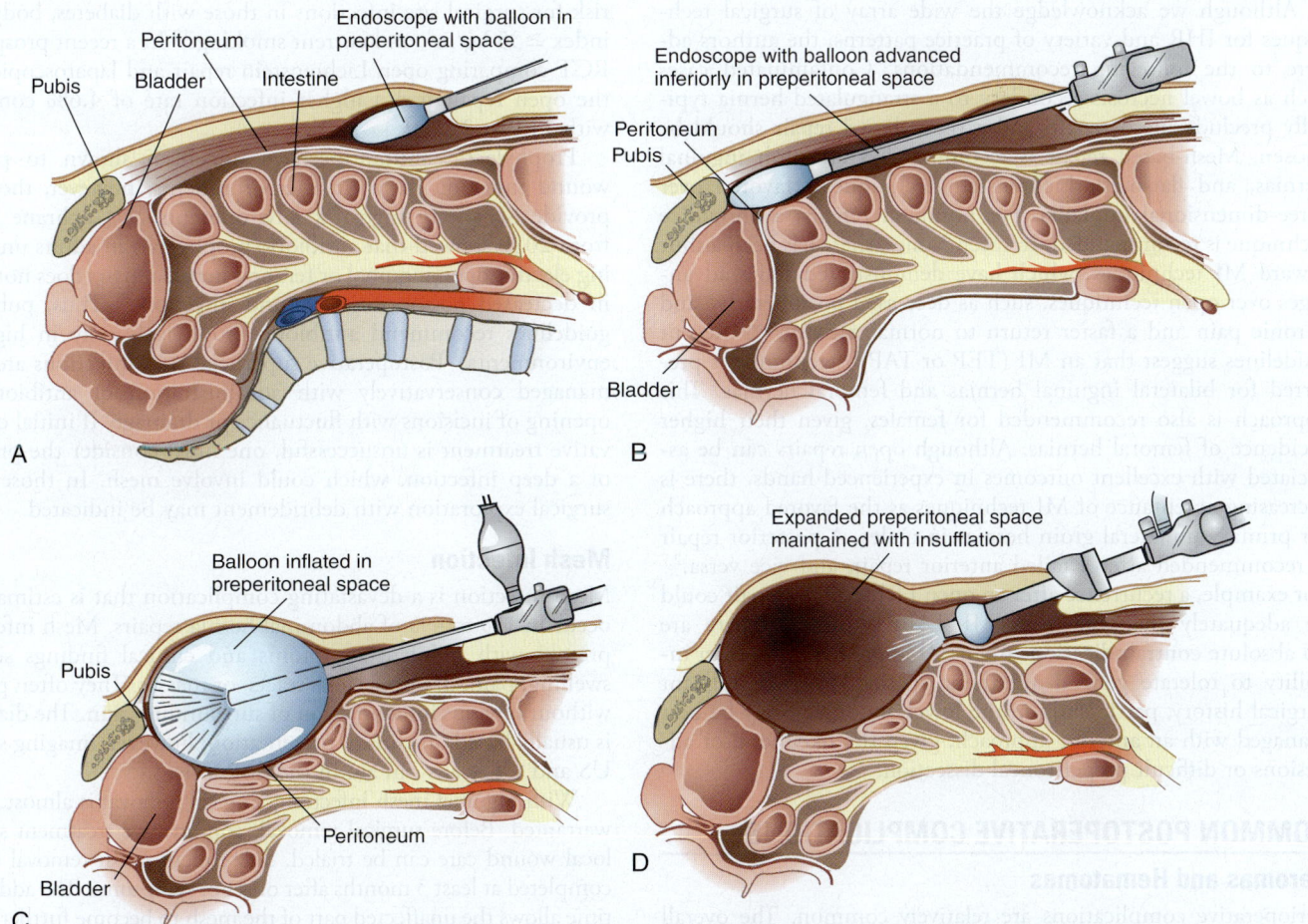

FIGURE 82.17 Totally extraperitoneal access using a balloon dissector. (A) The balloon dissector is placed in the retrorectus space. (B) Blunt dissection is performed to advance the balloon dissector into the space of Retzius. (C) The balloon dissector is insufflated to develop the preperitoneal space. (D) The balloon dissector is deflated and additional laparoscopic ports are placed to perform the procedure.

extraperitoneal approach.[14] The port placement between the pubis and the umbilicus in the TEP approach can pose ergonomic challenges to the surgeon. With division of either the medial or lateral aspect of the arcuate line, the preperitoneal space can be significantly increased for dynamic port placement.

During an extraperitoneal approach, especially TEP, it is critical to avoid creating holes in the peritoneum because CO_2 will otherwise escape from the preperitoneal space into the peritoneal cavity and significantly decrease the surgeon's working room. Breaches in the peritoneum should be controlled with either clips or suture. Another intraperitoneal port may be placed to vent the peritoneum. However, if the preperitoneal space is unable to be maintained, conversion to a transabdominal approach may be warranted. In addition, unrecognized large peritoneal defects increase the risk of an intraparietal hernia in which herniation of bowel contents occurs between the layers of the abdominal wall. This can present as early bowel obstruction. Please refer to Video 82.3 for further details.

Selection of Operative Technique

Selecting a surgical technique for IHR should be tailored to the patient and hernia characteristics, the surgeon's experience and preferences, and the resources available.[2] Surgeons desiring to offer comprehensive treatment for inguinal hernia should be proficient in both anterior and posterior approaches, mesh and nonmesh repairs, and open and MI techniques.

Although we acknowledge the wide array of surgical techniques for IHR and variety of practice patterns, the authors adhere to the following recommendations. Contaminated cases such as bowel necrosis secondary to a strangulated hernia typically preclude mesh repair, and a tissue-based repair should be chosen. Mesh-based repair is recommended for adult inguinal hernias, and flat-mesh Lichtenstein technique is favored over three-dimensional implants. For nonmesh repairs, a Shouldice technique is recommended. In recent times, there has been a shift toward MI techniques, which have demonstrated some advantages over open techniques, such as decreased postoperative and chronic pain and a faster return to normal activity.[15,16] Recent guidelines suggest that an MI (TEP or TAPP) technique is preferred for bilateral inguinal hernias and femoral hernias. This approach is also recommended for females, given their higher incidence of femoral hernias. Although open repairs can be associated with excellent outcomes in experienced hands, there is increasing acceptance of MI techniques as the favored approach for primary unilateral groin hernias in males. A posterior repair is recommended after a failed anterior repair, and vice versa.[2,7] For example, a recurrence after an open Lichtenstein repair could be adequately managed with MI TAPP. Although there are no absolute contraindications to an MI approach other than inability to tolerate general anesthesia, patients with significant surgical history, particularly in the lower abdomen, may be best managed with an anterior approach, given the likelihood of adhesions or difficult preperitoneal dissection.

COMMON POSTOPERATIVE COMPLICATIONS

Seromas and Hematomas

Perioperative complications are relatively common. The overall complication rate is estimated to range from 5% to 10%. Seromas and hematomas result from fluid or blood collecting in the dead space that remains after repair. A recent prospective randomized controlled trial (RCT) comparing open Lichtenstein repair and

laparoscopic TEP showed an increased seroma risk in TEP of 7.9% versus 3.4%.[17] At the end of the procedure, some surgeons opt to leave a drain in the preperitoneal space. A study from 2023 showed that closed-suction drainage led to decreased scrotal edema, seroma, and urinary retention at 3 months.[18] The benefits of routine drain placement should be balanced with the possible risk of a foreign body adjacent to the mesh. In our practice, drains are not routinely used and are reserved for complex or large inguinal hernias. Most small seromas and hematomas can be successfully managed conservatively with observation. Seromas that persist with time or cause significant discomfort may be aspirated. Rarely, seromas may need to be surgically excised if refractory to percutaneous drainage. Large hematomas should be evacuated to decrease clot burden because they can cause significant discomfort and take a long period of time to resolve on their own. This can be done with an MI or open approach, depending on the location of the hematoma. Acute postoperative hematoma formation with concerns of active bleeding or hemodynamic changes should be urgently explored in the operating room.

Surgical Site Infection

Surgical site infections are characterized as superficial, deep, or involving organ space. A recent study using the National Surgical Quality Improvement Program database found an infection rate of 0.4% in a cohort of unilateral, initial open hernia repairs. Like other surgical site infections, this study found a two-times-greater risk for surgical site infections in those with diabetes, body mass index ≥ 35 kg/m^2, and current smoking.[19] In a recent prospective RCT comparing open Lichtenstein repair and laparoscopic TEP, the open repair had a higher infection rate of 4.6% compared with TEP at 2.2%.[17]

Prophylactic antibiotics have not been shown to prevent wound infection in low-risk environments; however, they may provide benefit in high-risk environments. A Cochrane review from 2020 showed that antibiotic prophylaxis in adults undergoing elective open inguinal or femoral hernia repairs does not result in decreased postoperative wound infection.[20] Thus, published guidelines recommend antibiotic prophylaxis only in high-risk environments.[7] Postoperative superficial skin infections are often managed conservatively with administration of antibiotics or opening of incisions with fluctuance or drainage. If initial conservative treatment is unsuccessful, one must consider the presence of a deep infection, which could involve mesh. In those cases, surgical exploration with debridement may be indicated.

Mesh Infection

Mesh infection is a devastating complication that is estimated to occur in 1% to 4% of abdominal hernia repairs. Mesh infections present with indolent symptoms and clinical findings such as swelling, pain, draining sinus tracts, or masses. They often present without obvious inflammation of surrounding skin. The diagnosis is usually based on clinical presentation; however, imaging such as US and CT scans can aid in the diagnosis.

With inguinal mesh infection, surgical removal is almost always warranted. Before surgical removal, conservative treatment such as local wound care can be trialed. Subsequent mesh removal can be completed at least 3 months after onset of symptoms. The additional time allows the unaffected part of the mesh to become further incorporated into the surrounding tissue. Meanwhile, the infected part of the mesh separates secondary to the purulent exudate, allowing for easier mesh removal. Typically, the mesh is removed with the same surgical technique that was used for placement, such that TAPP or

TEP hernia repairs have mesh removed laparoscopically. However, if an open repair is complicated by peritoneum penetration or presence of a sinus, then surgeons may consider a laparoscopic approach to visualize the abdominal cavity. Studies suggest that complete removal of mesh results in less infection recurrence compared with partial mesh removal.[21] After explantation of the infected mesh, replacement with another synthetic mesh in the setting of infection is contraindicated. Hernia recurrence after removal of an infected mesh is not common because there is typically an inflammatory reaction that provides strength for the repair.

Postoperative Urinary Retention

Postoperative urinary retention (POUR) has a highly variable incidence of 0.4% to 41.6%. A recent large international multicenter prospective cohort study was developed to identify related risk factors. In the study's cohort of 4151 adults across 32 countries, the incidence was 5.8% in males, 3.0% in females, and 9.5% of male patients ≥65 years old.[22] The study found multiple risk factors, several of which are modifiable, including anticholinergic medication, history of prior urinary retention, constipation, involvement of bladder within hernia, temporary intraoperative urethral catheterization, longer operative times, and increasing age. Treatment for POUR is conservative. Most patients are managed with indwelling ureteral catheterization. Less commonly, patients undergo intermittent catheterization or, in even rarer circumstances, suprapubic catheterization. Of 30-day readmissions in the RETAINER I trial, 51.8% were a result of POUR, accounting for the majority of cases. Unplanned admissions and readmissions from POUR still occurred relatively infrequently, occurring in 1% to 3% of patients. Between 12% and 27% of patients admitted were discharged with indwelling catheters. By 30-day follow-up, most (65%) had successfully passed a void trial and no longer required catheterization. Results of this study suggest that POUR is not an uncommon complication and that although most patients can spontaneously void by 30 days postoperatively, many required catheterization, which can be uncomfortable and traumatic.

Additional studies have compared neuromuscular blockade agents and association with POUR. The use of the newer cyclodextrin agent sugammadex relative to the traditional anticholinesterase group was associated with reduced 30-day POUR by 66% overall. This was also significant in subsets of groups, including open, MI, unilateral, and bilateral repairs.[23] Additionally, research has shown an independent association between perioperative administration of dexamethasone and decreased urinary retention.[24]

Hernia Recurrences

Inguinal hernia recurrences are estimated to occur in 5% to 10% of patients. Mesh repairs are the standard of care in most cases and have been found to substantially reduce recurrence by 60%. Risks for recurrence include any condition that results in chronically elevated intraabdominal pressure (e.g., chronic cough, ascites, benign prostatic hyperplasia) or impairs wound healing, such as connective tissue disorders, tobacco use, and infection. There is also a higher frequency of recurrences with recurrent hernia repairs. Additionally, recurrence is seen more often after repair of direct hernias rather than indirect hernias that originate at the deep ring. If a recurrence occurs, the typical approach for repair of the recurrence is usually from the opposite side of the index procedure to prevent operating in the failed surgical plane. If an anterior repair, such as the Lichtenstein repair, fails, an MI posterior approach is typically used. Similarly, if a posterior repair fails, an anterior repair is recommended.[25]

Chronic Groin Pain

Chronic pain is estimated to affect approximately 10% of patients after IHRs and is defined as postoperative pain lasting over 3 months. Of these patients, 2% to 4% report pain that interferes with daily activity.[26] With mild symptoms, patients suffer a decrease in quality of life, whereas those with more severe symptoms may have an impaired ability to work or suffer from psychological conditions such as depression. Some have suggested that a waiting period of 3 months after hernia surgery is appropriate before making the diagnosis of chronic pain. This time frame is appropriate, except in the setting of severe new-onset postoperative pain that was not present before the hernia repair. This presentation suggests nerve entrapment, and prompt surgical reexploration should be performed to identify and treat the source of pain.

There is a wide array of causes of chronic pain after IHR, which will be discussed later in this chapter. The workup of chronic pain is very important, and patients should be referred to experts who are experienced in treating postoperative chronic pain. The ilioinguinal nerve, which provides sensation to skin of the groin, inner thigh, upper part of the scrotum, and root of the penis, has been implicated as a contributor to postoperative pain. This nerve is typically at risk of injury during open repairs because it is not exposed during MI posterior repairs, such as branches of the GF and lateral femoral cutaneous nerves. Although there have been studies advocating prophylactic ilioinguinal neurectomy, it is our practice to preserve this nerve if possible.[27,28] It is advised against dissecting these nerves from their muscular beds or placing them behind retractors to maintain the surgical field. Maneuvers such as these increase the chance of nerve injury. However, most experts agree that the ilioinguinal nerve and/or the iliohypogastric nerve should be resected if they are injured or interfere with mesh positioning, given the risk of nerve entrapment.[25]

Chronic pain has also been associated with penetrating mesh fixation. An RCT from 2023 compared mesh fixation with tacks versus no fixation and found similar recurrence rates with less acute and chronic pain without fixation.[29] Other independent risk factors for chronic postoperative pain include bilateral IHR, preoperative pain, preoperative anxiety, and relatively high intensity of acute pain for 1 week postoperatively.[30] For MI posterior approaches, the nerves at risk of injury are the lateral femoral cutaneous and both the genital and femoral branches of the GF nerve. Aggressive dissection and mesh fixation should be avoided below the IPT to avoid injury to these nerves. Chronic pain after IHR is initially managed conservatively with nonsteroidal antiinflammatory medications and analgesics. Local nerve blocks can also be pursued and, if successful, suggest that the patient may benefit from surgical exploration with neurectomy or mesh removal if the patient's pain recurs once the block wears off. The workup and treatment of chronic pain patients can be very time consuming and stressful for both the patient and the surgeon, highlighting the importance of multidisciplinary management.

SPECIAL CONSIDERATIONS

Sliding Hernias

A sliding hernia is one in which a retroperitoneal organ "slides" down posteriorly and herniates because it is part of the hernia sac. A recent study of the National Danish Hernia Database estimated the incidence of sliding hernias to be 13.5%. The risk of sliding inguinal hernias increases with age. Common involved organs include the cecum, ascending colon, appendix on the right side, and sigmoid colon on the left side. These hernias may also involve the uterus, fallopian tubes, ovaries, ureters, and bladder on either side. If a sliding hernia is present, the repair must be modified such that the hernia sac is opened with care not to injure the involved organ. Intraperitoneal structures should then be identified and reduced. Redundant sac management will differ depending on the chosen technique, either open or laparoscopic. In open repairs, the excess sac should be excised and the peritoneal defect closed. In laparoscopic repair, after complete reduction of contents, the excess sac should be separated from the spermatic cord and is often reduced. If the wall of the sac appears thick, care should be taken to confirm this is not, in fact, the wall of a retroperitoneal organ itself that is involved in the hernia. The presence of a sliding hernia likely does not result in a higher risk of postoperative complications, although there are few studies that report increased seroma, hematoma, and urinary retention. In terms of recurrence, there is a higher risk of recurrence, especially after open Lichtenstein repairs.[31]

Scrotal Hernias/Loss of Domain

Giant inguinal hernias, or "scrotal abdomen," are classified as those that extend past the midpoint of the inner thigh in the standing position. They are uncommon and develop in those who neglect their symptoms or do not have access to surgical services. Risk factors for massive scrotal hernias are similar to those for recurrence, including conditions that increase intraabdominal pressure or impair wound healing. In cases of large scrotal hernias or loss of domain, open repairs are typically preferred. Preoperatively, efforts should be made to decrease the bulk of contents in the hernia sac by altering the patient's diet to reduce intraluminal intestinal contents or by intraoperatively completing simultaneous intestinal resection. Repair of these large hernias can be morbid secondary to the rise in intraabdominal pressure that reduction causes, thereby decreasing diaphragmatic compliance. This postoperative rise in pressure can result in respiratory failure, pneumonia, wound dehiscence, or hernia recurrence. As a result, careful preoperative patient selection should be performed, including those with adequate pulmonary function. Adjuncts that can assist in decreasing intraabdominal pressure include Botox and progressive pneumoperitoneum.

INGUINODYNIA (GROIN PAIN) AS A CHIEF COMPLAINT

Workup

When investigating the source of chronic groin pain, a comprehensive history, physical exam, and review of prior radiographic studies must be performed. The SPORT acronym developed by the International Hernia Collaboration is a helpful framework for pursuing a thorough workup in these patients (Box 82.1).

When providing pain history, the patient should provide details such as the onset of the pain, quality of pain, radiation

patterns, and prior trials of medical therapies. If operative reports are available, it is helpful to note the type of mesh and which nerves, if any, were identified. It is important to investigate whether there were any complications intraoperatively or perioperatively. To document the starting event, the full pain history must include the following:

- Where is it located, exactly?
- When did it start (how, why)?
- Constant or intermittent?
- What makes it worse or better (medications/injections)?
- Does it radiate, and if so, to where?
- Severity (vas score 1–10)
- Mental health history (posttraumatic stress disorder [PTSD], depression, anxiety, etc.)

The differential diagnosis of chronic groin pain is vast:

- Mesh, meshoma, sutures, or tacks
- Trapped nerve (iatrogenic or anterior cutaneous nerve entrapment syndrome [ACNES]), with or without fascial tear
- Hernias (direct, femoral, obturator, or indirect), which includes occult (hidden) and recurrent hernias (lump not required)
- Lipoma (usually retained cord lipomas)
- Endometrioma, round ligament pain
- Osteitis, rectus sheath tear, aponeurotic plate avulsion, adductor tear, other
- Intraabdominal pathology (e.g., adhesions or appendicitis)
- Back/spine (sacroiliac joint dysfunction or thoracolumbar syndrome)
- Hip joint (femoral-acetabular impingement or labral tear)
- "Psychosomatic," "pain-body," or other previous unprocessed trauma or mental health conditions (conscious or unconscious)

A distinction also needs to be made between neuropathic and nociceptive pain. Pain mapping in the office can aid in this differentiation. The physician can simply mark a "+" along all the areas where the patient endorses pain and a "0" where there is none. Typically, a large area aligns with neuropathic pain, whereas a narrow area is more indicative of nociceptive pain (Figs. 82.18 and 82.19).

Relevant radiographic studies include dynamic sonograms, CT scans with radiopaque markers, MRI with radiopaque markers, and diagnostic laparoscopy. Dynamic sonograms are completed with the US probe placed at the point of pain with the patient

BOX 82.1	**SPORT Acronym for Groin Pain Assessment**
S	Starting event
P	Pain description and mapping with photos
O	Objective exam (back, hip, etc.)
R	Radiology (ultrasound, x-ray, CT or MRI with marking)
T	Treatment intervention

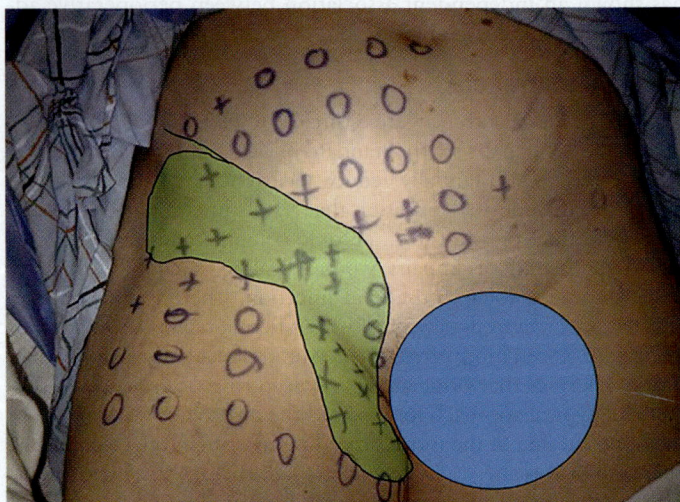

FIGURE 82.18 Pain mapping (neuropathic).

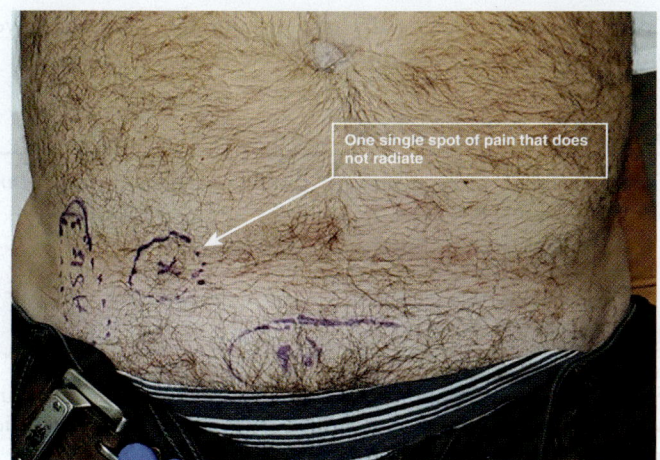

One single spot of pain that does not radiate

FIGURE 82.19 Pain mapping (nociceptive).

standing still and performing the Valsalva maneuver. These tests are relatively inexpensive and can effectively evaluate for a hernia or recurrence but depend on a good technician and experienced interpreter. Some hernias can be missed in inexperienced hands. If US is proven to be nondiagnostic, CT or MRI with a radiopaque marker at the point of pain are the next imaging modalities of choice.

Treatment

The treatment of inguinodynia, much like the treatment of other forms of chronic pain, is generally approached in a stepwise and tailored fashion. Noninvasive techniques such as rest, ice and heat, and over-the-counter antiinflammatory medication can provide relief to many patients, especially those with a clear inciting event for their pain, such as a sports injury or recent surgery. Certainly, a referral to a pain specialist to aid in the nonoperative workup and treatment is always helpful.

If conservative therapy does not manage the patient's pain, more aggressive pain management techniques are available. Patients with neuropathic pain may benefit from gamma-aminobutyric acid (GABA) modulators such as gabapentin. However, it is important to avoid prescribing narcotic pain medications before other methods have been exhausted. Inguinal or other nerve blocks administered by a surgeon or an interventional pain specialist can provide relief, but patients may need repeated nerve blocks to maintain pain control. If patients respond to the block but require repeated interventions, a surgical neurectomy may offer benefit. Adjunctive treatment options such as physical therapy and massage are available for patients who have a sports-related injury or other musculoskeletal complaint.

The surgical treatment for chronic pain will depend on the history and the etiology of pain, and sometimes multiple surgical interventions may be necessary. Despite surgical intervention, the pain-free success rate will approach around 70%, with the remaining 30% having some level of persistent chronic pain or discomfort.

Surgical Evaluation and Mesh Explantation

Surgical diagnosis and therapy with diagnostic laparoscopy can be helpful in patients who have failed nonsurgical management, particularly those who have a history of surgery associated with the onset of their groin pain. Laparoscopy can identify adhesions, recurrent or occult hernias, and issues with mesh placement or

fixation that may be contributing to a patient's pain. It is helpful to perform pain mapping preoperatively and postoperatively to assess the patient's response to the intervention.

During the procedure, the preperitoneal space can be explored to evaluate the cord structures and nerves that may be injured or inflamed. The triple neurectomy, performed through an open approach and targeting the ilioinguinal, iliohypogastric, and GF nerves, has proven to be one of the most effective options for patients with persistent postoperative neuropathic groin pain. If a hernia is present, the goal of the operation is to provide a durable hernia repair. If there is no hernia, the goal is to eliminate any adhesions from the groin and clear the groin of all foreign materials, which may include mesh and its fixation materials, thereby freeing up the cord structures and nerves.

If prior mesh is thought to be the source of pain, the approach in which the mesh was previously implanted (e.g., open anterior approach) should be used to remove it. Although mesh explantation alone or with neurectomy can provide improvement in foreign body sensation and neuropathic pain, approximately a third of patients will not have resolution of their symptoms. Thus, although mesh removal is a viable surgical option, it is not always the cure for chronic pain after a hernia repair.

Referral to a cognitive or behavioral therapist may provide benefit in some patients with chronic pain. Mental health can play a role in the onset of pain, and mental health issues can develop during the months or years of patients experiencing pain without being able to obtain an accurate diagnosis. In these situations, some patients may feel neglected. Posttraumatic stress, anxiety, depression, and suicidal ideation have been reported during the workup of chronic pain. It is important to determine if there are ongoing mental health issues or ruminations during the evaluation and treatment of chronic pain patients, and findings should be well documented.

Sports Hernias and Athletic Pubalgia

A sports hernia, otherwise known as *athletic pubalgia,* is a groin pain syndrome that typically involves the deep muscular layers of the abdominal wall and tendons as they interact with the bony pelvis and inguinal ligament. It typically affects athletes, especially those participating in high-impact sports (e.g., ice hockey, rugby, soccer, American football) that put strain on musculotendinous structures of the inguinal region. The pubic tubercle is the site of insertion of the rectus abdominis, the conjoint tendon, the pubic symphysis, the adductor longus, and the inguinal ligament. The characteristic sports hernia pain typically exists around the pubic tubercle and may extend to or be more significant at the point of insertion of the adductor longus tendon on the pubic bone or above the insertion point of the rectus abdominis. Pain can also be at the inguinal ligament or directly at the pubic symphysis. Symptoms typically worsen with sprinting or lateral or twisting movements. Unlike typical groin hernias, sports hernias do not present with a bulge.

On physical exam, there is usually point tenderness of the external ring, which may also be dilated. The patient may also have point tenderness present at the pubic tubercle where the conjoint tendon meets. Another helpful physical exam maneuver involves putting the patient in a "frog leg" position (supine, knees bent, heels touching) to assess for pain with forced adduction against the examiner. It is important to distinguish this pathology from an adductor muscle injury because muscle injury alone is best managed with physical therapy. MRI is the diagnostic imaging study of choice to help differentiate sports hernia pain from hip joint–specific pathology. It may be used to diagnose inflammation of one or both tendons of the rectus abdominis or adductor longus muscle near their insertion sites. In severe cases, these tendons may also be avulsed and cause fracture of the pubic bone. MRI may also show bone marrow edema within the pubic bone that results from chronic strain at the tendon insertion sites. US with Valsalva is helpful to assess the inguinal canal and rule out inguinal hernias.

Initial management for sports hernias is conservative and includes applying ice packs, typically for around 10 minutes three to four times per day, administration of nonsteroidal antiinflammatory medications, rest, and subsequent rehabilitation once symptoms subside. Surgical treatment often follows when initial conservative management fails. The aim of surgical intervention is to reduce tension and torque on the pubic joint and decompress the inguinal sensory nerves. This is often performed with suture or mesh reinforcement. Studies have demonstrated that physical therapy has overall similar outcomes to surgery; however, these patients are often athletes eager to return to their sports and are not willing to wait.[32] The standard repair is a laparoscopic preperitoneal or open anterior repair with synthetic mesh. The open technique has the advantage of better identifying specific abnormalities responsible for pain and more precise anatomy given exposure. The outcomes for laparoscopic and open approaches were similar in prior RCTs; however, patients had less pain in the first month and sooner return to activity after laparoscopic compared with open repairs.[33] Similar to IHRs, these MI repairs can be performed via a TAPP or TEP approach.

An open repair begins with an incision slightly more caudal than in typical open IHRs to allow visualization of insertion points of the lower rectus and adductor longus tendons on pubic bone. From this point, there are various repair techniques that can be used to recognize anatomy and help correct weaknesses in the inguinal floor. These can be performed with or without mesh. Mesh can decrease tension on repair; however, it can result in mesh infection or related pain. These repairs can also be performed at the same time as adductor longus tenotomy, which results in a change in the pulling vector on the pubic bone. The goal of an adductor longus tenotomy is to relieve pressure on the adductor compartment and potentially decompress the obturator nerve. Overall, surgical treatment via laparoscopic and open repairs is successful in the short term, and most athletes can return to sports within 3 months.[33]

Complications from repairs are uncommon. Postoperative physical therapy is recommended.

SELECTED REFERENCES

Daes J, Felix E. Critical view of the myopectineal orifice. *Ann Surg*. 2017;266(1):e1-e2.

> *Drs. Daes and Felix describe the widely adopted critical view of the myopectineal orifice for minimally invasive inguinal hernia repair.*

Fitzgibbons RJ Jr, Giobbie-Hurder A, Gibbs JO, et al. Watchful waiting vs repair of inguinal hernia in minimally symptomatic men: a randomized clinical trial. *JAMA*. 2006;295(3):285-292.

> *This is a large RCT that demonstrated safety of watchful waiting versus surgical repair in minimally symptomatic males. It also demonstrated that the majority of individuals with minimally symptomatic hernias went on to have surgical repair.*

HerniaSurge Group. International guidelines for groin hernia management. *Hernia*. 2018;22(1):1-165. doi:10.1007/s10029-017-1668-x

> *This work demonstrates guidelines for groin hernia management that are endorsed by five continental hernia societies.*

Lichtenstein IL, Shulman AG, Amid PK, Montllor MM. The tension-free hernioplasty. *Am J Surg*. 1989;157(2):188-193.

> *This is a description of the tension-free hernioplasty with onlay mesh.*

Zuckerbraun BS, Cyr AR, Mauro CS. Groin pain syndrome known as sports hernia: a review. *JAMA Surg*. 2020;155(4):340-348.

> *This work is a review of sports hernias and their clinical presentation, workup, and management.*

The full reference list appears on Elsevier eBooks+.

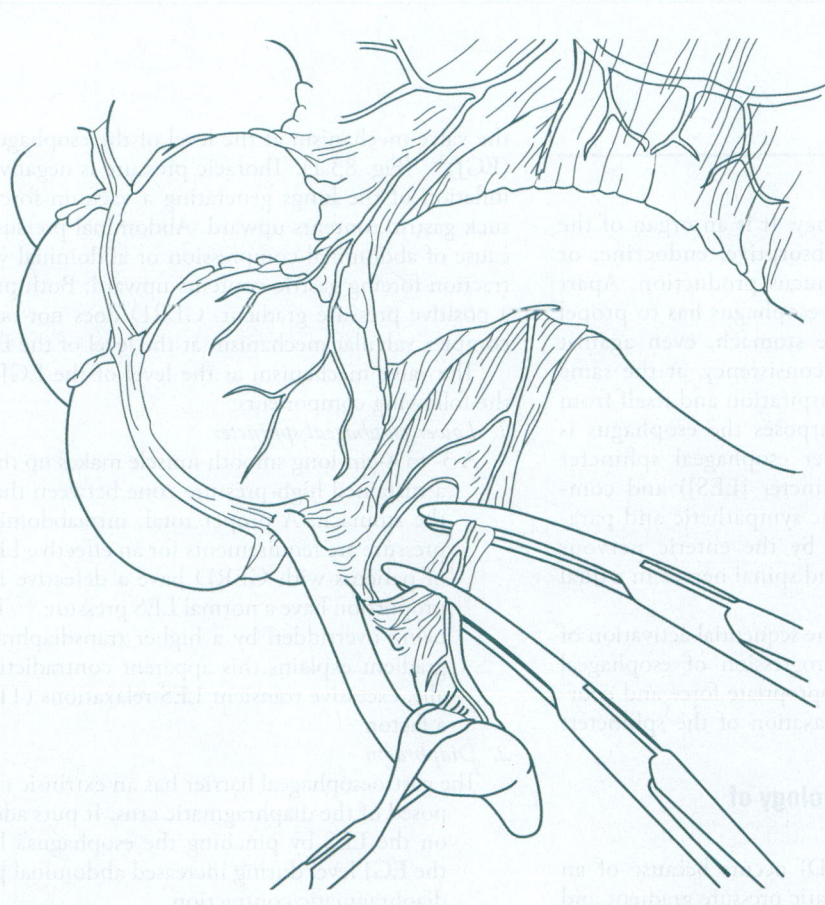

83 CHAPTER

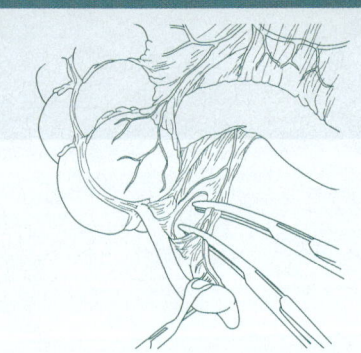

Benign Esophageal Disorders

Marco G. Patti, Fernando A. Herbella, Karan Chhabra, and Matthew M. Hutter

ESOPHAGEAL PHYSIOLOGY

Swallowing

The esophagus has a peculiar physiology. It is an organ of the digestive system without digestive, absorptive, endocrine, or exocrine functions and neglectable mucus production. Apart from peculiar, it is also complex. The esophagus has to propel food down from the pharynx to the stomach, even against gravity and irrespective of the bolus consistency, at the same time that it protects the airway from aspiration and itself from gastroesophageal reflux. For these purposes the esophagus is limited by two sphincters (the upper esophageal sphincter [UES] and the lower esophageal sphincter [LES]) and complexly innervated centrally by extrinsic sympathetic and parasympathetic nerves and peripherally by the enteric nervous system mediated by the vagus nerve and spinal nerves in a dual innervation.[1]

Peristaltic contraction results from the sequential activation of motor units innervating an aboral progression of esophageal muscle segments.[2] This will generate appropriate force and coordination for peristalsis. Opportune relaxation of the sphincters also occurs.

Antireflux Mechanism: Pathophysiology of Gastroesophageal Reflux Disease

Gastroesophageal reflux disease (GERD) occurs because of an imbalance between the transdiaphragmatic pressure gradient and the valve mechanism at the level of the esophagogastric junction (EGJ)[3–5] (Fig. 83.1). Thoracic pressure is negative because of the inflation of the lungs generating a vacuum force. This tends to suck gastric contents upward. Abdominal pressure is positive because of abdominal compression or abdominal wall muscle contraction forcing gastric contents upward. Both pressures generate a positive pressure gradient. GERD does not occur thanks to a complex valvular mechanism at the level of the EGJ.

The valve mechanism at the level of the EGJ is composed of the following components:

1. *Lower esophageal sphincter*

   A 3- to 4-cm-long smooth muscle makes up the LES. It creates a sustained high-pressure zone between the esophagus and the stomach. A proper total, intraabdominal, and resting pressure are requirements for an effective LES. The majority of patients with GERD have a defective LES, but a large proportion have a normal LES pressure.[6,7] The LES pressure being overridden by a higher transdiaphragmatic pressure gradient explains this apparent contradiction.[8,9] Additionally, excessive transient LES relaxations (TLESRs) could be a factor.

2. *Diaphragm*

   The gastroesophageal barrier has an extrinsic component composed of the diaphragmatic crus. It puts additional pressure on the LES by pinching the esophagus's lower portion at the EGJ level during increased abdominal pressure through diaphragmatic contraction.

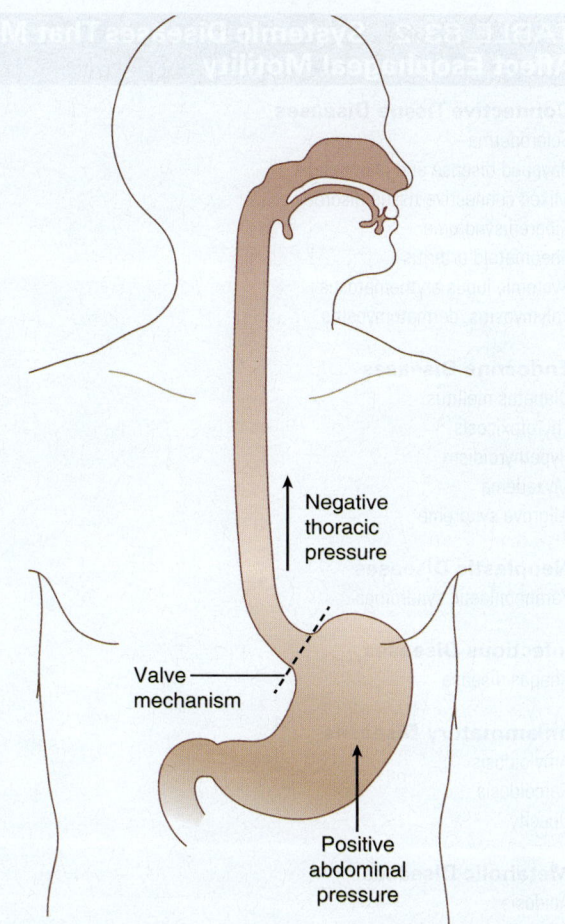

FIGURE 83.1 Gastroesophageal reflux disease pathophysiology is based on a balance between the transdiaphragmatic pressure gradient and the valve mechanism at the level of the esophagogastric junction.

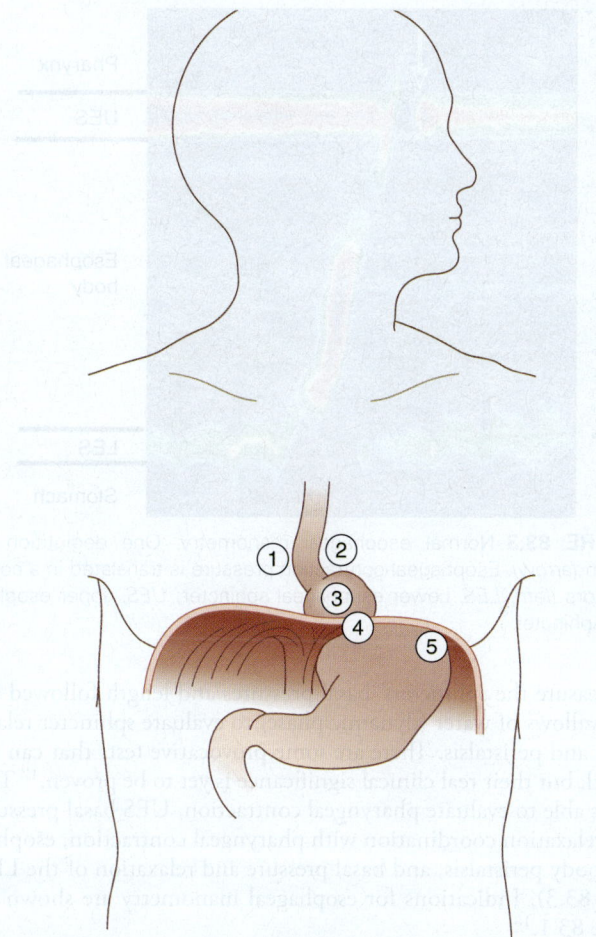

FIGURE 83.2 Disruption of natural antireflux mechanisms by a hiatal hernia. (1) Absence of intraabdominal esophagus length; (2) obtuseness of the angle of His; (3) lower esophageal sphincter in a negative pressure environment; (4) pressurization of the herniated stomach; (5) diaphragm does not pinch the lower esophageal sphincter.

3. *Angle of His*

The angle of His refers to the acute angle created by the esophagus and gastric fundus. The distance between the gastric fundus, where food is stored, and the EGJ increases with increasing angle, acting as a barrier to the rise of the refluxate.[10,11]

4. *Gubaroff valve*

Gubaroff valves consist of a thickening of the esophageal mucosa at the EGJ acting as a cushion keeping the area closed.[3]

5. *Intraabdominal portion of the esophagus*

Because the abdominal pressure has the effect of collapsing the esophageal wall, the presence of an intraabdominal portion of the esophagus contributes to the valve mechanism.[12]

GERD will occur in the following scenarios when there is an imbalance between the transdiaphragmatic pressure gradient and the valve mechanism.

1. *Increased abdominal pressure*

The clinical scenario where there is an increased abdominal pressure leading to GERD is in the setting of obesity, especially in males and females with central (opposed to peripheral) fat distribution.[13] It may occur also during pregnancy, in athletes with excessive abdominal training, and other situations.

2. *Decreased thoracic pressure*

Decreased thoracic pressure related to an increased respiratory effort and consequently more negative thoracic pressure

may occur in patients with obstructive pulmonary diseases or even professional glass blowers or singers.[14,15]

3. *Defective valve*

Hiatal hernias are the most common reason for a defective EGJ valve because they disrupt most of the natural antireflux mechanisms. There is a lack of intraabdominal esophageal length that is now in the mediastinal position, obtuseness of the angle of His shortening the path from the gastric fundus to the esophagus, pressurization of the herniated gastric pouch, enlargement of the hiatus, and the fact that the diaphragm pinches the stomach rather than the esophagus. TLESR is also more frequent in patients with hiatal hernias[16] (Fig. 83.2).

ESOPHAGEAL FUNCTION TESTS

Esophageal Manometry

Esophageal manometry is performed through a transnasal catheter that is positioned with the tip in the stomach. The test is done after fasting, and sedation is not possible because the patient's collaboration is necessary, and esophageal function may be compromised by the action of the drugs. Drugs that may affect motility must be stopped opportunely. The test consists of a static phase

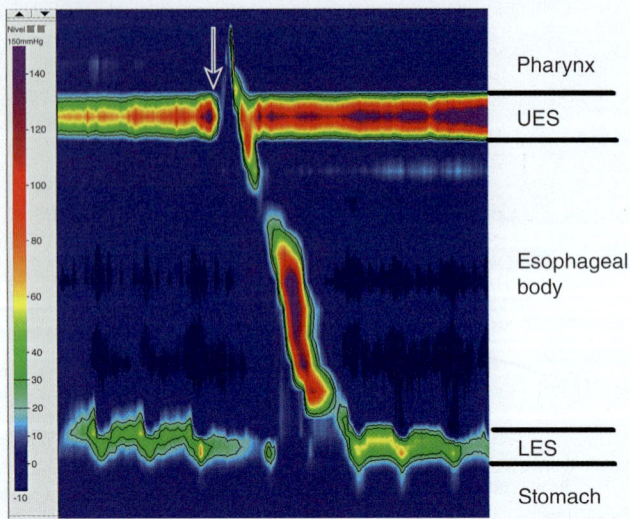

Pharynx

UES

Esophageal body

LES

Stomach

FIGURE 83.3 Normal esophageal manometry. One deglutition is shown *(arrow).* Esophageal contraction pressure is translated in a code of colors *(left). LES,* Lower esophageal sphincter; *UES,* upper esophageal sphincter.

to measure the sphincters' basal pressures and length followed by 10 swallows of water (dynamic phase) to evaluate sphincter relaxation and peristalsis. There are some provocative tests that can be added, but their real clinical significance is yet to be proven.[17] The test is able to evaluate pharyngeal contraction, UES basal pressure and relaxation coordination with pharyngeal contraction, esophageal body peristalsis, and basal pressure and relaxation of the LES (Fig. 83.3). Indications for esophageal manometry are shown in Table 83.1.[18]

The LES must be located using esophageal manometry in order to accurately determine the position of the pH monitoring catheter because other approaches are inaccurate. Esophageal manometry is useful to diagnose primary esophageal motility disorders (PEMDs) or the esophagus' involvement in systemic diseases (Table 83.2),[19,20] such as in patients with dysphagia or connective tissue diseases. Before esophageal operations at the EGJ, it is particularly crucial. Some believe that esophageal manometry findings may guide the type of antireflux operation, but it provides, nonetheless, a baseline comparison in case of unsuccessful outcomes. It may also classify achalasia according to the Chicago classification. It must be kept in mind that esophageal manometry cannot diagnose GERD. A normal LES does not rule out GERD because an abnormal transdiaphragmatic pressure gradient may overcome it, and an abnormal LES is not synonymous with GERD because other natural antireflux mechanisms may compensate for it. (see Table 83.2). Esophageal manometry interpretation is currently mostly guided by the Chicago classification.[21]

TABLE 83.1   Indications for Esophageal Manometry

- pH monitoring beforehand to determine the position of the catheter
- Evaluation of dysphagia
- Diagnosis of primary esophageal motility disorders
- Diagnosis of esophageal involvement in systemic diseases
- Determination of esophageal motility before antireflux surgery
- Evaluation of symptomatic patients after esophageal surgery

---

TABLE 83.2   Systemic Diseases That May Affect Esophageal Motility

Connective Tissue Diseases
Scleroderma
Raynaud disease and phenomena
Mixed connective tissue disorder
Sjögren syndrome
Rheumatoid arthritis
Systemic lupus erythematosus
Polymyositis, dermatomyositis

Endocrine Diseases
Diabetes mellitus
Thyrotoxicosis
Hypothyroidism
Myxedema
Allgrove syndrome

Neoplastic Diseases
Paraneoplastic syndromes

Infectious Diseases
Chagas disease

Inflammatory Diseases
Amyloidosis
Sarcoidosis
Obesity

Metabolic Diseases
Acidosis
Alkalosis
Electrolyte abnormalities
Hypomagnesemia

Drug Usage
Alcohol
Opioids
Calcium channel blockers
Vasodilators
Anticholinergics
Anxiolytics
Tricyclic antidepressants
Acetylcholine release inhibitors
PD5-inhibitors
Antiparasitic agents

PD5-inhibitors, Phosphodiesterase type 5 inhibitors.

Lower Esophageal Sphincter and Esophagogastric Junction

Esophageal manometry is able to measure LES basal (resting) pressure. It will also define a hypotensive or normal LES. LES length can also be measured. Shorter LES total length and intraabdominal length also make the LES effective. Relaxation (residual) pressure is measured by the integrated relaxation pressure (IRP)—the 4 seconds of lowest pressure in a 10-second measurement even if not consecutive. This will define a nonrelaxing LES.

Manometry can determine if there is a disjunction of the LES and diaphragm pressures (manometric hiatal hernia) (Fig. 83.4). In type I, diaphragmatic pressure and LES pressure components are coincident. In types II and III, there is a progressive separation of the components.

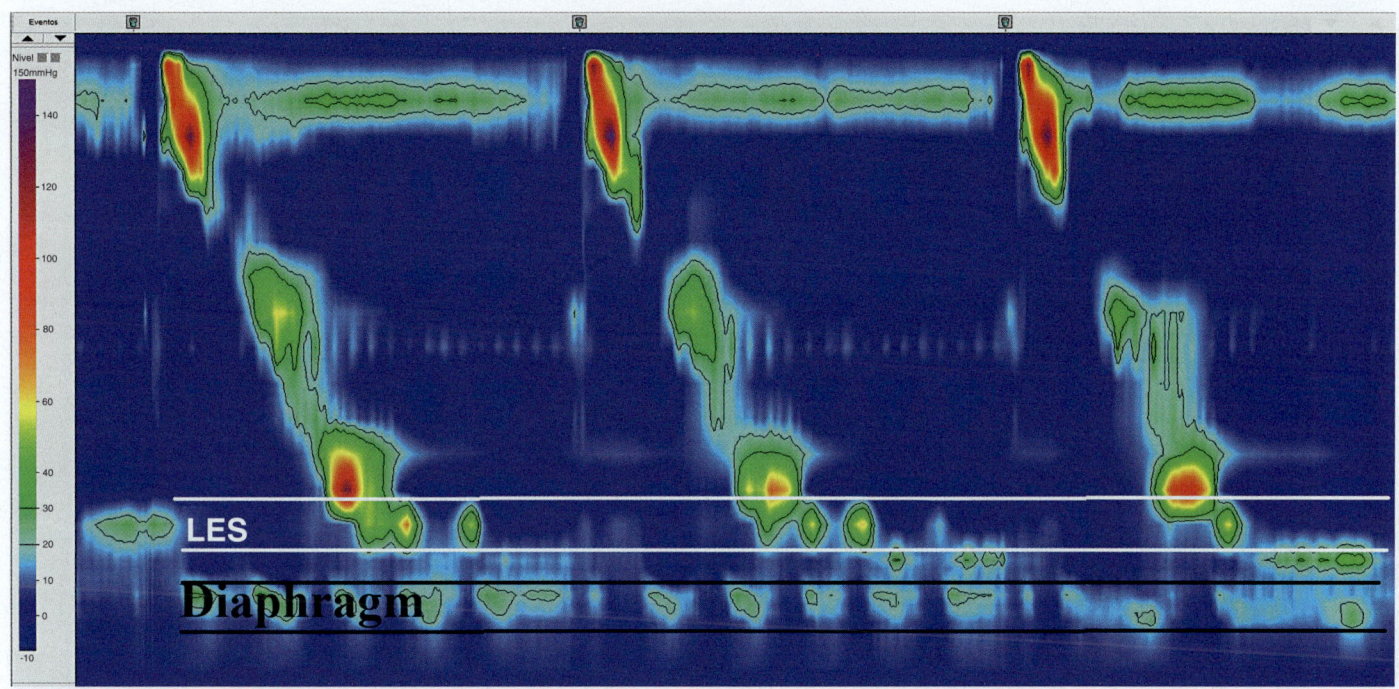

FIGURE 83.4 Esophagogastric junction type III by esophageal manometry. Note the separation of the lower esophageal sphincter *(LES)* pressure from the diaphragm.

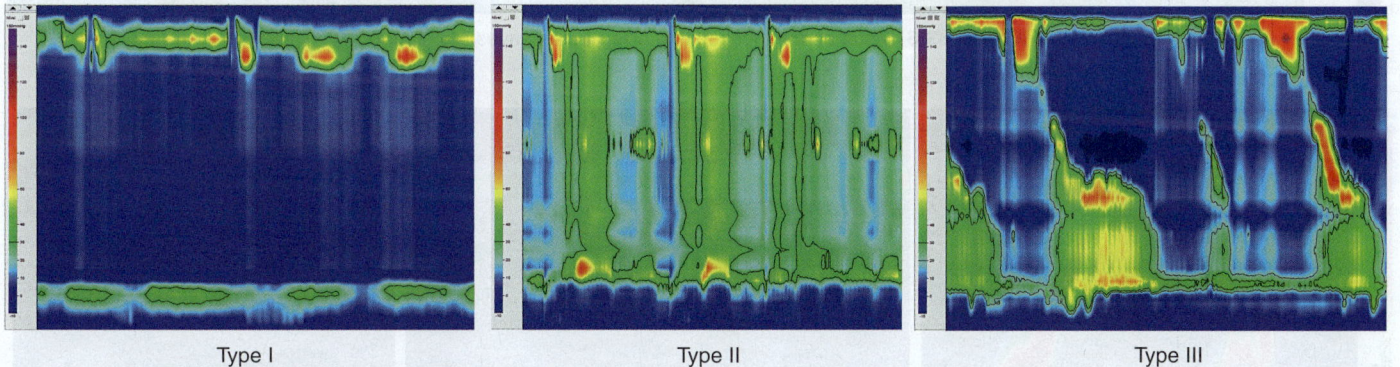

| Type I | Type II | Type III |

FIGURE 83.5 Achalasia types according to the Chicago classification.

Motility disorders associated with an abnormal LES relaxation are **achalasia** (in the absence of peristalsis) and **esophagogastric outflow obstruction** (in the presence of peristalsis). Achalasia is categorized into three groups according to esophageal pressurization[22,23] (Fig. 83.5):

Type I: incomplete LES relaxation, aperistalsis, and absence of esophageal pressurization

Type II: incomplete LES relaxation, aperistalsis, and panesophageal pressurization in at least 20% of swallows

Type III: incomplete LES relaxation, aperistalsis, and spastic contractions in at least 20% of swallows

Esophageal Body

When there is sufficient esophageal muscle force and coordination to push the bolus down to the stomach, esophageal body motility is normal.

An abnormal esophageal body characterizes the majority of motility disorders linked to GERD that can only be classified as primary disorders in the absence of GERD. The motility abnormality is regarded as secondary if GERD is present, and reflux should be the focus of treatment.

The distal latency (DL), which is measured as the period of time between the start of UES relaxation and the change from the esophageal body to the epiphrenic ampulla, is what determines coordination. Waves can be normal or premature. The disease of the lack of coordination is the distal esophageal spasm, defined as at least 20% of premature contractions with normal contractile vigor (Fig. 83.6). Symptoms of dysphagia or chest pain are necessary for a clinically significant diagnosis.[21]

The distal contractility integral (DCI), which is calculated as the product of the mean amplitude of contraction in the distal esophagus (mm Hg) times the contraction's duration(s) times the length of the distal esophageal segment (cm), determines force (contraction vigor). Depending on the DCI, waves can be failed, weak, normal, or hypercontractile.

The manometric disease defined by hypercontractile peristalsis is the **hypercontractile esophagus** (HE, previously nutcracker and jackhammer), defined by excessive contraction vigor in at

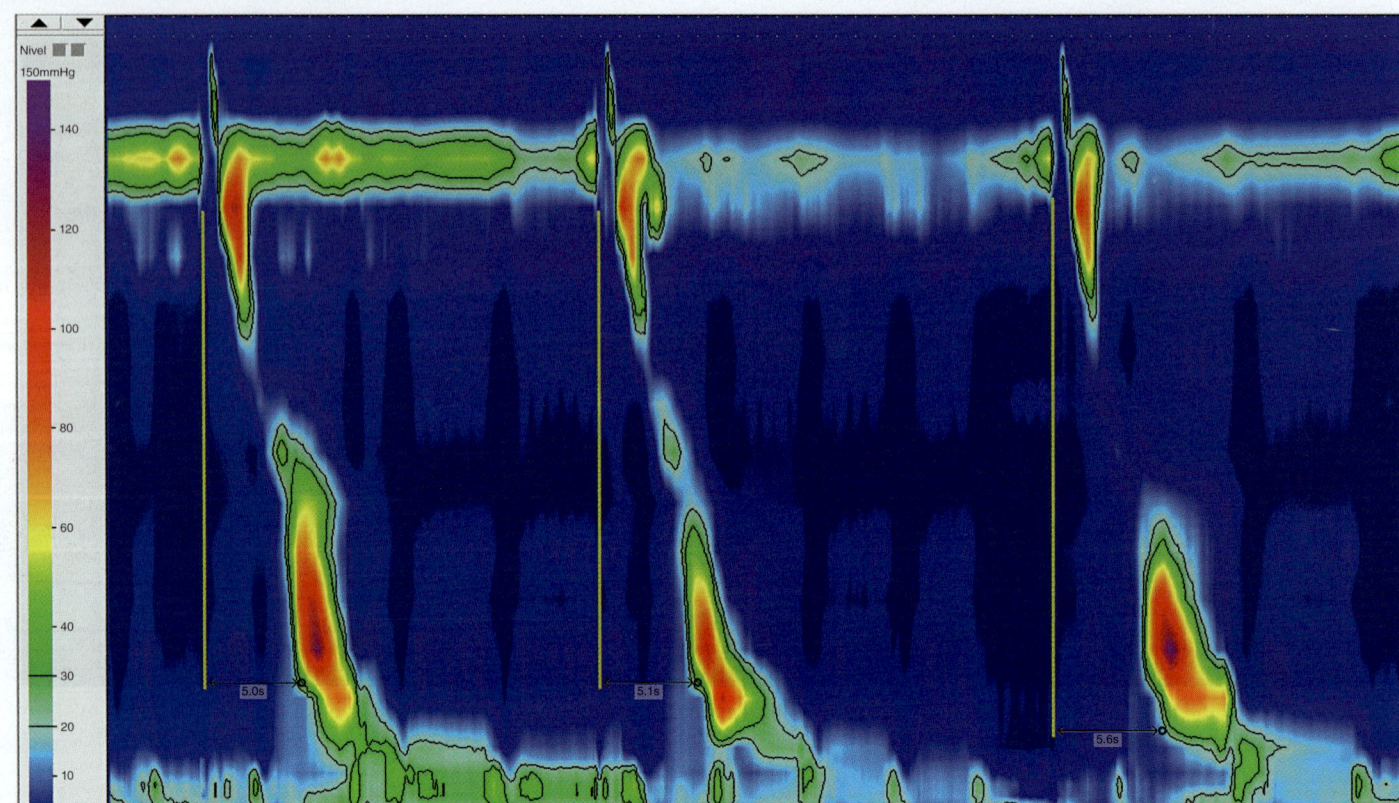

FIGURE 83.6 Distal esophageal spasm. Premature waves are shown.

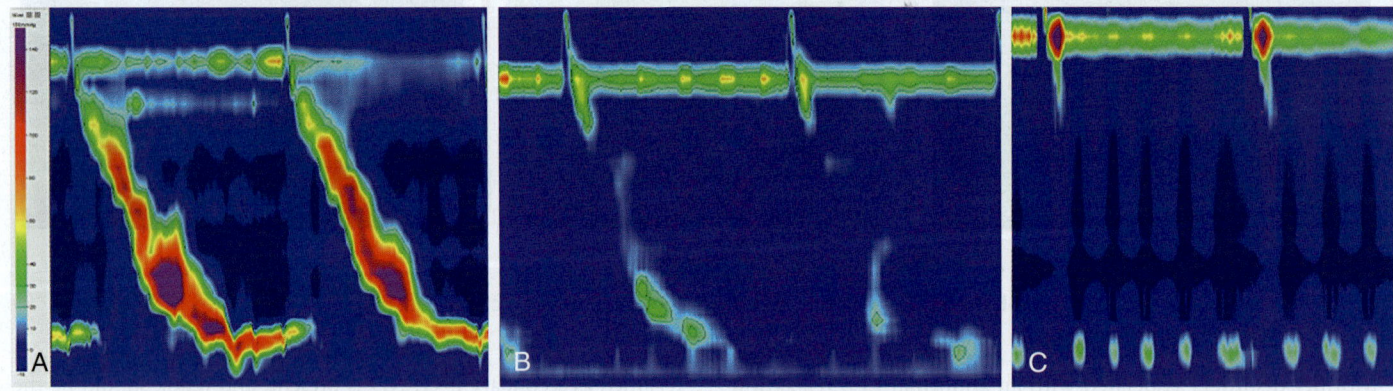

FIGURE 83.7 Diseases of the contraction vigor. Hypercontractile esophagus (A), ineffective esophageal motility (B), and absent contractility (C).

least 20 of the swallows. Similar to distal esophageal spams, the presence of symptoms is mandatory to distinguish between clinically relevant disease and clinically irrelevant manometric observations.[21]

The manometric disease defined by hypocontractile peristalsis is the **ineffective esophageal motility,** defined by presence of ≥70% ineffective swallows or ≥50% failed waves, and the **absent contractility,** defined by 100% failed peristalsis[21] (Fig. 83.7).

Upper Esophageal Sphincter

Because of technical limitations of manometry equipment, incomplete understanding of the anatomophysiology of the pharyngo-upper esophageal area,[24,25] and exclusion of the UES from the current guidelines, manometric evaluation of the UES has

been neglected, with only a few studies evaluating patients with oropharyngeal dysphagia.[26]

Ambulatory pH Monitoring

Transnasal catheters, wireless esophageal mucosa capsules, and intraluminal impedance measurements can all be used for ambulatory pH monitoring.[27,28] Catheters allow multiple sensors to detect the height of reflux and are more unconformable but cheaper and more dependable. Although wireless capsules are more expensive, there is a significant loss of data due to radio interference, the presence of the capsule may cause chest pain, and there is a chance that it will come off too soon or too late. However, they are more tolerable and enable monitoring for periods longer than 24 hours. The test is usually performed immediately

TABLE 83.3 Indications for Ambulatory pH Monitoring

Diagnose GERD	• Symptoms suggestive of GERD
	• Organs possibly damaged by GERD
Associate GERD and symptoms	• Extraesophageal symptoms
	• Visceral hypersensitivity
Evaluate GERD severity	• DeMeester score
	• Pattern (supine, upright, combined)
Preoperative workup	• Exclude other motility disorders
	• Baseline comparison in cases of unfavorable outcome
Postoperative workup	• Unfavorable outcome
	• Continued damage to organs despite the operation

GERD, Gastroesophageal reflux disease.

after the esophageal manometry. Fasting is necessary, and antacid medications must be stopped. There is no good reason to perform the test under the influence of acid blockade.

Clinical guidelines usually indicate pH monitoring only when GERD is not proven by specific findings at the upper digestive endoscopy or after failure of empirical pharmacologic treatment. pH monitoring, however, also reveals information about the severity, pattern, and temporal relationship between reflux and symptoms (Table 83.3).

GERD can be present in a myriad of clinical scenarios. It may occur from the "classic" presentation, with esophageal symptoms, to a silent presentation only noticed by damage to target organs. Thus, objective evaluation is mandatory.[29,30]

A certain amount of reflux is considered physiologic and does not define GERD. Pathologic (abnormal) acid exposure can be simply defined by the percentage of time that the esophagus was

acidic (pH <4) (acid exposure time [AET]) greater than 6%. Most surgeons, however, prefer the DeMeester score that accredits points to the following parameters: (1) total number of episodes of reflux; (2) % total time esophageal pH <4; (3) % upright time esophageal pH <4; (4) supine time esophageal pH <4; (5) number of reflux episodes ≥5 minutes; and (6) longest reflux episode (minutes). The DeMeester score is influenced by the pattern of reflux and esophageal clearance correlating clinically with GERD severity[31] (Fig. 83.8). GERD may occur predominantly in the orthostatic or supine position or in a combined pattern (bipositional).

The height that the reflux episodes reach can be estimated thanks to the inclusion of multiple sensors in the catheter. However, because there is no recognized reference value for proximal reflux, there is no standardization of technique, and few surgical studies addressed this; interpreting the height of reflux is very challenging.[32,33]

pH monitoring may calculate the temporal relationship between symptoms and reflux episodes. This association can be calculated using a variety of metrics. The most popular and simpler method uses the percentage of GERD-related symptoms compared with all other symptoms to define the symptom index (SI), which is positive when it is greater than 50%.[34]

PRIMARY ESOPHAGEAL MOTILITY DISORDERS

Esophageal motility disorders can be broadly subdivided into two categories:
1. PEMDs caused by esophageal diseases per se.
2. Secondary esophageal motility disorders caused by esophageal dysfunction that is part of more global disease, such as GERD or scleroderma.

The classification of PEMD is based on the findings of esophageal manometry. Traditionally, esophageal manometry was

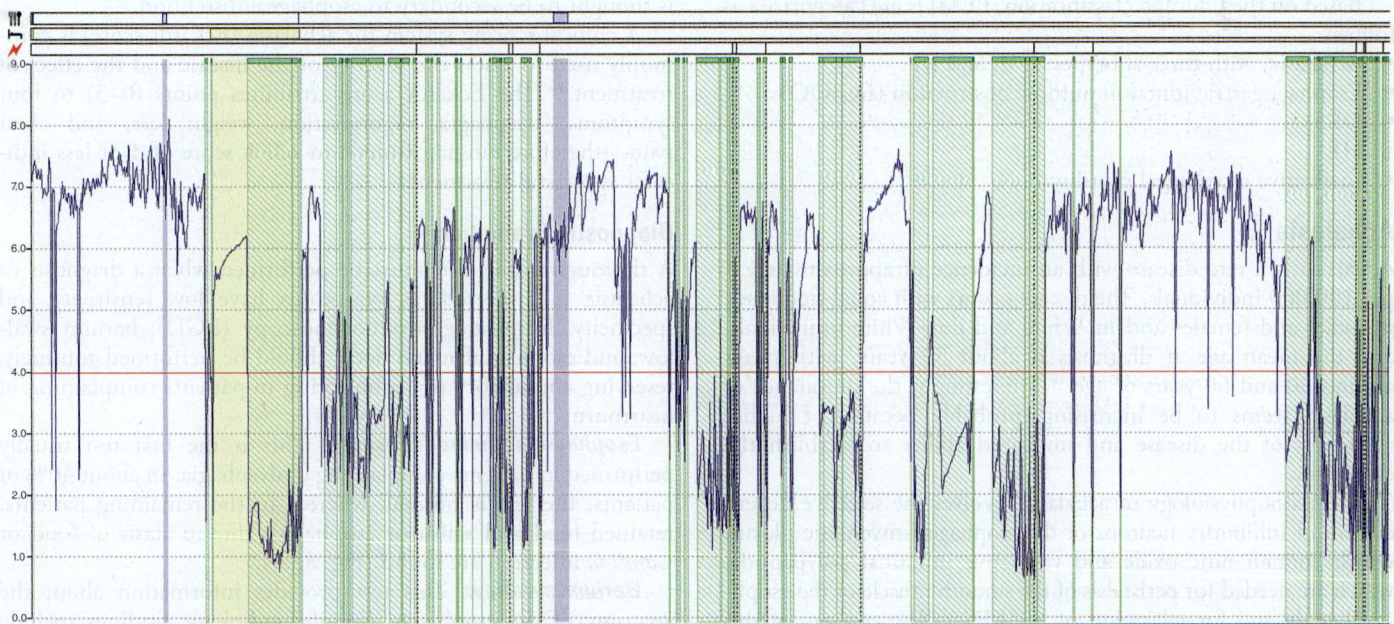

FIGURE 83.8 Example of pH monitoring traces. The *red horizontal line* represents pH = 4. All lines below the red line indicate an episode of reflux *(green rectangles)*. DeMeester score will be calculated based on the six parameters, including these episodes of reflux. *Vertical dotted lines* represent the moments symptoms were reported. The temporal correlation between symptoms and reflux can be calculated. Meal times are excluded because acid can be originated in the food *(blue rectangles)*.

performed with water-perfused catheters, often with a configuration with four distal circumferential sensors to measure the LES and four sensors spaced at intervals of 5 cm at 90-degree angles from each other (usually placed 3, 8, 13, and 18 cm above the upper border of the LES). Initially, the resting pressure, relaxation, total length, and abdominal length of the LES were assessed. Subsequently, 10 swallows of 5 mL of water were given at 30-second intervals for the evaluation of esophageal peristalsis (amplitude, duration, velocity, nontransmitted, or partially transmitted waves). Based on this test, four PEMDs were identified[35,36]: achalasia, diffuse esophageal spasm (DES), nutcracker esophagus, and hypertensive LES. Each disorder was characterized as follows:

- Achalasia: Partial or absent LES relaxation and absent esophageal peristalsis. Hypertensive LES (resting pressure >45 mm Hg) in about 50% of patients.[37]
- DES: Normal or elevated LES pressure. Simultaneous contractions after >20% but <100% of the wet swallows. Intermittent normal peristalsis. The contraction amplitude is usually >30 mm Hg.
- Nutcracker esophagus (hypercontracting esophagus): Normal or elevated LES pressure. Normal peristaltic progression with high-amplitude (>180 mm Hg) and long-duration (>6 seconds) waves in the distal esophagus.
- Hypertensive LES: Elevated LES resting pressure >45 mm Hg. The relaxation might be incomplete. Normal esophageal peristalsis.

Over the past 15 years, there have been significant advances in manometric device technology, manometric data display, and manometric data analysis.[38] In most centers, the water-perfused catheters have been substituted with solid-state catheters with 36 closely spaced pressure sensors, and data are displayed in the format of Clouse plots (color isobaric contours). Today high-resolution manometry (HRM) and the Chicago classification, now in version 4.0, are considered standard in clinical practice worldwide.[39]

Based on the Chicago classification, PEMDs are categorized as follows:

- Achalasia, with three subtypes: I, II, and III
- Esophagogastric junction outflow obstruction (EGJOO)
- DES
- HE
- Ineffective esophageal motility

Achalasia

Achalasia is a rare disease with an incidence of approximately 1 per 100,000 individuals. The disease occurs with equal frequency in males and females and in White and non-White individuals, and the mean age at diagnosis is about 50 years, with peaks around 30 and 60 years of age.[40] Interestingly, the prevalence of achalasia seems to be increasing, probably because of higher awareness of the disease and improved ability to establish the diagnosis.

The pathophysiology of achalasia involves the selective degeneration of inhibitory neurons of the esophageal myenteric plexus, which contain nitic oxide and vasoactive intestinal polypeptide, which are needed for peristalsis of the smooth muscle of the esophageal body and for relaxation of the LES.[41] The etiology of this degenerative process is still unknown. Some viruses such as varicella-zoster, human papilloma, and herpes have been implicated in initiating an inflammatory reaction. Interestingly, the excitatory neurons that contain acetylcholine are spared. Consequently, the LES does not relax properly, and it is often hypertensive.

In addition to the idiopathic form of achalasia, there are some secondary forms. One is Chagas disease, caused by the inoculation through a bug bite of a parasite, *Trypanosoma cruzi*. Organs other than the esophagus are also affected such as the heart, the brain, and the gastrointestinal tract. Another secondary form of achalasia known as *pseudoachalasia* is caused by malignancy, particularly cancer of the esophagus. Pseudoachalasia should be excluded in older patients (>60 years of age) who have been symptomatic for a short time and who have lost a considerable amount of weight.[42] Achalasia is also part of Allgrove syndrome (triple A) characterized by achalasia, alacrimia, and adrenal insufficiency.[43]

Clinical Presentation

Dysphagia, regurgitation, chest pain, heartburn, and aspiration are the most common symptoms experienced by patients with achalasia.[37] Because these symptoms can be caused by other diseases, there is often a delay between the onset of symptoms and the diagnosis of achalasia.

Dysphagia for solids and liquids is the most common symptom, present in approximately 95% of patients. Although some patients can make changes in their diet and maintain a stable weight, others experience progressive weight loss.

Regurgitation of undigested food occurs in about 70% of patients. It can cause aspiration with cough, hoarseness, and episodes of pneumonia.[44]

Heartburn is experienced by 40% to 50% of patients. It is not the result of esophageal reflux of gastric contents, but rather by stasis and fermentation of undigested food in the esophagus. Unfortunately, when heartburn is present, patients are often treated with acid reducing medications on the assumption that this symptom is caused by GERD. In the absence of a response to therapy, these patients are assumed to have "refractory GERD," delaying the correct diagnosis, and even referred for antireflux surgery.[45] Chest pain is present in 40% to 50% of patients, and it is thought to be secondary to esophageal distention.

A clinical scoring system for achalasia (Eckardt score) is commonly used to assess the severity of the disease and the effect of treatment.[46] The Eckardt score attributes points (0–3) to four symptoms—dysphagia, regurgitation, weight loss, and chest pain—therefore ranging from 0 to 12. A score of 3 or less indicates successful treatment.

Diagnostic Evaluation

A thorough evaluation must be performed when a diagnosis of achalasia is suspected, as symptoms have low sensitivity and specificity. Esophagogastroduodenoscopy (EGD), barium swallow, and esophageal manometry should be performed routinely, reserving ambulatory pH monitoring to patients complaining of heartburn.

Esophagogastroduodenoscopy. This is the first test usually performed in patients complaining of dysphagia. In about 40% of patients, the test is normal, whereas in the remaining patients, retained food and saliva or esophagitis due to stasis of food or *Candida* infection are found (Fig. 83.9).

Barium swallow. This test provides information about the anatomy of the esophagus. Specific radiologic findings include distal esophageal narrowing, an air-fluid level, slow emptying of the contrast into the stomach, and tertiary contractions (Fig. 83.10). Information about the axis (straight vs. sigmoid) and the amount of dilatation is very important for planning treatment (Fig. 83.11). In addition, the test can show additional and

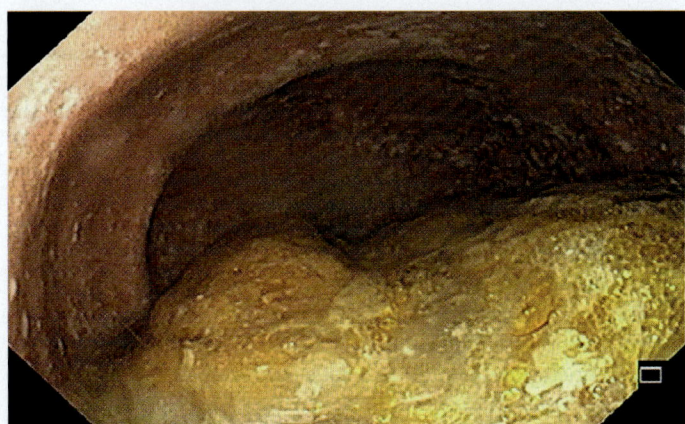

FIGURE 83.9 Endoscopy in a case of achalasia with food residues in the esophagus.

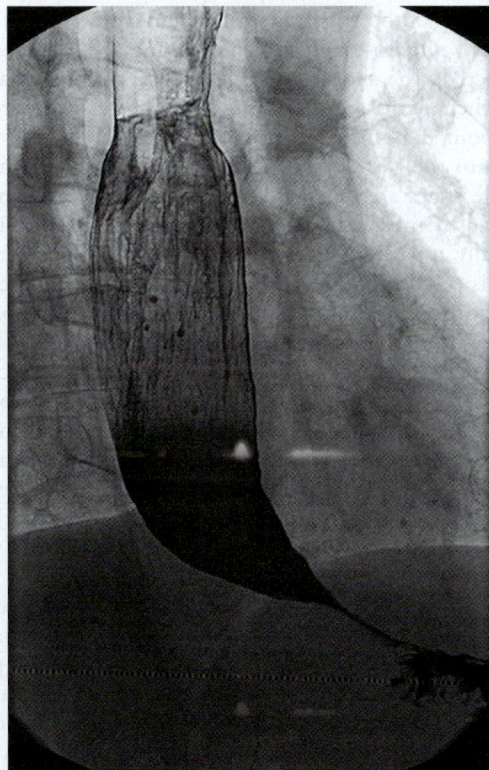

FIGURE 83.10 Barium swallow findings in a case of achalasia: distal esophageal narrowing, an air-fluid level, slow emptying of the contrast into the stomach, and tertiary contractions.

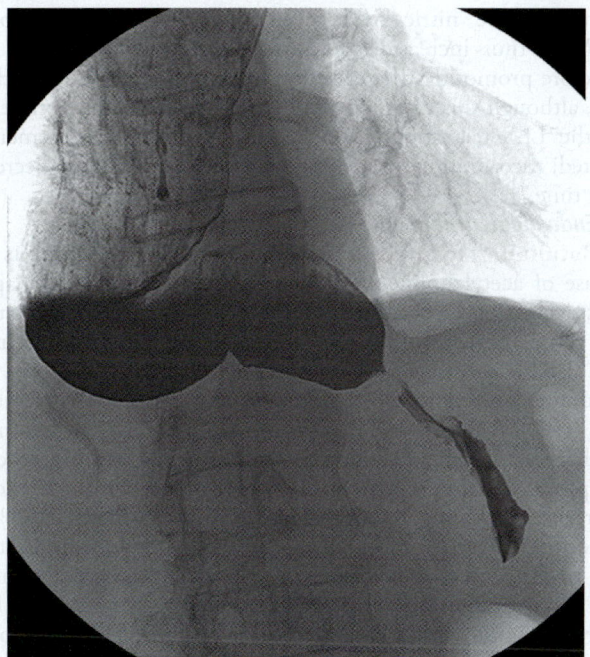

FIGURE 83.11 Dilated and sigmoid esophagus.

unexpected pathology such as an esophageal diverticulum. In early stages of the disease, the test can be normal in about 30% of patients.

Esophageal manometry. As mentioned before, high-resolution esophageal manometry is considered today the gold standard for the diagnosis of achalasia. In addition to establishing the diagnosis, this test defines the subtype of achalasia—type I, II, or III—with important implications for the choice and outcome of treatment.

Ambulatory pH monitoring. This test is recommended for patients who complain of heartburn to distinguish between GERD and achalasia. A recent study showed that 29% of patients whose final diagnosis was achalasia had been treated for an average of 29 months with proton pump inhibitors (PPIs) and eventually

referred for antireflux surgery, as they were considered to have "refractory GERD."[45]

When analyzing the pH monitoring test, it is important to look not only at the reflux score or percentage pH <4 but also at the tracing. A positive score can in fact be caused by real reflux (intermittent drop of the pH below 3 with subsequent return to values above 5) or by false reflux secondary to stasis and fermentation of food in the esophageal lumen, with slow and progressive drift of the pH below 4 and a very slow return to higher values.[47]

Functional lumen imaging probe. The functional lumen imaging probe (FLIP) is a catheter-based system used to evaluate esophageal compliance in patients with achalasia. This test uses impedance planimetry to calculate the esophageal lumen dimensions and distensibility. In addition, it is used to corroborate findings from HRM and/or barium swallow and assess the effect of treatment.[48]

This is a relatively new technology, complementary to other tests, and its usefulness is not fully determined.

Treatment

Treatment is palliative, as it does not cure the disease. The goal of treatment is to decrease the functional obstruction caused by a nonrelaxing and often hypertensive LES, therefore improving emptying of food from the esophagus into the stomach. Various treatment modalities are available today: pharmacologic (calcium channel blockers, phosphodiesterase inhibitors), endoscopic (botulinum toxin injection, pneumatic dilatation [PD], peroral endoscopic myotomy [POEM]), and surgical (laparoscopic Heller myotomy [LHM] with partial fundoplication).

Pharmacologic treatment. Nifedipine is the most frequently used calcium channel blocker. In a placebo-controlled, double-blind crossover study, it was shown that even though nifedipine and verapamil decreased the contraction amplitude in the distal esophagus and the LES pressure, there was no significant improvement in the symptomatology.[49] More recently, the use of sildenafil, normally used for erectile dysfunction, has been investigated. This is an inhibitor of phosphodiesterase type 5 that inactivates the nitric oxide cyclic guanosine monophosphate (cGMP), thus increasing the intracellular levels of cGMP and therefore promoting the relaxation of smooth muscle cells. However, although this drug reduces the LES pressure, it has no effect on the LES relaxation. Overall, the symptom improvement is limited, the duration of action is short, and the efficacy decreases over time.[50]

Endoscopic treatment

Botulinum toxin injection. Botulinum toxin inhibits the release of acetylcholine at the level of the cholinergic synapses, thus decreasing LES pressure. It has no effect on LES relaxation. The standard protocol for the endoscopic botulinum toxin injection (EBTI) consists of the injection of 100 units of toxin in four quadrants, approximately 1 cm above the gastroesophageal junction (GEJ). A review and meta-analysis of the different treatment modalities for achalasia showed that EBTI determines relief of symptoms in approximately 80% of patients within a month after the procedure, but its effect decreases over time: 70% at 3 months, 53% at 6 months, and 40% at 12 months.[51] In addition to the decreased efficacy over time, some studies have shown that this treatment may cause an inflammatory process at the level of the injection with loss of the normal anatomic planes. Consequently, in patients undergoing LHM for recurrent dysphagia after EBTI, the operation may be challenging, with an increased incidence of mucosal perforation and worse outcome.[52,53] Based on these considerations, EBTI should be considered only in patients who are not fit for PD, LHM, or POEM.

Pneumatic dilatation. PD is an effective option for the treatment of esophageal achalasia. A graded approach should be used, starting with a 30-mm balloon, and reserving larger balloons (35 and 40 mm) for patients with persistent or recurrent symptoms. Many studies have shown that the results of PD are comparable to those of LHM, even though PD needs to be repeated in about one-fourth of patients. Predictors of poor response are persistence of symptoms after the first or second dilatation, age less than 40 years, male sex, large esophageal diameter, type I and III according to the Chicago classification, pulmonary symptoms, and postprocedure LES pressure >10 mm Hg.[54]

A European prospective and randomized trial comparing PD (starting with a 30-mm balloon and reserving 35- and 40-mm balloons for persistent or recurrent dysphagia) and LHM with a Dor fundoplication was published in 2011.[55] The primary outcome was therapeutic success (a drop in the Eckardt score to ≤3) at the yearly follow-up assessment. The secondary outcomes included the need for retreatment, pressure of the LES, esophageal emptying on a timed barium esophagogram, quality of life, and the rate of complications. After 2 years, the therapeutic success of PD (86%) or LHM (90%) was similar. At 5-year follow-up there was still no significant difference between the two treatments—84% LHM and 82% PD—but 25% of patients undergoing PD required addition dilatations.[56] No differences in secondary outcome parameter were observed.

Even though these results suggest that these treatment modalities are equivalent, some limitations of this trial need to be stressed. First, the protocol was revised during the study period, changing the initial PD technique using a 35-mm balloon to a 30-mm balloon after the observation of a 31% perforation rate with the 35-mm balloon. Second, expert gastroenterologists performed the PD, whereas the skills and experience of the surgeons involved in the study were questionable, as they were required to have performed just five myotomies to participate, and the mucosal perforation rate during LHM was 11%—very high in general

and particularly in the absence of previous treatment. In addition, subgroup analysis showed that patients younger than 40 years had better results with LHM.

Finally, the applicability of the findings of this study to the practice in the United States is questionable. Because of the extensive use of LHM during the last 15 years, the expertise for PD has faded away considerably. Consequently, it seems that today the pendulum has swung toward either LHM or POEM as initial treatment for achalasia, reserving PD for the treatment of recurrent dysphagia after these two therapeutic modalities.

Surgical treatment.
The past three decades have witnessed major changes in the surgical treatment of achalasia, moving from an open operation through either a laparotomy or thoracotomy to a thoracoscopic approach and eventually to a laparoscopic myotomy with a partial fundoplication (Dor or Toupet).

Laparoscopic myotomy with partial fundoplication (Fig. 83.12). The operation is usually performed with four or five trocars placed in the upper abdomen. After opening the gastrohepatic ligament, the right pillar of the crus is identified and dissected and the peritoneum and phreno-esophageal membrane above the esophagus are transected. The short gastric vessels are divided to avoid any tension when performing the fundoplication. The myotomy is usually about 8.5 cm in length, with 6 cm above the GEJ and 2.5 cm onto the gastric wall. After completion of the myotomy, the muscle edges are separated so that the esophageal mucosa is not covered by muscle fibers for about 140 degrees of circumference. Finally, a partial anterior fundoplication (Dor) or posterior (Toupet) is performed.[57] Each procedure has pros and cons: The Dor anterior fundoplication does not need dissection posterior to the esophagus, therefore avoiding the risk of damaging the posterior vagus nerve. The Toupet requires the posterior dissection, but it might help keep the muscular edges separated, therefore avoiding recurrent dysphagia. The minimally invasive technique has evolved over time as it became clear that a fundoplication was necessary to control postoperative reflux, that a 360-degree wrap determined too much resistance at the level of the GEJ causing dysphagia, and that a longer myotomy onto the gastric wall gave better results.[58,59]

The LHM has shown excellent results over the years. The Padua group reported a 90% success rate among 407 patients at a median follow-up of 2.5 years, with a 5-year actuarial probability of being asymptomatic of 87%.[60] The European multicenter study showed a success rate of 84% after 5 years.[56] The long-term results of a prospective and randomized trial in Sweden comparing PD and LHM showed that after the LHM, 92% of patients had excellent results after 5 years and 80% at 10-year follow-up.[61]

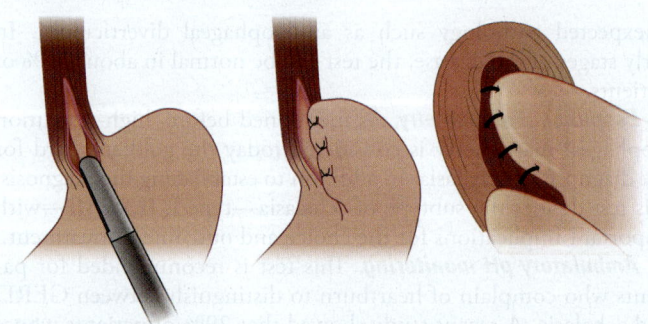

FIGURE 83.12 Laparoscopic Heller myotomy and partial fundoplication (Dor).

Recent years have shown an increasing use of robots to perform myotomy. The advantages of robotic surgery include improved visibility of the operative field with three-dimensional imaging, increased degrees of freedom of movements, and improved ergonomics. In addition, it might decrease the incidence of mucosal perforations, even though the long-term results are like those of an LHM.[62] Considering these findings, it seems that cost may remain a significant barrier to the widespread use of the robotic platform for the treatment of esophageal achalasia.

Peroral endoscopic myotomy. In 2010 Dr. Inoue published the results of a new endoscopic technique called *peroral endoscopic myotomy* (POEM) for the treatment of esophageal achalasia, showing clinical success in 100% of 17 patients with achalasia.[63] This initial report represents a milestone in the treatment of this disease, and today POEM is used in many centers across the world, either as primary treatment or for treating recurrent symptoms after PD or LHM.

The procedure is usually done under general anesthesia and consists of four steps: (1) submucosal injection and mucosal incision, usually 10 to 12 cm above the GEJ; (2) submucosal tunneling, extended past the GEJ for 2 to 3 cm onto the stomach; and (3) myotomy. The circular fibers are transected with preservation of the longitudinal fibers. The myotomy extends from 2 cm distal to the mucosal entry to 2 to 3 cm onto the gastric wall and (4) closure of the mucosal entry with clips or endoscopic sutures.

Many studies have shown that POEM is effective in relieving symptoms in more than 90% of patients, suggesting that it might be considered the primary treatment modality for patients with achalasia.[64-66] However, POEM has a clear "Achilles heel" due to a very high incidence of postprocedure GERD—around 50%—as the procedure is based on a myotomy alone without a fundoplication.[67,68] This finding reproduces the results of the prospective and randomized trial comparing a laparoscopic myotomy alone with a laparoscopic myotomy and Dor fundoplication.[69] Postoperative GERD was present in 48% of patients after myotomy alone but in 9% alone when a Dor fundoplication was added. The relief of dysphagia was similar in the two groups. A meta-analysis comparing the efficacy of POEM and LHM and the incidence of postprocedure reflux in patients with achalasia showed that the control of symptoms was excellent with either procedure (at 2-year follow-up, 92.7% after POEM and 90% after LHM). However, pH monitoring showed that the incidence of pathologic reflux was more than fourfold higher after POEM as compared with LHM (47.5% vs. 11.1%).[70] These findings have been recently confirmed in a multicenter, randomized controlled trial (RCT) comparing the endoscopic and the surgical myotomy in patients with esophageal achalasia.[71] A total of 221 patients were randomized to either POEM (112 patients) or LHM (109 patients). At 2-year follow-up, clinical success was observed in 83% of patients in the POEM group and in 81.7% in the LHM group. The incidence of pathologic reflux was 57% after POEM and 20% after LHM.

This high incidence of GERD must be considered when treatment is chosen, particularly in young patients, as a lifelong exposure to reflux can cause esophagitis, Barrett esophagus, and even adenocarcinoma.

The achalasia subtype, shown by HRM, must be taken into consideration when planning treatment. Both LHM and POEM can be chosen as primary treatment for type I and II achalasia, but POEM is superior to LHM for type III, probably because it allows a longer myotomy onto the esophageal wall.[72,73]

Evaluation and Treatment of Recurrent Symptoms After Prior Intervention

Particularly when treating young patients, it is quite common that some degree of dysphagia recurs, necessitating additional treatment. Scarring of the distal aspect of the myotomy is probably the most common cause. This can occur despite performing a long myotomy onto the gastric wall and separating the edges of the myotomy. Gastroesophageal reflux can also play a role, with the development of a peptic stricture. In addition, it is always important to confirm the diagnosis of achalasia and to rule out technical problems at the time of the first intervention.[74]

The first step should be to review the history and the tests performed to establish the diagnosis (did the patient really have achalasia?). It is important to review the operative report of the original procedure, as it can help understand the cause of failure: For instance, in case the initial treatment was an LHM, was the surgeon able to identify the anatomic planes? How long did the myotomy extend onto the gastric wall? Was a 360-degree fundoplication performed rather than a partial one?

A full workup is necessary to try to identify the cause of the recurrent symptoms. A barium swallow is probably the most useful test assessing the anatomy and the emptying of the barium from the esophagus into the stomach. An upper endoscopy should always be performed to rule out a stricture caused by reflux, *Candida* esophagitis, or cancer. If pseudoachalasia is suspected, an endoscopic ultrasound and a CT scan of chest and abdomen should be obtained. Esophageal manometry is essential to confirm the diagnosis and to measure pressure and length of the LES. Finally, a 24-hour pH monitoring should be obtained to see if pathologic reflux is present.

If the PD was used as a first step and dysphagia is still present after repeated dilatation, either POEM or LHM can be used.

If the initial treatment was POEM, PD, a repeat POEM, or LHM should be used depending on the expertise of the center. However, if POEM was performed on the anterior wall of the esophagus and stomach, an LHM might be very difficult.

In case of recurrent dysphagia after LHM, PD can alleviate the symptoms in most patients.[26] POEM avoids a challenging redo operation because of the presence of adhesions and scar tissue and can be done safely on the posterior wall of the esophagus.[75-77] An esophagectomy should be considered a last resort, only after the failure of all the other treatment modalities.

End-Stage Achalasia

An esophagectomy was traditionally recommended as primary treatment of patients with a dilated and sigmoid esophagus, so-called "end-stage achalasia," on the assumption that a myotomy could not improve the swallowing status.[78] However, some studies have shown that when the myotomy is performed by experienced surgeons, symptoms can be alleviated and an esophagectomy avoided in most patients.[79,80] In these patients, the operation is more challenging for the following reasons: (1) extensive dissection must be done in the posterior mediastinum in order to straighten the esophageal axis and bring more esophagus below the diaphragm; (2) the esophageal wall is usually very thick; (3) because of the extensive dissection, the esophageal hiatus can be enlarged, and stitches might be necessary to approximate the crura, usually posteriorly, avoiding angulation of the esophagus; and (4) if possible, a partial fundoplication should be added to the myotomy; however, if the esophagus is very dilated (8–10 cm), a fundoplication is not feasible.

Esophagectomy is more challenging than in patients with cancer, as the dilated esophagus occupies most of the posterior mediastinum and the feeding vessels are usually quite enlarged.

In 2001, a report of 93 patients who underwent an esophagectomy showed a very high incidence of complications: anastomotic leak (10%), recurrent laryngeal nerve injury (5%), bleeding requiring thoracotomy (2%), chylothorax (2%), and two patients died. In addition, 50% of patients developed an anastomotic stricture requiring dilatation.[78] A recent meta-analysis of eight studies comprising 1307 patients who had esophagectomy for achalasia (transthoracic 78.7%; transhiatal 21.3%) showed pneumonia in 10% of patients, anastomotic leak in 7%, and mortality in 2% of patients.[81] Overall, based on these results, a myotomy should be considered the first line of treatment, reserving an esophagectomy for patients who are still symptomatic after other interventions.

Considering the rarity and the complexity of this disease, the best results are obtained when patients are evaluated by a multidisciplinary group of experts and treatment is tailored to the individual patient.

Nonachalasia Esophageal Motility Disorders

Esophagogastric Junction Outflow Obstruction

A manometric diagnosis of EGJOO is defined as an elevated median IRP and ≥20% swallows with elevated intrabolus pressure in the supine position, with evidence of peristalsis (therefore not meeting the criteria for achalasia).[5] EGJOO can be idiopathic with normal anatomy or secondary to a hiatal hernia, a peptic stricture, or eosinophilic esophagitis. For this reason, a conclusive diagnosis requires relevant symptoms (dysphagia, regurgitation, chest pain) and additional tests such as a barium swallow, EGD, and/or FLIP.

When the EGJOO is secondary to other conditions such as a hiatal hernia, addressing them will alleviate the symptoms.[82] When EGJ is a primary problem, the same therapeutic approach for achalasia can be used to alleviate the distal esophageal obstruction. There are limited data about the effect of therapy in the idiopathic form of EGJOO, but it seems that both POEM and an LHM can be successful in alleviating symptoms in a high percentage of patients.[83,84]

Distal Esophageal Spasm

DES describes a specific abnormal esophageal motor pattern characterized by spastic or premature contractions in at least 20% of swallows in the distal esophagus and DL <4.5 seconds.[39] However, to define DES as PEMD, it is important to perform a pH monitoring study to rule out GERD. It has been shown that up to 40% of patients with GERD diagnosed by pH monitoring have a picture compatible with DES on HRM.[85] Clinically relevant symptoms for DES include dysphagia, noncardiac chest pain, regurgitation, and heartburn. Unlike achalasia, dysphagia is not progressive and weight loss is rare. Chest pain may mimic myocardial infarction, and it is usually described as a crushing or squeezing pain that can radiate to the jaw, arms, or back. In addition to the esophageal function tests, a barium swallow, an EGD, FLIP, and a cardiac evaluation are usually performed.

Once a solid diagnosis is established in a symptomatic patient, different therapeutic options are available. Overall, pharmacologic therapy has a limited role in the treatment because of limited efficacy and adverse side effects. Recently, peppermint oil has been used with some success in patients with DES, improving dysphagia and chest pain, although further studies are needed.[86]

In patients with persistent symptoms who do not respond to medical therapy, an LHM or POEM can achieve good results. A retrospective study involving 11 centers that included 17 patients with DES and 18 with jackhammer esophagus found that POEM improved chest pain in 87% with clinical success (based on Eckardt score) of 84.9% with median follow-up of 272 days.[87] Surgical myotomy has also been studied in a small prospective study of 20 patients with extended myotomy for DES (the myotomy extended upward for 12–16 cm above the cardia and downward for 2 cm below the EGJ) and found that both dysphagia and chest pain improved in 100% and 90%, respectively, over 50-month follow-up.[88]

Because of the lack of well-controlled, long-term randomized controlled trials (RCTs), POEM and LHM for treatment of spastic esophageal body disorders should be reserved for highly selected patients because long-term prognosis even without treatment seems to be good for these disorders.

Hypercontractile Esophagus

A clinically relevant diagnosis of HE (jackhammer esophagus) requires both the presence of dysphagia and noncardiac chest pain and HRM showing 20% or more hypercontractile supine swallows with DCI >8000 and normal DL.[39] Hypercontractility can be limited to the esophageal body or can include the LES. In addition to HRM, an EGD should be performed to rule out the presence of eosinophilic esophagitis, which can determine the same symptoms and findings on HRM, requiring treatment with acid-reducing medications and steroids.[89]

This is a rare disorder, with a low prevalence around 2%, and a standard treatment has not been established thus far.[90] A multicenter study from Japan provided important information about the need and the outcome of treatment.[91] It reported that 77% of patients (13 patients) did well without treatment; POEM was successful in 76% of 21 patients, and laparoscopic myotomy in 2 of 2 patients (100%). Patients who required invasive treatment usually had a higher DCI and more severe disability. A systematic review and meta-analysis have shown that POEM was very successful in patients with spastic esophageal disorders, determining good results in 92% of patients with type III achalasia, 88% for DES, and 72% for HE.[92]

Overall, nonachalasia esophageal disorders are quite rare, and the best results are obtained in specialized centers where a complete workup can be performed and treatment tailored to the individual patient based on the symptoms, diagnostic findings, and expertise of the physicians.

ESOPHAGEAL DIVERTICULA

Esophageal diverticula are classified based on their location within the esophagus:
- Pharyngoesophageal (Zenker's) diverticulum
- Midthoracic diverticulum
- Epiphrenic diverticulum

Pharyngoesophageal (Zenker's) Diverticulum

This is the most common of the esophageal diverticula. Most patients are over age 60, and it is more common in males than in females. This diverticulum originates from the posterior wall of the esophagus, in a triangular area (Killian triangle) limited inferiorly by the cricopharyngeal muscle and laterally by the oblique fibers of the inferior constrictor of the pharynx (Fig. 83.13). When the diverticulum gets bigger, it tends to deviate from the

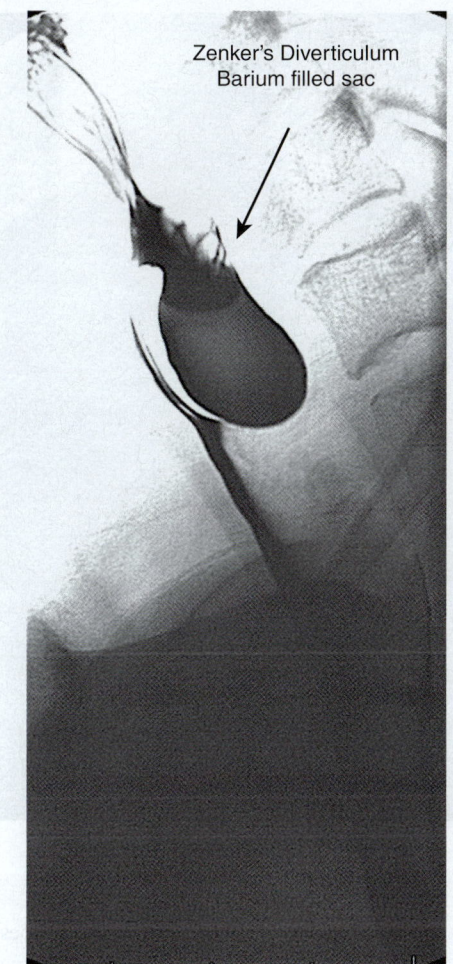

Zenker's Diverticulum
Barium filled sac

FIGURE 83.13 Zenker's diverticulum.

midline, mostly toward the left. A Zenker diverticulum is usually secondary to a lack of coordination between the pharyngeal contraction and the opening of the UES; therefore, it is a *pulsion* diverticulum secondary to increased intraluminal pressure. Only mucosa and submucosa herniate through the Killian triangle (false diverticulum).[93] Another area of potential weakness where a diverticulum can form is the so-called "Killian-Jamieson area" located just below the cricopharyngeal muscle.

Dysphagia is the most common symptom, present in about 80% to 90% of patients. Regurgitation of undigested food from the diverticular pouch occurs often and can lead to aspiration and pneumonia. Patients can also experience halitosis and hear gurgling sounds in the neck. About 30% have associated GERD.

A barium swallow shows the position (at the level of C5–C6) and size of the diverticulum or a prominent cricopharyngeal bar without an associated diverticulum. Endoscopy to rule out other pathology must be performed with great caution to avoid perforation. Esophageal manometry can show lack of coordination between the pharynx and UES and a hypertensive UES. It also locates the LES for ambulatory pH monitoring in patients suspected of having GERD—information especially useful to guide therapy.

Treatment consists of eliminating the functional obstruction of the UES with a myotomy of the cricopharyngeus muscle and the upper 3 cm of the posterior esophageal wall.[94] Traditionally, this approach was performed using a cervical incision, and the

myotomy was associated with either excision or suspension of the diverticulum. A diverticulum less than 2 cm rarely requires treatment. Today transoral alternatives to ablate the septum between the esophagus and the esophageal diverticulum are available with particularly good results.

Open Transcervical Approach

A left-sided incision in the neck is made, following the medial border of the sternocleidomastoid muscle. Dissection is continued until the prevertebral fascia is reached. Usually there is no need to divide muscles. Once the esophagus and the diverticulum are identified, the cricopharyngeus muscle is divided completely and the myotomy is extended onto the esophageal muscle wall, exposing the esophageal mucosa for 3 cm below the diverticulum. There is no need to dissect the esophagus circumferentially because it increases the risk of damage to the left recurrent laryngeal nerve.

Small diverticula (<2 cm) should not be resected. Large diverticula can be resected or fixed upward to the prevertebral fascia. Resection is usually accomplished using a stapling device. Before stapling the neck of the diverticulum, it is important to place a bougie inside the esophagus to avoid pulling too much mucosa with consequent narrowing of the esophageal lumen. Infection, leak and mediastinitis, esophageal stenosis, and recurrent laryngeal nerve damage are the most common complications and occur in about 2% to 3% of cases. The recurrence rate of the diverticulum is between 5% and 10%.

If the preoperative evaluation has shown the presence of pathologic gastroesophageal reflux, either medical or surgical therapy should be prescribed to avoid the risk of aspiration, as it is increased after the resection of the UES.

Endoscopic Approach

Two different approaches are available: rigid endoscopy or flexible endoscopy. To date, no controlled trials have been performed to compare the two techniques, and, consequently, there are no guidelines for the management of this rare esophageal disorder.

Rigid endoscopic technique. The procedure is performed under general anesthesia with the patient in supine position with the neck extended. A diverticuloscope is introduced through the mouth, placing one blade inside the esophagus and one inside the diverticular pouch. After suctioning any undigested food, saliva, and pills, two stay sutures are placed on each side of the septum to obtain traction and facilitate the insertion of a modified linear stapler with the jaws across the septum. Firing the stapler creates a common cavity between the esophagus and the diverticular pouch.[95,96]

Flexible endoscopic technique. The rigid endoscopic technique has some limitations such as the need for general anesthesia and the need for hyperextension of the neck. In addition, small diverticula (2–3 cm) do not allow proper positioning of the stapler. The flexible endoscopic technique is performed with the patient on a left lateral decubitus, and the transection of the septum is done under direct vision. Division of the septum can be performed with different devices such as a needle knife, a hook knife, or argon plasma coagulation. After septotomy is completed, one or more endoclips are placed to close the incision and avoid leaks or bleeding.[97,98] Both the rigid and flexible endoscopic techniques have a success rate of 90%.

Z–Peroral endoscopic myotomy. POEM has been used for more than 10 years for the treatment of esophageal achalasia, with excellent results. This technique has been recently applied successfully for the treatment of Zenker's diverticulum.[99] The procedure starts with a submucosal injection and mucosotomy about 3 cm proximal to the septum, and then a submucosal tunnel is created along both sides of the septum, ending in the normal esophagus 2 cm distally to the end of the septum. The fibers of the cricopharyngeus muscle are transected under direct vision, and the mucosotomy is then closed with clips. Good results are obtained in 90% of patients, with a complication rate around 6%, mostly due to perforation or bleeding. As this is a new procedure, long-term results are not available.

Midesophageal Diverticulum

A midesophageal diverticulum is in the midportion of the thoracic esophagus. This is considered a *traction* diverticulum, secondary to an inflammatory process in the mediastinum, most frequently from histoplasmosis or tuberculosis. They are most seen on the right because of the close association of the esophagus with the subcarinal lymph nodes in this area. As the entire esophageal wall forms the diverticulum, this is considered a true diverticulum.

These diverticula are generally small and asymptomatic and do not need treatment. Larger diverticula (>4 cm) can become symptomatic and cause dysphagia. The workup consists of a barium swallow to identify size and location and an endoscopy to rule out cancer. In addition, an esophageal manometry should be performed because it has been suggested that a motility disorder is often present.[100]

Treatment of the symptomatic diverticula consists of a diverticulectomy through either a thoracotomy or a thoracoscopic approach.[101] A myotomy should be added if a motility disorder is present.

Epiphrenic Diverticulum

Epiphrenic diverticulum is a pulsion diverticulum usually located in the distal 10 cm of the esophagus. It is caused by the herniation of mucosa and submucosa through the muscle layers of the esophageal wall. Almost 60 years ago Belsey suggested that this diverticulum is not a primary disorder, but it is rather secondary to an underlying esophageal motility disorder so that treatment must address not only the diverticulum but also the motility disorder by a myotomy.[102] This brilliant intuition was confirmed in the following decades and today constitutes the basis for the modern treatment of epiphrenic diverticula. Esophageal achalasia and DES are identified by conventional manometry in about 70% of cases; when ambulatory manometry is used, a motility abnormality is present in every patient.[103,104]

The symptoms experienced by the patients are secondary to the underlying motility disorder. Dysphagia and regurgitation are the most common, followed by chest pain and weight loss. Aspiration can cause nocturnal cough, laryngitis, and pneumonia. Some patients experience heartburn, which is not caused by real reflux, but rather by stasis and fermentation of undigested food in the esophageal lumen. Bleeding, perforation, and malignant transformation are rare.

The barium swallow is a key test in patients with epiphrenic diverticulum, as it defines the size of the diverticulum and its neck, the location (about two-thirds are located on the right side), and the distance of the diverticulum from the GEJ (Fig. 83.14). About 15% of patients have more than one diverticulum.[104]

Endoscopy should be performed in all patients with dysphagia to rule out cancer; in addition, it can help with the placement of the manometry catheter. Manometry identifies the motility disorder,

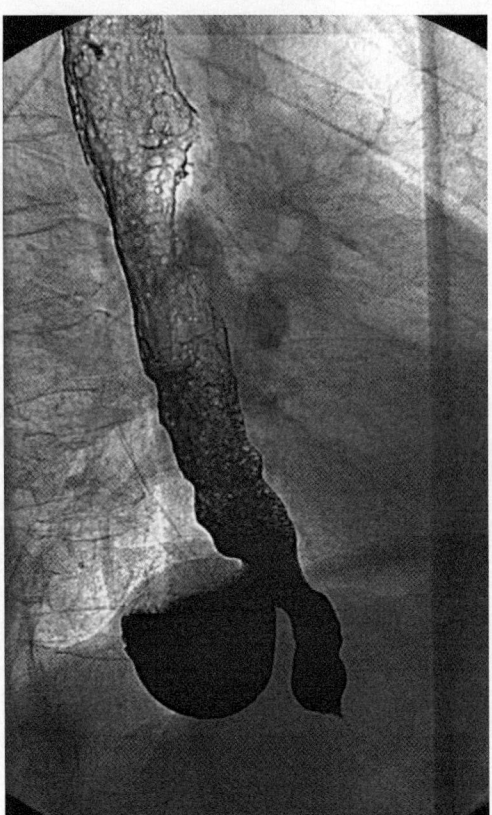

FIGURE 83.14 Epiphrenic diverticulum.

but it might be considered of academic interest, as it does not influence management.

Treatment is recommended for symptomatic patients only for two reasons: (1) fewer than 10% of asymptomatic patients eventually develop symptoms,[105] and (2) even in expert hands, the operation carries significant morbidity.[106]

The transthoracic approach through a left thoracotomy has been traditionally used to treat epiphrenic diverticulum. This approach provides excellent exposure for the dissection, for the resection of the diverticulum with oversewing of the staple line, for a myotomy, and for a partial fundoplication, either a Dor or a Belsey.[104,106] However, even in the hands of expert surgeons, this approach is associated with significant morbidity. For instance, Varghese et al. reported on 35 patients operated on between 1976 and 2005 and showed that although relief of symptoms occurred in 74% of patients, 21% required periodic dilatations for treating dysphagia, there were two leaks (6%), and one patient died (3%).[106]

In 1988, Rosati described the laparoscopic approach to epiphrenic diverticulum, consisting of diverticulectomy, myotomy, and partial fundoplication.[107] The same group later described the long-term results of this approach in 20 patients.[108] At a median follow-up of 52 months, the results were excellent in 16 patients (80%).

These are the steps of a laparoscopic operation:
1. Dissection of the diverticulum and the diverticular neck.
   It is particularly important to completely dissect the neck circumferentially and identify the muscle layers before firing the stapler.
2. Transection of the diverticular neck.
   A 50-Fr to 56-Fr bougie must be placed inside the esophagus to avoid narrowing of the lumen when the stapler is applied.

Using a reticulating stapler allows optimal positioning across the neck of the diverticulum. The staple line is covered with interrupted stitches using nonabsorbable sutures.

3. A myotomy is then performed on the contralateral side of the esophagus.

The myotomy extends from the level of the diverticular neck all the way down for 2 to 2.5 cm onto the gastric wall.

4. Closure of the crura, as often the hiatus is quite enlarged after an extensive dissection.

5. A partial fundoplication, either a Dor or a Toupet, is then performed.[109]

Sometimes the laparoscopic approach can be challenging if the diverticulum is very large (8–10 cm), if there is severe inflammation, or if it is not possible to safely dissect the neck circumferentially. In these cases, based on the consideration that the symptoms are mostly caused by the underlying motility disorder, it is reasonable to perform only a myotomy and partial fundoplication as described in patients with achalasia, without a diverticulectomy. The results of this approach are good in most cases, and very few patients eventually need a second operation to resect the diverticulum.[110,111]

Peroral endoscopic myotomy (D-POEM) has been used recently for the treatment of epiphrenic diverticulum with a remarkably high success rate.[112,113] Similar to laparoscopic myotomy alone, D-POEM can relieve the symptoms of dysphagia and regurgitation without the need for resection of the diverticulum. Compared with a surgical myotomy and fundoplication, D-POEM has the advantage of allowing a longer myotomy in patients with type III achalasia and DES. The major drawback of this technique is the absence of an antireflux procedure, with rates of pathologic reflux between 40% and 50%.

GASTROESOPHAGEAL REFLUX DISEASE

GERD is the most common benign gastroesophageal disorder. It carries significant implications for patients' quality of life and is inextricably linked with other medical conditions, including esophageal adenocarcinoma, pulmonary disease, and obesity. Though most patients with GERD benefit from medical therapy, surgery still has an essential role in patients with medically refractory disease. Given the complex interplay of factors underlying GERD, the surgical approach should be tailored to patients' anatomy and pathophysiology.

Pathophysiology

As described previously in this chapter, GERD may arise if GEJ pressure is lower than the transdiaphragmatic pressure gradient. GEJ pressure, however, is not determined by any one structure, but instead is a complex of anatomic features—including the intrinsic muscle of the LES, the gastric sling fibers, the diaphragmatic crura, and the angle of His.[114] Alterations to any of these anatomic structures can predispose to reflux.

Evaluation

Evaluation of patients with suspected GERD begins with a detailed history. Patients often complain of "reflux"; however, GERD is a diagnosis, not a symptom. It is important to elicit specific symptoms, such as heartburn, regurgitation, waterbrash, dysphagia, and chest or abdominal pain. Heartburn and regurgitation are the most common symptoms, with regurgitation indicating more severe disease. Waterbrash is an increase in saliva production in response to acid reflux. Dysphagia may signal an

underlying motility disorder or obstructing lesion. Bloating may signal an issue with gastric emptying. Patients may also have atypical or extraesophageal symptoms such as cough, shortness of breath, globus sensation, and throat clearing. Patients reporting chest or upper abdominal pain in the setting of cardiovascular risk factors must always have a cardiac cause excluded. It is essential to inquire about comorbid conditions, including pulmonary disease and obesity, as well as whether medical therapy has been tried and been effective. Relief of symptoms with PPIs predicts a good response from fundoplication. PPI therapy may successfully address heartburn in many patients but may not address regurgitation or dysphagia or eradicate the extraesophageal symptoms. Lack of response to PPI may also indicate an alternative disease process. In addition to the GERD workup described next, patients with extraesophageal symptoms require additional testing to rule out primary disorders of the lungs, airway, or oropharynx. Physical examination is often unrevealing in cases of GERD; however, in some cases, dental changes, throat clearing, or cough may be apparent. Central obesity is a major risk factor for GERD and should be assessed by, at a minimum, calculating the patient's BMI.

Diagnostic Workup

Often in the primary care setting, PPI therapy is initiated empirically for suspected GERD. However, if patients' symptoms are severe enough to warrant surgical evaluation, they generally ought to undergo four diagnostic tests before intervention, according to expert consensus guidelines.[115] This workup serves several purposes: (1) to establish that the patient's symptoms are caused by GERD rather than an alternate diagnosis, (2) to identify important conditions that must be addressed during or before any intervention for GERD, and (3) to rule out motility disorders that may mimic GERD or affect the success of antireflux surgery.[116]

Barium Swallow

A barium swallow (aka upper GI series) is commonly performed in the initial assessment of GERD. It can evaluate hiatal hernias in detail as well as obstructing lesions such as webs or strictures. It can also identify gastroesophageal reflux events, though it is not sufficient to establish the diagnosis of GERD. Barium swallow can also provide some information regarding esophageal motility, though it is not the gold standard test for this. If a paraesophageal hernia is found on barium swallow and it is causing classic symptoms, ambulatory pH monitoring and esophageal manometry might not be necessary before proceeding to definitive surgical treatment.

Upper Endoscopy

Upper endoscopy is essential before performing antireflux surgery. This may establish the diagnosis of Barrett esophagus or reflux esophagitis and rule out malignancy in the esophagus or stomach before proceeding to surgery. LA class C and D esophagitis, peptic strictures, and Barrett esophagus are pathognomonic for GERD. Assessing the GEJ on retroflexion may also provide information on the presence of a hiatal hernia and the integrity of the LES complex.

Ambulatory pH Monitoring

Ambulatory pH monitoring is the gold standard test for the diagnosis of GERD. Earlier in the chapter we discussed how it is performed and how to interpret the findings. pH monitoring is typically performed off acid suppression, but this topic is controversial, and the most recent consensus guidelines do suggest a role for pH monitoring while on acid suppression.[117] pH monitoring performed off PPI is typically used to make the diagnosis of GERD. Acid exposure calculations will be artificially decreased if the patient is on a PPI, and a diagnosis may be missed if testing is performed on a PPI. However, for patients who already have an established diagnosis of GERD, pH monitoring on a PPI may be useful to assess if acid suppression is adequate and/or if symptoms might be related to nonacid issues, which could be addressed nonoperatively.

Esophageal Manometry

Esophageal manometry is used to identify achalasia and other disorders of esophageal motility before antireflux surgery, as patients with poor motility may not tolerate a full fundoplication. However, prolonged acid exposure can also cause esophageal dysmotility that may improve with surgery. Distinguishing dysmotility that may preclude antireflux surgery from dysmotility that may benefit from antireflux surgery can be challenging. The multiple rapid swallows maneuver assesses esophageal "reserve"; patients with dysmotility but a normal multiple rapid swallows response tend to see improvement of dysmotility after antireflux surgery without worsening dysphagia. Esophageal manometry is not required before surgery in patients with paraesophageal hernias because they can make manometry testing unreliable.

Treatment

Medical Management

By the time patients present for surgical evaluation for GERD, they have often initiated medical therapy, typically in the form of a PPI. Surgeons should inquire about both lifestyle and medical treatments attempted during treatment for GERD because antireflux surgery is typically only indicated for patients refractory to maximal medical management. Lifestyle approaches include weight loss, avoiding dietary triggers, elevation of the head of the bed, tobacco, alcohol cessation, and avoiding late night meals.

Over-the-counter antacids such as Tums may offer temporary relief but are not effective in healing esophagitis. H_2 blockers such as famotidine may be useful for breakthrough symptoms and are stronger than antacids but can be limited by tachyphylaxis or tolerance with repeated dosing and low potency relative to PPIs.

PPIs are currently the most potent antisecretory therapy available. They have the highest rates of symptom control and healing of esophagitis. The various PPIs appear to be equally effective at equivalent doses, though some find certain formulations to be better than others. Guidelines by the American Gastroenterological Association recommend that patients with suspected uncomplicated GERD undergo a 4- to 8-week trial of a PPI, beginning at once-daily dosing and possibly escalating the dose to twice daily for a partial response to treatment. Those who do not have adequate relief after a 4- to 8-week PPI trial should undergo further testing before escalating the dose.[118,119]

Patients often inquire about adverse events from long-term PPI use. Most reports of adverse effects are from observational rather than randomized controlled studies.[6] The best evidence is for a slightly increased risk of worsening chronic kidney disease, *Clostridioides difficile* infection, and community-acquired pneumonia.[120–122] Some observational studies have also suggested that PPI use is a risk factor for osteoporosis, dementia, and gastric cancer, but the strength of this evidence is poor.[118,123,124]

Surgical Management

Antireflux surgery is indicated for patients who are intolerant of acid suppression, who are refractory to it, or who do not want to continue acid suppression in the long term. Two initial branch points when considering antireflux surgery are (1) the presence of obesity (BMI >35) and (2) the presence of a hiatal hernia. These conditions strongly predispose to reflux and influence its surgical decision-making, as detailed later in this chapter. For patients without obesity (BMI <35) or a large hiatal hernia, numerous treatment options are available that will be detailed in this section.

Operative Technique

Laparoscopic and robotic approaches have become the norm for antireflux surgery. Laparoscopy can be performed in the supine or French (low lithotomy) position, depending on surgeon preference, whereas robotic surgery is typically performed with the patient supine. Antibiotics and deep vein thrombosis (DVT) prophylaxis (unfractionated or low-molecular-weight heparin) are administered. Pneumoperitoneum can be achieved via a Veress needle or open technique. Steep reverse Trendelenburg positioning and a liver retractor enhance exposure of the hiatus. At least four ports (two for the surgeon, one for the camera, and one for the assistant) are used in addition to the liver retractor.

The hiatal dissection typically begins on the right crus by dividing the pars flaccida of the gastrohepatic ligament, noting any aberrant hepatic arteries. This plane is taken to the right crus, and then the right phrenoesophageal ligament is opened close to the crus and further opened anteriorly and posteriorly along the length of the crus. Care is taken to leave the diaphragmatic fascia on the crus to facilitate later closure and to stay close to the crus to avoid injuring nearby structures. This is followed by the left-sided dissection, which begins by dividing the short gastric vessels using an energy device, taking care to avoid thermal energy to the stomach and the spleen. This plane is carried around the fundus to the angle of His and then onto the left phrenoesophageal ligament, where the phrenoesophageal ligament is divided as it was on the right side. This dissection is typically taken anteriorly around the hiatus until it meets the right-sided dissection. After this, the esophagus is elevated anteriorly, and a tunnel is carefully made posterior to it. A Penrose is passed through this tunnel, around the esophagus, to retract the esophagus. To complete the circumferential dissection, the phrenoesophageal ligament dissection is continued posteriorly, connecting the left and right sides with a 360-degree clearance of the crura. If there is a hiatal hernia, the esophagus is mobilized in the mediastinum until at least 3 cm of intraabdominal esophageal length is obtained. The crura are closed posteriorly with interrupted permanent sutures, with or without pledgets depending on the surgeon's preference and the strength of the crura, taking care not to narrow the esophagus. After this, the fundoplication is constructed. Of note, some surgeons begin with the left-sided dissection and then connect this to the right-sided dissection; this is simply a matter of surgeon preference (Fig. 83.15).

Three Hundred and Sixty-Degree Total (Nissen) Fundoplication

We pass a large (56 Fr) bougie to calibrate the diameter of the fundoplication. The fundus must be generously mobilized and passed posterior to the esophagus without becoming distorted or flipped upon itself. This can be accomplished by passing a grasper posterior to the esophagus to a suitable point on the fundus and then pulling this posterior to the esophagus. It is important to maintain the correct orientation of the fundoplication, keeping the greater curve cephalad—this can be identified as the cut edge of the short gastric vessels. To perform the "shoeshine maneuver,"

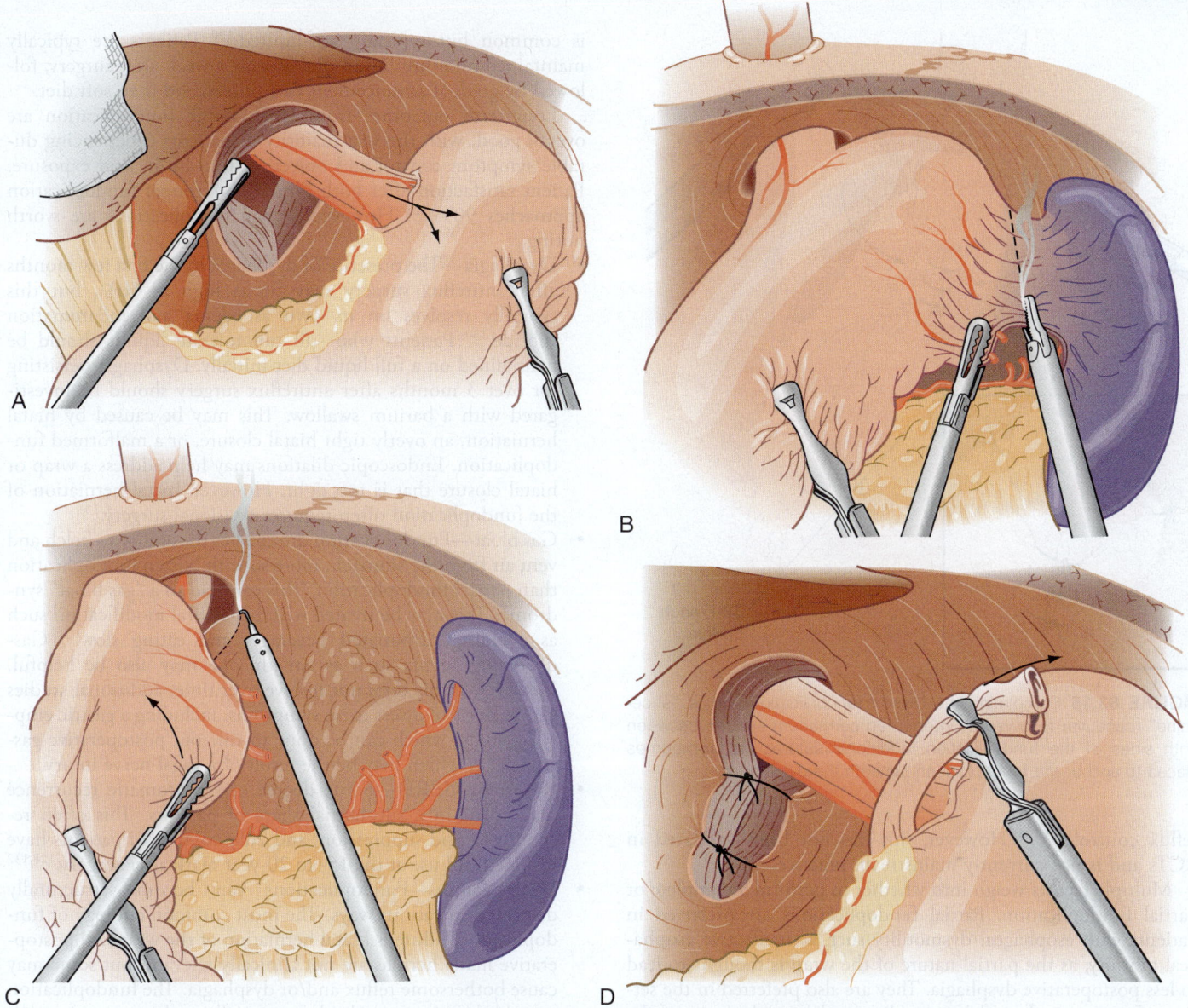

FIGURE 83.15 (A) The pars flaccida of the gastroesophageal ligament is opened onto the right crus, after which the phrenoesophageal ligament is opened. (B) To begin the left-sided dissection, the short gastric vessels are divided with an energy device. (C) The left-sided dissection is continued up to the phrenoesophageal ligament. (D) After the 360-degree mobilization is complete and an adequate length of esophagus is reduced into the abdomen, the crura are closed posteriorly with permanent suture.

the surgeon's left hand grasps the fundus that has been brought behind the esophagus, and the right hand grasps the proximal greater curvature, ensuring that there is enough fundus mobilized and that the two can be brought together anterior to the esophagus without tension. It is also intended to avoid too loose a fundoplication if the greater curvature of the stomach is grabbed too low. These are then sutured together with a permanent suture for a total length of 2 to 3 cm. Some surgeons suture the fundoplication to the esophagus to prevent slippage of the wrap. Some surgeons also place gastropexy sutures between the fundoplication and diaphragm to help prevent hiatal herniation (Fig. 83.16).

Partial Fundoplication

Partial fundoplications can be performed anteriorly (Dor fundoplication) or posteriorly (Toupet fundoplication). These partial fundoplications do not need to be performed over bougies because they are not circumferential. In a Toupet fundoplication, a shoeshine maneuver is performed similarly to a Nissen, but the fundus is sutured to the esophagus rather than to the fundus on the other side for a total of 240 to 270 degrees. The most cephalad sutures also incorporate the crura. A posterior suture from the wrap to the hiatal closure is also placed. A Dor fundoplication can be performed without dissecting the posterior attachments of the esophagus and without a shoeshine maneuver. It is performed by bringing the fundus over the anterior aspect of the esophagus and suturing it to the hiatus and esophagus (see "Achalasia" section).

Emerging evidence suggests that endoFLIP planimetry may help tailor the tightness of both complete and partial fundoplication. A postfundoplication distensibility index of 2.6 to 3.7 (for Toupet) and >2.2 (for Nissen) has been associated with decreased postoperative gas bloat and dysphagia and improved

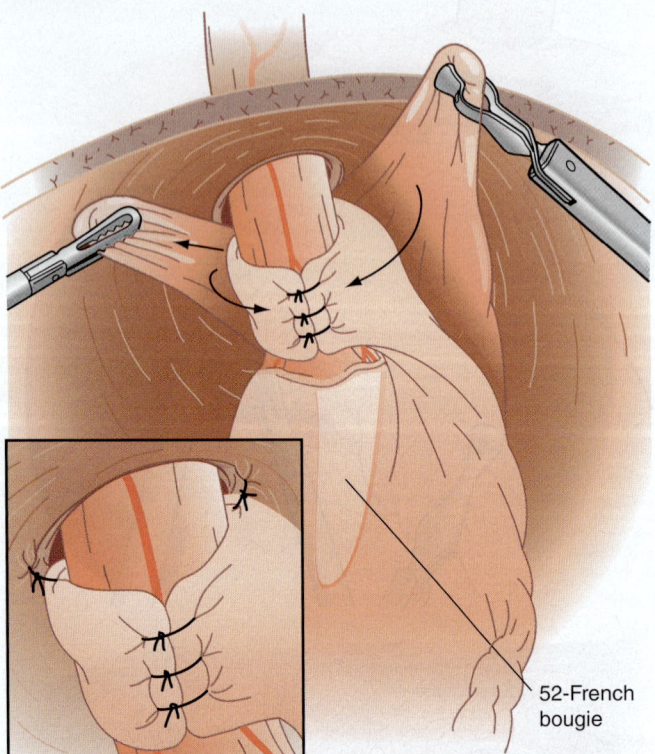

52-French
bougie

FIGURE 83.16 Completing the Nissen fundoplication with a "shoe-shine" maneuver followed by interrupted permanent sutures between both sides of the fundoplication. Additional sutures are sometimes placed to anchor the fundoplication beneath the diaphragm.

reflux control.[125,126] However, this has not been validated in RCTs and is not currently mainstream practice.

Multiple factors weigh into whether to perform a complete or partial fundoplication. Partial fundoplications are preferred in patients with esophageal dysmotility such as ineffective esophageal motility, as the partial nature of the wrap is thought to lead to less postoperative dysphagia. They are also preferred in the setting of a paraesophageal hernia (discussed later) because of the inability to obtain accurate preoperative manometry. A recent RCT compared the outcomes of Nissen and Toupet fundoplication and found equivalent reflux outcomes over a 3-year follow-up period, with slightly less dysphagia after Toupet in the short term.[127] Another recent RCT compared Nissen and Dor fundoplication over 15 to 20 years and found slightly improved reflux outcomes after Nissen but improved dysphagia and belching after Dor.[128] Multisociety consensus guidelines published in 2023 favor partial fundoplication over complete fundoplication because of decreased hiatal hernia recurrence, dysphagia, and inability to belch, with only a modest difference in long-term reflux control; this is a "conditional" recommendation based on "moderate" evidence.[129] Overall, the approach should be tailored to each individual patient's anatomy, physiology, and goals for surgery (Fig. 83.17).

Outcomes of Fundoplication

Short-term complications are rare, with perioperative mortality rates approaching 0.1% and the risk of bleeding, infection, and gastric or esophageal perforation approximately 1% each. Severe dysphagia with inability to manage oral secretions mandates immediate surgical revision. Mild to moderate short-term dysphagia

is common but typically self-limited.[130] Patients are typically maintained on a full liquid diet at least a week after surgery, followed by gradual advancement to a pureed and then soft diet.

Long-term outcomes from laparoscopic fundoplication are overall good, with the vast majority of patients experiencing durable symptom control and objective decrease in acid exposure. Patient satisfaction after both Nissen and Toupet fundoplication approaches 90%.[128] However, several complications are worth noting.

- Dysphagia—The presence of dysphagia in the first few months after antireflux surgery may be as high as 50%, but this typically resolves on its own as edema and inflammation subside.[130] Patients who still can tolerate liquids should be maintained on a full liquid diet initially. Dysphagia persisting for over 3 months after antireflux surgery should be investigated with a barium swallow. This may be caused by hiatal herniation, an overly tight hiatal closure, or a malformed fundoplication. Endoscopic dilations may help address a wrap or hiatal closure that is too tight. However, hiatal herniation of the fundoplication often requires revisional surgery.[131]
- Gas bloat—Fundoplication diminishes the ability to belch and vent air from the stomach, more so with Nissen fundoplication than partial fundoplication. This can lead to a "gas bloat" syndrome. This may be treated with behavioral modification such as avoiding carbonated beverages and eating slowly. Gas-dissolving agents such as simethicone may also be helpful. However, if this does not resolve over time, additional studies can be done to assess these symptoms, including a gastric emptying study, which can be done to rule out postoperative gastroparesis, which may be the result of a vagal nerve injury.
- Recurrent GERD—Some degree of symptomatic recurrence may occur in a substantial share of patients. This often responds to acid suppression, and 20% to 40% of patients have resumed PPI use at the 15- to 20-year mark after surgery.[128,132]
- Wrap failure—Fundoplications can become structurally disrupted in various ways. The most common etiology of fundoplication failure is hiatal herniation of the wrap. All postoperative hiatal hernias are not clinically relevant, but some may cause bothersome reflux and/or dysphagia. The fundoplication can also become completely or partially undone over time.[133]

Horgan et al. published a classification of fundoplication failures in 1999 that remains relevant today when evaluating suspected anatomic failures (see Fig. 83.16). According to this study, type IA failures (herniation of the GEJ and fundoplication) most often caused heartburn with or without a component of dysphagia, but other types of failures (e.g., type IB, herniation of the GEJ; type II, herniation of the fundoplication only; or type III, malpositioned fundoplication) were frequently associated with dysphagia only[131] (Fig. 83.18).

The long-term reoperation rate after fundoplication is 5% to 7%, primarily because of recurrent GERD symptoms and/or persistent dysphagia.[134,135] Patients presenting for revisional surgical evaluation should be comprehensively evaluated with manometry and ambulatory pH monitoring, EGD, and a barium swallow. The threshold to reoperate should be higher than to perform primary surgery given the increased technical difficulty of reoperative surgery and resultant complication rate and the increased likelihood that an alternate issue (e.g., dysmotility or hypersensitivity) may be underlying the patient's symptoms. Patient satisfaction decreases with each surgical attempt, from 91% at the primary operation to 76% at the first reoperation and 49% at the second reoperation.[136]

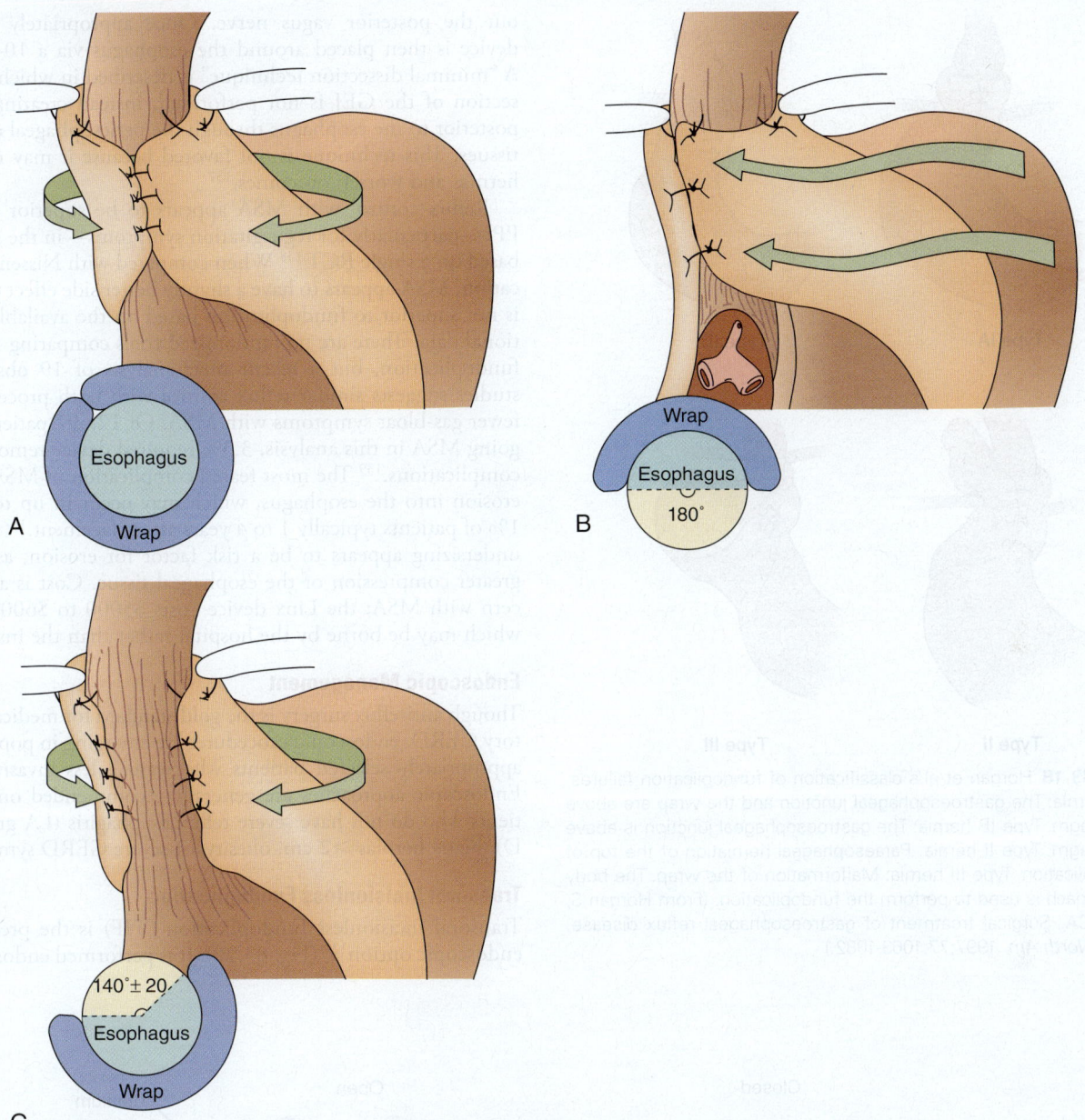

FIGURE 83.17 Three types of fundoplication. (A) 360-degree (Nissen) fundoplication. (B) Partial anterior (Dor) fundoplication. (C) Partial posterior (Toupet) fundoplication.

In 2012, the FDA approved the Linx (Ethicon) magnetic sphincter augmentation (MSA) device as an alternative surgical treatment for medically refractory reflux, with the promise of simpler, more reproducible surgical technique and fewer side effects than fundoplication. The device has a "Roman Arch" design that, when sized appropriately, does not exert any compressive force on the esophagus when the device is in the closed position. When closed, the magnetic force is highest, but the beads exert this force on each other rather than on the esophagus. When a food bolus passes, the ring expands and the magnetic force between the beads decreases to permit bolus passage (Fig. 83.19).

The device is recommended for use in patients with grade A or B esophagitis, no hiatal hernia larger than 3 cm, BMI less than 35, and adequate esophageal motility, defined as distal wave amplitude greater than 35 mm Hg and greater than 70% effective swallows. It is not indicated for patients with paraesophageal hernias,

grade C or D esophagitis, Barrett esophagus, dysphagia or inadequate esophageal motility, or the need for MRIs greater than 1.5 Tesla. Indications with emerging clinical evidence include the use of MSA rather than fundoplication in paraesophageal hernias and in patients with reflux status post sleeve gastrectomy, who do not have a fundus with which to perform fundoplication. Observational studies suggest reflux improvement and acceptable safety in these populations, but they have not been tested in RCTs against the standard of care.

The surgical technique for Linx implantation begins similar to that of fundoplication, typically involving full dissection of the hiatus and GEH, without taking down the short gastric vessels. If a hiatal hernia is noted, it must be repaired. After this, a tunnel is created between the posterior vagus nerve and the esophagus, and a sizing device is placed circumferentially around the esophagus through this tunnel, incorporating the anterior vagus but leaving

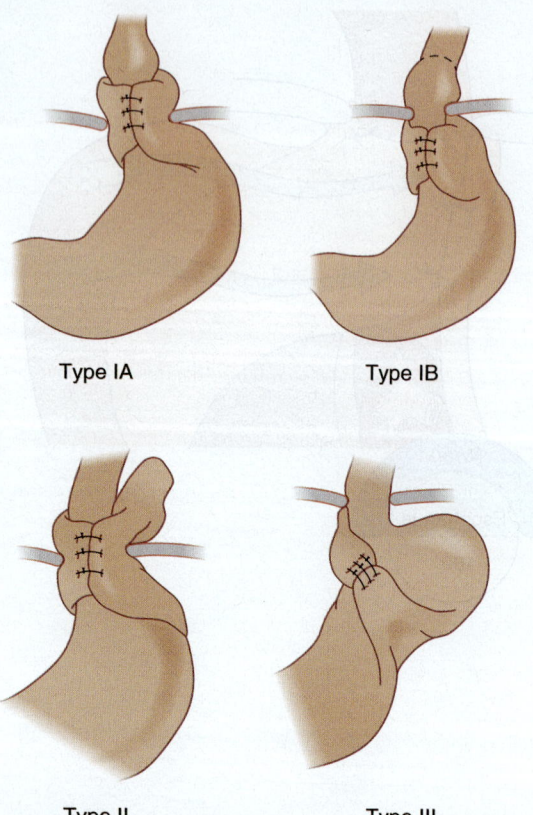

Type IA **Type IB**

Type II **Type III**

FIGURE 83.18 Horgan et al.'s classification of fundoplication failures. Type IA hernia: The gastroesophageal junction and the wrap are above the diaphragm. Type IB hernia: The gastroesophageal junction is above the diaphragm. Type II hernia: Paraesophageal herniation of the top of the fundoplication. Type III hernia: Malformation of the wrap. The body of the stomach is used to perform the fundoplication. (From Horgan S, Pellegrini CA. Surgical treatment of gastroesophageal reflux disease. *Surg Clin North Am.* 1997;77:1063-1082.)

out the posterior vagus nerve. Once appropriately sized, the device is then placed around the esophagus via a 10-mm port. A "minimal dissection technique" is described in which a full dissection of the GEJ is not performed, instead creating a tunnel posterior to the esophagus through the periesophageal connective tissues. This technique is not favored because it may miss hiatal hernias and worsen outcomes.[137]

Reflux control with MSA appears to be superior to that of PPI—particularly for regurgitation symptoms—in the short term based on a single RCT.[138] When compared with Nissen fundoplication, MSA appears to have a slightly better side effect profile but is not superior to fundoplication based on the available observational data. There are no randomized trials comparing MSA with fundoplication, but a recent meta-analysis of 19 observational studies suggests similar reflux control with both procedures and fewer gas-bloat symptoms with MSA. Of 12,697 patients undergoing MSA in this analysis, 3.3% required device removal due to complications.[139] The most feared complication of MSA is device erosion into the esophagus, which may occur in up to 0.3% to 1% of patients typically 1 to 4 years after placement.[137,140] Device undersizing appears to be a risk factor for erosion, as it causes greater compression of the esophageal tissue. Cost is also a concern with MSA; the Linx device costs $5000 to $6000 per use, which may be borne by the hospital rather than the insurer.[141]

Endoscopic Management

Though antireflux surgery is the gold standard for medically refractory GERD, endoscopic procedures are emerging in popularity for appropriately selected patients who want a less invasive option. Endoscopic approaches are generally recommended only for patients who do not have severe reflux esophagitis (LA grades C or D), hiatal hernias >2 cm, obesity, or severe GERD symptoms.

Transoral Incisionless Fundoplication

Transoral incisionless fundoplication (TIF) is the predominant endoscopic option[129] (Fig. 83.20). It is performed endoscopically,

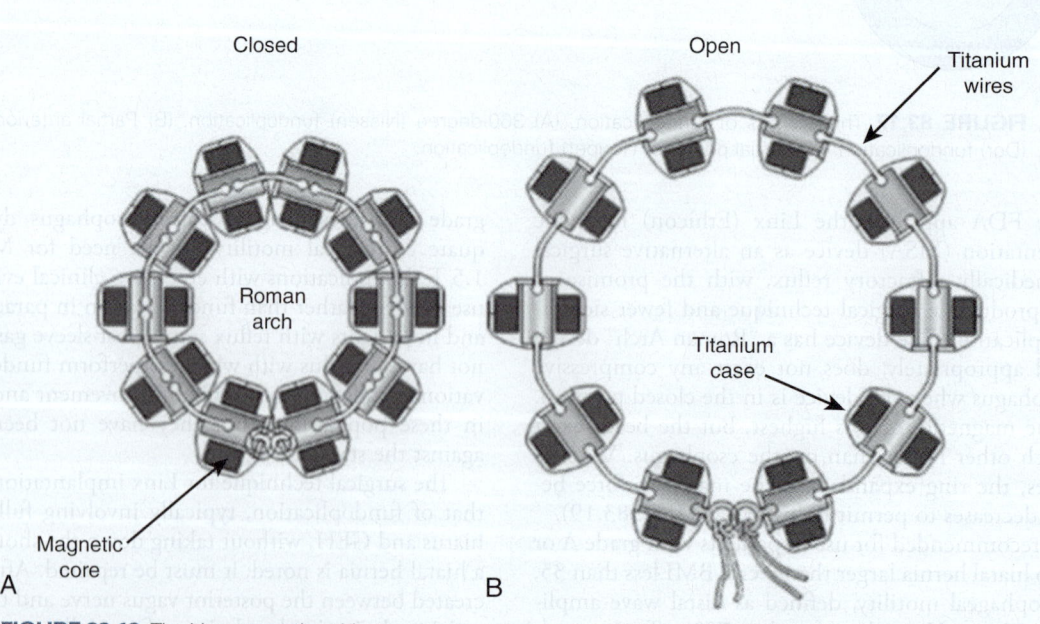

Closed Open

Titanium wires

Roman arch

Titanium case

Magnetic core

A B

FIGURE 83.19 The Linx magnetic sphincter augmentation device. (A) Illustration of closed implant. (B) Illustration of open implant.

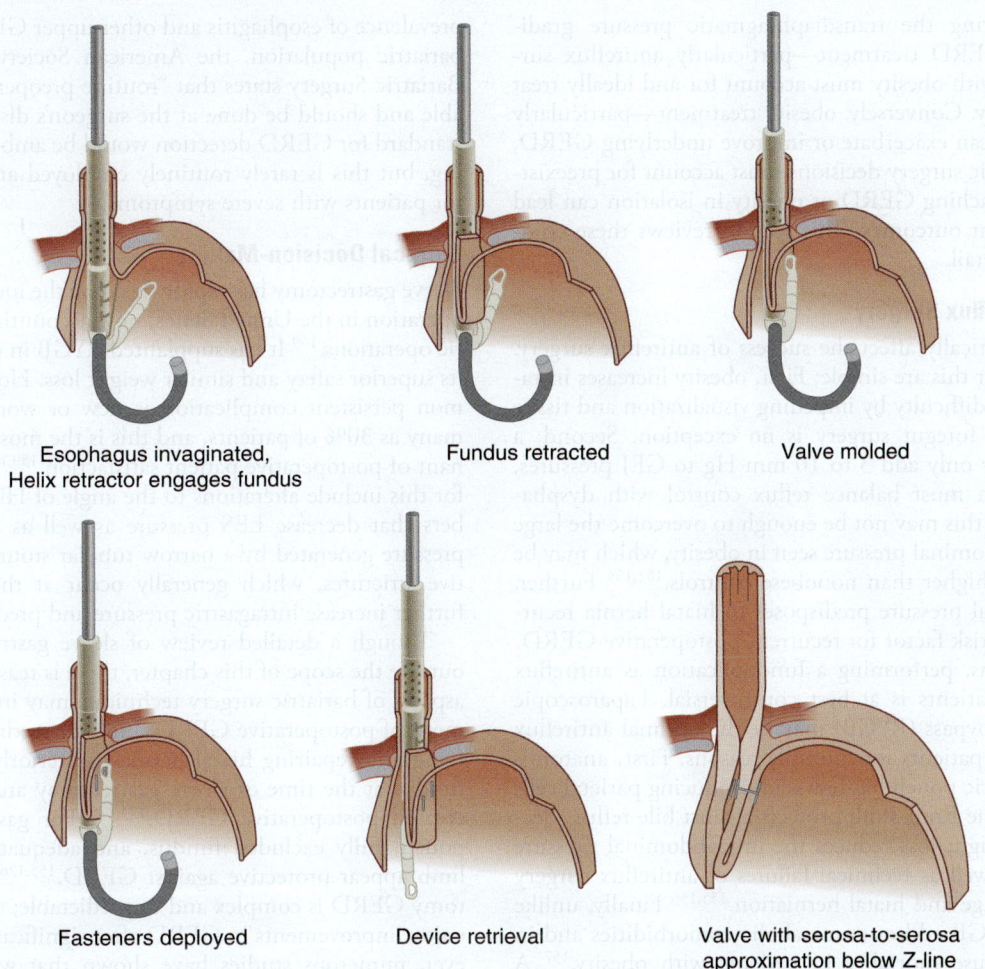

Esophagus invaginated,
Helix retractor engages fundus

Fundus retracted

Valve molded

Fasteners deployed

Device retrieval

Valve with serosa-to-serosa
approximation below Z-line

FIGURE 83.20 Illustration of the TIF 2.0 procedure (EndoGastric Solutions).

using one of two systems: the EsophyX device (EndoGastric Solutions, Redmond, WA) or Xylo Technologies system. Of these, the EsophyX TIF 2.0 device has the largest body of supporting evidence and has supplanted the TIF 1.0 technique first published in 2008. The EsophyX is an over-the-scope device that uses a helical retractor to pull the fundus into the gastric lumen, then deploys polypropylene H-fasteners between the fundus and esophageal lumen. These are carried circumferentially to create a 270-degree, 3-cm fundoplication. The technique requires general anesthesia and two skilled operators. TIF 2.0 has a 2.4% rate of severe complications, including perforations, bleeding, and pneumothorax.[142] In terms of outcomes, TIF 2.0 has shown superiority to PPI for subjective and objective reflux resolution in multiple RCTs.[142–146] However, evidence comparing TIF 2.0 to fundoplication is lacking, leading the most recent multispecialty consensus guidelines to favor fundoplication over TIF 2.0.[129] TIF may have a role in treating medically refractory heartburn or regurgitation in patients who wish to avoid surgery and do not have contraindications to endoscopic management.[129,147] It bears noting that some patients may have persistent symptoms after TIF, and performing a surgical fundoplication after TIF can be challenging.

The MUSE system consists of an endoscopic stapling device coupled with an ultrasound transducer. The technique involves retroflexing an endoscope within the stomach, with the stapler at the tip used to push the fundus toward the esophagus, where the ultrasound confirms correct alignment of the fundoplication. Staples are serially fired until an anterior fundoplication is created. Outside of small observational studies, evidence comparing MUSE with other antireflux treatment is lacking, and this procedure is not widespread in the United States.[148–150]

Stretta

Stretta (Mederi Therapeutics, Norwalk, CT) is another endoscopic antireflux device that delivers radiofrequency energy to the distal esophagus, thickening the muscular tissue, increasing LES pressure, and decreasing transient relaxations. Based on inconsistent efficacy, guidelines currently favor fundoplication over Stretta based on superior reflux control and patient satisfaction. According to the most recent guidelines of the American Gastroenterological Association, Stretta should not be considered in any scenario of PPI-refractory cases.[129,147]

Gastroesophageal Reflux Disease and Obesity

Obesity and reflux are deeply intertwined. For one, obesity is a key factor in the pathogenesis of GERD: Obesity increases intraabdominal pressure, thus augmenting the transdiaphragmatic pressure gradient driving GERD. Obesity is associated with increased GERD severity as well as rates of esophagitis and esophageal and gastric adenocarcinoma. This has numerous mechanisms, outlined earlier, including an increase in transient LES relaxations and, most notably, an increase in intraabdominal pressures exacerbating the transdiaphragmatic pressure gradient.[151] As such, GERD treatment—particularly antireflux surgery—in patients with obesity must account for and ideally treat obesity concurrently. Conversely, obesity treatment—particularly bariatric surgery—can exacerbate or improve underlying GERD, and as such, bariatric surgery decisions must account for preexisting GERD. Approaching GERD or obesity in isolation can lead to untenable patient outcomes. This section reviews these complex decisions in detail.

Obesity and Antireflux Surgery

Obesity can dramatically affect the success of antireflux surgery. The mechanisms for this are simple: First, obesity increases intraoperative technical difficulty by impeding visualization and tissue manipulation, and foregut surgery is no exception. Second, a fundoplication may only add 3 to 10 mm Hg to GEJ pressures, as a fundoplication must balance reflux control with dysphagia.[152,153] However, this may not be enough to overcome the large increase in intraabdominal pressure seen in obesity, which may be 15 to 20 mm Hg higher than nonobese controls.[151,154] Further, high intraabdominal pressure predisposes to hiatal hernia recurrence, another key risk factor for recurrent postoperative GERD.

For these reasons, performing a fundoplication as antireflux surgery in obese patients is at best controversial. Laparoscopic Roux-en-Y gastric bypass (RYGB) may be the optimal antireflux operation in obese patients for multiple reasons. First, anatomically, the short gastric pouch has few acid-producing parietal cells and the length of the Roux limb protects against bile reflux. Second, significant weight loss reduces the intraabdominal pressure driving GERD as well as technical failures of antireflux surgery such as wrap slippage and hiatal herniation.[155,156] Finally, unlike fundoplication, RYGB addresses metabolic comorbidities and in turn reduces all-cause mortality in patients with obesity.[157] A SAGES Foregut Task Force White Paper from 2020 stated that in patients with BMI >35, "RYGB is the [antireflux] procedure of choice for patients with GERD."[158] However, patients who undergo gastric bypass have a 10% to 30% risk of ongoing reflux symptoms or need for ongoing antireflux medications.[159–165] They also risk long-term complications including marginal ulceration, dumping syndrome, and internal hernias. Some patients are not good candidates for RYGB or may be unwilling to undergo such a complex procedure. As such, a subsequent multisociety consensus guideline softened the recommendation for RYGB, stating that patients with reflux and BMI >35 should be offered the choice between fundoplication and RYGB, but that with BMI >50, RYGB only should be offered as an antireflux procedure.[129]

Gastroesophageal Reflux Disease and Bariatric Surgery

Among patients seeking bariatric surgery, 20% to 40% may have preexisting GERD.[166] Bariatric surgery confers numerous benefits to patients' quality and quantity of life, but it may worsen GERD in a subset of patients. This section reviews best practice in evaluating, preventing, and managing GERD around bariatric surgery.

Preoperative Evaluation

A history inquiring about upper GI symptoms before proceeding with bariatric surgery is essential. However, as 20% of asymptomatic patients may have "silent" esophagitis and up to 40% may have abnormal acid exposure on pH monitoring, history alone is an insensitive screening test for GERD.[166–168] Many programs routinely use some form of objective evaluation before proceeding with bariatric surgery, but this is by no means universal. Given the prevalence of esophagitis and other upper GI abnormalities in the bariatric population, the American Society for Metabolic and Bariatric Surgery states that "routine preoperative EGD is justifiable and should be done at the surgeon's discretion."[166] The gold standard for GERD detection would be ambulatory pH monitoring, but this is rarely routinely employed and generally reserved for patients with severe symptoms.

Surgical Decision-Making

Sleeve gastrectomy has rapidly become the most common bariatric operation in the United States, now accounting for 70% of bariatric operations.[169] It has supplanted RYGB in popularity because of its superior safety and similar weight loss. However, its most common persistent complication is new or worsening GERD in as many as 30% of patients, and this is the most important determinant of postoperative patient satisfaction.[159,160,170,171] Mechanisms for this include alterations to the angle of His and gastric sling fibers that decrease LES pressure as well as the high intragastric pressure generated by a narrow tubular stomach.[172,173] Postoperative strictures, which generally occur at the incisura angularis, further increase intragastric pressure and predispose to reflux.

Though a detailed review of sleeve gastrectomy technique is outside the scope of this chapter, there is reasonable evidence that aspects of bariatric surgery technique may influence the development of postoperative GERD. Fully dissecting the hiatus, identifying and repairing hiatal hernias posteriorly, and excluding the fundus at the time of sleeve gastrectomy are associated with decreased postoperative GERD.[174,175] For gastric bypass, a small pouch, fully excluded fundus, and adequate (>100 cm) Roux limb appear protective against GERD.[155,176] Post–sleeve gastrectomy GERD is complex and unpredictable; many patients in fact enjoy improvements in GERD after significant weight loss. However, numerous studies have shown that when compared with sleeve gastrectomy, RYGB has a superior impact on GERD outcomes, and as such, it is the bariatric operation of choice in patients with medically refractory reflux.[129,158–160,171] However, given its long-term complication profile, some patients with GERD and obesity are not good candidates for RYGB, and bariatric decision-making in these cases needs to be individualized for each patient.

Managing Post–Bariatric Surgery Gastroesophageal Reflux Disease

As in the general population, behavioral modification and PPIs are the initial management of postoperative reflux. However, for refractory symptoms, we recommend a comprehensive workup akin to that of any patient considering antireflux surgery, including upper GI, EGD, pH monitoring, and esophageal manometry. In fact, the American Society for Metabolic and Bariatric Surgery (ASMBS) conditionally recommends routine EGD 3 to 5 years after sleeve gastrectomy to screen for Barrett esophagus even in asymptomatic patients.[166] This evaluation is needed to prove the diagnosis of GERD, identify complications of GERD, and assess for related pathology such as hiatal hernias and esophageal dysmotility.

Patients who have undergone sleeve gastrectomy cannot receive fundoplication, as they no longer have a fundus. The gold standard treatment for severe GERD in patients who have undergone sleeve gastrectomy is conversion to RYGB.[129,155,161,164] There is interest in revisional antireflux options that do not carry the risks of RYGB. If a hiatal hernia is present, some surgeons simply repair the hernia. Several small single-arm studies suggest this may be effective for several years.[177–179] MSA has also been used in the post–sleeve gastrectomy population, with a subjective response rate of 80.8% at 1 year.[180] However, the long-term durability of these approaches is unknown, and they are less likely to be effective in patients with BMI >35.

Patients with reflux after RYGB have few revisional options. Given the numerous antireflux mechanisms of RYGB, it is essential to objectively confirm the diagnosis of GERD in these patients using pH monitoring before considering revisional surgery. If patients with confirmed GERD have a significant hiatal hernia, repairing this may address symptoms. Fundoplication using the fundus of the remnant stomach has been described but is not mainstream practice. MSA has been employed in post-RYGB patients but has much less supporting evidence than post–sleeve gastrectomy.[181]

Gastroesophageal Reflux Disease and Idiopathic Pulmonary Fibrosis

Idiopathic pulmonary fibrosis (IPF) is a chronic and progressive form of usual interstitial pneumonia of unknown origin that leads to pulmonary fibrosis. IPF affects about 40,000 individuals every year in the United States. Median survival after the diagnosis is established is between 3 and 5 years, with approximately 80% of all deaths caused by respiratory failure. Because pharmacologic therapy is mostly ineffective, lung transplantation offers the only chance of survival.

Although the pathogenesis of this disease is probably multifactorial, there is evidence today that GERD might play a role in the genesis and/or progression of the disease through repeated episodes of microaspiration of gastric contents.

GERD is quite common in patients with IPF, with pH monitoring showing high rates of pathologic reflux: between 60% and 70% in the distal esophagus and 30% and 50% in the upper esophagus.[182,183] Esophageal manometry has shown that in patients with IPF, the LES is often hypotensive and esophageal peristalsis abnormal.[184] A hiatal hernia is frequently present and associated with a higher reflux score. In addition, an increased transdiaphragmatic pressure gradient caused by a more negative intrathoracic pressure might contribute to gastroesophageal reflux.[154,185] These findings suggest that patients with IPF are at high risk of aspiration of gastric contents.

Although the findings of these studies show a high prevalence of pathologic reflux in patients with IPF and potential for aspiration of gastric contents, the relationship of GERD and IPF is still uncertain, as it is not clear if these two diseases are independent from each other or if GERD contributes to the genesis and progression of IPF. This is of key importance, as it would influence both the diagnostic evaluation and treatment: Specifically, would the treatment of the abnormal reflux influence the progression of the disease?

Considering the elements that play a role in causing the abnormal reflux, it is doubtful that PPI can be an effective treatment, as it is known that although they can suppress the acid production by the parietal cells, therefore changing the pH of the refluxate, they are not able to stop the reflux through an incompetent LES. Only a fundoplication, by restoring the competence of the LES, can control any type of reflux, acidic or nonacidic.

As of today, there are only a few retrospective studies in the literature that have assessed the effect of antireflux treatment in patients with IPF and GERD. For instance, Lee et al. assessed the effect of antireflux treatment—PPI or Nissen fundoplication—in a large cohort of patients with IPF.[186] The study cohort consisted of 204 patients with IPF from the University of California San Francisco and the Mayo Clinic in Rochester. Mean forced vital

capacity (FVC) was 69% predicted, and the diffusing capacity for carbon monoxide (DLCO) was 47% predicted. Eighty-six patients were treated with PPI and 17 with H2-blocking agents. Eleven patients had a Nissen fundoplication. The study showed that use of acid-reducing medications or laparoscopic antireflux surgery (LARS) was associated with lower high-resolution CT fibrosis score and longer survival time in patients from both institutions, suggesting that gastroesophageal reflux and microaspiration may play an important role in the pathobiology of IPF.

To properly test the hypothesis that treatment of GERD in IPF could change the natural history of the disease by altering the progression, a prospective, randomized trial was designed—the WRAP-IPF trial.[187] In this phase II NIH trial, patients with IPF and GERD were recruited from six academic centers in the United States. The enrolled patients had abnormal acid exposure by 24-hour pH monitoring and preserved FVC. The primary end point was change in the FVC from randomization to week 48. Twenty-nine patients were randomly assigned to receive surgery and 29 to no surgery (treated with PPIs). All patients tolerated the LARS well with no complications. The results showed that there was no difference between the two groups in terms of FVC. Acute exacerbations, respiratory-related hospitalizations, nonelective hospitalization, and lung transplantation were less common in the surgery group but without statistical significance. In summary, this long-awaited controlled trial in patients with IPF and GERD showed that LARS was safe and well tolerated and suggested that antireflux surgery significantly did not slow the rate of FVC decline.[187] Unfortunately, a careful analysis of the methods and the results shows that this study had many severe flaws that compromise the validity of the conclusions: The study was very underpowered, as 400 patients rather than 58 were required to achieve 90% power. In addition, the effect of LARS on FVC decline and clinical events in patients with IPF and GERD might have been reduced by the near-universal use of antiacid medications in the nonsurgery group. Finally, when the authors did a post hoc exploratory analysis of the primary end point using Lachin worst rank analysis (an approach that assumes that missing values are informative and reflect poor outcomes), the difference between groups was significant ($p = 0.017$) and favored the surgical group.

Recently a bidirectional two-sample Mendelian randomization study demonstrated that GERD increases the risk of IPF but found no evidence that IPF increases the risk of GERD.[188] In addition, abnormal bolus reflux on impedance pH testing is associated with decreased time to poor pulmonary outcomes and death.[189]

Overall, these studies suggest that there is a subgroup of patients with IPF in whom pathologic reflux is documented who might benefit from antireflux therapy, particularly before a lung transplant: These are patients in whom proximal reflux is documented by pH monitoring or impedance, and pepsin or bile acids are detected in the bronchoalveolar lavage fluid (BALF), suggesting that aspiration of gastric contents is occurring. These patients might benefit from fundoplication before their functional status deteriorates.

HIATAL AND PARAESOPHAGEAL HERNIAS

Hiatal hernias have an important association with GERD; identifying and repairing these are key components of antireflux surgery. Paraesophageal hernias, a subset of hiatal hernias, are often themselves an indication for surgery, with unique symptomatology, evaluation, and treatment considerations (Fig. 83.21).

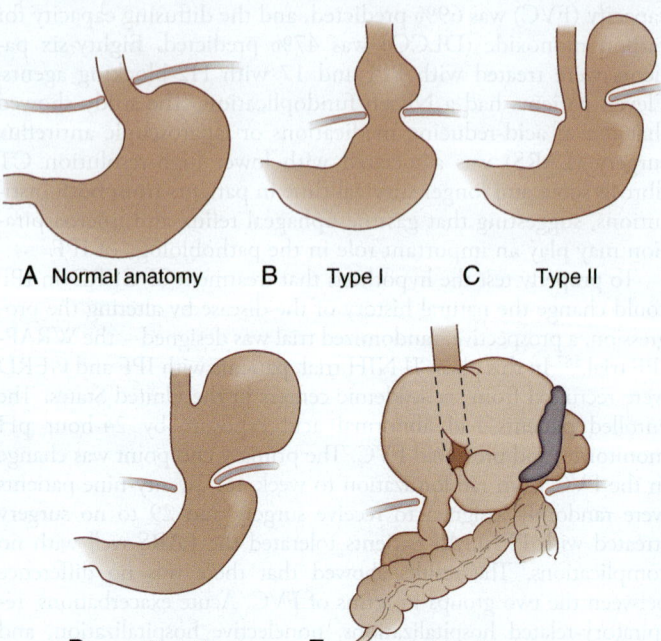

FIGURE 83.21 Hiatal hernia types. (A) normal anatomy. The stomach is completely in the abdomen. (B) Type I: esophagogastric juntion is above the diaphragm. (C) Type II: esophagogastric juntion is in the abdomen but the gastric fundus is herniated. (D) Type III: both esophagogastric juntion and the gastric fundus are herniated. (E) Type IV: another organ apart from the stomach is also herniated.

Classification and Pathophysiology

In normal anatomy, the GEJ and the entire stomach lie within the abdomen, below the diaphragmatic hiatus. Hiatal hernias are classified as follows, with type II, III, and IV considered "true" paraesophageal hernias. Overall, hiatal hernias may be present in 10% to 15% of adults based on radiologic studies.[190]

- *Type I* (aka "sliding" hiatal hernia)—The GEJ migrates through the hiatus into the mediastinum. These are the vast majority (70%–90%) of all hiatal hernias and may not be clinically significant unless they are associated with severe GERD or other symptoms.
- *Type II*—The fundus migrates into the mediastinum, but the GEJ remains intraabdominal. These are uncommon.
- *Type III*—The GEJ and a portion of the stomach have herniated. These are the most common "true" paraesophageal hernias.
- *Type IV*—The stomach and another intraabdominal organ (typically colon, pancreas, omentum, or spleen) form the hernia contents.

Hiatal hernias result from laxity of the diaphragmatic crura and the phrenoesophageal ligaments. They likely progress in part because of the transdiaphragmatic pressure gradient; as such, they are more common in patients with high intraabdominal pressure (e.g., obesity, weightlifters) and low intrathoracic pressure (e.g., chronic pulmonary disease). They are more common in females and with increasing age.[190,191]

Clinical Presentation

Because the diaphragmatic crura are a key component of the GEJ antireflux barrier, hiatal hernias (particularly sliding hernias) contribute to the development of GERD, esophagitis, and Barrett esophagus.[192] The prevalence of hiatal hernias may be as high as

75% in patients with objectively confirmed GERD.[193] Moreover, hiatal hernias may cause symptoms that do not resolve with acid suppression, such as regurgitation or dysphagia.

True paraesophageal hernias do more than undermine the antireflux barrier; they may compress the GEJ or the stomach and cause obstructive symptoms such as dysphagia, early satiety, pain, regurgitation, and/or bloating. They also have numerous non-GI implications. Paraesophageal hernias may cause dyspnea and pulmonary complications because of mass effect, cardiac compression, and/or microaspiration, which improve after repair.[191,194,195] They are also associated with anemia in 30% to 40% of patients; chronic gastric compression can lead to ischemic "Cameron ulcers" that resolve when the hernia is repaired.[196] Rarely, a paraesophageal hernia can cause acute gastric volvulus, resulting in obstruction, ischemia, and possible gastric perforation.

Evaluation and Decision-Making

When patients present for surgical consultation regarding a hiatal hernia, the initial history and physical are like those for GERD. Often the hiatal hernia is identified during the preoperative evaluation for GERD. In addition to these symptoms, surgeons should inquire about non-GI symptoms outlined earlier. Patients with paraesophageal hernias are often more frail and elderly than the typical general surgical population, so specific attention should be paid to cardiopulmonary risk factors and exercise tolerance. However, laparoscopic paraesophageal hernia repair remains safe even in these populations.

In terms of diagnostic workup, hiatal hernia is typically identified during an EGD or imaging such as CT scan or barium swallow. Chest x-ray may sometimes identify a large hernia, but it needs to be followed with dedicated imaging. Barium swallow does provide the highest degree of detail regarding the anatomy of the hernia and the presence of associated pathology (e.g., esophageal webs, strictures, dysmotility) but is not necessarily required if CT imaging clearly shows a large paraesophageal hernia. Upper endoscopy is strongly recommended before surgery to assess for mucosal pathology. The degree and size of herniation are assessed in retroflexion after the stomach is fully insufflated. Historically, the Hill grading system was used to classify the GEJ flap valve. In 2023 the American Foregut Society Endoscopic Classification of Esophagogastric Junction Integrity was described, and time will tell if this is more broadly adopted (Fig. 83.22).[197]

Additional testing such as esophageal manometry and ambulatory pH monitoring may be useful in patients with sliding hiatal hernias but is not necessary in patients with true paraesophageal hernias. Esophageal manometry is particularly unreliable with large paraesophageal hernias, and some degree of dysmotility should be presumed in these patients.

All sliding hiatal hernias do not require surgery; they should only be repaired if patients otherwise qualify for antireflux surgery (or bariatric surgery) based on objective physiologic testing and symptoms that persist after maximal medical therapy. Historically, all paraesophageal hernias were thought to require surgery, regardless of symptoms, based on the risk of acute gastric volvulus causing catastrophic outcomes. However, the risk of acute volvulus is low, currently estimated at 1% per year, and operative mortality after emergency repair is lower than previously thought—5.4% based on Nationwide Inpatient Sample data.[198] As such, paraesophageal hernia repair is currently recommended only for patients with associated symptoms or complications. Paraesophageal hernias may only cause atypical or subtle symptoms, though, and up to 90% of patients may disclose symptoms when carefully questioned.[199] Repair in asymptomatic patients remains

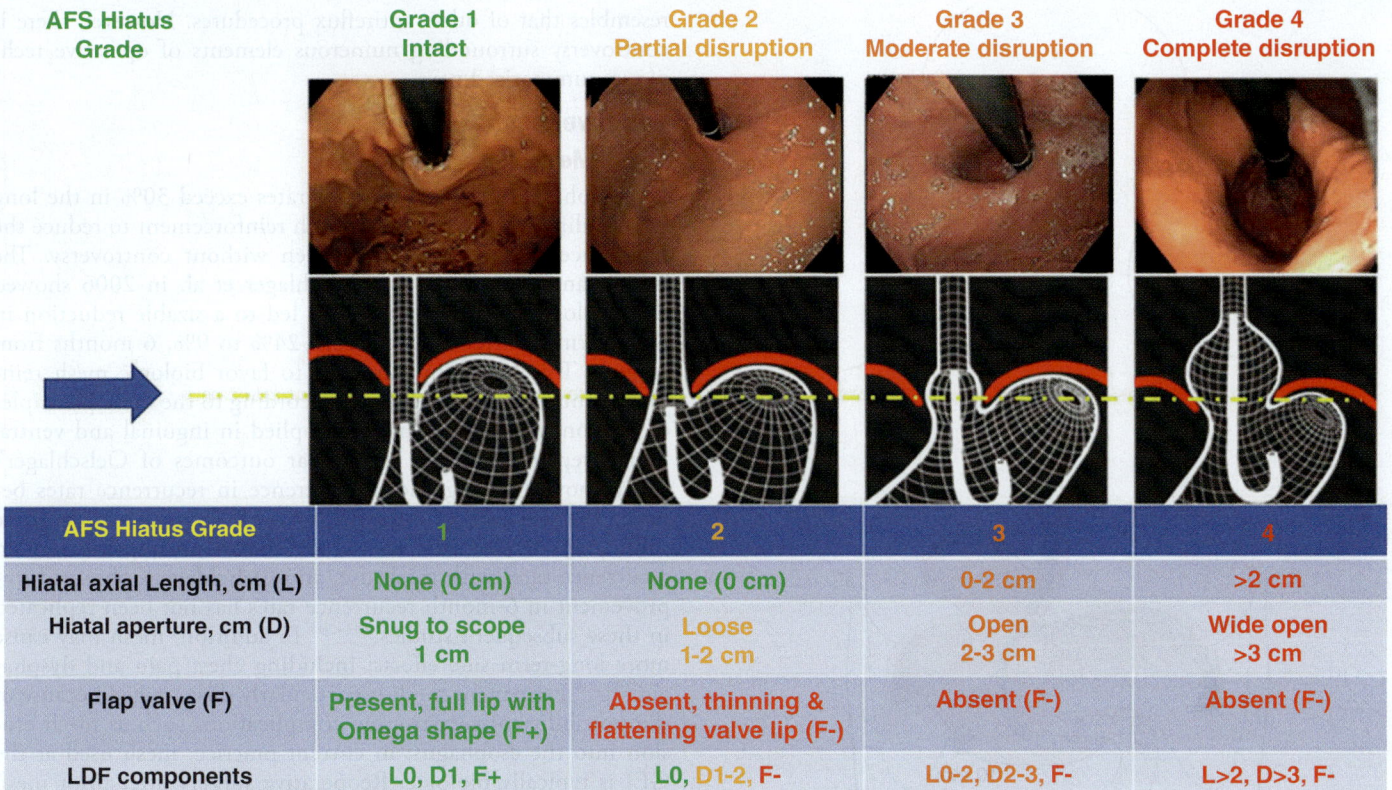

AFS Hiatus Grade	Grade 1 Intact	Grade 2 Partial disruption	Grade 3 Moderate disruption	Grade 4 Complete disruption
AFS Hiatus Grade	1	2	3	4
Hiatal axial Length, cm (L)	None (0 cm)	None (0 cm)	0-2 cm	>2 cm
Hiatal aperture, cm (D)	Snug to scope 1 cm	Loose 1-2 cm	Open 2-3 cm	Wide open >3 cm
Flap valve (F)	Present, full lip with Omega shape (F+)	Absent, thinning & flattening valve lip (F-)	Absent (F-)	Absent (F-)
LDF components	L0, D1, F+	L0, D1-2, F-	L0-2, D2-3, F-	L>2, D>3, F-

FIGURE 83.22 The American Foregut Society *(AFS)* Endoscopic Classification of Esophagogastric Junction Integrity. The "L" within the LDF components represents the hiatal hernia length, measured in centimeters between the Z line and the diaphragmatic pinch. The "D" represents the largest diameter of the hiatus measured in centimeters with 1 conventional scope diameter being approximately 1 centimeter; and the "F" represents the presence (F+) or absence (F−) of the gastroesophageal flap valve. (From Del Grande LM, Herbella FAM, Katayama RC, Schlottmann F, Patti MG. The role of the transdiaphragmatic pressure gradient in the pathophysiology of gastroesophageal reflux disease. *Arq Gastroenterol.* 2018;55[Suppl 1]:13-17.)

controversial and may be offered based on shared decision-making and patient fitness for surgery.[200]

Surgical Treatment

In current practice, laparoscopic and robotic transabdominal approaches dominate the treatment of paraesophageal hernia. Transthoracic approaches make up 2% or less of paraesophageal hernia repairs and will not be discussed here.[201] Positioning and setup for paraesophageal hernia resemble that of other antireflux operations; the authors' preferred port placement is illustrated in Fig. 83.23.

The surgical approach begins like that of fundoplication described earlier in this chapter. After obtaining laparoscopic access to the peritoneum and positioning the patient in steep reverse Trendelenburg, we reduce the hernia contents with manual traction and attempt to decompress the stomach via an orogastric tube. We then enter the lesser sac with an energy device either on the right (via the pars flaccida) or the left (via the short gastrics). Once this plane is carried to the crura, the key maneuver is to develop the plane between the hernia sac medially and the crura laterally. When done precisely, the fascia overlying the crura is left intact to facilitate crural closure, and the sac is divided close to the crura. This plane is carried circumferentially, first anteriorly to the opposite crus, until the sac is largely reduced into the abdomen. Though not intended, and especially during recurrent repairs, the pleural space may end up being opened, but this is generally inconsequential because the patient is being ventilated with positive pressure and the CO_2 used for

insufflation absorbs rapidly. If the patient has respiratory issues, the pleural tear can be enlarged to equalize the pressure with the abdomen, the insufflation pressure can be temporarily decreased, and the anesthesiologist can increase the respiratory rate to address CO_2 retention. After the sac is mobilized anteriorly, we typically carry the dissection posterior to the esophagus, encircling the esophagus with an elastic drain to facilitate retraction. The sac's attachments to the pleura and mediastinum must be completely mobilized out of the chest with blunt dissection or an energy device, and the esophagus is also fully mobilized. Excision of the hernia sac is important because its bulk may interfere with subsequent fundoplication or serve as a lead point for rehatation; however, one must take care not to injure the vagi, esophagus, or stomach during this step. As the stomach and esophagus are reduced into the abdomen, the vagus nerves will enter the field and must be identified and protected. We continue dividing attachments of the esophagus to the mediastinum until we obtain at least 2 to 3 cm of intraabdominal esophageal length off tension. This dissection can be carried up to the pulmonary veins or even the aortic arch if necessary; laparoscopic visualization is typically excellent and can be enhanced with a 0-, 30-, or even a 45-degree scope to look high in the mediastinum.

Hiatal Closure

Once we have adequate esophageal length, we proceed with hiatal closure. Numerous techniques exist for hiatal closure: interrupted, running, figure-eight, and mattress patterns are all used, with

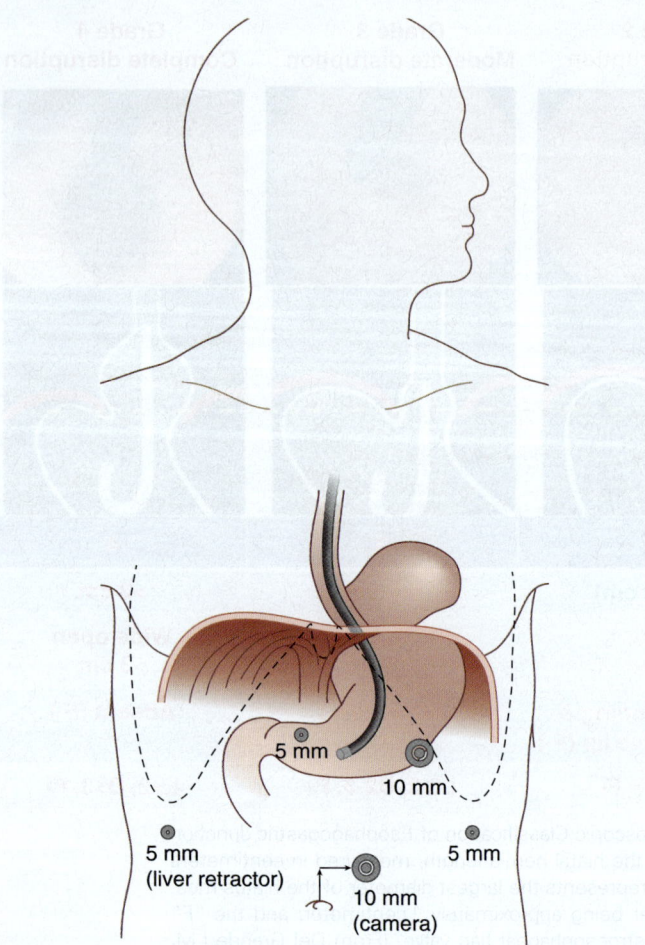

FIGURE 83.23 The authors' preferred port placement for paraesophageal hernia repair.

braided permanent sutures, which can be placed intracorporeally, using a free needle, Endo-Stitch, or extracorporeal knot-tying system. We generally use double pledgeted 0-Ethibond suture in an interrupted suture pattern. No suturing technique has proven superior to any other, but a posterior repair with permanent suture is generally preferred. It is critical to avoid aortic injury while passing the suture through the left crus at the bottom-most suture, which we do by passing the left-handed grasper between the aorta and the left crus before suturing; this creates distance between the aorta and the crus while also deflecting the path away from the aorta. When suturing the right crus, it is similarly critical to avoid injuring the inferior vena cava. Sutures begin posteriorly and are tied sequentially toward the esophagus. We generally include at least one hiatal stitch anterior to the esophagus to help minimize recurrence anteriorly and to avoid abnormally kinking the esophagus with repair of large hiatal hernias where numerous posterior sutures are required. We ensure that the hiatal closure is not overly tight by retracting the esophagus gently in multiple directions and assessing the ease with which an instrument will pass alongside the esophagus through the closure.

Generally, even large defects can be approximated primarily with sutures without excessive tension. If they cannot, relaxing incisions can be performed in the fascial covering of the right or left hemidiaphragm to reduce tension, with that defect closed with mesh. After hiatal closure, a partial fundoplication is generally performed to conclude the procedure. Postoperative care

resembles that of other antireflux procedures. However, there is controversy surrounding numerous elements of operative technique, summarized next.

Controversies

Use of Mesh

Paraesophageal hernia recurrence rates exceed 30% in the long run, leading many to propose mesh reinforcement to reduce the recurrence rate. This has not been without controversy. The initial randomized trial by Oelschlager et al. in 2006 showed that biologic mesh reinforcement led to a sizable reduction in short-term recurrence rates, from 24% to 9%, 6 months from surgery. This led many surgeons to favor biologic mesh reinforcement of the hiatal closure, according to the same principles of tension-free closure that are applied in inguinal and ventral hernia repair. However, the 5-year outcomes of Oelschlager's study showed no significant difference in recurrence rates between the two arms (mesh 54%, no mesh 59%, $p = 0.7$). Three subsequent randomized trials have shown no improvement in recurrence rates with mesh use, and Oelschlager's observed improvement in 6-month recurrence rates has not been replicated in these subsequent studies.[202–204] In addition, mesh may cause more long-term side effects, including chest pain and dysphagia.[202,203] Permanent mesh is particularly discouraged because of the possibility of catastrophic complications such as mesh erosion into the esophagus; in current practice, mesh used at the GEJ is typically biologic. Reoperative surgery after prior mesh repairs has a very high complication rate and may require esophagectomy. As such, we currently avoid mesh in paraesophageal hernia repair, with the rare exception of cases with very poor tissue quality or excessive tension despite relaxing incisions. With a relaxing incision, mesh can be used to cover the defect created, without having it right against the hiatal opening or the esophagus. Overall, whether or not to use mesh remains controversial, and practice varies considerably.[200]

Fundoplication

Fundoplication has been traditionally included in paraesophageal hernia repair to prevent the subsequent onset of reflux. Because esophageal manometry is unreliable in this population, and because this population is at risk of esophageal dysmotility because of age and long-standing reflux, a partial fundoplication is typically performed. This limits the risk of postoperative dysphagia relative to a complete (Nissen) fundoplication. A fundoplication is also thought to add bulk to the LES complex with additional suturing that may protect against hiatal hernia recurrence. However, evidence supporting fundoplication is limited. A recent meta-analysis did not identify any RCTs of fundoplication in the setting of paraesophageal hernia repair. In the retrospective studies reviewed, fundoplication was associated with lower risks of recurrent GERD (relative risk [RR] 0.64, $p = 0.07$) and hiatal hernia (RR 0.53, $p = 0.06$), but these findings were not statistically significant.[205] In emergency settings and in patients with severe esophageal dysmotility, omitting fundoplication may be reasonable.

Gastropexy

Some surgeons suture the stomach to the diaphragm to further anchor it in the abdomen. Some surgeons perform gastropexy routinely or preferentially instead of fundoplication. Many surgeons find gastropexy alone preferable in an emergency setting. When a fundoplication has not been performed, gastropexy sutures can be placed between the fundus and the left hemidiaphragm or between the greater or lesser curvature and the anterior abdominal wall. When a fundoplication has been performed, sutures can be placed posteriorly between the fundoplication and the hiatal closure. Gastrostomy tubes may also be placed in an acute setting to anchor the stomach, to provide decompression, or even for eventual feeding. The evidence to date on gastropexy is weak. Current guidelines do not recommend gastropexy in place of fundoplication in the elective setting because it may have inferior reflux outcomes.[206] However, performing gastropexy may be a benign adjunct to fundoplication as long as one does not abnormally kink the GEJ or injure an adjacent structure.[207]

Esophageal Lengthening Procedures

Surgeons generally agree that a 2- to 3-cm segment of intraabdominal esophagus is needed to prevent postoperative GERD and hiatal hernia recurrence. However, there is controversy surrounding the prevalence and management of a "short esophagus" precluding 2 to 3 cm intraabdominal length. Chronic inflammation, dysmotility, and a large hernia can foreshorten the esophagus. This has led some to employ esophageal lengthening procedures such as the Collis gastroplasty, in which linear staplers are used to perform a wedge resection of the fundus that brings the neo-GEJ 3 to 4 cm distally (Fig. 83.24).

Use of esophageal lengthening procedure varies widely by surgeon and center, likely because of practice pattern variation. The true incidence of "short esophagus" is thought to be approximately 10%, of which most cases do not require gastroplasty.[208] We find that in the vast majority of cases, with an adequate mediastinal mobilization, the GEJ will eventually reach into the abdomen off tension. Only 1% to 4% of cases are truly thought to require gastroplasty.[208]

Acute Gastric Volvulus

Acute gastric volvulus, incarceration, and/or obstruction are the feared sequelae of paraesophageal hernias. Gastric volvulus can occur in the organoaxial or mesoaxial plane (Fig. 83.25).

The classic presentation of gastric volvulus is "Borchardt triad": sudden chest or epigastric pain, dry heaving, and inability to pass a nasogastric tube. This is a surgical emergency, as it can progress to gastric ischemia and/or perforation. The first step in management is to pass a nasogastric tube for decompression; this has several benefits: (1) converting an emergent operation into one that can be performed in 24 to 48 hours; (2) facilitating hernia reduction and repair with healthy, decompressed tissue; and (3) allowing resuscitation and correction of electrolyte imbalances before surgery. If a nasogastric tube cannot be passed at bedside, it may be placed endoscopically. If this is unsuccessful, the patient must proceed immediately to surgery. If nasogastric tube placement is successful, the patient may be allowed a brief period of optimization before proceeding with paraesophageal hernia repair during the same hospital admission. Surgical technique during emergency repairs is like that in the elective situation; the stomach must be fully reduced into an intraabdominal position and the hernia must be closed. However, based on the patient's overall fitness and physiology at the time of surgery, some surgeons may defer extensive mediastinal dissection or fundoplication and simply reduce the acute herniation/volvulus and perform suture or double–percutaneous endoscopic gastrostomy (PEG) tube gastropexy instead.

Outcomes

Overall, paraesophageal hernia repair is safe and effective in high-volume centers, with a complication profile like that of other laparoscopic antireflux procedures. Short-term complications that may be more common with large paraesophageal hernias include pleural injury and capnothorax (which are typically inconsequential); injury to the esophagus, stomach, or vagus nerves; and dysphagia. The short-term mortality rate of laparoscopic repair is 0.5%.[201] In the long term, symptom relief is substantial and durable. The radiographic recurrence rate of large paraesophageal hernia repairs is high, approximately 30%, but these are typically small sliding recurrences that do not require reoperation.[201–203,209]

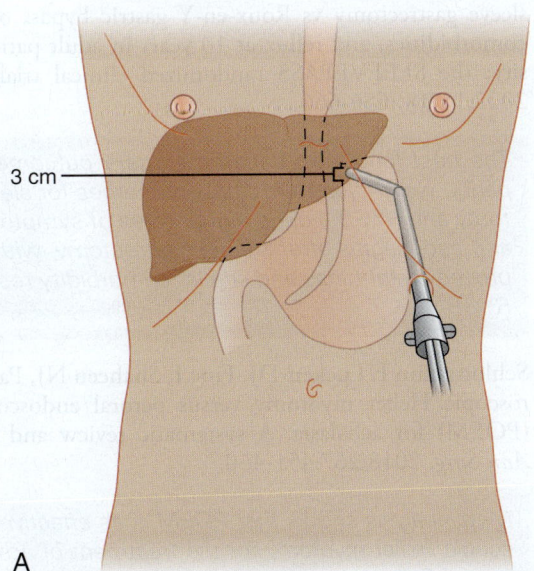
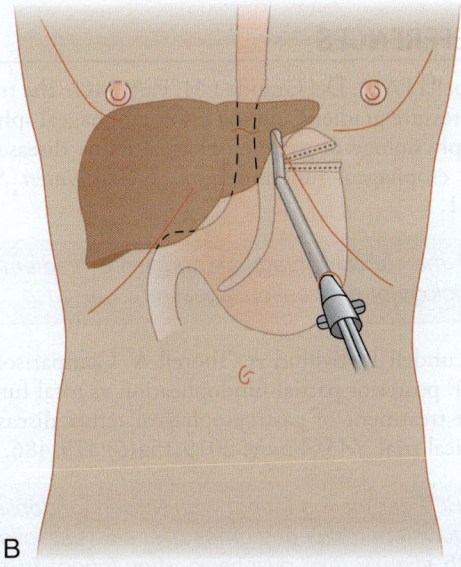

3 cm

A   B

FIGURE 83.24 Technique for laparoscopic Collis gastroplasty. (A) After placing a bougie into the stomach, a linear stapler is used to transect the fundus transversely, approximately 3 to 4 cm distal to the angle of His. (B) A second linear stapler fire is used to resect the fundus parallel to the bougie.

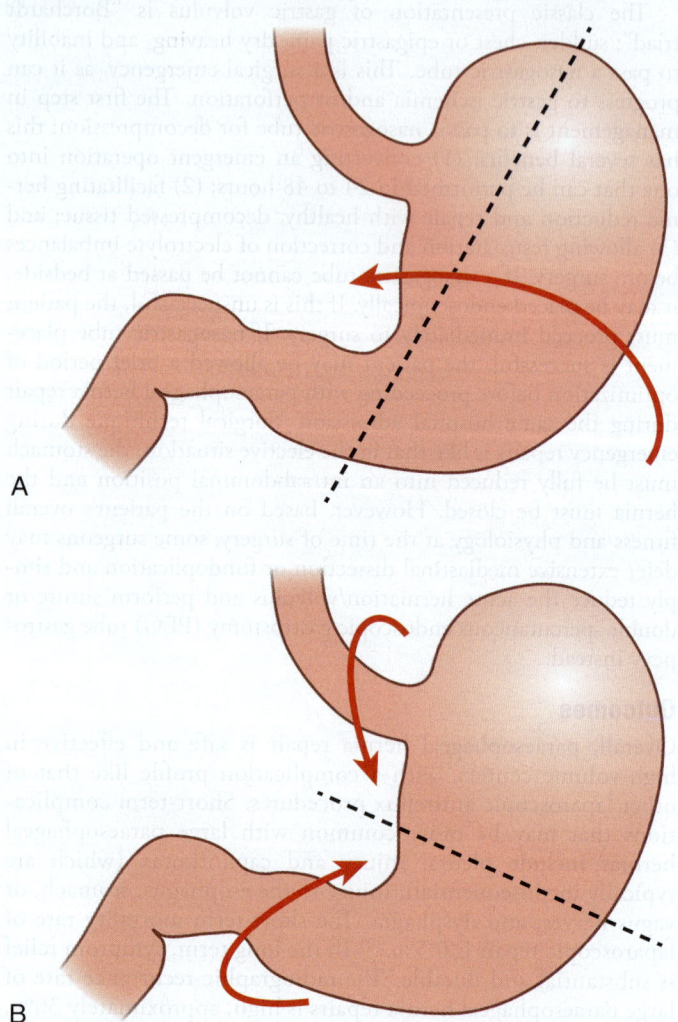

FIGURE 83.25 Classification of gastric volvulus. (A) Organoaxial volvulus. (B) Mesoaxial volvulus.

SELECTED REFERENCES

Dias NCB, Herbella FAM, Del Grande LM, Patti MG. The transdiaphragmatic pressure gradient and the lower esophageal sphincter in the pathophysiology of gastroesophageal reflux disease: an analysis of 500 esophageal function tests. *J Gastrointest Surg.* 2023;27:677-681.

Importance of the transdiaphragmatic pressure gradient in the pathophysiology of gastroesophageal reflux disease.

Håkanson BS, Lundell L, Bylund A, Thorell A. Comparison of laparoscopic 270° posterior partial fundoplication vs total fundoplication for the treatment of gastroesophageal reflux disease: a randomized clinical trial. *JAMA Surg.* 2019;154(6):479-486.

A high-quality RCT comparing Toupet with Nissen fundoplication, finding equivalent reflux outcomes over a 3-year follow-up period, with slightly less dysphagia after Toupet in the short term.

Horgan S, Pohl D, Bogetti D, Eubanks T, Pellegrini C. Failed antireflux surgery: what have we learned from reoperations? *Arch Surg.* 1999;134(8):809-817.

A classic review of laparoscopic fundoplication technique and a classification of anatomic failures with implications for revisional surgery.

Markar SR, Menon N, Guidozzi N, et al. EAES Multidisciplinary Rapid Guideline: systematic review, meta-analysis, GRADE assessment and evidence-informed recommendations on the surgical management of paraesophageal hernias. *Surg Endosc.* 2023;37(12):9013-9029.

The most recent expert guidelines on paraesophageal hernia repair, though these are admittedly based on a limited body of evidence.

Moonen A, Annese V, Belmans A, et al. Long-term results of the European achalasia trial: a multicentre randomized controlled trial comparing pneumatic dilation versus laparoscopic Heller myotomy. *Gut.* 2016;65:732-739.

Prospective and randomized trial comparing pneumatic dilatation with laparoscopic Heller myotomy in patients with esophageal achalasia.

Nguyen NT, Thosani NC, Canto MI, et al. The American Foregut Society white paper on the endoscopic classification of esophagogastric junction integrity. *Foregut.* 2022;2(4):339-348.

This paper describes a major revision to the Hill classification of the endoscopic appearance of the GEJ in the context of paraesophageal hernias, including factors like axial hiatal hernia length and flap valve, to enhance the endoscopic classification of hiatal hernias.

Salminen P, Grönroos S, Helmiö M, et al. Effect of laparoscopic sleeve gastrectomy vs Roux-en-Y gastric bypass on weight loss, comorbidities, and reflux at 10 years in adult patients with obesity: the SLEEVEPASS randomized clinical trial. *JAMA Surg.* 2022;157(8):656-666.

The best long-term bariatric surgery outcome data, comparing weight loss and reflux outcomes for sleeve gastrectomy and RYGB. Found higher rates of symptomatic GERD and esophagitis after sleeve gastrectomy, with slightly improved weight loss and similar comorbidity resolution after RYGB.

Schlottmann F, Luckett DJ, Fine J, Shaheen NJ, Patti MG. Laparoscopic Heller myotomy versus peroral endoscopic myotomy (POEM) for achalasia. A systematic review and meta-analysis. *Ann Surg.* 2018;267:451-460.

Meta-analysis shows that POEM is as effective as a laparoscopic Heller myotomy for the treatment of achalasia, but it is associated with a very high incidence of pathologic gastroesophageal reflux.

Slater BJ, Collings A, Dirks R, et al. Multi-society consensus conference and guideline on the treatment of gastroesophageal reflux disease (GERD). *Surg Endosc.* 2023;37(2):781-806.

> The most recent and authoritative guidelines for the multidisciplinary treatment of GERD, endorsed by SAGES, ASGE, ASMBS, EAES, SSAT, and STS. Primarily focused on procedural options, these discuss preoperative evaluation, endoscopic options, and management of GERD in the setting of obesity.

Watson DI, Thompson SK, Devitt PG, et al. Five-year follow-up of a randomized controlled trial of laparoscopic repair of very large hiatus hernia with sutures versus absorbable versus nonabsorbable mesh. *Ann Surg.* 2020;272(2):241.

> The most recent multicenter trial of mesh in large paraesophageal hernia repair, which concludes that there are no advantages to using mesh and potentially inferior symptom outcomes compared with suture repair.

Yadlapati R, Kahrilas PJ, Fox MR, et al. Esophageal motility disorders on high resolution manometry: Chicago classification version 4.0. *Neurogastroenterol Motil.* 2021;33:1-36.

> Most used classification of esophageal motility disorders based on high-resolution manometry.

The full reference list appears on Elsevier eBooks+.

84 | CHAPTER

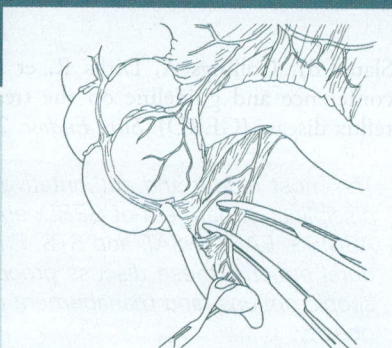

Esophageal Cancer

Ngoc-Quynh Chu, Betty Caroline Tong, Thomas D'Amico, David Harpole, and Daniela Molena

EPIDEMIOLOGY

Esophageal cancer is the seventh most common cancer in the world, with an incidence of 604,000 new cases in 2020 and accounting for 3.1% of all new cancer diagnoses. In the same year, it was the sixth leading cause of cancer mortality, with 544,000 deaths (5.5% of all cancer-related deaths).[1] In the United States, it is the 17th most common cancer, with 21,560 new diagnoses and 16,120 deaths estimated in 2023.[2] Over the past 40 to 50 years, esophageal cancer survival has markedly improved. From 1973 to 2010, 5-year overall survival (OS) increased from 3.6% to 21.1% for esophageal squamous cell carcinoma (SCC) and from 5.4% to 24.2% for esophageal adenocarcinoma.[3] Despite this, the 5-year OS rate remains only approximately 20%.[2] Because early disease is asymptomatic, most patients are usually diagnosed at an advanced stage when they present with dysphagia. At this point, most will have cancer that has already spread to regional lymph nodes (33%) or to distant sites (38%). Early-stage disease is diagnosed only in 18% of patients (Fig. 84.1).[4]

The global burden of esophageal cancer varies considerably geographically (Fig. 84.2). The highest incidence rates are found in the central Asian "esophageal cancer belt," which spans across the regions of Iran, central Asian republics, and China, followed by Southern and Eastern Africa and Northern Europe.[1] It is a disease of older age, with peak incidence in the sixth and seventh decades.[4] Males are more affected than females, with approximately 70% of cases occurring in males, and there is a twofold to threefold difference in incidence and mortality rates between the sexes.[1]

Esophageal cancer has two predominant histologic subtypes: adenocarcinoma and SCC. They differ in epidemiologic distribution, risk factors, pathogenesis, and clinical and prognostic consequences (Table 84.1). Esophageal SCC is the most common esophageal cancer worldwide, although there has been an overall decline in incidence in the last decade. The majority of cases occur

in southern Asia (from China to Mongolia, through India, and to the Middle East). At the same time, there has been an increase in the incidence of esophageal adenocarcinoma, especially in developed countries. Esophageal adenocarcinoma is the more common histology in North America and Western Europe. These trends are thought to reflect changes in the risk factors associated with each histologic subtype, namely, an increasing obesity epidemic and gastroesophageal reflux disease (GERD) contributing to adenocarcinoma, in conjunction with a global decline in alcohol and tobacco abuse, key risk factors for SCC.[1]

RISK FACTORS

The strongest risk factors for esophageal SCC are tobacco and alcohol use, with a synergistic threefold increased risk with both. The relative risk increases with the amount of alcohol consumed and the number of cigarettes smoked. The disease is three to four times more prevalent in males.[1] Dietary factors such as diets low in fruit and vegetables and vitamin and nutrient deficiencies may contribute to SCC. Consumption of foods containing N-nitrosamines, certain pickled vegetables, and high-temperature liquids or foods have also been implicated.[5] Although human papillomavirus (HPV) has been implicated in other SCC cancers, HPV-related SCC represents only a small subset of esophageal SCC, with unclear clinical implications. Disorders of the esophagus that contribute to a chronic inflammatory state, such as achalasia, Plummer-Vinson syndrome, and a history of caustic ingestion, can also increase the risk of SCC. Hereditary cancer syndromes associated with esophageal SCC include tylosis and Fanconi anemia.

As with SCC, esophageal adenocarcinoma has a male predominance. GERD is a major risk factor for esophageal adenocarcinoma. Adenocarcinoma arises in the setting of Barrett metaplasia, an acquired condition from chronic inflammation due to acid exposure. Obesity is another associated risk factor, as is tobacco use.[6] *Helicobacter pylori* infection has been found to be inversely correlated.

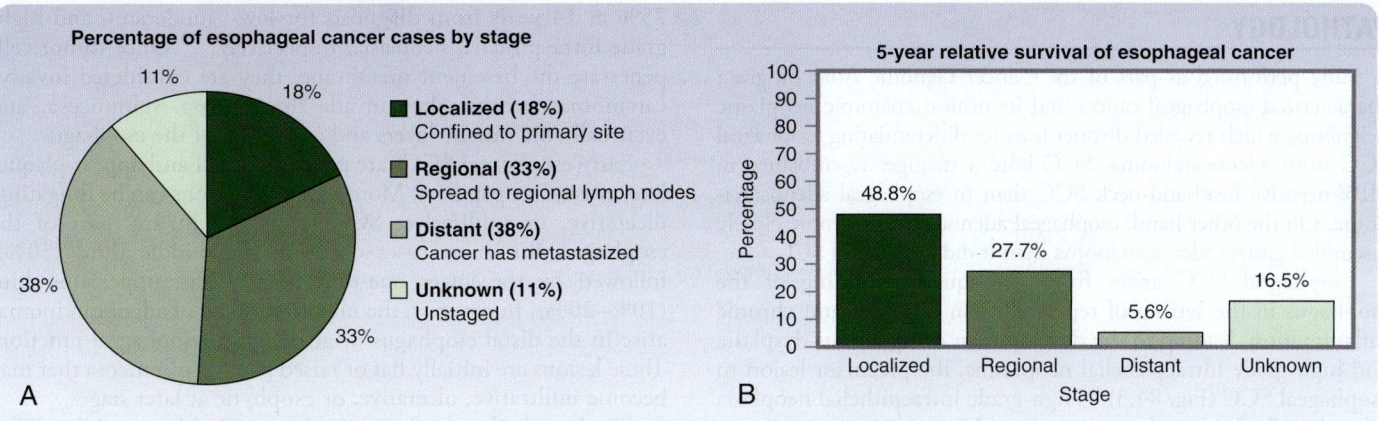

FIGURE 84.1 Stage and survival statistics for esophageal cancer in the United States. (A) Percentage of cases by stage. (B) Five-year relative survival. (From Surveillance, Epidemiology, and End Results Database. 2023. https://seer.cancer.gov/statfacts/html/esoph.html.)

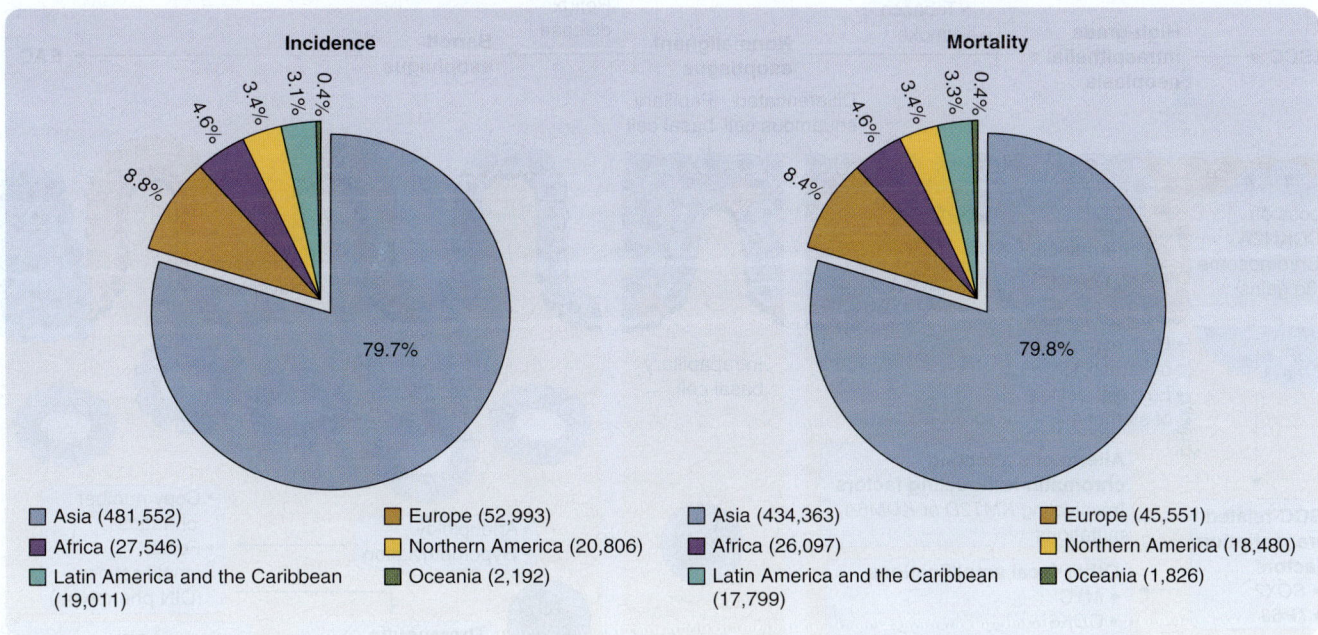

FIGURE 84.2 Incidence and mortality of esophageal cancer worldwide in 2020 distributed by continent. (From Liu CQ, Ma YL, Qin Q, et al. Epidemiology of esophageal cancer in 2020 and projections to 2030 and 2040. *Thorac Cancer.* 2023;14[1]:3-11.)

TABLE 84.1	**Differences Between the Two Predominant Histologic Subtypes of Esophageal Cancer**	
	ADENOCARCINOMA	**SQUAMOUS CELL CARCINOMA**
Epidemiology	Most common in North America and Western Europe	Most common worldwide
Sex predilection	Males	Males
Key risk factors (see Fig. 84.10)	GERD	Tobacco use
	Obesity	Alcohol use
Pathogenesis	Glandular differentiation	Squamous dysplasia
Location in esophagus	80% in distal esophagus or EGJ	Upper third (10%–20%)
		Middle third (50%)
		Lower third (40%)

EGJ, Esophagogastric junction; *GERD,* gastroesophageal reflux disease.

PATHOLOGY

A study performed as part of the Cancer Genome Atlas program characterized esophageal cancer and its nearest anatomic neoplastic neighbors, which revealed distinct features differentiating esophageal SCC from adenocarcinoma. SCC bore a stronger resemblance to HPV-negative head-and-neck SCC than to esophageal adenocarcinoma. On the other hand, esophageal adenocarcinoma more closely resembled gastric adenocarcinoma than it did esophageal SCC.[7]

Esophageal SCC arises from the squamous lining of the esophagus in the setting of repeated toxin exposure and chronic inflammation, leading to the development of squamous dysplasia and high-grade intraepithelial neoplasms, the precursor lesion to esophageal SCC (Fig. 84.3).[8] High-grade intraepithelial neoplasia (also described as moderate to severe dysplasia) is carcinoma in situ without violation of the basement membrane. The risk of progression to SCC has been estimated to be 24%, 50%, and

75% at 14 years from diagnosis for low-, moderate-, and high-grade intraepithelial neoplasia, respectively.[9-10] Once tumor cells penetrate the basement membrane, they are considered invasive carcinomas because they invade the mucosa, submucosa, and eventually the muscle layers and adventitia of the esophagus.

Early esophageal SCCs are generally small and appear plaque-like, erosive, or papillary. More advanced lesions can be fungating, ulcerative, or infiltrative. SCC may arise in any part of the esophagus, but most cases occur in the middle third (50%), followed by the lower one-third (40%) and upper one-third (10%–20%). In contrast, the majority (80%) of adenocarcinomas arise in the distal esophagus or at the gastroesophageal junction. These lesions are initially flat or raised patches of mucosa that may become infiltrative, ulcerative, or exophytic at later stages.

Esophageal adenocarcinoma is characterized by glandular differentiation that arises in the setting of Barrett esophagus (BE), a condition defined by the replacement of the normal stratified squamous

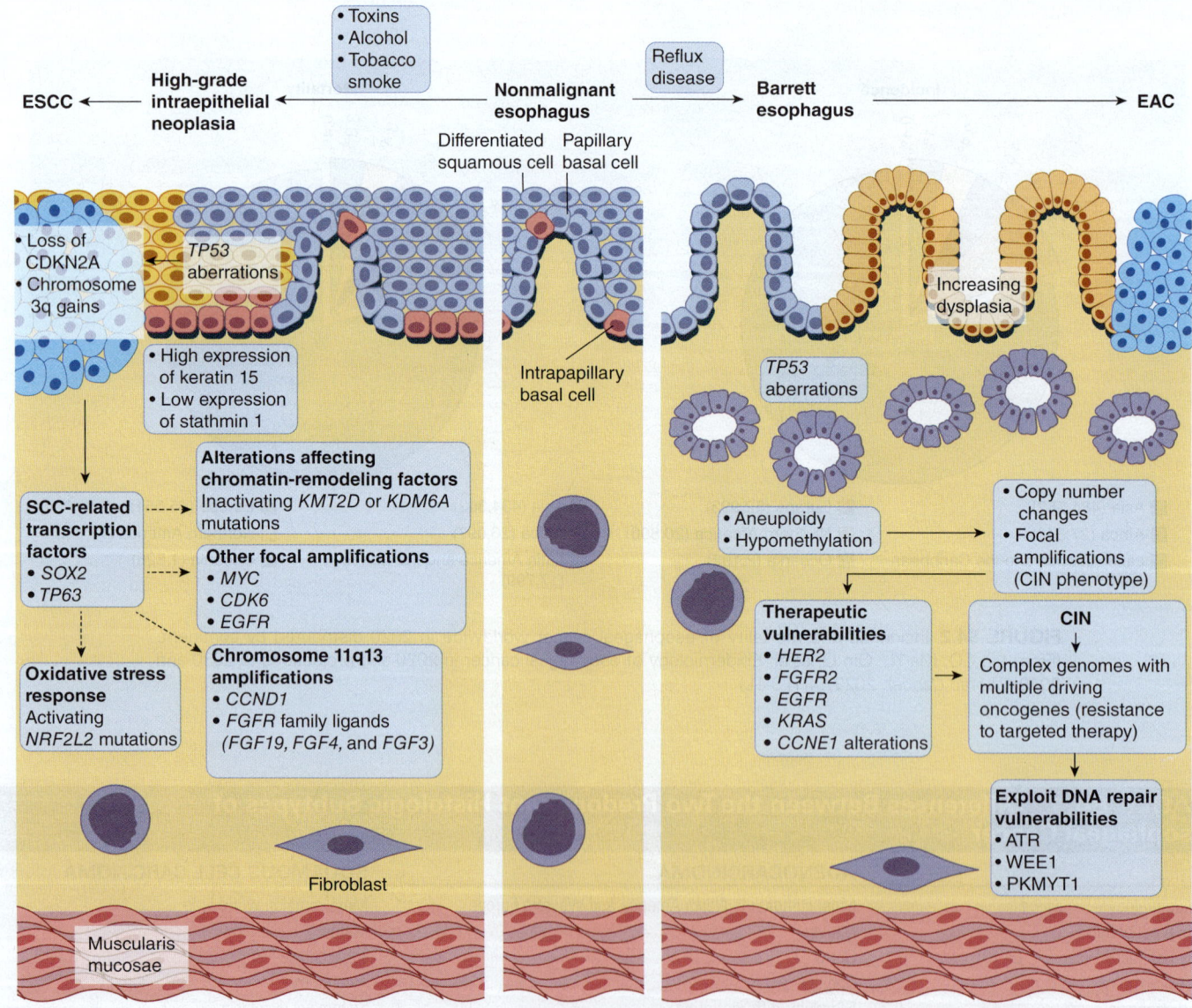

FIGURE 84.3 Pathogenesis and carcinogenesis of esophageal adenocarcinoma *(EAC)* and esophageal squamous cell carcinoma *(ESCC). CIN,* Chromosomal instability; *SCC,* squamous cell carcinoma. (From Shah MA, Altorki N, Patel P, et al. Improving outcomes in patients with oesophageal cancer. *Nature Reviews Clin Oncol.* 2023;20:390-407.)

epithelium of the distal esophagus by columnar metaplasia due to chronic inflammation secondary to acid exposure. Barrett metaplasia is a precursor to adenocarcinoma, and high-grade dysplasia seen on histopathology is the best predictor for progression to adenocarcinoma. A small subset of esophageal adenocarcinomas exhibit mucinous differentiation and diffuse signet ring cell morphology. There are patients who develop adenocarcinoma without antecedent BE. Carcinoma is thought to result from an accumulation of multiple genetic abnormalities, including inactivating mutations of the tumor suppressor *TP53* gene and subsequent overexpression of oncogenic drivers such as ERBB2 (encoding human epidermal growth factor 2 [HER2]), KRAS, and CCNE1 (see Fig. 84.3).[11,12]

Similar to esophageal adenocarcinoma, the most prevalent genomic aberration in esophageal SCC is *TP53* mutation. Oncogene activation also occurs via amplification of CCND1, MYC, CDK6, EGFR, and genes encoding FGFR ligands (see Fig. 84.3).[13,14]

Both esophageal SCC and adenocarcinoma spread via lymphatics. Lymphatic channels begin in the mucosa and drain into the submucosa of the esophageal wall, forming long collection channels with primarily longitudinal flow. Cervical, supraclavicular, and abdominal lymphadenopathy are seen in both upper and lower esophageal cancers. The incidence of lymphatic spread ranges from 30% to 70%. The deeper the tumor invasion, the higher the likelihood of nodal spread.[15] The two most common sites of distant metastasis are liver and lung; other less common sites are bone, kidney, adrenal glands, and brain.

CLINICAL PRESENTATION

The majority of esophageal cancers are symptomatic at the time of diagnosis. Regardless of histology, dysphagia is the most common symptom. Often, patients will report progressive dysphagia over a period of weeks to months, beginning with an initial episode after eating solid food, after which many patients will adapt by chewing more thoroughly, avoiding hard foods, or drinking liquids with swallows. Eventually, dysphagia with solid food progresses to dysphagia with liquids. Thus, it is only after dysphagia has worsened significantly that patients seek medical attention, by which point the majority have also experienced weight loss.

Unfortunately, dysphagia usually signifies locally advanced disease (at least T3). Other associated symptoms may include fatigue, regurgitation, retrosternal pain, dyspnea, and anemia. Locally advanced tumors may also manifest with hoarseness (suggesting laryngeal nerve involvement causing hoarseness) or cough (suggesting tracheoesophageal fistula).

Many, although not all, patients with adenocarcinoma will endorse a long history of reflux symptoms including heartburn and regurgitation. Early-stage tumors, which are usually asymptomatic, are often discovered during endoscopy for BE surveillance. Patients with BE have endoscopic examinations every 3 to 5 years with targeted biopsy samples taken of suspicious lesions and random four-quadrant biopsy sampling. Screening for esophageal squamous dysplasia and SCC is performed in East Asian regions where the incidence is high.[16] Outside of this, there are no defined screening programs.

Physical examination is usually unremarkable and does not generally aid with diagnosis. Weight loss and dehydration can be seen secondary to malnutrition from an obstructed esophageal lumen. However, attention should be paid to supraclavicular and cervical adenopathy. Laboratory evaluation may reveal anemia from chronic blood loss, hypoproteinemia from malnutrition, and hypercalcemia and abnormal liver function tests if there is distant metastatic spread.

DIAGNOSIS AND EVALUATION

The diagnosis of esophageal cancer is made by endoscopy with confirmation by biopsy. Tissue diagnosis is mandatory to determine the histologic subtype and for molecular characterization. If a barium esophagram is obtained, it may demonstrate irregular narrowing, ulceration, or an asymmetric bulge. However, endoscopy should be performed in any patient presenting with dysphagia, even if esophagram suggests a motility disorder.

Esophageal cancers appear as friable, ulcerated masses or as strictures, but the endoscopic appearance can vary (Fig. 84.4A). Early-stage tumors may appear as ulcerations, small nodules, or even flat mucosal irregularities. In many cases, the initial endoscopist may not recognize the presence of cancer, and a single biopsy may not

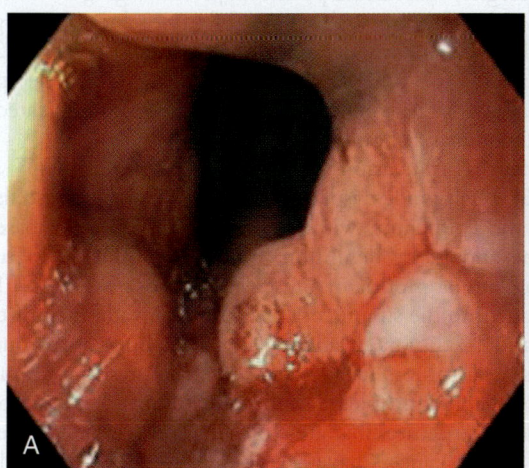

Partially obstructing esophageal tumor at the GEJ on upper endoscopy

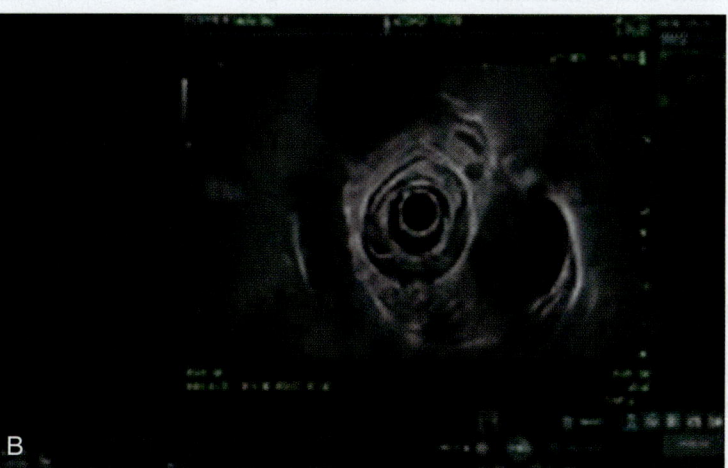

Endoscopic ultrasound image of esophageal tumor

FIGURE 84.4 (A) Endoscopic view of a partially obstructing esophageal tumor at the gastroesophageal junction *(GEJ)*. (B) Alternating layers of echogenicity as visualized on endoscopic ultrasound of the esophagus.

be diagnostic. Therefore, multiple biopsies should be performed for any suspicious lesions to attain accurate tissue diagnosis.

During endoscopy, it is essential to note the location of the tumor relative to the incisors and the esophagogastric junction (EGJ), the length of the tumor, and the degree of obstruction. The most proximal extent and circumferential extent of any BE should also be noted according to the Prague criteria.[17] For treatment planning, it is critical to know the upper border for cancers of the cervical and upper thoracic esophagus and the lower border for cancers of the lower thoracic esophagus and EGJ (Fig. 84.5). Adenocarcinomas at the EGJ require particular attention. Under current American Joint Committee on Cancer (AJCC) and National Comprehensive Cancer Network (NCCN) staging guidelines, EGJ adenocarcinomas are staged and classified as esophageal cancers if the tumor's epicenter is no more than 2 cm into the gastric cardia. Tumors with epicenters 2 cm below the EGJ are classified as gastric cancers and treated as such.[18,19]

Once tissue diagnosis is made, accurate clinical staging is essential to guide therapy. Esophageal cancer staging is based on tumor depth (T), nodal involvement (N), and distant metastasis (M). Clinical staging is performed using a combination of complementary modalities: esophagogastroduodenoscopy (EGD) with biopsy, endoscopic ultrasound (EUS), endoscopic ultrasound–fine-needle aspiration (EUS-FNA), endoscopic mucosal resection (EMR) or endoscopic mucosal dissection (ESD), computed tomography (CT), and/or positron emission tomography (PET)/CT.

There are two common strategies for staging that differ based on resources available, scheduling logistics, cost, and patient and physician preference. One strategy involves EGD (with biopsy and possibly endoscopic resection [ER]) and EUS (with or without FNA) to obtain upfront the grade, tumor, and nodal staging. This is followed by fluorodeoxyglucose (FDG)-PET/CT for additional N and M staging. This approach is efficient but costly.[20]

After tissue diagnosis, the second strategy begins with CT or FDG-PET/CT for M staging. No further testing is required if metastatic disease is confirmed. If there is no evidence of distant metastatic disease, then EUS should be done to assess T status and regional lymph nodes. Coupling EUS with FNA of any suspicious nodes further increases the accuracy of this test. Obtaining FDG-PET/CT before EUS has several advantages. FDG-PET/CT may demonstrate distant metastatic disease, eliminating the need for the patient to undergo EUS. FDG-PET/CT may also identify suspicious lymph nodes that can be specifically examined and sampled during the EUS procedure. EUS is superior to CT or PET for assessment of both T and N status.[20] It is highly accurate for celiac nodal status, although slightly lower for other regional lymph nodes because of difficulty accessing the node without traversing the tumor. Obstructing lesions may preclude EUS assessment. In these cases, dilatation to perform EUS is associated with a risk of perforation. Most tumors with such tight stenoses are locally advanced, and patients presenting with dysphagia generally have at least T3 disease. In these situations, practitioners may forego EUS altogether because this represents locally advanced disease for which treatment begins with neoadjuvant therapy regardless.

Although EUS provides information about invasion of adjacent structures, bronchoscopy should also be performed for proximal and middle-third esophageal tumors to assess for direct tracheal invasion. It is important to remember that for more superficial tumors (T1a–T2), the accuracy of EUS is significantly diminished, and EMR provides the most accurate staging information.[19,21]

STAGING AND PROGNOSIS

Staging of esophageal cancer is based on tumor-node-metastasis (TNM) categories (Table 84.2). The 8th edition AJCC staging system acknowledges differences in the biology of adenocarcinoma and SCC by creating separate stage groupings for each histology. Additionally, this is the first edition to separate staging into clinical (cTNM), pathologic (pTNM), and postneoadjuvant pathologic (ypTNM) staging groups. Clinical staging is based on imaging studies (EUS, CT, and PET/CT) (Table 84.3). Pathologic stage is based on microscopic examination of resected specimens (in patients who did not have neoadjuvant therapy) (see Table 84.3). The prognostication based on cTNM differs from that based on pTNM, reflecting the inaccuracies of characterizing tumors by current clinical staging modalities. ypTNM is based on resected specimens in patients who underwent neoadjuvant therapy before surgery (see Table 84.3). This staging was created in response to the increasing number of patients treated in this manner and to account for categories particular to the postneoadjuvant state (i.e., ypT0N0-3M0 and ypTisN0-3M0), dissimilar stage group compositions, and markedly different survival profiles compared with pTNM categories.[20]

Histopathologic cell type affects survival of cTNM-staged patients. SCC features squamous differentiation, whereas adenocarcinoma is characterized by glandular formation. Survival of early- and intermediate-stage patients is worse for SCC than with adenocarcinoma, necessitating separate staging groups for each histology. Additionally, tumor location affects pathologic stage for SCC but not for adenocarcinoma.[20] Tumor location is defined by distance from the incisors to the epicenter of the tumor. For adenocarcinomas located at the EGJ, tumors with epicenters no more than 2 cm into the gastric cardia are staged and treated as esophageal adenocarcinomas, and those extending distally (Siewert III) are staged and treated as gastric cancers.[18]

Tumor grade is included in the pathologic stage classification for early-stage tumors for both adenocarcinoma (pT1-2N0M0) and SCC (pT2N0M) because it is a predictor of survival. However, tumor grade is often inconsistently reported (and not mandated) in biopsy specimens because superficial biopsy samples may not provide enough material to accurately grade cancer differentiation. For both histologies, clinical and postneoadjuvant staging includes only the TNM classification without use of tumor location or grade. Low-grade (G1) and moderately differentiated cancers (G2) are likely subject to interobserver variability. However, poorly differentiated or signet ring cell morphology (G3) is associated with poorer outcome and should be noted.[20]

The depth of invasion of the tumor defines the T status (Fig. 84.6). High-grade dysplasia is defined by malignant cells confined to the epithelium without penetration into the basement membrane and is, by definition, noninvasive (Tis). T1a tumors invade the lamina propria or muscularis mucosa, whereas T1b tumors invade into the submucosa. T2 tumors invade the muscularis propria, and T3 tumors invade the adventitia but not surrounding structures. T4a tumors invade adjacent structures that are usually resectable (diaphragm, pleura, and pericardium). T4b tumors invade adjacent structures that are typically unresectable (trachea and aorta).[18] T3–T4 cancers have a very high (>80%) probability of nodal spread and require neoadjuvant therapy, whereas T1–T2 cancers are likely N0 and can be treated with upfront resection.[22]

T status is most commonly assessed by EUS, which provides a view of the esophageal wall as alternating hyperechoic (white) and hypoechoic (black) layers (Fig. 84.4B). Tumors appear hypoechoic

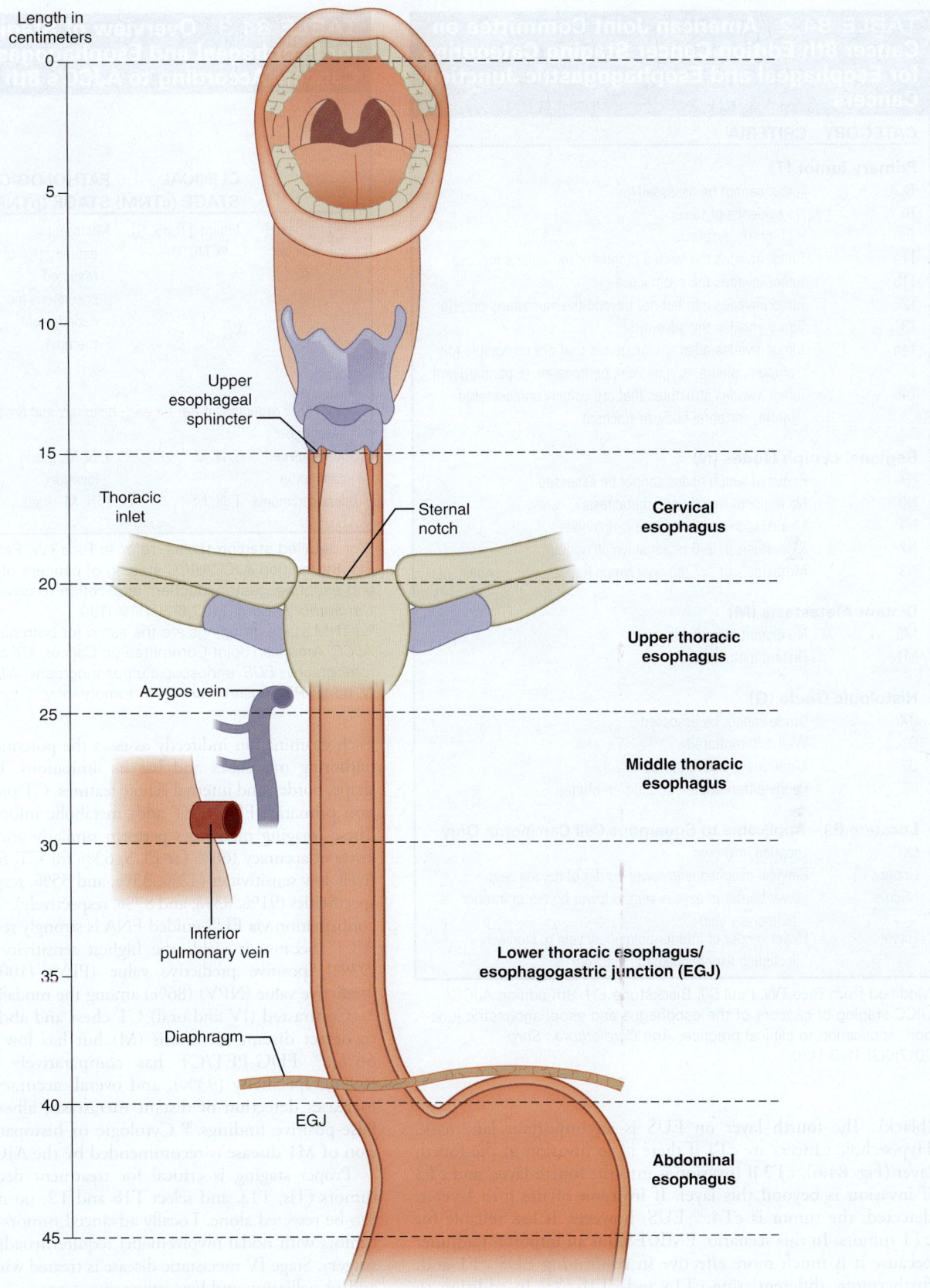

FIGURE 84.5 Regions of the esophagus. The cervical esophagus extends from the upper esophageal sphincter to the thoracic inlet. The upper thoracic esophagus extends from the thoracic inlet to the azygos vein. The midthoracic esophagus extends from the lower border of the azygous vein to the inferior pulmonary vein. The lower thoracic esophagus extends from the lower border of the inferior pulmonary vein to the gastroesophageal junction.

TABLE 84.2 American Joint Committee on Cancer 8th Edition Cancer Staging Categories for Esophageal and Esophagogastric Junction Cancers

CATEGORY	CRITERIA
Primary Tumor (T)	
TX	Tumor cannot be assessed
T0	No evidence of tumor
Tis	High-grade dysplasia
T1a	Tumor invades the lamina propria or muscularis mucosa
T1b	Tumor invades the submucosa
T2	Tumor invades into but not beyond the muscularis propria
T3	Tumor invades the adventitia
T4a	Tumor invades adjacent structures that are resectable (diaphragm, pleura, azygos vein, peritoneum, or pericardium)
T4b	Tumor invades structures that are usually unresectable (aorta, vertebral body, or trachea)
Regional Lymph Nodes (N)	
NX	Regional lymph nodes cannot be assessed
N0	No regional lymph node metastasis
N1	Metastasis in 1–2 regional lymph nodes
N2	Metastasis in 3–6 regional lymph nodes
N3	Metastasis in ≥7 regional lymph nodes
Distant Metastasis (M)	
M0	No distant metastasis
M1	Distant metastasis
Histologic Grade (G)	
GX	Grade cannot be assessed
G1	Well differentiated
G2	Moderately differentiated
G3	Poorly differentiated or undifferentiated
Location (L)—Applicable to Squamous Cell Carcinoma Only	
LX	Location unknown
Upper	Cervical esophagus to lower border of azygos vein
Middle	Lower border of azygos vein to lower border of inferior pulmonary vein
Lower	Lower border of inferior pulmonary vein to stomach, including esophagogastric junction

Modified from Rice TW, Patil DT, Blackstone EH. 8th edition AJCC/UICC staging of cancers of the esophagus and esophagogastric junction: application to clinical practice. *Ann Cardiothorac Surg.* 2017;6(2):1119-1130.

TABLE 84.3 Overview of Staging Schema for Esophageal and Esophagogastric Junction Cancers According to AJCC's 8th Edition

	CLINICAL STAGE (cTNM)	PATHOLOGIC STAGE (pTNM)	POSTNEOADJUVANT PATHOLOGIC STAGE (ypTNM)
Staging based on...	Imaging (EUS, CT, PET/CT)	Microscopic examination of resected specimens (no neoadjuvant therapy)	Microscopic examination of resected specimens (patient received neoadjuvant therapy)
Staging I–V groupings differ for each histology and are based on the listed categories[a]			
Squamous cell carcinoma	T, N, M	T, N, M, grade location	
Adenocarcinoma	T, N, M	T, N, M, grade	T, N, M[b]

[a]For detailed staging tables, refer to Rice TW, Patil DT, Blackstone EH. 8th edition AJCC/UICC staging of cancers of the esophagus and esophagogastric junction: application to clinical practice. *Ann Cardiothorac Surg.* 2017;6(2):1119-1130.
[b]ypTNM stage groupings are the same for both histologies.
AJCC, American Joint Committee on Cancer; *CT,* computed tomography; *EUS,* endoscopic ultrasonography; *M,* Metastasis; *N,* node; *PET,* positron emission tomography; *T,* tumor.

Each examination indirectly assesses the potential for lymph nodes harboring metastases and has its limitations. EUS evaluates size, shape, border, and internal echoic features. CT provides size information primarily. FDG/PET adds metabolic information (Fig. 84.7). These imaging modalities perform similarly and provide moderate levels of accuracy (66% for EUS, 63% for CT, 68% for PET), relatively low sensitivities (42%, 35%, and 35%, respectively), and high specificities (91%, 93%, and 87%, respectively).[26] As such, histologic confirmation via EUS-guided FNA is strongly recommended by the AJCC because it yields the highest sensitivity (92%), specificity (93%), positive predictive value (PPV) (100%), and negative predictive value (NPV) (86%) among the modalities.[27,28]

Contrasted (IV and oral) CT chest and abdomen can be used to detect distant metastasis (M) but has low sensitivity (37%–66%).[29] FDG-PET/CT has comparatively higher sensitivity (69%), specificity (93%), and overall accuracy (84%) and thus increases detection of distant metastasis, albeit with the risk of false-positive findings.[30] Cytologic or histopathologic confirmation of M1 disease is recommended by the AJCC.[18]

Proper staging is critical for treatment decisions. Early-stage tumors (Tis, T1a, and select T1b and T2; no nodal involvement) can be resected alone. Locally advanced tumors (T3 tumors or T2 tumors with nodal involvement) require neoadjuvant therapy and surgery. Stage IV metastatic disease is treated with systemic therapy and/or palliation and best supportive care.

BIOMARKERS

Biomarker testing of biopsy specimens has relevant treatment implications (especially for advanced disease) because the design of new

(black). The fourth layer on EUS is an important landmark. Hypoechoic cancers are cT1 if there is no invasion of the fourth layer (Fig. 84.6), cT2 if invasion is into the fourth layer, and cT3 if invasion is beyond this layer. If invasion of the fifth layer is detected, the tumor is cT4.[20] EUS, however, is less reliable for cT1 tumors. In this scenario, EMR/ESD is an important adjunct because it is much more effective in confirming EUS cT1 and, furthermore, differentiating cT1a and cT1b.[23–25] In addition to providing more accurate depth of involvement, EMR/ESD can also yield information regarding high-risk features (e.g., lymphovascular invasion) that may weigh heavily in treatment decisions.

Nodal classification (N) is based on the total number of involved regional nodes as assessed clinically by EUS, CT, and FDG/PET.

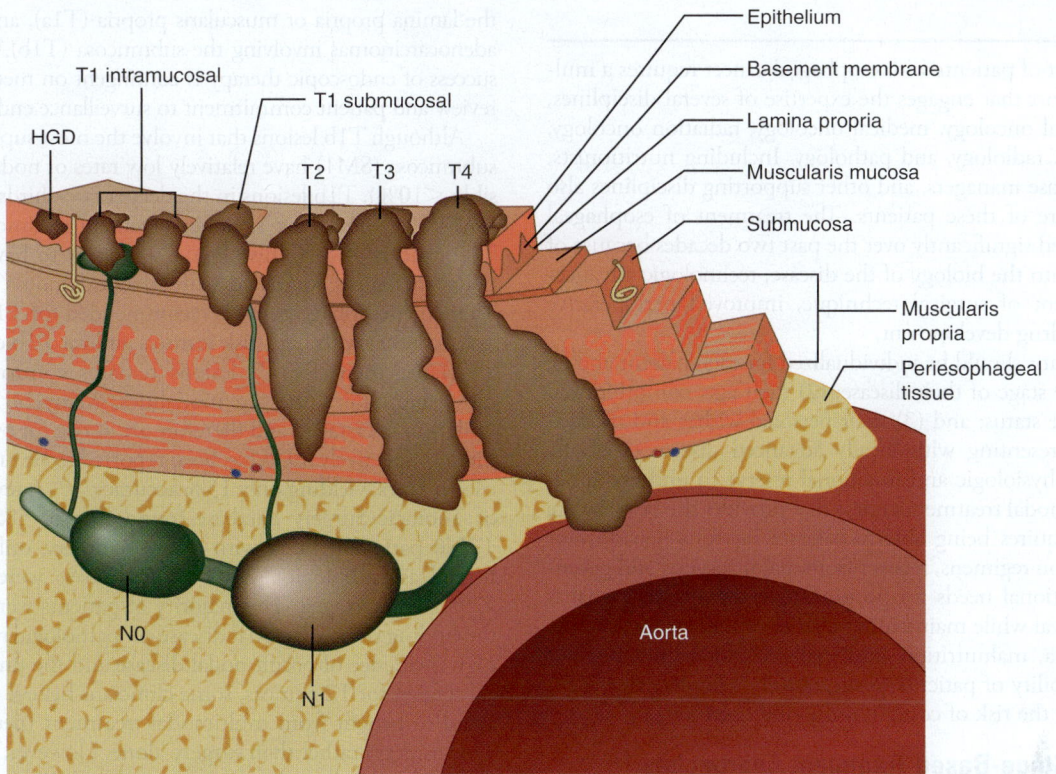

FIGURE 84.6 Tumor classification (T stage) for esophageal carcinoma as defined by depth of invasion. *HGD,* High-grade dysplasia. (Modified from Krill T, Baliss M, Roark R, et al. Accuracy of endoscopic ultrasound in esophageal cancer staging. *J Thorac Dis.* 2019;11(Suppl):S1602-S1609.)

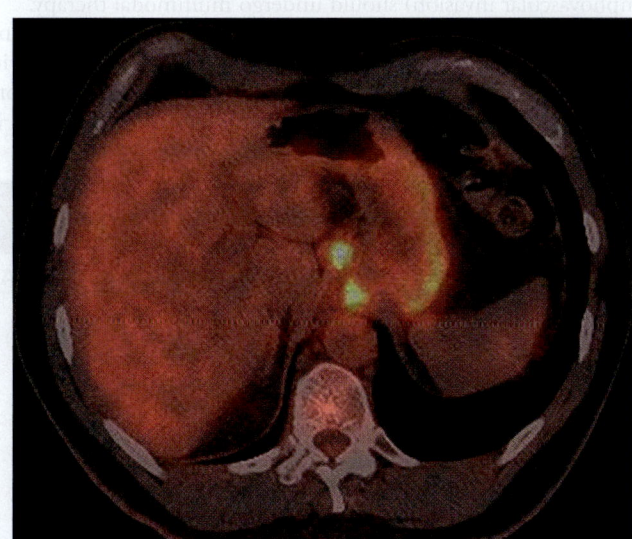

FIGURE 84.7 Fused transaxial PET/CT showing increased fluorodeoxyglucose-avidity of gastroesophageal junction tumor and celiac lymphadenopathy.

therapeutics has focused on the molecular features of esophageal carcinogenesis. Biomarker testing is achieved by immunohistochemistry and/or molecular testing. When tissue is limited, genomic profiling via validated next-generation sequencing (NGS) assays can also be used. Biomarkers of interest include HER2/ERBB2 status, microsatellite instability (MSI) or mismatch repair (MMR) status, programmed

cell death ligand 1 (PD-L1) expression, tumor mutational burden-high status, neurotrophic tropomyosin-related kinase *(NTRK)* gene fusions, rearranged during transfection *(RET)* gene fusions, and *BRAF* V600E mutations.

HER2 protein (encoded by the *ERBB2* gene) is the most frequently overexpressed and/or amplified growth receptor in esophageal cancer, more so in adenocarcinoma (15%–30%) than in SCC (5%–13%).[31] Although some studies suggest that HER2 positivity is correlated with tumor invasion, nodal metastasis, and poorer survival, the prognostic significance of HER2 status is still unclear.[32] Nevertheless, HER2 is a target for therapy, specifically with the monoclonal antibody drug trastuzumab.

Expression of the immune checkpoint protein PD-L1 has been correlated with unfavorable survival in esophageal cancer.[33] Approximately 60% of esophageal SCC and 40% of SCC are PD-L1 positive (i.e., have a combined positive score of ≥10).[34] Many immune checkpoint inhibitor (ICI) drugs targeting this pathway are under trial investigation, with some FDA approved. Although MMR deficiency is reported in <1% of esophageal cancers,[7] MSI and MMR status should be evaluated because MMR deficiency is associated with clinical efficacy of ICIs across solid tumors.

An emerging method of interrogating genomic alterations in solid cancers is the liquid biopsy, which evaluates circulating tumor DNA (ctDNA).[35] Liquid biopsy is being used in patients who are unable to have a clinical biopsy for disease surveillance and management. The detection of genetic alterations in DNA shed from esophageal carcinomas can identify targetable alterations or clones with altered treatment response profiles, such as in the case of disease recurrence.

TREATMENT

The management of patients with esophageal cancer requires a multidisciplinary effort that engages the expertise of several disciplines, including surgical oncology, medical oncology, radiation oncology, gastroenterology, radiology, and pathology. Including nutritionists, social workers, case managers, and other supporting disciplines also enhances the care of these patients. The treatment of esophageal cancer has evolved significantly over the past two decades because of greater insight into the biology of the disease, technologic advancements, refinement of surgical technique, improved perioperative care, and novel drug development.

Treatment plans should be individualized for each patient and be based on (1) the stage of their disease; (2) their age, comorbidities, and performance status; and (3) their personal wishes and motivation. Patients presenting with locally advanced disease especially must have the physiologic and functional reserve to undergo a demanding multimodal treatment course that provides the best chance of cure. This requires being able to tolerate rigorous neoadjuvant drug and radiation regimens, recover from major surgery, and potentially meet additional needs for postoperative therapy. The goal is enhancing survival while maintaining quality of life. Factors such as frailty, sarcopenia, malnutrition, and major comorbidities can not only limit the ability of patients to successfully complete treatment but also increase the risk of complications and morbidity.

Overview of Stage-Based Treatment Approaches

Current stage-based treatment algorithms (Table 84.4) are based on a better understanding of the behavior of esophageal cancer. The greater the depth of invasion, the higher the likelihood of lymphatic spread. The strategies employed thus are focused on local control and/or systemic eradication, depending on disease stage.

Historically, esophagectomy was offered for patients with superficial or early-stage disease. However, with the understanding that superficial cancers have a lower risk of nodal involvement and with the evolution of endoscopic technology, ER (endoscopic resection) and ablation are now accepted therapies for high-grade dysplasia (Tis), tumors involving the lamina propria or muscularis propria (T1a), and select superficial adenocarcinomas involving the submucosa (T1b).[19] Importantly, the success of endoscopic therapy is contingent on meticulous pathologic review and patient commitment to surveillance endoscopies.

Although T1b lesions that involve the most superficial third of the submucosa (SM1) have relatively low rates of nodal metastases (possibly <10%), T1b lesions in the deeper two-thirds of the submucosa (SM2/SM3) may have nodal involvement in almost 40% of cases.[36] T1b cancers of SCC histology also appear to have a higher risk of nodal metastasis compared with adenocarcinoma (45% vs. 26%).[37] Therefore, esophagectomy is recommended for T1b esophageal adenocarcinoma with high-risk features and for T1b esophageal SCC.

Management for T2 lesions remains controversial because of unreliable clinical staging modalities. Many of these patients are under- or overstaged and therefore are at risk for over- or undertreatment, respectively. EUS has been reported to be unreliable in staging cT2 cancers, yielding only 13% accuracy.[38,39] A review of the Society of Thoracic Surgery database found that of 482 clinically staged T2N0 patients treated with upfront surgery, only 27% were confirmed as pathologic T2N0, whereas 26% were downstaged and 47% were upstaged. The majority of patients were upstaged due to the finding of occult nodal disease on pathologic review.[40] Given the high incidence of occult nodal disease and the unreliability of clinical staging for T2 tumors, some clinicians believe that these patients stand to benefit from multimodal treatment (neoadjuvant therapy with surgery) rather than surgery alone. However, routine use of this approach may result in overtreatment with its associated morbidity and costs. As such, treatment decisions for these patients should factor in low- and high-risk pathologic features. The NCCN guidelines recommend that clinical T1b–T2, low-risk lesions <3 cm in diameter and well-differentiated can be surgically resected up front. Higher-risk lesions (poorly differentiation, ≥3 cm, positive lymphovascular invasion) should undergo multimodal therapy.

Approximately 32% of patients are found to have locoregional disease at diagnosis. Dysphagia generally signifies T3 disease with approximately 80% probability of lymph node metastasis. Therefore, patients with T3-4aN0 or any clinical nodal disease (cT1b–4aN+)

TABLE 84.4   Stage-Based Treatment Approaches and Strategies for Esophageal Cancer by Histologic Subtype

	STAGE	ADENOCARCINOMA	SQUAMOUS CELL CARCINOMA
Early-stage disease	pTis	ER ± ablation	ER ± ablation
	pT1a	or	or
	cT1bN0–cT2N0 low risk (well differentiated, no lymphovascular invasion, <3 cm)	Esophagectomy	Esophagectomy
	cT1bN0–cT2N0 high risk (moderate to poorly differentiated, lymphovascular invasion, invasion depth beyond superficial one-third or >500 um into submucosa)	Esophagectomy	Esophagectomy (noncervical esophagus)
Locally advanced, resectable disease	cT2N0	Neoadjuvant chemoRT + esophagectomy	Neoadjuvant chemoRT + esophagectomy
	cT1b–T2, N+	or	or
	cT3–T4a, N+	Perioperative chemotherapy + esophagectomy	Definitive chemoradiation (cervical esophagus)
		or	
		Definitive chemoradiation	
Locally advanced, unresectable disease	cT4b, N+	Definitive chemoradiation	Definitive chemoradiation
		or	or
		Systemic therapy	Systemic therapy
		and/or	and/or
		Palliation/best supportive care	Palliation/best supportive care

chemoRT, Chemoradiation; *ER,* endoscopic resection.

and who are medically fit require multimodal therapy (i.e., neoadjuvant therapy followed by esophagectomy). This approach has been shown in multiple large, randomized controlled trials to confer the best survival outcomes for this patient population.

Tumors that have invaded into the adjacent structures, such as the aorta, vertebral body, or trachea (T4b), are considered unresectable, for which definitive chemoradiation is recommended. Definitive chemoradiation is also an option for those who decline surgery or are not fit for surgery. Patients with stage IVA (T4b or unresectable N3) and stage IVB (metastatic disease) may be treated with systemic therapy and/or palliation and best supportive care.

Treatment Modalities

Treatment modalities employed for esophageal cancer include surgery, chemotherapy, radiation, and endoscopic therapy. Targeted therapies and immunotherapy are emerging strategies. Each modality plays a different role in eliminating cancer cells, and in most cases, they must be used in combination (multimodality therapy) to achieve the best oncologic outcome, especially for locoregional disease. The rationale for endoscopic therapy, surgery, and radiation is to control local disease, whereas chemotherapy, targeted therapy, and immunotherapy address disease at a systemic level.

Endoscopic Therapies

Because BE is a known precursor lesion to esophageal adenocarcinoma, a surgeon should be familiar with its management. BE is the result of metaplastic changes in the distal esophagus associated with chronic GERD whereby normal squamous epithelium is replaced by columnar epithelium with goblet cells (i.e., intestinal metaplasia). Therefore, diagnosis is made histologically on biopsies obtained above the Z line. Grossly, BE appears as salmon pink–colored extensions ("tongues") of mucosa from above the EGJ into the esophagus. Assessment of BE requires a high-quality endoscopic examination. Disease burden is quantified by the Prague C&M criteria, which characterize the circumferential ("C") and longitudinal ("M") extent of BE based on standardized landmarks.[40–42] For screening and surveillance, BE should be sampled according to the Seattle protocol, which dictates obtaining four-quadrant biopsies every 2 cm through the length of BE or every 1 cm in patients with a history of BE and dysplasia, in addition to targeted biopsies of all visible lesions (i.e., depressed, flat, raised mucosal abnormalities).[43]

Presence of dysplasia within BE requires confirmation by a second pathologist. The degree of dysplasia within BE is the best current marker to predict progression to esophageal adenocarcinoma and therefore determines management by continued surveillance or endoscopic eradication therapy (EET) (Fig. 84.8).[17] Surveillance involves endoscopy with biopsy at defined time intervals. EET offers an effective and minimally invasive alternative to esophagectomy and involves ER of any visible lesion within the BE segment followed by ablative techniques (e.g., radiofrequency ablation [RFA] and cryotherapy) to achieve complete eradication of dysplasia and intestinal metaplasia.

BE without dysplasia has a very low risk of progression to cancer, and therefore, surveillance is recommended. After the initial diagnosis, a repeat EGD with biopsy should be done within 1 year because of the relatively high incidence of missed cancer or inadequate sampling on initial endoscopy. If there are no findings of dysplasia, then EGD with biopsy can be repeated every 3 (for >3-cm BE segment) to 5 years (if <3-cm BE segment). For patients with *BE with low-grade dysplasia,* either endoscopic surveillance or EET is appropriate based on a risk-benefit discussion.

Management of BE with low-grade dysplasia is challenging because of high interobserver variability among pathologists, the variable natural history of the disease (including regression in some cases), and lack of well-defined risk stratification tools. EET is suggested, but if a patient should prefer to avoid the risks related to EET, surveillance is appropriate. Surveillance is recommended every 6 months for 1 year, followed by annual endoscopy (unless the degree of dysplasia changes). In the case of *BE with high-grade dysplasia* (or T1a intramucosal carcinoma), endoscopic eradication is strongly recommended over surveillance or surgical resection. After eradication therapy, patients must continue an endoscopic surveillance program.[17] Complete eradication of intestinal metaplasia is standardly considered as two endoscopic examinations at least 3 months apart during which no visible or histologic evidence of BE is found on biopsy.[44]

In terms of the role of chemoprevention and antireflux procedures to reduce the risk of neoplastic progression in BE, at least daily proton pump inhibitor (PPI) therapy is recommended to control associated GERD symptoms. Twice-daily dosing should be used during eradication to favor growth of normal squamous epithelium. Antireflux surgery is very effective at reducing reflux episodes, decreasing symptoms, and healing esophagitis. Although trials have shown equivalent effect as medical therapy to control GERD,[45] surgery should be considered for patients who have poor symptom control with medications, large hiatal hernias, or difficulty with BE eradication. Although there is some evidence that fundoplication may delay development of dysplasia in BE, the data do not convincingly show that patients with BE treated with antireflux surgery have a lower risk of progression to neoplasia than those treated with medical therapy. Moreover, the risk of progression to cancer in the setting of nondysplastic BE is so low that surgery and its inherent risks may not be merited in patients who otherwise do not need fundoplication for symptoms already controlled by medication. In other words, the guidelines currently suggest against the use of antireflux surgery as an antineoplastic strategy in BE.[17] However, antireflux surgery should be pursued for patients with symptoms or complications of GERD that fail medical management or for those noncompliant with or unable to take PPIs due to side effects.

Various endoscopic ablative (cryotherapy, RFA, photodynamic therapy) and resection (endoscopic mucosal resection [EMR], endoscopic submucosal dissection [ESD]) techniques have largely supplanted the role of esophagectomy for high-grade dysplasia and superficial esophageal cancers. High-grade dysplasia (pTis) and early-stage disease (pT1a, select small pT1b adenocarcinoma with low-risk features) can be effectively treated with ER and/or ablation. The goal of endoscopic therapy is complete removal of early-stage lesions and complete eradication of Barrett's mucosa.

Ablative therapy uses energy to generate extremes of heat to destroy tissue. RFA transmits radiofrequency energy via balloon or electrical plate to generate heat (Fig. 84.9). Cryotherapy uses cold liquid nitrogen to deliver extreme cold. Photodynamic therapy involves systemic administration of a photosensitizing drug with an affinity for tumors. A laser light directed at the lesion triggers a destructive photodynamic reaction. Multiple studies have shown the effectiveness of RFA and cryotherapy in eradicating BE and dysplasia. These ablative techniques also offer alternative treatment options when lesions are challenging to resect or as salvage therapy after prior failed RFA.

There are two important limitations of ablative therapies: limited depth of penetration and the lack of definitive pathologic analysis. Areas of BE with nodular or ulcerated features or with

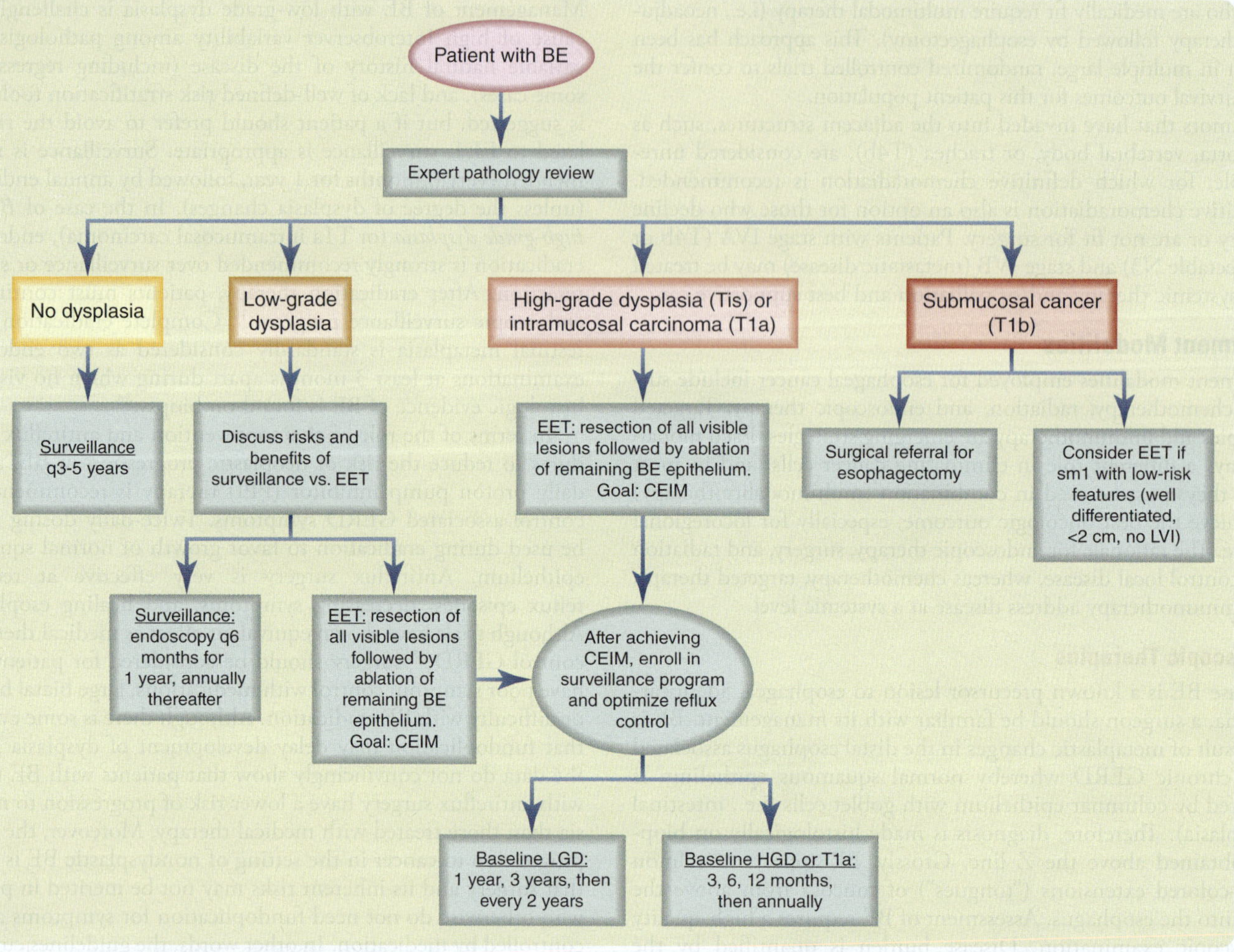

Patient with BE

↓

Expert pathology review

↓

No dysplasia | **Low-grade dysplasia** | **High-grade dysplasia (Tis) or intramucosal carcinoma (T1a)** | **Submucosal cancer (T1b)**

Surveillance q3-5 years

Discuss risks and benefits of surveillance vs. EET

EET: resection of all visible lesions followed by ablation of remaining BE epithelium. Goal: CEIM

Surgical referral for esophagectomy

Consider EET if sm1 with low-risk features (well differentiated, <2 cm, no LVI)

Surveillance: endoscopy q6 months for 1 year, annually thereafter

EET: resection of all visible lesions followed by ablation of remaining BE epithelium. Goal: CEIM

After achieving CEIM, enroll in surveillance program and optimize reflux control

Baseline LGD: 1 year, 3 years, then every 2 years

Baseline HGD or T1a: 3, 6, 12 months, then annually

FIGURE 84.8 Algorithm for consideration of endoscopic eradication therapy *(EET)*. *BE,* Barrett esophagus; *CEIM,* complete eradication of intestinal metaplasia; *HGD,* high-grade dysplasia; *LGD,* low-grade dysplasia; *LVI,* lymphovascular invasion; *PPI,* proton pump inhibitor. (Adapted from Shaheen NJ, Falk FW, Iyer PG, et al. Diagnosis and management of Barrett's esophagus: an updated ACG guideline. *J Am Coll Gastroenterol.* 2022;117[4]:559-587.)

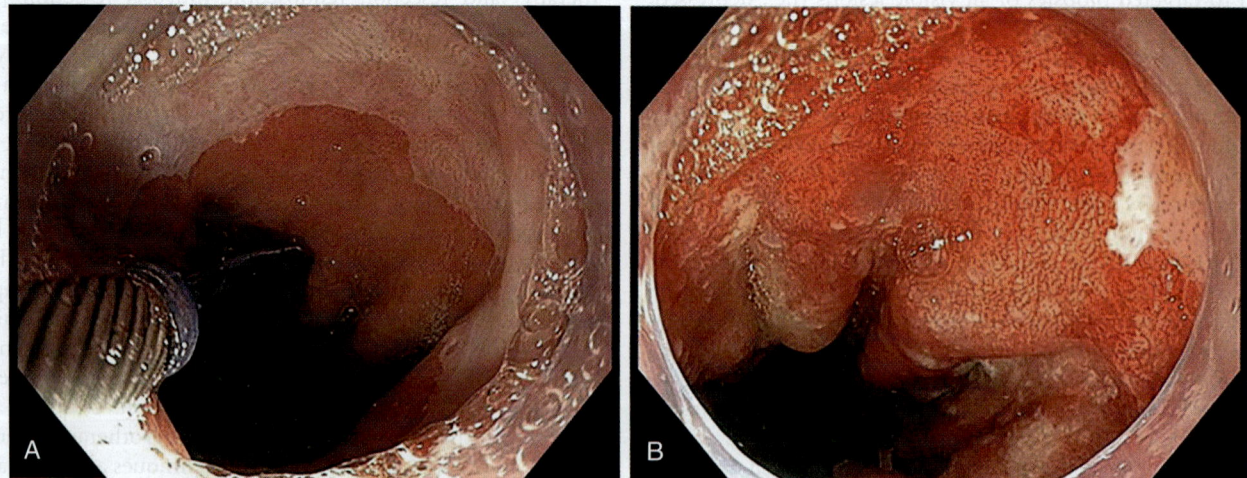

FIGURE 84.9 Radiofrequency ablation performed in a patient with Barrett esophagus. *(BE)*. (A) Preablation with catheter seen adjacent to area of metaplastic disease. (B) Posttreatment after radiofrequency ablation. *CEIM,* Complete eradication of intestinal metaplasia; *EET,* endoscopic eradication therapy. (From Rajaram R, Hofstetter WL. Mucosal ablation techniques for Barrett's esophagus and early esophageal cancer. *Thorac Surg Clin.* 2018;28:473-480.)

other abnormalities concerning for superficial invasive cancer should undergo ER rather than ablation to yield tissue for pathologic analysis of depth of invasion. EMR and ESD remove the full thickness of mucosa down into the submucosa. The basic technique of EMR is incising lesions by a through-the-scope snare with or without cautery. For flat lesions, adjunctive techniques, such as double-channel endoscope, submucosal injection, and cap- and ligation-assisted EMR, are needed. EMR can remove lesions <2 cm in size en bloc. Larger lesions require removal in piecemeal fashion, which may limit margin assessment. On the other hand, ESD allows en bloc dissection of a lesion regardless of size. It is performed by injection of fluid into the submucosa, creating an incision around the perimeter of the lesion, and carefully dissecting the lesion from the deeper layers using a specialized knife. It is labor intensive and has a greater risk of perforation but is favored over EMR for lesions larger than 15 mm, lesions with poor lifting (due to fibrosis), and better assessment of depth of invasion if there is concern for submucosal invasion. In Japan and Europe, there are guidelines that provide specific recommendations on the use of ESD, but no guidelines currently exist in the United States.[46,47]

The NCCN guidelines recommend EMR with or without ablation in patients with Tis and T1a tumors as well as superficial T1b adenocarcinomas with low-risk features (well or moderately differentiated, no lymphovascular invasion, mucosal penetration <500 micrometers) as preferred therapy over esophagectomy. EMR successfully eradicates 91% to 98% of T1a cancer.[47] A large retrospective analysis of the Surveillance, Epidemiology, and End Results (SEER) database that reviewed patients who underwent surgery versus endoscopic therapy for T1N0 esophageal cancer found that patients treated with endoscopic therapy had better cancer-specific survival and equivalent OS.[48] EMR is considered a relatively safe technique, with complications including bleeding (10%), perforation (3%), and stricture formation.[46,47]

Surgery

Esophagectomy is a key component of curative treatment for esophageal cancer. The first successful esophagectomy for cancer was performed by Franz Torek in 1913. Since that time, vast improvements in surgical techniques and perioperative care have contributed to a marked reduction in surgical morbidity and mortality. Esophagectomy should be offered for all patients with resectable esophageal cancer (>5 cm from the cricopharyngeus) who are medically fit. Enteral nutritional support should be considered for patients with significant dysphagia and/or weight loss before or during neoadjuvant therapy, with preference for jejunostomy feeding tube over gastrostomy tube to preserve the stomach as a conduit for reconstruction.

The NCCN guidelines emphasize that esophagectomies should be done at high-volume centers based on studies that showed a correlation between hospital volume and surgical mortality. In 2002, a study in the *New England Journal of Medicine* showed that mortality ranged from the single digits at high-volume centers to above 20% at low-volume centers.[49] A follow-up study in 2011 found that just over 30% of esophagectomies had moved to high-volume centers, with an associated 11% decrease in surgical mortality.[50]

Several approaches for esophageal resection exist and can be done open or with minimally invasive techniques. The types of esophagectomies include Ivor Lewis, McKeown ("three-hole"), transhiatal, and left transthoracic/thoracoabdominal—they differ in the types of incision and the location of the anastomosis (cervical or thoracic). The choice of operative approach depends on the tumor location and surgeon preference.

Minimally invasive esophagectomy (MIE) can be performed using video-assisted laparoscopy and thoracoscopy as well as robot-assisted approaches. These procedures are associated with a steep learning curve and higher technical complexity than open approaches.[51] Some surgeons use a hybrid open/minimally invasive approach as well. Nevertheless, MIE is becoming increasingly embraced by surgeons around the world. In the United States, use of MIE increased from 38% in 2010 to 57% in 2015.[52] Randomized trials comparing different MIE approaches to open esophagectomy suggest that MIE is associated with a lower incidence of pulmonary and major complications, shorter length of hospital stay, and faster functional recovery.[53,54] Furthermore, MIE is associated with similar survival outcomes to those observed with open surgery. A trial comparing robot-assisted MIE to non–robot-assisted MIE is ongoing.

Regardless of the type of resection or selected approach, the goal of surgery for curative intent is achieving complete resection with negative microscopic margins (R0) and adequate lymphadenectomy (of thoracic and abdominal fields) (Fig. 84.10). The extent of lymphadenectomy has significant prognostic implications; data from several large registry studies and multi-institutional retrospective studies indicate that extended nodal dissection might have survival benefit beyond the purpose of pathologic disease staging. The number of lymph nodes removed has been shown to be an independent predictor of survival. Although the total number of lymph nodes needed to ensure accurate staging and prognostication is not actually known, the evidence continues to suggest that more is better. Currently, the NCCN guidelines recommend thorough dissection to achieve at least 15 lymph nodes for pathologic examination in patients undergoing resection with and without preoperative therapy.[19]

After the resection phase of the operation, reconstruction to create a neoesophagus involves preparation of a well-perfused conduit and creating a tension-free esophagogastric end-to-side or side-to-side anastomosis either stapled or hand-sewn. A gastric conduit relying on blood supply from a preserved right gastroepiploic artery is preferred for esophageal reconstruction. In some centers, select patients at high risk for conduit ischemia undergo preoperative selective embolization of the right gastric, left gastric, and splenic arteries as a strategy for gastric conditioning to minimize the risk of anastomotic leak or conduit failure. If the stomach cannot be used, such as in patients who have had previous surgery or other procedures that may have devascularized the stomach, the colon or the jejunum are alternative conduit options.

A cervical anastomosis allows more extensive resection of the esophagus, possibly avoiding thoracic access and less severe reflux symptoms. An anastomotic leak in the neck is easier to control than one in the chest. However, advantages of a thoracic anastomosis may include lower incidence of anastomotic leak (presumably due to less tension), lower stricture rate, and lower rate of left recurrent nerve injury.[55] In a prospective randomized trial, cervical and thoracic anastomoses after esophageal resection were equally safe and had similar oncologic outcomes when performed in standardized fashion.[56] In the era of minimally invasive surgery, a randomized clinical trial showed much lower leak rates with intrathoracic (12.3%) than with cervical anastomosis (31.7%) in patients undergoing transthoracic MIE for mid- to distal and EGJ tumors.[57]

Whether done with an open or minimally invasive approach, the transthoracic Ivor Lewis esophagectomy involves intrabdominal and intrathoracic exposure and is the most commonly performed esophageal resection worldwide (see Fig. 84.10). It allows visualization of the entire intrathoracic esophagus and complete intrathoracic

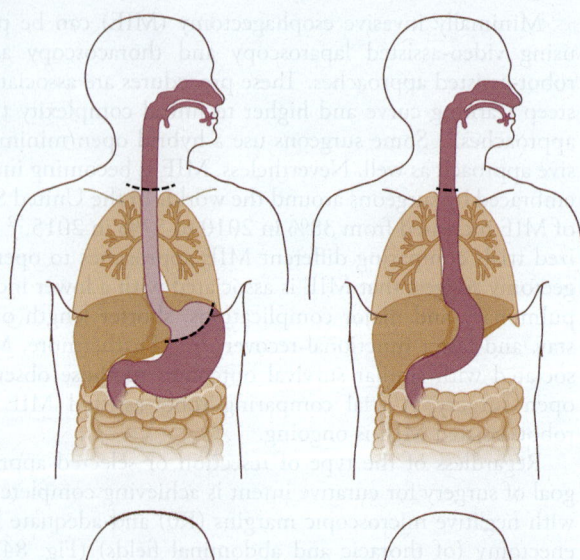

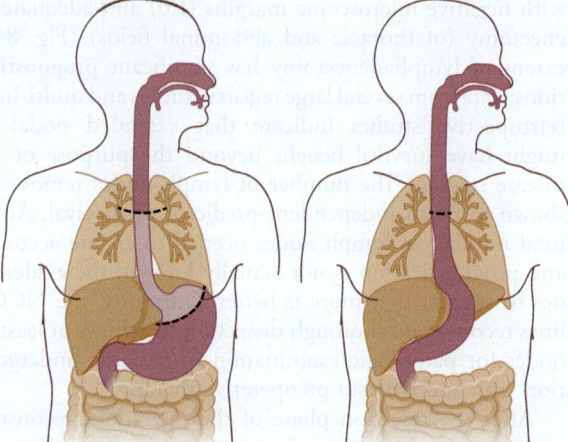

McKeown 3-hole esophagectomy

Exposures
1) Chest
2) Neck
3) Abdomen

Neck anastomosis

Ivor Lewis esophagectomy

Exposures
1) Abdomen
2) Chest

Intrathoracic anastomosis

Key Principles of Esophagectomy

Complete resection with microscopic margins (R0)

Adequate abdominal and thoracic lymphadenectomy (15 lymph nodes)

Reconstruction with well-perfused conduit (stomach most common)

Tension free esophagogastric anastomosis

FIGURE 84.10 Key principles of esophagectomy and key features of the two common approaches: (A) McKeown three-hole esophagectomy and (B) Ivor Lewis esophagectomy. (Adapted from Yassin E, van Workum, van den Wildenberg F, et al. European consensus on essential steps of minimally invasive Ivor Lewis and McKeown esophagectomy through Delphi methodology. *Surgical Endoscopy.* 2022;36[1]:446-460.)

---

lymphadenectomy. The operation begins with the abdominal portion (by laparotomy or laparoscopy), in which the stomach is mobilized with dissection of the celiac and left gastric lymph nodes, division of the left gastric artery, and preservation of the right gastroepiploic as the main blood supply for the gastric conduit. After tubularization of the stomach to be used as the conduit, the patient is repositioned for right chest access via thoracotomy or thoracoscopy. The thoracic portion involves circumferential mobilization of the esophagus, resection of the tumor (with the esophagus) to negative margins, and pulling the gastric conduit up into the chest for creation of the esophagogastric anastomosis at or above the azygos vein. The Ivor Lewis approach may be used for distal esophageal lesions but is inadequate to obtain an acceptable margin for lesions in the midesophagus.

In cases of more proximal tumors or when there is concern for attaining an adequate proximal margin, the McKeown (three-hole) esophagectomy is preferred (see Fig. 84.10). The McKeown esophagectomy is applicable for tumors in any part of the esophagus and situates the anastomosis in the neck. Similar to the Ivor Lewis esophagectomy, it also takes a transthoracic approach and is performed in a similar fashion, except that the thoracic portion is performed first, followed by the abdominal portion and finishing with the cervical portion. The esophagus is exposed via a left neck incision, with careful attention to avoid recurrent laryngeal nerve injury. The conduit is pulled up through the chest to create an esophagogastric anastomosis in the neck.

The transhiatal esophagectomy avoids opening the chest and is accomplished via abdominal and cervical incisions. The abdominal portion is done in a similar fashion to the Ivor Lewis esophagectomy. Mobilization of the thoracic esophagus and mediastinal dissection is done via the hiatus in "blinded" fashion, although visualization is improved if done laparoscopically. The gastric conduit is pulled up through the posterior mediastinum and exteriorized in the cervical incision for the anastomosis. This approach may be used for lesions at any location. Because it avoids opening the thoracic cavity, it is the least invasive of the approaches, requires less operative time, and yields lower pulmonary complications and morbidity.[58] With regard to oncologic outcome, a randomized clinical trial showed that although median overall, disease-free, and quality-adjusted survival did not differ statistically between transhiatal esophagectomy and transthoracic esophagectomy with extended en bloc lymphadenectomy, there was a trend toward improved long-term survival at 5 years with the latter approach. Still, many experts believe that the transhiatal approach is oncologically inadequate (by virtue of subpar nodal dissection), and transhiatal dissection of large, midesophageal tumors adjacent to the trachea may be challenging and hazardous. As such, transhiatal esophagectomy may then be more suitable for early-stage tumors.

Less common approaches are the left transthoracic or thoracoabdominal esophagectomy, which uses a contiguous abdominal and left thoracic incision through the eighth intercostal space. This approach may be useful for bulky lesions in the distal esophagus or for patients in which the right chest cannot be accessed. The anastomosis is placed in the left chest.

Esophagectomy is a complex procedure and is associated with major morbidity in 30% to 40% of patients. However, 30-day and in-hospital mortality have steadily declined from 8% to 10% in the 1990s down to 2% to 4% currently.[59,60] Common postoperative complications after esophagectomy are atrial fibrillation, respiratory compromise, anastomotic/conduit complications, and chyle leak. As with other thoracic procedures, atrial fibrillation is most common, especially in older patients. Postesophagectomy patients are also at high risk for respiratory complications, such as aspiration and pneumonia. Early ambulation and aggressive pulmonary toilet are thus critical in postoperative care. Anastomotic leak is a highly morbid complication. CT with oral contrast or endoscopy can confirm the diagnosis. Management depends on the location of the anastomosis, the patient's clinical stability, and the severity of the dehiscence. Cervical anastomoses can be managed with a bedside neck washout and negative-pressure therapy. If small, a thoracic anastomosis can be covered with a stent. A larger anastomotic breakdown may require reoperation. Endovac therapy is now also a viable option to manage these leaks. Anastomotic stricture is a late complication presenting with dysphagia and can be treated with endoscopic balloon dilatation.

To address perioperative morbidity, centers have implemented enhanced recovery or fast-track programs with results suggesting fewer intensive care unit (ICU) days, shorter length of stay, reduced costs, and fewer complications. There is now also growing interesting in implementation of "prehabilitation" programs for patients before surgery focused on preoperative exercise and nutrition regimens. Multiple ongoing studies are examining the impact of such programs on in-hospital complications as well as on postoperative morbidity and quality of life. Prospective studies have shown that most postesophagectomy patients return to baseline quality-of-life status at about 1 to 3 years.[61]

Radiation

Radiation was historically the first treatment modality for esophageal cancer. The method of delivery and particles used have evolved significantly. With improved surgical care, radiotherapy was then incorporated into multimodal treatment to gain additional local control within or around the operative field in an attempt to reduce local recurrence. It is now part of standard treatment for locally advanced esophageal cancer and used concurrently with chemotherapy in the preoperative setting for resectable disease and as definitive or palliative therapy for those with unresectable disease.

Modern advances in radiotherapy are related to overall reduction of irradiation volume as compared with historical standards and development of techniques to deliver a radiation dose that is conformational to the target. Technologies such as intensity-modulated radiotherapy (IMRT) and proton-beam therapy (PBT) substantially reduce irradiation of nontarget tissues, thereby resulting in fewer side effects, and are associated with fewer postoperative complications.[62]

For patients being treated with definitive chemoradiation, investigative efforts have focused on determining the optimal dose to address high rates of locoregional failure. So far, large trials (INT-0123 and ARTDECO) have not shown better locoregional disease control with higher radiation doses.[63,64] Accordingly, the current standard of care dictates delivery of at least 50 Gy for definitive chemoradiation. For neoadjuvant treatment, 41.4- to 50.4-Gy radiotherapy combined with chemotherapy is recommended. In the palliative setting, conventional modest dose (30–35 Gy) is effective for mitigating malignant dysphagia.[19]

Chemotherapy

Because esophageal cancer has likely spread systemically in most patients at time of diagnosis, chemotherapy plays an important role in treating both resectable locally advanced and unresectable disease. Chemotherapeutic drugs exert cytotoxic effects on tumor cells. Administered systemically, chemotherapy is intended to treat the primary tumor itself and disease that has spread beyond the primary site. Even in the setting of seemingly localized disease, chemotherapy has the potential to target clinically undetectable micrometastatic deposits. It can downstage marginally resectable tumors, improve the chance for R0 resection, and decrease the incidence of locoregional recurrence. It can also have a synergistic antitumor effect when used with radiation. Furthermore, when administered preoperatively, the biologic response can be evaluated and quantified pathologically in terms of tumor viability and inform prognosis. The challenge with chemotherapy has been determining the most synergistic combinations at doses to maximize antitumor effect while minimizing toxicity and side-effect profiles.

Early prospective randomized trials found an effective role for preoperative chemotherapy for both locally advanced adenocarcinoma and SCC. In 2002, the England Medical Research Council (MRC) trial studied 802 patients treated with neoadjuvant cisplatin/5-fluorouracil and surgery versus surgery alone. The results showed that neoadjuvant chemotherapy significantly enhanced the R0 resection rate (60% vs. 54%), increased the median survival time (16.8 months vs. 13.3 months), and prolonged the 2-year survival rate (43% vs. 34%) compared with surgery alone.[65] Subsequently, in 2009, a long-term update of the MRC trial (known as the UK OEO2 trial) was the first to show a significant OS benefit with neoadjuvant chemotherapy. Patients who had received neoadjuvant chemotherapy and surgery had a 5-year survival of 23.0% versus 17.1% in patients who had surgery alone.[66] In both studies, the survival benefit was observed for both adenocarcinoma and SCC. These initial studies launched a number of landmark randomized trials that helped establish preoperative and perioperative chemotherapy as standard of care (and will be discussed in the "Multimodal Therapy for Locally Advanced Disease" section).

Before 2000, the only FDA-approved drugs used for esophageal cancer included the platinums (cisplatin, carboplatin), anthracyclines (epirubicin, doxorubicin), and pyrimidine analogues (5-fluorouracil [5-FU]). In the early 2000s, oxaliplatin (a third-generation platinum) and capecitabine (a newer version of 5-FU) came into use, with similar efficacy and toxicity profiles. Later in that decade, taxanes (docetaxel, paclitaxel) were FDA approved for use in upper GI cancers.

Targeted Therapy

The role of targeted therapies is primarily in advanced metastatic disease, and they are used in combination with chemotherapy.

HER2 is an important biomarker and key driver of tumorigenesis in esophageal cancer. Based on the success of trastuzumab (an anti-HER2 monoclonal antibody) in breast cancer, the drug was also studied for gastric and EGJ adenocarcinomas. Although the majority (80%) of patients in the ToGA trial had gastric cancer, the results showed increased median OS with the addition of trastuzumab compared with chemotherapy alone (13.8 months vs. 11 months).[67] Trastuzumab deruxtecan (an antibody-drug conjugate) is now the standard second-line treatment option for patients with HER2-positive gastroesophageal adenocarcinoma after showing improvement in OS over chemotherapy alone (median 12.5 months vs. 8.4 months).[68] Another FDA-approved second-line therapy is ramucirumab, a monoclonal antibody targeting vascular endothelial growth receptor (VEGFR). The REGARD trial showed a survival benefit with this drug for patients who failed first-line chemotherapy for EGJ adenocarcinoma.[69]

Additionally, the FDA approved the use of select tropomyosin receptor kinase (TRK) inhibitors for *NTRK* gene fusion–positive tumors, selpercatinib for *RET* gene fusion–positive tumors, and dabrafenib/trametinib for tumors with *BRAF* V600E mutations.

Immunotherapy

Immunotherapy has emerged as a significant strategy across all fields of oncology. Specifically, therapies known as *immune checkpoint inhibitors* (ICIs) target pathways that allow cancers to evade immune attack. Binding of PD-L1 on the surface of cancer cells to the programmed cell death 1 (PD-1) on T and B lymphocytes activates a pathway that prevents T cells from recognizing cancer as foreign. ICIs are monoclonal antibodies that bind either to PD-L1 (atezolizumab, durvalumab) or PD-1 (nivolumab, pembrolizumab) and block this pathway, thereby facilitating T-cell–mediated antitumor response. Another set of ICIs targets the cytotoxic T-lymphocyte–associated protein 4 (CTLA-4) pathway (ipilimumab, tremelimumab). Treatment with ICIs is based on testing for MSI or MMR, PD-L1 expression, or high tumor mutational burden (TMB).

The effectiveness of ICIs has been demonstrated in many cancers, including malignant melanoma and non–small cell lung cancer. Numerous phase III trials have evaluated ICIs in patients with esophageal cancer, leading to FDA approvals across multiple lines of therapy. One key observation from these trials is that ICIs have greater efficacy against SCC than against adenocarcinoma. Furthermore, tumors with higher PD-L1 positivity (combined positive score [CPS] or tumor area positive ≥10) were associated with improved efficacy.[70] Thus far, anti–PD-1 drugs (nivolumab, pembrolizumab) are indicated in combination with chemotherapy or with ipilimumab in the first-line treatment of advanced-stage esophageal SCC and as monotherapy in the second-line setting. The benefit of ICIs for esophageal adenocarcinoma remains unclear.

The role of immunotherapy in multimodal treatment for locally advanced disease was most recently demonstrated in the phase III CheckMate 577 trial. Patients with locally advanced esophageal cancer (SCC and adenocarcinoma) treated with neoadjuvant chemoradiation with residual pathologic disease after resection were randomized to either adjuvant nivolumab or placebo. Patients in the nivolumab arm experienced a median disease-free survival (DFS) of 22.4 months as compared with 11.0 months with placebo. Adjuvant nivolumab also had longer metastasis-free survival. As such, nivolumab is FDA approved for patients with completely resected esophageal or EGJ tumors with residual pathologic disease who had received neoadjuvant chemoradiation.[71]

Studies are underway to investigate the role of immunotherapy in the neoadjuvant setting, such the as MATTERHORN trial

(durvalumab with fluorouracil, leucovorin, oxaliplatin, and docetaxel [FLOT]).[72] As the results of ongoing trials are reported, immunotherapy may change the landscape of multimodal treatment in the near future.

Multimodal Therapy for Locally Advanced Disease

Each treatment modality offers a different mechanism for eliminating cancer, but no treatment alone is sufficient for locoregional disease. Although surgical resection was the mainstay of esophageal cancer treatment in the past, it became clear that even the most radical resections with extensive lymph node dissection are not enough to cure locoregionally advanced disease. Distant recurrence or metastatic disease continues to be the primary cause of mortality. Therefore, adding other modalities of treatment to surgery is necessary.

Large randomized controlled trials investigating combining these modalities and the sequence of each have led to considerable progress in treating resectable locally advanced esophageal cancer, overall demonstrating that neoadjuvant therapy with surgery significantly increases survival compared with surgery alone. (*Neoadjuvant therapy* refers to all treatment before surgical resection, whereas treatment occurring after surgery is termed *adjuvant therapy*. The term *induction therapy* is sometimes used interchangeably with *neoadjuvant therapy*. However, *induction* specifically refers to delivery of chemotherapy before radiation therapy [RT], in contrast with concurrent chemoradiotherapy.)

For resectable locally advanced esophageal cancer, neoadjuvant therapy followed by surgery has become the standard of care. Neoadjuvant therapy aims to downsize tumors, increase local control, improve rates of R0 resection, and eradicate undetected metastatic disease. Two main strategies are supported: (1) neoadjuvant chemoradiation and (2) perioperative chemotherapy. Regimens within these schemes are variable. Therefore, treatment plans should be made in multidisciplinary fashion and tailored to each patient's specific disease and traits. Restaging FDG-PET/CT should be done at 5 to 8 weeks after completion of neoadjuvant therapy before proceeding with surgery.

A third option, definitive chemoradiation, exists for patients with resectable disease but deemed not medically fit to undergo surgery or who decline surgery. Definitive chemoradiation is also indicated for patients with unresectable (T4b) locally advanced disease.

Neoadjuvant Chemoradiation

For the treatment of locally advanced esophageal cancer, preoperative chemoradiation is associated with improved OS, DFS, and pathologic complete response (pCR) as compared with surgery alone (Table 84.5).[73–75]

The landmark multicenter phase III randomized Chemoradiotherapy for Oesophageal Cancer Followed by Surgery (CROSS) trial (2012) showed that preoperative chemoradiation significantly improved OS and DFS compared with surgery alone in patients with resectable locally advanced (T2–T3, N0–N1, M0) esophageal and EGJ cancer. The majority (75%) of patients had adenocarcinoma, and 23% had SCC. The chemoradiation regimen consisted of carboplatin and paclitaxel administered concurrently with RT (41.4 Gy in 23 fractions). Esophagectomy was performed within 4 to 6 weeks in the treatment group and immediately after randomization in the control group. A number of significant observations were made. In the preoperative chemoradiation arm, the rate of R0 resection was higher than in the surgery-alone group (92% vs. 69%). In patients with SCC, those who received preoperative chemoradiation experienced complete pathologic response

TABLE 84.5 Clinical Trials for Establishing the Role of Multimodal Therapy Versus Surgery Alone for Esophageal Cancer

A. NEOADJUVANT CHEMORADIATION PLUS SURGERY VERSUS SURGERY ALONE				
CLINICAL TRIAL	SIZE	HISTOLOGY	INTERVENTION/CONTROL	KEY OUTCOMES IN INTERVENTION GROUP
CROSS (2012)	366	Adenocarcinoma (75%) SCC (23%)	I: Carboplatin/paclitaxel with concurrent RT (41.4 Gy, 23 fractions), then surgery C: Surgery alone	• Higher rate of R0 resection (92% vs. 69%) • 49% rate of pathologic complete response for SCC, 29% for adenocarcinoma • Longer median OS (49.4 months vs. 24 months) • Higher 5-year OS (47% vs. 34%)
NEOCRTEC (2018)	451	SCC	I: Vinorelbine/cisplatin with concurrent RT (40 Gy, 20 fractions), then surgery C: Surgery alone	• Higher rate of R0 resection (98.4% vs. 91.2%) • 43.2% rate of pathologic complete response • Longer median OS (100.1 months vs. 66.5 months) • Prolonged DFS (100.1 months vs. 41.7 months) • Higher 5-year OS (59.9% vs. 49.1%) in long-term follow-up study (2021)
B. PERIOPERATIVE CHEMOTHERAPY PLUS SURGERY *VERSUS* SURGERY ALONE				
CLINICAL TRIAL	SIZE	HISTOLOGY	INTERVENTION/CONTROL	KEY OUTCOMES IN INTERVENTION GROUP
MAGIC (2006)	503	Adenocarcinoma (*majority stomach,* 25% esophageal and EGJ)	I: Pre- and post-op epirubicin, cisplatin, 5-FU C: Surgery alone	• Improved DFS • Improved 5-year OS (36% vs 23%)
FNCLCC ACCORD 07 (2011)	224	Adenocarcinoma (75% esophageal and EGJ)	I: Pre- and post-op cisplatin, 5-FU C: Surgery alone	• Improved 5-year OS (38% vs 24%) • 8% decrease in distant recurrence rates • Improved R0 resection rate (84% vs 74%)

C, Control; *CROSS*, Chemoradiotherapy for Oesophageal Cancer Followed by Surgery; *DFS*, disease-free survival; *I*, intervention; *NEOCRTEC*, Neoadjuvant Chemoradiotherapy for Esophageal Cancer; *OS*, overall survival; *RT*, radiation therapy; *SCC*, squamous cell carcinoma.

(ypT0N0M0) significantly more than patients with adenocarcinoma (49% vs. 29%). Expectedly, nodal positivity was higher in patients with surgery alone compared with the preoperative chemoradiation group (75% vs. 31%). At a median follow-up duration of 45 months, patients receiving preoperative chemoradiation had significantly longer median OS (49.4 months) than patients undergoing surgery alone (24 months). The 1-, 2-, 3-, and 5-year OS rates were 82%, 67%, 58%, and 47%, respectively, in the preoperative chemoradiation arm compared with 70%, 50%, 44%, and 34%, respectively, in the surgery-alone arm.[76] After a minimum follow-up of 24 months, the overall rate of recurrence was 35% in the preoperative chemoradiation arm compared with 58% with surgery alone. Additionally, preoperative chemoradiation significantly reduced locoregional recurrence from 34% to 14%.[77] Importantly, preoperative chemoradiation did not negatively affect postoperative health-related quality of life.[78]

Although the CROSS trial established the survival benefit for preoperative chemoradiation therapy with a paclitaxel and carboplatin regimen, subsequent trials examined other chemotherapy regimens. The single-arm SWOG trial demonstrated the efficacy and safety of preoperative FOLFOX (5-fluorouracil and oxaliplatin) combined with radiation. PROTECT is an ongoing randomized phase II trial that is directly comparing preoperative chemoradiation with FOLFOX versus carboplatin/paclitaxel regimens, both with concurrent RT (41.4 Gy). The Cancer and Leukemia Group B (CALGB) 9781 prospective phase III trial investigated the preoperative regimen of cisplatin and 5-FU (CF) and 50.4 Gy followed by surgery versus surgery alone, which also showed 5-year OS benefit (39% vs. 16%).[79]

Although the majority of patients in the previous trials had adenocarcinoma, the NEOCRTEC trial (2018) exclusively enrolled patients with locally advanced SCC and compared safety and survival outcomes of preoperative chemoradiation plus surgery versus surgery alone. The preoperative chemoradiation arm had a higher R0 resection rate (98.4% vs. 91.2%), improved median OS (100.1 months vs. 66.5 months), and prolonged DFS. Incidences of postoperative complications were similar between both groups.[80]

In summary, the collective findings of these randomized control trials consistently showed that preoperative chemoradiation improves OS compared with surgery alone among patients with locally advanced esophageal cancer for both adenocarcinoma and SCC.

Given that pCR was found in a substantial portion of patients who had undergone neoadjuvant chemoradiation and given the morbidity of esophagectomy, some have questioned the necessity of surgical resection. Two early studies that compared patients who received neoadjuvant chemoradiation followed by surgery versus additional chemoradiation found no difference in OS.[81,82] In a more recent study involving patients who achieved clinical complete response to chemoradiation, active surveillance was associated with similar progression-free survival and OS to that observed with immediate esophagectomy.[83] Several phase III studies are investigating variations of a selective surgery approach, including the most recently published SANO trial (2025), which investigated the option for active surveillance for patients with clinical complete response after neoadjuvant chemoradiation. Clinical complete response was defined by no tumor detected by endoscopic biopsies, EUS, and PET/CT at 6 and 12 weeks following completion of neoadjuvant therapy, after which patients were then randomized to active surveillance or esophagectomy. The study found that OS after active surveillance was noninferior compared with standard surgery after two years.[84] Despite these findings, active surveillance remains controversial as the ability to accurately determine complete clinical response remains limited: Concordance between clinical complete response and pCR is only ~30%.[85] Developing methods, such as ctDNA, for detecting minimal residual disease could help fill this knowledge gap.

Perioperative Chemotherapy

Since the initial trials that showed survival benefit with neoadjuvant chemotherapy (e.g., the MRC and UK OEO2 studies previously mentioned), several notable studies have established the effectiveness of perioperative chemotherapy (i.e., neoadjuvant and adjuvant) for the treatment of locally advanced esophageal cancer (see Table 84.5).

One of the first landmark trials was the phase III MRC Adjuvant Gastric Infusional Chemotherapy (MAGIC) trial (2006), which used a regimen of epirubicin, cisplatin, and 5-FU (ECF) pre- and postoperatively (three cycles each). It should be noted that the majority of enrolled patients had adenocarcinoma of the stomach, but there was a subgroup with EGJ and lower esophageal cancer. Moreover, only 50% of patients were able to complete the prescribed course of adjuvant therapy. Regardless, the results demonstrated improved DFS and OS, with better 5-year OS of 36% with perioperative chemotherapy versus 23% with surgery alone. Preoperative chemotherapy also reduced tumor size in all patients but had limited effects on R0 resection rates. The limitation of this trial was that only 25% of participants had EGJ or lower esophageal adenocarcinoma; therefore, the results could not be extrapolated to esophageal cancer with certainty.[86]

Therefore, the French FNCLCC ACCORD 07 FCCD 9703 trial (2011) randomized 224 patients, 75% of whom had adenocarcinoma of the distal esophagus or EGJ, to perioperative CF and surgery compared with surgery alone. The researchers found a significant OS benefit (38% vs. 24%) in the perioperative chemotherapy group compared with surgery alone and an 8% reduction in distant recurrence rates. This trial also showed a significantly improved R0 resection rate in the perioperative chemotherapy group compared with surgery alone (84% vs. 74%). Although this trial was prematurely terminated because of low accrual, it argued for CF as a viable neoadjuvant regimen.[87]

The phase II/III FLOT4 trial (2019) received significant attention because it compared two different perioperative chemotherapy regimens—FLOT (four cycles pre- and postoperative of fluorouracil, leucovorin, oxaliplatin, docetaxel) to standard ECF (the MAGIC trial regimen)—in patients with resectable gastric or EGJ adenocarcinoma (Table 84.6). The results showed that FLOT was associated with a significantly higher rate of pCR than ECF (16% vs. 6%). FLOT was also associated with a reduction in the percentage of patients who experienced at least one grade 3 or 4 adverse event (40% vs. 25% in the ECF group). The phase III portion of the trial showed that median OS was increased in the FLOT group compared with the ECF group (50 months vs. 35 months), as was 5-year OS (45% vs. 36%). The percentage of patients with serious chemotherapy-related adverse events was the same (27% in both groups).[88] Given these findings, FLOT is now considered the standard care for esophageal adenocarcinoma patients, with the NCCN recommending its use for patients with good performance status. FOLFOX is recommended for patients with good to moderate performance status.[19]

For esophageal SCC, the Japan Clinical Oncology Group (JCOG) 9907 trial (2012) confirmed the benefits of using perioperative CF-based chemotherapy regimen, which improved the R0 resection rate and OS (55% vs. 43%).[89] As a result, neoadjuvant CF-based chemotherapy has become the standard treatment for locally advanced esophageal SCC in Japan.

Based on these large clinical trials, neoadjuvant therapy, whether given as preoperative chemoradiation or perioperative chemotherapy, confers survival advantage compared with surgery alone for patients with locally advanced esophageal cancer. Which strategy is better (see Table 84.6)? The Neoadjuvant Trial in Adenocarcinoma

---

TABLE 84.6   Clinical Trials Comparing Different Multimodal Therapies for Esophageal Cancer

A. COMPARING DIFFERENT PERIOPERATIVE CHEMOTHERAPY REGIMENS

CLINICAL TRIAL	SIZE	HISTOLOGY	INTERVENTION/CONTROL	KEY OUTCOMES IN INTERVENTION GROUP
FLOT4 (2019)	265	Adenocarcinoma (gastric, GEJ)	I: FLOT (fluorouracil, leucovorin, oxaliplatin, docetaxel) C: Epirubicin, leucovorin, oxaliplatin (MAGIC regimen)	• Higher rate of pCR (16% vs. 6%) • Improved median OS (50 vs. 35 months) • Improved 5-year OS (45% vs. 36%)

B. NEOADJUVANT CHEMORADIATION VERSUS PERIOPERATIVE CHEMOTHERAPY

CLINICAL TRIAL	SIZE	HISTOLOGY	INTERVENTION/CONTROL	KEY OUTCOMES IN INTERVENTION GROUP
NEO-AEGIS (2023)	377	Adenocarcinoma (esophagus, GEJ)	C: Modified MAGIC or FLOT regimen (perioperative chemotherapy) I: CROSS regimen (preoperative chemoRT)	• Similar number of deaths in both arms • Similar 3-year OS (55% vs. 57%) • Pathologic endpoints (pathologic complete response, R0 resection, nodal downstaging) favored preoperative chemoRT
ESOPEC (2025)	438	Adenocarcinoma (esophagus, GEJ)	C: FLOT regimen (perioperative chemotherapy) I: CROSS regimen (preoperative chemoRT)	• Improved 3-year OS with FLOT (57.4%) compared to CROSS (50.7%) • Lower 90-day mortality after surgery with FLOT (3.1%) compared to CROSS (5.6%) • Higher rate of adverse events in FLOT group

C, Control; *chemoRT*, chemoradiation therapy; *CROSS*, Chemoradiotherapy for Oesophageal Cancer Followed by Surgery; *GEJ*, gastroesophageal junction; *I*, intervention; *MAGIC*, Medical Research Council Adjuvant Gastric Infusional Chemotherapy; *NEO-AGIS*, Neoadjuvant Trial in Adenocarcinoma of the Esophagus and Esophago-Gastric Junction International Study; *OS*, overall survival; *pCR*, pathologic complete response.

of the Esophagus and Esophago-Gastric Junction International Study (Neo-AEGIS, 2023) directly compared preoperative chemoradiation (CROSS regimen) to perioperative chemotherapy (modified MAGIC or FLOT regimen) in 377 patients with esophageal adenocarcinoma. At a median follow-up of 38.8 months, median OS was 48 months in the perioperative chemotherapy group and 49.2 months in the preoperative chemoradiation group with 3 year OS of 55% and 57%, respectively. All pathologic end points (pCR rate and R0 resection status) favored preoperative chemoradiation.[90] Though underpowered and incomplete, Neo-AEGIS suggested noninferiority of perioperative chemotherapy to preoperative chemoradiation. Subsequently, the ESOPEC trial (2025) made a similar comparison by evaluating the effectiveness of perioperative chemotherapy (using FLOT) versus preoperative chemoradiation (per the CROSS regimen) in 438 patients with esophageal adenocarcinoma. In contrast to Neo-AEGIS, this trial found a greater survival benefit with perioperative FLOT than with preoperative chemoradiation (CROSS), with 3-year OS being 57.4% compared to 50.7%, respectively. While longer term results are to be seen, both strategies remain viable options for patients of resectable locoregional adenocarcinoma.[91]

Definitive Chemoradiation

Definitive chemoradiation is indicated for nonsurgical candidates (patients who decline surgery or patients unable to tolerate major surgery). It is also recommended for patients with cT4b (unresectable) esophageal cancer and, in some cases, can facilitate surgical resection (salvage esophagectomy) in select patients who have good response.[19] For inoperable disease, although radiation is a method of local control, chemotherapy is thought to sensitize tumor cells to radiation while also contributing to control of micrometastatic disease. The Radiation Therapy Oncology Group (RTOG) 85-01 was an early randomized trial that compared chemoradiation (with CF) versus radiation alone at a standard 50.4-Gy dose.[92] Patients in the chemoradiation arm showed significant improvement in median survival (14 months vs. 9 months) and 5-year OS (27% vs. 0%) and also had a lower incidence of local failure (47% vs. 65%). Multiple trials (the follow-up INT-0123, ARTDECO, and CONCORDE) have shown no benefit of radiation dose escalation above 50 Gy.[64,93,94] Cisplatin with either docetaxel or paclitaxel is the recommended regimen for definitive chemoradiation.

Posttreatment Management and Outcomes

Postoperative management is based on surgical margins, pathologic tumor stage, histology, and previous treatment. Patients who received neoadjuvant chemotherapy as part of a perioperative protocol should complete the adjuvant cycles of chemotherapy once recovered from surgery. For patients who had undergone neoadjuvant chemoradiation and R0 resection found to have residual disease on final pathology, adjuvant nivolumab is recommended based on the CheckMate 577 trial.[68] Other than this, the components of postoperative management have not been established in randomized trials specifically for esophageal cancer. Instead, available evidence for the use of postoperative chemoradiation and chemotherapy is extrapolated from trials for gastric cancer. For patients who had not received neoadjuvant therapy, capecitabine/oxaliplatin or FOLFOX are acceptable options. The INT-0116 trial demonstrated effectiveness of postoperative chemoradiation in patients with resected gastric or EGJ adenocarcinoma who had not received preoperative therapy.[95–97]

All patients should be followed in a systematic manner after completion of multimodal therapy. However, surveillance strategies after successful therapy remain variable and controversial, with no high-level evidence to guide algorithms that balance benefits and risks. The NCCN guidelines provide stage-specific strategies based on currently available evidence from retrospective studies and expert consensus. Approximately 90% of recurrences occur within the first 2 years of local therapy, and most recurrences occur as distant disease. Although routine esophageal cancer-specific surveillance is generally not recommended for more than 5 years after end of treatment, exceptions should be considered based on risk factors.[19]

In general, follow-up for asymptomatic patients should include complete history and physical examination every 3 to 6 months in the first 2 years and then every 6 to 12 months for years 3 to 5. A complete blood count, chemistry profile, upper endoscopy with biopsy, and cross-sectional imaging should be performed based on stage of treated disease and as clinically indicated.[19]

Although Tis-T1aN0 disease have prognoses that approximate a noncancer cohort, T1b disease has comparatively worse prognosis. Thus, surveillance recommendations vary according to depth of invasion as well as the treatment modality. Endoscopic surveillance is recommended for early-stage disease (Tis, T1a, T1b) in patients treated with ER/ablation. Imaging studies should additionally be considered for T1b patients.[19]

Locoregional recurrence is relatively uncommon with neoadjuvant therapy followed by esophagectomy, so endoscopic surveillance is not indicated (although endoscopy should be considered if symptomatic). Instead, distant recurrence is the more common pattern.[98–99] Therefore, these patients are followed with cross-sectional imaging every 6 months for up to 2 years and annually for up to 5 years. On the other hand, locoregional recurrence is common after definitive chemoradiation, making upper endoscopy a logical surveillance strategy in these patients in addition to cross-sectional imaging.[100]

Unresectable Locally Advanced, Recurrent, and Metastatic Disease

In patients with locoregional recurrence after definitive chemoradiation therapy, salvage esophagectomy is an option if the patient is deemed medically fit for surgery and if the recurrence is resectable. For patients who have had prior esophagectomy with recurrent disease, treatment options include concurrent chemoradiation, reoperation, systemic therapy (chemotherapy, targeted therapy, or immunotherapy), or palliative management/best supportive care. For those who are medically unable to tolerate major surgery and those with unresectable or metastatic recurrence, palliative management and best supportive care are always indicated.[19]

Systemic therapy, which includes chemotherapy and targeted therapy or immunotherapy (depending on MSI or MMR, PD-L1, and HER2 status), is also an option but should only be offered to patients with good performance status. For both esophageal adenocarcinoma and SCC, cisplatin with 5-FU is the standard first-line treatment option for patients with locally advanced disease who are not candidates for surgery or definitive chemoradiation. Adding docetaxel and variants of this regimen have demonstrated better tolerability and outcomes. Oxaliplatin plus capecitabine is noninferior to CF, possibly with a more manageable toxicity profile. Nonetheless, chemotherapy has limited efficacy (OS less than 12 months) in most patients with advanced disease. In HER2-positive patients, trastuzumab combined with first-line chemotherapy has become standard therapy in advanced-stage esophageal adenocarcinoma. In patients with MMR deficiency and PD-L1–positive status, ICIs (anti-PD1 antibody drugs) are now indicated as first-line treatment for advanced-stage esophageal SCC in combination with chemotherapy or ipilimumab and as monotherapy in the second-line setting.[19]

Palliative and best supportive care are aimed at mitigating suffering and improving quality of life for patients and their caregivers, regardless of disease stage. In advanced or metastatic disease, such care can provide symptom relief and improve overall quality of life and may result in life prolongation, especially when a multimodality interdisciplinary approach is employed. Dysphagia and obstruction can be palliated with self-expanding metal stents. Palliative radiation is also an option. Additionally, enteral feeding access by jejunostomy or gastrostomy tube (if no resection is planned) may be needed to provide adequate nutrition and hydration.[19]

SUMMARY AND CONCLUSION

Esophageal cancer is a global disease with high mortality that remains a complex and challenging disease to treat. A multimodal therapeutic approach involving chemotherapy, surgery, and radiation has been shown by multiple large trials to confer the best chances for survival. Insight into the role of immunotherapy is forthcoming. Although survival outcomes have markedly improved over the past 40 to 50 years as a result of significant advances in treatment strategies and tools, OS remains low. There is still much to unravel about the biology of the disease and much to be distilled regarding which patients would benefit most from the armamentarium of treatment options and strategies.

SELECTED REFERENCES

Al-Batran SE, Homann N, Pauligk C, et al. Perioperative chemotherapy with fluorouracil plus leucovorin, oxaliplatin, and docetaxel versus fluorouracil or capecitabine plus cisplatin and epirubicin for locally advanced, resectable gastric or gastrooesophageal junction adenocarcinoma (FLOT4): a randomised, phase 2/3 trial. *Lancet.* 2019;393(10184):1948-1957.

In the footsteps of the MAGIC trial establishing a role for perioperative chemotherapy, this trial sought to compare a new regimen (FLOT) to the MAGIC regimen to see if it could also increase overall survival with potentially a better toxicity profile. Although the toxicity profiles were similar for both groups, overall survival proved to be better with the FLOT regimen than with the MAGIC regimen. As such, FLOT has become the standard-of-care regimen in patients with good functional status.

Cunningham D, Alum WH, Stenning SP, et al. Perioperative chemotherapy versus surgery alone for resectable gastroesophageal cancer. *N Engl J Med.* 2006;355(1):11-20.

Also known as the MAGIC trial, this is one of the early landmark trials establishing a role for perioperative chemotherapy in the treatment of resectable gastric and esophagogastric cancer, showing survival advantage in patients who received perioperative chemotherapy and surgery versus surgery

alone. *Although not definitively applicable to esophageal cancer at the time because that patient cohort was the minority population, it laid the foundation for subsequent trials of multimodal therapy with different drug regimens and majority esophageal cancer patients.*

Kelly RJ, Ajani JA, Kuzdzal J, et al. Adjuvant nivolumab in resected esophageal or gastroesophageal junction cancer. *N Engl J Med.* 2021;384(13):1191-1203.

This was an important trial for two reasons: (1) establishing a role for immunotherapy in the treatment of resectable esophageal cancer and (2) presenting an adjuvant option for patients treated with neoadjuvant chemoradiation and then surgery who had residual pathologic disease and thus were at higher risk of recurrence. This trial showed that this group of patients benefitted from adjuvant nivolumab in terms of improved DFS.

National Comprehensive Cancer Network. *NCCN Guidelines Version 2.2023 Esophageal and Esophagogastric Junction Cancers.* 2023. https://www.nccn.org/guidelines/guidelines-detail?category=1&id=1433

The NCCN provides guidelines and stage-based treatment algorithms that oncologists reference to help real-world decision-making. The guidelines are developed by a multi-institutional committee of oncologists from all fields and updated regularly. In addition to flowcharts, the guideline provides in-depth discussions of all aspects of cancer care.

Rice TW, Patil DP, Blackstone EH. 8th Edition AJCC/UICC staging of cancers of the esophagus and esophagogastric junction: application to clinical practice. *Ann Cardiothorac Surg.* 2017;6(2):1191-1130.

This article comprehensively reviews all aspects of the 8th edition AJCC/Union for International Cancer Control (UICC) staging for esophageal and esophagogastric junction cancers, including the rationale and data supporting the changes made from the previous edition. It elaborates on how the staging system can and should be applied in clinical practice.

van Hagen P, Hulshof MC, van Lanschot JJ, et al. Preoperative chemoradiotherapy for esophageal or junctional cancer. *N Engl J Med.* 2012;366:2074-2084.

Also known as the CROSS trial, this is an early landmark trial that established the now standard-of-care for neoadjuvant chemoradiation therapy for resectable esophageal cancer.

The full reference list appears on Elsevier eBooks+.

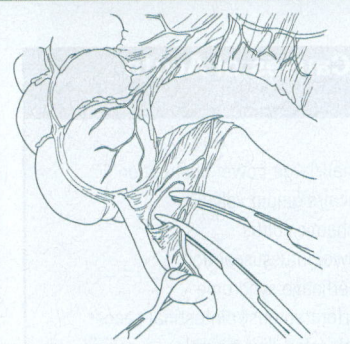

CHAPTER 85

The Acute Abdomen

Kaitlin A. Ritter, Mary I. Junak, John E. Scarborough, and Vanessa P. Ho

The abdomen is compartmentalized into intraperitoneal and retroperitoneal spaces. Critical to the acute abdomen, the intraperitoneal space houses organs such as the stomach, small intestines, transverse colon, liver, spleen, and appendix. In contrast, the retroperitoneal space contains the kidneys, pancreas, ascending and descending parts of the colon, and major vessels. Abdominal pain can originate from any of these organs because of varied etiologies such as inflammation, obstruction, perforation, or ischemia.

Vascular supply to the abdomen is primarily from the abdominal aorta, which bifurcates into the common iliac arteries at the level of the fourth lumbar vertebra. Emerging from the aorta to supply the abdominal organs are major branches: the celiac trunk, the superior mesenteric artery (SMA), and the inferior mesenteric artery (IMA). These vessels, in turn, branch out to supply blood to the abdominal organs (Fig. 85.1). Compromise in the perfusion from any of these arteries, as seen in conditions like mesenteric ischemia, can precipitate acute abdominal symptoms. Furthermore, the venous return is predominantly through the portal system into the inferior vena cava, and obstruction or thrombosis in these veins can also contribute to acute abdominal pathology.

The physiologic basis for abdominal pain is rooted in the intricate innervation of the peritoneum. The peritoneum is divided into the parietal and visceral components. The parietal peritoneum, lining the abdominal wall, is innervated by somatic nerves that correspond to the dermatomes of the overlying skin. As a result, any irritation or inflammation of this layer produces sharp, well-localized pain. In contrast, the visceral peritoneum, which envelops the abdominal organs, is supplied by autonomic nerves. Irritation of the visceral peritoneum yields dull, poorly localized pain, often described as "crampy" or "achy." Therefore, the nature and localization of abdominal pain can offer invaluable clues regarding the underlying pathology, be it arising from the abdominal wall or the internal organs themselves. Visceral inflammation can evolve to parietal inflammation, explaining the classic abdominal pain patterns in inflammatory diseases such as appendicitis: vague periumbilical pain that localizes to the right lower quadrant as the parietal peritoneum becomes involved in the inflammatory process.

DIFFERENTIAL DIAGNOSIS

The diagnosis of an "acute abdomen" is in and of itself not actually a specific medical or surgical condition, but rather a collection of symptoms, physical examination findings, and diagnostic workup that suggests an acute process within or even external to the abdominal cavity that frequently requires operative management. The threshold for labeling the onset of abdominal pain as acute (vs. subacute or chronic) is generally, though arbitrarily, set at 1 week. The differential diagnosis for an acute abdomen is broad and can involve multiple organ systems. A list of frequent causes of an acute abdomen can be seen in Table 85.1.

Narrowing of this differential relies heavily on thorough clinical history taking and physical examination. The history must include the patient age, sex, and associated signs and symptoms and must incorporate the patient's past medical and surgical history. Certain diagnoses are more common in specific age groups because the likelihood of developing various processes will change over the course of a patient's life. Diverticulitis, biliary tract disease, and peptic ulcers are common causes of acute pain in adults, but not in younger patients. Even within pediatric populations, disease frequency varies across childhood (Table 85.2). Females of childbearing age have a unique set of gynecologic-related conditions that must be considered (see the later section "Special

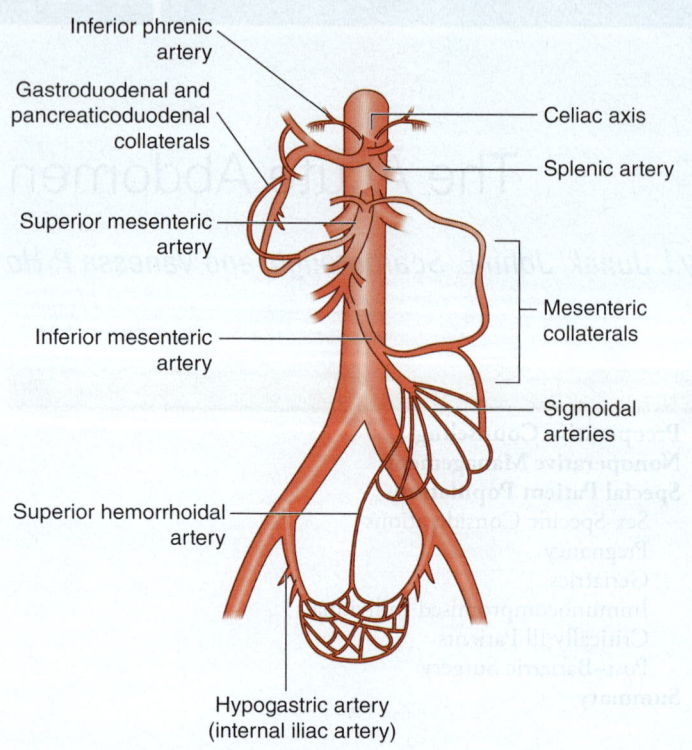

FIGURE 85.1 Vascular anatomy of the abdominal viscera. (From Jomha A, Schmidt M. Mesenteric vascular disease. In: Brzozowski T, ed. *New Advances in the Basic and Clinical Gastroenterology.* Intechopen; 2012.)

Inferior phrenic artery
Gastroduodenal and pancreaticoduodenal collaterals
Celiac axis
Splenic artery
Superior mesenteric artery
Mesenteric collaterals
Inferior mesenteric artery
Sigmoidal arteries
Superior hemorrhoidal artery
Hypogastric artery (internal iliac artery)

TABLE 85.1 Surgical Causes of Acute Abdomen in Adults

Gastrointestinal

Perforated gastric/duodenal ulcer	Small/large bowel obstruction
Cholecystitis	Cecal/sigmoid volvulus
Appendicitis	Ischemic colitis
Incarcerated/strangulated hernia	Bowel intussusception
Meckel diverticulitis	Boerhaave syndrome
Colonic/intestinal diverticulitis	Perforated gastrointestinal cancer
Internal hernia	Perforated diverticulitis

Solid Organ

Hepatic abscess	Acute pancreatitis/pancreatic necrosis
Splenic abscess	Pancreatic pseudocyst
Traumatic hepatic/splenic laceration	Spontaneous splenic rupture

Genitourinary

Nephrolithiasis	Tuboovarian abscess
Renal abscess	Pelvic inflammatory disease with abscess
Ectopic pregnancy	Endometriosis
Ovarian/testicular torsion	Hemorrhagic ovarian cyst
Uterine torsion/rupture	Placental abruption

Vascular

Aortoduodenal fistula	Hemoperitoneum
Abdominal aortic aneurysm	Aortic dissection
Arteriovenous malformation	Visceral aneurysms
Mesenteric arterial occlusion	Gastrointestinal bleeding

TABLE 85.2 Differential Diagnosis of Abdominal Pain in Pediatric Populations By Age

BIRTH TO 2 YEARS OLD	2–5 YEARS OLD	5–12 YEARS OLD	>12 YEARS OLD
Intussusception	Intussusception	Appendicitis	Appendicitis
Gastroenteritis	Appendicitis	Gastroenteritis	Gastroenteritis
Constipation	Gastroenteritis	Constipation	Constipation
Infantile colic	Constipation	Mesenteric adenitis	Ovarian/testicular torsion
Malrotation with midgut volvulus	Mesenteric adenitis	Functional abdominal pain	Dysmenorrhea
Incarcerated inguinal hernia	Malrotation with midgut volvulus	Pneumonia	Pelvic inflammatory disease
Obstruction due to Hirschsprung disease	Sickle cell crisis	Sickle cell crisis	Ectopic pregnancy
Urinary tract infection	Henoch-Schönlein purpura	Henoch-Schönlein purpura	
Meckel diverticulum	Urinary tract infection	Urinary tract infection	
Necrotizing enterocolitis	Trauma	Trauma	
	Meckel diverticulum		

Adopted from Yang WC, Chen CY, Wu HP. Etiology of non-traumatic acute abdomen in pediatric emergency departments. *World J Clin Cases.* 2013;1:276-284.

Patient Populations"). Similarly, geriatric populations are at risk for atypical presentation of common conditions because of age-related changes in muscle and nerve fibers, which can alter motor and sensory functions.[1] An understanding of a patient's prior abdominal procedures and operations may also provide clues to possible diagnoses because prior surgeries, infections, and cancers can change the differential.

Although a consult for an acute abdomen often sparks concern for an underlying surgical process, several medical conditions can also produce these findings.[2] Attention to potential medical confounders is equally important for the evaluating surgeon so as to avoid the unnecessary surgical intervention. Acute pancreatitis,

sickle cell crisis, diabetic ketoacidosis, spontaneous bacterial peritonitis, and pyelonephritis are just a few of the common medical processes that can mimic an acute surgical pathology (Table 85.3). Careful attention to a patient's history can often provide insight into these conditions.

EVALUATION

History

Although advances in laboratory studies and imaging help facilitate more accurate diagnoses, a comprehensive history remains the first key step in workup of the acute abdomen. Careful attention

TABLE 85.3 Nonsurgical Causes of Acute Abdomen in Adults

Metabolic/Endocrine
Diabetic ketoacidosis	Hypercalcemia
Hyperosmolar hyperglycemic state	Hypophosphatemia
Addison disease	Hypokalemia
Porphyria	Hyperthyroidism
Familial Mediterranean fever	Uremia

Hematologic/Immunologic
Sickle cell crisis	Henoch-Schönlein purpura
Thrombotic thrombocytopenic purpura	Mast cell activation syndrome
Hemolytic uremic syndrome	Hereditary angioneurotic edema
Acute leukemia	

Cardiopulmonary/Vascular
Myocardial infarction	Pulmonary embolus
Aortic dissection	Pneumonia

Infectious
Malaria	Yersinia enterocolitica
Staphylotoxin	Dengue fever
Tuberculosis mesenteritis	Spontaneous bacterial peritonitis
Pyelonephritis	

Drugs/Toxins
Salicylate	Anticholinergics
Tricyclic antidepressant overdose	Heavy metals
Cocaine	Narcotic

Neuropsychiatric
Herpes zoster	Abdominal migraine
Radiculopathy	Irritable bowel syndrome
Functional abdominal pain syndrome	

Vasculitis/Connective Tissue
Systemic lupus erythematosus	Scleroderma
Systemic vasculitis	

Adapted from Sapmaz F, Basyigit S, Basaran M, et al. Non-surgical causes of acute abdominal pain. In: Garbuzenko D, ed. *Actual Problems of Emergency Abdominal Surgery*. London: IntechOpen; 2016:95-107.

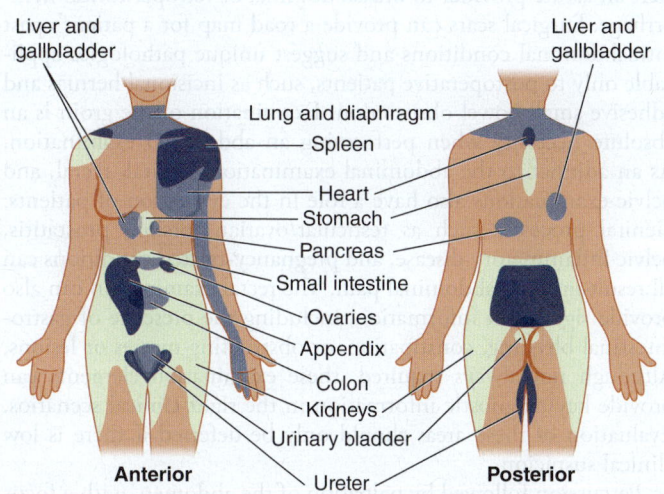

FIGURE 85.2 Cutaneous sites of referred pain from visceral structures. (From Anderson MK. *Foundations of Athletic Training*. 6th ed. Lippincott Williams & Wilkins; 2016, Figure 6-1.)

to the onset, character, location, quality, and duration of the abdominal pain can provide key clues to the underlying etiology. As discussed earlier, the two-part innervation of the abdominal cavity by the parietal and visceral peritoneum allows for often unique presentations of various pathologies[3] (Fig. 85.2). One such example includes irritation of the diaphragm by free intraperitoneal air resulting in referred pain to the shoulder because of the phrenic nerve's anatomic connections to the brachial plexus.[4,5] Thus, although the nature of the patient's abdominal pain is an important element of the history, other nonabdominal pain should be evaluated as well. In addition to abdominal pain referred to nonabdominal locations, it is also possible for extraabdominal processes to present with abdominal pain, such as occurs when acute myocardial infarction manifests as upper abdominal pain.[6]

Once an assessment of pain has been performed, the next step should include an evaluation of any other associated symptoms the patient is experiencing. Nausea, vomiting, diarrhea, or lack of bowel function can all provide important insight into an underlying gastrointestinal process. Fever, chills, and recent sick contacts can be suggestive of an infective process. Assessing for

accompanying symptoms can help guide the diagnostic workup, including the need for specific imaging adjuncts.

An understanding of the patient's past medical and surgical history is also important in the initial assessment. Certain causes of an acute abdomen are more likely with various medical conditions and can raise these diagnoses higher on the differential. Vascular processes such as ruptured abdominal aortic aneurysmal disease or acute mesenteric ischemia are of higher likelihood in a patient with chronic vasculopathy who remains an active smoker then in a healthy college student. Similarly, a patient's past surgical history can provide insight into the leading diagnosis. In the immediately postoperative patient, a unique set of causes of acute abdominal pain exist, such as a missed enterotomy or anastomotic leak. For females, questions regarding menstrual history, including last menstrual period, history of endometriosis, prior pregnancy/sexually transmitted diseases (STDs), recent sexual activity, and contraceptive use, are also essential.

Finally, a review of the patient's current medications, allergies, and social history (including tobacco, alcohol, and illicit drug use) should also be performed. Patients on steroids or immunosuppressive medications can often present with blunted physiologic responses to pain and infection and thus may require a higher degree of suspicion for more uncommon disease processes.[7] Potential noncompliance with prescribed medications may also suggest certain pathologies. The person with diabetes who has not been taking their insulin may present with diabetic ketoacidosis, whereas the patient with atrial fibrillation who has not been taking their prescribed anticoagulant may present with abdominal pain because of an embolic phenomenon.

Physical Examination

A thorough and complete physical examination, including abdominal inspection, palpation, percussion, and auscultation, can provide critical information in the assessment of a patient with an acute abdomen.[8] Inspection or visual assessment of the abdomen should pay attention to distention, scars/skin abnormalities, masses/hernias, or striae/enlarged veins. Skin changes such as periumbilical (Cullen sign) or flank (Grey Turner sign) bruising can alert an astute provider to intraabdominal or retroperitoneal hemorrhage. Surgical scars can provide a road map for a patient's past intraabdominal conditions and suggest unique pathologies applicable only to postoperative patients, such as incisional hernias and adhesive small bowel obstruction. Examination of the groin is an absolute necessity when performing an abdominal examination. As an adjunct to the abdominal examination, genital, rectal, and pelvic examinations also have a role in the evaluation of patients. Genital processes such as testicular/ovarian torsion, prostatitis, pelvic inflammatory disease, and pregnancy-related conditions can all result in acute abdominal pain. The rectal examination can also provide significant information, including the presence of gastrointestinal bleeding, constipation, or obstructing masses or lesions. Although not always required, these examination elements can provide key diagnostic information in the right clinical scenarios. Evaluation of these areas should only be deferred if there is low clinical suspicion.

Percussion followed by palpation of the abdomen, with a focus on areas of tenderness, referred pain, rebound, and involuntary guarding, can be instructive. Additionally, the surgeon should palpate for potential intraabdominal masses, abdominal wall defects, shifting dullness, or pulsative vascular structures. Palpable irreducible hernias with abdominal distention and tympany can reveal acute obstructive processes. Attention should be paid to the area of maximal tenderness because patients may initially endorse generalized abdominal pain but subsequently localize to a specific area upon careful examination. This localization and correlation with underlying anatomic structures can help narrow the differential diagnosis. Most patients with an acute abdomen will present with at least some of the classic findings of peritonitis, including involuntary guarding, abdominal rigidity, and rebound tenderness. Involuntary guarding can be difficult to determine, as patients will often voluntarily tense their abdominal wall muscles in response to palpation. Having the patient lie supine with their legs bent and soles of their feet on the bed will help to relax the abdominal musculature and allow for more accurate examination. Rebound tenderness, which occurs when the release of pressure from the abdominal wall causes worsening of the patient's pain, is caused by irritation of the parietal peritoneum and can thus be indicative of peritonitis. A special note should be made for complaints of severe pain without concomitant tenderness, referred to as *pain out of proportion to exam,* as this may herald organ ischemia rather than perforation. Careful assessment of vascular risk factors in these patients may raise the suspicion for acute mesenteric ischemia.

Auscultation, although a common examination maneuver taught in medical school, has limited utility in the assessment of the acute abdomen. Traditionally students are taught to listen for an absence of bowel sounds, or *high-pitched tinkling,* as indications of an obstruction. Studies of the accuracy of this maneuver have found poor sensitivity and specificity; consequently, its clinical use has gone by the wayside.[9] Auscultation for vascular abnormalities such as bruits, although technically possible, also has low specificity and sensitivity. Any data gathered from abdominal auscultation should be used in conjunction with the remainder of the physical examination.

In addition to the traditional abdominal examination, several eponymously named maneuvers and techniques have been developed, with variable correlation with specific disease processes (Table 85.4). One of the most commonly encountered (and often

TABLE 85.4   Eponymous Abdominal Examination Signs and Maneuvers

NAME	SIGN/MANEUVER	CLINICAL CORRELATION
Aaron sign	Pain or pressure in epigastrium with firm pressure applied to McBurney point	Referred pain in epigastrium from acute appendicitis
Balance sign	Dullness to percussion in the left upper quadrant/flank with shifting dullness in right flank	Splenic rupture/hematoma
Blumberg sign	Pain with removal of pressure rather than application of pressure to the abdomen	Peritoneal inflammation/peritonitis
Carnett sign	Continued or increased abdominal pain when abdominal wall muscles are tensed	Abdominal wall source of pain
Chandelier sign	Extreme pelvic pain with movement of the cervix	Pelvic inflammatory disease
Cullen sign	Periumbilical bruising	Hemoperitoneum
Danforth sign	Shoulder pain on inspiration	Irritation of the diaphragm by hemoperitoneum
Fothergill sign	Abdominal wall mass that does not cross midline and is palpable when rectus is contracted	Rectus sheath hematoma
Grey Turner sign	Discoloration/bruising of flanks between the last rib and the top of the hip	Retroperitoneal hemorrhage, severe acute pancreatitis
Hannington-Kiff sign	Absent adductor reflex in thigh with presence of positive patellar reflex	Compression of obturator nerve caused by obturator hernia
Howship-Romberg sign	Pain of inner thigh on internal rotation of the hip	Obturator hernia
Iliopsoas sign	Elevation of extended leg against resistance is painful	Retrocecal acute appendicitis
Murphy sign	Respiratory arrest during inspiration with palpation of the right upper quadrant	Acute cholecystitis
Obturator sign	Pain on passive internal rotation of the hip when the right knee is flexed	Pelvic abscess or inflammatory mass, pelvic appendicitis
Ransohoff sign	Yellow discoloration of umbilical region	Ruptured common bile duct
Rovsing sign	Pain felt in right lower quadrant when palpating the left lower quadrant	Acute appendicitis
Ten Horn sign	Pain in the right iliac fossa caused by gentle traction of right testicle	Acute appendicitis

misunderstood) findings is Murphy's sign of acute cholecystitis. With the patient supine, they are asked to exhale as the examiner palpates the right subcostal region. The patient is then asked to take a deep breath. As the diaphragm pushes the abdominal contents caudally during this inhalation, an acutely inflamed gallbladder will come in contact with parietal peritoneum underlying the examiner's hand. The pain of contact will result in the involuntary pausing of the patient's inhaled breath. Although potentially useful examination adjuncts, these eponymous findings must be used in the context of a complete history and physical examination because most do not provide sufficient sensitivity or specificity to allow for a definitive diagnosis on their own.[10]

Although the abdominal examination is a key feature of the physical examination for patients with a concern for an acute abdomen, evaluation of other body systems is also important. Patients with acute abdominal pain will often present with signs of systemic toxicity, including tachycardia, diaphoresis, and pallor. Increased work of breathing in the absence of pulmonary wheezing or rales can be suggestive of a compensatory respiratory process, and abdominal sepsis with acidosis can likewise manifest as a respiratory issue. Similarly, other nonabdominal examination findings can indicate an extraabdominal process masquerading as an acute abdomen. In a patient who presents with epigastric pain, the finding of distant heart sounds and diminished auscultation of bilateral lung bases may indicate the presence of an acute coronary syndrome rather than an intraabdominal process. To avoid such diagnostic errors, a full physical assessment should be performed in any patient who presents with acute abdominal pain.

Laboratory Studies

Laboratory results often help to provide additional clarity regarding the clinical condition of a patient who presents with an acute abdomen. In general, a complete blood count (CBC), basic metabolic panel (BMP), and serum lactate should be obtained in most patients who present with acute abdominal pain and whose history and physical examination support the existence of an acute abdominal disease process. The white blood cell count found on the CBC can be either elevated or reduced in many acute intraabdominal infectious processes. Further analysis of the white blood cell count using a cell differentiation test can demonstrate elevation of the neutrophil count (so termed *a left shift*), supporting the potential diagnosis of bacterial infection.[11] Low hematocrit or hemoglobin may suggest a hemorrhagic source of abdominal pathology, whereas elevation of the hematocrit/hemoglobin may alternatively suggest intravascular volume depletion caused by an intraabdominal process. Platelets are an acute-phase reactant that undergoes agonistic synergism with other acute-phase reactants such as C-reactive protein, and thus a reactive thrombocytosis may be found with many acute inflammatory/infectious conditions.[12] Similarly, the presence of acidosis on the BMP or an elevated serum lactate level can be indicative of a metabolic derangement with its own broad differential, ranging from dehydration, to evolving sepsis, to end-organ ischemia. The addition of an arterial blood gas in patients with lactic acidosis may help to further delineate underlying metabolic/respiratory disturbances.

Further laboratory evaluation should be based on the patient's clinical history, examination, and a differential diagnosis that has been narrowed by history and physical examination. Organ-specific tests such as liver function tests (LFTs) or serum amylase/lipase can be used to support the diagnosis of conditions such as cholecystitis, choledocholithiasis, or pancreatitis. A urinalysis can assist in the diagnosis of cystitis, pyelonephritis, or nephrolithiasis.

Clostridioides difficile toxin assay and an infectious stool panel, including ova/parasites, may be obtained in patients with the correct historical risk factors, such as recent antibiotic use or foreign travel. β–Human chorionic gonadotropin (β-HCG) is an important laboratory test in any females of reproductive age because pregnancy and pregnancy-related complications must always be considered in the differential of acute abdominal pain in sexually active females of childbearing age. In addition to the use of laboratory tests for diagnostic purposes, an active type and screen and updated coagulation studies are essential for patients in whom surgical intervention is anticipated.

DIAGNOSTIC STUDIES AND IMAGING

After a thorough medical history and physical examination, and in conjunction with laboratory studies, diagnostic imaging may be obtained. There are a wide variety of imaging options for the evaluation of abdominal pathology, ranging from noninvasive and low-cost to potentially harmful and expensive. A comprehensive but precise differential should be established before obtaining imaging so that the most appropriate modality can assist in establishing a definitive diagnosis. Although the initial instinct is to reflexively order cross-sectional imaging for any patient with a concerning abdominal examination, careful clinical workup and a thorough differential diagnosis can often spare these patients nondiagnostic tests and unnecessary radiation exposure. Relatively low-cost, low-risk, and time-saving imaging modalities such as ultrasound and plain film radiographs can offer significant information to narrow a differential diagnosis.

Ultrasound

Ultrasound uses high-frequency sound waves emitted from piezoelectric crystals in the transducer probe and allows for visualization of underlying structures because of the variable reflective and impedance properties of different tissues. This form of imaging does not require ionizing radiation and can provide rapid assessment for multiple acute intraabdominal pathologies. Ultrasound has moderate to excellent sensitivity for some disease processes and is the diagnostic gold standard for others.[13] Transabdominal, transthoracic, and transvaginal approaches all exist, each with their own unique set of views and identifiable pathologies. In the hands of an experienced operator, ultrasound can assess multiple organ systems, including the hepatic/biliary, vascular, gastrointestinal, and genitourinary systems (Fig. 85.3). Increasingly, point-of-care ultrasound (sometimes referred to as *POCUS*) has expanded within the emergency department and the intensive care unit, allowing for even more rapid image assessment of the acute abdomen.[14] Associated with high diagnostic accuracy, POCUS imaging has also been demonstrated to decrease the time to diagnosis and to be associated with a financial cost savings.[15,16] Limitations of ultrasound include the inability to penetrate bowel gas for visualization of deeper structures and the technical challenge for the patient with a larger body habitus, which reduces the ultrasound wave penetration and picture quality.

Plain Radiography

Plain film radiographs of the abdomen are another commonly used imaging modality. Although the diagnostic accuracy of plain film radiographs is significantly lower than that of other imaging studies, there are still several specific disease pathologies where they can provide significant information (Fig. 85.4). In the case of a perforated hollow viscus, an upright abdominal radiograph can

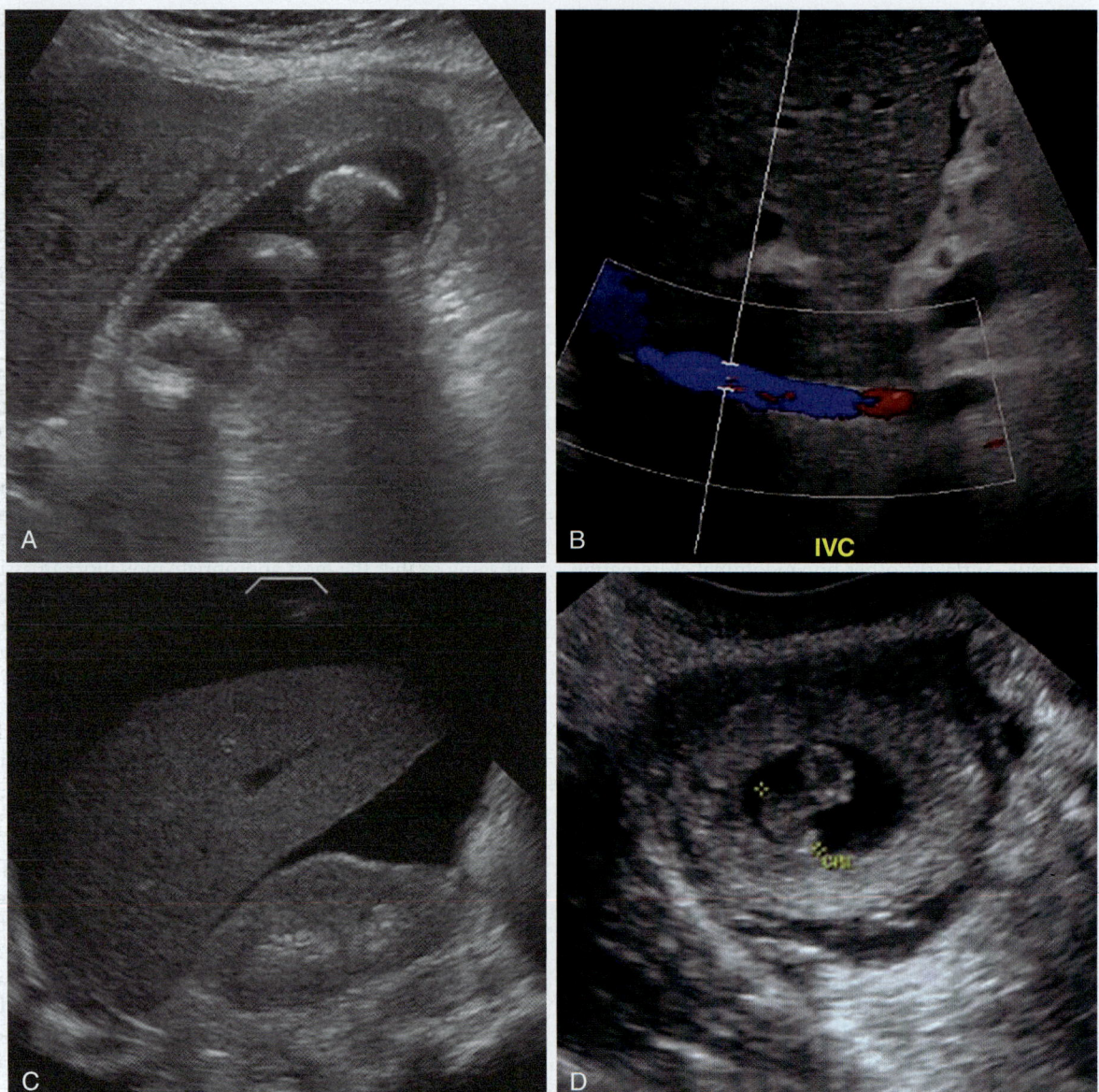

FIGURE 85.3 Ultrasound images of various abdominal structures. (A) Right upper quadrant ultrasound demonstrated gallbladder wall thickening, hyperechoic gallstones, and findings consistent with acute chole-cystitis. (B) Right upper quadrant ultrasound of liver and inferior vena cava *(IVC)* demonstrating cirrhotic liver morphology and calculation of IVC size for volume assessment. (C) Right upper quadrant ultrasound dem-onstrating free fluid between liver and kidney consistent with hemoperitoneum. (D) Pelvic ultrasound dem-onstrating ectopic pregnancy. (C, From American Institute of Ultrasound in Medicine; American College of Emergency Physicians. AIUM practice guideline for the performance of the focused assessment with sonography for trauma [FAST] examination. *J Ultrasound Med.* 2014;33:2047-2056; D, From Rizk B, Owens S, LaFleur J, Abuzeid M. Ectopic pregnancy: ultrasound diagnosis and management. In: Rizk B, Puscheck E, eds. *Ultrasonography in Gynecology.* Cambridge University Press; 2014:139-154.)

demonstrate free air under the diaphragm and allow for earlier surgical consultation and more timely intervention. A dilated stomach and small bowel loops with air-fluid levels and paucity of colonic gas can be demonstrated on abdominal radiograph and is suggestive of a small bowel obstruction. Although a patient with a bowel obstruction will still likely require cross-sectional imaging to determine the etiology, early abdominal radiography will allow for the placement of a nasogastric tube and help reduce the risk of potential aspiration while the patient lies flat for a CT scan. Similarly, massive colonic dilation with the classic radiographic

findings of the "bent inner tube" or "coffee bean sign" are heralds for cecal or sigmoid volvulus and result in prompt surgical/gastro-intestinal consult. An abdominal radiograph can also assist in identification of nephrolithiasis and gastrointestinal/rectal foreign bodies.

Computed Tomography

In the modern era, the CT scan has become the primary diagnos-tic tool in the workup of abdominal pain. Allowing for complete visualization of all intrathoracic and intraabdominal structures,

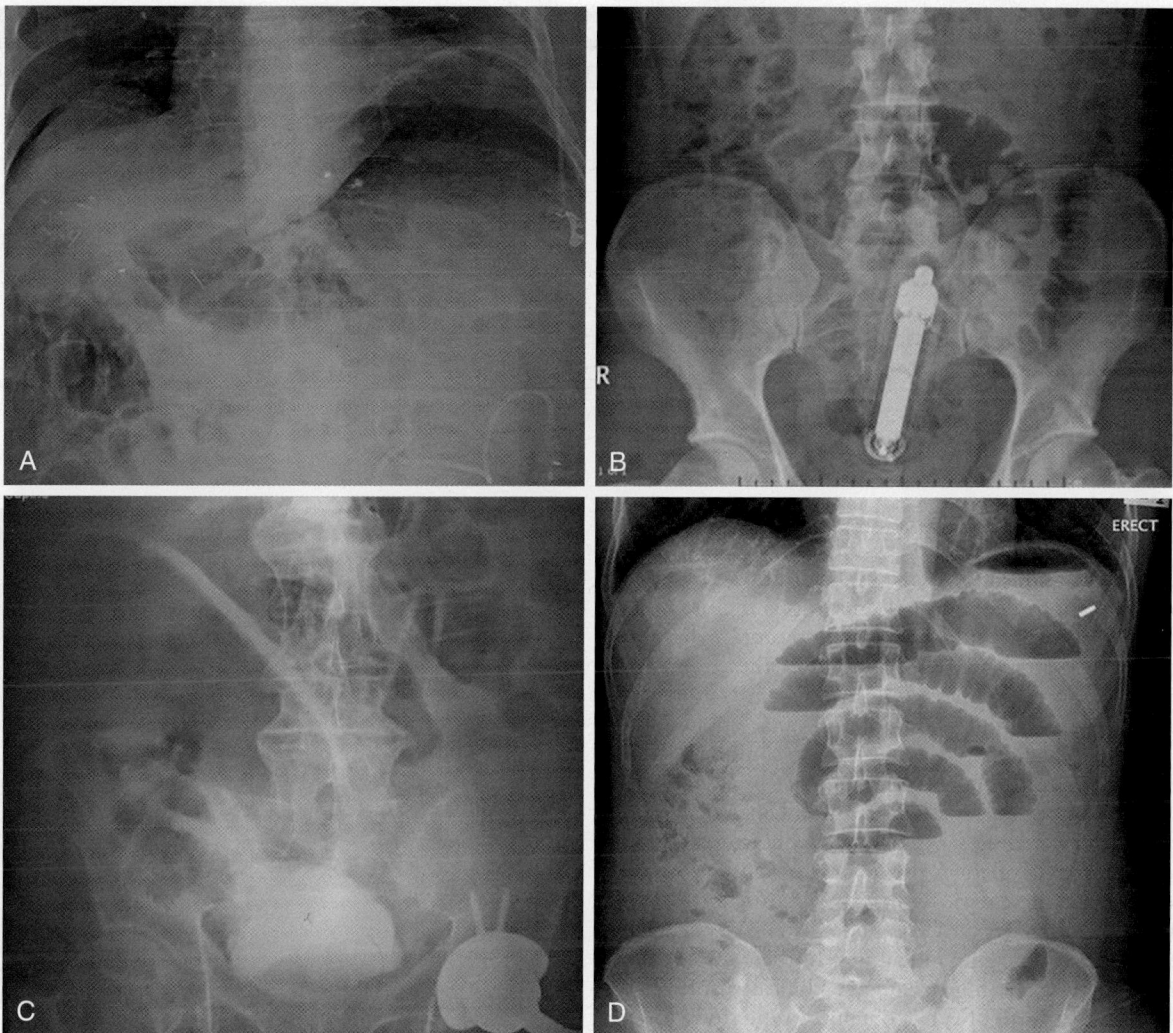

FIGURE 85.4 Plain film radiographs of acute abdominal pathologies. (A) Kidney, ureter, and bladder with free air under the diaphragm suggestive of a perforated viscus. (B) Radiograph with rectal foreign body. (C) Abdominal radiography with classic bent inner tube sign suggestive of colonic volvulus. (D) KUB with dilated small bowel loops and air-fluid levels suggestive of small bowel obstruction. (B, From Gaillard F. Rectal foreign body. Case study. Radiopaedia.org. Accessed on October 31, 2023.)

the CT scan trades the need for ionizing radiation with the benefit of high-quality pictures and less dependence on operator skill. Not all CT scans are created equal, however, and in the workup of the acute abdomen, an understanding of the various contrast options and timing protocols is critical to ensure your scan is maximally diagnostic while minimizing the radiation exposure to the patient. A table of the average radiation dosing from various imaging modalities can be seen in Table 85.5.

The simplest of CT scans includes a noncontrasted scan, which is useful for several disease processes including nephrolithiasis, acute stroke, and evaluation of chronic lung disease. In efforts to save patients the dose of IV contrast and the increasingly outdated fear of contrast-induced kidney injury,[17] workup of the acute abdomen in the emergency department often starts with a noncontrasted CT. Although noncontrasted studies have demonstrated moderate diagnostic accuracy,[18,19] a blinded retrospective review of contrasted versus noncontrasted CT scans in the emergency department for the workup of acute abdominal pain found a 30% reduction in diagnostic accuracy for noncontrasted scans.[20] Consequently, use of IV contrast and the theoretical risk of acute

kidney injury or potential hypersensitivity reactions should be weighed against the leading diagnoses and the additional radiographic information able to be obtained from a contrasted scan.

The addition of oral or rectal contrast is another consideration for a CT scan. Oral contrast can add a significant delay because the scans must be timed to allow for the contrast to be delivered to the patient, for the patient to ingest the contrast, and then a predetermined amount of time allotted to allow the contrast to pass from the stomach and through the gastrointestinal tract. Time delays of over an hour have been reported in some series with the addition of oral contrast,[21] and several large series evaluating the omission of oral contrast for workup of acute abdominal pain have found no significant loss in diagnostic accuracy.[22,23] The one exception in favor of the use of oral contrast is evaluation for a gastrointestinal perforation or concern for anastomotic leak. The presence of oral contrast leakage has a high specificity for a perforation and can aid in localization but has a low sensitivity.[24] Often other ancillary signs such as wall discontinuity, fat stranding, and extraluminal gas will accompany a perforation or leak, obviating the need for oral contrast. Rectal contrast, which is given in a

TABLE 85.5   Relative Radiation Dose Estimates for Abdominal Radiographic Imaging

	ADULT EFFECTIVE DOSE RANGE	PEDIATRIC EFFECTIVE DOSE RANGE
Ultrasound abdomen	0 mSv	0 mSv
Plain film radiograph abdomen	0.1–1 mSv	0.03–0.3 mSv
CT abdomen pelvis without IV contrast	1–10 mSv	0.3–3 mSv
CT abdomen pelvis with IV contrast	1–10 mSv	0.3–3 mSv
CT abdomen pelvis with and without IV contrast	10–30 mSv	3–10 mSv
MRI abdomen pelvis without IV contrast	0 mSv	0 mSv
MRI abdomen pelvis with and without IV contrast	0 mSv	0 mSv
Nuclear medicine scan gallbladder	0.1–1 mSv	0.03–0.3 mSv
Fluoroscopy upper GI series with follow-through	1–10 mSv	0.3–3 mSv
Fluoroscopy contrast enema	1–10 mSv	0.3–3 mSv

Abridged from Expert Panel on Gastrointestinal Imaging; Scheirey CD, Fowler KJ, Therrien JA, et al. ACR Appropriateness Criteria acute nonlocalized abdominal pain. *J Am Coll Radiol.* 2018;15(11S):S217-S231.

CT scan and administered through a temporary rectal tube under hydrostatic pressure, has no time delay but can lead to patient discomfort without significant increase in diagnostic accuracy.

A final consideration related to CT imaging is the use of IV contrast, which is specifically timed or phased to capture distribution throughout the vascular system. Timing of the contrast to allow for opacification of the mesenteric arterial and venous systems can be especially helpful for specific vascular etiologies of abdominal pain. CT angiography (CTA) is a technique used to visualize the vasculature throughout the body, as imaging is obtained at the time of peak arterial or venous enhancement. This can be useful when evaluating select patients with acute abdominal pain. For example, if a patient presents with signs and symptoms concerning for mesenteric ischemia or aortic dissection, prompt evaluation with CTA can help guide further management and is superior to other imaging modalities. In these instances, it is important to maintain a high degree of clinical suspicion to ensure the appropriate form of CT is obtained. One study found that for patients with acute SMA occlusion, in-hospital mortality was 42% for patients who underwent contrast-enhanced CT as opposed to 90% for those without contrasted imaging.[25] In addition to vascular abnormalities, CTA can visualize the health of the bowel, as diminished wall enhancement and mesenteric stranding can suggest bowel ischemia (Fig. 85.5).

Magnetic Resonance Imaging

Magnetic resonance imaging (MRI) is an additional technology available for the workup of an acute abdomen, but comes with several limitations. The benefits of MRI stem from its high-quality imaging of the entire abdominal cavity without the use of ionizing radiation, making it an attractive option for any patient but specifically for high-risk groups such as children and pregnant patients. For example, in pregnant patients with acute appendicitis, MRI was found to have a greater than 90% sensitivity and specificity for the diagnosis, which is far superior to other nonradiating imaging modalities such as ultrasound.[26] Furthermore, one study found that in the over 200 pregnant females with acute appendicitis who were enrolled, there was not a single instance where the appendix was not visualized on MRI.[27] Limitations include its relatively high cost compared with other cross-sectional imaging modalities; long scan time (30–90 minutes vs. seconds to minutes for a CT scan); inability to use for patients with specific metal implants, pacemakers/defibrillators, and history of retained metallic foreign bodies; and the need for patients to remain still for extended periods. It is for these reasons that

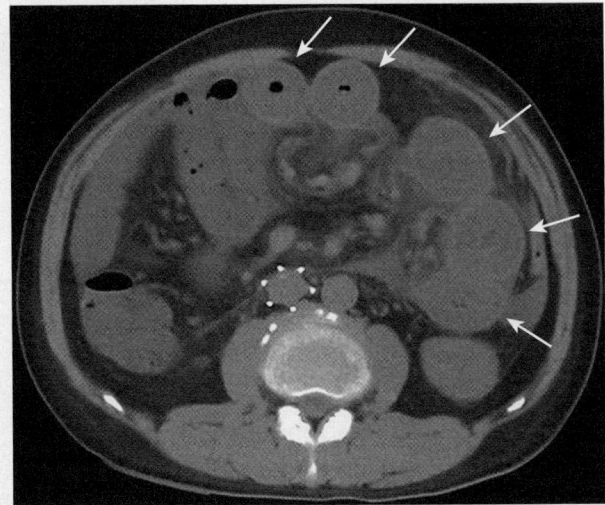

FIGURE 85.5 Contrast-enhanced computed tomography with hypoenhancement of the bowel wall concerning for intestinal ischemia. The *arrows* indicate segments of bowel wall with thickening and hypoenhancement concerning for intestinal ischemia.

the American College of Radiology recommends selective use of MRI in appropriate clinical scenarios for the workup of the acute abdomen.[28]

Diagnostic Procedures

In addition to laboratory and imaging evaluation, several diagnostic procedures can aid in determining the etiology of a patient's acute abdomen. Insertion of a nasogastric tube with saline lavage and aspiration of blood contents can guide a clinician to an upper gastrointestinal bleed. Although studies have found no difference in clinical patient outcomes for those who undergo lavage, this procedure was associated with a shorter time to endoscopy and can help guide management pathways.[29]

For a patient with concern for intraabdominal hypertension, using a bladder catheter hooked up to a pressure transducer can be used to measure intraabdominal pressure (IAP). With the bladder drained and the patient supine, 25 mL of saline is instilled into the bladder, and the pressure is then measured with the transducer zeroed at the iliac crest at the midaxillary line (for pediatric patients, 1 mL/kg up to 25 kg with a minimum of at least 3 mL saline is instilled). Normal IAP should be between 5 and 7 mm Hg in the supine and paralyzed patient. Elevations in pressures can be seen with abdominal obesity, pregnancy, upright positioning, and Valsalva maneuvers. Intraabdominal hypertension is diagnosed with sustained elevations of the IAP >12 mm Hg, and abdominal compartment syndrome is defined as sustained IAP >20 mm Hg with evidence of end-organ dysfunction.[30] Prompt diagnosis and intervention are necessary to avoid ongoing or permanent organ dysfunction in these patients.

With advances in the quality and technology of CT scanners, CTA has largely replaced the need for traditional catheter-based angiography to evaluate for intraabdominal vascular issues.[31] Although CTA has increasingly become the gold standard, use of catheter-based angiography does still play a role in diagnosis of acute pathologies. Patients who are hemodynamically unstable because of a suspected vascular lesion (such as a history of a known abdominal aortic aneurysm) may be taken emergently to the catheterization laboratory for dual diagnosis and therapeutic intervention. This approach, however, requires specific clinical scenarios and the rapid availability of an angiography operating room and team. Additionally, if the CTA is nondiagnostic in the setting of a suspicious lesion, angiography may be used as a second-line test to help confirm or disprove the diagnosis. In the modern era, however, catheter-based angiography is uncommonly used as a first-line diagnostic modality and is instead increasingly being reserved for therapeutic interventions.

In select situations, laparoscopy may be used as a diagnostic modality. The use of laparoscopy for diagnostic purposes has been explored for clinical situations where the diagnosis remains unclear, but most studies that have evaluated this topic did not use cross-sectional imaging as part of their diagnostic workup.[32-34] Laparoscopy may assist in situations where disease pathologies present similarly such as acute appendicitis and acute gynecologic issues in females of reproductive age. Diagnostic imaging in these scenarios can often be limited because of the adjacent nature of the appendix and gynecologic structures, with inflammation and fluid further confounding the identification of the offending organ.[35] Similarly, other clinical scenarios, such as an acute abdomen in a patient with a history of bariatric surgery, can often benefit from diagnostic laparoscopy in situations where the cross-sectional imaging is nondiagnostic.[36]

Trauma patients represent a unique cohort for whom the use of laparoscopy as a standard part of diagnostic workup has been well studied. In patients with blunt abdominal trauma, high rates of missed blunt bowel injury and diaphragmatic injury have been reported with CT imaging. In patients with the appropriate clinical symptoms, trauma mechanism, or presence of free fluid on CT imaging without concomitant injury, diagnostic laparoscopy should be considered.[37] For patients with penetrating trauma who are nonperitoneal and have equivocal peritoneal violation on local wound exploration, diagnostic laparoscopy can be used to help identify peritoneal violation. This allows for assessment of any intraabdominal injuries while reducing the risk of a negative laparotomy.[38]

PREPARATION FOR EMERGENCY OPERATION

Patients with an acute abdomen can vary tremendously in their hemodynamic stability and overall state of health. Unlike elective procedures where risk factors can be optimized preoperatively, the acute abdomen often requires emergent operative intervention, leaving little time for preparation for surgery. A preoperative assessment of a patient's cardiovascular and respiratory risk factors

is important, and simple tests such as an electrocardiogram or chest radiograph may provide relevant information without any significant delay in intervention. The benefits of further workup or optimization must be weighed against the increased morbidity and mortality associated with a delay in treatment.

All patients should undergo basic resuscitation while awaiting operative intervention, including the placement of sufficient intravenous (IV) access, infusion of IV fluids or blood products as required, and correction of electrolyte abnormalities. Obtaining a preoperative type and screen (and a crossmatch if significant blood loss is possible), coagulation panel, blood cultures, and lactate can assist with the intraoperative and postoperative resuscitation. Most patients with an acute abdomen will require antibiotic administration, and initial selection should be targeted at organisms most likely involved in the disease process. In acute abdominal emergencies, gram-negative enteric organisms and anaerobes represent the most common offenders, and broad-spectrum therapy is indicated for initial therapy. Guidance on antibiotic selection should be informed by your institution's microbiology and specific antibiogram and population studies.[39] Antibiotics should be narrowed based on intraoperative findings and organism sensitivities as soon as possible. Additional support devices such as nasogastric tubes, Foley catheters, and central/arterial lines should be placed as required depending on the clinical scenario.

The postoperative level of care, specifically the need for an intensive care unit (ICU) bed, should be anticipated and arranged to minimize postoperative delays in transfer and ongoing resuscitation. If possible, a preoperative discussion with the operating room nursing staff and anesthesiology team about the patient's clinical condition, anticipated interventions, and potentially required equipment/medications can help facilitate a smooth operative course.

PREOPERATIVE COUNSELING

Preoperative counseling is an essential part of preparing a patient for the operating room. Frequently, the exact diagnosis and extent of the required operation are not known preoperatively. Preparing the patient and their family for the wide potential of surgical interventions and postoperative issues before surgery can help streamline the patient's future care. Operative interventions such as open versus laparoscopic approaches, bowel resections, ostomies, need for temporary abdominal closure, and repeat operations are just some considerations to be discussed. Postoperative concerns such as need for prolonged ICU care, ventilator dependence, renal failure/dialysis, need for tracheostomy, and feeding tubes are also important issues to discuss because many patients have strong opinions about advanced life support devices.

These discussions are all an essential part of informed consent, which should include a review of the purpose, risks, benefits, and alternatives (including nonoperative management) of surgery. This process should be an open and engaged conversation, allowing for expression of any concerns or questions. If the patient has a living will or designated medical power of attorney, identifying this person before surgery or discussing the patient's desired code status can help guide your postoperative medical decision-making. For patients with an anticipated long postoperative or ICU admission, the preoperative consent may be the only opportunity to speak to a patient about the possibility of a prolonged intubation, and if appropriate, the patient's preferences about a tracheostomy or a feeding tube should be discussed and the patient's desired surrogate decision-maker should be identified. Discussing the potential operative and postoperative course and setting expectations with the patient and their family help build a therapeutic alliance and build a culture of patient-centered care.

NONOPERATIVE MANAGEMENT

Although most cases of an acute abdomen require surgical intervention, there are several distinct pathologies for which nonoperative management is a viable and sometimes preferred approach. The use of selective nonoperative management hinges on the patient's hemodynamic parameters. Any patient with hemodynamic instability from their abdominal process is unlikely to be successfully managed nonoperatively, and prompt surgical care should not be delayed in these cases. In medically complex patients who require further optimization before surgical intervention, nonoperative management can be a bridge while comorbidities are addressed.

In select cases, nonoperative management may entail only fluid resuscitation and antibiotic therapy. Treatment with antibiotics has become an appropriate alternative to surgery in some instances. The CODA trial followed adult patients with acute uncomplicated appendicitis, with and without an appendicolith, who were randomized to treatment with antibiotics versus appendectomy. The study found that antibiotics were noninferior to appendectomy for the treatment of appendicitis. Specifically, among the patients who received antibiotics, 29% ultimately underwent appendectomy within 90 days.[40] It should also be noted that nonoperative management of acute appendicitis has been associated with higher rates of abscess formation, readmission, and overall cost of care.[41] Acute uncomplicated diverticulitis is another common entity that is now often treated with a short course of oral antibiotics. The benefit of nonoperative management in patients with this condition is the avoidance of emergent surgery, which has up to a 40% complication rate.[42] For patients with a contained perforation of their sigmoid diverticulitis without peritonitis, management with nil per os and IV antibiotics was found to have a 71.4% to 94% success rate. This approach spared patients operative intervention, bowel resection, and need for stoma creation.[43]

Alternative options for nonoperative treatment of the acute abdomen include percutaneous drainage, often performed by an interventional radiologist. Cases of intraabdominal abscess from perforated appendicitis or diverticulitis can resolve with antibiotics and percutaneous drainage, which mitigates the risk of an often technically challenging emergency surgery. Percutaneous drainage is also a reasonable option in patients who are poor surgical candidates. For example, a percutaneous cholecystostomy tube is an appropriate treatment for critically ill patients with acute cholecystitis who would not withstand cholecystectomy. Although percutaneous drainage may be a reasonable option in some patients, it is associated with procedure-related pain, increased hospital length of stay, radiation from repeated imaging, and potential delayed diagnosis of malignancy.[44]

The selective use of nonoperative management should be predicated upon the patient's overall clinical condition and in discussion with the patient regarding their preferences and the risks of non-operative management and entered into with an understanding that failure of nonoperative management will require surgical intervention. For some patients, nonoperative management despite the high risk for failure is a purposeful choice to align their treatment with their overall goals of care. A trial of medical therapy is started, and if signs point to failure, patients may choose to pursue no further escalation of care and transition to hospice measures. Again, joint decision-making and open communication with the patient and their families are critical for these approaches.

SPECIAL PATIENT POPULATIONS

Sex-Specific Considerations

The presentation of the acute abdomen can be influenced by sex-specific anatomic structures and related pathologies. In female patients, understanding potential etiologies related to gynecologic structures is crucial. Factors such as menstrual and sexual history can offer diagnostic clues. Conditions can include endometriosis, ovarian torsion, and ectopic pregnancy. Endometriosis presents with cyclical pain, which corresponds to menstrual cycles; ovarian torsion can present with severe pelvic pain and adnexal mass; and ectopic pregnancy can present with a positive pregnancy test or a missed period along with abdominal pain and vaginal bleeding. Likewise, in male patients, pathologies of the testes and epididymis, such as testicular torsion or epididymitis, should be considered when evaluating acute abdominal and scrotal pain.

Pregnancy

Evaluation of the pregnant patient presents unique challenges, as acute abdominal pain in pregnancy can stem from both obstetric and nonobstetric causes. Differential conditions in the obstetric realm can include placental abruption, round ligament pain, HELLP (hemolysis, elevated liver enzymes, and low platelets) syndrome, uterine and ovarian torsion, and uterine rupture.[45] However, nonobstetric causes such as appendicitis and cholecystitis also occur during pregnancy, and anatomic changes that can occur with the growing uterus can change the location and characteristics of pain. For example, appendicitis occurs in approximately 100 of every 100,000 births; these patients have significantly higher rates of peritonitis, sepsis, septic shock, and postoperative complications.[46] However, operative management remains the preferred treatment because medical management in appendicitis is associated with a higher rate of adverse outcomes. A careful consideration of diagnostic testing should be employed in the pregnant patient, with preference for methods that reduce ionizing radiation such as ultrasound and MRI. However, if ionizing radiation is necessary to provide expeditious care for the mother, it is important to note that delays in diagnosis and treatment can lead to adverse outcomes in both the mother and fetus, and a CT scan should be performed if the benefits outweigh the risks. Radiation risk is dependent on two factors: the cumulative radiation dosage and the fetal age at exposure; fetal mortality is highest within the first 2 weeks of conception, and the fetus is most vulnerable to teratogenesis between 10 and 17 weeks. Expert consensus is that the risk of ionizing radiation–induced fetal harm is low at 50 mGy or less, and the usual fetal radiation dose of a routine CT scan of the abdomen and pelvis is around 25 mGy.[45]

Geriatrics

The older patient with acute abdominal pain also poses unique challenges. Concomitant with age and aging, patients are more likely to present with increased rates of comorbidities, more severe comorbidities, more functional limitations, and an increased risk of baseline frailty. Frailty is the increased vulnerability resulting from aging-related decline in reserve and function, which reduces an individual's ability to cope with stressors[47] and is a more superior predictor of outcomes than age alone.[48] In addition, the presence of polypharmacy and other preexisting medical conditions can cloud the diagnostic picture. Older patients have a higher risk of surgical complications and mortality when an operation is pursued compared with younger patients with the same diseases and presentations.[49]

Immunocompromised Individuals

Patients with compromised immune systems represent a particularly vulnerable group. An immunocompromised state can stem from underlying diseases such as human immunodeficiency virus (HIV), organ transplantation, chemotherapy, or other immunosuppressive medications. In these patients, common abdominal pathologies may present with muted or atypical presentations, leading to diagnostic delays. Recent or chronic steroid use can also alter the body's response to infection and mask peritonitis, requiring a higher level of suspicion. The immunocompromised patient is also more susceptible to postoperative complications, progression of sepsis, and infection from atypical pathogens.

Critically Ill Patients

In critically ill patients, rapid diagnosis is vital but can also be challenging. Patients may present with altered mental status, making the patient history unreliable, or may be intubated at the time of surgery consultation. Critical illness from other causes can also lead to abdominal pathologies. Examples of this include acalculous cholecystitis, bowel ischemia from high-dose vasopressors, or acute colonic pseudoobstruction (Ogilvie syndrome).

Post–Bariatric Surgery

Unique differential diagnoses need consideration in patients who have a history of bariatric surgery. The anatomy is often altered because of procedures such as gastric bypass, sleeve gastrectomy, or adjustable gastric banding, leading to nontraditional presentations of common abdominal conditions. Anastomotic leaks, internal hernias, and complications related to marginal ulceration (such as bleeding or perforation) must additionally be considered when evaluating the post–bariatric surgery patient. Postoperative gallstone formation can also occur as a side effect of rapid weight loss.

SUMMARY

Evaluation and treatment of the acute abdomen necessitates a systematic and methodical approach, combining a detailed history and physical examination, pertinent laboratory studies, and diagnostic imaging to narrow what often starts as a very broad list of differential diagnoses. Diagnostic and therapeutic strategies should be individualized, taking into consideration the specific diagnosis, the unique biology and physiology of the patient, and the wishes of the patient and their surrogate decision-makers if needed. Notably, special patient populations bring to the table distinct challenges and considerations. Evaluation of the acute abdomen remains the most fundamental and quintessential skill for the general surgeon.

SELECTED REFERENCES

Mazuski JE, Tessier JM, May AK, et al. The Surgical Infection Society revised guidelines on the management of intra-abdominal infection. *Surg Infect (Larchmt)*. 2017;18(1):1-76.

This Surgical Infection Society publication provides GRADE based recommendations regarding the infectious management of the acute abdomen. Guidelines include recommendations regarding timing, duration, and type of antibiotic use.

Scheirey CD, Fowler KJ, Therrien JA, et al. ACR appropriateness criteria acute nonlocalized abdominal pain. *J Am Coll Radiol*. 2018;15(suppl 11):S217-S231.

These practice management guidelines from the American College of Radiology provide recommendations regarding imaging type selection for patients presenting with the acute abdomen. Guidelines consider patient factors and clinical differentials to aid physicians in appropriate imaging selection balance risks of radiation exposure with diagnostic utility.

Kameda T, Taniguchi N. Overview of point-of-care abdominal ultrasound in emergency and critical care. *J Intensive Care*. 2016;4:53.

This review article summaries key disease processes and ultrasound findings which can air physicians in clinical diagnosis. The article reviews the sensitivity, specificity, benefits and limitations of ultrasound for various abdominal ultrasound findings.

De Simone B, Chouillard E, Ramos AC, et al. Operative management of acute abdomen after bariatric surgery in the emergency setting: the OBA guidelines. *World J Emerg Surg*. 2022;17:51.

This systematic meta-analysis used the PICO system to provide guidelines regarding management of the acute abdomen following bariatric surgery. These recommendations explore complications both acutely and remote from bariatric surgery and specific considerations providers must have when encounter a patient with an acute abdomen following bariatric surgery.

Golash C, Willson PD. Early laparoscopy as a routine procedure in the management of acute abdominal pain: a review of 1,320 patients. *Surg Endosc*. 2005;19(7):882-885.

This retrospective review of patients with acute abdominal pain undergoing laparoscopy as a diagnostic modality reports the findings of these procedures in over 1,000 patients. This intervention was posited to decrease the need for exploratory laparotomy and deemed to be both safe and efficacious.

The full reference list appears on Elsevier eBooks+.

86 | CHAPTER

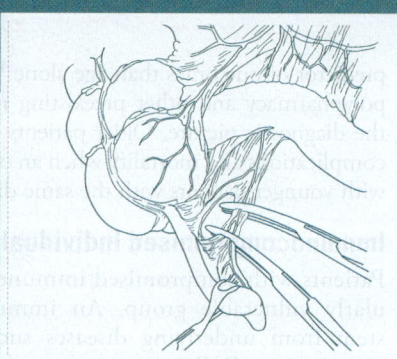

Stomach

David A. "Sasha" Mahvi and David M. Mahvi

ANATOMY

Gross Anatomy

Divisions

The stomach is derived from the embryonic primitive gut tube, beginning as a dilation during the fourth to fifth week of gestation in the caudal portion. The embryonic stomach is invested by two mesenteries: dorsal (which becomes the gastrosplenic, gastrocolic, and gastrophrenic ligaments) and ventral (which becomes the hepatoduodenal and gastrohepatic ligaments of the lesser omentum and the falciform ligament). By the seventh week of gestation, the stomach rotates 90 degrees in the clockwise direction along its longitudinal axis and dilates, with a disproportionate elongation of the greater curvature into its normal anatomic shape and position. The 90-degree rotation results in the left vagus nerve being ventral and the right vagus nerve being dorsal; rotation also creates the omental bursa (or lesser sac).

The stomach is fixed at the gastroesophageal (GE) junction and pylorus. The most proximal region of the stomach is the cardia. The cardiac orifice (or cardioesophageal junction) is the opening of the esophagus into the stomach. Immediately proximal to the cardia is the physiologically competent lower esophageal sphincter. The fundus is to the left of the cardia and represents the superior-most part of the stomach. The fundus is floppy and distensible. The angle of His, also referred to as the *esophagogastric angle,* is an important anatomic feature formed between the fundus and the left margin of the esophagus. The angle of His forms an anatomic sphincter, helping to prevent GE reflux. The body of the stomach represents the largest portion and is also referred to as the *corpus.* The body is bounded on the right by the relatively straight lesser curvature and on the left by the longer greater curvature. At the angularis incisura, the lesser curvature abruptly angles to the right. The body of the stomach ends here and the antrum begins. Distally, the pylorus connects the distal stomach (antrum) to the proximal duodenum (Fig. 86.1).

The left lateral section of the liver covers a large portion of the stomach anteriorly. The gastrohepatic ligament connects the liver to the lesser curve of the stomach and contains the right and left gastric arteries. Posteriorly, the stomach is bounded by the diaphragm, left kidney, pancreas, aorta, and celiac trunk. Inferiorly, the stomach is attached to the transverse colon via the gastrocolic ligament, which contains the right and left gastroepiploic vessels. Superiorly, the GE junction is found approximately 2 to 3 cm below the diaphragmatic esophageal hiatus in the horizontal plane of the seventh chondrosternal articulation. The gastrosplenic

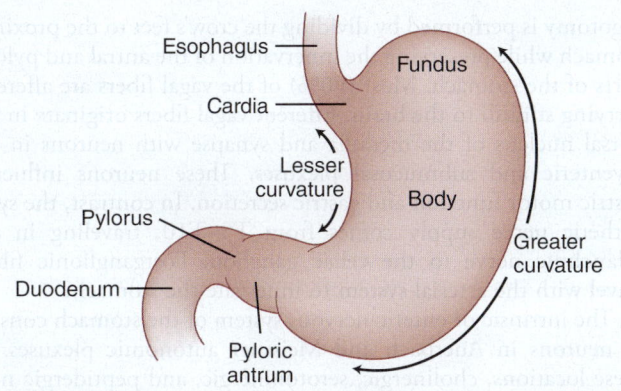

FIGURE 86.1 Divisions of the stomach. (From Yeo C, Dempsey DT, Klein AS, et al., eds. *Shackelford's Surgery of the Alimentary Tract*. 6th ed. Philadelphia: Saunders; 2007.)

ligament attaches the proximal greater curvature to the spleen and contains the short gastric arteries.

Blood Supply

The celiac artery provides the majority of the blood supply to the stomach (Fig. 86.2). There are four main arteries—the left and right gastric arteries along the lesser curvature and the left and right gastroepiploic arteries along the greater curvature, with the left gastric artery being the largest. In addition, a substantial quantity of blood may be supplied to the proximal stomach by the short gastric arteries (which arise from the splenic artery) and the inferior phrenic artery. The left gastric artery is one of the three branches of the celiac trunk, along with the common hepatic artery and splenic artery. The right gastric artery typically arises from the proper hepatic artery. The left gastroepiploic artery originates from the splenic artery, and the right gastroepiploic artery originates from the gastroduodenal artery. The extensive anastomotic connections between these major vessels ensure that, in most cases, the stomach will survive if three out of four arteries are ligated, provided that the arcades along the greater and lesser curvatures are not disturbed. In general, the veins of the stomach parallel the arteries. The left gastric (coronary) and right gastric veins usually drain into the portal vein or at the confluence of the superior mesenteric and splenic veins. The left gastroepiploic vein drains into the splenic vein. The right gastroepiploic vein typically joins with the superior right colic and anterior superior pancreaticoduodenal veins to form Henle's trunk, which then drains into the superior mesenteric vein, though multiple anatomic variations of Henle's trunk exist.[1]

Lymphatic Drainage

The lymphatic drainage of the stomach parallels the vasculature and drains into four zones of lymph nodes. The superior gastric group drains lymph from the upper lesser curvature into the left gastric and paracardial nodes. The suprapyloric group of nodes drains the antral segment on the lesser curvature of the stomach

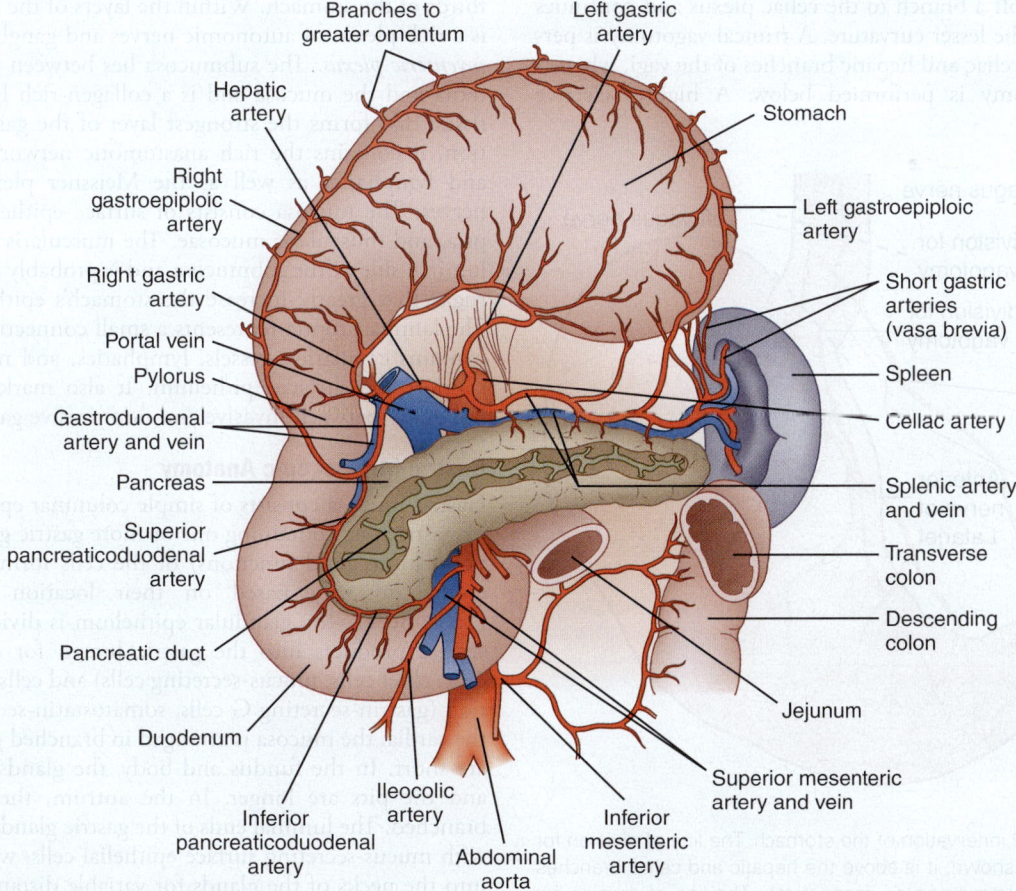

FIGURE 86.2 Blood supply to the stomach and duodenum showing anatomic relationships to the spleen and pancreas. The stomach is reflected cephalad. (From Yeo C, Dempsey DT, Klein AS, et al., eds. *Shackelford's Surgery of the Alimentary Tract*. 6th ed. Philadelphia: Saunders; 2007.)

into the right suprapancreatic nodes. The pancreaticolienal group of nodes drains lymph high on the greater curvature into the left gastroepiploic and splenic nodes. The inferior gastric and subpyloric group of nodes drains lymph along the right gastroepiploic vascular pedicle. All four zones of lymph nodes drain into the celiac nodes and eventually into the thoracic duct. Although these lymph nodes drain different areas of the stomach, gastric cancers may metastasize to any of the four nodal groups. In addition, the extensive submucosal plexus of lymphatics accounts for the fact that there is frequently microscopic evidence of malignant cells several centimeters from gross disease.

Innervation

As shown in Fig. 86.3, the extrinsic innervation of the stomach is both parasympathetic (via the vagus nerve) and sympathetic (via the celiac plexus). The vagus nerve originates in the vagal nucleus in the floor of the fourth ventricle and traverses the neck in the carotid sheath to enter the mediastinum, where it divides into several branches around the esophagus. These branches coalesce above the esophageal hiatus to form the left and right vagus nerves. It is not uncommon to find more than two vagal trunks at the distal esophagus. At the GE junction, the left vagus is anterior and the right vagus is posterior.

The left vagus gives off the hepatic branch to the liver and continues along the lesser curvature as the nerve of Latarjet. The so-called *criminal nerve of Grassi* is the first branch of the right posterior vagus nerve; it is recognized as a potential cause of recurrent ulcers when it is not divided during a vagotomy. The right vagus nerve gives off a branch to the celiac plexus and continues posteriorly along the lesser curvature. A truncal vagotomy is performed above the celiac and hepatic branches of the vagi, whereas a selective vagotomy is performed below. A highly selective

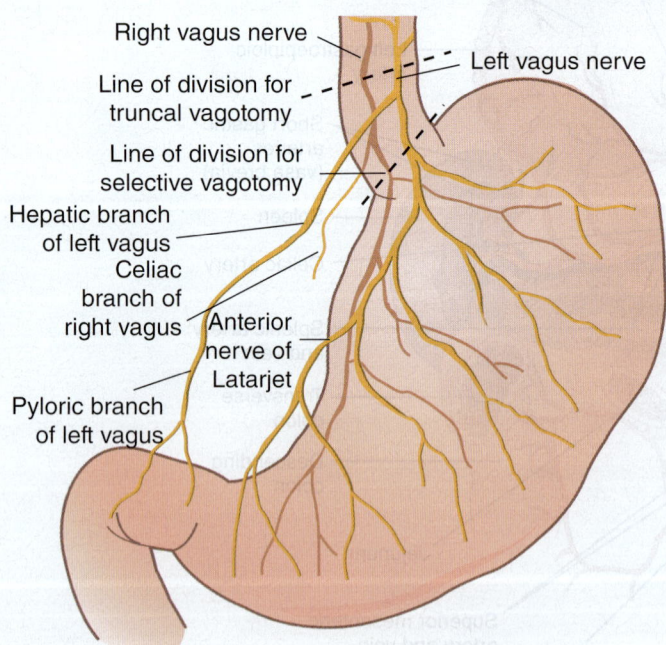

FIGURE 86.3 Vagal innervation of the stomach. The line of division for truncal vagotomy is shown; it is above the hepatic and celiac branches of the left and right vagus nerves, respectively. The line of division for selective vagotomy is shown; this is below the hepatic and celiac branches. (From Mercer D, Liu T. Open truncal vagotomy. *Oper Tech Gen Surg.* 2003;5:80-85.)

vagotomy is performed by dividing the crow's feet to the proximal stomach while preserving the innervation of the antral and pyloric parts of the stomach. Most (90%) of the vagal fibers are afferent, carrying stimuli to the brain. Efferent vagal fibers originate in the dorsal nucleus of the medulla and synapse with neurons in the myenteric and submucosal plexuses. These neurons influence gastric motor function and gastric secretion. In contrast, the sympathetic nerve supply comes from T5–T10, traveling in the splanchnic nerve to the celiac ganglion. Postganglionic fibers travel with the arterial system to innervate the stomach.

The intrinsic or enteric nervous system of the stomach consists of neurons in Auerbach and Meissner autonomic plexuses. In these locations, cholinergic, serotoninergic, and peptidergic neurons are present. The exact function of these neurons is not fully elucidated. Nevertheless, numerous neuropeptides have been localized to these neurons, including acetylcholine, serotonin, substance P, calcitonin gene–related peptide, bombesin, cholecystokinin (CCK), and somatostatin.

Gastric Morphology

The stomach is covered by peritoneum, which forms the outer serosa of the stomach. Below this is the thicker muscularis propria, or muscularis externa, which is composed of three layers of smooth muscles. The middle layer of smooth muscle is circular and is the only complete muscle layer of the stomach wall. At the pylorus, this middle circular muscle layer becomes progressively thicker and functions as a true anatomic sphincter. The outer muscle layer is longitudinal and predominates in the distal two-thirds of the stomach. Within the layers of the muscularis externa is a rich plexus of autonomic nerves and ganglia, called *Auerbach myenteric plexus.* The submucosa lies between the muscularis externa and the mucosa and is a collagen-rich layer of connective tissue that forms the strongest layer of the gastric wall. In addition, it contains the rich anastomotic network of blood vessels and lymphatics as well as the Meissner plexus of autonomic nerves. The mucosa consists of surface epithelium, lamina propria, and muscularis mucosae. The muscularis mucosae is on the luminal side of the submucosa and is probably responsible for the rugae that greatly increase the stomach's epithelial surface area. The lamina propria represents a small connective tissue layer and contains capillaries, vessels, lymphatics, and nerves necessary to support the surface epithelium. It also marks the microscopic boundary between invasive and noninvasive gastric carcinoma.

Gastric Microscopic Anatomy

Gastric mucosa consists of simple columnar epithelia interrupted by gastric pits containing one or more gastric glands. The cellular populations (and functions) of the cells forming this glandular epithelium vary based on their location in the stomach (Table 86.1). The glandular epithelium is divided into cells that secrete products into the gastric lumen for digestion (parietal cells, chief cells, mucus-secreting cells) and cells that control function (gastrin-secreting G cells, somatostatin-secreting D cells). In the cardia, the mucosa is arranged in branched glands and the pits are short. In the fundus and body, the glands are more tubular and the pits are longer. In the antrum, the glands are more branched. The luminal ends of the gastric glands and pits are lined with mucus-secreting surface epithelial cells, which extend down into the necks of the glands for variable distances. In the cardia, the glands are predominantly mucus-secreting. In the body, the glands are mostly lined from the neck to the base with parietal and chief cells. There are a few parietal cells in the fundus and

TABLE 86.1 Gastric Cell Types, Location, and Function

CELL TYPE	LOCATION	FUNCTION
Parietal	Body	Secretion of acid and intrinsic factor
Mucus	Body, antrum	Mucus
Chief	Body	Pepsin
Surface epithelial	Diffuse	Mucus, bicarbonate, prostaglandins
Enterochromaffin-like	Body	Histamine
G	Antrum	Gastrin
D	Body, antrum	Somatostatin
Gastric mucosal interneurons	Body, antrum	Gastrin-releasing peptide
Enteric neurons	Diffuse	Calcitonin gene–related peptide, others
Endocrine	Body	Ghrelin

proximal antrum, but none in the cardia or prepyloric antrum. The endocrine G cells are present in greatest quantity in the antral glands.

PHYSIOLOGY

The principal function of the stomach is to prepare ingested food for digestion and absorption in the small intestine. Receptive relaxation of the proximal stomach with ingestion of food enables the stomach to function as a storage organ. This relaxation enables liquids to pass easily from the stomach along the lesser curvature, whereas the solid food settles along the greater curvature of the fundus. In contrast to liquids, emptying of solid food is facilitated by the antrum, which propels solid food components into and through the pylorus. The antrum and pylorus function in a coordinated fashion, returning material to the proximal stomach until the size is suitable for delivery into the duodenum.

In addition to storing food, the stomach begins digestion of a meal. Starches undergo enzymatic breakdown through the activity of salivary amylase. Pepsin initiates protein digestion, though this hydrolysis is not completed in the stomach. The small intestine is primarily responsible for digestion of a meal and nutrient absorption.

Regulation of Gastric Function

Gastric function is under neural (sympathetic and parasympathetic) and hormonal (peptides or amines that interact with target cells in the stomach) control. An understanding of the roles of neural and hormonal regulation of digestion is critical to understanding gastric physiology and the resultant physiologic effects of gastric surgical procedures on digestion. We initially focus here on peptide regulation of gastric function and then describe the interactions of these peptides with neural inputs in regard to acid secretion and gastric function.

Gastric Peptides

Gastrin

Gastrin was initially discovered in 1905 and in 1964 became the first gastrointestinal (GI) peptide to be fully molecularly characterized. The vast majority of gastrin is produced by G cells located in the gastric antrum (see Table 86.1). It is synthesized as a prepropeptide and undergoes posttranslational processing to produce several biologically active gastrin peptides. The two major forms are gastrin-34 (big gastrin) and gastrin-17 (little gastrin). There are also relatively small percentages of gastrin-71, gastrin-14, and gastrin-6. Approximately 85% of antral gastrin is released as the 17–amino acid peptide, although gastrin-34 slightly predominates in plasma because its circulating half-life is 5 to 10 times longer. The pentapeptide sequence contained at the carboxy terminus of gastrin is identical to that found on another gut peptide, CCK. CCK and gastrin differ by their tyrosine sulfation sites. Gastrin initiates its biologic actions by activation of surface membrane receptors CCK1 and CCK2. These receptors are members of the G protein–coupled receptor family. The gastrin or CCK2 receptor has an equally high affinity for gastrin and CCK, whereas CCK1 receptors have a 1000-fold higher affinity for sulfated CCK analogues as compared with gastrin. CCK2 receptors are found on parietal and enterochromaffin-like (ECL) cells in the stomach. CCK1 receptors are more abundant in the pancreas and gallbladder.

The release of gastrin is regulated by multiple factors. Gastric distention, particularly in the antrum, leads to cholinergic activation, which in turn increases gastrin release. Cholinergic neurons also activate gastrin-releasing peptide (GRP, also referred to as *bombesin*), which directly stimulates the G cell to release gastrin. Bombesin also increases gastric mucosal blood flow both directly and by stimulating cyclooxygenase production of prostaglandins. The presence of amino acids in the stomach increases gastrin release both by direct stimulation of G cells and indirectly via GRP. G cells contain calcium receptors, so hypercalcemia can also stimulate gastrin release. Conversely, luminal acid inhibits the release of gastrin via somatostatin, particularly at intragastric pH of less than 3.0. Somatostatin inhibits gastrin by a paracrine mechanism, binding to the SSTR2 G protein–coupled receptor near antral G cells. In the antral location, somatostatin and gastrin release are functionally linked, and an inverse reciprocal relationship exists between these two peptides. Vasoactive intestinal peptide (VIP) also indirectly lowers gastrin levels by stimulating somatostatin release.

Gastrin is the major hormonal regulator of the gastric phase of acid secretion primarily by stimulating ECL cells to synthesize and release histamine. However, gastrin also exerts direct actions on the parietal cell to stimulate acid release. Gastrin has considerable trophic effects on both parietal cells and ECL cells. Prolonged hypergastrinemia from any cause leads to mucosal hyperplasia and an increase in the number of ECL cells. Gastrin is also the main hormonal regulator of the secretory response to protein-containing meals by stimulating pepsinogen release from chief cells. Pancreatic islet cells contain CCK2 receptors; thus, high levels of gastrin can increase insulin secretion.

The detection of hypergastrinemia may suggest a pathologic state of acid hypersecretion but most commonly is the result of treatment with agents to reduce acid secretion, such as proton pump inhibitors (PPIs) or chronic atrophic gastritis. Table 86.2 lists common causes of chronic hypergastrinemia. Hypergastrinemia that results from the administration of acid-reducing drugs is an appropriate physiologic response caused by loss of feedback inhibition of gastrin release by luminal acid. Lack of acid causes a reduction in somatostatin release, which causes increased release of gastrin from antral G cells. Hypergastrinemia can also occur in the setting of pernicious anemia or uremia or after surgical procedures such as vagotomy. In contrast, gastrin levels increase inappropriately in patients with gastrinoma (Zollinger-Ellison

TABLE 86.2   Causes of Hypergastrinemia

ULCEROGENIC CAUSES	NONULCEROGENIC CAUSES
Antral G cell hyperplasia or hyperfunction	Antisecretory agents (PPIs)
Retained gastric antrum	Atrophic gastritis
Zollinger-Ellison syndrome	Pernicious anemia
Gastric outlet obstruction	Acid-reducing procedure (vagotomy)
Short-gut syndrome	Gastric cancer
	Chronic renal failure

PPIs, Proton pump inhibitors.

syndrome [ZES]). These gastrin-secreting tumors are not located in the antrum and secrete gastrin autonomously. The trophic effect of gastrin on ECL cells can result in type II gastric neuroendocrine tumor development.

Somatostatin

Somatostatin in the GI system is produced by delta cells primarily in the stomach, duodenum, and pancreas. Posttranslational processing converts somatostatin into either a 14– or 28–amino acid peptide. The predominant molecular form in the stomach is somatostatin-14. It is produced by diffuse neuroendocrine cells located in the fundus and antrum. The principal stimulus for somatostatin release is antral acidification as well as GRP, whereas acetylcholine from vagal fibers inhibits somatostatin release. Somatostatin inhibits parietal cell acid secretion directly and also indirectly through inhibition of gastrin release from G cells and downregulation of histamine release from ECL cells. Somatostatin inhibits many other hormones in the GI system, including glucagon, insulin, motilin, secretin, CCK, and VIP.

Somatostatin receptors are G protein–coupled receptors. Binding of somatostatin with its receptors is coupled to one or more inhibitory guanine nucleotide–binding proteins. Parietal cell somatostatin receptors appear to be a single subunit of glycoproteins with equal affinity for somatostatin-14 and somatostatin-28. Somatostatin can inhibit parietal cell secretion through G protein–dependent and G protein–independent mechanisms. However, the ability of somatostatin to exert its inhibitory actions on cellular function is primarily thought to be mediated through the inhibition of adenylate cyclase, with a resultant reduction in cyclic adenosine monophosphate (cAMP) levels.

Histamine

Histamine plays a prominent role in parietal cell stimulation. Administration of H_2 receptor antagonists almost completely abolishes gastric acid secretion in response to gastrin and acetylcholine, suggesting that histamine may be a necessary intermediary of these pathways. Histamine is stored in the acidic granules of ECL cells and in resident mast cells. ECL cells are located in the oxyntic mucosa in close proximity to the parietal cell and play an essential role in parietal cell activation, possessing stimulatory and inhibitory feedback pathways. Histamine release is stimulated by gastrin, VIP, ghrelin, acetylcholine, and epinephrine through receptor-ligand interactions on ECL cells. In contrast, somatostatin inhibits gastrin-stimulated histamine release through interactions with somatostatin receptors located on the ECL cell. Other inhibitors of histamine release include peptide YY and prostaglandins.

Ghrelin

Ghrelin is a 28–amino acid peptide predominantly produced by the P/D1 endocrine cells of the oxyntic glands in the fundus and is a member of the motilin peptide family. Ghrelin appears to be under both endocrine and metabolic control, has a diurnal rhythm, and likely plays a major role in the neuroendocrine and metabolic responses to changes in nutritional status. Ghrelin also stimulates growth hormone release via the growth hormone secretagogue receptor. Ghrelin appears to be upregulated in times of negative energy balance and downregulated in times of positive energy balance, with high ghrelin levels during fasting and decreased levels after meals. Carbohydrates have the greatest suppressive effect on ghrelin release. Decreased ghrelin levels are associated with gastritis. Within the stomach, ghrelin increases gastric emptying and motility and increases gastric acid secretion.

In human volunteers, peripheral ghrelin administration enhances appetite and increases food intake. In patients who have undergone a gastric bypass or sleeve gastrectomy, ghrelin levels are lower.[2] Although the mechanism responsible for suppression of ghrelin levels after bariatric surgery is unknown, it is suggested that ghrelin may be responsive to the normal flow of nutrients across the stomach. Other studies have suggested that ghrelin leads to a switch toward glycolysis and away from fatty acid oxidation, which would favor fat deposition. Prader-Willi syndrome is the most common syndromic form of obesity, and these patients have been shown to have high circulating ghrelin levels that do not appropriately decrease after meals. Ghrelin antagonists may come to have a role in the treatment and prevention of obesity.

Gastric Acid Secretion

The hydrogen-potassium-ATPase (H^+/K^+-ATPase) acid–secreting pump is located in the parietal cell. Gastric acid secretion by the parietal cell is positively regulated mainly by three stimuli—acetylcholine, gastrin, and histamine. Acetylcholine is the principal neurotransmitter modulating acid secretion and is released from the vagus and parasympathetic ganglion cells; it mainly exerts effects on M3 receptors. Vagal fibers not only have a direct effect on parietal cells but also modulate peptide release from G cells and ECL cells as well as inhibit somatostatin secretion. Gastrin has direct hormonal effects on the parietal cell and also stimulates histamine release. Histamine has paracrine-like effects on the parietal cell and, as shown in Fig. 86.4, plays a central role in the regulation of acid secretion by the parietal cell after its release from ECL cells. Somatostatin exerts inhibitory actions on gastric acid secretion. Release of somatostatin from antral D cells is stimulated in the presence of low intraluminal pH as well as VIP and gastrin. After its release, somatostatin inhibits gastrin release through paracrine effects and modifies histamine release from ECL cells. Glucagon-like peptide 1 and peptide YY also inhibit gastric acid secretion. Consequently, the precise state of acid secretion by the parietal cell depends on the overall influence of the positive and negative stimuli.

Stimulated Acid Secretion

There is always a basal level of acid secretion that is approximately 2 mEq per hour. Ingestion of food is the physiologic stimulus for increasing acid secretion, with average maximal acid output of 30 mEq per hour. There are three interrelated phases of the acid secretory response to a meal: cephalic, gastric, and intestinal.

Cephalic phase. The cephalic phase originates with the sight, smell, thought, or taste of food. Although the exact mechanisms whereby these senses lead to increased acid secretion are not yet

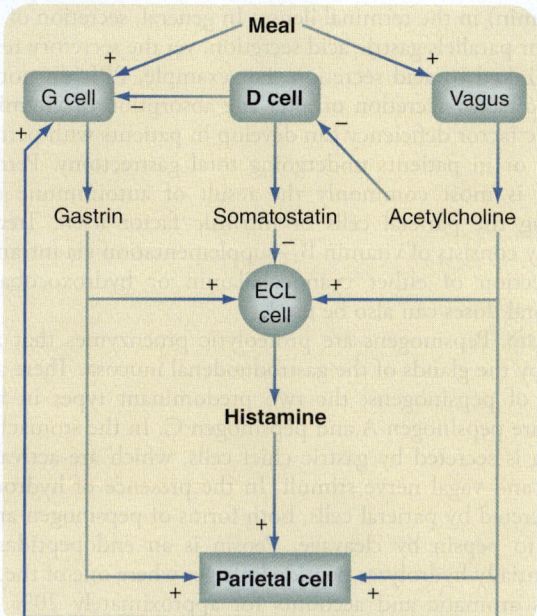

FIGURE 86.4 Central role of the enterochromaffin-like *(ECL)* cell in regulation of acid secretion by the parietal cell. As shown, ingestion of a meal stimulates vagal fibers to release acetylcholine (cephalic phase). Binding of acetylcholine to M3 receptors located on the ECL cell, parietal cell, and G cell results in the release of histamine, hydrochloric acid, and gastrin. Binding of acetylcholine to M3 receptors on D cells results in the inhibition of somatostatin release. After a meal, G cells are also stimulated to release gastrin, which interacts with receptors located on ECL cells and parietal cells to cause the release of histamine and hydrochloric acid (gastric phase). Release of somatostatin from D cells decreases histamine release and gastrin release from ECL cells and G cells. In addition, somatostatin inhibits parietal cell acid secretion (not shown). The principal stimulus for the activation of D cells is antral luminal acidification (not shown). (From Yeo C, Dempsey DT, Klein AS, et al., eds. *Shackelford's Surgery of the Alimentary Tract.* 6th ed. Philadelphia: Saunders; 2007.)

fully elucidated, it is hypothesized that several sites are stimulated in the brain, including neural centers in the hypothalamus. These higher centers transmit signals to the stomach via the vagus nerves, which release acetylcholine that activates muscarinic receptors located on target cells. Acetylcholine directly increases acid secretion by the parietal cells, stimulates ECL and G cells to release histamine and gastrin, respectively, and inhibits D cells from releasing somatostatin. Although the intensity of the acid secretory response in the cephalic phase surpasses that of the other phases, it accounts for only 20% to 30% of the total volume of gastric acid produced in response to a meal because of its short duration.

Gastric phase. The gastric phase of acid secretion begins when food enters the gastric lumen. Protein products of ingested food interact with microvilli of antral G cells to stimulate gastrin release. Food also stimulates acid secretion by causing mechanical distention of the stomach. Gastric distention as food enters the stomach, termed *receptive relaxation,* activates stretch receptors in the stomach to elicit the vagovagal reflex arc as well as local enteric nervous system acetylcholine release. The vasovagal reflex is abolished by proximal gastric vagotomy and is, at least in part, independent of changes in serum gastrin levels. Antral distention also causes gastrin release. The entire gastric phase accounts for most (60%–70%) of meal-stimulated acid output.

Intestinal phase. The intestinal phase of gastric secretion is initiated by entry of chyme into the duodenum, which initially stimulates gastrin release and suppresses gastric motility. It occurs after gastric emptying and lasts as long as partially digested food components remain in the proximal small bowel. It accounts for only 5% to 10% of the acid secretory response to a meal and does not appear to be mediated by serum gastrin levels. Chyme also stimulates release of CCK and secretin in the duodenum.

Activation and Secretion by the Parietal Cell

The two second messengers principally involved in stimulation of acid secretion by parietal cells are intracellular cAMP and calcium. These two messengers activate protein kinases and phosphorylation cascades. The intracellular events following ligand binding to receptors on the parietal cell are shown in Fig. 86.5. Histamine causes an increase in intracellular cAMP, which initiates a cascade of phosphorylation events that culminates in activation of the gastric proton pump (H^+/K^+-ATPase). In contrast, acetylcholine and gastrin stimulate phospholipase C, which converts membrane-bound phospholipids into inositol triphosphate to mobilize calcium from intracellular stores. Increased intracellular calcium activates other protein kinases that ultimately activate H^+/K^+-ATPase in a similar fashion to initiate the secretion of hydrochloric acid.

The H^+/K^+-ATPase is the final common pathway for gastric acid secretion by the parietal cell. It is a heterodimer composed of a catalytic α-subunit and a glycoprotein β-subunit. During the resting state, gastric parietal cells store H^+/K^+-ATPase intracellularly. Cellular relocation of the proton pump subunits through cytoskeletal rearrangements must occur for acid secretion to increase in response to stimulatory factors. The subsequent heterodimer assembly of the H^+/K^+-ATPase subunits and insertion into the microvilli of the secretory canaliculus allows an increase in gastric acid secretion. A KCl efflux pathway must exist to supply potassium to the extracytoplasmic side of the pump. Cytosolic hydrogen is secreted by H^+/K^+-ATPase in exchange for extracytoplasmic potassium (see Fig. 86.5), which is an electroneutral exchange and does not contribute to the transmembrane potential difference across the parietal cell. Secretion of chloride is accomplished through a chloride channel moving chloride from the parietal cell cytoplasm into the gastric lumen. The exchange of hydrogen for potassium requires energy in the form of adenosine triphosphate (ATP) because hydrogen is being secreted against a gradient of more than a millionfold. Because of this large energy requirement, the parietal cell has a mitochondrial compartment representing about one-third of its cellular volume. In contrast to stimulated acid secretion, cessation of acid secretion requires endocytosis of H^+/K^+-ATPase with regeneration of cytoplasmic tubulovesicles containing the subunits; this occurs through a tyrosine-based signal. The tyrosine-containing sequence is located on the cytoplasmic tail of the β-subunit.

Roughly 1 billion parietal cells are found in the normal human stomach and are responsible for secreting, on average, a maximum of 30 mEq per hour of hydrochloric acid in response to a meal. There is a linear relationship between maximal acid output and parietal cell number. Gastric acid secretory rates may be altered in patients with upper GI disease. For example, gastric acid is decreased in patients with pernicious anemia or atrophic gastritis. Gastric acid plays a critical role in the digestion of a meal. It is required to convert pepsinogen into pepsin, elicits the release of secretin from the duodenum, and limits colonization of the upper GI tract with bacteria.

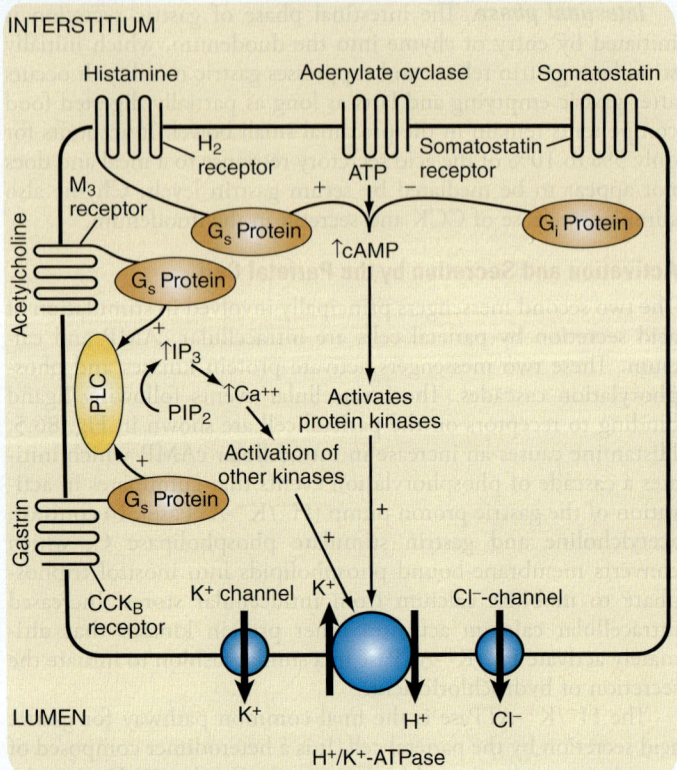

INTERSTITIUM

LUMEN

H⁺/K⁺-ATPase

FIGURE 86.5 Intracellular signaling events in a parietal cell. As shown, histamine binds to H₂ receptors, stimulating adenylate cyclase through a G protein–linked mechanism. Adenylate cyclase activation causes an increase in intracellular cyclic adenosine monophosphate *(cAMP)* levels, which activates protein kinases. Activated protein kinases stimulate a phosphorylation cascade, with a resultant increase in levels of phosphoproteins that activate the proton pump. Activation of the proton pump leads to extrusion of cytosolic hydrogen in exchange for extracytoplasmic potassium. In addition, chloride is secreted through a chloride channel located on the luminal side of the membrane. Gastrin binds to type B cholecystokinin receptors, and acetylcholine binds to M3 receptors. After the interaction of gastrin and acetylcholine with their receptors, phospholipase C is stimulated through a G protein–linked mechanism to convert membrane-bound phospholipids into inositol triphosphate *(IP₃)*. IP₃ stimulates the release of calcium from intracellular calcium stores, leading to an increase in intracellular calcium that activates protein kinases, which activate the H⁺/K⁺-ATPase. *ATP,* Adenosine triphosphate; *ATPase,* adenosine triphosphatase; *Gᵢ,* inhibitory guanine nucleotide protein; *Gₛ,* stimulatory guanine nucleotide protein; *PIP₂,* phosphatidylinositol 4,5-diphosphate; *PLC,* phospholipase C. (From Yeo C, Dempsey DT, Klein AS, et al., eds. *Shackelford's Surgery of the Alimentary Tract.* 6th ed. Philadelphia: Saunders; 2007.)

Other Gastric Secretory Products

Gastric juice. Gastric juice is the combined result of secretion by the parietal cells, chief cells, and mucous cells, in addition to swallowed saliva and duodenal refluxate. The two main components of gastric juice are hydrochloric acid and pepsin. The electrolyte composition varies with the rate of gastric secretion. Parietal cells secrete an electrolyte solution that is isotonic with plasma, with a pH of 0.8. The lowest intraluminal pH commonly measured in the stomach is approximately 2.0 because of dilution of the parietal cell secretion by other gastric secretions containing sodium, potassium, and bicarbonate. The acidity of gastric juice inactivates most ingested microorganisms.

Intrinsic factor. Intrinsic factor is a glycoprotein produced by the parietal cells that is essential for the absorption of vitamin B₁₂ (cobalamin) in the terminal ileum. In general, secretion of intrinsic factor parallels gastric acid secretion, yet the secretory response is not linked to acid secretion. For example, PPIs do not block intrinsic factor secretion or alter the absorption of vitamin B₁₂. Intrinsic factor deficiency can develop in patients with pernicious anemia or in patients undergoing total gastrectomy. Pernicious anemia is most commonly the result of autoimmune disease targeting the parietal cells or intrinsic factor itself. Treatment typically consists of vitamin B₁₂ supplementation via intramuscular injection of either cyanocobalamin or hydroxocobalamin. Large oral doses can also be used.

Pepsin. Pepsinogens are proteolytic proenzymes that are secreted by the glands of the gastroduodenal mucosa. There are five groups of pepsinogens; the two predominant types in human adults are pepsinogen A and pepsinogen C. In the stomach, pepsinogen is secreted by gastric chief cells, which are activated by gastrin and vagal nerve stimuli. In the presence of hydrochloric acid secreted by parietal cells, both forms of pepsinogen are converted to pepsin by cleavage. Pepsin is an endopeptidase that preferentially hydrolyzes peptide linkages where one of the amino acids is aromatic and accounts for approximately 20% of the protein digestion in the GI tract. Pepsins have optimal function at a pH of 1.5 to 2.0 and become inactive at a pH of 6.5, with irreversible inactivation above a pH of 8.0.

Mucus and bicarbonate. Mucus and bicarbonate combine to neutralize gastric acid at the gastric mucosal surface. They are secreted by the surface mucous cells and mucous neck cells in the antrum. Gastric mucin is a large glycoprotein; the mucus is a viscoelastic gel containing approximately 85% water and 15% mucin. It provides a mechanical barrier to injury, is relatively impermeable to pepsins, and also acts as an impediment to ion movement from the gastric lumen to the apical cell membrane. Stability of the mucin layer is largely the result of disulfide bonds. Mucus is in a constant state of flux because it is secreted continuously by mucosal cells while simultaneously being solubilized by luminal pepsin in the stomach. Mucus production is increased by vagal stimulation, cholinergic agonists, prostaglandins, and some bacterial toxins. In contrast, anticholinergic drugs and nonsteroidal antiinflammatory drugs (NSAIDs) inhibit mucus secretion. *Helicobacter pylori* secretes various proteases and lipases that break down mucin and impair the protective function of the mucus layer.

In the acid-secreting portion of the stomach, bicarbonate secretion is an active process, whereas in the antrum, active and passive secretion of bicarbonate occurs. However, the magnitude of bicarbonate secretion is considerably less than acid secretion. Although the luminal pH is 2, the pH observed at the surface epithelial cell level is usually 7. The pH gradient found at the epithelial surface is a result of the unstirred layer of water in the mucus gel and of the continuous secretion of bicarbonate by the surface epithelial cells.

Gastric Barrier Function

The stomach's barrier function depends on multiple physiologic and anatomic factors. Prostaglandins have several mucosal protection mechanisms including increasing mucosal blood flow and stimulating mucus, bicarbonate, and phospholipid secretion. Cyclooxygenase is the enzyme responsible for prostaglandin production. Thus, cyclooxygenase inhibitors such as NSAIDs and aspirin can result in gastric injury. Blood flow plays a critical role in gastric mucosal defense by providing nutrients and delivering oxygen to ensure that the intracellular processes that underlie mucosal resistance to injury can proceed unabated. Marked decreases in gastric blood flow can result in mucosal injury and ulcer formation, which is exacerbated in the presence of luminal acid. After damage occurs, injured surface epithelial cells are replaced rapidly by the migration of surface mucous cells located along the basement membranes. This process is referred to as *restitution* or *reconstitution*.

Exposure of the stomach to noxious agents causes a reduction in the potential difference across the gastric mucosa. In normal gastric mucosa, the potential difference across the mucosa is -30 to -50 mV and results from the active transport of chloride into the lumen and sodium into the blood by the activity of Na^+/K^+-ATPase. Disruption of the tight junctions between mucosal cells causes the epithelium to become leaky to ions (i.e., Na^+ and Cl^-) and a resultant loss of the high transepithelial electrical resistance normally found in gastric mucosa.

GASTRIC MOTILITY

Gastric motility is regulated on three main levels: extrinsic neural control, intrinsic neural control, and myogenic control. The extrinsic neural controls are mediated through parasympathetic (vagal) and sympathetic (splanchnic) pathways, whereas the intrinsic controls involve the enteric nervous system and interstitial cells of Cajal. Myogenic control resides in the excitatory membranes of the gastric smooth muscle cells.

Fasting Gastric Motility

The electrical basis of gastric motility begins with the depolarization of pacemaker cells located in the mid-body of the stomach along the greater curvature. Once initiated by the interstitial cells of Cajal, slow waves travel at three cycles per minute in a circumferential and antegrade fashion toward the pylorus. In addition to these slow waves, gastric smooth muscle cells are capable of producing action potentials, which are associated with larger changes in membrane potential than slow waves. During fasting, the stomach goes through a cyclical pattern of electrical activity composed of slow waves and electrical spikes, which has been termed the *migrating myoelectric complex (MMC)*. Motilin, released from the small intestine, is a key stimulant of MMC initiation. Each cycle of the MCC lasts 90 to 120 minutes and consists of four distinct phases. The MMC results in clearance of gastric contents during periods of fasting. The exact regulatory mechanisms of MCC activities are unknown, but these activities remain intact after vagal denervation.

Postprandial Gastric Motility

Ingestion of a meal results in an active decrease in the resting tone of the proximal stomach and fundus, termed *receptive relaxation;* this allows for gastric accommodation of the meal with minimal increase in luminal pressure. This reflex is mediated by the vagus nerve. Thus, interruption of vagal innervation to the proximal stomach via truncal vagotomy impairs receptive relaxation, with resultant early satiety and rapid emptying of ingested liquids. In addition to its storage function, the stomach is responsible for the mechanical mixing of ingested solid food particles. This activity involves repetitive forceful contractions of the mid-body and antral portions of the stomach, causing food particles to be propelled against a closed pylorus, with subsequent retropulsion of solids and liquids. The net effect is a thorough mixing of solids and liquids and sequential shearing of solid food particles to smaller than 1 mm before passage through the pylorus to the proximal duodenum.

The emptying of gastric contents is influenced by coordinated neural and hormonal mediators. Additionally, the chemical and mechanical properties and temperature of the intraluminal contents can influence the rate of gastric emptying. In general, liquids empty more rapidly than solids, and carbohydrates empty more readily than fats. Cold liquids tend to empty at a slower rate than those at ambient temperature. These responses to luminal stimuli are regulated by the enteric nervous system. CCK, stimulated by protein and fat in the small intestine, inhibits gastric emptying. Osmoreceptors and pH-sensitive receptors in the proximal small bowel have also been shown to be involved in the activation of feedback inhibition of gastric emptying.

Abnormal Gastric Motility

Gastroparesis is the combination of objectively delayed gastric emptying and resultant symptoms in the absence of mechanical obstruction.[3] Symptoms of gastroparesis are nausea/vomiting, early satiety, abdominal pain, and bloating. In the most severe cases, patients can suffer weight loss. The first steps in evaluating patients with suspected abnormal gastric motility after history and physical examination should be to exclude a mechanical obstruction with upper endoscopy and either a computed tomographic (CT), magnetic resonance (MR) enterography, or barium follow-through. The most common causes of gastroparesis are idiopathic, diabetes mellitus, viral infection (i.e., cytomegalovirus [CMV] and Epstein-Barr virus [EBV]), neurologic disease (i.e., multiple sclerosis, stroke, Parkinson disease), autoimmune disease, and certain medications such as narcotics, tricyclic antidepressants, calcium channel blockers, and cyclosporine. Additionally, gastric motility can be impaired after surgery because of either intentional or accidental vagotomy. Vagotomy results in loss of receptive relaxation and gastric accommodation in response to meal ingestion, with resultant early satiety, postprandial bloating, accelerated emptying of liquids, and delay in emptying of solids.

Clinical manifestations of diabetic gastropathy, which can occur in insulin-dependent or non–insulin-dependent patients, are thought to be related to a variety of factors. Up to 50% of patients with diabetes have objective delayed gastric emptying; however, many have no or minimal symptoms. Impaired neural control via the vagus nerve, myenteric nervous system, interstitial cells of Cajal, oxidative stress, and the underlying smooth muscle have been implicated. Additionally, hyperglycemia itself has been shown to cause a decrease in contractility of the gastric antrum and an increase in pyloric contractility, to relax the proximal stomach, and to suppress the MMC. Hyperinsulinemia, which is often associated with non–insulin-dependent diabetes, may play a role in the gastroparesis seen in this condition because it also leads to suppression of MMC activity.

Gastric-Emptying Studies

There are numerous ways to assess gastric emptying. The most commonly used is nuclear scintigraphy. Scans are obtained immediately after ingestion of a technetium-labeled meal and at 1, 2, and 4 hours after the meal. Standard upper normal limits for gastric retention are 90% at 1 hour, 60% at 2 hours, and 10% at 4 hours. The measurement of residual gastric contents at 4 hours is the most sensitive for diagnosing gastroparesis. At 4 hours, retention of 10% to 15% signifies mild gastroparesis, 15% to 35% is moderate, and greater than 35% is severe. There are multiple other diagnostic options; however, they are used less frequently. An upper abdominal x-ray series after barium swallow can provide information on gastric emptying and may reveal mechanical causes that could contribute to a delay, such as gastric outlet obstruction. Wireless motility capsules have also been investigated as an alternative to scintigraphy, which can measure the pH, temperature, and pressure amplitude during their transit through the GI tract. Noninvasive breath tests, such as ^{13}C-spirulina, measure the expiratory $^{13}CO_2$ concentration after an isotope-labeled meal. Antropyloroduodenal manometry can reveal excessive tonic pressure at the pylorus, and newer technology such as endoluminal functional lumen imaging probes can measure the pyloric dimensions, possibly identifying patients who would benefit from pyloric interventions. An electrogastrogram or autonomic testing can aid in identifying the underlying etiology of gastroparesis, though the resulting clinical implications are unclear at this time.

Treatment

Regardless of the cause of gastroparesis, initial first-line treatment of mild gastroparesis involves dietary modification.[4] Patients should be encouraged to eat multiple small meals low in fat and insoluble fiber. Acidic and spicy foods should also be avoided. In patients who cannot tolerate solid foods, a liquid diet can be used. Attention to hydration, vitamin deficiency, and electrolyte abnormalities is necessary in patients with recurrent vomiting. Medications that affect gastric motility, such as opioids, calcium channel blockers, tricyclic antidepressants, and dopamine agonists, should be stopped when possible. Glycemic control should be optimized in patients with diabetes.

Pharmacologic therapy is necessary for persistent symptoms despite conservative measures. First-line medical therapy is metoclopramide, a dopamine D2 receptor antagonist that stimulates antral contractions and decreases postprandial relaxation of the fundus. Metoclopramide also has central nervous system antinausea effects and is the only FDA-approved medication for gastroparesis. Outside of the United States, domperidone, another D2 antagonist, is an available option. Macrolide antibiotics (erythromycin and azithromycin) are motilin agonists that act by stimulating fundal contraction and have also shown benefit. However, their prokinetic effects are limited by tachyphylaxis and thus can be considered for second-line therapy. Other prokinetic agents (5-HT4 and ghrelin receptor agonists) can be considered in refractory cases. Antinausea medications should be prescribed for symptom management.

Endoscopic or surgical management can be considered in patients with refractory symptoms despite maximal medical therapy. Venting gastrostomy tubes can alleviate symptoms, and jejunostomy tubes can provide nutritional support for patients with severe gastroparesis. A trial of nasogastric (NG) decompression and nasojejunal feeding should be performed before either procedure. Gastrostomy and jejunostomy tubes are typically able to be placed endoscopically, though surgical placement is also possible. Enteral nutrition is preferred to parenteral nutrition for long-term management of severe gastroparesis when possible.

Gastric electric stimulation is currently approved as a humanitarian exemption use device by the FDA for refractory idiopathic and diabetic gastroparesis. Permanent stimulators are implanted surgically via either an open or laparoscopic approach. Two electrical leads are placed in the muscularis propria of the greater curvature approximately 10 cm proximal to the pylorus and connected to a subcutaneously positioned simulator that delivers high-frequency, low-energy current. Symptoms of nausea, vomiting, and pain are reported to improve in observational studies; however, these effects are much less in small blinded randomized trials. Pyloromyotomy and pyloroplasty are options for the surgical management of gastroparesis that function by lowering outflow resistance at the pylorus and enhancing any remaining gastric contractility. Measurements of pyloric function described earlier can be used to guide patient selection for these interventions. A systematic review of 38 studies reported that pyloric surgery improved nausea and abdominal pain more than gastric electrical stimulation[5]; however, patient selection criteria for intervention were heterogeneous, and robust comparative trials are lacking. Gastric peroral endoscopic myotomy (G-POEM) is being increasingly used in place of surgical pyloromyotomy. A prospective randomized trial comparing G-POEM with a sham procedure in patients with severe gastroparesis was stopped early after interim analysis after 41 patients showed significant improvement in symptoms and gastric emptying at 4 hours.[6] Trials evaluating pyloric measurement before the G-POEM procedure are ongoing. Endoscopic pyloric dilation and stenting can also be considered in select settings.

PEPTIC ULCER DISEASE

Peptic ulcers are erosions in the GI mucosa that extend through the muscularis mucosae. The most common symptom of peptic ulcer disease (PUD) is dyspepsia, though the majority of patients with peptic ulcers are asymptomatic. PUD can be complicated by bleeding, gastric outlet obstruction, and perforation. The two predominant causes of PUD are *H. pylori* and NSAIDs. Many other less common mechanisms exist as well, including ZES, other medication and infectious exposures, radiation therapy, and gastric bypass surgery.

Epidemiology

The incidence and prevalence of PUD worldwide have been declining in recent decades, as has the progression to complicated PUD. Both the age-standardized incidence and prevalence of PUD from the Global Burden of Disease study decreased worldwide by 31% from 1990–2019.[7] Although PUD remains an important cause of hospitalization and morbidity, the rates of hospitalization and mortality have also decreased over time.[8] Similarly, a composite index including mortality, disability, and prevalence-to-incidence ratios showed overall improved quality of care globally over the previous decades, though heterogeneity still exists.[7] Much of this decline in ulcer incidence and the need for hospitalization has stemmed from increased knowledge of ulcer pathogenesis. Specifically, the role of *H. pylori* has been clearly defined and the risks of long-term NSAID use have been better elucidated. The need for surgery in the treatment of ulcer disease has also decreased primarily as a result of a marked decline in elective surgical therapy for chronic disease.

Pathogenesis

Peptic ulcers are caused by decreased protective factors, increased damaging factors, or both. Protective (or defensive) factors include mucosal bicarbonate secretion, mucus production, adequate mucosal blood flow, growth factors, cell renewal, and endogenous prostaglandins. Damaging or aggressive factors include hydrochloric acid secretion, pepsins, ethanol ingestion, smoking, duodenal reflux of bile, ischemia, NSAIDs, hypoxia, and, most notably, *H. pylori* infection. Although it is now clear that most ulcers are caused by *H. pylori* infection or NSAID use, it is still important to understand all of the other protective and causative factors to optimize treatment and ulcer healing and prevent disease recurrence.

Helicobacter pylori Infection

The global prevalence of *H. pylori* infection is estimated to be approximately 43%, which is decreased from 58% in the 1980s.[9] This decrease is multifactorial, with improvements in diagnosis, treatment, and environmental factors playing a role. Approximately 80% of people with *H. pylori* are asymptomatic. *H. pylori* remains the predominant risk factor for PUD, associated with 90% of duodenal ulcers and 70% to 90% of gastric ulcers.[10] Infection with *H. pylori* has been shown to temporally precede ulcer formation, and when this organism is eradicated as part of ulcer treatment, ulcer recurrence is extremely rare. These observations have secured the place of *H. pylori* as a primary causative factor in the pathogenesis of PUD.

The interplay between bacterial and host factors determines the clinical outcome of *H. pylori* infection. *H. pylori* is a spiral-shaped, flagellate, microaerophilic, gram-negative bacteria that resides in gastric-type epithelium within or beneath the mucus layer. Its shape and flagella aid its movement through the mucus layer. Mucolytic enzyme production facilitates passage through the mucus layer and protects the bacteria from mucin's antibiotic effects. *H. pylori* is a potent producer of urease, which is capable of splitting urea into ammonia and bicarbonate. This creates an alkaline microenvironment in the setting of an acidic gastric milieu, allowing for the bacteria's survival in the stomach. The bacteria attach to the gastric epithelial cells by binding to surface adhesins and are able to enter the mucus layer via flagella-driven motility.

The exact mechanisms responsible for *H. pylori*–induced GI injury are still not fully understood, but the following four potential mechanisms have been proposed (and likely interact) to cause a derangement of normal gastric and duodenal physiology that leads to subsequent ulcer formation:

1. *Production of toxic products that cause local tissue injury.* Locally produced toxic mediators include breakdown products from urease activity (e.g., ammonia), cytotoxins, mucinase (which degrades mucus and glycoproteins), phospholipases that damage both epithelial and mucus cells, and platelet-activating factor (which is known to cause mucosal injury and thrombosis in the microcirculation). *H. pylori* strains that produce both CagA (cytotoxin-associated gene A) and VacA (vacuolating cytotoxin) virulence factors induce more inflammation; CagA-positive strains are also associated with gastric adenocarcinoma.[11]

2. *Induction of a local mucosal immune response.* The lipopolysaccharides of *H. pylori* have evolved to largely be unrecognized by the human innate immune system, allowing for immune evasion and colonization. *H. pylori* can cause a local inflammatory reaction in the gastric mucosa via multiple innate immune pathways, attracting neutrophils and monocytes, which then produce numerous proinflammatory cytokines and reactive oxygen metabolites.

3. *Increased gastrin levels and changes in acid secretion.* In patients with antral *H. pylori* infection, basal and stimulated gastrin levels are significantly increased secondary to a reduction in somatostatin release from antral D cells because of infection with *H. pylori*. During the acute phase of *H. pylori* infection, acid secretion is decreased. With chronic infection, *H. pylori* has trophic effects on ECL and G cells, which can result in acid hypersecretion. The decrease in serum levels of somatostatin also contributes to the gastric hyperacidity. However, if oxyntic glands are destroyed by the chronic infection, hypoacidity will result.

4. *Gastric metaplasia occurring in the duodenum.* Metaplastic replacement of duodenal mucosa with gastric epithelium likely occurs as a protective response to decreased duodenal pH resulting from the previously described acid hypersecretion. This allows for *H. pylori* to colonize these areas of the duodenum, which causes duodenitis and likely predisposes to duodenal ulcer formation. The presence of *H. pylori* in the duodenum is more common in patients with ulcer formation compared with patients with asymptomatic infections isolated to the stomach.

Peptic ulcers are strongly associated with antral gastritis. Studies performed before the *H. pylori* era demonstrated that almost all patients with peptic ulcers have histologic evidence of antral gastritis. In most cases, the infection tends to be confined initially to the antrum and results in antral inflammation. The causative role of *H. pylori* infection in the pathogenesis of gastritis and PUD was first elucidated by Marshall and Warren in Australia in 1984.[12] Marshall himself ingested inocula of *H. pylori*, and within days he developed abdominal pain, nausea, and histologically confirmed presence of gastric *H. pylori* infection. Acute inflammation was observed histologically on days 5 and 10. By 2 weeks, acute inflammation had been replaced by chronic inflammation with evidence of a mononuclear cell infiltration. For their pioneering work, Marshall and Warren were jointly awarded the Nobel Prize in Physiology or Medicine in 2005.

Evidence of infection can be seen in early childhood. There is an inverse relationship between infection rates and socioeconomic status. The reasons for this relationship are poorly understood, but it seems to be the result of environmental factors such as sanitation, familial clustering, lack of running water, and overcrowding. Such factors likely also explain why developing countries have a comparatively higher rate of *H. pylori* infection, especially in children. *H. pylori* infection is associated with many common upper GI disorders and is almost always present in the setting of active chronic gastritis, but most infected individuals are asymptomatic. In addition, up to 90% of patients with gastric cancer have current or past *H. pylori* infection; the WHO classified *H. pylori* as a class I carcinogen in 1994. The lifetime gastric cancer risk associated with *H. pylori* infection is estimated at 1% to 5% depending on other genetic, environmental, and patient risk factors. There is also a strong association between mucosa-associated lymphoid tissue (MALT) lymphoma and *H. pylori* infection. Regression of these lymphomas has been demonstrated after eradication of *H. pylori*.[13]

Invasive Diagnostic Tests for Helicobacter pylori

Urease assay. Endoscopic biopsy specimens should be taken from the gastric body and the antrum and then tested for urease. Sensitivity in diagnosing infection is 84% to 95%, and specificity is 95% to 100%. However, the sensitivity of the test is lowered in patients with acute bleeding or who are taking PPIs, H_2 receptor antagonists, or antibiotics. Rapid urease test kits are commercially available and can detect urease in gastric biopsy specimens within 1 hour with a similar level of diagnostic accuracy.

Histology. Endoscopy can also be performed with biopsy samples of gastric mucosa, followed by histologic visualization of *H. pylori* using either routine hematoxylin-eosin stains or special stains (e.g., Giemsa stain). Sensitivity is approximately 95% and specificity is 99%, making histology slightly more accurate than the urease assay testing. Similar to the urease assay, the sensitivity of histologic evaluation is lower in patients taking PPIs or H_2 antagonists, but it remains the most accurate test available even in this setting. Histology additionally affords the ability to assess the severity of gastritis and confirm the presence or absence of the organism; however, it is more expensive than the rapid urease assay.

Culture. Culturing of gastric mucosa obtained at endoscopy can also be performed to diagnose *H. pylori*. The sensitivity is approximately 80%, and specificity is 100%. However, culture requires laboratory expertise, is not widely available, and is relatively expensive, and diagnosis requires 3 to 5 days. The advantage of culture is that it provides the opportunity to perform antibiotic sensitivity testing especially given increasing antibiotic resistance.

Noninvasive Diagnostic Tests for *Helicobacter pylori*

Urea breath test. The carbon-labeled urea breath test is based on the ability of *H. pylori* to hydrolyze urea as a result of its production of urease and is the most commonly used noninvasive diagnostic test. Both sensitivity and specificity are greater than 95%. As with other testing modalities, the sensitivity of the urea breath test is reduced in patients taking PPIs and antibiotics. It is recommended that patients discontinue antibiotics for 4 weeks and PPIs for 2 weeks to ensure optimal test accuracy. The urea breath test is less expensive than endoscopy and samples the entire stomach. In evaluating treatment efficacy, false-negative results can occur if the test is performed too soon after treatment, so it is usually best to perform this test 4 weeks after therapy is completed.

Stool antigen. *H. pylori* bacteria are present in the stool of infected patients, and several assays have been developed that use monoclonal antibodies to *H. pylori* antigens to test fecal specimens. These tests have demonstrated sensitivities and specificities of greater than 95%. Several studies have shown that stool antigen testing has an accuracy of greater than 90% in detecting eradication of infection after treatment, on par with invasive histology and noninvasive urea breath testing.

Serology. Various enzyme-linked immunosorbent assay laboratory-based tests are available and some rapid office-based immunoassays that are used to test for the presence of IgG antibodies to *H. pylori*. There is heterogeneity between various serologic test kits, with sensitivity ranging from 57% to 100% and specificity from 58% to 96%. Test kits need to be locally validated based on the prevalence of specific bacterial strains. Furthermore, antibody titers can remain high for 1 year or longer after eradication; consequently, this test cannot be used to distinguish between active and prior infection or to assess response to therapy. Serologic testing can be helpful if trying to assess for prevalence of disease in a location. For these reasons, stool antigen and urea breath tests are the preferred noninvasive modalities for diagnosis and evaluation of treatment efficacy in patients with PUD and suspected *H. pylori* infection.

Nonsteroidal Antiinflammatory Drugs

NSAIDs, including aspirin, are absorbed through the stomach and small intestine and function as inhibitors of the cyclooxygenase enzymes. Cyclooxygenase enzymes form the rate-limiting step of prostaglandin synthesis in the GI tract. Prostaglandins (including thromboxane A2) promote gastric and duodenal mucosal protection from luminal acid and pepsin via numerous mechanisms, including increasing mucin and bicarbonate secretion, increasing blood flow to the mucosal endothelium, and promoting epithelial cell proliferation and migration to the luminal surface. NSAIDs disrupt these naturally protective mechanisms,

increasing the risk of peptic ulcer formation in the stomach and the duodenum.

The use of NSAIDs is associated with a threefold to fourfold higher risk of PUD independent of *H. pylori* status. NSAID use also increases the risk of complicated PUD (including bleeding, obstruction, and perforation). NSAID-induced ulcers are more often found in the stomach. *H. pylori* ulcers are also almost always associated with chronic active gastritis, whereas gastritis is not always seen with NSAID-induced ulcers. When NSAID use is discontinued, the ulcers usually do not recur unless there is an untreated *H. pylori* infection as well.

Gastric and Duodenal Ulcers
Gastric Ulcer Types

The modified Johnson anatomic classification system for gastric ulcers (types I–V, described in Table 86.3) was developed before the modern understanding that most ulcers are the consequence of *H. pylori* infection or NSAID usage. However, despite having an increased understanding of the mechanisms of how and why most ulcers develop, this historical classification system is still relevant to surgical treatment because it dictates what operation should be performed.

Gastric ulcers can occur at any location in the stomach, although they usually manifest on the lesser curvature near the incisura. Approximately 50% to 60% of gastric ulcers are in this location and are classified as type I gastric ulcers. These ulcers occur with low to normal gastric acid output. Most occur near the histologic transition zone between the fundic and antral mucosa. Type II gastric ulcers (accounting for approximately 15%–20%) are located in the body of the stomach in combination with a duodenal ulcer. Type II ulcers are associated with excess acid secretion. Type III gastric ulcers are prepyloric ulcers and account for approximately 20% of the lesions. They behave similar to duodenal ulcers and are associated with hypersecretion of gastric acid. Type IV gastric ulcers occur high on the lesser curvature near the GE junction. The incidence of type IV gastric ulcers is less than 10%, and they are not associated with excessive acid secretion. Type V gastric ulcers can occur at any location and are associated with long-term NSAID use.

Gastric ulcers rarely develop before the age of 40 years, and the peak incidence occurs in individuals 55 to 65 years old. Some risk factors that may predispose to gastric ulceration include chronic alcohol intake, smoking, radiation therapy, and long-term corticosteroid therapy. The presence of acid appears to be essential to the production of a gastric ulcer; however, the total secretory output appears to be less important. In contrast to the acidification of the duodenum leading to ulcer formation, patients with gastric ulcers caused by *H. pylori* can have normal or reduced total gastric acid production. Gastric ulcer formation is more likely caused by an inflammatory response to the bacterial infection itself.

TABLE 86.3   Gastric Ulcer Types

TYPE	LOCATION	ACID LEVEL
I	Lesser curve at incisura	Low to normal
II	Gastric body with duodenal ulcer	Increased
III	Prepyloric	Increased
IV	High on lesser curve	Normal
V	Anywhere	Normal, NSAID-induced

NSAID, Nonsteroidal antiinflammatory drug.

Gastric Ulcer Clinical Manifestations

One clinical challenge of gastric ulcer management is the differentiation between gastric carcinoma and a benign ulcer. This is in contrast to duodenal ulcers, in which malignancy is extremely rare. Similar to duodenal ulcers, gastric ulcers are also characterized by recurrent episodes of epigastric pain. Complications of gastric ulcer disease include bleeding, obstruction, and perforation. Occasionally, benign ulcers have also been found to result in spontaneous gastrocolic fistulas. Surgical intervention is required in patients who develop complications from gastric ulcer disease. The most frequent complication overall of gastric ulceration is bleeding, with the most common requiring surgery being perforation. Most perforations occur along the anterior aspect of the lesser curvature. Gastric outlet obstruction can also occur in patients with type II or III gastric ulcers. However, one must carefully differentiate between benign obstruction and obstruction secondary to carcinoma.

Duodenal Ulcer: Clinical Manifestations

Patients with duodenal ulcer disease can present in various ways. The most common symptom associated with duodenal ulcer disease is midepigastric abdominal pain that is usually well localized. The pain is generally tolerable and frequently relieved by food. When the pain becomes constant, this suggests that there is deeper penetration of the ulcer. Referral of pain to the back is usually a sign of penetration into the pancreas, whereas diffuse peritoneal irritation is the result of free perforation.

Diagnosis and Management of Gastric and Duodenal Ulcers

The diagnosis and treatment of gastric ulceration generally mirror that of duodenal ulcer disease. The significant difference is the possibility of malignancy in a gastric ulcer. This critical difference necessitates that cancer be ruled out in acute and chronic presentations of gastric ulcer disease. Acid suppression and *H. pylori* eradication are important aspects of any treatment and are further detailed next.

Intractable nonhealing ulcers are becoming increasingly less common with improvements in medical therapy. It is important to ensure that adequate time has elapsed and appropriate therapy has been administered to allow healing of the ulcer to occur; this includes confirmation that *H. pylori* has been eradicated and that NSAIDs have been eliminated. The presentation of a nonhealing gastric ulcer in the *H. pylori* era should raise serious concerns about the presence of an underlying malignancy. These patients should undergo a thorough evaluation with multiple biopsies to exclude malignancy (Fig. 86.6). The approach for a complicated gastric ulcer varies depending on the type of ulcer and its association with pathophysiologic acid levels. Type I and IV ulcers, which are not associated with increased acid levels, do not require acid-reducing vagotomy. Fig. 86.7 is an algorithm for surgical management of complicated gastric ulcers.

History and physical examination are of limited value in distinguishing between gastric and duodenal ulceration. Routine laboratory studies include complete blood count, liver chemistries, serum creatinine, serum amylase, and calcium levels. A serum gastrin level should also be obtained in patients with ulcers that are refractory to medical therapy or require surgery. The two principal means of diagnosing gastric and duodenal ulcers are upper GI radiography and flexible upper endoscopy.

Upper gastrointestinal radiography. Diagnosis of gastric or duodenal ulcer by upper GI radiography requires the demonstration of barium within the ulcer crater, which is usually round or

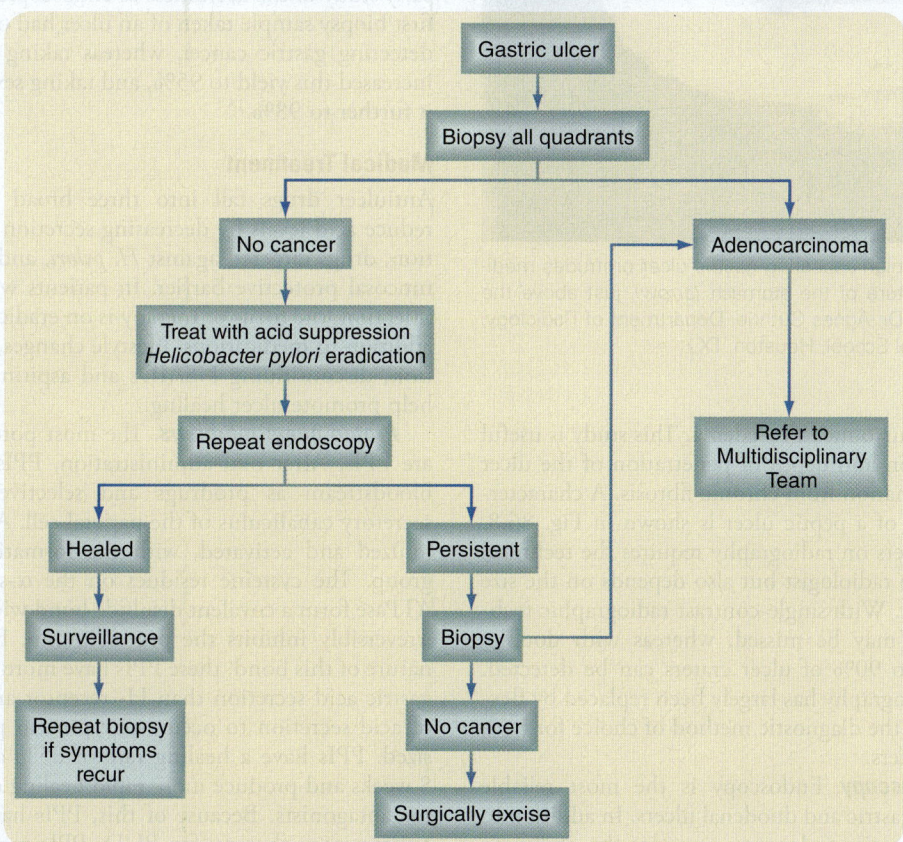

FIGURE 86.6 Algorithm for evaluation, treatment, and surveillance of a patient with a gastric ulcer.

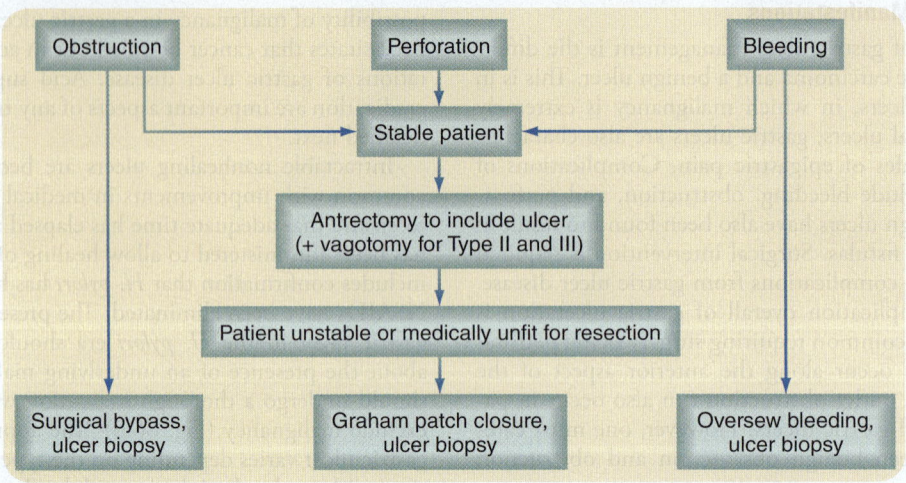

FIGURE 86.7 Algorithm for the surgical management of complicated gastric ulcer disease.

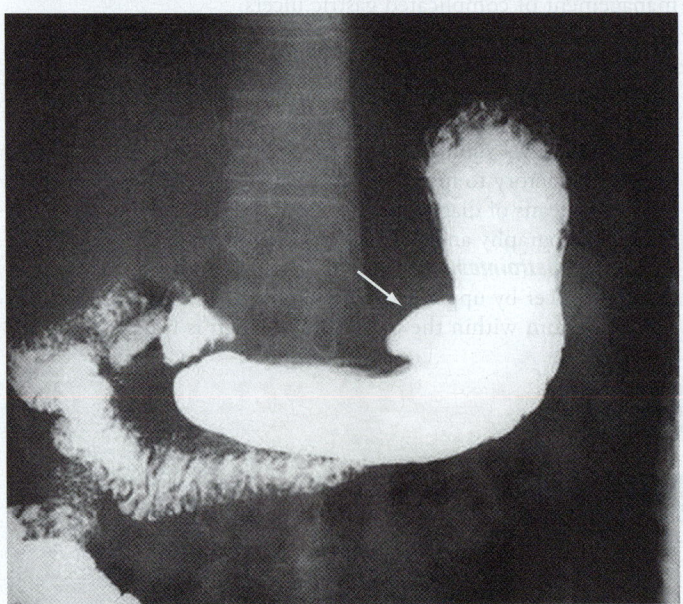

FIGURE 86.8 A large, benign-appearing gastric ulcer protrudes medially from the lesser curvature of the stomach *(arrow)*, just above the gastric incisura. (Courtesy Dr. Agnes Guthrie, Department of Radiology, University of Texas Medical School, Houston, TX.)

oval. The ulcer may be surrounded by edema. This study is useful to determine the location and depth of penetration of the ulcer and the extent of deformation from chronic fibrosis. A characteristic barium radiograph of a peptic ulcer is shown in Fig. 86.8. The ability to detect ulcers on radiography requires the technical skills and abilities of the radiologist but also depends on the size and location of the ulcer. With single-contrast radiographic techniques, 50% of ulcers may be missed, whereas with double-contrast studies, 80% to 90% of ulcer craters can be detected. However, upper GI radiography has largely been replaced by flexible upper endoscopy as the diagnostic method of choice for both gastric and duodenal ulcers.

Flexible upper endoscopy. Endoscopy is the most reliable method for diagnosing gastric and duodenal ulcers. In addition to providing a visual diagnosis, endoscopy provides the ability to sample tissue to evaluate for malignancy and *H. pylori* infection

and may be used for therapeutic purposes in the setting of GI bleeding or obstruction. Endoscopy also can evaluate for other pathologies of the esophagus, stomach, and duodenum that may be causing the patient's symptoms.

When a gastric ulcer has been detected endoscopically, biopsy is generally recommended in all cases to rule out malignancy. In very low-risk patients with benign-appearing ulcers, foregoing biopsy can be considered.[14] Larger ulcers and ulcers with irregular or heaped-up edges are more likely to harbor cancers. Multiple biopsy specimens should be taken of the ulcer for maximum diagnostic yield, preferably from all four quadrants if possible. An early study of the usefulness of endoscopic biopsy showed that the first biopsy sample taken of an ulcer had only a 70% sensitivity in detecting gastric cancer, whereas taking four biopsy specimens increased this yield to 95%, and taking seven specimens increased it further to 98%.[15]

Medical Treatment

Antiulcer drugs fall into three broad categories—drugs that reduce acid levels by decreasing secretion or chemical neutralization, drugs targeted against *H. pylori,* and drugs that increase the mucosal protective barrier. In patients with PUD and *H. pylori* infection, the focus of therapy is on eradication of the bacteria. In addition to medications, lifestyle changes, such as smoking cessation, discontinuing NSAIDs and aspirin, and avoiding alcohol, help promote ulcer healing.

Proton pump inhibitors. The most potent antisecretory agents are PPIs. After oral administration, PPIs are absorbed into the bloodstream as prodrugs and selectively concentrate in the secretory canaliculus of the parietal cell. At low pH, they become ionized and activated, with the formation of an active sulfur group. The cysteine residues on the α-subunit of the H^+/K^+-ATPase form a covalent disulfide bond with activated PPIs, which irreversibly inhibits the proton pump. Because of the covalent nature of this bond, these PPIs have more prolonged inhibition of gastric acid secretion than H_2 receptor antagonists. For recovery of acid secretion to occur, new protein pumps must be synthesized. PPIs have a healing rate of 85% at 4 weeks and 96% at 8 weeks and produce more rapid healing of ulcers than H_2 receptor antagonists. Because of this, PPIs have become the primary antisecretory therapy for PUD. PPIs require an acidic environment within the gastric lumen to become activated; thus, using antacids or H_2 receptor antagonists in combination with PPIs could have deleterious effects by promoting an alkaline environment. Maintenance PPI therapy is considered in patients with large (>2 cm) ulcers, refractory or frequent PUD, those who failed *H. pylori* eradication, or patients requiring continued NSAID/aspirin use.

Histamine H_2 receptor antagonists. The histamine H_2 receptor antagonists are structurally similar to histamine and function by inhibiting the H_2 receptors on parietal cells. Currently available H_2 receptor antagonists differ in their potency but only modestly in half-life and bioavailability. Famotidine is the most potent, and cimetidine is the weakest. However, as stated earlier, PPIs are preferred. In a meta-analysis of randomized controlled trials, PPIs showed significantly improved ulcer healing and rebleeding in patients who presented with a GI bleed as compared with H_2 receptor antagonists.[16]

Treatment of Helicobacter pylori infection. After it became clear that the majority of cases were caused by *H. pylori* infection, there was a paradigm shift that saw PUD as an infectious disease, rather than solely a consequence of pathologic acid secretion. Accordingly, treatment philosophy has shifted to focus on eradication of the infectious agent when present.

Current therapy is twofold in its approach, combining antibiotics against *H. pylori* with acid-reducing medications. The primary goal of the acid-reducing medication is to promote short-term healing by reducing pathologic acid levels and to improve patient symptoms. *H. pylori* eradication also helps with initial healing, but its primary efficacy is in preventing recurrence. There have been numerous trials comparing eradication therapy with ulcer-healing drugs alone or no treatment. Eradication of *H. pylori* has shown recurrence rates of 2%, with initial healing rates of 90%. However, eradication rates after an initial course of therapy have been decreasing, likely as a result of increased prevalence of antibiotic-resistant strains of *H. pylori;* approximately 20% to 30% of patients fail initial therapy. For this reason, monitoring for infection eradication with a urea breath test, stool antigen, or repeat endoscopy with biopsy at 4 to 6 weeks after therapy is important, as many patients will require further treatment with alternative regimens.

The treatment of *H. pylori*–positive PUD is triple or quadruple therapy aimed at the eradication of *H. pylori* (Box 86.1). This triple therapy includes a PPI and two antibiotics, with the addition of bismuth representing quadruple therapy. The choice of antibiotics should be guided by risk factors for macrolide resistance and presence of a penicillin allergy. When available, regional antibiotic susceptibility data should also help guide initial treatment regimen choice. Risk factors for macrolide resistance are prior exposure to a macrolide antibiotic or local clarithromycin resistance rates of greater than 15%. Patients who do not have risk factors for macrolide resistance and are not allergic to penicillin should receive standard triple therapy, consisting of clarithromycin, amoxicillin, and a PPI. The amoxicillin can be replaced with metronidazole if the patient has a penicillin allergy. Patients who have a risk factor for macrolide resistance should be given bismuth quadruple therapy, which consists of bismuth, tetracycline, metronidazole, and a PPI. Bismuth quadruple therapy should also be given to patients with a penicillin allergy and recent metronidazole use.

Clinical guidelines generally recommend treatment with a 14-day course of triple therapy and a 10- to 14-day course of bismuth quadruple therapy.[17] Side effects include diarrhea, nausea/vomiting, rash, and altered taste. The side effects are generally mild and resolve with cessation of treatment. Resistance to antibiotics is

---

> ### BOX 86.1 First-Line *Helicobacter pylori* Treatment Regimen
>
> *Patients without penicillin allergy, prior macrolide exposure, or in a region with >5% clarithromycin resistance:*
> - Clarithromycin triple therapy (PPI, clarithromycin, and amoxicillin)
> - Bismuth quadruple therapy (PPI, bismuth, tetracycline, metronidazole)
> - Concomitant regimen (PPI, clarithromycin, amoxicillin, nitroimidazole)
>
> *Patients without penicillin allergy with either prior macrolide exposure or in a region with >15% clarithromycin resistance:*
> - Bismuth quadruple therapy
> - Levofloxacin triple therapy (PPI, levofloxacin, amoxicillin)
>
> *Patients with a penicillin allergy but without prior macrolide exposure:*
> - Bismuth quadruple therapy
> - Clarithromycin triple therapy with metronidazole (PPI, clarithromycin, and amoxicillin)
>
> *Patients with both a penicillin allergy and either prior macrolide exposure or in a region with >15% clarithromycin resistance:*
> - Bismuth quadruple therapy

PPI, Proton pump inhibitor.
From Chey WD, Leontiadis GI, Howden CW, Moss SF. ACG Clinical Guideline: treatment of *Helicobacter pylori* infection. *Am J Gastroenterol.* 2017;112:212-238.

---

increasing and varies geographically. In a systematic review and meta-analysis from 2018, worldwide rates of clarithromycin resistance ranged from 20% to 35%, metronidazole from 29% to 60%, and levofloxacin from 12% to 31%.[18] For the 20% to 30% of patients with refractory disease, a treatment course with new antibiotics, such as metronidazole and tetracycline, is initiated, and quadruple therapy with the addition of bismuth is recommended if not previously used. Levofloxacin and rifabutin triple therapies represent other salvage therapeutic options.[19]

Antacids. Antacids are the oldest form of therapy for PUD. They reduce gastric acidity by reacting with hydrochloric acid, forming a salt and raising the gastric pH. Antacids differ greatly in their buffering ability, absorption, and side effects. Antacids typically contain aluminum hydroxide, calcium carbonate, or magnesium trisilicate and can be used to neutralize gastric acid and decrease acid delivery to the duodenum, though the exact mechanism of action is unclear. Magnesium antacids tend to be the best buffers but can cause significant diarrhea, whereas acids precipitated with phosphorus can occasionally result in hypophosphatemia and sometimes constipation. Aluminum hydroxide can bind growth factors and may increase their delivery to injured mucosa. The use of antacids has largely been replaced by the more efficacious antisecretory therapies (either H_2 receptor antagonists or PPIs) for the treatment of PUD.

Sucralfate. Sucralfate is structurally related to heparin but does not have any anticoagulant effects. It is an aluminum salt of sulfated sucrose that dissociates under the acidic conditions in the stomach. It is hypothesized that the sucrose polymerizes and binds to the ulcer crater to produce a protective coating that can last for 6 hours. Sucralfate has also been shown to stimulate angiogenesis and granulation tissue formation. The efficacy and role of sucralfate in healing peptic ulcers caused by *H. pylori* infection has not been clearly established, and sucralfate is not currently included as part of initial treatment guidelines for PUD.

Complicated Peptic Ulcer Disease

Ulcer surgery was previously a major part of general surgery practice. With the shift in understanding the pathophysiology of

---

> **BOX 86.2   Surgical Treatment Recommendations for Complications Related to Peptic Ulcer Disease**
>
> Bleeding:
> - Gastric: Partial gastrectomy or oversewing of bleeding vessel with treatment of *Helicobacter pylori*
> - Duodenal: Oversewing of bleeding vessel with treatment of *H. pylori*
>
> Perforation: Patch closure with treatment of *H. pylori*
>
> Obstruction: Rule out malignancy followed by gastrojejunostomy with treatment of *H. pylori*
>
> Intractable: Truncal vagotomy ± antrectomy

PUD and improved medical management, the surgeon's role now is primarily to treat the patients who have a complication from their disease. Complicated PUD includes hemorrhage, perforation, and obstruction (Box 86.2). Frequently included in discussions of complicated ulcer disease is an intractable ulcer. Although intractable disease no doubt exists, its definition is nebulous, and determining exactly when and what type of surgical intervention is required is primarily a matter of judgment. In the current era of excellent treatment options for *H. pylori* infection and acid suppression, few patients who are truly compliant with medical therapy develop intractable ulcer disease in the absence of malignancy or another underlying cause such as ZES. Early multidisciplinary management is imperative for patients with complicated PUD to ensure optimal patient outcomes.

Hemorrhage. PUD is the most common cause of upper GI bleeding, accounting for roughly 35% to 50% of cases; bleeding occurs in 15% to 20% of patients with PUD.[20] The predominant risk factor for PUD bleeding is NSAID use; *H. pylori* infection, older age, significant medical comorbidities, and anticoagulant use are other known risks. Patients can present with hematemesis, melena, or both. The initial approach to an upper GI bleed from PUD is similar to the approach to other patients presenting with acute hypovolemic blood loss. Large-bore intravenous (IV) access, rapid restoration of intravascular volume with fluid and blood products as the clinical situation dictates, and close monitoring of vital signs are all essential to effective management of these patients. Patients should be initiated on an IV PPI during their initial evaluation. The role of NG lavage is controversial and is no longer routinely recommended, as no clinical benefit has been shown with its use.[21] Additionally, the use of a prokinetic such as erythromycin before endoscopy can improve mucosal visualization as well as NG lavage.

Upper flexible endoscopy is the best initial procedure for diagnosis of the source of upper GI bleeding and for therapeutic intervention, including in the setting of bleeding peptic ulcers. Patients with an acute upper GI bleed should undergo endoscopy within 24 hours. Patients who are noted on endoscopy to have active bleeding or a visible vessel within the ulcer require endoscopic therapy. Patients without active bleeding, no visible vessel, and a clean ulcer base are low risk and do not require further intervention. There is no consensus on endoscopic intervention for patients with an adherent clot that does not dislodge after vigorous irrigation.[22] The most commonly used system for classifying the endoscopic appearance of bleeding ulcers is the Forrest classification (Table 86.4), which stratifies the risk of rebleeding based on observed "stigmata of recent hemorrhage."[23] All patients undergoing endoscopic examination should be tested for *H. pylori* status with either urease assay, histology, or culture. Endoscopic treatment options include hemostatic clips, electrocoagulation, argon plasma coagulation, heater probe, and absolute ethanol injection. Epinephrine injection should not be used as monotherapy but can be used in combination with another therapeutic method.

A randomized trial compared 241 patients with high-risk bleeding ulcers (defined in this study as 2 cm in size or greater, active bleeding during endoscopy, hemoglobin levels less than 9 g/dL, or hypotensive shock) after control endoscopically to receive either angiographic embolization or standard treatment. The primary end point was recurrent bleeding within 30 days. There was no significant difference in rebleeding rates with prophylactic embolization (10% vs. 11%). Mortality was also similar with an overall mortality in the study of 3%.[24]

Patients who have a second episode of bleeding after initially successful endoscopic therapy are typically treated with repeat endoscopy. Patients with recurrent bleeding can be considered for interventional angiography with transarterial embolization (Fig. 86.9) if they are hemodynamically stable and those resources and expertise are available.

All high-risk patients should be placed in a monitored setting. Although prior consensus guidelines advocated for continuous IV PPI infusion, a systematic review and meta-analysis showed intermittent high-dose PPI therapy was comparable to continuous infusion for patients with endoscopically treated high-risk bleeding ulcers.[25] IV PPI therapy should be initiated on patient presentation and is recommended for 3 days after endoscopy and then oral PPI for at least 2 weeks. A longer duration of PPI treatment may be needed depending on the underlying clinical scenario.[22]

TABLE 86.4   Forrest Classification of Stigmata of Recent Hemorrhage on Endoscopic Examination of Peptic Ulcers and Relative Prevalence

STIGMATA OF RECENT HEMORRHAGE	FORREST CLASSIFICATION	PREVALENCE	RISK OF REBLEEDING
Active bleeding			
Active spurting	IA	10%	90%
Active oozing	IB	10%	10%–20%
Recent hemorrhage			
Nonbleeding, visible vessel	IIA	25%	50%
Adherent clot	IIB	10%	25%–30%
Flat pigmented spot	IIC	10%	5%–10%
No signs of hemorrhage			
Clean-based ulcer	III	35%	3%–5%

Adapted from Katschinski B, Logan R, Davies J, et al. Prognostic factors in upper gastrointestinal bleeding. *Dig Dis Sci.* 1994;39(4):706-712.

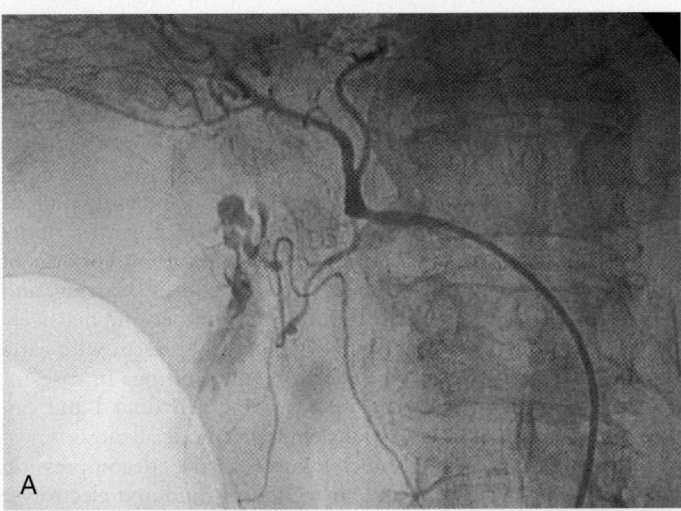

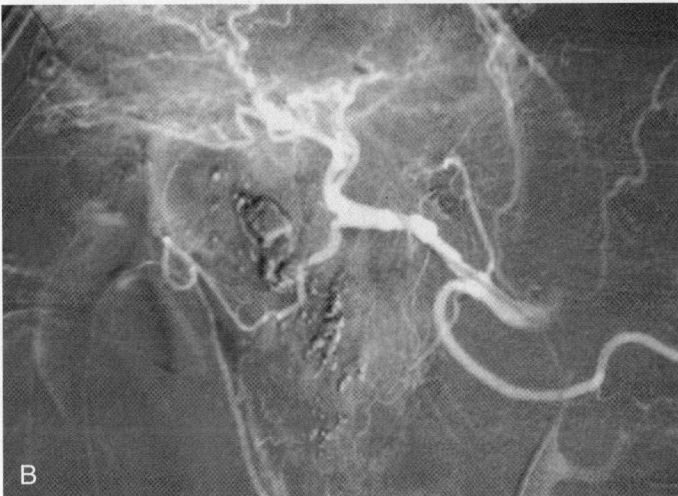

FIGURE 86.9 Endovascular control of a bleeding duodenal ulcer. (A) An angiogram is obtained, which shows extravasation from a branch off of the gastroduodenal artery. (B) A completion angiogram after glue embolization of the vessel shows resolution of the bleed with preservation of flow through the gastroduodenal artery. (From Loffroy R, Guiu B, Cercueil JP, et al. Refractory bleeding from gastroduodenal ulcers: arterial embolization in high-operative-risk patients. *J Clin Gastroenterol.* 2008;42:361-367.)

Despite the use of PPIs and improved methods of nonoperative control, some patients will require surgical intervention. Indications for surgical intervention include hemodynamic instability, failed endoscopic treatment, or recurrent hemorrhage after multiple endoscopic and/or interventional radiology treatments. The vessel most likely to be bleeding is the gastroduodenal artery because of a posterior duodenal ulcer erosion. Although bleeding duodenal ulcers can be treated laparoscopically, the more typical approach is through an upper midline laparotomy, especially in patients who are hemodynamically unstable. A Kocher maneuver is performed to mobilize the duodenum. The anterior wall of the duodenal bulb is opened longitudinally, and the incision can be carried across the pylorus if needed. The gastroduodenal artery is oversewn with a three-point U stitch technique, which effectively ligates the main vessel (superior and inferior stitches) and prevents back-bleeding from any smaller branches (medial stitch), such as the transverse pancreatic artery, that head to the patient's left toward the body of the pancreas. One must be careful to avoid

incorporating the common bile duct into the stitch. The course of the common bile duct can be identified by inserting a probe through the ampulla of Vater transduodenally or performing an intraoperative cholangiogram. Hemostasis should be confirmed before duodenal closure. The duodenotomy is closed transversely to avoid narrowing. Surgery for a bleeding gastric ulcer typically includes partial gastrectomy with either Billroth I or II reconstruction. If the patient is hemodynamically stable, a careful preoperative history should be taken to assess if the patient may benefit from concurrent truncal vagotomy, though this should not be performed in unstable patients. If the gastric ulcer is not resected and the bleeding is controlled with suture ligature, biopsy at the time of surgery is necessary to exclude malignancy.

Perforation. Patients with perforation from PUD typically report sudden-onset, severe epigastric pain. They frequently have free air visible on the chest radiograph and have localized peritoneal signs on examination. Patients with more widespread spillage will have diffuse peritonitis. Perforation is a less frequent complication of PUD, occurring at about one-sixth the incidence of bleeding. However, perforation has the highest mortality rate of any complication of ulcer disease, reported as high as 30%.[20]

Perforation necessitates emergent surgical consultation. Initial empiric antibiotic therapy should cover enteric gram-negative rods, anaerobes, and mouth flora and should be based on local susceptibility patterns when available. Upright x-ray can be obtained to assess for free air, but CT scan with oral and IV contrast has higher sensitivity for diagnosis. Patients with localized symptoms, in stable clinical condition, and with a water-soluble contrast study confirming a sealed leak can be considered for nonoperative management. An early description of nonoperative management of perforated PUD was made by Herman Taylor in the 1940s. At that time nonoperative treatment consisted of NG decompression, IV fluid resuscitation, and serial abdominal x-rays. Currently, nonoperative management (often referred to as *Taylor's method*) should consist of close hemodynamic monitoring, serial abdominal examinations, nil per os with NG tube, broad-spectrum IV antibiotics, and IV PPI. This can be effective in well-selected patients. For example, in a retrospective series of 64 patients managed nonoperatively with small-volume perforated peptic ulcers, 89% of patients successfully avoided intervention and only 4 required surgical drainage of the abscess.[26] Small series of patients treated endoscopically have been published but at this time is not standardly used.

At surgery, the perforation usually can easily be accessed through an upper midline incision. Perforations smaller than 2 cm can generally be closed primarily and buttressed with the omentum or falciform ligament. For larger perforations or ulcers with fibrotic edges that cannot be brought together without tension, a Graham patch repair with healthy omentum is performed. Multiple stay sutures are placed that incorporate healthy tissue on the proximal and the distal sides of the ulcer. The omentum is placed underneath these sutures, and they are tied to secure it in place and seal the perforation (Fig. 86.10). A modification of the Graham patch repair involves closing the perforation first with sutures, placing the omentum over the now closed perforation, and securing the omentum by tying knots a second time with the same suture. A meta-analysis of eight randomized trials including 615 patients compared laparoscopic omental patch repair with open repair. This showed that laparoscopic surgery was associated with less postoperative pain and fewer wound infections with equivalent leak rates and mortality.[27] In stable patients with small

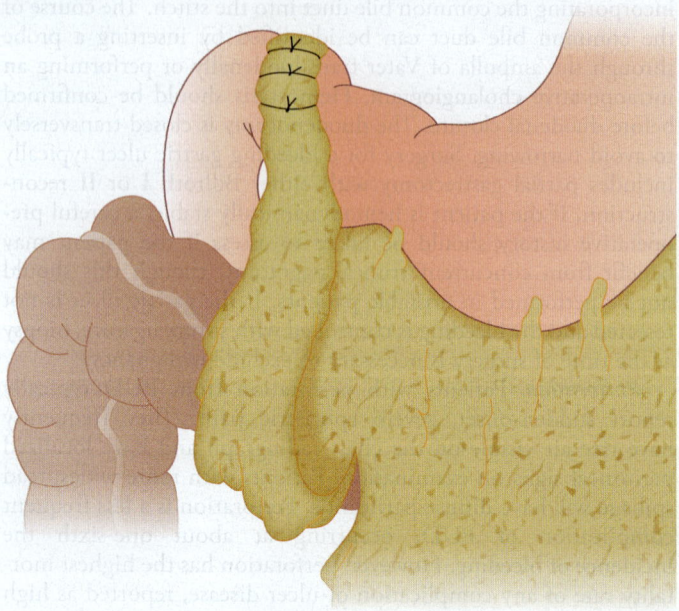

FIGURE 86.10 Graham patch repair of a perforated duodenal ulcer. A "tongue" of omentum is brought up to cover the ulcer defect and secured in position with a series of interrupted sutures. In Graham's original description, the ulcer defect is not closed, but if the tissue edges are healthy and come together without undue tension, a primary closure can be performed and reinforced with an omental patch. (From Baker RJ. Perforated duodenal ulcer. In: Baker RJ, Fischer JE, eds. *Mastery of Surgery.* London: Little, Brown, and Company; 2001:969.)

perforations, laparoscopic repair is thus preferred if the surgeon has adequate technical experience to perform this safely.

For very large perforations (>2 cm), control of a duodenal defect can be difficult and there is no standardized approach. The defect should be closed by the application of healthy tissue, such as omentum or jejunal serosa from a Roux-en-Y–type limb. In such cases, a pyloric exclusion is typically performed by oversewing the pylorus using absorbable suture or stapling across the pylorus using a noncutting linear stapler. A gastrojejunostomy is created to bypass the duodenum in a Billroth II or Roux-en-Y fashion. Over several weeks, the pyloric exclusion stitches or staples give way, restoring normal GI anatomy after the perforation site has been given time to heal. Alternatively, a duodenostomy tube can be placed through the perforation with wide peritoneal drainage. An alternative in this difficult situation is antrectomy and a Billroth II or Roux-en-Y reconstruction to include the duodenal ulcer if the duodenal stump has healthy tissue and there is sufficient distance from the ampulla of Vater. Feeding jejunostomy placement should be considered at time of operation for enteral nutrition access.

Perforated gastric ulcers are managed based on their location. Given their association with malignancy, resection is generally preferred when possible. Partial gastrectomy with reconstruction is performed if the patient is stable without significant comorbidities. Either wedge resection or patch closure can also be performed depending on the clinical situation; biopsies should be obtained in cases of patch closure to rule out malignancy.

For patients who are known to be negative for *H. pylori,* who are taking long-term NSAIDs that they cannot discontinue, or who have failed medical therapy in the past for their ulcer disease,

an acid-reducing procedure can be added at the time of repair if the patient is stable. These procedures are discussed elsewhere in this chapter and must be based on the clinical situation and comfort of the surgeon. All *H. pylori*–positive patients should undergo eradication postoperatively with appropriate triple or quadruple therapy regimens.

Gastric outlet obstruction. Acute and chronic inflammation of the duodenum or pylorus can lead to mechanical gastric outlet obstruction. Chronic inflammation leads to recurrent episodes of injury and healing. This ultimately leads to fibrosis, scarring, and stenosis of the outflow tract. The stomach can become massively dilated and lose its muscular tone. Patients will present with early satiety, anorexia, weight loss, nausea, and vomiting. In cases of prolonged vomiting, patients often become dehydrated and can develop a hypochloremic, hypokalemic metabolic alkalosis.

Initial management should involve gastric decompression with NG tube placement and correction of fluid and electrolyte abnormalities. Nutritional status should be assessed. Gastric outlet obstruction from PUD is not a surgical emergency, and full diagnostic workup before any surgical intervention is necessary, especially as gastric cancer is now a more common cause of this disorder. Upper endoscopy should be performed to rule out a malignancy and test for *H. pylori* infection.

Endoscopic dilation and *H. pylori* eradication are the mainstays of initial therapy for PUD gastric outlet obstruction. Other endoscopic techniques, including self-expanding metal stents, ultrasound-guided gastric bypass, and POEM, have also been reported; decisions between these endoscopic interventions and surgery should be done in a multidisciplinary fashion. Surgery entails primary antrectomy with resection of the obstructing portion and vagotomy. Another surgical option, especially when there is significant duodenal inflammation or scarring present, is vagotomy with a drainage procedure, typically either a Jaboulay gastroduodenostomy or a gastrojejunostomy.

Refractory peptic ulcer disease. Refractory PUD is defined as failure of an ulcer to heal after an initial trial of 8 to 12 weeks of PPI therapy or if patients relapse after therapy has been discontinued; it is estimated to occur in 5% to 10% of patients. Benign gastric ulcers that persist must be evaluated for malignancy. Additionally, other less common sources of ulceration such as ZES, Crohn disease, or sarcoidosis should be considered. For any refractory ulcer, adequate duration of antisecretory therapy, *H. pylori* eradication, and elimination of NSAID use must be confirmed. A fasting serum gastrin level should be obtained to rule out gastrinoma. Although rarely seen today, truly intractable ulcer disease that fails medical management should be treated with a vagotomy, with or without an antrectomy.

Surgical procedures for peptic ulcer disease. Elective operative intervention for PUD has become rare as medical therapy has improved. The recognition of *H. pylori* and its eradication suggest that the refractory indication for surgery may apply only to patients in whom the organism cannot be eradicated, who cannot be taken off NSAIDs, who cannot tolerate their medical regimen, or who have a rarer cause of PUD. Patients who are noncompliant with acid suppression therapy may also fall into this category, but this is more controversial.

The goal of operative ulcer therapy is to resect or promote ulcer healing and to reduce gastric acid secretion. Surgical gastric acid reduction can be accomplished by removing vagal stimulation via vagotomy, gastrin-driven secretion by performing an antrectomy, decreasing the number of parietal cells with a subtotal gastrectomy, or a combination procedure. Vagotomy decreases peak acid output by approximately 50% to 70%, whereas vagotomy plus antrectomy decreases peak acid output by approximately 85%. These surgeries can be performed either open or minimally invasively. Pathologic confirmation of resected vagal trunks should be performed.

Truncal vagotomy. Truncal vagotomy is performed by dividing the left and right vagus nerves above the hepatic and celiac branches, just above the GE junction (see Fig. 86.3). The vagal nerves should be clipped or ligated proximally and distally with at least 2 cm resected. Pyloric relaxation is mediated by vagal stimulation, and a vagotomy without a drainage procedure can cause delayed gastric emptying. Truncal vagotomy in combination with a Heineke-Mikulicz pyloroplasty is shown in Fig. 86.11. When the duodenal bulb is scarred, a Finney pyloroplasty or Jaboulay gastroduodenostomy may be a useful alternative. Significant scarring or inflammation may necessitate a gastrojejunostomy. In general, there is little difference in the side effects associated with the type of drainage procedure performed, although bile reflux may be more common after gastroenterostomy, and diarrhea is more common after pyloroplasty. The incidence of dumping syndrome is similar for both.

Selective vagotomy. Selective vagotomy divides the main right and left vagus nerves just distal to the celiac and hepatic branches (see Fig. 86.3). A pyloric drainage procedure is also performed. However, selective vagotomy results in higher ulcer recurrence rates than truncal vagotomy, with no advantage in terms of decreased postgastrectomy symptoms. For these reasons, selective vagotomy has largely been abandoned.

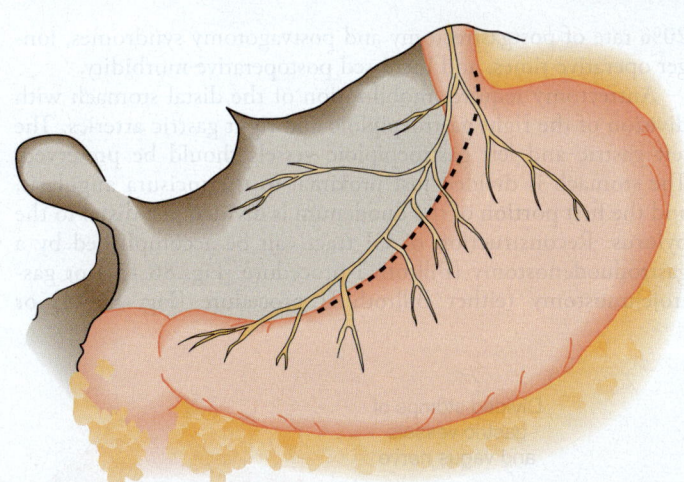

FIGURE 86.12 Anterior view of the stomach and anterior nerve of Latarjet. Note the line of dissection for parietal cell or highly selective vagotomy *(dashed line)*. The last major branches of the nerve are left intact, and the dissection begins 7 cm from the pylorus. At the gastroesophageal junction, the dissection is well away from the origin of the hepatic branches of the left vagus. (From Kelly KA, Teotia SS. Proximal gastric vagotomy. In: Baker RJ, Fischer JE, eds. *Mastery of Surgery.* Philadelphia: Lippincott Williams & Wilkins; 2001:943.)

Highly selective vagotomy. Highly selective vagotomy is also referred to as a *parietal cell vagotomy.* A highly selective vagotomy divides only the vagus nerve branches supplying the acid-producing portion of the stomach within the corpus and fundus. This procedure preserves the vagal innervation of the gastric antrum and pylorus, so there is no need for routine drainage procedures. In general, the nerves of Latarjet are identified anteriorly and posteriorly, and the crow's feet innervating the fundus and body of the stomach are divided. These nerves are divided up until approximately 7 cm proximal to the pylorus, the area in the vicinity of the gastric antrum. Superiorly, division of these nerves is carried to a point at least 5 cm proximal to the GE junction on the esophagus (Fig. 86.12). The criminal nerve of Grassi represents a very proximal branch of the posterior vagus trunk; great attention is needed to avoid missing this branch in the division process because it is frequently cited as a reason for ulcer recurrence if left intact.

The ulcer recurrence rates after highly selective vagotomy are variable and depend on the skill of the surgeon. Lengthy longitudinal follow-up is necessary to evaluate the results of this procedure. Recurrence rates of 10% to 15% have been reported for this procedure when performed by a skilled surgeon. These rates are slightly higher than the rates reported after truncal vagotomy in combination with pyloroplasty; however, highly selective vagotomy has lower rates of postvagotomy dumping syndrome and diarrhea. This operation is less frequently performed today given the decreasing need for elective PUD surgery.

Truncal vagotomy and antrectomy. Antrectomy is generally not performed for duodenal ulcers and is more commonly performed for gastric ulcers. Relative contraindications include cirrhosis, extensive scarring of the proximal duodenum that leaves a difficult or tenuous duodenal closure, and previous operations on the proximal duodenum. When done in combination with truncal vagotomy, it is more effective at reducing acid secretion and recurrence than truncal vagotomy in combination with a drainage procedure or highly selective vagotomy. The recurrence rate for ulceration after truncal vagotomy and antrectomy is 0% to 2%. However, this low recurrence rate needs to be balanced against the

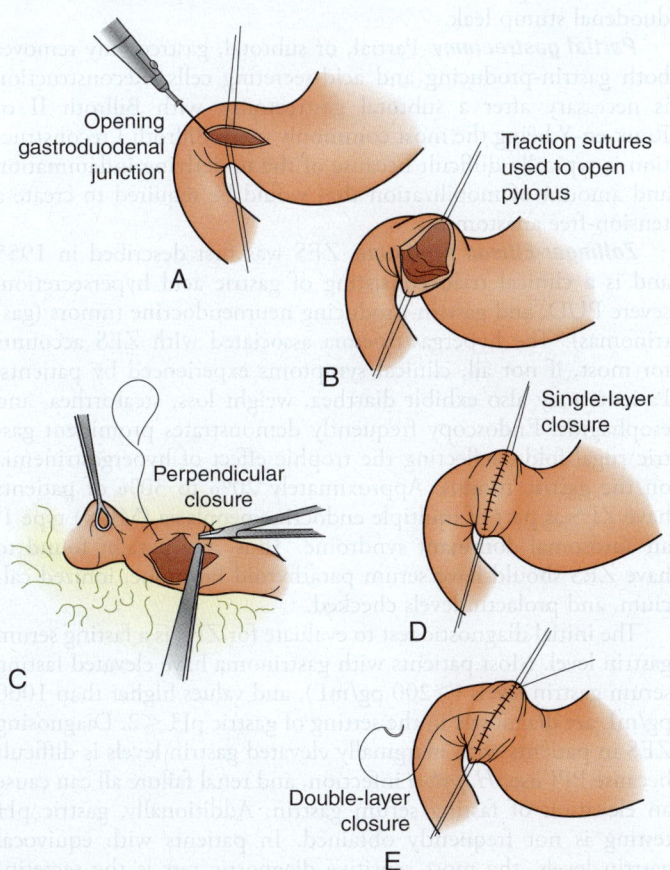

Opening gastroduodenal junction

Traction sutures used to open pylorus

Perpendicular closure

Single-layer closure

Double-layer closure

FIGURE 86.11 (A–E) Heineke-Mikulicz pyloroplasty. (From Soreide JA, Soreide A. Pyloroplasty. *Oper Tech Gen Surg.* 2003;5:65-72.)

20% rate of postgastrectomy and postvagotomy syndromes, longer operative times, and increased postoperative morbidity.

Antrectomy requires mobilization of the distal stomach with division of the right gastroepiploic and right gastric arteries. The left gastric and left gastroepiploic vessels should be preserved. The stomach is divided just proximal to the incisura angularis, and the first portion of the duodenum is divided just distal to the pylorus. Reconstruction of GI tract can be accomplished by a gastroduodenostomy (Billroth I procedure [Fig. 86.13]) or gastrojejunostomy (either Billroth II procedure [Fig. 86.14] or

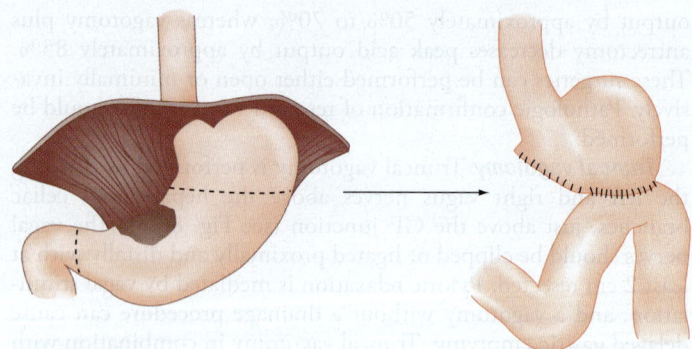

FIGURE 86.14 Subtotal gastrectomy with a Billroth II anastomosis.

Roux-en-Y reconstruction). For benign disease, gastroduodenostomy is generally favored because it avoids the risks of retained antrum syndrome, duodenal stump leak, and afferent loop obstruction associated with gastrojejunostomy after resection. Retained antrum syndrome is a result of incomplete antrectomy; residual G cells are no longer exposed to gastric acid, leading to hypergastrinemia with resultant stimulation of acid production and marginal ulceration at the gastrojejunostomy. If the duodenum is significantly scarred, gastroduodenostomy may not be technically feasible, necessitating a gastrojejunostomy. The gastric anastomosis is typically placed in a dependent portion of the stomach to facilitate drainage, often along the posterior wall of the greater curvature. A retrocolic anastomosis minimizes the length of the afferent limb and decreases the likelihood of twisting or kinking that could lead to afferent loop obstruction and duodenal stump leak.

Partial gastrectomy. Partial, or subtotal, gastrectomy removes both gastrin-producing and acid-secreting cells. Reconstruction is necessary after a subtotal gastrectomy, with Billroth II or Roux-en-Y being the most commonly used. Billroth I reconstruction is typically difficult because of the underlying inflammation and amount of mobilization that would be required to create a tension-free anastomosis.

Zollinger-Ellison syndrome. ZES was first described in 1955 and is a clinical triad consisting of gastric acid hypersecretion, severe PUD, and gastrin-producing neuroendocrine tumors (gastrinomas). The hypergastrinemia associated with ZES accounts for most, if not all, clinical symptoms experienced by patients. Patients may also exhibit diarrhea, weight loss, steatorrhea, and esophagitis. Endoscopy frequently demonstrates prominent gastric rugal folds, reflecting the trophic effect of hypergastrinemia on the gastric fundus. Approximately 20% to 30% of patients have ZES as part of multiple endocrine neoplasia (MEN) type 1, an autosomal dominant syndrome. Thus, any patient found to have ZES should have serum parathyroid hormone, ionized calcium, and prolactin levels checked.

The initial diagnostic test to evaluate for ZES is a fasting serum gastrin level. Most patients with gastrinoma have elevated fasting serum gastrin levels (>200 pg/mL), and values higher than 1000 pg/mL are diagnostic in the setting of gastric pH <2. Diagnosing ZES in patients with marginally elevated gastrin levels is difficult because PPI use, *H. pylori* infection, and renal failure all can cause an elevation of fasting serum gastrin. Additionally, gastric pH testing is not frequently obtained. In patients with equivocal gastrin levels, the most sensitive diagnostic test is the secretin-stimulated gastrin level. Serum gastrin samples are measured before and after IV secretin administration. An increase in the serum

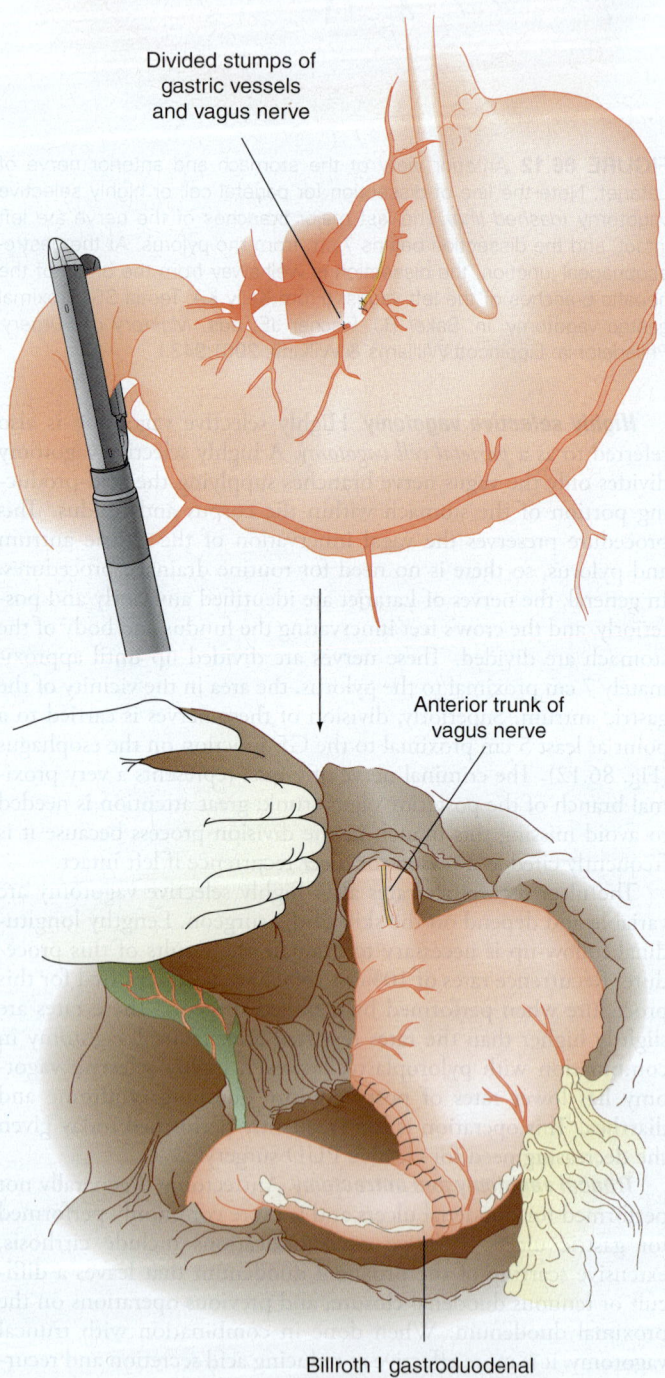

Divided stumps of
gastric vessels
and vagus nerve

Anterior trunk of
vagus nerve

Billroth I gastroduodenal
anastomosis completed

FIGURE 86.13 Hemigastrectomy with a Billroth I (gastroduodenal) anastomosis. (From Dempsey D, Pathak A. Antrectomy. *Oper Tech Gen Surg.* 2003;5:86-100.)

gastrin level of greater than 200 pg/mL above basal levels is suggestive of gastrinoma versus other causes of hypergastrinemia, which normally do not demonstrate this response. Other supportive tests include ^{68}Ga-DOTATATE PET/CT, known or suspected MEN1 syndrome, and a positive biopsy for neuroendocrine tumor.[28]

Acid suppression therapy is initiated after diagnosis of gastrinoma, preferably with a high-dose PPI. Medical management is indicated preoperatively and for patients with metastatic or unresectable gastrinoma. The next step in management is localization and staging of the tumor. Most ZES gastrinomas are located in the duodenum or pancreas, within the "gastrinoma triangle." The points of this triangle are made up of the cystic–common bile duct junction, the pancreas body-neck junction, and the junction between the second and third portions of the duodenum. The initial imaging study to localize the gastrin-secreting tumor is either triple-phase CT or MRI of the abdomen. Somatostatin receptor imaging, most often ^{68}Ga-DOTATATE PET/CT, is increasingly being used to aid in diagnosis and localization of neuroendocrine tumors, including gastrinomas. If cross-sectional imaging is nondiagnostic, endoscopic ultrasound (EUS) can be performed. If one is still unable to localize the tumor, patients can be offered a surgical exploration.

Localized gastrinomas should be resected whenever possible. The exception is gastrinomas less than 2 cm in patients with MEN1. Once the tumor is located intraoperatively, a resection according to oncologic principles should be performed (rather than a tumor enucleation) with at least 10 lymph nodes removed. Patients with advanced or metastatic disease can be treated with a variety of treatments, and there is no standardized algorithm at this time. Surgical re-resection can be considered in cases of recurrent disease. Systemic therapies include somatostatin analogs, everolimus, and cytotoxic chemotherapy. Peptide receptor radionuclide therapy (PRRT) delivers radiolabeled somatostatin analogs systemically. PRRT has been shown to have significantly improved progression-free survival and a nonsignificant trend toward improved overall survival in patients with advanced neuroendocrine tumors compared with octreotide alone, though this was not specifically studying patients with gastrinoma.[29] For patients with liver-only metastases, liver-directed therapies (radiofrequency ablation, cryoablation, transarterial embolization, resection/debulking, or liver transplantation) can be considered in a multidisciplinary setting.

STRESS GASTRITIS

Stress ulceration is defined as an upper GI tract ulcer occurring because of hospitalization and most commonly occurs in the stomach. Stress gastritis can occur after physical trauma, shock, sepsis, hemorrhage, or respiratory failure and may lead to life-threatening gastric bleeding. Stress gastritis is characterized by multiple superficial (nonulcerating) erosions that typically begin in the proximal portion of the stomach and progress distally. They may also occur in the setting of a central nervous system disease elevating intracranial pressure with resultant vagal nerve stimulation (Cushing ulcer) or as a result of thermal burn injury involving more than 20% to 30% of the body surface area leading to gastric ischemia (Curling ulcer).

Stress gastritis lesions can change over time. Early lesions are typically multiple and shallow, with discrete areas of erythema along with focal hemorrhage or adherent clot. These early lesions can develop within the first hours of major trauma or illness. If the lesion erodes into the submucosa, significant bleeding may result. They are almost always seen in the fundus or body of the stomach and only rarely in the distal stomach. Late lesions appear identical to regenerating mucosa around a healing gastric ulcer. Both early and late lesions can be seen endoscopically.

Pathophysiology

Although the precise mechanisms responsible for the development of stress gastritis remain to be fully elucidated, evidence suggests a multifactorial cause related to an imbalance between acid production and mucosal protection. Examples of impaired mucosal defense mechanisms against luminal acid are reduction in blood flow, mucus, or bicarbonate secretion by mucosal cells or decreased endogenous prostaglandins. All these factors render the stomach more susceptible to damage from luminal acid, with the resultant hemorrhagic gastritis. Stress is considered present when hypoxia, sepsis, or organ failure occurs. When stress is present, mucosal ischemia is thought to be the main factor responsible for the breakdown of these normal defense mechanisms. Although increased gastric acid secretion rarely occurs in this situation, the presence of luminal acid appears to be a prerequisite for this form of gastritis to evolve.

A seminal Canadian multicenter cohort study of patients admitted to the intensive care unit (ICU) sought to identify risk factors for clinically important stress ulceration, defined as overt bleeding associated with hemodynamic compromise or need for blood transfusion.[30] Of 2252 patients, only 30% received stress ulcer prophylaxis and 1.5% developed clinically important bleeding. Two risk factors were significant on multivariable regression: mechanical ventilation for over 48 hours (odds ratio 15.6) and coagulopathy (odds ratio 4.3). Coagulopathy was defined as platelet count less than 50,000, international normalization ratio (INR) greater than 1.5, or partial thromboplastin time (PTT) greater than two times normal. Other reported risk factors for stress gastritis include liver or kidney failure, shock, sepsis, trauma, severe burn, use of antiplatelets or NSAIDs, and prior history of GI bleeding. Initiation of enteral nutrition, along with its other beneficial effects in critically ill patients, has been shown to decrease the risk of stress ulceration.[31]

Presentation and Diagnosis

Stress gastritis develops within 1 to 2 days after a traumatic event or critical illness in more than 75% of patients historically,[30] though the majority of patients have minimal or no related symptoms. The only clinical sign may be painless upper GI bleeding or anemia. The bleeding is usually slow and intermittent. Overt bleeding is defined as hematemesis, frank blood in NG aspirate, or melena. Clinically significant or clinically important bleeding is defined as overt bleeding with the addition of either hypotension, transfusion requirement, or need for therapeutic intervention. The rate of clinically significant bleeding in critically ill patients from stress ulceration has been reported from 1% to 3%. Although upper endoscopy is required to definitively confirm the diagnosis and differentiate stress gastritis from other sources of GI hemorrhage, it is often unnecessary in patients with asymptomatic or minimally symptomatic manifestations.

Prophylaxis

Development of hemodynamically significant stress gastritis substantially increases mortality in critically ill patients. The decision whether or not to give stress ulcer prophylaxis in high-risk patients is being actively studied. Historically, stress ulcer prophylaxis was routinely given in the ICU, but more recent guidelines suggest only administering prophylaxis to those at high risk of developing stress ulceration. However, the precise definition of what features constitute high risk is also debated.

A European multicenter trial randomized 3298 patients admitted to the ICU to either receive 40 mg IV pantoprazole or placebo during their ICU stay. The primary outcome was 90-day mortality, which was statistically similar between the two groups (31.1% in the PPI group and 30.4% in the placebo group). Pantoprazole did have a lower rate of clinically important GI bleeding at 2.5% compared with 4.2%, but no p-values were reported on secondary outcomes to avoid adjustment for multiple comparisons. Infectious complications were also similar.[32] A multicenter trial that included 50 ICUs across five countries randomized 26,982 patients who required mechanical ventilation within 24 hours of ICU admission to either PPI or H_2 receptor antagonist stress ulcer prophylaxis. The primary outcome was 90-day mortality, which was similar at 18% in the PPI group and 17% in the H_2 receptor antagonist group. There was a slightly lower rate of clinically important upper GI bleeding in favor of the PPI group (1.3 vs. 1.8%, $p = 0.009$). However, this is difficult to interpret given that over 20% of the patients randomly assigned H_2 receptor antagonist therapy received a PPI.[33]

There have been multiple systematic reviews and meta-analyses assessing the efficacy of stress ulcer prophylaxis. One recent network meta-analysis included 72 randomized trials with 12,660 patients.[34] For patients at highest risk (>8%) or high risk (4%–8%) of bleeding, both PPIs and H_2 receptor antagonists reduced clinically important GI bleeding compared with placebo or no prophylaxis with odds ratios of 0.61 and 0.46, respectively. However, neither had an effect on mortality compared with placebo. Earlier data suggested that stress ulcer prophylaxis correlated with increased frequency of *Clostridioides difficile* and nosocomial pneumonia infections; however, more recent trials and meta-analyses are conflicting.

Patients at high risk for stress gastritis should be treated prophylactically to minimize their incidence of clinically significant bleeding, though the exact definition of what constitutes high risk is still debated and no clear guidelines exist. Because mucosal ischemia may alter many mucosal defense mechanisms that enable the stomach to withstand luminal irritants and protect itself from injury, every effort should be made to correct any perfusion deficits secondary to shock. If prophylaxis is deemed indicated, a PPI or H_2 antagonist should be used, with most institutions favoring PPI.

Treatment

Improvements in critical care resuscitation, prophylaxis for high-risk patients, and nonoperative interventions with endoscopy or angiography have significantly decreased the need for surgical intervention for gastric stress ulceration. Any patient with upper GI bleeding requires resuscitation with correction of any coagulation or platelet abnormalities, adequate IV access, blood availability, and close hemodynamic monitoring. Where available, thromboelastography (TEG) or rotational thromboelastometry (ROTEM) can be useful diagnostic adjuncts. An NG tube should be placed if not already present and IV PPI therapy started promptly. NG lavage can help remove blood and clots from the stomach, and NG decompression will decrease gastrin production. Sepsis is a common cause of stress gastritis, and if there is clinical concern, broad-spectrum antibiotics should be promptly initiated.

Upper endoscopy is typically the first-line intervention for upper GI bleeding and should be performed for both diagnosis and treatment. Treatment can include coagulation therapy, hemostatic clipping, or injection therapy depending on the clinical scenario and endoscopist expertise. Bleeding associated with stress gastritis is typically diffuse without a single discrete bleeding source; thus, rebleeding rates are high. In hemodynamically stable patients at centers with available resources, angiography is another diagnostic and therapeutic option. If a single arterial source of bleeding is identified, embolization can be performed. Catheter-directed vasopressin into the left gastric artery can temporize diffuse bleeding from stress gastritis. The usual dose is up to 0.4 pressor units/minute. The infusion is either continued in the ICU or embolization is performed given the risk of rebleeding after vasopressin discontinuation. Catheter-directed vasopressin can cause peripheral vasoconstriction and bradyarrhythmia and should be avoided in patients with a history of heart disease.

Surgical intervention for stress gastritis is required in patients with hemodynamic instability from hemorrhage, persistent bleeding not amenable to nonsurgical interventions, or in rare instances of gastric perforation from stress ulceration. The surgical intervention is individualized based on the patient's clinical status. Temporary abdominal closure followed by a second-look laparotomy can be used because many patients are coagulopathic. Because most lesions are in the proximal stomach or fundus, a long anterior gastrotomy should be made in this area. The gastric lumen is cleared of blood, and the mucosal surface is inspected for bleeding points. All bleeding areas are oversewn with figure-of-eight stitches taken deep within the gastric wall. Most superficial erosions are not actively bleeding and do not require ligation unless a blood vessel is seen at its base. In hemodynamically stable patients, the operation is completed by closing the anterior gastrotomy in two layers and performing a truncal vagotomy and pyloroplasty to reduce acid secretion. Less commonly, a partial gastrectomy is performed if persistent bleeding occurs from only a portion of the stomach. Before the advent of PPIs and nonsurgical therapies, total gastrectomy and gastric devascularization were described; however, these should rarely be performed in the present day and only considered in patients with life-threatening hemorrhage refractory to other forms of therapy. Gastric devascularization involves ligating the left and right gastric and the left and right gastroepiploic arteries. Because of collateral circulation, this does not always lead to full-thickness necrosis in patients who have not had prior foregut surgery. Patients with a perforation from stress ulceration should be managed with either closure or resection of the perforated region depending on intraoperative assessment and consideration of truncal vagotomy and pyloroplasty based on the patient's clinical stability.

POSTGASTRECTOMY SYNDROMES

Gastric surgery can result in numerous physiologic derangements caused by loss of reservoir function, interruption of the pyloric sphincter mechanism, and vagal nerve transection. The GI and cardiovascular symptoms may result in disorders collectively referred to as *postgastrectomy syndromes*. The physiologic changes are not specific to the underlying disease for which the surgery was indicated, occurring after gastrectomy for PUD, oncologic resection, or obesity surgery. Approximately 1% to 5% of patients become permanently disabled from their postgastrectomy symptoms.

Dumping Syndrome

Dumping syndrome is a constellation of symptoms caused by rapid postprandial gastric emptying that can be divided into two categories: early and late. This symptom complex can develop after any operation on the stomach but is most common after partial gastrectomy with the Billroth II reconstruction. It is less commonly observed after Billroth I or Roux-en-Y reconstruction or after vagotomy and drainage procedures. International consensus definition of early dumping syndrome is symptoms occurring within 1 hour of a meal, though most effects are seen within 30 minutes.[35] GI symptoms include abdominal pain, early satiety, nausea/vomiting, diarrhea, and bloating. Vasomotor systemic symptoms include diaphoresis, tachycardia, palpitations, headache, and syncope. Early dumping syndrome is a result of rapid passage of high-osmolarity food from the stomach into the small intestine. The hypertonic food bolus induces a rapid shift of extracellular fluid into the intestinal lumen to achieve isotonicity, leading to luminal distention. Several hormones are also stimulated for release, including neurotensin, VIP, glucagon-like peptide-1 (GLP-1), insulin, and glucagon.

Late dumping syndrome occurs 1 to 3 hours after a meal and is less common than early dumping syndrome.[35] The basic defect of late dumping is also rapid gastric emptying; however, its symptoms are related specifically to carbohydrates being delivered rapidly into the proximal intestine. An exaggerated GLP-1 response is the key mediator in late dumping syndrome. When carbohydrates are delivered to the small intestine, they are quickly absorbed, resulting in hyperglycemia. This triggers the release of large amounts of insulin to control the increasing blood sugar level, but overcompensation of this normal physiologic mechanism results in hypoglycemia. This hypoglycemia activates the adrenal glands to release catecholamines, which results in diaphoresis, tremulousness, lightheadedness, tachycardia, and confusion.

The diagnosis of dumping syndrome is primarily a clinical one. When indicated, a modified oral glucose tolerance test can support the diagnosis. Patients ingest 75 g of a glucose solution after an overnight fast. This test is considered positive for early dumping syndrome if after 30 minutes there is an increase of the hematocrit by at least 3% or increase in heart rate of at least 10 beats/minute. The test is positive for late dumping syndrome if blood glucose is less than 50 mg/dL between 1 and 3 hours after ingestion. Gastric emptying tests have low sensitivity and specificity for dumping syndrome diagnosis and are not typically used.

Dietary measures are usually sufficient to treat most patients. These include avoiding foods containing large amounts of sugar, frequent feeding of small meals rich in protein and fiber, and separating liquids from solids during a meal. In some patients without a response to dietary measures, pharmacologic treatments directed at specific symptoms can be effective, such as tincture of opium or Imodium for diarrhea and meclizine for nausea. Small studies have shown that acarbose can reduce the incidence of hypoglycemia when taken with meals. Somatostatin analogs, such as octreotide, are the most studied pharmacologic treatment for dumping syndrome. These peptides not only inhibit gastric emptying but also slow small bowel transit and inhibit release of GI hormones and insulin. Somatostatin analogs are the preferred treatment option for patients with established dumping syndrome who fail to respond to dietary modification (with or without acarbose treatment).[35]

Patients with severe symptoms may require a reoperation if conservative dietary and medical management is unsuccessful.

The choice of operation depends on the original gastric surgery. Pyloric reconstruction can sometimes be performed. For patients with a gastrojejunostomy without a gastrectomy, takedown of the gastrojejunostomy can be performed if the pylorus function is maintained. In patients with a prior Billroth II distal gastrectomy, converting the loop gastrojejunostomy to a Roux-en-Y reconstruction is recommended.

Metabolic Disturbances

Anemia is commonly seen in patients who have undergone a gastrectomy. Postgastrectomy anemia is related to iron or vitamin B_{12} deficiency. Iron is normally absorbed in the duodenum and proximal jejunum, so iron deficiency is more often seen after Billroth II and Roux-en-Y reconstruction than Billroth I. In general, the addition of iron supplements to the patient's diet corrects this problem. Vitamin B_{12} deficiency occurs secondary to poor absorption of dietary vitamin B_{12} because of the lack of intrinsic factor. Patients undergoing subtotal gastrectomy should be placed on lifelong vitamin B_{12} supplementation.

Osteoporosis has also been observed after gastric resection and is caused by deficiencies in calcium. If fat malabsorption is also present, the calcium malabsorption is aggravated further because fatty acids bind calcium. Bone disease generally develops approximately 5 years after surgery. Treatment of this disorder usually requires calcium supplements in conjunction with vitamin D. Patients with Billroth II or Roux-en-Y reconstruction that bypasses the duodenum should also receive supplementation of fat-soluble vitamins (vitamins A, D, E, and K).

Afferent Loop Syndrome

The afferent loop is the duodenojejunal loop proximal to the gastrojejunal anastomosis. Afferent loop syndrome is caused by mechanical obstruction of the afferent limb and often related to a long afferent limb. Pancreatic and hepatobiliary secretions accumulate within the limb, resulting in distention, epigastric discomfort, and cramping. The intraluminal pressure eventually increases enough to empty the contents of the afferent loop forcefully into the stomach, resulting in projectile bilious vomiting that offers immediate relief of symptoms. If the obstruction has been present for a long time, patients can develop blind loop syndrome. In this situation, bacterial overgrowth occurs in the static loop, and the bacteria bind with vitamin B_{12} and deconjugated bile acids; this results in a systemic deficiency of vitamin B_{12} (with the development of megaloblastic anemia), fat malabsorption, and deficiency in fat-soluble vitamins. Diagnosis of afferent loop syndrome is typically made with CT imaging showing a dilated afferent limb. Failure to visualize the afferent limb on upper endoscopy and failure of normal radionucleotide passage into the distal small bowel on hepatobiliary iminodiacetic acid (HIDA) scan are also suggestive of the diagnosis.

In the immediate postoperative setting, prompt correction is indicated to prevent bowel necrosis or duodenal stump blowout. A long afferent limb is usually the underlying problem, so treatment involves the elimination of this loop. Remedies include conversion of the Billroth II construction into a Billroth I anastomosis, enteroenterostomy between the afferent and efferent loops, and conversion to a Roux-en-Y reconstruction. Endoscopic enteroenterostomy or stenting are emerging options in centers with available expertise and in patients without concern for bowel ischemia.[36] Percutaneous enterostomy to drain the afferent limb has been described in patients with significant comorbidities in palliative settings.

Efferent Loop Obstruction

Obstruction of the efferent limb is rare. Efferent loop obstruction may occur at any time; however, the majority occur within the first postoperative month. Initial complaints may include left upper quadrant abdominal pain that is colicky in nature, bilious vomiting, and abdominal distention. The diagnosis is usually established by an upper GI series or CT with oral contrast, with failure of contrast to enter the efferent limb. Efferent obstructions can be caused by adhesions, strictures, jejunogastric intussusception, or retroanastomotic herniation. Operative intervention is almost always necessary and consists of reducing and closing the retroanastomotic hernia if this is the cause of the obstruction, anastomotic revision, or conversion to a Roux-en-Y reconstruction.

Alkaline Reflux Gastritis

After gastrectomy, reflux of bile is common. In a small percentage of patients, this reflux is associated with severe epigastric abdominal pain accompanied by bilious vomiting and weight loss. The diagnosis is typically made by careful history and exclusion of other causes. A technetium biliary scan can demonstrate reflux of bile into the stomach. Upper endoscopy demonstrates friable, beefy red mucosa.

Most patients with alkaline reflux gastritis have had gastric resection performed with a Billroth II anastomosis. Although bile reflux appears to be the inciting event, the exact pathogenesis is unclear. Most medical therapies that have been tried to treat alkaline reflux gastritis have not shown any consistent benefit. For patients with intractable symptoms, surgery is indicated. Revision options include Roux-en-Y reconstruction (with a Roux limb of 45–60 cm), Henley isoperistaltic jejunal interposition, or Braun enteroenterostomy.

Gastric Atony

Gastric emptying is delayed after truncal and selective vagotomies but not after a highly selective vagotomy. With selective or truncal vagotomy, patients lose their antral pump function and have a reduction in the ability to empty solids. In contrast, emptying of liquids is accelerated because of the loss of receptive relaxation in the proximal stomach. Although most patients undergoing vagotomy and a drainage procedure manage to empty their stomach adequately, some patients have persistent gastric stasis that results in retention of food within the stomach for several hours.

The diagnosis of gastric atony is confirmed by scintigraphic assessment of gastric emptying. However, other causes of delayed gastric emptying should be excluded. In addition, a mechanical cause of gastric outlet obstruction, such as postoperative adhesions, afferent or efferent loop obstruction, and internal herniation, must be ruled out. In patients with a functional gastric outlet obstruction and documented gastroparesis, pharmacotherapy is generally used. The agents most commonly used are prokinetic agents such as metoclopramide and erythromycin. In rare cases of persistent gastric atony refractory to medical management, subtotal or total gastrectomy may be required.

Roux Stasis Syndrome

Disordered motility of the Roux limb can result in stasis. Symptoms include vomiting, epigastric pain, and weight loss. Differentiation from gastric atony can be done with imaging showing a dilated Roux limb. Medical treatment is similar to gastric atony with either metoclopramide or erythromycin. In patients with Roux stasis syndrome and a large residual gastric remnant, surgical revision to create a smaller gastric remnant may be beneficial.

Postvagotomy Diarrhea

Episodic, significant diarrhea can result after vagotomy procedures. The mechanism is not fully understood but is thought to be partially related to rapid transit of unconjugated bile salts to the colon. It is most frequently seen after truncal vagotomy. Increased fiber intake and oral cholestyramine (a bile acid sequestrant) or an antidiarrheal agent are typically effective. Historically, surgery with a short antiperistaltic jejunal loop interposition was described, but this is not typically used today.

OTHER GASTRIC LESIONS

Atrophic Gastritis

Atrophic gastritis is a result of chronic inflammation leading to replacement of normal gastric glandular mucosa with connective tissue or intestinal-type cells. The two most common causes are *H. pylori* and autoimmune disease. Autoimmune gastritis can lead to pernicious anemia caused by vitamin B_{12} deficiency. On endoscopy, patients will have a pale mucosa. The updated Sydney protocol with biopsies from five specified sites in the stomach has high diagnostic accuracy for both atrophic gastritis and *H. pylori*. If *H. pylori* is diagnosed, it should be treated appropriately. Patients are recommended to undergo surveillance endoscopies after diagnosis of atrophic gastritis, as they are at increased risk of developing type 1 gastric neuroendocrine tumors and intestinal-type gastric adenocarcinoma, though the exact interval is not well defined.[37] Small gastric neuroendocrine tumors less than 1 cm can be managed with either endoscopic resection or active surveillance. Larger lesions should undergo EUS. Patients should undergo surgery if there is evidence of invasion beyond the submucosa, poor differentiation on biopsy, size greater than 2 cm, or positive margin after endoscopic resection.

Hypertrophic Gastritis (Ménétrier Disease)

Ménétrier disease is a rare disorder characterized by protein-losing gastropathy and massive gastric folds in the fundus and body of the stomach, giving the mucosa a cobblestone or cerebriform appearance. The antrum is typically spared in adults. Histologic examination reveals foveolar hyperplasia (expansion of surface mucus cells), with decreased or absent parietal cells. The condition is also associated with protein loss from the stomach, excessive mucus production, and decreased acid secretion. The pathogenesis of Ménétrier disease is poorly understood. It has been associated with CMV infection in children and *H. pylori* infection in adults. Increased levels of transforming growth factor-α have been noted in the gastric mucosa of patients with the disease, which can stimulate epithelial cell growth and inhibit gastric acid secretion. Patients often present with epigastric pain, vomiting, weight loss, decreased appetite, and peripheral edema caused by hypoalbuminemia. Typical gastric mucosal changes can be detected by radiographic or endoscopic examination. Biopsy should be performed to establish the diagnosis and to rule out malignant etiologies such as gastric adenocarcinoma or lymphoma. Patients with Ménétrier disease are at increased risk of gastric cancer, though the exact risk is not well known given the rarity of the disease. Medical treatment yields inconsistent results; however, some benefit has been shown with the use of acid suppression, octreotide, and CMV or *H. pylori* eradication. A small phase I trial of cetuximab (epidermal growth factor [EGF] receptor monoclonal antibody) showed clinical improvement in seven out of nine patients, with four achieving histologic remission.[38] Total gastrectomy should be considered in patients who continue to have massive protein loss despite optimal medical therapy and a high-protein diet or if they develop malignant changes.

Mallory-Weiss Tear

Mallory-Weiss tears are mucosal lacerations related to forceful vomiting, retching, coughing, or straining. These lacerations can cause acute upper GI bleeding from submucosal blood vessels. The most common risk factor is alcohol use. Patients present with hematemesis. Massive bleeding is more likely in patients with preexisting portal hypertension. Initial management is similar to other patients with acute upper GI bleed, with assessment of hemodynamic stability, PPI initiation, and antiemetics for nausea. Upper endoscopy is both diagnostic of Mallory-Weiss tears and therapeutic. Most patients with active bleeding can be treated with endoscopic methods, such as epinephrine injection, thermal coagulation, endoscopic band ligation, or endoscopic hemoclipping. Angiographic transarterial embolization may be useful in patients who have persistent or recurrent bleeding after endoscopy. Operative intervention is rarely needed. If surgery is required, an anterior gastrotomy is performed and the bleeding site is oversewn with several deep suture ligatures to reapproximate the gastric mucosa in an anatomic fashion.

Cameron Lesion

Cameron lesions are ulcers occurring as a result of a hiatal hernia and are seen as linear ulcers or erosions at the diaphragmatic impression. These are often discovered incidentally and rarely cause acute upper GI bleeding. They have been associated with chronic iron deficiency anemia. Acute bleeding is treated with standard endoscopic measures. Chronic iron deficiency anemia can initially be managed with PPI and iron repletion along with diagnostic workup to exclude other potential causes. Patients with persistent anemia with lack of another source and patients with symptoms of dysphagia should be evaluated for surgical hiatal hernia repair.

Dieulafoy Gastric Lesion

Bleeding from a gastric Dieulafoy lesion is caused by an abnormally large (1–3 mm), tortuous artery coursing through the submucosa without a primary ulcer. Erosion of the superficial mucosa overlying the artery occurs secondary to the pulsations of the large submucosal vessel. The artery is then exposed to the gastric contents, and further erosion and bleeding occur. The lesions generally occur near the GE junction along the lesser curvature. Dieulafoy lesions are more common in males, with associated comorbidities including cardiovascular disease, chronic kidney disease, and diabetes. The classic presentation of a patient with a Dieulafoy lesion is sudden onset of massive, painless hematemesis.

Detection and identification of the Dieulafoy lesion can be difficult. The diagnostic modality of choice is upper endoscopy, but because of the intermittent nature of the bleeding, repeat endoscopies may be needed in the absence of active bleeding. If the lesion can be identified endoscopically and is actively bleeding, endoscopic modalities such as bipolar electrocoagulation, heater probe thermocoagulation, injection sclerotherapy, or endoscopic hemoclipping can be applied. Angiography can be useful in cases in which endoscopy is unable to definitely identify the source of bleeding. Angiographic findings may include a tortuous ectatic artery in the distribution of the left gastric artery. Angiography can also show IV contrast extravasation in the setting of active bleeding. Embolization has been reported to control bleeding successfully in patients with Dieulafoy lesions. Surgery is rarely required and only indicated if patient fails less invasive interventions. Surgical management consists of gastric wedge resection to include the offending vessel, which can be facilitated by asking the endoscopist to tattoo the stomach when the lesion is identified or with intraoperative endoscopic localization.

Gastric Antral Vascular Ectasia

Gastric antral vascular ectasia (also referred to as GAVE or watermelon stomach) is an uncommon cause of acute upper GI bleeding, more often resulting in chronic iron deficiency anemia. The name watermelon stomach is derived from its endoscopic appearance of red stripes of ectatic mucosal vessels from the pylorus to the antrum. GAVE most commonly occurs in older females and is associated with cirrhosis and sclerosis. However, portal decompression has not been shown to decrease bleeding in GAVE. Endoscopic therapy is the preferred treatment modality for symptomatic patients. Antrectomy can be curative for patients who require intervention and fail more conservative measures.

Gastric Varices

Gastric varices are dilated submucosal veins commonly seen in patients with portal hypertension and cirrhosis, serving as a vascular shunt between the portal and systemic circulation. The prevalence of gastric varices is between 17% and 25% in patients with portal hypertension, and they are associated with more severe bleeding and higher mortality compared with the more common esophageal varices.[39] The Sarin classification characterizes two types: isolated gastric varices and GE varices.[40] Isolated gastric varices are further subclassified into type 1 varices, located in the fundus of the stomach, and type 2, isolated ectopic varices located anywhere in the stomach. GE varices are divided into type 1 along the lesser curvature of the stomach and type 2 along the greater curvature. Although GE varices are more common overall, isolated gastric varices are more prone to bleeding.

Gastric varices can develop secondary to portal hypertension, in conjunction with esophageal varices, or secondary to sinistral hypertension from splenic vein thrombosis. In generalized portal hypertension, the increased portal pressure is transmitted by the left gastric (coronary) vein to esophageal varices and by the short and posterior gastric veins to the fundic plexus and cardia veins. Isolated gastric varices tend to occur secondary to splenic vein thrombosis, which is most commonly the result of pancreatitis. Splenic blood flows retrograde through the short and posterior gastric veins into the varices and then through the coronary vein into the portal vein. Left-to-right retrograde flow through the gastroepiploic vein to the superior mesenteric vein can explain the development of ectopic varices in the stomach.

The incidence of bleeding from gastric varices has been reported to be between 3% and 30%. However, the incidence of bleeding can be much higher in patients with splenic vein thrombosis and fundic varices. Cardiofundal location, larger size of the varices, presence of discolored marks, and decompensated cirrhosis increase the risk for bleeding.[39]

Bleeding isolated gastric varices in the setting of splenic vein thrombosis are readily treated by splenectomy. Patients with bleeding gastric varices should have an imaging study to document splenic vein thrombosis before a splenectomy is performed because gastric varices are more often associated with generalized portal hypertension.

Acutely bleeding gastric varices in the setting of portal hypertension should be managed similarly to esophageal varices. The patient should have adequate vascular access and be volume-resuscitated, with attention paid to the correction of abnormal coagulation profiles. Temporary tamponade can be attempted with a Sengstaken-Blakemore tube, though this should be followed promptly by more definitive therapy to prevent mucosal erosion. Octreotide, a somatostatin analog, can be administered with bolus followed by continuous infusion. Prophylactic ceftriaxone should be administered if the patient is not allergic. When possible, CT with portal venous phase best defines the underlying vascular anatomy in patients with portal hypertension.

Management of gastric variceal bleeding should be done in a multidisciplinary setting. Endoscopy serves as the primary diagnostic and therapeutic tool and should be done urgently for actively bleeding varices; preprocedure erythromycin can be used to improve visualization. Endoscopic options to initially treat gastric variceal bleeding include sclerotherapy, band ligation, glue, or thrombin injection. A major problem with gastric varices after endoscopic treatment is rebleeding. The American Gastroenterological Association 2021 guidelines[39] for management of bleeding gastric varices recommend endoscopic cyanoacrylate injection in cases where definitive endoscopic therapy is favored; the guidelines also note that for lesser curvature gastric varices, band ligation can be definitive therapy. EUS can be used to improve the accuracy of cyanoacrylate injection, and this can be done with or without concomitant coil injection. When a gastrorenal shunt is present between the gastric varices and left renal vein, balloon-occluded retrograde transvenous obliteration can be performed with a sclerosant if local expertise is available. The major complication of this procedure is aggravation of esophageal varices secondary to an increase in portal pressure as a consequence of occluding the gastrorenal shunt. Repeat endoscopy should be performed within 48 hours to confirm obliteration of the gastric varices and evaluate for esophageal varix exacerbation. Transjugular intrahepatic portosystemic shunting (TIPS) can be effective in controlling gastric variceal hemorrhage that does not respond to endoscopic treatments or for patients with decompensated cirrhosis at high risk of failing endoscopic management. TIPS is more effective for lesser curvature gastric varices than cardiofundal greater curvature varices. Complications from TIPS include hepatic encephalopathy, liver failure, and heart failure.

Gastric Volvulus

Gastric volvulus is an uncommon condition. Torsion occurs along the stomach's long longitudinal axis (organoaxial) in approximately two-thirds of cases and along the short vertical axis (mesenteroaxial) in one-third of cases (Fig. 86.15). Rarely, a more complex form can occur with elements of both rotations. Rotation more than 180 degrees causes gastric outlet obstruction and can lead to ischemia, necrosis, and potentially perforation if left uncorrected. Primary gastric volvulus is caused by abnormalities of the gastric ligaments (i.e., gastrocolic, gastrohepatic). Secondary gastric volvulus is the result of other anatomic abnormalities, the most common being a paraesophageal hernia. In children, congenital defects such as the foramen of Bochdalek or diaphragmatic eventration are involved.

The sudden-onset severe upper abdominal pain, recurrent retching with limited vomiting, and the inability to pass an NG tube constitute the Borchardt triad for acute gastric volvulus. Plain films of the abdomen can reveal a spherical gas-filled viscus in the chest or upper abdomen with an air-fluid level. CT imaging will show a dilated stomach, a swirl sign of the esophagus and stomach, and possibly radiographic features of gastric necrosis such as pneumatosis or free air. CT also has the benefit of showing associated anatomic abnormalities (such as paraesophageal hernia)

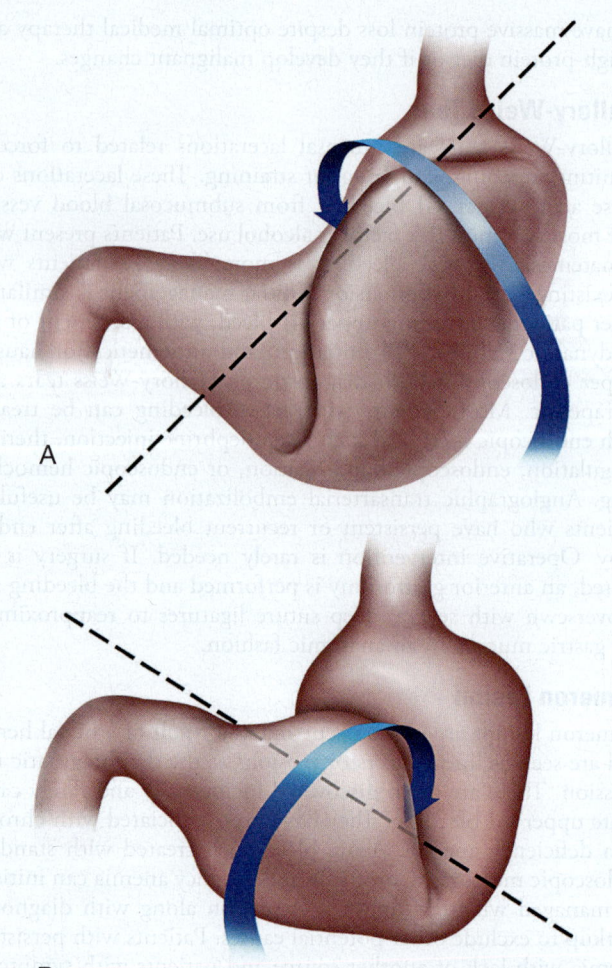

FIGURE 86.15 Torsion of the stomach along the longitudinal axis (organoaxial) (A) and along the short vertical axis (mesenteroaxial) (B). (From White RR, Jacobs DO. Volvulus of the stomach and small bowel. In: Yeo CJ, Dempsey DT, Klein AS, et al., eds. *Shackelford's Surgery of the Alimentary Tract.* 6th ed. Philadelphia: Saunders; 2007:1035-1040.)

and excluding other more common causes of abdominal pain or lower chest pain. Chronic volvulus symptoms are intermittent and less severe. Imaging should be obtained during symptomatic episodes.

Acute volvulus necessitates urgent treatment. IV fluids should be started and electrolyte abnormalities corrected. NG decompression should be performed immediately, which sometimes can detorse the stomach spontaneously. If bedside NG placement is unsuccessful, endoscopic decompression can be performed with care to limit insufflation. The distal stomach should be suctioned, the mucosa should be evaluated for ischemia, and an NG tube should be placed. Immediate surgical intervention is recommended for patients who fail NG or endoscopic decompression, have gastric perforation, or have severe sepsis or refractory hypotension. Patients that stabilize with decompression can delay definitive treatment until after appropriate preoperative workup.

If the patient is unstable, an urgent open operation is recommended. The stomach should be detorsed and then assessed for viability. Areas that remain ischemic should be resected. In the uncommon situation where the entire stomach is necrotic, a total gastrectomy can be performed with jejunostomy tube placement and esophagostomy with an elective reconstruction in the future. For stable patients with acceptable surgical risk, an open or laparoscopic approach can be undertaken. Primary gastric volvulus can be managed with suture gastropexy of the stomach to the anterior abdominal wall and is often combined with gastrostomy tube placement, though no technique is standardized. Secondary gastric volvulus should undergo repair of the anatomic defect rather than gastropexy alone when possible; typically, this involves repair of a paraoesophageal hernia. The diaphragmatic defect is repaired after the stomach hernia sac is reduced and the distal esophagus is mobilized; this is typically combined with a fundoplication. Patients with high surgical risk can instead undergo endoscopic detorsion with percutaneous endoscopic gastrostomy (PEG) tube placement to fixate the stomach. Two PEG tubes are used to prevent rotation. PEG tube placement can also be used as a temporizing measure in a hemodynamically unstable patient before definitive surgical repair.

Gastric Bezoars

A gastric bezoar is a collection of nondigestible materials found as a hard mass in the stomach. They are defined by their composition. The most common type of bezoar is composed of vegetable material, termed a *phytobezoar*. A subtype of phytobezoar, diospyrobezoars, are associated with ingestion of persimmon fruits, which contain a tannin that polymerizes in the acidic stomach environment. Bezoars can also contain hair (trichobezoar), medications (pharmacobezoars), or other substances.

Bezoars are most commonly found in patients who have underlying gastric dysmotility issues, such as prior gastric surgery, gastroparesis, or gastric outlet obstruction. Trichobezoars are often associated with psychiatric disorders. Impaired grinding mechanism of the stomach and migrating motor complexes have been implicated as pathogenic causes of bezoars, though some patients may have normal stomach function. Patients are often asymptomatic or have gradual symptom onset over years. The symptoms of gastric bezoars include early satiety, pain, nausea/vomiting, and weight loss. Gastric outlet obstruction from a bezoar is rare. Physical examination is usually unremarkable, although sometimes a large mass may be palpable. Abdominal radiographs or CT scans can show a bezoar as a mass or filling defect within the stomach; diagnosis is confirmed by upper endoscopy.

Initial management of symptomatic bezoars is attempted with chemical dissolution. This was first attempted in the 1950s using Adolph's Meat Tenderizer, which contains papain. There is currently a wide array of options, including soda (Coca-Cola being the most studied), cellulose, papain, and acetylcysteine; no randomized trials exist to suggest superiority of one dissolving agent compared with others. Of note, trichobezoars are typically resistant to chemical dissolution. Pharmacobezoars may require decontamination to prevent toxicity depending on the medication involved in the bezoar. If chemical dissolution is ineffective or contraindicated, endoscopic fragmentation with a water jet, forceps, or direct suction can be performed. The resulting fragments can either be removed via the endoscope, with an Ewald tube, or allowed to pass through the GI tract. Adjuvant prokinetics such as metoclopramide can be used in conjunction with either chemical dissolution or endoscopic therapy. Surgical removal is typically reserved for patients who fail more conservative management, present with a complication (i.e., gastric perforation or excessive bleeding), or if other therapies are contraindicated based on the bezoar's composition. Surgical removal of bezoars is typically done via an anterior gastrotomy. The stomach and small intestine should be fully evaluated for other bezoars at time of surgery.

SELECTED REFERENCES

Cook DJ, Fuller HD, Guyatt GH, et al. Risk factors for gastrointestinal bleeding in critically ill patients. Canadian Critical Care Trials Group. *N Engl J Med.* 1994;330(6):377-381.

This prospective multicenter cohort study of 2252 patients admitted to the ICU reported a 1.5% rate of clinically important bleeding. Two strong independent risk factors were identified: respiratory failure (odds ratio 15.6) and coagulopathy (odds ratio 4.3).

Laine L, Barkun AN, Saltzman JR, et al. ACG clinical guideline: upper gastrointestinal and ulcer bleeding. *Am J Gastroenterol.* 2021;116(5):899-917.

This 2021 American College of Gastroenterology Guideline was published for upper GI and ulcer bleeding. Systematic review and recommendations are given for which patients should undergo endoscopy, timing of endoscopy, endoscopic therapy, PPI therapy, and management of recurrent bleeding.

Malfertheiner P, Camargo MC, El-Omar E, et al. Helicobacter pylori infection. *Nat Rev Dis Primers.* 2023;9(19):1-24.

This article gives an excellent and comprehensive review of the current understanding of Helicobacter pylori infection. Specifically, the authors address current knowledge of the epidemiology, pathophysiology, cancer risk, diagnosis, and treatment of H. pylori infection.

Metz DC, Cadiot G, Poitras P, et al. Diagnosis of Zollinger-Ellison syndrome in the era of PPIs, faulty gastrin assays, sensitive imaging and limited access to acid secretory testing. *Int J Endocr Oncol.* 2017;4(4):167-185.

This paper first summarizes current guidelines for Zollinger-Ellison syndrome diagnosis. It then highlights current issues with the standard diagnosis in assay reliability as well as ancillary testing availability and also addresses newer more commonly used modalities in clinical practice such as DOTATATE scans. A new proposed diagnostic algorithm is made based on their review.

Scally B, Emberson JR, Spata E, et al. Effects of gastroprotectant drugs for the prevention and treatment of peptic ulcer disease and its complications: a meta-analysis of randomised trials. *Lancet Gastroenterol Hepatol.* 2018;3(4):231-241.

This study examined the effects of three classes of gastroprotectants (PPIs, H$_2$ receptor antagonists, and prostaglandin analogs) for prevention and treatment of peptic ulcer disease by doing meta-analyses from randomized trials that either compared a gastroprotectant with a control or another medication. Larger proportional reductions in upper GI bleeding were seen with PPIs, and PPIs were the most effective in ulcer healing. In trials of patients with acute bleeding, PPIs had a larger protective effect than H$_2$ blockers for further bleeding and blood transfusion, but there was no significant difference in mortality.

The full reference list appears on Elsevier eBooks+.

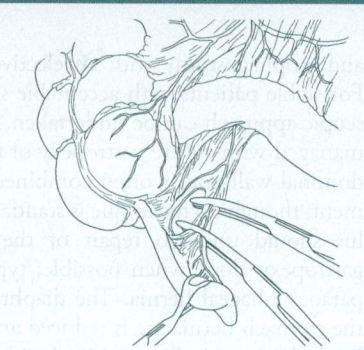

Gastric Cancer

Sam Yoon, Joshua Leinwand, and Vivian E. Strong

OUTLINE

Gastric Adenocarcinoma
    Epidemiology
    Pathology
    Diagnosis and Workup
    Staging
    Treatment
    Outcomes
Gastrointestinal Stromal Tumor
    Epidemiology and Mutational Patterns
    Diagnosis and Workup
    Treatment

Gastric Lymphoma
    Epidemiology
    Pathology
    Evaluation and Staging
    Treatment
Gastric Neuroendocrine Tumors
Heterotopic Pancreas
Hypertrophic Gastritis (Menetrier Disease)

GASTRIC ADENOCARCINOMA

Epidemiology

Incidence

Gastric cancer is one of the most common malignancies worldwide, with over 1 million cases per year and over 780,000 deaths per year.[1] The prevalence of gastric cancer is highest in Asia and Eastern Europe, with much lower rates in North America and Northern Europe. In the United States, there are an estimated 26,500 gastric cancer cases per year and 11,000 deaths per year. Within the United States, about 60% of gastric cancer cases and deaths occur in males; it is more common and has higher mortality in Blacks, Asian Americans, and Hispanics compared with Whites. Mortality rates also vary significantly throughout the world, with 5-year disease-specific survival over 80% in a Japanese national database compared with <50% in the United States; these differences are not fully explained by baseline differences in patient demographics and disease stage but may be related to differences in molecular subtypes of gastric cancer that predominate in different geographic regions.[2]

In addition, the prevalence of *Helicobacter pylori* infection (discussed later) explains much of the geographic variation in the global burden of gastric cancer. *H. pylori* infection can occur in infancy or childhood and causes chronic inflammation in the stomach that over years leads to cancer. The *H. pylori* seroprevalence rate varies markedly by country, ranging from 19% in Sweden to 88% in Nigeria; over half the world's population is infected.[3] Within the United States, the seroprevalence rate in Blacks and Hispanics is approximately 1.3 to 5.4 times higher than in Whites. It is thought that standards of living that provide better access to refrigeration and preservation of food and improved sanitation in industrialized countries have contributed to decreased *H. pylori* prevalence over time. Indeed, in the United States, gastric cancer was the leading cause of

cancer deaths in the early 20th century but dropped sharply after 1930 with the establishment of the FDA and government-imposed standards on food preparation, sanitization, and preservation.[4]

In contrast to distal (noncardia) gastric cancers, which are principally associated with chronic *H. pylori* infection, cancers of the gastric cardia share similar risk factors with Barrett esophagus and esophageal adenocarcinoma, specifically obesity and gastroesophageal reflux disease. As such, the incidence of cardia gastric cancers has remained stable or increased in Western countries.[5] Alarmingly, like other GI cancers, young-onset noncardia gastric cancers in patients age 25 to 40 years have increased significantly since the 1970s; the risk factors that have led to this remain uncertain.[6]

Risk Factors

The major risk factors for gastric cancer are discussed here, including both environmental and genetic factors (Box 87.1).

H. pylori, Epstein-Barr virus, and the microbiome. Globally, chronic *H. pylori* infection is by far the most important risk factor for gastric cancer. *H. pylori* is associated with approximately 75% of all gastric cancer cases worldwide and is classified by the World Health Organization (WHO) International Agency for Research on Cancer (IARC) as a group 1 (definite) carcinogen.[7] As such, stomach cancer is the most common infection-related cancer. *H. pylori* seropositivity confers an approximately sixfold increased risk of developing gastric cancer; even after *H. pylori* eradication, an increased risk of gastric cancer persists.

H. pylori infection is associated with a variety of gastric phenotypes; the vast majority of *H. pylori*–infected individuals do not go on to develop gastric cancer. The most common phenotype is mild pangastritis with largely normal gastric acid secretion. Next most common is the duodenal ulcer phenotype, characterized by antral gastritis with high gastrin and high acid secretion. In contrast, gastric cancer is typically associated with a gastric body–predominant gastritis with multifocal gastric atrophy and decreased gastric acid secretion. These changes are induced by chronic inflammation caused by *H. pylori* infection and increase the risk of gastric cancer. The progression of chronic *H. pylori* infection to invasive cancer is believed to develop sequentially from nonatrophic gastritis, to atrophic gastritis, then to intestinal metaplasia, dysplasia, and adenocarcinoma. *H. pylori*–associated stomach cancer is almost always seen in the context of intestinal metaplasia.

The best-characterized *H. pylori* virulence factors are cytotoxin-associated gene A (*cag*A) and vacuolating cytotoxin A (*vac*A), which co-opt the host inflammatory response to promote oncogenesis; this is illustrated by the finding that high-risk *H. pylori* genotypes act synergistically with proinflammatory interleukin-1 gene cluster variants in patients to increase the risk of gastric cancer up to 87-fold.[8] Epidemiologically, *cag*A-positive isolates comprise a higher percentage of *H. pylori* strains in East Asian countries than in Western countries, and *cag*A gene variants originating in East Asia induce gastric cancer more efficiently compared with those from the West.[9]

Latent Epstein-Barr virus (EBV) infection is also associated with the development of gastric cancers. In these tumors, the integrated viral genome, and consequently transcribed viral messenger RNA (mRNA) and translated viral proteins, can be detected. EBV alters host gene expression within infected cells both by EBV-encoded microRNAs and by inducing hypermethylation of host DNA. EBV-associated tumors comprise a unique molecular subtype of gastric cancer, as discussed later.

Microbes other than *H. pylori* and EBV may also contribute to gastric cancer. Various studies have shown differences between the gastric microbiome in patients with gastric cancer compared with controls or in resident microbes obtained from gastric cancer tissue versus benign gastric tissue from the same patient. In particular, microbes that contribute to the production of nitrite and *N*-nitroso compounds (which are known to contribute to gastric carcinogenesis; see "Dietary Factors") may be more prevalent in the stomachs of patients with gastric cancer.[10] *H. pylori* may perturb the gastric microbiome by increasing gastric pH via urease production, allowing overgrowth of nitrite- and *N*-nitroso–producing bacteria. A similar pH-dependent mechanism may underly epidemiologic findings linking long-term proton pump inhibitor (PPI) use with increased risk of gastric cancer.[11] Based on the potential for adverse effects from long-term PPI use, deprescribing PPIs is recommended for patients without an ongoing indication for PPI use. Patients with persistent dyspepsia on PPI therapy warrant surveillance for and eradication of *H. pylori*.

Dietary factors. *N*-nitroso compounds, either derived directly from dietary sources or by endogenous production from nitrates and nitrites, are the major dietary contributors to gastric carcinogenesis. Smoked, cured, and preserved meats and other foods are the primary dietary sources of these compounds. Consistent with epidemiologic data linking smoking with an increased risk of gastric cancer, *N*-nitroso species are also present in cigarette smoke. Salted and pickled food intake is also associated with gastric cancer, possibly because of mucosal injury to the stomach. Fresh fruits and vegetables are dietary sources of ascorbic acid, an antioxidant that inhibits the conversion of nitrites to *N*-nitroso compounds. Accordingly, low intake of fresh fruits and vegetables is associated with increased risk of developing gastric cancer.

The interactions between the gastric microbiome and dietary factors are complex, but there is evidence for synergistic effects of *H. pylori* infection with smoking or high salt intake to promote gastric carcinogenesis. Alongside improvements in sanitation that have reduced *H. pylori* infection, the widespread introduction of refrigeration, by reducing reliance on other meat preservation methods and allowing for increased consumption of fresh fruits and vegetables, has likely contributed to decreased gastric cancer incidence in industrialized countries. In 2015, the WHO IARC classified processed meats as a group 1 carcinogen.

Hereditary risk factors. Hereditary diffuse gastric cancer (HDGC), classically resulting from a germline mutation in the gene encoding the cell adhesion and signaling molecule E-cadherin, *CDH1*, is associated with an increased risk of developing diffuse gastric cancer. The original estimates of lifetime risk of developing HDGC in individuals with germline *CDH1* mutation were 55% to 70% or greater.[12,13] However, this estimate of lifetime risk was subject to ascertainment bias, as most identified cases were derived from kindreds with high burden of HDGC among multiple family members. As additional kindreds with weaker phenotypic expression (lower penetrance) have been reported among individuals undergoing germline *CDH1* testing for conditions other than diffuse gastric cancer, the risk estimates for HDGC in the setting of germline *CDH1* mutation have declined. Currently, the lifetime risk of HDGC in individuals with germline *CDH1* mutation is estimated at 37% to 42% for males and 25% to 33% for females.[14,15] The risk of developing gastric cancer may vary in each family depending on how many gastric cancer cases have been found. Roberts *et al.* estimated the risk in families with three or more gastric cancer cases as 64% in males and 47% for females.[14] This risk decreased to 27% for males and 24% for females in families with two or fewer gastric cancer cases. Females with germline *CDH1* mutation also carry a 39% to 55% risk of developing lobular breast cancer.

Prophylactic total gastrectomy should be considered for medically fit individuals with germline *CDH1* mutation who are deemed to have a significant risk of gastric cancer, typically between the ages of 20 and 30 years. In the vast majority of cases, microscopic foci of early gastric cancer will be seen in the gastrectomy specimen. In patients who refuse or wish to delay gastrectomy, annual endoscopy with Cambridge protocol biopsies (targeted biopsies of all identified lesions plus at least 6 random biopsies from each of 5 different anatomic regions) or Bethesda protocol biopsies (targeted biopsies of all identified lesions plus at least 4 random biopsies from each of 22 different sites) are recommended. The targeted biopsies of suspected clinical cancers may be the most important aspect of surveillance endoscopies. Many, if not most, microscopic foci of early gastric cancer in *CDH1* individuals will never go on to become a clinically significant cancer. Because 90% or more of those with germline *CDH1* mutation will have one or more microscopic foci of early gastric cancer on prophylactic total gastrectomy,[16] the clinical significance of such foci on random biopsy is unclear. For patients with HDGC with uncertain risk of gastric cancer, such as those with *CDH1* variants of unknown significance and the more recently described pathogenic *CTNNA1* variants, annual surveillance with endoscopy and Cambridge or Bethesda protocol biopsies is also recommended.

Patients with HDGC are also at higher risk for lobular breast cancer, and annual surveillance with breast MRI is thus recommended beginning at age 30.[17] Lobular breast cancer often does not form a discrete mass or form microcalcifications, so the utility of mammogram is lower than that for infiltrating ductal carcinoma.[18] Bilateral risk-reducing mastectomies can also be considered.

Other germline genetic conditions associated with gastric cancer are listed in Table 87.1. Among these, in familial adenomatous polyposis (FAP), most patients will have fundic or body sessile polyps, with 40% of these polyps having some degree of dysplasia. These polyps, combined with the much higher frequency of potentially malignant duodenal polyps, warrant upper GI surveillance. Gastric adenocarcinoma and proximal polyposis of the stomach (GAPPS) is characterized by fundic gland polyposis of the gastric fundus and body, classically with >100 polyps carpeting the proximal stomach, which can progress to dysplasia and invasive cancer. Because of its rarity, there are no comprehensive guidelines for patients with GAPPS, but gastroscopy should be performed annually starting at age 15, and risk-reducing total gastrectomy should be considered starting in the third decade of life. Lynch syndrome predisposes to microsatellite-unstable malignancies, including stomach cancer. As discussed later, these are more amenable to treatment with immunotherapy than conventional cytotoxic

chemotherapy. Upper GI screening with esophagogastroduodenoscopy (EGD) starting in the teenage years is recommended for patients with juvenile polyposis and Peutz-Jeghers syndromes.

Gastric polyps. Gastric polyps are identified in approximately 6% of gastroscopies in the United States and are usually asymptomatic. These comprise a variety of pathologic entities, including adenomas, fundic gland polyps, and hyperplastic polyps. All gastric polyps detected at endoscopy should be biopsied to determine malignancy risk and guide further management. Solitary polyps >1 cm in size should undergo complete polypectomy. In cases of multiple polyps, the largest should be removed endoscopically, if possible, and remaining polyps should be biopsied. In addition, normal antral and body mucosa should be biopsied to rule out atrophic gastritis and to diagnose *H. pylori*.

Adenomatous polyps often occur in the background of chronic or atrophic gastritis but also can occur in patients without preexisting gastritis and are most commonly found in the antrum. They can progress to atypia, dysplasia, and invasive carcinoma, with higher risk of invasive carcinoma correlating with increased size, villous contour, and degree of dysplasia. Complete endoscopic removal of gastric adenomas should be performed. In addition to the local risk of progression to invasive cancer, the risk of synchronous or metachronous gastric cancer is elevated in patients with an adenomatous polyp; as such, thorough endoscopic evaluation and endoscopic follow-up are mandatory after resection of gastric adenomas.

Hyperplastic polyps most commonly occur in the setting of chronic atrophic gastritis, resulting from chronic inflammatory conditions, including *H. pylori* infections and pernicious anemia. These can progress to carcinoma in a stepwise process via dysplasia. Foci of dysplasia are found in approximately 1% to 20% of hyperplastic polyps. The risk of malignancy is higher in pedunculated polyps and those >1 cm in size.

Fundic gland polyps are benign lesions that can occur sporadically, but are also associated with long-term PPI use and can be seen in adenomatous polyposis coli (APC), GAPPS, and *MUTYH*-associated polyposis syndromes, as discussed earlier. They occur in one-third of patients by 1 year of PPI treatment, and resolution of fundic gland polyps after cessation of PPIs has been described. Dysplasia is most common in patients with fundic gland polyps resulting from hereditary cancer syndromes and occurs only rarely in patients whose polyps result from PPI therapy. PPI-associated fundic gland polyps do not require excision, regular surveillance, or cessation of therapy. The finding of numerous fundic gland polyps or fundic gland polyps harboring

TABLE 87.1 Hereditary Cancer Syndromes Associated With Stomach Cancer

GENETIC LOCI	SYNDROME	GASTRIC CANCER RISK	OTHER CANCER RISKS
CDH1	Hereditary diffuse gastric cancer (HDGC)	Up to 70%	Lobular breast
CTNNA1	HDGC	Up to 57%	Lobular breast
STK11	Peutz-Jeghers syndrome	29%	Breast, GI, pancreas, ovarian, lung, GYN
SMAD4, BMPR1A	Juvenile polyposis	21%	Colon, pancreas, small bowel
MLH1, MSH2, MSH6, PMS2	Lynch syndrome	1%–13%	Colon, ovarian, uterine, urinary tract, other
APC	Familial adenomatous polyposis	1%–2%	Colon, duodenum, thyroid
APC promoter 1B	Gastric adenocarcinoma and proximal polyposis of the stomach (GAPPS)	12%–25%	Unknown, possibly colon
MUTYH	*MUTYH*-associated polyposis	2%	Colon, duodenal, ovarian, bladder, skin

Adapted from Slavin TP, Weitzel JN, Neuhausen SL, Schrader KA, Oliveira C, Karam R. Genetics of gastric cancer: what do we know about the genetic risks? *Transl Gastroenterol Hepatol.* 2019;4:55.

dysplasia in a patient under age 40 should prompt workup for cancer-polyposis syndromes, including colonoscopy.

Other risk factors. Patients with pernicious anemia are at increased risk for developing gastric cancer. Achlorhydria is the defining feature of this condition; it occurs when chief and parietal cells are destroyed by an autoimmune reaction. Obesity was determined by the IARC to be a risk factor for gastric cardia cancers.[19] Smoking is associated with an approximately 1.5-fold increase in gastric cancer risk. Prior abdominal irradiation, most commonly after testicular cancer or Hodgkin lymphoma, increases gastric cancer risk.

Pathology

Gross and Histologic Classification

Borrman classification. Numerous pathologic classification schemes of gastric cancer have been proposed. The Borrmann classification system was developed in 1926 based on the gross appearance of advanced tumors. This system divides gastric adenocarcinoma into four types: type I for polypoid, type II for fungating, type III for ulcerating, and type IV for diffusely infiltrating growths (also referred to as *linitis plastica in signet ring cell carcinoma*). This classifier may be useful for the description of endoscopic findings, but its prognostic significance is limited.

Lauren classification. In 1965, Lauren proposed classifying gastric adenocarcinoma based on histology into intestinal or diffuse types; subsequently, others have included mixed-type tumors in this scheme. The intestinal variant is more well differentiated and typically arises in the setting of a recognizable precancerous condition, such as gastric atrophy or intestinal metaplasia. Males are more commonly affected than females, and the incidence of intestinal-type gastric adenocarcinoma increases with age. These cancers tend to form glands. The intestinal type is also the dominant histology in areas in which gastric cancer is epidemic, suggesting an environmental cause. Local rates of *H. pylori* prevalence likely play a large part in this increased environmental risk, as infection has been linked to the development of intestinal variant gastric cancer specifically. The diffuse form of gastric adenocarcinoma consists of tiny clusters of small, uniform signet ring cells; is poorly differentiated; and lacks glands. It tends to spread submucosally, with early metastatic spread via transmural extension and lymphatic invasion. It is generally not associated with chronic gastritis, is equally frequent in both sexes, and affects a slightly younger age group. The diffuse form also has an association with blood type A. Diffuse-type tumors often metastasize to the peritoneal cavity as carcinomatosis, whereas intestinal-type tumors more frequently metastasize to the liver.[20] The prognosis for diffuse-type tumors is less favorable than for patients with intestinal-type tumors. Mixed-type gastric adenocarcinoma is characterized by both intestinal and diffuse components and has an intermediate to poor prognosis.[21] The combination of Lauren classification with tumor location, known as the *modified Lauren classification,* is used to classify tumors as diffuse, proximal nondiffuse, or distal nondiffuse.[22] Modified Lauren classification is a better predictor of survival than histologic classification alone, with distal nondiffuse cancers having the best prognosis and diffuse cancers having the worst prognosis.[23]

World Health Organization classification. The WHO classifies gastric cancer as tubular, papillary, mucinous, poorly cohesive (including signet ring cell carcinoma), or mixed carcinomas based on the microscopic morphology of the tumor. Tubular and papillary carcinomas generally correspond to Lauren intestinal type, whereas poorly cohesive carcinomas, including signet ring cell tumors, correspond to diffuse type. Although the WHO system provides a standardized framework that encompasses uncommon histologic variants, it does not add significant prognostic or therapeutic clinical utility.

Molecular Subtypes

Stomach cancers exhibit significant heterogeneity in terms of their genetic alterations. The molecular drivers of gastric cancer include mutations that are common across a variety of cancers, such as the tumor suppressor gene *TP53* and the oncogene *KRAS*. Other important pathways that can be dysregulated in oncogenesis include cell adhesion (most commonly via *CDH1* mutations in diffuse-type and signet ring cell gastric cancer), cell cycle, apoptosis, microsatellite instability (MSI), and epigenetic changes. An important molecular marker is HER2 (encoded by the *ERBB2* gene), as its amplification or overexpression predicts response to HER2 inhibition. To address the challenges presented by the genetic heterogeneity of gastric cancer, mRNA and protein expression-based classification systems have been proposed.

The Cancer Genome Atlas molecular classification. Based on transcriptomic and proteomic profiles of gastric cancers from The Cancer Genome Atlas (TCGA), four molecular subtypes of gastric cancer were proposed in 2014: EBV-positive, MSI, genomically stable (GS), and chromosomal instability (CIN).[24] These subtypes correlate, albeit imperfectly, with previously known gastric cancer characteristics. CIN tumors generally exhibit intestinal-type histology and have a high prevalence of *TP53*-inactivating mutations, whereas GS tumors are enriched for diffuse-type histology and accordingly have a higher prevalence of somatic *CDH1* mutations. TCGA-based molecular classification alone is not a strong prognostic indicator, but it can be used to predict response to therapy. As discussed later, MSI tumors are generally unresponsive to cytotoxic chemotherapy, but MSI and EBV tumors show greater response to immunotherapy.

Asian Cancer Research Group molecular classification. In 2015, using gene expression data from the Asian Cancer Research Group (ACRG), another classification scheme was proposed, dividing gastric cancers into four molecular subtypes: Microsatellite-unstable (MSI), microsatellite stable/TP53 active (MSS/TP53+), microsatellite stable/TP53 inactive (MSS/TP53−), and microsatellite stable/epithelial-mesenchymal transition (MSS/EMT). Compared with the TCGA-based molecular classification, MSI subtypes are generally concordant and MSS/EMT correlates with the GS subtype, but these classification schemes have significant heterogeneity. This may be attributable to different baseline characteristics in the cohorts used to derive the molecular signatures in each study.[25]

Diagnosis and Workup

Screening

Gastric cancer screening has been implemented for the general population in countries with high incidence, including Japan, South Korea, Venezuela, and Chile, via upper endoscopy or barium radiography. For example, the South Korean national healthcare system covers screening upper endoscopies every 2 years beginning at age 40. Upper endoscopy is more invasive and costly than barium radiography, but it is more sensitive. Recommendations for modality, interval, and age of screening vary between countries and have not been directly compared. In contrast to universal screening, selective screening of high-risk patients should be considered in areas with low gastric cancer incidence. Screening and surveillance in patients with hereditary cancer syndromes is discussed earlier.

Patients with extensive gastric atrophy or gastric intestinal metaplasia should undergo endoscopic surveillance every 1 to 3 years.

Signs and Symptoms

Patients with gastric cancer tend to have vague and nonspecific symptoms, most commonly weight loss and persistent abdominal pain. As a result, stomach cancers are frequently diagnosed at advanced stages. With tumor growth, gastric cancer may cause dysphagia when located near the gastroesophageal (GE) junction or gastric outlet obstruction when located in the distal stomach. GI bleeding is also common, with 40% of patients having some degree of anemia.

A complete history and physical examination should be performed, with special attention to any evidence of advanced disease, including metastatic nodal disease. Presence of supraclavicular (Virchow node), axillary (Irish node), or periumbilical (Sister Mary Joseph node) adenopathy should be assessed as well as any evidence of intraabdominal metastases such as hepatomegaly, jaundice, or ascites. Drop metastases to the ovaries (Krukenberg tumor) may be detectable on pelvic examination, and peritoneal metastases can be felt as a firm shelf (Blumer shelf) on rectal examination. Complete blood count, chemistry panel including liver function tests, and coagulation studies should be performed. The tumor markers CEA and CA19-9 are sometimes elevated.

Staging

The most widely used staging system is the American Joint Committee on Cancer (AJCC) TNM staging system. This system is based on the depth of tumor invasion (T), number of involved lymph nodes (N), and presence or absence of metastatic disease (M), with the 8th edition published in 2017 (Table 87.2). Before 1997, N stage was determined by the anatomic location of the nodes with respect to the primary tumor, rather than the absolute number of nodes. The current system determines N stage based on the number of positive nodes, which has greater prognostic value than the location of positive nodes, with the caveat that a minimum of 16 lymph nodes must be evaluated for accurate staging.[26] The current AJCC staging system also includes a separate staging section for patients who received

---

TABLE 87.2   Tumor, Node, Metastasis Classification of Carcinoma of the Stomach

		PATHOLOGIC STAGE	PROGNOSTIC GROUP		
Primary Tumor (T)					
TX	Primary tumor cannot be assessed	0	Tis	N0	MD
T0	No evidence of primary tumor	IA	71	N0	MO
Tis	Carcinoma in situ; intraepithelial tumor without invasion of the lamina propria, high-grade dysplasia	IB	71	N1	MO
			72	N0	MO
T1	Tumor invades lamina propria, muscularis mucosae, or submucosa	I1A	71	N2	MO
			T2	N1	MO
Tla	Tumor invades lamina propria or muscularis mucosae		T3	N0[1]	MO
T1b	Tumor invades submucosa	IB	T1	N3a	MO
T2	Tumor invades muscularis propria[a]		72	N2	MO
T3	Tumor penetrates subserosal connective tissue without invasion of visceral peritoneum or adjacent structures[b]		73	N1	MO
			T4a	N0	MO
T4	Tumor invades serosa (visceral peritoneum) or adjacent structures[b]	IIIA	72	N3a	MO
			T3	N2	MD
T4a	Tumor invades serosa (visceral peritoneum)		T4a	N1	MO
T4b	Tumor invades adjacent structures		Ha	N2	MD
			T4b	N0	MD
Regional Lymph Nodes (N)		DIE	T1	H3b	MD
NX	Regional lymph nodes cannot be assessed		T2	N3b	MD
N0	No regional lymph node metastasis[c]		T3	N3a	MD
N1	Metastasis in 1–2 regional lymph nodes		Ha	N3a	MD
N2	Metastasis in 3–6 regional lymph nodes		Hb	MI	MD
N3	Metastasis in 7 or more regional lymph nodes		Hb	N2	MD
N3a	Metastasis in 7–15 regional lymph nodes	me	T3	N3b	MD
N3h	Metastasis in 16 or more regional lymph nodes		Ha	N3b	MD
			Hb	N3a	MD
Distant Metastasis (M)			Hb	N3b	MD
MD	No distant metastasis	IV	AnyT	AnyN	MI
MI	Distant metastasis				

[a]A tumor may penetrate the muscularis propria with extension into the gastrocolic or gastrohepatic ligaments or into the greater or lesser omentum without perforation of the visceral peritoneum covering these structures. In this case, the tumor is classified T3. If there is perforation of the visceral peritoneum covering the gastric ligaments or the omentum, the tumor should be classified T4.

[b]The adjacent structures of the stomach include the spleen, transverse colon, liver, diaphragm, pancreas, abdominal wall, adrenal gland, kidney, small intestine, and retroperitoneum.

[c]A designation of pN0 should be used if all examined lymph nodes are negative, regardless of the total number removed and examined.

From Amin MB, Edge SB, Greene FL, et al. *AJCC Cancer Staging Manual.* 8th ed. New York: Springer International Publishing; 2017.

neoadjuvant therapy. Other parameters in addition to TNM have been proposed, including location of the primary tumor (as in the Japanese Research Society for Gastric Cancer system) or lymph node ratio (the percentage of all harvested lymph nodes that are positive), because these may provide additional prognostic information.

The Siewert classification is used for adenocarcinomas of the GE junction, defined as tumors with an epicenter with 5 cm proximal or distal to the GE junction. There are three Siewert types: Type I tumors are tumors of the distal esophagus, centered within 1 to 5 cm above the GE junction; type II tumors have a tumor center located from 1 cm above the GE junction to 2 cm below; type III tumors are centered between 2 and 5 cm caudad to the GE junction. In general, Siewert type I tumors are staged using the esophageal cancer staging system and treated similarly to esophageal adenocarcinoma, whereas type III tumors can be staged and treated according to the guidelines for gastric adenocarcinoma described here; these distinctions are reflected in the current AJCC TNM staging guidelines. Current AJCC guidelines stage Siewert II tumors as esophageal cancers. However, there are studies showing these tumors are better staged as gastric cancer.[27,28]

Although not part of the formal AJCC staging system, R status, first described by Hermanek in 1994, is used to describe tumor status after resection and is important for determining the adequacy of surgery. R0 describes a microscopically margin-negative resection in which no gross or microscopic tumor remains in the tumor bed. R1 indicates removal of all macroscopic disease, but microscopic margins are positive for tumor. R2 indicates gross residual disease. Because the extent of resection can influence survival, some include this R designation to complement the TNM system. R0 resection is associated with improved overall survival (OS) in patients with early stage disease, but not in patients with locally advanced disease.[29]

Staging Workup

The goals of preoperative staging are to gain information on prognosis, to counsel the patient effectively, and to determine the extent of disease to decide the most appropriate course of therapy. All patients should undergo endoscopic biopsy to confirm the diagnosis and CT imaging of the chest, abdomen, and pelvis. Based on these evaluations, if early disease (cT1-2/N0) is suspected (small tumor and normal gastric distensibility on endoscopy; no visible primary tumor, ascites, or metastatic disease on CT), endoscopic ultrasound (EUS) is the next step for locoregional staging. However, if locally advanced (cT3-4 and/or N+) or metastatic disease is suspected, PET/CT imaging and diagnostic laparoscopy are indicated (Fig. 87.1). PET/CT and laparoscopy will identify metastatic disease in about 25% to 30% of patients deemed to have locally advanced disease based on CT scans.

Endoscopy and biopsy. Flexible endoscopy is an essential tool for the diagnosis of gastric cancer. It allows visualization of the tumor, provides tissue for pathologic diagnosis, and can help treat patients with obstruction or bleeding (Fig. 87.2). The location of the tumor in the stomach and, in particular, its relation to the GE junction for proximal lesions (including Siewert classification) should be documented. On initial diagnostic endoscopy, if a suspicious mass or ulcer is encountered in the stomach, it is essential to obtain adequate tissue to confirm the correct diagnosis histologically. Current National Comprehensive Cancer Network (NCCN) guidelines recommend harvesting six to eight biopsy specimens from different areas of the lesion in order to maximize the diagnostic yield.[30] Small lesions (<2 cm in diameter) without ulceration can be resected endoscopically at the time of initial diagnostic endoscopy.[31] This resection can provide a more complete specimen to aid the pathologist in obtaining an accurate diagnosis and can potentially be curative for early stage cancers. Techniques of endoscopic resection are discussed in detail later.

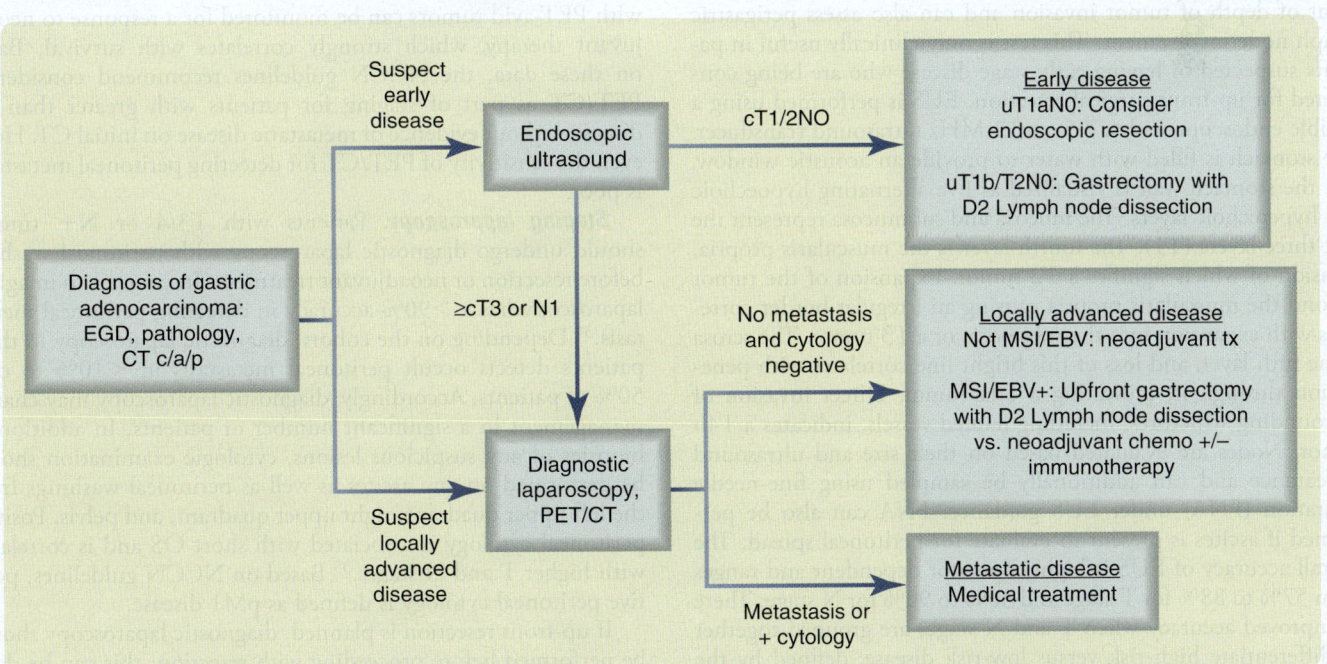

FIGURE 87.1 Algorithm for the workup and treatment of gastric adenocarcinoma. *CT c/a/p,* Computed tomography chest, abdomen, pelvis; *EBV,* Epstein-Barr virus; *EGD,* esophagogastroduodenoscopy; *MSI,* microsatellite instability; *PET,* positron emission tomography. *See Box 87.2 and Figure 87.6 for endoscopic resection criteria and guidelines.

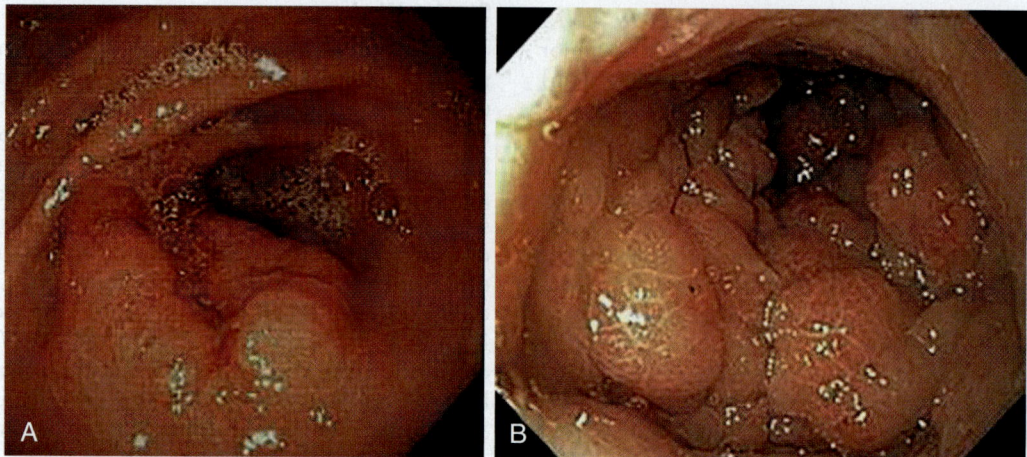

FIGURE 87.2 Endoscopic views of (A) small intestinal–type adenocarcinoma and (B) large diffuse-type adenocarcinoma. (From Dr. Yoon, Department of Surgery, Columbia University Medical Center, New York, NY.)

In addition to histologic assessment, tumors should be assessed for MSI or MMR protein expression status, HER2, programmed cell death ligand 1 (PD-L1), and EBV status. *H. pylori* testing and treatment should also be performed when the clinical picture is consistent with *H. pylori*–associated disease.

Computed tomography. All patients with gastric cancer should undergo CT of the chest, abdomen, and pelvis with IV contrast to evaluate the primary tumor and lymph nodes and to rule out metastatic disease. CT has limited accuracy for locoregional staging, with 43% to 82% accuracy in measuring depth of invasion and 78% accuracy in detecting local lymph node involvement.[32] As such, EUS should be performed for local staging if early stage disease is suspected or if early versus locally advanced disease needs to be determined.

Endoscopic ultrasound. EUS provides the most accurate assessment of depth of tumor invasion and can also assess perigastric lymph node involvement. This test is only clinically useful in patients suspected of having early stage disease who are being considered for up-front surgical resection. EUS is performed using a flexible endoscope with a 7.5- to 12-MHz ultrasound transducer. The stomach is filled with water to provide an acoustic window, and the stomach wall is visualized as five alternating hypoechoic and hyperechoic layers. The mucosa and submucosa represent the first three layers (T1). The fourth layer is the muscularis propria, invasion of which signifies a T2 tumor. Expansion of the tumor beyond the muscularis propria causing an irregular border correlates with expansion into the subserosa, or a T3 tumor. The serosa is the fifth layer, and loss of this bright line correlates with penetration through it, indicating a T4a tumor. Direct invasion of surrounding structures, including named vessels, indicates a T4b tumor. Nodes are evaluated based on their size and ultrasound appearance and can additionally be sampled using fine-needle aspiration (FNA) under EUS guidance. FNA can also be performed if ascites is present to evaluate for peritoneal spread. The overall accuracy of EUS is highly operator dependent and ranges from 57% to 88% for T stage and 30% to 90% for N stage. There is improved accuracy when T and N stages are grouped together to differentiate high-risk versus low-risk disease, defined by the presence of any subserosal or serosal (T3/T4) involvement or any nodal disease (>N0). A Cochrane meta-analysis found that the summary sensitivity and specificity of EUS for discriminating T1/T2 versus T3/T4 disease were 86% and 90%, respectively.[32] The

sensitivity and specificity for nodal involvement were 83% and 67%, respectively. As such, EUS is reliable in identifying patients with locally advanced tumors who should receive neoadjuvant treatment, as discussed later. However, given the importance of T staging to predict lymph node status in early stage gastric cancer, accurate EUS assessment is increasingly important to guide treatment decisions regarding neoadjuvant therapy and consideration for endoscopic resection (see later). A collaborative relationship with a skilled and experienced endoscopist is therefore critical for the surgeon who treats gastric cancer.

Positron emission tomography. Combined PET/CT is more accurate in preoperative staging (68%) than either PET (47%) or CT (53%) alone. It is particularly useful in patients with locally advanced disease and patients being considered for neoadjuvant therapy to better assess for occult metastasis.[33] Further, patients with PET-avid tumors can be monitored for a response to neoadjuvant therapy, which strongly correlates with survival. Based on these data, the NCCN guidelines recommend considering PET/CT as part of staging for patients with greater than T1 disease without evidence of metastatic disease on initial CT. However, the sensitivity of PET/CT for detecting peritoneal metastases is poor.

Staging laparoscopy. Patients with T3/4 or N+ tumors should undergo diagnostic laparoscopy with peritoneal washing before resection or neoadjuvant treatment. In contrast to imaging, laparoscopy has a >90% accuracy in detecting peritoneal metastasis.[34] Depending on the cohort, diagnostic laparoscopy in these patients detects occult peritoneal metastasis in <10% to over 50% of patients. Accordingly, diagnostic laparoscopy may change management in a significant number of patients. In addition to biopsies of any suspicious lesions, cytologic examination should be performed on any ascites as well as peritoneal washings from the left upper quadrant, right upper quadrant, and pelvis. Positive peritoneal cytology is associated with short OS and is correlated with higher T and N stages.[35] Based on NCCN guidelines, positive peritoneal cytology is defined as pM1 disease.

If up-front resection is planned, diagnostic laparoscopy should be performed before proceeding with resection; this can be done in a single-stage procedure. If neoadjuvant chemotherapy is planned, diagnostic laparoscopy should occur before initiating chemotherapy. Repeat diagnostic laparoscopy after neoadjuvant therapy is not currently part of the NCCN response assessment algorithm but should be considered in patients with evidence of disease progression on preoperative chemotherapy. A proportion of patients with initially positive peritoneal cytology will convert to negative cytology after neoadjuvant therapy; this group has an improved prognosis compared with those with persistently positive cytology, but the role of surgery after conversion to negative cytology is not well defined.[36]

Treatment

Surgical Therapy

For resectable gastric cancers, surgical excision remains the cornerstone of curative-intent treatment. Once staging is complete and resectability is established, the options are (1) endoscopic resection, (2) up-front resection with partial or total gastrectomy, or (3) preoperative chemotherapy or chemoradiation. Patient selection and technical aspects of resection options, including minimally invasive techniques and extent of lymphadenectomy, are discussed here. Patient selection for chemotherapy and radiation therapy and decision-making about treatment sequencing are discussed later.

Endoscopic resection. For select patients with early gastric cancer, endoscopic tumor resection can be performed for curative intent with adequate oncologic outcomes. The two primary modalities are endoscopic mucosal resection (EMR; Fig. 87.3) and endoscopic submucosal dissection (ESD; Fig. 87.4). The most significant advantage of endoscopic resection is avoiding the need for gastrectomy. The major disadvantages are risk of incomplete resection and unrecognized lymph node metastases. The standard criteria for endoscopic resection consideration are intestinal type adenocarcinoma, tumor confined to the mucosa, absence of lymphovascular invasion, nonulcerated, and less than 2 cm in diameter (Box 87.2). Meta-analyses have shown

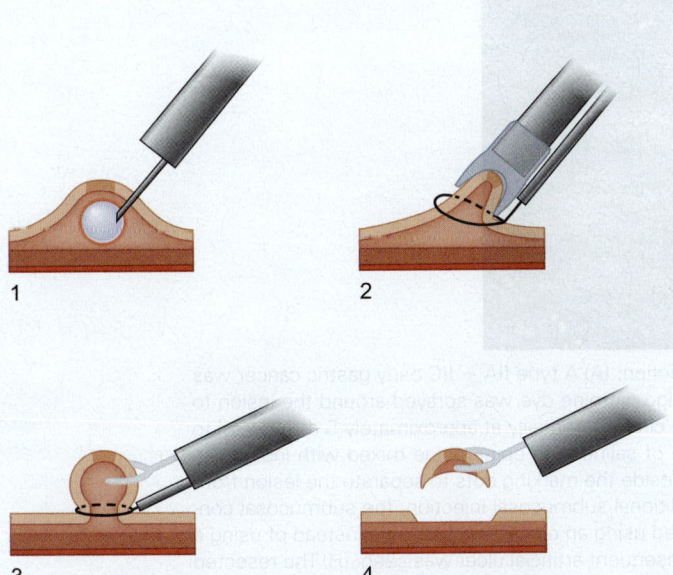

FIGURE 87.3 Endoscopic mucosal resection by strip biopsy. Saline is injected into the submucosal layer, and the area is elevated. *(1)* The top of the mound is pulled upward with forceps, and the snare is placed at the base of the lesion *(2 and 3)*. Electrosurgical current is applied through the snare to resect the mucosa, and the lesion is removed *(4)*. (From Tanabe S, Koizumi W, Kokotou M, et al. Usefulness of endoscopic aspiration mucosectomy as compared with strip biopsy for the treatment of gastric mucosal cancer. *Gastrointest Endosc.* 1990;50:819-822.)

> ### BOX 87.2 Standard Criteria for Endoscopic Resection of Gastric Adenocarcinoma
>
> Intestinal-type adenocarcinoma
> Tumor confined to the mucosa (Tis or T1a)
> Absence of lymphovascular invasion
> Nonulcerated tumor
> Less than 2 cm in diameter

that endoscopic resection is associated with higher rates of incomplete resection and recurrence but no differences in 5-year OS compared with conventional resection.[37] Some East Asian guidelines now suggest expanded indications for endoscopically resectable tumors >2 cm without ulceration and those ≤3 cm with ulceration that otherwise meet standard criteria and for nonintestinal and poorly differentiated tumors <2 cm confined to the mucosa without ulceration (Fig. 87.5). Risk of lymph node involvement in patients meeting expanded criteria is higher at 0.7% compared with 0.2% among patients meeting standard criteria, and expanded criteria have not been widely adopted in Western centers.[38]

EMR involves elevating the tumor using a saline injection, encircling the affected mucosa using a snare device or suction cap, and then excising it with electrocautery. Perforation rates are low, and bleeding rates are approximately 15%; these can generally be controlled endoscopically without the need for further intervention. En bloc resection is preferred, as piecemeal resection is associated with an increased risk of recurrence. Patients with positive lateral margins can be considered for repeat endoscopic therapy or close surveillance. Patients with positive vertical margins, lymphovascular invasion, or submucosal invasion should be referred for gastrectomy with lymphadenectomy

ESD is mostly used in East Asia and allows for resection of larger tumors and those with limited submucosal involvement. This technique begins by marking the borders of the lesion using electrocautery. A submucosal injection of epinephrine with indigo carmine hydrodissects the lesion, and an insulation-tipped knife is used to remove the lesion by dissecting a submucosal plane deep to the tumor and removing it en bloc. Any bleeding is controlled with electrocautery. ESD is more technically challenging than EMR, and there is a higher risk of perforation with ESD compared with EMR.

Extent of resection. Complete resection of a gastric tumor with a wide margin of normal stomach remains the standard of care for resection with curative intent. Patients without metastatic disease or invasion of unresectable vascular structures such as the aorta, celiac axis, or common hepatic artery are candidates for curative resection. The extent of resection depends on the location of the tumor in the stomach and size of the tumor. For T4 tumors, any organ with invasion should be removed en bloc with the gastrectomy specimen to achieve a curative resection.

For cancers of the distal stomach, including the body and antrum, a distal gastrectomy is the appropriate operation. The proximal stomach is transected with a margin of at least 2 cm for cT1 tumors, at least 3 cm for cT2-T4 tumors with noninfiltrative margins, and at least 5 cm for cT2-T4 tumors with infiltrative margins. Frozen section analysis on any close proximal and/or distal margin should be performed before reconstruction, and, if positive, a wider excision should be performed when possible.

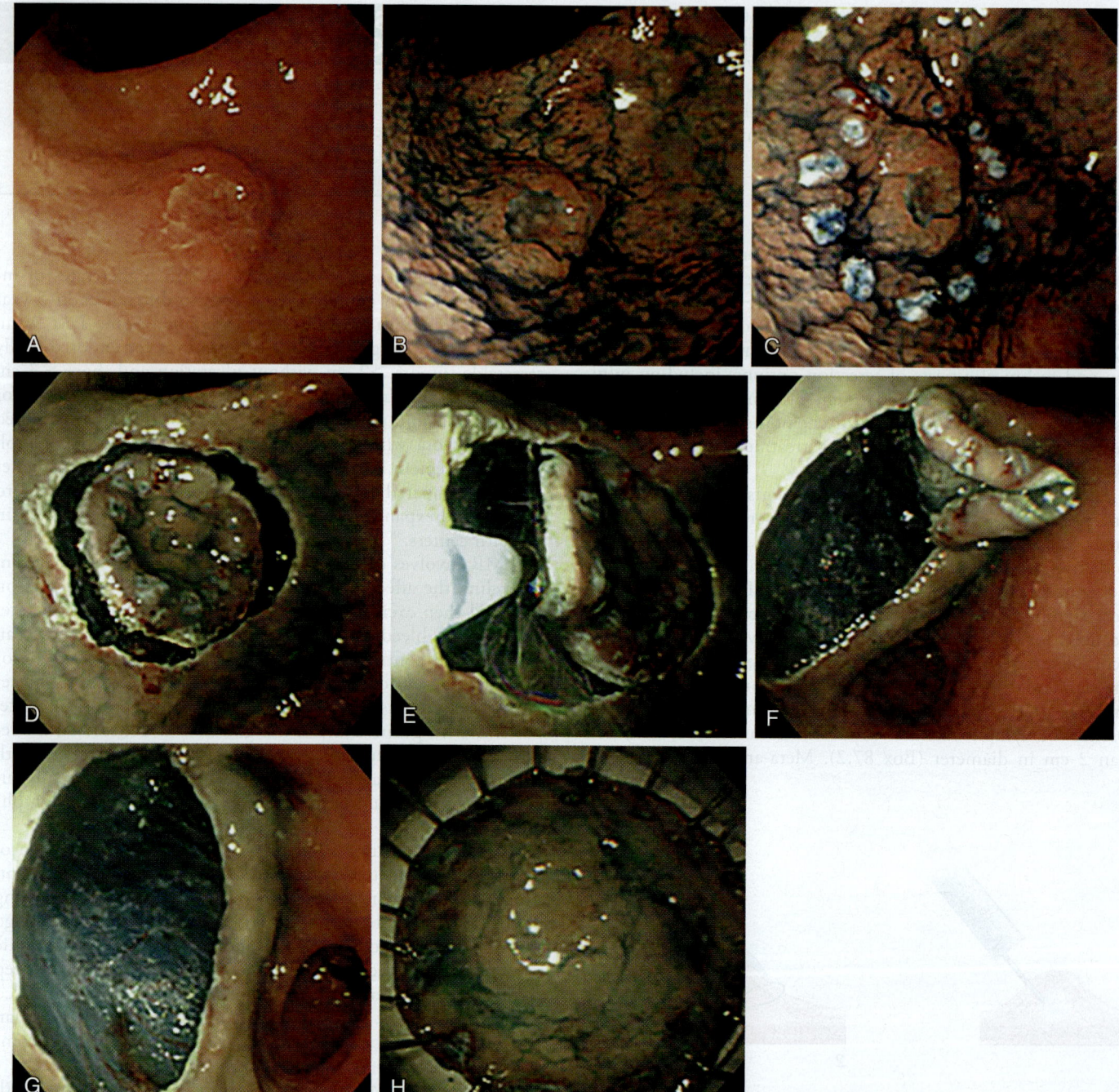

FIGURE 87.4 Procedure of endoscopic submucosal dissection. (A) A type IIA + IIC early gastric cancer was located at the lesser curvature side of the antrum. (B) Indigo carmine dye was sprayed around the lesion to define the margin accurately. (C) Marking dots were made circumferentially at approximately 5 mm lateral to the margin of the lesion. (D) After a submucosal injection of saline with epinephrine mixed with indigo carmine, a circumferential mucosal incision was performed outside the marking dots to separate the lesion from the surrounding nonneoplastic mucosa. (E–F) After an additional submucosal injection, the submucosal connective tissue just beneath the lesion was directly dissected using an electrosurgical knife instead of using a snare. (G) The lesion was completely resected, and the consequent artificial ulcer was seen. (H) The resected specimen with a central early gastric cancer. (From Min BH, Lee JH, Kim JJ, et al. Clinical outcomes of endoscopic sub-mucosal dissection [ESD] for treating early gastric cancer: comparison with endoscopic mucosal resection after circumferential precutting. [EMR-P]. *Dig Liver Dis.* 2009;41[3]:201-209.)

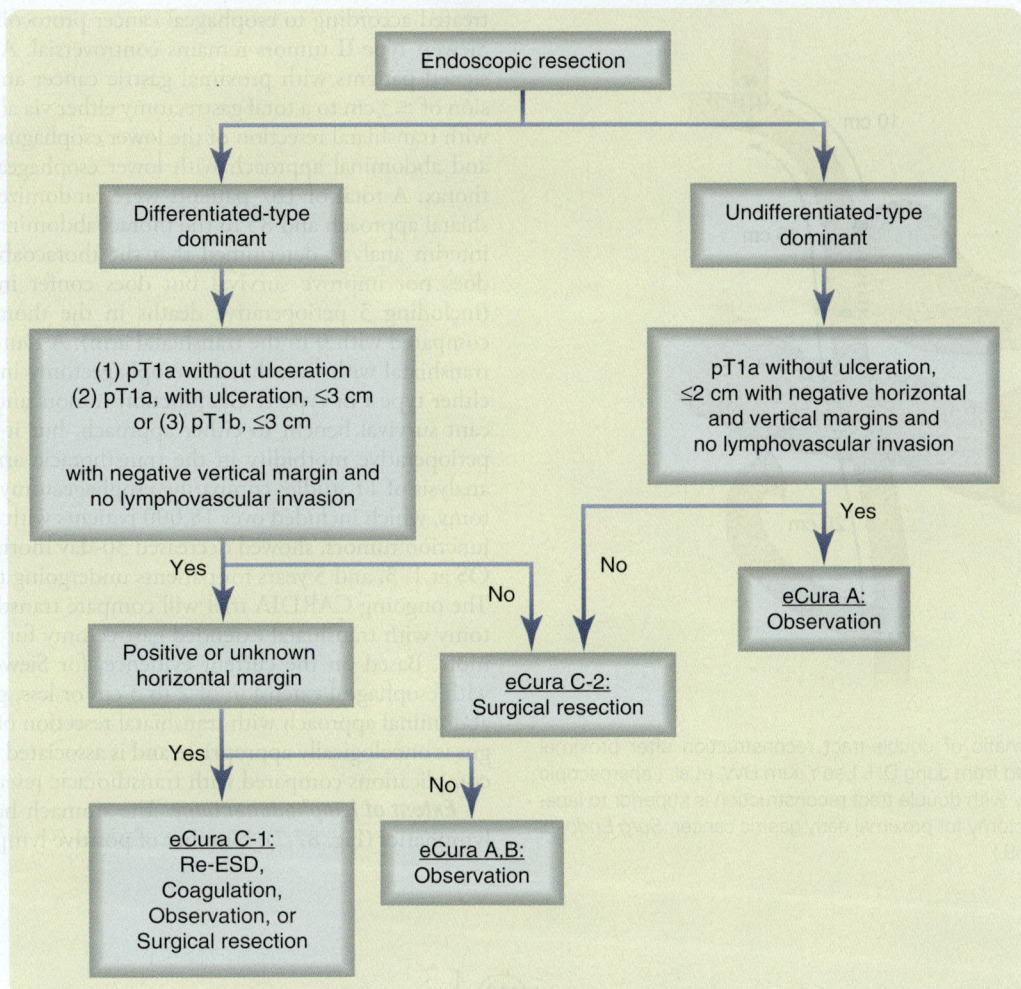

FIGURE 87.5 Japanese Gastric Cancer Treatment guidelines for endoscopic resection. Undifferentiated-type dominant tumors include poorly differentiated adenocarcinoma and signet ring cell carcinoma, whereas differentiated-type dominant tumors comprise all other adenocarcinoma types. *eCura,* Endoscopic curability classification; *ESD,* endoscopic submucosal dissection. (Adapted from Japanese Gastric Cancer Association. Japanese Gastric Cancer Treatment Guidelines 2021 [6th ed.]. *Gastric Cancer.* 2023;26[1]:1-25.)

The choice of reconstruction depends on the remnant anatomy with consideration of postgastrectomy physiology, although a Roux-en-Y reconstruction has been shown to result in less remnant gastritis and bile reflux esophagitis and improved quality of life at 1 year compared with Billroth reconstruction.[39]

In East Asian countries, where early gastric cancer is more common, a pylorus-preserving segmental gastrectomy can be performed for cT1N0M0 disease for cancers in the middle third of the stomach at least 5 cm from the pylorus. A Korean randomized controlled trial (RCT), the KLASS-04 trial, found no difference in overall complication rate with pylorus preservation; however, there was a 7% rate of pyloric stenosis requiring endoscopic intervention.[40] Antral cuff length in the pylorus preservation group averaged 4 cm. For early gastric cancers, the oncologic outcomes were similar between pylorus-preserving segmental gastrectomy and distal gastrectomy, with the former having lower rates of dumping syndrome, bile reflux, and malnutrition.

For proximal lesions of the fundus or cardia, a total gastrectomy with a Roux-en-Y esophagojejunostomy and proximal gastrectomy are equivalent from an oncologic perspective. The advantages of proximal gastrectomy include the preservation of the reservoir function and intrinsic factor production of the remnant distal stomach, pylorus preservation preventing reflux of duodenal contents, and decreased rate of dumping syndrome. On the other hand, additional care must be taken to ensure adequate lymph node harvest with proximal gastrectomy, and the incidence of anastomotic complications and reflux esophagitis may be higher with proximal esophagectomy depending on the method of reconstruction. Common reconstruction techniques after proximal gastrectomy include jejunal interposition, esophagogastrostomy, and double tract reconstruction consisting of three anastomoses: esophagojejunostomy, gastrojejunostomy, and jejunojejunostomy (Fig. 87.6). A Korean RCT, the KLASS-05 trial, compared laparoscopic total gastrectomy with laparoscopic proximal gastrectomy with double-tract reconstruction for early upper gastric cancer and showed similar perioperative morbidity without a significant difference in anastomotic complications and decreased vitamin B_{12} supplementation requirements in the double-tract reconstruction arm.[41]

As discussed earlier, Siewert type III GE junction tumors are treated as gastric cancers, whereas type I tumors are staged and

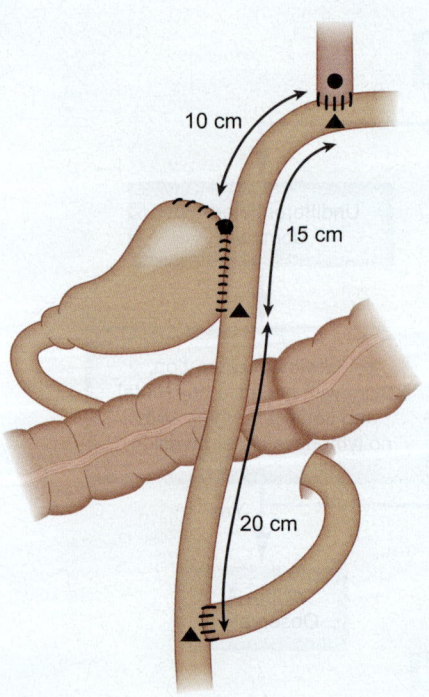

FIGURE 87.6 Schematic of double-tract reconstruction after proximal gastrectomy. (Adapted from Jung DH, Lee Y, Kim DW, et al. Laparoscopic proximal gastrectomy with double tract reconstruction is superior to laparoscopic total gastrectomy for proximal early gastric cancer. *Surg Endosc.* 2017;31[10]:3961-3969.)

treated according to esophageal cancer protocols. The approach to Siewert type II tumors remains controversial. A Japanese RCT assigned patients with proximal gastric cancer and esophageal invasion of ≤3 cm to a total gastrectomy either via abdominal approach with transhiatal resection of the lower esophagus or via left thoracic and abdominal approach with lower esophageal resection via the thorax. A total of 167 patients were randomized (82 to the transhiatal approach and 85 to the thoracoabdominal approach) before interim analysis determined that the thoracoabdominal approach does not improve survival but does confer increased morbidity (including 3 perioperative deaths in the thoracoabdominal arm compared with 0 in the transhiatal arm). A Dutch RCT compared transhiatal with transthoracic esophagectomy in 220 patients with either type I or type II GE junction tumors and found no significant survival benefit to either approach, but it did find increased perioperative morbidity in the transthoracic arm. A recent meta-analysis of 11 studies comparing esophagectomy with total gastrectomy, which included over 18,000 patients with Siewert type II GE junction tumors, showed decreased 30-day mortality and improved OS at 1, 3, and 5 years for patients undergoing total gastrectomy.[42] The ongoing CARDIA trial will compare transthoracic esophagectomy with transhiatal extended gastrectomy for Siewert type II tumors. Based on the current evidence, for Siewert type II tumors with esophageal extension of 2 to 3 cm or less, gastrectomy via the abdominal approach with transhiatal resection of the lower esophagus is oncologically appropriate and is associated with fewer surgical complications compared with transthoracic resection.

Extent of lymphadenectomy. The stomach has a rich supply of lymphatics (Fig. 87.7). Number of positive lymph nodes correlates

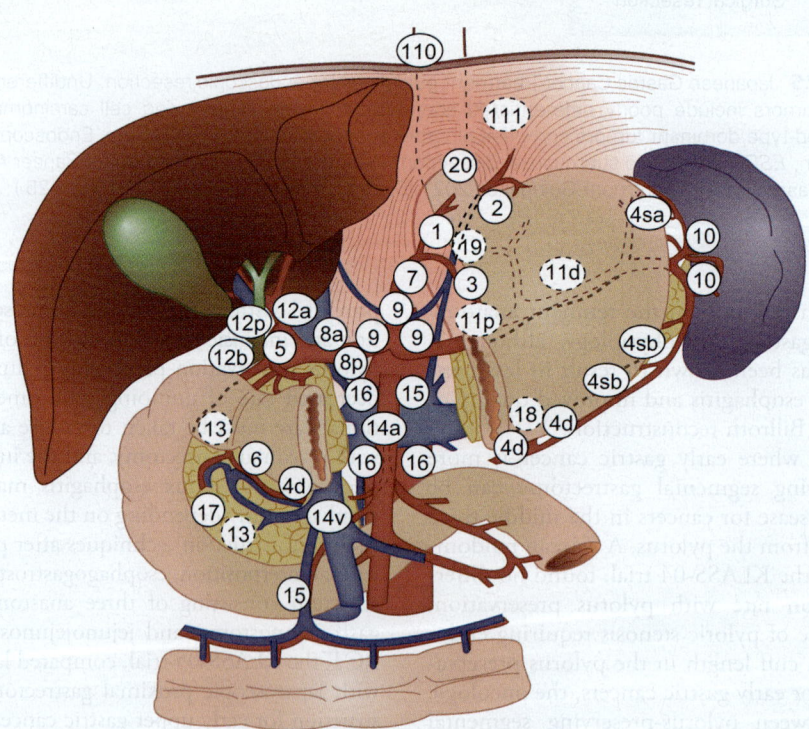

FIGURE 87.7 Lymph node station numbers as defined by the Japanese Gastric Cancer Association. (From Japanese Gastric Cancer Association. Japanese Classification of Gastric Carcinoma, 2nd English edition. *Gastric Cancer.* 1998:1:10-24.)

with survival in gastric cancer (Table 87.3). The extent of lymphadenectomy for gastric adenocarcinoma has been debated extensively. Historically, lymphadenectomy for gastric adenocarcinoma was defined by, and is still often discussed in terms of, the location of the nodes relative to the primary tumor. Various definitions have been proposed for extent of lymphadenectomy. The Japanese Gastric Cancer Association (JGCA) definitions of D1, D1+, and D2 lymphadenectomy are listed in Table 87.4.

More extensive lymphadenectomy certainly provides better staging in gastric cancer, but the relationship between lymph node dissection and clinical outcomes is complex.[43] Historically, more extensive lymphadenectomy has been standard in Asian centers, with less extensive lymph node dissections performed in Western practice. A Cochrane meta-analysis of European and Asian RCTs found an improvement in disease-specific survival with D2 compared with D1 lymphadenectomy, but with higher perioperative mortality.[44] Much of the morbidity and mortality is thought to be related to the practice of distal pancreatectomy and splenectomy as part of the D2 lymphadenectomy in these trials. Modification of the D2 lymphadenectomy to a D1+ dissection excluding distal pancreatectomy and splenectomy resulted in decreased postoperative morbidity with equivalent disease-free survival in an Italian RCT. The Cochrane review also found that in Asian RCTs there was no survival benefit to D3 over D2 lymphadenectomy. Based on these data, NCCN guidelines recommend modified D2 lymph node dissection without routine pancreatectomy or splenectomy

in centers experienced with this technique. For nonreferral centers, lymphadenectomy for gastric adenocarcinoma should incorporate at least a D1 lymphadenectomy. A D2 lymphadenectomy should only be performed if it can be done with low morbidity and almost no mortality. Western RCTs on extent of lymphadenectomy in gastric cancer are listed in Table 87.5.

In addition to the anatomic extent of lymph node dissection, the number of lymph nodes removed correlates with outcomes. Retrospective data show a trend toward improved survival with greater numbers of lymph nodes. It is not clear whether this is attributable directly to improved disease control from greater lymphadenectomy, from confounding because of stage migration (as patients who would otherwise be understaged are now classified as having node-positive disease status, improving the prognosis of both groups), or because it serves as a surrogate for overall surgical quality. Nevertheless, adequate lymphadenectomy is an indispensable staging tool. NCCN guidelines recommend pathologic analysis of a minimum of 16 nodes and suggest that over 30 lymph nodes is desirable. Minimally invasive approaches are associated with equivalent or higher rates of adequate lymphadenectomy.[45]

Minimally invasive surgery. Numerous retrospective propensity-matched studies and prospective RCTs have now established noninferior perioperative safety profiles and long-term survival outcomes with laparoscopic gastrectomy as compared with open gastrectomy in both Asian and Western cohorts and in both early and locally advanced disease.[46] Initial trials, including Japanese and Korean RCTs, did not identify differences in oncologic outcomes based on surgical approach for early-stage gastric cancer. Subsequent East Asian trials in locally advanced gastric cancer also showed noninferiority of the laparoscopic approach. Less prospective Western data have been reported, but data from European and North American series showed no differences in oncologic outcomes.[47–50] Much of the data for robotic-assisted gastrectomy is retrospective or too immature to assess long-term oncologic outcomes, but reported outcomes are generally equivalent between robotic-assisted and laparoscopic gastrectomy.[51] Two recent phase III prospective RCTs found that patients undergoing robotic-assisted gastrectomy had fewer postoperative complications and faster postoperative recovery than those undergoing

TABLE 87.3 Median Survival According to Location of Positive Nodes Versus Number of Positive Nodes

SIZE	MEDIAN SURVIVAL (MONTHS)		
	1–6 PN	7–15 PN	>15 PN
<3 cm (n = 402)	38.8 (n = 311)	20.8 (n = 82)	9.5 (n = 9)
>3 cm (n = 233)	35.5 (n = 81)	19.7 (n = 96)	12.5 (n = 56)

PN, Positive nodes.
Adapted from Karpeh MS, Leon L, Klimstra D, et al. Lymph node staging in gastric cancer: is location more important than number? An analysis of 1038 patients. *Ann Surg.* 2000;232:362-371.

TABLE 87.4 Definition of Extent of Lymphadenectomy by Resection Type (JGCA 6th edition)

DISSECTION	DISTAL GASTRECTOMY	TOTAL GASTRECTOMY	PROXIMAL GASTRECTOMY
D1	No. 1, 3, 4sb, 4d, 5, 6, 7	No. 1–7	No. 1, 2, 3a, 4sa, 4sb, 7
D1+	D1 plus No. 8a, 9	D1 plus No. 8a, 9, 11p	D1 plus No. 8a, 9, 11p
D2	D1 plus No. 8a, 9, 11p, 12a	D1 plus 8a, 9, 11p, 11d, 12a	

TABLE 87.5 Western Randomized Trials on Extent of Lymphadenectomy in Gastric Cancer

LEAD AUTHOR	YEAR	COUNTRY	N	ARMS	PERIOPERATIVE OUTCOMES	LONG-TERM OUTCOMES
Dent DM	1988	South Africa	43	D1 vs. D2	D2: ↑ LOS, ↑ operating time, ↑ transfusion	Not reported
Cuschieri A	1999	United Kingdom	400	D1 vs. D2	D2: ↑ post-op mortality, ↑ post-op morbidity, ↑ LOS	ND: 5-year OS, DSS, RFS
Songun I	2010	Netherlands	1078	D1 vs. D2	D2: ↑ post-op mortality, ↑ post-op morbidity, ↑ LOS	ND: 15-year OS
						D2: ↑ 15-year DSS, RFS
Degiuli M	2014	Italy	267	D1 vs. D2	ND: post-op morbidity, mortality	ND: 5-year OS, DSS
Galizia G	2015	Italy	73	D1+ vs. D2	D2: ↑ post-op morbidity	ND: 5-year DFS

DSS, Disease-specific survival; *LOS,* length of stay; *ND,* no difference; *OS,* overall survival; *RFS,* recurrence-free survival.
Adapted from Hu Y, Yoon SS. Extent of gastrectomy and lymphadenectomy for gastric adenocarcinoma. *Surg Oncol.* 2022;40:101689.

laparoscopic gastrectomy.[52,53] The prospective trials for minimally invasive gastrectomy generally excluded patients with T4b or N2 bulky disease; based on the characteristics of the disease and surgeon experience, open gastrectomy may be offered to these patients. It should be noted that prospective trials of minimally invasive techniques were performed in high-volume specialty centers. Laparoscopic and robotic gastrectomy and lymphadenectomy have a significant learning curve, and it can be difficult to achieve proficiency without high surgical volumes. Regardless of approach, the most important principle of surgery for gastric cancer is to perform an oncologically sound operation.

Postoperative management. Similar to other GI surgeries, Enhanced Recovery After Surgery (ERAS) protocols have been developed for perioperative care after gastrectomy. Specific recommendations from the ERAS society include no routine use of nasogastric (NG)/nasojejunal decompression, avoiding perianastomotic drains, and using minimally invasive approaches when possible.[54] A weak recommendation was also made for offering oral diet to patients undergoing a total gastrectomy starting on postoperative day 1. Randomized trials have generally shown small advantages with ERAS protocols in postoperative length of stay and pulmonary infections. However, there is a great deal of heterogeneity between trials in terms of patient populations, surgical techniques, and details of ERAS/fast-track protocols. For example, one trial found that ERAS benefited patients aged 45 to 74 years but resulted in worse outcomes for patients over 75 years old—specifically a higher readmission rate.[55] Moreover, much of the literature supporting ERAS protocols is retrospective, comparing the pre-ERAS era with current ERAS practice. A recent RCT in patients undergoing laparoscopic distal gastrectomy showed an advantage in clinical recovery of 15 hours, but this did not translate to any difference in actual hospital stay.[56] ERAS and other fast-track protocols after gastrectomy are an area of active research interest, and further optimization should elucidate ideal patient selection and balancing decreased length of stay with readmission rates.

Perioperative Therapy

Although surgical resection remains the cornerstone of curative-intent treatment for stomach cancer, perioperative multimodal treatment with chemotherapy and/or radiation has shown benefit, particularly for patients with stage II or higher disease, who are at significant risk of recurrence and mortality.[57] Recurrences are most commonly distant or peritoneal, but many patients also have locoregional recurrence, with a subset of 10% to 20% having only a local recurrence. Local recurrence rates are lower after D2 lymphadenectomy compared with D1 lymphadenectomy. For patients who recur, the prognosis is dismal, and there has been much focus on how to prevent recurrent disease with neoadjuvant and/or adjuvant therapies. A variety of approaches have been tested, and practices of multimodal therapy vary between countries and centers.

Chemotherapy. In Western countries, both pre- and postoperative chemotherapy is favored. The MAGIC and FLOT4-AIO studies were landmark RCTs establishing this paradigm. The MAGIC trial randomized patients with resectable gastric, GE junction, or distal esophageal cancer to surgery alone or perioperative chemotherapy with epirubicin, cisplatin and 5-fluorouracil (5-FU) (three cycles before and three cycles after resection), resulting in an improvement in OS for the perioperative chemotherapy group.[58] More recently, the FLOT4-AIL trial compared the MAGIC trial regimen with four cycles of preoperative and four

cycles of postoperative 5-FU, leucovorin, oxaliplatin, and docetaxel (FLOT), resulting in improved OS in the FLOT arm.[59] Based on these data, NCCN guidelines recommend the FLOT regimen for patients with good performance status. Of note, completion of all postoperative chemotherapy cycles was relatively low in both the MAGIC and FLOT4 trials (41% and 46%, respectively). As such, the less toxic FOLFOX (5-FU, leucovorin, and oxaliplatin) regimen is recommended for patients with moderate to good performance status who may not tolerate FLOT.

In Eastern countries, the practice for resectable gastric cancer tends toward up-front resection followed by adjuvant chemotherapy if deemed necessary. The ACTS-GC trial randomized patients to surgery alone or surgery followed by adjuvant S-1 (an oral fluoropyrimidine) for 1 year, resulting in an improvement in OS in the S-1 arm.[60] The CLASSIC trial compared surgery alone with surgery followed by eight 3-week cycles of capecitabine plus oxaliplatin, resulting in improved disease-free and OS in the adjuvant chemotherapy group.[61] These trials also had relatively low rates of chemotherapy completion (66% and 67%, respectively), though better than the Western trials encompassing pre- and postoperative chemotherapy.

Chemoradiotherapy. The US INT-0116 trial was an early milestone study that compared gastrectomy alone or combined with adjuvant 5-FU and radiotherapy, demonstrating improved overall and recurrence-free survival in the chemoradiotherapy group.[62] A major criticism of this trial is that the majority of patients did not receive even a D1 lymphadenectomy, and consequently, the survival advantage with chemoradiation appeared to be mainly through reduction of locoregional recurrence. As multiagent chemotherapy regimens were developed, additional RCTs compared chemotherapy alone with chemoradiotherapy. The ARTIST trial randomized South Korean patients after gastrectomy to adjuvant capecitabine and cisplatin with or without radiation therapy.[63] There was no overall or disease-free survival advantage in the cohort as a whole, although on subgroup analysis, node-positive patients appeared to have a disease-free survival benefit. Subsequently, the ARTIST 2 trial randomized only node-positive patients to adjuvant (1) S-1, (2) S-1 and oxaliplatin, or (3) S-1 and oxaliplatin with radiation therapy.[64] Disease-free survival was longer in the S-1 and oxaliplatin group compared with S-1 alone, but the addition of radiation therapy did not confer any further benefit. Based on these trials, which specified D2 lymph node dissection, NCCN guidelines recommend postoperative chemotherapy only after up-front gastrectomy with adequate lymphadenectomy; however, the addition of radiation therapy is recommended for patients who underwent less than a D2 lymphadenectomy.

The CRITICS trial randomized patients who received preoperative epirubicin, cisplatin or oxaliplatin, and capecitabine to either postoperative chemotherapy with the same drugs or chemoradiation with capecitabine and cisplatin.[65] In this context, there was no overall or disease-free survival benefit to the addition of radiation therapy. The CROSS trial included patients with esophageal or GE junction cancers (GEJCs, including 23% squamous cell cancers) and randomized to neoadjuvant chemoradiation (with carboplatin and paclitaxel) versus surgery alone.[66] There was an improvement in OS with chemoradiation, but this was most pronounced in patients with squamous histology. Nevertheless, based on this trial, NCCN guidelines include preoperative chemoradiation as an option for patients with gastric cancer.

Immunotherapy. The advent of checkpoint immunotherapy is an exciting recent development in oncology, but at this point only a minority of patients with gastric cancer have been shown to benefit significantly from this approach. In metastatic gastric cancer, MSI-high and mismatch repair-deficient (dMMR) tumors and those with high expression of PD-L1 are clinically approved indications for checkpoint inhibition. Additionally, as discussed earlier, EBV-associated tumors tend to respond well to immunotherapy.

Importantly, MSI-high tumors do not respond to conventional cytotoxic chemotherapy.[67] Currently, the standard approach for locally advanced, nonmetastatic MSI-H gastric cancer is up-front surgical resection without neoadjuvant or adjuvant therapy. MSI-H gastric cancers have a high response rate to checkpoint blockade, making perioperative immunotherapy a potentially attractive option. There is a lack of head-to-head data on choice of immunotherapy drugs or timing in relation to surgery. There are now two phase II trials (NEONIPIGA and INFINITY) showing an approximately 60% pathologic complete response rate in MSI-high/dMMR gastric cancer with neoadjuvant dual checkpoint inhibition (targeting both programmed cell death 1 [PD-1] and cytotoxic T-lymphocyte–associated protein 4 [CTLA-4]). Long-term data are lacking, but the possibility of nonoperative management with endoscopic and imaging surveillance may be feasible in a subset of MSI-high/dMMR gastric cancers that show clinical complete responses to immunotherapy.

Targeted therapy. In addition to MSI/MMR, PD-L1, and EBV status, pathologic analysis of gastric cancer should include HER2 analysis, as tumors that overexpress or have amplified HER2 are eligible for anti-HER2 therapy. Trastuzumab is a monoclonal anti-HER2 antibody that should be added to first-line chemotherapy for HER2-overexpressing gastric cancer. Based on the anti-HER2 antibody platform, trastuzumab deruxtecan (an antibody-drug conjugate that delivers targeted chemotherapy to HER2-positive cells) was recently FDA approved in the second-line setting for patients with unresectable or metastatic HER2-amplified gastric cancer.

In terms of HER2-positive blockade for locally advanced gastric cancer, the PETRARCA trial studied the effect of perioperative trastuzumab, pertuzumab, and FLOT compared with FLOT alone in patients with cT2-T4 and/or N+ gastric or GEJC and HER2-positive overexpression.[68] The pathologic complete response rate was significantly improved in the trastuzumab/pertuzumab group compared with that in the group receiving FLOT alone (35% vs. 12%, $p = 0.02$), as was the rate of pathologic lymph node negativity (65% vs. 39%). However, the trastuzumab/pertuzumab group experienced more grade 3 or greater adverse events, particularly diarrhea and leukopenia. Ultimately, the negative results of the JACOB trial, which evaluated the efficacy of dual-HER2 therapy and chemotherapy in metastatic GC/GEJC, led to a premature termination of the PETRARCA trial.[69]

The phase II INNOVATION trial is currently underway for patients with resectable GC/GEJC.[70] This trial is investigating whether neoadjuvant and adjuvant trastuzumab or trastuzumab and pertuzumab in combination with chemotherapy is more efficacious than chemotherapy alone. The chemotherapy backbone of this trial was modified from cisplatin + capecitabine to FLOT based on the FLOT4-AIO trial. Preliminary results show a trend toward increased major pathologic response with the addition of trastuzumab (37% vs. 23% with chemotherapy alone), which was more pronounced after protocol modification (53% vs. 33%), but no improvement with the addition of both trastuzumab and pertuzumab. Study completion with follow-up survival data is expected in 2028.

Outcomes

The overall incidence and mortality rate of gastric cancer in the United States have been declining since 1930, likely because of changes in diet such as decreased sodium intake, changes in food storage and preparation, decreased smoking, and improved treatment options. Nonetheless, the overall 5-year survival remains poor, at approximately 35%. More than 60% of patients present with locally advanced or distant disease. For patients who undergo a potentially curative resection, overall 5-year survival rates range from 25% to 75%; however, for the subset with early gastric cancer, cure rates are greater than 80%. For patients who present with distant disease, 5-year survival is only 5% to 10% (Fig. 87.8).

Recurrence and Surveillance

Recurrence rates after gastrectomy are high, from 30% to 90%, depending on the series. Most recurrences occur within the first

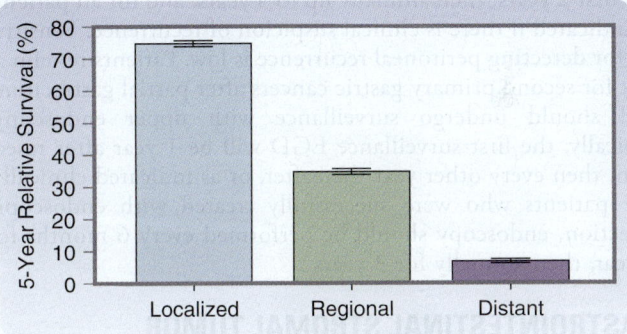

Stomach
SEER 5-Year Relative Survival Rates, 2013-2019
By Stage at Diagnosis, Both Sexes, All Races / Ethnicities, All Ages

Data source:
- SEER Incidence data, November 2022 submission (1975-2020) SEER 22 registries [https://seer.cancer.gov/registries/terms.html] (excluding Illinois and Massachusetts).
- Expected survival life tables [https//seer.cancer.gov/expsurvival/] by socioeconomic standards.

Methodology:
- The 5-year survival rates are calculated using monthly intervals.

Race/Ethnicity/Coding:
- For more details on SEER race/ethnicity groupings and changes made to the grouping for this year's data release, please see race and hispanic ethnicity changes [https://seer cancer gov/seerstat/variables/see/race-ethnicity/).
- Incidence data for Hispanics and non-Hispanics are based on the NAACCR Hispanic Latino Identification Algorithm (NHIA).
- Rates for American Indians/Alaska Natives only include cases that are in a purchased/referred care delivery area (PRCDA).

Cancer site coding:
- See SEER explore cancer site definitions (https://seer.cancer.gov/statistics-network/explore-cancer-sites.htm) for details about the cancer site coding used for SEER incidence data.

Created by https://seer.cancer.gov/statistics-network/explorer on Wed Oct 04 2023.

FIGURE 87.8 The 5-year relative survival rates in patients with stomach cancers by stage at diagnosis. *SEER,* The Surveillance, Epidemiology, and End Results Program. (From SEER database, seer.cancer.gov.)

2 years.[71] Locoregional recurrence is seen in about 40% of these patients. As stated earlier, the rate of locoregional recurrence depends on the extent of lymphadenectomy, with lower rates after D2 lymphadenectomy compared with D1. The most common sites of locoregional recurrence are the gastric remnant at the anastomosis, in the gastric bed, and in the regional nodal basins. The predominant sites of systemic recurrence are the liver and peritoneum.

Although all patients should be followed systematically, the evidence for how this should occur is unclear, and there is currently no evidence that more intensive follow-up improves long-term survival. The NCCN recommends a complete history and physical examination every 3 to 6 months for 1 to 2 years, then every 6 to 12 months for 3 to 5 years. Laboratory tests, including complete blood count and chemistry profile, should be performed as clinically indicated. Given the nutritional sequelae of gastrectomy, iron studies and levels of vitamin B_{12} and vitamin D can also be obtained. Postgastrectomy patients are at risk of calcium loss, so bone density tests should be performed for those at risk of osteopenia and osteoporosis. For patients with pathologic stage II or higher disease, CT chest/abdomen/pelvis should be obtained every 6 months for the first 2 years, then annually up to 5 years, and for all patients as indicated if there is clinical suspicion of recurrence. Sensitivity for detecting peritoneal recurrence is low. Patients remain at risk for second primary gastric cancers after partial gastrectomy and should undergo surveillance with upper endoscopy; typically, the first surveillance EGD will be 1 year after resection, then every other year thereafter, or as indicated clinically. For patients who were successfully treated with endoscopic resection, endoscopy should be performed every 6 months for 1 year, then annually for 3 years.

GASTROINTESTINAL STROMAL TUMOR

Epidemiology and Mutational Patterns

GI stromal tumors (GISTs) are the most common mesenchymal neoplasm of the GI tract. Gastric GISTs can manifest at any age, although they typically manifest in patients older than 50 years. Approximately 5% of GISTs are associated with an underlying heritable mutation such as familial GIST syndrome (mutation in KIT or PDGFRA), neurofibromatosis type 1, or Carney-Stratakis syndrome (GIST and paraganglioma with or without pulmonary chondroma). Originally thought to be a type of smooth muscle sarcoma, they are now known to be a distinct tumor derived from the interstitial cells of Cajal, GI pacemaker cells that reside in the muscularis propria layer. The incidence was difficult to assess previously given variable histologic definitions. However, since the discovery of KIT (CD117), DOG1, and CD34 expression in GIST, more accurate estimates range from 7 to 15 cases per million per year. KIT is a receptor tyrosine kinase, and approximately 95% of GISTs express KIT. KIT mutations are identified in 75% to 85% of GISTs. Most GISTs that lack a KIT mutation will have a mutation in platelet-derived growth factor receptor alpha (PDGFRA). Of the small KIT- and PDGFRA-wild-type subset, many are succinate dehydrogenase (SDH) deficient. Although GISTs can appear anywhere within the GI tract, they most commonly arise in the stomach (40%–60%), small intestine (20%–40%), and colon/rectum (5%–15%). GISTs vary considerably in their presentation and clinical course, ranging from small, very slow-growing tumors to massive lesions with necrosis, hemorrhage, and wide

metastases. Their pathology, presentation, and management as they relate to the stomach are discussed here.

Diagnosis and Workup

Most GISTs manifest with nonspecific symptoms, typically with early satiety, bloating, or vague abdominal pain. Bleeding can occur and is generally in the form of melena or, less frequently, frank hematemesis. Tumor rupture with intraabdominal hemorrhage is uncommon, but when it occurs, it may require emergent surgical intervention. Many patients remain asymptomatic, and their tumors are discovered incidentally with cross-sectional imaging performed for other indications.

Patients are evaluated with upper endoscopy, on which a smooth-appearing, round, submucosal tumor can be identified, occasionally containing an area of central ulceration. Upper endoscopy may be normal when tumors are exophytic. Because of the submucosal nature of the tumor, obtaining tissue for histologic and immunohistochemical analysis via conventional endoscopic forceps biopsy results in a low diagnostic yield. EUS-directed FNA or fine-needle biopsy (FNB) results in superior diagnostic accuracy, with a sensitivity of >80% and specificity of 100% in diagnosing GIST. Given the expense and specialized expertise involved in performing EUS-directed FNA, in addition to the fact that most submucosal GI tumors require surgical resection regardless of histology, some experts have argued that routine preoperative pathologic diagnosis is not needed for such tumors. Presently, preoperative biopsy is not recommended if there is a high suspicion for GIST and the patient is otherwise operable, but it is preferred if there is metastatic disease or if the patient is being considered for neoadjuvant therapy. CT of the abdomen and pelvis with IV contrast is used to assess for metastatic disease. MRI is preferred in patients who cannot receive IV contrast or for rectal GISTs. Pathologically, GISTs can either have a spindle cell or epithelioid appearance. Immunohistochemical staining for CD117, DOG1, CD34, and/or PDGFRA is used to confirm the diagnosis.

Treatment

Surgery

The mainstay of treatment is complete surgical resection. Tumors that are symptomatic or greater than 2 to 3 cm in diameter should be resected, but the treatment for smaller tumors is controversial. Tumors that are less than 2 to 3 cm but that have high-risk features on endoscopy and EUS, such as irregular borders, ulceration, echogenic foci, and heterogeneity, should be resected, whereas tumors without such features can be observed with repeat endoscopy and EUS at 6- to 12-month intervals. Depending on tumor size and location, resection can include wedge resection, sleeve gastrectomy, segmental, or, rarely, total gastrectomy, with or without en bloc resection of adjacent organs. GISTs generally have noninfiltrative margins; thus, a 1-cm gross margin of normal tissue almost always results in a negative margin. GISTs rarely metastasize to lymph nodes, so lymphadenectomy is not needed. These tumors are often friable and prone to rupture, so tumors should be handled carefully intraoperatively to avoid rupture and spillage of tumor cells.

As with gastric adenocarcinoma, minimally invasive approaches are acceptable for resection of GISTs provided that oncologic principles are not compromised. For gastric GISTs, size and location are the main factors affecting surgical approach. In particular, smaller tumors that are distant from the GE junction and from the pylorus are most amenable to laparoscopic or robotic resection. NCCN guidelines state that a minimally invasive approach may be considered for select GISTs in favorable anatomic locations by surgeons with appropriate minimally invasive experience.

Adjuvant and Neoadjuvant Therapy

GISTs can metastasize to the liver and to the peritoneal cavity. Locoregional recurrence after surgical resection is rare. Gastric GISTs carry a more favorable prognosis compared with GISTs in other locations in terms of recurrence. The two primary prognostic factors for gastric GISTs are tumor size and mitotic rate. Based on a long-term follow-up study of 1700 patients with gastric GISTs, metastatic potential based on the combination of these two factors has been established.[72] These factors also predict the likelihood of recurrence after surgery for gastric GISTs.[73]

Adjuvant therapy for GIST changed dramatically with the discovery of the tyrosine kinase inhibitor (TKI) imatinib (Gleevec). Originally designed to treat chronic myelogenous leukemia, it has proven in RCTs to be an effective treatment modality for patients with GIST. The ACOSOG Z9001 phase III, placebo-controlled, randomized trial of 713 patients with c-kit+ tumors 3 cm or larger who underwent complete resection found that patients treated with imatinib for 1 year had a significantly improved 1-year recurrence-free survival (98% vs. 83%, $P < 0.0001$).[74] This difference was even more pronounced for patients with larger tumors. The Scandinavian Sarcoma Group XVIII trial compared an extended 36-month course of adjuvant imatinib with a 12-month course after resection for 400 patients with high-risk GISTs (defined as >10 cm tumor, mitotic count >10/50 high-power field [HPF], both tumor >5 cm and mitotic count >5 per 50 HPF, or tumor rupture). In the second planned analysis of the trial, patients in the extended treatment arm had higher 5-year recurrence-free survival (71.1% vs. 52.3%, $P < 0.001$) and OS (91.9% vs. 85.3%, $P = 0.036$).[75] The results of these trials have established a 3-year course as the standard of care after surgical resection of high-risk GIST, though longer duration of therapy is being explored, as it appears the protective effect of imatinib does not persist after drug discontinuation. Imatinib appears to prevent microscopic residual disease from growing but does not eradicate it. Thus, some oncologists recommend lifelong therapy for those at moderate to high risk of harboring microscopic disease.

Imatinib has also been reported to be successful in the neoadjuvant treatment of patients with nonmetastatic but unresectable disease, in some cases resulting in conversion to resectability. Currently, patients with locally advanced, borderline resectable disease or in whom tumor shrinkage would increase the likelihood of organ preservation should also be considered for neoadjuvant therapy. As stated previously, patients with limited metastatic disease can be offered neoadjuvant imatinib followed by possible metastasectomy based on clinical response.

Patients presenting with recurrent or metastatic disease are primarily treated with imatinib or a second-line TKI (see later), but a subset of patients may benefit from surgical intervention. Two trials addressing this question were begun in Europe and in China, but both failed to recruit quickly enough to meet target accrual. In the absence of randomized trials, single-institution and multi-institutional retrospective studies document long-term disease control and longer OS for selected patients with limited metastatic disease who undergo metastasectomy. In general, resection appears to benefit responding patients (i.e., those who have a partial response, stable

disease, or focal progression and possibly those with isolated sites of progression) but has little to offer those who experience generalized or multifocal disease progression while receiving a TKI. A series of 323 patients found that response to neoadjuvant imatinib predicted clinical response after metastasectomy.[76] Among the patients receiving imatinib, radiographic response at the time of surgery was predictive of both progression-free survival (PFS) and OS after surgery:

- Responsive disease—Median PFS 36 months, median OS not reached
- Stable disease—Median PFS 30 months, median OS 110 months
- Unifocal progressive disease—11 months, median OS 59 months
- Multifocal progressive disease—6 months, median OS 24 months

Patients with responsive or stable disease had a median PFS of 30 to 36 months, whereas those with unifocal or multifocal progressive disease had median PFS of only 6 to 11 months. Some surgeons propose that patients be treated for 6 to 9 months with neoadjuvant systemic therapy and subsequently evaluated for surgery if the disease appears completely grossly resectable. Although it has been shown that tumor load continues to decrease even after 1 year of imatinib, the median time to best response is 3.5 months, and there is little incremental tumor shrinkage after 9 months. The timing of surgery in this setting is typically 6 to 9 months after initiation of neoadjuvant therapy. Restaging imaging is useful to plan for surgery at the time of maximal response. Patients with isolated liver metastases can be considered for liver metastasectomy, radiofrequency ablation, hepatic artery embolization, chemoembolization, or radioembolization using yttrium-90–tagged microspheres, radiofrequency ablation, or hepatic arterial embolization, which have shown some benefit in nonrandomized series.

Fig. 87.9 is an algorithm for using imatinib in the treatment of GISTs in the neoadjuvant, adjuvant, and palliative settings. Patients who progress on imatinib or are intolerant to the drug are typically offered second-line TKIs such as sunitinib or regorafenib, although the duration of PFS is shorter on subsequent-line TKIs compared with first-line imatinib.

Relative differences in sensitivity to TKIs based on KIT and PDGFRA mutational status have been recognized for over 20 years based on in vitro data and subgroup analyses of imatinib trials (Fig. 87.10). KIT exon 11 mutations are most common and are most sensitive to imatinib therapy, whereas KIT exon 9 mutations are rarer and more imatinib resistant; however, increased imatinib doses can improve response in KIT exon 9 mutant GISTs. Other KIT mutations, including those in exon 13 and 17, occur most commonly as secondary events in the setting of imatinib resistance. PDGFRA mutations tend to have poor responses to imatinib, particularly the D842V mutation. First-line TKI therapy in patients with PGDFRA D842V mutations should be avapritinib based on a phase I trial that achieved a 91% radiographic response rate in this population.[77] An algorithm for TKI treatment in advanced GIST is depicted in Fig. 87.10.

GASTRIC LYMPHOMA

Epidemiology

The stomach is the most common site of extranodal lymphoma. However, primary gastric lymphoma is still relatively uncommon, accounting for approximately 3% of gastric cancers. Patients often present with vague symptoms, such as epigastric pain, early satiety, and fatigue. Constitutional B symptoms (i.e., fevers, night

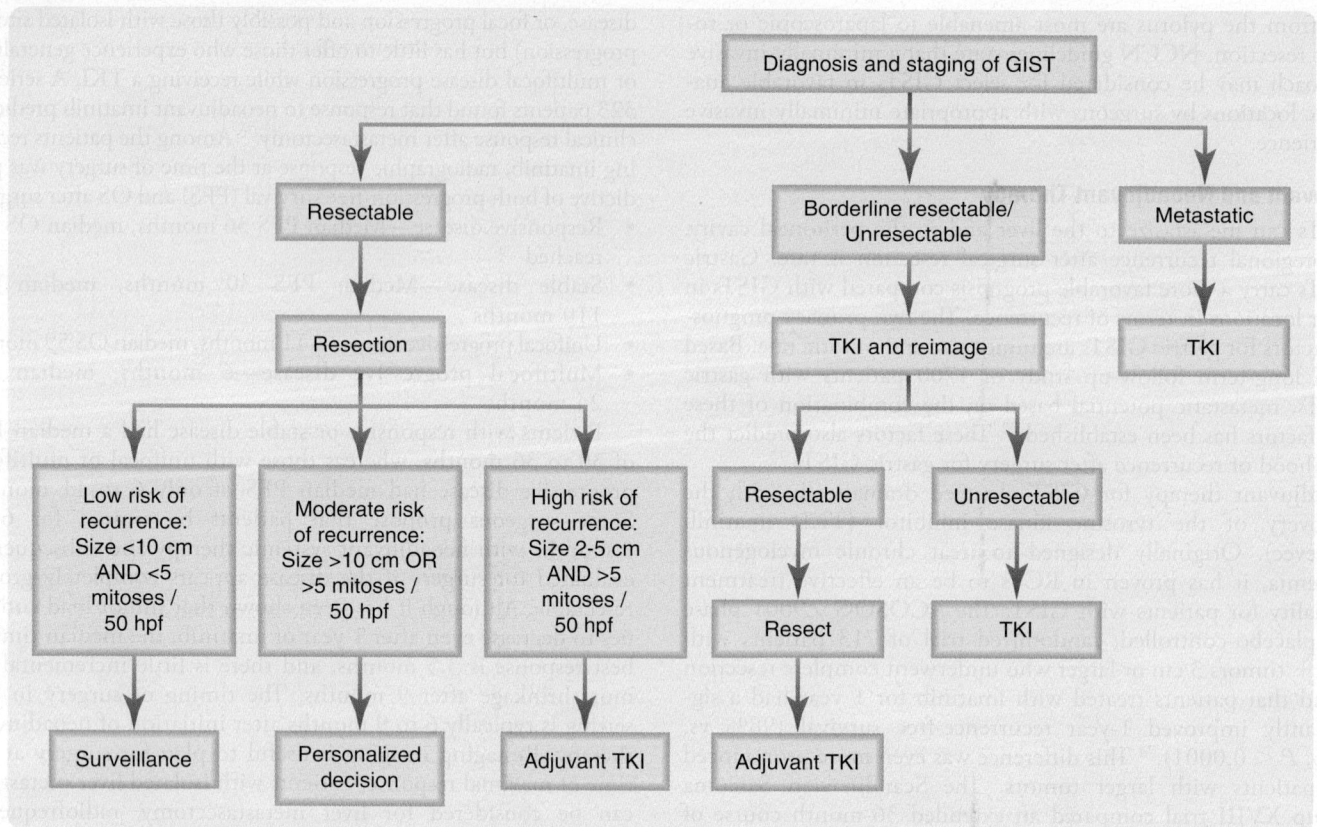

FIGURE 87.9 Algorithm for use of tyrosine kinase inhibitors *(TKIs)* in gastric GI stromal tumor *(GIST).* *hpf,* High powered field.

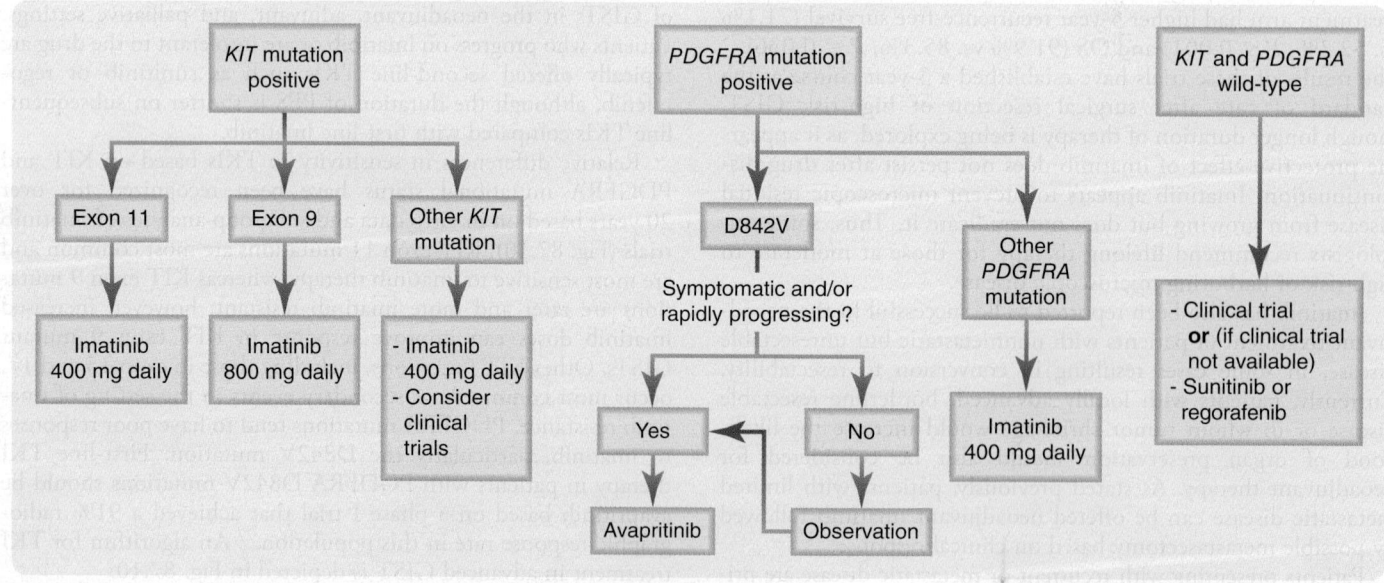

FIGURE 87.10 Tyrosine kinase inhibitor therapy for advanced gastrointestinal stromal tumors.

GASTRIC LYMPHOMA

Epidemiology

sweats) occur in only about 10% of patients. Lymphomas occur in older patients, with the peak incidence in the sixth and seventh decades, and there is a slight male predominance. Gastric lymphomas usually occur in the gastric alntrum but can arise from any part of the stomach. Patients are considered to have primary gastric lymphoma if the stomach is the exclusive or predominant site of disease. Several conditions have been shown to be associated with gastric lymphoma, including *H. pylori* infection, certain autoimmune diseases (i.e., rheumatoid arthritis, systemic lupus erythematous), immunosuppression, and celiac disease.

Pathology

In the management of gastric lymphomas, as in the management of nodal lymphomas, it is important to determine not only the stage of disease but also the subtype of lymphoma. There are many classification systems for lymphomas (Table 87.6). The most common gastric lymphoma is diffuse large B-cell lymphoma (DLBCL; 45%–60%), followed by gastric mucosa-associated lymphoid tissue (MALT) lymphoma (40%–50%). Less commonly, peripheral T-cell lymphoma (1%–4%) and mantle cell and follicular lymphomas (both <1%) are seen.

DLBCLs are generally primary lesions; however, they may also occur from progression of less aggressive lymphomas, such as chronic lymphocytic leukemia, small lymphocytic lymphoma, follicular lymphoma, and MALT lymphoma. Immunodeficiency and *H. pylori* infection are risk factors for the development of primary DLBCL.

Evaluation and Staging

Endoscopy with biopsy is indicated for workup of patients with suspected gastric lymphoma. Occasionally, a submucosal growth pattern renders endoscopic biopsies nondiagnostic. EUS is useful to determine the depth of gastric wall invasion and to evaluate for regional lymph node involvement. Evidence of distant disease should be sought through upper airway examination to evaluate the Waldeyer tonsillar ring, bone marrow biopsy, and PET/CT to detect lymphadenopathy. Biopsies should be performed of enlarged lymph nodes. Histologic *H. pylori* testing should be performed and, if negative, confirmed by serology. Staging is important both for prognosis and treatment decision-making. The modified Lugano staging system is the most widely used for gastric lymphoma (Table 87.7).

Treatment

Surgeons should be aware that gastric lymphoma rarely requires surgical resection either for diagnosis or treatment.

Diffuse Large B-Cell Lymphoma Oncologists use multiagent chemotherapy regimens for patients with gastric lymphoma. The most common chemotherapeutic combination is R-CHOP (rituximab, cyclophosphamide, hydroxydaunomycin [doxorubicin], Oncovin [vincristine], prednisone). A prospective randomized study evaluated several treatment strategies—surgical resection, resection plus radiation, resection plus chemotherapy, chemotherapy alone—in patients with early stage (stage IE or II1) disease.[78] The addition of chemotherapy was essential, with the surgery plus chemotherapy and chemotherapy-alone groups having significantly higher OS than the surgery-alone and surgery plus radiation groups. However, the addition of surgery to chemotherapy did not improve outcomes and increased morbidity. Thus, the primary role of surgery is currently limited to patients with symptomatic recurrence after treatment failure and patients who develop complications, such as bleeding, gastric outlet obstruction, or perforation. Chemotherapy for gastric lymphoma is associated with a 5% rate of gastric perforation and GI bleeding.

Mucosa-Associated Lymphoid Tissue Lymphoma

Gastric MALT lymphoma is lower grade than DLBCL and is usually preceded by *H. pylori*–induced gastritis. Evidence of *H. pylori* infection can be found in almost every case of gastric

TABLE 87.6 Comparison of Gastrointestinal Lymphoma Classifications

WHO CLASSIFICATION	REAL	WORKING	LUKES-COLLINS	KIEL	RAPPAPORT
Extranodal marginal zone lymphoma (MALT lymphoma)	—	Small-cleaved cell type	Small-cleaved cell type	Immunocytoma	Well-differentiated lymphocytic
Follicular lymphoma	Follicular center lymphoma	Small-cleaved cell type	Small-cleaved cell type	Centroblastic-centrocytic, follicular and diffuse	Nodular, poorly differentiated lymphocytic
Mantle cell lymphoma	—	—	—	Centrocytic	Intermediately or poorly differentiated lymphocytic, diffuse or nodular
Diffuse large B-cell lymphoma	Diffuse large B-cell lymphoma	Large-cleaved follicular center cell	Large-cleaved follicular center cell	Centroblastic, B-immunoblastic	Diffuse mixed lymphocytic and histiocytic
Burkitt lymphoma	Burkitt lymphoma	Small-noncleaved follicular center cell	Small-noncleaved follicular center cell	Burkitt lymphoma with intracytoplasmic immunoglobulin	Undifferentiated lymphoma, Burkitt type

TABLE 87.7 Lugano Staging System for Gastrointestinal Lymphoma

STAGE	DESCRIPTION
I	Tumor confined to gastrointestinal tract
IE1	Involvement of mucosa ± submucosa
IE2	Involvement of muscularis propria ± serosa
II	Tumor extension into abdomen
II$_1$	Involvement of local nodes (paragastric for gastric lymphoma)
II$_2$	Involvement of distal nodes (paraaortic, paracaval, pelvic, or inguinal)
IIE	Serosa penetration to involve adjacent organs/tissues
IV	Disseminated extranodal involvement or supradiaphragmatic nodal involvement

MALT lymphoma. Genetically, MALT lymphoma is characterized by four chromosomic translocations: t(1;14), t(3;14), t(11;18), and t(14;18). The t(1;14), t(11;18), and t(14;18) translocations result in increased nuclear factor-κB activity, with resultant enhanced cell survival. The t(3;14) translocation increases FOXP1 transcription factor levels, which has been shown to expand marginal zone B cells.

Given the strong association with *H. pylori* and the low-grade MALT lymphoma, patients should be evaluated for active infection. Patients with early stage MALT lymphomas and active *H. pylori* infection may be effectively treated by *H. pylori* eradication alone. Successful eradication results in remission in more than 75% of cases. However, careful follow-up is necessary, with repeat endoscopy in 2 months to document clearance of the infection and biannual endoscopy for 3 years to document regression. Some patients continue to demonstrate the lymphoma clone after *H. pylori* eradication, suggesting that the lymphoma became dormant rather than disappearing. The presence of transmural tumor extension, nodal involvement, transformation into a large cell phenotype, and nuclear BCL-10 expression all predict failure after *H. pylori* eradication alone. Additionally, some patients with MALT lymphoma are *H. pylori*–negative. In these patients, consideration should be given to radiation therapy (if all the involved sites can be encompassed in a single field) and chemotherapy. A recent MALT lymphoma prognostic index was developed that identified three primary risk factors: age of 70 or above, stage IV disease, and elevated lactate dehydrogenase (LDH) level. The 5-year OS rates were 98.7% for no risk factors, 93.1% for one risk factor, and 64.3% for two to three risk factors ($P < 0.0001$).[79]

GASTRIC NEUROENDOCRINE TUMORS

Gastric neuroendocrine tumors (NETs), also referred to as *carcinoid tumors,* are a rare malignancy that arise from neuroendocrine precursor cells and can manifest at any site in the body. The most common sites in the GI tract are the small intestine, rectum, and appendix. The stomach is becoming an increasing common site of NETs, now representing 8% of tumors. This increasing incidence is thought to be due to a combination of improved surveillance and the widespread use of PPIs. Unlike other GI tract NETs, gastric NETs are typically nonfunctioning and rarely cause carcinoid syndrome.

There are three distinct subtypes of gastric NETs (Table 87.8). Type I gastric NETs are the most common, accounting for 70% to 80% of cases. They are associated with chronic achlorhydria from atrophic gastritis or autoimmune gastritis, leading to chronically elevated gastrin levels. Type I gastric NETs are typically seen as multiple small tumors confined to the mucosa and submucosa with a relatively benign course and favorable prognosis.

The tumors are derived from enterochromaffin-like (ECL) cells. It is thought that ECL cells develop into NETs after chronic stimulation by high gastrin levels. This is supported by the observation that regression of gastric NETs can be achieved by antrectomy, which is occasionally recommended. Patients with type I gastric NETs are usually diagnosed in their 60s or 70s during endoscopic evaluation. They are more common in females. Endoscopically, the tumors are usually smaller than 1 cm, are often multiple, and may appear as polypoid lesions with a small central ulceration. These tumors are usually indolent and generally represent a benign condition. Type II gastric NETs are associated with hypergastrinemia in the setting of gastrinomas (Zollinger-Ellison syndrome), typically of the pancreas or duodenum, and often in the setting of multiple endocrine neoplasia type 1 (MEN1). They account for 5% to 10% of gastric NETs. These tumors are also thought to arise from ECL cells stimulated by elevated serum gastrin levels. Type III gastric NETs are known as *sporadic NETs* because they are independent of gastrin level. They account for 20% of gastric NETs and are the most aggressive. Nodal or hepatic metastases are present in up to 65% of patients who come to resection.

Diagnosis of gastric NET is established on EGD with biopsy of the lesion. EUS can be performed subsequently to assess for depth of invasion. Based on North American Neuroendocrine Tumor Society recommendations,[80] gastric pH and serum gastrin levels should be obtained; for type I, antiintrinsic factor and anti–parietal cell antibodies help confirm the diagnosis. Chromogranin A levels may be elevated and serve as a biomarker for type III tumors, but false positives can result from PPI use and renal insufficiency. CT or MRI should be used to evaluate for metastatic disease for type II and type III tumors. Somatostatin-receptor imaging (most commonly ^{68}Ga-DOTATATE PET/CT) can be useful in some instances, such as evaluation of metastatic disease, but need not be obtained routinely.

Management of type I gastric NETs is usually endoscopic resection and surveillance, and surgery is reserved only for tumors that cannot be managed endoscopically. For type II lesions <1 cm, surveillance or endoscopic removal is indicated. For those >1 cm in size, endoscopic removal with subsequent endoscopic surveillance is recommended. For large polyps (>2 cm in size), complete removal may not be possible endoscopically; in that case, or in cases of six or more large polyps, wedge resection or partial gastrectomy may be required. In patients with type II NETs, gastrinoma resection should be performed as well, if possible. Patients with localized type III NETs should undergo oncologic resection with lymphadenectomy. For patients with recurrent or metastatic disease, somatostatin analogues or chemotherapy can be used to decrease the burden of disease and treat carcinoid syndrome. Liver-directed therapies, including

TABLE 87.8	**Gastric Carcinoid Types**			
	TYPE I		**TYPE II**	**TYPE III**
Percentage of gastric NETs	70%–80%		5%–10%	10%–15%
Associated pathology	Pernicious anemia, prolonged PPI use		ZES, MEN1	n/a
Location	Fundus or body		Fundus, body, antrum	Fundus or antrum
Tumor number	Multiple		Multiple	Single
Gastric acid level	Low		High	Normal
Serum gastrin level	High		High	Normal
Prognosis	Excellent		Good	Poor

MEN1, Multiple endocrine neoplasia type 1; *NETs,* neuroendocrine tumors; *PPI,* proton pump inhibitor; *ZES,* Zollinger-Ellison syndrome.

ablation and embolization, may be useful in cases of liver-dominant metastasis. Peptide receptor radionuclide therapy (PRRT), which is a form of systemic radiotherapy using radionuclides coupled with a somatostatin analog, is a newer modality available for treatment of NETs expressing the somatostatin receptor and is useful in cases of metastatic disease and carcinoid syndrome.

HETEROTOPIC PANCREAS

Heterotopic pancreas (i.e., functioning pancreatic tissue is found in an abnormal anatomic location) is found in 0.5% to 14% of autopsy specimens. The most common location is within the stomach, typically along the antral greater curvature. Symptomatic patients generally present with vague abdominal pain. There have been reports of pancreatitis, islet cell tumors, and pancreatic adenocarcinoma within these lesions. On endoscopy and CT, they are frequently small submucosal masses and may be confused with a GIST or some other gastric neoplasm. The treatment is surgical excision, and the diagnosis is confirmed pathologically.

HYPERTROPHIC GASTRITIS (MÉNÉTRIER DISEASE)

Ménétrier disease (hypoproteinemic hypertrophic gastropathy) is a rare disease (<1000 reported cases) characterized by massive gastric folds in the fundus and body of the stomach, giving the mucosa a cobblestone or cerebriform appearance. The antrum is typically spared. Histologic examination reveals foveolar hyperplasia (expansion of surface mucus cells), with decreased or absent parietal cells. The condition is also associated with protein loss from the stomach, excessive mucus production, and hypochlorhydria or achlorhydria. The cause of Ménétrier disease is unknown, but it has been associated with cytomegalovirus infection in children and *H. pylori* infection in adults. Also, increased levels of transforming growth factor-α have been noted in the gastric mucosa of patients with the disease, which can stimulate epithelial cell growth and inhibit gastric acid secretion. Patients often present with epigastric pain, vomiting, weight loss, decreased appetite, and peripheral edema. Typical gastric mucosal changes can be detected by radiographic or endoscopic examination. Biopsy should be performed to establish the diagnosis and to rule out gastric carcinoma or lymphoma. Medical treatment yields inconsistent results; however, some benefit has been shown with the use of acid suppression, octreotide, and cytomegalovirus or *H. pylori* eradication. Total gastrectomy should be performed in patients who continue to have massive protein loss despite optimal medical therapy and high-protein diet, continue to have intractable pain, or if dysplasia or carcinoma develops. One series estimated 73% OS at 5 years and 65% at 10 years after diagnosis, with a 9% risk of gastric cancer after 10 years of follow-up. Given the increased risk of gastric neoplasms in patients with Ménétrier disease, patients should undergo endoscopic surveillance every 1 to 2 years.

SELECTED REFERENCES

Cancer Genome Atlas Research Network. Comprehensive molecular characterization of gastric adenocarcinoma. *Nature*. 2014;513(7517):202-209.

Cristescu R, Lee J, Nebozhyn M, et al. Molecular analysis of gastric cancer identifies subtypes associated with distinct clinical outcomes. *Nat Med*. 2015;21(5):449-456.

These two major transcriptomic studies used molecular classifiers to identify subgroups of gastric adenocarcinoma with distinct clinical features and outcomes. The Cancer Genome Atlas classification system identified Epstein-Barr virus–positive (EBV), microsatellite instability (MSI), genomically stable (GS), and chromosomal instability (CIN) subtypes. In the current era of immunotherapy, MSI status (and, to a lesser extent, EBV status, because of its relative rarity) is now used as a predictor of response to checkpoint inhibition therapy.

Cunningham D, Allum WH, Stenning SP, et al. Perioperative chemotherapy versus surgery alone for resectable gastroesophageal cancer. *N Engl J Med*. 2006;355(1):11-20.

Al-Batran SE, Homann N, Pauligk C, et al. Perioperative chemotherapy with fluorouracil plus leucovorin, oxaliplatin, and docetaxel versus fluorouracil or capecitabine plus cisplatin and epirubicin for locally advanced, resectable gastric or gastro-oesophageal junction adenocarcinoma (FLOT4): a randomised, phase 2/3 trial. *Lancet*. 2019;393(10184):1948-1957.

These two large randomized controlled trials established the benefit of perioperative chemotherapy on overall survival in gastric adenocarcinoma. The earlier MAGIC trial used pre- and postoperative epirubicin, cisplatin, and 5-FU (ECF), resulting in improved overall survival compared with surgery alone. The subsequent FLOT4 trial showed that pre- and postoperative 5-FU, leucovorin, oxaliplatin, and docetaxel (FLOT) resulted in improved overall survival compared with the ECF regimen.

DeMatteo RP, Ballman KV, Antonescu CR, et al. Adjuvant imatinib mesylate after resection of localised, primary gastrointestinal stromal tumour: a randomised, double-blind, placebo-controlled trial. *Lancet*. 2009;373(9669):1097-1104.

Joensuu H, Eriksson M, Sundby Hall K, et al. Survival outcomes associated with 3 years vs 1 year of adjuvant imatinib for patients with high-risk gastrointestinal stromal tumors: an analysis of a randomized clinical trial after 10-year follow-up. *JAMA Oncol*. 2020;6(8):1241-1246.

These two major randomized controlled trials established the role of adjuvant imatinib after surgical resection for the treatment of localized GIST. The first study by DeMatteo and colleagues showed significantly less recurrence in patients who received imatinib compared with patients who did not; this was especially pronounced for patients at high risk of developing metastatic disease. The second trial by Joensuu and colleagues showed that a 36-month course of adjuvant imatinib was superior to a 12-month course in terms of disease-free and overall survival. These studies established long-term adjuvant treatment with imatinib as the standard of care for patients with GISTs. The optimal length of adjuvant treatment for intermediate- and high-risk GISTs remains controversial.

Miettinen M, Sobin LH, Lasota J. Gastrointestinal stromal tumors of the stomach: a clinicopathologic, immunohistochemical, and molecular genetic study of 1765 cases with long-term follow-up. *Am J Surg Pathol*. 2005;29(1):52-68.

Gold JS, Gönen M, Gutiérrez A, et al. Development and validation of a prognostic nomogram for recurrence-free survival after complete surgical resection of localised primary gastrointestinal stromal tumour: a retrospective analysis. *Lancet Oncol.* 2009;10(11):1045-1052.

> These two retrospective studies in large cohorts identified prognostic factors associated with metastasis and recurrence of GISTs. Both studies identified tumor size and mitotic rate as negative prognostic factors. Currently, risk stratification and recommendation for or against adjuvant tyrosine kinase inhibitor therapy is based on these factors.

Mocellin S, McCulloch P, Kazi H, Gama-Rodrigues JJ, Yuan Y, Nitti D. Extent of lymph node dissection for adenocarcinoma of the stomach. *Cochrane Database Syst Rev.* 2015;2015(8):CD001964.

> The appropriate extent of lymphadenectomy for gastric adenocarcinoma was a subject of debate for many years, with most Western centers favoring D1 lymphadenectomy and East Asian centers favoring more extensive D2 or even D3 lymphadenectomy. Randomized clinical trials in both Western and Eastern centers, as described in this Cochrane review, have now converged on D2 lymphadenectomy as providing appropriate N staging with an acceptable safety profile. In long-term follow-up, D2 lymphadenectomy is associated with improved cancer-specific survival compared with D1.

The full reference list appears on Elsevier eBooks+.

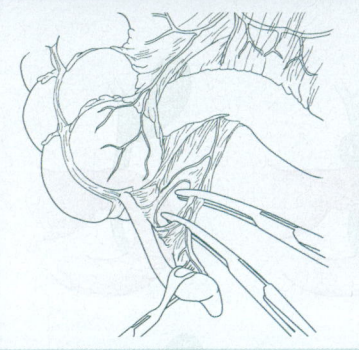

CHAPTER 88

Biliary System

Bryan Clary, Ryan Broderick, August B. Schaeffer, Jennifer Moffett, and Rebekah White

ANATOMY AND PHYSIOLOGY

Anatomic variations in biliary anatomy and of the vascular structures in the hepatoduodenal ligament are common, occurring in up to 30% of patients. The optimal management of patients with biliary tract diseases is highly dependent on a thorough understanding of both normal anatomy and the common variations.

The common bile duct (CBD) lies anterior to the hepatic arteries (proper hepatic artery and right hepatic artery) and portal vein in the duodenohepatic ligament (Fig. 88.1). At the level of the hilum the biliary bifurcation abuts the base of segment IVB of the liver and assumes a location superior to the intrahepatic branches of the portal vein and hepatic arteries. The left hepatic duct retains a longer transverse extrahepatic portion and travels under the edge of segment IVB from the umbilical fissure to the biliary bifurcation making it more surgically accessible. The left duct drains segments I, II, III, and IV, with the most distal branch draining segment IVA. Further superolateral, the ducts draining segment IVB arise, and yet further up the left duct are the ducts for segments II and III. These ducts can generally be found just posterior and lateral to the umbilical recess. The caudate lobe drains through smaller ducts that typically enter the right and left hepatic duct systems. In normal variant anatomy, there are two principal right hepatic duct systems (right anterior duct and right posterior duct) that join to form a short main right hepatic duct. The right anterior sectoral duct runs in a vertical direction to drain segments V and VIII, whereas the right posterior sectoral duct follows a horizontal course to drain segments VI and VII. In approximately 20% of patients the right posterior sectoral duct courses posterior to the right anterior duct to join the left

hepatic duct. The right posterior duct in a small minority of patients has a lower entry point into the CBD making it susceptible to injury during cholecystectomy. The common variations in the main hepatic duct are depicted in Fig. 88.2.

The gallbladder is a partially intraperitoneal structure that lies attached to the undersurface of the liver on segments IVB and V. It is 7 to 10 cm in length; holds 30 to 60 mL of bile as a reservoir; and is divided into neck, infundibulum with Hartmann pouch, body, and fundus (see Fig. 88.1). On the side of the gallbladder that is attached to the liver, there is no peritoneal covering; a fibrous lining known as the *cystic plate* occupies this space. Bile is drained via a cystic duct to the CBD. The cystic duct can range from 1 to 5 cm in length and drains at an acute angle into the CBD. There are numerous variations in this insertion all along the length of the CBD, even including into the right hepatic duct (Fig. 88.3). The valves of Heister, which are folds of mucosa oriented in spiral pattern within the neck of gallbladder, function to retain bile in the gallbladder until contraction in response to enteric stimulation.

The common hepatic duct is anatomically defined as the segment of the extrahepatic bile duct below the biliary bifurcation and above the cystic duct insertion. Given the variability of the insertion of the cystic duct as described earlier, it is often more practical to divide the common duct system into proximal (within 2 cm of the bifurcation), distal CBD (coursing behind the duodenum and intrapancreatic), and mid-CBD (between the proximal and distal CBD segments). The distal CBD courses behind the first portion of the duodenum to enter into a groove on the posterior surface of the superior pancreatic head before joining the pancreatic duct and ending in the ampulla. The pancreatic duct also joins the ampulla, although in variants it may have a separate orifice (Fig. 88.4).

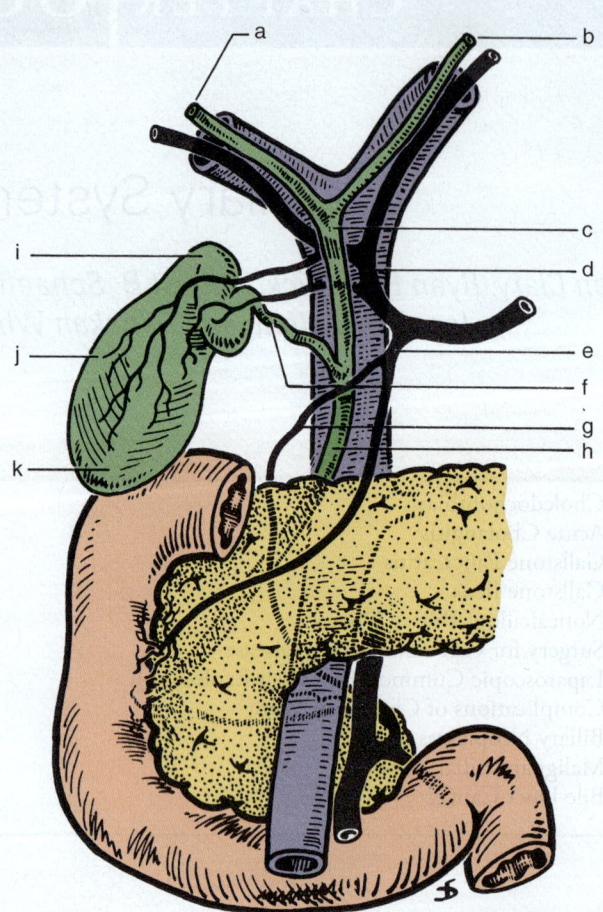

FIGURE 88.1 Extrahepatic biliary anatomy: *a*, right hepatic duct; *b*, left hepatic duct; *c*, common hepatic duct; *d*, hepatic artery; *e*, gastroduodenal artery; *f*, cystic duct; *g*, retroduodenal artery; *h*, common bile duct; *i*, neck of the gallbladder; *j*, body of the gallbladder; *k*, fundus of the gallbladder.

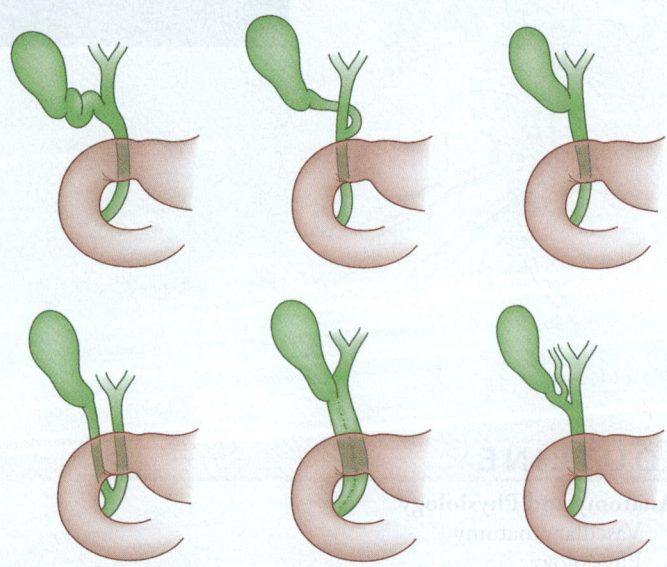

FIGURE 88.3 Variability in cystic duct anatomy. Knowledge of these variations is important to avoid inadvertent injury to the biliary tree during cholecystectomy.

Vascular Anatomy

As described by Couinaud,[1] the hepatic parenchyma is divided into lobes, each of which is divided into lobar segments to define the basic hepatic anatomic resections. The blood supply to the entire biliary tree is solely arterial in contrast with the hepatic parenchyma, where dual perfusion also comes from the portal vein, which makes the biliary tree susceptible to ischemic injury. The cystic artery normally arises from the right hepatic artery, and similar to the variability of the cystic duct, it may arise from the right hepatic, left hepatic, proper hepatic, common hepatic, gastroduodenal, or superior mesenteric artery. The cystic artery can pass posterior or anterior to the CBD to supply the gallbladder.

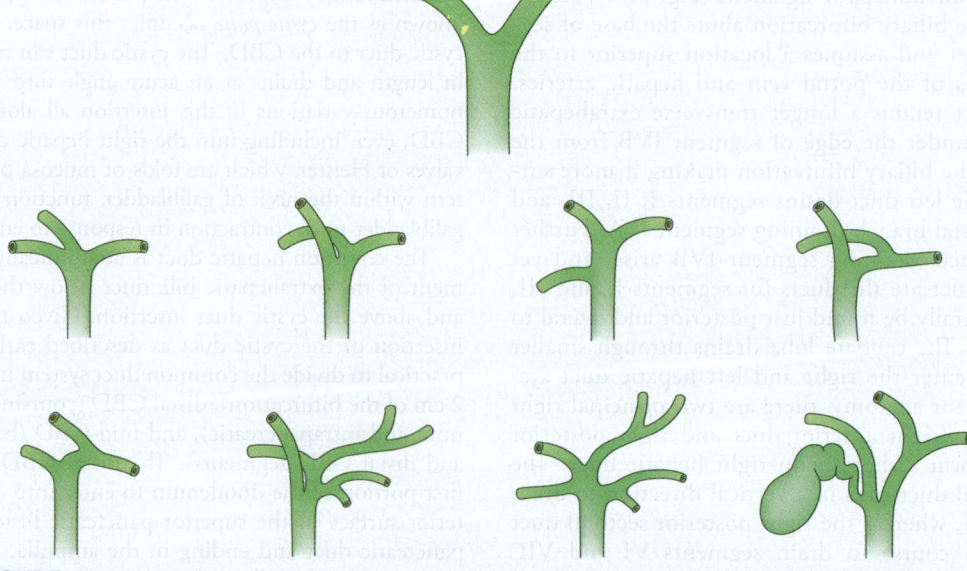

FIGURE 88.2 Variability in hepatic duct anatomy. Knowledge of these variations is important to avoid inadvertent injury to the biliary tree during liver resection.

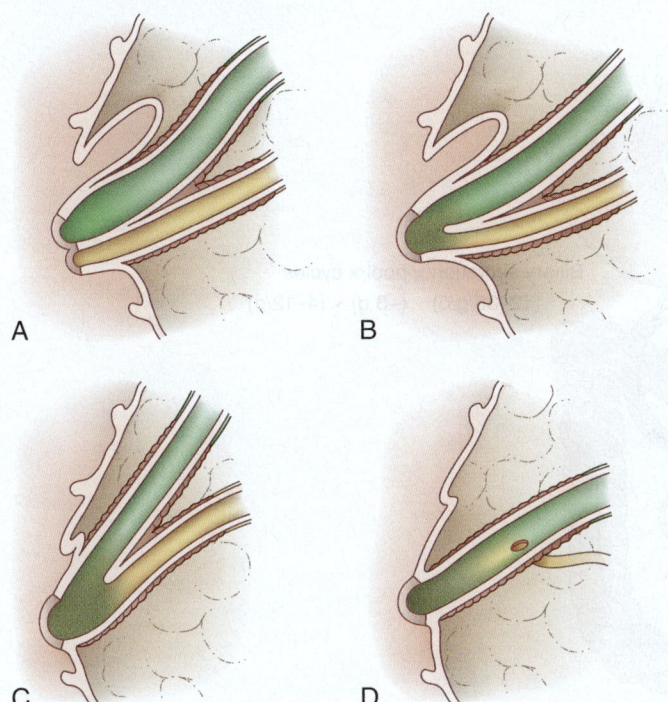

FIGURE 88.4 Patterns of biliary duct–pancreatic duct junction and insertion into the duodenal wall. (A) Separate common bile duct (CBD) and pancreatic duct (PD) entry. (B) Joining ducts at the ampulla. (C) Joining ducts before the ampulla. (D) PD entering the CBD.

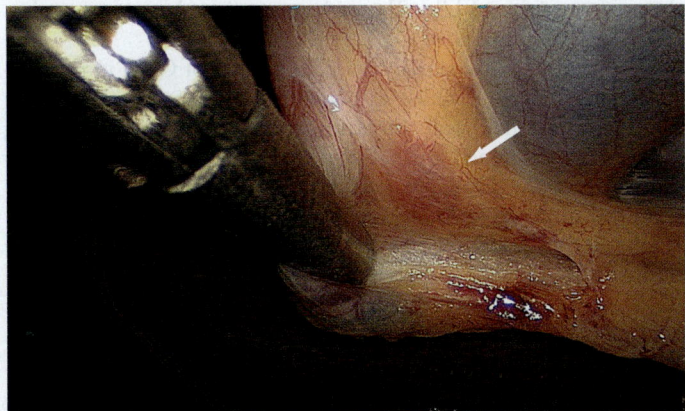

FIGURE 88.5 Operative photograph of Calot node. This node *(arrow)* is useful for identification of the common location of the cystic artery.

Although variable, the cystic artery generally lies superior to the cystic duct and is usually associated with a lymph node known as *Calot node* (Fig. 88.5). This node can be enlarged in the setting of gallbladder disease, whether inflammatory or neoplastic, because it provides the lymphatic drainage of the gallbladder.

The blood supply of the common hepatic duct and CBD comes from the right hepatic and cystic arteries. Typically, the right hepatic artery passes posterior to the common hepatic duct to supply the right lobe of the liver. It passes through the triangle of Calot (bordered by the cystic duct, common hepatic duct, and edge of the liver) after crossing the duct. The cystic artery takes off from the right hepatic artery in this triangle, which is at risk for injury during cholecystectomy. In performing a cholecystectomy, limiting the dissection to the right of the node of Calot helps minimize the risk of injury to the right hepatic artery and adjacent CBD.

It is important to remember that in 20% of the population, there is an accessory or replaced right hepatic artery passing through the portacaval space and ascending to the right lobe along the posterior and right lateral aspect of the CBD. A pulsatile structure palpated on the most lateral aspect of the porta during a Pringle maneuver identifies this anomaly. In addition, it can be noted on computed tomography (CT) as a vessel passing transversely between the portal vein and inferior vena cava behind the head of the pancreas.

The perfusion to the inferior bile duct, below the duodenal bulb, comes from tributaries of the posterosuperior pancreaticoduodenal and gastroduodenal arteries. The small branches coalesce to form the two vessels that run along the CBD at the 3- and 9-o'clock positions. These vessels can be damaged and leave the bile duct at risk for ischemic injury with close dissection of the areolar tissue surrounding the bile duct.

Physiology

The smallest functional unit of liver is the hepatic lobule. It is created by four to six portal triads and identified by its central terminal hepatic venule. Each hepatocyte is encircled by bile canaliculi, which coalesce to form small bile ducts. Bile salts, such as cholic acid and deoxycholic acid, are originally created from cholesterol and secreted into bile canaliculi as cholic acid and its metabolite, deoxycholic acid. The liver actually makes only a small amount of the total bile salt pool used on a daily basis because most bile salts are recycled after use in the intestinal lumen, known as the *enterohepatic circulation* (Fig. 88.6). Bile is secreted into canaliculi directly from hepatocytes. Once the bile components are secreted into the bile canaliculi, the tight junctions in the biliary tree keep these components within the bile secretory pathway. The secretion of bile components into the biliary tree is a major stimulus to bile flow, and the volume of bile flow is an osmotic process. Because bile salts combine to form spherical pockets, known as *micelles,* the salts themselves provide no osmotic activity. Instead, the cations that are secreted into the biliary tree along with the bile salt anion provide the osmotic load to draw water into the duct and to increase flow to keep bile electrochemically neutral. For this reason, bile maintains an osmolality approximately comparable to that of plasma.

After passage into the intestinal tract and reabsorption by the terminal ileum, bile acids are transported back to the liver for recycling bound to albumin. On the opposite side from the canalicular surface of the hepatocyte lies the sinusoidal surface, which contacts the space of Disse. In this contact area, the hepatocyte absorbs the circulating components of bile, an important step in the enterohepatic circulation. The passage of reabsorbed bile salts bound to albumin through the space of Disse allows uptake into the hepatocyte in an efficient process that involves sodium cotransport and sodium-independent pathways. In the less specific sodium-independent pathway, a number of organic anions are transported, including unconjugated and indirect bilirubin. The transport of bile salts across the canalicular membrane remains the rate-limiting step in bile salt excretion. Given the vast differences in concentration of bile salts, the transport of bile up an extreme concentration gradient is adenosine triphosphate dependent. Less than 5% of bile salts are lost each day in the stool. When sufficient quantities of bile salts reach the colonic lumen, the powerful detergent activity of the bile salts can cause inflammation and diarrhea. This can sometimes be seen after a cholecystectomy when the speed of the enterohepatic circulation of bile increases and may overwhelm the ability of the terminal ileum to absorb bile salts.

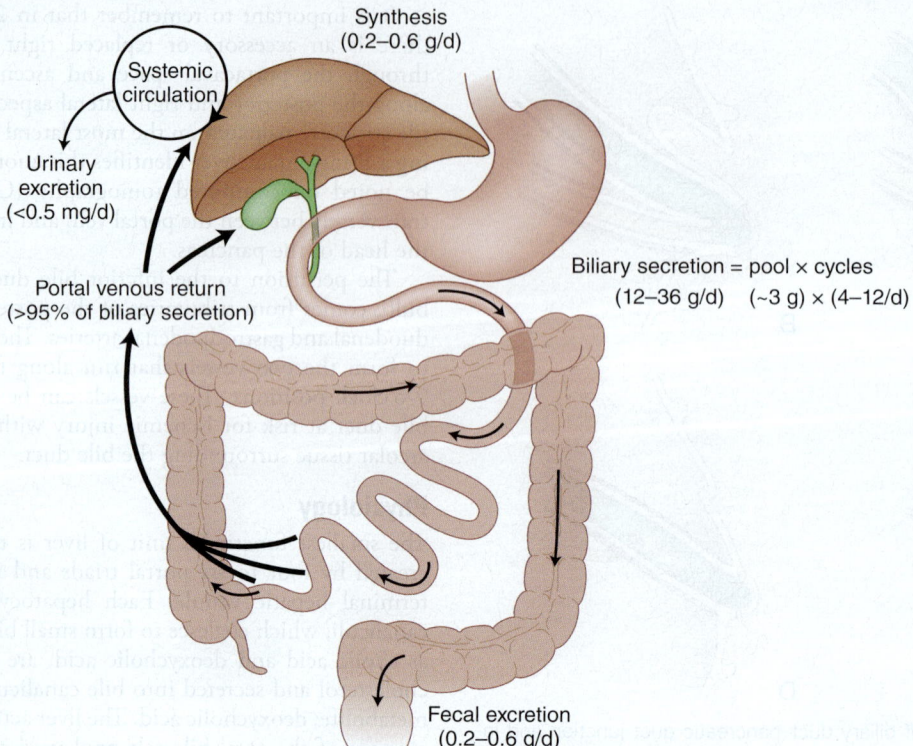

Synthesis
(0.2–0.6 g/d)

Systemic
circulation

Urinary
excretion
(<0.5 mg/d)

Portal venous return
(>95% of biliary secretion)

Biliary secretion = pool × cycles
(12–36 g/d)   (~3 g) × (4–12/d)

Fecal excretion
(0.2–0.6 g/d)

FIGURE 88.6 Enterohepatic circulation.

In addition to bile salts, bile contains proteins, lipids, and pigments. The major lipid components of bile are phospholipids and cholesterol. These lipids dispose of cholesterol from low- and high-density lipoproteins and serve to protect hepatocytes and cholangiocytes from the toxic nature of bile. The sources of most biliary cholesterol are circulating lipoproteins and hepatic synthesis. Therefore, the biliary secretion of cholesterol actually serves to excrete cholesterol from the body.

Aside from absorption of nutrients from the intestinal tract, bile secretion from the liver serves an opposing function, namely, excretion of toxins and metabolites from the liver. Bile pigments such as bilirubin are breakdown products of hemoglobin and myoglobin. These products are bound to albumin and transported in the blood to hepatocytes. Inside hepatocytes, they will be transferred into the endoplasmic reticulum and conjugated to form bilirubin glucuronides, known as *conjugated* or *direct* bilirubin. Bile pigment gives the color of bile and, when converted to urobilinogen by bacterial enzymes, gives stool its characteristic color.

Much of the bile flow is dependent on neural, humoral, and chemical stimuli. Vagal activity induces bile secretion as does the gastrointestinal hormone secretin. Cholecystokinin (CCK), secreted by the intestinal mucosa, serves to induce biliary tree secretion and gallbladder wall contraction, thereby augmenting excretion of bile into the intestines. Secreted bile will pass through the biliary tree into the intestine and be reabsorbed. The gallbladder serves as an extrahepatic storage site of bile, absorbing water and concentrating bile in an osmotic process performed through the active sodium transport. With the absorption of sodium and water across the gallbladder epithelium, the chemical composition of bile changes in the gallbladder lumen. Increases in cholesterol and calcium concentration lead to decreased stability of phospholipid cholesterol vesicles. The reduced vesicle stability predisposes to nucleation of this stagnant pool of cholesterol Tract, thus, to cholesterol stone formation. The gallbladder neck and cystic duct

also secrete glycoproteins to help protect the gallbladder from the detergent activity of bile. These glycoproteins also promote cholesterol crystallization.

An increase in the activity of the sphincter of Oddi in the fasting state (Fig. 88.7), whose musculature is independent from the duodenal intestinal wall, increases pressure in the CBD, filling the gallbladder, which is capable of storing up to 300 mL of daily bile production, through a retrograde mechanism. This muscular sphincter normally maintains high tonic and phasic activity, which is inhibited by CCK. The passage of fat, protein, and acid into the duodenum induces CCK secretion from duodenal epithelial cells.

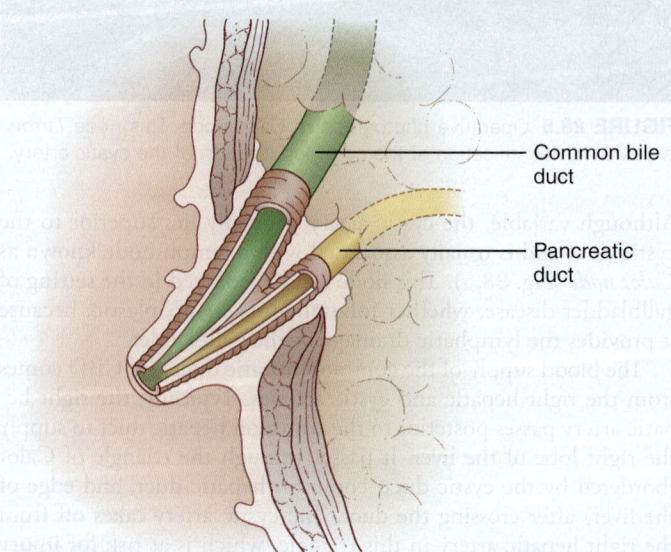

Common bile
duct

Pancreatic
duct

FIGURE 88.7 Sphincter of Oddi. Because the sphincter is responsible for control of most bile flow, this sphincter maintains a high tonic contraction but is inhibited by cholecystokinin.

CCK, as its name suggests, then causes gallbladder contraction, with intraluminal pressures up to 300 mm Hg. Vagal activity also induces gallbladder emptying but is a less powerful stimulus to gallbladder contraction than CCK. At the same time, CCK induces relaxation of the sphincter, causing bile flow more readily from the biliary tree. Coordinated with gallbladder contraction, the relaxation of this sphincter allows evacuation of up to 70% of the gallbladder contents within 2 hours of CCK secretion. During the fasting state, the oblique passage of the bile duct through the duodenal wall and the tonic activity of the sphincter prevent duodenal contents from refluxing into the biliary tree.

DIAGNOSTIC MODALITIES

Laboratory Tests

Laboratory studies are an integral part in the diagnosis and management of both benign and neoplastic pathologies. Both normal and abnormal results can illuminate the underlying disease process; however, it should be noted that there is no single laboratory test that can confirm or exclude a diagnosis, and adjunct tests including imaging should be considered.

Complete Blood Count

A complete blood count (CBC) is recommended for patients being evaluated for biliary disease. The diagnosis of cholecystitis is aided by the presence of leukocytosis, but it is not required. An elevated white blood cell count (WBC) serves as a systemic sign of inflammation, suggesting a diagnosis of acute cholecystitis or cholangitis when seen with biliary obstruction. When assessing the severity scores for a patient with acute cholecystitis, a WBC count of greater than 18,000/mm^3 is classified as grade II (moderate) acute cholecystitis per the 2018 Tokyo Guidelines and portends a worse prognosis.[2] In general, an elevated WBC in the setting of suspected biliary pathology should raise alarms.

Hepatic Function Panel

A hepatic function panel, or liver function test (LFT), investigates a number of metabolic and functional aspects of the liver and biliary system. Hyperbilirubinemia could be secondary to conjugated bilirubin, possibly due to obstruction, or secondary to unconjugated hyperbilirubinemia caused by increased synthesis, impaired hepatocyte uptake of unconjugated bilirubin, and decreased intracellular conjugation. Although this is an oversimplification of a complex process, derangements up to and including conjugation will be manifested as elevated unconjugated bilirubin levels. Elevation in serum bilirubin caused by obstruction of the biliary system will be identifiable first in the frenulum of the tongue, followed by the sclera (where the level of bilirubin must reach 2.5 mg/dL to be observed), and followed by the skin (minimum serum bilirubin of 5 mg/dL).

In cases of severe acute cholecystitis, pericholecystic and periductal inflammation can lead to mild elevations of total bilirubin (<3 mg/dL). Additionally, significant gallbladder distention can obstruct the extrahepatic biliary ducts leading to mild jaundice. The most common cause of biliary obstruction is choledocholithiasis, although Mirizzi syndrome, strictures, and malignancy should be considered in the differential.

Elevations in alkaline phosphatase (ALP) occur in response to cholestasis with minimal elevations in the parenchymal enzymes alanine aminotransferase (ALT) and aspartate aminotransferase (AST). This pattern is referred to as a *cholestatic pattern,* as opposed to a *hepatocellular pattern,* which is suggestive of a hepatocyte physiology where the derangement is primarily an elevation in AST and ALT. However, it is important to note that significant elevations (especially elevated ALT) can be observed in some instances of biliary obstruction due to choledocholithiasis.

Unique Markers

Additional tests in the diagnosis of biliary diseases include gamma-glutamyl transferase (GGT), which can aid in the diagnosis of choledocholithiasis with a sensitivity and specificity of 90% and 85%, respectively.[3] Unlike the traditional LFTs, GGT levels increase earlier and persist longer in diseases that cause a cholestatic process, which makes it a potentially useful screening test. Carbohydrate antigen 19-9 (CA 19-9) is a tumor marker used in the diagnosis and prognostication of pancreaticobiliary malignancies. It can also be elevated in benign obstructions of the bile duct and should be interpreted with caution when suspecting a benign process.[4]

Imaging Studies

Plain Films

Historically, findings of pneumobilia, intestinal obstruction, and a stone in the right lower quadrant on abdominal x-ray (Rigler's triad) were pathognomonic for gallstone ileus. Plain radiographic films are of limited use in the overall evaluation of biliary disease as gallstones are not regularly observed by this modality. Therefore, the role of plain radiographs in the evaluation of biliary disease is limited to the exclusion of other diagnoses, such as a gastric or duodenal ulcer with free air, small bowel obstruction, or right lower lobe pneumonia causing right upper quadrant pain.

Ultrasound

Transabdominal ultrasound (US) is a sensitive, inexpensive, reliable, and reproducible test and is recommended as the first-choice imaging method for the initial evaluation of jaundice or symptoms of biliary disease. Although US has a high specificity and sensitivity for detecting gallstones (>95%), a meta-analysis revealed a sensitivity of 81% and specificity of 83% in the diagnosis of acute cholecystitis.[2] The gallbladder is easily evaluated by US due to its superficial location with no overlying bowel gas. The density of gallstones allows crisp reverberation of the sound wave, showing an echogenic focus with a characteristic shadowing behind the stone (Fig. 88.8). Most gallstones, unless impacted, will move promptly with positional changes in the patient. This characteristic allows their differentiation from gallbladder polyps, which are fixed in position, and from sludge, which moves more slowly, and do not have the sharp echogenic pattern of gallstones.

Pathologic changes of gallbladder disease can be identified by US. For example, the stigmata of cholecystitis includes gallbladder wall thickening and pericholecystic fluid, which are visible by US (Fig. 88.9). The sonographer may elicit a Murphy sign during the examination by pressing the probe into the right upper quadrant during inspiration eliciting cessation of inspiration. US can also assess dilation of the CBD in the setting of jaundice, which suggests obstruction of the duct and can be seen with choledocholithiasis, cholangitis, and malignant obstructions like cholangiocarcinoma (Fig. 88.10). Unlike a CT scan, US only provides a single slice view of the CBD, and therefore may underestimate CBD dilation. Rarely, a CBD stone may be visualized by US in the setting of choledocholithiasis.

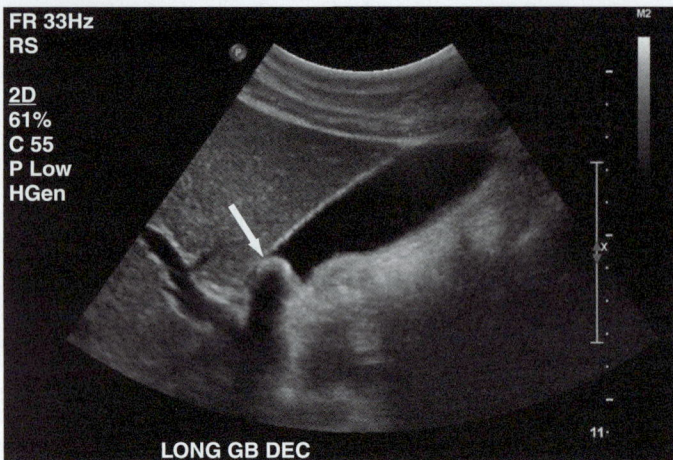

FIGURE 88.8 Ultrasound image of a gallstone in the gallbladder neck. The sharp echogenic wall of the gallstone *(arrow)*, with the characteristic posterior shadowing stripe under the stone, helps differentiate it from other intraluminal findings.

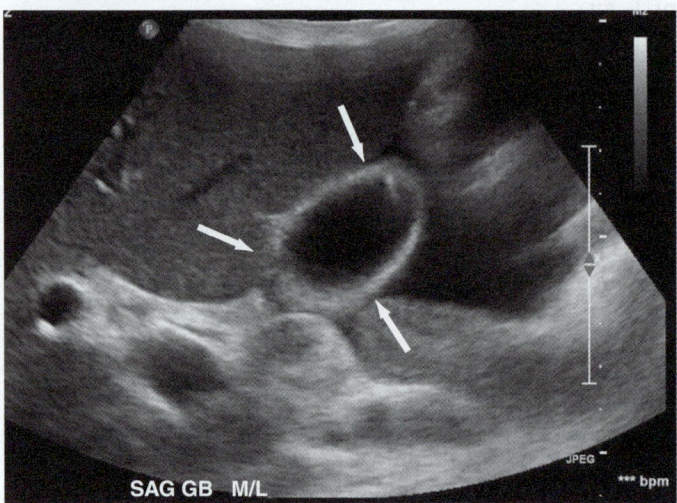

FIGURE 88.9 Ultrasound image with acute cholecystitis and thickened gallbladder wall *(arrows)*.

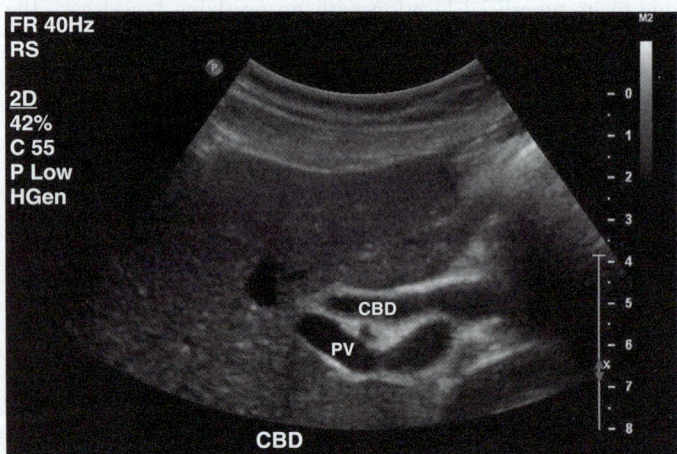

FIGURE 88.10 Ultrasound image of dilated biliary tree. The common bile duct *(CBD)* is dilated. As it travels parallel to the portal vein *(PV)*, it is easy to identify. The depiction of the parallel stripes of duct and vein helps ensure that the common duct diameter is not overestimated by a tangential view, which would artificially increase the anteroposterior diameter.

Computed Tomography

CT is an alternative imaging modality to evaluate biliary pathology. It provides superior anatomic detail given its ability to produce a high-resolution image of the surrounding anatomy. Because most gallstones are radiographically isodense to bile, many will be indistinguishable from bile. However, CT scans are more sensitive than US in the diagnosis of cholecystitis (90% vs. 80%).[5] As US provides no anatomic reconstruction of the biliary tree, CT can be used to identify the cause and site of biliary obstruction and is more sensitive when detecting ductal dilation seen with choledocholithiasis (Fig. 88.11).

CT should be strongly considered in the setting of obstructive jaundice when malignancy is suspected for the evaluation of hepatic and pancreatic parenchyma resulting in possible neoplastic processes. The addition of an arterial phase, portal venous phase, and delayed phase imaging, known as a *triple-phase CT*, is invaluable in preoperative planning for complex resections or reconstructions.

Cholescintigraphy

Although incapable of providing any precise anatomic delineation or ability to detect gallstones, cholescintigraphy, also known as a hepatic iminodiacetic acid (HIDA) scan, can be used to evaluate the physiologic secretion of bile. This test involves injection of the radiotracer iminodiacetic acid into the venous circulation, which is then processed in the liver and secreted into the biliary tree over several hours. Failure of the radiotracer to fill the gallbladder 2 hours after injection demonstrates obstruction of the cystic duct, as seen in acute cholecystitis, although false positives can occur in the fasting state (Figs. 88.12 and 88.13). Cholescintigraphy is extremely sensitive and specific (95% and 90%, respectively) for diagnosing acute cholecystitis. The HIDA scan can also help in confirming patency of the CBD and the presence of extraductal accumulation, indicating a leak of the biliary tree. Cholescintigraphy may also be useful in evaluating patients with biliary colic-type pain in the absence of stones. CCK is given during the

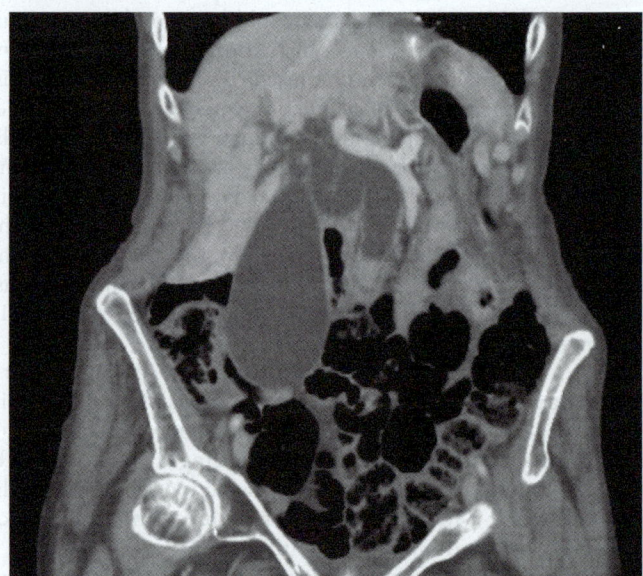

FIGURE 88.11 Computed tomography scan, coronal view, showing a dilated biliary tree and gallbladder with a distal filling defect of the common bile duct.

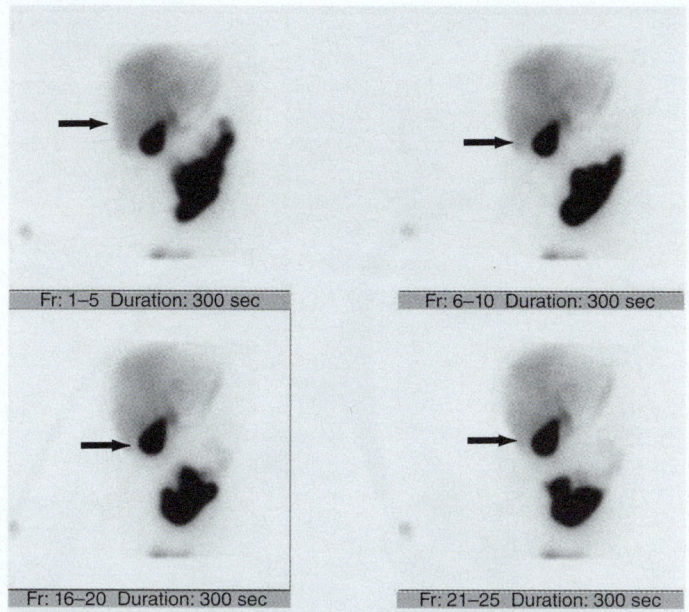

Fr: 1–5 Duration: 300 sec

Fr: 6–10 Duration: 300 sec

Fr: 16–20 Duration: 300 sec

Fr: 21–25 Duration: 300 sec

FIGURE 88.12 Hepatic iminodiacetic acid scan showing filling of the gallbladder. With gallbladder filling *(arrows)*, the diagnosis of acute cholecystitis is effectively eliminated.

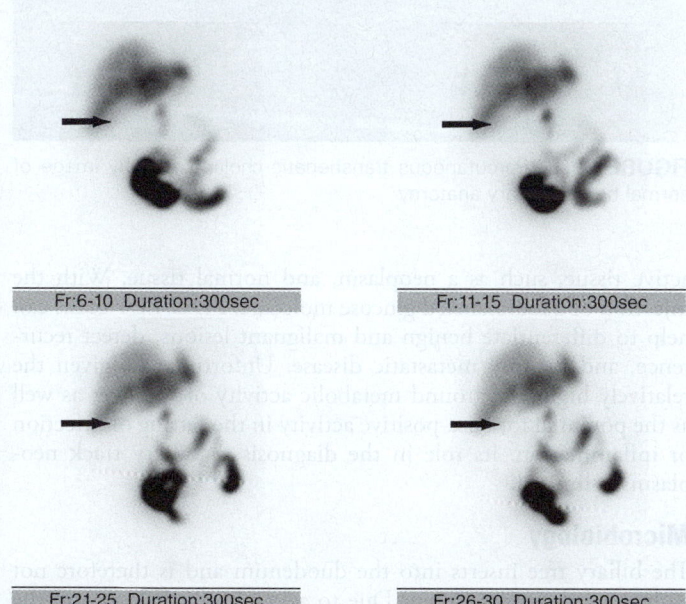

Fr:6-10 Duration:300sec

Fr:11-15 Duration:300sec

Fr:21-25 Duration:300sec

Fr:26-30 Duration:300sec

FIGURE 88.13 Hepatic iminodiacetic acid (HIDA) scan showing nonfilling of the gallbladder. With no filling of the gallbladder *(arrows)* even on delayed images, HIDA confirms occlusion of the cystic duct, the characteristic feature of acute cholecystitis.

scan to assess for physiologic ejection of the gallbladder, and a reduced ejection fraction (<35%) indicates impaired gallbladder emptying, known as *biliary dyskinesia*.

Magnetic Resonance Cholangiopancreatography

Magnetic resonance cholangiopancreatography (MRCP) is an imaging modality introduced in the early 1990s as a noninvasive method to create a high-resolution image of the biliary system. It uses water in bile to delineate the biliary tree, thus providing superior anatomic definition of the intrahepatic and extrahepatic

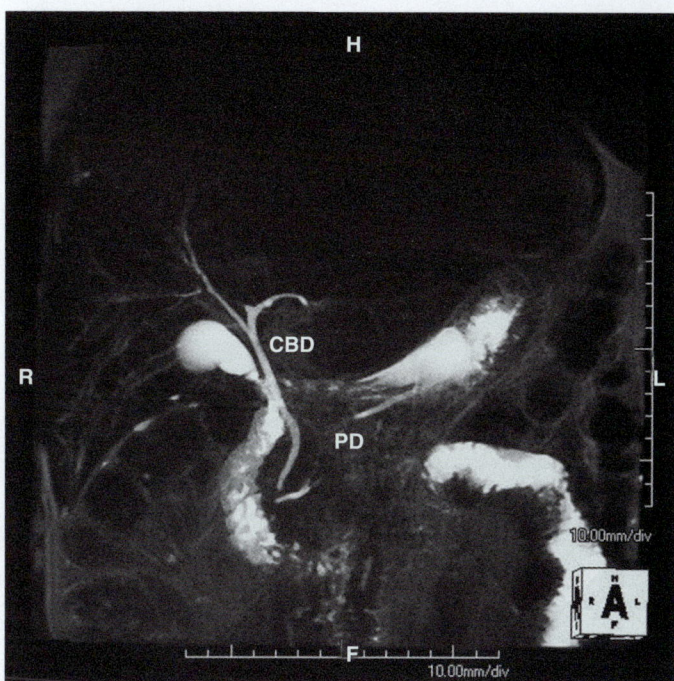

FIGURE 88.14 Normal magnetic resonance cholangiopancreatography image. Note the normal common bile duct *(CBD)* and pancreatic duct *(PD)*.

biliary tree and pancreas (Fig. 88.14). Unlike endoscopic retrograde cholangiopancreatography (ERCP), MRCP avoids ionizing radiation or an invasive procedure. For choledocholithiasis, it is a noninvasive option in patients with intermediate risk being considered for preoperative ERCP as it has significant diagnostic capacity (sensitivity of over 90% and specificity approaching 99%).[6] Its limitations include availability and inability to rule out a stone at the ampulla. This test is also useful in diagnosing and characterizing choledochal cysts, for planning resection of biliary or pancreatic neoplasms, and for the management of complex biliary disease.

Endoscopic Retrograde Cholangiopancreatography

ERCP, first described in 1968, is an invasive test using endoscopy and fluoroscopy to image the biliary tree (Fig. 88.15). A specialized endoscope with a side port is advanced into the duodenum to the ampulla of Vater. The ampulla is intubated, contrast is injected into the biliary tree, and fluoroscopic imaging is used to delineate biliary anatomy and identify biliary pathology. If stones are identified in the CBD, a sphincterotomy and/or sphincteroplasty may be performed with balloon sweeps to relieve obstruction. Although it does carry a complication rate of up to 10%, ERCP can diagnose and treat many diseases of the biliary tree and it has a greater than 90% stone clearance rate when treating choledocholithiasis. ERCP is also instrumental in the nonsurgical treatment of biliary duct injuries as the deployment of biliary stents diverts flow away from the injury to facilitate healing. For patients with a malignant obstruction, ERCP can provide tissue samples for diagnosis and temporize the obstruction with stenting. If biopsies are inconclusive and biliary malignancy remains highly suspected, retrograde cholangioscopy can be used to further evaluate the biliary tree and to obtain a tissue biopsy. When available, ERCP is a powerful tool in the treatment of biliary diseases.

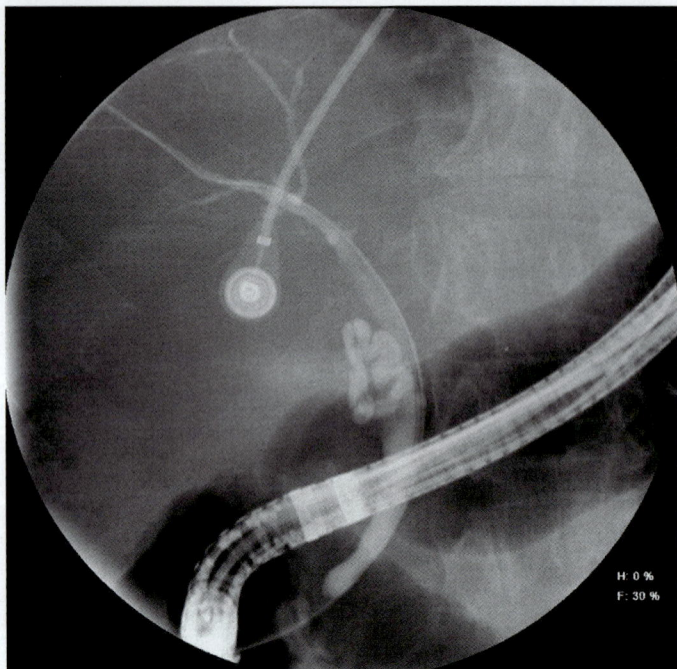

FIGURE 88.15 Normal endoscopic retrograde cholangiopancreatography image.

Endoscopic Ultrasound

Although of limited use in the evaluation of gallbladder disease or intrahepatic disease, endoscopic ultrasound (EUS) is a valuable tool to assess the distal CBD and ampulla. As it can be performed concurrently with ERCP, EUS is highly sensitive and specific (>95% and 90%, respectively) in the diagnosis of choledocholithiasis and can identify small and distal stones not seen on other imaging modalities such as MRCP.[7] It may also be used to assess neoplastic processes, including the degree of local invasion, in the distal biliary tree not well visualized with other techniques. Echoendoscopes are subdivided into those that scan perpendicular to the long axis of the endoscope, known as *radial echoendoscopes,* and those that scan parallel, known as *linear echoendoscopes.* Radial echoendoscopes are most useful for providing a tomographic evaluation, whereas linear echoendoscopes can guide interventions such as needle biopsies under real-time US guidance.

Percutaneous Transhepatic Cholangiography

Percutaneous transhepatic cholangiography (PTC) is an invasive radiologic procedure used to evaluate the biliary tree. Cannulation of the hepatic biliary ducts is performed by passing a needle percutaneously through the liver parenchyma into the biliary radicals under US guidance followed by contrast imaging of the biliary tree (Fig. 88.16). Image-guided access to the biliary tree can facilitate insertion of transhepatic catheters for drainage, biopsy, or stone extraction. This diagnostic and therapeutic technique can be instrumental in situations where decompression of the biliary tree is required and ERCP is not an option for anatomic, clinical, or resource reasons. However, in the setting of malignant obstruction and cholangitis, evidence suggests that endoscopic interventions have improved outcomes.[8]

Fluorodeoxyglucose Positron Emission Tomography

Fluorodeoxyglucose–positron emission tomography (FDG/PET) exploits the metabolic differences between a highly metabolically

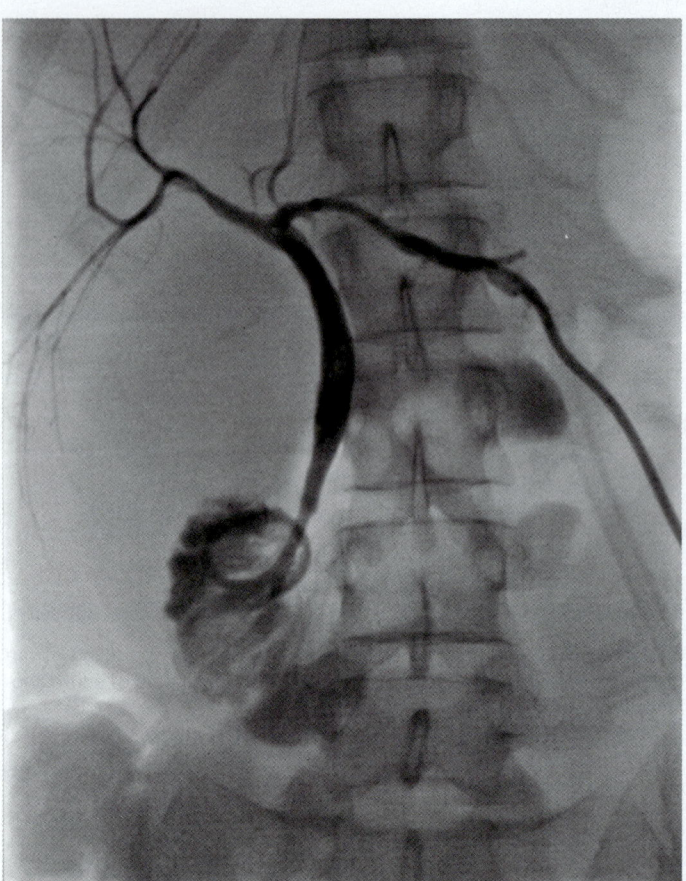

FIGURE 88.16 Percutaneous transhepatic cholangiography image of normal hepatic biliary anatomy.

active tissue, such as a neoplasm, and normal tissue. With the injection of a radiolabeled glucose molecule, FDG/PET scans can help to differentiate benign and malignant lesions, detect recurrence, and identify metastatic disease. Unfortunately, given the relatively high background metabolic activity of the liver as well as the potential for false-positive activity in the setting of infection or inflammation, its role in the diagnosis of biliary track neoplasms is limited.

Microbiology

The biliary tree inserts into the duodenum and is therefore not truly a sterile environment. Due to a low bacterial load and the flow of bile, infection in the absence of obstruction is rare, and the presence of stones or obstruction increases the likelihood of bacterial infection. There is a similarity in the microbiota of the duodenum and the biliary system, suggesting the bacteria that colonize the biliary tree arise from the upper enteric tract. Most bacteria isolated from the biliary tree are gram-negative or anaerobes. *Escherichia coli* followed by *Klebsiella* are the most common gram-negative bacteria isolated from the biliary tree and from blood cultures in cholangitis. The most common gram-positive bacteria associated with the biliary tract is *Enterococcus.*[9]

Biliary colic and choledocholithiasis do not have an infectious component to their pathology. Although cholecystitis is primarily an inflammatory process, cystic duct obstruction and biliary stasis can lead to a superimposed bacterial infection. Recommended regimens for antibiotic therapy include coverage for gram-negative bacteria and anaerobes, including piperacillin-tazobactam or a cephalosporin or fluoroquinolone with metronidazole for patients with a penicillin allergy. Even though there is no universally infectious process involved, the 2018 Tokyo Guidelines recommended antibiotic treatment before and at the time of cholecystectomy, whereas postoperative antibiotic use does not confer improved outcomes.[2]

BENIGN BILIARY DISEASE

Calculous Biliary Disease

Cholelithiasis is the most common disease of the gallbladder and biliary tree, affecting 10% to 15% of the population. Gallstones are generally classified into two major subtypes, cholesterol and pigment stones, depending on the principal solute that precipitates into a stone. More than 70% of gallstones in the United States are formed by precipitation of cholesterol and calcium, and pure cholesterol stones account for less than 10%. Pigment stones can be divided into black stones, as seen in hemolytic conditions and cirrhosis, and brown stones, which tend to be found in the bile ducts and are thought to be secondary to infection. The difference in color arises from incorporation of cholesterol into the brown stones. Because black pigment stones occur in hemolytic states from concentration of bilirubin, they are found almost exclusively in the gallbladder. Alternatively, brown stones can occur within the biliary tree and suggest a disorder of biliary motility and associated bacterial infection.

Four major factors explain most gallstone formation: supersaturation of secreted bile, concentration of bile in the gallbladder, crystal nucleation, and gallbladder dysmotility. High concentrations of cholesterol and lipid in bile secretion from the liver constitute one predisposing condition to cholesterol stone formation, whereas increased hemoglobin processing is seen in most patients with pigment stones. Once in the gallbladder, bile is concentrated further through the absorption of water and sodium, increasing the concentrations of the bile solutes and calcium. Bile salts act to solubilize cholesterol. With respect to cholesterol stones (Fig. 88.17), cholesterol precipitates out into crystals when the concentration in the gallbladder vesicles exceeds the solubility of cholesterol (Fig. 88.18).[10] Crystal formation is further accelerated by pronucleating agents, including glycoproteins and immunoglobulins. Finally, abnormal gallbladder motility can increase stasis in the gallbladder, allowing more time for solutes to precipitate in the gallbladder. Therefore, increased stone formation can be seen in conditions associated with impaired gallbladder emptying, such as in prolonged fasting states; with use of total parenteral nutrition; after vagotomy; with use of somatostatin analogues; and more recently with the use of GLP-1 receptor agonists for weight loss.[11]

Cholelithiasis is the most common disease of the gallbladder and biliary tree, affecting 10% to 15% of the population. Gallstones are generally classified into two major subtypes, cholesterol and pigment stones, depending on the principal solute that precipitates into a stone. More than 70% of gallstones in the United States are formed by precipitation of cholesterol and calcium, and pure cholesterol stones account for less than 10%. Pigment stones can be divided into black stones, as seen in hemolytic conditions and cirrhosis, and brown stones, which tend to be found in the bile ducts and are thought to be secondary to infection. The difference in color arises from incorporation of cholesterol into the brown stones. Because black pigment stones occur in hemolytic states from concentration of bilirubin, they are found almost

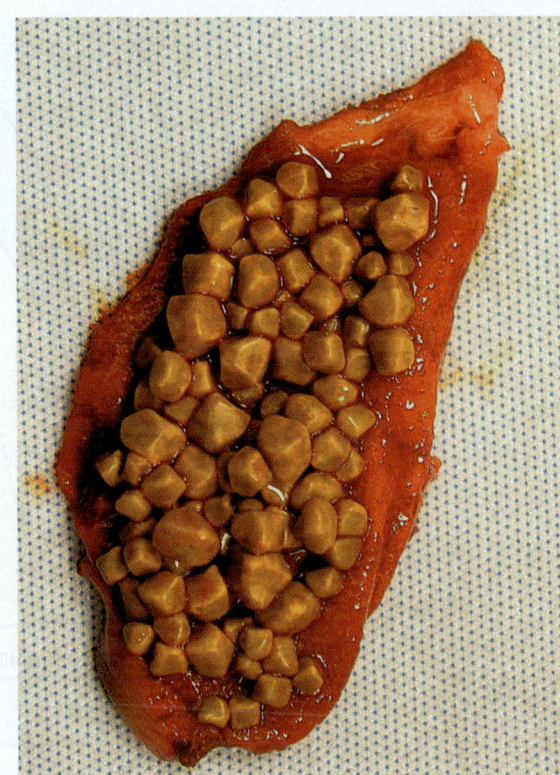

FIGURE 88.17 Gallbladder with characteristic yellow cholesterol stones.

exclusively in the gallbladder. Alternatively, brown stones can develop within the biliary tree and suggest a disorder of biliary motility and associated bacterial infection.

Natural History

Gallstones become symptomatic when they obstruct a visceral structure such as a cystic duct. More commonly, gallstones remain asymptomatic and are only found incidentally on imaging. Biliary colic, caused by temporary blockage of the cystic duct, tends to occur after a meal in which the secretion of CCK leads to gallbladder contraction. Stones that do not obstruct the cystic duct or pass through the entire biliary tree into the intestines without impaction do not cause symptoms. Only 20% to 30% of patients with asymptomatic stones will develop symptoms within 20 years, and because approximately 1% of patients with asymptomatic stones develop complications of their stones before onset of symptoms, prophylactic cholecystectomy is not warranted in asymptomatic patients.[12]

Certain subsets of patients, however, constitute a higher risk pool, so prophylactic cholecystectomy may be considered. Among these are patients with hemolytic anemias, such as sickle cell anemia. These patients have an extremely high rate of pigment stone formation, and cholecystitis can precipitate a crisis. Patients with a calcified gallbladder wall (known as *porcelain gallbladder*) and those with large (>3 cm) gallstones have a potentially higher risk of symptomatic disease or conversion to cancer and should consider cholecystectomy. Also, in diabetic patients with gallstones, one should have a lower threshold for cholecystectomy, considering higher rate of gangrene.

In the era of open Roux-en-Y gastric bypass, there was a higher incidence of prophylactic cholecystectomy for asymptomatic cholelithiasis due to technical considerations and complications with

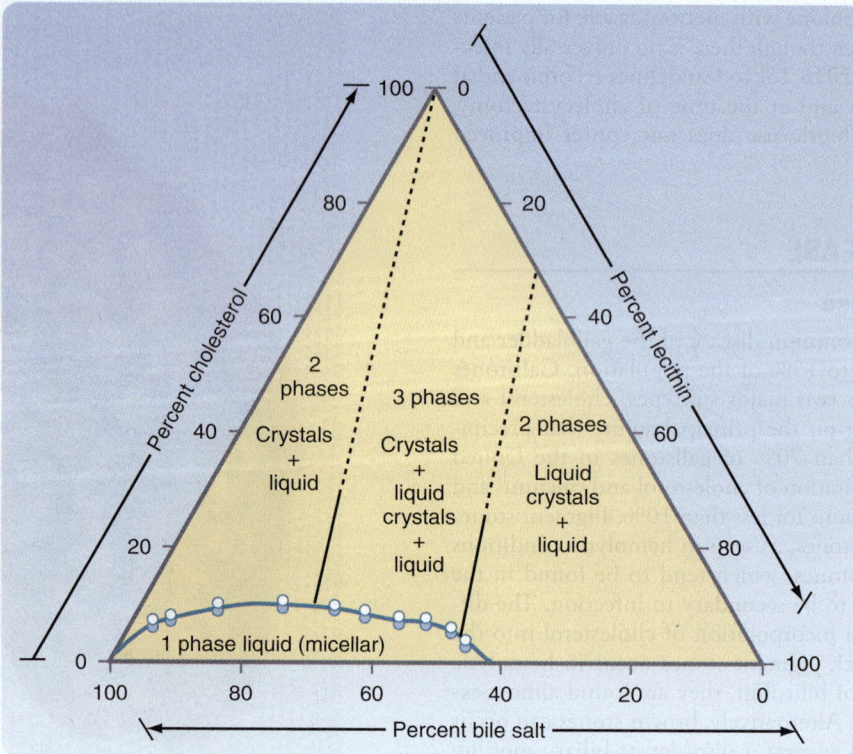

FIGURE 88.18 Triangle of solubility. With the three major components of bile that determine cholesterol solubility and stability, each can be quantified by molar percentage to show a relative ratio to the other two. Cholesterol is completely soluble in only the small area in the left lower corner, where a clear micellar solution exists, below the *closed circles*. Just above this, in the area between the *open* and *closed circles*, cholesterol is supersaturated but stable and thus crystallized only with stasis. In the remainder of the triangle, cholesterol is significantly supersaturated and unstable. In this region, crystals form immediately. (From Admirand WH, Small DM: The physicochemical basis of cholesterol gallstone formation in man. *J Clin Invest.* 1968;47:1043-1052.)

delayed cholecystectomy. There continues to be controversy over performing prophylactic concomitant cholecystectomy in patients undergoing minimally invasive bariatric surgery. In most cases, prophylactic cholecystectomy is not recommended. However, studies have shown that it is safe and effective for higher risk patients, or biliary colic patients, to have concomitant cholecystectomy at the time of metabolic bariatric surgery.[13] Rapid weight loss favors stone formation, but also, after gastric bypass, ERCP to remove CBD stones in ascending cholangitis can be challenging. Techniques for both laparoscopic and endoscopic management of CBD stones have improved over time, increasing success rates. Options for access to the biliary tree include laparoscopic-assisted access to the excluded stomach for which ERCP can be performed through a gastrotomy. Laparoscopic transcystic CBD exploration is described in detail later in the chapter. Newer endoscopic-only techniques include endoscopic stent placement between the pouch and gastric remnant to then perform ERCP through the stent (EUS-directed transgastric ERPC [EDGE procedure]).

Nonoperative Treatment of Cholelithiasis

Medical treatment of gallstones is mostly unsuccessful and includes oral bile salt therapy, contact dissolution that requires cannulation of the gallbladder and infusion of organic solvent, and extracorporeal shock wave lithotripsy. With the dissolution strategies, unacceptable recurrence rates of up to 50% limit their application to the most select group of patients. Extracorporeal

shock wave lithotripsy has a lower recurrence rate, approximately 20%, and can be used in patients with single stones 0.5 to 2 cm in size. Newer modalities include cystic duct embolization with chemical ablation of the gallbladder; studies on these techniques have low patient volumes but prove to be safe for patients who are not operative candidates.[14] The widespread use, safety, and efficacy of laparoscopic cholecystectomy have relegated nonoperative therapy to patients for whom general anesthesia presents a prohibitively high risk.

Chronic Cholecystitis

Recurrent attacks of biliary colic, with only temporary occlusion of the cystic duct, can cause inflammation and scarring of the neck of the gallbladder and cystic duct. This process causes fibrosis as histologic evidence of repeated self-limited episodes of inflammation, resulting in chronic cholecystitis. The diagnosis of chronic cholecystitis lies along a continuum with biliary colic because it results from recurrent attacks. Therefore, the presentation is usually that of symptomatic cholelithiasis, or biliary colic. Pain occurring after ingestion of a fatty meal, with the attendant increase in CCK secretion in response to duodenal intraluminal fat, is classic for biliary colic, although only 50% of patients will report an association with food. Pain from stones tends to locate in the epigastrium or right upper quadrant and may radiate around to the scapula. These attacks of pain generally last a few hours. Pain lasting longer than 24 hours or associated with fever is more suggestive of acute cholecystitis. The pain of biliary colic, even in the absence of cholecystitis, may also cause other gastrointestinal symptoms, such as bloating, nausea, and vomiting.

Symptomatic stones constitute a risk profile different from that of asymptomatic stones, with a higher likelihood of complications including acute cholecystitis, choledocholithiasis, gallstone pancreatitis, cholangitis, and more. Therefore, symptomatic cholelithiasis is an indication for cholecystectomy. Documented stones and symptoms are the most common indications to perform a cholecystectomy.

Diagnosis

The diagnosis of chronic cholecystitis relies on a history consistent with biliary tract disease. Transabdominal ultrasonography reliably documents the presence of cholelithiasis. US can provide other important information, such as CBD dilation, gallbladder polyps, porcelain gallbladder, or evidence of hepatic parenchymal processes. Cholesterolosis, or the accumulation of cholesterol found in gallbladder mucosal macrophages, can also be seen. Gallbladder "sludge" or microlithiasis can be found on US and, with appropriate symptoms, is consistent with symptomatic cholelithiasis.

Treatment

Patients with sufficient symptoms from gallstones should undergo elective cholecystectomy. Cholecystectomy carries a low-risk profile but is not without complications, so an analysis of risks and benefits is important. Because patients with mild symptoms have a low rate of complications from gallstones (1%–3% per year), observation and dietary and lifestyle changes can be appropriate in this population, especially in the patient who does not wish to have surgery. Patients with more severe or recurrent symptoms have a higher rate of complications of the disease (7% per year), so elective laparoscopic cholecystectomy is warranted and encouraged. In more than 90% of patients, cholecystectomy is curative, leaving them symptom free.

Acute Calculous Cholecystitis

Acute calculous cholecystitis is the result of blocking the cystic duct with a gallstone. The blockage does not resolve spontaneously, leading to inflammation, edema, and subserosal hemorrhage. Continued cystic duct obstruction can lead to infection of stagnant bile and may progress to ischemia, necrosis, or gangrenous versus emphysematous cholecystitis. Patients presenting with acute cholecystitis experience symptoms of upper abdominal pain (right upper quadrant and/or epigastric) that lasts more than 4 to 6 hours. Often, careful history taking can elicit previous episodes of similar symptoms of shorter duration and less severe pain. Nausea and vomiting are often concomitant symptoms. Fever may also be present, but objectively occurs less frequently. The patient may have a known history of gallstones from previous episodes or incidentally from earlier imaging, focusing the diagnostic workup.

Diagnosis

The most common physical examination finding is right upper quadrant tenderness to palpation; an inflammatory mass may also be palpated, depending on body habitus. Inspiratory arrest with palpation over the gallbladder (Murphy's sign) is a classic physical finding. Alternatively, biliary colic in the absence of infection and inflammation is not associated with Murphy's sign. Despite these classic signs and symptoms, the presentation can be highly variable, especially in patients who are obese, diabetic, elderly, or

immunosuppressed from various causes. There is also significant symptom overlap with other intraabdominal causes (e.g., peptic ulcer, gastritis, colitis).

Laboratory tests helpful in diagnosis are a CBC and complete metabolic profile including transaminases, ALP, and bilirubin. Mild elevations of ALP, bilirubin, and transaminase levels and leukocytosis support the diagnosis of acute cholecystitis. However, given that the CBD is not obstructed, profound jaundice in the setting of acute cholecystitis is rare and should raise the suspicion of cholangitis. Mirizzi syndrome should also be considered, in which inflammation or a stone in the gallbladder neck leads to inflammation of the adjoining biliary system causing obstruction of the common hepatic duct.

Imaging studies are standard in the diagnosis of cholecystitis. US, CT, HIDA, and MRI are all capable of diagnosing acute cholecystitis. Transabdominal ultrasonography is a sensitive, inexpensive, and reliable tool for the diagnosis of acute cholecystitis, with a sensitivity of 85% and specificity of 95%. In addition to identifying gallstones, US can demonstrate pericholecystic fluid, gallbladder wall thickening, and even a sonographic Murphy sign. US is therefore the diagnostic test of choice.

In atypical cases, or when ruling out other abdominal pathology, abdominal CT may be useful. CT is able to identify pericholecystic fluid, inflammation, and gallbladder thickening with high sensitivity. If the CT scan has characteristic findings, it is not necessary to perform an US even when stones are not radiographically visible. A HIDA scan may also be used to demonstrate obstruction of the cystic duct, which definitively diagnosis acute cholecystitis. Filling of the gallbladder during a HIDA scan eliminates the diagnosis of cholecystitis. MRI is highly sensitive for cholecystitis but is more expensive and less expeditious; therefore, it is typically reserved to rule out choledocholithiasis and malignancy when laboratory studies are suggestive of biliary obstruction.

There have been multiple grading systems evaluating severity of cholecystitis; the most widely used are the Tokyo Guidelines[15] and the American Association for the Surgery of Trauma (AAST) Emergency General Surgery (EGS) guidelines.[16] AAST EGS categorizes acute cholecystitis into five grades: Grade I is localized inflammation and grade V shows pericholecystic abscess, bilioenteric fistula, and peritonitis. The Tokyo Guidelines also grade the systemic effect of cholecystitis such as organ failure. Both classifications are helpful to categorize the management of these patients and consider treatment options relative to their severity of disease.

Treatment

In general, the ideal treatment for acute cholecystitis is cholecystectomy. However, treatment is often dependent on the severity of disease and the physiologic status of the patient. Therefore, treatment can vary from immediate surgical intervention to conservative management with interval cholecystectomy to nonoperative adjuncts. Patients with minimal medical comorbidity presenting early in the disease process should generally be managed with surgery. Those with significant, optimizable comorbidities but mild cholecystitis may merit a trial of medical therapy or "cool down" period followed by cholecystectomy after 6 to 12 weeks. Those who are critically ill or with severe comorbidities and severe acute cholecystitis are often best managed with early percutaneous cholecystostomy tube placement in conjunction with antibiotics and delayed cholecystectomy once their medical condition is satisfactory.

Although the primary pathophysiologic event in acute cholecystitis is the obstruction of the cystic duct and infection is a secondary event that follows stasis and inflammation, most cases of acute cholecystitis are complicated by superinfection of the inflamed gallbladder. Patients are given nothing by mouth, and intravenous (IV) fluids and parenteral antibiotics are started. Antibiotics are directed to treatment of common pathogens in bile cultures including *E. coli, Klebsiella, Enterobacter,* and *Bacteroides* species; broad-spectrum antibiotics are warranted. Parenteral narcotics are usually required to control the pain.

Cholecystectomy, whether open or laparoscopic, is the treatment of choice for acute cholecystitis. The timing of operative intervention in acute cholecystitis has long been, and continues to be, a source of debate. In the past, many surgeons advocated for delayed cholecystectomy with patients managed nonoperatively during their initial hospitalization and discharged home with resolution of symptoms. An interval cholecystectomy was then performed at approximately 6 weeks after the initial episode. More recent studies have shown that early in the disease process (within the first week), the operation can be performed laparoscopically with equivalent or improved morbidity, mortality, and length of stay as well as a similar conversion rate to open cholecystectomy.[17] In addition, approximately 20% of patients initially admitted for nonoperative management failed to respond to medical treatment before the planned interval cholecystectomy and required surgical intervention. No demonstrable difference is found in mortality rate, major bile duct injury, postoperative pain, or other significant complication in patients treated with early or delayed cholecystectomy. Multiple studies have shown the safety and efficacy of early, same-admission cholecystectomy in the management of cholecystitis.

Robotic cholecystectomy is an extension of the laparoscopic toolset and is preferred by some surgeons. Robotic port placement and technique is theoretically equivalent to laparoscopic cholecystectomy, as the robot is a laparoscopic device. Three-dimensional visualization and wristed instrument movement are described as advantages from frequent robotic users. Early studies suggested bile duct injury rates higher for robotic cholecystectomy than for laparoscopic approach, but meta-analyses of more recent studies have demonstrated similar outcomes except for longer operative times with the robotic approach.[18]

Indocyanine green (ICG) cholangiography during minimally invasive cholecystectomy (in both robotic and laparoscopic approaches) allows for real-time identification of biliary structures during cholecystectomy and in the current era is straightforward to perform. Selective intraoperative intraluminal contrast cholangiogram can also be useful in confirming difficult anatomy, and both modalities are discussed later.

Initial nonoperative therapy remains a viable option for patients who present in a delayed fashion or with prohibitive medical comorbidity and should be decided on an individual basis. If laparoscopic cholecystectomy is attempted, one must be prepared for significant inflammation in the porta hepatis. Early conversion to open cholecystectomy should be considered when delineation of anatomy is unclear; conversion to open rates approaches 10% is these cases. Alternatively, bailout options discussed later in this chapter may prove useful in the severely inflamed, difficult cholecystectomy.

For those patients in which up-front surgery is avoided, a course of antibiotics is attempted as "conservative" therapy. In the event of failed medical therapy, a percutaneously placed cholecystostomy tube may be necessary. Frequently performed with US or CT guidance under local anesthesia with some sedation, cholecystostomy can act as a temporizing measure by draining the infected bile. Percutaneous drainage results in improvement in symptoms and physiology, allowing a delayed cholecystectomy 3 to 6 months after medical optimization. In patients with cholecystostomy tubes, when fluoroscopy shows a patent cystic duct, the cholecystostomy tube can be removed and the decision for cholecystectomy determined by the patient's ability to tolerate surgical intervention. In patients who will not tolerate a general anesthetic due to severe medical comorbidity, interventional radiology (IR) or gastroenterology may offer long-term treatment options.[19] First, IR may be able to dilate the drain tract and remove residual stones, then on a separate procedure date embolize the cystic duct followed by chemical ablation of the gallbladder. A gastroenterologist, on the other hand, may be able to perform transcystic drainage or transduodenal drainage of the gallbladder for long-term decompression. These options are not to be considered lightly and are reserved for the highest surgical risk patients.

Choledocholithiasis

Choledocholithiasis, or gallstones within the CBD, is present in up to 20% of patients with cholelithiasis. Primary choledocholithiasis refers to de novo stone formation in the CBD and are usually brown pigmented stones due to a combination of precipitated bile pigments and cholesterol. Brown pigment stones, more common in Asian populations, are associated with bacterial infections where free bilirubin is formed by hydrolyzing enzymes released by bacteria and then precipitates forming a stone. Secondary choledocholithiasis, more commonly seen in the United States, is characterized by cholesterol or pigmented stones formed in the gallbladder that escape from the gallbladder into the CBD. Retained stones, which occur in 1% to 2% of patients, refer to secondary stones identified in the CBD within 2 years after cholecystectomy (Fig. 88.19).

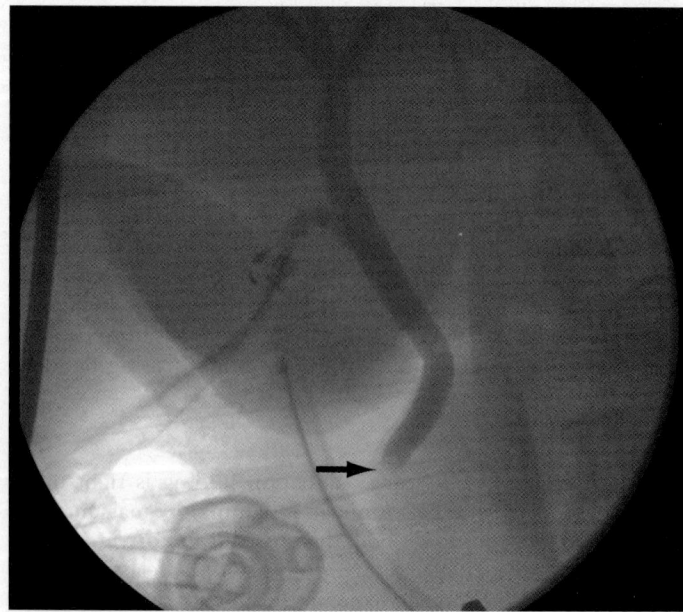

FIGURE 88.19 Intraoperative cholangiogram showing choledocholithiasis in an asymptomatic patient with no filling of duodenum and outline of stone *(arrow).*

Diagnosis

When symptomatic, clinical manifestations of common duct stones range from biliary colic to signs of obstructive jaundice, including darkening of the urine, scleral icterus, and lightening of the stools. Jaundice with choledocholithiasis is more likely to be painful because the onset of obstruction is acute, causing rapid distention of the bile duct and activation of pain fibers. The presence of pain is an important distinguishing factor between choledocholithiasis and malignant obstructions.

Although asymptomatic choledocholithiasis is usually an incidental finding, biliary type pain, jaundice, an abnormal liver function panel indicating cholestasis, and a dilated bile duct (usually more than 8 mm) are all highly suggestive of choledocholithiasis. Although certain laboratory derangements can suggest a diagnosis of choledocholithiasis, there are no specific lab findings that are pathognomonic for the diagnosis. An elevated total bilirubin carries a low sensitivity but a high specificity for choledocholithiasis. When elevated bilirubin is seen in conjunction with an abnormal US, the pretest probability of finding choledocholithiasis approaches 90%, whereas a patient with a normal US and LFTs has a probability of <5% for choledocholithiasis.[20] Elevations in AST, ALT, and ALP are also useful, but no consensus exists regarding their cutoff values. In general, LFTs should not be relied upon as the sole predictor for choledocholithiasis and the overall clinical picture with radiographic findings should be considered when diagnosing choledocholithiasis.

Other laboratory findings can suggest pathologies that are associated with choledocholithiasis. Leukocytosis, especially with other signs of systemic inflammatory response, warrants concern for cholangitis. Epigastric pain elicited on examination should also raise suspicion for concomitant pancreatitis and serum lipase levels should be investigated. Elevations in lipase greater than three times the upper limit of normal are diagnostic for pancreatitis. Dilation of the CBD on US is suggestive of choledocholithiasis, and in some cases an actual stone in the CBD can be visualized. US is more specific than sensitive for diagnosing choledocholithiasis, with values of roughly 90% and 80%, respectively. The cutoff value for CBD dilation in the average adult is greater than 5 to 6 mm. Normal CBD dilation can be seen in patients after cholecystectomy due to reservoir effect and in the elderly due to normal dilation related to age. In patients over 65 years old, a CBD greater than 8 mm is typically considered abnormally dilated. It is important to note that overreliance on ductal dilation may underestimate the presence of choledocholithiasis given the variation in technician skills and the single view of the duct generated by US. Furthermore, lack of CBD stone visualization on US does not rule out choledocholithiasis in patients with other findings consistent with the disease.

Although CT is not necessary for the diagnosis of choledocholithiasis, it is often obtained as part of a workup for abdominal symptoms and is highly sensitive with values upward of 90% versus 80% of US. Additionally, it gives a full anatomic view of the biliary system, pancreas, and liver and may identify anatomic or vascular anomalies, which can be advantageous for preoperative planning. Unlike the previous tests typically ordered when patients are first evaluated in the emergency department, MRCP is used as an ancillary test for the diagnosis of choledocholithiasis. MRCP is highly sensitive (>90%) and specific (>99%) in identifying CBD stones (Fig. 88.20). Limitations of MRCP are in its ability to detect small stones (i.e., <6 mm) in the distal duct or those impacted in the ampulla. As it only serves as a noninvasive, diagnostic test, a therapeutic procedure, such as ERCP or CBD

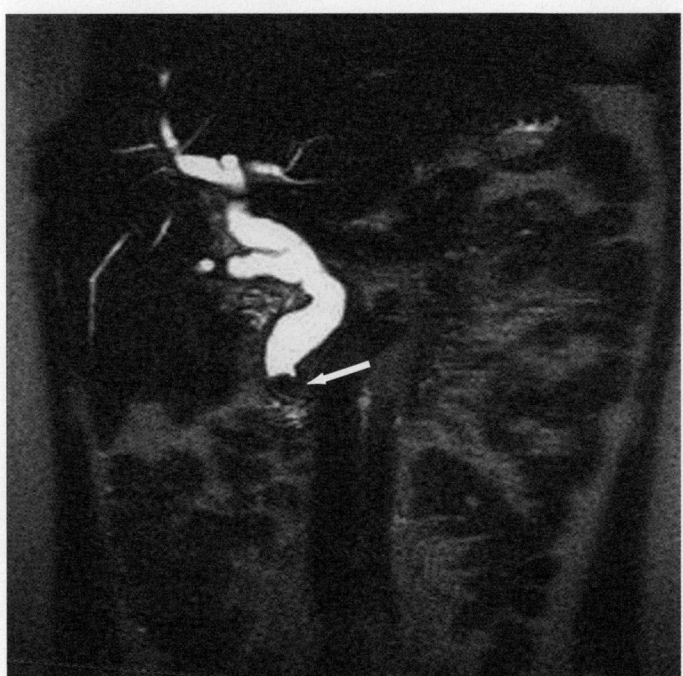

FIGURE 88.20 Magnetic resonance cholangiopancreatography with choledocholithiasis. The dilated common bile duct ends abruptly with a convex intraluminal filling defect *(arrow)* consistent with choledocholithiasis.

exploration (CBDE), is still required once the diagnosis in confirmed. When the operating surgeon does not have the technical skill or equipment to perform a CBDE at the time of cholecystectomy, and there is a moderate likelihood for choledocholithiasis, MRCP can aid in the decision to perform a preoperative ERCP.

ERCP is also highly sensitive and specific for choledocholithiasis (Fig. 88.21). It is often the therapeutic procedure used to clear the duct in more than 75% of patients during a first procedure and in 90% with repeated ERCP. A sphincterotomy with a balloon sweep is performed and stones are extracted, with a complication rate including pancreatitis of up to 10%. Indications for preoperative ERCP include cholangitis, ongoing biliary pancreatitis, and patients with multiple comorbidities that are high risk for surgery. However, some studies have suggested higher risk of surgical site infection in patients who receive preoperative ERCP before cholecystectomy.[21]

Findings of choledocholithiasis via intraoperative cholangiogram during cholecystectomy may be managed by either CBDE or postoperative ERCP. The use of CBDE exploration by surgeons has dramatically declined with the advent of laparoscopic surgery and with concomitant advances in endoscopy. However, it is a safe and feasible procedure with similar duct clearance rates to ERCP and will be discussed in the next section as a one-stage management for choledocholithiasis.

PTC can also be used to treat choledocholithiasis in case of unsuccessful ERCP or in the setting of anatomic difficulty for ERCP such as a previous history of Roux-en-Y gastric bypass. PTC is as effective as ERCP in patients with a dilated biliary system with similar complication rate, but less effective and more technically challenging in patients without intrahepatic ductal dilation.

Treatment

Treatment for choledocholithiasis is generally ERCP or CBDE, which can be performed via robotic-assisted laparoscopic, laparoscopic, or

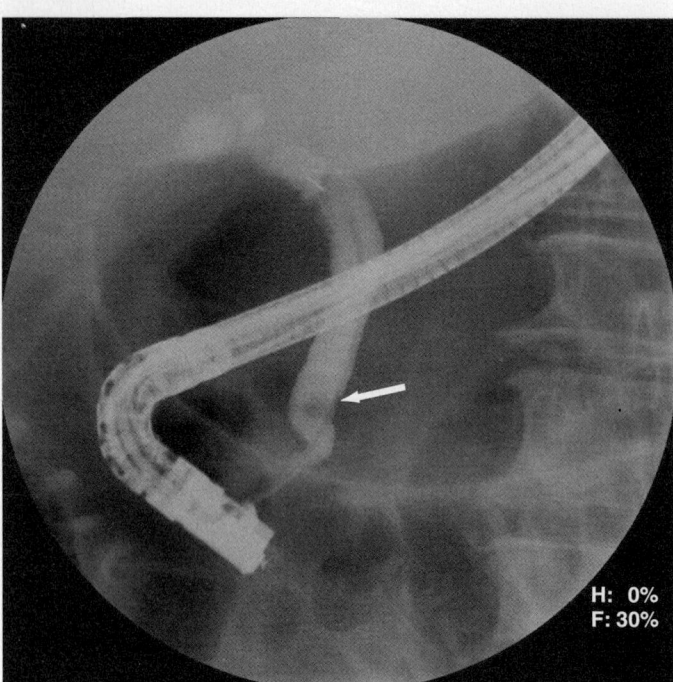

FIGURE 88.21 Endoscopic retrograde cholangiopancreatography (ERCP) with choledocholithiasis. With retrograde injection of contrast material, a filling defect noted within the lumen of the common bile duct *(arrow)* identifies choledocholithiasis. ERCP can also be used to remove the stone through sphincterotomy and balloons or baskets.

open technique. In patients with a low index of suspicion, a laparoscopic cholecystectomy can be performed with an intraoperative cholangiogram to confirm that the duct is clear of stones. In patients with a high index of suspicion, the surgeon should proceed with a plan to clear the duct. This can be done via a preoperative or postoperative ERCP or via a laparoscopic CBDE (LCBDE) with cholecystectomy. For patients with moderate risk for choledocholithiasis, the order of intervention may vary based on institutional policies and ERCP availability. Several medical societies have created algorithms to assist physicians in the diagnosis and management of choledocholithiasis, including the American Society for Gastrointestinal Endoscopy (ASGE)[22] and Society of American Gastrointestinal and Endoscopic Surgeons (SAGES).[6]

In the preoperative setting, endoscopic sphincterotomy with stone extraction by ERCP is effective for the treatment as it can clear the duct of stones. Because more than half of patients managed by ERCP without cholecystectomy will have recurrent symptoms of biliary tract disease, same-admission cholecystectomy is advised. When initial ERCP is unsuccessful at removal of all stones, a stent can be placed to temporize the obstruction and allows for serial attempts at duct clearance. Large stones (usually more than 2.5 cm), altered gastric or duodenal anatomy such as Roux-en-Y, impacted stones, intrahepatic stones, or multiple stones are the most common causes of ERCP failure. In these cases, operative CBDE, laparoscopic-assisted ERCP, or PTC drain placement to alleviate duct obstruction should be considered. With the advancement of technology for choledochoscopy that can be used as an adjunct to ERCP, PTC, or intraoperatively, visualization of the bile duct with options for lithotripsy and stone retrieval are more frequently employed in the management of complex choledocholithiasis.

Acute Cholangitis

Cholangitis, first described by Jean Martin Charcot in 1877, is an ascending infection of the CBD secondary to obstruction and increased intraluminal pressure. The classic Charcot triad of fever, jaundice, and right upper quadrant pain can be seen in less than 50% of all patients, with jaundice as the least common finding. Leukocytosis with an abnormal liver panel is more common. Hepatocellular injury from the infection and inflammation elevate serum transaminase and ALP levels. Symptoms may progress to septic shock with mental status changes, and hypotension (known as *Reynolds pentad*), which is an ominous sign, and mortality approaches 100% without prompt treatment.

Any obstructing phenomenon, from stones to neoplasms, can cause ascending bacterial infection of the biliary tree, but choledocholithiasis is the most common cause. A compelling reason to treat choledocholithiasis early is the risk of developing cholangitis, which is upward of 5% in admitted patients with choledocholithiasis. With obstruction from a stone, bactibilia can be identified in up to 90% of patients. The most common pathogens include *Klebsiella, E. coli, Enterobacter, Pseudomonas,* and *Citrobacter* spp.

US should be the first screening test and will commonly show dilation of the biliary tree. HIDA scans should be interpreted with caution because infection of the biliary tree reduces the secretion of these agents into the biliary tree. CT can be helpful in identifying the site of obstruction, although it is not always the case. The most valuable modalities are cholangiography through ERCP or PTC as they are not only diagnostic but also therapeutic.

Once the diagnosis of cholangitis is confirmed, the severity of the disease should be assessed, and adequate hydration and IV antibiotics should be started immediately. For patients with mild acute cholangitis, treatment with antibiotics alone is usually sufficient, but there should be a low threshold for immediate biliary drainage if the patient does not respond to initial treatment. For moderate acute cholangitis, early duct clearance via endoscopic or percutaneous techniques should be employed. For severe acute cholangitis, the patient will require stabilization of their acute hemodynamic and respiratory conditions followed by prompt biliary drainage.[23] Most patients will improve with medical therapy and either endoscopic or percutaneous biliary drainage. If endoscopic and percutaneous means are unavailable or unsuccessful, surgical drainage consists of common duct exploration with placement of a T-tube. Given the unstable nature of the patient, definitive surgical treatment of the cause is deferred until the patient is stabilized, the cholangitis is treated, and the diagnosis is confirmed.

Gallstone Pancreatitis

Gallstones are the most common cause of pancreatitis in the Western world and are present in 45% of cases.[24] When a stone passes from the bile duct through the ampulla into the duodenum, this may cause secondary injury to the pancreas. Temporary elevation of the pancreatic duct pressure causes inflammation and may result in severe pancreatic injury. Symptoms usually persist even after passage of the stone. US usually shows gallstones, choledocholithiasis, or a dilated CBD. The offending stone usually passes spontaneously, but the injury still can be severe. In most cases of gallstone pancreatitis, the pancreatic inflammation is self-limited. Early ERCP to remove a stone that may not have passed is indicated only for patients with concomitant cholangitis or complications from ongoing biliary obstruction. To prevent a future episode of gallstone pancreatitis, a cholecystectomy is warranted before discharge for mild to moderate cases and cholecystectomy should be delayed for patients with severe or complicated disease including necrotizing pancreatitis. Multiple studies have demonstrated that cholecystectomy within 2 days of admission was safe for patients with mild disease.[25] Given the suspicion of choledocholithiasis, intraoperative cholangiography should be performed at the time of cholecystectomy to confirm the passage of stones.

Gallstone Ileus

A misnomer, gallstone ileus is in fact a mechanical intestinal obstruction secondary to a gallstone. It occurs when a large stone in the dependent portion of the gallbladder fistulizes into the adjacent duodenum, passing directly into the intestine. This usually happens in older patients and can be caused by inflammation or pressure necrosis. The most common site for obstruction is in the terminal ileum before entering the cecum (Fig. 88.22) but can also occur in the duodenum leading to a gastric outlet obstruction called *Bouveret syndrome.*

Diagnosis

The common presentation for gallstone ileus is an elderly patient with some history of biliary tree disorder, with no past surgical history or hernia, who presents with a sudden mechanical small intestine obstruction.

Although most patients will have constant pain from the obstruction, others can present with only episodic discomfort because the gallstone only intermittently obstructs the intestinal tract. Historically, the diagnosis of gallstone ileus was made on plain abdominal film. The pathognomonic findings of pneumobilia from the fistula, signs of a high-grade small bowel obstruction, and a radiopaque stone in the right lower quadrant is called Rigler's triad. More often, emergency departments will perform an abdominal CT, which will still show these findings but with better anatomic detail. Pneumobilia, which may sometimes be identified only by CT scan, is a ubiquitous finding because the fistula that permitted a stone to pass into the duodenum allows air to enter the biliary tree.

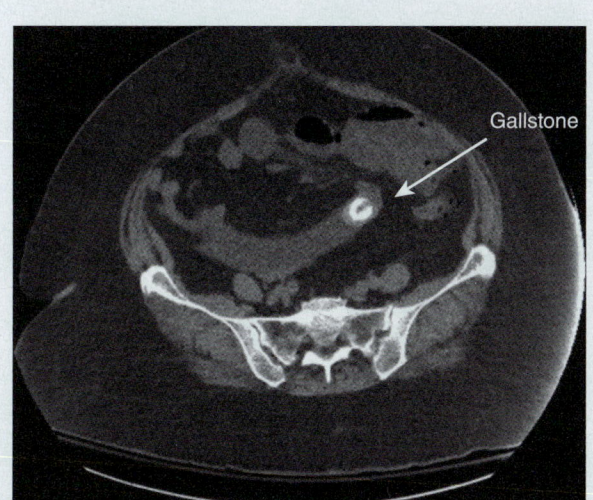

FIGURE 88.22 Computed tomography scan of stone *(arrow)* obstructing the distal ileum.

Treatment

Gallstone ileus is a surgical disease. Once the site of obstruction is identified, a longitudinal incision on the antimesenteric border of the ileum is made a few centimeters proximal to the stone. This site of impaction is at risk of perforation, so signs of ischemia may mandate resection. The stone is milked back through the enterotomy. Approximately 10% of patients have multiple large stones. Therefore, palpation of the remaining small intestine should be performed to exclude a second stone that could cause recurrent obstruction.

Concomitant cholecystectomy should be avoided at the time of stone extraction given the underlying intense inflammatory process that leads to formation of the biliary enteric fistula in the first case. Furthermore, because most of these patients are older, their overall physiologic status may not permit fistula repair in the emergent setting. One-stage repair should be reserved for healthy patients without severe inflammatory changes in the right upper quadrant. For patients with recurrent symptoms, an interval cholecystectomy can be considered to avoid the possibility of future biliary complications.

Noncalculous Biliary Disease

Acute Acalculous Cholecystitis

Blockage of the cystic duct in the absence of gallstones is called acalculous cholecystitis. The pathogenesis of acalculous cholecystitis is poorly understood, but is likely the result of biliary stasis, distention, inflammation, and ultimately superimposed infection and gangrene. Risk factors include old age, burns and trauma, prolonged use of *total parenteral nutrition,* critical illness, immunosuppression, and diabetes, and the presentation can be similar or more fulminant than calculous cholecystitis and may progress to gangrenous gallbladder. Critically ill patients with acalculous cholecystitis may not have right upper quadrant pain or any fever with unknown origin in critically ill patients, especially with pericholecystic fluid and gallbladder wall thickening on imaging, which should raise suspicion for this disorder. HIDA scan is diagnostic for acalculous cholecystitis but can have false-positive result.

Treatment of acalculous cholecystitis is similar to that of calculous cholecystitis, with cholecystectomy being therapeutic. However, unlike calculus cholecystitis, this disease process occurs in some of the most critically ill patients who are unable to tolerate surgical intervention and often require nonoperative strategies. Therefore, percutaneous cholecystostomy tube placement under imaging to drain the gallbladder is a much safer option. More than 90% of these patients improve with a cholecystostomy tube, and interval cholecystectomy is necessary only if follow-up imaging continues to demonstrate the positive findings. In the rare situation in which a patient undergoes a percutaneous cholecystostomy tube placement and fails to improve after 24 hours, exploration with cholecystectomy should be considered because these patients are likely to have perforated and drainage alone will be insufficient.

Biliary Dyskinesia

Biliary dyskinesia is a functional disorder of the biliary tree, generally defined by gallbladder dysmotility. Many hypotheses have been proposed, and it likely involves a malfunction in the normal motility response that leads to symptoms of biliary colic without cholelithiasis. It is usually a diagnosis of exclusion. Patients may present with classic symptoms of biliary colic but have no ultrasonographic evidence of stones or sludge. More vague symptoms, including nausea and oral intolerance, may also be present.

A confounding factor in these patients is that they often have other functional disorders including delayed colonic transit and gastric emptying. Thus, the amalgamation of symptoms may sometimes delay the diagnosis of these patients. The Rome foundation was developed with a mission to help diagnose and treat functional gastrointestinal disorders. They developed a diagnostic criterion to help rule out other frequent causes including gastroesophageal reflux disease (GERD) and inflammatory bowel syndrome.[26] Additional tests to help evaluate for other diagnoses include CT and endoscopy. Cholescintigraphy can be a useful tool in the diagnosis of biliary dyskinesia. The dysmotility of the gallbladder can be identified during a CCK-stimulated HIDA scan. The CCK stimulates the gallbladder to contract and an ejection fraction can be estimated. An ejection fraction less than ~35% is considered suggestive of biliary dyskinesia. More than 85% of patients show improvement in symptoms after cholecystectomy. Factors that predict a better response to cholecystectomy are typical biliary colic symptoms and a reduced ejection fraction. However, these do not guarantee a response. In patients with atypical symptoms, such as nausea as the primary symptom, response to cholecystectomy is less beneficial. In nonresponders, ERCP with sphincterotomy may prove useful.

Sphincter of Oddi Dysfunction

Sphincter of Oddi dysfunction (SOD) is a rare but clinically significant disease presentation. It is caused by a structurally or physiologically abnormal sphincter with higher tone and failure to relax, manifested by pain, and recurrent pancreatitis with a usually normal liver function panel. Risk factors include chronic pancreatitis or calculous disease, which can cause fibrosis due to inflammation, and, subsequently, failure of the sphincter to relax.

The disease's etiology is a failure of the sphincters to relax, increasing the pressures of the biliary tree. The two major types of disease presentations are the biliary and pancreatic subtypes. As the name suggests, the biliary subtype will present with classic biliary colic symptoms, whereas the pancreatic subtype will present with recurrent pancreatitis. The diagnosis of SOD should be suspected in patients with biliary pain and a common duct diameter of more than 12 mm. The bile duct in these patients tends to increase in diameter in response to CCK, as does the pancreatic duct after secretin administration. Initial diagnosis can be assisted through the presence of certain criteria. One of the most widely used is the Milwaukee classification.[27] Type I SOD has typical pain, abnormal pancreatic or hepatic enzymes, and CBD dilation. This is the most likely to respond to intervention. Type II has pain in addition to one of the other criteria. Type III has pain only and is the least likely to respond to intervention.

The intervention for SOD is ERCP with sphincterotomy and is highly effective with up to 90% resolution in symptoms. During ERCP, sphincter manometry can be performed and a pressure greater than 40 mm Hg is consistent with the diagnosis. However, manometry is not widely done as it is an invasive procedure that brings a real risk of pancreatitis. The successful use of botulinum toxin on the muscles of the sphincter predicts responsiveness to sphincterotomy. However, if nonprocedural interventions are desired, treatment with nitrates and calcium channel blockers have been attempted with moderate success.

Primary Sclerosing Cholangitis

Primary sclerosing cholangitis (PSC) is an idiopathic disorder and considered an autoimmune process affecting the biliary tree. PSC

is associated with other autoimmune disorders such as ulcerative colitis (in almost 70% of patients) and Riedel thyroiditis.[28] PSC can be categorized into four anatomic subtypes depending on the level of biliary tree it involves, including intrahepatic, extrahepatic, combined, or small ducts disease. The course of PSC is characterized by progressive chronic cholestasis and advances at an unpredictable rate to biliary cirrhosis and eventually death from liver failure. With improved understanding of the disease and early diagnosis, PSC outcomes have improved.

Clinical presentation. Most patients present with general symptoms such as fatigue and pruritus, but abnormal liver function studies are usually what prompts biliary imaging. Approximately 80% of patients have elevated perinuclear antineutrophil cytoplasmic antibodies, but the severity of disease does not correlate to titer levels. Abnormal LFTs in a patient observed for inflammatory bowel disease should suggest PSC.

Imaging with cholangiography demonstrates a multifocal diffuse dilation and stricturing of the intrahepatic and/or extrahepatic biliary trees. This pattern is called *beading* or *chain of lakes* and is characteristic of PSC. MRCP is useful in the diagnosis and surveillance of PSC patients, whereas ERCP is reserved for the treatment of dominant strictures and to exclude malignancy, namely, cholangiocarcinoma (Fig. 88.23).

Liver biopsy tends to show an onionskin concentric periductal fibrosis. With disease progression, periportal fibrosis occurs, progressing to bridging necrosis and, eventually, biliary cirrhosis. Unfortunately, PSC is associated with cholangiocarcinoma, and distinguishing the strictures of PSC fibrosis from those of cholangiocarcinoma can be challenging.

Treatment. Ursodeoxycholic acid is commonly used as medical therapy for PSC and has demonstrated some improvement in LFTs; however, it is controversial whether this alters the progression of disease. Ongoing trials in PSC include ursodeoxycholic acid homologs, antibiotics to alter the microbiome, and interruption of the enterohepatic bile circulation. However, none of these agents has shown a consistent clinical benefit. In the symptomatic patient, endoscopic therapy, consisting of balloon dilation of the dominant strictures, has been shown to alleviate pruritus, to reduce likelihood of cholangitis, and even to prolong survival.

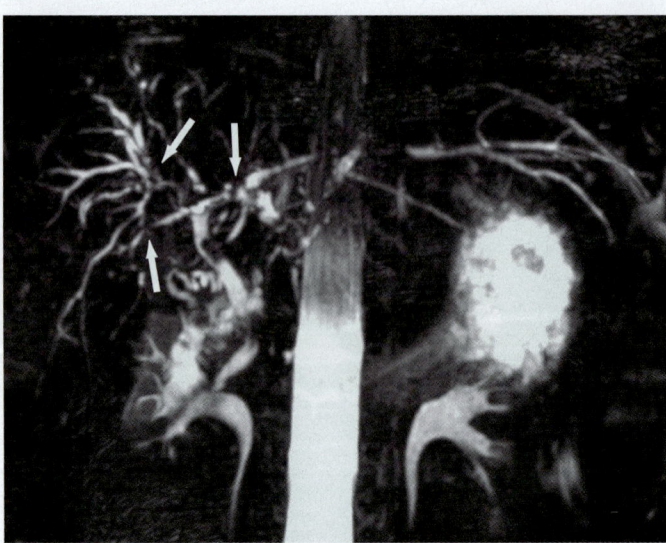

FIGURE 88.23 Magnetic resonance cholangiopancreatography showing primary sclerosing cholangitis. Note the multilevel strictures *(arrows)*.

Surgical treatment options include biliary reconstruction in symptomatic patients with focal extrahepatic disease in some cases. Such patients are rare, and repeated operations for drainage have been shown to complicate definitive treatment by liver transplantation. Therefore, the use of biliary reconstructive procedures has decreased for this indication. Although it is associated with ulcerative colitis, a proctocolectomy does not appear to affect biliary disease progression or survival in patients with both ulcerative colitis and PSC.

Orthotopic liver transplantation appears to be the only lifesaving option for patients with progressive hepatic dysfunction from PSC. The survival rate for patients undergoing liver transplantation for PSC is approximately equivalent to that of those undergoing transplantation for other causes of end-stage liver disease, with 5-year survival rates ranging from 75% to 85%. Although the development of cholangiocarcinoma in a PSC liver used to be considered a contraindication to transplantation, some centers have shown excellent survival rates, up to 70% at 5 years, for patients with limited hilar disease who undergo a neoadjuvant protocol of chemotherapy and radiation followed by transplantation.[29] After liver transplantation, 10% to 30% of PSC patients develop recurrent biliary strictures, suggestive of recurrence of disease in the donor liver. Even with the development of strictures, disease progression does not usually follow the aggressive course for which PSC is known. In cases where retransplantation is required, the morbidity and mortality are higher than for primary transplantation.

Recurrent Pyogenic Cholangitis

More common in East Asian populations, recurrent pyogenic cholangitis is caused by cholangiohepatitis or intrahepatic stones. Biliary pathogens such as *Clonorchis sinensis* and *Ascaris lumbricoides* populate the biliary tree. These and other pathogens secrete an enzyme that hydrolyzes water-soluble bilirubin glucuronides to form free bilirubin, which then precipitates to form brown pigment stones. These stones may partially or fully obstruct the biliary tree, causing recurrent episodes of cholangitis and, eventually, abscesses or even cirrhosis. The chronicity of the infection and inflammation places these patients at risk for the development of cholangiocarcinoma. It is unclear whether the primary inciting event is infection causing inflammatory stricture or inflammatory stricture with subsequent infection of stagnant bile.

Recurrent pyogenic cholangitis tends to occur in the third to fourth decade of life, affecting males and females equally. The clinical presentation is that of cholangitis with fever, right upper quadrant pain, and jaundice. Because the infection, inflammation, and stones commonly present in a segmental or lobar pattern, the jaundice tends to be mild. Serum studies are similar to other causes of cholangitis, with a leukocytosis and elevated bilirubin and high ALP levels. Diagnosis is usually made by a combination of CT or MRCP with ERCP (Fig. 88.24). Lobar or segmental atrophy or hypertrophy may be seen in chronic cases.

In the setting of an acute attack, conservative treatment with parenteral antibiotics, IV fluids, and analgesics will usually suffice. Failure of this approach, with clinical deterioration, mandates biliary drainage by ERCP or percutaneous methods. Once the attack has subsided, a thorough investigation of biliary tree anatomy will help direct treatment. Definitive operative treatment is almost always required. The goals of surgical therapy are threefold: (1) remove all stones; (2) bypass, enlarge, or resect the strictures; and (3) provide adequate biliary drainage. The variability of presentation and location of disease have spurred the development of

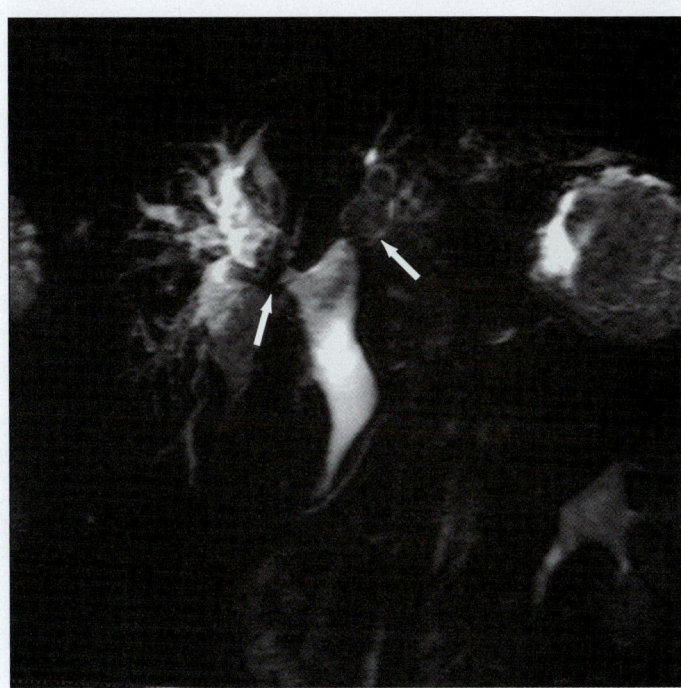

FIGURE 88.24 Magnetic resonance cholangiopancreatography of recurrent pyogenic cholangitis. Intraluminal filling defects from stones are noted in both lobes *(arrows)*.

a number of operations to achieve these goals. The presence of intrahepatic strictures connotes a complicated case and may warrant resection, strictureplasty, or hepaticojejunostomy. When clearance of all stones is not possible or future need for endoscopic therapy is anticipated, the terminal end of the Roux limb for a hepaticojejunostomy can be brought out as a stoma to provide easy access for choledochoscopy. Given the risk of cholangiocarcinoma, disease affecting predominantly one lobe should be resected in patients with adequate hepatic reserve. In the absence of the development of cholangiocarcinoma, surgical management is highly successful.[30]

Biliary Strictures

Benign strictures can occur anywhere along the intrahepatic or extrahepatic portions of the biliary tree. Intrahepatic strictures are usually a result of cholangiohepatitis and/or ischemic events. Any inflammatory ischemic process along the length of the CBD may cause an extrahepatic stricture. Chronic pancreatitis can cause strictures in the intrapancreatic portion of CBD and are usually long (2–4 cm) with gradually tapered narrowing. Stricturing at the middle portion of the CBD is usually associated with a gallbladder process. The most common reason is iatrogenic and postcholecystectomy, reported in up to 1% of postcholecystectomy patients. Alternatively, Mirizzi syndrome is a large stone in the Hartmann pouch of the gallbladder, compressing the adjacent bile duct and leading to biliary obstruction (Fig. 88.25). These patients often have a cystic duct parallel to the common hepatic duct and an impacted gallstone in the neck or cystic duct. The resultant inflammation can cause a cholecystocholedochal fistula. The treatment of Mirizzi syndrome is cholecystectomy, which may require repair of the common duct; when a large fistula exists, a choledochojejunostomy may be necessary.

Long-standing choledocholithiasis also can cause fibrosis and stricture. ERCP with sphincterotomy, balloon dilation, and stent

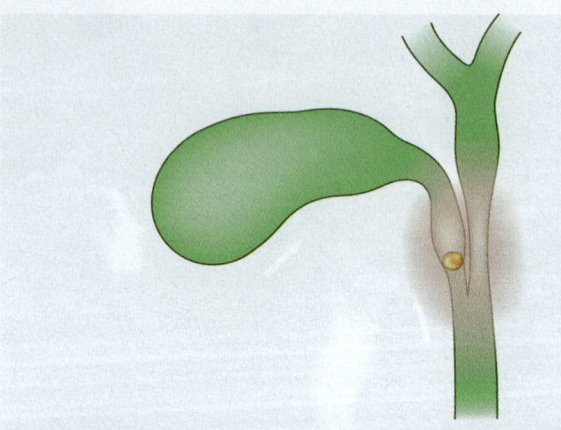

FIGURE 88.25 Mirizzi syndrome. Obstruction of the bile duct from an inflammatory process is the hallmark of this syndrome; the cholecystocholedochal fistula may or may not be apparent.

placement is generally regarded as primary treatment for benign bile duct strictures to make the diagnosis and potentially to treat the process. Endoscopic and percutaneous therapy can provide long-term success in more than 50% of patients. When this is unsuccessful, surgical management with anastomosis of the biliary tree to a Roux-en-Y jejunal limb has success rates of up to 90%.

Biliary Cysts

Choledochal cysts, or biliary cysts, are congenital intrahepatic and/or extrahepatic dilation anomalies. Due to new insights into epithelial markers, and different pathophysiology in different etiologic subtypes, now they are called biliary malformations rather than cysts. They are rare disorders, occurring in less than 1/100,000 patients. They occur more frequently in female patients and in Asian populations. These are considered premalignant conditions and are sometimes diagnosed in infancy; however, they can present in adulthood (Fig. 88.26).[31] Type I choledochal cyst is the

most common form and involves only the extrahepatic biliary tree with a fusiform dilation. Type II cysts appear as a saccular diverticulum off the CBD and may be mistaken for an accessory gallbladder. Type III cysts appear as a cystic dilation of the intramural CBD, within the wall of the duodenum, and are also known as choledochoceles. Cysts involving the intrahepatic and extrahepatic biliary tree are known as type IVA, with type IVB as they are multiple cysts limited to the extrahepatic biliary tree. Type V cysts, also known as *Caroli disease*, involve the intrahepatic ducts only. Type V cysts may be solitary but usually occur diffusely in all segments. Although classified as a single disease, there are multiple theories for etiology, but mostly accepted, especially for types I and IV, is the anomalous pancreatobiliary junction (APBJ; Figs. 88.27 and 88.28). With APBJ, the pancreatic duct and biliary tree fuse to form a common channel before passage through the duodenal wall. APBJ is seen in up to 90% of patients with choledochal cysts, but almost exclusively in types I and IV. The fused duct forms a long common channel, which allows pancreatic secretions to reflux into the biliary tree. Because the pancreatic duct has higher secretory pressures than the biliary tree, exocrine pancreatic secretions reflux up into the bile duct and can inflame and damage the biliary epithelium, leading to cystic degeneration. Types II and III almost never present with APBJ and are associated with minimal risk of malignancy.

Presentation. Jaundice is the most consistent symptom, sometimes accompanied with right upper quadrant pain and rarely a palpable mass. Patients may also suffer from nonspecific problems such as weight loss, nausea, and vomiting. Rarely, a long-standing malformation can cause liver injury and even cirrhosis. Diagnostic imaging is the only diagnostic confirmation test. With the current liberal use of CT, the diagnosis of a choledochal cyst is usually suspected on CT but further classified by MRCP or ERCP. Sometimes the distal bile duct is difficult to evaluate by MRCP, so ERCP is more useful for defining the distal biliary tree and pancreaticobiliary junction. Laboratory studies may identify cholestasis and jaundice. In late stages of

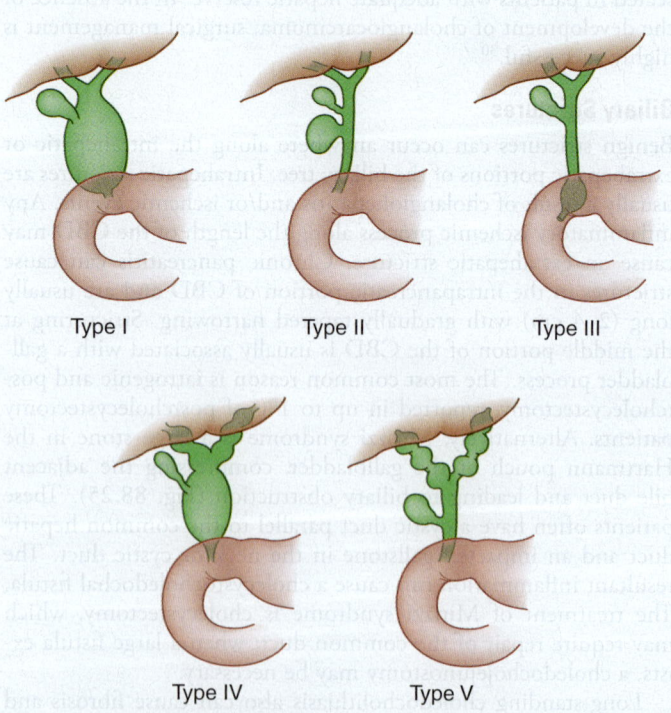

Type I   Type II   Type III

Type IV   Type V

FIGURE 88.26 Choledochal cyst classification.

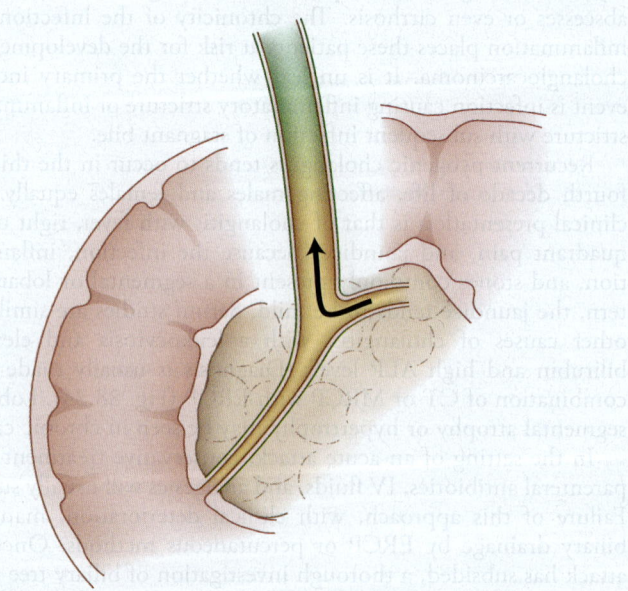

FIGURE 88.27 Anomalous pancreaticobiliary junction. With fusion of the common bile duct and pancreatic duct long before they pass through the duodenal wall, the pancreatic secretions can reflux into the common bile duct and may cause damage to the common duct through pressure or chemical injury.

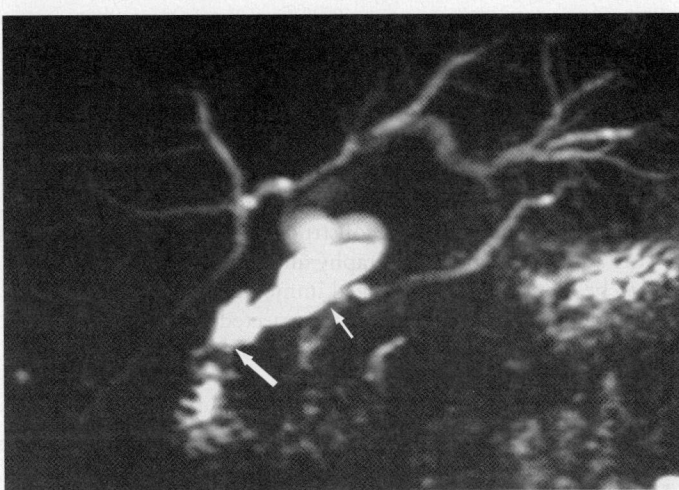

FIGURE 88.28 Magnetic resonance cholangiopancreatography showing anomalous pancreaticobiliary junction with long common channel. The pancreatic duct fuses with the common bile duct *(slender arrow)*, and the common channel enters the duodenum *(bold arrow)*. Also noted in this illustration is the fusiform dilation of only the extrahepatic bile duct, as seen in a type I choledochal cyst.

disease, secondary hepatic injury and evidence of cirrhosis may be seen. Rarely, first presentation is cholangiocarcinoma. The incident of malignancy ranges between 5% and 30% over a lifetime, most commonly occurring in the seventh decade and almost exclusively occurring in types I *and* IV.[32]

Treatment. Historically, enteric drainage of the cyst was performed without resection, but this approach is complicated by the development of malignancy, recurrent biliary stasis, and infection. Surgical management of choledochal cysts consists of resection of the entire cyst and appropriate surgical reconstruction. Type I cysts are treated by complete surgical excision, cholecystectomy, and Roux-en-Y hepaticojejunostomy. The proximal extent of resection should continue to the nondilated biliary tree and may require anastomosis to the left and right hepatic ducts. The distal duct is oversewn, with care taken not to injure the pancreatic duct. Type II cysts should be excised entirely. Type III cysts are uncommon and may be approached transduodenally. Because the pathogenesis of type III cysts is not clear and almost always does not involve APBJ, endoscopic drainage may suffice. In the setting of duodenal or biliary obstruction, transduodenal excision or sphincteroplasty can be performed. Surgical treatment of type IV cysts must be carefully individualized to the affected anatomy. Type IV cysts affecting only the extrahepatic bile ducts are managed similarly to type I cysts, with excision and hepaticojejunostomy. Those with intrahepatic extension involving only one lobe can be treated with partial hepatectomy and reconstruction. Surgical treatment of Caroli disease ranges from resection if the disease is unilobar to liver transplantation when diffuse disease is detected.

Surgery for Calculous Biliary Disease
Laparoscopic Cholecystectomy

Laparoscopic cholecystectomy, first done by Muhe in 1985 (using a direct scope) and later in 1987 by Mouret, is one of the most commonly performed general surgery procedures in the United States. Laparoscopic cholecystectomy has a 0.1% to 0.5% mortality and 2% to 3% morbidity.[33] Laparoscopic surgery results in

smaller incisions, less pain, and shorter hospitalization compared with traditional open cholecystectomy, which has significantly increased the number of these procedures done worldwide. Most cholecystectomies are performed for biliary colic, but the operation can be performed safely, and is the gold standard, in the setting of acute cholecystitis. Studies have shown that laparoscopic cholecystectomy for acute cholecystitis may carry longer operative times and a higher conversion rate to the open procedure than when it is performed in the elective setting, with possibly a higher risk of common duct injury. General anesthesia with muscle relaxation is required when a laparoscopic cholecystectomy is performed. Therefore, one contraindication to the procedure is the inability to tolerate general anesthesia. Other contraindications include end-stage liver disease with portal hypertension, precluding safe portal dissection, and coagulopathy. Relative contraindications to surgery include severe chronic obstructive pulmonary disease (poor ability for CO_2 gas exchange), congestive heart failure, and pulmonary hypertension.

The patient is positioned supine with an arm tucked to allow for potential intraoperative cholangiogram, although some prefer both arms out. A Foley catheter may be placed if concerned for prolonged operation or critical illness of the patient. An orogastric tube is placed to decompress the stomach for better view of the upper abdomen intraoperatively. The abdomen and lower chest should be prepped and draped in a manner that can accommodate a retractor system in the event of conversion to an open procedure. The patient should be well secured to the bed to allow for steep reverse Trendelenburg positioning.

Four laparoscopic ports are standard. A 12-mm port at or near the umbilicus is often used for extraction of the gallbladder specimen. The other three ports are 5-mm or even smaller for dissection placed in the right anterior axillary line, right midclavicular line, and subxiphoid location (Fig. 88.29). The lateral port at the anterior axillary line is used to elevate the fundus of the gallbladder toward the right shoulder. This retraction provides exposure to the infundibulum and porta hepatis. The midclavicular trocar is used to grasp the gallbladder infundibulum, retracting it inferolaterally to open the triangle of Calot. Alternative positioning is in the modified French position (split legs), with fundus retraction performed via a subxiphoid port and the 5-mm working ports in the left and right upper quadrants, respectively.

The gallbladder fundus is grasped and retracted cephalad, and the region of the infundibulum retracted laterally to provide exposure for dissection of the cystic structures until a critical view of safety is obtained. A key maneuver is for the surgeon's left operative instrument to distract the infundibulum/Hartmann pouch laterally.[34] The cystic duct and artery are identified by this inferolateral traction of the infundibulum while dissecting free the fibrofatty tissue attaching the infundibulum to the liver. A useful landmark for the cystic artery is the overlying lymph node, known as the Calot node. A high dissection at the infundibulum should be used. If the node of Calot is visible, then limiting the line of peritoneal/serosal division to the upside (gallbladder side) of this structure helps to minimize the risk of CBD injury. With rare exceptions, this lymph node lies immediately on top of the cystic artery. Also, useful to minimize bile duct injury is to obtain a view known as the critical view of safety. Critical view of safety is defined as two and only two structures entering the gallbladder, the lower third of the gallbladder dissected from the liver to expose cystic plate, and a cleared hepatocystic triangle (Fig. 88.30).

Clips are then placed on the cystic artery and duct. The clipped artery and duct are transected between the clips and the gallbladder is

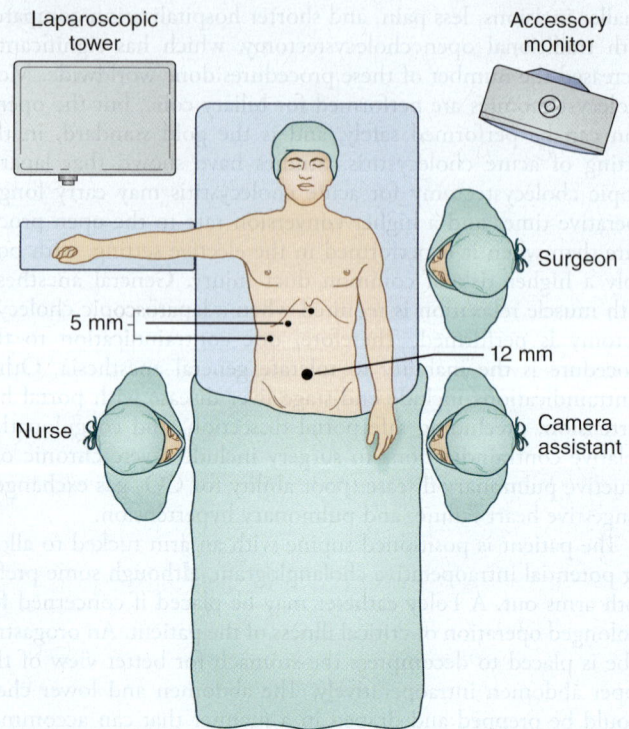

FIGURE 88.29 Laparoscopic cholecystectomy ports. The assistant uses the periumbilical port to provide access for the camera and the most lateral port to elevate the fundus and to expose the neck. The surgeon can then provide inferolateral traction on the infundibulum and open the critical view of safety.

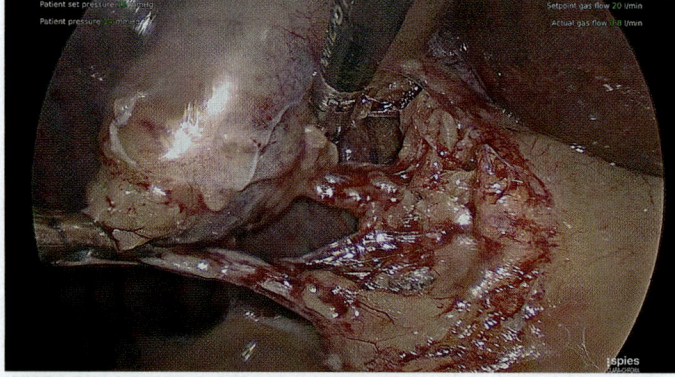

FIGURE 88.30 Critical view of safety. Two structures entering the retracted fundus of gallbladder (left side).

dissected off the liver bed using electrocautery. Because the venous drainage of the gallbladder is directly into the liver bed through venules, excellent hemostasis must be achieved during this dissection. The cystic duct and cystic artery clips are inspected just before completion of the dissection of the fundic attachments because the superior traction of the fundus has provided exposure to the porta and triangle of Calot. The gallbladder is then brought out of the abdominal cavity through the umbilical port with the aid of a specimen retrieval bag. Spillage of stones escaping the field must be searched for and retrieved to prevent the development of late perihepatic abscesses.

Intraoperative Cholangiography

Intraoperative cholangiography (IOC) is an essential tool in the armamentarium of the modern surgeon. It was first performed by

Dr. Mirizzi in 1932 using plain films and, other than the adoption of live fluoroscopy and change in dye, the technique has remained largely unchanged. A catheter is passed into the cystic duct via a ductotomy and water-soluble contrast is injected to opacify the biliary system (Fig. 88.31). This technique is commonly used to identify choledocholithiasis, help delineate anomalous biliary anatomy, confirm anatomy during a difficult operative dissection, or guide biliary reconstruction.

Intraoperative cholangiography allows CBD stones and injuries to be identified and managed immediately. However, routine cholangiography will identify unsuspected stones in less than 10% of patients, does not decrease the incidence of biliary injury, and can be misinterpreted. Because it adds operative time and fluoroscopic exposure to the operation, many surgeons use intraoperative cholangiography only selectively at the time of cholecystectomy. Although some surgeons still advocate for its use in the academic setting to ensure that trainees are facile in its performance, the Tokyo Guidelines do not encourage the routine use of cholangiography.[33] Indications for the selective use of cholangiography include a diagnosis of gallstone pancreatitis, anomalous or unclear biliary anatomy, and in patients with suspected choledocholithiasis where cholecystectomy is being performed to confirm the diagnosis before ERCP. Familiarity with this procedure is essential for surgeons who wish to manage choledocholithiasis in a one-stage manner with CBDE, which is discussed later this chapter.

Fluorescent Cholangiography

ICG is a water-soluble green dye with spectral absorption at 800 nm. When injected intravenously, ICG binds plasma proteins before being rapidly metabolized by hepatocytes and excreted exclusively into the bile; protein-bound ICG fluoresces green when illuminated with near-infrared (NIR) light and allows for fluorescent cholangiography (FC). The excretion of ICG into the biliary

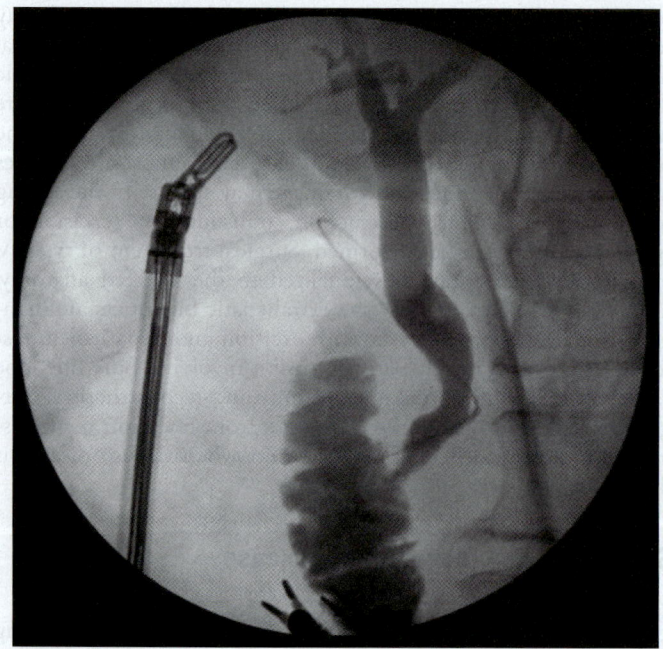

FIGURE 88.31 Intraoperative cholangiogram after retrieval of stone by common bile duct explorations showing filling of the duodenum, common bile duct, common hepatic duct, and left/right hepatic ducts with no filling defects.

tree peaks at 2 to 4 hours after IV injection but can be seen as early as 10 to 15 minutes after injection. FC offers a potentially detailed anatomic mapping of extrahepatic biliary structures and can be a useful adjunct to the critical view of safety technique. Dynamic, real-time NIR light capability is built into many modern laparoscopic and robotic cameras. It has the added benefit of not requiring cannulation of the biliary tree, such as with IOC, but can also be used in conjunction with IOC to help identify anatomy. No substantial contraindication for use of ICG exists, and it has been used safely in patients with iodine allergy. Anaphylactic reaction has been reported at a rate of 0.003%. ICG dye in patients with a history of anaphylactic reaction to shellfish is avoided. ICG is safe for use in pregnancy as maternal-to-fetal transfer is limited by the placental barrier. This is a tool that is growing in popularity. Its use is still actively being studied, but early systematic reviews show a trend toward reducing operative time, conversion to open, and injuries.[35]

Firm recommendations for routine use of ICG are limited by published study sizes. Early published data suggest both reduced operative time and conversion to open surgery in FC cases for both inflamed and noninflamed pathology. Additionally, there is a high success rate for identification of extrahepatic biliary structures. There are limited data on whether fluorescence cholangiography helps reduce major CBD injuries compared with historic techniques. Examples of ICG use in practice are seen in Fig. 88.32.

Laparoscopic Common Bile Duct Exploration

A survey of general surgery residents from 2000–18 demonstrated a precipitous decrease in the experience with both open and laparoscopic CBDE. At the turn of the millennium, the average general surgery resident participated in three open and one laparoscopic CBDE by graduation. Two decades later, the average experience was less than one procedure per resident.[36] This correlates with an overall decline in open and laparoscopic CBDE with concomitant increase in ERCP utilization for the management of choledocholithiasis. Common reasons surgeons choose not to perform CBDE include access to ERCP, lack of equipment, lack of comfort with the procedure, time constraints, and lack of trained staff.

Despite current practice patterns, numerous studies have demonstrated the benefits of one-stage management of choledocholithiasis with CBDE at the time of cholecystectomy over two-stage management with ERCP and cholecystectomy. The two techniques have equivalent stone clearance rates, but one-stage management is associated with decreased length of stay, decreased costs, and decreased rates of complications including pancreatitis.[37] Given these benefits, there has been a shift in the surgery community to reclaim the bile duct and to return to surgical management of choledocholithiasis as the standard of care.

The two laparoscopic approaches to CBDE for stone removal include a transcystic and transcholedochal approach. Techniques to clear the CBD via the cystic duct include sphincteroplasty under fluoroscopic guidance and choledochoscopy with basket retrieval of stones. Both approaches use the Seldinger technique and start with introducing a flexible guidewire through the cystic duct into the CBD. For sphincteroplasty, after the guidewire is positioned into the duodenum, a balloon is positioned across the ampulla and dilated. Stones are then cleared from the CBD into

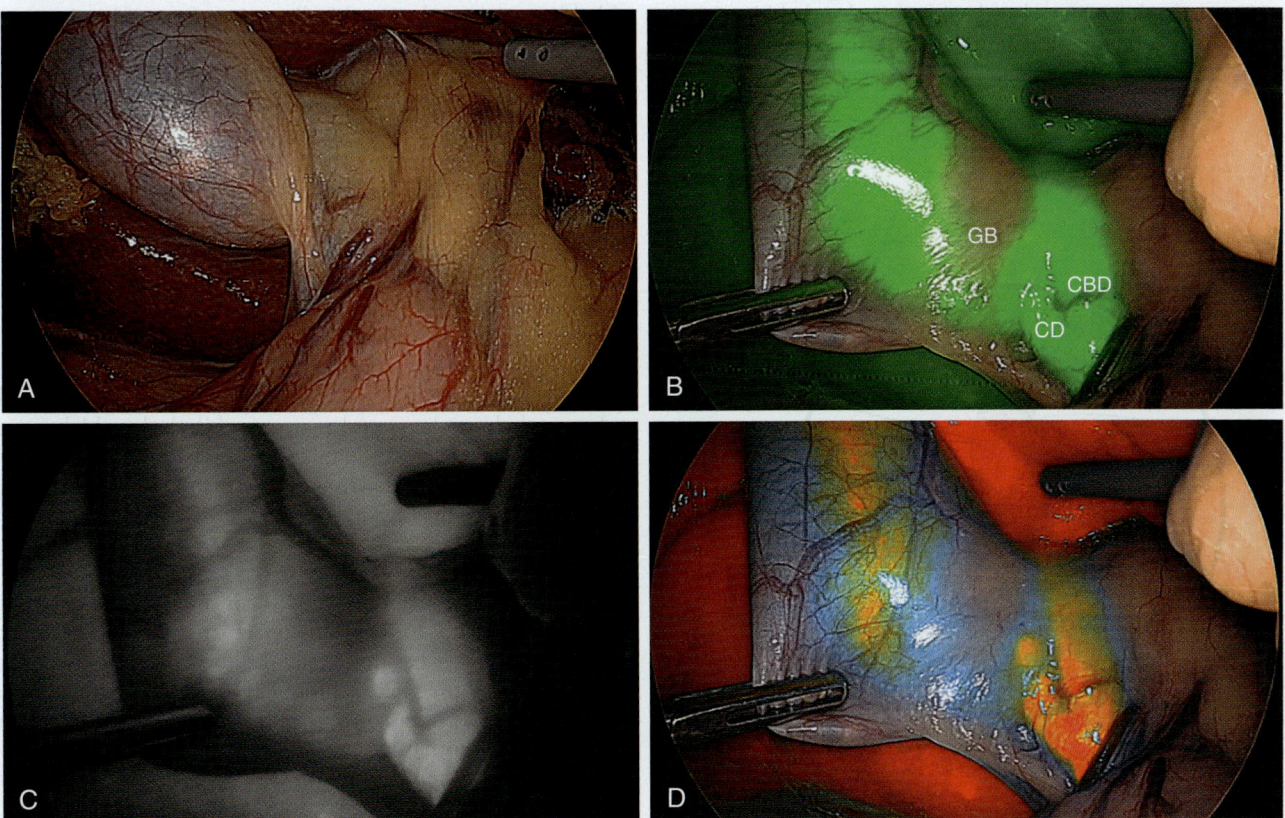

FIGURE 88.32 (A) Bright light/traditional laparoscopic view before peritoneal dissection. (B) Fluorescence cholangiography with "overlay" mode for the same image/patient as (A). (C) Fluorescence cholangiography with grayscale mode. (D) Fluorescence cholangiography with color segmented fluorescent mode. *CD,* Cystic duct; *CBD,* common bile duct; *GB,* gallbladder.

the duodenum with flushing maneuvers. Choledochoscopy requires CBD dilation of at least 6 to 8 mm to allow for passage of a flexible choledochoscope or ureteroscope. After the guidewire is passed through the cystic duct into the CBD, the valves of Heister along the cystic duct are lysed with balloon dilation. Choledochoscopy facilitates direct visualization of the bile duct and stones can either be pushed into the duodenum or captured with a basket under direct visualization and retrieved via the cystic duct.

For larger stones (>1 cm) or stones that are too big to be retrieved via the cystic duct, options for duct clearance include electrohydraulic lithotripsy or a transcholedochal approach. Electrohydraulic lithotripsy uses high-voltage electrical impulses, discharged in fluid, to produce hydraulic pressure waves, and these waves are able to fragment solid objects. Unlike extracorporeal shock wave lithotripsy, which uses sparks and shock waves generated outside the body to fragment stones, electrohydraulic lithotripsy requires close contact with the gallstone with a choledochoscope or endoscope. Once the stone is broken into fragments, they can be retrieved via the cystic duct in a wire basket.

In the transcholedochal approach, a longitudinal incision is made in the CBD after two stay sutures are placed on either side of the planned choledochotomy (Fig. 88.33). The size of the incision should be at least as large as the diameter of the largest stone. The choledochoscope can then be fed down into the distal bile duct and stone extraction performed as described earlier. At the completion of the exploration, larger diameter bile ducts (i.e., 1 cm and larger) can be closed primarily with interrupted 4-0 absorbable suture. For smaller diameter ducts, when there is a concern for stricture, or the CBD obstruction has not been entirely cleared, a T-tube should be placed through the choledochotomy and the bile duct closed with 4-0 absorbable sutures. Completion cholangiography should be routinely performed to document clearance of the CBD.

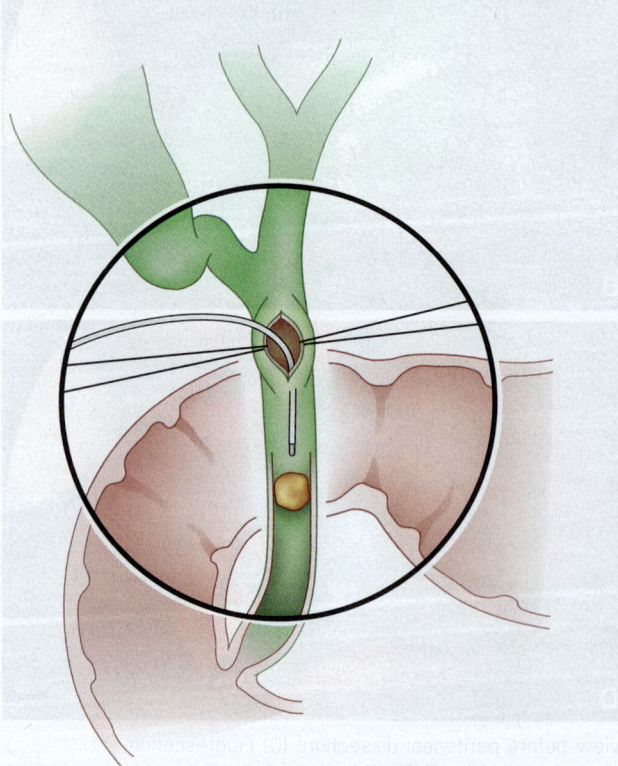

FIGURE 88.33 Laparoscopic choledochotomy for common bile duct exploration.

When feasible, the transcystic approach is preferred as it is technically easier and does not require advanced laparoscopic suturing. However, with the advent of the robotic platform, difficult dissection and advanced suturing in a minimally invasive fashion are within reach for the general surgeon. Relative contraindications to the transcystic approach include numerous (more than eight) stones, a stone larger than 1 cm, intrahepatic stones, and a cystic duct that does not permit dilation and choledochoscope passage.

Bailout Procedures

As the grade of cholecystitis increases from I to II or III, a laparoscopic procedure becomes increasingly difficult to complete safely. The Tokyo Guidelines on recommendations for surgical management of cholecystitis recommended a few bailout options, and a surgeon must be prepared to perform these, especially with a higher grade cholecystitis. As surgical training features fewer open cholecystectomy operations, it is becoming more common to see laparoscopic bailout options used.

Although crucial for safe anatomic dissection, grasping the fundus and infundibulum of an acutely inflamed, distended gallbladder may prove difficult. Decompression of the gallbladder with a laparoscopic needle aspirator (most common) or a 14-gauge angiocatheter can help suction the gallbladder contents and alleviate tension. A very inflamed gallbladder, even with decompression, may not be amenable to grasping with routine laparoscopic devices. In this scenario, claw or rat-tooth graspers may prove useful, but an early conversion to open surgery may be required. Alternatively, a dome-down (or retrograde) approach may be possible, but very close care and attention must be directed to gallbladder anatomy during this dissection. Loss of bearings medially can lead to high injury of the common hepatic duct, so early dissection away from the cystic plate is critical.

If the cystic structures cannot be safely dissected from the portal structures, a subtotal cholecystectomy can be performed. The gallbladder is surgically divided high on the infundibulum, all stones are removed, and the infundibulum is left in situ. Subtotal cholecystectomy such as this can be "fenestrating" or "reconstituting." Fenestrating leaves the cystic duct stump open and reconstituting is closure of the stump with stapler or suture. Data are limited on the whether fenestrating or reconstituting has better outcomes as sample size is low; however, patient anatomic factors often influence the decision (e.g., in a gangrenous gallbladder the tissue may be too friable for a suture). A drain is left in place to help evaluate and manage a bile leak, which is a somewhat common occurrence in these cases. If any of the previously mentioned techniques are not successful in aiding dissection, there should be no hesitation to convert to open cholecystectomy.

Open Cholecystectomy

Although open cholecystectomy is considered a safe alternative or bailout procedure for the difficult laparoscopic cholecystectomy, experience with it has drastically declined, making this procedure not necessarily the safer technique. Open cholecystectomy is generally performed after conversion from the laparoscopic approach, for patients who have a contraindication to the laparoscopic approach, or as a step during another operation, such as a pancreaticoduodenectomy. Open cholecystectomy can be performed through a midline or right subcostal incision. Early identification and ligation of the cystic artery limit the blood loss during the procedure but may prove difficult because of inflammation. This approach must be used with caution as the extension of the dissection continues inferiorly, putting portal vein and other portal structures at risk.[38] When it is performed for severe cholecystitis, the dissection of the gallbladder of the liver bed may be associated with substantial blood loss, but with removal of the infected gallbladder and packing of the area, the bleeding is usually well controlled.

Open Common Bile Duct Exploration

Clearance of choledocholithiasis or any other reason for CBDE is typically performed by open technique. Most surgeons prefer right upper quadrant incision; however, an upper midline incision can be used as well. Gentle palpation of the distal bile duct will frequently find the offending stone, which may be milked backward. Stay sutures are then placed and a choledochotomy is performed in the supraduodenal bile duct. Flushing of the duct with a soft rubber catheter will frequently remove the offending stones. Balloon catheters and, with fluoroscopic guidance, wire baskets may be useful to withdraw the stone. Flexible choledochoscopes

are used to visualize the distal bile duct. With complete removal of stones, a T-tube is placed, and a cholangiogram obtained before closure to document clearance.

With dilated bile ducts, multiple distal impacted stones, a distal duct stricture with stones, intrahepatic stones, or primary bile duct stones drainage procedures provide more successful long-term outcomes. Options in this setting include choledochoduodenostomy (Fig. 88.34) or Roux-en-Y hepaticojejunostomy (Fig. 88.35). A side-to-side or end-to-side choledochoduodenostomy allows future endoscopic intervention of the upper biliary tree, if necessary. An alternative to duodenostomy is a Roux-en-Y choledochojejunostomy.

Transduodenal sphincteroplasty must be the procedure of choice when impacted stones at the ampulla cannot be removed through choledochotomy or several stones are impacted in a *nondilated tree* (Figs. 88.36 and 88.37). After completion of the Kocher maneuver, a longitudinal duodenotomy is made on the lateral wall. Compression of the lateral wall against the medial

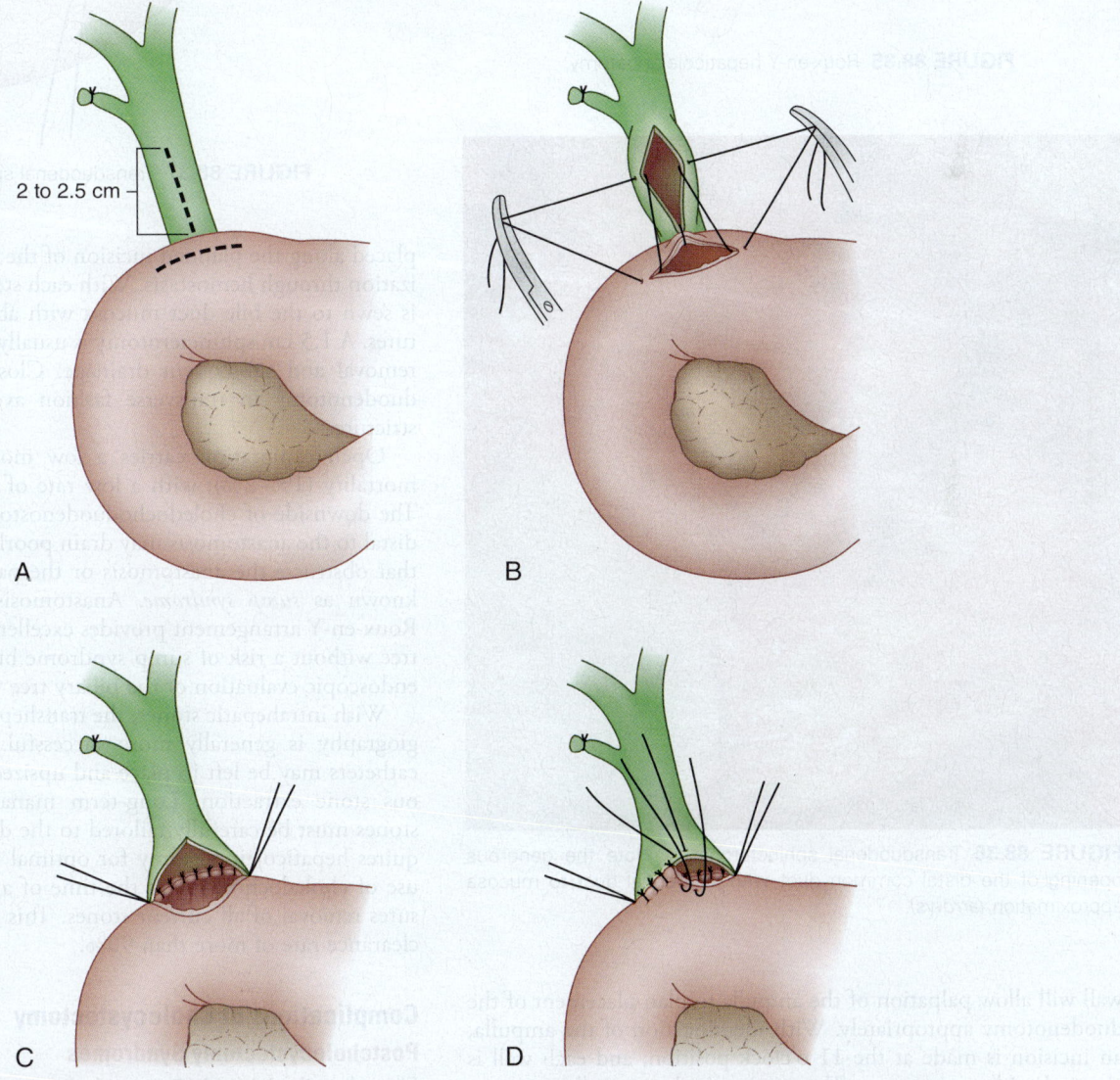

FIGURE 88.34 Choledochoduodenostomy. In the setting of a dilated common bile duct (CBD) with inability to clear all the stones from the distal duct, an anastomosis can be performed between the CBD and adjacent duodenum. Although maintaining the possibility of future endoscopic therapy, this arrangement risks sump syndrome in the undrained distal duct. (A) Vertical incision on CBD and horizontal incision on duodenum. (B) Stay sutures on corners, creating open anastomosis. (C) Suturing posterior wall. (D) Suturing anterior wall.

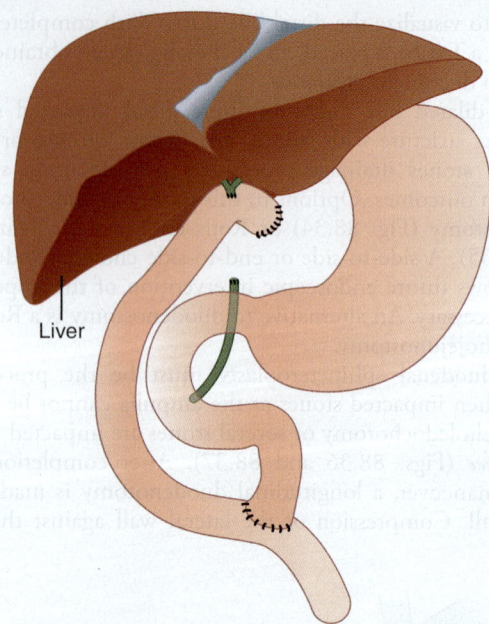

Liver

FIGURE 88.35 Roux-en-Y hepaticojejunostomy.

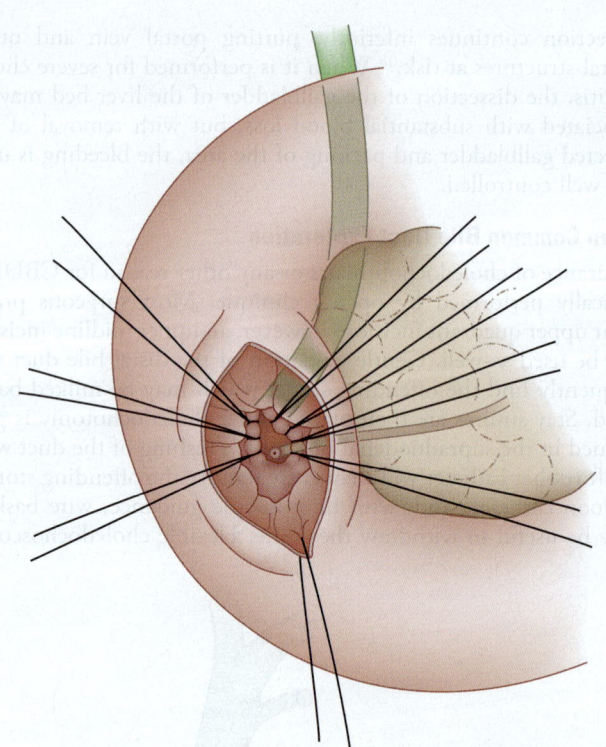

FIGURE 88.37 Transduodenal sphincteroplasty.

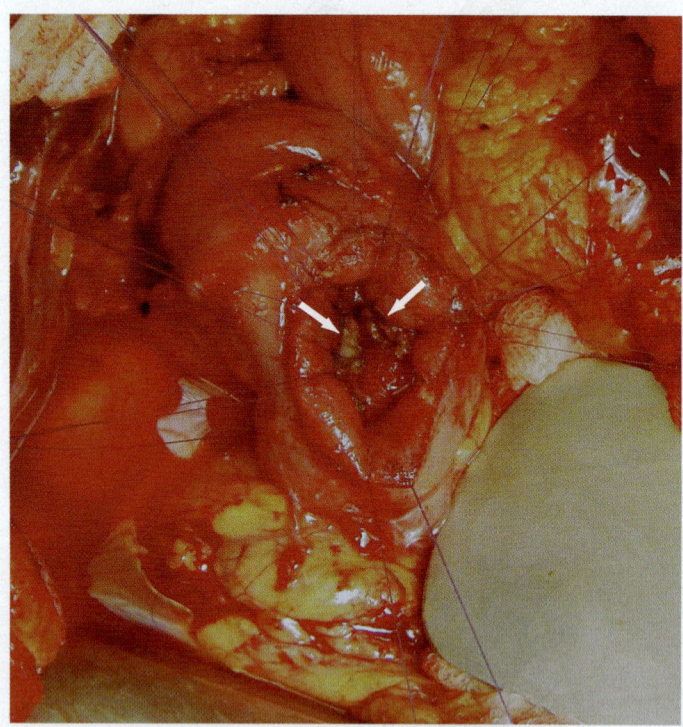

FIGURE 88.36 Transduodenal sphincteroplasty. Note the generous opening of the distal common duct with sequential duct to mucosa approximation *(arrows)*.

wall will allow palpation of the ampulla to plan placement of the duodenotomy appropriately. With identification of the ampulla, an incision is made at the 11 o'clock position, and each wall is elevated with stay sutures. The pancreatic duct usually enters at the 5 o'clock position on the ampulla and must be avoided. It is also imperative to remember that the inferior pancreaticoduodenal arcade is adjacent to the distal part of the ampulla and can be injured during sphincterotomy. Sequential straight clamps are

placed along the planned incision of the ampulla to guide visualization through hemostasis. With each step, the duodenal mucosa is sewn to the bile duct mucosa with absorbable 4-0 or 5-0 sutures. A 1.5-cm sphincterotomy is usually sufficient to allow stone removal and subsequent drainage. Closure of the longitudinal duodenotomy in transverse fashion avoids a future duodenal stricture.

Open exploration carries a low morbidity (8%–15%) and mortality (1%–2%), with a low rate of retained stones (<5%). The downside of choledochoduodenostomy is that the bile duct distal to the anastomosis may drain poorly and may collect debris that obstructs the anastomosis or the pancreatic duct, a process known as *sump syndrome*. Anastomosis to the jejunum in a Roux-en-Y arrangement provides excellent drainage of the biliary tree without a risk of sump syndrome but does not allow future endoscopic evaluation of the biliary tree (see Fig. 88.35).

With intrahepatic stones, the transhepatic approach to cholangiography is generally more successful. Percutaneous drainage catheters may be left in place and upsized to perform percutaneous stone extraction. Long-term management of intrahepatic stones must be carefully tailored to the disease but frequently requires hepaticojejunostomy for optimal biliary drainage. Liberal use of choledochoscopy at the time of a drainage procedure ensures removal of all current stones. This approach allows a stone clearance rate of more than 90%.

Complications of Cholecystectomy

Postcholecystectomy Syndromes

First described in 1947, postcholecystectomy syndrome, recurrence of heterogeneous symptoms similar to those experienced before a cholecystectomy, such as upper abdominal pain and dyspepsia, with or without jaundice, occurs in 10% to 15% of all cholecystectomies worldwide. These symptoms may manifest from days to years after cholecystectomy and are more common in females. The etiology ranges from surgical complications (in more severe forms) to primary unrelated etiology such as esophagitis, GERD, and more. Biliary etiologies specifically include, but are not limited to, a retained stone, bile salt–induced diarrhea, biliary leak, long remnant cystic duct, or functional problems with biliary tree and/or sphincter of Oddi.

Bile Duct Injury

More than 80% of bile duct injuries occur during cholecystectomy. Variable anatomy, porta hepatis inflammation, inappropriate exposure, inadequate experience or skill, and aggressive hemostasis have been cited as risk factors. Studies have suggested that misperception of the anatomy is a much more common factor in iatrogenic injury than surgical skill.[34] With sufficient cephalad retraction of the gallbladder fundus, the cystic duct overlies the common hepatic duct, running in a parallel path. Without inferolateral traction of the gallbladder infundibulum to dissociate these structures, dissection of the apparent cystic duct may actually include the common hepatic duct, placing it in jeopardy. By retraction of Hartmann pouch inferolaterally and opening of the triangle of Calot, the cystic duct is displaced from the porta, no longer collinear with the hepatic duct. The use of a 30-degree laparoscope provides adequate visualization of the critical view of safety during laparoscopic cholecystectomy. Also, in many of these cases, a confirmation bias occurs in which surgeons tend to rely on evidence that supports their perception while discounting visual cues that suggest an alternative explanation. Confirmation bias helps explain why most bile duct injuries are identified in the postoperative setting, not intraoperatively. Cholangiography does not completely avoid bile duct injury but may reduce the incidence and extent of injury and allow immediate recognition and management. The original analysis of biliary reconstruction was based on the Bismuth classification and has been modified by Strasberg. Classification of bile duct injuries is determined by location and helps guide later surgical reconstruction (Fig. 88.38).[39] Injury to the bile duct that does not leak bile will usually be manifested with jaundice, with or without pain. Among postoperative bile duct strictures, occurring roughly in less than 1% of all cases, types E1 and E2 involve the common hepatic duct but not the bifurcation, with type E1 maintaining more than 2 cm of common hepatic duct below the bifurcation and type E2 being within 2 cm of the confluence. Type E3 strictures occur at the confluence, preserving the extrahepatic ducts, and in type E4, the stricturing process includes the extrahepatic biliary tree. Type E5 strictures involve aberrant right hepatic duct anatomy, with injury to the aberrant duct and common hepatic duct.

Presentation. Bile duct injury can result in bile leakage or stricture. Leakage into the peritoneal cavity followed by peritonitis tends to manifest earlier than stricture. Less than 10% of strictures are found in first week postoperatively, and more than 70% are diagnosed within 6 months. In the setting of bile leakage, patients may present with fever, increasing abdominal pain, jaundice, or bile leakage from an incision. Regardless of timing or presentation, adequate repair and subsequent outcome depend on diagnosis, sufficient delineation of anatomy, creation of a tension-free anastomosis, and liberal use of transanastomotic stents.

Treatment

Recognized at the time of cholecystectomy. When bile duct injury is suspected intraoperatively, conversion to an open operation and use of cholangiography help delineate management. Goals for

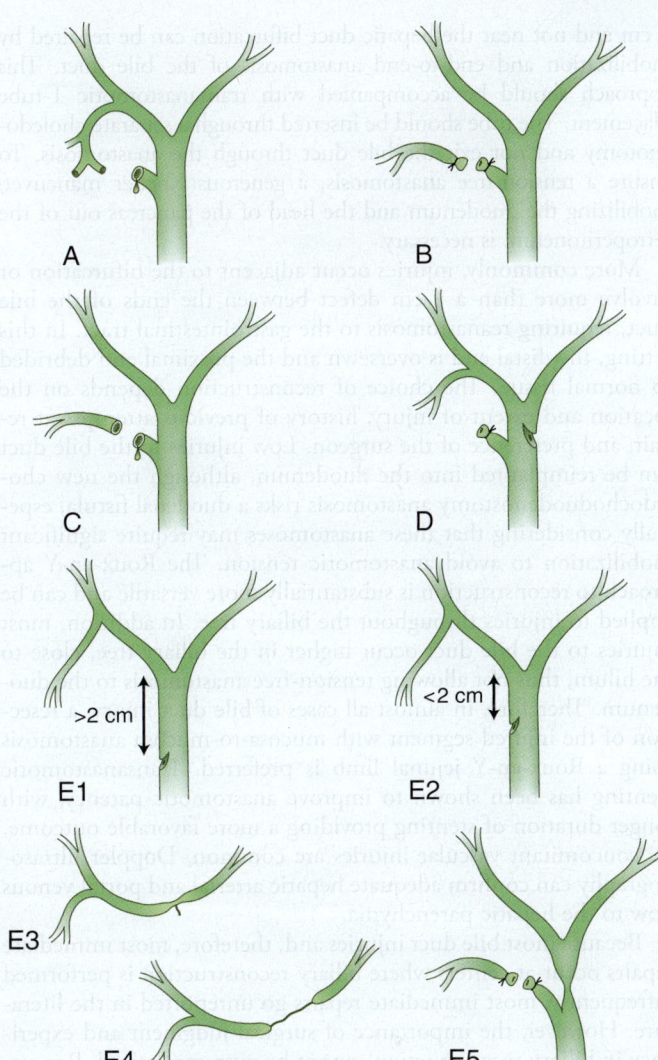

FIGURE 88.38 Strasberg classification of postoperative bile duct strictures. (A) Injury to small ducts in continuity with the biliary system with a leak in the duct of Luschka or the cystic duct. (B) Injury to a sectoral duct, causing obstruction of portion of the biliary system. (C) Injury to a sectoral duct with bile leak; the leak is from a duct and is not continuous with the biliary system. (D) Lateral injury to the extrahepatic biliary ducts. (E1) Bismuth type 1: injury more than 2 cm from the confluence. (E2) Bismuth type 2: injury less than 2 cm from the confluence. (E3) Bismuth type 3: injury at the confluence; confluence intact. (E4) Bismuth type 4: destruction of the biliary confluence. (E5) Complete occlusion of all bile ducts, including sectoral ducts.

the immediate treatment of bile duct injury include maintenance of ductal length, elimination of any bile leakage that would affect subsequent management, and creation of a tension-free repair. If the injury occurs to a larger than 3-mm duct but is not caused by electrocautery and involves less than 50% of the circumference of the wall, a T-tube is placed through the injury. This choledochotomy with T-tube usually will allow healing without the need for subsequent biliary-enteric anastomosis. Ducts smaller than 3 mm that by cholangiography drain only a single segment or subsegment of the liver and simple ligation may suffice for management. Any thermal injury in which the extent of thermal damage may not be manifested immediately or an injury involving more than 50% of the duct circumference requires resection of the injured segment with anastomosis to reestablish biliary-enteric continuity. Defects smaller than

1 cm and not near the hepatic duct bifurcation can be repaired by mobilization and end-to-end anastomosis of the bile duct. This approach should be accompanied with transanastomotic T-tube placement. The tube should be inserted through a separate choledochotomy and not exit the bile duct through the anastomosis. To ensure a tension-free anastomosis, a generous Kocher maneuver, mobilizing the duodenum and the head of the pancreas out of the retroperitoneum, is necessary.

More commonly, injuries occur adjacent to the bifurcation or involve more than a 1-cm defect between the ends of the bile duct, requiring reanastomosis to the gastrointestinal tract. In this setting, the distal end is oversewn and the proximal end debrided to normal tissue. The choice of reconstruction depends on the location and extent of injury, history of previous attempts at repair, and preference of the surgeon. Low injuries to the bile duct can be reimplanted into the duodenum, although the new choledochoduodenostomy anastomosis risks a duodenal fistula, especially considering that these anastomoses may require significant mobilization to avoid anastomotic tension. The Roux-en-Y approach to reconstruction is substantially more versatile and can be applied to injuries throughout the biliary tree. In addition, most injuries to the bile duct occur higher in the biliary tree, close to the hilum, thus not allowing tension-free anastomosis to the duodenum. Therefore, in almost all cases of bile duct injury, a resection of the injured segment with mucosa-to-mucosa anastomosis using a Roux-en-Y jejunal limb is preferred. Transanastomotic stenting has been shown to improve anastomotic patency, with longer duration of stenting providing a more favorable outcome. As concomitant vascular injuries are common, Doppler ultrasonography can confirm adequate hepatic arterial and portal venous flow to the hepatic parenchyma.

Because most bile duct injuries and, therefore, most immediate repairs occur at centers where biliary reconstruction is performed infrequently, most immediate repairs go unreported in the literature. However, the importance of surgical judgment and experience in biliary reconstruction cannot be overemphasized. Reports of previous failed attempts at reconstruction highlight the value of experience in the treatment of bile duct injuries. Therefore, when one is confronted with a bile duct injury and no surgeon with experience in biliary reconstruction is available, the most appropriate management strategy is placement of one or multiple drains in the right upper quadrant and immediate referral to an experienced center.[34]

Identified after cholecystectomy. The diagnosis of iatrogenic bile duct injury should be suspected in any patient who presents with new or increasing symptoms after a laparoscopic cholecystectomy. Leakage may be manifested as bilious drainage into a subhepatic drain placed at the time of operation or bilious drainage from a surgical incision. Without a site for external drainage, bile leakage can be manifested as a biloma, whether sterile or infected, or with biliary ascites. Persistent or worsening postprandial pain, shoulder pain, malaise, and/or fever must raise the suspicion of a bile duct injury.

Patients suspected of having an iatrogenic bile duct injury should undergo imaging to assess for a fluid collection and to evaluate the biliary tree. Ultrasonography can achieve both these goals, but because percutaneous drainage may be required and anatomic delineation is valuable, cross-sectional imaging by CT will generally provide more useful data. Some surgeons advocate the use of radionuclide scanning to confirm bile leakage, but with any documentation of a leak, CT will be necessary to plan management. Also, ischemia is a common cause of bile duct stricture.

In the setting of a bile duct injury, 20% or more of patients will have concomitant unrecognized vascular injuries.

In the delayed presentation of a bile duct injury, three major goals guide therapy (Box 88.1). First, control of infection with drainage of any fluid collections will minimize the inflammatory process. Inflammation in the porta hepatis leads to fibrosis, which acts only to increase stricture formation. Broad-spectrum antibiotics, decompression of the biliary tree, and drainage, whether percutaneous or operative, of any fluid collections will achieve this goal. With control of sepsis, there is no urgency for biliary reconstruction. In fact, with time, resolution of the periportal inflammation helps with the execution of a durable reconstruction. In addition, the retraction of an injured bile duct into the hilum of the liver, as well as inflammation in this region, makes successful repair in the immediate postoperative setting unlikely. Therefore, although immediate reexploration to manage the injury as expeditiously as possible is tempting, successful long-term management of bile duct injuries identified postoperatively depends on clear and deliberate preoperative planning of the reconstruction.

A second goal of management is clear and thorough delineation of the biliary anatomy with cholangiography. Without preoperative cholangiography, any attempts at repair are unlikely to be successful. The cholangiogram must indicate the intrahepatic anatomy and bile duct bifurcation. For patients with bile duct continuity, ERCP may be possible. However, PTC will demonstrate the intrahepatic biliary tree, identify the location of the injury, provide drainage of bile, and possibly even allow the leak to close (Fig. 88.39). Percutaneous biliary catheters can also be left in place during reconstruction to assist in dissection and to provide drainage perioperatively. PTC can be combined with ERCP as necessary, depending on the site and extent of injury. Small bile leaks with bile duct continuity and cystic duct stump leaks can be successfully managed by endoscopic stenting and sphincterotomy.

The third goal of management is to reestablish durable biliary-enteric drainage. Although a combination of percutaneous and endoscopic biliary dilations and stenting may establish continuity, surgical reconstruction has the highest patency rates. To achieve a successful and durable repair, the anastomosis must be performed between a minimally inflamed bile duct to intestines in a tension-free, mucosa-to-mucosa fashion. When the anastomosis is within 2 cm of the hepatic duct bifurcation or involves intrahepatic ducts, some evidence suggests that long-term stenting may improve patency. If the bifurcation is involved, stenting of both right and left ducts should be performed. When the reconstruction

---

BOX 88.1 Goals of Therapy in Iatrogenic Bile Duct Injury

1. Control of infection, limiting inflammation
   - Parenteral antibiotics
   - Percutaneous drainage of periportal fluid collections
2. Clear and thorough delineation of entire biliary anatomy
   - Magnetic resonance cholangiopancreatography or percutaneous transhepatic cholangiography
   - Endoscopic retrograde cholangiopancreatography (especially if cystic duct stump leak is suspected)
3. Reestablishment of biliary-enteric continuity
   - Tension-free, mucosa-to-mucosa anastomosis
   - Roux-en-Y hepaticojejunostomy
   - Long-term transanastomotic stents if bifurcation or higher is involved

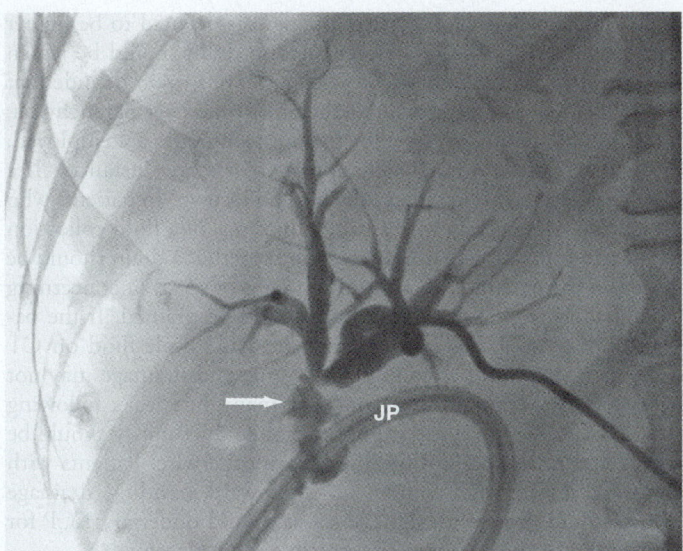

FIGURE 88.39 Percutaneous transhepatic cholangiogram of bile duct injury. Note the extravasation of contrast material *(arrow)* and the Jackson-Pratt *(JP)* drain placed at the time of initial operation.

involves the CBD or common hepatic duct more than 2 cm from the bifurcation, stenting is not necessary; therefore, a preoperatively placed transhepatic drain or intraoperatively placed T-tube will provide adequate decompression in the immediate postoperative period.

At the time of operation, the adhesions of the duodenum and colon to the liver should be separated. The porta hepatis can be encircled with a Penrose drain. Although the bile duct should lie on the lateral border of the porta hepatis, preoperatively placed percutaneous biliary drainage catheters can assist in the dissection, as the marked fibrosis and inflammatory process may make its identification difficult. If necessary, a small-caliber needle attached to a syringe can be used to aspirate and to identify the bile duct while avoiding inadvertent injury to a vascular structure. Once identified, above the stricture, only a limited segment of bile duct (<5 mm) is dissected free. Any further dissection of normal duct risks vascular compromise of the segment to be used in the anastomosis. Preservation of as much normal biliary tree as possible remains a goal of the reconstruction. Next, the bile duct can be opened and the percutaneously placed catheters advanced through the incision. At this point, a wire can be used to exchange the catheters for long-term Silastic stents, if appropriate, or the catheters can be left in place for transanastomotic decompression. The mucosa-to-mucosa anastomosis can be created in an end-to-side fashion to the Roux-en-Y jejunal limb. In the setting of substantial inflammation at the bifurcation, another reconstruction option involves anastomosis of the Roux limb to the left hepatic duct. As noted, the left hepatic duct retains a substantial extraparenchymal length, allowing an anastomosis in this portion of normal duct. Before this section is used for drainage of the entire liver, cholangiography must confirm that the biliary bifurcation is widely patent, thus ensuring drainage of the right lobe across the bifurcation to the left duct system.

Interventional radiologic and endoscopic techniques.
Fluoroscopic-guided management using percutaneous access to traverse the stricture can be used when the duct continuity of the duct is preserved. Balloon dilation can treat strictures, and this

approach is successful in up to 70% of patients.[40] Complications, although frequent, are generally manageable and include cholangitis, hemobilia, and bile leaks requiring repeated intervention. Endoscopic balloon dilation of bile duct strictures is generally reserved for those with primary bile duct strictures or patients who have undergone choledochoduodenostomy for reconstruction because the Roux limb does not usually allow endoscopic strategies. Therefore, series are limited, but results are encouraging, with 88% of patients responding to therapy and a complication rate of 8% from pancreatitis and cholangitis.

Outcomes. Successful outcomes can be achieved in patients undergoing biliary-enteric reconstruction after bile duct injury, with many series showing more than 90% of patients free of jaundice and cholangitis. High success rates are generally achieved when injuries are identified early, and patients are referred immediately to experienced centers. In several studies, referral to centers performing complex biliary surgery routinely was associated with better long-term success.[34] Surgical reconstruction provides a durable long-term management strategy. Management of these injuries requires a multidisciplinary management and may need percutaneous techniques as well as surgical reconstruction. Sepsis at the time of reconstruction and biliary cirrhosis are predictors of stricture. In some studies, results were generally better if transanastomotic stents were used during reconstruction.[41] Chronic liver disease and hepatic fibrosis are associated with higher operative mortality and lower success rates. Although a devastating complication, management is highly successful and restores health-related quality of life scores to preinjury levels.

Biliary Leak
After a cholecystectomy, patients may suffer a leak from the cystic duct or an unrecognized duct of Luschka. Fevers, chills, right upper quadrant pain, jaundice, leakage of bile from an incision or into a drain, or persistent anorexia or bloating are common signs and symptoms. Although it can be seen after any cholecystectomy, those performed for acute cholecystitis carry the greatest risk. With inflammation and fibrosis around an obstructed cystic duct, clips placed on the duct may not fully occlude it or may be dislodged as the inflammatory process resolves. Patients will generally present within 1 week of cholecystectomy as the bile collects. A CT, when performed, will show ascites or a right upper quadrant fluid collection consistent with a biloma. After drain placement and controlling the leak and infection, ERCP can be performed if the leak is high output (>300–500 mL/day). Some of these leaks may dry up on their own with sufficient external drainage. If there is high output or persistent bile leak, ERCP with sphincterotomy with stenting of the common duct will allow the leak to seal without need for surgical management.[41] Reexploration in this setting is rarely indicated, especially in patients with evidence of septic shock or those in whom the leakage is not percutaneously accessible. If percutaneous drainage is not feasible because of overlying bowel or the fluid is not localized and thus not amenable to percutaneous drainage, a laparoscopic washout of the abdomen and placement of subhepatic drains can be considered. No attempt should be made to fix the leak; any such intervention is almost always unsuccessful and risks further biliary tree injury. Persistence of a bile leak longer than 6 weeks should raise the suspicion of an unrecognized bile duct injury. Similar to CBD injuries, surgical treatment of a duct leak is most successful once the inflammatory process has resolved.

Lost Stones

Accidental opening of the gallbladder with spillage of stones occurs in 20% to 40% of cholecystectomies. Pigmented stones, a high number of stones, less experienced surgeons performing the surgery, and severe cholecystitis are all risk factors. Unfortunately, stones lost during a cholecystectomy can have significant and even substantially delayed consequences, such as chronic abscess, fistula, wound infection, and bowel obstruction. Most dropped stones settle into the Morison pouch or the retrohepatic space along the abdominal wall, which may develop into a chronic abscess in this location. The likelihood for the development of complications from lost stones is difficult to quantify because surgeon documentation of gallbladder perforation is variable and a substantial delay frequently exists between cholecystectomy and complication from lost stones. On the basis of available studies, lost stones do not necessitate conversion to an open operation; treatment should include extensive irrigation, significant attempt to retrieve lost stones, course of antibiotics, documentation of the perforation in the operative notes, and clear communication with the patient of the small possibility of delayed presentation from erosion or abscess.

Postcholecystectomy Pain

Although unusual, pain similar to biliary colic may persist or recur after cholecystectomy. A thorough evaluation of the biliary tree should be undertaken after cholecystectomy if the pain recurs. Recurrence of pain, if it is associated with other system findings of jaundice, fever, or chills within days to weeks after cholecystectomy, suggests a secondary choledocholithiasis or a bile leak. Other biliary tree phenomena may cause a similar picture, such as SOD. Postoperative bile duct strictures, which usually are manifested with jaundice, are generally identified within the first year after cholecystectomy and may be manifested with pain or fever if only one lobar duct is obstructed. In the setting of normal liver chemistries, other causes of right upper quadrant pain should be investigated.

Retained Biliary Stones

Retained stones or secondary stones, originating in the gallbladder and passing into the common duct, are usually cholesterol stones and frequently become symptomatic within weeks of a cholecystectomy but may be identified for up to 2 years after cholecystectomy. Hyperbilirubinemia and an elevated ALP level should raise the suspicion of a retained stone. US may not show intrahepatic biliary ductal dilation if the stone does not fully occlude the duct or the obstruction is early. Endoscopic removal of these stones through a generous sphincterotomy has very high success rates.

Other Postoperative Complications

The most common intraabdominal complications following laparoscopic cholecystectomy for acute cholecystitis are abscess formation, bleeding, and bile leak. These complications can usually be managed with the assistance of IR rather than return to the operating room; although in the setting of a bile leak causing diffuse peritonitis, operative washout and drain placement is indicated. Bile and gallstone spillage are common in cases of acute inflammation. Bile should be irrigated and aspirated and efforts should be made to retrieve all dropped gallstones. Larger dropped stones can result in abscess formation so every effort should be made to retrieve them.

Most bile leaks postoperatively are not related to major CBD injury, but due to leakage from the cystic duct or small subcapsular ducts (ducts of Luschka). When a patient is deemed to be higher than average risk of leak, a closed suction drain should be left in the operative field. Examples of when to leave a drain include that the gallbladder is exceptionally adherent to the liver parenchyma, poor cystic duct quality, or when bailout techniques are employed. Leaks may not be immediately apparent in many instances. If a small leak is present, it will usually heal on its own. In patients who present postoperatively with imaging findings of a fluid collection in the surgical bed, one must determine whether a drain should be placed. If the patient is demonstrating signs of sepsis or concerning lab and imaging findings, the fluid should be drained. If the patient appears well, has normal labs, and has simple fluid on CT scan, then the fluid may represent seroma, and drainage may not be necessary. Although it is true that many bile leaks following cholecystectomy are cystic stump leaks, bile duct injury should be considered unless clinical findings prove otherwise. Patients with abnormal LFTs, high-volume leaks, upward trending drainage volumes, and those with signs of sepsis should undergo ERCP for delineation of the anatomy and possible stent placement.

Biliary Neoplasms
Gallbladder Polyps

Benign masses of the gallbladder are common, occurring in up to 12% of the population. Polyps are nonmobile protrusions into the gallbladder lumen that can be divided into pseudopolyps and true polyps. Most polyps are pseudopolyps and can be further divided into cholesterol polyps, focal adenomyomatosis, hyperplastic polyps, and inflammatory polyps, none of which have malignant potential. Cholesterol polyps appear as pedunculated echogenic lesions of the gallbladder, are usually smaller than 1 cm, and are frequently multiple. Adenomyomatosis is seen as a sessile lesion, commonly in the fundus, with characteristic microcysts within the lesion, and is frequently larger than 1 cm (Fig. 88.40). True polyps are neoplastic growths in the wall of the gallbladder that have the potential to harbor or become gallbladder cancer. The risk of malignancy increases with polyp size, and expert consensus is that cholecystectomy should be recommended to all patients with polyps 10 mm or greater or symptoms potentially attributable to the gallbladder.[42] For patients with smaller polyps (6–9 mm), clinical risk factors, such as Asian race and PSC, and radiographic features, such as sessile morphology and vascularity,

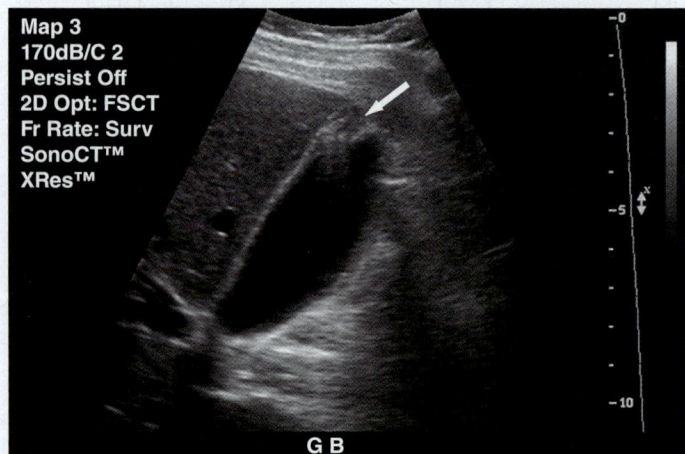

FIGURE 88.40 Ultrasound image of adenomyomatosis. Seen in the fundus of the gallbladder is a sessile thickening *(arrow)* with smaller microcysts within it, consistent with adenomyomatosis.

should also influence recommendation for cholecystectomy. Polyps smaller than 10 mm with no other risk factors and no ultrasonographic features suggesting malignant disease can be observed with serial ultrasonography.

Benign Biliary Masses

Benign intraluminal lesions of the biliary tract have been an evolving field. The most accepted categorization of benign biliary lesions distinguishes biliary intraepithelial neoplasms from intraductal papillary neoplasms.[43] Intraepithelial neoplasms are flat lesions that are not evident grossly and are usually incidental findings on resection for other indications. Their epidemiology and molecular features strongly suggest that they are precursors of bile duct malignancy (cholangiocarcinoma). In contrast, intraductal papillary neoplasms are grossly visible polypoid lesions that are the rarer counterparts to intraductal papillary mucinous neoplasms (IPMNs) of the pancreas and are also considered premalignant. The presentation is typically that of biliary obstruction with jaundice and sometimes right upper quadrant pain. Treatment consists of complete resection with a small rim of normal epithelium because incomplete excision of affected epithelium carries a high risk of recurrence. Like IPMNs of the pancreas, intraductal papillary neoplasms of the bile duct can affect multiple parts of the biliary tree synchronously or nonsynchronously.

Inflammatory lesions of the biliary tree, known as pseudotumors or benign fibrosing disease, may be mistaken for cholangiocarcinoma. When this process follows surgical intervention on the biliary tree, the masslike stricture may be the result of ischemia to the duct, with subsequent inflammation and fibrosis. Alternatively, pseudotumors may occur de novo; these commonly affect the extrahepatic biliary tree above the bifurcation.

Malignant Biliary Disease

Gallbladder Cancer

Gallbladder cancer is an aggressive malignant disease and carries an extremely poor prognosis. Patients have no specific presenting symptoms; therefore, presentation with late-stage disease is common. The poor prognosis corresponds to the high proportion of patients presenting with advanced disease. For patients with earlier stage disease, a more aggressive surgical approach is warranted.

Incidence

Gallbladder cancer generally occurs in the sixth and seventh decades of life and is two to three times more common in females than in males. Ethnicity plays an important role in the development of gallbladder cancer, with the highest incidences in South America and parts of Asia. Among North American populations, Native Americans and immigrants from Latin America have the highest rates. In the United States overall, gallbladder cancer is the most common cancer of the biliary tract and the fifth most common gastrointestinal cancer.[44]

Cause

The prevailing theory of gallbladder cancer focuses on chronic inflammation with subsequent development of neoplasia. The presence of gallstones is considered to be the primary risk factor, and risk of cancer development increases with longer history of gallstone disease. More than 70% of patients with gallbladder cancer have cholelithiasis, and gallbladder cancer is approximately five times more common in patients with gallstones than in those without stones. Extensive calcification of the wall of the gallbladder, termed

porcelain gallbladder, has historically been considered an indication for cholecystectomy due to the risk of cancer development. Whereas the risk of gallbladder cancer is higher in patients with focal gallbladder wall calcification, the finding of diffuse calcifications with modern CT imaging is common compared with the finding of calcifications on plain films, and is not associated with such a high risk of gallbladder cancer that resection in asymptomatic patients is required.[45] Other risk factors include entities that may also cause inflammation in the gallbladder wall, such as APBJ, choledochal cysts, and PSC. Genetic profiling of gallbladders with chronic cholecystitis and cancer, as well as preclinical models, strongly suggest that chronic inflammation leads to an accumulation of mutations (most commonly P53) in a metaplasia-dysplasia-neoplasia sequence.[46]

Pathology and Staging

Gallbladder cancer is generally adenocarcinoma. It is staged by the standard tumor-node-metastasis (TNM) staging system (Table 88.1[47]). Gallbladder cancer spreads via lymphatics, hematogenously, and notoriously into the peritoneal cavity or along biopsy or surgical wound tracts.

Gross descriptions of gallbladder cancer have been grouped into infiltrative, nodular, papillary, and combined forms. Most tumors have an infiltrative pattern and spread in a subserosal plane and can invade the entire gallbladder wall and even into the porta hepatis. Nodular types tend to grow as a more circumscribed mass and can invade the liver. A small subset of gallbladder cancers are of the papillary subtype and carry a better prognosis because they tend to have an indolent course and are commonly limited to the gallbladder wall at the time of diagnosis (Fig. 88.41).

The first draining nodal basin for gallbladder cancer includes the cystic and pericholedochal nodes. From these, the primary drainage areas are the retroportal and pancreaticoduodenal notes. Progressing from these lower portal areas, the lymphatics course to the celiac, superior mesenteric, and finally to aortocaval notes. Involvement of these more distant lymph node stations portends a poor prognosis. Suspicious lymph nodes outside the portal region seen on imaging can be sampled preoperatively by EUS or they should be explored intraoperatively before resection.[48] The gallbladder wall is thin, contains a narrow lamina propria, and is only a single muscular layer with no serosal covering between it and the liver. Thereby, gallbladder malignancies can invade the liver early in their progression. In addition, because the venous drainage of the gallbladder includes direct venous tributaries into the liver parenchyma, these tumors may spread directly into segment IV of the liver. Transperitoneal spread is also common and can progress to carcinomatosis.

Clinical Presentation

Because 90% of gallbladder cancers originate in the fundus or body of the gallbladder, most do not produce symptoms until the disease is advanced (Fig. 88.42). Most gallbladder carcinomas have systemic disease at the time of presentation, with grossly enlarged lymph nodes and/or visible distant metastases in over 50%. Symptoms of acute cholecystitis, with obstruction of the neck of the gallbladder, may portend a better prognosis because patients with these symptoms may present with earlier stages of disease. Some patients describe symptoms of chronic cholecystitis in which the pain has recently changed in quality or frequency. Presentation with jaundice can be difficult to distinguish from hilar cholangiocarcinoma and is a powerful negative prognostic

TABLE 88.1   AJCC Staging Systems for Biliary Tract Cancers[47]

		GALLBLADDER CANCER	INTRAHEPATIC CHOLANGIOCARCINOMA	PROXIMAL/HILAR CHOLANGIOCARCINOMA	DISTAL CHOLANGIOCARCINOMA
TX		Primary tumor cannot be assessed			
T0		No evidence of primary tumor			
Tis		Carcinoma in situ			
T1		Tumor invades the lamina propria or muscular layer	Solitary tumor without vascular invasion, ≤5 cm or >5 cm	Tumor confined to the bile duct, with extension up to the muscle layer or fibrous tissue	Tumor invades the bile duct wall with a depth <5 mm
	T1a	Tumor invades the lamina propria	Solitary tumor ≤5 cm without vascular invasion		
	T1b	Tumor invades the muscular layer	Solitary tumor >5 cm without vascular invasion		
T2		Tumor invades the perimuscular connective tissue	Solitary tumor with intrahepatic vascular invasion or multiple tumors, with or without vascular invasion	Tumor invades beyond the wall of the bile duct to surrounding adipose tissue, or tumor invades adjacent hepatic parenchyma	Tumor invades the bile duct wall with a depth of 5–12 mm
	T2a	Tumor invades the perimuscular connective tissue on the peritoneal side without involvement of the visceral peritoneum		Tumor invades beyond the wall of the bile duct to surrounding adipose tissue	
	T2b	Tumor invades the perimuscular connective tissue on the hepatic side with no extension into the liver		Tumor invades adjacent hepatic parenchyma	
T3		Tumor perforates the visceral peritoneum and/or directly invades the liver and/or one other adjacent organ or structure	Tumor perforating the visceral peritoneum	Tumor invades unilateral branches of the portal vein or hepatic artery	Tumor invades the bile duct wall with a depth >12 mm
T4		Tumor invades the main portal vein or hepatic artery or invades two or more extrahepatic organs or structures			
NX		Regional lymph nodes cannot be assessed			
N0		No regional lymph node metastasis			
N1		Metastases to one to three regional lymph nodes	Regional lymph node metastasis present	One to three positive lymph regional nodes	Metastasis in one to three regional lymph nodes
N2		Metastases to four or more regional lymph nodes		Four or more positive regional lymph nodes	Metastasis in four or more regional lymph nodes
M0		No distant metastasis			
M1		Distant metastasis			

AJCC PROGNOSTIC STAGE GROUPS				
I	T1N0M0	T1N0M0	T1N0M0	T1N0M0
II	T2N0M0	T2N0M0	T2N0M0	T2-3N0M0 or T1-3N1M0
III	T3N0M0 or T1-3N1M0	T3-4N0M0 or any TN1M0	T3-4N0M0 or any TN1M0	T4N0-1M0 or any TN2M0
IV	T4 or N2 or M1	M1	N2 or M1	M1

factor. Weight loss, abdominal mass, and ascites are associated with later stages of disease.

Diagnosis

Laboratory examination generally is not helpful except to identify signs of advanced disease, such as anemia, hypoalbuminemia, leukocytosis, and elevated ALP or bilirubin levels. Carcinoembryonic antigen and CA 19-9 may be elevated in gallbladder cancer.

Ultrasonography is generally the first examination used in the evaluation of right upper quadrant pain. Ultrasonographic findings of gallbladder cancer include an irregularly shaped lesion in the subhepatic space, heterogeneous mass in the gallbladder

lumen, and asymmetrically thickened gallbladder wall (Fig. 88.43). The finding of a polyp larger than 10 mm should also raise the suspicion of gallbladder cancer.

Cross-sectional imaging with CT or MRI is an important part of the preoperative assessment of gallbladder cancer and can provide critical information on the local extent of disease and whether distant metastases are present. CT and MRI may demonstrate peritoneal metastases, hepatic parenchymal metastases, lymphadenopathy, and adjacent vascular involvement (Fig. 88.44). Invasive diagnostic cholangiography has largely been replaced by MRI cholangiography in most high-volume centers. PET can also be a valuable adjunct in searching for metastatic disease or when CT or MRI provides limited information about the primary tumor.

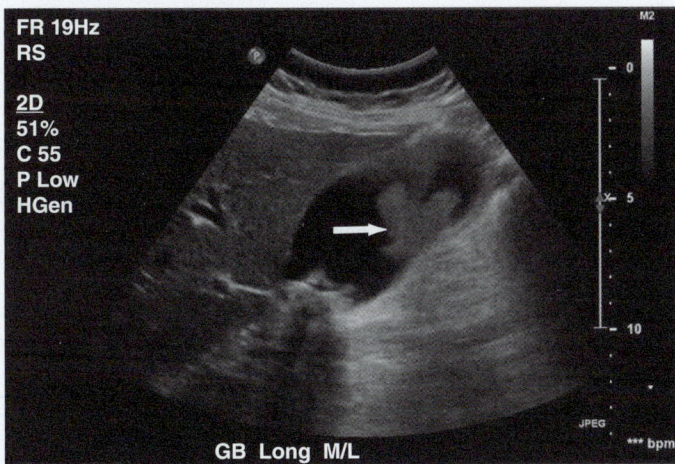

FIGURE 88.41 Ultrasound image showing intraluminal polypoid gallbladder wall mass *(arrow)* but without extraluminal extension.

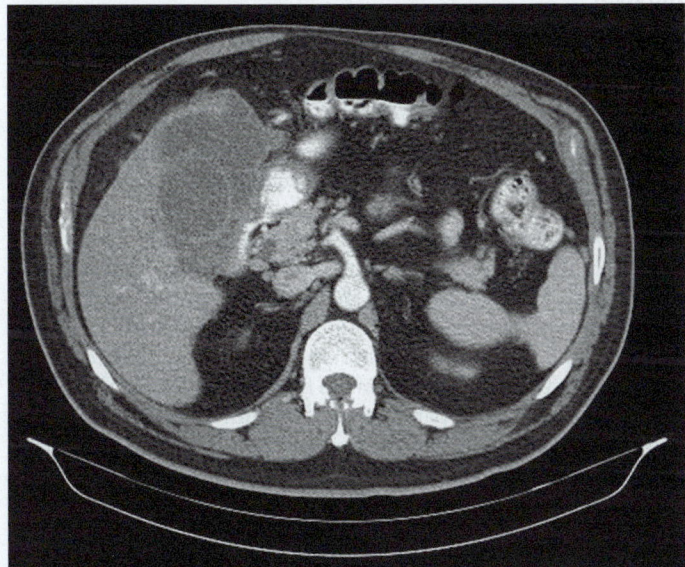

FIGURE 88.42 Computed tomography scan showing gallbladder cancer with invasion into the duodenum and liver parenchyma.

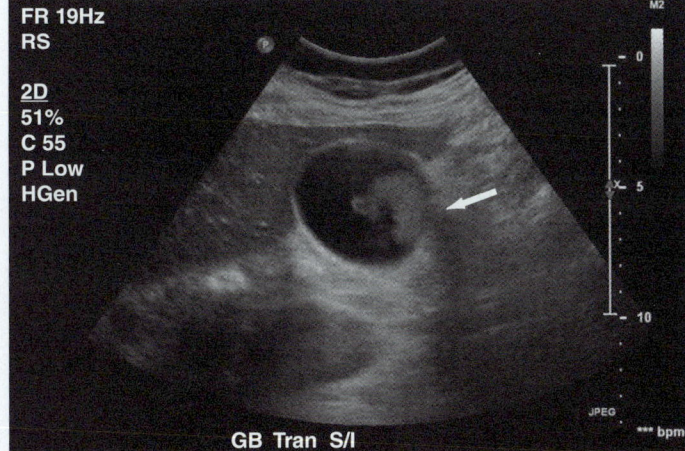

FIGURE 88.43 Ultrasound image of gallbladder mass with loss of continuity of gallbladder wall *(arrow)*, suggesting extraluminal growth.

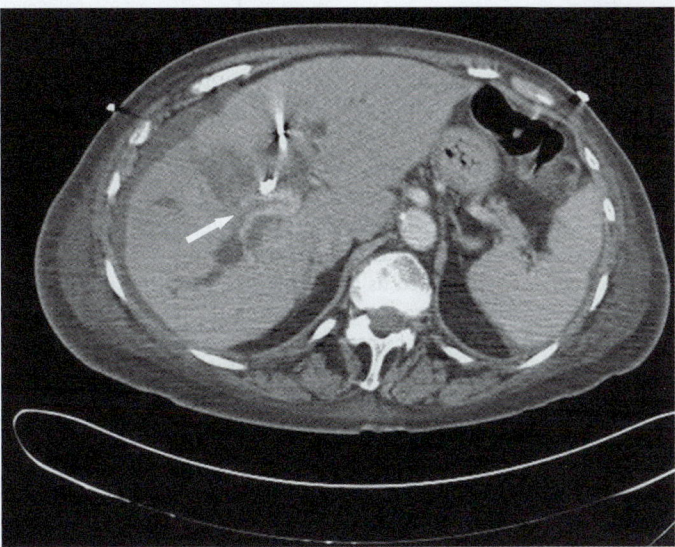

FIGURE 88.44 Computed tomography scan showing gallbladder mass with local invasion into portal vein *(arrow)*.

Gallbladder cancer has a tendency to seed biopsy tracts, and unnecessary biopsies simply increase this risk. If the diagnosis is suspected, the surgeon and patient must be prepared for a definitive operation. In the setting of unresectability (vascular encasement or extensive hepatic involvement) or incurability (hepatic or peritoneal metastases), a biopsy for confirmatory tissue diagnosis should be performed.

Treatment

Resection of gallbladder cancer remains the only potential for cure. Patients with gallbladder cancer can be divided into three specific subgroups of presentation: patients with an incidental finding of gallbladder cancer at the time of or after cholecystectomy, patients suspected of having gallbladder cancer preoperatively, and patients with advanced disease at presentation.

Gallbladder Cancer After Cholecystectomy

With the finding of carcinoma after cholecystectomy, subsequent treatment depends on depth of penetration of the gallbladder wall and surgical margins. With T1a lesions, in which the carcinoma penetrates the lamina propria but does not invade the muscle layer, cholecystectomy suffices for therapy. The likelihood of nodal disease in this setting is less than 3% and cholecystectomy cures 85% to 100% of patients. The cystic duct margin should be reviewed to ensure a negative margin, and sometimes, it is necessary to resect the CBD to obtain a negative margin. For T1b lesions, which penetrate the muscularis but not the deeper connective tissue or serosa, the likelihood of residual liver bed and/or nodal disease begins to increase significantly. Therefore, extended cholecystectomy is generally recommended for all patients who are medically fit with T1b or greater level of invasion but remains controversial.[48] Although re-resection has been associated with improved survival, patients with residual disease have such a poor prognosis that some surgeons regard it more as a staging than a therapeutic procedure.[49]

The extended cholecystectomy is directed at obtaining an R0 resection of the disease, including the draining lymph node basins. Therefore, removal of the hepatoduodenal, gastrohepatic, and retroduodenal lymph nodes should be included. Resection of the cystic duct margin to uninvolved mucosa may require resection of the CBD with Roux-en-Y reconstruction. Because local extension into the hepatic parenchyma is common, approximately 2 cm of apparently normal hepatic parenchyma from the gallbladder fossa is resected. As port site recurrences have been reported for patients with even early-stage disease, some surgeons previously recommended port site excision. However, port site recurrences rarely occur in isolation and generally represent aggressive disease. Port site resection has not been associated with improved survival and is no longer recommended as a routine practice. In patients with T2 lesions, in which the cancer extends past the muscularis but not beyond the serosa, a similar approach with radical cholecystectomy is indicated because more than 40% of these patients have lymph node metastases and up to 25% have positive margins when treated with standard cholecystectomy alone. Patients suspected of having gallbladder cancer preoperatively

Patients in whom preoperative evaluation suggests possibly resectable gallbladder cancer without metastatic disease should be offered an attempt at resection, even though survival is poor compared with those found incidentally. These patients tend to present with advanced locoregional disease and may require an extended liver resection. Because surgical intervention provides the only potential for cure or prolongation of life, radical resection should be considered for adequate operative candidates. The operation begins with a staging laparoscopy to identify small-volume peritoneal or hepatic metastases that would preclude a resection, thereby avoiding an unnecessary laparotomy. Staging laparoscopy should be considered in all patients due to its high yield, even for patients with suspected early stage disease (>10%), but especially for patients with suspected locally advanced disease (>25%).[50]

In the setting of metastatic disease, nonoperative strategies should be used to palliate symptoms. Radical resection in the setting of T3 and T4 lesions includes at least segments IVB and V but more often requires a central hepatectomy, including all of segments IV, V, and VIII. To achieve R0 margin status in large tumors, a right trisegmentectomy may be required. Direct extension of tumor into adjacent structures, such as the hepatic flexure, is not a contraindication to resection as long as negative margins can be obtained. Debulking without the possibility of complete resection has no role in the management of gallbladder cancer.

Patients With Advanced Disease at Presentation

Many patients with gallbladder cancer will present with advanced, incurable disease. The goal of therapy should be palliation of common symptoms, which include jaundice, pain, and intestinal obstruction. Jaundice can be managed by endoscopic biliary stenting, and self-expanding endobiliary metal stents can provide a durable solution, with less need for repeated interventions than with plastic stents. Pain is generally treated with oral narcotics but may progress to require parenteral opioids in the hospice setting. Percutaneous neurolysis of the celiac ganglion can help with the palliation of pain. Intestinal obstruction is usually gastric outlet obstruction from local extension of tumor and is generally managed by an endoscopic duodenal wall stent. In 2010, the landmark ABC-02 study established the combination of gemcitabine and cisplatin as standard of care for systemic therapy of advanced biliary cancer, including gallbladder cancer.[51] The survival benefit of chemotherapy is relatively less for gallbladder cancer than for cholangiocarcinoma, and molecular profiling also demonstrates fewer actionable mutations for targeted therapy in gallbladder cancer than in cholangiocarcinoma (see the following section).

Adjuvant Therapy

The majority of gallbladder cancer recurrences include distant sites as part of the recurrence pattern, highlighting the importance of systemic therapies. Several studies have attempted to extrapolate the benefit of gemcitabine-based chemotherapy from the metastatic setting to the adjuvant setting without success. The large BILCAP trial in 2019 was the first to demonstrate a significant survival benefit of capecitabine (oral 5-fluorouracil) in an adjuvant setting following resection of biliary cancers, including gallbladder cancer (T1b or higher).[52] Adjuvant capecitabine was therefore established as standard of care following complete (radical) resection of gallbladder cancer. However, the optimal sequencing of chemotherapy and radical re-resection in patients with incidentally identified gallbladder cancer remains controversial.

Survival

Survival of patients diagnosed with gallbladder cancer is dependent on the stage of disease at presentation and whether surgical resection is performed. Independent factors affecting survival include T status, N status, histologic differentiation, CBD involvement, and R0 resection. Advances in surgical management and extent of resection have led to improvements in survival in surgical patients, although most patients present with late-stage disease and are not candidates for resection. Patients with T1a lesions, limited to the mucosa and lamina propria, have an excellent prognosis. Complete resection of T1b lesions to negative margins also affords an excellent prognosis. Survival of patients with T2 lesions depends on nodal status and ability to achieve complete resection, with 5-year survival rates that range from 20% to more than 60%. The 5-year survival of patients with T3 tumors is less than 20%, and patients with T4 lesions or metastatic disease have a survival measured in months. Because most patients with gallbladder cancer present with advanced disease, the overall survival of gallbladder cancer is approximately 20%.

Bile Duct Cancer

Cholangiocarcinoma is a rare disease entity that carries a dismal prognosis. Cholangiocarcinoma can arise anywhere along the biliary tree and are best classified according to their anatomic location. Tumors arising beyond the second-order bile ducts within the liver are called intrahepatic or peripheral cholangiocarcinoma, whereas tumors involving the periampullary region are called distal cholangiocarcinoma. Tumors involving the extrahepatic proximal biliary tree near the bifurcation are referred to as proximal or hilar cholangiocarcinoma and as Klatskin tumors. The incidence of cholangiocarcinoma is rising worldwide, especially intrahepatic cholangiocarcinoma, which is the second most common primary cancer of the liver behind hepatocellular carcinoma. Some of this increase may be due to the previous misdiagnosis of intrahepatic cholangiocarcinoma as carcinoma of unknown primary.

Risk Factors

Although most patients with cholangiocarcinoma have no identifiable cause, the risk of development of cholangiocarcinoma appears to correlate with chronic inflammation in the biliary tree and compensatory cellular proliferation. Therefore, many predisposing disease states carry an increased risk for development of cholangiocarcinoma. Congenital lesions, such as choledochal cysts, predispose to the development of cholangiocarcinoma from exposure of the biliary epithelium to toxic pancreatic secretions (see earlier). Cholangiocarcinoma is more prevalent in Southeast Asia, where infection with the liver flukes *C. sinensis* and *Opisthorchis viverrini* creates chronic biliary inflammation, with obstructions and strictures. Recurrent pyogenic cholangitis is characterized by primary bile duct stone formation with infections and carries a risk of cholangiocarcinoma development. PSC, with its autoimmune multifocal strictures of the intrahepatic and extrahepatic biliary trees, also carries an increased risk of cholangiocarcinoma. PSC is the most common identified risk factor for cholangiocarcinoma in the West. PSC carries a cumulative annual risk for cholangiocarcinoma of 1.5% per year, and this risk is increased in those with associated inflammatory bowel disease. Although sporadic cases of cholangiocarcinoma tend to occur at the bifurcation, patients with PSC may have multifocal disease not amenable to resection. Medications and chemical carcinogens have been associated with the development of cholangiocarcinoma, including Thorotrast, oral contraceptives, asbestos, and cigarette smoke. Finally, cirrhosis, infection with hepatitis B and C, choledocholithiasis, and, to a lesser extent, diabetes mellitus are important risk factors for cholangiocarcinoma that may explain the rising incidence.[53]

Staging and Classification

The three distinct pathologic subtypes include nodular (or mass forming), sclerosing (or periductal infiltrating), and papillary cholangiocarcinoma. Intrahepatic cholangiocarcinoma is most commonly mass forming, and advanced tumors may develop satellite lesions. Most proximal (extrahepatic) cholangiocarcinomas are the sclerosing subtype causing periductal fibrosis in a concentric pattern and a circumferential duct occlusion. Both papillary and nodular subtypes occur in distal cholangiocarcinomas and are manifested with intraluminal growths. In the nodular subtype, a firm mass based in the duct wall can be seen growing into the duct lumen, whereas the more common papillary subtype appears as a polypoid lesion that is soft with less periductal fibrosis and a better prognosis.

The staging of cholangiocarcinoma relies on the TNM staging system but is slightly different based on anatomic location.[47] The three staging subdivisions include intrahepatic, proximal/hilar, and distal bile duct (see Table 88.1). Similar to many adenocarcinomas, direct local invasion and local lymph node spread are common and have a worse prognosis. Tumors confined to the bile duct (T1) and those extending outside the bile duct but not invading adjacent structures such as the hepatic artery or portal vein (T2) carry a significantly better prognosis than those invading any nearby structure. The two most important prognostic factors after resection are ability to achieve complete (R0) resection to negative margins and the presence or absence of lymph node metastases.

Clinical Presentation

The presentation of cholangiocarcinoma depends on the anatomic site of origin. Intrahepatic cholangiocarcinoma does not usually cause biliary obstruction and more typically presents with abdominal pain, weight loss, or as an incidental finding. Painless jaundice is a common symptom of proximal and distal cholangiocarcinoma, but patients with unilobar obstruction of a bile duct may present without jaundice but with unilateral lobar atrophy

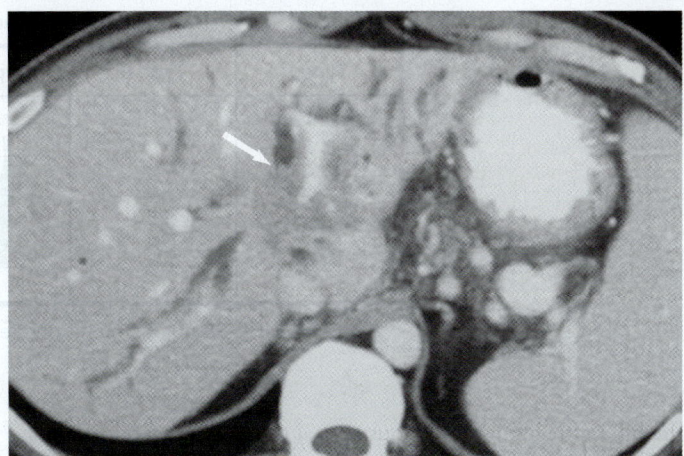

FIGURE 88.45 Computed tomography scan of cholangiocarcinoma with left lobar atrophy caused by obstruction of the left duct. Noted in the atrophied left lobe are dilated biliary radicals *(arrow)*.

and subsequent contralateral lobar hypertrophy (Fig. 88.45). The resultant hepatic compensation can delay presentation until the later stages of disease. Therefore, cholangiocarcinoma causing obstruction at or below the hepatic bifurcation tends to be manifested at earlier stages than intrahepatic cholangiocarcinoma. The common manifestations of biliary obstruction and hyperbilirubinemia, such as pruritus, dark urine, and acholic stools, can be seen. Other markers of hepatic synthetic function, such as prothrombin time and albumin level, are generally unaffected until later in the disease or when the biliary obstruction is longstanding. Cholangiocarcinoma tends to extend in a submucosal route, with associated perineural invasion, but constant pain on presentation suggests more advanced disease.

Diagnosis and Assessment of Resectability

The radiologic evaluation of jaundice includes a right upper quadrant US examination, which may show intrahepatic biliary ductal dilation but does not usually identify the actual site of obstruction. With hilar cholangiocarcinomas, the gallbladder and visualized extrahepatic biliary tree are usually decompressed, whereas distal lesions will have extrahepatic biliary ductal dilation and gallbladder distention. For intrahepatic and extrahepatic cholangiocarcinoma, cross-sectional imaging by triphasic CT allows not only assessment of metastatic disease but also initial evaluation of resectability. The location of the tumor can be identified, and its relationship to vascular structures also can be assessed. Identification of aberrant anatomy and determination of segmental or lobar involvement by CT are helpful for preoperative planning. Tumor markers, including carcinoembryonic antigen and CA 19-9, are unreliable for diagnosis of cholangiocarcinoma but, if elevated, may be useful postoperatively in the surveillance of recurrence.

Typically, CT alone is insufficient for the assessment of feasibility and appropriateness of resection for proximal (perihilar) cholangiocarcinoma. Cholangiography by MRCP, PTC, or ERCP helps determine the proximal extent of resection. For patients who are potential candidates for resection, PTC with percutaneous biliary drainage has advantages over ERCP in its ability to easily target specific ducts, drain longer stenoses, and maintain access to the biliary tree for repeated intervention. Endoscopic cholangiography also carries the additional risk of cholangitis by the introduction of enteric bacteria into an undrained portion of

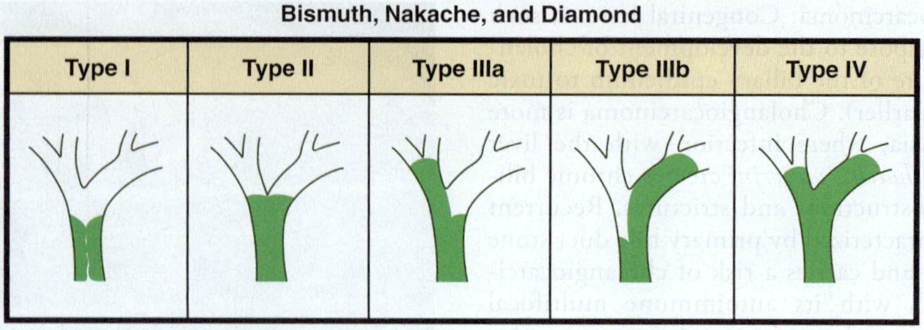

Bismuth, Nakache, and Diamond

Type I	Type II	Type IIIa	Type IIIb	Type IV

FIGURE 88.46 Bismuth-Corlette classification of tumor involvement.

the biliary tree but has obvious appeal over percutaneous drainage in the palliative setting. Bilobar intrahepatic metastases and any extrahepatic disease are contraindications to resection. Because complete (R0) resection is the only strategy that affords the possibility of cure, other contraindications to resection include encasement of the main portal vein (Fig. 88.46), bilateral hepatic lobar artery involvement, involvement of bilateral secondary biliary radicals, and lobar atrophy with involvement of the contralateral portal vein or biliary radicals. Involvement of unilobar vascular structures is managed with resection of the primary and affected lobe in continuity and therefore is not a contraindication.

Tissue diagnosis before resection in operative patients is unnecessary. With obstructive jaundice, bile cytology and brushings are unreliable, and a negative cytology report does not exclude malignant disease. Fluorescence in situ hybridization (FISH) for chromosomal polysomy increases the sensitivity of cytology and may be helpful in indeterminate lesions, but establishment of a tissue diagnosis is important only when the patient is not a candidate for resection. However, preoperative biliary drainage may be useful in select cases. In patients with distal cholangiocarcinoma, preoperative biliary drainage increases the rate of infectious complications of resection but is generally useful for those with preoperative hyperbilirubinemia (bilirubin level >10 mg/dL) and those with a prolonged time interval between presentation and resection. For patients with hilar cholangiocarcinoma, hepatic resection remains an important feature of the operative strategy. In the setting of complete biliary obstruction, hepatic resection carries an additional risk of bleeding, sepsis, and hepatic failure. Drainage of the obstructed but unaffected segments can enhance the postresection hypertrophy of the remaining liver but may increase perioperative infectious complications.

Patients with intrahepatic cholangiocarcinoma, in contrast, do not require cholangiography. Furthermore, a resectable solid liver mass in a noncirrhotic patient with no evidence of a primary malignancy outside of the liver does not require biopsy. However, preoperative biopsy and tumor markers (such as CA 19-9) can be useful in distinguishing intrahepatic cholangiocarcinoma from hepatocellular carcinoma and metastatic lesions, which are much more common than primary malignancies.

Treatment

Operative management. With the clinical suspicion of cholangiocarcinoma in adequate operative candidates without contraindications to resection, exploration should proceed, even in the absence of a confirmed tissue diagnosis. Up to 15% of patients undergoing resection for suspected biliary malignant disease will prove to have benign disease. More than 50% of patients undergoing exploration have historically had findings precluding

resection, such as peritoneal metastases, hepatic metastases, or locally advanced lesions. With advances in the quality of preoperative imaging, this rate is decreasing. However, staging laparoscopy still can be an important initial step at the time of resection to reduce the incidence of nontherapeutic laparotomy.

Distal cholangiocarcinoma. Distal cholangiocarcinoma is managed by pancreaticoduodenectomy. Because these lesions tend to grow in a submucosal plane, a frozen section of the proximal bile duct margin helps ensure an R0 resection. An R0 resection remains one of the most important prognostic factors for this disease, with 5-year survival rates of up to 50% in node-negative patients with an R0 resection.

Proximal cholangiocarcinoma. Surgical management of proximal cholangiocarcinoma involves resection of regional nodal tissue and en bloc resection of the CBD with hepatic parenchyma as necessary to achieve negative margins. The Blumgart preoperative staging system incorporates the longitudinal involvement of biliary radicals (the Bismuth-Corlette classification) as well as extent of vascular involvement and hepatic lobar atrophy to help with operative planning and prognosis (see Fig. 88.46).[54] Small mid-duct tumors can sometimes be completely resected with common duct resection and cholecystectomy, but most proximal cholangiocarcinomas also require partial hepatic resection, which commonly includes resection of the caudate lobe. Resection of the bile duct and nodal tissue requires skeletonization of the hepatic artery and portal vein. Reconstruction is performed using a Roux limb of jejunum. More advanced tumors may involve complex resection and reconstruction of the portal vein, hepatic artery, or both. With resection to secondary biliary radicals, transanastomotic stenting may allow healing and confirmation of anastomotic integrity. Improvements in long-term survival over time have correlated with the increasing use of hepatic resection to achieve negative margins. Intraoperative assessment of margins by frozen section is important, as negative margin status is the most important variable associated with outcome after resection. Five-year survival rates greater than 50% have been reported in selected series, and, with vascular resection and reconstruction techniques, resectability rates have also increased. Although the importance of achieving an R0 resection is clear, the role of routine lymph node dissection is debated. There has been no demonstrable therapeutic benefit of routine lymph node dissection. However, lymph nodes are one of the most important prognostic factors in cholangiocarcinoma and may help direct adjuvant therapy.

With high rates of local unresectability and its frequent association with primary sclerosis cholangitis, liver transplantation has been explored for proximal cholangiocarcinoma since the 1980s. An extensive neoadjuvant therapy protocol that includes high-dose chemoradiation followed by transplantation has shown excellent results (>60% 5-year survival) in highly selected patients that have small (<3 cm) but unresectable tumors without evidence of lymph node metastases.[29] In spite of these findings, the role of transplantation in the management of cholangiocarcinoma remains controversial, and there is substantial debate over the routine use of an extremely limited resource in this disease process.

Intrahepatic cholangiocarcinoma. Intrahepatic cholangiocarcinoma is managed with partial hepatectomy with the goal of negative margins. Multifocal disease is common and associated with poor prognosis as are regional lymph node metastases. Preoperative evidence of multifocal disease and/or regional lymph node metastases should be considered contraindications to resection except in selected patients. With more effective systemic agents (see the following), there is increasing interest in neoadjuvant therapy for such high-risk patients. In patients that undergo resection, portal lymph node dissection (with goal of at least six lymph nodes) is recommended for adequate staging and may help guide the use of adjuvant therapy.[55]

Palliation. In patients found to have unresectable or incurable disease preoperatively, all attempts to palliate their symptoms nonoperatively should be used. The goals of palliation should include relief of jaundice, alleviation of pain, and relief of duodenal obstruction, if necessary. Surgical palliation has not been shown to prolong survival or to reduce complication rates and thus should be reserved for candidates found to be unresectable or metastatic at time of operation. Depending on the location of the biliary obstruction, endoscopic or percutaneous routes of drainage can be used, and placement of a self-expandable metallic stent provides a durable solution. When plastic stents are used, additional manipulation or placement of subsequent stents may be required. For distal cholangiocarcinomas, ERCP is the preferred route of nonoperative biliary drainage, whereas PTC is more useful for proximal lesions. Drainage of atrophic lobes with stents does not improve palliation of disease. Percutaneous destruction of the celiac plexus has demonstrated some benefit for pain relief. For distal cholangiocarcinomas, in which duodenal obstruction may occur, endoscopic duodenal stenting can relieve obstruction in this preterminal condition.

Medical treatment. As described earlier, the ABC-02 study established the combination of gemcitabine and cisplatin as standard of care for systemic therapy of advanced biliary cancer, with the greatest benefit seen in patients with intrahepatic cholangiocarcinoma. Cholangiocarcinoma has a high incidence of somatic genetic alterations, including isocitrate dehydrogenase (IDH) and fibroblast growth factor receptor (FGFR), which are considered actionable with associated targeted therapies. The high tumor mutational burden of cholangiocarcinoma likely explains its relative responsiveness to immunotherapy. In 2022, the TOPAZ-1 trial demonstrated a significant benefit of adding a programmed cell death ligand 1 (PD-L1) checkpoint inhibitor to gemcitabine and cisplatin for unselected patients with advanced biliary cancer, establishing checkpoint inhibition as part of first-line therapy.[56]

In the adjuvant setting, as described previously, the BILCAP trial established capecitabine (oral 5-fluorouracil) as the preferred agent following resection of biliary cancers.[52] Radiation therapy has not been proven in prospective randomized studies to affect survival in cholangiocarcinoma in any setting. However, some nonrandomized studies have suggested that adjuvant radiation may provide a small survival advantage as an adjunct to resection when microscopic residual disease remains, such as patients with R1 resections. Furthermore, radiation therapy is often used in the palliative setting, especially for proximal cholangiocarcinoma, since many patients will experience pain and other local symptoms from unresectable or recurrent tumors

Survival

Long-term survival is highly dependent on stage at presentation and complete surgical resection to negative margins. Most patients present with advanced disease that is not amenable to resection, but the anatomic location of cholangiocarcinoma greatly affects presentation and ability to achieve negative margins. Intrahepatic cholangiocarcinoma is more likely than extrahepatic cholangiocarcinoma to present with distant metastatic disease. Patients with intrahepatic and distal cholangiocarcinoma are more likely to undergo R0 resection than patients with proximal cholangiocarcinoma. Although postoperative morbidity rates of 35% to 50% are still common, mortality rates are generally low (<5%) in modern series. Five-year overall survival rates following resection of cholangiocarcinoma range from 20% to 50% in most series. Variability in overall survival appears to be the related to the incidences of lymph node metastases and R1 resections in various studies, which in turn are likely related to differences in patient selection and surgical technique. However, the landscape of systemic therapy for cholangiocarcinoma is changing so rapidly that these overall survival outcomes are moving targets that will certainly improve in the coming years.

SELECTED REFERENCES

Aloia TA, Jarufe N, Javle M, et al. Gallbladder cancer: expert consensus statement. *HPB (Oxford).* 2015;17(8):681-690.

This article summarizes the consensus of experts from the Americas Hepatobiliary Pancreatic Association on many aspects of the the management of gallbladder cancer, including diagnosis, surgical therapy, and nonsurgical therapy.

Broderick RC, Li JZ, Huang EY, et al. Lighting the way with fluorescent cholangiography in laparoscopic cholecystectomy: reviewing 7 years of experience. *J Am Coll Surg.* 2022;235(5):713-723.

This manuscript describes one of the largest single-institution experiences with fluorescent cholangiography with ICG during laparoscopic cholecystectomy.

Brunt LM, Deziel DJ, Telem DA, et al. Safe cholecystectomy multi-society practice guideline and state-of-the-art consensus conference on prevention of bile duct injury during cholecystectomy. *Surg Endosc.* 2020;34(7):2827-2855.

This article summarizes the consensus of experts from multiple surgical societies on prevention and management of bile duct injuries during cholecystectomy.

Matsuo K, Rocha FG, Ito K, et al. The Blumgart preoperative staging system for hilar cholangiocarcinoma: analysis of resectability and outcomes in 380 patients. *J Am Coll Surg.* 2012; 215(3):343-355.

This article describes one of the largest single-institutional experiences with hilar cholangiocarcinoma as well as the Blumgart modification of the Bismuth-Corlette system for determining resectability.

Strasberg SM, Hertl M, Soper NJ. An analysis of the problem of biliary injury during laparoscopic cholecystectomy. *J Am Coll Surg.* 1995;180:101-125.

This is the most cited article for classification of iatrogenic bile duct injuries and is considered the seminal article on the topic.

The full reference list appears on Elsevier eBooks+.

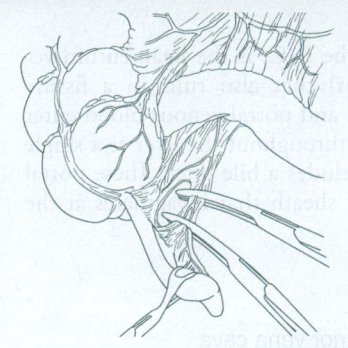

CHAPTER 89

The Liver

Laleh Melstrom, Kevin Labadie, and Yuman Fong

OUTLINE

HISTORICAL PERSPECTIVE

The surface anatomy of the liver was described as early as 2000 BCE by the ancient Babylonians. Even Hippocrates understood and described the seriousness of liver injury. In 1654, Francis Glisson was the first physician to describe the essential anatomy of the blood vessels of the liver accurately. The beginnings of liver surgery are described as rudimentary excisions of eviscerated liver from penetrating trauma. The first documented case of a partial hepatectomy is credited to Berta, who amputated a portion of protruding liver in a patient with a self-inflicted stab wound in 1716.

In the late 1800s, the first gastrectomies and cholecystectomies were being performed in Europe. At that time, surgery on the liver was regarded as dangerous, if not impossible. European surgeons began to experiment with techniques of elective liver surgery on animals in the late 1800s. The credit for the first elective liver resection is a matter of debate, and many surgeons have been given credit, but it certainly occurred during this period.

The early 1900s saw some small but significant advances in liver surgery. Techniques for suturing major hepatic vessels and using cautery for small vessels were applied and reported. The most significant advance of that time was probably that of J. Hogarth Pringle. In 1908, he described digital compression of the hilar vessels to control hepatic bleeding from traumatic injuries. The modern era of hepatic surgery was ushered in by the development of

a better understanding of liver anatomy and formal anatomic liver resection. Credit for the first anatomic liver resection is usually given to Lortat-Jacob, who performed a right hepatectomy in 1952 in France. Pack from New York and Quattelbaum from Georgia performed similar operations within the next year and were unlikely to have had any knowledge of Lortat-Jacob's report. Descriptions of the segmental nature of liver anatomy by Couinaud, Goldsmith, and Woodburne in 1957 opened the door even wider and introduced the modern era of liver surgery.

Despite these improvements, hepatic surgery was plagued by tremendous operative morbidity and mortality from the 1950s into the 1980s. Operative mortality rates over 20% were common and usually related to massive hemorrhage. Many surgeons were reluctant to perform hepatic surgery because of these results, and understandably, many physicians were reluctant to refer patients for hepatectomy. With the courage of patients and their families, as well as the persistence of surgeons, safe hepatic surgery has now been realized. A complete list is not possible here, but courageous hepatic surgeons such as Blumgart, Bismuth, Longmire, Fortner, Schwartz, Starzl, and Ton deserve mention.

Advances in anesthesia, intensive care, antibiotics, and interventional radiologic techniques have also contributed tremendously to the safety of major hepatic surgery. Total hepatectomy with liver transplantation and live donor partial hepatectomy for transplantation are now performed routinely in specialized transplantation centers. Partial hepatectomy for many indications is now performed throughout the world in specialized centers, with mortality rates of 5% or less. Partial hepatectomy on normal livers is now consistently performed, with mortality rates of 1% to 2%.

Safely performed open hepatic surgery, with its liberal use in the management of a wide variety of diseases, is now a reality. Moreover, minimally invasive approaches to liver surgery have been developed and are now being used in significant numbers. However, the learning curve remains steep, and the indications for this technique are being carefully defined. Using robotics in liver surgery may help address the issues with the learning curve with laparoscopy. The addition of robotics offers advanced suturing and articulation that closely approximate open surgery. This allows a greater proportion of cases to be performed in a total, minimally invasive fashion.[1] The role of robotics in liver surgery is rapidly evolving. Thermal ablative techniques to treat hepatic tumors, including radiofrequency and microwave ablation, have exploded in popularity. Finally, techniques to improve the safety of liver resection, such as portal vein embolization to induce preoperative hypertrophy of the future liver remnant (FLR), are being developed and used.

ANATOMY AND PHYSIOLOGY

Anatomy

Gross Anatomy

Precise knowledge of the liver anatomy is a prerequisite to performing surgery on the liver or biliary tree. Over the last several decades, a greater appreciation for complex anatomy beyond the misleading minimal external markings has been realized. The anatomic contributions of Couinaud (see later) and the description of the segmental nature of the liver should be embraced and studied by students of hepatic surgery.

General description and topography. The liver is a solid gastrointestinal organ whose mass (1.2–1.6 kg) largely occupies the right upper quadrant of the abdomen. The costal margin coincides with the lower margin of the liver, and the diaphragm drapes over its superior surface. The thoracic cage covers most of the right and left liver. The posterior surface straddles the inferior vena cava (IVC). A wedge of the liver extends to the left of the abdomen. The liver is invested in the peritoneum except for the gallbladder fossa, porta hepatis, and posterior aspect of the liver on either side of the IVC in two wedge-shaped areas. This region of the liver to the right of the IVC, devoid of peritoneal coverage, is called the *bare area*. The peritoneal duplications on the liver surface are referred to as *ligaments*. The diaphragmatic peritoneal duplications are referred to as the *coronary ligaments*, whose lateral margins are the right and left triangular ligaments on either side. From the center of the coronary ligament emerges the falciform ligament, which extends anteriorly as a thin membrane connecting the liver surface to the diaphragm, abdominal wall, and umbilicus.

The ligamentum teres (the obliterated umbilical vein) runs along the inferior edge of the falciform ligament from the umbilicus to the umbilical fissure. The umbilical fissure is on the inferior surface of the left liver and contains the left portal pedicle. In early descriptions of hepatic anatomy, the falciform ligament, the most apparent surface marker of the liver, was used as the division of the right and left lobes of the liver. However, this description is inaccurate and not useful to the hepatobiliary surgeon (see later for detailed segmental anatomy). On the posterior surface of the left liver, running from the left portal vein in the porta hepatis

toward the left hepatic vein and the IVC, is the ligamentum venosum (obliterated sinus venosus) that also runs in a fissure (Fig. 89.1). Hepatic arterial blood and portal venous blood enter the liver at the hilum and branch throughout the liver as a single portal pedicle unit, which also includes a bile duct. These portal triads are invested in a peritoneal sheath that invaginates at the

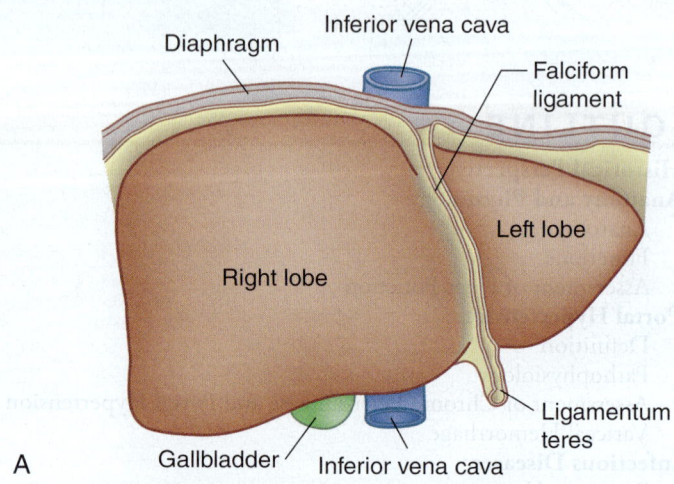

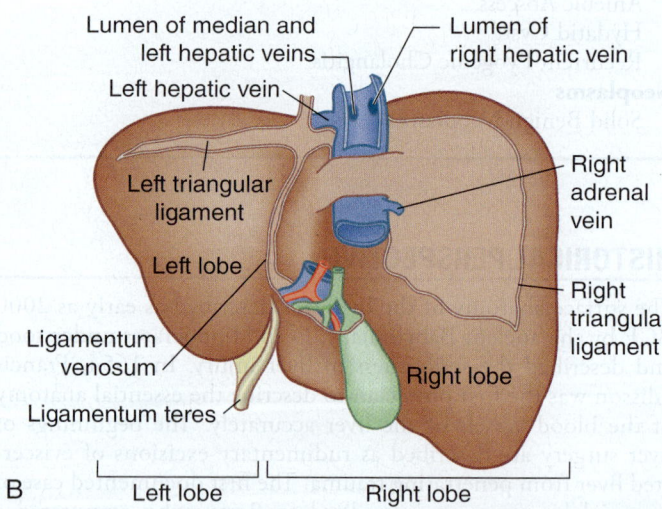

FIGURE 89.1 (A) Historically, the liver was divided into right and left lobes by the external marking of the falciform ligament. On the inferior surface of the falciform ligament, the ligamentum teres can be seen entering the umbilical fissure. (B) The posterior and inferior surface of the liver is shown. The liver embraces the inferior vena cava (IVC) posteriorly in a groove. The lumens of the three major hepatic veins and right adrenal vein can be seen directly entering the IVC. The bare area, bounded by the right and left triangular ligaments, is illustrated. To the left of the IVC is the caudate lobe, which is bounded on its left side by a fissure containing the ligamentum venosum. The lesser omentum terminates along the edge of the ligamentum venosum, and thus, the caudate lobe lies within the lesser sac and the rest of the liver lies in the supracolic compartment. A layer of fibrous tissue can be seen bridging the right lobe to the caudate lobe posterior to the IVC, thus encircling it. This ligament of tissue must be divided on the right side in mobilizing the right liver off the IVC. (From Blumgart LH, Hann LE. Surgical and radiologic anatomy of the liver and biliary tract. In: Blumgart LH, Fong Y, eds. *Surgery of the Liver and Biliary Tract.* London: WB Saunders; 2000:3-34.)

hepatic hilum. Venous drainage is through the right, middle, and left hepatic veins that empty directly into the suprahepatic IVC.

Normal development and embryology. The developing liver shares a common progenitor with the biliary tree and pancreas. During embryogenesis, signals are transmitted from the cardiac mesenchyme and septum transversum. The molecules regulating this (e.g., fibroblast growth factor, bone morphogenetic protein, Wnt, transforming growth factor-β) are being elucidated. The liver primordium begins to form in the third week of development as an outgrowth of endodermal epithelium, known as the *hepatic diverticulum* or *liver bud.* The connection between the hepatic diverticulum and the future duodenum narrows to form the bile duct, and an outpouching of the bile duct forms into the gallbladder and cystic duct. Hepatic cells develop cords and intermingle with the vitelline and umbilical veins to form hepatic sinusoids. Simultaneously, hematopoietic cells, Kupffer cells, and connective tissue form from the mesoderm of the septum transversum that connects the liver to the ventral abdominal wall and foregut. As the liver protrudes into the abdominal cavity, these structures are stretched into thin membranes, forming the falciform ligament and lesser omentum. The mesoderm on the surface of the developing liver differentiates into visceral peritoneum, except superiorly, where contact between the liver and mesoderm (future diaphragm) is maintained, forming a bare area devoid of visceral peritoneum (Fig. 89.2).

The primitive liver plays a central role in fetal circulation. The vitelline veins carry blood from the yolk sac to the sinus venosus, forming a network of veins around the foregut (future duodenum) that drain into the developing hepatic sinusoids. These vitelline veins eventually fuse to form the portal, superior mesenteric, and splenic veins. The sinus venosus empties into the fetal heart and becomes the hepatocardiac channel and then the hepatic veins and retrohepatic IVC. The umbilical veins, paired early on, carry oxygenated blood to the fetus. Initially, the umbilical veins drain into the sinus venosus, but at week 5 of development,

they drain into the hepatic sinusoids. The right umbilical vein ultimately disappears, and the left umbilical vein later drains directly into the hepatocardiac channel, bypassing the hepatic sinusoids through the ductus venosus. In the adult liver, the remnant of the left umbilical vein becomes the ligamentum teres, which runs in the falciform ligament into the umbilical fissure, and the remnant of the ductus venosus becomes the ligamentum venosum at the termination of the lesser omentum under the left liver (Fig. 89.3).

The adult liver is a complex system of numerous cell types, including hepatocytes, cholangiocytes, neuroendocrine cells, hepatic progenitors (oval cells), myofibroblastic mesenchymal cells (hepatic stellate cells and portal myofibroblasts), resident macrophages (Kupffer cells), and vascular endothelial cells.

Functional Anatomy

Historically, the liver was divided into left and right lobes by the obvious external landmark of the falciform ligament. Not only was this description oversimplified, but it was anatomically incorrect in relation to the blood supply to the liver. Our understanding of functional liver anatomy has become more sophisticated.

The functional anatomy of the liver (Figs. 89.4 and 89.5) is composed of eight segments, each supplied by a single portal triad (also called a *pedicle*) composed of a portal vein, hepatic artery, and bile duct. These segments are further organized into four sectors separated by scissurae containing the three main hepatic veins. The four sectors are even further organized into the right and left liver. The terms *right liver* and *left liver* are preferable to the terms *right lobe* and *left lobe* because there is no external mark that allows the identification of the right and left liver. This system was originally described in 1957 by Goldsmith and Woodburne and by Couinaud. It defines hepatic anatomy because it is most relevant to surgery of the liver. The functional anatomy is more often seen as cross-sectional imaging (Fig. 89.6).

The main scissura contains the middle hepatic vein, which runs in an anteroposterior direction from the gallbladder fossa to the left side of the vena cava. It divides the liver into right and left hemilivers. The line of the main scissura is also known as the *Cantlie line.* The right liver is divided into anterior (segments V and VIII) and posterior (segments VI and VII) sectors by the right scissura, which contains the right hepatic vein. The right portal pedicle is composed of the right hepatic artery, portal vein, and bile duct. It splits into right anterior and right posterior pedicles, which supply the segments of the anterior and posterior sectors.

The left liver has a visible fissure along its inferior surface called the *umbilical fissure.* The ligamentum teres, containing the remnant of the umbilical vein, runs into this fissure. The falciform ligament is contiguous with the umbilical fissure and ligamentum teres. The umbilical fissure is not a scissura and does not contain a hepatic vein; it contains the left portal pedicle, which contains the left portal vein, hepatic artery, and bile duct. This pedicle runs in this fissure and branches to feed the left liver. The left liver is split into anterior (segments III and IV) and posterior (segment II, the only sector composed of a single segment) sectors by the left scissura. The left scissura runs posterior to the ligamentum teres and contains the left hepatic vein.

At the hilum of the liver, the right portal triad has a short extrahepatic course of approximately 1 to 1.5 cm before entering the substance of the liver and branching into anterior and posterior sectoral branches. The left portal triad, however, has a long extrahepatic course of up to 3 to 4 cm and runs transversely along the

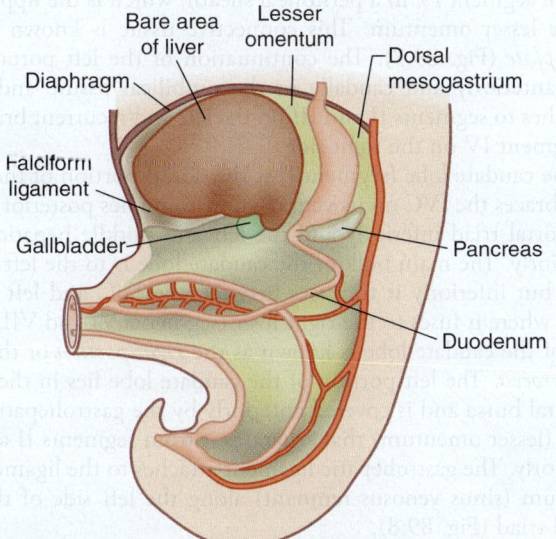

FIGURE 89.2 An approximately 36-day-old embryo is shown. The extensions of the septum transversum can be seen developing as the liver protrudes into the abdominal cavity, stretching out and forming the lesser omentum and the falciform ligament. The liver is completely invested in visceral peritoneum, except for a portion next to the diaphragm known as the bare area. (From Sadler TW. *Langman's Medical Embryology.* 5th ed. Baltimore: Williams & Wilkins; 1985.)

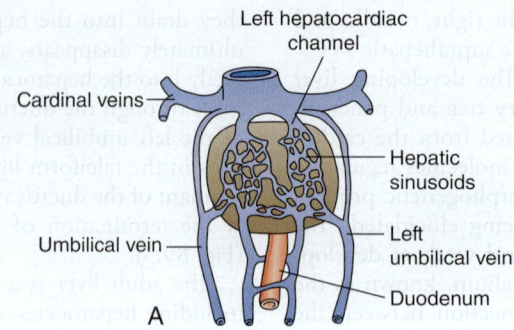

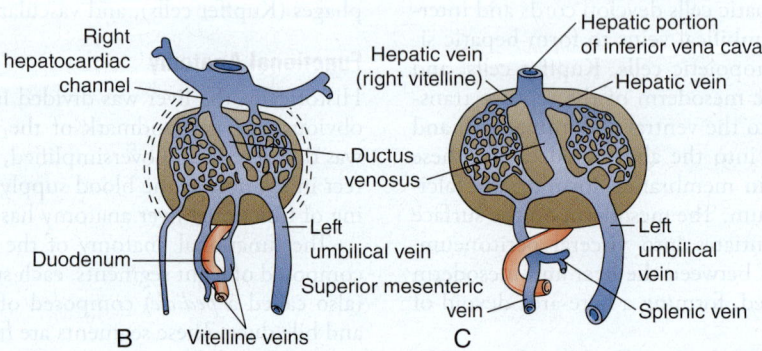

FIGURE 89.3 (A) Umbilical and vitelline vein development of a 5-week-old embryo. The hepatic sinusoids have developed, and although there are channels that bypass these sinusoids, the vitelline and umbilical veins are beginning to drain into them. (B) In the second month, the vitelline veins drain directly into the hepatic sinusoids. The ductus venosus has formed and accepts oxygenated blood from the left umbilical vein, bypasses the hepatic sinusoids, and directly enters the hepatocardiac channel. (C) By the third month, the vitelline veins have formed into the portal system (splenic, superior mesenteric, and portal veins). The right umbilical vein has disappeared, and the left umbilical vein (future ligamentum teres) drains into the sinus venosus, bypassing the hepatic sinusoids. Note the development of the inferior vena cava and hepatic veins. (From Sadler TW. *Langman's Medical Embryology.* 5th ed. Baltimore: Williams & Wilkins; 1985.)

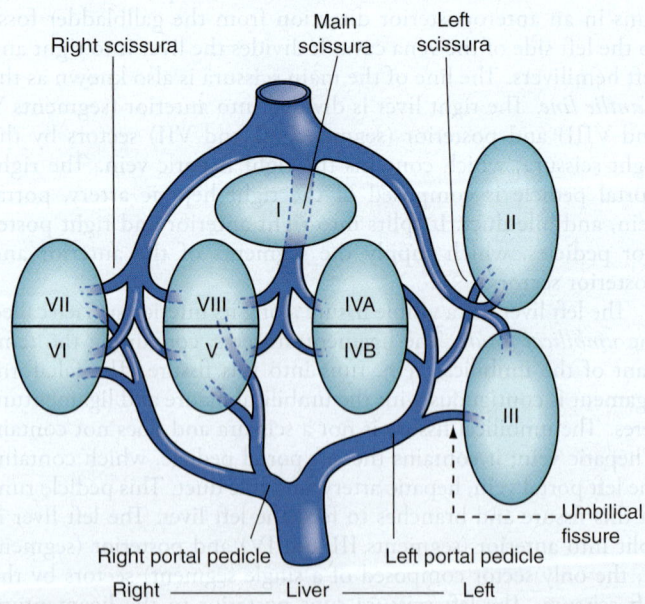

FIGURE 89.4 Schematic depiction of the segmental anatomy of the liver. Each segment receives its own portal pedicle (triad of portal vein, hepatic artery, and bile duct). The eight segments are illustrated, and the four sectors, divided by the three main hepatic veins running in scissurae, are shown. The umbilical fissure (not a scissura) is shown to contain the left portal pedicle. (From Blumgart LH, Hann LE. Surgical and radiologic anatomy of the liver and biliary tract. In: Blumgart LH, Fong Y, eds. *Surgery of the Liver and Biliary Tract.* London: WB Saunders; 2000:3-34.)

base of segment IV in a peritoneal sheath, which is the upper end of the lesser omentum. This connective tissue is known as the *hilar plate* (Fig. 89.7). The continuation of the left portal triad runs anteriorly and caudally in the umbilical fissure and gives branches to segments II and III on the left and recurrent branches to segment IV on the right side.

The caudate lobe (segment I) is the dorsal portion of the liver. It embraces the IVC on its ventral surface and lies posterior to the left portal triad inferiorly and the left and middle hepatic veins superiorly. The main bulk of the caudate lobe is to the left of the IVC, but inferiorly it traverses between the IVC and left portal triad, where it fuses to the right liver (segments VI and VII). This part of the caudate lobe is known as the *right portion* or the *caudate process.* The left portion of the caudate lobe lies in the lesser omental bursa and is covered anteriorly by the gastrohepatic ligament (lesser omentum) that separates it from segments II and III anteriorly. The gastrohepatic ligament attaches to the ligamentum venosum (sinus venosus remnant) along the left side of the left portal triad (Fig. 89.8).

The vascular inflow and biliary drainage to the caudate lobe come from both the right and left pedicles. The caudate process largely derives its portal venous supply from the right portal vein or the bifurcation of the main portal vein. The left portion of the caudate derives its portal venous inflow from the left main portal vein. The arterial supply and biliary drainage are generally through the right posterior pedicle system for the right portion and through the left main pedicle for the left portion. The hepatic

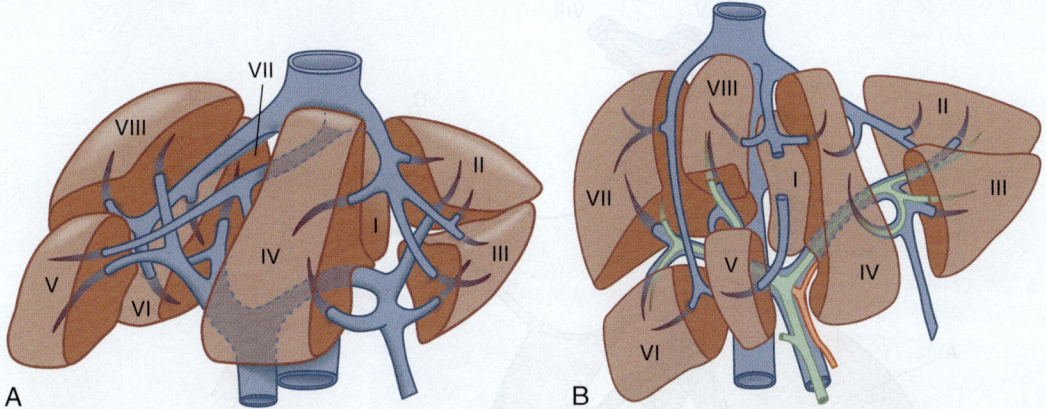

FIGURE 89.5 Segmental anatomy of the liver. (A) As seen at laparotomy in the anatomic position. (B) In the ex vivo position. (From Blumgart LH, Hann LE. Surgical and radiologic anatomy of the liver and biliary tract. In: Blumgart LH, Fong Y, eds. *Surgery of the Liver and Biliary Tract*. London: WB Saunders; 2000:3-34.)

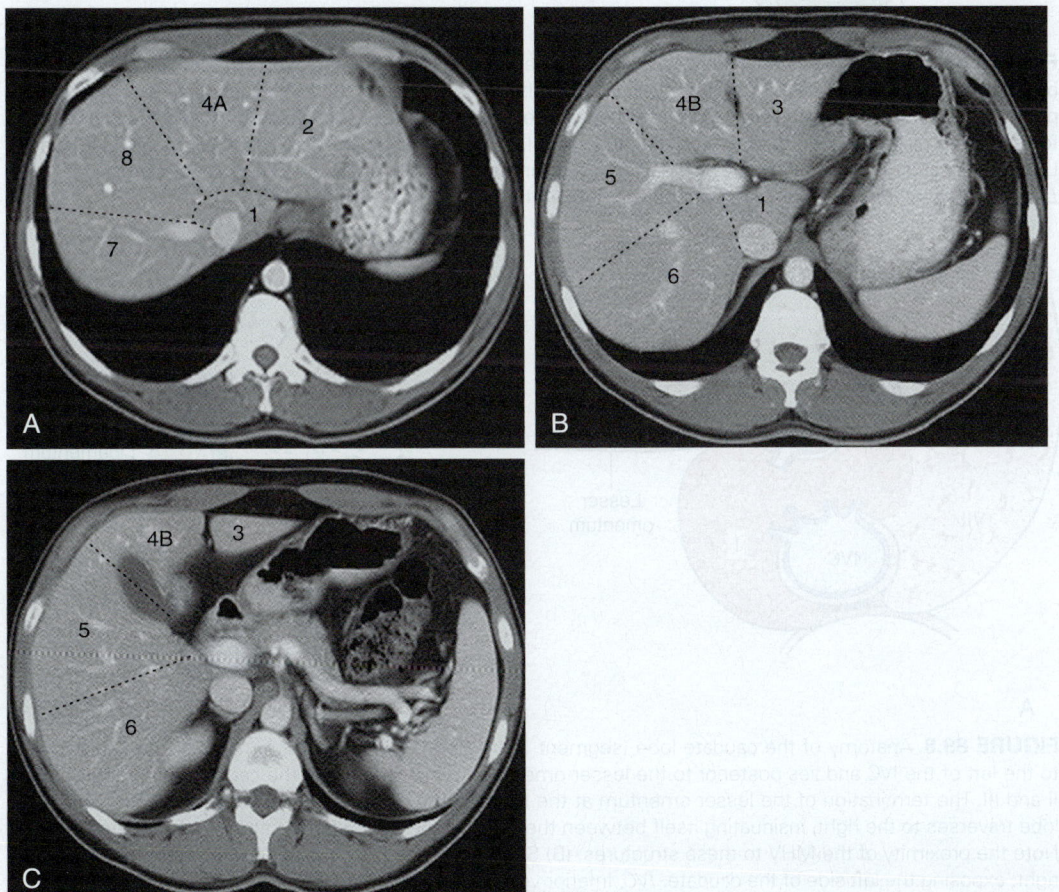

FIGURE 89.6 Segmental anatomy of the liver is demonstrated at three levels on contrast-enhanced computed tomography images. (A) At the level of the hepatic veins, the caudate lobe (segment 1) is seen posteriorly embracing the vena cava. Segment 2 is separated from segment 4A by the left hepatic vein. Segment 4A is separated from segment 8 by the middle hepatic vein, and segment 8 is separated from segment 7 by the right hepatic vein. (B) At the level of the portal vein bifurcation, segment 3 is visible as it hangs inferiorly in its anatomic position and is separated from segment 4B by the umbilical fissure. Note that segment 2 is not visible at this level. Terminal branches of the middle hepatic vein separate segment 4B from segment 5, and terminal branches of the right hepatic vein separate segment 5 from segment 6. Note that segments 4A, 8, and 7 are not visible at this level. Segment 1 is seen posterior to the portal vein and embracing the vena cava. (C) Below the portal bifurcation, one can see the inferior tips of segments 3 and 4B. The terminal branches of the middle hepatic vein and the gallbladder mark the separation of segment 4B from segment 5. Segments 5 and 6 are separated by the distal branches of the right hepatic vein. Note how the right liver hangs well inferior to the left liver.

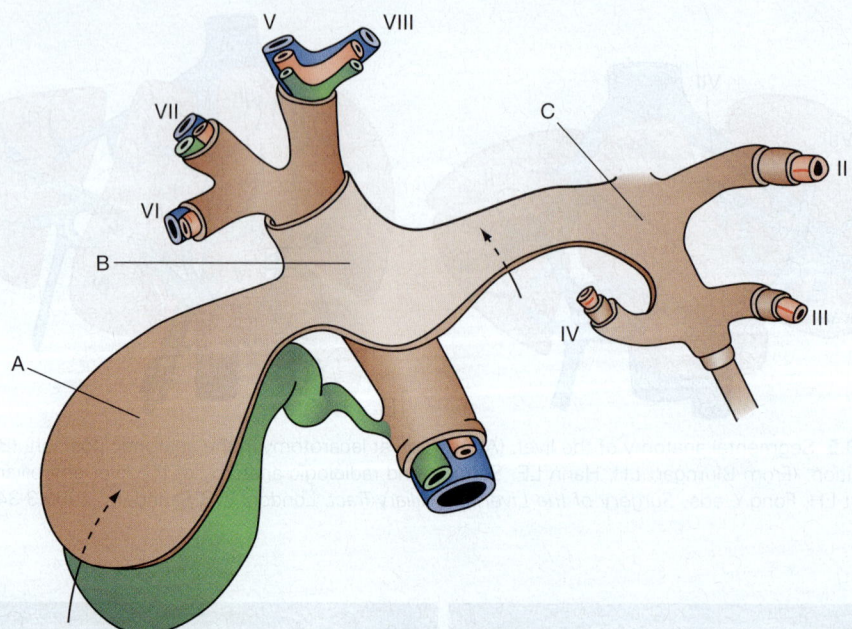

FIGURE 89.7 The plate system: The cystic plate between the gallbladder and liver *(A)*, the hilar plate at the biliary confluence at the base of segment IV *(B)*, and the umbilical plate above the umbilical portion of the portal vein *(C)*. Shown are the plane of dissection of the cystic plate for cholecystectomy and the hilar plate for exposure of the hepatic duct confluence and main left hepatic duct *(arrows)*. (From Blumgart LH, Hann LE. Surgical and radiologic anatomy of the liver and biliary tract. In: Blumgart LH, Fong Y, eds. *Surgery of the Liver and Biliary Tract*. London: WB Saunders; 2000:3-34.)

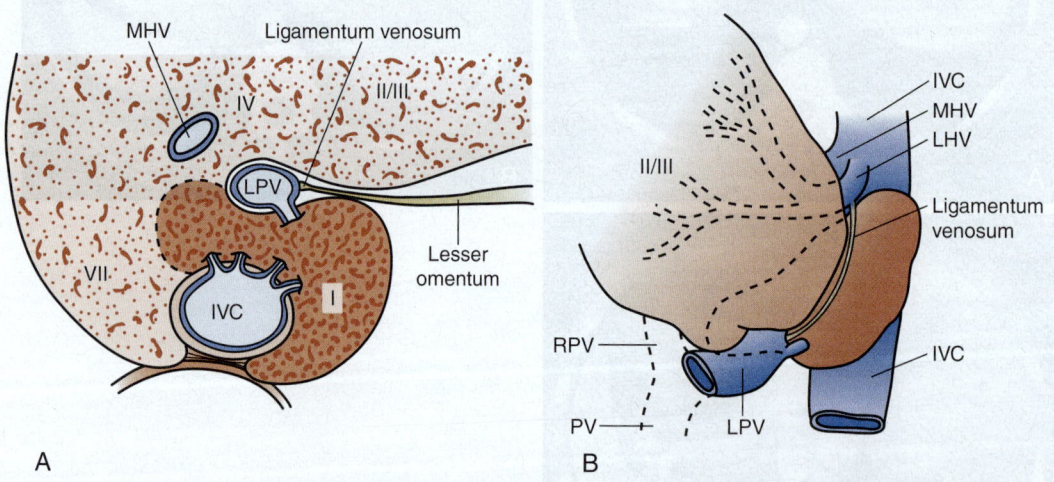

FIGURE 89.8 Anatomy of the caudate lobe (segment I). (A) Seen in cross-section, most of the caudate is to the left of the IVC and lies posterior to the lesser omentum, which separates the caudate from segments II and III. The termination of the lesser omentum at the ligamentum venosum is demonstrated. The caudate lobe traverses to the right, insinuating itself between the IVC and the LPV, where it attaches to the right liver. Note the proximity of the MHV to these structures. (B) Segments II and III have been rotated to the patient's right, exposing the left side of the caudate. *IVC*, Inferior vena cava; *LHV*, left hepatic vein; *MHV*, middle hepatic vein; *PV*, portal vein: *RPV*, right portal vein. (From Blumgart LH, Hann LE. Surgical and radiologic anatomy of the liver and biliary tract. In: Blumgart LH, Fong Y, eds. *Surgery of the Liver and Biliary Tract*. London: WB Saunders; 2000:3-34.)

venous drainage of the caudate is unique because several posterior small veins drain directly into the IVC.

The posterior edge of the left side of the caudate terminates as a fibrous component that attaches to the crura of the diaphragm and runs posteriorly, wrapping behind the IVC and attaching to segment VII of the right liver. In up to 50% of people, this fibrous component is composed partially or entirely of liver parenchyma. Thus, liver tissue may completely encircle

the IVC. This structure is known as the *caval ligament* and is important to recognize in mobilizing the right liver or the caudate lobe off the vena cava.

Anomalous development of the liver is uncommonly encountered. Complete absence of the left liver has been reported. A tongue of tissue extending inferiorly off the right liver has been described (Riedel lobe). Rare cases of supradiaphragmatic liver in the absence of a hernia sac have been noted.

Portal vein. The portal vein provides approximately 75% of the hepatic blood inflow. Despite being postcapillary and largely deoxygenated, its high flow rate provides 50% to 70% of the liver's oxygen requirement. The lack of valves in the portal venous system provides a system that can accommodate high flow at low pressure. This also allows the measurement of portal venous pressure at any point along the system.

The portal vein forms behind the neck of the pancreas at the confluence of the superior mesenteric and splenic veins. The length of the main portal vein ranges from 5.5 to 8 cm, and its diameter is approximately 1 cm. Cephalad to its formation behind the neck of the pancreas, the portal vein runs behind the first portion of the duodenum and into the hepatoduodenal ligament, where it runs along the right border of the lesser omentum, usually posterior to the common bile duct and proper hepatic artery. The left gastric or coronary vein can variably drain into the portal vein, splenic vein, or the junction of the two.

The portal vein divides into main right and left branches at the hilum of the liver. The portal vein is the only vein with both tributaries and branches. The left branch of the portal vein runs transversely along the base of segment IV and into the umbilical fissure, where it gives off branches to segments II and III and feedback branches to segment IV. The left portal vein also gives off posterior branches to the left side of the caudate lobe. The right portal vein has a short extrahepatic course; it usually enters the substance of the liver, where it splits into anterior and posterior sectoral branches. These sectoral branches can occasionally be seen extrahepatically and can come off the main portal vein before its bifurcation. There is usually a small caudate process branch off the main right portal vein or at the right portal vein bifurcation that comes off posteriorly to supply this portion of liver (Fig. 89.9).

There are several connections between the portal and systemic venous systems. Under conditions of high portal venous pressure, these portosystemic connections may enlarge secondarily to collateral flow. This concept is reviewed in more detail later in the chapter, but the most significant portosystemic collateral locations are the following: the submucosal veins of the proximal stomach and distal esophagus receive portal flow from the short gastric veins and the left gastric vein and can result in varices, with the potential for hemorrhage; the umbilical and abdominal wall veins recanalize from flow through the umbilical vein in the ligamentum teres, resulting in caput medusae; the superior hemorrhoidal plexus receives portal flow from inferior mesenteric vein tributaries and can form large hemorrhoids; and other retroperitoneal communications yield collaterals that can make abdominal surgery hazardous.

The anatomy of the portal vein and its branches is relatively constant and has much less variation than the biliary ductal and hepatic arterial systems. The standard configuration, where main portal vein divides into the left and right branches and the right portal vein then divides into right anterior and right posterior portal vein, is found in up to 70% of individuals. The most common variant of this configuration is the so-called portal vein trifurcation where the main portal vein divides into three branches: the left portal vein, the right anterior portal vein, and the right posterior portal vein. The second most common variant is the right posterior portal vein, which originates as the first branch of the portal vein. This can also be envisioned as the right anterior portal vein arising from the left portal vein. These two variations account for most of the variations from the so-called normal anatomy. The portal vein is rarely found anterior to the neck of the pancreas and duodenum. Entrance of the portal vein directly

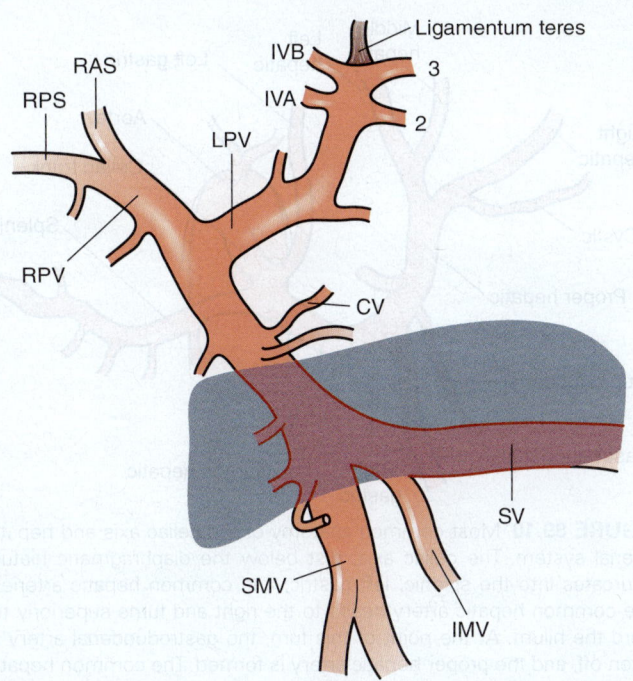

FIGURE 89.9 Anatomy of the portal vein. The superior mesenteric vein *(SMV)* joins the splenic vein *(SV)* posterior to the neck of the pancreas *(shaded area)* to form the portal vein. Note the entrance of the inferior mesenteric vein *(IMV)* into the splenic vein, the most common anatomic arrangement. In its course superiorly in the edge of the lesser omentum posterior to the common bile duct and hepatic artery, the portal vein receives venous effluent from the coronary vein *(CV)*. At the hepatic hilum, the portal vein bifurcates into a larger right portal vein *(RPV)* and a smaller left portal vein *(LPV)*. The LPV runs transversely at the base of segment IV and enters the umbilical fissure to supply the segments of the left liver. Just before the umbilical fissure, the LPV usually gives off a sizable branch to the caudate lobe. The RPV enters the substance of the liver and splits into right anterior sectoral *(RAS)* and right posterior sectoral *(RPS)* branches. It also gives off a posterior branch to the right side of the caudate lobe–caudate process. (From Blumgart LH, Hann LE. Surgical and radiologic anatomy of the liver and biliary tract. In: Blumgart LH, Fong Y, eds. *Surgery of the Liver and Biliary Tract.* London: WB Saunders; 2000:3-34.)

into the vena cava has also been described. Very rarely, a pulmonary vein may enter the portal vein. Finally, there may be a congenital absence of the left branch of the portal vein. In this situation, the right branch courses through the right liver and curves around peripherally to supply the left liver, or the right anterior sectoral vein can arise from the left portal vein.

Hepatic artery. The hepatic artery, representing high-volume oxygenated systemic arterial flow, provides approximately 25% of the hepatic blood flow and 30% to 50% oxygenation. The common description of the arterial supply to the liver and biliary tree is present only approximately 60% of the time (Fig. 89.10). The celiac trunk originates directly off the aorta, just below the aortic diaphragmatic hiatus, and branches into the splenic artery, left gastric artery, and common hepatic artery. The common hepatic artery passes forward and to the right along the superior border of the pancreas. It runs along the right side of the lesser omentum, where it ascends toward the hepatic hilum, lying anterior to the portal vein and the left of the bile duct. At the point where the common hepatic artery begins to head superiorly toward the hepatic hilum, it gives off the gastroduodenal artery, followed by the supraduodenal artery and right gastric artery. The common

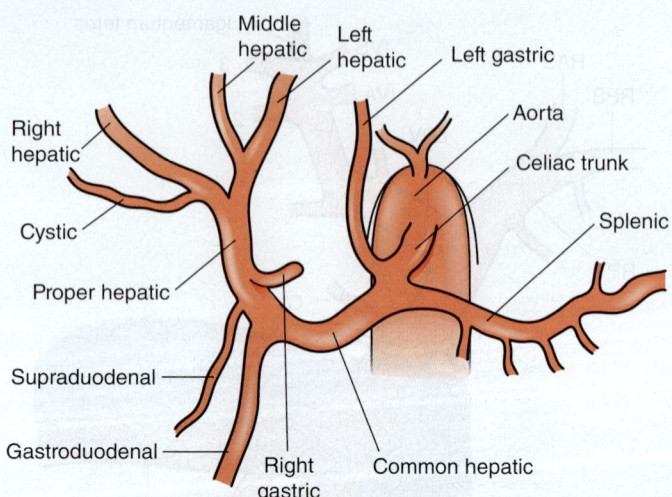

FIGURE 89.10 Most common anatomy of the celiac axis and hepatic arterial system. The celiac axis, just below the diaphragmatic hiatus, trifurcates into the splenic, left gastric, and common hepatic arteries. The common hepatic artery heads to the right and turns superiorly toward the hilum. At the point of this turn, the gastroduodenal artery is given off, and the proper hepatic artery is formed. The common hepatic artery gives off right and left hepatic arteries in the hilum. Note the middle hepatic artery off the proximal left hepatic artery, which goes on to supply segment IV. The cystic artery usually comes off the right hepatic artery within the triangle of Calot. (From Blumgart LH, Hann LE. Surgical and radiologic anatomy of the liver and biliary tract. In: Blumgart LH, Fong Y, eds. *Surgery of the Liver and Biliary Tract*. London: WB Saunders; 2000:3-34.)

hepatic artery beyond the takeoff of the gastroduodenal is called the *proper hepatic artery;* it divides into right and left hepatic arteries at the hilum. The left hepatic artery heads vertically toward the umbilical fissure to supply segments II, III, and IV. The left hepatic artery usually also gives off a middle hepatic artery branch that heads toward the right side of the umbilical fissure and supplies segment IV. The right hepatic artery usually runs posterior to the common hepatic bile duct and enters the Calot triangle, bordered by the cystic duct, common hepatic duct, and liver edge, where it gives off the cystic artery to supply the gallbladder and then continues into the substance of the right liver.

Unlike portal vein anatomy, hepatic arterial anatomy is extraordinarily variable (Fig. 89.11). An accessory vessel is described as an aberrant origin of a branch that is in addition to the normal branching pattern. A replaced vessel is described as an aberrant origin of a branch that substitutes for the lack of the normal branch. The hepatic artery usually originates off the celiac trunk. However, branches or the entire hepatic arterial system can originate off the superior mesenteric artery. The right and left hepatic arteries can also arise separately off the celiac axis. Replaced or accessory right hepatic arteries come off the superior mesenteric artery and are present approximately 11% to 21% of the time. Hepatic vessels replaced to the superior mesenteric artery run behind the head of the pancreas, posterior to the portal vein in the portacaval space. This is evident on cross-sectional imaging as well as during operative exploration by feeling hepatic artery pulsation in the lateral border of the hepatoduodenal ligament behind the portal vein and bile duct. The right hepatic artery, in its usual branching pattern, can also course anterior to the common hepatic duct. A replaced or accessory left hepatic artery is present

approximately 3.8% to 10% of the time, originates from the left gastric artery, and courses within the lesser omentum, heading toward the umbilical fissure. Other important variations include the origin of the gastroduodenal artery, which originates from the right hepatic artery and is occasionally duplicated. The anatomy of the cystic artery is also variable; knowledge of these variations is of particular importance in the performance of cholecystectomy (Fig. 89.12). An accessory cystic artery can originate from the proper hepatic artery or gastroduodenal artery, where it runs anterior to the bile duct. A single cystic artery can originate anywhere off the proper hepatic artery or gastroduodenal artery or directly from the celiac axis. These variant cystic arteries can run anterior to the bile duct and are not necessarily present in the triangle of Calot. All these variations in hepatic arterial anatomy are of obvious importance during hepatic resection, hepatic arterial pump placement, cholecystectomy, and hepatic interventional radiologic procedures.

Hepatic veins. The three major hepatic veins drain from the superior-posterior surface of the liver directly into the IVC (see Figs. 89.4–89.6). The right hepatic vein runs in the right scissura between the anterior and posterior sectors of the right liver and drains most of the right liver after a short (1-cm) extrahepatic course into the right side of the IVC. The left and middle hepatic veins usually join intrahepatically and enter the left side of the IVC as a single vessel, although they may drain separately. The left hepatic vein runs in the left scissura between segments II and III and drains segments II and III; the middle hepatic vein runs in the portal scissura between segment IV and the anterior sector of the right liver, composed of segments V and VIII, and drains segment IV and some of the anterior sector of the right liver. The umbilical vein is an additional vein that runs under the falciform ligament, between the left and middle veins, and usually empties into the left hepatic vein. Several small posterior venous branches from the right posterior sector and caudate lobe drain directly into the IVC. A substantial inferiorly located accessory right hepatic vein is commonly encountered. There is also often a venous tributary from the caudate lobe that drains superiorly into the left hepatic vein.

Biliary system. The intrahepatic bile ducts are the terminal branches of the right and left hepatic ductal branches that invaginate the Glisson capsule at the hilum, along with their corresponding portal vein and hepatic artery branches, forming the peritoneal covered portal triads also known as *portal pedicles.* Along these intrahepatic portal pedicles, the bile duct branches are usually superior to the portal vein, whereas the hepatic artery branches run inferiorly. The left hepatic bile duct drains segments II, III, and IV, which constitute the left liver. The intrahepatic ductal branches of the left liver join to form the main left duct at the base of the umbilical fissure, where the left hepatic duct courses transversely across the base of segment IV to join the right hepatic duct at the hilum. In its transverse portion, the left hepatic duct drains one to three small branches from segment IV. The right hepatic duct drains the right liver and is formed by the joining of the anterior sectoral duct (draining segments V and VIII) and the posterior sectoral duct (draining segments VI and VII). The posterior sectoral duct runs in a horizontal and posterior direction; the anterior sectoral duct runs vertically. The main right hepatic duct bifurcates just above the right portal vein. The short right hepatic duct meets the longer left hepatic duct to form the confluence anterior to the right portal vein, constituting the common hepatic duct. The caudate lobe (segment I) has its own

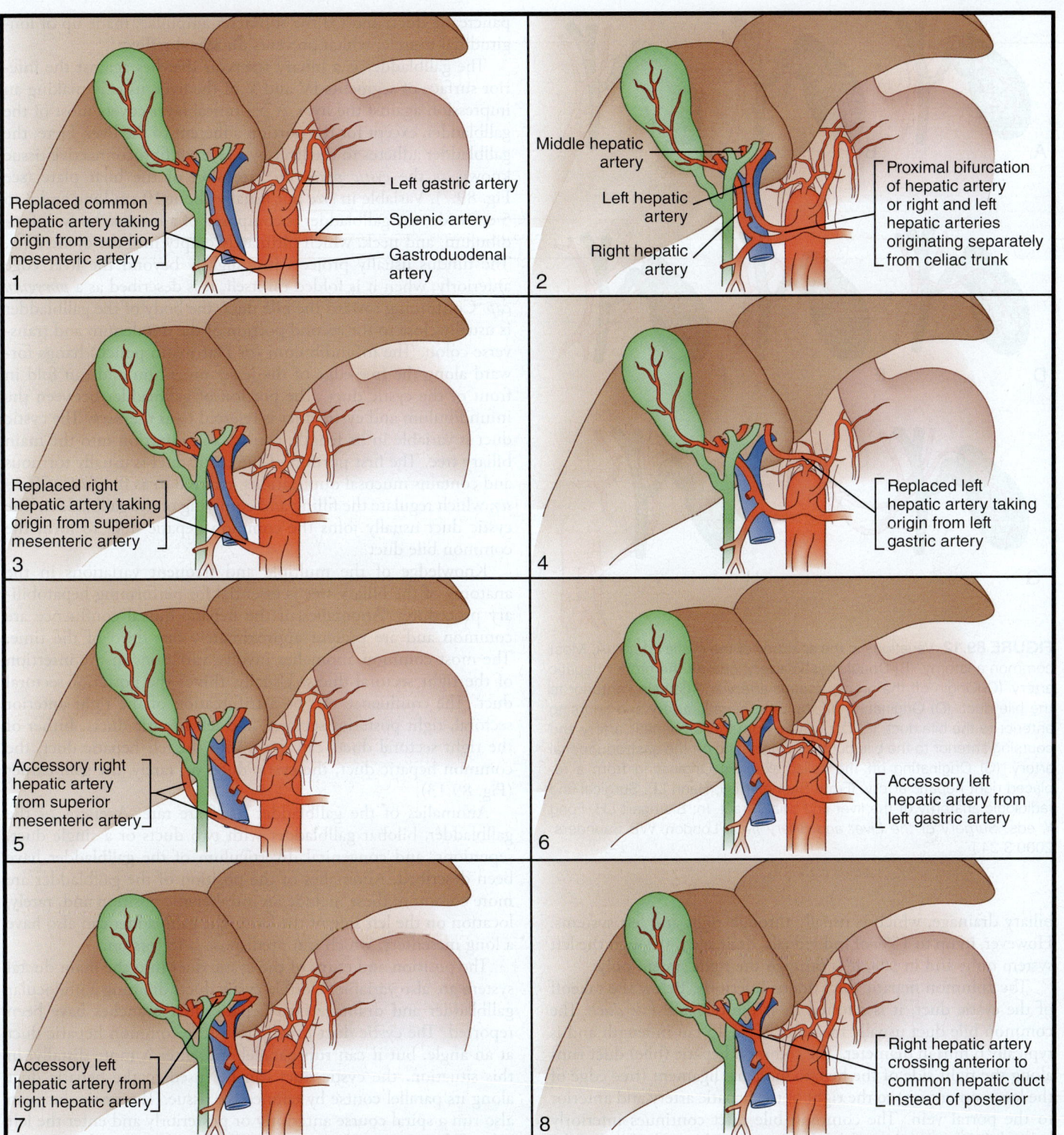

1 — Replaced common hepatic artery taking origin from superior mesenteric artery — Left gastric artery — Splenic artery — Gastroduodenal artery

2 — Middle hepatic artery — Left hepatic artery — Right hepatic artery — Proximal bifurcation of hepatic artery or right and left hepatic arteries originating separately from celiac trunk

3 — Replaced right hepatic artery taking origin from superior mesenteric artery

4 — Replaced left hepatic artery taking origin from left gastric artery

5 — Accessory right hepatic artery from superior mesenteric artery

6 — Accessory left hepatic artery from left gastric artery

7 — Accessory left hepatic artery from right hepatic artery

8 — Right hepatic artery crossing anterior to common hepatic duct instead of posterior

FIGURE 89.11 Variable anatomy of the hepatic artery. The common hepatic artery can originate off the superior mesenteric artery instead of the celiac axis. A replaced or accessory right hepatic artery comes off the superior mesenteric artery and runs posterior to the head of the pancreas, to the right of the portal vein, and behind the common bile duct into the hilum. A replaced or accessory left hepatic artery originates off the left gastric artery and runs through the lesser omentum into the umbilical fissure. (From Netter FH. Netter Anatomy Collection. www.netterimages.com. Copyright Elsevier, Inc. All rights reserved.)

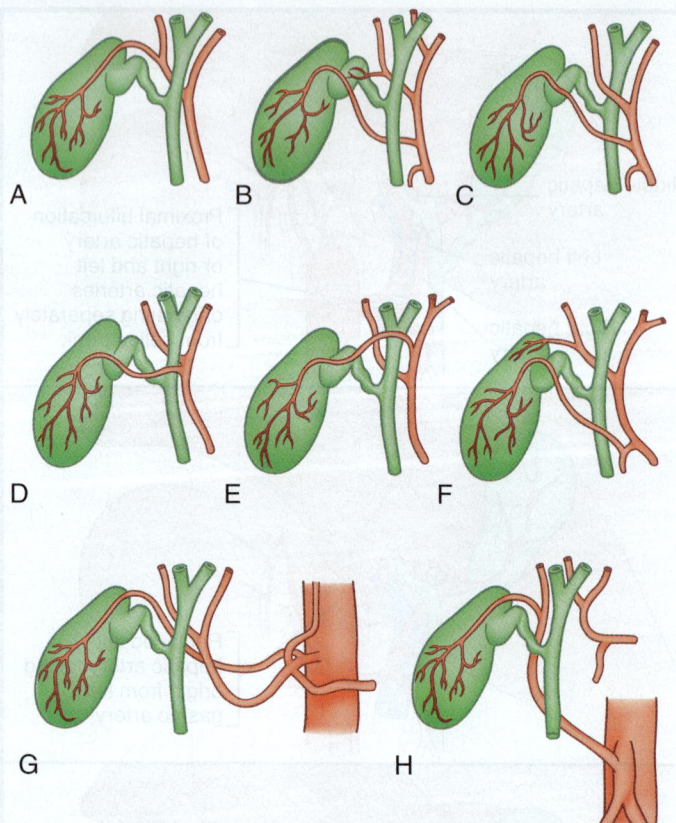

FIGURE 89.12 Variations in the anatomy of the cystic artery. (A) Most common anatomy. (B) Double cystic artery, one off the proper hepatic artery. (C) Origin off the proper hepatic artery and coursing anterior to the bile duct. (D) Originating off the right hepatic artery and coursing anterior to the bile duct. (E) Originating from the left hepatic artery and coursing anterior to the bile duct. (F) Originating off the gastroduodenal artery. (G) Originating off the celiac axis. (H) Originating from a replaced right hepatic artery. (From Blumgart LH, Hann LE. Surgical and radiologic anatomy of the liver and biliary tract. In: Blumgart LH, Fong Y, eds. *Surgery of the Liver and Biliary Tract*. London: WB Saunders; 2000:3-34.)

biliary drainage, which is usually through right and left systems. However, in up to 15% of individuals, drainage is through the left system only, and in 5%, it is through the right system only.

The common hepatic duct drains inferiorly. Below the takeoff of the cystic duct, it is referred to as the *common bile duct*. The common bile duct usually measures 10 to 15 cm in length and is typically 6 mm in diameter. The common hepatic (bile) duct runs along the right side of the hepatoduodenal ligament (free edge of the lesser omentum) to the right of the hepatic artery and anterior to the portal vein. The common bile duct continues inferiorly behind the first portion of the duodenum and into the head of the pancreas in an inferior and slightly rightward direction. The intrapancreatic distal common bile duct then joins with the main pancreatic duct (of Wirsung), with or without a common channel, and enters the second portion of the duodenum through the major papilla of Vater. At the choledochoduodenal junction, a complex muscular complex known as the *sphincter of Oddi* regulates bile flow and prevents reflux of duodenal contents into the biliary tree. There are three major parts to this sphincter: (1) the sphincter choledochus, a circular muscle that regulates bile flow and the filling of the gallbladder; (2) the pancreatic sphincter, present to variable degrees, which surrounds the intraduodenal

pancreatic duct; and (3) the sphincter ampullae, made up of longitudinal muscle, which prevents duodenal reflux.

The gallbladder is a biliary reservoir that lies against the inferior surface of segments IV and V of the liver, usually making an impression against the liver. A peritoneal layer covers most of the gallbladder, except for the portion adherent to the liver. Here, the gallbladder adheres to the liver by a layer of fibroconnective tissue known as the *cystic plate,* an extension of the hilar plate (see Fig. 89.7). Variable in size but usually about 10 cm long and 3 to 5 cm wide, the gallbladder is composed of a fundus, body, infundibulum, and neck, which ultimately empty into the cystic duct. The fundus usually projects just slightly beyond the liver edge anteriorly; when it is folded on itself, it is described as a *phrygian cap.* Continuing toward the bile duct, the body of the gallbladder is usually close to the second portion of the duodenum and transverse colon. The infundibulum (or Hartmann pouch) hangs forward along the free edge of the lesser omentum and can fold in front of the cystic duct. The portion of gallbladder between the infundibulum and cystic duct is referred to as the *neck.* The cystic duct is variable in its length, course, and insertion into the main biliary tree. The first portion of the cystic duct is usually tortuous and contains mucosal duplications, referred to as the *folds of Heister,* which regulate the filling and emptying of the gallbladder. The cystic duct usually joins the common hepatic duct to form the common bile duct.

Knowledge of the multiple and frequent variations in the anatomy of the biliary tree is essential for performing hepatobiliary procedures. Anomalies of the hepatic ductal confluence are common and are present approximately one-third of the time. The most common anomalies involve variations in the insertion of the right sectoral ducts. Usually, this is the posterior sectoral duct. The confluence can be a trifurcation of the right anterior sectoral, right posterior sectoral, and left hepatic ducts. Either of the right sectoral ducts can drain into the left hepatic duct, the common hepatic duct, the cystic duct, or, rarely, the gallbladder (Fig. 89.13).

Anomalies of the gallbladder itself are rare. Agenesis of the gallbladder, bilobar gallbladder with two ducts or a single duct, septations, and congenital diverticulum of the gallbladder have been described. Anomalies of the position of the gallbladder are more common; these include an intrahepatic position and, rarely, location on the left side of the liver. The gallbladder can also have a long mesentery, which can predispose it to torsion.

The position and entry of the cystic duct into the main ductal system are also variable. Double cystic ducts draining a unilocular gallbladder and drainage into hepatic duct branches have been reported. The cystic duct usually joins the common hepatic duct at an angle, but it can run parallel and enter it more distally; in this situation, the cystic duct can be fused to the hepatic duct along its parallel course by connective tissue. The cystic duct can also run a spiral course anteriorly or posteriorly and enter the left side of the common hepatic duct. Finally, the cystic duct can be very short or even absent (Fig. 89.14).

The supraduodenal and infrahilar bile ducts are predominantly supplied by two axial vessels that run at 3-o'clock and 9-o'clock positions. These vessels are derived from the superior pancreaticoduodenal, right hepatic, cystic, gastroduodenal, and retroduodenal arteries. It has been estimated that only 2% of the arterial supply to this portion of the bile duct is segmental, arising directly from the proper hepatic artery. The bile duct and its bifurcation in the hilum derive their arterial blood supply from a rich network of multiple small branches from surrounding vessels. Similarly, the retropancreatic bile duct derives its arterial supply between each terminal portal triad by terminal portal triad branches. In between each terminal portal triad is the central hepatic venule. These are arranged in a manner which places, surrounded on each side by endothelium-lined, blood-filled sinusoids. Blood flow from the terminal portal triad through the sinusoids into the hepatic venule. In the venous within the in-processes and empties into terminal canaliculi, which form on the lateral walls of interlobular hepatocytes. These ultimately coalesce into bile ducts and flow toward the portal triads. This functional lobule unit provides the anatomy for the many metabolic and secretory functions of liver.

Between the periportal triad and central hepatic venule are three zones. Differ in their oxygen supply as well as exposure to nutrients and oxygenated blood. There is debate about the shape of these zones and their relationship to the basic lobular unit, but in general, zone 1 through 3 may run from the terminal portal venule, the central hepatic venule. Zone 1 (periportal zone) rich in nutrients, while Zone 2 (intermediate zone) and 3 (perivenular zone) exposed to environments that are more poor in oxygen and nutrients. The cells of the different zones are enzymatically and vary correspondingly to oxygen exposure and hypoxia. This anatomic arrangement also explains the mechanism of centrilobular necrosis from hypoperfusion because it is the most vulnerable cells to oxygen delivery.

Hepatic arterial and portal venous and hepatic arterial blood supply the hepatic parenchyma with blood. The portal blood provides a constant blood flow into this

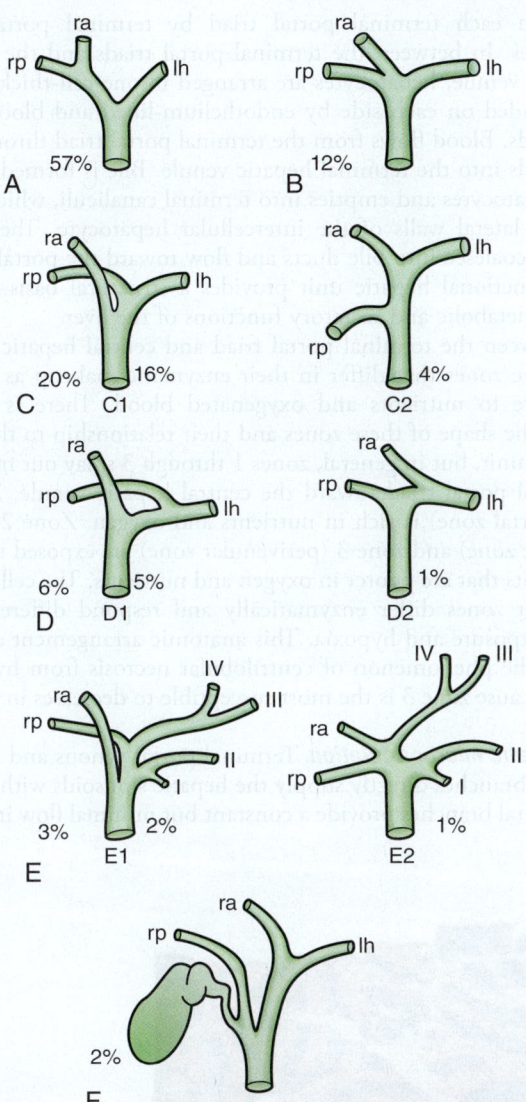

FIGURE 89.13 Variations of the hepatic duct confluence. (A) Most common anatomy. (B) Trifurcation at the confluence. (C) Either of the right sectoral ducts drains into the common hepatic duct. (D) Either of the right sectoral ducts drains into the left hepatic duct. (E) Absence of a hepatic duct confluence. (F) Absence of right hepatic duct and drainage of right posterior sectoral duct into the cystic duct. (From Blumgart LH, Hann LE. Surgical and radiologic anatomy of the liver and biliary tract. In: Blumgart LH, Fong Y, eds. *Surgery of the Liver and Biliary Tract*. London: WB Saunders; 2000:3-34.)

from the retroduodenal artery, which provides a rich network of multiple small branches (Fig. 89.15). Venous drainage of the bile duct parallels the arterial supply and drains into the portal venous system. The venous drainage of the gallbladder empties into the veins that drain the bile duct and does not flow directly into the portal vein.

Nerves. The innervation of the liver and biliary tract is through sympathetic fibers originating from T7–T10 as well as parasympathetic fibers from both vagal nerves. The sympathetic fibers pass through celiac ganglia before giving off postganglionic fibers to the liver and bile ducts. The right-sided celiac ganglia and right vagal nerve form an anterior hepatic plexus of nerves that runs along the hepatic artery. The left-sided celiac ganglia and left vagal nerve form a posterior hepatic plexus that runs posterior to the

bile duct and portal vein. The bile ducts are supplied by sympathetic fibers as well. Parasympathetic and extrahepatic bile ducts receive sympathetic and parasympathetic fibers. The functional significance of these nerves is still not well understood. Arterial denervation of the liver and thus the liver capsule can result in right upper quadrant pain, which may be referred to right shoulder through phrenic afferent nerve innervation of the diaphragm and peritoneum.

Lymph. Lymph node drainage generally closest to the hepatoduodenal ligament. From here lymph drains usually common along the hepatic artery to the celiac ganglia and then to the cisterna chyli. Lymphatic drainage can also follow the hepatic veins to paracaval nodes near the area of the suprahepatic IVC and through the diaphragm in hiatus. The lymphatic drainage of the gallbladder and most of the extrahepatic biliary tract is generally into the lymph nodes around the cystic duodenal ligament. This drainage may follow along superiorly to the celiac lymph nodes, but it can also flow to lymph nodes behind the head of the pancreas or within the periportal groove.

Microscopic Anatomy. Functional microscopic organization of hepatic parenchyma chyme into microscopic and lobular units has been described in several ways referenced over an interval as described in several works. That was originally described by Rappaport and thereafter by Matz.

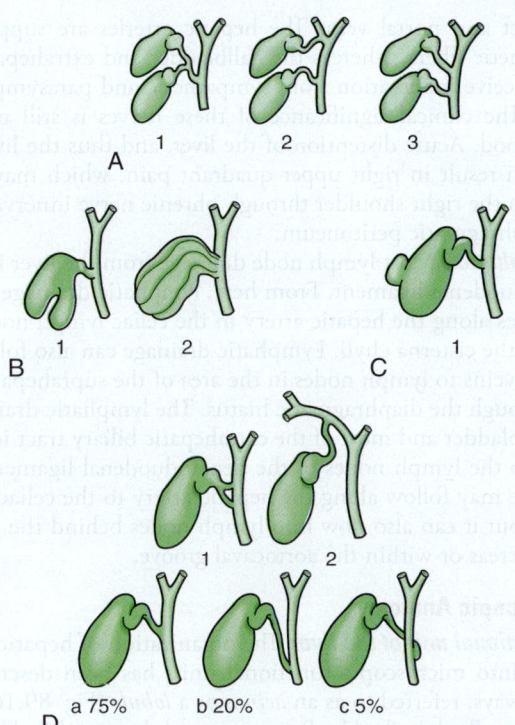

FIGURE 89.14 Variations in the anatomy of the gallbladder and cystic duct. (A) Bilobar gallbladder. (B) Septations of the gallbladder. (C) Diverticulum of the gallbladder. (D) Variations in cystic duct anatomy. The three types of union of the cystic duct and common hepatic duct are illustrated. (From Blumgart LH, Hann LE. Surgical and radiologic anatomy of the liver and biliary tract. In: Blumgart LH, Fong Y, eds. *Surgery of the Liver and Biliary Tract*. London: WB Saunders; 2000:3-34.)

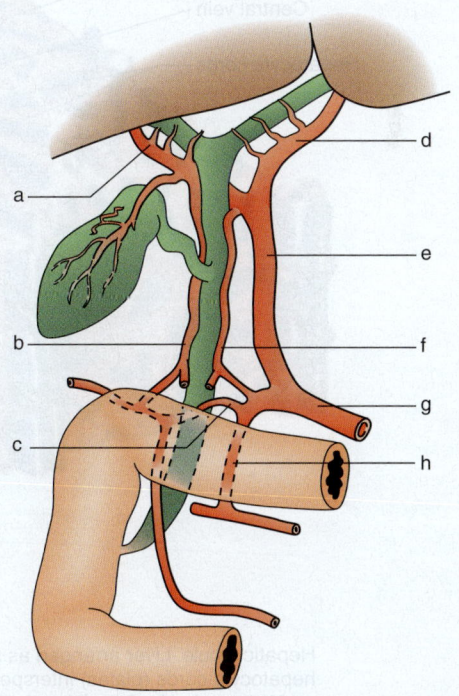

FIGURE 89.15 Blood supply to the common bile duct and common hepatic duct: right hepatic artery (a); 9:00 artery (b); retroduodenal artery (c); left hepatic artery (d); proper hepatic artery (e); 3:00 artery (f); common hepatic artery (g); gastroduodenal artery (h). (From Blumgart LH, Hann LE. Surgical and radiologic anatomy of the liver and biliary tract. In: Blumgart LH, Fong Y, eds. *Surgery of the Liver and Biliary Tract*. London: WB Saunders; 2000:3-34.)

bile duct and portal vein. The hepatic arteries are supplied by sympathetic fibers, whereas the gallbladder and extrahepatic bile ducts receive innervation from sympathetic and parasympathetic fibers. The clinical significance of these nerves is still not well understood. Acute distention of the liver, and thus the liver capsule, can result in right upper quadrant pain, which may be referred to the right shoulder through phrenic nerve innervation of the diaphragmatic peritoneum.

Lymphatics. Most lymph node drainage from the liver is to the hepatoduodenal ligament. From here, lymphatic drainage usually continues along the hepatic artery to the celiac lymph nodes and then to the cisterna chyli. Lymphatic drainage can also follow the hepatic veins to lymph nodes in the area of the suprahepatic IVC and through the diaphragmatic hiatus. The lymphatic drainage of the gallbladder and most of the extrahepatic biliary tract is generally into the lymph nodes of the hepatoduodenal ligament. This drainage may follow along the hepatic artery to the celiac lymph nodes, but it can also flow into lymph nodes behind the head of the pancreas or within the aortocaval groove.

Microscopic Anatomy

Functional unit of the liver. The organization of hepatic parenchyma into microscopic functional units has been described in several ways, referred to as an *acinus* or a *lobule* (Fig. 89.16). This was originally described by Rappaport and then modified by Matsumoto and Kawakami. A lobule is made up of a central terminal hepatic venule surrounded by four to six terminal portal triads that form a polygonal unit. This unit is lined on its periphery

between each terminal portal triad by terminal portal triad branches. In between the terminal portal triads and the central hepatic venule, hepatocytes are arranged in one-cell-thick plates, surrounded on each side by endothelium-lined and blood-filled sinusoids. Blood flows from the terminal portal triad through the sinusoids into the terminal hepatic venule. Bile is formed within the hepatocytes and empties into terminal canaliculi, which form on the lateral walls of the intercellular hepatocyte. These ultimately coalesce into bile ducts and flow toward the portal triads. This functional hepatic unit provides a structural basis for the many metabolic and secretory functions of the liver.

Between the terminal portal triad and central hepatic venule are three zones that differ in their enzymatic makeup as well as exposure to nutrients and oxygenated blood. There is debate about the shape of these zones and their relationship to the basic lobular unit, but in general, zones 1 through 3 splay out from the terminal portal triad toward the central hepatic venule. Zone 1 (periportal zone) is rich in nutrients and oxygen. Zone 2 (intermediate zone) and zone 3 (perivenular zone) are exposed to environments that are poorer in oxygen and nutrients. The cells of the different zones differ enzymatically and respond differently to toxin exposure and hypoxia. This anatomic arrangement also explains the phenomenon of centrilobular necrosis from hypotension because zone 3 is the most susceptible to decreases in oxygen delivery.

Hepatic microcirculation. Terminal portal venous and hepatic arterial branches directly supply the hepatic sinusoids with blood. The portal branches provide a constant but minimal flow into this

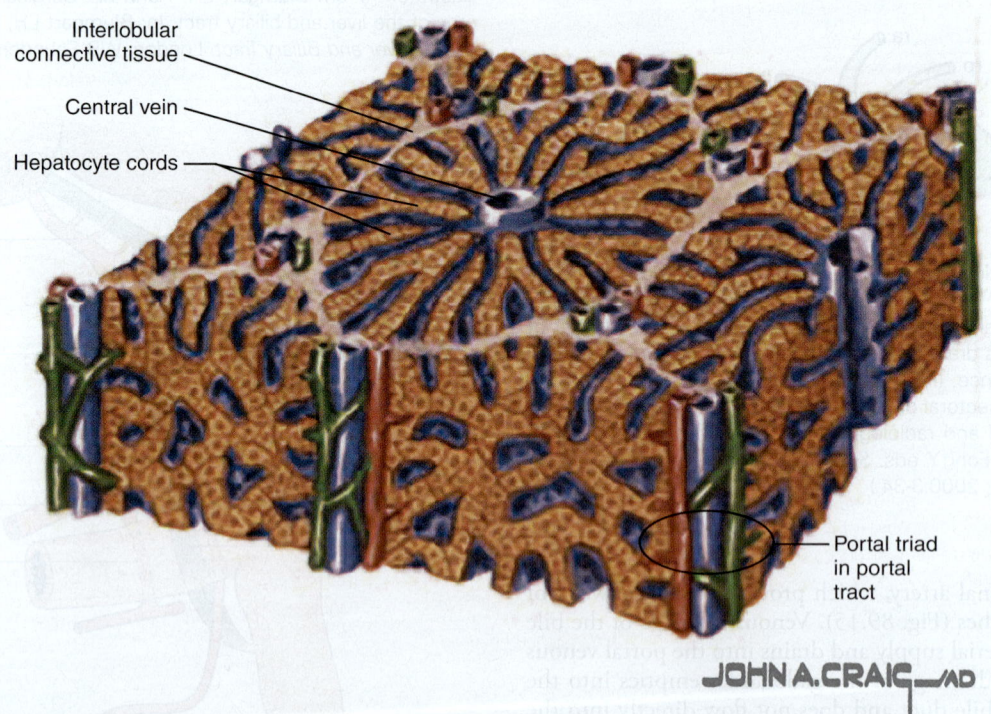

Interlobular connective tissue

Central vein

Hepatocyte cords

Portal triad in portal tract

JOHN A. CRAIG—AD

Hepatic lobule. Liver arranged as series of hexagonal lobules, each composed of series of hepatocyte cords (plates) interspersed with sinusoids. Each lobule surrounds a central vein and is bounded by 6 peripheral portal triads (low magnification).

FIGURE 89.16 Schematic illustration of a hepatic lobule seen as a three-dimensional polyhedral unit. The terminal portal triads (hepatic artery, portal vein, and bile duct) are at each corner and give off branches along the sides of the lobule. Hepatocytes are in single-cell sheets with sinusoids on either end aligned radially toward a central hepatic venule. (From Netter FH. Netter Anatomy Collection. www.netterimages.com. Copyright Elsevier, Inc. All rights reserved.)

low-volume system; the arterial branches provide the sinusoids with pulsatile but low-volume flow that enhances flow in the sinusoids. Hepatic arterial branches terminate in a plexus around the terminal bile ductules and provide nutrients. Arterial and portal vein flow varies inversely in the sinusoids and can be compensatory. Local control of blood flow in the sinusoids likely depends on arteriolar sphincters and contraction of the sinusoidal lining by endothelial cells and hepatic stellate cells or portal myofibroblasts. Blood within the sinusoids empties directly into terminal hepatic venules at the center of a functional lobule. This process results in the unidirectional flow of blood in the liver from zone 1 to zone 3.

The endothelium-lined sinusoids of the hepatic lobule represent the functional unit of the liver, where afferent blood flow is exposed to functional hepatic parenchyma before being drained into hepatic venules (Fig. 89.17). The hepatic sinusoids are 7 to 15 μm wide but can increase in size by up to tenfold. This yields a low-resistance and low-pressure (generally 2–3 mm Hg) system. The sinusoidal endothelial cells account for 15% to 20% of the total hepatic cell mass.

Sinusoidal endothelial cells are separated from hepatocytes by the space of Disse (perisinusoidal space). This is an extravascular fluid compartment into which hepatocytes project microvilli, which allows proteins and other plasma components from the sinusoids to be taken up by the hepatocytes. Within this space, the endothelial cells are specialized in that they lack intercellular junctions and a basement membrane but contain multiple large fenestrations. This arrangement provides for the maximal contact of hepatocyte membranes with this extravascular fluid compartment and blood in the sinusoidal space. Thus, this system permits bidirectional movement of solutes (high- and low-molecular-weight substances) into and out of hepatocytes, providing tremendous filtration potential. On the other hand, the fenestrations of the endothelial cells restrict movement of molecules between the sinusoids and hepatocytes and vary in response to exogenous and endogenous mediators.

Other cell types are found along the sinusoidal lining. Kupffer cells, derived from the macrophage-monocyte system, are irregularly shaped cells that also line the sinusoids insinuating between endothelial cells. Kupffer cells are phagocytic, can migrate along sinusoids to areas of injury, and play a major role in the trapping of foreign substances and initiating inflammatory responses. Major histocompatibility complex II antigens are expressed on Kupffer cells but do not confer efficient antigen presentation compared with macrophages elsewhere in the body. Other lymphoid cells also exist in hepatic parenchyma, such as natural killer, natural killer T, CD4 T, and CD8 T cells. These provide the liver with an innate immune system. Hepatic stellate cells, previously known as *Ito cells,* are cells high in retinoid content (accounting for their phenotypic identification) found in the space of Disse. They have dendritic processes that contact hepatocyte microvilli and wrap around endothelial cells. The major functions of these stellate cells include vitamin A storage and the synthesis of extracellular collagen and other extracellular matrix proteins. In acute and chronic hepatic liver injuries, hepatic stellate cells are activated to a myofibroblastic state associated with morphologic changes, cellular contractility, decreases in intracellular vitamin A, and production of extracellular matrix. Ultimately, stellate cells play a central role in the development and progression of hepatic fibrosis to cirrhosis and are the target for the development of antifibrotic treatments.

Hepatocytes. Hepatocytes are complex multifunctional cells that make up 60% of the hepatic cellular mass and 80% of the

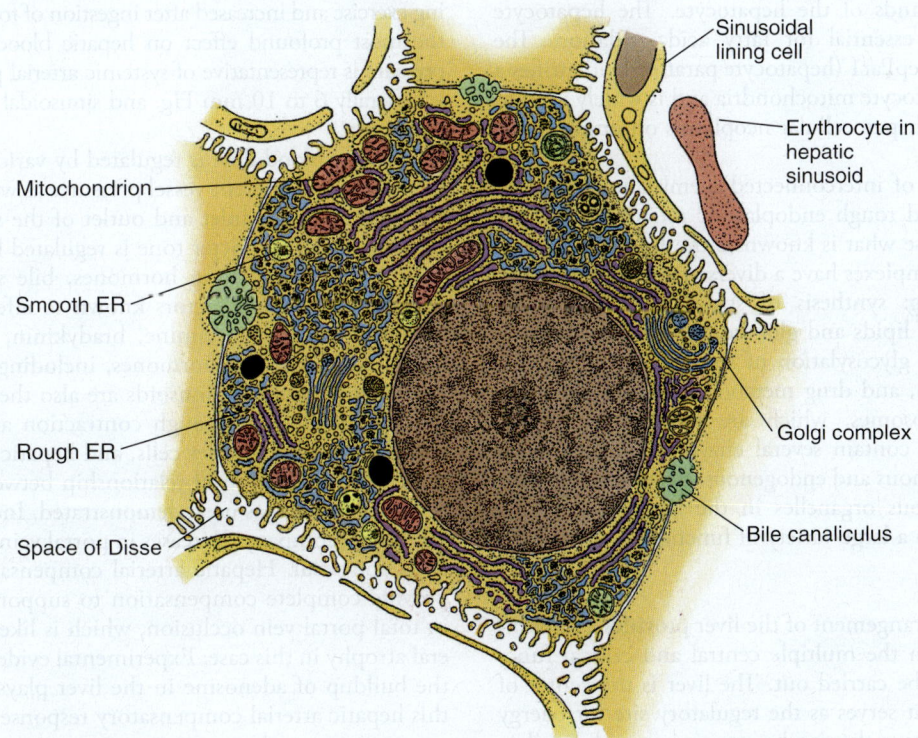

FIGURE 89.17 A hepatocyte and its sinusoidal and lateral domains. *ER,* Endoplasmic reticulum. (From Ross MH, Reith EJ, Romrell LJ. The liver. In: Ross RH, Reith EJ, Romrell LJ, eds. *Histology: A Text and Atlas.* Baltimore: Williams & Wilkins; 1989:471-478.)

cytoplasmic mass of the liver (see Fig. 89.17). The hepatocyte is a polyhedral cell with a central spherical nucleus. As noted, hepatocytes are arranged in single-cell-layer plates lined on either side by blood-filled sinusoids. Every hepatocyte has contact with adjacent hepatocytes, the biliary space (bile canaliculus), and the perisinusoidal space, enabling these cells to perform their broad range of functions. Among the many essential functions of the hepatocyte are uptake, storage, and release of nutrients; synthesis of glucose, fatty acids, lipids, and numerous plasma proteins (including C-reactive protein and albumin); production and secretion of bile for digestion of dietary fats; and degradation and detoxification of toxins.

To carry out these functions, the plasma membrane of the hepatocyte is organized in a specific manner into three specific domains. The sinusoidal membrane is exposed to the space of Disse and has multiple microvilli that provide a surface specializing in the active transport of substances between the blood and hepatocytes. The lateral domain exists between neighboring hepatocytes and contains gap junctions that provide for intercellular communication. The canalicular membrane is a tube containing microvilli formed by two apposed hepatocytes. These bile canaliculi are sealed by zonula occludens (tight junctions), which prevent the escape of bile. The bile canaliculi form a ring around the hepatocyte that drains into small bile ducts known as *canals of Hering*, which empty into a bile duct at a portal triad. The canalicular membrane contains adenosine triphosphate (ATP)-dependent active transport systems that enable solutes to be secreted into the canalicular membrane against large concentration gradients.

The hepatocyte is one of the most diverse and metabolically active cells in the body, as reflected by its abundance of organelles. There are 1000 mitochondria/hepatocytes, occupying approximately 20% of the cell volume. Mitochondria generate energy (ATP) through oxidative phosphorylation and provide the energy for the metabolic demands of the hepatocyte. The hepatocyte mitochondria are also essential for fatty acid oxidation. The monoclonal antibody HepPar1 (hepatocyte paraffin 1) identifies a unique antigen on hepatocyte mitochondria and is widely used to identify hepatocytes or hepatocellular neoplasms on immunohistochemical examination.

An extensive system of interconnected membrane complexes made up of smooth and rough endoplasmic reticulum and the Golgi apparatus compose what is known as the *hepatocyte microsomal fraction*. These complexes have a diverse range of functions, including the following: synthesis of structural and secreted proteins, metabolism of lipids and glucose, production and metabolism of cholesterol, glycosylation of secretory proteins, bile formation and secretion, and drug metabolism. Finally, hepatocytes also contain lysosomes, which are intracellular single-membrane vesicles that contain several enzymes. These vesicles store and degrade exogenous and endogenous substances. Coordination of these numerous organelles in the hepatocyte allows these cells to accomplish a large variety of functions.

Functions

The unique anatomic arrangement of the liver provides a remarkable landscape on which the multiple central and critical functions of this organ can be carried out. The liver is the center of metabolic homeostasis; it serves as the regulatory site for energy metabolism by coordinating the uptake, processing, and distribution of nutrients and their subsequent energy products. The liver also synthesizes many proteins, enzymes, and vitamins that participate in a broad range of body functions. Finally, the liver detoxifies and eliminates many exogenous and endogenous substances, serving as the major filter of the human body. The following sections summarize the functions.

Energy

The liver is the critical intermediary between dietary sources of energy and the extrahepatic tissues that require this energy. The liver receives dietary byproducts through portal circulation and sorts, metabolizes, and distributes them into the systemic circulation. The liver also plays a major role in regulating endogenous sources of energy, such as fatty acids and glycerol from adipose tissues and lactate, pyruvate, and certain amino acids from skeletal muscle. The two major sources of energy that the liver releases into the extrahepatic circulation are glucose and acetoacetate. Glucose is derived from the glycogenolysis of stored glycogen and from gluconeogenesis from lactate, pyruvate, glycerol, propionate, and alanine. Acetoacetate is derived from the β-oxidation of fatty acids. Also, storage lipids such as triacylglycerols and phospholipids are synthesized and stored as lipoproteins by the liver. These can be circulated systemically for uptake by peripheral tissues. These complex and essential functions are regulated by hormones, overall nutritional state of the organism, and requirements of obligate glucose-requiring tissues.

Blood Flow

There is a dual blood supply to the liver that comes from the portal vein and hepatic artery. The portal vein provides approximately 75% of the blood flow to the liver, which is oxygen poor but rich in nutrients. The hepatic artery provides the other 25% of the blood flow, which is oxygen rich and represents systemic arterial blood flow. The large flow rate of the portal vein is still able to provide 50% to 70% of the afferent oxygenation to the liver. Overall, hepatic blood flow represents about 25% of the cardiac output, demonstrating its central role in whole-body metabolism. Hepatic blood flow is decreased during exercise and increased after ingestion of food. Carbohydrates have the most profound effect on hepatic blood flow. Hepatic arterial pressure is representative of systemic arterial pressure. Portal pressure is generally 6 to 10 mm Hg, and sinusoidal pressure is usually 2 to 4 mm Hg.

Hepatic blood flow is regulated by various factors. Differences in afferent and efferent vessel pressures as well as muscular sphincters located at the inlet and outlet of the sinusoids play a major role. Muscular sphincter tone is regulated by the autonomic nervous system, circulating hormones, bile salts, and metabolites. Specific endogenous factors known to affect hepatic blood flow include glucagon, histamine, bradykinin, prostaglandins, nitric oxide, and many gut hormones, including gastrin, secretin, and cholecystokinin. The sinusoids are also the primary regulators of hepatic blood flow through contraction and expansion of their endothelial cells, Kupffer cells, and hepatic stellate cells.

A one-way reciprocal relationship between hepatic artery and portal vein flow has been demonstrated. Increases in hepatic arterial flow accompany decreases in portal vein flow, but the opposite does not occur. Hepatic arterial compensation, however, cannot provide complete compensation to support hepatic parenchyma in total portal vein occlusion, which is likely the cause of ipsilateral atrophy in this case. Experimental evidence has suggested that the buildup of adenosine in the liver plays an important role in this hepatic arterial compensatory response.

Bile Formation

One of the primary functions of the liver is bile production and secretion. The physiologic role of bile is twofold. The first is to

TABLE 89.1 Solute Concentrations of Hepatic Bile

SOLUTE	CONCENTRATION
Na+	132–165 mEq/L
K+	4.2–5.6 mEq/L
Ca2+	1.2–4.8 mEq/L
Mg2+	1.4–3.0 mEq/L
Cl−	96–126 mEq/L
HCO3−	17–55 mEq/L
Bile acids	3–45 mM
Phospholipid	25–810 mg/dL
Cholesterol	60–320 mg/dL
Protein	300–3000 mg/L

dispose of substances secreted into bile; the second is to provide enteric bile salts to aid in the digestion of fats. Bile is a substance containing organic and inorganic solutes produced by an active process of secretion and subsequent concentration of these solutes. The concentration of inorganic solutes in bile in the main biliary tree resembles that of plasma (Table 89.1). In the case of bile loss (e.g., from an external biliary fistula), the high concentrations of protein and electrolytes must be considered in replacing the losses. The osmolality of bile is approximately 300 mOsmol/kg and is accounted for by the inorganic solutes. The major organic solutes in bile are bile acids, bile pigments, cholesterol, and phospholipids.

The contents of bile are generally absorbed from the bloodstream through sinusoids into the hepatocyte through the sinusoidal membrane. Bile is initially secreted by hepatocytes into the canaliculi through specialized microvilli containing lateral membranes of the hepatocytes that form the canaliculi. Tight junctions along the canalicular membranes prevent leakage of bile in the normal state. This also provides a route for paracellular secretion of solutes and water into bile. The canaliculi coalesce into larger bile ductules containing biliary epithelium, which then form the intrahepatic and extrahepatic biliary tree. Thus, the liver, in part, serves as an epithelial structure that moves solutes from the blood to the bile and provides a route of secretion for bile into the intestines.

Approximately 1500 mL of bile is secreted daily, and about 80% is secreted by hepatocytes into canaliculi. Such canalicular bile flow is largely the result of water flow in response to active solute transport. Bile acids are transported from the sinusoidal blood into the hepatocyte by an ATP-requiring active transport system. Intracellular transport to the canalicular membrane is through bile acid–binding proteins that are transported by a vesicular system derived from the Golgi apparatus. The bile acids are then actively pumped into the canaliculus through an ATP-requiring active transport system. It is well recognized that bile flow has a linear association with bile acid secretion, known as *bile acid–dependent flow*. Because bile acids form micelles in the bile and do not provide osmotic potential, it is likely that flow related to bile acid secretion is secondary to ions that accompany the bile acids (counterions). Bile flow can also occur in the near-absence of bile acid secretion, known as *bile acid–independent flow*. Experimental evidence has suggested that bile acid–independent flow is at least partially the result of biliary glutathione secretion.

Once bile has passed from the canaliculi to the biliary ductules and then to main bile ducts, bile undergoes further reabsorption

and secretion. The epithelial cells of the biliary tract actively reabsorb and secrete water and electrolytes. Secretion is generally through a chloride channel activated by secretin, its most powerful activator, and its subsequent activation of cyclic adenosine monophosphate production. There is usually a net secretion of water and electrolytes, accounting for the other 20% of biliary secretion. Ultimately, bile becomes highly enriched in bicarbonate ions. Many organic substances, such as glutathione, are degraded in the biliary tree. Many drugs can be secreted into the biliary tree in a highly concentrated form (e.g., ceftriaxone). The gallbladder acts as the reservoir of the biliary tree; its function is to store bile in the fasting state. The gallbladder reabsorbs water, concentrating stored bile, and secretes mucin. Contraction of the gallbladder is mediated hormonally, largely through cholecystokinin, in response to a meal, with the simultaneous relaxation of the sphincter of Oddi and release of bile into the duodenum.

Enterohepatic Circulation

Bile salts are primarily produced in the liver and secreted to be used in the biliary tree and intestine. The primary bile salts cholic acid and chenodeoxycholic acid are produced in the liver from cholesterol and subsequently conjugated with glycine or taurine in the hepatocyte. Once secreted in the gut, the primary bile acids are modified by intestinal bacteria to form the secondary bile acids deoxycholic acid and lithocholic acid. Bile acids are reabsorbed passively into the jejunum and actively into the ileum. Thus, the bile acids reenter the portal venous system, and up to 90% of the bile acids are extracted by hepatocytes. Only a small fraction spills over into the systemic circulation because of efficient hepatic extraction, which accounts for low levels of plasma bile acids. After hepatic extraction, bile acids are recirculated into the canaliculi and back into the biliary tree, completing the circuit. A small amount of intestinal bile acids is not absorbed by the portal system and is excreted in the stool. Thus, the active secretion of bile salts from hepatocytes into bile and from ileal enterocytes into the portal vein is the engine behind the enterohepatic circulation.

The enterohepatic circulation is more than a unique mechanism for reusing physiologically valuable bile acids. This circulation of bile constitutes the primary mechanism for eliminating excess cholesterol because cholesterol is consumed during the production of bile salts and is excreted in the feces by mixed micelles formed by organic biliary solutes. Bile salts also play a critical role in the absorption of dietary fats, fat-soluble vitamins (i.e., vitamins A, D, E, and K), and lipophilic drugs. Water movement from hepatocytes into bile and water absorption through the small bowel are also regulated by bile salts. The enterohepatic circulation is therefore central to a number of solubilization, transport, and regulatory functions.

Bilirubin Metabolism

Bilirubin is the result of heme breakdown. An early phase of heme breakdown, accounting for 20% of bilirubin, is from hemoproteins (heme-containing enzymes) and occurs within 3 days of labeling with radioactive heme. A late phase of heme breakdown, accounting for 80% of bilirubin, is from senescent red blood cells. This occurs approximately 110 days after administration of radioactively labeled heme and is consistent with the life span of red blood cells. Heme is initially broken down into green biliverdin by heme oxygenase, which is then broken down into the orange bilirubin by biliverdin reductase.

Circulating bilirubin is bound to albumin, which protects many organs from the potentially toxic effects of this compound.

The bilirubin-albumin complex enters hepatic sinusoidal blood, where it enters the space of Disse through the large sinusoidal fenestrations. The bilirubin-albumin complex is disassociated in this space. Free bilirubin is internalized into the hepatocyte, where it is conjugated to glucuronic acid. Conjugated bilirubin is then secreted in an energy-dependent fashion into canalicular bile against a large concentration gradient. Bilirubin is secreted with bile into the gastrointestinal tract. Within the gastrointestinal tract, bilirubin is deconjugated by intestinal bacteria to a group of compounds known as *urobilinogens*. These urobilinogens are further oxidized and reabsorbed into the enterohepatic circulation and secreted into bile. A small percentage of the reabsorbed urobilinogens is excreted into urine. These oxidized urobilinogens account for the colored compounds that contribute to the yellow color of urine and the brown color of stool.

Bilirubin has long been known to be a toxic compound and is the agent responsible for neonatal encephalopathy and cochlear damage secondary to severe unconjugated hyperbilirubinemia (kernicterus). The binding of serum bilirubin to albumin protects the tissues from exposure to bilirubin. However, binding sites can be overwhelmed by increasing amounts of bilirubin or displaced by other binding agents (e.g., various drugs). The mechanism of bilirubin toxicity appears to be related to several of its effects. Free bilirubin can uncouple oxidative phosphorylation, inhibit ATPases, decrease glucose metabolism, and inhibit a broad spectrum of protein kinase activities.

Portosystemic shunts, such as those seen with cirrhosis and portal hypertension, decrease the first-pass hepatic clearance of bilirubin, resulting in a mildly increased serum unconjugated hyperbilirubinemia. Several disorders can result in an unconjugated serum hyperbilirubinemia, including neonatal hyperbilirubinemia, an increased bilirubin load caused by hemolytic syndromes, and inherited enzymatic deficiencies such as Crigler-Najjar and Gilbert syndromes. Disorders presenting with serum conjugated hyperbilirubinemia include cholestasis, Dubin-Johnson, and Rotor syndromes.

Carbohydrate Metabolism

The liver is the center of carbohydrate metabolism because it is the primary regulator of storage and distribution of glucose to the peripheral tissues and, in particular, to glucose-dependent tissues such as the brain and erythrocytes. Both the liver and muscle can store glucose in the form of glycogen, but only the liver can break down glycogen to provide glucose for systemic circulation. Glycogen that is broken down can be used only in muscle and is therefore not a source of systemically circulated glucose.

In the fed state, carbohydrates absorbed through the intestines (mostly glucose) are circulated systemically. Carbohydrates reaching the liver are rapidly converted to glycogen for storage. The liver contains up to 65 g of glycogen per kilogram of liver tissue. Excess carbohydrates are mostly converted to fatty acids and stored in adipose tissue. In the postabsorptive state (between meals, nonfasting), there is no further systemic glucose coming directly from the gut, and the liver becomes the primary source of circulating glucose by the breakdown of glycogen. This is crucial for the brain and erythrocytes, which rely on glucose for their metabolism. In the postabsorptive state, most other tissues begin to rely on fatty acids derived from adipose tissue as their primary fuel. Highly active muscle may deplete its own glycogen and depend on liver-derived glucose for its substrate in the postabsorptive state. After 48 hours of fasting, hepatic glycogen is depleted, and the liver shifts from glycogenolysis to gluconeogenesis.

The substrate for hepatic gluconeogenesis is mostly from amino acids (mainly alanine) derived from muscle breakdown, but they also come from glycerol derived from adipose breakdown. During a prolonged fast, fatty acids from adipose breakdown are β-oxidized in the liver, which releases ketone bodies that then become the primary fuel for the brain.

Transitions in and out of these various metabolic states and regulation of carbohydrate metabolism are mostly influenced by glucose concentration in sinusoidal blood and hormonal influences (e.g., insulin, catecholamines, glucagon). In the fasting state, during anaerobic metabolism, lactate is produced largely from muscle. The liver uses this lactate, which is converted to pyruvate that enters the gluconeogenic pathways to produce glucose. This cycle is known as the *Cori cycle*.

Derangements of carbohydrate metabolism are common in liver disease. People with cirrhosis often demonstrate abnormal glucose tolerance. Its mechanism is unclear but is probably related to associated insulin resistance. This phenomenon is not caused by shunting of glucose-containing blood away from the liver. Hypoglycemia is distinctly uncommon in chronic liver disease because of the remarkable resilience of the liver and its metabolic function. Only with massive hepatocyte loss in fulminant hepatic failure does gluconeogenesis fail and hypoglycemia ensue.

Lipid Metabolism

Fatty acids are synthesized in the liver during states of glucose excess when the liver's ability to store glycogen has been exceeded. Adipocytes have a limited ability to synthesize fatty acids. Therefore, the liver is the predominant source of synthesized fatty acids, although they are largely stored in adipose tissue. During lipolysis, free fatty acids are transported to the liver, where they are metabolized. Fatty acids in the liver undergo esterification with glycerol to form triglycerides for storage or transportation, or they undergo β-oxidation, yielding energy in the form of ATP and ketone bodies. In general, this process is regulated by the nutritional state; starvation favors oxidation, and the fed state favors esterification.

There is a constant cycling of fatty acids between the liver and adipose tissue that is under a delicate balance, which can easily be offset, resulting in fatty infiltration of the liver. A few factors influence this balance; for example, hepatic uptake of fatty acids is a function of plasma concentrations. Although there is no limit to the liver's ability to esterify fatty acids, its ability to dispose of or break down fatty acids is limited, as is its ability to secrete triglycerides in the form of lipoproteins. Therefore, conditions of increased circulating fatty acids can easily override the liver's ability to handle them, resulting in fatty accumulation in the liver. This is known as *steatosis* or, when it is associated with chronic inflammation in more advanced cases, *steatohepatitis*. Many conditions have been associated with hepatic steatosis, such as diabetes, steroid use, starvation, obesity, and extensive administration of cytotoxic chemotherapeutic agents. Fatty liver associated with alcohol intake has several causes; it is related to increased lipolysis, reduced oxygenation, and augmented esterification of hepatic fatty acids and may also be related to relative starvation in the chronic alcoholic.

Protein Metabolism

The liver is also a central site for the metabolism of proteins and is involved in synthesis of protein, catabolism of proteins into energy or storage forms, and management of excess amino acids and nitrogen waste. Ingested protein is broken down into amino acids that are circulated throughout the body, where they are used as the building blocks for proteins, enzymes, and hormones. Excess amino acids not used in peripheral tissues are generally handled by the liver, in which they are oxidized for energy—providing 50% of the liver's energy needs—or converted into glucose, ketone bodies, or fats. When amino acids are catabolized for energy production throughout the body, ammonia, glutamine, glutamate, and aspartate are produced. These products are largely processed in the liver, where the waste nitrogen is converted to urea through the urea cycle, and the urea is generally excreted in the urine. Thus, the liver is central and critical to the body's nitrogen balance and amino acid metabolism.

Although the liver can catabolize most amino acids, yielding energy or other storable energy forms such as glucose and fats, notable exceptions are the branched-chain amino acids. Branched-chain amino acids cannot be catabolized in the liver and are mostly dealt with by muscle. It has been postulated that this may act as a so-called safety net that helps spare the liver some of the demands of protein and amino acid metabolism.

The liver is also the main site of synthesis for many proteins involved in such wide-ranging and critical functions as coagulation, transport, copper and iron binding, and protease inhibition. These proteins include ceruloplasmin, iron storage and binding proteins, and α_1-antitrypsin. Albumin is made exclusively in the liver and is the predominant serum binding protein. Hepatic insufficiency or specific genetic abnormalities can result in altered amounts and functions of these proteins, with wide-ranging pathologic effects.

The liver is also responsible for the so-called acute-phase response, a synthetic response by protein to trauma or infection. Its purpose is to restrict organ damage, maintain vital hepatic function, and control defense mechanisms. The response is incited by proinflammatory cytokines such as interleukin-1 (IL-1), IL-6, and tumor necrosis factor, which induce acute-phase protein gene expression in the liver. Some of the well-known hepatic acute-phase proteins are α_1-, α_2-, and β-globulin as well as C-reactive protein and serum amyloid A. An equally important part of this response is its termination. Antiinflammatory cytokines such as IL-1 receptor antagonist, IL-4, and IL-10 appear to play important roles. The acute-phase response is usually completed in 24 to 48 hours but can be prolonged in the context of ongoing injury.

Vitamin Metabolism

Along with the intestine, the liver is responsible for the metabolism of the fat-soluble vitamins A, D, E, and K. These vitamins are obtained exogenously and absorbed in the intestine. Their adequate intestinal absorption is critically dependent on adequate fatty acid micellization, which requires bile acids.

Vitamin A is from the retinoid family and is involved in normal vision, embryonic development, and adult gene regulation. Storage of vitamin A is solely in the liver and occurs in the hepatic stellate cells. Overingestion of vitamin A can result in hepatic toxicity. Vitamin D is involved in calcium and phosphorus homeostasis. One of vitamin D's activation steps (25-hydroxylation) occurs in the liver. Vitamin E is a potent antioxidant and protects membranes from lipid peroxidation and free radical formation. Finally, vitamin K is a critical cofactor in the posttranslational γ-carboxylation of the hepatically synthesized coagulation factors II, VII, IX, and X as well as of protein C and protein S, the so-called vitamin K–dependent cofactors. Cholestasis syndromes can result in the inadequate absorption of these vitamins secondary to poor micellization in the intestine. The associated vitamin

deficiency syndromes, such as metabolic bone disease (vitamin D deficiency), neurologic disorders (vitamin E deficiency), and coagulopathy (vitamin K deficiency), can subsequently occur.

The liver is also involved in the uptake, storage, and metabolism of several water-soluble vitamins, including thiamine, riboflavin, vitamin B_6, vitamin B_{12}, folate, biotin, and pantothenic acid. The liver is responsible for converting some of these vitamins to active coenzymes, transforming some to storage metabolites, and using some for enterohepatic circulation (e.g., vitamin B_{12}).

Coagulation

The liver is responsible for synthesizing almost all the identified coagulation factors as well as many of the fibrinolytic system components and several plasma regulatory proteins of coagulation and fibrinolysis. As noted, the liver is critical for the absorption of vitamin K, synthesizes the vitamin K–dependent coagulation factors, and contains the enzyme that activates these factors. Also, the reticuloendothelial system of the liver clears activated clotting factors, activated complexes of the coagulation and fibrinolytic systems, and end products of fibrin degradation. Diseases of the liver are often associated with thrombocytopenia, qualitative platelet abnormalities, vitamin K deficiency with impaired modulation of vitamin K–dependent coagulation factors, and disseminated intravascular coagulation. It is no surprise that liver disease is firmly associated with coagulation disorders that are often challenging to deal with.

Warfarin, one of the most dispensed anticoagulants, acts in the liver by blocking vitamin K–dependent activation of factors II, VII, IX, and X. Factor VII has the shortest half-life of the coagulation factors; its deficiency is manifested clinically as abnormalities of the measured prothrombin time (PT) or international normalized ratio (INR). Patients with hepatic synthetic dysfunction similarly have an abnormal PT.

Metabolism of Drugs and Toxins (Xenobiotics)

The human body is exposed to an inordinate amount of foreign chemicals during a lifetime. This poses a challenge to our ability to detoxify and eliminate these potentially harmful chemicals. Many of these chemicals are not incorporated into cellular metabolism and are referred to as xenobiotics. The liver plays a central role in handling them through complex enzymes and reaction pathways, which are increasingly recognized as new chemicals are discovered.

Hepatic-based reactions to xenobiotics are broadly classified into phase I and phase II reactions. Through oxidation, reduction, and hydrolysis, phase I reactions increase the polarity and thus water solubility of compounds. This, in turn, allows easier excretion. Phase I reactions do not necessarily detoxify chemicals and may, in fact, create toxic metabolites. Phase I reactions occur in the cytochrome P450 system. Phase II reactions generally act to create a less toxic or less active byproduct. This is generally accomplished through transferase reactions, in which a compound is usually coupled to a conjugate, rendering the xenobiotic more innocuous.

Regeneration

The liver possesses the unique quality of adjusting its volume to the needs of the body. This is observed clinically in its regeneration after partial hepatectomy or after toxic liver injury. It is also seen in liver transplantation, in that donor liver size mismatches adjust to the new host. This quality is highly conserved evolutionarily because of the critical functions of the liver and the fact that the liver is the first line of exposure to ingested toxic agents.

Liver regeneration is a hyperplastic response of all cell types of the liver, in which the microscopic anatomy of the functional liver is maintained. Much information about the regenerative response of the liver is based on experimental evidence in rodents. Normally quiescent hepatocytes rapidly enter the cell cycle after partial hepatectomy. Maximal hepatocyte DNA synthesis occurs 24 to 36 hours after partial hepatectomy, and maximal DNA synthesis occurs in the other cell types 48 to 72 hours later. Most of the increase in hepatic mass in rodents is seen 3 days after partial hepatectomy, and it is usually almost complete after 7 days.

In the late 1960s, it was recognized that circulating factors were responsible, in part, for the regenerative response, and much research has focused on the humoral and genetic control of hepatic regeneration. The major circulating factors identified, largely from rodent studies, are hepatocyte growth factor, epidermal growth factor, transforming growth factors, insulin, glucagon, and the cytokines tumor necrosis factor-α, IL-1, and IL-6. These factors, when infused into a normal host, do not result in hepatic growth, indicating that hepatocytes must be primed in some way before responding to these growth factors. Remarkable progress in the understanding of liver regeneration has been made because of the development of improved genetic and molecular biology techniques. Hundreds of genes involved at all stages of regeneration have been identified by RNA microarray techniques. Also, numerous cytokine-dependent and growth factor–independent pathways have been further defined. A complete description is beyond the scope of this chapter, however, and many questions remain.

Assessment of Liver Function

A wide variety of tests are available to evaluate hepatic diseases. Screening for hepatic disease, assessing hepatic function, diagnosing specific disorders, and prognosticating are critical in the management of hepatic disease. For the surgeon, assessment of hepatic function and estimation of the ability of a hepatic remnant to be sufficient after liver resection are also of obvious importance. Unfortunately, most measures of hepatic disease are gross indicators and lack sensitivity, specificity, and accuracy. We have divided these hepatic function tests into three categories: routine screening, specific diagnostic, and quantitative tests.

Routine Screening Tests

Screening blood tests are often used to determine whether there is disease in the hepatobiliary system. Standard liver function tests (LFTs) are generally not tests of function and are not always specific to hepatic disease. Nonetheless, they are a valuable screening tool to provide basic indications to recognize the presence of hepatic disease and yield clues about the cause of that disease. Total bilirubin, direct bilirubin (conjugated), and indirect bilirubin (unconjugated) levels can be affected by several processes related to bilirubin metabolism. Unconjugated hyperbilirubinemia can reflect increased bilirubin production (e.g., hemolysis), drug effects, inherited enzymatic disorders, or physiologic jaundice of the newborn. Conjugated hyperbilirubinemia is generally a result of cholestasis or mechanical biliary obstruction but can also be seen in some inherited disorders or hepatocellular disease.

The transaminases alanine aminotransferase (ALT) and aspartate aminotransferase (AST) are the most common serum markers of hepatocellular necrosis, with subsequent leak of these intracellular enzymes into the circulation. AST is found in other organs, such as the heart, muscle, and kidney, but ALT is liver specific. However, the degree of elevation of these enzyme levels has never

been shown to be of prognostic value. Alkaline phosphatase (ALP) is expressed in liver, bile ducts, bone, intestine, placenta, kidney, and leukocytes. Isoenzyme determinations can sometimes help distinguish the source of an elevated ALP level. Elevations of ALP levels in hepatobiliary diseases are generally secondary to cholestasis or biliary obstruction. Such elevations are caused by increased production of this enzyme. The ALP level can also be increased in malignant disease of the liver. Gamma-glutamyl transpeptidase (GGT) is an enzyme in many organs in addition to the liver, such as the kidneys, seminal vesicles, spleen, pancreas, heart, and brain. Its level can be elevated in diseases affecting any of these tissues. It is also induced by alcohol intake and is elevated in biliary obstruction. Thus, it is also a nonspecific marker of liver disease but can help determine whether an elevated ALP level is from hepatic disease. 5′-Nucleotidase is found in a wide variety of organs in addition to the liver, but increased levels are specific to hepatic disease. Like GGT, it can help determine whether an elevated ALP level is secondary to hepatic disease.

Albumin is synthesized exclusively in the liver and can be used as a general measure of hepatic synthetic function. Because chronic malnutrition and acute injury, infection, and/or inflammation can decrease albumin synthesis, these factors must be considered in evaluating a low serum albumin level. Because of the remarkable protein synthetic capacity of the liver, hypoalbuminemia is a marker of severe liver disease. However, it lacks sensitivity, and large decreases in hepatic function are required to be reflected in albumin levels. In general, it is most helpful in chronic liver disease.

Clotting factors are largely synthesized in the liver; abnormalities of coagulation can be a marker of hepatic synthetic dysfunction. Measurement of specific clotting factors, such as factors V and VII, has been used to evaluate hepatic function in the transplantation population. PT or INR is the best test to measure the effects of hepatic disease on clotting, and prolonged PT or elevated INR is usually a marker of advanced chronic liver disease. Hepatic disease can also affect clotting through intravascular coagulation and vitamin K malabsorption. Patients with liver disease have thrombocytopenia. Although platelets are not incorporated in any measure of liver function and thrombocytopenia may be multifactorial, platelet levels provide insight into severity of portal hypertension in patients with liver disease.

Specific Diagnostic Tests

Once screening tests, along with clinical findings, have suggested liver disease, specific tests can help elucidate the cause and guide treatment, if necessary. Hepatitis serologies are important to determine the presence of viral hepatitis. Autoimmune antibodies are used to diagnose primary biliary cirrhosis (e.g., antimitochondrial), primary sclerosing cholangitis (e.g., antineutrophil), and autoimmune hepatitis. α1-Antitrypsin and ceruloplasmin levels assist in the diagnosis of α1-antitrypsin deficiency and Wilson disease, respectively. Tumor markers such as α-fetoprotein (AFP) and carcinoembryonic antigen (CEA) are helpful in the diagnosis and management of primary and metastatic tumors of the liver.

In general, the LFTs discussed in this section are gross, nonspecific, and of little, if any, prognostic value. Many attempts have been made to formulate dynamic and quantitative tests of hepatic function based on the liver's ability to clear various exogenously administered substances. Despite many years of research, it remains unclear whether these tests of hepatic function are any better than scoring systems derived from simple blood tests and clinical observations. For example, the aminopyrine breath test is based on cytochrome P450 clearance of radiolabeled aminopyrine. A breath test measuring radiolabeled CO_2 as a breakdown product of aminopyrine is performed after administration at a specified time. The results largely depend on the functional hepatic mass, which is generally not depleted until end-stage liver disease has developed. There are varying results of studies comparing the aminopyrine breath test with standard LFTs and scoring systems; its main value appears to be prognosis in chronic liver disease, but it is clearly not an effective test to detect subclinical hepatic dysfunction.

Substances such as antipyrine and caffeine can evaluate liver function in a similar way, with similar results. The lidocaine clearance test yields similar information to the aminopyrine test because it is based on its clearance by the hepatic cytochrome P450 test. Lidocaine clearance depends on blood flow and a complex distribution process, but measurement of one of its metabolites, monoethylglycinexylidide, has greatly simplified the test. It has been shown to have some prognostic value in the transplantation population. The galactose elimination test is based on the liver's role in phosphorylating galactose and converting it to glucose. The rate at which galactose is eliminated from the bloodstream can be used as a measure of hepatic function. Problems related to this test are that the enzymes involved are genetically heterogeneous, and considerable extrahepatic metabolism occurs. Also, multiple blood draws are necessary, which makes the test cumbersome. The value of this test is probably in assessing the prognosis of patients with chronic liver disease rather than in screening. Indocyanine green is a dye removed by the liver by a carrier-mediated process and excreted into bile. This dye is rapidly cleared from the bloodstream and is not metabolized. This is the only test that has been shown to have some prognostic ability in patients with cirrhosis undergoing liver resection, although this is not universally demonstrated in studies, nor is it universally accepted.

Nuclear imaging studies overcome some of the limitations of the lidocaine and indocyanine green tests described earlier and have the advantage of providing simultaneous morphologic (visual) and physiologic (quantitative functional) information about the liver. This not only helps quantitate the liver function but also in determining the distribution of that function. Thus, regional (segmental) differentiation allows specific functional assessment of the future remnant liver. Technetium-99m (99mTc)–galactosyl human serum albumin scintigraphy and 99mTc-mebrofenin hepatobiliary scintigraphy potentially identify patients at risk for postresectional liver failure who might benefit from liver-augmenting techniques.

Quantitative Tests

Many scoring systems based on clinical observation and standard blood tests have been proposed. The most used system is Pugh's modification of the Child score (Table 89.2). Although all these

systems are less than perfect and not universally accepted, the Child-Pugh score is commonly used for patients with cirrhosis who require liver surgery. Mortality and survival rates after hepatectomy correlate with this score but are not always related to liver failure. Child-Pugh class B and C patients have higher perioperative mortality after any partial hepatectomy than Child-Pugh class A patients, who can generally withstand a major hepatectomy. The presence of portal hypertension has been shown to predict poor outcome after partial hepatectomy. Portal hypertension in patients with cirrhosis is usually manifested as thrombocytopenia, splenomegaly, and presence of intraabdominal varices on imaging or at endoscopy. The best evidence for portal hypertension is a hepatic vein wedge pressure higher than 10 mm Hg, which has been shown to correlate strongly with postoperative liver failure.

PORTAL HYPERTENSION

Cirrhosis is the result of a healing response initiated by chronic liver injury. It is characterized by development of fibrous septa surrounding regenerating hepatocellular nodules. Besides development of synthetic deficiencies, cirrhosis is associated with development of portal hypertension. At present, effective treatments for cirrhosis are nonexistent. As a result, its treatment has largely been focused on the treatment of resultant portal hypertension and its complications. The major challenge for the hepatologist or surgeon treating patients with cirrhosis and end-stage liver disease is determining when definitive treatment (e.g., liver transplantation) rather than palliative treatment (e.g., interventions to prevent recurrent variceal hemorrhage) should be applied. Cirrhosis can be classified as compensated or decompensated based on the absence or presence of clinically evident decompensating events (variceal hemorrhage, encephalopathy, ascites). This classification provides important prognostic information, as patients with compensated cirrhosis have a median survival exceeding 12 years, whereas patients with decompensated cirrhosis have a median survival of only 1.8 years.

Definition

Portal hypertension is defined by a portal pressure gradient (the difference in pressure between the portal vein and the hepatic veins) higher than 5 mm Hg. The best method to estimate this gradient is by transfemoral-hepatic vein catheterization with a balloon tip catheter. However, higher pressures (8–10 mm Hg) are typically required to begin stimulating the development of portosystemic collateralization. Collateral vessels usually develop where the portal and systemic venous circulations are in close apposition (Fig. 89.18). The collateral network through the coronary and short gastric veins to the azygos vein is clinically the most important because it results in formation of esophagogastric varices. However, other sites include a recanalized umbilical vein from the left portal vein to the epigastric venous system (caput medusae), retroperitoneal collateral vessels, and hemorrhoidal venous plexus. In addition to extrahepatic collateral vessels, a significant fraction of portal venous flow passes through anatomic and physiologic (e.g., capillarization of hepatic sinusoids) intrahepatic shunts. As hepatic portal perfusion decreases, hepatic arterial flow generally increases (buffer response).

Pathophysiology

Portal hypertension usually occurs because of increased portal venous resistance that is prehepatic, intrahepatic, or posthepatic in location. Several factors may contribute to this, including the

TABLE 89.2 Child-Pugh Classification

FACTOR	NO. OF POINTS		
	1	2	3
Bilirubin (mg/dL)	<2	2–3	>3
Albumin (g/dL)	>3.5	2.8–3.5	<2.8
Prothrombin time (increased seconds)	1–3	4–6	>6
Ascites	None	Slight	Moderate
Encephalopathy	None	Minimal	Advanced

Class A, 5–6 points; class B, 7–9 points; class C, 10–15 points.

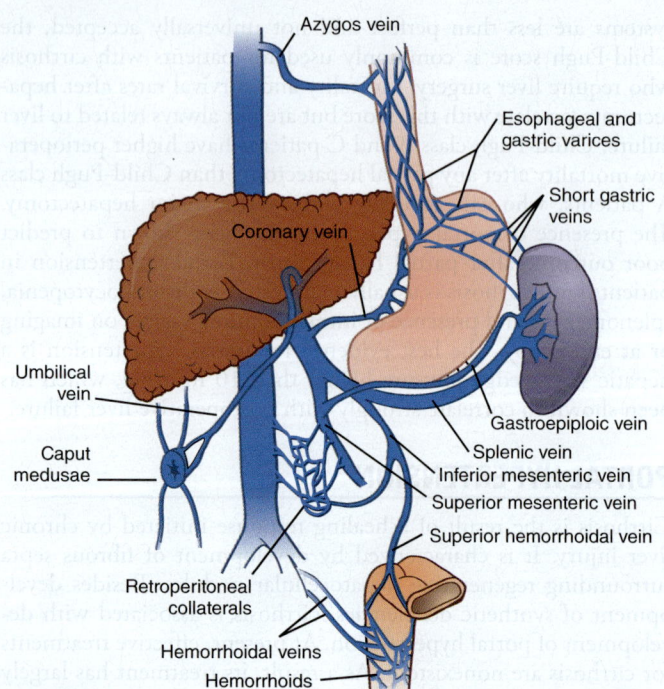

Azygos vein

Esophageal and gastric varices

Short gastric veins

Coronary vein

Umbilical vein

Caput medusae

Gastroepiploic vein

Splenic vein

Inferior mesenteric vein

Superior mesenteric vein

Superior hemorrhoidal vein

Retroperitoneal collaterals

Hemorrhoidal veins

Hemorrhoids

FIGURE 89.18 Portosystemic collateral pathways develop where the portal venous and systemic venous systems are in close apposition. (From Rikkers LF. Portal hypertension. In: Miller TA, ed. *Physiologic Basis of Modern Surgical Care*. St Louis: Mosby; 1988:417-428.)

following: increased passive resistance secondary to fibrosis and regenerative nodules; increased hepatic vascular resistance caused by active vasoconstriction by norepinephrine, endothelin, and other humoral vasoconstrictors; and increased portal venous inflow secondary to a hyperdynamic systemic circulation and splanchnic hyperemia. The last one is a major contributor to the maintenance of portal hypertension as portal systemic collaterals develop. Unfortunately, the exact causes remain unknown, but splanchnic hormones, decreased sensitivity of the splanchnic vasculature to catecholamines, and increased production of nitrous oxide and prostacyclin may be involved. Understanding the pathophysiology of portal hypertension may have therapeutic implications because these factors may represent targets for treatment.

The most common cause of prehepatic portal hypertension is portal vein thrombosis (PVT). This accounts for approximately 50% of cases of portal hypertension in children. When the portal vein is thrombosed in the absence of liver disease, hepatopetal (to the liver) portal collateral vessels develop to restore portal perfusion. This combination is termed *cavernomatous transformation of the portal vein*. Isolated splenic vein thrombosis (left-sided portal hypertension) is usually secondary to pancreatic inflammation or neoplasm. The result is gastrosplenic venous hypertension, with superior mesenteric and portal venous pressures remaining normal. The left gastroepiploic vein becomes a major collateral vessel, and gastric rather than esophageal varices develop. This variant of portal hypertension is important to recognize because it is easily reversed by splenectomy alone.

The site of increased resistance in intrahepatic portal hypertension may be at the presinusoidal, sinusoidal, or postsinusoidal level. Frequently, more than one level may be involved. The most common cause of intrahepatic presinusoidal hypertension is schistosomiasis. In addition, many causes of nonalcoholic cirrhosis result in presinusoidal portal hypertension. In contrast, alcoholic

cirrhosis, the most common cause of portal hypertension in the United States, usually causes increased resistance to portal flow at the sinusoidal (secondary to deposition of collagen in the space of Disse) and postsinusoidal (secondary to regenerating nodules distorting small hepatic veins) levels.

Posthepatic or postsinusoidal causes of portal hypertension are rare; they include Budd-Chiari syndrome (hepatic vein thrombosis), constrictive pericarditis, and heart failure. Rarely, increased portal venous flow alone, secondary to massive splenomegaly (e.g., idiopathic portal hypertension) or a splanchnic arteriovenous fistula, causes portal hypertension.

Assessment of Chronic Liver Disease and Portal Hypertension

The key aspects of assessing a patient with suspected chronic liver disease or complications of portal hypertension are the following: diagnosis of the underlying liver disease; estimation of functional hepatic reserve; definition of portal venous anatomy and hepatic hemodynamic evaluation; and identification of the site of upper gastrointestinal hemorrhage, if present. These diagnostic categories take on varying degrees of importance, depending on the clinical situation. For example, estimation of functional hepatic reserve is useful in determining the risk associated with therapeutic intervention and whether definitive (e.g., hepatic transplantation) or palliative (e.g., endoscopic variceal ligation or a shunt procedure) treatment is indicated.

Variceal Hemorrhage

Bleeding from esophagogastric varices is the single most life-threatening complication of portal hypertension. It is responsible for approximately one-third of all deaths in patients with cirrhosis. Approximately 50% of these deaths are caused by uncontrolled bleeding. The risk for death from bleeding is mainly related to the underlying hepatic functional reserve. Patients with extrahepatic portal venous obstruction and normal hepatic function rarely die of bleeding varices, whereas those with decompensated cirrhosis (e.g., Child-Pugh class C) may face a mortality rate of more than 50%. Once bleeding is controlled, the greatest risk for rebleeding from varices is within the first few days after the onset of hemorrhage; the risk declines rapidly between that point and 6 weeks. Subsequently, the risk returns to the prehemorrhage rate.

Treatment

In a patient with upper gastrointestinal bleeding, general measures are instituted; these include securing the airway (especially in an encephalopathic patient), ensuring adequate access (two large-bore intravenous [IV] lines), fluid infusion, type and cross-match of blood, and judicious blood and products transfusion. A randomized controlled trial comparing liberal transfusion (transfusion when the hemoglobin fell below 9 g/dL) with restrictive transfusion (transfusion when the hemoglobin levels fell below 7 g/dL) demonstrated that the restrictive strategy led to better survival at 6 weeks and reduced risk of rebleeding. Therapy for portal hypertension and variceal bleeding has evolved over time and now encompasses a spectrum of treatment modalities in which sequential therapies are often necessary. For acutely bleeding patients with portal hypertension, nonoperative treatments are generally used as a first-line approach, as these patients are at high operative risk because of decompensated hepatic function. Endoscopic treatment (e.g., sclerosis or ligation) has become the mainstay of nonoperative treatment of acute hemorrhage because bleeding can be controlled in more than 85% of patients. This allows an interval of medical management for improvement of hepatic function, resolution of ascites and encephalopathy, and enhancement of nutrition before definitive treatment for prevention of recurrent bleeding is instituted. Pharmacotherapy can also be initiated, and trials have suggested that it may be as effective as endoscopic treatment. Balloon tamponade, which is infrequently used, can be lifesaving in patients with exsanguinating hemorrhage when other nonoperative methods are not successful. A transjugular intrahepatic portosystemic shunt (TIPS) is another treatment option whereby a percutaneous connection is created within the liver, between the portal and systemic circulations, to reduce portal pressure in patients with complications related to portal hypertension. TIPS has replaced operative shunts for managing acute variceal bleeding when pharmacotherapy and endoscopic treatment fail to control bleeding. As a result, emergency surgical intervention in most centers is reserved for select patients who are not TIPS candidates.

Endoscopy. About 80% to 90% of acute variceal bleeding episodes are successfully controlled by endoscopic measures. Sclerotherapy and band ligation of varices are the two main options available for control of acute variceal bleeding. Data suggest that band ligation is better than sclerotherapy in the initial control of bleeding and is associated with fewer complications. The literature also suggests that sclerotherapy, but not band ligation, may increase portal pressures. Thus, currently, band ligation is the modality of choice for initial control of variceal bleeding. Endoscopic sclerotherapy may be used if technology for band ligation is not available. Early endoscopy, preferably within 12 hours of admission, with an attempt at control of bleeding is recommended. Patients should be started on vasoactive drugs early, and endoscopy with band ligation is performed after initial resuscitation.

Pharmacotherapy. Pharmacotherapy works by reducing variceal blood flow, which in turn reduces variceal pressure. Medical therapy should be initiated at the onset of variceal bleeding. Because infections are common in patients with variceal bleeding, antibiotic prophylaxis should be initiated. This has been shown to decrease the infection rate by more than 50%, to decrease rebleeding, and to improve survival. Randomized trials have also shown that somatostatin and its longer-acting analogue octreotide are as efficacious as endoscopic treatment for control of acute variceal bleeding. Because of the minimal adverse effects and ease of administration, octreotide is now commonly used as an adjunct to endoscopic therapy. In fact, the combination of octreotide and endoscopic therapy is more effective than octreotide alone in controlling bleeding and is the preferred treatment for most patients. In severe cases of hemorrhage, vasopressin can be used to diminish splanchnic blood flow. However, because of the adverse systemic effects of vasopressin, nitroglycerin should be simultaneously infused and then titrated to achieve blood pressure control.

Variceal tamponade. Controlled trials have demonstrated that balloon tamponade is as effective as pharmacotherapy and endoscopic therapy in controlling acute variceal bleeding. The major advantages of variceal tamponade using the Sengstaken-Blakemore tube are immediate cessation of bleeding in more than 85% of patients and the widespread availability of this device (Fig. 89.19). However, there are also significant disadvantages of balloon tamponade, including frequent recurrent hemorrhage in up to 50% of patients after balloon deflation, considerable discomfort for the patient, and a high incidence of serious complications when it is used incorrectly by an inexperienced healthcare provider.

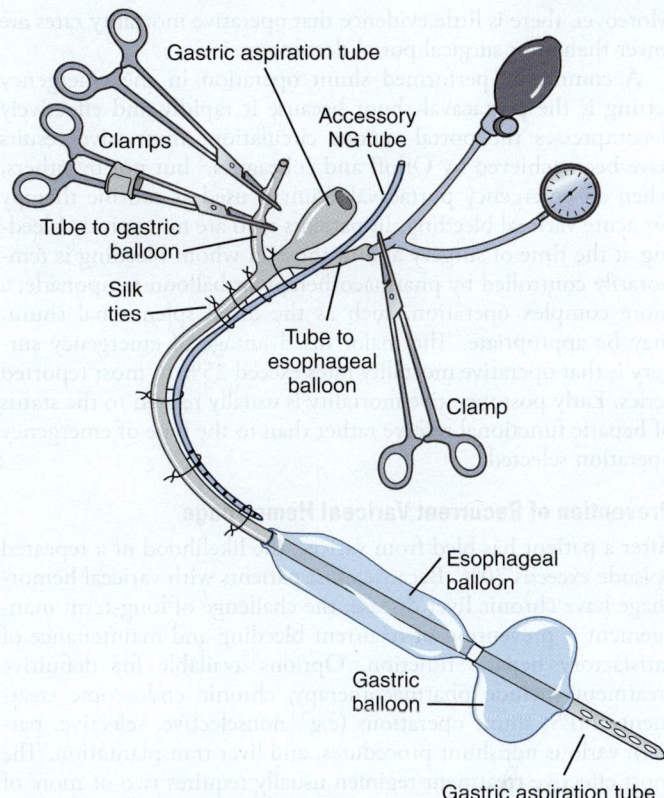

FIGURE 89.19 Modified Sengstaken-Blakemore tube. Note the accessory nasogastric *(NG)* tube for suctioning of secretions above the esophageal balloon and the two clamps, one secured with tape, to prevent inadvertent decompression of the gastric balloon. (From Rikkers LF. Portal hypertension. In: Goldsmith H, ed. *Practice of Surgery.* Philadelphia: Harper & Row; 1981:1-37.)

Interventional approaches. In most institutions, TIPS has become the preferred treatment for acute variceal bleeding when pharmacotherapy and endoscopic treatment fail. With TIPS, a functional portacaval side-to-side shunt is established. TIPS can control bleeding in almost all patients, but it is associated with risk of encephalopathy. Furthermore, in the case of shunt dysfunction, there is risk of recurrent bleeding. Use of polytetrafluoroethylene (PTFE)-covered stents has been a major step forward. PTFE stents have higher patency rates over time and reduced mortality rates.[2] Use of TIPS in patients with multiorgan failure or in patients with decompensated liver disease is associated with high 30-day mortality. In such patients, early use of TIPS, rather than after failure of other therapies, may be associated with better outcomes.

Operative approaches. Operative procedures are typically reserved for those situations in which TIPS is not indicated or is not available. Selection of the appropriate emergency operation should mainly be guided by the experience of the surgeon. Although nonoperative therapies are effective in most patients with acute variceal bleeding, an emergency operation should be promptly carried out when less invasive measures fail to control hemorrhage or are not indicated. The most common situations requiring urgent or emergency surgery are failure of acute endoscopic treatment, failure of long-term endoscopic therapy, hemorrhage from gastric varices or portal hypertensive gastropathy, and failure of TIPS placement.

Esophageal transection with a stapling device is rapid and relatively simple, but rebleeding rates after this procedure are high.

Moreover, there is little evidence that operative mortality rates are lower than after surgical portal decompression.

A commonly performed shunt operation in the emergency setting is the portacaval shunt because it rapidly and effectively decompresses the portal venous circulation. Impressive results have been achieved by Orloff and colleagues,[3] but not by others, when an emergency portacaval shunt is used as routine therapy for acute variceal bleeding. In patients who are not actively bleeding at the time of surgery and in those in whom bleeding is temporarily controlled by pharmacotherapy or balloon tamponade, a more complex operation, such as the distal splenorenal shunt, may be appropriate. The major disadvantage of emergency surgery is that operative mortality rates exceed 25% in most reported series. Early postoperative mortality is usually related to the status of hepatic functional reserve rather than to the type of emergency operation selected.

Prevention of Recurrent Variceal Hemorrhage

After a patient has bled from varices, the likelihood of a repeated episode exceeds 70%. Because most patients with variceal hemorrhage have chronic liver disease, the challenge of long-term management is prevention of recurrent bleeding and maintenance of satisfactory hepatic function. Options available for definitive treatment include pharmacotherapy, chronic endoscopic treatment, TIPS, shunt operations (e.g., nonselective, selective, partial), various nonshunt procedures, and liver transplantation. The most effective treatment regimen usually requires two or more of these therapies in sequence. In most centers, initial treatment consists of pharmacotherapy or endoscopic therapy, with portal decompression by means of TIPS or an operative shunt reserved for failures of first-line treatment. Hepatic transplantation is used for patients with end-stage liver disease.

Pharmacotherapy. A meta-analysis of controlled trials of nonselective β-adrenergic blockade has shown that this treatment significantly decreases the likelihood of recurrent hemorrhage and demonstrates a trend toward decreased mortality. The combination of a β-blocker and long-acting nitrate (e.g., isosorbide 5-mononitrate) has been shown to be more effective than variceal ligation.[4] Combination therapy is also more effective than β-blockade alone. Long-term pharmacotherapy should be used only in compliant patients who are observed closely by their physician.

Endoscopic therapy. Several controlled trials and a meta-analysis comparing endoscopic sclerotherapy with variceal ligation have shown a significant advantage to variceal ligation. Complications are less frequent after variceal ligation, and fewer treatment sessions are required to eradicate varices (Fig. 89.20). Rebleeding and mortality rates also appear to be lower after variceal ligation. The combination of variceal ligation and pharmacotherapy with nonselective β-blockade is more effective than variceal ligation alone. This result has been confirmed in a meta-analysis that included the data from 17 randomized controlled trials.[5] In this trial, a combination of β-blocker and endoscopic treatment significantly reduced rebleeding rates at 6, 12, and 24 months. Furthermore, mortality at 24 months was significantly lower for the combined treatment group. Thus, at this time, combination therapy should be recommended as the first line of treatment for secondary prophylaxis of variceal bleeding.

Several controlled trials comparing chronic endoscopic therapy with conventional medical management have been completed. Although fewer patients receiving endoscopic treatment than medical treatment experienced rebleeding in all the investigations, recurrent bleeding still occurred in approximately 50% of endoscopic therapy

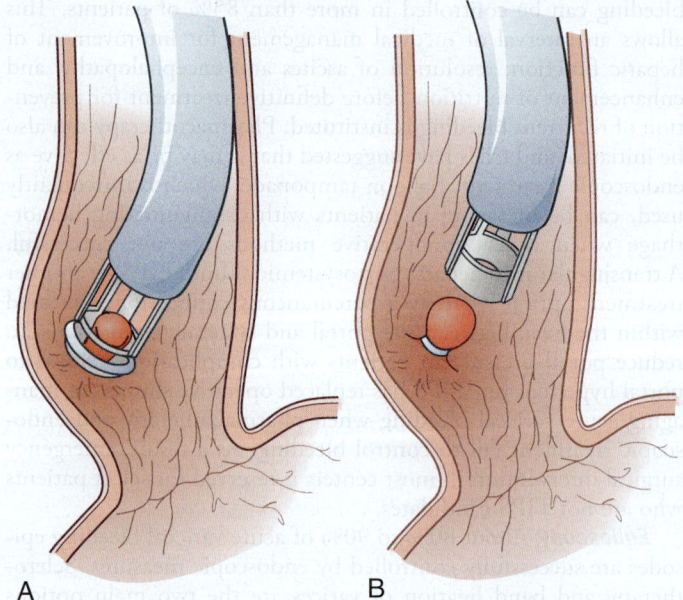

FIGURE 89.20 Endoscopic ligation of esophageal varices. (A) The varix is drawn into the ligator by suction. (B) An O ring is applied. (From Turcotte JG, Roger SE, Eckhauser FE. Portal hypertension. In: Greenfield LJ, Mulholland MW, Oldham KT, eds. *Surgery: Scientific Principles and Practice.* Philadelphia: JB Lippincott; 1993:899.)

patients. Rebleeding is most frequent during the initial year, but the rate decreases by about 15% annually thereafter. Although a single episode of recurrent hemorrhage does not signify failure of therapy, uncontrolled hemorrhage, multiple major episodes of rebleeding, and hemorrhage from gastric varices and hypertensive gastropathy all require that endoscopic therapy be abandoned and another treatment modality substituted. Endoscopic treatment failure secondary to rebleeding occurs in as many as one-third of patients. Thus, chronic endoscopic therapy is a rational initial treatment for many patients who bleed from esophageal varices, but subsequent treatment with TIPS, a shunt procedure, a nonshunt operation, or liver transplantation should be anticipated for a significant percentage of patients. Because of its relatively high failure rate, a course of chronic endoscopic therapy should not be undertaken for noncompliant patients and those living a long distance from advanced medical care.

Interventional therapy. TIPS is being increasingly used for definitive treatment of patients who bleed from portal hypertension (Fig. 89.21). A major limitation of TIPS, however, is a high incidence (up to 50%) of shunt stenosis or shunt thrombosis within the first year. Shunt stenosis, which is usually secondary to neointimal hyperplasia, is more common than thrombosis and can often be resolved by balloon dilation of the TIPS or, in some cases, by placement of a second shunt. Total shunt occlusion occurs in 10% to 15% of patients. Shunt stenosis and shunt thrombosis are often followed by recurrent portal hypertensive bleeding. TIPS stenosis and occlusion have become less frequent with use of PTFE-covered stents.

TIPS has been compared with chronic endoscopic therapy in 11 randomized controlled trials. Fewer patients rebled after TIPS (19%) than after endoscopic treatment (47%), but encephalopathy was significantly more common in patients undergoing TIPS (34%). TIPS dysfunction developed in 50% of patients. The major advantage of TIPS is that it is a nonoperative approach.

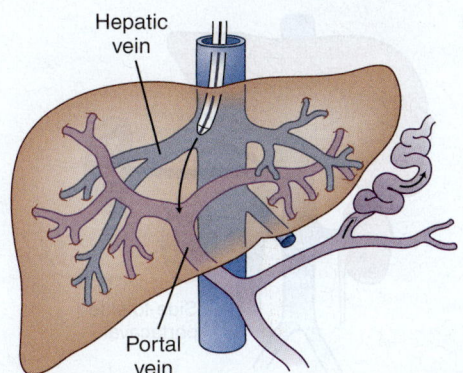
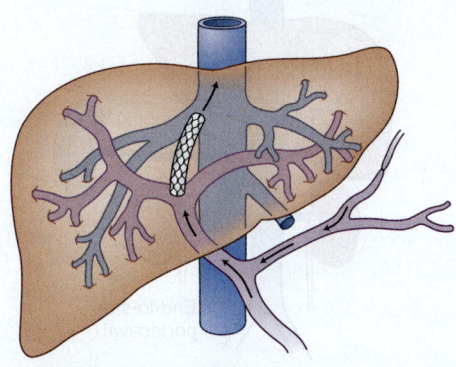

Hepatic vein

Portal vein

FIGURE 89.21 Transjugular intrahepatic portosystemic shunt placement. The inferior vena cava is accessed through the right internal jugular vein. If the right internal jugular vein is unsuitable, the left internal jugular vein may also be used. Through this access, a 5-Fr catheter is placed into the right hepatic vein and wedged into a peripheral branch. Wedged hepatic venography is then performed with CO_2 gas to opacify the portal venous system. Using the wedged hepatic venogram image as a guide, a needle is advanced through the wall of the right hepatic vein and directed in an anteroinferior direction to access the right portal vein. Once the portal vein is cannulated, CO_2 is injected into the parenchymal tract to exclude transgression of the bile duct or hepatic artery. Once proper placement is confirmed, TIPS endoprosthesis is deployed, which creates a shunt between the portal vein and the hepatic vein, thus decreasing resistance and decompressing varices. *TIPS,* Transjugular intrahepatic portosystemic shunt.

Thus, it would appear to be the ideal therapy when only short-term portal decompression is required. Liver transplantation candidates who fail to respond to endoscopic therapy or pharmacotherapy are therefore well suited for TIPS followed by transplantation when a donor organ becomes available. As a result, the patient is protected from bleeding in the interim, and the transplantation procedure may be facilitated by the lower portal pressure. Another group of patients in whom TIPS may be advantageous includes those with advanced hepatic functional decompensation who are unlikely to survive long enough for the TIPS to malfunction. Because it functions as a side-to-side portosystemic shunt, TIPS is also effective for the treatment of medically intractable ascites.

Surgical therapy. Portosystemic shunts are the most effective at preventing recurrent hemorrhage in patients with portal hypertension. These procedures are effective because they all decompress the portal venous system to varying degrees by shunting portal flow into the lower-pressure systemic venous system. However, diversion of portal blood, which contains hepatotropic hormones, nutrients, and cerebral toxins, is also responsible for the adverse consequences of shunt operations, namely, portosystemic encephalopathy and accelerated hepatic failure. Depending on whether they completely decompress, compartmentalize, or partially decompress the portal venous circulation, portosystemic shunts can be classified as nonselective, selective, or partial. In addition to variceal decompression, selective and partial portosystemic shunts aim to preserve hepatic portal perfusion and therefore to prevent or to minimize the adverse consequences of these procedures.

Nonselective shunts. Commonly used nonselective shunts, all of which completely divert portal flow, include the end-to-side portacaval shunt (Eck fistula), side-to-side portacaval shunt, large-diameter interposition shunts, and conventional splenorenal shunt (Fig. 89.22). The end-to-side portacaval shunt is the prototype of nonselective shunts and is the only shunt procedure that has been compared with conventional medical treatment in randomized controlled trials.

All the other nonselective shunts in Fig. 89.22 maintain continuity of the portal vein, thereby connecting the portal and systemic venous systems in a side-to-side fashion. Therefore, these procedures decompress the splanchnic venous circulation and intrahepatic sinusoidal network. Because the liver and intestines are both important contributors to ascites formation, side-to-side portosystemic shunts are the most effective for relieving ascites and preventing recurrent variceal bleeding. Because they completely divert portal flow, like the end-to-side portacaval shunt, however, side-to-side shunts also accelerate hepatic failure and lead to frequent postshunt encephalopathy.

The conventional splenorenal shunt consists of anastomosis of the proximal splenic vein to the renal vein. Splenectomy is also performed. Because the smaller proximal rather than the larger distal end of the splenic vein is used, shunt thrombosis is more common after this procedure than after the distal splenorenal shunt. Although early series noted that postshunt encephalopathy was less common after the conventional splenorenal shunt than after the portacaval shunt, subsequent analyses have suggested that this low frequency of encephalopathy was probably a result of restoration of hepatic portal perfusion after shunt thrombosis developed in many patients. A conventional splenorenal shunt that is of sufficient caliber to remain patent gradually dilates and eventually causes complete portal decompression and portal flow diversion. A purported advantage of the procedure is that hypersplenism is eliminated by splenectomy. The thrombocytopenia and leukopenia that accompany portal hypertension, however, are rarely of clinical significance, making splenectomy an unnecessary procedure in most patients.

In summary, nonselective shunts effectively decompress varices. Because of complete portal flow diversion, however, they are complicated by frequent postoperative encephalopathy and accelerated hepatic failure. Side-to-side nonselective shunts effectively relieve ascites and prevent variceal hemorrhage. Presently, nonselective shunts are only rarely indicated. TIPS, also a nonselective shunt, is the preferred therapy for most situations in which nonselective shunts were previously used (e.g., patients with both variceal bleeding and medically

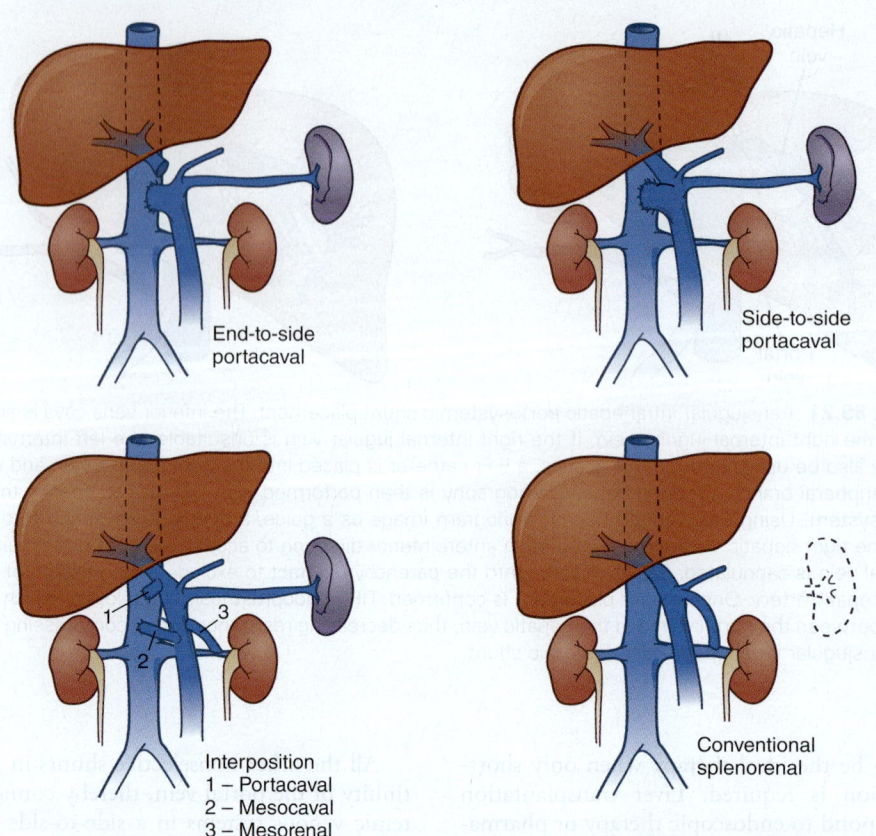

End-to-side
portacaval

Side-to-side
portacaval

Interposition
1 – Portacaval
2 – Mesocaval
3 – Mesorenal

Conventional
splenorenal

FIGURE 89.22 Nonselective shunts completely divert portal blood flow away from the liver. (From Rikkers LF. Portal hypertension. In: Moody FG, Carey LC, Scott Jones RS, et al., eds. *Surgical Treatment of Digestive Disease.* Chicago: Year Book Medical; 1986:409-424.)

intractable ascites). In general, a nonselective shunt is constructed only when a TIPS cannot be performed or when a TIPS fails.

Selective shunts. The hemodynamic and clinical shortcomings of nonselective shunts stimulated development of the concept of selective variceal decompression. In 1967, Warren and colleagues introduced the distal splenorenal shunt. In the following year, Inokuchi and associates reported their initial results with the left gastric–vena cava shunt, which consists of interposition of a vein graft between the left gastric (coronary) vein and IVC. Therefore, it directly and selectively decompresses esophagogastric varices. However, only a minority of patients with portal hypertension have appropriate anatomy for this operation; experience with it has been limited to Japan, and no controlled trials have been conducted.

The distal splenorenal shunt consists of anastomosis of the distal end of the splenic vein to the left renal vein and interruption of all collateral vessels (e.g., coronary vein and gastroepiploic veins) that connect the superior mesenteric vein and gastrosplenic components of the splanchnic venous circulation (see Fig. 89.23). This results in separation of the portal venous circulation into a decompressed gastrosplenic venous circuit and high-pressure superior mesenteric venous system that continues to perfuse the liver. Although the procedure is technically demanding, it can be mastered by most well-trained surgeons who are knowledgeable in the principles of vascular surgery.

Not all patients are candidates for the distal splenorenal shunt. Because sinusoidal and mesenteric hypertension is maintained and important lymphatic pathways are transected during dissection of the left renal vein, the distal splenorenal shunt tends to aggravate rather than to relieve ascites. Thus, patients with medically intractable ascites should not undergo this procedure. However, the

larger population of patients who develop transient ascites after resuscitation from a variceal hemorrhage are candidates for a selective shunt. Another contraindication to a distal splenorenal shunt is prior splenectomy. A splenic vein diameter less than 7 mm is a relative contraindication to the procedure because the incidence of shunt thrombosis is high when a small-diameter vein is used. Although selective variceal decompression is a sound physiologic

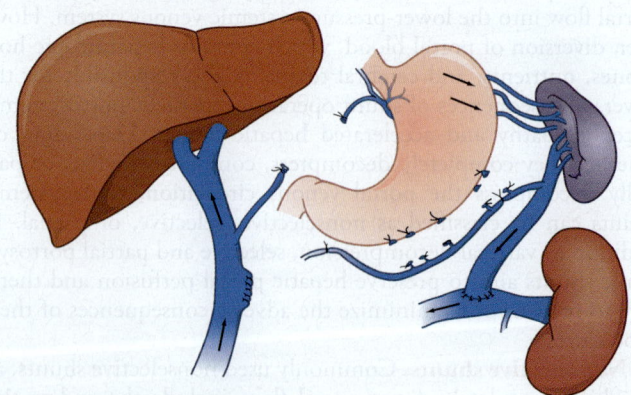

FIGURE 89.23 The distal splenorenal shunt provides selective variceal decompression through the short gastric veins, spleen, and splenic vein to the left renal vein. Hepatic portal perfusion is maintained by interrupting the umbilical vein, coronary vein, gastroepiploic vein, and any other prominent collaterals. (From Salam AA. Distal splenorenal shunts: hemodynamics of total versus selective shunting. In: Baker RJ, Fischer JE, eds. *Mastery of Surgery.* 4th ed. Philadelphia: Lippincott Williams & Wilkins; 2001:1357-1366.)

concept, the distal splenorenal shunt remains controversial after an extensive clinical experience spanning almost 40 years.

Although the distal splenorenal shunt results in portal flow preservation in more than 85% of patients during the early postoperative interval, the high-pressure mesenteric venous system gradually collateralizes to the low-pressure shunt, resulting in loss of portal flow in approximately 50% of patients by 1 year. The degree and duration of portal flow preservation depend on the cause of portal hypertension and the technical details of the operation (the extent to which mesenteric and gastrosplenic venous circulations are separated). Although portal flow is maintained in most patients with nonalcoholic cirrhosis and noncirrhotic portal hypertension (e.g., PVT), portal flow rapidly collateralizes to the shunt in patients with alcoholic cirrhosis.

Modification of the distal splenorenal shunt by purposeful or inadvertent omission of coronary vein ligation results in early loss of portal flow. Even when all major collateral vessels are interrupted, portal flow may be gradually diverted through a pancreatic collateral network (pancreatic siphon). This pathway can be discouraged by dissecting the full length of the splenic vein from the pancreas, splenopancreatic disconnection, which results in better preservation of hepatic portal perfusion, especially in patients with alcoholic cirrhosis. However, this extension of the procedure makes it technically more challenging and a significant disadvantage in an era when fewer shunts are being placed because of increased use of endoscopic therapy, TIPS, and liver transplantation.

Six of the seven controlled comparisons of the distal splenorenal shunt and nonselective shunts have included predominantly patients with alcoholic cirrhosis. None of these trials has demonstrated an advantage to either procedure with respect to long-term survival. Three of the studies found a lower frequency of encephalopathy after the distal splenorenal shunt, whereas the other trials showed no difference in the incidence of this postoperative complication. In contrast to survival, encephalopathy is a subjective end point that was assessed with various methods in the trials. Another important end point in comparing treatments for variceal hemorrhage was the effectiveness with which recurrent bleeding was prevented. In almost all uncontrolled and controlled series of the distal splenorenal shunt, this procedure was equivalent to nonselective shunts in preventing recurrent hemorrhage. Mainly because of these inconsistent results of the controlled trials, there is no consensus as to which shunting procedure is superior in patients with alcoholic cirrhosis. Because the quality of life (e.g., lower encephalopathy rate) was significantly better in the distal splenorenal shunt group in three of the trials, there appears to be an advantage to selective variceal decompression, even in this population.

Considerably fewer data are available regarding selective shunting in nonalcoholic cirrhosis and noncirrhotic portal hypertension. Because hepatic portal perfusion after the distal splenorenal shunt is better preserved in these disease categories, one might expect improved results. A single controlled trial in patients with schistosomiasis (presinusoidal portal hypertension) has demonstrated a lower frequency of encephalopathy after the distal splenorenal shunt than after a conventional splenorenal shunt (nonselective). Another large series from Emory University has shown that distal splenorenal shunt is associated with better survival in patients with nonalcoholic cirrhosis than in those with alcoholic cirrhosis. However, this has not been a consistent finding in all centers in which the distal splenorenal shunts have been performed.

Several controlled trials have also compared the distal splenorenal shunt with chronic endoscopic therapy. In these investigations, recurrent hemorrhage was more effectively prevented by selective shunting than by sclerotherapy. However, hepatic portal perfusion was maintained in a significantly higher fraction of patients undergoing sclerotherapy. Despite this hemodynamic advantage, encephalopathy rates were similar after both therapies.

The two North American trials were dissimilar with respect to the effect of these treatments on long-term survival. Sclerotherapy with surgical rescue for one-third of sclerotherapy failures resulted in significantly better survival than selective shunt alone, whereas 85% of sclerotherapy failures could be salvaged by surgery. In contrast, a similar investigation conducted in a sparsely populated area (Intermountain West and Great Plains) showed superior survival after the distal splenorenal shunt. Only 31% of sclerotherapy failures could be salvaged by surgery in this trial. The survival results of these two studies suggest that endoscopic therapy is a rational initial treatment for patients who bleed from varices if sclerotherapy failure is recognized, and these patients promptly undergo surgery or TIPS. However, patients living in remote areas are less likely to be salvaged by shunt surgery when endoscopic treatment fails; therefore, a selective shunt may be preferable initial treatment for such patients.

In one nonrandomized comparison to TIPS, the distal splenorenal shunt had lower rates of recurrent bleeding, encephalopathy, and shunt thrombosis. Ascites was less prevalent after TIPS. A multicenter randomized trial comparing TIPS and the distal splenorenal shunt for the elective treatment of variceal bleeding in good-risk patients with cirrhosis has shown generally equivalent results for these two procedures. Rebleeding rates were not significantly different between the distal splenorenal shunt (6%) and TIPS (11%), but this represents the lowest reported rate of rebleeding after TIPS. This was likely secondary to meticulous surveillance of TIPS patency by duplex ultrasound and angiography. Frequent reintervention in TIPS patients (82% compared with 11% for distal splenorenal shunt patients) was necessary to achieve these results. In this trial, postshunt encephalopathy and survival were similar after the two procedures.

Hepatic transplantation. Liver transplantation is not a treatment for variceal bleeding, but rather needs to be considered for all patients who present with end-stage hepatic failure, whether or not it is accompanied by bleeding. Transplantation in patients who have bled secondary to portal hypertension is the only therapy that addresses the underlying liver disease in addition to providing reliable portal decompression. Because of economic factors and a limited supply of donor organs, liver transplantation is not available to all patients. Also, transplantation is not indicated for some of the more common causes of variceal bleeding, such as schistosomiasis (normal liver function) and active alcoholism (noncompliance).

There is accumulating evidence that variceal bleeders with well-compensated hepatic functional reserve (Child-Pugh class A and B+) are initially better served by nontransplantation strategies. The first-line treatment for such patients should be pharmacologic and endoscopic therapy. For those who fail to respond to first-line therapy, an operative shunt or TIPS can be performed. These can also be applied when pharmacologic or endoscopic treatment would be risky, such as patients with gastric varices and those geographically separated from tertiary medical care.

Patients with variceal bleeding who are transplantation candidates include nonalcoholic cirrhotic patients and abstinent alcoholic cirrhotic patients with limited hepatic functional reserve (Child-Pugh class B and C) or a poor quality of life secondary to the disease (e.g., encephalopathy, fatigue, bone pain). In these patients, the acute hemorrhage should be treated with endoscopic therapy and pharmacotherapy and the patient's transplantation candidacy immediately activated. If endoscopic treatment and pharmacotherapy are ineffective, a TIPS should be inserted as a short-term bridge to transplantation.

If a nontransplantation procedure (e.g., operative shunt or TIPS) is performed initially, these patients should be carefully assessed at regular intervals of 6 to 12 months. Hepatic transplantation should be considered when other complications of cirrhosis develop or when hepatic functional decompensation is evident clinically or by careful assessment with quantitative LFTs.

Algorithm for Management of Variceal Hemorrhage

Definitive management of variceal hemorrhage is based on several factors, including cause of portal hypertension, abstinence for patients with alcoholic cirrhosis, presence or absence of other diseases, and physiologic rather than chronologic age. Transplantation candidates with decompensated hepatic function or a poor quality of life secondary to their liver disease should undergo transplantation as soon as possible.

Most future transplantation and nontransplantation candidates should undergo initial endoscopic treatment or pharmacotherapy unless they bleed from gastric varices or portal hypertensive gastropathy or live in a remote geographic location and have limited access to emergency tertiary care. Patients who live in remote locations and those who fail to respond to endoscopic and drug therapy should receive a selective shunt or TIPS. A controlled trial has shown that if careful surveillance of TIPS patency and frequent TIPS reinterventions are done, these procedures are equally efficacious.

Until improvements in TIPS technology are fully realized, the distal splenorenal shunt is likely to remain a more durable long-term solution and a reasonable alternative for TIPS failure. However, a TIPS is more commonly done, and few surgeons who are experienced in shunt surgery remain. Therefore, it is likely that operative shunts will play an even smaller role in the management of variceal bleeding in the future than they do now. Patients with medically intractable ascites in addition to variceal bleeding are best treated with TIPS when less invasive measures fail to control bleeding. If the TIPS eventually fails, an open side-to-side shunt can then be constructed if the patient has reasonable hepatic function and is not a transplantation candidate. On the other hand, TIPS is clearly indicated for patients with endoscopic treatment failure who may require transplantation soon and for nontransplantation candidates with advanced hepatic functional deterioration. Future transplantation candidates should be carefully monitored so that they undergo transplantation at the appropriate time before they become poor operative risks.

The treatment algorithm for variceal bleeding has changed considerably since the 1970s, during which time endoscopic therapy, liver transplantation, and TIPS have become available to these patients. Nontransplantation operations are now less

frequently necessary, the survival results are better because patients at high operative risk are managed by other means, and emergency surgery has almost been eliminated.

INFECTIOUS DISEASES

Pyogenic Abscess

Epidemiology

Ochsner and DeBakey, in their classic paper on pyogenic liver abscess in 1938, described 47 cases and reviewed world literature. This was the largest experience at that time and the first serious attempt to study this disease. In that era, pyogenic liver abscess was largely a disease of people in their 20s and 30s, mostly the result of acute appendicitis. With the marked changes in medical care since then, notably effective antibiotics and prompt effective treatments for acute inflammatory disorders, and an aging population, the spectrum of this disease has changed. Pyogenic liver abscess is now mostly seen in patients in their 50s to 60s and is more often related to biliary tract disease or is cryptogenic in nature (Table 89.3). There are no significant sex, ethnic, or geographic differences in disease frequency; the male-to-female ratio is approximately 1.5:1. Comorbid conditions associated with pyogenic abscess are cirrhosis, diabetes, chronic renal failure, and a history of malignant disease.

Pathogenesis

The liver is probably exposed to portal venous bacterial loads on a regular basis and usually clears this bacterial load without problems. The development of a hepatic abscess occurs when an inoculum of bacteria, regardless of the route of exposure, exceeds the liver's ability to clear it. This results in tissue invasion, neutrophil infiltration, and formation of an organized abscess. The potential routes of hepatic exposure to bacteria are the biliary tree, portal vein, hepatic artery, direct extension of a nearby nidus of infection, and trauma. The relative contribution of these routes to the formation of hepatic abscess is summarized in Table 89.3.

Along with cryptogenic infections, infections from the biliary tree are the most common identifiable cause of hepatic abscess. Biliary obstruction results in bile stasis with the potential for subsequent bacterial colonization, infection, and ascension into the liver. This process is known as *ascending suppurative cholangitis*. The nature of biliary obstruction is mostly related to stone disease or malignant disease. In Asia, intrahepatic stones and cholangitis (recurrent pyogenic cholangitis [RPC]; see later) are common causes, whereas in the West, malignant obstruction has become a more predominant cause. Other factors associated with increased risk include Caroli disease, biliary ascariasis, and biliary tract surgery. The common link between all causes of hepatic abscesses from the biliary tree is obstruction and bacteria in the biliary

TABLE 89.3   Pyogenic Abscesses Attributable to Specific Cause

| YEAR OF REPORT | NO. OF PATIENTS | CAUSE (%) | | | | | |
		PORTAL VEIN	HEPATIC ARTERY	BILIARY TREE	DIRECT EXTENSION	TRAUMA	CRYPTOGENIC
1927–38 (one study[a])	622	42	—	—	17	4	20
1945–82 (eight studies)	521	17	9	38	10	4	16
1970–99 (eight studies)	1264	5	3	38	1	2	43

[a]From Ochsner A, DeBakey M, Murray S. Pyogenic abscess of the liver. *Am J Surg.* 1938;40:292-319. This is the classic study of Ochsner and DeBakey that reviewed 286 previously reported cases and 47 new cases.

tract. Prior biliary-enteric anastomosis has also been associated with hepatic abscess formation, likely because of unimpeded exposure of the biliary tree to enteric organisms.

The portal venous system drains the gastrointestinal tract; therefore, any infectious disorder of the gastrointestinal tract can result in an ascending portal vein infection (pylephlebitis), with exposure of the liver to large amounts of bacteria. Historically, untreated appendicitis was considered the most common cause of hepatic abscess, but with the advent of antibiotics and the development of prompt and effective treatment of acute intraabdominal infections, portal venous infections of the liver have become less frequent. The most common causes of pylephlebitis are diverticulitis, appendicitis, pancreatitis, inflammatory bowel disease, pelvic inflammatory disease, perforated viscus, and omphalitis in the newborn. Hepatic abscess has also been associated with colorectal malignant disease. In a case-control study from Taiwan, the incidence of gastrointestinal cancers was increased fourfold among patients with pyogenic liver abscess compared with controls.[6]

Any systemic infection (e.g., endocarditis, pneumonia, osteomyelitis) can result in bacteremia and infection of the liver through the hepatic artery. Microabscess formation is a relatively common finding at autopsy in patients dying of sepsis, but these patients are generally not included in analyses of pyogenic liver abscess. Hepatic abscess from systemic infections may also reflect an altered immune response, such as in patients with malignant disease, AIDS, or disorders of granulocyte function. Children with chronic granulomatous disease are particularly susceptible.

Hepatic abscess can be the result of direct extension of an infectious process. Common examples include suppurative cholecystitis, subphrenic abscess, perinephric abscess, and even perforation of the bowel directly into the liver.

Penetrating and blunt trauma can also result in an intrahepatic hematoma or an area of necrotic liver, which can subsequently develop into an abscess. Bacteria may have been introduced from the trauma, or the affected area may have been seeded from systemic bacteremia. Hepatic abscesses associated with trauma can be manifested in a delayed fashion up to several weeks after injury. Other mechanisms of iatrogenic hepatic necrosis, such as hepatic artery embolization or, more recently, thermal ablative procedures, can be complicated by abscess. This is an uncommon complication of these procedures but is seen more often when there has been a previous biliary-enteric anastomosis.

Usually, no cause for a hepatic abscess is found. Cryptogenic abscesses predominate in many series and are more common in some case reports. Possible explanations for cryptogenic hepatic abscess are undiagnosed abdominal disease, resolved infectious process at the time of presentation, and host factors such as diabetes or malignant disease rendering the liver more susceptible to transient hepatic artery or portal vein bacteremia. In patients with cryptogenic hepatic abscess who have undergone computed tomography (CT) and ultrasonography, it has been argued whether a diligent search for a cause should ensue. In a series evaluating colonoscopy and endoscopic retrograde cholangiopancreatography (ERCP) in patients with cryptogenic abscess, the yield has been low and often is only fruitful in patients with some objective finding that might have suggested a subclinical abnormality (e.g., mildly elevated bilirubin level). In general, these patients should undergo a thorough history, physical examination, and laboratory workup in search of abnormalities in the intestinal tract or biliary tree. Further invasive procedures or imaging studies should be based on clinical suspicions raised by this workup.

Pathology and Microbiology

Most hepatic abscesses involve the right hemiliver, accounting for about 75% of cases. The explanation for this is not known, but preferential laminar blood flow to the right side has been postulated. The left liver is involved in approximately 20% of the cases; the caudate lobe is rarely involved (5%). Bilobar involvement with multiple abscesses is uncommon. Approximately 50% of hepatic abscesses are solitary. Hepatic abscesses can vary in size from less than 1 mm to 3 or 4 cm in diameter and can be multiloculated or a single cavity. At abdominal exploration, hepatic abscesses appear tan and are fluctuant to palpation, although deeper abscesses may not be visible and can be difficult to palpate. Surrounding inflammation can cause adhesions to local structures.

Studies of the microbiology of hepatic abscesses have had variable results, for several reasons. In early series, sterile abscesses were commonly reported but probably reflected inadequate culture techniques, whereas in modern series, few abscesses are sampled before the administration of antibiotics. Also, the heterogeneity of the routes of infection makes the microbiology variable. Abscesses from pylephlebitis or cholangitis tend to be polymicrobial, with a high preponderance of gram-negative bacilli. Systemic infections, on the other hand, usually cause infection with a single organism.

Although the rate of sterility reported by Ochsner's review in 1938 was approximately 50%, series in the 1990s reported sterile abscess rates in approximately 10% to 20% of cases. Many hepatic abscesses are polymicrobial in nature and account for approximately 40% of cases. Some have suggested that solitary abscesses are more likely to be polymicrobial. Anaerobic organisms are involved approximately 40% to 60% of the time. The most common organisms cultured are *Escherichia coli* and *Klebsiella pneumoniae*. Other commonly encountered organisms are *Staphylococcus aureus, Enterococcus* spp., viridans streptococci, and *Bacteroides* spp. *Klebsiella* is frequently associated with gas-forming abscesses. Enterococci and viridans streptococci are generally found in polymicrobial abscesses, whereas staphylococcal infections are typically caused by a single organism. Uncommonly encountered organisms (<10% of cultures) include species of *Pseudomonas, Proteus, Enterobacter, Citrobacter, Serratia,* β-hemolytic streptococci, microaerophilic streptococci, *Fusobacterium, Clostridium,* and other rare anaerobes. Blood cultures are positive in approximately 50% to 60% of cases. Of note, highly resistant organisms in patients with indwelling biliary catheters, multiple episodes of cholangitis, and repeated use of antibiotics are being encountered as the use of these catheters becomes more common. Fungal and mycobacterial hepatic abscesses are rare and are almost always associated with immunosuppression, usually from chemotherapy.

Clinical Features

The classic description of the presenting symptoms of hepatic abscess is fever, jaundice, and right upper quadrant pain, with tenderness to palpation. Unfortunately, this presentation is seen in only 10% of cases. Fever, chills, and abdominal pain are the most common presenting symptoms, but a broad array of nonspecific symptoms can be present (Table 89.4). A study from Taiwan of 133 patients found fever in 96% of patients, chills in 80%, abdominal pain in 53%, and jaundice in 20%. Many of the symptoms, such as malaise and vomiting, were constitutional in nature. Involvement of the diaphragm may result in symptoms of cough or dyspnea. Rarely, patients can present with peritonitis secondary to rupture. Cases of rupture into the pleural space or

TABLE 89.4 Pyogenic Abscesses With Noted Symptoms

YEAR OF REPORT	NO. OF PATIENTS	SYMPTOM (%)								
		FEVER, CHILLS	NIGHT SWEATS	MALAISE	ANOREXIA, WEIGHT LOSS	NAUSEA, VOMITING	DIARRHEA	ABDOMINAL PAIN	CHEST PAIN	COUGH
1927–38 (one study[a])	333	94	—	—	—	33	—	92	—	—
1945–82 (eight studies)	494	88	8	58	62	40	17	66	14	13
1970–95 (ten studies)	1314	72	9	25	33	30	14	59	16	6

[a]From Ochsner A, DeBakey M, Murray S. Pyogenic abscess of the liver. *Am J Surg.* 1938;40:292-319. This is the classic study of Ochsner and De-Bakey that reviewed 286 previously reported cases and 47 new cases.

pericardium have been reported but are distinctly uncommon. The duration of symptoms is variable, ranging from an acute presentation to a chronic illness lasting months. It has been suggested that acute presentation is associated with identifiable abdominal disease, whereas chronic presentation is often associated with a cryptogenic abscess. A rare complication specific to *Klebsiella* hepatic abscesses is endogenous endophthalmitis, occurring in approximately 3% of cases. This serious complication is more common in patients with diabetes. The best chance to preserve visual function is with early diagnosis and treatment.

On physical examination, fever and right upper quadrant tenderness are the most common findings. Tenderness is present in 40% to 70% of patients. Jaundice is also found in approximately 25% of cases and is often secondary to underlying biliary disease. Chest findings are often found in approximately 25% of patients, and hepatomegaly is also commonly noted in approximately 50%. Ascites, splenomegaly, and severe sepsis are uncommon signs of hepatic abscesses.

Nonspecific abnormalities of blood tests are common in pyogenic abscesses. Leukocytosis is present in 70% to 90% of patients, and anemia is commonly encountered. Abnormalities of LFT results are generally present. The ALP level is mildly elevated in 80% of patients, whereas total bilirubin concentration is elevated 20% to 50% of the time. Transaminases are mildly elevated in approximately 60% of patients. Severe abnormalities of liver function are almost always associated with underlying biliary disease. Hypoalbuminemia or mild elevations of the PT and INR can be present and reflect a degree of chronicity. None of these blood tests specifically help diagnose a hepatic abscess. However, together, they may suggest a liver abnormality that often leads to imaging studies.

The most essential element to establishing the diagnosis of hepatic abscess is radiographic imaging. Chest radiographs are abnormal approximately 50% of the time, and findings generally reflect subdiaphragmatic disease, such as an elevated right hemidiaphragm, right pleural effusion, or atelectasis. On occasion, these can be left-sided findings in the case of an abscess involving the left liver. Plain abdominal radiographs, in rare cases, can be helpful. They can show air-fluid levels or portal venous gas (Fig. 89.24).

Ultrasound and CT are the mainstays of diagnostic modalities for hepatic abscess. Ultrasound usually demonstrates a round or oval area less echogenic than the surrounding liver. Ultrasound can reliably distinguish solid from cystic lesions. The limitations of ultrasound are in its ability to visualize lesions high up in the dome of the liver and that it is a user-dependent modality. The sensitivity of

ultrasound in diagnosing hepatic abscess is 80% to 95%. CT demonstrates similar findings to ultrasound, and lesions are of lower attenuation than surrounding hepatic parenchyma. High-quality CT scans can demonstrate very small abscesses and can more easily identify multiple small abscesses. The abscess wall usually has an intense enhancement on contrast-enhanced CT. The sensitivity of CT in diagnosing hepatic abscess is 95% to 100%. Both CT and ultrasound are useful in diagnosing other intraabdominal pathologic processes, such as biliary disease (ultrasound) and inflammatory disorders such as appendicitis and diverticulitis (CT). Magnetic resonance imaging (MRI) can help distinguish the cause of many hepatic masses and in evaluating the biliary tree for pathologic changes, but it does not appear to have any distinct advantage over CT in diagnosing hepatic abscess.

Differential Diagnosis

Differentiating pyogenic abscess from other cystic infective diseases of the liver, such as amebic abscess or echinococcal cyst, is important because of differences in treatment. Pyogenic abscess (see later) is largely treated by antibiotics and drainage. Amebic abscess is mainly treated by antibiotics, whereas echinococcal cysts

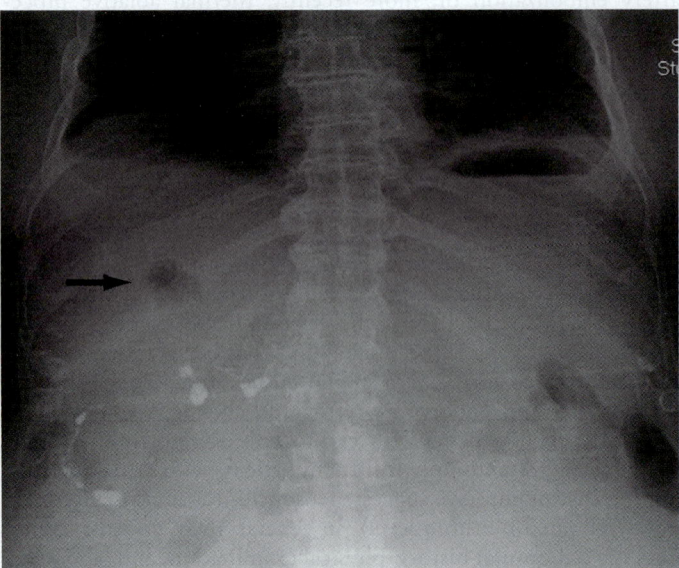

FIGURE 89.24 Plain abdominal radiograph demonstrating an abnormal collection of air in the right upper quadrant consistent with a pyogenic hepatic abscess *(arrow)*.

TABLE 89.5   Features of Amebic Versus Pyogenic Liver Abscess

CLINICAL FEATURES	AMEBIC ABSCESS	PYOGENIC ABSCESS
Age	20–40 years	>50 years
Male-to-female ratio	≥10:1	1.5:1
Solitary versus multiple	Solitary 80%[a]	Solitary 50%
Location	Usually right liver	Usually right liver
Travel in endemic area	Yes	No
Diabetes	Uncommon (~2%)	More common (~27%)
Alcohol use	Common	Common
Jaundice	Uncommon	Common
Elevated bilirubin	Uncommon	Common
Elevated alkaline phosphatase	Common	Common
Positive blood culture	No	Common
Positive amebic serology	Yes	No

[a]In acute amebic abscess, 50% are solitary.

often require surgical management. Fortunately, echinococcal cysts can usually be diagnosed by history and characteristic radiologic findings (see later). The presentations of amebic and pyogenic abscess, however, are more similar, with some notable exceptions that are critical in distinguishing the two (Table 89.5). Amebic abscesses generally occur in young Hispanic males, whereas pyogenic abscess tends to occur in patients 50 to 60 years of age, with no predominant sex or race. Fever is common in both, but chills and symptoms of severe acute bacteremia are more common in pyogenic abscess. On serologic testing, *Entamoeba histolytica* antibodies are almost always present in amebic abscesses but are uncommon in patients with pyogenic abscess. A study comparing 471 patients with amebic abscess with 106 patients with pyogenic abscess found age older than 50 years, pulmonary findings on physical examination, multiple abscesses, and low amebic serology titers to be independently predictive of pyogenic abscess. On occasion, differentiating the two is not possible, and diagnostic aspiration or a trial of antiamebic antibiotics may be necessary. Unfortunately, aspiration is diagnostic in amebic abscess only approximately 10% to 20% of the time.[7]

Treatment

Before the availability of antibiotics and the routine use of drainage procedures, untreated hepatic pyogenic abscess was almost uniformly fatal. It was not until the classic review by Ochsner and DeBakey in 1938 (see earlier) that routine surgical drainage was used and dramatic reductions in mortality were noted. Open surgical drainage of pyogenic abscesses was the sole treatment (with the addition of antibiotics eventually) for hepatic abscess until the 1980s. Since then, less invasive percutaneous drainage techniques and IV antibiotics have been used. Laparotomy is generally reserved for failures of percutaneous drainage.

Once the diagnosis of pyogenic hepatic abscess is suspected, broad-spectrum IV antibiotics should be started immediately to control ongoing bacteremia and its associated complications. Blood samples and specimens of abscess from aspiration should be sent for aerobic and anaerobic cultures. In immunosuppressed patients, mycobacterial and fungal cultures of the aspirate should be considered. Patients who are at risk for amebic infections should have blood samples drawn for amebic serology. Until cultures have specifically identified the offending organisms,

broad-spectrum antibiotics covering gram-negative, gram-positive, and anaerobic organisms should be used. Combinations such as ampicillin, an aminoglycoside, and metronidazole or a third-generation cephalosporin with metronidazole are appropriate. The optimal duration of antibiotic treatment is not well defined and must be individualized, depending on the success of the drainage procedure. Antibiotics should certainly be continued while there is evidence of ongoing infection, such as fever, chills, or leukocytosis. Beyond this, it is unclear how long to continue antibiotics, but recommendations are usually for 2 weeks or more.

Percutaneous drainage for pyogenic hepatic abscesses was first reported in 1953 but did not gain widespread acceptance until the 1980s with the development of high-quality imaging and expertise in interventional radiologic techniques. During the past 25 years, percutaneous catheter drainage has become the treatment of choice for most patients (Fig. 89.25). Success rates range from 66% to 90%. The obvious advantages are the simplicity of treatment (usually at the time of radiologic diagnosis) and avoidance of general anesthesia and a laparotomy. Relative contraindications to percutaneous catheter drainage include the presence of ascites, coagulopathy, and proximity to vital structures. Percutaneous drainage of multiple abscesses is usually met with a higher failure rate, but reports have demonstrated a high enough success rate that percutaneous approaches should be made first, reserving surgery for failures. A retrospective study comparing surgical with percutaneous drainage for large abscesses (>5 cm) has shown a better success rate with surgical drainage. Despite this, two-thirds of percutaneous treatments were successful, and the overall morbidity and mortality rates were similar. There has never been a randomized prospective comparison between percutaneous and surgical therapy for hepatic abscess. However, case series have suggested that for most cases, there are similar success and mortality rates. Modern series attempting to compare these two techniques retrospectively must be read with caution because most patients treated surgically have failed to respond to other, less invasive techniques. In general, surgery should be reserved for patients who require surgical treatment of the primary pathologic process (e.g., appendicitis) or for those who have failed to respond to percutaneous techniques. Laparoscopic drainage procedures have been reported with some success, and this can be considered a reasonable option to pursue in select cases.

Percutaneous aspiration without the placement of an indwelling drain has been investigated by several groups. Success rates are generally 60% to 90% and somewhat similar to percutaneous catheter drainage.[8] Most patients, however, require more than one aspiration, and 25% of patients require three or more aspirations. One randomized trial has evaluated percutaneous aspiration versus percutaneous catheter drainage. Success rates were 60% in the aspiration group and 100% in the catheter group. All but one patient in the aspiration group had a single aspiration. Another randomized trial of 64 patients has compared aspiration alone with catheter drainage. There were similar outcomes in terms of treatment success rate, hospital stay, antibiotic duration, and mortality. In the aspiration-only group, 40% required two aspirations and 20% required three aspirations. In general, catheter drainage remains the treatment of choice, although a trial of a single aspiration is reasonable to consider.

Some investigators have reported success with antibiotics alone. Most of these patients, however, have had a diagnostic aspiration and thus at least a partial drainage. Also, other series have reported that antibiotic treatment without drainage carries a prohibitively high mortality (59%–100%). In patients who are not

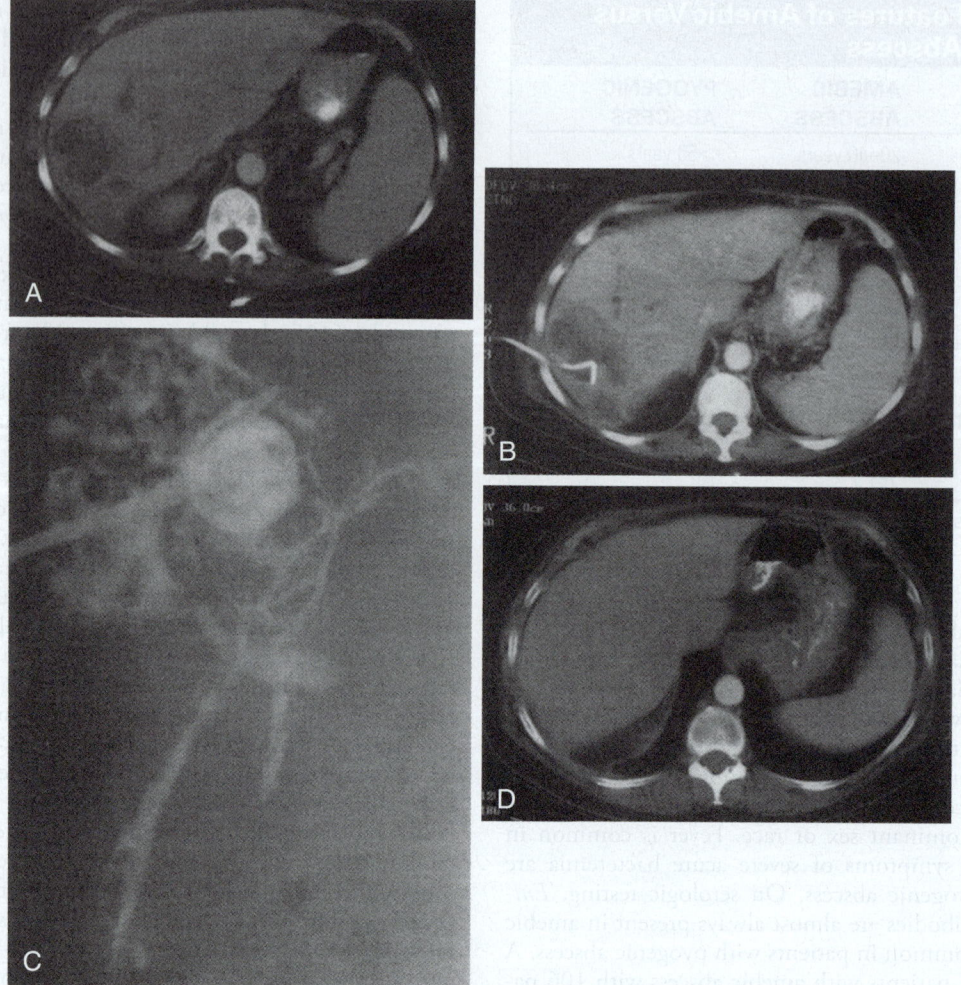

FIGURE 89.25 (A) Computed tomography (CT) scan demonstrating multiloculated hepatic abscess in the right liver. (B) CT scan at the time of percutaneous drainage. (C) Contrast study through the drainage catheter demonstrating typical irregular loculated appearance as well as communication with biliary tree. (D) Follow-up CT scan 3 months after treatment demonstrating complete resolution of abscess. (From Brown KT, Getrajdman GI. Interventional radiologic techniques in the liver and biliary tract. In: Blumgart LH, Fong Y, eds. *Surgery of the Liver and Biliary Tract*. London: WB Saunders; 2000:575-594.)

surgical candidates or who refuse any invasive procedure, an attempt at antibiotic treatment is reasonable. However, this is not recommended in other situations.

Liver resection is occasionally required for hepatic abscess. This may be required for an infected hepatic malignant neoplasm, hepatolithiasis, or intrahepatic biliary stricture. If hepatic destruction from infection is severe, some patients may benefit from resection.

Outcomes

Mortality from pyogenic hepatic abscess has dramatically improved during the past 70 years. Before the routine use of surgical drainage, pyogenic abscess was uniformly fatal. With the routine use of surgical drainage and the use of IV antibiotics, mortality was reduced to approximately 50%, a figure that stayed relatively constant from 1945 until the early 1980s. Since then, the mortality has been reported from 10% to 20%, and series from the 1990s have demonstrated a mortality rate below 10%.[8] The most recent series from Memorial Sloan Kettering Cancer Center (MSKCC) has reported a 3% mortality. Several studies have analyzed factors predictive of a poor outcome in patients with hepatic pyogenic

abscess. The presence of malignant disease, factors associated with malignant disease (e.g., jaundice, markedly elevated LFT results), and signs of sepsis appear to be consistent markers of poor prognosis. Signs of chronic disease, such as hypoalbuminemia, are also often associated with a poor outcome. Finally, signs of severe infection, such as marked leukocytosis, APACHE II (Acute Physiology and Chronic Health Evaluation II) scores, abscess rupture, bacteremia, and shock, are also associated with mortality.

Amebic Abscess

Epidemiology

Amebiasis is largely a disease of tropical and developing countries but is also a significant problem in developed countries because of immigration and travel between countries. *E. histolytica* is endemic in Mexico, India, Africa, and parts of Central and South America. In 1995, the World Health Organization estimated that 40 to 50 million people suffer from amebic colitis or amebic liver abscess worldwide, resulting in 40,000 to 100,000 deaths each year.[7] Before this, estimates of amebiasis were unreliable because *E. histolytica* (the pathogenic form) was not differentiated from

Entamoeba dispar (the nonpathogenic form). Male homosexuals with diarrhea, previously thought to harbor *E. histolytica,* were found to be infected with *E. dispar,* which requires no treatment. Epidemiologic studies specifically addressing *E. histolytica* infections have estimated that 55% of those in endemic regions are infected, although less than 50% are symptomatic.

In contrast to pyogenic hepatic abscesses, patients with amebic liver abscesses tend to be Hispanic males 20 to 40 years of age with a history of travel to (or origination from) an endemic area. Poverty and cramped living conditions are associated with higher rates of infection. A male preponderance of more than 10:1 has been reported in almost all studies. For unclear reasons, menstruating females have a low incidence of invasive amebiasis, and pregnancy appears to abrogate this resistance. Heavy alcohol consumption is commonly reported and may render the liver more susceptible to amebic infection. Patients with impaired host immunity also appear to be at higher risk of infection and have higher mortality rates. Patients with amebic liver abscess without a history of travel to an endemic area often have associated immunosuppression, such as human immunodeficiency virus (HIV) infection, malnutrition, chronic infection, or chronic steroid use.

Pathogenesis

E. histolytica is a protozoan and exists as a trophozoite or a cyst. All other species in the genus *Entamoeba* are considered nonpathogenic, and not all strains of *E. histolytica* are considered virulent. Ingestion of *E. histolytica* cysts through a fecal-oral route is the cause of amebiasis. Humans are the principal host, and the main source of infection is human contact with a cyst-passing carrier. Contaminated water and vegetables are also sources of human infection. Once ingested, the cysts are not degraded in the stomach and pass to the intestines, where the trophozoite is released and passed on to the colon. In the colon, the trophozoite can invade mucosa, resulting in disease.

It is thought that the trophozoites reach the liver through the portal venous system. There is no evidence for trophozoites passing through lymphatics. As implied by its name, *E. histolytica* trophozoites can lyse tissues through complex events, including cell adherence, cell activation, and subsequent release of enzymes, resulting in necrosis. The principal mechanism is probably enzymatic cellular hydrolysis. Amebic liver abscesses are formed by progressing, localized hepatic necrosis producing a cavity containing acellular proteinaceous debris surrounded by a rim of invasive amebic trophozoites. Early development of an amebic liver abscess is associated with an accumulation of polymorphonuclear leukocytes, which are then lysed by the trophozoites.

Antiamebic antibodies develop rapidly in patients with invasive disease or an amebic hepatic abscess. Secretory immunoglobulin A (IgA) antibodies have been shown to inhibit adherence to colonic epithelium in vitro. However, the development of these antibodies does not halt the progression of disease. Interestingly, children who lack antiamebic IgG have innate resistance to invasive infection, suggesting an alternative immune-mediated response. There is now evidence that a cell-mediated helper T-cell response is probably the major mechanism of resistance.

Pathology

Hepatic amebic abscess is essentially the result of liquefaction necrosis of the liver, producing a cavity full of blood and liquefied liver tissue. The appearance of this fluid is typically described as resembling anchovy sauce; the fluid is odorless unless secondary bacterial infection has taken place. The progressive hepatic necrosis

continues until the Glisson capsule is reached because the capsule is resistant to hydrolysis by the amebae. Thus, amebic abscesses tend to abut the liver capsule. Because of the resistance of the Glisson capsule, the cavity is typically crisscrossed by portal triads protected by this peritoneal sheath. Early on, the formed cavity is ill-defined, with no real fibrous response around the edges. However, a chronic abscess can ultimately develop a fibrous capsule and may even calcify. Like pyogenic abscesses, amebic abscesses tend to occur mainly in the right liver.

Clinical Features

Approximately 80% of patients with amebic liver abscess present with symptoms lasting from a few days to 4 weeks. The duration of symptoms has been found to be typically less than 10 days. The presenting clinical signs and symptoms are summarized in Table 89.6. The typical clinical picture is a patient 20 to 40 years of age who has recently traveled to an endemic area, with fever, chills, anorexia, right upper quadrant pain and tenderness, and hepatomegaly. The abdominal pain is typically constant, dull, and localized to the right upper quadrant. Although some studies report higher numbers, approximately 25% of patients have diarrhea despite an obligatory colonic infection. Synchronous hepatic abscess is found in one-third of patients with active amebic colitis. Jaundice, as a result of a large abscess compressing the biliary tree, is not as rare as was once thought, with an average 22% of patients presenting with this feature worldwide. Weight loss and myalgias may occur when symptoms have been present for weeks. Pleuritic or right shoulder pain can occur if there is irritation of the right hemidiaphragm. Symptoms and tenderness may be epigastric or left sided if the abscess is in the left liver. Rupture into the peritoneum with peritonitis occurs infrequently; when it does occur, it is more often with left-sided

TABLE 89.6 Signs, Symptoms, and Laboratory Findings in Amebic Liver Abscess[a]

PARAMETER	AVERAGE	RANGE	NO. OF CASES REVIEWED
Symptoms and Signs			
Abdominal pain (%)	92	73–100	1701
Fever (%)	90	72–100	2192
Abdominal tenderness (%)	78	40–100	1424
Hepatomegaly (%)	62	20–100	1539
Anorexia (%)	47	28–89	499
Weight loss (%)	39	11–83	871
Diarrhea (%)	23	12–40	1426
Jaundice (%)	22	5–50	1630
Laboratory Tests			
Stool cysts, trophozoites (%)	12	4–30	4908
Amebae in cyst aspirate (%)	42	30–76	1402
Hemoglobin (g/dL)	12.1	10.2–12.8	229
Alkaline phosphatase (% >120 U/L)	76	65–91	589
Total bilirubin (g/dL)	1.4	0.8–2.4	509
Albumin (g/dL)	2.8	2.3–3.4	404
AST (× upper limit normal)	1.7	1.0–2.5	459

[a]In an extensive literature review.

abscesses. Rare cases of rupture into the pleural space, pericardium, and other intraabdominal organs have also been reported.

Patients presenting acutely (symptoms <10 days) versus those with a chronic presentation (>2 weeks) differ clinically. Acute presentations are typically more dramatic, with high fevers, chills, and significant abdominal tenderness. In the acute presentation, 50% of patients have multiple lesions, whereas with the chronic presentation, more than 80% of patients have a single right-sided lesion. A more complicated course tends to ensue in the acute presentation, but response to therapy is similar in both groups.

Laboratory abnormalities are common in amebic abscess (see Table 89.6). Patients typically have mild to moderate leukocytosis, without eosinophilia. Anemia is common. Mild abnormalities of LFT results, including albumin, PT-INR, ALP, AST, and bilirubin levels, are typical. The most common LFT abnormality is an elevated PT-INR. Because more than 70% of patients with amebic liver abscess do not have detectable amebae in their stool, the most useful laboratory evaluation is the measurement of circulating antiamebic antibodies, which are present in 90% to 95% of patients. Many serologic tests have been devised over the years. An indirect hemagglutinin test was used extensively in the past and has a sensitivity of 90%. This test has largely been replaced by enzyme immunoassays, which detect presence of antibodies against the parasite and are simple, rapidly performed, and inexpensive. An enzyme immunoassay has a reported sensitivity of 99% and specificity higher than 90% in patients with hepatic abscess. Unfortunately, the presence of antibodies may reflect prior infection, and interpretation can be difficult in endemic areas. Ongoing studies are focusing on identifying specific *E. histolytica* antigens to identify acute infection. The antigen detection kits have been evaluated in endemic areas. These kits can detect the *E. histolytica* lectin antigen in the serum and liver abscess pus and in small studies have been shown to have high sensitivity. However, the sensitivity may decrease if the test is performed after treatment with metronidazole.

Radiologic studies are a critical element in the diagnosis of amebic liver abscess. Plain chest radiographs are abnormal in approximately 50% of cases, usually demonstrating an elevated right diaphragm, pleural effusion, or atelectasis. Abdominal ultrasound has a reported accuracy of approximately 90% when combined with a typical history and clinical presentation. Typical findings on abdominal ultrasound are a rounded lesion abutting the liver capsule (see earlier) without significant rim echoes, interpreted as an abscess wall. The contents of the cavity are usually hypoechoic and nonhomogeneous (Fig. 89.26). These findings on ultrasound are found in 40% to 70% of cases. Abdominal CT scanning is probably more sensitive than ultrasound and is helpful in differentiating amebic from pyogenic abscess, with rim enhancement noted in the pyogenic abscess (Fig. 89.27). CT can also help identify simple cysts and necrotic tumors. MRI of the liver has no distinct advantages over CT or ultrasound in typical cases but may be helpful in differentiating atypical lesions. Nuclear medicine studies, such as gallium scanning or technetium-99m liver scans, can be helpful in differentiating pyogenic from amebic abscesses because the amebic abscesses typically do not contain leukocytes and therefore do not light up on these scans.[9]

When this workup is still not definitive and diagnostic uncertainty persists, two options should be considered. First, a therapeutic trial of antiamebic drugs can be used. If a rapid improvement occurs, this supports the diagnosis. In situations in which amebic serology is inconclusive and a therapeutic trial of antibiotics is deemed inappropriate or has failed to improve symptoms, the second

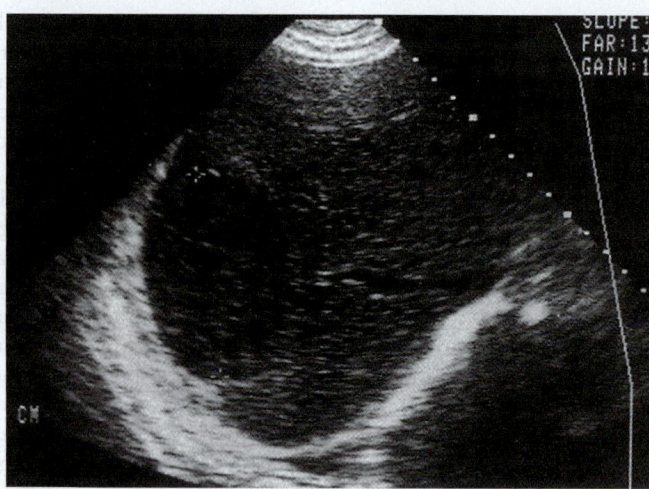

FIGURE 89.26 Typical ultrasound image of an amebic hepatic abscess. Note the peripheral location, rounded shape with poor rim, and internal echoes. (From Thomas PG, Ravindra KV. Amebiasis and biliary infection. In: Blumgart LH, Fong Y, eds. *Surgery of the Liver and Biliary Tract*. London: WB Saunders; 2000:1147-1166.)

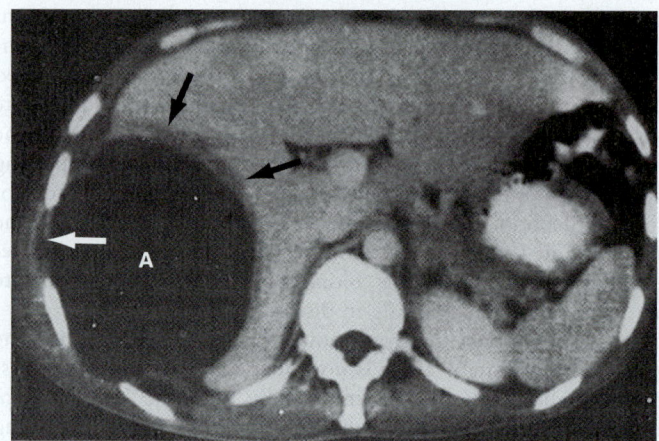

FIGURE 89.27 Computed tomography scan of amebic abscess (*A*). The lesion is peripherally located and round. The rim is nonenhancing but shows peripheral edema (*black arrows*). Note the extension into the intercostal space (*white arrow*).

option, a diagnostic aspiration, should be considered. A pyogenic abscess would have bacteria and leukocytes, whereas an amebic abscess would contain the typical so-called anchovy sauce. Cultures of amebic abscess are usually negative and do not contain leukocytes. In patients for whom neoplasm or hydatid disease is in the differential diagnosis, aspiration should not be performed.

Differential Diagnosis

The differential diagnosis of an amebic liver abscess can be broad and include diseases such as viral hepatitis, echinococcal disease, cholangitis, cholecystitis, and even other inflammatory abdominal disorders, such as appendicitis. Malignant lesions of the liver can also have similar presentations in atypical situations. On occasion, primary pulmonary disorders must be considered. Usually, the most important distinction to be made is between pyogenic and amebic abscess. The essential elements of this distinction are summarized in Table 89.5 and in the earlier section on pyogenic abscess.

Treatment

The mainstay of treatment for amebic abscesses is metronidazole (750 mg orally, three times daily for 10 days), which is curative in more than 90% of patients. Clinical improvement is usually seen within 3 days. Other nitroimidazoles (e.g., secnidazole, tinidazole) are also as effective and are commonly used outside the United States. If response to metronidazole is poor or the drug is not tolerated, other agents can be used. Emetine hydrochloride is effective against invasive amebiasis, particularly in the liver, but requires intramuscular injections and has serious cardiac side effects. A more attractive option is chloroquine, but this is a less effective agent. After treatment of the liver abscess, it is recommended that luminal agents such as iodoquinol, paromomycin, and diloxanide furoate be administered to treat the carrier state.

Therapeutic needle aspiration of amebic abscesses has been proposed. However, a Cochrane systematic review did not support any benefit of therapeutic aspiration in addition to metronidazole treatment over metronidazole treatment alone to hasten clinical or radiologic resolution of amebic liver abscesses.[10] In general, aspiration is recommended for diagnostic uncertainty (see earlier), with failure to respond to metronidazole therapy in 3 to 5 days, or in abscesses thought to be at high risk for rupture. Abscesses larger than 5 cm in diameter and in the left liver are thought to carry a higher risk of rupture, and aspiration should be considered.

Outcomes

Although amebic liver abscesses usually respond rapidly to treatment, there are uncommon complications of which one must be aware. The most frequent complication of amebic abscess is rupture into the peritoneum, pleural cavity, or pericardium. The size of the abscess appears to be the most important risk factor for rupture, and the overall incidence of rupture ranges from 3% to 17%. Most peritoneal ruptures tend to be contained by the diaphragm, abdominal wall, or omentum, but rupture can fistulize into a hollow viscus. A peritoneal rupture usually is manifested as abdominal pain, peritonitis, and a mass or generalized distention. Laparotomy was advocated in the past for this complication, but now many patients are treated successfully with percutaneous drainage. Laparotomy is indicated in cases of doubtful diagnosis, hollow viscus perforation, fistulization resulting in hemorrhage or sepsis, and failure of conservative therapy. Rupture into the pleural space usually results in a large and rapidly accumulating effusion that collapses the involved lung. Treatment consists of thoracentesis, but if secondary bacterial infection ensues, more aggressive surgical approaches may be necessary. Rupture can occur into the bronchi and is usually self-limited with postural drainage and bronchodilators. Rarely, a left-sided abscess may rupture into the pericardium and can be manifested as an asymptomatic pericardial effusion or even tamponade. This must be treated with aspiration or drainage through a pericardial window. Other complications include compression of the biliary tree or IVC from a very large abscess and the development of a brain abscess.

The mortality for all patients with amebic liver abscess is approximately 5% and does not appear to be affected by the addition of aspiration to metronidazole therapy or by chronicity of symptoms. When an abscess ruptures, mortality ranges from 6% to as high as 50%. Factors independently associated with poor outcome are elevated serum bilirubin level (>3.5 mg/dL), encephalopathy, hypoalbuminemia (<2.0 g/dL), multiple abscess cavities, abscess volume larger than 500 mL, anemia, and diabetes. Although clinical improvement after adequate treatment with

antiamebic agents is the rule, radiologic resolution of the abscess cavity is usually delayed. The average time to radiologic resolution is 3 to 9 months, and in some patients, it can take years. Studies have shown that more than 90% of the visible lesions disappear radiologically, but a small percentage of patients are left with a clinically irrelevant residual lesion.

Hydatid Cyst

Hydatid disease, or echinococcosis, is a zoonosis that occurs primarily in sheep-grazing areas of the world but is common worldwide because the dog is a definitive host. Echinococcosis is endemic in Mediterranean countries, the Middle East, Far East, South America, Australia, New Zealand, and east Africa.[11] Humans contract the disease from dogs, but there is no human-to-human transmission.

Three species cause hydatid disease. *Echinococcus granulosus* is the most common, and *Echinococcus multilocularis* and *Echinococcus ligartus* account for a small number of cases.[11] Dogs are the definitive host of *E. granulosus;* the adult tapeworm is attached to the villi of the ileum. Up to thousands of ova are passed daily and deposited in the dog's feces. Sheep are the usual intermediate host, but humans are an accidental intermediate host. Humans are an end stage to the parasite. In the human duodenum, the parasitic embryo releases an oncosphere containing hooklets that penetrate the mucosa, allowing access to the bloodstream. In the blood, the oncosphere reaches the liver (most commonly) or lungs, where the parasite develops its larval stage—the hydatid cyst.

Three weeks after infection, a visible hydatid cyst develops, which then slowly grows in a spherical manner. A pericyst, or fibrous capsule derived from host tissues, develops around the hydatid cyst. The cyst wall itself has two layers: an outer gelatinous membrane (ectocyst) and an inner germinal membrane (endocyst). Brood capsules are small, intracystic cellular masses in which future worm heads develop into scoleces. In a definitive host, the scoleces develop into an adult tapeworm; in the intermediate host, they can differentiate only into a new hydatid cyst. Freed brood capsules and scoleces are found in the hydatid fluid and form the so-called hydatid sand. Daughter cysts are true replicas of the mother cyst. Hydatid cysts can die with degeneration of the membranes, development of cystic vacuoles, and calcification of the wall. Calcification of a hydatid cyst, however, does not always imply that the cyst is dead.

Hydatid cysts are diagnosed in equal numbers of males and females at an average age of about 45 years. Approximately 75% of hydatid cysts are located in the right liver and are solitary. The clinical presentation of a hydatid cyst is largely asymptomatic until complications occur. The most common presenting symptoms are abdominal pain, dyspepsia, and vomiting. The most frequent sign is hepatomegaly. Jaundice and fever are each present in approximately 8% of patients. Bacterial superinfection of a hydatid cyst can occur and manifest like a pyogenic abscess. Rupture of the cyst into the biliary tree or bronchial tree or free rupture into the peritoneal, pleural, or pericardial cavities can occur. Free ruptures can result in disseminated echinococcosis or a potentially fatal anaphylactic reaction. In cases of diagnostic uncertainty, a battery of serologic tests are available to evaluate antibody response, but all are plagued by low sensitivity and specificity.

Ultrasound is most commonly used worldwide for the diagnosis of echinococcosis because of its availability, affordability, and accuracy. Several findings on ultrasound can be diagnostic but depend on the stage of the cyst at the time of the examination. A simple hydatid cyst is well circumscribed with budding signs on the cyst membrane and may contain free-floating hyperechogenic hydatid sand. A rosette appearance is seen when daughter cysts are present. The cyst can be filled with an amorphous mass, which can be diagnostically misleading. Calcifications in the wall of the cyst are highly suggestive of hydatid disease and can be helpful in the diagnosis (Fig. 89.28). Similar findings are seen on CT or MRI scans. These cross-sectional imaging studies can also evaluate extrahepatic disease and demonstrate detailed hepatic anatomic relationships to the cyst. In patients with suspected biliary involvement, ERCP or percutaneous transhepatic cholangiography may be necessary.

Although the treatment of hepatic hydatid cysts is primarily surgical, alternative options are in evolution.[12] In general, most cysts should be treated, but in older patients with small, asymptomatic, densely calcified cysts, conservative management is appropriate. In preparation for an operation, preoperative steroids have been recommended but are not universally used. The anesthesiologist should have epinephrine and steroids available in case of an anaphylactic reaction. Many operations have been used, but in general, the abdomen is completely explored, the liver mobilized, and the cyst exposed. Packing off the abdomen is important because rupture can result in anaphylaxis and diffuse seeding. The cyst is usually then aspirated through a closed suction system and flushed with a scolicidal agent, such as hypertonic saline. It is then unroofed, which can be followed by several possibilities, including excision (or pericystectomy), marsupialization procedures, leaving the cyst open, drainage of the cyst, omentoplasty, and partial hepatectomy to encompass the cyst. Total pericystectomy or formal partial hepatectomy can also be performed without entering the cyst (Fig. 89.29). Both radical (resection) and conservative (drainage and evacuation)

surgical approaches appear to be equally effective at controlling disease, although a prospective comparison has never been performed. When bile duct communication is diagnosed preoperatively or at operation, it must be meticulously sought after. Simple suture repair is often sufficient, but major biliary repairs, approaches through the common bile duct, or postoperative ERCP may be necessary. Laparoscopic techniques for drainage and unroofing of cysts have been reported in many series, with encouraging results.[13] Recurrence rates after surgical treatment range from 1% to 20% but are generally 5% or less in experienced centers.

In the past, percutaneous aspiration of hydatid cysts was contraindicated because of the risk of rupture and uncontrolled spillage. However, percutaneous aspiration with injection of scolicidal agents has been reported with high success rates in highly selected patients.[14] This technique, known as *PAIR* (puncture, aspiration, injection, and reaspiration), has become more accepted in some centers. Two randomized trials, one comparing PAIR with surgery ($N = 50$) and one comparing PAIR with medical therapy, have shown similar success rates. These trials were small and had significant methodologic problems, limiting the ability to draw firm conclusions. Although surgery remains the treatment of choice, further prospective trials are clearly indicated to address this interesting and potentially useful technique. Treatment of echinococcosis with albendazole or mebendazole is effective at shrinking cysts in many patients with *E. granulosus* infection, but cyst disappearance occurs in well below 50% of patients. Preoperative treatment may decrease the risk of spillage and is a reasonable and safe practice. Medical therapy without definitive resection or drainage should be considered only for widely disseminated disease or poor surgical candidates.

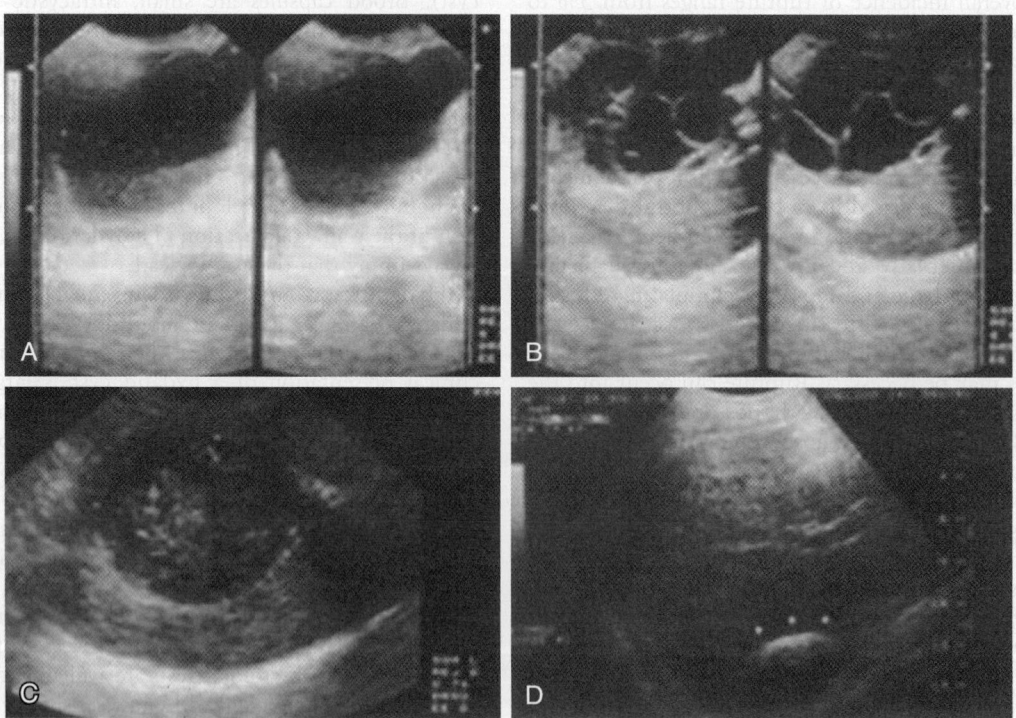

FIGURE 89.28 Ultrasound image demonstrating typical characteristics of a hydatid cyst at varying stages. (A) Simple hydatid cyst with hydatid sand. (B) Daughter and granddaughter cysts and typical rosette appearance. (C) Hydatid cyst filled with amorphous mass, giving a solid or semisolid appearance. (D) Calcified cyst with eggshell appearance. (From Thomas PG, Ravindra KV. Amebiasis and biliary infection. In: Blumgart LH, Fong Y, eds. *Surgery of the Liver and Biliary Tract*. London: WB Saunders; 2000:1147-1166.)

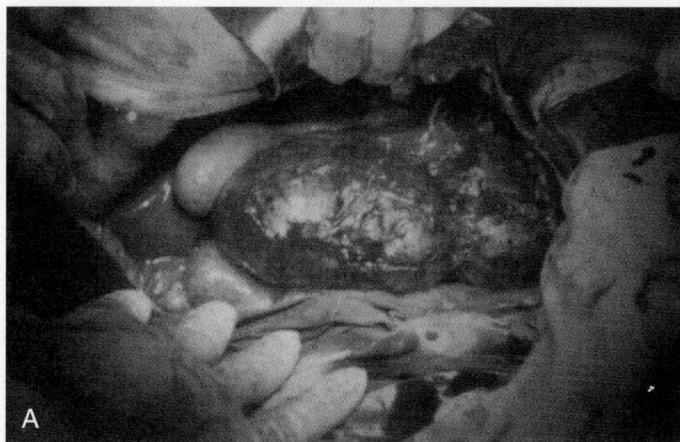

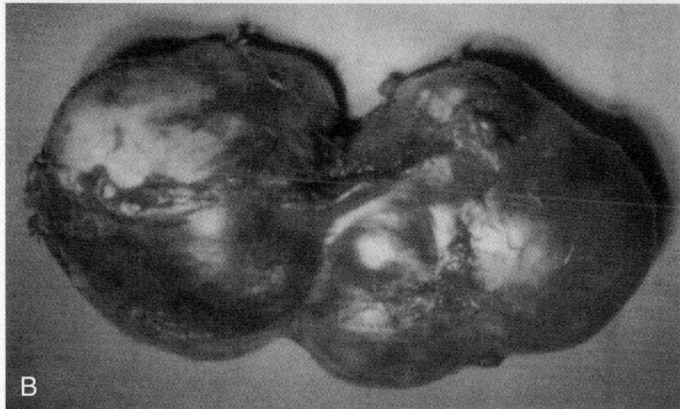

FIGURE 89.29 (A) Peripheral hydatid cyst of the left liver. (B) Intact specimen after pericystectomy. Note that the entire pericyst has been removed. (From Milicevic MN. Hydatid disease. In: Blumgart LH, Fong Y, eds. *Surgery of the Liver and Biliary Tract.* London: WB Saunders; 2000:1167-1204.)

Recurrent Pyogenic Cholangitis

Recurrent pyogenic cholangitis (RPC) is a syndrome of repeated attacks of cholangitis secondary to biliary stones and strictures that involve the extrahepatic and intrahepatic ducts. The condition has many names but is often referred to as Oriental cholangiohepatitis or hepatolithiasis. The disease is almost exclusively found in Asians and Asian medical centers. However, it is also seen in Asian immigrants throughout the world. Males and females are equally affected, and historically, the disease strikes at an early age (20–40 years) in patients from lower socioeconomic classes.

The cause of RPC is unknown but is related to recurrent infection of biliary radicals with gut bacteria. Ultimately, stones and strictures develop in the biliary tree, but it is not known which occurs first. The stones are bilirubinate stones; in some patients, no stones are found and only biliary sludge is demonstrated. An association between RPC and *Clonorchis sinensis* and *Ascaris lumbricoides* infection has been noted, but a true causal relationship has never been proven.[15]

Strictures can be found anywhere in the biliary tree but usually involve the intrahepatic main hepatic ducts, most often the left hepatic duct. The gallbladder is involved in approximately 20% of cases. Cirrhosis and liver failure are seen only in long-standing disease, usually after multiple operations. Other complications include choledochoduodenal fistulas and acute pancreatitis from common bile duct stones. An increased incidence of

cholangiocarcinoma has been noted, but a causal relationship is difficult to prove.

The typical patient with RPC is a young Asian of a lower socioeconomic background who presents with repeated bouts of cholangitis. The symptoms and presentation are those of cholangitis. These include fever, right upper quadrant abdominal pain, and jaundice. Biliary obstruction is usually incomplete; therefore, marked jaundice and pruritus are not common. There is usually leukocytosis and abnormal LFT results consistent with biliary obstruction. Evaluation of the anatomic distribution of disease is critical to formulation of a sound therapeutic plan. A combination of ultrasound, CT, and direct cholangiography is often necessary to evaluate these patients. Direct cholangiography is performed endoscopically or transhepatically and is considered an important study complementing the cross-sectional imaging. Magnetic resonance cholangiopancreatography can combine cross-sectional imaging and cholangiography in one noninvasive test and may ultimately replace direct cholangiography.

In an acute presentation, most patients improve with conservative management, allowing time for radiologic studies and planning of a definitive operation, which is the treatment of choice. If intervention is necessary during the acute phase, it must focus on adequate decompression of the biliary tree through open common bile duct exploration or endoscopic papillotomy with stenting. Although nonoperative approaches, such as percutaneous transhepatic cholangioscopic lithotomy, have been developed, surgical treatment remains the treatment of choice. Percutaneous transhepatic cholangioscopic lithotomy is generally used for poor-risk surgical patients and those who have failed to respond to surgical treatment. Stone clearance rates are high (>80%) and necessary for a successful long-term outcome. Unfortunately, stone recurrence is common and is mostly related to the presence of biliary strictures.

The goal of operative approaches is to clear the biliary tree of stones and to bypass, resect, or enlarge strictures.[16] Many cases require only exploration of the common bile duct, with or without hepaticojejunostomy. In complicated cases, providing permanent access to the biliary tree for interventional radiologic procedures by extending the end of the Roux-en-Y hepaticojejunostomy to the skin or subcutaneous space has been a successful approach (Fig. 89.30). Other potentially necessary procedures include stricturoplasty and partial hepatectomy. Partial hepatectomy is advocated for patients with intrahepatic strictures, hepatic atrophy, liver abscess, or suspicion of cholangiocarcinoma.

In a large series from Asia, where surgery and hepatectomy are liberally applied, surgical mortality rates are 1%. Moreover, with aggressive treatment, there is almost a 100% stone clearance rate. Long-term outcome is excellent, with a less than 5% stone recurrence rate. Long-term survival is mostly related to the presence of cholangiocarcinoma, which is found in approximately 10% of patients. Particularly complicated cases can have a higher rate of recurrent symptoms. In some cases, liver transplantation may be necessary.[17]

NEOPLASMS

Solid Benign Neoplasms

It is estimated that benign focal liver masses are present in approximately 10% to 20% of the population in developed countries. With the increasing use of rapidly improving radiologic examinations, these entities have been encountered more frequently. Familiarity with the clinical characteristics, natural history, imaging

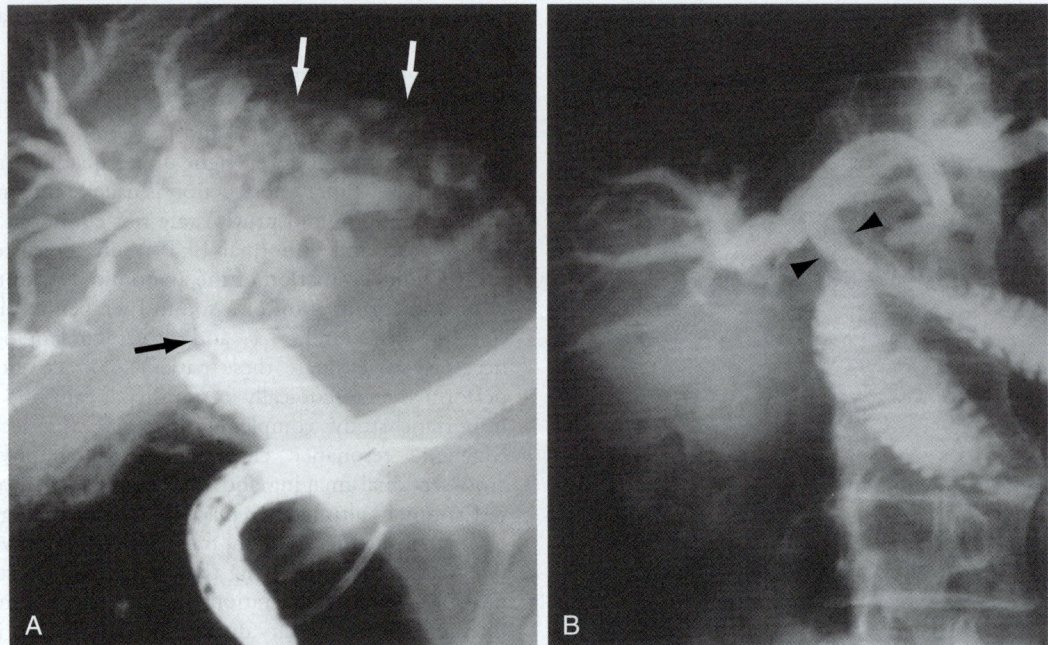

FIGURE 89.30 (A) Cholangiogram of a patient with recurrent pyogenic cholangitis and a common hepatic duct stricture *(black arrow)*. There are numerous stones inside dilated left ducts *(white arrows)*. (B) A hepaticojejunostomy to the segment III duct *(arrowheads)* has been performed, and a flexible choledochoscope is shown passing through the anastomosis into the peripheral left ducts. All stones have been cleared. (From Fan ST, Wong J. Recurrent pyogenic cholangitis. In: Blumgart LH, Fong Y, eds. *Surgery of the Liver and Biliary Tract*. London: WB Saunders; 2000:1205-1225.)

characteristics, and indications for surgery in these tumors is essential. Many benign lesions can be adequately characterized by modern imaging studies, such as CT, ultrasound, and MRI. In unclear cases, serum tumor markers (e.g., AFP, CEA) and a search for a primary tumor in the case of suspected metastases should be carried out. A resection might be necessary to make a definitive diagnosis. Laparoscopy for assessment, biopsy, or resection has become an important diagnostic technique as well.[18,19]

Liver Cell Adenoma

Liver cell adenoma (LCA) is a relatively rare benign proliferation of hepatocytes in the context of a normal liver. It is predominantly found in young females (aged 20–40 years) and is often associated with steroid hormone use, such as long-term oral contraceptive pill (OCP) use. Increased prevalence of LCA was observed in the 1970s, after the introduction of oral contraceptives. Male anabolic hormone use can also predispose to development of LCA. The female-to-male ratio is approximately 11:1. Other risk factors for LCA include vascular liver diseases, glycogenosis type 1A, and familial adenomatous polyposis. LCAs are usually singular, but multiple lesions have been reported in 12% to 30% of cases. Liver adenomatosis is defined by the presence of more than 10 LCAs in the liver. Interestingly, cases with multiple adenomas are not associated with OCP use and do not have as dramatic a female preponderance. On histologic evaluation, LCAs are composed of cords of benign hepatocytes containing increased glycogen and fat. Bile ductules are not observed histologically, and the normal architecture of the liver is absent in these lesions. Hemorrhage and necrosis are commonly seen.[20] On the basis of detailed molecular pathology correlation studies, a French collaborative group has recently proposed a molecular-pathologic classification whereby the adenomas are classified as β-catenin mutated adenoma, *HNF1A* mutated

adenoma, inflammatory adenoma, and not otherwise specified adenoma. Molecular studies have also identified genetic signatures associated with a higher risk of malignant transformation. Specifically, the highest risk of malignant transformation is observed in LCA with β-catenin activation.[21,22] With further research, new pathways driving the formation of adenomas are being identified and the "not otherwise specified adenoma" group is becoming smaller. For example, recently sonic hedgehog activation has been observed in 5% of LCAs.[23] Interestingly, these LCAs with sonic hedgehog activation are associated with obesity and bleeding. Furthermore, LCA with β-catenin mutations can be classified by the nature of the mutation. For example, those with exon-3 mutation have increased risk of hepatocellular carcinoma (HCC) degeneration, whereas mutation in exon 7/8 leads to only weak activation of β-catenin and no risk of malignant transformation.

Patients with LCA present with symptoms approximately 50% to 75% of the time. Upper abdominal pain is common and may be related to hemorrhage into the tumor or local compressive symptoms. The physical examination is usually unrevealing, and tumor markers are normal. Dramatic presentations with free intraperitoneal rupture and bleeding can occur. Imaging tends to be characteristic and obviates the need for tissue diagnosis most of the time. Because of intratumoral hemorrhage, the necrosis and fat component of LCA tends to be heterogeneous on CT. On contrast-enhanced CT, LCA tends to have peripheral enhancement with centripetal progression. MRI scans of LCA also have specific imaging characteristics, including a well-demarcated heterogeneous mass containing fat or hemorrhage. Despite high-quality imaging, resection may sometimes be necessary to secure a diagnosis in difficult cases. Intriguingly, studies are elucidating a correlation between the molecular subtypes described and imaging characteristics.[24]

The two major risks of LCA are rupture, with potentially life-threatening intraperitoneal hemorrhage, and malignant transformation. Quantifying the risk of rupture is difficult, but it has been estimated to be as high as 30% to 50%, with all instances of spontaneous rupture occurring in lesions 5 cm and larger.[25] Although there are numerous reports of transformation of LCA into HCC, the true risk of transformation is probably low. Hepatic adenomas with β-catenin activation should be considered for early surgical intervention, as malignant transformation most commonly occurs in this subtype.[22,26]

Patients who present with acute hemorrhage need emergent attention. If possible, hepatic artery embolization is a helpful and usually effective temporizing maneuver. Once the patient is stabilized and appropriately resuscitated, a laparotomy and resection of the mass are required. Symptomatic masses should be similarly resected. Patients with asymptomatic LCAs taking OCPs can be watched for regression after stopping of the OCPs, although progression and rupture have been observed in this setting. Behavior of LCAs during pregnancy has been unpredictable, and resection before a planned pregnancy is usually recommended. Overall, the surgeon must compare the risks of expectant management with serial imaging studies and AFP measurements against those of resection. Resection is usually recommended because of low mortality in experienced hands and the risks of observation. Margin status is not important in these resections, and limited resections can be performed. The management of adenomatosis is controversial, but large lesions should probably be resected because of the risk of rupture, whereas the risk of malignancy is low in lesions smaller than 5 cm. On occasion, liver transplantation is necessary for aggressive forms of adenomatosis.[27,28]

Focal Nodular Hyperplasia

Focal nodular hyperplasia (FNH) is the second most common benign tumor of the liver after hemangioma and is predominantly discovered in young females.[25] FNH is characterized by a central fibrous scar with radiating septa, although no central scar is seen in approximately 15% of cases (Fig. 89.31). On microscopic examination, FNH contains cords of benign-appearing hepatocytes divided by multiple fibrous septa originating from a central scar. Typical hepatic vascularity is not seen, but atypical biliary epithelium is found scattered throughout the lesion. The central scar often contains a large artery that branches out into multiple smaller arteries in a spoke wheel pattern. The cause of FNH is not known, but the most common theory is that FNH is related to a developmental vascular malformation. Female hormones and OCPs have been implicated in the development and growth of FNH, but the association is weak and difficult to prove.

In most patients, FNH is an incidental finding at laparotomy or, more commonly, on imaging studies. If symptoms are noted, vague abdominal pain is most often present, but various nonspecific symptoms have been described. It is often difficult to ascribe these reported symptoms to the presence of FNH; therefore, other possible causes must be sought. Physical examination is usually unrevealing, and mild abnormalities of liver function may be found. Serum AFP levels are normal.

With advances in hepatobiliary imaging, most cases of FNH can be diagnosed radiologically with reasonable certainty. Contrast-enhanced CT and MRI have become accurate methods of diagnosing FNH. FNH typically shows strong hypervascularity in the arterial phase of CT or MRI with a central nonenhancing scar. The enhancement fades over time, and the lesion becomes isointense to the liver parenchyma in the portal and delayed phases. When no central scar is seen, however, radiologic diagnosis is difficult, and

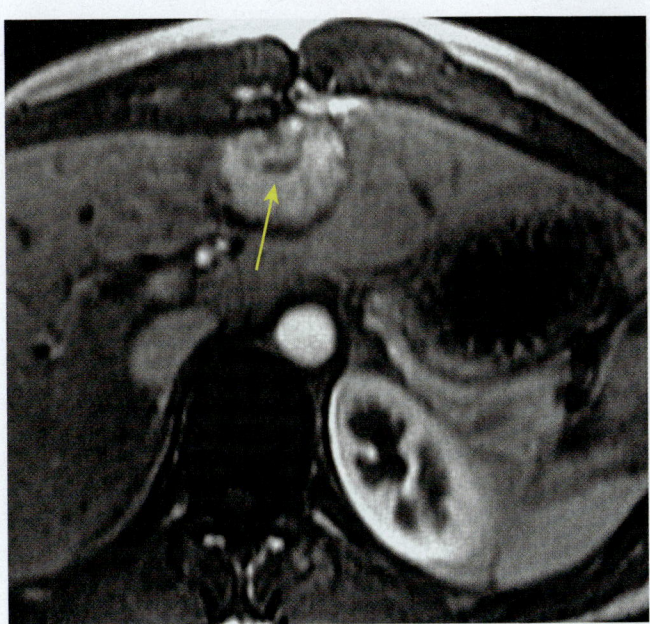

FIGURE 89.31 CT scan of a focal nodular hyperplasia. Note homogenous arterial enhancement with central scar *(arrow)*.

differentiation from LCA or a malignant mass, especially fibrolamellar HCC, can sometimes be impossible. On occasion, histologic confirmation is necessary, and resection is recommended for definitive diagnosis. Fine-needle aspiration for the diagnosis of FNH has been recommended but is often unrevealing.

Most FNH tumors are benign and indolent. Rupture, bleeding, and infarction are exceedingly rare, and malignant degeneration of FNH has never been reported. The treatment of FNH therefore depends on diagnostic certainty and symptoms. Asymptomatic patients with typical radiologic features do not require treatment.[25] If diagnostic uncertainty exists, resection may be necessary for histologic confirmation. Symptomatic patients should be thoroughly investigated to look for other pathologic processes to explain the symptoms. Careful observation of symptomatic FNH with serial imaging is reasonable because symptoms may resolve in a significant number of cases. Patients with persistent symptomatic FNH or an enlarging mass should be considered for resection. Because FNH is a benign diagnosis, resection must be performed, with minimal morbidity and mortality.

Hemangioma

Hemangioma is the most common benign tumor of the liver.[25] It occurs in females more than in males (3:1 ratio) and at a mean age of approximately 45 years. Small capillary hemangiomas are of no clinical significance, whereas larger cavernous hemangiomas more often come to the attention of the liver surgeon (Fig. 89.32). Cavernous hemangiomas have been associated with FNH and are also theorized to be congenital vascular malformations. The enlargement of hemangiomas is by ectasia rather than by neoplasia. They are usually solitary and less than 5 cm in diameter, and they occur with equal incidence in the right and left hemilivers. Lesions larger than 5 cm are arbitrarily called *giant hemangiomas*. Involution or thrombosis of hemangiomas can result in dense fibrotic masses that may be difficult to differentiate from malignant tumors. On microscopic examination, they are endothelium-lined, blood-filled spaces separated by thin fibrous septa.

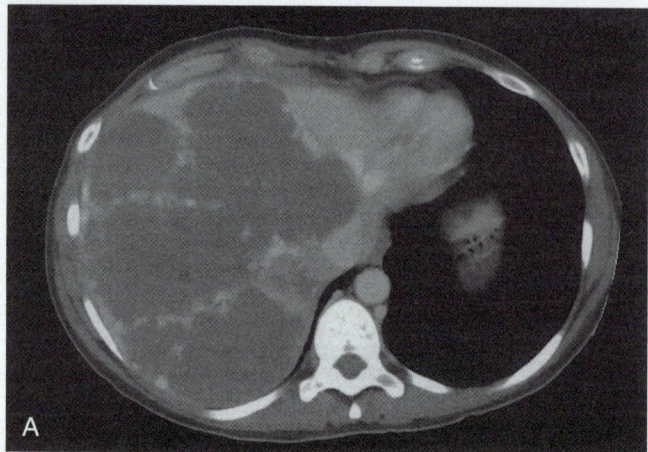
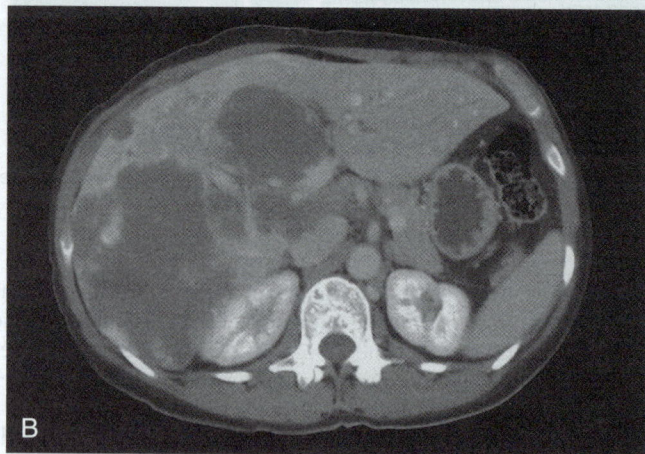

FIGURE 89.32 (A–B) Computed tomography scans of a large cavernous hemangioma showing displacement of left and middle hepatic veins and abutment of the left portal vein. The mass was symptomatic and required an extended right hepatectomy for removal.

Hemangiomas are usually asymptomatic and found incidentally on imaging studies. Large compressive masses may cause vague upper abdominal symptoms. Symptoms ascribed to liver hemangioma, however, mandate a search for other disease because an alternative cause of symptoms will be found in approximately 50% of cases. Rapid expansion or acute thrombosis can occasionally cause symptoms. Spontaneous rupture of liver hemangiomas is exceedingly rare. An associated syndrome of thrombocytopenia and consumptive coagulopathy known as *Kasabach-Merritt syndrome* is rare but well described.

LFT results and tumor markers are usually normal in liver hemangiomas. Radiologic investigation can reliably make the diagnosis in most cases. CT and MRI are usually sufficient if a typical peripheral nodular enhancement pattern is seen. Isotope-labeled red blood cell scans are an accurate test but are rarely necessary if high-quality CT and MRI are available. Percutaneous biopsy of a suspected hemangioma is potentially dangerous and inaccurate. Therefore, biopsy is not recommended.

The natural history of liver hemangioma is generally benign; it appears that most remain stable for a long time, with a low risk of rupture or hemorrhage.[25] Growth and development of symptoms do occur, however, occasionally requiring resection. There has never been a report of malignant degeneration of a liver hemangioma. An asymptomatic patient with a secure diagnosis can therefore be simply observed.[25] Symptomatic patients should undergo a thorough evaluation looking for alternative explanations for the symptoms but are candidates for resection if no other cause is found. Rupture, significant change in size, and development of the Kasabach-Merritt syndrome are indications for resection. In rare cases of diagnostic uncertainty, resection may be necessary for a definitive diagnosis. Resection of liver hemangiomas should be performed, with minimal morbidity and mortality. The preferred approach to resection is enucleation with arterial inflow control, but anatomic resections may be necessary in some cases. Surgery on large central hemangiomas can be associated with significant morbidity.

Liver hemangiomas in children are common, accounting for approximately 12% of all childhood hepatic tumors. They are usually multifocal and can involve other organs. Large hemangiomas in children can result in congestive heart failure secondary to arteriovenous shunting. Untreated symptomatic childhood hemangiomas are associated with high mortality. On the other hand, almost all small capillary hemangiomas resolve. Symptomatic childhood hemangiomas may be treated with therapeutic embolization; medical therapy should be initiated for congestive heart failure. Radiation and chemotherapeutic agents have been used, but experience has been limited. Resection may be necessary for symptomatic lesions or rupture.

Other Benign Tumors

Most benign solid liver tumors are LCAs, FNHs, or hemangiomas, but there are other benign hepatic tumors. However, these are rare and can be difficult to differentiate from malignant neoplasms. Macroregenerative nodules, previously known as adenomatous hyperplasia, are single or multiple well-circumscribed, bile-stained, bulging surface nodules that occur primarily in people with cirrhosis and result from the hyperplastic response to chronic liver injury. These lesions have malignant potential and can be difficult to distinguish from HCC. Nodular regenerative hyperplasia is a benign, diffuse, micronodular (usually <2 cm) process associated with lymphoproliferative disorders, collagen vascular diseases, and the use of steroids or chemotherapy. Nodular regenerative hyperplasia has no malignant potential and is not associated with cirrhosis. Biopsy may be necessary to distinguish these focal nodules from malignant neoplasms.

Mesenchymal hamartomas are rare solitary tumors of childhood that account for 5% of pediatric liver tumors. They are usually large cystic masses found in the right liver that present as progressive, painless abdominal distention. Resection of mesenchymal hamartomas may be necessary in the case of large lesions causing a mass effect.

Fatty tumors of the liver are rarely encountered but can usually be distinguished by typical characteristics on CT or MRI scans. Fatty tumors of the liver include primary lipomas, myelolipomas (which contain hematopoietic tissue), angiolipomas (which contain blood vessels), and angiomyolipomas (which contain smooth muscle). Focal fatty change in the liver can be confused with a neoplastic process and is becoming more common with improved imaging and the increasing incidence of hepatic steatosis.

Benign fibrous tumors of the liver can become large and symptomatic, requiring resection. Inflammatory pseudotumors of the liver are localized masses of inflammatory cells that can mimic a neoplasm. The cause of these inflammatory lesions is unknown but may be related to thrombosed vessels or old abscesses. Other extremely rare benign hepatic tumors include leiomyomas, myxomas, schwannomas, lymphangiomas, and teratomas.

Intrahepatic biliary cystadenomas or bile duct adenomas are rare but can cause biliary symptoms. Biliary hamartomas and biliary hyperplasia are common and are often seen as small white surface lesions that can mimic small metastatic tumors at abdominal exploration. Adrenal and pancreatic rests have also been found in the liver.

Primary Solid Malignant Neoplasms

Hepatocellular Carcinoma

Epidemiology. Liver cancer is the fifth most common cancer and the second most frequent cause of cancer-related death globally.[29] HCC is the most common primary malignant neoplasm of the liver and one of the most common malignant neoplasms worldwide. The epidemiology of HCC varies around the world, being affected by the varying etiologies in different parts. Hepatitis B is the most common cause of HCC. Thus, the highest incidence of HCC occurs in geographic areas where hepatitis B is rampant, namely sub-Saharan Africa and Southeast Asia (>10–20 cases/100,000). The lowest incidence (1–3 cases/100,000) is found in Australia, North America, and Europe. Epidemiologic evidence strongly suggests that HCC is largely related to environmental factors; the incidence of HCC in immigrants eventually approaches that of the local population after several generations. An exception to this is that Whites living in high-prevalence areas tend to have a low incidence of HCC. This is likely related to the continuation of the lifestyle and environment of their home country. It is probable that the variation in incidence rates among immigrants is related to hepatitis B virus (HBV) carrier rates.

A significant rise in the incidence of HCC in the United States and other Western countries has been noted during the past 35 years. However, recent data suggest that at least in the United States, the epidemic may have peaked, as the incidence rates have stabilized in the last few years.[30,31] The explanation for the observed increase during the past few decades is not understood, but the emergence of hepatitis C virus (HCV) infection and immigration patterns have been suggested, as has the increase in obesity and nonalcoholic steatohepatitis (NASH).[32] Given that obesity and its ensuing complications are increasing at epidemic proportions in the Western world, obesity as the cause of HCC is becoming more important. Recent data also suggest that addressing the environmental factors can lead to reduction in incidence of HCC. In Taiwan, treatment of chronic hepatitis B and C under the auspices of a national viral hepatitis therapy program has met with a reduction in incidence and mortality related to HCC.[33]

HCC is two to eight times more common in males than in females in low- and high-incidence areas. Although sex hormones may play a minor role in the development of HCC, the higher incidence in males is probably related to higher rates of associated risk factors, such as HBV infection, cirrhosis, smoking, alcohol abuse, and higher hepatic DNA synthesis in cirrhosis. In general, the incidence of HCC increases with age, but a tendency to develop HCC earlier in high-incidence areas has been noted. For example, in Mozambique, 50% of patients with HCC were found to be younger than 30 years. This may be related to differing ages at infection and the natural histories of hepatitis B and C.

Causative factors. A large number of associations between hepatic viral infections, environmental exposure, alcohol use, smoking, genetic metabolic diseases, cirrhosis, and OCP use and the development of HCC have been recognized. Overall, 75% to 80% of HCC cases are related to HBV (50%–55%) or HCV (25%–30%) infections. Research also shows that the development of HCC is a complex and multistep process that involves any number of these risk factors.

Hepatitis C has been discovered to be a major cause of chronic liver disease in Japan, Europe, and the United States, where there is a relatively low rate of HBV infection. Two percent of the world's population is infected with HCV. Antibodies to HCV are found in 76% of patients with HCC in Japan and Europe and 36% of patients in the United States. HBV and HCV infections are both independent risk factors for the development of HCC but probably act synergistically when an individual is infected with both viruses. Although the natural history of HCV infection is not completely understood, it appears to be one of chronic infection, with a benign early course. However, the ultimate development of cirrhosis with increased risk of HCC may ensue. The rate of HCC among HCV-infected persons ranges from 1% to 3% over 30 years, and in individuals with HCV-related cirrhosis, HCC develops at an annual rate of 1% to 4%. Studies on the rates of progression to cirrhosis estimate a median time of 30 years, but differing progression rates yield a range of less than 20 years to more than 50 years. Factors associated with a more rapid progression include male sex, chronic alcohol use, and older age at the time of infection. HCV is an RNA virus that does not integrate into the host genome; therefore, the pathogenesis of HCV-related HCC may be connected more to chronic inflammation and cirrhosis than to direct carcinogenesis.[34,35] Data from era of interferon-based therapy suggest that the patients who achieved a sustained viral response had up to 75% reduction in their risk of HCC. This is exciting and has immense global health significance, especially now, as many effective HCV treatments are available. However, future studies will determine if these new treatments will change the incidence and course of HCC.

The true relationship between cirrhosis and HCC is difficult to ascertain, and suggestions of causation remain speculative. Cirrhosis is not required for the development of HCC, and hepatocarcinogenesis is not an inevitable result of cirrhosis. The relationship between cirrhosis and HCC is further complicated by the fact that they share common associations. Furthermore, some associations (e.g., HBV infection, hemochromatosis) are associated with higher risk of HCC, whereas others (e.g., alcohol, primary biliary cirrhosis) are associated with a lower risk of HCC. Research has demonstrated that cirrhotic livers with higher DNA replication rates are associated with the development of HCC.

Chronic alcohol abuse has been associated with an increased risk of HCC, and there may be a synergistic effect with HBV and HCV infection. Alcohol causes cirrhosis but has never been shown to be directly carcinogenic in hepatocytes. Thus, alcohol likely acts as a cocarcinogen. Cigarette smoking has been linked to the development of HCC, but the evidence is not consistent, and the contributing risk independent of viral hepatitis is likely to be small. Aflatoxin, produced by *Aspergillus* spp., is a powerful hepatotoxin. With chronic exposure, aflatoxin acts as a carcinogen and increases the risk of HCC. The offending fungi grow on grains, peanuts, and food products in tropical and subtropical regions. Ingestion of contaminated foods results in aflatoxin exposure. Levels of aflatoxin in these implicated foods are regulated in the United States.

Other chemicals have also been implicated as carcinogens related to HCC. These include nitrites, hydrocarbons, solvents, pesticides, and vinyl chloride. Thorotrast (colloidal thorium dioxide) is an angiographic medium that was used in the 1930s. It emits high levels of long-lasting radiation and has been associated with hepatic fibrosis, angiosarcoma, cholangiosarcoma, and HCC. Associations with inherited metabolic liver diseases, such as hereditary hemochromatosis, α_1-antitrypsin deficiency, and Wilson disease, have also been implicated as risk factors for HCC. Associations with hormonal manipulations, such as the use of OCPs and anabolic steroids, have been suggested but are weak and are probably better linked specifically to adenoma and well-differentiated HCC. Research has been focusing on relationships of HCC with diabetes, obesity, and metabolic syndrome.[32,36-38]

Clinical presentation. Most commonly, patients presenting with HCC are males 50 to 60 years of age who complain of right upper quadrant abdominal pain and weight loss and have a palpable mass. In countries endemic for HBV, presentation at a younger age is common and probably related to childhood infection. Unfortunately, in unscreened populations, HCC tends to be manifested at a later stage because of the lack of symptoms in early stages. Presentation at an advanced stage is often with vague right upper quadrant abdominal pain that sometimes radiates to the right shoulder. Nonspecific symptoms of advanced malignant disease, such as anorexia, nausea, lethargy, and weight loss, are also common. Another common presentation of HCC is hepatic decompensation in a patient with known mild cirrhosis or even in patients with unrecognized cirrhosis.

HCC can rarely be manifested as a rupture, with the sudden onset of abdominal pain followed by hypovolemic shock secondary to intraperitoneal bleeding. Other rare presentations include hepatic vein occlusion (Budd-Chiari syndrome), obstructive jaundice, hemobilia, and fever of unknown origin. Less than 1% of cases of HCC are manifested with a paraneoplastic syndrome, usually hypercalcemia, hypoglycemia, and erythrocytosis. Small, incidentally noted tumors have become a more common presentation because of the knowledge of specific risk factors, screening programs for diagnosed HBV or HCV infection, and increasing use of high-quality abdominal imaging.

Diagnosis. Radiologic investigation is a critical part of the diagnosis of HCC. In the past, liver radioisotope scans and angiography were common methods of diagnosis, but ultrasound, CT, and MRI have replaced these studies. Ultrasound plays a significant role in screening and early detection of HCC, but definitive diagnosis and treatment planning rely on CT or MRI. Contrast-enhanced CT and MRI protocols aimed at diagnosing HCC take advantage of the hypervascularity of these tumors, and arterial-phase images are critical to assess the extent of disease adequately. Unlike many other cancers, the diagnosis of HCC can be established based on imaging findings alone. Typical imaging criteria for HCC include rapid arterial enhancement followed by washout in the delayed phase. An enhancing capsule supports the diagnosis of HCC. CT and MRI also evaluate the extent of disease in terms of peritoneal metastases, nodal metastases, and extent of vascular and biliary involvement. Detection of bland or tumor thrombus in the portal or hepatic venous system is also important and can be diagnosed with any of these modalities (Fig. 89.33).

AFP measurements can be helpful in the diagnosis of HCC. However, AFP measurement is associated with multiple problems. First, AFP measurements have low sensitivity and specificity. The specificity and positive predictive values of AFP improve with higher cutoff levels (e.g., 400 ng/mL) but at the cost of sensitivity. False-positive elevations of serum AFP levels can be seen in inflammatory disorders of the liver, such as chronic active viral hepatitis. Furthermore, AFP is not specific to HCC and can be elevated with intrahepatic cholangiocarcinoma (IHC) and colorectal metastases. With improvements in imaging technology and the ability to detect smaller tumors, AFP is largely used as an adjunctive test in patients with liver masses. AFP levels are

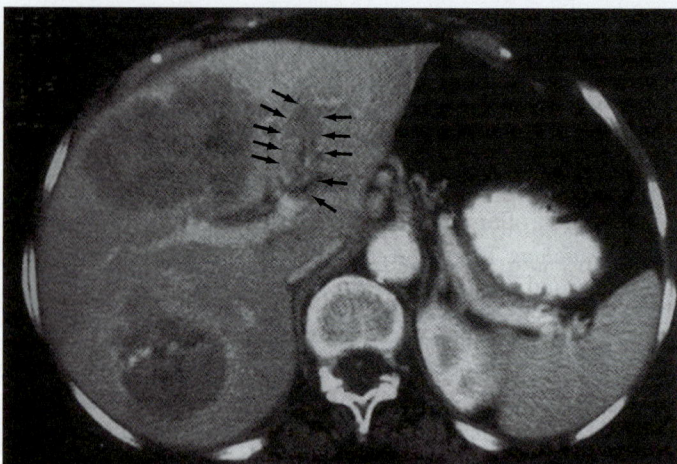

FIGURE 89.33 Contrast-enhanced computed tomography scan demonstrating multifocal hepatocellular carcinoma. The left portal vein is invaded and expanded by tumor *(arrows)*. (From Roddie ME, Adam A. Computed tomography of the liver and biliary tree. In: Blumgart LH, Fong Y, eds. *Surgery of the Liver and Biliary Tract.* London: WB Saunders; 2000:309-340.)

particularly useful in monitoring treated patients for recurrence after normalization of levels.

Since the proposal of guidelines for the diagnosis of HCC by the Barcelona-2000 European Association for the Study of the Liver conference and the American Association for the Study of Liver Disease,[39] new data have accumulated and the recommendations have evolved. AFP used to play a major role in the diagnosis of HCC larger than 2 cm.[39] However, given the excellent performance of contrast-enhanced imaging modalities, AFP does not play a critical role in the diagnosis of HCC anymore.[40,41] For hepatic nodules 1 to 2 cm in size on a background of cirrhosis, a contrast-enhanced triple-phase CT and MRI scan is now recommended.[40,41] If typical features of HCC on imaging (arterially enhancing mass with washout of contrast material in delayed phases) are observed, diagnosis of HCC is presumed. For lesions larger than 2 cm, a single study may suffice. However, for lesions 1 to 2 cm in size, contrast-enhanced CT and MRI have a sensitivity of 53% to 62%, specificity of approximately 100%, positive predictive value of 95% to 100%, and negative predictive value of 80% to 84%.[42] Performance of both MRI and CT in a sequential fashion can increase the sensitivity and may be required for difficult cases.[42]

Patients with appropriate risk factors and suggestive radiologic features, with or without an elevated AFP level, who are candidates for potentially curative surgical therapy do not require preoperative biopsy unless the diagnosis is in question. Percutaneous fine-needle aspiration of HCC does run a small risk of tumor cell spillage (estimated to be ~1%) and rupture or bleeding, especially in cirrhotic livers and subcapsular tumors. Once the diagnosis of HCC has been made, the disease must be staged to develop an appropriate treatment plan. Most patients with HCC have two diseases, and survival is as much related to the tumor as it is to cirrhosis. Staging includes extent of disease and extent of cirrhosis workup.

In assessing the extent of disease, the common sites of metastases must be considered. HCC largely metastasizes to the lung, bone, and peritoneum. Preoperative history should focus on symptoms referable to these areas. Extent of disease in the liver, including macrovascular invasion and the presence of multiple liver masses, must also be considered. Cross-sectional abdominal imaging, including arterial-phase images (see earlier), yields information on the extent of disease in the liver as well as peritoneal disease. Preoperative chest CT is mandatory because lung metastases are usually asymptomatic. Routine bone scans are not performed unless there are suggestive symptoms or signs.

Assessment of liver function is absolutely critical when considering treatment options for a patient with HCC. Liver resection is considered the treatment of choice for HCC, and the risk of postoperative liver failure and death must be considered. This risk is related to the degree of cirrhosis, portal hypertension, amount of liver resected (functional liver reserve), and regenerative potential response. Other successful treatments are available for HCC, such as ablative techniques, embolization techniques, and liver transplantation. Therefore, a complete assessment of tumor and liver function must be carried out. Several LFTs are available, generally divided into clinical assessment and functional tests, and there are many clinical assessment schemes (see earlier). However, Child-Pugh status is used most often. Child-Pugh class C patients are not candidates for resectional therapy, whereas Child-Pugh class A patients can usually tolerate some extent of liver resection. Many consider Child-Pugh class B patients to be candidates for operation, but they are generally borderline, and therapy must be individualized. Major resections are not well tolerated by a patient with class B cirrhosis.

Outside of scoring systems, it has been demonstrated that significant portal hypertension, regardless of biochemical assessments, is highly predictive of postoperative liver failure and death. Portal hypertension can be assessed directly through hepatic vein wedge pressures, but it is usually obvious on high-quality imaging in the form of splenomegaly, a cirrhotic-appearing liver, and intraabdominal varices. Blood work usually demonstrates marked cytopenias. Most typically, patients have thrombocytopenia. Functional tests of liver function have been well described but are not routinely used in most Western centers because the results of studies evaluating their predictive value have been mixed.

Laparoscopy has been used as a staging tool in HCC and spares about one in five patients a nontherapeutic laparotomy. Laparoscopy yields additional information about the extent of disease in the liver, extrahepatic disease, and cirrhosis. The yield of laparoscopy is dictated by the extent of disease and is only selectively used. The presence of clinically apparent cirrhosis, radiologic evidence of vascular invasion, or bilobar tumors increases the yield to 30%, whereas without these factors, the yield is 5%.[43]

There are a number of staging systems for HCC, but none are particularly superior; they probably depend on the specific population in which the disease is being staged as well as the cause of HCC in that particular population of patients. The tumor-node-metastasis (TNM) staging system is not routinely used for HCC because it does not accurately predict survival; it does not take liver function into account. Moreover, the TNM staging system relies on pathology that is frequently unavailable preoperatively. The Okuda staging system is an older but simple and effective system that takes liver function and tumor-related factors into account. It adds up a single point for the presence of tumor involving more than 50% of the liver, presence of ascites, albumin level less than 3 g/dL, and bilirubin level higher than 3 mg/dL. The Okuda staging system reliably distinguishes patients with a prohibitively poor prognosis from those with potential for long-term survival. The most well-validated staging system is the Cancer of the Liver Italian Program (CLIP), which was rigorously developed and prospectively

TABLE 89.7 Cancer of the Liver Italian Program Score[a]

CLINICAL PARAMETERS	CUTOFF VALUES	POINTS
Child-Pugh class	A	0
	B	1
	C	2
Tumor morphology	Uninodular, <50% extension	0
	Multinodular, <50% extension	1
	Massive or extension >50%	2
AFP level	<400 ng/dL	0
	>400 ng/dL	1
Portal vein thrombosis	No	0
	Yes	1

[a]Score ranges from 0 to 6; a score of 4 to 6 is generally considered advanced disease, whereas a score of 0 to 3 has the potential for long-term survival.
AFP, α-Fetoprotein.

validated (Table 89.7). An example of a scoring system that is probably population specific is the Chinese University Prognostic Index (CUPI), which takes into account TNM stage, symptoms, and ascites and the levels of AFP, bilirubin, and ALP; it appears to apply mainly to HBV-related HCC in China.

Pathology. On histologic evaluation, HCC is graded as well, moderately, or poorly differentiated. The grade of HCC, however, has never been shown to predict outcome accurately. In gross appearance, the growth patterns of HCC have been classified in a number of ways. The most useful scheme divides HCC into three distinct growth patterns that have specific relationships to outcome. The hanging type of HCC is connected to the liver by a small vascular stalk and is easily resected without sacrificing a significant amount of adjacent nonneoplastic liver tissue and can grow to substantial size. The pushing type of HCC is well demarcated and often contains a fibrous capsule. It is characterized by growth that displaces vascular structures rather than invading them and is usually resectable. The last type is called the infiltrative type of HCC, which tends to invade vascular structures, even at a small size. Resection of the infiltrative type is often possible, but positive histologic margins are common. Small tumors (<5 cm) usually do not fall into any of these groups and are often discussed as a separate entity.

Finally, HCC can manifest in a multifocal manner. Most HCC probably starts as a single tumor, but ultimately multiple satellite lesions can develop secondary to portal vein invasion and metastases. Multifocal tumors throughout the liver probably represent the end stage of HCC, with multiple metastases and multiple primary tumors.

Treatment. There are a large number of treatment options for patients with HCC, reflecting the heterogeneity of this disease and the lack of a proven superior treatment, except complete resection (Box 89.1). Deciding on a treatment regimen for any one patient must take into consideration the stage of malignancy, condition of the patient and of the liver, and experience of the treating physician.

Surgical Management

Resection. Complete excision of HCC by partial hepatectomy or by total hepatectomy and liver transplantation is the treatment of choice, when possible, because it has the highest chance of long-term

BOX 89.1 Treatment Options for Hepatocellular Carcinoma

Surgical
Resection
Orthotopic liver transplantation

Ablative
Ethanol injection
Acetic acid injection
Thermal ablation (cryotherapy, radiofrequency ablation, microwave)

Transarterial
Embolization
Chemoembolization

Radiotherapy
Combination transarterial and ablative: external beam radiation

Systemic
Chemotherapy
Hormonal
Immunotherapy

survival. In general, however, only 10% to 20% of patients are considered to have resectable disease. Historically, mortality rates for partial hepatectomy have ranged from 1% to 20%, but if it is performed in healthy patients without advanced cirrhosis, most series have a mortality rate of less than 5%. Advances in surgical technique have also allowed the development of limited segmental resections when appropriate, which preserves liver function and improves early postoperative recovery. Selection of the appropriate patient for resection is critical and must take into account the condition of the liver and extent of disease. Hepatic resection is indicated as a potentially curative option in patients with adequate liver function (Child-Pugh class A without portal hypertension) and solitary HCC without major vascular invasion. Patients with Child-Pugh class B or C cirrhosis or portal hypertension do not tolerate resection. The volume of the FLR is also an important consideration and is associated with postoperative complications and mortality. Preoperative PVT is an effective strategy to increase the volume and function of the FLR and should be used liberally in patients with Child-Pugh class A cirrhosis with a small FLR (i.e., <30%–40% of the total liver volume) who are being considered for a major resection. The overall postresection survival rates for HCC are 58% to 100% at 1 year, 28% to 88% at 3 years, 11% to 75% at 5 years, and 19% to 26% at 10 years. These results obviously depend on the tumor stage and degree of cirrhosis in each series. Together, they give a sense of the possibilities.

Various prognostic factors predictive of survival after resection have been identified, but none are universally agreed on. The most cited negative prognostic factors are tumor size, cirrhosis, infiltrative growth pattern, vascular invasion, intrahepatic metastases, multifocal tumors, lymph node metastases, margin less than 1 cm, and lack of a capsule. The best outcomes are found in patients with single small tumors, but size alone should not contraindicate resection. Especially for patients with large tumors that are outside the criteria for transplantation, not many therapeutic options are available. In such patients with adequate liver function, adequate functional liver remnant, and resectable tumors, surgical resection may offer the best possible outcomes. Multifocal

tumors and major vascular invasion are generally associated with a poor outcome, but some groups advocate resection in highly select patients. A randomized controlled trial corroborated these findings. In this study, patients with multifocal HCC outside Milan criteria were randomized to resection or transarterial chemoembolization.[44] In this study, resection provided better overall survival for patients with multifocal HCC compared with transarterial chemoembolization, suggesting that resection may be an option for these patients. For potentially resectable tumors that have high-risk features, various neoadjuvant strategies may help select patients for resection. For instance, a period of observation and tumor control with intraarterial therapies (e.g., transarterial chemoembolization/radioembolization) may help select patients that will benefit most from resection.

Transplantation. Theoretically, orthotopic liver transplantation is the ideal treatment for HCC because it addresses the liver dysfunction and cirrhosis and the HCC. The limitations of transplantation are the need for chronic immunosuppression and the lack of organ donors. There has been growing interest in the use of partial hepatectomy from live donors, which addresses the lack of organ donors but remains a somewhat controversial approach. Early series of transplantation for HCC had high recurrence rates and relatively poor long-term survival, largely attributed to the fact that most of these patients were undergoing transplantation for advanced disease. Refinements in patient selection—namely, patients with single tumors smaller than 5 cm or no more than three tumors 3 cm in size—have resulted in improved outcomes. Long-term survival rates with more stringent selection criteria have ranged from 50% to 85%. Studies have begun to expand the indications for orthotopic liver transplantation without a major effect on long-term survival but likely an increase in overall recurrence rates. While the enlisted patient with HCC and cirrhosis awaits organ availability, the progression of HCC is typically controlled with locoregional therapy, including ablation and transarterial therapies. Comparison of results of resection with transplantation is difficult, as the patients considered for transplantation have a period of observation during which the patients with aggressive disease progress and drop out from the transplant list. As such, these two strategies should be viewed as complementary rather than competitive. Patients with advanced cirrhosis (Child-Pugh class B and C) and early-stage HCC should be considered for transplantation, whereas those with Child-Pugh class A cirrhosis have similar results with transplantation and resection and should probably be resected.

Locoregional Therapies

Ablation. A number of other nonsurgical local ablative therapies are available for the treatment of small tumors. Percutaneous ethanol injection (PEI) is a useful technique for ablating small tumors. The tumor is killed by a combination of cellular dehydration, coagulative necrosis, and vascular thrombosis. Most tumors smaller than 2 cm can be ablated with a single application of PEI, but larger tumors may require multiple injections. Long-term survival after PEI for tumors smaller than 5 cm has been reported to range from 24% to 40%. Percutaneous injection of acetic acid is a technique similar to PEI but has stronger necrotizing abilities, making it more useful in septated tumors.

Thermal ablative techniques that freeze or heat tumors to destroy them have become popular. Cryotherapy uses a specialized cryoprobe to freeze and thaw tumor and surrounding liver tissue, with resulting necrosis. Cryotherapy is usually performed at laparotomy or laparoscopically, but it has been performed with percutaneous techniques. One advantage is that the ice ball formed is easily monitored with ultrasound. Disadvantages include a heat sink effect limiting the usefulness of freezing near major blood vessels and a relatively high complication rate of 8% to 41%. Reported 2-year survival rates for cryoablation of HCC range from 30% to 60%, but no comparative studies to resection have been carried out. Radiofrequency ablation (RFA) uses high-frequency alternating current to create heat around an inserted probe, resulting in temperatures higher than 60°C (140°F) and immediate cell death. Although initially limited to smaller tumors, technologic improvements have created RFA probes reportedly able to ablate tumors as large as 7 cm. Nonetheless, the efficacy of RFA for HCCs larger than 3 cm is limited because of increased local recurrence rates. RFA is also limited by the protective effect of blood vessels and does not ablate well in these areas. The procedure can easily be performed percutaneously, with low complication rates, and optimal guidance systems are being developed. Recent data suggest that resection may be superior to RFA for small HCCs in terms of both disease-free and overall survival.[45] Microwave ablation has emerged as a commonly used thermoablative procedure with durable disease control for small tumors.[46]

Arterially directed therapies. Transarterial therapy for HCC is based on the fact that most of the tumor's blood supply is from the hepatic artery. Today, transarterial therapy is applied in a percutaneous fashion, thus avoiding morbidity and mortality of laparotomy. Percutaneous transarterial embolization can induce ischemic necrosis in HCC, resulting in response rates as high as 50% (Fig. 89.34). Attempts to improve the efficacy of arterial embolization have included adding chemotherapeutic agents (chemoembolization) to the bland embolization particles and oils, such as ethiodized oil (Ethiodol), that are selectively taken up by HCCs. Seven randomized trials have compared embolization or chemoembolization with conservative management. Two of these trials and a meta-analysis have confirmed an overall survival advantage from the embolization strategies.[47] The selection of appropriate candidates for embolization is important, and treatment should generally be limited to patients with preserved liver function and asymptomatic multinodular tumors without vascular invasion. Poor selection will result in a higher incidence of treatment-induced liver failure, offsetting the potential benefits. Intraarterial injections of iodine-131 with Ethiodol or yttrium-90 in glass microspheres have also been used to deliver localized radiation to HCCs, with reports of dramatic response rates. Transarterial radiotherapy is a potentially promising therapy for HCC as a primary or adjuvant therapy.

Radiation. External beam radiation therapy (EBRT) has a limited role in the treatment of HCC, although occasional dramatic responses are seen. EBRT is limited by damage to normal liver parenchyma and to surrounding organs, but newer methods of conformal radiotherapy and breath-gated techniques are improving the usefulness of this treatment modality.

Systemic Therapies

Chemotherapy. Systemic chemotherapy with a variety of agents (e.g., cisplatin, doxorubicin, etoposide, 5-fluorouracil [5-FU], mitomycin C, amsacrine, mitoxantrone, picibanil, tamoxifen, uracil, VM-26) has been ineffective and has had a minimal role in the treatment of HCC. Response rates are generally below 20% and of short duration. Hormonal therapy has been used in small numbers of patients with HCC, with some early promising results, but have not yet demonstrated superiority to standard regimens.

Most recently, sorafenib, a molecular targeted therapy that inhibits the serine-threonine kinases Raf-1 and B-Raf and the receptor tyrosine kinase activity of vascular endothelial growth factor (VEGF) receptors 1, 2, and 3 and platelet-derived growth factor β, was evaluated. Llovet and colleagues[48] randomized 599 patients with advanced-stage HCC and Child-Pugh level A cirrhosis to oral sorafenib or placebo. The median overall survival was 10.7 months in the sorafenib group and 7.9 months in the placebo group ($P < 0.001$), a difference of 2.8 months. The median time to radiologic progression was 5.5 months in the sorafenib group and 2.8 months in the placebo group ($P < 0.001$), a difference of 2.7 months. Neither group demonstrated any complete responses by radiologic criteria. Although the adverse event profile of sorafenib was similar to the placebo group, this and earlier studies have shown that sorafenib is best tolerated in patients with Child-Pugh class A cirrhosis. With better understanding of the molecular pathogenesis, there is hope that novel therapeutics will be increasingly evaluated in this disease.[48]

Immunotherapy for primary liver cancers. The liver hosts a complex immune microenvironment that is naturally immunosuppressive and tolerogenic. Physiologically, this immunotolerant environment is essential for normal hepatic function as the primary metabolic organ for digested, non–self-material from the gastrointestinal tract. The environment is maintained by a host of immune cells including resident tissue macrophages (Kupffer cells), myeloid-derived suppressor cells, and regulatory T cells. Dysregulation of these cells contributes to suppression of antitumor immune cells, such as CD8+ T cells, creating a milieu that is predisposed to hepatocarcinogenesis and metastasis. Reactivation of these antitumor immune cells is the primary goal of immunotherapy.[49]

Immunotherapy plays a major role in the treatment of advanced primary liver cancers. Although vaccine and cellular-based therapies are in clinical development, immune checkpoint inhibitors (ICIs) targeting programmed cell death 1 (PD-1), programmed cell death ligand 1 (PD-L1), and cytotoxic T-lymphocyte–associated protein 4 (CTLA-4) are mainstays of treatment for HCC and biliary tract cancers (BTCs). Used in combination with antiangiogenic agents (anti-VEGF), tyrosine kinase inhibitors, and traditional cytotoxic chemotherapies such as gemcitabine and cisplatin, ICI therapy is now used in the first-line setting for HCC and BTC. The approved PD-1, PD-L1, and CTLA-4 inhibitors for HCC and BTCs are listed in Table 89.8.

As described elsewhere in this chapter, HCC most commonly develops in the setting of chronic hepatic inflammation. This chronic inflammation leads to dysregulation of the immunologic network through sustained hepatocellular DNA damage and cell death, compensatory hepatic regeneration, and liver fibrosis. Persistent viral infection and nonviral chronic liver diseases such as nonalcoholic fatty liver disease (NAFLD)/NASH and alcoholic

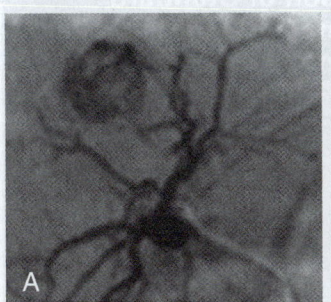
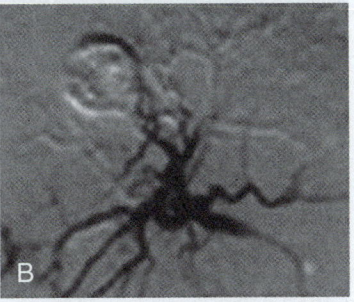

FIGURE 89.34 Angiograms demonstrating hypervascular hepatocellular carcinoma before (A) and after (B) embolization.

TABLE 89.8 Immunotherapy Options for HCC and Cholangiocarcinoma

DRUG	TARGET	HCC	BILIARY TRACT CANCERS	REFERENCE TRIAL
Atezolizumab	PD-L1	1L for advanced/unresectable disease (combined with bevacizumab)	n/a	HCC - IMbrave150
Dostarlimab	PD-1	2L for advanced/unresectable disease (monotherapy)	2L for metastatic/unresectable disease (MSI-H tumors)	HCC - GARNET Study
Durvalumab	PD-L1	1L for advanced/unresectable disease (monotherapy or combined with tremelimumab)	1L for metastatic/unresectable disease (combined with gemcitabine, cisplatin)	HCC - HIMALAYA Cholangiocarcinoma - TOPAZ
Ipilimumab	CTLA-4	2L for advanced/unresectable disease (combined with nivolumab)	2L for metastatic/unresectable disease (combined with nivolumab in MSI-H tumors)	HCC - Checkmate 040 trial
Nivolumab	PD-1	2L for advanced/unresectable disease (monotherapy or combined with ipilimumab)	2L for metastatic/unresectable disease (monotherapy, combined with ipilimumab in MSI-H tumors)	HCC - Checkmate 040 trial Cholangiocarcinoma
Pembrolizumab	PD-1	2L for advanced/unresectable disease secondary to HBV (monotherapy)	1L for metastatic/unresectable disease (combined with gemcitabine, cisplatin)	HCC - KEYNOTE-224, KEYNOTE-240, KEYNOTE-394 Cholangiocarcinoma – KEYNOTE-966
Tremelimumab	CTLA-4	1L for advanced/unresectable disease (combined with durvalumab)	n/a	HCC – HIMALAYA

1L, First-line; *2L,* second/subsequent-line; *CTLA-4,* cytotoxic T-lymphocyte–associated protein 4; *HCC,* hepatocellular carcinoma; *MSI-H,* microsatellite instability, high; *PD-1,* programmed cell death 1; *PD-L1,* programmed cell death ligand 1.

steatohepatitis (ASH) induce liver inflammation and uniquely affect the liver immune microenvironment, which significantly influences the efficacy of immunotherapy. Indeed, nonviral-induced HCC is associated with worse responses to ICI. In a meta-analysis of the three large studies evaluating ICI in treatment of HCC, patients with NAFLD/NASH did not respond to ICI; therefore, ICI treatment selection based on etiology of HCC has been advocated.[50]

BTC arises in a desmoplastic tumor microenvironment with a heterogeneous, immunosuppressive cellular milieu. Cancer-associated fibroblasts, tumor-associated macrophages, and myeloid-derived suppressor cells are abundant in the tumor microenvironment and function to exclude and exhaust antitumor T cells. Pharmacologic modification of this microenvironment with ICI has proven efficacious in a subset of patients with BTC in combination with gemcitabine and cisplatin. Along with identification of targetable mutations in BTC (i.e., IDH1, FGFR), the systemic therapeutic options for treatment of BTC are rapidly evolving.

Postoperative adjuvant treatment. Currently, there is no definitive recommendation for adjuvant treatment after HCC resection. This is largely because of a lack of effective chemotherapy for HCC. In a phase III double-blind placebo-controlled study evaluating the efficacy of sorafenib in decreasing recurrence of HCC in patients who underwent complete radiologic response after resection or ablation, sorafenib treatment was not able to decrease recurrence.[51] However, antiviral treatment in patients with HBV infection has been shown to decrease the risk of HCC recurrence and HCC-related deaths.[52,53] With availability of newer and effective antivirals for treatment of HCV, similar results are hoped for in patients infected with this virus. Although a lower level of evidence does suggest that sustained viral response is associated with improved overall survival and better recurrence-free survival after resection or locoregional therapy for HCV-related HCC, this needs to be confirmed in better-designed trials. A recent trial (IMbrave 050 trial) demonstrated adjuvant atezolizumab plus bevacizumab provided a benefit in recurrence-free survival but not overall survival in patients with a high risk of

relapse after resection or local ablation.[54] Combinations of immunotherapy, small molecule therapies, and chemotherapies continue to be tested in this setting.

Distinct variants of hepatocellular carcinoma. Fibrolamellar HCC[55] is a variant of HCC with remarkably different clinical features, summarized in Table 89.9. This tumor generally occurs in younger patients without a history of cirrhosis. The tumor is usually well demarcated and encapsulated and may have a central fibrotic area. The central scar can make distinguishing this tumor from FNH difficult. On histologic evaluation, fibrolamellar HCC is composed of large polygonal tumor cells embedded in a fibrous stroma, forming lamellar structures (Fig. 89.35). Fibrolamellar HCC does not produce AFP but is associated with elevated neurotensin levels. In general, fibrolamellar HCC has a better prognosis than HCC, probably related to high resectability rates, lack of chronic liver disease, and a more indolent course (see Table 89.9). Long-term survival can be expected in approximately 50% to 75% of patients after complete resection, but recurrence is common and occurs in at least 80% of patients. The presence of lymph node metastases predicts a worse outcome. Resection of lymph node metastases and recurrent disease has been advocated because of a lack of alternative therapy and the possibility

TABLE 89.9 Comparison of Standard Hepatocellular Carcinoma and Fibrolamellar Hepatocellular Carcinoma

PARAMETER	HCC	FIBROLAMELLAR HCC
Male-to-female ratio	2:1–8:1	1:1
Median age	55 years	25 years
Tumor	Invasive	Well circumscribed
Resectability	<25%	50%–75%
Cirrhosis	90%	5%
AFP positive	80%	5%
Hepatitis B positive	65%	5%

AFP, α-Fetoprotein; *HCC,* hepatocellular carcinoma.

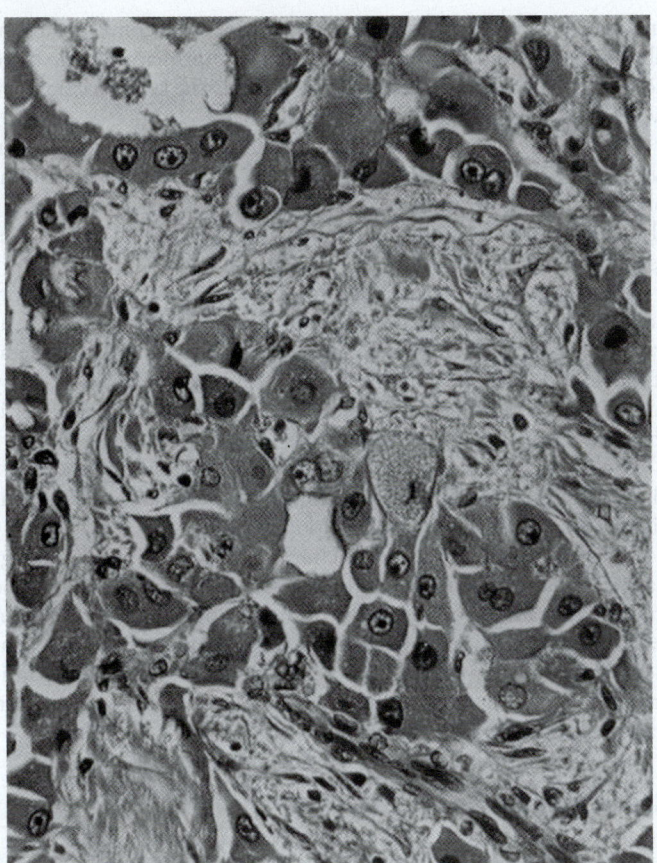

FIGURE 89.35 Fibrolamellar hepatocellular carcinoma. Abundant collagen is evident interconnecting clusters of cells. The cells are often in single-layer sheets. An acinus is present in the left upper field.

of long-term survival. A study identified a chimeric transcript that is expressed in fibrolamellar HCC but not in the adjacent normal liver.[56] The study also suggested that this transcript codes for a chimeric protein containing the catalytic domain of protein kinase A, thus suggesting that this gain of kinase activity may have a role in the pathogenesis of fibrolamellar HCC. Elucidation of such novel processes can lead to development of novel targeted therapies against this disease, which typically strikes young, healthy people.

Rarely, HCC can manifest as a mixed hepatocellular-cholangiocellular tumor, with cellular differentiation of both types present. Whether this is two separate tumors growing into each other or mixed differentiation of the same tumor is not known. These mixed tumors tend to have a prognosis that is worse than for standard HCC but better than expected for IHC.

A clear cell variant of HCC also exists, in which the cells contain a clear cytoplasm. These tumors can resemble renal cell neoplasms. The clear cell variant may have a better prognosis than standard HCC, but this is debatable. A pleomorphic or giant cell variant of HCC has also been reported. Cells of this type are multinucleated, pleomorphic, and large and likely to originate from primary hepatic cells. Some HCCs show evidence of sarcomatoid differentiation and are referred to as a *sarcomatoid variant* or *carcinosarcoma*. These tumors tend not to produce AFP and have a higher incidence of metastases at presentation.

Childhood HCC is a distinct entity that represents almost 25% of pediatric liver tumors but rarely occurs in infancy. Viral hepatitis is associated with childhood HCC in Asia but less so in

the United States. Other inherited metabolic liver diseases (see earlier) are often associated with childhood HCC. As in adult HCC, complete resection is the only potentially curative treatment. There is a high incidence of multifocality, vascular invasion, and extrahepatic metastases, resulting in relatively poor long-term survival rates of 10% to 20%.

Intrahepatic Cholangiocarcinoma

Cholangiocarcinoma is an uncommon neoplasm, with an incidence of 1 to 2/100,000 in the United States, and can develop anywhere along the biliary tree, from the ampulla of Vater to the peripheral intrahepatic bile ducts. Most of these tumors (40%–60%) involve the biliary confluence (Klatskin tumor), but approximately 10% emanate from intrahepatic ducts and are known as IHC. IHC is the second most common primary hepatic neoplasm. Studies on the incidence and natural history of IHC have been confused by the fact that in the past, many of these tumors were mistaken for metastatic adenocarcinoma because biopsy is unable to differentiate the two.

IHC is associated with diseases that cause biliary inflammation and fibrosis. Historically, the most common risk factors for the development of cholangiocarcinoma (all types) were primary sclerosing cholangitis, choledochal cyst disease, hepatolithiasis,[57] and RPC. Recent epidemiologic evidence has now linked IHC to HBV infection,[58] HCV infection, cirrhosis, NASH, and diabetes.[59] Increases in the diagnosis of IHC in the United States are likely related to better recognition of the disease, changed classification, and perhaps the rise in HCV infections in the 1960s and 1970s.

The clinical presentation of IHC is similar to that of HCC. These tumors are asymptomatic in early stages. When present, the most common symptoms are right upper abdominal pain and weight loss. Jaundice occurs less commonly, as these tumors tend to arise in the periphery of the liver. More commonly, patients present with incidentally found liver masses on cross-sectional imaging. Unlike in HCC, the AFP levels are normal, although CEA or carbohydrate antigen 19-9 (CA 19-9) levels can be elevated in some cases. Because metastatic adenocarcinoma to liver is more common, IHC is a diagnosis of exclusion, and a search for a primary tumor with upper and lower gastrointestinal endoscopy and cross-sectional imaging of the chest, abdomen, and pelvis should be carried out. If a biopsy has been performed, it is often read as adenocarcinoma. Although special stains may suggest diagnosis of IHC, they are not conclusive. On CT and MRI, IHC is seen as a focal hepatic mass that may be associated with peripheral biliary dilation. The mass typically has peripheral or central enhancement on contrast-enhanced scans. Furthermore, unlike HCC, there is persistent enhancement on delayed phases because of the fibrotic nature of cholangiocarcinoma, in contrast with the vascular nature of HCC. Hepatic capsular retraction is also frequently observed. Intrahepatic metastases, lymph node metastases, and growth along the biliary tree are often encountered.

Complete resection is the treatment of choice for IHC. The concept of optimal surgical margins in the treatment of IHC is evolving. However, surgeons should strive for R0 margins. Because of large tumor size and invasion into the surrounding structures, major hepatectomies with or without resection of surrounding organs may be required for achieving a margin-negative resection. Resectability rates generally range up to 60%, and long-term survival in unresected patients is rare. If it is completely resected, 3-year survival rates range from 16% to 61%, and 5-year survival rates range from 24% to 44%. Factors associated with a poor outcome include multifocality, lymph node metastases, vascular invasion, and positive margins. These factors have now been included in the American Joint Committee on Cancer (AJCC) staging system. A review of prospectively evaluated patients with IHC who underwent resection suggested that although patients with R0 resection did better when compared with R1 resection, width of margin did not influence outcomes. Because of the rarity of IHC, little is known about the effectiveness of radiation therapy and chemotherapy in the adjuvant setting. Thus, their application is not routine.

Use of chemotherapy as an adjuvant strategy is controversial. Because of the overall low incidence of biliary cancers, studies of adjuvant therapy have typically grouped various disease sites to include both intrahepatic and extrahepatic cholangiocarcinoma as well as gallbladder cancer. In a recently reported clinical trial from the United Kingdom (phase III BILCAP study), patients with completely resected gallbladder and cholangiocarcinoma were randomized to receive adjuvant capecitabine or observation. Although on intention-to-treat analysis, adjuvant capecitabine did not improve survival, when comparing patients who received adjuvant therapy per protocol, adjuvant capecitabine was associated with 25% reduced risk of death. Retrospective studies have provided conflicting evidence regarding the benefits of adjuvant therapy. Regional hepatic artery chemotherapy is currently under study and may be a promising approach.

For nonresectable disease, combination chemotherapy of gemcitabine and cisplatin and the anti–PD-L1 agent durvalumab has been considered the most effective first-line regimen (see Table 89.8).[60]

This regimen is often used in the adjuvant setting for patients at high risk for recurrence or in attempts to downstage patients with initially unresectable disease to resectable.

Other Primary Malignant Neoplasms

Hepatoblastoma is the most common primary hepatic tumor of childhood. There are approximately 50 to 70 new cases per year in the United States. Rare cases of adult hepatoblastoma have been reported, but overall, the median age at presentation is 18 months, and almost all cases occur before the age of 3 years. Hepatoblastoma has been associated with familial polyposis syndrome. There are several histologic subtypes, but in general, the tumor is derived from fetal or embryonic hepatocytic progenitors, and mesenchymal elements are often present. This tumor generally is manifested as an asymptomatic mass. Mild anemia and thrombocytosis are commonly found at presentation. Serum AFP levels are elevated in 85% to 90% of patients and can serve as a useful marker for therapeutic response. Most studies have supported the use of chemotherapy followed by resection, and survival appears to be dependent on complete resection. Chemotherapy can serve to downstage tumors, which facilitates resection. In patients without metastatic disease or the anaplastic variant, long-term survival rates of 60% to 70% can be expected with complete resection. Interestingly, 50% of patients with pulmonary metastases can be cured with resection of the hepatic tumor and chemotherapy or resection of the pulmonary metastases.

A variety of sarcomas can rarely be manifested as primary liver tumors, but they must always be considered metastatic lesions until proven otherwise. Angiosarcoma is probably the best-described primary hepatic sarcoma because of its well-known association with vinyl chloride or Thorotrast exposure. Angiosarcoma typically manifests as multiple hepatic masses and can appear in childhood. Long-term survival is uncommon with primary hepatic angiosarcoma. Other sarcomas, including leiomyosarcoma, malignant fibrous histiocytoma, embryonic sarcoma, and primary hepatic rhabdoid tumors, have been described but are rare. The last two lesions are typically seen in the pediatric population.

Non-Hodgkin lymphoma can manifest primarily in the liver, with or without extrahepatic disease. Primary hepatic lymphoma should be treated in the same manner as lymphoma elsewhere in the body if the diagnosis can be made before a liver resection.

Primary hepatic neuroendocrine tumors or carcinoid tumors have been described but are probably extremely rare. Distinguishing the rare primary hepatic neuroendocrine tumor from a metastatic lesion can be difficult because the extrahepatic primary tumor can be radiologically occult for many years, and the liver is the most common site of metastases.

Malignant germ cell tumors of the liver, including teratomas, choriocarcinomas, and yolk sac tumors, are very rare and are principally described in the pediatric population.

Epithelioid hemangioendothelioma of the liver is a rare malignant vascular tumor that manifests with multiple bilateral hepatic masses. Extrahepatic metastases occur in approximately 25% of patients, and clinical behavior is unpredictable, with some patients having a prolonged indolent course. Most patients ultimately die of liver failure, but cases of successful transplantation have been reported.

Cystic Neoplasms

Simple Cyst

Simple cysts of the liver contain serous fluid, do not communicate with the biliary tree, and do not have septations. They are generally spherical or ovoid and can be as large as 20 cm. Large cysts can compress normal liver, inducing regional atrophy and sometimes compensatory contralateral hypertrophy. In 50% of cases, the cysts are singular. On histologic evaluation, a single layer of cuboidal or columnar cells without atypia lines these cysts. Simple cysts are generally regarded as congenital malformations.

Simple cysts are a relatively common finding in adults and are mostly asymptomatic incidental radiologic findings. On occasion, a large cyst will cause symptoms. Although CT demonstrates anatomic relationships, ultrasound is a helpful test of choice to confirm a single thin-walled simple cyst. Hydatid disease, cystadenoma, and metastatic neuroendocrine tumor are the most important differential diagnoses to consider. A thick or nodular wall raises the suspicion of a cystadenoma but can also represent hemorrhage within the cyst. The most common complication is intracystic bleeding, but overall, complications are rare. The treatment of simple hepatic cysts is indicated only if they are symptomatic or there is diagnostic uncertainty. Because most cysts are asymptomatic, a thorough evaluation of the cause of the symptoms must be carried out before attributing them to the cyst. Nonsurgical treatment consists of aspiration and injection of a sclerosing agent. Few studies have documented long-term follow-up of sclerotherapy for hepatic cysts. Surgical therapy is achieved by fenestration or unroofing of the portion of the cyst that is extrahepatic. This can be performed at laparotomy with good long-term results or through laparoscopic approaches. The laparoscopic approach is favored, but long-term efficacy has not been well documented. A meta-analysis including nine retrospective case-control studies involving 657 patients comparing laparoscopic fenestration with the open approach demonstrated that the laparoscopic approach was associated with shorter operative time, shorter hospital stay, and less operative blood loss with no difference in cyst recurrence rates.[61]

Cystadenoma and Cystadenocarcinoma

Cystadenoma of the liver is a rare neoplasm that generally is manifested as a large cystic mass, usually 10 to 20 cm. The cyst has a globular external surface with multiple protruding cysts and locules of various sizes. The fluid contained in these cysts is usually mucinous. On microscopic examination, atypical cuboidal or columnar cells resting on a basement membrane, with ovarian-like stroma, line the cysts. The epithelium often forms polypoid or papillary projections.

Cystadenoma of the liver mainly affects females older than 40 years. Although many cystadenomas are asymptomatic, symptoms can include abdominal pain, anorexia, nausea, and abdominal distention. The diagnosis is usually suspected by a combination of cross-sectional imaging (CT or MRI) and ultrasound. Ultrasound usually demonstrates a cystic structure with varying wall thickness, nodularity, septations, and fluid-filled locules. Importantly, contrast-enhanced CT demonstrates enhancement of the cyst wall and septa. Hydatid disease must always be considered in the differential diagnosis. Cystadenomas tend to grow slowly but can eventually progress to their malignant counterpart, cystadenocarcinomas.

Cystadenocarcinoma is an extremely rare malignant neoplasm with little documentation of its natural history and outcome after resection. Malignant degeneration is typically suggested on imaging, with large projections and a markedly thickened wall. The treatment of cystadenoma or cystadenocarcinoma is complete excision, which can be done with an enucleation if there is no evidence of invasive malignant disease. Incomplete resection risks recurrence or the development of cystadenocarcinoma.

Polycystic Liver Disease

Liver cysts are commonly seen in patients with the autosomal dominant inherited adult polycystic kidney disease.[62] The cysts are histologically similar to simple cysts (see earlier). The main difference between the two entities is the number of cysts. When liver cysts are present in patients with adult polycystic kidney disease, they are always multiple in number. Also, there are usually numerous microscopic hepatic cysts as well as the grossly visible macrocysts. Despite the large number of liver cysts, hepatic parenchyma and function are usually preserved. When polycystic liver disease is associated with polycystic kidney disease, liver cysts are always preceded by kidney cysts, and their prevalence in adult polycystic kidney disease increases with age. Molecular diagnostic tests of autosomal dominant mutations causing the disease (PKD1 and PKD2) can be used to confirm the clinical diagnosis. In those younger than 20 years, the prevalence of liver cysts is 0%, whereas in those older than 60 years, it is 80%.

Liver cysts in patients with adult polycystic kidney disease are generally asymptomatic, but in a few patients, numerous large cysts may cause abdominal pain and distention. LFT results are almost always normal. Rare complications can occur; these include infection and intracystic bleeding. Ultrasound and CT reveal multiple simple cysts throughout the liver and kidneys. Treatment of polycystic liver disease is reserved for severe symptoms related to large cysts and complications. Treatment includes percutaneous aspiration with or without sclerotherapy, cyst fenestration (by laparotomy or laparoscopy), hepatic resection, and orthotopic liver transplantation. Liver transplantation is used only with progressive disease after fenestration or resection with liver or renal dysfunction.

In the context of renal failure, a combined kidney and liver transplantation may be appropriate.

Bile Duct Cysts

Bile duct cysts or choledochal cysts are congenital dilations of the biliary tree that are usually diagnosed in childhood but can present in adulthood. Because of the risk of malignancy and recurrent cholangitis, treatment is excision with reestablishment of biliary-enteric continuity. Most bile duct cysts involve the extrahepatic biliary tree, but in type IV cysts, there is involvement of the extrahepatic bile duct and intrahepatic ducts. In contrast, Caroli disease (type V) is characterized by multiple intrahepatic cysts. Thus, bile duct cysts must be considered in the differential diagnosis of a patient with multiple hepatic cystic lesions. The intrahepatic lesions of type IV bile duct cysts and Caroli disease are multifocal dilations of the segmental bile ducts separated by portions of normal-caliber bile ducts. Approximately 50% of cases of Caroli disease are associated with congenital hepatic fibrosis; the cysts are diffusely located throughout the liver. In the other 50% of cases, the dilations may be confined to a portion of the liver, usually the left hemiliver. Recurrent bacterial cholangitis usually dominates the clinical course of these diseases, and death generally ensues within 5 to 10 years without adequate treatment. When intrahepatic bile duct cysts are localized, hepatic resection, with or without biliary reconstruction, is the treatment of choice. Treatment of diffuse hepatic involvement is poor; in complicated cases, the only probably effective treatment is transplantation.

Principles of Hepatic Resection

Although liver resections were performed in the late 1800s, it was not until 1952 that Lortat-Jacob was given credit for the first true anatomic right hepatectomy. This event ushered in the modern era of hepatic surgery. However, early series were plagued by high morbidity and mortality, which were largely related to massive intraoperative blood loss. Series from the 1970s and 1980s often reported mortality rates in excess of 10%, often as high as 20%, especially for major resections. This high mortality limited the use of liver resection, and there was reluctance to refer patients for such operations. During the past three decades, a number of advances have improved perioperative outcomes dramatically for patients undergoing major hepatic surgery. The understanding that most blood loss during a liver resection comes from the hepatic veins has prompted surgeons to perform these operations with a low central venous pressure. We perform partial hepatectomy with a central line in place, with the patient in a mild Trendelenburg position, and fluid restriction and venodilators if necessary to maintain a central venous pressure lower than 5 mm Hg. The other major advance has been an improved understanding of the segmental anatomy of the liver, making intrahepatic dissection safer and more precise. There are numerous techniques to transect liver tissue and many methods to coagulate and to control vessels. The most important concept, however, is that dividing liver tissue is a dissection done by a surgeon with complete understanding of the liver's vascular anatomy.

In experienced centers, perioperative mortality is routinely 5% or less and depends on a number of factors. The three most critical factors related to perioperative morbidity are blood loss, the amount of normal liver resected, and the condition of the liver itself (e.g., cirrhosis). A partial hepatectomy must be performed with these factors in mind to minimize morbidity. In a review of more than 1800 liver resections during a 10-year period from MSKCC, the operative mortality was 3.1%.[63] The median blood loss was 600 mL, and two-thirds of patients did not require a red blood cell transfusion. Overall, postoperative morbidity was 45%, but the median hospital stay was 8 days. Morbidity was mostly related to blood loss and the extent of resection. Minor resections were associated with a mortality of 1%. Most complications and deaths were seen in complex biliary tumors, people with cirrhosis and HCC, and extensive resections. Improving outcomes after partial hepatectomy continues, and experienced hepatobiliary centers have reported mortality rates that approach 1% to 2%, with fewer patients now requiring perioperative blood transfusions. As a result of the increasing safety of hepatic surgery, liver resection has become the treatment of choice for many malignant and benign hepatic conditions.

Bile leaks are a problem in cases requiring complex biliary reconstruction but can also occur in approximately 10% to 20% of hepatectomies without biliary reconstruction. Careful ligation of biliary radicals is of obvious importance in minimizing this complication. Because of the regenerative capacity of the liver, resections of up to 80% of normal noncirrhotic livers can be performed, with functional compensation within a few weeks. Because many resections encompass tumors and normal liver, the concepts of functional liver parenchyma and FLR volume are important because there is often compensatory hypertrophy of normal liver when tumors occupy a significant amount of the liver volume. The risk of hepatic dysfunction is minimal if the reduction of functional liver parenchyma is less than 50% but begins to rise when this figure approaches 20% to 25%. Patients with cirrhosis have much higher rates of postoperative liver dysfunction because of impaired regenerative capacity and impaired primary liver function. Liver failure, extrahepatic multiorgan failure, and death are serious hazards to performance of major liver resections in patients with cirrhosis. In general, patients with Child-Pugh class B or C cirrhosis or portal hypertension do not tolerate liver resections, and selection of patients is therefore critical. Ascites and infectious complications are also common problems after major liver resection. One strategy to minimize postoperative liver dysfunction and morbidity after major hepatectomy is to embolize the portal vein percutaneously on the side of the liver to be resected. In approximately 4 weeks, this induces atrophy of the liver parenchyma to be resected and hypertrophy of the FLR. In turn, this increases the relative volume of the FLR.

Techniques of liver resection differ according to the disease being treated. In benign hepatic diseases requiring resection, the indications for operation are usually symptoms or infection. Removal of normal liver should be kept to a minimum in these cases, and techniques such as enucleation are appropriate, although a major resection is occasionally necessary. For malignant

disease, a margin of normal tissue is important, and formal anatomic resections yield the best results. Techniques such as wedge resection often result in higher rates of margin involvement and disease recurrence and should therefore be used carefully and sparingly. It must be noted that for colorectal liver metastases, parenchymal-sparing nonanatomic resection provides comparable oncologic outcomes with marked reduction in complications when compared with major hepatic resections.

Detailed knowledge of liver anatomy is essential to the practice of safe hepatic surgery (see earlier). Unfortunately, detailed and complicated descriptions of liver anatomy and common liver resections can be confusing to the student. A 2000 consensus conference conducted in Brisbane, Australia, with the assistance of the Americas Hepato-Pancreato-Biliary Association has published guidelines for this terminology (Table 89.10 and Fig. 89.36). In general, the term *lobectomy* is not preferred because there are no external markings on the liver denoting a lobe. When in doubt, one should always revert to the numeric segments of the liver if there is any confusion about the description of a liver resection. Recall that the right liver is composed of segments V through VIII, and *right hepatectomy* and *right hemihepatectomy* are appropriate terms for resection of these segments. Segments II through IV compose the left liver, and *left hepatectomy* and *left hemihepatectomy* are appropriate terms for resection of these segments. A right hepatectomy can be extended farther to the left to include segment IV, and a left hepatectomy can be extended farther to the right to include segments V and VIII. Terms such as *extended right-left hepatectomy*, *right-left trisectionectomy*, and *trisegmentectomy* are appropriate to describe these resections. Resection of segments II and III is a commonly performed sublobar resection and is often referred to as a *left lateral segmentectomy* or *left lateral sectionectomy*. Other common sublobar resections, such as that of the right posterior sector (segments VI and VII) or the right anterior sector (segments V and VIII), are referred to as a *right posterior sectorectomy-sectionectomy* and *right anterior sectorectomy-sectionectomy*, respectively. Single or bisegmental resections can always be simply referred to by a numeric description of the segments to be resected.

A detailed discussion of the techniques of liver resection is beyond the scope of this chapter; in general, it requires specialty training, but general principles can be discussed. A liver resection must consider the disease to be treated and the goal of the operation, whether that is a margin-negative resection of a malignant neoplasm or the removal of benign tissue to alleviate symptoms. The most basic steps can be distilled down to inflow control (portal vein, hepatic artery, bile duct), outflow control (hepatic veins), and parenchymal transection, with preservation of a liver remnant

TABLE 89.10	Nomenclature for Most Common Major Anatomic Hepatic Resections[a]		
SEGMENTS[b]	**COUINAUD, 1957**	**GOLDSMITH AND WOODBURNE, 1957**	**BRISBANE, 2000**
V–VIII	Right hepatectomy	Right hepatic lobectomy	Right hemihepatectomy
IV–VIII[c]	Right lobectomy	Extended right hepatic lobectomy	Right trisectionectomy
II–IV	Left hepatectomy	Left hepatic lobectomy	Left hemihepatectomy
II, III	Left lobectomy	Left lateral segmentectomy	Left lateral sectionectomy
II, III, IV, V, VIII[c]	Extended left hepatectomy	Extended left lobectomy	Left trisectionectomy

[a]The original terminology is based on the anatomic descriptions of Couinaud and of Goldsmith and Woodburne.
[b]See Figure 89.5.
[c]Another common name for these operations is right or left trisegmentectomy.
Adapted from the Terminology Committee of the International Hepato-Pancreatico-Biliary Association: The Brisbane 2000 Terminology of Liver Anatomy and Resections, 2000. http://www.ahpba.org/assets/documents/Brisbane_Article.pdf.

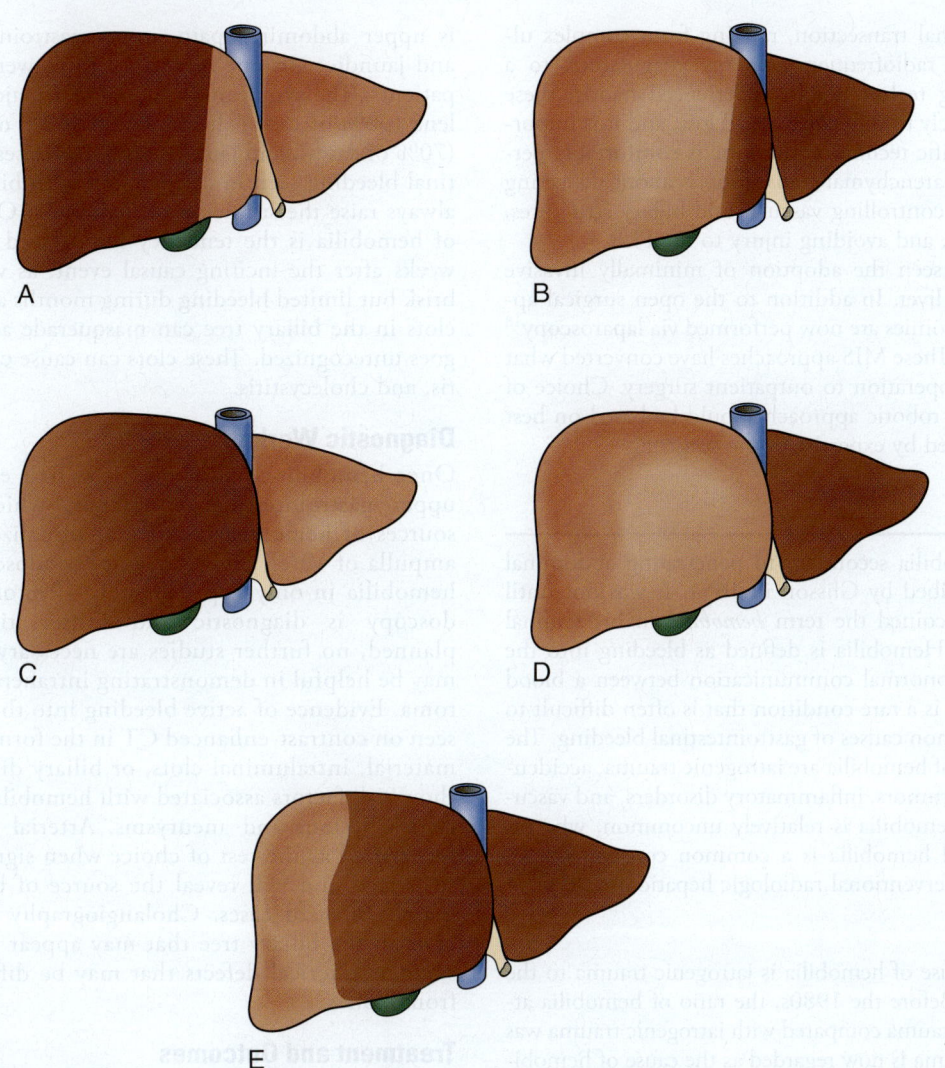

FIGURE 89.36 Commonly performed major hepatic resections are indicated by the *shaded areas*. (A) Right hepatectomy, right hepatic lobectomy, or right hemihepatectomy (segments V–VIII). (B) Left hepatectomy, left hepatic lobectomy, or left hemihepatectomy (segments II–IV). (C) Right lobectomy, extended right hepatic lobectomy, or right trisectionectomy (trisegmentectomy; segments IV–VIII). (D) Left lobectomy, left lateral segmentectomy, or left lateral sectionectomy (segments II–III). (E) Extended left hepatectomy, extended left lobectomy, or left trisectionectomy (trisegmentectomy; segments II–V and VIII). See Table 54.11. (From Blumgart LH, Jarnagin W, Fong Y. Liver resection for benign disease and for liver and biliary tumors. In: Blumgart LH, Fong Y, eds. *Surgery of the Liver and Biliary Tract*. London: WB Saunders; 2000:1639-1714.)

of adequate size with intact inflow, biliary drainage, and venous outflow.

The most common approach to an anatomic resection, in the most common order, is mobilization of the liver to be resected, dissection of inflow and outflow structures, division of the inflow, division of the outflow, and parenchymal transection. Mobilization of the liver involves division of the right or left triangular ligaments, freeing up the liver from the diaphragm. Often, the liver must be mobilized completely off the vena cava, which it straddles, and this requires careful dissection and division of multiple retrohepatic caval venous branches. For major resections, the hepatic vein of the resected portion of liver is often encircled before the resection. There are various techniques to dissect, control, and divide inflow vessels. Classic inflow control is obtained by dissection of the liver hilum, with control of the portal vein and hepatic artery to the hemiliver to be resected. These can be suture

ligated or divided with vascular staplers. Unless tumor proximity mandates, we advocate dividing the bile duct within the liver substance to minimize absolutely contralateral biliary injuries related to anatomic anomalies. Inflow control can also be obtained by dissection of the intrahepatic inflow pedicle to the anatomic section of liver to be resected. Recall that the inflow structures invaginate peritoneum at the hepatic hilum and run intrahepatically as an invested pedicle of the three inflow structures. The inflow pedicles can be encircled by making flanking hepatotomies or by splitting parenchyma down to the pedicle of interest. The pedicle can usually be divided with a vascular stapler, but suture ligation is sometimes necessary. Typically, the hepatic vein is divided in its extrahepatic position, which can also usually be done with a vascular stapler.

The hepatic vein can also be divided within the substance of the liver during parenchymal transection. There are a number of methods of parenchymal transection, ranging from complex ultrasonic irrigators, to radiofrequency energy coagulators, to a simple clamp-crushing technique. In experienced hands, these can all be used effectively to minimize blood loss, and it is important to develop a specific technique that one is comfortable performing. Ultimately, parenchymal transection is about dissecting intrahepatic anatomy, controlling vascular and biliary structures, minimizing blood loss, and avoiding injury to the FLR.

Recent years have seen the adoption of minimally invasive surgery (MIS) for the liver. In addition to the open surgical approach, many hepatectomies are now performed via laparoscopy[18] or robotic assistance.[1] These MIS approaches have converted what once was a daunting operation to outpatient surgery. Choice of open, laparoscopic, or robotic approach should be based on best patient outcome, guided by expertise of the surgeon.

HEMOBILIA

A case of lethal hemobilia secondary to penetrating abdominal trauma was first described by Glisson in 1654. It was not until 1948 that Sandblom coined the term *hemobilia* in his seminal paper on the subject. Hemobilia is defined as bleeding into the biliary tree from an abnormal communication between a blood vessel and bile duct. It is a rare condition that is often difficult to distinguish from common causes of gastrointestinal bleeding. The most common causes of hemobilia are iatrogenic trauma, accidental trauma, gallstones, tumors, inflammatory disorders, and vascular disorders. Major hemobilia is relatively uncommon, whereas minor inconsequential hemobilia is a common consequence of gallstone disease or interventional radiologic hepatic procedures.

Causes

The most common cause of hemobilia is iatrogenic trauma to the liver and biliary tree. Before the 1980s, the ratio of hemobilia attributed to accidental trauma compared with iatrogenic trauma was 2:1, but iatrogenic trauma is now regarded as the cause of hemobilia in 40% to 60% of cases. Percutaneous liver biopsy results in hemobilia in less than 1% of cases, but percutaneous transhepatic biliary drainage procedures have an incidence of 2% to 10%. Similarly, surgical exploration of the biliary tree can result in hemobilia from direct injury or arterial pseudoaneurysm. A number of cases of hemobilia after cholecystectomy have been reported. Hemobilia secondary to accidental trauma is more common with blunt than with penetrating abdominal trauma and occurs with a reported incidence of 0.2% to 3%. Risk factors for the development of hemobilia after accidental trauma are central hepatic rupture with a cavity, the use of packs, and inadequate drainage. The gallbladder can be a source of bleeding from trauma, gallstones, or acalculous cholecystitis. Primary vascular diseases, such as aneurysms, angiodysplasia, and hemangiomas, are rare causes of hemobilia. Malignant tumors of the liver, biliary tree, gallbladder, and pancreas as well as parasitic infections, hepatic abscesses, and cholangitis are uncommon causes of hemobilia.

Clinical Presentation

Portal venous bleeding into the biliary tree is rare and often self-limited unless the portal pressure is elevated. Minor hemobilia generally runs an uneventful asymptomatic clinical course. However, arterial hemobilia, the most common source, can be dramatic. Clinical sequelae of hemobilia are related to blood loss and the formation of potentially occlusive blood clots in the biliary tree. The classic triad of symptoms and signs of hemobilia

is upper abdominal pain, upper gastrointestinal hemorrhage, and jaundice. In one report, all three were present in 22% of patients. The symptoms and signs of major hemobilia are melena (90% of cases), hematemesis (60% of cases), biliary colic (70% of cases), and jaundice (60% of cases). Upper gastrointestinal bleeding seen in conjunction with biliary symptoms must always raise the suspicion of hemobilia. One interesting aspect of hemobilia is the tendency for delayed presentations, up to weeks after the inciting causal event, as well as recurrent and brisk but limited bleeding during months and even years. Blood clots in the biliary tree can masquerade as stones if hemobilia goes unrecognized. These clots can cause cholangitis, pancreatitis, and cholecystitis.

Diagnostic Workup

Once hemobilia is suspected, the first evaluation should be upper gastrointestinal endoscopy, which rules out other sources of hemorrhage and may visualize bleeding from the ampulla of Vater. However, upper endoscopy is diagnostic of hemobilia in only approximately 10% of cases. If upper endoscopy is diagnostic and conservative management is planned, no further studies are necessary. Ultrasound or CT may be helpful in demonstrating intrahepatic tumor or hematoma. Evidence of active bleeding into the biliary tree may be seen on contrast-enhanced CT in the form of pooling contrast material, intraluminal clots, or biliary dilation. CT may also show risk factors associated with hemobilia, such as cavitating central lesions and aneurysms. Arterial angiography is now recognized as the test of choice when significant hemobilia is suspected and will reveal the source of bleeding in approximately 90% of cases. Cholangiography demonstrates blood clots in the biliary tree that may appear as stringy defects or smaller spherical defects that may be difficult to distinguish from stones.

Treatment and Outcomes

The treatment of hemobilia must be focused on stopping the bleeding and relieving biliary obstruction. Most cases of minor hemobilia can be managed conservatively with correction of coagulopathy, adequate biliary drainage (only if necessary), and close observation. In a review of 171 reported cases from 1996–99, 43% were successfully managed conservatively. The first line of therapy for major hemobilia was transarterial embolization, and success rates of 80% to 100% were reported. Angiography with transarterial embolization is indicated for major hemobilia requiring blood transfusion (Fig. 89.37).

Surgery is indicated when conservative therapy and transarterial embolization have failed. Surgical treatment of hemobilia is rarely necessary, and even in cases in which a laparotomy may be mandated for other reasons, transarterial embolization is still the therapy of choice for hemobilia because of its lower morbidity. Surgical approaches generally involve ligation of bleeding vessels, excision of aneurysms, or nonselective ligation of a main hepatic artery. Hepatic resection may be necessary for failed arterial ligation or for cases of severe trauma or tumor. Hemorrhage from the gallbladder or hemorrhagic cholecystitis mandates cholecystectomy. There have been isolated reports of successful management of hemobilia with endoscopic coagulation, somatostatin, and vasopressin. The management of hemobilia after percutaneous transhepatic biliary drainage usually consists of removal of the catheter or replacement with larger catheters but may require transarterial embolization.

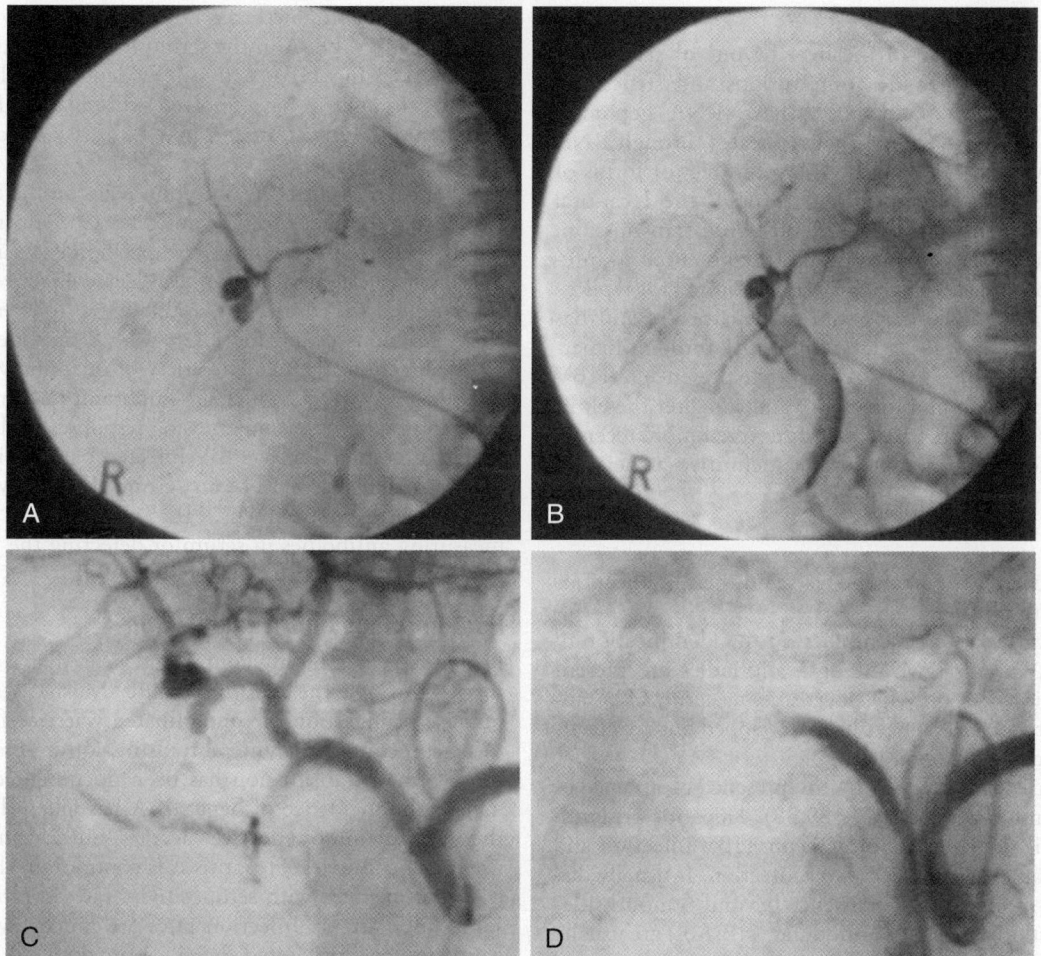

FIGURE 89.37 Classic findings of hemobilia. After a complicated cholecystectomy, an iatrogenic pseudoaneurysm developed and ruptured into the biliary tree. Exsanguinating hemobilia ensued; the diagnosis was made by endoscopy and then treated by arterial embolization. (A) Arteriogram demonstrating a pseudoaneurysm of the hepatic artery at the hilum. (B) A few seconds later, the contrast material is seen flowing down the hepatic duct, with evidence of clot in the biliary tree. (C–D) The same aneurysm before (C) and after (D) successful embolization. (From Sandblom JP. Hemobilia and bilhemia. In: Blumgart LH, Fong Y, eds. *Surgery of the Liver and Biliary Tract*. London: WB Saunders; 2000:1319-1342.)

At the time of Sandblom's report from the early 1970s, the mortality for hemobilia was at least 25%. A report from 1987 noted a mortality of 12%. In a review of cases from 1996 through 1999, only four deaths were reported. There has clearly been a reduction in mortality from hemobilia, which is probably related to two factors. First, the incidence of minor self-limited hemobilia has increased secondary to the rising number of percutaneous hepatic procedures. Second, improvements in selective angiography and transarterial embolization have greatly improved the treatment of major hemobilia.

BILHEMIA

Bilhemia is an extremely rare condition in which bile flows into the bloodstream through the hepatic veins or portal vein branches. This flow occurs in the context of a high intrabiliary pressure exceeding that of the venous system. The cause can be gallstones eroding into the portal vein or accidental or iatrogenic trauma. The condition can be fatal secondary to embolization of large amounts of bile into the lungs. Usually, however, bile flow is low,

and the fistulas close spontaneously. The clinical presentation is that of rapidly increasing jaundice, marked direct hyperbilirubinemia without elevation of hepatocellular enzyme levels (e.g., AST, ALT), and septicemia. This diagnosis is best determined by ERCP. Treatment is directed at lowering intrabiliary pressures through stents or sphincterotomy.

VIRAL HEPATITIS AND THE SURGEON

Viral hepatitis is a major health problem and is the most common cause of liver disease worldwide.[64] More than 5 million people suffer from chronic hepatitis, and it is estimated that more than 1.1 million patients die each year of viral hepatitis globally. Viral hepatitis is not a surgical disease, but it can lead to the development of cirrhosis and HCC, two diseases that can be amenable to surgical therapy. Furthermore, for any surgeon performing hepatic surgery, the functional state of the liver is extremely important, and patients with chronic viral hepatitis may experience declines in synthetic and metabolic function. Finally, the risk of transmission from patient to surgeon and vice versa is an issue with which all surgeons should be familiar.

Definition

Viral hepatitis is an infection of the liver by one of six known viruses that have diverse genetic compositions and structures. HAV, HCV, HDV, HEV, and HGV have RNA genomes, whereas HBV has a DNA genome that replicates through RNA intermediates. HAV and HEV are both responsible for forms of epidemic hepatitis and are transmitted through the fecal-oral route. The remainder are spread via blood-borne transmission. HBV has a circular DNA genome and has the potential to integrate into host genomes, although this is not required for replication. HCV replicates in the cytoplasm of hepatocytes and has complex mechanisms of evading host immunity through hypervariable areas in its genome. HDV requires the presence of HBV coinfection for replication and infectivity and can alter the clinical course of HBV infection. HGV was discovered more recently and has similarities to HCV but has no definitive association with clinical hepatitis.

Diagnosis

Table 89.11 summarizes the serologic tests and their implications for HAV, HBV, and HCV.

The diagnosis of HAV infection relies on the identification of antibodies to HAV. Both IgM and IgG antibodies are present early in the infection, but only IgG persists long-term. HAV antigens and tests for HAV RNA have been developed but are generally restricted to research laboratories.

HBV infection is characterized by the presence or absence of several antigens and antibodies (Fig. 89.38). Hepatitis B serum antigen (HBsAg) is the hallmark of an acute HBV infection and appears in the serum 1 to 10 weeks after infection. It usually disappears in 4 to 6 months, but persistence beyond 6 months defines chronic infection. Anti-HBs antibodies (HBsAbs) are usually present in the serum after the disappearance of serum HBsAg and indicate recovery from acute HBV infection. HBsAbs are also induced by the HBV vaccine and indicate prior immunization or infection. The hepatitis core antigen (HBcAg) is an intracellular antigen that is not detectable in serum. On the other hand, anti-HBc antibodies are detectable early after infection and persist after recovery and in chronic infections. Therefore, the presence of HBcAb and HBsAb indicates prior HBV infection, whereas the presence of HBsAb alone indicates prior HBV vaccination. Hepatitis B e antigen (HBeAg) is a secretory protein that is a marker of HBV replication and infectivity. It is usually present early and may persist for years in chronic infection but generally disappears within months in the absence of chronic infection. Seroconversion to anti-HBe antibodies is usually associated with resolution of infection. Determining the presence of HBeAg or anti-HBe antibodies helps decipher the phases of infection described later. It has also been shown that many patients who have seroconverted

often have measurable HBV DNA, albeit at low levels. Quantification of HBV DNA in the serum has become the most accurate way of assessing HBV activity. Evidence has shown that many patients thought to have resolved acute HBV infection may have persistent viral infection and may be at risk for ongoing hepatitis or reactivation.

The diagnosis of HCV infection relies on the detection of antibodies to a number of HCV antigens. Current immunoassays are highly specific and sensitive. No specific HCV antigen tests exist, but in patients at high risk for HCV, screening for chronic infection is performed with anti-HCV antibody test followed by polymerase chain reaction testing for HCV RNA. In patients with known HCV infection, there are a variety of quantitative and qualitative tests for HCV RNA, which are important in confirming the diagnosis in unclear cases and assessing responses to therapy.

HDV coinfection of HBV-infected patients is best diagnosed by measuring HDV RNA in serum. The HDV antigen can be detected in liver specimens. HEV infection can be diagnosed by measuring antibodies in serum or detecting the virus or its components in feces, serum, or the liver itself.

Epidemiology and Transmission

Hepatitis A is a highly contagious virus that is transmitted primarily through the fecal-oral route. Most cases of HAV occur because of ingestion of contaminated water or food and person-to-person contact. Parenteral transmission is possible but uncommon. Sexual transmission has been documented in homosexual males. The incidence of hepatitis A has fallen dramatically since the introduction of effective vaccines, but vaccination is not routine in all countries. Hepatitis A is common in third-world countries and overlaps with seropositivity rates approaching 100% in some populations. Infection rates are much lower in developed countries. In the United States, approximately 10% of children and 35% of adults have been infected with HAV. Despite vaccination availability, 5700 cases were reported in the United States in 2021, four times higher than in 2015.

Hepatitis B is a major worldwide health problem with approximately 296 million people affected. Hepatitis B contributes to an estimated 820,000 deaths every year, and 25% of chronic hepatitis B infections can progress to liver cancer. The prevalence of HBV infection has considerable geographic variation. Low-prevalence areas such as the United States and Western Europe have carrier rates of 0.1% to 2%. Carrier rates in intermediate-prevalence areas such as Japan and Singapore range from 3% to 5%. In high-prevalence areas such as Southeast Asia and sub-Saharan Africa, carrier rates range from 10% to 20%. Transmission in high-prevalence areas is largely perinatal and horizontal during childhood. In low-prevalence areas, transmission is generally through sexual intercourse or IV drug abuse. In the United

TABLE 89.11 Serologic Evaluation of the Most Common Viral Hepatitides

VIRUS	ANTIGEN NAME	INTERPRETATION	ANTIBODY NAME	INTERPRETATION
HAV	HAV antigen	Acute infection	Anti-HAV IgM	Acute infection
			Anti-HAV IgG	Immunity
HBV	HBsAg	Acute or chronic infection	Anti-HBs	Immunity
	HBeAg	HBV replication, infectivity	Anti-HBc	All phases of infection
			Anti-HBe	Late convalescence
HCV	None	—	Anti-HCV	Late convalescence or chronic infection

HAV, Hepatitis A virus; *HBc,* hepatitis B core; *HBe,* hepatitis e-antigen; *HBeAg,* hepatitis Be antigen; *HBs,* hepatitis surface antigen; *HBsAg,* hepatitis B surface antigen; *HBV,* hepatitis B virus; *HCV,* hepatitis C virus; *IgG,* immunoglobulin G; *IgM,* immunoglobulin M.

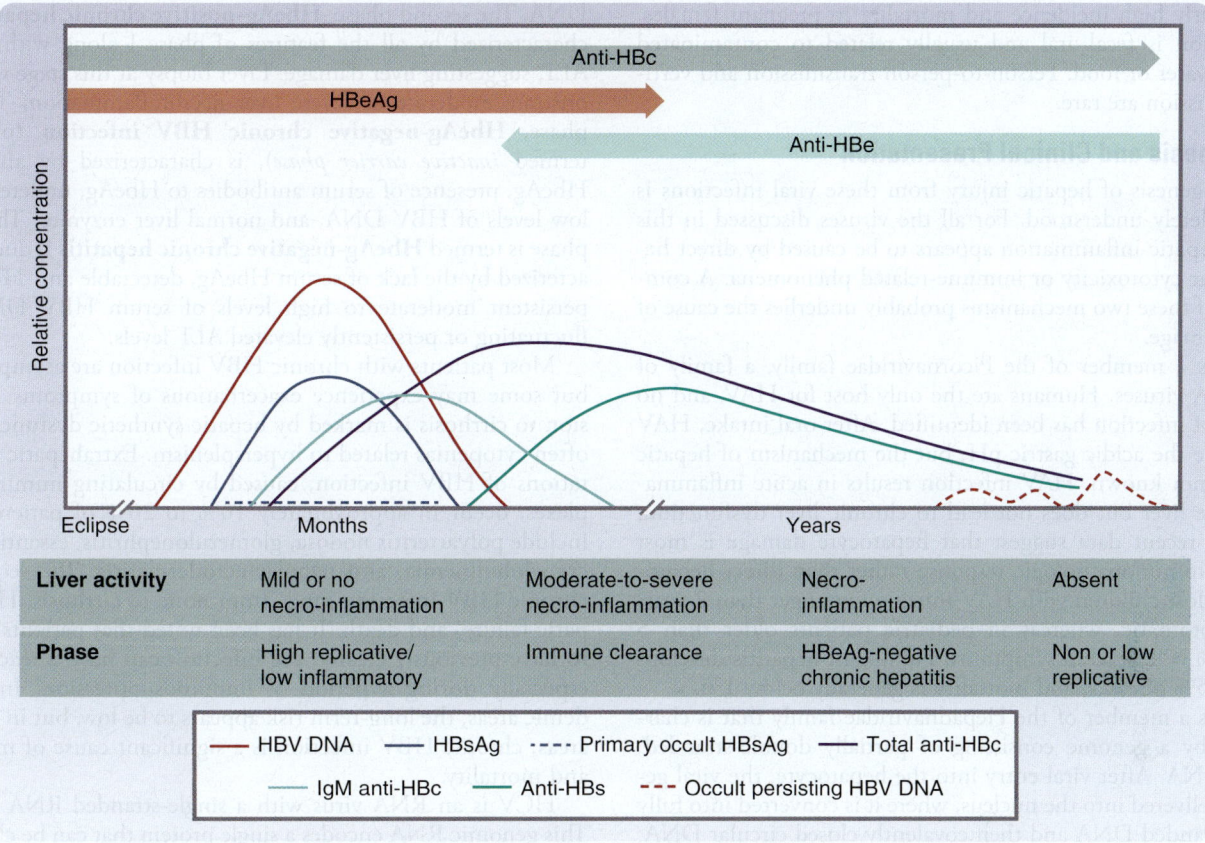

FIGURE 89.38 Serologic biomarkers for HBV over time. *HBV,* Hepatitis B virus. (Adapted from Kramvis A, Chang KM, Dandri M, et al. A roadmap for serum biomarkers for hepatitis B virus: current status and future outlook. *Nat Rev Gastroenterol Hepatol.* 2022;19[11]:727-745.)

States, racial and ethnic disparities exist regarding HBV infection. In 2019, the rate of HBV infection among non-Hispanic Black adults was triple that of Asian or Pacific Islander adults and twice that of Hispanic adults.

Transfusion-associated HBV infection was common in the 1960s, and the risk has been estimated to be as high as 50% at that time. Currently, HBV nucleic acid testing and blood donor screening have decreased the risk of acquiring HBV from a blood transfusion to 1 in 63,000. Percutaneous transmission through the use of any contaminated needle is a major route of HBV infection and is common in IV drug abusers. Sexual transmission is common in low-prevalence countries and is estimated to account for approximately 30% of cases in the United States. There is a particularly high incidence in male homosexuals and heterosexuals with multiple sexual partners. Perinatal HBV infection accounts for less than 10% of cases in the United States but is common in endemic regions, with rates of transmission of 90% in some areas. Horizontal transmission among children is common and is probably related to minor breaks in the skin and mucous membranes. HBV is the most commonly transmitted virus among healthcare personnel, and transmission is usually patient to patient or patient to worker. Needle-stick risk has been related to HbeAg positivity. Rare cases of physician-to-patient transmission have been reported.

Hepatitis C is the most common cause of chronic liver disease in the United States, with an estimated prevalence of 1.8% accounting for 3.9 million infected people. New infections typically occur at a younger age (20–39 years), and the most common risk

factor is IV drug abuse. Healthcare workers have higher carrier rates than the general public. Transmission among healthcare workers is usually related to needle-stick incidents, and the risk of transmission is higher than that of HBV and HIV. In the past, blood transfusion was the major cause of HCV infection, accounting for at least 85% of cases. Currently, less than 2% of acute infections are caused by transfusions, and the risk of transfusion-associated transmission is estimated to be about 1 in 10,000. Although HCV has never been documented in semen, it is estimated that approximately 20% of HCV infections are caused by sexual transmission. Risk of sexual transmission appears to be related to the number of partners and presence of other sexually transmitted diseases. Monogamous sexual partners of HCV-infected people occasionally test positive for HCV in the absence of other risk factors, but this appears to be rare. Perinatal transmission has been documented but is also rare. No identifiable risk factors are found in 30% to 40% of HCV cases. The introduction of direct-acting antiviral (DAA) agents has dramatically improved treatment of HCV and will be discussed later.

HDV infection occurs worldwide, with a variable distribution that parallels that of HBV infection. Approximately 5% of HbsAg-positive patients also harbor HDV infection. Transmission of HDV is parenteral and can occur only in patients previously infected with HBV.

HEV is endemic in Southeast Asia and Central Asia and occurs with low frequency in other areas of the world. HEV infection outbreaks are usually large, affecting hundreds to thousands of people at once, and often follow large rains and flooding. There is a particularly high incidence and mortality in pregnant females. Transmission is fecal-oral and usually related to contaminated drinking water or food. Person-to-person transmission and vertical transmission are rare.

Pathogenesis and Clinical Presentation

The pathogenesis of hepatic injury from these viral infections is not completely understood. For all the viruses discussed in this section, hepatic inflammation appears to be caused by direct hepatocellular cytotoxicity or immune-related phenomena. A combination of these two mechanisms probably underlies the cause of hepatic damage.

HAV is a member of the Picornaviridae family, a family of small RNA viruses. Humans are the only host for HAV, and no reservoir of infection has been identified. After oral intake, HAV can survive the acidic gastric pH, but the mechanism of hepatic uptake is not known. HAV infection results in acute inflammation of the liver but does not lead to chronic liver dysfunction. The most recent data suggest that hepatocyte damage is most likely an immunopathologic response rather than direct hepatotoxicity. Most children with HAV infection younger than 2 years are asymptomatic, whereas in pediatric patients older than 5 years, 80% will develop symptoms. Fulminant hepatitis develops in 1% to 5% of cases, and mortality is generally below 1%.

HBV is a member of the Hepadnaviridae family that is characterized by a genome consisting of partially double-stranded, circular DNA. After viral entry into the hepatocyte, the viral genome is delivered into the nucleus, where it is converted into fully double-stranded DNA and then covalently closed circular DNA. This stable form of HBV DNA is responsible for its persistence in infected hepatocytes. HBV also has the ability of integrating into the hepatocyte genome.

Approximately 70% of patients with acute HBV infection have subclinical or anicteric hepatitis; the other 30% have icteric hepatitis. The incubation period for HBV infection ranges from 1 to 4 months. A prodromal serum sickness–like syndrome may develop, followed by a multitude of constitutional symptoms, such as malaise, anorexia, and nausea. The constitutional symptoms last about 10 days and are followed by jaundice in 30% of patients. Clinical symptoms usually disappear within 3 months. Fulminant hepatic failure develops in 0.1% to 0.5% of patients. Almost 80% of patients with fulminant HBV-related hepatitis will die unless liver transplantation is performed.

Risk of chronic HBV infection is related to immunocompetence and age. Immunocompetent adults have a risk of less than 5%, whereas 30% of children and 90% of infants will develop chronic disease. The effect of age on HBV persistence is most likely caused by differences in immune maturity between adults and young children. The natural history and disease course of chronic HBV infection are the result of complex interactions between the virus and host immune response. A substantial proportion of patients will develop liver injury, cirrhosis and its complications, and HCC, whereas others will harbor the virus with limited, if any, injury.

Different phases of HBV infection, each with unique viral and biochemical profiles, have been described (see Table 89.11)[65] However, it must be noted that these phases are not necessarily sequential and can be reversed. The first phase, **HBeAg-positive chronic infection** (previously known as *immune tolerant phase*), is characterized by high serum HBV DNA but normal liver enzymes. There is a high serum level of HbeAg, and patients in this phase are highly contagious because of the high level of HBV

DNA. The second phase, **HbeAg-positive chronic hepatitis B,** is characterized by all the features of phase I along with elevated ALT, suggesting liver damage. Liver biopsy at this stage will demonstrate moderate or severe liver necroinflammation. The third phase, **HbeAg-negative chronic HBV infection** (previously termed *inactive carrier phase*), is characterized by absence of HbeAg, presence of serum antibodies to HbeAg, undetectable or low levels of HBV DNA, and normal liver enzymes. The fourth phase is termed **HbeAg-negative chronic hepatitis B** and is characterized by the lack of serum HbeAg, detectable anti-Hbe levels, persistent moderate to high levels of serum HBV DNA, and fluctuating or persistently elevated ALT levels.

Most patients with chronic HBV infection are asymptomatic, but some may experience exacerbations of symptoms. Progression to cirrhosis is marked by hepatic synthetic dysfunction and often cytopenias related to hypersplenism. Extrahepatic manifestations of HBV infection, caused by circulating immune complexes, occur in approximately 10% to 20% of patients; these include polyarteritis nodosa, glomerulonephritis, essential mixed cryoglobulinemia, and papular acrodermatitis. The sequelae of chronic HBV infection range from none to cirrhosis, HCC, hepatic failure, and death. It has been noted that patients thought to have previously cleared the infection can have a reactivation, especially during a period of immunosuppression. In nonendemic areas, the long-term risk appears to be low, but in endemic areas, chronic HBV infection is a significant cause of morbidity and mortality.

HCV is an RNA virus with a single-stranded RNA genome. This genomic RNA encodes a single protein that can be cleaved by a protease enzyme into its components. HCV replicates in the hepatocyte cytoplasm. The components of viral replication are targeted by the recently successful DAAs. For instance, protease inhibitors target the protease responsible for cleaving the initial protein into the various viral components. Acute HCV infection generally is manifested with mild elevation of hepatocellular enzyme levels. In general, 80% of cases occur 5 to 12 weeks after infection. Symptoms occur in less than 30% of patients and are usually so mild and nonspecific that they do not affect daily life. Jaundice occurs in less than 20% of patients, and fulminant hepatic failure caused by HCV is extremely uncommon. Chronic HCV infection develops in approximately two-thirds of patients; the other third appear to clear the infection. Most patients with chronic HCV infection are asymptomatic without evidence of overt liver disease and present with only mildly elevated hepatocellular enzyme levels. Despite this quiet clinical course, patients with chronic HCV infection are at risk for development of cirrhosis and HCC. Estimates place the risk of cirrhosis at 2% to 20% at a 20- to 30-year interval. The risk for development of HCC from that point has been estimated at 1% to 4% per year. Progression of liver damage can be variable, and several factors appear to affect its rate. Factors associated with a more rapid progression include male sex, older age at infection, immunosuppression (e.g., HIV infection), coinfection with HBV, moderate alcohol intake, and obesity. Extrahepatic manifestations, such as autoimmune disorders and lymphoma, can occur with HCV infection and are likely related to circulating immune complexes.

The clinical presentation of HDV infection is related to a complex relationship between the degree of HBV and HDV infection. Simultaneous coinfection with high expression of HBV and HDV results in higher rates of acute fulminant hepatitis. Superinfection in a previous HBV carrier generally results in more rapidly progressive chronic liver damage. Some milder forms of acute HDV infection are associated with decreased expression of HDV and repression of HBV infection.

Hepatitis E has a histologic picture different from that of the other viral hepatitides in that a cholestatic type of hepatitis is seen in more than 50% of patients. HEV is introduced orally, and it is not known how the virus travels to the liver. The incubation period of HEV infection ranges from 2 to 9 weeks. The most common form of illness is acute icteric hepatitis; most series report jaundice in more than 90% of patients. Asymptomatic forms of the disease occur and are probably more common than the icteric form, but the actual frequency is unknown. The disease is usually self-limited, but fulminant hepatic failure can occur in a small percentage of patients. Overall, the mortality rate is probably significantly less than 1%. Pregnant females tend to have a more severe clinical course; mortality rates range from 5% to 25%.

Prevention

HAV infection prophylaxis relies on sanitary measures and administration of serum immunoglobulin. The development of safe and effective HAV vaccines, however, has made the use of preexposure immunoglobulin unnecessary. Serum immunoglobulin is still the therapy of choice for postexposure prophylaxis and may be safely given, along with active immunization. In the United States, the Centers for Disease Control and Prevention (CDC) has recommended universal vaccination of children on the basis of the safety and efficacy of the vaccine in high-risk populations. Public health researchers are investigating vaccination schemes to eradicate HAV infection in high-risk populations throughout the world. However, cost-benefit analyses have not supported universal vaccination worldwide. Similarly, HEV infection prophylaxis has focused on sanitary measures, particularly strategies aimed at drinking water. Unfortunately, HEV immunoglobulin has not been successful in preexposure or postexposure prevention of HEV infection, whereas anti-HEV antibodies appear to be effective at attenuating the clinical syndrome. Vaccines for HEV infection have been developed and evaluated in clinical trials.

Remarkable advances have been made in the prevention of HBV infection. In the past, prevention of HBV infection was limited to passive immunization with immunoglobulin containing high titers of antibody to HBsAg. Currently, immunoglobulin immunization is used only in postexposure prophylaxis. HBsAg-containing vaccines have been developed, with good safety and efficacy profiles. These vaccines are used primarily for preexposure prophylaxis but can also be used in a postexposure setting along with immunoglobulin. Currently, CDC recommends a three-dose HBV vaccination for all children, with the first dose being administered preferably within 24 hours after birth followed by two subsequent booster doses. Universal adult HBV vaccination through age 59 and in adults greater than 60 years of age is also advocated by the CDC. Revaccination is generally not indicated but can be considered in certain patients who are at high risk for reinfection including healthcare workers, persons on hemodialysis, and nonresponder infants born to persons testing positive for HBsAg. Although no vaccine is available for HDV infection, effective prevention of HBV infection prevents HDV infection.

The only effective way to prevent HCV infection is to avoid behaviors that can spread the disease and to expand public health strategies mitigating major risk factors for transmission. Conventionally prepared anti-HCV immunoglobulin has been evaluated in a number of trials and has not been demonstrated to prevent transfusion-related non-A, non-B hepatitis. Screening of blood donors has rendered this issue irrelevant today. Unfortunately, because of various obstacles, a successful HCV vaccine has not been developed.

Treatment

Treatment of HAV or HEV infection is supportive in nature and is generally aimed at correcting dehydration and providing adequate calorie intake. Although fatigue may mandate significant periods of rest, hospitalization is usually not necessary, except in cases of fulminant liver failure.

The treatment of HBV infection is largely aimed at patients with chronic active disease. Interferon alfa and the nucleoside analogue lamivudine used to be the only two approved therapies for the treatment of HBV. Now, many nucleoside analogues for the treatment of HBV infection have been developed and probably work through inhibition of DNA synthesis. Interferon alfa is an immunomodulatory agent with some antiviral properties that can induce a virologic response in 35% to 40% of patients. However, long-term benefits with interferon therapy have not been proven. Oral nucleoside analogues are currently the main form of anti-HBV treatment, which include entecavir and two prodrugs of tenofovir. These three drugs are very effective in inducing virologic suppression in a high proportion of patients with favorable safety and tolerability profiles. Long-term viral suppression with nucleoside analog therapy leads to significant histologic improvement, including regression of cirrhosis,[66] reduced complications of cirrhosis, and decreased risk of developing HCC. Indication for treatment of HBV infection is based on three parameters: serum HBV DNA, serum ALT levels, and severity of liver disease. All experts agree that patients with cirrhosis, with or without decompensation, should be treated when serum HBV DNA is detectable. Most experts will also suggest treatment with higher levels of HBV DNA with ALT elevations or with moderately elevated levels of HBV DNA with evidence of liver fibrosis.

During the last 20 years, tremendous advances in the treatment of HCV infection have occurred. Interferon alfa and ribavirin were the recommended treatment for hepatitis C for decades after a benefit for interferon-α in the treatment of non-A, non-B hepatitis was originally demonstrated in 1986, before the discovery of HCV. With interferon-α treatment regimens, complete viral response, defined as sustained loss of serum viral RNA, occurs in 12% to 20% of patients. The addition of ribavirin to interferon-α resulted in response rates of 35% to 45%. In the most recent trials, treatment with pegylated interferon-α and ribavirin for 48 weeks resulted in viral clearance in 55% of patients. The specific genotype appears to be predictive of response, with some types resulting in response rates of 80% and others of 45%. Relapse can occur, but it usually occurs with monotherapy and shortened courses of therapy. Interferon-α regimens had significant side effects.

Over the past 10 years, the treatment of chronic HCV infection has been revolutionized by the introduction of DAAs (e.g., ledipasvir, sofosbuvir, glecaprevir, pibrentasvir, velpatasvir) (Table 89.12) that target specific nonstructural proteins of HCV and thus disrupt viral replication and infection. First developed in 2014, combinations of these medications have now become the first-line treatment and have replaced prior regimens containing pegylated interferon-α and ribavirin where available. The current all-oral treatments are of shorter duration and have fewer side effects and higher cure rates. By tailoring the combination of DAA agents to patient factors and the specific HCV genotype, a sustained virologic response can be achieved in more than 90% of patients.

TABLE 89.12   Treatments Available for Hepatitis C

DAA TRADE NAME	DAA GENERIC NAME	TREATMENT CLASS
Harvoni	Ledipasvir/sofosbuvir	NS5A, NS5B Inhibitor
Mavyret	Glecaprevir/pibrentasvir	NS5A, NS3/4A Inhibitor
Vosevi	Sofosbuvir/velpatasvir/voxilaprevir	NS5A, NS5B Inhibitor
Epclusa	Sofosbuvir/velpatasvir	NS5A, NS5B Inhibitor
Zepatier	Elbasvir/grazoprevir	NS5A, NS3/N4a Inhibitor

DAA, Direct-acting antiviral.

The therapeutic efficacy of DAAs has resulted in dramatic declines in the incidence of decompensated cirrhosis and, to a lesser extent, HCC secondary to HCV infection.[67] This has led to a decrease in the number of liver transplants performed for HCV-related decompensated cirrhosis and HCC.[68,69] In the United States, the proportion of liver transplants for HCV-related disease has declined to 7% in 2020, from 27% in 2010 (Fig. 89.39). In Europe, it has been estimated that at least 600 liver grafts can be allocated to patients with indications other than HCV each year, such as NASH, which is increasing in incidence. Furthermore, availability of DAA has shifted attitudes toward accepting HCV-positive donor liver grafts, with 60% of liver transplant candidates willing to accept HCV-positive donor grafts in 2020 compared with 21% in 2015, thus increasing the liver graft donor pool.

Needle-Stick Injuries and Viral Hepatitis

Exposure to hepatitis viruses remains an occupational risk for surgeons and healthcare personnel. Viral transmission may occur after percutaneous or mucocutaneous exposure to the blood or body fluids of an infected patient. Hepatitis B virus is one of the most readily transmissible viruses after percutaneous exposure. In patients with

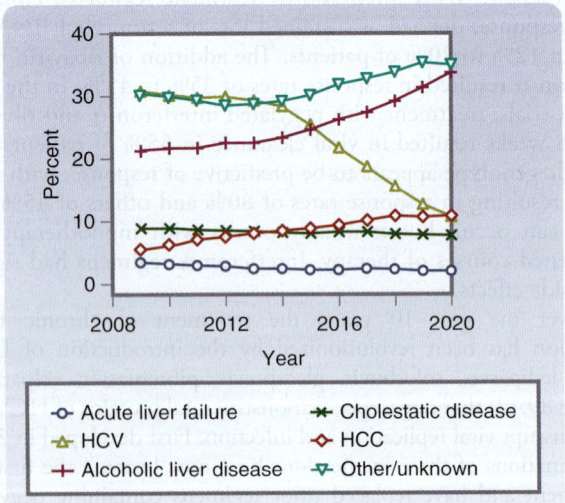

FIGURE 89.39 Liver transplant waitlist by diagnosis. *HCC*, Hepatocellular carcinoma; *HCV*, hepatitis C virus. (From Kwong AJ, Ebel NH, Kim WR, et al. OPTN/SRTR 2020 annual data report: liver. *Am J Transplant.* 2022;22[Suppl 2]:204-309.)

HBeAg-positive blood, the rate of transmission via needle stick is nearly 20%. If exposed, HBV vaccination and hepatis B immune globulin are typically used together for postexposure treatment.

HCV is less readily transmitted than HBV, and the risk of acquiring the infection after exposure is low. In a source patient with anti-HCV–positive blood, the risk of transmission after percutaneous or mucocutaneous exposure is 0.2% and 0%, respectively. If an occupational exposure is sustained, baseline testing of the healthcare personnel and source patient is recommended to detect the presence of HCV RNA or anti-HCV antibodies. This will determine subsequent testing and treatment. Routine postexposure prophylaxis is not currently recommended by the CDC.

SELECTED REFERENCES

Bioulac-Sage P, Laumonier H, Couchy G, et al. Hepatocellular adenoma management and phenotypic classification: the Bordeaux experience. *Hepatology.* 2009;50(2):481-489.

This study classifies hepatocellular adenomas based on their phenotypic characteristics and provides specific treatment recommendations for each. It emphasizes the role of molecular classification and highlights the importance of individualized treatment plans based on the subtype of hepatocellular adenoma.

Bruix J, Takayama T, Mazzaferro V, et al. Adjuvant sorafenib for hepatocellular carcinoma after resection or ablation (STORM): a phase 3, randomised, double-blind, placebo-controlled trial. *Lancet Oncol.* 2015;16(13):1344-1354.

The STORM trial was a phase 3, double-blind, placebo-controlled trial evaluating the efficacy of sorafenib in the adjuvant setting for patients after complete resection or ablation of HCC. The study found no significant idfference in median recurrence free survival about concluded that sorafenib is not an effective adjuvant therapy for HCC.

European Association for the Study of the Liver. EASL 2017 Clinical Practice Guidelines on the management of hepatitis B virus infection. *J Hepatol.* 2017;67(2):370-398.

This clinical practice guidelines provides a contemparory update to the optimal management of hepatitis B virus infection. It discusses current and future treatment strategies and its impact on HCC risk.

European Association for the Study of the Liver, European Organisation for Research and Treatment of Cancer. EASL-EORTC clinical practice guidelines: management of hepatocellular carcinoma. *J Hepatol.* 2012;56(4):908-943.

This clinical practice guidelines provides an update on the management of hepatocellular carcinoma and the defines the use of surveillance, diagnosis, and therapuetic strategies in HCC. It provides specific treatment recommendations, and uses the GRADE system to examine the quality of evidence and strength of recommendations.

Huang G, Lau WY, Wang ZG, et al. Antiviral therapy improves postoperative survival in patients with hepatocellular carcinoma: a randomized controlled trial. *Ann Surg.* 2015;261(1):56-66.

This study evaluated the effect of antiviral therapy with adefovir on long-term survival and recurrence rates in patients with hepatitis B related HCC after complete surgical resection. The study found that antiviral therapy significantly improved postoperative survival and reduces recurrence in patients with HBV related HCC.

Jarnagin WR, Gonen M, Fong Y, et al. Improvement in perioperative outcome after hepatic resection: analysis of 1,803 consecutive cases over the past decade. *Ann Surg.* 2002;236(4):397-407.

This study analyzes the perioperative outcomes of over 1,800 patients after hepatectomy and demonstrated improvements in perioperative outcomes, noting a significant decrease in intra-operative blood loss and use of blood products with newer techniques, such as parencyhmal sparing resection.

Llovet JM, Castet F, Heikenwalder M, et al. Immunotherapies for hepatocellular carcinoma. *Nat Rev Clin Oncol.* 2022;19(3):151-172.

This review discusses the role of immunotherapy in the treatment of hepatocellular carcinoma. It reviews the different immune-checkpoint inhibitors used in the treatment of HCC and discusses future challenges and directions for immunotherapy in HCC.

Marrero JA, Ahn J, Rajender Reddy K. ACG clinical guideline: the diagnosis and management of focal liver lesions. *Am J Gastroenterol.* 2014;109(9):1328-1348.

This American College of Gastroenterology clinical guideline provides an evidence-based approach for the diagnosis and management of both benign and malignant liver lesions. The guideline provides specific recommendations for the follow-up and treatment of different liver lesions, and uses the GRADE system to examine the quality of evidence and strength of recommendations.

Mezhir JJ, Fong Y, Jacks LM, et al. Current management of pyogenic liver abscess: surgery is now second-line treatment. *J Am Coll Surg.* 2010;210(6):975-983.

This review discusses the current and future management landscape for intrahepatic chilangiocarcinoma including advances in immunotherapy, targeted, combination and locoregional therapies. It reviews ongoing clincal trials and highlights future directions for the treatment of ICC.

Njei B, Rotman Y, Ditah I, et al. Emerging trends in hepatocellular carcinoma incidence and mortality. *Hepatology.* 2015;61(1):191-199.

This study examines the incidence, mortatlity and survival of patients with hepatocellular carcinoma in the United States over 40 years. It demonstrated a significant improvement in survival in spite of increased HCC incidence, suggesting earlier detection and curative treatment options are improving.

The full reference list appears on Elsevier eBooks+.

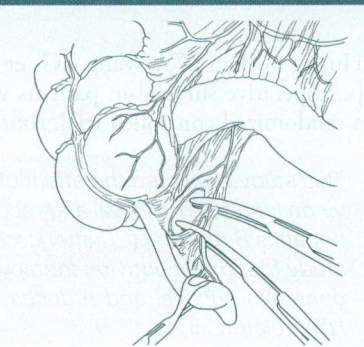

90 CHAPTER

Secondary Tumors of the Liver

Reed I. Ayabe, Mengyuan Liu, Michael I. D'Angelica, and Yun Shin Chun

OUTLINE

The liver is the solid organ most frequently affected by metastases, due to its rich blood supply, anatomy, and immunosuppressive environment.[1] Liver metastases will develop in up to 50% of all cancer patients throughout the course of their disease, resulting in significant reduction in survival and quality of life (Fig. 90.1).[2] Among patients with primary tumors in the gastrointestinal tract, the liver is the second most common site of metastases after lymph nodes, likely due to hematogenous dissemination via the portal venous system. Colorectal cancer is the leading cause of liver metastases, followed by lung, pancreas, and breast cancer.[3]

Most patients with liver metastases are not candidates for metastasectomy due to disseminated disease and poor tumor biology. However, well-selected patients with colorectal liver metastases (CLMs) may derive significant benefit and even cure from hepatic resection. In fact, CLM is the most frequent indication for liver resection in the United States. Although relatively uncommon, neuroendocrine liver metastases (NELMs) are also managed surgically in appropriately selected patients. Both diseases represent exceptions to the historical dogma that stage IV disease should be managed nonoperatively. Indeed, advances in systemic and regional therapies and an improved understanding of the natural history of these tumors have expanded the pool of patients who are candidates for surgery. This chapter will review pathogenesis, clinical presentation and diagnosis, and perioperative considerations, particularly for CLMs and NELMs. In addition, we summarize treatment strategies for CLMs used by two high-volume,

tertiary cancer centers, highlighting the complexity and diversity of surgical management of liver metastases.

PATHOGENESIS OF LIVER METASTASES

The pathogenesis of liver metastases involves a multistep process of invasion, extravasation, and colonization necessary for metastasis formation in any organ (see Chapter 60). After cancer cells from the primary organ invade through the extracellular matrix into the blood or lymphatic vessels, these circulating tumor cells (CTCs) must arrest and extravasate between endothelial cells of a distant organ to form micrometastatic colonies.[4] The liver provides a particularly hospitable environment for metastatic seeding due to direct hematogenous access for cancers of the gastrointestinal tract via the portal venous system, microscopic anatomy, and immunotolerogenic milieu.

The liver's microscopic anatomy is conducive to extravasation and metastasis formation (see Chapter 89). The liver is organized into lobules, which are centered around the terminal tributaries of the hepatic vein, termed *central veins* (Fig. 90.2). Portal tracts lie at the periphery of the lobule. Within each lobule, hepatocytes are organized into plates that extend from the portal tracts to the central vein. Sinusoids are unique capillaries of the liver located between the plates of hepatocytes that carry a mixture of arterial and venous blood from the portal tract to the central vein. Liver sinusoidal endothelial cells (LSECs) lining the sinusoids are fenestrated and, therefore, highly permeable to extravasation of CTCs.[5]

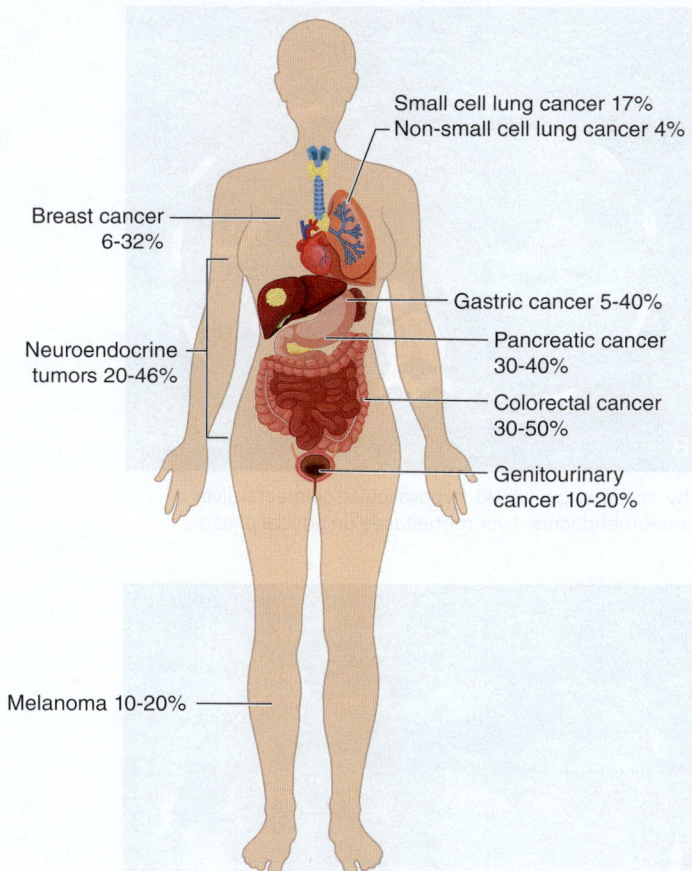

FIGURE 90.1 Incidence of liver metastases from primary tumors.

Small cell lung cancer 17%
Non-small cell lung cancer 4%

Breast cancer 6-32%

Neuroendocrine tumors 20-46%

Gastric cancer 5-40%

Pancreatic cancer 30-40%

Colorectal cancer 30-50%

Genitourinary cancer 10-20%

Melanoma 10-20%

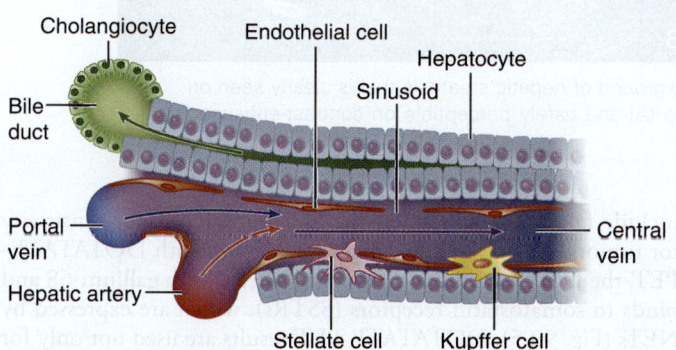

FIGURE 90.2 Microscopic anatomy of the liver. (From Trefts E, Gannon M, Wasserman DH. The liver. *Curr Biol.* 2017;27:R1147-R1151.)

Cholangiocyte
Endothelial cell
Hepatocyte
Sinusoid
Bile duct
Portal vein
Central vein
Hepatic artery
Stellate cell
Kupffer cell

In addition to its rich blood supply and fenestrated LSECs, the liver is a frequent site of metastases due to its favorable microenvironment, which provides a fertile "soil" for the "seeds" of cancer cells. In 1889, Paget proposed in his seed-and-soil hypothesis that CTCs from a particular primary site will form metastases only in organs with specific tumor-permissive environments.[6] More recently, emerging evidence suggests that primary tumors can release circulating factors that induce a favorable microenvironment for metastatic growth in secondary organs, termed *premetastatic niches*.[7] The liver microenvironment is geared toward immune tolerance due to the constant exposure to circulating nutrients

and endotoxins entering from the gut via the portal circulation.[8] This tolerogenic milieu promotes the survival of disseminated tumor cells and metastatic outgrowth. The highly complex and multifactorial response of the liver microenvironment is orchestrated by various resident and recruited cells that have both prometastatic and antimetastatic effects.[9] An increasing understanding of the role of the liver microenvironment may elucidate novel approaches to prevent and treat liver metastases.

CLINICAL PRESENTATION AND DIAGNOSIS

Symptoms in patients with liver metastases arise more often from their primary tumors, such as bleeding or obstruction from a colorectal cancer. The liver metastases themselves typically do not cause symptoms unless the tumor burden is extensive or there is underlying liver disease, such as portal hypertension and cirrhosis. An important exception is NELMs, which can cause carcinoid syndrome or other symptoms of hormone excess from functional islet cell tumors. Patients with extensive hepatic metastases may present with abdominal pain, weight loss, and malaise. Tumors obstructing the biliary tree can cause jaundice.

Laboratory evaluation should include a complete blood count, comprehensive metabolic panel, and coagulation panel. Increases in bilirubin and prothrombin time should prompt suspicion for hepatic dysfunction, whereas thrombocytopenia may be indicative of portal hypertension. Tumor markers pertinent for liver metastases are carcinoembryonic antigen (CEA) in patients with known or suspected colorectal cancer, chromogranin A for neuroendocrine tumor (NET), CA 19-9 for pancreatobiliary tumors, CA 15-3 for breast cancer, and CA 125 for ovarian cancer. Clinical correlation is needed when interpreting tumor marker levels because of potential false-positive and false-negative results.[10,11] CEA may be elevated in epithelial cancers other than colorectal cancer as well as nonneoplastic processes, including chronic inflammation and smoking.

High-quality cross-sectional imaging is critical for accurate assessment of liver metastases and their relationship to hepatic vasculature, presence of extrahepatic disease (EHD), and anticipated volume of the remnant liver after resection. Multidetector contrast-enhanced computed tomography (CT) scan is the preferred imaging modality to evaluate liver metastases due to the ability to capture high-resolution images of the liver and extrahepatic organs and tissues, wide availability, and fast scanning speed. At a minimum, CT scans to evaluate liver metastases should include arterial and portal venous phases with a slice thickness of 5 mm or less. For preoperative planning and indeterminate lesions, quadruple-phase CT, which includes unenhanced and delayed phases, is preferred.[12] Most hepatic metastases are hypovascular and appear dark relative to background liver on the portal venous phase (Fig. 90.3). On the arterial phase, metastases may exhibit a peripheral rim of enhancement due to desmoplastic reaction, vascular proliferation, and/or abundant cancer cells at the tumor-normal interface.[13,14] The most common causes of hypovascular liver metastases are colon, lung, breast, and gastric cancer. Hypervascular liver metastases, which appear bright relative to surrounding liver on the arterial phase, occur with NETs, renal cell carcinoma, and melanoma.

Magnetic resonance imaging (MRI) with diffusion-weighted sequences may be appropriate for patients with abnormal renal function, extensive hepatic steatosis, or significant contrast allergy. The sensitivity of MRI compared with CT in the detection and characterization of liver metastases depends upon underlying

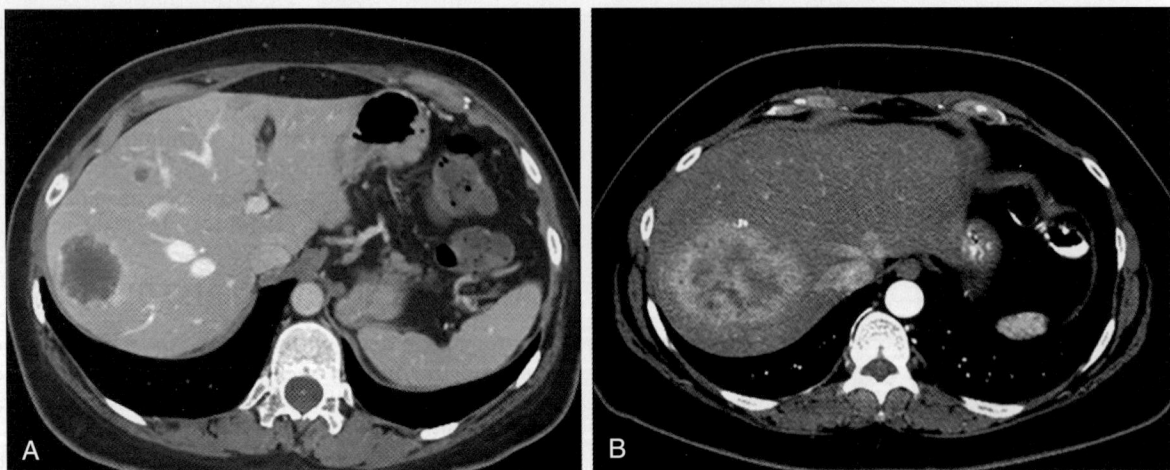

FIGURE 90.3 Contrast-enhanced computed tomography scans showing (A) hypovascular colorectal liver metastases on portal venous phase and (B) hypervascular neuroendocrine liver metastases on arterial phase.

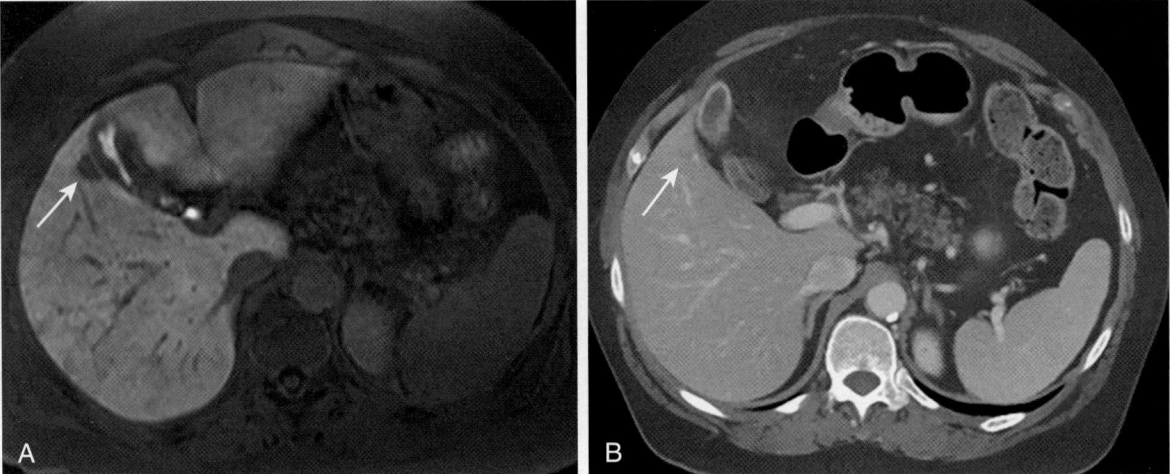

FIGURE 90.4 Colorectal liver metastasis *(arrows)* in background of hepatic steatosis that is clearly seen on delayed hepatobiliary phase magnetic resonance imaging (A) and barely perceptible on contrast-enhanced computed tomography (B).

liver disease, imaging techniques and protocols, and use of hepatocyte-specific contrast agents.[15,16] On T2-weighted images, liver metastases tend to be mildly hyperintense, in contrast with cysts and hemangiomas, which are markedly hyperintense. On contrast-enhanced MRI, patterns of enhancement are similar to those seen on CT scans. Gadoxetic acid (Eovist, Bayer Healthcare LLC, Whippany, NJ) is a hepatocyte-specific MRI contrast agent available in the United States. After administration of Eovist, 50% is taken up by hepatocytes and eliminated by biliary excretion. Liver metastases, which lack functioning hepatocytes, do not take up Eovist and appear as hypoattenuating lesions in the delayed hepatobiliary phase of the MRI (Fig. 90.4). In patients with significant hepatic steatosis, liver metastases may be difficult to detect with CT; therefore, MRI with hepatobiliary contrast agents is the preferred imaging modality.

Commonly used nuclear medicine scans to evaluate liver metastases include fluorodeoxyglucose–positron emission tomography (FDG/PET) for diverse tumor types and gallium-68 DOTATATE-PET, specifically for NETs. FDG/PET is not routinely indicated for liver metastases but may be used to characterize indeterminate lesions that may alter the course of care. Limitations of PET

include false-positive results with inflammation, poor sensitivity for tumors <1 cm, and low anatomic detail. With DOTATATE-PET, the DOTA-conjugate peptide is labeled with gallium-68 and binds to somatostatin receptors (SSTRs), which are expressed by NETs (Fig. 90.5). DOTATATE-PET results are used not only for tumor detection but also for assessment of response to SSTR-targeted therapy.

Percutaneous biopsy is not mandatory to diagnose liver metastases, particularly when the primary tumor site is known and the clinical and imaging features are consistent with metastatic disease. However, tissue diagnosis of either the primary and/or metastasis may be helpful to assess disease biology by analyzing factors such as tumor grade and molecular/genomic markers. This, in turn, can help select effective systemic therapy regimens.

PERIOPERATIVE CONSIDERATIONS

Perioperative principles for resection of liver metastases are similar to surgery for primary liver cancer, as described in Chapter 89. These include assessment of patient fitness and liver function, low central venous pressure anesthesia, and intraoperative techniques

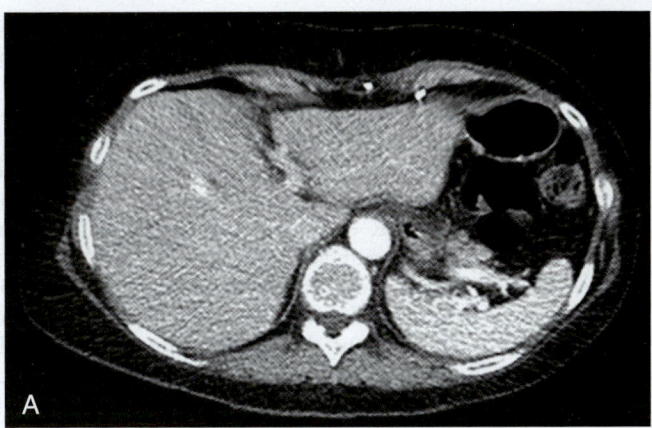
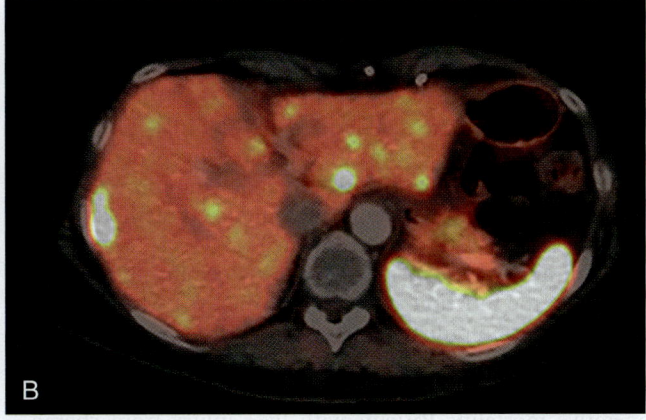

FIGURE 90.5 Contrast-enhanced gallium-68 DOTATATE positron emission tomography–computed tomography (B) delineates neuroendocrine liver metastases compared to computed tomography (A).

to reduce blood loss and bile leak. Technical resectability of liver metastases is defined as the ability to resect all intrahepatic disease while preserving adequate biliary drainage and vascular inflow and outflow, and sparing at least two contiguous hepatic segments with adequate remnant liver volume.[17] Important perioperative considerations for resection of liver metastases include parenchymal-sparing hepatectomy, systematic intraoperative ultrasound (IOUS), and assessment of remnant liver volume.

Parenchymal-Sparing Hepatectomy

Wide resection margins are typically not necessary for liver metastases, and thus, nonanatomic resections that spare nontumoral liver parenchyma are favored when possible over major hepatectomy.[18,19] A systematic review of over 2500 patients undergoing resection of CLM found that parenchymal-sparing hepatectomy resulted in similar rates of R0 resection and overall survival (OS) compared with anatomic resection.[20] For NELMs, a microscopically positive R1 margin is not associated with worse outcomes compared with R0 margin.[21]

Ablation can be used for small, deep metastases that would require sacrifice of a large volume of liver parenchyma to resect. Depending on institutional practice, ablation can be performed intraoperatively under ultrasound or percutaneously under CT guidance. Microwave is preferred over radiofrequency ablation (RFA) due to more efficient heat generation and less susceptibility

to the heat sink effect near major blood vessels.[22,23] The efficacy of ablation over resection depends upon tumor size, ablation margin, and tumor type, with NELMs having lower local recurrence after ablation than CLMs.[24]

Intraoperative Ultrasound

IOUS is critical to define intrahepatic anatomy, identify metastases missed on preoperative imaging, and to guide resection margins for parenchymal-sparing hepatectomy. For metastases located deep in the parenchyma, IOUS is necessary to localize the tumor and guide the lines of transection (Fig. 90.6). While visualizing the tumor with ultrasound, the capsule of the liver is scored with cautery, marking the intended lines of transection. The ultrasound probe is placed perpendicular to the cautery line to confirm sufficient margin from the tumor to the transection line. As parenchymal transection progresses, IOUS is repeated to evaluate intrahepatic vessels and adequacy of margins.

Remnant Liver Volume

Accurate assessment of the volume of the liver that will remain after surgery, termed the *future liver remnant (FLR)*, is critical to avoid hepatic insufficiency and liver failure, which occur in 3% to 8% of patients after major hepatectomy.[25,26] The FLR is calculated using contrast-enhanced CT or MRI images and involves outlining the contours of each hepatic segment in cross section,

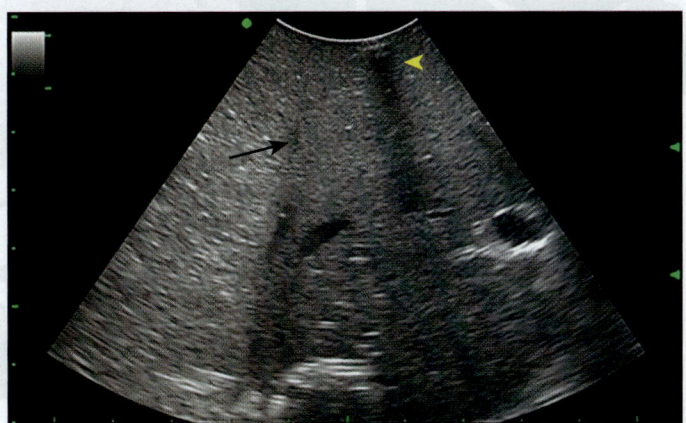

FIGURE 90.6 Intraoperative ultrasound showing hyperechoic tumor *(black arrow)* and intended transection line marked by cautery on the liver capsule, resulting in hypoechoic line *(yellow arrowhead)*.

calculating the enclosed area, and multiplying by the thickness of each slice. Tumor volumes are subtracted.[27] This measurement can be performed manually or with specialized software (Fig. 90.7). The calculated FLR is standardized to the total liver volume (TLV) to yield the standardized FLR (sFLR). TLV can be measured directly on CT scans or estimated by patients' body weight or body surface area (BSA). The following formula based on BSA has been found to be a precise, unbiased method to calculate TLV: TLV = 1267.28 × BSA (m^2) − 794.41.[28,29]

The minimum sFLR to avoid posthepatectomy liver failure depends upon the function and health of the liver. Most patients undergoing resection of liver metastases do not have cirrhosis but may have chemotherapy-induced hepatotoxicity. In patients without chronic liver disease, sFLR <20% predicts liver failure and postoperative mortality. Patients with liver injury from chemotherapy require sFLR of 30%, whereas those with cirrhosis require at least 40%.

Strategies to Increase Future Liver Remnant Volume

For patients with insufficient sFLR, strategies to induce liver hypertrophy for safe hepatectomy include portal vein embolization (PVE) and liver venous deprivation (LVD). First described in 1984 by Makuuchi et al., PVE is the most well-established method for inducing FLR hypertrophy.[30] During PVE, the portal system supplying the hemiliver intended for resection is embolized, which leads to atrophy of the embolized liver and compensatory hypertrophy of the nonembolized liver (see Fig. 90.7). The choice of embolic agent depends upon cost, availability, and operator preference. A combination of microspheres for embolization of distal portal branches and coils proximally has been shown to be safe and effective.[31]

After PVE, the FLR volume is expected to increase significantly the first 3 weeks, followed by a plateau.[32] Comparing the sFLR before and after PVE allows a dynamic assessment of the capacity of the liver to regenerate The kinetic growth rate (KGR) is calculated by dividing the difference in sFLR before and after PVE by the elapsed time in weeks after PVE.[33] KGR provides a powerful predictor of liver regenerative capacity and posthepatectomy liver failure. KGR ≥2% per week is associated with 0% postoperative hepatic insufficiency.

PVE alone fails to induce adequate hypertrophy in approximately 5% of patients.[34] For these patients, hepatic vein embolization (HVE) can augment the hypertrophy induced by PVE. HVE can be used as a salvage procedure following inadequate hypertrophy from PVE, as well as up front in patients with a particularly limited sFLR, a procedure known as *liver venous deprivation* (Fig. 90.8). A retrospective comparison of patients who underwent LVD (*n* = 37) and PVE (*n* = 36) in preparation for right or extended right hepatectomy found that LVD was associated with superior increase in liver volume (61% vs. 29%, *p* < 0.0001) and a reduced rate of postoperative liver failure.[30] A recent retrospective analysis suggests that patients with a starting sFLR <19% or those that need staged hepatectomy for bilateral CLM may benefit from upfront LVD.[35]

Bilateral Liver Metastases

Two-stage hepatectomy involves a sequential approach for bilateral liver metastases that cannot be safely removed in a single procedure. In the first stage, tumors are removed from the FLR, typically the left liver. If needed, PVE is performed after the first-stage hepatectomy. The second-stage hepatectomy, typically right

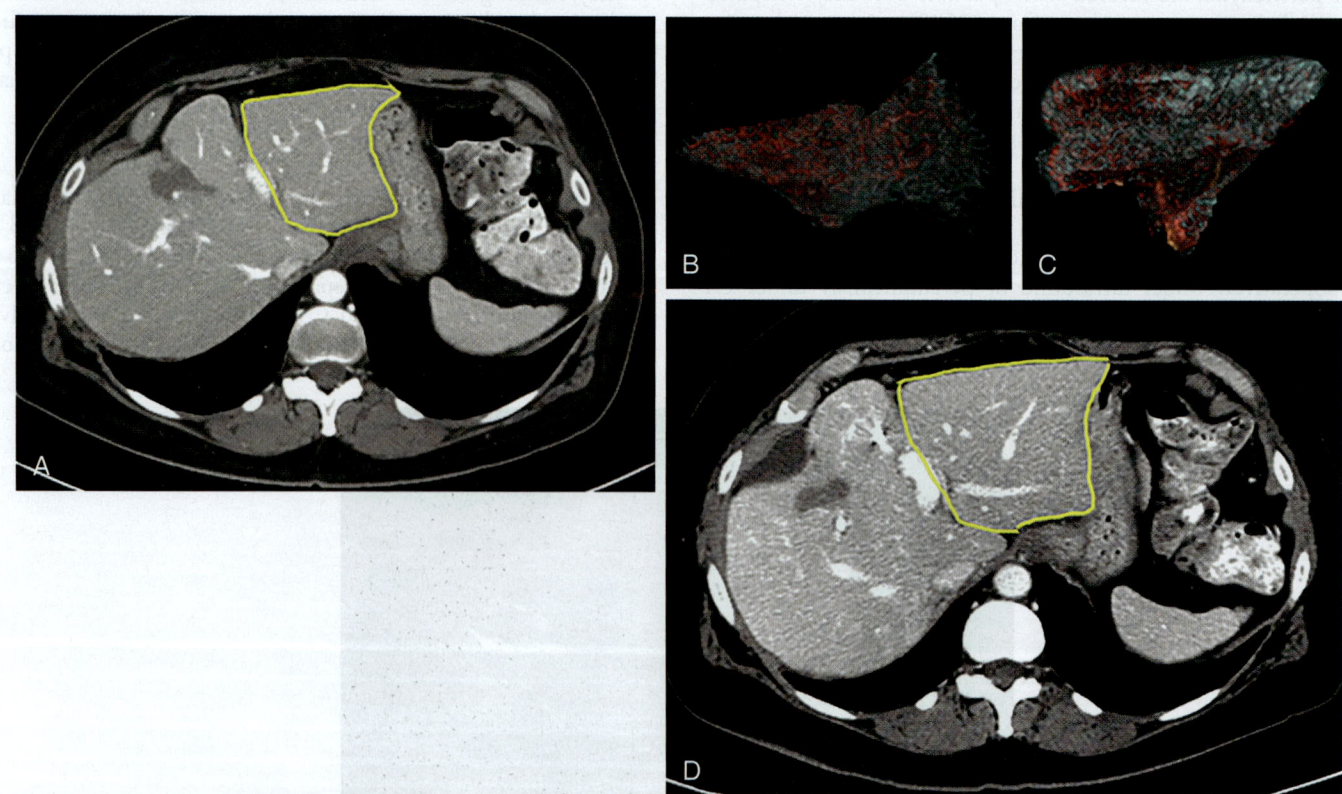

FIGURE 90.7 The volume of the future liver remnant, outlined in *yellow*, is measured on computed tomography (CT) scan (A) using specialized software to calculate the volumes of segments 2 and 3 (B–C). CT after portal vein embolization (D) shows hypertrophy of segments 2 and 3.

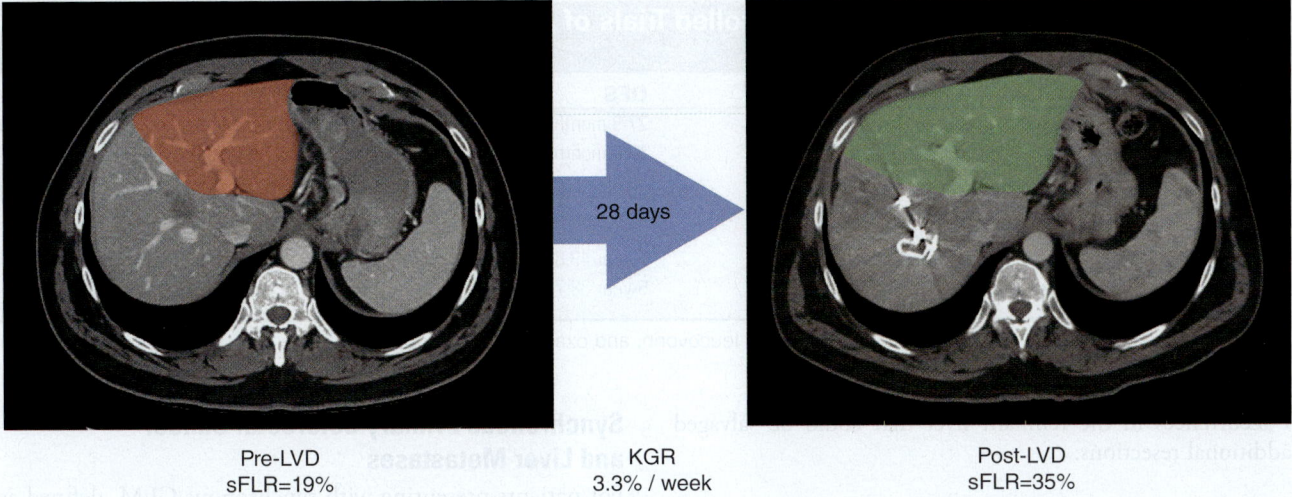

Pre-LVD
sFLR=19%

KGR
3.3% / week

Post-LVD
sFLR=35%

FIGURE 90.8 Example of future liver remnant hypertrophy after liver venous deprivation. *KGR*, Kinetic growth rate; *LVD*, liver venous deprivation; *sFLR*, standardized future liver remnant.

or extended right hepatectomy, is performed 6 to 8 weeks after the first stage.

The associating liver partition and portal vein ligation for staged hepatectomy (ALPPS) procedure has been proposed as an alternative to conventional two-stage hepatectomy. In the first stage of ALPPS, as initially described, the right portal vein is ligated and the liver parenchyma transected, leading to rapid FLR hypertrophy.[36] A median of 9 days later completion hepatectomy is performed, including arterial, biliary, and hepatic vein division. ALPPS remains a controversial procedure due to high rates of major morbidity and mortality and unclear survival benefit over conventional two-stage hepatectomy.

COLORECTAL LIVER METASTASES

In patients with colorectal cancer, the liver is the most common site of distant metastases, developing in nearly 50% of patients.[1] One in four patients with colorectal cancer present with synchronous liver metastases, and another quarter go on to develop metachronous disease. Liver disease is directly linked to mortality in over 50% of patients with CLMs.[37] Complete resection is the cornerstone of curative-intent treatment for CLM and is associated with 5-year OS rates between 51% and 58% in well-selected patients.[38,39] Historically, liver resection carried a significant risk of morbidity and mortality, with 30-day mortality rates exceeding 5%. However, with improvements in understanding of hepatic anatomy, surgical technique, and perioperative fluid management, mortality rates after major hepatectomy have fallen to less than 2%.[40] Unfortunately, surgery is underutilized in the treatment of CLM on a national level, with population-based studies reporting resection rates as low as 10%.[41]

Systemic Therapy

Survival for patients with metastatic colorectal cancer has increased significantly due to advances in systemic therapy. First-line chemotherapy regimens are 5-fluorouracil, leucovorin, and oxaliplatin (FOLFOX) and 5-fluorouracil, leucovorin, and irinotecan (FOLFIRIee), resulting in response rates exceeding 50%.[42] The addition of vascular endothelial growth factor (VEGF) blockade with bevacizumab is associated with improved survival when added to oxaliplatin or irinotecan-based regimens.[43] For patients whose tumors do not have mutations in the *KRAS* gene, targeted therapies against epidermal growth factor receptor (anti-EGFR), such as cetuximab and panitumumab, can improve response rates and extend progression-free survival (PFS) when added to standard chemotherapy.[44]

In patients with initially unresectable CLM, response to chemotherapy correlates with future resectability. In a 2004 retrospective series by Adam et al. of 1439 consecutive patients with CLM, 77% were initially unresectable.[45] Among those with unresectable disease, 12.5% had sufficient response to chemotherapy to undergo hepatic resection. Their 5-year OS was 33%, which was significantly lower than that of patients with initially resectable disease (48%) but higher than patients treated with chemotherapy alone during the same era (16%).

For patients with resectable CLM, the addition of perioperative and adjuvant chemotherapy is controversial (Table 90.1). The EORTC intergroup 40983 trial recruited 364 patients from 78 institutions and randomized patients to receive either surgery alone or surgery with preoperative and postoperative FOLFOX.[46] The majority of patients had only one CLM, and 43% had an objective response to chemotherapy with an average 25% reduction in tumor diameter. Analysis of randomized patients showed a nonstatistically significant higher 3-year PFS with chemotherapy (28% vs. 35%, P = 0.06). When adjusted for patients who underwent resection, the difference in 3-year PFS was significant, favoring the chemotherapy group (33% vs. 42%, P = 0.03). The long-term 5-year results showed no difference in OS between the groups (49% vs. 51%, P = 0.34).[47] Together, these results suggest that perioperative chemotherapy does not influence OS.

More recently, a large prospective trial from Japan randomized 300 patients to observation or 12 cycles of FOLFOX after complete resection of CLM.[49] The primary end point was disease-free survival (DFS), and there was a significant difference favoring adjuvant chemotherapy at 3 years (43% vs. 53%) and 5 years (39% vs. 50%, P = 0.006). However, the OS analysis favored the hepatectomy-only group at 3 years (92% vs. 87%) and 5 years (83% vs. 71%, P = 0.42). These contradictory results may be explained by the pattern of recurrence. The chemotherapy group experienced later recurrences that were more prevalent in the lungs or other distant sites, whereas the observation group had

TABLE 90.1   Selected Randomized Controlled Trials of Adjuvant Systemic Therapy After Resection of Colorectal Liver Metastases

AUTHOR (YEAR)	ARMS	DFS	P	OVERALL SURVIVAL	P
Mitry (2008)[48]	Surgery + adjuvant 5-FU/LV (N = 138)	27.9 months	0.058	62.2 months	0.095
	Surgery alone (N = 140)	18.8 months		47.3 months	
Nordlinger (2008)[46]	Perioperative FOLFOX (N = 151)	20.0 months	0.068	61.3 months	0.34
	Surgery alone (N = 152)	12.5 months		54.3 months	
Kanemitsu (2021)[49]	Surgery + adjuvant FOLFOX (N = 151)	5-year 49.8%	0.006	3-year 71.2%	0.42
	Surgery alone (N = 149)	5-year 38.7%		3-year 83.1%	

5-FU, 5-Fluorouracil; *DFS*, disease-free survival; *FOLFOX*, 5-FU, leucovorin, and oxaliplatin; *LV*, leucovorin.

earlier recurrences in the remnant liver that could be salvaged with additional resections.

Chemotherapy-Associated Hepatotoxicity

When treating CLM patients with perioperative chemotherapy, it is important to note that chemotherapy causes liver damage. Oxaliplatin injures LSECs, leading to hepatic sinusoidal obstruction syndrome, whereas irinotecan is associated with steatosis and steatohepatitis.[50] These patterns of injury can be recognized intraoperatively as a "blue" liver with sinusoidal injury and "yellow" liver with steatohepatitis and significant steatosis (Fig. 90.9). Steatohepatitis has been associated with increased mortality after CLM resection, whereas sinusoidal injury can progress to clinically significant portal hypertension. FOLFOXIRI, a regimen that combines 5-fluorouracil (5-FU) with both oxaliplatin and irinotecan, is associated with high response rates but increased hepatotoxicity. Among 37 patients who underwent hepatectomy after FOLFOXIRI for initially unresectable CLM, rates of sinusoidal injury and steatohepatitis were 100% and 76%, respectively.[51] Chemotherapy-associated hepatotoxicity can be mitigated by limiting the duration of preoperative therapy to 2 to 3 months and by waiting >4 weeks after chemotherapy before liver resection.[52] A study from Memorial Sloan Kettering Cancer Center (MSKCC) showed that maximum radiologic response occurs after 2 to 4 months of chemotherapy, with little therapeutic benefit when continued beyond 4 months.[53] In addition, for patients receiving FOLFOX, the addition of bevacizumab has been shown to have a protective effect from oxaliplatin-induced sinusoidal injury.[54]

Synchronous Primary Colorectal Cancer and Liver Metastases

For patients presenting with synchronous CLM, defined as liver metastases detected at the time of primary colorectal cancer diagnosis, the sequencing of liver and primary tumor resection must be decided on a case-by-case basis.[2] No series has demonstrated superiority of combined or staged resection, either primary-first or liver-first. The combined approach is attractive because it reduces the number of operations patients must undergo and, thus, decreases both hospital costs and time off systemic chemotherapy. However, it may be associated with increased complication rates.[55] A recent multicenter trial randomized 85 patients with resectable CLM to simultaneous or staged, primary-first resection and found comparable rates of major complications (49%, simultaneous vs. 46%, staged, *P* = 0.70). Limitations of this trial include patients in the staged group having more advanced disease and long study duration of 10 years. An analysis of the American College of Surgeons National Surgical Quality Improvement Program database reported that patients undergoing combined major hepatectomy and high-risk colectomy had major morbidity and mortality rates of 55% and 5%.[56] However, at high-volume centers, combined resection can be performed safely, with a series from MSKCC of simultaneous rectal and major liver resection having a grade 3 to 4 morbidity rate of 23% and 0% mortality.[57,58] Thus, simultaneous high-risk colorectal and hepatic resections must be approached with caution or referred to high-volume centers.

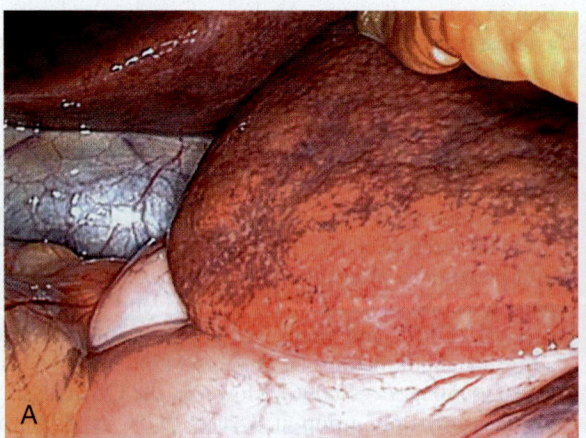
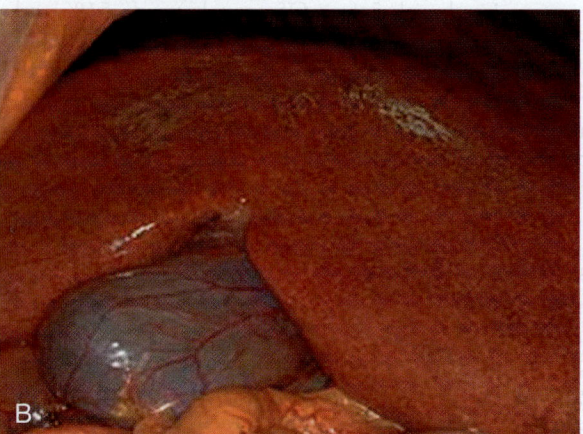

FIGURE 90.9 Intraoperative photos showing (A) blue liver from oxaliplatin-induced sinusoidal injury and (B) yellow liver due to steatosis and steatohepatitis, associated with irinotecan. (From Chun YS, Kawaguchi Y, and Vauthey JN. Hepatic metastasis from colorectal cancer. In: Jarnagin WR, ed. *Blumgart's Surgery of the Liver, Biliary Tract and Pancreas.* Elsevier; 2023:1226-1238.)

For patients undergoing staged resection, factors to consider include primary tumor symptoms, extent of liver disease, and sequencing of radiotherapy for rectal tumors. Patients who have bleeding or obstruction from their primary tumors and limited liver disease may benefit from primary resection first. However, for patients with extensive hepatic metastases, the liver-first approach is favored because their hepatic disease drives prognosis.[59] For patients with obstructing primary tumors, laparoscopic diversion will allow early initiation of systemic therapy. Bleeding from primary tumors can be treated with transfusions as indicated and will usually improve with systemic therapy. The liver-first approach is particularly important for patients with low rectal tumors, given the high incidence of complications and quality of life concerns associated with low anterior and abdominoperineal resections, and the potential for complete response after neoadjuvant chemoradiation.[60]

Role of Diagnostic Laparoscopy

Diagnostic laparoscopy allows for direct visual inspection of the liver and peritoneal cavity, and use of IOUS to evaluate for underlying liver disease or occult metastases not appreciated on CT scans. Although early reports found that staging laparoscopy helped circumvent unnecessary laparotomy in a significant proportion of CLM cases, more contemporary series suggest that the role of laparoscopy is limited due to improvements in preoperative cross-sectional imaging.[61,62] Thus, diagnostic laparoscopy is used selectively in patients with high burdens of systemic disease felt by the surgeon to be at risk of peritoneal dissemination and in patients who have received extensive preoperative chemotherapy and may have more severe chemotherapy-associated liver injury than is apparent on imaging and laboratory studies.

Prognostic Factors

A number of prognostic indicators based on clinicopathologic variables have been defined and validated in the literature (Table 90.2). One of the earliest and most well-known prognostic scores, the clinical risk score, was published by Fong and colleagues in 1999.[63] The authors evaluated 1001 consecutive patients undergoing CLM resection and identified seven factors that were independently predictive of shorter OS. These factors are positive hepatectomy margin, node-positive primary tumor, disease-free interval between primary resection and presentation of liver metastasis <12 months, more than one hepatic metastasis, liver metastasis size >5 cm, CEA >200 ng/mL, and extrahepatic disease (EHD). For patients receiving preoperative chemotherapy, pathologic and radiologic response to therapy are strong predictors of survival after CLM resection.[64,65]

Biomarkers

Biopsy is not mandatory before resection of CLM. However, tissue acquisition, often from the primary tumor via endoscopy, is helpful in assessing disease biology and selecting systemic therapy regimens. Genotyping can be performed from either the primary colorectal cancer or liver metastasis due to >90% concordance in mutation status of *RAS*, *BRAF*, and *TP53* between the primary tumor and CLM.[71] Advances in next-generation sequencing have led to the discovery of distinct molecular subtypes of colorectal cancer that drive prognosis and response to therapy. Assessment of microsatellite instability (MSI) and molecular testing for somatic mutations in the genes *KRAS*, *NRAS*, *BRAF*, and *ERBB2* are standard of care for metastatic colorectal cancer.[72] With the widespread availability of next-generation sequencing, it is becoming

TABLE 90.2 Clinicopathologic and Molecular Prognostic Factors After Resection of Colorectal Liver Metastases

AUTHOR (YEAR)	N	PROGNOSTIC INDICATORS
Nordlinger (1996)[66]	1568	Age Tumor size CEA Primary tumor stage Disease-free interval Number of metastases Resection margin
Iwatsuki (1999)[67]	305	≥3 tumors Size >8 cm Time to hepatic recurrence ≤30 months Bilateral metastases
Fong (1999)[63]	1001	Node-positive primary Disease-free interval <12 months >1 metastasis CEA >200 ng/mL Size >5 cm
Margonis (2018)[68]	502	*KRAS* mutation CEA ≥20 ng/mL Node-positive primary Tumor burden score Extrahepatic disease
Kawaguchi (2021)[69]	579	*RAS* mutation Tumor size Number of metastases
Berardi (2023)[70]	783	Primary tumor location, T stage, and nodal status Disease-free interval Number and size of liver metastases

CEA, Carcinoembryonic antigen.

increasingly important for surgeons to be familiar with these molecular determinants of prognosis, both to guide multidisciplinary clinical decision-making and patient expectations (see Table 90.2).

Tumors with deficient DNA mismatch repair are characterized by numerous insertions and deletions in microsatellites, which are short tandem repeats of DNA prone to mismatch errors (see Chapter 61). MSI-high (MSI-H) tumors, occurring in 15% of all colorectal cancers, are associated with a high mutational burden, a more robust inflammatory response, and potential sensitivity to immune checkpoint blockade. Patients with MSI-H colorectal cancer are less likely to present with liver metastases and comprise <2% of CLM resection series. When CLM occur in the setting of MSI, they may carry a worse prognosis.[73,74]

The *RAS* genes, *KRAS*, *NRAS*, and *HRAS*, are the most frequently mutated family of genes in cancer.[75] They encode small GTPases in the mitogen-activated protein kinase (MAPK) signaling pathway to regulate cell proliferation, differentiation, and apoptosis. *RAS* mutations are identified in 40% to 50% of patients undergoing CLM resection and cause constitutive activation of the Ras protein, leading to resistance to therapies that block EGFR, which lies upstream of Ras in the MAPK pathway (Fig. 90.10). In addition to predicting resistance to therapy with the EGFR inhibitors, cetuximab and panitumumab, *RAS* mutations have been found to predict worse outcome after CLM resection. In 2013, Vauthey et al. evaluated 193 patients undergoing

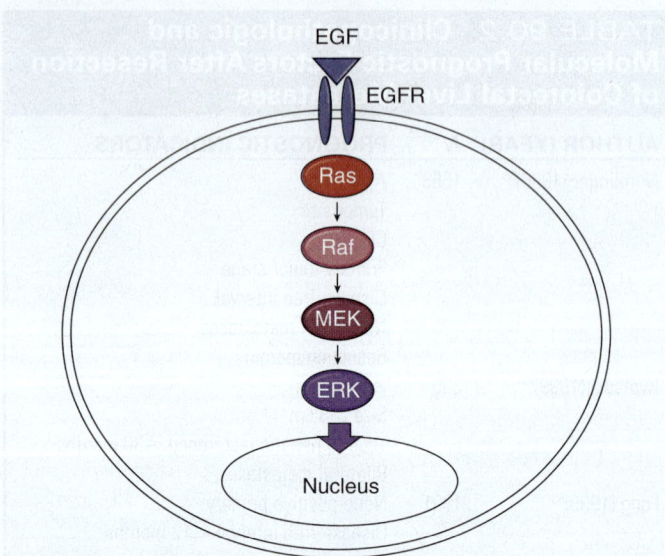

FIGURE 90.10 Schematic of mitogen-activated protein kinase pathway. *EGF,* Epidermal growth factor; *EGFR,* epidermal growth factor receptor. (From Chun YS, Kawaguchi Y, and Vauthey JN. Hepatic metastasis from colorectal cancer. In: Jarnagin WR, ed. *Blumgart's Surgery of the Liver, Biliary Tract and Pancreas.* Elsevier; 2023:1226-1238.)

CLM resection who did not receive anti-EGFR therapy and found significantly lower 3-year OS with a *RAS* mutation, compared with wild type (52% vs. 81%, *P* = 0.002).[76] Subsequent studies have shown that co-mutation of *RAS/TP53* portends even worse survival.[77,78] Other gene mutations associated with worse survival after CLM resection are *FBXW7* and *SMAD4.*[79,80]

BRAF encodes a member of the rapidly accelerated fibrosarcoma (Raf) family of protein kinases, and mutated *BRAF* leads to activation of the MAPK signaling cascade downstream of Ras. The most common *BRAF* mutation, V600E, results in a substitution of glutamic acid for valine at codon 600. *BRAF V600E* mutations are identified in 8% to 12% of metastatic colorectal cancer patients and associated with a median OS of only 11 months.[81] Patients with *BRAF* mutations are less likely to present with liver-limited disease and, thus, comprise <5% of the population in hepatectomy series. In a multicenter study of 1497 patients undergoing CLM resection, *BRAF* mutations were identified in 2% of patients and associated with significantly worse median OS, compared with *BRAF* wild type (40 vs. 81 months, *P* < 0.001).[82]

Extrahepatic Disease

The presence of EHD is associated with higher recurrence rates and worse prognosis but not an absolute contraindication to CLM resection. Studies have demonstrated favorable outcomes after CLM resection in selected patients with EHD, particularly when complete resection of all sites of disease is possible. A retrospective evaluation of 219 patients who underwent resection of CLM and synchronous EHD reported a 28% 5-year OS rate and 8 actual 10-year survivors.[83] Metastases to portal and retroperitoneal nodes, CLM size >3 cm, and progression on chemotherapy were independently associated with worse survival. Another series of 109 patients undergoing concurrent resection of CLM and EHD found that peritoneal metastases and *RAS/TP53* co-mutation were associated with worse survival on multivariable analysis.[84] Patients with EHD isolated to the lung had the longest median OS of 78 months.

Resection Margin

The optimal width of resection margin and prognostic impact of residual microscopic disease (R1 resection) is under debate. In the 1980s, published studies demonstrated improved survival with resection margins of ≥1 cm.[85] More recently, a multi-institutional report of over 500 patients found that the width of negative margin, from 1 mm to ≥1 cm, did not affect recurrence rates.[86] Fueling the controversy, De Haas et al. reported in 2008 similar OS rates after R1 and R0 resection.[87] Multiple studies have shown that the prognostic impact of a positive margin depends upon other factors such as response to systemic therapy, suggesting that the R1 margin represents a surrogate marker of worse tumor biology.[88,89] Based on available evidence, the goal of CLM resection should be a margin-negative resection with preservation of as much nontumoral liver parenchyma as possible.

Liver-Directed Therapies

Most patients with CLM will present with unresectable disease, and only 10% to 30% will have sufficient downstaging after systemic therapy to undergo resection.[45] When liver resection is not possible due to anatomic or biologic constraints, multiple liver-directed therapies are available to achieve local disease control.

Ablation

For tumors <3 cm, RFA can achieve durable tumor eradication. RFA uses high-frequency alternating currents (300–500 kHz) to heat and induce tissue coagulation necrosis. Blood vessels act as heat sinks and limit RFA effectiveness. Care should be employed around portal pedicles as potential complications include bile duct injuries, hemorrhage, and liver infarction. Subcapsular ablations have a risk for capsular rupture and bleeding. The phase II EORTC-CLOCC trial evaluated the additional benefit of RFA to chemotherapy in patients with unresectable CLM and found improved survival with RFA compared with chemotherapy alone (median OS 46 vs. 41 months, *P* = 0.01).[90] However, the trial results are confounded by half the patients in the RFA arm also undergoing hepatic resections. Microwave ablation (MWA) uses higher energy waves (900–2450 MHz) that disrupt water molecules to generate friction and heat, causing necrosis of surrounding tissue. It is less sensitive to heat sink and can propagate a larger ablation zone than RFA.[23]

Hepatic Artery Infusion Pump

The concept of delivering regional liver-directed chemotherapy dates back to the 1950s, when nitrogen mustard gas was injected directly into the hepatic artery. Around the same time, rationale for regional therapy was strengthened by the discovery that hepatic tissues mainly derive their blood supply from the portal vein, but metastases are perfused almost entirely by the hepatic artery. Modern day hepatic artery infusion chemotherapy (HAIC) is refined by two additional innovations. First, fluorodeoxyuridine (FUDR) is found to be the ideal chemotherapy agent because it is converted to the active metabolite 5-FU in the liver. It has a hepatic extraction rate of 94% to 99%, meaning most of the drug remains in the liver and very little circulates systemically. Second, the development of an implantable hepatic artery infusion pump (HAIP) allows for continuous administration of HAIC.[91]

In patients with unresectable disease, HAIC can convert half to resectable disease, even in patients who have been heavily treated previously with chemotherapy. In a prospective phase II trial at MSKCC, 47% of patients with initially unresectable CLM were able to undergo complete resection after HAIC and systemic therapy.[92] The overall response rate was 76%, and median OS was 38 months, with significantly longer survival in patients who had complete resections than those who did not undergo resection (3-year OS: 80% vs. 26%, $P = 0.005$). Those with completely resected CLM after HAIC had survival comparable to those presenting with up-front resectable disease.

After complete resection of CLM, the use of adjuvant systemic chemotherapy has not been shown to improve OS.[47] For this reason, the addition of HAIC has been investigated as an adjunct. There have been two prospective trials in which HAIC was studied in conjunction with systemic chemotherapy. The first was a prospective randomized trial from MSKCC, where patients were randomized to receive systemic 5-FU/leucovorin, with or without HAIC FUDR, after CLM resection.[93] The HAIC group showed significant improvement in 2-year OS (86% vs. 72%, $P = 0.03$) and hepatic recurrence-free survival (90% vs. 60%, $P < 0.0001$). This single-center trial was followed by a randomized multicenter trial in which adjuvant HAIC FUDR and systemic 5-FU were compared with no further therapy.[94] Although the 4-year OS was not statistically different in the adjuvant therapy arm (62% vs. 53%, $P = 0.6$), a significant difference in 4-year DFS was observed (46% vs. 25%, $P = 0.04$).

There are few contraindications to the placement of HAIP, namely the presence of multiple sites of EHD, extensive hepatic replacement by tumor, impaired liver function or evidence of portal hypertension, and main portal vein thrombus. High-quality CT angiography is required to ensure the patency of the hepatic artery, gastroduodenal artery (GDA), and assess for aberrant hepatic arterial anatomy. In most cases, the HAIP catheter is placed in the GDA (Fig. 90.11). Accessory/replaced hepatic arteries can be ligated, as flow to the contralateral lobe is maintained via cross-perfusion. HAIP can be safely placed in combination with colorectal or liver resection with minimal added morbidity. In selected patients, it can also be placed robotically with shorter recovery time.[16] After catheter placement, a methylene blue test is performed intraoperatively to evaluate for bilobar perfusion and the absence of extrahepatic perfusion. Postoperatively, a nuclear medicine perfusion scan provides additional confirmation, and sometimes angiography may be needed to address extrahepatic perfusion.

Because bile ducts also derive their blood supply from the hepatic artery, biliary complications can occur after HAIC, requiring careful monitoring of liver function. Usually, liver enzyme elevation can be mitigated by FUDR dose reduction and filling the pump with dexamethasone but rarely can progress to biliary sclerosis and cholangitis. Other HAIP complications can be categorized as those related to the pump pocket (hematomas, infections), catheter (dislodgements, erosions), or those related to the vasculature (arterial dissections, pseudoaneurysms). The majority of early pump complications are salvageable.[95]

Radioembolization

Radioembolization entails delivery of yttrium-90 microspheres, which emit β particles, through hepatic tumor-feeding arteries. It is also called transarterial radioembolization (TARE) or selective internal radiation therapy (SIRT). Yttrium-90 resin microspheres are approved in the United States for the treatment of CLM, whereas glass microspheres are approved for treatment of hepatocellular carcinoma. Because radiation is emitted, this technique is limited by tumor proximity to adjacent bowel and stomach. Randomized phase III trials of patients with liver-only or

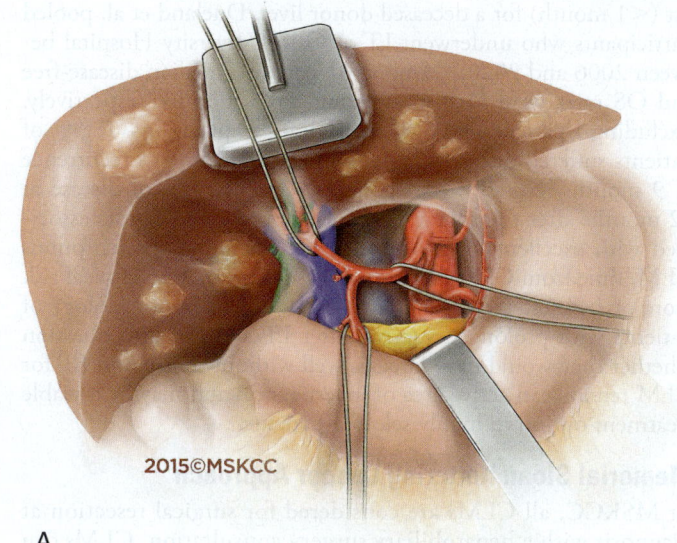

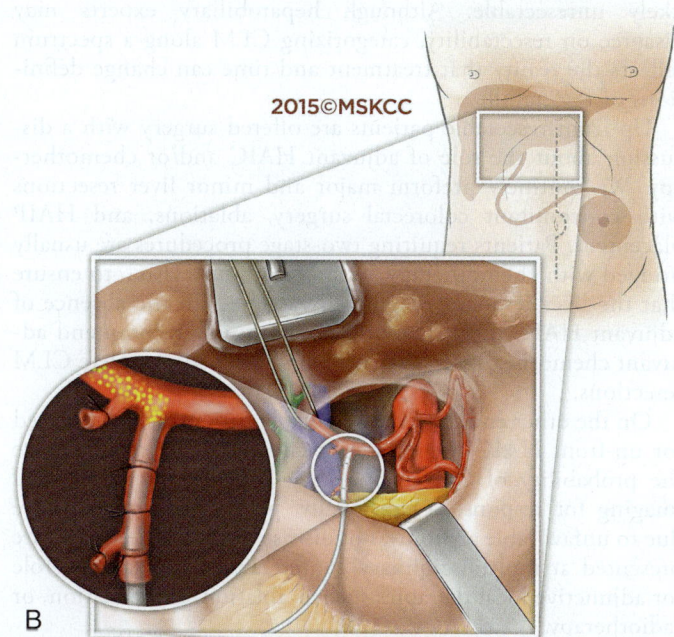

FIGURE 90.11 Placement of hepatic artery infusion pump in the gastroduodenal artery (A) and secured in place with ties (B). (From Qadan M, D'Angelica MI, Kemeny NE, Cercek A, Kingham TP. Robotic hepatic arterial infusion pump placement. *HPB*. 2017;19:429-435.)

liver-dominant metastatic colorectal cancer have failed to demonstrate a survival benefit with radioembolization when added to first-line chemotherapy.[96] The benefit of radioembolization in a second-line or salvage setting remains undetermined.

Liver Transplantation

The role of liver transplantation (LT) for metastatic colorectal cancer isolated to the liver is controversial and currently undergoing investigation in multiple randomized controlled trials.[97] Metastatic cancer was traditionally considered a contraindication to LT. In the 1980s and 1990s LT for CLM was attempted, but due to a dismal 5-year OS of 18%, it was largely abandoned. However, interest in LT was rekindled by studies from Norway, which has a surplus of liver grafts and short time on the waiting list (<1 month) for a deceased donor liver. Dueland et al. pooled participants who underwent LT at Oslo University Hospital between 2006 and 2020.[98] Among 61 patients, median disease-free and OS rates were 11.8 months and 60.3 months, respectively. Excluding 1 patient who died of surgical complications, 78.3% of patients suffered disease relapse, with median time to recurrence of 9 months. Notably, four patients remained free of disease at 72 months after transplant. The authors presented factors associated with excellent prognosis after LT, including metachronous CLM, time from CLM diagnosis to LT >3 years, and clinical risk score of 1. These factors highlight the indolent tumor biology of patients with prolonged survival after LT and call into question whether they would have fared as well without transplant. LT for CLM remains an active area of investigation and may be a viable treatment option in highly selected patients.

Memorial Sloan Kettering Cancer Approach

At MSKCC, all CLMs are considered for surgical resection at diagnosis with a hepatobiliary surgery consultation. CLMs can be categorized as up-front resectable, potentially resectable, or likely unresectable. Although hepatobiliary experts may disagree on resectability, categorizing CLM along a spectrum reflects the reality that treatment and time can change definitions of resectability.

Up-front resectable patients are offered surgery with a discussion about the role of adjuvant HAIC and/or chemotherapy. We routinely preform major and minor liver resections with concomitant colorectal surgery, ablations, and HAIP placement. Patients requiring two-stage procedures are usually bridged with chemotherapy, with or without HAIC, to ensure that the liver remnant remains disease free. In the absence of adjuvant HAIC therapy, we do not routinely recommend adjuvant chemotherapy to patients who have had complete CLM resections.

On the other end, likely unresectable patients are considered for up-front HAIC with systemic chemotherapy to maximize the probability of conversion. They are followed with serial imaging for response. Occasionally, patients are unresectable due to unfavorable anatomy, not disease burden. These cases are presented at multidisciplinary conferences to discuss the role for adjunctive local therapies such as ablation, embolization, or radiotherapy.

Potentially resectable patients require detailed planning that starts with identifying the barriers to resectability. If tumor size and insufficient FLR are the main deterrents, then preoperative chemotherapy is considered, along with PVE. If disease burden and bilobar disease are the major concerns, then we would perform two-staged procedures with HAIP placement. To decide which tumors to resect in the first procedure, we identify the tumors near inflow/outflow vessels, as those lesions define the liver remnant. Typically, we clear the tumors in the FLR with a combination of resections and ablations and place an HAIP in the first procedure. Then, we wait for a period on HAIC and chemotherapy to allow for liver remnant growth and resect if disease does not progress to be unresectable.

Patients with unresectable CLM and extensive liver-only disease will die of liver failure due to tumor burden; therefore, curbing the progression of liver disease with palliative regional therapy is also of interest. In a retrospective study from MSKCC, the median survival from time of HAIP placement in patients with unresectable CLM was 32 months.[99] This included patients who had been pretreated with and progressed on first-line chemotherapy.

Even patients with a single site of EHD may benefit from HAIC, with median survival of 18 months after HAIP placement. These data suggest that there is a role for HAIC in the palliative setting for unresectable patients as well.

MD Anderson Cancer Center Approach

The majority of MD Anderson Cancer Center (MDACC) patients with CLM are treated with neoadjuvant systemic therapy, typically consisting of 5-FU combined with oxaliplatin or irinotecan. The VEGF inhibitor, bevacizumab, is often included in the neoadjuvant regimen to potentially increase response to therapy and protect from oxaliplatin-associated sinusoidal injury.[54,64] Although pretreatment with systemic chemotherapy bears the risk of chemotherapy-induced liver injury, there are several important advantages to this approach. First, patients with CLMs already have disseminated disease, evidenced by the presence of micrometastases and CTCs that are not apparent on gross examination or cross-sectional imaging.[100] In theory, systemic therapy can help eliminate some or all of these cells, increasing the likelihood of cure after R0 liver resection. Second, treatment with neoadjuvant therapy serves as a valuable test of disease biology. Radiologic and pathologic response to preoperative therapy are important surrogates of tumor biology.[64,65] Patients with tumors that progress through systemic chemotherapy have aggressive biology and are unlikely to benefit from an extensive liver operation. In fact, the systemic inflammatory milieu induced by surgery may hasten the progression of their disease in the early postoperative setting.[101] Third, neoadjuvant chemotherapy affords an opportunity to test a tumor's sensitivity to cytotoxic and targeted agents. This allows for better tailoring of adjuvant regimens following surgery. Fourth, response to neoadjuvant therapy may allow for parenchymal-sparing operations in patients who might otherwise require a major hepatectomy to clear their disease.

For patients with extensive bilateral CLM and an initially insufficient FLR, our preferred approach is neoadjuvant systemic therapy followed by two-stage hepatectomy. This typically involves surgical clearance of left-sided liver lesions followed by PVE, with or without hepatic vein occlusion. After a 4-week period of hypertrophy after PVE, patients undergo a right or extended right hepatectomy to clear the remainder of their disease. We have reported favorable outcomes with this approach, even in patients with extensive bilateral disease.[102] One disadvantage to this approach is that some patients may develop disease progression while awaiting FLR hypertrophy. A strategy to minimize tumor progression between the two stages is to treat patients with systemic chemotherapy during the period of hypertrophy after PVE. It should be noted that patients who develop disease progression during the short 4-week period of hypertrophy generally have aggressive biology and may not benefit from completion of the second-stage hepatectomy.

From a technical standpoint, we generally use the Cavitron ultrasonic surgical aspirator (CUSA; Integra, Princeton, NJ) to divide the liver parenchyma and saline-linked monopolar sealer (DS3.5-C Dissecting Sealer, Medtronic, Minneapolis, MN) to seal small vessels and bile ducts. Larger vessels and bile ducts are controlled with surgical clips, suture ligature, or vascular staplers depending on the size and quality of the structure being divided. Inflow occlusion with the Pringle maneuver is used liberally, as we have found that intermittent Pringle does not increase the risk of posthepatectomy liver insufficiency. After specimen removal, intraoperative air cholangiogram is performed to detect bile leaks.[103]

Discussion

Complete resection remains indispensable for curative-intent treatment of CLM. However, treatment paradigms and, in particular, the timing of resection differs between our institutions. Although MDACC generally favors a neoadjuvant approach to test biology and potentially eliminate micrometastatic disease before surgery, patients with resectable tumors at MSKCC are commonly offered up-front surgery with consideration for adjuvant systemic or HAIC therapy. No randomized trial has demonstrated definitive superiority of one strategy over the other.

Although our institutional practices differ, both MDACC and MSKCC support the management of CLM by a multidisciplinary team, including surgeons with hepatobiliary expertise. We agree that complete resection should be the goal of every CLM operation and provides the best chance for long-term survival. Our approaches also place paramount importance on the assessment of disease biology, considering tumor burden, time (disease-free interval), mutation profile, and response to previous therapy in every treatment decision. As molecular diagnostic techniques and our understanding of CLM biology continue to evolve, so too will our ability to individualize treatment and provide a more nuanced approach to the multimodal management of this disease.

NEUROENDOCRINE LIVER METASTASES

NETs are well-differentiated, slow-growing tumors that can arise from neuroendocrine cells present throughout the body. NETs should be differentiated from neuroendocrine carcinomas, which are poorly differentiated and highly aggressive. The most common sites of primary NETs are the gastrointestinal tract (48%), lung (25%), and pancreas (9%).[104] The potential for distant metastases depends upon the primary site, with appendiceal and lung NETs having lower rates. In contrast, small bowel and pancreatic NETs (PNETs) frequently develop distant metastases, 90% in the liver, which represent the dominant driver of prognosis.

NETs are categorized by grade, based on mitotic rate and Ki-67 index, and hormone secretion.[105] Carcinoid syndrome occurs in patients with small bowel NETs that have metastasized to the liver, resulting in production of vasoactive hormones, including serotonin. Symptoms include diarrhea, flushing, and wheezing from bronchospasm. Carcinoid syndrome is rare in the absence of liver metastases due to first pass metabolism in the liver and degradation of secreted vasoactive substances. In patients with carcinoid syndrome, plasma or 24-hour urine 5-hydroxyindoleacetic acid (5-HIAA) will be elevated. A quarter of PNETs are associated with hormone secretion, such as insulinomas, glucagonomas, somatostatinomas, and VIPomas. Insulinomas have a low risk of metastasis, whereas glucagonomas and somatostatinomas frequently metastasize to the liver (80%–90%). Nonfunctional PNETs will often have elevations in pancreatic polypeptide or chromogranin A; both can be nonspecifically elevated and should not be used to guide treatment decisions.

Surgical Cytoreduction

Given the prolonged natural history of NELMs, management of liver metastases is based on careful evaluation of treatment goals. Surgical cytoreduction is a critical consideration for patients with NELMs who are fit for surgery and have resectable disease. Although cure without recurrence is uncommon, resection is associated with improved OS and quality of life for patients with functional tumors through reduction of hormone load. Resection of NELMs has been associated with excellent 10-year survival

TABLE 90.3 Selected Studies Evaluating Cytoreductive Surgery for Neuroendocrine Liver Metastases

AUTHOR (YEAR)	N	GOAL % CYTOREDUCTION	SURVIVAL
Sarmiento (2003)[109]	170	90%	5-year OS 61%
Chambers (2008)[110]	30	70%	5-year OS 74%
Graff-Baker (2014)[111]	52	70%	5-year PFS 64%
Maxwell (2016)[107]	108	70%	Median PFS 3.2 years Median OS not reached after 4.1 years
Gudmundsdottir (2023)[108]	546	>90%	Median OS, 122 months Median PFS, 17 months

OS, Overall survival; *PFS*, progression-free survival.

rates as high as 79%.[106] However, the data supporting cytoreduction are all retrospective and highly confounded. Although anatomic hepatectomy may be required for lesions inseparable from vital structures, a parenchymal-sparing approach, including enucleation, is strongly preferred.

The amount of cytoreduction necessary for the associated prolongation of survival is a matter of ongoing debate. All available data are retrospective and subject to both selection bias and subjectivity pertaining to the degree of cytoreduction achieved. Various series suggest that 70% to 90% cytoreduction of tumor burden may provide a survival benefit (Table 90.3). A series from the University of Iowa of 108 patients who underwent NELM resection, many with concomitant ablation, found improved OS and PFS for patients undergoing ≥70% reduction, compared with <70%.[107] In a study from the Mayo Clinic of 546 patients undergoing cytoreductive hepatectomy, 37% had functional disease.[108] Symptom-free interval was significantly worse for patients undergoing incomplete cytoreduction, defined as <90% debulking (median, 21 vs. 62 months, $P = 0.021$). On multivariable analysis, the Ki-67 index was the strongest predictor of OS, with markedly worse survival with Ki-67 >20%.

The biology of NELM spans a wide spectrum from indolent disease to progressive liver replacement, but the majority will fall on the indolent end. Most institutions would agree that surgery for functional tumors can mitigate symptoms and is recommended when somatostatin analogues (SSAs) are ineffective. Surgery for nonfunctional NELMs is debatable because complete debulking is rarely possible and often leaves residual nonvisible disease. At both MSKCC and MDACC, the role for surgery is considered in the context of multiple adjuncts such as systemic and liver-directed therapies, as reviewed in the following sections.

Perioperative Considerations

Patients with carcinoid syndrome undergoing hepatectomy and other procedures are at risk for release of high levels of vasoactive substances and carcinoid crisis, characterized by life-threatening hemodynamic instability, with or without bronchospasm and arrhythmias. Perioperative octreotide prophylaxis is recommended, although the optimal timing and dose are not well established.[112] In addition to intravenous octreotide, aggressive treatment with intravenous fluids and vasopressors, either phenylephrine or vasopressin, is required to treat a carcinoid crisis.

Carcinoid heart disease develops in approximately 20% of patients with carcinoid syndrome due to vasoactive substances released by NETs, leading to plaquelike deposits in the right heart, tricuspid and pulmonic regurgitation, and right heart failure.[113] First-line treatment of carcinoid heart disease is SSAs, with valve replacement reserved for patients with refractory disease. It is critical to obtain an echocardiogram preoperatively in patients with carcinoid syndrome who are considered for surgery. For the rare patient who is a candidate for cytoreductive hepatectomy but needs cardiac surgery, the sequence of operations should be individualized. Increased right atrial pressure and hepatic congestion represent contraindications to liver surgery.

Nonsurgical Management

Nonsurgical management of NELMs has been investigated in randomized trials (see Chapters 76 and 77). Given the indolent nature of low-grade NETs, most therapies have been found to improve PFS but not OS. SSAs inhibit the receptor in SSTR-avid tumors and are effective in managing hormone excess. Octreotide long-acting release (LAR) is a long-acting SSA that was shown in the PROMID trial to delay progression in metastatic midgut NETs compared with placebo (14 vs. 6 months, $P < 0.001$).[114] Most patients had liver involvement (86%) but low liver tumor burden (<10% of liver volume). Long-term results of this trial, however, failed to show an OS benefit secondary to either crossover after progression or prolonged survival even in those with progressive disease.[115] Similar results were seen in the CLARINET trial with the SSA lanreotide, suggesting that while SSAs suppress hormone hypersecretion and are cytostatic, this does not translate to improved long-term survival.[116]

Systemic therapies are also available in progressing disease. Everolimus inhibits the mTOR pathway and is approved for the treatment of PNETs based on the RADIANT-3 trial, which showed improved PFS compared with placebo alone (11 vs. 5 months, $P < 0.001$), but no difference in OS.[117] It is also approved for advanced gastrointestinal tract NETs based on the RADIANT-4 trial, in which everolimus was superior to placebo for PFS (11 vs. 4 months, $P < 0.001$).[118] Long-term survival data from this trial are not yet mature, but there may be a trend toward improved survival. More recently, the multicenter, prospective randomized trial ECOG-ACRIN E2211 showed superiority of temozolomide and capecitabine to temozolomide alone in metastatic PNETs for the primary end point of PFS (23 vs. 14 months, $P < 0.02$).[119] The majority of these patients had already progressed on SSAs. Unlike SSAs, which are mostly cytostatic, there was a 34% to 40% response rate in both cohorts, raising the possibility of tumor shrinkage with chemotherapy before cytoreduction.

For SSTR-avid tumors, radiotherapy can be added to SSAs to achieve higher response rates. Lutetium-177 (^{177}Lu)-DOTATATE is a radiolabeled SSA that delivers systemic radiotherapy to SSTR-avid tumors in a method called peptide receptor radionuclide therapy (PRRT). NETTER-1 was a phase III trial that randomized patients to receive PRRT and octreotide LAR or octreotide LAR alone in midgut NETs.[120] It met the primary end point of improved PFS in the group also receiving PRRT (not reached vs. 8 months, $P < 0.001$). There was an 18% overall response rate with the addition of PRRT, which is significant given that SSA alone is cytostatic. Long-term results showed a nonstatistically significant improvement in OS (48 vs. 36 months, $P = 0.3$). Currently, the NETTER-2 trial is accruing patients to study the benefit of PRRT in midgut NETs with higher proliferation index.

Similar to CLM, NELMs that are not amenable to surgical resection can be treated with liver-directed therapies. These tumors respond well to arterially directed therapies because they are hypervascular. In a large, multicenter retrospective analysis comparing surgery ($N = 339$) versus arterially directed therapies ($N = 414$) for NELMs, surgery was associated with improved 5-year OS (74% vs. 30%, $P < 0.001$), although patients undergoing surgery had less advanced disease.[121] In a propensity-adjusted multivariate Cox model, surgery provided a survival benefit over intraarterial therapy for symptomatic patients with >25% liver involvement but not for patients without symptoms.

NONCOLORECTAL NONNEUROENDOCRINE LIVER METASTASES

Data on outcomes after hepatectomy for noncolorectal nonneuroendocrine (NCNN) liver metastases are limited to small case series or retrospective analyses with heterogeneous patient populations. In 2006, a retrospective review of 1452 patients undergoing resection of NCNN liver metastases at 41 centers in France reported that the most common primary tumors were breast (32%), gastrointestinal (16%), genitourinary (14%), and melanoma (10%).[122] Factors independently associated with worse survival were age >60; nonbreast primary, melanoma, or squamous histology; disease-free interval <12 months; extrahepatic metastases; R2 resection; and major hepatectomy. More recently, a multicenter study from Japan by Sano et al. evaluated 1539 patients undergoing NCNN resection.[123] The most common primary tumors were gastric (35%), gastrointestinal stromal tumor (GIST) (13%), biliary (10%), and ovarian (7%). This study found that prognostic factors differed by primary tumor type.

The divergent findings in the reports from France and Japan likely reflect different patient populations and selection criteria. Patients who will derive benefit from hepatic resection for NCNN are those with favorable tumor biology, as indicated by the absence of EHD, solitary liver metastasis, and long disease-free interval from primary resection. Given the improvement in morbidity of hepatectomy and the emergence of novel therapeutics across tumor types, NCNN liver metastases are being increasingly considered for resection, including prospective randomized trials, as described in the following section.

Gastric and Gastroesophageal Junction

The role of surgical resection of metastatic gastric and gastroesophageal junction adenocarcinoma was investigated in a phase II, multicenter trial in Germany (AIO-FLOT3).[124] Patients were stratified into three arms: (A) resectable, nonmetastatic, (B) limited metastasis, and (C) extensive metastasis. Patients in arms A and B received perioperative chemotherapy and resection of all disease sites if feasible. In arm B, 18.3% of patients had liver-confined metastasis, fewer than five in number. Among 36 patients with limited metastasis undergoing surgery, those with liver metastasis had worse median OS compared with retroperitoneal nodal metastases (13.6 months vs. not reached). There are two ongoing randomized phase III trials in Europe investigating the role of metastasectomy, including liver-confined metastases, up to five in number.[125]

Breast Cancer

Hepatectomy for breast cancer liver metastases is controversial. Only 10% of patients with breast cancer have metastases isolated to the liver; thus, the role of hepatectomy is limited. Factors associated with higher survival after resection of breast cancer liver metastases include response to systemic therapy, hormone receptor status, hepatectomy margin, and number of metastases.[126,127]

Gastrointestinal Stromal Tumor

GISTs are rare mesenchymal tumors of the gastrointestinal tract that metastasize to the liver in approximately one-third of patients. A retrospective study of 239 patients who underwent resection of metastatic GIST and received imatinib therapy demonstrated 5-year OS exceeding 80% for patients with liver-limited metastases responsive to imatinib therapy.[128] However, whether hepatic resection offers a survival benefit over imatinib alone remains unclear. A randomized study of patients with metastatic GIST to the liver showed that surgery was associated with improved 3-year overall OS compared with imatinib alone (89.5% vs. 60%, $P = 0.03$).[129] However, this trial was limited by small sample size of 39 patients. Based on available evidence, hepatic resection in selected patients responding to systemic therapy with tyrosine kinase inhibitors improves outcomes. Adjuvant therapy should be continued postoperatively due to high rates of recurrence.[130]

Pancreas

Historically considered an absolute contraindication to surgery, improvements in systemic therapy and surgical outcomes have sparked interest in complete resection of pancreatic adenocarcinoma and hepatic metastasis. A retrospective study from Heidelberg University analyzed 173 patients with metastatic pancreas cancer who received preoperative chemotherapy followed by surgical exploration; 67% had liver-confined metastasis. Among patients who underwent resection of the primary tumor and metastasis, 48% of patients had a complete pathologic response in the metastasis and median OS of 25.5 months. These results raise the question whether patients with complete pathologic response to systemic therapy derive benefit from surgery. Multiple prospective trials are ongoing in China and Europe investigating the role of surgery or ablation for patients with limited hepatic metastases from pancreas cancer.[131] However, liver metastasectomy for pancreatic adenocarcinoma remains highly controversial.

Melanoma

Cutaneous melanoma represents an extremely rare indication for hepatic resection, due to widespread metastatic disease and poor tumor biology.[132] Uveal melanoma has a high predilection for liver metastasis, identified in 90% of patients with metastatic disease. Due to diffuse intrahepatic metastases, <10% of patients with liver-confined uveal metastases are candidates for surgery.[133]

Gynecologic Malignancies

Ovarian cancer often seeds the surface of the liver, but intrahepatic metastasis is uncommon. Liver resection for ovarian and other gynecologic malignancies has been shown to be safe. However, high-level evidence on patient selection criteria and survival benefit of hepatectomy is lacking.

SELECTED REFERENCES

Fong Y, Fortner J, Sun RL, Brennan MF, Blumgart LH. Clinical score for predicting recurrence after hepatic resection for metastatic colorectal cancer: analysis of 1001 consecutive cases. *Ann Surg.* 1999;230(3):309-321.

This is a landmark series from Memorial Sloan Kettering Cancer Center of hepatectomy for metastatic colorectal cancer. A subset of patients will be cured after complete resection of colorectal liver metastases, with 10-year survival rate of 22%. Clinicopathologic factors that predict prognosis include primary tumor margin and lymph node status, disease-free interval, extrahepatic disease, size and number of liver metastases, and CEA.

Li X, Ramadori P, Pfister D, Seehawer M, Zender L, Heikenwalder M. The immunological and metabolic landscape in primary and metastatic liver cancer. *Nat Rev Cancer.* 2021;21(9): 541-557.

Detailed review of the role of the liver metabolic and immunosuppressive environment in the development of liver metastases.

Mise Y, Aloia TA, Brudvik KW, Schwarz L, Vauthey JN, Conrad C. Parenchymal-sparing hepatectomy in colorectal liver metastasis improves salvageability and survival. *Ann Surg.* 2016;263(1): 146-152.

This study from MD Anderson Cancer Center demonstrated that parenchymal-sparing hepatectomy for colorectal liver metastases is noninferior to major hepatectomy with respect to liver recurrences and overall survival. Parenchymal-sparing resection has the advantage of allowing options for additional salvage operations in the event of future liver recurrence.

Nordlinger B, Sorbye H, Glimelius B, et al. Perioperative FOLFOX4 chemotherapy and surgery versus surgery alone for resectable liver metastases from colorectal cancer (EORTC 40983): long-term results of a randomised, controlled, phase 3 trial. *Lancet Oncol.* 2013;14(12):1208-1215.

Randomized trial of patients with resectable colorectal liver metastases demonstrating no significant overall survival difference with the addition of perioperative chemotherapy over surgery alone.

Tsilimigras DI, Brodt P, Clavien PA, et al. Liver metastases. *Nat Rev Dis Primers.* 2021;7(1):27.

Comprehensive primer of pathophysiology, clinical presentation, and treatment of liver metastases.

The full reference list appears on Elsevier eBooks+.

Small Intestine

B. Mark Evers

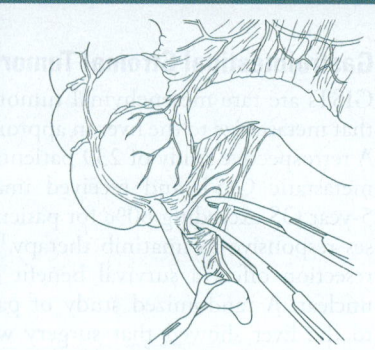

EMBRYOLOGY

The primitive gut is formed from the endodermal lining—the yolk sac, which is enveloped by the developing embryo as a result of cranial and caudal folding during the fourth week of human fetal gestation.[1] The endodermal layer gives rise to the epithelial lining of the digestive tract, and the splanchnic mesoderm surrounding the endoderm gives rise to the muscular connective tissue and all the other layers of the intestine. The splanchnic mesoderm wraps around the gut tube to form the mesenteries that suspend the gut within the body cavity; the mesoderm immediately adjacent to the endodermal tube also contributes to most of the wall of the gut tube. Nerves and neurons found in the wall are derived from the neural crest. Except for the duodenum, which is a primitive foregut structure, the small intestine is derived from the midgut. During the fifth to sixth week of fetal development, when the intestinal length is rapidly increasing, herniation of the midgut occurs through the umbilicus (Fig. 91.1). This midgut loop has a cranial and caudal limb, with the cranial limb developing into the distal duodenum, jejunum, and proximal ileum, and the caudal limb becoming the distal ileum and proximal two-thirds of the transverse colon. The juncture of the cranial and caudal limbs is

where the vitelline duct joins to the yolk sac. This duct structure normally becomes obliterated before birth; however, it can persist as a Meckel diverticulum in approximately 2% of the population. As the gut tube develops, the endoderm proliferates rapidly and temporarily occludes the lumen of the tube around the fifth week of gestation. Growth and expansion of mesoderm components in the wall, coupled with apoptosis of the endoderm during the seventh week, result in recanalization of the tube, and by the ninth week of gestation, the tube is again patent. This midgut herniation persists until about 10 weeks of fetal gestation, when the intestine returns to the abdominal cavity. Before reentering the abdomen, the midgut loop rotates 90 degrees counterclockwise around the superior mesenteric artery axis. As the small and large intestine return to the abdominal cavity, they continue to rotate in this direction for a complete 270-degree rotation from the initial starting point. Congenital anomalies of gut malrotation and fixation can occur during this process. Intestinal nonrotation occurs when the midgut loop only completes the first 90-degree rotation and returns to the abdomen without further rotation, thus leaving the small intestine in the right abdomen and large intestine in the left abdomen. When the intestine fails to complete the final 90-degree rotation, the cecum is fixed just below the stomach

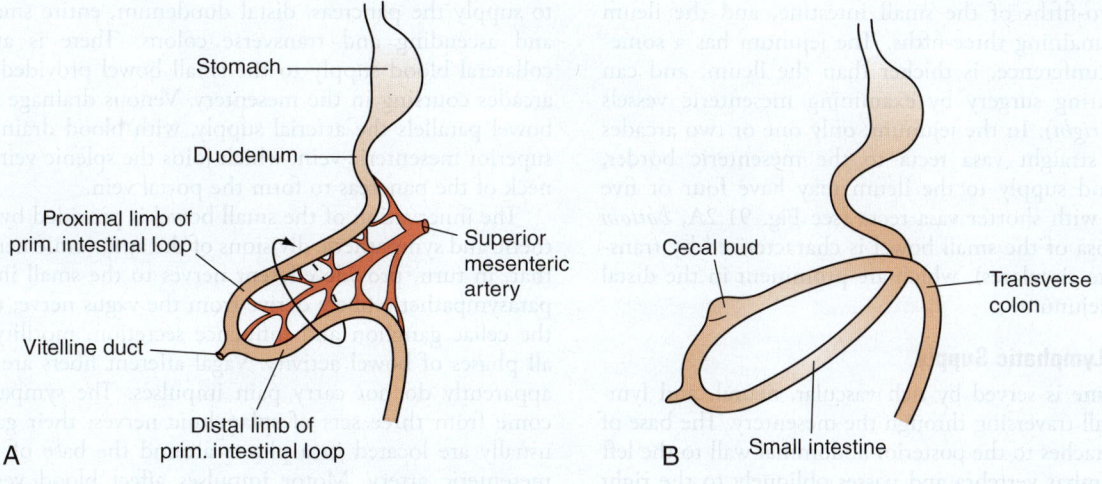

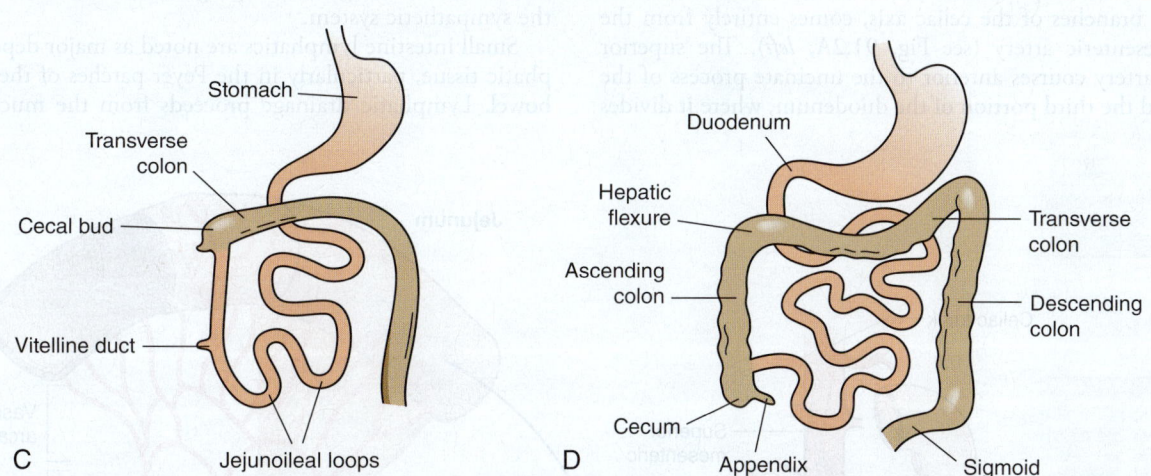

FIGURE 91.1 Rotation of the intestine. (A) The intestine after a 90-degree rotation around the axis of the superior mesenteric artery, the proximal loop on the right and the distal loop on the left. (B) The intestinal loop after a further 180-degree rotation. The transverse colon passes in front of the duodenum. (C) Position of the intestinal loops after reentry into the abdominal cavity. Note the elongation of the small intestine, with formation of the small intestine loops. (D) Final position of the intestines after descent of the cecum into the right iliac fossa. (From Podolsky DK, Babyatshy MW. Growth and development of the gastrointestinal tract. In: Yamada T, ed. *Textbook of Gastroenterology.* Vol 2. Philadelphia: JB Lippincott; 1995.)

and the root of the mesentery is narrowed, leaving the bowel susceptible to midgut volvulus.

The primitive small bowel is lined by a sheet of cuboidal cells until about the ninth week of gestation, when villi begin to form in the proximal intestine and then proceed in a caudal fashion until the entire small bowel, and even the colon, for a time are lined by these finger-like projections. Crypt formation begins in the 10th to 12th weeks of gestation. The crypt layer of the small bowel is the site of continual cell renewal and proliferation. As the cells ascend the crypt-villous axis, proliferation ceases, and cells differentiate into one of the four main cell types: absorptive enterocytes, which compose about 95% of the intestinal cell population; goblet cells; Paneth cells; and enteroendocrine cells. An important distinction regarding Paneth cells is that they remain in the crypt bases, where they protect intestinal stem cells from damage by releasing signaling molecules that affect the host tissues and influence the microbial populations to maintain homeostasis in the intestine.[2] The other differentiating cells ascending the crypt-villous axis are eventually extruded into the intestinal lumen. Amazingly, with the exception of Paneth cells, epithelial cell turnover occurs rapidly, with a life span of 3 to 5 days in humans.

ANATOMY

Gross Anatomy

The entire small intestine, which extends from the pylorus to the cecum, measures differently in everyone and can range from 250 to over 800 cm, with duodenal length estimated at approximately 20 cm, jejunal length at 100 to 110 cm, and ileal length at 150 to 160 cm. The jejunum begins at the duodenojejunal angle, which is supported by a peritoneal fold known as the *ligament of Treitz.* There is no obvious demarcation between the jejunum and the ileum; by convention, the jejunum comprises the proximal two-fifths of the small intestine, and the ileum makes up the remaining three-fifths. The jejunum has a somewhat larger circumference, is thicker than the ileum, and can be identified during surgery by examining mesenteric vessels (Fig. 91.2A, *top right*). In the jejunum, only one or two arcades send out long, straight vasa recta to the mesenteric border, whereas the blood supply to the ileum may have four or five separate arcades with shorter vasa recta (see Fig. 91.2A, *bottom right*). The mucosa of the small bowel is characterized by transverse folds (plicae circulares), which are prominent in the distal duodenum and jejunum.

Neurovascular-Lymphatic Supply

The small intestine is served by rich vascular, neural, and lymphatic supplies, all traversing through the mesentery. The base of the mesentery attaches to the posterior abdominal wall to the left of the second lumbar vertebra and passes obliquely to the right and inferiorly to the right sacroiliac joint. The blood supply of the small bowel, except for the proximal duodenum, which is supplied by branches of the celiac axis, comes entirely from the superior mesenteric artery (see Fig. 91.2A, *left*). The superior mesenteric artery courses anterior to the uncinate process of the pancreas and the third portion of the duodenum, where it divides

to supply the pancreas, distal duodenum, entire small intestine, and ascending and transverse colons. There is an abundant collateral blood supply to the small bowel provided by vascular arcades coursing in the mesentery. Venous drainage of the small bowel parallels the arterial supply, with blood draining into the superior mesenteric vein, which joins the splenic vein behind the neck of the pancreas to form the portal vein.

The innervation of the small bowel is provided by parasympathetic and sympathetic divisions of the autonomic nervous system that, in turn, provide efferent nerves to the small intestine. The parasympathetic fibers derive from the vagus nerve; they traverse the celiac ganglion and influence secretion, motility, and likely all phases of bowel activity. Vagal afferent fibers are present but apparently do not carry pain impulses. The sympathetic fibers come from three sets of splanchnic nerves; their ganglion cells usually are located in a plexus around the base of the superior mesenteric artery. Motor impulses affect blood vessel motility and, to some extent, gut secretion and motility. Pain from the intestine is transmitted through general visceral afferent fibers of the sympathetic system.

Small intestine lymphatics are noted as major deposits of lymphatic tissue, particularly in the Peyer patches of the distal small bowel. Lymphatic drainage proceeds from the mucosa through

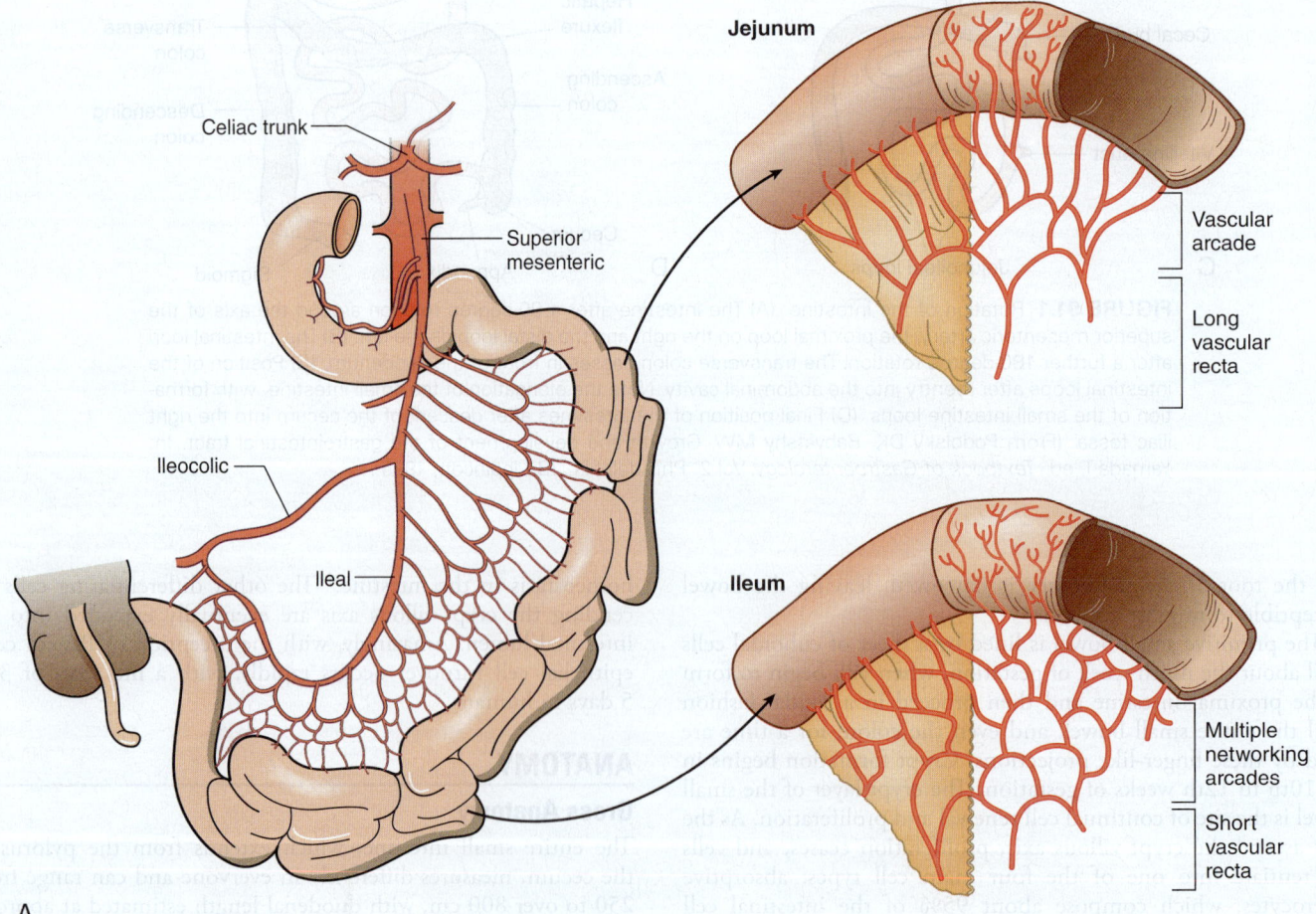

FIGURE 91.2 (A) Vascular supply of the small intestine. *(Top right)* The jejunal mesenteric vessels form only one or two arcades with long vasa recta. *(Bottom right)* The mesenteric vessels of the ileum form multiple vascular arcades with short vasa recta. *(Left)* The superior mesenteric artery, which courses anterior to the third portion of the duodenum, provides blood supply to the jejunoileum and distal duodenum. The celiac artery supplies the proximal duodenum.

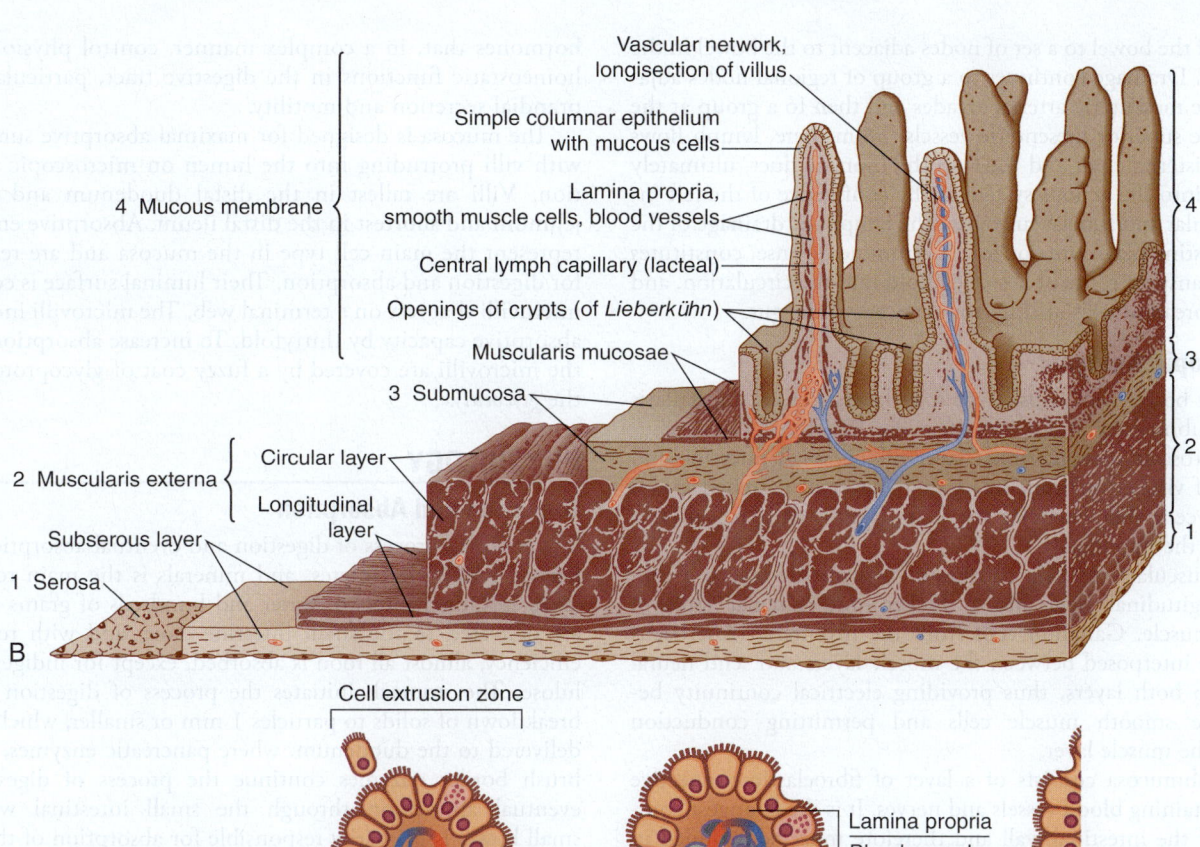

Vascular network, longisection of villus

Simple columnar epithelium with mucous cells

4 Mucous membrane

Lamina propria, smooth muscle cells, blood vessels

Central lymph capillary (lacteal)

Openings of crypts (of *Lieberkühn*)

Muscularis mucosae

3 Submucosa

Circular layer

2 Muscularis externa

Longitudinal layer

Subserous layer

1 Serosa

B

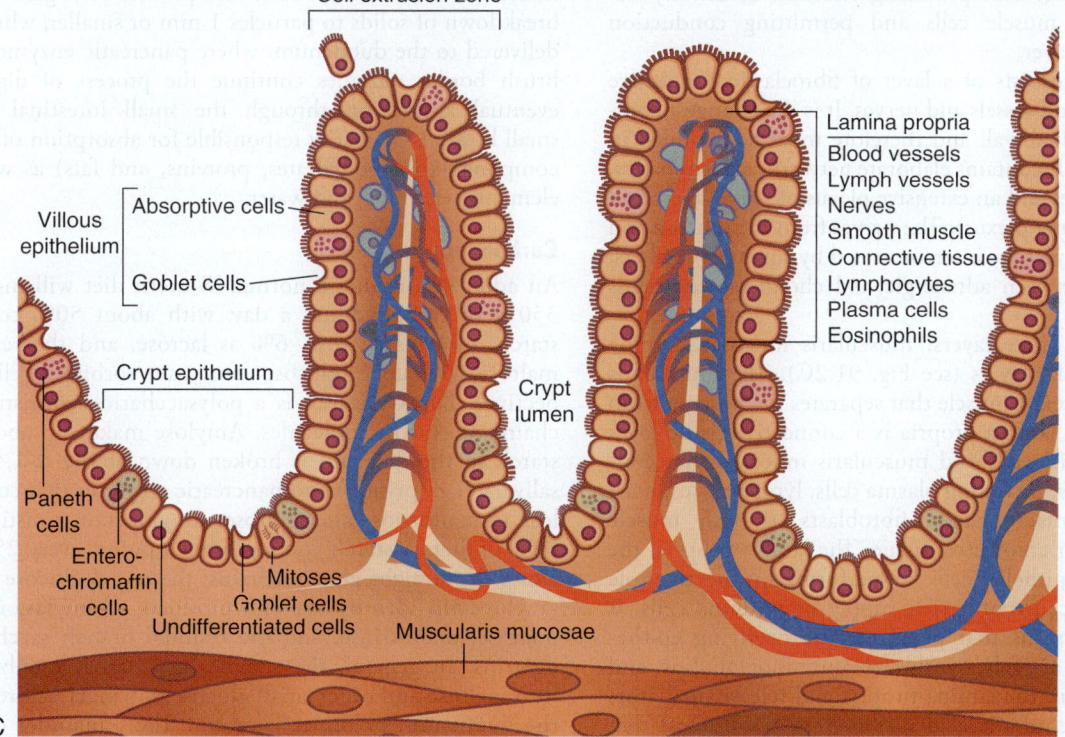

Cell extrusion zone

Villous epithelium

Absorptive cells

Goblet cells

Crypt epithelium

Crypt lumen

Lamina propria
Blood vessels
Lymph vessels
Nerves
Smooth muscle
Connective tissue
Lymphocytes
Plasma cells
Eosinophils

Paneth cells

Entero-chromaffin cells

Mitoses

Goblet cells

Undifferentiated cells

Muscularis mucosae

C

FIGURE 91.2, cont'd (B) Layers of the small intestine. A large surface is provided by villi for the absorption of required nutriments. The solitary lymph follicles in the lamina propria of the mucous membrane are not labeled. In the stroma of both sectioned villi are shown the central chyle (lacteal) vessels or villous capillaries. (C) Schematic diagram of the histologic organization of the small intestinal mucosa. (A, Adapted from Keljo DJ, Gariepy CE. Anatomy, histology, embryology, and developmental anomalies of the small and large intestine. In: Feldman M, Scharschmidt BF, Sleisenger MH, eds. *Sleisenger and Fordtran's Gastrointestinal and Liver Disease: Pathology, Diagnosis, Management.* Philadelphia: Saunders; 2002:1646; illustration courtesy Matt Hazzard, University of Kentucky Medical Center, Lexington, KY. B, From Sobotta J, Figge FHJ, Hild WJ. *Atlas of Human Anatomy.* New York: Hafner. C; 1974. Adapted from Keljo DJ, Gariepy CE. Anatomy, histology, embryology, and developmental anomalies of the small and large intestine. In: Feldman M, Scharschmidt BF, Sleisenger MH, eds. *Sleisenger and Fordtran's Gastrointestinal and Liver Disease: Pathology, Diagnosis, Management.* Philadelphia: Saunders; 2002:1646.)

the wall of the bowel to a set of nodes adjacent to the bowel in the mesentery. Drainage continues to a group of regional nodes adjacent to the mesenteric arterial arcades and then to a group at the base of the superior mesenteric vessels. From there, lymph flows into the cisterna chyli and then up the thoracic duct, ultimately to empty into the venous system at the confluence of the left internal jugular and subclavian veins. The lymphatic drainage of the small intestine plays a major role in immune defense, constitutes a major transport route of absorbed lipid into the circulation, and aids the spread of cells arising from cancers of the gut.

Microscopic Anatomy

The small bowel wall consists of four layers: serosa, muscularis propria, submucosa, and mucosa (see Fig. 91.2B).

The serosa is the outermost layer of the small intestine and consists of visceral peritoneum, a single layer of flattened mesoepithelial cells that encircles the jejunoileum, and the anterior surface of the duodenum.

The muscularis propria consists of two muscle layers: a thin outer longitudinal layer and a thicker inner circular layer of smooth muscle. Ganglion cells from the myenteric (Auerbach) plexus are interposed between the muscle layers and send neural fibers into both layers, thus providing electrical continuity between the smooth muscle cells and permitting conduction through the muscle layer.

The submucosa consists of a layer of fibroelastic connective tissue containing blood vessels and nerves. It is the strongest component of the intestinal wall and therefore must be included in anastomotic sutures. It contains elaborate networks of lymphatics, arterioles, and venules and an extensive plexus of nerve fibers and ganglion cells (Meissner plexus). The nerves from the mucosa and submucosa muscle layers are interconnected by small nerve fibers; cross-connections between adrenergic and cholinergic elements have been described.

The mucosa has three layers: muscularis mucosae, lamina propria, and epithelial layers (see Fig. 91.2C). The muscularis mucosae is a thin layer of muscle that separates the mucosa from the submucosa. The lamina propria is a connective tissue layer between the epithelial cells and muscularis mucosae that contains a variety of cells, including plasma cells, lymphocytes, mast cells, eosinophils, macrophages, fibroblasts, smooth muscle cells, and noncellular connective tissue. The lamina propria, the base on which the epithelial cells lie, performs a protective role in the intestine; because of a rich supply of immune cells, it combats microorganisms that penetrate the overlying epithelium. Plasma cells actively synthesize immunoglobulins and other immune cells in the lamina propria and release mediators (e.g., cytokines, arachidonic acid metabolites, histamines) that can modulate the cellular functions of the overlying epithelium. The epithelial layer is a continual sheet of epithelial cells covering the villi and lining the crypts. The main functions of the crypt epithelium are cell renewal as well as exocrine, endocrine, water, and ion secretion; the main functions of the villous epithelium are digestion and absorption. Four main cell types are contained in the mucosal layer: (1) absorptive enterocytes; (2) goblet cells, which secrete mucus; (3) Paneth cells, which secrete lysozyme, tumor necrosis factor (TNF), and cryptdins, which are homologues of leukocyte defensin peptides thought to be related to the host mucosal defense system; and (4) enteroendocrine cells, of which there are more than 15 distinct populations that produce the gastrointestinal hormones. The enteroendocrine cells also secrete a wide range of peptide hormones that, in a complex manner, control physiologic and homeostatic functions in the digestive tract, particularly postprandial secretion and motility.

The mucosa is designed for maximal absorptive surface area, with villi protruding into the lumen on microscopic examination. Villi are tallest in the distal duodenum and proximal jejunum and shortest in the distal ileum. Absorptive enterocytes represent the main cell type in the mucosa and are responsible for digestion and absorption. Their luminal surface is covered by microvilli that rest on a terminal web. The microvilli increase the absorptive capacity by thirtyfold. To increase absorption further, the microvilli are covered by a fuzzy coat of glycoprotein called the *glycocalyx*.

PHYSIOLOGY

Digestion and Absorption

The complex process of digestion and eventual absorption of nutrients, water, electrolytes, and minerals is the main role of the small intestine. Liters of water and hundreds of grams of chyme are delivered to the small intestine daily, and with remarkable efficiency, almost all food is absorbed, except for indigestible cellulose. The stomach initiates the process of digestion with the breakdown of solids to particles 1 mm or smaller, which are then delivered to the duodenum, where pancreatic enzymes, bile, and brush border enzymes continue the process of digestion and eventual absorption through the small intestinal wall.[3] The small bowel is primarily responsible for absorption of the dietary components (carbohydrates, proteins, and fats) as well as trace elements, vitamins, and water.

Carbohydrates

An adult consuming a normal Western diet will ingest 300 to 350 g of carbohydrates a day, with about 50% consumed as starch, 30% as sucrose, 6% as lactose, and the remainder as maltose, trehalose, glucose, fructose, sorbitol, cellulose, and pectins.[3] Dietary starch is a polysaccharide consisting of long chains of glucose molecules. Amylose makes up about 20% of starch in the diet and is broken down at the α-1,4 bonds by salivary (i.e., ptyalin) and pancreatic amylases that convert amylose to maltotriose and maltose. Amylopectin constitutes about 80% of dietary starch and has branch points every 25 molecules along the straight glucose chains; the α-1,6 glucose linkages in amylopectin identify the end products of amylase digestion—maltose, maltotriose, and the residual branch saccharides, the dextrins. In general, the starches are almost totally converted into maltose and other small glucose polymers before they reach the duodenum or upper jejunum. The remainder of carbohydrate digestion occurs as a result of brush border enzymes of the luminal surface.

The brush border of the small intestine contains the enzymes lactase, maltase, sucrase-isomaltase, and trehalase, which split the disaccharides as well as other small glucose polymers into their constituent monosaccharides (Table 91.1). Lactase hydrolyzes lactose into glucose and galactose. Maltase hydrolyzes maltose to produce glucose monomers. Sucrase-isomaltase is a complex with two subunits: sucrase hydrolyzes sucrose to yield glucose and fructose, and isomaltase hydrolyzes the α-1,6 bonds in α-limit dextrins to yield glucose. Glucose represents more than 80% of the final product of carbohydrate digestion, with galactose and fructose usually representing no more than 10% of the products of carbohydrate digestion.

TABLE 91.1 Characteristics of Brush Border Membrane Carbohydrases

ENZYME	SUBSTRATE	PRODUCTS
Lactase	Lactose	Glucose
	Galactose	
Maltase (glucoamylase)	α-1,4-linked oligosaccharides, up to nine residues	Glucose
Sucrase-isomaltase (sucrose-α-dextrinase)		
Sucrase	Sucrose	Glucose Fructose
Isomaltase	α-Limit dextrin	Glucose
Both enzymes	α-Limit dextrin	
	α-1,4-link at nonreducing end	Glucose
Trehalase	Trehalose	Glucose

From Marsh MN, Riley SA. Digestion and absorption of nutrients and vitamins. In: Feldman M, Scharschmidt BF, Sleisenger MH, eds. *Sleisenger and Fordtran's Gastrointestinal and Liver Disease: Pathophysiology, Diagnosis, Management.* Vol 2. Philadelphia: Saunders; 1998:1480.

Carbohydrates are absorbed as monosaccharides. Transport of the released hexoses (glucose, galactose, and fructose) is by specific mechanisms involved in active transport. The major routes of absorption are by three membrane carrier systems (Fig. 91.3A): sodium-glucose cotransporter-1 (SGLT1), glucose transporter 5 (GLUT5), and glucose transporter 2 (GLUT2).[3] Glucose and galactose are absorbed by a carrier-mediated active transport mechanism that involves the cotransport of sodium (SGLT1). As sodium diffuses into the cell, it pulls the glucose or galactose along with it, thus providing the energy for transport of the monosaccharide. The exit of glucose from the cytosol into the intracellular space is achieved predominantly by a sodium-independent carrier (GLUT2) located at the basolateral membrane of enterocytes. Fructose, the other significant monosaccharide, is also absorbed from the intestinal lumen through facilitated diffusion. This carrier, GLUT5, is located in the apical membrane of the enterocytes. In contrast to SGLT1, this transport process does not depend on sodium or energy. Fructose exits the basolateral membrane by another facilitated diffusion process involving the GLUT2.

Protein

Protein digestion is initiated in the stomach, where gastric acid denatures proteins.[3] Digestion continues in the small intestine, where protein comes into contact with pancreatic proteases. Pancreatic trypsinogen is secreted in the intestine by the pancreas in an inactive form but becomes activated by the enzyme enterokinase (a brush border enzyme in the duodenum) to an activated form of trypsin. Trypsin then activates the other pancreatic proteolytic enzyme precursors. The endopeptidases, which include trypsin, chymotrypsin, and elastase, act on peptide bonds at the interior of the protein molecule, producing peptides that are substrates for the exopeptidases (carboxypeptidases), which serially remove a single amino acid from the carboxyl end of the peptide (Table 91.2). This process results in splitting of the complex proteins into dipeptides, tripeptides, and some larger proteins, which are absorbed from the intestinal lumen by a sodium-mediated active transport mechanism and digested further by enzymes in the brush border and in the cytoplasm of enterocytes (see Fig. 91.3B). These peptidase enzymes include aminopeptidases and several dipeptidases, which split the remaining larger polypeptides into tripeptides, dipeptides, and some amino acids. The amino acids, dipeptides, and tripeptides are easily transported through the microvilli into the epithelial cells where, in the cytosol, additional peptidases hydrolyze the dipeptides and tripeptides into single amino acids; these molecules then pass through the epithelial cell membrane into the portal venous system. In normal humans, digestion and absorption of protein are usually 80% to 90% completed in the jejunum.

Fats

Emulsification. Most adults in North America consume 60 to 100 g/day of fat. Triglycerides, the most abundant fats, are composed of a glycerol nucleus and three fatty acids; small quantities of phospholipids, cholesterol, and cholesterol esters are also found in the normal diet. Essentially all fat digestion occurs in the small intestine, where the first step is the breakdown of fat globules into smaller sizes to facilitate further breakdown by water-soluble digestive enzymes, a process termed *emulsification*.[3] This process is facilitated by bile from the liver, which contains bile salts and the phospholipid lecithin. The polar regions of bile salts and the lecithin molecules are soluble in water, whereas the remaining portions are soluble in fat. Therefore, the fat-soluble portions interact with the surface layer of the fat globules, and the polar portions, projecting outward, are soluble in the surrounding aqueous fluids. This arrangement renders the fat globules more accessible to fragmentation by agitation in the small intestine. Therefore, a major function of bile salts, and especially lecithin, is to allow the fat globules to be fragmented by agitation in the intestinal lumen, which increases the fat globule surface area. With the increase in surface area, the fats are readily attacked by pancreatic lipase, the most crucial enzyme in the digestion of triglycerides, which splits triglycerides into free fatty acids and 2-monoglycerides.

Micelle formation. Fat digestion is accelerated by bile salts, which, secondary to their amphipathic nature, can form micelles. Micelles are small spherical globules composed of 20 to 40 molecules of bile salts with a sterol nucleus that is highly fat soluble and a hydrophilic polar group that projects outward. The mixed micelles thus formed are arrayed so that the insoluble lipid is surrounded by the bile salts oriented with their hydrophilic ends facing outward. Therefore, as quickly as the monoglycerides and free fatty acids are formed by lipolysis, they become dissolved in the central hydrophobic portion of the micelles, which then act to carry these products of fat hydrolysis to the brush borders of the epithelial cells, where absorption occurs.

Intracellular processing. The monoglycerides and free fatty acids, which are incorporated into the central lipid portion of the bile acid micelles, are absorbed through the brush border because of their highly lipid-soluble nature, then simply diffuse into the interior of the cell.[3] After disaggregation of the micelle, bile salts remain within the intestinal lumen to repeat the process by forming new micelles and carrying more monoglycerides and fatty acids to the epithelial cells. Inside the cell, the released fatty acids and monoglycerides re-form into triglycerides. This re-formation of a triglyceride occurs through the interactions of intracellular enzymes that are associated with the endoplasmic reticulum. The major pathway of triglyceride reconstruction involves 2-monoglycerides and coenzyme A (CoA)–activated fatty acids. Microsomal acyl-CoA lipase is necessary to cleave acyl-CoA from the

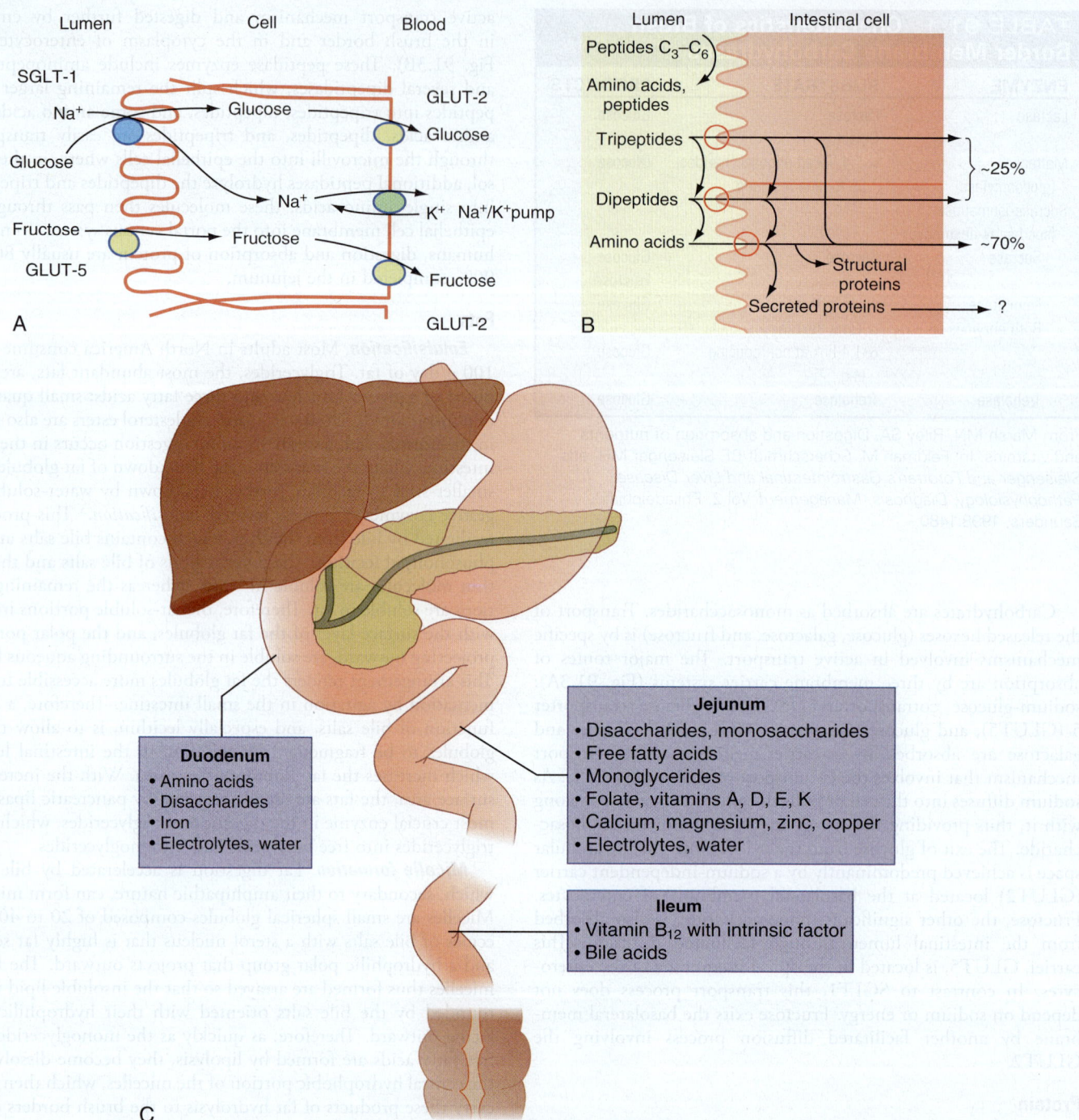

FIGURE 91.3 (A) Model for glucose, galactose, and fructose transport across the intestinal epithelium. Glucose and galactose are transported into the enterocyte across the brush border membrane by the sodium-glucose cotransporter *(SGLT1)* and then transported out across the basolateral membrane down their concentration gradients by glucose transporter *(GLUT)*-2. The low intracellular sodium concentration driving uphill sugar transport across the brush border is maintained by the Na^+,K^+ pump on the basolateral membrane. Glucose and galactose therefore stimulate sodium absorption across the epithelium. Fructose is transported across the cell down the concentration gradient across the brush border and basolateral membranes. GLUT5 is the brush border fructose transporter, whereas GLUT2 handles fructose transport across the basolateral membrane. (B) Digestion and absorption of proteins. Endopeptidases and exopeptidases split complex proteins into dipeptides and tripeptides that are absorbed from the intestinal lumen by a sodium-mediated active transport mechanism. These peptides are further digested by enzymes in the brush border and within enterocytes. (C) Absorption of water, electrolytes, and nutrients in the small bowel. Each segment of small intestine plays different roles in the absorption of micro- and macronutrients.

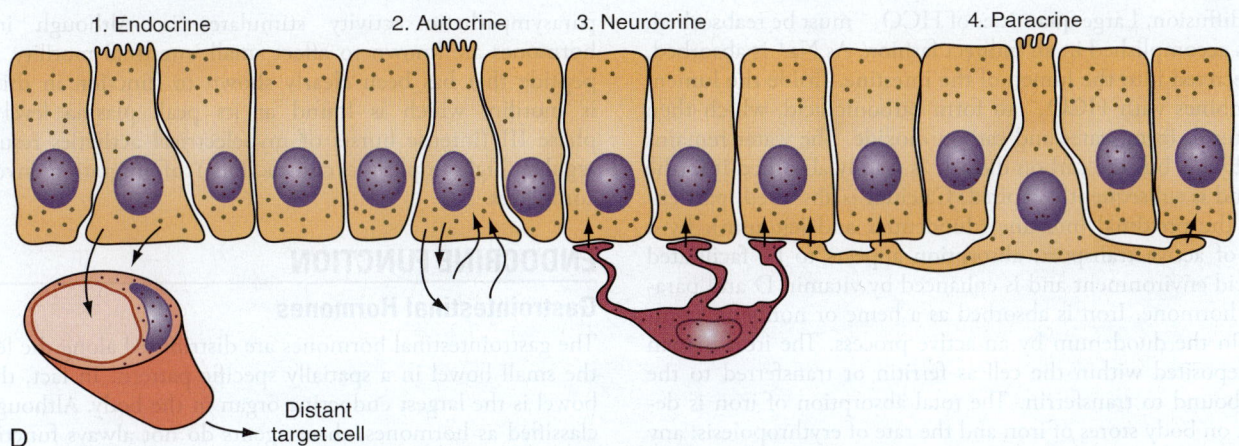

FIGURE 91.3, cont'd (D) Mechanisms of hormonal action in the intestinal epithelium. Intestinal hormones may act through endocrine, autocrine, neurocrine, or paracrine effects. (A, From Wright EM, Hirayama BA, Loo DDF, et al. Intestinal sugar transport. In: Johnson LR, Alpers DH, Christensen J, et al., eds. *Physiology of the Gastrointestinal Tract*. 3rd ed. Vol 2. New York: Raven Press; 1994:1752. B, Adapted from Alpers DH. Digestion and absorption of carbohydrates and proteins. In: Johnson LR, Alpers DH, Christensen J, et al., eds. *Physiology of the Gastrointestinal Tract*. 3rd ed. Vol 2. New York: Raven Press; 1994:1733. C, Adapted from Westergaard H. Short bowel syndrome. In: Feldman M, Scharschmidt BF, Sleisenger MH, eds. *Sleisenger and Fordtran's Gastrointestinal and Liver Disease: Pathology, Diagnosis, Management*. Philadelphia: Saunders; 2002:1549. D, Adapted from Miller LJ. Gastrointestinal hormones and receptors. In: Yamada T, Alpers DH, Laine L, et al., eds. *Textbook of Gastroenterology*. 3rd ed. Vol 1. Philadelphia: Lippincott Williams & Wilkins; 1999:37.)

TABLE 91.2   Principal Pancreatic Proteases

ENZYME	PRIMARY ACTION
Endopeptidases	Hydrolyze interior peptide bonds of polypeptides and proteins
Trypsin	Attacks peptide bonds involving basic amino acids; yields products with basic amino acids at carboxyl-terminal end
Chymotrypsin	Attacks peptide bonds involving aromatic amino acids, leucine, glutamine, and methionine; yields peptide products with these amino acids at carboxyl-terminal end
Elastase	Attacks peptide bonds involving neutral aliphatic amino acids; yields products with neutral amino acids at carboxyl-terminal end
Exopeptidases	Hydrolyze external peptide bonds of polypeptides and protein
Carboxypeptidase A	Attacks peptides with aromatic and neutral aliphatic amino acids at carboxyl-terminal end
Carboxypeptidase B	Attacks peptides with basic amino acids at carboxyl-terminal end

From Castro GA. Digestion and absorption. In: Johnson LR, ed. *Gastrointestinal Physiology*. St. Louis: Mosby; 1991:108-130.

fatty acid before esterification. These reconstituted triglycerides then combine with cholesterol, phospholipids, and apoproteins to form chylomicrons, which consist of an inner core containing triglycerides and a membranous outer core of phospholipids and apoproteins. The chylomicrons pass from the epithelial cells into the lacteals and then through the lymphatics into the venous system. About 80% to 90% of all fat absorbed from the gut is absorbed in this manner and transported to the blood by way of the thoracic lymph in the form of chylomicrons. Small quantities of short- to medium-chain fatty acids may be absorbed directly into the portal blood rather than being converted into triglycerides and absorbed into the lymphatics. These shorter-chain fatty acids are more water soluble, which allows direct diffusion into the bloodstream.

Enterohepatic circulation. The proximal intestine absorbs most of the dietary fat. Although unconjugated bile acids are absorbed into the jejunum by passive diffusion, the conjugated bile acids that form micelles are absorbed in the ileum by active transport and then reabsorbed from the distal ileum and passed

through the portal venous system to the liver for secretion as bile. The total bile acid pool (approximately 2–3 g) recirculates about six times every 24 hours through the enterohepatic circulation.[3] Almost all the bile salts are reabsorbed, with only about 0.5 g lost in the stool every day; this loss is replaced by newly synthesized bile acids from cholesterol.

Water, Electrolytes, and Vitamins

Every day, 8 to 10 L of water enter the small intestine. Much of this is absorbed, with approximately 500 mL or less leaving the ileum and entering the colon (see Fig. 91.3C).[3] Water may be absorbed by the process of simple diffusion. In addition, water may be drawn in and out of the cell through a process of osmotic pressure, resulting from active transport of sodium, glucose, or amino acids into cells.

Electrolytes can be absorbed in the small bowel by active transport or by coupling to an organic solute.[3] Na^+ is absorbed by active transport through the basolateral membranes. Cl^- is absorbed in the upper part of the small intestine by a process of passive diffusion. Large quantities of HCO_3^- must be reabsorbed, which is accomplished in an indirect fashion. As Na^+ is absorbed, H^+ is secreted into the lumen of the intestine. Inside the lumen, H^+ combines with HCO_3^- to form carbonic acid, which then dissociates to form water and carbon dioxide. The water remains in the chyme, but the carbon dioxide is readily absorbed into the blood and is subsequently expired. Calcium is absorbed, particularly in the proximal intestine (duodenum and jejunum), by a process of active transport; absorption appears to be facilitated by an acid environment and is enhanced by vitamin D and parathyroid hormone. Iron is absorbed as a heme or nonheme component in the duodenum by an active process. The iron is then either deposited within the cell as ferritin or transferred to the plasma bound to transferrin. The total absorption of iron is dependent on body stores of iron and the rate of erythropoiesis; any increase in erythropoiesis increases iron absorption. Potassium, magnesium, phosphate, and other ions also can be actively absorbed throughout the mucosa.

Vitamins are either fat soluble (e.g., vitamins A, D, E, and K) or water soluble (e.g., ascorbic acid [vitamin C], biotin, nicotinic acid, folic acid, riboflavin [vitamin B_2], thiamine [vitamin B_1], pyridoxine [vitamin B_6], and cobalamin [vitamin B_{12}]).[3] The fat-soluble vitamins are carried in mixed micelles and transported in chylomicrons of the lymph to the thoracic duct and into the venous system. The absorption of water-soluble vitamins appears to be more complex than originally thought. Vitamin C is absorbed by an active transport process that incorporates a sodium-coupled mechanism as well as a specific carrier system. Vitamin B_6 appears to be rapidly absorbed by simple diffusion into the proximal intestine. Vitamin B_1 is rapidly absorbed in the jejunum by an active process similar to the sodium-coupled transport system for vitamin C. Vitamin B_2 is absorbed in the upper intestine by facilitated transport. The absorption of vitamin B_{12} occurs primarily in the terminal ileum. Vitamin B_{12} is derived from cobalamin, which is freed in the duodenum by pancreatic proteases. The cobalamin binds to intrinsic factor, which is secreted by the stomach and is protected from proteolytic digestion. Specific receptors in the terminal ileum take up the cobalamin–intrinsic factor complex, probably by translocation. In the ileal enterocyte, free vitamin B_{12} is bound to an ileal pool of transcobalamin II, which transports it into the portal circulation.

MOTILITY

Food particles are propelled through the small bowel by a complex series of muscle contractions.[3] Peristalsis consists of intestinal contractions passing aborally at a rate of 1 to 2 cm/sec. The major function of peristalsis is the movement of intestinal chyme through the intestine. Motility patterns in the small bowel vary greatly between the fed and fasted states. Pacesetter potentials, which are thought to originate in the duodenum, initiate a series of contractions in the fed state that propel food through the small bowel.

During the interdigestive (fasting) period between meals, the bowel is regularly swept by cyclical contractions that move aborally along the intestine every 75 to 90 minutes. These contractions are initiated by the migrating myoelectric complex, which is under the control of neural and humoral pathways. Extrinsic nerves to the small bowel are vagal and sympathetic. The vagal fibers have two functionally different effects; one is cholinergic and excitatory, and the other is peptidergic Irand probably inhibitory. Sympathetic activity inhibits motor function, whereas

parasympathetic activity stimulates it. Although intestinal hormones are known to affect small intestinal motility, the one peptide that has been clearly shown to function in this regard is motilin, which is found at its peak plasma level during phase III (intense bursts of myoelectrical activities resulting in regular, high-amplitude contractions) of migrating myoelectric complexes.

ENDOCRINE FUNCTION

Gastrointestinal Hormones

The gastrointestinal hormones are distributed along the length of the small bowel in a spatially specific pattern. In fact, the small bowel is the largest endocrine organ in the body. Although often classified as hormones, these agents do not always function in a true endocrine fashion (i.e., discharged into the bloodstream, where an action is produced at some distant site; see Fig. 91.3D). Sometimes, these peptides are discharged and act locally in a paracrine or autocrine manner. In contrast, some of these peptides may serve as neurotransmitters (e.g., vasoactive intestinal peptide). Gastrointestinal hormones play a major role in pancreaticobiliary and intestinal secretion, absorption, and motility. In addition, certain gastrointestinal hormones exert a trophic effect on normal and neoplastic intestinal mucosa and the pancreas. Moreover, recent studies show that certain hormones (e.g., neurotensin), when secreted in excess, can contribute to obesity, diabetes, and cardiovascular disease.[4] The location, major stimulants of release, and primary effects of the more important gastrointestinal hormones are summarized in Table 91.3. In addition, the diagnostic and therapeutic uses of gastrointestinal hormones are listed in Table 91.4.

Receptors

The gastrointestinal hormones interact with their cell surface receptors to initiate a cascade of signaling events that eventually culminate in their physiologic effects. These hormones primarily signal through G protein–coupled receptors that traverse the plasma membrane seven times and represent the largest group of receptors found in the body. The heterotrimeric G proteins, which are composed of α, β, and γ subunits, are the molecular switches for signal transduction. Agonist binding to the seven-transmembrane domain receptor is thought to cause a conformational change in the receptor that allows it to interact with the G proteins. Intracellular second messengers that are activated include cyclic adenosine monophosphate, Ca^{2+} cyclic guanosine monophosphate, and inositol phosphate.

In addition to the gastrointestinal hormones, receptors for a number of other peptides and growth factors are located in the gastrointestinal mucosa, including those for epidermal growth factor, transforming growth factor α and β, insulin-like growth factor (IGF), fibroblast growth factor, and platelet-derived growth factor (PDGF). These peptides play a role in cell growth and differentiation and act through tyrosine kinase receptors, which have a single membrane-spanning domain.

A third class of surface receptors, the ion channel–linked receptors, is found most commonly in cells of neuronal lineage and usually bind specific neurotransmitters. Examples include receptors for excitatory (acetylcholine and serotonin) and inhibitory (γ-aminobutyric acid and glycine) neurotransmitters. These receptors undergo a conformational change on binding of the mediator that allows passage of ions across the cell membrane and results in changes in voltage potential.

TABLE 91.3 Gastrointestinal Hormones

HORMONE	PRODUCED BY	MAJOR STIMULANTS OF PEPTIDE SECRETION	PRIMARY EFFECTS
Gastrin	Antrum, duodenum (G cells)	Peptides, amino acids, antral distention, vagal and adrenergic stimulation, gastrin-releasing peptide (bombesin)	• Stimulates gastric acid and pepsinogen secretion • Stimulates gastric mucosal growth
Cholecystokinin	Duodenum, jejunum (I cells)	Fats, peptides, amino acids	• Stimulates pancreatic enzyme secretion • Stimulates gallbladder contraction • Relaxes sphincter of Oddi • Inhibits gastric emptying
Secretin	Duodenum, jejunum (S cells)	Fatty acids, luminal acidity, bile salts	• Stimulates release of water and bicarbonate from pancreatic ductal cells • Stimulates flow and alkalinity of bile • Inhibits gastric acid secretion and motility and inhibits gastrin release
Somatostatin	Pancreatic islets (D cells), antrum, duodenum	• Gut: fat, protein, acid, other hormones (e.g., gastrin, cholecystokinin) • Pancreas: glucose, amino acids, cholecystokinin	• Universal "off" switch • Inhibits release of gastrointestinal hormones • Inhibits gastric acid secretion • Inhibits small bowel water and electrolyte secretion • Inhibits secretion of pancreatic hormones
Gastrin-releasing peptide (mammalian equivalent of bombesin)	Small bowel	Vagal stimulation	• Universal "on" switch • Stimulates release of all gastrointestinal hormones (except secretin) • Stimulates gastrointestinal secretion and motility • Stimulates gastric acid secretion and release of antral gastrin • Stimulates growth of intestinal mucosa and pancreas
Gastric inhibitory polypeptide	Duodenum, jejunum (K cells)	Glucose, fat, protein adrenergic stimulation	• Inhibits gastric acid and pepsin secretion • Stimulates pancreatic insulin release in response to hyperglycemia
Motilin	Duodenum, jejunum	Gastric distention, fat	• Stimulates upper gastrointestinal tract motility • May initiate the migrating motor complex
Vasoactive intestinal peptide	Neurons throughout the gastrointestinal tract	Vagal stimulation	• Primarily functions as a neuropeptide • Potent vasodilator • Stimulates pancreatic and intestinal secretion • Inhibits gastric acid secretion
Neurotensin	Small bowel (N cells)	Fat	• Stimulates growth of small and large bowel mucosa • Facilitates absorption of fats in the intestine • Stimulates growth of cancer with neurotensin receptors
Enteroglucagon	Small bowel (L cells)	Glucose, fat	• Glucagon-like peptide-1 • Stimulates insulin release • Inhibits pancreatic glucagon release • Glucagon-like peptide-2 • Potent enterotrophic factor
Peptide YY	Distal small bowel, colon	Fatty acids, cholecystokinin	• Inhibits gastric and pancreatic secretion • Inhibits gallbladder contraction

Adapted from Rao JN, Wang JY. Role of GI hormones on gut mucosal growth. In: *Regulation of Gastrointestinal Mucosal Growth*. San Rafael, CA: Morgan & Claypool Life Sciences; 2010:19-29.

TABLE 91.4 **Diagnostic and Therapeutic Uses of Gastrointestinal Hormones**

HORMONE	DIAGNOSTIC AND THERAPEUTIC USES
Gastrin	Pentagastrin (gastrin analogue) used to measure maximal gastric acid secretion
Cholecystokinin	Biliary imaging of gallbladder contraction
Secretin	Provocative test for gastrinoma
	Measurement of maximal pancreatic secretion
Glucagon	Suppresses bowel motility for endocrine spasm
	Relieves sphincter of Oddi spasm
	Provocative test for insulin, catecholamine, and growth hormone release
	Intraoperative relaxation of sphincter of Oddi to stimulate passage of common bile duct stone
Somatostatin analogues	Treat carcinoid diarrhea and flushing
	Decrease secretion from pancreatic and intestinal fistulas
	Ameliorate symptoms associated with hormone-overproducing endocrine tumors
	Treat esophageal variceal bleeding
	Used in imaging studies to localize somatostatin sensitive neuroendocrine tumors

Adapted from Townsend CM Jr, Thompson JC. The clinical use of gastrointestinal hormones for alimentary tract disease. *Adv Surg.* 1996;29:79-92; and Brubaker PL. Gut hormones fulfill their destiny: from basic physiology to the clinic. *Annu Rev Physiol.* 2014;76(1): 515-517.

IMMUNE FUNCTION

During the course of a normal day, we ingest a number of bacteria, parasites, and viruses. The intestinal epithelium is a single layer of cells and serves as a major immunologic barrier in addition to its important role in digestion and endocrine function. The small intestine has epithelial-lined villi that are absent in the colon; these villi significantly increase the surface area for interaction with foreign pathogens. As a result of constant antigenic exposure, the intestine possesses abundant lymphoid cells (e.g., B and T lymphocytes) and myeloid cells (e.g., macrophages, neutrophils, eosinophils, and mast cells). To deal with the constant barrage of potential toxins and antigens, the gut has evolved a highly organized and efficient mechanism for antigen processing, humoral immunity, and cellular immunity. The gut-associated lymphoid tissue is localized in four areas: Peyer patches, lamina propria lymphoid cells, Paneth cells, and intraepithelial lymphocytes.

Peyer patches are unencapsulated lymphoid nodules that constitute an afferent limb of the gut-associated lymphoid tissue, which recognizes antigens through a specialized sampling mechanism by the microfold (M) cells contained within the follicle-associated epithelium (Fig. 91.4). Antigens that gain access to Peyer patches activate and prime B and T cells in that site. The M cells cover the lymphoid follicles in the gastrointestinal tract and provide a site for selective sampling of intraluminal antigens. Activated lymphocytes from the intestinal lymphoid follicles then migrate into afferent lymphatics that drain into mesenteric lymph

nodes. Furthermore, some of these cells migrate into the lamina propria to interact with intestinal epithelial cells to generate the mucosal immune response. The B lymphocytes become surface IgA. IgA-bearing lymphoblasts also serve a critically important role in mucosal immunity.

B lymphocytes and plasma cells, T lymphocytes, macrophages, dendritic cells, eosinophils, and mast cells are scattered throughout the connective tissue of the lamina propria. Approximately 60% of the lymphoid cells are T cells. These T lymphocytes are a heterogeneous group of cells and can differentiate into one of several types of T effector cells. Cytotoxic T effector cells damage the target cells directly. Helper T cells are effector cells that help mediate the induction of other T cells or the induction of B cells to produce humoral antibodies. T suppressor cells perform just the opposite function. Approximately 40% of the lymphoid cells in the lamina propria are B cells, which are primarily derived from precursors in Peyer patches. These B cells and their progeny, plasma cells, are predominantly focused on IgA synthesis and, to a lesser extent, IgM, IgG, and IgE synthesis.

Paneth cells, like M cells, are unique to the small intestine. Paneth cells line the base of crypts and release antimicrobial factors to protect adjacent stem cells.[5] The intraepithelial lymphocytes are located in the space between the epithelial cells that line the mucosal surface and lie close to the basement membrane. Most of the intraepithelial lymphocytes are a unique subtype of T cells. On activation, the intraepithelial lymphocytes may acquire cytolytic functions that can contribute to epithelial cell death through apoptosis. These cells may be important in the immunosurveillance against abnormal epithelial cells.

As noted, one of the major protective immune mechanisms for the intestinal tract is the synthesis and secretion of IgA. The intestine contains more than 70% of the IgA-producing cells in the body. IgA is produced by plasma cells in the lamina propria and is secreted into the intestine, where it can bind antigens at the mucosal surface. The IgA antibody traverses the epithelial cell to the lumen by means of a protein carrier (the secretory component) that not only transports the IgA but also protects it against the intracellular lysosomes. IgA does not activate complement and does not enhance cell-mediated opsonization or destruction of infectious organisms or antigens, which is in sharp contrast to the role of other immunoglobulins. Secretory IgA inhibits the adherence of bacteria to epithelial cells and prevents their colonization and multiplication. In addition, secretory IgA neutralizes bacterial toxins and viral activity and blocks the absorption of antigens from the gut.

Recent studies demonstrated a symbiotic relationship between the intestinal microbiome and intestinal growth and function. The intestinal mucosa in germ-free mice has decreased epithelial proliferation and decreased production of mucin and immunologic mediators that result in thinning of the mucosa with decreased tissue protection and repair. In addition, microbial metabolites from anaerobes generate much of the luminal butyrate, which is a fuel source for colonic cells, and luminal lactate, which promotes small intestinal stem cell proliferation and differentiation. Essentially, a functional molecular "crosstalk" occurs between intestinal epithelial cells and the gut microbiome. Disruption of this crosstalk can lead to adverse changes to the microbiome, a process called *dysbiosis*. Enteric microbial dysbiosis has been identified in certain intestinal pathologies such as in inflammatory bowel disease.[5] Current studies focusing on the importance

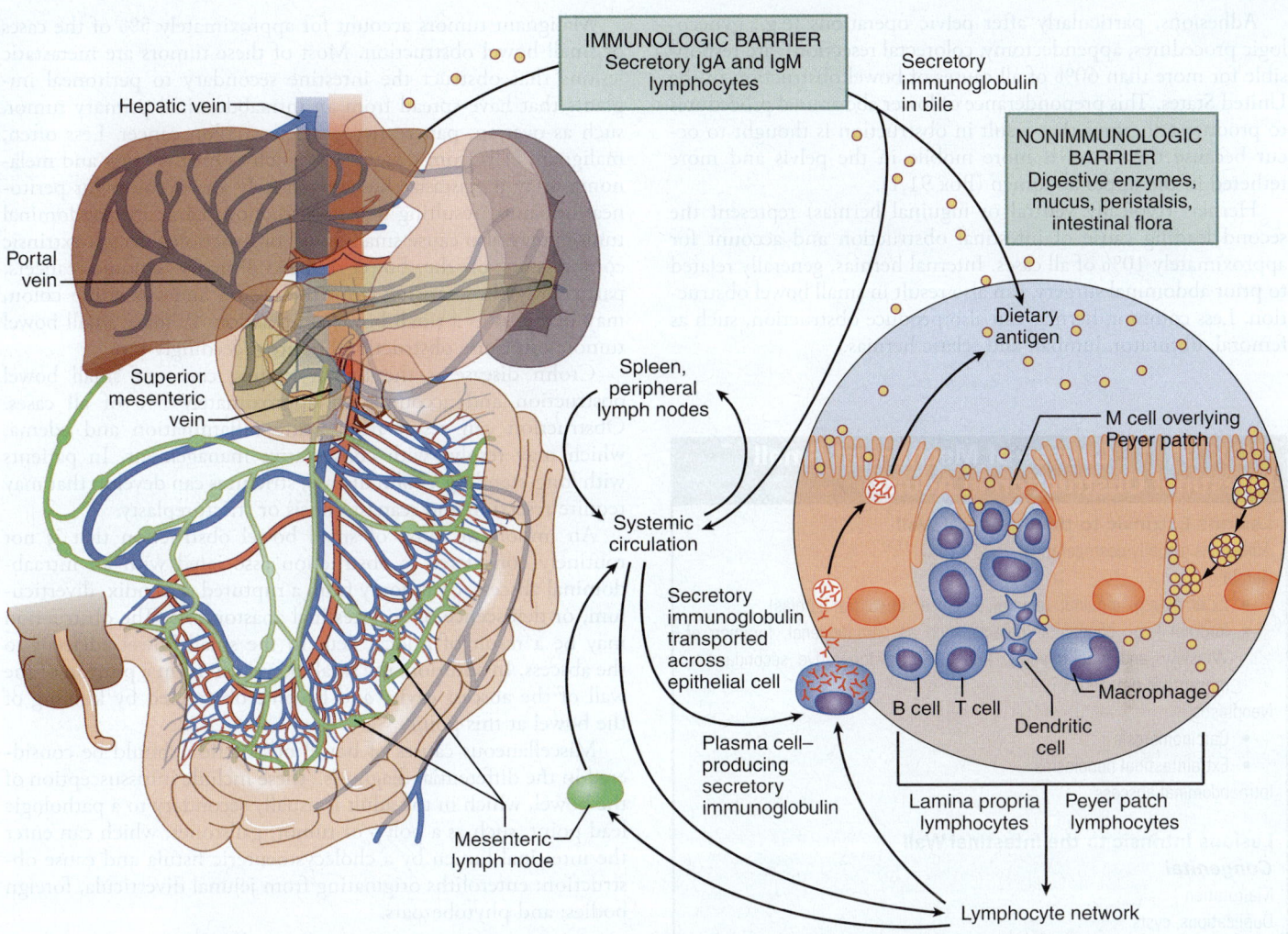

FIGURE 91.4 Mucosal barrier of the gut. Antigens contact specialized microfold *(M)* cells that overlie Peyer patches, which then process and present the antigen to the immune system. When B lymphocytes are stimulated by antigenic material, the cells develop into antibody-forming cells that secrete various types of immunoglobulins *(Ig)*, the most important of which is IgA. (Adapted from Duerr RH, Shanahan F. Food allergy. In: Targan SR, Shanahan F, eds. *Immunology and Immunopathology of the Liver and Gastrointestinal Tract.* New York: Igaku-Shoin; 1990:510; illustration courtesy Matt Hazzard, University of Kentucky Medical Center, Lexington, KY.)

of the intestinal epithelium and crosstalk with the microbiome will lead to a better understanding of many small bowel diseases and are the source of many ongoing investigational efforts.

OBSTRUCTION

The description of patients presenting with small bowel obstruction dates back to the 3rd or 4th century BCE, when Praxagoras created an enterocutaneous fistula to relieve a bowel obstruction. Despite this success with operative therapy, the nonoperative management of these patients with attempted reduction of hernias, laxatives, ingestion of heavy metals (e.g., lead, mercury), and leeches to remove toxic agents from the blood was common practice until the late 1800s, when antiseptic and aseptic surgical techniques made operative intervention safer and more acceptable. A better understanding of the pathophysiologic process of bowel obstruction, surgical advances, antibiotics, intestinal tube decompression, and use of isotonic fluid resuscitation have greatly reduced the mortality rate for patients with a mechanical bowel obstruction. However,

patients with a bowel obstruction still represent some of the most difficult and vexing problems that surgeons face with regard to accurate diagnosis, optimal timing of therapy, and appropriate treatment. Ultimately, a clinical decision about the management of these patients requires a thorough history and workup with a heightened awareness of potential complications.

Causes

Small bowel obstructions continue to be a significant cause of morbidity and mortality in the United States. The most common cause of intestinal obstruction in the Western countries is adhesive disease.[6] Other causes of small bowel obstruction are many, but as a group, they can be effectively divided into three major categories:

1. Obstruction arising from extraluminal causes (e.g., adhesions, hernias, carcinomas, abscesses)
2. Obstruction intrinsic to the bowel wall (e.g., primary tumors)
3. Intraluminal obturator obstruction (e.g., gallstones, enteroliths, foreign bodies, bezoars)

Adhesions, particularly after pelvic operations (e.g., gynecologic procedures, appendectomy, colorectal resection), are responsible for more than 60% of all causes of bowel obstruction in the United States. This preponderance of lower abdominal procedures to produce adhesions that result in obstruction is thought to occur because the bowel is more mobile in the pelvis and more tethered in the upper abdomen (Box 91.1).

Hernias (typically ventral or inguinal hernias) represent the second leading cause of intestinal obstruction and account for approximately 10% of all cases. Internal hernias, generally related to prior abdominal surgery, can also result in small bowel obstruction. Less common hernias can also produce obstruction, such as femoral, obturator, lumbar, and sciatic hernias.

BOX 91.1 Causes of Mechanical Small Intestinal Obstruction in Adults

Lesions Extrinsic to the Intestinal Wall
Adhesions (usually postoperative)
Hernia
- External (e.g., inguinal, femoral, umbilical, or ventral hernias)
- Internal (e.g., congenital defects such as paraduodenal, foramen of Winslow, and diaphragmatic hernias or postoperative secondary to mesenteric defects)
Neoplastic
- Carcinomatosis
- Extraintestinal neoplasms
Intraabdominal abscess

Lesions Intrinsic to the Intestinal Wall
Congenital
Malrotation
Duplications, cysts

Inflammatory
Crohn disease
Infections
- Tuberculosis
- Actinomycosis
- Diverticulitis

Neoplastic
Primary neoplasms
Metastatic neoplasms

Traumatic
Hematoma
Ischemic stricture

Miscellaneous
Intussusception
Endometriosis
Radiation enteropathy/stricture

Intraluminal, Obturator Obstruction
Gallstone
Enterolith
Bezoar
Foreign body

Adapted from Tito WA, Sarr MG. Intestinal obstruction. In: Zuidema GD, ed. *Surgery of the Alimentary Tract*. Philadelphia: WB Saunders; 1996:375-416.

Malignant tumors account for approximately 5% of the cases of small bowel obstruction. Most of these tumors are metastatic lesions that obstruct the intestine secondary to peritoneal implants that have spread from an intraabdominal primary tumor, such as ovarian, pancreatic, gastric, or colon cancer. Less often, malignant cells from distant sites, such as breast, lung, and melanoma, may metastasize hematogenously and account for peritoneal implants, resulting in an obstruction. Large intraabdominal tumors may also cause small bowel obstruction through extrinsic compression of the bowel lumen. Primary colonic cancers, particularly those arising from the cecum and ascending colon, may manifest as a small bowel obstruction. Primary small bowel tumors can cause obstruction but are exceedingly rare.

Crohn disease is the fourth leading cause of small bowel obstruction and accounts for approximately 5% of all cases. Obstruction can result from acute inflammation and edema, which may resolve with conservative management. In patients with long-standing Crohn disease, strictures can develop that may require resection and reanastomosis or strictureplasty.

An important cause of small bowel obstruction that is not routinely considered is obstruction associated with an intraabdominal abscess, commonly from a ruptured appendix, diverticulum, or dehiscence of an intestinal anastomosis. The obstruction may be a result of a local ileus in the small bowel adjacent to the abscess. In addition, the small bowel can form a portion of the wall of the abscess cavity and become obstructed by kinking of the bowel at this point.

Miscellaneous causes of bowel obstruction should be considered in the differential diagnosis. These include intussusception of the bowel, which in the adult is usually secondary to a pathologic lead point, such as a polyp or tumor; gallstones, which can enter the intestinal lumen by a cholecystoenteric fistula and cause obstruction; enteroliths originating from jejunal diverticula; foreign bodies; and phytobezoars.

Pathophysiology

Early in the course of an obstruction, intestinal motility and contractile activity increase in an effort to propel luminal contents past the obstructing point. The increase in peristalsis that occurs early in the course of bowel obstruction is present above and below the point of obstruction; this process can account for the finding of diarrhea that may accompany partial or even complete small bowel obstruction in the early period. Later in the course of obstruction, the intestine becomes fatigued and dilates, with contractions becoming less frequent and less intense.

As the bowel dilates, water and electrolytes accumulate intraluminally and in the bowel wall itself. This massive third-space fluid loss accounts for the dehydration and hypovolemia. The metabolic effects of fluid loss depend on the site and duration of the obstruction. With a proximal obstruction, dehydration may be accompanied by hypochloremia, hypokalemia, and metabolic alkalosis associated with increased vomiting. Distal obstruction of the small bowel may result in large quantities of intestinal fluid into the bowel; however, abnormalities in serum electrolyte levels are usually less dramatic. Oliguria, azotemia, and hemoconcentration can accompany the dehydration. Rarely, hypotension and shock can ensue. Other consequences of bowel obstruction include increased intraabdominal pressure, decreased venous return, and elevation of the diaphragm, compromising ventilation. These factors can serve to potentiate the effects of hypovolemia.

As the intraluminal pressure increases in the bowel, a decrease in mucosal blood flow can occur. This alteration is particularly noted in patients with a closed loop obstruction, in which greater intraluminal pressures are attained. A closed loop obstruction, produced commonly by a twist of the bowel, can progress to arterial occlusion and ischemia if it is left untreated and may potentially lead to bowel perforation and peritonitis.

In the absence of intestinal obstruction, the jejunum and proximal ileum have only 10^3 to 10^5 colony-forming units per milliliter (CFU/mL) of bacteria. With obstruction, however, the flora of the small intestine changes dramatically in both the type of organism (most commonly *Escherichia coli*, *Streptococcus faecalis*, and *Klebsiella* spp.) and the quantity, with organisms reaching concentrations of 10^9 to 10^{10} CFU/mL. Studies have shown an increase in the number of indigenous bacteria translocating to mesenteric lymph nodes and even systemic organs. Bacterial translocation amplifies the local inflammatory response in the gut, leading to intestinal leakage and subsequent increase in systemic inflammation. This inflammatory cascade may result in systemic sepsis and multiorgan failure if it is unrecognized and untreated.

Clinical Manifestations and Diagnosis

The major challenge in the diagnosis of intestinal obstruction is the identification of bowel incarceration or strangulation. Although a thorough history and physical examination are important, neither is sensitive nor specific to the diagnosis of ischemia. In some patients, a meticulous history and physical examination complemented by plain abdominal radiographs are all that is required to establish the diagnosis and to devise a treatment plan. More sophisticated radiographic studies, such as a computed tomography (CT) scan of the abdomen, represent invaluable tools in the identification of complications and potential causes.

History

The cardinal symptoms of intestinal obstruction include colicky abdominal pain, nausea, vomiting, abdominal distention, and obstipation. These symptoms may vary with the site and duration of obstruction. The typical crampy abdominal pain associated with intestinal obstruction occurs in paroxysms at 4- to 5-minute intervals and occurs less frequently with distal obstruction. Nausea and vomiting are more common with a higher obstruction and may be the only symptoms in patients with gastric outlet or high intestinal obstruction. An obstruction located distally is associated with less emesis; the initial and most prominent symptom is cramping abdominal pain. Abdominal distention occurs as the obstruction progresses and the proximal intestine becomes increasingly dilated. Obstipation is a later development. It must be reiterated that patients, particularly in the early stages of bowel obstruction, may relate a history of diarrhea that is secondary to increased peristalsis. Therefore, the important point to remember is that a complete bowel obstruction cannot be ruled out on the basis of a history of loose bowel movements. The character of the vomitus is also important to obtain in the history. As the obstruction becomes more complete with bacterial overgrowth, the vomitus becomes more feculent, indicating a late and established intestinal obstruction.

Physical Examination

The patient with intestinal obstruction may present with tachycardia and hypotension, demonstrating the severe dehydration that is present. Fever suggests the possibility of strangulation. Abdominal examination demonstrates a distended abdomen, with the amount of distention somewhat dependent on the level of obstruction. Previous surgical scars should be noted. Early in

the course of bowel obstruction, peristaltic waves can be observed, particularly in thin patients, and auscultation of the abdomen may demonstrate hyperactive bowel sounds with audible rushes associated with vigorous peristalsis (borborygmi). Late in the obstructive course, minimal or no bowel sounds are noted. Mild abdominal tenderness may be present, with or without a palpable mass; however, localized tenderness, rebound, and guarding suggest peritonitis and the likelihood of strangulation. A careful examination must be performed to rule out incarcerated hernias in the groin, femoral triangle, and obturator foramen. A rectal examination should *always* be performed to rule out a distal colonic obstruction by intraluminal masses and to examine the stool for occult blood, which may be an indication of malignant disease, intussusception, or infarction.

Laboratory and Radiologic Studies

With a high suspicion of intestinal obstruction after a thorough history and physical examination, further studies are necessary to confirm the diagnosis. Laboratory tests are usually not helpful in the actual diagnosis of patients with small bowel obstruction but are extremely important in assessing the degree of dehydration and may help indicate signs of ischemic changes. Patients with a bowel obstruction should routinely have laboratory measurements of serum sodium, chloride, potassium, bicarbonate, and creatinine levels. The serial determination of serum electrolyte levels should be performed to assess the adequacy of fluid resuscitation. Dehydration may result in hemoconcentration, as noted by an elevated hematocrit value. This level should be monitored because fluid resuscitation results in a decrease in the hematocrit, and some patients (e.g., those with intestinal malignant neoplasms) may require blood transfusions before surgery. In addition, the white blood cell count should be assessed. Leukocytosis may be found in patients with strangulation; however, an elevated white blood cell count does not necessarily denote strangulation. Conversely, the absence of leukocytosis does not eliminate strangulation as a possibility. Elevated lactic acid levels suggest intestinal ischemia or necrosis.

Radiographic studies can be helpful in the diagnosis of small bowel obstruction. Characteristic findings on supine radiographs are dilated loops of small intestine, without evidence of colonic distention (Box 91.2). Upright radiographs demonstrate multiple air-fluid levels, which often layer in a stepwise pattern. Paucity of

---

BOX 91.2 Plain Abdominal Film Signs of Small Bowel Obstruction

Supine or Prone:
  Dilated gas or fluid filled small bowel >3 cm
  Dilated stomach
  Small bowel dilated out of proportion to colon
  Stretch sign
  Absence of rectal gas
  Gasless abdomen
  Pseudotumor sign
Upright or Left Lateral Decubitus:
  Multiple air fluid levels
  Air fluid levels longer than 2.5 cm
  Air fluid levels in same loop of small bowel of unequal lengths
  String of beads sign

Adapted from Paulson EK, Thompson WM. Review of small-bowel obstruction: the diagnosis and when to worry. *Radiology*. 2015;275: 332-342.

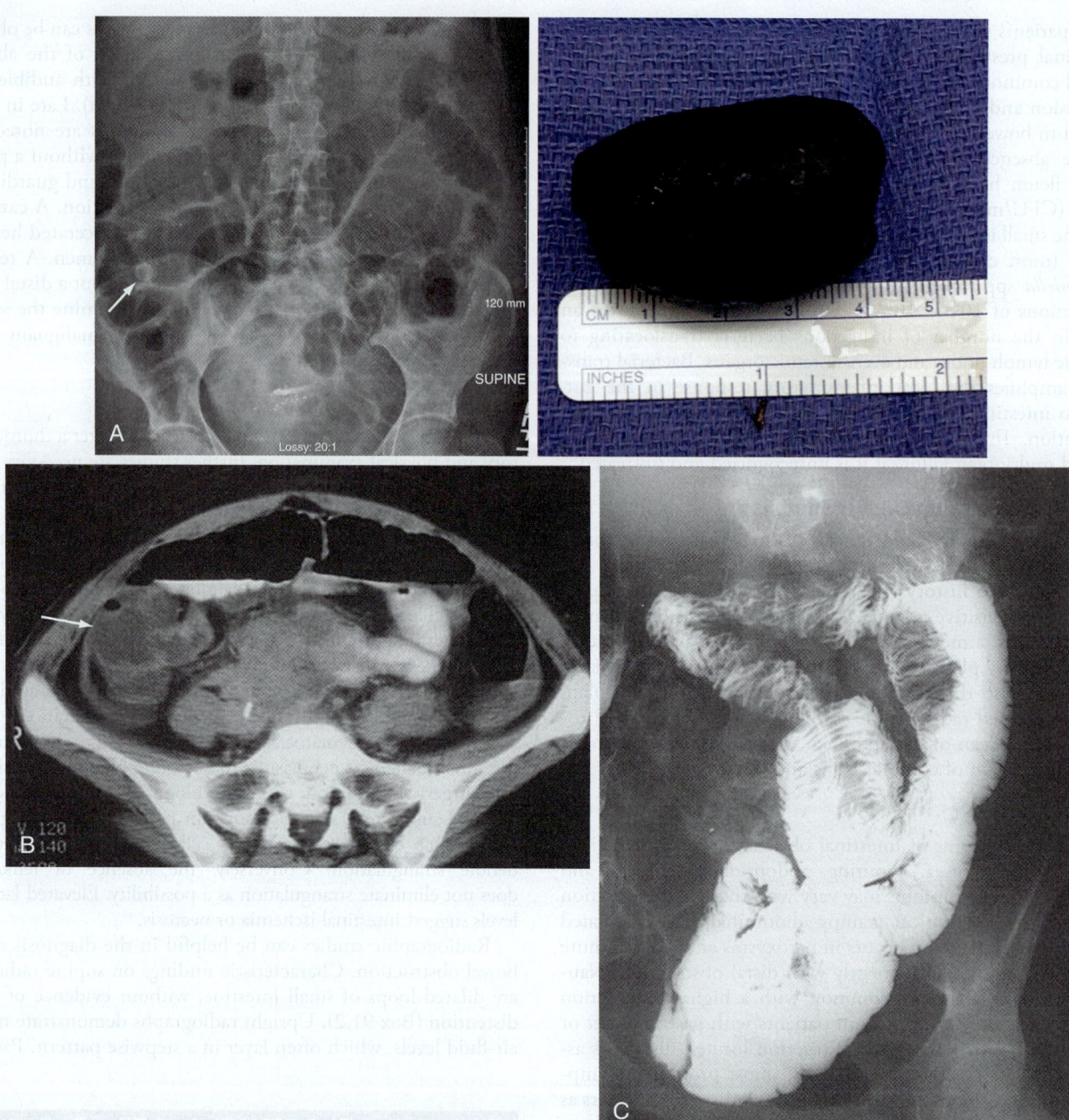

FIGURE 91.5 (A) Patient presents with gallstone ileus. *(Left)* Plain abdominal film shows complete bowel obstruction caused by a large radiopaque gallstone *(arrow)* obstructing the distal ileum. *(Right)* The large gallstone responsible for the obstruction seen in the corresponding plain abdominal film. (B) Intraabdominal abscess causing small bowel obstruction. CT scan of the abdomen of a patient with a mechanical bowel obstruction secondary to an abscess in the right lower quadrant *(arrow)*. Multiple dilated and fluid-filled loops of small bowel are noted. (C) Barium study demonstrates jejunojejunal intussusception. (A, Courtesy Dr. Kristin Long, University of Kentucky Medical Center, Lexington, KY. B, Courtesy Dr. Melvyn H. Schreiber, The University of Texas Medical Branch, Galveston, TX. C, Courtesy Dr. Melvyn H. Schreiber, The University of Texas Medical Branch, Galveston, TX.)

gas when supine and small pockets of air appearing like a string of beads when upright is more concerning for high-grade or closed loop obstruction. Plain abdominal films (Fig. 91.5A, *left*) may also demonstrate the cause of the obstruction (e.g., foreign bodies, gallstones; see Fig. 91.5.A, *right*). In uncertain cases or when one is unable to differentiate partial from complete obstruction, further diagnostic imaging is required.

Although plain radiographs can be diagnostic, abdominal CT imaging is the standard imaging modality for diagnosis of small bowel obstruction. CT is particularly sensitive and specific for diagnosing complete or high-grade obstruction of the small bowel and for determining the location and cause of obstruction. However, a CT scan is less sensitive in patients with partial small bowel obstruction. A dilated bowel loop of more than

2.5 cm is very concerning for high-grade small bowel obstruction. In addition, CT is helpful in identifying transition zones and extrinsic causes of bowel obstruction (e.g., abdominal tumors, inflammatory disease, or abscess; see Fig. 91.5B). CT has also been described as useful for determining bowel strangulation, most commonly seen in the presence of a hernia. Unfortunately, CT findings associated with strangulation are those of irreversible ischemia and necrosis. Importantly, the emergent surgical management of a toxic patient with a bowel obstruction identified by a thorough history and physical examination should not be delayed to perform unnecessary and costly radiographic studies.

Barium studies, namely, enteroclysis, were previously often used in certain patients with a presumed obstruction. This procedure involves the continued infusion of 500 to 1000 mL of thin barium sulfate and methylcellulose suspension into the intestine through a duodenal tube. The suspension is then viewed continuously with use of either fluoroscopy or standard radiographs taken at frequent intervals; therefore, this technique is a double-contrast procedure that allows detailed imaging of the entire small intestine, which can precisely demonstrate the level of the obstruction as well as the cause of the obstruction in certain cases (see Fig. 91.5C). The main disadvantages of enteroclysis are the need for nasoenteric intubation, slow transit of contrast material in patients with a fluid-filled hypotonic small bowel, and enhanced expertise required by the radiologist to perform this procedure. Barium studies have largely been replaced by the increasingly used Gastrografin small bowel follow-through study. Gastrografin is a water-soluble contrast agent that is similarly administered via nasogastric tube or by mouth. Radiographs are taken at timed intervals to observe the transit of the contrast and can both aid in locating the obstruction and, in some cases, expediting nonoperative resolution of an obstruction that is thought to be secondary to its osmotic effect on decreasing bowel wall edema.[6]

Ultrasound has been reported to be useful for pregnant patients because radiation exposure is a concern. Magnetic resonance imaging (MRI) has been described in patients with obstruction; however, it is not typically used in the standard diagnostic workup of patients with small bowel obstruction.

To summarize, plain abdominal radiographs can be used in the diagnostic workup of obstruction, but CT is the standard diagnostic imaging modality for small bowel obstruction. Contrast-enhanced radiograph studies can be used in tandem with bowel rest and decompression to aid in both identifying the location of the obstruction and, for some, accelerate resolution of the obstruction.

Simple Versus Strangulating Obstruction

Most patients with small bowel obstruction are classified as having simple obstructions that involve mechanical blockage of the flow of luminal contents without compromised viability of the intestinal wall. In contrast, a strangulated obstruction, which usually involves a closed loop obstruction with a compromised vascular supply to a segment of intestine, can lead to intestinal infarction. A strangulated obstruction is associated with an increased morbidity and mortality risk; therefore, recognition of early strangulation is important. In differentiating from the simple intestinal obstruction, classic signs of strangulation have been described; these include tachycardia, fever, leukocytosis, lactic acidosis, and a constant, noncramping abdominal pain. However, a number of studies have convincingly shown that no clinical parameters or laboratory measurements can accurately detect or exclude the presence of strangulation in all cases. This reinforces

the dictum that a careful history and physical examination are key for an accurate and timely diagnosis.

Closed loop obstructions occur when both ends of a segment of bowel are obstructed either by an adhesive band or from an internal hernia, which may result in ischemia and necrosis. Ischemia may worsen when this loop twists, creating a volvulus (mesenteric whirl). CT examination is useful for detecting evidence of closed loop obstruction (U loop or coffee bean sign with tapering of both ends of bowel) and volvulus. CT scans also demonstrate evidence of ischemia, such as bowel wall thickening (>3 mm), mesenteric edema, fluid trapped in between loops, decreased bowel wall enhancement, pneumatosis intestinalis, and mesenteric or portovenous gas.[6] Serum levels, including lactate dehydrogenase, amylase, alkaline phosphatase, ammonia, D-lactate, creatinine kinase isoenzyme, and intestinal fatty acid–binding protein, have been investigated as predictive values for bowel ischemia in obstruction. Although outstanding values may increase a provider's clinical suspicion for ischemia, none can definitively rule in or rule out ischemia. Thus, it is important to remember that bowel ischemia and strangulation cannot be reliably diagnosed or excluded preoperatively in all cases by any known clinical parameter, combination of parameters, or current laboratory and radiographic examinations.

Treatment

Patients with symptoms of a bowel obstruction usually present to the emergency department for evaluation and often require a surgical consultation. Patients identified to have small bowel obstruction should be primarily managed by a surgical service. A large population-based study demonstrated significantly shorter length of stay, lower cost, readmission rate, and mortality rate when adhesive bowel obstruction was managed by a surgical service compared with being managed by a medicine service.[7]

Fluid Resuscitation and Antibiotics

Patients with intestinal obstruction are usually dehydrated and depleted of sodium, chloride, and potassium, requiring aggressive intravenous (IV) replacement with an isotonic saline solution such as lactated Ringer solution or normal saline. Urine output should be monitored with placement of a Foley catheter or external collection device to limit risk of catheter-associated infection. After the patient has formed adequate urine, potassium chloride can be added to the infusion, if needed. Serial electrolyte level measurements as well as hematocrit and white blood cell count are performed to assess the adequacy of fluid repletion. Broad-spectrum antibiotics are given prophylactically by some surgeons on the basis of the reported findings of bacterial translocation occurring even in simple mechanical obstructions; however, there is no substantial evidence to support the use of antimicrobial therapy in nontoxic-appearing patients or those without suspected bacterial overgrowth of the small intestine. Antibiotics should only be administered preoperatively in the event that the patient requires surgery.

Tube Decompression

In addition to IV fluid resuscitation, another important adjunct to consider in the supportive care of patients with intestinal obstruction is nasogastric decompression. Suction with a nasogastric tube empties the stomach, reducing the hazard of pulmonary aspiration of vomitus and minimizing further intestinal distention from swallowed air. Nasogastric decompression in a patient with small bowel obstruction has long been the standard of care.

However, recently, studies have been questioning the utility and benefit of nasogastric tube decompression. The evidence to support or refute the universal use of nasogastric decompression in the management of small bowel obstructions remains inconclusive. As such, although the use of tube decompression is still typically recommended, use should be determined on case-by-case basis.

The use of long intestinal tubes (e.g., Cantor or Baker tube) has been advocated by some. However, prospective randomized trials have demonstrated no significant difference regarding the decompression achieved, success of nonoperative treatment, or incidence of postoperative morbidities compared with the use of nasogastric tubes. Furthermore, the use of these long tubes has been associated with a significantly longer hospital stay, duration of postoperative ileus, and postoperative complications in some series. Therefore, it appears that long intestinal tubes offer no benefit in the preoperative setting over nasogastric tubes.

Patients with a partial intestinal obstruction may be treated conservatively with resuscitation and tube decompression alone. Resolution of symptoms and discharge without the need for surgery have been reported in up to 85% of patients with a partial obstruction. Although an initial trial of nonoperative management of most patients with partial small bowel obstruction is warranted, clinical deterioration of the patient or increasing small bowel distention on abdominal radiographs during tube decompression warrants prompt operative intervention. The decision to continue to treat a patient nonoperatively with a presumed bowel obstruction is based on clinical judgment and requires constant vigilance and reevaluation to ensure that the clinical course has not changed.

Contrast Challenge

As previously mentioned, water-soluble contrast has become more regularly used in the diagnosis and treatment of adhesive small bowel obstruction. The challenge requires 100 mL of water-soluble contrast given through the nasogastric tube or orally and follow-up radiographs obtained at timed intervals such as at 8 and 24 hours. If contrast material still has not passed into the colon after 24 hours, conservative management will probably fail and surgical intervention is likely needed.[6] Studies continue to investigate the optimal timing of administration, but, typically, it is given 24 to 48 hours after adequate decompression. Although improved outcomes with use of water-soluble contrast are evident in adhesive bowel obstructions, there is not similar evidence to support its use in nonadhesive obstructive disease.

Operative Management

As the management of intestinal obstruction has shifted more to conservative care with nasogastric tube decompression and rehydration, operative intervention is reserved for those who fail conservative management or have evidence of vascular compromise, strangulation, or perforation. A nonoperative approach for selected patients with complete small intestinal obstruction has been proposed by some surgeons, who argue that prolonged gastrointestinal decompression is safe in these patients, provided that no fever, tachycardia, tenderness, or leukocytosis is noted. Nevertheless, one must weigh the risks and benefits of nonoperative management in overlooking an underlying strangulated obstruction. Retrospective studies report that a 12- to 24-hour delay is safe but that the incidence of strangulation and other complications increases significantly after this period.

The nature of the problem dictates the approach for the obstructed patient. Patients with intestinal obstruction secondary to an adhesive band may be treated with lysis of adhesions. Great care should be used in the gentle handling of the bowel to reduce serosal trauma and to avoid unnecessary dissection and inadvertent enterotomies. Incarcerated hernias can be managed by manual reduction of the herniated segment of bowel and closure of the defect.

The treatment of patients with an obstruction and history of malignant tumors can be particularly challenging. In the terminal patient with widespread metastasis, nonoperative management, if successful, is usually the best course; however, only a small percentage of cases with complete obstruction can be successfully managed nonoperatively. In this case, an intestinal bypass of the obstructing lesion, by whatever means, may offer the best option rather than a long and complicated operation that might entail bowel resection.

An obstruction secondary to Crohn disease will often resolve with conservative management if the obstruction is acute. If a chronic fibrotic stricture is the cause of the obstruction, a bowel resection or strictureplasty may be required.

Patients with an intraabdominal abscess can present in a manner indistinguishable from those with mechanical bowel obstruction. CT is particularly useful in diagnosing the cause of the obstruction in these patients. Percutaneous drainage of the abscess may be sufficient to relieve the obstruction. Laparoscopic drainage is also an option in cases not amenable to image-guided percutaneous drainage; this procedure is associated with reduced wound morbidity, is useful in multiloculated collections, and allows a washout of the peritoneal cavity at the same time. Otherwise, laparotomy and abdominal washout may be required for large and established abscesses.

Radiation enteropathy, as a complication of radiation therapy for pelvic malignant neoplasms, may cause bowel obstruction. Most cases can be treated nonoperatively with tube decompression and the potential addition of corticosteroids, particularly during the acute setting. In the chronic setting, nonoperative management is rarely effective; laparoscopy or laparotomy will be required with possible resection of the irradiated bowel or bypass of the affected area.

At the time of exploration, it can sometimes be difficult to evaluate bowel viability after the release of a strangulation. If intestinal viability is questionable, the bowel segment should be completely released and placed in a warm, saline-moistened sponge for 15 to 20 minutes and then reexamined. If normal color has returned and peristalsis is evident, it is safe to retain the bowel. Doppler flow probe can be used to identify flow in the mesentery but has not typically added to the conventional clinical judgment of the surgeon. In difficult borderline cases, fluorescence with fluorescein or indocyanine green can help discriminate viability of bowel intraoperatively. If there remains question as to the viability of the bowel, the provider can elect to perform a temporary abdominal closure with planned second-look laparotomy 18 to 24 hours after the initial procedure. This decision should be made at the time of the initial operation. A second-look laparotomy is clearly indicated for a patient whose condition deteriorates after the initial operation.

Multiple studies have evaluated the efficacy of laparoscopic management of acute small bowel obstruction. Laparoscopic treatment of small bowel obstruction is effective and leads to lower morbidity and mortality, shorter length of stay, shorter operating time, lower reoperation rate, and reduced overall complications.[8] The patient profile appropriate for consideration of laparoscopic management includes those with the following clinical presentation: mild abdominal distention, proximal or partial obstruction, anticipated single-band obstruction, and low risk of strangulation or perforation. Patients with matted adhesions or carcinomatosis or who remain distended after nasogastric intubation may be better managed with conventional laparotomy. This is dependent on the laparoscopic skill of the surgeon, and increasingly more surgeons elect to proceed, at least initially, laparoscopically.

Management of Specific Problems
Recurrent Intestinal Obstruction

All surgeons can readily remember the complicated patient with multiple previous abdominal operations and a frozen abdomen who presents with yet another bowel obstruction. An initial nonoperative trial is usually desirable and often safe. In patients who do not respond conservatively, reoperation is required. This can often be a long and arduous procedure, with great care taken to prevent enterotomies or adjacent organ injury. In these difficult patients, various surgical procedures and pharmacologic agents have been tried in an effort to prevent recurrent adhesions and obstruction.

External plication procedures have been described in which the small intestine or its mesentery is sutured in large, gently curving loops. Common complications include the development of fistulas, gross leakage, peritonitis, and death. Because of frequent complications and low overall success rate, these procedures have largely been abandoned. Several series have reported moderate success with internal fixation or stenting procedures using a long intestinal tube inserted through the nose, a gastrostomy, or even a jejunostomy that is left in place for 2 weeks or longer. However, complications associated with these tubes include prolonged drainage of bowel contents from the tube insertion site, intussusception, and difficult removal of the tube, which may require surgical reexploration. Such means to prevent recurrent obstruction are not typically employed today.

Pharmacologic agents, including corticosteroids and other antiinflammatory agents, cytotoxic drugs, and antihistamines, have been used with limited success. The use of anticoagulants, such as heparin, dextran solutions, dicumarol, and sodium citrate, may modify the extent of adhesion formation, but their side effects far outweigh their efficacy. Investigations into intraperitoneal instillation of various proteinases (e.g., trypsin, papain, pepsin), which cause enzymatic digestion of the extracellular protein matrix, have been largely unsuccessful. Hyaluronidase has been of questionable value, and conflicting results were obtained with fibrinolytic agents such as streptokinase, urokinase, and fibrinolytic snake venoms. The use of a hyaluronate-based, bioresorbable membrane is debatable. A meta-analysis demonstrated reduced risk of adhesive bowel obstruction and less severe adhesions when they do occur, but its use may also increase the risk of anastomotic leak.[9] Therefore, the use of such a membrane may be beneficial in some patients but should be thoughtfully considered given the risk.

To date, the most effective means of limiting the number of adhesions is a good surgical technique. This includes the gentle handling of the bowel to reduce serosal trauma, avoidance of unnecessary dissection, exclusion of foreign material from the peritoneal cavity (the use of absorbable suture material when possible, avoidance of excessive gauze sponge use, and the removal of starch from gloves), adequate irrigation with removal of infectious and ischemic debris, and preservation and use of the omentum around the site of surgery or in the denuded pelvis.

Acute Postoperative Obstruction

Small bowel obstruction that occurs in the immediate postoperative period presents a challenge with regard to diagnosis and treatment. Diagnosis is often difficult because the primary symptoms of abdominal pain and nausea or emesis may be attributed to a postoperative ileus. Electrolyte deficiencies, particularly hypokalemia, can be a cause of ileus and should be corrected. Plain abdominal films are usually not helpful to distinguish an ileus from obstruction. Where there is high concern for obstruction, CT may be useful. More than 90% of early postoperative obstructions are partial and will resolve spontaneously, given ample time. Conservative management in the form of bowel rest, fluid resuscitation, electrolyte replacement, and parenteral nutrition, if necessary, is routinely successful. However, the development of complete obstruction or signs of strangulation mandates reoperative intervention. Postoperative bowel obstruction after laparoscopic surgery is more commonly associated with a definitive obstruction point, such as a port site, hernia, or an internal hernia, and should prompt a high index of suspicion for the need for operative intervention.

Ileus

An ileus is defined as intestinal distention and the slowing or absence of passage of luminal contents without a demonstrable mechanical obstruction. An ileus can result from a number of causes, including those that are drug induced or from metabolic, neurogenic, and infectious factors (Box 91.3).

Pharmacologic agents that can produce an ileus include anticholinergic drugs, autonomic blockers, antihistamines, and various psychotropic agents, such as haloperidol and tricyclic antidepressants. One of the more common causes of drug-induced ileus in the operative patient is the use of opiates, such as morphine or meperidine. Metabolic causes of ileus are common and include hypokalemia, hyponatremia, and hypomagnesemia. Other metabolic causes include uremia, diabetic coma, and hypoparathyroidism. Neurogenic causes of an ileus include postoperative ileus, which occurs after abdominal operations. Spinal injury, retroperitoneal irritation, and orthopedic procedures on the spine or pelvis can result in an ileus. Finally, infections can result in an ileus; common infectious causes include pneumonia, peritonitis, and generalized sepsis from a nonabdominal source.

Patients often present in a manner similar to those with a mechanical small bowel obstruction. Abdominal distention, usually without the colicky abdominal pain, is the typical and most notable finding. Nausea and vomiting may occur but may also be absent. Patients with an ileus may continue to pass flatus and

---

BOX 91.3 Causes of Ileus

After laparotomy
Metabolic and electrolyte derangements (e.g., hypokalemia, hyponatremia, hypomagnesemia, uremia, diabetic coma)
Drugs (e.g., opiates, psychotropic agents, anticholinergic agents)
Intraabdominal inflammation
Retroperitoneal hemorrhage or inflammation
Intestinal ischemia
Systemic sepsis

Adapted from Turnage RH, Bergen PC. Intestinal obstruction and ileus. In: Feldman M, Scharschmidt FG, Sleisenger MH, eds. *Sleisenger and Fordtran's Gastrointestinal and Liver Disease: Pathophysiology, Diagnosis, Management.* Philadelphia: Saunders; 1998:1799-1810.

diarrhea, which may help distinguish these patients from those with a mechanical small bowel obstruction.

Radiologic studies may help distinguish ileus from small bowel obstruction. Plain abdominal radiographs may reveal distended small bowel as well as large bowel loops. In cases that are difficult to differentiate from obstruction, CT imaging and enteral contrast studies may be beneficial.

The treatment of an ileus is entirely supportive, with nasogastric decompression and IV fluids. The most effective treatment to correct the underlying condition may be aggressive treatment of the sepsis, correction of any metabolic or electrolyte abnormalities, and discontinuation of medications that may produce an ileus. Pharmacologic agents have been used but for the most part have been ineffective. Drugs that block sympathetic input (e.g., guanethidine) or stimulate parasympathetic activity (e.g., bethanechol, neostigmine) have been tried. Hormonal manipulation, using cholecystokinin or motilin, has been evaluated, but the results have been inconsistent. Erythromycin has been ineffective, and cisapride, although apparently beneficial in stimulating gastric motility, does not appear to alter intestinal ileus. Chewing gum has been shown to be an easy and inexpensive method to stimulate the cephalic phase of digestion (e.g., vagal cholinergic stimulation and the release of gastrointestinal hormones) and therefore a potential adjunct to prevent and to treat ileus.

INFLAMMATORY AND INFECTIOUS DISEASES

Crohn Disease

Crohn disease is a chronic, transmural inflammatory disease of the gastrointestinal tract for which the definitive cause is unknown, although a combination of genetic and environmental factors has been implicated. Crohn disease can involve any part of the alimentary tract from the mouth to the anus but most commonly affects the small intestine and colon. The most common clinical manifestations are abdominal pain, diarrhea, and weight loss. Crohn disease can be complicated by intestinal obstruction or localized perforation with fistula formation. Medical and surgical treatments are palliative; however, operative therapy can provide effective symptomatic relief for patients with complications from Crohn disease and produces a reasonable long-term benefit.

History

The first documented case of Crohn disease was described by Morgagni in 1761. In 1913, the Scottish surgeon Dalziel described nine cases of intestinal inflammatory disease. However, it was the landmark paper by Crohn and colleagues in 1932 that provided, in eloquent detail, the pathologic and clinical findings of this inflammatory disease in young adults.[10] This classic paper crystallized the description of this inflammatory condition. Although many different (and sometimes misleading) terms have been used to describe this disease process, Crohn disease has been universally accepted as its name.

Incidence and Epidemiology

Crohn disease is the most common primary surgical disease of the small bowel. The annual incidence of Crohn disease, which is rising in the United States, is 6 to 24 cases per 100,000 individuals.[11] Crohn disease primarily attacks young adults in the second and third decades of life. However, all ages can be affected, and a bimodal distribution, with a second smaller peak occurring in the sixth decade of life, has classically been described. Although earlier reports suggested a somewhat higher female predominance, males and females are affected equally. The risk for development of Crohn disease is almost twice as high in smokers as in nonsmokers. Several studies indicate an increased incidence of Crohn disease in females using oral contraceptives. The condition is predominately seen in industrialized nations, and incidence increases with Westernized diets. Certain ethnic groups, particularly Ashkenazi Jews, have a higher incidence of Crohn disease than age- and sex-matched control subjects. Of note, within one generation, migrants moving from a low-risk region to a high-risk region develop Crohn disease at similar rates to those in the high-risk region. There is a strong familial association, with the risk for development of Crohn disease increased about thirtyfold in siblings and fourteenfold to fifteenfold for all first-degree relatives. Intestinal microflora and epigenetic changes induced by environmental factors play an important role in disease development and progression in genetically susceptible individuals.[12]

Etiology

The causes of Crohn disease remain unknown. A number of potential causes have been proposed, with the most likely possibilities being infectious, immunologic, and genetic. Other possibilities that have met with various levels of enthusiasm include environmental and dietary factors, smoking, and psychosocial factors. Although these factors may contribute to the overall disease process, it is unlikely that they represent the primary etiology for Crohn disease.

Infectious agents. Although a number of infectious agents have been proposed as potential causes of Crohn disease, the two that have received the most attention are mycobacterial infections, particularly *Mycobacterium paratuberculosis* and enteroadherent *E. coli*. The existence of atypical mycobacteria as a cause for Crohn disease was proposed by Dalziel in 1913. Subsequent studies using polymerase chain reaction (PCR) techniques have confirmed the presence of mycobacteria in intestinal samples of patients with Crohn disease. Transplantation of tissue from patients with the condition has resulted in ileitis, but antimicrobial therapy directed against mycobacteria has not been effective in ameliorating the established disease process. Strains of enteroadherent *E. coli* are in higher abundance in patients with Crohn disease compared with the general population based on PCR analysis. Studies using fluorescent in situ hybridization have demonstrated increased numbers of *E. coli* in the lamina propria of patients with active Crohn disease compared with those with inactive disease. Furthermore, an increased number of *E. coli* has been associated with a shorter time before relapse of the disease.

Immunologic factors. Humoral and cell-mediated immune reactions directed against intestinal cells in Crohn disease suggest an autoimmune phenomenon. Attention has focused on the role of cytokines, such as interleukin (IL)-1, IL-2, IL-8, and TNF-α, as contributing factors in the intestinal inflammatory response. The role of the immune response remains controversial in Crohn disease and may represent an effect of the disease process rather than an actual cause.

Genetic factors. Genetic factors play an important role in the pathogenesis of Crohn disease because the single strongest risk factor for its development is having a first-degree relative with the disease. Several genome-wide association sequencing studies have been performed and have identified more than 200 alleles associated with Crohn disease (Table 91.5).

More recent genome-wide association sequencing studies in monozygotic twins have shown no reproducible differences within

TABLE 91.5 Genetic Polymorphisms Related to Crohn Disease

Genes and the Diagnosis of Crohn Disease

Genes related to innate pattern recognition receptors	*NOD2/CARD15, OCTN, TLR*
Genes related to epithelial barrier homeostasis	*IBD5, DLG5*
Genes related to molecular mimicry and autophagy	*ATG16L1, IRGM, LRRK2*
Genes related to lymphocyte differentiation	*IL23R, STAT3*
Genes related to secondary immune response and apoptosis	*MHC, HLA*

Genes and the Prognosis of Crohn Disease

Genes related to age at Crohn disease onset	*TNFRSF6B, CXCL9, IL23R, NOD2, ATG16L1, CNR1, IL10, MDR1, DLG5, IRGM*

Genes Related to Crohn Disease Behavior

Stenotic/structuring behavior	*NOD2, TLR4, IL12B, CX3CR1, IL10, IL6*
Penetrating/fistulizing behavior	*NOD2, IRGM, TNF, HLADRB1, CDKAL1*
Inflammatory behavior	*HLA*
Granulomatous disease	*TLR4/CARD15*

Genes Related to Crohn Disease Location

Upper gastrointestinal	*NOD2, MIF*
Ileal	*IL10, CRP, NOD2, ZNF365, STAT3*
Ileocolonic	*ATG16L1, TCF4 (TCF7L2)*
Colonic	*HLA, TLR4, TLR1, TLR2, TLR6*

Other Genes Related to Crohn Disease

Genes related to Crohn's disease activity	*HSP702, NOD2, PAI1, CNR1*
Genes related to surgery	*NOD2, HLAG*
Genes related to dysplasia and cancer	*FHIT*
Genes related to extraintestinal manifestations	*CARD15, FcRL3, HLADRB103, HLAB27, HLA-B44, HLA-B35, TNFa-308A, TNF-1031C, STAT3*
Pharmacogenetics in Crohn disease	*CARD15, NAT, TPMT, MDR1, MIF, DLG5, TNF, LTA*

Adapted from Tsianos EV, Katsanos KH, Tsianos VE. Role of genetics in the diagnosis and prognosis of Crohn's disease. *World J Gastroenterol.* 2012;18:105-118.

twin pairs in comparing whole genome sequences and tissue-specific variants in the intestinal mucosa directly affected by the inflammation of Crohn disease. These findings suggest that it is unlikely that somatic mutations have a substantial impact on the development of the disease, and simple Mendelian inheritance cannot account for the pattern of occurrence. Therefore, it is likely that multiple causes (e.g., environmental factors) contribute to the origin and pathogenesis of this disease.

Environmental factors. Low-risk countries in Asia that have adopted a more Western lifestyle have noted a significant rise in the incidence of Crohn disease. Smoking is the single largest environmental factor, with a twofold increase in risk of Crohn disease. A genetic predisposition to smoking is associated with an increased risk, identifying a genetic disposition for an environmental risk factor.[13] Other factors that increase the risk of Crohn disease include medications (oral contraceptives, aspirin, nonsteroidal antiinflammatory drugs [NSAIDs], antibiotics), decreased dietary fiber, and increased fat intake. In addition, dysbiosis with a decrease in intraluminal *Bacteroides* and *Firmicutes* and an increase in *Gammaproteobacteria* and *Actinobacteria* are associated with higher risk. Specifically, an increase of mucosal—adherent—invasive *E. coli* survive within macrophages and induce higher TNF-α production. There are numerous studies evaluating the therapeutic benefits of microbiota manipulation.[14]

Pathology

The most common sites of Crohn disease are the small intestine and colon. The location of disease involvement is biologically

defined by the genetic variation. As such, a large multi-institutional study proposed a three-category model to better characterize inflammatory bowel disease into ileal Crohn disease, colonic Crohn disease, and ulcerative colitis. These categories provide risk stratification for surgical complications and genetic risk score based on location.[15] Ileal involvement has been shown with mutations of *IL10, CRP, NOD2, ZNF365,* and *STAT3;* ileocolonic involvement has been shown with mutations of *ATG16L1, TCF4,* and *TCF7L2;* and colonic involvement has been associated with mutations of *HLA, TLR4, TLR1, TLR2,* and *TLR6.* The involvement of the large and small intestine has been noted in about 55% of patients. Thirty percent of patients present with small bowel disease alone, and in 15%, the disease appears limited to the large intestine. The disease process is discontinuous and segmental. In patients with colonic disease, rectal sparing is characteristic of Crohn disease and helps distinguish it from ulcerative colitis. Perirectal and perianal involvement occurs in about one-third of patients with Crohn disease, particularly those with colonic involvement. The disease can also involve the mouth, esophagus, stomach, duodenum, and appendix. Involvement of these sites can accompany disease in the small or large intestine, but in rare cases these locations have been the only apparent sites of involvement.

Gross pathologic features. At exploration, thickened gray-pink or dull purple-red loops of bowel are noted, with areas of thick gray-white exudate or fibrosis of the serosa. Areas of diseased bowel separated by areas of grossly appearing normal bowel, called *skip areas,* are commonly encountered. A striking finding of Crohn disease is the presence of extensive fat wrapping caused by the circumferential growth of the mesenteric fat around the bowel wall, also known as *creeping fat* (Fig. 91.6A). As the disease progresses, the bowel wall becomes increasingly thickened, firm, rubbery, and almost incompressible (see Fig. 91.6B). The uninvolved proximal bowel may be dilated secondary to obstruction of the diseased segment. Involved segments often are adherent to adjacent intestinal loops or other viscera, with internal fistulas common in these areas. The mesentery of the involved segment is usually thickened, with enlarged lymph nodes often noted.

On opening of the bowel, the earliest gross pathologic lesion is a superficial aphthous ulcer noted in the mucosa. With increasing disease progression, the ulceration becomes pronounced, and complete transmural inflammation results. The ulcers are characteristically linear and may coalesce to produce transverse sinuses with islands of normal mucosa in between, thus giving the characteristic cobblestone appearance.

Microscopic features. Mucosal and submucosal edema may be noted microscopically before any gross changes. A chronic inflammatory infiltrate appears in the mucosa and submucosa and extends transmurally. This inflammatory reaction is characterized by extensive edema, hyperemia, lymphangiectasia, intense infiltration of mononuclear cells, and lymphoid hyperplasia. Characteristic histologic lesions of Crohn disease are noncaseating granulomas

with Langerhans giant cells. Granulomas appear later in the course and are found in the wall of the bowel or in regional lymph nodes in 60% to 70% of patients (see Fig. 91.6C).

Clinical Manifestations

Crohn disease can occur at any age, but the typical patient is a young adult in the second or third decade of life. The onset of disease is often insidious, with a slow and protracted course. Characteristically, there are symptomatic periods of abdominal pain and diarrhea interspersed with asymptomatic periods of varying lengths. With time, the symptomatic periods gradually become more frequent, more severe, and longer lasting. The most common symptom of Crohn disease is chronic diarrhea, followed by intermittent and colicky abdominal pain, most commonly noted in the lower abdomen. The pain, however, may be more severe and localized in the right lower quadrant and may mimic the signs and symptoms of acute appendicitis.[11] In contrast to ulcerative colitis, patients with Crohn disease typically have fewer bowel movements, and the stools rarely contain mucus, pus, or blood. Systemic nonspecific symptoms include a low-grade fever present in about one-third of the patients, weight loss, loss of strength, and malaise.

Clinically, Crohn disease is often classified on the basis of age at onset, behavior, and site of origin. The Montreal classification

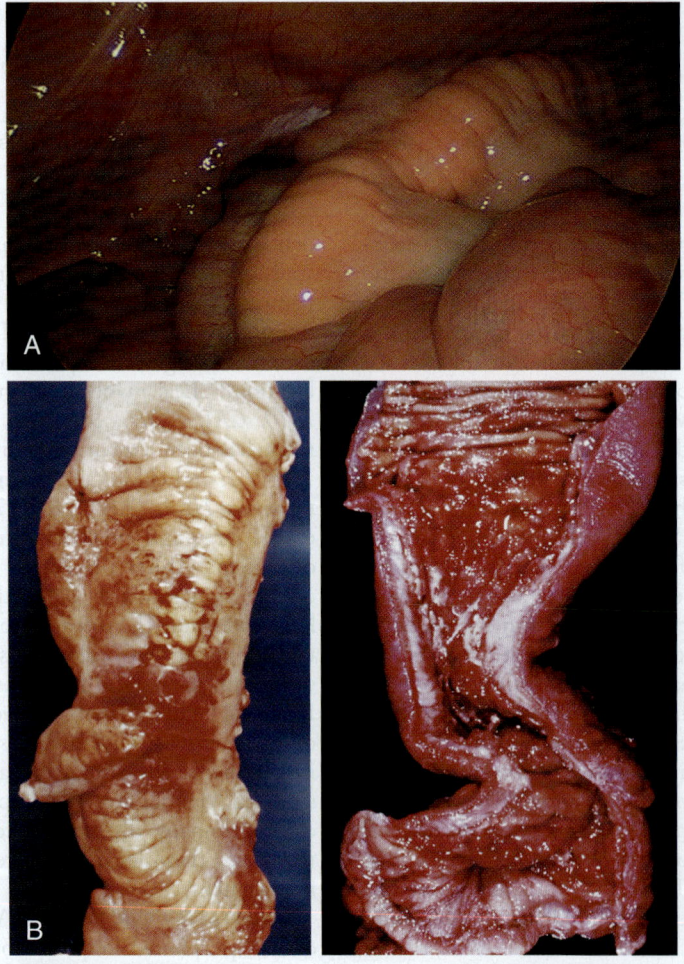

FIGURE 91.6 (A) Crohn disease with evidence of creeping fat. Laparoscopic evaluation of extensive fat wrapping caused by the circumferential growth of the mesenteric fat around the bowel wall. (B) Gross pathologic features of Crohn disease. *(Left)* Serosal surface demonstrates extensive fat wrapping and inflammation. *(Right)* Resected specimen demonstrates marked fibrosis of the intestinal wall, stricture, and segmental mucosal inflammation.

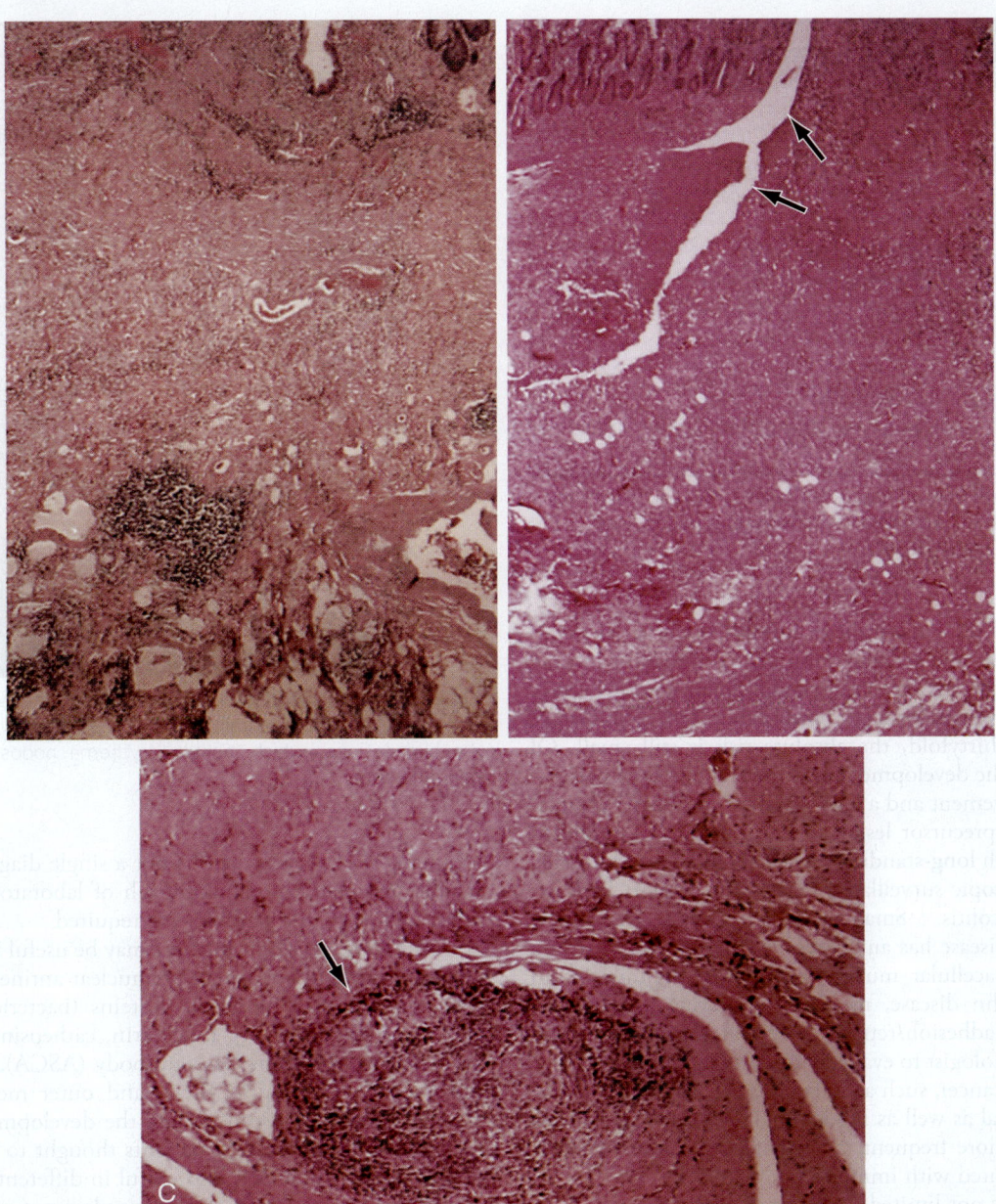

FIGURE 91.6, cont'd (C) Microscopic features of Crohn disease. *(Upper left)* Transmural inflammation. *(Upper right)* Fissure ulcer *(arrows)*. *(Bottom)* Noncaseating granuloma located in the muscular layer of the small bowel *(arrow)*. (A, Courtesy Dr. John Draus, University of Kentucky Medical Center, Lexington, KY. B–C, Courtesy Dr. Mary R. Schwartz, Baylor College of Medicine, Houston, TX.)

(Table 91.6) divides all patients into distinct categories based on symptom onset (before or after the age of 40 years), disease behavior (nonstricturing/nonpenetrating, stricturing, or penetrating), and disease site (terminal ileum, colon, ileocolonic, upper gastrointestinal tract). This classification was developed to provide a reproducible staging of the disease, to help predict remission and relapse, and to direct therapy. The main intestinal complications of Crohn disease include obstruction and perforation. Obstruction can occur as a manifestation of an acute exacerbation of active disease or as the result of chronic fibrosing lesions, which eventually narrow the lumen of the bowel, producing partial or near-complete obstruction. Free perforations into the peritoneal cavity leading to a generalized peritonitis can occur in patients

with Crohn disease, but this presentation is rare. More commonly, fistulas occur between the sites of perforation and adjacent organs, such as loops of small and large intestine, urinary bladder, vagina, stomach, and sometimes the skin, usually at the site of a previous laparotomy. Localized abscesses can occur near the sites of perforation. Patients with Crohn colitis may develop toxic megacolon and present with a marked colonic dilation, abdominal tenderness, fever, and leukocytosis. Bleeding is typically indolent and chronic, but massive gastrointestinal bleeding can occasionally occur, particularly in duodenal Crohn disease associated with chronic ulcer formation.

Long-standing Crohn disease predisposes the patient to cancer of the small intestine and colon. These carcinomas typically arise

TABLE 91.6   Montreal Classification of Crohn Disease

Age at diagnosis (yr)	A1: ≤16
	A3: 17–40
	A2: >40
Behavior	B1: Nonstricturing/nonpenetrating
	B2: Stricturing
	B3: Penetrating
	P: Perianal disease modifier (can add to B1–B3)
Location	L1: Ileal
	L2: Colonic
	L3: Ileocolonic
	L4: Isolated upper gastrointestinal tract (can add to L1–L3)

Adapted from Spekhorst LM, Visschedijk MC, Alberts R, et al. Performance of the Montreal classification for inflammatory bowel diseases. *World J Gastroenterol.* 2014;20:15374-15381.

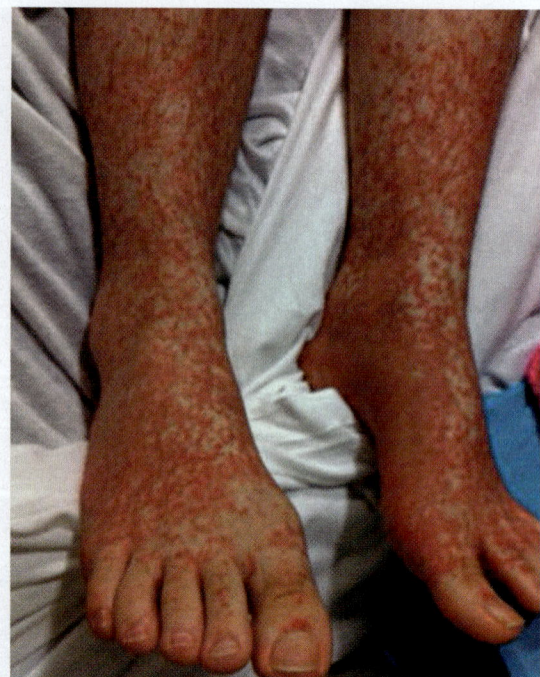

FIGURE 91.7 Patient with Crohn disease with erythema nodosum. The most common extraintestinal presentations of Crohn disease are skin lesions, which include erythema nodosum and pyoderma gangrenosum.

at sites of chronic disease and more commonly occur in the ileum as a result of the chronic inflammation of the mucosa. Most are not detected until the advanced stages, and the prognosis is poor. Although the relative risk for small bowel cancer in Crohn disease is approximately thirtyfold, the absolute risk is still small. Of greater concern is the development of colorectal cancer in patients with colonic involvement and a long duration of disease. Dysplasia is the putative precursor lesion for Crohn disease–associated cancer. Patients with long-standing disease should have an equally aggressive colonoscopic surveillance regimen as patients with extensive ulcerative colitis.[11] Small bowel adenocarcinoma associated with Crohn disease has an aggressive behavior and a strong probability of extracellular mucin. In surgical specimens from patients with Crohn disease, mucinous-appearing anal fistulas and ileal areas of adhesion/retraction should always be closely examined by a pathologist to evaluate for dysplasia or malignancy.

Extraintestinal cancer, such as squamous cell carcinoma of the vulva and anal canal as well as Hodgkin and non-Hodgkin lymphomas, may be more frequent in patients with Crohn disease, especially those treated with immunomodulators.

Crohn disease is not limited to the small intestine, with 41% of patients presenting with ileocolitis and 48% of patients with colonic involvement alone. Perianal disease (fissure, fistula, stricture, or abscess) is common and occurs in 25% of patients with the disease. Perianal disease may be the sole presenting feature in 5% of patients and may precede the onset of intestinal disease by months or even years. In 10% to 30% of patients, perianal disease will be the first presenting symptom. Crohn disease should be suspected in any patient with multiple chronic perianal fistulas.[16]

Extraintestinal manifestations of Crohn disease may be present in 30% of patients. Common findings are skin lesions (Fig. 91.7), which include erythema nodosum and pyoderma gangrenosum, arthritis and arthralgias, uveitis and iritis, hepatitis, pericholangitis, and aphthous stomatitis. In addition, amyloidosis, pancreatitis, and nephrotic syndrome may occur in these patients. These symptoms may precede, accompany, or appear independently of the underlying bowel disease.

Diagnosis

A diagnosis of Crohn disease should be considered in patients with chronic recurring episodes of abdominal pain, diarrhea, and

weight loss. However, there is not a single diagnostic test for the condition; a multimodal approach of laboratory testing, endoscopy, radiology, and pathology is required.

Laboratory. Serologic markers may be useful in the diagnosis of Crohn disease. In particular, perinuclear antineutrophil cytoplasmic antibody and its target proteins (bactericidal/permeability increasing protein [BPI], lactoferrin, cathepsin G, and elastase), anti–*Saccharomyces cerevisiae* antibody (ASCA), outer membrane porin of flagellin (anti-CBir1), and outer membrane porin of *E. coli* (OmpC-IgG) can predict the development of inflammatory bowel disease even in patients thought to be at low risk for developing it.[17] ASCA is also useful in differentiating Crohn disease from ulcerative colitis as well as playing a role in determining patients who will require surgery in the future.

Noninvasive inflammatory markers (historically, C-reactive protein and erythrocyte sedimentation rate) were used to aid in the initial diagnosis, to rule out exacerbations, to monitor response to systemic therapy, and to predict relapse; however, these markers were generally nonspecific and have largely been abandoned. Stool lactoferrin, an iron-binding protein in the secretory granules of neutrophils, and fecal calprotectin, a protein with antimicrobial properties released by squamous cells in response to inflammation, are inflammatory markers specific to the intestine that have shown promising results for the detection and surveillance of Crohn disease. A prospective study showed that both calprotectin and lactoferrin levels correlate well with CT enterography (CTE) images of small bowel inflammation (mucosal irregularity, hyperdensity, stenosis, prestenotic dilation, and mesenteric hypervascularity [i.e., comb sign]). Elevated fecal calprotectin is predictive of small bowel inflammation with a sensitivity of 87% and specificity of 67%. Fecal lactoferrin (>6 ng/mL) has been found to be similarly predictive with a lower sensitivity but higher specificity for small bowel inflammation. Together, these findings identify fecal calprotectin and lactoferrin as helpful screening tools for detecting early small bowel Crohn disease.[11]

Radiology. CTE or magnetic resonance enterography (MRE) are often used as the initial assessment of Crohn disease to complement direct ileocolonoscopy. Imaging studies can provide information regarding severity of inflammation, length, and focality and can identify complications (e.g., obstruction or fistula). In addition, these studies support surgical planning and the evaluation of response to medical therapy. Previously, barium enema was commonly used to identify features of Crohn disease. For example, long lengths of narrowed terminal ileum (Kantor string sign) may be present with long-standing disease (Fig. 91.8A). Segmental and irregular patterns of bowel involvement may be noted. Fistulas between adjacent bowel loops and organs may be apparent (see Fig. 91.8B).

CTE may be useful in demonstrating the marked transmural thickening; it can also greatly aid in diagnosing extramural complications of Crohn disease, especially in the acute setting (see Fig. 91.8C). MRE and CTE are equally accurate in assessing disease activity and bowel damage; however, MRE may be superior to CTE in detecting intestinal strictures and ileal wall enhancement.[18] Recent studies suggest limiting the use of CTE in patients with long-standing Crohn disease because of its significant radiation exposure and need for numerous studies during the course of the disease. MRE is a useful adjunct to determine intestinal strictures as well as fistulas and sinus tracts; however, the relatively high cost, prolonged examination time, and limited availability may preclude many patients from receiving this procedure. Intestinal ultrasound is increasing in utility for the diagnosis and assessment of severity of Crohn disease, with the

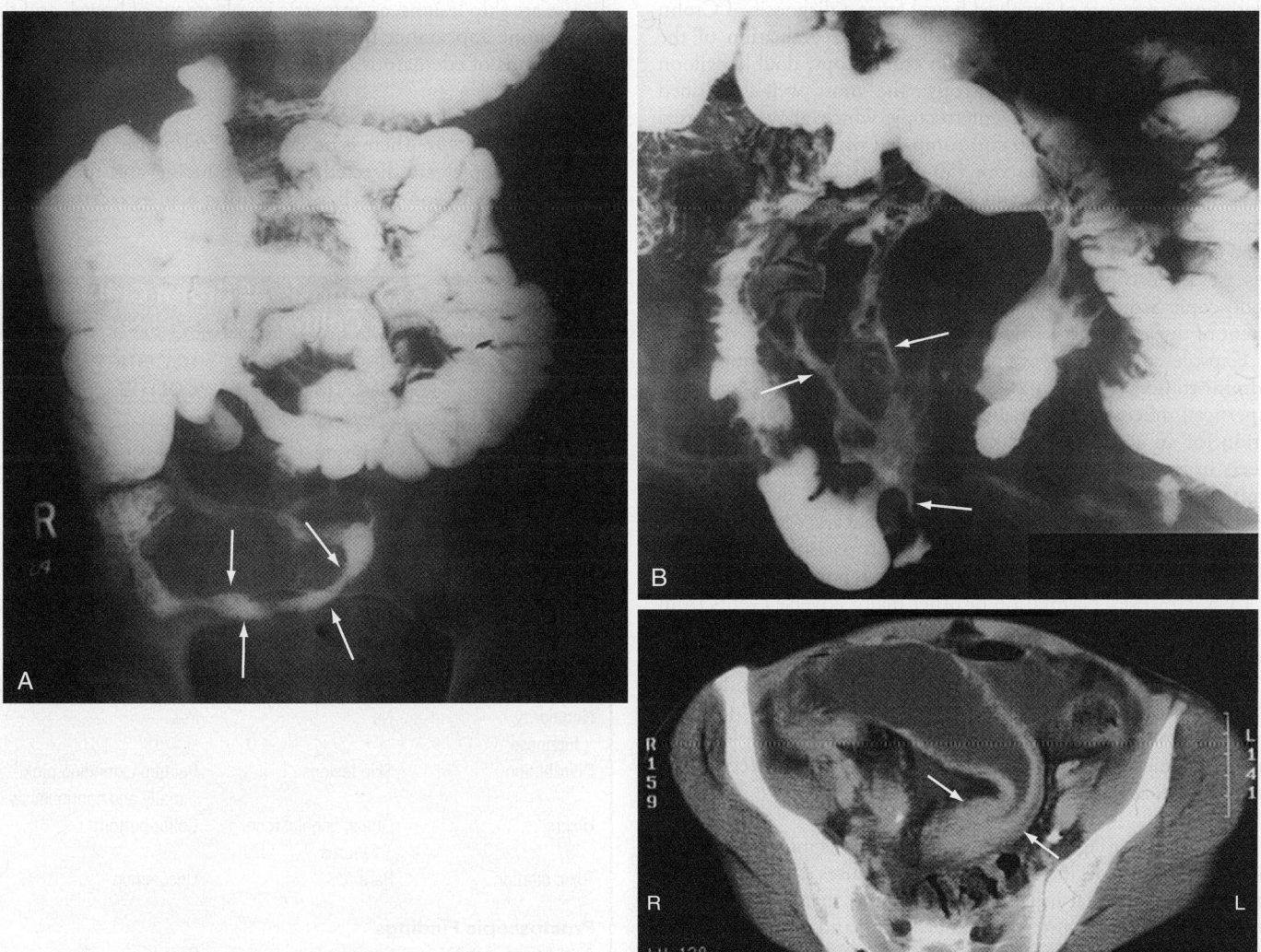

FIGURE 91.8 (A) Small bowel obstruction secondary to Crohn disease. Small bowel series in a patient with Crohn disease demonstrates a narrowed distal ileum *(arrows)* secondary to chronic inflammation and fibrosis. (B) Intraabdominal fistulas in Crohn disease. Multiple short fistulous tracts communicating between the distal loops of ileum and the proximal colon in a patient with Crohn disease *(arrows)*. (C) Mechanical small bowel obstruction secondary to chronic structuring disease. CTE of a patient with Crohn disease demonstrates marked thickening of the bowel *(arrows)* with a high-grade partial small bowel obstruction and dilated proximal intestine. *CTE,* CT enterography. (A, Courtesy Dr. Melvyn H. Schreiber, The University of Texas Medical Branch, Galveston, TX. B–C, Adapted from Evers BM, Townsend CM Jr, Thompson JC. Small intestine. In: Schwartz SI, ed. *Principles of Surgery.* 7th ed. New York: McGraw-Hill; 1999:1233.)

recent development of scoring systems based on ultrasound findings. Being noninvasive, low cost, and accessible makes ultrasound a potentially advantageous tool in the management of these patients. However, its use is new, and validation studies are ongoing.

Endoscopy. Ileocolonoscopy with biopsies of the terminal ileum are the gold standard for the diagnosis of Crohn disease. When the colon is involved, sigmoidoscopy or colonoscopy may reveal characteristic aphthous ulcers with granularity and a normal-appearing surrounding mucosa. Intubation of the ileocecal valve during colonoscopy allows examination and biopsy of the terminal ileum but fails to evaluate other segments of the small intestine. With more advanced and severe disease, the ulcerations involve progressively more of the bowel lumen, and it may be difficult to distinguish Crohn disease from ulcerative colitis. However, the presence of discrete ulcers and cobblestoning as well as the discontinuous segments of involved bowel favor a diagnosis of Crohn disease. Endoscopic advances that allow better evaluation of the small intestine include single-balloon enteroscopy, double-balloon enteroscopy, and spiral enteroscopy; the most well-established technique is double-balloon enteroscopy, which allows increased enteral intubation (240–360 cm) compared with push enteroscopy (90–150 cm) or ileocolonoscopy (50–80 cm). Limitations include specialized examiner skills and equipment, prolonged procedure times, and a 1% risk of complications (e.g., pancreatitis, perforation, or bleeding). After the diagnosis is confirmed, the Crohn's Disease Endoscopic Index of Severity (CDEIS) or the Simple Endoscopic Score for Crohn's Disease (SES-CD) is used to define extent of disease and severity.

Capsule endoscopy was approved by the US Food and Drug Administration (FDA) in 2001 and is helpful in the diagnosis of superficial mucosal abnormalities. The most commonly used criterion for an abnormal finding is the presence of three or more ulcers in the absence of NSAID use. The use of this modality is limited because of concern for capsule retention, defined as the presence of the capsule in the gastrointestinal tract for more than 2 weeks. The risk of retention is higher in patients with Crohn disease, averaging about 3%, but has been reported to be as high as 13%. However, perforation or other major adverse events from retention are rare. Capsule endoscopy has been found to be superior to any other modality in the identification of intestinal ulceration.[19] Severity can be measured using the Capsule Endoscopy Crohn's Disease Activity Index (CECDAI or Niv score). As endoscopic technology advances, studies continue to be developed to further characterize Crohn disease throughout the entirety of the gastrointestinal tract.

Histology

Differential diagnosis. The differential diagnosis of Crohn disease includes specific and nonspecific causes of intestinal inflammation. Bacterial inflammation (such as that caused by *Salmonella* and *Shigella*), intestinal tuberculosis, and protozoan infections (such as amebiasis) may manifest as an ileitis. In the immunocompromised host, rare infections, particularly mycobacterial and cytomegalovirus (CMV) infections, have become more common and may cause ileitis. Acute distal ileitis may be a manifestation of early Crohn disease, but it also may be unrelated, such as when it is caused by a bacteriologic agent (e.g., *Campylobacter, Yersinia*). Patients usually present in a similar fashion to those with acute appendicitis, with a sudden onset of right lower quadrant pain, nausea, vomiting, and fever. These entities normally resolve spontaneously, and when they are noted during surgery, no biopsy or resection should be performed.

In most cases, Crohn disease of the colon can be readily distinguished from ulcerative colitis; however, in 5% to 10% of patients, the delineation between Crohn disease and ulcerative colitis may be difficult, if not impossible, to make (see Table 91.7). Ulcerative colitis almost always involves the rectum most severely, with lessening inflammation from the rectum to the ileocolic area. In contrast, Crohn disease may be worse on the right side of the colon than on the left side, and sometimes the rectum is spared. Ulcerative colitis also demonstrates continuous involvement from rectum to proximal segments, whereas Crohn disease is segmental. Although ulcerative colitis involves the mucosa of the large intestine, it does not extend deep into the wall of the bowel as does Crohn disease. Bleeding is a more common symptom in ulcerative colitis. Perianal involvement and rectovaginal fistulas are unusual in ulcerative colitis but are more common in Crohn disease. Other endoscopic features of Crohn disease are skip lesions, asymmetric involvement of bowel, and the cobblestone appearance that results from ulcerations interspersed with islands of edematous mucosa.

Management

Medical therapy. There is no cure for Crohn disease. Therefore, medical therapies are directed toward inducing and maintaining steroid-free remission as well as preventing acute exacerbations or

---

TABLE 91.7 Diagnosis of Crohn Colitis Versus Ulcerative Colitis

PARAMETER	CROHN COLITIS	ULCERATIVE COLITIS
Symptoms and Signs		
Diarrhea	Common	Common
Rectal bleeding	Less common	Almost always
Abdominal pain (cramps)	Moderate to severe	Mild to moderate
Palpable mass	At times	No (unless large cancer)
Anal complaints	Frequent (>50%)	Infrequent (<20%)
Radiologic Findings		
Ileal disease	Common	Rare (backwash ileitis)
Nodularity, fuzziness	No	Yes
Distribution	Skip lesions	Rectum extending proximally and continuously
Ulcers	Linear, cobblestone, fissures	Collar-button
Toxic dilation	Rare	Uncommon
Proctoscopic Findings		
Anal fissure, fistula, abscess	Common	Rare
Rectal sparing	Common (50%)	Rare (5%)
Granular mucosa	No	Yes
Ulceration	Linear, deep, scattered	Superficial, universal

Adapted from Waugh N, Cummins E, Royle P, et al. *Faecal Calprotectin Testing for Differentiating Amongst Inflammatory and Non-Inflammatory Bowel Diseases: Systematic Review and Economic Evaluation*. Southampton, UK: NIHR Journals Library; 2013 Nov. (Health Technology Assessment, No. 17.55.) Appendix 1, Comparison of ulcerative colitis, Crohn's disease, irritable bowel syndrome and coeliac disease.

complications of the disease. However, it is important to note that endoscopic healing has emerged as the therapeutic goal because of poor association of inflammation with symptoms. Surgery is advocated for neoplastic and preneoplastic lesions, obstructing stenoses, suppurative complications, or medically intractable disease. Narcotic analgesia should be avoided except during the perioperative period because of the potential for tolerance and abuse in the setting of chronic disease. Drugs that have demonstrated efficacy in the induction or maintenance of remission in Crohn disease include aminosalicylates, such as sulfasalazine and mesalamine; corticosteroids; TNF antagonists, such as infliximab, adalimumab, and certolizumab; immunosuppressive agents, such as azathioprine (AZT), 6-mercaptopurine (6-MP), methotrexate (MTX), and tacrolimus (FK-506); antiadhesion molecules such as vedolizumab, etrolizumab, and natalizumab; the IL inhibitor ustekinumab; and antibiotics. The recent increase in the use of immunomodulators and biologic agents has significantly reduced surgery rates. The primary target of medical treatment is reduction of the Crohn's Disease Activity Index (CDAI), which uses eight major clinical factors to evaluate disease severity (Box 91.4). Clinical remission is achieved when CDAI is below 150, and clinical response to therapy occurs with a drop of 100 points.[17] A score between 150 and 220 is considered mild to moderate disease and can be followed by outpatient visits; a score between 220 and 450 is considered moderate to severe disease and occurs after failure with first-line therapy; a score greater than 450 is considered severe fulminant disease with failed medical therapy and complications of obstruction, peritonitis, and abscess. Other innovative therapies such as MadCAM-1 (mucosal addressin cell adhesion molecule 1 inhibitor), tofacitinib (JAK3 pathway inhibitor), mongersen (SMAD7 inhibitor), and ozanimod (S1P1 inhibitor) continue to be investigated in clinical trials with variable results thus far. Upadacitinib, a JAK inhibitor, has demonstrated promising results in two phase III induction trials (U-EXCEL and U-EXCEED) with increased remission rates and endoscopic response in patients with moderate to severe Crohn disease when compared with placebo.[20]

Aminosalicylates. Sulfasalazine (azulfidine) is an aminosalicylate with 5-aminosalicylic acid as the active moiety. Although a clear benefit has been noted in patients with colonic involvement, the effectiveness of sulfasalazine alone in the treatment of small

bowel Crohn disease is controversial, and its use in maintenance therapy has fallen out of favor. Mesalamine, which is also an aminosalicylate, provides a slow release of 5-aminosalicylic acid with passage through the small bowel and colon. However, high-dose mesalamine has not been shown to be more effective than placebo at achieving remission and is not typically employed in treating patients with Crohn disease.[11]

Corticosteroids. Steroids are fast acting and effective at inducing remission but are not ideal as maintenance therapy. Given advances in alternative treatment options with improved efficacy in steroid-sparing therapies, the use of steroids is declining. Budesonide, a corticosteroid, has a high first-pass hepatic metabolism, which allows targeted delivery to the intestine while mitigating the systemic effects of steroid therapy. Controlled ileal-release budesonide (9 mg/day) is effective when active disease is confined to the ileum or right colon and has been shown to be more effective than either placebo or mesalamine.[21] Given a relatively good response and its relative safety, budesonide is recommended as the preferred primary treatment over mesalamine for patients with mild to moderately active Crohn disease with localized ileal disease.

An alternative corticosteroid, prednisone, can be beneficial in moderate to severe Crohn disease. Patients with moderate to severe disease should be treated with high-dose (40–60 mg daily) prednisone until resolution of symptoms and resumption of weight gain. Parenteral corticosteroids are indicated for patients with severe disease once the presence of an abscess has been excluded. Steroids should be tapered once the patient experiences clinical improvement. Currently, there are no standards for corticosteroid taper, but doses are generally tapered by 5 to 10 mg/week until 20 mg and then by 2.5 to 5 mg weekly until cessation. Dual-energy x-ray absorptiometry scan, calcium and vitamin D supplementation, and consideration of bisphosphonate therapy are warranted once corticosteroid therapy is initiated to identify baseline bone density and to prevent steroid-induced loss of bone mineral density.[11]

Antibiotics. Antibiotics are useful as an adjunct therapy in the treatment of Crohn disease. Although initially thought to help promote remission, antibiotics were found to be no more effective than placebo for inducing remission and are no longer considered as the primary therapy for induction of remission. Classically, metronidazole and ciprofloxacin are used in the treatment of complications from Crohn disease. Other antibiotics that have been used with varying success include rifaximin, clofazimine, ethambutol, isoniazid, and rifabutin. Antibiotic therapy has a clear role in the septic complications associated with Crohn disease, perianal disease, and fistulizing disease.[21] However, antibiotics are associated with side effects (i.e., *Clostridioides difficile* infection) and should not be used for long-term maintenance or as the primary treatment to induce remission.

Immunosuppressive agents. The immunosuppressive agents AZT, 6-MP, and MTX are effective in maintenance therapy and for the treatment of moderate to severe Crohn disease. AZT and 6-MP are effective for maintaining steroid-induced remission, and weekly IV MTX is effective for both induction and maintenance therapy but is less effective than biologics.[11] Because of the slow onset of action of immunosuppressive agents and to prevent flares, steroids are needed from induction until the transition to immunosuppressive agents is complete. Despite their potential toxicity, these drugs have proved to be relatively safe in patients with Crohn disease; the most common side effects are pancreatitis, hepatitis, fever, and rash. The more disconcerting complications of immunosuppressants include chronic liver disease, bone

---

BOX 91.4 Crohn Disease Activity Index (CDAI)

Number of liquid or soft stools (each day for 7 days)

Abdominal pain, sum of 7 daily ratings (0 = none, 1 = mild, 2 = moderate, 3 = severe)

General well-being, sum of 7 daily ratings (0 = generally well, 1 = slightly under par, 2 = poor, 3 = very poor, 4 = terrible)

Number of listed complications (arthritis or arthralgia, iritis, uveitis, erythema nodosum or pyoderma gangrenosum, aphthous stomatitis, anal fissure, fistula or abscess, fever greater than 37.8°C [100°F]).

Use of diphenoxylate or loperamide for diarrhea (0 = no, 1 = year)

Abdominal mass (0 = no, 2 = questionable, 5 = definite)

Hematocrit (males >47% or females >42%)

Body weight (1 − weight/standard weight) × 100 (add or subtract according to sign)

Adapted from Sandborn WJ, Feagan BG, Hanauer SB, et al. A review of activity indices and efficacy endpoints for clinical trials of medical therapy in adults with Crohn's disease. *Gastroenterology.* 2002; 122:512-530.

marrow suppression, and the potential for malignant transformation. Genetic polymorphisms for thiopurine methyltransferase (TPMT), which is the primary enzyme that metabolizes AZT and 6-MP, have been identified and suggested for use to regulate therapy according to the measurement of their metabolites (6-thioguanine nucleotides). Patients with decreased TPMT activity have a significantly increased risk of fatal bone marrow suppression. Previous studies reported severe myelosuppression in patients who are wild-type or heterozygous carriers for TPMT variant alleles; these findings suggest that TPMT genotype testing may be a safe screening tool to determine which patients may have a genetic predisposition to adverse outcomes. MTX also has side effects of hepatotoxicity, can cause myelosuppression, and should not be used in pregnant females.

Anti–tumor necrosis factor therapy. The introduction of anti-TNF therapy for Crohn disease was considered a breakthrough in medical management. The first anti-TNF agent introduced was infliximab, a chimeric monoclonal antibody to TNF-α. Infliximab is efficacious and safe as a monotherapy in the treatment of moderate to severe Crohn disease and is effective as an induction and maintenance agent. Multiple studies demonstrated that treatment with infliximab results in perineal fistula closure in approximately two-thirds of patients. Although it is highly effective in certain patients with penetrating and extraintestinal disease, not every patient responds to infliximab. Other FDA-approved TNF antagonists include adalimumab (humanized IgG1 monoclonal antibody), which is an effective maintenance agent that can be self-administered, and certolizumab (humanized antibody fragment), which is ideal in pregnant and nursing females, as it is linked to a polyethylene glycol moiety, does not cross the placenta, and is not excreted in breast milk. Safety profiles for these three anti-TNF medications are similar. There is an increased risk for tuberculosis reactivation, invasive fungal and other opportunistic infections, demyelinating central nervous system lesions, activation of latent multiple sclerosis, exacerbation of congestive heart failure, and concerns for increased risk of melanoma. Patients who develop a flare while on anti-TNF agents require measurement of serum drug concentrations and antidrug antibodies (antibodies binding to competitive and noncompetitive sites to inhibit drug function). Measured levels would indicate the need to increase dosage (if low drug concentration and low antibodies), switch to another anti-TNF agent (high antidrug antibodies), or switch to another drug class (normal drug concentration). Because of the potential for immunogenicity of monoclonal antibodies, the combination of an anti-TNF agent and an immunosuppressive provides optimal drug levels and low antidrug antibodies.[11]

Novel therapies. Other therapeutic agents for Crohn disease include leukocyte trafficking inhibitors, IL inhibitors, and antibodies to antiadhesion molecules. These agents are often used if the patient has failed or is unable to tolerate anti-TNF therapy. Natalizumab, a recombinant humanized monoclonal antibody against α4 integrin, showed effectiveness in the induction and maintenance of remission in patients with active Crohn disease. It was removed from the market after several patients developed progressive multifocal leukoencephalopathy but was later reinstated for refractory Crohn disease and approved for use in 2008. Similarly, vedolizumab is a humanized monoclonal antibody that specifically binds to α4β7 integrin and blocks its interaction with MadCAM-1; this action inhibits the translocation of memory T lymphocytes into inflamed gastrointestinal parenchymal tissues. Vedolizumab can be used for induction of remission, but it has a very slow onset of action. Because MadCAM-1 is preferentially

expressed on blood vessels in the gastrointestinal tract, vedolizumab is more gut specific and therefore a more targeted form of immunosuppression.[11] Also, vedolizumab prevents the gastrointestinal mucosal or transmural inflammation without the nonspecific neurologic side effects seen in less selective α4 integrin inhibitors, such as natalizumab. Ustekinumab is a humanized IgG1 monoclonal antibody that inhibits IL-12/23 through targeting of a shared p40 subunit that has been shown to be effective in severe Crohn disease that is refractory to anti-TNF therapies with similar efficacy.

Nutritional therapy. Nutritional therapy in patients with Crohn disease has been used with varying success. The use of chemically defined elemental diets has been shown in some studies to reduce disease activity, particularly in patients with disease localized to the small bowel, and they can reduce corticosteroid-induced toxicities. Liquid polymeric diets may be as effective as elemental feedings and are more acceptable to patients. With few exceptions, standard elemental diets have not been effective to prevent relapse of Crohn disease. Total parenteral nutrition (TPN) was also useful in patients with active Crohn disease; however, complication rates exceed those for enteral nutrition. There remains interest in investigating different modified diets to improve outcomes in patients with Crohn disease. Although the primary role of nutritional therapy is questionable in patients with inflammatory bowel disease, there is definitely a secondary role for nutritional supplementation to replenish depleted nutrient stores, to allow intestinal protein synthesis and healing, and to prepare patients for surgery.[17]

Smoking cessation. Although the implication of tobacco abuse as a causative factor in the development of Crohn disease has been difficult to prove, smoking clearly affects the disease course. Smoking is associated with the late bimodal onset of disease and has been shown to increase the incidence of relapse, failure of maintenance therapy, and increased need for surgery. It also appears to be associated with the severity of disease in a linear dose-response relationship. Tobacco exposure is an independent predictor of the need for maintenance treatment, specifically biologic therapy. Therefore, smoking cessation therapy is an important component of medical therapy.

Surgical treatment. Although medical management is indicated during acute exacerbations of disease, most patients with chronic Crohn disease will require surgery at some time during the course of their illness. The goals are to preserve bowel length while minimizing postoperative complications and disease recurrence. With the advancements made in the management of patients with Crohn disease, the rate of surgical intervention has decreased. However, approximately 75% of patients will require surgical resection within their lifetime. Indications for surgery include failure of medical treatment, bowel obstruction, perforation, fistula or abscess formation, steroid dependence, dysplasia, or malignancy. Most patients can be treated with elective surgery, especially with the improvement of medical management in the past decade. However, patients with intestinal perforation, peritonitis, excessive bleeding, or toxic megacolon require urgent surgery.[22] Children with Crohn disease and resulting systemic symptoms, such as growth retardation, may benefit from resection. The extraintestinal complications of Crohn disease, although not primary indications for operation, often subside after resection of the involved bowel; exceptions are that problems may continue with ankylosing spondylitis and hepatic complications.

The aim of surgery for Crohn disease has shifted from a radical operation to one that achieves inflammation-free margins with minimal surgery, intended to remove just grossly inflamed tissue or to increase the luminal diameter of the bowel (i.e., dilation or strictureplasty). Even if adjacent areas of bowel are clearly diseased, they should be ignored. Fistulizing disease rarely requires operative intervention unless the fistula involves the bladder, vagina, or skin. A bowel resection with fistulotomy may be needed. Early in the history of surgical therapy for Crohn disease, surgeons tended to perform wider resections with the hope of cure or significant remission. However, recurring wide resections resulted in neither cure nor a greater incidence of remissions and led to short bowel syndrome, a devastating surgical complication. Frozen sections to determine microscopic disease are unreliable and should be performed only when malignant disease is suspected. It must be emphasized that operative treatment of a complication must be limited to that segment of bowel involved with the complication, and no attempt should be made to resect more bowel, even though grossly evident disease may be apparent.

Laparoscopic surgery for patients with Crohn disease is most used today. The advantages of minimally invasive approaches and the advances in this technology have made laparoscopy feasible for the operative treatment of Crohn disease. Studies reveal only a 10% conversion rate of laparoscopic to open for ileocolic resections in Crohn disease. Advantages to laparoscopy include shorter median operative time, earlier return of bowel function, less pain, and shorter hospital stays. Multiple randomized clinical trials verified that laparoscopic surgery is associated with a more rapid recovery of bowel function and shorter hospital stay; importantly, the rate of disease recurrence is similar when compared with open procedures. Randomized controlled trials with long-term follow-up have demonstrated that patients undergoing laparoscopic ileocolonic resection for Crohn disease had improved body image and satisfaction with cosmesis of surgery and less incidence of incisional hernia compared with the open surgery group. Additional options that have shown similar outcomes to laparoscopic intervention include hand-assisted laparoscopic surgery, single-incision laparoscopic surgery, and robot-assisted laparoscopic surgery. Each patient should be carefully evaluated for appropriate operative technique, as not every patient is appropriate for minimally invasive techniques. In general, the rate of open intervention is decreasing as laparoscopy has become favored, even in the treatment of complex Crohn disease.[23]

Another difficult surgical decision important in Crohn disease involves performing a primary anastomosis versus initial ostomy formation with delayed reconstruction. Patients with this condition are often malnourished and receive intensive immunosuppressive therapy or present with an element of intraabdominal sepsis. In general, standard surgical principles should direct this decision. Patients with adequate nutrition and minimal intraabdominal sepsis can safely undergo primary anastomosis at the initial operation, whereas malnourished and septic patients are best served by diversion, if possible. Although caution should be exercised in performing an anastomosis in the setting of high-dose immunosuppression, large series have confirmed that surgery is safe for patients with Crohn disease while they are receiving perioperative infliximab or immunosuppressive therapy. Regarding the anastomotic technique, previous studies suggested that creating a wider anastomosis with a stapled functional end-to-end anastomosis may decrease fecal stasis and subsequent bacterial overgrowth, which are implicated in anastomotic recurrence in Crohn disease. However, a randomized controlled trial comparing side-to-side anastomosis versus end-to-end anastomosis determined that there was no difference in overall complication rates,

anastomotic leak rates, or rates of symptomatic recurrence, with only a slight increase in endoscopic recurrence seen in the end-to-end anastomosis group (43% vs. 38%). Additionally, a new antimesenteric, functional, end-to-end, hand-sewn anastomosis (known as *Kono-S anastomosis*) was created to minimize anastomotic restenosis in Crohn disease. This technique was demonstrated to have a significantly lower rate of stenosis and recurrence compared with conventional end-to-end anastomosis. Although further randomized control trials are needed, these findings demonstrate a promising novel surgical approach that may decrease the need for additional biologic therapy.[24]

An evolving consideration in surgical resection is the management of the mesentery of the diseased bowel. Although still under investigation, the mesentery, as a site of inflammatory cells and nerves, is proposed as a source for recurrent and spreading disease. As such, during any resection for diseased bowel, the surgeon should also consider what the appropriate mesenteric resection should be to reduce future disease.[22]

Specific Problems

Acute ileitis (nonstricturing, nonpenetrating). Patients can present with acute abdominal pain localized to the right lower quadrant, signs and symptoms consistent with a diagnosis of acute appendicitis. At exploration, the appendix is found to be normal, but the terminal ileum is edematous and beefy red with a thickened mesentery and enlarged lymph nodes. This condition, known as *acute ileitis,* is a self-limited disease. Acute ileitis may be a manifestation of early Crohn disease but is most often unrelated. Bacteriologic agents such as *Campylobacter* and *Yersinia* may cause acute ileitis. Intestinal resection should not be performed. In the absence of acute inflammatory involvement of the appendix or the cecum, appendectomy has been recommended to eliminate the appendix as a source of abdominal pain in the future. However, this continues to be controversial, and each patient should be evaluated individually for risk from surgery versus leaving the appendix in situ.

Stricturing disease. Intestinal obstruction is the most common indication for surgical therapy in patients with Crohn disease. Obstruction in these patients is often partial, and nonoperative management is initially indicated. The success of nonoperative management can often be predicted on the basis of the chronicity of symptoms at the affected site. In patients for whom it is difficult to determine whether the site of obstruction is caused by an acute exacerbation or a chronically strictured segment, stool lactoferrin and calprotectin levels may help identify acute inflammation, whereas certain genetic markers (e.g., *NOD2, TLR4, CX3CR1*) may predict potential success of medical therapy. In the case of a chronically strictured segment, medical therapy is rarely effective. Operative intervention is required for patients with complete obstruction and partial obstruction whose condition does not resolve with nonoperative management. The treatment of choice for intestinal obstruction in patients with Crohn disease is segmental resection of the involved segment with primary anastomosis. This may involve segmental resection and primary anastomosis of a short segment of ileum or an ileocecectomy if both the ileum and cecum are involved (Fig. 91.9A).

In selected patients with obstruction caused by strictures (single or multiple), one option is to perform a strictureplasty that effectively widens the lumen but avoids intestinal resection. Strictureplasty is performed by making a longitudinal incision through the narrowed area of the intestine, followed by closure in a transverse fashion, termed a *Heineke-Mikulicz strictureplasty*

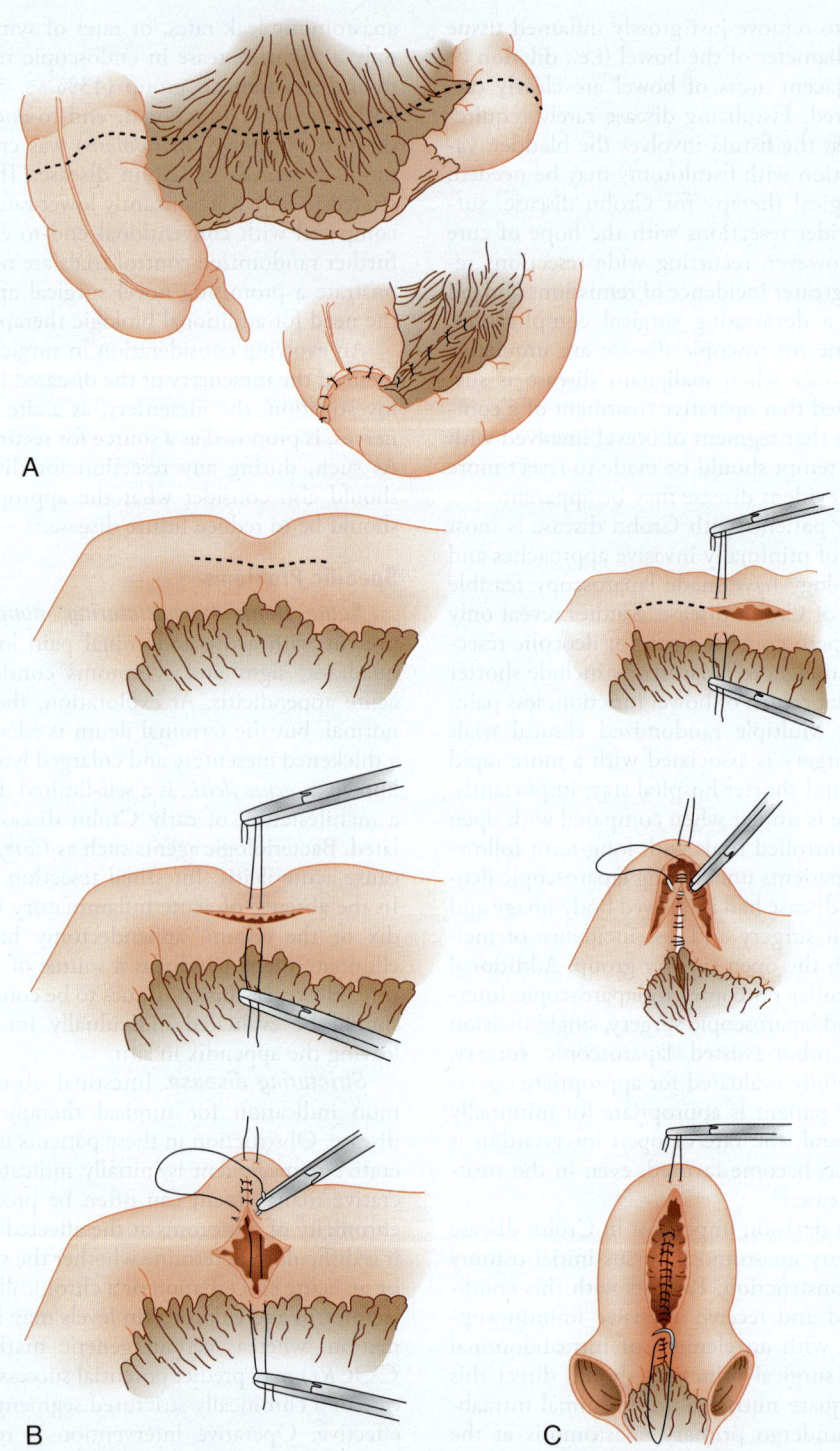

FIGURE 91.9 (A) Ileocecal resection secondary to Crohn disease. Resection of the ileum, ileocecal valve, cecum, and ascending colon for Crohn disease of the ileum. Intestinal continuity is restored by end-to-end anastomosis. (B) Technique of short strictureplasty in the manner of a Heineke-Mikulicz pyloroplasty. (C) For longer diseased segments, strictureplasty may be performed in a manner similar to Finney pyloroplasty. (Adapted from Alexander-Williams J, Haynes IG. Up-to-date management of small-bowel Crohn's disease. In: Mannick JA, ed. *Advances in Surgery*. St. Louis: Mosby; 1987:245-264.)

(see Fig. 91.9B). For longer diseased segments (10–25 cm), a Finney strictureplasty can be performed, which involves folding the diseased segment on itself and creating a common channel of the strictured segment. For longer strictures, the Michelassi strictureplasty can be performed, which involves creating a side-to-side

isoperistaltic strictureplasty (see Fig. 91.9C).[25] Strictureplasty is best used in patients with multiple short areas of narrowing present over long segments of intestine, in those who have already had several previous resections of the small intestine, and in patients with chronic fibrous obstruction. This procedure preserves intestine and is associated with complication and recurrence rates comparable to those of resection and anastomosis. Given the concerns for development of carcinoma at chronically strictured segments, full-thickness biopsy with a frozen section of the stricture site has been advocated at the time of surgery to rule out malignant disease before strictureplasty is performed (Box 91.5).

In the past, bypass procedures were commonly used. There are two types of bypass operations: exclusion bypass and simple (continuity) bypass. For certain types of ileocecal disease associated with an abscess or phlegmon densely adherent to the retroperitoneum, the proximal transected end of the ileum is anastomosed to the transverse colon in an end-to-side fashion, with or without construction of a mucous fistula, using the distal transected end of the ileum (exclusion bypass), or an ileotransverse colonic anastomosis is made in a side-to-side fashion (continuity bypass). Currently, bypass with exclusion is most useful for patients with severe gastroduodenal Crohn disease that is not amenable to strictureplasty. Rarely, but remaining a consideration, bypass can be used in older, poor-risk patients; patients who have had several prior resections and cannot afford to lose any more bowel; and those in whom resection would necessitate entering an abscess or endangering a normal structure.

Penetrating disease. Fistula and abscess in patients with Crohn disease are relatively common and usually involve adjacent small bowel, colon, or other surrounding viscera (e.g., bladder). The presence of a radiographically demonstrable enteroenteric fistula with no signs of sepsis or other complications is not in itself an indication for surgery. Furthermore, penetrating disease is particularly sensitive to anticytokine therapy, and a conservative, surgical approach to Crohn disease–related fistula is most appropriate.[26] Enterocutaneous fistulas may develop but are rarely spontaneous and are more likely to follow resection or drainage of intraabdominal abscesses. These fistulas may close spontaneously, and treatment should entail outflow reduction, preventing infection and maximizing nutrition and optimal skin care. If conservative management fails, excision of the fistula tract and primary anastomosis is preferred. Note that preoperative optimization is necessary, as patients with penetrating disease tend to have longer operative times, higher reoperation rates, increased length of stay, and postoperative complications. If the fistula forms between two or more adjacent loops of diseased bowel, the involved segments should be excised. Alternatively, if the fistula involves an adjacent normal organ, such as the bladder or colon, only the segment of the diseased small bowel and fistulous tract should be resected, and the defect in the normal organ should simply be closed. Most patients with ileosigmoid fistulas do not necessarily require resection of the sigmoid because the disease is usually confined to the

small bowel. However, if the segment of sigmoid is also found to have Crohn disease, it should be resected along with the segment of diseased small bowel. All patients presenting with more aggressive disease characterized with fistulas and/or abscesses should have treatment tailored and individualized to the patient.

Perforation. Penetrating disease in the form of free perforation into the peritoneal cavity is uncommon in patients with Crohn disease. Typically, penetration manifests with a localized abscess densely adherent to the diseased segment of bowel. Patients with small abscesses (typically less than 3 cm) who are hemodynamically stable and have not been on biologics or have an associated fistula can be treated with antibiotics alone. Abscesses that do not meet these criteria should undergo percutaneous drainage. In fact, early treatment of an abscess is key regardless of percutaneous or surgical drainage in terms of time to resolution. In cases of free perforation, the segment of involved bowel should be resected, and in the presence of minimal contamination, a primary anastomosis can be performed. If generalized peritonitis is present, a safer option may be to create an ostomy until the intraabdominal sepsis is controlled and then have the patient return for restoration of intestinal continuity after a period of 4 to 6 weeks. Abscesses can be treated with percutaneous drainage and antibiotics; however, fistula or uncontrolled sepsis may develop, requiring resection with or without primary anastomosis.

Gastrointestinal bleeding. Although anemia from chronic blood loss is common in patients with Crohn disease, life-threatening gastrointestinal hemorrhage is rare. The incidence of hemorrhage is more common in patients with Crohn disease involving the distal colon rather than the small bowel. As with the other complications, the segment involved should be resected and intestinal continuity restored. In hemodynamically unstable hemorrhage, colectomy with end ileostomy is appropriate. Arteriography may be useful to localize the bleeding before surgery. In cases of bleeding associated with duodenal disease, endoscopic intervention is usually successful. However, in cases of failure, duodenotomy with oversewing of the bleeding ulcerative area is indicated. However, there remains a scarcity of data on the appropriate management of gastroduodenal disease, as medically refractory disease can progress to cancer.[22]

Urologic complications. Genitourinary complications occur in up to one-third of patients with Crohn disease. Such complications include ureteral obstruction and recurrent urinary tract infections (enterovesical fistulas). Ureteral obstruction is usually secondary to ileocolic disease with retroperitoneal inflammatory compression. Surgical treatment of the primary intestinal disease is adequate in most patients. In a few cases of long-standing inflammatory disease, periureteric fibrosis may be present and require ureterolysis with or without ureteral stenting.

Cancer. Patients with long-standing Crohn disease of the small bowel and, in particular, the colon have an increased incidence of cancer. The management of these patients is the same as that for any patient—resection of the cancer with appropriate margins, lymphadenectomy, and perioperative chemotherapy/radiation. Patients with cancer associated with Crohn disease commonly have a worse prognosis than those who do not have Crohn disease, largely because the diagnosis in these patients is often delayed. In addition, a strictureplasty should not be performed if malignant disease is suspected.

Colorectal disease. The same principle applies to patients with Crohn disease limited to the colon as to those with disease to the small bowel; that is, surgical resection should be limited to the main segment involved. Indications for surgery include a lack of response to medical management and complications of Crohn colitis, which include obstruction, hemorrhage, perforation, and toxic megacolon. Depending on the diseased segments, procedures commonly include segmental colectomy with colocolonic anastomosis; total abdominal colectomy with ileorectal anastomosis; total proctocolectomy with ileoanal anastomosis; and in patients with extensive perianal and rectal disease, abdominoperineal resection with end ileostomy. In the case of acute illness, temporizing colectomy with end ileostomy is a consideration. Strictureplasty has limited usefulness in colonic Crohn disease, and concerns of malignant transformation at an area of colonic obstruction should limit its application.

A particularly troubling problem after abdominoperineal resection in patients with Crohn disease is delayed healing of the perineal wound. More than half of perineal wounds are open 6 months after surgery in these patients. Persistent nonhealing wounds require excision with secondary closure. Large cavities or sinuses may be filled by using well-vascularized pedicles of muscle (e.g., gracilis, semimembranosus, rectus abdominis) or omentum or by using an inferior gluteal myocutaneous graft.

Although controversial, continence-preserving operations, such as ileal pouch–anal anastomosis or continent ileostomies (Kock pouch), may be considered in very carefully selected patients with Crohn disease isolated to the colon who undergo thorough counseling about the increased risk of anastomotic failure and wound complication. However, these procedures should never be considered in patients with evidence of terminal ileal or perianal disease, as these patients have a significantly increased rate of recurrence of Crohn disease in the pouch, fistulas to the anastomosis, and peripouch abscesses.

Perianal disease. Diseases involving the perianal region include fissures and fistulas and are common in patients with Crohn disease, particularly those with colonic involvement. The treatment of perianal disease should be nonoperative unless an abscess or complex fistula develops, and even in these cases, surgery should be approached cautiously and limited to addressing the specific problem with minimal tissue loss. Nonsuppurative, chronic fistulization or perianal fissuring is treated with antibiotics, immunosuppressive agents (e.g., AZT or 6-MP), and anti-TNF therapy, which is the most widely supported therapy as it has shown the best results in fistula closure. Additionally, there is some evidence to support the use of cyclosporine, FK-506, or IL-12/23 inhibition treatment for fistula management.[16]

Wide excision of abscesses or fistulas is not indicated, but more conservative interventions, including the liberal placement of drainage catheters and noncutting Setons, are preferable. Definitive fistulotomy is indicated for most patients with superficial, low transsphincteric, and low intersphincteric fistulas, although one must recognize that some degree of anal stenosis may occur as a result of chronic inflammation. High transsphincteric, suprasphincteric, and extrasphincteric fistulas are usually treated with noncutting Setons. Fissures are usually lateral, relatively painless, large, and indolent and often respond to conservative management. Abscesses should be drained, but large excisions of tissue *should not* be performed. Advancement flap closure of perineal fistulas may be required in certain cases. Selective construction of diverting stomas has good results in combination with optimal medical therapy to induce remission of inflammation. Proctectomy is infrequent but required in a subset of patients who have persistent and unremitting disease despite conservative medical and surgical therapy.

Duodenal disease. Crohn disease of the duodenum occurs in less than 5% of patients and occurs most commonly in the duodenal bulb. Operative intervention is uncommon. The primary indication for surgery in these patients is duodenal obstruction that does not respond to medical therapy, with endoscopic balloon dilation and surgery being the mainstays of treatment. Antrectomy with Roux-en-Y bypass and laparoscopic bypass with gastrojejunostomy without resection are surgical options. Strictureplasties for short segments have been performed with success in selected patients and may avoid the marginal ulceration and diarrhea associated with gastrojejunostomy. For disease refractory to medical management, surgical resection should be considered, as the disease can progress to dysplasia and cancer.[22]

Prognosis

Crohn disease is a chronic inflammatory disorder that is not medically or surgically curable; therefore, therapeutic approaches are required to induce and to maintain symptomatic control, to improve quality of life, and to minimize long-term complications. Thanks to improvements in medical management, surgery in these patients is decreasing; however, over half will require at least one operation in their lifetime.[27] Symptomatic recurrence varies from 40% to 80%. Endoscopic recurrence is an effective temporizing procedure; however, eventual recurrence requiring surgical intervention is inevitable. The only clearly modifiable risk factor is smoking cessation. Surgery is generally indicated when the patient fails to respond to medical therapy or develops complications, and multiple studies have shown that patients report significant improvement in quality-of-life scores after surgical intervention. Although postsurgical recurrence is high, algorithms using careful endoscopic surveillance combined with maintenance immunomodulators, anti-TNF antibodies, antiintegrin therapy, and even investigational traditional Chinese medicine all play a role in the prevention of postoperative recurrence of Crohn disease. Although there is currently no cure, advances in medical and surgical therapies have clearly increased quality of life and disease-free progression.

Long-term survival studies suggest that patients with Crohn disease have a death rate approximately two to three times higher than that of the general population. Mortality has been associated with cardiovascular disease, wound complications, sepsis, cancer, thromboembolic complications, and electrolyte disorders.

Typhoid Enteritis

Typhoid fever remains a significant problem in developing countries, most commonly in areas with contaminated water supplies and inadequate waste disposal. Roughly 9 million people worldwide develop typhoid fever, with an estimated 110,000 deaths per year. Children and young adults are most often affected. Improvements in sanitation have decreased the incidence of typhoid fever in industrialized countries. Most cases of typhoid fever in the United States arise in international travelers; however, unrecognized and untreated typhoid fever is a life-threatening illness with significant long-term morbidity.

Typhoid enteritis is an acute systemic infection caused primarily by *Salmonella typhi*. The pathologic events of typhoid fever are initiated in the intestinal tract after oral ingestion of the typhoid bacillus. These organisms penetrate the small bowel mucosa, make their way rapidly to the lymphatics, and then spread systemically. Hyperplasia of the reticuloendothelial system, including lymph nodes, liver, and spleen, is characteristic of typhoid fever. Peyer patches in the small bowel become hyperplastic and may subsequently ulcerate, complicated by hemorrhage or perforation.

The diagnosis of typhoid fever is confirmed by isolating the organism from blood, bone marrow, and stool cultures. In addition, the finding of high titers of agglutinins against O and H antigens (Widal test) was used historically but is nonspecific and is no longer an acceptable clinical method. Assays for the diagnosis of *S. typhi* using PCR analysis are unpredictable and too costly for many endemic areas. Skin biopsies of active lesions, indirect enzyme-linked immunosorbent assay for IgM and IgG antibodies to *S. typhi* polysaccharide, and urine cultures can detect active or prior disease but are not typically used today. Using a combination of tests can achieve sensitivity and specificity as high as 83% and 100%, respectively.

Typhoid fever and uncomplicated typhoid enteritis are treated by antibiotic administration. If a patient presents with clinical symptoms and has been in an endemic area, broad-spectrum empirical antibiotics should be started immediately. Treatment should not be delayed for confirmatory tests because prompt treatment drastically reduces the risk of complications and fatalities. Antibiotic therapy should be narrowed once more information is available. Chloramphenicol was initially the mainstay of treatment in the 1950s, but widespread antibiotic resistance occurred. Currently, the most widely used agents are fluoroquinolones, mainly ciprofloxacin. Alternatively, amoxicillin, trimethoprim-sulfamethoxazole, and third-generation cephalosporins can be used. Vaccination against typhoid has decreased disease burden and is used in endemic areas.

Complications requiring potential surgical intervention include hemorrhage and perforation. The incidence of hemorrhage was reported to be as high as 20%, but with the availability of antibiotics, this figure has decreased. When hemorrhage occurs, transfusion is indicated and usually suffices. Rarely, laparotomy must be performed for uncontrollable, life-threatening hemorrhage. Intestinal perforation through an ulcerated Peyer patch occurs in approximately 2% of cases. Typically, it is a single perforation in the terminal ileum, and simple closure of the perforation is the treatment of choice. Multiple perforations, which occur in about 25% of patients, may require resection with primary anastomosis or exteriorization of the intestinal loop.

Enteritis in the Immunocompromised Host

The acquired immunodeficiency syndrome (AIDS) epidemic, as well as the widespread use of immunosuppressive agents after organ transplantation, has resulted in a number of rare and exotic pathogens infecting the gastrointestinal tract. Almost all patients with AIDS have gastrointestinal symptoms during their illness, the most common of which is diarrhea. A surgeon may be asked to evaluate the immunocompromised patient with abdominal pain, acute abdomen, or gastrointestinal bleeding; a number of protozoal, bacterial, viral, and fungal organisms may be responsible.

Protozoa

Protozoa (e.g., *Cryptosporidium, Isospora,* and *Microsporidium*) are the most frequent class of pathogens causing diarrhea in patients with AIDS. The small bowel is the most common site of infection. Diagnosis may be established by acid-fast staining of the stool or duodenal secretions, and the introduction of specific antigen tests for stool examination has improved diagnostic capabilities. Immunochromatography cards for the rapid detection of protozoal proteins from a small sample of stool are available from several different commercial sources and are more sensitive and specific (>90%) than traditional microscopic examinations.

Symptoms are most commonly related to diarrhea, which may be intractable at times. Current treatment regimens in immunocompromised patients have not been entirely effective, but drugs such as prophylactic cotrimoxazole and a highly active antiretroviral therapy appear to elicit a response to human immunodeficiency virus (HIV)–related diarrheal illnesses.

Bacteria

Infections by enteric bacteria are more frequent and more virulent in individuals infected with HIV than in healthy hosts. *Salmonella, Shigella,* and *Campylobacter* are associated with higher rates of bacteremia and antibiotic resistance in the immunocompromised patient. The diagnosis of *Shigella* or *Salmonella* infection may be established by stool cultures. The diagnosis of *Campylobacter* infection is not as easily established because stool cultures are often negative, but PCR techniques evaluating stool and serum have shown promising diagnostic results in patients with negative cultures. These enteric infections are manifested clinically with high fever, abdominal pain, and diarrhea that may be bloody. Abdominal pain may mimic an acute abdomen. Bacteremia and serious infections should be treated by IV administration of antibiotics. Antibiotic resistance has been growing in *Campylobacter* strains, but most commonly can be treated with ciprofloxacin or erythromycin.

Diarrhea caused by *C. difficile* is more common in patients with AIDS because of the increased antibiotic use in this population compared with healthy hosts. Diagnosis is by standard assays of stool for *C. difficile* enterotoxin. Treatment with metronidazole or vancomycin is usually effective.

Mycobacteria

Mycobacterial infection is a frequent cause of intestinal disease in immunocompromised hosts. This can be secondary to *Mycobacterium tuberculosis* or *Mycobacterium avium complex* (MAC), which is an atypical mycobacterium related to the type that causes cervical adenitis (scrofula). The usual route of infection is by swallowed organisms that directly penetrate the intestinal mucosa. The luminal gastrointestinal tract is affected by MAC infection, with massive thickening of the proximal small intestine often noted. Clinically, patients with MAC present with diarrhea, fever, anorexia, and progressive wasting.

The most frequent site of intestinal involvement of *M. tuberculosis* is the distal ileum and cecum, with approximately 90% of patients demonstrating disease at this site. The gross appearance can be ulcerative, hypertrophic, or ulcerohypertrophic. The bowel wall appears thickened, and an inflammatory mass often surrounds the ileocecal region. Acute inflammation is apparent, as are strictures and even fistula formation. The serosal surface is normally covered with multiple tubercles, and mesenteric lymph nodes are frequently enlarged and thickened; on sectioning, caseous necrosis is noted. The mucosa is hyperemic, edematous, and, in some cases, ulcerated. On histologic evaluation, the distinguishing lesion is a granuloma, with caseating granulomas found most commonly in the lymph nodes. Most patients complain of chronic abdominal pain that may be nonspecific, weight loss, fever, and diarrhea.

The diagnosis of mycobacterial infection is made by identification of the organism in tissue by direct visualization with an acid-fast stain, culture of the excised tissue, or PCR assay. Radiographic examinations usually reveal a thickened mucosa with distorted mucosal folds and ulcerations. CT may be useful and shows a thickening of the ileocecal valve and cecum.

The treatment of *M. tuberculosis* is similar in the immunocompromised or nonimmunocompromised host. The organism is usually responsive to multidrug antimicrobial therapy. The therapy for MAC infection is evolving; drugs that have been successfully used in vivo and in vitro include amikacin, ciprofloxacin, cycloserine, and ethionamide. Clarithromycin has also been successfully used in combination with other agents. Surgical intervention may be required for intestinal tuberculosis, particularly *M. tuberculosis*. Obstruction and fistula formation are the leading indications for surgery; however, with current treatment, most fistulas now respond to medical management. Surgery may be necessary for ulcerative complications when free perforation, perforation with abscess, or massive hemorrhage occurs. The treatment is usually resection with anastomosis.

Viruses

CMV is the most common viral cause of diarrhea in immunocompromised patients. Clinical manifestations include intermittent diarrhea accompanied by fever, weight loss, and abdominal pain. The manifestations of enteric CMV infection result from mucosal ischemic ulcerations, which account for the high rate of perforations noted with CMV. As a result of the diffuse ulcerating involvement of the intestine, patients may present with abdominal pain, peritonitis, or hematochezia. Diagnosis of CMV is made by demonstrating viral inclusions. The most characteristic form is an intranuclear inclusion, which is often surrounded by a halo, producing a so-called *owl's eye appearance*. There may also be cytoplasmic inclusions. Cultures for CMV are usually positive when inclusion bodies are present, but these cultures are less sensitive and specific than histopathologic identification. Once CMV infection is diagnosed, treatment is usually effective with ganciclovir. An alternative to ganciclovir is foscarnet, a pyrophosphate analogue that inhibits viral replication. Infections with other less common viruses, including adenovirus, rotavirus, and novel enteric viruses such as astrovirus and picornavirus, have been reported.

Fungi

Fungal infections of the intestinal tract have been recognized in patients with AIDS. Gastrointestinal histoplasmosis occurs in the setting of systemic infection, often in association with pulmonary and hepatic disease. Diagnosis is made by fungal smear and culture of infected tissue or blood. The infection is most commonly treated by the administration of amphotericin B followed by itraconazole. Coccidioidomycosis of the intestinal tract is rare and, like histoplasmosis, occurs in the context of systemic infection.

NEOPLASMS

General Considerations

Despite composing 75% of the length and 90% of the surface area of the gastrointestinal tract, the small bowel develops relatively few primary neoplasms and less than 3% of gastrointestinal malignant neoplasms. Small bowel cancers encompass around 40 different disease entities, with an ever-increasing incidence comprising both malignant (i.e., adenocarcinoma) and benign (i.e., stromal tumors, adenomas) entities. In general, most benign lesions go undiagnosed in a lifetime and are only detected at autopsy, whereas most symptomatic lesions are of a malignant origin. Distribution, epidemiologic risk factors, and survival all depend on the type of small bowel cancer.[28]

The risk factors and associated conditions related to small bowel neoplasms have been described. These include patients with familial adenomatous polyposis (FAP), juvenile polyposis syndrome, hereditary nonpolyposis colorectal cancer, Peutz-Jeghers syndrome, Crohn disease, gluten-sensitive enteropathy (i.e., celiac sprue), prior peptic ulcer disease, cystic fibrosis, and biliary diversion (i.e., previous cholecystectomy). Controversial factors that may contribute to small bowel neoplasms include smoking, heavy alcohol consumption (>80 g/day of ethanol), and consumption of red meat or salt-cured foods.

Although the molecular genetics of small bowel neoplasms have not been entirely characterized, similar to colorectal cancers, mutations of the *KRAS* gene are commonly identified. Allelic losses, particularly involving tumor suppressor genes at chromosome locations 5q (*APC* gene), 17q (*p53* gene), and 18q (*DCC* [deleted in colon cancer] and *DPC4* [*SMAD4*] genes), have been noted in some small bowel cancers. Approximately 15% of small intestinal adenocarcinomas have an inactivated DNA mismatch gene repair and display a high level of microsatellite instability (MSI-H). Interestingly, MSI-H is typical of small bowel carcinomas associated with celiac disease, which is potentially linked by an aberrant CpG island methylation. Other genetic mutations of clinical interest include human epidermal growth factor receptor 2 (HER2) and programmed cell death ligand 1 (PD-L1). Microarray analyses demonstrate a high percentage of small bowel tumors expressing both epidermal growth factor receptor and vascular endothelial growth factor (VEGF), which may contribute to carcinogenesis.

Clinical Manifestations

Symptoms associated with small bowel neoplasms are often vague and nonspecific and may include dyspepsia, anorexia, malaise, and dull abdominal pain, often intermittent and colicky. These symptoms may be present for months or years before diagnosis. Most patients with benign neoplasms remain asymptomatic, and the neoplasms are only discovered at autopsy or as incidental findings at laparotomy or upper gastrointestinal radiologic studies. Of the remainder, pain, obstruction, and bleeding are the most frequent complaints. Usually, obstruction is the result of intussusception, and benign, small tumors are the most common cause of this condition in adults. Bleeding is usually occult; hematochezia or hematemesis may occur, although life-threatening hemorrhage is uncommon.

Diagnosis

Because of the insidious nature of many small bowel neoplasms, a high index of suspicion must be present for these neoplasms to be diagnosed. In most series, a correct preoperative diagnosis is made in only 50% of symptomatic patients. Plain films may show dilated loops of small bowel suspicious for an obstruction; however, for the most part, plain films are not helpful in making a diagnosis of small bowel neoplasms. An upper gastrointestinal tract series with small bowel follow-through can sometimes yield an accurate diagnosis with malignant neoplasms of the small intestine but is not as accurate or specific as more advanced imaging modalities. Small bowel capsule endoscopy has a negative predictive value of 90%, but it can fail to detect more proximal tumors. Ultrasonography has not proved effective for preoperative diagnosis of small bowel neoplasms. CT of the abdomen can prove particularly useful in detecting extraluminal tumors, such as malignant gastrointestinal stromal tumors (GISTs), and can provide helpful information about the staging of malignant cancers

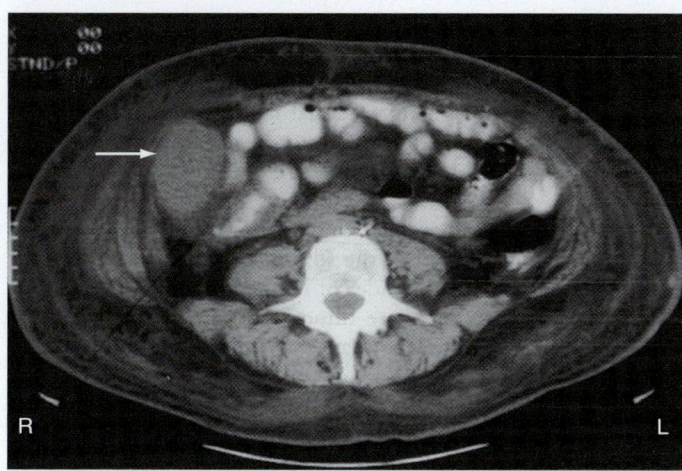

FIGURE 91.10 Small bowel neoplasm. CT scan of abdomen demonstrates a small bowel neoplasm *(arrow)*. (Courtesy Dr. Melvyn H. Schreiber, The University of Texas Medical Branch, Galveston, TX.)

(Fig. 91.10). CTE appears to be a more sensitive technique, with sensitivity of 90% and positive predictive value of 98%, whereas MRE has a sensitivity and specificity of 98% and 97%, respectively.

Flexible endoscopy may be useful, particularly in diagnosing duodenal lesions, and the colonoscope can be advanced into the terminal ileum for visualization and biopsy of ileal neoplasms. Push enteroscopy has not been used routinely to evaluate lesions in the small bowel because this test may take up to 8 hours to perform and may not visualize the entire small bowel. Double-balloon enteroscopy can be a helpful adjunct; however, it should be reserved for cases in which biopsy or preoperative tattoo is required, as it carries a risk of perforation, and for cases where less invasive and more accurate diagnostic tools are unavailable. Angiography is of value in diagnosing and localizing tumors of vascular origin. Despite these sophisticated imaging and diagnostic modalities, diagnosis of a small bowel tumor is often achieved only at the time of surgical exploration.

Benign Neoplasms

The most common benign neoplasms include benign stromal tumors, adenomas, and lipomas. In general, when a benign tumor is identified at operation, resection is indicated because symptoms are likely to develop over time. At operation, a thorough search of the remainder of the small bowel is warranted because multiple tumors are not uncommon.

Stromal Tumors

GISTs are most prevalent in the stomach (60%) and jejunum and ileum (30%) and rarely in duodenum (5%). Stromal tumors arise from the interstitial cell of Cajal, an intestinal pacemaker cell of mesodermal descent. The median age of diagnosis is 65 years of age, with slight male predominance. GISTs can be very large, with a median size of 6 cm at diagnosis; some GISTs can even be larger than 20 cm. With the advances in noninvasive imaging technology, many GISTs are being identified earlier, when they are small and asymptomatic. GISTs can be malignant tumors, and nearly 20% of patients are found to have metastatic disease, most commonly in the liver. Symptoms of GIST include abdominal pain, fullness, bowel obstruction, or tumor hemorrhage resulting in anemia, melena, or hematemesis. The workup of GIST is often

initiated with a CT scan. MRI may provide more information for tumors in the rectum, duodenum, and liver metastases. After identification on imaging, CT-guided or endoscopic core-needle biopsy can be used to obtain tissue. Tissue samples undergo immunohistochemical staining for KIT, which is positive in 95% of GISTs. DOG-1 (anoctamin-1) is positive in approximately 88% of GISTs.[29] More than 95% of stromal tumors express CD117, the KIT proto-oncogene protein that is a transmembrane receptor for the stem cell growth factor, and 70% to 90% express CD34, the human progenitor cell antigen. These tumors infrequently stain positive for actin (20%–30%), S100 (2%–4%), and desmin (2%–4%). In gross appearance, stromal tumors are firm, gray-white lesions with a whorled appearance noted on cut surface; microscopic examination demonstrates well-differentiated smooth muscle cells. These tumors may grow intramurally and cause obstruction. Alternatively, the tumors demonstrate intramural and extramural growth, sometimes achieving considerable size and eventually outgrowing their blood supply, resulting in bleeding manifestations.

Surgical resection is necessary for appropriate treatment. GIST malignancy risk and prognosis are stratified based on the number of mitoses per high-power field (hpf) and tumor size. The mitotic index is classified as low (<5 mitoses/50 hpf) or high (>5 mitoses/50 hpf). Although benign tumors generally show a low mitotic index (<5 mitoses/50 hpf), the size of the tumor also must be considered. Tumors larger than 5 cm, regardless of mitotic index, have higher rates of metastasis and recurrence, whereas those with a high mitotic index have a higher risk of metastasis and recurrence regardless of size. Higher-risk GIST lesions may require adjuvant therapy after resection.

Adenomas

Adenomas account for approximately 15% of all benign small bowel tumors and are of three primary types: tubular adenomas, villous adenomas, and Brunner gland adenomas. The majority of adenomas are found in the duodenum near the ampulla of Vater. Most of these lesions are asymptomatic; most occur singly and are found incidentally at autopsy. When symptoms do occur, they are most commonly bleeding and obstruction. Both true and villous adenomas have malignant potential, but villous adenomas have a particular propensity for malignant degeneration and may be relatively large (>3 cm) in diameter.[30] Treatment is determined by location and adenoma type. The majority are able to be removed endoscopically, with piecemeal resection emerging as a viable option. If endoscopic resection is not possible, segmental resection is indicated. Endoscopic resection is heavily favored for duodenal lesions given the potential morbidity (about 40%) associated with duodenal resection by pancreaticoduodenectomy or pancreas-preserving duodenectomy. However, invasive changes or a recurrence after polypectomy necessitates a more definitive approach (e.g., pancreaticoduodenectomy). Endoscopic ultrasound is a useful modality in the preintervention evaluation and may help guide in therapeutic planning, particularly if there are malignant concerns. Duodenal adenomas are associated with colonic polyps, and colonoscopy is necessary for evaluation after detection of a duodenal adenoma.

Familial adenomas typically occur in the presence of FAP syndrome and require a different algorithm. Extracolonic manifestations of FAP have significant consequences. Numerous studies have shown that adenomas in the duodenum can be found in 50% to 90% of cases, and increasing age was identified as an independent risk factor for adenoma development. Although these neoplasms grow slowly, patients with FAP carry a 5% lifetime risk for development of duodenal adenocarcinoma, which represents the leading cause of cancer-related mortality in these patients; therefore, routine lifelong surveillance is a priority. To direct surveillance and treatment, patients are classified by the Spigelman classification (Table 91.8). Screening endoscopy with a forward- and side-viewing endoscope is performed at regular intervals with biopsy of all suspicious, villous, or large (>3 cm) adenomas. The frequency of endoscopic screening ranges from 1 to 5 years, depending on the Spigelman classification (Box 91.6). Random sampling of the duodenum was previously recommended, but now duodenal/ampullary surveillance with lesion management is based on endoscopic findings; however, different guidelines have different recommendations, with optimal surveillance still under investigation.[31] Endoscopic mucosal resection and cold snaring are typically used to remove polyps, with surgical polypectomy as a valid alternative should the lesions not be amenable to endoscopic intervention. Ablative therapy in the form of argon beam coagulation or photodynamic therapy has been attempted for these patients but is not widely used because of suboptimal results. The presence of high-grade dysplasia, invasive cancer, or a Spigelman stage IV classification should be considered for pancreaticoduodenectomy or pancreas-preserving duodenectomy. Adenomas of the remaining small bowel also occur more frequently in patients with FAP but are not as prevalent as duodenal disease in this population of patients.

Brunner gland adenomas represent benign hyperplastic lesions arising from the Brunner glands of the proximal duodenum. These adenomas may produce symptoms mimicking those of peptic ulcer disease. Diagnosis can usually be accomplished by endoscopy and biopsy, and symptomatic lesions in an accessible region can be resected by simple excision, preferably endoscopic, with surgery reserved for those not amenable to endoscopic resection. There is no malignant potential for Brunner gland adenomas, and a radical resection should not be used.

Lipomas

Lipomas are most common in the ileum and manifest as single intramural lesions located in the submucosa. They usually occur in the sixth and seventh decades of life and are more frequent in males. Less than half of these tumors are symptomatic and are often found incidentally. They can grow to be large and manifest as obstruction and bleeding from superficial ulcerations. The treatment of choice for symptomatic lesions is excision. Lipomas do not have malignant potential and, therefore, if found incidentally, should be removed only if the resection is simple.

Peutz-Jeghers Syndrome

Hamartomas of the small bowel occur as part of Peutz-Jeghers syndrome, an inherited syndrome of mucocutaneous melanotic pigmentation and gastrointestinal polyps. The pattern of inheritance is autosomal dominant, with a high degree of penetrance. The classic pigmented lesions are small, 1 to 5 mm, as brown or black spots located in the circumoral region of the face, buccal mucosa, forearms, palms, soles, digits, and perianal area. Hamartomas are most commonly found in the jejunum and ileum. However, 50% of patients may also have rectal and colonic lesions, and 25% of patients have gastric lesions. The most common symptom is recurrent colicky abdominal pain, usually the result of intermittent intussusception. Lower abdominal pain associated with a palpable mass has been reported in one-third of patients. Hemorrhage as a result of autoamputation of the polyps occurs, but infrequently, and is most commonly manifested by anemia. Acute life-threatening hemorrhage is uncommon but may occur. Although once considered a purely benign disease, adenomatous changes have been reported in 3% to 6% of hamartomas. Extracolonic cancers are common, occurring in 50% to 90% of patients (small intestine, stomach, pancreas, ovary, lung, uterus, and breast). The most frequent site for cancer is the colon and rectum. The treatment for complications of Peutz-Jeghers syndrome is directed at bowel obstruction or persistent gastrointestinal bleeding. Resection should be limited to the segment of bowel that is producing complications. Because of the widespread nature of intestinal involvement, cure is not possible; therefore, extensive resection is not indicated.

TABLE 91.8   Spigelman Classification for Duodenal Adenomatosis

PARAMETER	POINTS		
	1	2	3
No. of polyps	1–4	5–20	>20
Polyp size (mm)	1–4	5–10	>10
Histology	Tubular	Tubulovillous	Villous
Degree of dysplasia	Mild	Moderate	Severe

Stage 0, 0 points; stage I, 1–4 points; stage II, 5–6 points; stage III, 7–8 points; stage IV, 9–12 points.
From Johnson MD, Mackey R, Brown N, et al. Outcome based on management for duodenal adenomas: sporadic versus familial disease. *J Gastrointest Surg.* 2010;14:229.

BOX 91.6   Recommended Surveillance Interval for Upper Gastrointestinal Endoscopic Examination in Relation to Spigelman Classification

Spigelman Classification (Surveillance Interval in Years)
0 (4–5 years)
I (3–5 years)
II (2–3 years)
III (0.1–1 year)
IV (consider surgery)

Adapted from Campos FG, Sulbaran M, Safatle-Ribeiro AV, Martinez CA. Duodenal adenoma surveillance in patients with familial adenomatous polyposis. *World J Gastrointest Endosc.* 2015;7:950-959.

Hemangiomas

Hemangiomas are developmental malformations consisting of submucosal proliferation of blood vessels. They can occur at any level of the gastrointestinal tract; the jejunum is the most commonly affected small bowel segment. Hemangiomas account for 3% to 4% of all benign tumors of the small bowel and are multifocal in 60% of patients. In addition, hemangiomas of the small bowel may occur as part of an inherited disorder known as Osler-Weber-Rendu disease. Hemangiomas may also occur in the lung, liver, and mucous membranes. Patients with Turner syndrome are likely also to have cavernous hemangiomas of the intestine. The most common symptom of small bowel hemangiomas is intestinal bleeding. Angiography and technetium-99m (Tc-99m) red blood cell scanning are the most useful diagnostic studies. If a hemangioma is localized preoperatively, resection of the involved intestinal segment is warranted. Intraoperative transillumination and palpation may help to identify a nonlocalized hemangioma.

Malignant Neoplasms

Population-based analyses have shown that the incidence of malignant neoplasms of the small intestine have increased steadily during the past three decades. A large retrospective study evaluating the Surveillance, Epidemiology, and End Results (SEER) and Medicare database from 1976 to 2016 showed that small bowel carcinoma incidence has more than doubled.[32] This increase has mirrored the increase in diagnosis of small bowel neuroendocrine neoplasms (NENs), which have increased nearly fourfold (3.7–14.6 cases per million population) during the past four decades, whereas changes in the frequency of adenocarcinomas, stromal tumors, and lymphomas are less pronounced. Some theorize that the increase in detection is the result of advancements and increased use of cross-sectional imaging subsequently leading to increased detection of tumors that may have previously gone undiagnosed. Although the incidence of small bowel malignancies has increased, mortality rates have remained relatively stable, particularly for adenocarcinoma and neuroendocrine tumors (NETs).

In contrast to benign lesions, malignant neoplasms almost always produce symptoms, the most common of which are pain and weight loss. Obstruction develops in 15% to 35% of patients and, unlike the intussusception produced by benign lesions, is usually the result of tumor infiltration and adhesions. Diarrhea with tenesmus and passage of large amounts of mucus may occur. Gastrointestinal bleeding, manifested by anemia and guaiac-positive stools or occasionally by melena or hematochezia, occurs to varying degrees with malignant lesions and is more common with GISTs. A palpable mass may be felt in 10% to 20% of patients, and perforations develop in approximately 10%, usually secondary to lymphomas and sarcomas. Although presentation may be similar, each tumor type has a distinct biology that dictates management and prognosis.

Neuroendocrine Neoplasms

Intestinal NENs arise from enterochromaffin cells (Kulchitsky cells), which are considered neural crest cells situated at the base of the crypts of Lieberkühn. These cells are also known as *argentaffin cells* because of their staining by silver compounds. These tumors were first described by Lubarsch in 1888; in 1907, Oberndorfer coined the term *karzinoide* to indicate the carcinoma-like appearance and the presumed lack of malignant potential. However, the term *carcinoid* has become a misnomer, as all NENs have malignant potential. These tumors have been reported in a number of organs, including lungs, bronchi, and the gastrointestinal tract. Most patients with small bowel NENs are in their seventh decade of life, with a median age for gastroenteric NEN of 63 years. The classification of NENs is based predominately on tumor grade and differentiation. NENs are divided into NETs and neuroendocrine carcinomas (NECs). NETs may be benign or of the well-differentiated malignant type and are further subdivided into three groups—low-grade (grade 1, G1), intermediate-grade (grade 2, G2), or high-grade (grade 3, G3) tumors—based on the appearance, mitotic rates, behavior (invasion of other organs, angioinvasion), and Ki-67 proliferative index. On the other hand, NECs are all G3, poorly differentiated malignant tumors. The distinction between a G3 well-differentiated NET and a G3 poorly differentiated NEC can be difficult and may require additional pathologic confirmation or immunohistochemical staining.[33]

NENs are also categorized based on the embryologic site of origin and secretory product. These tumors may derive from the foregut (respiratory tract, thymus), midgut (jejunum, ileum and right colon, stomach, proximal duodenum), and hindgut (distal colon, rectum). Foregut NENs characteristically produce low levels of serotonin (5-hydroxytryptamine) but may secrete 5-hydroxytryptophan or adrenocorticotropic hormone. Midgut NENs are characterized by having high serotonin production. Hindgut NENs rarely produce serotonin but may produce other hormones, such as somatostatin and peptide YY. In adults, the gastrointestinal tract is one of the most common sites for NENs. In the small intestine, NENs are most frequently found within the last 2 feet of the ileum, but many patients have multifocal disease. NENs have a variable malignant potential and are composed of multipotential cells with the ability to secrete numerous humoral agents, the most prominent of which are serotonin and substance P (Table 91.9). In addition to these substances, NENs have been found to secrete corticotropin, histamine, dopamine, neurotensin, prostaglandins, kinins, gastrin, somatostatin, pancreatic polypeptide, calcitonin, and neuron-specific enolase.

The primary importance of NENs is the malignant potential of the tumors themselves. Additionally, carcinoid syndrome, secondary to serotonin or tachykinin production, is characterized by episodic attacks of cutaneous flushing, bronchospasm, diarrhea, and vasomotor collapse. Because of the liver's ability to metabolize these analytes, most patients who present with carcinoid syndrome have hepatic metastases, where the substances are secreted directly into the systemic vasculature, bypassing hepatic metabolism. Similarly, primary tumors that secrete directly into the venous system, bypassing the portal system (e.g., ovary, lung), give rise to carcinoid syndrome without metastasis.

Pathology. About 70% to 80% of NETs are asymptomatic and found incidentally at the time of surgery.[33] The malignant potential (ability to metastasize) is related to location, size, depth of invasion, and growth pattern. Only approximately 9% of appendiceal NENs metastasize, but about 80% to 90% of small bowel NENs are associated with liver metastasis. Similar to other malignancies, larger size is associated with a higher likelihood of metastatic disease.

In gross appearance, these tumors are small, firm, submucosal nodules that are usually yellow on the cut surface (see Fig. 91.11A).

TABLE 91.9 Secretory Products of Neuroendocrine Tumors[a]

AMINES	TACHYKININS	PEPTIDES	OTHER
5-HT	Kallikrein	Pancreatic polypeptide (40%)	Prostaglandins
5-HIAA (88%)	Substance P (32%)	Chromogranins (100%)	
5-HTP	Neuropeptide K (67%)	Neurotensin (19%)	
Histamine		HCG-α (28%)	
Dopamine		HCG-β	
		Motilin (14%)	

[a]Values in parentheses represent percentage frequency.
HCG, Human chorionic gonadotropin; *5-HIAA,* 5-hydroxyindoleacetic acid; *5-HT,* 5-hydroxytryptamine; *5-HTP,* 5-hydroxytryptophan.
Compiled with help of Zandee WT, Kamp K, van Adrichem RC, et al. Effect of hormone secretory syndromes on neuroendocrine tumor prognosis. *Endocr Relat Cancer.* 2017;24(7):R261-R274.

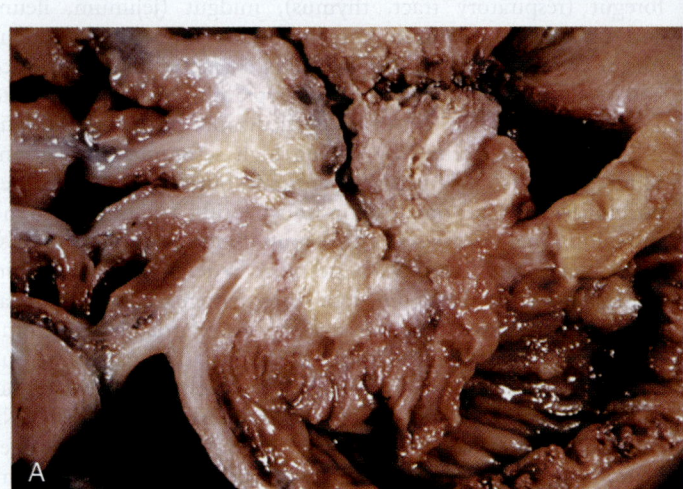

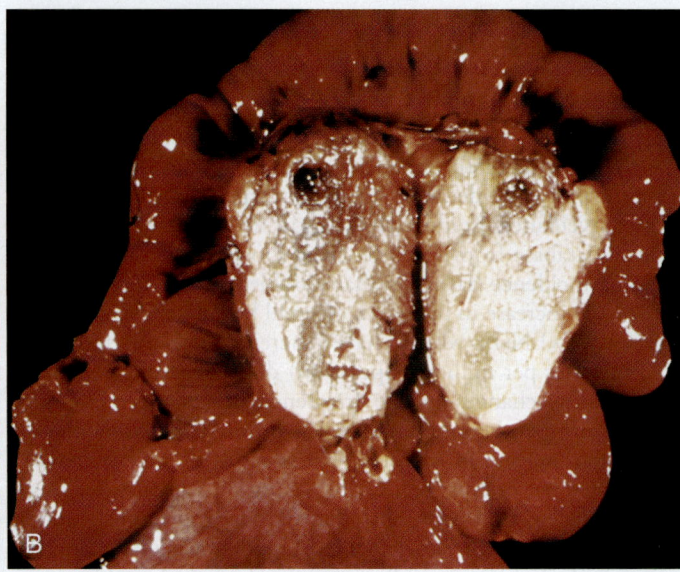

FIGURE 91.11 Gross pathologic characteristics of neuroendocrine tumor (NET). (A) NET of the distal ileum demonstrates the intense desmoplastic reaction and fibrosis of the bowel wall. (B) Mesenteric metastases from a NET of the small bowel. (Adapted from Evers BM, Townsend CM Jr, Thompson JC. Small intestine. In: Schwartz SI, ed. *Principles of Surgery.* 7th ed. New York: McGraw-Hill; 1999:1245.)

They may be as subtle as a small whitish plaque seen on the antimesenteric border of the small intestine (see Fig. 91.11B). Typically, they are associated with a larger mesenteric mass caused by nodal disease and desmoplastic invasion of the mesentery, which is often mistaken for the primary tumor. They tend to grow very slowly, but after invasion of the serosa, the intense desmoplastic reaction produces mesenteric fibrosis, intestinal kinking, and intermittent obstruction. Small bowel NENs are multicentric in 20% to 30% of patients. This tendency toward multicentricity exceeds that of any other malignant neoplasm of the gastrointestinal tract. Another unusual observation is the frequent coexistence of a second primary malignant neoplasm of a different histologic type. This is usually a synchronous adenocarcinoma (most commonly in the large intestine) that can occur in 10% to 20% of patients with NENs. Multiple endocrine neoplasia type 1 is associated with NENs in approximately 10% of cases.

Clinical manifestations. In the absence of carcinoid syndrome, symptoms of patients with NENs of the small bowel are similar to those of patients with small bowel tumors of other histologic types. The most common symptom is abdominal pain, which is variably associated with partial or complete small intestinal obstruction. Obstructive symptoms can be caused by intussusception but usually occur secondary to a local desmoplastic reaction, apparently produced by humoral agents elaborated by the tumor. Diarrhea and weight loss may also occur. The diarrhea is a result of a partial bowel obstruction rather than the secretory diarrhea noted in patients with malignant carcinoid syndrome. As mesenteric and nodal extension progresses, local venous engorgement and, ultimately, ischemia of the affected segment of intestine contribute to most symptoms and complications related to the tumor.

Malignant Carcinoid Syndrome

Malignant carcinoid syndrome is a relatively rare disease, occurring in less than 10% of patients with NENs. The syndrome is usually associated with NENs of the gastrointestinal tract, particularly from the small bowel, but NENs in other locations, such

as the bronchus, pancreas, ovary, and testes, have also been described in association with the syndrome. Because of the first-pass metabolism of the vasoactive peptides responsible for carcinoid syndrome, hepatic metastasis or extraabdominal disease is necessary to elicit the syndrome. The classic description of carcinoid syndrome includes vasomotor, cardiac, and gastrointestinal manifestations. A number of humoral factors are produced by NENs, but those considered to contribute to carcinoid syndrome include serotonin, 5-hydroxytryptophan (a precursor of serotonin synthesis), histamine, dopamine, tachykinin, kallikrein, substance P, prostaglandin, and neuropeptide K. Most patients who exhibit malignant carcinoid syndrome have massive hepatic replacement by metastatic disease. However, tumors that bypass the liver, specifically ovarian and retroperitoneal NETs, may produce the syndrome in the absence of liver metastasis.

Common symptoms and signs include cutaneous flushing (80%); diarrhea (76%); hepatomegaly (71%); cardiac lesions, most commonly right-sided heart valvular disease (41%–70%); and asthma (25%). Cutaneous flushing in carcinoid syndrome may be of four varieties:

1. Diffuse erythematous, which is short-lived and normally affects the face, neck, and upper chest
2. Violaceous, which is similar to a diffuse erythematous flush except that the attacks may be longer and patients may develop a permanent cyanotic flush, with watery eyes and injected conjunctivae
3. Prolonged flushes, which may last up to 2 or 3 days and involve the entire body and may be associated with profuse lacrimation, hypotension, and facial edema
4. Bright-red patchy flushing, typically seen with gastric NENs

The diarrhea associated with carcinoid syndrome is episodic (usually occurring after meals), watery, and often explosive. Increased circulating serotonin levels are thought to be the cause of the diarrhea because the serotonin antagonist methysergide effectively controls the symptom. Cardiac lesions usually involve the right side of the heart, but left-sided lesions are present in 15% of patients and can lead to congestive heart disease and symptomatic left-sided heart failure. The three most common cardiac lesions are pulmonary stenosis (90%), tricuspid insufficiency (47%), and tricuspid stenosis (42%). Asthmatic attacks are usually observed during the flushing symptom, and serotonin and bradykinin have been implicated in this. Malabsorption and pellagra (dementia, dermatitis, and diarrhea) are occasionally present and are thought to be caused by excessive diversion of dietary tryptophan.

Diagnosis. The elevation of various humoral factors forms the basis for diagnostic tests in patients with NENs and carcinoid syndrome. NENs produce serotonin, which is then metabolized in the liver and the lung to the pharmacologically inactive 5-hydroxyindoleacetic acid (5-HIAA). Elevated urinary levels of 5-HIAA measured during 24 hours with high-performance liquid chromatography are highly specific although not sensitive. For the last decade, chromogranin A (CgA) has been a well-established marker for carcinoid disease; it is elevated in more than 80% of patients with NENs. CgA alone may be used for the diagnosis of NENs, given its specificity of 95%, but some investigators suggest that other tests should be used in conjunction with CgA for diagnostic purposes because its sensitivity is as low as 60%. A combination of serum CgA measurement with 24-hour urine 5-HIAA is an acceptable diagnostic combination with increased sensitivity. Studies suggest that serum CgA and N-terminal pro-brain natriuretic peptide may also be used in combination for both diagnosis and surveillance because patients with increased N-terminal pro-brain natriuretic peptide and CgA levels show worse overall survival than patients with elevated CgA alone. In terms of surveillance after resection or as a prognostic marker to monitor response to therapy, CgA levels have proven efficacy over urine 5-HIAA levels.

Plasma serotonin, substance P, neurotensin, neurokinin A, and neuropeptide K levels can be measured, but these peptides may not be elevated in all patients. Provocative tests using pentagastrin, calcium, or epinephrine may be used to reproduce the symptoms of NENs. More recently, pentagastrin has been used to differentiate between NENs and chronic atrophic gastritis but is generally not used for the diagnosis of NENs, given the diagnostic reliability of 5-HIAA, CgA, and N-terminal pro-brain natriuretic peptide.

NENs of the small intestine are rarely diagnosed preoperatively. Barium radiographic studies of the small bowel may exhibit multiple filling defects as a result of kinking and fibrosis of the bowel but are not typically used today in the workup of suspected small intestinal NENs. A combination of anatomic and functional imaging techniques is routinely performed to optimize sensitivity and specificity.

Traditionally, CT scanning was the imaging modality of choice for identifying the site of disease and the presence of lymphatic or hematogenous metastases. CT scan findings depend on the size, the degree of mesenteric invasion and desmoplastic reaction, and the presence of regional lymph node invasion. If these entities are not well defined, CT has limited diagnostic capabilities in this disease. However, when CT scanning reveals a solid mass with spiculated borders and radiating surrounding strands that are associated with linear strands within the mesenteric fat and kinking of the bowel, a diagnosis of gastrointestinal NENs can be made fairly confidently. CT angiography may be useful in cases associated with a large mesenteric process to identify encasement and pseudoaneurysm formation, typical of a malignant process in the mesentery. In general, MRI is not used in the diagnosis of gastrointestinal NENs but can be helpful in diagnosing metastatic disease, especially in the liver. Liver metastases are well demonstrated with MRI and usually have low signal intensity on T1-weighted images and high signal intensity on T2-weighted images. After the administration of a gadolinium-based contrast agent, liver metastases enhance peripherally in the hepatic arterial phase and appear as hypointense defects in the portal venous phase. Diffusion-weighted MRI and dynamic contrast-enhanced techniques have become increasingly capable of detecting liver metastases from intestinal NENs.[34]

Octreotide is a synthetic analogue of somatostatin, and indium (^{111}In)-labeled pentetreotide specifically binds to somatostatin receptor subtypes 2 and 5. Functional nuclear imaging studies capitalize on the concept of somatostatin receptor positivity, and these techniques are used to image many NENs, including those with somatostatin-binding sites. Scintigraphic localization has a higher sensitivity than CT for delineating and localizing NENs and is particularly useful in the identification of extraabdominal metastatic disease or in cases in which the primary tumor cannot be identified by CT scan. With this modality of imaging, there is an 84% positive predictive value and 50% negative predictive value. Another imaging modality, ^{18}F-fluorodeoxyglucose positron emission tomography (^{18}FDG PET) scanning, alone has limited capabilities because ^{18}FDG is taken up only in high-grade NENs (e.g., high Ki-67 expression), whereas most NENs have low Ki-67 expression and are not apparent with this imaging modality. However, the addition of newer isotopes, such as ^{18}F-L-dihydroxyphenylalanine (^{18}F-DOPA), has dramatically improved the sensitivity of PET for the diagnosis and surveillance of neuroendocrine malignant neoplasms.

Somatostatin receptor imaging with gadolinium ^{68}Ga–DOTATATE PET/CT is increasingly used for the preoperative staging for patients with NENs. DOTATATE is an amide of 1,4,7,10-tetraazacyclododecane-1,4,7,10-tetraacetic acid (DOTA) and the octreotide-derived radionuclide tyrosine-3-octreotate (TATE). The latter binds to somatostatin receptors and thus directs the radioactivity into the tumor. ^{68}Ga-DOTATATE PET/CT is a clinically useful imaging technique to localize primary tumors in patients with neuroendocrine metastases of unknown origin as well as to define the existence and extent of metastatic disease. Combining the two modalities may be even more helpful in diagnosing and managing NENs. Studies have demonstrated a 95% detection rate with the use of ^{68}Ga-DOTATATE PET/CT, with a sensitivity of 93.5%. Additionally, it is a shorter study with less radiation. There continues to be investigational studies into different hybrid chelators to further maximize detection, including ^{68}Ga-DOTA-peptides and ^{64}Cu-DOTATATE.[35] The benefits of ^{64}Cu-DOTATATE imaging include better true positive lesion detection, longer shelf life, and longer scanning window when compared with ^{68}Ga-DOTATATE, making it an ideal diagnostic tool. Lastly, the peptide receptor radionuclide therapy agent lutetium-177 (^{177}Lu) is both diagnostic and therapeutic and belongs to a new class of drugs known as *theranostics.* The reason for developing compounds with high affinity for somatostatin receptors 2, 3, and 5 is to improve diagnostic sensitivity. Because resection is the only curative treatment in patients with small intestinal NENs, accurate preoperative imaging is critical to guide surgical management.

Treatment

Surgical therapy. Currently, surgery is the only curative treatment for NENs, regardless of their location. Patients should undergo segmental intestinal resection with regional lymph node excision. Lesions of the terminal ileum are best treated by right hemicolectomy. Small duodenal tumors can be excised endo-scopically; however, more extensive lesions may require pancreati-coduodenectomy. Outcomes between laparoscopic and open surgery are comparable. However, guidelines recommend bidigital palpation of the entirety of the small bowel, which is not feasible in a purely laparoscopic case. As such, many guidelines recommend open surgical resection as the standard of care. Alternatively, laparoscopic procedures with hand-assist or an extraction point to run the bowel would allow for palpation of the bowel. Determination of surgical technique should weigh the risks and benefits of both techniques for the individual patient and the extent of their disease.[36]

Caution should be exerted in the anesthetic management of patients with NENs because anesthesia may precipitate a carcinoid crisis characterized by hypotension, bronchospasm, flushing, and tachyarrhythmias. Carcinoid crisis is treated with IV octreotide given as a bolus of 500 to 1000 μg, which may be continued as an infusion at 50 μg/h. In patients with liver lesions, prophylactic perioperative administration of IV octreotide should be considered.

In addition to treating the primary tumor, the abdomen must be thoroughly explored for multicentric lesions. There often is a large desmoplastic reaction causing shortening, folding, and pleating of the small bowel mesentery resulting in intestinal angina and obstruction. In cases in which the mesenteric disease appears to involve a large portion of the mesentery, dissection of the tumor off the mesenteric vessels, with preservation of the blood supply to unaffected bowel, is appropriate, albeit technically demanding. Extensive mobilization of the small bowel mesentery is required to perform a difficult resection. All guidelines emphasize the need to preserve bowel when able and only consider tumors with their desmoid reactions unresectable if they involve vessels at the root of the mesentery.

In patients with NENs and widespread metastatic disease, surgery may still be indicated. In contrast to metastases from other tumors, there is a definite role for surgical debulking, which often provides beneficial symptomatic relief. In patients with limited hepatic involvement, metastasectomy provides the most durable survival benefit compared with other treatment modalities. For patients with liver metastases, surgical resection is an option as long as there are no extrahepatic metastases, liver function is not compromised, and hepatic disease burden is less than 70%. Patient performance status should also be an important consideration in deciding on surgical intervention. Unfortunately, most patients are not candidates for liver resection because of extensive disease at diagnosis. Even with liver metastasectomy, there is still a high recurrence rate of 75%. In these cases, transarterial chemoembolization or radioembolization has been shown to provide liver-directed control of disease. Furthermore, resection of the primary tumor, with or without mesenteric resection, has been shown to improve survival and to slow progression of hepatic metastases in patients with unresectable disease. Although some small studies have evaluated hepatic transplantation for extensive liver metastases from NENs, unacceptably high recurrence rates limit this approach. Overall, because of the complexity of treatment regimens, all surgical resections should be performed at a high-volume center.

Medical therapy. Medical therapy for patients with malignant carcinoid syndrome is primarily directed toward the relief of symptoms caused by the excess production of humoral factors. Table 91.10 summarizes medical therapies for NEN treatment. Somatostatin analogs (SSAs) are the standard of care for controlling symptoms of

TABLE 91.10	Medical Therapies for Neuroendocrine Tumor Treatment
Approved Therapeutics	
Somatostatin analogues	Octreotide (Sandostatin; Sandostatin LAR)
	Lanreotide (Somatuline depot)
Cytotoxic therapies	Streptozotocin (pancreatic NET only)
mTOR inhibitor	Everolimus (Afinitor; gastrointestinal, pancreatic, lung NET)
Tyrosine kinase inhibitors	Sunitinib (Sutent; pancreatic NET only)
Peptide receptor radionuclide therapy	^{177}Lu isotopes conjugated with somatostatin analogues (Lutathera)
Serotonin synthesis inhibitors	Telotristat etiprate (Xermelo)
Used Off-Label	
Pan-receptor somatostatin agonists	Pasireotide (Signifor); approved indication for Cushing disease only
Interferons	Interferon alfa-2b (Intron A)
Cytotoxic therapies	5-Fluorouracil (5-FU)
	Capecitabine (Xeloda); oral 5-FU
	Temozolomide (Temodar)
Investigational	
Peptide Receptor Radiotherapy	^{177}Lu-OPS 201
	^{177}Lu-DOTA JR11
Dopamine agonists	Dopastatins
Checkpoint Inhibitor	JS001
Somatostatin Drug Conjugate	PEN-221

mTOR, Mammalian target of rapamycin; *NET*, neuroendocrine tumor.
Compiled with assistance of Lowell B. Anthony, MD, University of Kentucky.

patients with functional gastrointestinal NENs, and they control symptoms in more than 70% of patients with carcinoid syndrome. SSAs such as octreotide and lanreotide and their depot formulations (Sandostatin LAR and Somatuline, respectively) relieve symptoms of carcinoid syndrome (e.g., diarrhea, flushing, antisecretory effect) in most patients and delay cancer progression (antiproliferative effect). The antiproliferative effect was demonstrated in two randomized phase III trials. First, the PROMID trial of 85 patients confirmed that tumor burden is an important predictor of survival, and octreotide LAR provided delayed tumor progression compared with placebo.[37] Octreotide LAR is recommended for grade 1 and 2 NENs and is not recommended in grade 3 disease. Second, the landmark controlled study of Lanreotide Antiproliferative Response In Neuro-Endocrine Tumors (CLARINET) trial found that lanreotide, an SSA, was associated with prolonged progression-free survival among patients with metastatic grade 1 or 2 enteropancreatic NENs.[38] Octreotide LAR and lanreotide are both appropriate as first-line therapy. The treatment of asymptomatic patients with low-volume and unresectable disease requires a personalized decision regarding observation or initiation of SSAs. However, observation requires close monitoring with diagnostic imaging every 3 to 6 months.[39]

For patients who have disease progression on SSA therapy, several treatment options remain. Everolimus, a mammalian target of rapamycin (mTOR) inhibitor initially developed as an immunosuppressant therapy, is approved for the treatment of nonfunctional gastrointestinal NENs with unresectable, locally advanced or metastatic disease. A randomized controlled trial

(RADIANT-4) demonstrated that with everolimus treatment, progression-free survival improved from 3.9 months to 11 months. Although everolimus can slow tumor progression, significant tumor reduction is rarely obtained. Targeting multiple signaling pathways is a treatment strategy that may provide better tumor control and overcome resistance mechanisms involved with simply targeting a single pathway. There are many ongoing studies investigating combinational therapy, including the addition of mTOR inhibitors, VEGF pathway inhibitors, cytotoxic chemotherapy, immunotherapy, and combination therapy with radiation treatments.[39]

Peptide receptor radionuclides are another class of therapy used in progressive disease. The NETTER-1 randomized control trial demonstrated that treatment with radionuclide ^{177}Lu-DOTATATE had a 79% improvement in progression-free survival when compared with high-dose octreotide. ^{177}Lu-DOTATATE can be used for PET imaging and to determine the distribution and the dosimetry of the tumor. Given the success of peptide receptor radionuclide therapy (PRRT), it continues to gain support for the treatment of NENs and is considered second-line therapy if somatostatin analogues fail. There are investigational studies looking at combination therapies to maximize therapeutic effect. Another second-line therapy is pasireotide, a second-generation SSA developed to address the limitations of the current regimens. Pasireotide has been shown to provide a 25% reduction in diarrhea and 42% reduction in flushing.[39]

Other treatment options include interferon-α, which was used as monotherapy for NENs in 1983. Interferon binds to two different receptors to elicit effects that include cell cycle inhibition at G_1/S, antiangiogenesis effects through downregulation of VEGF, and upregulation of somatostatin receptors. Although some series showed tumor regression in 20% to 40% of patients and tumor stabilization in 40% to 70% of patients, side effects, which included chronic fatigue, pancytopenia, thyroiditis, and systemic lupus erythematosus, were not tolerable. Thus, interferon-α has declined in use. Some series showed that given the upregulation of somatostatin receptors by interferon-α, its combination with SSAs may be efficacious. However, the literature is not consistent in these findings. Prospective randomized controlled trials have demonstrated variable findings, with resultant improved progression-free survival in some studies and no difference observed in other trials. Interferon is less expensive than the SSAs, but the increased incidence of side effects and variable outcomes preclude the widespread use of this drug.[39]

Patients with carcinoid syndrome resistant to SSAs have limited treatment options, which include increasing the dose of SSA or adding a short-acting octreotide and starting antidiarrheals. An extensive workup is needed to rule out other causes of diarrhea, but few treatment options remain. Currently, the serotonin synthesis inhibitor telotristat etiprate is indicated for somatostatin-refractory diarrhea in the setting of carcinoid syndrome. In the TELESTAR trial, telotristat treatment reduced daily bowel movements by 35%.[39] Methysergide is no longer used because of the increased incidence of retroperitoneal fibrosis.

Historically, the only available treatment for metastatic NENs was cytotoxic chemotherapy, most frequently combinations that included streptozotocin, 5-fluorouracil (5-FU), and cyclophosphamide. These treatments resulted in a median survival of around 2 years. Currently, the role of chemotherapy is confined predominantly to patients who have failed all other therapeutic options. The duration of response, however, is short-lived. Temozolomide as monotherapy has acceptable toxicity and provided

antitumoral effects in a small series of patients with advanced NENs, and in combination with capecitabine, it was shown to prolong survival in patients with well-differentiated, metastatic NENs who experienced progression with previous therapies. Capecitabine-temozolomide in combination with PRRT studied in patients who had already failed single therapy demonstrated disease control in 38% to 55% of patients with progression-free survival of 7.1 months.[39] The use of cisplatin and etoposide has shown some promise, but only in patients with poorly differentiated NECs.

The treatment of metastatic NENs requires a multidisciplinary approach; combined modalities may be the best option, including surgical debulking, hepatic artery embolization, chemoembolization, or radioembolization and medical therapy. In addition, newer and more targeted therapies are being developed that may be useful in the future.

Prognosis. Although the incidence of NETs has increased, the mortality rate has remained stable. Other small bowel tumors, such as lymphomas and GISTs, have demonstrated improvements in survival that are likely secondary to advances in therapeutic options. This emphasizes the need for further investigations into effective treatments for NETs.[32] Survival in small intestinal NENs depends on the grade and stage of the disease. Resection of a NET localized to its primary site approaches a 100% survival rate. Five-year survival rate in metastatic disease is 35% to 80%. Given their indolent nature and delays in diagnosis, up to 90% of patients present with disease that has already metastasized to the liver. When widespread metastatic disease precludes cure, extensive resection for palliation may be indicated. In fact, long-term palliation often can be obtained because these tumors are relatively slow growing. Many factors have been evaluated to identify patients with NENs who have a poor prognosis. However, there are currently no reliable markers for prognosis beyond grade (including Ki-67 and mitotic rate) and stage. CgA is widely used to assist in the diagnosis of NENs and may indicate more aggressive disease, but it remains controversial in its ability to predict aggressive disease.

Adenocarcinomas

Adenocarcinomas constitute approximately 30% to 45% of the malignant tumors of the small bowel. The median age at diagnosis is in the seventh decade of life, and most series show a slight male predominance. Most of these tumors are located in the duodenum and proximal jejunum (Fig. 91.12A).[40] Those arising in association with Crohn disease or other familial syndromes tend to occur at a somewhat younger age and have an increased risk of developing multiple lesions. Small bowel adenocarcinoma may have important gene mutations (APC, β-CATENIN, EGFR, VEGF-A, KRAS, HER2, TP53). Familial syndromes associated with small bowel adenocarcinomas include FAP, Lynch syndrome, and Peutz-Jeghers syndrome. Tumors of the duodenum tend to manifest somewhat earlier than those in the jejunum and ileum because of the earlier presentation of symptoms, which are usually jaundice and chronic bleeding. Adenocarcinomas of the jejunum and ileum usually produce more nonspecific symptoms that include vague abdominal pain and weight loss. Intestinal obstruction and chronic bleeding may also occur. Perforation is uncommon. As with adenocarcinomas in other organs, survival of patients with small bowel adenocarcinomas is related to the stage of disease at the time of diagnosis. Unfortunately, diagnosis is often delayed, and the disease is advanced at the time of surgery secondary to a variety of factors (e.g., vagueness of symptoms, absence of

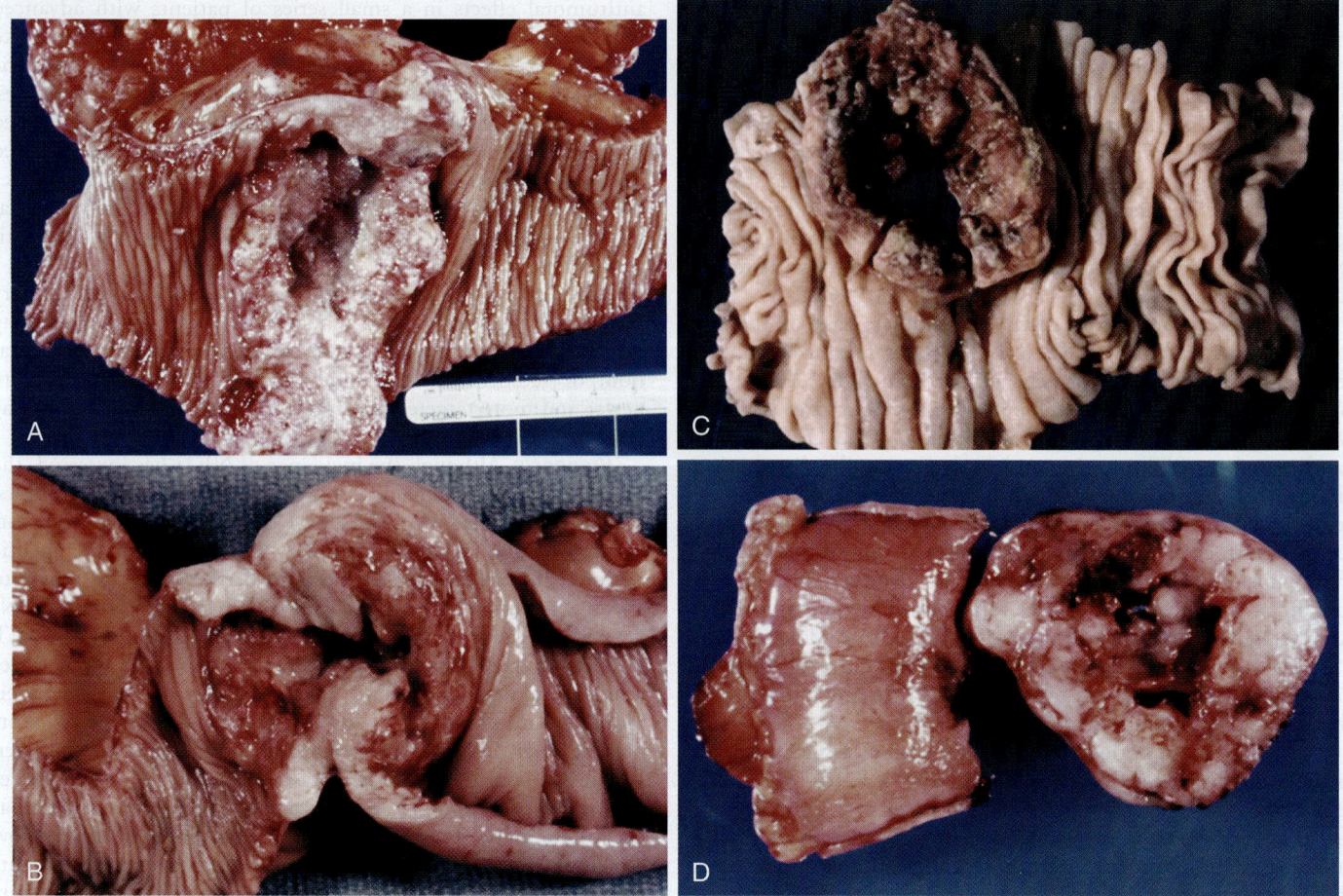

FIGURE 91.12 (A) Jejunal adenocarcinoma. Large circumferential mucinous adenocarcinoma of the jejunum. (B) Lymphoma of the small intestine. Gross photograph of primary lymphoma of the ileum shows replacement of all layers of the bowel wall with tumor. (C) Lymphoma of the small intestine. Small bowel lymphoma manifests as perforation and peritonitis. (D) Small intestine gastrointestinal stroma tumor (GIST). Small bowel GIST with hemorrhagic necrosis. (A–D, Courtesy Dr. Mary R. Schwartz, Baylor College of Medicine, Houston, TX.)

physical findings, lack of clinical suspicion because of the rarity of these lesions). A variety of radiologic and endoscopic techniques such as CT of the abdomen and pelvis, esophagogastroduodenoscopy with endoscopic ultrasound, MRI, video capsule endoscopy, and double-balloon enteroscopy (for biopsy and diagnosis) may be very useful in establishing the diagnosis before surgery.

Treatment of small bowel adenocarcinoma is determined by location and stage. An R0 resection of the primary tumor with locoregional lymph node resection is the only curative treatment. Neoadjuvant chemotherapy is appropriate to consider if there is unresectable disease, such as tumor invasion into adjacent structures. Duodenal resection can be performed for a noninfiltrating tumor if it is located in the first, third, or fourth portion of the duodenum, but this is not recommended if an expected R0 resection (no microscopic tumor at margin) is not possible. Residual microscopic tumor (R1 status) and grossly visible tumor after resection (R2 status) are associated with poor prognosis. Resectable adenocarcinomas in the second portion of the duodenum are treated with pancreaticoduodenectomy. In addition, regional lymphadenectomy of the periduodenal, peripancreatic, and hepatic lymph nodes as well as involved vascular structures is necessary. Jejunal and ileal adenocarcinomas require surgical resection with regional lymphadenectomy and jejunojejunal or ileoileal anastomosis. If the terminal ileum is involved, an ileocecectomy with right hemicolectomy should be performed with ligation of the ileocolic artery and subsequent regional lymphadenectomy.

There is currently no standard adjuvant protocol for small bowel adenocarcinoma, with clinical trials being the optimal route for medical therapy. Most guidelines suggest that patients with poorly differentiated cancers or those who had incomplete lymph node resections (<10 nodes identified) should at least be considered for adjuvant chemotherapy. Adjuvant regimens are often dictated by location, although studies have suggested that fluoropyrimidine and oxaliplatin may increase overall survival in patients with advanced disease. A prospective international phase III trial (BALLAD study) comparing observation with adjuvant chemotherapy in patients with an R0 resection is currently ongoing. This trial proposes that adjuvant chemotherapy will result in an improvement in disease-free survival and overall survival compared with observation alone after potentially curative surgery for patients with stage I, II, and III small bowel adenocarcinoma. Guidelines currently recommend adjuvant therapy with agents such as FOLFOX (oxaliplatin, 5-FU, and leucovorin), capecitabine plus oxaliplatin, 5-FU/leucovorin, and capecitabine. FOLFIRI (irinotecan, 5-FU, and leucovorin) can also be used as a second-line therapy for advanced and metastatic disease. Unresectable metastatic disease may require surgical intervention for uncontrolled bleeding, bowel obstruction, or perforation.

The prognosis of small bowel adenocarcinoma is poor, probably because of the delayed presentation and presence of advanced disease at diagnosis. Five-year survival rates for localized disease are much higher at 85% compared with stage IV disease, with a 5-year survival of 42%. Those with peritoneal carcinomatosis have a median overall survival of only about 6 months. Lymph node invasion is the main prognostic factor for local small bowel adenocarcinoma; moreover, the number of lymph nodes assessed and the number of positive lymph nodes are of prognostic value. Guidelines recommend obtaining at least eight regional lymph nodes during surgical resection with the possibility that greater lymph node resection may improve survival.[40]

Lymphoma

Malignant lymphomas involve the small bowel primarily or as a manifestation of systemic disease. Lymphomas constitute 20% of small bowel malignant tumors in the adult; in children younger than 10 years, they are the most common intestinal neoplasm. Lymphomas are commonly found in the ileum, where there is the greatest concentration of gut-associated lymphoid tissue. An increased risk for development of primary small bowel lymphomas was reported in patients with celiac disease and immunodeficient states (e.g., AIDS). Grossly, their appearance is variable, but they have a tendency to grow to large sizes (see Fig. 91.12B). Symptoms of small bowel lymphoma include pain, weight loss, nausea, vomiting, and change in bowel habits. Patients may also present with perforation or obstruction (see Fig. 91.12C). Fever is uncommon and suggests systemic involvement.

The treatment of small bowel lymphoma remains controversial. Traditionally, a combination of surgery, chemotherapy, and radiation therapy was used for all small bowel tumors. However, in the absence of symptoms, small bowel lymphomas are often chemoresponsive and do not require surgery. This can typically be predicted by cell type because B-cell lymphomas are more chemosensitive than T-cell lymphomas and have high remission rates with or without surgery. T-cell lymphomas are traditionally more resistant to therapy and will progress to symptoms of obstruction or perforation if not resected. Regardless of cell type, resection is indicated at any onset of symptoms because progression to life-threatening hemorrhage or perforation portends a dismal prognosis. Survival also depends on the type of lymphoma and extent of disease, but it is also largely dependent on response to systemic therapy rather than by the success of surgical resection.[41]

Gastrointestinal Stromal Tumors

Malignant GISTs arise from mesenchymal tissue, with the small bowel being the second most common location behind the stomach (see Fig. 91.12D). These tumors are more common in the jejunum and ileum and typically are diagnosed in the fifth and sixth decades of life. The most common indications for surgery include bleeding and obstruction, although free perforation may occur as a result of hemorrhagic necrosis in large tumor masses. Typically, GISTs tend to invade locally and to spread by direct extension into adjacent tissues and hematogenously to the liver, lungs, and bone; lymphatic metastases are unusual. The most useful indicators of survival and the risk for metastasis include the size of the tumor at presentation, mitotic index, and evidence of tumor invasion into the lamina propria.[29]

Treatment of GISTs continues to evolve and represents one of the first breakthroughs in signal transduction manipulation. The treatment regimen is based on localized versus metastatic disease. Surgical management includes complete resection for localized GISTs, with extreme care to avoid rupture of the tumor capsule, which results in one of the highest risk factors for disease recurrence. If capsule rupture occurs, these patients should receive adjuvant therapy regardless of the extent of the tumor before surgery. It is advisable to perform an en bloc resection to include adjacent organs for prevention of tumor capsule rupture. A laparoscopic approach in patients with large tumors is discouraged if it places the patient at risk for tumor rupture. Radiologic criteria for unresectability include large tumors with nonrecoverable infiltration of surrounding organs, which would cause significant comorbidity, and can include infiltration of the celiac trunk, superior mesenteric artery, or portal vein. Lymphadenectomy is unnecessary, given the low frequency of lymph node metastasis. The management of small GISTs (<2 cm) is controversial. Where surgical resection has classically been recommended for GISTS found on endoscopy, some now suggest that if there are no high-risk features, endoscopic surveillance may be appropriate. For similarly small GISTs identified incidentally in a surgical specimen, no further treatment is typically required. Before the development of tyrosine kinase inhibitors, adjuvant strategies for GISTs were lacking, and recurrence rates after resection were as high as 70%. However, the development of imatinib mesylate (Gleevec) has significantly altered previous treatment strategies. Imatinib mesylate is a tyrosine kinase inhibitor that blocks the unregulated mutant c-kit tyrosine kinase and inhibits the BCR-ABL and PDGF tyrosine kinases. Multiple randomized trials have confirmed its efficacy as a first-line agent in the treatment of GIST. Current guidelines suggest that patients with high-risk disease should receive 3 years of adjuvant treatment with imatinib, but it is not recommended for low-risk patients after an R0 resection. Neoadjuvant imatinib should be considered for patients requiring extensive surgery to allow for tumor shrinkage before resection.[29]

Relapse-risk assessment for a primary GIST is critical, as it provides prognostic information as well as estimates of the potential benefits of medical therapy. There are a multitude of risk stratification systems, including the National Institutes of Health (NIH) GIST consensus criteria, the American Forces Institute of Pathology criteria, the Joensuu risk criteria, prognostic nomograms, and mutational analysis. The modified NIH risk stratification system separates tumors into four groups ranging from very low risk to high risk based on tumor size, mitotic rate, and tumor site. In addition to staging information, several mutations are found to have implications on prognosis. For example, deletions affecting CD117 exons 9, 11, 13, or 17 and D842V PDGFR-α mutations have a higher risk of recurrence within the first 3 to 4 years after surgery. In fact, adjuvant imatinib therapy is not recommended in patients with D842V PDGFR-α mutations, given its known resistance to this agent.

Imatinib is also a first-line treatment for unresectable and metastatic GISTs with characteristic tumor biology. Genotyping is standard of care for patients with advanced or metastatic GIST. Standard-dose therapy (400 mg daily) is recommended. Unfortunately, there is a growing resistance to imatinib in metastatic GISTs. Tumors with CD117 mutations in exons 9, 13, or 14 should be treated with sunitinib, whereas ponatinib is useful for the treatment of tumors with exon 17 mutations.[29]

New molecular-targeted therapies may provide better treatments for patients with genetic mutations and GISTs. In phase III clinical trials evaluating imatinib dosing in patients with metastatic GIST, there was no objective response in patients who carry the D842V PDGFR-α mutation. Other medications are available as second- and third-line therapy, including dasatinib, an oral tyrosine kinase inhibitor of c-kit, PDGFR, ABL (Abelson murine leukemia viral oncogene homologue), and the proto-oncogene Src with a distinct binding affinity for c-kit and PDGFR. Regorafenib is a second-generation tyrosine kinase inhibitor that targets c-kit, RET, BRAF, VEGFR, PDGFR, and fibroblast growth factor receptor. Nilotinib is a second-generation tyrosine kinase inhibitor active in chronic myeloid leukemia and has an inhibitory effect on c-kit and PDGF. Sorafenib is a VEGF, c-kit, PDGFR, and BRAF inhibitor. All these agents may be useful in tumors resistant to imatinib but have shown variable results.

Metastatic Neoplasms

Metastases to the small intestine usually arise from other intraabdominal organs, including the uterine, cervix, ovaries, kidneys, stomach, colon, and pancreas. Small intestinal involvement is by direct extension or implantation of tumor cells. Metastases from extraabdominal tumors are rare but may be found in patients with adenocarcinoma of the breast and carcinoma of the lung. Cutaneous melanoma is the most common extraabdominal source to involve the small intestine and should always be a consideration when presented with a patient with advanced melanoma and gastrointestinal symptoms. Common symptoms of metastatic disease include anorexia, weight loss, anemia, bleeding, and partial bowel obstruction. Treatment is often palliative to relieve symptoms or, occasionally, a bypass if the metastatic tumor is extensive and not amenable to resection. Nonoperative palliation of malignant bowel obstruction includes endoscopic or radiologic placement of self-expandable metal stents, especially in patients with very poor performance status who may not tolerate a surgical procedure. Gastrostomy and jejunostomy tubes also may be placed to provide decompression when other palliative methods are not possible.

DIVERTICULAR DISEASE

Diverticular disease of the small intestine is relatively common. It may manifest as true or false diverticula. A true diverticulum contains all layers of the intestinal wall and is usually congenital. False diverticula consist of mucosa and submucosa protruding through a defect in the muscle coat and are usually acquired defects. Small bowel diverticula may occur in any portion of the small intestine. Duodenal diverticula are the most common acquired diverticula of the small bowel, and Meckel diverticulum is the most common true congenital diverticulum of the small bowel.

Duodenal Diverticula
Incidence and Cause

First described by Chomel, a French pathologist, in 1710, diverticula of the duodenum are relatively common, representing the second most common site for diverticulum formation after the colon, representing 60% to 79% of all small bowel diverticula.[42] The incidence of duodenal diverticula varies, depending on the age of the patient and method of diagnosis. Upper gastrointestinal

radiographic studies may show pooling of contrast in the diverticula but are not commonly used for diagnosis, given only a 1% to 5% identification rate. Endoscopic retrograde cholangiopancreatography has an increased ability to identify diverticula. Diverticula are classified as congenital or acquired, true or false, and intraluminal or extraluminal. Extraluminal duodenal diverticula are considerably more common than intraluminal diverticula, are acquired, and consist of mucosal or submucosal outpouchings herniated through a muscle defect in the bowel wall. Intraluminal duodenal diverticula (also known as windsock diverticula) are congenital and occur as a single saccular structure that is connected to the entire circumference or part of the wall of the duodenum to create a duodenal web. Incomplete recanalization of the duodenum during fetal development leads to intraluminal diverticula, which are exceedingly rare. In general, extraluminal diverticula usually occur within the second portion of the duodenum (62%) and less commonly in the third (30%) and fourth (8%) portions. They rarely occur in the first part of the duodenum (<1%). When they occur in the second portion, most (88%) are noted on the medial wall around the ampulla (i.e., periampullary), 8% are seen posteriorly, and 4% occur on the lateral wall.

Clinical Manifestations

Importantly, the overwhelming majority of duodenal diverticula are asymptomatic and were previously noted incidentally by an upper gastrointestinal series for an unrelated problem. These studies have become less commonly used with the increased use of CT. CT can identify large diverticula by the presence of a masslike structure interposed between the duodenum and pancreatic head, containing air, air-fluid levels, fluid contrast material, or debris. However, CT has been shown to identify only 7% of known diverticula. Arguably, this is a reflection of both the technology and the ability to identify diverticula from surrounding tissue. Upper gastrointestinal endoscopy identifies approximately 75% of duodenal diverticula, and the use of a side-viewing scope further increases the success rate. Magnetic resonance cholangiopancreatography is particularly helpful to demonstrate the relationship of the diverticulum to the biliary and pancreatic ducts and associated pathologic changes in the biliary system and pancreas. Hemorrhage in duodenal diverticula is less common than jejunal and ileal diverticula. It can be diagnosed via triple-phase CT imaging, Tc-99m-labeled red blood cell scan, or endoscopy for duodenal and very proximal jejunal lesions; however, surgery should not be delayed to obtain imaging in the event of hemorrhage in a hemodynamically unstable patient. Less than 5% of duodenal diverticula will require surgery because of a complication from the diverticulum itself. Major complications of duodenal diverticula include obstruction of the biliary or pancreatic ducts that may contribute to cholangitis and pancreatitis, hemorrhage, perforation, and, rarely, blind loop syndrome. Iatrogenic injuries, most commonly acquired during endoscopic instrumentation of an asymptomatic diverticulum, can result in perforation or hemorrhage.

Only diverticula associated with the ampulla of Vater are significantly related to complications of cholangitis and pancreatitis. In these patients, the ampulla usually enters the duodenum at the superior margin of the diverticulum rather than through the diverticulum itself. Perivaterian diverticulum, defined as within 3 cm of the ampulla of Vater, may distort the common bile duct as it enters the duodenum, resulting in partial obstruction and stasis. However, other causes of biliary obstruction should be investigated before determining a diverticulum to be the causative entity. In addition, hemorrhage can be caused by inflammation, leading to erosion of a branch of the superior mesenteric artery. Perforation of duodenal diverticula has been described but is rare. Finally, stasis of intestinal contents within a distended diverticulum can result in bacterial overgrowth, malabsorption, steatorrhea, diarrhea, and megaloblastic anemia, essentially producing a blind loop syndrome. Symptoms related to duodenal diverticula in the absence of any other demonstrable disease usually are nonspecific epigastric complaints that can be treated conservatively and may actually prove to be the result of another problem not related to the diverticulum itself.

Treatment

Most duodenal diverticula are asymptomatic and benign; when they are found incidentally, no intervention is indicated. For symptomatic duodenal diverticula, treatment consists of removal of the diverticulum, which can be accomplished endoscopically or surgically. Appropriate classification of these diverticula guides management. All intraluminal duodenal diverticula typically require treatment, as recurrence of symptoms is certain. Curative treatment consists of removal of the intraluminal diverticulum by laparotomy and duodenotomy or by endoscopic resection. A large (>3 cm) or obstructing intraluminal duodenal diverticulum does not preclude endoscopic resection, but an endoscopic approach in the setting of massive hemorrhage or perforation with intraabdominal contamination secondary to intestinal contents is discouraged. These entities are relatively rare and often require a multidisciplinary approach to determine the best treatment strategy.

Extraluminal duodenal diverticula should be resected in the setting of symptomatic disease or need for urgent surgery, such as free perforation or hemorrhage. Several operative procedures have been described for treatment of the symptomatic extraluminal duodenal diverticula. The most common and effective treatment is diverticulectomy, which is most easily accomplished by performing a wide Kocher maneuver that exposes the duodenum. The diverticulum is then excised, and the duodenum is closed in a transverse or longitudinal fashion, whichever produces the least amount of luminal obstruction. Careful identification of the ampulla is essential to prevent injury to the common bile duct and pancreatic duct. For diverticula embedded deep within the head of the pancreas, a duodenotomy is performed, with invagination of the diverticulum into the lumen, which is then excised, and the wall is closed. An alternative method that has been described for duodenal diverticula associated with the ampulla of Vater is an extended sphincteroplasty through the common wall of the ampulla in the diverticulum. Laparoscopic duodenal diverticulectomy is safe and effective in patients with symptomatic and noncomplicated (i.e., not perforated or bleeding) diverticula. An endoscopic stapler is most commonly used to traverse and to resect the diverticulum at its base, and an omental patch reinforcement can be placed over the staple line.

The treatment of a perforated diverticulum may require procedures similar to those described for patients with massive trauma-related defects of the duodenal wall. The perforated diverticulum should be excised and the duodenum closed in a manner that limits luminal obstruction. This can include the use of a serosal patch from a jejunal loop. If the surrounding inflammation is severe, it may be necessary to divert the enteric flow away from the site of the perforation with a gastrojejunostomy or duodenojejunostomy. Interruption of duodenal continuity proximal to the perforated diverticulum may be accomplished by pyloric closure

with suture or a row of staples in conjunction with a diversion procedure. If the diverticulum is posterior and perforates into the substance of the pancreas, operative repair may be difficult and dangerous. Wide drainage with duodenal diversion may be all that is feasible in such cases. Great care should be taken if the perforation is adjacent to the ampulla of Vater. Surgical jejunostomy should also be a consideration for all patients with acute perforation to ensure nutrition repletion. Lastly, stable patients with a contained perforation, without active enteric leak, may be able to be managed nonoperatively in the acute setting. However, such patients should be monitored closely and considered for future intervention to prevent recurrence.

Jejunal and Ileal Diverticula
Incidence and Cause

Diverticula of the small bowel are much less common than duodenal diverticula, with 20% to 25% found in the jejunum and approximately 5% in the ileum. These are false diverticula, occurring mainly in an older age group (after the sixth decade of life). These diverticula are multiple, usually protrude from the mesenteric border of the bowel, and may be overlooked at surgery because they are embedded within the small bowel mesentery (Fig. 91.13A). The cause of jejunoileal diverticulosis is thought to be a motor dysfunction of the smooth muscle or the myenteric plexus, resulting in disordered contractions of the small bowel, generating increased intraluminal pressure and herniation of the mucosa and submucosa through the weakest portion of the bowel (i.e., the mesenteric side).

Clinical Manifestations

Jejunoileal diverticula are usually found incidentally at laparotomy or during an upper gastrointestinal study (see Fig. 91.13B); the great majority remain asymptomatic. Acute complications, such as intestinal obstruction, hemorrhage, and perforation, can occur but are rare. Chronic symptoms include vague chronic abdominal pain, malabsorption, functional pseudoobstruction, and chronic low-grade gastrointestinal hemorrhage. Acute complications are diverticulitis with or without abscess or perforation, gastrointestinal hemorrhage, and intestinal obstruction. Stasis of intestinal flow with bacterial overgrowth (blind loop syndrome), caused by the jejunal dyskinesia, may lead to deconjugation of bile salts and uptake of vitamin B_{12} by the bacterial flora, resulting in steatorrhea and megaloblastic anemia, with or without neuropathy.

Treatment

For incidentally noted, asymptomatic jejunoileal diverticula, no treatment is required. Treatment of complications of obstruction, bleeding, and perforation is usually by intestinal resection and end-to-end anastomosis. Patients presenting with malabsorption secondary to blind loop syndrome and bacterial overgrowth in the diverticulum can typically use antibiotics for symptom resolution. Obstruction may be caused by enteroliths that form in a jejunal diverticulum and are subsequently dislodged and obstruct the distal intestine. This condition may be treated by enterotomy and removal of the enterolith, or sometimes the enterolith can be milked distally into the cecum. When the enterolith causes obstruction at the level of the diverticulum, bowel resection is necessary. When a perforation of a jejunoileal diverticulum is encountered, resection with reanastomosis is required because lesser procedures, such as simple closure, excision, and invagination, are associated with greater mortality and morbidity rates. Laparoscopic bowel resection with reanastomosis is a safe option

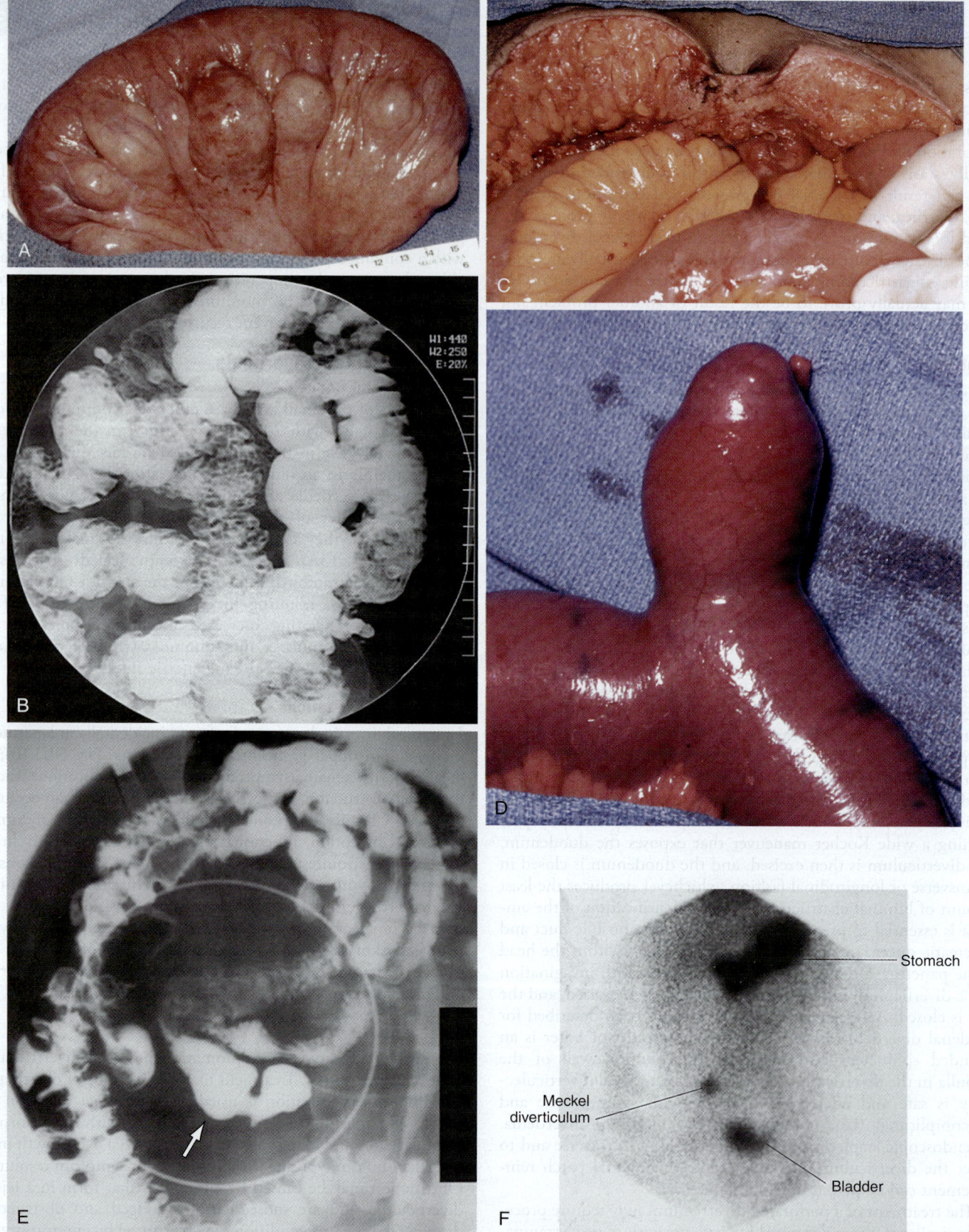

FIGURE 91.13 (A) Jejunal diverticulum. Multiple large jejunal diverticula located in the mesentery in an older patient presenting with obstruction secondary to an enterolith. (B) Contrasted radiograph demonstrating jejunal diverticula. Multiple jejunal diverticula demonstrated by a barium contrast upper gastrointestinal study. (C) Persistent omphalomesenteric remnant. Omphalomesenteric remnant persisting as a fibrous cord from the ileum to the umbilicus. (D) Meckel diverticulum. Common presentation of a Meckel diverticulum projecting from the antimesenteric border of the ileum. (E) Contrasted radiograph of Meckel diverticulum. Barium radiograph demonstrates an asymptomatic Meckel diverticulum *(arrow)*. (F) Nuclear imaging of Meckel diverticulum. A Tc-99m-pertechnetate scintigram from a child demonstrates a Meckel diverticulum clearly differentiated from the stomach and bladder. (A, Adapted from Evers BM, Townsend CM Jr, Thompson JC. Small intestine. In: Schwartz SI, ed. *Principles of Surgery*. 7th ed. New York: McGraw-Hill; 1999:1248. B, E, F, Courtesy Dr. Melvyn H. Schreiber, The University of Texas Medical Branch, Galveston, TX.)

in minimally contaminated surgical fields. In extreme cases, such as diffuse peritonitis, enterostomies may be required if judgment dictates that reanastomosis is not feasible.

Meckel Diverticulum

Incidence and Cause

Meckel diverticulum is the most commonly encountered congenital anomaly of the small intestine, occurring in about 2% of the population. It was reported initially in 1598 by Hildanus and then described in detail by Johann Meckel in 1809. Meckel diverticulum is located on the antimesenteric border of the ileum 45 to 60 cm proximal to the ileocecal valve and results from incomplete closure of the omphalomesenteric, or vitelline, duct. Meckel diverticulum may exist in different forms, ranging from a small bump that may be easily missed to a long projection that communicates with the umbilicus by a persistent fibrous cord (see Fig. 91.13C) or, much less commonly, a patent fistula. The usual manifestation is a relatively wide-mouthed diverticulum measuring about 3 to 6 cm in length (see Fig. 91.13D). Cells lining the vitelline duct are pluripotent; therefore, about half contain heterotopic tissue. The most common ectopic tissue identified is gastric mucosa, followed by pancreatic mucosa and, in rare cases, colonic mucosa.

Clinical Manifestations

Most Meckel diverticula are benign and are incidentally discovered during autopsy, laparotomy, or barium studies (see Fig. 91.13E). The most common clinical presentation of Meckel diverticulum is gastrointestinal bleeding; hemorrhage is the most common symptomatic presentation in children 2 years of age or younger. This complication may manifest as acute massive hemorrhage, anemia secondary to chronic bleeding, or a self-limited recurrent episodic event. The usual source of the bleeding is a chronic acid-induced ulcer in the ileum adjacent to a Meckel diverticulum that contains gastric mucosa.

Another common presenting symptom of Meckel diverticulum is intestinal obstruction. Obstruction may result from a volvulus of the small bowel that surrounds the diverticulum and is associated with a fibrotic band attached to the abdominal wall, intussusception, or, rarely, incarceration of the diverticulum in an inguinal hernia (Littre hernia). Volvulus is usually an acute event and, if allowed to progress, may result in strangulation of the involved bowel. In intussusception, a broad-based diverticulum invaginates and then is carried forward by peristalsis. This may be ileoileal or ileocolic and manifest as acute obstruction associated with an urge to defecate, early vomiting, and occasionally passage of the classic currant jelly stool. A palpable mass may be present. Although reduction of an intussusception secondary to Meckel diverticulum can sometimes be performed by air enema, the patient should still undergo resection of the diverticulum to negate subsequent recurrence of the condition.

Meckel diverticulitis is more common in adult patients. Meckel diverticulitis, which is clinically indistinguishable from appendicitis, should be considered in the differential diagnosis of a patient with right lower quadrant pain. Progression of the diverticulitis may lead to perforation and peritonitis. When the appendix is found to be normal during exploration for suspected appendicitis, the distal ileum should be inspected for the presence of an inflamed Meckel diverticulum.

Neoplasms can also occur in 0.5% to 3.2% of Meckel diverticulum, with NET the most common malignant neoplasm (33%–44%). Other histologic types include leiomyosarcoma (18%–25%); adenocarcinoma (12%–16%), which generally originates from the gastric mucosa; GIST (12%); and, less frequently, lymphoma and pancreatic malignancies.[43]

Diagnostic Studies

The diagnosis of Meckel diverticulum may be difficult. Plain abdominal radiography, CT, and ultrasonography are rarely helpful. In children, the single most accurate diagnostic test for Meckel diverticula is with sodium Tc-99m-pertechnetate scintigraphy. The Tc-99m-pertechnetate is preferentially taken up by the mucus-secreting cells of gastric mucosa and ectopic gastric tissue in the diverticulum (see Fig. 91.13F). The diagnostic sensitivity of this scan has been reported as high as 85%, with a specificity of 95% and an accuracy of 90% in the pediatric age group.

In adults, however, the sensitivity of Tc-99m-pertechnetate scan falls to 63% because of the smaller presence of gastric mucosa in the diverticulum compared with that noted in the pediatric age group. The sensitivity and specificity can be improved by the use of pharmacologic agents. Cimetidine may be used to increase the sensitivity of scintigraphy by decreasing the peptic secretion while not affecting radionuclide uptake, which may be caused by the release of pertechnetate from the diverticular lumen. Therefore, cimetidine treatment results in higher radionuclide concentrations in the wall of the diverticulum. False-negative results can occur because of absent gastric mucosal cells, inflammatory changes causing edema or necrosis, presence of outlet obstruction of the diverticulum, or anemia. In false-negative cases, barium contrast imaging, mesenteric arteriography, or double-balloon endoscopy can be helpful. In patients with acute hemorrhage, angiography is sometimes useful. Nevertheless, surgical intervention should not be delayed to obtain imaging for a patient with signs and symptoms of hemorrhage and hemodynamic instability.

Treatment

The treatment of a symptomatic Meckel diverticulum requires prompt surgical intervention with diverticulectomy or segmental resection of ileum containing the diverticulum. Segmental small bowel resection is required for treatment of patients with hemorrhage because the bleeding site is usually adjacent to the diverticulum. Diverticulectomy for nonbleeding Meckel diverticula can be performed with a hand-sewn technique or stapling across the base of the diverticulum in a diagonal or transverse line to minimize the risk for subsequent stenosis. Retrospective studies have demonstrated equivalent outcomes in laparoscopic resection as compared with open resection of Meckel diverticulum.

Although the treatment of a complicated or symptomatic Meckel diverticulum is straightforward, the optimal treatment of an asymptomatic diverticulum found incidentally is still debated. It is generally recommended that asymptomatic diverticula found in children during laparotomy should be resected. The treatment of Meckel diverticula encountered in the adult patient, however, remains controversial. A landmark paper by Soltero and Bill[44] formed the basis of the surgical management of asymptomatic Meckel diverticula in adults for many years. In this study, the likelihood of a Meckel diverticulum becoming symptomatic in the adult patient was estimated to be 2% or less, and given that the morbidity rates from incidental removal were 12% at the time, the recommendation was to not remove the incidental Meckel diverticulum. Recent studies have argued for surgical resection because of their propensity for harboring malignancies.[43] The factors associated with a higher risk of complications, and warranting consideration of resection, include age younger than 50 years, male sex, diverticulum length >2 cm, and ectopic tissue or palpable abnormalities. Taken together, the decision for surgical resection of Meckel diverticulum needs to be made on a personalized basis, weighing the risk and benefits of malignancy, age, and complications. Future prospective trials are needed to clarify this controversy.

MISCELLANEOUS PROBLEMS

Small Bowel Ulcerations

Ulcerations of the small bowel are relatively uncommon and may be attributed to Crohn disease, typhoid fever, tuberculosis, lymphoma, and gastrinoma (Table 91.11). Drug-induced ulcerations can occur and were, in the past, attributed to enteric-coated potassium chloride tablets and corticosteroids. In addition, ulcerations of the small intestine in which no causative agent can be identified have been described. Currently, many different drugs are linked to small bowel injury, including certain NSAIDs, biologic therapies, immunosuppressive medications, and blood pressure medications (i.e., olmesartan). NSAID-induced ulcers occur more commonly in the ileum, with single or multiple ulcerations noted. Complications necessitating operative intervention include bleeding, perforation, and obstruction. In addition to ulcerations, NSAIDs are known to induce an enteropathy characterized by increased intestinal permeability leading to protein loss and hypoalbuminemia, malabsorption, and anemia. Treatment of complications from small bowel ulcerations is segmental resection and intestinal reanastomosis.[45]

Ingested Foreign Bodies

Ingested foreign bodies, which can lead to subsequent perforation or obstruction of the gastrointestinal tract, are swallowed, usually accidentally, by children or adults. These include glass and metal fragments, pins, needles, toothpicks, fish bones, coins, whistles, toys, and broken razor blades (Fig. 91.14). Intentional ingestion of foreign bodies is sometimes seen in the prison population and those who have a psychiatric illness. For most patients, treatment is observation to permit safe passage of these objects through the intestinal tract. If the object is radiopaque, progress can be

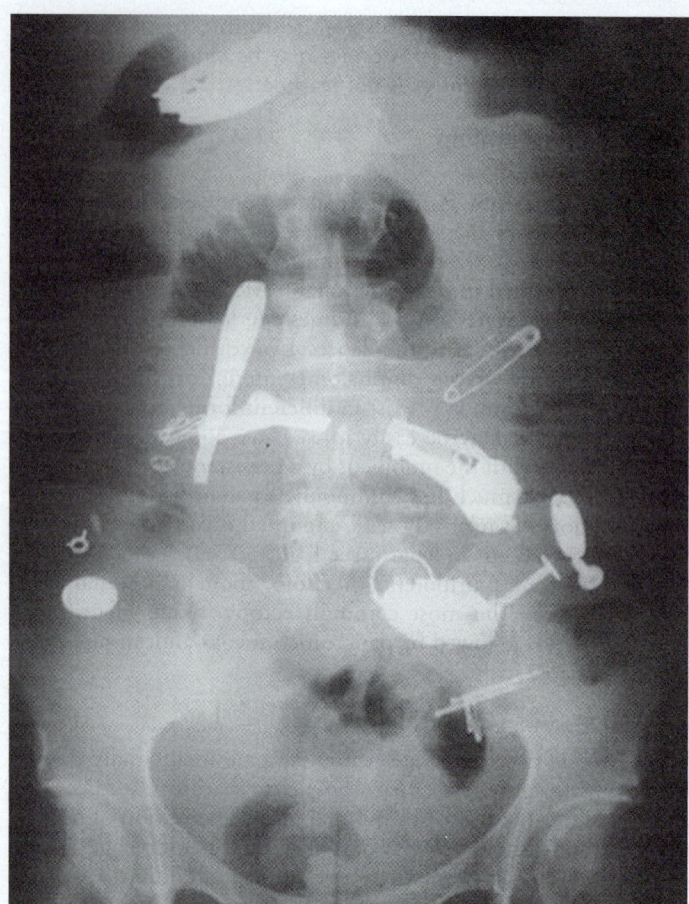

FIGURE 91.14 Intestinal foreign bodies. Plain abdominal film demonstrates a number of ingested foreign bodies in a patient presenting with a small bowel obstruction. (Courtesy Dr. Melvyn H. Schreiber, The University of Texas Medical Branch, Galveston, TX.)

followed by serial abdominal films. Cathartic agents are contraindicated. Sharp pointed objects such as needles, razor blades, or fish bones may penetrate the bowel wall. If abdominal pain, tenderness, fever, or leukocytosis occurs, immediate surgical intervention with removal of the offending object(s) is indicated. Similarly, if obstruction occurs, surgery should be performed to remove the object(s).

Small Bowel Fistulas

Despite improvements in surgical nutrition and critical care, mortality from enterocutaneous fistulas remains high at 10% in recent reports. Improvements in outcome focus on prevention and, when fistulas occur, prompt recognition and intervention. Multidisciplinary care is critical for improving fistula outcomes. Enterocutaneous fistulas are most commonly iatrogenic after surgical intervention (e.g., anastomotic leakage, injury of the bowel or blood supply, erosion by suction catheters, laceration of the bowel by wire mesh or retention sutures). Additional causes include predisposing conditions such as Crohn disease, malignant disease, radiation enteritis, diverticulitis, intraabdominal sepsis, or trauma.

Clinical Manifestations

Recognition of enterocutaneous fistulas is usually not difficult. The typical clinical presentation is that of a febrile postoperative patient with an erythematous wound. When a few skin sutures are

	STAGE					
	I	IIA	IIB	IIIA	IIIB	IV
Primary tumor size[a]	T1 or T2	T3	T4	Any T		
Regional lymph node metastasis[b]	N0			N1	N2	Any N
Distant metastasis[c]	M0					M1

TABLE 91.11 Small Intestinal Gastrointestinal Tumor Classification

[a]**T1,** Tumor invades the lamina propria or submucosa; **T2,** Tumor invades the muscularis propria; **T3,** Tumor invades into the subserosa or extends into nonperitonealized perimuscular tissue (mesentery or retroperitoneum) without serosal penetration; **T4,** Tumor perforates the visceral peritoneum or directly invades other organs/structures (other loops of small bowel, mesentery of adjacent bowel, abdominal wall, invasion of pancreas or bile duct [for duodenum]).
[b]**N0,** No regional lymph node metastasis; **N1,** One or two regional lymph node metastasis; **N2,** Three or more regional lymph node metastasis.
[c]**M0,** No distant metastasis; **M1,** Distant metastasis.

TABLE 91.12   Causes of Small Intestine Ulceration

CAUSE	EXAMPLES
Infections	Tuberculosis, syphilis, cytomegalovirus, typhoid, parasites, *Strongyloides* hyperinfection, *Campylobacter, Yersinia*
Inflammatory	Crohn disease, systemic lupus erythematosus, celiac disease, ulcerative enteritis
Ischemia	Mesenteric arterial insufficiency or venous thrombosis
Idiopathic	Primary ulcer, Behçet syndrome
Drug induced	Potassium, indomethacin, phenylbutazone, salicylates, antimetabolites
Radiation	Therapeutic, accidental
Vascular	Vasculitis, giant cell arteritis, amyloidosis (ischemic lesion), angiocentric lymphoma
Metabolic	Uremia
Hyperacidity	Zollinger-Ellison syndrome, Meckel diverticulum, stomal ulceration
Neoplastic	Lymphoma, adenocarcinoma, melanoma
Toxic	Acute jejunitis (β-toxin–producing *Clostridium perfringens*), arsenic
Mucosal lesions	Lymphocytic enterocolitis

Adapted from Rai R, Bayless TM. Isolated and diffuse ulcers of the small intestine. In: Feldman M, Scharschmidt BF, Sleisenger MH, eds. *Gastrointestinal and Liver Disease: Pathophysiology, Diagnosis, Management.* Philadelphia: WB Saunders; 1998:1771-1778.

removed, a purulent or bloody discharge is noted; leakage of enteric contents then occurs, sometimes immediately but often within 1 or 2 days. Small bowel fistulas can also be manifested with generalized peritonitis, although this is less common. Recently, the popularization of damage control laparotomy and staged management of the open abdomen has led to a more virulent form of small bowel fistula referred to as an *enteroatmospheric fistula*. These patients typically present with an open segment of intestine exposed through a large fascial defect, without a surrounding epidermal margin.

Enterocutaneous fistulas are classified according to their location and volume of daily output (Tables 91.12 and 91.13). These factors dictate treatment and morbidity and mortality rates. Proximal fistulas are associated with higher output, greater fluid and electrolyte loss, and greater loss of digestive capacity. Distal fistulas tend to have lower output, making them easier to manage and more likely to close spontaneously. Multiple factors prevent the spontaneous closure of fistulas, including retained **F**oreign body, **R**adiation enteritis, **I**nflammatory bowel disease or infection, **E**pithelialization of the fistula tract, **N**eoplasm, and **D**istal obstruction (FRIENDS). Once a fistula is identified, management

TABLE 91.13   Factors Predictive of Nonoperative Fistula Closure

FAVORABLE	UNFAVORABLE
Surgical etiology	Ileal, jejunal, nonsurgical etiology
Appendicitis or diverticulitis	Inflammatory bowel disease, cancer, radiation
Transferrin >200 mg/dL	Transferrin <200 mg/dL
No evidence of bowel obstruction, discontinuity, infection, inflammation	Distal small bowel obstruction, bowel is in discontinuity, adjacent infection, adjacent inflammation
Length >2 cm, end fistula	Length <2 cm, lateral or multiple fistulas
Output <200 mL/24 hours	Output >500 mL/24 hours
No sepsis, balanced electrolytes	Sepsis, electrolyte disturbances
Initial referral to tertiary care center and subspecialty care	Delay getting to tertiary care center and subspecialty care

Adapted from Gribovskaja-Rupp I, Melton GB. Enterocutaneous fistula: proven strategies and updates. *Clin Colon Rectal Surg.* 2016;29:130-137.

should focus on prompt IV fluid resuscitation and consideration of potential factors that could prevent spontaneous closure. Successful management of patients with intestinal fistulas requires a coordinated staged approach that can be defined in three phases: (1) stabilization, (2) staging and supportive care, and (3) definitive management.

Treatment

Stabilization. Historically, malnutrition and fluid losses were the leading causes of death in patients with small bowel fistula. However, with better nutritional supplementation and critical care support, sepsis has become the most common cause of death in affected patients. Nevertheless, the fluid losses and volume depletion associated with small bowel fistula cannot be marginalized. Therefore, prompt fluid resuscitation and electrolyte replacement should occur on recognition of a fistula. Sepsis control is critical, and in the early period, CT scanning may be invaluable in identifying undrained abscesses, complete distal obstructions, or generalized intraabdominal sepsis with peritonitis. Numerous treatment options are available for enterocutaneous fistulas (Box 91.7). All infections should be adequately drained percutaneously or operatively, if necessary, along with appropriate antibiotic administration. Once sepsis is controlled and the patient is resuscitated, effluent control with skin protection and adequate nutrition are necessary. Fistula output can be controlled by intubation of the fistula tract with a drain. Protection of the skin around the fistulous opening is important to prevent excoriation and destruction of the skin. This can be accomplished by using a Stomahesive product with applications of zinc oxide, aluminum paste, or karaya powder. The suction catheter can be brought out through the end of the Stomahesive appliance, which is cut to just fit the fistulous opening. This will allow collection and accurate measurement of the output. The use of TPN has been an important advance in the management of patients with high-output enterocutaneous fistulas and significantly decreases the incidence of malnutrition. TPN is particularly valuable in the stabilization period to help minimize high-output fistula losses and for immediate nutritional repletion while the fistula is being delineated. However, if the patient can meet calorie goals without the use of TPN, especially when a high-output fistula is not present, enteral feeding is preferable and recommended.

BOX 91.7 Treatment Strategy in Patients With an Enterocutaneous Fistula

Sepsis Control
Radiologic drainage of abscess
Relaparotomy on demand, minimally invasive if possible
Consider other infectious foci: intravenous line, urinary tract infection, pulmonary

Optimization of Nutritional Status
Rehydration and electrolyte supplementation
Enteral nutrition is preferred
Parenteral nutrition to meet calorie requirements, small bowel ECF
Allow 500 mL/day clear liquids orally

Wound Care
Gauzes for low-output ECF
Collect ECF fluids with bag (wound manager, fistula bag), paste to protect the skin
Drainage of excessive ECF fluid with sump suction
Proton pump inhibitors

Anatomy of ECF
Macroscopic
Biochemical analysis of ECF fluid (bilirubin/amylase)
Methylene blue
Preoperatively: fistulography or contrast CT; length of intestine and localization of origin of ECF, stenosis, obstruction, and fluid collection

Timing of Surgery
Clinically stable (above)
Psychologically willing to undergo surgery
Albumin >25 g/L
Period of convalescence >6 weeks

Surgical Strategy
One-stage procedure
Careful adhesiolysis
Wedge excision of intestinal resection
Limit number of anastomoses to minimum
Cover sutures with healthy, viable tissue
Keep away from compromised area

ECF, Enterocutaneous fistula.
Adapted from Visschers RG, van Gemert WG, Winkens B, et al. Guided treatment improves outcome of patients with enterocutaneous fistulas. *World J Surg.* 2012;36:2341-2348.

Staging and supportive care. When sepsis has been controlled and nutritional therapy has been instituted, the fistula must be adequately staged. The combined use of fluoroscopic contrast studies, fistulography if necessary, and CT, along with the patient's clinical behavior, will characterize the anatomy and underlying pathology of the fistula. Some have advocated conservative management for up to 3 months to allow spontaneous closure. However, others have shown that after sepsis is controlled, more than 90% of small intestinal fistulas that closed did so within 1 month. Less than 10% of the fistulas closed after 2 months, and none closed spontaneously after 3 months. In one large retrospective study, the majority of enterocutaneous fistulas closed spontaneously (54%), whereas 18% needed definitive surgery at a later time. Operative mortality was 9.8%, and recurrence rate was 8%. Uncomplicated proximal fistulas have higher spontaneous closure

rates, with duodenal fistulas closing within 2 to 4 weeks. Therefore, a reasonable management plan would be to follow a 6-week period of convalescence, at which time, if closure has not been obtained, surgical management should be considered if the preoperative albumin level is above 25 g/L. However, knowledge that spontaneous closure is unlikely should not prompt immediate reexploration at 8 weeks. In general, a period of 3 to 6 months is beneficial to allow the profound inflammatory response associated with intraabdominal sepsis to subside completely and for the adhesion formation to stabilize. This period will provide a better opportunity for safe and successful operative intervention. Furthermore, as is the case with enteroatmospheric small bowel fistulas, it may take several months to stabilize the complex abdominal wound associated with the fistula.

Several adjuncts have been proposed to help assist in spontaneous fistula closure and management of the associated abdominal wound, although none are supported by vigorous level I data. Studies suggest that bowel rest with TPN therapy improves fistula closure rates and time to closure in patients with high-output fistulas. Low-output fistulas can successfully be managed with enteral therapy while avoiding the known complications of parenteral therapy. Dysmotility agents such as loperamide and codeine can also assist with attempts at enteral therapy. Furthermore, newer techniques, such as fistuloclysis, in which the distal limb of a proximal fistula is intubated and enteral therapy is delivered to the distal bowel, have proved effective. Several randomized trials have evaluated the role of octreotide in the management of fistulas. Although octreotide has been shown to decrease fistula output, which can be useful in the presence of a high-output fistula, it has not convincingly provided an improvement in spontaneous closure rates. Vacuum devices are valuable in the setting of enteroatmospheric fistulas to help contract the open abdominal wound around the associated fistula. Care should be given to avoid direct contact with visceral contents, as this can cause new fistulas. Skin grafting up to the fistula has also been used in cases associated with an open abdomen, with a graft success rate of up to 80% in some series. Importantly, patients who could not be discharged before definitive repair also have higher mortality risk.

Definitive management. If the fistula persists despite adequately addressing the patient's nutritional, fluid, and wound care needs, reoperative intervention will ultimately be necessary for some patients. Surgery is most easily accomplished by entering the previous abdominal wound, with great care taken to avoid further damage to adherent bowel. The preferred operation is fistula tract excision and segmental resection of the involved segment of intestine and reanastomosis. Simple closure of the fistula after removal of the fistula tract almost always results in fistula recurrence. If an unexpected abscess is encountered or if the bowel wall is rigid and distended over a long distance, thus making primary anastomosis unsafe, exteriorization of both ends of the intestine should be accomplished. Various bypass procedures have also been described as part of a staged approach in which exclusion of the segment containing the fistula is accomplished in the first reoperation, and then another operation is required for resection of the involved segment and fistula tract. Although this may be necessary in extreme circumstances, this is certainly not the preferred surgical management. Basic surgical considerations include attempting a one-stage procedure, careful adhesiolysis, addressing compromised tissues with wedge excision or intestinal resection, covering sutures with viable tissues, and avoiding friable areas that are not directly involved with the fistula.

In summary, enterocutaneous fistulas occur most commonly as a result of a previous operative procedure. Once identified, a three-phase approach of stabilization, staging, and supportive care and, in some cases, definitive surgical intervention is necessary. Most of these fistulas heal spontaneously within 6 weeks. If closure is not achieved after 6 weeks, surgery is indicated.

Pneumatosis Intestinalis

Pneumatosis intestinalis is an uncommon condition manifesting as multiple gas-filled cysts of the gastrointestinal tract. The cysts may be located in the subserosa, submucosa, and, rarely, muscularis layer and vary in size from microscopic to several centimeters in diameter. They can occur anywhere along the gastrointestinal tract, from the esophagus to the rectum; however, they are most common in the jejunum, followed by the ileocecal region and colon. Extraintestinal structures such as mesentery, peritoneum, and the falciform ligament may also be involved. There is an equal incidence in males and females, and the condition usually occurs in the fourth to seventh decades of life. Pneumatosis in neonates is usually associated with necrotizing enterocolitis. The cause of pneumatosis intestinalis has not been completely delineated. A number of theories have been proposed; mechanical, mucosal damage, bacterial, and pulmonary hypotheses seem to be the most plausible.

There are two forms of pneumatosis intestinalis. Primary pneumatosis (15%) is a benign idiopathic condition that is not associated with any other conditions or symptoms and is found incidentally. The majority of pneumatosis intestinalis cases (85%) are "secondary" and can be associated with a multitude of other local and systemic factors such as chronic obstructive pulmonary disease, autoimmune diseases, malignancies, obstructive pathologies, infections, and trauma.

Upon gross inspection, the cysts resemble cystic lymphangiomas or hydatid cysts. On histologic section, the involved portion has a honeycomb appearance. The cysts are thin walled and break easily. Spontaneous rupture gives rise to pneumoperitoneum.

Symptoms are nonspecific and, in pneumatosis associated with other disorders, may be those of the associated disease. Symptoms in primary pneumatosis intestinalis are rare, but when present, usually include diarrhea, abdominal pain, abdominal distention, nausea, vomiting, weight loss, and mucus in stools. Hematochezia and constipation have also been described. Pneumatosis intestinalis represents one of the few cases of sterile pneumoperitoneum and should be considered in the patient with free abdominal air but no evidence of peritonitis. However, pneumatosis intestinalis is an ominous sign when associated with peritonitis, mesenteric gas, or portovenous gas, as this is most concerning for life-threatening small bowel ischemia.

The diagnosis is usually made radiographically by plain abdominal or CT studies. On plain films, pneumatosis intestinalis appears as radiolucent areas within the bowel wall, which must be differentiated from luminal intestinal gas (Fig. 91.15A). The radiolucency may be linear or curvilinear or appear as grapelike clusters or tiny bubbles. CT is the gold standard for diagnosis and can help elucidate any causative etiology (see Fig. 91.15B). Visualization of intestinal cysts has also been described by ultrasound.

No treatment is necessary unless one of the complications supervenes, such as small bowel ischemia, rectal bleeding, cyst-induced volvulus, or tension pneumoperitoneum. Prognosis in most patients is that of the underlying disease, but in most studies the presence of peritonitis is a strongly negative predictive factor. The important point is to recognize that pneumatosis intestinalis is a radiographic finding and not a diagnosis. Treatment should be directed at the underlying cause of the pneumatosis, and surgical intervention should be predicated on the clinical course of the patient.[46]

Blind Loop Syndrome

Blind loop syndrome is a rare condition manifested by diarrhea, steatorrhea, megaloblastic anemia, weight loss, abdominal pain, and deficiencies of the fat-soluble vitamins as well as neurologic disorders. The underlying cause of this syndrome is bacterial

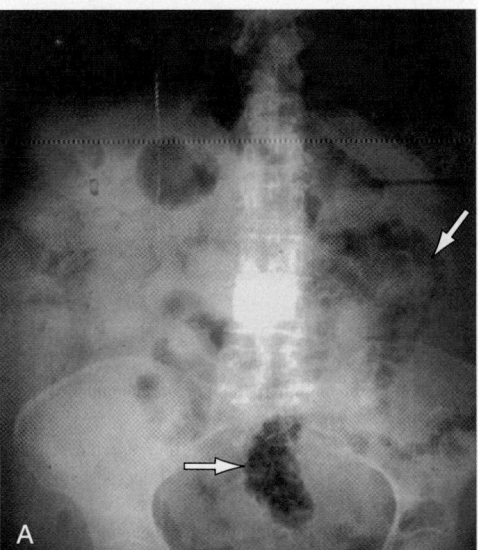
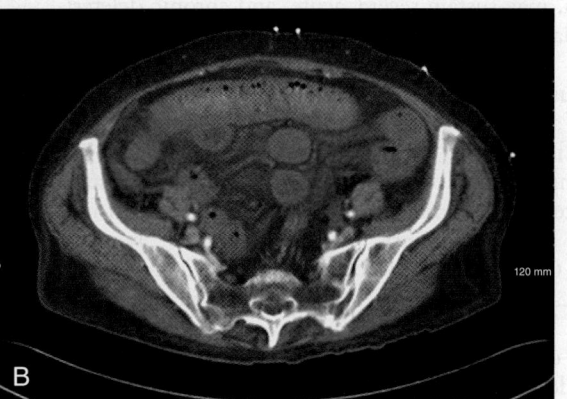

FIGURE 91.15 Pneumatosis intestinalis. (A) Plain abdominal film demonstrates pneumatosis intestinalis *(arrows)*. (B) CT findings consistent with curvilinear radiolucency appearing as tiny bubbles in the antimesenteric border of the bowel consistent with pneumatosis intestinalis. (A, Courtesy Dr. Melvyn H. Schreiber, The University of Texas Medical Branch, Galveston, TX. B, Courtesy Dr. Kristin Long, University of Kentucky Medical Center, Lexington, KY.)

overgrowth in stagnant areas of the small bowel produced by stricture, stenosis, fistulas, or diverticula (e.g., jejunoileal or Meckel diverticulum). Under normal circumstances, the upper gastrointestinal tract contains fewer than 10^3 bacteria/mL, mostly gram-positive aerobes and facultative anaerobes. However, with stasis, the number of bacteria increases, with excessive proliferation of aerobic and anaerobic bacteria; *Bacteroides,* anaerobic lactobacilli, coliforms, and enterococci are likely to be present in varying numbers. The bacteria compete for dietary vitamin B_{12}, producing a systemic deficiency of vitamin B_{12} and megaloblastic anemia.

The syndrome can be confirmed by a series of laboratory investigations. Bacterial overgrowth can be diagnosed with cultures obtained through an intestinal tube or by indirect tests such as carbohydrate breath tests, which detect substrates produced by bacteria, such as hydrogen from lactulose. Historically, after bacterial overgrowth and steatorrhea were confirmed, the Schilling test (^{57}Co-labeled vitamin B_{12} absorption) would be performed, which would reveal a pattern of urinary excretion of vitamin B_{12} resembling that of pernicious anemia (a urinary loss of 0%–6% of vitamin B_{12} compared with the normal of 7%–25%). In patients with blind loop syndrome, vitamin B_{12} excretion is not altered by the addition of intrinsic factor, but a course of a broad-spectrum antibiotic (e.g., tetracycline) should return vitamin B_{12} absorption to normal. Although previously in common use, the Shilling test is no longer used today.

Treatment of patients with blind loop syndrome includes parenteral vitamin B_{12} therapy and broad-spectrum antibiotics. Tetracyclines have been the mainstay of treatment, but studies have shown that rifaximin and metronidazole demonstrate less resistance and are also effective. For most patients, a single course of therapy (7–10 days) is sufficient, and the patient may remain symptom free for months. Prokinetic agents have been used without real success. Surgical correction of the condition causing stagnation and blind loop syndrome produces a permanent cure and is indicated for patients who require multiple rounds of antibiotics or are receiving continuous therapy.

Radiation Enteritis

Radiation therapy is generally used as adjuvant therapy for various abdominal and pelvic cancers. In addition to tumor cells, however, other rapidly dividing cells in normal tissues may be affected by radiation. Surrounding normal tissue, such as the small intestinal epithelium, may sustain severe, acute, and chronic deleterious effects. Radiation injury to the small bowel can be subdivided into acute and chronic forms. Acute radiation-induced small bowel disease usually manifests with colicky abdominal pain, bloating, loss of appetite, nausea, diarrhea, and fecal urgency during or shortly after a course of radiotherapy. Most patients notice symptoms during the third week of treatment, and these resolve 2 to 6 weeks after completion of radiation. Symptoms consistent with chronic radiation injury typically develop between 18 months and 6 years after a completed course of radiotherapy, but symptoms can be present up to 30 years after the treatment course.

The amount of radiation appears to correlate with the probability for the development of radiation enteritis. Serious late complications are unusual if the total radiation dosage is less than 4000 cGy; morbidity risk increases with dosages exceeding 5000 cGy. Other factors, including previous abdominal surgeries, preexisting vascular disease, hypertension, diabetes, and adjuvant treatment with certain chemotherapeutic agents (such as 5-FU,

doxorubicin, dactinomycin, and MTX), contribute to the development of enteritis after radiation treatments. A previous history of laparotomy increases the risk for enteritis, presumably because of adhesions that fix portions of the small bowel into the irradiated field. Radiation damage leads to symptoms of diarrhea, abdominal pain, and malabsorption. The late effects of radiation injury are the result of damage to small submucosal blood vessels, with a progressive obliterative arteritis and submucosal fibrosis; these events eventually result in thrombosis and vascular insufficiency. This injury may produce necrosis and perforation of the involved intestine, but more commonly leads to stricture formation with symptoms of obstruction or small bowel fistulas.

Multiple strategies are used to reduce radiation injury to the small bowel (Box 91.8). Radiation enteritis may be minimized by adjusting ports and dosages of radiation to deliver optimal treatment specifically to the tumor and not to surrounding tissues. Placement of radiopaque markers, such as titanium clips, at the time of the original operation facilitates better targeting of the radiation treatment. A reduction in field size, multiple field arrangements, conformal radiotherapy techniques, and intensity-modulated radiotherapy can reduce toxicity related to radiotherapy. Methods designed to exclude the small bowel from the irradiated field include reperitonealization, omental transposition, and placement of absorbable mesh slings.

Various pharmacologic interventions have also been described to reduce the side effects of radiation enteritis. Angiotensin-converting enzyme inhibitors and statins significantly reduce acute gastrointestinal symptoms during radical pelvic radiotherapy. Sucralfate, a highly sulfated polyanionic disaccharide thought to stimulate epithelial healing and thereby form a protective barrier over damaged mucosal surfaces, may help in the treatment of bleeding from radiation proctitis, but no evidence exists supporting its use in the prevention of radiation-induced small bowel disease. Superoxide dismutase, a free radical scavenger, has been used successfully to reduce complications. Other compounds that have been evaluated include glutathione, antioxidants (e.g., vitamin A, vitamin E, beta-carotene), histamine antagonists, and the combination of pentoxifylline and tocopherols, a class of chemical compounds with vitamin E activity. There is currently a double-blind randomized controlled trial investigating the use of probiotics as a radioprotective agent for the gut. Amifostine (WR-2721), a sulfhydryl compound that is converted intracellularly to an active metabolite, WR-1065, which in turn binds to free radicals,

---

> ### BOX 91.8 Prevention of Radiation-Induced Small Bowel Disease
>
> **Clinical Guidance**
>
> Use of modern imaging and radiotherapy techniques to minimize radiation exposure to normal tissues
>
> Consideration of circadian rhythm effects and use of evening radiotherapy sessions
>
> Continuation of angiotensin-converting enzyme inhibitors and statins and consideration of their introduction if appropriate
>
> Consideration of the use of probiotics
>
> Consideration of surgical techniques to minimize radiation exposure to the small bowel if appropriate and surgical team is experienced and competent at the procedure involved

Adapted from Stacey R, Green JT. Radiation-induced small bowel disease: latest developments and clinical guidance. *Ther Adv Chronic Dis.* 2014;5:15-29.

has also been used to protect the cell from radiation injury. Glutamine has been found to offer little benefit, even when it is used before or during radiation therapy.

The treatment of acute radiation enteritis is directed at controlling symptoms. Antispasmodics and analgesics may alleviate abdominal pain and cramping, and diarrhea usually responds to opiates or other antidiarrheal agents. The use of corticosteroids for acute radiation enteritis is of uncertain value. Dietary manipulation, including oral elemental diets, has also been advocated to ameliorate the acute effects of radiation enteritis; however, results are conflicting. Antibiotics are frequently used in the setting of bacterial overgrowth. Bile acid malabsorption, thought to be partially responsible for diarrheal symptoms in some patients with radiation-induced small bowel disease, responds well to cholestyramine, but it is not well tolerated, and many patients voluntarily discontinue use.

Approximately 30% of patients with radiation enteritis will require operative intervention.[47] Indications for operation include obstruction, fistula formation, perforation, and bleeding, with obstruction being the most common presentation. Operative procedures include a bypass or resection with reanastomosis. Previously, bypass was strongly advocated for as a safer procedure and reduces the risk of anastomotic leaks. However, recent studies have demonstrated resection with reanastomosis is safe if an appropriate resection of diseased bowel is performed. In patients presenting with obstruction, extensive lysis of adhesions should be avoided. Obstruction caused by rigid, fixed intestinal loops in the pelvis is best bypassed. If resection and reanastomosis are planned, at least one end of the anastomosis should be from intestine outside the irradiated field. Macroscopic inspection may not be accurate in evaluating the full extent of radiation damage. Frozen section and laser Doppler flowmetry techniques have been used to assist resection and anastomosis. Perforation of the intestine should be treated with resection and anastomosis. When reanastomosis is thought to be unsafe, the ends should be exteriorized.

Short Bowel Syndrome

Short bowel syndrome results from a total small bowel length that is inadequate to support nutrition. Short bowel syndrome occurs mostly from massive intestinal resection (i.e., midgut volvulus, mesenteric occlusion, traumatic disruption of the superior mesenteric vessels) or multiple sequential resections (i.e., patients with Crohn disease). In neonates, the most common causes of short bowel syndrome are bowel resection secondary to necrotizing enterocolitis and intestinal malformations. The clinical hallmarks of short bowel syndrome include diarrhea, fluid and electrolyte deficiency, and malnutrition. Other complications include an increased incidence of gallstones caused by disruption of the enterohepatic circulation and of nephrolithiasis from hyperoxaluria. Specific nutrient deficiencies must be prevented, and levels must be monitored closely; these nutrients include iron, magnesium, zinc, copper, and vitamins. The likelihood that a patient with short bowel syndrome will be permanently dependent on TPN is thought to be primarily influenced by the length, location, and health of the remaining intestine. In patients with short bowel syndrome, postabsorptive levels of plasma citrulline, a nonprotein amino acid produced by intestinal mucosa, may provide an indicator to differentiate transient from permanent intestinal failure.

The bowel has a remarkable capacity to adapt after small bowel resection; in many cases, this process of intestinal adaptation, termed *adaptive hyperplasia,* effectively prevents severe complications that result from the markedly decreased surface area available for absorption and digestion. However, any adaptive mechanism can be overwhelmed, and adaptation can be inadequate if too much small bowel is lost. Although there is considerable individual variation, resection of up to 70% of the small bowel usually can be tolerated if the terminal ileum and ileocecal valve are preserved. Length alone, however, is not the only determining factor of complications related to small bowel resection. For example, if the distal two-thirds of the ileum, including the ileocecal valve, is resected, significant abnormalities of absorption of bile salts and vitamin B_{12} may occur, resulting in diarrhea and anemia, although only 25% of the total length of the small bowel has been removed. Proximal bowel resection is tolerated better than distal resection because the ileum can adapt and increase its absorptive capacity more efficiently than the jejunum.

Treatment

The most important issue to remember about short bowel syndrome is prevention. In patients with Crohn disease, limiting bowel resections to only segments with a particular complication should be performed. In addition, during surgery for problems related to intestinal ischemia, the smallest possible resection should be performed, and if necessary, second-look operations should be carried out to allow the ischemic bowel to demarcate, thus potentially preventing unnecessary extensive resection of the bowel.

After massive small bowel resection, the treatment course may be divided into early and late phases. In its early phase, treatment is primarily directed at the control of diarrhea, replacement of fluid and electrolytes, and prompt institution of TPN in patients who cannot safely tolerate enteral feedings. Volume losses may exceed 5 L/day, and vigorous monitoring of intake and output with adequate replacement must be carried out. Diarrhea in this early phase can be caused by a multitude of sources. For example, hypergastrinemia and gastric hypersecretion occur after massive small bowel resection and can significantly contribute to diarrhea after a massive small bowel resection. Acid hypersecretion can be managed by H_2 receptor antagonists or proton pump inhibitors, such as omeprazole. Diarrhea may also be caused by ileal resection, resulting in disruption of the enterohepatic circulation and excessive amounts of bile salts entering the colon. Cholestyramine may be beneficial when diarrhea is related to the cathartic effects of unabsorbed bile salts in the colon. In addition, the judicious use of agents that inhibit gut motility (e.g., codeine, diphenoxylate) may be helpful. The long-acting SSA octreotide also appears to reduce the amount of diarrhea during the early phase of short bowel syndrome; however, it has an inhibitory effect on gut adaptation and is not generally recommended, particularly early during the gut adaptation period.

As soon as the patient has recovered from the acute phase, enteral nutrition should be started. Controversy exists about the optimal diet for these patients. Many different restrictive diets have been trialed, including purely elemental diets, high-carbohydrate, high-protein, and low-fat, without universal success. It is recommended to tailor the diet to the patient with consideration of their remaining anatomy, as different resections will have different absorptive deficits.[48] For example, in patients who retained their colon, a high-carbohydrate and low-fat diet is beneficial, whereas for patients without their colon (i.e., end jejunostomy), a low-fat diet is not beneficial. Guidelines suggest a focus on maintaining a patient's compensatory hyperphagia with at least a 50% increase in their estimated caloric needs split into small meals throughout the day. Vitamins, especially fat-soluble vitamins, as well as calcium, magnesium, and zinc supplementation should be provided. The roles of hormones administered systemically and glutamine administered enterally have been evaluated. The hormones neurotensin, growth hormone, bombesin, and glucagon-like peptide-2 (GLP-2) have demonstrated marked mucosal growth in a variety of experimental studies and have been shown to prevent gut atrophy associated with TPN in experimental studies; combination therapy appears more efficacious than single-agent administration. Randomized controlled trials showed that teduglutide, a GLP-2 analogue that is resistant to degradation by the proteolytic enzyme dipeptidyl peptidase 4 and therefore has a longer half-life than natural GLP-2, is well tolerated and led to the restoration of intestinal functional and structural integrity through significant intestinotrophic and proabsorptive effects. It is the first targeted therapeutic agent to gain approval for use in short bowel syndrome in both pediatric and adult patients with intestinal failure.

Two other hormones, not derived from the gut, that have been evaluated extensively in various experimental and limited clinical trials include growth hormone. Although trials demonstrated the use of growth hormone may show some benefit in terms of body weight, lean body mass, and absorptive capacity, it is no longer recommended for use in this population because of side effects and poor long-term efficacy.

The first step in terms of surgical intervention is to restore digestive continuity, which can be accomplished by the reversal of a proximal stoma to reduce rates of dehydration. A number of surgical strategies have been attempted in patients who are chronically TPN dependent, with limited success; these include procedures to delay intestinal transit time, methods to increase absorptive area, and small bowel transplantation. Methods to delay intestinal transit time include the construction of various valves and sphincters, with inconsistent results reported. Antiperistaltic segments of small intestine have been constructed to slow the transit, thus allowing additional contact time for nutrient and fluid absorption. Moderate successes have been described with this technique. Other procedures, including colonic interposition, recirculating loops of small bowel, and retrograde electrical pacing, have been tried but were found to be unsuccessful in humans and were largely abandoned. Surgical procedures to increase absorptive area include the intestinal tapering and lengthening procedure (e.g., Bianchi procedure), which improves intestinal function by correcting the dilation and ineffective peristalsis of the remaining intestine and by doubling the intestinal length while preserving the mucosal surface area. Serial transverse enteroplasty creates staple lines parallel to the mesenteric blood supply on alternating sides to create a channel of intestine that is both longer and smaller in diameter. This technique also increases the surface area of bowel for nutritional absorption. Although beneficial in selected patients, potential complications can include necrosis of divided segments because of poor vasculature, stenosis from smaller caliber of bowel, and anastomotic leaks.

Intestinal transplantation remains the standard of care for patients for whom intestinal rehabilitation attempts have failed and who are at risk of life-threatening complications of TPN; these include impending liver failure, thrombosis of more than two major access veins, frequent severe line infections, and dehydration. Patient survival after intestinal transplantation has significantly improved with the use of the immunosuppressive agents alemtuzumab and tacrolimus and transplantation at a high

volume center (≥10 grafts per year). The 5-year survival rates for isolated intestinal transplantation are over 65%. The challenges of small bowel transplantation continue to require better immunosuppression and earlier detection of rejection.

Vascular Compression of the Duodenum

Vascular compression of the duodenum, also known as *superior mesenteric artery syndrome* or *Wilkie syndrome,* is a rare condition characterized by compression of the third portion of the duodenum by the superior mesenteric artery as it passes over this portion of the duodenum. Symptoms include profound nausea and vomiting, abdominal distention, weight loss, and postprandial epigastric pain, which varies from intermittent to constant, depending on the severity of the duodenal obstruction. Weight loss usually occurs before the onset of symptoms and contributes to the syndrome.

This syndrome is most commonly seen in young asthenic individuals, with females more commonly affected than males. Predisposing factors for vascular compression of the duodenum, aside from weight loss, include supine immobilization, scoliosis, and placement of a body cast, sometimes called the *cast syndrome.* An association between vascular compression of the duodenum and peptic ulcer has been observed. Vascular compression of the duodenum has been reported in association with anorexia nervosa and after proctocolectomy and J-pouch anal anastomosis, resection of an arteriovenous malformation of the cervical cord, abdominal aortic aneurysm repair, and orthopedic procedures, usually spinal surgery.

Diagnosis of this condition is made by a barium upper gastrointestinal series, which demonstrates abrupt or near-total cessation of flow of barium from the duodenum to the jejunum. CT imaging is used to establish the angle of the superior mesenteric artery coming off the aorta. Conservative measures should be tried initially and have been increasingly successful as definitive treatment. The main component of conservative management is nutrition. Operative management may include duodenojejunostomy, gastrojejunostomy to bypass the obstructing segment, or duodenal derotation (Strong procedure).

SELECTED REFERENCES

Aka AA, Wright JP, DeBeche-Adams T. Small bowel obstruction. *Clin Colon Rectal Surg.* 2021;34:(4):219-226.

> This article provides an extensive review of the diagnosis and management of small bowel obstructions, a clinical phenomenon that is common in all surgical practices.

Caplin ME, Pavel M, Cwikla JB, et al. Lanreotide in metastatic enteropancreatic neuroendocrine tumors. *N Engl J Med.* 2014;371 (3):224-233.

> The landmark CLARINET trial (Lanreotide Antiproliferative Response in patients with GEP-NET) is the largest phase III, randomized, double-blind, placebo-controlled, multinational study that evaluated the antiproliferative effect of the somatostatin analogue lanreotide in patients with GEP-NETs. Lanreotide was associated with significantly prolonged progression-free survival among patients with grade 1 or 2 metastatic enteropancreatic NETs.

Crohn BB, Ginzburg L, Oppenheimer GD. Regional ileitis - a pathologic and clinical entity. *JAMA*. 1932;99:1323-1329.

This landmark paper succinctly crystallizes the clinical course, differential diagnosis, and pathologic findings of regional ileitis in young adults. Although other terms have been applied to this disease process, based on the descriptions in this classic paper, Crohn disease has been universally accepted as the name.

Cushing K, Higgins PDR. Management of Crohn disease – reply. *JAMA*. 2021;325 (17):1794-1795.

This is a comprehensive yet concise review of Crohn disease, including presentation, diagnostic evaluation, induction, and maintenance therapy.

Tropeano G, Di Grezia M, Puccioni C, et al. The spectrum of pneumatosis intestinalis in the adult. A surgical dilemma. *World J Gastrointest Surg*. 2023;15(4):553-565.

This review highlights the diagnostic evaluation of patients with the radiographic finding of pneumatosis intestinalis, a finding that ranges from completely benign to a life-threatening disease process. As such, every surgeon should be familiar with the evaluation of a patient with this finding.

The full reference list appears on Elsevier eBooks+.

92 CHAPTER

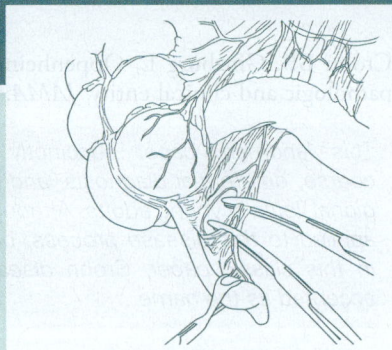

Exocrine Pancreas

Alykhan M. Premji and Timothy R. Donahue

▶ **Please access Elsevier eBooks+ to view the videos for this chapter.**

ANATOMY

The average pancreas weighs around 100 g and, in the adult, measures 14 to 20 cm in length. It lies in the retroperitoneum just anterior to the first lumbar vertebra and is anatomically divided into five sections, the head, uncinate, neck, body, and tail. The head lies to the right of midline within the C loop of the duodenum, immediately anterior to the vena cava at the confluence of the renal veins. The uncinate process extends from the head of the pancreas behind the superior mesenteric vein (SMV) and terminates adjacent to the superior mesenteric artery (SMA). The neck is the short segment of pancreas that immediately overlies the SMV. The body and tail of the pancreas then extend across the midline, anterior to Gerota fascia and slightly cephalad, terminating within the splenic hilum (Fig. 92.1).

Arterial Blood Supply

The pancreas is supplied by a complex arterial network arising from the celiac trunk and SMA. It can be divided into two main regions: the head and the body/tail of the pancreas. There can be several arterial variations, with the conventional anatomy being the most common. The gastroduodenal artery (GDA) provides the main arterial supply to the pancreatic head. The tributaries of the gastroduodenal artery, the anterior and posterior superior pancreatoduodenal arteries, supply the respective aspects of the pancreatic head. They branch and form arcades with tributaries of

the SMA (the anterior and posterior inferior pancreatoduodenal arteries). These arterial arcades are located in the soft tissue of the pancreatoduodenal groove, at the bottom of the natural crevice between the duodenal wall and the anterior or posterior pancreatic surface, respectively. The inferior pancreaticoduodenal artery arises from SMA and also divides into anterior and posterior branches as it runs superiorly within the pancreaticoduodenal groove. It is often visible as a plexus of arterial vessels in the mediocaudal aspect of the pancreatic head.

The splenic artery provides the blood supply to the body and tail of the pancreas. It has several main branches (dorsal, inferior, and greater pancreatic arteries), which form an anastomosing network around the pancreatic body and tail up to the neck of the pancreas. At the neck, communicating anastomoses between the splenic and pancreatoduodenal arterial systems commonly occur. The greater pancreatic artery, a large tributary of the splenic artery, penetrates the pancreas and provides branches that run parallel to the main pancreatic duct (MPD) and form anastomoses with the other tributaries of the splenic artery. The interlobular and intralobular arteries extend as branches of the greater pancreatic artery.

Venous Drainage

The venous drainage parallels the arterial supply, with blood flow from the head of the pancreas draining into the anterior and posterior pancreaticoduodenal veins. The posterior superior pancreaticoduodenal vein enters the SMV laterally at the superior border of the neck of the pancreas. The anterior superior pancreaticoduodenal vein enters the right gastroepiploic vein just before its confluence with the SMV at the inferior border of the pancreas. The

Blood supply of the pancreas

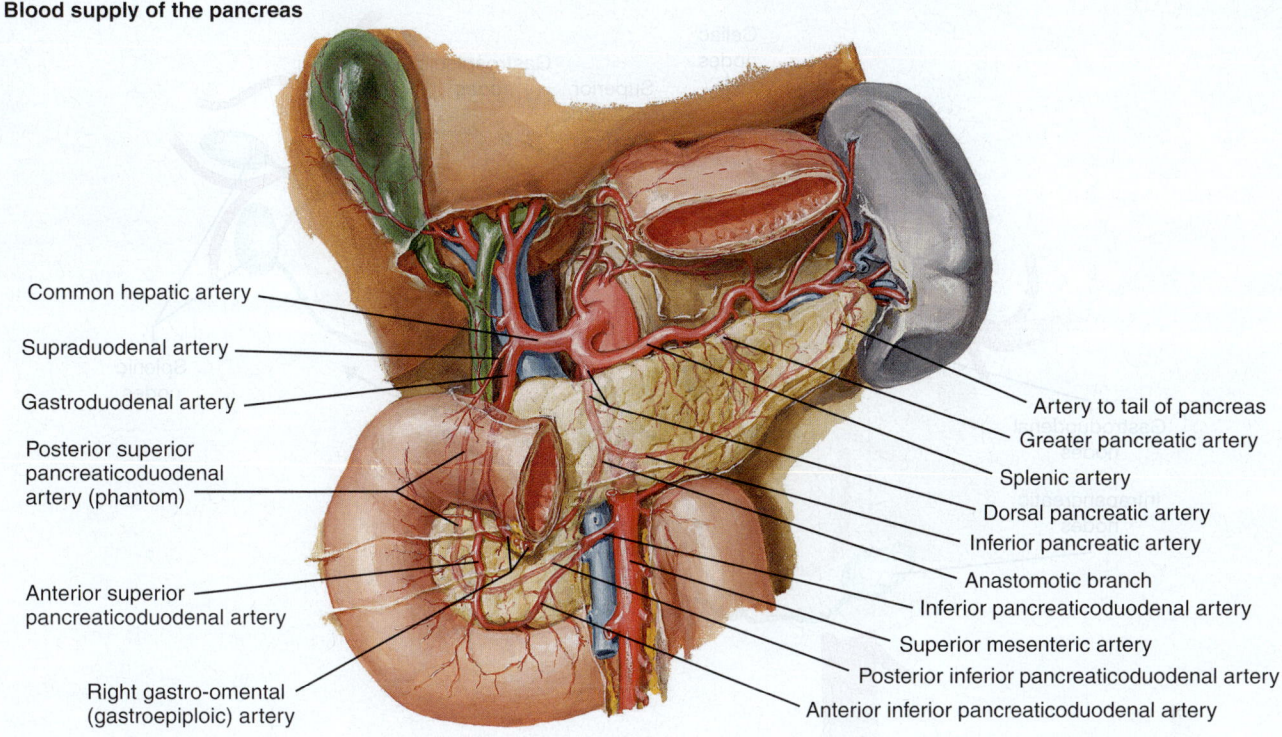

FIGURE 92.1 Anatomy. (Netter illustration from www.netterimages.com. Copyright Elsevier Inc. All rights reserved.)

anterior and posterior inferior pancreaticoduodenal veins enter the SMV along the inferior border of the uncinate process. The remaining body and tail are drained through the splenic venous system.

Lymphatic Drainage

Understanding the lymphatic drainage of the pancreas is paramount to performing an appropriate oncologic resection. The pancreas can be thought of as having four quadrants of primary drainage. The tissue in the left side of the gland drains to lymph nodes in the splenic hilum or gastrosplenic omentum via lymphatics along the superior and inferior border of the pancreas. Small lymph nodes are present along this drainage pathway. Tissue in the right side of the gland drains superiorly to gastroduodenal lymph nodes and inferiorly to infrapancreatic lymph nodes. Again, small lymph nodes are present along these lymphatic channels. These four pathways form a "ring" around the border of the pancreas. A secondary drainage pathway occurs via retropancreatic lymph nodes located anterior to the aorta between the celiac and SMA. These lymph nodes can receive drainage either directly from the pancreatic tissue (first-order lymph nodes) or from the "ring" (second order).[1] A schematic of this drainage is shown in Fig. 92.2.

Innervation

The pancreas is innervated by both the sympathetic (through splanchnic nerves) and parasympathetic (via the vagus nerve) nervous systems. The sympathetic nerve fibers originate from the neural bodies in the thoracic region of the spinal cord and connect with neurons in the abdominal plexus (e.g., the celiac node). The postganglionic fibers from these neurons follow the arterial routes to the pancreas. Meanwhile, the parasympathetic vagal efferent nerves end at nodes within the pancreatic tissue, where their postganglionic fibers extend to the acinar cells, islets of Langerhans, and pancreatic ducts.

To alleviate pain associated with pancreatic cancer that infiltrates the celiac plexus, a local anesthetic (e.g., xylocaine) is administered directly via celiac node infiltration during endoscopic ultrasound (EUS).

Embryology

The exocrine pancreas begins development during the fourth week of gestation. Pluripotent pancreatic epithelial stem cells give rise to exocrine and endocrine cell lines as well as the intricate pancreatic ductal network. Initially, dorsal and ventral buds appear from the primitive duodenal endoderm (Fig. 92.3A). The dorsal bud typically appears first and ultimately develops into the superior head, neck, body, and tail of the mature pancreas. The ventral bud develops as part of the hepatic diverticulum and maintains communication with the biliary tree throughout development. The ventral bud will become the inferior part of the head and uncinate process of the gland. Between the fourth and eighth weeks of gestation, the ventral bud rotates posteriorly in a clockwise fashion to fuse with the dorsal bud (see Fig. 92.3B). At approximately 8 weeks of gestation, the dorsal and ventral buds are fused (see Fig. 92.3C).

The initiation of pancreas bud formation and differentiation of the ventral bud from the hepatic-biliary fates is dependent on the expression of pancreatic duodenal homeobox 1 (PDX1) protein and pancreas-specific transcription factor 1 (PTF1). In the absence of PDX1 expression in mice, pancreatic agenesis occurs, indicating its importance in the early phases of organogenesis. PTF1 expression is first detectable shortly after PDX1 in cells of the early endoderm, which will become the dorsal and ventral pancreas. By lineage analysis, 95% of acinar cells express PTF1. In PTF1 null mice, acini do not form. The notch signaling pathway

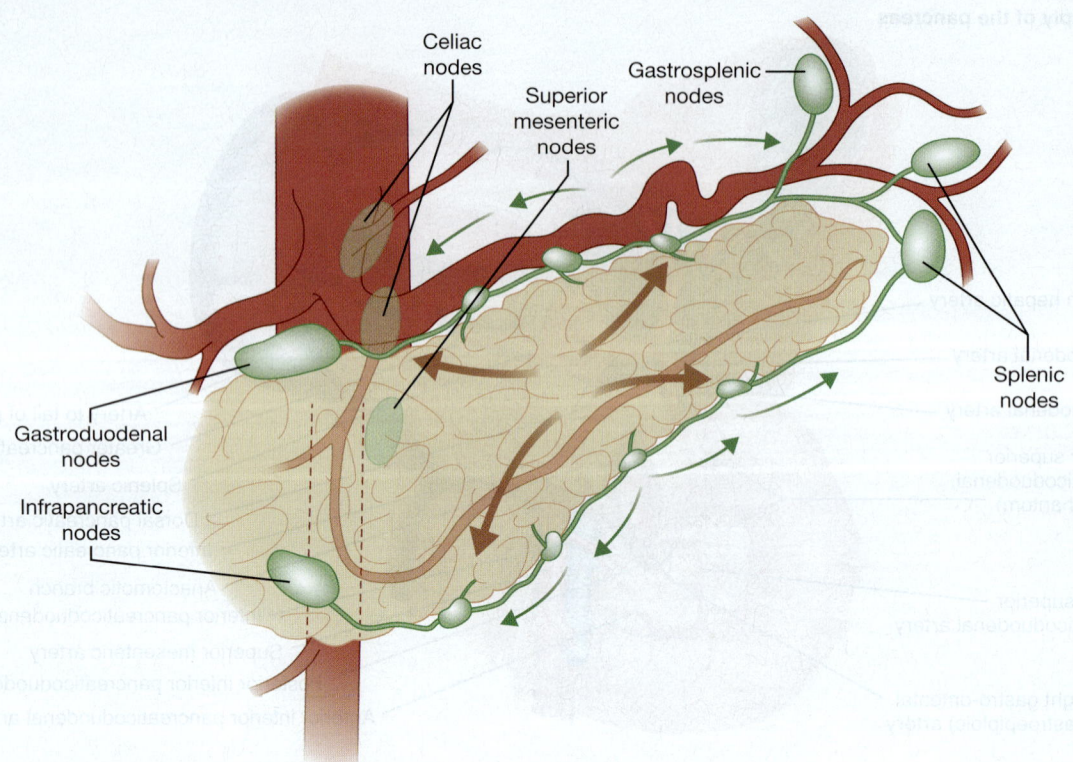

FIGURE 92.2 Lymphatic drainage of the pancreas. (Adapted from Strasberg SM, Drebin JA, Linehan D. Radical antegrade modular pancreatosplenectomy. *Surgery.* 2003;133:521-527.)

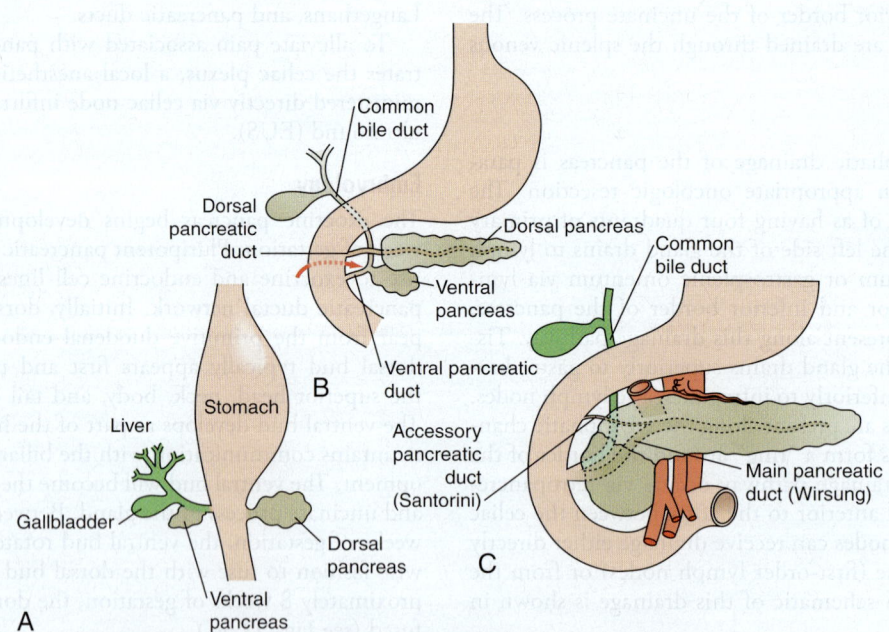

FIGURE 92.3 Embryologic development of the pancreas.

is also critical to duct and acinar differentiation. In the absence of notch signaling, embryonic cells commit to endocrine lineage, suggesting that notch signaling is vital to exocrine differentiation. In addition to PDX1, PTF1, and notch signaling, complex interactions between mesenchymal growth factors, such as transforming growth factor-β (TGF-β), and other signaling pathways, including hedgehog and Wnt, seem to play critical roles in

pancreas development.[2] The precise interactions that lead to normal organogenesis continue to be defined. Table 92.1 summarizes the factors and pathways that affect pancreas development.[2]

Pancreas Divisum

During normal organogenesis, the primitive ducts of both the dorsal and ventral buds contribute to the mature ductal system of

TABLE 92.1 Molecular Factors and Pathways Associated With Pancreatic Organogenesis

GENE	RELEVANCE
PDX1	Critical role in exocrine differentiation; knockout mice develop primitive pancreatic buds but agenesis of the organ
PTF1	Coexpression with PDX1 determines progenitor cells to pancreatic fate
Notch signaling pathway	Suppresses endocrine differentiation, promoting exocrine development via induction of Hes1 transcription factor; prolonged notch expression prevents acinar formation via RBP-Jκ binding of Ptf1a
Hedgehog	Inhibition of hedgehog in PDX1-positive cells leads to initiation of endoderm differentiation into pancreas lineage
Wnt	Complex Wnt signaling is important in all aspects of pancreas development; lack of Wnt signaling results in varying levels of pancreatic agenesis
Neurogenin 3	Repressed by notch signaling, drives endocrine lineage differentiation.
Arx and Pax-4	Arx expression favors α/PP cell differentiation, whereas Pax-4 expression favors β versus δ cell differentiation, depending on length of exposure.

Arx, Aristaless-related homeobox; Pax-4, paired box gene 4; PDX1, insulin promoter factor 1; PTF1, pancreas-specific transcription factor 1.

the pancreas. These ducts fuse together such that the proximal aspect of the dorsal duct forms the duct of Santorini, whereas the distal aspect combines with the duct of the ventral bud to form the duct of Wirsung. The duct of Wirsung is generally the major exocrine drainage pathway of the pancreas, joins the common bile duct at the ampulla of Vater, and enters the duodenum through the major papilla. The duct of Santorini may drain through a minor papilla that is more proximal in the duodenum. Failure of the dorsal and ventral ducts to fuse during embryogenesis leads to pancreas divisum, the most common congenital anomaly of the pancreas. This condition is identified by a ventral pancreatic duct and common bile duct that enter the duodenum through a major papilla, whereas a dorsal pancreatic duct enters through a minor papilla that is slightly proximal (Fig. 92.4). Because most pancreatic exocrine secretions exit through the dorsal duct, pancreas divisum can lead to a condition of partial obstruction caused by a small minor papilla, leading to chronic backpressure in the duct. This relative outflow obstruction has been implicated in the development of relapsing acute or chronic pancreatitis. Although 10% of the population is affected by pancreas divisum, only rarely do affected individuals develop pancreatitis.

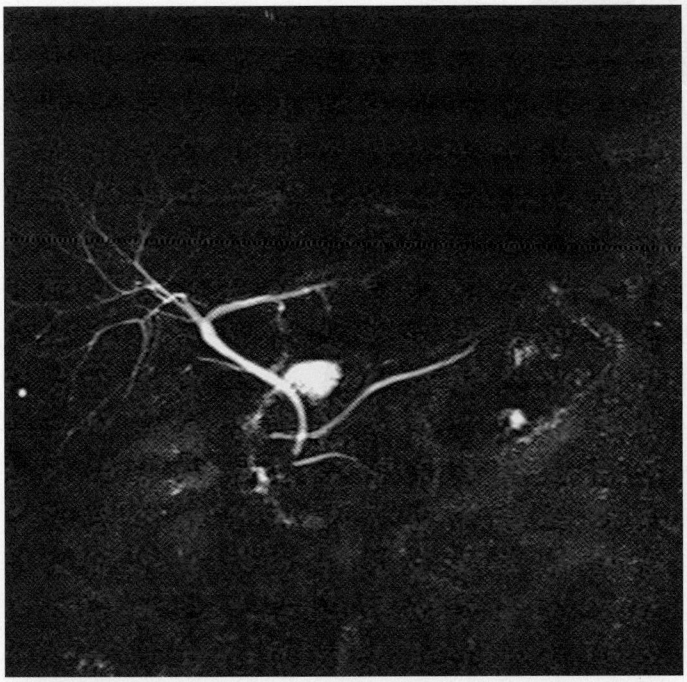

Annular Pancreas

Annular pancreas results from aberrant migration of the ventral pancreas bud, which leads to circumferential or near-circumferential pancreas tissue surrounding the second portion of the duodenum. This abnormality may be associated with other congenital defects, including Down syndrome, malrotation, intestinal atresia, and cardiac malformations. At a molecular level, formation of annular pancreas may result from reduced hedgehog signaling.[3] If symptoms of obstruction occur, surgical bypass through duodenojejunostomy is performed instead of dividing the pancreatic tissue because this annular pancreas has a pancreatic duct, and its division will likely lead to pancreatic fistula formation.

Ectopic Pancreas

Ectopic pancreas may arise anywhere along the primitive foregut but is most common in the stomach, duodenum, and Meckel diverticulum. Clinically, ectopic nodules may result in bowel obstruction caused by intussusception, bleeding, or ulceration. They can sometimes be found incidentally as firm yellow nodules that arise from the submucosa. Although there have been rare case reports of adenocarcinoma arising in ectopic pancreas tissue, resection is not necessary unless symptoms occur.

PHYSIOLOGY

The human pancreas is a complex gland with endocrine and exocrine functions. It is mainly composed of acinar cells (85% of the gland) and islet cells (2%) embedded in a complex extracellular matrix, which composes 10% of the gland. The remaining 3% to 4% of the gland is composed of the epithelial duct system and blood vessels.

Major Components of Pancreatic Juice

The main function of the exocrine pancreas is to provide most of the enzymes needed for alimentary digestion. The cells responsible for the synthesis and secretion of these enzymes are grouped into an acinus. These acinar cells have a characteristic pyramidal shape, with a wide basophilic basal portion in contact with vessels and nerves and a narrow acidophilic apical portion that opens onto a duct where enzymes can be released. Acinar cells synthesize many enzymes that digest food proteins, such as trypsin, chymotrypsin, carboxypeptidase, and elastase. Under physiologic conditions, acinar cells synthesize these proteases as inactive proenzymes that are

FIGURE 92.4. MRCP showing pancreas divisum, with the dorsal pancreatic duct draining through the minor papilla and the ventral pancreatic duct joining the biliary tree draining through the major papilla. MRCP, Magnetic resonance cholangiopancreatography.

stored as intracellular zymogen granules. With stimulation of the pancreas, these proenzymes are secreted into the pancreatic duct and, eventually, the duodenal lumen. The duodenal mucosa expresses enterokinase on its brush boarder, which catalyzes the enzymatic activation of trypsin from trypsinogen.[4] Trypsin also plays an important role in protein digestion by propagating pancreatic enzyme activation through autoactivation of trypsinogen and other proenzymes, such as chymotrypsinogen, procarboxypeptidase, and proelastase. Fig. 92.5 summarizes the mechanisms of pancreatic exocrine secretion.

In addition to protease production, acinar cells also produce pancreatic amylase and lipase, also known as *glycerol ester hydrolase,* as active enzymes. With the exception of cellulose, pancreatic amylase hydrolyzes major polysaccharides into small oligosaccharides, which can be further digested by the oligosaccharidases present in the duodenal and jejunal epithelium. Pancreatic lipase hydrolyzes ingested fats into free fatty acids and 2-monoglycerides. In addition to pancreatic lipase, acinar cells produce other enzymes that digest fat, but they are secreted as proenzymes, like the proteases previously mentioned. These include colipase, cholesterol ester hydrolase, and phospholipase A2. The main function of colipase is to stabilize the activity of pancreatic lipase in the presence of bile salts. Pancreatic acinar cells also secrete deoxyribonuclease and ribonuclease, enzymes required for the hydrolysis of DNA and RNA, respectively.

Pancreatic enzymes are inactive inside acinar cells because they are synthesized and stored as inactive enzymes. In addition to this autoprotective mechanism, acinar cells synthesize pancreatic

secretory trypsin inhibitor, which also protects acinar cells from autodigestion because it counteracts premature activation of trypsinogen inside acinar cells. Pancreatic secretory trypsin inhibitor is encoded by the serine protease inhibitor Kazal type 1 *(SPINK1)* gene. *SPINK1* gene mutations are associated with the development of chronic pancreatitis, especially in childhood.

The primary function of pancreatic duct cells is to provide the water and electrolytes required to dilute and deliver the enzymes synthesized by acinar cells. Although the concentrations of sodium and potassium are similar to their respective concentrations in plasma, the concentrations of bicarbonate and chloride vary significantly according to the secretion phase.

The mechanism responsible for the secretion of bicarbonate was first described in 1988 on the basis of in vitro studies. According to this model, extracellular CO_2 diffuses across the basolateral membrane of ductal cells. Once CO_2 is inside pancreatic duct cells, it is hydrated by intracellular carbonic anhydrase; as a result of this reaction, HCO_3^- and H^+ are generated. The apical membrane of pancreatic duct cells contains an anion exchanger that secretes intracellular HCO_3^- into the lumen of the cell and favors the exchange of luminal Cl^- inside the ductal epithelium. Studies have shown that this exchanger interacts with the cystic fibrosis transmembrane conductance regulator (CFTR); mutations in the *CFTR* gene have been linked to chronic pancreatitis. This may correlate with the inability of patients with cystic fibrosis to secrete water and bicarbonate. Although the nature of this exchanger has not been completely elucidated, it is possible that this anion exchanger is an SLC26 family member. This family

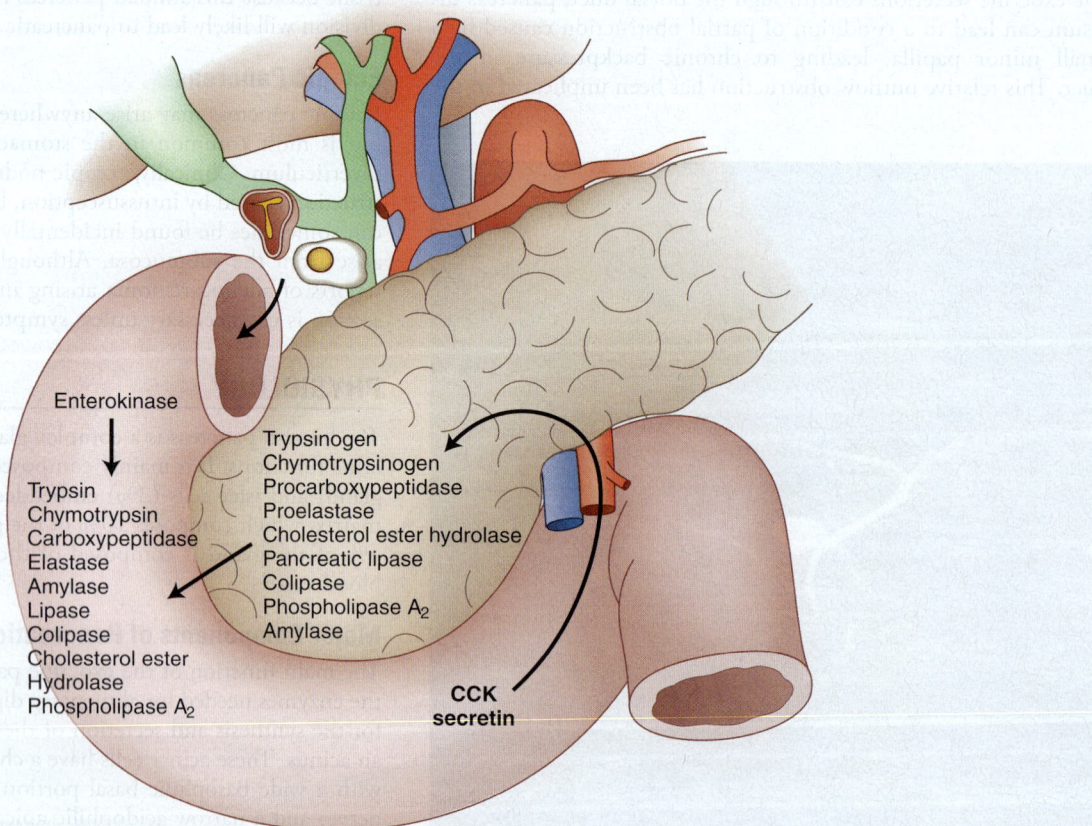

FIGURE 92.5 Physiology of the secretion of pancreatic enzymes. The presence of peptides and fatty acids from food triggers the release of cholecystokinin *(CCK)*. CCK induces the release of pancreatic enzymes into the duodenal lumen. Conversely, S cells located in the duodenum release secretin in response to the acidification of the duodenum. Secretin induces the secretion of HCO_3^- from pancreatic cells into the duodenum.

contains different anion exchangers that transport monovalent and divalent anions, such as Cl^- and HCO_3^-. Some of these exchangers are known to interact with CFTR. Thus, HCO_3^- level in the pancreatic juice varies inversely to the Cl^- level. Secretin hormone is the major stimulator of the HCO_3^- secretion. Cholecystokinin (CCK) weakly stimulates HCO_3^- secretion and also synergizes with the effect of secretin.

In addition to HCO_3^- CO_2 hydration also generates H^+ ions, which are secreted by Na^+ and H^+ exchangers present in the basolateral membrane of ductal cells. These exchangers belong to the *SLC9* gene family. The main function of these exchangers is to maintain the intracellular pH within a physiologic range. In addition, the basolateral membrane of duct cells contains multiple Na^+,K^+-ATPases that provide the primary force that drives HCO_3^- secretion; the Na^+,K^+-ATPase maintains the Na^+ gradient used to extrude H^+ as well. Finally, K^+ channels present in the basolateral membrane of acinar cells maintain the membrane potential to allow recirculation of K^+ ions brought by the Na^+,K^+ pump inside the cell. Fig. 92.6 illustrates HCO_3^- secretion inside pancreatic duct cells. The level of Na^+ and K^+ in pancreatic juice remains relatively constant, without much variation with the secretory rate.

Once the HCO_3^- secreted by pancreatic duct cells reaches the duodenal lumen, it neutralizes the hydrochloric acid secreted by gastric parietal cells. Pancreatic enzymes are inactivated at a low pH; therefore, pancreatic bicarbonate provides an optimal pH for pancreatic enzyme function. The optimal pH for the function of chymotrypsin and trypsin is 8.0 to 9.0; for amylase, the optimal pH is 7.0; and for lipase, it is 7.0 to 9.0.

Phases and Regulation of Pancreatic Secretion

Pancreatic exocrine secretion occurs during the interdigestive state and after the ingestion of food, which is also known as the *digestive state*. The same phases of secretion that have been identified in the stomach during the digestive state have also been described in pancreatic secretion. The first phase is the cephalic phase, in which the pancreas is stimulated by the vagus nerve in response to the sight, smell, or taste of food. This phase is generally mediated by the release of acetylcholine at the terminal endings of postganglionic fibers. The main effect of acetylcholine is to induce acinar cell secretion of enzymes. This phase accounts for 20% to 25% of the daily secretion of pancreatic juice. Every day, 1.5 to 2 L of pancreatic juice is released into the duodenum.

The second phase of pancreatic secretion is known as the *gastric phase*. It is mediated by vagovagal reflexes triggered by gastric distention after the ingestion of food. These reflexes induce acinar cell secretion. It accounts for 10% of the pancreatic juice produced daily.

The most important phase of pancreatic secretion is the intestinal phase, which accounts for 65% to 70% of the total secretion of pancreatic juice. It is mediated by secretin and CCK. Acidification of the duodenal lumen induces the release of secretin by S cells. Secretin was the first polypeptide hormone identified and was first discovered more than 100 years ago. It is the most important mediator of the secretion of water, bicarbonate, and other electrolytes into the duodenum. Secretin receptors are located in the basolateral membrane of all pancreatic duct cells but cannot be identified in other pancreatic components, such as islet cells, blood vessels, or extracellular matrix. The most important effect of secretin stimulation is an increase of intracellular cyclic adenosine monophosphate, which activates the HCO_3^--Cl^- anion exchanger in the apical membrane of pancreatic duct cells. It also increases the activity of the enzyme carbonic anhydrase, the excretion of H^+ outside the duct cell, and the activity of the CFTR.

The presence of lipid, protein, and carbohydrates inside the duodenum induces the secretion of CCK-releasing factor and monitor peptide. Both peptides induce release of CCK by I cells present in the duodenal mucosa. Whereas secretin is the main mediator of the secretion of water and bicarbonate in the intestinal phase, CCK is the main mediator of the secretion of pancreatic enzymes. CCK exerts a number of effects:

1. CCK travels through the bloodstream and induces the release of pancreatic enzymes by acinar cells.
2. CCK induces local duodenal vagovagal reflexes that cause the release of acetylcholine, vasoactive intestinal peptide, and gastrin-releasing peptide, which promotes the release of pancreatic enzymes.
3. CCK induces the relaxation of the sphincter of Oddi. Also, CCK potentiates the effects of secretin, and vice versa.

ACUTE PANCREATITIS

The incidence of acute pancreatitis (AP) has increased during the past 20 years. AP is responsible for more than 300,000 hospital admissions annually in the United States. Most patients develop a mild and self-limited course; however, 10% to 20% of patients have a rapidly progressive inflammatory response associated with prolonged length of hospital stay and significant morbidity and mortality. Patients with mild pancreatitis have a mortality rate of less than 1%, but in severe pancreatitis, this increases up to 10% to 50%.[5] The highest mortality rates in this group of patients are those who present with multiple organ dysfunction syndrome. Mortality in pancreatitis has a bimodal distribution. In the first 2 weeks (early phase), it is a result of multiple organ dysfunction caused by the intense inflammatory cascade triggered by pancreatic inflammation. Mortality after 2 weeks (late phase) is often caused by septic complications.[4]

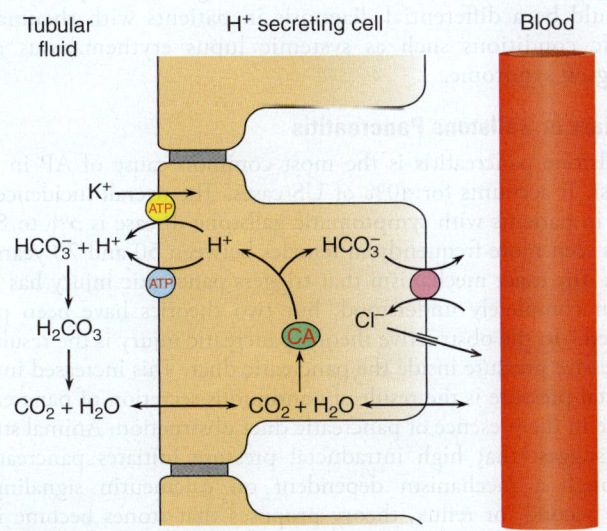

FIGURE 92.6 Concentration, dilution, and acidification of urine. Cellular mechanism for secretion of H^+ and reabsorption of HCO_3^- by intercalated cells of the late distal tubule and collecting ducts. (From Khurana I, Khurana A, Kowlgi NG. *Textbook of Medical Physiology.* 4th ed. Elsevier; 2025: Fig. 6.3.)

Pathophysiology

The exact mechanism whereby predisposing factors such as ethanol and gallstones produce pancreatitis is not completely known. Most researchers believe that AP is the final result of abnormal pancreatic enzyme activation inside acinar cells. Immunolocalization studies have shown that after 15 minutes of pancreatic injury, both zymogen granules and lysosomes colocalize inside the acinar cells. The fact that zymogen and lysosome colocalization occurs before amylase level elevation, pancreatic edema, and other markers of pancreatitis are evident suggests that colocalization is an early step in the pathophysiologic process and not a consequence of pancreatitis. Studies also suggest that lysosomal enzyme cathepsin B activates trypsin in these colocalization organelles. In vitro and in vivo studies have elucidated an intricate model of acinar cell death induced by premature activation of trypsin. In this model, once cathepsin B in lysosomes and trypsinogen in zymogen granules are brought in contact by colocalization induced by pancreatitis-inciting stimuli, activated trypsin then induces leak of colocalized organelles, releasing cathepsin B into the cytosol. It is the cytosolic cathepsin B that then induces apoptosis or necrosis, leading to acinar cell death. Thus, acinar cell death and, to a degree, the inflammatory response seen in AP can be prevented if acinar cells are pretreated with cathepsin B inhibitors. In vivo studies have also shown that cathepsin B knockout mice have a significant decrease in the severity of pancreatitis.[6]

Intraacinar pancreatic enzyme activation induces autodigestion of normal pancreatic parenchyma. In response to this initial insult, acinar cells release proinflammatory cytokines, such as tumor necrosis factor-α (TNF-α) and interleukin (IL)-1, IL-2, and IL-6, and antiinflammatory mediators, such as IL-10 and IL-1 receptor antagonist. These mediators do not initiate pancreatic injury but propagate the response locally and systemically. As a result of TNF-α, IL-1, and IL-6, neutrophils and macrophages are recruited into the pancreatic parenchyma and cause the release of more TNF-α, IL-1, and IL-6; reactive oxygen metabolites; prostaglandins; platelet-activating factor; and leukotrienes.[7] The local inflammatory response further aggravates the pancreatitis because it increases vascular permeability and damages the microcirculation of the pancreas. In severe cases, the inflammatory response causes pancreatic necrosis and hemorrhage in the pancreas or retroperitoneum. In addition, some of the inflammatory mediators released by neutrophils aggravate the pancreatic injury because they cause pancreatic enzyme activation. The dead, necrotic pancreatic tissue can become infected. The pathophysiology is from translocation of gut bacteria into the portal system, which seeds the pancreas. Accordingly, antibiotics should be selected for gram negatives and GI flora, with Imipenem considered the most effective because of its favorable pharmacokinetic pancreatic tissue perfusion. Long-lasting functional impairments, such as exocrine and endocrine deficiencies, can result from necrosis of pancreatic tissue.

In addition to the local pancreatic inflammation and destruction, there can be a massive release of inflammatory mediators to the systemic circulation. Systemic consequences such as sepsis, renal failure, and acute lung injury contribute to the high mortality in this group. A summary of the inflammatory cascade seen in AP is shown in Fig. 92.7.

Risk Factors

Gallstones and ethanol abuse account for 70% to 80% of AP cases.[8] In pediatric patients, abdominal blunt trauma and systemic diseases are the two most common conditions that lead

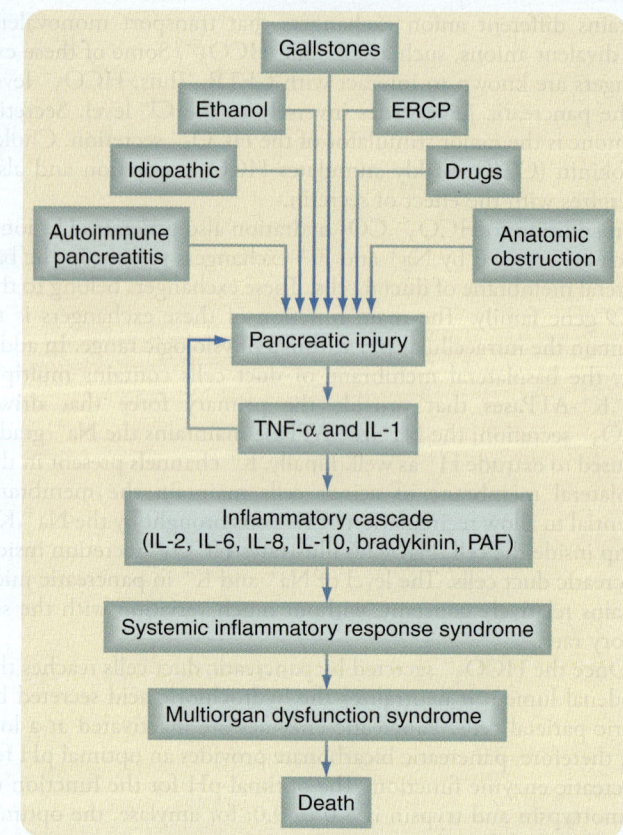

FIGURE 92.7 Pathophysiology of severe acute pancreatitis. The local injury induces the release of tumor necrosis factor-α *(TNFα)* and interleukin-1 *(IL-1)*. Both cytokines produce further pancreatic injury and amplify the inflammatory response by inducing the release of other inflammatory mediators, which cause distant organ injury. This abnormal inflammatory response is responsible for the mortality seen during the early phase of acute pancreatitis. *ERCP,* Endoscopic retrograde cholangiopancreatography; *PAF,* platelet-activating factor.

to pancreatitis. Autoimmune and drug-induced pancreatitis should be a differential diagnosis in patients with rheumatologic conditions such as systemic lupus erythematosus and Sjögren syndrome.

Biliary or Gallstone Pancreatitis

Gallstone pancreatitis is the most common cause of AP in the West. It accounts for 40% of US cases. The overall incidence of AP in patients with symptomatic gallstone disease is 3% to 8%. It is seen more frequently in females between 50 and 70 years of age. The exact mechanism that triggers pancreatic injury has not been completely understood, but two theories have been proposed.[9] In the obstructive theory, pancreatic injury is the result of excessive pressure inside the pancreatic duct. This increased intraductal pressure is the result of continuous secretion of pancreatic juice in the presence of pancreatic duct obstruction. Animal studies suggest that high intraductal pressure initiates pancreatitis through a mechanism dependent on calcineurin signaling.[10] The second, or reflux, theory proposes that stones become impacted in the ampulla of Vater and form a common channel that allows bile salt reflux into the pancreas. Animal models have shown that bile salts cause direct acinar cell necrosis because they increase the concentration of calcium in the cytoplasm; however, this has never been proven in humans.[4]

Alcohol-Induced Injury

Excessive ethanol consumption is the second most common cause of AP worldwide. It accounts for 35% of cases and is more prevalent in young males (30–45 years of age) than in females. However, only 5% to 10% of patients who drink alcohol develop AP. Factors that contribute to ethanol-induced pancreatitis include heavy ethanol abuse (>100 g/day for at least 5 years), smoking, and genetic predisposition. Compared with nonsmokers, the relative risk of alcohol-induced pancreatitis in smokers is 4.9.[11]

Alcohol has a number of deleterious effects on the pancreas, and its mechanism of injury is likely multifaceted. It has been shown to (1) trigger proinflammatory pathways via upregulation of nuclear factor κB (NF-κB), TNF-α, and IL-1; (2) cause inappropriate basolateral exocytosis of pancreatic zymogens; (3) result in increased autophagy, possibly as a result of dysregulation of cathepsin L and B; (4) cause increased oxidative stress, leading to mitochondrial dysfunction; (5) cause activation of pancreatic stellate cells (PSCs), leading to increased secretion of matrix metalloproteases; (6) cause impaired pancreatic cell repair as a result of dysregulation in developmental factors PDX1, PTF1a, and Notch; and (7) result in a shift in cell death from apoptosis to necrosis by decreasing caspase 3/8 activity and through loss of adenosine triphosphate (ATP) production via mitochondrial depolarization.[12]

Anatomic Obstruction

Abnormal flow of pancreatic juice into the duodenum can result in pancreatic injury. AP has been described in patients with pancreatic tumors, parasites, and congenital defects.

Pancreas divisum is an anatomic variation present in 10% of the population. Its association with AP is controversial. Patients with this variation have a 5% to 10% lifetime risk for development of AP caused by relative outflow obstruction through the minor papilla. Endoscopic retrograde cholangiopancreatography (ERCP) with minor papillotomy and stenting may be beneficial for such patients.

Infrequent anatomic obstructions that have been associated with AP include *Ascaris lumbricoides* infection and annular pancreas. Although pancreatic cancer can also cause ductal obstruction and should be considered in the differential diagnosis, patients with pancreatic cancer usually do not develop AP.

Endoscopic Retrograde Cholangiopancreatography–Induced Pancreatitis

AP is the most common complication after ERCP, occurring in up to 5% of patients. However, the incidence of this complication after ERCP can be as high as 15% in high-risk patients. Post-ERCP pancreatitis is more common in female patients, young individuals, and patients with prior history of ERCP-induced pancreatitis. AP occurs more frequently in patients who have undergone therapeutic procedures compared with diagnostic procedures. It is also more common in patients who have had multiple attempts of cannulation, sphincter of Oddi dysfunction, and abnormal visualization of the secondary pancreatic ducts after injection of contrast material. The clinical course is mild in 90% to 95% of patients. ERCP-induced pancreatitis is one of the rare opportunities where primary prevention of development of AP may be possible. First, ERCP should only be performed when absolutely necessary. With improvement in other diagnostic modalities, including magnetic resonance cholangiopancreatography (MRCP), the use of diagnostic ERCP with its associated complications, including ERCP-induced pancreatitis, has decreased.

Among pharmacologic agents to prevent ERCP-induced pancreatitis, use of indomethacin has gained the most traction. Technique-related and interventional strategies that have been shown to reduce the risk of post-ERCP pancreatitis include use of pancreatic stents and use of minimal pressure while performing ERCP.

Drug-Induced Pancreatitis

Up to 2% of AP cases are caused by medications. The most common agents include sulfonamides, metronidazole, erythromycin, tetracyclines, didanosine, thiazides, furosemide, 3-hydroxy-3-methylglutaryl-coenzyme A (HMG-CoA) reductase inhibitors (statins), azathioprine, 6-mercaptopurine, 5-aminosalicylic acid, sulfasalazine, valproic acid, and human immunodeficiency virus antiretroviral agents.

Metabolic Factors

Hypertriglyceridemia and hypercalcemia can also lead to pancreatic damage. Direct pancreatic injury can be induced by triglyceride metabolites. It is more common in patients with type I, II, or V hyperlipidemia. It should be suspected in patients with a triglyceride level higher than 1000 mg/dL. A triglyceride level higher than 2000 mg/dL confirms the diagnosis. Hypertriglyceridemia secondary to hypothyroidism, diabetes mellitus, and alcohol does not typically induce AP.

Hypercalcemia is postulated to induce pancreatic injury through the activation of trypsinogen to trypsin and intraductal precipitation of calcium, leading to ductal obstruction and subsequent attacks of pancreatitis. Approximately 1.5% to 13% of patients with primary hyperparathyroidism develop AP.

Miscellaneous Conditions

Blunt and penetrating abdominal trauma can be associated with AP in 0.2% and 1% of cases, respectively. Prolonged intraoperative hypotension and excessive pancreatic manipulation during abdominal surgery can also result in AP. Pancreatic ischemia in association with acute pancreatic inflammation can develop after splenic artery embolization. Other rare causes include scorpion venom stings and perforated duodenal ulcers.

Clinical Manifestations

The cardinal symptom of AP is epigastric or periumbilical pain that radiates to the back. Up to 90% of patients have nausea or vomiting that typically does not relieve the pain. The nature of the pain is constant; therefore, if the pain disappears or decreases, another diagnosis should be considered.

Dehydration, poor skin turgor, tachycardia, hypotension, and dry mucous membranes are commonly seen in patients with AP. Severely dehydrated and older patients may also develop mental status changes.

The physical examination findings of the abdomen vary according to the severity of the disease. With mild pancreatitis, the physical examination findings of the abdomen may be normal or reveal only mild epigastric tenderness. Significant abdominal distention associated with generalized rebound and abdominal rigidity is present in severe pancreatitis. The nature of the pain described by the patient may not correlate with the physical examination findings or the degree of pancreatic inflammation.

Rare findings include flank and periumbilical ecchymosis (Grey Turner and Cullen signs, respectively). Both are indicative of retroperitoneal bleeding associated with severe pancreatitis. Patients with concomitant choledocholithiasis or significant edema in the head of the pancreas that compresses the intrapancreatic portion of the common bile duct can present with jaundice. Dullness to percussion and decreased breathing sounds in the left or, less commonly, in the right hemithorax suggest pleural effusion secondary to AP.

Diagnosis

The diagnosis of AP requires two of the following three features to be present according to the Revised Atlanta Classification (RAC): (1) abdominal pain consistent with AP (acute onset of a persistent, severe epigastric pain, often radiating to the back), (2) a threefold or higher elevation of serum amylase or lipase levels above the upper laboratory limit of normal, or (3) characteristics findings of pancreatitis by imaging.[13] The serum half-life of amylase (10 hours) is shorter than that of lipase (6.9–13.7 hours), and it therefore normalizes faster (3–5 vs. 8–14 days, respectively). In patients who do not present to the emergency department within the first 24 to 48 hours after the onset of symptoms, determination of lipase levels is a more sensitive indicator to establish the diagnosis. Lipase is also a more specific marker of AP because serum amylase levels can be elevated in a number of conditions, such as peptic ulcer disease, parotitis, cholecystitis, mesenteric ischemia, renal failure salpingitis, and macroamylasemia.

Patients with AP are typically hyperglycemic; they can also have leukocytosis and abnormal elevation of liver enzyme levels. Increased levels of hemoglobin and hematocrit suggest hypovolemia in the vascular space resulting from "third-spacing," or the leakage of fluid into the retroperitoneum. The elevation of alanine aminotransferase levels in the serum in the context of AP confirmed by high pancreatic enzyme levels has a positive predictive value of 95% in the diagnosis of acute biliary pancreatitis.[9]

Imaging Studies

Imaging studies are not required for diagnosis but may be helpful in determining need for intervention in severe AP or elucidating an elusive etiology. Although simple abdominal radiographs are not useful for diagnosis of pancreatitis, they can help rule out other conditions, such as perforated ulcer disease. Nonspecific findings in patients with AP include air-fluid levels suggestive of ileus, cutoff colon sign as a result of colonic spasm at the splenic flexure, pleural effusions, and widening of the duodenal C loop caused by severe pancreatic head edema. Additionally, pancreatic calcifications can be indicative of underlying chronic pancreatitis.

The usefulness of ultrasound for diagnosis of pancreatitis is limited by intraabdominal fat and increased intestinal gas as a result of ileus. Nevertheless, this test should always be ordered in patients with AP because of its high sensitivity (95%) in diagnosing gallstones. Combined elevations of liver transaminase, elevated pancreatic enzyme levels, and the presence of gallstones on ultrasound have an even higher sensitivity (97%) and specificity (100%) for diagnosing acute biliary pancreatitis.

Contrast-enhanced computed tomography (CT) is currently the best modality for evaluation of the pancreas, especially if the study is performed with a multidetector CT scanner. Indications for CT include diagnostic uncertainty, confirmation of severity based on clinical predictors, failure to respond to conservative treatment, or clinical deterioration. The most valuable contrast phase in which to evaluate the pancreatic parenchyma is the portal venous phase (65–70 seconds after injection of contrast material), which allows evaluation of the viability of the pancreatic parenchyma, amount of peripancreatic inflammation, and presence of intraabdominal free air or fluid collections. Noncontrast

CT scanning may also be of value in the setting of renal failure by identifying fluid collections or extraluminal air.

Abdominal magnetic resonance imaging (MRI) is also useful to evaluate the extent of necrosis, inflammation, and presence of free fluid. However, its applicability is limited by the higher cost, lower availability, and the fact that patients requiring imaging are more likely to be critically ill and in intensive care units. Although MRCP is not indicated in the acute setting of AP, it has an important role in the evaluation of patients with unexplained or recurrent pancreatitis because it allows complete noninvasive visualization of the biliary and pancreatic duct anatomy. For difficult-to-view pancreatic ducts, IV administration of secretin before imaging can cause a transient distention of the pancreatic duct by stimulating pancreatic juice secretion. Any pain associated with the timing of secretin stimulation should be noted because it may help in confirming an uncertain etiology of epigastric pain. For example, secretin-stimulated MRCP is useful in patients with AP and no evidence of a predisposing condition to rule out pancreas divisum, intraductal papillary mucinous neoplasm (IPMN), or a small tumor in the pancreatic duct.

In the setting of gallstone pancreatitis, EUS may play an important role in the evaluation of persistent choledocholithiasis. Several studies have shown that routine ERCP for suspected gallstone pancreatitis reveals no evidence of persistent obstruction in most cases and may actually worsen symptoms because of manipulation of the gland. EUS has been proven to be sensitive for identifying choledocholithiasis; it allows examination of the biliary tree and pancreas with no risk of worsening of the pancreatitis. In patients in whom persistent choledocholithiasis is confirmed by EUS, ERCP can be used selectively as a therapeutic measure.

Assessment of Severity of Disease

Several risk scores have been developed to predict outcome. The earliest scoring system designed to evaluate the severity of AP was introduced by Ranson and colleagues in 1974. It predicts the severity of the disease on the basis of 11 parameters obtained at the time of admission or 48 hours later. The mortality rate of AP directly correlates with the number of parameters that are positive. Severe pancreatitis is diagnosed if three or more of the Ranson criteria are fulfilled. The Ranson score has a low positive predictive value (50%) and high negative predictive value (90%). Therefore, it is mainly used to rule out severe pancreatitis or to predict the risk of mortality. The main disadvantage is that it does not predict the severity of disease at the time of the admission because six parameters are assessed only after 48 hours of admission. The original scoring symptom designed to predict the severity of the disease and its modification for acute biliary pancreatitis are shown in Boxes 92.1 and 92.2.

AP severity can also be addressed by the Acute Physiology and Chronic Health Evaluation (APACHE II) score. Based on the patient's age, previous health status, and 12 routine physiologic measurements, APACHE II provides a general measure of the severity of disease. An APACHE II score of 8 or higher defines severe pancreatitis. The main advantage is that it can be used on admission and repeated at any time. However, it is complex, not specific for AP, and based on the patient's age, which easily upgrades the AP severity score. Additionally, the required 12 variables are not routinely obtained in patients who are not critically ill. APACHE II has a positive predictive value of 43% and a negative predictive value of 89%.

The Bedside Index for Severity in Acute Pancreatitis (BISAP) score, created in 2008, gauges the risk of death from AP using five

BOX 92.1   Ranson Prognostic Criteria for Nongallstone Pancreatitis

At presentation
- Age >55 years
- Blood glucose level >200 mg/dL
- White blood cell count >16,000 cells/mm³
- Lactate dehydrogenase level >350 IU/L
- Aspartate aminotransferase level >250 IU/L

After 48 hours of admission
- Hematocrit[a]: decrease >10%
- Serum calcium level <8 mg/dL
- Base deficit >4 mEq/L
- Blood urea nitrogen level: increase >5 mg/dL
- Fluid requirement >6 L
- PaO₂ <60 mm Hg

Ranson score ≥3 defines severe pancreatitis.

[a]Compared with admission value.

BOX 92.2   Ranson Prognostic Criteria for Gallstone Pancreatitis

At presentation
- Age >70 years
- Blood glucose level >220 mg/dL
- White blood cell count >18,000 cells/mm³
- Lactate dehydrogenase level >400 IU/L
- Aspartate aminotransferase level >250 IU/L

After 48 hours of admission
- Hematocrit[a]: decrease >10%
- Serum calcium level <8 mg/dL
- Base deficit >5 mEq/L
- Blood urea nitrogen level: increase >2 mg/dL
- Fluid requirement >4 L
- PaO₂: Not available

Ranson score ≥3 defines severe pancreatitis.

[a]Compared with admission value.

TABLE 92.2   Computed Tomography Severity Index (CTSI) for Acute Pancreatitis

FEATURE	POINTS
Pancreatic Inflammation	
Normal pancreas	0
Focal or diffuse pancreatic enlargement	1
Intrinsic pancreatic alterations with peripancreatic fat inflammatory changes	2
Single fluid collection or phlegmon	3
Two or more fluid collections or gas in or adjacent to the pancreas	4
Pancreatic Necrosis	
None	0
≤30%	2
30%–50%	4
>50%	6

CTSI 0–3, mortality 3%, morbidity 8%; CTSI 4–6, mortality 6%, morbidity 35%; CTSI 7–10, mortality 17%, morbidity 92%.

Although many prognostic indices have been developed to predict severity of disease, most are hindered by complexity, need for imaging, or inability to be calculated at admission. This has led to multiple professional societies recommending the use of the SIRS scoring system (Box 92.3) as a fast, inexpensive, and reliable replacement.[14,15] Having a persistent SIRS throughout hospital admission, having a transient SIRS, or never meeting SIRS criteria has been associated with mortality rates of 25%, 8%, and 0%, respectively.

In 1992, the International Symposium on Acute Pancreatitis defined *severe pancreatitis* as the presence of local pancreatic complications (necrosis, abscess, or pseudocyst) or any evidence of organ failure. Severe pancreatitis is diagnosed if there is any evidence of organ failure or a local pancreatic complication (Box 92.4). In 2012, the International Symposium on Acute Pancreatitis updated its three-tiered grading schema of pancreatitis severity. Mild pancreatitis has no organ dysfunction or local/systemic complications, moderate pancreatitis can have organ failure lasting less than 48 hours and/or local/systemic complications, and severe pancreatitis is characterized by organ failure lasting beyond 48 hours. With increasing severity comes increased rates of morbidity and mortality.[8]

Treatment

Regardless of the cause or the severity of the disease, the cornerstones of treating AP are aggressive fluid resuscitation with isotonic crystalloid solution to restore tissue perfusion, early nutrition to counteract the catabolic state and decrease the rate of infectious complications, and pain control.

criteria: elevated blood urea nitrogen (BUN) levels, altered mental state, systemic inflammatory response syndrome (SIRS), age over 60, and pleural effusion within 24 hours of admission. The lowest score is associated with <1% mortality risk, and the highest is associated with over 20% mortality risk. High BISAP scores also correlate with increased risks of organ failure and pancreatic necrosis. Its widespread use stems from its straightforwardness and easy computation.

C-reactive protein (CRP) is an inflammatory marker that peaks 48 to 72 hours after the onset of pancreatitis and correlates with the severity of the disease. A CRP level of 150 mg/mL or higher defines severe pancreatitis. The major limitation is that it cannot be used on admission; the sensitivity of the assay decreases if CRP levels are measured within 48 hours after the onset of symptoms. In addition to CRP, a number of studies have shown other biochemical markers (e.g., serum levels of procalcitonin, IL-6, IL-1, elastase) that correlate with the severity of the disease. However, their main limitation is their cost, and they are not widely available.

Using imaging characteristics, Balthazar and associates have established the CT severity index. This index correlates CT findings with the patient's outcome. The CT severity index is shown in Table 92.2.

BOX 92.3   Definition of Systemic Inflammatory Response Syndrome (SIRS)

Two or more of the following conditions must be met:
- Temperature >38.3°C (100.9°F) or <36.0°C (96.8°F)
- Heart rate of >90 beats/minute
- Respiratory rate of >20 breaths/minute or PaCO₂ of <32 mm Hg
- White blood cell count of >12,000 cells/mL, <4000 cells/mL, or >10% immature (band) forms

From Annane D, Bellissant E, Cavaillon JM. Septic shock. *Lancet.* 2005;365:63-78.

> ### BOX 92.4   Atlanta Criteria for Acute Pancreatitis
>
> **Organ Failure, as Defined By**
> Shock (systolic blood pressure <90 mm Hg)
> Pulmonary insufficiency (PaO$_2$ <60 mm Hg)
> Renal failure (creatinine level >2 mg/dL after fluid resuscitation)
> Gastrointestinal bleeding (>500 mL/24 hour)
>
> **Systemic Complications**
> Disseminated intravascular coagulation (platelet count ≤100,000)
> Fibrinogen <1 g/L
> Fibrin split products >80 μg/dL
> Metabolic disturbance (calcium level ≤7.5 mg/dL)
>
> **Local Complications**
> Necrosis
> Abscess
> Pseudocyst
> Severe pancreatitis is defined by the presence of any evidence of organ failure or a local complication.

IV fluid replacement is necessary to compensate for a reduced oral intake as well as for losses resulting from vomiting or creation of a third space in the abdominal cavity (intraabdominal or retroperitoneal). Hypovolemia is recognized as an unfavorable prognostic factor, and its treatment is essential. Although the nature of the fluid that should be used for initial resuscitation is still being debated, some evidence suggests that lactated Ringer (LR) may be best for initial resuscitation because of an association between an apparent antiinflammatory effect and decreased odds of developing SIRS at 24 hours compared with normal saline.[16] The American College of Gastroenterology (ACG) Acute Pancreatitis Task Force on Quality guideline cites a meta-analysis reporting decreased odds of developing SIRS with LR compared with normal saline when used for the initial resuscitation in AP (OR 0.38 [95% CI 0.15–0.98]).[17]

The rate of fluid administration should be individualized and adjusted on the basis of age, comorbidities, vital signs, mental status, skin turgor, and urine output, titrating to specific measures of perfusion. In 2022, findings of the WATERFALL trial challenged the concept of aggressive fluid resuscitation.[18] In this international, multicenter randomized controlled trial (RCT), adults with AP were randomly assigned to receive either aggressive (bolus 20 mL/kg, maintenance 3 mL/kg) or moderate (bolus 10 mL/kg or no bolus with normovolemia, maintenance 1.5 mL/kg) resuscitation with LR solution. The primary outcome was development of moderately severe or severe pancreatitis during the hospitalization, and the main safety outcome was fluid overload. The study was stopped early because fluid overload occurred in 21% of patients in the aggressive treatment compared with just 6% in the moderate group. There was no statistically significant difference in the primary outcomes; however, there was a trend toward fewer complications with the moderate strategy. Patients who do not respond to initial fluid resuscitation or have significant renal, cardiac, or respiratory comorbidities often require invasive monitoring with central venous access and a Foley catheter.

In addition to fluid resuscitation, patients with AP require continuous pulse oximetry because one of the most common systemic complications of AP is hypoxemia caused by the acute lung injury associated with this disease. Patients should receive supplementary oxygen to maintain arterial saturation above 95%.

It is also essential to provide effective analgesia. Narcotics are usually preferred, especially morphine. One of the physiologic effects described after systemic administration of morphine is an increase in tone in the sphincter of Oddi; however, there is no evidence that narcotics exert a negative impact on the outcome of patients with AP.

Nutritional support is vital in the treatment of AP. The intense inflammatory response in moderate and severe AP incites a catabolic state with subsequent higher caloric requirements. The main options to provide this nutritional support are enteral feeding and total parenteral nutrition (TPN). Evidence overwhelmingly supports enteral feeding over TPN because it reduces the risk of death, organ failure, and systemic infections, especially for severe AP. The mechanisms by which enteral nutrition improves outcomes are likely related to replenishing caloric losses, increasing splanchnic blood flow to preserve the integrity of the bowel mucosa, and stimulating intestinal motility. Current recommendations advise starting enteral feeding within 24 to 72 hours.[19,20] Evidence supporting immediate enteral feeding upon admission was provided in a recent RCT by a Spanish group. In this trial, 131 patients with mild-moderate AP were given a low-fat, solid diet immediately after admission, regardless of symptoms or laboratory parameters, or conventional feeding with progressive diet as clinical and laboratory parameters improved. The results indicated that immediate feeding is safe and feasible, with significantly decreased complications (4.2% vs. 18.3%) and shorter length of stay (LOS) (3.4 d vs. 8.8 d) at 50% of the cost.[21]

If patients are unable to tolerate oral intake within 72 hours, nasoentera—via either nasogastric or nasojejunal tubes—should be initiated. For those who are unable to undergo enteral feeding because of conditions like paralytic ileus or obstruction, TPN can be considered within 72 hours. Although TPN provides most nutritional requirements, it is associated with mucosal atrophy, decreased intestinal blood flow, increased risk of bacterial overgrowth in the small bowel, antegrade colonization with colonic bacteria, and increased bacterial translocation. In addition, patients with TPN have more central line infections and metabolic complications (e.g., hyperglycemia, electrolyte imbalance).

Given the significant increase in mortality associated with septic complications in severe pancreatitis, a number of physicians advocated the use of prophylactic antibiotics in the 1970s. Recent meta-analyses and systematic reviews that have evaluated multiple RCTs have proven that prophylactic antibiotics do not decrease the frequency of surgical intervention, infected necrosis, or mortality in patients with severe pancreatitis. In addition, they are associated with gram-positive cocci infection, such as by *Staphylococcus aureus,* and *Candida* infection, which is seen in 5% to 15% of patients. Current recommendations are to only administer antibiotics if a preexisting infection is present on presentation or radiographic imaging suggests infected peripancreatic fluid collections (e.g., gas within collection or rim enhancement).

Special Considerations

Endoscopic retrograde cholangiopancreatography. Early ERCP, with or without sphincterotomy, was initially advocated to reduce the severity of biliary pancreatitis because the obstructive theory of AP states that pancreatic injury is the result of pancreatic duct obstruction by gallstones. However, multiple randomized trials have evaluated the use and efficacy of early ERCP in the management of acute biliary pancreatitis. The results of these trials do not support the use of early ERCP in the management of acute biliary pancreatitis, regardless of the severity. Routine use of ERCP is not indicated for patients with mild pancreatitis because the bile duct obstruction is usually transient and resolves within 48 hours after the onset of symptoms. Based on a meta-analysis of these clinical trials as well as two major society guidelines based on these clinical trials, ERCP is only indicated for patients who develop cholangitis and those with persistent bile duct obstruction demonstrated by other imaging modalities, such as EUS.[14,22] Finally, in older patients with poor performance status or severe comorbidities that preclude surgery, ERCP with sphincterotomy is a safe alternative to prevent recurrent biliary pancreatitis.

Laparoscopic cholecystectomy. In the absence of definitive treatment, 30% of patients with acute biliary pancreatitis will have recurrent disease. With the exception of older patients and those with poor performance status, laparoscopic cholecystectomy is indicated for all patients with mild acute biliary pancreatitis. Studies have shown that early laparoscopic cholecystectomy, defined as laparoscopic cholecystectomy during the initial admission to the hospital, is a safe procedure that decreases recurrence of the disease.[8] Choledocholithiasis can be excluded by intraoperative cholangiography, EUS, or MRCP. For patients with severe pancreatitis, early surgery may increase the morbidity and length of stay. Current recommendations suggest conservative treatment for at least 6 weeks before laparoscopic cholecystectomy is attempted in this setting. This approach has significantly decreased morbidity.[9]

Complications

Sterile and Infected Peripancreatic Fluid Collections

Discussion regarding appropriate management of pancreatic and peripancreatic fluid collections requires an understanding of the current classification of these entities, as defined in Table 92.3. Fluid collections are divided into acute (present for less than 4 weeks) and chronic (lasting past 4 weeks) and either simple or complex in nature. Acute peripancreatic fluid collections are simple in nature and, after 4 weeks, are referred to as a pseudocyst. Fluid collections associated with necrotizing pancreatitis are referred to as an *acute necrotic collection* (ANC) before 4 weeks and as *walled-off pancreatic necrosis* (WOPN) after that period. The presence of acute peripancreatic fluid collections during an episode of AP has been described in 30% to 57% of patients. In contrast to pseudocysts and cystic neoplasias of the pancreas, fluid collections are not surrounded or encased by epithelium or fibrotic capsule. Treatment is supportive because most fluid

collections will be spontaneously reabsorbed by the peritoneum. All of these fluid collections may become infected. The usual signs and symptoms of infection (e.g., fever, elevated white blood cell count, and abdominal pain) may also be present without an infection in AP due to a robust SIRS response in many of these patients, making diagnosis of infection difficult. Evidence of gas within a fluid collection on imaging without prior instrumentation is diagnostic. Acute decompensation or failure to improve after 10 to 14 days may suggest infection, and consideration should be given to CT-guided fluid sampling. Drainage (percutaneous or endoscopic) and IV administration of antibiotics should be instituted if infection is present. Antibiotics known to penetrate pancreatic necrosis include carbapenems, quinolones, metronidazole, and high-dose cephalosporins.

Pancreatic Necrosis and Infected Necrosis

Necrosis is the presence of nonviable pancreatic parenchyma or peripancreatic fat and can manifest as a focal area or diffuse involvement of the gland. Contrast-enhanced CT is the most reliable technique to diagnose ANC, which is typically seen as areas of low attenuation (<40–50 HU) after the IV injection of contrast material. Normal parenchyma usually has a density of 100 to 150 HU. Up to 20% of patients with AP develop ANCs. It is important to identify and provide proper treatment of these complications because most patients who develop multiorgan failure have necrotizing pancreatitis; pancreatic necrosis has been documented in up to 80% of the autopsies of patients who died after an episode of AP.[6]

The main complication of ANC is infection. The risk is directly related to the amount of necrosis; in patients with pancreatic necrosis involving less than 30% of the gland, the risk of infection is 22%. The risk is 37% for patients with pancreatic necrosis that involves 30% to 50% of the gland and up to 46% if more than 70% of the gland is affected.[4] This complication is associated with bacterial translocation, usually involving enteric flora, such as gram-negative rods (e.g., *Escherichia coli*, *Klebsiella*, and *Pseudomonas* spp.) and *Enterococcus* spp.

An infected necrotic collection should be suspected in patients with prolonged fever, elevated white blood cell count, or progressive clinical deterioration. It should also be suspected if the patient develops sepsis, SIRS, and/or organ failure later in the course of the disease (>7 days after the onset of the AP). Evidence of gas

TABLE 92.3	Atlanta Classification of Morphological Features of Acute Pancreatitis	
SUBTYPE	**≤4 WEEKS**	**>4 WEEKS**
Interstitial edematous[a]	**Acute Peripancreatic Fluid Collection (APFC)** • Homogeneous collection with fluid density • No definable wall or capsule • Confined to pancreatic fascial planes • No intrapancreatic extension	**Pseudocyst** • Homogeneous fluid • Encapsulated, round or oval • No nonliquid component • Well-defined wall
Necrotizing[b]	**Acute Necrotic Collection (ANC)** • Heterogeneous with nonliquid densities • No definable wall or capsule • Located intra-/extra-pancreatic	**Walled-Off Necrosis (WON)** • Mixed liquid and nonliquid content • Encapsulated with well-defined wall • Varying loculations • Located intra-/extra-pancreatic

[a]Interstitial edematous pancreatitis: characterized by inflammation and enlargement of the pancreas and surrounding tissues without any evidence of necrosis on imaging.

[b]Necrotizing pancreatitis: nonviable pancreatic tissue and/or peripancreatic fat necrosis, often seen as areas lacking contrast enhancement on CT.

within the pancreatic necrosis seen on a CT scan confirms the diagnosis but is a rare finding. If infected necrosis is suspected, fine-needle aspiration (FNA) may be performed if the diagnosis is equivocal; from the aspirate, a positive Gram stain or culture establishes the diagnosis. Although positive cultures are confirmatory, a review has demonstrated that despite negative preoperative cultures, 42% of patients with so-called persistent unwellness will have infected necrosis.[23] Fig. 92.8 illustrates the pathophysiologic process of pancreatic necrosis infection.

With decades of experience in treatment of pancreatic necrosis, few general concepts have emerged. First, all sterile necrotic collections do not need to be intervened upon. Indications for intervening in sterile necrotizing pancreatitis include persistent pain, failure to improve clinically with conservative management, and/or symptomatic biliary or enteric obstruction. Intervention for these indications should be delayed as much as possible to allow development of walled-off necrosis (WON). Second, clinical suspicion of or documented infected necrotic collection with clinical deterioration is a clear indication for intervention. Even in this situation, the intervention should be delayed as much as possible to allow the collection to become walled off.

Once infection has been demonstrated, IV antibiotics should be given. Because of their penetration into the pancreas and spectrum coverage, carbapenems are the first option for treatment. Alternative therapy includes quinolones, metronidazole, third-generation cephalosporins, and piperacillin. Historically, the definitive treatment of infected pancreatic necrosis is surgical debridement with necrosectomy, closed continuous irrigation, or open packing (Fig. 92.9). The overall mortality rate after open necrosectomy has

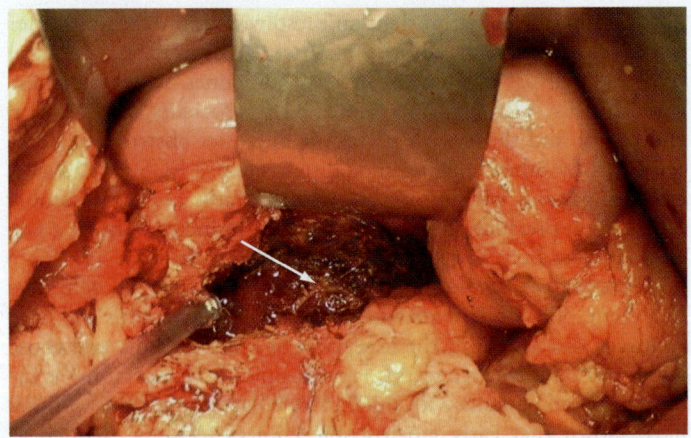

FIGURE 92.9 Infected pancreatic necrosis. This 45-year-old male had severe ethanol-induced pancreatitis. Four weeks after the initial episode, the patient developed fever (39.5°C [103°F]), hypotension, and leukocytosis (19,000 cells/mm³). The computed tomography scan documented pancreatic necrosis involving 35% of the gland. After fine-needle aspiration, Gram staining documented the presence of gram-negative rods. The exploratory laparotomy indicated pancreatic necrosis involving mainly the body of the gland *(arrow)*. The patient was treated with necrosectomy, closed drainage, and intravenous meropenem. Final culture documented the presence of *Escherichia coli*. The patient was discharged home 56 days after the initial episode.

been as high as 25% to 30%[12] because of the severe nature of the disease as well as the high complication rate of an open debridement. Outcomes are time dependent; patients who undergo surgery in the first 14 days have a mortality rate of 75%, and those who undergo surgery between 15 and 29 days and after 30 days have mortality rates of 45% and 8%, respectively.[24] As a result of the elevated morbidity and mortality rates with open debridement, percutaneous, endoscopic, and laparoscopic techniques with an anterior or retroperitoneal approach have been employed as alternatives.

In 2010, the Dutch Pancreatitis Study Group performed a randomized trial evaluating open necrosectomy versus a "step-up approach" consisting of percutaneous drainage followed by minimally invasive video-assisted retroperitoneal debridement for necrotizing and infected necrotizing pancreatitis. The results showed that long-term end-point complications (e.g., exocrine and endocrine insufficiency) and mortality rates were better in the group using the step-up approach compared with the group undergoing early open necrosectomy.[14] A companion study to this was published in 2018 wherein endoscopic management was compared with the step-up approach. Although the endoscopic approach was nonsuperior to the minimally invasive surgical approach regarding mortality and most secondary end points, it was associated with fewer pancreatic fistulae, reduced cumulative hospital length of stay, and lower cost.[25]

Recent findings have led to a significant change in the approach to treating infected necrotizing pancreatitis, now favoring the use of antibiotics alone with delayed drainage over the previously standard practice of combining antibiotics with immediate drainage for infections that develop after AP. This change is supported by evidence from the Postponed or Immediate Drainage of Infected Necrotizing Pancreatitis (POINTER) trial, an RCT conducted in the Netherlands that evaluated the outcomes of immediate versus delayed drainage in patients with infected necrotizing pancreatitis diagnosed within 35 days from the initial symptoms of AP. The study,

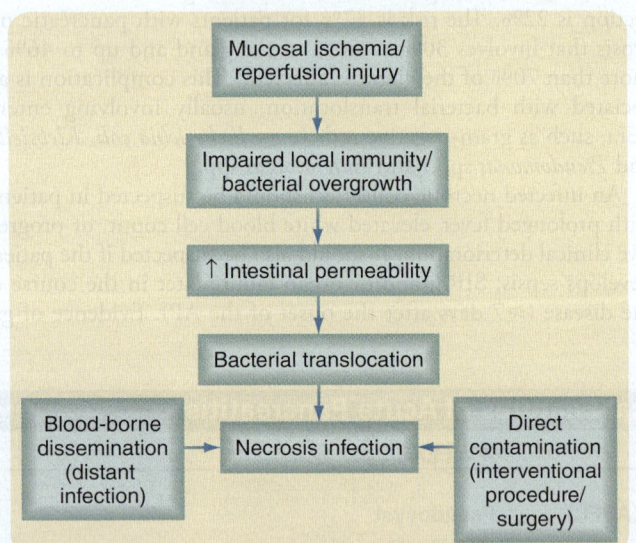

FIGURE 92.8 Pathophysiology of pancreatic necrosis infection. The acute inflammatory injury that occurs during the first 48 to 72 hours causes mucosal ischemia and reperfusion injury. Both effects favor bacterial overgrowth because they alter local immunity. Mucosal ischemia also produces an increase in the permeability of intestinal cells, which is initiated 72 hours after the acute episode but typically peaks 1 week later. These transient episodes of bacteremia are associated with pancreatic necrosis infection. Less frequently, distant sources of infection, such as pneumonia and vascular or urinary tract infection associated with central lines and catheters, are associated with bacteremia and pancreatic necrosis. Finally, local contamination after surgery or interventional procedures, such as endoscopic retrograde cholangiopancreatography, is responsible for necrosis infection.

which included 104 patients with documented infection, found no difference in complications and mortality rates between the two groups, but it did find that the group that underwent immediate drainage had an average of 4.4 interventions, in contrast to just 2.6 interventions in the delayed-drainage group. Notably, 37% (19 out of 52) of patients in the delayed-drainage group avoided the need for drainage altogether, and their hospital stays were 15% shorter.[26]

Currently, an endoscopic drainage with a large-bore stent and possible endoscopic debridement with or without percutaneous drainage can avoid an operation in most patients. If the endoscopic and/or percutaneous management fails, a minimally invasive operation will usually be more straightforward, and the results will be improved. Occasionally, when there is a large amount of necrosum, the surgical approach may be preferred to the endoscopic approach, which would require several repeat procedures to clear the debris. These points highlight the complexity of treating this disease and the importance that patients be managed at high-volume centers and discussed at multidisciplinary conferences with all relevant expert physicians present. Regardless of which route is taken, physiologic and nutritional support of the patient will have a large impact on outcome.

Pancreatic Pseudocysts

Pancreatic pseudocysts occur in 5% to 15% of patients who have peripancreatic fluid collections after AP. By definition, the capsule of a pseudocyst is composed of collagen and granulation tissue, and it is not lined by epithelium. The fibrotic reaction typically requires at least 4 to 8 weeks to develop. Fig. 92.10 shows CT scans of a large pseudocyst arising in the tail of the pancreas.

Up to 50% of patients with pancreatic pseudocysts will develop symptoms. Persistent pain, early satiety, nausea, weight loss, and elevated pancreatic enzyme levels in plasma suggest this diagnosis. The diagnosis is corroborated by CT or MRI. EUS with FNA is indicated for patients in whom the diagnosis of pancreatic pseudocyst is not clear. Characteristic features of pancreatic pseudocysts include high amylase levels associated with the absence of mucin and low carcinoembryonic antigen (CEA) levels.

Observation is indicated for asymptomatic patients because spontaneous regression has been documented in up to 70% of cases; this is particularly true for patients with pseudocysts smaller than 4 cm in diameter, located in the tail, and no evidence of pancreatic duct obstruction or communication with the MPD. Invasive therapies are indicated for symptomatic patients or when the differentiation

between a cystic neoplasm and pseudocyst is not possible. Because most patients are treated with decompressive procedures and not with resection, it is imperative to have a pathologic diagnosis. Surgical drainage had been the traditional approach for pancreatic pseudocysts. However, modern evidence suggests that transgastric and transduodenal endoscopic drainage are safe and effective approaches for patients with pancreatic pseudocysts in close contact (defined as <1 cm) with the stomach and duodenum, respectively. In addition, transpapillary drainage can be attempted in pancreatic pseudocysts communicating with the MPD. For patients in whom a pancreatic duct stricture is associated with a pancreatic pseudocyst, endoscopic dilation and stent placement are indicated.

Surgical drainage is generally reserved for patients with pancreatic pseudocysts that cannot be treated with endoscopic techniques for anatomic reasons and for patients who fail to respond to endoscopic treatment. Definitive treatment depends on the location of the cyst. Pancreatic pseudocysts closely attached to the stomach should be treated with a cystogastrostomy. In this procedure, an anterior gastrostomy is performed.[25] Once the pseudocyst is located, it is drained through the posterior wall of the stomach using a linear stapler (Video 92.1). The defect in the anterior wall of the stomach is closed in two layers. Pancreatic pseudocysts located in the head of the pancreas that are in close contact with the duodenum are treated with a cystoduodenostomy. Finally, some pseudocysts are not in contact with the stomach or duodenum. The surgical treatment for these patients is a Roux-en-Y cystojejunostomy. Surgical cyst enterostomy is successful in achieving immediate cyst drainage in more than 90% of cases. After initial resolution, pseudocyst formation may recur in up to 12% of cases during long-term follow-up, depending on the location of the cyst and underlying cause of the disease.

Complications of pancreatic pseudocysts include bleeding and pancreaticopleural fistula secondary to vascular and pleural erosion, respectively; bile duct and duodenal obstruction; rupture into the abdominal cavity; and infection. Percutaneous drainage is indicated only for septic patients secondary to pseudocyst infection because it has a high incidence of external fistula.

Pancreatic Ascites and Pancreaticopleural Fistulas

Although very rare, complete disruption of the pancreatic duct can lead to significant accumulation of fluid. This condition should be suspected in patients who have an episode of AP, develop significant abdominal distention, and have free intraabdominal fluid. Diagnostic paracentesis typically demonstrates

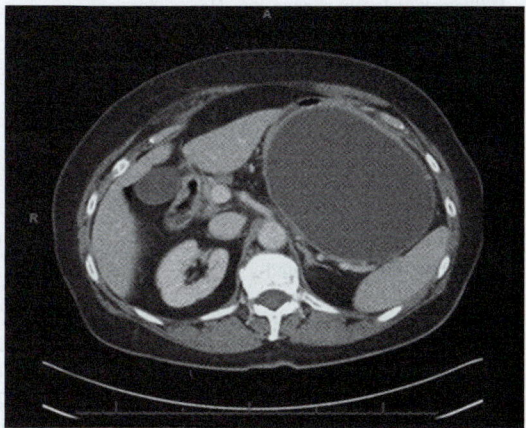
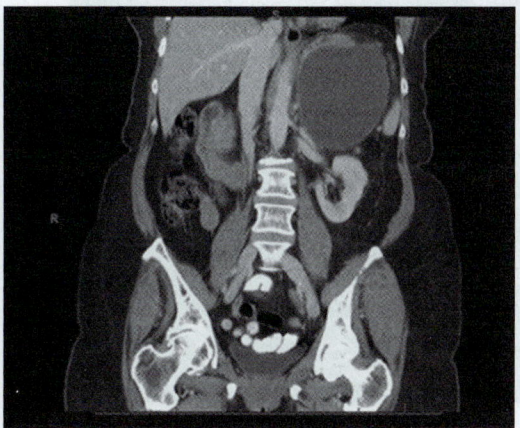

FIGURE 92.10 Computed tomography scans showing a large pseudocyst arising in the tail of the pancreas.

elevated amylase and lipase levels. Treatment consists of abdominal drainage combined with endoscopic placement of a pancreatic stent across the disruption. Failure of this therapy may require surgical treatment; it consists of distal resection and closure of the proximal stump. Pancreatic leak or pancreatic fistula is also a frequent complication after pancreatic operations, defined by the International Study Group on Pancreatic Surgery (ISGPS) as drain output (intraoperative or percutaneous) with amylase > 3 times normal serum value. In 2016 ISGPS guidelines redefined Grade A fistula as "biochemical leak," a indicating amylase-rich fluid without any clinical impact. Grade B fistula require ongoing drainage and active mangaement after 3 weeks, while Grade C includes severe outcomes such as reoperation, organ failure, or death (Table 92.4). Most fistulas are controlled by operatively placed drainage catheters, though uncontrolled fistulas may require additional drain placement or operative exploration, sometimes mandating complete pancreatectomy.

Posterior pancreatic duct disruption into the pleural space has been described rarely—a pancreatic-pleural fistula. Symptoms that suggest this condition include dyspnea, abdominal pain, cough, and chest pain. The diagnosis is confirmed with chest radiography, thoracentesis, and CT scan. Fig. 92.11 demonstrates a large, left-sided pleural effusion caused by a pancreatic-pleural fistula. Amylase levels above 50,000 IU in the pleural fluid confirm the diagnosis. It is more common after alcoholic pancreatitis, and in 70% of patients, it is associated with pancreatic pseudocysts. Iatrogenic pancreaticopleural fistulas may also be seen after placement of percutaneous drainage catheters that traverse the diaphragm. Initial treatment requires chest drainage, parenteral nutritional support, and administration of octreotide. Up to 60% of patients respond to this therapy. Persistent drainage should also be treated with endoscopic sphincterotomy and stent placement. Patients who do not respond to these measures require surgical treatment of the source of the fistula from the pancreas, similar to that described for pancreatic ascites.

Vascular Complications

AP is rarely associated with arterial vascular complications. The most common vessel affected is the splenic artery, but the SMA, cystic artery, and GDA have also been found to be affected. It has been proposed that pancreatic elastase damages the vessels, leading to pseudoaneurysm formation. Spontaneous rupture results in massive bleeding. Clinical manifestations include sudden onset of abdominal pain, tachycardia, and hypotension. If possible, arterial embolization should be attempted to control the bleeding. Refractory cases require ligation of the affected vessel. The mortality ranges from 28% to 56%.

Pancreatic inflammation can also produce vascular thrombosis; the vessel usually affected is the splenic vein, but in severe cases, it can extend into the portal venous system. Imaging demonstrates splenomegaly, gastric varices, and splenic vein occlusion. Thrombolytics have been described in the acute early phase; however, most patients can be managed with conservative treatment. Anticoagulation for splanchnic vein thrombosis related to pancreatitis has not been shown to improve recanalization rates compared with expectant management.[27]

Recurrent episodes of upper gastrointestinal bleeding caused by short gastric venous hypertension in the wall of the fundus of the stomach should be treated with splenectomy.

Pancreatocutaneous Fistula

The frequency of pancreatic fistulas is low. Only 0.4% of patients have this complication after an acute episode. However, the incidence of this complication increases in patients with other complications after AP: 4.5% in patients with pancreatic pseudocysts (4.5%) and 40% in patients with infected necrosis after surgical debridement.[23] Treatment is conservative for most patients.

CHRONIC PANCREATITIS

In contrast to AP, the histologic hallmark of chronic pancreatitis is the persistent inflammation and irreversible fibrosis associated with atrophy of the pancreatic parenchyma. These histologic

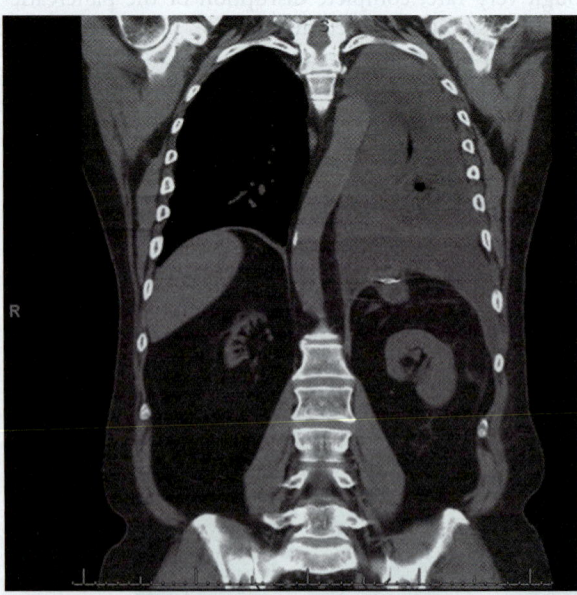

FIGURE 92.11 Massive left-sided pleural effusion secondary to a pancreaticopleural fistula.

TABLE 92.4 International Study Group on Pancreatic Surgery Classification of Pancreatic Fistulas

PARAMETER	GRADE		
	BL	B	C
Increased amylase >3× upper normal limit	Yes	Yes	Yes
Persistent peripancreatic drainage >3 weeks	No	Yes	Yes
Clinically relevant change in management of POPF	No	Yes	Yes
POPF percutaneous or endoscopic interventions for collections	No	Yes	Yes
Angiographic procedures for POPF-related bleeding	No	Yes	Yes
Reoperation	No	No	Yes
POPF-related organ failure	No	No	Yes
Signs of infections related to POPF	No	Yes, without organ failure	Yes, with organ failure
Death related to POPF	No	No	Yes

BL, Biochemical leak; *POPF,* postoperative pancreatic fistula.
From Bassi C, Marchegiani G, Dervenis C, et al. The 2016 update of the International Study Group (ISGPS) definition and grading of postoperative pancreatic fistula: 11 years after. *Surgery.* 2017;161(3):584-591.

features are associated with chronic pain and endocrine and exocrine insufficiency that significantly decrease the quality of life of these patients. Chronic pancreatitis affects between 5 to 8 per 100,000 adults, two-thirds of patients with chronic pancreatitis are males, and risk is higher among Blacks than among Whites.[28]

Risk Factors

The specific cause and frequency of each condition vary among countries, hospital populations, and referral practices. In general, heavy alcohol consumption is the most common cause of chronic pancreatitis (70%–80% of cases), especially in urban hospitals. Conditions such as chronic duct obstruction, trauma, pancreas divisum, cystic dystrophy of the duodenal wall, hyperparathyroidism, hypertriglyceridemia, autoimmune pancreatitis, tropical pancreatitis, and hereditary pancreatitis are rare and account for less than 10% of all cases. However, hereditary, chronic, and autoimmune pancreatitis are more common in referral centers. In up to 20% of patients, a clear cause cannot be documented, and cases are considered to be idiopathic. The natural history of chronic pancreatitis is not well understood but is currently being studied in a prospective cohort study in the United States (Prospective Evaluation of Chronic Pancreatitis for Epidemiologic and Translational Studies [PROCEED] trial).[29]

Alcohol Abuse

Prolonged alcohol abuse is the most important risk factor associated with chronic pancreatitis. The fact that only 3% to 7% of heavy drinkers develop chronic pancreatitis suggests that alcohol is only a cofactor and that other factors are required for development of this complication. Alcohol exerts multiple noxious effects in the pancreas: It increases the total protein concentration in the pancreatic juice, it promotes the synthesis and secretion of lithostathine by acinar cells, and it increases glycoprotein 2 secretion in pancreatic juice. These factors lead to protein precipitation and subsequent formation of protein plugs and, eventually, stones inside the pancreatic duct. As a result of the obstruction, acinar cells are no longer able to secrete pancreatic enzymes and are predisposed to autodigestion. In addition, several products of alcohol metabolism, such as fatty acid ethyl esters and reactive oxygen species, cause fragility of intraacinar organelles, such as zymogen granules and lysosomes, which leads to abnormal pancreatic enzyme activation inside acinar cells. Acetaldehyde, another alcohol metabolite, causes direct acinar injury. Chronic alcohol consumption is associated with enhanced NF-κB activity, decreased perfusion in the microcirculation of the pancreas, and increased intracellular calcium levels.

The identification of PSCs in the late 1990s is one of the most important discoveries in the pathophysiology of chronic pancreatitis.[30] PSCs are specialized quiescent fibroblasts found at the base of acinar cells. Once stimulated, PSCs differentiate into activated myofibroblasts, which synthesize proteins that form the extracellular matrix. Examples of these proteins include collagen I and III, fibronectin, laminin, and matrix metalloproteinases. PSCs have responses similar to hepatic stellate cells; chronic necrosis and inflammation (necroinflammation) induce the release of inflammatory mediators, such as platelet-derived growth factor, TGF-β, TNF-α, IL-1, and IL-6, which are known to activate PSCs. Consequently, the synthesis of collagen and other components of pancreatic fibrosis is increased. It has been postulated that the chronic necroinflammation induced by ethanol activates PSCs and induces pancreatic fibrosis. Interestingly, it has also been shown that alcohol and some of its metabolites (e.g., acetaldehyde) cause activation of PSCs.

Although they have been evaluated only in preclinical studies, novel therapies that target the activation of PSCs are being investigated. It has been reported that antioxidants, angiotensin-converting enzyme inhibitors, peroxisome proliferator-activated receptor gamma ligands, and vitamin A inhibit the activity of PSCs.

Smoking

Epidemiologic studies have shown that smoking increases the risk of alcohol-induced chronic pancreatitis. Active smokers develop chronic pancreatitis at a younger age compared with nonsmokers. In addition, the risk of pancreatic calcifications and diabetes mellitus is increased in patients who smoke compared with nonsmokers.

Gene Mutations

Under physiologic conditions, pancreatic enzyme activation is strictly controlled. Mutations in proteins that regulate this activation increase the risk of chronic pancreatitis. Mutations in the cationic trypsinogen gene, also known as the *protease serine 1 (PRSS1)* gene, are common in hereditary chronic pancreatitis. *PRSS1* is located on chromosome 7 and regulates trypsinogen production; mutations in this gene are associated with intraacinar trypsinogen activation. *PRSS1* mutations have been documented in hereditary pancreatitis but are uncommon in other forms of chronic pancreatitis.

SPINK-1 is a peptide secreted by acinar cells that regulates the premature activation of trypsinogen. Because *SPINK1* mutations are present in 1% to 2% of healthy patients but the prevalence of chronic pancreatitis is much lower, it has been hypothesized that *SPINK1* mutations are not enough to trigger pancreatic inflammation. However, they lower the threshold for its development and influence the severity of the disease. *SPINK1* mutations are more prevalent in alcoholic, hereditary, and idiopathic pancreatitis.

The secretion of bicarbonate and chloride in respiratory and pancreatic secretions is regulated by the *CFTR* gene. *CFTR* mutations affect the normal secretion of bicarbonate, decrease pancreatic juice volume, and augment the concentration of pancreatic enzymes inside the pancreatic duct. Homozygous *CFTR* mutations result in cystic fibrosis; heterozygous mild mutations predispose to pancreatic exocrine insufficiency and chronic pancreatitis. The prevalence of *CFTR* gene mutations is higher in patients with alcoholic, idiopathic, and hereditary pancreatitis compared with the general population. Similarly, mutation in human chymotrypsin C gene has been found to be associated with development of chronic pancreatitis. It seems that chymotrypsin C protects against pancreatitis by degrading trypsinogen and thereby curtailing harmful intrapancreatic trypsinogen activation.[31]

Although our understanding of the pathogenesis of chronic pancreatitis has evolved in a largely trypsin-centric fashion, animal studies in trypsin knockout mice suggest that even in the absence of trypsin, chronic noxious stimuli can induce chronic pancreatitis.[32] These results suggest that alternative pathways independent of trypsin may exist that can lead to chronic injury in pancreatitis, and elucidation of these pathways may lead to development of novel therapeutics.

Types of Chronic Pancreatitis
Autoimmune Pancreatitis

Autoimmune pancreatitis is a chronic inflammatory disorder that involves the pancreas. At least two different histologic variants have been defined: (1) type 1, which is the pancreatic manifestation of an immunoglobulin G4-related disease, and (2) type 2, a pancreatic-specific disorder that is not associated with immunoglobulin G4. Type 1 is the most common; it is characterized by dense, periductal lymphoplasmacytic infiltrates, storiform fibrosis, and obliterative venulitis. Plasmatic cells typically stain positive for immunoglobulin G4. In type 2, the pancreas is infiltrated by neutrophils, lymphocytes, and plasma cells that destroy and obliterate the epithelium in the pancreatic duct. Autoimmune pancreatitis is more common in males than in females. Up to 80% of patients are older than 50 years. Typical imaging findings include a "sausage-shaped" pancreas due to the edema and inflammation. Patients with autoimmune pancreatitis can develop acute symptoms, such as jaundice, or AP, closely mimicking patients with pancreatic adenocarcinoma. Similarly, patients with focal autoimmune pancreatitis may have a pseudomass on imaging that appears like a hypoenhancing mass in pancreatic cancer.[33]

Tropical Pancreatitis

Tropical pancreatitis is not common in the United States; it is more common in tropical areas within 30 degrees of the equator, particularly in India. Its pathophysiology has not been completely delineated, but it has been associated with cassava ingestion and *SPINK1* mutations. Up to 45% to 50% of patients with tropical pancreatitis have *SPINK1* mutations.

Idiopathic Pancreatitis

In up to 10% to 20% of patients with chronic pancreatitis, a clear cause that predisposed to the disease is not evident. Future identification of genetic defects associated with chronic pancreatitis may allow the identification of individuals at highest risk for development of this disease.

Clinical Manifestations

Pain is the primary manifestation of chronic pancreatitis. Initially precipitated by oral intake, the intensity, frequency, and duration of pain gradually increase with worsening disease. Quality of life of these patients is significantly affected because of

decreased oral intake, interference with daily activities, and dependence on narcotic pain medications. Nausea and vomiting are not common early on; however, they may appear as the disease progresses.

Pancreatic inflammation and fibrosis not only affect the pancreatic ducts but also decrease the number and function of acinar cells. At least 90% of the gland needs to be dysfunctional before pancreatic exocrine insufficiency, as evidenced by steatorrhea, diarrhea, and other symptoms of malabsorption, develops. In severe cases, diseases associated with fat-soluble vitamin deficiency, such as bleeding, osteopenia, and osteoporosis, develop. Exocrine insufficiency occurs in 80% to 90% of patients with long-standing chronic pancreatitis.

Chronic pancreatitis also affects islet cell populations. As a result, 40% to 80% of patients will have clinical manifestations of diabetes mellitus, typically occurring years after the onset of abdominal pain and pancreatic exocrine insufficiency.

Jaundice or cholangitis occurs in 5% to 10% of patients because of fibrosis of the distal common bile duct. Extensive scarring in the head of the pancreas can also obstruct the duodenum, leading to severe nausea, vomiting, and abdominal pain. Upper gastrointestinal bleeding secondary to portal or splenic vein thrombosis is a rare manifestation of chronic pancreatitis.

Diagnosis

Imaging Studies

Cross-sectional imaging plays an important role in the diagnosis of chronic pancreatitis; however, a standardized approach to the diagnosis and assessment of disease is lacking. The most common CT findings in chronic pancreatitis include dilated pancreatic duct (68%), parenchymal atrophy (54%), and pancreatic calcifications (50%; Fig. 92.12). Other findings include peripancreatic fluid, focal pancreatic enlargement, biliary duct dilation, and irregular pancreatic parenchyma contour. CT has a sensitivity of 56% to 95% and a specificity of 85% to 100% for the diagnosis of chronic pancreatitis. In addition to establishing the diagnosis, CT is particularly useful for assessing complications, such as

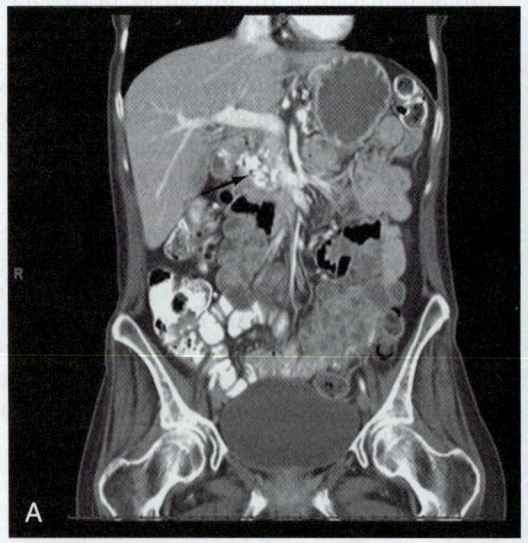
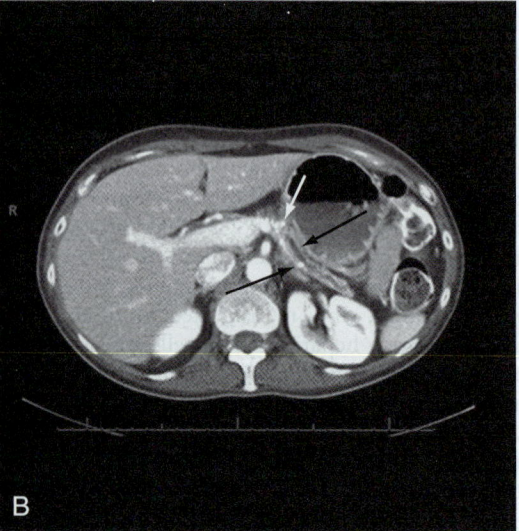

FIGURE 92.12 Typical computed tomography findings associated with chronic pancreatitis. Shown are pancreatic duct dilation *(long arrow)* and intrapancreatic calcifications, which are also typical of chronic pancreatitis *(short arrow)*.

pancreatic duct disruption, pseudocysts, portal and splenic vein thrombosis, and splenic and pancreaticoduodenal artery pseudoaneurysms.

MRI is a reliable alternative to evaluate patients with chronic pancreatitis. The sensitivity for the diagnosis of pancreatic calcifications is lower, but MRI is useful to detect changes in the pancreatic parenchyma suggestive of chronic inflammation, such as changes in intensity, pancreatic atrophy, and irregularities in the contour. In addition, MRCP with secretin injection is particularly useful to evaluate intraductal strictures and pancreatic duct disruption. Efforts to standardize imaging evaluation of chronic pancreatitis patients are underway.

Although ERCP was historically considered the "gold standard" for the diagnosis of chronic pancreatitis, current indications include patients for whom other diagnostic tests, including CT and MRCP, are contraindicated or have failed to corroborate the diagnosis. ERCP should be considered a therapeutic modality in patients who develop pancreatic duct complications amenable to endoscopic therapy, such as stricture, stone, pseudocysts, and biliary stenosis.

EUS has emerged as the most accurate technique to diagnose chronic pancreatitis in patients with minimal-change disease or in the early stages. The criteria required for diagnosis of chronic pancreatitis based on EUS are known as the *Rosemont criteria* (Box 92.5). Histologic evidence of inflammation, atrophy, and fibrosis is the gold standard for the diagnosis of chronic pancreatitis; however, current evidence does not support the use of EUS-guided FNA or Tru-Cut biopsies to diagnose this disease. Although positive Rosemont criteria are predictive of histologic pancreatitis, a finding of Rosemont "normal" has a poor negative predictive value, with as many as 55% of cases ultimately found to have chronic pancreatitis on histopathologic exam.[28]

Functional Tests

Measurement of the fecal elastase 1 level is the preferred noninvasive study to diagnose pancreatic exocrine insufficiency. It quantifies the amount of fecal elastase 1 using monoclonal or polyclonal anti–human elastase 1 antibodies. A fecal elastase 1 concentration above 200 μg/g feces is normal, a fecal elastase 1 concentration between 100 and 200 μg/g defines mild to moderate pancreatic insufficiency, and a fecal elastase 1 concentration below 100 μg/g establishes the diagnosis of severe pancreatic exocrine insufficiency.

The fecal fat and weight estimation test measures the stool content of fat after a nutritional fat intake of 100 g/day for 3 days. If the stool fat content exceeds 7 g/day, the diagnosis of steatorrhea is established.

Treatment

Medical Treatment

The main goal in the treatment of chronic pancreatitis is palliation of symptoms and removal of predisposing factors. Optimal treatment requires that a multidisciplinary team follow a systematized and well-structured therapeutic plan. Patient counseling is an important component because current evidence suggests that this disease is irreversible, but disease progression can be delayed if the predisposing condition is eradicated. Patients should

---

BOX 92.5 Rosemont Consensus-Based Endoscopic Ultrasound Features for Diagnosis of Chronic Pancreatitis

Parenchymal Features
Major A Criteria
- Hyperechoic foci with postacoustic shadowing

Major B Criteria
- Honeycombing lobularity[a]

Minor Criteria
- Hyperechoic, nonshadowing foci ≥3 mm in length and width
- Lobularity including three or more noncontiguous lobules in the body or tail
- Pancreatic cysts ≥2 mm in short axis
- At least three strands[b]

Ductal Features
Major A Criteria
- Main pancreatic duct calculi[c]

Minor Criteria
- Irregular main pancreatic duct contour
- Dilated side branches[d]

- Main pancreatic duct dilation (≥3.5 mm in the body or ≥1.5 mm in the tail)
- Hyperechoic main pancreatic duct margin >50% of the main pancreatic duct in the body and tail[e]

Diagnosis of Chronic Pancreatitis
Consistent With Chronic Pancreatitis
- 1 major A criterion + ≥3 or more minor criteria
- 1 major A criterion + major B criterion
- 2 major A criteria

Suggestive of Chronic Pancreatitis[f]
- 1 major A criterion + <3 minor criteria
- 1 major B criterion + ≥3 minor criteria
- ≥5 minor criteria

Indeterminate for Chronic Pancreatitis[f]
- 3 to 4 minor criteria in the absence of major criteria
- Major B criterion + <3 minor criteria

Normal
- <3 minor criteria

[a]Defined as lobularity that includes at least three contiguous lobules in the body or tail. It should be assessed in the body and tail.
[b]Strands are defined as hyperechoic lines ≥3 mm in length seen in at least two different directions in the body or tail of the pancreas.
[c]The presence of calculi in the main pancreatic duct, regardless of location, is the most predictive finding of chronic pancreatitis.
[d]Defined as at least three tubular anechoic structures, each one ≥1 mm in width, budding from the main pancreatic duct.
[e]With suggestive and indeterminate chronic pancreatitis, the diagnosis needs to be confirmed with another imaging modality.
Adapted from Catalano MF, Sahai A, Levy M, et al. EUS-based criteria for the diagnosis of chronic pancreatitis: the Rosemont classification. *Gastrointest Endosc.* 2009;69:1251-1261.

be strongly encouraged to stop drinking and smoking. Furthermore, other risk factors, such as hypertriglyceridemia, should be treated, and diet modification (i.e., low-fat diet) may benefit some patients.

Pain Management

Because most patients develop pain during the natural history of the disease, analgesic selection is a cornerstone of treatment. Nonsteroidal antiinflammatory drugs are the first line of treatment. Moderate to severe pain that does not respond to nonsteroidal antiinflammatory drugs should be treated with tramadol. Patients with severe pain that does not respond to these recommendations should be treated with potent, long-acting narcotics. It cannot be overemphasized that adjuvant measures to prevent addiction, depression, and poor quality of life should be considered for patients with severe pain who require narcotics. Alternative drugs useful in the treatment of other conditions associated with chronic pain, such as tricyclic antidepressants, selective serotonin reuptake inhibitors, combined serotonin and norepinephrine reuptake inhibitors, gabapentin, and $\alpha 2\delta$ inhibitors, may also be considered. RCTs have shown that nonnarcotic medications can reduce pain and reduce the need for opioids in chronic pancreatitis patients, highlighting the need for a multidisciplinary team that includes pain management experts. For patients with unrelenting pain, celiac neurolysis has been attempted but without sustained success in those with chronic pancreatitis. A recent randomized surgical study of 88 patients with weak to strong pain of less than 6 months in duration compared early pancreatic ductal drainage versus conventional medical/endoscopic therapy (Early Surgery Compared to Endoscopy-First Approach in Patients with Chronic Pancreatitis [ESCAPE] trial) and found a lower pain score in the surgical group (37 vs. 49, $p = 0.02$).[34] This study supported two previous RCTs that showed superiority of surgery over endoscopic therapies for pain relief with similar complication rates and mortality and a greater use of reinterventions in the endoscopic group.[35,36]

Pancreatic Exocrine Insufficiency

There is no question about the digestive benefits of pancreatic enzyme replacement in patients with pancreatic exocrine insufficiency. In the absence of pancreatic enzyme replacement therapy, patients with chronic pancreatitis may suffer from steatorrhea or diarrhea, leading to malabsorption, malnutrition, and vitamin and mineral deficiencies. A thorough nutritional evaluation should be performed before initiation of therapy; however, generally, 90,000 USP of lipase per day, usually divided by 30,000 USP per meal, is required to avoid malabsorption. Therapeutic trials with pancreatic enzymes should last at least 6 weeks and should be given along with proton pump inhibitors because acid suppression improves the effects of uncoated pancreatic enzymes.

Endocrine Insufficiency

Endocrine insufficiency and resulting diabetes are not always present early on but may develop in patients with chronic pancreatitis. Unlike more common type 1 or type 2 diabetes, patients with chronic pancreatitis may develop diabetes, which includes deficiency of insulin and other regulatory hormones such as glucagon. These patients are at higher risk of suboptimal glucose control, particularly severe hypoglycemia related to insulin use, and should be managed by an endocrinologist with experience in managing these complex patients.

Interventional Therapy: Endoscopic Treatment

ERCP is the primary modality for treating symptomatic pancreatic duct obstruction with dilation and polyethylene stent placement. Note that the differential diagnosis of pancreatic duct strictures includes pancreatic cancer. Only after a thorough evaluation that includes CT, MRCP, or EUS has completely ruled out the possibility of malignant disease should endoscopic treatment be considered. Surgical resection is indicated if any concern of malignant disease exists.

Endoscopic stone extraction should be considered for patients with pain and pancreatic duct dilation secondary to stones. Extracorporeal shock wave lithotripsy followed by therapeutic ERCP may be required for the treatment of large, impacted stones. The success rate varies from 44% to 77% for this technique. In conjunction with stone extraction, pancreatic duct stenting may benefit patients by relieving obstruction. Although this relief may be temporary, during the interim, a patient may be able to improve nutritional and functional status before further, perhaps more invasive therapy.

Biliary obstruction caused by chronic pancreatitis occurs in 10% of patients and is best treated with surgical bypass. Temporary relief of the obstruction with plastic stents is indicated for patients with cholangitis or for those who are severely malnourished.

Surgical Treatment

Several factors, including intractable pain, biliary or pancreatic duct obstruction, duodenal obstruction, pseudocyst or pseudoaneurysm formation, and the inability to rule out malignant disease, may prompt surgical intervention. The choice of surgical procedure depends on the symptoms requiring palliation and the presence or absence of pancreatic ductal dilation. In general, patients with a dilated pancreatic duct (defined as diameter >7 mm), or large duct disease, require a decompressing procedure; patients with a nondilated pancreatic duct, or small duct disease, require a resectional procedure. Several clinical scenarios that require surgical intervention are described here.

Pancreatic duct dilation secondary to duct stones or strictures. *Pancreatic duct dilation* is defined as a MPD measuring at least 7 mm in diameter. Pancreatic duct dilation can be secondary to a single stone or stricture; however, it is often caused by multiple strictures and stones in the pancreatic duct. The pancreatic duct dilation observed on pancreatography for chronic pancreatitis is classically described as a chain of lakes, which reflects the presence of multiple dilations and stenoses. When it is accompanied by intractable pain, this condition is best treated with side-to-side Roux-en-Y pancreaticojejunostomy, also known as the *modified Puestow procedure* or *lateral pancreaticojejunostomy.*

The anterior surface of the pancreatic duct is opened, and the anterior surface of the duct is completely unroofed. This tissue should be sent for frozen section analysis to rule out underlying malignant disease. The proximal extent of tissue resection can extend to the ampulla and medial duodenal wall, and the distal limit is within 1 to 2 cm of the end of the pancreas. Failure to cross the GDA into the neck and head of the pancreas may leave undrained pancreatic head or uncinate process ducts obstructed by stones or strictures, which may give incomplete relief or early recurrence of symptoms. After all stones are extracted, a standard Roux-en-Y is used to create a lateral pancreaticojejunostomy. The main advantage offered by this procedure is parenchymal conservation, which preserves endocrine and exocrine function. The modified Puestow procedure provides palliation of pain in 80% of cases; however,

30% of cases will recur, usually 3 to 5 years after surgery. Decompressive procedures temporarily relieve the ductal obstruction, but in most cases, they do not modify the natural history of the disease, and chronic pancreatitis progresses. Other factors associated with recurrence include smoking and alcohol ingestion after surgery, failure to decompress the head and uncinate process properly, and length of the pancreaticojejunostomy.

In 1987, Andersen and Frey described the local resection of the pancreatic head (i.e., "coring") with longitudinal pancreaticojejunostomy as an alternative procedure for patients in which the pancreatic head is enlarged (≥5 cm in transverse diameter). The surgical approach is similar to the Puestow procedure; however, once the anterior surface of the pancreatic duct has been completely exposed, the anterior portion of the head of the pancreas is also resected, leaving a 1-cm rim of pancreatic tissue along the duodenal margin. Fig. 92.13 shows intraoperative images of a Frey procedure. This procedure is also an alternative for patients with a dilated pancreatic duct secondary to a benign stricture in the head of the pancreas associated with severe inflammation, scarring, or portal hypertension surrounding the head of the pancreas that precludes a safe pancreaticoduodenectomy. The main disadvantage is the removal of pancreatic parenchyma. A study has demonstrated that after this procedure, 62% of patients are completely free of pain, and 95% of patients have satisfactory pain control. In the same series, 34% of patients developed endocrine or exocrine pancreatic insufficiency.[37]

Pancreatic duct dilation secondary to a single stricture or stone. On occasion, a single stricture that is proximal to the papilla produces pancreatic duct dilation. As an alternative to a Puestow or Frey procedure, a pancreaticoduodenectomy (or pancreatoduodenectomy) can be performed to relieve the obstruction. This procedure is described further in the chapter focusing on the surgical treatment of pancreatic adenocarcinoma. It must be emphasized that this procedure is absolutely contraindicated if more than one obstruction is present in the duct. Single distal obstructions can occasionally be treated with a distal pancreatectomy. The main disadvantage of both procedures is that they can be associated with pancreatic insufficiency because normal parenchyma is removed. This issue may be ameliorated with autotransplantation of islet cells derived from the resected parenchyma, further discussed later in the chapter.

Focal inflammatory mass without significant dilation of the pancreatic duct. In a small percentage of patients with chronic pancreatitis, a predominant mass in the head or, less commonly,

in the tail of the pancreas without any evidence of pancreatic duct dilation is seen. Long-standing chronic pancreatitis is also a risk factor for development of pancreatic cancer; therefore, even in patients with a known history of chronic pancreatitis, finding a focal mass is concerning because it may represent an area of pancreatic adenocarcinoma that has developed in the setting of chronic pancreatitis. An EUS-guided biopsy should be obtained before any other treatment.

Once malignant disease is ruled out, resection of the pancreatic head may be done with either of two operations: pancreaticoduodenectomy or duodenum-preserving pancreatic head resection, otherwise known as the *Beger procedure.* The Beger procedure was designed to remove the pancreatic head while preserving the remainder of the foregut anatomy and therefore function. Once the pancreatic head is removed, a Roux-en-Y is created and anastomosed to the rim of pancreas or duodenum, pancreatic duct, and body—and perhaps the bile duct if it was entered. RCTs have demonstrated that the Beger procedure offers symptomatic relief that is equivalent to the pancreaticoduodenectomy and Frey procedure in appropriately selected patients.

Diffuse glandular involvement without dilation of the pancreatic duct. These patients can be treated with a Whipple resection, which removes the head of the pancreas. Despite involvement of the total gland, the head is thought to be the so-called "pacemaker" with the greatest density of nerve fibers. Although this treatment can yield durable pain relief, the most effective treatment to eliminate pain in patients without dilation of the pancreatic duct is total pancreatectomy. However, this procedure is invariably associated with diabetes mellitus. In contrast to type 1 diabetes mellitus, the severity and risk of hypoglycemia are increased in these patients. In 1977, researchers at the University of Minnesota described islet autotransplantation after total pancreatectomy to prevent the effects of surgically induced diabetes. In the largest experience there, one-third of patients who underwent this procedure were insulin independent, an additional one-third required insulin intermittently, and the other third was fully dependent. According to this study, 90% had pain relief or reduction, and 50% were able to discontinue narcotics. Similar results were demonstrated at the University of Cincinnati; up to two-thirds of patients had complete or partial islet function, and 40% were insulin independent. Narcotics were discontinued in 66% of patients.[38] Although preliminary results have been encouraging, routine implementation of this operative intervention has been controversial. Major limitations

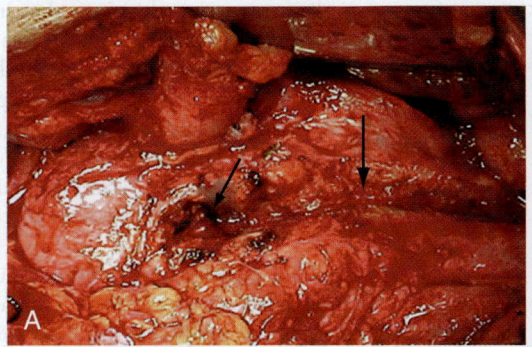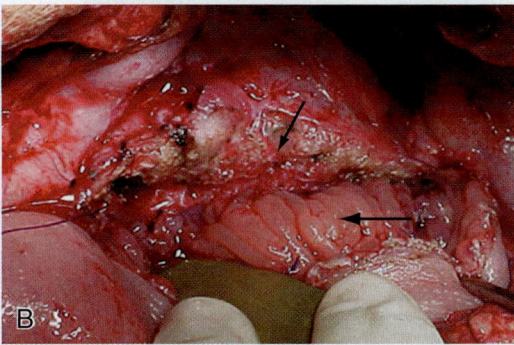

FIGURE 92.13 Frey procedure, intraoperative photographs. (A) Significant dilation of the main pancreatic duct at the level of the head *(short arrow)* and body of the pancreas *(long arrow)* after the anterior surface of the pancreas has been opened. (B) Side-to-side anastomosis between the pancreatic duct *(short arrow)* and jejunum *(long arrow).*

associated with this procedure include the cost and lack of islet-processing facilities.

As several other centers have established islet autotransplantation programs and laboratories, it has become clear that the treatment of patients with severe diffuse chronic pancreatitis should be coordinated by a multidisciplinary team. This should include a pancreatic surgeon, pancreatologist, interventional endoscopist, radiologist, anesthesia pain specialist, endocrinologist, nutritional expert, and perhaps a neuropsychologist or psychiatrist. A multi-faceted approach to the decision and the type of treatment is crucial to long-term success. Groups at the Medical University of South Carolina and the University of Alabama at Birmingham have shown that patients with depression or substance abuse, such as alcoholism, have a poor outcome compared with patients without depression or alcoholism.

In pediatric patients with genetic predisposition to pancreatitis, early pancreatectomy and islet autotransplantation are highly effective at improving quality of life.

Biliary strictures. Chronic scarring and fibrosis of the head of the pancreas result in external compression of the intrapancreatic portion of the common bile duct. Up to one-third of patients with chronic pancreatitis develop radiologic evidence of bile duct dilation; however, significant biliary obstruction occurs in 6% of patients. Biliary strictures typically appear as a long symmetric narrowing that involves the intrapancreatic portion of the common bile duct in MRCP or ERCP (Fig. 92.14). IV fluid and antibiotic therapy and temporary bile duct decompression with plastic stents are indicated for patients who present with cholangitis. Pancreaticoduodenectomy is indicated for patients in whom malignant disease cannot be excluded before surgery. A Roux-en-Y hepaticojejunostomy is an alternative treatment for patients without evidence of malignant disease or significant scarring that precludes resection of the head of the pancreas. A Frey or Beger procedure can often relieve the biliary obstruction by removing the pancreatic head parenchyma that causes compression, thus avoiding the need for a separate biliary bypass.

Duodenal stenosis. Up to 1.2% of patients with chronic pancreatitis develop duodenal strictures. Clinical manifestations include abdominal pain, nausea, vomiting, and significant weight loss. Differential diagnoses include other causes of gastric outlet obstruction secondary to upper gastrointestinal malignant neoplasms and gastroparesis. Severely malnourished patients require IV hydration, nutritional support, and gastric decompression with a nasogastric tube. Permanent treatment requires a gastrojejunostomy.

Pancreatic pseudocyst. Pancreatic pseudocysts develop more frequently in patients with chronic pancreatitis compared with AP. Up to 30% to 40% of patients develop pseudocysts during the course of their disease. Only 10% of patients have spontaneous pancreatic pseudocyst regression. Spontaneous regression is less likely to occur in these patients because pancreatic pseudocysts arise more frequently in the setting of pancreatic duct obstruction. Indications for treatment include symptoms secondary to gastric, duodenal, or biliary compression or associated complications, such as bleeding, pancreaticopleural fistulas, rupture, or spontaneous bleeding. Alternative modalities in the treatment include endoscopic and surgical drainage (see earlier).

Traditionally, management of a symptomatic or persistent pseudocyst has been open operation and, depending on location, drainage through either cystogastrostomy or Roux-en-Y cystojejunostomy. With advancements in interventional endoscopy, drainage has proven successful with ERCP. More recently, drainage with EUS has been shown to be more successful because of improved visualization of vasculature as well as fluid collections and necrosis. Small-caliber plastic stents may be used for simple pancreatic fluid collections or larger metal stents for complex collections or those with infection or necrosis. At the University of Alabama at Birmingham, a prospective randomized trial of endoscopic versus operative cystogastrostomy showed equal efficacy but quicker improvement in quality of life and less hospital expenditure from the endoscopic approach for simple pancreatic pseudocysts.[39]

CYSTIC NEOPLASMS OF THE PANCREAS

Second only to adenocarcinoma, pancreatic cystic neoplasms (PCNs) have become an increasingly recognized entity, with sometimes complex treatment decision algorithms to balance cancer prevention with the risk of (surgical) overtreatment. Currently, there are three widely recognized guidelines providing recommendations for the surveillance and management of PCNs: the American Gastroenterological Association (AGA) guidelines issued in 2015, the International Association of Pancreatology (IAP) guidelines last revised in 2017, and the guidelines from the European Study Group on Cystic Tumors of the Pancreas, last updated in 2018.[40]

PCNs are classified broadly into nonmucinous and mucinous types. Nonmucinous PCNs, such as serous cystic neoplasms (SCNs) and solid pseudopapillary neoplasms (SPNs), are lined by simple cuboidal epithelium, whereas mucinous PCNs, which include IPMNs and mucinous cystic neoplasms (MCNs), are lined by endoderm-derived columnar epithelium.[41] Table 92.5 summarizes the distinguishing features of cystic neoplasms of the pancreas.

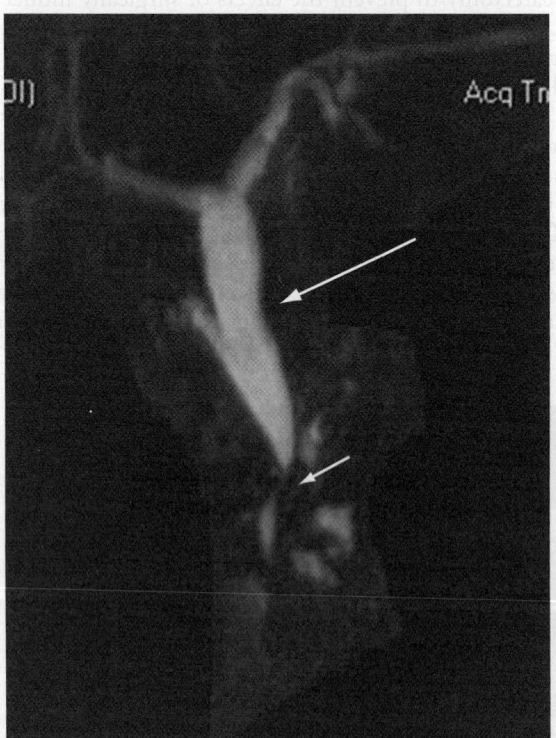

FIGURE 92.14 Bile duct stricture secondary to chronic pancreatitis. Magnetic resonance cholangiopancreatography indicates common bile duct dilation *(large arrow)* secondary to a stricture at the level of the intrapancreatic portion of the common bile duct *(small arrow).*

TABLE 92.5	Defining Characteristics of Pseudocysts and Pancreatic Cystic Neoplasms				
CHARACTERISTICS	**PSEUDOCYST**	**SCN**	**MCN**	**IPMN**	**SPN**
Epidemiology					
Sex	F = M	F ≫ M (4:1)	F ≫> M (10:1)	F = M	F >> M
Age (years)	40–60	60–70	50–60	60–70	25–40
Imaging Findings					
Location	Evenly distributed	Evenly distributed	Head ≪ body/tail	Head > diffuse > body/tail	Body/tail
Appearance	Round, thick-walled large cyst; gland atrophy ± calcification	Multiple small cysts separated by internal septations with central starburst calcifications	Thick-walled, septated macrocyst with smooth contour; ± solid component, eggshell calcifications	Poorly demarcated, lobulated, polycystic mass with dilation of main or branch ducts	Thick-walled encapsulated structures with peripheral solid and central cystic components
Communication with ducts	Yes	No	Very rare	Yes	No
Cyst Fluid Analysis					
Cytology	Inflammatory cells	Scant glycogen-rich cells, with positive periodic acid–Schiff stain	Sheets and clusters of columnar, mucin-containing cells	Tall, columnar, mucin-containing cells	Papillary clusters with central capillaries, myxoid stroma, monomorphism, cercariform cells, and hyaline globules
Mucin stain	Negative	Negative	Positive	Positive	Negative
Amylase	Very high	Low	Low	High	Low
CEA	Low	Low	High	High	Low

CEA, Carcinoembryonic antigen; *F*, female; *M*, male; *IPMN*, intraductal papillary mucinous neoplasm; *MCN*, mucinous cystic neoplasm; *SCN*, serous cystic neoplasm.
From Tran Cao HS, Kellogg B, Lowy AM, et al. Cystic neoplasms of the pancreas. *Surg Oncol Clin N Am*. 2010;19:267-295.

Distinguishing between different types of PCNs is essential because of their varying malignant potential. SCNs are mostly benign and usually do not require surveillance, whereas IPMNs, MCNs, and SPNs are premalignant and need either surveillance or surgical resection. PCNs are known precursors for invasive pancreatic cancer; therefore, patients with premalignant PCNs are routinely monitored.[42] A multidisciplinary approach that incorporates clinical findings, cyst fluid analyses, radiologic findings, and ancillary studies is necessary to ensure accurate classification. The primary goal is to prevent malignancy and alleviate symptoms while avoiding unnecessary surgery.

Subtypes of Cystic Neoplasms

Solid Pseudopapillary Neoplasm

SPN, or Frantz tumor, is a low-grade epithelial neoplasm primarily found in young females (25–35 years). Many lesions are diagnosed incidentally, but a palpable mass is the most common presentation in symptomatic patients. The majority of SPNs have a mean size of 8 cm and are located in the body and tail of the pancreas.[43] Cyst fluid analysis typically shows low CEA and amylase. Macroscopically, they can vary from pure solid to entirely cystic or be composed of a mixture of solid and cystic areas, and they are large, round, and well circumscribed. Analysis of resection specimens has shown a characteristic mutation in the β-catenin gene and the absence of other common mutations, such as *KRAS, SMAD4*, and *TP53*.[44] SPNs are classified as malignant because of the potential for lymphatic spread, recurrence, and distant metastases and ought to be resected.[45]

After complete surgical resection, the long-term outcome for patients with SPN is generally excellent, with 95.6% of patients remaining disease-free over long-term follow-up. However, around 6% of patients present with locally advanced tumors, such as vascular involvement or lymph node metastases, and 8% have distant metastases; therefore, annual lifelong follow-up is essential.[43]

Serous Cystic Neoplasm

SCNs have a predilection for the head of the pancreas and occur in patients with a higher median age. Patients commonly present with vague abdominal pain and less frequently with weight loss and obstructive jaundice. On gross inspection, SCNs are large, well-circumscribed masses. Microscopic examination reveals multiloculated, glycogen-rich small cysts. Central calcification, with radiating septa giving the sunburst appearance, is a radiographic sign on CT in 10% to 20% of patients (Fig. 92.15). With the advent of EUS, these features can now be better delineated. Recently, differential cyst fluid protein expression was observed between SCNs and IPMNs, with low CEA and amylase noted in SCNs compared with IPMNs.[23] Although serous cystic tumors are generally considered benign, pancreatectomy is suggested when the diagnosis of malignant disease is uncertain or in symptomatic serous cystadenomas. Patients with a tumor larger than 4 cm are more likely to be symptomatic and to display a more rapid median growth rate than patients with tumors smaller than 4 cm. Thus, in select patients with large (>4 cm) or rapidly growing lesions, resection of an SCN is appropriate.[46]

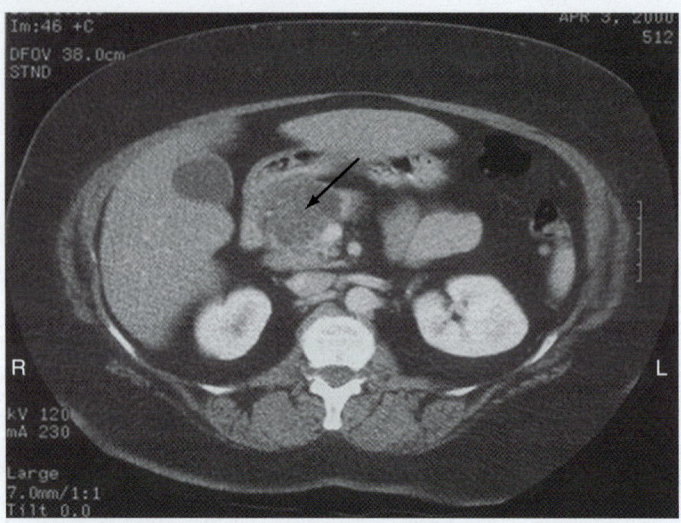

FIGURE 92.15 Computed tomography scan of serous cyst neoplasm. The *arrow* depicts the sunburst appearance and central calcification.

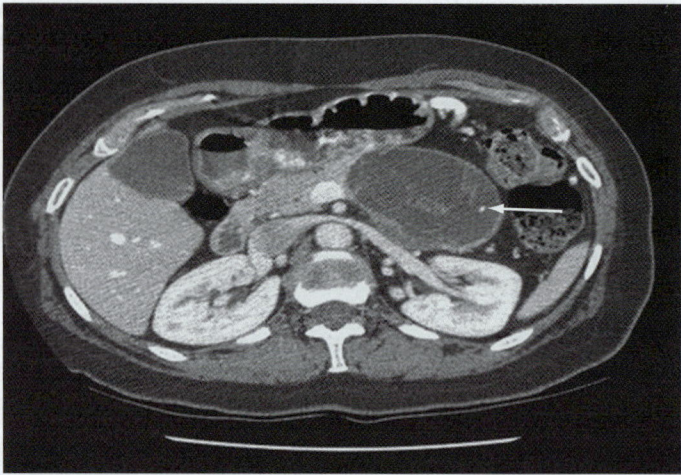

FIGURE 92.17 Computed tomography scan of the tail of the pancreas mucinous cystic neoplasm showing a large multiloculated cyst *(arrow)* in the absence of pancreatic ductal communication.

Mucinous Cystic Neoplasm

MCNs are mucin-producing cyst tumors that, unlike IPMNs (described later), lack communication with the pancreatic duct. These tumors span the histologic spectrum from benign to invasive carcinomas. MCNs contain mucin-producing epithelium and are identified histologically by the presence of mucin-rich cells and ovarian-like stroma surrounding the cyst (Fig. 92.16). Staining for estrogen and progesterone receptors is positive in most cases. Frequently seen in young females, the mean age at presentation is in the fifth decade. Males are rarely affected. MCNs are typically found in the body and tail of the pancreas but infrequently can occur in the head. Although incidental MCN is becoming increasingly common, up to 50% of patients present with vague abdominal pain. A history of pancreatitis may be found in up to 20% of patients, which explains the common misdiagnosis of pseudocyst.

The radiologic characteristic of an MCN on a CT scan is the presence of a solitary cyst, which may have fine septations and be surrounded by a rim of calcification (Fig. 92.17). Cross-sectional imaging may not be able to distinguish between benign and

malignant MCNs; however, the presence of eggshell calcification, larger tumor size, or a mural nodule on cross-sectional imaging is suggestive of malignancy.

EUS and cyst fluid analyses play an important role in the diagnosis of MCN and other cystic neoplasms. FNA with cyst fluid analysis of MCNs demonstrates mucin-rich aspirate, high CEA levels (>192 ng/mL; log scale), and low amylase. Fig. 92.18 illustrates the sensitivity and specificity of CEA in identifying mucinous neoplasms on the basis of fine-needle fluid aspiration. These fluid analyses provide accurate diagnosis in up to 80% of cases.[24]

Pancreatic resection is the standard treatment for MCNs, given the potential for malignant transformation. In the absence of invasive malignant disease, resection is curative, and no further surveillance is required. The prognosis of patients who undergo pancreatectomy for invasive MCNs is poor, although more favorable than that of patients with ductal adenocarcinoma of the pancreas that develops from other precursor lesions. Invasive

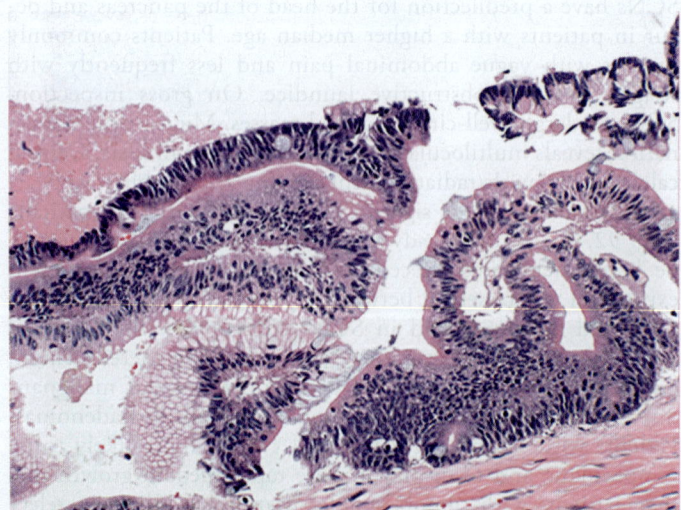

FIGURE 92.16 Ovarian-like stroma is a histologic feature often seen in mucinous cystic neoplasms.

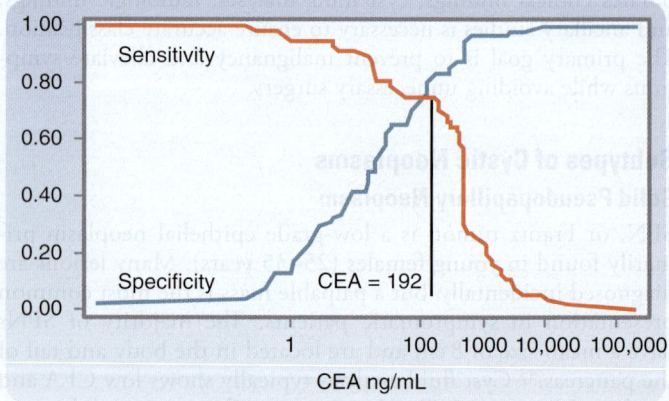

FIGURE 92.18 Sensitivity and specificity curves of cyst fluid carcinoembryonic antigen *(CEA)* concentrations (ng/mL; log scale) for differentiating between mucinous and nonmucinous cystic lesions. An optimal cutoff value of 192 ng/mL correlated with the crossover of the sensitivity and specificity curves. (From Brugge WR, Lewandrowski K, Lee-Lewandrowski E, et al. Diagnosis of pancreatic cystic neoplasms: a report of the cooperative pancreatic cyst study. *Gastroenterology.* 2004;126:1330-1336.)

MCNs exhibit slower growth, less frequent nodal involvement, and less aggressive clinical behavior compared with IPMNs or pancreatic intraepithelial (PanIN)-derived ductal adenocarcinoma; a 5-year survival of 50% to 60% can be expected after resection. Despite limited experience with invasive MCNs, most centers offer adjuvant systemic chemotherapy after surgical resection, especially when node-positive disease is present.

Intraductal Papillary Mucinous Neoplasm

IPMNs of the pancreas are mucinous epithelial neoplasms that arise from the MPDs, branch ducts, or both. IPMNs were first described by Ohashi and typically manifest in the sixth to seventh decade of life. As with other PCNs, because of the increasing use of cross-sectional imaging (CT and MRI), this entity is being increasingly diagnosed. IPMNs encompass a wide spectrum of epithelial changes. Recent efforts to standardize nomenclature for IPMN have been critical to allow for better study of diagnosis, management, and outcomes for IPMN. The terms *adenoma* and *carcinoma in situ* have been abandoned in order to standardize reporting. Current histopathologic grading includes low, moderate, or high-grade dysplasia and presence or absence of invasive malignancy.

There are three subtypes of IPMN, which are defined by the pattern of ductal involvement that is present. Neoplasia that affects only the small side branches is termed *side branch* or *branch duct IPMN* (BD-IPMN), whereas involvement of the MPD is termed *main duct IPMN* (MD-IPMN). Side branch IPMNs that extend into the main duct, often leading to upstream dilation, are termed *mixed-type IPMNs*.

Management Strategies for Intraductal Papillary Mucinous Neoplasm

Risk of malignant transformation has been described in IPMN and is related to multiple factors that have been stratified as worrisome and high risk. These factors have been identified through international consensus and are reported in the international consensus guidelines for the management of IPMN of the pancreas, most recently updated in 2017.[47]

Worrisome features of IPMN based on imaging include BD-IPMN cyst size larger than 3 cm, enhancing mural nodule smaller than 5 mm, thickened enhancing cyst wall, MPD size of 5 to 9 mm, abrupt change in caliber of MPD with distal pancreatic atrophy, and lymphadenopathy. In addition, patients who present with clinical signs of pancreatitis, an elevated carbohydrate antigen 19-9 (CA 19-9) level, or cyst growth of more than 5 mm over 2 years should be considered to have worrisome features. These features are summarized in Table 92.6.

High-risk features of IPMN include the presence of an enhancing nodule larger than 5 mm within the cyst and MPD dilation of more than 1 cm. Patients who present with clinical signs of jaundice should also be considered at high risk.

Numerous genetic mutations that may lead to malignant transformation of IPMN have been evaluated, including *GNAS, KRAS, p53, MUC,* and others. To date, genetic analysis of cyst fluid has failed to improve our ability to predict malignancy or select patients for surgical resection over existing clinical guidelines.

Branch duct intraductal papillary mucinous neoplasm. As the name implies, BD-IPMN involves dilation of the pancreatic duct side branches that communicate with but do not involve the MPD. BD-IPMNs may be focal, involving a single side branch, or multifocal, with multiple cystic lesions throughout

TABLE 92.6 Summary of Worrisome and High-Risk Features of Intraductal Papillary Mucinous Neoplasm

WORRISOME FEATURES	HIGH-RISK FEATURES
Main duct 5–9 mm	Main duct >1 cm
Enhancing mural nodule <5 mm	Enhancing mural nodule >5 mm
Thickened, enhancing cyst wall	Jaundice
BD-IPMN >3 cm	
Abrupt caliber change in main duct with upstream atrophy	
Lymphadenopathy	
Pancreatitis	
Increased serum 19-9	
Cyst growth >5 mm over 2 years	

BD-IPMN, Branch duct intraductal papillary mucinous neoplasm.

the length of the pancreas. Multiplicity of cysts favors a diagnosis of BD-IPMN.

All cysts with worrisome features on CT or MRI should undergo EUS; all cysts with high-risk features should be resected. Recommendations for management of suspected BD-IPMN are summarized in Fig. 92.19.[46] For asymptomatic patients with BD-IPMN who have no worrisome or high-risk features, surveillance may be a reasonable initial strategy; however, multiple variables, including patient age and comorbidities, also play a role in decision-making. In BD-IPMN, new European guidelines suggest that cyst diameter over 4 cm is a relative indication for surgery, alongside factors like cytology positive for malignancy/HGD, solid masses, jaundice, enhancing mural nodules (≥5 mm), and MPD dilation over 10 mm. Relative indications also include fast cyst growth (≥5 mm/year), elevated serum CA 19-9 levels (>37 U/mL), MPD dilation of 5 to 10 mm, and symptomatic lesions (e.g., IPMN-related AP or new-onset diabetes).[48]

Any patient with symptoms or high-risk features related to BD-IPMNs (e.g., jaundice, enhancing mural nodule, and dilated MPD) should undergo surgical resection because the risk of malignant disease in symptomatic patients is heightened. Overall, the risk of invasive malignant disease in the setting of BD-IPMN is approximately 10% to 15%; however, it is increasingly clear that not all patients with IPMNs require surgery. Overall, for BD-IPMN, the risk of invasive malignant disease is approximately 2% to 3% per year. A plan for watchful surveillance with delayed intervention in these patients is reasonable because the risk for malignant transformation with small and asymptomatic branch duct tumors is low, most patients are older, and the time required for development of invasive malignant disease may be longer than the patient's life expectancy.

Main duct intraductal papillary mucinous neoplasm. In contrast to BD-IPMN, MD-IPMN indicates abnormal cystic dilation of the MPD with columnar metaplasia and thick mucinous secretions, which can be seen oozing from a patulous papilla, often described as a "fish mouth" appearance, on endoscopic evaluation (Fig. 92.20). Involvement of the MPD may be focal or diffuse; it is most relevant because of the significantly increased risk of malignant degeneration. Individuals with MD-IPMN have a 30% to 50% risk of harboring invasive pancreatic cancer at the time of presentation. Thus, surgical resection is the cornerstone of treatment. Fig. 92.21 demonstrates MD-IPMN with dilation of the entire pancreatic duct.

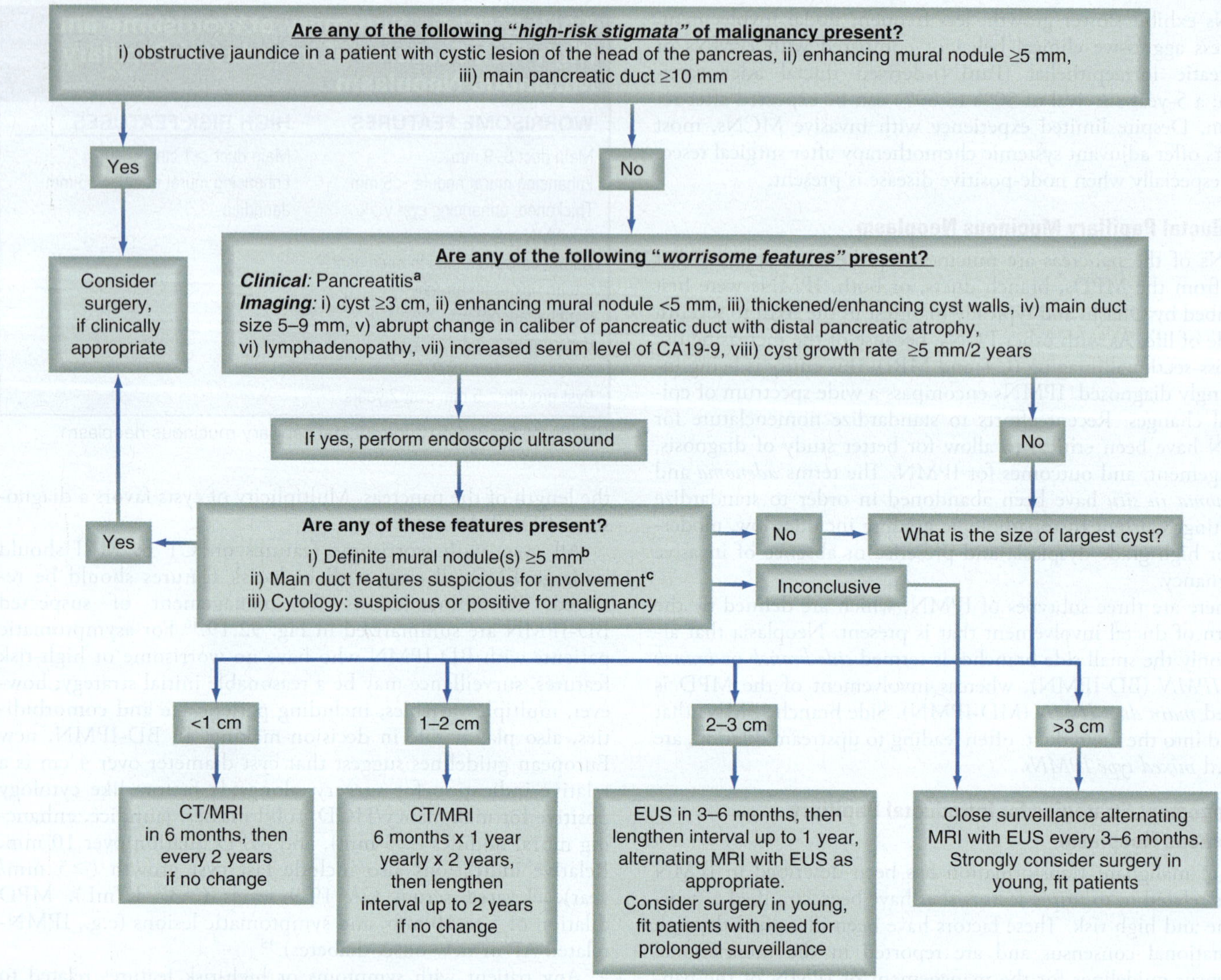

Are any of the following _"high-risk stigmata"_ of malignancy present?
i) obstructive jaundice in a patient with cystic lesion of the head of the pancreas, ii) enhancing mural nodule ≥5 mm,
iii) main pancreatic duct ≥10 mm

Yes → No →

Are any of the following _"worrisome features"_ present?

Clinical: Pancreatitis[a]
Imaging: i) cyst ≥3 cm, ii) enhancing mural nodule <5 mm, iii) thickened/enhancing cyst walls, iv) main duct size 5–9 mm, v) abrupt change in caliber of pancreatic duct with distal pancreatic atrophy, vi) lymphadenopathy, vii) increased serum level of CA19-9, viii) cyst growth rate ≥5 mm/2 years

Consider surgery, if clinically appropriate

If yes, perform endoscopic ultrasound

No →

Are any of these features present?
i) Definite mural nodule(s) ≥5 mm[b]
ii) Main duct features suspicious for involvement[c]
iii) Cytology: suspicious or positive for malignancy

Yes

No

Inconclusive

What is the size of largest cyst?

<1 cm	1–2 cm	2–3 cm	>3 cm
CT/MRI in 6 months, then every 2 years if no change	CT/MRI 6 months x 1 year yearly x 2 years, then lengthen interval up to 2 years if no change	EUS in 3–6 months, then lengthen interval up to 1 year, alternating MRI with EUS as appropriate. Consider surgery in young, fit patients with need for prolonged surveillance	Close surveillance alternating MRI with EUS every 3–6 months. Strongly consider surgery in young, fit patients

FIGURE 92.19 Recommendations for management of suspected branch duct intraductal papillary mucinous neoplasm. *CA 19-9,* Carbohydrate antigen 19-9; *EUS,* endoscopic ultrasound. (From Tanaka M, Fernandez-del Castillo C, Adsay V, et al. International consensus guidelines 2012 for the management of IPMN and MCN of the pancreas. *Pancreatology.* 2012;12:183-197.)

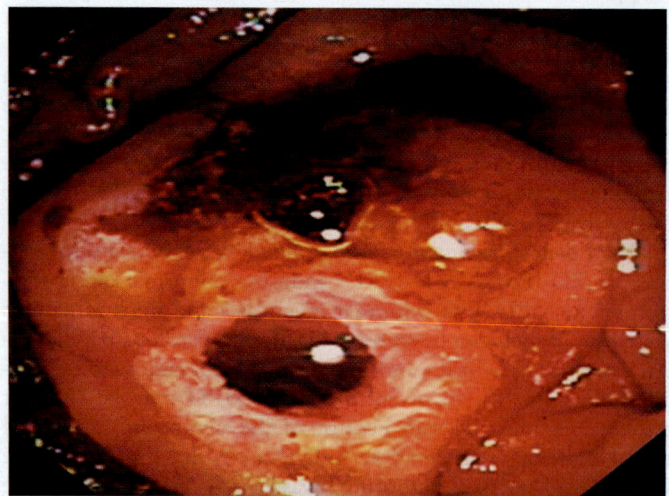

FIGURE 92.20 Classic endoscopic view of intraductal papillary mucinous neoplasm showing viscous fluid oozing from a patulous ampulla of Vater.

Unlike patients with pancreatic ductal adenocarcinomas (PDACs), 50% of patients with IPMNs of the pancreas present with abdominal pain, and up to 25% present with AP, which, not surprisingly, has led to the diagnosis of chronic pancreatitis in many series. Several investigators have studied clinical and pathologic markers as predictors of malignancy and found that jaundice, elevated serum alkaline phosphatase level, mural nodules, diabetes, and MPD diameter of 7 mm or larger are strongly associated with invasive IPMNs. Current guidelines suggest that main duct dilation of more than 5 mm is consistent with a diagnosis of MD-IPMN and a worrisome feature, whereas more than 1 cm is considered high risk. Given the overall high risk of malignant transformation, all patients with evidence of MD-IPMN should be considered for surgical resection if they are surgically fit.

The radiographic features of IPMNs on pancreatic CT scans may include a dilated MPD, cysts of varying sizes, and possibly mural nodules (see Fig. 92.21). MRCP and EUS are important secondary diagnostic studies for the evaluation of patients with suspected IPMN. MRCP may allow localization of mural nodules and pretreatment classification of suspected side branch or main

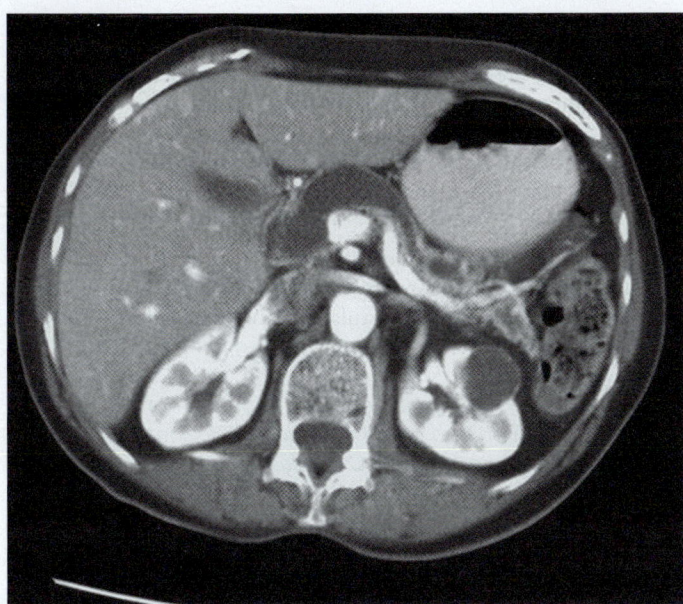

FIGURE 92.21 Cross-sectional imaging of main duct intraductal papillary mucinous neoplasm throughout the entire pancreatic gland and a prominent ampulla of Vater.

duct types of IPMN. EUS can evaluate the pancreatic duct and assess the fluid and solid components of the neoplasm. Aspirated fluid is typically viscous and clear and contains mucin. Cytology studies demonstrate mucin-rich fluid with variable cellularity; columnar mucinous cells with variable atypia may also be seen. As in MCNs and BD-IPMNs, fluid aspirates characteristically reveal an elevated CEA level (>192 ng/mL; log scale). This elevation of the CEA level is not predictive of invasive malignant disease, only the presence of mucinous metaplasia.

Mixed-type intraductal papillary mucinous neoplasm. Mixed-type IPMN denotes a side branch IPMN that has extended to involve the MPD to a varying degree. Concern for mixed-type IPMNs should be raised in individuals with side branch cysts who exhibit upstream dilation of the pancreatic duct because this is an indication of main duct involvement. The biologic behavior of mixed-type IPMNs most closely resembles that of MD-IPMNs, with a significant risk of invasive malignant disease at the time of presentation (30%–50%). As for MD-IPMN, surgical resection is indicated for the treatment of mixed-type IPMN.

Treatment: Surgical Resection for Intraductal Papillary Mucinous Neoplasm

Partial pancreatectomy is the primary treatment for high-risk lesions; however, the optimal extent of pancreatic resection for some patients remains unknown. For BD-IPMN, resection should target the lesion of concern, and therefore, surgical decision-making is usually straightforward. For MD-IPMN, however, it is not always possible to determine the extent of microscopic abnormality within the duct. In the absence of diffuse polyps or enhancing nodules in the main duct, a right-sided pancreatectomy is preferred. Intraoperative frozen section of the pancreas neck margin is obtained, and total pancreatectomy is reserved for those cases with high-grade dysplasia or invasive carcinoma identified at the margin. Although some investigators continue to advocate total pancreatectomy for the treatment of any IPMN, the evidence supporting this approach is decreasing with longer follow-up of patients treated by R0 and R1 partial

pancreatectomy. It is appropriate to recommend partial pancreatectomy and discuss management of the pancreatic margin preoperatively, advising the patient that approximately 15% of patients will require conversion to total pancreatectomy to achieve negative parenchymal resection margins.

Survival outcomes are significantly better in patients with IPMNs than in patients with PDACs. Sohn and associates have analyzed a series of 136 patients with IPMNs; survival rates for patients with noninvasive IPMNs are 97% at 1 year, 94% at 2 years, and 77% at 5 years.[49] When the group of patients with noninvasive IPMNs was analyzed further, no survival differences were found between patients with IPMNs and those with borderline IPMNs. On the contrary, there was a significant difference in survival rate between patients with noninvasive IPMNs and those with invasive IPMNs. The 1-, 3-, and 5-year survival rates for patients with invasive IPMNs were 72%, 58%, and 43%, respectively. Therefore, survival is clearly dependent on the invasive component of the lesion.[50]

Patients diagnosed with invasive cancer associated with their IPMN on pathology should adhere to follow-up schedules akin to those established for PDAC, following the National Comprehensive Cancer Network (NCCN) guidelines. Individuals with high-grade dysplasia are advised to undergo surveillance every 6 months during the first year, shifting to once a year thereafter. Continued monitoring is also advocated for those with low- to moderate-grade dysplasia or benign conditions because the likelihood of developing a new IPMN after surgery is 25% at 5 years and 63% at 10 years.[51]

The decision to terminate surveillance should depend on the age and condition of the patient. Reoperation should be considered for patients who present with recurrence or progression of disease in the pancreas remnant.[52]

Minimally Invasive Approaches to Resection of Cystic Neoplasms

Resections of PCNs must balance the risk of malignant transformation with potential complications and long-term pancreatic insufficiency, deciding between oncologic resection, parenchyma-sparing techniques, and surveillance. If high-grade dysplasia or malignancy is suspected, oncologic resections with radical margins and lymphadenectomy are necessary, regardless of PCN etiology. Recent evidence suggests that minimally invasive approaches may benefit patients with PCNs. Most PCNs are detected in a premalignant stage, allowing for prophylactic surgical treatment.[53] Unlike patients with PDAC, those with PCNs are often younger and curable with resection, making long-term quality of life a priority. Therefore, surgery with minimal morbidity is desirable. However, the specific biology of PCNs must be considered, and minimally invasive resections should adhere to oncologic principles similar to open approaches.

The first laparoscopic pancreaticoduodenectomy was performed in 1994 by Gagner and Pomp. Since then, minimally invasive pancreaticoduodenectomy (MIPD) has seen a rise in popularity. In recent years, at least four randomized control trials have been conducted to compare laparoscopic pancreaticoduodenectomy (LPD) and open pancreaticoduodenectomy (OPD) (Video 92.2; Video 92.3). The results from the single-center, nonblinded RCTs PLOT and PADULAP showed that MIPD has significant benefits over OPD in terms of reduced blood loss, quicker recovery, and shorter LOS, despite longer operating times and having similar postoperative complications.[54–56] However, the LEOPARD-2 trial, a multicenter patient-blinded phase II/III

RCT, was closed early because of significantly increased mortality seen in the MIPD group. After enrolling 99 patients, the risk of mortality after minimally invasive surgery was 10% (five patients) versus 2% (one patient) for open surgery.[57] Debate continues as to the appropriateness of minimally invasive pancreaticoduodenectomy, and the DIPLOMA-2 trial, an RCT performed in 14 high-volume pancreatic centers in Europe, is currently underway to assess outcomes between MIPD and open PD.[58] Additionally, although postoperative outcomes have been well published, data regarding oncologic outcomes are limited. Systematic reviews and single-center retrospective analyses show no major differences between LPD and OPD.[59,60]

Given the limitations of current laparoscopic technology and the need for meticulous vascular control and complex reconstruction in pancreatic surgery, robotic pancreaticoduodenectomy (RPD) has been proposed as an alternative to LPD. The robotic approach has been gaining popularity in the United States, with most high-volume centers offering the technique. The most extensive report on RPD outcomes is from the University of Pittsburgh group, which shared insights from a decade of experience, including 500 consecutive RPDs.[61] This group observed an 8% rate of clinically relevant postoperative pancreatic fistula (CR-POPF), major complications in 24% of cases, median LOS of 8 days, and 90-day mortality rates of 3.1%. Further retrospective propensity-matched analysis of single-center and large databases has supported the association of RPD with decreased rate of CR-POPF.[62–64] Currently underway are two RCTs comparing RPD to OPD: the Dutch DIPLOMA-2 trial, as mentioned before, and the Chinese phase 3 multicenter RCT Robotic Versus Open Pancreaticoduodenectomy for Pancreatic and Periampullary Tumors (PORTAL) study using time to functional recovery as a main outcome. The EUROPA trial, a single-center phase 2b exploratory trial, was just recently published with 62 total patients (RPD, $n = 29$) and only surgeons who had conducted at least ≥40 OPDs and RPDs. Most outcomes, including complications, recovery, and oncologic metrics, were similar. Notably, there was increased delayed gastric emptying in the RPD group and, as expected, increased intraoperative time and cost.[65] RPD presents potential benefits compared with the conventional open method, including enhanced visibility, magnification, and maneuverability, all of which could lead to increased surgical accuracy. However, a critical factor to consider is the learning curve associated with this technically challenging procedure. Defining the point at which a surgeon overcomes the learning curve for RPD remains somewhat unclear, with the reported number of procedures needed ranging widely.[66,67] Looking ahead, as experience grows and robotic technology becomes more widely embraced, it is anticipated that the learning curve for RPD will become more manageable, rendering it an accessible choice for a broader range of pancreatic surgeons.

SELECTED REFERENCES

Andersen DK, Frey CF. The evolution of the surgical treatment of chronic pancreatitis. *Ann Surg.* 2010;251:18-32.

A review of the pathophysiology of chronic pancreatitis and clinical management strategies.

Bassi C, Marchegiani G, Dervenis C, et al. The 2016 update of the International Study Group (ISGPS) definition and grading of postoperative pancreatic fistula: 11 Years After. *Surgery.* 2017;161(3):584-591.

Clinical update to the management of postoperative pancreatic fistula that shifted grade A to biochemical leak and more strictly defined grade B and C fistulas.

Gittes GK. Developmental biology of the pancreas: A comprehensive review. *Dev Biol.* 2009;326:4-35.

A comprehensive review of pancreatic embryology and development.

Mederos MA, Reber HA, Girgis MD. Acute pancreatitis: a review. *JAMA.* 2021;325(4):382-390.

This article provides evidence-based guidelines addressing multiple issues in the management of acute pancreatitis, including the role and timing of endoscopic retrograde cholangiopancreatography and use of antibiotics.

Tanaka M, Fernandez-Del Castillo C, Kamisawa T, et al. Revisions of international consensus Fukuoka guidelines for the management of IPMN of the pancreas. *Pancreatology.* 2017;17:738-753.

The latest version of the consensus guidelines (2017) for diagnosis and management of cystic neoplasms of the pancreas points out the issues and provides guidelines and the evidence behind the guidelines.

van Santvoort HC, Besselink MG, Bakker OJ, et al. A step-up approach or open necrosectomy for necrotizing pancreatitis. *N Engl J Med.* 2010;362:1491-1502.

Clinical trial showing minimally invasive step-up approach for infected necrotizing pancreatitis had fewer major complications and mortalities than open necrosectomy.

The full reference list appears on Elsevier eBooks+.

CHAPTER 93

Pancreatic Cancer

Susan Tsai and Douglas B. Evans

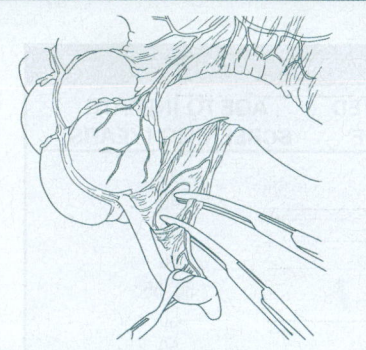

INTRODUCTION

Pancreatic ductal adenocarcinoma (PDAC) is the third leading cause of cancer death in the United States (behind lung and colorectal cancer) and is the tenth most common cancer among males and seventh most common cancer among females.[1] As screening for colorectal cancer continues to expand, we anticipate pancreatic cancer becoming the second leading cause of adult cancer death very soon. The general population's lifetime risk of PDAC is estimated to be 1.7%.[1] The rates of the most common cancers have generally declined over the past 30 years as a result of the implementation of screening guidelines. In contrast, the annual incidence of PDAC has grown by approximately 1%, in part because of a lack of effective early detection.[2] Population-based screening for PDAC is not currently justified because of its relatively low incidence in the United States as compared with breast (30%), colon (8%), or lung cancer (12%). Unfortunately, over 80% of patients with PDAC present with metastatic disease at the time of diagnosis. Although the prognosis of patients with PDAC remains guarded, with a 5-year overall survival rate of 11.5% among all stages, the adoption of alternative treatment sequencing for the management of operable disease and expanding systemic therapies for patients with metastatic disease fuel new optimism for meaningful advancements in this disease.[2] This chapter provides an overview of the pathogenesis, diagnosis, staging, and treatment of this disease, with a focus on the historical context and latest understanding of the genetics and molecular biology of PDAC.

EPIDEMIOLOGY

The biology of PDAC is uniquely different from that of other solid tumors, with several unique features, including, at the molecular level, a near-universal presence of *KRAS* mutations and, at the histologic level, the overabundance of a desmoplastic stroma. Over two decades ago, the molecular drivers of PDAC were identified, and a conceptual framework was proposed that included the accumulation of a series of acquired mutations over years, ultimately leading to the development of invasive carcinoma. More recently, catastrophic rearrangements of the genome have been described that greatly accelerate the time to malignant conversion. This section provides an overview of the multifactorial pathogenesis of PDAC and contributions from associated risk factors, including familial risk from susceptibility gene mutations, chronic pancreatitis, pancreatic cysts, and diabetes mellitus.

Hereditary Risk Factors

The majority of patients with PDAC develop a sporadic tumor as a result of acquired molecular alterations and population-level risk factors. However, approximately 10% to 15% of patients with PDAC have a pathologic germline variant identified.[3] Current National Comprehensive Cancer Network (NCCN) guidelines recommend that all individuals diagnosed with PDAC receive a comprehensive cancer family history.[4] Any proband and their first-degree relatives are recommended to undergo genetic testing. Increased risk of PDAC has been associated with several well-described *hereditary* cancer syndromes, including breast-ovarian cancer syndromes *(BRCA1, BRCA2, PALB2)*, familial atypical mole and melanoma syndrome *(CDKN2A)*, and Peutz-Jeghers syndrome *(STK11)*.[3] Patients with known hereditary syndromes (Table 93.1) are recommended to undergo PDAC screening and may benefit from a comprehensive screening approach to address all other at-risk sites for other associated cancers as well. Although genetic testing can identify underlying genetic susceptibility, the genetic basis of inherited susceptibility to PDAC remains largely unknown.

TABLE 93.1 **High-Risk PDAC Syndromes**

	PATHOGENIC VARIANT	GENETIC SYNDROME	LIFETIME RISK	PDAC IN AFFECTED BLOOD RELATIVE	AGE TO INITIATE SCREENING (YEARS)
High risk	CDKN2A	FAMM	10%–17%	None	40
	P16 Leiden Variant	FAMM	17%–58%	None	40
	PRSS1	Hereditary pancreatitis	24%–40%	None	40
	STK11/LKB1	Peutz-Jeghers	30%–60%	None	30
	Unknown	Familial PDAC	8%–12%	2 FDR	50–55
Moderate risk	BRCA1	Breast-ovarian	1.2%	>1 FDR or 2+	50
	BRCA2	Breast-ovarian	2%–5%	>1 FDR or 2+	50
	PALB2	Breast-ovarian	Unknown	>1 FDR or 2+	50
	ATM		Unknown	>1 FDR or 2+	50
	MLH1, MSH2, MSH6	Lynch	3.7%	>1 FDR or 2+	50
	Unknown	Familial PDAC	8%–12%	2 FDR	50

FAMM, Familial atypical multiple mole melanoma syndrome; *FDR,* first-degree relative; *PDAC,* pancreatic adenocarcinoma.

Therefore, in addition to genetic testing, individuals with an extensive family history of PDAC (in the absence of an identified high-risk germline mutation) are identified as having *familial* pancreatic cancer and are considered to be at high risk as well. Individuals with familial PDAC syndromes are defined as having at least two affected blood relatives with PDAC, including at least one being a first-degree relative.[5] Interestingly, the risk of PDAC is not uniform across individuals with hereditary versus familial PDAC syndromes. Two large, well-characterized, high-risk cohorts with long-term follow-up of more than 411 patients demonstrated a significantly greater risk of neoplastic progression to high-grade dysplasia or PDAC in individuals with hereditary cancer syndromes as compared with patients with familial pancreatic cancer syndromes.[6,7]

In addition, patients with familial pancreatitis have an increased risk of PDAC. Mutations in the *PRSS1* gene, which encodes cationic trypsinogen, are responsible for 80% of the cases of hereditary pancreatitis. Mutations in *PRSS1* result in inappropriate intrapancreatic activation of trypsin, either by enhanced autoactivation or impaired inactivation, leading to pancreatic tissue destruction. Patients with constitutional mutations in the *PRSS1* gene have a 50% risk of PDAC by age 75. The *SPINK1* gene codes for a serine protease inhibitor, which prevents the premature intrapancreatic activation of trypsinogen. Cumulative rates of PDAC by age 70 for patients with inherited pancreatitis have been estimated to be as high as 28%.[8]

Multiple different approaches have been described for surveillance, including imaging-based or endoscopic-based approaches.[5] Imaging-based PDAC screening has been demonstrated to be cost-effective among high-risk individuals. In contrast, the average lifetime risk of developing pancreatic cancer in the United States is 1.5%, which is too low for general population-based screening.[9] A meta-analysis of prospective studies on surveillance included 7085 high-risk individuals and estimated that the number needed to screen in order to identify 1 patient with either high-grade dysplasia or PDAC was 135.[6] Furthermore, high-risk screening was associated with a stage shift in those found to have invasive cancer; 60% to 80% of PDACs were resectable, and only 20% of PDACs were diagnosed with metastatic disease.[6,10,11] In addition, over the long term, individuals who underwent high-risk screening experienced decreased psychological distress and cancer worry.[12]

Acquired Risk Factors

Studies in large patient cohorts have revealed several environmental and chronic disease–related factors that increase the risk of

PDAC. In particular, tobacco, alcohol, and obesity have been associated with an increased risk of PDAC. Tobacco use is associated with a 1.74-fold increased odds of cancer among smokers as compared with nonsmokers. Heavy alcohol consumption (>6 drinks/day) is also associated with a 1.60-fold increased odds of cancer when compared with nondrinking controls.

Obesity has been correlated with PDAC and has been associated with a 1.72-fold increased risk of cancer among patients with a body mass index (BMI) >30 kg/m² as compared with those with a BMI of less than 30 kg/m².[13] Patients with diabetes have an increased risk of PDAC, but this varies based on the onset of the disease. Patients with long-standing diabetes (>3 years) have a 1.5- to 2.4-fold increased risk of PDAC, whereas those with new-onset diabetes (<2 years) have a 1.5-fold increased risk. In addition, patients with new-onset diabetes in the setting of at least an 8-pound weight loss have an age-adjusted hazard ratio (HR) for PDAC of 6.75 (95% CI 4.55–10.00) as compared with those with neither.[14] In older adults, the hemoglobin A1c usually rises in response to weight gain. A PDAC diagnosis can often be associated with an elevation in hemoglobin A1c despite weight loss.

PATHOGENESIS

The pancreas contains two epithelial cell types: exocrine and endocrine cells. The majority of the gland is composed of exocrine cells, which line an organized ductal network. Acinar cells line the smallest ducts and synthesize and secrete digestive enzymes. Larger ducts are lined by intercalated duct cells and secrete bicarbonate and water. Ultimately, the ducts converge into the main pancreatic ducts, which drain into the duodenum. The endocrine cells make up only 1% of the pancreas and include the islets of Langerhans. These hormone-producing cells are primarily involved in glucose homeostasis. The principal endocrine cells include A, B, and D cells, which synthesize glucagon, insulin, and somatostatin, respectively. Although the anatomic location of PDAC supports a ductal cell of origin, studies in murine models have shown that acinar cells can give rise to premalignant lesions after pancreatic injury and metaplasia, adding controversy to the cell of origin of PDAC.

Precursor Lesions

PDAC arises from noninvasive precancerous lesions that are thought to acquire successive mutations leading to malignant transformation. Most PDACs arise from microscopic pancreatic intraepithelial neoplasia (PanIN), a neoplasm involving the pancreatic ducts. It is not uncommon to develop PanIN with age; in autopsy series, over 75% of sampled pancreata had evidence of PanINs.[15] Although these lesions have a risk for progression into PDAC, most will not progress to cancer. Morphologically, these lesions are categorized as low grade or high grade based on architectural and cytologic atypia.[16] Low-grade precancers have basally oriented nuclei and mild to moderate cytologic atypia, whereas high-grade precancers have marked architectural alterations (cribriforming micropapillae, budding), loss of nuclear polarity, and severe cytologic atypia. PanINs are rarely detected clinically. The anatomic location of precancerous lesions in the ductal system could suggest a ductal cell of origin, but numerous studies in murine models have shown that acinar cells can give rise to PanINs after pancreatic injury and metaplasia.

A much smaller proportion of PDAC (<10%) arises from intraductal papillary mucinous neoplasms (IPMNs), which are macrocystic lesions that involve the pancreatic ductal system. The least common precancerous neoplasm, mucinous cystic neoplasms (MCNs), are clinically and pathologically distinct.[17] MCNs do not involve the ductal system and have a characteristic ovarian-type stroma. They are characteristically seen in females and are more likely to involve the body and tail of the pancreas. Both IPMNs and MCNs are usually first identified as incidental findings on abdominal imaging studies. In IPMN, the grade of dysplasia is correlated with the tissue subtype, with gastric-type IPMN being enriched for low-grade dysplasia and intestinal and pancreatobiliary subtypes more likely to have high-grade dysplasia. Associated carcinomas are much more frequently associated with high-grade rather than low-grade IPMNs.[18]

Pathologically, PDAC consists of malignant glands with haphazard architecture embedded in a dense desmoplastic stroma. This pauci-cellular matrix complicates the molecular analysis of PDAC because most of the cells are nonneoplastic, and fewer than 10% of the cells may be malignant. There are also several morphologic variants, including adenosquamous carcinoma and undifferentiated carcinoma with osteoclast-like giant cells. Most PDACs are not confined to the pancreas at diagnosis, and over 50% of patients will have metastatic disease. The most common sites of metastases are the liver and peritoneum; however, a subset of patients may have lung-only metastases, which is associated with a more favorable prognosis as compared with other sites. Autopsy studies have suggested that distinct molecular alterations may increase the likelihood of local versus systemic disease progression, with distant metastases being more common in patients with somatic mutations in the gene *SMAD4*.

Molecular Alterations

PDAC is thought to arise from the accumulation of somatic mutations. The most common pathogenic variant identified involves the oncogene *KRAS,* which occurs in over 90% of PDACs. Among the *KRAS* mutations associated with PDAC, the *G12D* and *G12V* mutations are found most frequently.[19] As the most common activating mutation in PDAC, KRAS impairs the intrinsic GTPase activity of *KRAS* and prevents GTPase-activating proteins from converting the active GTP bound form to the inactive form. Recently, there is growing evidence that *KRAS* mutations affect diverse signaling pathways, leading to distinct functional consequences, and may be vulnerable to mutant-specific targeted therapies.[20] Other genes, including the tumor-suppressor genes *TP53, CDKN2A,* and *SMAD4,* are also frequently mutated in PDAC.[21] Approximately 50% to 70% of

PDACs have inactivating mutations in *TP53,* which impairs DNA damage recognition and blocks cell cycle arrest. Mutations in *CDKN2A* are detected in 40% to 60% of PDACs and can lead to loss of regulation of cyclin-dependent kinase (CDK)4 and CDK6 cell cycle checkpoints. Approximately a third of PDACs have mutations in *SMAD4,* which negatively affects transforming growth factor-β (TGF-β) and promotes noncanonical TGF-β signaling. Further comprehensive whole genomic sequencing performed using samples from the Cancer Genome Atlas and the International Cancer Genome Consortium identified other genes involved in DNA repair, chromatic remodeling, and axon guidance at frequencies below 20%, including *ARID1A, BRAF, TGFBR2, SWI/SNF,* and *SMARCA4*. Remarkably, large chromosomal alterations, including copy-number alterations, chromosomal rearrangements, and chromothripsis, have also been described.[22] *Chromothripsis* refers to a phenomenon in which one or a few chromosomes contain hundreds of clustered genomic rearrangements. Investigators propose that these alterations are acquired through catastrophic DNA damage events, resulting in punctuated rather than gradual genetic evolution.

On the transcriptomic level, two predominant molecular subtypes of PDAC have been validated across multiple studies: the classical and basal-like subtypes, with the latter being associated with more aggressive tumor biology and worse prognosis.[23] In nonrandomized data, basal-like subtype has been associated with poor response to multimodality fluorouracil (5-FU)–based regimens (5-FU, irinotecan, and oxaliplatin; FOLFIRINOX). The predictive ability of RNA subtypes is being investigated in several clinical trials in patients with operable disease (PANCREAS trial, NCT: 04683315) and metastatic disease (PASS-01 trial, NCT: 04469556).

CLINICAL MANAGEMENT

Clinical Presentation

The majority of PDACs occur in the head of the pancreas, and the most common associated symptoms are jaundice, upper abdominal or back pain, and weight loss. A history of significant unintentional weight loss is not uncommon and can be a result of exocrine insufficiency, which manifests as steatorrhea, or simply resolution of chronic constipation, which is quite common in older adults. The presence of intractable nausea or vomiting may be a result of a concomitant gastric outlet obstruction and can be corroborated by radiographic findings of extreme gastric distention. Approximately 40% of patients with PDAC present with new-onset diabetes (pancreatogenic, type 3c diabetes) in the setting of weight loss. Although physical exam is often unrevealing, the presence of palpable periumbilical or left supraclavicular lymph nodes may be indicative of metastatic disease, which can be confirmed with a positron emission test (PET) scan or biopsy.

All patients with PDAC should undergo a thorough review of family history, with particular emphasis on a history of PDAC; breast, ovarian, or colon cancers; or melanoma. Routine genetic counseling and genetic testing should be offered to all patients with PDAC regardless of age or stage of disease. Identification of germline pathogenic variants may also have therapeutic implications for the patient because some genetic variants may be predictive of specific chemotherapeutic sensitivities (e.g., patients with *BRCA* pathogenic variants may have increased sensitivity to platinum agents and poly-ADP ribose polymerase inhibitors).

Diagnostic Studies

Because the majority of patients with PDAC present with jaundice, there is an impulse to perform an endoscopic retrograde cholangiopancreatography (ERCP) as the first diagnostic study because it may be both diagnostic and therapeutic. In contrast to biliary obstruction secondary to choledocholithiasis, which can occur acutely and is often associated with significant pain and cholangitis, PDAC in the head of the pancreas usually presents with gradual painless jaundice that is uncommonly associated with cholangitis. For this reason, although patients may present with jaundice and symptomatic pruritis, emergent therapeutic endoscopic intervention is rarely needed. An emphasis should be placed on obtaining a computed tomography (CT) scan in patients suspected of having PDAC before any invasive endoscopic or radiologic procedure. The incidence of ERCP-associated pancreatitis is approximately 4%, and procedure-related complications can result in significant peripancreatic inflammation, which can obscure the relationship between the primary tumor and adjacent vasculature, resulting in inaccurate assessment of the initial clinical stage (Fig. 93.1). Prioritizing a high-quality CT scan before any invasive intervention ensures accurate initial staging of the disease.

CT scan is the preferred diagnostic study for PDAC to assess the location of the primary tumor in relation to adjacent vascular structures and to assess for distant metastases. The CT scan should include the chest as well as a pancreatic-protocol CT scan. The latter includes thin (1-mm slice thickness) image acquisition of the pancreas through both late-arterial and venous phases. The late-arterial phase is usually the best phase to identify PDAC because the timing provides the maximum contrast difference between normally enhancing pancreatic parenchyma and the PDAC, which is generally hypoenhancing. In addition, this is the best phase for analyzing the tumor-artery relationships and noting the presence of any aberrant arterial anatomy. The portal-venous phase is valuable for assessing variant venous anatomy and tumor-vessel abutment or encasement. In addition, metastatic lesions in the liver are often best appreciated in the venous phase. Additional diagnostic studies, such as a magnetic resonance imaging (MRI) study or

PET scan, may be helpful if indeterminate liver lesions or suspicious nodal involvement are detected on CT imaging.

In addition to delineating tumor-vessel anatomy, cross-sectional imaging provides additional valuable information as to the origin of the periampullary tumor. In general, PDAC of the periampullary region is associated with (1) a mass in the head of the pancreas; (2) a double duct sign, involving dilation of both the common bile duct and the main pancreatic duct; and (3) distal pancreatic atrophy. The absence of any or all of these findings may suggest that the tumor may be caused by a periampullary tumor other than PDAC. For example, ampullary adenocarcinomas, duodenal adenocarcinomas, or distal cholangiocarcinomas can cause biliary obstruction without concomitant pancreatic ductal obstruction or atrophy. Ampullary and duodenal adenocarcinomas may be associated with a luminal mass involving the duodenum and may be best appreciated on coronal CT reformats or by direct endoscopic evaluation. Distal cholangiocarcinoma often results in biliary obstruction with subtle enhancement of the bile duct in the absence of an anatomic mass (duodenal, ampullary, or pancreatic). Importantly, most periampullary cancers are pancreatic in origin and, as discussed in this chapter, will be most effectively treated with combined modality therapy, most often with a neoadjuvant approach.

Clinical Staging

Accurate clinical/radiographic staging provides the framework for multidisciplinary management and shared decision-making with patients. Although consensus among clinicians may not exist (Table 93.2), all published guidelines generally agree upon two overarching clinical stages of PDAC: potentially operable (resectable and borderline resectable disease) and likely inoperable (locally advanced and metastatic disease).[24] Resectable disease (Fig. 93.2) is defined by an absence of tumor extension to the superior mesenteric artery (SMA), celiac axis, or hepatic artery with limited abutment/encasement of the superior mesenteric vein (SMV)/portal vein (PV) confluence on CT imaging. Lack of arterial abutment is characterized by the presence of a normal soft tissue plane between the tumor and the visceral arteries. SMV/PV abutment/encasement also can distinguish resectable

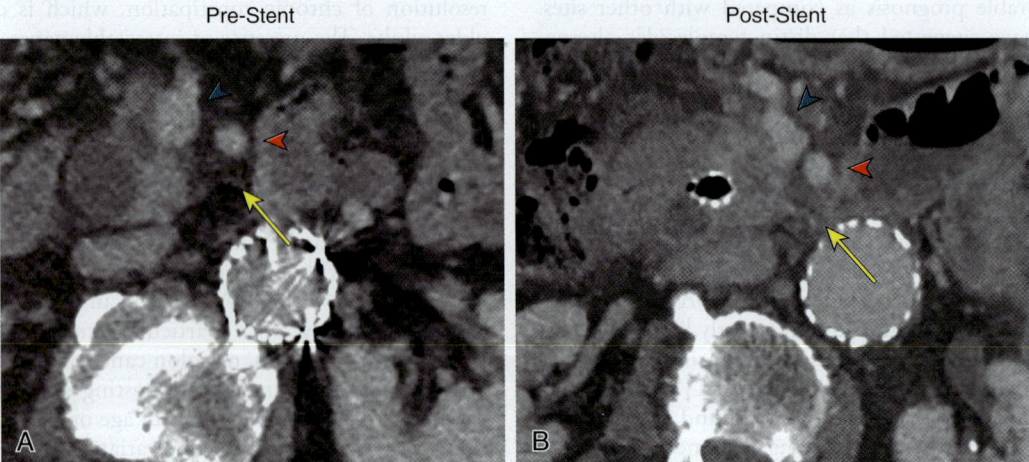

FIGURE 93.1 (A) Tumor in the pancreatic head causing pancreatic ductal dilation. SMV without narrowing *(blue arrowhead)*, SMA with no soft tissue abutment *(red arrowhead)*, preserved fat plane between head of pancreas and SMA *(yellow arrow)*. (B) After ERCP with pancreatitis, there is now contour abnormality of SMV *(blue arrow)* and haziness of the soft tissue between the head of pancreas and SMA *(yellow arrow)*. *ERCP,* Endoscopic retrograde cholangiopancreatography; *SMA,* superior mesenteric artery; *SMV,* superior mesenteric vein.

TABLE 93.2 Comparison of Radiographic Differences Between Clinical Stages of Pancreatic Cancer

	COMMONALITY	NCCN	AHPBA/SSO/SSAT	MDA/MCW
Resectable				
SMA, celiac artery, CHA	No abutment	No abutment	No abutment, with clear fat planes	No abutment
SMV/PV	No abutment	No abutment, or ≤180 degree contact without contour irregularity	No abutment, distortion, thrombus, or encasement	No abutment, or <50% narrowing
Borderline Resectable				
SMV/PV	Abutment	Abutment, ≤180 degree with contour irregularity, or thrombosis	Abutment, impingement, encasement, or short segment occlusion	>50% narrowing or short segment occlusion with reconstruction possible
SMA	Abutment	Abutment	Abutment	Abutment
Celiac artery	Abutment	Abutment	Abutment	Abutment
CHA	Abutment or short segment encasement	Abutment or short segment encasement	Abutment or short segment encasement	Abutment or short segment encasement
Locally Advanced				
SMV/PV	Involvement or occlusion without reconstruction options	Unreconstructable SMV/PV	Major extensive thrombosis	Occlusion without reconstruction options
SMA	Encasement	Encasement	Circumferential encasement	Encasement
Celiac artery	Encasement	Encasement	Circumferential encasement	Encasement without reconstruction options
CHA	Encasement	Encasement	Circumferential encasement	Encasement without reconstruction options

Abutment = tumor involves ≤180 degree vessel circumference.
Encasement = tumor involves >180 degree vessel circumference.
AHPBA/SSO/SSAT, Americas Hepato-Pancreato-Biliary Association/Society of Surgical Oncology/Society for Surgery of the Alimentary Tract; *CHA*, common hepatic artery; *MDA/MCW*, MD Anderson/Medical College of Wisconsin; *NCCN*, National Comprehensive Cancer Network; *SMA*, superior mesenteric artery; *SMV/PV*, superior mesenteric vein/portal vein.

Late-Arterial Phase   Portal-Venous Phase

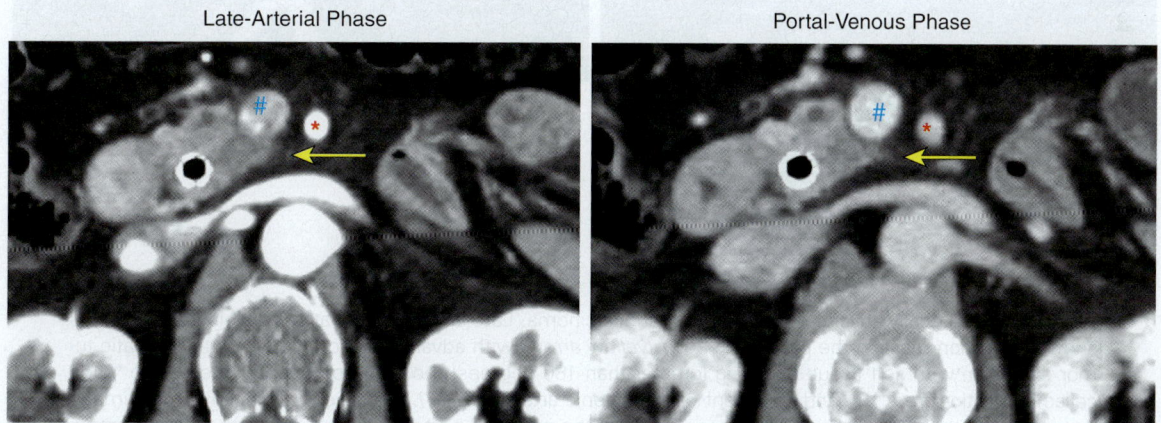

FIGURE 93.2 Resectable pancreatic adenocarcinoma. Computed tomography in the late-arterial and portal-venous phases demonstrates a low-attenuation mass completely confined to the pancreas with no tumor contact of the superior mesenteric artery *(red *)* and vein *(blue #)*, with primary tumor seen best in the arterial phase. Note that the tumor is more easily identified in the late-arterial phase *(yellow arrow)*.

from borderline resectable disease and often varies between staging systems used at different centers. For patients with venous encasement or occlusion, there must be adequate inflow and outflow targets for venous reconstruction to remain operable (borderline resectable). The distinction between borderline resectable (Fig. 93.3) and locally advanced disease (Fig. 93.4) is most often determined by the degree of tumor-artery interface (abutment is defined as ≤180 degrees and encasement as

>180 degrees). Borderline resectable disease is defined as tumor-artery abutment (≤180 degrees) of the SMA or celiac axis. This was based on the understanding that neoadjuvant therapy may successfully sterilize at least the periphery of the tumor, thereby facilitating a margin negative (R0) resection. As the tumor-artery interface progresses from abutment to encasement, a complete gross resection of all disease is likely not possible without arterial resection. The borderline resectable

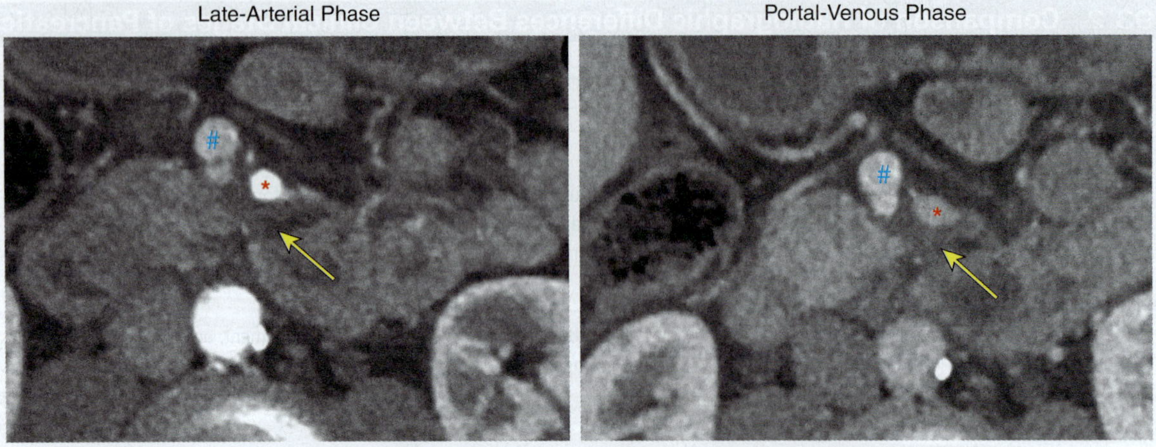

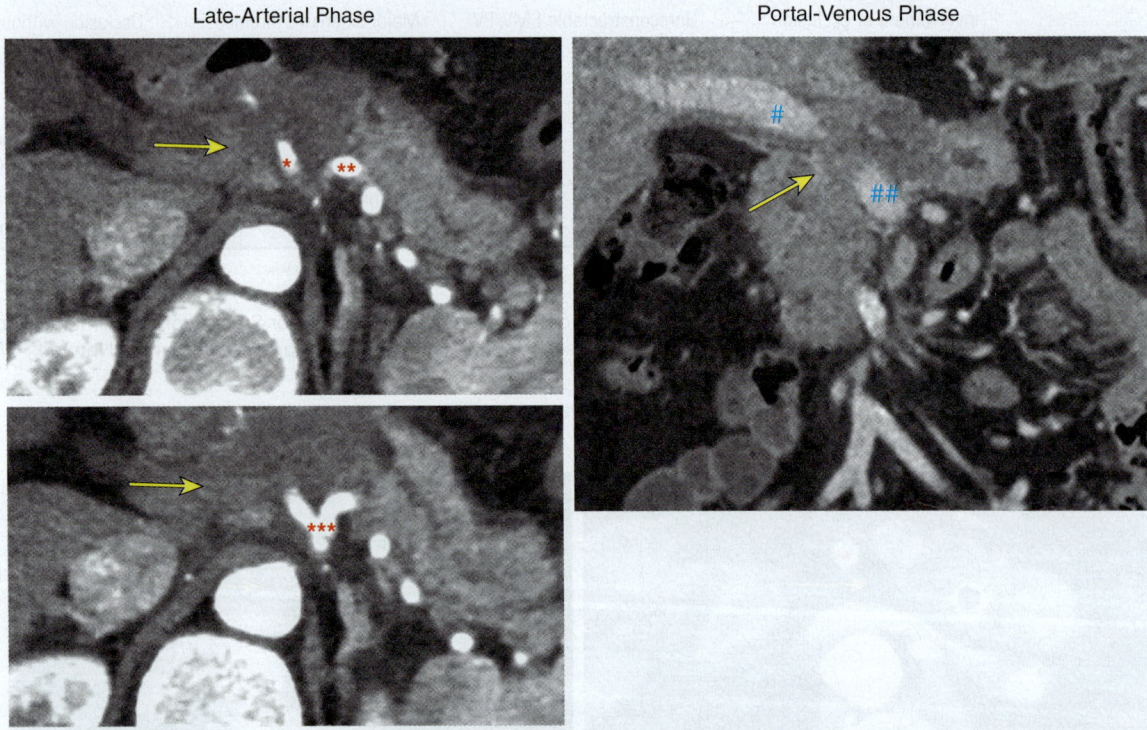

Late-Arterial Phase | Portal-Venous Phase

FIGURE 93.3 Borderline resectable pancreatic adenocarcinoma. Late-arterial and portal-venous phases demonstrate a mass in the uncinate process. The media margin of the tumor abuts (less than 180 degrees) the posterior walls of the superior mesenteric artery *(red *)* and vein *(blue #)*.

Late-Arterial Phase | Portal-Venous Phase

FIGURE 93.4 Locally advanced pancreatic adenocarcinoma. Late-arterial phase at two levels demonstrates a low-attenuation mass in the pancreatic body *(yellow arrow)* with advanced locoregional extrapancreatic tumor extension with soft tissue encasing (greater than 180 degrees) the common hepatic artery *(red *)* and celiac bifurcation *(red ***)* and abutment of the splenic artery *(red **)*. Portal-venous phase coronal image demonstrates the mass causing severe narrowing of the cephalad portal vein *(blue #)* and the superior mesenteric vein *(blue ##)*, with a "gap" below the portal–splenic–superior mesenteric vein venous confluence *(yellow arrow)*.

category also includes tumor abutment/encasement of a short segment of the hepatic artery, usually at the origin of the gastroduodenal artery (GDA), or an occluded SMV/PV, amenable to reconstruction. In contrast, locally advanced tumors are characterized by arterial encasement ≥180 degrees of the celiac artery or SMA. The locally advanced category also includes patients with SMV/PV occlusion with no technical option for reconstruction. Finally, metastatic disease is defined by the presence of extrapancreatic metastases.

Endoscopic Procedures

After CT imaging, an endoscopic ultrasound (EUS) with fine-needle aspiration (FNA) or FNA biopsy is preferred to facilitate a tissue diagnosis. EUS is preferred over percutaneous CT-guided biopsy, which has been associated with up to a 16% rate of peritoneal carcinomatosis, presumably related to dissemination of malignant cells along the biopsy tract. For tissue diagnosis, rapid on-site cytopathologic evaluation increases the diagnostic success of EUS/FNA biopsies by allowing for additional endoscopic sampling to be performed until an adequate cytologic specimen can be obtained. Once a preliminary cytologic diagnosis is obtained, the placement of a decompressive metal stent can be performed during the same endoscopic anesthesia and alleviates the need for two separate procedures. Ideally, this "one-stop-shop" approach facilitates simultaneous diagnosis and therapeutic intervention for the obstructive jaundice. In general, uncovered metal endobiliary stents are preferred over plastic stents for their higher patency rates (104 days vs. 83 days) and lower rates of complications (12% vs. 35%). Covered metal stents have higher rates of stent migration and higher rates of stent-related cholecystitis because the stents can cover and occlude the cystic duct orifice. Covered stents are most often employed in patients who do not have a gallbladder (prior cholecystectomy) or when a tissue diagnosis has not been obtained because they can be removed at a subsequent endoscopy (unlike uncovered stents, which usually cannot be removed).

Laboratory Studies

Standard laboratory testing for PDAC should include complete blood count, comprehensive metabolic panel, albumin, hemoglobin A1c, and tumor markers, including carbohydrate antigen (CA) 19-9, CA 125, and carcinoembryonic antigen (CEA). CA 19-9 is a sialylated Lewis blood antigen that is elevated in approximately 75% of patients with PDAC at the time of diagnosis. It can be falsely elevated in the setting of hyperbilirubinemia and should be considered evaluable only when the total bilirubin is less than 2 mg/dL. Trends in CA 19-9 levels have been correlated with treatment response and are considered an important clinical adjunct to radiographic response. Among patients who are CA 19-9 nonproducers, 25% may have an elevated CEA, and changes in CEA have been similarly observed to correlate with treatment response and prognosis. It is important to remember that CEA levels are significantly higher in smokers (to include tobacco and cannabis products) as compared with nonsmokers, and therefore, the trend in results over time is more important than an isolated value. In other solid tumors, alternative blood-based biomarkers, such as cell-free DNA, are being evaluated as quantitative biomarkers of disease burden. In general, recurrent disease can be detected by a rise in cell-free DNA approximately 3 months before traditional protein-based biomarkers or diagnostic imaging. The utility of cell-free DNA and other blood-based biomarkers is under active investigation in PDAC.

TREATMENT

The treatment of PDAC is stage specific, emphasizing the importance of accurate initial staging. Nonmetastatic PDAC often requires a concerted multidisciplinary approach that involves a multidisciplinary team, including surgeons, medical oncologists, radiation oncologists, advanced gastroenterologists, body imaging specialists, pathologists, genetic counselors, dietitians, physical therapists, and palliative care specialists. Efficient communication and care coordination are essential to provide timely and appropriate care for patients with PDAC to optimize their clinical outcomes while minimizing delays and toxicities.

Multimodality Approach to Operable Pancreatic Adenocarcinoma

Patients with operable PDAC are at risk for both local and systemic recurrence, with over 75% of patients developing recurrent disease within 1 year of surgery.[25] The high risk of both local and distant disease recurrence may be predicted by the advanced pathologic stage of most patients with PDAC. If taken directly to surgery, over 70% of patients will have node-positive (N1 or N2) disease, and 40% will have a margin-positive (R1) resection.[26,27] Of patients with recurrent disease after potentially curative surgery, the majority of patients develop metastatic disease recurrence; however, up to 25% to 33% of patients experience local-only disease recurrence.[28,29] Given the high rates of recurrent disease, adjuvant therapy is recommended for all patients with PDAC who undergo surgery first, independent of pathologic stage. Although a recent randomized controlled trial comparing adjuvant gemcitabine versus 5-fluorouracil/irinotecan/oxaliplatin (PRODIGE-24) demonstrated historic improvements in median overall survival (54 months) with the triple-therapy arm, it is important to remember that adjuvant clinical trials have an inherent selection bias in their design because patients who are enrolled in adjuvant trials must have recovered from a pancreatectomy with minimal complication, have preserved performance status, and have no evidence of disease progression on postoperative restaging before initiating adjuvant therapy.[30] When accounting for all patients who undergo surgical resection for PDAC, the delivery of any adjuvant therapy after pancreatectomy is unpredictable. Among multiple retrospective analyses of large institutional experiences, approximately 50% of patients with PDAC may never receive adjuvant therapy after surgery because complications related to surgery, the inability to fully recover from surgery, or patient refusal.[31,32] This finding was recapitulated in the results of another recent randomized controlled trial that compared perioperative (neoadjuvant and adjuvant) therapy to surgery followed by adjuvant therapy (PREOPANC trial) in patients with localized PDAC.[33] Only 65 (51%) of the 128 patients in the surgery-first arm received any adjuvant therapy. In addition, in the adjuvant setting, the primary tumor has been removed, so the ability to assess treatment response to the chemotherapy prescribed is limited or impossible. Because response to chemotherapeutic regimens is not uniform across all patients (response rates from 30% to potentially as high as 50%), at least half of the patients who receive adjuvant therapy receive no benefit and incur unnecessary toxicity.

In contrast to a surgery-first approach, neoadjuvant therapy has several advantages: (1) early delivery of systemic therapy for presumed micrometastases, which are likely present in the majority of patients at diagnosis; (2) the ability to identify aggressive tumor biology, which may be resistant to available systemic therapies; (3) assessment of treatment response in the primary tumor; and (4) improved selection of patient for surgery according to stage of disease and response to therapy. For patients with an elevated CA 19-9 level at the time of diagnosis, changes in CA 19-9 levels have been demonstrated to correspond to treatment response and be prognostic of overall survival. Among patients who receive neoadjuvant therapy, approximately one-third of patients will normalize their CA 19-9 levels before surgery, one-third of patients will normalize their CA 19-9 levels after surgery, and one-third of patients will never normalize their CA 19-9 levels even after neoadjuvant therapy and surgery.[34] Approximately 70% of patients who initiate neoadjuvant therapy will be able to complete neoadjuvant therapy and surgical resection.[35,36] Of the 30% of patients who do not undergo resection, approximately 92% of those patients have metastatic disease progression during/after neoadjuvant therapy, and in 5% of patients, performance status and medical comorbidities that argue strongly against a trip to the operating room become apparent. Local disease progression during/after neoadjuvant therapy, which precludes surgical resection, occurs in 3% or less of patients; it is a very uncommon event.

Trials Comparing Neoadjuvant Therapy Versus Surgery First

The first randomized trial to compare a neoadjuvant therapy (given as pre- and postoperative therapy) to up-front surgical resection and adjuvant therapy was the PREOPANC trial. The long-term results of the PREOPANC trial were recently published and demonstrated improved overall survival for patients with resectable and borderline resectable PDAC who received perioperative therapy as compared with a surgery-first approach (5-year overall survival: 20.5% vs. 6.5%; HR 0.73; $p = 0.025$).[37] Several institutions have also reported their outcomes with neoadjuvant therapy, and among patients who are able to complete neoadjuvant therapy and surgery, the median overall survival exceeds 40 months at most centers.[38,39] In contrast, the Norwegian Pancreatic Cancer Trial-1 (NORPACT 1) trial included 130 patients with resectable PDAC in the head of the pancreas. Patients were randomized to up-front surgical resection versus neoadjuvant chemotherapy with 5-fluorouracil, oxaliplatin, and irinotecan (FOLFIRINOX). There was no difference in median overall survival (38 mo vs. 25 mo; HR 1.52; 95% CI 1.00–2.33).[40] It is important to note that 21% of patients in the neoadjuvant arm were unable to achieve biliary drainage and underwent up-front surgical resection. In addition, only 46% of patients in the neoadjuvant arm received the full 2 months of neoadjuvant therapy. Currently, there are two ongoing clinical trials (Alliance A021806 [NCT 04340141], PREOPANC 3 [NCT 04927790]) that will further evaluate neoadjuvant versus surgery-first treatment approaches using a similar clinical trial design of 4 months of contemporary chemotherapy before surgery.

Trials Comparing Neoadjuvant Therapeutic Approaches

Many centers have already adopted neoadjuvant therapy for patients with localized PDAC based on promising outcome data from phase II and III clinical trials. Currently, all consensus guidelines recommend neoadjuvant therapy for borderline resectable disease, and an increasing number of centers advocate neoadjuvant therapy for resectable disease as well. Future investigations will be focused on defining the optimal neoadjuvant therapy for patients, including the best chemotherapeutic regimen, duration of treatment, and whether to include radiation/chemoradiation. The Southwestern Oncology Group (SWOG) S1505 trial randomized 102 patients to receive perioperative modified FOLFIRINOX (mFOLFIRINOX) versus gemcitabine/nab-paclitaxel (GnP).[35] The trial confirmed the safety of both treatment regimens, with over 84% of each arm able to complete all intended preoperative chemotherapy. However, there was no difference in efficacy observed between the two regimens (2-year overall survival: 42% vs. 49%). Currently, the selection of which chemotherapy regimen to include in neoadjuvant therapy is primarily driven by patient factors.

Although early neoadjuvant trials for patients with PDAC included radiation, the value of neoadjuvant radiation has come into question after the report of the Alliance A012501 trial.[41] This was a phase II randomized trial of 126 patients with borderline resectable PDAC who received neoadjuvant mFOLFIRINOX with or without hypofractionated radiation. There was minor variability in the radiation dose given on trial; however, the majority of patients received stereotactic body radiotherapy of 33 to 40 Gy in

5 fractions. At a planned interim analysis, the radiation arm was closed to accrual because of a larger proportion of patients who had disease progression. It is important to note that the patients in the radiation arm had an increased proportion of patients who experienced distant disease progression, not local progression, and a number of patients in both arms failed to complete intended therapy. The results of all recent trials for patients with operable PDAC have demonstrated the importance of managing treatment-associated toxicity and providing direction for physicians when an adaptive trial design is implemented. Although the value of local control for patients with operable PDAC has come under question, the patterns of first recurrence, nonetheless, suggest that 30% to 40% of patients will have local-only recurrence as the first site of recurrence. In single-institution series of patients with operable PDAC, the addition of neoadjuvant chemoradiation to surgery has been associated with less than 10% local recurrence rates, suggesting that radiation can provide a meaningful reduction in local recurrences and potentially improve long-term survival.[42] At the Medical College of Wisconsin, patients with operable PDAC (resectable, borderline resectable, and locally advanced type A) are currently being treated with a total neoadjuvant therapy approach. This consists of 4 months of neoadjuvant chemotherapy with an adaptive trial design to include interval restaging at 2 months to assess for treatment response, and in the absence of response, a change in chemotherapy is implemented. Systemic therapy is followed by preoperative radiation/chemoradiation, and we are exploring alternate fractionation schedules to include the use of stereotactic body radiation therapy as well.

SURGICAL MANAGEMENT

Preoperative Preparation

Preoperative evaluation should include a detailed history and physical exam. A pancreatic-protocol CT scan is the cornerstone of staging, and we always have a new scan within 1 month of the planned date of surgery. Reassessment of the tumor-vessel relationship is essential and should include a careful evaluation of the tumor's relationship to the SMA, SMV-PV, celiac axis, and hepatic artery. It is important to evaluate for the presence of aberrant arterial anatomy (replaced right or left hepatic artery) and the presence of median arcuate ligament compression of the celiac artery. Assessment of the venous anatomy should also note the insertion of the inferior mesenteric vein (into the splenic vein or SMV) and the location of the first jejunal branch (either anterior or posterior to the SMA). Depending on the extent of the tumor-vessel involvement, the need for autologous conduits, such as the saphenous vein or internal jugular vein, can be anticipated based on preoperative imaging. Often, it is helpful to reference the CT at the time of diagnosis to evaluate for the presence of venous narrowing or contour irregularity (bird's beak or teardrop deformity). If present, even after a robust radiographic response to neoadjuvant therapy, vascular resection and reconstruction may be necessary.

Pancreaticoduodenectomy

Pancreaticoduodenectomy is the most common operation for tumors of the periampullary region, and it involves removal of the pancreatic head, duodenum, gallbladder, and bile duct with or without removal of the gastric antrum. Before an extended abdominal incision, at the time of anesthesia induction, we recommend a diagnostic laparoscopy because up to 10% of patients will have small-volume metastatic disease that is not detected on preoperative imaging. After careful laparoscopic inspection of the liver and all visceral and parietal surfaces, we generally use an upper midline incision. The round ligament is carefully taken down from the abdominal wall and preserved as a pedicled flap upon entering the abdomen, to be used at the conclusion of the operation as a physical barrier to cover the GDA stump. The subsequent surgical resection can be broken down into six steps.

Resection of the Head of Pancreas

1. The purpose of the first step is to define the infrapancreatic SMV. The greater omentum is elevated from the transverse colon, and the hepatic flexure of the colon is mobilized to the level of the duodenum. The lesser sac is entered, and the visceral peritoneum along the inferior border of the pancreas is incised medially to laterally to expose the infrapancreatic SMV and the junction of the middle colic vein and the SMV. The middle colic vein may enter directly into the anterior surface of the infrapancreatic SMV or arise as a common trunk with the gastroepiploic vein (gastrocolic trunk). If the middle colic vein and gastroepiploic vein share a common trunk, the common trunk can be preserved (and the gastroepiploic vein divided) or the entire trunk divided. When there is extensive inflammatory change or scarring at the root of mesentery, it may not be possible to identify the infrapancreatic SMV early in the operation. In such cases, the SMV will be exposed during step 6 after the pancreatic neck is divided in a caudal direction from the level of the PV. Occasionally, when there is a large tumor in the uncinate process, it may be necessary to divide the middle colic vein and resect a portion of transverse colon mesentery en bloc with the pancreatic head. For tumors that additionally extend inferiorly and posteriorly to involve the third or fourth portions of the duodenum, a Cattell-Braasch maneuver may be necessary to allow adequate visualization of the root of mesentery. When completed, this maneuver allows cephalad retraction of the right colon and small bowel to expose the third and fourth portions of the duodenum.

2. The purpose of the second step is to mobilize the duodenum and head of pancreas. A Kocher maneuver is begun at the transverse portion (third portion) of the duodenum by identifying the inferior vena cava. The duodenum and pancreatic head are mobilized medially to the level of the left renal vein and the left lateral aspect of the aorta. It is particularly helpful to divide the leaf of visceral peritoneum that extends from the retroperitoneum to the posterior aspect of the mesenteric vessels. There are often a number of lymphatics in this tissue, which are best ligated if possible. With the head of the pancreas rotated medially, this visceral peritoneum is located at the most posterior aspect (medial to the head of pancreas). Releasing the tissue at this level from the third portion of the duodenum to the level of the foramen of Winslow greatly facilitates the subsequent dissection of the SMA.

3. The third step involves the portal dissection and defining the superior border of the pancreatic head. To begin, the common hepatic artery is identified, and the hepatic artery lymph node is removed. This will facilitate visualization of the common hepatic artery as it gives off the GDA and proper hepatic artery and often exposes the medial border of the PV. A small right gastric artery is usually anterior to the GDA, arising from the left hepatic or proper hepatic artery, and should be ligated. The origin of the GDA can be dissected, but before ligation, it is often helpful to first expose the lateral aspect of the porta hepatis, especially if there is variant arterial anatomy suspected. If the foramen of Winslow was initially obliterated as a result of adhesions, it should be reestablished in order to palpate the porta hepatis and appreciate the pulsation of an anomalous hepatic artery. If a cholecystectomy has not previously been performed, the gallbladder is taken down in a retrograde fashion, and the common hepatic duct is transected at the level of the cystic duct (Fig. 93.5). In cases where an anomalous location of the right hepatic artery has been identified on preoperative CT, we often isolate the aberrant

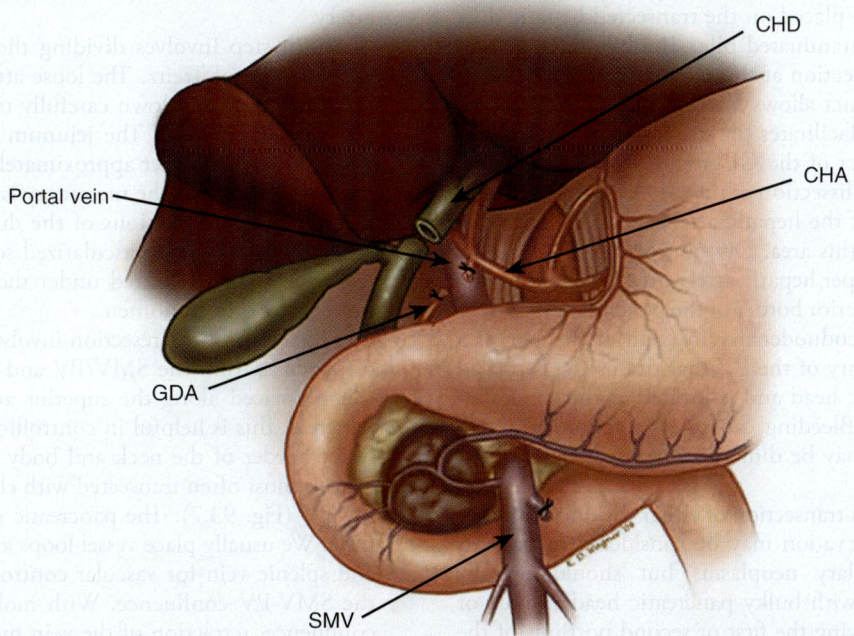

FIGURE 93.5 Step 3: Top-down cholecystectomy to identify the junction of the cystic duct to the common hepatic duct. Division of the common hepatic duct above the level of the cystic duct. *CHA,* Common hepatic artery; *CHD,* common hepatic duct; *GDA,* gastroduodenal artery; *SMV,* superior mesenteric vein.

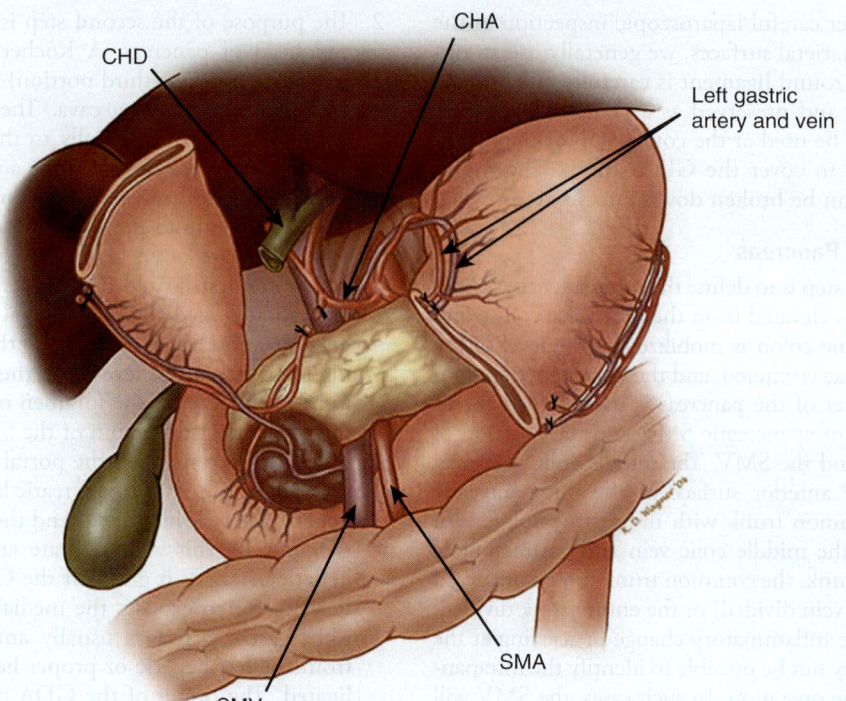

FIGURE 93.6 Step 3: Portal dissection involves identification of the common hepatic artery *(CHA)* and the origin of the gastroduodenal artery *(GDA)*. Division of the common hepatic duct *(CHD)* facilitates the exposure of the origin of the GDA for ligation. *SMA,* Superior mesenteric artery; *SMV,* superior mesenteric vein.

arterial anatomy before division of the common hepatic duct because the artery is often in close proximity of the duct and can be injured. A replaced or an accessory right hepatic artery arising from the proximal SMA usually courses posterolateral to the PV. After transection of the bile duct, biliary fluid cultures may be sent, and any indwelling endobiliary stents are removed if possible. Intraoperative bile cultures may be used to guide therapeutic antibiotic treatment postoperatively, and a bulldog clamp can be placed on the transected hepatic duct to limit spillage of contaminated bile. The bile duct margin can be sent for frozen section at this time as well. Division of the common hepatic duct allows for exposure of the anterior surface of the PV and facilitates the dissection and mobilization of the lateral aspect of the GDA and proper hepatic artery. Overly aggressive dissection at the GDA origin can result in intimal dissection of the hepatic artery. Careful sharp dissection is preferred in this area. Division of the GDA allows mobilization of the proper hepatic artery off of the underlying PV and exposes the superior border of the pancreas (Fig. 93.6). The superior pancreaticoduodenal vein (vein of Belcher) is a constant venous tributary of the PV that drains the cephalad aspect of the pancreatic head and is located at the superolateral aspect of the PV. Bleeding caused by traction injury to this venous tributary may be difficult to control at this time in the operation.

4. The fourth step involves transection of either the duodenum or stomach. Pylorus preservation may be considered in patients with small periampullary neoplasms but should not be performed in patients with bulky pancreatic head tumors or duodenal tumors involving the first or second portions of the duodenum. To ensure adequate blood supply to the duodenojejunostomy, the duodenum is generally divided approximately 2 cm distal to the pylorus. In the setting of preoperative

radiation, we usually favor removal of the antrum because this area is usually within the radiation field. The stomach is transected with a gastrointestinal stapler at the level of the third or fourth transverse vein on the lesser curvature and at the confluence of the gastroepiploic veins on the greater curvature, completing a standard/modest antrectomy. When opening pars flaccida, one should specifically look for and preserve an accessory or replaced left hepatic artery arising from the left gastric artery.

5. The fifth step involves dividing the jejunum and mobilizing the ligament of Treitz. The loose attachments of the ligament of Treitz are taken down carefully to avoid injury to the inferior mesenteric vein. The jejunum is then transected with a gastrointestinal stapler approximately 10 cm distal to the ligament of Treitz, and the mesentery is divided to the level of the fourth and third portions of the duodenum, usually with an energy device. The devascularized segment of duodenum and jejunum is then reflected under the mesenteric vessels to the right side of the abdomen.

6. The final step of the resection involves the removal of the head of pancreas from the SMV/PV and SMA. Hemostatic sutures can be placed along the superior and inferior borders of the pancreas; this is helpful in controlling the vessels along the inferior border of the neck and body of the pancreas. The pancreas is most often transected with electrocautery at the level of the PV (Fig. 93.7). The pancreatic margin can be sent at this time. We usually place vessel loops around the distal SMV, PV, and splenic vein for vascular control and medial retraction of the SMV-PV confluence. With mobilization of the SMV-PV confluence, retraction of the vein medially facilitates the identification of the SMA posteriorly. Direct exposure of the SMA avoids iatrogenic injury and ensures direct ligation of the inferior pancreaticoduodenal arteries (IPDAs). Failure to fully

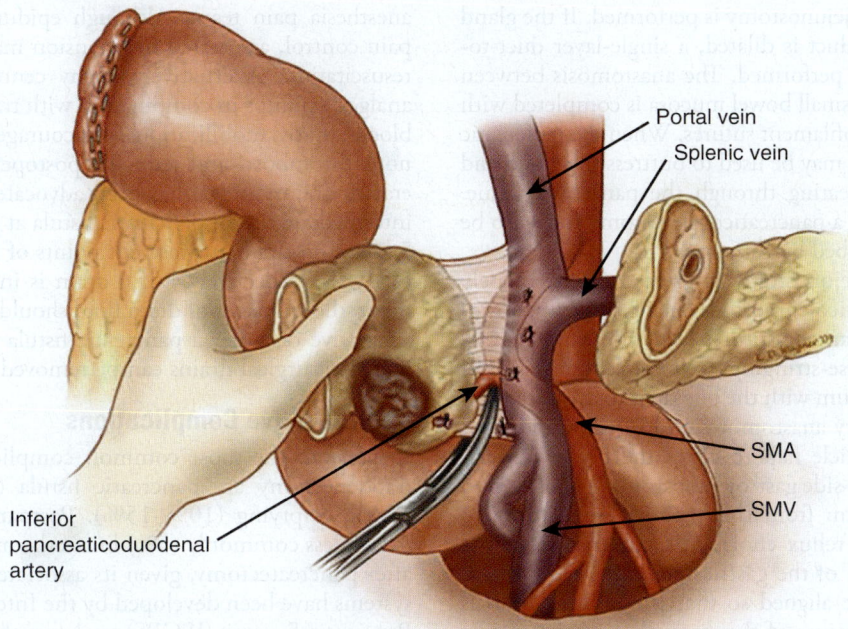

Portal vein
Splenic vein
SMA
SMV
Inferior pancreaticoduodenal artery

FIGURE 93.7 Step 6: Division of the neck of the pancreas and separation of the head of the pancreas from the superior mesenteric vein *(SMV)* and superior mesenteric artery *(SMA)*.

mobilize the SMV-PV confluence risks injury to the SMA and often will result in a positive SMA resection margin. The specimen is separated from the SMV by ligation and division of the small venous tributaries to the uncinate process and pancreatic head. The first jejunal branch is usually encountered at the caudal aspect of the pancreatic head. The jejunal branch can usually be preserved by ligating small tributaries to the uncinate process. Injury to the distal SMV at this level, or a tangential laceration in its jejunal branch (as it courses posterior to the SMA), is difficult to control and probably represents the most frequent cause of iatrogenic SMA injury as one attempts to suture a venous injury before full exposure of the SMA. Once the uncinate process is separated from the distal SMV, medial retraction of the SMV-PV confluence allows one to expose the SMA. Once the first jejunal branch is released, the more distal IPDA is usually encountered immediately cranially. The specimen is then separated from the right lateral wall of the SMA and sent to pathology. Direct visual exposure of the IPDAs allows for their individual ligation, which will largely eliminate early postoperative intraabdominal hemorrhage.

Vascular Resection

Resection of the SMV and/or PV may need to be performed if tumor extension precludes the safe dissection of the SMV and PV off of the pancreatic head and uncinate process. Generally, this can be predicted based on preoperative imaging because deformity of the SMV/PV resulting from tumor abutment/encasement usually portends the need for vascular resection. Importantly, preoperative anticipation of the need for vascular resection facilitates the intraoperative management as a planned event rather than an emergent response to a vascular injury. When vascular resection is anticipated, it is helpful to have included the upper thigh or neck in the sterile field to facilitate access to the saphenous vein or internal jugular vein. Historically, division of the splenic vein was considered standard practice because this facilitates exposure of the SMA medial to the SMV and allows for

greater mobility of the SMV and PV for reconstruction. When possible, the splenic vein–PV confluence should be preserved because ligation of the splenic vein can result in future sinistral hypertension, especially if the left coronary vein is not preserved. A generous 2-cm segment of SMV-PV confluence can often be resected without the need for interposition grafting if the splenic vein is divided. When performing venous resection, we usually incorporate inflow occlusion of the SMA with systemic heparinization because this will minimize small bowel ischemia and edema. Marking the anterior surface of the SMV and PV before venous resection assists in maintaining the orientation of the anastomosis. The proximal and distal targets are circumferentially dissected; vascular clamps are placed 2 to 3 cm proximal (on the PV) and distal (on the SMV) to the involved venous segment; and the vein is transected, allowing tumor removal. If the resection cannot be reconstructed with a tension-free anastomosis, an autologous vein graft (e.g., internal jugular vein) can be used as an interposition graft. Autologous conduits are preferred over synthetic grafts because of the potential for infection and superior long-term patency rates. Currently, the role of major arterial resection for PDAC remains controversial, and it should only be performed in highly selected patients who have completed an extensive course of neoadjuvant therapy. Given the surgical morbidity and mortality with such procedures, arterial resections should be limited to carefully selected patients and be performed at centers with the institutional volume and experience to support these patients.

Reconstruction

Reconstruction usually starts with the pancreaticojejunostomy followed by the hepaticojejunostomy and gastrojejunostomy or duodenojejunostomy. For the pancreaticojejunostomy, mobilization of approximately 2 cm of the pancreatic remnant facilitates exposure and placement of sutures. We prefer to pass the jejunal limb through the transverse mesocolon to the left of the middle colic vessels. If the pancreatic gland is soft, a two-layer, end-to-side, duct-to-mucosa pancreaticojejunostomy is performed. If the gland is firm and the pancreatic duct is dilated, a single-layer duct-to-mucosa anastomosis can be performed. The anastomosis between the pancreatic duct and the small bowel mucosa is completed with interrupted 4-0 or 5-0 monofilament sutures. When the pancreatic parenchyma is soft, pledgets may be used to buttress the gland and prevent the sutures from tearing through the pancreatic tissue. With such high-risk glands, a pancreaticogastrostomy may also be employed, as recently described by Kazantsev.[43]

A single-layer hepaticojejunostomy is created approximately 10 cm distal to the pancreaticojejunostomy using interrupted 4-0 or 5-0 absorbable monofilament sutures. An interrupted technique is used to avoid purse-stringing of the anastomosis. It is important to align the jejunum with the bile duct to avoid tension on the pancreatic and biliary anastomoses and to allow room for the falciform ligament pedicle flap to cover the hepatic artery. Finally, an antecolic, end-to-side gastrojejunostomy is constructed in two layers at least 50 cm from the hepaticojejunostomy to minimize the risk for bile reflux cholangitis. Starting from the greater curvature, a portion of the gastric staple line is removed. The jejunal limb should be aligned so that the efferent limb is adjacent to the greater curvature of the stomach, and the gastrojejunostomy is usually constructed with an interrupted outer layer of sutures and a running inner layer. The use of drains remains an active area of controversy in the field of pancreatic surgery, and many surgeons still drain both the hepaticojejunostomy and the pancreaticojejunostomy. Finally, the previously mobilized falciform ligament is placed over the GDA stump to minimize the risk of pseudoaneurysm formation at the site of the GDA stump in the event of a pancreatic anastomotic leak.

Minimally Invasive Approaches

Pancreaticoduodenectomy is increasingly being performed with laparoscopic or, more commonly, robotic approaches. A minimally invasive approach has been associated with decreased pain, fewer wound complications, and a shorter length of hospital stay.[44,45] There is a significant learning curve for minimally invasive pancreaticoduodenectomy, requiring approximately 80 cases for proficiency, although in the setting of a formal training program with mentorship and formal skills curriculum, this learning curve can be greatly reduced.[46,47] Patient selection is key when deciding between a minimally invasive or open approach because the former approach can be challenging in the setting of chronic pancreatitis. At this time, execution of minimally invasive pancreaticoduodenectomy should be performed in carefully selected patients with favorable anatomy at an institution with surgeons experienced in this technique.

POSTOPERATIVE CARE

After surgery, a standardized approach to postoperative care can improve surgical outcomes and reduce hospital stay. Various programs have implemented protocols for enhanced recovery after surgery that emphasize avoidance of hyperglycemia, maintaining a near-zero fluid balance, early drain removal, early oral intake, minimization of narcotics, and mobilization. In general, in the absence of significant gastroparesis or preoperative gastric outlet obstruction, nasogastric tubes can be removed on postoperative day 1 or 2 with the introduction of limited clear liquids. The diet can be advanced over the next few days in the absence of nausea or vomiting. Optimal perioperative pain management may vary from center to center depending on the expertise and availability of the

anesthesia pain team. Although epidurals can provide excellent pain control, associated hypotension may require additional fluid resuscitation. Alternatively, many centers use patient-controlled analgesia pumps in combination with transversus abdominis plane blocks. Early mobilization is encouraged in preventing deep venous thrombosis and reducing postoperative ileus. Early postoperative drain removal has been advocated in patients with low or intermediate risk of pancreatic fistula at postoperative days 1, 3, or 5 based on drain amylase cut points of 300 IU/L, 150 IU/L, and 50 IU/L, respectively.[48] If a drain is in place after diet advancement, the character of drain fluid should be monitored for changes suggestive of either a pancreatic fistula or a chyle leak. For most patients, surgical drains can be removed before discharge.

Postoperative Complications

In general, the most common complications after pancreaticoduodenectomy are pancreatic fistula (10%–30%) and delayed gastric emptying (10%–15%). Postpancreatectomy hemorrhage occurs less commonly (5%) but is the most dreaded complication after pancreatectomy, given its associated high mortality. Scoring systems have been developed by the International Study Group of Pancreatic Surgery (ISGPS) to define the severity of each of these complications and are summarized in Table 93.3.[49–51]

Pancreatic Fistula

Pancreatic fistula rates are related to the gland texture, main pancreatic duct diameter, and intraoperative blood loss. Based on the aforementioned features, a Fistula Risk Score Calculator was developed to predict postoperative risk of pancreatic fistula and guide the management of perianastomotic drains.[48,52] Pancreatic fistulas are generally detected by the presence of amylase-rich fluid from the surgical drains or the presence of a peripancreatic fluid collection on CT imaging. Pancreatic fistula can be associated with signs of infection (leukocytosis, fever) and can cause delayed gastric emptying or postpancreatectomy hemorrhage. If a deep-space infection is present, it is important to obtain adequate drainage not only for source control but also to prevent the fluid from necessitating out the surgical site, leading to fascial dehiscence. ISGPS grade B fistulas can usually be managed with drainage, antibiotics, and the use of somatostatin analogues. On rare occasions, patients with severe disruption of the pancreaticojejunostomy may require surgical reexploration for definitive management; in our personal experience, this is very uncommon, having only been considered in a handful of patients with a very large denominator.

Delayed Gastric Emptying

Delayed gastric emptying remains a troublesome complication after pancreaticoduodenectomy, the pathophysiology of which is not fully understood and is likely multifactorial. Differences in surgical technique have been analyzed. The incidence of delayed gastric emptying appears to be lower with antecolic as compared with retrocolic gastrojejunostomy.[53] Rates of delayed gastric emptying do not appear to be different when comparing standard pancreaticoduodenectomy with pylorus-preserving pancreaticoduodenectomy. However, it is possible that surgical technique may affect delayed gastric emptying; a recent review of robotic pancreaticoduodenectomies identified an acute angle (<30 degrees) between the stomach and the efferent jejunal limb as a risk factor for delayed gastric emptying.[54] A CT scan is often helpful to rule out a subclinical pancreatic fistula or an intraabdominal abscess as a cause of delayed gastric emptying. An upper gastrointestinal series may be helpful to assess gastric emptying. With significant stasis,

TABLE 93.3 International Study Group of Pancreatic Surgery Consensus Definitions of Postoperative Complications

COMPLICATION	GRADE		
	A	B	C
Delayed Gastric Emptying[a]			
Nasogastric tube requirement, reinsertion on POD	4–7 days, >POD 3	8–14 days, >POD 7	>14 days, >POD 14
Days of oral intolerance	7	14	21
Vomiting and gastric distention	±	+	+
Use of prokinetics	±	+	+
Postoperative Pancreatic Fistula[b]			
	Biochemical leak	Persistent drainage >3 weeks, clinically relevant change in management, percutaneous/endoscopic drainage, angiographic procedures, infection without organ failure	Reoperation, organ failure, death
Postoperative Pancreatic Hemorrhage[c]			
Onset (early ≤24 h, late >24 h)/severity	Early/Mild	Early/Severe or late/mild	Late/Severe
Location	Intraluminal/Extraluminal	Intraluminal/Extraluminal	Intraluminal/Extraluminal
Clinical condition	Good	Good to moderately impaired	Severely impaired, life threatening

[a]Delayed gastric emptying definition: functional gastroparesis after surgery without mechanical obstruction as determined by upper gastrointestinal contrast series or endoscopic evaluation.
[b]Postoperative pancreatic fistula definition: amylase >3 times upper limit of institutional normal serum amylase value.
[c]Postpancreatectomy hemorrhage definition: all postoperative episodes of hemorrhage after pancreatic resection, including gastrointestinal or intraabdominal hemorrhage, and early or delayed postoperative bleeding.
POD, Postoperative day.

nasogastric tube decompression and initiation of prokinetics (erythromycin or metoclopramide) are the mainstays of therapy. Upper endoscopy can be considered to rule out an associated marginal ulcer. In rare cases, refractory delayed gastric emptying may require percutaneous gastrostomy tube placement and parental nutrition, but it is most often self-limited and will resolve with time and supportive care. In the experience of the authors, how the gastrojejunostomy is completed is important, and the overwhelming majority of patients with delayed gastric emptying have a pancreatic leak responsible for this complication.

Postpancreatectomy Hemorrhage

Postpancreatectomy hemorrhage can be either early (within 24 hours of surgery) or late (usually postoperative day 7–14 or later). Early postpancreatectomy hemorrhage is caused by technical failures related to inadequate hemostasis and generally requires reoperation. Late postpancreatectomy hemorrhage is most commonly related to either bleeding from a pseudoaneurysm (frequently associated with a pancreatic fistula) or ulceration at the site of the gastrojejunostomy. Patients who suffer from early postpancreatectomy hemorrhage present with postoperative hypotension and blood in the surgical drains; return to the operating room is in order. Patients who present with late postpancreatectomy hemorrhage often have a herald gastrointestinal bleed in the setting of a complicated postoperative course that invariably includes a pancreatic anastomotic leak/fistula. The hemorrhage (hematemesis and occasionally melena) is often acute and sometimes can be catastrophic. Regardless of presentation, late postpancreatectomy hemorrhage requires rapid recognition, controlled resuscitation, and mobilization of the interventional radiology team. Bleeding can be controlled with either endovascular embolization of the pseudoaneurysm or stenting across the involved artery. When

possible, if the bleeding is related to a GDA pseudoaneurysm and coil embolization of the aneurysm sac is not possible, stenting of the common hepatic artery is preferred over embolization. Mortality rates are high, and for those who survive the initial bleed postembolization, patients may have additional complications related to the intrabdominal abscess (present in most patients) as well as hepatic abscess and/or hepatic insufficiency.

SUMMARY

We are in an exciting time in surgical oncology, and advances in early diagnosis and the treatment of pancreatic cancer are poised to occur at a very rapid pace over the next 5 to 10 years. In the absence of an accurate blood-based test for early diagnosis, pancreatic cancer will likely become the second leading cause of adult cancer death very soon. Treatment strategies for all stages of disease emphasize early systemic therapy. Such treatment is only successfully implemented if we are able to effectively manage biliary and gastric outlet obstruction, nutrition challenges, and pain control. As therapeutic advances continue, their benefits will only be realized if we are able to deliver them successfully to the patient—likely the major challenge for healthcare and the study of healthcare disparities in the next decade. Potentially curative surgery for patients with pancreatic cancer should be completed with a close to 0% mortality and should be performed only in those who have a reasonable chance of cure. Despite the failure of past attempts to regionalize cancer surgery to high-volume centers, consolidation of health systems holds promise for the future. Although we have made significant advances in surgical care, we will be seeing more and more patients with unique toxicities from new and emerging systemic therapies, making the surgical management of this disease (and others) ever more complicated.

SELECTED REFERENCES

Conroy T, Desseigne F, Ychou M, et al. FOLFIRINOX versus gemcitabine for metastatic pancreatic cancer. *N Engl J Med.* 2011;364(19):1817-1825.

> *Phase III trial comparing gemcitabine to mFOLFIRINOX in the adjuvant setting, which demonstrated significant improvement in overall survival in the mFOLFIRINOX arm. Important to consider that the trial was highly selective, as evidenced by the average number of patients enrolled per center per year (average 1.4 patients/center/yr) across the 77 international sites and the duration of overall survival in the gemcitabine-alone arm, which greatly exceeded that of prior historical controls.*

Evans DB, Varadhachary GR, Crane CH, et al. Preoperative gemcitabine-based chemoradiation for patients with resectable adenocarcinoma of the pancreatic head. *J Clin Oncol.* 2008; 26(21):3496-3502.

> *Seminal phase II trial to use neoadjuvant therapy in patients with operable pancreatic ductal adenocarcinoma (PDAC). Demonstrated that neoadjuvant therapy can select for patients who have early metastatic disease progression for whom surgical resection may have limited oncologic value.*

Goggins M, Overbeek KA, Brand R, et al. Management of patients with increased risk for familial pancreatic cancer: updated recommendations from the International Cancer of the Pancreas Screening (CAPS) Consortium. *Gut.* 2020;69(1):7-17.

> *Often-cited updated consensus guidelines on the management of cystic disease of the pancreas with guidelines for management of side branch, main duct intraductal papillary mucinous neoplasms, (IPMNs) and mucinous neoplasms.*

Sohal DPS, Duong M, Ahmad SA, et al. Efficacy of perioperative chemotherapy for resectable pancreatic adenocarcinoma: a phase 2 randomized clinical trial. *JAMA Oncol.* 2021;7(3):421-427.

> *Multicenter cooperative group neoadjuvant trial for patients with resectable pancreatic ductal adenocarcinoma (PDAC) that compared the two most commonly used first-line chemotherapeutic regimens. Neither regimen was superior to a prespecified end point. Demonstrated that either neoadjuvant regimen could be delivered safely, with approximately 70% of patients completing neoadjuvant therapy and surgery.*

Versteijne E, van Dam JL, Suker M, et al. Neoadjuvant chemoradiotherapy versus upfront surgery for resectable and borderline resectable pancreatic cancer: long-term results of the Dutch Randomized PREOPANC Trial. *J Clin Oncol.* 2022;40(11): 1220-1230.

> *Landmark phase III trial comparing neoadjuvant chemoradiation to up-front surgical resection. Initial report of the trial demonstrated no difference at 18 months in overall survival. However, long-term follow-up demonstrated a significant increase in overall survival among patients who received neoadjuvant therapy, suggesting that local control may improve long-term overall survival in PDAC.*

The full reference list appears on Elsevier eBooks+.

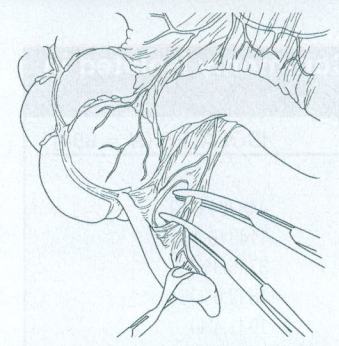

CHAPTER 94

The Appendix

Sabrina E. Sanchez, Daniel Counihan, Elishana Kanu, and Dan G. Blazer 3rd

Please access Elsevier eBooks+ to view the videos for this chapter.

Appendicitis is the most common urgent or emergent general surgical operation performed in the United States and is responsible for as many as 300,000 hospitalizations annually.[1] It is estimated that as much as 6% to 7% of the general population in the United States will develop appendicitis during their lifetime, with the incidence peaking in the second decade of life.[2] Appendicitis is much less common in underdeveloped countries, suggesting that elements of the Western diet, specifically a low-fiber, high-fat intake, may play a role in the development of the disease process.[3]

ANATOMY AND EMBRYOLOGY

The appendix is a midgut organ first identified at 8 weeks of gestation as a small outpouching of the cecum. As gestation progresses, the appendix becomes more elongated and tubular as the cecum rotates medially and becomes fixed in the right lower quadrant of the abdomen. The appendiceal mucosa is of the colonic type, with columnar epithelium, neuroendocrine cells, and mucin-producing goblet cells.[3] Lymphoid tissue is found in the submucosa of the appendix, leading some to hypothesize that the appendix may play a role in the immune system. In addition, evidence suggests that the appendix may serve as a reservoir of "good" intestinal bacteria and may aid in recolonization and maintenance of the normal colonic flora.[4] Although historically, removal of the appendix was not felt to result in any adverse sequelae, this has recently been challenged. For example, patients who have had previous appendectomy have been demonstrated to have a more

difficult clinical course and overall poorer outcomes in recurrent cases of *Clostridioides difficile* infection when compared with patients who have not undergone appendectomy. The theory is that the microbiome of the appendix has a protective function and that the loss of this eliminates an element of beneficial immunologic redundancy.[5] In addition, a recently published epidemiologic study found a significant link between appendectomy before age 20 and the development of prostate cancer, although a precise causative mechanism could not be elucidated.[6]

The blood supply of the appendix is through the appendiceal artery, a branch of the ileocolic artery, which is in turn a branch of the superior mesenteric artery. The appendix can be of variable size (5–35 cm in length) but averages 8 to 9 cm in length in adults. Its base can be reliably identified by defining the area of convergence of the taeniae at the tip of the cecum and then elevating the appendiceal base to define the course and position of the tip of the appendix. The appendiceal tip may be found in a variety of locations: it is retrocecal (but intraperitoneal) in approximately 60% of individuals, pelvic in 30%, and retroperitoneal in 7% to 10%. Agenesis of the appendix has been reported, as has duplication and even triplication.[3–7]

OVERVIEW OF APPENDICITIS

History

Some of the earliest descriptions of the appendix date back to 1522 by Jacopo Berengario da Capri.[8] Since then, many anatomists have struggled with the role and purpose of the appendix, a debate that continues today.[9] The first appendectomy was reported in 1735 by a French surgeon, Claudius Amyand, who identified and successfully removed the appendix of an 11-year-old male that was found within an inguinal hernia sac and that had been perforated by a pin. Although autopsy findings consistent with perforated appendicitis appeared sporadically thereafter in the literature, the first formal description of the disease process, including the common clinical features and a recommendation for prompt surgical removal, was in 1886 by Reginald Heber Fitz of Harvard University.[3]

Notable advances in surgery for appendicitis include McBurney's description of his classic muscle-splitting incision and technique for removal of the appendix in 1894 and the description of the first laparoscopic appendectomy by Kurt Semm in 1982.[3] Finally, but of no less significance, was the development of broad-spectrum antibiotics, interventional radiologic techniques, and better surgical critical care strategies, all of which have resulted in substantial improvements in the care of patients with appendiceal pathology.

Pathophysiology and Bacteriology

Appendicitis is caused by luminal obstruction.[3] The causes of the luminal obstruction are many and varied, including fecal stasis, fecaliths, lymphoid hyperplasia, neoplasms, fruit and vegetable material, ingested barium, and parasites such as ascaris or pinworm. Obstruction of the proximal lumen of the appendix leads to elevated pressure in the distal portion because of ongoing mucus secretion and production of gas by bacteria within the lumen. With progressive distention of the appendix, the venous drainage becomes impaired, resulting in mucosal ischemia. If there is persistent obstruction, full-thickness ischemia may ensue, which has the potential to lead to perforation. Bacterial stasis distal to the obstruction can lead to bacterial overgrowth within the appendix.[3] This is significant because this overgrowth results in the release of a larger bacterial inoculum in cases of perforated appendicitis. The most common sequela from appendiceal perforation is the formation of an abscess in the periappendiceal region or pelvis. On occasion, however, free perforation occurs that results in diffuse peritonitis.[3]

The flora within the appendix is similar to that found within the colon. Infections associated with appendicitis should be considered polymicrobial, and antibiotic coverage should include agents that address the presence of both gram-negative bacteria and anaerobes. Common isolates include *Escherichia coli, Bacteroides fragilis,* enterococci, *Pseudomonas aeruginosa,* and *Klebsiella pneumoniae* (Table 94.1).[10]

Differential Diagnosis

Appendicitis must be considered in every patient who has not had an appendectomy and presents with acute abdominal pain.[11,12] Consideration of the patient's age and sex may help narrow the list of possible diagnoses. In children, other considerations include but are not limited to mesenteric adenitis (often seen after a recent viral illness), acute gastroenteritis, intussusception, Meckel diverticulitis, inflammatory bowel disease, and (in males) testicular torsion. Nephrolithiasis and urinary tract infection may be manifested with right lower quadrant pain in either sex.[3,11,13] In females of childbearing age, the differential diagnosis is expanded even further. Gynecologic pathology may be mistaken for appendicitis, including ruptured ovarian cysts, *mittelschmerz* (midcycle abdominal pain occurring with ovulation), endometriosis, ovarian torsion, ectopic pregnancy, and pelvic inflammatory disease.[3,11,13] In the elderly, consideration must be given to acute diverticulitis and malignant disease as possible causes of lower abdominal pain. In the neutropenic patient, *typhlitis* (also known as *neutropenic enterocolitis*) should also be considered.[14,15] Appendicitis in these special populations is discussed in greater detail later in the chapter.

TABLE 94.1   Bacteria Commonly Isolated in Perforated Appendicitis

TYPE OF BACTERIA	ISOLATES (*N* = 694)
Gram-Negative Bacteria	
Escherichia coli	448 (64.6%)
Pseudomonas aeruginosa	114 (16.4%)
Klebsiella pneumoniae	37 (5.3%)
Citrobacter species	18 (2.6%)
Enterobacter species	10 (1.4%)
Serratia marcescens	3 (0.4%)
Raoultella planticola	3 (0.4%)
Comamonas testosterone	2 (0.3%)
Aeromonas species	2 (0.3%)
Proteus species	2 (0.3%)
Acinetobacter species	1 (0.1%)
Yersinia species	1 (0.1%)
Morganella species	1 (0.1%)
Gram-Positive Bacteria	
Enterococcus species	27 (3.9%)
Streptococcus species	20 (2.9%)
Staphylococcus species	5 (0.7%)

Adapted from Song DW, Park BK, Suh SW, et al. Bacterial culture and antibiotic susceptibility in patients with acute appendicitis. *Int J Colorectal Dis.* 2018;33:441-447.

Presentation

History

Patients presenting with acute appendicitis typically complain of vague abdominal pain that is most commonly periumbilical in origin. This reflects the stimulation of visceral afferent pathways through the progressive distention of the appendix. As the distension of the appendix progresses and the appendiceal tip becomes inflamed, it irritates the adjacent parietal peritoneum. This leads to somatic pain localized to the position of the appendiceal tip, typically the right lower quadrant. This phenomenon remains a reliable symptom of appendicitis[3,11] and should serve to further increase the clinician's index of suspicion for appendicitis.[3,11] Anorexia is often present, as is nausea with or without associated vomiting. Either diarrhea or constipation may be present as well.

Although these symptoms represent the "classic" presentation of appendicitis, the clinician must be aware that the disease may be manifested in an atypical fashion. For example, patients with a retroperitoneal appendix may present in a more subacute manner, with flank or back pain, whereas patients with an appendiceal tip in the pelvis may have suprapubic pain suggestive of urinary tract infection.[3,11]

Physical Examination

Patients with appendicitis typically appear ill. They frequently lie still because of the presence of localized peritonitis, which makes movement painful. Tachycardia and mild dehydration are often present to varying degrees. Fever is frequently present, ranging from low-grade temperature elevations (<38.5°C) to more impressive elevations of body temperature, although absence of fever does not exclude a diagnosis of appendicitis.[1,3,11]

Abdominal examination typically reveals a quiet abdomen with tenderness and guarding on palpation of the right lower quadrant. The location of the tenderness is classically over McBurney point, which is located one-third the distance between the anterior superior iliac spine and the umbilicus. The pain and tenderness are typically accompanied by localized peritonitis, as evidenced by the presence of rebound tenderness. Diffuse peritonitis or abdominal wall rigidity resulting from involuntary spasm of the overlying abdominal wall musculature is strongly suggestive of perforation.[1,3]

A number of signs have been described to aid in the diagnosis of appendicitis. These include the Rovsing sign (right lower quadrant pain on palpation of the left lower quadrant), the obturator sign (right lower quadrant pain on internal rotation of the hip), and the psoas sign (pain with extension of the ipsilateral hip), among others.[1] Although these are of historical interest, it is important to realize that they are simply indicators of localized peritonitis rather than a diagnostic of a specific disease process.

Rectal examination findings are typically normal. However, a palpable mass or tenderness may be present if the appendiceal tip is located within the pelvis or if a pelvic abscess is present. In female patients, pelvic examination is important to exclude pelvic disease. However, cervical motion tenderness, a finding typically associated with pelvic inflammatory disease, may be present in appendicitis because of irritation of the pelvic organs from the adjacent inflammatory process.[3,11]

Laboratory Studies

Laboratory studies should be interpreted with caution in cases of suspected appendicitis and used to support the clinical picture rather than to definitively prove or exclude the diagnosis. Leukocytosis, often with a predominance of neutrophils and sometimes an increase in bands, is present in 90% of cases. A normal white blood cell count is found in 10% of cases, however, and it should not be used as an isolated test to exclude the presence of appendicitis.[16–19] Urinalysis is typically normal as well, although the finding of trace leukocyte esterase or pyuria is not unusual and is presumably due to the proximity of the inflamed appendix to the bladder or ureter. Ketonuria has also been associated with appendicitis in recent studies.[20,21]

In addition to the white blood cell count, several biomarkers have been investigated as additional diagnostic clues to the diagnosis. These have included C-reactive protein, procalcitonin, interleukin-6, and others. Although C-reactive protein appears to be the most sensitive of these, none provides sufficient specificity to definitively diagnose appendicitis.[10,12]

Ultimately, no symptom, sign, or laboratory test has been demonstrated to be uniquely predictive of appendicitis.[1,16–18] Rather, it is the assessment of the collective body of information that allows more precise diagnosis.[1,16–18] Several clinical scoring systems have been developed to serve as predictive models for appendicitis. These have included the Alvarado score, the pediatric appendicitis score, the appendicitis inflammatory response (AIR) score, and the adult appendicitis score (AAS)—to name a few.[22–24] In the most recent consensus guidelines, use of the AIR or AAS score is recommended over the use of the Alvarado score, which can be useful in ruling out appendicitis but is not sufficiently specific.[17,18]

Imaging Studies

Imaging studies in patients suspected to have acute appendicitis can reduce the negative appendectomy rate, which can be as high as 15%.[17,25] A variety of radiographic studies may be used to diagnose appendicitis. These consist of plain radiographs, ultrasound (US), computed tomography (CT) scanning, and magnetic resonance imaging (MRI).

Plain radiographs may be obtained in the emergency department setting for the evaluation of acute abdominal pain but lack both sensitivity and specificity for the diagnosis of appendicitis and are rarely helpful. A calcified fecalith in the right lower quadrant may support the diagnosis, but this finding must be placed into the appropriate clinical context and is typically present in only 5% of cases.[26] Pneumoperitoneum, if present, should alert the clinician to other causes of a perforated viscus (e.g., a perforated ulcer or diverticulitis) because this is not typically observed in cases of appendicitis, even with perforation.[26,27]

US has been used for diagnosis of appendicitis since the 1980s. As US technology has become more advanced, so has its ability to visualize the appendix. The inflamed appendix is typically enlarged, immobile, and noncompressible (Fig. 94.1). If the appendix cannot be visualized, the study is inconclusive and cannot be relied on to guide treatment, although secondary signs such as free fluid, hyperemia of adjacent bowel loops, induration of mesenteric fat, and regional adenopathy may be considered in the overall picture and serve to increase the diagnostic accuracy of US.[28] Although US is time efficient and provides the advantage of avoiding ionizing radiation, the success of the study depends greatly on the skill of the sonographer and is, thus, highly operator dependent. The sensitivity is reported to range from 71% to 94%, whereas the specificity ranges from 81% to 98%, although again, this varies greatly based on the skill and experience of the sonographer.[17,29] Its greatest utility appears to be in the evaluation of the pediatric or pregnant patient, in whom the associated radiation exposure from CT is especially undesirable.[26] It has recently been suggested that a standardized reporting method or "template" might improve the overall results of US in this clinical setting.[18,29,30]

CT scanning is the most common imaging study used to diagnose appendicitis and is highly effective and accurate.[17,26] A recent systematic review has reported the sensitivity of CT scan to be 95%, with a specificity of 94%.[31] Contrast administration (IV, PO, or rectal) has been shown to confer a higher sensitivity in the diagnosis of acute appendicitis without affecting specificity.[31] Further, a randomized trial from 2018 showed that low-dose CT

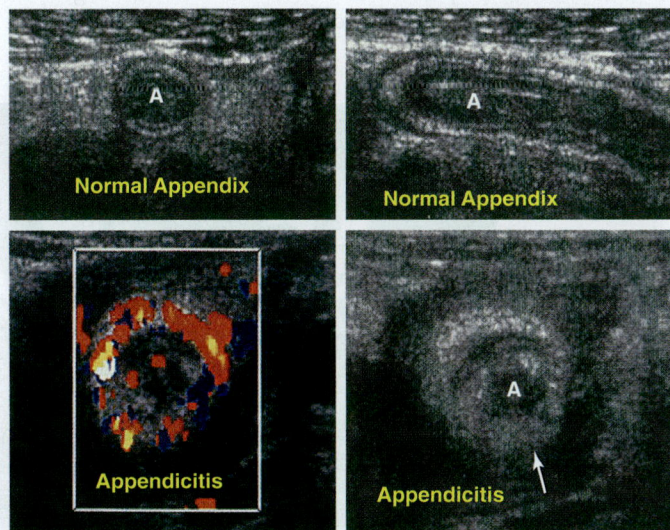

FIGURE 94.1 Ultrasound image of a normal appendix *(top)* illustrating the thin wall in coronal *(left)* and longitudinal *(right)* planes. In appendicitis, there is distention and wall thickening *(bottom, right)*, and blood flow is increased, leading to the so-called ring-of-fire appearance. *A,* Appendix.

imaging was not inferior to standard CT in diagnosing acute appendicitis.[32] Currently, contrast-enhanced low-dose CT imaging is the recommended technique for evaluation of acute appendicitis.[18]

The diagnosis of appendicitis on CT is based on the appearance of a thickened, inflamed appendix with surrounding "stranding" indicative of inflammation. The appendix is typically more than 7 mm in diameter, with a thickened, inflamed wall and mural enhancement or "target sign" (Fig. 94.2). Periappendiceal fluid or air is also highly suggestive of appendicitis and suggests perforation. In cases in which the appendix is not visualized, the absence of inflammatory findings on CT suggests that appendicitis is not present.[18,26] CT scans are recommended in any adult patient with suspected appendicitis for operative planning and ruling out other causes of peritoneal symptoms, especially given the existence of multiple pathologies with overlapping symptomatology.[31,33]

MRI is typically reserved for use in the pregnant patient and should be performed without contrast.[34,35] Criteria for MRI diagnosis include appendiceal enlargement (>7 mm), thickening (>2 mm), and the presence of inflammation.[26] A recent meta-analysis found the sensitivity of MRI to be 97%, with a specificity of 95%.[17,36,37] Drawbacks associated with the use of MRI include its higher cost; motion artifact; greater difficulty in interpretation by nonradiologists, who may have limited experience with the technology; and limited availability (especially in the after-hours emergency setting).[17,18,26,37]

Classification of Appendicitis

There are several different ways of classifying appendicitis. The first differentiation comes between acute and chronic appendicitis, with acute appendicitis evolving over the course of hours to days and chronic appendicitis referring to a chronicity that usually spans weeks to months, even years.[38]

Within acute appendicitis, the most common classification system separates the condition into "uncomplicated" and "complicated," although establishing what this means can be challenging. Traditional surgical teaching has purported that uncomplicated appendicitis will inevitably progress to complicated appendicitis without treatment; however, this is no longer believed to be the case. Multiple recent studies have made the argument that complicated and uncomplicated appendicitis have different

pathophysiologic mechanisms, and as such, the traditional dogma of putting them in a continuum of disease is increasingly being shown to be erroneous.[39,40]

Uncomplicated appendicitis refers to an inflamed appendix without evidence of necrosis or perforation, whereas *complicated appendicitis* has focal or transmural necrosis that has led to or can eventually lead to perforation.[41] Complicated appendicitis can progress to appendicitis with an abscess or phlegmon, whereas uncomplicated appendicitis does not.[41] This distinction is key because patients with uncomplicated appendicitis may be able to forego emergent surgical treatment (and potentially, even surgical treatment at all), whereas patients with complicated appendicitis should be managed with appendectomy.[41] Thus, differentiating between these two entities is essential to determining appropriate management. Specifically, it is important to rule out complicated appendicitis so that patients with this pathology are not inappropriately treated with only antibiotics.[41] Unfortunately, the differentiation between complicated and uncomplicated appendicitis is not something that we are yet able to gather with great certainty before deciding on a management strategy. Certain imaging features, such as abscess, appendicolith, free air, and free fluid, have been associated with complicated appendicitis, and diagnosing a patient with a significant periappendiceal abscess or free air with complicated appendicitis is not difficult (Fig. 94.3). However, the absence of these features does not mean that complicated appendicitis is not present.[42] Atema et al. have described two new scoring systems where clinical, laboratory, and imaging characteristics can be evaluated to determine whether a patient has uncomplicated or complicated appendicitis; one uses US imaging, the Scoring System for Appendicitis Severity-US (SAS-US), and the other uses CT imaging, the Scoring System for Appendicitis Severity-CT (SAS-CT).[43] As noted by Born et al., the SAS-US and SAS-CT perform well in ruling out complicated appendicitis but are yet to be externally validated in prospective studies.[41]

TREATMENT OF APPENDICITIS

Treatment for appendicitis has been debated frequently as less invasive therapies, including nonoperative therapies, have been shown to be effective. For decades, the mainstay treatment for acute

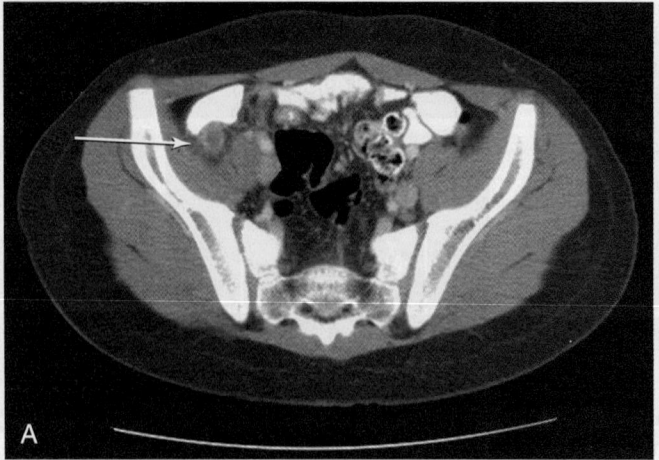
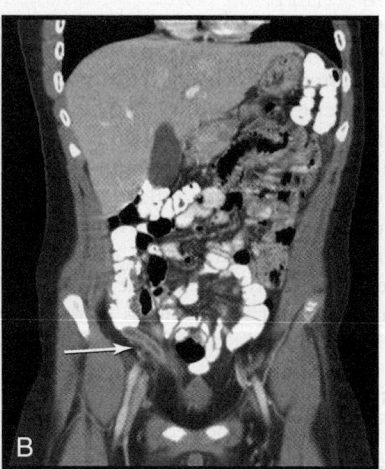

FIGURE 94.2 Computed tomography scan of the abdomen demonstrating classic findings of acute appendicitis. (A) Sagittal view with *arrow* demonstrating a thickened, inflamed, and fluid-filled appendix (target sign). (B) Coronal view of same patient. The *arrow* points to the thickened, elongated appendix with periappendiceal fat stranding and fluid around the appendiceal tip.

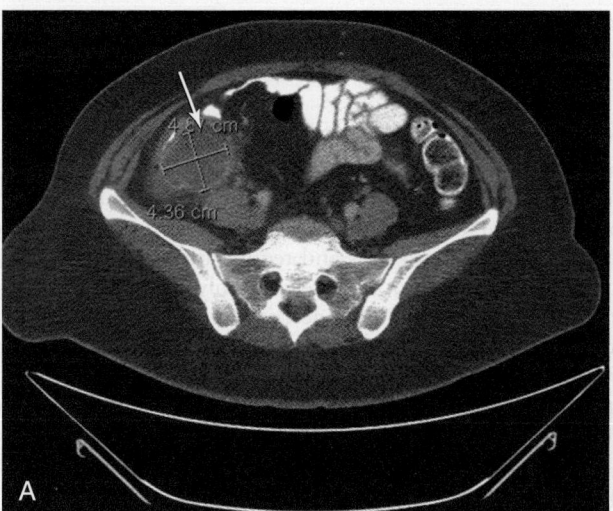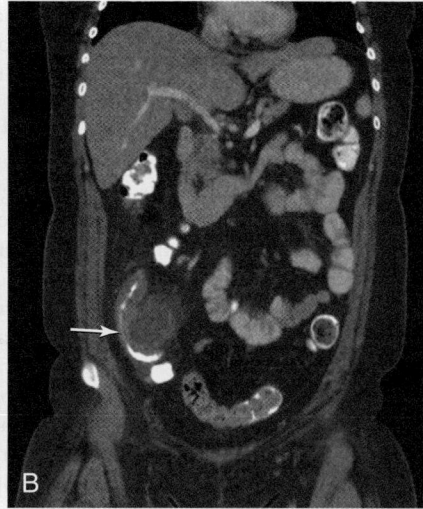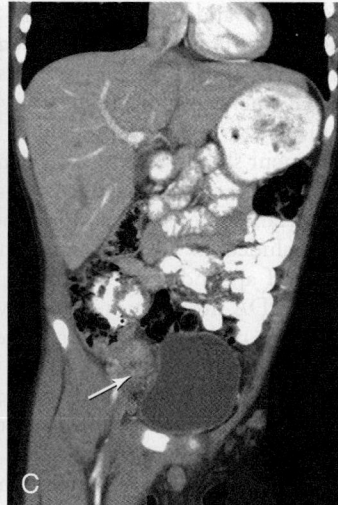

FIGURE 94.3 Computed tomography scan of the abdomen demonstrated complicated appendicitis. Sagittal (A) and coronal (B) computed tomography images demonstrate an appendiceal abscess in a patient who presented with a 2-week history of abdominal pain and was found to have a palpable mass on examination. The *arrows* point to a periappendiceal abscess cavity. The patient was successfully managed with percutaneous drainage and antibiotic therapy. (C) A similar case in which the patient presented with an appendiceal phlegmon and was successfully treated with antibiotics alone. The *arrow* points to the phlegmon. (Note the mass effect on the bladder.)

appendicitis was open appendectomy. However, newer strides in research have opened the door for a larger set of options in the management of acute appendicitis, including laparoscopic appendectomy, robotic appendectomy, single-incision appendectomy, percutaneous and transrectal drainage, and nonoperative management with only antibiotics.[44,45] As discussed earlier, determining the best strategy for management is highly dependent on the type of appendicitis being treated. For patients presenting acutely, however, the mainstay of treatment consists of fluid resuscitation and administration of broad-spectrum antibiotics targeting intraabdominal pathogens until further management plans are established based on appendicitis severity and patient preference.[17,18,44]

Acute Uncomplicated Appendicitis

Although appendectomy has traditionally been considered the gold standard in management of acute appendicitis without the presence of a phlegmon or abscess, multiple large trials over the past decade have questioned the absolute necessity for surgical intervention versus management with only antibiotics for this population. Results from the first of these large trials were published in 2015 by the Appendicitis Acuta (APPAC) multicenter clinical trial researchers. In this trial, 530 patients with acute uncomplicated appendicitis confirmed by CT imaging were randomized to early appendectomy or antibiotic treatment. The study investigators found that antibiotic treatment efficacy was –27%, which failed to meet their prespecified criteria for noninferiority (efficacy of –24%). Importantly, however, the trial did demonstrate no complications in the participants who underwent appendectomy after originally being placed in the antibiotic group.[46] Follow-up studies on quality of life for study participants at 5 and 7 years did not show a difference in satisfaction between treatment groups as long as the treatment was successful. However, they did show lower satisfaction for patients who failed treatment in the antibiotics-alone treatment group.[47,48] A meta-analysis published shortly after exploring the management of acute appendicitis nonoperatively found an initial failure rate of antibiotics

of 9% (95% confidence interval [CI] 4.00%–13.0%) and a 1-year recurrence rate of 25% (95% CI 12.0%–35%).[49] Most significantly, however, the authors also noted a statistically significant increase in the likelihood of progressing to complicated appendicitis in the failed nonoperative group.[49] The authors also reported a longer length of stay with antibiotic therapy but an overall lower cost of the initial treatment. However, the subsequent downstream cost of reintervention for recurrence was not considered.[49] More recently, the Comparison of Outcomes Between Drugs and Appendectomy (CODA) investigators have published findings on their multicenter, randomized control trial comparing antibiotics versus appendectomy in patients with uncomplicated appendicitis. The original study published in 2020 found that based on a standardized measure of health status, the European Quality of Life–5 Dimensions questionnaire, at 30 days, antibiotics were a noninferior treatment option to appendectomy. However, it was found that 29% of patients did undergo a subsequent appendectomy within 90 days. Additionally, the study found that patients with appendicolith treated nonoperatively were at higher risk for appendectomy and complications than those without.[50] A smaller single-institution trial published shortly after, the Conservative Versus Open Management of Acute Uncomplicated Appendicitis (COMMA) trial, found a similar rate of recurrence of appendicitis after nonoperative treatment of 25%. The authors reported a similar quality of life between both groups early on but found a significantly lower quality of life in patients treated nonoperatively at 1 year.[51]

Based on these data, antibiotics are now considered an acceptable first-line treatment for acute uncomplicated appendicitis, and given there are two safe and effective treatment options for the disease, patient preference has become an important factor in informing the decision of whether to proceed with appendectomy or antibiotic treatment.[44,50] As such, the risks and benefits of operative intervention versus antibiotic management should be discussed with patients using a shared decision-making model to optimize patient-centered treatment for this disease. Risk of recurrence and risk of neoplasm should be presented as part of the risks of nonoperative treatment, whereas risk of surgical complications should be presented as part of the risks of operative management. Importantly, however, the patient's preferences and values with regard to pursuing operative versus nonoperative treatment should also be considered in the decision-making process. Of note, the presence or absence of an appendicolith is an important factor that modifies their risks, and as such, it should be included in any conversation about nonoperative management of appendicitis.[44,50] To help facilitate these conversations, the CODA investigators have developed a decision-aid tool that can help patients and their surgeons make treatment decisions about appendicitis care.[52]

Once a decision is made regarding whether to pursue surgical or nonsurgical intervention, these treatments can ensue in different ways. If operative intervention is chosen, an open versus laparoscopic approach may be used, with the laparoscopic approach now being significantly more common, as will be discussed in detail later. For patients managed nonoperatively, treatment consists of 10 days of antibiotics to cover gastrointestinal flora, also as described earlier, with the first 24 hours administered intravenously.[53]

Acute Complicated Appendicitis

Although antibiotic treatment is a safe and effective option for the management of acute uncomplicated appendicitis, proven or suspected complicated appendicitis without an abscess or phlegmon should be treated surgically.[41] The technique of appendectomy for complicated appendicitis is the same as for uncomplicated appendicitis; however, the level of difficulty encountered in removing a friable, gangrenous, and/or perforated appendix can be a challenge and requires gentle, meticulous handling of the appendix and inflamed periappendiceal tissues to avoid injury. Cultures are not necessary unless there is a significant concern for encountering resistant bacteria (patient with exposure to a healthcare environment or recent antibiotic therapy.)[54] In fact, intraoperative cultures have not been shown to decrease the incidence of postoperative intraabdominal abscesses or modify their treatment.[55] Once the appendix is successfully removed, careful attention should be given to the clearance of infectious material from the abdomen. This task may be accomplished by suction and irrigation, with special attention given to removal of any obvious fecaliths or spilled fecal material. Recent data suggest that simple suction aspiration of gross purulence may be just as effective as large-volume irrigation in cases of appendiceal rupture.[18] Drains are not routinely placed unless a discrete abscess cavity is present, in which case a single closed suction drain can be placed within its base. Recent data, however, suggest that prophylactic drain placement does not decrease the rate of postoperative complications in this population but can increase length of stay.[56,57] Postoperative antibiotic management in this population should continue for a maximum of 4 days after appendectomy, with recent data supporting a duration of only 2 days.[58–62] Knowledge of regional and institutional bacterial resistance patterns should be considered when choosing empiric coverage until culture results, if collected, are available.[63]

If the patient develops fever, leukocytosis, pain, and delayed return of bowel function, the possibility of a postoperative abscess must be entertained. Abscess complicates perforated appendicitis in 10% to 20% of cases and represents the major source of morbidity related to perforation.[1,3] A CT scan with IV administration of a contrast agent is diagnostic. Once an abscess is diagnosed, treatment usually consists of antibiotics and percutaneous

drainage.[17,18] If CT drainage is not technically possible because of the location of the abscess, laparoscopic, transrectal, or transvaginal drainage is an alternative.

Acute Appendicitis With Abscess or Phlegmon

In patients presenting with acute appendicitis with an abscess or phlegmon, treatment should be individualized based on the nature of the presentation (Fig. 94.4). Although rare, a patient may present with diffuse peritonitis and require urgent surgical intervention for management. More commonly, however, patients present similarly to the previous description. Immediate exploration and attempted appendectomy in these patients may result in substantial morbidity, including failure to identify the appendix, postoperative abscess or fistula, and unnecessary extension of the operation to include ileocecectomy, all due to the extreme induration and friability of the involved tissues. Furthermore, nonoperative treatment is often successful and has fewer complications than immediate operative management.[64–66] That being said, there is some evidence to support immediate operative management with regard to decreased length of stay, fewer readmissions, fewer additional interventions, and lower rates of eventual bowel resection.[67–69] The current World Society of Emergency Surgeons (WSES) Jerusalem guidelines recommend nonoperative management if laparoscopic expertise is not available but support operative management in experienced hands.[18]

If a localized abscess is identified, imaging-guided percutaneous drainage should be performed for source control. Once source control is obtained, antibiotics should be continued for 4 days.[62] The drainage catheter is typically left in place until the drainage

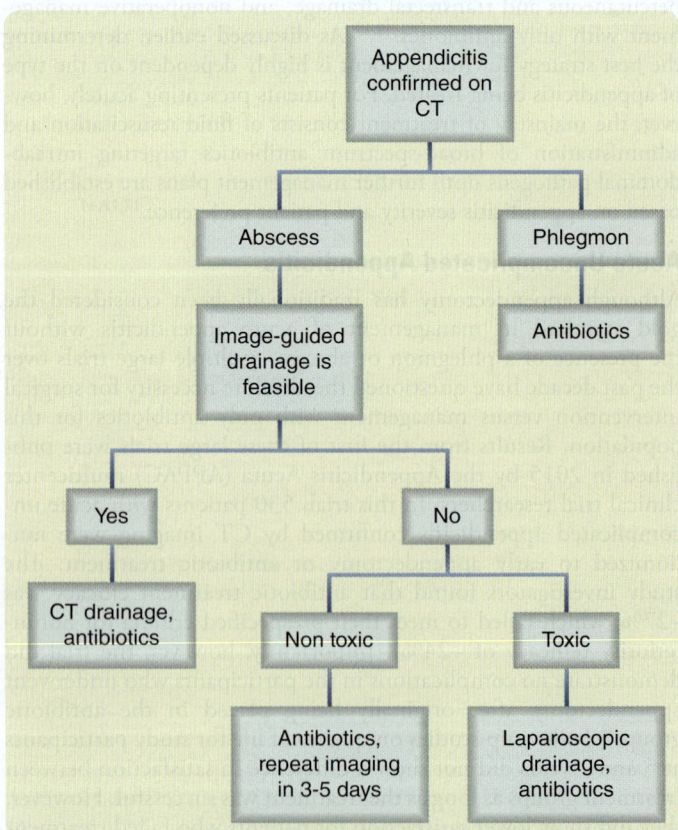

FIGURE 94.4 Suggested algorithm for managing the patient with acute appendicitis with an abscess or phlegmon. *CT*, Computed tomography; *OR*, operating room.

stops or slows down to institutional standard amounts.[70,71] If percutaneous drainage is not technically feasible, laparoscopic drainage may be necessary. Postoperative management for these patients is identical to that of patients who are successfully drained percutaneously. If a periappendiceal phlegmon is present or if the amount of fluid present is not sufficient to drain, the patient may be treated with antibiotics alone, typically for 4 to 7 days, as recommended by Infectious Diseases Society of America (IDSA) guidelines for treatment of intraabdominal infection.[54] If a patient with a phlegmon fails to improve with antibiotic treatment alone, reimaging is warranted to evaluate for the interval development of a drainable abscess.

After successful nonoperative treatment of complicated appendicitis, interval appendectomy, where patients undergo removal of the appendix several weeks to months later, should be considered. The rationale for interval appendectomy is based on the potential for development of recurrent appendicitis and the subsequent risks associated with emergent removal or reperforation of the appendix. On the other hand, interval appendectomy can be challenging and consequently yield a higher risk of postoperative complications when performed.[64,72] Multiple studies have investigated the recurrence rate of appendicitis after nonoperative management, which ranges from 8% to 31.8%.[73–77] The findings in these studies as well as similar results reported by others and the costs associated with operative intervention to prevent recurrence have led to the WSES Jerusalem guideline recommendation against routine interval appendectomy.[18] However, the presence of an appendicolith on CT has been shown to be predictive of a higher risk of recurrent appendicitis and may be used as a justification to proceed with interval appendectomy in that subgroup of patients.[50,78] This selective approach to interval appendectomy has also been demonstrated to be more cost-effective than its routine performance in all affected patients.[72] On the other hand, the risk of appendiceal neoplasms in patients presenting with complicated appendicitis with phlegmon or abscess treated nonoperatively is significant, and there are population-level data to support an association between tumor risk and complicated appendicitis.[76,79–82] Importantly, the Peri-Appendicitis Acuta randomized clinical trial, a multicenter, noninferiority trial comparing interval appendectomy to MRI after initial successful nonoperative treatment of complicated appendicitis with abscess, had to be stopped early because of the high rate of neoplasm in the interval appendectomy group, with all neoplasms in patients older than 40 years.[18,81,83,84] For this reason, if no interval appendectomy is performed, colonoscopy and full-dose contrast-enhanced CT should be performed in all adult patients 40 and older as routine follow-up after nonoperative management of complicated appendicitis.[18]

The Normal-Appearing Appendix at Operation

In cases of "negative appendectomy," in which a normal appendix is identified at operation for suspected acute appendicitis, there is controversy as to whether the appendix should be removed.[85,86] First, the abdomen should be thoroughly evaluated for other causes of pain severe enough to warrant an operation; this is easiest if the operation is laparoscopic. The terminal ileum should be examined for a Meckel diverticulum and the serosa of the small bowel for any stigmata of Crohn disease, such as inflammation, stricture formation, or the characteristic "creeping fat" appearance of the mesentery. The ileal mesentery should also be inspected for enlarged lymph nodes suggestive of mesenteric adenitis. The uterine adnexa should be examined for any evidence of tuboovarian or salpingeal disease, such as ovarian torsion, tuboovarian abscess,

endometriosis, or ruptured ovarian cysts. The sigmoid colon should be examined for evidence of acute diverticulitis, especially in cases in which a redundant sigmoid colon is found in the right lower quadrant. If these are all normal, attention should be turned to the upper abdomen for examination of the gallbladder and duodenum.

If everything looks normal, including the appendix, during an operation for suspected appendicitis, appendectomy should be strongly considered. This is mainly because many causes of right lower quadrant pain mentioned earlier may be recurrent, and removal of the appendix removes appendicitis from the differential diagnosis if the patient re-presents with pain. In cases of Crohn disease suggested by findings at operation, appendectomy is advisable unless the base of the appendix and cecum are involved (in this scenario, appendectomy is deferred to avoid breakdown of the inflamed stump and subsequent fistula formation) for the same reason. In addition, abnormalities of the appendix not apparent on gross inspection at the time of operation are sometimes identified on pathologic examination.[85]

Stump Appendicitis

Stump appendicitis occurs when residual appendiceal tissue at the base of the cecum, resulting from incomplete resection at the time of appendectomy, develops recurrent inflammation. It is a relatively rare diagnosis with an incidence between 0.002% and 0.15%.[87,88] Patients with stump appendicitis usually present with similar symptoms as patients with appendicitis without prior appendectomy. Imaging is nonspecific and includes cecal wall thickening, fluid in the right paracolic gutter, infiltration of the surrounding fat, and if the stump is long enough, similar findings to those of primary acute appendicitis.[89] Stump appendicitis has been reported after both open and laparoscopic appendectomy and is associated with difficulty in visualization and, thus, identification of the actual appendiceal base during appendectomy. Appendectomy in the setting of perforation, necrosis, or abscess makes this visualization more challenging and, thus, increases the risk of stump appendicitis at a later date.[90] Stump appendicitis should be managed as recurrent appendicitis and, thus, warrants surgical resection of the remnant appendix.[91]

Chronic Appendicitis as a Cause of Abdominal Pain

On occasion, patients will present with a history of recurrent right lower quadrant pain, and a surgical opinion will be sought as to the benefit of elective appendectomy for treatment of this condition. Studies suggest that uncomplicated appendicitis may occasionally resolve without intervention, so it is conceivable that appendicitis may wax and wane in some patients.[92,93] In addition, some patients with pain are found to have a thickened appendix or an appendicolith on CT despite no evidence of a systemic illness or acute periappendiceal inflammation. In some of these cases, appendectomy will produce relief of symptoms, and in these cases, examination of the appendix will sometimes reveal findings consistent with chronic inflammation.[94,95]

More complex, however, is the patient with nonspecific lower abdominal pain in the absence of radiographic evidence of appendiceal disease. This typically requires a multidisciplinary workup involving input from specialists in gastroenterology and gynecology as well as surgery. Appendectomy is typically not offered unless disease is demonstrated radiographically. However, if diagnostic laparoscopy is performed to investigate or exclude other disease (typically by a gynecologist), it is reasonable to offer the patient an appendectomy to be performed at that time.[96,97]

This should be approached through a shared decision-making model, where the risks of appendectomy are weighed against the possible resolution of the patient's symptoms (if the appendix was the source) and the ability to remove the appendix from consideration as a source in the future and, thus, potentially avoid unnecessary imaging and facilitate the search for other sources of pain.

Incidental Appendectomy

Incidental appendectomy is the term applied when a grossly normal appendix is removed at the time of an unrelated procedure. Once commonly performed, incidental appendectomy is no longer recommended. Wen and coworkers actually demonstrated that incidental appendectomy is associated with an increase in both morbidity and mortality.[93,98] Other investigators have demonstrated that incidental appendectomy does not appear to be cost-effective as a preventive measure.[99] Finally, the recent finding that the appendix may actually have a role in the maintenance of healthy colonic flora makes the practice of incidental appendectomy even more controversial.[4,5,39] For these reasons, we advocate careful inspection of the appendix for abnormalities during abdominal operations as part of a thorough exploration but do not advocate appendectomy unless an abnormality is detected.

Laparoscopic Versus Open Appendectomy

The debate about the choice of open versus laparoscopic appendectomy for the treatment of appendicitis was historically a major point of controversy among surgeons. However, the literature now strongly supports performing appendectomy laparoscopically, including in complicated appendicitis, elderly patients, and pregnant patients.[100–103] Laparoscopic appendectomy is associated with a lower risk of complications in both complicated and uncomplicated appendicitis, including lower overall morbidity, reduced wound complications, reduced postoperative pain, and a slightly shorter recovery time, with only a slightly higher versus similar rate of postoperative intraabdominal abscess development.[104–107] Thus, although both open and laparoscopic approaches are acceptable, there are significant advantages with laparoscopy. Furthermore, laparoscopy allows examination of the entire peritoneal space, making it exceptionally useful to exclude other intraabdominal disease that may be manifested in a similar fashion, such as diverticulitis or tuboovarian abscess. Although debate remains regarding the cost-effectiveness of a laparoscopic versus open approach, the advantages of the laparoscopic approach appear to outweigh the marginally increased hospital costs associated with it.[108,109]

For open appendectomy the patient is placed in the supine position, and the appendix is approached through an oblique muscle-splitting incision (McArthur-McBurney), a transverse incision (Rockey-Davis), or a conservative midline incision. The cecum is grasped by the taeniae and delivered into the wound, allowing visualization of the base of the appendix and delivery of the appendiceal tip. The appendix is divided with the use of a stapler or crushed just above the base and ligated with an absorbable ligature. The stump is then either cauterized or, if desired, inverted by a purse-string or "Z" suture technique, although simple ligation is preferred (Fig. 94.5).[110]

For laparoscopic appendectomy, the patient is placed in the supine position with the right arm out and the left arm tucked. The bladder is emptied by a straight catheter or by having the patient void immediately before the procedure. The abdomen is entered via an open access (Hasson) or optical trocar technique

(Fig. 94.6). Two additional working ports are then placed, typically in the left lower quadrant and in either the suprapubic area or supraumbilical midline, based on surgeon preference. With both the surgeon and assistant on the left side of the patient, atraumatic graspers are used to elevate the appendix. The appendix can then be divided using a laparoscopic stapler or Endoloop,[111–113] and the mesoappendix can also be divided with a laparoscopic stapler, a LigaSure, or a harmonic scalpel.[111–113] Retrieval of the appendix is accomplished using a plastic retrieval bag. The pelvis is suctioned and irrigated as needed, the trocars are removed, and the wounds are closed. Laparoscopic appendectomy may also be performed with single-site laparoscopic surgical techniques based on the experience and preferences of the surgeon. Laparoscopic appendectomy is demonstrated in Video 94.1. Video 94.2 demonstrates a single-incision laparoscopic approach (SILS) to several variants of appendiceal pathology.

APPENDICITIS IN SPECIAL POPULATIONS

Appendicitis in the Pregnant Patient

Appendicitis is the most common nonobstetric emergency in pregnancy and, consequently, the most frequent reason for general surgical intervention in this group of patients (Fig. 94.7).[114,115] In pregnancy, appendicitis has a typical clinical presentation in only 50% to 60% of cases.[114,115] The common symptoms of early appendicitis, such as nausea and vomiting, are nonspecific and are also often associated with normal pregnancy. Also, the normal febrile response to illness may be blunted and physical examination possibly altered because of the displacement of the appendix to a more cephalad location within the abdomen as a result of the gravid uterus. Finally, biochemical and laboratory indicators used to support the diagnosis of appendicitis in the nonpregnant patient are unreliable in pregnancy. For example, mild leukocytosis and elevated C-reactive protein levels may be physiologically normal findings in pregnancy. In addition, the surgeon must be concerned about the possibility of obstetric emergencies as a cause of abdominal pain, such as preterm labor, placental abruption, or uterine rupture.[114]

The impact of appendicitis on the pregnant patient is severe. The risk of preterm labor has been shown to be 11% and fetal loss 6% with complicated appendicitis.[116] On the other hand, negative appendectomy has also been associated with preterm labor and fetal loss (10% and 4%, respectively).[116] The lowest rates of preterm labor and fetal loss (6% and 2%, respectively) were seen in cases of uncomplicated appendicitis.[116] For these reasons, preoperative accuracy of diagnosis is crucial in the pregnant patient with suspected appendicitis; thus, routine imaging is recommended.

The initial study of choice for the diagnosis of appendicitis in pregnant patients is US with graded compression.[18] The criteria for US diagnosis are the same as in the nonpregnant patient. Unfortunately, the sensitivity and specificity (83%) of US are reduced in pregnancy because of the presence of the gravid uterus.[117] If US examination findings are equivocal, MRI without gadolinium contrast is the best next imaging study to pursue, given its excellent preserved sensitivity and specificity in the pregnant patient (Fig. 94.8).[18] Routine use of MRI in pregnant patients has been demonstrated to reduce the negative appendectomy rate by 47% without a significant increase in the perforation rate, and it has been shown to be a cost-effective study.[117] If US is inconclusive and MRI scanning is not immediately available, CT scanning may be used. Despite the risks associated with radiation

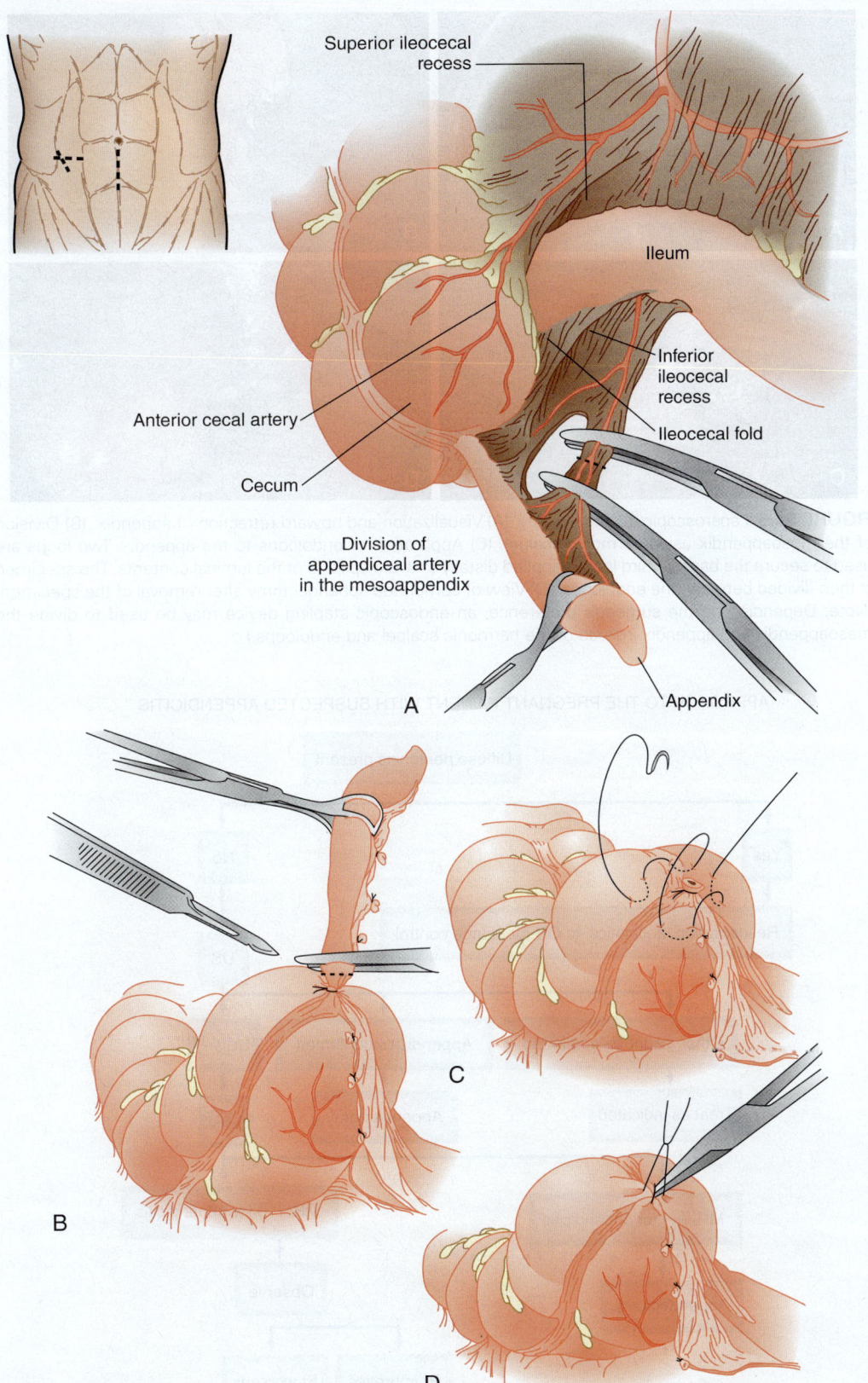

FIGURE 94.5 (A) *Left,* Location of possible incisions for an open appendectomy. *Right,* Division of the mesoappendix. (B) Ligation of the base and division of the appendix. (C) Placement of purse-string suture or Z stitch. (D) Inversion of the appendiceal stump. (From Ortega JM, Ricardo AE. Surgery of the appendix and colon. In: Moody FG, ed. *Atlas of Ambulatory Surgery.* WB Saunders; 1999.)

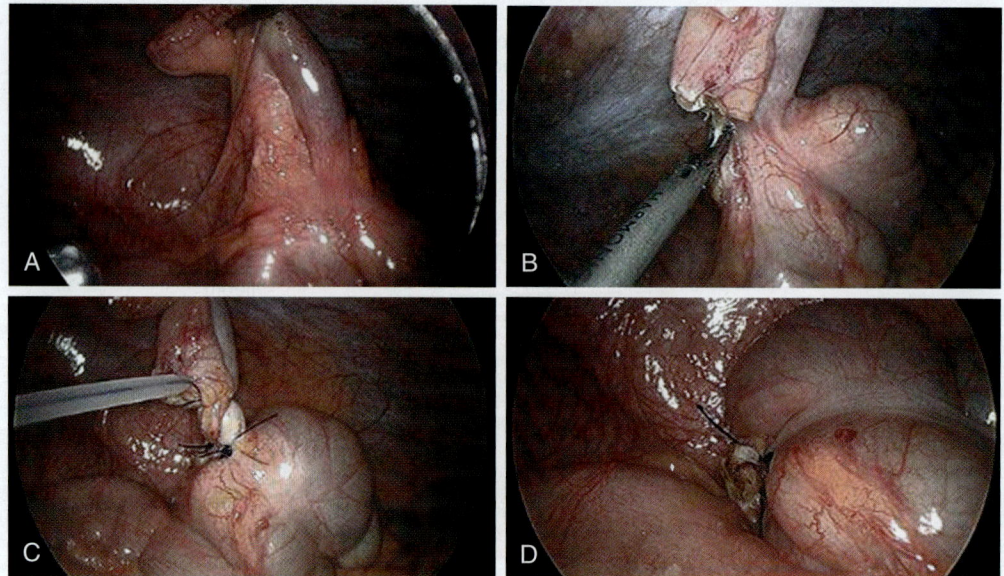

FIGURE 94.6 Laparoscopic appendectomy. (A) Visualization and upward retraction of appendix. (B) Division of the mesoappendix using harmonic scalpel. (C) Application of endoloops to the appendix. Two loops are used to secure the base; a third loop is applied distally to avoid spillage of the luminal contents. The specimen is then divided between the endoloops. (D) View of completed appendectomy after removal of the specimen. (Note: Depending on the surgeon's preference, an endoscopic stapling device may be used to divide the mesoappendix and appendix instead of the harmonic scalpel and endoloops.)

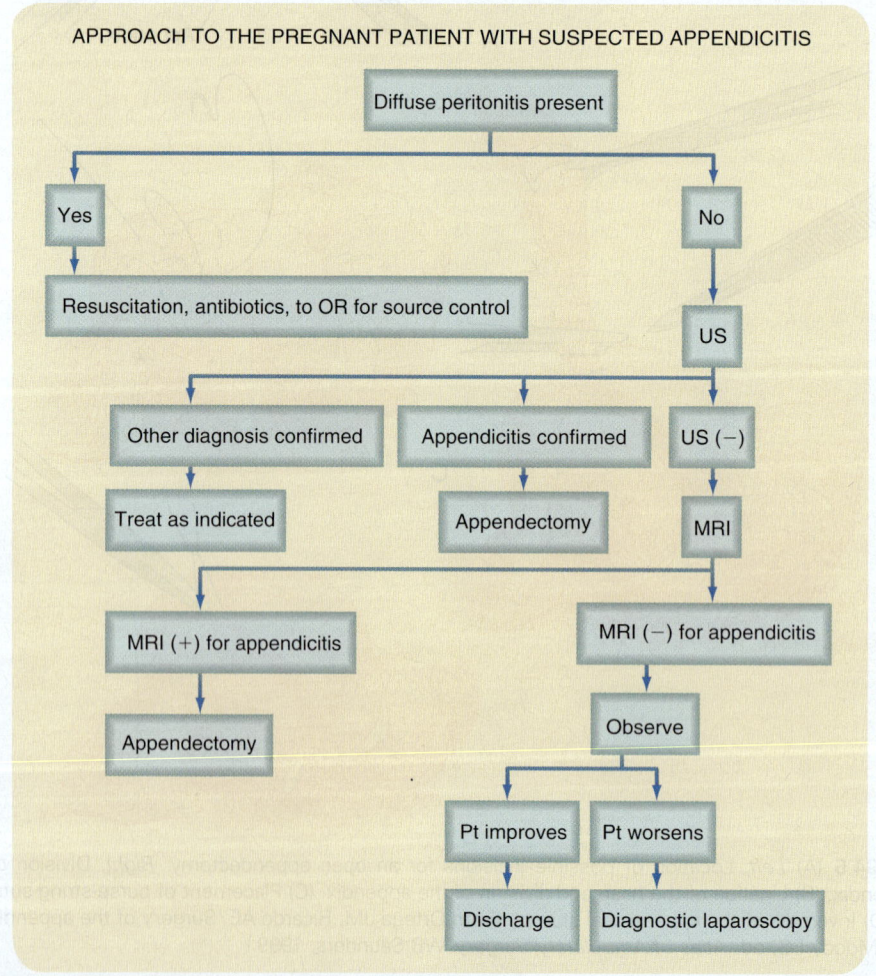

FIGURE 94.7 Suggested algorithm for managing the pregnant patient with possible appendicitis. *MRI*, Magnetic resonance imaging; *OR*, operating room; *Pt*, patient; *US*, ultrasound.

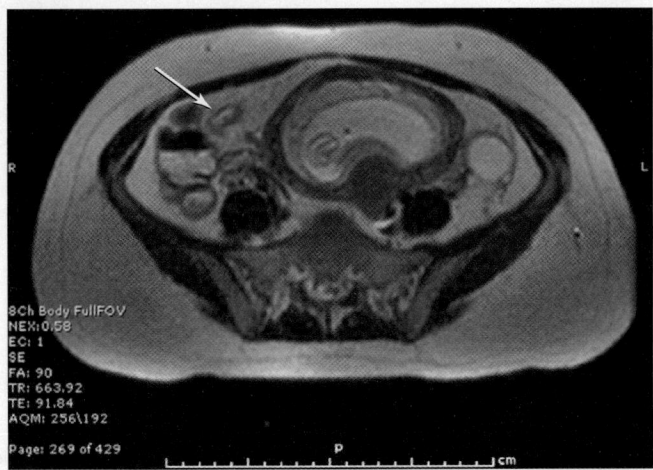

FIGURE 94.8 Magnetic resonance imaging scan with T1-weighted axial image of the abdomen in a gravid patient. The *arrow* highlights the thickened appendix. (From Parks NA, Schroeppel TJ. Update on imaging for acute appendicitis. *Surg Clin North Am.* 2011;91:141-154.)

exposure to the fetus, this can still be offered if the study is in the best interest of the pregnant patient and the patient understands the risks, which are minimal.[118] Although protocols vary, if CT is used during pregnancy, care should be taken to perform as limited a study as possible using a technique with the lowest possible radiation exposure and with avoidance of IV administration of contrast material.

Laparoscopic appendectomy is the most common approach currently used in pregnant patients[119] and is safe, provided that the surgeon has adequate experience with laparoscopy. Video 94.3 demonstrates a safe technique for appendectomy in a pregnant patient. At operation, consideration should be given to the height of the gravid uterus in choosing sites for trocar placement and entry technique to avoid inadvertent puncture of the uterus.

Appendicitis in the Elderly

Appendicitis is not infrequently seen in elderly patients and should remain in the differential diagnoses of any elderly patient presenting with acute abdominal pain who has not had an appendectomy. Data suggest that the reduced physiologic reserves and impaired immunologic and inflammatory responses in the elderly result in higher morbidity with a diagnosis of appendicitis.[17] The most important aspect when dealing with an elderly patient with abdominal pain is to realize the expanded differential diagnosis that must be considered, including but not limited to acute diverticulitis (uncomplicated or complicated), malignant disease, intestinal ischemia, ischemic colitis, complicated urinary tract infection, and perforated ulcer. Appendicitis may also be manifested in an atypical manner, so a high index of suspicion must be maintained in patients with an appendix. The higher perforation rate in the elderly population, as high as 40% to 70%, combined with the frequent coexistence of comorbidities resulting in higher morbidity, makes the diagnosis and treatment of appendicitis in the elderly a challenge, to say the least.[3,17,120]

Laparoscopic appendectomy is safe in the elderly and is the procedure of choice in this group of patients.[17] For patients too ill to undergo surgery, selective use of nonoperative therapy for appendicitis has shown success, as discussed previously. Certainly, when dealing with the elderly and the infirm, the approach must be individually tailored to the specific challenges presented by the patient.

Appendicitis in the Immunocompromised Patient

Immunocompromised patients with a concern for appendicitis should be evaluated promptly with CT imaging. This allows confirmation of the diagnosis of appendicitis as well as the exclusion of diagnoses, such as neutropenic enterocolitis (typhlitis), that may be amenable to nonoperative treatment.[14] A high index of suspicion in the management of this population is key because of their blunted ability to mount an immune response, which may result in the absence of fever, leukocytosis, and peritonitis. Appendicitis in the immunocompromised patient should be managed with appendectomy.

NEOPLASMS OF THE APPENDIX

Neoplasms of the appendix, although rare entities, are an important consideration for the practicing clinician. The annual incidence is estimated at 6 per 1,000,000 people.[121] Most cases are diagnosed incidentally because the majority of patients initially present with signs and symptoms concerning for appendicitis. Diagnosis is often achieved only after pathologic review of the appendectomy specimen. However, occasionally, these neoplasms may be detected on imaging as "incidentalomas"—including suspicion of underlying mass or mucocele. Despite their low incidence, these tumors present a management challenge for clinicians, and most general surgeons will encounter appendiceal neoplasms at some point in their careers. Their broad and diverse nature is reflected in their varying tumor biology and histopathology and the wide range of reported long-term survival, between 10% and 90%.[122] Altogether, this diversity creates confusion for practicing clinicians regarding classification, terminology, and management strategies.

In 2016, the Peritoneal Surface Oncology Group International (PSOGI) Modified Delphi Process[123] created a consensus for the terminology and classification of appendiceal neoplasms, which has been further expounded on by the 8th edition of the American Joint Committee on Cancer (AJCC) *Cancer Staging Manual*[124] in 2017 and by the World Health Organization (WHO) classification of digestive system tumors[125] in 2019. Appendiceal neoplasms are classified into "epithelial" versus "nonepithelial" tumors (Table 94.2). Epithelial tumors, as defined by PSOGI, include adenomas, serrated polyps, low-grade appendiceal mucinous neoplasms (LAMNs), high-grade appendiceal mucinous neoplasms (HAMNs), mucinous adenocarcinomas, poorly differentiated (mucinous) adenocarcinomas with signet ring cells, (mucinous) signet ring cell carcinomas, and adenocarcinomas. Nonepithelial tumors include lymphomas and sarcomas. Neuroendocrine neoplasms (NENs), although originally classified as "nonepithelial" by PSOGI, have been designated as *epithelial tumors* by the WHO. This section provides an overview of the approach to and management of appendiceal neoplasms.

Clinical Presentation

A common presentation for appendiceal neoplasms may mimic the classic symptoms of acute appendicitis: right lower quadrant pain and tenderness, nausea, anorexia, fever, and leukocytosis. An incidental mass may also be noted during radiographic workup for presumed appendicitis; however, most often, these tumors are detected postoperatively during evaluation of the appendectomy specimen. A previous retrospective study found that up to 3.7% of appendectomy specimens contained appendiceal neoplasms, with a higher frequency found in patients undergoing interval

TABLE 94.2	Classification of Appendiceal Neoplasms
SUBTYPE	**NEOPLASM**
Noncarcinoid epithelial tumors	• Adenoma • Serrated polyp • Low-grade appendiceal neoplasm (LAMN) • High-grade appendiceal neoplasm (HAMN) • Mucinous adenocarcinoma • Poorly differentiated (mucinous) adenocarcinoma with signet ring cells • (Mucinous) signet ring cell carcinoma • (Nonmucinous) adenocarcinoma • Goblet cell adenocarcinoma
Neuroendocrine neoplasms	• Neuroendocrine tumor (NET) • Neuroendocrine carcinoma (NEC) • Mixed neuroendocrine–nonneuroendocrine neoplasm (MiNEN)

Nonepithelial tumors	• Lymphoma
	  • Burkitt
	  • Diffuse large B-cell
	  • Non-Hodgkin
	• Myeloid sarcoma

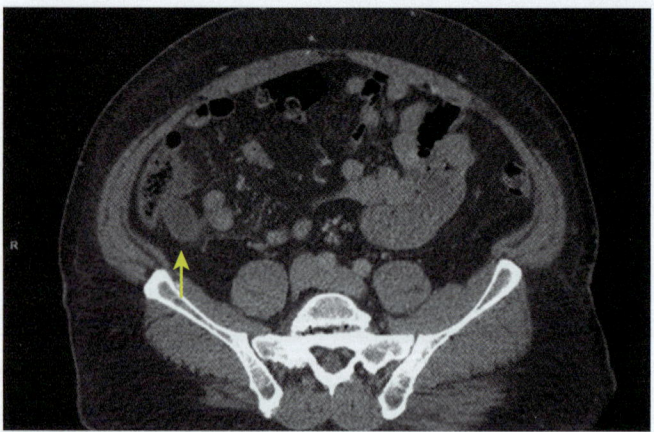

FIGURE 94.9 Computed tomography scan of the abdomen depicting a dilated, mucus-filled appendix, representative of a mucocele (arrow).

appendectomy.[79] Intraoperatively, the diagnosis may be masked by inflammation and distortion of the surrounding anatomy. Thus, all appendectomy specimens should be sent for pathologic review, and adequate review is critical for diagnosis and subsequent management decision-making.

Efforts to distinguish features of appendicitis secondary to a neoplasm from primary appendicitis have been limited by the rarity of such masses. However, certain factors, such as age greater than 40, immunocompromised status, and presence of a periappendiceal abscess or phlegmon, have been associated with increased risk of harboring a neoplasm.[126] Studies have identified radiographic features thought to portend a higher risk of an underlying appendiceal neoplasm, such as increased soft tissue thickening and wall irregularity,[127] focal dilatation, lack of periappendiceal fat stranding, mural calcification, and luminal diameter greater than 2 cm.[128] Nevertheless, the low incidence of this condition limits the ability to draw truly definitive conclusions.

Often, an incidental mucocele—a distended, mucus-filled appendix (Fig. 94.9)—may be identified on cross-sectional imaging or encountered during appendectomy or colonoscopy. Like other appendiceal neoplasms, mucoceles are rare, and symptoms may mimic those of appendicitis. The term *mucocele* is a broad and nonspecific descriptive term, however, and not a formal diagnosis because it can present secondary to both benign and neoplastic obstructive processes. Mucoceles can be subdivided into mucinous retention cysts, mucosal hyperplasia, mucinous cystadenoma (now an outdated term largely referring to LAMN), and mucinous cystadenocarcinoma.

Most appendiceal mucinous neoplasms begin as mucoceles; however, it is difficult to differentiate between a malignant versus benign mucocele when visualized grossly intraoperatively. Therefore, upon resection, every effort must be taken to avoid rupture and inadvertent peritoneal seeding.[129] In addition, the surgeon should carefully look for any evidence of peritoneal dissemination, which may include peritoneal mucin deposits or nodularities. If any suspicious nodules or mucin deposits are identified, they should be biopsied and sent for pathologic evaluation, in addition to careful evaluation of the appendectomy specimen.

Once the diagnosis of an appendiceal neoplasm has been made by an experienced pathologist, additional management strategies can include focused oncologic history and physical examination, follow-up colonoscopy to detect the presence of synchronous colonic pathology, and cross-sectional imaging of the abdomen and pelvis with either CT or MRI (and possible chest CT based on underlying histologic subtype).[130] Most importantly, all treatment plans should involve multidisciplinary discussion in a tumor board at a high-volume treatment center.

Management of Primary Appendiceal Neoplasms by Histologic Classification

Herein, we discuss basic management principles of appendiceal neoplasms according to histologic subtype.

Epithelial Neoplasms

Appendiceal adenomas and serrated polyps are similar in behavior to their colonic counterparts. Occasionally, patients may present with obstructive symptoms, but like most appendiceal lesions, adenomas and serrated polyps are most often found incidentally after postappendectomy pathology review. These lesions, typically confined to the muscularis mucosa and lamina propria and without evidence of invasion, are sufficiently managed with a simple appendectomy. However, they are associated with an increased risk of synchronous colonic pathology and can be a manifestation of serrated polyposis syndrome.[126] Therefore, such patients should be counseled to undergo a full colonoscopy.[126,131,132]

Appendiceal mucinous neoplasms are the most common noninvasive epithelial lesions. These are adenomas marked by prominent mucin production and can be associated with extraappendiceal deposits. They can be further divided into LAMNs and HAMNs based on cytologic atypia. LAMN was previously referred to as a *mucinous cystadenoma,* now an extinct terminology. Both LAMN and HAMNs can be safely managed with simple appendectomy, but if high-grade atypia is present, careful pathologic examination must be undertaken to rule out any invasive component. In the absence of invasion, disease recurrence is low if complete resection is achieved. The presence of extraappendiceal mucin deposits or perforation is associated with an increased risk of recurrence.[121,126]

Mucinous adenocarcinomas are largely composed of mucin-producing cells, such that >50% of the tumor is composed of extracellular mucin. However, unlike LAMNs or HAMNs, these tumors are additionally characterized by infiltrative invasion.[123] They can be further subdivided based on differentiation (well, moderately, and poorly differentiated) and the presence of signet ring cells. Well-differentiated mucinous adenocarcinomas have a greater association with peritoneal spread, whereas moderately and poorly differentiated adenocarcinomas are more associated with lymphatic spread and distant metastasis.[133] Adenocarcinomas with signet ring cells portend an even worse prognosis and are considered poorly differentiated by nature.[133] When disease is localized and identified on an appendectomy specimen, interval right colectomy is typically recommended. Complete staging with imaging and tumor markers (carcinoembryonic antigen [CEA], carbohydrate antigen [CA]125, and CA19-9 have all been advocated for appendiceal neoplasms) should precede planned colectomy.

Nonmucinous adenocarcinomas of the appendix are similar in nature to adenocarcinomas of the colon and rectum and are traditionally treated as such. For all appendiceal adenocarcinomas, treatment recommendations include complete staging with cross-sectional imaging and tumor markers (CEA, CA125, and CA19-9), followed by interval right hemicolectomy, with sufficient lymph node sampling for staging, and consideration of adjuvant chemotherapy.[134]

In recent years, some studies have posited that in select patients with T1, well-differentiated tumors without evidence of lymphovascular invasion, less extensive surgical resection (i.e., simple appendectomy or ileocecectomy) may suffice,[135,136] but the rarity of this disease limits the ability to further investigate with prospective studies. Ultimately, prognostic biomarkers such as circulating tumor DNA (ctDNA) may provide further clarity on this issue.

Goblet cell adenocarcinoma, previously termed *goblet cell carcinoid,* demonstrates both neuroendocrine and mucinous features. However, the neuroendocrine component is considered relatively minor, as reflected in the updated terminology in the most recent WHO classifications.[130,137,138] In general, this histologic subtype is managed similarly to nonmucinous (colonic type) adenocarcinomas, with cross-sectional imaging for complete staging, tumor markers (including the addition of chromogranin A at some centers), interval right hemicolectomy, lymph node staging, and consideration of adjuvant therapy.[126,134]

Neuroendocrine Neoplasms

NENs originate from subepithelial neuroendocrine cells, which are largely concentrated in the tip of the appendix, explaining the propensity for NENs to arise from this region most commonly. As per WHO classifications, NENs can be subdivided into well-differentiated neuroendocrine tumors (NETs), poorly differentiated neuroendocrine carcinomas (NECs), and mixed neuroendocrine–nonneuroendocrine neoplasms (MiNENs; previously termed *mixed adenoneuroendocrine neoplasms* [MANECs]).[138] Somatostatin receptor imaging, such as ^{68}Ga-DOTATATE–positron emission tomography/CT (PET/CT), can be useful in identifying occult and distant disease, susceptibility to somatostatin receptor antagonists, and response to treatment. However, these benefits should be weighed against the tremendous costs of such imaging, and it is, therefore, not currently recommended for routine use.[126,130,137]

NETs represent the majority of appendiceal NEN cases, and although associated with an overall favorable prognosis, they have a high incidence of lymph node spread. A retrospective Surveillance, Epidemiology, and End Results (SEER) database study reported a correlation between tumor size and lymph node spread as follows: 15% of tumors measuring 1 cm or smaller, 47% of tumors between 1 and 2 cm, and 86% of tumors larger than 2 cm. The corresponding 10-year survival rates for each tumor size subgroup were as follows, respectively: 100% with either positive or negative lymph nodes, 92% with node-positive disease versus 100% with negative nodes, and 91% with node positivity versus 100% without nodal disease.[139]

National Comprehensive Cancer Network (NCCN) guidelines recommend surgical resection as the gold standard of treatment and offer the following guidance.[140] For tumors less than 2 cm in size and tumors located in the distal one-third of the appendix, simple appendectomy is sufficient. However, in cases of incomplete resection, node positivity, or positive margins, completion right hemicolectomy should be considered. For proximal NETs located at the base of the appendix or for tumors greater than 2 cm, a formal right hemicolectomy with lymph node staging is indicated. In these patients for whom colectomy is considered, complete staging with cross-sectional imaging is also recommended. The North American Neuroendocrine Society (NANETS) and European Neuroendocrine Tumor Society (ENETS) additionally recommend completion hemicolectomy if any of the following characteristics are present: positive mesenteric nodes, invasion at the base of the appendix or of the mesoappendix, a Ki-67 (proliferation) index greater than 20%, or mixed tumor histology.[141,142] It should be noted that data on survival benefit with interval colectomy are limited.

Nonepithelial Neoplasms

The nonepithelial appendiceal neoplasms are lymphomas and sarcoma. With these neoplasms being extremely rare, there is little information published in the literature. This classification includes Burkitt lymphoma; diffuse large B-cell, non-Hodgkin lymphoma; and myeloid sarcoma. As with other appendiceal neoplasms, these are typically incidental findings after appendectomy for presumed appendicitis.[143]

Management of Peritoneal Dissemination From Appendiceal Neoplasms

Pseudomyxoma Peritonei

Pseudomyxoma peritonei (PMP) (Fig. 94.10) occurs when a mucin-producing tumor of the appendix perforates through the appendix, leading to intraabdominal spread of tumor cells and mucinous ascites. Most commonly, it is associated with LAMN. PSOGI classifies PMP according to three histologic subtypes: PMP with low-grade histologic features (low cellularity with mild atypia), PMP with high-grade histologic features (more cellularity with features of invasion), and PMP with signet ring cells.[133] Standard treatment recommendations include surgical cytoreduction (CRS) with hyperthermic intraperitoneal chemotherapy (HIPEC).[134] Although the adoption of combination CRS/HIPEC has greatly improved survival compared with historical controls, outcomes after treatment vary widely and are primarily determined by underlying histologic subtype, burden of disease, and completeness of cytoreduction. Systemic therapy may also play a significant role in patients with higher-grade disease. PMP with low-grade features has the highest reported survival after CRS/HIPEC, with 5-year survival at 62.5%,[144] although it may be as high as 80% to 90%[145–148] in patients with favorable biology and complete cytoreduction. On the other hand, high-grade PMP has a reported 5-year survival of 37.7%.[144]

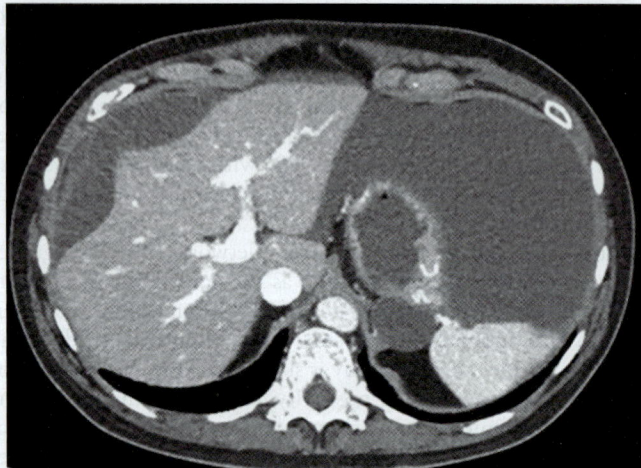

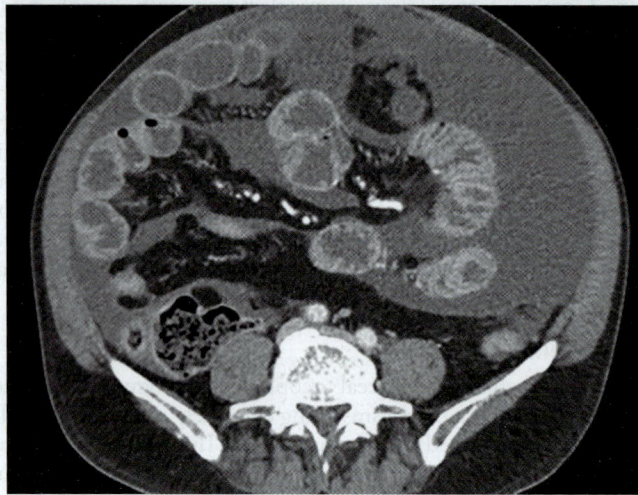

FIGURE 94.10 Computed tomography scan of the abdomen depicting mucinous ascites and disseminated peritoneal disease consistent with pseudomyxoma peritonei.

Patients with PMP should be referred to a high-volume center with expertise in the treatment of peritoneal surface malignancies. In patients who have undergone CRS/HIPEC, surveillance guidelines can vary. The American Society of Colon and Rectal Surgeons recommends that patients with low-grade PMP who have undergone CRS with HIPEC should be surveilled with CT or MRI of the abdomen and pelvis 2 months after surgery and then annually for at least 5 years. For patients with high-grade PMP, obtaining additional chest imaging and more frequent surveillance every 6 months for at least 6 years may help detect recurrent disease earlier.[130]

Peritoneal Carcinomatosis

In patients whose peritoneal disease burden has a lower degree of mucin-producing tumor, *peritoneal carcinomatosis* (PC) is the more appropriate terminology. Again, outcomes for these patients vary widely based on histologic subtype, disease burden, symptomatology, and candidacy for CRS/HIPEC. Diagnosis and determination of candidacy for CRS/HIPEC often require careful assessment with diagnostic laparoscopy because peritoneal metastases, especially lesions of small size, can be missed on standard imaging, and disease burden is frequently underestimated by cross-sectional imaging. Furthermore, systemic therapy is often a critical component for patients with PC, and surgical management frequently may center around palliative efforts rather than the ability to completely cytoreduce a patient. Moreover, treatment centers with experience in the management of peritoneal surface malignancies are important in making the best decisions around the role of systemic therapy, candidacy for CRS/HIPEC, and palliative treatment options.

CONCLUSION

Diagnosis and decision-making around the treatment of appendiceal neoplasms can be challenging because of the rarity and heterogeneous nature of these neoplasms. The histologic features of these neoplasms are complex and varied, giving rise to diverse tumor behavior. Decision-making should involve multidisciplinary tumor board discussions, and patients should be referred to high-volume treatment centers specializing in peritoneal surface malignancies. Overall, management centers around complete surgical resection with careful pathologic review. Patients with more advanced disease should be considered for systemic therapy and CRS/HIPEC.

SELECTED REFERENCES

Bom WJ, Scheijmans JCG, Salminen P, Boermeester MA. Diagnosis of uncomplicated and complicated appendicitis in adults. *Scand J Surg.* 2021;110(2):170-179.

This is an excellent review emphasizing the importance of differentiating between complicated and uncomplicated appendicitis and the challenges involved.

Davidson GH, Flum DR, Monsell SE, et al. Antibiotics versus appendectomy for acute appendicitis—longer-term outcomes. *N Engl J Med.* 2021;385(25):2395-2397.
Flum DR, Davidson GH, Monsell SE, et al. A randomized trial comparing antibiotics with appendectomy for appendicitis. *N Engl J Med.* 2020;383(20):1907-1919.

These two recently published articles include the short- and long-term results of the largest randomized controlled trial to date comparing antibiotic treatment versus appendectomy in the management of uncomplicated appendicitis.

Di Saverio S, Podda M, De Simone B, et al. Diagnosis and treatment of acute appendicitis: 2020 update of the WSES Jerusalem guidelines. *World J Emerg Surg.* 2020;15(1):27.
Gorter RR, Eker HH, Gorter-Stam MA, et al. Diagnosis and management of acute appendicitis. EAES Consensus Development Conference 2015. *Surg Endosc.* 2016;30:4668-4690.

These two consensus statements provide a comprehensive review of the current literature and expert opinion relating to all aspects of the diagnosis and treatment of appendicitis.

The full reference list appears on Elsevier eBooks+.

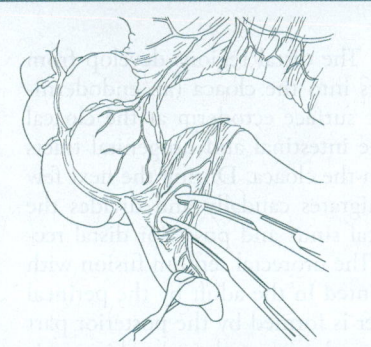

CHAPTER 95

Colon and Rectum

Nir Horesh, Sameh Emile, and Steven D. Wexner

OUTLINE

EMBRYOLOGY OF THE COLON AND RECTUM

A sound knowledge base of the gastrointestinal (GI) tract embryologic development is important in understanding colon and rectal anatomy and pathophysiology. The primitive gut tube is formed from the endodermal roof of the yolk sac. Early in the development process, beginning in the third week of gestation, the gut tube divides into three sections: the foregut, midgut, and hindgut (Fig. 95.1).

The foregut forms the oral (buccopharyngeal) membrane, esophagus, stomach, and proximal duodenum (to the duodenal ampulla) and is supplied by the celiac artery. The midgut, including the distal part of the duodenum, small intestine, right colon,

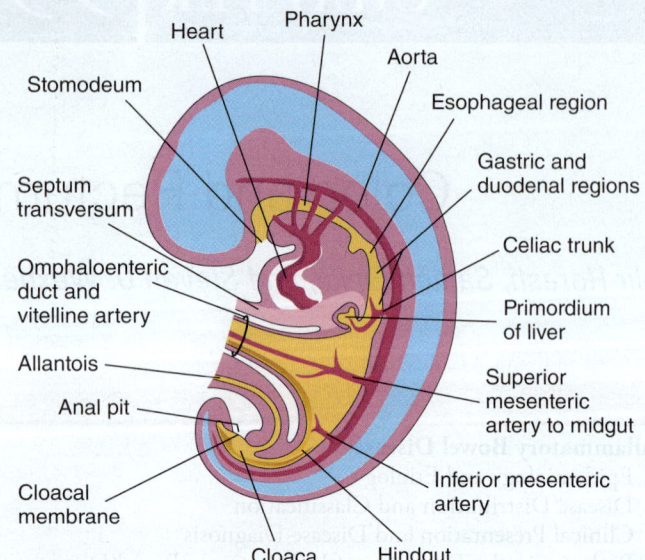

FIGURE 95.1 Median section of the embryo showing the early alimentary system and its blood supply (week 4). (From Moore KL, Persaud TVN, Torchia MG. Alimentary system. In: *The Developing Human.* 11th ed. Philadelphia: Elsevier; 2020:193-221.)

and the proximal two-thirds of the transverse colon, receives its blood supply from the superior mesenteric artery (SMA). The midgut temporarily herniates ventrally out of the abdomen, a key step in the physiologic development progress for acquiring length and correct positioning of its structures (Fig. 95.2). The hindgut develops into the distal third of the transverse colon, descending colon, sigmoid, and rectum all the way to the upper anal canal. It is supplied by the inferior mesenteric artery (IMA). The venous and lymphatic networks develop parallel to their corresponding sectional arteries.

The embryologic development of the rectum is complex and prone to developmental complications. The proximal rectum

develops similarly to the colon. The distal regions develop from the terminal hindgut that enters into the cloaca (an endoderm-lined cavity in contact with the surface ectoderm at the cloacal membrane). Before 5 weeks, the intestinal and urogenital tracts terminate at a common cavity in the cloaca. During the next few weeks, the urorectal septum migrates caudally and divides the cloaca into an anterior urogenital sinus and posterior distal rectum and anal sinus (Fig. 95.3). The urorectal septum fusion with the cloacal membrane is represented in the adult by the perineal body. The external anal sphincter is formed by the posterior part of the cloacal sphincter, whereas the internal anal sphincter is formed from enlarging circular fibers of the rectum. The upper two-thirds of the anal canal is derived from the hindgut, and the lower third is derived from the proctodeum. The dentate line marks the fusion of endodermal (hindgut) and ectodermal depression (proctodeum). The anal transition zone is formed from the cloacal part of the anal canal. The hindgut part of the anal canal is supplied by the IMA, whereas the lower third is supplied by the internal pudendal artery.

ANATOMY OF THE COLON, RECTUM, AND PELVIC FLOOR

The large bowel, including the colon and rectum, is a tube of variable diameter, approximately 150 cm in length (Fig. 95.4).

Colon Anatomy

The cecum is the saccular beginning of the colon, with an average diameter of 7.5 cm and a length of 10 cm. It has no mesentery and is completely covered with peritoneum and is therefore considered an intraperitoneal structure. The cecum is variably connected to the posterior abdominal wall by a peritoneal reflection. Patients with an abnormally mobile cecum and ascending colon, found in a small proportion of patients, can be predisposed to volvulus (torsion) or cecal bascule (intermittent anterior and superior folding of the cecum associated with obstructive symptoms). The cecum has a thin wall compared with the rest of the

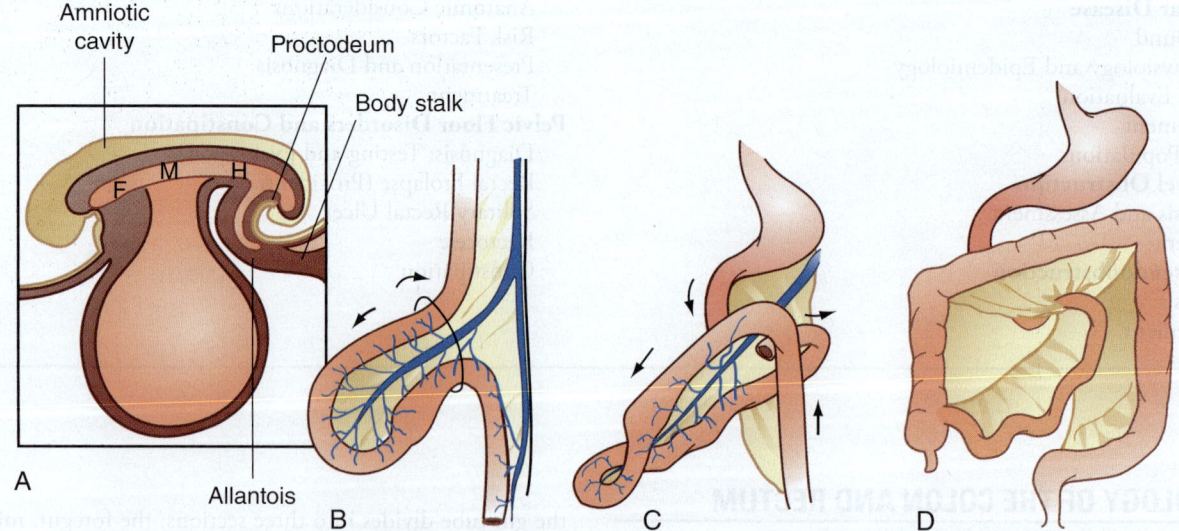

FIGURE 95.2 At the third week of development, the primitive tube can be divided into three regions (A): the foregut *(F)* in the head fold, the hindgut *(H)* with its ventral allantoic outgrowth in the smaller tail fold, and the midgut *(M)* between these two portions. Stages of development of the midgut are physiologic herniation (B), return to the abdomen (C), and fixation (D). (From Corman ML, ed. *Colon and Rectal Surgery.* 4th ed. Philadelphia: Lippincott-Raven; 1998:2.)

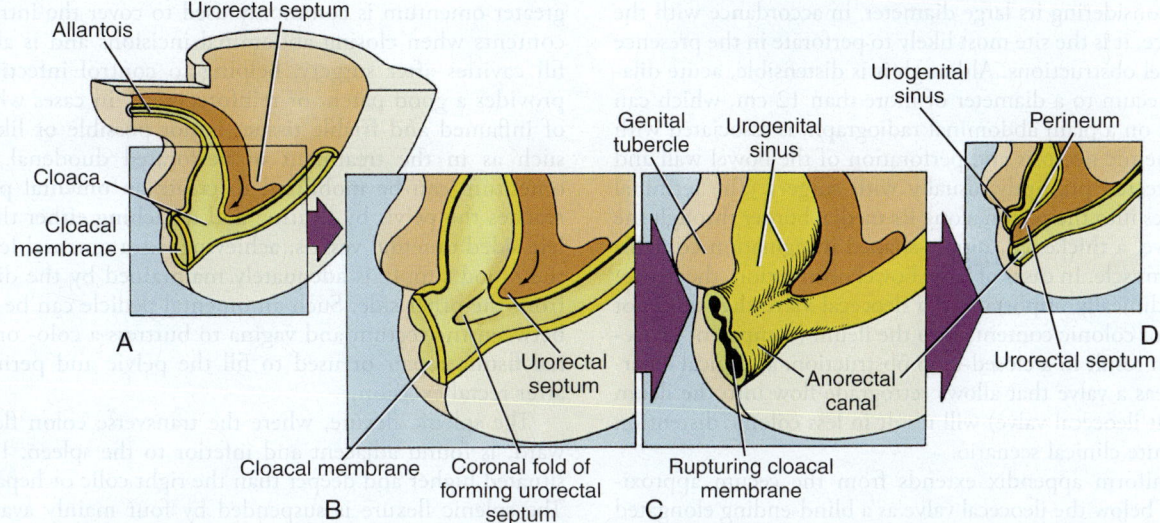

FIGURE 95.3 Development of the distal rectum and anus. Progressive steps between 4 and 6 weeks in subdivision of the cloaca into a ventral primitive urogenital sinus and a dorsal anorectal canal (A–D). The urorectal septum is formed by the fusion of yolk sac extraembryonic mesoderm and allantois mesoderm, which produces a tissue wedge between the hindgut and urogenital sinus during craniocaudal folding of the embryo. As the tip of the urorectal septum approaches the cloacal membrane dividing the cloaca into the urogenital sinus and anorectal canal, the cloacal membrane ruptures, thereby opening the urogenital sinus and dorsal anorectal canal to the exterior. The tip of urorectal septum forms the perineum. (A–B, D) Sections through the cloacal and related endoderm-derived structures. (C) Surface view of the caudal endoderm to better depict its three-dimensional shape. *Curved arrows* indicate the direction of growth of the developing urorectal septum. (From Schoenwolf GC, Bleyl SB, Brauer PR, et al. *Larsen's Human Embryology*. 5th ed. Philadelphia: Churchill Livingstone, an imprint of Elsevier; 2015.)

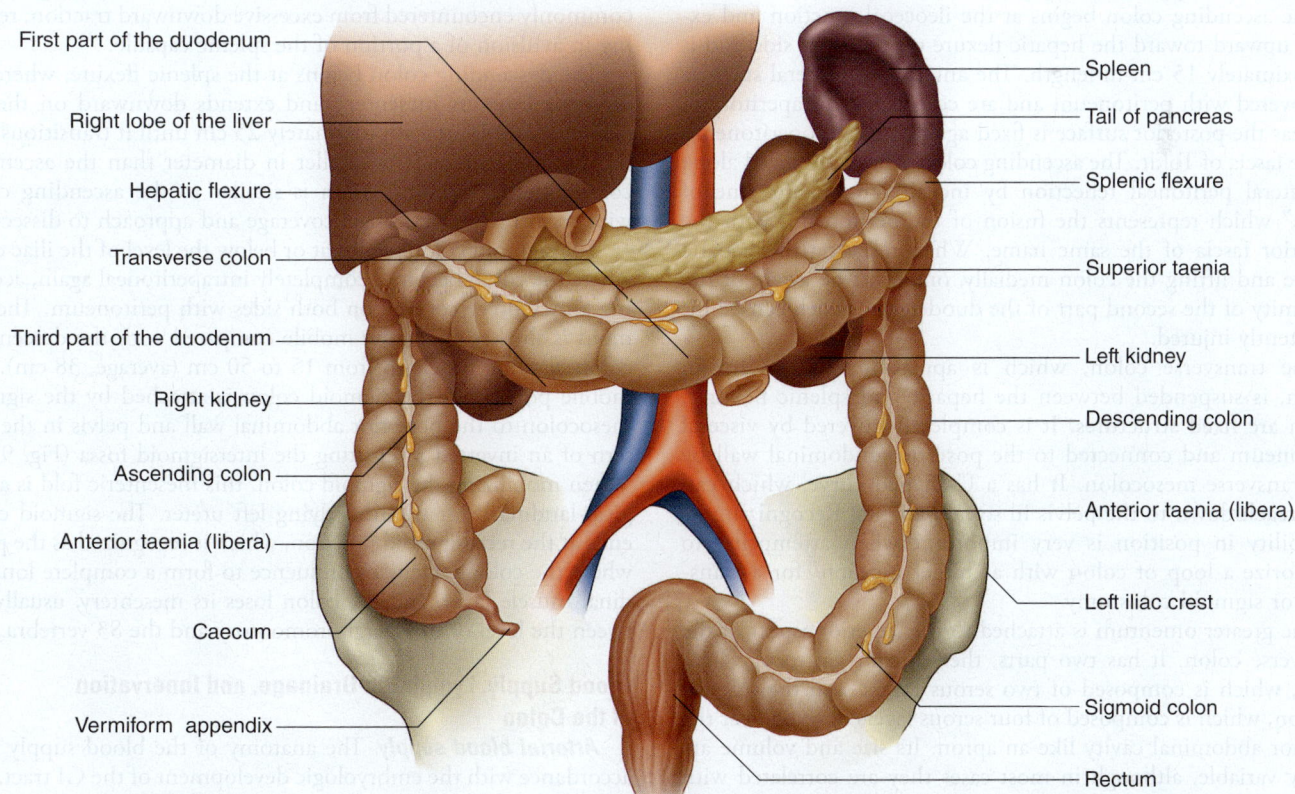

FIGURE 95.4 The large bowel includes the colon, consisting of ascending, transverse, descending, and sigmoid colon and the rectum, shown here in relation to neighboring anatomic structures. (From Standring S, Anand N, Rolfe B, et al. *Gray's Anatomy*. 41st ed. Philadelphia: Elsevier; 2016.)

colon, and considering its large diameter, in accordance with the law of Laplace, it is the site most likely to perforate in the presence of large bowel obstructions. Although it is distensible, acute dilation of the cecum to a diameter of more than 12 cm, which can be measured on a plain abdominal radiograph, is associated with a risk of ischemic necrosis and perforation of the bowel wall and should be treated promptly, usually with surgery. The terminal ileum empties into the cecum along its medial border through the ileocecal valve, a thickened, nipple-shaped invagination containing circular muscle. In cases of large bowel obstruction, the ileocecal valve is clinically important. An ileocecal valve that does not allow reflux of colonic contents into the ileum (competent ileocecal valve) can result in a closed-loop obstruction, a surgical emergency, whereas a valve that allows retrograde flow into the ileum (incompetent ileocecal valve) will result in less colonic distention and a less acute clinical scenario.

The vermiform appendix extends from the cecum approximately 3 cm below the ileocecal valve as a blind-ending elongated tube, 8 to 10 cm in length (Fig. 95.5). It is most commonly found in a retrocecal position (65%), followed by pelvic (31%), subcecal (2.3%), preileal (1.0%), and retroileal (0.4%) locations. In the setting of inflammation and adhesions, locating the appendix can be difficult. One can reliably reach its base by following the anterior taenia of the cecum to the convergence with the other two taeniae. The bloodless fold of Treves extends from the antimesenteric border of the terminal ileum to the base of the appendix or the anterior surface of the mesoappendix, or to both areas. This fold contains no sizable blood vessels. Because it is the only part of the ileum that has a fold on the antimesenteric side of the bowel, it can help in the recognition of the ileocecal region and the base of the appendix.

The ascending colon begins at the ileocecal junction and extends upward toward the hepatic flexure on the right side and is approximately 15 cm in length. The anterior and lateral surfaces are covered with peritoneum and are considered intraperitoneal, whereas the posterior surface is fixed against the retroperitoneum by the fascia of Toldt. The ascending colon is best mobilized along the lateral peritoneal reflection by incising the "white line of Toldt," which represents the fusion of the peritoneum with the posterior fascia of the same name. When releasing the hepatic flexure and lifting the colon medially, one must be aware of the proximity of the second part of the duodenum, which can be inadvertently injured.

The transverse colon, which is approximately 45 cm in length, is suspended between the hepatic and splenic flexures, which are fixed structures. It is completely covered by visceral peritoneum and connected to the posterior abdominal wall by the transverse mesocolon. It has a U-shaped curve, which can even reach down to the pelvis in some patients. Recognizing its variability in position is very important when attempting to exteriorize a loop of colon with a "target incision" for a transverse or sigmoid colostomy.

The greater omentum is attached to the superior aspect of the transverse colon. It has two parts, the superior gastrocolic ligament, which is composed of two serous layers, and the inferior portion, which is composed of four serous layers draping over the anterior abdominal cavity like an apron. Its size and volume are highly variable, although in most cases they are correlated with body weight. Lifting the greater omentum upward with downward traction of the transverse colon will reveal an avascular plane adjacent to the colon, most easily identified close to the midline. This plane is useful when separating these two structures. The greater omentum is commonly used to cover the intraperitoneal contents when closing abdominal incisions and is also used to fill cavities after surgery, helping to control infection. It also provides a good patch, or reinforcement, in cases when closure of inflamed and friable tissues is not possible or likely to fail, such as in the treatment of perforated duodenal ulcer. The omentum can be mobilized to create an omental pedicle that reaches the pelvis by ligating and detaching either the right- or left-sided omental vessels, achieving extra omental length while the blood supply is adequately maintained by the distal arcade from the other side. Such an omental pedicle can be positioned between the rectum and vagina to buttress a colo- or rectovaginal fistula repair or used to fill the pelvic and perineal spaces after rectal excision.

The splenic flexure, where the transverse colon flexes downward, is found adjacent and inferior to the spleen. It is usually situated higher and deeper than the right colic or hepatic flexure. The splenic flexure is suspended by four mainly avascular ligaments: the phrenicocolic ligament to the diaphragm; the splenocolic ligament to the lower pole of the spleen; the renocolic ligament to the Gerota fascia, which surrounds the left kidney; and the pancreaticocolic ligament to the tail of the pancreas. Pancreatic injuries are rare but can carry significant sequela and occur mainly during splenic flexure mobilization, with a 0.6% incidence rate reported in a recent study.[1] The splenic flexure can be released or mobilized without dividing any major blood vessels if one is separating the correct plane (Fig. 95.6). Surgeons commonly dissect the descending colon along the line of Toldt from below and then enter the lesser sac by lifting the omentum above the transverse colon. This maneuver allows mobilization of the flexure to be achieved, with minimal traction. Bleeding is most commonly encountered from excessive downward traction, resulting in avulsion of a portion of the splenic capsule.

The descending colon begins at the splenic flexure, where the intestine loses its mesentery and extends downward on the left side of the abdomen approximately 25 cm until it transitions into the sigmoid colon. It is smaller in diameter than the ascending colon. The descending colon is similar to the ascending colon with regard to its peritoneal coverage and approach to dissection.

The sigmoid colon begins at or below the level of the iliac crest, where the colon becomes completely intraperitoneal again, acquiring a mesentery covered on both sides with peritoneum. The sigmoid is thicker and more mobile compared with the descending colon, varying in length from 15 to 50 cm (average, 38 cm). The mobile portion of the sigmoid colon is attached by the sigmoid mesocolon to the posterior abdominal wall and pelvis in the pattern of an inverted V, creating the intersigmoid fossa (Fig. 95.7). When mobilizing the sigmoid colon, this mesenteric fold is a surgical landmark for the underlying left ureter. The sigmoid colon ends at the rectosigmoid junction, which is recognized as the point where the colonic taeniae confluence to form a complete longitudinal muscle layer, and the colon loses its mesentery, usually between the level of the sacral promontory and the S3 vertebra.

Blood Supply, Lymphatic Drainage, and Innervation of the Colon

Arterial blood supply. The anatomy of the blood supply is in accordance with the embryologic development of the GI tract. The celiac artery supplies the foregut, the SMA supplies the midgut, and the IMA supplies the hindgut. The colon receives its blood supply from the SMA and the IMA, both anterior branches of the abdominal aorta (Fig. 95.8).

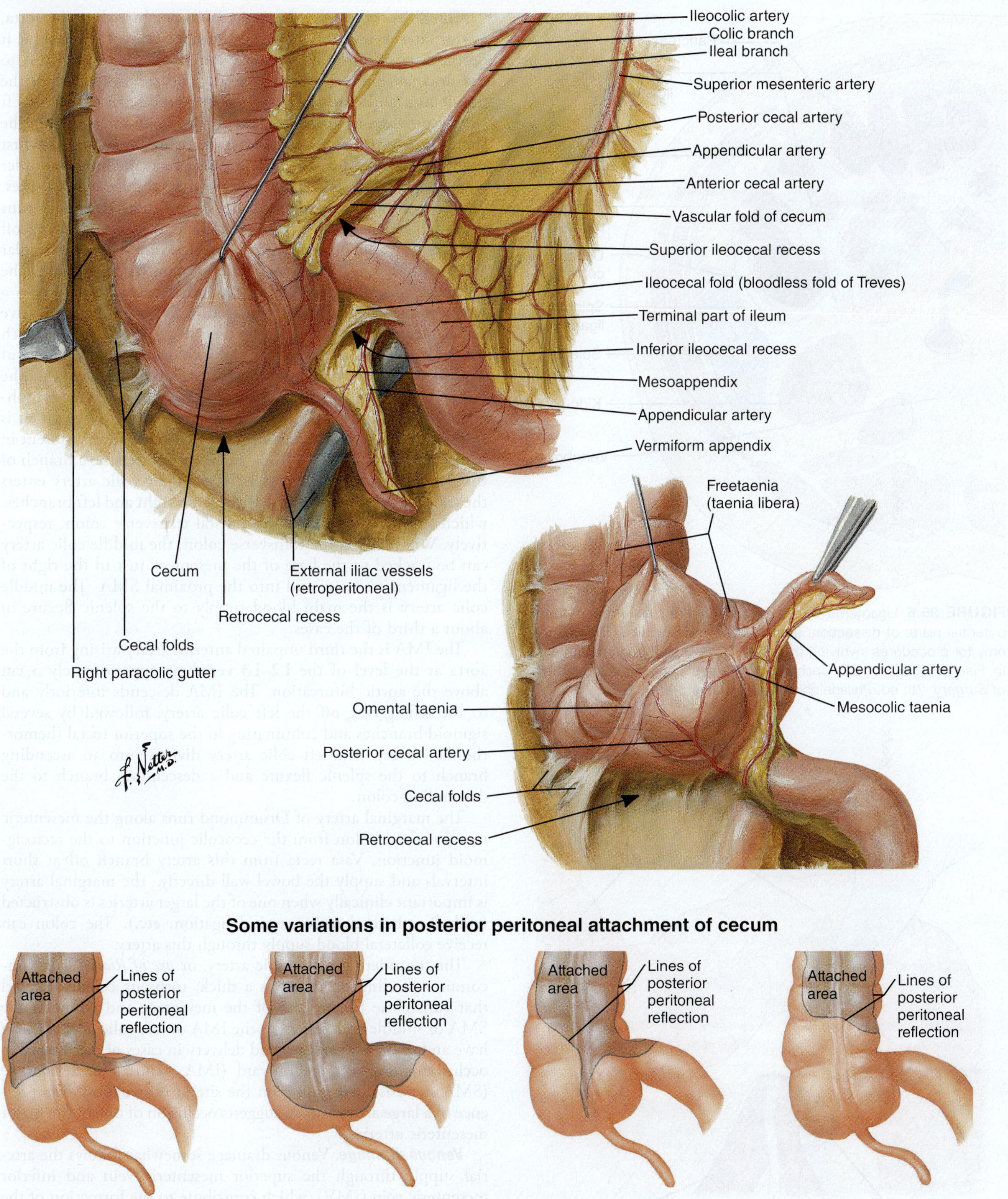

Ileocolic artery

Colic branch

Ileal branch

Superior mesenteric artery

Posterior cecal artery

Appendicular artery

Anterior cecal artery

Vascular fold of cecum

Superior ileocecal recess

Ileocecal fold (bloodless fold of Treves)

Terminal part of ileum

Inferior ileocecal recess

Mesoappendix

Appendicular artery

Vermiform appendix

Freetaenia (taenia libera)

Appendicular artery

Mesocolic taenia

Cecum

External iliac vessels (retroperitoneal)

Retrocecal recess

Cecal folds

Right paracolic gutter

Omental taenia

Posterior cecal artery

Cecal folds

Retrocecal recess

Some variations in posterior peritoneal attachment of cecum

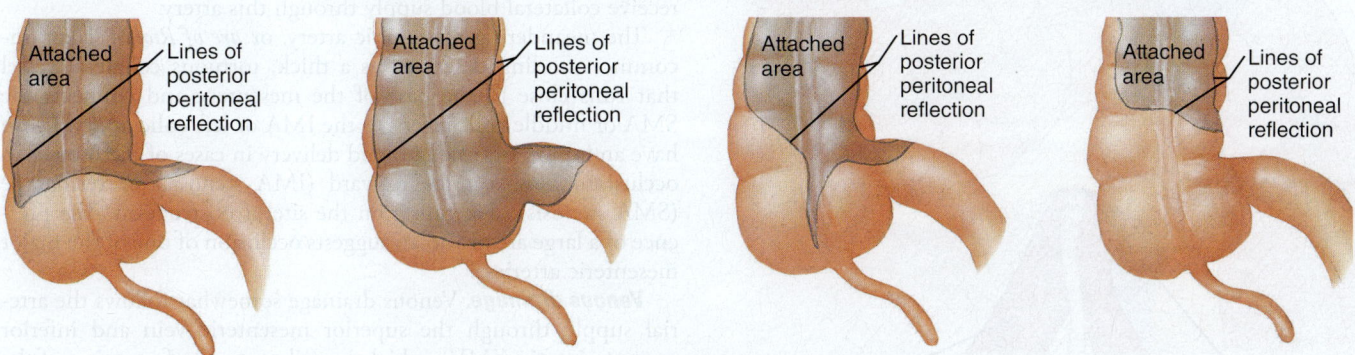

Attached area — Lines of posterior peritoneal reflection

Attached area — Lines of posterior peritoneal reflection

Attached area — Lines of posterior peritoneal reflection

Attached area — Lines of posterior peritoneal reflection

FIGURE 95.5 The appendix and mesoappendix in relation to the cecum and surrounding structures. (From Netter FH. *Atlas of Human Anatomy*. Philadelphia: Elsevier; 2019.)

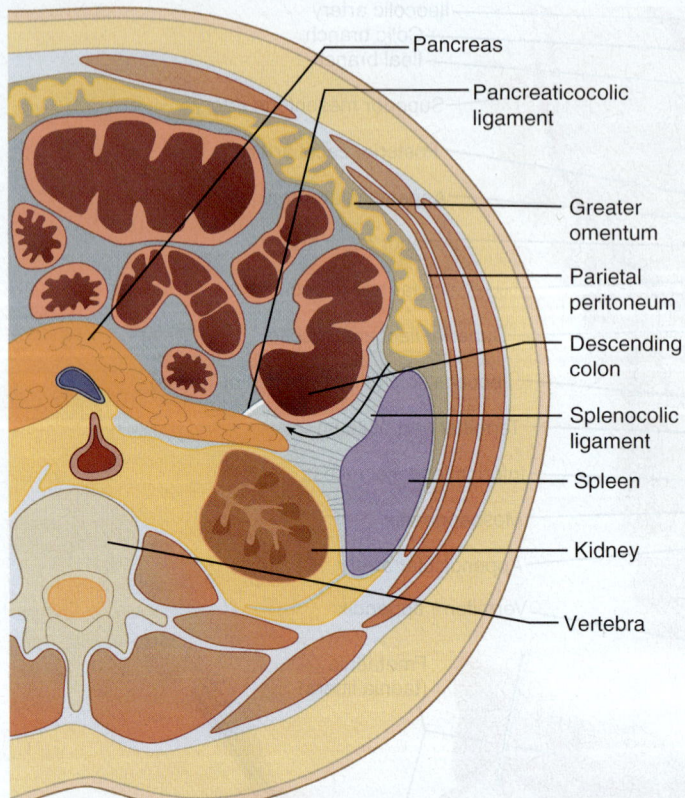

FIGURE 95.6 Ligaments of the splenic flexure; the *arrow* indicates potential plane of dissection. (From Netz U, Galandiuk S. Clinical anatomy for procedures involving the small bowel, colon, rectum and anus. In: Fischer JE, Ellison EC, Upchurgh Jr GR, et al., eds. *Fischer's Mastery of Surgery.* 7th ed. Philadelphia: Wolter Kluwer; 2019.)

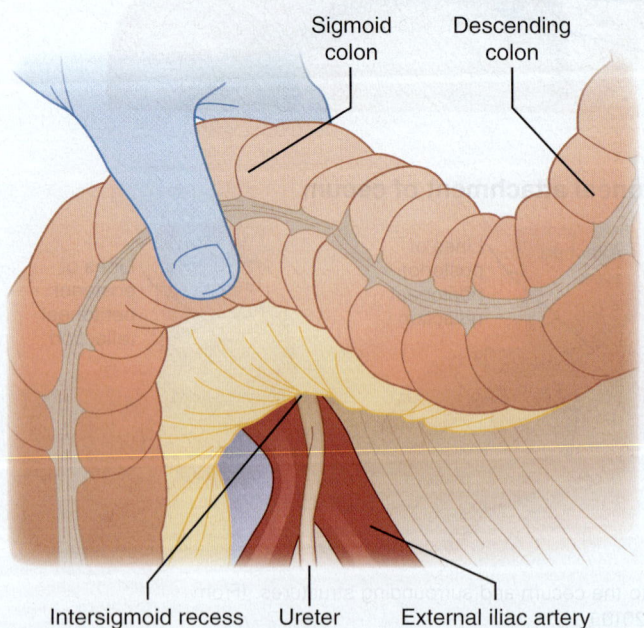

FIGURE 95.7 The intersigmoid recess, the sigmoid colon being retracted upward and to the right. (From Hollinshead WH. *Anatomy for Surgeons.* Vol 2. 2nd ed. New York: Harper and Row; 1971.)

The SMA is the second unpaired anterior branch of the aorta, arising at the level of the lower border of the L1 vertebra; it descends posterior to the pancreas and then crosses anteriorly to the uncinate process of the pancreas and the third part of the duodenum and enters the mesentery of the bowel. On the left side, it provides up to 20 branches to the small intestine. On the right, it gives off three major branches to the colon. The first branch is the middle colic artery, arising near the inferior border of the pancreas, followed by the right colic and ileocolic arteries. The ileocolic artery is the most constant of these arteries. It runs toward the ileocecal junction within the mesentery, giving off the anterior and posterior cecal arteries and the appendicular artery, supplying the terminal ileum, cecum, and appendix. The avascular space between the SMA and the ileocolic artery is a safe region to begin vascular dissection in a minimally invasive right colectomy and can also be used as a space through which one can pull the transverse or right colon through in cases of "retroileal" colorectal anastomoses to gain bowel length. The same plane along the SMA is also followed in extended lymphadenectomy (D3 lymphadenectomy) right colectomy, which is recommended in selected cases.[2] The right colic artery, absent in up to 20%, usually arises from the SMA but may be a branch of the ileocolic or left colic vessels. The middle colic artery enters the transverse mesocolon and divides into right and left branches, which supply the proximal and distal transverse colon, respectively. When lifting the transverse colon, the middle colic artery can be tracked to the base of the mesentery just to the right of the ligament of Treitz and into the proximal SMA. The middle colic artery is the main blood supply to the splenic flexure in about a third of the cases.

The IMA is the third unpaired anterior artery arising from the aorta at the level of the L2–L3 vertebrae approximately 3 cm above the aortic bifurcation. The IMA descends inferiorly and to the left, giving off the left colic artery, followed by several sigmoid branches and culminating in the superior rectal (hemorrhoidal) artery. The left colic artery divides into an ascending branch to the splenic flexure and a descending branch to the descending colon.

The marginal artery of Drummond runs along the mesenteric margin of the colon from the cecocolic junction to the rectosigmoid junction. Vasa recta from this artery branch off at short intervals and supply the bowel wall directly. The marginal artery is important clinically when one of the larger arteries is obstructed (emboli, atherosclerosis, surgical ligation, etc.). The colon can receive collateral blood supply through this artery.

The meandering mesenteric artery, or *arc of Riolan*, is an uncommon finding described as a thick, tortuous collateral vessel that runs close to the base of the mesentery and connects the SMA or middle colic artery to the IMA or left colic artery. It can have an important role in blood delivery in cases of SMA or IMA occlusion. Flow can be forward (IMA stenosis) or retrograde (SMA stenosis), depending on the site of obstruction. The presence of a large arc of Riolan suggests occlusion of one of the major mesenteric arteries.

Venous drainage. Venous drainage somewhat follows the arterial supply through the superior mesenteric vein and inferior mesenteric vein (IMV), which contribute to the formation of the portal vein. It is important to note that the IMV continues beyond the IMA along the base of the mesentery to the left of the ligament of Treitz and into the portal vein (Fig. 95.9). The IMV can be divided to achieve extra colonic length for low pelvic anastomoses.

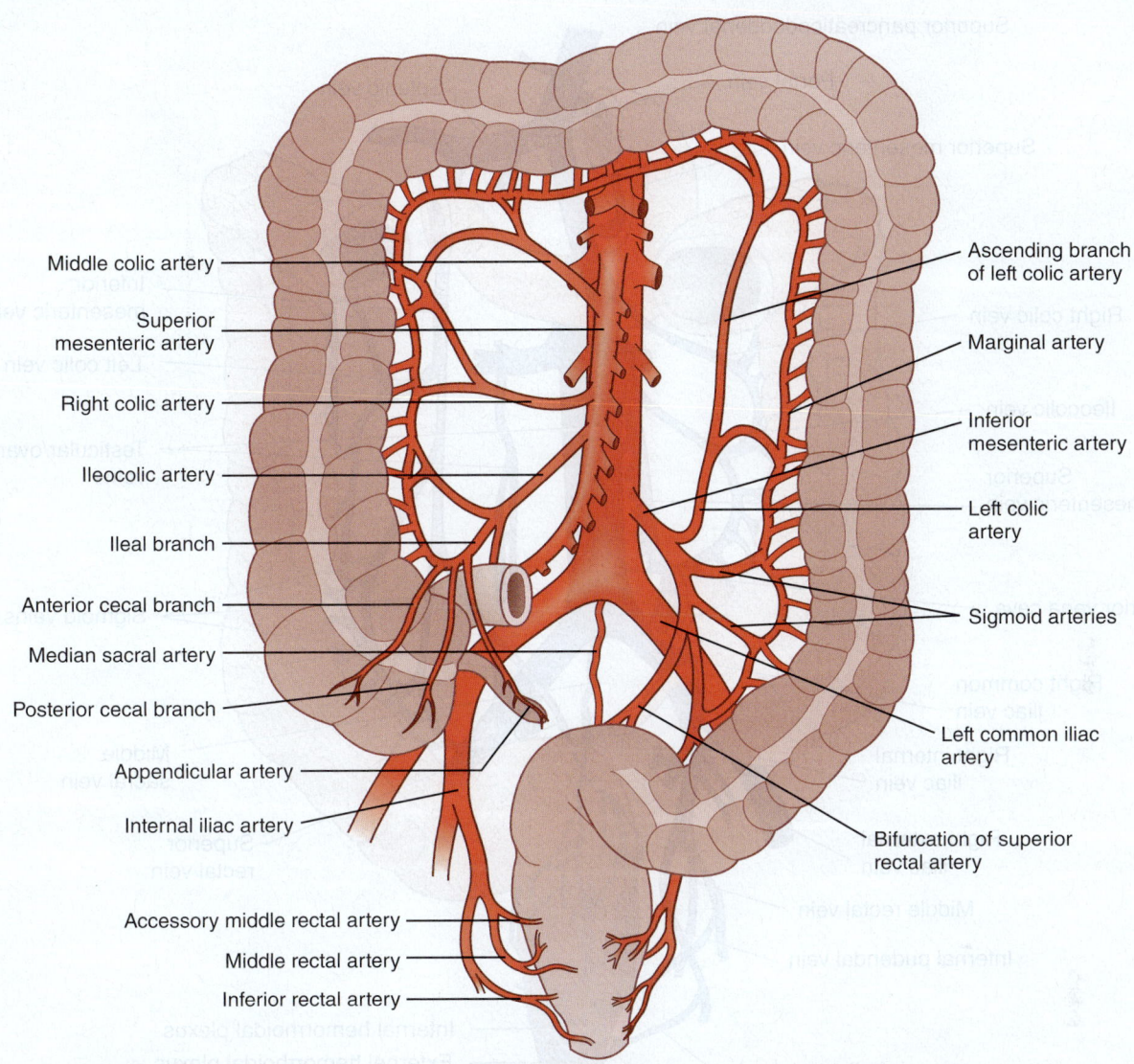

FIGURE 95.8 The arterial blood supply to the colon is from the superior and inferior mesenteric arteries. (From Gordon PH, Nivatvongs S, eds. *Principles and Practice of Surgery for the Colon, Rectum and Anus.* 2nd ed. St. Louis: Quality Medical Publishing; 1999:23.)

Lymphatic system. Lymphatic drainage generally follows the vascular supply. The wall of the large bowel is supplied with a rich network of lymphatic capillaries that drain to groups of lymph nodes, paralleling the arterial supply. Most of the lymphatic drainage goes in this direction, but communications are found between groups of lymph nodes, especially at the level of the paracolic groups at the level of the marginal arteries. There is also some dual drainage from the distal transverse and splenic flexure into both the superior and inferior mesenteric lymph nodes.

Innervation. The innervation of the large intestine has both sympathetic and parasympathetic components, which generally follow the blood supply.

Rectal Anatomy

The rectum begins at the rectosigmoid junction and ends at the level of the anus. Anatomists define the distal border as the dentate (pectinate) line based on the mucosal surface, whereas surgeons define it as the proximal border of the anal sphincter complex at the level of the levator ani (about 2 cm above the

dentate line). The rectum, with a total length of around 15 to 20 cm, is divided into thirds based on its peritoneal relationships. The upper rectum is covered by peritoneum anteriorly and laterally, and its lower limit extends to approximately 10 cm above the dentate line. The middle third is covered by peritoneum only anteriorly and extends from 5 to 10 cm above the dentate line. The lower third of the rectum is totally extraperitoneal, extending from 1 to 5 cm above the dentate line. The rectum has three lateral curves or valves of Houston; the proximal and distal valves fold to the right, and the middle folds to the left. They are lost after full surgical mobilization of the rectum, providing approximately 5 cm of additional length, assisting the surgeon's ability to fashion an anastomosis deep in the pelvis. Structurally, the rectum lacks taeniae coli, epiploic appendices, and haustra. The anterior peritoneal reflection between the rectum and anterior structures, the rectovesicular pouch in males and rectouterine or Douglas pouch in females, is 7 to 9 cm from the anal verge in males and 5 to 7.5 cm in females (Fig. 95.10). The anterior peritoneal reflection is the lowest dependent part of the peritoneal cavity. It is

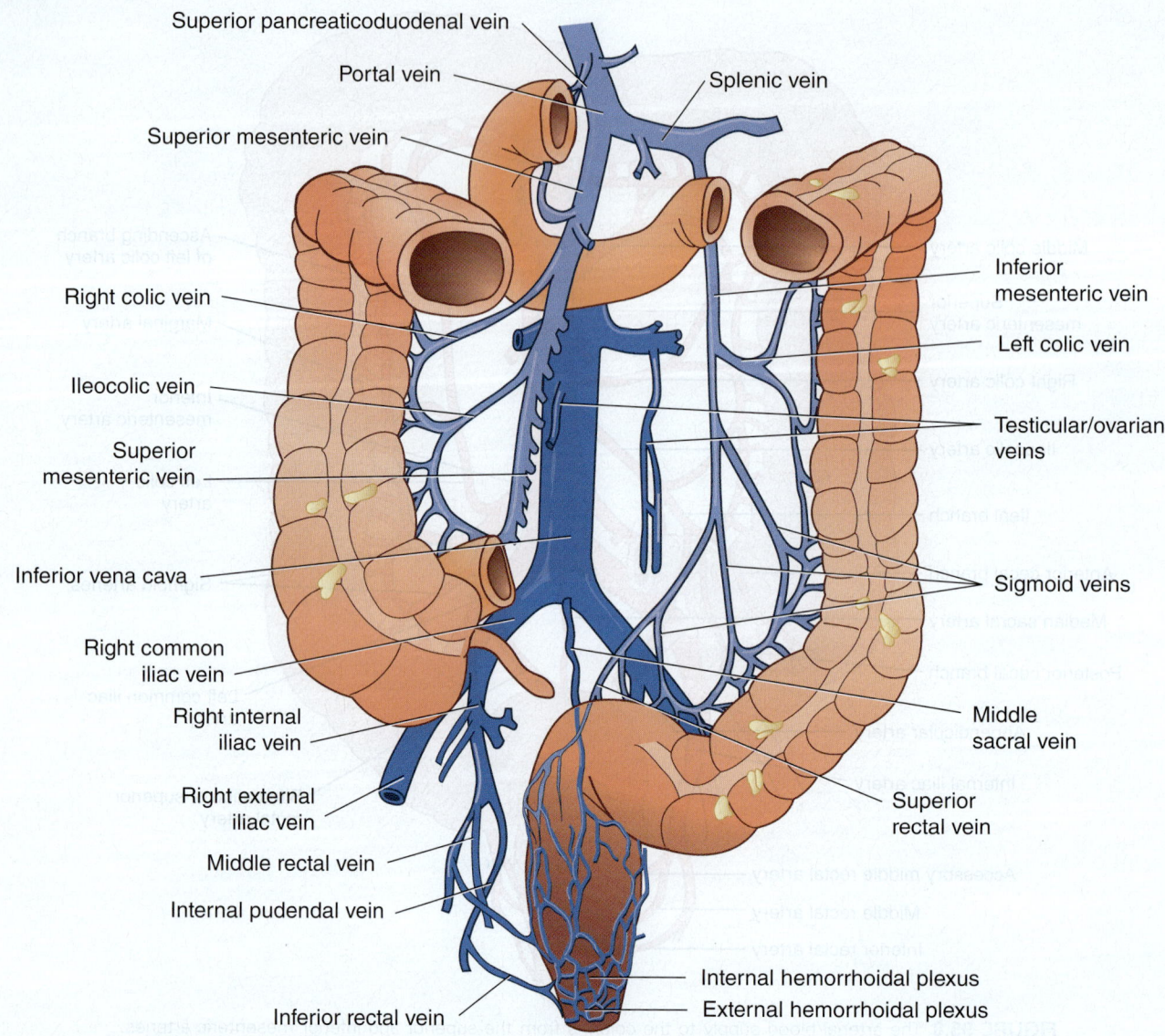

FIGURE 95.9 Venous anatomy of the colon and rectum. (From Gordon PH, Nivatvongs S, eds. *Principles and Practice of Surgery for the Colon, Rectum and Anus.* 2nd ed. St. Louis: Quality Medical Publishing; 1999:30.)

clinically important as a common location of fluid and pus accumulation and may serve as a site of peritoneal metastases from visceral tumors. These "drop" metastases can form a mass in the cul-de-sac (Blumer shelf) that can be recognized on digital rectal examination. *Mesorectum* refers to the visceral mesentery of the rectum. Recognition of mesorectal planes during rectal surgery is extremely important because it allows for a relatively bloodless dissection with consistent excision of relevant lymphatic tissues, adhering to the basic surgical oncologic principle of removing the cancer in continuity with its blood and lymphatic supply.

Total Mesorectal Excision

Pioneered by Prof. Richard J. "Bill" Heald and colleagues in the 1970s,[3] total mesorectal excision (TME) involves meticulous dissection along the mesorectal plane (also known as the *holy plane*) during rectal cancer surgery, ensuring complete tumor removal while preserving pelvic autonomic nerves and thus increasing the preservation of urinary and sexual function. This revolutionary technique has significantly improved oncologic outcomes, lowered

local recurrence rates, and become a standard in modern rectal cancer surgery. The mesorectum is relatively thick posteriorly, thinner along the sides, and very thin anteriorly.

Anatomic structures adjacent to the rectum are clinically important with regard to dissection planes and direct extension of tumors and/or fistulas. In males, the rectum is adjacent anteriorly and extraperitoneally to the urinary bladder, ureters, vas deferens, seminal vesicles, and prostate. Although injuries to these structures are uncommon, intraoperative identification of these injuries may be facilitated when a bladder Foley catheter and ureteric stents are placed at the beginning of the operation. Such consideration is especially important in patients with significant inflammation (diverticular disease, inflammatory bowel disease [IBD]), prior abdominal surgery, prior radiation, obesity, and other reasons and/or anticipated unclear anatomy. In females, intraperitoneally, the ureters are adjacent to the uterus, tubes, ovaries, and the upper part of the posterior vaginal wall. Careful dissection of the vaginal wall is needed in distal bulky anterior tumors to try to avoid injury and the possible formation of a rectovaginal fistula. Extraperitoneally,

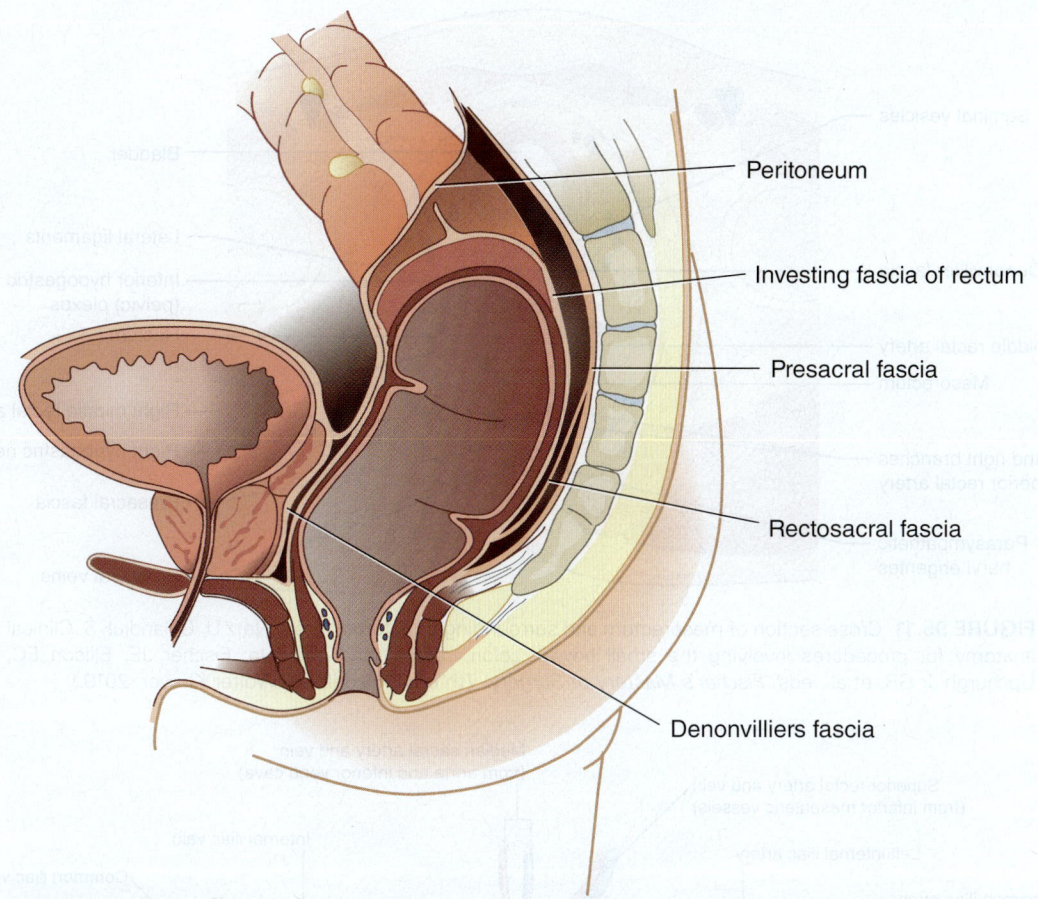

FIGURE 95.10 Fascial relationships of the rectum. (From Gordon PH, Nivatvongs S, eds. *Principles and Practice of Surgery for the Colon, Rectum and Anus.* 2nd ed. St. Louis: Quality Medical Publishing; 1999:10.)

the rectum is adjacent to the uterine cervix and posterior vaginal wall. In both sexes, the intraperitoneal cul-de-sac is commonly filled with small bowel and colon. The sacrum, sacral vessels, and sacral nerve roots are located posterior to the rectum.

The posterior aspect of the rectum is invested with a thick, closely applied mesorectum (Fig. 95.11). A thin layer of investing fascia (fascia propria) coats the mesorectum and represents a distinct layer from the presacral fascia against which it lies. During proctectomy for rectal cancer, mobilization and dissection of the rectum proceed between the presacral fascia and fascia propria. The presacral fascia covers the anterior sacrum and coccyx. A group of veins, on the presacral periosteum, the presacral veins, drains into the sacral foramina. Dissection deep to the presacral fascia can cause severe bleeding from the underlying presacral venous plexus. Such bleeding can be very difficult to control because the torn vessels tend to withdraw into the sacral foramina. The rectosacral fascia, or Waldeyer fascia, is a thick condensation of endopelvic fascia connecting the presacral fascia to the fascia propria at the level of S4 that extends to the posterior-inferior rectum. Dividing Waldeyer fascia during dissection from an abdominal approach provides access to the deep retrorectal pelvis. Laterally, the rectum is connected to the pelvic sidewall by the "lateral stalks" or ligaments. These are found in the low pelvis at the level of the prostate or midvagina. It is important to remember that in about a quarter of the cases, a branch of the middle rectal artery traverses them and may cause bleeding when cutting through them. Denonvilliers fascia, located anterior to the rectum, is a membranous layer that is an extension of the inferior

peritoneal reflection and extends to the perineal body. This fascial layer separates the rectum from the previously mentioned anterior structures and is considered the anterior border of a TME.

Blood Supply, Lymphatic Drainage, and Innervation of the Rectum

The blood supply to the rectum is derived from the superior, middle, and inferior rectal (hemorrhoidal) arteries. All three rectal arteries are connected with a strong anastomotic network, which helps avoid rectal ischemia after dividing the superior rectal arteries during anterior resections (Fig. 95.12). The superior rectal artery is the end branch of the IMA. It usually divides into left and right branches that run posteriorly downward. The middle rectal arteries are paired vessels derived from the internal iliac arteries to the lower rectum through the lateral columns. They are not considered a major blood supply to the rectum and are found inconstantly. They can be inadvertently injured when dissecting the lateral ligaments. The inferior rectal arteries are branches of the internal pudendal arteries and generally supply the anus distal to the dentate line.

The superior rectal vein drains the upper two-thirds of the rectum, draining into the IMV and portal system. The lower rectum and anus drain into the middle and inferior rectal veins, which are connected to the internal iliac and systemic circulation. This drainage pattern explains the higher rate of lung metastases observed with low rectal cancers as compared with midrectal and upper rectal cancers, which are much more likely to metastasize to the liver.

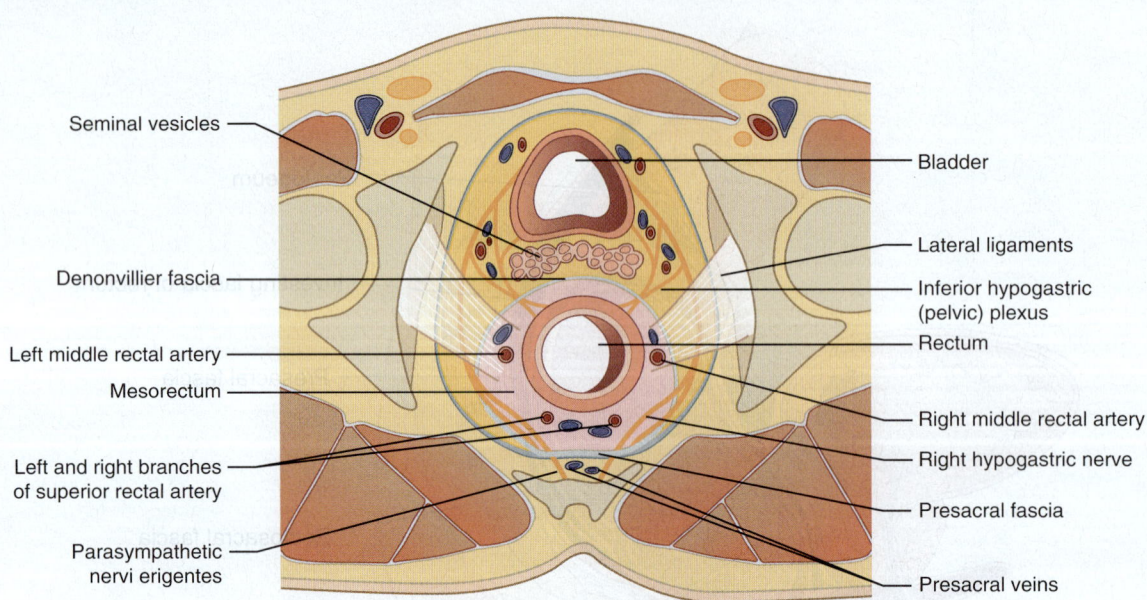

Seminal vesicles

Denonvillier fascia

Left middle rectal artery

Mesorectum

Left and right branches of superior rectal artery

Parasympathetic nervi erigentes

Bladder

Lateral ligaments

Inferior hypogastric (pelvic) plexus

Rectum

Right middle rectal artery

Right hypogastric nerve

Presacral fascia

Presacral veins

FIGURE 95.11 Cross-section of mesorectum and surrounding structures. (From Netz U, Galandiuk S. Clinical anatomy for procedures involving the small bowel, colon, rectum and anus. In: Fischer JE, Ellison EC, Upchurgh Jr GR, et al., eds. *Fischer's Mastery of Surgery.* 7th ed. Philadelphia: Wolter Kluwer; 2019.)

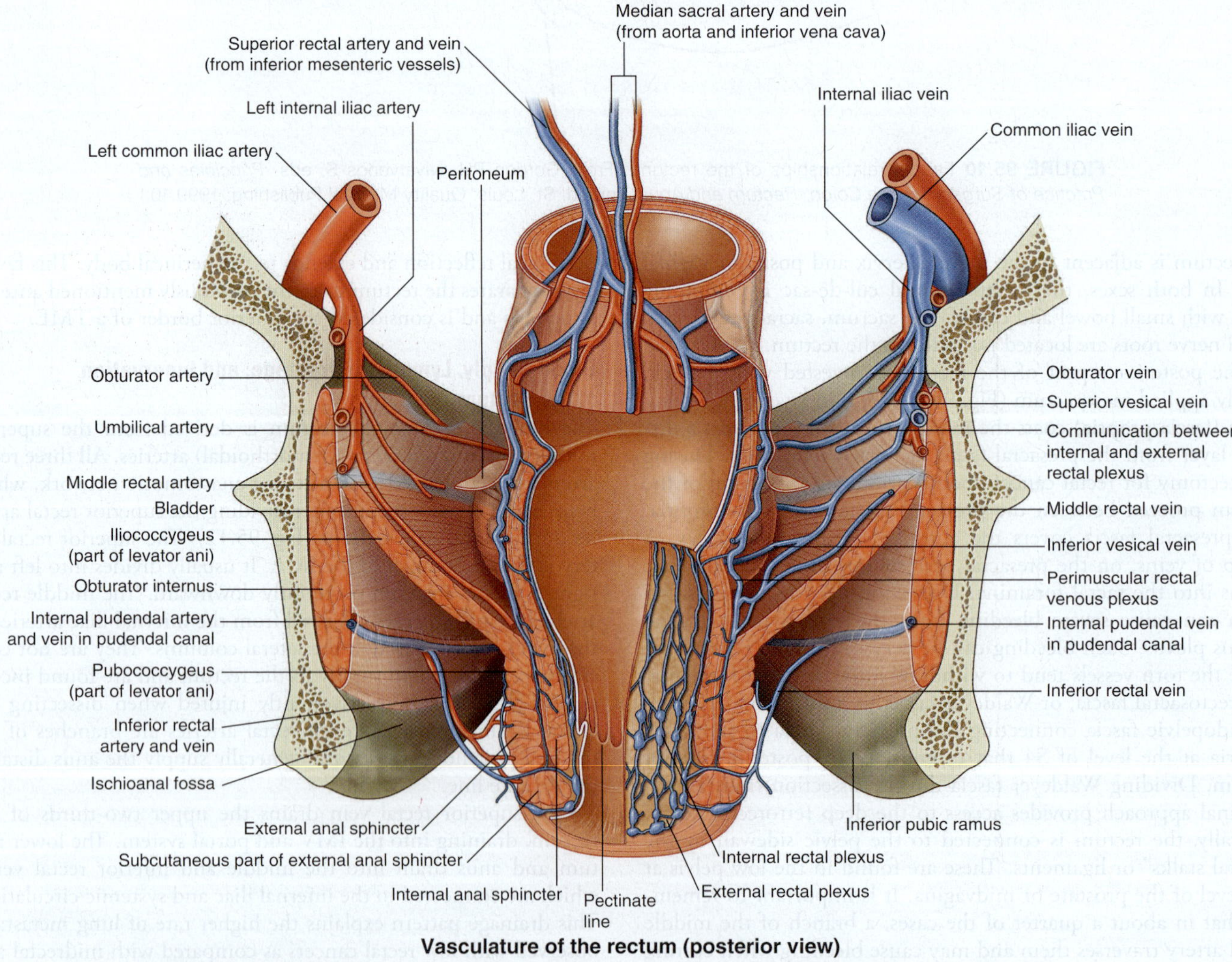

Superior rectal artery and vein (from inferior mesenteric vessels)

Left internal iliac artery

Left common iliac artery

Peritoneum

Median sacral artery and vein (from aorta and inferior vena cava)

Internal iliac vein

Common iliac vein

Obturator artery

Umbilical artery

Middle rectal artery

Bladder

Iliococcygeus (part of levator ani)

Obturator internus

Internal pudendal artery and vein in pudendal canal

Pubococcygeus (part of levator ani)

Inferior rectal artery and vein

Ischioanal fossa

External anal sphincter

Subcutaneous part of external anal sphincter

Internal anal sphincter

Pectinate line

Obturator vein

Superior vesical vein

Communication between internal and external rectal plexus

Middle rectal vein

Inferior vesical vein

Perimuscular rectal venous plexus

Internal pudendal vein in pudendal canal

Inferior rectal vein

Inferior pubic ramus

Internal rectal plexus

External rectal plexus

Vasculature of the rectum (posterior view)

FIGURE 95.12 Vasculature of the rectum, posterior view. (From Drake RL, Vogl AW, Mitchell AWM, et al. *Gray's Atlas of Anatomy.* 2nd ed. Philadelphia: Churchill Livingstone, an imprint of Elsevier; 2015.)

The lymph from the upper two-thirds of the rectum drains upward toward the inferior mesenteric and paraaortic nodes. The lower part of the rectum drains in two directions, cephalad toward the inferior mesenteric nodes and laterally and inferiorly toward the internal iliac nodes. Below the dentate line, lymph drains toward the inguinal lymph nodes. In recent years, the removal of the lateral lymph node compartments in patients with rectal cancer (lateral pelvic lymph node dissection [LPLND]) with clinically suspected lateral pelvic lymph nodes has become somewhat popular. An International Consortium for LPLND recently found that patients with lateral pelvic nodes of more than 7 mm on pretreatment MRI experienced significantly less local recurrence when treated with neoadjuvant chemoradiation, TME, and LPLND (5.7%) in comparison with neoadjuvant chemoradiation and TME alone (19.5%).[4] However, LPLND requires technical skills and is associated with increased male urinary and sexual dysfunction after surgery.[5]

The sympathetic innervation of the rectum is derived from sympathetic nerves exiting at the level of L1–L3, forming the superior hypogastric plexus (Fig. 95.13). At the level of the sacral promontory, they divide into left and right hypogastric nerves, traveling on both sides of the pelvis. These nerves supply the rectum and send branches to supply the genitourinary system anteriorly. When performing pelvic operations, it is important to be aware of these nerves and try to avoid injuring them. A high IMA ligation injuring the superior hypogastric plexus or severing the hypogastric nerves near the sacral promontory may result in sympathetic dysfunction characterized by retrograde ejaculation in males. Division of the lateral stalks too close to the pelvic sidewall may injure the pelvic plexus and nervi erigentes and cause erectile dysfunction, impotence, and atonic bladder. Injury to the periprostatic plexus when dissecting anteriorly can also cause sexual and bladder dysfunction.

Pelvic Floor Anatomy

The pelvic floor or diaphragm supports the pelvic organs and, together with the anal sphincter, regulates defecation. The pelvic diaphragm resides between the sacrum, obturator fascia, ischial spines, and pubis. The levator ani muscle, which makes up the floor, consists of three subdivisions: the pubococcygeus, iliococcygeus, and the puborectalis (Fig. 95.14). The pubococcygeus forms the levator hiatus, which ellipses the top of the anal canal, urethra, and vagina in females and the dorsal vein in males. The puborectalis originates in the lower part of the symphysis pubis and courses parallel to the anorectal junction, forming a U-shaped sling of striated muscle posterior to the rectum. The puborectalis is in a state of constant contraction, increasing the anorectal angle, a factor critical to the maintenance of fecal continence. Relaxation of the puborectalis straightens the anorectal angle and permits defecation. Puborectalis dysfunction is an important cause of defecation disorders.

PHYSIOLOGY OF THE COLON

Absorption of Fluid and Electrolytes

The major functions of the colon are water absorption and electrolyte exchange. This process converts succus from the terminal ileus into formed stool that is stored in the rectal reservoir until it can be excreted at a convenient time. The body has the ability to adapt and sustain life without a colon, making it uniquely different from small bowel. The problems associated with colonic patients provide a simplistic view of colonic function—individuals

with a diverting ileostomy are at particular risk for dehydration and electrolyte derangement.

The colon, with its large surface area, is the most efficient site of absorption in the GI tract, capable of absorbing up to 5 L of fluid daily, although usually only 1 to 2 L are excreted from the ileum. By the time the digestive fluid, or succus, reaches the terminal ileum, most nutrients have been absorbed, leaving a mix of electrolyte-rich fluid, bile salts, and some undigested proteins and starches, with about 90% of the fluid in succus being reabsorbed in the colon.

Secretion

Colon secretion plays a vital role in patients with chronic renal failure, where uremic patients can maintain normal potassium levels before requiring dialysis as a result of an increase in colonic potassium secretion and fecal excretion. Aldosterone promotes colonic potassium secretion, whereas spironolactone can block this effect. Various colitis conditions, such as IBD, cholera, and shigellosis, are associated with increased potassium secretion, and other forms of colitis impair colonic absorption or induce chloride secretion. Colonic secretion of H+ and bicarbonate is linked to systemic acid-base metabolism through carbonic anhydrase, allowing the colon to regulate pH levels as needed.

Urea Recycling

Colonic bacteria are rich in urease, which is important for urea recycling. Because mammalian cells do not produce urease, this process relies on the symbiotic relationship found in a healthy colonic lumen. Ammonia is the byproduct of urea metabolism, and its absorption depends on the concentration of bacteria present and the intraluminal pH. Antibiotics and lactulose decrease the amount of ammonia absorbed by lowering the concentration of bacteria and reducing the pH, respectively. Absorbed ammonia is transported to the liver.

Recycling Bile Salts

The colon absorbs bile acids that escape absorption by the terminal ileum. Bile acids are passively transported across the colonic epithelium by nonionic diffusion. When the colonic absorptive capacity is exceeded, colonic bacteria deconjugate bile acids. Deconjugated bile acids can then interfere with sodium and water absorption, leading to secretory, or choleretic, diarrhea. Choleretic diarrhea is seen early after right hemicolectomy as a transient phenomenon and more permanently after extensive ileal resection.

Colonic Flora, Fermentation, and Short-Chain Fatty Acids

Large bowel contents have a concentration of 10^{11} to 10^{12} bacterial cells per gram, contributing approximately 50% of fecal mass. Over 400 bacterial species, mostly anaerobic, are present in the colon. Bacteroides species are obligate anaerobes that comprise two-thirds of the total colonic bacteria. Other species commonly found in the colonic flora are the following facultative anaerobes: *Escherichia, Klebsiella, Proteus, Lactobacillus,* and *Enterococci.* These bacteria feed on proteins sloughed from the bowel wall and undigested complex carbohydrates. In turn, colonocytes and gut-associated lymphoid tissue rely on the colonic flora for nutrients.

The main source of energy for intestinal bacteria is dietary fiber, composed of complex carbohydrates (including starches and non-starch polysaccharides). However, not all complex carbohydrates are

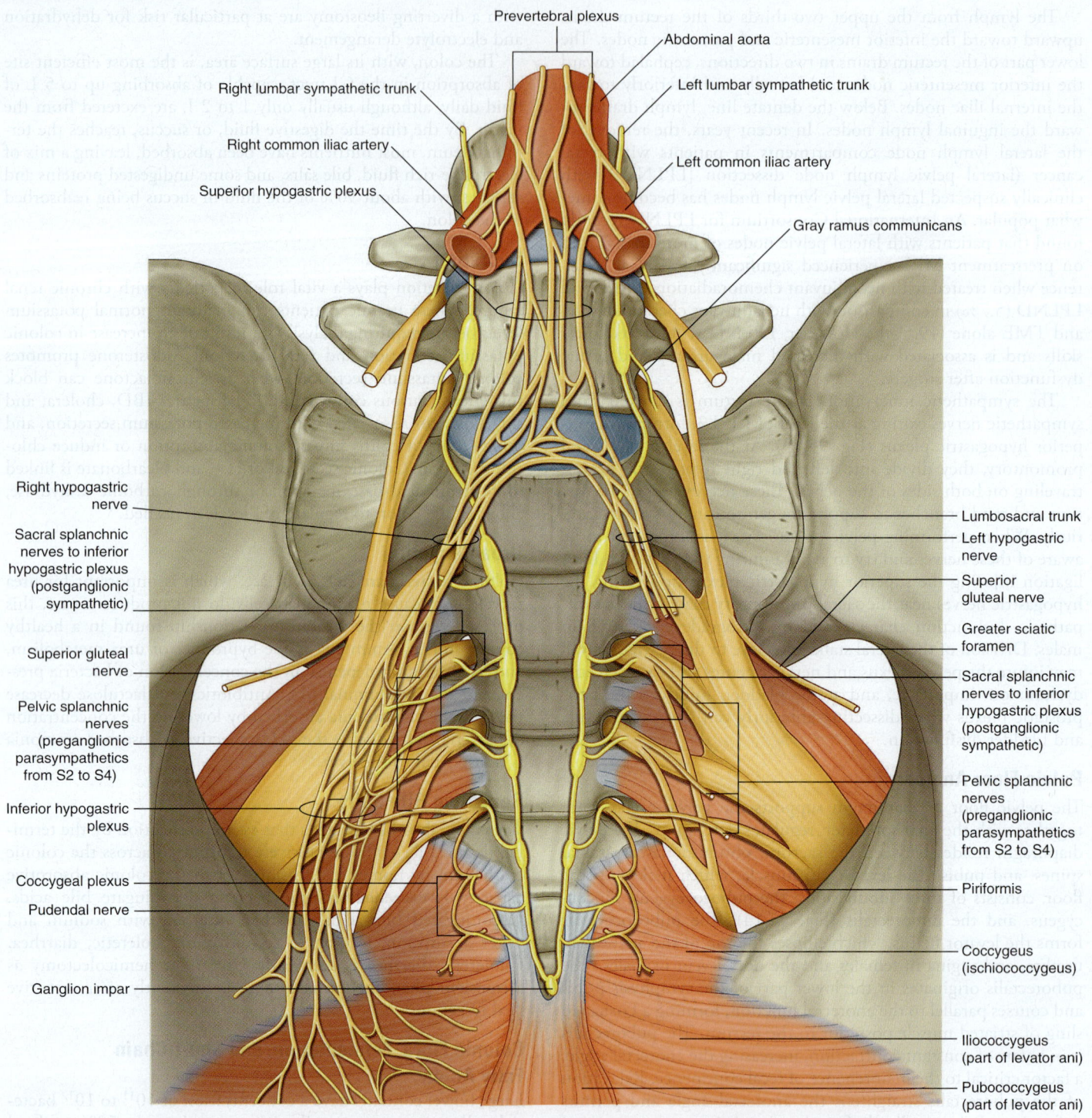

Pelvic extensions of the prevertebral nerve plexus (anterior view)

FIGURE 95.13 Pelvic nerve plexus. (From Drake RL, Vogl AW, Mitchell AWM, et al. *Gray's Atlas of Anatomy.* 2nd ed. Philadelphia: Churchill Livingstone, an imprint of Elsevier; 2015.)

fermented in the same manner. Dietary recommendations ("adding fiber," for example) generally refer to bulking agents, such as lignin and psyllium, which are nonabsorbable and nonfermentable by colonic bacteria. Bulking agents decrease intracolonic pressures and increase colonic transit time, which help prevent the formation of colonic diverticula and minimize colonic exposure to toxins.

For the fermentable complex carbohydrates available, colonic flora produce short-chain fatty acids (SCFAs). Butyrate, an SCFA, is the principal source of nutrition for the colonocyte. Because mammalian cells do not produce butyrate, the colonic epithelium and luminal bacteria form an essential and elegant symbiotic relationship. Antibiotics disrupt this cohabitation—decreased

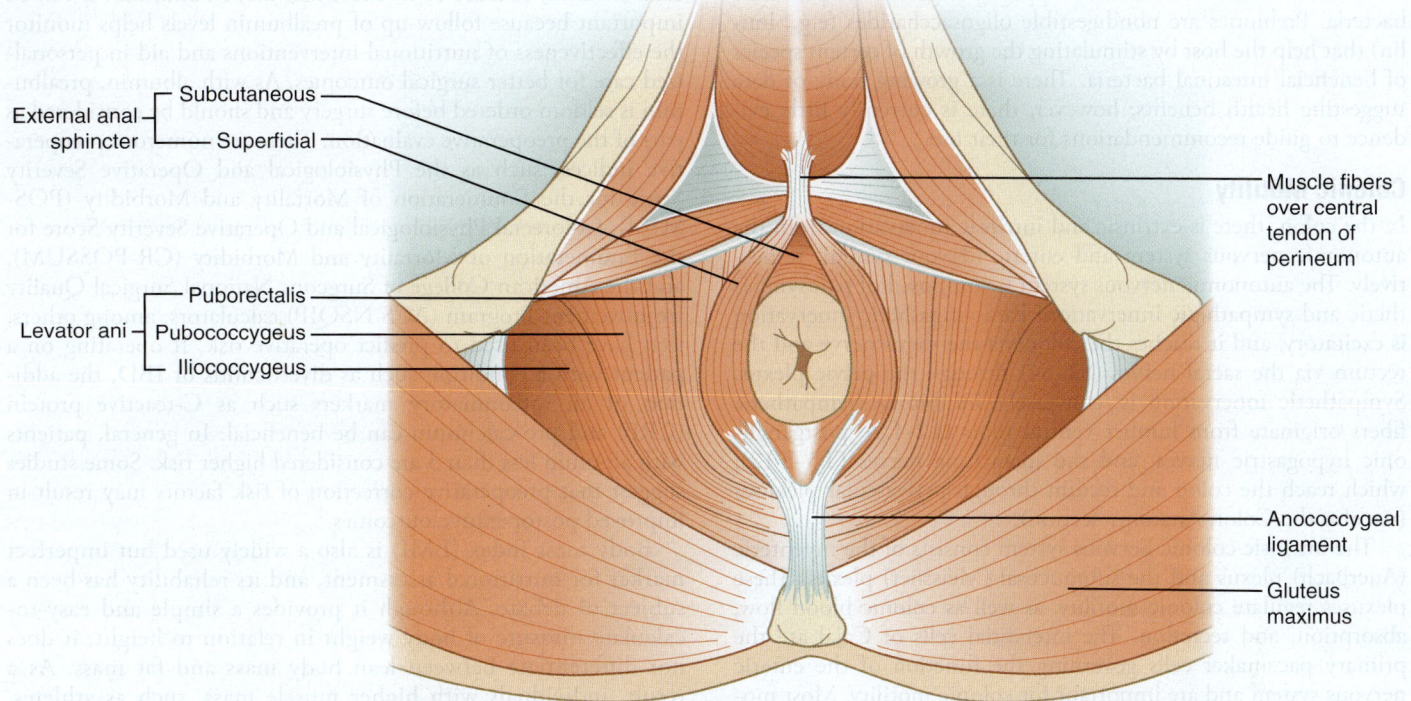

FIGURE 95.14 The pelvic musculature and innervation from below. The deep anal sphincter muscles are hidden under the superficial part. (From Netz U, Galandiuk S. Clinical anatomy for procedures involving the small bowel, colon, rectum and anus. In: Fischer JE, Ellison EC, Upchurgh Jr GR, et al., eds. *Fischer's Mastery of Surgery.* 7th ed. Philadelphia: Wolter Kluwer; 2019.)

Labels (from figure): External anal sphincter — Subcutaneous; Superficial; Puborectalis; Levator ani — Pubococcygeus; Iliococcygeus; Muscle fibers over central tendon of perineum; Anococcygeal ligament; Gluteus maximus

bacteria leads to less butyrate, which, in turn, negatively affects colonocyte function, leading to diarrhea. Likewise, mucosal atrophy is seen after fecal diversion (e.g., diversion colitis). The other physiologic effects of SCFAs on the colon include stimulation of blood flow, mucosal cell renewal, and regulation of intraluminal pH for homeostasis of the bacterial flora.

The role of SCFAs in homeostasis extends beyond the colon. Besides butyrate, two other SCFAs, acetate and propionate, are produced in the colon, with acetate being the most common of all three. Over 90% of the SCFAs produced are absorbed. Hepatocytes metabolize SCFAs for use in gluconeogenesis, and muscle cells oxidize acetate to generate energy. Additionally, acetate is the primary substrate for cholesterol synthesis. The production of acetate is reduced by nonabsorbable, nonfermentable dietary fiber, such as psyllium, which in turn has a beneficial effect on cholesterol levels. Similarly, propionate, which has a glycolytic role in the liver, may also lower serum lipid levels by inhibiting cholesterol synthesis. Butyrate may also play an important role in maintaining cellular health by arresting the proliferation of neoplastic colonocytes while paradoxically being trophic for normal colonocytes.

The end products of fermentation are SCFAs and gas—carbon dioxide, methane, and hydrogen.

Probiotics and Prebiotics

Colorectal surgery can have various effects on the composition of the gut microbiota. Factors that contribute to these changes include stress and disruption of homeostasis, exposure to oxygen during surgery, tissue ischemia, the type of surgical reconstruction, and chemo-/radiotherapy. Stress can influence the gut microbiota composition, and the gut microbiota can in turn affect the host's response to stress. Exposure to oxygen during surgery

can deplete beneficial anaerobic species in the gut microbiota. Tissue ischemia, caused by bowel and vascular sections, can lead to significant changes in the gut microbiota. Different types of surgical reconstruction can affect food digestion, nutrient absorption, and the gut microbiota. Chemo-/radiotherapy before surgery can also affect the gut microbiota. The hypothesis is that these factors can impair the return to a healthy gut microbiota composition, potentially leading to surgical complications and compromised immune function.

Researchers have investigated the manipulation of gut microbiota using probiotics, prebiotics, and synbiotics to achieve a healthier balance between harmful and beneficial bacteria. Probiotics, live microorganisms offering health benefits primarily in the colon, have shown various positive properties, including antiinflammatory effects and the ability to counteract harmful bacteria growth. Probiotics have been shown to prevent *Clostridioides difficile*–associated diarrhea, but there are insufficient data to recommend probiotics for the primary prevention of *C. difficile* infection (CDI).[6] Additionally, prebiotics, nonviable components promoting the growth of beneficial microbiota, have also been explored. Recent meta-analyses have shown that the administration of probiotics and synbiotics resulted in a significant reduction in postoperative infectious complications, especially in colorectal surgery patients. The use of these interventions was also associated with a shorter hospital stay and improved postcolectomy quality of life. Moreover, no significant adverse effects were reported.[7] Currently, the routine use of probiotics is not supported in clinical guidelines except for certain pathologies, including necrotizing enterocolitis in neonates, ulcerative colitis (UC), pouchitis, and constipation. Further research is needed, but the evidence for probiotic use in various settings is encouraging.

Prebiotics are nutrients that support the growth of probiotic bacteria. Prebiotics are nondigestible oligosaccharides (e.g., inulin) that help the host by stimulating the growth of certain species of beneficial intestinal bacteria. There is a growing body of data suggesting health benefits; however, there is currently little evidence to guide recommendations for their use.

Colonic Motility

In the colon, there is extrinsic and intrinsic innervation from the autonomic nervous system and enteric nervous system, respectively. The autonomic nervous system is composed of parasympathetic and sympathetic innervation. Parasympathetic innervation is excitatory, and it reaches the colon via the vagus nerve and the rectum via the sacral nerves (S2–S4) through the pelvic plexus. Sympathetic innervation is, conversely, inhibitory. Sympathetic fibers originate from lumber ventral roots (L2–L5), postganglionic hypogastric nerves, and the splanchnic nerves (T5–T12), which reach the colon and rectum through perivascular plexuses (see also the Colon Anatomy section).

The intrinsic colonic nervous system consists of the myenteric (Auerbach) plexus and the submucosal (Meissner) plexus. These plexuses regulate colonic motility, as well as colonic blood flow, absorption, and secretion. The interstitial cells of Cajal are the primary pacemaker cells governing the function of the enteric nervous system and are important for colonic motility. Most motility is involuntary and is divided into two primary patterns[1]: low-amplitude propagated contractions (LAPCs)[2] and high-amplitude propagated contractions (HAPCs). LAPCs allow mixing, which promotes optimal absorption, and are bursts of short-duration contractions. HAPCs propagate colonic contents distally in a coordinated fashion, and their role lies in shifting large quantities of contents through the colon one to three times per day. Other factors affecting motility are circadian rhythms and food ingestion.

Defecation

Normal defecation requires adequate colonic transit time, stool consistency, and fecal continence. The frequency of defecation is just as variable among individuals as their perception of abnormal stool frequency. The definitions of diarrhea and constipation differ by individual patients and providers; therefore reporting stool frequency and consistency provides a clearer understanding of defecation patterns.

Many factors influence colonic transit rate. Colonic transit is longer in females than in males and longer in premenopausal than in postmenopausal females. Supplementation with nonstarch polysaccharides shortens colonic transit time in individuals with idiopathic constipation.

PREOPERATIVE EVALUATION

Nutritional and Risk Assessment

Over the past 20 years, since the original work on the National Veterans Administration Surgical Risk Study, few parameters have been as reliable at predicting postoperative complications as preoperative serum albumin level. Unfortunately, this laboratory value is seldom obtained preoperatively in elective surgery patients and therefore needs to be explicitly ordered. Another important tool in the preoperative assessment of patients before surgery is prealbumin. Prealbumin is a small protein produced primarily in the liver. It has a short half-life of 2 to 3 days, making it a responsive indicator of nutritional status and more accurate

than albumin because of its short half-life. In addition, it can be important because follow-up of prealbumin levels helps monitor the effectiveness of nutritional interventions and aid in personalized care for better surgical outcomes. As with albumin, prealbumin is seldom ordered before surgery and should be considered as part of the preoperative evaluation. There are numerous preoperative indices, such as the Physiological and Operative Severity Score for the Enumeration of Mortality and Morbidity (POSSUM), Colorectal Physiological and Operative Severity Score for the Enumeration of Mortality and Morbidity (CR-POSSUM), and the American College of Surgeons National Surgical Quality Improvement Program (ACS NSQIP) calculators, among others, that have been used to predict operative risk. If operating on a patient with a condition such as diverticulitis or IBD, the addition of an inflammatory markers such as C-reactive protein (CRP) and pro-calcitonin can be beneficial. In general, patients with albumin less than 3 are considered higher risk. Some studies suggest that preoperative correction of risk factors may result in improved postoperative outcomes.

Body mass index (BMI) is also a widely used but imperfect marker for nutritional assessment, and its reliability has been a subject of debate. Although it provides a simple and easy-to-calculate measure of body weight in relation to height, it does not differentiate between lean body mass and fat mass. As a result, individuals with higher muscle mass, such as athletes, may have a higher BMI but not necessarily be malnourished. Conversely, older adults or individuals with muscle wasting may have a lower BMI but could still be malnourished. Additionally, BMI does not take into account the distribution of body fat, which can be relevant in assessing surgical risk. Visceral fat, located in the abdominal cavity, is associated with a higher risk of surgical complications compared with subcutaneous fat. To obtain a more comprehensive understanding of the patient's nutritional status before surgery, healthcare providers often use BMI in conjunction with other nutritional markers and clinical assessments, recognizing its limitations as a standalone measure.

There is a growing field of immunonutrition suggesting that consumption of nutritional supplements rich in arginine may, in fact, boost the immune system and lead to a reduction in postoperative infectious complications, such as surgical site infection (SSI).[8]

Patients who are at particularly high risk are those who have chronic partial bowel obstruction and cancer and those who have lost a significant amount of weight (greater than 10% of body weight) in unintentional weight loss.

Preoperative Bowel Preparation

Because human feces can have as much as 10^{12} bacteria/gram, colon surgery has been associated with a higher rate of SSI than small bowel and upper GI surgery. Issues of antibiotic prophylaxis have focused on the choice of an antibiotic with an appropriate spectrum, administration before making the surgical incision, and discontinuation of the antibiotic postoperatively. Over the past 20 years, performing or omitting preoperative bowel preparation has been a cyclical phenomenon.

Studies suggest that mechanical bowel preparation alone is not beneficial before *colon* resection. These recommendations were based on findings that bowel preparation generally led to fluid and electrolyte abnormalities that, in turn, led to large volumes of fluid administration during surgery and subsequent bowel edema and ileus. In addition, bowel preparation is poorly tolerated in the elderly and in those with multiple medical comorbidities.

Lower-volume bowel preparations generally have higher patient compliance. Higher rates of spillage of liquid as opposed to more formed stool at the time of surgery after mechanical bowel preparation were thought to be the cause of the higher observed rates of SSI. However, for many surgeons performing rectal resection, either with minimally invasive or open techniques, particularly when inserting intraluminal staplers for the purpose of creating intestinal anastomoses, it was felt to be more convenient and safer to have the large bowel free of solid particulate matter. Recently, large administrative database studies have demonstrated that the combination of a mechanical and an oral antibiotic bowel preparation is associated with a very low rate of postoperative infectious complications in patients undergoing colorectal surgery. Mechanical bowel preparation and oral antibiotics are used before colorectal surgery to reduce the risk of SSIs and complications. Mechanical bowel preparation involves cleansing the colon to decrease the bacterial load, minimizing the chances of contamination during surgery. Oral antibiotics further target specific bacteria in the colon that could lead to infections. Although these practices have been routine in the past, their benefits have been debated recently, and some centers adopt a selective approach based on individual patient risk factors and surgeon preference.

Preoperative nutritional optimization and infection prevention strategies also play a vital role in enhancing surgical outcomes for colorectal surgery patients. The decision to use these measures should be carefully considered, weighing the potential benefits against the risk of adverse effects.

Therefore preoperative oral antibiotics alone without mechanical bowel preparation may be a safe alternative in patients who cannot tolerate full bowel preparation. A large-scale multicenter randomized study performed in Spain examined the role of oral antibiotics alone in reducing the rate of SSIs and found that administering oral antibiotics the day before surgery significantly reduced the occurrence of SSIs without the use of mechanical bowel preparation.[9] Generally, many surgeons believe that a formal mechanical bowel preparation is not required for patients undergoing surgery for IBD because these patients are already having numerous liquid bowel movements. Bowel preparation is also not used for patients with partial obstruction.

Planning Intestinal Stomas

When operating on a patient in whom there may be a need for a diverting stoma (e.g., patients with Crohn disease, diverticular disease, intestinal obstruction, and low rectal cancer), it is *always* wise to mark the patient for a preoperative stoma site. *Most* patients do not have an ideal abdomen. The area of the abdomen that usually is chosen for a stoma, the infraumbilical fat mound (Fig. 95.15), may not look the same in a patient who is sitting up as it does when they are recumbent. In many patients, there are skin folds that may prevent a stoma bag from sealing properly. It is essential to mark the patients in a sitting position and to avoid old scars and any skin folds that may interfere with adherence of a stoma appliance. Fig. 95.16 shows how important it is to avoid skin folds that would interfere with normal adherence of a stoma appliance and how this can be underestimated if the patient is supine (Fig. 95.17).

Stoma Types

Many different types of stoma configurations can be chosen at the time of surgery (Fig. 95.18). Stomas can be differentiated by whether they:
- Are small bowel stomas or colostomies
- Drain stool or urine

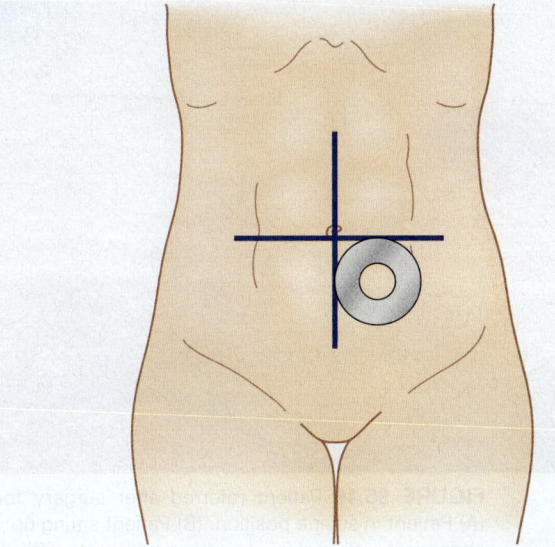

FIGURE 95.15 Demonstration of the infraumbilical fat mound that is the ideal stoma site in many patients, here showing marking for a descending colostomy.

- Are temporary or permanent
- Are end, loop, end-loop, or double-barrel stomas
- Are continent or incontinent stomas

Temporary stomas are often chosen to aid in anastomotic healing or in the presence of sepsis or other conditions when it is not considered safe to perform an unprotected anastomosis. Loop ileostomies are often chosen for temporary diversion because of their lack of odor, ease of care, and ease of closing. Loop descending or sigmoid colostomies can be similarly easily closed. Transverse loop colostomies should seldom be used because they are large and are very prone to prolapse, and it can be difficult to maintain pouch adherence because they are frequently located in an area around the patient's belt line or mid-upper abdomen. In some cases, a double-barrel ostomy is needed to divert fecal matter away from a specific area in order to allow healing, prevent disease progression, or avoid complications. A double-barrel ostomy is typically needed in emergency cases, cases with significant inflammation, or during complex surgical procedures, and the decision to perform a double-barrel ostomy is often made intraoperatively based on clinical judgment.

Temporary diversion can be performed for a number of situations. Most often, temporary diversion is used to aid in healing of distal anastomosis. Alternatively, diversion of the fecal stream is sometimes recommended in patients undergoing treatment of distal pathology, such as obstructing rectal cancer. In these scenarios, a diverting stoma is anticipated to be closed after healing of the anastomosis or after conclusion of treatment. Unlike a standard ileostomy, a ghost ileostomy involves preparing and marking a loop of the ileum (part of the small intestine) that is sutured beneath the abdominal wall but not immediately functional. It acts as a safety net, allowing for a quick conversion into a functioning ileostomy if an anastomotic leak occurs after surgery.[10]

Permanent stomas are often required when a section of the bowel (either the colon or rectum) has to be removed because of diseases like colorectal cancer (CRC), IBD (e.g., Crohn disease or UC), certain types of injuries, or obstructions. In addition, patients with significant incontinence and/or bedridden patients should be consulted for permanent ostomy, which can potentially

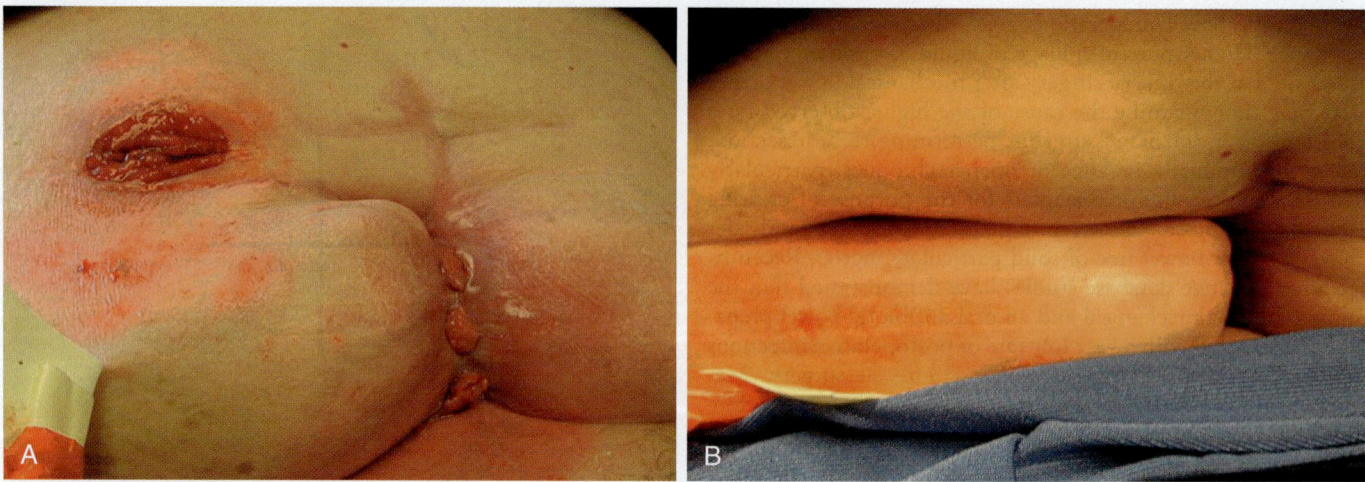

FIGURE 95.16 Patient referred after surgery for ischemic colitis without preoperative stoma marking. (A) Patient in supine position. (B) Patient sitting up. Note that the colostomy "disappears" within folds of the abdominal wall, making pouching extremely difficult.

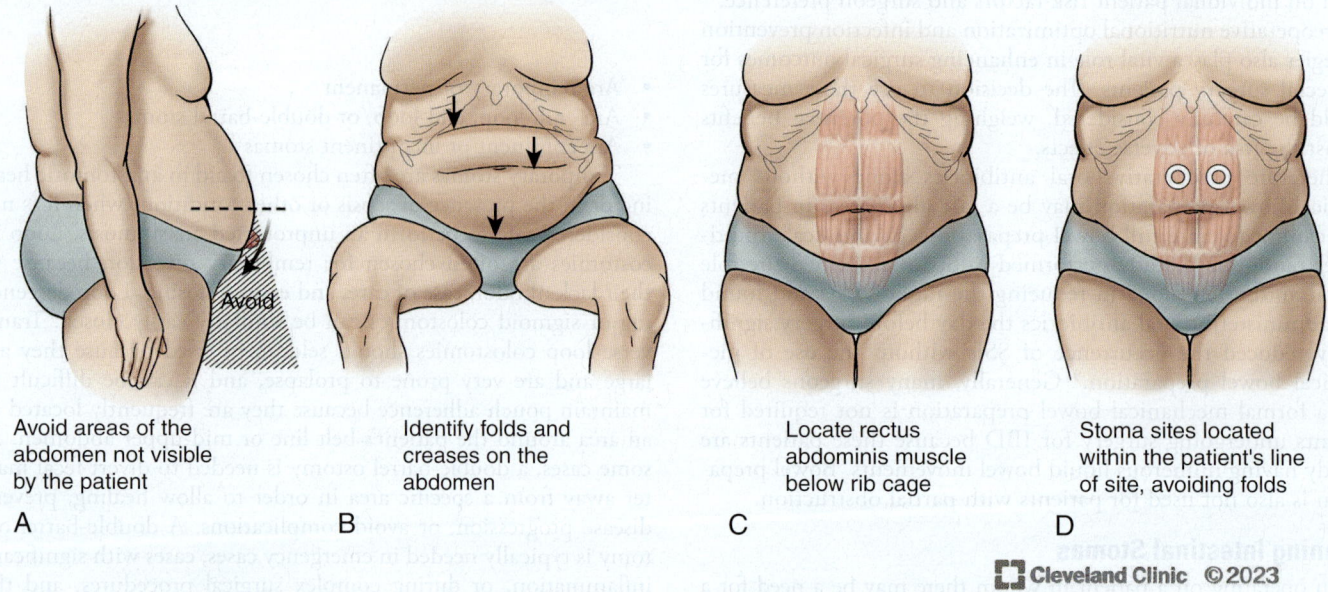

Avoid areas of the abdomen not visible by the patient

A

Identify folds and creases on the abdomen

B

Locate rectus abdominis muscle below rib cage

C

Stoma sites located within the patient's line of site, avoiding folds

D

Cleveland Clinic ©2023

FIGURE 95.17 Illustration of the method used for stoma planning. (Reprinted with permission, Cleveland Clinic Foundation ©2024. All Rights Reserved.)

improve their quality of life. When planning a permanent stoma, surgeons should opt for a comfortable and discreet location to allow patients better handling of their ostomy in daily life. Caregivers should be aware of the psychological and emotional impacts of a permanent stoma. Professional stoma care nurses, support groups, and counseling can all help someone adjust to life with a stoma. It is also important for people with stomas to receive regular follow-up care to monitor for potential complications, such as skin irritation, infection, herniation, stenosis, or prolapse.

The stoma nurse, often referred to as an *ostomy* or *enterostomal therapist,* is a specialized healthcare professional who guides patients through the process of ostomy surgery. Their responsibilities encompass preoperative education about the procedure and postoperative stoma care, including hygiene, pouch system management, and potential complications. They also offer invaluable emotional support because adapting to life with a stoma can be

emotionally taxing, and they keep patients updated on the latest in stoma care resources and products.

During the preoperative phase, the stoma nurse determines the optimal stoma site by considering the patient's anatomy and daily activities. This process involves assessing the abdomen in various positions, including sitting, standing, and bending, to avoid natural creases or folds. Additionally, the nurse inquires about the patient's clothing preferences, such as the type of attire they wear and their use of belts, to ensure the stoma's placement does not interfere with their lifestyle or cause discomfort.

Each of the three different types of stomas (end, loop, and end loop) has advantages and disadvantages. The **consistency** and **amount** of stoma effluent can differ significantly depending on the following:

- Whether the small bowel or the colon is selected for stoma construction

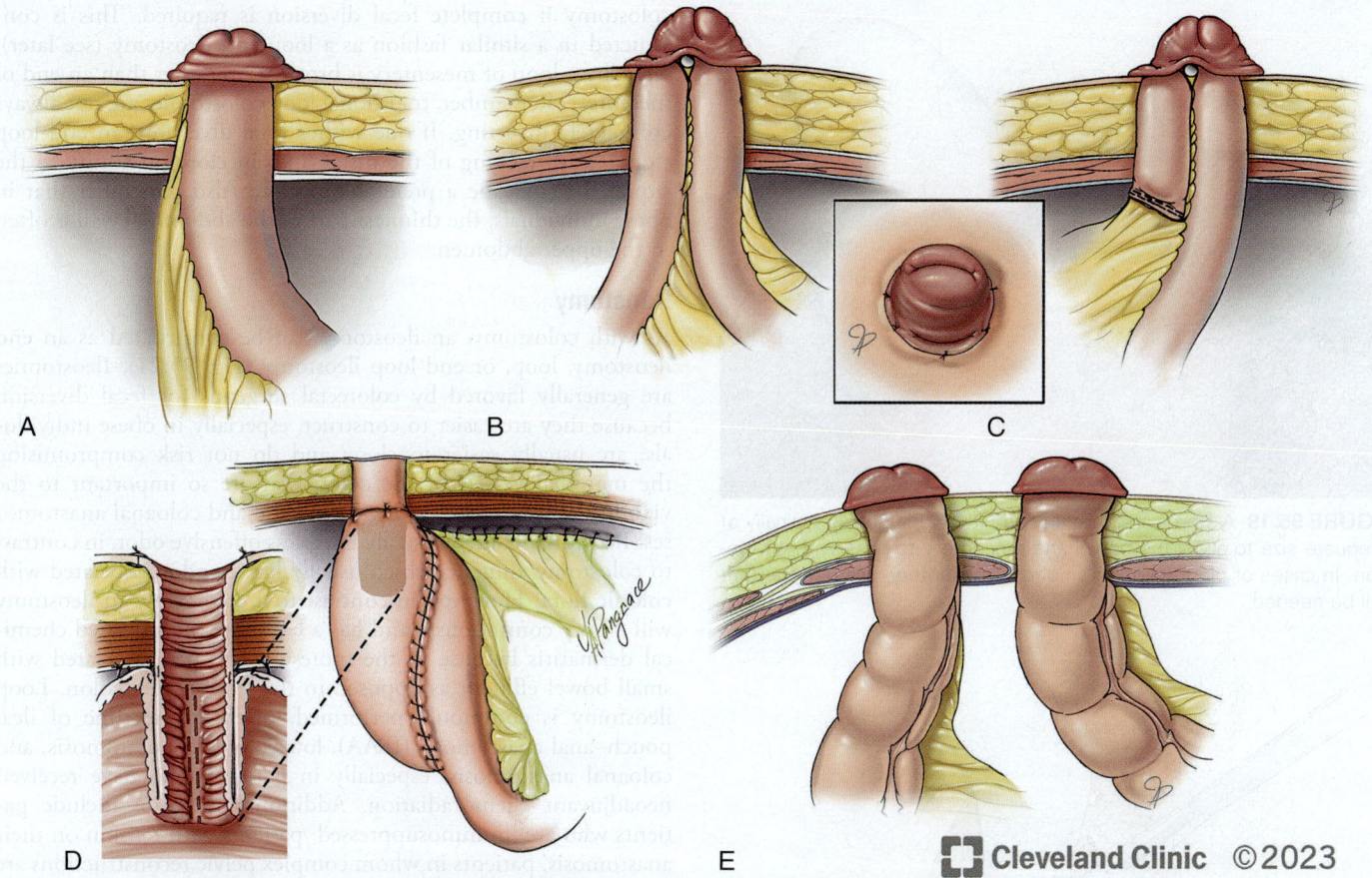

FIGURE 95.18 Different types of intestinal stoma. (A) End stoma. (B) Loop stoma. (C) End loop stoma. (D) Continent ileostomy. (E) Double-barrel stoma. (Reprinted with permission, Cleveland Clinic Foundation ©2024. All Rights Reserved.)

- If the colon is selected, which site of the colon is selected for stoma construction
- What types of treatment (e.g., radiation) the patient has undergone
- Previous bowel resection(s) the patient may have undergone

It is imperative that every **stoma must be well made.** Proper stoma construction as a prophylactic maneuver is vastly superior to any therapeutic options to attempt to improve upon a suboptimally constructed stoma. Any questions about viability can be addressed with indocyanine green perfusion assessment. The solution for an inadequately perfused intended stoma is to use a more proximal segment of well-perfused intestine. A key aspect of creating a good stoma is to create a large enough aperture in the abdominal wall to allow the stoma to reach the skin without tension but not to create such a wide opening that the patient will develop a hernia at the site.

Prophylactic mesh in ostomy construction surgery serves as a potentially preventive measure against parastomal hernias, a common postoperative complication where the intestine protrudes near the stoma site. By reinforcing the abdominal wall, the mesh aims to reduce hernia risk, thereby enhancing patient comfort and overall quality of life. The choice of mesh type, whether synthetic or biologic, and the surgical technique employed are pivotal for its success. However, although the mesh offers notable benefits, it is essential to weigh these against potential complications, such as infections, mesh erosion, or allergic reactions, ensuring that its application is both judicious and tailored to individual patient needs. A recent meta-analysis of 12 randomized controlled trials determined that the preventive use of mesh decreases the risk of a parastomal hernia by 40%. Yet, when the authors examined randomized controlled trials conducted in the past 5 years, no advantages were observed. Additionally, postoperative complications and mortality rates remained comparable.[11]

Colostomy

Ascending colostomies tend to have a higher amount of liquid effluent, whereas descending and left-sided colostomies are usually preferable because most of the colon is in circuit, allowing for more colonic water absorption, with a more formed effluent, while still providing proximal diversion.

With the increasing BMI of patients in the United States today, creating a well-functioning stoma can be a challenge. Both early and late complications can occur with stoma construction. Typically, creating an aperture that will admit two fingers is adequate (Fig. 95.19). In addition, one should ensure that the patient is marked for a stoma site preoperatively, as discussed earlier. It is important to create a muscle-splitting stoma aperture within the rectus muscle and sharply divide the rectus sheath (Fig. 95.20). In creating a colostomy in an obese patient, especially with the left side of the colon, one frequently has to perform the same central vascular ligation as one does for a cancer resection merely to achieve the same degree of mobilization and mobility to enable the colon to reach to the abdominal wall in a tension-free manner. This can be particularly true with patients who have a very rigid

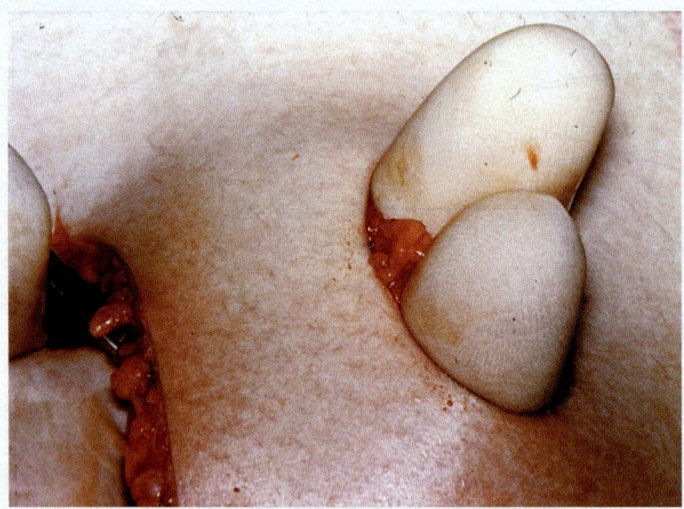

FIGURE 95.19 A stoma aperture that admits two fingers is typically of adequate size to allow the bowel and mesentery to pass without tension. In cases of obstruction or an obese mesentery, a larger aperture will be needed.

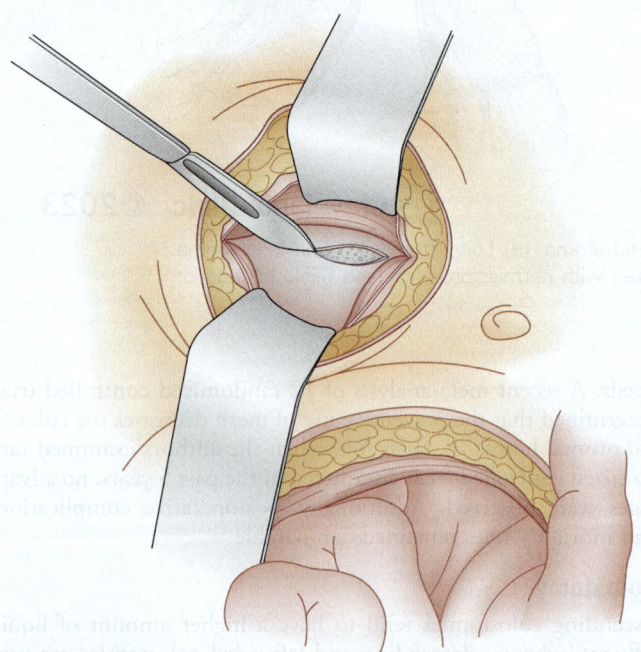

FIGURE 95.20 In making the stoma aperture in the abdominal wall, the rectus muscle is split and the rectus sheath is divided sharply. In laparoscopic cases, one can cut down directly on the trocar inserted through this site.

abdominal wall and those with a very thick layer of subcutaneous tissue. In constructing an end colostomy, this typically does not need to protrude more than 0.5 to 1 cm above the level of the abdominal skin. However, there are some circumstances where the patient may be expected to have a more liquid effluent (e.g., as a result of receiving chemotherapy), and one may wish to have the stoma protrude more to permit easier pouch placement and adherence. In the presence of a liquid effluent, a protruding "spoutlike" stoma is always easier to maintain pouch adherence compared with a flatter stoma. In the obese patient, it is sometimes easier to construct an end-loop colostomy than an end

colostomy if complete fecal diversion is required. This is constructed in a similar fashion as a loop-end ileostomy (see later), whereby a loop of mesentery is brought up rather than an end of mesentery. Remember, traditional loop colostomies are not always completely diverting. If one wishes total diversion, an end-loop stoma, with tacking of the distal limb in close proximity to the stoma site, may be a preferable option. Also remember that in obese individuals, the thinnest part of the abdominal wall is often in the upper abdomen.

Ileostomy

As with colostomy, an ileostomy can be constructed as an end ileostomy, loop, or end-loop ileostomy (Fig. 95.21). Ileostomies are generally favored by colorectal surgeons for fecal diversion because they are easier to construct, especially in obese individuals; are usually easier to close; and do not risk compromising the marginal vessels of the colon that are so important to the viability of low and ultra-low colorectal and coloanal anastomoses. Ileostomy effluent usually has a less offensive odor, in contrast to colostomy effluent, which usually has an odor associated with colonic flora. However, in contrast to a colostomy, an ileostomy will empty continuously and has a high rate of associated chemical dermatitis because of the more alkaline pH associated with small bowel effluent as opposed to the stool of the colon. Loop ileostomy is commonly performed, often at the time of ileal pouch–anal anastomosis (IPAA), low colorectal anastomosis, and coloanal anastomosis, especially in patients who have received neoadjuvant chemoradiation. Additional scenarios include patients who are immunosuppressed, patients with tension on their anastomosis, patients in whom complex pelvic reconstructions are planned, and situations in which fecal diversion is performed when trying to avoid total proctocolectomy. Examples include patients with severe perianal Crohn disease and patients in whom perineal reconstructive operations are planned. Minimally invasive diversion is particularly convenient for these cases.

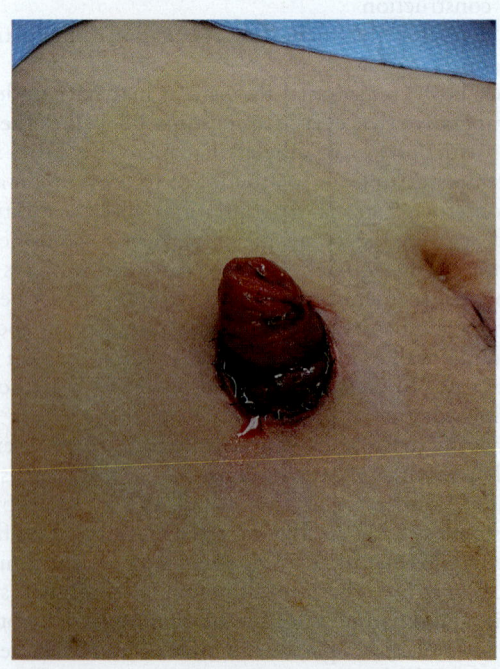

FIGURE 95.21 The intraoperative photo showing the "matured" loop ileostomy protruding 2 to 3 cm above the abdominal wall. The distal limb at skin level is located inferiorly.

BOX 95.1 Interventions to Reduce Readmissions for Ileostomy Patients

- Patient education: Comprehensive guidance on stoma care and potential complications.
- Follow-up appointments: Regular postoperative checks.
- Nutritional counseling: Dietary guidance to regulate stoma output.
- Hydration management: Emphasis on staying hydrated and recognizing dehydration signs.
- Home care services: Access to professional care at home.
- Support groups: Connection to peer support and advice.
- Telemedicine: Virtual consultations for minor concerns.

An end-loop ileostomy, a configuration in which the small bowel is transected and the proximal diversion is brought up as a loop with the staple line immersed in the stoma site, can be used when there is difficulty maturing an end stoma, typically because of an elevated BMI. There is also a much higher risk of dehydration with an ileostomy, which is a frequent reason for hospital readmission after elective colorectal surgery. Before hospital discharge, one should ensure that the 24-hour stoma output is less than 1000 mL. If the output is greater than this amount, the patient is at high risk of hospital readmission (Box 95.1).

Reducing readmissions for patients with ileostomies requires a multifaceted approach. Comprehensive preoperative education can ensure patients and caregivers understand how to manage the ileostomy, identify signs of complications, and adjust solid and liquid alimentation. Regular prompt postdischarge follow-ups, preferably with a stoma care nurse and/or visiting nurses, can facilitate early identification and management of issues. Easy access to outpatient care or telemedicine for minor concerns can prevent these issues from escalating into major problems requiring hospital readmission. High-output ileostomies, characterized by a large volume of stool output (>1200 mL), require strategies to prevent dehydration, electrolyte imbalances, and malnutrition. Dietary modifications to lower fiber intake and include stool-thickening foods can help control output. Adequate hydration and electrolyte intake are crucial to maintain balance. Medications that slow the movement of food through the digestive tract can reduce stool volume, and supplemental nutrition may be required in severe cases. Regular follow-ups with the healthcare team and patient education on recognizing signs of complications, such as dehydration, are key to early intervention and management. The management plan should always be personalized to the patient's individual needs and circumstances.

The timing of ileostomy closure, the reconnection of the bowel after a temporary ileostomy, traditionally occurs several months after initial surgery, typically between 3 and 6 months. However, recent research has proposed early ileostomy closure, within 2 months of the initial surgery, as a safe, feasible option for selected patients. Early closure advantages include a reduced period with a stoma, lowering the overall risk of stoma-related complications and potentially improving the patient's quality of life. Early closure is not suitable for all individuals; careful patient selection, considering factors such as nutritional status, overall health, healing of the initial surgical site, and complicating factors (e.g., ongoing chemotherapy), is crucial. Optimal closure timing should involve patient preferences and circumstances, determined through shared decision-making.

Continent Ostomies

A continent ileostomy, or Kock pouch, facilitates controlled waste drainage through a catheter rather than continuous drainage into an external bag, as with the conventional ileostomy. Despite the benefits of increased control and discretion, continent ileostomies are more complex procedures associated with higher rates of complications, such as pouchitis, valve slippage, and stoma obstruction. A recent meta-analysis found a pooled complication rate of over 60% for Kock pouches with a revision rate of 46% and a failure rate of 12.9%, with increased BMI and previous IPAA, correlated with increased risk for complications.[12] These recurrent complications often necessitate multiple surgical interventions. Indeed, many patients eventually undergo stoma pouch resection because of these persistent issues, leading to the conversion of their ostomy to a noncontinent variant. Although continent ileostomies have declined in use because of alternatives like IPAA, they remain an option for certain patients when IPAA is not possible or desired. A potential alternative to avoid the need for an external appliance are continence devices, which are designed to allow the ostomates to selectively empty intestinal contents. A variety of both externally fixed and internally implanted alternatives have been devised during the last several decades. A recent meta-analysis evaluated the effectiveness of these devices, focusing on their ability to improve continence and quality of life. The findings indicated that these devices can significantly improve both continence and quality of life for ostomates, with patients often reporting a preference for them over traditional pouching systems. Additionally, the devices were associated with relatively low leakage rates, although some complications were noted.[13]

Another type of continent ostomy is the Malone antegrade continence enema (MACE) procedure, a surgical intervention primarily developed to manage chronic constipation and fecal incontinence, particularly in pediatric patients with spina bifida or other congenital anomalies and trauma patients. Surgically creating a conduit, usually using the appendix, allows for the antegrade introduction of fluids into the large bowel, facilitating regular and predictable bowel evacuations. However, similar to other continent ostomies, the MACE procedure has limitations, including the risk of valve malfunction, the requirement for routine catheterization, and an increased susceptibility to infections and surgical revisions.

ENHANCED RECOVERY PROTOCOLS

Enhanced Recovery Protocols (ERPs) (Box 95.2), or Enhanced Recovery After Surgery (ERAS) protocols, are evidence-based strategies aimed at optimizing patient recovery after surgical procedures, including colorectal surgery.[14] These protocols incorporate a range of perioperative interventions to minimize surgical stress, maintain postoperative physiologic function, and expedite recovery. Key elements of ERAS protocols in colorectal surgery involve preoperative counseling to educate patients about the surgical procedure, the expected recovery process, and the significance of early mobilization and nutrition after surgery. Preoperative nutrition is also a crucial aspect, often involving carbohydrate loading before surgery to mitigate postoperative insulin resistance. In many ERAS protocols, there is an avoidance of mechanical bowel preparation preoperatively because research suggests it may not enhance outcomes and could potentially worsen them. Anesthetic management generally encompasses a multimodal approach to analgesia, including regional techniques, and a focus on maintaining euvolemia rather than administering excessive intravenous fluids.

Encouraging patients to mobilize and begin oral intake of fluids and food soon after surgery stimulates gut function and can

---

BOX 95.2   Interventions

Preoperative Interventions
- Patient education
- Nutritional screening
- Preoperative carbohydrate loading
- Bowel preparation (minimal or none)
- Avoidance of preoperative fasting
- Optimization of comorbidities
- Thromboprophylaxis
- Antibiotic prophylaxis

Intraoperative Interventions
- Goal-directed fluid therapy
- Minimally invasive techniques
- Avoidance of drains and nasogastric tubes
- Regional anesthesia/transversus abdominis plane (TAP) block
- Maintenance of normothermia
- Short-acting anesthetic agents

Postoperative Interventions
- Early mobilization
- Early oral feeding
- Multimodal analgesia
- Avoidance of nasogastric tubes
- Stimulating bowel function
- Early removal of catheters
- Postoperative nausea and vomiting (PONV) prophylaxis
- Structured follow-up

---

improve patient morale and well-being. The use of drains and nasogastric tubes is often avoided whenever possible because they can cause discomfort and delay recovery.

ERAS protocols have been associated with reduced lengths of hospital stay and postoperative complications without increasing readmission rates. However, successful implementation requires a multidisciplinary team approach, significant efforts in patient education, staff training, and process redesign. Patient adherence to the protocol is also vital for achieving desired outcomes. Prehospitalization education is essential for the patient and family to help ensure compliance.

Although these protocols generally are not intended for nonelective cases, components of ERPs can be applied to urgent/emergent patients. ERPs have shown efficacy in reducing morbidity rates and length of hospital stay without increasing readmission rates in colorectal surgery. ERPs are also associated with reduced healthcare costs, improved patient satisfaction, lower complication rates, and decreased mortality. They improve outcomes irrespective of laparoscopic or open surgery and are safe and effective in elderly patient populations. However, their implementation should not be dogmatic, but requires ongoing compliance evaluation and continuous quality improvement. Better adherence to ERPs is linked with decreased complications and shorter hospital stays.[15]

Preoperative Interventions

Counseling before surgery to set expectations on milestones and discharge criteria is considered a cornerstone of successful ERPs. This education helps to set patient expectations, reduce anxiety, and increase compliance with the ERP pathway. In addition, chronic conditions such as diabetes, hypertension,

and heart disease should be optimally managed before surgery. This might involve working closely with primary care doctors or specialists to ensure the patient is in the best possible health before surgery. Furthermore, some medications may need to be adjusted or temporarily stopped before surgery, especially those that could increase the risk of surgical complications. If an ostomy is a part of the planned operation, marking, education, and counseling on dehydration should be started in the preoperative period.

Prehabilitation before surgery is also a fairly new concept that aims to enhance a patient's functional capacity before surgery, which is particularly beneficial for deconditioned patients or those with multiple comorbidities. Pre-habilitation can involve physical exercises, nutritional optimization, mental health support, and patient education, with the goal of reducing postoperative complications and promoting more efficient recovery. The underlying premise is that patients with higher preoperative fitness levels possess more physiologic reserves, enabling them to better withstand surgical stress and recover more efficiently. The evidence supporting prehabilitation is still evolving but suffers from lack of standardization and outcome reporting bias. Studies have suggested potential benefits, including improved physical fitness and reduced postoperative complications in patients undergoing abdominal or colorectal surgery. However, a recent meta-analysis focusing on high quality randomized controlled trials examining the impact of excercise-based prehabilitation on postoperative outcomes in colorectal surgery found that, while prehabilitation was associated with shorter length of stay and improved preoperative functional outcomes (e.g., better walking distance), it did not reduce post operative complication or readmission rates compared to standard care.[16] Further research is needed to identify specific patient populations that would benefit most from pre-habilitation with optimization of intervention protocols.

Preadmission Nutrition and Bowel Preparation

There is strong evidence to support the recommendation of a clear liquid diet up until 2 hours before the induction of anesthesia. However, there is weaker evidence to support the use of per os carbohydrate loading before surgery.

Mechanical bowel preparation alone has not been shown to be beneficial (strong recommendation based on high-quality evidence, 1A). In the United States, mechanical bowel preparation plus oral antibiotics preparation has become the preferred preparation to reduce complications, including SSIs, especially when left-sided and rectal resections are anticipated. In the American Society of Colon and Rectal Surgeons Clinical Practice Guidelines for the Use of Bowel Preparation in Elective Colon and Rectal Surgery, this practice was given a strong recommendation based on moderate-quality evidence (1B). Interestingly, a recent randomized controlled trial found no evidence to support this practice for elective colon resection compared with no bowel preparation as a mechanism to reduce SSIs or postoperative morbidity.[17] It is important to note that the majority of reported studies, including this one, were performed in patients undergoing colon as opposed to rectal resections.

Perioperative Interventions

ERPs commonly involve preset orders for the preoperative, intraoperative, and postoperative care for all patients. These pathways can typically include 20 or more individual components that span the entire surgical process, from preoperative preparation through intraoperative management to postoperative care.

However, the exact number can vary based on the specific ERAS protocol in use, the type of surgery, and the individual hospital's policies and guidelines. Standardization requires collaborative buy-in from different stakeholders, which helps avoid confusion and promotes timely adherence to care.

Colorectal surgery patients have up to a 20% risk of developing a postoperative SSI. Bundles of care aimed at SSI reduction have shown SSI rates to be significantly reduced. These bundles include some, if not all, of the following measures: preoperative chlorhexidine shower; mechanical bowel preparation with oral antibiotics; prophylactic antibiotic administration within 1 hour of incision; the use of wound protectors during surgery; changing gown, gloves, and instruments before fascial closure; euglycemia; and normothermia. The degree to which each element affects the reduction of SSIs is unclear. A recent meta-analysis found that although larger bundles were not associated with a larger effect, perioperative care bundles that contained a high proportion of evidence-based interventions showed a more substantial impact in preventing SSIs.[18]

There is strong evidence to support the use of multimodal, opioid-sparing pain management plans starting before the induction of anesthesia. Minimizing opioids is associated with earlier return of bowel function and shorter length of stay. Acetaminophen, nonsteroidal antiinflammatory drugs (NSAIDs), and gabapentin have all been incorporated into various ERPs. Transverse abdominis plane (TAP) block with local anesthetic, including liposomal bupivacaine, has shown promising results for short-term pain. A recent meta-analysis revealed that the TAP block significantly reduced the need for opioids and pain intensity within 24 hours of both laparoscopic and combined surgeries, but it did not significantly affect the overall opioid consumption during the hospital stay. Epidural analgesia is generally recommended for open, but is not commonly performed for laparoscopic surgery.

The use of goal-directed fluid therapy in the intraoperative and postoperative phases of care is associated with a reduction in time to return of bowel function and length of stay. Lastly, minimally invasive surgical (MIS) approaches should be used, when possible, with avoidance of routine use of intraabdominal drains and nasogastric tubes.

Postoperative Interventions

Postoperative interventions in the ERP occupy a crucial role in accelerating recovery and mitigating the risks of complications. These tenets include a multimodal approach to pain management to minimize opioid use, promoting early mobilization postsurgery, and reintroducing a normal diet within 24 hours to stimulate gut function and provide essential nutrition. Proactive management of postoperative nausea and vomiting as well as the prevention of ileus are other key aspects to ensure patient comfort and facilitate early feeding.

Further postoperative interventions include careful fluid management to prevent fluid overload and electrolyte imbalances; early catheter removal to reduce urinary tract infection risk and promote patient mobilization; prophylactic measures against deep vein thrombosis (DVT), such as medication and compression stockings; and avoidance or early removal of drains. Regular patient follow-ups are performed to monitor recovery, manage complications, and provide ongoing support. Although these ERAS interventions are widely accepted to enhance recovery, reduce complications, and shorten hospital stays, it is crucial that they be personalized to each patient's unique needs and supervised

by a healthcare professional. In summary, ERPs are evidence-based protocols that benefit colorectal surgery patients. Local implementation involves buy-in for a range of stakeholders that may be in opposition to the preferences of individual healthcare professionals. Adherence to the constellation of ERP components and the outcomes of interest should be continually monitored and evaluated.

DIVERTICULAR DISEASE

Background

Diverticular disease is used to describe a spectrum of manifestations associated with colonic diverticulosis. Diverticula are saccular outpouchings of the bowel wall. They are described as "true" diverticula when they contain all layers of the bowel wall; these are rare and usually congenital. The vast majority of diverticula in the colon are "false" diverticula (pulsion, pseudodiverticula), containing only the mucosa and muscularis mucosa. Diverticulitis is thought to be mainly a disease of the modern world, coinciding with dietary changes after the Industrial Revolution. Additionally, as the average life span has steadily increased over the past several decades, the incidence of diverticular disease, which predominantly presents in older individuals, has also been on the rise.

Pathophysiology and Epidemiology

Hypertrophy of the muscular layers of the colon wall, combined with a narrowed lumen and disordered colonic motility, causes localized high-pressure zones in which the mucosa herniates through areas of relative weakness. Diverticula are classically formed on the mesenteric side of the colonic wall in regions where vasa recta traverse through the muscular layer to provide blood to the mucosa (Fig. 95.22). These small blood vessels supplying the colon are considered potential weak spots in the bowel wall. When increased pressure, inflammation, impaired blood supply, or trauma occurs at these weak points, it can lead to a perforation in the diverticulum, which leads to infection and, as a result, a significant local inflammatory response. When perforations occur on the mesenteric side, as they do in most cases, the surrounding mesentery often serves as a natural barrier, helping to contain the

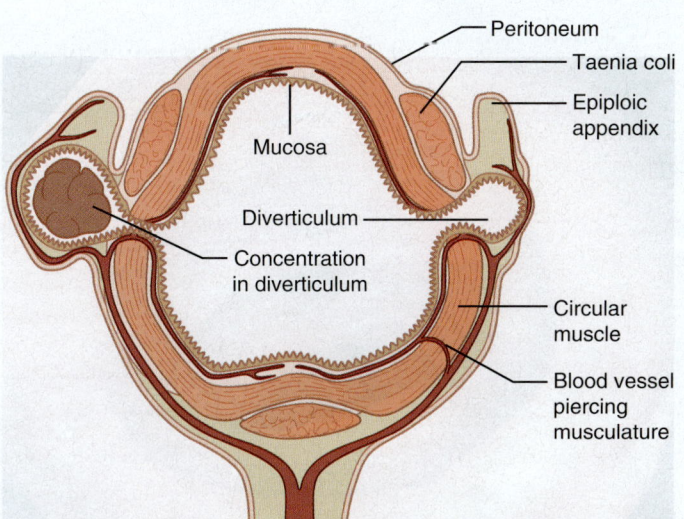

FIGURE 95.22 Pathogenesis of diverticulosis. (From Netter FH. *Netter Collection of Medical Illustrations.* Vol 9. Philadelphia: Elsevier Saunders; 2016:145.)

infection or inflammation to a localized area. The infected diverticulum can then form an abscess or walled-off area of infection within the confines of the mesenteric tissues, preventing further spread of bacteria into the peritoneal cavity, which could lead to peritonitis, a more serious and widespread infection. Therefore, the majority of diverticulitis cases are "contained" or localized because of this protective effect of the mesentery. However, if the infection or inflammation is not adequately controlled or treated, it could potentially spread beyond these barriers, leading to more serious complications, such as a generalized peritonitis and sepsis.

The sigmoid and descending colon are typically affected, whereas the rectum, having an extra layer of muscle, is generally not affected (Fig. 95.23). This has implications for surgery and is why the distal anastomosis margin in operations for diverticulitis should always be within the rectum, to reduce the likelihood of recurrence. Diverticulosis increases with age and is relatively rare in young adults. Colonic diverticula are noted in approximately 40% of individuals between the ages of 50 and 60 years and in over 60% of individuals over the age of 80 years (Fig. 95.24). The mechanism for developing diverticulitis is thought to be a result

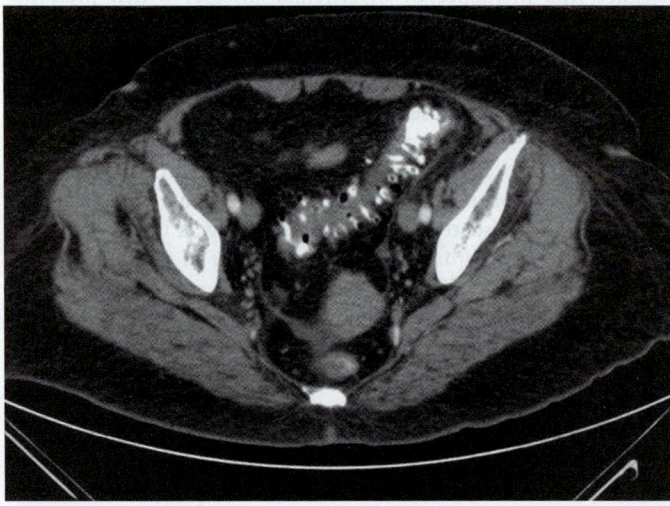

FIGURE 95.23 Computed tomography scan of the pelvis showing extensive sigmoid diverticulosis.

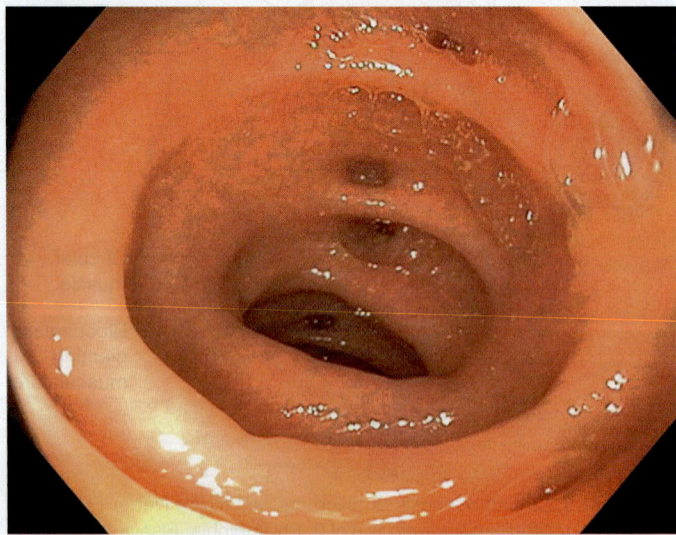

FIGURE 95.24 Endoscopic view of diverticulosis.

of obstruction of the orifice of a diverticulum, with stasis leading to bacterial overgrowth, inflammation, and increased pressure within the diverticulum, causing ischemia and microperforation. Interestingly, only a small proportion of patients with diverticulosis develop diverticulitis. Modern estimates indicate that fewer than 5% of patients with diverticulosis will develop diverticulitis; however, because of the high prevalence of diverticulosis, it has become a significant clinical and financial burden, accounting for more than 2.7 million outpatient visits in the United States annually and more than 200,000 inpatient admissions for diverticulitis at an estimated cost of more than $2 billion.

Diet and lifestyle factors play an important role in diverticular disease. Western dietary patterns high in red meat, fat, and refined grains are associated with an increased risk of the disease, whereas increased fiber intake, with abundant fruit, vegetables, and whole grains, reduces the risk of diverticulitis.[19] Intake of nuts, seeds, and popcorn does not appear to increase the risk. Central obesity and smoking increase the risk, whereas physical activity, such as running, has been correlated with a decreased risk. The European Prospective Investigation into Cancer and Nutrition (EPIC) study, a prospective cohort analysis, found that a vegetarian diet and high fiber intake significantly reduce the risk of diverticular disease. After 11.6 years of follow-up, vegetarians showed a 31% lower risk, and participants with the highest fiber intake (≥25.5 g/day for females and ≥26.1 g/day for males) showed a 41% lower risk of hospital admission or death from the disease compared with meat eaters and those individuals with low fiber intake.[20]

Clinical Evaluation

Diverticular disease can manifest as diverticulitis, but it is also the most common reason for massive lower GI bleeding. Because diverticulitis is caused by inflammation and perforation of a colonic diverticulum, signs and symptoms will generally result from the pericolonic inflammation. Patients will commonly present with abdominal pain localized to the left lower quadrant (following the location of the inflamed sigmoid colon). Additionally, fever, change in bowel habits, anorexia, and urinary urgency (in cases where the bladder is secondarily inflamed) are frequent. On physical examination, localized tenderness is noted, commonly with moderate abdominal distention. A tender mass can be palpable if there is a significant phlegmon. Rectal bleeding is rare in the presentation of acute diverticulitis and should raise suspicion of another diagnosis, such as ischemic colitis or IBD. Leukocytosis and other elevated inflammatory markers are common laboratory findings.

Several imaging modalities have been used to evaluate patients with suspected diverticular disease. Flat and upright plain films can be used to diagnose obstruction or free intraperitoneal air but are generally nonspecific. Contrast studies, ultrasound, and magnetic resonance imaging (MRI) have also been used, but, currently, computed tomography (CT) has become the most useful tool to confirm the diagnosis, exclude other diagnoses, and classify the severity of the disease. Signs of diverticulitis on CT include the presence of diverticula, colonic wall thickening, pericolic fat stranding, and abscess formation. CT studies have the capacity to localize abscesses and fistulas and define the extent of the disease. The modified Hinchey classification[21] is the most commonly used tool to describe the severity of diverticulitis (Table 95.1).

Grade 0, not included in the original publication, is commonly used to describe mild clinical diverticulitis. If CT is performed,

TABLE 95.1 Modified Hinchey Classification System

Stage 0	Mild clinical diverticulitis
Stage Ia	Confined pericolic inflammation—phlegmon
Stage Ib	Confined pericolic abscess (within sigmoid mesocolon)
Stage II	Pelvic, distant intraabdominal or intraperitoneal abscess
Stage III	Generalized purulent peritonitis
Stage IV	Fecal peritonitis

From Klarenbeek BR, de Korte N, van der Peet DL, et al. Review of current classifications for diverticular disease and a translation into clinical practice. *Int J Colorectal Dis.* 2012;27:207-214.

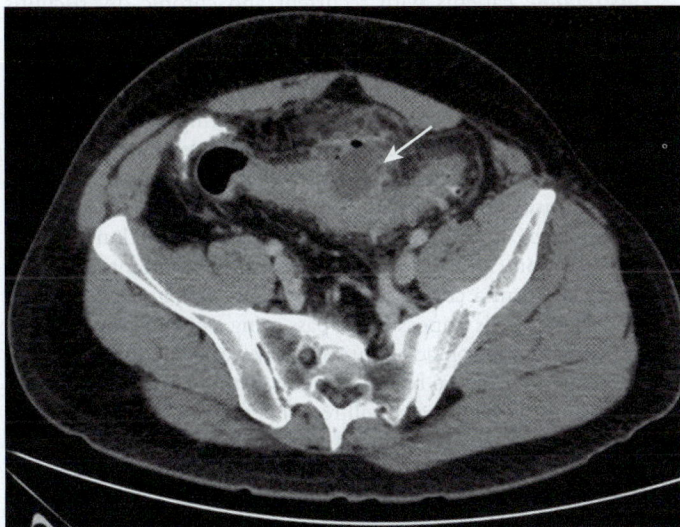

FIGURE 95.25 Computed tomography of the pelvis demonstrating sigmoid diverticulitis with a thickened bowel wall, fat stranding a pericolonic abscess *(arrow)*, modified Hinchey grade 1b.

colonic wall thickening without pericolonic fat stranding can be seen. Grade 1a presents with a phlegmon with colonic wall thickening and pericolonic fat stranding, whereas grade 1b also includes a pericolonic or mesocolic abscess (Fig. 95.25). Patients with grade 2 disease have distant intraabdominal or pelvic abscesses. Patients with grade 3 disease have generalized purulent peritonitis, and those with grade 4 disease have fecal peritonitis. The ability of a CT scan to distinguish between grade 3 and grade 4 is limited, and in these cases, accurate diagnosis is usually made in the operating room.

Flexible endoscopy during the acute setting should be approached with caution because distention of the colon may result in worsening perforation. Colonoscopy has traditionally played a pivotal role in the evaluation of diverticulitis by confirming the presence of diverticular disease, assessing its extent and severity, and crucially, excluding other colorectal conditions. By visualizing the diverticula in the colon and other potential abnormalities, endoscopy helps to exclude diagnoses like CRC, IBD, and ischemic colitis. This evaluation typically follows a 6- to 8-week period after an acute diverticulitis episode to minimize the risk of complications, such as bowel perforation.

However, recent studies have clearly demonstrated a shift in perspective, suggesting that a routine colonoscopy may not be necessary for all patients after acute diverticulitis, particularly in cases of uncomplicated diverticulitis diagnosed via a CT scan. Research demonstrates that the risk of CRC in these patients is low and comparable to that of the general population. Consequently, the necessity for endoscopy should be decided on an individual basis, considering factors such as diagnostic certainty, the presence of ongoing symptoms, patients' CRC risk factors, and the potential risks of the procedure itself.[22,23]

Management
Uncomplicated Diverticulitis

The treatment of uncomplicated diverticulitis depends on the severity of symptoms, and the approach is thus individualized. The majority of these patients can be managed as outpatients. The mainstay of treatment is based on pain medications, short-term alteration of diet, and antibiotics. Commonly, patients are initially prescribed clear liquids, followed by a low-residue diet until the inflammation subsides. Antibiotics have traditionally been prescribed to cover colonic bacteria. A systematic review and meta-analysis assessing the effect of antibiotic administration in patients with uncomplicated diverticulitis has not shown the use of antibiotics to accelerate recovery or prevent complications or subsequent surgery.[24] As a result, some physicians have stopped prescribing antibiotics for uncomplicated diverticulitis. Outpatient treatment of uncomplicated diverticulitis has also been investigated in recent years. A recent meta-analysis found that outpatient management of uncomplicated diverticulitis is safe and cost-effective, leading to low readmission rates and minimal complications while also providing substantial healthcare cost savings.[25]

A small proportion of patients diagnosed with diverticulitis will actually have a colonic neoplasm mimicking diverticulitis. Overall, this finding is currently estimated at around 1% to 3%, with significantly higher rates observed in the background of complicated disease.[26] Upon recovery, it is recommended that patients undergo a colonoscopy after 4 to 8 weeks to exclude malignancy.

After the initial episode of acute, uncomplicated diverticulitis, only 10% to 35% of individuals will have another episode.[27] After more episodes, the chances of recurrence increase significantly. In an attempt to avoid severe complicated diverticulitis, elective surgery was previously suggested after uncomplicated diverticulitis, depending on the number of episodes, with the thought that more episodes would lead to more chances of recurrence and a higher chance of severe complicated diverticulitis. However, recurrences generally tend to follow the severity of the initial episode. As a result, the number of attacks of uncomplicated diverticulitis has fallen out of favor as an indication for surgery. In addition, the traditional approach to elective surgery for diverticular disease, which considered young age (under 50 years old) as an indication, has been challenged by recent evidence. Contrary to previous assumptions, studies suggest that younger patients do not necessarily have a more aggressive disease course and often respond well to conservative management. Moreover, elective surgery carries inherent risks, such as infections, bleeding, potential damage to nearby organs, and the possible need for a permanent colostomy. This, coupled with potential impacts on quality of life, particularly for active younger individuals, has led to a more conservative approach, favoring surgery primarily for complicated disease or disease unresponsive to medical treatment. Personalization of care, considering individual risk factors, disease characteristics, lifestyle, and patient preferences, remains vital in management decisions. The DIRECT trial, which aimed to examine the long-term benefit on quality of life in patients suffering from recurrent disease, showed that elective sigmoidectomy improved quality of life in patients with recurring diverticulitis and/or ongoing complaints compared with conservative management.

Despite surgical risks, nearly half of conservatively managed patients eventually required surgery because of severe complaints.[28] Currently, an individual assessment is performed that includes the frequency of attacks, ongoing symptoms, and their effect on quality of life versus the age and medical condition of the patient and their surgical risk.[29]

The aim of elective surgery is to remove the affected segment of the colon (usually the sigmoid colon) and perform a primary anastomosis of the healthy remaining bowel. When removing the sigmoid colon, the proximal margin should be in soft, pliable bowel, but it is not necessary to include all proximal diverticula. The distal anastomosis, however, should be to the upper rectum because leaving a section of distal sigmoid colon is associated with a higher risk of recurrent diverticulitis. Surgery can be performed by either an open, laparoscopic, hand-assisted, or robotic approach. MIS for diverticular disease has been shown to be safe, with advantages of more rapid recovery of bowel function, less pain, and shorter hospitalization. Ureteric stents are often used to mitigate ureteric injury risk by serving as guides amid inflamed tissues, with their usage being case specific and dependent on such factors as disease severity and surgical complexity.

Complicated Diverticulitis

Patients with complicated diverticulitis are characterized by the presence of an abscess, fistula, obstruction, or free perforation.

Abscess. Signs and symptoms will depend on the size and location of the abscess, with diagnosis usually provided on imaging. Smaller abscesses can often be treated successfully with antibiotics alone. Larger abscesses will require drainage. After recovery, patients who present with a diverticular abscess often experience recurring episodes. Although substantial data suggest that many of these recurrences can be nonoperatively managed, the risks of recurrence and complications are increased in patients who present with a diverticular abscess. However, even with this recurrence risk, some studies suggest that surgery might not always be required, and nonoperative management can lead to acceptable outcomes in certain situations. Despite these findings, the most recent guidelines from the American Society of Colon and Rectal Surgeons (ASCRS) recommend considering elective resection after successful nonoperative treatment of a diverticular abscess. This recommendation is based on moderate-quality evidence, recognizing the balance between managing recurrence risk and avoiding unnecessary surgery. Patients with abscesses not amenable to percutaneous drainage and unresponsive to treatment require urgent surgery.

Fistula. Fistulas are abnormal connections to surrounding epithelial-lined organs and are a relatively common complication of diverticulitis. They are a result of the local inflammation and development of an abscess that decompresses into a neighboring organ. The most common type, especially in males, is a colovesical fistula to the dome of the bladder. Patients will present with recurrent urinary tract infections, which are, in many cases, polymicrobial. Pneumaturia and fecaluria may also be present. CT can reveal air or contrast in the bladder in the absence of prior instrumentation. Cystoscopy will usually disclose inflammation at the site of the fistula. Colovaginal fistulas occur almost exclusively in females who have undergone previous hysterectomy and present with vaginal discharge and passing of air per vagina. Colocutaneous fistulas usually present at a previous drain site in patients who have undergone percutaneous drainage. Patients with fistulas usually do not need emergency surgery because the abscess has usually decompressed through the

fistula. Initial management includes broad-spectrum antibiotics to decrease the inflammation. Patients are then investigated with colonoscopy and appropriate imaging (e.g., cystoscopy) to exclude malignancy and Crohn disease. Surgical principles then encompass resection of the involved colon and fistula tract with primary anastomosis. If possible, the fistula opening into the secondarily involved organ is primarily suture repaired; however, in many cases, the opening is small and difficult to recognize. In the case of the bladder, with small fistula openings, drainage of the bladder with a Foley catheter for 7 to 10 days will usually allow for healing. A cystogram can be done to confirm fistula healing before Foley removal. Fistulas to the small bowel will characteristically require resection and primary anastomosis.

Obstruction. Patients with recurrent and chronic diverticulitis can develop fibrosis of the colonic wall, leading to stricture formation. In most cases, these patients will present with insidious symptoms and a partial obstruction. Small bowel obstruction may also be seen as a result of a small bowel loop adhering to an area of inflamed colonic tissue or abscess. Management depends on the degree and type of obstruction. Patients with a partial obstruction can usually be initially treated with a nasogastric tube for decompression, antibiotics, fluids, and bowel rest. If the obstruction resolves, elective resection can be planned. It is usually important before resection to perform a colonoscopy to rule out malignancy. In cases where the stricture is impossible to pass using a colonoscope, virtual colonoscopy or a retrograde contrast study can be helpful to visualize the remainder of the bowel. Patients with a complete obstruction unresponsive to therapy will require emergency surgery.

Perforation. Patients with a free intraabdominal perforation with widespread contamination will present with diffuse peritonitis with rebound tenderness and guarding. Signs of sepsis, including fever, tachycardia, and hemodynamic instability, are frequently seen. Imaging can demonstrate free abdominal fluid, signs of peritonitis, and free intraabdominal air. In very few carefully selected, completely stable patients with diverticular perforation and distant pneumoperitoneum, nonoperative management with IV antibiotics, bowel rest, and possible percutaneous abscess drainage may be an option. This approach requires exceptionally careful selection and very close skilled monitoring to try to avoid complications, such as worsening peritonitis and sepsis, necessitating emergency surgery. The ability to distinguish between purulent and fecal diverticulitis before surgery is limited. Hinchey grades 3 and 4 are considered a surgical emergency. After initial resuscitation, patients are taken to the operating room, with the goal of controlling the source of infection by resection and washing out the abdominal contamination.

The mainstay of treatment in these cases has traditionally been Hartmann's procedure,[30] which removes the involved colon and exteriorizes an end colostomy. Reversing the colostomy, however, requires a second major surgical procedure with its own significant morbidity and mortality. Practically, up to 50% of patients will never be reversed, with even higher rates in the elderly. Given these implications, several studies have investigated alternatives to Hartmann's procedure.

Laparoscopic lavage. Laparoscopic lavage[31] is an MIS procedure for which there was some initial enthusiasm to treat perforated diverticulitis, generally presenting as purulent peritonitis (Hinchey grade 3). The technique involves cleaning the peritoneal cavity laparoscopically without removing the diseased colon segment. This aims to control the immediate infection, minimize surgical stress, and potentially allow for a more planned, less morbid procedure later if needed.

Several randomized controlled trials, including the DILALA and the LOLA arm of the LADIES trials, have investigated laparoscopic lavage's effectiveness and safety. The DILALA trial indicated that lavage was linked to a shorter initial hospital stay and fewer stoma formations compared with sigmoidectomy, with no significant difference in major morbidity and mortality rates in patients with Hinchey III disease. The LADIES trial (LOLA arm), however, was prematurely terminated because of high postoperative complications and surgical reinterventions in the lavage group.[32,33] A recent meta-analysis investigating long-term outcomes of different treatment methods for diverticulitis underscored several significant benefits of laparoscopic lavage. As opposed to resection procedures, lavage notably decreased the chances of long-term stoma by 87% and reduced the odds of subsequent operations by 42%, largely by obviating complications linked to Hartmann's procedure that may culminate in permanent colostomies. However, lavage isn't without its problems: It is associated with a nearly sixfold increase in the risk of disease recurrence because it is a damage control strategy that leaves the disease-riddled colon segment intact. Despite this, the long-term complications and mortality rates were on par between lavage and resection, vouching for the enduring safety of the laparoscopic lavage procedure.[34]

Primary resection and anastomosis (with/without proximal diversion). Primary resection and anastomosis have emerged as a promising alternative to the traditional Hartmann's procedure in the management of perforated diverticulitis. Early studies indicated a notable reduction in morbidity rates after ostomy reversal when primary anastomosis with a covering loop ileostomy was used compared with Hartmann's reversal. Furthermore, primary anastomosis saw significantly higher rates of ostomy closure.

Confirming these results, long-term outcome reports from the French DIVERTI trial and the Dutch LADIES trial's DIVA arm showed superior outcomes for resection and primary anastomosis over Hartmann's procedure. The analyses from these trials suggested that primary anastomosis could decrease the chance of a long-term ostomy by a remarkable 98%, reduce long-term complications and the need for reoperation by 80%, and lower incisional hernia rates by 82% when compared with Hartmann's procedure. The data imply that, for hemodynamically stable patients with perforated diverticulitis and peritonitis, primary anastomosis may offer superior long-term outcomes and be the preferred surgical approach.[34] However, these results must be viewed carefully, as recruitment issues and selection bias of these trials raised some concern for nonapplicability.

Damage control strategy. The "damage control" strategy, a concept borrowed from trauma surgery, has also emerged as an alternative approach in managing patients presenting with generalized peritonitis resulting from perforated diverticulitis who require urgent surgical intervention. This strategy, described by Kafka-Ritsch et al., involves an initial surgery that includes abdominal washout and resection without restoring bowel continuity, leaving closed intestinal stumps with an open or temporarily closed abdomen.[35] The decision of whether to anastomose is then deferred to a second-look intervention, typically 24 to 48 hours after the initial surgery. Although this approach still requires large-scale validation studies, it is seen as a positive step toward individualized surgical intervention based on the patient's clinical characteristics and operative findings.

Surgical decision-making in complex septic patients resulting from diverticular perforation involves considering multiple patient-related factors, such as hemodynamic stability, symptom severity, and the extent of perforation, along with factors related to the caregiver, such as surgical capability, experience level, and available resources. With these considerations in mind, it is suggested that fit and hemodynamically stable patients be considered for resection with primary anastomosis or laparoscopic lavage in Hinchey 3 perforations and considered for primary resection and anastomosis with a diverting loop ileostomy in Hinchey 4 perforations. Hartmann's procedure should be mainly reserved for unstable patients or cases where a colostomy could significantly improve quality of life, such as in bedridden patients or those suffering from fecal incontinence. Damage control strategy might be appropriate in unstable patients; however, further research is needed to evaluate the safety of this surgical approach. A suggested treatment algorithm can be seen in Fig. 95.26.

Special Populations

Right-Sided Diverticulitis

Right-sided diverticulitis is common in Asian countries but rare in Western populations. This typically affects younger patients and may be challenging to diagnose because signs and symptoms are very similar to those of acute appendicitis. Other differential diagnoses to be considered include Meckel diverticulitis, cholecystitis, ischemic colitis, mesenteric adenitis, pyelonephritis, and pelvic inflammatory disease. The recommended approach should generally be similar to that for diverticulitis in other sites. Patients who have recurrent episodes or complicated disease and patients with an uncertain diagnosis should be considered for resection with a right hemicolectomy.

Immunocompromised Patients

Immunocompromised patients include transplant patients; patients with diabetes mellitus, renal failure, or cirrhosis; and patients being treated with systemic steroids and/or chemotherapy. The most updated recommendation from the most recent ASCRS guidelines states that after recovery from uncomplicated acute diverticulitis in immunosuppressed patients, the decision to perform elective surgery needs to be individualized. Immunosuppressed patients constitute a unique cohort that requires careful consideration when it comes to recommending elective surgery after medical treatment for diverticulitis. A review of the NSQIP database revealed comparable mortality rates between immunosuppressed and immunocompetent patients who underwent elective sigmoidectomy. However, the rates of major morbidity and wound dehiscence were significantly higher in the immunosuppressed group. Therefore, the decision to proceed with colectomy in this setting should consider these increased risks.

Different studies presented varying viewpoints regarding the recurrence rates of diverticulitis in immunosuppressed patients, challenging the recommendation for interval elective sigmoidectomy in this group. Although one study found that immunosuppressed patients who experienced a severe initial episode were more likely to have a recurrence, the necessity for emergency surgery was similar to the incidence in immunocompetent patients. A review of patients who underwent renal transplant found high recurrence rates but claimed that nonoperative management is safe for this group. It should be noted that the literature advocating for elective resection after a single episode of uncomplicated diverticulitis in immunosuppressed patients is not universally convincing, and the specific cause of immunosuppression might need to be considered when making treatment recommendations.[29]

Young Patients

Historically, patients younger than 50 years of age were considered to have a more virulent form of diverticulitis and were recommended to

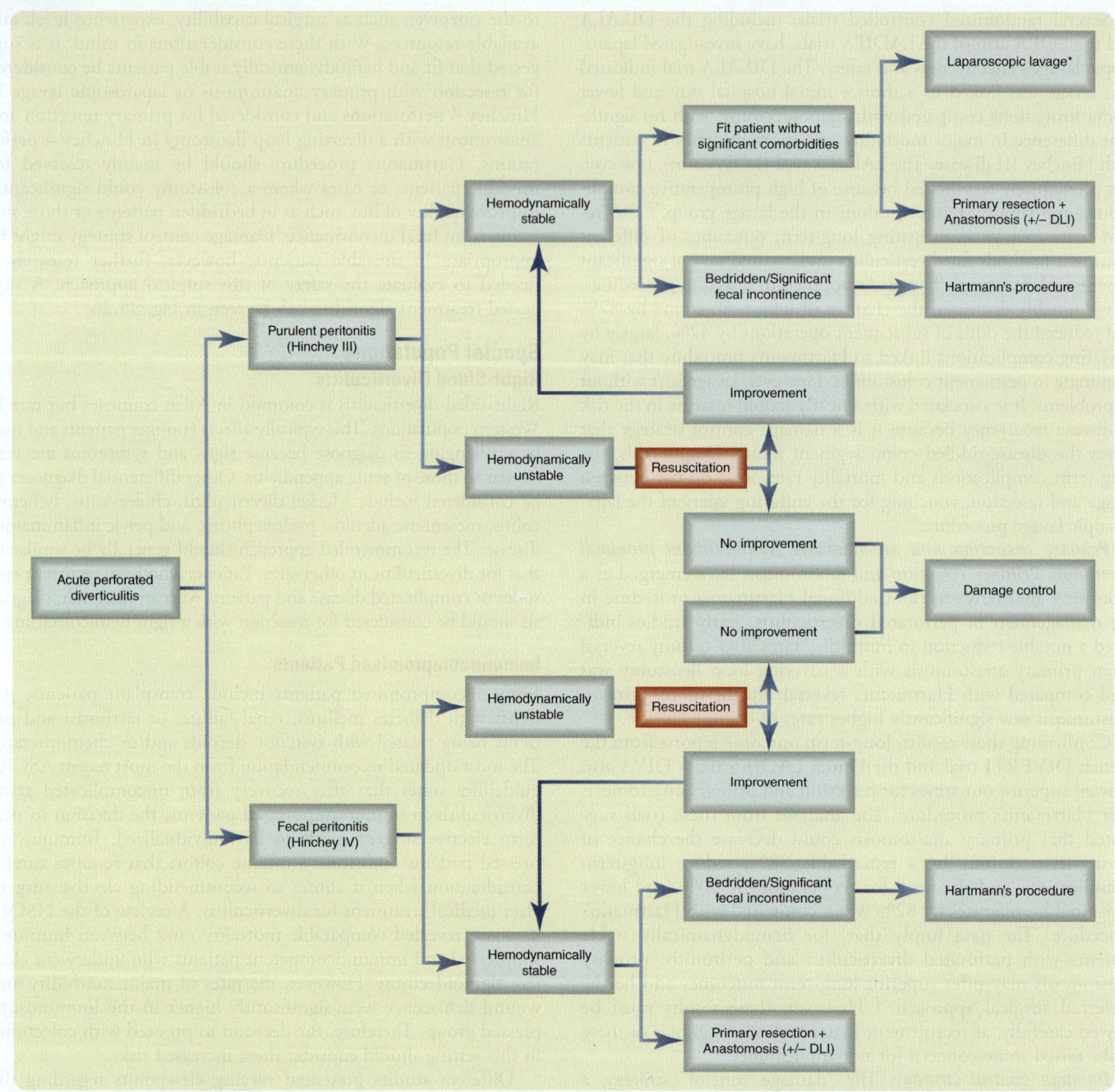

FIGURE 95.26 Suggested algorithm for the treatment of acute perforated diverticulitis in patients with Hinchey III and IV perforations. (Reused with permission from Horesh N, Emile SH, Khan SM, et al. Meta-analysis of randomized clinical trials on long-term outcomes of surgical treatment of perforated diverticulitis. *Ann Surg.* 2023;78[5]:e966-e972. Copyright Wolters Kluwer.)

undergo resection after one episode of uncomplicated disease. Although current evidence does demonstrate higher rates of recurrence, young patients do not have a higher rate of emergency surgical intervention. Current guidelines do not support treating young patients differently than others.

LARGE BOWEL OBSTRUCTION

Large bowel obstruction, defined as bowel obstruction distal to the ileocecal valve, can occur as a result of a variety of etiologies. Broadly, it is classified into mechanical (dynamic) obstruction and functional (adynamic or pseudoobstruction). Mechanical obstruction can be further characterized into endoluminal, mural, and extraluminal causes (Box 95.3).

The most common etiology of mechanical obstruction in the United States is CRC, whereas colonic volvulus is more common in Russia, Eastern Europe, Africa, the Middle East, and India. Presentation and symptoms depend on whether it is an acute obstruction or a more chronic progressive change, as well as partial obstruction, in which some gas/fecal contents are able to pass, versus complete obstruction, in which nothing passes distally. It is thought that, worldwide, volvulus is responsible for roughly one-third of the cases

BOX 95.3 Large Bowel Obstruction Common Etiologies

Mechanical
Intraluminal
Intrinsic mass—neoplasm
Foreign body
Bezoar
Fecal impaction

Mural
Diverticular stricture
Crohn disease stricture
Ischemic stricture
Radiation stricture
Infectious (including lymphogranuloma venereum, tuberculosis, schistosomiasis)
Hirschsprung disease

Extraluminal
Sigmoid volvulus
Cecal volvulus
Hernia (inguinal, ventral, internal)
Metastatic/intraabdominal tumor
Abdominal abscess
Retroperitoneal fibrosis
Adhesions (rare in large bowel)

Functional
Colonic pseudoobstruction (Ogilvie)
Toxic megacolon
Paralytic ileus

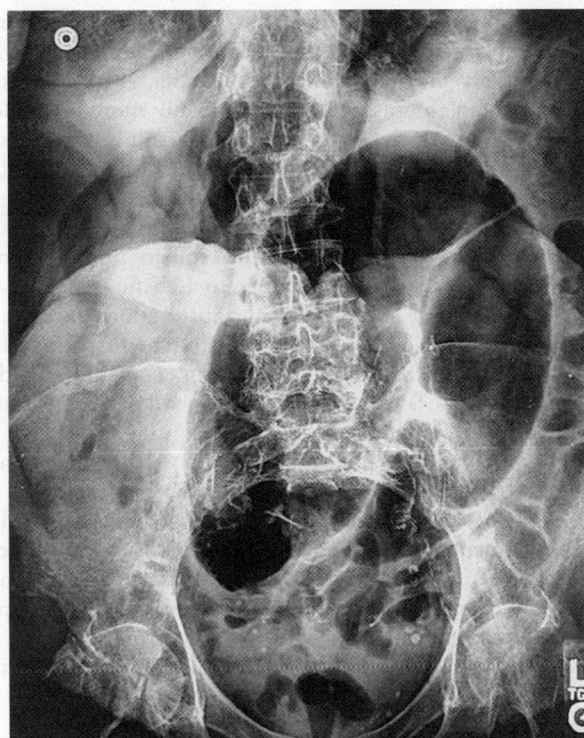

FIGURE 95.27 Plain film of sigmoid volvulus. Note bent inner-tube appearance.

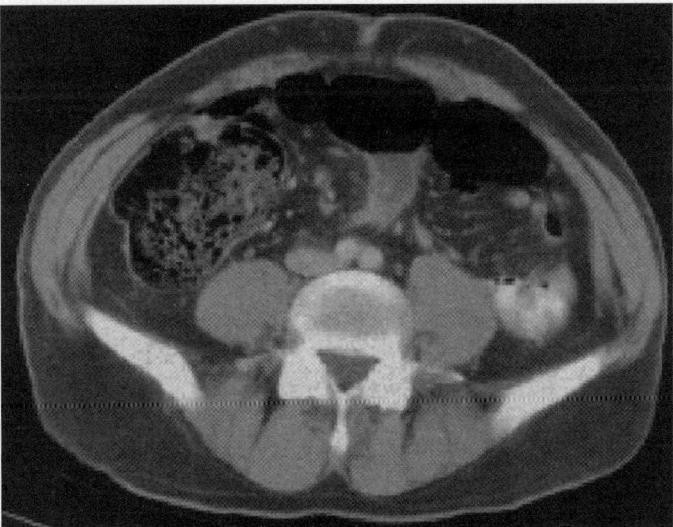

FIGURE 95.28 Computed tomography scan of the abdomen in a patient with sigmoid volvulus. Note characteristic whorl in mesentery.

of large bowel obstruction. The most common site of volvulus is the sigmoid colon; however, cecal volvulus can also occur. Any portion of the colon that is not fixed to the retroperitoneum and that has an elongated mesentery has the potential for volvulus. In these cases, there is an axial twisting of the colon around the mesentery, resulting in an obstruction.

Mechanical obstruction will generally present with increased peristalsis and low-grade colicky pain, but late, long-lasting obstruction may have decreased bowel sounds. In addition, patients will fail to pass stool and flatus and demonstrate increasing abdominal distention. Acute obstructions tend to present more dramatically, with rapid onset of pain, distention, and abdominal tenderness, whereas patients with progressive obstruction may present with increasing constipation, pencil-thin stools, and intermittent abdominal pain. Functional obstruction usually presents with distention, vague abdominal pain, and weak or absent bowel sounds.

Patients with a closed-loop obstruction in which both the proximal and distal parts of a segment of bowel are blocked must be promptly recognized and treated because they have the potential for ischemia and perforation with rapid deterioration. Closed-loop obstruction is commonly encountered in cases such as volvulus and strangulated hernias. Fig. 95.27 shows a plain film of a patient with a sigmoid volvulus. Note the bent, inner-tube appearance of the colon. A plain abdominal x-ray of colonic volvulus typically reveals a large, gas-filled loop of colon, often termed the *coffee-bean sign* because to its distinctive shape. This image suggests a significantly distended loop of colon twisted on its mesentery. The volvulus has resulted in a closed-loop obstruction. In these situations, the colon becomes progressively

distended, with pressure increasing to the point of ischemic necrosis and perforation. Fig. 95.28 shows a CT scan illustrating the characteristic mesenteric whorl seen in patients with a volvulus.

In patients with competent ileocecal valves, obstructing colon cancers can lead to a closed-loop obstruction because the valve does not permit the backflow of intestinal contents. This condition usually results in a more acute presentation. However, when the ileocecal valve is incompetent, the presentation tends to be less severe and immediate because intestinal contents can flow back into the small bowel. This scenario often manifests as a progressively bloating abdomen accompanied by feculent nausea and vomiting, with a decreased risk of perforation. It is worth noting that most obstructions tend to occur in the left colon, where tumors typically grow circumferentially. This is in contrast to right-sided colon tumors, which are generally more polypoid in nature. Distention of the colon occurs as a result of gas and stool that gather proximal to the obstruction. The gas originates both from swallowed air (around two-thirds) and bacterial fermentation. In segments that undergo increasing distention, the pressure within the bowel wall can rise above the capillary pressure, diminishing adequate oxygenation, leading to ischemic necrosis and perforation. Although most malignant obstructions occur in the distal parts of the colon, the necrosis and perforation usually occur in the cecum because it has the largest diameter and, in accordance with the law of Laplace, will distend more under lower pressures and develop higher wall stress.

In cases such as incarcerated hernias and volvulus, pressure on the mesentery can compromise the blood supply, initially obstructing venous return and, with increasing edema and inflammation, eventually occluding the arterial blood supply. The resultant ischemia can also lead to early necrosis and perforation. In closed-loop obstructions, distention initially involves the trapped or incarcerated segment, but with time, the proximal bowel will also distend as a result of ongoing accumulation of gas and stool.

Diagnosis and Assessment

A thorough history and physical examination are critical in the diagnosis of large bowel obstruction. The onset and progression of symptoms, background illnesses, medications, and recent endoscopic evaluations can provide important clues. The abdomen should be palpated for masses, tenderness, and previous incisions; the groin should be examined for hernias; and a digital rectal examination should be performed to inspect for neoplasia and the presence of fecal impaction (Fig. 95.29).

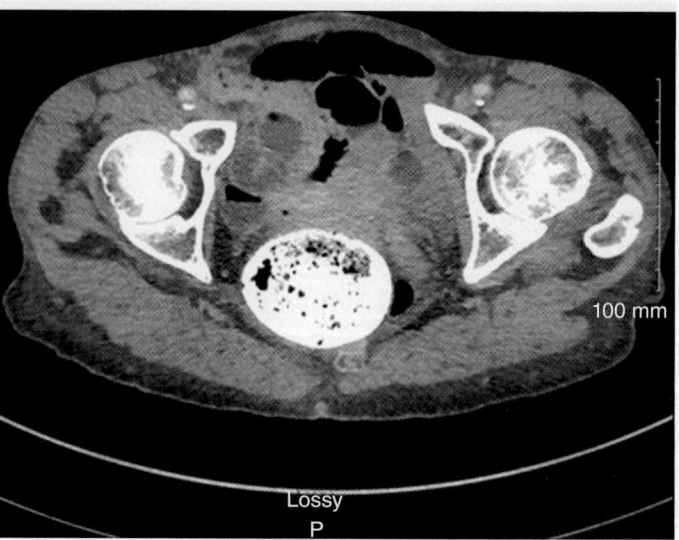

FIGURE 95.29 Computed tomography scan of the pelvis showing a sizable barium impaction after a barium enema resulting in a large bowel obstruction. This patient required disimpaction in the operating room.

Plain films of the abdomen can help in localizing the obstruction, demonstrating the degree of distention and the status of the ileocecal valve (competent vs. incompetent), and in some cases, provide the diagnosis. Water-soluble and IV contrast-enhanced CT scans provide significant information revealing the location and etiology of the obstruction, such as diverticulitis, IBD, and extraluminal causes (e.g., abscesses and inflammation) (Fig. 95.30). CT can also provide clues regarding tissue ischemia and impending perforation. CT with rectal contrast is often preferred in suspected colonic obstruction because of its ability to provide detailed, quick, and safe imaging of

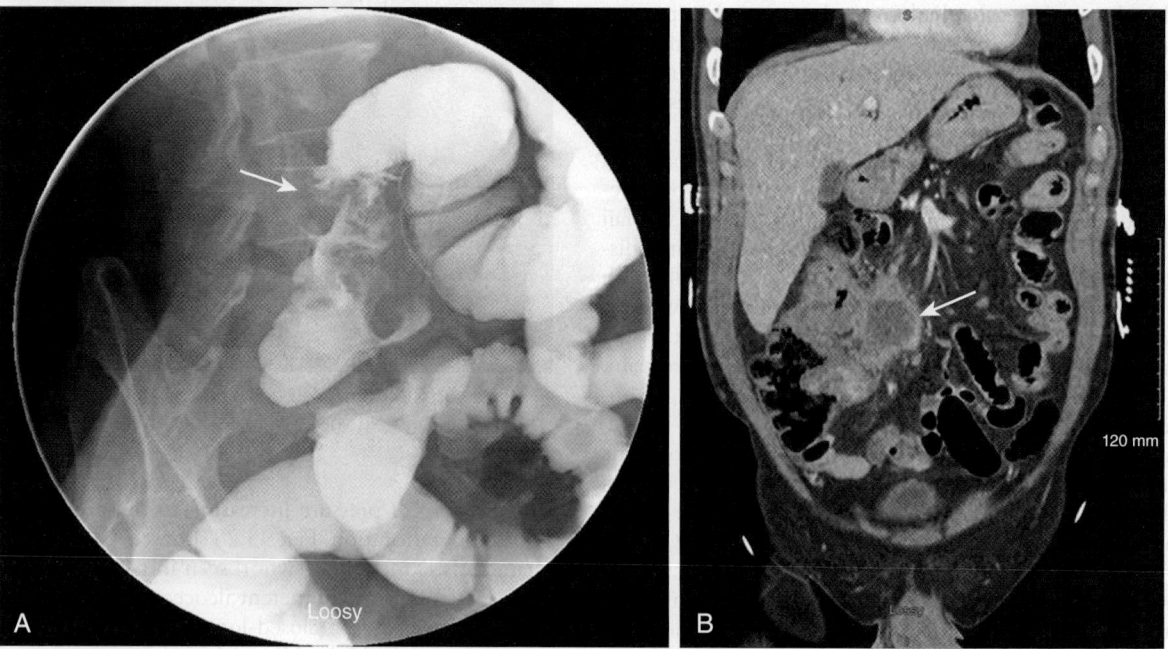

FIGURE 95.30 (A) Gastrografin enema in a patient presenting with obstructing symptoms revealing an "apple-core"–type lesion in the vicinity of the hepatic flexure *(arrow)*. (B) Computed tomography scan of the abdomen and pelvis in the same patient showing a large hepatic flexure carcinoma with perforation into the mesentery and associated mesenteric abscess *(arrow)*. Computed tomography–guided abscess drainage was not possible. This patient underwent extended right hemicolectomy with exteriorization of his ileocolic anastomosis as a loop ileostomy.

the obstruction site and cause as well as evaluate the competence of the ileocecal valve. A standard water-soluble contrast enema is another option for both diagnostic and occasionally even therapeutic purposes. Flexible endoscopy can assist in the diagnosis of the obstruction and permit biopsies to be collected for further investigation. Endoscopy can also allow for treatment such as detorsion of a sigmoid volvulus and insertion of stents in cases of malignant or benign obstruction. Basic blood analyses are also important in the initial workup. Electrolyte abnormalities can be diagnosed, which are important both as a cause for adynamic nonfunction and a consideration in the operative and perioperative care. Increased white blood cell counts and CRP, as well as increased lactate, base excess, and decreased pH, are all generally associated with a more severe state and can help guide the aggressiveness of treatment.

Treatment

The treatment of large bowel obstruction is tailored to the etiology of the obstruction, several of which are discussed in detail later in the chapter. Treatment options vary considerably depending on the cause of obstruction, suspicion of bowel ischemia, and impending perforation, as well as the patient's general condition and comorbidities. Patients who present with peritonitis, signs of perforation, or ischemic bowel should be taken immediately to surgery.

It is imperative to promptly relieve mechanical obstructions, particularly those with complete and closed-loop obstructions, before compromise of the blood supply results in necrosis and perforation. Patients who do not present with immediate, ominous signs can be managed according to the cause of obstruction. In patients with sigmoid volvulus, endoscopic decompression is often successful using either a rigid or flexible sigmoidoscope with placement of a rectal tube proximal to the point of torsion. If this is unsuccessful, patients require surgery with resection, colostomy, and Hartmann's procedure. If decompression is successful, elective sigmoid resection with primary anastomosis should be performed because of the high rate of recurrence. With cecal volvulus, primary resection and anastomosis can typically be performed unless the patient is at increased risk of anastomotic leak (e.g., nonviable bowel, sepsis, hypotension, and other conditions). Patients with obstruction as a result of active IBD will commonly respond initially to steroids. Paracolic abscesses can be drained percutaneously. Foreign bodies can usually be removed endoscopically. Fecal impaction is commonly relieved with a combination of stool softeners and laxatives from above and manual disimpaction at the bedside or in the operating room under anesthesia. Hernias causing mechanical large bowel obstruction usually require surgery. Adult colonic intussusceptions, in contrast to pediatric intussusceptions, are almost always associated with a pathologic lead point, such as a polyp, cancer, or Meckel or colonic diverticulum. A recent meta-analysis found malignancy as the causative factor in 36.9% of ileocolonic and 46.5% of colonic intussusceptions.[14,36] Most authors recommend surgical resection adhering to oncologic principles without reduction.

Patients with malignant obstruction of the low and midrectum usually require an initial diverting stoma to allow for neoadjuvant chemoradiation before definitive surgery. Colonic stents offer a nonsurgical intervention to manage obstructing colon cancer, enabling symptom relief and providing time for patient optimization and preoperative chemotherapy if needed. Particularly beneficial for high-risk surgical candidates, unfit patients, or those requiring palliation, they may also serve as a bridge to surgery, potentially enabling single-stage operations and stoma avoidance. However, complications such as stent migration, perforation, and reobstruction can occur. Trials and meta-analyses provide mixed results on morbidity, mortality, stoma rates, and long-term survival, indicating the need for case-by-case evaluation considering patient health, tumor location and stage, and available resources and expertise.[2] Surgical options include segmental resection with Hartmann's operation (end colostomy with internal closure of the rectal stump) or primary anastomosis with or without a diverting stoma. If the cecum is ischemic or nonviable, a subtotal colectomy is performed. In cases of right-sided obstruction, a right hemicolectomy is typically performed with primary anastomosis. Patients who are unstable with a high risk for anastomotic failure should undergo creation of a temporary diverting stoma or exteriorization of the anastomosis as a loop ileostomy.

COLONIC PSEUDOOBSTRUCTION

Acute colonic pseudoobstruction, also termed *Ogilvie syndrome*, was initially described by Sir William Heneage Ogilvie in 1948. It is characterized by acute colonic dilatation in the absence of a mechanical obstruction. Ogilvie syndrome is rare, with an estimated incidence of 100/100,000 admissions.[37] Dysregulation of the colonic autonomic innervation is hypothesized to play an important part. Several mechanisms have been implicated, including autonomic imbalance with a relative excess of sympathetic over parasympathetic activity, disrupted colonic reflex arcs, chronic disease, and medications.[37]

It is most commonly encountered among elderly and comorbid patients, classically after an acute illness on a background of neurologic, cardiac, or respiratory diseases. Common associated conditions are depicted in Table 95.2.

Diagnosis

The typical patient is elderly, has multiple comorbidities, and is hospitalized for an acute medical event or has undergone recent surgery (abdominal or nonabdominal). The presenting symptoms of the condition commonly include abdominal distention, pain, nausea, and vomiting. Obstipation is common, but some patients will have diarrhea as a result of hypersecretion of water. Lack of intestinal contractility is often associated with decreased or absent bowel sounds, but high-pitched, tinkling bowel sounds may also be encountered. Systemic toxicity and peritoneal signs

TABLE 95.2 Conditions Associated With Pseudoobstruction

CATEGORY	RISK FACTORS
Postsurgical	After major orthopedic and/or spinal surgery, solid organ transplants, cardiac procedures
Neurologic disease	Parkinson disease, Alzheimer disease, stroke, spinal cord injury
Cardiac	Congestive heart failure, myocardial infarction
Pulmonary	Chronic obstructive pulmonary disease
Trauma	Major trauma, shock, burns
Metabolic	Diabetes mellitus, renal failure, electrolyte disturbances
Infectious	Cytomegalovirus, varicella-zoster virus
Obstetric/ gynecologic	Cesarean section, normal and instrumental delivery
Miscellaneous	Lupus, scleroderma
Drugs	Opiates, chemotherapy, anti-Parkinson drugs, anticholinergics, antipsychotic drugs, clonidine

are uncommon and should raise suspicion of ischemia and perforation. Initial evaluation should include a complete blood count, serum electrolytes, renal function assessment, and diagnostic imaging. Plain abdominal radiographs typically demonstrate a distended colon, with the largest diameter usually encountered in the cecum and right colon, which can reach 10 to 12 cm in diameter (Fig. 95.31). Dilation and gas continuing all the way down to the distal rectum support the suspicion of pseudoobstruction in contrast to a mechanical obstruction, in which a paucity of gas is commonly encountered distal to the obstruction. A water-soluble contrast enema can reliably distinguish between a mechanical obstruction and pseudoobstruction. Currently, however, abdominal CT is typically used as the standard confirmatory test; it has the ability to commonly distinguish the type of obstruction and assess for signs of ischemia and impending perforation (Fig. 95.32). Abdominal tenderness, leukocytosis, fever, and cecal dilation of more than 12 cm are signs that may be indicative of colon ischemia, perforation, or impending perforation.

The differential diagnosis includes mechanical obstruction, toxic megacolon due to *C. difficile*, or toxic megacolon resulting from other causes.

Management

The treatment of colonic pseudoobstruction comprises a series of escalating interventions contingent on the degree of distention, risk for perforation, and the patient's response. Treatment options include supportive care, pharmacologic therapy (neostigmine), endoscopic decompression (colonoscopy), and surgery. A rectal tube can be used as an initial step to decompress the dilated colon, providing temporary relief while addressing the underlying cause. The insertion of a rectal tube can be done at the bedside, but it must be very carefully inserted to try to avoid injury to the rectal mucosa.

Nonoperative, supportive care is initiated for patients with a cecal diameter that is less than 12 cm without evidence of ischemia or perforation. This includes nothing by mouth (NPO); correction of electrolyte disturbances; and discontinuation of

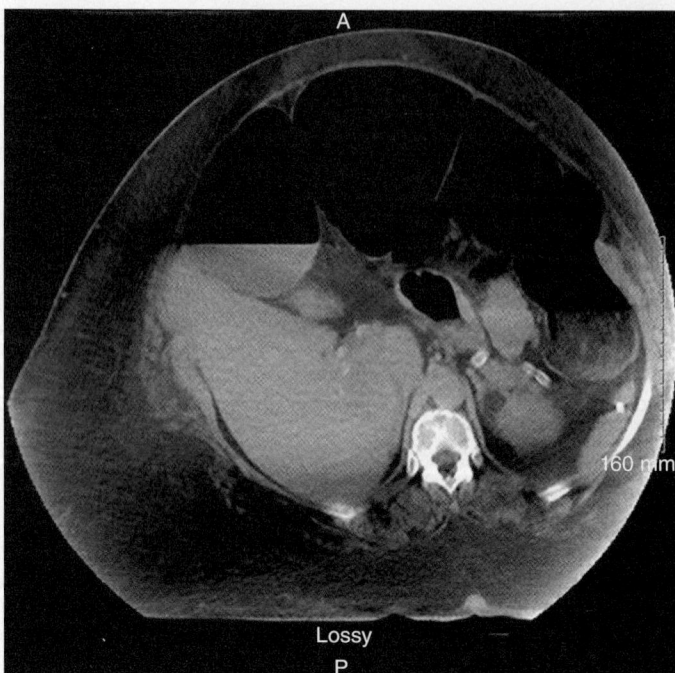

FIGURE 95.32 Computed tomography scan showing massively distended colon without sign of ischemic change.

medications that may be contributing, such as opiates, anticholinergics, anti-Parkinson agents, antidepressants, neuroleptics, clonidine, atropines, and antihypertensives. Insertion of a nasogastric tube and rectal tube for decompression may be of help. Osmotic and stimulant laxatives should be avoided because they can worsen colonic dilation. Ambulation, prone positioning, and knee-chest position to encourage passage of flatus can assist. Patients should be monitored with serial physical exams and abdominal x-rays to assess for response or deterioration. Ischemia or perforation of the colon is the most feared complication and has been reported in the range of 3% to 15% of cases, leading to an associated mortality rate of close to 50%. In cases that do not improve with supportive care or with a cecal diameter of more than 12 cm but without systemic toxicity and abdominal tenderness, colonic decompression is indicated.

Neostigmine is the keystone of pharmacologic decompression therapy. It is an acetylcholinesterase inhibitor that stimulates the muscarinic receptors and enhances colonic motor activity. Neostigmine is given as a 2- to 2.5-mg IV bolus injected over 3 to 5 minutes and results in significant parasympathetic stimulation, causing strong colonic peristalsis that usually leads to subsequent flatus and bowel movements. It has been found to be a safe and effective option for patients with acute colonic pseudoobstruction who have failed conservative management. Success rates for neostigmine treatment range from 60% to 94%, with recurrences observed in up to 31% of patients, with some patients requiring multiple drug administrations. Neostigmine is contraindicated in mechanical bowel obstruction and in patients with signs of ischemia or perforation. It should be used with caution among patients with asthma, chronic obstructive lung disease, bradycardia, and recent acute coronary syndrome and in those with renal failure. Neostigmine should be given in a monitored setting with atropine immediately available. Common side effects include vomiting, crampy abdominal pain, excessive salivation, and bradycardia. Colonoscopic decompression should be considered in

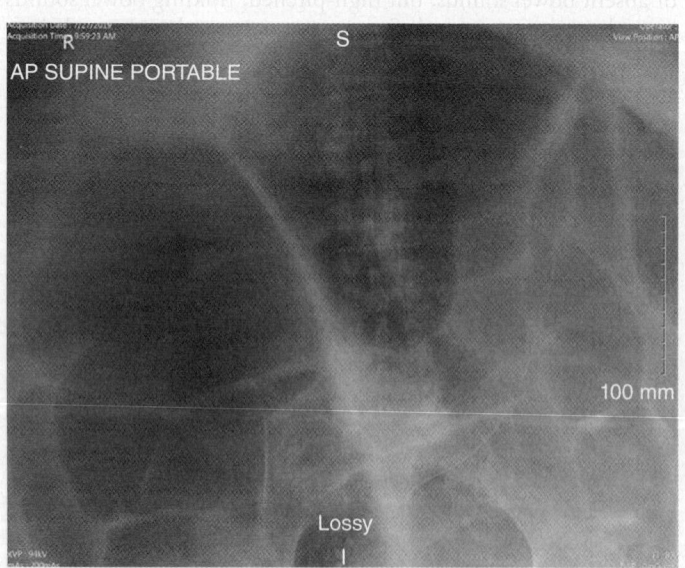

FIGURE 95.31 Massive transverse colon distention due to Ogilvie syndrome in a female with multiple comorbidities, including a body mass index of 69, severe pulmonary hypertension, and cardiac disease.

patients with contraindications to neostigmine or for those who are unresponsive to it. The aim of endoscopic decompression is to advance the scope to the right colon with minimal insufflation and use of narcotics and place a colonic decompression tube while removing as much gas as possible from the colon. Endoscopic decompression has a high success rate of 61% to 95% for initial decompression and 70% to 90% for sustained decompression. Colonoscopic perforation rates after decompression for pseudoobstruction are in the range of 1% to 3%.

Patients who do not respond to other lines of treatment or those who demonstrate signs of systemic toxicity, ischemia, or perforation require surgery. Surgical options are determined according to the condition of the colon and the patient. If the colon is viable, tube cecostomy or cecostomy can be performed, with high rates of success. For patients with signs of ischemia or perforation, a resection, usually with a diverting stoma, is recommended.

INFLAMMATORY BOWEL DISEASE

Epidemiology and Etiology

IBD, which includes both UC and Crohn disease, is largely a disease of the Western world. As Asian countries are adopting a more Western diet, the incidence of these disorders is increasing in these countries as well. The prevalence of IBD in Western countries is approximately 0.5% of the general population.[38] In the United States, over 1 million individuals are estimated to have IBD, with over 200,000 Canadians affected and 2.5 to 3 million individuals in Europe having these disorders.[38] The highest incidence of UC has been reported in Europe, followed by the United States, whereas for Crohn disease, the highest incidence was observed in the United States, followed by Europe. Europe was noted to have the highest prevalence of IBD. Over time, the incidence of both disorders appears to be increasing. Both disorders appear to have a genetic predisposition, with many contributing environmental factors. Over 10% of patients with IBD have a family history of IBD. To date, genome-wide association studies have linked to over 230 IBD susceptibility loci.[39] Cigarette smoking is the most studied environmental factor, having opposite effects in UC and Crohn disease. In UC, smoking tends to suppress symptoms, whereas in Crohn disease, smoking tends to exacerbate symptoms. Antibiotic use in early life has also been thought to predispose to IBD, as has NSAID use.

Disease Distribution and Classification

The extent of UC can also be graded with respect to the extent of inflammation within the colon. It can be limited only to the rectum and sigmoid colon (proctitis or proctosigmoiditis), restricted to the left side of the colon, or extended to involve the entire colon (pancolitis).

There are many classification schemes for Crohn disease. However, one of the most popular was initially the Vienna Classification, which was later updated to the Montreal Classification. With these classification schemes, patients are classified according to age of onset of disease, bowel location of their Crohn disease, and type of disease behavior. In addition to the different ages of onset, the Vienna Classification divided patients into whether or not they develop inflammatory Crohn disease at the age of 40 or later. The Montreal Classification subdivides this into less than 20 or greater than 20 years old. In addition, the Montreal Classification adds a further subdivision of whether the patients have perianal Crohn disease. The three different types of behavior classifications for Crohn disease that are possible include inflammatory Crohn disease, fibrostenotic Crohn disease, and fistulizing Crohn disease. Many people feel that these three types of disease behaviors represent different time points in the progression of disease. In other words, a patient is initially diagnosed with inflammatory Crohn disease, which, over time, progresses to fibrostenotic Crohn disease. This, in turn, will frequently progress to an obstruction, with perforation proximal to the obstruction and abscess formation. When this abscess spontaneously drains into an adjacent structure or organ, fistula formation ensues. In this manner, there is a progression from inflammatory to fibrostenosing to fistulizing Crohn disease. It is with this thought in mind that the progression to "top-down" medical therapy has evolved (see the section "Medications for Treatment of IBD"). The goal is to interrupt this natural progression or cycle in the course of Crohn disease to prevent the progressive fibrosis that results in many of the complications leading to surgery.

Clinical Presentation and Disease Diagnosis
Clinical Presentation

Clinical presentation of both diseases can be similar. Diarrhea can be a presenting symptom in both diseases; however, this is typically more prevalent and severe in UC, where the diarrhea is characteristically bloody. Significant hemorrhage is much more common with UC than with Crohn disease. Typical UC symptoms also include tenesmus and urgency as well as associated anemia. In Crohn disease, symptoms of abdominal pain may predominate. In any patient initially presenting with diarrhea, stool cultures should first be obtained to exclude the presence of infectious causes of diarrhea, such as *Salmonella, Giardia,* or community-acquired *C. difficile,* which is now increasingly seen. Patients with Crohn's disease may present with a palpable abdominal mass resulting from an intraabdominal abscess or have an external fistula. Roughly 25% of patients with Crohn disease will have associated perianal disease. This can include a variety of problems, including anal fissure, which, in contrast to patients without Crohn, is often not painful and may be multiple and/or in atypical locations (lateral and not posterior/anterior location). In addition, these patients can present with large anal skin tags (Fig. 95.33), which are not true external hemorrhoids. As a rule, these should not be excised because they may lead to very delayed wound healing. These patients may also present with anorectal abscesses, fistula(s) (Fig. 95.34), and anal stenosis. Digital rectal examination should always be performed.

Extraintestinal manifestations. Extraintestinal manifestations can occur in many IBD patients, and it is estimated that up to half of IBD patients will have one or more extraintestinal manifestations. Data suggest the prevalence of at least one joint, ocular, or skin extraintestinal manifestation to be 24% in all cases of IBD, 27% in UC, and 35% in Crohn disease. Arthritis is by far the most common extraintestinal manifestation. One of the most common manifestations is sacroiliitis. One of the most serious joint manifestations is ankylosing spondylitis, which runs a course independent of the bowel disease. These patients are HLA-B27 positive and may present in advanced cases with decreased cervical flexion, which has important anesthetic implications for intubation. These patients may require fiberoptic intubation and will require specific preoperative anesthesia evaluation.

Cutaneous extraintestinal manifestations include erythema nodosum and pyoderma gangrenosum. From the long experience of treating surgical patients with IBD, pyoderma is much more frequent than erythema nodosum. Erythema nodosum (Fig. 95.35) is characterized by red, painful, swollen nodules that can occur and

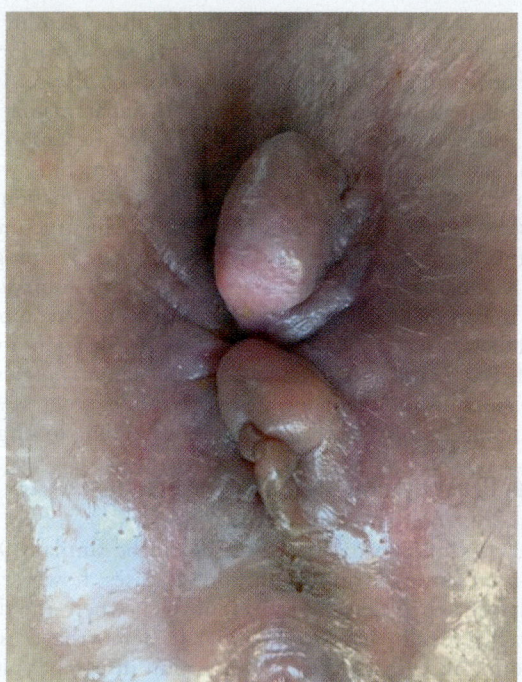

FIGURE 95.33 Large anal Crohn tags. Note the bluish coloring and waxy appearance of the perianal skin.

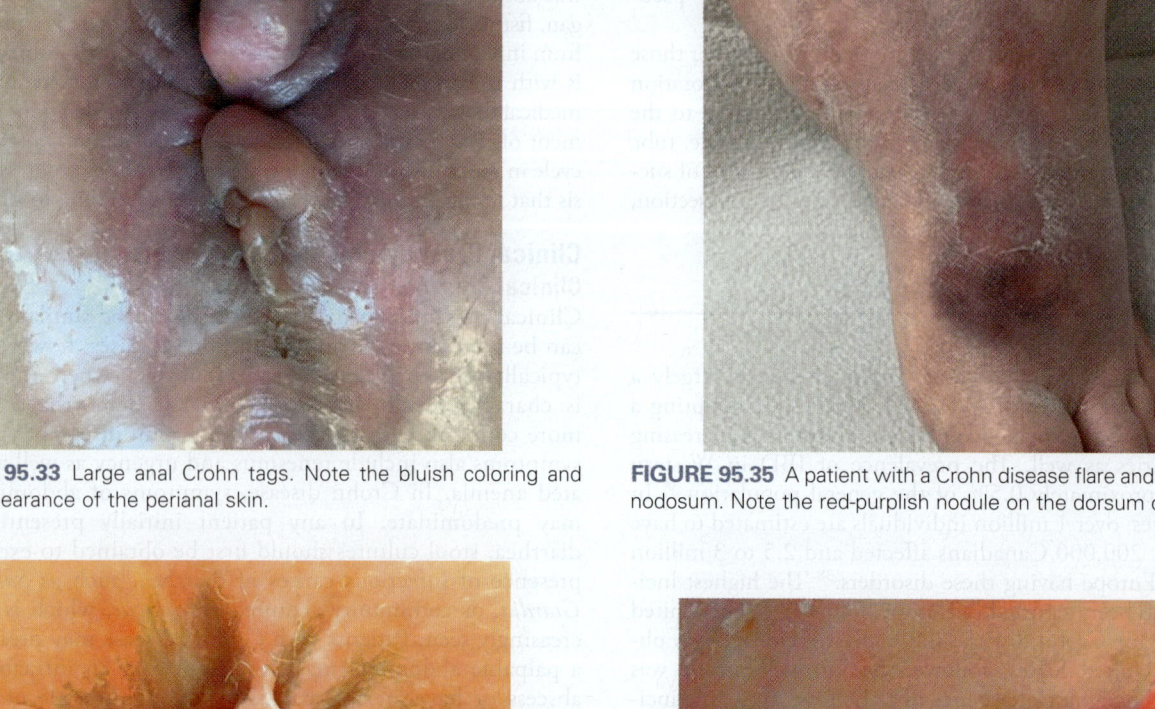

FIGURE 95.35 A patient with a Crohn disease flare and active erythema nodosum. Note the red-purplish nodule on the dorsum of the foot.

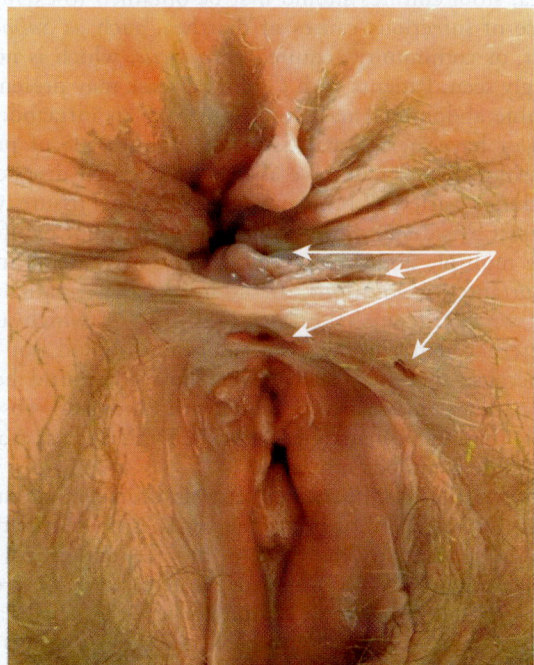

FIGURE 95.34 A female with significant fistulizing perianal Crohn disease. Note the multiple external fistula openings shown by the *white arrows*. These all had a common internal opening in the anterior midline, which was also associated with a rectovaginal fistula. This patient ultimately elected to undergo ileostomy diversion.

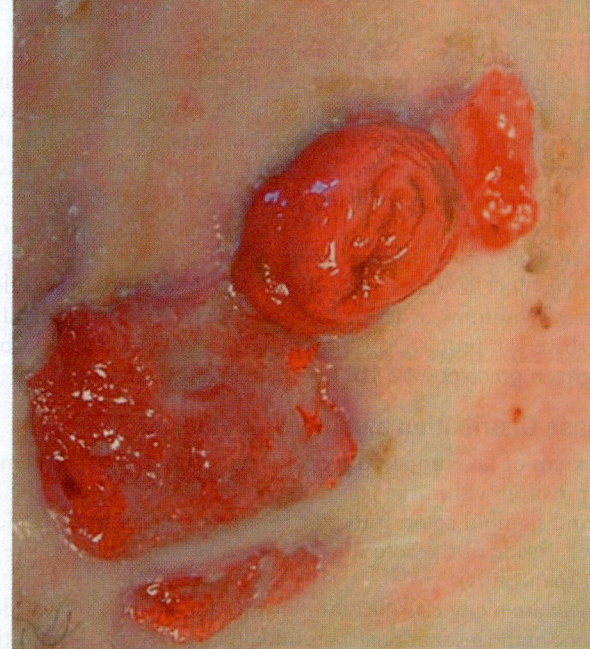

FIGURE 95.36 Pyoderma gangrenosum adjacent to an end ileostomy in a patient with Crohn disease. Here, the lesions have started to heal with granulation tissue.

usually will respond to systemic steroid administration, whereas pyoderma gangrenosum is characterized by typically extremely painful ulcerating lesions that frequently occur at sites of repeated trauma, such as in the vicinity of surgical incisions or, more frequently, around intestinal stomas (Fig. 95.36). There is a phenomenon called *pathergy*, which refers to a worsening of the pyoderma with any type of surgical manipulation or debridement. These lesions are therefore best treated by nonoperative means, which can include intralesional steroid injections (e.g., triamcinolone), topical (tacrolimus 0.1%), or systemic biologic therapy (anti–tumor necrosis factor

[TNF] antibodies or similar agents). Such treatment will typically result in symptom resolution.

Ocular manifestations of UC can include uveitis, iritis, and episcleritis. Some of these can lead to significant irritation and require referral to an ophthalmologist.

Sclerosing cholangitis is estimated to affect approximately 2.16% of patients with IBD. Pooled prevalence in patients with UC, Crohn disease, and IBD-unclassified is 2.47%, 0.96%, and 5%, respectively.[40] It has a course that is curiously independent of the IBD. At its worst, it can progress to cirrhosis, result in liver failure, and require hepatic transplantation. Patients with sclerosing cholangitis are at higher risk for developing colorectal neoplasia, as will be discussed later, and are also at higher risk of developing pouchitis, as will be discussed in the section on IPAA and surgical treatment.

Disease Diagnosis

Endoscopy. The diagnosis of IBD is usually made by endoscopy. This can be accomplished by either rigid proctoscopy, flexible sigmoidoscopy, or colonoscopy. Generally, a complete evaluation of the colon with colonoscopy is performed to both evaluate the extent of the disease and examine the terminal ileum.

With UC, inflammation begins at the level of the dentate line and extends proximally, whereas in Crohn disease, in many cases, the inflammation is patchier, and there can be discontinuous inflammation (skip), with areas of intervening normal-appearing mucosa. In some cases, differentiation between the two diseases can be difficult, both endoscopically and histologically. A typical endoscopic view of UC is shown in Fig. 95.37. Note the more roughened or granular appearance of the colonic mucosa. One of the most common scoring systems for endoscopic assessment of UC is the Mayo Clinic Scoring System, which grades the endoscopic findings based on the severity of the mucosal ulceration or the absence thereof. Grade 1 refers to a normal endoscopic appearance, grade 2 refers to slightly more erythematous, grade 3 refers to even more erythematous area with touch bleeding, and grade 4 refers to significant bleeding and friability. As the disease becomes more severe, there is an increasingly erythematous appearance of the mucosa with progressive mucosal ulceration.

With respect to endoscopy, Crohn disease is more characterized by deeper, punched-out-appearing ulcerations. In these cases, there are often longer serpiginous ulcerations covered with fibrin. These can oftentimes extend longitudinally along the lumen of the bowel, in which case they are sometimes referred to as *bear claw* ulcerations (Fig. 95.38). In many cases, Crohn disease ulcers are worse on the mesenteric side of the bowel. Regarding the distribution of Crohn disease, the most common site of involvement in nearly half of patients is ileocolic, followed by colonic involvement. Crohn disease can also affect the small bowel or upper GI tract.

Histologic evaluation. In UC, colonic mucosal biopsies will typically show significant inflammation with the presence of multiple polymorphonuclear leukocytes within the lamina propria. There may be depletion of mucin in goblet cells. One can also identify crypt abscesses, although this is somewhat of a nonspecific finding. As a rule, inflammation in UC is restricted to the surface epithelium (Fig. 95.39). The disease process is limited to the large intestine. Proximal colonic disease occurs in continuity with an involved rectum (no gross or histologic skip lesions). The inflammation is characterized by the absence of mural sinus tracts, deep fissural ulcers, and granulomas, as well as by the absence of transmural lymphoid aggregates in an area not deeply ulcerated.

In contrast, in patients with Crohn disease, there is often transmural inflammation, which is seen in histologic evaluation of resected specimens. In approximately one-third of patients, there are noncaseating granulomas (Fig. 95.40). In biopsy specimens, the diagnosis of Crohn disease is made in the presence of non-necrotizing granulomas or the presence of transmural lymphoid aggregates in an area not deeply ulcerated. In patients with Crohn disease, just as one can macroscopically see "skip" disease with patchy inflammation, the same is true on microscopic evaluation. The term *focal active enteritis* is used. The differential diagnosis frequently includes infectious colitis or drug-induced colitis, and pathology reports often include this differential diagnosis when areas are biopsied during GI endoscopy. In patients who are suspected of having Crohn disease, it is important to make an effort to intubate the terminal ileum because this is a common site of disease involvement.

IBD undetermined refers to a subset of patients who have overlapping characteristics of both Crohn disease and UC on endoscopic biopsy. It is thought that up to 10% to 15% of patients fall into this category. The diagnosis of **indeterminate colitis** is made in patients in whom there is uncertainty of the diagnosis on evaluation of the colectomy specimen because histologic features of both Crohn and UC are seen. Overall, this diagnosis is more likely in patients with fulminant disease, where the significant amount of inflammation interferes with precise disease diagnosis.

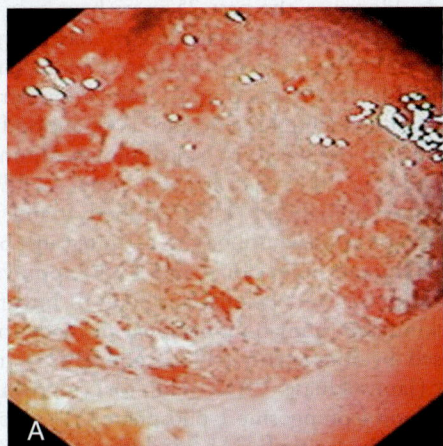
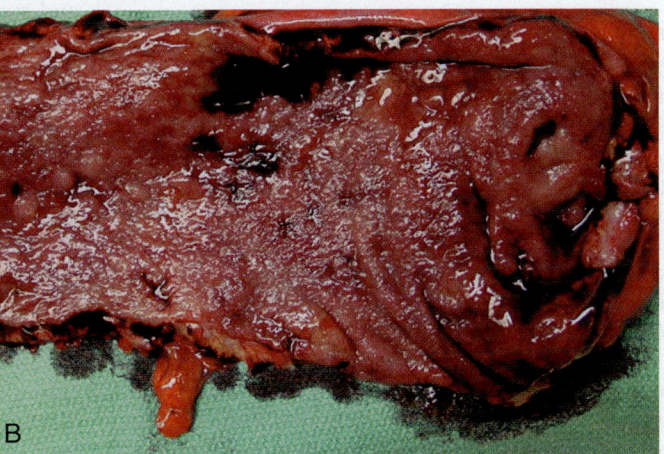

FIGURE 95.37 (A) Endoscopic view of moderately severe ulcerative colitis. Note the bleeding and ulceration. (B) Macroscopic view of right colon after total proctocolectomy for fulminant ulcerative colitis.

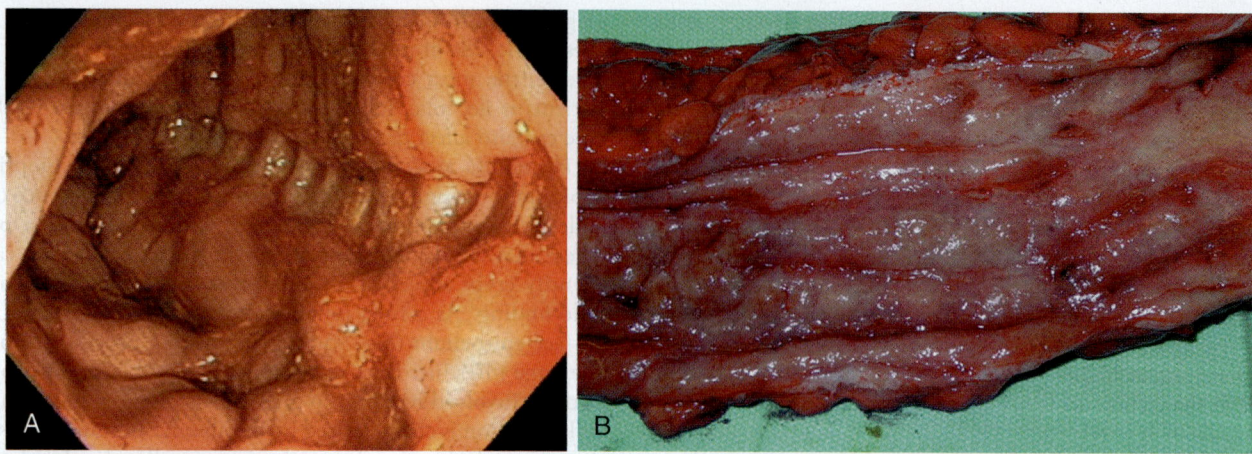

FIGURE 95.38 Bear claw ulcers in Crohn colitis. (A) Endoscopic view. (B) Macroscopic view.

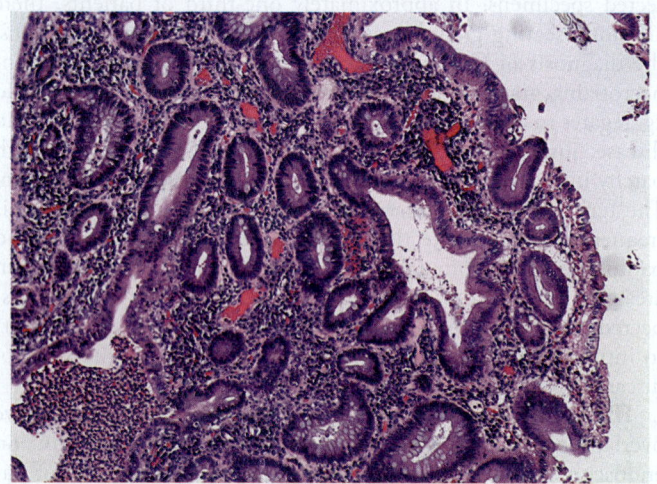

FIGURE 95.39 Histologic section of active ulcerative colitis. There is glandular architectural distortion manifested by irregular branching and orientation of glands relative to the surface. The lamina propria is expanded with inflammatory cells, and intraepithelial neutrophils are present. A crypt abscess is noted *(lower left)*. (Courtesy Dr. Jeffrey P. Baliff, Thomas Jefferson University, Philadelphia.)

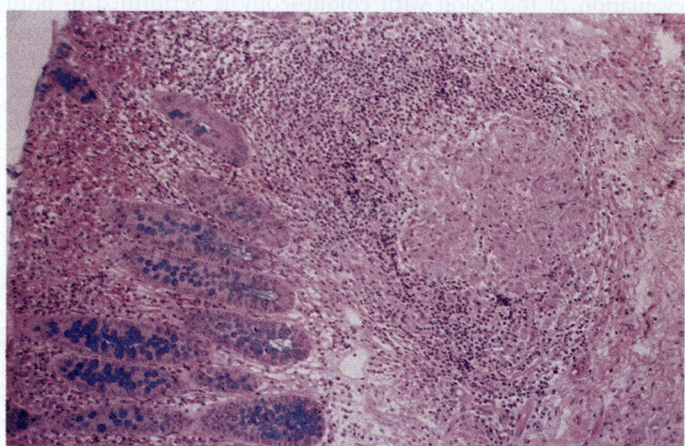

FIGURE 95.40 Crohn colitis with noncaseating granuloma.

Medical Treatment

Changing medical treatment philosophy. The past two decades have seen a tremendous change in medical treatment for IBD. There has been a gradual evolution from a *bottom-up* approach to what is termed a *top-down* approach. The bottom-up approach begins with the safest, least expensive medications first and only proceeds to the more potent, more expensive medications with a higher side-effect profile once these have failed. This treatment approach has been largely replaced by the top-down approach, whereby patients are initially treated with the stronger, more potent medications, which may, in turn, have a greater side-effect profile and are associated with higher costs. Many of these drugs have been implicated in the higher rate of postoperative complications in patients undergoing surgery, and their use has also been associated with reactivation of certain remote infections. It is important for the surgeon to be aware of these medications and knowledgeable about their mechanism of action. Table 95.3

lists some of the medications more commonly used in the treatment of IBD. The surgeon will find that these medications are being used increasingly not only in patients with IBD but also in patients with rheumatoid arthritis and psoriasis. Medical therapy formerly was based largely on medications such as sulfasalazine and steroids. However, the past 25 years have seen a revolution with the introduction of "biologic therapy," based largely on treatment with antibodies directed against TNF-α (anti–TNF-α). This began with the US Food and Drug Administration (FDA) approval for infliximab (chimeric anti-TNF antibody) for Crohn disease in 1998; followed by adalimumab (humanized anti-TNF antibody) in 2007; certolizumab pegol (a PEGylated Fab' fragment of a humanized TNF antibody) and natalizumab (humanized monoclonal antibody to α4-integrin), both in 2008; golimumab (human monoclonal anti-TNF) approval for UC in 2013; vedolizumab (monoclonal antibody to integrin α4β7) in 2014; ustekinumab (human monoclonal antibody to p40 protein subunit used by interleukin [IL]-12 and IL-23) in 2016; and tofacitinib (Janus kinase [JAK] inhibitor) approval for UC in 2018, ozanimod (sphingosine 1-phosphate [S1P] receptor modulator) in 2021, upadacitinib (JAK inhibitior) in 2023 and risankizumab (human monoclonal antibody binding the p19 subunit of IL-23) in 2024. Currently, there is a wide assortment of drugs to

TABLE 95.3	Different Types of Medical Treatment Used for Inflammatory Bowel Disease		
DRUG CLASS	**EXAMPLES**	**INDICATION**	**ADMINISTRATION**
Biologics	Infliximab	UC, CD	IV
	Adalimumab	UC, CD	SC
	Cetrolizumab	CD	SC
	Golimumab	UC	IV
	Natalizumab	UC, CD	IV
	Risankisumab	UC	SC
	Upadacitinib	UC	PO
	Ozanimod	UC	PO
	Vedolizumab	UC, CD	IV
	Ustekinumab	UC, CD	IV, SC
Antiinflammatory	Sulfasalazine	UC, CD	PO
	Mesalamine	UC, CD	PO, enema, suppository
Immunosuppressives	Conventional steroids	UC, CD	PO, IV, suppository
	Budesonide	UC, CD	PO, rectal foam
	Antimetabolites	UC, CD	PO
	Tofacitinib	UC	PO
Probiotics	*Lactobacillus*	UC, CD	Food, tablets, capsules, powders
	Bifidobacterium		
Antibiotics	Ciprofloxacin	UC, CD	PO, IV
	Metronidazole	UC, CD	PO, IV
	Rifaximin	Off-label	PO

CD, Crohn disease; *IV*, intravenous; *PO*, per os; *SC*, subcutaneous; *UC*, ulcerative colitis.

choose from. There has also been a change in the philosophy of treatment with respect to IBD.

Medications for treatment of IBD

Aminosalicylates. Sulfasalazine has long been used for the treatment of colonic IBD. Originally used as a treatment for arthritis, it was noted that many arthritis patients with coexisting IBD noted an improvement in the latter when taking this medication. Use of this drug was limited by its sulfapyridine ring, which excludes use in patients with sulfa allergies. When this medication is used, patients require folic acid supplementation. Eventually, the sulfapyridine ring is cleaved, leaving the active 5-aminosalicylate (5-ASA) moiety. Pharmacologists rapidly realized that depending on how this drug was formulated, its delivery could be targeted to different portions of the GI tract. For example, mesalamine (Pentasa) begins to dissolve in the stomach and releases drug throughout the GI tract, whereas Asacol begins to be released in the terminal ileum by means of a pH-dependent mechanism and coats the entire colon. Drugs manufactured with an "MMX technology" are designed as once-a-day preparations and formulated so that they slowly dissolve, thus releasing medication throughout the colon. For this reason, they are thought to have greater patient compliance. There are also topical formulations of these medications for distal disease. Suppository formulations are administered at bedtime. While the patient sleeps, the suppositories melt and coat the rectum with mesalamine, which has a very potent antiinflammatory effect. The most popular brand of suppository is Canasa. The same medication in small-volume enema form (Rowasa enemas) can also be administered at bedtime. The patient is advised to lie on their left side, allowing the small volume of fluid to be delivered not only to the rectum but also the sigmoid and, in some cases, the left colon. These medications are most effective for mild to moderate disease.

Corticosteroids. If the patient has severe disease, steroids still play a prominent role in the treatment of IBD. Although they have numerous side effects, they are inexpensive, act quickly, and are

readily available, not requiring lengthy insurance preauthorizations as with the more expensive biologic medication alternatives. The recognized side effects of steroids include:

- Cushingoid appearance that is very unpopular, particularly among young patients
- Feared complication of aseptic necrosis of the hips
- Hypertension
- Mood changes that can escalate up to actual psychiatric conditions
- Hyperglycemia
- Increased risk of infectious complications after surgery
- Cataract formation
- Striae and others

Because of these complications, as well as the growth retardation seen when these drugs are used for prolonged periods in children, these medications should be used sparingly for as short a period as possible. Steroids are usually started at a high dose and then tapered quickly. Their main uses are either in the outpatient setting in the form of pulse therapy, as high doses that are tapered quickly, or intravenously in patients who are hospitalized with flares of their disease. In the outpatient setting, pulse therapy is usually given in the form of prednisone at doses starting at 40 to 60 mg/day, tapering by 5 to 10 mg at 2-week intervals until 10 mg/day is reached and then tapering by 5 mg every 2 weeks, at which time the drug is discontinued. In the hospital setting, 100 mg of hydrocortisone can be given intravenously every 6 to 8 hours, depending on disease severity.

Immunomodulators

Thiopurines. Thiopurines are a "steroid-sparing" class of medication that are usually begun once patients are placed on steroids and perhaps have been unsuccessful in weaning off steroids after one or two attempts at pulse therapy. Thiopurines have been used for many decades in the treatment of Crohn disease and have long been used in the organ transplant population. Two drugs fall into this category: azathioprine and its metabolite 6-mercaptopurine. The side effects of this therapy include leukopenia and pancreatitis. These side effects are largely seen in individuals who are homozygous for a variant of the enzyme thiopurine methyltransferase, which is responsible for metabolizing these drugs poorly. For this reason, many physicians now routinely perform thiopurine methyltransferase genotyping of patients to see whether they will be able to metabolize these drugs properly before initiating thiopurine treatment. These drugs have several advantages in that they are readily available and are an oral medication taken once a day, and dosing is based on body weight. On the downside, once a patient begins therapy, there is usually a 3- to 4-month lag time until these medications exert their therapeutic effect. For this reason, these medications cannot be used to treat a flare. Long-term thiopurine use is also associated with a higher risk of developing non-Hodgkin lymphoma compared with the general population.

Methotrexate. Methotrexate is another commonly used immunosuppressive for the treatment of IBD. This medication, which has long been used, particularly in the treatment of patients with arthritis, can be dosed either orally or intramuscularly. Intramuscular dosing is particularly convenient in patients who have problems with significant diarrhea or absorption issues (e.g., short bowel syndrome). The side effects of methotrexate include elevations in liver function tests, as well as pulmonary fibrosis. When methotrexate is given, patients require folic acid supplementation.

Biologics in the Treatment of Inflammatory Bowel Disease

The term *biologics* as it pertains to drugs used for IBD initially referred to monoclonal antibodies.[41] The first such agent, infliximab, a targeted therapy against TNF-alpha, was approved by the FDA for use in 1998. Since then, there has been a continued increase in both the number and type (based on mechanism of action) of medications that have been approved (see Table 95.3). The side effects of these drugs include reactivation of infections, including tuberculosis, histoplasmosis, actinomycosis, and hepatitis. For this reason, a careful patient history regarding these infections should be taken before consideration of treatment. In addition, before starting these drugs, the patient should either have a tuberculin skin test or undergo testing with QuantiFERON gold assay, and a hepatitis profile should be obtained. There is currently no accurate test for past exposure to histoplasmosis. In addition, these types of agents, similar to the thiopurines, can be associated with a higher risk of developing non-Hodgkin lymphoma compared with the general population. In addition, anti–TNF-α antibody has been associated with a low risk of hepatosplenic T-cell lymphomas, particularly in young males who have been taking anti-TNF antibody therapy in combination with other immunosuppressive therapy, such as a thiopurine.

In the past decade, new therapies have emerged as alternatives to traditional anti-TNF medications, including (JAK inhibitors, anti-α4 integrins, and anti-ILs). Commonly known JAK inhibitors include tofacitinib and upadacitinib. These drugs target the JAK-STAT signaling pathway, which plays a pivotal role in immune cell function and inflammatory responses. By inhibiting JAK enzymes, these medications modulate the immune response, offering relief from inflammation. Another class of drugs, the anti-α4 integrins, such as vedolizumab, specifically target cell adhesion molecules involved in leukocyte migration to the inflamed gut tissue, thereby reducing gut-specific inflammation without compromising systemic immunity. Lastly, anti-IL agents, which include such drugs as ustekinumab and risankizumab,

target specific interleukins, namely, IL-12 and IL-23. These cytokines are involved in cell signaling of immune responses, and by inhibiting their action, anti-IL agents help modulate the immune response and reduce inflammation in IBD.

Assessment of Symptom Severity

The Truelove and Witts is a popular classification scheme that characterizes patients by the severity of their diarrhea and the presence of blood in stool, fever, tachycardia, anemia, or an elevated erythrocyte sedimentation rate. Many similar classification schemes are used, in addition to analyzing stool samples for either fecal calprotectin or lactoferrin, which can be used as an inflammatory marker to assess disease activity. With Crohn disease, both the Crohn's Disease Activity Index (CDAI) and the Harvey Bradshaw Index have been used to quantitate symptoms.[42] The CDAI is made up of eight clinical and laboratory variables, including the number of bowel movements per day, the presence of abdominal pain, hematocrit, and weight loss. A score of less than 150 indicates clinical remission, and a score of more than 450 denotes severe disease. Because the CDAI requires a 7-day patient symptom diary, the Harvey-Bradshaw Index was proposed as a modification of this scheme that only uses clinical data.

Indications for Surgery for Ulcerative Colitis

There are several indications for surgery for UC, the foremost of which is failure to respond to maximum medical therapy. The frequency of surgery for UC has actually decreased over the last several decades with the improvement in efficacy and the number of new and more effective medical options, such as the entire class of biologic therapies. However, despite these new therapies, patients still present with a failure to respond. Patients falling into this category include those patients who have severe disease, namely, those patients with multiple bowel movements, poor nutritional status, "failure to thrive," and a need for surgery in order to regain their good physical health. These patients have a very poor quality of life with urgency, tenesmus, and low body weight; surgery represents a significant improvement in the quality of life. The second group of patients failing to respond to maximum medical therapy includes patients with fulminant colitis. These patients have such severe disease that they need to be hospitalized and placed on IV steroids. In some cases, they have received in-hospital biologic therapy; in rare cases, these patients may be receiving IV cyclosporine as an attempt to avert colectomy. In these patients with fulminant colitis, toxic megacolon may be present (Fig. 95.41). Fulminant colitis has been arbitrarily defined as having three or more of the following criteria present: tachycardia greater than 100, leukocytosis greater than $12,000/dL^3$, hypoalbuminemia less than 3 g/dL^3, a temperature greater than 38°C, or a diameter of the transverse colon greater than 5 cm on a plain abdominal radiograph. Three or more of these criteria meet the definition of toxic megacolon; note that a "megacolon" does not need to be present in order to meet this definition. Thus, the definition of toxic megacolon merely refers to a patient who is septic as a result of very severe colitis. Toxic megacolon can be present not only from severe UC but also from severe Crohn colitis or severe infectious or ischemic colitis. When the colitis is severe enough, it is associated with a significant colonic ileus, and in these cases, the colon becomes dilated, and there is a significant risk of colonic perforation. The next category of indication for surgery occurs in patients in whom there is significant GI bleeding. Recalling basic anatomy, the vessels located underneath the colonic vessels are located underneath the mucosa. If the mucosa

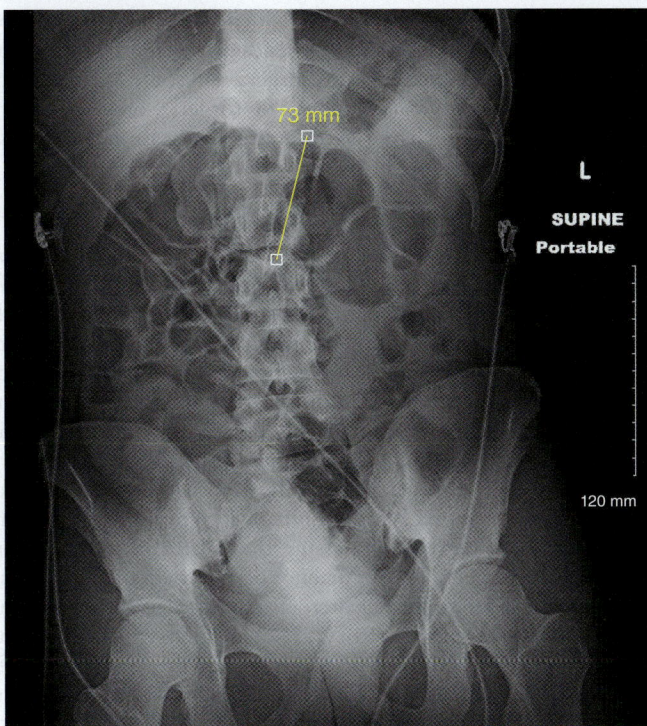

FIGURE 95.41 Toxic megacolon. Abdominal film shows significant distention of the transverse colon in a 20-year-old male with toxic megacolon. (From Rojas-Khalil Y, Galandiuk S. Management of chronic ulcerative colitis. In: Cameron JL, Cameron A, eds. *Current Surgical Therapy.* 13th ed. Philadelphia: Elsevier; in press.)

sloughs, this will, in effect, expose the underlying blood vessels of the colon and can result in massive GI hemorrhage if an ulcer erodes into these vessels. Significant hemorrhage can be one of the reasons for urgent surgery with UC, although the frequency of this complication has decreased over time. Another indication for surgery in children with UC is failure to grow, which is also an

indication for surgery in patients with Crohn disease. The presence of dysplasia or cancer is also an indication for surgery. Patients with longstanding UC (>8 years) have a high risk of developing dysplasia or cancer, as do those who have sclerosing cholangitis. Once the disease has been present longer than 8 years, patients are advised to undergo regular (yearly) colonoscopic surveillance with or without chromoendoscopy. If multiple areas of low-grade dysplasia or areas of high-grade dysplasia (Fig. 95.42) are found, a colectomy is recommended to prevent the development of invasive adenocarcinoma. The finding of colonic dysplasia in patients with longstanding UC is an indication for surgery that has undergone significant change over the last 20 years. Whereas past reports estimated a 2%, 8%, and 18% cumulative risk of CRC at 10, 20, and 30 years post-UC diagnosis, respectively, recent meta-analyses suggest a reduced cumulative risk of 1%, 3%, and 7%, respectively, at the same intervals.[43] There is currently somewhat of a controversy as to exactly who requires surgery and who requires continued observation with close surveillance. The current guidelines from the ASCRS published in 2021 state that patients with visible polypoid or nonpolypoid dysplasia that is completely excised endoscopically should undergo endoscopic surveillance. Patients with visible dysplasia not amenable to endoscopic excision, invisible dysplasia in the flat mucosa surrounding a visible dysplastic lesion, or colorectal adenocarcinoma should typically undergo total proctocolectomy with or without IPAA. The changes in the management strategy for dysplasia in UC patients depend on the visibility of the dysplasia and the complete excision of visible lesions. Endoscopic excision is preferred when expertise is available, with en bloc removal favored for thorough histologic evaluation. After dysplasia identification, patients face a heightened risk of recurrent dysplasia, necessitating close endoscopic surveillance. In certain scenarios, total proctocolectomy is recommended because of the increased risk of CRC.

The current guidelines recommend referral of patients with invisible dysplasia (detected with random biopsies) to an experienced endoscopist for repeat endoscopy using high-definition

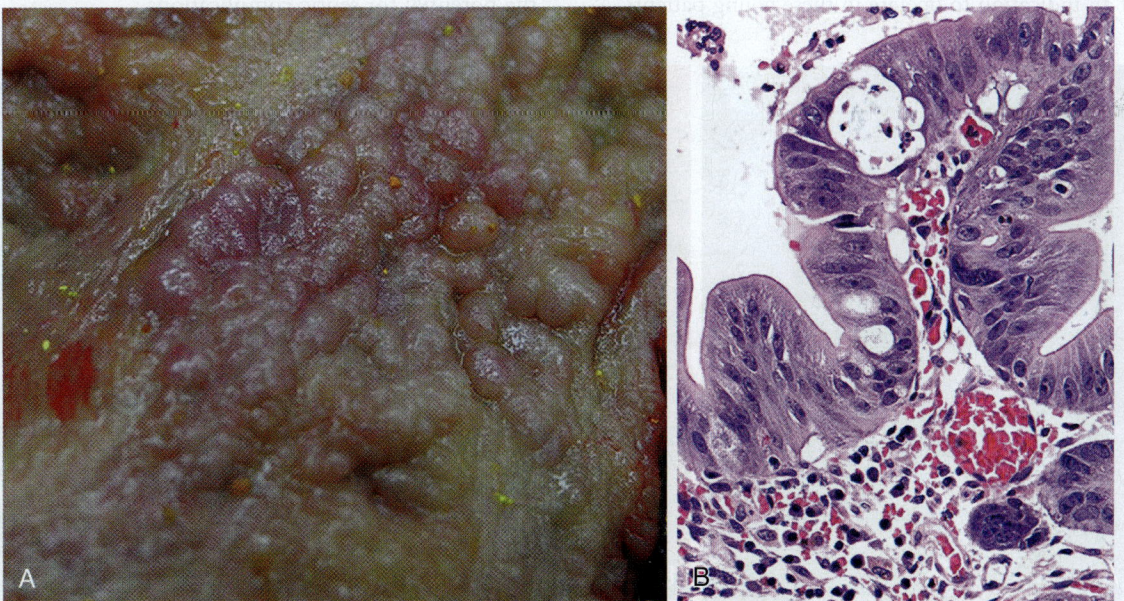

FIGURE 95.42 (A) A dysplasia-associated lesion or mass (DALM) in a patient with long-standing ulcerative colitis and sclerosing cholangitis. (B) High-grade dysplasia within a DALM in a patient with long-standing ulcerative colitis and sclerosing cholangitis.

colonoscopy with chromoendoscopy, with targeted and repeat random biopsies within 3 to 6 months. Patients confirmed to have invisible multifocal, low-grade dysplasia or any invisible high-grade dysplasia should typically be considered for total proctocolectomy.[44] Much of this has arisen as a result of the development of high-definition colonoscopy, as well as the development of techniques of surveillance such as chromoendoscopy. Chromoendoscopy involves the performance of colonoscopy with the spraying of dyes, such as methylene blue or indigo carmine, onto the colonic mucosa at the time of colonoscopy to highlight areas suspicious for dysplasia to permit targeted biopsies rather than just performing the random biopsies that were previously the standard of care. In addition to this, there has been recognition that there are different types of dysplasia. The flat dysplasia that is difficult to detect and blends in with the surrounding mucosa is very different from the "polypoid" dysplasia that is apparent and can be treated in many cases like a polyp and removed using techniques similar to those used for removal of a conventional polyp during colonoscopy. In some studies, patients with UC have undergone "polypectomy" removal of dysplastic lesions and have been followed long term without interval development of cancer.[45] What is important to stress is that patients must have very close follow-up colonoscopy and that meticulous colonoscopy and pathology expertise are vital to this process, as is excellent patient compliance. If any one of these three factors is lacking, this is clearly not a viable treatment alternative. There is, however, still agreement that if there are multiple areas of flat dysplasia within the colon, colectomy is indicated. There is still much to be learned regarding the actual risk of cancer in patients with IBD. Overall, it is felt that approximately one-fifth of the world's cancers arise in the setting of chronic inflammation. This mirrors the problem with hepatitis, anal cancer, gastric cancer, and many others. With the advent of better medications and interruption in this chronic cycle of inflammation, it will be interesting to see whether the incidence of cancer and IBD begins to decline compared with historical data. The same is true regarding the indication for failure to grow in children. As more effective medications are identified and are able to be instituted at earlier ages, it is anticipated that there will be less of an indication to operate in these young patients.

Similarly, if an adenocarcinoma is identified, colectomy is indicated. In certain patients, the presence of severe extraintestinal disease is also an indication for surgery. In some cases, severe extraintestinal disease will respond to surgery; however, there are some cases in which the extraintestinal disease has a course relatively independent of the colon.

Indications for Surgery for Crohn Disease

Unlike indications for surgery for UC, indications for surgery for Crohn disease are generally reserved for complications of the disease. Similar to UC, surgery is also performed in children with Crohn disease when they show failure to grow. In addition, surgery is frequently performed for symptoms of obstruction secondary to fibrostenosing Crohn disease (Fig. 95.43). In addition, if patients have a perforating Crohn disease associated with abscess or fistula, surgery may be indicated. The presence of many types of fistulas is also a relative indication for surgery. For example, the presence of a symptomatic ileal sigmoid fistula resulting in significant diarrhea bypassing the entire colon can be an indication for surgery. The occurrence of enterocutaneous fistulas is an indication for surgery. Enteroenteric fistulae are not an indication for surgery unless they are associated with significant symptoms of obstruction or discomfort. The presence of significant abdominal pain associated with obstruction is considered an indication for surgery. Patients with Crohn disease who have associated cancer or dysplasia, as with patients with UC, are an indication for surgery. In patients with UC, areas of dysplasia in the colon can be multifocal, and for this reason, if this occurs in the colon, a total proctocolectomy is considered preferable to a segmental resection.

Optimizing patients with Crohn disease before surgery plays a pivotal role in enhancing postoperative results. Antibiotics are often administered to control any active infection or abscess, as well as to decrease intestinal bacterial load, leading to a reduction in postoperative infection rates. In the event of an abscess formation, percutaneous drainage under radiologic guidance typically acts as the first-line treatment, helping manage the infection and bolstering the patient's condition presurgery, thereby minimizing the potential for septic complications.

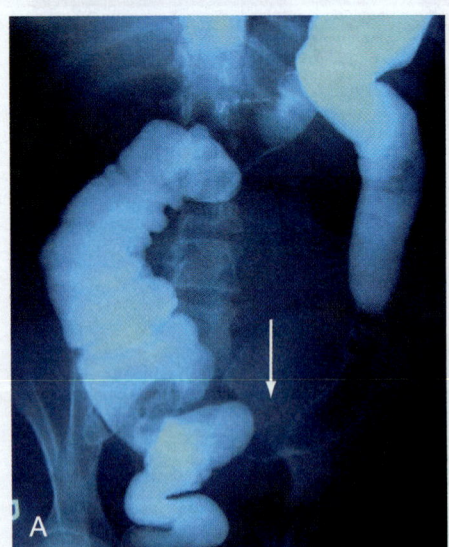
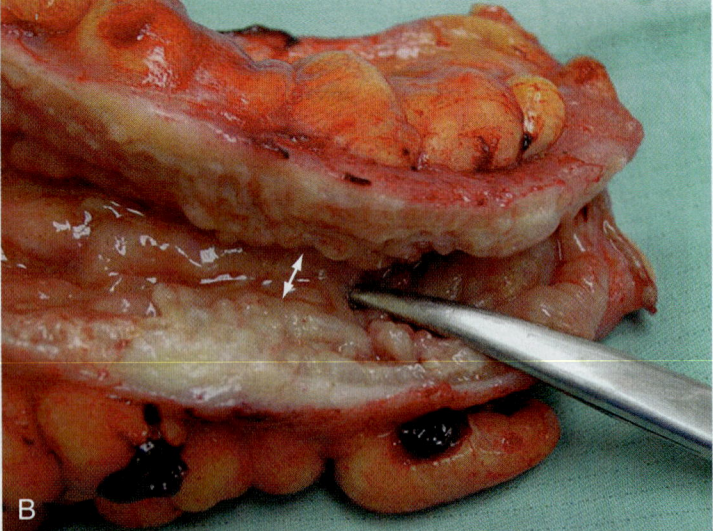

FIGURE 95.43 (A) Gastrografin enema showing significant stricture *(arrow)* of sigmoid colon secondary to Crohn disease. (B) Segmental colonic resection for fibrostenotic disease. Note the significant wall thickening and narrowed lumen *(arrow)* and its size compared with the tip of the scissors.

Malnutrition, a frequent issue with Crohn disease resulting from malabsorption and active disease, necessitates preoperative nutritional support. Both enteral and parenteral nutrition can boost nutritional status presurgery, promoting wound healing, immune function, and overall patient outcomes. Biologic agents and corticosteroids often used for Crohn disease management may increase postoperative complication risks, necessitating careful preoperative management. Biologics usually need to be discontinued for a period before surgery, whereas a gradual tapering is recommended for corticosteroids to avoid adrenal insufficiency. Lastly, patients with Crohn disease, and even more so in patients with UC, as a result of inflammation-induced hypercoagulability, are at elevated risk for DVT. Hence, DVT prophylaxis should be started before surgery to mitigate this risk. This multifaceted preoperative care requires careful management tailored to the patient's specific clinical scenario, involving a multidisciplinary team encompassing gastroenterologists, surgeons, radiologists, and dietitians.[46]

Surgical Options for Ulcerative Colitis

There are several operations that are currently performed for UC. These possibilities include subtotal colectomy, ileostomy, and Hartmann's procedure, frequently performed for fulminant disease. Total proctocolectomy with end ileostomy and proctocolectomy with either stapled or hand-sewn IPAA are commonly performed in the elective setting. Subtotal colectomy and ileal rectal anastomosis and total proctocolectomy with continent ileostomy are less commonly performed procedures. We discuss these in order next.

Subtotal/Total Colectomy With End Ileostomy

Subtotal/total colectomy and ileostomy and Hartmann's procedure is the treatment for patients with fulminant colitis not responding to maximal medical therapy. The term *toxic megacolon* has long been used to refer to a condition arising when patients become toxic from colitis irrespective of its etiology (e.g., whether this be UC, Crohn colitis, infectious, or ischemic). In any of these conditions, as the mucosa sloughs, the endotoxins within the bowel lumen are absorbed, leading to a septic state characterized by leukocytosis, tachycardia, fever, and in severe cases, hemodynamic instability. Many of these patients have protein-losing enteropathy and have associated hypoalbuminemia. If the colitis is severe enough to have an associated colonic ileus, this is apparent on an abdominal film with an increased diameter of the transverse colon (>5 cm). The definition of toxic megacolon is made when any three of these five factors are present. It is important to realize that a patient can have toxic megacolon without having a "megacolon" (specifically, patients can be "toxic" or septic from their colitis). When patients begin exhibiting symptoms of toxic megacolon, prompt surgery is indicated in order to prevent colonic perforation. With the improved medical therapy, this clinical scenario is becoming less common. In performing this operation, whether performed open or in a minimally invasive fashion, it is important to be gentle with the colon because ordinary manipulation can result in perforation. If the colon is very dilated and there is loss of domain, the procedure may not be able to be safely performed in a minimally invasive fashion. One of the common complications of this procedure postoperatively is a "blowout" of the Hartmann stump, resulting in a pelvic abscess. This complication can often be avoided simply by leaving a long Hartmann stump and incorporating this into the fascial closure of the midline abdominal laparotomy

wound or the specimen extraction site, depending on whether it is an open or minimally invasive procedure, and closing the incision over this. In this manner, if the stump dehisces and a wound infection develops, the wound is opened, and there is a controlled mucous fistula rather than a deep pelvic infection. Once the patient has stabilized and been weaned off immunosuppressant medications, usually after a period of 3 months, another procedure for restoration of intestinal continuity can be performed. It is important to realize that although the mid- and distal sigmoid colon may be delivered as a mucus fistula, the rectum cannot, for anatomic reasons, be extracorporealized and matured in this fashion.

Total Colectomy and Ileorectal Anastomosis

The option of ileal rectal anastomosis for the treatment of UC avoids complications of pelvic dissection, such as disturbances of sexual function in males and reduced fertility seen in females, because there is no pelvic dissection. The key to good function after this operation is proper patient selection. Patients with limited rectal involvement do best; however, that is uncommon in UC, where the worst disease is usually located distally. In addition, because the patient retains the rectum with this procedure, these patients need to undergo continued surveillance for dysplasia because they have an increased risk of cancer in the retained rectum over time.

Ileal Pouch–Anal Anastomosis

IPAA has become the most popular procedure for UC not responding to medical therapy as well as for patients requiring colectomy for the presence of dysplasia. It has several advantages over ileal-rectal anastomosis in that it removes the entire colon as well as the majority of the at-risk mucosa, depending on how the operation is performed (including stapled or hand-sewn anastomosis). IPAA was described in the mid- to late-1970s and involves removing the entire colon and the majority of the rectum. It has two essential components: proctocolectomy and creation of a small bowel reservoir using the terminal ileum. This reservoir is then either sewn or sutured to the anal canal or lower rectum. Many different configurations of pouches or reservoirs have been proposed in the past, including S pouches, W pouches, and H pouches, all with relative advantages and disadvantages. However, by far, the simplest and easiest pouch and the one with the least complications is the J pouch, which has withstood the test of time. This is created using 15-cm limbs of terminal ileum and two firings of a GIA stapler, preferably with a large caliber of 100 mm (Fig. 95.44). The apex of this J pouch is then either stapled to the distal rectum, leaving a very short rectal cuff (Fig. 95.45), or hand-sewn to the distal rectum after a 2-cm mucosectomy is performed (Fig. 95.46). Currently, the stapled approach is preferred simply because it provides superior continence and is much quicker to perform. However, in cases of dysplasia or cancer, hand-sewn approaches may still be warranted.

IPAA generally yields good functional results in patients with UC. Because many patients who are undergoing this operation are on immunosuppressives at the time of surgery or in a poor nutritional state, this operation is commonly performed with temporary fecal diversion (temporary loop ileostomy). This is in place for 2 to 3 months, during which these immunosuppressant medications are weaned and the patient regains their normal nutritional state. The temporary ileostomy can then be closed, typically without requiring a laparotomy. In patients who are *not* on immune suppression and in a good nutritional state (this usually

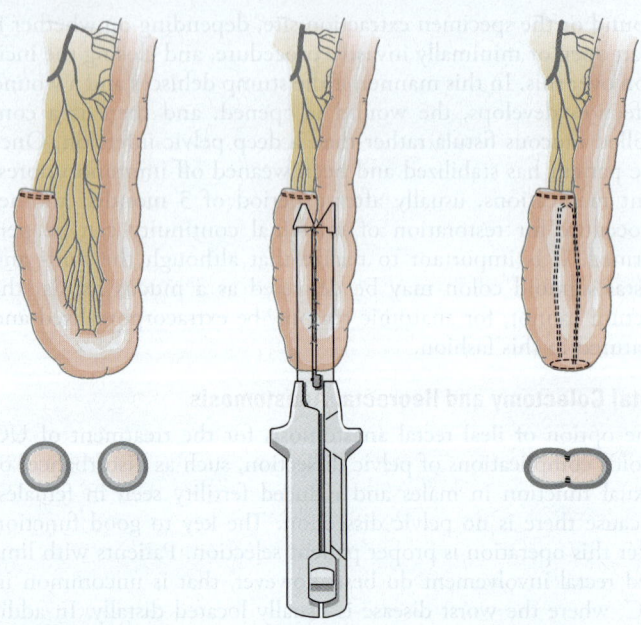

FIGURE 95.44 Creation of an ileal J pouch using a cutting linear stapler. For replacement of the rectum, a reservoir is created from the distal ileum. The stapler joins two limbs of intestine with staples while dividing the intervening wall. The diameter of the pouch is created twice as large as the original diameter of the ileum. The limbs of the J pouch should be 15 cm in length. Two fires of a linear stapler are required; either a 75- or 100-mm stapler can be used.

refers to patients undergoing surgery for the findings of colonic dysplasia), the operation can safely be done in one stage *without* fecal diversion, provided that there is no tension on the IPAA. Several technical maneuvers can be performed to lessen the tension on the IPAA, including mobilization of the small bowel mesentery to the level of the pancreas (Fig. 95.47). When dividing the right colon mesentery, the ileocolic vessels should be preserved in their entirety. If distal traction is placed on the apex of

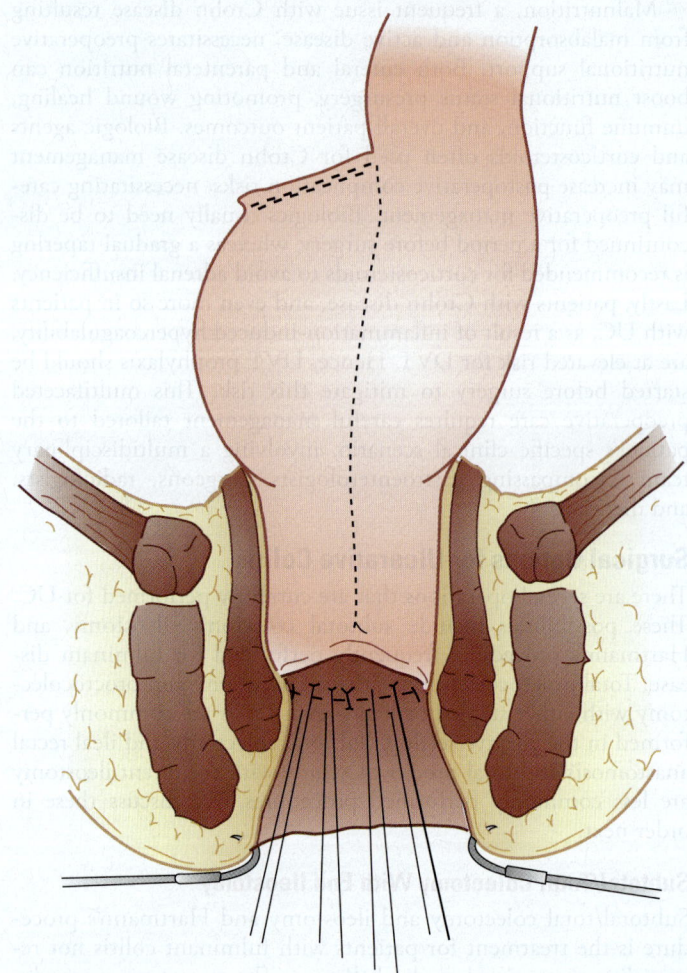

FIGURE 95.46 Hand-sewn ileal pouch–anal anastomosis after anorectal mucosectomy.

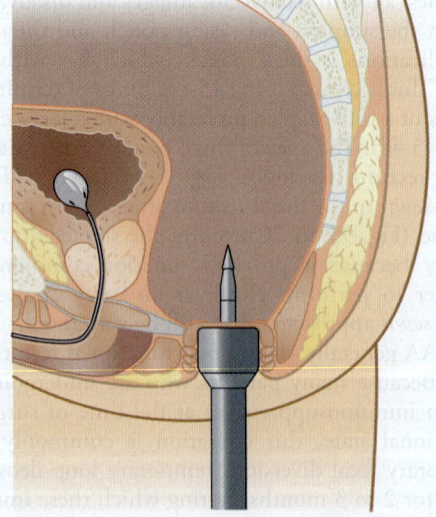

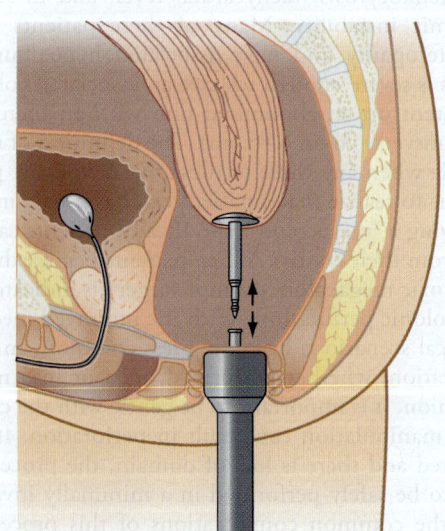

FIGURE 95.45 Fashioning of stapled ileal pouch–anal anastomosis. A circular stapler is used; typically a 29-mm stapler is selected. A common error is to leave too long a segment of rectum, resulting in the persistent symptoms from this retained segment of mucosa affected with inflammatory bowel disease (cuffitis).

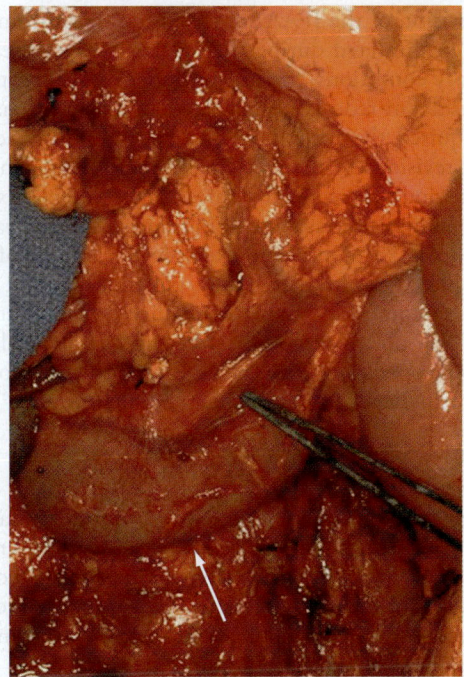

FIGURE 95.47 Mobilization of the small bowel mesentery to the third portion of the duodenum. Here the small bowel mesentery has been retracted cephalad, exposing the third portion of the duodenum *(arrow)*.

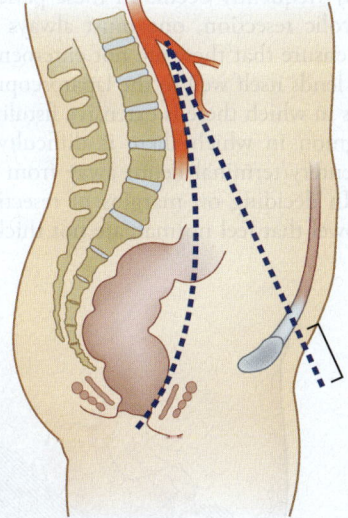

FIGURE 95.48 Estimation of J-pouch length. The apex of the J pouch should be able to be brought down below the level of the symphysis pubis. This is a good estimate of a tension-free reach to the anal canal.

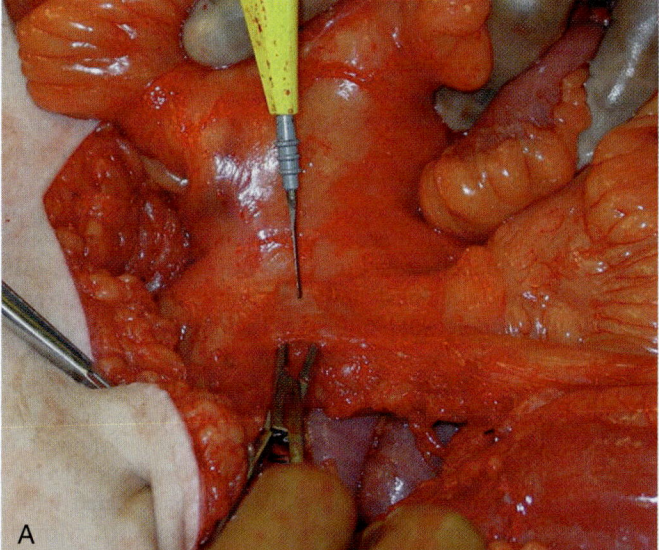

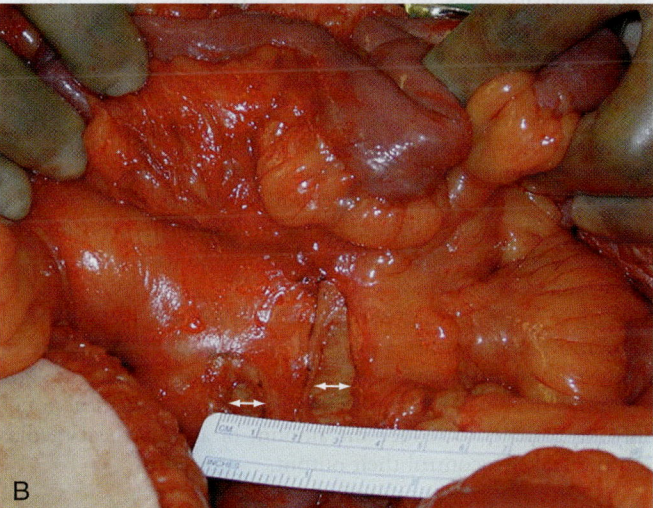

FIGURE 95.49 Peritoneal windowing. (A) The mesenteric peritoneum is lifted away from the superior mesenteric artery by lifting it up with a hemostat and then divided using the electrocautery. (B) The mesenteric peritoneum has been divided perpendicular to the axis of the superior mesenteric artery. Note that at each area where the peritoneum has been divided, an additional 1 cm of mesenteric length has been obtained.

the J pouch, it should easily reach just below the symphysis pubis (Fig. 95.48). When this maneuver is performed, one can either feel or visualize which small bowel mesenteric vessel is under more tension—the superior mesentery vessels or the ileocolic vessels. The vessel with the greater amount of tension can be divided, allowing greater length on the small bowel mesentery. "Peritoneal windowing" can also provide mesenteric length. This is a maneuver whereby small slits are created in the anterior and posterior peritoneum covering the mesenteric vessels. These horizontal slits in the peritoneum, in most cases, provide for 1 or 2 extra centimeters of mesenteric length (Fig. 95.49). Needless to say, the more obese an individual is, the more difficult it can be to obtain

sufficient mesenteric length for the small bowel to reach tension-free to the pelvis. In addition to this, with very tall individuals and those with a long torso, tension can also be an issue.

There are a few ongoing debates on the surgical practice of creating an IPAA. First, when considering the creation of an ileo-anal pouch, surgeons have several strategic options, each tailored to specific patient conditions and potential risks. The one-stage procedure offers efficiency by condensing the process into a single surgery. However, this approach has an elevated risk of anastomotic leakage because of the absence of a temporary ostomy diversion, which can aid in healing. The more prevalent two-stage procedure is favored for elective cases, particularly for patients without pronounced inflammation. This method involves a total proctocolectomy paired with pouch creation, subsequently followed by a temporary ileostomy diversion. In contrast, the three-stage procedure adopts a phased approach, commencing with a total abdominal colectomy. The subsequent stages involve a completion proctectomy, IPAA creation with a temporary diversion, and ultimately, closure of the ileostomy. This strategy is especially reserved for patients in dire need of surgery for acute UC symptoms, such as severe inflammation or bleeding. By postponing the elective IPAA creation, it offers these patients a safer and more staggered surgical experience, allowing for periods of recovery between each stage. Second, there are two predominant types of anastomosis debated: mucosectomy with hand-sutured anastomosis and the double-stapled method. The former involves complete rectal mucosa removal, aiming to reduce disease recurrence, but can affect anorectal physiology, leading to increased stool frequency. The double-stapled technique, although faster and technically simpler, raises concerns about incomplete mucosectomy and potential disease recurrence. Modified two-stage IPAA involves subtotal colectomy with end ileostomy, followed by completion proctectomy and pouch creation without diverting ileostomy. The modified two-stage IPAA was associated with a significantly lower rate of anastomotic leak compared with the traditional two-stage procedure.[47] A three-stage IPAA has been described in patients with acute colitis and high-risk patients with malnutrition or under steroid therapy (Fig. 95.50).

Common early complications of IPAA include those associated with nonhealing of the IPAA: pelvic sepsis, ileal pouch–anal anastomotic fistulae, ileal pouch–vaginal fistulae, ileal pouch–anal anastomotic sinuses, and IPAA strictures (often a reflection of anastomotic tension). Late complications include the diagnosis of Crohn disease, which is more common in patients who undergo emergent colectomy and in those patients who have a diagnosis of indeterminate colitis.

With a "good" result, patients with IPAA will have up to six bowel movements within a 24-hour period, usually including one nocturnal bowel movement. In the majority of patients, at about 6 months, there will be significant enlargement of the ileal pouch, allowing patients to reduce the amount of antidiarrheal medication they take to control their output.

Redo/revision of the IPAA surgery often stems from technical challenges encountered during the initial surgery or results from inflammatory conditions, mainly pelvic sepsis. A long-term study after the results of redo IPAA surgery demonstrated that 41% of patients required the formation of a new pouch, whereas 59% underwent revisions to their original pouch. Although the postoperative period was generally safe, some patients experienced significant complications, including anastomotic leaks. Over time, around 21% of patients experienced failures of the redo IPAA. Despite these hurdles, many patients reported improved functional outcomes and a better quality of life after the redo surgery.[48] Redo pouch surgery may be successfully undertaken as a laparoscopic operation, with the caveat that the surgeon must be extensively experienced in laparoscopic pouch surgery.[49]

Surgery for Crohn Disease
Ileocolic Resection

Ileocolic resection is one of the most common operations performed for patients with Crohn disease because it is estimated that the ileocecal area is the site of involvement in nearly half of patients. Indications for surgery in these patients are usually either fibrostenosing disease with obstruction or associated fistulizing disease/mass/abscess or phlegmon. Because the terminal ileum lies in the pelvis in close proximity to a number of pelvic structures, if there is a significant obstruction and a proximal perforation occurs, the resulting abscess can perforate into the sigmoid colon or bladder. The sigmoid colon is by far the more common, and the resulting ileosigmoid fistula fairly frequently occurs in these patients. When performing an ileocolic resection, one must always be alert to any "adhesions" and ensure that these are not enteroenteric fistulas. Ileocolic resection lends itself well to the laparoscopic approach. Exceptions are cases in which there is extensive fistulizing disease or a significant phlegmon in which there is difficulty separating the right colon mesentery/terminal ileum away from the retroperitoneal structures. In deciding on margins of resection, one should select areas of bowel that feel normal, are not thickened, and have

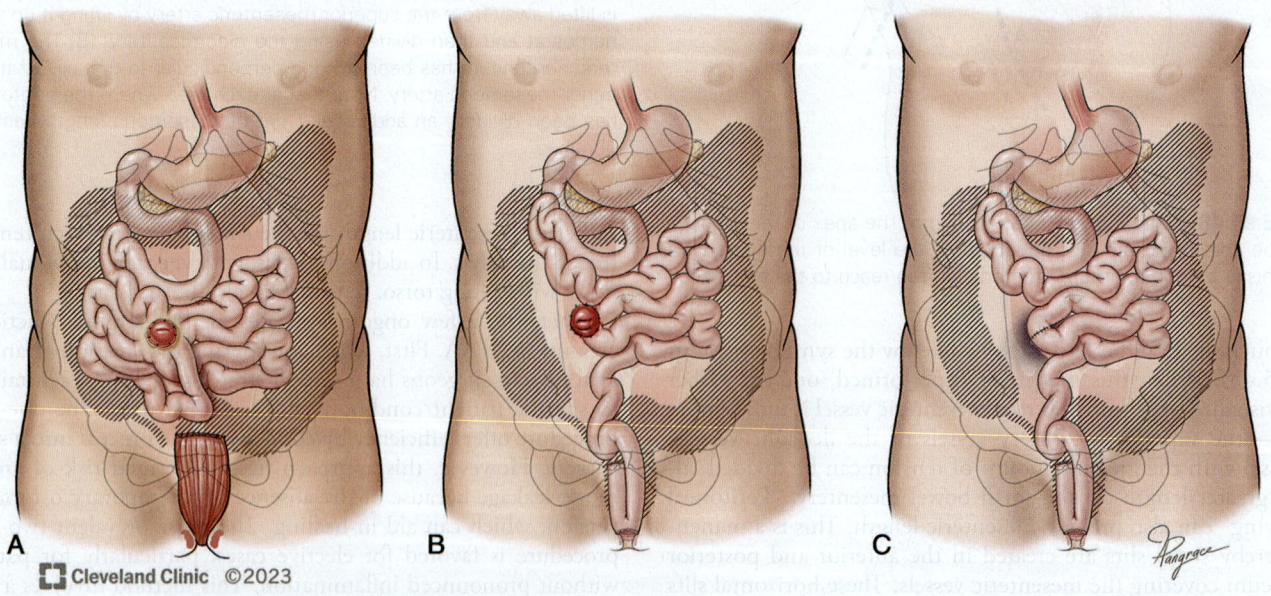

FIGURE 95.50 Three-stage ileal pouch anal anastomosis. (A) Total colectomy with ileostomy creation. (B) Completion proctectomy and creation of the J-pouch. (C) Closure of the ileostomy. (Reprinted with permission, Cleveland Clinic Foundation ©2024. All Rights Reserved.)

a normal thickness of the bowel-mesenteric junction. The ability to palpate a discrete small bowel–mesenteric junction is usually a good indicator that the lumen is free of significant Crohn inflammation. Documenting the residual bowel length in Crohn disease patients is vital for surgeons, given that up to 50% of these patients may require additional surgery within a decade. This information significantly informs future clinical decisions.[50] Although there are many ways to construct the ileocolic anastomosis, a stapled side-to-side anastomosis seems to be the most popular anastomosis. Recently, there has been increased interest in the Kono-S anastomosis, where the diseased bowel is resected and then the surgeon performs a functional end-to-end, side-to-side, hand-sewn anastomosis using a noncutting linear stapler to avoid narrowing at the anastomotic site (Fig. 95.51). This type of anastomosis creates a wide, antitension, antiangulation connection that enhances flow and prevents stasis of fecal content. The first randomized controlled study about the Kono S anastomosis (SUPREME CD trial) showed that this anastomosis significantly reduced both endoscopic and clinical recurrence rates compared with conventional side-to-side anastomosis in Crohn disease, without posing any safety issues.[51] However, a larger scale study published recently found comparable rates of endoscopic recurrence rates between the Kono S and the traditional side-to-side functional end anastomosis.[52] One possible advantage

of the Kono S anastomosis is that, postoperatively, these anastomoses are very easy to evaluate endoscopically and to dilate in the event of recurrent disease, which is not true of side-to-side stapled anastomoses. Further studies are ongoing, but in any case, it is paramount that however the anastomosis is constructed, it is made fairly wide.

Segmental Colon Resection

Segmental colonic resection has increasingly been used in the treatment of Crohn disease over the last two decades. This has been performed for two reasons: (1) recognition of the important role of water absorption (see section on colonic physiology) performed by the colon and recognition that many of these patients will undergo repeated operations and (2) availability of newer and more potent medications for Crohn disease allowing more effective suppression of recurrent disease. Segmental resection for colonic Crohn disease can be performed in patients who have isolated areas of colonic stricture with relatively normal areas of "skipped" normal-appearing colon with normal colonic distensibility. In these patients, performing a segmental resection is associated with a much higher risk of recurrence, so this should always be accompanied by some type of postoperative chemoprophylaxis to reduce the risk of recurrence of the disease.

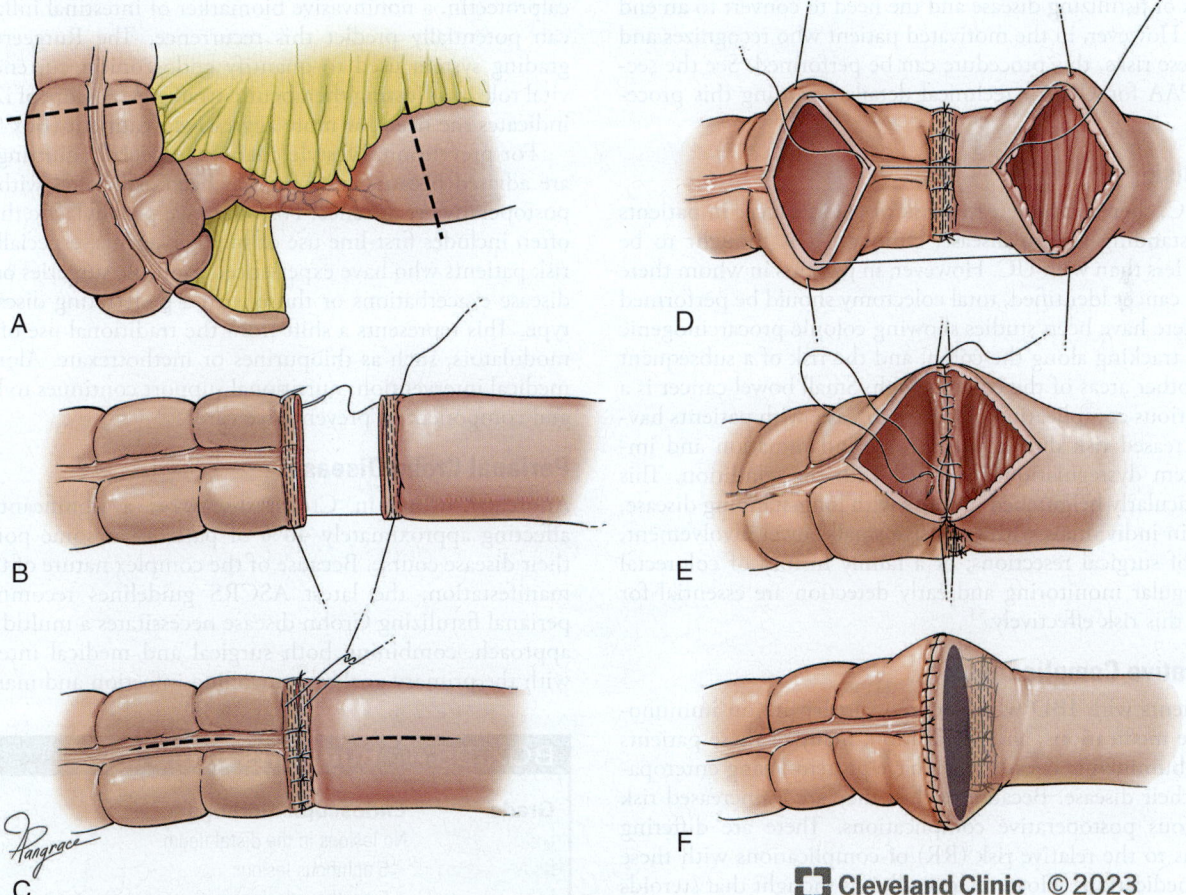

FIGURE 95.51 Technique of Kono-S anastomosis. (A) Division of the mesentery of the ileocecal region. (B) Transection of the bowel with linear stapler at 90-degree angle. (C) Staple lines sutured together transversely to create supporting columns. (D) Three-inch enterotomies are made at the antimesenteric edge. (E) A transverse hand-sewn anastomosis is created. (F) Pale line showing the mesenteric side below the anastomosis with supporting columns. (Reprinted with permission, Cleveland Clinic Foundation ©2024. All Rights Reserved.)

Subtotal Colectomy and Ileorectal Anastomosis

This is an operation that is well suited to patients with Crohn disease if they have a relative rectal-sparing and an otherwise diseased colon. Segmental resection is preferable if there are areas of normal intervening colon. However, this operation also, as with segmental colectomy, is associated with a much higher rate of recurrence. Options for this, if there is a smaller amount of retained rectum, are to perform an ileal pouch–rectal anastomosis in order to lessen the number of bowel movements that the patient has after surgery. Depending on the height of the anastomosis and the circumstances of the surgery (redo, associated immunosuppression, patient's nutritional state), this may require temporary fecal diversion (temporary loop ileostomy) to facilitate healing.

Proctocolectomy and Ileal Pouch–Anal Anastomosis

In previous editions of the Sabiston textbook, there perhaps was only a passing mention of this procedure; however, every year, this is more frequently considered a possibility for patients with Crohn disease, provided that they do not have obvious perianal disease. With the advent of newer and more potent immunosuppressive drugs, this procedure is considered an option in an educated patient who is aware of the increased risk of morbidity and the less favorable functional results (including a greater number of bowel movements) as compared with when this operation is performed for patients with UC. In addition, there is, of course, a higher risk of fistulizing disease and the need to convert to an end ileostomy. However, in the motivated patient who recognizes and accepts these risks, this procedure can be performed. See the section on IPAA for UC for technical details regarding this procedure.

Cancer Risk

As with UC, there is an increased risk of colon cancer in patients with longstanding Crohn disease, although it is thought to be somewhat less than with UC. However, in patients in whom there has been a cancer identified, total colectomy should be performed because there have been studies showing colonic procarcinogenic mutations tracking along the colon, and the risk of a subsequent cancer in other areas of the colon is high. Small bowel cancer is a rare but serious complication of Crohn disease, with patients having an increased risk due to the chronic inflammation and immune system dysregulation associated with the condition. This risk is particularly heightened in those with long-standing disease, especially in individuals with extensive small bowel involvement, a history of surgical resections, or a family history of colorectal cancer. Regular monitoring and early detection are essential for managing this risk effectively.[53]

Postoperative Complications

Many patients with IBD who undergo surgery are on immunosuppressive medications, and in addition, many of these patients are hypoalbuminemic because they have protein-losing enteropathy from their disease. Because of this, they are at increased risk for infectious postoperative complications. There are differing opinions as to the relative risk (RR) of complications with these different medications. However, overall, it is thought that steroids pose an increased risk for infectious complications. Perioperative use of biologics in Crohn disease is a nuanced issue. Although there were initial concerns about the increased risk of postoperative complications because of their immunosuppressive effects, large-scale studies and meta-analyses have indicated that there is no significant increase in such risks. Timing for discontinuation

and resumption of therapy should be personalized, considering disease severity and individual patient recovery. The latest guidelines from the European Crohn and Colitis Organization (ECCO) suggest that preoperative treatment with anti-TNF therapy, vedolizumab, or ustekinumab does not increase the risk of postoperative complications in patients with Crohn disease having abdominal surgery. Small scale studies showed lower risks of postoperative complications in patients undergoing re-do surgery while treated with biologic therapy.[54] Cessation of these medications before surgery is not mandatory.[55] IBD patients are at a notably increased risk of venous thromboembolism (VTE) after surgery, with the RR nearly doubled compared with non-IBD individuals. Even after adjusting for factors such as smoking and BMI, the elevated risk persists, signaling a critical need for vigilant postoperative VTE prophylaxis.[56]

Postoperative Recurrence

Surveillance and preventative measures are pivotal in the postoperative management of patients with Crohn disease.[57] Clinical follow-ups, fecal calprotectin monitoring, and endoscopic investigations form the backbone of surveillance strategy. Regular assessments are essential for early detection of recurrent disease because endoscopic recurrence often precedes clinical manifestations. It is recommended to perform ileocolonoscopy within 6 to 12 months after surgery to spot any signs of endoscopic recurrence. Fecal calprotectin, a noninvasive biomarker of intestinal inflammation, can potentially predict this recurrence. The Rutgeerts score, a grading system used to quantify endoscopic recurrence, plays a vital role in adjusting therapeutic strategies. A score of i2 or higher indicates the need for more aggressive treatment (Box 95.4).

For prevention, lifestyle changes, especially quitting smoking, are advised because smoking has been associated with increased postoperative recurrence. Postoperative prophylactic therapy now often includes first-line use of biologic agents, especially in high-risk patients who have experienced multiple surgeries or recurrent disease exacerbations or those with a penetrating disease phenotype. This represents a shift from the traditional use of immunomodulators, such as thiopurines or methotrexate. Alongside this medical intervention, nutritional support continues to be an integral component of preventative care.

Perianal Crohn Disease

Anorectal fistula in Crohn disease is a significant concern, affecting approximately 40% of patients at some point during their disease course. Because of the complex nature of this disease manifestation, the latest ASCRS guidelines recommend that perianal fistulizing Crohn disease necessitates a multidisciplinary approach, combining both surgical and medical interventions, with the primary goal of controlling infection and managing the

BOX 95.4	Rutgeerts Score
Grade	**Endoscopic findings**
i₀	No lesions in the distal ileum
i₁	<5 aphthous lesions
i₂	>5 aphthous lesions with normal mucosa between the lesions, or skip areas of larger lesions or lesions confined to ileocolonic anastomosis
i₃	Diffuse aphthous ileitis with diffusely inflamed mucosa
i₄	Diffuse inflammation with already larger ulcers, nodules, and/or narrowing

underlying Crohn disease effectively.[58] As with most conditions, the use of a scoring system is useful to quantify the severity of disease and monitor the response to therapy. The Perianal Disease Activity Index (PDAI) is a tool designed to measure the severity of perianal disease in patients with Crohn disease. It considers various clinical parameters, such as the number and type of active fistulas, the intensity of pain, the degree to which daily activities are restricted, and the patient's overall well-being. Each component is scored individually, and the total PDAI score is the sum of these, with higher values indicating increased disease severity. This index is crucial for monitoring disease progression in individuals and evaluating the effectiveness of treatments in research settings (Box 95.5).[59]

Over the past decade, biologic therapy has become the mainstay of medical management. Although immunosuppressants like azathioprine and cyclosporine have shown some efficacy, with a success rate of around 30%, infliximab, a type of biologic, has demonstrated fistula healing rates of up to 60% in randomized controlled trials. Other biologics, such as adalimumab and certolizumab, have also been tested, with success rates ranging from 50% to 55%.

A draining seton is often employed, especially during the initial stages of treatment, with a success rate of about 70% in controlling infection and promoting healing. The approach to definitive fistula surgery is highly individualized, considering such factors as the severity of symptoms, fistula tract anatomy, and the overall status of Crohn disease. Postsurgical challenges are frequent, with nearly 25% of Crohn disease patients requiring additional interventions because of complications such as nonhealing wounds or recurrent fistula.

In cases where drainage is not the primary concern, antibiotics, especially metronidazole and fluoroquinolones, have shown symptom improvement in 80% of patients. Interestingly, not all fistulas in Crohn disease patients are symptomatic. Asymptomatic fistulas, accounting for about 15% of all cases, can remain dormant for years. Surgical intervention in such cases might introduce unnecessary risks, so a conservative approach is often recommended.

For severe, refractory cases, proctectomy and permanent fecal diversion might be the only options. These drastic measures are considered for less than 5% of patients but can be lifesaving. Recent advancements have introduced the local administration of mesenchymal stem cells (MSCs) as a potential treatment. Preliminary clinical trials have shown that MSCs have a success rate of 65% in treating refractory fistulizing anorectal Crohn disease, but long-term outcomes were lower. The recently published ADMIRE-CD phase 3 randomized trial found that 56% of patients treated with MSC for complex perianal Crohn disease were in clinical remission for two years following treatment.[60] Although still in the early stages, the potential of MSCs offers hope for those who have exhausted other treatment options. However, these treatments often require multiple applications and are assoicated with significantly increased costs compared to traditional theraputic measures.

INFECTIOUS COLITIS

Infectious colitis may be diagnosed among patients with acute diarrhea and colonic inflammation. Its importance for the surgeon arises from its capacity to mimic surgical conditions such as an acute abdomen or IBD and, in some cases, to deteriorate to the point where it requires surgical treatment.

Clostridioides difficile Infection

C. difficile infection (CDI) is a common inhabitant of the GI tract that can manifest in a spectrum of symptoms ranging from that of an asymptomatic carrier to fulminant colitis.

Epidemiology

C. difficile is the most common cause of healthcare-associated diarrhea and is considered to be a major source of healthcare-associated

---

BOX 95.5 Perianal Crohn Disease Index (PCDI)

Feature	Score	Feature	Score
Abscess		Single ulcer/fissure or	1
None or	0	Multiple ulcers/fissures	2
First occurrence, single abscess or	1	Maximum ulcer/fissure score	4
First occurrence, multiple abscesses or	3	**Stenosis**	
First recurrence, single or multiple abscesses or	4	None	0
Multiple recurrence, single or multiple abscesses	5	Short-term (<30 d) stenosis or	1
Maximum abscess score	a	Long-term (>30 d) stenosis	2
		Recurrent stenosis	4
Fistula		Maximum stenosis score	6
None	0	**Incontinence score**	
Short-term (<30 d) fistula or	1	No incontinence or	0
Long-term (>30 d) fistula or	2	Incontinence score of 1–6 or	1
Persistent postsurgery fistula or	3	Incontinence score of 7–14 or	3
Recurrent fistula	3	Incontinence score >14	5
Multiple fistulas	3	Maximum incontinence score	5
Rectovaginal/rectourethral fistula or	4	**Concomitant disease**[a]	
Recurrent rectovaginal/rectourethral fistula	6	None or	0. 0.0
Maximum fistula score	14	Moderate or	3, 2,1
		Severe	4. 3.2
Ulcer and fissure		Active fistula	4. 3.2
None	0	Maximum concomitant disease score	18
Short-term (<30 d) ulcer/fissure or	1		
Long-term (>30 d) ulcer/fissure or	2		

[a]Scores are for rectal, colonic, and small bowel disease, respectively.

morbidity, occurring in 2% of all hospital discharges for all diseases. The prevalence of asymptomatic colonization of *C. difficile* among adult hospitalized patients ranges from 3% to 26% in different studies. Around 453,000 new cases of CDI are diagnosed annually in the United States, of which 83,000 are recurrent cases, with 29,300 attributed deaths.[61] Interestingly, after plateauing at historically high rates, some regions have begun to show a decline in incidence attributed to specific prevention and treatment programs. In participating Canadian hospitals, for example, the incidence of CDI decreased from 7.9/10,000 patient-days in 2011 to 4.3/10,000 patient-days in 2015.[62]

Microbiology and Transmission

C. difficile is an anaerobic, spore-forming, gram-positive bacillus. Transmission routes include person-to-person spread through the fecal-oral route or through exposure to a contaminated environment by ingestion of spores from other patients and transmission via healthcare personnel's hands. Toxicogenic *C. difficile* pathogens can produce A and B toxins, both of which have been associated with colitis. Binding of toxin A or B to colonocyte glycoprotein receptors leads to colonocyte death and release of inflammatory mediators. The emergence of the *C. difficile* Ribotype 027 strain in the mid-2000s resulted in significant outbreaks across the Western world associated with more severe disease outcomes and deaths.

Risk Factors

The most important risk factor for the development of a clinical infection is recent exposure to antibiotics. Antibiotics affect the natural bowel flora, decreasing the natural ability to suppress the growth and spread of *C. difficile*. Virtually all antibiotics have been associated with *C. difficile*, but particularly third- and fourth-generation cephalosporins, fluoroquinolones, clindamycin, and carbapenems have been linked to a higher risk of CDI. Other risk factors include immunodeficiency (including HIV infection); chemotherapy treatment; use of acid-suppressing medications, such as proton pump inhibitors; GI surgery or manipulation of GI tract, including tube feeding; and prolonged hospitalization or lengthy stay in nursing homes or rehabilitation units. Patients with IBD have increased rates of CDI, along with worse outcomes (e.g., HIV) and higher rates of colectomy. These patients are more likely to receive immunosuppressants and antibiotics and have a different intestinal flora compared with healthy subjects. Differentiating between an IBD exacerbation and CDI can be difficult because the symptoms overlap, and a high index of suspicion must be maintained. Patients with an increased risk for death from CDI include those with advanced age, multiple comorbidities, hypoalbuminemia, leukocytosis, or acute renal failure and those infected with Ribotype 027.

Clinical Presentation

Symptoms of CDI commonly begin 4 to 9 days after initiation of antibiotics but can commence 10 weeks or more after antibiotic treatment. Patients presenting with new-onset, unexplained, watery diarrhea (with three or more unformed stools in 24 hours) should be suspected of having CDI. Patients may also have abdominal pain, fever, and an associated ileus. Patients with CDI can be categorized into asymptomatic colonization, nonsevere disease, severe disease, and fulminant disease. Various scores have been used to assess clinical severity and treatment response. Leukocytes of at least 15,000 cells/μL and/or serum creatinine of at least 1.5 cells/μL are predictors of severe disease, according to the Infectious Disease Society of America. Fulminant or severe CDI is diagnosed in patients demonstrating hypotension or shock, ileus, or megacolon. The ATLAS criteria is a simple clinical bedside score that includes age, temperature, leukocytosis, albumin, and systemic antibiotic treatment and has been used to assess response to treatment.[63]

Diagnosis

The diagnosis of CDI is based on typical symptoms in combination with stool testing. Laboratory testing is based on detection of *C. difficile* toxins, *C. difficile* antigen, or the bacteria itself. Various commercial tests are used, including enzyme-linked immunosorbent assay for toxin detection, glutamate dehydrogenase immunoassay for *C. difficile* antigen detection, nucleic acid amplification test, polymerase chain reaction testing, and stool cultures.

Flexible sigmoidoscopy may be helpful as a diagnostic modality for CDI. Although it is not a first-line modality for diagnosis, it can be helpful in cases of inconclusive stool testing or to help exclude other etiologies. Classically, raised, yellowish-white small (2- to 10-mm) plaques (pseudomembranes) can be observed in approximately half of patients with CDI (Fig. 95.52). Nonspecific

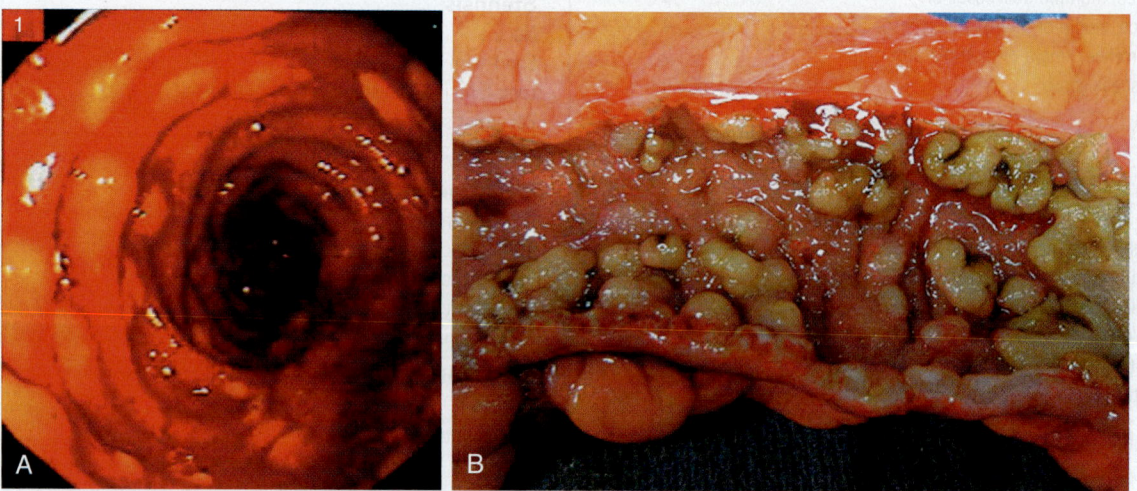

FIGURE 95.52 (A) Endoscopic view of pseudomembranes associated with *Clostridioides difficile*. (B) Pseudomembranes overlying the colon mucosa at the time of colectomy. The patient had active *C. difficile* colitis with coexisting Crohn colitis.

colitis can be found in an additional 25%. Histologic findings from the plaques reveal an inflammatory exudate with mucinous debris, fibrin, necrotic epithelial cells, and polymorphonuclear cells. In fulminant colitis, colonoscopy may increase the risk of perforation and should be considered only when the benefit is higher than the risk of complications.

Imaging is not very useful for diagnosis because it is not specific, but it can assist in assessing disease severity and response to treatment. Typical CT findings include significant colonic wall thickening, bowel dilation, pericolonic fat stranding, high-attenuation oral contrast in the colonic lumen alternating with low-attenuation inflamed mucosa (accordion sign), and ascites. Ultrasound may also be useful, especially among critically ill patients who cannot be transported to the CT scanner in radiology. Ultrasonography may show bowel wall thickening; narrowing of the lumen; and pseudomembranes, which are seen as hyperechoic lines covering the mucosa.

Treatment

Initial treatment includes stopping or minimizing previous antibiotics, parenteral fluids, and correction of electrolytes. The use of antiperistaltic agents for the treatment of CDI should be avoided. Antibiotic treatment of CDI is determined according to the clinical setting and can be divided into the initial episode, recurrent episode, severe disease, and fulminant disease. Table 95.4 summarizes current antibiotic treatment recommendations for initial episodes and for severe and fulminant disease.

Treatment options for recurrent episodes generally include changing antibiotics (from metronidazole to vancomycin or fidaxomicin from vancomycin). In addition, tapered and pulsed regimens are used.

Fecal Microbiota Transplant

Fecal microbiota transplant (FMT) for patients with recurrent episodes of CDI is a relatively new treatment. Patients with CDI lack protective colonic microbiota to resist replication and colonization of *C. difficile*. Reimplantation of normal gut bacteria, particularly bacteria resistant to *C. difficile*, from healthy donors can help restore normal gut biodiversity and correct the imbalance. Different routes of administration have been described in the literature, including nasogastric, oral (frozen fecal microbial capsules), rectal enema, and colonic per colonoscopy. A recent comparison between upper and lower methods of delivery demonstrated the lower approaches being more effective.[64] The efficacy of FMT ranges from 77% to 100%, with multiple FMTs needed to achieve a good clinical response. Current guidelines recommend FMT for patients with multiple recurrences of CDI in whom antibiotic treatment has failed.

Monoclonal Antibodies

Bezlotoxumab and actoxumab are monoclonal antibodies directed against *C. difficile* toxins B and A, respectively. These antibodies limit colonic damage by neutralizing the toxin and blocking the binding to host cells.[65] They can be used as coadjuvant treatment with antimicrobial therapy to help prevent recurrence, especially among patients infected by Ribotype 027, in severe CDI, and in immunocompromised patients.

Surgery

Patients with fulminant CDI who develop signs of systemic toxicity, toxic megacolon, or perforation should be operated on emergently. Emergency colectomy for patients with fulminant colitis provides a survival advantage compared with continuing antibiotics. Among severely ill patients, a total or subtotal abdominal colectomy with preservation of the rectum has traditionally been performed. A newer option with similar results for patients without necrosis or perforation is exteriorization of a diverting loop ileostomy with on-table colonic lavage followed by antegrade vancomycin flushes.[66]

OTHER COLONIC INFECTIONS

Diarrhea and colitis can be caused by other pathogens. Most of these will not require surgery. A careful history can discover the source in many cases, such as polluted drinking or recreational water or consumption of contaminated fruits and vegetables, unpasteurized milk, undercooked meat and fish, shellfish, and eggs. International travel as well as contact with animals and their feces should also be queried. Table 95.5 summarizes the important characteristics of common bacteria causing diarrhea and colitis.

The initial approach includes a careful history, evaluation for dehydration and electrolyte disturbances, and stool testing for ova and parasites and for culture and sensitivity. Patients with signs of sepsis or those who have traveled from enteric fever–endemic

TABLE 95.4	Antibiotic Treatment of *Clostridioides difficile* Infection	
CLINICAL CONDITIONS	**TREATMENT**	**TREATMENT DURATION**
First episode	1. Oral vancomycin 125 mg 4 times daily OR 2. Fidaxomicin 200 mg twice daily If vancomycin and fidaxomicin are not available, metronidazole 500 mg 3 times daily can be given for nonsevere disease.	10 days
First episode—fulminant (hypotension, shock, ileus, megacolon)	Vancomycin, 500 mg 4 times daily (oral or by nasogastric tube) In case of ileus: 1. Consider adding rectal instillation of vancomycin. 2. Intravenously administered metronidazole (500 mg every 8 hours) should be administered together with oral or rectal vancomycin.	At least 10 days, duration should be individualized

Adopted from McDonald LC, Gerding DN, Johnson S, et al. Clinical practice guidelines for *Clostridium difficile* infection in adults and children: 2017 update by the Infectious Diseases Society of America (IDSA) and Society for Healthcare Epidemiology of America (SHEA). *Clin Infect Dis.* 2018;66:987-994.

TABLE 95.5 **Clinical Characteristics of Common Enteric Infections**

PATHOGEN	CHARACTERISTICS AND CLINICAL PRESENTATION
Campylobacter jejuni	Spiral, microaerophilic gram-positive rod
	Exposure to improperly prepared chicken or beef
	Fever, watery diarrhea, and abdominal pain
	Commonly involves the cecum and terminal ileum
	May mimic appendicitis or Crohn disease
Yersinia enterocolitica	Gram-negative coccobacillus
	Exposure to contaminated water or food
	Abdominal pain and bloody diarrhea, may mimic appendicitis or Crohn disease
Shigella	Gram-negative, facultative anaerobe
	Common cause for dysentery in developing countries
	Often affects rectum and sigmoid colon
	Fever, abdominal pain, watery diarrhea that can progress to bloody diarrhea
Salmonella typhi or Salmonella enterica serotypes Paratyphi	Gram-negative, facultatively anaerobic bacilli
	Recent travel to an endemic area, consumption of foods prepared by a traveler to an endemic area
	Fever with or without diarrhea, abdominal pain, cramping and vomiting

Adapted from Shane AL, Mody RK, Crump JA, et al. 2017 Infectious Diseases Society of America clinical practice guidelines for the diagnosis and management of infectious diarrhea. *Clin Infect Dis*. 2017;65: 1963-1973.

regions and immunocompromised patients should also have blood cultures obtained.

Initial treatment includes rehydration and correction of electrolyte disturbances. Oral rehydration solution is recommended for mild to moderate disease. Nasogastric administration of oral rehydration solution may be considered for patients who do not tolerate oral intake. Patients with signs of severe dehydration or ileus should be treated with isotonic IV fluids (normal saline or lactated Ringer solution). The majority of patients who present with acute watery diarrhea and those without recent international travel *do not require* antimicrobial therapy. Immunocompromised or septic patients, as well as those suspected of enteric fever, should be treated with empirical, broad-spectrum antimicrobial therapy, usually with fluoroquinolones, such as ciprofloxacin, or macrolides, such as azithromycin, depending on local susceptibility patterns. Surgical intervention is rarely required apart from those cases developing severe fulminant disease that leads to perforation or toxic megacolon.

Viruses can also cause acute diarrhea and colitis. Cytomegalovirus (CMV) is an important etiology to consider in immunocompromised hosts, particularly in advanced HIV infection, transplant patients, patients with IBD, and those receiving chemotherapy. CMV colitis commonly presents with watery or bloody diarrhea, fever, and abdominal pain. Diagnosis is established by serology and by determining viral load in the blood. Endoscopy demonstrates patchy mucosal erythema in the colon.

Inclusion bodies seen on biopsy are pathognomonic for CMV. CMV colitis can progress to sepsis, toxic megacolon, and colonic perforation. Treatment is usually supportive with the addition of ganciclovir. Patients with severe, complicated disease may require surgery.

ISCHEMIC COLITIS

Ischemic colitis is a common disorder that develops when the arterial blood supply to the colon is insufficient to support cellular metabolic demands. It is the most common form of GI ischemia, with rates of 7.1 to 22.9/100,000 person-years.[67] Severity varies within a wide spectrum, from mild, self-limiting disease to severe, life-threatening colonic ischemia. Considering the wide range of clinical findings, with most patients presenting with mild, nonspecific symptoms, the true incidence is likely much higher. It is important to differentiate ischemic colitis from situations of acute mesenteric ischemia, in which a major vessel of the bowel is obstructed, wherein patients commonly present with severe pain out of proportion to physical findings and require immediate vascular intervention. Ischemic colitis is considered a disease of small blood vessels and typically presents less dramatically, seldom requiring vascular intervention. Most cases, when recognized and managed promptly, do not require surgery. Delays in diagnosis and treatment, however, can result in the need for emergency colectomy, with high morbidity and mortality.

Anatomic Considerations

The arterial blood supply to the colon is derived from the SMA and the IMA. The SMA gives off the ileocolic, right colic, and middle colic arteries. The IMA gives rise to the left colic and sigmoid arteries and ends as the superior rectal (hemorrhoidal) artery (see Fig. 95.8). There are two well-described collateral networks that aid in preventing colonic ischemia by providing "backup" both within the territories of the two major arteries and between them. The main collateral vessel is the marginal artery of Drummond, which runs parallel and close to the mesenteric margin of the colon from the cecocolic junction to the rectosigmoid junction. The marginal artery was found to be absent at the splenic flexure in up to 18% of people.[68] The colon can receive collateral blood supply through this artery when one of the larger arteries is obstructed. It is important, when resecting a section of colon, to preserve this artery because only the vasa recta are located between it and the colon. When it is compromised, ischemia of that section of colon may result. The second collateral circulation can be found in the proximal region of the large arteries. The "arc of Riolan" (meandering mesenteric artery) is an infrequent finding, traversing close to the mesenteric root and connecting the SMA or middle colic artery to the IMA or left colic artery (Fig. 95.53). It can have a critical role in situations of SMA or IMA occlusion. The presence of a large arc of Riolan commonly indicates an obstruction of one of the major mesenteric arteries.

Watershed areas of the colon are potentially found at the edge of the region supplied by the two main arteries, the SMA and the IMA, zones that are frequently dependent on collateral circulation (Fig. 95.54). There are two well-described watershed areas where the collateral circulation is classically inconsistent and vulnerable to ischemia. The first is the area of the splenic flexure (Griffiths point). In some studies, up to 50% of specimens were found to lack a marginal artery in the region

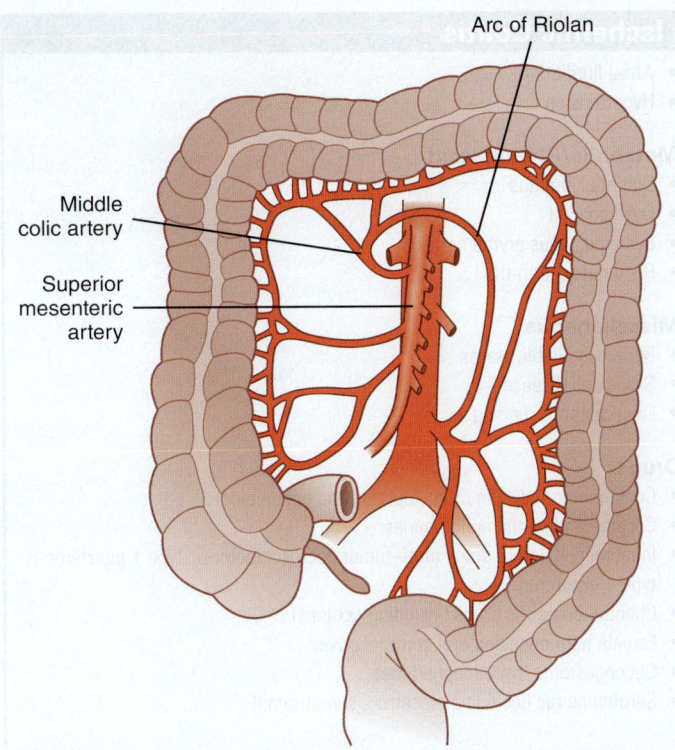

FIGURE 95.53 The arc of Riolan. (From Gordon PH, Nivatvongs S, ed. *Principles and Practice of Surgery for the Colon, Rectum and Anus.* 2nd ed. St. Louis: Quality Medical Publishing; 1999:27.)

where the SMA and IMA circulations meet. Commonly, surgeons avoid making anastomoses in this area for fear that the impaired blood supply will not be sufficient to permit anastomotic healing, leading to anastomotic leaks. A second potential watershed area is the rectosigmoid junction (Sudeck's point). This region receives its blood supply from the superior hemorrhoidal artery and distal sigmoid branches, both terminal branches of the IMA and prone to atherosclerotic changes. The right colon, although not classically considered a watershed area, is also vulnerable to ischemia from embolic occlusion because the ileocolic artery is the terminal branch of the SMA. For this reason, the right colon is also particularly prone to low-flow conditions, such as heart failure, hemorrhage, and sepsis. The rectum, which has a good blood supply from both the IMA and the iliac circulation, as well as a strong collateral network, is rarely the victim of ischemic injury.

Risk Factors

Ischemic colitis may occur in all ages but is significantly more common in elderly patients, in females, and in patients with multiple comorbidities. Several medical conditions and medications have been associated with ischemic colitis (Box 95.6).[69]

Patients with low-flow states, as a result of heart failure or sepsis, are especially prone to develop ischemic colitis. Diabetes mellitus, hypertension, chronic obstructive pulmonary disease, peripheral vascular disease, and renal disease have also been associated with this disorder. Recently, COVID-19 was found to be associated with ischemic colitis in some patients.[70] Patients

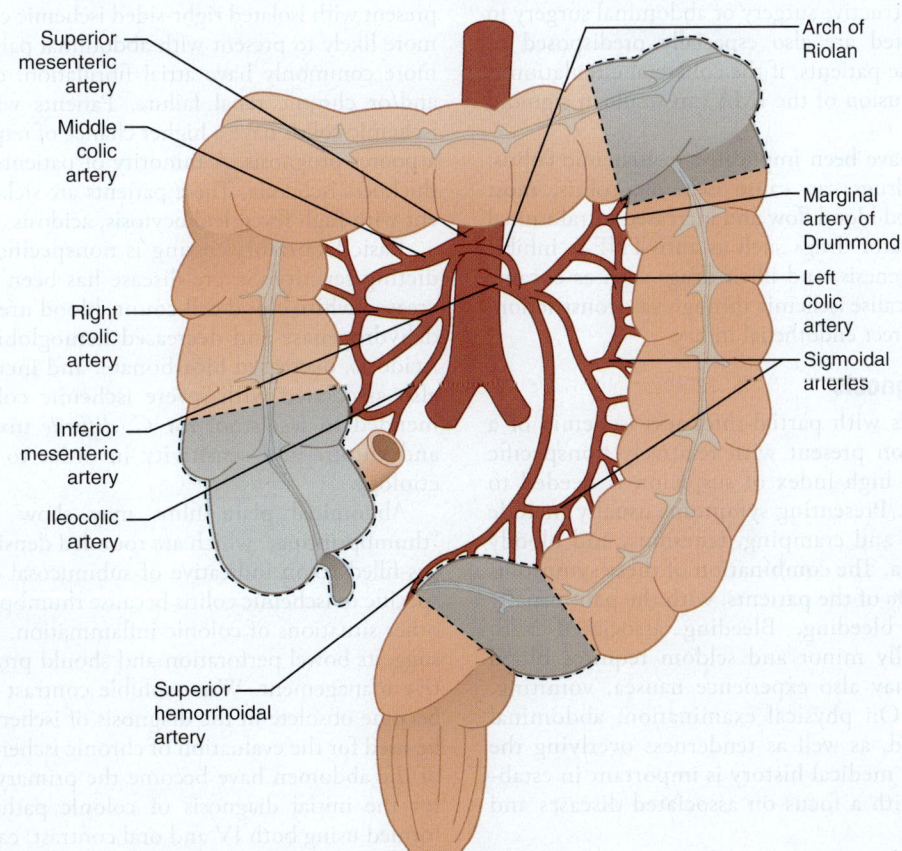

FIGURE 95.54 Lightly shaded colonic regions especially vulnerable to ischemia. (From Netz U, Galandiuk S. Management of ischemic colitis. In: Cameron JL, Cameron A, eds. *Current Surgical Therapy.* 12th ed. Philadelphia: Elsevier; 2017:171-176.)

BOX 95.6 Conditions and Drugs Associated With Ischemic Colitis

Low-Flow State
- Septic shock
- Congestive heart failure
- Hemorrhagic shock
- Hypotension

Atherosclerosis
- Ischemic heart disease
- Cerebrovascular disease
- Peripheral vascular disease

Gastrointestinal
- Constipation
- Diarrhea
- Irritable bowel syndrome

Surgery and Invasive Interventions
- Abdominal surgery
- Aortic surgery (especially abdominal aortic aneurysm repair)
- Cardiovascular surgery
- After endovascular abdominal manipulations (including chemoembolization)
- Postcolonoscopy

Cardiovascular/Pulmonary
- Chronic obstructive pulmonary disease

- Atrial fibrillation
- Hypertension

Metabolic/Rheumatoid
- Diabetes mellitus
- Dyslipidemia
- Systemic lupus erythematosus
- Rheumatoid arthritis

Miscellaneous
- Hypercoagulable states
- Sickle cell disease
- Long-distance running

Drugs
- Constipation-inducing drugs (opioids and nonopioids)
- Cocaine and methamphetamines
- Immunomodulatory drugs (anti–tumor necrosis factor-α, type 1 interferon-α, type 1 interferon-β)
- Chemotherapeutic drugs (including taxanes)
- Female hormones and oral contraceptives
- Decongestants (pseudoephedrine)
- Serotoninergic (including alosetron, sumatriptan)

undergoing aortic reconstructive surgery or abdominal surgery in which the IMA is ligated are also especially predisposed to colonic ischemia. In these patients, if the collateral circulation is not sufficient, acute occlusion of the IMA can result in sigmoid and left colon ischemia.

Several medications have been implicated in ischemic colitis. Constipation-inducing drugs can cause ischemic colitis, most likely as a result of reduced blood flow and increased intraluminal pressure. Immunomodulator drugs such as anti–TNF-α inhibitors can affect thrombogenesis, and illicit drugs such as cocaine and methamphetamines cause ischemia through vasoconstriction, hypercoagulation, and direct endothelial injury.

Presentation and Diagnosis

The majority of patients with partial-thickness ischemia of a localized section of colon present with relatively nonspecific signs and symptoms. A high index of suspicion is needed to make an early diagnosis. Presenting symptoms usually include sudden abdominal pain and cramping, tenesmus, and bloody diarrhea or hematochezia. The combination of these symptoms is present in close to 50% of the patients, with the pain usually beginning before the bleeding. Bleeding associated with ischemic colitis is usually minor and seldom requires blood transfusions. Patients may also experience nausea, vomiting, and a low-grade fever. On physical examination, abdominal distention may be noted, as well as tenderness overlying the involved region. A good medical history is important in establishing the diagnosis, with a focus on associated diseases and medications.

The most common affected region is the left colon (including the splenic flexure), followed by the sigmoid colon, based on the affected blood supply. Pancolitis resulting from ischemia is associated with a worse prognosis. About a quarter of the patients

present with isolated right-sided ischemic colitis. These patients are more likely to present with abdominal pain without bleeding and more commonly have atrial fibrillation, coronary artery disease, and/or chronic renal failure. Patients with isolated right-sided ischemic colitis have a higher chance of requiring surgery and have a poorer prognosis. A minority of patients will present with full-thickness ischemia. These patients are sicker and commonly present with high fever, leukocytosis, acidosis, and peritonitis.

Basic laboratory testing is nonspecific but can assist in predicting severity. Severe disease has been associated with an increased white blood cell count, blood urea nitrogen, and lactate dehydrogenase and decreased hemoglobin and albumin levels. Acidosis, decreased bicarbonate, and increased lactate levels are also associated with severe ischemic colitis. It is also recommended to test stool for *C. difficile* toxin, ova and parasites, and culture and sensitivity in order to exclude an infectious etiology.

Abdominal plain films may show bowel distention and "thumbprinting," which are rounded densities along the sides of a gas-filled colon indicative of submucosal edema. These are nonspecific to ischemic colitis because thumbprinting can be found in other situations of colonic inflammation. Free intraperitoneal air suggests bowel perforation and should prompt immediate operative management. Water-soluble contrast enemas have generally become obsolete in the diagnosis of ischemic colitis but may still be used for the evaluation of chronic ischemic strictures. CT scans of the abdomen have become the primary noninvasive modality for the initial diagnosis of colonic pathology. CT scans, performed using both IV and oral contrast, can assist in determining the location of involved areas to assess the severity, identify complications, and exclude the presence of other diseases. Findings suggestive of ischemic colitis, although relatively nonspecific, include segmental bowel thickening, pericolonic fat stranding, and thumbprinting. Pneumatosis intestinalis (the presence of gas in the colonic wall), portal venous gas, and the absence of large bowel enhancement on contrast-enhanced CT usually indicate severe transmural disease favoring immediate surgical intervention. Vascular imaging is usually not indicated in cases of ischemic colitis because this is usually a disease of small vessels; however, in cases of pain of sudden onset that is out of proportion to physical and laboratory findings and in isolated right colon ischemic colitis, multiphasic CT angiography should be performed to exclude acute proximal mesenteric ischemia. MRI may be used as an alternative to invasive procedures in diagnosis and grading of acute ischemic colitis, enabling the early identification of pathologic changes.[71]

The gold standard for the diagnosis of ischemic colitis is flexible endoscopy. Early colonoscopy should be performed (within 48 hours), except in cases of acute peritonitis or in cases of suspected severe transmural ischemia. In contrast to the expected increased risk of perforation resulting from endoscopy in the evaluation of ischemic colitis, current published literature does not demonstrate a higher rate of perforation compared with other patients. It is recommended, however, to refrain from overinsufflation and avoid advancing the scope beyond the most distal extent of disease. Common endoscopic findings characteristic of ischemic colitis include edematous and friable mucosa, erythema, petechial hemorrhage, and mucosal ulceration. The "single-stripe sign," a single linear ulcer running along the longitudinal axis of the colon, is rare but considered specific for ischemic colitis. Segmental distribution, with abrupt transition between injured and noninjured mucosa, and sparing of the rectum support ischemia over IBD. It is important to note that diagnostic endoscopy usually cannot distinguish between partial-thickness and full-thickness ischemia. Fig. 95.55 depicts a recommended algorithm for diagnosis and treatment of ischemic colitis.

Treatment

The majority of patients, nearly 80%, will respond to conservative nonoperative treatment, with significant improvement within a few days. The mainstay of treatment includes bowel rest, IV fluids, and broad-spectrum antibiotics. A nasogastric tube should be inserted if ileus is present. Medications including phosphodiesterase type 5 inhibitors, pentoxifylline, and prostaglandin E1 may improve blood flow to the ischemic colon and promote mucosal healing.[72]

Efforts should be made to correct low-flow states and hypotension with aggressive fluid resuscitation and optimal treatment of associated conditions, such as heart failure and sepsis. Colonic ischemia can result in failure of the intestinal epithelial barrier with bacterial translocation, leading to overt sepsis. For this reason, empiric broad-spectrum antibiotics against both anaerobic and aerobic coliform bacteria are prescribed in ischemic colitis to cover the normal colonic bacterial flora. Cathartics are not recommended because they may lead to colon perforation. Glucocorticoids should be avoided unless treating a preexisting disorder such as lupus or rheumatoid arthritis.

Most episodes of ischemic colitis are mild and self-limiting. Patients who fail to improve or have worsening symptoms within a few days should raise the concern for the development of full-thickness ischemia and should have repeat imaging or endoscopy to help guide treatment.

A small proportion of patients with mild to moderate symptoms will develop a chronic colitis, with ongoing or recurrent bouts of symptoms of abdominal pain, bloody diarrhea, and sepsis. These patients have a higher rate of complications and commonly require surgical resection of the involved segment. Some patients who initially recover from partial-thickness ischemic colitis will eventually develop a chronic stricture at the involved segment. These patients may complain of constipation, narrowed stools, and abdominal pain. Diagnosis can be confirmed with a contrast enema, CT, or endoscopy. Symptomatic patients or those in which malignancy cannot be excluded should undergo elective resection.

Patients who present with or develop signs of transmural ischemia and perforation—including peritonitis; hemodynamic instability; free peritoneal air; and ominous signs on CT, as mentioned earlier, such as portal venous gas—require emergent surgical exploration. A recent large database study identified a 25% 30-day postoperative mortality rate for ischemic colitis,[73] with other studies reporting up to 47% mortality after acute surgical intervention. Risk factors independently identified as associated with perioperative mortality after colectomy for ischemic colitis include elderly age, poor functional status, multiple comorbidities, preoperative septic shock, preoperative blood transfusions, preoperative acute renal failure, and delay from hospital admission to surgery.

During surgery, it is important to visualize and assess the entire small and large intestine for signs of ischemia and gangrene. Ischemia commonly affects a recognizable segment of the colon, frequently in watershed areas. In these cases, an anatomic resection should be performed to allow sufficient blood supply to the remaining colon with minimal reliance on stressed collaterals. Deciding how much to resect or whether a specific segment is likely to survive can be difficult. Visual examination tends to be inaccurate, especially when the bowel is ischemic but still viable. Intraoperative infrared angiography is a relatively new technique that has been gaining popularity as an adjunct for determining bowel viability and for determining the integrity of intestinal anastomoses. In this technique, indocyanine green is injected intravenously and distributes throughout the circulation. Then, using a variety of commercially available imaging systems, the indocyanine green undergoes laser excitation, demonstrating real-time tissue perfusion (Fig. 95.56). Creation of an anastomosis is usually not recommended in the acute setting because of the concern for evolving ischemia and the existence of hemodynamic instability and sepsis commonly encountered in these situations. A temporary abdominal closure with a planned second look after 24 hours may be prudent to determine the need for further resection. Staple the ends and leave them in the abdomen, avoiding complications of a stoma, as in very obese patients. Pancolic ischemia is rare, but such cases require total colectomy with ileostomy. In contrast to mesenteric ischemia of the small intestine, there is usually no indication for revascularizing the large bowel in primary colonic ischemia, which is not generally related to large artery obstruction.

PELVIC FLOOR DISORDERS AND CONSTIPATION

Disorders of the pelvic floor include multiple conditions, often involving colorectal, urologic, and gynecologic specialists. Constipation is a dysfunction of colonic motility and of the defecation process. It can be present with several medical and colorectal conditions, including colon obstruction and pelvic floor diseases. Functional constipation is an entity that must be differentiated from distinct anatomic problems during patient evaluation and

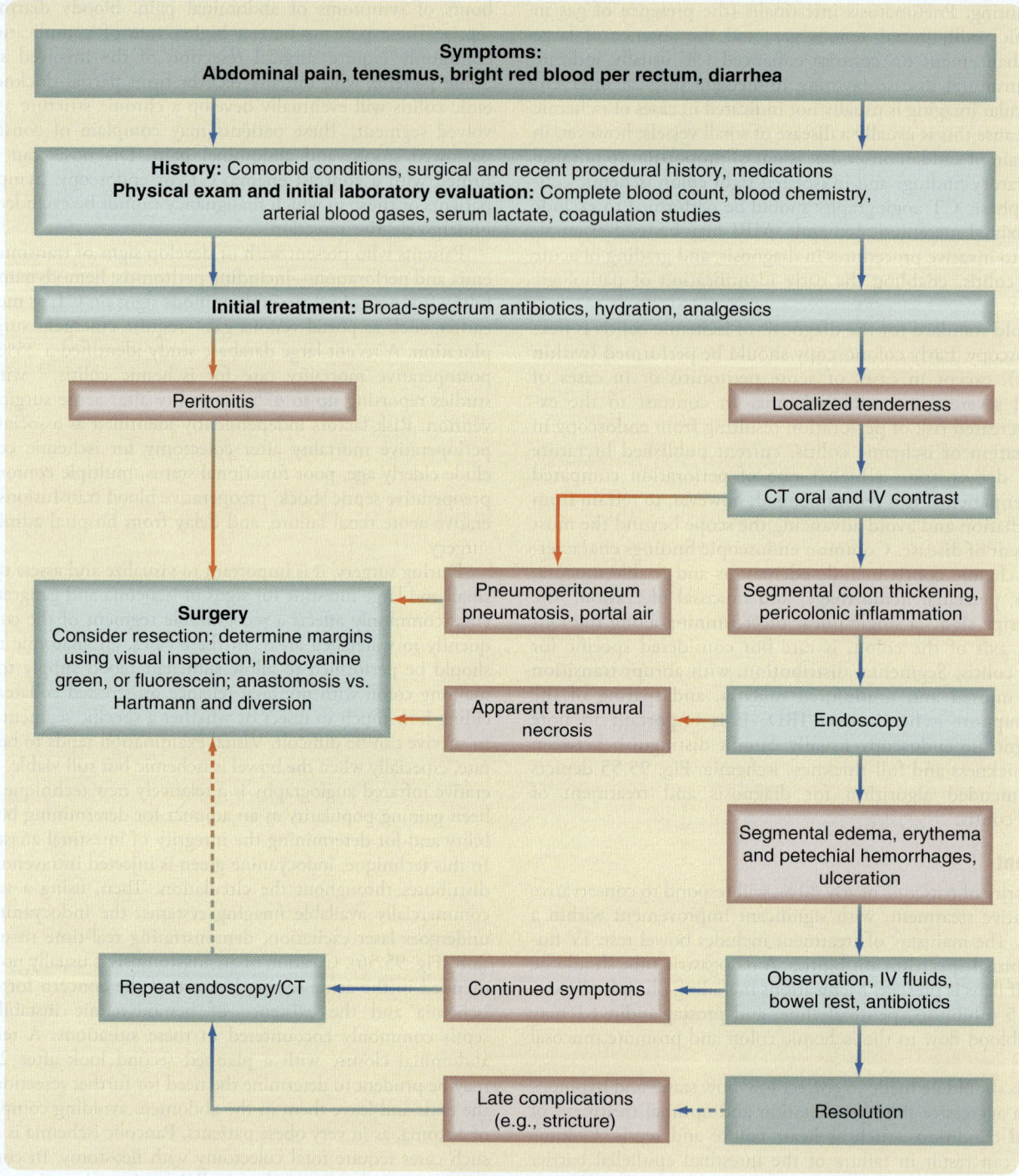

FIGURE 95.55 Algorithm for investigation and treatment for ischemic colitis. *CT,* Computed tomography; *IV,* intravenous. (From Netz U, Galandiuk S. Management of ischemic colitis. In: Cameron JL, Cameron A, eds. *Current Surgical Therapy.* 12th ed. Philadelphia: Elsevier; 2017:171-176.)

may be considered for surgical treatment if unresponsive to active medical therapy. The reader is referred to the ASCRS Consensus Statement of Definitions for Anorectal Physiology Testing and Pelvic Floor Terminology, Clinical Practice Guidelines for the Treatment of Rectal Prolapse, and Clinical Practice Guideline for the Evaluation and Management of Constipation.

The pelvic floor disorders that present to the surgeon include:
- Rectal prolapse or procidentia: a circumferential, full-thickness intussusception of the rectum

- Rectocele: a bulging of the rectum into the posterior wall of the vagina
- Cul-de-sac hernia: a protrusion of the peritoneum between the rectum and the vagina, referred to as *enterocele* if it contains the small bowel and as *sigmoidocele* if it contains the sigmoid colon.
- Anismus: the failure of the puborectalis and the external anal sphincter to relax during defecation (simple nonrelaxation or paradoxical contraction)

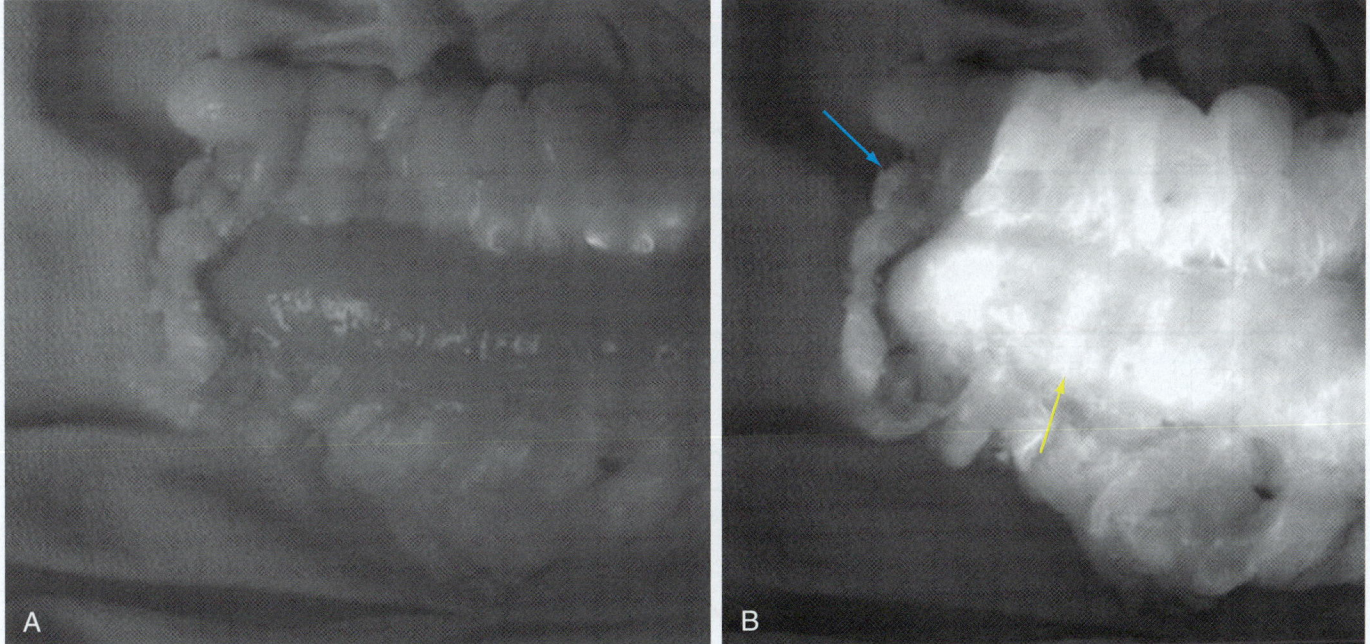

FIGURE 95.56 Indocyanine green–based infrared angiography. (A) Colon before injection. (B) Colon after injection: ischemia of resection margin *(blue arrow)*; normal perfusion of colon *(yellow arrow)*. (From Netz U, Galandiuk S. Management of ischemic colitis. In: Cameron JL, Cameron A, eds. *Current Surgical Therapy.* 12th ed. Philadelphia: Elsevier; 2017:171-176.)

Even if functional disorders do not always require surgical operation, the surgeon is almost always involved in the evaluation of these patients and in establishing a treatment plan.

Diagnosis: Testing and Evaluation

Anorectal Physiology Laboratory Tests

Anorectal physiology tests are performed to evaluate anal canal pressures to determine the presence of anal reflexes, anal sensation, and electromyography recruitment.

Anorectal manometry evaluates the high-pressure zone (including the length of the anal canal); the resting pressure, mostly due to the internal sphincter; the maximum voluntary pressure; and the squeeze pressure, due to the external anal sphincter (Fig. 95.57). The test is performed by placing a manometry catheter with a water-filled balloon at its tip in the anal canal so that the balloon at the tip lies within the rectal lumen. Normal resting pressure values are 40 to 80 mm Hg. Anorectal manometry also provides information on intrarectal pressures, reflexes, rectal sensation, and rectal compliance. High-resolution manometry can provide greater physiologic resolution and minimizes motion artifacts.

The balloon expulsion test evaluates the ability of the patient to expel a balloon inflated with 50 to 60 cc of water/gas/air that simulates stool.

Pudendal nerve terminal motor latency measures the conduction of the pudendal nerve from its emergence at the level of the ischial spines to the internal anal sphincter by the use of a transducer. Normal pudendal nerve terminal motor latency times are 2.0 ± 0.2 milliseconds. Prolonged values are seen in traumatic injuries (spinal cord) or with stretch injury from obstetric trauma resulting from prolonged labor, chronic stretch injury as seen in long-standing defecation disorders, sacral nerve root damage, or chronic diseases such as diabetes. This is typically measured with a special electrode taped to the index finger of the examiner, whereby the tip of the finger electrode stimulates the pudendal nerve, and the recording electrode at the base of the finger measures anal sphincter contraction.

Electromyography records the change from basal electrical activity of motor units of the external sphincter and puborectalis muscle during activity. Patients with inappropriate or paradoxical puborectalis contraction fail to show a relaxation of the muscles when asked to push.

Imaging to Evaluate the Pelvic Floor and Colonic Transit

Endoanal ultrasound (Fig. 95.58) can be used to evaluate the integrity, thickness, and possible abnormalities (scars, fistulas) of the internal and external anal sphincter.

Defecography is a dynamic study of the anorectum and the pelvic floor during defecation. It provides information regarding anatomic abnormalities, such as rectocele, rectal prolapse, internal rectal intussusception, and cul-de-sac hernia, as well as about functional disorders, such as nonrelaxation or paradoxical puborectalis contraction, perineal descent, and the degree of rectal emptying. Dynamic images are captured with fluoroscopy, with the rectum and the vagina opacified with radiographic contrast and the patient in the sitting position on a radiolucent commode. If magnetic resonance defecography is performed, the rectum is opacified with a mixture of ultrasonography gel and gadolinium. The advantages of MRI are high-quality images of the pelvic soft tissues and viscera and avoiding use of ionizing radiation. It is, however, limited by the supine position of the patient, which does not reproduce normal conditions of defecation (Fig. 95.59). Furthermore, a recent study showed that magnetic resonance defecography seems equivalent to traditional x-ray video defecography in the assessment of defecation disorders.[74]

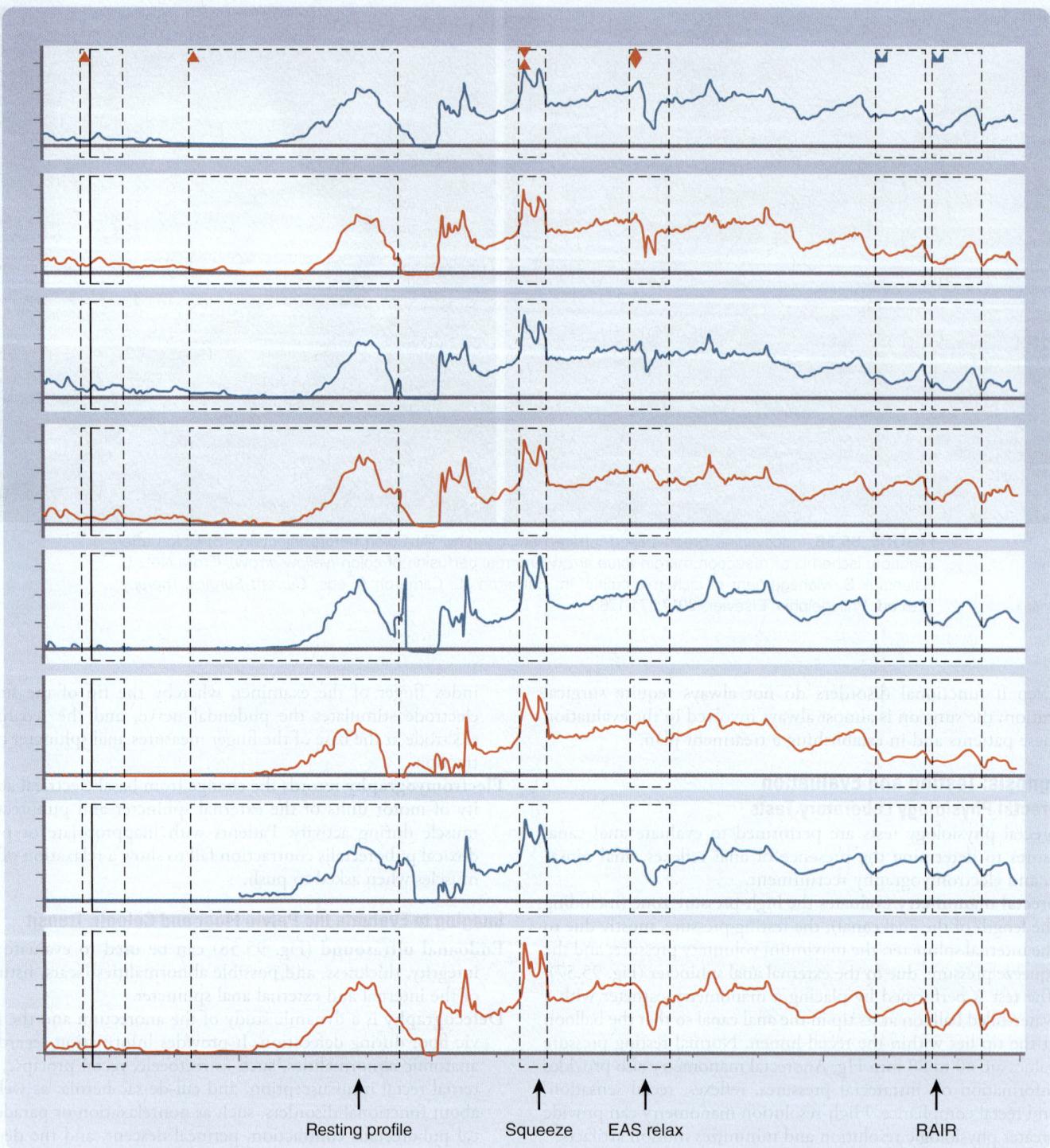

Resting profile   Squeeze   EAS relax   RAIR

FIGURE 95.57 A normal anorectal manometry: resting and squeeze pressure curves are evident, and the external anal sphincter relaxation when the patient is asked to push. The rectoanal inhibitory reflex is present. *EAS,* External anal sphincter.

Colonic transit time is a test that studies colonic inertia. The patient is asked to ingest 24 radio-opaque markers contained in a capsule (Sitzmarks®) and to refrain from using laxatives and any other mechanical measures that might interfere with colonic function. The progression of the markers through the three areas of the colon (right, left, and rectosigmoid) is studied with plain abdominal films that are taken every other day until day 7. In the healthy population, 80% of the markers

should be expelled by day 5. Patients with slow transit constipation or colonic inertia retain a significant portion of the markers during the entire time of the study (Fig. 95.60).

Rectal Prolapse (Procidentia)
Anatomy and Pathophysiology
Rectal prolapse is a circumferential, full-thickness intussusception of the rectal wall. The degree of prolapse can vary from intrarectal

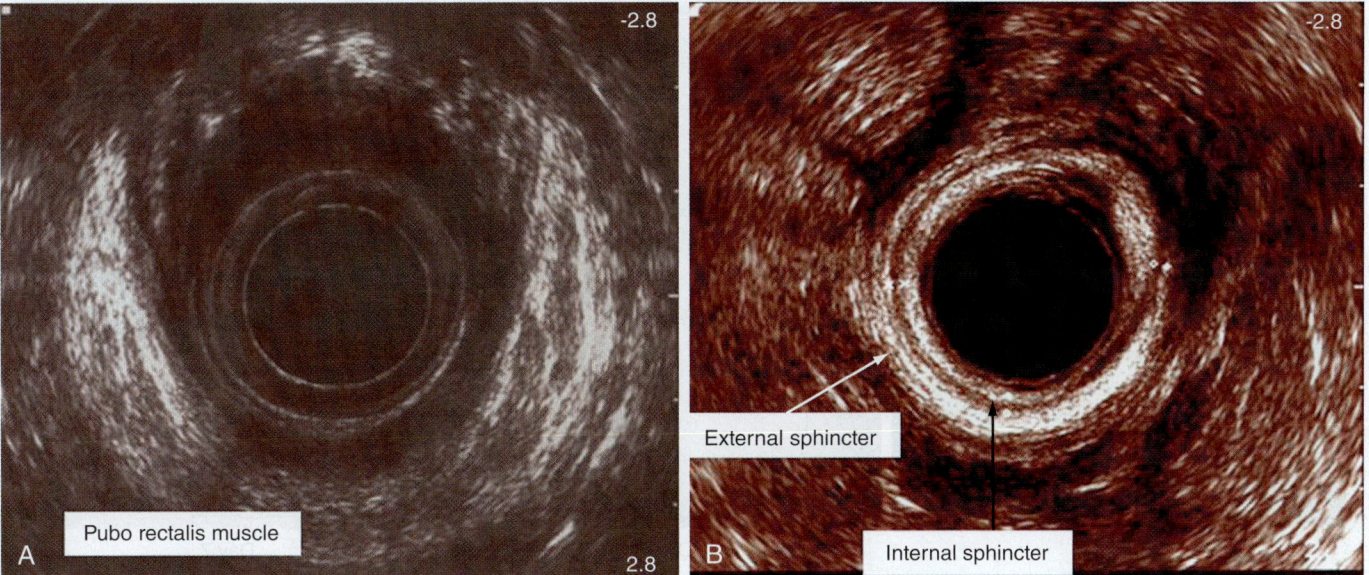

FIGURE 95.58 Endoanal ultrasound. (A) The arch-shaped hyperechoic puborectalis muscle appears as a whitish structure. (B) The hypoechoic internal sphincter *(black arrow)* and the hyperechoic external sphincter *(white arrow)* are shown.

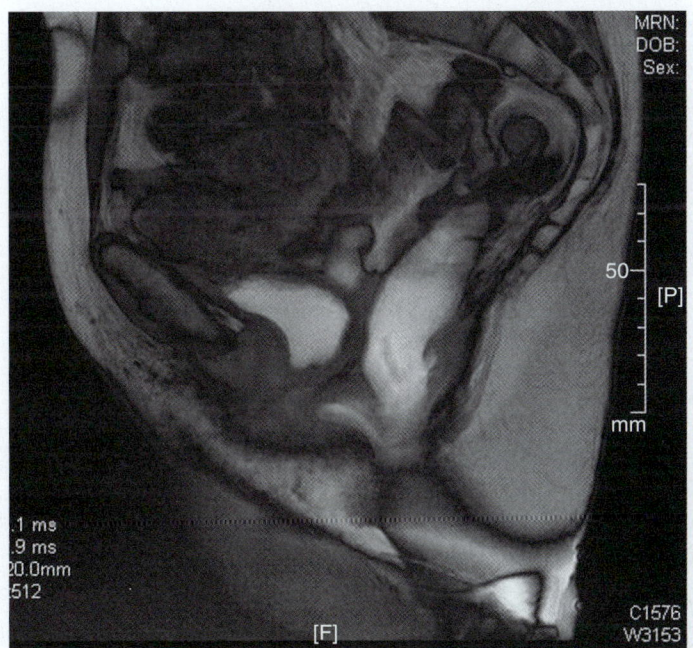

FIGURE 95.59 A magnetic resonance imaging image of rectal prolapse.

constipating medications. The cause of rectal prolapse is still unknown, but some anatomic defects are commonly found in patients with total rectal prolapse. These defects include a diastasis of the levator ani muscle, an abnormally deep cul-de-sac, a redundant sigmoid colon, a patulous anus, and a lack of fascial attachments of the rectum against the sacrum. Risk factors of rectal procidentia include age over 40 years, female sex, prior pelvic surgery, chronic straining and constipation, chronic diarrhea, vaginal delivery and multiparity (however, one-third of the female rectal prolapse patients are nulliparous), pelvic floor dysfunction and/or anatomic defects, neurologic diseases/injuries, and psychiatric diseases that require constipating medications. Rectal prolapse usually has a progressive course from transient self-reducing prolapse during defecation to prolapse requiring digital self-reduction, then to stable prolapse that may present with ulceration and even nonreducible, incarcerated prolapse with necrosis in the most advanced and complicated cases.

Symptoms

Symptoms include discomfort from the prolapsed tissue, incontinence with drainage of mucus or blood, and constipation. The majority (50%–75%) of patients with evident rectal prolapse complain of fecal incontinence (passive or urge incontinence) that is caused by the presence of a direct conduit and by the chronic stretching of the sphincter resulting from the prolapse, which may induce an anal sphincter injury graded into four grades by endoanal ultrasound.[75] Also, the persistent stimulation of the rectoanal inhibitory reflex caused by the prolapsed rectum is one of the contributing factors to continence impairment. Up to one-half of patients with incontinence also have pudendal neuropathy, with a prolonged pudendal nerve terminal motor latency. The other 25% to 50% of the patients, and in particular those with intrarectal prolapse, report constipation or obstructed defecation (feeling of an incomplete rectal evacuation during defecation) that results from the "telescoping" of the bowel on itself, creating a functional blockage that worsens with straining (Fig. 95.61), or by the presence of a concomitant rectocele.

or internal rectal prolapse (Fig. 95.61) to intraanal prolapse to external rectal prolapse (Fig. 95.62). Rectal prolapse is an uncommon condition that occurs in about 0.5% of the general population, with females older than 50 years being six times more likely than males to develop rectal prolapse. The few males who present with rectal prolapse are usually younger than 40 years. Rectal prolapse in young males may have a special geographic predilection because certain countries, including Egypt and India, tend to have a higher incidence of rectal prolapse in young males. Young patients (males and females) with prolapse often suffer from psychiatric diseases, such as autism or developmental delay, and take

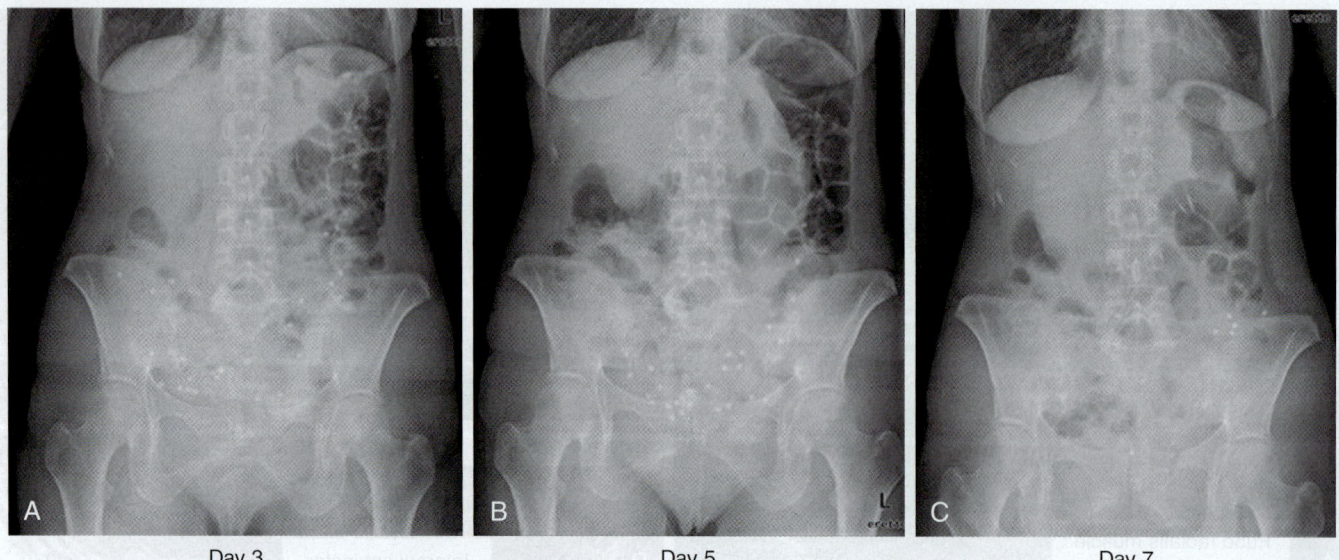

Day 3   Day 5   Day 7

FIGURE 95.60 Colonic transit study: plain abdominal films at 3, 5, and 7 days after ingestion of radiopaque markers. Note that at day 5, the majority of the radiopaque markers are within the pelvis; however, by day 7, most markers have passed.

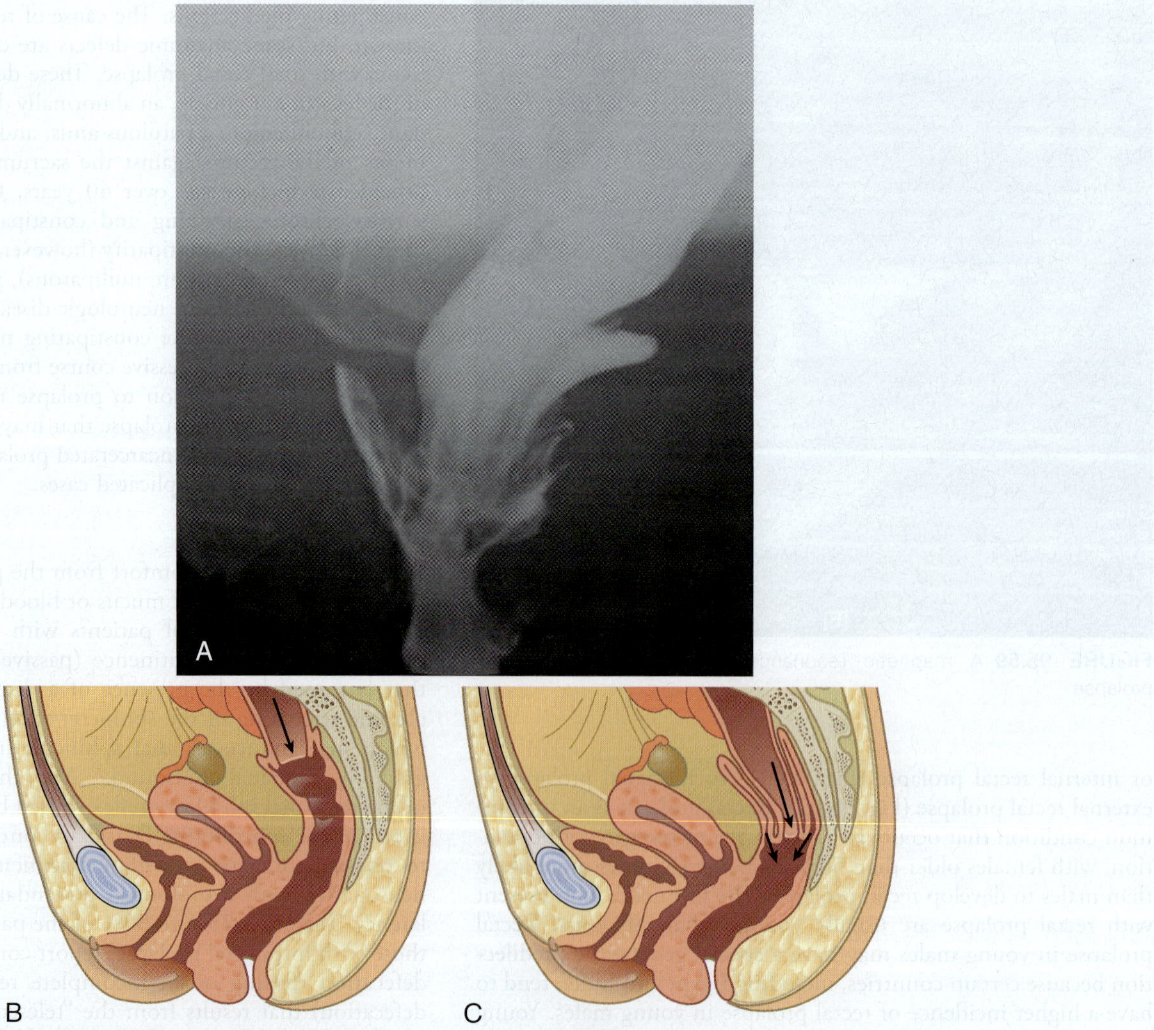

FIGURE 95.61 (A) The internal rectal prolapse of a male patient is nicely demonstrated by defecography. (B–C) Progression of the internal rectal prolapse.

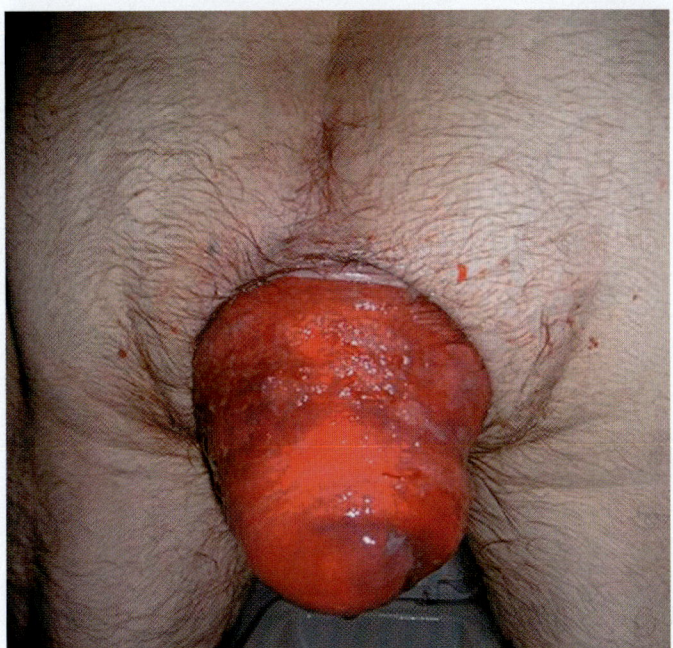

FIGURE 95.62 A patient with a large external rectal prolapse. (Courtesy G. Sarzo, MD, Hospital Sant Antonio, Department of Surgery, Padova Italy.)

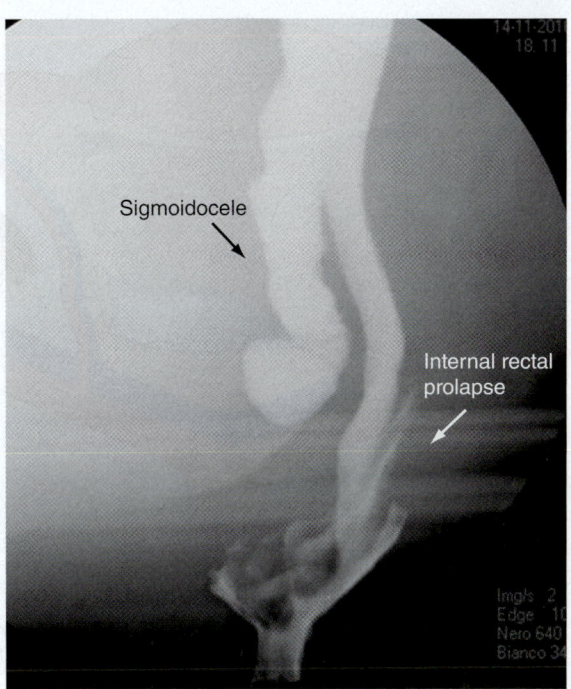

FIGURE 95.63 Defecography of a young male patient who presents with internal rectal prolapse *(white arrow)* and sigmoidocele *(black arrow)*.

Diagnosis and Differential Diagnosis

On physical exam, true rectal prolapse must be differentiated from prolapsed rectal mucosa or prolapsed hemorrhoids: the full-thickness rectal prolapse has concentric folds, whereas prolapsed hemorrhoids or rectal mucosa is characterized by radial folds, with grooves along hemorrhoid cushions. At rest, typical findings include a patulous anus with a lax sphincter. Examination is performed in the office with the patient in standard left lateral decubitus or in the sitting or squatting position during straining. If the prolapse cannot be observed in the office setting, the patient can be asked to take a "selfie" at home to document the prolapse. Proctoscopic examination demonstrates redundant tissue and, in 10% to 15% of patients, an anterior solitary rectal ulcer. Proctoscopy may indicate erythema at 5 to 6 cm, which is the leading edge of the prolapse. Fluoroscopic or MRI defecography is an additional test to confirm the diagnosis of rectal prolapse and provides more information regarding coexisting disorders, such as rectocele, cystocele, vaginal vault prolapse, enterocele, and sigmoidocele (see Figs. 95.62 and 95.63). Colonoscopy should always be performed to exclude the presence of CRC or other colonic pathology. A colonic transit study is performed in patients with a lifelong history of constipation in order to differentiate constipation resulting from obstructed defecation from constipation resulting from slow colonic transit. The two frequently coexist. Endoanal ultrasound usually shows a thickening of the internal anal sphincter.

Nonoperative Management

Prolapse-associated symptoms of constipation and fecal incontinence can be palliated with medical treatment to improve quality of life. Adequate fluid intake, fiber supplements, and stool softeners can treat constipation. Sugar or salt can be used topically to reduce rectal mucosal edema and facilitate reduction of the prolapsed tissue. Enemas and suppositories may be helpful to assist in defecation.

Operative Repair

The goals of surgery are to eliminate the prolapse and correct the anatomic and functional abnormalities. The approach can be transabdominal or transperineal. Perineal procedures are followed by a relatively high incidence of recurrence, yet an acceptably low complication rate as compared to the abdominal procedures.[76] The choice of procedure is based on the patient's comorbidities, the patient's age and bowel function, and the surgeon's preference. A network meta-analysis concluded that posterior mesh rectopexy was associated with the lowest recurrence while perineal procedures ranked worst with the highest recurrence rates. There were no significant differences between the abdominal and perineal procedures in complications and improvement in incontinence.[77]

Abdominal procedures. The rationale of the intraabdominal approach is to perform a fixation of the rectum with the goal of providing adequate upward tension to prevent a recurrence but at the same time allowing appropriate evacuatory movements during defecation. The abdominal approach can be performed via open or minimally invasive approaches (laparoscopic or robotic). Both have equivalent clinical and functional results, recurrence rates (4%–8%), and morbidity (10%–33%). Laparoscopy offers benefits in terms of pain control, hospital stay, and recovery time. The advantages offered by robotic rectal prolapse repair are the ease of suturing and tying and improved visualization of the deep pelvis. The rectum must be dissected, retracted intraabdominally, and fixed to the presacral fascia with sutures (posterior rectopexy). In these cases, a simultaneous resection of the redundant sigmoid can be performed in selected patients with coexisting constipation. A mesh can be used to increase scarring and improve fixation of the rectum posteriorly or anteriorly. With the posterior mesh rectopexy, the rectum is mobilized posteriorly and laterally down to the levator ani muscles, and a mesh is fixed to the presacral fascia, below the sacral promontory, and to the rectum laterally (Fig. 95.64). This technique is associated with significant improvement in fecal incontinence in 20% to 60% of patients but has a 20% rate of

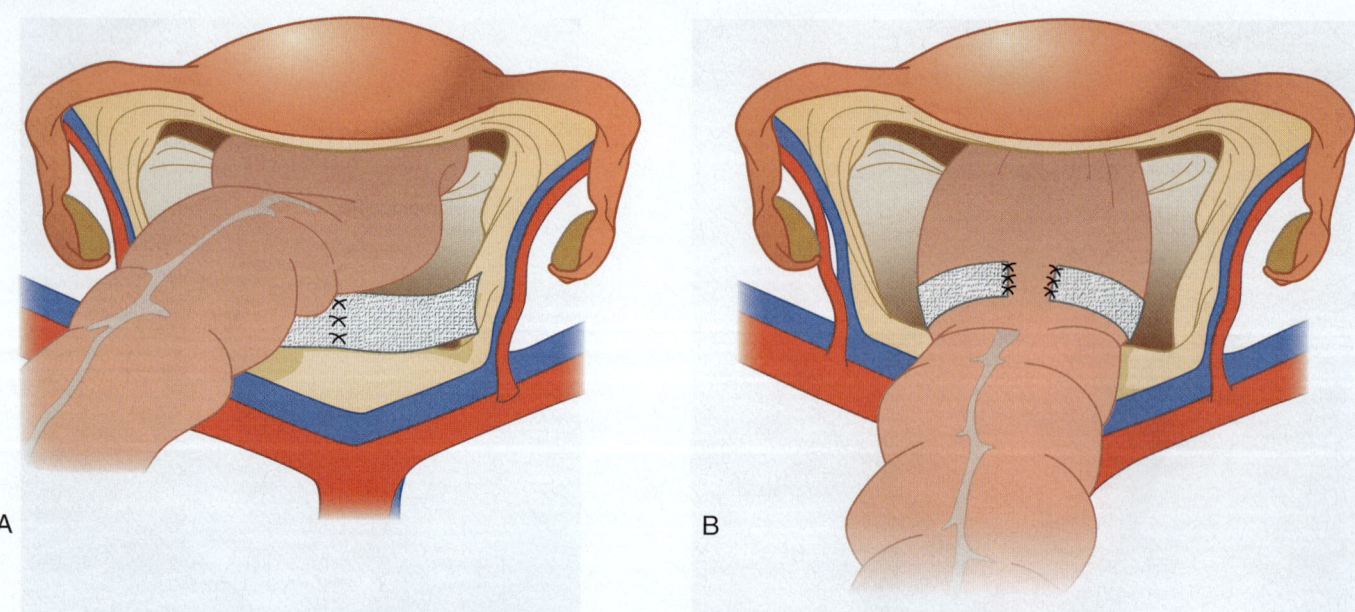

FIGURE 95.64 The posterior mesh rectopexy (modified Ripstein operation). (A) The rectum is mobilized, and the mesh is fixed to the presacral fascia. (B) The mesh is fixed to both sides of the rectum.

postoperative complications and is associated with a 2% to 5% recurrence rate. The more recently described ventral mesh rectopexy is a technique that involves a limited anterior rectal mobilization and a mesh suspension to the sacral promontory. The mesh is fixed to the anterior wall of the rectum and suspended to the sacral promontory (Fig. 95.65). Advantages of this technique are the improvement in postoperative incontinence and constipation,

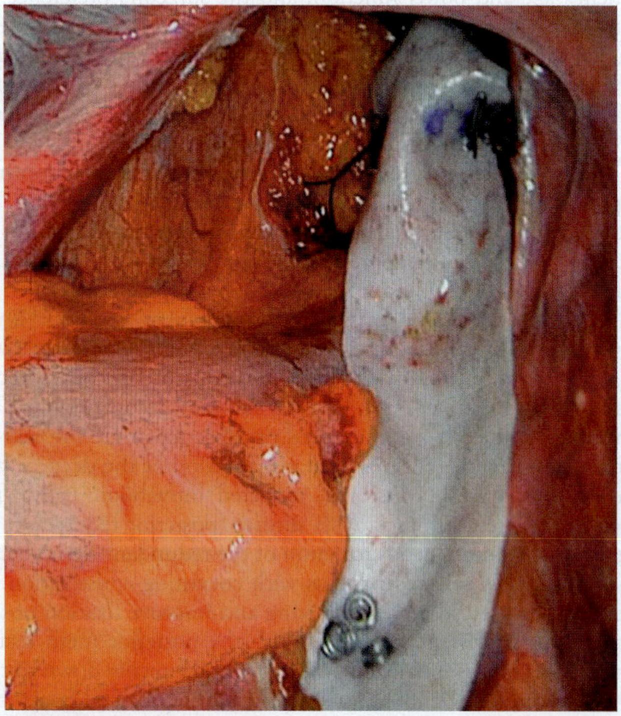

with few cases of de novo postoperative constipation, and low complication and recurrence rates (3%–5%).[78,79] In published series, many different types of mesh and fixation devices are used: nonabsorbable or biologic grafts, tacks, sutures, or staples to fix the mesh. Mesh-related complications include erosion, usually into the vagina; infection and pelvic sepsis; bowel obstruction; and mesh detachment and/or migration. In theory, with the use of biologic mesh, the risk of infection or erosion may be lower, and the risk of recurrence may be higher, but recent literature[78] shows no statistical improvement in recurrence and complication rates between biologic and nonabsorbable mesh. The follow-up for studies using biologic mesh is, however, short. One meta-analysis with a meta-regression analysis showed that male sex and the length of mesh used were significantly associated with full-thickness recurrence of rectal prolapse after ventral mesh rectopexy.[79] Concomitant pelvic organ prolapse (POP) and rectal prolapse repair with isolated apical prolapse repair or rectopexy may offer a comprehensive treatment for patients with multicompartmental prolapse without increasing the risk of postoperative complications.[80]

Perineal approach. Perineal procedures allow for the resection of the prolapse without concomitant fixation. They are recommended for the elderly or medically unfit patients and are thought to be associated with lower operative morbidity and mortality but with higher recurrence rates. Recent reviews and trials have, however, concluded that there are no significant differences in recurrence and reoperation rates between perineal and abdominal approaches. Therefore perineal procedures may have to be considered an option for all patients with rectal prolapse. The "Altemeier procedure," or perineal proctectomy or proctosigmoidectomy, is a true rectosigmoidectomy. The prolapse is exteriorized, it is grasped with Allis clamps, and a full-thickness circumferential incision is made through the rectum 1 cm above the dentate line. The peritoneal cavity is entered anteriorly, and the redundant sigmoid colon is extracted transanally (Fig. 95.66). The levator muscles are visualized and can be plicated posteriorly in order to reinforce the pelvic floor and restore the anorectal angle (levatorplasty, or Parks postanal repair). A hand-sewn or stapled coloanal anastomosis is then performed. The operation can be done under epidural anesthesia, with

FIGURE 95.65 Ventral mesh rectopexy. The mesh is attached to the anterior rectal wall and the sacral promontory. (Courtesy G. Sarzo, MD, Hospital Sant Antonio, Department of Surgery, Padova, Italy.)

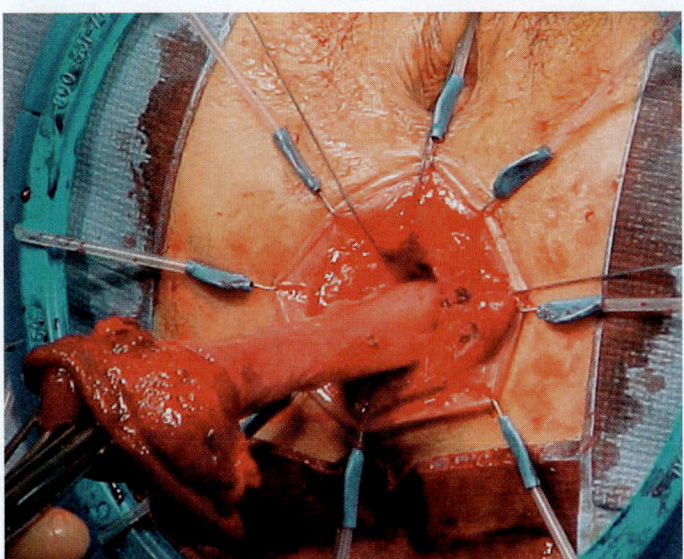

FIGURE 95.66 The Altemeier procedure or perineal proctectomy. The redundant rectosigmoid colon is resected through a transperineal approach, and a hand-sewn coloanal anastomosis is performed.

minimal postoperative pain. This technique allows for the resection of redundant bowel, it has low complication rates, and especially when levator plication is done, it is associated with low recurrence rates (10%). For patients with a short (<5 cm) rectal prolapse, the Delorme procedure can be appropriate. A circumferential incision within the submucosal plane is made 1 cm proximal to the dentate line, and the mucosa is stripped away from the muscularis propria of the rectum to the most proximal portion of prolapse. The stripped mucosa is then excised. A longitudinal suture plication of the muscularis propria is then performed. Finally, an anastomosis is performed between the proximal and distal mucosal edges (Fig. 95.67). This technique is very safe, entails a short hospital stay, and has lower complication rates than the abdominal approach. Incontinence and constipation are improved. Overall recurrence rates range from 7% to 27% and are comparable to the Altemeier or abdominal procedures. For symptomatic intrarectal prolapse, the stapled transanal rectal resection (STARR) has been proposed as an alternative possible technique. It consists of a full-thickness rectal resection, including the internal prolapse, with a circular stapler (STARR) or a specific curved-shape stapler (Transtar). These techniques have initially shown good results in cases of obstructed constipation, but the onset of chronic proctalgia and stool urgency with postoperative incontinence have often been reported. Other complications of transrectal stapled repair are staple-line bleeding and, rarely, staple-line disruption and rectovaginal fistula (overall morbidity rate from 7% to 21%). Because of the high rate of serious complications and poor functional outcome, this is not recommended by the ASCRS Clinical Practice Guidelines.

Solitary Rectal Ulcer

Solitary rectal ulcer syndrome (SRUS) is a rare chronic benign disorder characterized by a combination of symptoms, clinical findings, and histologic abnormalities. Twenty percent of patients have a single ulcer, whereas 40% of patients have multiple ulcers. The remainder have nonspecific lesions such as hyperemic mucosa or pseudopolyps.

SRUS is a disorder of young adults (30–40 years), with a slight female predominance. The cause is multifactorial and includes

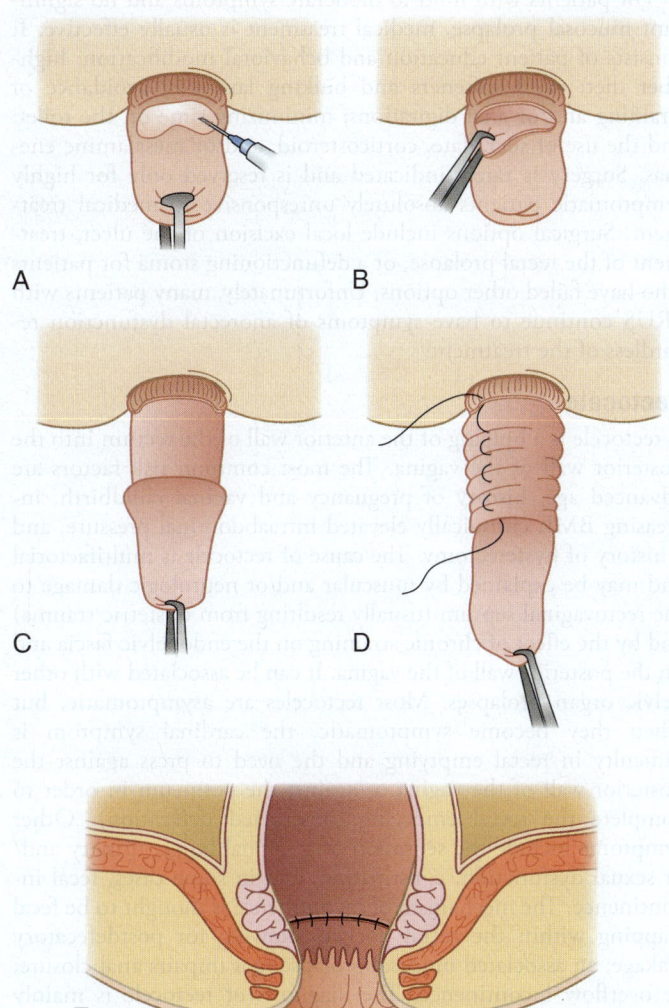

FIGURE 95.67 The Delorme procedure. The mucosal layer is infiltrated with epinephrine-containing solution (A), incised (B), and stripped off the underlying muscularis (C). Plication of the muscularis propria is performed (D). The operation concludes with an anastomosis between the proximal and distal mucosal edges (E).

internal rectal prolapse and abnormal/paradoxical contraction of the puborectalis muscle. These two conditions result in trauma and compression of the anterior rectal wall on the upper anal canal during straining and defecation, with resulting mucosal ischemia and, in some cases, ulceration. Symptoms reported by patients with SRUS include rectal bleeding, prolonged excessive straining, incomplete defecation/tenesmus, mucous discharge, perineal and abdominal pain, and constipation. Up to one-quarter of patients are asymptomatic.

Physical examination and anoscopy demonstrate an intrarectal prolapse and a 1- to 1.5-cm ulcer of the anterior rectal wall 3 to 10 cm from the anal verge that is sometimes difficult to differentiate from a rectal cancer. Histologic examination of biopsies shows characteristic findings: fibromuscular obliteration of the lamina propria, hypertrophied muscularis mucosae with muscular fibers between the crypts, and glandular crypt abnormalities. These specific findings differentiate SRUS from cancer and other inflammatory lesions such as IBD, ischemic colitis, and infectious proctitis.

For patients with mild to moderate symptoms and no significant mucosal prolapse, medical treatment is usually effective. It consists of patient education and behavioral modification: high-fiber diet; stool softeners and bulking laxatives; avoidance of straining and/or anal digitations; minimizing time on the toilet; and the use of sucralfate, corticosteroid, and/or mesalamine enemas. Surgery is rarely indicated and is reserved only for highly symptomatic patients absolutely unresponsive to medical treatment. Surgical options include local excision of the ulcer, treatment of the rectal prolapse, or a defunctioning stoma for patients who have failed other options. Unfortunately, many patients with SRUS continue to have symptoms of anorectal dysfunction regardless of the treatment.

Rectocele

A rectocele is a bulging of the anterior wall of the rectum into the posterior wall of the vagina. The most common risk factors are advanced age, history of pregnancy and vaginal childbirth, increasing BMI, chronically elevated intraabdominal pressure, and a history of hysterectomy. The cause of rectocele is multifactorial and may be explained by muscular and/or neurologic damage to the rectovaginal septum (usually resulting from obstetric trauma) and by the effect of chronic straining on the endopelvic fascia and on the posterior wall of the vagina. It can be associated with other pelvic organ prolapses. Most rectoceles are asymptomatic, but when they become symptomatic, the cardinal symptom is difficulty in rectal emptying and the need to press against the posterior wall of the vagina or against the perineum in order to complete the rectal emptying (obstructed defecation). Other symptoms include the sensation of a vaginal bulge, urinary and/or sexual dysfunction, constipation, and in some cases, fecal incontinence. The mechanism of incontinence is thought to be fecal trapping within the rectal pocket, allowing for postdefecatory leakage; an associated mucosal prolapse that impairs anal closure; or overflow incontinence. The diagnosis of rectocele is mainly clinical and based on physical examination. Digital vaginal and rectal examinations show a bulging in the posterior vaginal wall and in the anterior rectal wall during straining that can be associated with the prolapse of other pelvic organs and with anterior cystocele. Associated stress urinary incontinence is assessed by making the patient cough or perform the Valsalva maneuver with a full bladder.

On defecography, the rectocele appears as a bulging of the rectal wall toward the vagina. A rectocele is graded as small if it is less than 2 cm, moderate if it is between 2 and 4 cm, and large if it is larger than 4 cm in size (Fig. 95.68). This test also gives information about the possible trapping of contrast within the rectocele during defecation and about the possible association with an enterocele or sigmoidocele. It is important to realize that the degree of anatomic distortion often does *not* correlate with the degree of functional impairment and symptoms. Dynamic MRI and MRI defecography are limited by the fact that they are performed with the patient in the supine position (not in the normal upright position for defecation). The balloon expulsion tests can identify the inability to expel an inflated balloon from the rectum after 4 minutes of sitting on a commode. Asymptomatic rectoceles do not need treatment, whereas patients with a symptomatic rectocele are initially managed with a bowel regimen and fiber products in order to improve defecation. Only selected patients with markedly symptomatic rectoceles unresponsive to medical treatment are candidates for surgery. The goal of surgery is to remove the

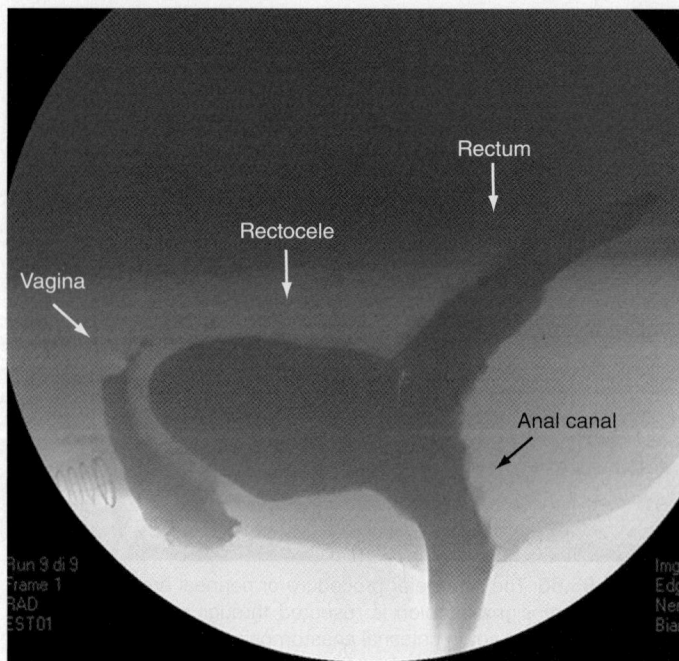

FIGURE 95.68 A defecating proctogram. Both the vagina and the rectum are opacified. The rectocele is clearly evident.

redundant tissue of the rectocele and strengthen the rectovaginal septum.

The transvaginal approach, preferred by gynecologists, allows for better visualization of and access to the levator muscles. A local anesthetic with epinephrine or vasopressin is injected below the vaginal mucosa to dissect the tissue and for hemostasis. The vaginal epithelium is opened in the posterior midline to the upper level of the defect; the fibromuscular layer is exposed and plicated in the midline with vertically or transversely placed sutures. The puborectalis can be reapproximated. The surplus vaginal epithelium is cut off if necessary and sutured with absorbable sutures.

An endorectal repair is performed by colorectal surgeons, with the patient in prone jackknife position. A local anesthetic plus epinephrine or vasopressin is injected into the submucosal plane to dissect the tissue and for hemostasis. A T-shaped or midline incision is made in the rectal mucosa just above the dentate line. Two lateral mucosal flaps are developed on either side of the midline to a level proximal to the rectocele. The excess rectal mucosa is excised. The underlying muscularis layer is exposed and plicated with transversely placed absorbable sutures, and the mucosal edges are then approximated with absorbable sutures. The transperineal rectocele repair is performed by a transverse incision across the bulbocavernosus and transverse perineal muscles; the two limbs of the puborectalis muscle are reapproximated. Transvaginal repair of rectocele was found to confer a better improvement in constipation and sexual-related quality of life than transperineal repair, without an increased incidence of dyspareunia.[81] A mesh can be placed in order to reinforce the plasty. This approach is indicated especially in patients with associated fecal incontinence because a concomitant sphincteroplasty or levatorplasty can be performed.

Constipation

Constipation is a frequent condition that can affect more than 50% of the population over age 65, but in a small subset of patients, constipation may present at a younger age. Several medical conditions can contribute to constipation, including metabolic, endocrine, neurologic, and psychiatric disorders. In adults, new-onset constipation is always a worrisome symptom, and the primary cause must be excluded. Hypothyroidism and medication-induced constipation are common causes. The presence of colorectal malignancies and other causes of colonic obstruction must be excluded with colonoscopy. Patients should be counseled to increase fluid intake up to 1.5 to 2 L/day and to increase the fiber content in the diet. Polyethylene-based solutions (e.g., MiraLAX), probiotics, and over-the-counter products may be helpful. Stimulant laxatives such as bisacodyl or senna should not be used long term. A locally acting chloride channel activator (lubiprostone; Amitiza), a guanylate cyclase agonist (Linzess), and/or a serotonin 5-HT4 agonist (Motegrity) can all be used to treat symptoms of constipation. Long-term constipation, resistant to medical treatment and laxatives, should be further investigated. According to Rome IV criteria, functional constipation is diagnosed if (1) there are at least two of the following symptoms, during at least 25% of defecations, for at least 3 months[82]: straining, lumpy or hard stools, a sensation of incomplete evacuation, sensation of anorectal obstruction/blockage, need for manual maneuvers to facilitate defecation (e.g., digital evacuation, support of the pelvic floor), or fewer than three spontaneous bowel movements per week; (2) loose stools are rarely present without the use of laxatives; and (3) there are insufficient criteria for irritable bowel syndrome. In the presence of obstructed defecation symptoms, defecography, anorectal manometry, balloon expulsion testing, and electromyography can exclude the presence of pelvic floor disorders. Measuring the colonic transit time with the use of radiopaque markers (Sitzmark) can establish the diagnosis of slow transit constipation or colonic inertia. Slow transit constipation can have a neuropathic origin, even if a specific histologic change has not yet been demonstrated. The frequency of bowel movements varies in these patients from one to two per week to one per month. Some patients are unable to have a complete bowel movement in the absence of laxatives or colonic enemas. Severe constipation is associated with abdominal distention, abdominal pain, and nausea, and these symptoms can so affect the quality of a patient's life that they can be absolutely miserable. Chronic symptoms can be present from childhood or adolescence. Slow transit constipation can present with a megacolon on plain x-ray (Fig. 95.69); a water-soluble enema or colon CT can show a redundant, hypotonic colon, and colonoscopy similarly demonstrates a dilated hypotonic colon. In a subset of patients, the colon can be normal and not dilated at radiologic examination. In these patients, the diagnosis and the decision to initiate surgical treatment can be challenging. In highly symptomatic patients with slow transit constipation who failed aggressive medical therapy and whose quality of life is severely impaired, surgical treatment is indicated. Abdominal colectomy with IRA (total abdominal colectomy with ileorectal anastomosis or colectomy with ileorectal anastomosis) can be performed with minimally invasive techniques. Despite postoperative diarrhea (5%–15%), abdominal pain (30%–50%), small bowel obstruction (10%–20%), fecal incontinence, and recurrence of constipation (10%–30%) that have been reported in long-term follow-up, single-center series have demonstrated acceptable results. A systematic review concluded that although colectomy may offer benefits for some patients with chronic constipation, it entails considerable short-term and long-term morbidity, highlighting the paucity of current evidence to guide patient or procedural selection.[83]

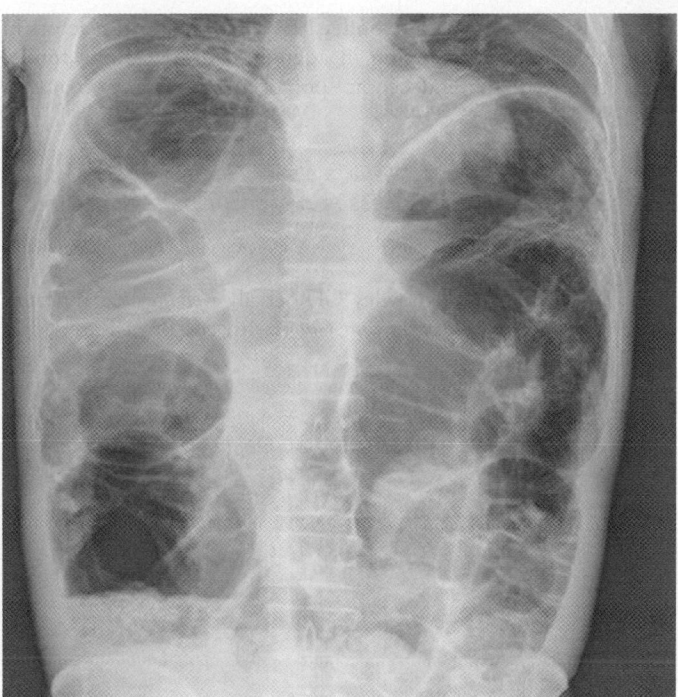

FIGURE 95.69 Plain abdominal film of a patient with slow transit constipation and megacolon.

Segmental colon resections based on transit time measurements are no longer recommended. The extreme therapeutic solution proposed to patients with intractable constipation is a permanent ostomy, usually an ileostomy.

SELECTED REFERENCES

American Society of Colon and Rectal Surgeons. Clinical practice guidelines published in *Diseases of the Colon & Rectum*. Available through a link to the clinical practice guidelines on the journal website: https://journals.lww.com/dcrjournal/pages/default.aspx

Specifically referred to in this chapter are the clinical practice guidelines for (1) Enhanced Recovery After Colon and Rectal Surgery, (2) the Use of Bowel Preparation in Elective Colon and Rectal Surgery, (3) Colon Volvulus and Acute Colonic Pseudo-Obstruction, (4) the Management of Inherited Polyposis Syndromes, (5) the Surgical Treatment of Patients With Lynch Syndrome, (6) the Treatment of Colon Cancer, (7) the Management of Rectal Cancer, (8) the Surveillance of Patients After Curative Treatment of Colon and Rectal Cancer, (9) the Treatment of Rectal Prolapse, (10) the Evaluation and Management of Constipation, and (11) the Consensus Statement of Anorectal Physiology Testing and Pelvic Floor Terminology.

Beck DE, Wexner SD, Rafferty RF, eds. *Gordon and Nivatvongs' Principles and Practice of Surgery for the Colon, Rectum, and Anus.* 4th ed. New York: Thieme Publishers; 2018.

This text provides excellent anatomic illustrations and detailed descriptions of all aspects of diseases of the colon, rectum, and anus.

Haggitt RC, Glotzbach RE, Soffer EE, et al. Prognostic factors in colorectal carcinomas arising in adenomas: implications for lesions removed by endoscopic polypectomy. *Gastroenterology.* 1985;89:328-336.

> Description of Haggitt criteria, a classification for polyps with adenocarcinoma that assesses malignant potential according to the depth of invasion.

Sagar PM, Hill AG, Knowles CH, et al. *Keighley & Williams' Surgery of the Anus, Rectum and Colon.* 4th ed. Boca Raton, FL: CRC Press; 2019.

> The most recently published two-volume textbook of colon and rectal surgery, with an international list of contributors.

Steele SR, Hull TL, Hyman N, et al. *The ASCRS Textbook of Colon and Rectal Surgery.* 3rd ed. New York: Springer; 2016.

> This text is sponsored by the ASCRS, with chapters written by recognized authorities in their field, including an excellent chapter on the molecular basis of colorectal cancer and inherited syndromes written by Dr. Matthew Kalady.

The full reference list appears on Elsevier eBooks+.

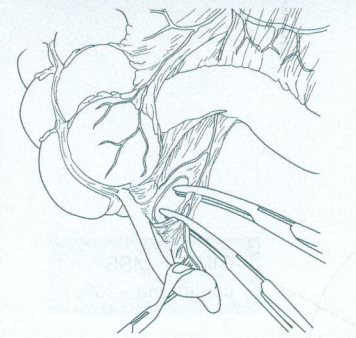

CHAPTER 96

Cancers of the Colon, Rectum, and Anus

Matthew Kalady, David Liska, and Mohammad Abbass

OUTLINE

COLORECTAL CANCER

Colorectal Cancer Genetics

Life requires continual cell division and reproduction, a process that must maintain integrity and has a series of checks and balances. Changes in cellular DNA may occur in a variety of ways and is tightly controlled by oncogenes, tumor suppressors, and DNA repair mechanisms. Multiple genetic and epigenetic events need to happen for normal tissue to become dysplastic, expand, and invade. Defining the genomic landscape and etiologies of colorectal cancer (CRC) provides a better understanding of the varied CRC phenotypes and the differences in the clinical spectrum. Genetic changes may occur via somatic mechanisms and occur within local cells or can exist within the germline and may be inherited, causing an inherent predisposition to developing cancer.

Distinct Colorectal Cancer Pathways

In general, three distinct but potentially overlapping pathways lead to CRC development: chromosomal instability (CIN), methylation, and microsatellite instability (MSI) (Fig. 96.1).

Chromosomal instability pathway. CIN is the most common pathway observed in CRC (65%–70%). It involves a mutation that causes the loss of one allele as a result of insertion, deletion, amplification, aneuploidy, or loss of heterozygosity. Although this can happen in any part of the genome, when it includes a tumor-suppressor gene or driver gene, it provides an initiating event. In

the CIN pathway, which was initially described by Fearon and Vogelstein,[1] the first hit includes abnormality in the adenomatous polyposis coli *(APC)* gene and leads to activation of the wnt signaling pathway, which produces accumulation of nuclear β-catenin and resultant proliferation signals. The initial manifestation of this is an accumulation of dysplastic cells, which can form a tubular adenoma. This pathway's activation has been identified in all CIN tumors, and 80% of these tumors have an *APC* mutation.[2–4] A subsequent *KRAS* mutation initiates extension and promotes growth, and then a third genetic change in genes such as *TP53, SMAD4, PIK3CA,* or *FBXW7* promotes invasion of surrounding tissue. The resultant lesions in this pathway include adenomas and follow the classic adenoma-to-carcinoma sequence.

The serrated or methylator pathway. The recognition of serrated polyps as precancerous lesions has led to the elucidation of the serrated or methylator pathway to CRC. Mutations in the *BRAF* gene are often the inciting event in this pathway. Subsequent increased DNA methylation in the promoter region of key tumor-suppressor genes and DNA repair genes leads to silenced expression of these genes and lack of protein transcription. Because the methylation tends to occur in the promoter regions that are rich in cysteine and guanine, these cancers have been termed the *CpG-island methylator phenotype* (CIMP).[5] CpG islands of CG dinucleotides are present in the 5′ region of almost half of human genes, and methylation leads to silencing or loss of gene expression of the downstream genes.[6] Approximately 15% to 20% of all CRCs evolve from serrated preneoplastic lesions. Some

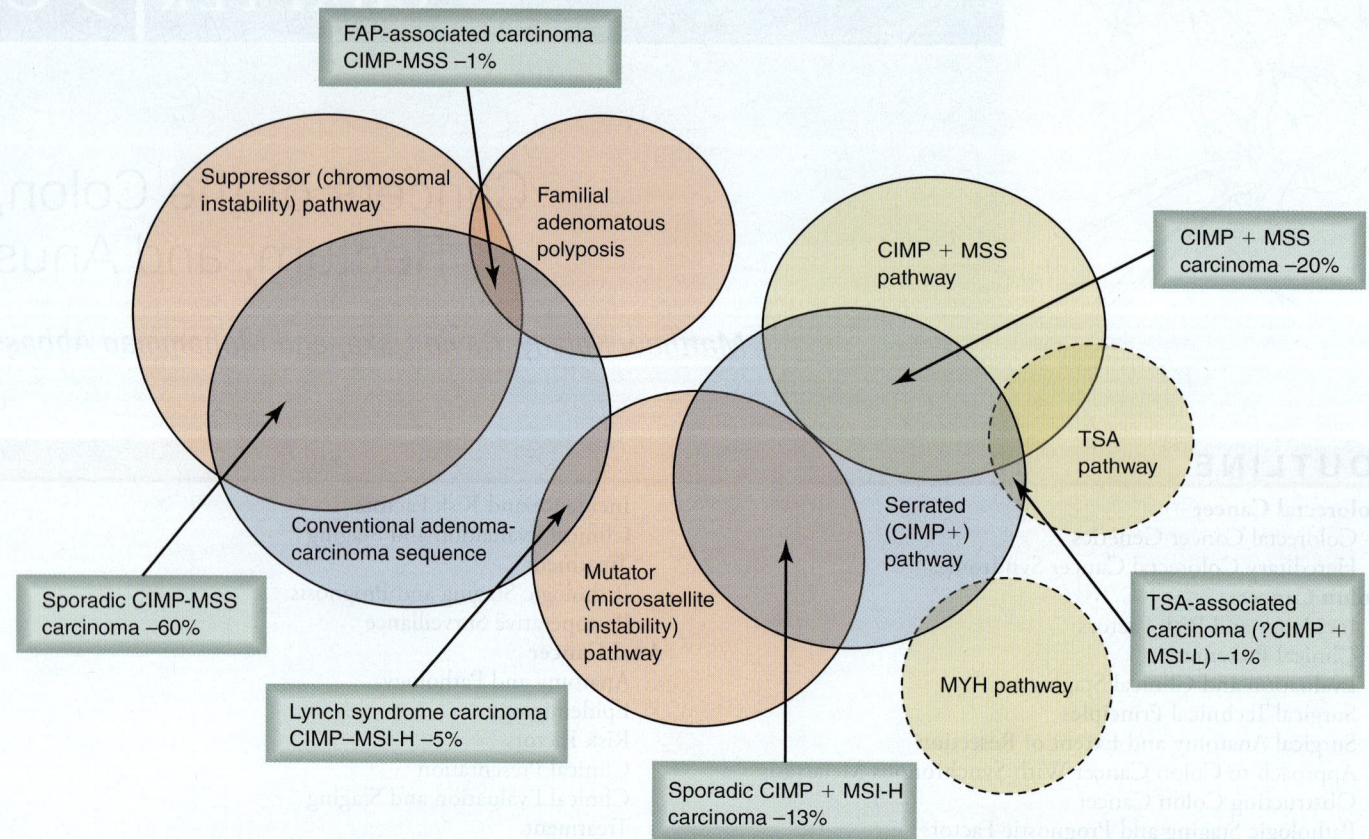

FIGURE 96.1 Schematic represents several overlapping ways to describe the development of colorectal carcinoma. The *red circles* represent mechanisms based on suppressor and mutator pathways. The *blue circles* represent mechanisms based on the precursor lesion (the conventional adenoma-carcinoma sequence and serrated pathways). The *yellow circles* represent poorly characterized pathways. *CIMP–,* CpG-island methylator phenotype negative; *CIMP+,* CpG -island methylator phenotype positive; *FAP,* familial adenomatous polyposis; *MSI-H,* high degree of microsatellite instability; *MSI-L,* low degree of microsatellite instability; *MSS,* microsatellite stable; *TSA,* traditional serrated adenoma. (From Snover DC. Update on the serrated pathway to colorectal carcinoma. *Hum Pathol.* 2011;42:1-10.)

authors suggest that most interval cancers (i.e., cancers that are found between routine screening examinations) are a result of the failure to detect serrated lesions during colonoscopy because these lesions can be flat and subtle.[7,8] Methylated CRCs tend to be more common in patients of older age, tend to be located in the right colon, and are more common in females.

Microsatellite instability pathway. The MSI pathway results from a loss of mismatch repair (MMR) function, usually secondary to loss of one of the four MMR genes (mutL homolog 1 *[MLH1]*, mutS homolog 2 *[MSH2]*, mutS homolog 6 *[MSH6]*, or PMS1 homolog 2 *[PMS2]*). There are three main etiologies for the development of MSI tumors[9]: (1) a germline pathogenic variant in one of the MMR genes (i.e., the cause of Lynch syndrome); (2) hypermethylation of the promoter region of *MLH1* with the subsequent loss of MLH1 expression; and (3) double somatic mutation loss of one of the MMR genes in the tumor. Regardless of the cause, loss of MMR function leads to the inability to fix DNA base-pair mismatches during transcription and thus the accumulation of errors in the DNA that can be incorporated and reproduced. Because DNA mismatches tend to occur in repeating areas of DNA sequences called *microsatellites,* these tumors are called *microsatellite instability-high* (MSI-H). MSI-H tumors have distinct pathologic features, such as a Crohnlike reaction, presence of

mucin, lymphocytic infiltration, and high tumor mutational burden. Approximately 12% to 15% of CRCs are MMR deficient.

Colorectal Cancer Molecular Subtypes

A significant collaborative effort has been made to establish a common ground for classifying CRC based on molecular features. Four CRC subtypes based on gene expression, signaling pathways, and molecular and transcriptome-wide analysis have been proposed[10,11]:

1. CMS1: Immune, characterized by MSI, high CIN, and *BRAF* mutations.
2. CMS2: Canonical, characterized by CIN and downstream targeting of the wnt and MYC pathways.
3. CM3: Metabolic, characterized by a distinct genomic and epigenomic profile with mixed metabolic reprogramming. This subtype includes dysregulated pathways enriched with *KRAS* mutations, a low mixed state of MSI, and intermediate CIMP.
4. CMS4: Mesenchymal, characterized by overexpression of proteins involved in stromal infiltration and mesenchymal activation.

Understanding these subtypes allows for more uniform classification and the ability to collaborate on prospective clinical trials that could help evolve more precise prognosis and treatment. It has been shown that CMS4 tumors have a twofold increased risk of relapse after curative treatment, and CMS1 MSI-H tumors have a worse prognosis in the metastatic setting.[4,12] Fig. 96.2 provides an overview of the different CRC subtypes.

Colorectal Polyps

Most CRCs develop through intermediary lesions called *polyps*. Colorectal polyps are any growth of cells noted in the colorectal lumen, and some may progress to CRC. Polyps can be characterized according to their endoscopic appearance but, more importantly, by their histologic classification. It is important to understand and recognize the different types of polyps in the context of potential advanced neoplasia and the necessary management. Traditionally, nonneoplastic polyps include hamartomas and inflammatory polyps. Hamartomas are accumulations or abnormal growths of normal cells. In the colorectum, hamartomas are rare. They can be sporadic or found in hereditary syndromes (see later). Hamartomas do not have intrinsic malignant potential. Removal is indicated for obstructive symptoms, often as a result of intussusception, or bleeding. Inflammatory polyps are areas of inflamed or healing tissue and are not premalignant. Inflammatory polyps often occur in inflammatory bowel disease and represent areas of normal or healing mucosa in a field of ulcerated or acutely inflamed tissue. The fact that these are usually normal tissue gives them the term *pseudopolyps*.

Polyps with malignant potential include adenomas and serrated polyps. All adenomas have potential for malignant transformation, but only a small percentage actually become cancerous. The risk of cancer depends on size and histology. Patients with an advanced adenoma, defined as size at least 1 cm, high-grade dysplasia, or tubulovillous or villous histology, are at a significantly increased risk of developing CRC. Polyps felt to be adenomas should be removed endoscopically.[13] Serrated polyps are defined

histologically by a sawtooth crypt pattern and nuclear atypia. As discussed earlier, recent research has demonstrated a serrated pathway to carcinoma. Sessile serrated lesions include hyperplastic polyps, sessile serrated adenomas (SSAs), and traditional serrated adenomas (TSAs). Hyperplastic polyps are a result of proliferation in the basal portion of the crypts, are composed of standard cellular components, and are not considered to have a risk of cancer. SSAs (also called *sessile serrated polyps* or *sessile serrated lesions*) are usually larger than hyperplastic polyps and have distorted architecture of the serrated crypts. They typically show one of the following histologic features: horizontal growth along the muscularis mucosa, dilation of the crypt base, serrations extending into the crypt base, or asymmetric proliferation. These polyps can harbor or develop dysplasia and thus have the potential to develop into invasive cancer.[14–16] TSAs histologically show distorted villous or tubulovillous architecture, and the villi have bulbous tips in many cases. These polyps can acquire adenoma-like or serrated dysplasia, thus having neoplastic potential.

Hereditary Colorectal Cancer Syndromes

Understanding and characterization of hereditary CRC syndromes have evolved vastly over the past three decades. The initial classification and understanding of these syndromes were based on phenotypic observation of the colorectum during endoscopy, that is, polyposis versus nonpolyposis syndromes. This understanding evolved as the genetic causes of these syndromes were discovered and defined. Timely identification of individuals at risk for hereditary CRC syndromes offers an opportunity for diagnosis and intervention to prevent cancer development. The development of next-generation multigene panel testing has made genetic diagnosis readily and widely available and has allowed for more precise diagnosis of patients. A summary of the different hereditary syndromes and their associated gene variant is provided in Table 96.1.

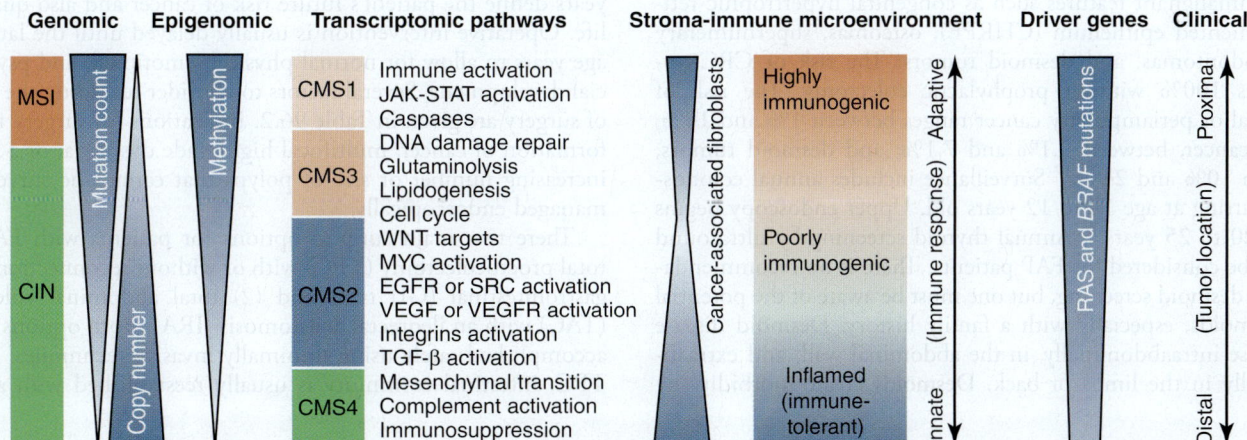

FIGURE 96.2 Schematic representation of colorectal cancer (CRC) subtypes. Microsatellite instability is linked to hypermutation, hypermethylation, immune infiltration, activation of RAS, *BRAF* mutations, and locations in the proximal colon. Tumors with chromosomal instability *(CIN)* are more heterogeneous at the gene-expression level, showing a spectrum of pathway activation ranging from epithelial canonical (consensus molecular subtype 2 *[CMS2]*) to mesenchymal (CMS4). Tumors with CIN are mainly diagnosed in left colon or rectum, and their microenvironment is either poorly immunogenic or inflamed, with marked stromal infiltration. A subset of CRC tumors enriched for RAS mutations has strong metabolic adaptation (CMS3) and intermediate levels of mutation, methylation, and copy number events. *EGFR*, Epidermal growth factor receptor; *JAK*, Janus kinase; *SRC*, steroid receptor coactivator; *STAT*, signal transducer and activator of transcription; *TGF-β*, transforming growth factor-β; *VEGF*, vascular endothelial growth factor; *VEGFR*, VEGF receptor. (From Dienstmann R, Vermeulen L, Guinney J, et al. Consensus molecular subtypes and the evolution of precision medicine in colorectal cancer. *Nat Rev Cancer*. 2017;17:79-92.)

TABLE 96.1   Inherited Colorectal Cancer Syndromes

SYNDROME	GENES	CLINICAL FINDINGS	CRC RISK
Familial adenomatous polyposis	APC	Colonic tubular adenomas, duodenal adenomas, gastric fundic gland polyps, desmoid tumors, epidermoid cysts, osteomas	100%
MUTYH-associated polyposis	MUTYH	Colonic tubular adenomas, CRC <50 years, gastric fundic gland polyps, duodenal adenomas and carcinomas	80%
NTLH1-associated polyposis	NTLH1	Adenomas, skin hemangiomas, seborrheic keratosis, intradermal nevi, ovarian and hepatic cysts, breast papilloma	—
Polymerase proofreading-associated polyposis	POLD1, POLE	Adenoma, meningioma, severe cases: café au lait, pediatric brain tumors	—
MSH3-associated polyposis	MSH3	Adenomas, scarce data	—
MBD4-associated polyposis	MBD4	Adenomas, acute myeloid leukemia, uveal melanoma, schwannoma	—
JPS	SMAD4, BMPR1A	≥5 Juvenile polyps; any juvenile polyp and JPS family history	40%
PJS	STK11	Peutz-Jeghers polyps (PJPs)	40%
		Orocutaneous pigmentation	
		Family history of PJP; cancer of small bowel, colon, stomach, pancreas, breast, ovary, testis	
PTHS	PTEN	Hamartomas, lipomas, fibromas, ganglioneuromas	9%–32%
Lynch syndrome	MLH1, MSH2, MSH6, PMS2, EPCAM	Microsatellite-unstable CRC, advanced adenomas, gastric, duodenal, small bowel, transitional cell, gallbladder, pancreas, endometrial, ovarian	60%–80%

AD, Autosomal dominant; *AR*, autosomal recessive; *CRC*, colorectal cancer; *JPS*, juvenile polyposis syndrome; *PJS*, Peutz-Jeghers syndrome; *PTHS*, PTEN hamartoma tumor syndrome.

Polyposis Syndromes

Familial adenomatous polyposis. Familial adenomatous polyposis (FAP) is an autosomal dominant syndrome resulting from a pathogenic variant in the *APC* gene. The incidence of FAP is approximately 1 in 10,000. This syndrome has a 20% reported incidence of de novo mutations, and thus, the absence of family history does not exclude this diagnosis. The known neoplastic features of this syndrome include colorectal polyps and CRC; gastric polyps; duodenal and periampullary polyps and cancer; medulloblastoma; papillary thyroid carcinoma; hepatoblastoma; and nonmalignant features such as congenital hypertrophic retinal pigmented epithelium (CHRPE), osteomas, supernumerary teeth, odontomas, and desmoid tumors. The risk of CRC approaches 100% without prophylactic colectomy. The risk of duodenal or periampullary cancer ranges between 1% and 10%; gastric cancer, between 0.1% and 7.1%; and desmoid tumors, between 10% and 24%.[17] Surveillance includes annual colonoscopy starting at age 10 to 12 years old. Upper endoscopy begins at age 20 to 25 years.[18] Annual thyroid screening by ultrasound should be considered for FAP patients. There is no recommendation for desmoid screening, but one must be aware of the potential for desmoids, especially with a family history. Desmoid disease may arise intraabdominally, in the abdominal wall, and extraabdominally in the limbs or back. Desmoids create morbidity by

local extension into surrounding structures, and complications of intraabdominal desmoids include bowel obstruction, enterocutaneous fistula, and ureteric obstruction. Asymptomatic or small desmoids may be observed, whereas growing or symptomatic desmoids may be treated with escalating therapies. Surgical management of desmoid disease should be planned in expert centers to balance the extent of the intervention with maintaining the patient's quality of life.

Judicious operative management of the colon and rectum in FAP patients is critical because those decisions made in the early years define the patient's future risk of cancer and also quality of life. Operative intervention is usually delayed until the late teenage years to allow for normal physical, emotional, and psychosocial development. Several factors to consider regarding the timing of surgery are given in Table 96.2. Indications for surgery include formation of cancer, multifocal high-grade dysplasia, or a rapidly increasing number or size of polyps that cannot be surveyed or managed endoscopically.

There two main surgical options for patients with FAP: (1) total proctocolectomy (TPC) with or without reconnection of the gastrointestinal (GI) tract and (2) total abdominal colectomy (TAC) with an ileorectal anastomosis (IRA). Both options can be accomplished safely using minimally invasive techniques. After a TPC, intestinal continuity is usually reestablished with an ileal

TABLE 96.2   Surgical Decision-Making in Patients With Familial Adenomatous Polyposis

SURGICAL RECOMMENDATION	INDICATION	COMMENT
Total abdominal colectomy	• Colon cancer • Uncontrolled colon polyp burden • Rectum <20 polyps	• Rectum polyp burden has to be manageable endoscopically
Total proctocolectomy	• Profuse polyposis • Rectal cancer • Rectal polyp burden >20	• Stapled anastomosis if the anal transitional zone is clear of polyps, otherwise will need mucosectomy and hand-sewn pouch-anal anastomosis
Pancreas-sparing duodenectomy (PSD)	• Spigelman stage IV on upper endoscopy findings	• Whipple procedure if cancer is present
Thyroidectomy	• Papillary thyroid cancer	—

pouch–anal anastomosis (IPAA). Each option has advantages and disadvantages in terms of cancer risk reduction and quality of life. In general terms, TPC/IPAA is associated with longer surgical times and increased complications, including sexual and urinary dysfunction, decreased fecundity, and more frequent bowel movements and incontinence, compared with a TAC/IRA. However, removing the rectum during TPC removes future rectal cancer risk, which remains after TAC/IRA. The main advantage of TAC/IRA is decreased daily bowel movements and better overall quality of life, but again, this is weighed against cancer risk. The main decision point relies on the rectal polyp burden, and most surgeons use 20 or fewer polyps in the rectum as a threshold to preserve the rectum. Following these guidelines, the risk of rectal cancer is approximately 3% at a median follow-up of 13 years, and the need for completion proctectomy is 8%.[19]

Another consideration regarding choice of TAC/IRA or TPC includes desmoid risk. Because most desmoid disease presents after surgery, patients with desmoid tumor or those at high risk of developing desmoid tumors should defer surgery as long as safely able. When surgery is indicated, these high-risk patients should be considered for TAC/IRA (if safe to survey the rectum), given that TPC/IPAA is more desmoidogenic than IRA.[20] For patients who undergo TPC/IPAA, the extent of the distal dissection is dependent on the extent of the polyposis in the anal transition zone (ATZ). The standard approach is to divide the rectum at the anorectal junction (top of the anal canal) and perform a double-stapled anastomosis, leaving a 2- to 3-cm segment of ATZ that will need to be surveyed. If there is diffuse polyposis or high-grade dysplasia in the ATZ, then mucosectomy should be performed with a hand-sewn IPAA. This decreases future neoplasia risk but also results in worse bowel function. Regardless of what surgery is done, any remaining anorectal mucosa, ATZ, and/or ileal pouch should be surveyed annually for neoplasia.

MUTYH-associated polyposis.
MUTYH-associated polyposis (MAP) is an autosomal recessive disease; thus, biallelic pathogenic variants in *MUTYH* are needed for diagnosis. About 1% to 2% of the general population carries a monoallelic *MUTYH* pathogenic variant, and less than 1% of all CRC diagnoses are due to MAP. Patients develop anywhere between 10 and 100 colorectal adenomas by the fifth or sixth decade, and up to 60% of those patients have CRC at presentation.[21,22] Some patients may present only with CRC and not have any other polyps. Duodenal polyps have been reported in patients with MAP and some rare occasions of duodenal cancer.[23] Surveillance includes colonoscopy every 1 to 2 years starting at diagnosis, a baseline upper endoscopy at age 30 to 35 years, and follow-up surveillance based on the Spigelman classification.[18] Surgical management of patients with MAP follows the same general guidelines used for decision-making in FAP. TAC/IRA is recommended if colon cancer develops or if endoscopic management of polyp burden is no longer feasible. Rectal cancer is uncommon in MAP, but patients with rectal cancer should be considered for proctocolectomy and IPAA.

Juvenile polyposis syndrome.
Juvenile polyposis syndrome (JPS) is an autosomal dominantly inherited syndrome caused by pathogenic variants in the *SMAD4* or *BMPR1A* genes and characterized clinically by hamartomatous polyps. There is a 25% chance of de novo mutations in JPS patients. The incidence of JPS is 1 per 100,000 in the general population. The clinical criteria of diagnosis have been set for any individual who meets at least one of the following: (1) ≥5 juvenile polyps in the colon, (2) multiple juvenile polyps throughout the GI tract, and (3) any number of juvenile polyps in an individual with a family history of JPS.[24]

SMAD4 mutations in JPS are associated with hereditary hemorrhagic telangiectasia (HHT).[25] JPS patients commonly present with GI bleeding or obstruction as a result of prolapsing polyps. Patients with JPS exhibit a 10% to 38% lifetime risk of colon cancer, and the average age at diagnosis is 34 years. For the pediatric population, upper endoscopy and colonoscopy should start at 12 to 15 years and be repeated every 1 to 3 years based on findings or every 5 years if no polyps were found.[26] Colectomy is recommended if a patient develops CRC or the polyp burden prevents adequate surveillance.

Peutz-Jeghers syndrome.
Peutz-Jeghers syndrome (PJS) is an autosomal dominant syndrome resulting from a pathogenic mutation in the *STK11 (LKB1)* gene. It is characterized by multiple hamartomatous polyps in the GI tract and mucocutaneous pigmentation and has a prevalence of 1 in 8000 to 200,000 in the general population. PJS has high penetrance by the third decade of life and has a de novo rate of 10% to 20%. Thus, the absence of family history should not exclude the diagnosis or referral to genetic testing. A clinical diagnosis can be made if individuals meet two or more of the following criteria: (1) two or more PJS hamartomatous polyps in the GI tract; (2) mucocutaneous hyperpigmentation of the mouth, lips, nose, eyes, genitalia, or fingers; or (3) family history of PJS.[27] Because of the increased risk of ovarian sex cord tumors and Sertoli cell testicular cancers, an annual physical examination is recommended for observation of precocious puberty in females or feminizing changes in male patients.[17]

Adult surveillance is intensive for this patient population because of the increased risk of breast cancer (32%–54%), colon cancer (39%), gastric cancer (29%), small intestine cancer (13%), pancreatic cancer (11%–36%), cervical and endometrial cancer (9%–10%), ovarian and testicular cancer (9%), and lung cancer (7%–17%). Thus, the following surveillance is recommended[28,29]:

- Mammogram and breast MRI at age 30; repeated every 6 months
- Colonoscopy at age 18; repeated every 2 to 3 years
- Upper endoscopy at age 18; repeated every 2 to 3 years
- Small bowel visualization with either video capsule endoscopy or CT/MRI enterography at age 18; repeated every 2 to 3 years
- Annual pancreatic endoscopic ultrasound (EUS) or magnetic resonance cholangiopancreatography at age 30 to 35
- Annual pelvic examination with pelvic ultrasound or biopsy if any abnormal bleeding, starting at age 18 to 20 years
- Annual testicular examination

Colectomy is recommended for the development of CRC or uncontrolled polyp burden. Small bowel polyps often cause obstruction. Those patients should be referred to expert centers that can focus on bowel preservation and perform a "clean-sweep" procedure with removal of all small and large bowel polyps to decrease future risk of malignancy and obstruction.[30]

PTEN hamartoma tumor syndrome.
There are multiple phenotypic variations of syndromes under the PTEN hamartoma tumor syndrome (PTHS) nomenclature. They follow an autosomal dominant inheritance and result from a pathogenic mutation in the *PTEN* gene. Cowden syndrome (CS) is the most thoroughly described phenotype in this syndrome thus far and has a prevalence of 1 in 200,000 to 250,000. There is a 10% to 30% de novo rate. Phenotypically, there are many characteristic findings in patients with CS:

- Mucocutaneous (trichilemmomas, acral keratoses, facial blemishes, and clear cell acanthomas)
- Breast cancer (up to 85% lifetime risk)
- Nonmedullary thyroid cancer

- Genitourinary manifestations, such as uterine fibroids, bilateral hyperechoic testicular lesions, lipomatosis of the testes, endometrial cancer (13%–30%), and renal cell carcinoma (13%–34%)
- Esophageal glycogen acanthosis
- Gastric, duodenal polyps: hyperplastic, hamartomas, ganglioneuromas, adenomas, and inflammatory polyps[31]
- Colorectal polyps: hamartomas, inflammatory, ganglioneuromas, lipoma, leiomyomas, and hyperplastic polyps. CRC has been reported in up to 13% of PTHS patients by the age of 50 years[31]
- Macrocephaly has been described in 21% to 38% of patients with CS, in addition to many other neurologic abnormalities, intellectual disability, developmental delay, and autism

The International Cowden Consortium has set testing criteria for PTHS. A clinical operational diagnosis is established in a family where one individual meets revised PTHS clinical diagnostic criteria or has a *PTEN* mutation.[32] Diagnosis and management of patients with potential PTHS is complex and requires multidisciplinary communication and management, and diagnosis and surveillance should be done in expert centers. National Comprehensive Cancer Network (NCCN) recommendations are to be followed: an annual physical examination; annual breast examination, mammogram, and MRI; colonoscopy starting at age 35 or 5 to 10 years before the earliest CRC in the family; renal ultrasound; psychomotor assessment in children; annual dermatology evaluation; annual thyroid ultrasound; and consideration of transvaginal ultrasound and endometrial biopsy.[33]

TAC/IRA is recommended for CRC patients with PTEN. Other phenotypes in PTHS are Bannayan-Riley-Ruvalcaba syndrome and Proteus syndrome.

Serrated polyposis syndrome. Serrated polyposis syndrome (SPS) is a clinical diagnosis. The World Health Organization has recently updated its diagnostic criteria for SPS as the following[34]:

- At least five serrated lesions or polyps proximal to the rectum >5 mm, with two or more larger than 10 mm
- More than 20 serrated lesions or polyps of any size distributed throughout the colorectum, with at least 5 proximal to the rectum

The lifetime CRC risk has been reported to be approximately 15% to 30% overall but also varies based on the patient's age, the number of polyps present, and the histologic type of polyps.[35,36] The current recommended surveillance is with high-quality colonoscopy and polypectomy of all polyps ≥5 mm and repeated every 1 to 3 years based on the number and size of polyps.[17] Total colectomy is recommended for CRC or high polyp burden that is not able to be effectively managed endoscopically.

Other polyposis syndromes. The advancement and accessibility of genetic testing of patients with polyposis phenotype has facilitated the description of other syndromes with CRC predisposition. The management of these syndromes follows the primary recommendations for oncologic resection and polyp burden management.

- NTLH1-associated polyposis (NAP) is an autosomal recessive inheritance in the *NTLH1* gene.[37]
- Polymerase proofreading-associated polyposis (PPAP) follows a dominant inheritance pattern in the *POLE* or *POLD1* genes.[38]
- MSH3-associated polyposis follows an autosomal recessive inheritance pattern in the *MSH3* gene.[39]

Nonpolyposis Syndromes

Lynch syndrome. Definitions of Lynch syndrome have evolved from phenotypic description and family history criteria to a more complex genetic characterization. Lynch syndrome was previously referred to as *hereditary nonpolyposis colorectal cancer* (HNPCC), a term that was initially established to distinguish the hereditary predisposition from FAP. HNPCC is a clinical diagnosis based on the Amsterdam criteria. For a family to meet Amsterdam II criteria, the following conditions must be met: (1) at least three relatives with an HNPCC-associated cancer (colorectum, endometrium, ovaries, small bowel, stomach, ureter or renal pelvis, pancreas, brain, skin), one of whom is a first-degree relative of the other; (2) two or more successive generations should be affected; and (3) at least one cancer should be diagnosed before age 50. The discovery of the underlying inherited variants in MMR genes led to a more precise definition of Lynch syndrome that is dependent on the presence of a pathogenic variant in a DNA MMR gene.

Lynch syndrome is an autosomal dominant inherited syndrome resulting from a pathogenic mutation in one of the four known MMR genes (*MLH1, MSH2, MSH6, PMS2*) and *EPCAM*. The incidence is 1/279 in the general population[40] and about 3% of all CRCs.[41] Patients with Lynch syndrome are at an increased risk of colorectal, endometrial, ovarian, urothelial, gastric, small bowel, pancreas, biliary tract, prostate, and skin cancer (sebaceous adenocarcinoma). The cumulative risk of cancer varies based on each gene mutation.[17] The cumulative risk of CRC by age 80 is 46% to 61% in patients with *MLH1* mutations, 33% to 52% in *MSH2*, 10% to 44% in *MSH6*, and 8.7% to 20% in patients with *PMS2* mutations.[17] Annual colonoscopy starting at age 20 to 25 is the cornerstone of surveillance and decreases both CRC formation and death from cancer in Lynch syndrome patients. Annual transvaginal ultrasound with endometrial biopsy beginning at age 30 to 35 should be considered, and prophylactic hysterectomy after childbearing is completed should also be discussed. Other screening includes annual physical examination and dermatology examination for detection of sebaceous tumors. Of note, *EPCAM* gene deletions can lead to silencing of the *MSH2* gene; thus, patients with *EPCAM* mutations should follow the same guidelines that patients with *MSH2* mutations follow.

CRC tumor testing for MSI or expression of MMR proteins is a common means of screening for Lynch syndrome. Patients with either a microsatellite-unstable tumor or whose tumor lacks expression of one of the MMR proteins (without *MLH-1* promoter hypermethylation indicating a sporadic tumor) should then be referred for genetic counseling and testing.[42] Historically, family history meeting Amsterdam criteria and tumor histologic characteristics for Bethesda criteria were used to identify and screen individuals for Lynch syndrome.[43] Because next-generation multigene panel testing has demonstrated a higher yield of detecting pathogenic variants than more focused testing, there is consideration for genetic germline testing of all patients with CRC.[42,44]

Surgery for Lynch syndrome is based on therapeutic resection of the tumor as well as prophylactic extended resection to reduce future CRC risk. Future cancer risk should be balanced against quality of life, and decisions should be individualized. The risk of metachronous CRC after segmental resection alone is 12% to 20% at 10 years and as high as 72% at 40 years.[45–49] The American Society of Colon and Rectal Surgeons recommends total colectomy as opposed to segmental colectomy for patients with colon cancer and Lynch syndrome to reduce future cancer risk.[50] The extent of resection for rectal cancer is more challenging and debated. Extended prophylactic resection would include TPC/IPPA, which has more significant functional implications. Based on small retrospective studies, the risk of metachronous colon cancer after proctectomy is 19% at 10 years, 47% at 20 years, and 69% at 30 years.[51,52] The decision for proctectomy alone versus TPC/IPAA should be discussed in the context of risk reduction and quality of life and be individualized after informed discussion. Regardless of the procedure performed, any remaining colon or rectum should be surveilled by endoscopy annually.

Recent advances in neoadjuvant immunotherapy in patients with DNA MMR deficiency (dMMR) rectal cancer are redefining the treatment paradigm for patients with Lynch syndrome. dMMR rectal cancer patients treated with neoadjuvant immunotherapy in a prospective trial have shown a 100% clinical response rate and yielded a nonsurgical approach.[53] Longer follow-up and more patients are needed before to better define these outcomes.

Constitutional mismatch repair deficiency. Constitutional mismatch repair deficiency (CMMRD) is a highly penetrant syndrome resulting from the inheritance of biallelic pathogenic mutations in one of the MMR genes *(MLH1, MSH2, MSH6, PMS2)*. The resultant phenotype involves formation of multiple cancers at a young age. Most cases are diagnosed in childhood. The surveillance and management of these patients are complex and done with an experienced center.[54]

Familial colorectal cancer type X. CRC patients from families who meet Amsterdam I criteria but have MMR proficiency are defined as having familial colorectal cancer type X (FCCX).[55] The CRC risk is twice that of the general population but less than those with Lynch syndrome. The mean age of CRC is also between that of the general population and Lynch syndrome, at age 61. Colonoscopy should start at age 45, or 10 years younger than the youngest CRC in that family. If colonoscopy is normal, it should be repeated every 5 years. For FCCX patients who develop CRC, a segmental rather than total colectomy is recommended because the risks of metachronous CRC are not as well defined, and there is an absence of evidence that extended resection reduces cancer risk. Recent data suggested that the risk of extracolonic cancers might also be present in this patient population, such as gastric cancer, urothelial cancer, breast cancer, ocular melanoma, and pancreatic cancer.[56] Surveillance in this patient population should be individualized based on family history and age of cancer presentation in families as well.

COLON CANCER

Incidence and Risk Factors

Colon cancer is among the top three cancers in both males and females in the United States. There are approximately 100,000 new cases nationally each year. The overall incidence has been declining as a result of the widespread adoption of CRC screening, but younger age groups (less than 50 years old) have had an increasing incidence.[57] From the mid-1980s through 2013, there was a 2.4% increase per year in people aged 20 to 29 years, a 1.0% increase in people aged 30 to 39, a 1.3% increase in people aged 40 to 49 years, and a 0.5% increase for people aged 50 to 54 years. In patients above the age of 50 years, 6% to 10% of all CRCs are the result of an inherited gene pathogenic variation, whereas 20% of all CRCs in patients younger than 50 years old have an inherited predisposition.[58-60] In patients with CRC younger than 50 years old, up to 10% of those patients have Lynch syndrome, and this increases to 23% in patients younger than age 35 years.[61]

There is an increased risk of CRC in patients with inflammatory bowel disease.[62] Beyond germline pathogenic mutations and inflammatory bowel disease, many other risk factors are documented to increase the risk of CRC but do not change the screening recommendation regarding age or frequency, such as obesity, diabetes mellitus and insulin resistance, tobacco use, alcohol use, red and processed meat intake, and lack of exercise and sedentary lifestyle.

Clinical Presentation

The most common presenting symptoms of colon cancer include change in bowel habits, blood per rectum, and abdominal pain. Symptoms also vary depending on tumor location. Right-sided tumors present with iron-deficiency anemia, whereas left-sided tumors more commonly present with a change in stool caliber or hematochezia. It is important to note that many colon cancers are asymptomatic, and screening at appropriate times and intervals is indicated.

Evaluation and Clinical Staging

Most colon cancers are diagnosed at colonoscopy. This examination should document the location of the tumor, including relationship to anatomic landmarks, and an endoscopic tattoo should be placed. It should be noted that the entire colon was evaluated for other lesions and that the examination was complete. The lesion should be biopsied because definitive diagnosis is made by histology. The biopsy should also undergo evaluation for MMR deficiency[63] to identify patients who qualify for genetic counseling to diagnose Lynch syndrome or qualify for treatment with checkpoint inhibitor immunotherapy.[64] Laboratory evaluation includes a complete blood count, chemistry, and the tumor marker carcinoembryonic antigen (CEA) testing. Evaluation for distant metastases incudes CT of chest, abdomen, and pelvis with intravenous and oral contrast unless the patient has any contraindications. Positron emission tomography (PET)/CT scan is not routinely recommended and should be used only to evaluate equivocal findings on contrast imaging.

Surgical Technical Principles

The most important surgical principles for primary colon cancer are to ensure negative margins and adequate lymphadenectomy for pathologic staging. The recommended resection margin is 5 to 7 cm proximal and distal to the tumor.[65-67] Regional lymph nodes are located in the mesocolon along the main vascular pedicles, and removal provides staging information and removes potential lymph node metastases. Evaluation of more than 12 lymph nodes harvested is associated with a survival benefit in stage II and III colon cancer,[68] and achieving this lymph node yield is facilitated by high vascular ligation. Evaluation of fewer than 12 lymph nodes is associated with an increased risk of recurrence.[69-71] Recent data from the National Cancer Database (NCDB) showed a survival benefit in patients with T3N0 disease who receive adjuvant chemotherapy when there is an inadequate lymph node harvest.[70] After the resection, the anastomosis must be constructed without tension, using healthy, well-vascularized segments of bowel. It is important to preserve the marginal artery to the segments of reconnected bowel to avoid ischemia and complications.

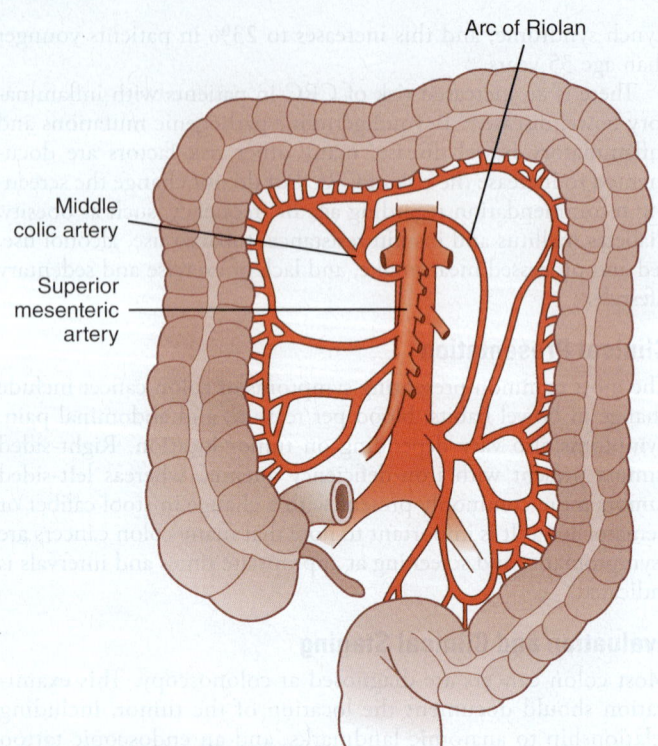

FIGURE 96.3 The arterial blood supply to the colon is from the superior and inferior mesenteric arteries. (From Gordon PH, Nivatvongs S, eds. *Principles and Practice of Surgery for the Colon, Rectum and Anus.* 2nd ed. Quality Medical Publishing; 1999:23.)

Surgical Anatomy and Extent of Resection

The extent of resection and name of the operation are usually dictated by the location of the primary tumor and the vascular supply of the resected colon segment. Understanding the vascular anatomy is essential for safe and effective colon cancer resection. The arterial supply to the colon is shown in Fig. 96.3. The main branches from the aorta that supply the colon include the superior mesenteric artery and its branches to the right colon, including the ileocolic artery, right colic artery, and middle colic artery, and the inferior mesenteric artery (IMA) with its branches to the rectum and left colon, including the superior rectal artery, sigmoid artery, and left colic artery. There is an arcade of collateral vascularization via the marginal artery running parallel to and near the colon wall.

Right-Sided Tumors

Tumors of the cecum and ascending colon are treated by right colectomy. This operation includes high ligation of the ileocolic artery, right colic artery (when present), and the right branch of the middle colic artery (Fig. 96.4). The lymph nodes associated with these vessels are harvested en bloc. The operation can be done using a medial-to-lateral or a lateral-to-medial approach. In either approach, the plane between the mesocolon and the duodenum under the ileocolic pedicle is dissected and developed, exposing the head of the pancreas and allowing access to the transverse colon mesentery to ligate the right branch of the middle colic artery. The terminal ileum is divided approximately 5 cm from the ileocecal valve and the transverse colon at its proximal third. The omentum should be resected en bloc with the specimen. An ileocolic anastomosis is performed and may be done

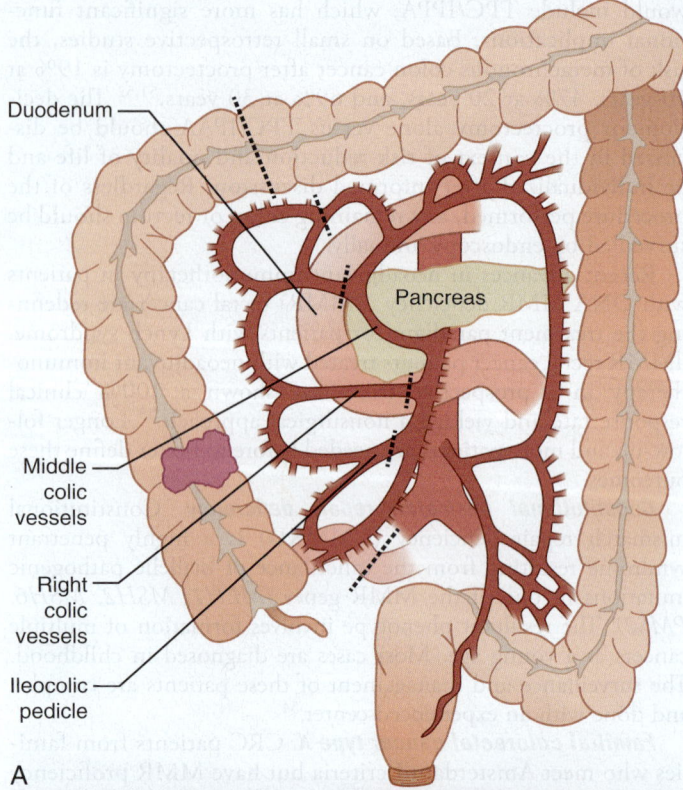

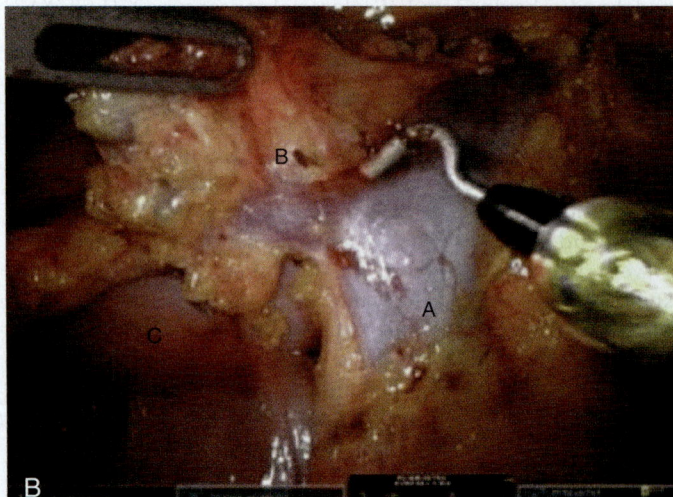

FIGURE 96.4 Resection for a right-sided cancer. The ileocolic, right colic, and right branch of the middle colic vessels are ligated. The terminal ileum and the transverse colon are divided as shown in (A). (B) Lapascopic view of a right-sided colon dissection from a medial approach. The duodenum *(A)*, right colon mesentery *(B)*, and cecum *(C)* are shown.

using a variety of techniques and configurations, including side-to-side antiperistaltic, side-to-side isoperistaltic, end-to-end, or end-to-side techniques. This can be constructed using staplers or hand-sewn techniques.

Transverse Colon Tumors

Most tumors in the transverse colon are treated with an extended right colectomy, which includes ligation of the ileocolic artery as in a right colectomy but also includes division of the middle colic

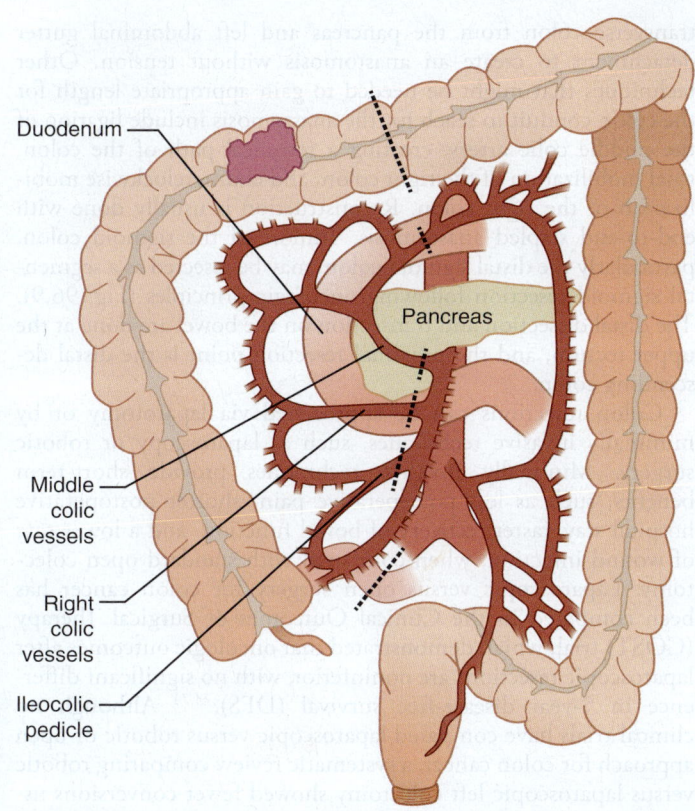

FIGURE 96.5 Resection for cancers of the proximal transverse colon. The ileocolic, right, and middle colic vessels are ligated. The terminal ileum and the transverse colon are transected as shown.

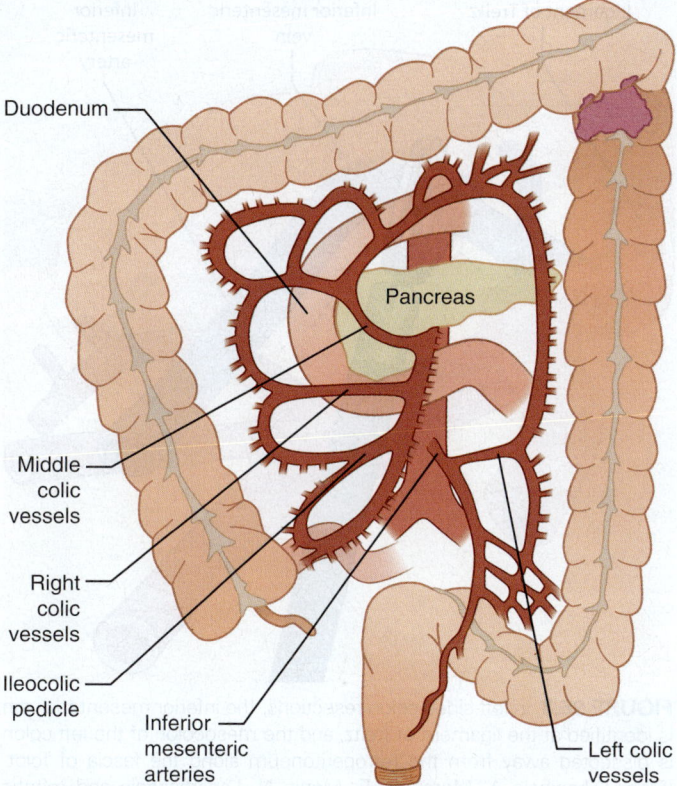

FIGURE 96.6 Segmental resection for cancers of the splenic flexure. The left colic artery and the left branch of the middle colic artery are ligated as shown.

artery at its base (Fig. 96.5). An ileocolic anastomosis is constructed in the distal transverse colon according to the same principles as described earlier.

Splenic Flexure Tumors

Some debate exists about the ideal surgical resection of splenic flexure tumors. Options include an extended right colectomy or subtotal colectomy with inclusion of the splenic flexure and ileo–descending colon anastomosis. Blood flow to the anastomosis is dependent on the marginal artery. Segmental resection of the splenic flexure alone has been described (Fig. 96.6). In this surgery, the left colic artery is divided at its origin from the IMA, and the inferior mesenteric vein is divided at the inferior border of the pancreas. The omentum in this region should be resected en bloc with the colon. The colocolonic anastomosis is often best suited for an end-to-end or isoperistaltic side-to-side configuration. Recent data suggest segmental resections have similar oncologic and survival outcomes to extended resections.[72]

Left-Sided Tumors

Tumors of the descending colon are generally treated with left colectomy, which includes high ligation of the IMA. The base of the inferior mesenteric is surrounded by the mesenteric and hypogastric nervous plexus and should be avoided during dissection (Fig. 96.7). The inferior mesenteric vein is also ligated lateral to the ligament of Treitz (Fig. 96.8), which increases lymph node harvest and also allows for increased mobilization of the colon for the anastomosis. The splenic flexure must be fully mobilized with detachment of the mesocolon of the splenic flexure and distal

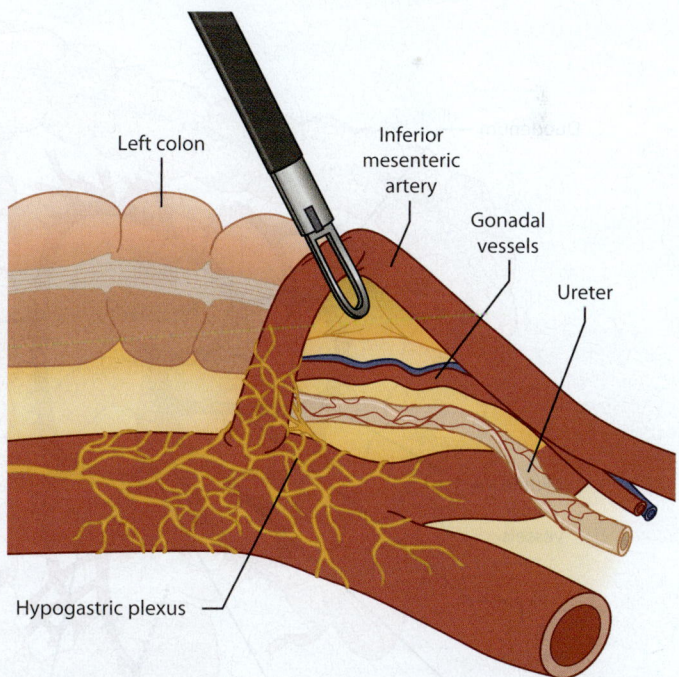

FIGURE 96.7 The inferior mesenteric artery originates from the aorta, 2 to 3 cm caudal from the area where the inferior mesenteric vein is identified; its origin is surrounded by the mesenteric and hypogastric nervous plexus. (From D'Annibale A, Morpurgo E, Menin N. Laparoscopic and robotic surgery in rectal cancer. In: Delaini GG, ed. *Rectal Cancer. New Frontiers in Diagnosis, Treatment and Rehabilitation.* Springer; 2005:167-176.)

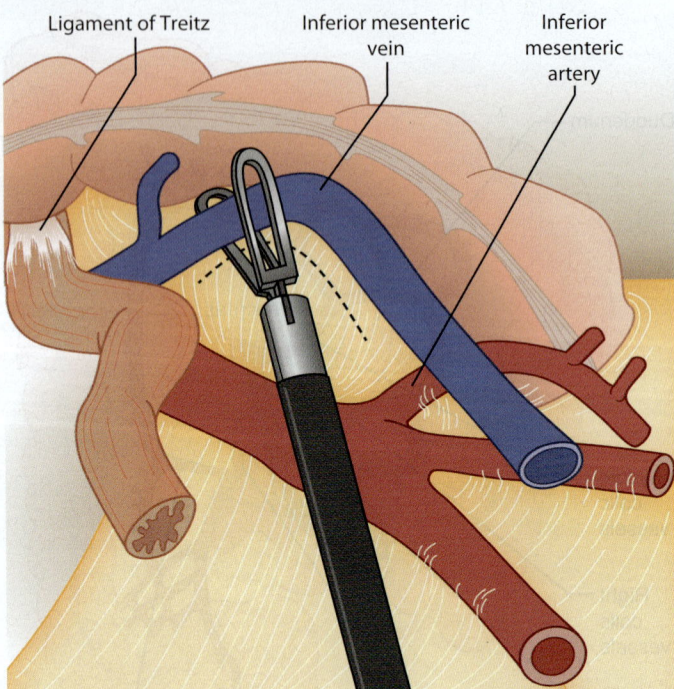

FIGURE 96.8 In left-sided colon resections, the inferior mesenteric vein is identified at the ligament of Treitz, and the mesocolon of the left colon is dissected away from the retroperitoneum along the fascia of Toldt. (From D'Annibale A, Morpurgo E, Menin N. Laparoscopic and robotic surgery in rectal cancer. In: Delaini GG, ed. *Rectal Cancer. New Frontiers in Diagnosis, Treatment and Rehabilitation.* Springer; 2005:167-176.)

transverse colon from the pancreas and left abdominal gutter detachment to create an anastomosis without tension. Other techniques that might be needed to gain appropriate length for the colon conduit to reach for the anastomosis include ligation of the middle colic artery, creating a retroileal path of the colon, total mobilization of the right colon, and counterclockwise mobilization of the right colon. Reconstruction is usually done with end-to-end stapled anastomosis. Tumors of the sigmoid colon, particularly the distal sigmoid colon, may be resected as a segmental sigmoid resection following oncologic principles (Fig. 96.9). The distal dissection and transection on the bowel are done at the upper rectum, and the proximal resection point is the distal descending colon.

Colon resections can be approached via laparotomy or by minimally invasive techniques, such as laparoscopy or robotic surgery. Minimally invasive techniques provide short-term benefits, such as less postoperative pain, shorter postoperative hospital stay, faster recovery of bowel function, and a lower rate of wound infection, when compared with standard open colectomy. Laparoscopic versus open surgery for colon cancer has been compared in the Clinical Outcomes of Surgical Therapy (COST) trial, which demonstrated that oncologic outcomes after laparoscopic resections are noninferior, with no significant difference in 5-year disease-free survival (DFS).[73,74] Although no clinical trials have compared laparoscopic versus robotic or open approach for colon cancer, a systematic review comparing robotic versus laparoscopic left colectomy showed fewer conversions using a robotic approach and no difference in other postoperative outcomes.[75]

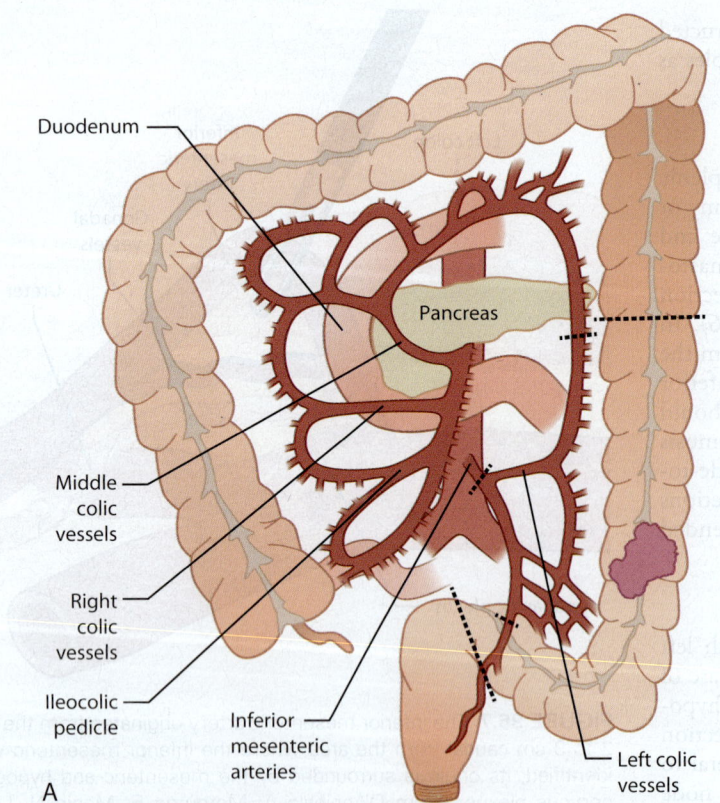

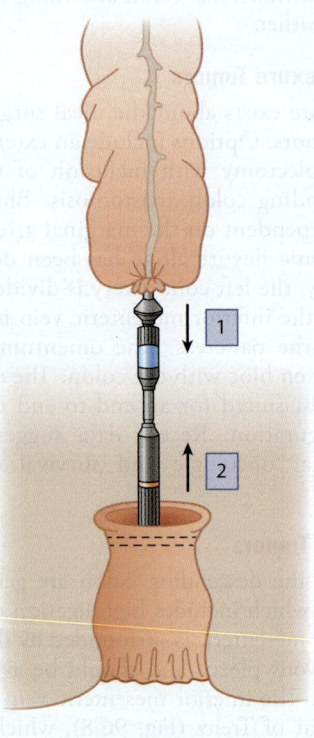

FIGURE 96.9 Left hemicolectomy. (A) The inferior mesenteric artery is ligated, and the marginal artery is ligated just distal to the level of transection of the colon. The hemorrhoidal vessels are ligated within the proximal mesorectum. (B) A double stapled technique is used to create an end-to-end anastomosis.

Approach to Colon Cancer With Synchronous Metastasis

For patients with synchronous metastatic disease, management depends on the extent of distant disease and on whether the primary tumor is symptomatic. If the primary is symptomatic, it is usually addressed first for palliation of symptoms before moving on to treatment of distant disease. With an asymptomatic primary, systemic treatment is the first line of therapy. Neoadjuvant chemotherapy before surgery improves progression-free survival in patients with liver metastasis.[76] Patients with colon cancer and resectable liver disease can be considered for a combined approach for low-complexity operations or a staged approach for more complex scenarios.[77] In patients with resectable lung metastasis, surgical resection allows improved survival.[78] In select cases with colon cancer and peritoneal metastasis, in-depth evaluation in a multidisciplinary conference should be done, and a recommendation of cytoreductive surgery with hyperthermic intraperitoneal chemotherapy can be considered.[79]

Obstructing Colon Cancer

Obstructing colon cancer changes the management of patients because of the time-sensitive nature of treating symptoms and potentially impending perforation. Significant bowel obstruction complicates 8% to 29% of colon cancers and accounts for most emergency presentations.[80] Patients with obstructing tumors of the colon may present indolently with pencil-thin stools, increasing constipation, and an increasingly distended abdomen or acutely with obstipation, complete obstruction, abdominal pain, and vomiting that may be feculent. Diagnosis is commonly confirmed with imaging, such as plain films or abdominal computed tomography. Treatment objectives entail relief of the obstruction, resection of ischemic or nonviable bowel, and resection of the tumor when able. Management depends on the location of tumor and clinical situation. Treatment of right-sided obstructions generally includes an oncologic segmental resection. In most cases, a primary ileocolic anastomosis can be performed safely, but for patients with a high risk of anastomotic failure, a temporary stoma can be created. The approach to left-sided obstructions is tailored according to the location of obstruction, viability of the proximal bowel, and general stability of the patient. In sigmoid and left colon obstructions, patients are commonly referred for urgent surgery. A segmental resection of the primary tumor is typically performed. If the proximal large bowel has perforated or is showing signs of ischemia, a subtotal colectomy is indicated. Historically, primary anastomosis has been avoided, with the distal stump closed and a proximal stoma exteriorized. However, more recent evidence supports the option of a primary anastomosis in appropriate patients who are hemodynamically stable and in whom a tension-free anastomosis with a good blood supply can be achieved. Endoscopic stenting as a bridge for surgery is an option to relieve obstructions and permit elective surgery under more favorable conditions. Stenting has been shown to result in higher rates of primary anastomosis, decreased wound infections, and a higher rate of completion of surgery laparoscopically. Stenting is contraindicated in suspected ischemic or perforated bowel.

Pathologic Staging and Prognostic Factors

The American Joint Committee on Cancer (AJCC) outlines a staging system based on the tumor-node-metastases (TNM) staging system.[81] Table 96.3 details and defines the stages. The staging system has been implemented to predict survival, the need for adjuvant therapy, and prognosis. The AJCC reports other prognostic factors:

- **Serum CEA levels:** Patients with CEA levels greater than 5 ng/mL both before and after surgical resection have lower DFS.[82]
- **Lymphovascular invasion (LVI):** Patients with LVI have an increased risk of death compared with those without LVI.[83] In addition, patients with resected stage II colon cancer with LVI had worse DFS and overall survival (OS).[84]
- **Perineural invasion (PNI):** PNI is an independent poor prognostic factor for 5-year DFS and OS.[84]
- **Tumor budding:** Tumor budding is the presence of single or small clusters of tumor cells in the tumor stroma. Intermediate and high tumor budding are more strongly associated with worse OS and DFS than low tumor budding in stage III colon cancer.[85]
- **Mucinous histology and the presence of signet ring cells:** Colon adenocarcinomas with mucinous features have worse progression-free survival and OS compared with nonmucinous cancers.[86,87] Signet cell colon cancer has an overall poor prognosis, with 5-year survival reported between 9% and 36% and an average survival time of 20 to 45 months.[88,89]
- **Somatic profile (KRAS, BRAF, and MSI status):** BRAF and KRAS mutant CRCs have a worse prognosis.[90,91] MSI predicts a better survival rate, even 15% more, than patients with microsatellite stable (MSS) CRC.[92–94]

Adjuvant Therapy

According to the NCCN guidelines,[44] adjuvant chemotherapy is recommended for stage III and IV patients and those with stage II who are at high risk for systemic recurrence. High-risk factors for systemic recurrence in stage II patients include the following: poorly differentiated histology; LVI; PNI; bowel obstruction from the tumor; less than 12 lymph nodes sampled after resection; localized perforation; close, indeterminate, or positive margin; and high tumor budding. Treatment regimens that use CAPEOX (capecitabine and oxaliplatin) or FOLFOX (leucovorin, fluorouracil, oxaliplatin) are superior to using the combination of 5-fluorouracil (5-FU) and leucovorin in patients with stage III colon cancer.[95,96] The addition of oxaliplatin to 5-FU and leucovorin has not shown any survival benefit in patients with high-risk stage II disease or patients older than 70 years old.[97,98] In low-risk stage III patients, defined as T1-3 N1, 3 months of CAPEOX is noninferior to 6 months of CAPEOX in terms of DFS and is associated with less toxicity. However, in high-risk stage III colon cancer, defined as T4 N1-2 or T any N2, 3 months of FOLFOX was inferior to 6 months of FOLFOX.[99] The International Duration Evaluation of Adjuvant Therapy (IDEA) collaboration did not show noninferiority of 3 months versus 6 months of treatment in stage II patients and showed a slight difference in DFS in stage III patients.[100] These recommendations have been made for patients with MMR proficient tumors or MSS cancer (MSS/MMR). For patients with dMMR, observation without adjuvant therapy is recommended for patients with stage I and stage II disease.[44] For high-risk stage III patients, the recommendation is for 3 to 6 months of CAPEOX or 6 months of FOLFOX, and further options include capecitabine or 5-FU for 6 months.

Although the concept of neoadjuvant treatment has not been introduced as a standard of care, dMMR tumors have a high response rate to checkpoint inhibitors, such as ipilimumab and nivolumab, as shown in the NICHE study.[101] The authors reported a major pathologic response rate of 95% and a complete

TABLE 96.3 Colorectal Cancer AJCC Staging (TNM)

AJCC STAGE	STAGE GROUPING	STAGE DESCRIPTION
0	Tis N0 M0	The cancer is in its earliest stage. This stage is also known as *carcinoma in situ* or *intramucosal carcinoma* (Tis). It has not grown beyond the inner layer (mucosa) of the colon or rectum.
I	T1 or T2 N0 M0	The cancer has grown through the muscularis mucosa into the submucosa (T1), and it may also have grown into the muscularis propria (T2). It has not spread to nearby lymph nodes (N0) or to distant sites (M0).
IIA	T3 N0 M0	The cancer has grown into the outermost layers of the colon or rectum but has not gone through them (T3). It has not reached nearby organs. It has not spread to nearby lymph nodes (N0) or to distant sites (M0).
IIB	T4a N0 M0	The cancer has grown through the wall of the colon or rectum but has not grown into other nearby tissues or organs (T4a). It has not yet spread to nearby lymph nodes (N0) or to distant sites (M0).
IIC	T4b N0 M0	The cancer has grown through the wall of the colon or rectum and is attached to or has grown into other nearby tissues or organs (T4b). It has not yet spread to nearby lymph nodes (N0) or to distant sites (M0).
IIIA	T1 or T2 N1/N1c M0	The cancer has grown through the mucosa into the submucosa (T1), and it may also have grown into the muscularis propria (T2). It has spread to 1 to 3 nearby lymph nodes (N1) or into areas of fat near the lymph nodes but not the nodes themselves (N1c). It has not spread to distant sites (M0).
	T1 N2a M0	The cancer has grown through the mucosa into the submucosa (T1). It has spread to 4 to 6 nearby lymph nodes (N2a). It has not spread to distant sites (M0).
IIIB	T3 or T4a N1/N1c M0	The cancer has grown into the outermost layers of the colon or rectum (T3) or through the visceral peritoneum (T4a) but has not reached nearby organs. It has spread to 1 to 3 nearby lymph nodes (N1a or N1b) or into areas of fat near the lymph nodes but not the nodes themselves (N1c). It has not spread to distant sites (M0).
	T2 or T3 N2a M0	The cancer has grown into the muscularis propria (T2) or into the outermost layers of the colon or rectum (T3). It has spread to 4 to 6 nearby lymph nodes (N2a). It has not spread to distant sites (M0).
	T1 or T2 N2b M0	The cancer has grown through the mucosa into the submucosa (T1), and it might also have grown into the muscularis propria (T2). It has spread to 7 or more nearby lymph nodes (N2b). It has not spread to distant sites (M0).
IIIC	T4a N2a M0	The cancer has grown through the wall of the colon or rectum (including the visceral peritoneum) but has not reached nearby organs (T4a). It has spread to 4 to 6 nearby lymph nodes (N2a). It has not spread to distant sites (M0).
	T3 or T4a N2b M0	The cancer has grown into the outermost layers of the colon or rectum (T3) or through the visceral peritoneum (T4a) but has not reached nearby organs. It has spread to 7 or more nearby lymph nodes (N2b). It has not spread to distant sites (M0).
	T4b N1 or N2 M0	The cancer has grown through the wall of the colon or rectum and is attached to or has grown into other nearby tissues or organs (T4b). It has spread to at least one nearby lymph node or into areas of fat near the lymph nodes (N1 or N2). It has not spread to distant sites (M0).
IVA	Any T Any N M1a	The cancer may or may not have grown through the wall of the colon or rectum (Any T). It might or might not have spread to nearby lymph nodes (Any N). It has spread to 1 distant organ (e.g., the liver or lung) or distant set of lymph nodes but not to distant parts of the peritoneum (the lining of the abdominal cavity) (M1a).
IVB	Any T Any N M1b	The cancer might or might not have grown through the wall of the colon or rectum (Any T). It might or might not have spread to nearby lymph nodes (Any N). It has spread to more than 1 distant organ (e.g., the liver or lung) or distant set of lymph nodes but not to distant parts of the peritoneum (the lining of the abdominal cavity) (M1b).
IVC	Any T Any N M1c	The cancer might or might not have grown through the wall of the colon or rectum (Any T). It might or might not have spread to nearby lymph nodes (Any N). It has spread to distant parts of the peritoneum (the lining of the abdominal cavity) and may or may not have spread to distant organs or lymph nodes (M1c).

AJCC, American Joint Cancer Committee; *TNM,* tumor-node-metastasis.

pathologic response of 67% in patients with high-risk stage III dMMR colon cancer. Larger studies with long-term follow-up are needed to define the role of immunotherapy in the neoadjuvant treatment of colon cancer.

Postoperative Surveillance

Colon cancer survival is reported to be 91% for localized cases, 72% for regional disease, and 13% for cases with distant disease,

with an overall Surveillance, Epidemiology, and End Results Program (SEER) 5-year survival rate of 63%.[102] Although those numbers combine all patients with similar stages without differentiating between high-risk features and MMR status, the risk of recurrence is still concerning. Thus, surveillance protocols should be followed to ensure patient safety and early diagnosis of any disease recurrence. According to the NCCN guidelines,[44] all patients with colon cancer need a complete colonoscopy 1 year after surgery. If there is a presence of any advanced adenoma, repeat colonoscopy in 1 year. If there are no advanced adenomas, then repeat colonoscopy in 3 years. For stage II or III patients, a history and physical examination are recommended every 3 to 6 months for 2 years, then every 6 months for a total of 5 years. CEA tumor markers will also follow the same frequency of physical examination visits. CT chest, abdomen, and pelvis are recommended every 6 to 12 months for 5 years. No imaging or tumor marker follow-up is recommended in patients with stage I disease. For patients with stage IV disease having undergone curative-intent resection, the recommendation is for a similar frequency of physical examination and CEA as for patients with stage II or III disease, with imaging studies to be repeated every 3 to 6 months for the first 2 years and every 6 to 12 months for a total of 5 years.

RECTAL CANCER

Incidence and Risk Factors

There were an estimated 46,050 new cases of rectal cancer diagnosed in the United States in 2023.[57] The proportion of CRCs occurring in the rectum has steadily increased over the past two decades, from 27% in 1995 to 31% in 2019. The trend of increasing rectal cancer is especially notable in people under the age of 50, where an increase of approximately 2% per year has been noted over the past decade.[57] Risk factors for rectal cancer are similar to those for colon cancer, as discussed earlier.

Clinical Evaluation and Staging

Initial evaluation of a patient with rectal cancer includes a cancer-specific history and physical examination. Eliciting symptoms such as nausea, vomiting, bloating, or constipation can provide important information regarding an impending large bowel obstruction and the potential need for more urgent intervention. Pain, especially neuropathic pain, can be indicative of a locally invasive tumor involving sacral nerve roots. It is also critically important to discuss the patient's baseline urinary, sexual, and bowel function. Imperfect stool continence before surgery will often predict poor bowel function and associated decreased quality of life after low anterior resection with sphincter preservation. Patients reporting tenesmus and rectal pain are often found to have low tumors with sphincter invasion. The patient's medical history, fitness, and frailty can guide preoperative optimization and risk stratification and predict the ability of the patient to tolerate neoadjuvant therapies and surgery. As discussed earlier for colon cancer, it is important to obtain a detailed family history to determine the likelihood of an underlying hereditary syndrome predisposing to CRC that could affect treatment and surveillance and therefore call for genetic counseling and testing.

In addition to general physical examination, the digital rectal examination (DRE) supplemented by flexible and/or rigid proctoscopy performed by the evaluating surgeon is of critical importance to guide further workup and treatment. The distance of the tumor from the anal verge and dentate line should be carefully assessed and documented. For tumors that are within the surgical anal canal, potential sphincter or adjacent structure invasion should be determined by assessing mobility of the lesion in relationship to the prostate, vagina, and sphincter complex. For early lesions or malignant polyps, endoscopic evaluation with assessment of polyp morphology and pit pattern provides important information that can guide appropriateness of local excision. If the tumor has not yet been histologically confirmed to be an invasive adenocarcinoma, further biopsies should be obtained that can confirm the diagnosis and also allow for immunohistochemical (IHC) analysis of MMR protein expression, if not already performed.

Routine laboratory examinations should include a baseline CEA level. In the absence of an obstructing rectal lesion, patients should undergo a complete colonoscopic evaluation to assess for synchronous cancers or premalignant neoplastic lesions, which have a reported incidence of approximately 3% and 30%, respectively.[103,104] If an obstructing tumor does not allow for complete colonoscopic evaluation, CT colonography can be used to assess the proximal colon. Alternatively, in patients receiving neoadjuvant therapy, a repeat full colonoscopy can be attempted after completion of neoadjuvant therapy, assuming downsizing of the obstructing tumor. If a complete colonoscopy still cannot be performed before surgery, it should be planned to be done in the early postoperative period.

Before considering treatment, rectal cancers should be clinically staged according to the AJCC TNM staging system (see Table 96.3). Similar to colon cancer, contrast-enhanced CT of the chest, abdomen, and pelvis should be obtained to assess for any metastatic disease. Although endorectal ultrasound has historically had an important role in locoregional staging of rectal cancer, pelvic MRI is currently the preferred imaging modality to determine T and N stage and also provide critical information regarding the location of the tumor in relationship to the anterior peritoneal reflection, the circumferential resection margin (CRM), and potential invasion of adjacent structures.[105,106] Fig. 96.10 provides an example of tumor staging of rectal cancer by pelvic MRI.

After completion of diagnostic evaluation and staging, all findings should be reviewed in the setting of a multidisciplinary tumor board composed of experts in colorectal surgery, medical and radiation oncology, surgical oncology, pathology, and radiology. A multidisciplinary tumor board discussion is one of the central quality metrics for rectal cancer care as recommended by the National Accreditation Program for Rectal Cancer (NAPRC) and other national guidelines.[107] Multidisciplinary tumor board review and discussion often change the initial management plan, even for experienced practitioners.[108] One of the key questions to

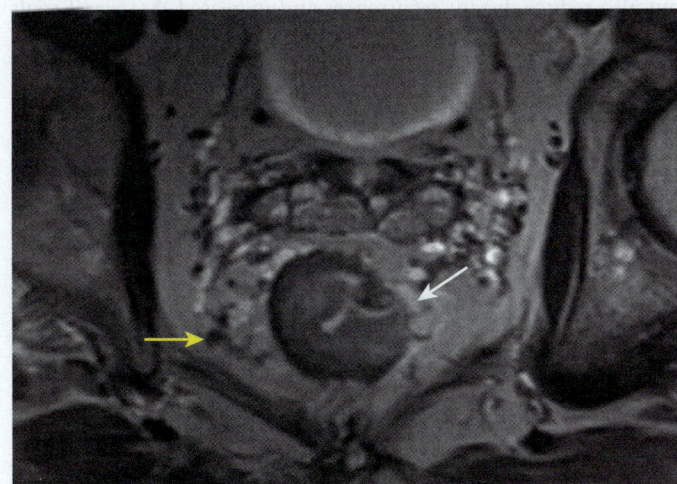

FIGURE 96.10 MRI image of pelvis that shows a T3 tumor penetrating through the rectal wall and into the mesorectal fat *(white arrow)*. There is enlarged and abnormal adenopathy in the mesorectum *(yellow arrow)*. This rectal cancer would be clinically staged as a T3N1 tumor.

be addressed during multidisciplinary review is whether the patient should be treated with surgery first or would benefit from neoadjuvant therapy.

Treatment

The treatment of rectal cancer has dramatically changed over the past 20 to 30 years and continues to rapidly evolve. Historically, rectal cancer was generally treated surgically with abdominoperineal resection (APR) and was plagued by high rates of postoperative morbidity and local recurrence. However, the modern treatment of rectal cancer, including neoadjuvant therapies, organ preservation, and minimally invasive restorative surgery strictly adhering to oncologic surgical principles, including total mesorectal excision (TME), has demonstrated significant improvement in outcomes with low local recurrence rates. To achieve optimal outcomes, the treatment of rectal cancer calls for a multidisciplinary approach provided by a team of experts, including surgeons, oncologists, radiation oncologists, radiologists, and pathologists, starting from the time of initial patient presentation and rectal cancer diagnosis and continuing through treatment, surveillance, and survivorship.

Neoadjuvant Therapy

At the beginning of the 21st century, several seminal trials evaluated the role of neoadjuvant radiotherapy in reducing rectal cancer local recurrence rates. It is important to note that neoadjuvant therapy is usually reserved for locally advanced tumors (T3-4 and/or N+) in the extraperitoneal rectum because of the historically high rates of local recurrence found with these tumors. The German Rectal Cancer Study[109] compared pre- and postoperative long-course chemoradiotherapy (CRT) in 823 patients with clinically staged locally advanced rectal cancer (LARC). The 5-year local recurrence rate was significantly lower in the neoadjuvant treatment group, 6% versus 13% ($p = 0.006$), whereas OS and the frequency of distant metastases were not significantly different. Furthermore, preoperative CRT was associated with a lower risk of severe toxicities (27%) compared with postoperative CRT (40%). Based on this and other similar prospective trials,[110,111] neoadjuvant CRT became the standard of care for LARC in the United States.

More recently, in an effort to not only optimize local control but also reduce distant recurrences and increase OS, several trials investigated the role of administering systemic chemotherapy (beyond the radiosensitizing dose of 5-FU given during CRT) in the neoadjuvant setting. *Total neoadjuvant therapy* (TNT) is the term used to describe a treatment algorithm where all chemotherapy and radiotherapy are given in the neoadjuvant setting. Promising results from recent prospective randomized controlled trials (RCTs) show that TNT improves DFS, pathologic complete response (pCR) rates, and chemotherapy completion rates.[112,113] The PRODIGE-23 trial, which randomized patients to traditional long-course neoadjuvant CRT followed by surgery and adjuvant therapy versus neoadjuvant TNT with FOLFIRINOX (leucovorin calcium, fluorouracil, irinotecan hydrochloride, and oxaliplatin) and CRT followed by surgery, showed that patients in the TNT arm had superior 3-year DFS (hazard ratio [HR] 0.69, 95% CI 0.49–0.097; $p = 0.034$), metastasis-free survival (HR 0.69, 95% CI 0.54–0.90; $p = 0.0048$), and increased rates of pCR (27.8% vs. 12.1%; $p < 0.001$). Of patients treated with TNT, 81% completed chemotherapy, compared with 75% in the standard arm.[112] Another randomized trial evaluated the use of short-course neoadjuvant radiation along with neoadjuvant

chemotherapy as an alternative TNT regimen. In the RAPIDO trial, patients with LARC were randomized to the experimental arm and received short-course radiotherapy (5 × 5 Gy) followed by six cycles of CAPEOX or nine cycles of FOLFOX4 before TME surgical resection, whereas the standard-of-care group had traditional long-course radiation (28 × 60.4 Gy) followed by TME surgery with adjuvant therapy.[113] Three-year treatment failures, defined as the first occurrence of locoregional failure, distant metastasis, new primary colorectal tumor, or treatment-related death, were lower in the experimental group (23.7%) than the standard-of-care group (30.4%) mostly as a result of a decrease in distant metastasis. A higher pCR (28% vs. 14%) was observed in the experimental group as well. Both of these RCTs demonstrated that TNT followed by TME improved DFS compared with standard CRT before TME and adjuvant therapy. Current guidelines from the NCCN therefore consider TNT as a standard-of-care neoadjuvant treatment for patients with LARC.[114]

Organ Preservation

Before the advent of TNT, the finding of a pCR in approximately 20% to 25% of patients who had surgery after neoadjuvant CRT had already triggered an interest in nonoperative management (NOM) of rectal cancer. Professor Habr-Gama's group first published long-term outcome data on NOM in a group of patients with a complete clinical response (cCR) to neoadjuvant CRT in 2004.[115] In this groundbreaking observational study, a group of patients ($n = 71$) with cCR was managed nonoperatively with close observation, including frequent DRE, proctoscopy, and imaging. In this "watch-and-wait" protocol, there was a 5-year OS of 100% and DFS of 92%. Although initially controversial, this study challenged the dogma that all patients with rectal cancer needed surgery by demonstrating that in complete responders, surgical resection may not be required to achieve excellent long-term outcomes. With growing evidence for NOM from multicenter cohorts[116] and strong patient interest in organ preservation, recent guidelines call for a selective approach to NOM for patients with a cCR as long as it is provided by an experienced multidisciplinary team in the context of defined protocols.[107,114] The prerequisite of a cCR for NOM requires comprehensive restaging after the completion of neoadjuvant therapy with CT scan of the chest and abdomen, MRI of the pelvis, and DRE with flexible proctoscopy performed by a surgeon with experience in NOM. Findings consistent with a cCR include no mass or nodularity on DRE, a smooth white or pale scar with or without telangiectasia and no ulceration, mucosal irregularity or stricture on high-definition endoscopy, and no mass or lymph nodes on diffusion-weighted MRI.[117,118] An example of an endoscopic cCR to treatment is shown in Fig. 96.11. MRI findings of a cCR may include a fibrotic scar with low signal intensity on T2-weighted imaging and no restriction of diffusion. Although optimal surveillance modalities and intervals for NOM still require further study, current protocols call for digital examination with flexible endoscopy and CEA levels every 3 to 6 months, MRI of the pelvis every 6 months, and CT of the chest and abdomen every 6 to 12 months for the first 2 years after the completion of treatment. After 2 years, with significantly decreasing rates of tumor regrowth,[119] surveillance intervals can be extended, but ongoing close monitoring is required for at least 5 years.

Considering the higher rates of pCR found with TNT protocols, the multicenter randomized Organ Preservation for Rectal Adenocarcinoma (OPRA) trial set out to examine the optimal sequence of therapies in patients with LARC. Patients were

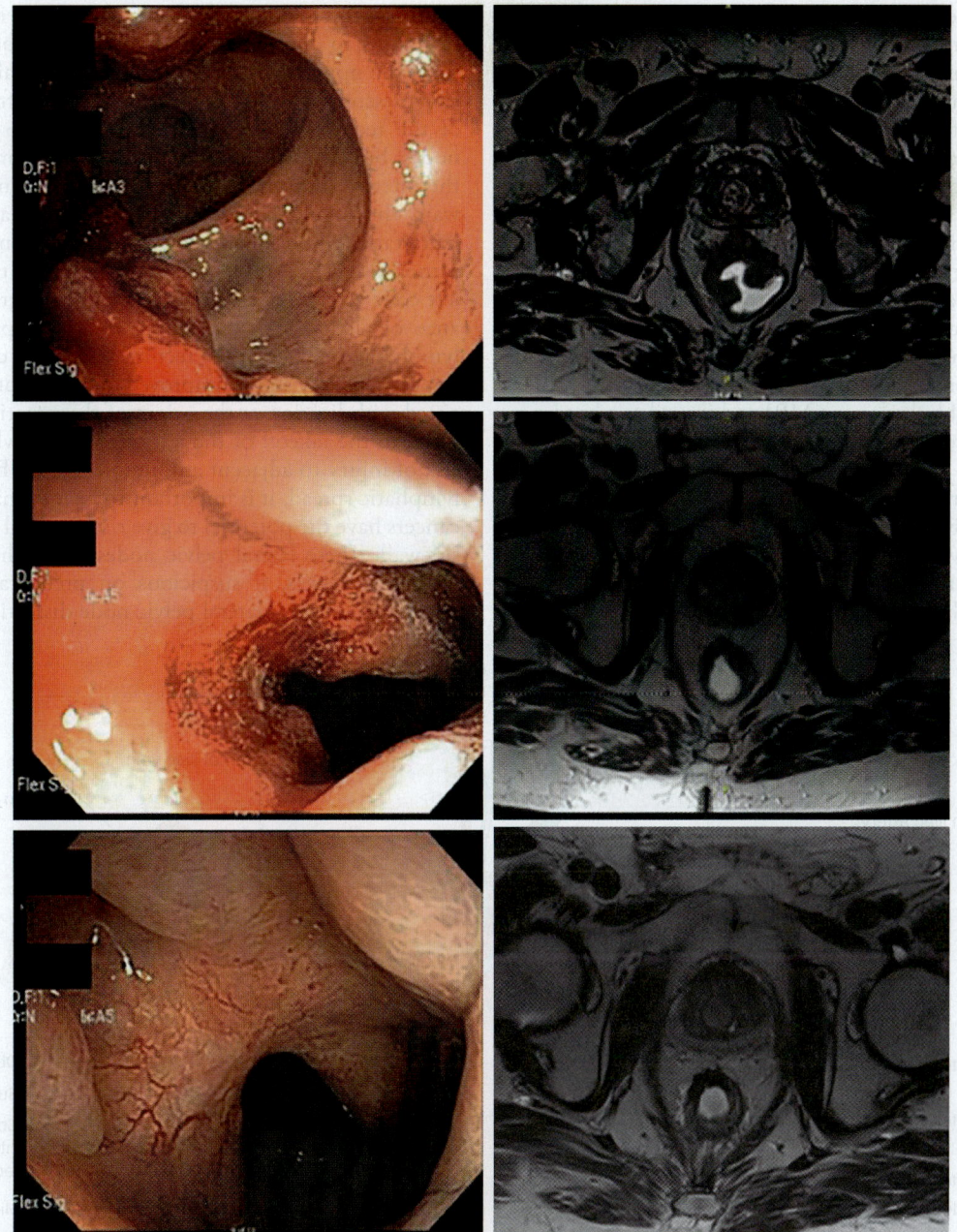

FIGURE 96.11 Clinical evaluation of rectal cancer with flexible endoscopy and MRI before and after neoadjuvant treatment. At the time of diagnosis, an oozing tumor is seen at the top of the anal canal, with MRI demonstrating a T3 tumor abutting the prostate. Restaging 6 to 8 weeks after the completion of neoadjuvant chemoradiotherapy demonstrates a partial tumor response on flexible sigmoidoscopy and MRI. Restaging evaluation after completion of total neoadjuvant therapy, including consolidation chemotherapy, shows a flat white scar with telangiectasia on endoscopy and a T2 dark scar on MRI, indicating a complete clinical response.

randomized to start with induction chemotherapy followed by chemoradiation (INCT-CRT) or to start with CRT followed by consolidation chemotherapy (CRT-CNCT), with patients who achieved a cCR after TNT being offered NOM.[120] The three-year DFS was 76% in both arms, but CRT-CNCT resulted in a higher rate of cCR and 3-year organ preservation rates of 53% compared with 41%for INCT-CRT. Patients who experienced tumor regrowth while on the watch-and-wait protocol proceeded directly to surgery (40% in the INCT-CRT arm and 28% in the CRT-CNCT arm), with no demonstrable survival detriment resulting

from delayed surgery. This trial demonstrated that TNT with selective use of NOM achieves similar long-term outcomes as historical controls treated with CRT followed by surgery and adjuvant chemotherapy and also that use of a consolidation chemotherapy protocol for TNT maximizes the percentage of patients eligible for organ preservation.[121]

Surgical Anatomy and Principles of Surgical Technique

Although advances in neoadjuvant therapies and NOM have revolutionized the modern treatment of rectal cancer, high-quality surgery with strict adherence to oncologic surgical principles remains the cornerstone to cure and optimizing quality of life for most patients. A thorough understanding of rectal and pelvic anatomy is critical to achieve excellent surgical outcomes. The distal limit of the rectum is surgically defined by the anorectal ring, an anatomic landmark palpable on physical examination or visible radiographically as the upper border of the anal sphincter and puborectalis muscles. The proximal extent of the rectum is somewhat more challenging to define because of variations in the distance between the peritoneal reflection and the distance from the anal verge. A recent consensus conference defined the junction of the sigmoid mesocolon and mesorectum as seen intraoperatively or on cross-sectional imaging as the upper limit of the rectum.[122] In practice, the anterior peritoneal reflection is a landmark that is consistently identifiable on staging MRI and is used as a border to select patients at increased risk for local recurrence for neoadjuvant therapy. The rectum proximal to the anterior peritoneal reflection is considered the intraperitoneal rectum.

The rectum receives its blood supply from the IMA via the superior rectal artery and the internal iliac artery via the middle and inferior rectal arteries (Fig. 96.12). The venous drainage of the rectum is via the inferior mesenteric vein, which is often ligated at the inferior border of the pancreas in the setting of low resections to allow for a tension-free anastomosis. Lymph flow from the upper two-thirds of the rectum drains toward the inferior mesenteric nodes. Lymphatic drainage from the lower third of the rectum occurs cephalad, toward the inferior mesenteric nodes, but also laterally along the middle hemorrhoidal vessels to the internal iliac nodes. Below the dentate line, lymph drains toward the inguinal lymph nodes. This explains the patterns of metastatic lymph node involvement based on the location of the tumor. High ligation of the IMA, proximal to the takeoff of the left colic artery, is performed by many centers to allow for clearance of all locoregional lymph nodes comprising the cephalad lymphatic drainage of the rectum. However, current evidence has not conclusively shown improved oncologic outcomes when compared with ligation at the origin of the superior rectal artery, just distal to the takeoff of the left colic artery, which can reduce the risk of injury to adjacent autonomic nerves. Besides the cephalad lymphatic spread, it is important to bear in mind that distal rectal cancers have the potential to give rise to nodal disease in the pelvic sidewall. These lateral pelvic nodes along the internal iliac and obturator vessels, if suspicious on preoperative MRI, warrant consideration for a lateral pelvic node dissection.[123]

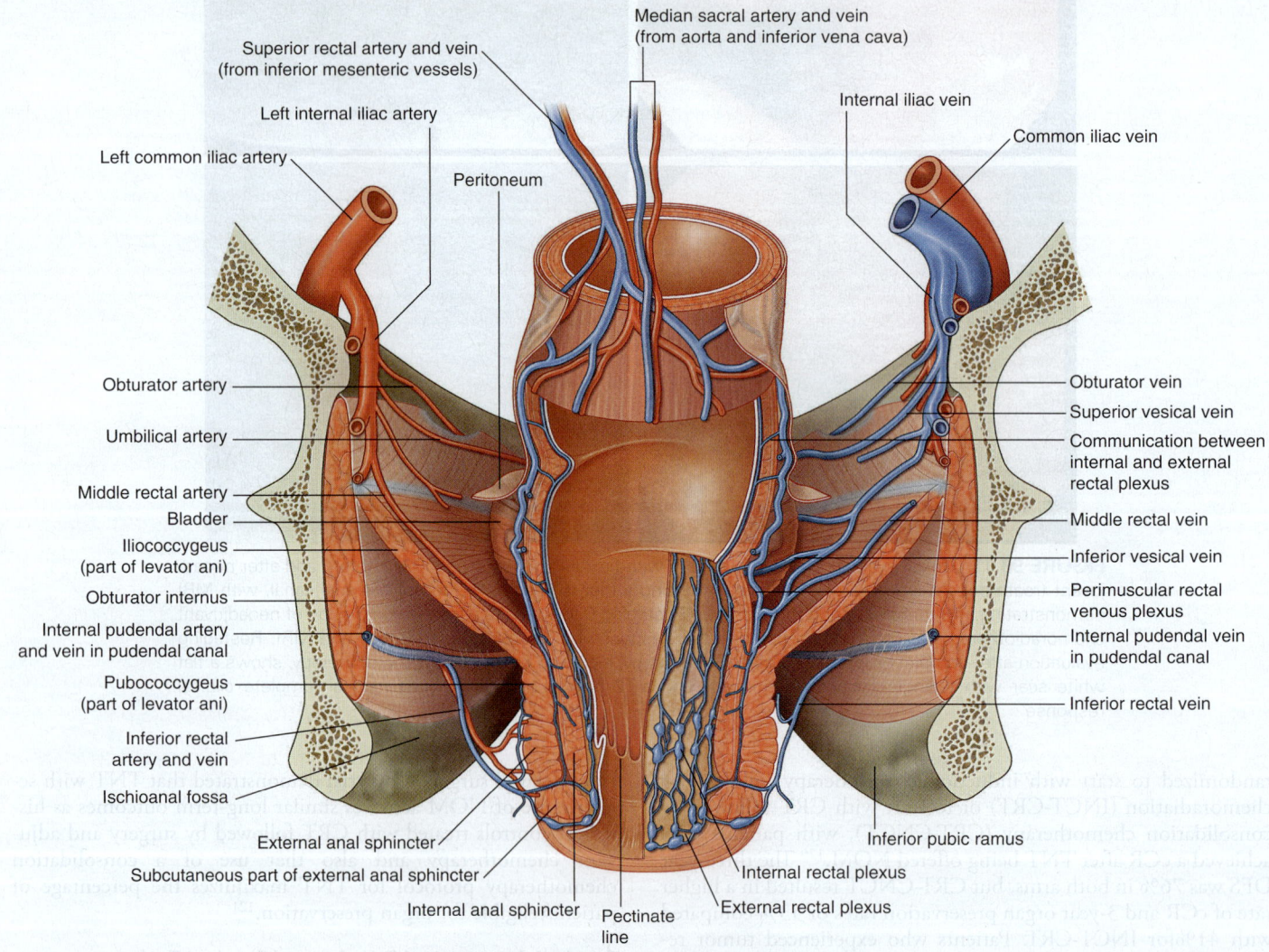

Vasculature of the rectum (posterior view)

FIGURE 96.12 Vasculature of the rectum, posterior view. (From Drake RL, Vogl AW, Mitchell AWM, et al. *Gray's Atlas of Anatomy.* 2nd ed. Churchill Livingstone, an imprint of Elsevier; 2015.)

Recognition of fascial planes in the pelvis that separate structures derived from different embryologic origins has dramatically changed the surgical approach to rectal cancer, resulting in improved oncologic and functional outcomes. The endopelvic fascia lines the pelvis and internal organs as a visceral fascia. The mesorectum is thus surrounded circumferentially by a thin "fascia propria" and contains the terminal branches of the IMA and the rectal lymphatics (Fig. 96.13). A TME, as emphasized and promoted by Bill Heald as the "holy plane" of rectal cancer surgery,[124] is performed just outside of the fascia propria of the rectum and anterior to the presacral fascia, thereby removing the rectum en bloc with its mesorectum, blood vessels, lymphatics, and lymph nodes (Fig. 96.14). The impact of performing a TME in the correct plane on long-term oncologic outcomes cannot be overstated. Traditional blunt dissection resulted in a 25% rate of positive CRM with high rates of recurrence and mortality. In an observational national cohort study of 3319 patients in Norway, implementation of TME resulted in a decrease in local recurrence from 12% to 6% and an increase in survival rates to 73% compared with 60% with conventional surgery.[125] In addition, surgical dissection outside the TME plane, such as deep to the presacral fascia, can cause severe bleeding from the underlying presacral venous plexus. Such bleeding can be very difficult to control because the torn vessels tend to withdraw into the sacral foramina. In cases where the CRM remains involved even after neoadjuvant therapies, a dissection plane beyond the TME plane must be followed to ensure negative margins, including the en bloc resection of involved adjacent organs, such as prostate or vagina.

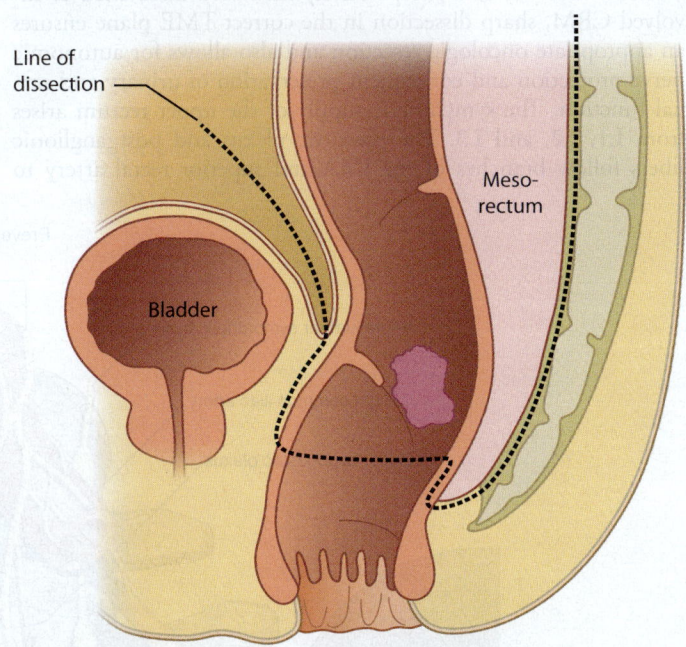

FIGURE 96.14 Low anterior resection for cancer of the upper rectum. *Dotted line* of dissection of the rectum en bloc with the mesorectum.

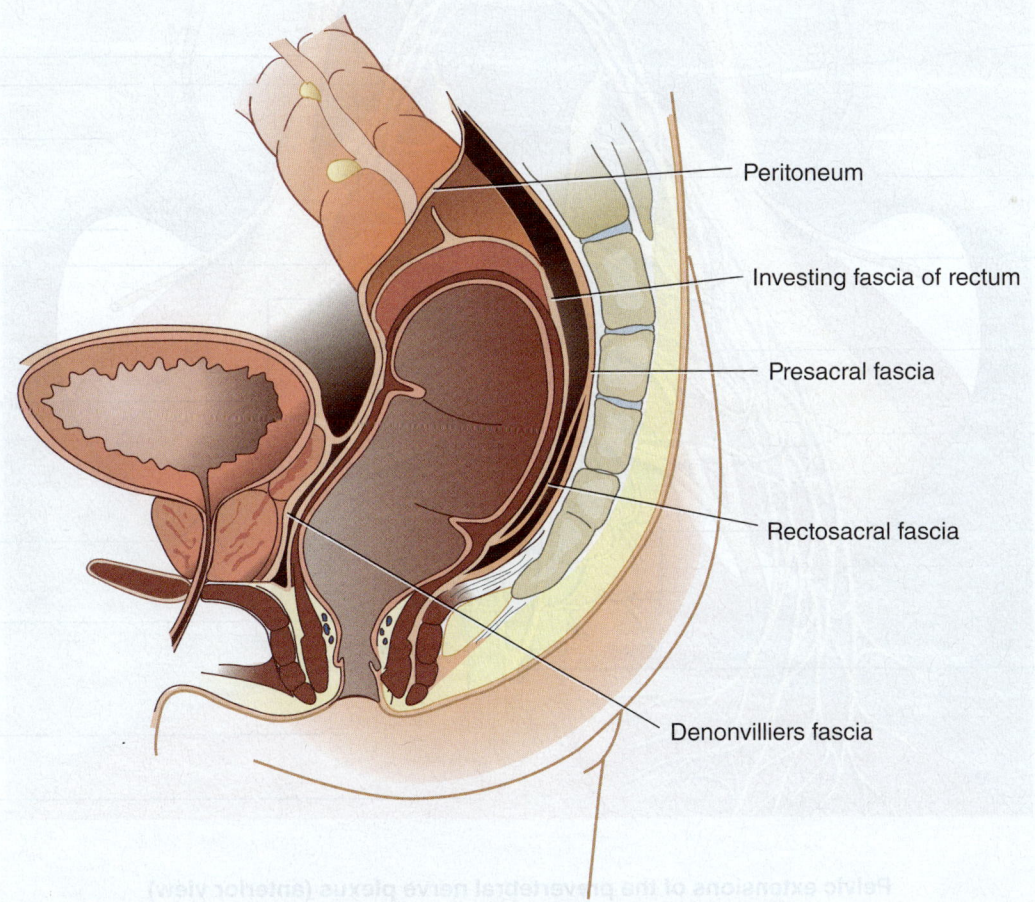

FIGURE 96.13 Fascial relationships of the rectum. (From Gordon PH, Nivatvongs S, ed. *Principles and Practice of Surgery for the Colon, Rectum and Anus.* 2nd ed. Quality Medical Publishing; 1999:10.)

In the absence of a preoperatively identified threatened or involved CRM, sharp dissection in the correct TME plane ensures an appropriate oncologic resection and also allows for autonomic nerve protection and consequent preservation of urinary and sexual function. The sympathetic supply of the upper rectum arises from L1, L2, and L3. The preaortic plexus and postganglionic fibers follow branches of the IMA and superior rectal artery to form the hypogastric plexus, which in turn forms two main trunks on either side posterior to the rectum. The parasympathetic fibers to the rectum, or nervi erigentes, originate from the sacral foramina (S2, S3, and S4). They join the sympathetic hypogastric nerves at the pelvic plexus, giving rise to broadly distributed combined sympathetic and parasympathetic fibers (Fig. 96.15). During oncologic proctectomy, injury to these nerves can occur at several

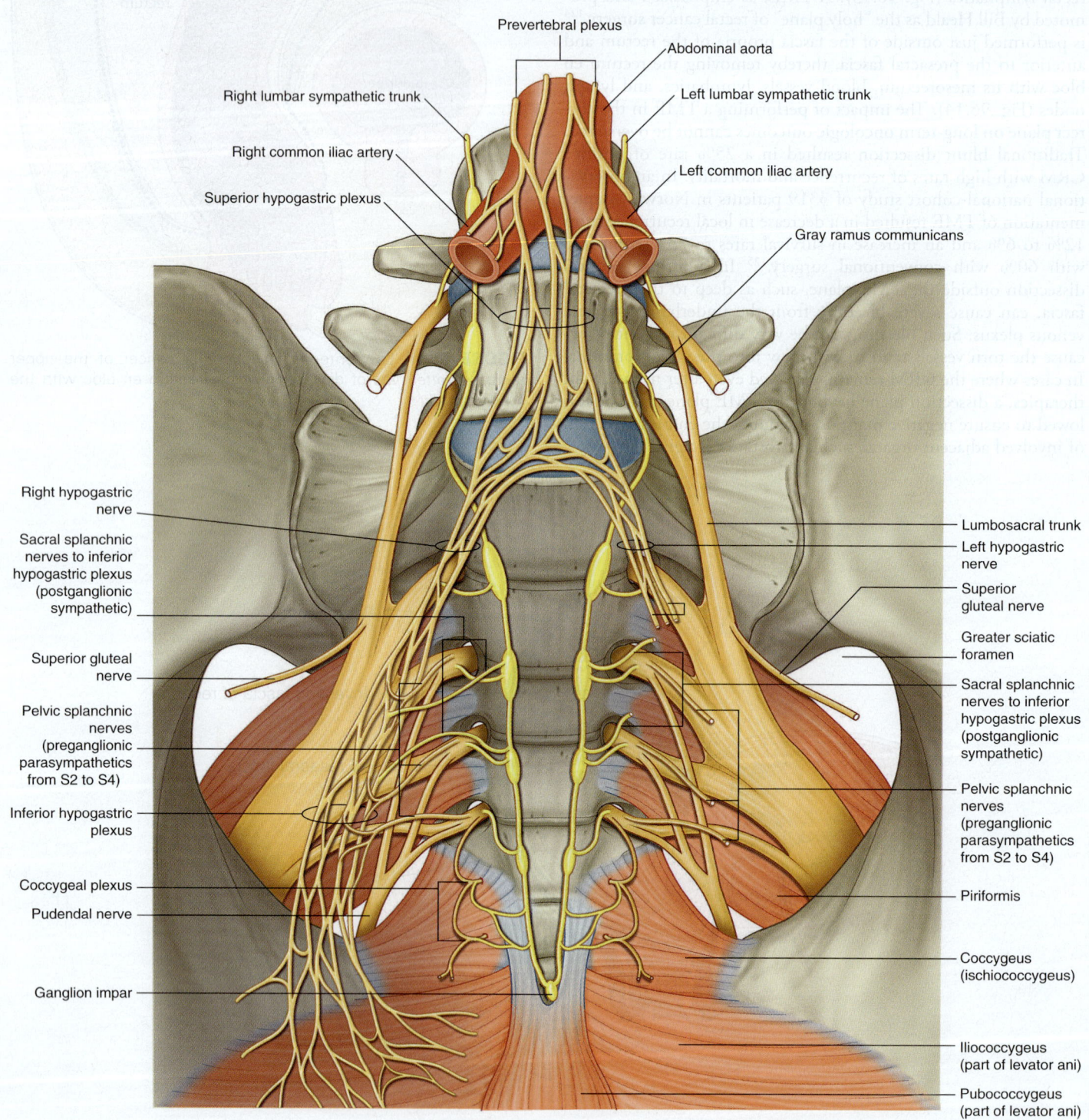

Pelvic extensions of the prevertebral nerve plexus (anterior view)

FIGURE 96.15 Pelvic nerve plexus. (From Drake RL, Vogl AW, Mitchell AWM, et al. *Gray's Atlas of Anatomy.* 2nd ed. Churchill Livingstone, an imprint of Elsevier; 2015.)

points during the dissection. The hypogastric plexus is at risk when performing a high ligation of the IMA and when dissecting behind the superior rectal artery over the sacral promontory. Injury to the hypogastric plexus at these points may result in sympathetic dysfunction characterized by retrograde ejaculation in males. A second point of caution is during lateral mesorectal dissection, where division of the lateral stalks too close to the pelvic sidewall may injure the pelvic plexus and nervi erigentes and cause erectile dysfunction, impotence, and atonic bladder. Lastly, injury to the periprostatic plexus when dissecting anteriorly can also cause sexual and bladder dysfunction.

For upper rectal tumors and rectosigmoid tumors, the distal extent of the dissection and inclusion of the mesorectum should be 5 cm distal to the tumor. Therefore, the dissection does not need to go to the top of the sphincter complex, and a partial or tumor-specific mesorectal excision may be done. This technique still adheres to the principles of not violating the fascia propria of the rectum around the tumor, but the mesorectum is thinned to the level of the bowel wall at least 5 cm distal to the most distal aspect of the tumor. An example of this is shown in Fig. 96.16.

If the tumor involves the sphincter, complex complete excision of both the rectum and the anus, en bloc with the sphincter apparatus, must be performed, with creation of a permanent colostomy. Because this is done via an abdominal and perineal approach, the procedure is called an *abdominoperineal resection* (APR) (Fig. 96.17). This might also be a choice for elderly patients with distal rectal cancer with poor sphincter function because an end colostomy offers a better quality of life compared with an ultra-low coloanal anastomosis (CAA) that could further compromise continence. The same principles as performed in a

low anterior resection are followed for the abdominal approach, adhering to the TME planes to the level of the pelvic floor muscles posterolaterally and the prostate or rectovaginal septum anteriorly. Care must be taken to avoid dissection close to the rectum and avoid narrowing or coning of the specimen, which can lead to involved circumferential margins. Attention is then turned to the perineal dissection. A purse-string suture is placed around the anus, and an elliptical incision is made around the anus that is then excised en bloc with the sphincter. Dissection continues cephalad until the abdominal plane of dissection is reached. The specimen is removed through the perineal incision, and the perineum is closed in layers. The empty space in the pelvis can often be filled with an omental pedicle flap and thereby keep the small bowel out of the proctectomy bed. Rotational tissue flaps (e.g., a vertical rectus abdominus myocutaneous or gracilis muscle flap) can be used selectively to decrease perineal wound complication rates, which are more common in patients treated with radiotherapy.

Sphincter Preservation and Bowel Function

The decision about whether a patient is a candidate for sphincter preservation with a LAR or requires APR with a permanent ostomy should generally be made in conjunction with the patient before surgery. As discussed earlier, this decision should be based on history, DRE, imaging studies, and the ability to obtain clear surgical margins. Patient factors, including age, comorbidities, body habitus, continence status, and patient desires, should also be considered. Because involved distal and CRMs are the most important risk factors for local recurrence, the relationship of the tumor to the anal verge and the internal and external sphincters

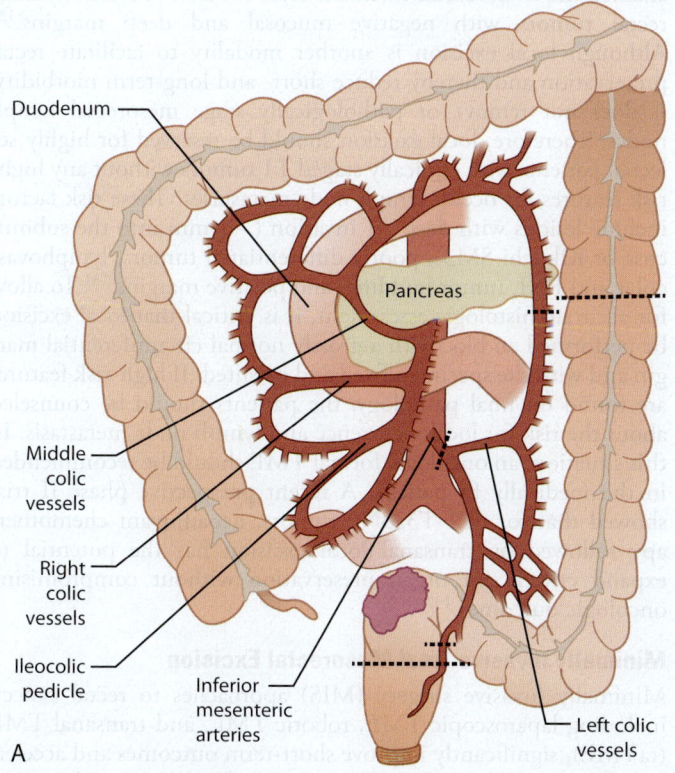

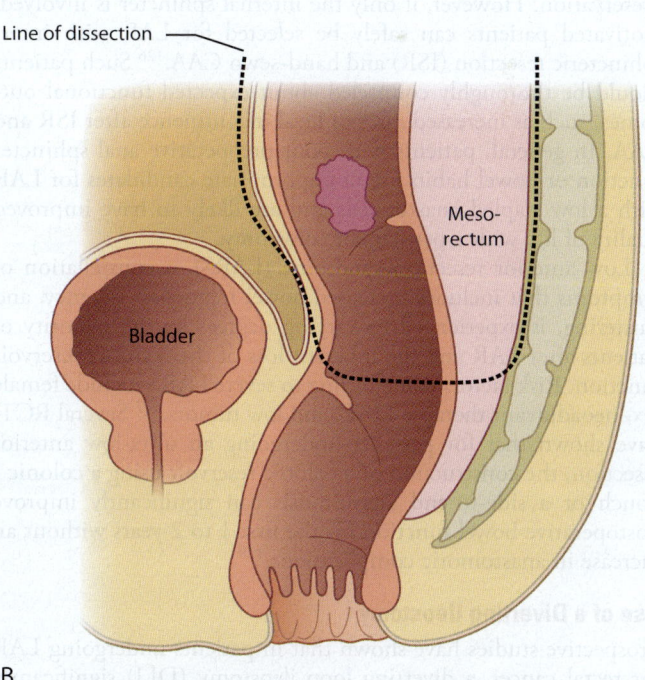

FIGURE 96.16 Low anterior resection for cancer of the upper rectum. (A) The inferior mesenteric artery is ligated. The marginal artery is ligated just distal to the level of colon transection; the hemorrhoidal vessels are ligated in the mesorectum. (B) For upper rectal cancer tumors, the distal margin in the mesorectum should be at least 5 cm.

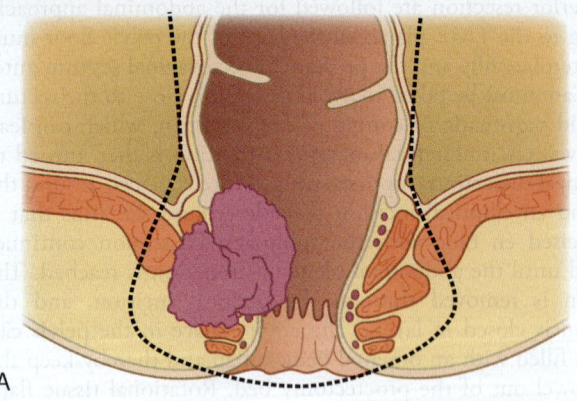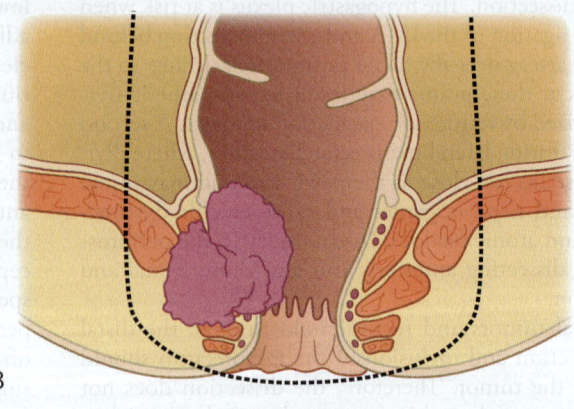

------ Line of
dissection

FIGURE 96.17 Abdominoperineal resection. Attention must be taken to avoid narrowing or coning of the specimen in the area around the levators (A). This can lead to higher rates of circumferential margin positivity and higher rates of local recurrence. The more oncologic techinque involves creating a cylindrical abdomino-perineal resection with en bloc removal of the levator ani (B).

must be carefully examined and documented on preoperative MRI. For tumors in the distal rectum, a 2-cm distal margin should generally be the goal, although a clear margin that is less than 1 cm may be acceptable for low rectal tumors, particularly after CRT. However, there is a higher risk of local recurrence for very close distal margins, especially in tumors that did not show a good response to CRT. In cases of sphincter involvement at the time of diagnosis, after neoadjuvant therapy, it can often be difficult to discern between fibrosis and residual tumor that may still be involving the sphincters. Therefore, when residual viable tumor is suspected, it is generally oncologically safer to assume that the sphincter is still involved rather than relying on intraoperative findings to guide this important decision. Patients with levator or external sphincter involvement are not candidates for sphincter preservation. However, if only the internal sphincter is involved, motivated patients can safely be selected for LAR with inter-sphincteric resection (ISR) and hand-sewn CAA.[126] Such patients should be thoroughly counseled about expected functional outcomes, such as increased rates of fecal incontinence after ISR and CAA. In general, patients with poor preoperative anal sphincter function or bowel habits are not appropriate candidates for LAR with a low stapled anastomosis and are likely to have improved quality of life with a permanent colostomy.

Low anterior resection syndrome (LARS), a constellation of symptoms that includes increased bowel frequency, urgency, and clustering, is experienced to varying degrees by the majority of patients after LAR and the inherent loss of the rectum's reservoir function. Risk factors contributing to severe LARS include female sex, neoadjuvant therapy, TME, and low tumors.[127] Several RCTs have shown that for patients undergoing an ultra-low anterior resection, the construction of a colonic reservoir using a colonic J pouch or a side-to-end anastomosis can significantly improve postoperative bowel function for the first 1 to 2 years without an increase in anastomotic complications.[128]

Use of a Diverting Ileostomy

Prospective studies have shown that in patients undergoing LAR for rectal cancer, a diverting loop ileostomy (DLI) significantly reduces the rate of clinical anastomotic leaks and reoperations. This protective effect of the DLI, however, comes at the expense of higher stoma-related morbidity, such as dehydration.[129] Risk factors for anastomotic leak include a low rectal anastomosis, male

sex, and neoadjuvant radiotherapy. In patients at increased risk for anastomotic leak and its dreaded consequences, construction of a DLI should be strongly considered. It is critical that this is discussed with the patient before surgery and that the patient is seen by a trained wound ostomy continence nurse (WOCN) for preoperative counseling and marking of an optimal anatomic location for a potential ostomy.

Role of Local Excision

Technical advances, including transanal endoscopic microsurgery (TEM) and transanal minimally invasive surgery (TAMIS), have enabled the en bloc, full-thickness local excision of relatively large rectal tumors with negative mucosal and deep margins.[130] Although local excision is another modality to facilitate rectal preservation and thereby reduce short- and long-term morbidity, it does not remove or pathologically stage mesorectal lymph nodes. Therefore, local excision should be reserved for highly selected patients with clinically staged T1 tumors without any high-risk features for occult lymph node metastases. These risk factors include lesions with deep T1 invasion (>1 mm into the submucosa or Kikuchi SM3), poorly differentiated tumors, lymphovascular and PNI, tumor budding, and positive margins.[131] To allow for accurate histologic assessment, it is critical that local excision be performed en bloc with a grossly normal circumferential margin and with the specimen fixed and oriented. If high-risk features are found on final pathology, the patients should be counseled about the risk for local recurrence and lymph node metastasis. In this situation, an oncologic formal TME should be recommended in the medically fit patient. A recent prospective phase II trial showed that for cT1-T3abN0 tumors, neoadjuvant chemotherapy followed by transanal local excision has the potential to expand criteria for organ preservation without compromising oncologic outcomes.[132]

Minimally Invasive Total Mesorectal Excision

Minimally invasive surgery (MIS) approaches to rectal cancer, including laparoscopic TME, robotic TME, and transanal TME (taTME), significantly improve short-term outcomes and accelerate recovery from surgery.[133] However, despite the wide acceptance of MIS approaches to rectal cancer, RCTs have failed to demonstrate that, from an oncologic perspective, laparoscopic TME is noninferior to open surgery.[134,135] The ambiguity related to oncologic outcomes after MIS TME is related to the technical challenge of obtaining a pathologic specimen with negative circumferential and distal resection margins and intact mesorectum within the confines of the bony pelvis. Current guidelines therefore recommend that MIS approaches to TME can be considered but should be performed by experienced surgeons with technical expertise.[107]

Adjuvant Therapy

Patients who received TNT with pathologic stage II or III disease should not receive adjuvant chemotherapy. Patients with clinical or pathologic stage II or III tumors who did not receive a full course of neoadjuvant chemotherapy are usually recommended to receive chemotherapy in the adjuvant setting. Although the evidence for the benefit of adjuvant therapy after neoadjuvant CRT is not strong, the NCCN recommends oxaliplatin-containing 5-FU regimens, such as FOLFOX for eight cycles, as the preferred adjuvant regimen, except for clinical T3N0 patients, in whom oxaliplatin can potentially be omitted. Studies have shown that early initiation of chemotherapy after resection was associated with improved outcomes.[136] Current guidelines recommend giving adjuvant radiotherapy selectively to patients with pathologic stage II or III cancers who did not receive any neoadjuvant radiotherapy and who are at increased risk for local recurrence. However, this needs to be carefully balanced with the potential risk of pelvic radiation negatively affecting postsurgical bowel function and wound healing.

Management of Rectal Cancer With Synchronous Metastases

Approximately 20% of patients with rectal cancer are diagnosed with synchronous metastatic disease. Although lung metastases are significantly more common in rectal cancer compared with colon cancer, the liver is still the most common site of disseminated disease found in rectal cancer, with about half of stage IV patients presenting with liver-only metastases. Retrospective studies have demonstrated superior outcomes for patients selected for surgical treatment of stage IV CRC. Patients with solitary liver metastases can have a 5-year OS rate as high as 71% if treated with a combination of chemotherapy and surgery. Therefore, for a rectal cancer patient presenting with synchronous metastases, it is critical to assess if all disease is resectable in a multidisciplinary setting that includes hepatic and/or thoracic surgeons. Metastatic disease is only considered resectable if margin-negative removal of all known tumor is realistically possible while maintaining adequate liver (or lung) reserve. In the absence of symptoms, there is no proven benefit to incomplete resection or debulking (R1/R2 resection), and these patients should typically be treated with systemic chemotherapy to extend survival. However, in symptomatic patients, palliative intervention should be strongly considered, even in the setting of unresectable metastases. Potential palliative interventions include radiotherapy, endoscopic self-expanding metal stent placement, fecal diversion, or resection of the primary tumor, depending on the presenting symptoms (e.g., bleeding, obstruction, pain), metastatic burden and prognosis, the morbidity and efficacy of the proposed palliative intervention, and impact of interrupting systemic chemotherapy. Shared decision-making regarding the optimal palliative intervention should be made in conjunction with the multidisciplinary team, including oncology, radiation oncology, surgery, and palliative medicine.

Rectal cancer patients with resectable or potentially resectable liver metastases should be treated with an individualized approach. Generally, initiating treatment with 3 to 4 months of systemic therapy can help assess disease biology, facilitate resectability, and potentially reduce the risk for early postoperative disease progression.[76] However, it is important to keep in mind that oxaliplatin and irinotecan regimens are associated with liver injury, which can then impair the liver functional reserve after resection. If follow-up imaging demonstrates good (or at least partial) treatment response and resectable disease, several surgical algorithms can be considered, including a "combined" approach where the primary and metastatic liver disease are resected jointly or a "rectum-first" or "liver-first" approach. The optimal approach depends on the comparative and cumulative disease burden in the rectum and liver, complexity of surgery required, symptoms related to the primary tumor, and medical fitness of the patient. Scenarios that favor a combined approach include healthy patients with upper rectal tumors and liver metastases that don't require major hepatic resections.[137] For low rectal tumors with threatened CRM, short-course radiotherapy should be strongly considered to reduce the risk of local recurrence while minimizing the interruption of systemic chemotherapy.[138]

Immunotherapy

Immunotherapy with checkpoint inhibitors has significantly changed the outcomes for dMMR or MSI-H CRC in the metastatic setting and is currently well established as a first-line therapy for stage IV patients.[139] Unfortunately, dMMR is only present in approximately 3% to 7% of rectal cancer patients because most dMMR tumors occur in the right colon. In this subgroup of patients, recent small studies have demonstrated that immunotherapy used in the neoadjuvant setting has a dramatic response. One important prospective study with 12 patients found a 100% cCR rate to neoadjuvant immunotherapy, without the need for subsequent CRT or surgery.[53] Long-term follow-up is required to establish the durability of these response rates and evaluate the risk for metachronous cancers in this patient population enriched in Lynch syndrome patients. Further maturation of data from prospective trials on neoadjuvant immunotherapy will likely change current neoadjuvant treatment paradigms for patients with dMMR LARC.[140]

Pathologic Staging and Prognosis

Pathologic assessment and staging of the resected specimen are critical in postoperative prognosis and risk stratification. Guidelines established by the College of American Pathologists (CAP) delineate the Protocol for the Examination of Specimens From Patients With Primary Carcinoma of the Colon and Rectum.[141] A synoptic pathology report developed by the CAP ensures standardized and comprehensive documentation of critical findings besides histologic grade, margins, and TNM stage that are specific to rectal cancer specimens, including macroscopic intactness of the mesorectum, relationship of the tumor to the peritoneal reflection, and the response to preoperative therapy, also known as the AJCC tumor regression grade (TRG), ranging from 0 (complete pathologic response with no viable cancer cells) to 3 (no treatment effect with extensive residual cancer). A summary of AJCC pathologic staging is shown in Table 96.3. If not already performed on the initial biopsy specimen, IHC analysis should be performed on the resected specimen to assess for MMR deficiency. In cases of metastatic disease, tumor genomic sequencing can guide the selection of targeted therapies.

Although clinical stage at presentation is an important prognosticator and guides the selection of multimodal therapies, for LARC patients receiving neoadjuvant therapy, the posttreatment pathologic stage (given a yp designation) and TRG is a more accurate predictor of survival and recurrence.[142,143] Patients with a TRG 0 (pCR) have the best prognosis, with 5-year OS rates of approximately 90%. TRG is directly correlated with OS.[144] In patients with margin-negative resections and residual tumor on final pathology, ypT and N stage, TRG, tumor distance from the anal verge, LVI, and PNI are all factors that predict survival.

Postoperative Surveillance

The goal of surveillance after the curative-intent treatment of rectal cancer is the early identification of recurrences that could potentially be cured by further surgical intervention and to detect and prevent the development of metachronous cancers. In general, surveillance regimens for stage II to III rectal cancer mirror those for colon cancer discussed earlier, including regular clinical encounters; CEA levels; cross-sectional imaging of the chest, abdomen, and pelvis; and colonoscopies at predetermined intervals for at least 5 years. For patients at increased risk for local recurrence (e.g., after local excision, patients treated without neoadjuvant CRT, or resections with positive margins), proctosigmoidoscopy every 6 months for at least 2 years is an important adjunct to other surveillance examinations.[145,146] In patients at high risk for local recurrence, proctosigmoidoscopy should be supplemented by pelvic MRI or EUS.

ANAL CANCER

Anatomy and Pathology

The anal canal is the most distal part of the GI tract. The average length is about 4 to 5 cm, and it extends proximally from the top of the anorectal ring to the anal verge. The anal canal contains both rectal columnar epithelium proximally and squamous epithelium distally. The area where these cells tend to overlap and transition in histology is called the *ATZ*, which starts about 1 cm proximal to the dentate line and extends for approximately 0.5 to 1.5 m in length. The anal margin extends from the anal verge to the area of hair-bearing and appendage skin (Fig. 96.18). Dysplastic and malignant cells can arise in the anal canal and anal margin. The most common cancer arising in this area is anal squamous cell carcinoma (SCC). Additional nonsquamous malignancies that occur in the anal canal are extremely less common and include adenocarcinoma, neuroendocrine tumors, melanomas, and rarely, lymphomas and sarcomas. It should be noted that histology is generally more important than location within the anal canal and usually dictates overall patient management.

Epidemiology

Anal carcinoma is rare and accounts for approximately 1% to 2% of all cancers of the large bowel. Nearly 10,000 people are affected annually in the United States, and anal carcinoma accounts for 1870 deaths annually.[147] It occurs more frequently in females compared with males, at a ratio of 2:1. The highest incidence is in White females and Black males. There has been increasing incidence and mortality over the past few decades, an increase of approximately 2.7% and 3.1%, respectively, per year.[148] The average age of diagnosis is approximately 61 years, and it is rare before age 35 years.

Risk Factors

The main risk factor for developing anal cancer is human papillomavirus (HPV) infection, with HPV being detected in nearly 90% of anal SCCs. The vast majority of anal SCCs demonstrate the presence of multiple HPV genotypes, and the high-risk genotypes are HPV-16 and HPV-18. HPV is usually sexually transmitted, and the risk of HPV-related SCC is greatly elevated in those who participate in anoreceptive intercourse, both males and females. Human immunodeficiency virus (HIV) infection is also a risk factor for anal cancer, and SCC rates are increased 30 times in people with HIV compared with the general population.[149] Other risk factors include age, cervical cancer, tobacco smoking, and immunosuppression.

Clinical Presentation

The most common presentation of anal cancer is bleeding, but patients often also report feelings of a mass or fullness, itching, pain, or anal discharge. Presenting symptoms may be mistaken for

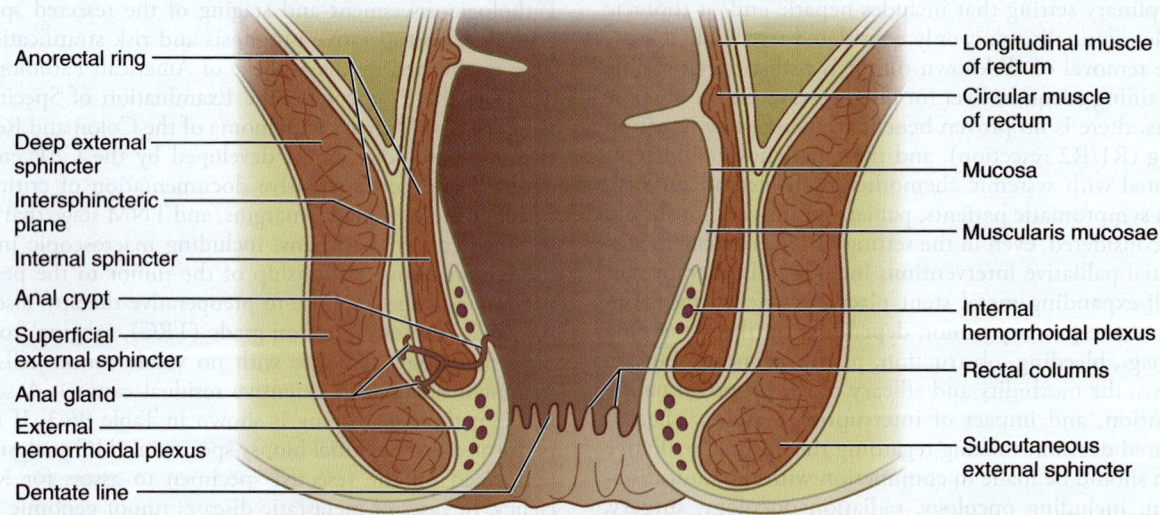

FIGURE 96.18 Anatomy of the anal canal and perianal area.

Anorectal ring

Deep external sphincter

Intersphincteric plane

Internal sphincter

Anal crypt

Superficial external sphincter

Anal gland

External hemorrhoidal plexus

Dentate line

Longitudinal muscle of rectum

Circular muscle of rectum

Mucosa

Muscularis mucosae

Internal hemorrhoidal plexus

Rectal columns

Subcutaneous external sphincter

TABLE 96.4 Anal SCC AJCC Staging Table

AJCC STAGE	PRIMARY TUMOR SIZE (cm)	T STAGE	LYMPH NODES	METASTASES
1	<2	1	—	–
2	2–5	2	—	–
	>5	3	—	–
3A	—	Any	Perirectal (N1)	–
3A	Invasion of adjacent organ	4	—	–
3B	Invasion of adjacent organ	4	Perirectal (N1)	–
3B	—	Any	Unilateral internal iliac and/or inguinal regions (N2)	–
3B	—	Any	Perirectal and inguinal or bilateral internal iliac and/or inguinal regions (N3)	–
4	—	Any	Any	+

AJCC, American Joint Cancer Committee; *SCC,* squamous cell carcinoma.

benign etiologies, such as hemorrhoids, and it is important that symptoms are further evaluated. More advanced lesions may cause bowel obstruction, incontinence, rectovaginal fistula, or inguinal adenopathy. Any suspicious mass or lesion should be biopsied for diagnosis.

Clinical Evaluation and Staging

Evaluation and staging are performed with a combination of clinical examination, endoscopy, and imaging (Table 96.4). A clinical history, including symptoms and risk factors, should be documented. Physical examination should evaluate for primary tumor size, location, and relationship to the anal sphincters; involvement of surrounding structures, such as prostate or vagina; and inguinal lymphadenopathy. Anoscopy or flexible proctosigmoidoscopy in the office can delineate the relationship to the dentate line and allows for biopsy as needed. A full colonoscopy should be performed to evaluate for synchronous CRC, which occurs in up to 15% of cases.[150,151] For females, a gynecologic examination should be conducted, including screening for cervical cancer. HIV testing should be done for both males and females. Cross-sectional imaging is recommended for chest, abdomen, and pelvis to evaluate both local and distant disease.[152] Pelvic MRI may be considered for additional evaluation of the primary tumor. PET scan has been suggested by some groups to help detect distant disease and nodal disease, but this does not replace cross-sectional imaging. Clinically suspicious inguinal nodes should undergo biopsy, particularly if they are not flude-oxyglucose F18 (FDG) avid.[153]

Treatment

Anal Margin Squamous Cell Carcinoma

The anal margin is generally defined as the area extending from the anal verge radially for 5 cm onto the perianal skin. SCC in the anal margin may be managed like SCC skin tumors in other parts of the body, depending on size and location. Wide local excision with 1-cm margins may be appropriate if adequate margins can be obtained without encroaching on the anal canal or musculature and there are no high-risk histologic features. For larger tumors or those with high-risk features or suspicion of lymph node involvement, CRT is the first line of treatment.

Anal Canal Squamous Cell Carcinoma

Local excision. Local excision of anal canal SCC is limited to early lesions without high-risk features. These early lesions are often superficial SCCs that are found incidentally after excision of presumed benign lesions, such as hemorrhoids, condylomas, or skin tags. If margins are negative and there are no high-risk features or evidence of nodal disease, only surveillance may be needed. Early discrete T1 well or moderately differentiated lesions that do not involve the sphincter complex can be resected with 1-cm margins, and if there is no regional involvement, they may be adequately treated with wide local excision alone.

Radiation and chemotherapy. Radiation with chemotherapy is the primary treatment for anal SCC and can be the definitive treatment in the majority of cases. Initially described by Nigro, CRT that includes concurrent pelvic external-beam radiation and 5-FU with mitomycin C[154] is the standard regimen. In a randomized trial, anal SCC patients treated with radiation therapy (45 Gy, with a boost dose of 15 to 20 Gy after a 6-week break) with concurrent infusional 5-FU and mitomycin C resulted in an 80% complete response rate and a 72% colostomy-free rate.[155] Current standard approaches include 5-FU, mitomycin C, and radiation therapy. Cisplatin may be substituted for mitomycin C without detriment to overall oncologic outcomes. Clinically or histologically positive lymph nodes should be included in the radiation fields.

Initial evaluation for response to treatment and persistent disease should be at approximately 12 weeks after completion of therapy and include anoscopy/proctoscopy and DRE. If there is no residual disease on clinical examination, patients can enter into surveillance protocols as described later. If they have had a good but incomplete response, it is reasonable to reassess in an additional 6 weeks. If there is no evidence of progression, surveillance without surgery may continue for up to 6 months. In one study, at initial assessment (11 weeks), 64% were found to have had a clinical complete response, and the complete response rate increased to 85% at 26 weeks. Of patients who experienced a good but not complete response at 11 weeks, 72% went on to achieve a complete response by 26 weeks. Patients who failed to achieve a complete response at 26 weeks had a significantly inferior 5-year OS (87% vs. 48%).[156] If a lesion persists at that time or if there is progression in the interval, the tumor should be biopsied for confirmation of SCC and then treated with salvage APR, as described later.

Posttreatment Evaluation and Surveillance

For those patients with a complete remission after CRT, NCCN guidelines recommend DRE and examination of the inguinal nodes by palpation every 3 to 6 months for 5 years; anoscopy every 6 to 12 months for 3 years; and a CT scan of the chest, abdomen, and pelvis (or pelvic MRI) annually for 3 years for patients who had stage II or stage III.[153] If local recurrence occurs without metastatic disease, an APR should be performed.

Salvage Surgery

Patients who have chronically persistent disease after CRT or those who develop local recurrence are recommended surgical treatment with APR. Preoperative evaluation should include cross-sectional imaging with either pelvic CT or MRI to define the local extent of disease and determine the need for en bloc resection of other organs, such as prostate, bladder, or vagina. General surgical oncology principles for APR using TME like those described for rectal cancer should be used (see Fig. 96.17). For patients who failed CRT, those who underwent surgery with curative intent had a 5-year OS of 66% compared with only 13.5% for those who had palliative treatment.[157] For pathologically proven or clinically suspected positive inguinal lymph nodes, a formal groin dissection should be performed. Negative margins remain the most important prognostic factor after surgical resection. Patients with an R0 resection may experience up to 75% 5-year OS.[158] Because radiation therapy and often-extensive surgery leave a large soft tissue defect, wound healing and morbidity are significant issues. A rotational tissue flap decreases complication rates. Commonly employed flaps include a vertical rectus abdominis myocutaneous flap, a gracilis muscle flap, or an omental pedicle flap.

Anal Adenocarcinoma and Anal Melanoma

Anal canal adenocarcinoma is rare and accounts for less than 5% of anal canal tumors. Because the histology is that of rectal adenocarcinoma, treatment is the same as rectal cancer, with neoadjuvant CRT followed by APR for those with persistent disease. Patients with anal adenocarcinoma have worse OS rates than those with rectal adenocarcinoma or anal SCC.[159] Best outcomes are achieved with CRT followed by APR. Anal melanoma is also an extremely rare disease and accounts for 0.5% of all anal canal tumors. Anal canal melanomas are usually pigmented lesions, but they can be amelanotic in as many as 29% of cases. Prognosis is generally poor, with 5-year survival rates of about 14% to 31%.[160,161] Surgery has traditionally been the standard treatment, with no significant difference in survival between wide local excision and APR; thus, local excision is the preferred approach when able to technically achieve negative margins. The advent of immunotherapy for anorectal melanoma has modified treatment paradigms, and its role continues to evolve. Early studies suggest improved short-term OS.

SELECTED REFERENCES

Nelson H, Sargent DJ, Wieand HS, et al. A comparison of laparoscopically assisted and open colectomy for colon cancer. *N Engl J Med.* 2004;350(20):2050-2059. doi:10.1056/NEJMoa032651

This was the first randomized controlled trial comparing open to laparoscopic partial colectomy for colon cancer. This was a multicenter trial designed to demonstrate noninferiority of the laparoscopic approach in terms of time to recurrence. The overall 3-year survival rate and time to recurrence was similar in the two groups, while the laparoscopic group had a shorter hospital length of stay and less narcotic use.

André T, Boni C, Mounedji-Boudiaf L, et al. Oxaliplatin, fluorouracil, and leucovorin as adjuvant treatment for colon cancer. *N Engl J Med.* 2004;350(23):2343-2351. doi:10.1056/NEJMoa032709

This is the key adjuvant trial that established the addition of oxaliplatin to 5-FU and leucovorin as a standard for adjuvant chemotherapy for surgically treated stage II and III colon cancer. The FOLFOX group had a statistically better 3-year recurrence and disease-free survival.

Habr-Gama A, Perez RO, Nadalin W, et al. Operative versus non-operative treatment for stage 0 distal rectal cancer following chemoradiation therapy: long-term results. *Ann Surg.* 2004;240(4):711-718. doi:10.1097/01.sla.0000141194.27992.32

This article was one of the earliest to establish and demonstrate safety and effectiveness of non-operative management for rectal cancer after neoadjuvant therapy in patients with a complete clinical response. This concept and approach were slow to be adopted but eventually has been reproduced in randomized controlled trials and is an acceptable approach to rectal cancer according to National Comprehensive Cancer Network guidelines.

Verheij FS, Omer DM, Williams H, et al. Long-term results of organ preservation in patients with rectal adenocarcinoma treated with total neoadjuvant therapy: the randomized phase II OPRA trial. *J Clin Oncol.* 2024;42(5):500-506. doi:10.1200/jco.23.01208

This was a randomized multicenter trial that examined oncologic outcomes after total neoadjuvant therapy for clinically stage II and III rectal cancers. It compared long course chemoradiation followed by consolidation chemotherapy vs. Induction chemotherapy followed by chemoradiation. This manuscript provided long term results of organ preservation. In the trial, patients who achieved a complete clinical response after finishing neoadjuvant therapy were offered non-operative management with active surveillance. The 5-year disease-free survival rates were similar, but the total mesorectal excision-free survival was greater in the group treated with chemoradiation first (54% vs 39%).

Le DT, Uram JN, Wang H, et al. PD-1 Blockade in tumors with mismatch-repair deficiency. *N Engl J Med.* 2015;372(26):2509-2520. doi:10.1056/NEJMoa1500596

This was the first major trial to demonstrate the clinical effectiveness of an anti-programmed death 1 immune checkpoint inhibitor, pembrolizumab in progressive metastatic colorectal cancer with mismatch repair deficiency. Patients treated with pembrolizumab demonstrated improved immune-related objective response rates and better progression-free survival. This study provided the foundation for additional studies of immune checkpoint inhibitors in colorectal cancer.

The full reference list appears on Elsevier eBooks+.

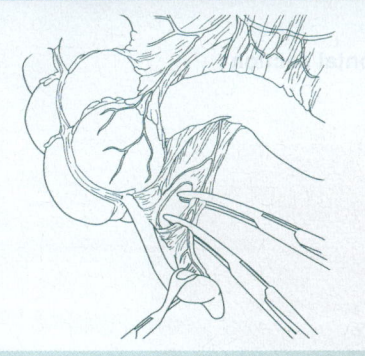

CHAPTER 97

Benign Anorectal Disorders

Joshua I.S. Bleier, Paul Tarver Hernandez, and Lea Lowenfeld

ANATOMY

The anal canal is approximately 4 cm in length, extending from the anal verge to the top of anorectal ring (Fig. 97.1). The proximal anal canal is lined by columnar epithelium, and the distal anal canal is lined by modified squamous epithelium. The junction between the columnar and squamous epithelium, located at the midpoint of the anal canal, appears as an undulating demarcation referred to as the *dentate line* and represents the division between the embryonic endoderm (proximal) and ectoderm (distal). Notably, the modified squamous epithelium in the distal anal canal, called *anoderm,* differs from the squamous epithelium of the skin because it is devoid of hair follicles and glands. The innervation of the anoderm distal to the dentate line is via somatic nerves, whereas the innervation of the mucosa proximal to the dentate line is via the sympathetic and parasympathetic systems. At the anal verge, the anoderm transitions to normal skin containing hair follicles and sweat and sebaceous glands.

The mucosa above the dentate line appears pleated with longitudinal folds, known as the *columns of Morgagni.* There is a small pocket or crypt at the base of most columns, in the region of the dentate line, that communicates with the anal glands. The glands themselves reside in the intersphincteric plane. These anal glands secrete lubricating fluid to assist with defecation. The glands number from 6 to 12 and are mostly concentrated in the posterior aspect of the anus. The anal gland duct traverses the submucosal plane, and its branches terminate within the internal anal sphincter or extend into the intersphincteric plane.

The submucosa in the distal anal canal is formed by a discontinuous layer of thickened tissue, creating hemorrhoidal "cushions," typically found in the left lateral, right anterior, and right posterior positions. These cushions generally receive their blood supply from six hemorrhoidal arteries distributed along the circumference of the distal rectum and anus.[1] The venous drainage is provided by the superior, middle, and inferior hemorrhoidal vessels, allowing for communication between the portal and systemic circulations. These vessels form direct arteriovenous communications within the cushions, and for this reason, hemorrhoidal bleeding is arterial rather than venous in nature. Venous and lymphatic drainage above the dentate line flows into the internal iliac vessels; below the dentate line, blood supply and drainage are provided by the inferior hemorrhoidal system.

The sphincter complex of the anus can be thought of as two concentric cylinders of muscle. The inner cylinder, the internal anal sphincter, is a thickened continuation of the circular layer of the muscularis propria of the distal rectum. This autonomically innervated smooth muscle occupies the distal 2 to 4 cm of the anal canal. The outer cylinder, the external anal sphincter, is a downward extension of skeletal muscle extending from the levator ani to the anoderm. The puborectalis muscle, often referred to as the *rectal sling,* is one of the main muscles contributing to the external anal sphincter. It originates at the pubis, passes around the rectum posteriorly, and returns to the pubis.

The internal anal sphincter is supplied by sympathetic (L5) and parasympathetic (S2, S3, and S4) nerves. The external anal sphincter is innervated on each side by the inferior rectal branch of the pudendal nerve (S2 and S3) and by the perineal branch of S4. There is considerable redundancy in innervation of the anal sphincter; therefore, unilateral interruption of the pudendal nerve will not result in external anal sphincter dysfunction, but the loss of bilateral S3 nerve roots (e.g., by surgical transection) will result in fecal incontinence. If the S1 through S3 nerve roots remain intact only on one side, the patient is still expected to maintain control of the anal sphincters and control continence.

Frontal section

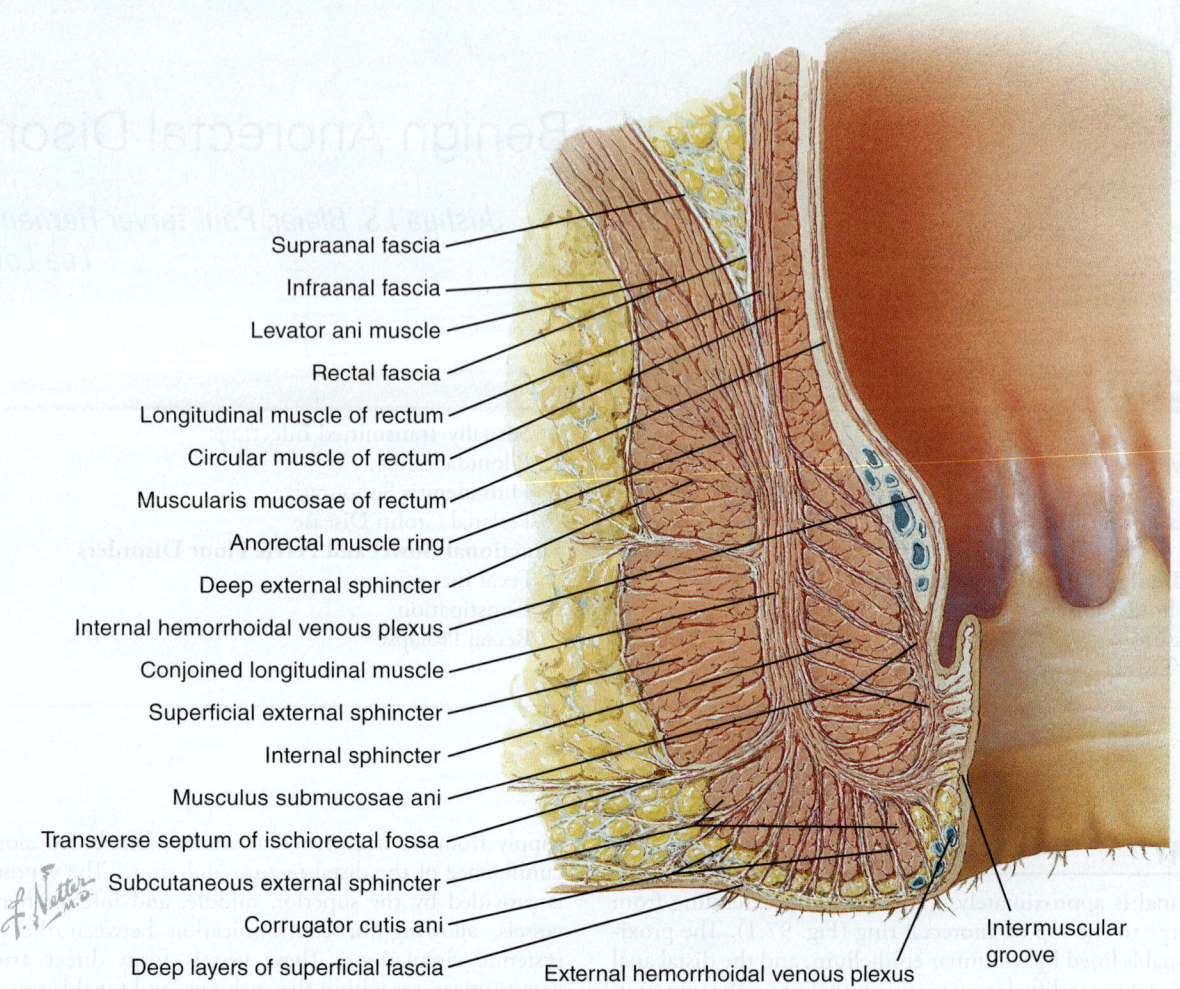

Supraanal fascia

Infraanal fascia

Levator ani muscle

Rectal fascia

Longitudinal muscle of rectum

Circular muscle of rectum

Muscularis mucosae of rectum

Anorectal muscle ring

Deep external sphincter

Internal hemorrhoidal venous plexus

Conjoined longitudinal muscle

Superficial external sphincter

Internal sphincter

Musculus submucosae ani

Transverse septum of ischiorectal fossa

Subcutaneous external sphincter

Corrugator cutis ani

Deep layers of superficial fascia

Intermuscular groove

External hemorrhoidal venous plexus

FIGURE 97.1 Anal canal. (From Bai JC, Bosworth BP, Cruz-Correa M, et al. Colon. In: Reynolds JC, Ward PJ, Rose S, et al., eds. *The Netter Collection of Medical Illustrations: Digestive System: Part II—Lower Digestive Tract.* St. Louis: Elsevier; 2017:Plate 3-12.)

The rectal branch of the pudendal nerve transmits anal sensation, and it is thought to play a role in maintenance of anal continence. The anal canal contains a rich supply of free and organized sensory nerve endings. Organized nerve endings include Meissner corpuscles (touch), Krause bulbs (temperature sensation), Golgi-Mazzoni bodies (pressure), and genital corpuscles (friction). Because of the robust concentration of nerves, the anus is extremely sensitive.

PHYSIOLOGY

Normal continence requires rectal wall compliance to accommodate fecal material, appropriate neurogenic control of the pelvic floor muscles, and properly functioning internal and external sphincter muscles. At rest, the puborectalis muscle creates a sling around the distal rectum, forming a relatively acute anorectal angle that distributes intraabdominal forces onto the pelvic floor rather than along the axis of the rectum and anus. The internal and external anal sphincters, together with the hemorrhoidal cushions, provide a complete airtight and watertight seal, with the pressure in the anal canal at rest measuring 25 to 120 mm Hg compared with 5 to 20 mm Hg in the rectum.[2] This pressure

gradient is a dynamic process in which rapid increases in intraabdominal pressure or intrarectal pressure lead to a reflexive and voluntary contraction of the external anal sphincter and puborectalis to prevent fecal leakage during rapid filling of the distal rectum with gas or with sneezing or coughing.

The process of defecation is a complex, coordinated event involving increased intraabdominal pressure, rectal contraction, and synchronized relaxation of the anal sphincters and pelvic floor musculature. This coordination is innervated by both the somatic and autonomic nervous systems and involves both conscious and unconscious responses to sensory input from nerves originating in the rectum and the anal canal. Distention of the rectum results in reflexive relaxation of the internal anal sphincter. This is known as the *rectoanal inhibitory reflex* (RAIR). This allows sensory epithelium of the anus to sample the fecal material in order for the individual to consciously distinguish between solid stool, liquid stool, and gas. If defecation is deemed appropriate, the external anal sphincter is voluntarily relaxed, together with the puborectalis muscle, which allows for straightening of the anorectal angle, descent of the pelvic floor, and opening of the anal canal, resulting in evacuation of the contents of the rectum.

HISTORY

Patients with diseases of the anus may present with various non-specific complaints, including rectal pain, bleeding, tissue prolapse, seepage, or anal itching. The skilled provider asks focused questions that elucidate the nature of the problem. Patient history is the cornerstone of diagnosis, and asking discerning questions will almost always lead to a presumptive or even definitive diagnosis. When the provider has an impression of the likely diagnosis, it leads to a more focused examination of the anus.

In addition to questions about the character of the symptoms, time of onset, and exacerbating and relieving factors, the history includes detailed questioning about defecation. It is important to ask specific questions regarding the number of daily bowel movements, straining with defecation, time spent on the toilet, caliber of stool and consistency of bowel movements (soft, formed, or liquid), incontinence episodes, seepage, and soiling. Regarding pain, differentiating the type of pain can help accurately diagnose many conditions before examining the patient because the common diagnoses typically present in distinct ways. Sharp, razor-like pain that occurs with bowel movements, sometimes followed by prolonged hours of painful spasm, will almost always indicate an anal fissure. Acute onset of anal pain with a palpable firm perianal lump may suggest a thrombosed hemorrhoid. Acute worsening pain associated with fever and malaise may suggest that a perianal or ischiorectal abscess is a likely culprit. Pain occurring even without defecation, especially with bleeding, could indicate malignancy. Patients may complain of anal itching rather than pain. Itching is often worse at night and may wake patients from sleep because the associated nerve fibers are more sensitive based on the circadian rhythm. Regarding bleeding, a provider must inquire about the presence or absence of blood per anus, the character of the bleeding (bright vs. dark, amount of blood, presence or absence of blood clots), association with bowel movements, blood mixed within the fecal material or present as streaks of blood on the surface of the stool, and whether blood is noted with wiping. Patients may report prolapsing tissue that reduces spontaneously, may require manual reduction, or may not be reducible. The patient should be asked about the presence or absence of anal seepage or drainage, fecal soilage, or perianal moisture. Tactful questioning regarding sexual history, particularly anoreceptive intercourse, should be obtained from both males and females. Questions may include the number of partners, use of protection, and sex without a partner as well as a detailed history of prior abnormal Pap smears, sexually transmitted infections (STIs), and human immunodeficiency virus (HIV). Focused surgical history should include previous anorectal surgeries, interventions for drainage of perirectal abscesses, fistulas, hemorrhoid surgery, or sphincterotomy. A history of radiation exposure for treatment of malignancy should be elicited. Females should be asked about number of pregnancies, vaginal deliveries, any tears or interventions during delivery, and a history of episiotomy. Urinary symptoms and dyspareunia may suggest pelvic floor dysfunction.

PHYSICAL EXAMINATION

Anorectal examination may be very sensitive or uncomfortable for the patient. Communication with the patient is critical. The provider should describe the proposed examination and ensure the patient is comfortable with proceeding. It is important to have a chaperone present in the room throughout the examination, to protect both the patient and the provider irrespective of the sex of the patient and the provider.[3]

Examination is generally conducted in either the left lateral position or in the prone jackknife position, depending on the availability of a proctology table and provider preference. The examination begins by inspecting the perianal skin and anal margin. Gentle spreading of the buttocks will reveal the anal verge and anoderm. The patient can be asked to squeeze and relax their sphincter muscle, which can reveal asymmetric contraction or abnormal recruitment of the gluteus muscles to aid with anal squeeze. When asked to bear down, the patient is expected to reflexively relax their anal sphincter, which may reveal rectal prolapse and/or abnormal pelvic floor descent. If prolapse is not present or produced on the exam table, it may be elicited by having the patient sit on the commode/toilet. Before inserting the examining finger into the anal canal, systematic palpation of the perianal skin and anal verge assesses for tenderness and allows the patient an opportunity to prepare for digital rectal examination.

Digital rectal examination should always use lubrication gel. The exam begins with evaluation of the length of the surgical anal canal to the top of puborectalis sling posteriorly, followed by a sweep around the sacrum with palpation of the tip of the coccyx and evaluation of the levator muscles on the posterolateral aspect of the rectal vault. In males, the prostate is palpated anteriorly; in females, the presence of a rectocele may be determined by gently flexing the examining finger anteriorly. Particular attention should be paid to digital examination of the anus, which can be overlooked if the provider palpates only the rectal vault. Using the first phalanx of the examining finger, a sweep of the anal canal should be performed. If a mass is detected within the rectum or anal canal, its location and relationship to the anterior-posterior or lateral aspect of the rectum should be noted, its size should be estimated, and the provider should observe if it is fixed or mobile and soft or firm. Care should be taken to specifically assess the relationship of the mass to the top of the anorectal ring to clinically ascertain involvement of the internal sphincter.

Before concluding the digital rectal examination, the patient is asked to squeeze in order to assess function of the pelvic floor musculature and to perform a Valsalva maneuver, during which the muscles of the internal and external sphincters should relax, indicating appropriate coordination of the anal sphincter complex.

Anoscopy is an important modality for the complete evaluation of any anorectal complaint and provides direct visualization of the anoderm, dentate line, internal and external hemorrhoids, and distal rectal mucosa. Although there are many varieties of anoscopes, they generally consist of a lighted, hollow scope fitted with an obturator. After generous lubrication, the anoscope is gently inserted into the anal canal, and then the obturator is removed. The anoscope should be gently rotated to spread the anal mucosa to provide a complete and thorough circumferential evaluation.

For patients with a reported history and visual external examination suggestive of an anal fissure, digital rectal examination and anoscopy may need to be deferred because of patient discomfort. Close monitoring of symptoms and examination after improvement of symptoms is reasonable. Patients presenting with pain, bleeding, or other concerning symptoms and in whom the diagnosis is less certain or whose symptoms do not improve should be evaluated by anorectal examination in the operating room under anesthesia. Until evaluation of the anal canal is completed, a complete assessment cannot be rendered.

IMAGING

Imaging can play an important role in the assessment of some benign anorectal disorders, including abscesses, fistula-in-ano, and pelvic floor dysfunction. Endoanal ultrasound may be used to evaluate the layers of

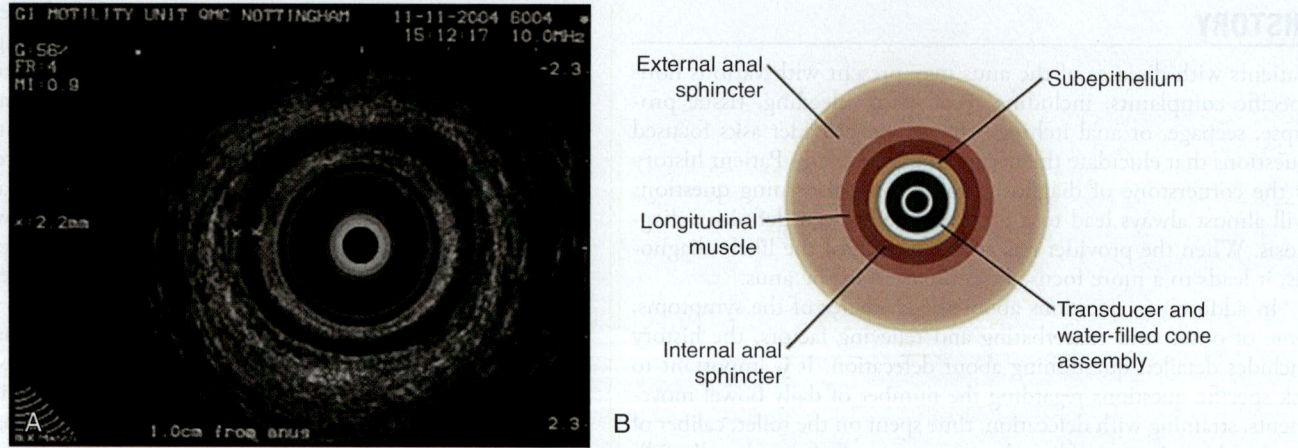

FIGURE 97.2 (A–B) Normal endoanal ultrasound. Axial image of the anal canal. The outer edge of the plastic transducer cone is seen. The subepithelium is hyperechoic and is surrounded by the dark hypoechoic internal anal sphincter, which has a thickness of 2.2 mm (indicated by x-x on the scan). The longitudinal muscle is moderately hyperechoic and is bordered by the mixed echogenicity of the external anal sphincter. (From Wright JW. Endoanal ultrasound. *Surgery.* 2008;26[6]:247-249. Copyright 2008 Elsevier Ltd.)

the anal canal, internal anal sphincter, external sphincters, and puborectalis muscle. Ultrasound can be used to accurately estimate the degree of anal sphincter disruption and outline the anatomy of a complex anal fistula. Although endoanal ultrasound is less costly than alternative imaging modalities and does not expose patients to radiation, it is often less available and is operator dependent (Fig. 97.2). Computed tomography (CT) of the pelvis can be a useful imaging modality to assess for the presence of anorectal abscess in the emergency department when physical exam findings are equivocal. Magnetic resonance imaging (MRI) can provide much higher resolution when evaluating the anorectal anatomy and is more sensitive than CT for the detection and delineation of a complex fistula-in-ano, especially when dedicated protocols, termed *MRI fistulography,* are performed (Fig. 97.3).

For patients suspected of defecatory dysfunction or fecal incontinence, functional studies, including anal manometry and defecography, provide a dynamic assessment. Anorectal manometry

measures the pressures generated by the anal sphincter muscles, sensation in the rectum, and the neural reflexes that are needed for normal defecation and continence. Defecography studies, performed under fluoroscopy or MRI, demonstrate the dynamic changes in and around the rectum, anal canal, vagina, and pelvic floor during the process of defecation. These studies demonstrate functional and anatomic causes for obstructive defecation, which results in excessive straining and incomplete rectal emptying and may include rectocele (or the anterior bulging of the rectal wall), enterocele, cystocele, rectal intussusception/prolapse or other pelvic organ prolapse, abnormal perineal descent, and paradoxical contraction of the puborectalis.

Evaluation of colonic transit/motility is an important part of evaluation of the constipated patient. The most common transit study involves the ingestion of radiopaque Sitz markers followed by serial abdominal radiographs to assess transit of the markers

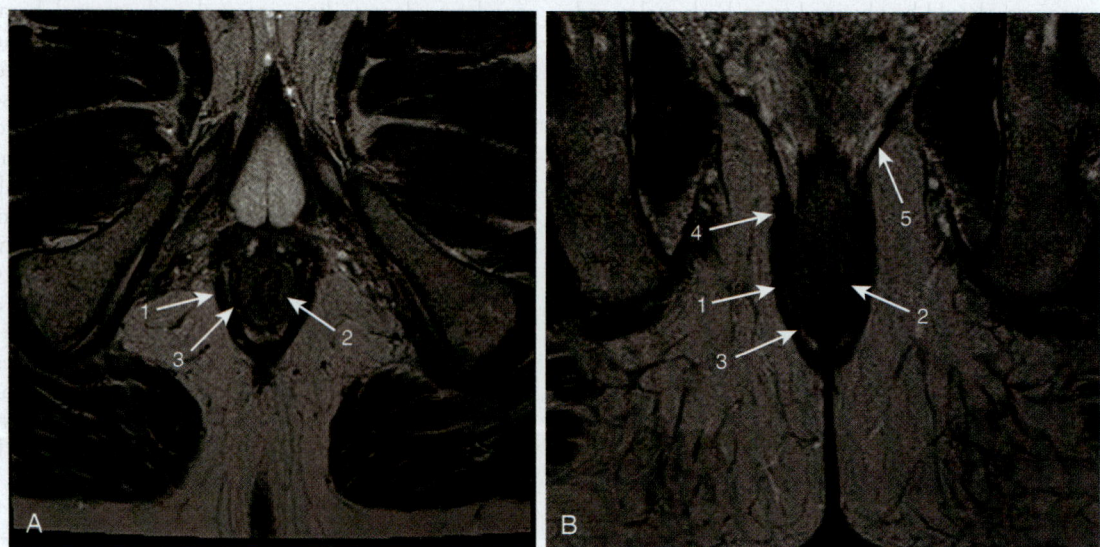

FIGURE 97.3 Normal MRI anal canal. (A) Axial T2 MRI of the anal canal: (1) external anal sphincter, (2) internal anal sphincter, (3) intersphincteric space. (B) Coronal T2 MRI of the anal canal: (1) external anal sphincter, (2) internal anal sphincter, (3) intersphincteric space, (4) puborectalis muscle, (5) levator ani complex.

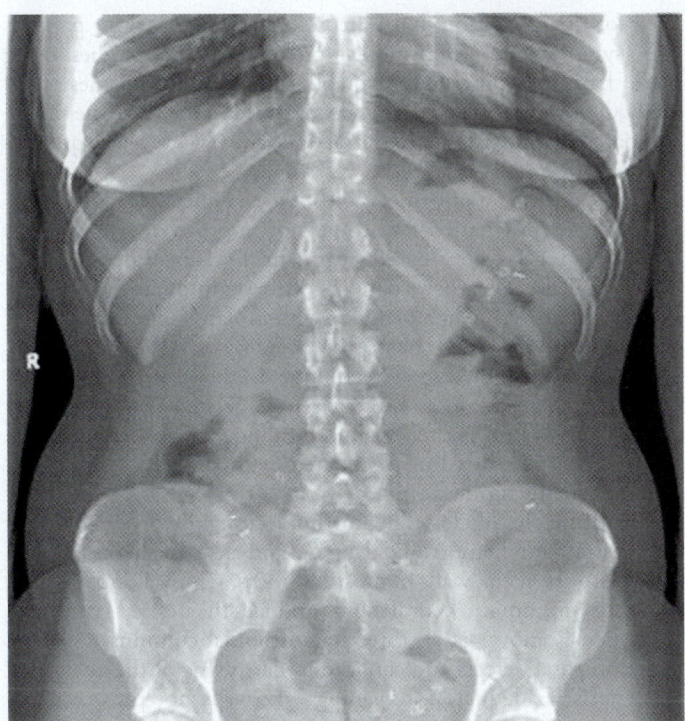

FIGURE 97.4 Example of Sitz marker study consistent with slow-transit constipation. (From Savitt L, Thurler A. biofeedback for constipation and fecal incontinence. *Semin Colon Rectal Surg.* 2011;22[1]:56-62. Copyright 2011 Elsevier Inc.)

through the gastrointestinal (GI) tract (Sitz marker study). With normal motility, at least 80% of the markers should pass within 5 days. If more than 20% of the markers are retained in the colon, the transit study is considered abnormal (Fig. 97.4). The position of the markers within the colon may distinguish between a defecatory disorder in which the markers pass through the colon normally, but accumulate in the rectum, and slow-transit constipation in which the markers may accumulate in the right colon or may be scattered throughout the colon. Colonic scintigraphy studies can provide similar information after the ingestion of an isotope (indium 111 or technetium 99) and serial measurements with gamma cameras. Scintigraphy studies and wireless motility capsules can be used to assess gastric, small bowel, and colon transit times if whole gut dysmotility is suspected.

COMMON BENIGN DISORDERS OF THE ANUS

Hemorrhoidal Disease

Internal Hemorrhoids

Symptomatic internal hemorrhoids result from enlargement and/or protrusion of the hemorrhoidal cushions in the proximal anal canal, which can lead to bleeding per rectum or prolapse. The most common etiologic factors contributing to the development of symptomatic internal hemorrhoids include constipation, prolonged straining, and excessive toilet time. Increased intraanal pressure leads to abnormal dilatation and engorgement of vascular channels, followed by chronic changes in the supporting connective tissue within the anal cushions.[4] This process can be further exacerbated by normal aging; starting as early as the second or third decade of life, the tissue supporting hemorrhoids can deteriorate or weaken, leading to further distal displacement of the

cushions and venous distention, bleeding, and tissue prolapse. Subsequent inflammatory reactions and vascular hyperplasia further contribute to the pathophysiology of symptomatic hemorrhoids.[5,6] Painless bleeding associated with bowel movements with or without intermittent tissue protrusion is the most common complaint of patients with symptomatic internal hemorrhoids.

When eliciting a history from a patient presenting with symptomatic internal hemorrhoids, focus should be on the extent, severity, and duration of symptoms; bleeding and prolapse; difficulty with perineal hygiene; and the presence or absence of pain. Bleeding may be dramatic, "splatter the toilet bowl," "look like a crime scene," stain clothing/furniture, or result in anemia, especially for patients taking anticoagulating medications or patients with coagulopathy (e.g., cirrhosis). A detailed review of fiber intake and bowel habits, including frequency, consistency, change in caliber of stool, and difficulty with evacuation, should also be sought. A baseline assessment of fecal continence is important before any anorectal procedure is undertaken. Anorectal examination should include visual inspection of the anus, digital rectal examination, and anoscopy to evaluate the extent of hemorrhoidal disease and evaluate for other abnormalities. Internal hemorrhoids can be assigned a grade based on the classification in Table 97.1.

The initial approach to a patient with symptomatic internal hemorrhoids should always be conservative and focus on optimizing bowel and toilet habits. This usually includes the recommendation to increase fluid intake to at least 64 ounces per day and start on fiber supplementation to achieve at least 20 to 35 g of dietary fiber consumed daily, with the goal of maintaining soft, formed, easy-to-pass stools.[7] Even those patients who regularly consume dietary fiber and report having "normal" bowel movements will benefit from additional fiber intake and hydration. Patients should also be counseled regarding defecation habits, such as avoidance of straining and limiting time on the toilet to no more than 2 to 3 minutes at a time. Patients should be cautioned against reading or using electronic devices while on the toilet because this can significantly increase toileting time.[8]

Sitz baths with warm water can help decrease pain, burning, and itching when performed after bowel movements. Additionally, there are many over-the-counter topical treatments for symptomatic internal hemorrhoids, although there are scarce data to support their efficacy. These therapies generally come in the form of either creams or suppositories and typically include a barrier compound combined with an antiinflammatory agent or astringent. Although there are scarce data to support the efficacy of these agents, some patients may report symptomatic relief.[9] A 6- to 8-week trial of medical management is usually indicated before considering more invasive interventions.

TABLE 97.1	Classification of Internal Hemorrhoids	
GRADE OF INTERNAL HEMORRHOIDS	**DESCRIPTION**
Grade I	No prolapse; hemorrhoidal bleeding
Grade II	Hemorrhoids with bleeding and protrusion; reduce spontaneously
Grade III	Hemorrhoids with bleeding and protrusion; manual reduction required
Grade IV	Prolapsed hemorrhoids that cannot be reduced

Most patients with grade I and II (and select patients with grade III) internal hemorrhoidal disease who remain symptomatic despite medical management can be offered an office-based procedure, such as rubber band ligation (RBL), sclerotherapy, or infrared coagulation (IRC).

Hemorrhoidal RBL is the most common and effective option and has been shown to be superior to sclerotherapy and IRC.[10] RBL strangulates hemorrhoidal tissue, which results in ischemia and necrosis of the prolapsing mucosa, followed by scar fixation to the rectal wall. This procedure alleviates symptoms of bleeding and prolapse by decreasing the size of the hemorrhoidal cushion and increasing the fixation of the hemorrhoidal tissue to the rectal wall (Fig. 97.5). RBL is generally well tolerated because the rubber band is placed proximal to the dentate line, in the area of the anus that is devoid of somatic pain fibers. Significant pain after RBL typically results from misplacement of the band below the dentate line and requires immediate band removal. RBL should be avoided (or considered cautiously) in therapeutically anticoagulated patients or in patients taking antiplatelet medications, given an increased risk for serious bleeding from the resultant ulcer when the hemorrhoidal cushion necroses and sloughs off, often days after the procedure.[9]

Sclerotherapy is accomplished by injection of a sclerosing agent directly into the hemorrhoidal cushion, which results in fibrosis of the submucosa and fixation of the hemorrhoidal tissue. The most common sclerosing agents are 5% phenol in almond or vegetable oil and 1% sodium tetradecyl sulfate. Injection is performed into the submucosa at the apex of a hemorrhoidal cushion, using approximately 1 mL of the sclerosing agent. Sclerotherapy is appropriately offered to anticoagulated patients or those receiving antiplatelet therapy, who are often not optimal candidates for RBL or surgical excision.

IRC uses direct application of infrared light, resulting in protein coagulation within the hemorrhoid. This is most commonly used for grade I and II hemorrhoids.

Doppler-guided hemorrhoid artery ligation (HAL) uses the current understanding of the arterial blood supply of hemorrhoids to identify and ligate selected feeding vessels. There is no need for tissue excision, but mucosal pexy is required for patients with symptomatic hemorrhoidal prolapse. Several studies using HAL have demonstrated favorable short-term outcomes. This method, however, is expensive and was not found to be cost-effective compared with RBL in terms of incremental cost per quality-adjusted life-year.[11]

Surgical excision of hemorrhoids is a very effective, albeit painful, approach for patients who did not improve or who are not candidates for an office-based treatment. Excisional hemorrhoidectomy can be offered to patients with symptomatic combined internal and external hemorrhoids with prolapse (grades III–IV).[9] Either open or closed hemorrhoidectomy can be performed. The most commonly used technique is the closed (Ferguson) hemorrhoidectomy. This approach is associated with decreased postoperative pain, faster wound healing, and a reduced risk of postoperative bleeding compared with an open (Milligan-Morgan) hemorrhoidectomy.[12]

The principles of closed hemorrhoidectomy involve removal of only redundant hemorrhoidal tissue and pexy of hemorrhoidal mucosa to the rectal wall. In most instances, removal of the largest or most symptomatic hemorrhoid produces the desired symptomatic relief. Removal of all three hemorrhoidal columns results in larger mucosal defects and can lead to narrowing of the anal canal or stenosis if adequate intervening mucosa is not preserved between the suture lines, or incontinence if the underlying sphincter muscles is injured. The procedure can be performed under general anesthesia, local with monitored anesthesia, or spinal anesthesia in either lithotomy position or prone jackknife position. Prophylactic antibiotics are not indicated.[13] An anal block is induced with local anesthetic, and exposure may be achieved with a Hill-Ferguson or other operating anoscope. The hemorrhoid is excised with a diamond-shaped excision with the distal apex at the base of the external hemorrhoid extending onto the anoderm and then narrowing to the proximal apex at the internal hemorrhoidal pedicle. The hemorrhoidal cushion is then dissected off the internal sphincter in what is typically an avascular plane. The hemorrhoidal pedicle at the proximal apex of the diamond can then be controlled with suture ligation using a braided, absorbable suture.

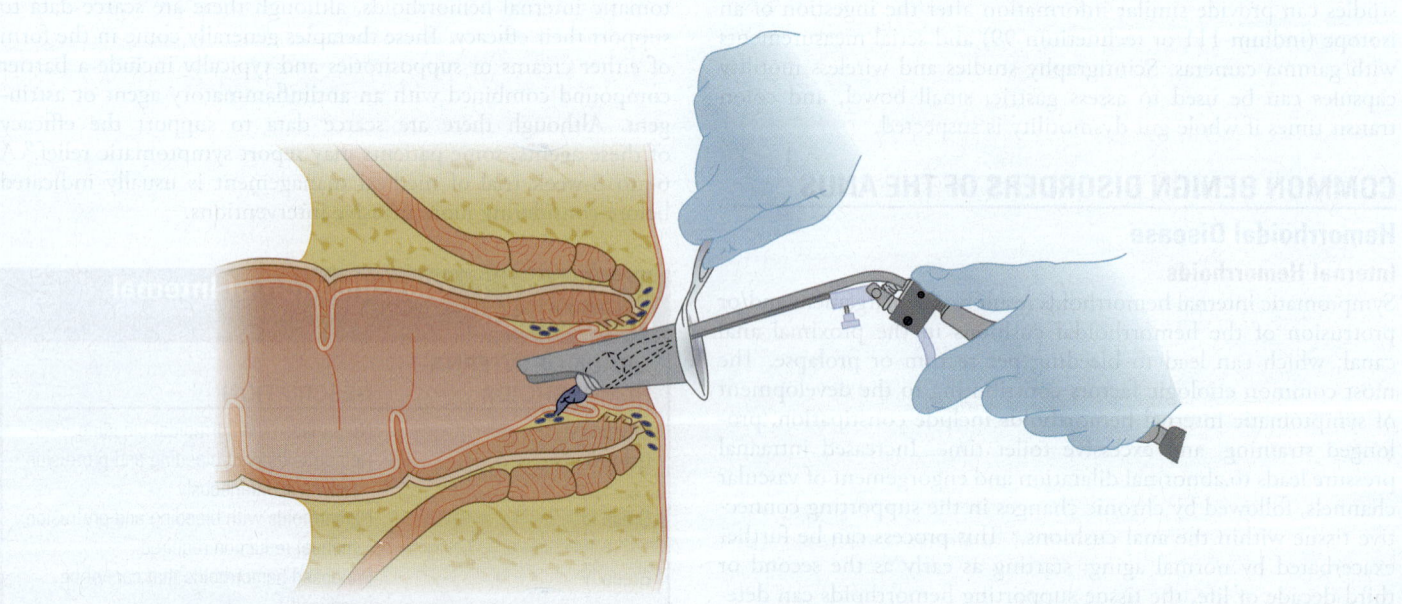

FIGURE 97.5 Diagram of suction ligator. Placement of band on hemorrhoid using specially designed application.

The edges of the hemorrhoidectomy wound are reapproximated with continuous locking stitches of the braided absorbable suture. Complete hemostasis should be achieved with suture closure of the defect. If suture line bleeding is present, additional figure-of-eight sutures can be placed as needed. The use of several bipolar or ultrasonic energy devices during excisional hemorrhoidectomy has also been described. The use of a bipolar energy device has been demonstrated to be faster and to cause less postoperative pain when compared with the traditional closed hemorrhoidectomy described previously.[14,15] Regardless of the excision technique, the internal sphincter fibers should be identified and preserved. There is no benefit in packing the anal canal at the completion of the operation because it is unlikely to stop postoperative bleeding, and large quantities of blood can accumulate above the packing, preventing early diagnosis of a postoperative bleed (Fig. 97.6).

Postoperative care should be aimed at maintaining regular bowel function with liberal use of stool softeners and laxatives to prevent constipation. Sitz baths are an important adjunct that can help with postoperative pain and itching. All patients should be prescribed a multimodal pain regimen to reduce narcotic use and promote a faster recovery.[9]

Complications after surgical hemorrhoidectomy are relatively uncommon; the most common is postoperative hemorrhage, ranging in incidence between 1% and 2%.[12] Acute urinary retention occurs in 1% to 15% of cases. A rare, but feared, complication of hemorrhoidectomy is pelvic sepsis. It can develop after excisional hemorrhoidectomy or office-based procedures. Patients with urinary retention (dysfunction), worsening anal or pelvic pain, or fever must be evaluated emergently for this potentially life-threatening complication. Immediate examination under anesthesia with debridement of any necrotic tissue is required.

Stapled hemorrhoidopexy uses a specially designed stapling device to create a mucosa-to-mucosa anastomosis while removing redundant mucosa proximal to the dentate line; the procedure also disrupts the feeding hemorrhoidal arteries and displaces the hemorrhoidal cushions into the proximal anal canal. Unlike excisional hemorrhoidectomy, this technique does not address external hemorrhoids. Patients undergoing stapled hemorrhoidopexy generally have less pain, pruritus ani, and fecal urgency but are significantly more likely to have recurrent symptoms requiring additional operative procedures compared with those who undergo excisional hemorrhoidectomy.[16] Stapled hemorrhoidopexy is also associated with several unique complications, such as rectovaginal fistula (RVF), staple line bleeding, chronic pain, and stricture at the staple line. Rectal perforation requiring fecal diversion or low anterior resection has also been reported as a rare, severe complication.[17]

Occasionally, patients may present acutely with strangulated, ischemic, gangrenous, or acutely thrombosed internal hemorrhoids. These patients generally have a previous history of prolapsing hemorrhoids (grade III or IV) and will present with an acute-episode prolapse that is no longer reducible (incarceration). If the presentation is delayed, incarcerated hemorrhoids may become necrotic and drain bloody or malodorous material (Fig. 97.7). For those patients with incarceration without strangulation or signs of sepsis, efforts can focus on reducing the prolapsed hemorrhoids to allow for resolution of the acute crisis and future evaluation if needed for a less invasive treatment modality, such as hemorrhoid banding, or a less extensive resection once the degree of swelling has subsided. Applying table sugar as an osmotic agent and ice packs to the prolapsed, edematous hemorrhoids as well as performing an anal block can facilitate reduction. Use of hyaluronidase injected directly into incarcerated edematous hemorrhoids can result in a prompt and dramatic resolution.[18] Patients who fail a limited trial of nonoperative management or those with strangulation and necrosis on presentation require prompt operation. In patients suffering from circumferential fourth-degree hemorrhoids with extensive thrombosis and inflammation, the anal canal is markedly distorted; special attention must be paid to anatomic planes, internal sphincter preservation, and meticulous hemostasis. Unless the tissue is necrotic, mucosa and anoderm should be preserved as much as possible to prevent postoperative anal stricture or incontinence, which is a very real risk in this setting.

External Hemorrhoids

External hemorrhoids are the portion of the hemorrhoidal vascular plexus located below the dentate line and are therefore covered by anoderm and have somatic innervation. The external hemorrhoids drain mostly via the inferior rectal veins into the pudendal vessels and then into the internal iliac vein. External hemorrhoids commonly become symptomatic when the vessels become acutely dilated, leading to stasis and thrombus formation. Thrombosed hemorrhoids can occur in patients who have had minimal hemorrhoidal symptoms in the past and may be preceded by an episode

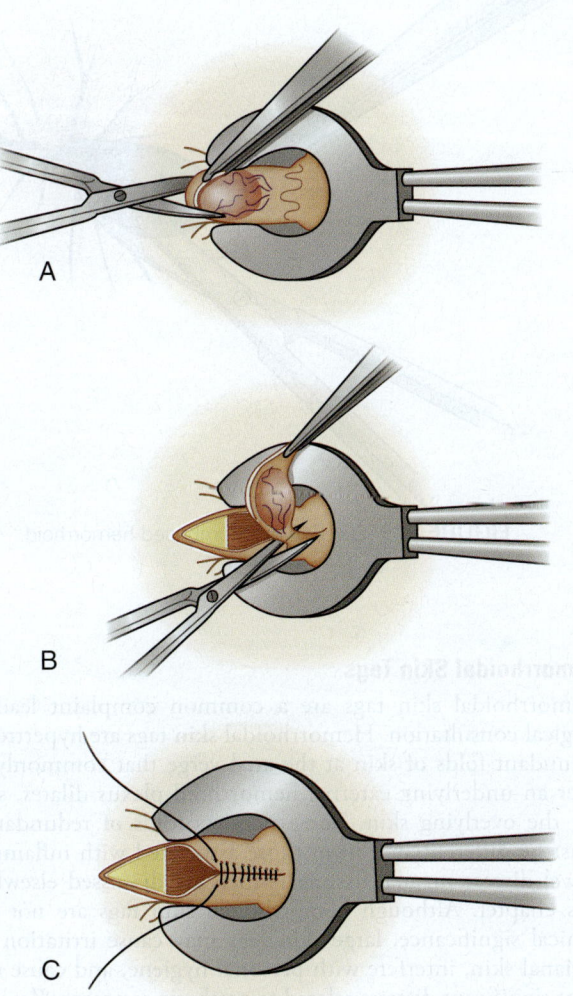

FIGURE 97.6 Open hemorrhoidectomy.

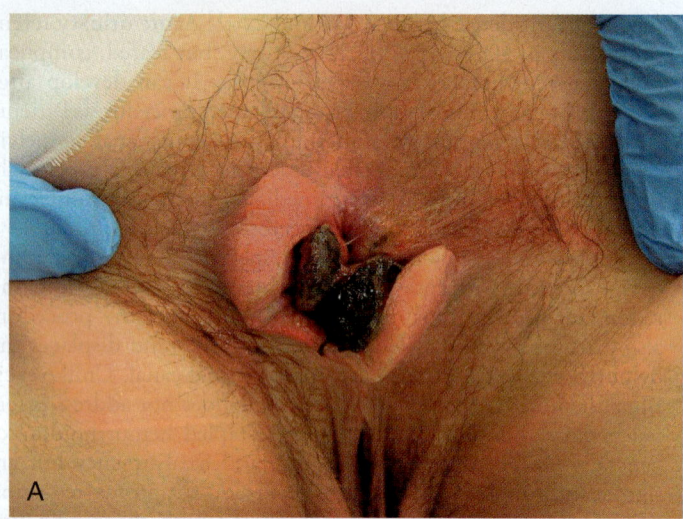

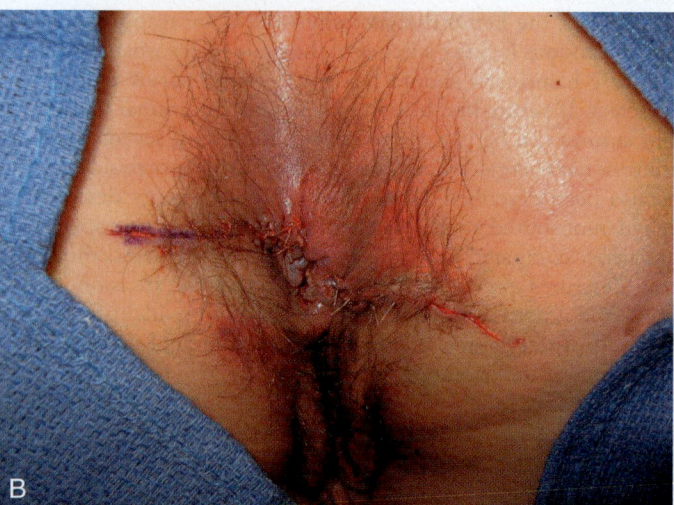

FIGURE 97.7 (A) Strangulated, fourth-degree internal hemorrhoids. (B) Perianal region after urgent excision of strangulated internal hemorrhoids.

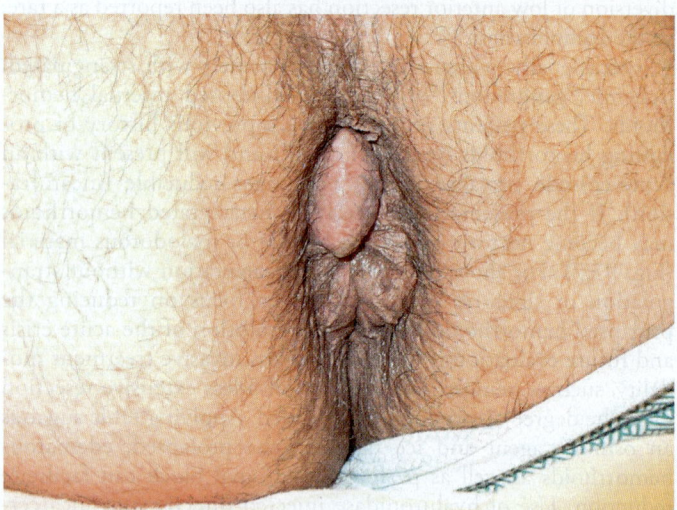

FIGURE 97.8 Thrombosed external hemorrhoid.

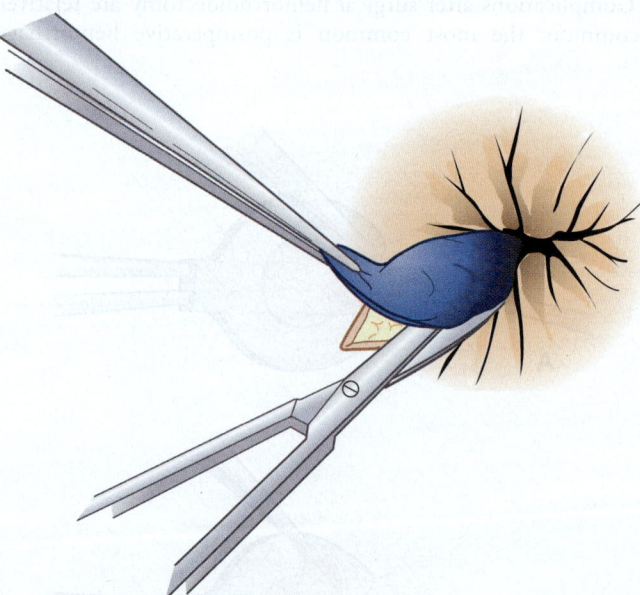

FIGURE 97.9 Excision of thrombosed hemorrhoid.

of constipation or diarrhea. Frequently, they may be associated with antecedent straining during exercise, lifting, or long-distance running. Patients with thrombosed external hemorrhoids typically present with acute onset of severe anal pain that may be exacerbated by sitting or defecation and a palpable round, firm perianal bulge (Fig. 97.8).

Most patients will experience gradual improvement of their symptoms within 48 to 72 hours after the onset with conservative measures, such as sitz baths, application of lidocaine ointment, and stool softeners. Acutely tender, thrombosed external hemorrhoids can be surgically treated when pain is excessive and/or fails to respond to expectant management. Thrombectomy with evacuation of clot is often performed in the emergency setting; however, excision of the hemorrhoid is usually a far better option because it results in faster resolution of symptoms and a greatly decreased chance of recurrence.[19] Both procedures may be readily accomplished with local anesthesia in an outpatient setting (Fig. 97.9).

Hemorrhoidal Skin Tags

Hemorrhoidal skin tags are a common complaint leading to surgical consultation. Hemorrhoidal skin tags are hypertrophied, redundant folds of skin at the anal verge that commonly occur after an underlying external hemorrhoid plexus dilates, stretching the overlying skin. These painless folds of redundant skin must be differentiated from those associated with inflammatory bowel disease or anal fissures, which are discussed elsewhere in this chapter. Although hemorrhoidal skin tags are not of any clinical significance, large skin tags may cause irritation of the perianal skin, interfere with personal hygiene, and cause the patient significant distress related to aesthetic concerns. Removal of anal skin tags can be safely and easily performed in the outpatient setting under local anesthesia. It is important to set realistic

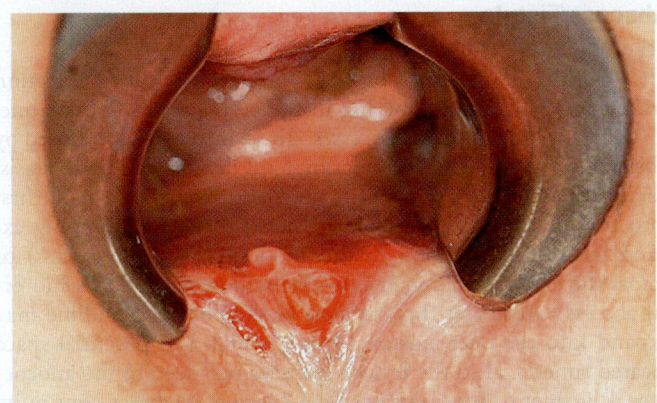

FIGURE 97.10 Acute anal fissure. (From Tiernan JP, Brown SR. Benign anal conditions: haemorrhoids, fissures, perianal abscess, fistula-in-ano and pilonidal sinus. *Surgery*. 2011;29:382-386.)

expectations in terms of postoperative pain (which can be significant) and postoperative aesthetic outcomes because the perianal skin may still not be perfectly smooth after skin tag removal and may recur.

Anal Fissure

An anal fissure is an elliptical or oval-shaped tear in the anal canal starting at the anal verge and extending proximally for a varying length toward the dentate line (Fig. 97.10). Acute fissures appear as a shallow tear in the anoderm. The most common presenting symptom is sharp anal pain with defecation, often described by patients as the feeling of passing "pieces of glass" or "razor blades." The sharp pain can be followed by throbbing and anal spasm, which can persist for minutes to hours after bowel movements. Anal bleeding is typically mild but can present as bright-red blood streaking on the stool or on the toilet paper.

Anal fissures that are present for more than 6 to 8 weeks are considered chronic. Features of a chronic fissure include the presence of exposed internal sphincter fibers at the base, a hypertrophied anal papilla proximally, and a skin tag or sentinel pile distally. Pain with defecation tends to be less severe than with an acute fissure, but the symptoms are nonetheless unrelenting, and in the most severe instances, patients will dread having bowel movements and may avoid oral intake and therefore report associated weight loss.

Fissures may occur as a result of a tear caused by passage of a hard stool, episodes of diarrhea, anal receptive intercourse, or anal trauma. The pain from the fissure leads to anal sphincter spasm, which further decreases blood flow to the anal mucosa, leading to relative ischemia at the site of the fissure. The most common location of an anal fissure is the posterior midline (75%), where there is a relatively less robust blood supply. The anterior midline is also a frequent location for fissures to develop, especially in females. Anal fissures found off the midline are considered atypical, and a broader differential diagnosis should be considered, including Crohn disease, anal cancer, tuberculosis, HIV, syphilis, herpes, and leukemia.

The diagnosis of an anal fissure can often be made based on the patient's reported history alone. Gentle separation of the buttocks can reveal the fissure or the sentinel tag; however, just spreading the buttocks may cause intolerable pain, and the examination may need to be terminated at this point. If the fissure is not clearly visible, focal gentle pressure with the examiner's fingertip or a cotton-tip applicator at the posterior or anterior aspect of the anal canal can reproduce the pain. Digital and anoscopic examinations are often deferred to avoid exacerbating the patient's pain, but if the diagnosis is unclear or the patient has other symptoms concerning for malignancy, an examination under anesthesia should be performed to confirm the diagnosis.

The majority of acute anal fissures resolve with medical management alone. The initial step in management should be to increase fluid and fiber ingestion in order to maintain soft, formed stools as well as sitz baths, which have been demonstrated to provide significant pain relief in over 90% of patients with acute fissures.[20]

Chronic fissures, however, are less likely to heal with exclusively conservative measures. The goals of treatment are aimed at (1) addressing the inciting factors, such as constipation or other causes of anal trauma; (2) addressing the symptoms of pain and bleeding; and (3) relaxation and dilation of the internal anal sphincter to improve blood flow and allow healing.

In addition to maintaining healthy bowel habits, topical nitrates or calcium channel blockers act to relax the internal anal sphincter and promote vasodilation, leading to improved blood flow to the anal mucosa and healing of the fissure. Topical application of nitrates is associated with healing in approximately 50% of chronic fissures, although severe headache is a common side effect that can limit efficacy and leads to cessation of therapy in up to 20% of patients.[21,22] Topical calcium channel blockers, including diltiazem and nifedipine, have demonstrated similar rates of healing chronic fissures when compared with topical nitrates with significantly better side-effect profile regarding headaches, making calcium channel blockers the preferred first-line topical agent.[23] Obtaining topical diltiazem or nifedipine can be challenging, however, because there is no readily available commercial formulation in the United States, and creams or ointments must be sought from specialized compounding pharmacies.

Botulinum toxin (BT) can produce potent and sustained relaxation of the anal sphincter by inducing temporary paralysis of the anal sphincter muscle. BT has similar results compared with topical therapies as first-line therapy for chronic anal fissures and modest improvement in healing rates as second-line therapy after failed treatment with topical therapies.[24] A typical dose of 20 to 100 IU of BT will produce relaxation lasting approximately 3 months. Injection can be done safely in the office or may be performed as an outpatient procedure with sedation. The most common side effects of BT injection are temporary incontinence to flatus. Other side effects include increased urinary residual volume, heart block, skin irritation, and allergic reactions.

A limited, lateral internal sphincterotomy (LIS) induces sustained partial relaxation of the internal anal sphincter and reduces anal sphincter tone, enabling healing of the anal fissure. LIS has shown to be superior to topical nitrates, calcium channel blockers, or BT, with healing rates of 88% to 100%. Reported rates of fecal incontinence after LIS rates range from 8% to 30%, usually limited to minor episodes of incontinence to flatus, most often in the first 30 days after the procedure. LIS is considered the treatment of choice for chronic anal fissure, although care should be taken to identify those patients at higher risk for postoperative fecal incontinence, in whom this procedure should be avoided, including patients with baseline incontinence, females with prior obstetrical injuries, patients who have undergone

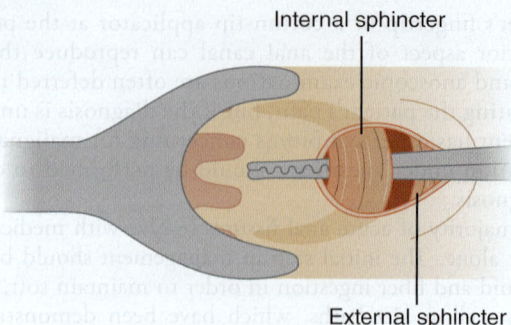

FIGURE 97.11 Open lateral internal sphincterotomy.

previous anorectal operations, and patients with a documented anal sphincter injury.[24]

LIS can be performed using either an open or a closed technique, with similar results. In the open technique, a radial incision in the anoderm exposes the distal internal sphincter muscle fibers (Fig. 97.11). The distal segment of the internal anal sphincter muscle is divided sharply for the length corresponding to that of the anal fissure. The wound can be left open or closed primarily. A closed LIS can be performed by inserting a narrow-bladed scalpel directly into the intersphincteric groove and dividing a length of the distal internal sphincter corresponding to the length of the fissure laterally to medially toward the surgeon's finger within the anal canal (Fig. 97.12).

Abscess/Fistula

Cryptoglandular Abscesses

The majority of perianal abscesses form as a result of infection arising in anal glands emptying in the crypts at the dentate line, so-called cryptoglandular abscesses. These infections are caused by obstruction of the draining duct by fecal debris, leading to stasis, bacterial overgrowth, and, ultimately, abscesses that expand first into the intersphincteric space.[25] These abscesses commonly expand by caudal extension to the anoderm (perianal abscess) or across the external sphincter into the ischiorectal fossa (ischiorectal abscess). Abscesses that develop in the posterior midline may expand into the deep postanal space, which is a potential space located superficial to the levator muscles but deep to the anococcygeal ligament. The deep postanal space is in direct continuity with the bilateral ischiorectal fossae, and lateral spread of infection in the deep postanal space commonly leads to the formation of a "horseshoe" ischiorectal abscesses. Less common routes of spread are cephalad along the intersphincteric space into supralevator space or within the submucosal plane (Fig. 97.13). Approximately 10% of perianal and perirectal abscesses occur as a result of other etiologies, such as Crohn disease, trauma, HIV, STIs, radiation therapy, or foreign body (Box 97.1).

A patient presenting with a cryptoglandular abscess typically presents with the indolent onset of a constant, throbbing anal pain associated with localized swelling, erythema, and fluctuance. Larger perianal abscesses or delayed presentation can lead to systemic signs and symptoms of infection in some patients, although this is less common. Perianal abscesses can be differentiated from other causes of acute anal pain, such as anal fissure and thrombosed external

Lateral Internal Sphincterotomy

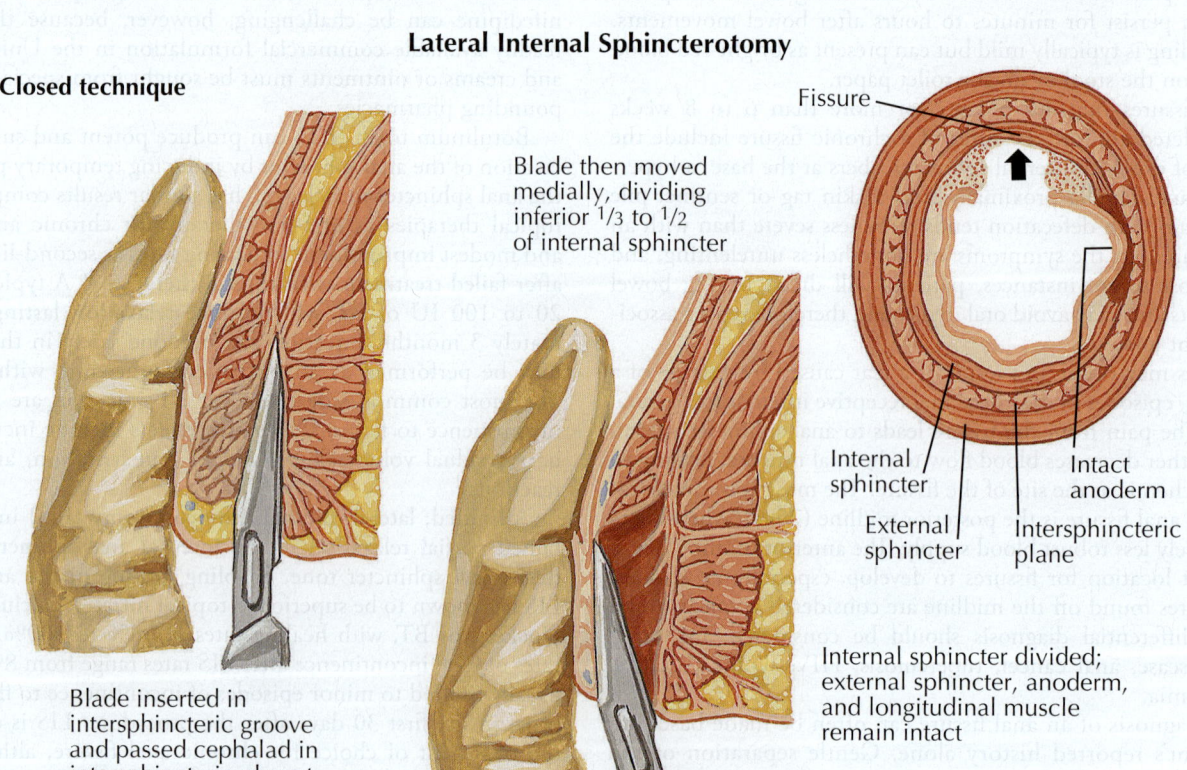

Closed technique

Blade then moved medially, dividing inferior 1/3 to 1/2 of internal sphincter

Blade inserted in intersphincteric groove and passed cephalad in intersphincteric plane to level of dentate line

Fissure

Internal sphincter

External sphincter

Intact anoderm

Intersphincteric plane

Internal sphincter divided; external sphincter, anoderm, and longitudinal muscle remain intact

FIGURE 97.12 Closed lateral internal sphincterotomy technique. (From https://www.netterimages.com/lateral-internal-sphincterotomy-labeled-gastroenterology-john-a-craig-22350.html)

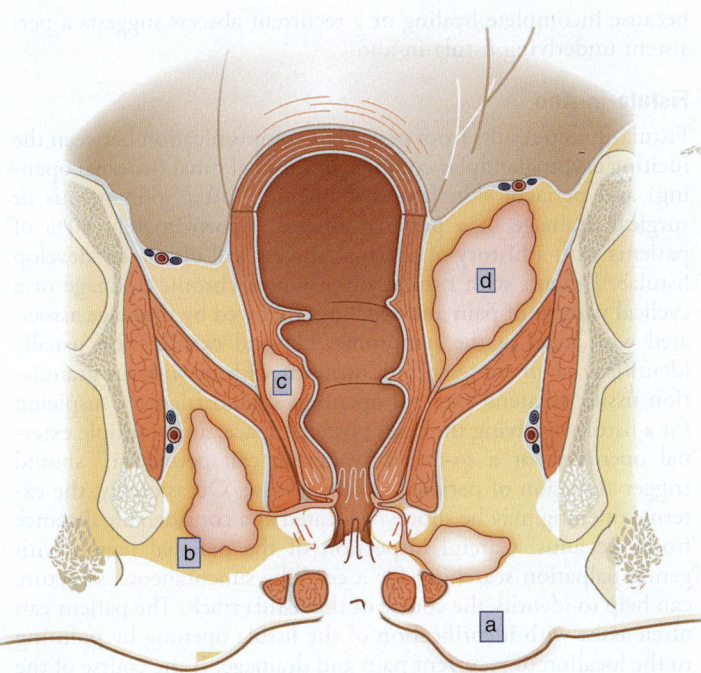

FIGURE 97.13 Common extensions of anorectal abscesses: *(a)* superficial perianal, *(b)* ischiorectal, *(c)* intersphincteric, and *(d)* supralevator. (From McAneny D. Anorectal disorders. In: Noble J, ed. *Textbook of Primary Care Medicine*. 3rd ed. Philadelphia: Mosby; 2001.)

BOX 97.1 Etiology of Anorectal Abscess

Nonspecific etiology
  Cryptoglandular
Specific etiology
  Inflammatory condition
  Crohn disease
  Tuberculosis
  Actinomycosis
  Lymphogranuloma venereum
Traumatic etiology
  Impalement
  Foreign body
  Anal fissure
  Iatrogenic
  Episiotomy
  Hemorrhoidectomy
  Prostatectomy
  Radiation
Malignancy
  Rectal or anal carcinoma
  Leukemia
  Lymphoma

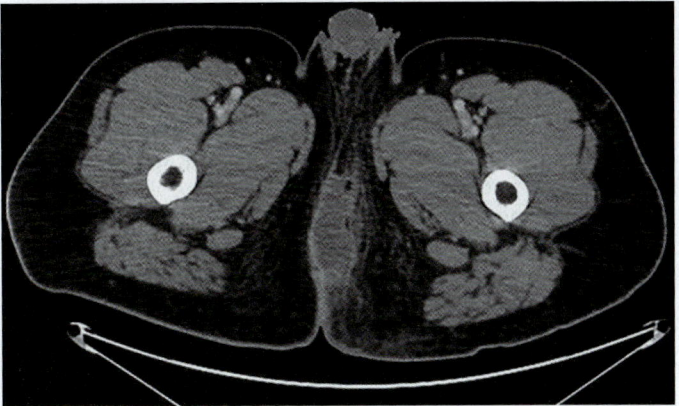

FIGURE 97.14 CT image of left perianal abscess.

more compelling; antibiotics alone in this situation will usually be insufficient. Routine use of diagnostic imaging is not typically necessary for patients with anorectal abscesses, but CT of the pelvis can be helpful if the diagnosis is in question (Fig. 97.14).

Perianal abscesses should be treated promptly by incision and drainage.[26] This can be done either in an ambulatory setting under local anesthesia or in the operating room as appropriate. The drainage should be performed starting at the most fluctuant aspect of the abscess, staying as close to the anus as possible to shorten the length of any subsequent fistula tract. The size of the incision should be tailored to the size of the abscess and large enough to ensure adequate drainage. This is accomplished by probing the cavity with the examining finger or an instrument to assess its extent. A cruciate incision with subsequent removal of the corners is a reliable way to ensure ongoing drainage and prevent premature closure of the skin and recurrent abscess accumulation. Loculations within the abscess cavity may be carefully broken up to achieve adequate drainage of the entire cavity. The practice of aggressive digital disruption of loculations, however, should be avoided because this maneuver may cause injury to the sphincter complex or pudendal nerve as well as cause hemorrhage from bridging vessels in the ischiorectal space. If the abscess cavity is larger than 5 cm, one may consider placing counter incisions and bridge them with Penrose drains or vessel loops. This technique avoids large, gaping perineal wounds that may result in prolonged healing, scarring, and distortion of the perianal anatomy. For a deeper abscess cavity, a drainage catheter (e.g., Pezzer or Malecot) can be left in place for several days to weeks until the abscess resolves and then is removed in the outpatient setting.

For those patients presenting with abscesses that do not have obvious external fluctuance, external drainage should be avoided to prevent the iatrogenic creation of a fistula. Low-lying intersphincteric abscesses should be drained through the intersphincteric groove or into the anal canal via an incision of the internal sphincter. Supralevator abscesses originating from the complicated extension of an intersphincteric abscess should also be drained internally by incising the rectal wall.

Horseshoe abscesses can also be challenging to manage. As described previously, these abscesses typically arise from a source at the posterior midline and track in the deep postanal space, extending laterally into one or bilateral ischiorectal spaces, so effective drainage of both the deep postanal space and one or both of the ischiorectal spaces is necessary. A modified Hanley

hemorrhoid, by history and gentle examination. Thorough digital rectal examination or anoscopic examination is often deferred in the acute setting because of pain. A common error is diagnosing "cellulitis" when patients present with pain, erythema, and tenderness but are not found to have fluctuance. Many of these patients simply have a deeper abscess, making the need for drainage even

technique involves posterior midline drainage of the deep post-anal space by incising the anococcygeal ligament as well as seton placement after identification of a posterior midline fistula tract. Counterincisions are also made to effectively drain the bilateral ischiorectal spaces. Commonly, additional Penrose drains are placed between the posterior midline incision and each of the anterior-lateral counter incisions.

Packing of the abscess cavity is not necessary but can be helpful in selected patients to provide hemostasis of the inflamed, hypervascular tissue. Any packing should be removed when hemostasis is confirmed, when soiled or saturated, when the patient is urinating/defecating or bathing/showering, or the following day. A well-drained abscess cavity does not require wet-to-dry dressing changes or packing to achieve debridement and prevent premature closure of the skin. Packing can be very challenging and uncomfortable for the patient, and patients can unwittingly retain the packing in the abscess cavity for days or weeks, despite being instructed to remove it. Packing does not reduce the risk of abscess recurrence or fistula formation.

A well-drained perirectal abscess also does not typically require treatment with antibiotics because they have not been shown to improve healing times or reduce the recurrence rates.[27] Antibiotics may be used selectively in patients whose abscesses are complicated by cellulitis or systemic illness or in patients with underlying immunosuppression.[26]

After successful drainage of the abscess, the patient should experience immediate improvement in pain. The patient may be instructed to perform warm sitz baths, use bulk-forming fiber supplements, and use multimodal analgesia with sparing narcotic medications only for breakthrough pain. Minor bleeding is common and usually subsides within a few days, but ongoing drainage of serosanguinous fluid is to be expected to continue for 1 to 2 weeks as the cavity heals, with most wounds healing completely within 6 to 8 weeks (depending on the size of the wound). Close surgical follow-up is recommended until complete healing

because incomplete healing or a recurrent abscess suggests a persistent underlying fistula-in-ano.

Fistula-in-Ano

Fistula-in-ano results from persistent communication between the inciting cryptoglandular complex in the anal canal (internal opening) and perianal skin (external opening) after spontaneous or surgical drainage of a perianal abscess. Approximately 50% of patients with a history of perianal abscess will ultimately develop fistulae. Patients with fistulae often report chronic drainage or a cyclical pattern of pain and swelling, followed by drainage associated with relief of the symptoms. Physical examination usually identifies one or more chronic wounds with or without granulation tissue. Bilateral external openings should trigger a suspicion for a fistula involving the deep postanal space, and multiple external openings, or a so-called "watering can perineum," should trigger suspicion of perianal Crohn disease. Occasionally, the external opening may be subtle or located at a considerable distance from the anus. Careful inspection of the perianal region with gentle palpation searching for a cordlike subcutaneous structure can help to identify the course of the fistula track. The patient can often assist with identification of the fistula opening by pointing to the location of recurrent pain and drainage. If the course of the fistulous track remains unclear, a pelvic MRI with anal fistula protocol can be useful to delineate the anatomy of the fistula tracks (Fig. 97.15).

Fistula-in-ano can be classified as superficial/subcutaneous, intersphincteric, transsphincteric, suprasphincteric, and extrasphincteric based on the Parks classification (Fig. 97.16). The goals for treatment of an anal fistula are to (1) treat any undrained infection, (2) define fistula anatomy, (3) remove or ablate epithelialized tracts, (4) avoid or minimize the risk of fecal incontinence, and (5) prevent recurrence.

Surgical treatment of fistula-in-ano carries a high risk of impaired continence; however, there is not a perfect linear relationship

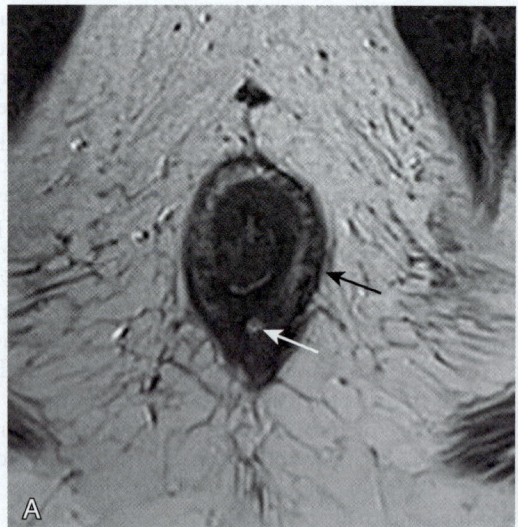
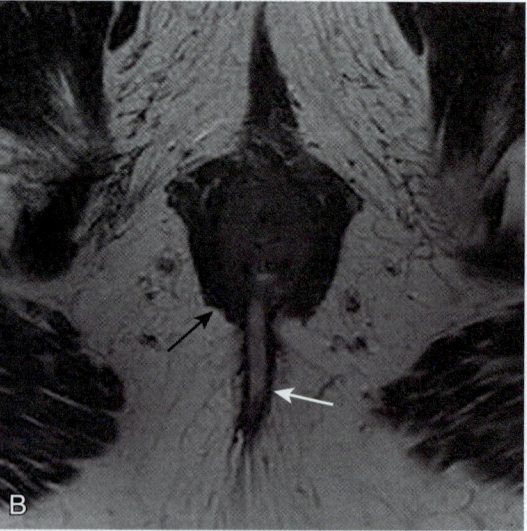

FIGURE 97.15 Anal fistula MRI. (A) Axial T2-weighted scan in a patient with an intersphincteric fistula *(white arrow)*. The fistula lies within the intersphincteric plane. The lateral margin of the external sphincter *(black arrow)* is appreciated easily on MRI. (B) Axial T2-weighted scan in a patient with a transsphincteric fistula *(white arrow)*. The fistula track clearly lies lateral to the external sphincter boundary *(black arrow)* and penetrates the sphincter to reach a posterior internal opening at 6 o'clock, at dentate-line level. (From Halligan S. Magnetic resonance imaging of fistula-in-ano. *Magn Reson Imaging Clin N Am.* 2020;28[1]:141-151.)

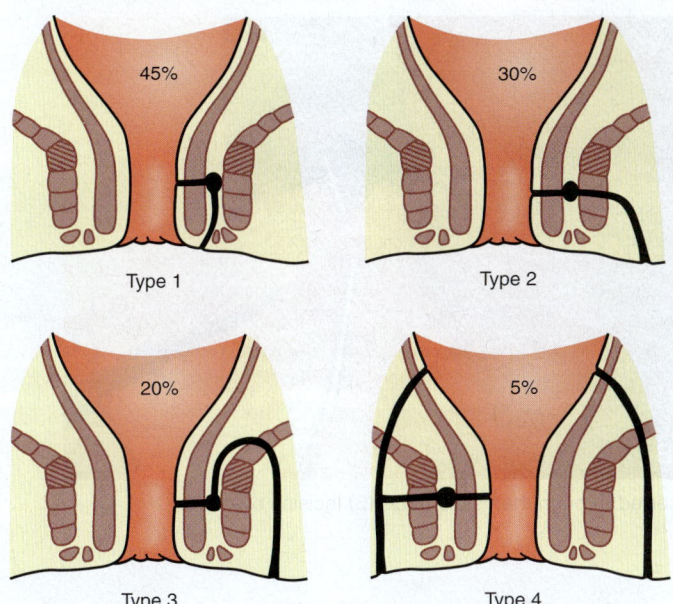

FIGURE 97.16 Park classification of fistula-in-ano: *type 1*, intersphincteric; *type 2*, transsphincteric; *type 3*, suprasphincteric; and *type 4*, extrasphincteric.

between the extent of operative intervention and continence impairment, with some patients reporting no or minimal incontinence despite division of a significant portion of sphincter muscle and some patients reporting significant incontinence despite division of no or minimal sphincter muscle.[28] Preoperative planning should consider preexisting continence, stool consistency, history of sphincter injury or surgery, the amount of sphincter that is likely to be divided, anterior location in females, and the patient's attitude toward potential imperfections in continence.

Intraoperative evaluation begins with identification of the fistula tracks. Goodsall's rule predicts the course of the fistula tract and the location of the internal opening (Fig. 97.17). Fistulas with an external opening anterior to the transverse bisection of the anus typically track in a radial fashion directly into the

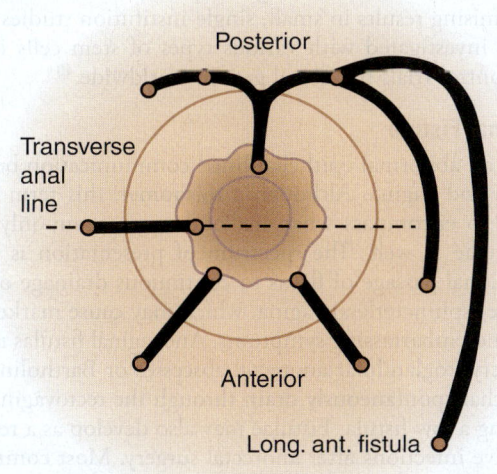

FIGURE 97.17 Goodsall rule of fistula-in-ano tracks extension.

anal canal, except for those located at a distance greater than 3 cm from the anal verge, which may be an anterior extension of a horseshoe fistula originating posteriorly. Fistulas with an external opening posterior to the transverse bisection of the anus often track in a curvilinear fashion to a posterior midline internal opening.

Anoscopy allows direct inspection of the dentate line and may reveal an erythematous crypt or a visible internal opening. Gentle pressure on the skin over the fistula tract may induce drainage from the offending crypt. In the operating room, an anal fistula probe may be passed gently through the external opening into the fistula tract and through the internal opening to demonstrate the anatomy. If the probe does not pass easily, extreme care should be taken to avoid creating a false passage and creating an iatrogenic fistula. The external opening can also be injected with dilute hydrogen peroxide, methylene blue, or milk when identification of the internal opening of the fistula in the anal canal is challenging. The anorectal mucosa should be evaluated to exclude a different origin of the perianal sepsis, such as Crohn disease, atypical ulcers, or cancer.

Simple, low-lying fistulae, commonly defined as those involving less than one-third of the external anal sphincter (intersphincteric or low transsphincteric), may be treated by lay-open fistulotomy (Fig. 97.18).[26] Multiple prospective, multicenter studies have shown that clinically significant fecal incontinence after simple fistulotomy in low-lying fistulae occurs in less than 5% of patients with normal preoperative sphincter function.[29–31] The recurrence rate for treatment of simple anal fistulas with fistulotomy is 2% to 8%.[28,32,33]

For patients in whom a fistula is diagnosed at the time of abscess drainage, primary fistulotomy remains controversial. Although fistulotomy would effectively address the offending crypt and decrease the risk of abscess recurrence and chronic fistula formation, inflammation and edema can make it difficult to accurately assess the anatomy, potentially leading to an underestimation of sphincter involvement.

In fistulas involving larger amounts of sphincter muscle, and in those patients in whom the degree of sphincter involvement cannot be accurately determined because of inflammation, the initial treatment is often focused on controlling the fistula with a draining seton using a silastic vessel loop or a rubber band (Fig. 97.19). This allows for formation of a narrow fistula tract and prevents the recurrent cyclical symptoms of swelling, pain, and drainage from closure of the external opening. This also affords the opportunity to "shorten" a fistula tract by performing a partial fistulotomy through soft tissue, up to the external sphincter. A seton can also be progressively tightened and used in a cutting manner, enabling a slow, controlled division of the fistula tract; alternatively, the cutting seton may shorten the tract over time and allow for a safe lay-open fistulotomy of a more superficial fistula. For a cutting seton to work, the epithelium along the fistula must be divided. Cutting setons should be used with caution because the incidence of incontinence approaches that of lay-open fistulotomy of the tract.[34,35]

The preferred treatment of anal fistulas would ideally result in obliteration of the internal opening and all associated tracts without the need to divide any of the sphincter muscle. Several techniques have been developed in the hopes of achieving this goal, but none has proven to provide a universally reliable cure. The fistula track may be plugged with a bioresorbable substance or filled with a fibrin glue that obliterates the tract and theoretically provides a scaffold on which native tissue can deposit collagen and

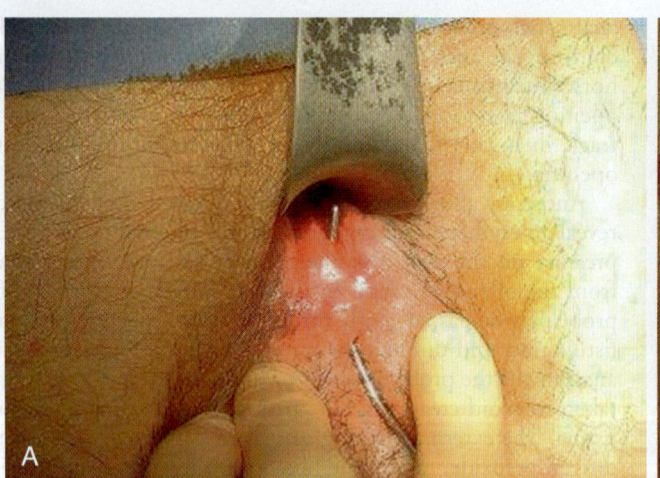
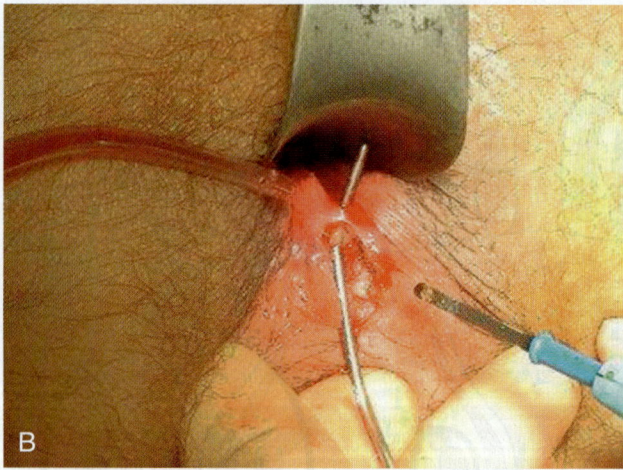

FIGURE 97.18 Lay-open fistulotomy. (A) Fistula probe inserted through the fistula track. (B) Incision over the fistula probe to lay open the fistula track.

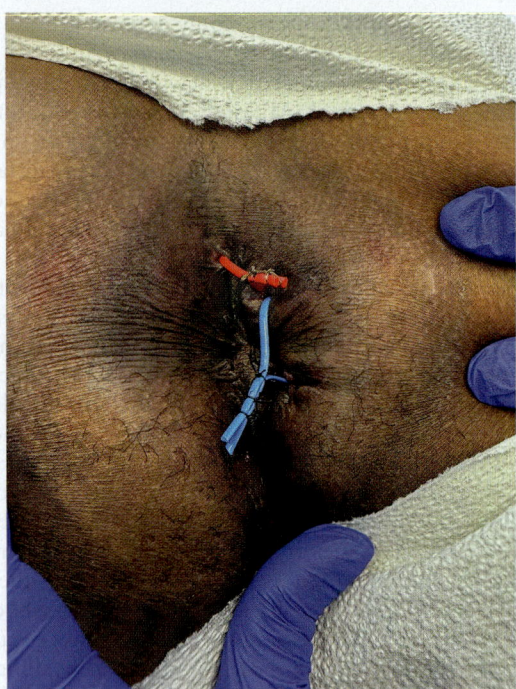

FIGURE 97.19 Seton.

seal the fistula tract. These devices have not been demonstrated to achieve long-term success. Ligation of the intersphincteric fistula tract (LIFT) involves accessing the fistula tract through the intersphincteric plane and ligating/interrupting the fistula tract.[36] Failure of this procedure may favorably result in an intersphincteric fistula that is then amenable to fistulotomy (Fig. 97.20). Endorectal advancement flaps have also been shown to effectively treat cryptoglandular fistula-in-ano, with healing rates between 66% and 87%.[37–39] This repair is often used to treat transsphincteric fistulae. This repair involves excision of the fistula tract and closure of the rectal portion of the fistula with a vascularized mucosal flap from proximal in the rectum (Fig. 97.21). The classic description involves raising a flap containing mucosa and submucosa off the internal sphincter muscle; some surgeons advocate including internal anal sphincter fibers to create a more robust flap and preserve the blood supply, although this approach has

been shown to increase rates of mild to moderate incontinence with concomitant decreased manometric resting and squeeze pressures in up to 35% of patients.[40–43]

In recent years there has been significant interest, although scarce robust data, in several minimally invasive approaches to treat fistula-in-ano. Video-assisted anal fistula treatment (VAAFT) uses a specially designed fistulascope that is inserted into the external fistula opening to precisely define the fistula tract and identify any branches. Once precisely identified, the internal opening is closed with suture ligation or stapling. Granulation tissue in the tract is debrided, an electrode is introduced via a working channel in the endoscope, and the fistula tract is ablated under direct vision without dividing any sphincter muscle. The technique has demonstrated encouraging short-term results, with reported healing rates after VAAFT ranging from 71% to 85% and minor or no fecal incontinence reported at a follow-up of up to 2 year.[44–46] The fistula laser closure (FiLaC) uses a conceptually similar technique of ablating the fistula tract along its length from the inside using a radially emitting laser probe rather than an electrode. A recent metanalysis demonstrated similarly promising short-term results, with healing in 65% of patients at a median of 24 months of follow-up.[47] Transplantation of mesenchymal stem cells into the tissue surrounding complex perianal fistulae has shown promising results in small, single-institution studies and is now being investigated with various types of stem cells in randomized control trials by several groups worldwide.[48]

Rectovaginal Fistula

An RVF is an abnormal epithelial-lined communication between the rectum and vagina. Although a misnomer, this term is also often used to encompass what are (and more commonly) anovaginal fistulae as well. The spectrum of presentation is broad, from occasional passage of flatus to continuous drainage of stool through the (sphincterless) vagina, which may cause marked skin irritation and embarrassing symptoms. Anovaginal fistulas may be caused by cryptoglandular anorectal abscesses or Bartholin gland infections that spontaneously drain through the rectovaginal septum, causing a low fistula. Fistulae may also develop as a result of postoperative infections after anorectal surgery. Most commonly, anovaginal fistulae develop after obstetric injuries or postpartum as a result of prolonged labor with necrosis of the rectovaginal septum, traumatic injury from instrumented delivery, third- or

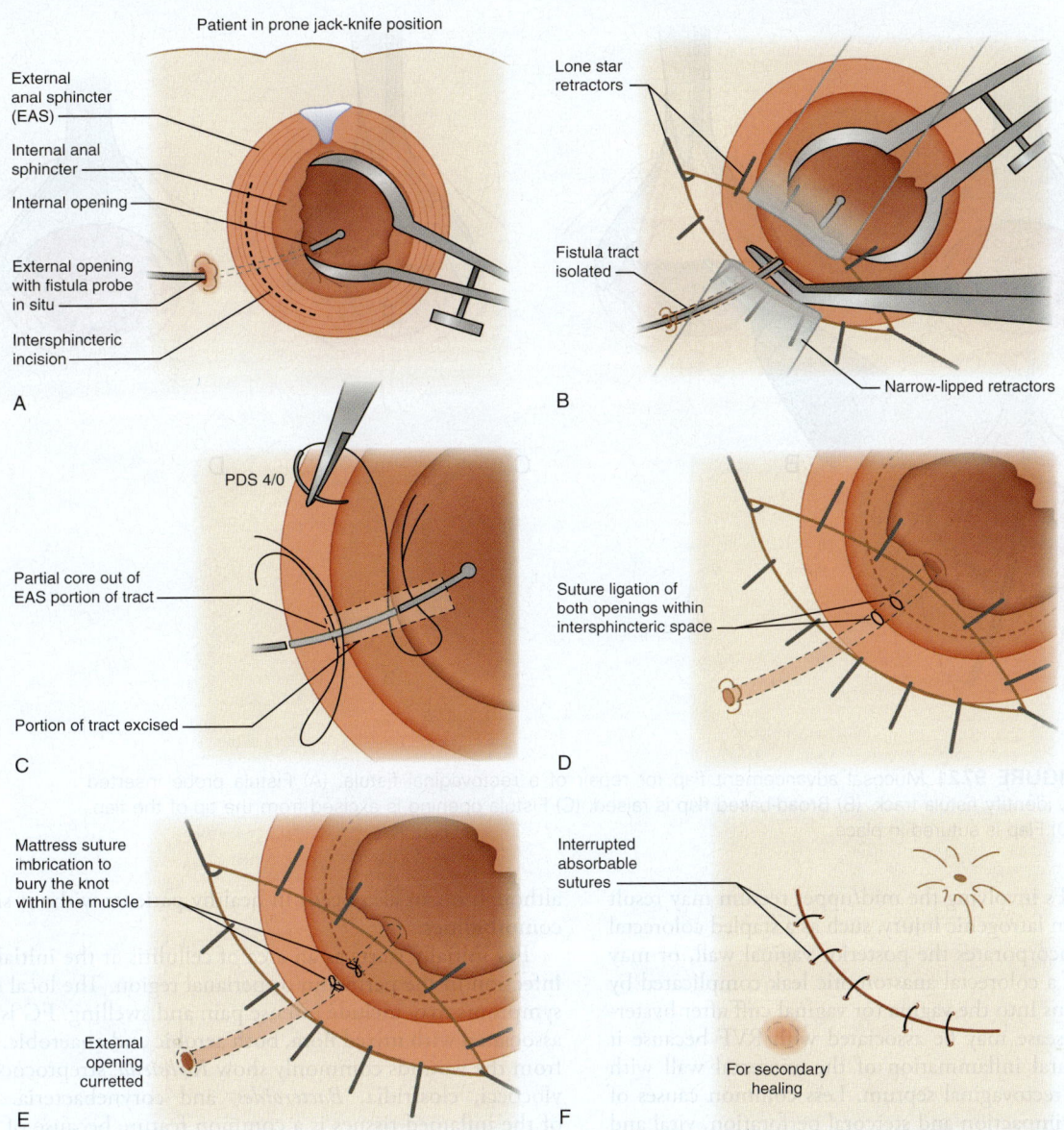

Patient in prone jack-knife position

External anal sphincter (EAS)

Internal anal sphincter

Internal opening

External opening with fistula probe in situ

Intersphincteric incision

A

Lone star retractors

Fistula tract isolated

Narrow-lipped retractors

B

PDS 4/0

Partial core out of EAS portion of tract

Portion of tract excised

C

Suture ligation of both openings within intersphincteric space

D

Mattress suture imbrication to bury the knot within the muscle

External opening curretted

E

Interrupted absorbable sutures

For secondary healing

F

FIGURE 97.20 Ligation of intersphincteric fistula tract procedure. (A) Fistula probe inserted into the fistula track: internal opening and external opening. (B) Intersphincteric plane is opened, and fistula track is identified within the intersphincteric space. (C) Fistula track is divided within intersphincteric space. (D) Both ends of divided track are suture ligated. (E) Sphincter muscle fibers are approximated to obliterate the intersphincteric space. (F) Perianal skin is closed. (From Koh SZ, Tsang CB. The LIFT procedure. *Semin Colon Rectal Surg.* 2014;25:190-199.)

fourth-degree perineal tear, or episiotomy after breakdown of the repair.[49,50]

For RVFs caused by benign disease, especially those related to obstetric injuries, nonoperative management for a period of 3 to 6 months can be considered because spontaneous healing rates ranging from 52% to 65% have been reported.[51,52] Nonoperative management frequently focuses on treating any associated infection or inflammation to optimize healing conditions and includes sitz baths, local wound care, and stool-bulking fiber supplements.[53] For fistulae with significant inflammation or troubling symptoms, draining seton, antibiotics, or fecal diversion may be necessary.

Endorectal advancement flap, as described earlier, is the most common treatment of choice for most anovaginal fistulae, with

success rates ranging from 41% to 78%. This procedure is well tolerated by patients and can be repeated if the initial repair is unsuccessful. A diverting stoma is not necessary before performing endorectal advancement flap because it has not been shown to significantly improve outcomes.[26] Nevertheless, it is sometimes considered to address intolerable symptoms or after failed prior attempts at repair. Anovaginal fistulae with a concomitant sphincter defect may be treated with perineal repair with overlapping sphincteroplasty or levatorplasty. Tissue transposition repair adds healthy, well-perfused tissue between the vagina and the anus, increasing the distance and adding new blood supply. The tissue used for interposition is most commonly the gracilis muscle or the bulbocavernosus and labial fat pad (Martius flap).

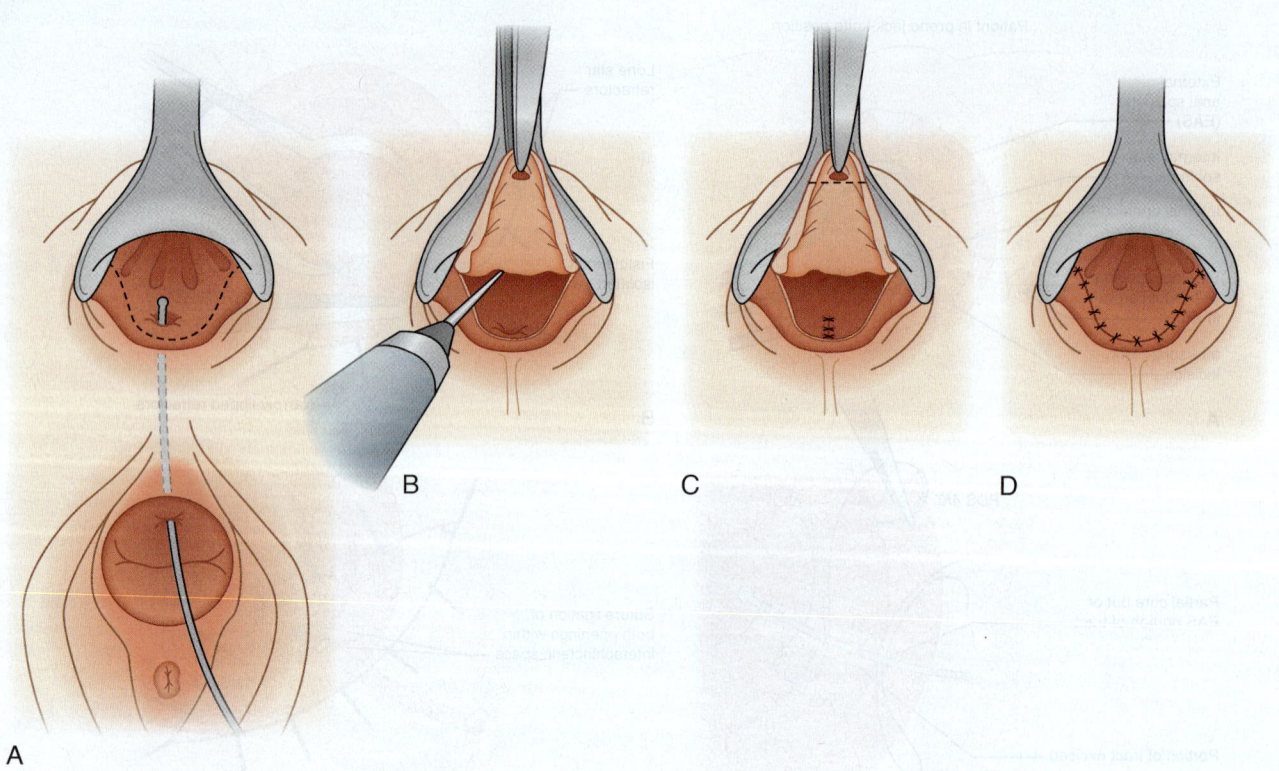

A

B

C

D

FIGURE 97.21 Mucosal advancement flap for repair of a rectovaginal fistula. (A) Fistula probe inserted to identify fistula track. (B) Broad-based flap is raised. (C) Fistula opening is excised from the tip of the flap. (D) Flap is sutured in place.

Higher true RVFs involving the mid/upper rectum may result postoperatively from iatrogenic injury, such as a stapled colorectal anastomosis that incorporates the posterior vaginal wall, or may occur as a result of a colorectal anastomotic leak complicated by an abscess that drains into the vagina (or vaginal cuff after hysterectomy). Crohn disease may be associated with RVF because it may cause transmural inflammation of the anorectal wall with extension into the rectovaginal septum. Less common causes of RVFs include fecal impaction and stercoral perforation, viral and bacterial infections (in immunocompromised patients), and trauma from sexual assault. Malignancies, particularly anal cancer or rectal cancer, may present as an RVF or may develop a fistula after radiation therapy. If suspicion for an undiagnosed malignancy is present, biopsy of the fistula should be performed. Higher RVFs in the midrectum, involving the fornix of the vagina, are difficult to access via a perineal approach and require a transabdominal repair. Repair typically involves a low anterior resection of the area of the rectum involved in the fistula with a colorectal or coloanal anastomosis and primary closure of the vagina. With limited disease, some have demonstrated successful healing by excision of the fistula with placement of omentum in the rectovaginal septum.[54]

Fournier Gangrene

Severe perianal abscesses and pelvic infections, or infections of the genitourinary tract, can progress to a rare but life-threatening form of necrotizing fasciitis involving the perineal, genital, or perianal regions called *Fournier gangrene* (FG). Less commonly, FG can result from an intrabdominal infection that tracks to the perineum via the inguinal canals.[55] FG has been associated with male sex, diabetes, chronic alcohol abuse, and immunosuppression, although it can also occur in healthy patients without significant comorbidities.

FG initially starts as an area of cellulitis at the initial focus of infection in the perineum or perianal region. The local signs and symptoms may include intense pain and swelling. FG is typically associated with mixed flora, both aerobic and anaerobic. Cultures from the wounds commonly show *Klebsiella*, streptococci, staphylococci, clostridia, *Bacteroides,* and corynebacteria. Crepitus of the inflamed tissues is a common feature because of the presence of gas-forming organisms. Bacterial infection results in microthrombosis of the small subcutaneous vessels, leading to tissue necrosis.

Necrotic patches appear in the overlying skin and progress to more extensive necrosis; purple/black bullae are classically described in FG and other necrotizing infections (Fig. 97.22). The patient is likely to demonstrate signs of severe systemic illness, which are commonly out of proportion to the visible local extent of the disease because the disease progresses deep along the fascial planes. Laboratory values generally demonstrate nonspecific findings of elevated inflammatory markers, making individual lab values largely unhelpful in distinguishing between necrotizing soft tissue infections, such FG, and severe cellulitis. The Laboratory Risk Indicator for Necrotizing Infection (LRINEC) score has been advocated as a clinical tool that can help determine which patients require further diagnostic testing. The scoring system assigns points for abnormalities in six common laboratory values: serum C-reactive protein level (>150 mg/L), white blood cell (WBC) count (>15,000/μL), hemoglobin level (<13.5 g/dL), serum sodium level (<135 mmol/L), serum creatinine level (>1.6 mg/dL), and serum glucose level (>180 mg/dL). A score of 6 points or higher has been shown to have a positive predictive

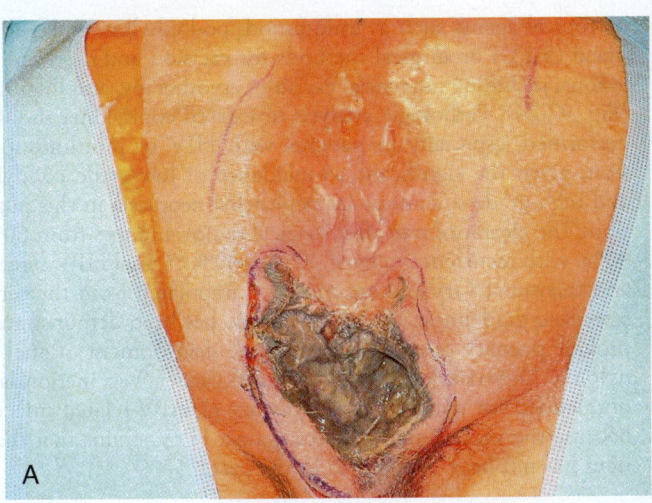 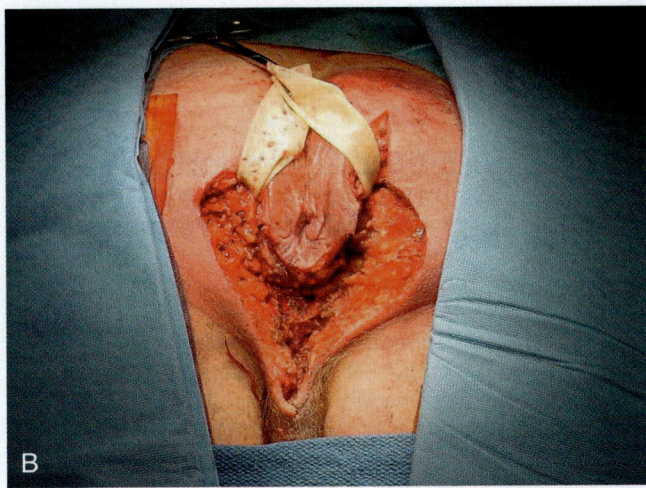

FIGURE 97.22 (A) Fournier gangrene. (B) Perineum after excision of Fournier gangrene.

value of 92% and a negative predictive value of 96% for the presence of a necrotizing infection (Table 97.2).[56,57]

FG is a surgical emergency. It is rapidly progressive and quickly leads to sepsis, potentially with multiple organ failure and even death. Spread of infection occurs along the fascial planes and is usually far more extensive than initially anticipated based on external appearance. Necrotizing fasciitis can extend to involve the scrotum and penis and can spread through the anterior abdominal wall and up all the way to the clavicles.[58] Urogenital infections tend to extend posteriorly along Bucks and Dartos fascia up to the Colles fascia but are often limited from the anal margin by the attachment of the Colles fascia to the perineal body. In contrast, anorectal sources of infection usually involve the perianal skin. The location and the spread of infection can serve as a guide to identifying the initial focus of infection.

Regardless of the cause of FG, the testes are usually spared because the blood supply originates intraabdominally.

Treatment of FG requires an aggressive multimodal approach, including hemodynamic stabilization, fluid resuscitation, and broad-spectrum antibiotics; the cornerstone of management, however, is early aggressive surgical debridement. Unnecessary delay in surgical debridement has a negative impact on prognosis. All nonviable and necrotic tissue must be excised until well-perfused, healthy tissue is reached. As noted earlier, the full extent of the disease may be far greater than estimated by the areas of cutaneous involvement. Urinary or fecal diversion may be necessary depending on the location and degree of tissue loss but is seldom necessary at the initial debridement. Multiple trips to the operating room are typically required, with an average of three to four procedures before complete debridement can be achieved. After controlling the infection and preserving healthy viable tissue, healing may be a prolonged course. The use of vacuum-assisted closure systems dressings has markedly improved wound care in these patients and accelerates wound healing. Split-thickness skin grafts can be used to provide coverage of the perineal and scrotal skin defects. Long-term, more extensive tissue coverage techniques may be necessary for reconstruction.

Sexually Transmitted Infections

Anorectal STIs may be transmitted by anoreceptive intercourse, oroanal sexual contact, contiguous spread from a genital infection, or any skin-to-skin contact. Symptoms of STIs are often nonspecific and latent, with some infected (and transmitting) individuals being completely asymptomatic. Complaints may include anal pain, tenesmus, urgency, purulent/mucus drainage, and bleeding. When evaluating a patient with an anorectal complaint, it is important to keep the diagnosis of STI in the differential when abnormalities such as ulcerations, vegetations, and proctitis are seen on examination (Table 97.3).

Human Papillomavirus/Condyloma Acuminata

Human papillomavirus (HPV) is the most common STI in the United States, with 5.5 million new infections occurring every year. The classic lesion is the condyloma acuminatum or anal wart. Serotypes 6 and 11 are found in benign warts, whereas serotypes 16 and 18 are more commonly seen in dysplasia and malignancies, as discussed in the chapter on anorectal malignancy (see Chapter 96).[59]

TABLE 97.2	**LRINEC Score**	
SCORE MARKER	**LEVELS**	**SCORING**
C-reactive protein	<150 mg/L	0
	>150 mg/L	4
White blood cells	<15 per mm³	0
	15–25 per mm	1
	>25 per mm³	2
Hemoglobin	>13.5 g/dL	0
	11–13.5 g/dL	1
	<11 g/dL	2
Sodium	>135	0
	<135	2
Creatinine	<1.6 mg/dL	0
	>1.6 mg/dL	2
Serum glucose	<180 mg/dL	0
	>180 mg/dL	1
STAGE	**SCORE**	**PROBABILITY OF NECROTIZING FASCIITIS (%)**
Low	<5	50
Moderate	6–7	50–75
High	>8	>75

LRINEC, Laboratory Risk Indicator for Necrotizing Infection.

TABLE 97.3 Etiology and Symptoms of Sexually Transmitted Proctitis

SEXUALLY TRANSMITTED INFECTION	COMMON SIGNS AND SYMPTOMS
Gonorrhea	Asymptomatic. If symptoms present: pruritus ani, constipation, mucopurulent anal discharge, rectal pain, and tenesmus.
Chlamydia	Asymptomatic. If symptoms present: pruritus ani, mucous discharge, anal pain.
Chlamydia (lymphogranuloma venereum)	Generalized illness: fever and malaise. Anal symptoms: purulent or bloody discharge. Anal pain and tenesmus. May mimic inflammatory bowel disease.
Syphilis	Primary: anorectal chancre commonly asymptomatic. If symptomatic: pain or discomfort, itching, bleeding, and/or tenesmus. Secondary: ulcers and mucous patches. Perianal condylomata lata. Generalized manifestations: rash, fever, and lymphadenopathy.
Herpes simplex virus	Vesicular lesions, severe pain, and tenesmus; difficulty with bowel movements. Generalized symptoms: fever and lymphadenopathy.

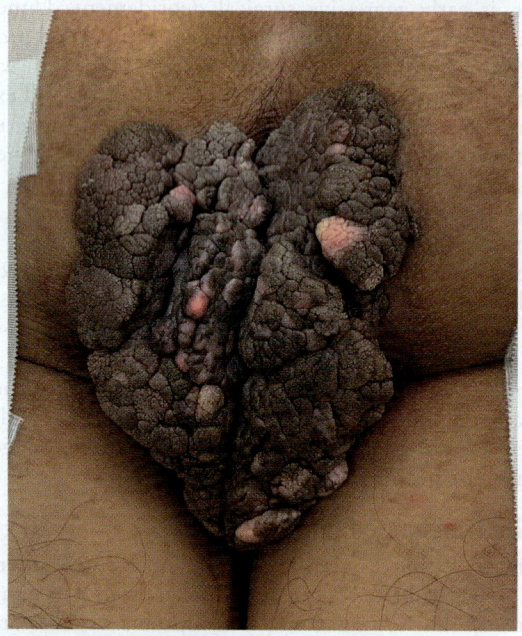

FIGURE 97.23 Buschke-Lowenstein tumor.

Anal HPV is transmitted by anoreceptive intercourse or skin-to-skin contact and may be associated with immunosuppression caused by HIV infection or immunosuppressant medications, especially in solid organ transplantation recipients. The use of condoms lowers the risk of sexual transmission, although infection can still be transmitted through the skin beyond the area covered by a condom. Lesions begin as small, raised, wartlike lesions. Other symptoms are uncommon but may develop as the lesion grows and may include anorectal bleeding or discharge, pain, and itching. Anoscopy may reveal disease present in the anal canal. An aggressive variant of HPV infection, Buschke-Lowenstein disease, results in a giant condyloma (Fig. 97.23). Anal condyloma can be treated by topical agents such as imiquimod, podophyllin, and 5-fluorouracil (5-FU) or surgical methods for excision and destruction of lesions, including tangential excision, cryotherapy, and fulguration (Fig. 97.24). Pathologic analysis of excised condyloma should be performed, especially in patients with HIV or immunosuppression, given the significant co-incidence of low-grade condyloma and high-grade squamous intraepithelial neoplasia in this population. The clearance rate after surgical removal ranges from 60% to 90%, with recurrence rates of 20% to 30%.[60] Anal HPV screening and treatment vary and are mostly extrapolated from the cervical screening guidelines. The HPV vaccine has been demonstrated to provide primary protection against the development of anal condyloma, high-risk lesions, and cervical cancer. Vaccination is recommended for patients with a history of HPV-related infections because the vaccine may protect against HPV strains that the patient has not been exposed to in the past.[61]

Herpes Simplex Virus

Herpes simplex virus (HSV) is highly prevalent in the United States. Both HSV types 1 and 2 (HSV-1 and HSV-2) may cause anogenital herpes infection. Over 90% of patients with genital herpes may be asymptomatic and unaware that they carry the virus.[62] When symptomatic, HSV proctitis is associated with anorectal pain, constipation, tenesmus, anal itching, difficulty with initiating urination, fever, and inguinal adenopathy.[63] Typical lesions are small vesicles that involve the perianal skin and anal canal but may also extend to the rectum. HSV testing can be performed with cell culture or polymerase chain reaction (PCR), although a negative result may be attributed to intermittent viral shedding. Type-specific HSV serologic assays are also available and can be used to evaluate patients with symptoms of anorectal herpes but with negative HSV cultures. Treatment is with acyclovir, famciclovir, or valacyclovir for 7 to 10 days.

Gonorrhea and Chlamydia

Anogenital gonorrhea is transmitted by anoreceptive intercourse with an infected partner. Symptoms may include pruritus ani, constipation, mucopurulent or bloody anal discharge, anal pain, and tenesmus.[64] However, 84% of asymptomatic males who engage in anal receptive intercourse are found to have rectal gonorrhea.[65] On anoscopic examination, the rectal mucosa can appear normal or erythematous and friable with pus. Nucleic acid amplification tests are the preferred testing modality and have significantly higher sensitivity and specificity than bacterial culture.[66] Given a high incidence of coinfection with chlamydia, treatment of patients testing positive for gonorrhea is directed toward both gonorrhea and chlamydia, even if chlamydia testing is negative. The recommended regimen is ceftriaxone 250 mg in a single intramuscular dose plus azithromycin 1 g orally in a single dose, or doxycycline 100 mg orally twice daily for 7 days.

Chlamydial infection can cause a mild form of proctitis, but most infections are asymptomatic. On physical examination, the rectal mucosa can range from normal appearing to erythematous and friable. Patients occasionally present with perirectal abscesses, anal fissures, and fistula formation mimicking Crohn disease. As with gonorrhea, nucleic acid amplification assays are the preferred diagnostic test. Recommended treatment is with azithromycin 1 g orally in a single dose or doxycycline 100 mg orally twice a day for 7 days.

Syphilis

Anorectal syphilis appears within 2 to 10 weeks of exposure after anal intercourse. Infections can be asymptomatic or manifest with

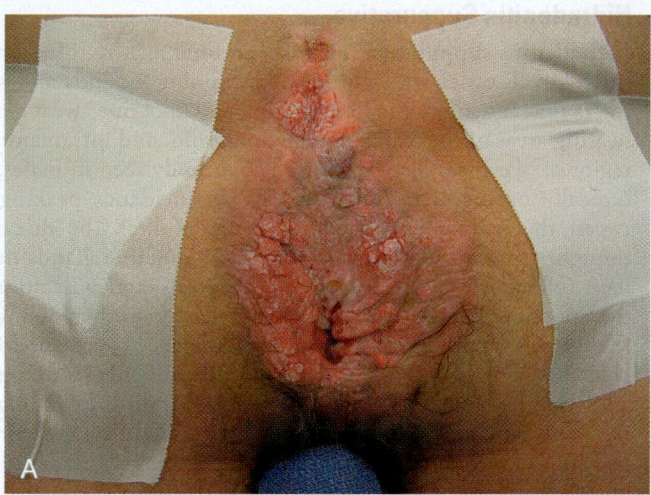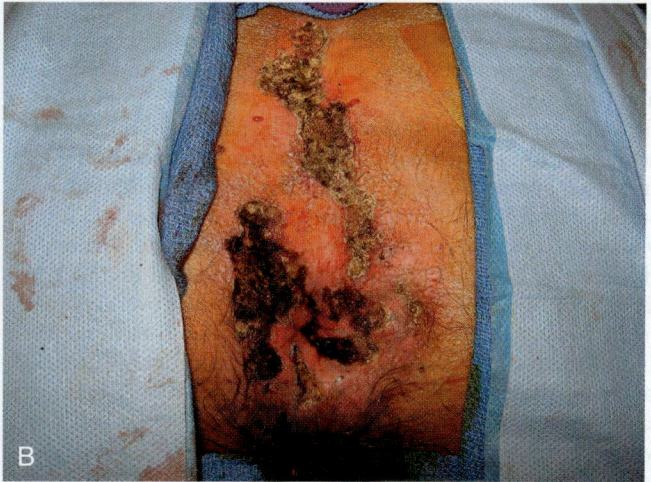

FIGURE 97.24 (A) Extensive anal condyloma. (B) Perianal region after ablation of condyloma.

proctitis, ulcers, and pseudotumors. Anal ulcers are frequently painful, in contrast to the classically described painless genital chancre. Anal lesions usually heal within several weeks, even if untreated. Secondary syphilis may present with a rectal mass, condylomata lata and mucous patches, generalized rash, fever, and lymphadenopathy. Tertiary syphilis presents many years after infection, with debilitating ulcerating gummas as well as damage to other organs and death.

Two types of serologic tests are used to make a presumptive diagnosis of syphilis. The nontreponemal tests, the Venereal Disease Research Laboratory (VDRL) and the rapid plasma reagin (RPR) tests, are used for screening because they become positive within weeks of the primary chancre. Treponemal tests include the fluorescent treponemal antibody absorbed tests, *Treponema pallidum* passive particle agglutination assay, and other immunoassays. These tests usually remain reactive for life in patients who have had a reactive test. Patients with a positive nontreponemal test should undergo a confirmatory treponemal test.

Primary or secondary syphilis is treated with benzathine penicillin G 2.4 million units intramuscularly in a single dose. Doxycycline or tetracycline can be used in patients who have a penicillin allergy.

Human Immunodeficiency Virus

Patients with an STI should be recommended to undergo testing for HIV. STI can coexist, and the immunosuppression associated with HIV can worsen or make patients more susceptible to other STIs. HIV-specific anorectal disorders include idiopathic anal ulcers that are diagnosed after ruling out other STIs and malignancy. Clinical characteristics include a broad-based appearance, localization to the posterior midline and more proximally in the anal canal, erosion into the submucosa, and sphincters with decreased anal sphincter tone. Treatment is with intralesional steroid injection and/or surgical debridement.

Pilonidal Sinus

Pilonidal disease is a common perianal/intergluteal problem affecting young people, typically in their middle to late 20s. Pilonidal disease is estimated to affect approximately 70,000 patients annually in the United States.[67] As the Latin origin of the name suggests—"hair" (*pilus*) and "nest" (*nidus*)—pilonidal disease is caused by shed hair drawn into the natal cleft as a result of the

anatomy of the cleft and the motion from the buttocks. This motion creates a vacuum effect, forcing loose hair into the skin through cutaneous pits in the midline of the gluteal cleft. The presence of pits along the midline of the natal cleft and sinus openings is the hallmark finding in pilonidal disease (Fig. 97.25). Some pilonidal pits are noted incidentally without any inflammation or infection. The foreign body reaction produced by trapped hair may lead to local inflammation and may further become superinfected, leading to a hair-filled abscess cavity. The abscess can drain spontaneously through the skin at the midline or to either side of the gluteus through sinus tracts. The location of the abscess is distinctly different from a perirectal abscess,

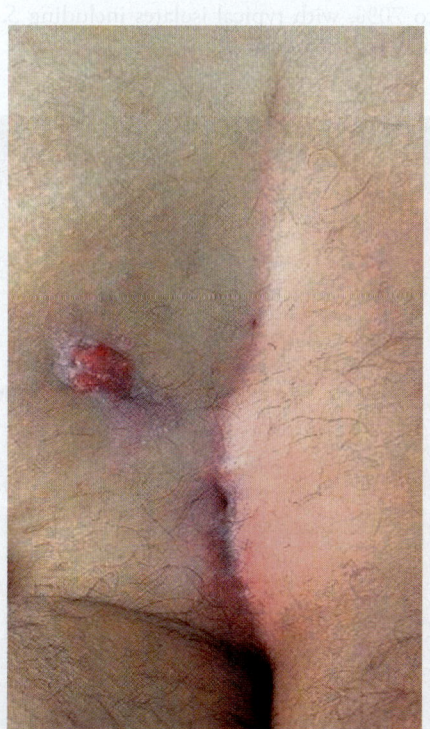

FIGURE 97.25 Pilonidal sinus. (From de Parades V, Bouchard D, Janier M, et al. Pilonidal sinus disease. *J Visc Surg*. 2013;150:237-247.)

which is typically found near the anus. Males are at higher risk because they tend to be more hirsute. Other associations with pilonidal disease are obesity, sedentary occupation, and local irritation or trauma.[67]

Treatment of pilonidal disease should be tailored to the severity of the disease. Antibiotics may be an important adjunct in surgical treatment of pilonidal disease because bacterial colonization was found to range from 50% to 70%, with typical isolates including *Staphylococcus aureus* and anaerobes such as *Bacteroides*. Acute pilonidal abscesses should be treated with incision and drainage. A lateral incision avoiding the midline should be made over the most fluctuant portion of the cavity whenever possible to facilitate the healing of the wound. The cavity should be thoroughly curetted, removing all the embedded hair and devitalized tissue. Hair removal by trimming, shaving, waxing, or laser depilation has been shown to be effective in decreasing recurrence rates.[68]

For recurrent infections or incomplete wound healing, surgical treatment may be considered. Excision of the pilonidal pits and debridement of the abscess cavity and sinus tracts is a less invasive procedure, also known as the *Gips procedure*, developed by Dr. Moshe Gips. Alternatively, the pits and the tracking sinuses may be completely excised. The cavity may then be left open to heal by secondary intention, dressed with a wound vac or negative-pressure dressing, or closed using a variety of different techniques. The importance of avoiding midline closure was popularized by Dr. John Bascom, who advocated lateral incision over the sinus cavity, together with excision of the midline pits and sinus tracts.[69] Complex, extensive pilonidal disease may require transposition of healthy, well-vascularized tissue to close the defect. Several reconstructive techniques have been proposed to cover the defect, including the Bascom cleft lift, Z-plasty, V-to-Y advancement flap, and Limberg flap (Figs. 97.26 and 97.27), note drain left to prevent postoperative seroma/hematoma. As noted, antibiotics may be an important adjunct in surgical treatment of pilonidal disease because bacterial colonization was found to range from 50% to 70%, with typical isolates including *S. aureus* and anaerobes such as *Bacteroides*.

Hidradenitis Suppurativa

Hidradenitis suppurativa (HS) is a chronic recurrent inflammatory skin disorder with chronically draining wounds and sinus tracts that can affect the hair-bearing and apocrine sweat gland–bearing areas of the axillae, perineum, groin, and inframammary regions.[70] Perineal disease is more commonly seen in males. HS typically occurs after puberty, with an incidence peaking between the second and fourth decades of life. The disease is thought to result from occlusion of the apocrine glands or the hair follicular duct. This results in stasis and dilatation of the apocrine gland, followed by bacterial superinfection. When the glands rupture into the subcutaneous space, superficial abscesses form that may lead to complex subcutaneous sinuses and draining tracks (Fig. 97.28). Long-standing inflammation may result in subcutaneous scarring, contractures, and chronic painful induration of the skin. Perianal HS may extend onto the buttocks, to the upper thighs, and medially to the anal verge. Although perianal HS should be differentiated from cryptoglandular abscess and fistula, HS may coexist with other inflammatory disorders, such as Crohn disease.[71]

The differential diagnosis may be challenging, but the distribution of disease, characteristic subcutaneous "pitlike" scarring, distorting contractures, and induration of the skin should be considered pathognomonic for advanced HS. Treatment is based on the Hurley stage of disease at presentation and ranges from medical therapy (antibiotics, antiandrogens, and immunosuppression) to more extensive excision of all affected apocrine sweat gland areas (Table 97.4).

Perianal Crohn Disease

Patients with Crohn disease can have inflammation of the distal rectum that manifests as fistula-in-ano, anal fissure, anal canal stricture, RVF, or abscess. Perianal involvement affects as many as 20% to 35% of patients with Crohn disease.[72,73] For some patients, perianal disease may be the first (or only) site of Crohn disease. The diagnosis should be considered in those patients

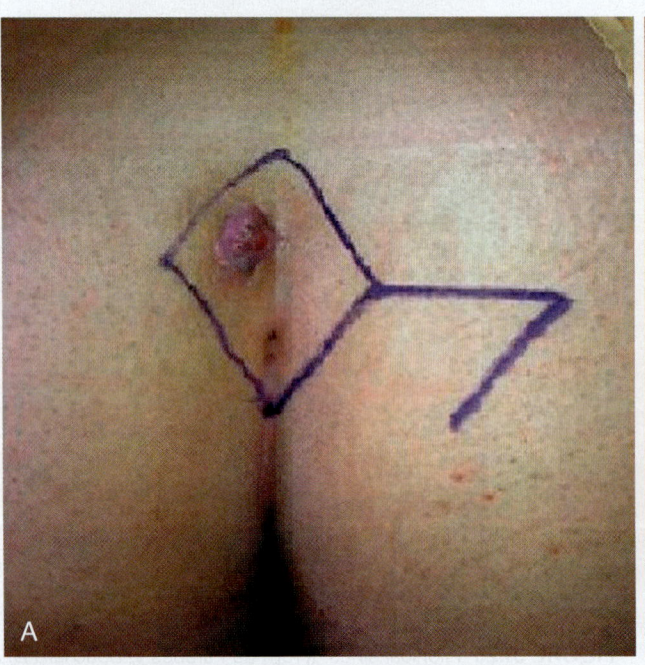
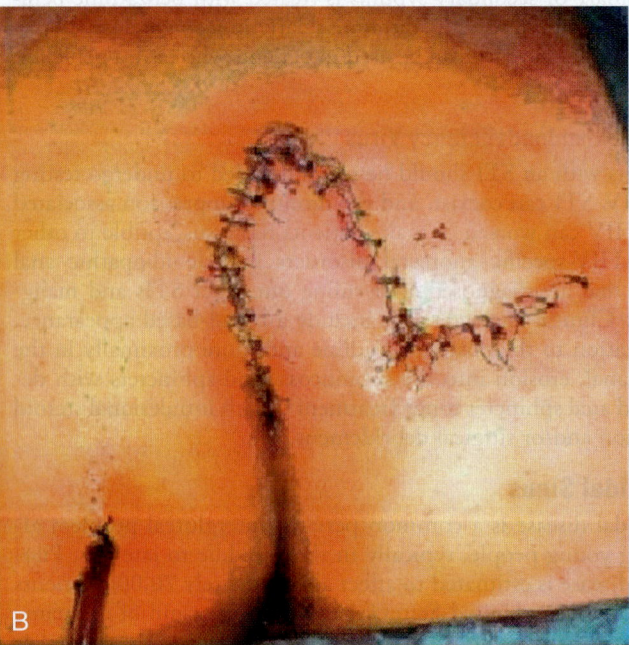

FIGURE 97.26 Limberg flap. (A) Initial marking of a proposed incision. (B) Completed rotation of the flap.

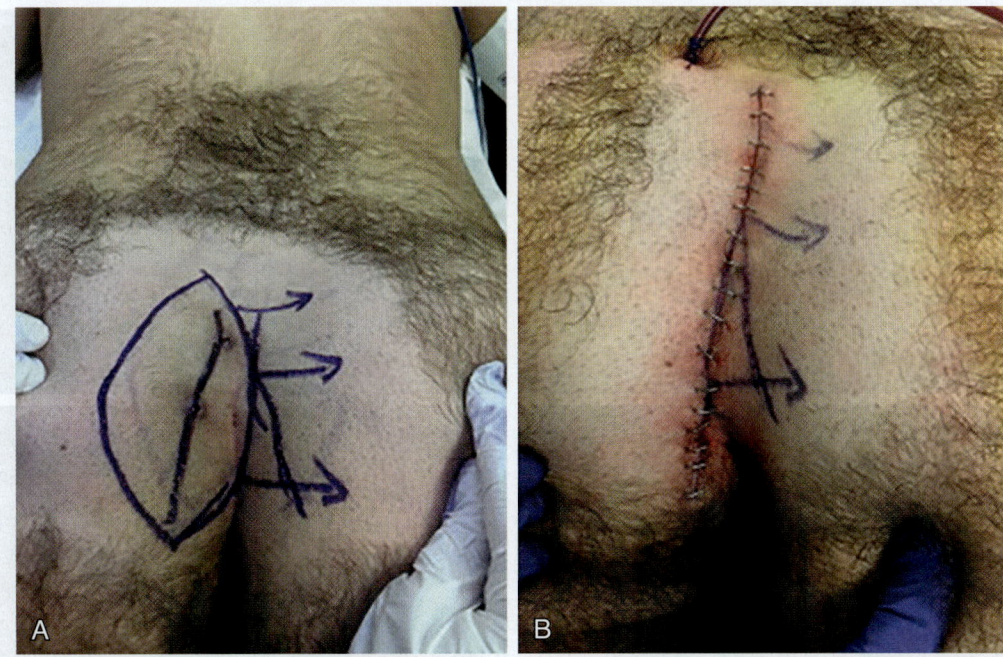

FIGURE 97.27 Bascom cleft lift. (A) The edges of the natal cleft have been marked and an "eccentric" ellipse is planned, which includes all primary midline sinuses and secondary sinuses (two are seen here to left of midline). The skin to the right is undermined in the direction of the arrows. (B) Result at completion of surgery. The ellipse has been excised, the natal cleft is flattened, and the staple line is out of the natal cleft. (From Umesh V, Sussman RH, Smith J, Whyte C. Long term outcome of the Bascom cleft lift procedure for adolescent pilonidal sinus. *J Pediatr Surg.* 2018;53[2]:295-297.)

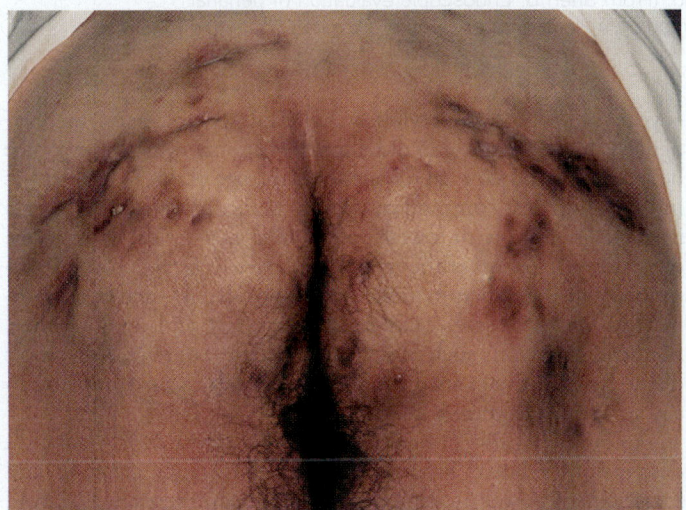

FIGURE 97.28 Hidradenitis suppurativa.

TABLE 97.4	Hurley Stage and Treatment Options	
HURLEY STAGE	DISEASE DESCRIPTION	TREATMENT
I	Abscess formation without sinus tracts or scarring	• Lifestyle modifications • Topical/oral antibiotics • Intralesional steroids • Unroofing
II	Recurrent abscesses with skin tunnels and scarring, single or multiple widely separated lesions	• Oral antibiotics • Oral antiandrogenic agents • Oral retinoids • Metformin • Systemic steroids
III	Diffuse involvement or multiple interconnected skin tunnels and abscesses across the entire area	• Anti-TNF • Wide excision

TNF, Tumor necrosis factor.

who have multiple or complex fistulas, especially located bilaterally; large "elephant ear"–type skin tags; or broad-based anal fissures, especially those located off the midline (Fig. 97.29). A history of chronic diarrhea, abdominal pain, and weight loss (or delayed growth in children) should increase the level of suspicion in patients with atypical fistulas/fissures. Colonoscopy with ileal intubation should be performed for all patients presenting with perianal complaints in whom Crohn disease is suspected.

The evaluation of patients with anorectal Crohn disease should include a careful anorectal examination and may be supplemented by MRI. The priority is to address any uncontrolled infection by draining any abscess, with or without placement of draining setons. This should provide control of perineal sepsis and enable medical therapy, which is the mainstay of management in perianal Crohn disease. Medical therapy for perianal Crohn typically includes antibiotics, particularly metronidazole; immunomodulators; and biologic agents. The antitumor necrosis factor-α agents (i.e., infliximab, adalimumab, certolizumab) have been shown to be particularly effective in preventing the progression of fistulizing Crohn disease band, in select cases, may result in successful closure of the fistula tract.[73]

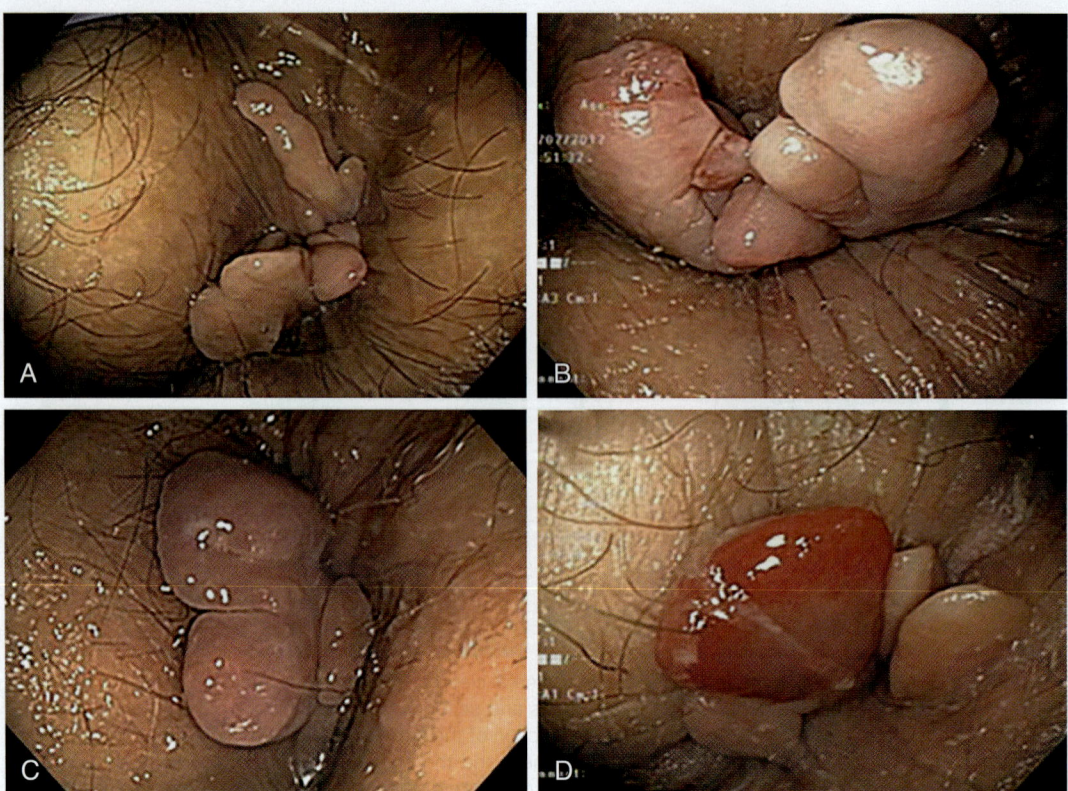

FIGURE 97.29 Crohn disease skin tags. Various forms of skin tags, mostly with an "elephant ear" appearance. (A–D) The skin tags can be single or multiple, thin or thick, flat or cylindrical. The surgical excision of Crohn disease–associated skin tags is not recommended. (From Shen B. Endoscopic evaluation of perianal Crohn's disease. In: Shen B, ed. *Atlas of Endoscopy Imaging in Inflammatory Bowel Disease.* Academic Press; 2020:77-95.)

Surgical management of perianal Crohn disease differs somewhat from the management of pathology not related to inflammatory bowel disease. Because of the risk of poor wound healing and fecal incontinence in these patients, who often suffer from frequent and loose stools, excision of asymptomatic tags and fistulotomy is typically avoided. In patients with long-standing perianal Crohn disease or unusual-appearing fistulas, strictures, or ulcerations, malignancy may develop, and biopsies should be performed. Anovaginal fistula in Crohn disease presents a particularly challenging problem and may require early fecal diversion. An attempt at endoanal mucosal advancement flap repair may be considered when the disease is well controlled and the rectal mucosa appears to be relatively healthy and is without active inflammation. Anal strictures are typically located at the top of anorectal ring and may be dilated if symptomatic. This can be done either by gentle dilation with an examining finger, self-dilation using anal dilators in an outpatient setting, or dilation under anesthesia. Patients with severe perianal disease that does not respond to optimal medical management may ultimately require proctectomy. These patients are often treated in a staged manner, starting with fecal diversion because proctectomy in the setting of significant perianal inflammation may result in a large perineal defect requiring complex reconstruction.[74]

FUNCTIONAL BOWEL AND PELVIC FLOOR DISORDERS

Fecal Incontinence

Fecal incontinence is defined as the uncontrolled passage of feces or gas for greater than 1 month's duration in an individual over

4 years old who had previously achieved control. Fecal incontinence is most common in older female patients, with a prevalence between 9% and 20% in females over the age of 45.[75,76] Obstetric injury is the most common cause of fecal incontinence.[77] Changes in rectal sensation or rectal compliance can result in urgency, diminished capacity of the rectum, and loss of fecal control. Conditions causing inflammation of the anorectum, such as inflammatory bowel disease, can result in urgency and incontinence. Medical conditions such as diabetes, diarrhea, obesity, neurologic diseases, and urinary incontinence may result in or contribute to the symptoms of fecal incontinence.[78]

A comprehensive evaluation of fecal incontinence includes a description of bowel habits, including consistency of stools and frequency of bowel movements, type of incontinence (gas, liquid stool, solid stool, urge, passive, or postdefecation), associated urgency symptoms, awareness of incontinence versus complete lack of sensation, concomitant urinary incontinence, diet, and medications (Fig. 97.30). Patient questionnaires, including the Cleveland Clinic Fecal Incontinence Score and the Fecal Incontinence Severity Index, can help better assess the nature and severity of patient symptoms and can help quantify the response to therapy.[79,80] Patients should be asked about prior anal surgery, anal trauma or sexual instrumentation, obstetric history, prior radiation therapy, and systemic conditions such as diabetes and neurologic diseases. Colorectal cancer must be ruled out in those individuals with a recent change in bowel habits, particularly when blood per rectum is present.

The physical examination should focus on the perineum and perianal region, evaluating for normal musculature, bulk of the

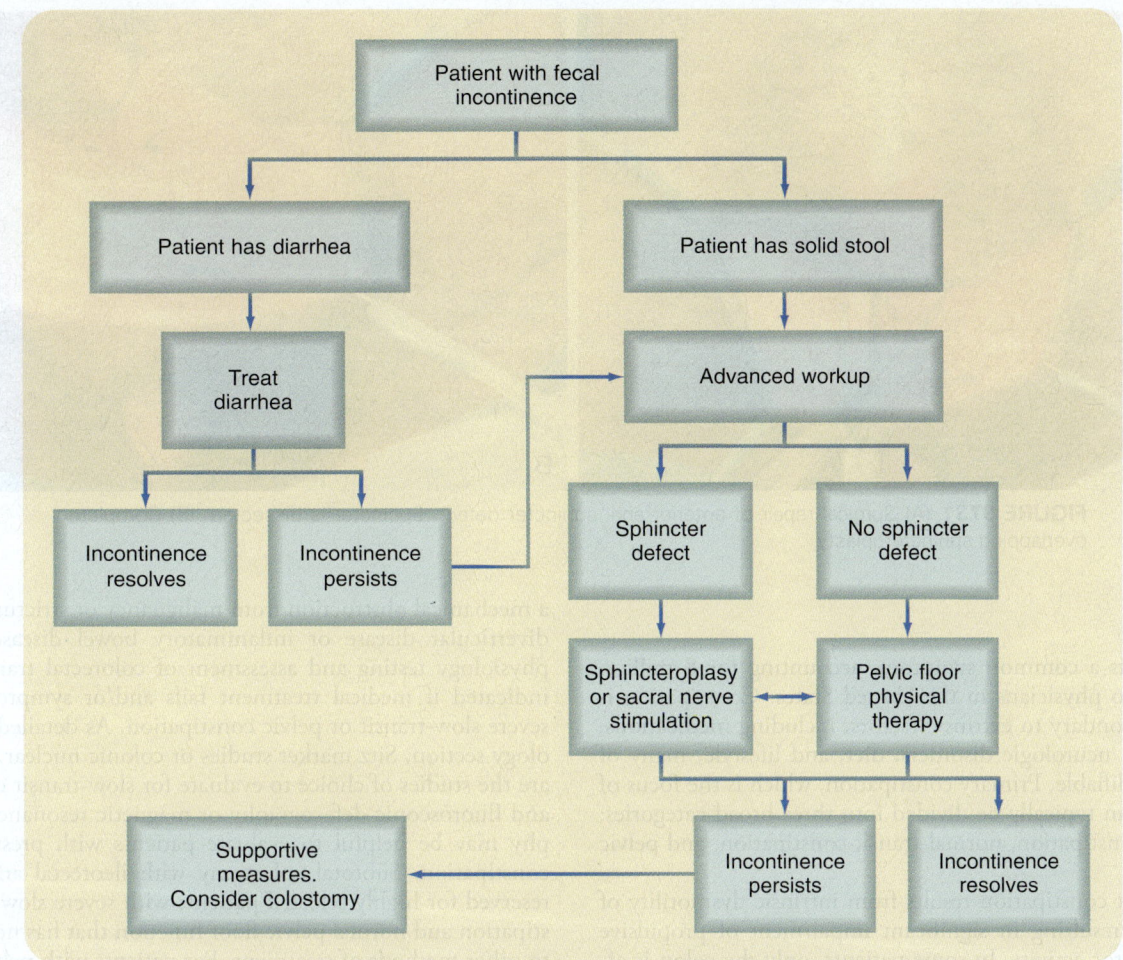

FIGURE 97.30 Evaluation and management of fecal incontinence.

perineal body, the perianal skin, and presence of any prolapsing tissue from the anus. Digital rectal examination may identify fecal impaction and the consistency of the stool and also evaluates resting tone of the anal canal and strength of the squeeze.

Pelvic floor physiologic testing, including anal manometry, anorectal sensation testing, rectal volume tolerance, and compliance testing, can be very helpful in patients when medical management has failed and in those being considered for surgical intervention. Endoanal ultrasound can also be useful to evaluate sphincter anatomy if there is a suspected sphincter injury.

Initial management is typically focused on dietary modification and fiber supplementation, which is used to bulk and firm stool consistency. Medical therapy may include antidiarrheal agents, such as loperamide, which can slow down transit time and decrease the frequency of loose stools. Biofeedback training performed by a pelvic floor physiotherapist is a noninvasive treatment option for patients who have not had sufficient improvement with diet modification and medical therapy. The goals of a comprehensive biofeedback program are to improve sensation, coordination, and strength and provide supportive counseling and practical advice regarding diet, bowel habits, behavior modification, and skin care.[81,82]

Surgical intervention is usually reserved for highly selected patients in whom conservative management has failed. Anal sphincter repair can be beneficial in patients with anal sphincter disruption secondary to traumatic childbirth or prior anal surgery

(Fig. 97.31). Although most patients report improvement in continence shortly after surgery, continence may deteriorate again over time. Sacral nerve stimulation has changed the paradigm for the treatment of fecal incontinence and is largely considered a first-line treatment in those patients who have not responded to conservative therapy; although the mechanism of action is not entirely clear, patients report fewer episodes of incontinence and decreased urgency.

Placement of sacral nerve stimulators is generally performed in two stages. The first stage involves placement of an electrode into either the right or left S3 sacral foramen via a posterior approach under fluoroscopic guidance. Adequate placement is confirmed by measuring electrical impedance and observation of robust motor response to stimulation, including dorsiflexion of the ipsilateral great toe and contraction of the perineum and anus, called the *bellows reflex*. The electrode is then connected to an external pulse generator, which is worn externally for a trial period of 7 to 14 days. If a patient experiences at least 50% improvement in fecal incontinence episodes during this trial period, the second stage exchanges the external pulse generator for an internal pulse generator, which is implanted in a subcutaneous pocket in the gluteus. Complications of sacral nerve stimulation include pain, infection, seroma formation, bleeding, and scarring. When alternative therapies are not appropriate or have failed, a colostomy may allow patients with fecal incontinence to resume normal activities and improve their quality of life.[83,84]

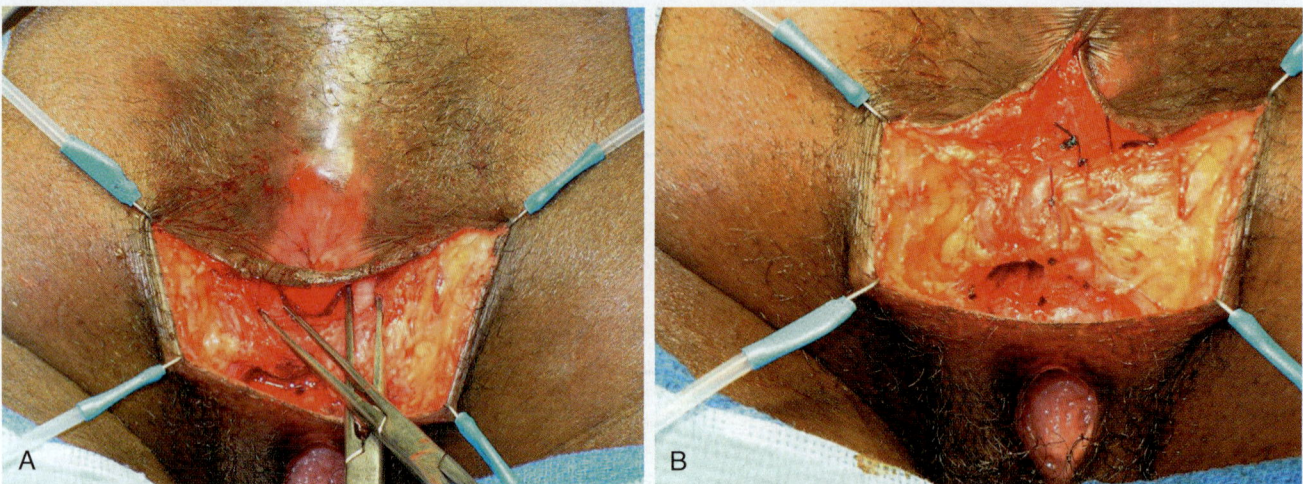

FIGURE 97.31 (A) Surgical repair of anterior anal sphincter defect. Sphincter is dissected. (B) Completed overlapping sphincteroplasty.

Constipation

Constipation is a common symptom, accounting for 8 million annual visits to physicians in the United States. Constipation is commonly secondary to extrinsic factors, including medications, endocrine and neurologic disorders, diet, and lifestyle, many of which are modifiable. Primary constipation, which is the focus of this section, can typically be divided into three broad categories: slow-transit constipation, normal-transit constipation, and pelvic constipation.

1. Slow-transit constipation results from intrinsic dysmotility of the colon, resulting in significant impairment of propulsive colonic motor activity. In some patients, only the colon is affected, whereas others have involvement of other parts of the GI tract as well. Patients with slow-transit constipation may not have bowel movements for days to weeks at a time despite using laxatives and enemas.

2. In normal-transit constipation, stool traverses the colon at a normal rate, and stool frequency may be normal, but patients feel constipated. Patients typically report that stools are hard and defecation is difficult; these patients may also report bloating, abdominal pain, and discomfort that is relieved by defecation. A significant overlap exists between this subgroup of constipation and constipation-predominant irritable bowel syndrome.

3. Pelvic constipation results from a lack of coordination of the pelvic floor during defecation or constipation from external compression or distortion of the rectum by rectocele, enterocele, and sigmoidocele. Additional causes of pelvic constipation include full-thickness rectal prolapse, rectal intussusception, and solitary rectal ulcer syndrome, all of which can disrupt the coordinated transit of stool through the rectum.

Initial management includes lifestyle modifications, including increased intake of dietary fiber, fiber supplementation, increased fluid intake, and exercise (Fig. 97.32). Use of polyethylene glycol solutions is typically safe and effective when these measures are inadequate. Stimulant laxatives such as senna and bisacodyl may be used judiciously in patients in whom lifestyle modification is inadequate. Prokinetics and secretagogues should be restricted to those not responding to simpler treatments.

For all patients with recent changes in bowel habits or those due for routine screening, colonoscopy is appropriate to rule out a mechanical obstruction from malignancy or strictures related to diverticular disease or inflammatory bowel disease. Anorectal physiology testing and assessment of colorectal transit time are indicated if medical treatment fails and/or symptoms indicate severe slow-transit or pelvic constipation. As detailed in the radiology section, Sitz marker studies or colonic nuclear scintigraphy are the studies of choice to evaluate for slow-transit constipation, and fluoroscopic defecography or magnetic resonance defecography may be helpful to evaluate patients with presumed pelvic constipation. Subtotal colectomy with ileorectal anastomosis is reserved for highly selected patients with severe slow-transit constipation and normal pelvic floor function that has not responded to other methods of treatment. For patients with pelvic constipation, rectopexy may address symptomatic rectocele and internal rectal intussusception (see description of these procedures in the next section). Ventral mesh rectopexy involves mobilization of the rectum anteriorly without division of the lateral ligaments. The pelvic floor musculature and anterior aspect of the rectum are suspended using a mesh sling sutured to the sacrum. Compared with traditional suture rectopexy, which completely circumferentially mobilizes the rectum to the pelvic floor, ventral mesh rectopexy has demonstrated lower rates of postoperative constipation, presumably as a result of preservation of rectal innervation via splanchnic nerves traveling in the lateral rectal stalks.[85]

Rectal Prolapse

Rectal prolapse is characterized by a full-thickness intussusception of the rectal wall that protrudes externally through the anus. Full-thickness rectal prolapse can be identified on physical examination by the characteristic appearance of concentric folds of rectal mucosa compared with the radial invaginations seen in prolapsing internal hemorrhoids and rectal mucosal-only prolapse (Fig. 97.33). Females are six times more likely than males to present with rectal prolapse, with a peak incidence in the seventh decade of life.[86] Symptoms of rectal prolapse may include the feeling of a bulge, mucus drainage, fecal incontinence, constipation, tenesmus, rectal pressure, pelvic pressure and pain, and rectal bleeding. Concomitant anterior compartment prolapse is also common, with 20% to 35% of patients complaining of urinary symptoms and 15% to 30% with vaginal vault or uterine prolapse.[87,88] There are several known anatomic risk factors for rectal prolapse, including laxity of rectal attachments, a

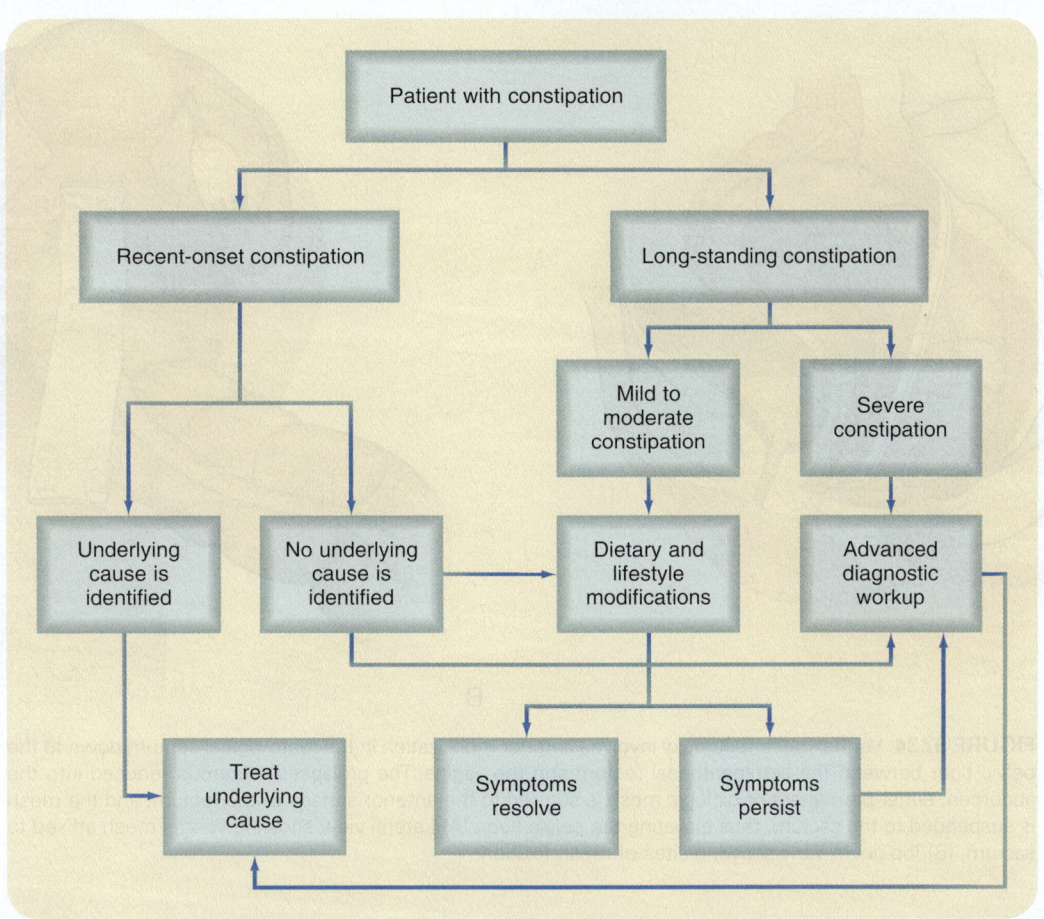

FIGURE 97.32 Evaluation and management of constipation.

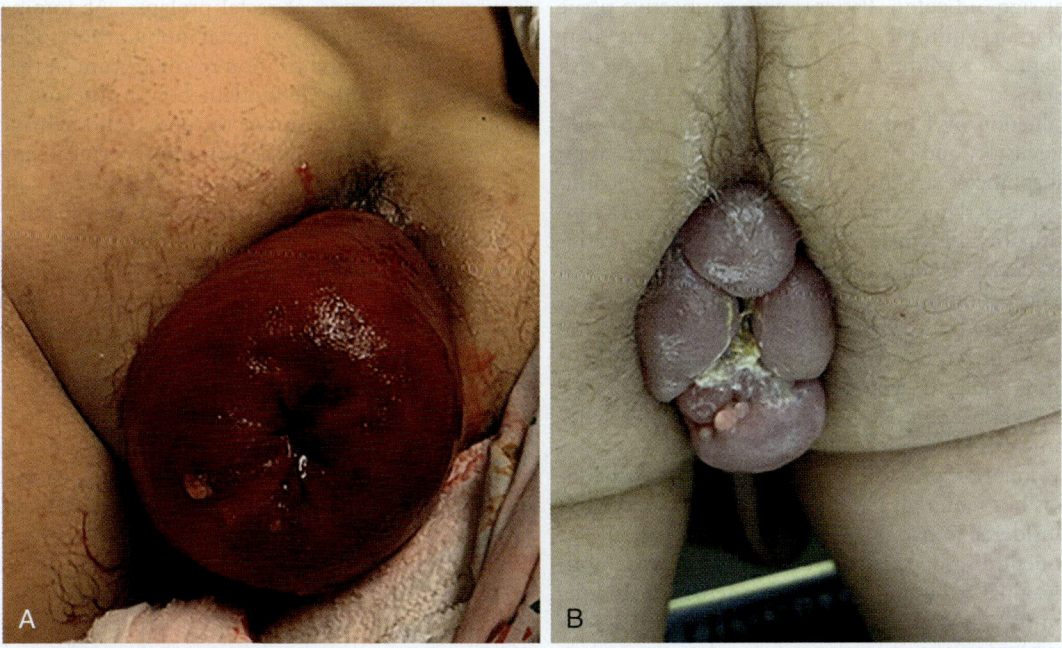

FIGURE 97.33 Rectal prolapse versus prolapsed hemorrhoids (A) Congested rectal prolapse with circumferential fold. (B) Incarcerated prolapse hemorrhoids with radial folds.

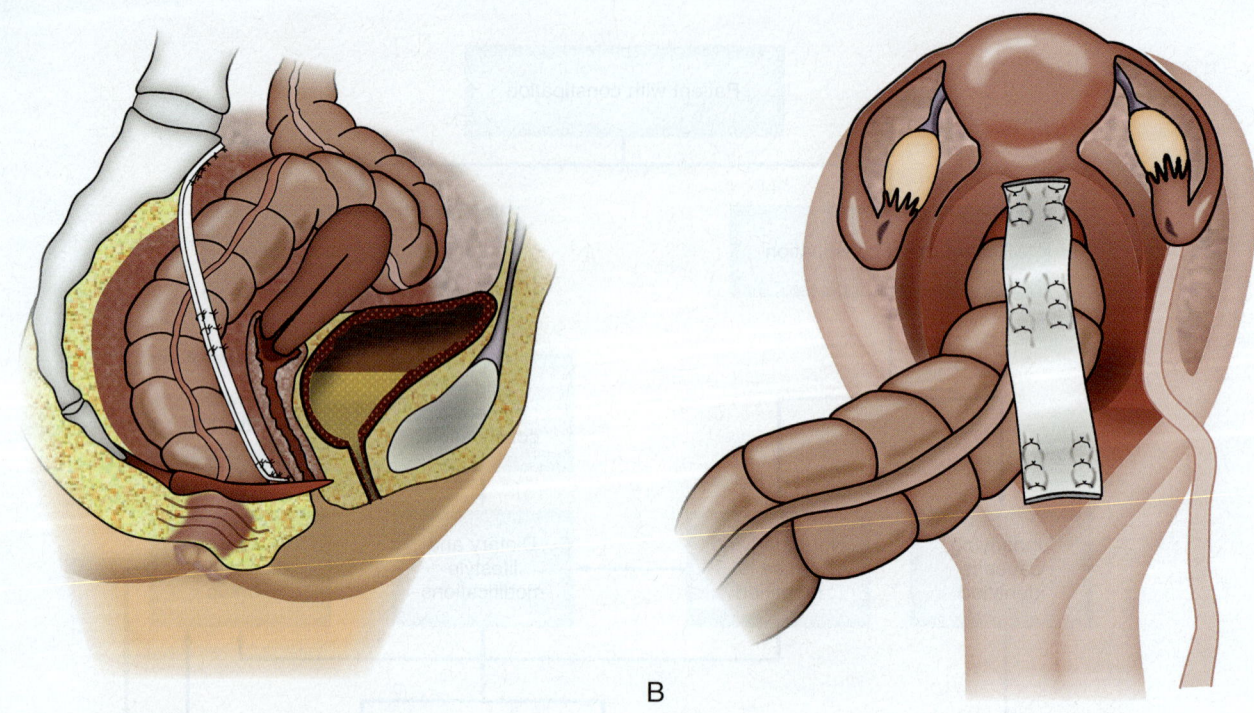

A   B

FIGURE 97.34 Ventral mesh rectopexy involves anterior mobilization in the rectovaginal septum down to the pelvic floor between the extraperitoneal rectum and the vagina. The prolapsed rectum is reduced into the abdomen; either permanent or biologic mesh is sutured to the anterior surface of the rectum; and the mesh is suspended to the sacrum, thus elevating the pelvic floor. (A) Lateral view showing ventral mesh affixed to sacrum. (B) Top-down view showing sites of mesh fixation.

deep cul-de-sac, lack of fixation of the rectum to the sacrum, and a large redundant sigmoid colon. Patients with connective tissue disorders (e.g., Marfan syndrome, Ehlers-Danlos syndrome) may present with prolapse at a younger age and may be at higher risk for recurrent prolapse.

The initial evaluation of a patient with rectal prolapse should include a complete history and physical examination, with focus on the prolapse; anal sphincter structure and function; and concomitant symptoms and underlying conditions, including chronic constipation and multiparity. In female patients, symptoms of anterior compartment disorders, including vaginal or uterine prolapse and urinary incontinence, should also be elicited. If the diagnosis of rectal prolapse is suspected but no prolapse is detected on physical examination, the patient can be asked to reproduce the prolapse in the office by straining while on a commode, with or without the use of an enema or a rectal balloon. Rectal examination frequently reveals a patulous anus with decreased sphincter tone.

If prolapse is evident on physical examination, additional confirmatory testing is not required. Fluoroscopic or MRI defecography should be considered in patients with symptoms suggestive of anterior compartment disorders because these studies can demonstrate cystocele, vaginal vault prolapse, and enterocele. Patients with anterior compartment disorders may benefit from urodynamics and urogynecologic examination to complete the evaluation and allow for concomitant surgical intervention to address both the anterior and posterior pelvic compartments. Rarely, a rectal mass may form the lead point to a rectal prolapse, so colonoscopy should be performed before surgery.

Both transabdominal and perineal approaches exist for the surgical correction of rectal prolapse. Abdominal approaches involve varying degrees of rectal mobilization followed by reduction of the prolapse and fixation of the rectum in the pelvis to prevent telescoping of the redundant bowel. The most common operations are posterior suture rectopexy and ventral mesh rectopexy (Fig. 97.34). The most common perineal approaches are the perineal proctosigmoidectomy (Altemeier) and the Delorme procedures (Figs. 97.35 and 97.36). In general, for patients with acceptable surgical risk (able to tolerate general anesthesia and pneumoperitoneum), transabdominal rectal fixation is preferred because of the lower recurrence rates (<10% at 10 years with transabdominal rectal fixation vs. 16%–30% perineal prolapse repair).[89–91]

Occasionally, patients present emergently with incarcerated rectal prolapse. Incarceration typically results from obstruction of venous return from the prolapsed rectum, leading to a bulky edematous rectum that cannot be reduced back into the anal canal. Mucosal ischemia and ulcerations may occur and may progress to full-thickness necrosis of the rectum. Initial conservative methods should be aimed at reducing the edema by the liberal application of sugar as an osmotic agent and relaxation, sedation, perianal nerve block, or general anesthesia to allow for attempts at manual reduction of the prolapse. If the rectal prolapse cannot be reduced or if there is rectal necrosis that should not be reduced, the patient needs to be taken to the operating room without delay for a perineal rectosigmoidectomy (Altemeier procedure) (Fig. 97.37).

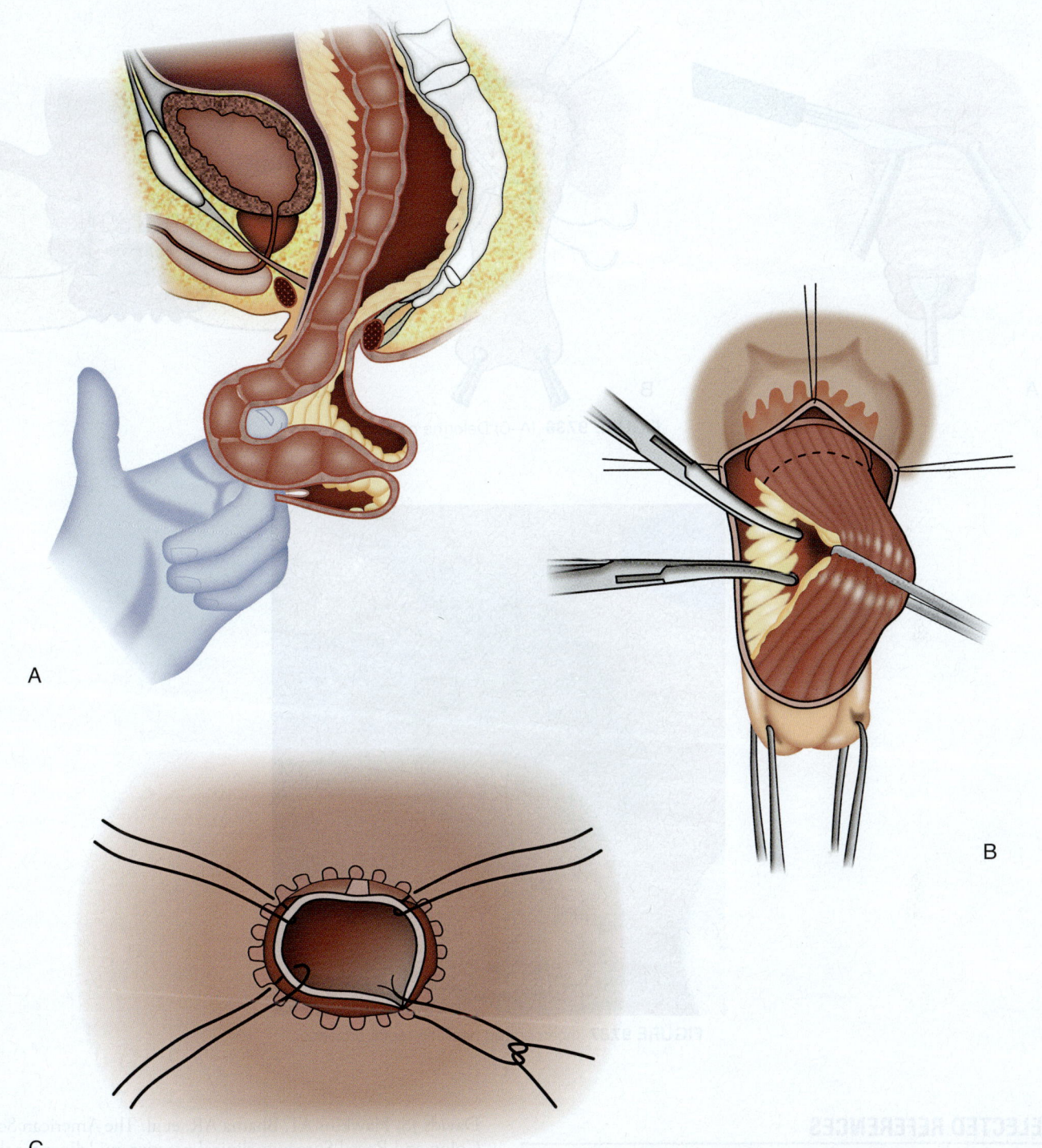

FIGURE 97.35 The perineal proctosigmoidectomy, or Altemeier procedure, involves the full-thickness excision of the prolapsed bowel with a coloanal anastomosis. (A) Sigmoid mesentery in prolapse. (B) Division of sigmoid mesentery adjacent to bowel wall. (C) Completed coloanal anastomosis after transection of redundant rectum and sigmoid.

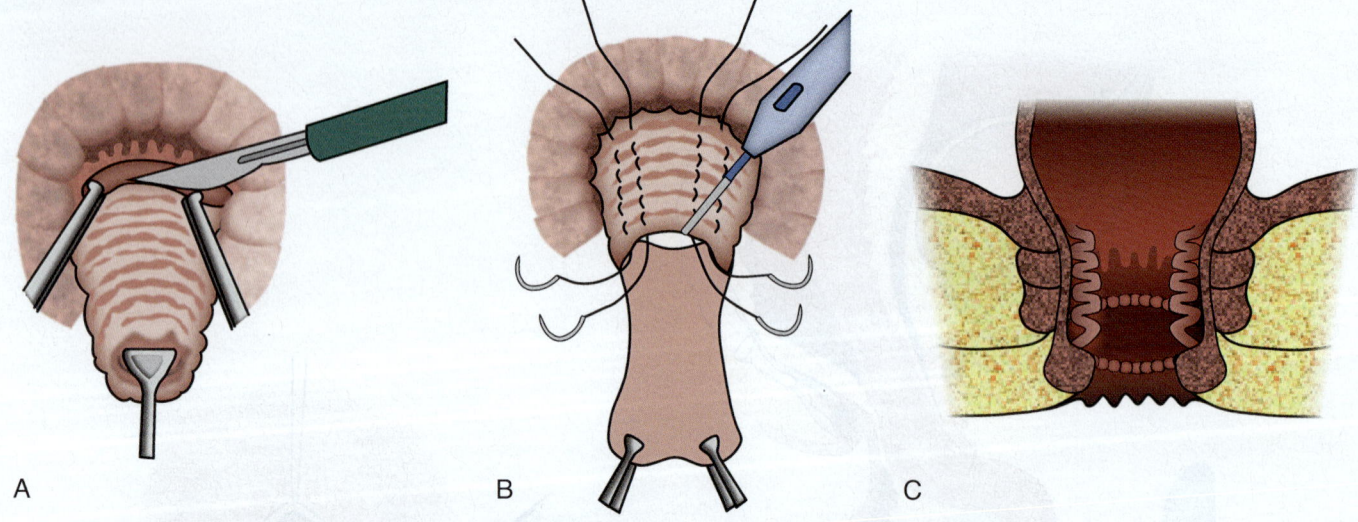

A B C

FIGURE 97.36 (A–C) Delorme procedure.

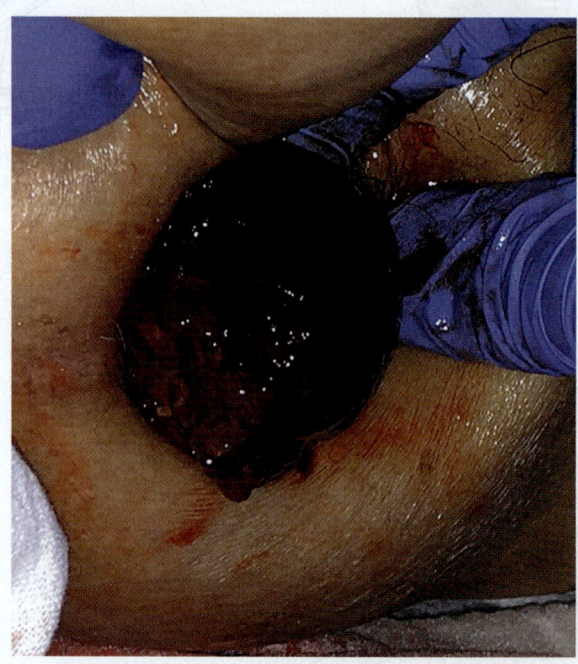

FIGURE 97.37 Incarcerated necrotic rectal prolapse.

SELECTED REFERENCES

Bordeianou LG, Thorsen AJ, Keller DS. The American Society of Colon and Rectal Surgeons clinical practice guidelines for the management of fecal incontinence. *Dis Colon Rectum.* 2023;66(5):647-661.

This is the most recently published clinical practice guideline from the American Society of Colon and Rectal Surgeons (ASCRS) on the management of fecal incontinence. It contains the most up-to-date, evidence-based guidelines for management and is freely accessed from the Diseases of the Colon & Rectum *journal website.*

Davids JS, Hawkins AT, Bhama AR, et al. The American Society of Colon and Rectal Surgeons clinical practice guidelines for the management of anal fissures. *Dis Colon Rectum.* 2023;66(2):190-199.

This is the most recently published clinical practice guideline from the ASCRS on the management of anal fissure. It contains the most up-to-date, evidence-based guidelines for management and is freely accessed from the Diseases of the Colon & Rectum *journal website.*

Gaertner WB, Burgess PL, Davids JS, et al. The American Society of Colon and Rectal Surgeons clinical practice guidelines for the management of anorectal abscess, fistula-in-ano, and rectovaginal fistula. *Dis Colon Rectum.* 2022;65(8):964-985.

This is the most recently published clinical practice guideline from the ASCRS on the management of cryptoglandular anorectal disease and RVFs. It contains the most up-to-date, evidence-based guidelines for management and is freely accessed from the Diseases of the Colon & Rectum *journal* website.

Hawkins AT, Davis BR, Bhama AR, et al. The American Society of Colon and Rectal Surgeons clinical practice guidelines for the management of hemorrhoids. *Dis Colon Rectum.* 2024;67(5): 614-623.

This is the most recently published clinical practice guideline from the ASCRS on the management of hemorrhoidal disease. It contains the most up-to-date, evidence-based

guidelines for management and is freely accessed from the Diseases of the Colon & Rectum *journal* website.

Johnson EK, Vogel JD, Cowan ML, et al. The American Society of Colon and Rectal Surgeons' clinical practice guidelines for the management of pilonidal disease. *Dis Colon Rectum.* 2019;62(2): 146-157.

This is the most recently published clinical practice guideline from the ASCRS on the management of pilonidal disease. It contains the most up-to-date, evidence-based guidelines for management and is freely accessed from the Diseases of the Colon & Rectum *journal* website.

The full reference list appears on Elsevier eBooks+.

98 CHAPTER

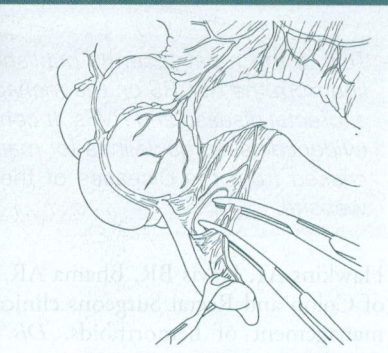

Acute Gastrointestinal Hemorrhage

Dimitrios Moris, Jacob Greenberg, and Theodore N. Pappas

OUTLINE

INTRODUCTION

Gastrointestinal (GI) diseases account for considerable healthcare use and expenditures. GI bleeding (GIB) is one of the most common GI diagnoses, requiring hospital admission in the United States, with more than 500,000 cases annually.[1] Upper GI bleeding (UGIB) refers to bleeding originating from sites in the esophagus, stomach, or duodenum (GI tract proximal to ligament of Treitz). Nearly 80% of patients visiting emergency departments for UGIB are admitted to the hospital with that principal diagnosis.[1] Lower GI bleeding (LGIB) refers to blood loss of recent onset distal to the ligament of Treitz, most commonly originating from the colon.[2] UGIB, with an incidence of 67 per 100,000 population, is more common than LGIB, which carries an incidence of 36 per 100,000 population.[3] LGIB is more common in males than females because vascular diseases and diverticulosis are more common in males.[2] Although the incidence of GIB increases with age, the overall incidence of GIB is decreasing in the United States annually.

Symptoms and Initial Evaluation of Gastrointestinal Bleeding

Causes of UGIB are as follows:
- Peptic ulcer disease (excess gastric acid, *Helicobacter pylori* infection, NSAID overuse, or physiologic stress)
- Esophagitis
- Gastritis and duodenitis
- Varices
- Portal hypertensive gastropathy
- Angiodysplasia
- Dieulafoy lesion (bleeding dilated vessel that erodes through the GI epithelium but has no primary ulceration)
- Gastric antral valvular ectasia (known as *watermelon stomach*)
- Mallory-Weiss tears
- Cameron lesions (bleeding ulcers occurring at the site of a hiatal hernia)
- Aortoenteric fistulas
- Foreign-body ingestion
- Postsurgical bleeds (postanastomotic bleeding, postpolypectomy bleeding, postsphincterotomy bleeding)

- Upper GI tumors
- Hemobilia (bleeding from the biliary tract)
- Hemosuccus pancreaticus (bleeding from the pancreatic duct)

Patients with acute UGIB commonly present with hematemesis (vomiting of blood or coffee-ground–like material) and/or melena (black, tarry stools). The initial evaluation of a patient with a suspected clinically significant acute UGIB includes a detailed pertinent history and physical examination, including vitals, as well as laboratory tests. The main goal of this initial assessment is to evaluate the severity of bleeding and potentially guide subsequent management (both medical and interventional), such as triage, hemodynamic stability, appropriate resuscitation, empiric medical therapy, and diagnostic testing.

A thorough history and physical examination are of critical importance because they can provide clinically important information in the setting of suspected UGIB that can help guide the appropriate diagnostic approach and management. Symptoms such as patient-reported melena (likelihood ratio [LR] 5.1–5.9), melenic stool on examination (LR 25), blood detected during nasogastric lavage (LR 9.6), and prerenal acute kidney injury (ratio of blood urea nitrogen to serum creatinine greater than 30, LR 7.5) are commonly encountered. Conversely, the presence of blood clots in the stool makes an upper GI source less likely (LR 0.05).

Hematemesis (either red blood or coffee-ground emesis) suggests bleeding proximal to the ligament of Treitz. The presence of frankly bloody emesis suggests moderate to severe bleeding that may be ongoing, whereas coffee-ground emesis suggests more limited bleeding that may have already stopped. Similarly, the presence of melena indicates bleeding originating proximal to the ligament of Treitz (90%), although it may also originate from the oropharynx or nasopharynx, small bowel, or colon.[4] Melena may be seen with variable degrees of blood loss, being seen with as little as 50 mL of blood.[5] Finally, hematochezia (red or maroon blood in the stool) is usually due to LGIB. However, it can occur with massive UGIB,[6] which is typically associated with orthostatic hypotension.

A thorough assessment of the patient's past medical history can also provide important information to help determine potential causes of bleeding. Patients should be asked about prior episodes of UGIB because up to 60% of patients with a history of UGIB are bleeding from the same lesion.[7] In addition, the patient's past medical history should be reviewed to identify important comorbid conditions that may lead to UGIB or may influence the patient's subsequent management, such as gastritis or peptic ulcer disease (*H. pylori*, NSAIDs, smoking, steroids), portal hypertension (varices), prior aortic aneurysm repair (aortoenteric fistula), angiodysplasia (in the setting of renal failure, aortic stenosis a patient with renal disease and aortic stenosis), malignancy (weight loss, obstruction, perforation in the setting of smoking or excess alcohol use), and marginal ulcers (in the setting of known bariatric surgery or prior gastroenteric anastomosis).[8] Finally, medications such as antiplatelets (e.g., P2Y12 inhibitors and aspirin), anticoagulants (including warfarin and direct oral anticoagulants), selective serotonin reuptake inhibitors (SSRIs), calcium channel blockers, and aldosterone antagonists can increase the bleeding diathesis and risk. Moreover, medications such as iron, licorice, charcoal, and bismuth can turn stool black and might alter the clinical presentation.

The presence of accompanying symptoms can facilitate the evaluation of the severity of bleeding. For example, orthostatic lightheadedness, altered mental status (confusion), and clammy extremities can indicate hemodynamically significant and potentially life-threatening bleeding. Abdominal pain, with rebound or guarding, might indicate perforation of hollow viscus in the setting of peptic ulcer disease. Dysphagia or odynophagia can indicate esophageal disease as the source of bleeding, whereas the presence of emesis or retching before hematemesis can be seen in Mallory-Weiss tears. A history of ascites, jaundice, and clinical findings of liver failure can be found in cases of hemorrhage due to esophageal varices and portal hypertensive gastropathy. A history of cachexia, weight loss, early satiety, or obstructive symptoms can be seen in the setting of malignancy.[9]

Physical examination is a key component of the assessment of hemodynamic stability and the estimated blood loss. Patients with less than 15% of blood volume lost (up to 750 mL) might have normal vitals. In patients with blood volume loss of 15% to 30% (750–1500 mL), pulse pressure will be widened, urine output will be decreased (<30 mL/h), and patients will very likely be tachycardic (heart rate >100 beats/minute). When the estimated blood loss is 30% to 40% of the total blood volume (1500–2000 mL), patients are generally hypotensive, tachycardic to 120 beats/minute, and confused, with low urine output (<20 mL/h). Finally, when more than 40% of the total blood volume is lost (>2000 mL), patients are hypotensive, tachycardic to 140 beats/minute, tachypneic, and lethargic, with negligible urine output.[10]

Laboratory tests that should be obtained in patients with acute UGIB include a complete blood count, serum chemistries, type and screen, liver tests, and coagulation studies. In addition, electrocardiogram and cardiac enzymes may be indicated in patients who are at risk for a cardiac event. The initial hemoglobin level in a patient with acute UGIB may be similar to the patient's baseline because the patient is losing whole blood and will take time to equilibrate. With time, the hemoglobin level will decline as the blood is diluted by the influx of extravascular fluid into the vascular space and by fluid administered during resuscitation. The hemoglobin level should initially be monitored every 2 to 8 hours, depending on the severity of the bleed. On the contrary, active hemorrhage will not change the mean corpuscular volume (MCV). If the MCV is low, it may suggest iron deficiency, which could be caused by chronic bleeding. Because blood is absorbed as it passes through the small bowel and patients may have

decreased renal perfusion, patients with acute UGIB typically have an elevated blood urea nitrogen (BUN)-to-creatinine or urea-to-creatinine ratio. Values of this ratio >30:1 or >100:1, respectively, suggest UGIB as the cause,[11,12] and the higher the ratio, the more likely the bleeding is from an upper GI source.[11]

Causes of LGIB are as follows:
- Diverticulosis
- Angiodysplasia
- Infectious colitis
- Ischemic colitis
- Inflammatory bowel disease
- Colon cancer
- Hemorrhoids
- Anal fissures
- Rectal varices
- Radiation-induced damage after treatment of abdominal or pelvic cancers
- Postsurgical (postpolypectomy bleeding, postbiopsy bleeding)

Patients with acute LGIB typically present with hematochezia (passage of maroon or bright-red blood or blood clots per rectum), although hematochezia may also be seen in patients with massive upper GI or small bowel bleeding. Although bleeding originating in the colon tends to present with the passage of bright-red blood per rectum, rarely, patients with right-sided colonic bleeding will present with melena. LGIB will stop spontaneously in 80% to 85% of patients, and the mortality rate is 2% to 4%.[13] The causes of acute LGIB may be grouped into several categories: anatomic (diverticulosis), vascular (angiodysplasia, ischemic, radiation induced), inflammatory (infectious, inflammatory bowel disease), and neoplastic. In addition, acute LGIB can occur after therapeutic interventions such as polypectomy. In patients suspected of having acute LGIB, the initial management is similar to the one in UGIB (obtaining adequate intravenous [IV] access, triaging the patient to the appropriate level of care, and providing supportive measures such as supplemental oxygen and resuscitation). Also, exclusion of acute UGIB is also required (e.g., in a patient with massive hematochezia and signs of hemodynamic compromise) because an upper GI source can be the cause of hematochezia in 10% to 15% of cases.[14] Past medical history, including prior episodes of LGIB, medications, and concomitant symptoms that may suggest the underlying etiology of the LGIB (e.g., painless hematochezia with diverticular bleeding, change in bowel habits with malignancy, abdominal pain with colitis), should be evaluated.

DIAGNOSIS AND MANAGEMENT OF GASTROINTESTINAL BLEEDING

Nonsurgical Management of Upper Gastrointestinal Bleeding

Although the principles behind the management of all patients with UGIB are similar, there are some special considerations when it comes to patients presenting with hemodynamic instability (shock, orthostatic hypotension). Of paramount importance is the establishment of adequate peripheral access, which should be attained with either two 18-gauge or larger IV catheters and/or a large-bore, single-lumen central cordis. Elective endotracheal intubation in patients with ongoing hematemesis or altered respiratory or mental status may facilitate endoscopy and decrease the risk of aspiration. However, among patients who are critically ill, elective endotracheal intubation has been associated with worse outcomes.[15] All patients with hemodynamic instability or active bleeding (manifested by hematemesis, bright-red blood per nasogastric tube [NGT], or hematochezia) should be admitted to an intensive care unit for resuscitation and close observation. Fluid resuscitation should begin immediately and should not be delayed pending transfer of the patient to an intensive care unit. For patients with active/brisk bleeding and hypovolemia, transfusion should be guided by hemodynamic parameters, the pace of the bleeding, estimated blood loss, and the ability to stop the bleeding, rather than by serial hemoglobin measurements. If the initial hemoglobin level is low (<7 g/dL), transfusions should be initiated.[16,17] In a patient with acute and ongoing hemorrhage, however, transfusion support should not be delayed while awaiting laboratory test results and should begin at the time of evaluation. Patients without active bleeding who become hemodynamically stable with fluid resuscitation alone may be managed without an initial transfusion but should be watched closely because the need for transfusion may develop as they clinically equilibrate. For most stable patients, a restrictive transfusion strategy is appropriate (transfuse if hemoglobin is <7 g/dL rather than at a higher hemoglobin) because it has been shown to be related to lower all-cause mortality and rebleeding rates compared with a liberal transfusion strategy.[18,19] Another crucial component of the management of UGIB is acid suppression, such as proton pump inhibitors (PPIs). Options include giving IV PPIs every 12 hours or starting a continuous infusion. For patients who may have stopped bleeding (e.g., patients who are hemodynamically stable), IV PPIs every 12 hours are preferred. In the setting of active UGIB from an ulcer, acid-suppressive therapy with H_2 receptor antagonists has not been shown to significantly lower the rate of ulcer rebleeding.[20-22] On the contrary, high-dose antisecretory therapy with an IV infusion of PPIs significantly reduces the rate of rebleeding compared with standard treatment in patients with bleeding ulcers.[23] Oral and IV PPI therapy also decreases the length of hospital stay, rebleeding rate, and need for blood transfusion in patients with high-risk ulcers treated with endoscopic therapy. PPIs may also promote hemostasis in patients with lesions other than ulcers. This likely occurs because neutralization of gastric acid leads to the stabilization of blood clots.[24]

Prokinetics, such as erythromycin and metoclopramide, have been studied in patients with acute UGIB. The goal of using a prokinetic agent is to improve gastric visualization at the time of endoscopy by clearing the stomach of blood, clots, and food residue. A reasonable dose is 250 mg intravenously over 20 to 30 minutes. Endoscopy is performed 20 to 90 minutes after completion of the erythromycin infusion. Patients receiving erythromycin need to be monitored for QTc prolongation. In addition, drug-drug interactions should be evaluated before giving erythromycin because it is a cytochrome P4503A inhibitor. Erythromycin promotes gastric emptying based on its ability to be an agonist of motilin receptors. The use of erythromycin was found to improve gastric visualization (77% vs. 51%, odds ratio [OR] 4.14, 95% CI 2.01–8.53), was less likely to require second-look endoscopy (15% vs. 26%, OR 0.51, 95% CI 0.34–0.77), and resulted in shorter hospital stays (mean difference –1.75 days, 95% CI –2.43 to –1.06). There were no differences in units of blood transfused, endoscopy duration, or need for emergent surgery between those who received erythromycin and those who did not.[25,26]

Vasoactive medications, such as somatostatin (analog octreotide) and terlipressin, are used in the treatment of variceal bleeding and may also reduce the risk of bleeding resulting from nonvariceal causes. In patients with suspected variceal bleeding, octreotide is given as an IV bolus of 50 μg, followed by a continuous infusion at a rate of 50 μg/h. Octreotide is not recommended for routine use in patients with acute nonvariceal UGIB, but it can be used as adjunctive therapy in some cases. Its role is generally limited to settings in which endoscopy is unavailable or to help stabilize patients before definitive therapy can be performed.[27] In patients with cirrhosis, a special consideration is the use of prophylactic antibiotics because bacterial infections are present in up to 20% of patients with cirrhosis who are hospitalized with GIB. Even for those cirrhotic patients who do not present initially with an infectious source, up to an additional 50% develop an infection while hospitalized. Not surprisingly, these patients have an increased rate of mortality. Multiple trials evaluating the effectiveness of prophylactic antibiotics in cirrhotic patients hospitalized for GIB suggest an overall reduction in infectious complications and possibly decreased mortality.[28] Antibiotics may also reduce the risk of recurrent bleeding in hospitalized patients who bled from esophageal varices.[29,30]

As a general rule, the management of UGIB should be primarily medical (gastroenterology) and should begin with an upper endoscopy. Surgical and interventional radiology consultation should be considered if endoscopic therapy is found to be unsuccessful; if the patient is deemed to be at high risk for rebleeding or there are complications associated with endoscopy; if there is concern that the patient may have a complicated intraabdominal process, such an aorto-enteric fistula; and in all patients with severe UGIB, such as those presenting with hemodynamic instability that fails to respond to resuscitation.[31] The role of routine use of NGT placement in patients with suspected acute UGIB is not recommended because studies have failed to demonstrate a benefit regarding clinical outcomes.[32-34] Early NGT placement is associated with shorter time to endoscopy but offers no benefit in terms of mortality, length of hospital stay, surgery, or transfusion requirement. It might be considered in cases of unclear diagnosis or unclear acuity of bleeding where patients might benefit from an early endoscopy. In addition, NGT lavage can be used to remove particulate matter, fresh blood, and clots from the stomach to facilitate endoscopy. An alternative to NGT lavage in this situation is to use prokinetics such as erythromycin or metoclopramide. The presence of red blood or coffee-ground material in the nasogastric aspirate also confirms an upper GI source of bleeding and predicts whether the bleeding is caused by a lesion at increased risk for ongoing or recurrent bleeding.[35] However, lavage may not be positive if bleeding has ceased or arises beyond a closed pylorus. Nasogastric aspiration of nonbloody bilious fluid suggests that the pylorus is open and that there is no active UGIB distal to the pylorus (Table 98.1).

Upper endoscopy is the diagnostic modality of choice for acute UGIB,[36] and early endoscopy (within 24 hours) is recommended for most patients with acute UGIB. Endoscopy has a high sensitivity and specificity for locating and identifying bleeding lesions in the upper GI tract. In addition, once a bleeding lesion has been identified, therapeutic endoscopy can achieve acute hemostasis and prevent recurrent bleeding in most patients. For patients with suspected variceal bleeding, endoscopy should be performed within 12 hours of presentation. Endoscopic findings in patients with bleeding peptic ulcers are described using the modified Forrest classification.[37] Findings include spurting hemorrhage (class Ia), oozing hemorrhage (class Ib), a nonbleeding visible vessel (class IIa), an adherent clot (class IIb), a flat pigmented spot (class IIc), and a clean ulcer base (class III). The endoscopic

---

TABLE 98.1   Overview of Upper Gastrointestinal Bleeding

Causes

Peptic ulcer, esophagogastric varices, arteriovenous malformation, tumor, Mallory-Weiss tear

Clinical Features

History: Medications (NSAIDs, aspirin, anticoagulants/antiplatelets), previous GI bleed, liver failure, coagulopathy
Symptoms and signs: Abdominal pain, hematemesis or coffee-ground emesis, passing melena/tarry stool
Examination: Tachycardia, orthostatic blood pressure, hypotension, rectal exam, abdominal tenderness, peritonitis

Diagnostic Testing

Type and screen, CBC, coagulation screen, LFTs, BUN, Cr
Nasogastric lavage may be helpful if the source of bleeding is unclear (upper or lower GI tract) or to clean the stomach before endoscopy.

Treatment

Continuous monitoring, resuscitation, oxygen, transfusion

• For severe, ongoing bleeding, immediately transfuse blood products in 1:1:1 ratio of RBCs, plasma, and platelets, as for trauma patients.
• For hemodynamic instability despite crystalloid resuscitation, transfuse 1 to 2 units RBCs.
• For hemoglobin <8 g/dL (80 g/L) in high-risk patients (e.g., older adult, coronary artery disease), transfuse 1 unit RBCs and reassess the patient's clinical condition.
• For hemoglobin <7 g/dL (70 g/L) in low-risk patients, transfuse 1 unit RBCs and reassess the patient's clinical condition.

Consult with gastroenterologist; obtain surgical and interventional radiology consultation for any large-scale bleeding.

Give a proton pump inhibitor:

   If evidence of active bleeding (e.g., hematemesis, hemodynamic instability), give esomeprazole or pantoprazole, 80 mg IV.
   If no evidence of active bleeding, give esomeprazole or pantoprazole, 40 mg IV.
   If endoscopy is delayed beyond 12 hours, give second dose of esomeprazole or pantoprazole, 40 mg IV.

Known or suspected esophagogastric variceal bleeding and/or cirrhosis: Somatostatin or an analog (e.g., octreotide 50 μg IV bolus followed by 50 μg/h continuous IV infusion)

   Give an IV antibiotic (e.g., ceftriaxone or fluoroquinolone).

   Balloon tamponade may be performed as a temporizing measure for patients with uncontrollable hemorrhage likely due to varices using any of several devices (e.g., Sengstaken-Blakemore tube, Minnesota tube); tracheal intubation is necessary if such a device is to be placed; ensure proper device placement before inflation to avoid esophageal rupture.

BUN, Blood urea nitrogen; *CBC,* complete blood count; *Cr,* creatinine; *GI,* gastrointestinal; *IV,* intravenous; *LFT,* liver function test; *RBC,* red blood cell.

TABLE 98.2   Endoscopic Predictors of Recurrent Peptic Ulcer Hemorrhage

FORREST CLASSIFICATION	PREVALENCE (%)	RISK OF REBLEEDING ON MEDICAL MANAGEMENT (%)
Forrest Ia (active arterial bleeding)	12% (arterial bleeding + oozing)	55 (arterial bleeding + oozing)
Forrest Ib (oozing without visible vessel)		
Forrest IIa (nonbleeding visible vessel)	8	43
Forrest IIb (adherent clot)	8	22
Forrest IIc (flat spot)	16	10
Forrest III (clean ulcer base)	55	5

---

appearance helps determine which lesions may require further management beyond endoscopic therapy (Table 98.2). In patients in whom blood obscures the source of bleeding, a second endoscopy may be required to establish a diagnosis and to potentially apply therapy, but routine second-look endoscopy is not recommended.

Other diagnostic tests for acute UGIB include CT angiography (CTA; using an occult GIB protocol) and angiography, which can detect active bleeding[38,39]; deep small bowel enteroscopy; and rarely, intraoperative enteroscopy. Upper GI barium studies are contraindicated in the setting of acute UGIB because they will interfere with subsequent endoscopy, angiography, or surgery.[40] There is also interest in using wireless capsule endoscopy for patients who have presented to the emergency department with suspected UGIB. An esophageal capsule (which has a recording time of 20 minutes) can be given in the emergency department and

reviewed immediately for evidence of bleeding. Confirming the presence of blood in the stomach or duodenum may aid with patient triage and identify patients more likely to benefit from early endoscopy.[41,42] Small bowel capsule endoscopy has also been employed to help localize bleeding in patients with acute GIB without hematemesis. A colonoscopy is generally required for patients with hematochezia and a negative upper endoscopy unless an alternative source for the bleeding has been identified. In addition, patients with melena and a negative upper endoscopy frequently undergo colonoscopy to rule out a colonic source for the bleeding because right-sided lesions may present with melena (Fig. 98.1).

Surgical Management of Upper Gastrointestinal Bleeding

The surgical management of UGIB will depend entirely on the source of the UGIB and the failure of nonsurgical options to

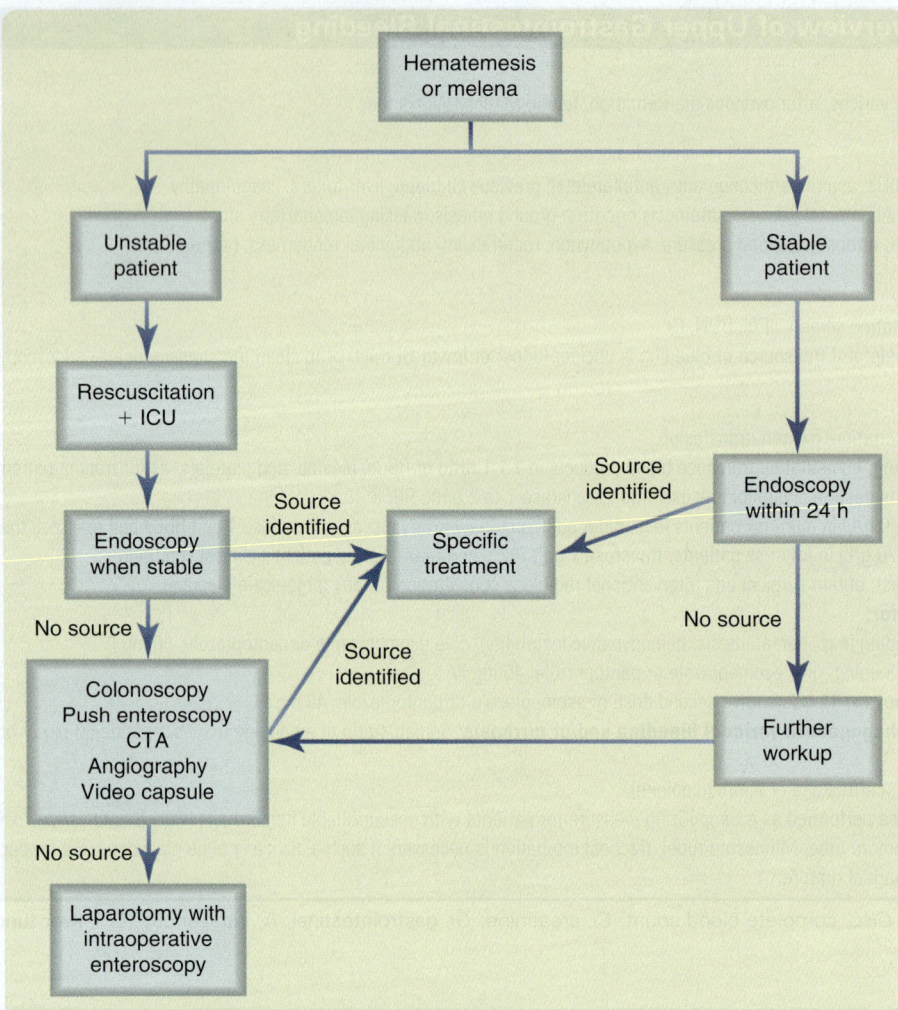

FIGURE 98.1 Algorithm for diagnosis and management of upper gastrointestinal bleed. *CTA*, Computed tomography angiography; *ICU*, intensive care unit.

control bleeding. In the case of malignancies, the management has dual intent, both controlling the bleeding and performing an appropriate oncologic procedure.

For Mallory-Weiss tears, surgery is rarely necessary and is considered only after the failure of endoscopic or angiographic procedures. Laparoscopic or open oversewing of the tear under endoscopic guidance has been performed with excellent results.[43]

In patients with esophageal varices who had failed medical/endoscopic management (unsuccessful 10%–20% of cases), the next step should be rescue therapy in the form of emergent transjugular intrahepatic portosystemic shunt (TIPS) or surgical portocaval shunt creation.[44] TIPS is typically preferred over surgery because operative mortality may be high in cirrhotic patients, although acute emergent variceal hemorrhage may be associated with significant mortality irrespective of treatment modality.[45] Surgical management of esophageal varices includes shunting and nonshunting operations. Nonshunting operations include esophagogastric devascularization, esophageal transection, and splenectomy. The idea of transthoracic ligation of esophageal varices was first proposed by Crile (1950), with many modifications of the procedure after its initial conception. In 1973, Sugiura and Futagawa formulated the Sugiura procedure, which included extensive transthoracic paraesophageal devascularization, esophageal

transection combined with an abdominal component consisting of splenectomy, devascularization of the upper stomach, vagotomy, and pyloroplasty.[46] Devascularization procedures are rarely the treatment of choice in the emergency setting; the operative mortality has been as high as 100% in Child C patients in some series. Nevertheless, when nonsurgical procedures fail, devascularization procedures can salvage critical situations of variceal bleeding. Also, in the elective setting, when the vascular anatomy is unsuitable for shunt procedures because of extensive portal, splenic, and superior mesenteric vein thrombosis and when other modalities have failed, devascularization procedures should be considered.[47] These procedures are related to a perioperative mortality of 12.7%. Long-term survival rates are dependent on the Child-Pugh classification at the time of the procedure. The survival rate was 44% in Child A patients, 22.5% in Child B patients, and 0% in Child C patients. In other series, the 5-year overall survival rate ranged from 58% to 93%.[48,49]

Shunting operations include total or portosystemic shunts, and they can be classified as nonselective or selective.[50] Total shunts may be an end-to-side shunt where the portal vein is divided at its bifurcation and the proximal end anastomosed to the inferior vena cava or a side-to-side anastomosis between the portal vein or a tributary greater than 10 mm in diameter and the inferior vena cava. All diverted-portal-flow and side-to-side shunts also decompress the liver sinusoids. Bleeding control is excellent, but portal flow is diverted, which may cause hepatocellular dysfunction. Partial portal systemic shunt is achieved with a portacaval anastomosis. This reduces portal pressure to 12 mm Hg while maintaining forward portal flow in 83% of patients.[51] The operative exposure is similar to that of total portal systemic shunts.

The selective shunts are further classified as follows:

- Distal splenorenal shunt (distal splenic vein to the left renal vein, with or without spleno-pancreatic and spleno-gastric connection).
- Small-diameter H-graft shunt (8-mm polytetrafluorethylene reinforced grafts anastomosing the superior mesenteric vein or portal vein to inferior vena cava)

The nonselective shunts are further classified as follows:

- Portocaval shunt (portal vein to the inferior vena cava directly)
- Mesocaval shunt (superior mesenteric vein to the inferior vena cava directly)
- Central (proximal) splenorenal shunt (proximal splenic vein to the left renal vein, with or without spleno-pancreatic and spleno-gastric connection or splenectomy)
- Large-diameter H-graft shunt (16-mm polytetrafluorethylene reinforced grafts anastomosing superior mesenteric vein or portal vein to the inferior vena cava)

Overall, the literature showed a superiority of selective shunts in terms of controlling bleeding (and bleeding prevention), maintaining portal flow, maintaining liver function, decreased postoperative encephalopathy, and overall survival, especially in nonalcoholics.[52]

In cases of bleeding gastric ulcer, the primary goal of any operation is hemorrhage control, with a secondary goal of definitively treating the underlying ulcer pathology. Bleeding gastric ulcers are generally best treated by excision of the ulcer and repair of the stomach. Excision or biopsy of the ulcer is important because 4% to 5% of benign-appearing ulcers are malignant ulcers.[53] For ulcers along the greater curvature of the stomach, antrum, or body of the stomach, wedge resection and primary closure can easily be achieved in most cases. For distal gastric ulcers along the lesser curvature in the area of the incisura angularis, a distal gastrectomy with reconstruction (Billroth I or Billroth II or Roux-en-Y [RY]) is often the easiest method of excising the ulcer and restoring GI continuity. In cases of gastroesophageal junction (GEJ) bleeding, wedge resection will often result in compromise of the GEJ and leak; thus, anterior gastrotomy with biopsy and oversewing of the ulcer from inside the gastric lumen is effective and relatively straightforward. In the event that ulcer excision is necessary, a Csendes procedure, a distal gastrectomy with tongue-shaped extension of the lesser curve resection margin to include the ulcer and subsequent RY esophagogastrojejunostomy, is an excellent option.[54]

In cases of bleeding duodenal ulcer, the standard approach is to perform an anterior longitudinal duodenotomy extending across the pylorus to the distal stomach. The bleeding vessel, often the gastroduodenal artery, is ligated in the ulcer crater by placing a figure-of-eight suture at the top and the bottom of the ulcer crater to control the artery proximally and distally. A third suture is placed as a U-stitch underneath the ulcer to control the transverse pancreatic branches that enter the gastroduodenal artery posteriorly. The transverse duodenal incision is then closed vertically to construct a Heineke-Mikulicz pyloroplasty. Classically, a truncal vagotomy is then performed to reduce the risk of recurrent ulceration if the patient is hemodynamically stable.[55,56] More extensive operation that includes gastric resection combined with ulcer resection is found to have lower rebleeding rates without significant differences in overall mortality. However, morbidity rates, mostly duodenal leaks, are significantly higher after gastric resection.[57]

Nonsurgical Management of Lower Gastrointestinal Bleeding

Similar to UGIB management, the goals are to determine if the bleeding is coming from the lower GI tract, determine the severity of bleeding, triage patients to the appropriate level of care, provide general supportive measures, and initiate resuscitation. Once these steps are complete, additional diagnostic studies can be obtained.[14] The approach to subsequent treatment depends on the source of the bleeding. If bleeding or stigmata of recent hemorrhage are identified during colonoscopy or angiography, attempts can be made to control the bleeding. However, frequently, active bleeding is not seen, and a presumptive diagnosis is made regarding the source of the bleeding (e.g., diverticular bleeding in a patient with diverticula). In those cases, the management approach will vary depending on the type of lesion (e.g., endoscopic treatment is appropriate for angiodysplasia but not for nonbleeding diverticula). If no source is identified, the patient may need to be evaluated for upper and mid-GI bleeding. In cases of blood per rectum, evaluation is warranted that includes gastroenterology consultation.[58] General surgery and interventional radiology consults are required in cases of massive hematochezia or those who are at high risk for complications. Other diagnostic procedures that may be useful include radionuclide imaging, CTA (multidetector row helical CT), and mesenteric angiography. These radiographic procedures require active bleeding at the time of examination in order to identify a bleeding source and are, therefore, reserved for the subset of patients with severe, ongoing bleeding.

Colonoscopy is the diagnostic test of choice for hemodynamically stable patients with LGIB because it allows the precise localization of the bleeding site as well as the ability to collect biopsy and provide therapeutic interventions. However, high-quality colonoscopy (colonic mucosa evaluation during both insertion and withdrawal, terminal ileum intubation, etc.) requires adequate bowel preparation and anesthesia, with its attendant risks, and incurs the risk of postprocedural bleeding or perforation.[59,60] Colonoscopy may not be needed in patients with previous presumptive or definitive diverticular bleeding who present with modest blood loss that stops spontaneously and who have had a high-quality colonoscopy within 12 months with adequate bowel preparation and no colorectal neoplasia.[59,60] A definitive or potential bleeding source is visualized in 45% to 90% of patients undergoing colonoscopy for LGIB.[61] Visualization of a potential bleeding site that is not actively bleeding does not exclude the presence of a more proximal source. The identification of more than one potential bleeding site is common (e.g., diverticulosis and hemorrhoids). Furthermore, a bleeding site is not always identified.[62] Colonoscopy should be performed on a next-available basis after adequate colon preparation because there is no difference in identification of stigmata of recent hemorrhage, rebleeding, or blood transfusions in patients undergoing colonoscopy in less than 24 hours of presentation versus within 24 to 96 hours (Table 98.3).[63]

TABLE 98.3   Overview of Lower Gastrointestinal Bleeding

Causes
Diverticular disease (most common), angiodysplasias, colon polyps, tumors (benign or malignant), inflammatory bowel disease, hemorrhoids, anal fissures

Clinical Features
History: Medications (NSAIDs, aspirin, anticoagulants/antiplatelets), previous GI bleed, liver failure, coagulopathy
Symptoms and signs: Abdominal pain, hematochezia
Examination: Tachycardia, orthostatic blood pressure, hypotension, rectal exam, abdominal tenderness, peritonitis

Diagnostic Testing
Type and screen, CBC, coagulation screen, LFTs, BUN, Cr
Nasogastric lavage may be helpful if the source of bleeding is unclear (upper or lower GI tract).

Treatment
Continuous monitoring, resuscitation, oxygen, transfusion
- For severe, ongoing bleeding, immediately transfuse blood products in 1:1:1 ratio of RBCs, plasma, and platelets, as for trauma patients.
- For hemodynamic instability despite crystalloid resuscitation, transfuse 1 to 2 units RBCs.
- For hemoglobin <8 g/dL (80 g/L) in high-risk patients (e.g., older adult, coronary artery disease), transfuse 1 unit RBCs and reassess the patient's clinical condition.
- For hemoglobin <7 g/dL (70 g/L) in low-risk patients, transfuse 1 unit RBCs and reassess the patient's clinical condition.
Consult with gastroenterologist; obtain surgical and interventional radiology consultation for any large-scale bleeding.

Colonoscopy
Computed tomographic angiography, angiography, radionuclide scan, push enteroscopy for small bowel bleeding

BUN, Blood urea nitrogen; *CBC,* complete blood count; *Cr,* creatinine; *GI,* gastrointestinal; *LFT,* liver function test; *RBC,* red blood cell.

Imaging for GIB can facilitate the diagnosis of bleeding throughout the GI tract, including small bowel sources. In addition, treatment of the bleeding site can be attempted during angiography (but not radionuclide imaging or CTA). However, these studies all require active bleeding at the time of the study to detect a bleeding site. In patients with severe bleeding who are unstable for colonoscopy or those with ongoing bleeding despite colonoscopy, CTA may be used to select patients with active bleeding for subsequent angiography or, less commonly, to localize the source before surgery. It is important that angiography be performed promptly after a positive CTA.[64] Otherwise, the patient may stop bleeding by the time the angiography is completed, thereby missing the opportunity for embolization. In patients with ongoing hemodynamically significant hematochezia, CTA is the initial diagnostic test of choice.[59] Patients with extravasation on a CTA should undergo prompt (ideally within 90 minutes) transcatheter arteriography and possible embolization.[65] CTA is an appealing diagnostic modality because it is widely available, fast, and minimally invasive. In addition, it provides anatomic detail that may be helpful for subsequent interventions such as angiography. Bleeding at a rate of 0.3 to 0.5 mL/minute can be detected with CTA.[66] CTA has a sensitivity of 85% and a specificity of 92% for detecting active GIB, and the accuracy of CTA is almost 100%.[67] CTA was found to be similar to radionuclide imaging for detecting bleeding on subsequent angiography (sensitivity of 90%, specificity of 20%), but it was more precise when it came to localizing the site of the bleeding. However, CTA lacks therapeutic capability, requires radiation exposure, and uses IV contrast, which can be associated with nephropathy and allergic reactions.[68] Like the other radiographic tests for GI bleeding, a positive scan requires active bleeding. Angiography requires active blood loss of 0.5 to 1.0 mL/minute under optimal conditions for a bleeding site to be visualized.[69] Angiography is

typically reserved for patients in whom endoscopy is not feasible because of severe bleeding with hemodynamic instability. CTA is commonly used to identify and localize the bleeding source before angiography.[64] Angiographies performed within 90 minutes of positive CT angiograms are more likely to detect bleeding than those that are delayed beyond this time frame. In the absence of prior localization (e.g., radionuclide imaging), the superior mesenteric artery is generally examined first in patients with presumed LGIB because bleeding sources tend to occur in bowel supplied by this artery.[70] If this test is negative, the inferior mesenteric and celiac vessels are studied. The success rate varies widely from 25% to 70%, depending on the timing relative to the episode of bleeding and local expertise.[71] The advantages of angiography over other tests for LGIB are that it does not require bowel preparation, and anatomic localization is accurate. Additionally, angiography also permits the opportunity for therapeutic intervention. Transcatheter embolization is a means of controlling hemorrhage and has largely replaced other temporizing interventions, such as vasopressin infusion. Superselective embolization of distal vessels using coaxial catheters decreases the risk of bowel infarction. A meta-analysis found that in patients with active bleeding, superselective embolization is feasible in 98%, and complications occur in 4.6%, most commonly bowel infarction or ulceration.[71,72] Radionuclide scanning detects bleeding that is occurring at a rate of 0.1 to 0.5 mL/minute, and it is the most sensitive radiographic test for GI bleeding.[73] It is important that angiography be performed promptly after a positive radionuclide scan to localize the source of bleeding. However, a major disadvantage of radionuclide imaging is that it can only localize bleeding to a general area of the abdomen. Accuracy rates have varied substantially across reports, ranging from 24% to 91%.[74] Poor localization occurs because blood can move in either a peristaltic or antiperistaltic direction.

TABLE 98.4 Procedures Used for Evaluation of Lower Gastrointestinal Bleeding

TECHNIQUE	ADVANTAGES	DISADVANTAGES
Radionuclide imaging	• Noninvasive • Sensitive to low rates of bleeding	• Has to be performed during active bleeding • Poor localization of bleeding site • Not therapeutic • Not widely available
CT angiography	• Noninvasive • Accurately localizes bleeding source • Provides anatomic detail • Widely available	• Has to be performed during active bleeding • Not therapeutic • Radiation and IV contrast exposure
Angiography	• Accurately localizes bleeding source • Therapy possible with superselective embolization • Does not require bowel preparation	• Has to be performed during active bleeding • Invasive
Colonoscopy	• Precise diagnosis and localization regardless of active bleeding or type of lesion • Allows endoscopic therapy	• Need colon preparation for optimal visualization • Risk of sedation and perforation in acutely bleeding patient • Definite bleeding source (stigmata) infrequently identified

CT, Computed tomographic; *IV,* intravenous.

A bleeding site may not be evident in some patients despite lower GI evaluation. If not already done, an upper endoscopy or push enteroscopy should be considered in those with severe, ongoing bleeding because up to 15% of such patients have a bleeding site in the upper digestive tract.[75] Push enteroscopy (endoscopy using a pediatric colonoscope or a dedicated enteroscope) allows visualization of approximately the proximal 60 cm of the jejunum.[76] Bleeding sites can also arise in more distal segments of the small bowel. There are several methods to evaluate the small intestine, such as capsule endoscopy and deep small bowel enteroscopy. In some patients, bleeding may have stopped, making efforts to identify the site more difficult. Such patients should be observed for 24 to 48 hours. An urgent CT angiogram/tagged red blood cell scan can be obtained to localize the region of bleeding if bleeding resumes (Table 98.4). Provocative challenges with vasodilators, anticoagulants, and/or thrombolytics have been reported to aid in the diagnosis of elusive bleeding. However, the risk of serious complications, including refractory bleeding and death, is substantial, and these methods should be used extremely rarely and only by expert centers after careful planning.[77]

Surgical Treatment of Lower Gastrointestinal Bleeding

The surgical treatment of LGIB depends on the source of the bleeding. In many cases, the bleeding can be controlled with therapies applied at the time of colonoscopy or angiography. Rarely, patients with exsanguinating LGIB will need immediate surgery. The morbidity and mortality associated with colectomy in the absence of preoperative localization of a bleeding site are higher than those in patients who have a bleeding site identified before surgery.[78] Thus, all efforts should be made to identify the bleeding source before surgery. In patients with significant, early (during the initial hospitalization) recurrent LGIB, a repeat colonoscopy should be performed with endoscopic hemostasis if indicated.[2]

The indications for surgery in LGIB include persistent hemodynamic instability with active bleeding; persistent, recurrent bleeding; and transfusion of more than 4 units of packed red bloods cells in a 24-hour period with active or recurrent bleeding. In these patients, the operation type is dependent on the patient's hemodynamic and overall performance status, the background preexisting disease, and the preoperative successful localization. Segmental bowel resection after precise localization of the bleeding point is a well-accepted surgical practice in hemodynamically stable patients. Subtotal colectomy is the procedure of choice in patients who are actively bleeding from an unknown source. The latter has an associated morbidity rate of around 37% and a mortality rate of about 11% to 33%. In those patients who have nonlocalized disease and are unstable, a two-stage procedure is preferred: temporary end ileostomy and delayed ileoproctostomy. In those patients who are hemodynamically stable with minimal medical comorbidities, this procedure can be performed as a single-stage procedure with ileoproctostomy (Fig. 98.2).[79]

OUTCOMES IN GASTROINTESTINAL BLEEDING

UGIB in-hospital mortality reaches 10%. This rate holds steady up to 1 month after hospitalization for GIB. Long-term follow-up of patients with UGIB shows that at 3 years after admission, mortality rates from all causes approach 37%. Mortality rates are higher in females than in males. Patients with multiple hospitalizations for GIB carry higher mortality rates. The long-term prognosis was the worst in patients who suffered from malignancies and variceal bleeding.[80]

For LGIB, all-cause in-hospital mortality is less than 4%. Death from LGIB itself is rare, with most in-hospital mortality occurring from other comorbid conditions. Increased risk of death corresponded to increasing age and comorbid conditions. Other negative prognostic factors include secondary bleeding (onset of bleed after being hospitalized for a different condition), patients with preexisting coagulopathies, hypovolemia, transfusion requirement, and male sex. The lowest risks of mortality are associated with more benign causes of LGIB, such as hemorrhoids, anal fissures, and colon polyps.[81]

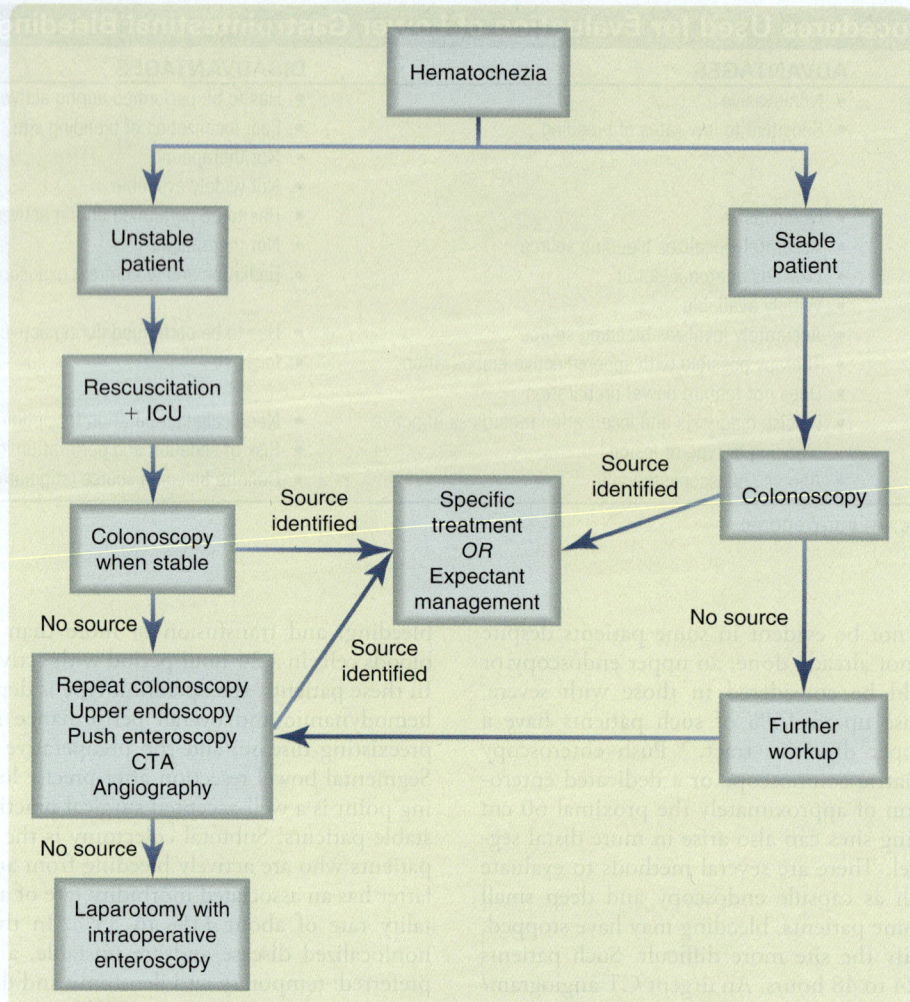

FIGURE 98.2 Algorithm for diagnosis and management of patients with lower gastrointestinal bleed. *CTA,* Computed tomography angiography; *ICU,* Intensive care unit.

SELECTED REFERENCES

Forrest JA, Finlayson ND, Shearman DJ. Endoscopy in gastrointestinal bleeding. *Lancet.* 1974;2(7877):394-397.

The results of early endoscopy in patients with upper-gastrointestinal-tract bleeding was successful in identifying the site of bleeding fell rapidly from 78% within 24 hours of admission to 32% after 48 hours.

Gralnek IM, Stanley AJ, Morris AJ, et al. Endoscopic diagnosis and management of nonvariceal upper gastrointestinal hemorrhage (NVUGIH): European Society of Gastrointestinal Endoscopy (ESGE) guideline—update 2021. *Endoscopy.* 2021;53(3):300-332.

This Guideline is an official statement from the European Society of Gastrointestinal Endoscopy (ESGE). It is an update of the previously published 2015 ESGE Clinical Guideline addressing the role of gastrointestinal endoscopy in the diagnosis and management of acute nonvariceal upper gastrointestinal hemorrhage.

Orloff MJ. Fifty-three years' experience with randomized clinical trials of emergency portacaval shunt for bleeding esophageal varices in cirrhosis: 1958–2011. *JAMA Surg.* 2014;149(2):155-169.

Summary of randomized clinical trials showing that emergency portacaval shunt permanently stopped variceal bleeding, almost never became occluded, accomplished 5 times the long-term survival than sclerotherapy or TIPS.

Schroder VT, Pappas TN, Vaslef SN, De La Fuente SG, Scarborough JE. Vagotomy/drainage is superior to local oversew in patients who require emergency surgery for bleeding peptic ulcers. *Ann Surg.* 2014;259(6):1111-1118.

Retrospective analysis compairing early postoperative outcomes of patients undergoing different types of emergency procedures for bleeding or perforated gastroduodenal ulcers.

Strate LL, Gralnek IM. ACG clinical guideline: management of patients with acute lower gastrointestinal bleeding. *Am J Gastroenterol.* 2016;111(4):459-474.

Updated guidelines in the management of lower GI bleed.

Strate LL. Lower GI bleeding: epidemiology and diagnosis. *Gastroenterol Clin North Am.* 2005;34(4):643-664.

Comprehensive review on the epidemiology and diagnosis of lower GI bleeding.

Sung JJ, Chan FK, Lau JY, et al. The effect of endoscopic therapy in patients receiving omeprazole for bleeding ulcers with non-bleeding visible vessels or adherent clots: a randomized comparison. *Ann Intern Med.* 2003;139(4):237-243.

Randomized trial showing that combination of endoscopic therapy and omeprazole infusion is superior to omeprazole infusion alone for preventing recurrent bleeding from ulcers with nonbleeding visible vessels and adherent clots.

Villanueva C, Colomo A, Bosch A, et al. Transfusion strategies for acute upper gastrointestinal bleeding. *N Engl J Med.* 2013;368(1):11-21.

Randomized clinical trial showing that compared with a liberal transfusion strategy (hb<9), a restrictive strategy (hb<7) significantly improved outcomes in patients with acute upper gastrointestinal bleeding.

Wang A, Yerxa J, Agarwal S, et al. Surgical management of peptic ulcer disease. *Curr Probl Surg.* 2020;57(2):100728.

Comprehensive review on the surgical management of peptic ulcer disease.

The full reference list appears on Elsevier eBooks+.

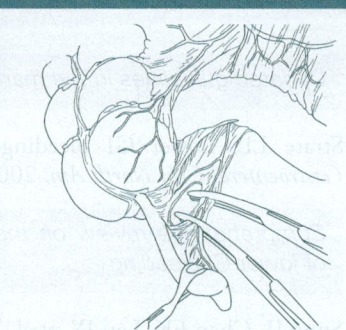

99 CHAPTER

Morbid Obesity

Alfonso Torquati, Nicholas J. Skertich, Philip Omotosho, and William O. Richards

OUTLINE

 Please access Elsevier eBooks+ to view the videos for this chapter.

OBESITY: THE MAGNITUDE OF THE PROBLEM

Until very recently, obesity was not recognized as a disease, which confounded the ability of physicians to be compensated for treatment they delivered and to treat the condition effectively. The American Medical Association (AMA) officially recognized obesity as a disease in 2013 and, in 2014, voted to approve the resolution "that our AMA, advocate for patient access to the full continuum of care of evidence-based obesity treatment modalities (including surgical interventions)."

Morbid obesity is defined as being 100 lb above ideal body weight, twice ideal body weight, or body mass index (BMI; measured as weight in kilograms divided by height in meters squared)

of 40 kg/m^2 or greater. The last definition is more accepted internationally and has essentially replaced the former ones for all practical and scientific purposes. A consensus conference by the National Institutes of Health (NIH) in 1991 suggested that the term *severe obesity* as perhaps a more appropriate terminology. This term is used interchangeably with *morbid obesity* in the remainder of this chapter.

The obesity epidemic in the United States is evidenced by the fact that over 40% of the US adult population is considered obese, and the prevalence of obesity in adolescents has increased to 22.2% in the most recent National Health and Nutrition Examination Survey (NHANES). The percentage of obese adults (BMI >30) in the United States increased 16% from 1980–2000 and by another 9% from 2000–16.[1] There are also significant differences in the prevalence of obesity in adults by sex, race, and Hispanic origin. Non-Hispanic Asians (16.1%) had significantly lower rates of obesity than all other race and non–Hispanic-origin groups. Non-Hispanic Whites (41.4%) had a lower prevalence of obesity than non-Hispanic Blacks (49.9%) and Hispanic adults (45.6%). Hispanic males (45.2%) had a greater prevalence of obesity compared with non-Hispanic Asian (17.6%) and non-Hispanic Black males (40.4%).[1]

The prevalence of morbidly obese adults (BMI $\geq$40 kg/m^2) has increased to 9.2% of the adult population, and morbid obesity is the second leading cause of preventable death in the United States. Morbid obesity is second only to smoking on the list of preventable factors responsible for increased healthcare costs. It is a sobering thought to realize that a 40-year-old male with morbid obesity has a 12.4% reduction in life expectancy, or 9.1 years of life lost, compared with a male who is nonobese. Moreover, the cost of care is staggering and may be as high as 9% of annual medical expenditures, or $147 billion per year. There appears to be significant population heterogeneity between BMI and mortality that is attenuated by increasing age of the individual. Mortality also increases significantly even for individuals with minimal increases in BMI greater than 30.0. Thus, it appears that age, sex, race, and income level all play a role in the development of obesity and obesity-related mortality.[2]

PATHOPHYSIOLOGY AND ASSOCIATED MEDICAL PROBLEMS

The pathophysiology of severe obesity is multifactorial and has as its basis a genetic predisposition. There is a clear familial predisposition, and it is rare for a single family member to have severe obesity. Specific genes associated with obesity have been identified, including the *FTO* gene (fat mass and obesity related), which plays a role in controlling feeding behavior and energy expenditure, and the *MC4R* deficiency gene (melanocortin 4 receptor), which is associated with obesity, increased fat mass, and insulin resistance.[3]

Single gene mutations causing obesity are rare and are expressed during early childhood (Table 99.1). The most common single gene etiology of severe obesity is the *MC4R* gene, which induces appetite-suppression (anorexigenic) effects on the hypothalamus in the regulation of energy homeostasis.[3] Recent studies have suggested that the cilium of MC4R neurons in the hypothalamus is the most common pathway underlying the genetic causes of human obesity (see Table 99.1).[3]

Another theory suggests that bacteria within the gut, known as the *microbiome,* play an essential role in the metabolism and immune system. Simply giving subtherapeutic antibiotic treatment to mice for 4 weeks increases adiposity and plasma levels of insulin, leptin, and triglycerides when the mice are later fed a high-fat diet. The predilection to obesity is transferrable to other mice when the low-dose penicillin-selected gut bacteria are transferred to germ-free hosts, thus

identifying that it is the action of the altered gut bacteria, not the antibiotics, that causes the obesity.[4] Recent studies have demonstrated that the gut microbiome circadian rhythm is disrupted by lifestyle differences in developed countries (shift work or jet lag), which provokes the development of altered microbial community, thus predisposing the host to obesity and glucose intolerance. Other studies have shown that degradation of dietary flavonoids through the altered microbiome results in diminished energy expenditure, which leads to obesity. It is fascinating to hypothesize that the current epidemic of obesity relates to changes in the microbiome created by the lifestyle changes and increased use of antibiotics in childhood seen in people who reside in developed countries.

Although there is no definitive answer to the pathophysiology of severe obesity, it is clear that a severely obese individual has, in general, persistent hunger that is not satiated by amounts of food that satisfy the nonobese. This lack of satiety or maintenance of hunger with corresponding increases in calorie intake may be the single most important factor in the process. There appear to be fundamental differences in the satiety and appetite hormonal control of eating that have created the current epidemic. This is hypothesized to occur when the brain's energy "set point" rises to increase energy intake through modulation of the individual's appetite.

We know that hormones, peptides, and vagal afferents to the brain have a major influence on satiety, appetite, and energy intake. Ghrelin, the only known orexigenic gut hormone, is also known as the *hunger hormone* and is secreted by P/D1 cells of the gastric fundus. Ghrelin stimulates release of various neuropeptides, such as neuropeptide Y (NPY) and growth hormone, from the hypothalamus, which creates an orexigenic, or increased appetite, state.[5] Increased levels of ghrelin produce increased food intake, and increased levels of ghrelin develop in individuals after low-calorie diets, thus suggesting that one possible mechanism for the failure of most diets after 6 months is the increase in the appetite hormone ghrelin.

One evolving concept is that the environment causes heritable change in gene function without modification of DNA sequences, termed *gene-environment interactions*. The changes in the epigenome lead to the development of obesity and are much more common than either the monogenetic or the syndromic forms of obesity.[5]

Morbid obesity is a metabolic disease associated with numerous medical problems, some of which are virtually unknown in the absence of obesity. Box 99.1 lists the most common. These problems must be carefully considered when one is contemplating offering a patient weight-reduction surgery. The most frequent problem is the combination of arthritis and degenerative joint disease, present in at least 50% of patients seeking surgery for severe obesity. The incidence of sleep apnea is high. Asthma is present in more than 25%, hypertension in more than 30%,

TABLE 99.1 Gene Mutations Associated With Obesity

GENE	EFFECT	ACTION ON	INHERITANCE	LINKED TO
Leptin/leptin receptor	Appetite stimulant	Hypothalamus	Autosomal recessive	Severe childhood obesity
Ghrelin receptor	Appetite stimulant	Hypothalamus	Autosomal recessive	Short stature and obesity
Melanocortin 4 receptor	Appetite inhibitor	Hypothalamus	Autosomal dominant	Increased fat mass, insulin resistance
Proopiomelanocortin (POMC)	Appetite inhibitor	Melanocortin 4 receptor in hypothalamus	Autosomal recessive	Severe early-onset obesity by age 1 and excessive eating caused by insatiable hunger
Neuropeptide Y (NPY)	Appetite stimulant	Hypothalamus	Autosomal recessive	Hypertension, high low-density lipoprotein cholesterol and triglycerides, increased food intake and hunger

BOX 99.1   Medical Conditions Associated With Severe Obesity

Cardiovascular
Hypertension
Sudden cardiac death myocardial infarction
Cardiomyopathy
Venous stasis disease
Deep venous thrombosis
Pulmonary hypertension
Right-sided heart failure

Pulmonary
Obstructive sleep apnea
Hypoventilation syndrome of obesity
Asthma

Metabolic
Metabolic syndrome (abdominal obesity, hypertension, dyslipidemia, insulin resistance)
Type 2 diabetes mellitus
Hyperlipidemia
Hypercholesterolemia
Nonalcoholic steatotic hepatitis (NASH) or nonalcoholic fatty liver disease (NAFLD)

Gastrointestinal
Gastroesophageal reflux disease
Cholelithiasis

Musculoskeletal
Degenerative joint disease
Lumbar disk disease

Osteoarthritis
Ventral hernias

Genitourinary
Stress urinary incontinence
End-stage renal disease (secondary to diabetes and hypertension)

Gynecologic
Menstrual irregularities

Skin/Integumentary System
Fungal infections
Boils, abscesses

Oncologic
Cancer of the thyroid, prostate, esophagus, kidney, stomach, colon, rectum, gallbladder, pancreas, female cancers of the breast, ovaries, cervix, and endometrium

Neurologic/Psychiatric
Pseudotumor cerebri
Depression
Low self-esteem
Stroke

Social/Societal
History of physical abuse
History of sexual abuse
Discrimination for employment
Social discrimination

---

diabetes in more than 20%, and gastroesophageal reflux in 20% to 30% of patients. The incidence of these conditions increases with age and the severity and duration of severe obesity.

The *metabolic syndrome* includes type 2 diabetes mellitus (insulin resistance), dyslipidemia, and hypertension. Patients with this constellation of problems are obese, with central body obesity being the primary essential feature (waist circumference >35 inches in females or >40 inches in males). The syndrome is characterized by impaired hepatic uptake of insulin, systemic hyperinsulinemia, and tissue resistance to insulin. Patients with metabolic syndrome are at high risk for early cardiovascular death.

Obesity has been shown to increase the risk of developing cancer of the thyroid, colon, rectum, esophagus, stomach, kidney, prostate, gallbladder, pancreas, breast (postmenopausal), endometrium, ovaries, and cervix.[5] There are several mechanisms that may be responsible for the increased risk of cancer. Obesity increases chronic inflammation, which is linked to the development of esophageal adenocarcinoma through chronic inflammation from gastroesophageal reflux disease (GERD). Fat produces excess levels of estrogen, which is linked to increased risk of endometrial, ovarian, and postmenopausal breast cancer. Increased levels of insulin and insulin-like growth factor-1 are hypothesized to be linked to the development of colon, prostate, kidney, endometrial, and postmenopausal breast cancer.[5]

Not listed in Box 99.1 are the associated societal discriminatory problems that severely obese individuals face. Public facilities, in terms of seating, doorways, and restroom facilities, often make access to events held in such settings unavailable to a severely obese person. Travel on public transportation is sometimes difficult, if not impossible. Employment discrimination clearly exists for these individuals. Finally, low self-esteem, a frequent history of sexual or physical abuse, and these social difficulties coalesce to create a very high incidence of depression in the population of patients with morbid obesity.

MEDICAL VERSUS SURGICAL THERAPY

Medical therapy for severe obesity historically has had limited short-term success and almost nonexistent long-term success. However, with the introduction of incretin-based therapies, which are becoming rapidly available, that may change. Nevertheless, once severely obese, the likelihood that a person will lose enough weight by dietary means alone and remain at a BMI below 35 kg/m^2 is estimated at 3% or less. The 1991 NIH consensus conference recognized that for this population of patients, medical therapy has been largely unsuccessful in treating the problem. Review of the clinical trials of lifestyle interventions for prevention of obesity demonstrated that the majority of trials were completely ineffective, and the few that were marginally effective had an extremely small impact on BMI. As the understanding of the disease of obesity has changed, and due to significant advances in medicine, the leadership of the American Society of Metabolic and Bariatric Surgery (ASMBS) and the International Federation for Surgery of Obesity and Metabolic Disorders (IFSO) reconvened in

TABLE 99.2 Results of Bariatric Surgery Compared With Medically Treated Controls

STUDY	SURGERY MORTALITY RATE	MEDICAL MORTALITY RATE	HAZARD RATIO SURGICAL REDUCTION IN MORTALITY	NOTES
Adams[10]	2.7%	4.1%	0.63 HR	Retrospective matched cohort of 7925 RYGB and 7925 severely obese control patients, mean follow-up 7.1 years
Aminian[9]	10.0%	17.8%	0.59 HR	Retrospective matched cohort of patients with diabetes, 2287 bariatric surgery and 11,435 matched control patients, 10-year follow-up
Arteburn[11]	13.8%	23.9%	0.47 HR	Veterans Affairs multisite cohort of 2500 bariatric surgery patients and 74,62 matched control patients, 10-year follow-up
Kauppilia[12]	3.6%	15.2%	0.74 HR	5 Nordic countries, population-based study of 49,977 bariatric surgery patients and 494,842 who did not have surgery, 15-year follow-up
Swedish Obesity Study[8]	22.8%	26.4%	0.77 HR	Prospective trial of 2007 bariatric surgery and 2040 matched control patients, with median 24- and 22-year follow-up, respectively

HR, Hazard ratio; *RYGB*, Roux-en-Y gastric bypass.

2022 to revise the criteria for surgery. Based on the large volume of new trials available, ASMBS and IFSO reasserted the safety, efficacy, durability, and resultant decrease in mortality associated with metabolic and bariatric surgery compared with nonoperative treatments.[6]

Although medical treatments are significantly improving, one of the most remarkable stories in modern medicine has been the absolute superiority of bariatric surgery over medical therapy for the treatment of morbid obesity and its comorbidities. In a 2021 meta-analysis, metabolic-bariatric surgery was associated with a reduction in the hazard rate of death of 49.2%, and median life expectancy increased by 6.1 years.[7] Multiple long-term follow-up trials comparing patients with morbid obesity who underwent bariatric surgery with those who did not have shown decreased mortality long term (Table 99.2).

The Swedish Obese Subjects (SOS) study is the first prospective controlled trial to provide long-term data on the effects of bariatric surgery on diabetes, cardiovascular events, cancer, and overall mortality. The study enrolled 2010 bariatric surgery patients (gastric bypass, 13%; banding, 19%; vertical banded gastroplasty, 68%) and 2037 matched controls who received standard medical treatment, and the subjects have now been observed for over 20 years. The SOS study was able to obtain follow-up on nearly 100% of the patients and found that at 20 years after initiation of the surgery, patients had a BMI reduction of 7 compared with baseline versus a small gain in the control group. The long-term sustained weight loss and reduction in comorbid conditions after bariatric surgery resulted in a 30% reduction in mortality in the bariatric surgery patients (adjusted hazard ratio [HR] = 0.70, 95% confidence interval [CI] 0.61–0.81, $p < 0.001$). The most common cause of death in the SOS study was cardiovascular diseases and cancers. The incidence of myocardial infarction was significantly reduced in the surgery group compared with the control group (HR = 0.51), and the surgery group had a lower number of first-time cardiovascular events (HR = 0.70).[8] As can be seen in Table 99.2, there are multiple studies with long-term follow-up comparing bariatric surgery to matched control groups, and these studies have found that the surgical groups have significant survival advantage (all cause, cancer, cardiovascular), associated with improvement in diabetes, obstructive sleep apnea, dyslipidemia, and hypertension.[8–12] These studies are convincing evidence that bariatric surgery provides long-term weight loss, resolution of comorbidities, and improvement

in mortality. Although the SOS study found improvement in all-cause mortality after 20 years of follow-up, most procedures performed were vertical banded gastroplasty, whereas only 13% were the much more effective Roux-en-Y gastric bypass (RYGB).[8] Therefore, it is not surprising that the Adams[7] and Aminian[9] studies, which compared RYGB to medical treatment, showed convincing mortality differences as early as 3 to 5 years after surgery, much earlier than the SOS.[8] Similarly, Kauppila[12] studied 49,977 patients undergoing bariatric surgery, of which RYGB made up 73.4% of the operative procedures, compared with a cohort of obese persons in five Nordic countries and found that all-cause mortality was reduced by 4 years and improved further at 15 years. Moreover, the Arterburn study[11] was from the Veterans Affairs (VA) hospitals in the United States, so it had a predominance of males (74% male) as opposed to all of the other reported trials having a majority of females, but it also identified a reduction in all-cause mortality at 5 years. These results also hold true for older patients, who may have a higher operative mortality and shorter time to see long-term benefits (HR = 0.75, 95% CI 0.65–0.85 for patients 55–80 years of age).[13]

The driving force behind the improved mortality is likely a reduction in health-related comorbidities, particularly cardiovascular disease, cancer, and diabetes, as discussed later. A large, retrospective cohort study with 5-year postoperative follow-up demonstrated significantly lower rates of lung, ovarian, and uterine cancer in obese patients undergoing sleeve gastrectomy or RYGB compared with bariatric patients without any surgical intervention (odds ratio [OR] 0.74, 95% CI 0.643–0.859; OR 0.778, 95% CI 0.674–0.898 for sleeve gastrectomy and gastric bypass, respectively).[14] Similarly, a large retrospective study with a matched cohort of nearly 15,000 patients demonstrated that at a median follow-up of 3.9 years, surgical intervention had an absolute risk reduction in composite all-cause mortality, coronary artery events, cerebrovascular events, heart failure, nephropathy, and atrial fibrillation of 16.9% (adjusted HR = 0.61, 95% CI 0.55–0.69). On secondary analysis, the composite of all-cause mortality, myocardial infarction, and ischemic stroke was also significantly lower in the surgical group, 17.0% versus 27.6% (HR = 0.62, $p < 0.001$).[9]

Despite the objective health benefits, one perception of bariatric surgery is that it may induce profound, unalterable changes in eating that negatively affect the patients' health-related quality of life (HRQOL). A well-done 12-year prospective study by

Kolotkin et al. evaluated HRQOL changes after gastric bypass surgery compared with two nonsurgical groups matched for similar demographics. The patients who underwent bariatric surgery had greatly improved quality of life (QOL) in the physical component compared with before surgery. There were also significant differences between the surgery patients and both nonsurgical groups for both the weight-related HRQOL and the physical HRQOL. The magnitude of improvement 12 years after gastric bypass surgery compared with before surgery and between matched control groups supports the conclusion that bariatric surgery improves the patients' QOL.[15] These QOL improvements were also seen in the Swiss Multicenter Bypass or Sleeve Study (SM-BOSS) and SLEEVEPASS trials.[16,17]

However, the Kolotkin study,[15] SOS,[8] and Utah long-term study[13] all identified an increase in suicides and self-harm in patients undergoing bariatric surgery. In all studies, the numbers remain low, and the authors concluded that the absolute risk and numbers of patients do not support not offering bariatric surgery to patients. We recommend that preoperative psychiatric mental health assessment and postoperative monitoring for mental health, particularly substance abuse, are needed.

Metabolic Surgery Versus Medical Therapy for Diabetes

The Surgical Treatment and Medications Potentially Eradicate Diabetes Efficiently (STAMPEDE) trial[18] is the preeminent randomized controlled trial (RCT) to demonstrate the superiority of bariatric surgery over intensive medical therapy in type 2 diabetes mellitus. However, multiple trials have shown bariatric surgery to be more effective in glycemic control, weight loss, medication reduction, improvement in lipids, and QOL, as shown in Fig. 99.1 and summarized in Table 99.3.[18–20] Metabolic surgery reduced hemoglobin A1c (HgbA1c) by 2% to 3.5%, whereas medical therapy was only able to reduce HgbA1c by 1% to 1.5%. The short- and long-term (2- to 5- year) results shown in Table 99.3 demonstrate that a significant number of patients (29%–43%) undergoing laparoscopic RYGB (LRYGB) achieved HgbA1c levels of less than 6 compared with only 5% to 7% of medically treated patients.[18–20] These results were further corroborated in the Alliance of Randomized Trials of Medicine Versus Metabolic Surgery in Type 2 Diabetes (ARMMS-T2D) study, which included patients from multiple prior randomized trials.[21] It again demonstrated superior glycemic control, more diabetes remission, and greater change in BMI than medical/lifestyle intervention. It is even more remarkable that the medically treated patients still required intensive medical therapy, whereas the surgery patients had reduced or eliminated diabetic medications. Weight loss for both LRYGB and laparoscopic sleeve gastrectomy (LSG) was far superior to that for medical therapy.

LRYGB also improves the other associated medical conditions of the metabolic syndrome, including improvements in hypertension and high-density lipoprotein (HDL) cholesterol, which results in reduced cardiovascular events/deaths. Specifically, diabetic patients who undergo bariatric surgery have a lower rate of developing microvascular diseases. The reduced incidence of microvascular disease was largest in the reduction of retinopathy (71% reduction, OR 0.29), followed by end-stage renal disease (ESRD; 69% reduction, OR 0.31) and nephropathy (59% reduction, adjusted odds ratio [AOR] 0.31). In pooled analysis, it did not reduce diabetic neuropathy.[22] The authors of this systematic review and meta-analysis concluded that bariatric surgery significantly reduced the incidence of microvascular disease, specifically retinopathy, ESRD, and nephropathy. We argue that the additional evidence of improvement in microvascular disease encourages primary care providers to discuss the benefits of bariatric surgery with their patients with diabetes and obesity.

Glucagon-Like Peptide-1 Receptor Agonists

Medical treatment of obesity is rapidly evolving with the introduction of incretin-mimetic–based treatments, which include glucagon-like peptide-1 receptor agonists (GLP-1 RAs). These medications were initially developed to treat diabetes because they were found to stimulate insulin release in the pancreas while increasing the insulin sensitivity of pancreatic cells and inhibiting glucagon secretion. Incidentally, they have increased appetite suppression via slowed gastric emptying and act on the hypothalamus, which is involved in regulation of appetite.[23] As of May 2024, 13 GLP-1 RAs are FDA approved, 3 of which are approved specifically for obesity (liraglutide, semaglutide, and tirzepatide). Tirzepatide is also a glucose-dependent insulinotropic polypeptide (GIP) receptor agonist that can also stimulate insulin release.

Incretin-based therapies, compared with placebo, have shown promise for the treatment of obesity, with semaglutide and tirzepatide faring best. In a systematic review and meta-analysis that included the Semaglutide Treatment Effect in People with Obesity (STEP) and Study of Tirzepatide in Participants With Obesity or Overweight (SURMOUNT) trials, the placebo-subtracted difference on body weight was –15.0%; it was –12.9% with semaglutide (95% CI –14.7 to –11.1) and –19.2% (95% CI –22.2 to –16.2) with tirzepatide.[24] It is important to note that these trials were industry sponsored; that weight regain occurs after stopping medications (two-thirds of prior weight loss within 1 year); and that these medications do have side effects, most commonly nausea, vomiting, and diarrhea.[24]

The place of incretin-mimetics in our armamentarium against obesity has yet to be fully elucidated. They are indeed an excellent option in nonsurgical candidates who meet indications for use or for patients who do not desire surgery. In our practice, they are also advantageous in bridging high-BMI patients to surgery as well as in postoperative patients with inadequate weight loss or recurrent weight gain.

A recent meta-analysis evaluating liraglutide and semaglutide in post–bariatric surgery patients found that postoperative GLP-1 RA use can lead to additional weight loss. This adjuvant effect is superior with semaglutide compared with liraglutide. Semaglutide led to a mean weight loss of nearly 10%, with over 60% of patients achieving greater than 10% weight loss at 12 months.[25] As GLP-1 RA continue to get FDA approval for treatment of obesity and as new drugs hit the market, additional and improved studies will be needed to further elucidate the benefits of perioperative use of GLP-1 RA.

BARIATRIC SURGERY MECHANISM OF ACTION

The first study reporting on the effectiveness of surgery in treating obesity and related comorbid conditions, published in 1955, reported observing "the amelioration of diabetes mellitus following subtotal gastrectomy." A few decades later, the wide acceptance of bariatric surgery as treatment for severe obesity has given significant momentum to study the physiology of bariatric surgery. The initial prevailing theory behind bariatric surgery was based on two primary mechanisms for surgically induced weight loss: caloric restriction and nutrient malabsorption. There is little question that the reduction in caloric intake and resulting postoperative energy deficit is one of the factors responsible for the

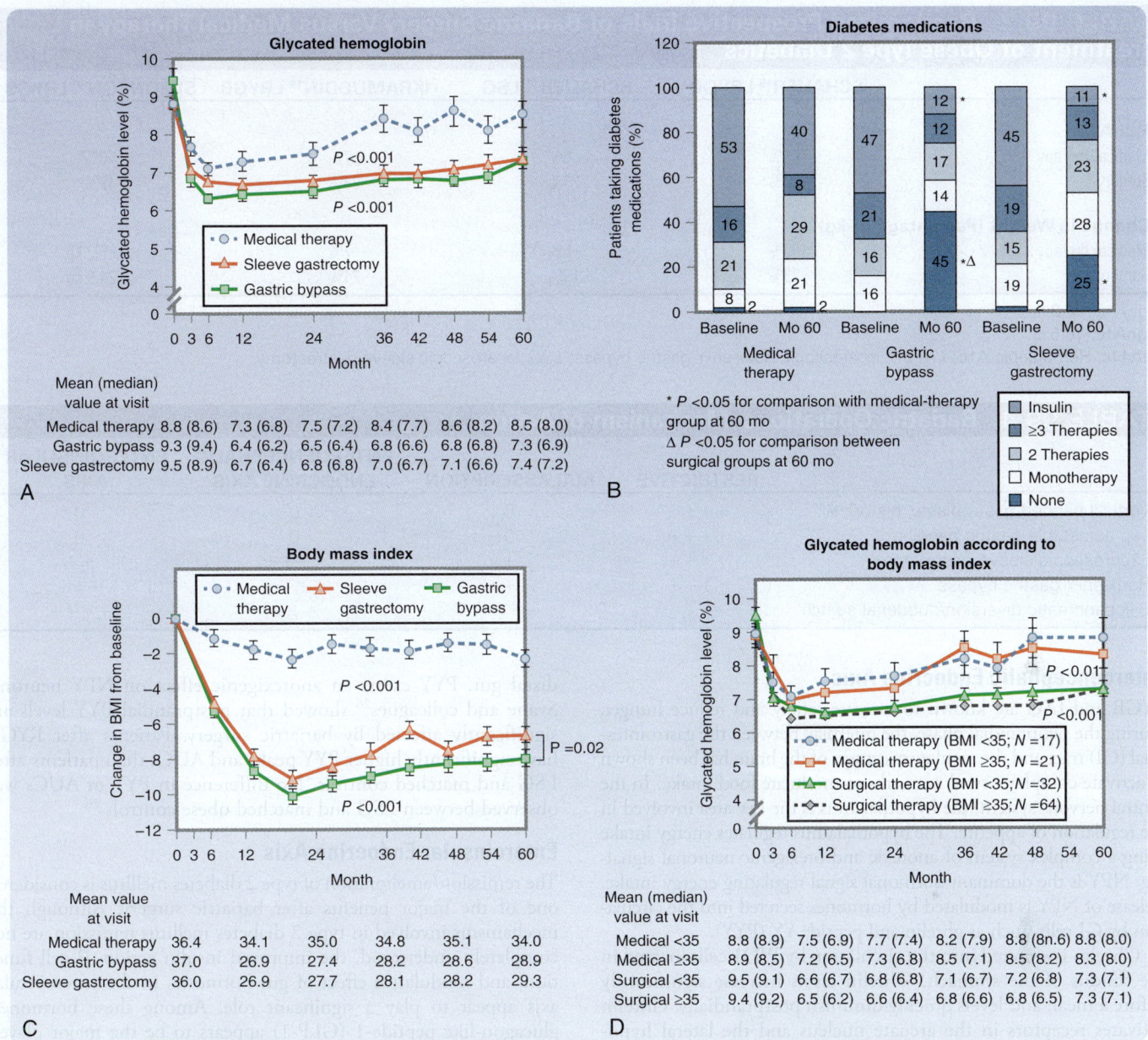

FIGURE 99.1 Mean changes in measures of diabetes control from baseline to 5 years in medical and surgically treated subjects. Shown are the mean glycated hemoglobin levels (A), the percent change in diabetes medications during the study period (B), the changes in body-mass index (BMI, the weight in kilograms divided by the square of the height in meters) (C), and the mean glycated hemoglobin levels according to BMI (D) over a 5-year period among patients receiving intensive medical therapy alone, those who underwent sleeve gastrectomy, and those who underwent a gastric bypass procedure. I bars indicate standard errors. Mean values in each group are provided below the graphs; in A and D, median values are also provided in parentheses. P values for the comparison between each surgical group and the medical-therapy group in A, C, and D were derived from overall treatment effect in the repeated measurements model. In D, P<0.001 for the comparison between the surgical groups and the medical-therapy group for the subgroup of patients with a BMI of less than 35; P<0.01 for the comparison for the subgroup with a BMI of 35 or more. *BMI*, Body mass index. (From Schauer PR, Bhatt DL, Kirwan JP, et al. Bariatric surgery versus intensive medical therapy for diabetes—5-year outcomes. *N Engl J Med*. 2017;376:641-651.)

rapid improvement in insulin sensitivity observed after RYGB and LSG. However, after taking into account the more recent scientific evidence, the concepts of restriction and malabsorption do not fully explain the metabolic effects of bariatric surgery. In fact, the mechanisms seem to extend beyond the magnitude of weight loss alone to include effects on central nervous system

regulation of appetite and metabolism and improvements in insulin secretion and insulin sensitivity. Long-term weight loss, improvement in glucose metabolism, and other metabolic effects clearly result from significant postoperative changes in the **enteroencephalic** and the **enteroinsular** endocrine axes, as shown in Table 99.4.

TABLE 99.3   Randomized Prospective Trials of Bariatric Surgery Versus Medical Therapy in Treatment of Obese Type 2 Diabetics

	SCHAUER[18] LRYGB	SCHAUER[18] LSG	IKRAMUDDIN[19] LRYGB	SIMONSON[20] LRYGB
HgbA1c				
Medical therapy	5%[a]	5%[a]	7%	0%[b]
Surgery	29%[a]	23%[a]	38%	42%[b]
Change in Weight (Percentage or kg)				
Medical therapy	−5%	−5%	−7%	−5.2 kg
Surgery	−23%	−19%	−24%	−24.9 kg

[a]HgbA1c <6.0%.
[b]HgbA1c <6.5%.
HgbA1c, Hemoglobin A1c; *LRYGB*, laparoscopic Roux-en-Y gastric bypass; *LSG*, laparoscopic sleeve gastrectomy.

TABLE 99.4   Bariatric Operations: Mechanism of Action

	RESTRICTIVE	MALABSORPTION	ENTEROENCEPHALIC ENDOCRINE AXIS	ENTEROINSULAR AXIS
Vertical banded gastroplasty, historical	++++	0	0	0
Lap adjustable gastric banding	++++	0	0	0
Laparoscopic sleeve gastrectomy	++++	+	++++	++
Roux-en-Y gastric bypass	++++	+++	++++	+++
Biliopancreatic diversion/duodenal switch	++	++++	+++	++++

Enteroencephalic Endocrine Axis

RYGB and LSG are known to increase satiety and reduce hunger. During the periprandial phase, the interplay between the gastrointestinal (GI) tract and the regulatory centers of the brain has been shown to activate complex neural networks to modulate food intake. In the central nervous system, the hypothalamus is the key area involved in the regulation of appetite. The hypothalamus regulates energy intake using a complex system of anorexic and orexigenic neuronal signaling. NPY is the dominant hormonal signal regulating energy intake. Release of NPY is modulated by hormones secreted into the circulation by GI cells, such as ghrelin and peptide YY (PYY).

Ghrelin is secreted into the circulation by P/D1 cells located in the fundus of the stomach. Ghrelin levels increase significantly before a meal, and levels quickly diminish postprandially. Ghrelin activates receptors in the arcuate nucleus and the lateral hypothalamus, stimulating the synthesis of NPY and agouti-related protein. This activation creates an orexigenic signal. The role of ghrelin in the post–bariatric surgery regulation of appetite has been extensively studied, sometimes with controversial results. Most studies show that ghrelin levels fall significantly after LSG. In patients who undergo RYGB, the results of various studies are contradictory, especially when they compare fasting levels. A recent cross-sectional study performed by Svane and colleagues[26] has finally provided more definitive data regarding ghrelin levels during the periprandial period in post–bariatric surgery patients. In this study, the postprandial areas under the curve (AUCs) for total and acylated ghrelin were significantly lower after LSG as compared with RYGB and controls. In addition, total ghrelin AUC was significantly lower after RYGB as compared with controls. This study provides significant evidence that anatomic changes after bariatric surgery reduce the postprandial secretion of ghrelin and thereby reduce hunger signals.

PYY is another hormone that acts on NPY neurons. L-cells found throughout the small and large intestines secrete PYY in response to the presence of nutrients within the lumen of the distal gut. PYY exerts an anorexigenic effect on NPY neurons. Svane and colleagues[26] showed that postprandial PYY levels are significantly affected by bariatric surgery. Patients after RYGB have significantly higher PYY peaks and AUCs than patients after LSG and matched controls. No difference in PYY or AUCs was observed between LSG and matched obese controls.[26]

Enteroinsular Endocrine Axis

The remission/amelioration of type 2 diabetes mellitus is considered one of the major benefits after bariatric surgery. Although the mechanisms involved in type 2 diabetes mellitus remission are not completely understood, the improved insulin action, β-cell function, and modulative effect of gut hormones in the enteroinsular axis appear to play a significant role. Among these hormones, glucagon-like peptide-1 (GLP-1) appears to be the major player. GLP-1 is released by L-cells in the distal GI tract, and levels increase in response to the presence of nutrients in the lumen of the distal or hindgut intestines. In obese subjects, there is a delay in the postprandial release of GLP-1 and, overall, significantly reduced circulating levels of the peptide.[27] GLP-1 is known to exert anorexigenic effects in obese subjects secondary to a reduction in gastric emptying. However, GLP-1 action is more predominant in the enteroinsular axis. GLP-1 is part of a family of peptides involved in the synthesis, secretion, and regulation of insulin: the incretins. In the enteroinsular axis, GLP-1 has many physiologic functions, including the stimulation of insulin secretion by the pancreas, an increase in the insulin sensitivity of pancreatic cells (α cells and β cells), and inhibition of glucagon secretion. Many studies have shown that GLP-1 is a major driver of insulin secretion after bariatric surgery. GLP-1 has been found to be consistently elevated (peak and postprandial AUC) in response to both RYGB and LSG, with significantly higher magnitude in RYGB than LSG. More important, the effect of both RYGB and LSG on postprandial GLP-1 secretion is not observed in subjects with an equivalent degree of weight loss achieved only by caloric restriction.[23] The pivotal role of GLP-1 in the metabolic changes observed after bariatric surgery was reaffirmed in a recent study focused on mechanisms of recurrent weight gain after RYGB.[28] The study demonstrated that the weight-regain group had less augmented postprandial GLP-1 response but exaggerated hyperinsulinemia compared with the sustained weight loss group. These results provide further evidence of a metabolic effect for bariatric surgery that is independent of weight loss.

PREOPERATIVE EVALUATION AND SELECTION

Eligibility

Selection of patients for bariatric surgery is based on currently accepted NIH and American Heart Association/American College of Cardiology/Obesity Society (AHA/ACC/OS) guidelines. Patients must have a BMI greater than 40 kg/m² without associated comorbid medical conditions or a BMI greater than 35 kg/m² with an associated comorbid medical problem. The ASMBS and IFSO recently updated their recommendations in 2022 to include all individuals with a BMI greater than 35 kg/m² regardless of presence, absence, or severity of comorbidities and noted that it should be considered in patients with a BMI of 30 to 34.9 kg/m² with associated comorbidity, although insurance companies have yet to adopt approval based on these newly recommended BMI parameters.[6]

In addition to BMI and comorbidities, patients must have also failed dietary and behavioral therapy. Several criteria must also be used as guidelines for indications for surgery, including psychiatric stability, motivated attitude, and ability to comprehend the nature of the operation and its resultant changes in eating behavior and lifestyle. Criteria for eligibility for bariatric surgery are given in Box 99.2. An inability to fulfill these criteria is a contraindication to bariatric surgery.

One criterion not listed in Box 99.2 that, unfortunately, is often a significant issue for a severely obese patient is insurance coverage for the operation. The Affordable Care Act (ACA) mandates that patients covered under the ACA Marketplace health plans must receive obesity screening and counseling without charging of copayment or coinsurance even if the patient has not met the yearly deductible. Remarkably, the ACA does not mandate coverage for bariatric surgery, and most federal Marketplace insurance coverage does not cover bariatric surgery, despite that the writers of the ACA wanted to prevent bias against preexisting conditions and the overwhelming evidence that bariatric surgery is the only effective modality of long-term treatment in this population. Meanwhile, medical societies recognize the need to refer severely obese individuals to bariatric surgeons, particularly for the care of patients with type 2 diabetes mellitus. In the most recent guidelines, the American

Diabetes Association states: "Consider metabolic surgery as a weight and glycemic management approach in patients with BMI > 30.0 kg/m²."[29]

The Centers for Medicare and Medicaid Services (CMS), the federal agency that sets Medicare guidelines, established criteria for coverage of bariatric surgery in 2006. The ruling required that only surgeons in hospitals that are designated Centers of Excellence perform bariatric surgery. As outcomes improved, in 2013 CMS removed this requirement. Yet today, the majority of bariatric procedures are performed at Metabolic and Bariatric Accredited and Quality Improvement Programs (MBSAQIPs). Accreditation, improvement in communication, and structured quality programs have been important in the improvements in quality of care. The ASMBS has recently published recommendations on credentialing of bariatric surgeons by hospitals that include the need for active participation within a structured bariatric surgery program and quality improvement program. Although hospital-wide coordination of care, communication, and multidisciplinary teams must function well to achieve best results in bariatric surgery, the technical skill of the individual surgeon is highly correlated with significantly fewer complications, readmissions, reoperations, and visits to the emergency department as well. Overall, bariatric operative mortality has declined around the world to remarkably low levels, and mortality in the United States is only 0.07%.[30] In summary, these studies show that the surgeon not only must achieve technical proficiency but also must engage the entire operative and hospital team to achieve excellent outcomes.

Medical contraindications to bariatric surgery are relative, and all patients with comorbid conditions are at greater risk. The surgeon must ensure that these risks are well understood by all patients before bariatric surgery, especially those at high risk. Ideally, several family members are included in these discussions. Surgery is also contraindicated in patients who are unable to ambulate because their level of debility precludes recovery during the phase of rapid weight loss after surgery. Prader-Willi syndrome is another absolute contraindication because no surgical therapy affects the hyperphagia that often characterizes this syndrome.

Patients who weigh more than 500 lb are at increased risk for mortality and have more complications. Many options for diagnostic testing, such as computed tomography (CT), are exceeded by this weight limit. At this weight, operating room tables, moving and lift equipment and teams, blood pressure cuffs, sequential compression device (SCD) boots, and any sort of invasive bedside procedures such as central venous catheters become extraordinarily difficult. It has been our practice to require patients weighing more than 500 lb to lose weight down to that level by nonoperative methods.

Age is a controversial consideration in bariatric surgery. For adolescents, most pediatric and bariatric surgeons recommend that the operation be performed after the major growth spurt (mid- to late teens), thus allowing increased maturity on the part of the patient. The Teen–Longitudinal Assessment of Bariatric Surgery (Teen-LABS) and multiple other studies demonstrated that severely obese teens (<19 years) had multiple comorbid conditions and could undergo one of three commonly performed operations (LRYGB, LSG, and laparoscopic adjustable gastric banding [LAGB]) with no mortality and a favorable short-term complication profile. Follow-up after LRYGB or LSG in the Teen-LABS study showed excellent and sustained weight loss and resolution of diabetes in 88% of patients who had type 2 diabetes mellitus at baseline at 5 years, a figure far higher than the 50% to 70% of adult bariatric surgery patients. The authors hypothesize

---

BOX 99.2 Indications for Bariatric Surgery

Patients must meet the following criteria for consideration for bariatric surgery:

- Body mass index (BMI) >35 kg/m² or BMI >30 kg/m² with an associated medical comorbidity worsened by obesity
- Failed dietary therapy
- Psychiatrically stable and without alcohol dependence or illegal drug use
- Knowledgeable about the operation and its sequelae
- Motivated individual
- Medical problems not precluding probable survival from surgery

that adults accumulate pounds-years that are less reversible than in the adolescent population. They conclude that bariatric surgery is effective at 5 years in adolescents.[31]

Although, in our practice, we have generally set the age of 65 years as a rough cutoff for performing gastric bypass and 70 years for LSG, patients older than 70 years have been individually evaluated. Such evaluations focus on the patient's level of frailty and potential for longevity rather than chronologic age. The duration and degree of obesity are the most important factors in evaluating an older patient. In general, the duration and the severity of obesity and the number of comorbid medical problems that exist lower the potential for such individuals to benefit from bariatric surgery.

General Bariatric Preoperative Evaluation and Preparation

Preoperative assessment of a bariatric surgical patient involves two distinct areas. One is a specific preoperative assessment of candidacy for bariatric surgery and evaluation for comorbid conditions. The second is a general assessment and preoperative preparation, just as for any major abdominal surgery, which is discussed in depth in Chapter 19. A team approach is required for optimal care of the patient, as shown in Box 99.3. Box 99.4 summarizes the steps and tests routinely performed for the preoperative evaluation of bariatric patients in the authors' clinics. Proper preoperative patient education is essential, and attendance at educational sessions is mandatory. After preoperative testing is completed, a final counseling session with the surgeon and an education session with the nurse educator and dietician are held.

Data support the use of preoperative antibiotics and deep venous thrombosis (DVT) prophylaxis. A first-generation cephalosporin, in a dose appropriate for weight, is given preoperatively. Bariatric surgery patients are at moderate to high risk for venous thromboembolism (VTE), and they should receive mechanical prophylaxis, such as early ambulation and use of SCDs. Most patients are at moderate or high risk for VTE, and the preponderance of data suggests that both chemoprophylaxis and mechanical measures be used based on individual assessment of clinical judgment and risk of bleeding. The Michigan Bariatric Surgery Collaborative (MBSC) identified that preoperative and postoperative use of low-molecular-weight heparin was associated with significantly lower rates of VTE compared with patients given unfractionated heparin. High-risk patients (e.g., those with history of DVT, venous stasis ulcers, known or highly suspected pulmonary hypertension, hypoventilation syndrome of obesity, or need for reoperation during

---

BOX 99.4   Preoperative Evaluation and Postoperative Care

Before the Clinic Visit
- Documented, medically supervised diet
- Counseling and referral from the primary care physician
- Reading a comprehensive written brochure and/or attendance at a seminar regarding operative procedures, expected results, and potential complications

Initial Clinic Visit
- Group presentation on information in the booklet
- Group presentation on preoperative and postoperative nutritional issues by the nutritionist
- Individual assessment by the surgeon's team
- Individual counseling session with the surgeon
- Individual counseling session with the nutritionist
- Screening blood tests

Subsequent Events/Evaluations
- Full psychological assessment and evaluation as indicated
- Medical specialist evaluations as indicated
- Insurance approval for coverage of the procedure
- Screening flexible upper endoscopy as indicated
- Screening ultrasound of the gallbladder (if present) as indicated
- Arterial blood gas analysis as indicated

Subsequent Clinic Visits
- Counseling session with the surgeon (including selection of the date for surgery)
- Education session with the nurse educator
- Preoperative evaluation by the anesthesiologist
- Final paperwork by the preadmissions center

BOX 99.3   The Bariatric Multidisciplinary Team

- Surgeon
- Assisting surgeon
- Nutritionist
- Anesthesiologist
- Operating room nurse
- Operating room scrub tech or nurse
- Nurse care coordinator or educator
- Secretary/administrator
- Psychiatrist/psychologist
- Primary care physician
- Medical specialists for cardiac, pulmonary, gastrointestinal, endocrine, musculoskeletal, and neurologic conditions as indicated

---

the initial hospitalization) are given low-molecular-weight heparin administered twice daily for a full 2-week course.

Evaluation of Specific Comorbid Conditions

Cardiovascular evaluation of a bariatric patient must include a history of recent chest pain and functional assessment of activity in relation to cardiac function. Patients with a history of recent chest pain or a change in exercise tolerance need to undergo a formal cardiology assessment, including stress testing as indicated.

The prevalence of obstructive sleep apnea diagnosed using sleep studies in patients with morbid obesity ranges between 35% and 94%, and the majority of the studies identified a prevalence of greater than 60%. A history of falling asleep while driving or while at work or a history of feeling tired after a night's sleep, coupled with a history of snoring or even witnessed apnea, is strongly suggestive of the condition. Patients with suggestive histories of clinically significant sleep apnea should undergo a preoperative sleep study. If the patient is found to have sleep apnea, use of a continuous or bilevel positive airway pressure apparatus postoperatively while sleeping can eliminate the stressful periods of hypoxia that would otherwise result and has been found to reduce perioperative complications. Although tolerated under normal circumstances, these hypoxic episodes in the immediate postoperative period are more treacherous because of the enhanced effect of narcotic pain medications and postoperative fluid shifts that affect hemodynamic stability.

Reactive asthma is another common problem in this patient population and one that is underrecognized. It requires less preoperative preparation in terms of testing than sleep apnea does and is less dangerous.

Because there is an increased incidence of hypertension and diabetes in patients with concomitant renal disease, the serum creatinine value is an excellent preoperative screening test for baseline renal function.

Musculoskeletal conditions, especially arthritis and degenerative joint disease, are the most common group of comorbid diseases found in patients with severe obesity. More than half the patients have some form of these conditions, often to an advanced degree. Limited ambulation, joint replacement, severe back pain, and other sequelae are not uncommon. Before surgery, it is important for patients to understand that any preexisting structural damage cannot be reversed by weight loss. Fortunately, significant weight loss often alleviates or even eliminates the chronic pain or disability from such conditions. Significant weight loss after bariatric surgery will make subsequent knee and hip replacement surgery more effective and safer.

Metabolic problems are common in severely obese patients, particularly hyperlipidemia, hypercholesterolemia, and type 2 diabetes mellitus. All are easily screened for by simple blood tests. Of patients undergoing bariatric surgery, 20% to 30% have clinically significant type 2 diabetes mellitus. Diabetes needs to be controlled preoperatively to reduce the risk of perioperative morbidity.

The skin must be examined for fungal infection and venous stasis changes, which are associated with a greatly increased incidence of postoperative DVT. Umbilical or ventral hernias may be present. It has been our practice to postpone repair of ventral and incisional hernias until after significant weight loss. Repair of the hernias at the time of abdominoplasty enables the surgeon to complete physical reconstruction of the abdominal wall and to place prosthetic mesh to reinforce the abdominal wall, something that often cannot be accomplished during the initial bariatric procedure.

Cholelithiasis is the most prevalent of the several GI conditions, and if a history of symptomatic cholelithiasis is present, most surgeons agree that cholecystectomy needs to be performed simultaneously with the bariatric surgery. However, we do not routinely perform screening ultrasounds. Of note, the incidence of gallstone or sludge formation after gastric bypass is approximately 30%. Ursodeoxycholic acid, 300 mg twice daily for 6 months postoperatively, reduces the incidence of gallstone formation to 3% in patients who follow this treatment plan. Our current recommendations for patients undergoing laparoscopic bariatric surgery are simultaneous cholecystectomy if a history of symptomatic gallstones is present and ursodiol therapy for 6 months after surgery if the gallbladder is normal.

GERD is also common in these patients because of the increased abdominal pressure and shortened lower esophageal sphincter. Preoperative upper endoscopy is indicated in all patients who have GERD symptoms to detect Barrett esophagus and the presence of hiatal hernias and to evaluate the distal stomach in patients undergoing RYGB.

A patient with nonalcoholic steatotic hepatitis (NASH) presents a potential problem. The size of the left lobe of the liver often interferes with the surgeon's ability to complete an operation laparoscopically. Patients with known enlarged fatty livers may benefit from calorie restriction, especially carbohydrate restriction, for a period of 5 to 10 days preoperatively. Bariatric surgery is beneficial for NASH because weight loss improves the prognosis. NASH is not a contraindication to bariatric surgery if there is no cirrhosis and portal hypertension or hepatocellular decompensation. Liver biopsy should be performed at the time of bariatric surgery in any patient whose liver appears abnormal.

Special Equipment

Clinic

The clinic for evaluating bariatric patients must be constructed with the needs of the patient in mind. The waiting area must contain comfortable benches with backs, not standard-size chairs. Doorways must be extra wide to accommodate wheelchairs. This is true for bathrooms as well, which must be equipped with toilets on the floor, not mounted on the wall. A scale that can weigh up to 800 lb is necessary. Large-sized gowns, wide examining tables stable enough for large patients, and wide blood pressure cuffs are needed. A large room with appropriate seating is needed for the patient group education session.

Operating Room

The operating room should contain a hydraulically operated table that can accommodate up to 800 lb. Side attachments to widen the table as needed are required. Foam cushioning, extra-large SCD stockings, wide and secure padded straps for the abdomen and legs, and a footboard for the operating room table are all essential to safely secure the patient for placement in a steep reverse Trendelenburg position during surgery. Video telescopic equipment, as used for any laparoscopic abdominal procedure, is necessary. Two monitors, one near each shoulder, and high-flow insufflators able to maintain pneumoperitoneum are essential.

A 45-degree telescope, extra-long staplers, atraumatic graspers, extra-long trocars, and ultrasonic scalpel or other energy source instruments are essential for laparoscopic operations. A fixed retractor device secured to the operating room table for clamping and holding the liver retractor is essential. This can pose one of the most difficult technical challenges in patients with a large, thick liver.

OPERATIVE PROCEDURES

Laparoscopic Adjustable Gastric Banding

The LAGB procedure may be performed with any of multiple types of adjustable bands with similar technique; only the locking mechanisms, band shape and configuration, and adjustment schedules vary somewhat for the different types of bands. Their advantage over other bariatric procedures is individualized adjustability and a markedly lower initial operative morbidity and mortality.

Trocar placement for LAGB may vary, but typically, an 11-mm trocar is placed supraumbilically, a 15-mm trocar in the left upper quadrant, a 5-mm trocar in the left upper quadrant, and a 12-mm trocar in the right upper quadrant, with a Nathanson retractor in the epigastric region. The surgeon stands to the patient's right; the assistant and the camera operator are to the patient's left. Most surgeons place the patient in the supine position, but some prefer to have the patient's legs spread so that the surgeon can stand between the legs. The peritoneum at the angle of His is divided to create an opening in the peritoneum between the angle of His and the top of the spleen.

The pars flaccida technique has become the approach of choice for placing the adjustable band; it begins with dividing the gastrohepatic ligament in its thin area just over the caudate lobe of the liver. The anterior branch of the vagus nerve is spared, and any aberrant left hepatic artery is preserved. The base of the right crus of the diaphragm is identified. Care must be taken to definitively identify the crus because, occasionally, the vena cava can lie close to the caudate lobe. The surgeon gently follows the surface of the right crus posterior and inferior to the esophagus while aiming for the angle of His (Fig. 99.2A). A gentle spreading and pushing technique is used to create a tunnel along this generally avascular plane. Once the tip of the tunneling instrument is seen near the superior pole of the spleen, it is gently pushed through any remaining peritoneal layers to complete the tunnel. The adjustable band has already been placed in the peritoneal cavity through the large 15-mm trocar located in the right upper quadrant before dissection of the pars flaccida. The narrow end of the band itself is grasped by the tunneling instrument and pulled through the tunnel from the greater to the lesser side of the stomach (see Fig. 99.2B). That end is then threaded through the locking mechanism of the band, after which the band is locked. Once the band has been locked in place, the buckle is adjusted to lie on the lesser curvature side of the stomach (see Fig. 99.2C). A 5-mm grasper inserted between the band and stomach ensures that the band is not too tight.

The anterior gastric wall is plicated over the band with three or four interrupted, nonabsorbable sutures (see Fig. 99.2D). There needs to be just enough stomach above the level of the band for incorporating that tissue into the suture. Suturing is carried as far

posterolaterally as possible because this region has been the most frequent area of fundus herniation through the band. The band is thus ideally secured about 1 cm below the gastroesophageal junction with this technique.

The Silastic tubing leading from the band is pulled through the 15-mm trocar site in the right upper quadrant paramedian area to complete the laparoscopic portion of the operation. The trocar site incision is enlarged to reveal the anterior rectus fascia, which is exposed approximately 2 to 4 cm lateral to the existing fascial defect for the trocar, and the access port is connected to the inflation tubing. Four sutures inserted through the four holes on the access port are placed in the fascia, after which the port is tied to the fascia. The redundant tubing is replaced in the abdominal cavity, with care taken to avoid kinking.

Roux-en-Y Gastric Bypass

The gastric bypass first described by Mason and Ito in 1969 incorporated a loop of jejunum anastomosed to a proximal gastric pouch.

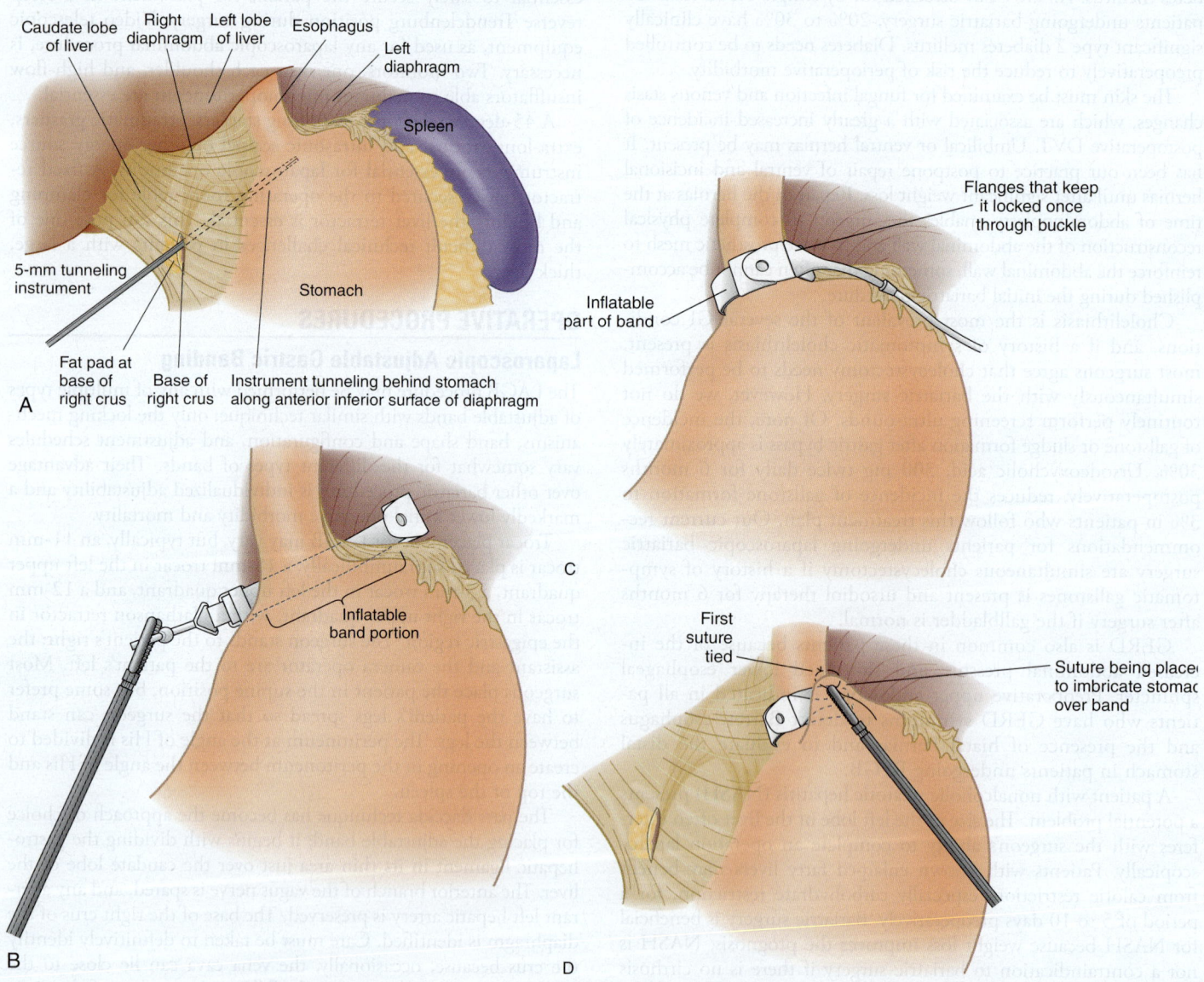

FIGURE 99.2 (A) Pars flaccida technique in which the fat pad is divided at the base of the right crus. (B) Pulling the lap band through the tunnel. (C) Locking the lap band. (D) Imbricating the anterior aspect of the stomach over the lap band.

This operation proved unacceptable because of bile reflux, and RYGB, which eliminates bile reflux, has become one of the most commonly performed bariatric operations in the United States.

Described here is one technique that incorporates many of these modifications. There are certainly many variations of this technique, and many, if not most, will give excellent results. The essential principles of the operation are listed in Table 99.5.

The left subcostal region, near the midclavicular line, is an ideal location for the first trocar. Either a bladed trocar (United States Surgical Corporation, Norwalk, CT) or an optical trocar (Optiview, Ethicon Endo-Surgery, Cincinnati, OH) that dilates a tract under direct vision is placed. Subsequent trocars are placed under laparoscopic vision to achieve the configuration shown in Fig. 99.3.

Once the omentum is mobilized, the ligament of Treitz is identified. A location approximately 50 cm distal to the ligament is chosen for division of the jejunum with an endoscopic stapler (Fig. 99.4). The mesentery is then further divided with staples or a harmonic scalpel.

The length of the Roux limb is influenced in our practices by the patient's weight. Patients with a BMI in the 40s will be well served with a Roux limb of 100 cm, whereas a Roux limb of approximately 150 cm is constructed for patients with a BMI in excess of 50. The

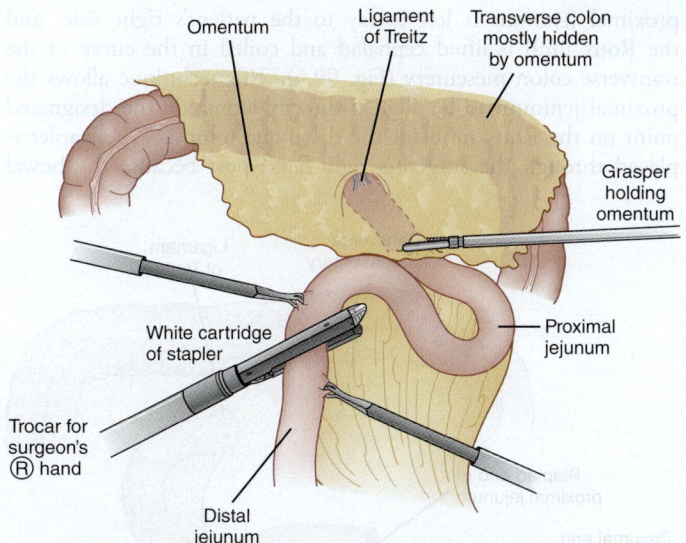

FIGURE 99.4 Trocar configuration for laparoscopic Roux-en-Y gastric bypass and for laparoscopic sleeve gastrectomy.

TABLE 99.5	Technical Considerations During Laparoscopic Roux-en-Y Gastric Bypass	
TECHNIQUE	**RECOMMENDATION**	**RATIONALE**
Pouch size	15–20 mL	Smaller pouch reduces marginal ulceration and is associated with improved long-term weight loss
Method of gastrojejunostomy	No difference in techniques between circular stapler, linear cutter, or hand-sewn	Although the circular stapler is the most common technique, all have similar outcomes. Biggest difference is skill and efficiency of the surgeon.
Operative time	Faster surgical procedures associated with reduced complications	Surgical skill and efficiency trump all other factors when comparing, adjusting for patient characteristics.
Mesenteric defects	Closure of all mesenteric defects with nonabsorbable sutures	Marked reduction in internal hernia formation requiring surgical correction
Antecolic or retrocolic Roux limb	Antecolic	The antecolic is technically easier and reduces the number of mesenteric defects from three to one; the Roux limb is at least 75 cm in length
Fibrin sealant	Use fibrin sealant	Associated in some studies with reduced leak rates

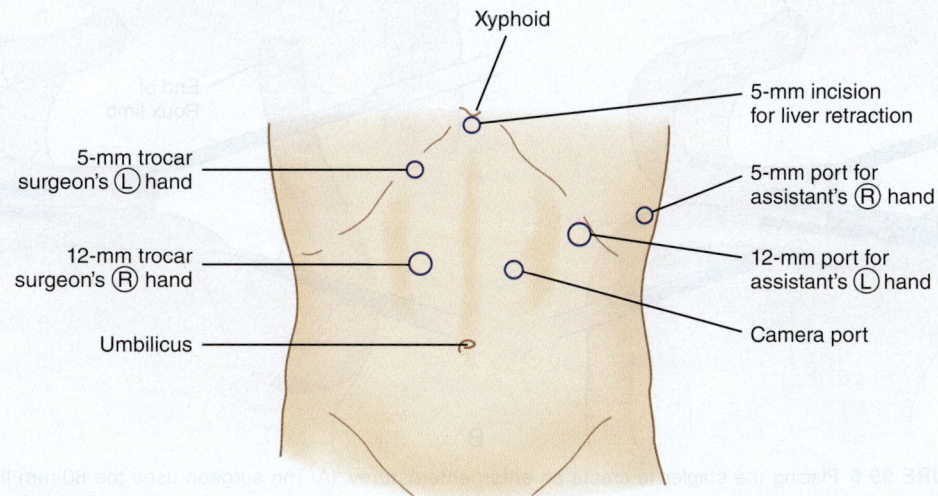

FIGURE 99.3 Trocar configuration for laparoscopic Roux-en-Y gastric bypass and for laparoscopic sleeve gastrectomy.

proximal jejunum is left to lay to the patient's right side, and the Roux limb is lifted cephalad and coiled in the curve of the transverse colon mesentery (Fig. 99.5). This technique allows the proximal jejunum to be aligned directly alongside the designated point on the Roux limb for the distal anastomosis. The stapler is placed through the surgeon's right-hand port because the bowel

segments are easily aligned to facilitate placement of the stapler into enterotomies created in each segment of bowel at the desired location of the anastomosis (Fig. 99.6). Another firing of the stapler, this time from the left side of the patient, creates a large side-to-side anastomosis. Once the anastomosis is created, the stapler defect is closed with another fire of the stapler.

The left lobe liver retractor is now placed, and the patient is placed in the reverse Trendelenburg position. Exposure of the angle of His allows division of the peritoneum between the top of the spleen and the gastroesophageal junction with the ultrasonic scalpel. The lesser sac is entered through the gastrohepatic ligament, 3 to 4 cm below the gastroesophageal junction. The linear stapler is now fired multiple times to create a 20- to 30-mL proximal gastric pouch based on the upper lesser curvature of the stomach (Fig. 99.7). Once the gastric pouch is created, the Roux limb may be passed toward the proximal gastric pouch through a retrocolic or antecolic pathway. The antecolic, antegastric approach is preferred to prevent the risk of an internal hernia through the transverse mesocolon or a hernia formed by the transverse mesocolon and the mesentery of the Roux limb in the retrocolic approach. The gastrojejunostomy may be performed with a circular stapler (Fig. 99.8), a hand-sutured technique, or a linear stapler oversewing the common enterotomy. The entire anastomosis is irrigated with saline, and a member of the operative team uses the endoscope to monitor occlusion of the Roux limb with an atraumatic 10-mm bowel clamp. Even the smallest leaks of air can be identified and closed with this technique. Studies have shown that use of this technique can dramatically reduce the incidence of postoperative leaks to very low levels. The mesenteric defect in the jejunojejunostomy is closed with a purse-string suture of 2-0 polypropylene, and Petersen's defect (between the Roux limb mesentery and the transverse mesocolon) is closed

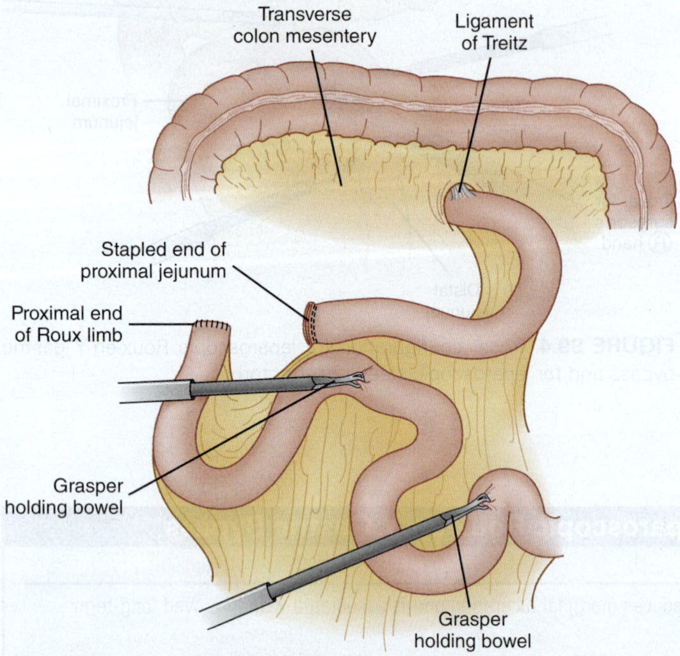

FIGURE 99.5 Measuring and laying out the jejunum to set up a distal anastomosis for the length of the Roux-en-Y gastric bypass.

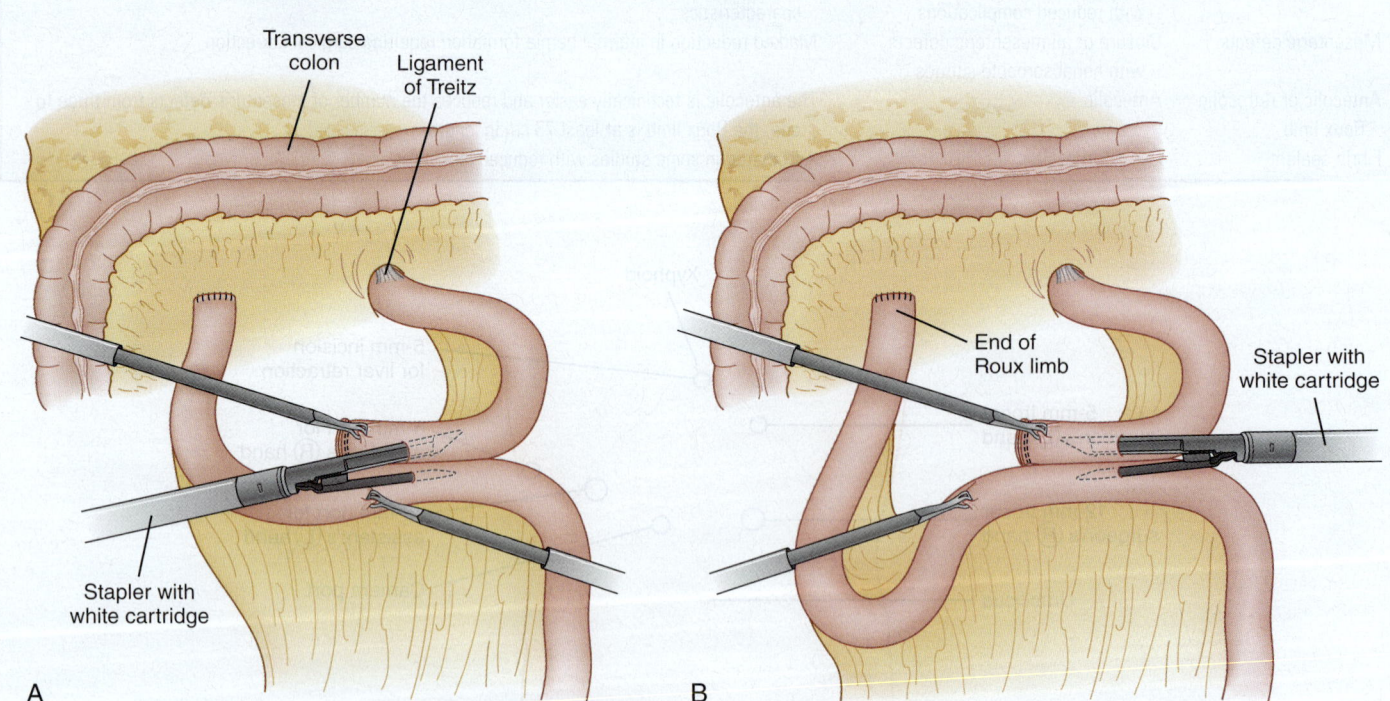

FIGURE 99.6 Placing the stapler to create an enteroenterostomy. (A) The surgeon uses the 60-mm linear stapler to create the jejunojejunostomy between the biliopancreatic limb and the Roux limb. (B) The first assistant uses the 60-mm linear stapler to create a larger jejunojejunostomy. Not shown is the closure of the enterotomy using the 60-mm linear cutter as the final step.

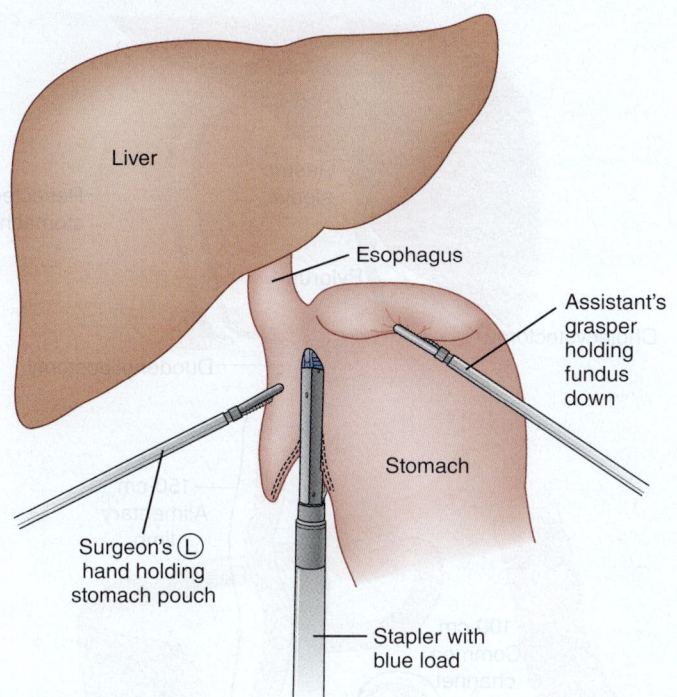

FIGURE 99.7 Firing the stapler to create the proximal gastric pouch.

with a purse-string suture of 2-0 silk; defect closure has significantly reduced internal hernia rates (Fig. 99.9; see Table 99.5).

Biliopancreatic Diversion

Biliopancreatic diversion (BPD), like most bariatric operations that had been performed through an open approach, can be performed through a laparoscopic approach. BPD produces weight loss primarily based on malabsorption, but it does have a restrictive component as well.

The anatomic configuration of BPD is shown in Fig. 99.10. The intestinal tract is reconstructed to allow only a short, so-called common channel of the distal 50 cm of terminal ileum for absorption of fat and protein. The alimentary tract beyond the proximal part of the stomach is rearranged to include only the distal 200 cm of ileum, including the common channel. The proximal end of this ileum is anastomosed to the proximal end of the stomach after a distal hemigastrectomy is performed. The ileum proximal to the end that is anastomosed to the stomach is in turn anastomosed to the terminal ileum within the 50- to 100-cm distance from the ileocecal valve, depending on the surgeon's preference and the patient's size. This procedure is very rarely performed today and is included for historical and educational context.

Biliopancreatic Diversion With Duodenal Switch

The biliopancreatic diversion with duodenal switch (BPD-DS) configuration is shown in Fig. 99.11. This modification was developed to help lessen the high incidence of marginal ulcers after BPD. The mechanism of weight loss is similar to that of BPD.

The first step is measurement of the terminal ileum. Notably, in the BPD-DS procedure, the common channel is 200 cm, and the entire alimentary tract is 350 cm. However, the major difference between BPD-DS and BPD is the gastrectomy and pyloric preservation. Instead of a distal hemigastrectomy, a sleeve gastrectomy is performed. This procedure is done as the initial part of the operation

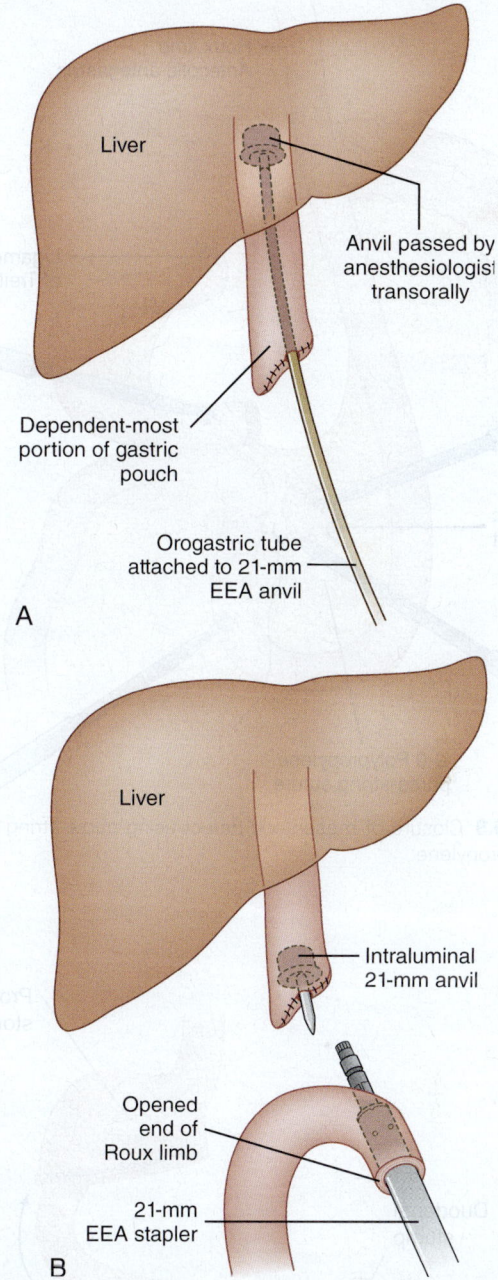

FIGURE 99.8 Creating the proximal anastomosis. (A) Insertion of anvil transorally. (B) Insertion of stapler through Roux and creation of stapled anastomosis using the circular end-to-end anastomosis *(EEA)* stapler.

because if the patient exhibits any intraoperative instability, the operation can be discontinued after the LSG alone. A two-stage BPD-DS has been used in patients who have an extremely high BMI and are high operative risks. The LSG alone usually produces enough weight loss to make the second stage of the operation technically easier. This approach lowers the mortality rate despite the need to undergo two operative procedures. The first step of a laparoscopic BPD-DS is to perform the LSG with a stapling technique that begins at the mid-antrum, and a staple line is created parallel to the lesser curvature of the stomach with a 40- to 60-Fr Maloney dilator placed along the lesser curve to prevent narrowing. The staple line is created with multiple firings of the stapler until the angle of His is reached. The goal is to produce a lesser curvature gastric sleeve with a volume of 150 to 200 mL.

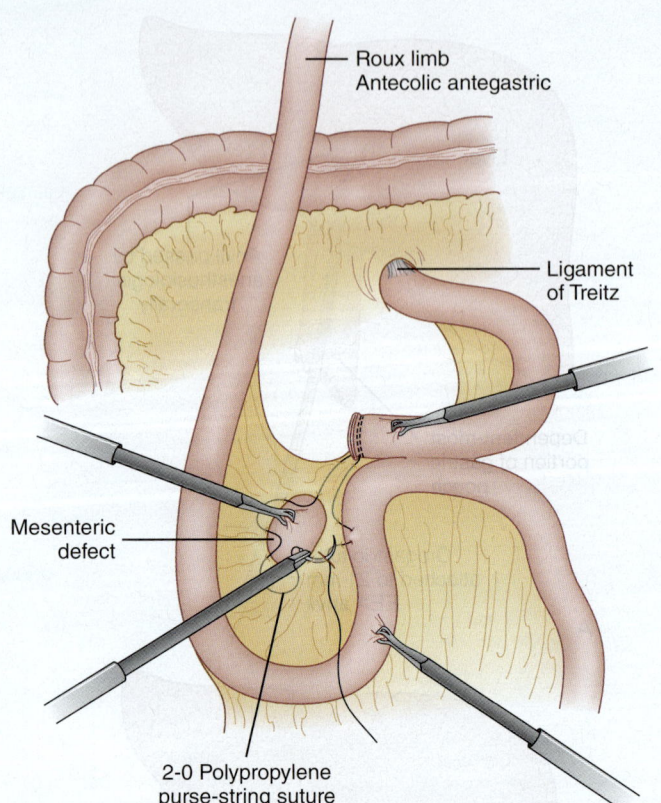

FIGURE 99.9 Closure of mesenteric defect using purse-string suture of 2-0 polypropylene.

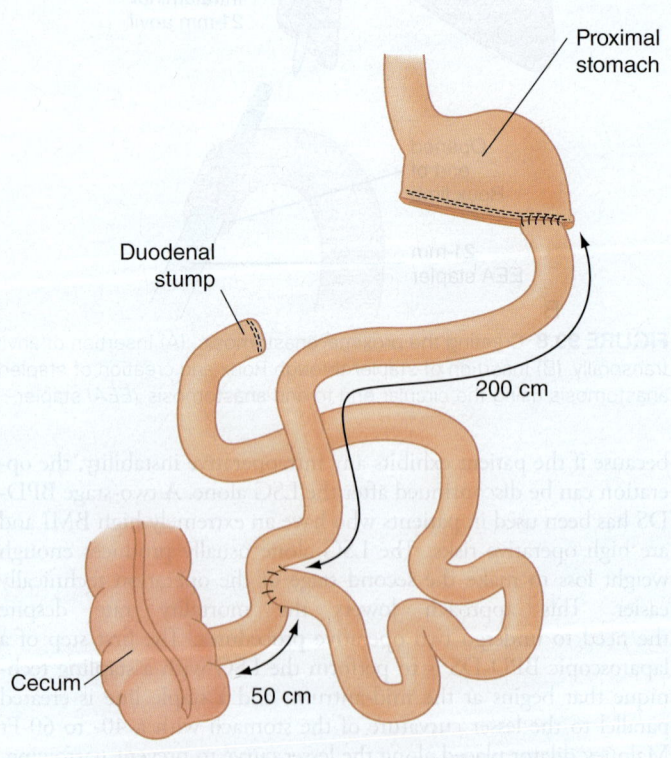

FIGURE 99.10 Anatomic configuration of biliopancreatic diversion.

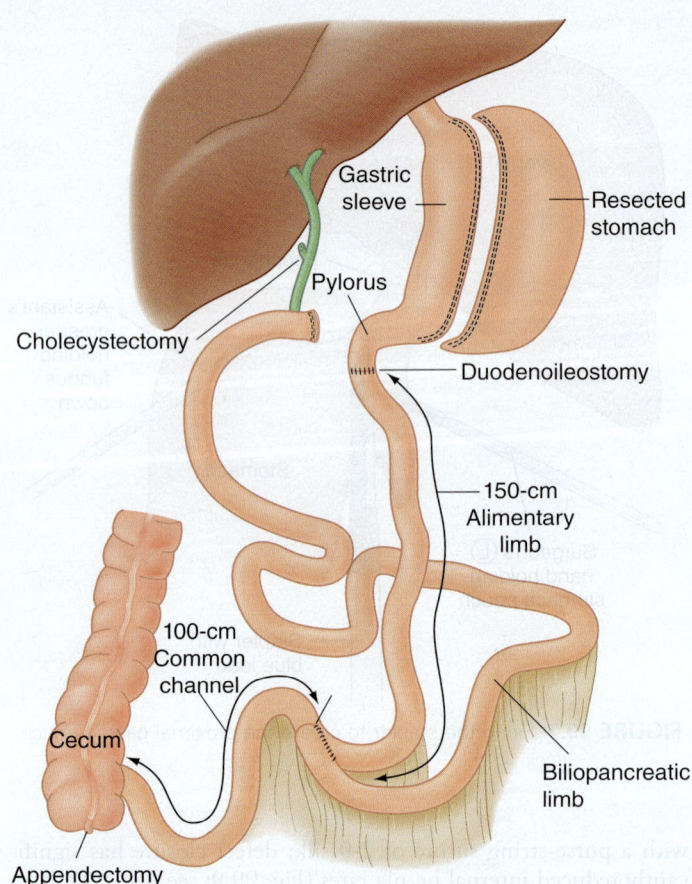

FIGURE 99.11 Anatomic configuration of the biliopancreatic diversion with duodenal switch.

After LSG, the duodenum is divided with the stapler approximately 2 cm beyond the pylorus. The distal connections are performed as for BPD. The distal anastomosis is created at the 200-cm point proximal to the ileocecal valve. The proximal anastomosis is created between the proximal end of the 350 cm of terminal ileum and the first portion of the duodenum (creating a 150-cm alimentary limb, a 100- to 200-cm common channel, and an unmeasured biliopancreatic limb). The duodenoileostomy is an antecolic end-to-side anastomosis. This anastomosis is one of the most critical parts of the operation and can be performed either with a circular stapler or using a hand-sewn technique. If the end-to-end anastomosis (EEA) stapler is used, the anvil is directly inserted through the staple line of the duodenal stump through a gastrostomy under suture guidance or through an oral approach with a nasogastric tube.

Single Anastomosis Duodenal-Ileal Bypass With Sleeve Gastrectomy

The single anastomosis duodenal-ileal bypass with sleeve gastrectomy (SADI-S) is shown in Fig. 99.12. This modification was developed to help decrease the postoperative complications of vitamin deficiencies and malnutrition that can occur with the BPD-DS.

Port placement depends on whether a laparoscopic or robotic-assisted technique is used. For robotic-assisted SADI-S, which is our approach, we use a 12-mm port in the right mid-abdomen, 8-mm port in the left periumbilical position for the camera, 8-mm port in the left lateral abdomen, 12-mm port in the left

size the sleeve, and the stomach is divided from 5 cm proximal to the incisura to the angle of His by sequential firings of a reinforced stapling device. The greater omentum is then taken down distally past the antrum. The first part of the duodenum is circumferentially dissected and transected approximately 3 cm distal to the pylorus. The marked ileum is then brought up into the duodenum, and enterotomies are made in both the duodenum and ileum. It is important to ensure there is no twisting of the ileal mesentery before the anastomosis is completed. An antecolic end-to-side duodenoileostomy is then created. We hand-sew the anastomosis with absorbable suture (posteriorly in two layers, anteriorly in one layer). This can alternatively be completed with a circular or linear stapler. We perform an upper endoscopy and air-leak test to ensure the integrity of the anastomosis.

Laparoscopic Sleeve Gastrectomy

LSG is now recognized as a primary procedure, and a *Current Procedural Terminology* code was assigned to the procedure in 2010. From 2008–17, there was a precipitous increase in the number of LSG procedures (0.9%–59.4% of the total number of bariatric procedures), which is approximately the current percentage of bariatric procedures performed in the United States (Table 99.6).[32] Advantages of LSG are the technical simplicity of the procedure, preservation of the pylorus (avoidance of dumping), metabolic reduction of ghrelin levels, no need for serial adjustments (as for LAGB), reduction in internal hernias (seen after LRYGB, BPD-DS, and SADI-S), reduction in malabsorption (seen with LRYGB, BPD-DS, and SADI-S), and ability to later modify the gastric sleeve to either an LRYGB or a BPD-DS configuration in a second stage of the operation. The trocar placement can be identical to that of LRYGB (see Fig. 99.3). We now often use a 5-mm trocar in the left upper quadrant, a 5-mm trocar left of the umbilicus, a 15-mm trocar right of the umbilicus, and a 5-mm trocar in the right upper quadrant, with a Nathanson retractor placed via an epigastric incision. As a primary procedure, the surgeon takes down the entire greater curvature, leaving intact the tissue within 3 to 5 cm of the pylorus and up to the angle of His and exposing the left crus of the diaphragm. Then, using a 38- or 40-Fr bougie, the stomach is divided from the antrum to

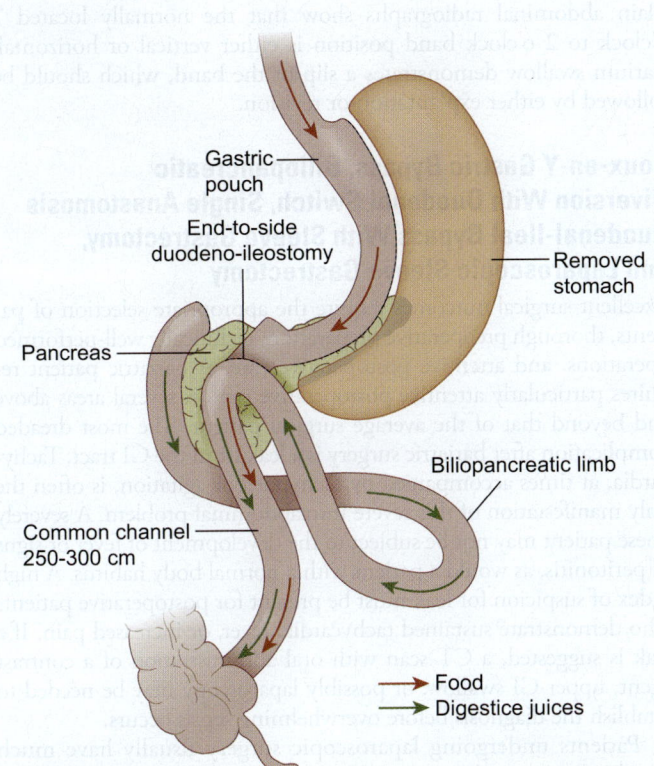

FIGURE 99.12 Anatomic configuration of the single anastomosis duodenal-ileal bypass with sleeve gastrectomy. (https://www.summahealth.org/medicalservices/weight-loss/weight-loss-surgery-options.)

hemi-abdomen between the two 8-mm ports, and a 12-mm port in the right lateral abdomen for assistance. The first step of the procedure is measurement from the terminal ileum. In the SADI-S, the common channel is typically 250 to 350 cm, and the biliopancreatic limb is unmeasured. Next, the sleeve gastrectomy is performed as described earlier. This is done by first taking down the omentum from the greater curve of the stomach with a vessel sealing device. A 38- to 40-Fr bougie is then used to loosely

TABLE 99.6	ASMBS Total Bariatric Procedures Performed in the United States, Published June 2024												
	2011	2012	2013	2014	2015	2016	2017	2018	2019	2020	2021	2022
Total	158,000	173,000	179,000	193,000	196,000	216,000	228,000	253,000	256,000	199,000	263,000	280,000
Sleeve	17.8%	33.0%	42.1%	51.7%	53.6%	58.1%	59.4%	61.4%	59.4%	61.4%	58.1%	57.5%
RYGB	36.7%	37.5%	34.2%	26.8%	23.0%	18.7%	17.8%	17.0%	17.8%	20.8%	21.5%	22.2%
Band	35.4%	20.2%	14.0%	9.5%	5.78%	3.4%	2.8%	1.1%	0.9%	1.2%	0.4%	0.9%
BPD-DS	0.9%	1.0%	1.0%	0.4%	0.6%	0.6%	0.7%	0.8%	0.9%	1.8%	2.1%	2.2%
SADI	—	—	—	—	—	—	—	—	—	0.2%	0.4%	0.6%
Revision	6.0%	6.0%	6.0%	11.5%	13.6%	13.9%	14.1%	15.4%	16.7%	11.1%	11.8%	11.0%
Other	3.2%	2.3%	2.7%	0.1%	3.2%	2.6%	2.5%	2.3%	2.4%	0.6%	2.8%	2.2%
Balloons	—	—	—	—	0.4%	2.7%	2.8%	2.0%	1.8%	1.4%	1.6%	1.6%

The ASMBS total bariatric procedure numbers are based on the best estimation from available data (Bariatric Outcomes Longitudinal Database, ACS/MBSAQIP, National Inpatient Sample Data, and outpatient estimations).
ACS/MBSAQIP, American College of Surgeons/Metabolic and Bariatric Surgery Accreditation and Quality Improvement Program; *ASMBS,* American Society for Metabolic and Bariatric Surgery; *Band,* adjustable gastric banding; *BPD-DS,* biliopancreatic diversion-duodenal switch; *SADI,* single anastomosis duodenal-ileal bypass; *Sleeve,* sleeve gastrectomy; *RYGB,* Roux-en-Y gastric bypass.
From Clapp B, Ponce J, Corbett J, et al. American Society for Metabolic and Bariatric Surgery 2022 estimate of metabolic and bariatric procedures performed in the United States. *Surg Obes Relat Dis.* 2024;20(5):425-431.

the angle of His by sequential firings of the stapler (Fig. 99.13). It is vitally important in this procedure to preserve the left gastric vessels and lesser curve blood supply and prevent twisting or spiraling of the gastric tube. Major controversy exists about techniques to reinforce the staple line to prevent bleeding or leaks from the staple line (Table 99.7).

POSTOPERATIVE CARE AND FOLLOW-UP

Laparoscopic Adjustable Gastric Banding

Patients undergoing LAGB experience an operation that may last as little as 1 hour in experienced hands. Same-day discharge is the norm. The band is initially placed without adding any saline to distend it. Saline is added in 1.0- to 1.5-mL increments to produce a desired weight loss of 1 to 2 kg/week. Excess weight loss (EWL) may lead to actual removal of a small amount of saline, whereas inadequate weight loss is an indication for the addition of more saline to the system to increase the restriction of the band. The incidence of nutritional deficiencies is low after LAGB because there is no disruption of the normal GI tract. Slippage of the lap band can result in acute strangulation of the stomach, necessitating emergency surgical removal of the band, but is more likely to present with symptoms of dysphagia, regurgitation, heartburn, and aspiration.

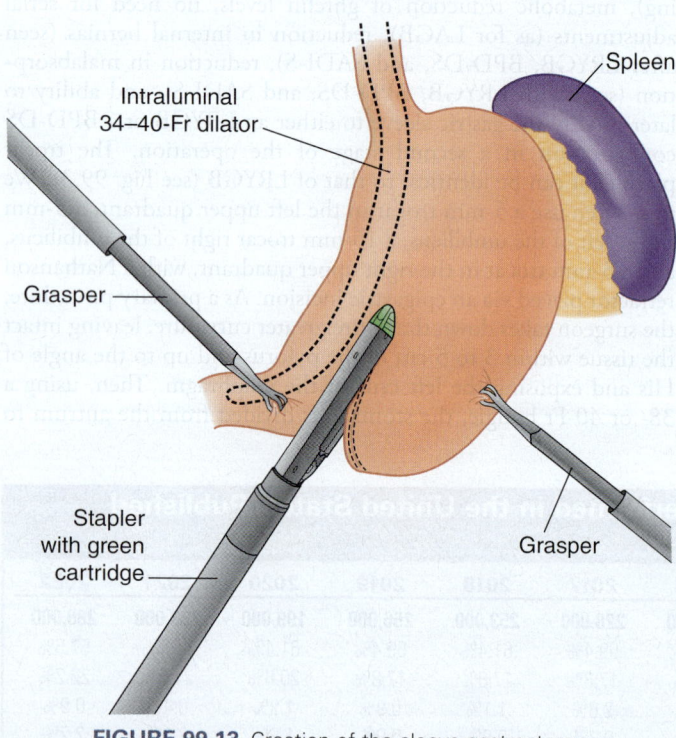

FIGURE 99.13 Creation of the sleeve gastrectomy.

Labels on figure: Spleen; Intraluminal 34–40-Fr dilator; Grasper; Stapler with green cartridge; Grasper

Plain abdominal radiographs show that the normally located 7 o'clock to 2 o'clock band position is either vertical or horizontal. Barium swallow demonstrates a slip of the band, which should be followed by either explantation or revision.

Roux-en-Y Gastric Bypass, Biliopancreatic Diversion With Duodenal Switch, Single Anastomosis Duodenal-Ileal Bypass With Sleeve Gastrectomy, and Laparoscopic Sleeve Gastrectomy

Excellent surgical outcomes require the appropriate selection of patients, thorough preoperative preparation, technically well-performed operations, and attentive postoperative care. A bariatric patient requires particularly attentive postoperative care in several areas above and beyond that of the average surgical patient. The most dreaded complication after bariatric surgery is a leak from the GI tract. Tachycardia, at times accompanied by tachypnea or agitation, is often the only manifestation of this severe intraabdominal problem. A severely obese patient may not be subject to the development of fever or signs of peritonitis, as would a patient with a normal body habitus. A high index of suspicion for leak must be present for postoperative patients who demonstrate sustained tachycardia, fever, or increased pain. If a leak is suggested, a CT scan with oral administration of a contrast agent, upper GI swallow, or possibly laparoscopy may be needed to establish the diagnosis before overwhelming sepsis occurs.

Patients undergoing laparoscopic surgery usually have much less third space and operative blood loss than patients undergoing open surgery and can be managed with 4 mL/kg/hour of intravenous (IV) fluids. Urine output intraoperatively is normally low because of the pneumoperitoneum and usually improves in the recovery room area. Some patients who have been taking diuretics chronically may not produce adequate urine output without diuretic use, but the surgeon must ensure that the patient is adequately volume resuscitated before giving diuretics. Higher-than-expected fluid requirements, oliguria, and tachycardia are a constellation of postoperative findings suggesting intraabdominal problems.

Adequate pain control is essential via a multimodal approach. An Enhanced Recovery After Surgery (ERAS) protocol is recommended. We use IV acetaminophen followed by a scheduled PO regimen. We also use an additional scheduled nonnarcotic agent, such as pregabalin or gabapentin, and an as-needed (pro re nata [PRN]) narcotic (e.g., oxycodone). We recommend avoiding a patient-controlled analgesia pump.

Care pathways and ERAS protocols have been implemented in bariatric surgery, emphasizing nonnarcotic multimodality pain control, limitation of IV fluids, and early ambulation. One-night hospitalization and discharge on a bariatric full liquid diet are routine for patients undergoing LSG and RYGB and for some experienced clinicians performing BPD-DS and SADI-S.

TABLE 99.7	Technical Considerations During Laparoscopic Sleeve Gastrectomy	
TECHNIQUE	**RECOMMENDATION**	**RATIONALE**
Bougie size	34–40 Fr	Smaller bougie size associated with gastroesophageal reflux disease
		Larger associated with weight regain
Staple line extent	5 cm proximal to the pylorus	Improved long-term weight loss; do not narrow the incisura
Staple line reinforcement	Surgeon preference	Some studies show increase in leak rate with staple line reinforcement but decrease in bleeding complications

BARIATRIC SURGERY RESULTS

Across the world, bariatric surgery has improved results, with declines over time in operative mortality, hospital stay, and postoperative morbidity. In the United States, Europe, and Asia, operative mortality is nil for LAGB, and the operative mortality for LRYGB and sleeve gastrectomy has fallen to under 0.1%, coming up against operative mortality associated with many other common procedures, such as laparoscopic cholecystectomy or joint replacement (Table 99.8).[33–35] Moreover, a large series reviewing the outcomes in countries or healthcare systems shows that there are significant reductions in comorbidities (diabetes, hypertension, dyslipidemia, sleep apnea, asthma, arthritis, and GERD) and an increase in weight-related QOL and physical HRQOL scores.[11,12,15,36,37]

Laparoscopic Adjustable Gastric Banding

As can be seen in Table 99.6, lap band operations rapidly increased in the early 2000s, peaked in 2011, and declined to 2.8% in 2017, largely secondary to a high rate of reinterventions and inadequate weight loss.[32] During the early 2000s, laparoscopic gastric bypass was associated with high mortality and complication rates, so a number of surgeons adopted the lap band procedure as a much simpler procedure with a dramatically lower morbidity and mortality rate. The early results with lap band were almost uniformly excellent, with modest weight loss and very little morbidity or mortality. Results of the LAGB procedure show no 30-day mortality and reasonable weight loss, as shown in Table 99.8, in select centers.[33,34]

Roux-en-Y Gastric Bypass

RYGB has an established record of accomplishment that is longer than that of any other bariatric operation. Its performance

TABLE 99.8 Results of the Four Major Bariatric Procedures

	O'BRIEN[34]	LAZZATI[33]	FINNO[35]
LAGB			
EWL (%)	45.9	44	NR
Mortality (%)	0.0 Single center (8378 patients)	0.0 (6506 patients)	NR
LSG			
EWL (%)	53–62	56	NR
Mortality (%)	NR	0.08 (17,960 patients)	NR
RYGB			
EWL (%)	56.7	67	NR
Mortality (%)	NR	0.11 (10,526 patients)	NR
BPD/DS			
EWL	74.1	NR	74.0, SADI-S, 78.2 BPD/DS
Mortality (%)	NR	NR	0.4 SADI-S, 0.6 BPD/DS

BPD, Biliopancreatic diversion; *DS*, duodenal switch; *EWL*, excess weight loss; *LAGB*, laparoscopic adjustable gastric banding; *LSG*, laparoscopic sleeve gastrectomy; *NR*, not reported; *RYGB*, Roux-en-Y gastric bypass; *SADI-S*, single anastomosis duodenal-ileal bypass with sleeve gastrectomy.

TABLE 99.9 Results of Roux-en-Y Gastric Bypass

CRITERIA	COURCOULAS[37]	ADAMS[36]
Number of patients	1738	418
Age (years)	19–75, median 45	18–72
BMI (kg/m^2)	47%	45.9%
Follow-up (years)	7	12
Excess weight loss	52%	NR
Reduction in BMI (kg/m^2)	NR	−11.5
Percentage of baseline weight loss	−28.4% at 7 years	—
Diabetes	58.9% at 7 years	51%
Hypertension	39.3% at 7 years	36%
Dyslipidemia	85.8% at 7 years[a]	59%–94%[b]

[a]High triglycerides
[b]At 12 years after surgery for high triglycerides, low high-density lipoprotein cholesterol, and high low-density lipoprotein cholesterol levels.
BMI, Body mass index; *NR*, not reported.

has been modified over the years, and the results presented in Table 99.9 reflect data from studies in the era of its performance as a laparoscopic procedure. Resolution of comorbid conditions after LRYGB has been excellent and sustained in long-term studies, as demonstrated in Table 99.9.[36,37] It has been commonly thought that gastric bypass has been associated with higher morbidity and mortality in older individuals and that older individuals would not benefit from surgery long term. However, Adams and colleagues identified a reduction in long-term mortality in older patients (55–80 years of age) when the patients were operated on at a center specializing in bariatric surgery. The demonstration of acceptable morbidity and mortality in older individuals, coupled with improvements in long-term survival, has led most bariatric surgeons to consider operating on older individuals if they meet criteria for operation.

Another important advantage of LRYGB is a decrease in the incidence of wound complications and incisional hernia seen after open RYGB. Long-term follow-up of a prospective randomized trial comparing laparoscopic and open gastric bypass found a much higher rate of incisional hernias in the open-surgery group. There was, however, no difference in the rate of resolution of comorbid conditions or weight loss between the two procedures. The duration of hospitalization has decreased in all patients undergoing RYGB. Patients undergoing LRYGB are usually hospitalized for, on average, 1 night.

RYGB has also been shown to resolve the symptoms of pseudotumor cerebri as well as to cure the difficult problem of venous stasis ulcers. Immediate resolution of symptoms of GERD occurs in more than 90% of cases. The extremely small gastric pouch has a limited reservoir for holding gastric juice, and the cardia is a low-acid-producing area of the stomach, so the Roux-en-Y reconstruction diverts gastric acid away from the esophagus immediately after surgery, thus accounting for its efficacy in alleviating heartburn.

Age has been shown previously to be an important determinant of operative morbidity and mortality. However, a matched-pair analysis of the MBSAQIP database of 3371 patients older than age 60 years matched to 3371 patients younger than 60 with similar BMI and comorbidities showed that there was comparable mortality between older individuals and younger individuals in both LSG and LRYGB. These data should not be misinterpreted to mean that older individuals have the same mortality risk as younger ones but to suggest that the surgeon can identify older patients most likely to benefit from bariatric surgery and can expect good short- and long-term outcomes.[38]

Biliopancreatic Diversion With Duodenal Switch and Single Anastomosis Duodenal-Ileal Bypass With Sleeve Gastrectomy

Most malabsorptive procedures performed in the United States are the DS modification of BPD or the SADI-S, so this section discusses the results of both operations. EWL (65%–80%) after BPD/DS and SADI-S is the highest of the bariatric operations discussed in this chapter, with a slightly higher EWL in the BPD/DS group. BPD/DS and SADI-S have been highly effective in treating comorbid conditions, including hypertension (remission >80%), diabetes (remission >85%%), lipid disorders (remission >75%), GERD (remission >75%), and obstructive sleep apnea (remission >80%).[35,39]

Thus, some surgeons argue that superobese patients maintain weight loss better in the long term after undergoing BPD/DS or SADI-S than after other bariatric operations. Others point out that serious complications, such as deficiency in vitamin D, vitamin K, and zinc; reoperation for correction of protein malnutrition, hernia, or bowel obstruction; and overall morbidity are much higher with BPD/DS; therefore, the incremental improvements in EWL are not justified. However, many of these complications are slightly lower with the SADI-S. Outcomes between BPD/DS and SADI-S are compared in Table 99.10.

After BPD/DS and SADI-S, patients typically have between two and four bowel movements per day. Excessive flatulence and foul-smelling stools are common. Malabsorption of starch and fat provides the major mechanism of weight loss and creates vitamin deficiencies in fat-soluble vitamins (K, A, D, and E).

Surgeons caring for these patients must be alert to measure protein levels for confirmation of adequate absorption. When protein malnutrition does occur, the common channel may need to be lengthened with a reoperation. This is less common with the SADI-S because of the longer common channel. Patients must also be aware that their ability to absorb simple sugars, alcohol, and short-chain triglycerides is good and that overindulgence in sweets, milk products, soft drinks, alcohol, and fruit may produce excess weight gain.

Major considerations for achieving excellent results in patients offered BPD/DS include the ability to monitor these patients and to confirm that they are compliant with the recommendations to take appropriate vitamin supplements. Supplements include multivitamins as well as at least 2 g of oral calcium per day. Supplemental fat-soluble vitamins, including D, K, and A, are indicated monthly as well.

Laparoscopic Sleeve Gastrectomy

Advantages of LSG are the technical ease of the procedure, induction of satiety through reduction in ghrelin levels, reduced need for postoperative adjustments as opposed to LAGB, preservation of the pylorus and avoidance of dumping, reduced risk of malabsorption, and apparent safety of the procedure in high-risk individuals. Use of LSG is advantageous for some populations of patients, as outlined in Table 99.11.[16–18]

TABLE 99.10 Results of Duodenal Switch and Single Anastomosis Duodenal-Ileal Bypass With Sleeve Gastrectomy

CRITERIA	FINNO[35] 2-YEAR FOLLOW-UP		SURVE[39] 6-YEAR FOLLOW-UP	
Procedure	BPD/DS (n = 259)	SADI-S (n = 181)	BPD/DS (n = 133)	SADI-S (n = 133)
Age (years)	48.2	50.8	51.5	55.6
Excess weight loss	78.2%	74.7%	79.7%	74.5%
Remission of type 2 diabetes mellitus	84.8%	85.7%	88.2%	86.6%
Remission of hypertension	62.4%	66.0%	86.6%	80.0%
Remission of dyslipidemia	80.5%	72.9%	NR	NR
Remission of OSA	83.0%	85.7%	89.4%	64.7%
Remission of GERD	NR	NR	80.0%	73.3%

BMI, Body mass index; BPD, biliopancreatic diversion; DS, duodenal switch; GERD, gastroesophageal reflux disease; NR, not recorded; OSA, obstructive sleep apnea; SADI-S, single anastomosis duodenal-ileal bypass with sleeve gastrectomy.

TABLE 99.11 Results of Laparoscopic Sleeve Gastrectomy

CRITERIA	STAMPEDE[18]	SLEEVEPASS[17]	SM-BOSS[16]
Number of patients	49	121	107
Age (years)	Mean = 48	Mean = 48.5	Mean = 43
BMI (kg/m^2)	36.1	45.5	43.9
Follow-up (years)	5	5	5
Excess weight loss	NR	49%	61.1% (excess BMI loss)
Percentage BMI loss	NR	NR	61.1%
Percentage of baseline weight loss	−18.6%	NR	NR
Remission diabetes	23.4%	12%	61.5%
Remission hypertension	NR	29%	62.5%
Remission dyslipidemia	NR	20%	42.6%

BMI, Body mass index; NR, not reported.

TABLE 99.12 Comparison of Laparoscopic Sleeve Gastrectomy Versus Laparoscopic Roux-en-Y Gastric Bypass: 5-Year Outcomes in the SLEEVEPASS and SM-BOSS Randomized Trials

MEASURE	LSG	LRYGB	COMMENTS
Percentage excess weight loss	49%	57%	LRYGB had more weight loss but not statistically significant
BMI at 5 years (kg/m²)	31.6–36.5	32.5–35.4	No significant difference between procedures
Remission of type 2 diabetes mellitus	12%–61.5%	25%–67.9%	No significant differences
Remission of hypertension	29%–62.5%	51%–70.3%	LRYGB in the SLEEVEPASS trial had increased remission rate
LDL cholesterol (mg/dL)	104.3–116.1	96.5–101.1	LDL level significantly lower after LRYGB
Quality of life (QOL)	Improved	Improved	Both procedures improved QOL
Remission of GERD	25%	60.4%	LRYGB associated with greater remission of GERD; in the SLEEVEPASS trial, 7/10 reoperations were done for severe reflux
Late complications	14.9%–19%	17.3%–26%	No difference between techniques

BMI, Body mass index; *GERD*, gastroesophageal reflux disease; *LDL*, low-density lipoprotein; *LRYGB*, laparoscopic Roux-en-Y gastric bypass; *LSG*, laparoscopic sleeve gastrectomy; *SM-BOSS*, Swiss Multicentre Bypass or Sleeve Study.

LSG was developed because of a high incidence of morbidity and mortality (23% and 7%, respectively) in patients with a BMI greater than 60 kg/m² undergoing laparoscopic DS. Surgeons developed the two-stage DS, with sleeve gastrectomy alone performed as the first stage to decrease morbidity in this population of superobese patients. The Clinical Issues Committee of the ASMBS performed a comprehensive review of the subject, which demonstrated a lower rate of complications for DS in this population of high-risk patients (leak rate of 1.2%, bleeding rate of 1.6%, and mortality of 0.24%). The ASMBS concluded that LSG could be used in high-risk patients to reduce perioperative complications and also to induce weight loss as a standalone procedure. Modifications to LSG, including reduced bougie size and extension of the LSG into the antrum, made LSG a primary bariatric procedure.

Five-year results after LSG in the STAMPEDE trial show good weight loss (−18.6% baseline) and remission of diabetes in 23.4% (Table 99.12).[18] O'Brien reported the collective series of LSG across the globe and reported a weighted mean of 58.3% EWL after LSG.[34] Two excellent RCTs give us comparative data on the outcomes 5 years after LSG and LRYGB, as shown in Table 99.12. The SLEEVEPASS trial shows that LRYGB has a greater percentage of weight loss than LSG (57% vs. 49%), but there was no statistically significant difference in HgbA1c (6.6% vs. 6.6%), dyslipidemia, QOL improvement, and late morbidity. There was a significant improvement in the resolution of hypertension based on medication use in LRYGB (51% vs. 29% resolution).[17] The Swiss Multicentre Bypass or Sleeve Study (SM-BOSS) randomized trial found no significant difference in percentage of BMI loss (68.3% vs. 61.1%), complete remission of type 2 diabetes mellitus (67.9% vs. 61.5%), hypertension remission (70.3% vs. 62.5%), improvement in QOL, or late complications (see Table 99.12).[16]

COMPLICATIONS OF BARIATRIC SURGERY

The various procedures are associated with complications that can occur with any intraabdominal operation. However, each operation has unique complications as well as different incidences of some of the shared common complications seen after any abdominal operation.

It is now well accepted that laparoscopic and robotic procedures are much safer than open gastric bypass in 30-day mortality (e.g., overall complication rates, surgical site infection, and pulmonary complications). The benefits touted for laparoscopic surgery go beyond the cosmetic benefits and really do influence postoperative complication rates, which makes the laparoscopic or robotic technique our preferred approach in every patient, including reoperative operations.

Laparoscopic Adjustable Gastric Banding

Although many centers have shown a very low (approaching zero) 30-day morbidity and mortality rate, long-term complications such as esophageal dilation, lap band slippage, lap band erosion, and failure to lose weight have been the Achilles heel of this operation. High-resolution manometry of the esophagus in patients who present for LAGB removal has shown that three-fourths of patients have abnormal esophageal peristalsis, including simultaneous or failed peristalsis. It has been noted that removal of the lap band in patients who have developed pseudoachalasia or megaesophagus will improve; therefore, surgeons should be vigilant regarding patients with lap bands who might have either a slip or significant esophageal motility disorders who need deflation and/or explantation of the band.

The 10-year outcomes of a prospective randomized trial of LAGB versus LRYGB demonstrated poor long-term weight loss with the LAGB procedure (LAGB 27.4 kg vs. LRYGB 42.4 kg), higher reoperation rate (LAGB 31.4% vs. LRYGB 8.1%), and lower rate of remission of comorbidities.[40] The natural history of LAGB was defined by a study of the French standardized national database of 53,000 patients, which demonstrated that 20% of the 52,868 patients underwent removal of the band, and by 7 years, 71% of the patients underwent revisional surgery. Many of the revisional procedures were conversions to either LSG or LRYGB for either lap band slippage or failure of weight loss with LAGB. The authors of the French study questioned whether the lap band was a viable procedure given the high rate of removal and complications.[41]

Although a few centers that specialize in LAGB have demonstrated much lower reoperation rates with much improved durable weight loss, the authors of this chapter no longer offer LAGB in their practices because the current surgical practices of LSG and LRYGB have low morbidity, much improved long-term weight loss, and improved resolution of comorbidity.

Roux-en-Y Gastric Bypass

The laparoscopic revolution has fundamentally changed the outcomes of many surgical procedures, but in particular, it has reduced operative mortality and morbidity significantly. The

TABLE 99.13   Complications After Laparoscopic Roux-en-Y Gastric Bypass

CRITERIA	COURCOULAS[37]	KUMAR[42]	CLAPP[43]
Number of patients	1738	41,080	134,188
Age	19–75	Median = 45	Median = 44.3
Mortality	0.17%	0.2%	0.1%
Leak/major wound complications	NR	1.6%	0.1%
Surgical site infection	NR	0.9%	0.8%
Pulmonary embolus/ venous thromboembolism	NR	0.15	0.1%
Reoperation	2.5%	3.2%	2.1%
Revision	0.06%	NR	NR
Reversal	0.02%	NR	NR
Bleeding	NR	1.2%	1.0%

NR, Not reported.

most recently reported mortality rates after LRYGB have generally been in the 0.1% to 0.3% range for a large series, as shown in Table 99.13.

Mortality rates are influenced heavily by patient selection. Male sex was associated with an increased risk for morbidity and mortality in older series but not in the most recent experience. Almost all studies have identified BMI and history of VTE as independent predictors of complications.

Complications specific to RYGB include anastomotic leaks from the proximal or distal anastomosis. They typically present early with signs of shock, including tachycardia, tachypnea, and abdominal pain. They can be diagnosed clinically or with CT with PO contrast. Leaks from the gastrojejunostomy are more common and are generally the cause of a significant percentage of the life-threatening complications and deaths. Whereas the older studies found a leak rate of 2.2% in open and LRYGB, the more recent LRYGB studies report anastomotic leak rates of under 1.0%.[38,44] These investigators found no difference in leak rates by type of anastomosis or stapling instrument used. Leak rate may be slightly higher in the buttressing group but with lower postoperative bleeds.[44] Early leaks are treated with sepsis control, which often means operative management, whereas later leaks in clinically stable patients can be managed nonoperatively.

Pulmonary embolism is one of the most feared complications after any form of bariatric surgery, and its incidence in large reported series of open RYGB sometimes exceeds 1%. Thrombotic complications such as DVT and pulmonary embolism are less frequently associated with laparoscopic surgery than with open gastric bypass but still account for 17% of deaths, and up to 80% of patients who die after bariatric surgery have evidence of VTE. Emphasis on DVT prophylaxis using SCDs, early ambulation, and low-molecular-weight heparin has reduced the incidence of VTE to 0.23% in both LSG and LRYGB, as evidenced by the latest reports from the MBSAQIP.[42]

Although nausea and vomiting are not unusual in isolated circumstances after RYGB, especially in relation to a patient's adaptation to food restriction, if persistent, these symptoms can lead to the obvious problem of dehydration. This must be aggressively treated in the postoperative period or in association with a viral or other GI illness compounding the problem and further limiting oral intake. IV fluids are adicated when in doubt. This is the case for all bariatric operations, not just RYGB.

One specific problem that may arise with persistent vomiting after *any* of the bariatric operations and that is *imperative* for the surgeon to treat is Wernicke's encephalopathy. This neurologic deficit is preventable with appropriate administration of parenteral thiamine (vitamin B_1) when the patient has persistent and severe vomiting. If the neurologic symptoms become significant, they may often not be fully reversed despite thiamine therapy.

Because depression is so frequent in the population of patients undergoing bariatric surgery, severe postoperative depression may develop after any of the bariatric operations as well. When it does occur, the patient may completely stop eating, thereby producing what at first seems like a wonderful response, but if unrecognized, can progress to loss of critical visceral and musculoskeletal protein mass, which can be life threatening.

Another specific life-threatening complication that may result after RYGB is bowel obstruction. Patients who have a clinical or radiographic picture of small bowel obstruction after RYGB need a reoperation. The potential for internal hernias after this operation makes strangulation obstruction a frequent presentation. Patients with bowel obstruction are best diagnosed by an oral and IV contrast-enhanced CT scan of the abdomen to visualize the bypassed stomach and small bowel that may be obstructed or the mesenteric twist with volvulus of the Roux limb. These patients *must* be promptly treated before retrograde distention of the biliopancreatic limb and distal part of the stomach results in rupture of the distal gastric staple line with subsequent peritonitis. Closure of the mesenteric defects has been shown to reduce the incidence of internal hernia from 4% to 17% to 0% to 7% or by approximately 70% and adds only minimal operative time.[45] It is our practice to perform antecolic LRYGB, and we close both the jejunojejunostomy and Petersen's defect.

Stenosis of the gastrojejunostomy may occur after RYGB and has been reported in 2% to 7% of patients in various series. The higher incidence seems to be associated with a circular stapler versus sutured anastomoses. Postoperative anastomotic stenosis is usually manifested at 4 to 6 weeks postoperatively as progressive intolerance to solids and then liquids. The problem is successfully treated with endoscopic balloon dilation. Unless a marginal ulcer is associated with the stenosis, the problem does not usually require a reoperation.

A marginal ulcer occurs after 2% to 14% of RYGB procedures. The incidence can be decreased by preoperative treatment of patients for *Helicobacter pylori* colonization of the stomach. Patients with a marginal ulcer typically have continuous boring epigastric pain. Larger pouch size was associated with increased marginal ulceration. For each 5-cm^3 increase in pouch size, patients had 2.4 times the odds of increase in marginal ulcer formation.[46] Presumably, the additional size of the pouch had more parietal cells secreting acid, which increased the risk of marginal ulceration. Treatment of marginal ulcer consists of medical therapy with proton pump inhibitors and avoidance of nonsteroidal anti-inflammatory drugs and smoking. Medical treatment resolves most of the marginal ulcers unless a fistula has formed to the lower part of the stomach, which creates an ongoing source of acid, thus exacerbating the ulcer. Surgery to divide the fistula is necessary to effect healing of the ulcer.

Iron and vitamin B_{12} deficiencies are the two most common long-term metabolic complications of RYGB. The incidence of iron insufficiency varies among reported series. Iron is preferentially absorbed in the duodenum and proximal jejunum. Hence, RYGB bypasses the area of maximal iron absorption in the gut.

The iron deficiency, based on serum values, is between 15% and 40%, whereas actual iron deficiency anemia occurs in as many as 20% of patients after RYGB. This problem is treated in most cases with oral iron supplements. The gluconate form of iron is best absorbed in a nonacid environment.

The incidence of vitamin B_{12} deficiency after RYGB is reported as being 15% to 20%, although it rarely causes anemia. Vitamin B_{12} deficiency is a result of inefficient absorption because of delayed mixing with intrinsic factor. Thus, B_{12} deficiency can develop despite plentiful oral administration. Several preparations include intrinsic factor, which maximizes absorption in the terminal ileum. Other routes of vitamin B_{12} administration include sublingual medication, nasal spray, and parenteral injections.

Biliopancreatic Diversion With Duodenal Switch and Single Anastomosis Duodenal-Ileal Bypass With Sleeve Gastrectomy

The most significant and specific long-term complication seen after BPD/DS is protein malnutrition, which occurs in 8% of patients. Treatment is hospitalization with 2 to 3 weeks of parenteral nutrition. This particular problem is usually manifested within the first few months after surgery, but it can occur sporadically, although less frequently, and may even require reoperation to lengthen the common channel. This occurs more frequently in BPD/DS patients because the common channel is shorter.

Malabsorption of fat-soluble vitamins is one of the major problems associated with BPD/DS and SADI-S. However, one of the main benefits of SADI-S is a lower rate of vitamin deficiencies. In one single institution study comparing BPD/DS to SADI-S, the rates of vitamin A (36.4% vs. 13.5%,), vitamin D (55.3% vs. 36.5%), calcium (36% vs. 12.4%), iron (41.1% vs. 19.1%), and copper (6% vs. 1.7%) deficiency were all significantly higher in the BPD/DS group. The overall rate of long-term complications was also higher in the BPD/DS group (13.1% vs. 4.4%), with higher rates of incisional hernia and internal hernias but lower rates of symptomatic GERD. Diarrhea may also be less frequent after SADI-S.[35,39]

Although the complication of protein malnutrition and poor intake is theoretically most likely to occur soon after BPD/DS, the fact that late deaths occur from protein malnutrition and Wernicke's encephalopathy suggests that these patients are always at risk for these problems. Marginal ulcers are a distinct problem of BPD, which has been addressed with the DS modification and SADI-S preserving the pylorus. Finally, mortality rates in recent studies are also low for both BPD/DS and SADI (0.3%–0.5%) but still higher than those of LSG and LRYGB.[35,39,43]

Although still low in total procedures performed, the rates of DS and SADI-S are slowly on the rise, reaching 2.8% of bariatric operations nationally in 2021. Further studies are needed to elucidate long-term outcomes and assess whether the excitement for SADI-S as a safer alternative to BPD/DS with better weight loss and comorbidity resolution than LRYGB is merited.

Laparoscopic Sleeve Gastrectomy

The mortality rate after LSG (~0.1%) is slightly lower than that of LRYGB (Table 99.14).[38,42,47] The morbidity associated with LSG, including infections and reoperation rates, is slightly below that of LRYGB but with similar rates of VTE. Malabsorption of vitamins and nutrients is much less for LSG compared with LRYGB or the laparoscopic DS and makes LSG ideally suited for patients with preexisting vitamin disorders or those who need full absorption of

CRITERIA	KUMAR[42]	JANIK[38]	ABOUEISHA[47]
Number of patients	93,062	3371	513,354
Age	Median = 44	>60	Median = 44.2
Mortality	0.1%	0.12%	<0.1%
Leak perforation	0.8%	0.5%	0.4%
Surgical site infection	0.2%	0.2%	0.2%–0.3%
Pulmonary embolus/venous thromboembolism	0.1%	0.1%	0.2%
Reoperation	1.2%	0.9%	0.8%–0.9%
Bleeding	0.6%	1.0%	0.5%–0.6%

TABLE 99.14 Complications After Laparoscopic Sleeve Gastrectomy

lifesaving medications. Moreover, studies of 30-day morbidity and mortality show that there has been a continual decline in postoperative complications associated with increased surgical experience.

The long-term morbidity of LSG is related to reoperation, primarily conversion to RYGB for severe GERD, which is exacerbated by the high-pressure system created by LSG in addition to decreased gastric compliance, disruption of gastric sling fibers, and increased transient lower esophageal sphincter relaxations. The SLEEVEPASS 10-year follow-up study showed that there was a high incidence of GERD in patients who underwent LSG, with 11.6% requiring conversion to RYGB. Moreover, of the 90 patients who underwent endoscopy postoperatively, 20% never experienced GERD symptoms, 18% had symptoms similar to preoperatively, and 13% had symptoms alleviated, but 49% had worsened symptoms.[48]

The most feared complications postoperatively after LSG are stenosis and leak. Stenosis occurs in less than 1% of cases but is most typically at the incisura. It typically presents with obstructive symptoms and may be diagnosed on esophagogastroduodenoscopy (EGD) or upper GI series. It is often treated with serial endoscopic dilation but may require revision to RYGB.[17,47] Leaks occur in approximately 0.3% to 0.5% of cases and typically present 1 to 4 weeks after surgery. They may present more indolently with infection and abscess but without frank shock and can be diagnosed by CT scan with oral contrast. Sleeve leaks are often a result of stricture or narrowing at the incisura, leading to proximal leak. Early leaks (within 48 hr) are more often related to stapler misfires or tissue trauma (and behave more like a post-RYGB anastomotic leak), whereas late leaks are related to ischemia and high intragastric pressure, particularly when there is a distal stenosis. Management of leaks includes sepsis control with adequate drainage and antibiotics as well as initial nil per os (NPO) with supplemental nutrition. They may require a combination of drainage (externally and intraluminally), stenting, or intraluminal wound vacuum placement, as discussed later.

REOPERATIVE SURGERY

A controversial topic is the appropriateness of performing repeated bariatric operations for recurrent weight gain or inadequate weight loss. It is well established that there is heterogeneity in postoperative weight loss outcomes. Long-term recurrent weight gain is also possible despite attention to diet and physical activity; thus, long-term follow-up is recommended. The absolute definition of a failure is unclear, but most surgeons would accept the criteria listed in

Box 99.2 as appropriate when considering reoperation in patients with inadequate weight loss (<50% EWL at 18 months), recurrent weight gain (>10%), or recurrence of comorbidities. Complications of procedures, such as stenosis causing gastric outlet obstruction after vertical banded gastroplasty or metabolic complications after jejunoileal bypass, are obvious indications for revisional surgery.

In assessing a patient for the appropriateness of reoperative surgery, the surgeon must determine whether the original bariatric operation is intact and anatomically still appropriate for maintaining weight loss. If not, consideration for reoperation is appropriate. The incidence of infection, organ ischemia, anastomotic leakage, blood transfusion, and other severe intraabdominal complications is increased in revisional surgery.

All bariatric operations have some incidence of failure, which includes inadequate weight loss, inadequate resolution of medical comorbid conditions, development of side effects negatively influencing lifestyle and satisfaction, development of complications requiring medical or surgical intervention, and complications requiring alteration or reversal of the operation. Analysis of the 449,753 bariatric operations in the Bariatric Outcomes Longitudinal Database (BOLD) showed that 4.4% were corrective operations (i.e., operations that addressed complications or incomplete treatment effect of the primary bariatric operation), and 1.9% were conversions (i.e., operations in which the primary bariatric procedure was converted to another bariatric procedure).[49] Only 6.3% of bariatric operations needed reoperation, and even fewer needed conversion to another bariatric procedure, which points out the relative efficacy of the common bariatric procedures being performed currently. Moreover, the reoperations had a low mortality rate of 0.12% to 0.21% and a 1-year EWL of 36% to 39%.[49] The data suggest that reoperations for failure are not that common; the clinical results are acceptable, albeit less predictable with less EWL; and have similar mortality rates. This should negate the bias among some primary care providers as well as insurance companies that reoperative bariatric surgery is risky and not worth the benefits. Nevertheless, appropriate counseling is necessary to set patient expectations.

ENDOSCOPIC PROCEDURES IN BARIATRIC SURGERY

Endoscopy has become an important part of management of complications after bariatric surgery, and in addition, a plethora of endoscopic weight loss procedures are being used or are in development.

Preoperative Use of Endoscopy

The ASMBS published guidelines on this topic in 2021 and concluded that EGD in preoperative patients may indeed guide treatment of modifiable conditions or identify anatomic abnormalities or conditions that would alter treatment. Moreover, clinical evaluation by symptoms alone does not reliably diagnose or rule out GERD. A comprehensive review of 28 studies and 12,385 patients identified that the majority (92.4%) of preoperative endoscopic findings did not alter management; however, 7.6% of patients had findings that delayed or altered surgery.[50] Therefore, the ASMBS states that EGD before bariatric surgery should be done at the surgeon's discretion. We recommend endoscopy for symptomatic patients before bariatric surgery, and consideration should be given to preoperative endoscopy in asymptomatic patients.

Intraoperative Endoscopy

Many surgeons will do an intraoperative leak test in the operating room at the time of the procedure to prevent complications after

the procedure. The method of leak test varies from using methylene blue through an orogastric tube to air insufflation with a tube or an endoscope. When using an insufflation test, the staple line of the stomach and any proximal anastomosis is submerged under sterile saline, and air is insufflated into the gastric pouch. One then looks for air bubbles to assess whether the staple lines are airtight under hyperdistention. The benefit of the endoscope is that it can be both diagnostic and therapeutic at the time of surgery. If a leak is noted, it may be able to be managed with endoscopic clips or externally placed sutures under endoscopic guidance. In addition, if bleeding is noted along any staple lines, it can be managed immediately rather than with a potential return to the operating room later once the bleed becomes clinically evident. Finally, endoscopy allows the surgeon to assess the postsurgical anatomy more thoroughly to ensure it looks as intended.

Postoperative Endoscopy

Once a patient has had altered anatomy for a weight loss procedure, endoscopy is invaluable in evaluating patients who return with abdominal complaints, suffer from weight regain, or develop a complication of their procedure. Understanding the postsurgical anatomy after a bariatric procedure can be challenging, especially if the surgery was many years ago. The most common procedures one should recognize are the gastric bypass, LSG, gastric banding, DS, and SADI-S.

Endoscopic Management of Complications After Bariatric Surgery

Leaks after bariatric surgery are one of the most dreaded complications, as discussed earlier, and carry a high mortality. One of the most commonly used interventions for a leak is the use of a fully covered stent. This endoscopically placed stent traverses the perforation, thereby decreasing ongoing contamination. However, a major issue with this treatment method is stent migration. To avoid this, multiple methods of prevention have been described, including suturing it or clipping the stent in place. Stents are left in place for 4 to 6 weeks. Sutures can be placed endoscopically, but these devices are sometimes bulky in this small space. Fluoroscopy is essential to ensure proper stent placement. Leaks after LSG can be particularly challenging because the stents available in the United States are not long enough to traverse the entire sleeve. Many use two stents placed overlapping to mitigate this problem.

Another approach to leak management is the use of over-the-scope clips. This technology generally does not work for these leaks in the acute setting unless the hole is very small with fresh edges. Usually, this technology works better for chronic leaks that are small or fistulas that are less than 1 cm.

Endoscopic vacuum-assisted closure is now being used for the closure of large leaks. This technique involves placing the vacuum sponge on the end of an orogastric tube into the cavity external to the leak. Over time, this allows closure of this area. This works for encapsulated leaks. This technique is very labor intensive because the device must be changed every few days, similar to any external wound vacuum device. Generally, patients will require 8 to 12 procedures over a period of weeks. The benefit is this can actually shorten the healing time compared with traditional methods.

If the hole is small but the external cavity of the leak is on the larger side, internal drainage with a double pigtail stent can also be used. This allows internal drainage of the extraluminal cavity. This is very helpful, particularly when the placement of an external drain is difficult. If the opening is small, an endoscopic septotomy has also been performed to allow better drainage of an extraluminal cavity.

Strictures After Bariatric Surgery

Strictures can occur at the outlet of a pouch after gastric bypass procedures or at the incisura angularis after LSG. After a gastric bypass, the anastomotic strictures can often be managed with through-the-scope balloons. These range from 5 to 20 mm in diameter. They are placed through the scope and across the stricture. If the scope cannot traverse the stricture, the balloon can be placed over a wire or with fluoroscopic guidance to avoid perforation. These strictures may require multiple dilations because one should not try to dilate the stricture more than 3 to 5 mm at any one sitting. In addition, the underlying cause of the stricture should be identified and addressed to avoid recurrence. Common causes include smoking and nonsteroidal medication use. Strictures after LSG are most often at the incisura angularis. These have been managed with endoscopic balloon dilation and stent placement. Unfortunately, these methods are not always successful, and conversion to a gastric bypass for management may be necessary.

Recurrent Weight Gain After Bariatric Surgery

Recidivism after bariatric surgery occurs around 10% to 15% of the time. Conversion of a primary procedure such as LAGB to sleeve or RYGB, conversion from sleeve to RYGB or DS, or revising an RYGB to a distal bypass can be done. Endoscopic suturing for pouch outlet reduction after gastric bypass procedure is another described procedure but has yet to demonstrate substantial results. An endoscopic suturing device that allows full-thickness bites is used to decrease the size of the gastrojejunostomy. The smaller-diameter anastomosis allows for longer retention of food within the pouch, leading to greater satiety and reduced food intake. The endoscopic procedure is accompanied by lifestyle counseling to improve dietary and exercise habits and has been able to obtain marginal weight loss at 6 months, but longer-term studies are needed.

Primary Endoscopic Weight Loss Procedures

Currently, for those overweight, diet and exercise are recommended. For those with severe obesity, weight loss surgery is an option. For those in between, few interventions were available before the introduction of GLP-1 RAs. In addition, many patients do not wish to undergo an anatomically altering weight loss surgery. Now there are several endoscopic options for weight loss that work in various ways, which include space filling devices and the endoscopic sleeve gastroplasty.

Space filling devices can come in single- and multiple-balloon systems. The most common is the Orbera balloon (Apollo Endosurgery, Inc., Austin, TX). Over 300,000 of these balloons have been placed, with reasonable success. This balloon is placed endoscopically, remains in place for 6 months, and then is removed endoscopically. Throughout this time and the ensuing 6 months, the patient receives dietary and lifestyle counseling. Patients learn how much food they can live on while the balloon is in place, and the ongoing counseling is to help them maintain that lifestyle once the balloon is removed. Patients can lose up to 30 to 50 lb, but this weight loss is often not sustained. Other balloon systems are air filled or use multiple balloons to minimize the nausea that is encountered at initial placement. Newer balloons are on the horizon that do not require endoscopy for placement or removal.

The other endoscopic procedure that has gained popularity is the endoscopic sleeve gastroplasty. The stomach walls are sutured together to collapse the stomach using an endoscopic suturing device.

By doing so, the only lumen left behind emulates a sleeve gastroplasty. The weight loss reported in the short term in small series is greater than that from medical therapy, and long-term controlled trials are needed to evaluate the potential of this approach.

Other endoscopic procedures include liners that decrease absorption or reduce gastric emptying, thereby inducing fullness in the patient. In addition, even magnets are being used to create bypasses endoscopically. All these procedures have minimal data, and their durability is unclear. Their long-term use may be further challenged by the success of incretin-mimetic drugs like GLP-1 RAs that are now flooding the market. These endoscopic procedures will likely not attain the effectiveness of surgery; however, they can provide a bridge to surgical procedures. They can also be an intervention that some patients can accept to facilitate weight loss that is less invasive than surgery.

CONCLUSION

Surgical treatment of morbid obesity is now a component of surgical residency training programs and represents the fastest-growing area of general surgery. Although patient demand for the procedure has vastly increased, at present, surgeons operate annually on less than 2% of the eligible patients who would benefit from bariatric surgery. This chapter has discussed all aspects of the performance of bariatric surgery in current surgical practice, including the most commonly performed procedures at this time. The disease process of morbid obesity is unfortunately incompletely understood, but morbid obesity is increasing in prevalence worldwide. Surgical therapy has been shown to reduce long-term mortality and aid in control of diabetes largely because surgery has proven to be a more effective intervention for weight loss than nonsurgical options. Recent randomized clinical trials of bariatric surgery versus medical treatment in obese diabetic patients have shown bariatric surgery to be more effective in the treatment of severe obesity, type 2 diabetes mellitus, hypertension, and dyslipidemia. With the positive results of bariatric surgery becoming more widely known, there has been a movement by multiple medical societies to recognize the need for referral to a bariatric surgeon for evaluation. It is hopeful that these data will also encourage the government and insurance companies to add or expand bariatric and metabolic surgery coverage.

SELECTED REFERENCES

Aminian A, Zajicheck A, Arterburn DE, et al. Association of metabolic surgery with major adverse cardiovascular outcomes in patients with type 2 diabetes and obesity. *JAMA*. 2019;322:1271-1282.

This study involved a 1:5 matched cohort of patients with type 2 diabetes and obesity and compared major adverse cardiovascular events (MACEs) between patients undergoing metabolic surgery (2287 patients) and nonsurgical patients (11,435) in the Cleveland Clinic Health System. The primary end point was incidence of extended MACE (composite of six outcomes), defined as first occurrence of all-cause mortality, coronary artery events, cerebrovascular events, heart failure, nephropathy, and atrial fibrillation, and secondary end points were the three-component MACE (i.e., myocardial infarction, ischemic stroke, and mortality) and the six individual *components of the primary end point. The study found that the surgical group experienced a primary end point in only 30.8% of patients compared with 47.7% in the nonsurgical group (p <0.001), with an absolute risk reduction of 16.9%. Surgical patients had a lower three-component MACE compared with nonsurgical patients as well (17.0% vs. 27.6%, HR 0.62, 95% CI 0.53–0.72). Metabolic surgery was also associated with significantly lower incidence of each individual primary component, including heart failure (HR 0.38), coronary artery disease (HR 0.69), cerebrovascular disease (HR 0.67), nephropathy (HR 0.40), and atrial fibrillation (HR 0.78). Therefore, among patients with type 2 diabetes and obesity, metabolic surgery was associated with significantly lower risk of incident MACE.*

Carlsson LMS. Sjoholm K, Jacobson P, et al. Life expectancy after bariatric surgery in the Swedish Obese Subjects Study. *N Engl J Med.* 2020;383:1535-1543.

This study compared a group of patients undergoing bariatric surgery with a group of matched control subjects and monitored them for 10.9 years. This is the long-term follow-up at median 22 and 24 years for the surgical and control groups. The study found a significant decrease in the weight and risk of death in individuals in the surgical weight loss group compared with control patients not undergoing surgery (HR 0.77, 95% CI 0.68–0.87). The corresponding HR for death from cardiovascular disease was 0.7 (95% CI 0.57–0.85), and that from cancer was 0.77 (95% CI 0.31–0.96). The median life expectancy in the surgery group was 3.0 years longer than in the control.

Khalid SI, Maasarani S, Wiegmann J, et al. Association of bariatric surgery and risk of cancer in patients with morbid obesity. *Ann Surg.* 2022;275:1-6.

This study compared 28,908 patients who underwent vertical sleeve gastrectomy (VSG) or RYGB or who met bariatric surgery eligibility criteria between 2010 and 2018 in a 1:1:1 matched cohort. It found that patients who underwent VSG or RYGB had a significantly lower risk of developing any cancer compared with bariatric surgery–eligible patients who did not undergo an intervention (VSG OR 0.74, 95% CI 0.64–0.86; RYGB OR 0.78, 95% CI 0.67–0.90). Bariatric surgery patients also had lower odds of developing lung cancer, ovarian cancer, and uterine cancer compared with nonsurgical patients. Moreover, compared with nonsurgical patients, patients undergoing an RYGB had lower odds of colorectal cancer (OR 0.47, 95% CI 0.30–0.75), and those undergoing VSG had lower odds of liver cancer (OR 0.44, 95% CI 0.22–0.89). The authors conclude that bariatric surgery may lower the postoperative cancer rates in obese patients compared with bariatric-eligible patients who do not undergo surgical intervention.

Salminen P, Helmio M, Ovaska J, et al. Effect of laparoscopic sleeve gastrectomy vs laparoscopic Roux-en-Y gastric bypass on weight loss at 5 years among patients with morbid obesity: the SLEEVEPASS Randomized Clinical Trial. *JAMA.* 2018;319:241-254.

Comparison of laparoscopic LRYGB to LSG in an RCT demonstrated that weight loss was slightly better (57% vs. 49%, respectively) and resolution of hypertension was improved after LRYGB compared with LSG. The difference in weight loss between procedures did not have clinical significance. The study also noted that both procedures had improved HRQOL and no difference in late complications. The majority (7/10) of reoperations after LSG were performed for severe reflux. The results of this trial and the SM-BOSS RCT show LSG to be an effective bariatric procedure that compares favorably to LRYGB at 5 years after surgery.

Schauer PR, Bhatt DL, Kirwan JP, et al. Bariatric surgery versus intensive medical therapy for diabetes—5-year outcomes. *N Engl J Med.* 2017;376:641-651.

The authors randomized 150 obese (BMI 27–43) uncontrolled diabetics (HbA1c >7.0%) to intensive medical therapy or to LSG or laparoscopic RYGB. Surgical groups had significant improvement in HbA1c, weight loss, and dyslipidemia and a reduction in the number of antihypertensive, lipid-lowering, and diabetic medications used at 1, 2, 3, and 5 years after randomization. The surgical patients also had a significant improvement in QOL, whereas there was no change in the QOL for the medically treated patients. They concluded, "Bariatric surgery represents a potentially useful strategy for the management of type 2 diabetes, allowing many patients to reach and maintain therapeutic targets of glycemic control that otherwise would not be achievable with intensive medical therapy alone." This study, now with a 5-year follow-up showing sustained improvements for the surgical groups, adds to the strong evidence supporting bariatric surgery as a safe and effective therapy for treatment of type 2 diabetes.

The full reference list appears on Elsevier eBooks+.

Vascular Surgery

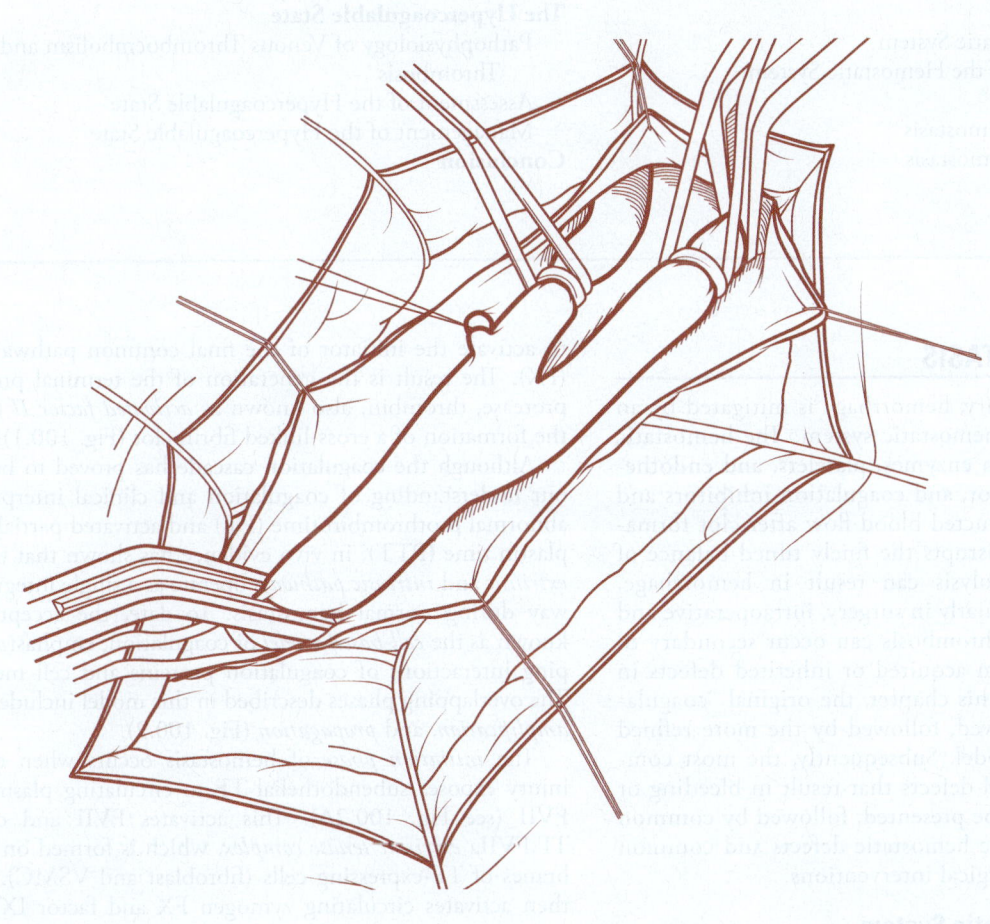

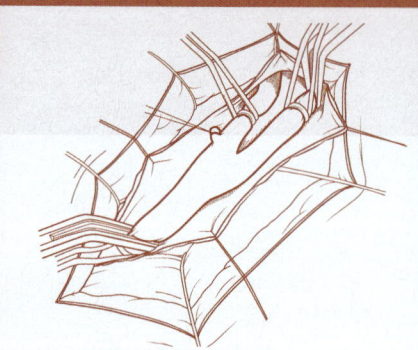

100 | CHAPTER

Hemostasis and Thrombosis

Ashley A. Peters, Sarah A. Loh, Alan Dardik, and Vivian Gahtan

OVERVIEW OF HEMOSTASIS

In response to vascular injury, hemorrhage is mitigated by an appropriately functioning hemostatic system. The hemostatic system relies on coagulation enzymes, platelets, and endothelial cells to form a blood clot, and coagulation inhibitors and fibrinolysis prevent unobstructed blood flow after clot formation. Any substance that disrupts the finely tuned balance of clot formation and fibrinolysis can result in hemorrhage, thrombosis, or both. Particularly in surgery, intraoperative and postoperative bleeding or thrombosis can occur secondary to technical challenges or from acquired or inherited defects in the hemostatic system. In this chapter, the original "coagulation cascade" will be reviewed, followed by the more refined and nuanced cell-based model. Subsequently, the most common inherited and acquired defects that result in bleeding or thrombosis in surgery will be presented, followed by common screening tools to determine hemostatic defects and common medical management or surgical interventions.

Activation of the Hemostatic System

In the mid-20th century, the original and renowned coagulation cascade proposed that coagulation could be triggered by one of two independent pathways, the *intrinsic* and *extrinsic* pathways. The *extrinsic pathway* is initiated when endothelial damage exposes plasma to tissue factor (TF), a subendothelial transmembrane glycoprotein that is abundantly expressed in adventitial tissues, such as fibroblast and vascular smooth muscle cells (VSMC).[1] The extrinsic pathway is complete when TF activates factor VII (FVIIa) and creates the TF:FVIIa complex. The *intrinsic pathway* was first described when clotting factors normally present in plasma were activated by artificial surfaces in vitro.[1] Subsequently, activated clotting factors activated downstream factors via limited proteolysis, which initiated an amplification cascade that proceeded in a stepwise manner. Although through different processes, the *extrinsic* and *intrinsic* pathways converged

to activate the initiator of the final common pathway, factor X (FX). The result is the generation of the terminal procoagulant protease, thrombin, also known as *activated factor II* (FIIa), and the formation of a cross-linked fibrin clot (Fig. 100.1).

Although the coagulation cascade has proved to be useful in our understanding of coagulation and clinical interpretation of abnormal prothrombin time (PT) and activated partial thromboplastin time (PTT), in vivo evidence has shown that the distinct *extrinsic* and *intrinsic pathways* operate as a single integrated pathway during normal hemostasis. To date, the accepted model, known as the *cell-based model* of coagulation, emphasizes overlapping interactions of coagulation proteins and cell membranes.[2] The overlapping phases described in this model include *initiation, amplification,* and *propagation* (Fig. 100.2).

The *initiation phase* of hemostasis occurs when endothelial injury exposes subendothelial TF to circulating plasma clotting FVII (see Fig. 100.2A). This activates FVII and creates the TF:FVIIa *extrinsic tenase complex,* which is formed on the membranes of TF-expressing cells (fibroblast and VSMC). TF:FVIIa then activates circulating zymogen FX and factor IX (FIX) via enzymatic cleavage. FIX is found in the subendothelial space bound to type IV collagen and in plasma, where it exists in a dynamic equilibrium.[3] Reversibly bound and activated FX (FXa) then combines with activated cofactor V (FVa) on the surface of negatively charged cell membranes in the presence of calcium ions to form the *prothrombinase complex.*[4] This complex converts prothrombin (factor II) to thrombin (FIIa) and is responsible for the trace amounts of thrombin that trigger coagulation.

As the *initiation phase* of coagulation is occurring, platelets begin to aggregate and activate at the site of injury by binding to endothelial-derived von Willebrand factor (vWF) and subendothelial collagen fibers via receptors glycoprotein (GP)Ib and GPIa/IIa or GPVI, respectively. Together, the stimulation of platelets with subendothelial collagen fibers and thrombin generated from the *prothrombase complex* enables platelet structural alterations.[2,5] One feature of this alteration is the outer membrane of the

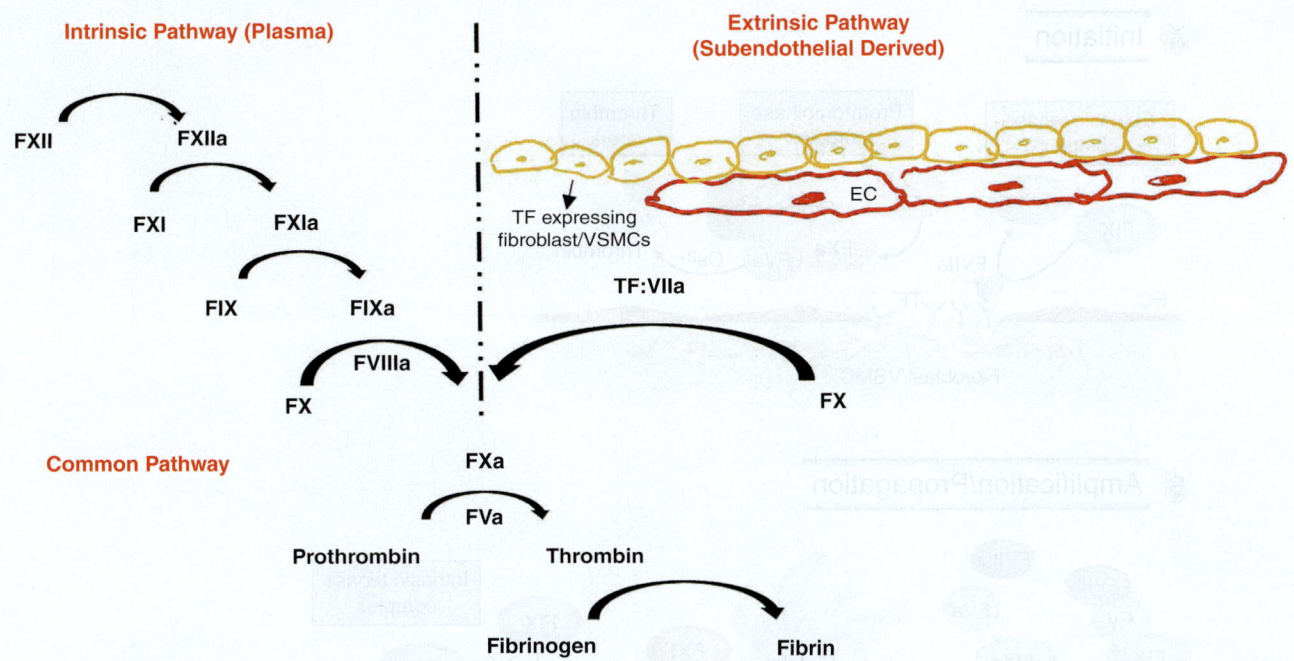

FIGURE 100.1 Classic coagulation cascade of the hemostatic system. *EC*, Endothelial cells; *F*, factor; *F#a*, activated factor; *VSMC*, vascular smooth muscle cells.

platelet becoming net negatively charged. Platelet structural change then initiates the *amplification phase* as the negatively charged membrane surface provides the platform for the activation of coagulation factors and creation of enzyme complexes (see Fig. 100.2B). Some of the plasma factors that negatively charged platelets activate are factor XII (FXII) and prekallikrien, via limited proteolysis.[1] FXII, prekallikrien and high-molecular-weight kininogen are responsible for propagating the *contact pathway*, initially referred to as the *intrinsic pathway*.[5] In the *contact pathway*, activated FXII (FXIIa) activates factor XI (FXIa), which in turn activates FIX (FIXa). While this is occurring, thrombin generated on TF-expressing cells (the thrombin spark) is further catalyzing the activation of FIX, FVIII, and FV. FIXa generated from the TF:FVIIa complex in the *initiation phase* and from the thrombin spark complexes with FVIIIa to form the *intrinsic tenase complex*. The *intrinsic tenase complex* then greatly accelerates FXa generation and therefore thrombin generation. As a reminder, thrombin generated from FXa is possible through the formation of the *prothrombinase complex* (FXa, FVa, and prothrombin). The overall net effect is a positive feedback loop amplification.

The *propagation phase* of coagulation follows the amplification phase in which accumulated enzyme complexes (*intrinsic tenase complex* and *prothrombinase*) on the platelet surface support large-scale thrombin generation (see Fig. 100.2B). As thrombin is being generated, fibrinogen binds to cell membrane receptor GPIIb/IIIa on activated platelets, serving as a molecular link to mediate platelet aggregation.[6] Generated thrombin then cleaves the soluble glycoprotein fibrinogen to insoluble fibrin and activates FXIII to FXIIIa. FXIIIa covalently links fibrin polymers, which gives the platelet clot shape, strength, flexibility, and stability.

Although platelets are demonstrated to be the cornerstone of thrombus, their role in hemostasis extends even further. To begin, platelets are small (~2–4 μm), short-lived (~8–10 days), anucleated cell fragments derived from the megakaryocyte lineage.[7] The platelet surface is covered by a layer of glycolipid and glycoprotein molecules containing receptors for various soluble and fixed ligands.

These ligands mediate adhesion, signaling, activation, spreading, and aggregation. However, the multifaceted function of platelets comes from the release of numerous intracytoplasmic granules (alpha, dense, and lysosomal) after platelet activation. More than 300 proteins from their intracytoplasmic granules are released in response to different agonists at different degrees of stimulation.[5] Activation of platelets can occur via thrombin stimulation (as previously described) or by adenosine diphosphate (ADP), adenosine triphosphate (ATP), and prostanoids such as thromboxane A2 (a mediator of vasoconstriction). Once activated, platelets undergo shape change (creating a negatively charged surface to provide the platform for the activation of clotting factors), degranulation, aggregation, and increased sensitivity to other agonists. Some factors released by platelets include platelet activators (platelet-activating factor, thromboxane A2), growth and angiogenic factors, cytokines and chemokines, adhesion molecules, coagulation factors (vWF, FV, FXIII, high-molecular-weight kininogen, fibrinogen), anticoagulation factors (TF pathway inhibitor, protein S), fibrinolytic factors (plasmin, plasminogen), antifibrinolytic factors (α2-antiplasmin, thrombin activatable fibrinolysis inhibitor, plasminogen activator inhibitor-1 [PAI-1]), ADP, ATP, and other molecules.[7] In sum, platelets play a key role not only in primary hemostasis but also in thrombosis and even inflammation.

Endogenous Inhibitors of the Hemostatic System

In an appropriately functioning coagulation system, inappropriate activation is regulated at various stages by inhibitors (Fig. 100.3). In *the initiation phase* of coagulation, tissue factor plasma inhibitor (TFPI) is bound to glycosaminoglycans on uninjured endothelium and prevents excessive fibrin clot formation down or upstream of injury by inhibiting TF:FVIIa as well as directly inhibiting FXa activity.[1,2] TFPI, a serine protease inhibitor, is also released by activated platelets. When TFPI binds to cofactor protein S, a circulating and platelet-stored vitamin K–dependent protein, TFPI's anti-FXa activity is enhanced.[8] Protein S is also known to be an important cofactor in inhibition

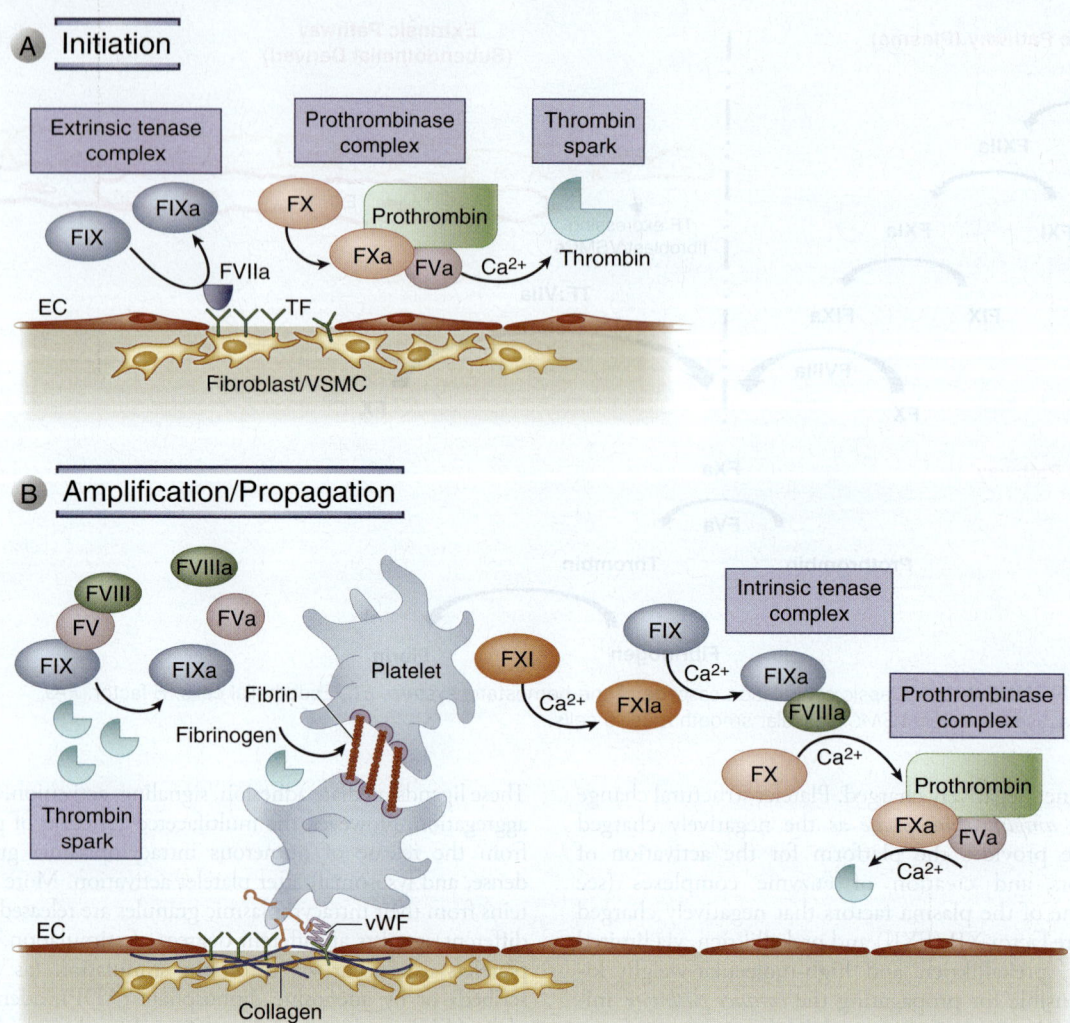

FIGURE 100.2 (A–B) Cell-based model of coagulation. In the cell-based model, there is an *initiation phase, amplification phase,* and *propagation phase.* (A) In the initiation phase, vascular injury results in the TF:FVIIa complex, also known as the *extrinsic tenase complex,* which activates FV, FIX, and FX and subsequently generates the *prothrombinase complex* (FXa:FVa). The *prothrombinase complex* then generates the thrombin spark. (B) The thrombin spark initiates the activation of platelets and other clotting factors, including FVa, FVIIIa, and FIXa. Once platelets are activated, amplification ensues as platelets behave as a platform for the activation of clotting factors. The result is the formation of the *intrinsic tenase complex,* which greatly accelerates FXa generation and therefore thrombin via the *prothrombinase complex. Ca²⁺* refers to the steps that require calcium. *Red cells* indicate endothelial cells *(EC); orange cells* indicate fibroblast/vascular smooth muscle cells. *GP,* Glycoprotein; *F,* factor; *TF,* tissue factor; *vWF,* von Willebrand factor.

during the *propagation phase* of coagulation. In this phase, protein S interacts with activated protein C. Protein C is a serine protease that is activated in response to thrombin binding to endothelial cofactor receptor thrombomodulin. Together, protein S and activated protein C inactivate FVa and FVIIIa, cofactors in the *prothrombinase* and *intrinsic complexes,* respectively.

Antithrombin is another serine protease inhibitor synthesized in the liver that regulates the *intrinsic and extrinsic complexes.* The liver synthesizes two isoforms of antithrombin: α and β. The α-isoform is more abundant (90%–95%) but demonstrates lower affinity for heparin than the β-isoform, therefore making the β-isoform more important for regulating anticoagulation.[9] Antithrombin's anticoagulant activity is activated once it binds to therapeutic heparins, heparan sulfate proteoglycans, and glycosaminoglycans on vascular endothelial cells.[10] The

activated antithrombin then undergoes a conformational change that creates a reactive loop site and covalent bonds between serpin and proteases, which leads to the irreversible binding of antithrombin-thrombin and antithrombin-FX complexes (FXa and, to a lesser degree, FIXa, XIa, XIIa, tissue-type plasminogen activator [t-PA], urokinase, trypsin, plasmin, and kallikrein).[9] The irreversibly bound factors are then excreted via the kidneys.

Although there are several inhibitors to the hemostatic system, the cornerstone for the removal of fibrin blood clots is via the fibrinolytic system. In this system, plasmin acts as the active fibrinolytic protease. Plasmin is derived from plasminogen. Plasminogen is a glycoprotein that circulates in blood and is activated to form plasmin on a needs-only basis by t-PA or urokinase-type plasminogen activator (u-PA).[11] Activation occurs when plasminogen binds fibrin, unfolding plasminogen and exposing

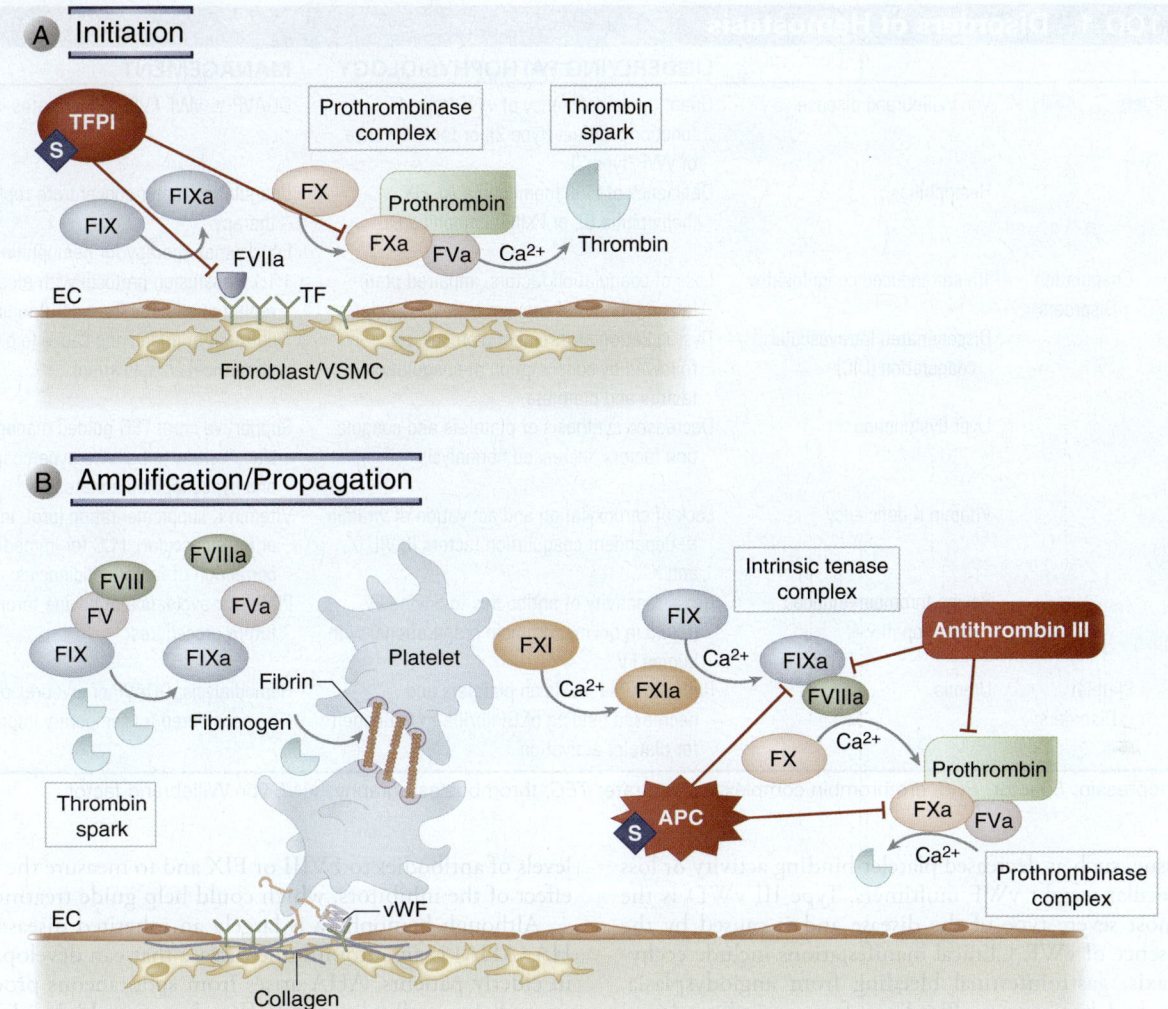

A Initiation

B Amplification/Propagation

FIGURE 100.3 (A–B) Inhibitors of coagulation. (A) Tissue factor plasma inhibitor *(TFPI)* inhibits the TF:FVIIa complex as well as directly inhibits FXa. Its inhibitory effect is enhanced when cofactor protein S is bound *(blue diamond)*. (B) Protein C is activated by thrombin binding to endothelial cofactor receptor thrombomodulin. Activated protein C then binds to cofactor protein S, and together, they inhibit cofactors FVa and FVIIIa. Antithrombin III is then activated by binding to heparan sulfate proteoglycans on vascular endothelial cells. Antithrombin III's role is preferentially to inhibit the common pathway by inhibiting FXa and inhibiting the intrinsic tenase complex by inhibiting FIXa. *F,* Factor; *TF,* tissue factor; *vWF,* von Willebrand factor.

plasminogen's cleavage sites to the cellularly secreted serine proteases t-PA or u-PA.[11] The activation to plasmin then causes degradation of FV and FVIII (disrupting the *prothrombinase complex* and *intrinsic tenase complex*) while cleaving cross-linked fibrin, dissolving the fibrin clot. Given plasmin's role in fibrinolysis, excessive plasmin formation can lead to excessive bleeding. In normal physiologic conditions, plasmin inhibition is controlled by t-PA and u-PA inhibitors, PAI-1, PAI-2, α_2-antiplasmin, thrombin activatable fibrinolysis inhibitor, α_2-macroglobulin, or C1 inhibitor.

DISORDERS OF HEMOSTASIS

Inherited Disorders of Hemostasis

Von Willebrand Disease (Types I-III)

Von Willebrand disease (vWD) is the most common inherited disorder of hemostasis, with an estimated population prevalence

of 0.6% to 1.3%.[12] The underlying etiology can be either a quantitative deficiency of vWF or a functional deficiency of vWF, depending on the type of vWD. vWF is a complex polypeptide with two primary functions for hemostasis. First, vWF activates platelets, as previously described. Additionally, vWF binds FVIII and prevents its degradation by proteases, thus stabilizing FVIII and prolonging FVIII half-life while circulating in plasma.[13] Thrombin later cleaves the vWF-FVIII complexes so that FVIIIa can contribute to the common pathway of the coagulation cascade. Without vWF, there would be decreased availability of FVIII for hemostasis (Table 100.1).

There are three main types of vWD, which follow an autosomal inheritance pattern. Type I vWD is the most common type, estimated to be 80% of vWD cases, with the mildest clinical manifestations.[12] Type I vWD is caused by a quantitative deficiency of circulating vWF with otherwise functional vWF. In comparison, type II vWD is caused by a dysfunctional vWF. The various subtypes of type II vWD are distinguished by the specific

TABLE 100.1 Disorders of Hemostasis

			UNDERLYING PATHOPHYSIOLOGY	MANAGEMENT
Inherited Disorders		Von Willebrand disease	Quantitative deficiency of vWF (type 1), functional defect (type 2), or total absence of vWF (type 3)	DDAVP ± vWF-FVIII concentrates
		Hemophilias	Deficiency of FVIII (hemophilia A), FIX (hemophilia B), or FXIII (hemophilia C)	Coagulation factor concentrate replacement therapy Emicizumab therapy for hemophilia A
Acquired Disorders	Coagulation Disorders	Trauma-induced coagulopathy	Loss of coagulation factors, impaired platelets, inhibition of calcium cofactor, acidosis	1:1:1 transfusion protocol with electrolyte repletion and stabilization of injuries
		Disseminated Intravascular coagulation (DIC)	Dysregulation of thrombotic processes followed by consumption of coagulation factors and platelets	Treatment of underlying cause (e.g., sepsis, obstetrical complication)
		Liver dysfunction	Decreased synthesis of platelets and coagulation factors; increased fibrinolysis	Supportive care; TEG-guided management of transfusions to balance hypercoagulable and hypocoagulable states
		Vitamin K deficiency	Lack of carboxylation and activation of vitamin K–dependent coagulation factors II, VII, IX, and X	Vitamin K supplementation (oral, intravenous, or intramuscular); PCC for immediate correction of factor deficiencies
		Bovine thrombin–induced coagulopathy	Cross-reactivity of antibodies to bovine FV (found in bovine thrombin preparations) with human FV	Platelets; avoidance of bovine thrombin in future procedures
	Platelet Disorders	Uremia	Reduced GPIa levels on platelets and decreased binding of GPIIb/IIIa to fibrinogen for platelet activation	Hemodialysis; DDAVP or cryoprecipitate can be considered for temporary improvement

DDVAP, Desmopressin; *F,* factor; *PCC,* prothrombin complex concentrate; *TEG,* thromboelastography; *vWF,* von Willebrand factor.

functional issue, such as decreased platelet-binding activity or loss of high-molecular-weight vWF multimers. Type III vWD is the rarest and most severe type of the disease and is caused by the complete absence of vWF. Clinical manifestations include ecchymosis, epistaxis, gastrointestinal bleeding from angiodysplasia, menorrhagia, and hematomas. Bleeding after surgical or dental procedures is very common in patients with vWD, and prophylactic treatment should be considered to aid with hemostasis in patients undergoing procedures.

Hemophilia

Hemophilia is a group of rare X-linked inherited diseases that result in deficiency of coagulation factors. Given its inheritance pattern, a meta-analysis of international registries focusing on hemophilia prevalence in males was performed in 2019. The results demonstrated an overall prevalence of 17.1 cases of hemophilia A (HA) per 100,000 males and 3.8 cases of hemophilia B (HB) per 100,000 males.[14] Specifically, HA is a deficiency of FVIII, and HB is a deficiency of FIX. Hemophilia C (HC) is even less common than HA and HB and is an autosomal recessive disorder with a deficiency of FXI.[15] Deficiency of coagulation factors results in delayed hemostasis and prolonged bleeding. Severity of the disease is dependent on the patient's baseline levels of coagulation factors. Therefore, clinical manifestations range from prolonged bleeding from minor injury or dental procedures to spontaneous hemorrhage into muscles, joint spaces, or intracranially.

Hemophilias are diagnosed and monitored using coagulation tests such as PT. Mixing studies can be performed to assess whether the prolonged PT is corrected with the addition of normal plasma and coagulation factors to the patient's plasma sample. Patients receiving factor replacement therapy may develop neutralizing antibodies that reduce the therapeutic effect in hemophilia patients.[16] Further testing can be performed to assess the levels of antibodies to FVIII or FIX and to measure the functional effect of the inhibitors, which could help guide treatment.[17]

Although hemophilia is largely an inherited disease, acquired HA (AHA) is an autoimmune disease that can develop, primarily in elderly patients. AHA arises from spontaneous production of neutralizing antibodies to FVIII and carries a high risk of mortality.[18] The occurrence of AHA may be preceded by malignancy, other autoimmune conditions, or infections. Human FVIII is ineffective in AHA, so porcine or recombinant FVIII may be used to aid in hemostasis. Emicizumab is hypothesized to be effective in the setting of AHA; however, further clinical trials are needed to support the safety and efficacy of this drug in this patient population.[19]

Acquired Disorders of Hemostasis

Trauma-Induced Coagulopathy

Trauma-induced coagulopathy (TIC) typically involves multiple factors, such as hypovolemia, metabolic derangements, liver dysfunction, and hypothermia. Hemorrhage after trauma is a major cause of death worldwide, and identifying the underlying issues for each patient is critical to correct the coagulopathy.[20] There are two phases of TIC. The early phase is characterized by diffuse endothelial trauma leading to altered thrombin production, loss of coagulation factors by hemorrhage, and hyperfibrinolysis. The protein C system is also activated, resulting in diminished FV and FVIII as well as increased fibrinolysis resulting from inhibition of PAI-1.[21] Platelets are commonly dysfunctional in TIC, preventing successful primary hemostasis and clot formation. This phenomenon has been termed *platelet exhaustion* because platelet levels may be normal, but platelet function is impaired.[22] With resuscitation and transfusions, the coagulopathy can worsen as a result of the dilutional effect on coagulation factors and decreased levels of calcium as a coagulation cofactor from citrate-containing blood products. More recent investigations also demonstrate inflammatory and immunomodulatory components of TIC.[22] As the trauma patient progresses through the resuscitative and stabilization phases, they move toward a more hypercoagulable state that resembles a consumptive coagulopathy state, such as in disseminated intravascular coagulation (DIC).[23] Early thromboprophylaxis is initiated in the late phase once hemostasis and supportive measures are in place.

Disseminated Intravascular Coagulation

DIC is a complex, systemic process that involves disorders of both coagulation and fibrinolysis and is associated with high (31%–86%) morbidity and mortality rates.[24] Most commonly, DIC is caused by infection; however, other etiologies include malignancy, severe bleeding after trauma, and obstetrical complications such as placental abruption or amniotic fluid embolism.[23] In the early phase of DIC, there is increased TF expression that leads to increased activation of prothrombin and thrombin.[25] Furthermore, the normal anticoagulant processes involving inhibitors such as TFPI, antithrombin, and protein C are impaired.[26] Additionally, normal fibrinolysis processes are interrupted by elevated levels of PAI-1, the primary inhibitor of fibrinolysis.[27] PAI-1 is increased during acute inflammatory phases and released by activated platelets, producing a prothrombotic state in which platelet activation and fibrin formation are elevated, with limited regulation.

The later phase of DIC involves a state of "consumptive coagulopathy" in which the liver cannot synthesize enough coagulation factors to compensate for the number of factors that were activated and used during the prothrombotic phase.[24] In this phase, the patient is subject to both bleeding and thrombotic complications as a result of competing processes of coagulation and fibrinolysis.

A defining feature of DIC is the "loss of localized activation of coagulation."[23] As part of this systemic process, dysregulated platelet aggregation and fibrin formation in the microvasculature result in microthrombus formation that can lead to organ failure. Other symptoms include mucosal bleeding, petechiae, and purpura secondary to thrombocytopenia. There are various scoring systems based on laboratory testing and symptoms that intend to detect DIC in the earlier phase; however, their predictive value has not yet been validated.[24] Laboratory abnormalities seen in DIC include thrombocytopenia, prolonged coagulation time, and increased fibrin degradation products (e.g., D-dimer).[27] Ongoing studies of biomarkers for DIC are investigating the potential utility of antithrombin, protein C, D-dimer, PAI-1, and vWF.[26]

Management of DIC is centered on treatment of the underlying cause. Once stabilized from obstetrical complications, patients may resolve within hours, whereas sepsis-induced DIC frequently persists and progresses.[26] Sequelae of failure of various organs should be recognized and addressed. Often, replacement of coagulation factors or platelets is given to help with hemostasis. However, transfusion of these products can also be challenging in the later phase of DIC because transfusion of blood products may worsen the thrombotic burden.

Liver Dysfunction

Traditionally, patients with liver dysfunction were believed to be in a hypocoagulable state as a result of decreased synthesis of platelets and coagulation factors. Although this is true to some extent, more recent investigations suggest there is also a hypercoagulable component with hepatic dysfunction. As a result of diffuse endothelial damage, there are increased vWF and FVIII

levels, leading to a higher risk of hypercoagulability.[28] Additionally, the liver is not able to synthesize normal levels of disintegrin and metalloproteinases that are responsible for the breakdown of vWF, further amplifying the prothrombotic effects of vWF. Fibrinolysis is also increased in hepatic dysfunction because FXIII synthesis is decreased and hepatic clearance of factors such as t-PA is diminished. Thus, hepatic dysfunction puts the patient in a balance between hypocoagulable and hypercoagulable states. Patients with end-stage liver disease are often at higher risk of deep venous thrombosis (DVT), portal venous thrombosis, and pulmonary embolism (PE) while also having an increased risk of excessive bleeding.

Standard laboratory testing may not accurately reflect the tenuous balance of coagulability in patients with end-stage liver disease. The PT, international normalized ratio (INR), and platelet levels are often abnormal with hepatic dysfunction. However, the American Gastroenterological Association best clinical practice guidelines for cirrhotic patients suggest that standard transfusion protocols based on INR levels are not supported by evidence, especially because excessive transfusions can lead to elevated portal pressures and volume overload.[29] Instead, recent studies suggest thromboelastography (TEG) as a better test to assess the overall hemostasis profile for patients with hepatic dysfunction because TEG-guided resuscitation versus standard laboratory tests led to reduced transfusions of platelets and fresh frozen plasma (FFP) without differences in postprocedural bleeding or complication rates (Fig. 100.1).[30,31] These findings suggest TEG may be a better test for patients with hepatic dysfunction because of its more comprehensive assessment of the phases of hemostasis.

Vitamin K Deficiency

Vitamin K is a fat-soluble vitamin that plays a role in multiple systems in the body, including bone development and cardiovascular disease. Vitamin K exists in different forms; vitamin K_1 is primarily found in leafy green plant sources, whereas vitamin K_2 is found in dietary sources such as fish, chicken, or dairy products and can also be biologically activated by gut flora of the distal small bowel and colon.[32] Vitamin K_2 has a longer half-life and a greater effect on vitamin K–dependent proteins compared with vitamin K_1. Notably, vitamin K serves as a cofactor to the enzyme gamma-glutamyl carboxylase, which adds carboxyl groups to various calcium-dependent proteins. Particularly in hemostasis, vitamin K helps activate the calcium-dependent proteins FII, FVII, FIX, and FX and proteins C and S[33]; therefore, vitamin K deficiency can prevent their normal functioning. Vitamin K deficiency can arise from inadequate dietary intake, malabsorption in the small bowel, and loss of storage sites in liver disease.[34] In preparation for surgery, individuals with vitamin K deficiency and prolonged PT or INR should be supplemented with oral or parental vitamin K. In the setting of acute bleeding with vitamin K deficiency, prothrombin complex concentrate (PCC) can also be administered to increase levels of vitamin K–dependent factors and improve hemostasis.

Vitamin K deficiency is also seen in the neonatal and postnatal periods as a result of certain medications given to the mothers during pregnancy, low placental transfer of vitamin K, low absorption in the newborn intestines, or low concentration of vitamin K in breast milk.[35] Therefore, the American Academy of Pediatrics recommends intramuscular administration of vitamin K to all newborn infants.[36] Additional redosing can be considered for infants who show signs of late-onset vitamin K–deficiency bleeding.

Uremia and Bleeding in End-Stage Renal Disease

Patients with end-stage renal disease (ESRD) have a higher tendency to bleed. This is attributed to not only lower levels of blood and coagulation factors resulting from anemia of chronic disease but also platelet dysfunction secondary to uremia.[34] In uremic patients, the cytoskeletal proteins are deficient, impairing platelet motility and adhesion.[37] Platelet activation is dependent on the binding of vWF to GPIb on platelets as well as the binding of fibrinogen to GPIIb/IIIa on platelets. Decreased levels of GPIb have been noted in patients with uremia, which may explain the impaired primary hemostasis for uremic patients.[37]

Additionally, toxins circulating in uremic plasma contribute to platelet dysfunction; however, the specific contributing components have not yet been identified. However, although the number of GPIIb/IIIa receptors is normal in uremia, their binding activity is diminished. The impaired binding of GPIIb/IIIa receptors is a reversible process that improves with dialysis.[38] Thus, although hemodialysis does not fully correct the platelet dysfunction, the clearance of potential toxins and reversal of abnormal GPIIb/IIIa binding to fibrinogen helps manage bleeding in patients with ESRD. Timing of hemodialysis sessions should be considered when scheduling patients with ESRD for surgery. Other adjuncts such as cryoprecipitate and desmopressin (DDAVP) may be considered to temporarily increase vWF, FVIII, or fibrinogen to overcome the platelet impairment.

Bovine Thrombin–Induced Coagulopathy

Bovine thrombin–induced coagulopathy is a rare disorder of hemostasis that has been described in various postoperative settings. The etiology is believed to be caused by development of antibodies to coagulation FV after prior exposure to topical bovine thrombin during surgery.[39] Thrombin is frequently used as a topical hemostatic agent in cardiovascular surgery, neurosurgery, and pediatric surgery. Different thrombin preparations exist, including bovine thrombin, plasma-derived human thrombin, and recombinant human thrombin. Although the thrombin is purified and processed, traces of bovine factors, such as FV, can remain.[40] Some patients may develop an immune response to these proteins during a second procedure, leading to development of antibodies to bovine FV. Cross-reactivity with human FV then results in destruction of the patient's own FV, leading to bleeding. Therefore, thrombin-induced coagulopathy is also referred to as *immune-mediated coagulopathy*.

Not all patients who develop antibodies to bovine thrombin preparations will develop bleeding complications; multiple exposures to bovine thrombin increase the risk of antibody development and the risk of bleeding complications.[41] Although rare, bovine thrombin–induced coagulopathy should be considered in the differential diagnosis of a patient with persistent postoperative bleeding that does not respond to surgical reexploration, blood products, or coagulation factor transfusions. If suspected, plasmapheresis or platelet transfusions have been suggested as management. Platelets contain FV that are released upon platelet activation. Platelet-derived FV is believed to be protected from anti-FV antibodies, as opposed to FV delivered from FFP.[40] Bovine thrombin should also be avoided in future procedures to prevent reexposures that could trigger antibody formation.

Iatrogenic Coagulopathies Secondary to Anticoagulant/Antiplatelet Use

There are a variety of medical conditions that require patients to be prescribed antiplatelet or anticoagulation therapy. The benefits

of the therapeutic agent should be weighed against the risk of bleeding in each patient. For example, the annual incidence of bleeding while on warfarin is estimated to be 15% to 20%, with an annual life-threatening bleeding rate of 1% to 3%.[42] This highlights the need to understand the underlying mechanism of each medication and its reversal agent to rapidly correct the hypercoagulable state in an emergency. Tables 100.2 and 100.3 show the most commonly prescribed anticoagulation and antiplatelet drugs, along with their corresponding mechanisms of actions and reversal agents.[43]

Diagnosis

Testing

Initial assessment of coagulation status involves measuring the PT, PTT, INR, and thrombin time. The PT evaluates the extrinsic and common pathway of coagulation, whereas the PTT evaluates the intrinsic and common pathway. When prolonged, the PT and PTT suggest a deficiency in coagulation factor(s) or whether an inhibitor to coagulation factors is present.[44] The PT is useful in monitoring the efficacy of vitamin K antagonists, such as warfarin, because it involves measurement of vitamin K–dependent factors II, VII, IX, and X.[45] The INR is calculated using the PT value and is therefore also commonly used for monitoring vitamin K–antagonist levels. The PTT is useful in testing for inherited diseases of coagulation, such as hemophilia, because the PTT measures include factors VIII and IX. Additionally, PTT is used to monitor and titrate unfractionated heparin for inpatients receiving continuous anticoagulation infusions. Unfractionated heparin inhibits prothrombin and FX, both of which are measured by the PTT. The activated clotting time (ACT) is a point-of-care test that is commonly used during procedures such as vascular surgeries or cardiopulmonary bypass to titrate anticoagulant doses to reach a desired threshold.

Quantification of blood components, such as a complete blood count, is also useful to determine the presence of thrombocytopenia that could be contributing to lack of hemostasis. Notably, pseudothrombocytopenia occurs when platelets clump in the laboratory sample as a result of anticoagulants such as ethylenediaminetetraacetic acid (EDTA) or cold agglutinins, leading to a falsely low platelet count.[44] Performing the test in tubes with other anticoagulants or with the sample kept at a different temperature can confirm the presence or absence of thrombocytopenia.

Fibrinogen is critical for the formation of stable clots for hemostasis. Fibrinogen levels can be measured from plasma samples directly, whereas the functional status of fibrinogen can be assessed using viscoelastic testing, such as rotational thromboelastometry (ROTEM).[46] Plasmin later breaks down the clot into fibrin degradation products that can be quantified by various immunoassay tests. These fibrin and fibrinogen degradation products are of varying sizes and molecular masses. One such fibrin degradation product is the D-dimer complex, which consists of two "D domains" that are connected by a central "E domain."[47] D-dimer levels can be measured via immunoassays that detect the D-dimer motifs that arise from fibrin degradation by plasmin. Measuring fibrin and fibrinogen degradation products can be particularly helpful with consumptive disease pathologies such as DIC.[48]

Additional testing for vWD includes measurement of the vWF antigen level, the vWF-Ristocetin assay, and measurement of FVIII activity. Low levels of vWF suggest type I vWD or type III vWD. These two types can be distinguished by extremely low

TABLE 100.2 Common Anticoagulation Therapies

	MEDICATION	ROUTE	MECHANISM	HALF-LIFE	CLEARANCE	REVERSAL AGENT
Anticoagulant	Heparin	Parenteral	Binds to antithrombin, then binds to and inhibits prothrombin	30–90 min	Reticuloendothelial System	Protamine
	Low-molecular-weight heparin (LMWH)	Parenteral	Activates antithrombin complex, which then inactivates factor Xa and prothrombin	3–6 h	Renal	Protamine Andexanet alfa[a]
	Fondaparinux	Parenteral	Highly selective binding to antithrombin to inhibit factor Xa	17–21 h	Renal	Recombinant factor VII PCC
	Bivalirudin, argatroban	Parenteral	Direct thrombin inhibitor, typically used for HIT	Bivalirudin: 25 min Argatroban: 40-50 min	Bivalirudin: renal Argatroban: Hepatic	N/A
	Warfarin (Coumarin)	Enteral	Vitamin K antagonists that inhibit activation of vitamin K–dependent coagulation factors (II, VII, IX, and X)	~35 h	Hepatic	Vitamin K therapy PCC or FFP
	Dabigatran (Pradaxa)	Enteral	Thrombin inhibitor	12–17 h	Renal	Idarucizumab (Praxbind)[b] Cryoprecipitate PCC
	DOACs (rivaroxaban [Xarelto], apixaban [Eliquis]; edoxaban [Savaysa])	Enteral	Bind directly to factor Xa or prothrombin without first binding to antithrombin	Apixaban: 12 h Rivaroxaban: 5–13 h Edoxaban: 10–14 h	*Apixaban:* 25% renal, 75% feces *Rivaroxaban:* hepatic, renal, minimal fecal *Edoxaban:* renal, fecal, minimal hepatic	Andexanet alfa PCC

[a]Andexanet alfa is recombinant factor Xa.
[b]Idarucizumab (Praxbind) is a monoclonal antibody that binds dabigatran.
DOAC, Direct oral anticoagulation; *FFP,* fresh frozen plasma; *HIT,* heparin-induced thrombocytopenia; *N/A,* not applicable; *PCC,* prothrombin complex concentrate.
From Yee J, Kaide CG. Emergency reversal of anticoagulation. *West J Emerg Med.* 2019;20(5):770-783; Dornbos D III, Nimjee SM. Reversal of systemic anticoagulants and antiplatelet therapeutics. *Neurosurg Clin N Am.* 2018;29(4):537-545.

TABLE 100.3 Common Antiplatelet Therapies

	MEDICATION	MECHANISM	REVERSAL AGENT
Antiplatelet	Acetylsalicylic acid/aspirin	Inhibits cyclooxygenase (COX)-1 → prevents generation of prostaglandin H2 and thromboxane A2 → impaired platelet activation and aggregation	No specific reversal agent • Stop aspirin 7–10 days before planned procedure • Consider platelet transfusion or DDAVP for acute bleeding
	Clopidogrel, ticagrelor, prasugrel, cangrelor	Thienopyridines that irreversibly block P2Y12 ADP receptors on platelets → preventing aggregation	No specific reversal agent • Stop clopidogrel 5 days before planned procedure • Consider platelet transfusion or DDAVP for acute bleeding
	Dipyridamole	Inhibits cAMP phosphodiesterase → increased cAMP levels within platelets and decreased thromboxane A2 activity → impaired platelet function	No specific reversal agent • Consider platelet transfusion or DDAVP for acute bleeding
	Cilostazol	Phosphodiesterase 3 inhibitor; similar mechanism to dipyridamole	No specific reversal agent • Consider platelet transfusion or DDAVP for acute bleeding
	Abciximab, eptifibatide, tirofiban	Inhibit GPIIb/IIIa receptors on platelets → platelets unable to bind fibrin and aggregate	No specific reversal agent • Consider platelet transfusion or DDAVP for acute bleeding

ADP, Adenosine diphosphate; *cAMP,* cyclic adenosine monophosphate; *DDVAP,* desmopressin.
From Popescu NI, Lupu C, Lupu F. Disseminated intravascular coagulation and its immune mechanisms. *Blood.* 2022;139(13):1973-1986; Yee J, Kaide CG. Emergency reversal of anticoagulation. *West J Emerg Med.* 2019;20(5):770-783.

levels of vWF antigen (<5 IU/dL) or by measuring the vWF propeptide, which is formed during the synthesis of vWF.[12] Type I vWD will have normal or slightly decreased vWF propeptide levels, whereas type III vWD will have absent or significantly decreased vWF propeptide levels. The vWF-Ristocetin assay evaluates the platelet-binding activity of vWF. Ristocetin is a cofactor that binds to vWF and platelets to trigger platelet aggregation.[49] Therefore, patients with vWD will have decreased platelet aggregation on the vWF-Ristocetin assay. Similarly, because vWF is an essential carrier for FVIII, patients with vWD will have decreased FVIII activity.

Rotational Thromboelastometry/Thromboelestography

TEG is a whole blood assay that evaluates all phases of hemostasis, including aggregation, clot strengthening, and fibrinolysis (Fig. 100.4). A sample is mixed with buffered sodium citrate and then placed into a cup in which there is a pin suspended in the center. The cup is oscillated around the pin, and the movement of the pin is recorded.[50,51] The TEG tracing is thus a reflection of the viscosity of blood as it progresses through hemostasis. A "rapid TEG" involves adding TF to the sample to accelerate the clotting process and provide results within 15 minutes, which can be particularly helpful in an acute setting.[50] The variables recorded in

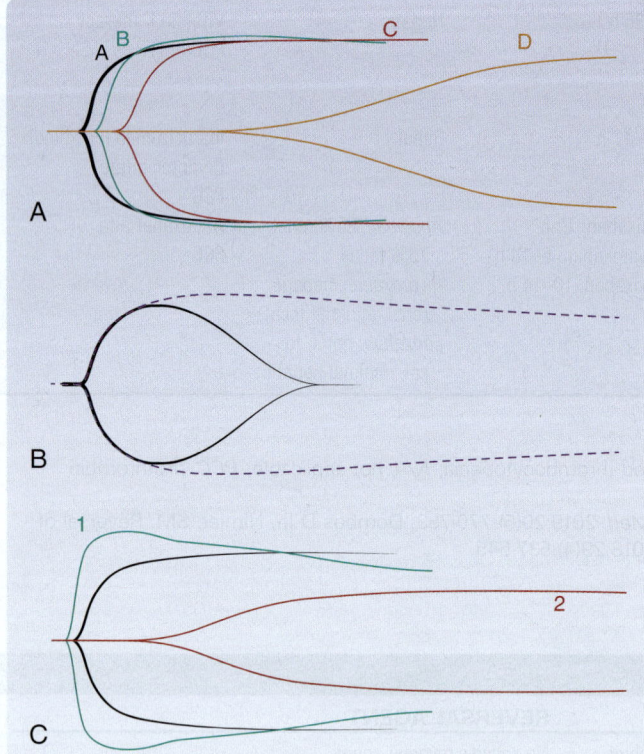

FIGURE 100.4 (A–C) Thromboelastography (TEG) tracings for disorders of hemostasis. (A) Hemophilia. The R-value will be prolonged when the coagulation factor level becomes significantly low. In mild cases, the parameters may be normal *(curve A)*, but the R time will get progressively longer with decreasing levels of the factor (as seen from *curve B to C to D*). In more severe cases, the thrombin may be low enough to affect the clot strength. (B) Primary fibrinolysis. The LY30 will be elevated significantly, and the maximum amplitude (MA) will be lower than normal. This is because the clot is breaking down faster than it can finish forming. The *black* curve peaks earlier and with a lower MA than the baseline *dashed purple curve;* however, the R and K times in the two curves are overlapping and roughly equal. (C) In stage 1 disseminated intervascular coagulation (DIC) *(blue curve)*, the patient will be hypercoagulable (both enzymatic and platelet), with moderately elevated LY30, elevated MA, and elevated alpha angle. The R time and K time are also decreased. The lysis is a physiologically appropriate response to an underlying thrombotic condition. If this hypercoagulable state is not treated effectively, the patient transitions into stage 2 DIC *(red curve)*, which involves consumptive coagulopathy. In stage 2 DIC, all parameters become hypocoagulable, reflected by prolonged R and K times and decreased MA and alpha angles. *K time,* Kinetical time; *LY30,* percentage of lysis 30 minutes after maximal clot strength; *R time,* reaction time. (Courtesy Anahita Dua, MD, MBA, MSC and Haemonetics Corporation.)

the TEG provide information on different factors that contribute to clot formation and degradation.

The reaction time, or R time, measures the time to develop clot formation. The R time is an assessment of coagulation factor activity in secondary hemostasis and the formation of thrombin. The kinetical time, or K time, measures the time until the clot has reached a specific viscosity. The K time reflects fibrin cross-linking and fibrin levels. Similarly, the alpha angle is a measurement of the slope or rate of the fibrin polymerization during the K time. The maximum amplitude (MA) is the highest amplitude of the TEG curve and represents the peak viscosity or strength of the clot.[51] The last variable measured with TEG is the LY30, which evaluates the percentage of clot breakdown or fibrinolysis over 30 minutes.

Abnormalities of the values recorded with TEG are helpful in guiding management of the bleeding patient. For example, a prolonged R time may prompt transfusion of FFP to supplement deficient or dysfunctional coagulation factors.[50] A prolonged K time or a decreased alpha angle may prompt cryoprecipitate transfusion to correct low fibrin levels and improve clot strengthening. Decreased MA suggests low platelet function, so platelet transfusion or DDAVP may be initiated. An elevated LY30 value may trigger TXA administration to decrease fibrinolysis. However, the accuracy of TEG may be worse for patients taking anticoagulants or antiplatelet therapy, which should be taken into consideration for each individual patient.

Several variations of TEG exist and can be used to test specific components of hemostasis. ROTEM is similar to TEG because ROTEM measures the viscosity of whole blood to create a profile of hemostasis. However, ROTEM is different in that the cup with the blood sample remains fixed, and the pin within the cup oscillates. The tracing from a ROTEM provides similar information on clot formation, strengthening, and lysis, but the measurements are not interchangeable with those of a TEG. Different reagents can be added to the ROTEM sample to focus on specific parts of the coagulation cascade (e.g., intrinsic or extrinsic pathways).[50] TEG is used more often than ROTEM in trauma centers in North America because of its availability.

Management

Common Hemostatic Medications

Plasma. Human plasma is commonly used to replace coagulation factors in several coagulopathies. Plasma is separated from erythrocytes, platelets, and leukocytes in whole blood and then stored in various ways. Plasma contains all coagulation factors as well as fibrinogen, albumin, proteins C and S, antithrombin, and TFPI. Plasma from a single donor can be stored individually or combined into "pooled plasma."[52] FFP is the most common way to store plasma, and FFP must be thawed before transfusion. Plasma is frequently given empirically for reversal of vitamin K antagonists when PCC is not available, in emergency surgery, or for patients with consumptive coagulopathies.[49] Abnormal lab values such as prolonged INR or prolonged R time on a TEG often trigger plasma transfusion. However, individual response to FFP may vary based on severity of illness and sex, making it difficult to determine how aggressive providers should be with transfusion.[53]

Additionally, plasma transfusions are not without risk. Higher levels of plasma transfusion are associated with increased risk of infection, sepsis, multiple organ failure, transfusion-related acute lung injury, and acute respiratory distress syndrome.[54] Additionally, there have not been many trials demonstrating benefit of plasma in hemostasis because plasma is commonly given in conjunction with other blood products.[55] Therefore, plasma is often used in the setting of coagulopathy and as part of massive transfusion protocols; however, providers should be cautious and intentional with its use.

Prothrombin complex. PCC contains plasma-derived coagulation factors II, VII, IX, and X, along with proteins C and S. Because these concentrates consist of vitamin K–dependent factors, they are the first-line treatment for emergent reversal of vitamin K antagonists. Compared with plasma, PCC has a lower rate of transfusion reactions and are more readily available. Additionally, the high concentration of factors in PCC requires less volume to deliver the factors, reducing the risk of volume overload.[56] Thus far, there remains a need for randomized controlled studies to assess the use of PCC in the perioperative or acute blood loss settings.[49] Various studies have investigated the use of PCC in the setting of major trauma, in end-stage liver disease, and as a reversal agent for anti-Xa inhibitors and suggest benefit from PCC in correcting deficiencies of vitamin K–dependent factors and improving survival after major trauma; however, further investigation is needed to assess the risk of venous thromboembolic events with PCC and the individual benefit of PCC as part of a transfusion protocol.[56]

Cryoprecipitate. Cryoprecipitate contains FVIII and FXIII, fibrinogen, fibrinonectin, anti-thrombin, and vWF. Fibrinogen is the first coagulation factor to be depleted during acute bleeding.[55] Hypofibrinogenemia after trauma is associated with the highest risk of massive transfusion requirements and mortality.[57] Therefore, cryoprecipitate is often considered for management of hypofibrinogenemia. Compared with FFP, cryoprecipitate is transfused in lower fluid volumes and contains higher concentrations of fibrinogen.[46] The Prospective Observational Multicenter Major Trauma Transfusion (PROMMTT) study was a multicenter observational study of transfusions given to adult trauma patients. As part of a secondary analysis, the use of cryoprecipitate and in-hospital mortality at 6 hours, 24 hours, and 30 days were also investigated. Patients who received cryoprecipitate were more injured and had higher physiologic abnormalities than those who did not receive cryoprecipitate; however, no significant survival benefit with cryoprecipitate transfusion was found.[58] However, the incorporation of cryoprecipitate in institutions' massive transfusion protocols varied greatly in the PROMMTT study, making conclusions regarding the true effect of early or structured cryoprecipitate transfusion protocols difficult. Thus, further studies are warranted to guide indications, timing, and quantity of cryoprecipitate transfusion.

As with many blood transfusion products, adverse reactions secondary to cryoprecipitate infusions include acute hemolytic transfusion reaction, anaphylactic response, transfusion-associated circulatory overload, febrile nonhemolytic transfusion reaction, and transfusion-related acute lung injury.[46] Patients receiving transfusions should be monitored closely, and the infusion should be stopped immediately if there is concern for any adverse reaction.

Desmopressin. Desmopressin, also known as *1-deamino-8-D-arginine vasopressin* or *DDAVP,* is a synthetic compound that mimics some of the functions of autogenous vasopressin. DDAVP stimulates V2 receptors, leading to release of endothelial vWF and increased FVIII.[59] DDAVP can be delivered to the patient intravenously, intranasally, or subcutaneously. Because DDAVP is a vasopressin analog, it also has antidiuretic hormone effects, which can lead to severe hyponatremia or seizures. Additional potential

side effects of DDAVP include flushing or cardiovascular complications.[60] However, evidence indicates that DDAVP is useful in hemostasis for patients with hemophilia, vWD, and even chronic liver or renal disease.[59] However, this response is transient and needs to be timed with the planned surgery in order to have the desired effects on hemostasis in the perioperative period.[13] Repeat doses of DDAVP can be administered to maintain desired vWF and FVIII activity levels. Close monitoring of fluid status and sodium levels should be maintained while patients are receiving DDAVP.

Tranexamic acid. TXA is administered to reduce bleeding by inhibiting fibrinolysis. TXA binds to plasminogen to inhibit the conversion of plasminogen into plasmin, therefore preventing the degradation of fibrin. TXA also plays an antiinflammatory role by inhibiting complement production.[61,62] For these reasons, TXA may be given in the setting of hyperfibrinolysis, such as when the LY30 is elevated on a TEG or fibrin degradation products are increased.

TXA has been used in multiple settings, including obstetrical bleeding, traumatic hemorrhage, and major surgeries. The Clinical Randomization of an Antifibrinolytic in Significant Hemorrhage (CRASH) Trials investigated 28-day mortality of trauma patients who received TXA within 3 hours of injury and those who did not receive TXA.[63] The CRASH trials support the use of TXA within the first 3 hours after injury; however, the dosage and interval of administration remain unclear.[64] The Pre-hospital Antifibrinolytics for Traumatic Coagulopathy and Hemorrhage (PATCH-Trauma) trial was a randomized, placebo-controlled trial investigating the effects of TXA given before hospital admission on survival and functional outcomes.[63] There was no significant difference in 6-month survival, with favorable functional outcomes between patients who received TXA and those who did not. However, TXA risks include thromboembolic events and seizures.[62] Therefore, further studies will be important to understand the impact of TXA and the risks of thromboembolic events associated with TXA administration.

Special Considerations

Von Willebrand disease. For patients with vWD, the specific type of vWD drives the choice of therapy. Patients with type I vWD respond well to DDAVP because it triggers the release of endothelial vWF that has already been synthesized. On the other hand, patients with type III vWD have complete absence of vWF synthesis and therefore will not be able to release any vWF even with stimulation from DDAVP. Instead, direct replacement of vWF and FVIII can be administered for treatment of type III vWD and most type II vWD patients.[13] Particularly in vWD patients with active bleeding or who are undergoing surgery, it is recommended that their vWF and FVIII activity levels are normalized and maintained within normal range within the first 5 to 10 days postprocedure, depending on the type of procedure.[60]

Hemophilias. The mainstay of therapy for hemophilia is replacement of the deficient coagulation factors. Traditionally, products such as cryoprecipitate, PCC, and plasma were administered to replete coagulation factors. However, more targeted therapies, such plasma-derived or recombinant FVIII and FIX concentrates, have been developed for these patients.[16] Prophylactic regimens have been developed to prevent bleeding episodes and involve intravenous infusions of replacement factor concentrates several times weekly. Replacement factors with longer half-lives have been developed to reduce the frequency of prophylactic infusions.[65] DDAVP can also be considered for patients with mild

HA to help boost endogenous FVIII; however, DDAVP is not adequate for acute bleeding episodes. Novel gene transfer therapies involving viral vectors have also been studied to increase circulating coagulation factor levels; however, sustained increases in plasma factor levels have not yet been demonstrated.[15]

Emicizumab is a bispecific monoclonal antibody that simulates FVIII by binding activated FIX with FX.[66] Most importantly, because this compound is distinct from FVIII, it is not affected by FVIII inhibitors. The HAVEN 1 trial was a randomized study of patients with HA and inhibitors who were treated with or without emicizumab and showed that once-weekly subcutaneous delivery of emicizumab had 87% lower treated bleeding rates compared with patients who did not receive emicizumab. Thus, emicizumab may be used in prophylactic treatment regimens for congenital HA patients with and without inhibitors.[19]

Trauma-induced coagulopathy. In the setting of TIC, it is recommended to transfuse in a 1:1:1 ratio (plasma:platelets:red blood cells) in the early resuscitation phase to minimize the dilutional effect of crystalloid fluids and to replete coagulation factors. The Pragmatic, Randomized Optimal Platelet and Plasma Ratios (PROPPR) trial was designed to compare the safety and effectiveness of a 1:1:1 transfusion ratio with a 1:1:2 ratio.[58] This trial showed no difference in mortality at 24-hour or 30-day time points between the two groups; however, more hemostasis was achieved in the 1:1:1 group, with fewer deaths secondary to exsanguination. Other studies suggest that the TEG may have a beneficial role in guiding transfusion management compared with standard laboratory tests.

Surgical Management

Electrocautery and suture ligation are first-line therapies for active bleeding within a surgical field. The electrocautery sends a current through the tissue to induce hemostasis by sealing vessels using heat. Methods such as suture ligation or clip placement provide physical barriers to small branches of arteries and veins to stop bleeding. Topical agents and biologically active agents may be used to control bleeding from microvasculature or diffuse ooze from impaired coagulation systems (Fig. 100.5).

Topical agents. Strategies for hemostasis intraoperatively include topical agents with several different underlying functions. Some agents, such as bone wax, act as a physical barrier to assist with tamponade in the surgical field and prevent further bleeding.[67] Overall, these rely on relatively normal-functioning coagulation factors and platelets. Bone wax is a nonabsorbable compound and has potential to become a source of infection as a foreign body. Ostene is a novel hemostatic compound that is used as an alternative to bone wax because it is absorbable and does not affect bone healing or cause an inflammatory response.[68]

Gelatin-based compounds (e.g., Gelfoam or Surgifoam) made from porcine skin are activated on contact with blood and then act as a matrix to promote platelet aggregation and clot formation. Similarly, collagen-based compounds (e.g., Avitene) increase platelet function and activate the intrinsic coagulation pathway for hemostasis.[69] Therefore, microfibrillar collagen agents are more successful in hemostasis for heparinized patients; however, these agents may be less effective for patients with thrombocytopenia. These agents exist in various preparation forms, such as powder, dry sheets, or paste, and may be left in situ to break down over the course of 4 to 6 weeks.

Cellulose-based agents (e.g., Surgicel) are made from oxidized cellulose and lead to hemostasis via multiple factors. First, activation of the agent promotes platelet aggregation and adherence.

Second, the low pH of the product has a caustic effect that results in coagulative necrosis and hemostasis. Third, the product expands when hydrated, leading to hemostasis by tamponade. Cellulose-based agents also have antimicrobial properties and can be left in the surgical field until breakdown in several weeks.

Caustic agents, such as silver nitrate or zinc chloride, induce hemostasis by causing "protein precipitation and vessel occlusion."[68] These are primarily used on superficial wounds and should be avoided in larger, open wounds. Additional benefits of these compounds include antimicrobial properties and the ease of application in a clinic setting.

Microporous polysaccharide hemospheres (MPH) are a newer option for topical hemostasis. MPH are hydrophilic and easily bind to platelets and factors needed to form a fibrin clot. The structure of the MPH also acts as a matrix for clot development once they contact blood.[67]

Synthetic sealants, such as cyanoacrylate or polyethylene glycol polymers, can also be used as physical barriers in the setting of bleeding. These compounds contain monomers that rapidly polymerize upon contact, creating an adhesive to seal a wound. BioGlue is made of glutaraldehyde and bovine albumin and is another alternative for topical hemostasis. It quickly transforms into an adherent scaffold that seals tissue or synthetic grafts, making it an option for sealing larger vessels or anastomoses.[67]

Biologically active agents. Thrombin can be prepared from bovine, human, or recombinant sources. Thrombin is applied directly to the surgical field and triggers the conversion of fibrinogen to fibrin, creating a clot. Thrombin also upregulates its own production via activation of factors V, VIII, and XI.[68] Thrombin is often used in conjunction with gelatin-based topical agents to further promote local hemostasis.[67] As previously discussed, rare cases of bovine thrombin–induced coagulopathy have been documented after exposure to bovine thrombin preparations.

Fibrin sealants (e.g., Tisseal, Artiss) contain fibrinogen, thrombin, calcium, and FXIII to enhance the common pathway of the coagulation cascade.[69] Some mixtures also include an antifibrinolytic, such as TXA or aprotinin, to further stabilize a nascent fibrin clot.[67] These sealants are biodegradable and are generally reabsorbed in the first 2 weeks after application. Fibrin sealants are kept frozen and then thawed into a liquid or spray at the time of use. Of note, this type of agent is not recommended in higher-volume arterial or venous bleeding because the developing thrombus could be dislodged by blood flow, resulting in an embolic event.[68]

"Flowable agents" describes a class of hemostatic products that combine active with passive hemostatic agents, combining a gelatin-based agent to serve as a scaffold for clot formation with an active biologic agent, such as topical thrombin, to activate the coagulation cascade.[67] This multifactorial mechanism is used in products like Floseal and Surgiflo.

Spontaneous intramuscular hematomas. Spontaneous intramuscular hematomas are relatively rare events. Most are managed conservatively; however, some can have severe sequela requiring additional interventions.[70,71] The pathophysiology of spontaneous intramuscular hematomas is not fully elucidated, although associated risk factors include advanced age, anticoagulation or antiplatelet therapy, hematologic disorders, and chronic kidney disease.[70–72] Clinical presentation is dependent on anatomic location of the hematoma. Rectus sheath hematomas are associated with damage to the superior or inferior epigastric arteries or their branches, which can result in abdominal pain, distention, ecchymosis, or peritonitis.[70,73] Retroperitoneal or iliopsoas muscle hematomas may be difficult to diagnose initially because of their

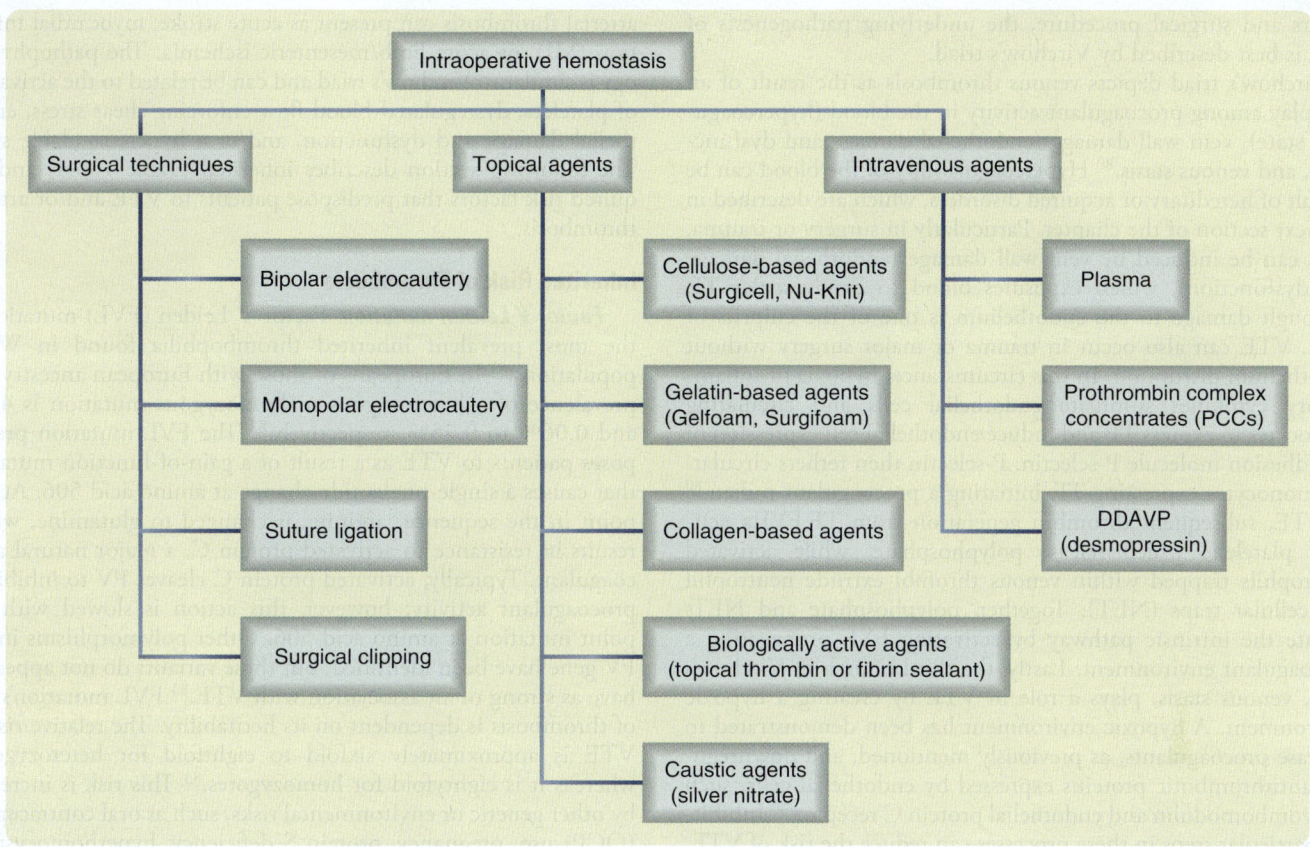

FIGURE 100.5 Options to consider for intraoperative hemostasis.

location. When large, iliopsoas hematomas can cause groin pain, muscle dysfunction, or compression of the femoral nerve, resulting in paresthesia or paralysis.[71]

Because of the deeper location of intramuscular hematomas, computed tomography (CT) imaging is the gold standard to evaluate size and location of hematomas.[70,73] Specifically, CT angiography is advantageous in identifying any vessels actively bleeding into the hematoma.[73] Initial management involves fluid resuscitation, pain control, reversal of anticoagulation, and blood transfusion if necessary. If the patient develops hemodynamic instability, ongoing transfusion requirements, neurologic symptoms, persistent pain, or compartment syndrome, further intervention may be warranted. Percutaneous arterial embolization is commonly the first-line therapy to stop further bleeding into the hematoma.[70,72,73] More invasive surgical decompression with ligation of bleeding vessels can be considered for severe cases without obvious target vessels for embolization.

Postoperative hematomas. Postoperative hematomas are a common complication in all surgical subspecialties. Contributing factors include inadequate hemostasis, sustained capillary bed bleeding from raw surfaces, surgical dead space, and coagulopathy.[74] Hypertension (described as a mean postoperative systolic blood pressure of 160 mm Hg) has also been found to be associated with hematoma formation after panniculectomy.[75] In patients with hematomas, risks and benefits should be weighed regarding cessation of anticoagulation or antiplatelet therapy. Commonly, these agents are discontinued until stabilization or resolution of the hematoma.

The management of postoperative hematomas is determined by the hematoma's anatomic location, size, and effect on surrounding tissues. Small postoperative hematomas generally self-resolve and do not require surgery. Larger hematomas can cause pain, wound dehiscence, and ischemic necrosis of overlying skin. These larger hematomas also pose a risk of infections that could result in additional complications. Special care should be taken for neck hematomas. Expanding hematomas in the neck region can compromise the airway and therefore require immediate surgical decompression.[76] For hematomas that pose a risk of skin necrosis and/or infection, evacuation should be performed. Evacuation of a hematoma involves reopening the wound, followed by mechanical expression, suctioning, or curettage.[77] The wound can then be reclosed or left open with packing or negative-pressure vacuum therapy. Temporary drains may be placed in the surgical bed to prevent reaccumulation of fluid and eliminate dead space; however, the drains have potential to become sources of infection and prolong hospitalization.[78] Further studies are warranted to determine the risks and indications for prophylactic surgical drain placement.

THE HYPERCOAGULABLE STATE

Pathophysiology of Venous Thromboembolism and Arterial Thrombosis

Venous thromboembolism (VTE), which includes DVT and PE, is a common source of morbidity and mortality in trauma patients and in patients undergoing major surgery. Overall, it is estimated to cause >50,000 deaths per annum in the United States, with ~25% of VTEs occurring in the perioperative period.[79] Although risk of VTE varies depending on patient risk factors and surgical procedure, the underlying pathogenesis of VTE is best described by Virchow's triad.

Virchow's triad depicts venous thrombosis as the result of an interplay among procoagulant activity in the blood (hypercoagulable state), vein wall damage (endothelial damage and dysfunction), and venous stasis.[80] Hypercoagulability of the blood can be a result of hereditary or acquired disorders, which are described in the next section of the chapter. Particularly in surgery or trauma, VTE can be induced by vein wall damage (endothelial damage and dysfunction), which exposures blood to extravascular TF. Although damage to the endothelium is one of the culprits of VTE, VTE can also occur in trauma or major surgery without endothelium disruption. In this circumstance, hypoxia or inflammatory cytokines stimulate endothelial cells and circulating monocytes to express TF and induce endothelial cell expression of the adhesion molecule P-selectin. P-selectin then tethers circulating monocytes expressing TF, initiating a procoagulant milieu.[80] In VTE, subsequent thrombin generation from TF:FVIIa activates platelets, which release polyphosphate, while activated neutrophils trapped within venous thrombi extrude neutrophil extracellular traps (NET). Together, polyphosphate and NETs initiate the intrinsic pathway by activating FXI, propagating a procoagulant environment. Lastly, the third branch of Virchow's triad, venous stasis, plays a role in VTE by creating a hypoxic environment. A hypoxic environment has been demonstrated to increase procoagulants, as previously mentioned, and downregulate antithrombotic proteins expressed by endothelial cells, such as thrombomodulin and endothelial protein C receptor.[80] Inhibiting particular steps in these processes can reduce the risk of VTE.

Arterial thrombosis can also occur in our perioperative surgical patients but is much less common. Risk of arterial thrombosis is largely dependent on type of surgery and coexisting risk factors, such as cardiovascular disease, inherited thrombophilia, and other acquired hypercoagulable disorders. In our surgical patients,

arterial thrombosis can present as acute stroke, myocardial infarction (MI), or acute limb/mesenteric ischemia. The pathophysiology is similar to Virchow's triad and can be related to the activation of platelets, dysregulated blood flow enforcing shear stress, endothelial damage and dysfunction, and/or a hypercoagulable state. The following section describes inherited (Table 100.4) and acquired risk factors that predispose patients to VTE and/or arterial thrombosis.

Inherited Risk of Thrombosis

Factor V Leiden mutation. Factor V Leiden (FVL) mutation is the most prevalent inherited thrombophilia found in White populations.[81] In Europeans or those with European ancestry, the prevalence of a heterozygous or homozygous mutation is 4.7% and 0.06% to 0.25%, respectively.[82] The FVL mutation predisposes patients to VTE as a result of a gain-of-function mutation that causes a single-nucleotide change at amino acid 506. At this point in the sequence, arginine is changed to glutamine, which results in resistance to activated protein C, a major natural anticoagulant. Typically, activated protein C cleaves FV to inhibit its procoagulant activity; however, this action is slowed with the point mutation at amino acid 506. Other polymorphisms in the FV gene have been identified, but these variants do not appear to have as strong of an association with VTE.[83] FVL mutation's risk of thrombosis is dependent on its heritability. The relative risk of VTE is approximately sixfold to eightfold for heterozygotes, whereas it is eightyfold for homozygotes.[83] This risk is increased by other genetic or environmental risks, such as oral contraceptive (OCP) use, pregnancy, protein S deficiency, hyperhomocysteinemia, and/or increasing age. Particularly in pregnancy, FVL mutation has been associated with recurrent pregnancy loss. FVL mutation has also been associated with increased risk of recurrent VTE. In a meta-analysis including 31 prospective observational cohort studies and 24 publications summarizing 13,571 patients

TABLE 100.4	Inherited Thrombophilias	
INHERITED THROMBOPHILIA	**UNDERLYING PATHOPHYSIOLOGY**	**DIAGNOSTIC MODALITIES**
Factor V Leiden mutation	Gain-of-function missense mutation of arginine to guanine at position 506 causing APC resistance	Functional assay of APC resistance using plasma or direct DNA-based tests[a]
Prothrombin gene mutation	Missense mutation of guanine to adenine at position 20210 causing increased thrombin synthesis	DNA-based methods[b]
Protein C deficiency	Monoallelic mutations in long arm of chromosome 2. Over 500 mutations have been identified.	Functional assays (clot-based or chromogenic). To minimize false positives, cease vitamin K–antagonism treatment.[c]
Protein S deficiency	*PROS1* gene mutation on chromosome 3 causing disrupted interaction with APC and TFPI	Immunoassay or functional clot-based methods. To minimize false positives, cease oral contraceptive or vitamin K–antagonism treatment.[d]
Antithrombin deficiency	*SERPINC1* gene mutation causing inability to clear thrombin and factor Xa	Functional chromogenic assay or immunoassay. DOAC can falsely increase antithrombin levels if using thrombin-based functional assay.[e]
Antiphospholipid antibody syndrome	Autoimmune systemic disorder causing persistent antiphospholipid antibodies, including LA, aCL, and aB2GPI.	Testing for presence of LA, aCL, and aB2GPI[f]

[a]DNA-based tests may not capture rare variants; therefore recommend using plasma.
[b]Functional assays not performed because there is variability in plasma prothrombin levels.
[c]Immunoassays not performed because not able to detect type II deficiencies.
[d]Diagnosis can be difficult because of variations in levels of protein S related to age (lower at birth), sex (females with 15% less protein S), and acquired conditions (pregnancy, oral contraceptive use). Need confirmation with second blood sample because of variations in protein S levels.
[e]Suspect with antithrombin activity <80%. Can use functional chromogenic assays measuring thrombin or FXa.
[f]Retest blood after 12-week interval to confirm diagnosis.
aB2GPI, Anti-*B2*Glycoprotein I antibodies; *aCL,* anticardiolpin; *APC,* activated protein C; *DOAC,* direct oral anticoagulation; *LA,* lupus anticoagulant; *TFPI,* tissue factor plasma inhibitor.

with provoked, unprovoked, or mixed VTE, FVL heterozygous mutations increased the risk of recurrent VTE by 42%.[81] Meanwhile, homozygous FVL mutation significantly increased risk of recurrence, with an odds ratio of 2.65.[83] Although not as common, FVL mutation is also associated with arterial thrombi presenting as ischemic stroke. In a 2019 meta-analysis using 68 eligible studies that described patients with arterial ischemic stroke with concomitant inherited thrombophilia, a total of 11,916 patients were identified to demonstrate that FVL was associated with a 1.25 odds ratio of acute ischemic stroke.[84]

Prothrombin gene mutation. Prothrombin G20210A gene mutation is the second most common inherited thrombophilia. Overall prevalence of heterozygous prothrombin gene mutation is estimated at 2%, whereas reports of homozygous mutations are clinically rare.[85] Prothrombin gene mutation develops from a missense mutation (guanine to adenine) at position 20210 of the prothrombin gene, which results in increased prothrombin synthesis.[86] The gain-of-function mutation leads to increased synthesis of thrombin and therefore increased risk of thromboembolic events. In patients with prothrombin gene mutation, the proposed increased risk of developing a first episode of VTE is threefold.[85] Typically, those who are carriers of the prothrombin gene mutation and have a thrombotic event will present most commonly with a DVT of the lower extremities or PE; however, thromboses in atypical sites, including portal, hepatic, or cerebral veins, have been reported. In these patients, prothrombin gene mutation carriers have a fourfold increased risk of developing portal vein thrombosis.[82] Interestingly, prothrombin gene mutation carriers do not have an increased risk of recurrent DVT in comparison to patients who do not carry this mutation but have a history of DVT.[82] Furthermore, polymorphisms of this gene defect do not have a clear association with VTE. In regard to arterial thrombi, prothrombin gene mutation has been associated with an increased risk of acute ischemic stroke in young patients, regardless of zygosity.[87] Depending on the study, the odds of an acute stroke in patients with PTM have ranged from 1.48 to 7.19.[87]

Protein C deficiency. Protein C is a vitamin K–dependent zymogen that is activated by the endothelial thrombomodulin-thrombin complex and protein C receptor. Its activation leads to its anticoagulant property, inhibiting FV and FVIII. The deficiency of protein C disturbs the hemostasis between procoagulant and anticoagulant proteins, thereby predisposing individuals to predominately VTE. Protein C deficiency results from pathologic mutations in the long arm of chromosome 2.[88] Monoallelic heterozygous deficiencies occur in 0.2% to 0.5% of the population and are inherited in an autosomal dominant manner.[88] Homozygous or compound heterozygous protein C deficiency is extremely rare. So far, >500 mutations in protein C have been identified.[89] Given the large quantity of mutations, protein C deficiencies have been further categorized into type 1 or type 2 deficiencies. Type 1 mutation is described as reduced concentration of protein C antigen and activity. Type 2, which is less common, results in dysfunctional protein C but normal protein levels.[90] The risk of VTE varies among patients with mutations in the protein C gene and is likely related to the degree of deficiency and whether other coexisting VTE risk factors exist. For example, the clinical presentation of protein C deficiency varies from asymptomatic patients to VTE to acute life-threatening complications such as purpura fulminans or DIC.[89] In regard to VTE alone, risk can be increased as high as tenfold to fifteenfold, with the first VTE usually occurring under the age of 50.[88,91] These patients are also at increased

risk of recurrent VTE. Protein C deficiency has been associated with multilocation arterial thrombosis, with patients presenting with acute stroke, MI, and critical limb ischemia.

Protein S deficiency. The incidence of protein S deficiency is rare, occurring in 0.03% to 0.13% of patients, with prevalence higher in the Southeast Asian population.[92,93] Protein S interacts with TFPI and is a vitamin K–dependent cofactor for activated protein C that is synthesized in the liver, vascular endothelium, monocytes, and megakaryocytes.[92] Protein S exists in the plasma in two forms: Approximately 60% is bound to complement component C4b-binding protein, and 40% is free.[86] The free component of protein S is the active anticoagulant. Protein S deficiency is inherited in an autosomal dominant fashion with mutations in the *PROS1* gene on chromosome 3. More than 200 mutations have been reported in the *PROS1* gene, and their effect can manifest in one of three forms: reduced levels of total and free protein (type I), normal levels of protein but reduced activity (type II), or normal total protein but reduced active (free) protein (tyle III).[86] All three subtypes have a similar clinical phenotype.

Patients with protein S deficiency have a higher risk of VTE and arterial thromboembolism (ischemic stroke). This risk is compounded by other genetic and acquired thrombophilic deficiencies. Acquired deficiencies include OCP, surgery, infection, pregnancy, and liver disease.[93] Particularly during inflammation, pregnancy, or usage of OCP, C4b-binding protein will increase, thereby redistributing protein S into a quiescent state.[86] In patients with arterial thromboembolism from protein S deficiency, the levels of protein S are variable, suggesting different mutations could exist that elicit a stronger thrombotic effect.[92] Protein S deficiency has also been linked to excessive blood clotting and immune hyperactivation seen in COVID-19 disease.[94] This hypercoagulability has been hypothesized to be the result of the SARS-CoV-2 papain-like protease cleaving protein S and thereby disrupting its ability to interact with both activated protein C and TFPI. In summary, any disruption of protein S, from inherited or acquired states, can increase patient risk of VTE or arterial thrombosis.

Antithrombin deficiency. Antithrombin is an anticoagulant that irreversibly binds thrombin; FX; and to a lesser degree, FIXa, XIa, XIIa, tPA, urokinase, trypsin, plasmin, and kallikrein. Inherited antithrombin deficiency is a rare autosomal dominant disorder, affecting 0.02% to 0.2% of the population.[9] Antithrombin deficiency is predominately caused by genetic defects in *SERPINC1* and is considered the most severe form of thrombophilia.[95] To date, 364 variants have been identified. When diagnosing congenital antithrombin deficiency, two types can be distinguished. *Type I* deficiency describes a reduction in antithrombin production, whereas *type II* describes a defect in protein function.[91] These distinctions are relevant because homozygous type I deficiency is thought to be incompatible with life. Homozygous type II is thought to cause severe VTE, whereas heterozygous type II is less virulent.

Patients with antithrombin deficiency compatible with life enter a hypercoagulable state with risk of venous and arterial thrombosis as a result of the inability to clear thrombin and FXa from the circulation.[9] However, the risk of arterial thrombosis is weaker than that for VTE. Risk of VTE has been reported to be as high as a fiftyfold increase.[95] VTE in these patients typically occurs as DVT of the legs, arms, and pulmonary arteries. VTE can also occur in unusual sites, including cerebral or sinus, mesenteric, portal, hepatic, renal, and retinal veins. Given exogenous heparin functions to promote antithrombin activity, patients with antithrombin deficiency have varying degrees of heparin resistance. Although antithrombin deficiency is certainly an inherited thrombophilic disorder, an acquired disorder is also seen with certain disease processes, including (1) transient or permanent reductions in hepatic synthesis and (2) consumption of plasma antithrombin at a faster rate than it can be produced. Some disease processes that reduce antithrombin include liver disease, DIC, active thrombosis, and proteinuria.

Antiphospholipid antibody syndrome. Antiphospholipid (aPL) syndrome is an autoimmune systemic disorder characterized by arterial, venous, or small vessel thrombosis and pregnancy complications in the setting of documented persistent antiphospholipid antibodies, including lupus anticoagulant (LA), moderate-high titer anticardiolipin (aCL), or *anti-B2*Glycoprotein I antibodies (aB2GPI).[96] The estimated prevalence is 0.05%, which is based on a cohort from Olmsted County, Minnesota.[97] The pathogenesis of aPL-mediated coagulation and fibrinolysis disruption is recognized to be related to aPL antibodies engaging with cell surface phospholipids and phospholipid-binding proteins, which activate platelets, monocytes, and endothelial cells. aPL antibodies are also recognized to upregulate TF and activate adhesion molecules, proinflammatory cytokines, neutrophils, and complement.[97]

The clinical manifestations are broad and include VTE in the lower extremities; arterial thrombosis in the cerebral arteries; and microvascular thrombi in the skin, eyes, heart, lungs, kidneys, and other organs. Obstetric complications include recurrent early miscarriages (<10 weeks), preterm delivery for preeclampsia with severe features of placental insufficiency, and fetal growth restrictions.[98] aPL syndrome can also manifest as catastrophic aPL syndrome, which is rapid-onset thrombosis in multiple vascular beds leading to multiorgan failure. Catastrophic aPL syndrome usually occurs in a small subgroup of patients and can be precipitated by a triggering event, such as infection, neoplasm, or surgery. Other manifestations of aPL syndrome can present as livedo reticularis, thrombocytopenia, cardiac valve damage, or nephropathy.

Risk of venous, arterial, or obstetric complications depends on antibody characteristics and other clinical factors.[96] Recent recommendations define high risk as the persistent presence of LA, double-aPL syndrome (any combination of LA, aCL, and aB2GPI), or triple-aPL syndrome (LA, aCL, aB2GPI) or the presence of persistently high titers.[99] Risk is further compounded by transient or acquired factors, such as smoking, prolonged immobilization, surgery, OCP, and so forth. In the prospective multicenter observational study Predictors of Pregnancy Outcomes: Biomarkers in Antiphospholipid Antibody Syndrome and Systemic Lupus Erythematosus (PROMISSE), the researchers identified LA as the strongest independent predictor of adverse pregnancy outcomes beyond 12 weeks' gestation.[96] Because of the relevance of each of these antibodies, testing includes identifying the presence of LA, aCL, and B2GPI with repeated testing at least once after an interval of 12 weeks. Repeated testing is recommended to monitor for transient elevations that can occur from infection, inflammation, or pregnancy.

Hyperhomocysteinemia. Hyperhomocysteinemia can be an inherited or acquired disorder that leads to cardiovascular, cerebrovascular, and thromboembolic disease. The most common genetic mutation resulting in elevated levels of homocysteine occurs in the enzyme methylenetetrahydrofolate reductase (MTHFR). The missense mutation results in MTHFR deficiency, dysregulating folate metabolism and homocysteine synthesis.[100] Another genetic mutation resulting in elevated levels of homocysteine involves defects in the transsulfuration pathway (cystathionine b-synthase deficiency). Acquired hyperhomocysteinemia can occur from deficiencies of folic acid, vitamin B_6, vitamin B_{12}, or chronic diseases (e.g., high blood pressure, diabetes mellitus, obesity, kidney failure, medications such as atorvastatin, and hypothyroidism). Approximately 5% to 7% of the general population is expected to have at least mild elevations in homocysteinemia, defined as a homocysteine level greater than 15 μmol/L.[101]

It is proposed that hyperhomocysteinemia leads to arterial and venous thrombosis by damaging endothelial cells, promoting inflammation, and increasing oxidative stress. At this time, data are controversial regarding whether hyperhomocysteinemia results in recurrent VTE.[102] In regard to treatment, reduction of homocysteine levels and its effect on cardiovascular and thromboembolic diseases is dependent on the type of disease. For example, studies have only demonstrated homocysteine-lowering therapies (folic acid, vitamin B_{12}, and vitamin B_6) to have a benefit in patients with homocystinuria; otherwise, homocysteine-lowering therapies remain controversial.[103]

Acquired Risk of Thrombosis

Cardiovascular disease. In this section, the pathophysiology of arterial thrombi in patients with atherosclerosis and atrial fibrillation is discussed. In patients with atherosclerosis, activated platelets play a significant role in the pathophysiology of arterial thrombosis. In this setting, acute thrombosis is initiated from plaque rupture or erosion, resulting in exposure of collagen and chronic inflammatory cells. Although the pathology of plaque rupture and erosion differ and are outside the scope of this chapter, in both circumstances, high shear conditions induced from blood flowing through luminal irregularities at the site of plaque disruption result in the aggregation and activation of platelets.[104] The coagulation cascade is then initiated by the milieu of activated platelets and TF deposited within and expressed by macrophages and VSMC in the atherosclerotic lesion. Together, these processes create a unique thrombus rich in platelets and fibrin.

In patients with valvular heart disease, cardiomyopathies, or arrhythmias such as atrial fibrillation, the pathophysiology of arterial thrombosis also involves the key elements of blood stasis, endothelial dysfunction, and a hypercoagulable state. Studies have demonstrated that about 14% to 20% of patients who underwent transesophageal echocardiogram, cardiac surgery, or autopsy had left atrial thrombi.[105] Particularly in atrial fibrillation, insufficient atrial systolic function leads to blood stasis in the long and narrow left atrial appendage, which provides a site for intraatrial thrombus formation.[105] The stagnant blood flow also causes atrial endothelial microinjury/dysfunction, leading to the recruitment of immune cells.[106] These immune cells then secrete systemic inflammatory mediators, including C-reactive protein and interleukin (IL)-6, that invigorate a hypercoagulable state by initiating TF production in monocytes.[105] Patients with atrial fibrillation are also known to have elevated levels of vWF, fibrinogen, and P-selectin, factors associated with a hypercoagulable state.[105]

Infection. Infections, such as sepsis and COVID-19, induce a thromboinflammatory state that contributes to organ damage and thrombotic complications. Particularly in patients with COVID-19, observational studies demonstrated that the robust thromboinflammatory milieu induced macrovascular thrombosis in 10% to 30% of patients, which included those receiving standard-dose anticoagulation.[107] *Thromboinflammation,* in general, describes the complex interactions between inflammation and hemostasis, involving proinflammatory cytokines, chemokines, adhesion molecules, TF expression, and platelet and endothelial activation. The cells particularly relevant in thromboinflammation are platelets and neutrophils.

At the site of inflammation, platelets are the first cellular component adhering to the inflamed endothelium. Adherent platelets promote inflammation and organ damage by recruiting leukocytes, increasing vascular permeability, and promoting edema.[108] Of these functions, platelet-leukocyte interactions dictate the outcome of the thromboinflammatory state. The initiating step in thromboinflammation includes platelet recruitment of leukocytes and regulation of leukocyte function through multiple mechanisms, including direct and indirect receptor-ligand pairs; platelet secretion of inflammatory cytokines, chemokines, and growth factors (PF4, IL-1, RANTES, B-thromboglobulin, platelet-derived growth factor [PDGF], platelet-activating factor, CXCL7, migration inhibiting factor [MIF], TXA_2, serotonin); and platelet activation of the complement system.[108] Some of the receptor-ligand pairs include P-selectin glycoprotein ligand-1 (PSGL-1), GP1bα-macrophage 1 antigen (MAC-1), GPIIbIIIa-MAC-1 through fibrinogen, and CD40-CD40L. Furthermore, platelet activation of complement promotes endothelial cell activation, upregulation of TF, and further release of inflammatory cytokines.

Once leukocyte recruitment is initiated, neutrophils are the first at the scene. Neutrophils adhere to the endothelium and transmigrate through cell-cell interactions, where they then operate to phagocytose pathogens, degranulate, and release NET (NETosis). NET are netlike complexes consisting of chromatin DNA, histones, and neutrophil granule proteins, which are released into the extracellular space.[109] They function to bind pathogens and prevent their spread as well as ensure their elimination though antimicrobial and toxic factors. Although NET trap and kill pathogens, they can become pathogenic. In the recent literature, NET and activated platelets are observed in patients with sepsis and COVID-19, with high levels of NET-derived damage-associated molecular patterns (DAMP) correlating with thrombotic complications.[110] Thus, NET from recruited neutrophils are an important influencer of thromboinflammation. One example of NET influence on thromboinflammation is the effect of histones. Histones are one of the DAMP that propagate thromboinflammation as a result of activation of platelets, endothelial cells, and coagulation while impairing fibrinolysis.[110] Another NET-derived protein discussed in thromboinflammation is calprotectin (S100A8/A9). Calprotectin has been shown to have a prothrombotic effect by interacting with endothelial cells, activating platelets, and promoting fibrin generation as well as supporting immune cell recruitment and migration.

In summary, the reciprocal interactions between platelets and neutrophils propagate the inflammatory and thrombotic complications seen in thromboinflammatory disease states, such as sepsis and COVID-19. Not discussed in this section, other thromboinflammatory states that demonstrate this reciprocal interaction include DVT, sickle cell disease, stroke, and ischemia/reperfusion injury.

Neoplasia. Cancer is associated with an increased risk of VTE in multiple venous systems and arterial thrombosis. These disease processes are associated with worsened survival in cancer patients.[111] The incidence of cancer-associated VTE is increasing over time, with recent data estimating incidence to be 3.4%, whereas incidence of VTE in the general population remains around 0.36%.[112] This increase is likely a result of improved treatment options prolonging survival as well as increased surveillance imaging capturing incidental VTE. Although all cancer types predispose patients to VTE and arterial thrombosis, risk is largely influenced by type and stage of cancer, underlying comorbidities, and treatment-related factors (chemotherapy, protein kinase inhibitors, antiangiogenic therapy, and immunotherapy). Of all cancers, the highest thrombotic risk is observed in pancreas, stomach, and primary brain tumors. Other important risk factors include younger age, distant metastasis, prior history of VTE, and use of two-agent immunotherapy.[111–113] Recently, certain germline single-nucleotide polymorphisms (SNP) were also identified as risk factors for cancer-associated VTE. Cancer-driven mutations, such as *STK11, KRAS, CTNNB1, KEAP1, CDKN2B,* and *MET,* have also been implicated.[111] Although each cancer patient is unique in their risk of VTE and arterial thrombosis, mechanistically, cancer-associated thrombosis is likely driven by a combination of different pathways. These pathways include altering host biologic systems and tumor expression of procoagulant proteins that are released into the circulation.

Cancer has also been known to cause thrombocytosis, which is an independent risk factor for VTE. Although high platelet count increases risk of thrombosis, certain cancers increase levels of vWF and biomarkers associated with platelet activation (P-selectin, soluble CD40 ligand, thrombospondin-1, and platelet factor 4), which are associated with VTE.[111] Cancer is also associated with leukocytosis, which can be detected in 14% to 30% of cancer patients.[111] Leukocytosis is particularly relevant because activated monocytes express TF, whereas neutrophils in some cancers release NET that increase the prothrombotic milieu and proteases that degrade anticoagulant TFPI. Although many cancers affect host systems, tumor cells also express their own procoagulant proteins. Particularly, many cancer cells express high levels of TF and secrete extracellular vesicles with TF, creating a prothrombotic environment. Taken together, cancer-associated VTE and arterial thrombosis result from an interplay between the alteration of host defenses and tumor-specific expression of proteins that create a prothrombotic environment.

Pregnancy. Pregnant females are at four times greater risk of VTE than nonpregnant females of similar age from the time of conception through 6 weeks postpartum.[114] VTE is particularly concerning in this patient population because acute PE is one of the leading causes of maternal death in the Western world, with incidence of PE reported to be 1.72 cases per 1000 deliveries.[114,115] The hypercoagulable state induced by pregnancy is generally believed to be an evolutionary adaptation to reduce hemorrhage at the time of childbirth and prevent pregnancy loss. The risk of VTE in pregnant patients is compounded by prior history of VTE, hospitalization for an acute illness or cesarean-section delivery, and presence of an inherited thrombophilia. Mechanistically, pregnancy follows Virchow's triad. The hypoxic or inflammatory state created during early pregnancy triggers endothelial cell activation and adhesion receptors and leads to the activation of circulating leukocytes. Furthermore, increased estrogen levels elevate vWF through direct stimulation of endothelial cells and induce elevated plasma levels of clotting factors (FII, FVII, FVIII, FX, fibrinogen, and PAI-1) while reducing anticoagulants (protein S, protein C, and antithrombin).[116] Venous stasis in pregnancy occurs through the enhanced responsiveness of the vessel wall to hormonal changes and by the mechanical pressure of the gravid uterus. Thus, pregnancy induces a hypercoagulable state as a result of endothelial activation, alterations in procoagulant proteins, and venous stasis.

Smoking. Smoking is a known risk factor for the development of atherosclerosis and VTE. In regard to VTE, a retrospective analysis using 1.1 million participants from the Emerging Risk Factors Collaboration and the UK biobank found smoking to be associated with VTE, with a hazard ratio (HR) of 1.38.[117] The association was similar in magnitude for PE and DVT outcomes and similarly associated with provoked and unprovoked VTE. This study mitigated the previous thought that VTE risk was secondary to increased hospitalization for smoking-related diseases. Mechanistically, nicotine and other additives in cigarettes increase the percentage of reactive oxygen species; they reduce nitric oxide availability and generate an inflammatory and prothrombotic microenvironment.[82] The loss of nitric oxide–related protective effects (endothelial cell stability, vascular homeostasis, antiinflammatory and antioxidant properties) and increased reactive oxygen species work together to increase platelet activation. Thus, smoking is an independent risk factor for unprovoked VTE by increasing platelet activation and generating an inflammatory microenvironment.

Obesity. Obesity and other metabolic disorders are closely linked to chronic systemic inflammation and cardiovascular complications, including arterial and venous thrombosis. With regard to VTE, obesity is demonstrated to be an independent risk factor in males and females, with risk increased 6.2-fold. This risk is further increased when another acquired risk factor is present.[118] The relationship between obesity and arterial or venous thrombosis is dependent on adipose tissue's central role in both immunity and vascular homeostasis. Adipose tissue secretes bioactive peptides known as *adipokines*.[119] These molecules reach different organs and have a wide range of functions, including appetite control and pro- and antiinflammatory actions. Particularly in obesity, the adipokine leptin is elevated as a result of the body's resistance to leptin's function. Hyperleptinemia then upsets the endothelial leptin signaling, leading to a proinflammatory microenvironment and predisposing obese patients to VTE. Furthermore, increased visceral fat is associated with a prothrombotic state by increasing expression of PAI-1, an inhibitor of t-PA and u-PA. Increased visceral fat is also associated with decreased levels of the adipokine adiponectin, which is associated with increased inflammatory mediators, including monocyte chemoattract protein-1 (MCP-1). MCP-1 contributes to cardiovascular disease, such as atherosclerosis, by recruiting monocytes and macrophages into arterial vessel walls, thereby increasing obese patients' risk for arterial thrombosis. Additional mechanisms that increase the risk of VTE include hypoxemia induced by hypoperfusion of an expanding fat mass. In summary, obesity increases inflammatory mediators that create a prothrombotic environment, increasing the risk of both VTE and arterial thrombosis in the setting of endothelial damage or hyperactivation.

Warfarin-induced skin necrosis. Warfarin-induced skin necrosis is a rare but severe complication occurring in 0.01% to 0.1% of patients who receive the drug warfarin.[120] Warfarin is an anticoagulant that inactivates vitamin K–dependent clotting factors II, VII, IX, and X; protein C; and protein S. Patients at highest risk of this rare complication include those who have an underlying thrombophilia, those with an acquired prothrombotic risk factor, and those who have not been pretreated with an anticoagulant that is non–vitamin K dependent. Of the thrombophilias, protein C deficiency is the highest risk factor for warfarin-induced skin necrosis. Other thrombophilias observed in warfarin-induced skin necrosis include hyperhomocysteinemia, congenital deficiency of protein S, antithrombin III deficiency, and FVL mutation.

The pathogenic mechanism underlying warfarin-induced skin necrosis relies on the rapid fall of protein C compared with the other vitamin K–dependent clotting factors. The rapid fall of protein C induces a hypercoagulable state that promotes microthrombi in the cutaneous and subcutaneous venules.[121] Warfarin-induced skin necrosis is associated with higher loading doses and typically occurs in the first 10 days of initiation; however, case reports have described late-onset presentation, varying from months to years.[120] Clinically, skin lesions develop in areas of high amounts of subcutaneous fat and appear as poorly demarcated erythematous eruptions that are generally preceded by paresthesias. Next, edema develops in the dermis and subcutaneous tissues, with progression to hemorrhagic bullae within 24 hours. The hemorrhagic bullae signify irreversible injury and full-thickness coagulative skin necrosis. Diagnosis is generally from clinical suspicion. Laboratory workup may be performed to exclude other potential causes because protein C and S concentrations are not recommended for diagnostic workup given their poor sensitivity and specificity.[121]

Heparin-induced thrombosis. Heparin-induced thrombosis (HIT) occurs in 0.5% to 1% of patients exposed to unfractionated heparin and 0.1% to 0.5% of patients exposed to low-molecular-weight heparin (LMWH).[122] It is an immune disorder that results in IgG antibodies that complex to platelet factor 4/heparin and result in arterial and venous thrombosis, with a predilection for venous thrombosis.[123] The platelet factor 4–heparin–IgG (PF4-H-IgG) complex then binds to platelets, monocytes, and neutrophils. Platelet binding results in platelet activation, and monocytes begin to produce TF, thrombin, and inflammatory mediators.[123] Neutrophil activation leads to the release of NETs. The PF4-H-IgG typically binds the Fcγ receptor on these differing cell types to elicit a robust thrombotic response.

Clinically, HIT manifests as a drop in platelet count greater than 30% from baseline about 5 to 10 days after heparin administration. HIT more commonly occurs after orthopedic surgeries, cardiac surgery, and extracorporeal circulation. Presentation of thrombosis includes skin necrosis, venous limb gangrene, bilateral adrenal hemorrhage, and cerebral vein thrombosis.[122] Diagnosis can be achieved using platelet activation assays such as 14C-serotonin release assay, platelet aggregation assay, and flow cytometric assay (>95% high specificity but lower sensitivity, 56%–100%). High-sensitivity tests with lower specificity (30%–70%) include immunoassays.[123] Once HIT is confirmed, heparin should be stopped immediately.

Assessment of the Hypercoagulable State

The Inherited Hypercoagulable Disorders

Inherited thrombophilia should be suspected in patients with VTE at a young age (<50), disease in first-degree relatives (at least one parent or sibling), VTE in unusual locations, idiopathic or recurrent VTE, or history of recurrent miscarriage.[124] Historically, testing for inherited thrombophilia is controversial because testing can lead to overdiagnosis, defined as labeling an individual with the disease who would have otherwise been asymptomatic while causing physical, psychological, or financial harm if the condition is discovered.[125] In 2023, evidence-based guidelines from the American Society of Hematology intended to support decision-making about thrombophilia testing were developed. The guidelines discussed recommendations for testing thrombophilias most consistently associated with VTE, which include FVL mutation, prothrombin G20210A mutation, protein C or protein S deficiency, antithrombin deficiency, and antiphospholipid syndrome. Recommendations were labeled as "strong" or "conditional" according to the GRADE (grading of recommendations assessment, development and evaluation) approach. In summary, the panel issued a strong recommendation against testing the general population before starting OCP therapy. Conditional recommendations were made for the following scenarios: (1) patients with VTE associated with nonsurgical major transient or hormonal risk factors; (2) patients with cerebral or splanchnic venous thrombosis, in settings where anticoagulation would otherwise be discontinued; (3) individuals with a family history of antithrombin mutation or protein C or protein S deficiency when considering thromboprophylaxis for minor provoking risk factors and for guidance to avoid contraceptive therapy or hormonal therapy; (4) pregnant females with a family history of high-risk thrombophilia types; and (5) patients with cancer at low or intermediate risk of thrombosis and with a family history of VTE.[125] Further recommendations outlined by Middeldorp et al. can be found in Tables 100.5A and 100.5B.

Management of the Hypercoagulable State

Risk Assessment in Hospitalized Patients

Risk assessment models (RAM) have been developed to predict future risk of VTE in hospitalized patients and guide type, duration, and strength of prophylaxis.[126] One such model is the Caprini RAM. Since its introduction in 1991, Caprini RAM has been validated in over 250,000 patients in more than 100 clinical trials. It is a dynamic scoring tool that allows ongoing evaluation of surgical patients during their hospital course to determine risk of 30- and 60-day VTE. Risk factors included in this scoring system are age,

medical history (including inherited/acquired thrombophilias), personal or family history of VTE, and surgery-related variables (type and length). The points allocated to each risk factor range from 1 to 5 and are determined by their association with VTE (Table 100.6).[127] Since its development, the Caprini RAM has proven to be consistent, thorough, and efficacious for risk stratification and selection of prophylaxis in postoperative surgical patients.

Medical Management—Role of Anticoagulation

The medical management of acute thromboembolism in patients with inherited or acquired thrombophilias is similar to that for the general population. Particularly for VTE, management consists of three phases: the initiation phase, treatment phase, and extended phase.[128] The initiation phase begins after the diagnosis of VTE and lasts 5 to 21 days. Treatment during this period is with parenteral or high-dose oral anticoagulation. The *treatment phase* describes the period after initiation and is considered complete after 3 months of standard therapeutic doses of anticoagulation. The *extended phase* describes the use of anticoagulants at full or reduced doses for the goal of secondary prevention. In the extended phase, there is no preplanned stop date. The decision to continue or stop anticoagulation is patient dependent. For patients with an inherited thrombophilia, the decision to continue or discontinue treatment should be guided by the 2023 ASH guidelines by Middeldorp et al. (see Tables 100.5A and 100.5B).[125] Anticoagulation for the hypercoagulable state includes parenteral anticoagulation (unfractionated heparin, LMWH, fondaparinux), direct oral anticoagulants (DOAC), parenteral anticoagulation followed by a DOAC, or parenteral anticoagulation overlapped by

TABLE 100.5A Recommendations Derived From the 2023 American Society of Hematology Guidelines for Management of Venous Thromboembolism: Thrombophilia Testing (Part 1)

QUESTION	RECOMMEND TESTING	TREATMENT
Should thrombophilia testing be performed in the following cases?		
Unprovoked symptomatic VTE	No	Short term
VTE provoked by surgery	No	Short term
Splanchnic VTE without cirrhosis, planning to continue anticoagulation indefinitely	No	Short term
Cerebral VTE planning to continue anticoagulation	No	Short term
Unspecified type of VTE	No	Short term
VTE by a nonsurgical major transient risk factor	Yes.	Indefinite
Females with VTE provoked by pregnancy	Yes	Indefinite
Females with VTE associated with COC	Yes	Indefinite
Cerebral VTE, planning to discontinue anticoagulation	Yes	Indefinite
Splanchnic VTE without cirrhosis, planning to discontinue anticoagulation	Yes	Indefinite
Should testing be performed to guide use of thromboprophylaxis for minor provoking risk factor?		**Treatment recommendation if tested and positive:**
Family hx of VTE and unknown thrombophilia status	No. Consider if multiple family members with VTE or if family member was young or patient preference.	
Family hx of VTE and thrombophilia	Yes[a]	Start thromboprophylaxis.
Family hx of thrombophilia but no VTE	Yes[a]	Start thromboprophylaxis.

Further remarks regarding recommendations can be found in the original guidelines. *Thrombophilia testing* refers to testing for antiphospholipid antibodies and all hereditary thrombophilia types. A positive family history is defined as having a first- or second-degree relative with VTE. These recommendations do not address homozygous defects or combinations of thrombophilia types, unless specified. Most recommendations are conditional based on GRADE approach.
[a]Designates if patient has family with history of antithrombin, protein C, or protein S deficiency.
COC, Combined oral contraceptive; *hx,* history; *VTE,* venous thromboembolism.
From Middeldorp S, Nieuwlaat R, Baumann Kreuziger L, et al. American Society of Hematology 2023 guidelines for management of venous thromboembolism: thrombophilia testing. *Blood Adv.* 2023;7(22):7101-7138.

TABLE 100.5B   Recommendations Derived From the 2023 American Society of Hematology Guidelines for Management of Venous Thromboembolism: Thrombophilia Testing (Part 2)

QUESTION	RECOMMEND TESTING	TREATMENT
Should testing be performed in females with a family hx of VTE and/or family hx of thrombophilia?		
To guide use of COC[a]	No	
To guide HRT	No	
Selective testing to guide COC use	Yes[b]	Avoid COC.
Selective testing to guide HRT	Yes[b]	Avoid COC.
Selective testing to guide thromboprophylaxis during pregnancy	Yes, if known family hx of homozygous FVL, combination FVL and PGM, or antithrombin deficiency. Either testing if family hx of protein C or S deficiency.	Start antepartum thromboprophylaxis.
Selective testing to guide thromboprophylaxis postpartum	Yes, if first-degree family hx of VTE and homozygous FVL; combination FVL and PGM; antithrombin, protein C, or protein S deficiency. Yes, if second-degree family hx of VTE and combination FVL and PGM or antithrombin deficiency. Either testing if second-degree family hx of VTE and protein C or S deficiency.	Start antepartum thromboprophylaxis.
Should testing be performed in females with family hx of VTE but unknown thrombophilia?		
To guide OCP use	No	
To guide HRT	No	
Cancer-associated testing:		
In ambulatory cancer patients receiving systemic therapy with a family hx of VTE	Yes	Start antepartum thromboprophylaxis.

Further remarks regarding recommendations can be found in the original guidelines.[116] *Selective testing* refers to testing for a specific thrombophilia type. A positive family history is defined as having a first- or second-degree relative with VTE. These recommendations do not address homozygous defects or combinations of thrombophilia types, unless specified. *Either testing* refers to testing or not testing the patient. These recommendations are conditional based on GRADE approach.
[a]Indicates strong recommendation.
[b]Designates if patient has family with history of antithrombin, protein C, or protein S deficiency.
COC, Combined oral contraceptive; *FVL*, factor V Leiden mutation; *HRT*, hormonal replacement therapy; *Hx*, history; *PGM*, prothrombin gene mutation; *VTE*, venous thromboembolism.
From Middeldorp S, Nieuwlaat R, Baumann Kreuziger L, et al. American Society of Hematology 2023 guidelines for management of venous thromboembolism: thrombophilia testing. *Blood Adv.* 2023;7(22):7101-7138.

warfarin until INR is between 2.0 and 3.0 (see Table 100.3).[124] DOAC include oral direct factor Xa inhibitors (rivaroxaban, apixaban, edoxaban, and betrixaban) and direct thrombin inhibitors (dabigatran).[129] Currently, DOAC are the recommended treatment modality for VTE, including patients with homozygous FVL, combined prothrombin gene mutation and FVL, protein C or S deficiency, and antithrombin deficiency or mutation.[130]

Special considerations. In pregnant patients with or at risk of VTE, LMWH is preferred because it does not cross the placenta and is associated with a lower risk of HIT and osteoporosis.[114] In cancer-associated VTE, LMWH was considered the standard of care.[124,128] However, recent guidelines recommend an oral Xa inhibitor (apixaban, edoxaban, rivaroxaban) over LMWH in cancer-associated DVT. In patients with HIT, heparin should be stopped immediately, and direct parenteral thrombin inhibitors (bivalirudin, argatroban) or DOAC should be initiated (see Table 100.2).

Warfarin, a vitamin K antagonist, was previously the standard oral anticoagulant for patients with VTE. Patients on warfarin require bridging with parenteral anticoagulation 5 days earlier to mitigate the risk of warfarin-induced skin necrosis. Currently, warfarin is the recommended first-line oral therapy for patients who are unable to adhere to DOAC and for patients with aPL syndrome.[128] For patients with high-risk aPL syndrome, INR should remain between 2 and 3. These patients should not be

transitioned to DOAC because DOAC-treated aPL patients have a higher risk of recurrent thrombosis.[97] For aPL patients with arterial thrombosis, target INR can be increased to 3 to 4. Low-risk aPL patients who have been started on a DOAC may remain on a DOAC if no complications have occurred.[97] Given warfarin is contraindicated in pregnancy, aPL pregnant females should be transitioned to a low-dose aspirin and prophylactic heparin. If the pregnant patient has a history of thrombotic aPL syndrome, then therapeutic heparin and low-dose aspirin should be started. Patients prescribed warfarin who experience warfarin-induced skin necrosis should be treated immediately. Treatment begins with immediate withdrawal of warfarin. Next, parenteral anticoagulation can be given as well as vitamin K and/or FFP.[120] If warfarin-induced skin necrosis is secondary to protein C deficiency, monoclonal antibody-purified concentrates of protein C can be administered.

Special consideration should also be taken in patients with antithrombin deficiency or COVID-19 and pregnant patients with FVL, prothrombin mutation, or antithrombin deficiency. Patients with antithrombin deficiency derived from inherited or acquired states may display resistance to heparin products, defined as inadequately increased aPTT values despite robust efforts at anticoagulation (using >35,000 units of heparin daily).[9] To anticoagulate these patients, they can receive a DOAC or be given antithrombin replacement therapy. Antithrombin replacement therapy induces sensitivity to heparin products and is particularly

TABLE 100.6 Caprini Risk Assessment

Risk Factor Representing 1 Point

Age 41–60 years	Medical patient on bed rest
Minor surgery	Past medical hx: BMI >25, acute MI, COPD, other risk factors
Recent events <1 month: major surgery, CHF, sepsis, pneumonia	COC or HRT
Venous disease or clotting disorder: varicose veins, current swollen legs	Pregnancy or postpartum
Infant that is premature with toxemia or growth restriction	

Risk Factor Representing 2 Points

Age 61–74 years	Current central venous access
Type of surgery: major >45 min, laparoscopic >45 min, or arthroscopic surgery	Patient confined to bed > 72 hours
Recent events <1 month: immobilizing plaster cast	Present or previous malignancy

Risk Factor Representing 3 Points

Age ≥75 years

Venous disease or clotting disorder: history of DVT/PE, family hx of thrombosis, positive FVL, elevated serum homocysteine, positive LA, elevated anticardiolipin antibody, HIT, other congenital acquired thrombophilia

Hx of unexplained stillborn infant, recurrent spontaneous abortion

Risk Factor Representing 5 Points

Type of surgery: elective major lower extremity arthroplasty

Recent events <1 month: hip, pelvis or leg fracture, stroke, multiple trauma, acute spinal cord injury causing paralysis

Recommended Prophylaxis[a]

SCORE (RISK)	MANAGEMENT
0–4 (low-moderate)	Early ambulation
5–8 (high–very high)	Early ambulation, intermittent pneumatic compression + 7–10 days anticoagulation,
> 9 (highest)	Intermittent pneumatic compression + 30 days anticoagulation

Points allocated to risk factors addressed in the Caprini Risk Assessment and the recommended prophylaxis in postoperative surgical patients. Anticoagulation options include unfractionated heparin or low-molecular-weight heparin.

[a]Recommended prophylaxis not including patients undergoing total joint replacement. Recommendations for total joint replacement include the following: score of <10—early ambulation, intermittent pneumatic compression, and aspirin for 30 days postoperatively; score >10—early ambulation, intermittent pneumatic compression, and anticoagulation (low-molecular-weight heparin or fondaparinux or direct oral anticoagulation [DOAC]) for 30 days postoperatively.

BMI, Body mass index; *CHF*, congestive heart failure; *COC*, combined oral contraceptive; *COPD*, congestive obstructive pulmonary disease; *DVT*, deep vein thrombosis; *FVL*, factor V Leiden mutation; *HIT*, heparin-induced thrombocytopenia; *HRT*, hormonal replacement therapy; *hx*, history; *LA*, Lupus anticoagulant; *MI*, myocardial infarction; *PE*, pulmonary embolism.

From Cronin M, Dengler N, Krauss ES, et al. Completion of the updated Caprini Risk Assessment Model (2013 version). *Clin Appl Thromb Hemost.* 2019;25:1076029619838052.

helpful in patients who are going to the operating room and need rapid discontinuation of anticoagulation for mitigation of bleeding risk. If the decision is to anticoagulate with a DOAC, plasma antithrombin activity should be repeated for confirmation during the transition away from heparin. Furthermore, these patients should be discharged on therapeutic anticoagulation and followed up by hematology.[129] Patients with COVID-19 are at risk for both macrothrombotic events (DVT, PE) and immunothrombosis. Non–critically ill hospitalized COVID-19 patients should receive *at least* standard-dose thromboprophylaxis, using LMWH or unfractionated heparin. However, therapeutic-intensity LMWH or unfractionated heparin demonstrated a decreased risk of major thromboembolic event or death, suggesting therapeutic intensity may be preferred over standard dose in non–critically ill COVID-19 patients.[131] Meanwhile, critically ill COVID-19 patients should receive standard-dose thromboprophylaxis instead of therapeutic dosing. If COVID-19 patients who meet criteria

are discharged on anticoagulation, they should receive rivaroxaban 10 mg daily for 35 days.[131] COVID-19–positive patients who develop VTE should be treated with anticoagulation for 3 to 6 months, in accordance with guidelines for VTE with a transient provoking risk factor. Our last special consideration includes pregnant patients with FVL, antithrombin deficiency, or PTM. These pregnant patients are at increased risk of recurrent pregnancy loss. Although no guidelines are available, studies have demonstrated that these patients may benefit from treatment with LMWH or unfractionated heparin, with or without aspirin.[132]

Medical Management—Role of Antiplatelets

Antiplatelet therapy is indicated for primary or secondary prevention of arterial disease, including acute ischemic stroke, MI, or peripheral arterial disease (see Table 100.3). For individuals with inherited thrombophilia, guidelines recommend aspirin in addition to heparin for pregnant patients with aPL syndrome.

Antiplatelet therapy has also been investigated in pregnant patients with FVL, antithrombin deficiency, or PTM who experience recurrent pregnancy loss. However, the results are debatable, with no guideline specifically endorsing the addition of aspirin to mitigate pregnancy loss in these patients. Antiplatelet therapy has also been investigated in prophylaxis for COVID-19 VTE. Randomized controlled trials (RECOVERY, ACTIVE-4a) demonstrated that the use of antiplatelet therapy (aspirin or ticagrelor) plus therapeutic-intensity heparin provided no difference in thromboembolic outcomes compared with therapeutic heparin alone.[131] In this section, we briefly discuss commonly used antiplatelets for the inherited or acquired risk factors for thromboembolism, which include aspirin, clopidogrel, and ticagrelor.

Aspirin exhibits its effects by irreversibly inhibiting cyclooxygenase (COX), thereby reducing platelet aggregation by inhibiting the synthesis of thromboxane A2.[133] Restoration of thromboxane A2 levels requires platelet turnover, which takes approximately 10 days. Aspirin has been recommended by the American Heart Association and American Stroke Association as the primary protective agent in cardiovascular disease in patients with a 10-year cardiovascular risk score above 10%.[133] Aspirin treatment failure, defined by vascular events during treatment, has been described in the literature with a frequency of 12.9%. Failure can be explained by poor medication adherence, poor absorption, drug interactions, insufficient dosing, and alternate pathways of platelet activation. Alternate pathways include upregulation of COX expression during times of inflammation and polymorphisms of COX, platelet membrane glycoproteins, the *P2Y1* gene, and/or vWF.

Clopidogrel (brand name Plavix) is a second-generation thienopyridine antiplatelet agent that reduces platelet aggregation by irreversibly inhibiting the $P2Y_{12}$ ADP receptors on the surface of platelets.[133] Subsequently, ADP-mediated activation of the glycoprotein IIb/IIIa complex is prevented. The benefits of clopidogrel have been demonstrated in multiple RCT. For example, clopidogrel has been shown to be more efficacious than aspirin in preventing adverse cardiovascular outcomes (Clopidogrel Versus Aspirin in Patients at Risk of Ischemic Events [CAPRIE] study) and beneficial when added to aspirin (dual-antiplatelet therapy) in patients with acute coronary syndrome (Clopidogrel in Unstable Angina to Prevent Recurrent Events [CURE] trial).[134] When ingested, clopidogrel starts as a prodrug and therefore requires metabolization to activate. Metabolism is mediated by the hepatic cytochrome P450 system. Hyporesponders or resistance to clopidogrel has been linked to genetic polymorphisms in the cytochrome P450 enzyme. Currently, the American College of Cardiology/American Heart Association guidelines state there is no randomized evidence to support routine genetic testing;

however, the decision to perform genotyping can be made on a selective basis.[134]

Ticagrelor reversibly binds to and inhibits the $P2Y_{12}$ platelet receptor. This drug is approved for the prevention of cardiovascular events in patients with atherosclerotic cardiovascular disease and may be beneficial in patients with clopidogrel resistance. In additional to its antiplatelet activity, ticagrelor has known antiinflammatory properties.[135] Particularly, ticagrelor-treated patients have demonstrated reduced risk of infection-related death and improved lung function in patients hospitalized with pneumonia.

Surgical or Endovascular Management

Acute thromboembolism has the potential to be managed through surgical or endovascular interventions. Management of thrombosis depends on type of thrombosis, anatomic location, extent of disease, and hemodynamic status of the patient. Treatment options include medical anticoagulation, surgical embolectomy, catheter-based interventions using fibrinolytic agents, percutaneous mechanical thrombectomy or pharmacomechanical thrombolysis, endovascular stenting, and/or systemic thrombolysis. In this section, we discuss fibrinolytics.

Fibrinolytic agents use plasminogen activators to activate plasmin. Activating plasmin leads to the cleavage of cross-linked fibrin, thereby dissolving the clot. There are three generations of plasminogen activators, which include streptokinase, urokinase, alteplase, reteplase, and tenecteplase.[136] Streptokinase and urokinase are both considered to be first-generation fibrinolytic agents. Unfortunately, the first-generation fibrinolytics lack fibrin specificity because they bind circulating systemic plasminogen and fibrin-bound plasminogen with similar affinity. Given this lack of affinity and streptokinase's high risk of allergic reactions in patients, these fibrinolytics have limited use. Alteplase, on the other hand, is a second-generation agent enzymatically manufactured to resemble t-PA, making it fibrin specific. By localizing to plasminogen on fibrin, there is a reduced risk of digestion of systemic soluble fibrinogen. Lastly, the third-generation agents, tenecteplase and reteplase, are modified versions of enzymatically manufactured t-PA with increased specificity to fibrin. The half-life of these third-generation agents is longer because they have been modified to evade binding of PAI-1 and therefore require reduced dosing. Absolute contraindications to the use of these various systemic fibrinolytics include active bleeding, prior history of intracerebral hemorrhage, brain or spinal surgery within the past month, ischemic stroke within the past 3 months, suspected aortic dissection, cerebrovascular disease or central nervous system neoplasia, recent head trauma with fracture or brain injury, and abdominal surgery (Table 100.7).[136]

TABLE 100.7	**Abbreviation Key**			
aB2GPI	Anti-B2Glycoprotein I		FXIIa	Activated factor XII
aCL	Anticardiolipin		FVL	Factor V Leiden
ACT	Activated clotting time		GP	Glycoprotein
ADP	Adenosine diphosphate		HA	Hemophilia A
ATP	Adenosine triphosphate		HB	Hemophilia B
AHA	Acquired hemophilia A		HC	Hemophilia C
APC	Activated protein C		HIT	Heparin-induced thrombocytopenia
aPL	Antiphospholipid		INR	International normalized ratio
CBC	Complete blood count		LA	Lupus anticoagulant
DAMP	Damage-associated molecular patterns		MCP-1	Monocyte chemoattract protein-1
DDAVP	Desmopressin		MI	Myocardial infarction

TABLE 100.7 Abbreviation Key—cont'd

DIC	Disseminated intravascular coagulation	MPH	Microporous polysaccharide hemospheres
DVT	Deep venous thrombosis	NET	Neutrophil extracellular trap
EDTA	Ethylenediaminetetraacetic acid	OCP	Oral contraceptive
ESRD	End-stage renal disease	PAI	Plasminogen activator inhibitor
FFP	Fresh frozen plasma	PCC	Prothrombin complex concentrate
FII	Factor II, prothrombin	PE	Pulmonary embolism
FIIa	Activated factor II, thrombin	PT	Prothrombin time
FV	Factor V	PTT	Partial thromboplastin time
FVa	Activated factor V	ROTEM	Rotational thromboelastometry
FVII	Factor VII	TEG	Thromboelastography
FVIIa	Activated factor VII	TF	Tissue factor
FVIII	Factor VIII	TFPI	Tissue factor plasma inhibitor
FVIIIa	Activated factor VIII	TIC	Trauma-induced coagulopathy
FIX	Factor IX	t-PA	Tissue-type plasminogen activator
FIXa	Activated factor IX	TXA	Tranexamic acid
FX	Factor X	u-PA	Urokinase-type plasminogen activator
FXa	Activated factor X	VTE	Venous thromboembolism
FXI	Factor XI	vWD	von Willebrand disease
FXIa	Activated factor XI	vWF	von Willebrand factor
FXII	Factor XII		

CONCLUSION

In conclusion, bleeding or thrombosis intraoperatively or postoperatively is a result of the complex interplay between coagulation enzymes, platelets, endothelial cells, and even immune cells. Understanding the molecular mechanisms in the hemostatic system is necessary to elucidate whether pathologic bleeding or thrombosis is related to inherited or acquired disorders. By understanding the mechanism of the disorder, an effective medical or surgical intervention can be used.

SELECTED REFERENCES

Adelborg K, Larsen JB, Hvas AM. Disseminated intravascular coagulation: epidemiology, biomarkers, and management. *Br J Haematol*. 2021;192(5):803-818.

Adelborg et al. provide a thorough review of the pathophysiology and etiology of DIC, along with current diagnostic testing, principles of management, and prospective biomarkers that may be used in the future.

Dornbos D III, Nimjee SM. Reversal of systemic anticoagulants and antiplatelet therapeutics. *Neurosurg Clin N Am*. 2018;29(4):537-545.

Dornbos et al. provide a comprehensive review of the most common anticoagulants and antiplatelet therapies, including the mechanisms of action, potential side effects, dosages, and reversal agents.

Erdoes G, Faraoni D, Koster A, Steiner ME, Ghadimi K, Levy JH. Perioperative considerations in management of the severely bleeding coagulopathic patient. *Anesthesiology*. 2023;138(5):535-560.

Erdoes et al. provide a comprehensive review of the perioperative patient with severe bleeding. The article then focuses on pathophysiology, testing, and management of specific disease processes, such as trauma, inherited bleeding disorders, and drug-related bleeding disorders.

Leebeek FW, Eikenboom JC. Von Willebrand's disease. *N Engl J Med*. 2016;375(21):2067-2080.

Leebeek et al. provide a comprehensive review of the diagnosis, treatment, and clinical manifestations of each type of vWD. The article goes in-depth into the pathophysiology of vWD and potential treatments in the future.

Middeldorp S, Nieuwlaat R, Baumann Kreuziger L, et al. American Society of Hematology 2023 guidelines for management of venous thromboembolism: thrombophilia testing. *Blood Adv*. 2023;7(22):7101-7138.

Middeldorp et al. provide the updated screening guidelines and management of venous thromboembolism secondary to inherited thrombophilia.

O'Donnell JS, O'Sullivan JM, Preston RJS. Advances in understanding the molecular mechanisms that maintain normal haemostasis. *Br J Haematol*. 2019;186(1):24-36.

O'Donnell et al. provide an updated overview of the "cascade" hypothesis of blood coagulation and then incorporate new accumulating data to reveal how the cascade model has been transformed into the cell-based model.

Pastori D, Cormaci VM, Marucci S, et al. A Comprehensive review of risk factors for venous thromboembolism: from epidemiology to pathophysiology. *Int J Mol Sci*. 2023;24(4):3169.

Pastori et al. provide an updated comprehensive review of risk factors for venous thromboembolism. The article goes in-depth regarding the pathophysiology of important inherited and acquired factors that are outlined in this book chapter.

Raval JS, Griggs JR, Fleg A. Blood product transfusion in adults: indications, adverse reactions, and modifications. *Am Fam Physician.* 2020;102(1):30-38.

Raval et al. provide a review of the current guidelines for transfusions, including the contents of each blood product and potential adverse effects.

Tompeck AJ, Gajdhar AUR, Dowling M, et al. A comprehensive review of topical hemostatic agents: the good, the bad, and the novel. *J Trauma Acute Care Surg.* 2020;88(1): e1-e21.

Tompeck et al. provide a comprehensive review of available topical hemostatic agents used intraoperatively, including benefits, contraindications, and mechanisms of action of each agent.

The full reference list appears on Elsevier eBooks+.

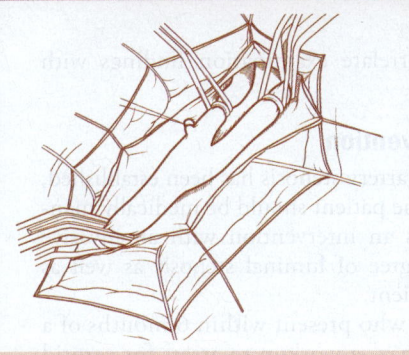

CHAPTER 101

Contemporary Management of Carotid Disease

Rohini J. Patel, Jesse A. Columbo, David H. Stone, and Mahmoud B. Malas

OUTLINE

INTRODUCTION

Carotid artery stenosis remains a major underlying risk factor for stroke, which is the fifth-leading cause of death in the United States.[1] Currently, it is estimated that extracranial carotid occlusive disease affects approximately 1.5% of individuals worldwide, with increasing prevalence among older patients.[2] Risk factors that predispose toward carotid artery stenosis are those commonly associated with atherogenesis and peripheral arterial disease, including smoking, hypertension, dyslipidemia, and diabetes.[3] In this setting, the American Heart Association (AHA) currently recommends ongoing surveillance for patients with moderate carotid stenosis and consideration of revascularization for those with severe disease.[4] Consequently, approximately 100,000 carotid artery interventions are performed annually in the United States alone, with many more patients followed on a longitudinal basis.[5]

PATHOPHYSIOLOGY

Evidence of early-stage atherosclerotic arterial disease can be detected as early as the third decade of life.[6,7] Damage of the arterial intima by free radicals or lipoproteins leads to fatty streak formation, the precursor to an arterial plaque.[8] Areas of the arterial tree that are subject to turbulent blood flow, such as the carotid artery bifurcation, are particularly prone to plaque formation.[9,10]

Infiltration of lipoproteins, accompanying proinflammatory cytokines, and turbulent blood flow at such anatomic locations collectively predispose to the physiologic environment where an atherosclerotic plaque may develop.[8,11] Over time, such plaque formation can evolve to frank luminal encroachment with ensuing arterial stenosis or occlusion.[11] For the carotid artery in particular, plaque formation can additionally serve as a nidus for thrombus formation, placing a patient at risk for thromboembolic complications, such as transient ischemic attack (TIA) or stroke.[12,13]

CLINICAL PRESENTATION

The clinical presentation for patients with carotid artery stenosis has historically been divided into symptomatic and asymptomatic disease. Symptomatic carotid stenosis is commonly defined as a patient who has experienced amaurosis fugax (transient monocular blindness), cortical TIA, or stroke within the 6 months before presentation, thought to be attributable to an ipsilateral carotid lesion. This definition is predicated on landmark randomized controlled trials (RCTs) that form the historical foundation for current evidence-based guidelines on the management of extracranial carotid disease.[14,15] Accurate designation of patients as either asymptomatic or symptomatic remains a critical diagnostic distinction with requisite therapeutic sequelae, most notably including the thresholds and benefits of revascularization, based on the presence or absence of adjudicated focal neurologic symptoms.[4]

Patients can be diagnosed with asymptomatic carotid disease in a variety of ways. Notably, the United States Preventative Services Task Force does not currently recommend routine screening for asymptomatic carotid disease, and consequently, most asymptomatic disease is detected on studies performed for alternative indications.[16] Deviations from this guidance occur not uncommonly and often transpire in the setting of an audible neck bruit, documented multifocal vascular disease, or the presence of multiple atherosclerotic risk factors. However, even under these considerations, most asymptomatic carotid disease is detected incidentally in current practice.

The presentation and diagnosis of patients with symptomatic carotid disease is accordingly more urgent. Patients with thromboembolic complications from an underlying associated carotid stenosis, including amaurosis fugax, TIA, or stroke, will commonly present acutely to the emergency room or clinic for urgent evaluation. Symptoms that resolve within 24 hours are historically categorized as TIA, whereas those lasting beyond this time interval or remaining beyond this interval are consistent with a stroke. Likewise, radiographic abnormalities on dedicated cerebral imaging such as magnetic resonance imaging (MRI) may confirm a diagnosis of stroke. As may be expected, TIA and stroke symptoms can vary widely in their severity. Patients with less severe symptoms may not always present to an emergency room for evaluation. Rather, some may present less acutely to their primary care provider, as may often be the case among patients with vision changes that may not be immediately apparent as amaurosis fugax. In other situations, patients may initially present to an ophthalmologist or other vision professional, which may subsequently prompt further evaluation of the carotid arteries. Although it may initially seem that the diagnosis of symptomatic carotid stenosis would be straightforward, a high index of clinical suspicion is paramount, considering the wide range of possible symptoms.

DIAGNOSIS

Carotid artery disease is diagnosed through a combination of the clinical history and physical examination in combination with imaging findings. The next part of this chapter focuses on the diagnosis of carotid artery atherosclerotic disease.

History

A thorough history is elucidated from the patient. This includes medical history, such as atrial fibrillation, which can make a patient more susceptible to a TIA or stroke. The Vascular Quality Initiative defines *history of neurologic event* as either stroke or TIA in the right or left eye, cortex, or vertebrobasilar region.

Physical Examination

Carotid artery disease can be identified by listening for a bruit on examination. A bruit is the sound of turbulent blood flow in a vessel and can be recognized on physical examination with a stethoscope. In patients with carotid artery stenosis, the luminal narrowing causes turbulent blood flow. However, not all diseased arteries produce a bruit, especially the ones with critical stenosis not allowing enough blood to flow through to cause turbulence (false-negative bruit). One the other hand, you could hear a bruit from a stenotic external carotid artery (ECA; false-positive bruit).

Thus, it is important to correlate examination findings with imaging.

Surveillance Versus Intervention

Once the diagnosis of carotid artery stenosis has been established, the next decision is whether the patient should be medically managed with surveillance versus an intervention with an invasive procedure. This varies by degree of luminal stenosis as well as symptomatic status of the patient.

For symptomatic patients who present within 6 months of a stroke, TIA, or amaurosis fugax, a workup to assess for carotid artery disease is performed. Initial presentation relies on carotid duplex ultrasound as a quick, efficient, and reliable method to diagnose carotid disease. Adjuncts to carotid duplex that will be discussed include computed tomography angiography (CTA), MRI/magnetic resonance angiography (MRA), and traditional angiography. Each modality has its own benefits and risks associated.

The threshold for intervention in both asymptomatic and symptomatic patients has been well studied, and guidelines have been created by the Society for Vascular Surgery as clinic practice guidelines for the management of extracranial cerebrovascular disease.[17] Level 1B evidence supports surgical intervention in combination with maximum medical therapy as opposed to medical therapy alone for individuals with asymptomatic carotid artery disease and greater than 70% stenosis. This comes from the results of RCTs, including both the Asymptomatic Carotid Atherosclerosis Study (ACAS) and the Asymptomatic Carotid Surgery Trial (ACST).[14,18] These RCTs found that combined stroke and death at 5 years in those who underwent carotid endarterectomy (CEA) for asymptomatic ≥60% stenosis was 4.1% compared with 10% in those who underwent medical therapy alone.

For symptomatic patients, guidelines are based on two RCTs, the European Carotid Surgery Trial (ECST) and the North American Symptomatic Carotid Endarterectomy Trial (NASCET). Both these trials found that for symptomatic patients with less than 50% stenosis, surgical intervention with CEA did not decrease the rate of future neurologic events compared with medical therapy alone.[19,20] However, for symptomatic patients with over 50% luminal stenosis, both the ECST and NASCET RCTs have found a benefit in CEA over maximal medical therapy alone. NASCET demonstrated that symptomatic patients with ≥70% stenosis have a 9% risk of stroke at 2 years compared with a 26% risk in the group with medical therapy alone.[20]

Regardless of symptomatic status, a patient's true degree of luminal stenosis must be ascertained before determining an intervention plan—whether this be surgical or medical therapy. The next part of this chapter focuses on the various modalities available to vascular surgeons to identify carotid artery disease.

Carotid Duplex Ultrasound

Duplex ultrasound is a relatively fast, cost-effective, and easy way to assess a patient's carotid artery in the outpatient setting, at inpatient bedside, or in the emergency department (Fig. 101.1). This modality was proven to be effective in the United Kingdom Health Technology Assessment meta-analysis in 2006, which found that duplex ultrasound should be used as a first-line imaging modality to identify patients with 70% to 99% internal carotid artery (ICA) stenosis, but that benefit is less prominent in patients with 50% to 69% stenosis.[21]

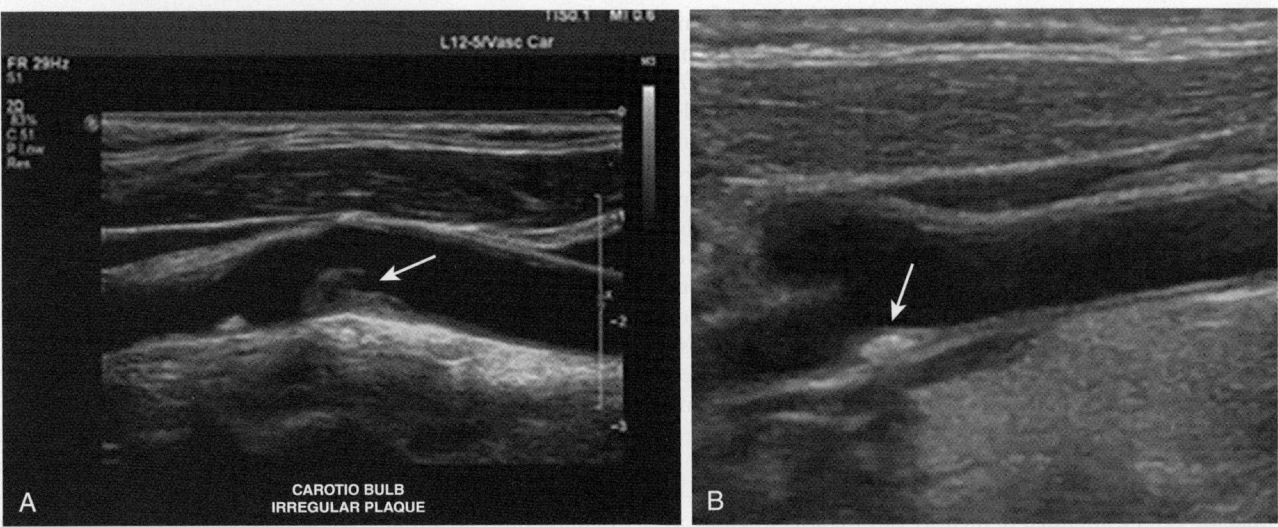

FIGURE 101.1 (A–B) Duplex ultrasound with plaque *(arrows)* in carotid artery. (From Al-Nouri O, Malas MB. Cerebrovascular disease. In: Dimick JB, ed. *Mulholland and Greenfield's Surgery Scientific Principles & Practice.* 7th ed. Philadelphia: Wolters Kluwer; 2021.)

Carotid duplex diagnosis of ICA stenosis is shown in Table 101.1. The findings in Table 101.1 have been proven and supported by the idea that duplex ultrasound can be used to diagnose greater than 70% stenosis.[22] According to the Society for Vascular Surgery, screening the base population of asymptomatic individuals is not recommended unless the individual has significant risk factors for carotid artery disease.[17]

Overall, the biggest limitation of carotid artery duplex ultrasound is the operator's skill and experience. When measuring the carotid artery, the information is delivered using either the ECST or the NASCET. The ECST multicenter RCT involved 3200 patients; percentage of stenosis was measured from the estimated original diameter at the site of the stenosis minus the narrowest ICA diameter divided by the estimated original diameter.[23] On the other hand, NASCET estimated percentage of stenosis from the normal distal cervical ICA minus the narrowest ICA diameter divided by the distal ICA diameter.[24] This historically was determined from angiographic data, whereas duplex is based on velocity, however, correlated to angiographic definitions.

Carotid duplex ultrasound provides an efficient means of carotid artery disease and is able to be incorporated into many medical settings. Although operator ability is the biggest drawback, its advantages, including cost and speed of use, have allowed many patients to be both surveilled over time as well as expeditiously transitioned from medical management to surgical treatment based on the results. It is critical to have well-trained technologists who are certified to do arterial studies and not only

gray-imaging ultrasound and are supervised by certified vascular surgeons. One of the limitations of duplex ultrasound is its inability to penetrate through calcified lesions, which could mask high-grade stenosis.

Computed Tomography Angiography

CTA of the head and neck can also be used to diagnose carotid artery disease. CTA scans involve an intravenous administration of a contrast agent followed by a spiral CT scan and, in the head and neck region, can identify carotid artery disease both in an extracranial and intracranial location. CTA has been found to mimic the results of luminal stenosis found on duplex ultrasound; however, it has less reliability when distinguishing moderate and severe stenosis.[25]

One of the strongest benefits of the use of CTA imaging is the ability to image and assess the soft tissue, bony structures, and vasculature simultaneously in a quick and efficient manner. CTA also provides imaging of the aortic arch, for example, tortuosity, aberrant anatomy, and degree of calcification. CTA also provides valuable information on lesion length, extent, and level of disease to identify high lesions not amendable to standard CEA. It allows identification of tandem lesions distally as well as proximal common carotid artery (CCA) orifical lesions at the arch—both of which can increase the risk of CEA and might change the surgical plan. In our practice, we routinely evaluate the circle of Willis to understand cerebral collateral flow. This is important in planning a shunt for CEA and flow reversal for transcarotid artery revascularization (TCAR). Limitations of CTA involve contrast exposure

TABLE 101.1 Carotid Duplex Diagnosis of Internal Carotid Artery (ICA) Stenosis

PERCENTAGE STENOSIS	ICA PSV (cm/s)	PERCENTAGE PLAQUE	ICA/CCA PSV (RATIO)	ICA EDV (CM/S)
Normal	<125	None	<2	<40
<50	<125	<50	<2	<40
50–69	125–230	≥50	2–4	40–100
>70	>230	≥70	>4	>100

CCA, Common carotid artery; *EDV,* end-diastolic velocity; *PSV,* peak systolic velocity.

for those with chronic kidney disease, radiation exposure, and cost compared with duplex ultrasound.[26] Additionally, patients with intravenous contrast allergy are unable to undergo a CTA. Given these limitations, the Society for Vascular Surgery has determined level 1B evidence for duplex over CTA in the screening modality for asymptomatic individuals.

CTA imaging is an important adjunct when patients are being planned for carotid artery stent (CAS). This is because of the valuable information obtained from the aortic arch to the circle of Willis involving vessel anatomy.[26] Additionally, in small-volume analyses, CTA was found to be helpful in assessing carotid plaque morphology and identifying both geometry and tissue composition.[27] The overall use for plaque characteristics is yet to be determined, but it could pave an avenue toward identifying high- and low-risk patients based on more than luminal stenosis.

Magnetic Resonance Angiography

MRA imaging can be obtained to identify carotid artery disease as well. MRA has been found to have high sensitivity and specificity, but with high variation in quality of studies. Additionally, the time for completion can be a limiting factor; however, software improvements have led to increased use for diagnosis.[28] MRA is advantageous because it avoids radiation exposure to the patient and does not require complex postprocessing to account for bony structures. MRA currently does not have a role in screening for carotid disease because of the cost.

As an adjunct tool, MRA can identify vessel anomalies, but occluded vessels or calcification is not well elucidated.[26] However, plaque morphology using MRA has been found to be helpful for monitoring the fibrous cap and lipid core.[29] Additionally, MR detection of intraplaque hemorrhage has been used to predict recurrent ischemia, stroke, and embolization after CEA.[30,31] MRA, however, cannot be performed in individuals with metal implants or those who are easily claustrophobic.

Digital Subtraction Angiography

Conventional angiography, or digital subtraction angiography (DSA), had been considered the gold standard for carotid artery disease identification. However, it can come with added risks. A review of almost 20,000 patients found that 2.6% of patients had

a neurologic complication, and 4% had an access site hematoma; the increased risk was found to be related to atherosclerotic disease, frequent TIA, and intracranial hemorrhage (subarachnoid).[32] Currently, these is no role for routine DSA as a diagnostic tool because of the improved imaging capability of both CTA and MRA. Limitations to DSA include risk of radiation exposure and patients with contrast allergy. The only indication is two conflicting studies comparing duplex ultrasound and CTA, in which case one found DSA to be the most accurate method to confirm the degree of stenosis.

TREATMENT

Medical Therapy

All patients with carotid disease, both symptomatic and asymptomatic, should receive optimal medical therapy. Once the diagnosis of underlying carotid occlusive disease is established, patients should be initiated on antiplatelet therapy, most commonly with daily aspirin.[4] High-intensity statin therapy has been demonstrated to reduce the long-term risk of stroke in patients with symptomatic carotid stenosis and should also be considered for asymptomatic patients based on their individual risk profile.[4,33]

Risk factor mitigation is also an important mainstay in the treatment of carotid artery stenosis. In addition to the management of dyslipidemia described earlier, several other risk factors warrant mentioning. Smoking cessation should certainly be strongly advised to all patients with active tobacco use.[34,35] Management of hypertension can both slow the progression of carotid disease and help to improve perioperative blood pressure management should revascularization be undertaken.[35] The management of diabetes, coronary disease, obesity, and pulmonary disease, among other comorbidities, remains integral to achieving optimal outcomes for patients.[4]

Carotid revascularization remains one of the most heavily studied procedures in vascular surgery, with more than a dozen randomized clinical trials investigating the efficacy of procedures versus medical therapy (Table 101.2) and comparing CEA to transfemoral stenting (Table 101.3). This high-quality evidence forms the foundation for clinical practice guideless by the AHA and Society for Vascular Surgery.[4]

TABLE 101.2 Trials of Carotid Endarterectomy (CEA) Versus Medical Therapy

TRIAL	YEAR	POPULATION	OUTCOME	ARM 1	ARM 2	RISK	ARR	RR
NASCET: high grade	1991	Symptomatic, >70%	Any ipsilateral stroke at 2 years	Aspirin	CEA	26% vs. 9%	17%	0.33
NASCET: moderate	1998	Symptomatic, 50%–69%	Any ipsilateral stroke at 5 years	Aspirin	CEA	22.2% vs. 15.7%	6.50%	0.7
NASCET: mild	1998	Symptomatic, <50%	Any ipsilateral stroke at 5 years	Aspirin	CEA	18.7% vs. 14.9%	p = 0.16	
ECST	1998	Symptomatic, >80% (ECST)	Major stroke or death at 3 years	Aspirin	CEA	26.5% vs. 14.9%	11.6%	0.56
ACAS	1995	Asymptomatic, >60%	Perioperative stroke/ death, ipsilateral stroke at 5 years	Aspirin	CEA	11.0% vs. 5.1%	6.9%	0.46
ACST	2004	Asymptomatic, >60%	Any stroke or perioperative death at 5 years	Aspirin ± statin	CEA	11.8% vs. 6.4%	5.4%	0.54
VA Trial	1993	Asymptomatic, >50%	Ipsilateral TIA or stroke under follow-up	Aspirin	CEA	20.6% vs. 8.0%	12.6%	0.39

ACAS, Asymptomatic Carotid Artery Surgery Trial; *ACST*, Asymptomatic Carotid Surgery Trial; *ARR*, absolute risk reduction; *ECST*, European Carotid Surgery Trial; *NASCET*, North American Symptomatic Carotid Endarterectomy Trial; *RR*, relative risk; *VA*, Veterans Association.

TABLE 101.3 Trials of Carotid Endarterectomy (CEA) Versus Transfemoral Carotid Artery Stenting (TFCAS)

TRIAL	YEAR	POPULATION	OUTCOME	ARM 1	ARM 2	RISK	ARR	RR
SAPPHIRE	2004	"High-risk" symptomatic, >50%; asymptomatic, >80%	Perioperative stroke/death/MI, ipsilateral stroke at 1 year	CEA	TFCAS	20.1% vs. 12.2%	7.9% P = 0.05	—
EVA-3S	2008	Symptomatic, >60%	Perioperative stroke/death, ipsilateral stroke at 4 years	CEA	TFCAS	6.2% vs. 11.1%	−4.9% P = 0.03	HR: 1.97
SPACE	2008	Symptomatic, >70%	Perioperative stroke/death, ipsilateral stroke at 2 years	CEA	TFCAS	8.8% vs. 9.5%	P = 0.62	—
ICSS	2015	Symptomatic, >50%, but mostly >70%	Any stroke at 5 years	CEA	TFCAS	9.4% vs. 15.2%	P = 0.77	—
CREST	2016	Symptomatic/asymptomatic, >70%	Perioperative stroke/death/MI, ipsilateral stroke at 10 years	CEA	TFCAS	9.9% vs. 11.8%	P = 0.51	—
ACT-1	2016	Asymptomatic, >70%	Perioperative stroke/death/MI, ipsilateral stroke at 1 year	CEA	TFCAS	3.4% vs. 3.8%	P = NS	—

ACT-1, Carotid Angioplasty and Stenting Versus Endarterectomy in Asymptomatic Subjects; *ARR*, absolute risk reduction; *CREST*, Carotid Revascularization Endarterectomy Versus Stenting Trial; *EVA-3S*, Endarterectomy Versus Angioplasty in Patients With Symptomatic Severe Carotid Stenosis; *HR*, hazard ratio; *ICSS*, International Carotid Stenting Study; *MI*, myocardial infarction; *RR*, relative risk; *SAPPHIRE*, Stenting and Angioplasty With Protection in Patients at High Risk for Endarterectomy; *SPACE*, Stent-Protected Angioplasty Versus Carotid Endarterectomy.

However, despite the abundance of data to support carotid revascularization, there remains persistent debate surrounding its utility in achieving long-term stroke risk reduction. This stems primarily from advances in medical therapy that have been made since these trials were conducted. In fact, some experts now claim that the results of these seminal trials no longer apply and that surgical revascularization for asymptomatic patients is not necessary.[36] Conversely, proponents of surgical therapy continue to cite a high longitudinal risk of stroke among patients with severe carotid stenosis, despite their asymptomatic status.[37] Accordingly, there remains persistent controversy on how best to manage patients with carotid stenosis, particularly among those who are asymptomatic.

The Carotid Revascularization and Medical Management for Asymptomatic Carotid Stenosis Trial (CREST-2) seeks to add evidence to this growing debate. CREST 2 is two parallel trials that are enrolling patients with asymptomatic carotid stenosis and randomizing them to either intervention with CEA or transfemoral carotid artery stenting (TFCAS), or best medical therapy.[38,39] This trial, sponsored by the National Institutes of Health, will provide important results that will likely help to optimally define which patients will derive benefit from carotid revascularization in contemporary practice.

Carotid Endarterectomy
Considerations
CEA remains the historical gold-standard procedure for revascularization of the extracranial carotid artery. Since its first description in 1953, CEA has been tested in over a dozen RCTs and rigorously compared against best medical therapy and TFCAS among symptomatic and asymptomatic patients.[40–42] To date, it remains one of the most comprehensively studied procedures in vascular surgery.

The choice of carotid revascularization strategy remains contingent on several important factors. Currently, three primary

therapeutic options exist. CEA is described in this section; TFCAS and TCAR are described elsewhere.[43] Before the development of TFCAS and TCAR, CEA was the only available carotid revascularization option. As such, CEA remains an option for most patients considered for revascularization. This is particularly prudent when considering TFCAS or TCAR in patients who may not be ideal for these stent-based therapies. Although these newer revascularization procedures may have nuanced benefits in certain clinical and/or anatomic situations, CEA remains a central component of the vascular surgeon's armamentarium in treating carotid occlusive disease.

There are some clinical indications where CEA may carry increased surgical risk. These include patients with hostile neck anatomy, such as those with a prior neck dissection, where the potential risk of cranial nerve injury is increased; patients with a tracheostomy, where wound infection rates may be higher; patients with a contralateral laryngeal nerve injury, where even the anticipated low risk of nerve injury could have a significant consequence; patients with anatomic disease extending above C2, which could make adequate surgical exposure technically difficult; and patients who cannot tolerate general or regional anesthesia. In these situations, patients may be considered for an alternate method of carotid revascularization.

Carotid Endarterectomy Technique
Anesthetic and support devices. CEA is most often performed under general anesthesia. Evidence suggests that local/regional anesthesia can also achieve similar outcomes in appropriate patients with an experienced anesthesia and surgical team.[44] Ultimately, the type of anesthesia that is administered should be selected at the discretion of the operating surgeon in collaboration with the attending anesthesiologist.

Commonly placed support devices include two peripheral intravenous lines for the administration of anesthetic and blood pressure management medications, an arterial line for invasive blood pressure monitoring and measuring anticoagulation parameters during the operation (e.g., the activated clotting time [ACT]), and a Foley catheter that may be removed at the end of the procedure.

Intraoperative blood pressure management is an important consideration that should be discussed with the anesthesia team. Clamping the carotid artery during endarterectomy will require the brain to rely on either contralateral and/or collateral circulation, or flow through a shunt if one is used. During this part of the operation, it is prudent to ensure that there is adequate perfusion pressure and be vigilant to avoid hypotensive episodes that could result in hypoperfusion to the brain or ischemic stroke. Preoperative and intraoperative communication between the surgeon and anesthesiologist on blood pressure goals as the operation progresses is critical for a successful outcome.

Positioning. Appropriate positioning is an important component of a successful CEA procedure because it can facilitate or hinder the exposure of the distal ICA. The patient should be positioned supine on the operating room table with both arms tucked at the patient's side. A gel shoulder support or rolled towel should be placed under the upper back at the level of the shoulder blades to facilitate neck extension. The patient should then have their neck rotated to the contralateral side. Depending on the flexibility of the patient's cervical spine, support for the head may be needed, using either additional towels, a gel pad, or both. A balance should be found that maximizes cervical spine extension and contralateral rotation, which will best facilitate the surgical exposure of the carotid artery.

It is the authors' preference to have the patient on an operating room table that articulates at the knees, hips, and neck. The "beach chair" position optimally facilitates the technical dissection/exposure. This position has the patient's knees slightly bent, hips flexed, and the neck extended. Securing straps are then placed around the patient to facilitate secure rotation to the contralateral side so that both the operating surgeon and assistant have optimal visibility of the surgical field. The neck should then be draped so that the sternal notch, angle of the mandible, and earlobe all remain visible.

Exposure of the carotid artery. An incision is made over the anterior border of the sternocleidomastoid muscle. The length of the incision is tailored to the extent of the carotid lesion and planned endarterectomy site. This can be lengthened during the procedure if the initial incision is inadequate. The platysma is next encountered and divided. Meticulous hemostasis should be kept throughout the incision and ensuing dissection. The robust lymphatic drainage and circulation to the tissues of the neck make the liberal use of electrocautery on the superficial tissues a useful option.

Next, the sternocleidomastoid muscle should be reflected laterally. The tissues medial and just overlying the muscle make up a bloodless plane that can be followed to the carotid sheath. Superficial branches of the external jugular vein can be ligated. Cranially, there is a superficial nerve that is often encountered in the subcutaneous tissue. This nerve provides sensory innervation to the upper neck. This can be divided, if necessary, but will cause a permanent area of sensory loss on the upper neck near the incision.

The internal jugular vein is next visible and should be carefully mobilized and gently retracted laterally. If a small venotomy is made during dissection, repair should be performed using polypropylene suture. The facial vein branch is often notable and frequently marks the level of the carotid bifurcation and can be

used as an initial guide as to whether the length of the incision and exposure are sufficient. The facial vein should be divided with silk ties, and then the jugular vein is gently retracted laterally along with the sternocleidomastoid muscle. Commonly during dissection of the jugular vein, the surgeon will encounter the omohyoid muscle, which typically marks the inferior aspect of the surgical exposure. The muscle can either be retracted inferiorly, divided with electrocautery, or tied and cut.

The carotid sheath is incised sharply, exposing the carotid artery. It is most often easiest to identify the CCA in the inferior aspect of the surgical exposure. The authors prefer to doubly loop the CCA with a silastic vessel loop to aid in proximal inflow control and if a shunt is needed during the procedure.

The vagus nerve is frequently found posterior and lateral to the carotid artery but occasionally may be found on its anterior surface. Care should be taken not to injure the vagus nerve during the dissection and, ultimately, clamping of the artery. The vagus nerve can sometimes be confused with branches of the ansa cervicalis that lie over the carotid artery. Branches of the ansa cervicalis are generally smaller and can be ligated with impunity.

An important anatomic variant is a nonrecurrent laryngeal nerve, which appears as a large branch off the vagus nerve overlying the carotid artery (rather than in the chest, where it generally originates). Identifying the vagus nerve will help delineate whether any branches arise from it, allowing the surgeon to avoid injuring this anatomic variant.

The exposure then progresses cranially over the carotid artery. Care should be taken not to extensively manipulate the carotid bulb, especially in symptomatic patients, to avoid potential disruption of the carotid plaque and inadvertently causing an embolic event with manipulation. Dissection of the tissue near the carotid bulb can also result in profound bradycardia as a result of stimulation of the carotid baroreceptors. If this occurs, the surgeon may anesthetize the carotid bulb with a small amount of 1% lidocaine.

The carotid bifurcation is next identified, exposing both the external and internal branches. The ECA generally branches toward the face, whereas the ICA progresses cranially and posteriorly toward the skull base. The ICA can be carefully dissected sharply, freeing it from surrounding tissue. The hypoglossal nerve is often apparent and typically encountered in the more cranial extent of the exposure. Once identified, the hypoglossal nerve should be carefully preserved to avoid injury. During this part of the dissection, a fixed retractor to assist in cranial exposure is often very helpful.

Once the exposure is satisfactory, the surgeon can proceed with the endarterectomy. Before clamping, systemic anticoagulation should be administered, most commonly with heparin, if no allergy is present. ACTs can be targeted to reach 250 or 300 seconds, depending on the preference of the surgeon and institutional norms. Particularly for symptomatic patients, it may be prudent to administer anticoagulation earlier in the operation, during the time of dissection of the carotid bulb and ICA. This should be left to the discretion of the operating surgeon because it can increase bleeding in the surgical exposure during dissection.

Endarterectomy. There are two commonly used techniques to perform the endarterectomy. One uses a longitudinal arteriotomy and patch angioplasty closure. The other approach is an eversion endarterectomy.

Longitudinal arteriotomy and patch angioplasty. The most common method of CEA is endarterectomy and patch angioplasty closure. The authors prefer to use a combination of angled clamps for the common and ECAs and atraumatic cerebral aneurysm clips to control the ICA. The ICA should be clamped first to avoid any thromboembolic events from clamping the common or ECAs. An arteriotomy is optimally made in a disease-free segment of the CCA. Angled fine scissors are used to extend the arteriotomy on the anterolateral surface of the carotid onto the ICA, extending just past the disease so that the endarterectomy can be ended in healthy carotid artery.

With the carotid opened, the endarterectomy can be performed. A plane is most often developed in the arterial media, and care should be taken not to allow the remaining carotid wall to be too thin. An assistant can retract the carotid plaque with a forceps while the surgeon uses a plaque elevator to gently push the arterial wall away from the plaque.

With the plaque removed from the artery, the surgeon then inspects the endarterectomy site. If the distal end point on the ICA has residual disease or any evidence of a flap is present, then fine-tacking sutures with 7-0 polypropylene suture should be considered to secure any end points and prevent dissection after restoration of antegrade flow. Meticulous care should be taken to remove any remaining debris from the endarterectomized site to avoid the potential for thromboembolic complications once perfusion is restored.

With the endarterectomy complete, the artery can then be closed. Patch angioplasty, with either bovine pericardium, vein, or polytetrafluoroethylene, is most often performed (Fig. 101.2). For large or redundant ICAs, primary closure may be considered, although this risks restenosis of the carotid upon closure and should be reserved for unusually large arteries.

Eversion endarterectomy. A less common but useful reconstruction option is eversion endarterectomy. To perform this, after arterial clamping, the carotid is opened transversely at the base of the internal carotid. Once transected, the plaque is focally endarterectomized and subsequently everted from the ICA by invaginating the ICA on itself, allowing for the entire plaque to

be removed across its extent. The carotid artery is then closed with running polypropylene suture.

Cerebral protection. There are a variety of modalities to ensure that the brain tolerates carotid clamping. Placing a shunt from the CCA to the ICA is the only method that preserves ipsilateral blood flow through the carotid artery. To perform this, after the arteriotomy has been created, a vessel shunt is placed from the common carotid to the ICA, and the vessel is either looped or clamped around the shunt. Shunt flow should be confirmed with a handheld Doppler. Other methods to ensure that the brain has adequate collateral circulation include intraoperative electroencephalogram (EEG); carotid stump measurement, whereby the back pressure of the ICA is determined with the external and CCAs clamped; and finally, local/regional anesthesia, whereby the patient is awake and able to be monitored in real time. If any of these cerebral monitoring techniques demonstrate impaired perfusion, a shunt can then be placed to restore flow to the ipsilateral ICA.

Completion imaging. Completion studies are often a useful adjunct to detect any technical deficiencies after the endarterectomy is completed and antegrade flow is restored. It is the authors' practice to perform a completion duplex ultrasound before reversal of anticoagulation. Duplex ultrasound offers the ability to measure the waveforms in the ICA, ensure low-resistance flow, and visualize any remaining mobile debris at the endarterectomy site with B-mode imaging. Large debris or high-resistance flow should prompt consideration to reopen the patch to inspect the endarterectomy site. Alternatively, conventional angiography can be performed to ensure the integrity of the reconstruction at the surgeon's discretion or if a dedicated duplex study is not available. In the absence of a completion imaging study, auscultating the distal ICA with a sterile handheld Doppler probe can help to reassure that there is requisite flow, although it has the potential to miss a more nuanced technical defect at the endarterectomy or clamp sites.

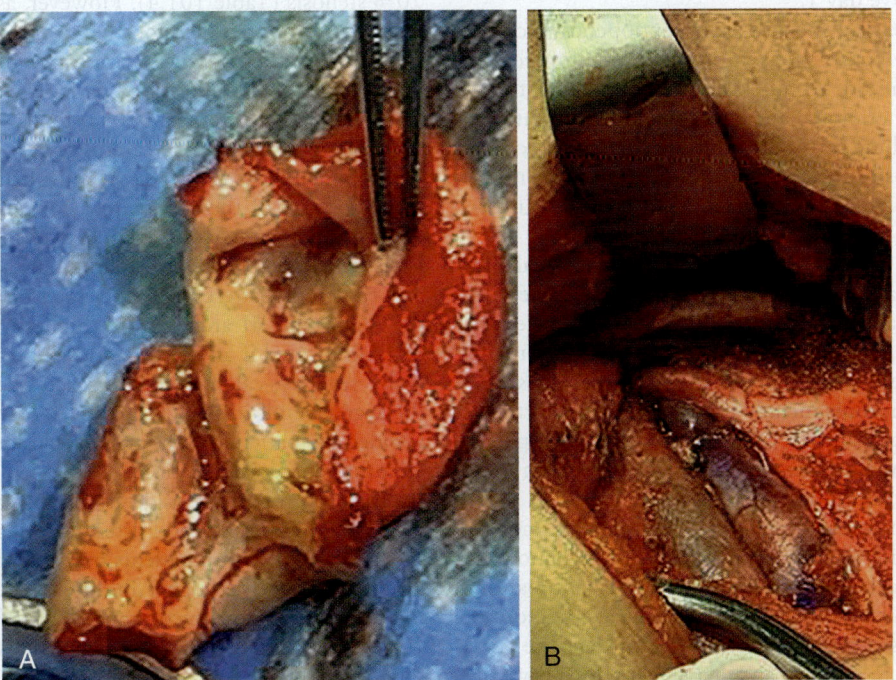

FIGURE 101.2 Carotid endarterectomy. (A) Endarterectomy sample. (B) Patch angioplasty.

Closure. After reversal of anticoagulation with protamine, hemostasis must be obtained at the patch and surgical field.[45,46] Additional polypropylene sutures can be used as needed, as well as topical hemostatic. When satisfied, the sternocleidomastoid can be approximated loosely to the more medial tissues. The platysma layer is then closed with braided absorbable sutures. The skin is then closed with absorbable monofilament suture. In patients who are on dual antiplatelet therapy (DAPT) or in whom there is a concern for hematoma development, a drain may be left in the surgical field at the surgeon's discretion.

Perioperative Care and Complications

Immediate postoperative course. After completion of the surgical procedure, the patient should be awakened from anesthesia in the operating room, and a neurologic examination should be completed before transferring the patient to the recovery unit. Dense hemiplegia with concern for intraoperative stroke should prompt immediate intervention. If no completion imaging was performed after arterial closure, then surgical reexploration should be considered. If completion imaging was performed, then immediate CTA may be considered versus reexploration to identify a potential source of the new-onset neurologic deficits.

If the patient's neurologic examination is back to baseline after extubation, then transfer to the recovery area is warranted. The recovery unit should be equipped to perform frequent neurologic and blood pressure monitoring via invasive measurements and intervene as needed. It is the authors' practice to keep patients in the postanesthesia care unit (PACU) for 4 hours before transfer to a regular ward bed if recovery has gone well. Practice patterns vary, and patients are commonly transferred to the intensive care unit (ICU) for their early recovery course. Patients may experience fluctuations in blood pressure postoperatively, and these should be managed with vasopressors or vasodilators as needed until the carotid baroreceptors have had the opportunity to reset, with corresponding normalization of the blood pressure. Refractory hypotension should prompt an evaluation for myocardial ischemia.

Most patients can expect an uneventful recovery course and discharge on postoperative day 1.

Perioperative stroke. The most dreaded perioperative complication is stroke. New neurologic symptoms in the immediate postoperative period should be quickly followed with a thorough workup for the etiology and neurologic consultation. Common etiologies include carotid thrombosis, distal dissection flap, or thromboembolism during the procedure. Each of these is potentially treatable, and prompt imaging with duplex ultrasound and/or CTA can guide an expedited intervention.

Neck hematoma. An expanding hematoma at the surgical site after CEA constitutes a potential emergency that can be life threatening. Reversal of anticoagulation during the procedure can reduce this risk but not eliminate it.[47] The surgeon must remain vigilant for neck hematoma, especially in the immediate postoperative course. Early symptoms include new hoarseness, shortness of breath, neck deviation, and of course, a new large palpable hematoma. Left untreated, an expanding neck hematoma can quickly lead to airway compromise and death.

Treatment of a neck hematoma therefore requires quick action. Clear communication with the anesthesiology team is paramount. If reoperation is required because of neck hematoma, intubation can be difficult as a result of tracheal deviation. Awake fiberoptic intubation is often advised by an experienced provider. The surgeon should be prepared to perform an emergent surgical airway if necessary, should the airway be lost during attempted intubation.

Once the airway is secured, the surgical incision can be reopened in a controlled fashion, and the hematoma is then evacuated. A meticulous inspection should then be conducted for the underlying etiology.

Acute coronary syndrome. The risk factors for carotid artery stenosis overlap substantially with those for coronary artery disease. As such, persistent hypotension, new angina, or an anginal equivalent should result in an immediate electrocardiogram, possible echocardiogram, and consideration of serum cardiac enzymes, with further interventions guided by the results of these studies in concert with cardiology consultation.

Reperfusion syndrome. Patients with severe carotid stenosis develop dilation of the cerebral vasculature to correct for the decreased flow across the carotid lesion. Once the carotid lesion is removed, it can take time for the cerebral vasculature to regain its normal vasoconstriction/vasodilation response to cerebral blood flow. It is difficult to predict how long it may take for the brain to regain this normal regulatory response. Unchecked cerebral blood flow into a very dilated arterial bed can lead to hyperperfusion, seizure, and cerebral hemorrhage, which carries a very high rate of mortality. It is therefore prudent to assess for this syndrome early and often. The first manifestation is often ipsilateral headache, although the headache can also be more generalized. Patients with headache after CEA should be fully investigated. Imaging options include transcranial Doppler, which can quantify the cerebral blood flow with established thresholds for reperfusion, or with noncontrast head computed tomography, which can evaluate for intracerebral hemorrhage. Any abnormalities should lead to close neurologic monitoring and meticulous blood pressure control, and discussion with a neurologist should be considered.

Transfemoral Carotid Artery Stenting

Considerations

TFCAS was initially approved for reimbursement by the Centers for Medicare and Medical Services (CMS) for high-risk medical or high-risk anatomic patients with symptomatic status and over 70% stenosis (Table 101.4). However, as of July 2023, CMS has released a proposed decision memo that approves TFCAS for the following: patients with symptomatic carotid artery stenosis greater than 50% stenosis and patients with asymptomatic carotid artery stenosis greater than 70% stenosis.[48]

If planning a TFCAS, careful review of preoperative imaging, including either CTA or MRA, must be undertaken to determine characteristics of the aortic arch (tortuosity, calcification, disease burden) and patency of the circle of Willis. Aortic arch characteristics can lead to excessive manipulation of the arch with wires and catheters that creates higher rates of embolization and stroke, of which type III arches are at highest risk.[49] Finally, TFCAS is contraindicated if any of the following are present: type III aortic arch, severely calcified arch, severely atherosclerotic arch, or 90-degree bends in the CCA or ICA. Stenting generally should be avoided in patients with unstable lesions, thrombus, or severe circumferential calcification.

There are several considerations that should be accounted for when planning for carotid artery stenting. A Cochrane review of 16 trials found that in patients over the age of 70 years, the rate of death or stroke was higher in TFCAS compared with CEA, and the review therefore recommends TFCAS in patients less than 70 years.[50] Additionally, a study using the Vascular Quality Initiative found that TFCAS stroke risk was related to age, whereas CEA was stable across age groups.[51] In terms of sex, a meta-analysis found no

TABLE 101.4 Criteria for Transfemoral Stent	
MEDICAL CRITERIA— HIGH RISK	**ANATOMIC CRITERIA— HIGH RISK**
Age greater than 75	Contralateral carotid artery occlusion
Greater than 2-vessel coronary artery disease	Tandem stenosis greater than 70%
Unstable angina	Lesion above C2
New York Heart Association class III or class IV congestive heart failure	Restenosis after carotid endarterectomy
Left ventricular ejection failure less than 35%	History of neck radiation
Myocardial infarction in past 6 months	Decreased cervical spine mobility
Severe pulmonary disease	Tracheostomy
Contralateral recurrent laryngeal nerve injury	Previous neck surgery

difference in outcomes in TFCAS between males and females.[52,53] Treating combined carotid disease and coronary artery disease was assessed in a meta-analysis of 11 studies, which found no difference in death, stroke, or myocardial infarction (MI) based on timing between TFCAS and coronary artery bypass graft.[54] The overall goal of TFCAS is to stabilize the plaque against the vessel wall with the stent. Patients who are deemed candidates for TFCAS must be optimized with at least 1 week of aspirin and clopidogrel or other DAPT and statin therapy. A large national study has shown a reduction in mortality from stroke or MI after TFCAS if the patient was on statin therapy (11.4%) compared with nonstatin users (30.8%).[55]

Technique

TFCAS should be performed in a procedure room with high-quality imaging. An arterial line is placed by the anesthesia team to monitor intraoperative and postprocedural blood pressure. Prophylactic glycopyrrolate administration can be done because of the risk of bradycardia and hypotension. Other anesthesia concerns include access to vasopressor agents and local anesthesia technique. These procedures should be performed under local anesthesia to allow for neurologic monitoring through both speech and fine motor skills in the contralateral upper extremity. In addition, either EEG or transcranial Doppler can be performed. Given the high medical and anatomic risk with patients undergoing TFCAS, local anesthesia is necessary to frequently assess neurologic function and decrease cardiac complications in the perioperative period.[56]

Patients are placed supine with access to bilateral groins. Ultrasound guidance is used to obtain common femoral artery access with microneedle and sheath. Although less common, transbrachial or transradial access can be used. Upper extremity access is reserved for patients with a highly diseased aorta, and a large study found that if transbrachial or transradial access is necessary, it can have lower access site complications; however, it also has a higher risk of MI and technical failure.[57] Heparin is administered by anesthesia for a goal ACT between 250 and 300 seconds. We prefer to exchange our initial 5-Fr sheath for a 90-cm shuttle select 6-Fr sheath (Cook Medical, Bloomington, IL) parked in the descending aorta under fluoroscopic guidance. Angiogram is performed to evaluate the aortic arch with a 120-cm diagnostic catheter in the proximal descending thoracic aorta to perform an arch angiogram.

The CCA is selected with one of the following catheters based on arch, innominate, and CCA anatomy: H1, JB1, JB2, Vert, VTK, or SIM. The catheter is placed proximal to the carotid bifurcation. The shuttle select sheath is telescoped over the catheter and wire to the mid-CCA. A carotid angiogram is then performed to identify the location of the stenosis, degree of stenosis, ECA patency, distal carotid artery flow, and ipsilateral intracerebral circulation.

The lesion is then crossed with an embolic protection device (EPD) placed in the distal ICA. With the EPD wire in place, rapid exchange is performed. Generally, the lesion is predilated with a balloon 3 to 4 mm smaller than the diameter of the artery. At this time, careful monitoring for bradycardia and hypotension must be undertaken. Balloon angioplasty is performed with slow inflation not to exceed 8 atmospheres, followed by immediate and slow deflation to minimize the embolic load. CASs are self-expanding and either straight or tapered with open or closed cells. Open-cell stents are conformable to tortuous anatomy or complex lesions, whereas closed stents have a decreased risk of embolization. However, data have shown no difference between closed- and open-cell stents in terms of stroke or death.[58,59] A multi-institutional study identified an increase in the risk of stroke with closed-cell stents if crossing the carotid bifurcation into the CCA.[60] The stent is sized 1 mm larger than the diameter of the CCA. The selected stent is advanced over the EPD wire and deployed to cover the entire lesion plus at least 5 mm proximal and distal to healthier vessels. It is our practice to use a 4-cm-long stent and extend it into the CCA on almost every patient to mimic CEA because we often extend the endarterectomy onto the CCA (Fig. 101.3). Postdilation has been found to be associated

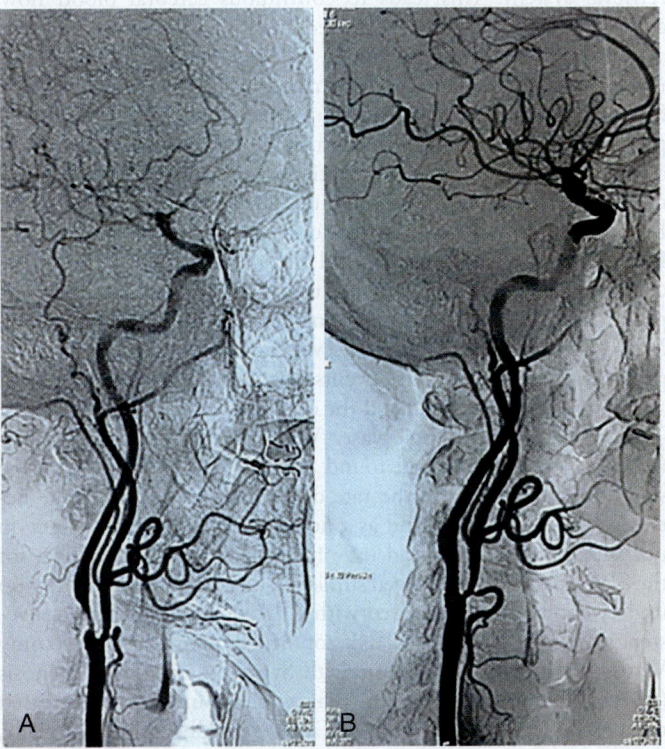

FIGURE 101.3 Transfemoral carotid artery stenting. (A) Prestent carotid angiogram. (B) Poststent carotid angiogram. (From Al-Nouri O, Malas MB. Cerebrovascular disease. In: Dimick JB, ed. *Mulholland and Greenfield's Surgery Scientific Principles & Practice.* 7th ed. Philadelphia: Wolters Kluwer; 2021.)

with increased risk of embolization, stroke/death, and hemodynamic instability.[61,62] It is our practice to postdilate only calcified and severely stenotic lesions with residual waste in the stent. Otherwise, these stents are self-expanding and will continue to expand postoperatively.[63] In patients who develop hypotension or bradycardia after dilation, they can be treated with volume expansion, atropine, or even vasopressor agents.

Completion cerebral angiogram is performed to confirm the absence of distal embolization and a patent stent. The EPD wire is retrieved, and the femoral access site sheath is removed with closure device deployment. Protamine can be administered per provider preference. There is no evidence of increased stroke with protamine administration, and we use it routinely to minimize the risk of access bleeding. The patient is then taken to the ICU for close monitoring of neurologic status and hemodynamics. Generally, patients are admitted for 24 hours and then discharged on aspirin and clopidogrel. Postoperative surveillance involves a duplex ultrasound within 6 weeks of the procedure, followed by 6-month ultrasound and then annually.

Perioperative Complications

Traditionally, the greatest complication after TFCAS is the risk of stroke. The introduction of EPDs has helped reduce the stroke risk. Initially introduced as a distal occlusion balloon, antegrade blood flow is stopped during stent deployment, and once deployment is complete, blood and embolic debris are suctioned endovascularly.[64] However, this has been abandoned because of distal ICA damage and plaque rupture as a result of the need to pass the lesion before balloon placement. These EPDs have largely been replaced with a filter. The filter allows antegrade blood flow, is passed across the lesion with a wire, and is recaptured with a filter-retrieval system. This leads to continuous cerebral blood flow, angiography access, and decreased manipulation of the carotid artery. However, there remains a risk of plaque disruption as a result of passing across the lesion before filter deployment. The final type of EPD is a proximal protection version, which deploys balloons in the common and ECAs to cause flow stasis, and intermittent syringe aspiration for debris. However, this device requires a larger 9-Fr sheath. The Prevention of Cerebral Embolization by Proximal Balloon Occlusion Compared to Filter Protection During Carotid Artery Stenting (PROFI) trial compared proximal balloon occlusion to filter and found that proximal occlusion had a lower incidence of ischemic lesions on MRI compared with filter; however, no significant difference in perioperative major adverse events was found.[65]

Many trials have compared the outcomes after TFCAS to CEA. The Stent-Protected Angioplasty Versus Carotid Endarterectomy (SPACE) randomized trial found that at 30 days, there were no significant differences in the rate of death or ipsilateral stroke between TFCAS or CEA, and as a noninferiority trial, the results do not support the widespread use of stenting.[66] The 2-year data for the SPACE trial again showed similar results; however, patients who underwent TFCAS compared with CEA were at higher risk of restenosis.[67] The results are further confirmed by the Endarterectomy Versus Angioplasty in Patients with Symptomatic Severe Stenosis (EVA-3S) randomized clinical trial, which found a 2.5 increased risk of stroke and death in the TFCAS versus CEA group.[68] Finally, the Carotid Revascularization Endarterectomy versus Stenting Trial (CREST) study found a higher rate of stroke in the TFCAS group but no difference between stroke and death at 10 years between TFCAS and CEA.[69,70] Table 101.3 summarizes the landmark randomized clinical trials comparing TFCAS to CEA.

Periprocedural stroke can be a result of arch or lesion embolization, EPD wire thrombosis, stent thrombosis, kinking, dissection, or hyperperfusion injury. Neuro-rescue techniques involve stent retrieval, aspiration thrombectomy, or catheter-directed thrombolysis. This is why it is critical to have the patient awake for neuromonitoring and when performing a cerebral angiogram before and after lesion treatment. Outcome of stroke can be dramatically improved with immediate recognition and rescue procedures. Additional complications include MI; however, CREST found lower rates of MI in TFCAS compared with CEA, likely because of lower rates of general anesthesia in TFACS.[69] Stent thrombosis has been identified in patients with densely calcified plaque and requires stent explantation and subsequent CEA.[71] Carotid dissections after stent placement are generally treated with either stent extension or antiplatelet therapy. Finally, because of groin access, complications can additionally include hematoma or infection and, in rare cases, fistula or pseudoaneurysm.

Transcarotid Artery Revascularization
Considerations

TCAR is a hybrid procedure that combines direct carotid artery access with stent placement. TCAR allows neuroprotection with flow reversal before any lesion manipulation. TCAR has several advantages over TFCAS by avoiding the atherosclerotic aortic arch and establishing CEA-like protection with clamping of the CCA, and TCAR has been found to have a lower learning curve than TFCAS, with most operators reaching technical proficiency after 10 to 15 procedures.[72] Similar to CEA and TFCAS, patients must first undergo medical therapy with dual antiplatelet agents, statins, antihypertensive medications, smoking cessation, and glycemic control.

TCAR was originally tested in Europe in 2009 with the Silk Road Medical Embolic Protection System: First-in-Man (PROOF) study, which found that TCAR had comparable embolic rates to CEA identified on diffusion-weighed MRI.[73] The safety of TCAR was confirmed in the Food and Drug Administration Investigation Device Exemption trial—Investigation of Transcarotid CAS With Dynamic Flow Reversal in Subjects With Significant Extracranial Carotid Stenosis (ROADSTER I). The stroke rates in this trial were 1.4% compared with 4.1% in TFCAS patients in the CREST trial. These data allowed TCAR to be approved in the United States in 2015.[74]

CMS requires that hospitals be enrolled in the Vascular Quality Initiative CAS registry as a condition for reimbursement. Patients are eligible for TCAR if they are symptomatic with greater than 50% stenosis of the carotid artery or asymptomatic with greater than 80% stenosis. Initially, at least one high-risk medical or anatomic criteria was required for TCAR eligibility (Table 101.5).

Additionally, certain anatomic criteria are needed in order to perform TCAR safely and need to be confirmed on duplex ultrasound and CTA. The CCA must be equal to or greater than 6 mm in diameter, the landing zone must be equal to or greater than 5 cm (defined as the distance between the clavicle and carotid bifurcation), the proximal CCA or access site should be free of calcification and significant atherosclerosis, and the ICA diameter should be between 4 and 9 mm. Additional criteria include a CCA depth of less than 4 cm from the skin surface and a ratio of the CCA depth to the clavicle-carotid bifurcation of less than 1. Patients undergoing TCAR must be on DAPT, including full-dose aspirin, clopidogrel, or other DAPT combination, in

TABLE 101.5 Criteria for Transcarotid Artery Revascularization

MEDICAL CRITERIA	ANATOMIC CRITERIA
Age over 75	Contralateral carotid artery occlusion
History of angina or greater than 2-vessel coronary artery disease	Tandem stenosis greater than 70%
Unstable angina	High cervical carotid artery stenosis
New York Heart Association class III or IV heart failure	Restenosis after CEA
Left ventricular ejection fraction less than 30%	Bilateral carotid artery stenosis
Myocardial infarction 72 hours to 6 weeks before procedure	Hostile neck
Chronic obstructive pulmonary disease with FEV₁ less than 50%	
Contralateral cranial nerve injury	
Renal insufficiency	

CEA, Carotid endarterectomy; *FEV₁*, forced expiratory volume in 1 second.

addition to a statin for at least 5 days before the procedure. It is our practice to test all patients for clopidogrel response, and if no adequate response is documented, the patient can be switched to another P2Y12 inhibitor.

Technique

One of the most unique features of TCAR is cerebral blood flow reversal, which allows neuroprotection. Additionally, direct cutdown and access to the carotid artery allow a stent to be placed without aortic arch manipulation. Neuroprotection is achieved when carotid blood and debris are shunted away from the brain through the carotid arterial sheath to the common femoral vein across an ENROUTE Flow Reversal System (Silk Road Medical, Sunnyvale, CA) that includes a filter and dual channels to allow for low- and high-flow reversal rates.[75] Flow reversal is achieved through the pressure gradient between the arterial and venous systems.

TCAR is generally performed in a room with high-quality imaging under either general, regional, or local anesthesia. There have been lower rates of reported MI with local or regional anesthesia compared with general anesthesia.[76] Similar to both CEA and TFCAS, an arterial line must be placed for close hemodynamic monitoring. Patients are positioned similar to CEA: supine with bilateral arms tucked in, a shoulder roll, and head/neck turned to the contralateral side. The procedure begins with an intraoperative ultrasound to confirm patent ICA, disease-free CCA, and distance between the clavicle and bifurcation.

An incision is made at the base of the neck to identify and isolate the CCA. The landmark for identifying the CCA is the triangular space between the sternal and clavicular heads of the sternocleidomastoid muscle (Fig. 101.4). A 3- to 4-cm segment of the CCA is isolated circumferentially, and a vessel loop or umbilical tape is placed proximally. Generally, a 5-0 Prolene suture is then used to create a purse string on the anterior surface of the CCA. Simultaneously, under ultrasound guidance, femoral vein access is obtained, and an 8-Fr venous sheath is placed for adequate flow reversal (Fig. 101.5).[75]

The patient is heparinized with a goal ACT of over 250 seconds. The Silk Road ENROUTE system includes an arterial sheath with dilator, venous sheath with dilator, flow controller with 200-um filter, 0.035 stiff guidewire, and floppy-tip wire. The set also

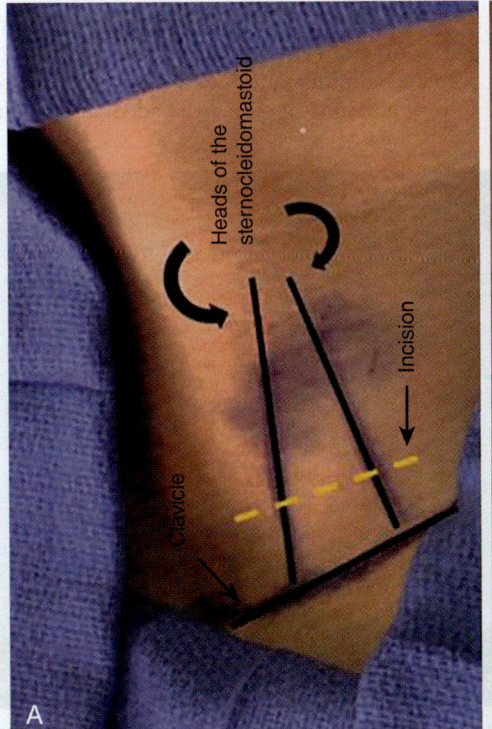
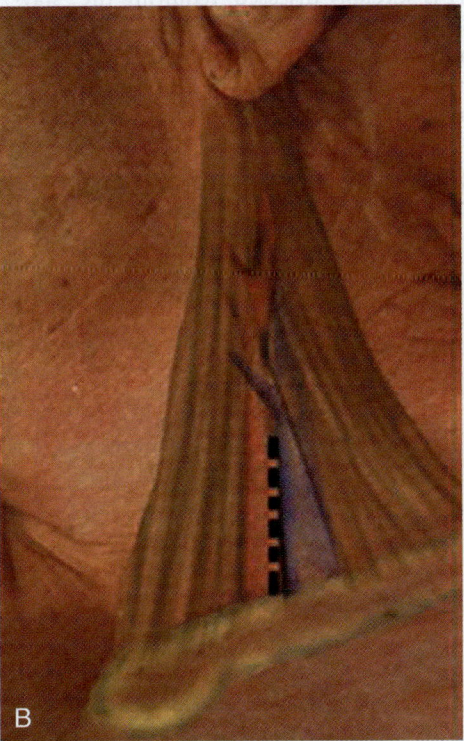

FIGURE 101.4 (A) The anatomic landmarks for cut-down of common carotid artery during transcarotid artery revascularization. (B) Longitudinal incision. (Courtesy Silk Road Medical, Inc.; Silk Road Medical, Inc. retains and reserves all rights, including copyrights.)

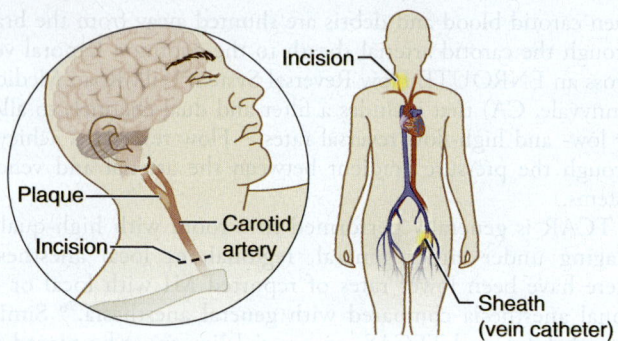

FIGURE 101.5 Overview of transcarotid artery revascularization access points. (Courtesy Silk Road Medical, Inc.; Silk Road Medical, Inc. retains and reserves all rights, including copyrights.)

includes an 0.018 guidewire to mark when 3 to 5 cm of the wire is in the vessel, and a short 0.014 wire is used to deliver the stent.

Heparin is bolused based on weight (80 units per kg) and given intravenously to achieve an ACT between 250 and 300. Gentle traction with the vessel loop on the CCA is applied to superficialize the artery and allows a 21-gauge micropuncture needle access through the purse-string suture. It is imperative not to advance the microneedle into the back wall of the vessel to avoid dissection. It is our practice to advance the microwire under direct fluoroscopic visualization to ensure free movement and confirm luminal access. There are two techniques for access: (1) stop short of the bifurcation, and (2) engage the ECA (Fig. 101.6). The authors' preference is to engage the ECA whenever free of significant disease. This allows for more wire purchase when advancing the arterial sheath (10-Fr outer diameter) to avoid dissection. Less often, the lesion is at the bifurcation, or the ECA is severally diseased, requiring the "staying-short technique."

The microwire is advanced 3 to 4 cm into the CCA. The microsheath with dilator is advanced over the wire 2 to 3 cm into the CCA using the marking on the sheath. Pulsatile backflow after the

wire and dilator are removed confirms proper positioning. An angiogram is performed to determine the location of the carotid bifurcation. We require at least a two-view angiogram to confirm intraluminal position of the sheath. If appropriate to engage the ECA, the wire is advanced 2 to 3 cm into the ECA with mask imaging guidance, followed by advancing the microsheath with the dilator. If the sheath is advanced without the dilator, there is a risk of dissection of the CCA. We like to perform another angiogram to ensure ECA selection. All angiograms should be hand-injected with 50% low-density contrast and 50% heparinized saline; a total of 4 to 6 cc is adequate. Care must be taken to inject the contrast gently to avoid embolization. Transcranial Doppler (TCD) has shown embolization even with contrast injection. A stiff wire is placed in the ECA through the microsheath. Advancing the stiff wire without sheath protection can cause dissection of the CCA. If stopping short, the same technique is used to get the stiff wire just proximal to the carotid bifurcation. We found that dilating the anterior wall of the CCA with the venous sheath dilatator helped advance the arterial sheath smoothly. Only 0.5 cm of the tip of the dilator is advanced into the anterior wall of the CCA with proper back tension on the wire. We prefer the incision to be along the longitudinal axis of the CCA and at least long enough to allow the operator to control the CCA directly after dilating the arterial hole with a two-finger hold on the wire. The Silk Road ENROUTE 8-Fr sheath is placed in the CCA over the wire and secured to the skin with silk sutures. The wire and dilator are withdrawn, and the arterial sheath is flushed gently with heparinized saline, ensuring no air in both the side port and connector. Next, the tubing is connected to the sheath and back-bled by holding the tubing up and then connected to the venous sheath in the common femoral vein to allow for passive flow reversal via a dynamic flow controller and filter. Two-view angiograms are performed to ensure an intraluminal position of the sheath.

Before proceeding, a specific TCAR time-out is performed. The time-out is performed to confirm adequate ACT; glycopyrrolate administration to prevent bradycardia and hypotension during lesion angioplasty; adequate mean arterial pressure to

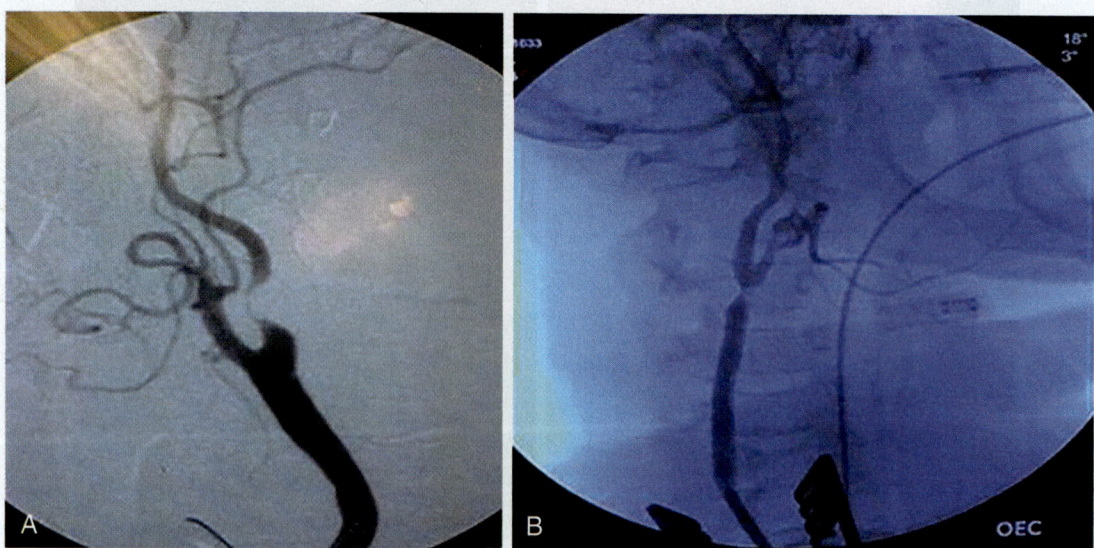

FIGURE 101.6 (A) When proximal external carotid artery (ECA) is free of disease, the engage-the-ECA technique is used. (B) When disease is present in distal common carotid artery or bifurcation, the stop-short technique is used.

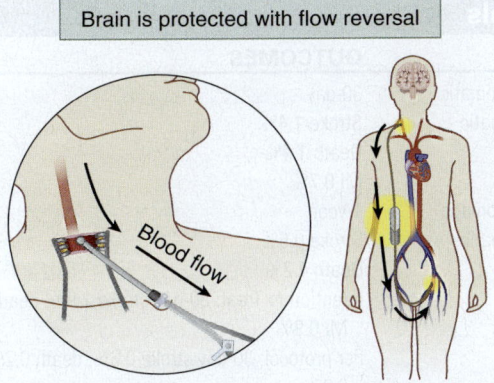

Brain is protected with flow reversal

Blood flow

FIGURE 101.7 Transcarotid arterial revascularization flow reversal. (Courtesy Silk Road Medical, Inc.; Silk Road Medical, Inc. retains and reserves all rights, including copyrights.)

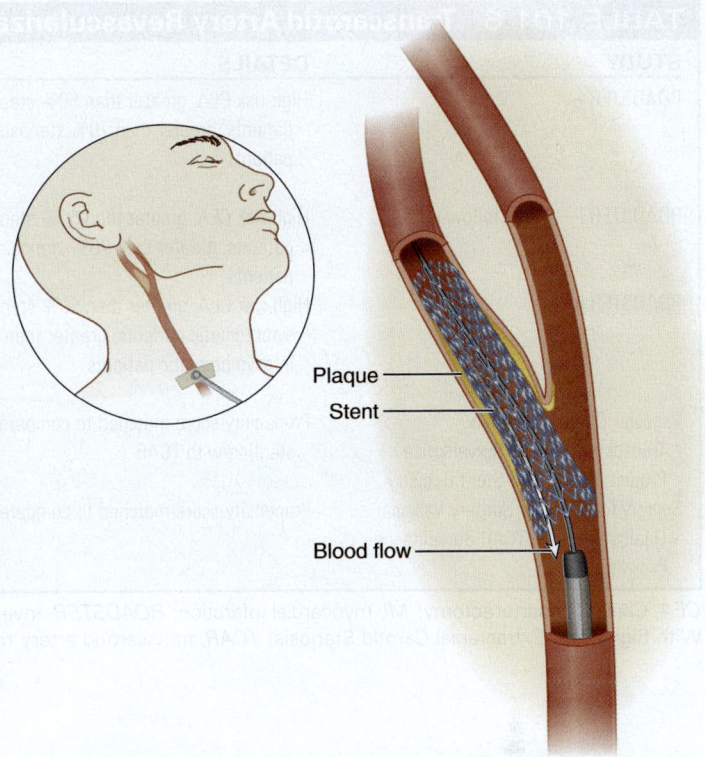

Plaque

Stent

Blood flow

FIGURE 101.8 Transcarotid arterial revascularization stent placement. (Courtesy Silk Road Medical, Inc.; Silk Road Medical, Inc. retains and reserves all rights, including copyrights.)

achieve flow reversal; and wire, balloon, and stent preparation to minimize clamp time. The CCA is then clamped under direct visualization to avoid vagus nerve injury and achieve active flow reversal. We have avoided Rummel technique in clamping because it can cause vessel injury and have resorted to using atraumatic vascular clamps.

At this point, any debris from lesion manipulation is flushed from the carotid artery to the filter and trapped (Fig. 101.7). The blood is then returned through the femoral vein. Angiogram is performed to mark the bifurcation because the bed was moved to allow direct visualization of CCA clamping. The ICA lesion is then crossed with a 0.014 wire placed in the distal ICA. One advantage of the TCAR is the ability to use a curved catheter to help cross difficult lesions under flow reversal protection. This is more cumbersome with TFCAS with long distance for travel and all tortuosity applied to the catheter from a femoral approach through the iliacs, aorta, and arch. It is also more difficult to use guiding catheters to advance the wires, which are usually attached to an EPD. Once the lesion is crossed, we redilate with a 3- to 5-mm balloon. Slow and careful inflation and deflation of the balloon are performed, not exceeding 8 atmospheres. It is our preference to use smaller balloon in standard lesions and larger balloon in calcified lesions. The Silk Road ENROUTE stent is then delivered and deployed to cover at least 1 cm proximal and distal to the lesion (Fig. 101.8). An angiogram is then performed to confirm stent placement in the appropriate position. The stent is a nitinol self-expanding stent that is delivered through an 8-Fr sheath. The delivery system is 57 cm in length, and stent sizes include 20, 30, and 40 mm in length, with a diameter between 5 and 10 mm. The stent is sized 1 to 2 mm larger than the diameter of the CCA and tapers in the ICA. Poststenting dilation is debated; however, a study found that, unlike post dilation after TFCAS, post dilation in TCAR does not increase the risk of stroke but has a slight increase in the risk of TIA.[77] We tend to balloon calcified lesions where we see a significant residual stenosis of the stent. We always obtain multiple-view angiograms to ensure patency of the stent (Fig. 101.9).

IICA spasm can occur distal to the stent and, if not self-limiting, can be treated with nitroglycerin. Acute carotid occlusion is an emergency requiring treatment with oxygen, blood pressure support, and clot aspiration versus thrombolytic. In the case of dissection, an additional stent can be placed. The CCA is

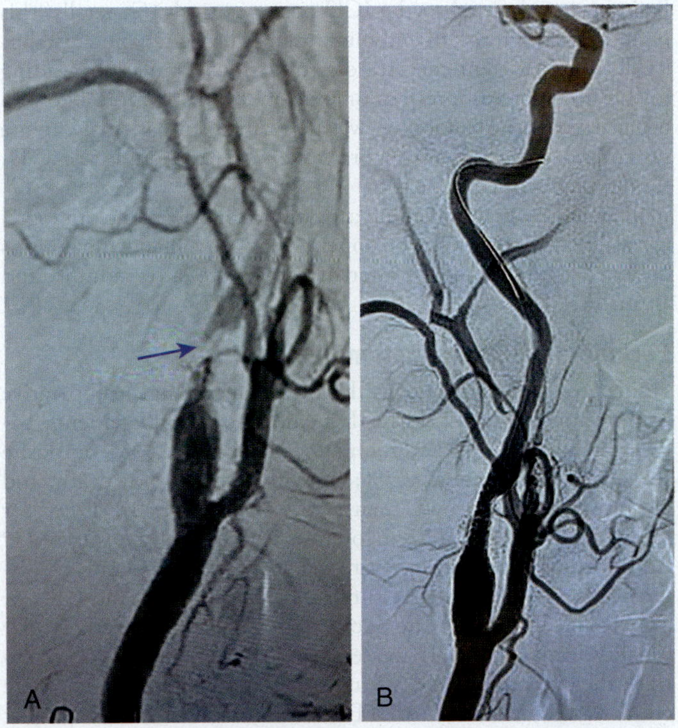

FIGURE 101.9 (A) Transcarotid artery revascularization prestent. (B) Transcarotid artery revascularization poststent.

TABLE 101.6 Transcarotid Artery Revascularization Trials

STUDY	DETAILS	OUTCOMES
ROADSTER I	High-risk CEA, greater than 50% stenosis in symptomatic patients, greater than 70% stenosis in asymptomatic patients	30-day Stroke 1.4% Death 1.4% MI 0.7%
ROADSTER I—1-year follow-up	High-risk CEA, greater than 50% stenosis in symptomatic patients, greater than 70% stenosis in asymptomatic patients	1-year Stroke 0.6% Death 4.2%
ROADSTER II	High-risk CEA, greater than 50% stenosis in symptomatic patients, greater than 80% stenosis in asymptomatic patients	Intention to Treat: 30-day stroke 1.9%, death 0.4%, MI 0.9% Per protocol: 30-day stroke 0.6%, death 0.2%, MI 0.9%
Vascular Quality Initiative Transcarotid Artery Surveillance Project and Carotid Stent Registry	Propensity-score-matched to compare transfemoral stenting with TCAR	TCAR in-hospital stroke/death: 1.6% TFCAS in-hospital stroke/death: 3.1%
Society for Vascular Surgery Vascular Quality Initiative TCAR Surveillance Project	Propensity-score-matched to compare CEA with TCAR	Stroke/death: CEA 1.6%, TCAR 1.6% MI: TCAR 0.5%, CEA 0.9%

CEA, Carotid endarterectomy; *MI*, myocardial infarction; *ROADSTER*, Investigation of Transcarotid CAS With Dynamic Flow Reversal in Subjects With Significant Extracranial Carotid Stenosis; *TCAR*, transcarotid artery revascularization; *TFCAS*, transfemoral carotid artery stenting.

unclamped, the arterial sheath is removed, and a purse string is tied while the venous sheath is removed and manual pressure is held. The neck incision is generally closed in multiple layers, and the patient is transferred to the ICU. Protamine administration is shown to reduce the risk of bleeding after TCAR, with no increase in MI, stroke, death, or pulmonary embolism.[78]

Postoperative Care

Patients are admitted to the ICU postoperatively. Generally, this period has a high risk of embolic stroke or hemodynamic instability. The TCAR stent can create carotid sinus simulation, leading to the need for vasopressors or inotropes. This is more likely to occur if poststent ballooning was performed. In patients who are recognized as having a TIA or stroke, a carotid duplex or CTA should be obtained.

Patients are maintained on aspirin indefinitely and clopidogrel for at least 4 to 6 weeks postoperatively. Surveillance imaging is obtained within 1 month after the procedure, at 6 months, and annually.

Perioperative Complications

Similar to TFCAS, stroke is the most concerning postoperative complication. ROADSTER II included over 600 patients between 2015 and 2019 and found a stroke rate of 1.9%; composite stroke and death rate of 2.3%; and composite stroke, death, and MI rate of 3.2%, all lower than TFCAS from CREST.[79] One-year results from ROADSTER I found a 96% stroke-free survival.[80] Additionally, a propensity-score-matched analysis found no difference in stroke/death-free survival between TCAR and CEA or TCAR and TFCAS.[81] The Society for Vascular Surgery Vascular Quality Initiative (VQI) created a TCAR Surveillance Project to track the outcomes of TCAR in order to provide data to compare with traditional CEA or TFCAS.[82] Data from this project have found a significantly decreased risk of stroke and death in TCAR compared with TFCAS and similar rates compared with

CEA.[83–86] Finally, other complications include wound infections, hematoma, and access site issues.

Stroke rates after TCAR have been studied extensively and found to be 1.4% in the ROADSTER study and 1.6% in the VQI surveillance project.[74,86] CCA dissection can occur if the CCA depth is over 4 cm or if a floppy guidewire is used. Our technique described previously has been effective in avoiding dissection in our practice. A rare complication can be intolerance to flow reversal, which can be relieved with oxygen, elevated blood pressure, changing the flow to low, or ischemic preconditioning.[75] High-risk lesions for embolization include an ulcerated symptomatic lesion with thrombus.

Cerebral hyperperfusion and intracranial hemorrhage manifest as a headache and can be seen in patients who are hypertensive or have bilateral carotid artery stenosis.[87,88] Cervical hematoma can also occur, and risk can be reduced with use of protamine. Cranial nerve injury can occur with both carotid dissection and clamping.

Overall, the goal of TCAR is to provide an acceptable alternative to TFCAS in patients who are unable to undergo CEA. ROADSTER I and II have shown comparable rates of stroke and death to CEA; however, there currently are no clinical trials comparing TCAR and CEA directly (Table 101.6). Next steps for TCAR would involve high-level clinical evidence data to support the use of TCAR outside of high-risk patients. Preliminary data from the VQI found that in a propensity score matching between standard-risk patients undergoing CEA or TCAR, there was no difference in stroke, death, or MI even up to 1 year postprocedure.[89] This has led to recent expansion of TCAR for standard-risk patients as well.

In terms of cost-effectiveness, TCAR was found to be more expensive than CEA after 5 years but had higher quality-adjusted life years than CEA, and ultimately, after 6 years, TCAR was also more cost-effective.[77] Overall, once a patient is determined to meet criteria for operative intervention for carotid artery stenosis, the decision between CEA, TFCAS, and TCAR is based on patient physiologic and anatomic factors. TCAR has been introduced as a novel hybrid therapy that has outcomes similar to the gold-standard CEA.

LONG-TERM FOLLOW-UP AND COMPLICATIONS

Follow-Up

Patients who undergo carotid revascularization should be followed longitudinally to assess for long-term sequelae. It is the authors' practice to obtain an ipsilateral carotid duplex at 30 days postprocedure to ensure no early abnormalities are apparent at the endarterectomy site. A bilateral carotid duplex is then performed at 6 months, then at every 12 months thereafter. Any abnormal findings identified on duplex are then often followed with a CTA scan to better characterize the lesion.

Restenosis

Approximately 10% to 15% of patients will experience restenosis of the carotid revascularization site under long-term follow-up. This may be slightly higher for stenting than for CEA, but rates of neurologic sequelae are similar. Patients presenting with focal neurologic symptoms and restenosis should be considered for repeat revascularization, the mode of which should be complementary to the index procedure. There is persistent debate on how patients with asymptomatic restenosis should be treated, and management remains individualized.

NONATHEROSCLEROTIC CAROTID DISEASE

Fibromuscular Dysplasia

Fibromuscular dysplasia (FMD) is a nonatherosclerotic, noninflammatory disease process classically described on imaging as a string of beads. It typically affects medium-sized arteries in the media, and the majority of cases are in females. If symptomatic in the carotid artery, patients typically describe headaches, TIA, stroke, or pulsatile tinnitus.[90] The US Registry, which tracks individuals with FMD, found that almost half of these individuals will present with either aneurysms or dissections.[91]

Clinical presentation is highly variable, and FMD can even be an incidental finding. Physical examination can be significant for Horner syndrome, cranial nerve abnormalities, or bruits.[92,93] Additionally, patients are diagnosed based on carotid duplex imaging, with typical disease pattern occurring in the distal carotid artery, and sometimes additional imaging with angiography is warranted to better assess the carotid artery distal to the lesion.[94] In terms of noninvasive imaging, both CTA and MRI can be used; however, CTA has been found to be more closely correlated to angiography.

Treatment for FMD can be either medically managed or surgically managed. Medical management consists of antiplatelet therapy. Surgical management consists of dilation with angioplasty and, less likely, stent placement. When FMD is treated in the renal arteries, balloon angioplasty is performed without stent placement. There is a paucity of literature on carotid FMD treatment.

Carotid Dissection

Dissection of the carotid artery is generally uncommon but occurs when blood is able to permeate through the vessel layers through intimal tear and can lead to stenosis or occlusion in the acute setting and aneurysm in the chronic setting. Causes can be iatrogenic, traumatic, or spontaneous. Spontaneous dissection has been associated with bony structure contact of the carotid artery, chiropractic manipulation, or underlying vascular anomalies. Clinical symptoms may either mimic a headache or can present as Horner syndrome. Traumatic dissection can occur after blunt injury in approximately 1% of patients.[95]

The gold standard for diagnosis is four-vessel cerebral angiography, which allows the lesion and artery to be identified. Dissection is identified with an intimal flap or two lumens, which can also be found on ultrasound. Occlusions are described as tapered and occur proximally in the artery. Additional diagnosis modalities include ultrasound, CTA, and MRA. Filling defects, luminal irregularities, contrast extravasation, and occlusion can all be identified.

In patients who present with carotid artery dissection, up to 50% can present with ischemic stroke or TIA.[96] After blunt trauma, patients with carotid dissection can have a 25% mortality risk and a 50% risk of permanent neurologic damage.[95] The Cervical Artery Dissection in Stroke Study (CADISS) studied over 200 patients randomized to either antiplatelet agents or anticoagulants and found that individuals with dissecting aneurysms had the same risk for a stroke in both groups. The overall main treatment strategy for carotid dissection is antithrombotic therapy. For surgical management, options include either endovascular or open surgical.

In terms of overall treatment for carotid artery dissection, there are no clinical trials that compare antiplatelet therapy with anticoagulation or open surgical intervention with endovascular intervention. In general, surgical intervention is pursued in patients with a change in clinical neurologic examination or inability to tolerate or respond to medical therapy. Given the distal nature of carotid dissections, surgical exposure can be challenging. Surgical management includes ligation, saphenous vein interposition, or patch angioplasty. Endovascular management includes stenting, coiling, and embolization (Fig. 101.10).

Carotid Aneurysm

Carotid aneurysms are a rare entity that can be caused by infectious processes, pseudoaneurysms secondary to trauma, atherosclerotic degeneration, or previous carotid surgery. In terms of clinical findings, aneurysms can be identified by a painless pulsatile mass, TIA, stroke, cranial nerve dysfunction, dysphagia, or rupture.[97] They are confirmed on imaging with ultrasound, CTA, or MRA. The imaging modalities also help determine the treatment approach and accessibility of the aneurysm.

Carotid aneurysms, unlike other carotid pathologies, are treated once identified because of the high rate of TIA, stroke, or rupture.[97] Treatment involves either open surgical or endovascular therapies. Open techniques involve ligation or resection with interposition bypass reconstruction. Endovascular treatment involves covered stent placement, thrombin injection, or coil embolization. We have described the first two carotid aneurysms treated with covered stent through a TCAR approach with flow reversal. This technique minimizes the risk of embolization from the aneurysm and dramatically reduces the technical challenges of a transfemoral approach for delivering covered stents (Fig. 101.11).[98] Mycotic aneurysms are treated with antibiotic therapy followed by open surgical intervention.

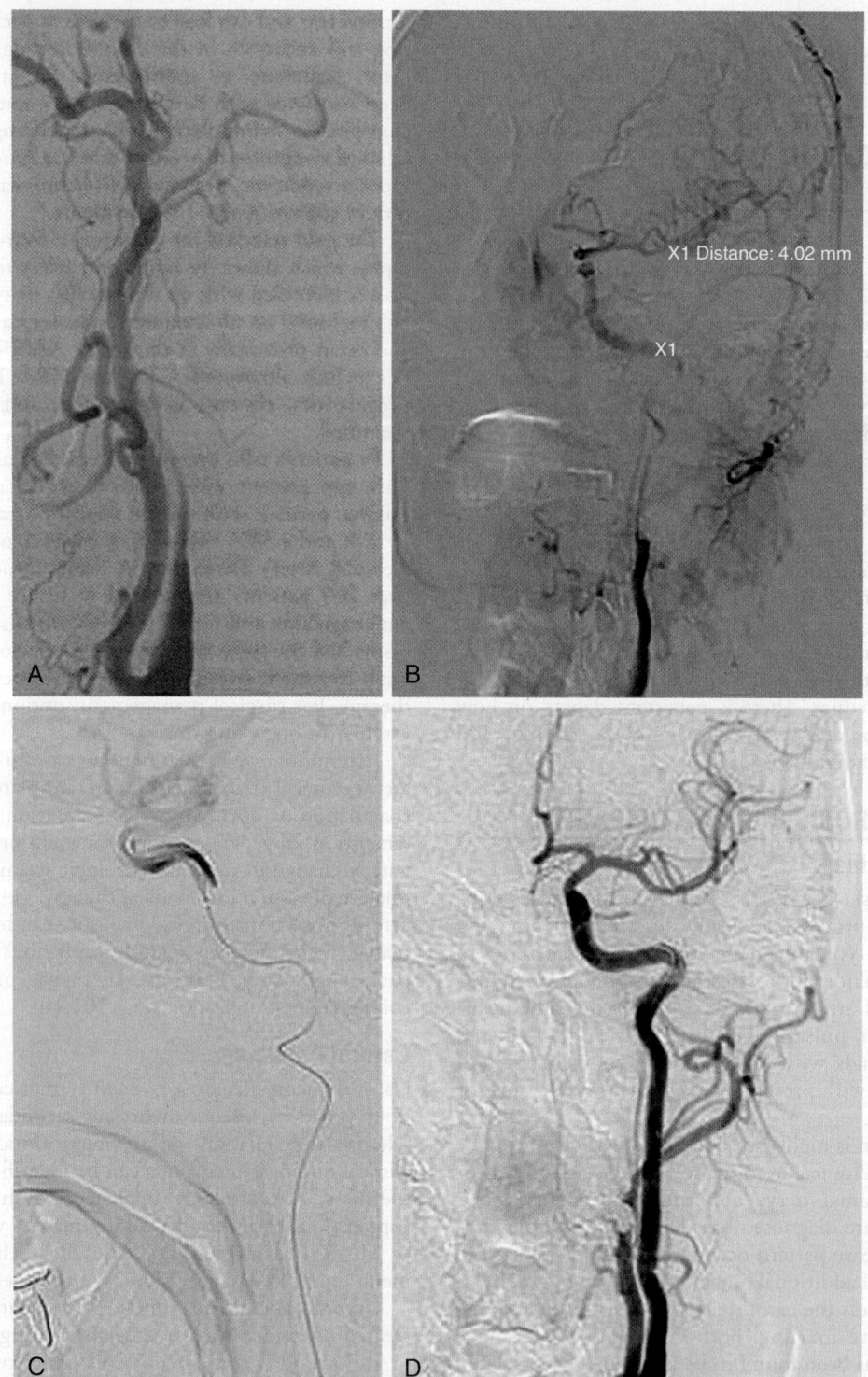

FIGURE 101.10 (A) Flame taper in distal carotid artery. (B) Occlusion of the internal carotid artery with distal reconstitution. (C) Wire across the lesion. (D) Stent deployment with distal flow. (From Elsayed N, Dakour-Aridi H, Malas MB. Cerebrovascular disease: carotid artery dissection. In: *Rutherford's Vascular Surgery and Endovascular Therapy*. 10th ed. Philadelphia: Elsevier; 2018.)

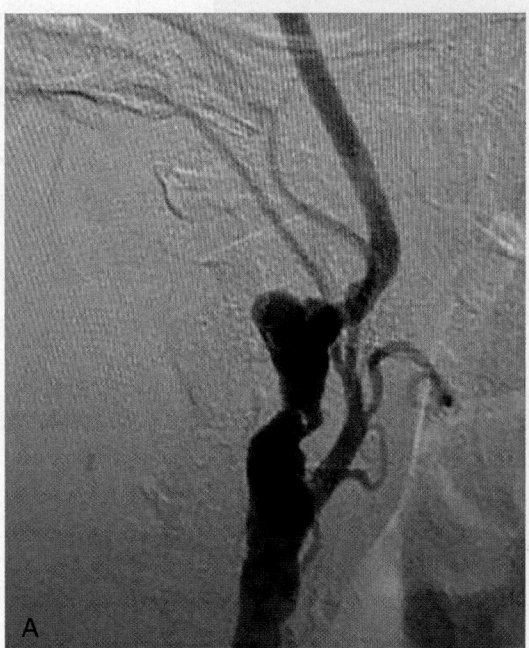 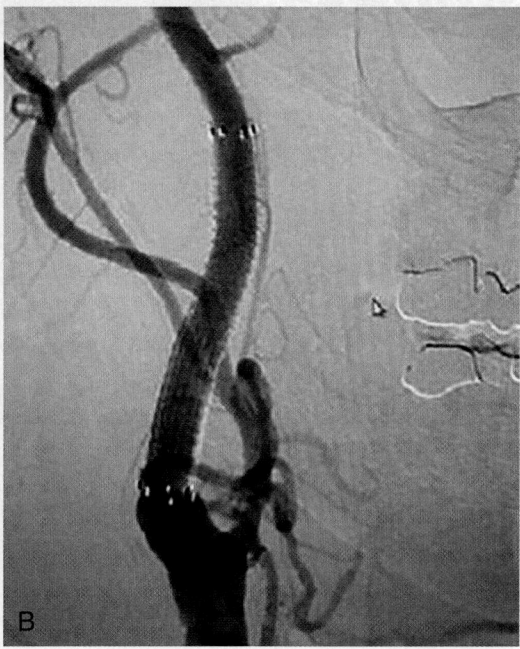

FIGURE 101.11 Transfemoral carotid artery stenting in a pseudoaneurysm. (A) Preoperative. (B) Postoperative. (From Rizwan M, Smith C, Faro S, Malas MB. Transcarotid artery stenting for carotid artery pseudoaneurysm using flow reversal technique. *J Vasc Surg Cases Innov Tech.* 2018;4[2]:115-118.)

SELECTED REFERENCES

AbuRahma AF, Avgerinos EM, Chang RW, et al. Society for Vascular Surgery clinical practice guidelines for management of extracranial cerebrovascular disease. *J Vasc Surg.* 2022;75(suppl 1):4S-22S.

> *Overview of the Society of Vascular Surgery's guidelines on the management of carotid artery disease*

Brott TG, Halperin JL, Abbara S, et al. 2011. ASA/ACCF/AHA/AANN/AANS/ACR/ASNR/CNS/SAIP/SCAI/SIR/SNIS/SVM/SVS guideline on the management of patients with extracranial carotid and vertebral artery disease: executive summary. A report of the American College of Cardiology Foundation/American Heart Association Task Force on Practice Guidelines, and the American Stroke Association, American Association of Neuroscience Nurses, American Association of Neurological Surgeons, American College of Radiology, American Society of Neuroradiology, Congress of Neurological Surgeons, Society of Atherosclerosis Imaging and Prevention, Society for Cardiovascular Angiography and Interventions, Society of Interventional Radiology, Society of NeuroInterventional Surgery, Society for Vascular Medicine, and Society for Vascular Surgery. *Circulation.* 2011;124(4):489-532.

> *American College of Cardiology and American Heart Association guidelines on management of carotid disease*

Kwolek CJ, Jaff MR, Leal JI, et al. Results of the ROADSTER multicenter trial of transcarotid stenting with dynamic flow reversal. *J Vasc Surg.* 2015;62(5):1227-1234.

> *30-day results of the transcarotid artery revascularization technique*

Mott M, Koroshetz W, Wright CB. CREST-2: identifying the best method of stroke prevention for carotid artery stenosis: National Institute of Neurological Disorders and Stroke organizational update. *Stroke.* 2017;48(5):e130-e131.

> *Clinical trial comparing carotid revascularization methods to best medical treatment*

North American Symptomatic Carotid Endarterectomy Trial Collaborators, Barnett HJM, Taylor DW, et al. Beneficial effect of carotid endarterectomy in symptomatic patients with high-grade carotid stenosis. *N Engl J Med.* 1991;325(7):445-453.

> *Benefit of carotid endarterectomy in symptomatic patients*

SPACE Collaborative Group, Ringleb PA, Allenberg J, et al. 30 day results from the SPACE trial of stent-protected angioplasty versus carotid endarterectomy in symptomatic patients: a randomised non-inferiority trial. *Lancet Lond Engl.* 2006; 368(9543):1239-1247.

> *Short-term results between stent placement and carotid endarterectomy*

Timaran CH, Mantese VA, Malas M, et al. Differential outcomes of carotid stenting and endarterectomy performed exclusively by vascular surgeons in the Carotid Revascularization Endarterectomy Versus Stenting Trial (CREST). *J Vasc Surg.* 2013;57(2):303-308.

> *Short-term results of carotid endarterectomy and stenting when performed by vascular surgeons*

The full reference list appears on Elsevier eBooks+.

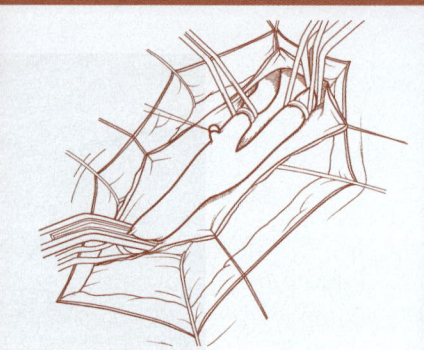

Aortic Disease

Abe DeAnda, Mitchell W. Cox, and Matthew J. Eagleton

▶ **Please access Elsevier eBooks+ to view the video for this chapter.**

DISSECTION/INTRAMURAL HEMATOMA

Classification

There are two major classification schemes for aortic dissections (AD; Fig. 102.1). The DeBakey classification was the first attempt to distinguish two clinically different scenarios—that is, dissections limited to the descending aorta versus those involving the ascending aorta. When the ascending aorta is involved, the dissection is either a type I (involving the entire ascending aorta, arch, and to some extent, descending aorta) or a type II (limited to the ascending aorta only). Dissection of the descending aorta alone is a DeBakey type III, with further subdivisions of IIIa (tear only in the descending thoracic aorta) and IIIb (tear extending below the diaphragm). The Stanford classification scheme is limited to type A, which encompasses dissections with *any* involvement of the ascending aorta, and type B, which is for dissections distal to the left subclavian artery (SCA). The original Stanford scheme thus distinguished between surgical management (type A) and medical management (type B), although there were exceptions. With the advent of endovascular therapy, there has been a shift away from medical management and toward endovascular intervention for type B dissections. The DeBakey scheme can also be separated into surgical (type I and II) and nonsurgical (type III), but in contrast to the Stanford classification, it also provides information on the extent of the disease process. More recently, there has been an interest in a modification of the Stanford scheme with a non-A, non-B subgroup. By convention, the classical separation between an acute and chronic dissection occurs at the 2-week mark, but a recent modification includes four domains: hyperacute (<24 hours), acute (2–7 days), subacute (8–30 days), and chronic (>30 days).[1] The DeBakey and Stanford classification schemes remain the most used designations clinically and in the literature.

Pathology, Management, and Outcomes

Aortic Dissection, Intramural Hematoma, and Penetrating Ulcers

We consider AD, intramural hematoma (IMH), and penetrating aortic ulcers (PAUs) together because of the interplay between these three disease states, and each may be representative of the same disease within a spectrum and, in fact, may occur together. What separates the three, in part, is the level of involvement of the aortic wall. Whereas aneurysmal disease involves all three layers of the aorta, PAU is a disease of the intima and media, and AD and IMH are diseases of the media, with significant overlap between the three.

Aortic Dissection

Acute AD is the most common clinical emergency involving the aorta, but the incidence is only an estimate for a number of reasons, including difficulties in making the diagnosis antemortem. Various prospective population studies and retrospective registries give estimates of the incidence range from 3.5 to 16.3 cases per 100,000 patient-years. Males are more frequently diagnosed with an AD compared with females (16 per 100,000 compared with 7.9 per 100,000), and females present later, are older, and have worse in-hospital and surgical mortalities. Type A ADs (TAADs) occur more commonly than type B ADs (TBADs) by 2:1; TBAD is more common than TAAD among Black patients (52.4% vs. 47.6%). Compared with aneurysmal disease, dissections occur in all age groups, although there is a bimodal pattern, with older patients having associated risk factors of hypertension and atherosclerosis and younger patients having connective tissue and genetic disorders as well as bicuspid aortic valve disease.

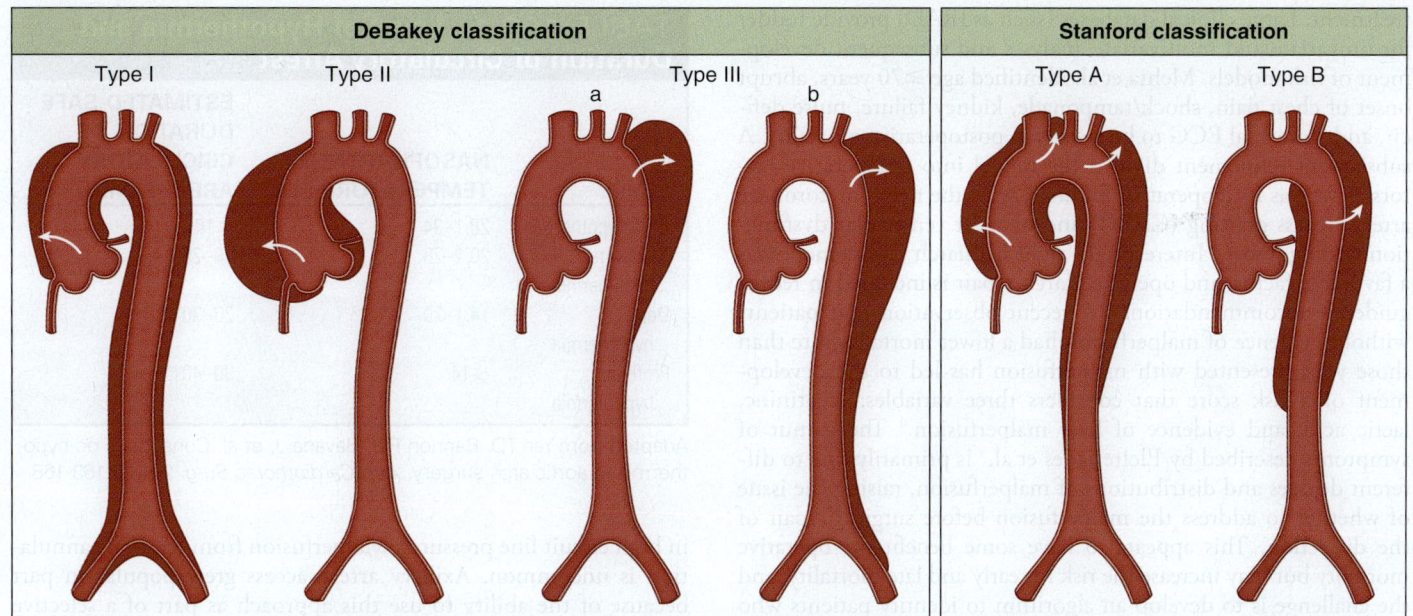

FIGURE 102.1 DeBakey *(left)* and Stanford *(right)* aortic dissection classifications.

Predisposing risk factors of hypertension, connective tissue disorders, vascular inflammation, and disruption of the intima and media (e.g., PAU and IMH) may play a role in the mechanisms leading to the initiation of an AD. Syndromes associated with AD include those with well-known genetic markers and mutations, such as Marfan syndrome (mutation of *FBN1*) and Loeys-Dietz (mutation of *TGFB1, TGFBR2,* and *TGFB*), as well as less commonly affected genes, such as *MYH11, ACTA2,* and *SMAD3*. Some of these mechanisms may also play a role in the development of aneurysmal disease and IMHs. When illicit drug use, including cocaine and methamphetamines, is present or suspected, patients tend to be younger and have type B dissections. It may not be the acute use of cocaine and associated hypertension but rather the long-term atherogenic effects of cocaine that predispose to AD. Finally, there are potential environmental and social factors that may transcend genetic factors alone. The Registry of Aortic Dissection in China (Sino-RAD), in comparison to the International Registry of Acute Aortic Dissection (IRAD), describes acute TAADs in the Chinese population to occur at an earlier age (mean age 50.5 vs. 61.1 years), with less hypertension (51.4% vs. 67%) and greater predominance of males (76.3% vs. 66.9%).

AD can mimic a variety of other medical problems, including acute coronary syndrome, stroke, paraplegia, lower extremity ischemia, acute renal failure, and an abdominal catastrophe, with each of these problems being attributable to malperfusion. In a review of 526 patients who ultimately had the diagnosis of an acute TAAD, although 90% of these patients had pain as a presenting symptom, in slightly over 20%, the pain was localized in the abdomen.[2] In the same study, the so-called pathognomonic sign of absent or differential pulses was present in only 139 of the 526 patients, and only 31% of patients had normal electrocardiograms (ECGs), with more than 25% of patients having ECG findings of myocardial ischemia, infarction, new Q waves, or ST-segment deviations. Such ECG findings could lead to the misdiagnosis of an acute coronary syndrome. Putting the difficulty in diagnosis in perspective, the incidence of AD is up to

16 per 100,000, which is lower in comparison to acute coronary syndromes (440 per 100,000) and pulmonary embolism (69 per 100,000), both of which can present similarly to AD.

Before the widespread introduction and implementation of computed tomography (CT), the diagnosis of an AD was made at autopsy in >25% of patients with the disease. Both CT and magnetic resonance imaging (MRI) are useful in the diagnostic confirmation of a dissection, with sensitivities and specificities reported to be as high as 100%. CT imaging has the added benefit of providing the "triple rule-out"—that is, specific protocols regarding the timing of contrast to rule out (or rule in) dissection, pulmonary embolism, or coronary artery calcification. Transthoracic echocardiography (TTE) is of limited utility for TAAD and has no utility in type B. For TAAD, TTE has a sensitivity range of 35% to 80% and a specificity range of 35% to 96%, depending on the location of the tear, and a normal TTE cannot exclude the possibility of a dissection. Transesophageal echocardiography (TEE) is more specific (63%–96%) and sensitive (98%) in diagnosing TAAD and will detect a flap in the descending thoracic aorta as well. Shiga et al. demonstrated that pooled sensitivities (98%–100%) and specificities (95%–98%) were comparable between TEE, contrast CT, and MRI.

TAADs are surgical emergencies requiring, with rare exceptions, open surgical repair. Current guideline recommendations include surgical management for TAADs, with the caveat that stable patients can potentially be transferred to centers with expertise. Medical management with impulse control therapy can be used either as a temporizing measure or for palliation in patients not deemed to be surgical candidates, but although surgical outcomes have improved with time, medical-management mortality remains unchanged.[3]

A frequently quoted risk of mortality is 1% to 2% per hour in the first 24 hours. Although this is likely true for untreated TAAD, medical management with blood pressure and antiimpulse therapy will reduce the 24-hour mortality rate. Subsequently, with surgical intervention, hospital and operative mortality becomes more of a function of patient characteristics than time to diagnosis and treatment. Large clinical databases (such as IRAD) provide fodder for univariate and multivariate analyses and subsequent development of risk models. Mehta et al. identified age ≥70 years, abrupt onset of chest pain, shock/tamponade, kidney failure, pulse deficit, and abnormal ECG to be factors in postoperative mortality. A subsequent refinement divided the model into preoperative factors as well as intraoperative findings, with the need for coronary artery bypass grafting (CABG) and/or right ventricular dysfunction boding poorly. Interestingly, right hemiarch replacement was a favorable factor, and open hemiarch repair is included in recent guideline recommendations.[3] A recent observation that patients without evidence of malperfusion had a lower mortality rate than those who presented with malperfusion has led to the development of a risk score that considers three variables: creatinine, lactic acid, and evidence of liver malperfusion.[4] The gamut of symptoms described by Elefteriades et al.[5] is primarily due to different degrees and distributions of malperfusion, raising the issue of whether to address the malperfusion before surgical repair of the dissection. This appears to have some benefit for operative mortality but may increase the risk for early and late mortality, and the challenge is to develop an algorithm to identify patients who will benefit from revascularization before central repair. Overall operative mortality rates for acute TAAD are typically reported in the range of 15% to 25% and are in single digits in specialized, multidisciplinary aortic surgery programs.[6]

Surgical Management of Acute Type A Aortic Dissection

Open surgical repair of an acute TAAD remains the standard of care when the patient is a surgical candidate. As reported by IRAD, in tertiary medical centers with expertise in the treatment of acute TAAD in the years from 1995 to 2013, the proportion of patients relegated to medical management declined from 21% to 10%, with a corresponding decline in surgical mortality rate from 25% to 18%.[7] Relative contraindications to surgery include advanced age, multiple comorbidities, and neurologic status. Stamou et al. did not see a difference in operative mortality or major morbidity in a comparison between patients ≥70 years and those younger,[8] but octogenarians do not fare as well. IRAD data have shown no difference in outcomes for octogenarians treated with surgical versus medical intervention. The presence of cerebrovascular accident (CVA) or coma has a significant impact on hospital survival, but for patients who undergo surgical repair, there is improved survival compared with medical management, and it remains a recommended strategy.[3] In 84.3% of patients presenting with CVA who underwent surgical repair, there was resolution of the neurologic deficit.

Once the decision is made to proceed with surgery, the primary goal of surgery is the elimination of the entry tear and obliteration of the false lumen in the aortic root and ascending aorta. Successful completion of these goals will often address secondary issues such as aortic valve insufficiency and distal visceral malperfusion. Specific considerations are the cannulation strategy, cerebral protection, conduct of cardiopulmonary bypass (CPB), and the proximal and distal extent of resection and repair.

Traditionally, femoral cannulation was the primary access for establishing arterial inflow for CPB, in part because of the ability to rapidly establish access via either surgical cut-down or percutaneously. The decision as to which vessel to approach is paradoxical in the sense that the femoral artery most likely to be in continuity with the true lumen is the one without the pulse (due to true lumen collapse). The clinical situation where true lumen collapse was occurring and the wrong vessel was cannulated would result

TABLE 102.1	Level of Hypothermia and Duration of Circulatory Arrest	
LEVEL	**NASOPHARYNGEAL TEMPERATURE (°C)**	**ESTIMATED SAFE DURATION OF CIRCULATORY ARREST (MIN)**
Mild hypothermia	28.1–34	<10
Moderate hypothermia	20.1–28	10–20
Deep hypothermia	14.1–20	20–30
Profound hypothermia	≤14	30–40

Adapted from Yan TD, Bannon PG, Bavaria J, et al. Consensus on hypothermia in aortic arch surgery. *Ann Cardiothorac Surg.* 2013;2:163-168.

in high circuit line pressures. Malperfusion from femoral cannulation is uncommon. Axillary artery access grew popular in part because of the ability to use this approach as part of a selective cerebral perfusion technique during periods of circulatory arrest as well as avoidance of atheroembolization and false lumen perfusion.[3] Other approaches include arterial access via the apex of the left ventricle with the cannula traversing the aortic valve, direct cannulation of the true lumen after transection of the ascending aorta, and echo-guided cannulation of ascending aorta/arch using a Seldinger technique.

With some exceptions, acute TAAD repair is performed with a period of hypothermic circulatory arrest. The initial approach to the arch reported by DeBakey et al. included a multicatheter approach to the great vessels and one of the femoral arteries to provide arterial inflow without circulatory arrest. Hypothermic circulatory arrest (Table 102.1) allows the establishment of a bloodless field, allowing for the evaluation of the distal ascending aorta and arch to confirm intimal integrity; ensures graft continuity to the true lumen; and assists in obliteration of the false lumen. Profound hypothermic circulatory arrest provides 30 to 40 minutes of protective cerebral time; deep hypothermia alone should be sufficient for open-distal and hemiarch repairs. The use of unilateral selective antegrade cerebral perfusion (SACP) or bilateral antegrade cerebral circulatory perfusion extends this protective time. With the adjunct of SACP, moderate hypothermia has been shown to be safe and effective. Cerebral perfusion during SACP (with right axillary cannulation) is via the right carotid and assumes the absence of right carotid stenosis and an intact circle of Willis. Concern for coagulopathy secondary to hypothermia has been raised, but adequate rewarming should be sufficient to address this concern.

Once the patient is successfully cannulated and CPB initiated, systemic cooling is started with the target temperature based on surgeon preference, experience, and patient characteristics. Topical ice on the patient's head is typically included, although evidence of its efficacy is limited. There is currently no consensus regarding the rate of cooling or the acid-based management strategy (alpha stat versus pH stat) during cooling, and the surgeon should discuss the target temperature with the anesthesia and perfusion team as part of the operative plan. Routine clamping of the ascending aorta during cooling is not necessary. Distention of the left ventricle may occur because of the presence of aortic valve insufficiency. If the distention is significant, the ventricle can be vented in several ways, including catheters inserted via the right superior pulmonary vein, the pulmonary artery, or directly via the apex of the ventricle. If unsuccessful in reducing the distention, the ascending aorta can be clamped and transected proximally with concomitant myocardial protection via retrograde or direct antegrade cardioplegia. When the distal anastomosis is completed first, the anastomosis can be tested with direct vision of the entire suture line, and rewarming is then initiated while the proximal aorta is dealt with.

If selective cerebral perfusion and circulatory arrest is used, when the target temperature is achieved, the patient is placed in a Trendelenburg position, and the surgical field can be flooded with CO_2 to minimize cerebral microbubbles when the arch is opened. The ascending aorta is then opened, and the arch is examined. Once the extent of repair has been decided, the base of the innominate artery is clamped, and SACP is started with a typical rate of 10 to 15 cc/kg and perfusion pressure of 40 to 50 mm Hg. The extent of repair, both proximally and distally, has also been a subject of debate. The aortic root is not infrequently involved, and resuspension of the aortic valve commissures in addition to reapproximating the walls of the sinuses is often sufficient to provide integrity to the aorta and correct aortic valve insufficiency. Barring this, the root should be addressed at the time of repair.

Management of Type B Dissection

Medical management of type B dissections is favored initially unless there is evidence of rupture or malperfusion (complicated TBAD). Selective β-blockade remains the preferred first-line treatment and has the dual ability to lower blood pressure and reduce aortic tension from the pressure impulse (dP/dt). The goal is a reduction of pulse pressure while maintaining end-organ perfusion, with an appreciation that some antihypertensive medications may increase pulse pressure while reducing mean arterial pressure secondary to their preferential impact on lowering diastolic pressure. With the development of endovascular techniques, thoracic endovascular aortic repair (TEVAR) has emerged as the treatment of choice for complicated TBAD (i.e., with rupture or malperfusion) and as an option for noncomplicated dissections with high-risk features.[3] Medical management remains the recommended standard of care for acute and chronic noncomplicated TBAD.[3] The primary goals of endovascular therapy include coverage of the primary intimal tear and obliteration and/or thrombosis of the false lumen. Fattori et al. showed that in-hospital mortality for open surgical repair of acute TBAD was almost 34%, whereas TEVAR and medical management were both in the range of 10%.[9] Most patients (68.3%) in this study were medically managed with open surgical repair, with TEVAR reserved for complicated dissections; the mortality rate for open surgically managed patients seen was substantially higher than in other studies, as noted in a subsequent meta-analysis, where the pooled mortality rate was 17.5%. The disparity in results may reflect the paucity of studies that directly and randomly compare TEVAR with open surgery or medical management as well as clear distinctions between complicated versus uncomplicated designations and acuity.

The first prospective trial to investigate TEVAR for uncomplicated acute TBAD was the INSTEAD (Investigation of Stent Grafts in Aortic Dissection) trial.[10] At 2 years, there was no difference in all-cause or aortic-related deaths, but remodeling was favorable in the TEVAR group compared with the medical-management cohort.[11] These results were attributed to an underpowered study. The ADSORB (Acute Dissection: Stent Graft OR Best Medical Therapy)[12] trial was a small trial prospectively comparing best

medical therapy (BMT; $n = 31$) with BMT and TEVAR ($n = 30$) in patients with uncomplicated TBAD. The end point was a composite of completeness of false lumen thrombosis, continued aortic growth ≥ 5 mm or a maximum aortic diameter ≥ 55 mm, or descending or abdominal aortic rupture at 1 year. At 1 year, the results favored BMT and TEVAR, chiefly because of completeness of false lumen thrombosis in the BMT and TEVAR group (57% vs. 3%, $p < 0.001$). The clinical significance of the findings from ADSORB, which was not powered to detect differences in aortic-related and all-cause mortality, remains unclear. An extension of the INSTEAD trial (INSTEAD-XL) did find a benefit in aortic-related mortality in the TEVAR cohort at 5 years.[13]

The provisional extension to induce complete attachment (PETTICOAT) technique was initially described as an adjunct to TEVAR for complicated acute type B dissection.[14] The original report noted that in 12 of 100 patients treated with TEVAR, there was persistent flow in the distal false lumen with true lumen collapse. With the subsequent deployment of an uncovered stent distal to the previously implanted stent graft, there was reperfusion of the true lumen and abolishment of malperfusion. These results persisted at 1 year, and there was evidence of improved aortic remodeling. This technique has been modified further to address the distal aorta in open repair of acute TAAD (DeBakey type I) as part of a frozen elephant trunk technique. An "extended" technique (e-PETTICOAT) has been proposed to preemptively address the entire descending thoracic and abdominal aorta, with the anticipated benefits being complete aortic remodeling and prevention of aneurysmal progression. The IMPROVE-AD (Improving Outcomes in Vascular Disease–Aortic Dissection) study will hopefully shed light on the optimal approach to TBAD and endovascular surgery.

Intramural Hematoma

IMH is a subadventitial lesion usually involving the outer third of the media. The nomenclature of IMH follows the Stanford dissection classification, so IMH involving the ascending aorta is type A IMH, and that confined to the descending aorta is type B IMH. One common hypothesis for the development of IMH is the rupture of a vaso-vasorum with subsequent intramural bleeding and hematoma formation, but others have suggested that IMH may reflect an unrecognized AD subsequently seen on pathologic examination or demonstrated using submillimeter-spatial-resolution contrast-enhanced multidetector CT.

IMH accounts for approximately 10% of acute aortic syndromes (AASs) in Western countries, and the rate may be higher in Asian countries. The incidence may be underestimated due to either misclassification of IMH as a discrete dissection or the evolution of IMH into an AD during transfer to a tertiary center for treatment. In contrast to AD, there is a slight predominance of IMH seen in females compared with males, type B IMH occurs more frequently than type A IMH, and patients with IMH tend to be older and more likely hypertensive.[15] Marfan syndrome or other connective tissue disorders do not appear to play a role in the development of IMH. Like AD and PAU, patients present with chest or back pain, but in contrast, the pain in IMH does not often radiate. In contrast to TAAD, with type A IMH, aortic valve insufficiency, distal malperfusion, and ECG abnormalities are not as frequent, but the presence of a pericardial effusion is increased in incidence.

The *sine qua non* for diagnostic noninvasive imaging requires the presence of a thickened aortic wall (localized or circumferential)

>5 mm with no detectable blood flow on CT imaging, and the combination of CT imaging with and without contrast has reported sensitivities of >95%.[16] TEE has been shown to have both a high sensitivity (100%) and specificity (91%) for IMH.

Management of IMH is similar to that of AD, with medical management generally limited to type B IMH, with a selective β-blocker as the therapy of choice. Medical-management failure includes persistent pain, uncontrollable hypertension, progressively enlarging wall thickness >11 mm, and recurrent pleural effusions.[16] Interestingly, in contrast to AD, Falconi et al. demonstrated that medical and surgical management of type B IMH had similar mortality rates (19% vs. 17%, respectively),[17] and because of this, type B IMH is more likely to be managed medically than TBAD.

Emergent or urgent management of type A IMH is typically recommended, especially in the setting of a pericardial effusion and ongoing pain, although in a selected group of patients, initial medical management and optimization have been reported. Open surgical repair of type A IMH proceeds similar to that of TAAD, with two caveats. First, "normal" aorta may not be identified distally, so surgical judgment as to the extent of resection is important, and second, clamping of the aorta may convert the IMH into a dissection upon release of the cross clamp, presumably because of the creation of intimal tears with the placement of the clamp.

Like TBAD, endovascular repairs have emerged as a treatment option for type B IMH. For an uncomplicated type B IMH, the European Consensus Guidelines recommend initial medical management and surveillance with noninvasive imaging (class I recommendation). With expansion of the hematoma, development of a periaortic hematoma, recurrent pain, or conversion to a frank dissection, TEVAR (class IIa) or open repair (class IIb) is recommended.[16] Bischoff et al. compared TEVAR with medical management and, in support of the equipoise seen by Falconi et al., found no difference in early or late mortality, incidence of complete remodeling, or regression between the two groups.[18] The results suggest that TEVAR might be reserved for specific cases of type B IMH. The difficulty with TEVAR in type B IMH is determining the extent of coverage, similar to determining the extent of open repair. Because there (by definition) is no primary intimal tear, coverage territory becomes either presumptive of where the process started or targeted in the case of a periaortic hematoma or associated PAU.

Penetrating Aortic Ulcer

PAU involves both the intima and media, arising from an ulceration of an atherosclerotic plaque that has penetrated the elastic lamina. PAU can be associated with IMH, serve as a nidus for AD, or lead to the development of a saccular pseudoaneurysm. Coady et al. found that 7.6% of their patients treated for either TAAD or TBAD had an associated PAU.[19] Isolated PAU accounts for 2% to 7% of AAS, and although there is an overall slight predominance in males,[19] PAU occurs more frequently in the thoracic aorta in females and more frequently in the abdominal aorta in males. When considering only the thoracic aorta in PAU, for both males and females, the descending aorta is the predominant site of occurrence 90% of the time.

In contrast to AD and IMH, pain may not be a component of PAU, and often the ulcer is detected incidentally. In a Mayo Center study, 87% of patients with PAU were asymptomatic at the time of diagnosis.[20] PAU is defined by a distinct, focal outpouching through an area of intimal calcification or in an area

with associated diffuse atherosclerosis when contrast-enhanced CT scanning is performed.

Asymptomatic PAU may be managed medically with antiimpulse therapy and routine surveillance noninvasive imaging, but early intervention has been suggested for large PAUs, specifically when the greatest diameter is >20 mm or the neck is >10 mm.[3] With open surgical repair, the involved segment is resected and replaced with a prosthetic graft or homograft. Because PAU is associated with, and defined by the presence of, severe atherosclerosis and calcification, finding normal aorta proximally and/or distally to sew to may be difficult. Although studies on the efficacy of endovascular repair for PAU are lacking, limited data have shown good results for TEVAR in the setting of PAU and pseudoaneurysm formation or rupture. The same challenge for open repair of PAU, namely, extensive atherosclerosis, may pose problems if the atherosclerotic disease extends into the peripheral (and therefore access) vessels or if the presence of laminated thrombus associated with PAU makes achieving a safe landing zone difficult.

AORTIC ANEURYSM

Pathophysiology

Aneurysms, typically defined as an increase in size of more than 50% above the normal arterial diameter, may occur anywhere along the aorta, from the aortic root to the bifurcation. Because the mean aortic diameter differs between the ascending, descending, and infrarenal aorta, the absolute size criteria for aneurysm changes. Normal values will also vary due to methods of measurement, the patient's age and sex, and other factors. Anatomy or etiology may also be the basis for characterization of aneurysms. Anatomically, fusiform aneurysms exhibit smooth, circumferential dilatation across the entire vessel, as opposed to saccular aneurysms, which appear as a focal outpouching of the arterial wall. Whereas true aneurysms involve all three layers of the vessel wall, *false aneurysm* or *pseudoaneurysm* describes a focal defect in the artery with an associated collection of blood contained by surrounding connective tissue. Pseudoaneurysms may be degenerative, infectious, or traumatic in etiology. These pseudoaneurysms may occur at sites of prior surgical anastomosis and represent anastomotic disruption. The majority of aneurysms addressed in this chapter are degenerative in nature. Less frequently, aneurysms may be associated with infection, inflammation, or autoimmune or connective tissue disease. These cases merit special consideration in their evaluation and management.

Aneurysmal enlargement of the aorta is associated with factors that result in weakening of the arterial wall and increased local hemodynamic forces. These may include heritable conditions, such as Marfan syndrome, familial thoracic aortic aneurysm and dissection, and vascular-type Ehlers-Danlos as well as less well-defined entities that contribute to the significantly elevated incidence of aneurysm in patients with a family history of aneurysm. Factors that contribute to the degradation of extracellular matrix and reduction of elastin concentration are also associated with aneurysmal disease, and research in this area has focused on the role of matrix metalloproteinases, both their presence in the aneurysm specimens and for deficits of antiproteolytic enzymes that normally inhibit metalloproteinases. Ongoing avenues of investigation in this area also include the role of the immune response and hormone milieu. Finally, aneurysmal dilatation may also occur as a degenerative complication after AD.

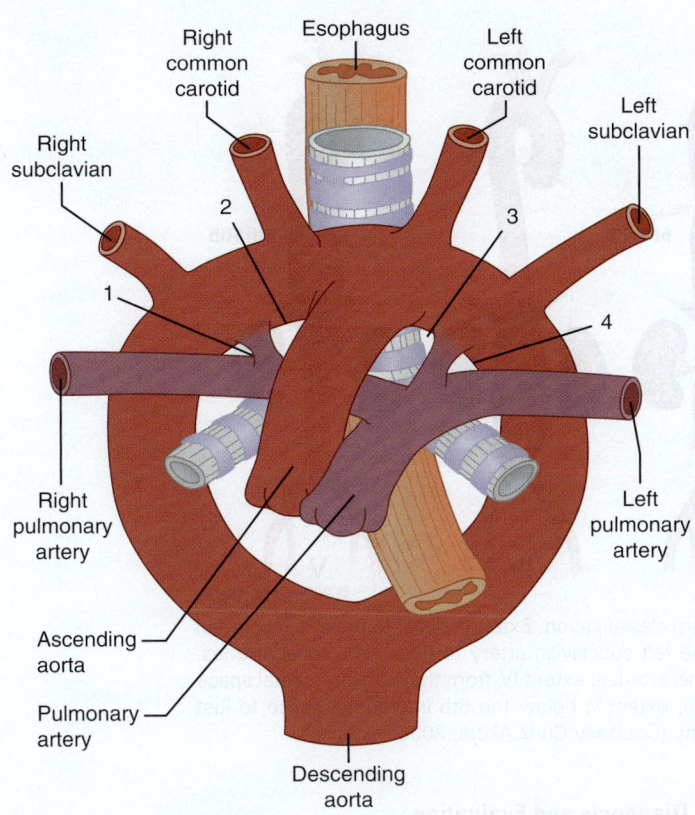

FIGURE 102.2 Edwards theoretical arch.

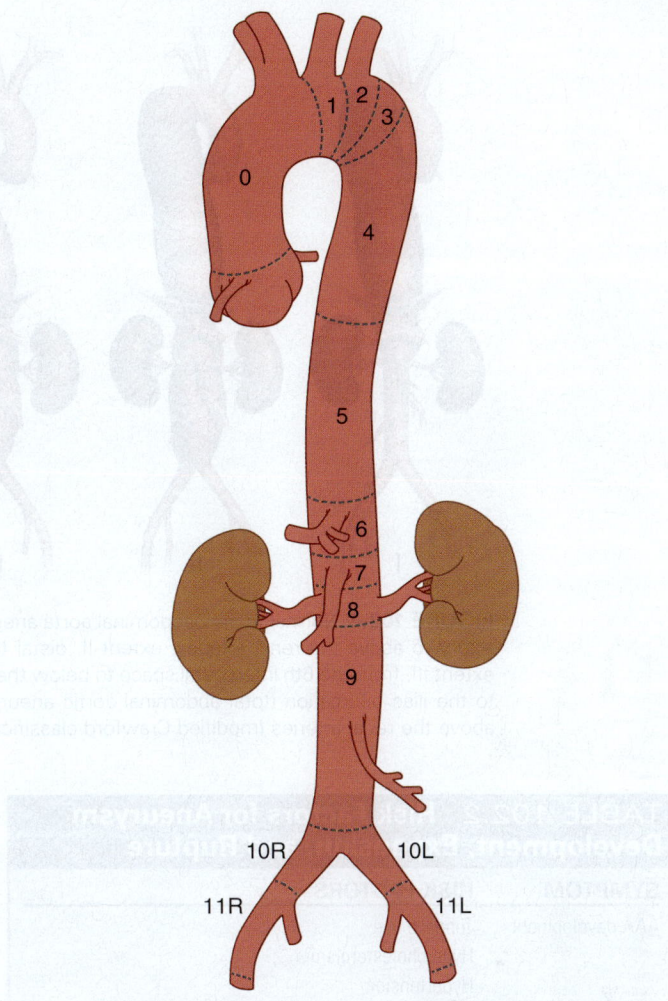

FIGURE 102.3 Aortic endograft attachment zones.

Clinical Presentation

Aortic pathologic conditions have their own unique nomenclature. Aneurysmal disease is perhaps the easiest to describe because typically, the label is simply the location (e.g., root aneurysm, arch aneurysm), with some exceptions. For example, Estrera and colleagues subdivide the descending thoracic aorta into three subtypes (A: proximal to the sixth rib, B: distal to the sixth rib, C: entire descending thoracic aorta) because this has implications for the risk of postoperative paraplegia (Fig. 102.2).[21] The Society for Vascular Surgery (SVS) divides the aorta into "zones," which pertain to endograft attachment sites rather than to disease extent (Fig. 102.3).[22] In the case of thoracoabdominal aortic aneurysms (TAAAs), first catalogued and subsequently refined by Crawford and colleagues, the original groupings attempted to describe the aneurysm in relationship to the extent of thoracic and abdominal involvement. The label "group" later evolved into "extent" or "type." Extent I involved the descending thoracic aorta and abdominal aorta to the level of the celiac artery. Extent II involved the entire thoracic and abdominal aorta, and extent III had lesser involvement of the thoracic aorta and most of the abdominal aorta. Extent IV involved the entire abdominal aorta. In the original classification scheme, there was also an extent V, which involved the lower abdominal aorta and renal arteries. This classification scheme was refined to four groups, or extents, and later modified to five extents to account for aneurysms involving only a portion of the thoracic aorta with sparing of the infrarenal aorta (Fig. 102.4). The Crawford classification system remains as an important tool in comparing procedural outcomes for TAAAs.

Determining the incidence and prevalence of aneurysmal disease is difficult, in part because of the tendency for aneurysms to be asymptomatic and found incidentally during imaging for unrelated medical issues. The incidence of abdominal aortic aneurysm (AAA), based on large screening studies, is estimated to range from 3% to 10%. Numerous risk factors, in addition to genetic or familial disorders, for the development, expansion, and rupture of AAAs have been identified (Table 102.2). Risk factors for development of an AAA include age, male sex, concurrent aneurysms, family history, tobacco use, hypertension, hyperlipidemia, and height. Female sex, Black race, and diabetes appear to be protective.[23] Recent studies have suggested that in first-world countries, the incidence has been decreasing over the past two decades, most likely related to the decreased tobacco burden in those countries. Sex differences extend to the presentation, associations, and natural history of aneurysms. Males with AAA, for instance, are more likely to present with concurrent iliac or femoropopliteal aneurysms. Females are more likely to experience rupture and consistently demonstrate poorer outcomes after repair, perhaps because of a significantly higher incidence of challenging anatomy. With screening of an at-risk population, specifically for the 65- to 89-year-old demographic, the incidence of AAA is 5% to 7%, with a male-to-female ratio of roughly 4:1. Estimates of the prevalence of thoracic aortic aneurysms are 400 per 100,000 patients in 65-year-olds and 670 per 100,000 in 80-year-olds, and in contrast to AAA, there does not appear to be a sex difference.

Although aneurysms may be asymptomatic, an acutely enlarging or inflamed aorta may present with pain. Depending on the

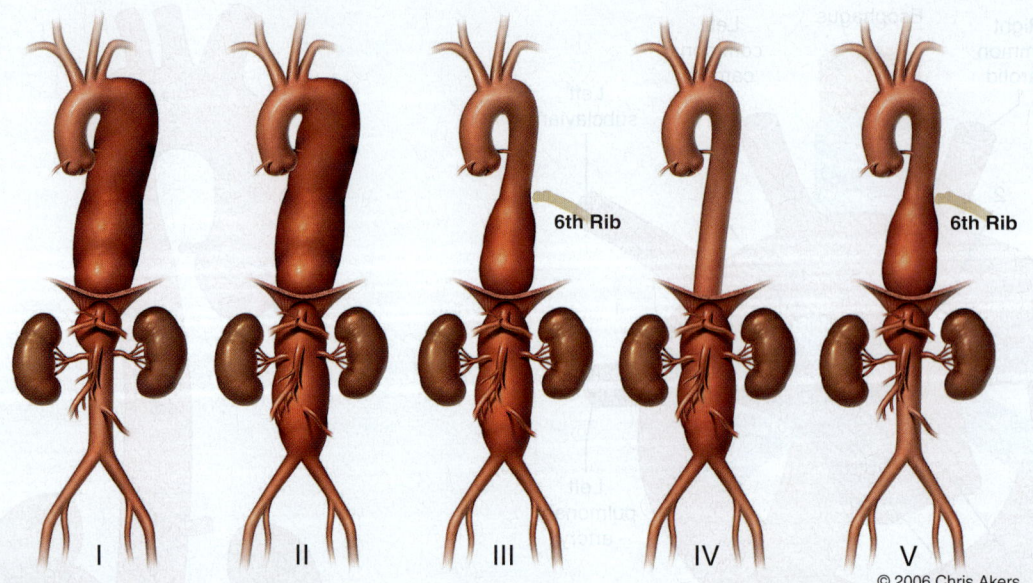

FIGURE 102.4 Normal thoracoabdominal aorta aneurysm classification. Extent I, distal to the left subclavian artery to above the renal arteries; extent II, distal to the left subclavian artery to below the renal arteries; extent III, from the 6th intercostal space to below the renal arteries; extent IV, from the 12th intercostal space to the iliac bifurcation (total abdominal aortic aneurysm); extent V, below the 6th intercostal space to just above the renal arteries (modified Crawford classification). (Courtesy Chris Akers, 2006.)

TABLE 102.2 Risk Factors for Aneurysm Development, Expansion, and Rupture	
SYMPTOM	**RISK FACTORS**
AAA development	Tobacco use
	Hypercholesterolemia
	Hypertension
	Male sex
	Family history (male predominance)
AAA expansion	Advanced age
	Severe cardiac disease
	Previous stroke
	Tobacco use
	Cardiac or renal transplantation
AAA rupture	Female sex
	↓ FEV$_1$
	Larger initial abdominal aortic diameter
	Higher mean blood pressure
	Current tobacco use (length of time smoking ≫ amount)
	Cardiac or renal transplantation
	Critical wall stress–wall strength relationship

AAA, Abdominal aortic aneurysm; *FEV$_1$,* forced expiratory volume in 1 second. Adapted from Chaikof EL, Brewster DC, Dalman RL, et al. The care of patients with an abdominal aortic aneurysm: the Society for Vascular Surgery practice guidelines. *J Vasc Surg.* 2009;50:S2-S49.

location of the aneurysm, other less common signs or symptoms may occur. For example, an enlarged ascending aorta or proximal arch may result in superior vena cava syndrome. An expanding proximal descending aorta can impinge on the left recurrent laryngeal nerve, leading to hoarseness (Ortner syndrome) or pulmonary embarrassment from extrinsic compression of the left main stem bronchus. Large AAAs may give a feeling of fullness or early satiety after small meals.

Diagnosis and Evaluation

Imaging of aortic disease is necessary to define its exact anatomic location, extent, and size. A number of imaging modalities can be used, with each having its own specific limitations and benefits. Chest x-ray (CXR) studies may detect incidental thoracic aneurysms due to abnormalities in aortic contour, size, or calcifications, but CXR is not a good screening tool. Ultrasound is an important tool in AAA management because it is accurate, noninvasive, and cost-effective. Contrast-enhanced ultrasound may be particularly useful in detecting, localizing, and quantifying endoleaks in patients after endovascular aneurysm repair (EVAR). Echocardiography is ultrasonography when performed on the chest and its contents, and the noninvasive technique is TTE. TTE is useful for measuring certain segments of the ascending aorta and assessing the degree of aortic valve insufficiency, if present. TEE, although more invasive, is useful for visualizing the thoracic aorta from the aortic annulus to the celiac axis, with the exception of a short segment of the ascending aorta proximal to the innominate artery. Intravascular ultrasound (IVUS) is an additional modality for imaging of the aorta, and although it is not typically used for diagnostic purposes, it is invaluable as an adjunct in endovascular procedures, particularly in the treatment of AD.

CT provides excellent imaging of the aorta and remains an important tool in the diagnosis, management, and surveillance of aortic disease. CT, particularly with the adjunctive use of iodinated contrast agents to perform CT angiography (CTA), provides a wealth of anatomic information; it detects vessel calcification, thrombus, and concurrent arterial occlusive disease and permits multiplanar and three-dimensional reconstruction and analysis for operative planning. Drawbacks include substantial radiation exposure, particularly in the setting of serial examinations, and the use of iodinated contrast media in a population with a high incidence of comorbid kidney disease.

MRI provides a reasonable alternative to CT for imaging of the aorta, with the benefits being the elimination of ionizing radiation and iodinated contrast. Spin-echo black blood and gradient echo sequences provide an intrinsic contrast between the blood flow and aortic wall to provide dimensional and geometric information. With the addition of intravenous gadolinium as a contrast agent, magnetic resonance angiography (MRA) provides rapid three-dimensional (3D) imaging of the aorta without the need for ECG gating. The ability to acquire dynamic images throughout the cardiac cycle allows physiologic parameters, such as estimates of wall shear stress, to be determined, which may lead to clinical applications. Unlike CT, MRI does not demonstrate aortic wall calcification, which may be important in operative planning, especially for endovascular approaches. MRI does not necessarily use iodinated contrast material but instead can use gadolinium, which has been associated with the development of nephrogenic systemic fibrosis in patients with low glomerular filtration rate. Additionally, a contraindication for MRI is the presence of incompatible metallic implants or foreign bodies. Mechanical valves, pacemakers, and implantable cardioversion devices currently marketed in the United States are MRI compatible. Newer ferrous-based contrast agents coupled with MRA may provide a viable alternative to vascular imaging when iodinated contrast or gadolinium is contraindicated.

Medical Management and Screening

Size and symptoms play a large role in determining the management of aortic aneurysms (Table 102.3). For aneurysms that do not meet criteria or appropriateness for surgical intervention, medical management is a mainstay. Lifestyle modifications may be necessary, such as tobacco use cessation. Current smoking has been associated with significantly increasing the expansion rate of

AAA (~0.4 mm/yr). Although moderate levels of exercise have a beneficial impact on patient cardiopulmonary health and progression of atherosclerosis, patients should avoid vigorous levels of activity and contact sports. Activities that cause a sudden spike in blood pressure may lead to aortic rupture or dissection in the presence of underlying aortic pathology. Blood pressure management, in the reduction of both systolic pressure and pulse pressure (an indirect measure of dP/dt and wall stress), may require multiple medications. β-blockers, both selective and nonselective, are useful in accomplishing both goals.

Prevention of aneurysmal dilatation or even regression would be an ideal consequence of medical therapy.[3] This has been shown to be the case in the specific clinical scenario of the patient with Marfan syndrome treated with β-blockers, angiotensin II receptor blockers, and angiotensin-converting enzyme inhibitors. None of these drugs has been shown to be effective in patients who do not have Marfan syndrome. HMG–coenzyme A reductase inhibitor (statin) therapy has been associated with reduced rates of AAA enlargement and is otherwise appropriate in a population with a high prevalence of concurrent atherosclerotic disease. Statin therapy improves survival after open and endovascular repair of AAAs and has been shown to decrease the incidence of major cardiovascular events (stroke, myocardial infarction, and death) for patients with the diagnosis of AAA. Finally, antiplatelet therapy using aspirin offers a secondary preventive benefit in this population.

Screening recommendations for aneurysms are informed by the sensitivity and specificity of ultrasound screening (or other imaging modality), the detection yield of screening based on various risk factor selection criteria, and cost. Screening for thoracic aneurysms is generally not done without a pretest high probability (e.g., suspicion of an aortic syndrome). The caveat is that when an AAA is diagnosed, it is a general recommendation that the thoracic aorta should be screened to rule out metasynchronous disease. Current consensus guidelines recommend one-time screening of all males aged 65 years and older or males 55 years and older with a family history of AAA. In 2014, the US Preventive Services Task Force (USPSTF) issued a more limited recommendation for one-time screening for AAA using ultrasonography of males between 65 and 75 years of age who have a personal smoking history and selective screening for nonsmokers. For females, the recommendations remain controversial. The USPSTF concluded that there was insufficient evidence to recommend routine screening in females who smoke and recommended against routine screening in nonsmoking females. One issue that may have biased these results is the paucity of females in large screening trials. In one meta-analysis that looked at a combination of four studies with over 125,000 patients enrolled, less than 10,000 subjects were females.[24] Payer policies regarding reimbursement may not track either of these recommendations. Medicare, for instance, because of the Screening Abdominal Aortic Aneurysms Very Efficiently (SAAAVE) Act, reflects an intermediate approach in offering a screening benefit for males with a personal smoking history and males or females with a family history of AAA, although only as a part of the initial Welcome to Medicare physical examination.

After the initial detection of a nonsurgical aneurysm, surveillance is necessary in addition to optimal medical management. Ideally, surveillance should be low cost, have high sensitivity, and pose minimal harm to the patient. For the abdominal aorta, ultrasound follow-up is advisable. Those patients with a known AAA who do not have appropriate surveillance may have up to a sixfold increase in rate of rupture. The SVS Clinical Practice Council

---

TABLE 102.3 Recommended Size for Intervention of Asymptomatic Aortic Aneurysm

LOCATION	SIZE CRITERIA	COMMENT
Ascending/root	≥55 mm	All patients, including BAV
	≥50 mm	Patients with Marfan syndrome BAV with risk factors for dissection
	≥45 mm	Selected patients with Marfan syndrome
	>45 mm	When aortic valve is being intervened on
	>27.5 mm/m²	For patients with a small body size
Arch	≥55 mm	All patients
	Any size	Signs or symptoms of local compression
Descending	≥55 mm	When TEVAR possible
	≥60 mm	Open repair (less for Marfan syndrome)
Abdominal	≥55 mm	All patients

BAV, Bicuspid aortic valve; *TEVAR,* thoracic endovascular aortic repair. Adapted from Erbel R, Aboyans V, Boileau C, et al. 2014 ESC guidelines on the diagnosis and treatment of aortic diseases: document covering acute and chronic aortic diseases of the thoracic and abdominal aorta of the adult. The Task Force for the Diagnosis and Treatment of Aortic Diseases of the European Society of Cardiology (ESC). *Eur Heart J.* 2014;35:2873-2926.

recommends the following screening intervals based on aneurysm size (maximum external aortic diameter) and associated risk of rupture:

- <2.6 cm: no further screening recommended
- 2.6 to 2.9 cm: reexamination at 5 years
- 3 to 3.4 cm: reexamination at 3 years
- 3.5 to 4.4 cm: reexamination at 12 months
- 4.5 to 5.4 cm: reexamination at 6 months

These recommendations, as is the case for thoracic aortic aneurysms, stem from our understanding of growth rates of normal and abnormal aortas as well as published rates of rupture at given sizes. No large, prospective studies that compare surveillance intervals exist. For the abdominal aorta, although the SVS recommends no further screening for aneurysms less than 2.6 cm, others have suggested 3 cm as the cutoff. Countering this are the findings that a significant proportion of 65-year-old males (13.8%) with an initial aortic diameter of 2.6 to 2.9 cm developed aneurysms exceeding 5.5 cm at 10 years. Given current life expectancy projections, it is evident that a subset of patients deemed "normal" at screening will go on to develop clinically significant aneurysms.

With the exception of the aortic root, visible with TTE, the thoracic aorta generally requires CT or MRI contrast imaging. For the ascending aorta, arch, and descending aorta, after the initial diagnosis, a second study at 6 months should suffice to determine if there is measurable growth in the aortic diameter. This is followed with yearly scans until there is reasonable certainty of stability in size, at which time extending surveillance to a 2- to 3-year interval is tolerable. Conversion to MRI for surveillance avoids exposure of the patient to ionizing radiation.

Prevention of rupture of the growing aorta is the rationale for surveillance imaging, and risk models for rupture do exist. Juvonen and colleagues[25] developed a model that included risk factors of age, presence of pain, chronic obstructive pulmonary disease, and maximal diameters of the thoracic and abdominal aorta. Based on this model, surgery was recommended when the calculated risk of rupture within 1 year exceeded the anticipated mortality risk of an elective procedure, even if the recommended aortic diameter for intervention was not reached.

Operative Management

When the risk of continued observation exceeds the risk of operative repair, surgery is warranted. There are two main approaches to surgical repair: conventional (or open) surgery and endovascular surgery. Hybrid repair, which calls on the strengths of both open and endovascular repair in order to obtain a durable result, is also frequently a viable approach. Endovascular repair offers a less invasive approach but has limitations based on anatomic location.

Open Surgical Aortic Repair

Aortic root replacement. Aortic root replacement is primarily for aneurysmal disease or TAAD but is also performed in certain cases of aortic valve endocarditis as well as reoperative aortic valve replacement. There are three standard approaches to replacement of the aortic root: composite valve grafts (CVGs; mechanical or biologic), complete tissue replacement (either cadaveric homograft or autograft [Ross procedure]), and valve-sparing root replacement (remodeling, reattachment, and Florida sleeve).

As noted earlier, the boundaries of the aortic root are the aortic annulus proximally and the sinotubular junction distally; components of the root include the aortic valve and ostia of the coronary

arteries. Thus, when the aortic root is repaired or replaced, with few specific exceptions, the coronaries are always reimplanted or bypassed, the valve is addressed (replaced or spared), and circulatory arrest is not needed unless the ascending aorta is also affected and needs to be replaced.

Modifications to the procedure, as originally described by Bentall and colleagues,[26] have made the term *Bentall procedure* an anachronism. The original description was a CVG with an inclusion technique to deal with the coronaries (i.e., sewing the coronaries onto the graft not as Carrel buttons but rather in a side-to-side fashion). Wheat preceded Bentall in an earlier publication describing a technique where the valve and graft were separate, and the coronaries were reimplanted on "tongues of aortic wall" extending from the annulus. Subsequent work by Kouchoukos and colleagues incorporated the now-familiar coronary button technique. The CVG concept evolved into preconstructed composites, initially with a mechanical valve, followed by biologic valves as an option. With a mechanical and tissue option, the indications for the type of CVG used are the same as those for a valve replacement (e.g., mechanical valves favored in younger patients because of durability, tissue valves in older patients or when lifelong anticoagulation is not a reasonable option).

Balancing the desire for a durable valve or root replacement with avoidance of lifelong anticoagulation led to a number of innovative techniques. Work by Lower and Shumway and promoted by Ross resulted in the eponymous Ross procedure. This technique is an autotransplantation of the pulmonary valve into the aortic position and subsequent replacement of the pulmonary artery root with a cadaveric homograft. Although the procedure never gained popularity in adult patients, it remains a viable alternative, especially when performed in high-volume environments. An alternative to the Ross procedure is replacement of the aortic root with a cadaveric homograft, notably in the setting of aortic valve endocarditis with destruction of the aorta annulus. Both of these procedures have the theoretical advantage of the lack of need for anticoagulation as well as an increase in durability compared with a tissue valve. However, both procedures are technically challenging, and the outcomes are dependent on the experience of the surgeon.

Dilatation of the aortic root or of the sinotubular junction because of an ascending aortic aneurysm may result in valve insufficiency in the face of normal valve leaflets. In this setting, the replacement of the normal valve while addressing the aortic root or ascending aorta seems like overkill. With sinotubular junction dilatation alone, replacement of the ascending aorta with a downsized graft may be sufficient to restore the aortic valve competency. With root dilatation and an anatomically normal valve, two valve-sparing approaches have been popularized: the remodeling technique and the reimplantation technique, championed respectively by Yacoub and David. Miller has summarized the techniques, referenced as David I through V (Table 102.4). Although expansion on each of the valve-sparing techniques is beyond the scope of this chapter, Miller summarizes the differences between the Yacoub remodeling and David reimplantation technique by the number of suture lines; remodeling employs two aortic suture lines, and reimplantation employs three. Both techniques use a Dacron graft as the neoaorta, and both, as previously mentioned for root replacements, require reimplantation of the coronary ostia. There is an exception to the comment that the coronaries are always reimplanted (i.e., the Florida sleeve technique where "slots" are made on the Dacron graft to accommodate the coronaries).

TABLE 102.4 Miller Classification of David Valve-Sparing Root Replacement

NAME	CLASSIFICATION	DESCRIPTION
David I	Reimplantation	Implantation in cylindric tube graft
David II	Remodeling	Classic Yacoub
David III	Remodeling	David II combined with aortic annuloplasty
David IV	Reimplantation	David I with 4-mm larger graft and plication at the sinotubular junction
David V	Reimplantation	David I with 6- to 8-mm larger graft and plication at sinotubular junction and annulus to create pseudosinuses

Adapted from Miller DC. Valve-sparing aortic root replacement in patients with the Marfan syndrome. *J Thorac Cardiovasc Surg.* 2003;125:773-778.

Open surgery of the descending thoracic aorta. Open surgical repair of thoracic aortic pathology has changed dramatically since the introduction of endovascular techniques. Although TEVAR has a predominant role in the management of thoracic aortic disease, there remain clinical scenarios in which knowledge of open approaches to the thoracic aorta is an important part of the surgeon's armamentarium. As mentioned previously, TEVAR may not always be appropriate or doable for some TBADs and, with a few exceptions, is not applicable to patients with Marfan disease or other connective tissue disorders. Issues regarding spinal cord protection and intraoperative monitoring are pertinent to open and endovascular techniques. Considerations specific to open surgery include the need and approach to distal perfusion ("clamp and sew," left heart bypass, CPB) as well as access. Many of the issues and considerations with open thoracic aortic surgery also pertain to TAAAs (see later).

Hemodynamic monitoring, specifically invasive arterial lines, during open repair of thoracic aneurysms and dissections is required and may necessitate transducing from both upper and lower body sites, depending on the surgical plan. Pulmonary artery catheterization is not typically helpful during the intraoperative period but can be useful in postoperative management. Use of TEE is reasonable in open surgery (as well as TEVAR) and carries a class IIa recommendation. A second class IIa monitoring recommendation relates to spinal cord perfusion, acknowledging the potential for the devastation of spinal cord ischemia after surgery on the thoracic aorta. Although not a therapeutic modality, motor or somatosensory evoked potential monitoring can help guide therapy and alterations in intraoperative management.

Avoidance of spinal cord injury secondary to ischemia is paramount in surgery of the thoracic and thoracoabdominal aorta for both open and endovascular approaches. Adjuncts used include cerebrospinal fluid (CSF) drainage, distal perfusion (either left heart bypass or CPB with femorofemoral cannulation), hypothermia, and pharmacotherapeutics. The rationale for CSF drainage is to increase spinal cord perfusion pressure (SCPP) by lowering CSF pressure. By definition, SCPP is as follows:

$$SCPP = \text{Mean distal aortic pressure} - \\ (\text{CSF pressure} + \text{Central venous pressure})$$

Thus, SCPP can be favorably increased with increases in distal aortic pressure, decreases in CSF pressure (by drainage), and decreases in central venous pressure. Management of the CSF drain varies between setting a limit of CSF pressure (e.g., 10–15 mm Hg)

to draining at a constant rate (e.g., 10–20 cc/h). Whichever approach is used, two things must be remembered. First, in instances of acute changes in neurologic status, an immediate drainage of 10 to 20 cc of CSF may salvage the spinal cord. Second, the two other variables related to SCPP—namely, mean aortic pressure and central venous pressure—can also be manipulated to maximize SCPP. CSF drainage is not innocuous, with almost 10% of patients developing a postdural puncture headache and a 2.8% reported risk of intracranial hemorrhage, the majority being subdural hematomas.[27]

Maintenance of distal aortic pressure and perfusion of visceral branches (including collaterals to the spinal cord) can be supplemented with circulatory support. For procedures of the thoracic aorta associated with dissection, CPB may be preferable because it provides not only circulatory support but also a mechanism for temperature regulation and rapid volume infusion. For both thoracic and thoracoabdominal procedures, the use of hypothermic circulatory arrest has been championed because of the elimination of the need for proximal and sequential aortic clamping (and the periaortic dissection required), easy proximal access to the arch, a bloodless field, and the ability to return all shed blood back to the perfusion circuit.

Open surgical repair of thoracoabdominal aortic aneurysms. For TAAA repair, an incision entering both the thoracic and abdominal compartments is required, representing a significant physiologic stress. For this reason, preoperative workup may be more extensive, including pulmonary function tests and more intense evaluation of cardiac function. Although repair can be performed with a clamp-and-sew technique, most high-volume centers perform repair with either left heart bypass or full CPB with hypothermic arrest. This approach is specifically advantageous for extent II TAAAs that do not have a safe location for clamping the most proximal aorta.

As in descending thoracic aortic procedures, paraplegia is an uncommon but feared complication of TAAA repair. Mortality after TAAA repair is significantly increased should paraplegia develop. The risk of paraplegia is increased with extent II TAAA, TAAA associated with AD, acute presentations, or previous infrarenal aortic surgery. Increase in SCPP, as previously discussed, may be protective. Other approaches to maximize spinal cord perfusion include intercostal artery reimplantation and maintenance of central perfusion. Strategies to decrease the metabolic rate of the spinal cord may include preoperative steroids, the use of a naloxone drip, moderate hypothermia (to 34°C), and injection of propofol just before clamping.

Construction of the visceral component of the graft may depend on the underlying cause for repair. For patients with degenerative TAAA, a Carrel patch may be considered for the reimplantation of the visceral vessels. This approach many simplify the operation and decrease the visceral ischemia time but may run the risk of future degeneration of the residual aorta and subsequent pseudoaneurysm formation. For those with connective tissue disorders or aneurysmal degeneration of a previous dissection, most would consider individual branch grafts to each visceral artery, thereby eliminating any suspect aortic tissue in the repair.

Open infrarenal abdominal aortic aneurysm repair. Open repair of AAA can be performed through a transabdominal or retroperitoneal approach. Advantages of the transabdominal approach include the ability to inspect the abdominal contents, supraceliac control without entering the thorax, and better exposure of the right iliac bifurcation and external iliac arteries. Potential disadvantages may include hernia formation, increased risk of bowel obstruction, and perhaps an increased risk of late aortoenteric fistula. With this approach, after the abdominal contents are inspected, the omentum and transverse colon are retracted cephalad, and the small intestines are retracted to the patient's right to expose the retroperitoneum and the ligament of Treitz. The ligament is taken down, and the duodenum is retracted to the right. A slip of tissue should be left attached to the duodenum for closure of this space after the repair. A self-retaining retractor can be helpful to maintain optimal exposure.

The posterior parietal peritoneum is incised to expose the aorta, and the dissection is carried proximally to expose the neck. The inferior mesenteric vein is generally encountered and should be identified, retracted, or ligated. As the dissection is carried cephalad, the left renal vein is encountered. This vein can be duplicated or travel behind the aorta; its course can and should be identified on preoperative imaging. The left renal vein can be retracted, and if needed, the adrenal and gonadal veins can be divided to provide more mobility of the left renal vein. Some have advocated for division of the left renal vein; if this is considered, the adrenal and gonadal veins must be left intact because they will subsequently provide the venous drainage of the left kidney. Proximal aortic control should be obtained at healthy aorta and with enough room to safely place sutures. Control can be either circumferential, which may allow a transversely oriented aortic occlusion clamp, or anterior and on either side of the aorta with the dissection carried down to the spine.

The dissection is then carried distally. If a tube graft is considered, it is safer to control the bilateral proximal iliac arteries to avoid injury to the iliac veins that travel directly behind the arteries and may be more densely adherent at the aortic bifurcation. If dissection and arterial control are required at or past the iliac bifurcation, care should be taken to avoid the ureters because they traverse anteriorly at this level.

Once the dissection is complete, the patient should be given heparin at 10 units/kg before clamping, with a goal activated clotting time (ACT) of 250 to 300 seconds. Once clamped, the aneurysm is opened and thrombus is removed. Back-bleeding from lumbar vessels should be controlled with suture ligatures. The origin of the inferior mesenteric artery (IMA) should be inspected. If back-bleeding is absent or brisk, it can also be suture-ligated; however, if back-bleeding is scant, the IMA should be preserved for possible reimplantation.

Appropriately sized polyester or polytetrafluoroethylene graft is then sewn into place, first proximally and then distally. The vessels are flushed to remove all debris, and then flow is slowly reestablished, making certain that the blood pressure remains stable. If a bifurcated graft is required, flow should be reestablished to one limb at a time. Heparin is then reversed if needed, hemostasis is secured, and then the sigmoid colon is interrogated for ischemia visually and with a Doppler probe; if present, the IMA should be reimplanted with either a Carrel patch or interposition graft. The wound is closed in layers, starting with the aneurysm sac and then posterior parietal peritoneum to protect the repair from the intestines. The remainder of the incision is then closed in a standard fashion.

Retroperitoneal exposure is generally performed with the patient in a semilateral position and through an oblique incision to the tip of the 11th rib. The incision can be extended into the chest for more proximal control if needed. With this approach, the left kidney is usually left down for infrarenal exposure but can be retracted upward with the peritoneum for more proximal exposure.

Endovascular Aortic Repair

Endovascular abdominal aortic aneurysm repair. EVAR has nearly become the gold standard for repair for AAA since first reported in the English literature by Parodi and colleagues in 1991.[28] A number of generations of devices have been developed, tested, and replaced with updated versions throughout the world. The success of EVAR for the treatment of AAA rests heavily on the interaction of the aortic stent graft and its seal and fixation zone within the aorta. For all endovascular procedures, certain principles apply, beginning with careful planning and correct sizing based on device-specific manufacturer instructions for use (IFU). Evaluation of access vessels (typically the common femoral or external iliac arteries) ensures adequate diameter as well as noting the presence of tortuosity and calcification. Verifying healthy arteries will allow for percutaneous access, performed by accessing the anterior noncalcified surface of the common femoral artery. Deployment of closure devices (if used) occurs before placement of the larger-bore sheaths required for stent graft delivery. Questionable access vessels may require open femoral exposure, with or without a conduit to the more proximal iliac artery. If a conduit is used, a 10-mm diameter will generally ensure passage of the delivery device. Once open access is obtained, stiff wires should be placed and used for endograft delivery. Limiting radiation exposure is paramount, and the recent implementation of image fusion (projection of preoperative CTA scan onto two-dimensional [2D] intraoperative fluoroscopic images [2D-3D fusion imaging]) demonstrates a reduction in exposure. Device configurations will vary by manufacturer. Many devices will have a bare-metal component that crosses the renal/visceral aortic segment and assists in device fixation (prevention of distal device migration). Devices can be constructed of woven polyester or polytetrafluoroethylene, with either a stainless-steel or nitinol-metal framework. Many devices will have a bare-metal component that crosses the renal/visceral aortic segment and assists in device fixation (prevention of distal device migration). Devices are typically Y-shaped and will require placement of at least one additional iliac extension piece. The devices are inserted in a delivery system and then deployed once their location in the correct portion of the aorta is ensured. When the endograft placement is complete and balloon molding is performed, a final angiogram is obtained to investigate the presence of endoleaks. Closure of open incisions is standard after reversal of heparin. For percutaneous access, sheaths are removed over a wire as the sutures are secured. Maintaining wire access at this point is important should there be either an iliac artery injury requiring vascular control and/or endovascular repair or the need for placement of an additional closure device. Wires can then be removed after satisfactory hemostasis.

Postoperative evaluation of a successful EVAR includes serial CT scans and/or color duplex ultrasonography, looking for aortic sac diameter or volume, graft migration, and endoleaks. Surveillance imaging is generally recommended at 1 month, 6 months, 12 months, and yearly thereafter provided a stable examination. Because of the need for ongoing surveillance, patients who may be unwilling or unable to undergo postoperative imaging may not be appropriate candidates for EVAR.

When identified, endoleaks are classified as follows:
- Type 1A (proximal seal zone)
- Type 1B (distal seal zone)
- Type 2 (retrograde flow from lumbar and/or IMAs)
- Type 3 (component separation)
- Type 4 (fabric porosity)
- Type 5 (expanding aneurysm without demonstrable blood flow)

Type 1 and 3 endoleaks require repair. Type 2 endoleaks are common early after EVAR, with most resolving by 1 to 12 months. Management of persistent type 2 endoleaks is controversial, with most favoring observational management in the absence of sac growth. If sac growth occurs after EVAR with an otherwise stable type 2 endoleak, delayed type 1 or 3 endoleak may be the underlying culprit.

For infrarenal AAA, reported outcomes for open abdominal aortic repair vary from 1% to 4% for infrarenal repair performed in centers of excellence to 4% to 8% noted in statewide or nationwide databases.[23] Complications associated with open repair occur in 15% to 30% of patients. Both early mortality and complication rates are better with an endovascular approach to AAAs, although this may represent a selection bias. The UK EVAR trial investigators randomized 1252 patients with AAAs larger than 5.5 cm for elective open repair versus EVAR, and although the 30-day mortality rate was favorable for EVAR (1.8% vs. 4.3%, $P = 0.02$), this benefit was lost by the end of the study.[29] Additionally, EVAR was more costly, in part due to increased rates of graft-related complications and need for reintervention. A similar study by the Dutch Randomized Endovascular Aneurysm Management (DREAM) trial group found that early advantages of EVAR had disappeared by the 2-year follow-up mark.[30]

More recent long-term outcomes, though, have begun to call into question the durability of EVAR. The long-term follow-up from most of the randomized prospective trials evaluating open and EVAR has demonstrated that patients undergoing EVAR are at risk for having a higher reintervention rate than those who underwent open surgery. In fact, the early outcomes favoring EVAR resolved by 6 months postoperatively, and an increase in aneurysm-related mortality was observed at 4 years.[31] Crossover occurred at 6 to 8 years and was partially due to an increase in the rate of ruptured AAA.[32]

Endovascular approaches to the thoracic aorta. There have not been any randomized controlled trials to compare endovascular to open repair of the thoracic aorta, but nonrandomized studies, meta-analyses, and comparisons to historical data have suggested a decreased incidence of perioperative mortality and morbidity, including paraplegia. In the FDA phase II trial of the GORE TAG device, Makaroun and colleagues documented mortality rates of 1.5%, 1.5%, and 0% at 30 days, 1 year, and 2 years, respectively.[33] Early major adverse events included stroke (4%) and paraplegia (3%), which compared favorably with historical numbers. At 5 years, the aneurysm-related mortality was 2.8% in the endovascular patients versus 11.7% in the open controls, although there was no difference when considering all-cause mortality (68% survival in the endovascular group vs. 67% in the open group). A meta-analysis by Cheng and colleagues of TEVAR versus open surgical repair showed a reduction in 30-day and 1-year all-cause mortality (odds ratio of 0.44 and 0.73, respectively), with this reduction in all-cause mortality lost beyond 1 year.[34] The overall stroke rate was similar between the two groups. This meta-analysis revealed the primary benefit of TEVAR over open surgery to be a significant reduction in the risk of paraplegia and paraparesis. Thus, at least in the early follow-up period, reductions in all-cause mortality and complications favor TEVAR, especially in high-surgical-risk patients with suitable anatomy.

Considerations for suitable anatomy include appropriate landing zones with possible coverage of the left SCA, vertebral artery anatomy, angulation and tortuosity of the aorta, size and amount of disease in the planned access arteries, and concurrent AAA. For landing zones, it is usually adequate to obtain a 2- to 3-cm seal zone proximally with extension if the aorta is particularly tortuous or angulated. As shown in Fig. 102.3, there are five potential landing zones for the ascending aorta, arch, and proximal descending thoracic aorta:

- Zone 0: proximal to the innominate artery
- Zone 1: proximal to the left common carotid artery
- Zone 2: proximal to the origin of the left SCA
- Zone 3: proximal descending thoracic aorta less than 2 cm from the left SCA
- Zone 4: greater than 2 cm from the left SCA and extends to the proximal portion of the descending aorta (level of T6 vertebral body)

Proximal lesions of the thoracic aorta may require coverage of the left SCA (i.e., zone 2 landing). In patients with previous coronary revascularization where an in situ left internal mammary was used as a conduit, it is essential to perform left SCA revascularization before zone 2 coverage to prevent myocardial ischemia. The overall reported incidence of left SCA coverage in single-center studies ranges from 23% to over 40% incidence with or without left SCA revascularization. In a multicenter study, the European Collaborators on Stent/Graft Techniques for Aortic Aneurysm Repair (EUROSTAR) reported 26% of 606 requiring left SCA coverage.[35] In the EUROSTAR study, there was a 2.5% incidence of paraplegia or paraparesis and a 3.1% incidence of stroke. Multivariate regression analysis demonstrated a correlation between spinal cord ischemia and SCA coverage without revascularization (odds ratio 3.9, $P = 0.027$). Paraplegia or stroke occurred in 8.4% of patients with left SCA coverage when prophylactic revascularization was not performed, compared with 0% when it was performed. Feezor and colleagues found that in their TEVAR patients who had strokes, 78% of strokes were in the posterior circulation territory, highlighting the importance of evaluating the vertebral artery anatomy preoperatively to determine those who might be at a higher risk for posterior circulation strokes with acute coverage of the left SCA.[36] All of the patients in the Feezor and colleagues study had coverage of zones 0 to 2, and only one of the six patients had preemptive carotid-subclavian bypass.

Buth and colleagues also found that in addition to SCA coverage, the use of three or more stents had a significant impact on the development of spinal cord ischemia (odds ratio 3.5, $P = 0.43$).[35] A meta-analysis by Cooper and colleagues reported an incidence of spinal cord ischemia of 2.3% without SCA coverage versus 2.8% with SCA coverage (pooled odds ratio 2.39).[37] Because the thyrocervical trunk branches and vertebral artery contribute to the anterior spinal artery, revascularization may be important for prevention of spinal cord ischemia. Woo and colleagues reported that their indications for left subclavian revascularization included a dominant left vertebral artery; a stenotic, atretic, hypoplastic, or absent right vertebral artery; an incomplete vertebrobasilar system; a history of arm ischemia; and a patent left internal mammary artery–left anterior descending artery (LIMA-LAD) bypass. In a single-center comparison, the reported incidence of spinal cord ischemia with TEVAR was less compared with open repair (6.7% vs. 8.6%, respectively), although it did not reach statistical significance.[38]

Other proposals to reduce the risk of spinal cord ischemia, other than selective left SCA revascularization, as mentioned earlier, include avoiding intraoperative and postoperative hypotension, spinal fluid drainage, and naloxone infusion. It is important to have both preoperative and postoperative protocols in conjunction with your anesthesia team to achieve this. If the patient needs treatment of both abdominal and thoracic aortic pathology, staging the procedures should allow adequate collateralization to develop. The EUROSTAR study found that concomitant open abdominal aorta surgery had a significant impact on the development of spinal cord ischemia (odds ratio 5.5), presumably from interruption of the IMA and/or intercostal and lumbar artery branches.

Finally, another consideration to determine the feasibility of TEVAR is adequacy of access vessels. Ideally, an access vessel measuring at least 8 mm in diameter will be adequate for most device delivery systems. The size of the thoracic aorta generally requires larger endograft devices compared with EVAR and will therefore require larger sheath access. It is important to have imaging of the abdominal aorta and iliac arteries to determine the best access vessel based on size, disease, and tortuosity. If the femoral and/or external iliac arteries are not adequate, then a common iliac conduit graft can be considered. In rare cases, if neither iliac system is adequate, then an aortic conduit may be feasible. A dreaded complication of TEVAR is disruption of the iliac vessel upon removal of the access sheath, requiring either endovascular or open repair, usually with temporary endovascular balloon inflation for control of hemorrhage.

Fenestrated and branched aortic endografts. Endovascular treatment of aortic disease in regions of the aorta that abut or cross significant vessels becomes more difficult and has led to the development of fenestrated aortic endografts and branched aortic endografts. This nomenclature defines a structural addition to conventional endografts that allows for a reinforced hole to be "cut" into the stent graft, known as a fenestration, or an actual branch to be attached to the endograft. The use of these modifications was first employed to treat short-neck infrarenal aortic aneurysms. This device, called the Z-Fen device (Cook Medical, Bloomington, IN), was the first commercially available, custom-designed stent graft available in the United States. It allowed for custom-placed fenestrations to be placed on a stent graft in order to allow for continuous perfusion of the renal arteries and superior mesenteric artery—extending the proximal landing and seal zone of an EVAR device. Five-year outcomes for these devices showed excellent durability with continued 5-year renal artery patency of 98%, freedom from mortality of 91%, and no aneurysm ruptures or conversion to open repair. Unfortunately, as we have observed in most aortic endograft treatments, there was only a 63% rate of freedom from reintervention. Based on the success of this technology, the extent of treatment has been significantly advanced. Treatment of more extensive AAAs and TAAAs has been possible. Technologic approaches to this have been based on concepts that involved custom-made devices as well as off-the-shelf options. There has been tremendous success using these types of grafts worldwide, with some of the greatest experience arising within the United States through physician-sponsored research programs. Similar to the 5-year outcomes for the Z-Fen trial, outcomes from the physician-sponsored programs have demonstrated excellent long-term results with regard to aneurysm exclusion and branch patency but high rates of reintervention to achieve these results.[39,40] At the time of writing this chapter, no commercially available option is available within the United States, but the Gore TAMBE (Gore Medical, Flagstaff, AZ), a four-vessel off-the-shelf option, has completed enrollment and is awaiting final data collection before submission to the FDA.

Similar to the visceral segment of the aorta, fenestrated and branched technology is actively being evaluated for treatment of aortic disease that involves the aortic arch. The device designs have varied to incorporate anywhere from one to three arch branches. Single-branch and dual-branch designs require a hybrid approach with revascularization of the left subclavian or both the left carotid and SCAs. Early experience with multibranch designs demonstrates a significant learning curve, with anatomic constraints and risk of stroke limiting some of their clinical applicability.[41] Various graft designs and deployment systems are currently under investigation globally. Within the United States at the time of writing of this chapter, the Gore TBE single-branch device is commercially available for incorporation of the left SCA. Expansion of this approval to zone 0 landing with incorporation of the innominate artery and debranching of the other great vessels is anticipated.

Ruptured abdominal aortic aneurysms. Ruptured AAAs deserve special attention. Approximately 15,000 annual deaths from ruptured AAAs occur in the United States. In ruptured AAAs where it would be ideal to treat with an endovascular approach, there has not been any statistical evidence of a short-term benefit of one approach versus another. In one European trial, comparison between open and EVAR showed no difference in operative mortality (39% vs. 35%, respectively) or 90-day mortality (42% vs. 40%).[42] In the IMPROVE (Immediate Management of the Patient With Ruptured Aneurysm: Open Versus Endovascular Repair) trial, there was no difference in 30- or 90-day mortality, but there was an advantage for EVAR at 4 years (42% vs. 54%); once again, however, this advantage was gone by 7 years.[43] Interpreting these trials is challenging because intention to treat and treatment received may not align, thereby biasing the conclusions. Post hoc analysis of these data suggests that those who were able to receive an endovascular repair enjoyed better outcomes; therefore, it is the recommendation of many to consider an "endovascular-first approach."

Rapidly and effectively treating ruptured AAA requires trained personnel, access to endovascular inventory, and standard standardized protocols. Examples of such may include systems for rapid transport to an operating room (OR) with both open surgical and endovascular capability, minimal preoperative testing and imaging, and placement of an aortic occlusion balloon. The latter should be placed before induction of anesthesia because it may support blood pressure regardless of the type of repair offered. For patients amenable to EVAR for ruptured AAA, outcomes may be improved if general anesthesia is avoided altogether and the procedure is performed under local anesthesia.

Of note, many patients with ruptured AAA present with significant comorbidities or severe acutely deteriorating clinical condition. For this reason, over the past two to three decades, many scoring systems have been proposed to predict nonsurvivability and therefore consider comfort care instead of attempts at definitive repair. These scoring systems either were developed before the advent of EVAR or have not been validated with contemporary care. The University of Washington scoring system is one of the few that predicts futility rather than increased mortality risk and therefore may be more useful.[44] A recent institutional study demonstrated that only a very small proportion of patients met futility criteria with this scoring system. Additionally, outcomes outperformed all predictive models, thereby raising concerns about the clinical usefulness of such scoring systems.[45] Thus, each patient should be judged individually to determine suitability for intervention and definitive repair.

With increasing specialization of vascular surgery and expansion of EVAR for ruptured AAA, many hospitals are no longer equipped to provide care, thereby necessitating the need for transfer of these critically ill patients. Use of transfer appears to be increasing, creating additional challenges for timely intervention. When available, local care may represent the best treatment because although operative mortality is better for transferred patients, overall mortality is worse. This paradox is most likely explained by selection bias of those who are clinically stable to receive treatment once they arrive at the receiving hospital. In fact, approximately one in seven patients who are transferred does not receive treatment, which may be a result of clinical deterioration, severe comorbidities that may not have been recognized at the sending hospital, or patient refusal. To address this, current guidelines[23] provide recommendations for transferring patients with ruptured AAA to optimize the transfer process and provide the greatest opportunity for definitive repair in transferred patients.

OCCLUSIVE DISEASE OF THE AORTA

Symptomatic arterial occlusive disease is much more common in small- and medium-sized arteries; however, unusual variants of occlusive disease in the thoracic and abdominal aorta should be recognized and treated appropriately to avoid substantial morbidity and mortality. Although typical lower extremity symptoms such as claudication, ischemic rest pain, or ischemic tissue loss may be present in patients with aortic occlusive disease, the symptoms can be much more protean and are easily misdiagnosed or inappropriately treated. There are unique disease patterns and clinical scenarios with occlusive disease of the aorta that can be managed successfully with excellent long-term results if diagnosed promptly and addressed expeditiously. The widespread availability and use of CTA has made diagnosis of these aortic conditions more common, and medical, endovascular, and traditional open surgical options may be employed in treatment, depending on the severity and acuity of the disease.

Coral Reef Aorta

Coral reef aorta is defined by the presence of irregular, heavily calcified aortic plaques that protrude into the aortic lumen. These plaques may be up to 70% calcium, whereas atherosclerotic plaques more generally are typically less than 15% calcium. There is a slight female predominance in the literature, with 62% of reported cases involving females. The cause of these calcified lesions is unknown; however, the appearance is characteristic and unmistakable on CT angiogram (Fig. 102.5). Coral reef plaques may appear anywhere in the thoracic or abdominal aorta but are most commonly localized to the visceral or infrarenal aorta.

Diagnosis is often delayed by a symptom complex that can be rather vague, and patients can present with claudication, renovascular hypertension, intestinal angina, or emboli to the lower extremities (Table 102.5). Acute presentations with renal or visceral infarction or acute limb ischemia may be particularly challenging to manage, given the urgency of revascularization and the complexity of treating the lesion. An initial ankle-brachial index (ABI) or arterial duplex is often obtained but is typically nonspecific, demonstrating only arterial occlusive disease localized to the aortoiliac segment. After noninvasive testing, patients with evidence of severe occlusive disease in the abdominal aorta should typically undergo CTA of the abdomen and pelvis as the next step in evaluation. CTA with an appropriately timed contrast load will demonstrate the extent of the calcified plaque and is almost always adequate for planning definitive treatment.

As routine abdominal CT scanning becomes standard for evaluations of vague abdominal pain and major trauma, coral reef

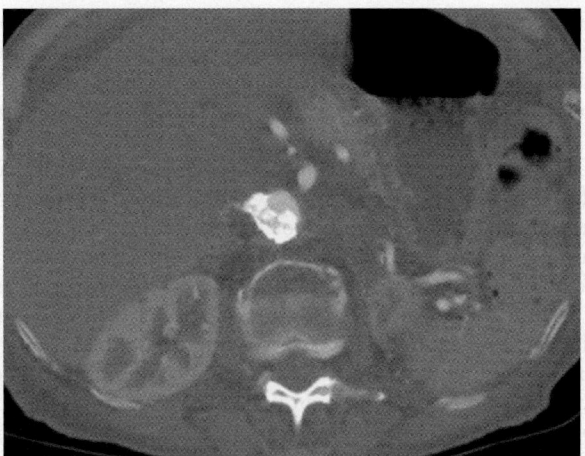

FIGURE 102.5 A large coral reef plaque is seen at the level of the renal arteries. This patient presented with renovascular hypertension and was treated with an ilio-renal bypass.

TABLE 102.5	Symptoms of Coral Reef Aorta
Presenting Symptoms	
Intermittent claudication	44%
Ischemic rest pain	8%
Ischemic tissue loss	2%
Refractory hypertension	36%
Renal insufficiency	12%
Intestinal angina	22%

plaques may be noted as incidental findings in asymptomatic patients. The majority of reports in the literature, however, have focused on patients with severe symptoms, and on this basis, the coral reef plaque is assumed to have a more malignant course. Although an asymptomatic coral reef plaque can certainly be treated conservatively with observation, antiplatelets, and statins, presenting symptoms are often severe enough that surgical or endovascular treatment is warranted.

Treatment algorithms in the past have focused exclusively on open surgical options, employing either extraanatomic bypass or aortic endarterectomy; however, endovascular adjuncts may certainly be employed, particularly in patients with multiple comorbidities who may not tolerate an open surgical approach to the visceral segment. Addressing the coral reef aorta is particularly complicated because it usually involves multiple vessels in the visceral segment. A treatment plan must restore flow to all of the compromised visceral vessels as well as the lower extremities. And although endovascular options may be appealing from the standpoint of a quick postoperative recovery, they typically play an adjunctive role. Bulky, rock-hard coral reef plaques do not usually angioplasty well, potentially leaving residual narrowing, a crushed stent, or a catastrophically ruptured aortic wall. Much of the existing literature has focused on aortic endarterectomy as the primary treatment for coral reef plaques. This approach has the potential to completely clear the disease process from the aorta and all of the involved visceral vessels with a durable result that may last the remainder of the patient's life. The surgical approach is, however, quite challenging and should be attempted only by surgeons who have extensive experience with open surgical reconstruction of the visceral aorta and mesenteric vessels. In practice, however, there is probably not a one-size-fits-all approach to these lesions, and some combination of endarterectomy, bypass, or even angioplasty and stenting may be employed.

Endarterectomy is most easily applied in patients with plaques confined to the infrarenal aorta, where a direct transperitoneal approach can provide exposure of the entire involved aortic segment to facilitate clamping, aortotomy, and endarterectomy.[46] Unfortunately, most of these plaques involve the visceral vessels, and a more complicated retroperitoneal approach to this portion of the aorta is required. This is most often described as a thoracoabdominal incision with complete mobilization of the abdominal contents to the patient's right to gain exposure from the supradiaphragmatic aorta to the bifurcation. A trapdoor aortotomy is then created to facilitate endarterectomy and complete clearance of the plaque from each of the visceral orifices (Fig. 102.6). In practice, endarterectomy may be combined with bypass to the visceral vessels or even replacement of a segment of the aorta if adequate end points cannot be obtained or the remaining aorta is too friable to close securely.

Alternative strategies can be considered in patients who are poor candidates for thoracoabdominal exposure with its attendant prolonged visceral ischemia, blood loss, and cardiopulmonary complications. These approaches may involve extraanatomic bypass to the visceral vessels or lower extremities or employ endovascular

adjuncts.[47] Axillofemoral bypass, for instance, may be a sound, if imperfect solution for frail patients presenting primarily with lower extremity occlusive symptoms. Operative debranching with retrograde bypass to one or more of the visceral vessels with stent grafting through the primary aortic lesion may offer another somewhat less definitive but also less morbid approach that can avoid long visceral ischemic times in patients with appropriate anatomy.

Not all patients necessarily require revascularization of all four visceral vessels, and a targeted approach to the most severe disease in the most salvageable vessels can allow for a limited operation that is still durable enough for an older patient with multiple comorbidities. For instance, in a patient with severe hypertension and declining renal function with heavily calcified renal involvement, an extraanatomic renal artery bypass can alleviate the short-term problem. Fig. 102.5 illustrates a patient with a coral reef plaque involving the renal arteries but with preserved flow through the visceral segment. In this case, a right ilio-renal bypass restored flow and eliminated the immediate risk of renal failure. Hepato-renal or spleno-renal bypass could also be considered if the celiac artery is patent and uninvolved. A similar approach may be considered for the superior mesenteric artery in patients with chronic mesenteric ischemia, with antegrade or retrograde bypass configurations.

Stent grafting through the affected segments of the aorta can restore flow; however, rupture of the treated segment or poor expansion of the graft are real risks, and balloon-expandable stent

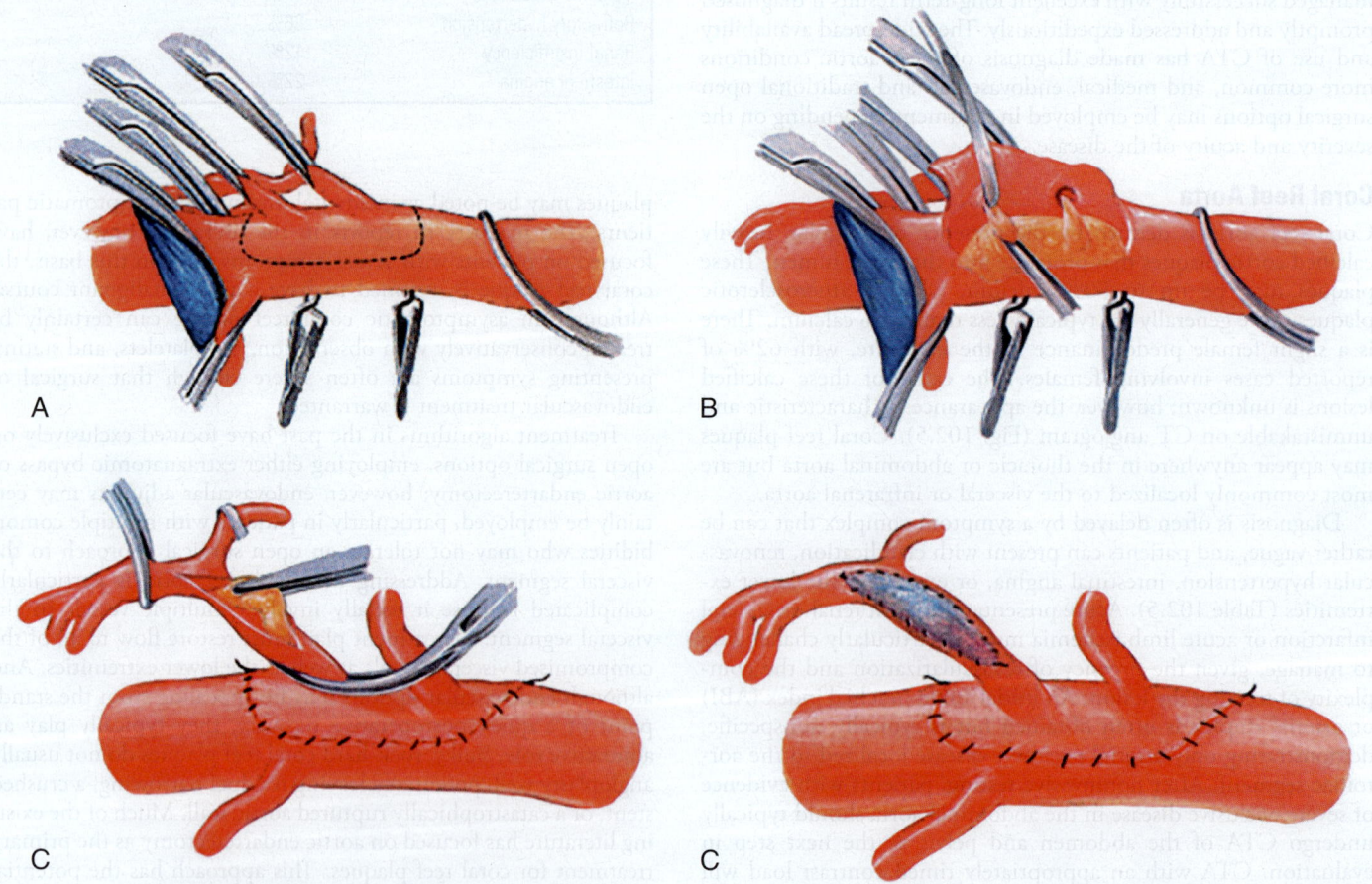

FIGURE 102.6 Steps involved with trapdoor aortotomy are illustrated. (A) Isolation of visceral branches of the thoracoabdominal aorta. (B) Endarterectomy of the visceral segments. (C) Visceral endarterectomy and closure of trapdoor aortotomy. (From Wylie EJ, Stoney RJ, Ehrenfeld WK. *Manual of Vascular Surgery*. Vol 1. New York: Springer-Verlag; 1980:215.)

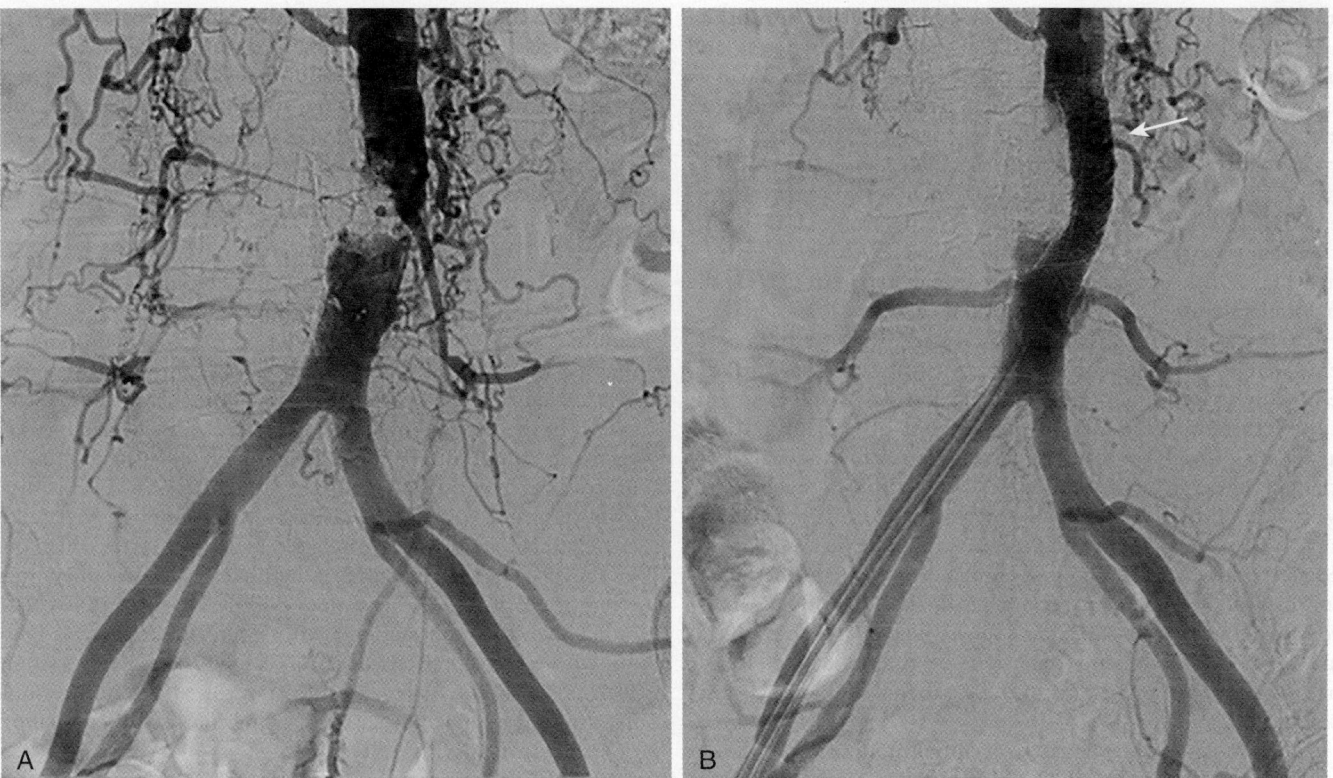

FIGURE 102.7 Stent grafting through a coral reef plaque in the infrarenal aorta is illustrated. (A) Coral Reef aorta involving the infrarenal aorta. (B) Stent graft in place with reconstitution of distal perfusion *(arrow)*.

grafts are often employed to obtain maximal radial force and seal off any perforations caused by angioplasty. Aggressive attempts to restore a completely normal aortic lumen with a stent graft are not warranted, and the goal would be to create a channel through the involved segment that is large enough to alleviate the symptoms and perfuse the viscera (Fig. 102.7).

Shaggy Aorta

Extensive irregular thrombus lining the aorta, the so-called "shaggy aorta," is not infrequently a source of acute embolic events to both the viscera and the lower extremities. Typically, shaggy aorta occurs in patients with extensive aortic atherosclerosis and surface degeneration, resulting in exposure of friable plaques or the accumulation of irregular, chronic thrombus (Fig. 102.8). This pathology may involve any segment of the aorta but more commonly is diffuse, with involvement of multiple segments. It may occur in isolation or accompany aneurysmal disease, which can significantly complicate an aneurysm repair. Diagnosis of this entity is increasing as more contrasted CT scans are ordered as a part of the workup for nonspecific chest and abdominal pain.

Shaggy aorta may be the source of spontaneous emboli to any of the aortic branches, depending on the areas of involvement. Showers of cholesterol microemboli can cause blue toe syndrome, but these microembolic events can also result in acute renal failure or bowel ischemia. Accumulated mobile thrombus may result in large-vessel occlusion of major visceral or lower extremity branches and result in an acute presentation with bowel or limb ischemia. Microembolic events may be treated expectantly, but larger macroembolic events need to be treated expeditiously with open embolectomy or percutaneous mechanical thrombectomy. Postevent,

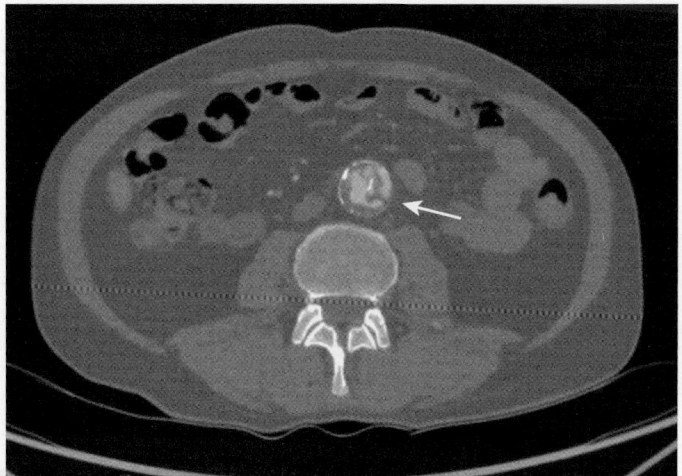

FIGURE 102.8 This patient demonstrates a severe shaggy aorta syndrome in the infrarenal segment *(arrow)*.

most patients will be systemically anticoagulated; however, longer term, only dual-antiplatelet treatment is recommended for prophylaxis against secondary events. Statins are indicated both from the standpoint of preventing progression of atherosclerosis generally and for plaque stabilization.

Most of the literature regarding shaggy aorta is, however, concerned with its potential for complications during either open or EVAR or other percutaneous procedures that may traverse the aorta. Aneurysm repair in any segment of the aorta is fraught with complications in patients with a shaggy aorta. Open TAAA repair in the presence of a shaggy aorta has an approximately 30% risk of major complication or death. Risks of spinal cord ischemia and acute renal failure, in particular, are markedly increased in the presence of shaggy aorta. Infrarenal aortic repair is also a higher risk in the presence of shaggy aorta. A recent large institutional series demonstrated a roughly 11% rate of shaggy aorta syndrome in 447 patients presenting for elective AAA repair.[48] This series documented a fourfold increase in morbidity and mortality for patients with a shaggy aorta. One might assume that EVAR would carry a much higher risk in patients with a shaggy aorta because of the intraarterial manipulation with wires and catheters; however, open aortic repair carried a substantially increased risk as well. Embolic events were much more common in patients with a shaggy aorta, presumably accounting for much of the increased overall mortality.

The substantially increased risk profile of patients with a shaggy aorta should be considered carefully before advising any patient to undergo aneurysm repair. Patients with a shaggy aorta have a significantly reduced life expectancy overall, regardless of which type of repair is chosen. Given the increased risk of immediate perioperative embolic events and the overall poor long-term survival of the patient cohort, repair should only be considered when the risk of rupture is substantial in the short term. Some authors recommend that the size threshold for elective repair of infrarenal aneurysms in these patients should be at least 6 cm and possibly larger.

If open repair is considered, procedural modifications should be made to minimize the risk of a catastrophic embolic shower. The clamp site should be chosen to avoid the worst areas of mobile thrombi. This may involve a supraceliac clamp if the pathology is mainly confined to the visceral segment, and care should be taken to minimize any movement of the clamp after initial application. Once the repair is completed, the proximal aorta should be flushed out onto the field to remove any debris around the clamp and back-flushed to remove as much distal debris as possible.

If CPB or left heart bypass is implemented for more extensive aortic arch or thoracoabdominal repairs, the site for arterial cannulation must be chosen carefully to avoid areas with extensive atherosclerotic plaque. A shaggy aorta should not be directly accessed, and axillary cannulation is generally preferable to femoral cannulation because retrograde flow across a shaggy aorta and into the cerebral circulation may result in a devastating stroke.

Atypical Aortic Thrombus

Patients with either inherited or acquired hypercoagulability may also develop more localized thrombus within the thoracic or abdominal aorta, which has a distinct appearance and presentation that is different from the shaggy aorta. This has been termed *atypical aortic thrombus* (AAT). This pathology almost always occurs in the descending aorta or visceral segment and has a characteristic appearance with a noncalcified eccentric thrombus protruding into the aortic lumen (Fig. 102.9A). AAT is distinct from thrombus with a cardiac origin or thrombus associated with aneurysmal disease and is unrelated to shaggy aorta, which occurs in the presence of extensive atherosclerosis. This phenomenon often occurs in a younger patient population in their 40s and 50s rather than the older patients with severe atherosclerosis presenting with either coral reef aorta or shaggy aorta. AAT is often associated with a hypercoagulable state or a significant smoking history, and malignancy should be high on the differential of patients presenting with AAT.

AAT almost always presents with macroembolization to large branch vessels and is identified on CTA as a part of a comprehensive embolic workup. It is often manifest as an eccentric plaque in the descending or visceral aorta that protrudes significantly into the lumen. Acute limb ischemia, renal emboli, or bowel ischemia must be addressed promptly with any number of surgical options, which may include embolectomy, bowel resection, percutaneous mechanical thrombectomy, or covered stenting, depending on the location, degree of ischemia, and the overall patient condition.

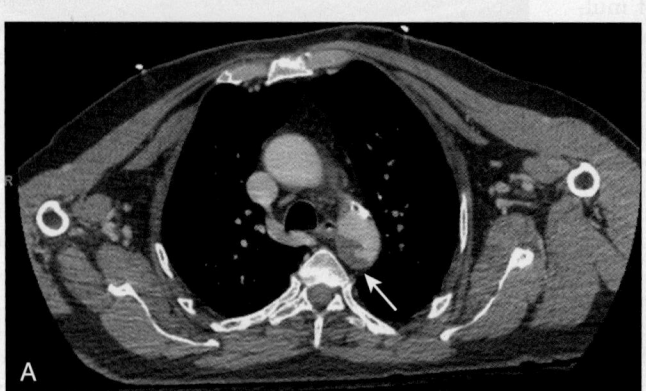
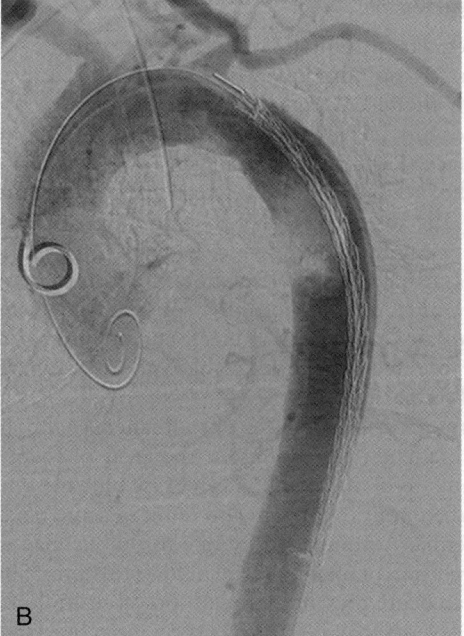

FIGURE 102.9 A patient with atypical aortic thrombus of the proximal descending aorta (A) underwent bilateral femoral-popliteal embolectomy followed by stent grafting over the aortic thrombus (B).

Once the acute ischemia has been dealt with, the source must be addressed, and various approaches have been described. The most obvious solution is trapping the thrombus behind an aortic stent graft (see Fig. 102.9B). However, this may not be applicable with thrombi that are near major visceral branches. Endovascular manipulation may risk additional embolic events, and thrombus may be displaced directly into nearby branches as the graft is expanded. For this reason, various treatments have been employed, ranging from simple systemic anticoagulation to systemic tissue plasminogen activator (tPA) or even aortotomy with direct thrombus extraction. Although a potentially morbid operation, aortotomy and thrombus removal eliminates any further risk of embolus. For a patient with a visceral-level thrombus and mesenteric and renal emboli, aortotomy with visceral embolectomy may offer the only chance to remove the offending aortic thrombus and restore visceral perfusion.

Aortoiliac Occlusive Disease

Atherosclerotic disease of the infrarenal aorta resulting in lower extremity symptoms such as claudication or ischemic tissue loss is more properly considered as aortoiliac disease because the atherosclerosis is rarely isolated to the abdominal aorta. Aortoiliac disease that develops chronically may be well tolerated because collateral networks can be extensive, and patients may have severe occlusive disease or aortic occlusion with only mild to moderate claudication.

This disease pattern is almost always localized below the visceral segment and develops over a period of years to decades. Risk factors mirror those for atherosclerotic disease more generally, including diabetes, hypertension, and hyperlipidemia; however, severe aortoiliac occlusive disease is most strongly associated with a smoking history.

A combination of physical examination findings and noninvasive vascular testing will usually identify patients with an aortoiliac pattern of disease, but a suggestive history and weak or absent femoral pulses may be sufficient to make a diagnosis. Symptomatology often includes buttock or thigh claudication and impotence, which, along with absent femoral pulses, constitutes the Leriche syndrome. Although moving straight to aortography is an option, most practitioners prefer cross-sectional imaging with CTA to plan a treatment course, which may be endovascular intervention, surgical bypass, or some combination of the two. Recommendations for treatment should be based on the extent of the disease and the patient's fitness to undergo a major surgical procedure. Although iliac atherosclerotic disease can almost always be addressed with an endovascular approach, extensive aortic involvement is often most durably treated with direct aortic reconstruction or extraanatomic bypass.

Traditionally, an aortobifemoral bypass was considered the gold standard for treatment of aortoiliac occlusive disease and was frequently performed for almost any pattern of disease involving the aorta or bilateral iliac arteries. More recently, iliac stenting has largely replaced aortobifemoral bypass for most iliac disease, including atherosclerosis that involves the distal aorta. Extension of the stents into the distal aorta, so-called "kissing stents," will address distal aortic pathology as well as iliac disease. Both balloon-expandable and self-expanding stents or stent grafts have been used successfully; however, stent grafts are increasingly used to both limit in-stent restenosis and avoid free rupture of the vessel, which can occur with angioplasty of heavily calcified arteries.

Total occlusion of the infrarenal aorta is the end point of severe atherosclerosis and represents the most challenging clinical scenario (Fig. 102.10). Endovascular approaches can be considered in patients who are poor surgical candidates, and an initial attempt to cross extensive occlusions and deliver a stent is not unreasonable. Stents can be extended up to near the level of the renal arteries, effectively raising the aortic flow divider to just below the renal arteries.

Ideally, a patient with an occluded infrarenal aorta should undergo aortic replacement with an aortobifemoral or aorto-biliac graft. The surgical procedure is somewhat more complicated because the occlusion often extends to the level of the renal arteries. Clamp application is at the suprarenal or, more commonly, the supraceliac location, and the aorta is opened, followed by removal of intraluminal thrombus with or without endarterectomy of bulky, calcified plaque. End-to-end anastomosis is then created for the inflow, and the distal anastomoses are commonly to the common femoral or profundafemoral arteries. If a transabdominal procedure is considered high risk because of cardiopulmonary issues or previous surgeries, an axillo-bifemoral bypass can be a lower-risk option. Although the long-term patency is not as good as with an aortobifemoral graft, the procedure is generally lower risk because it avoids a laparotomy, major blood loss, and a period of visceral ischemia.

Hypoplastic Aortic Syndrome

Hypoplastic aortic syndrome, or small aorta syndrome, is a variant of aortoiliac disease found in females with a relatively small distal aorta and iliac arteries characterized by early onset of ischemic symptoms in patients with a small-diameter distal aorta

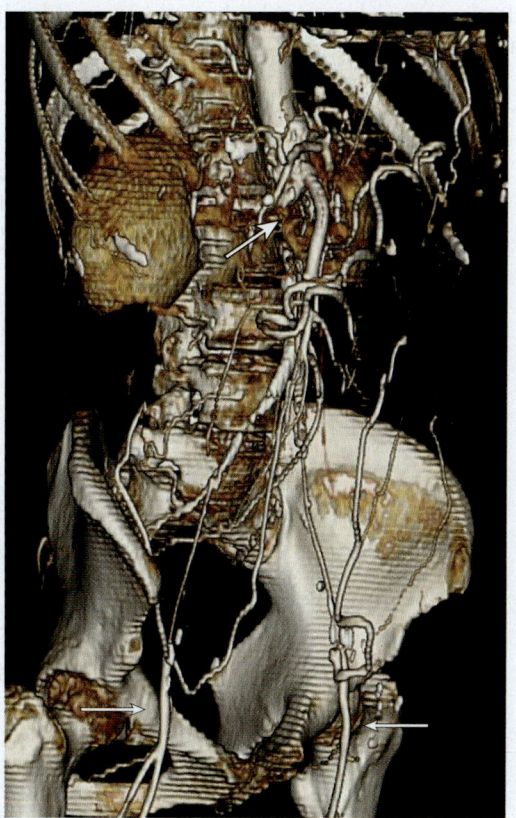

FIGURE 102.10 Chronic occlusion of the aorta just below the renal arteries is shown *(large arrow)*. There is reconstitution of the common femoral arteries via extensive collaterals *(small arrows)*.

and iliac arteries. These patients present in their fourth and fifth decades with severe symptoms and almost universally have an extensive smoking history. Whether this represents a truly separate pathologic entity or simply one end of a continuum in the size of the aorta and iliac vessels is unclear; however, it should be recognized that successful treatment may be much more challenging in these young patients.

Endovascular techniques are often employed initially but may lack durability, given the small size of the vessels, the extensive stenting that may be required, and the persistence of a smoking habit. Aorto-femoral bypass is often recommended as the preferred option in a patient population that is younger and presumably able to tolerate a more extensive operation. Bypass results may, however, also be suboptimal, given the small graft sizes needed to accommodate the smaller inflow and outflow vessels. Aggressive antismoking interventions, antiplatelet and statin therapy, and long-term graft surveillance are all key to a long-term successful outcome.

Aortic Sarcoma

Aortic sarcoma is a rare entity with a literature dominated by single case reports of patients presenting with advanced disease. It is instructive that 26% of patients with the disease are diagnosed postmortem, and 5-year survival is estimated at a dismal 9%. Larger pooled analysis of available cases, however, can shed some light on this challenging pathology.[49]

Patients with aortic sarcoma typically present with a constellation of symptoms that are often ascribed to other diagnoses. The most common is embolization to the extremities or visceral vessels; however, less specific complaints, such as constitutional symptoms, claudication, abdominal discomfort, hypertension, back pain, and anemia, are almost as frequent. Early diagnosis is rare in this setting, and even with adequate imaging, the diagnosis may not be obvious.

The most common histology is angiosarcoma, but there is a wide variety of histologic subtypes (Fig. 102.11), and the overall outlook is typically grim, with poor overall survival (Fig. 102.12) regardless of subtype. Ideally, complete resection with adjuvant radiation and/or chemotherapy may offer the best chance of long-term survival, but resection of a large segment of the aorta may require an extensive procedure. Sternotomy and circulatory arrest or thoracoabdominal exposure with aortic resection and replacement are very unappealing in a patient with aggressive disease and likely poor long-term outcome, but they can be considered in young patients with localized disease who are felt to be excellent surgical candidates. In most cases, however, palliation is the only option, and in this context, prevention of repeat embolic episodes will be helpful. Systemic anticoagulation with or without stent grafting over the embolizing lesion will typically be better tolerated than an open surgical resection, and patients may proceed with palliative chemotherapy or radiation shortly postoperatively.

CONGENITAL AORTOPATHY

Heritable thoracic aortic disease (HTAD) accounts account for approximately 20% of thoracic aortic aneurysms and can alter the recommendations for treatment and/or the expected clinical outcomes. Some of these are associated with multisystem features (known as *syndromic HTAD*), whereas other presentations are limited to the aorta (*nonsyndromic HTAD* or *familial TAA*).[3] Diseases involving HTAD can affect the entire aorta but most commonly present in the more proximal portions of the aorta. They can also present with either AD or aneurysm formation. There is a growing list of different HTADs that have been identified, and describing all of them is beyond the scope of this chapter. In addition, treatment guidelines for all of these are similarly outside

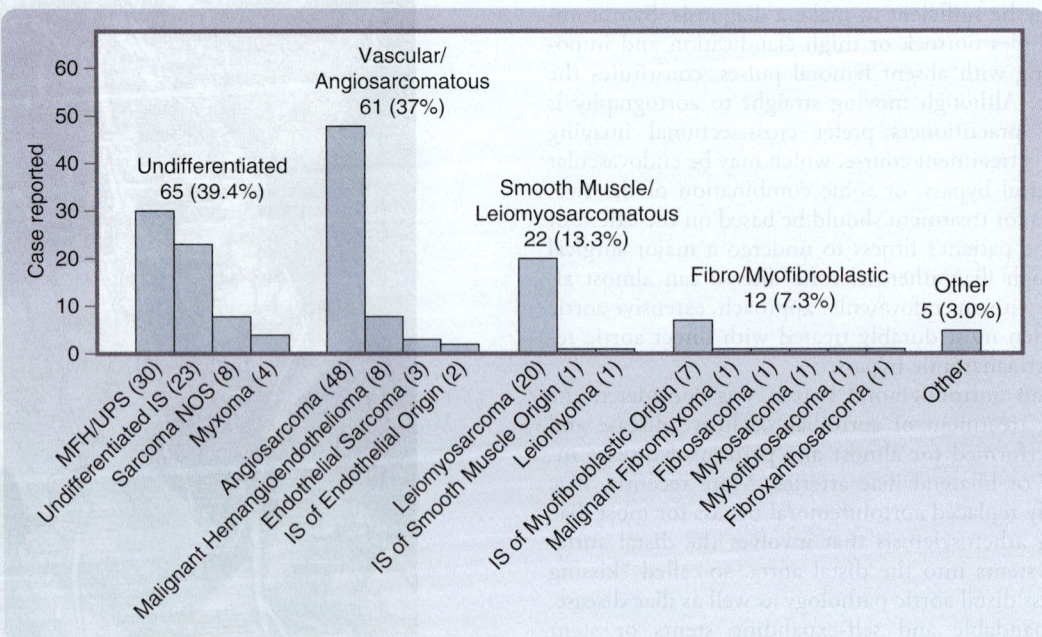

FIGURE 102.11 Cases reported by histology. "Other" includes two cases of chondrosarcoma, two cases of hemangiopericytoma, and one case of intimal sarcoma of rhabdomyosarcomatous differentiation. *IS,* Intimal sarcoma; *MFH,* malignant fibrous histiocytoma; *NOS,* not otherwise specified; *UPS,* undifferentiated pleomorphic sarcoma.

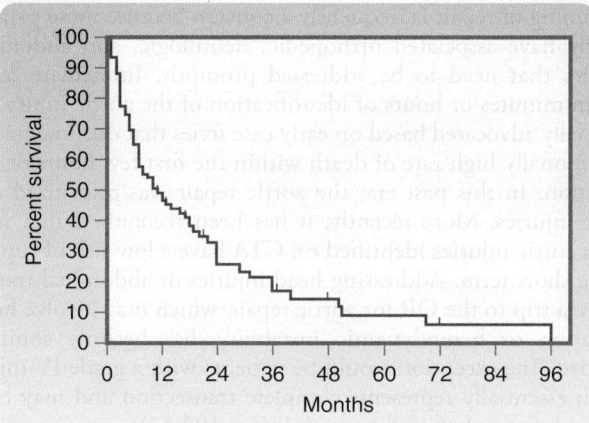

FIGURE 102.12 Kaplan-Meier overall survival estimate. Graph includes data for patients diagnosed antemortem (*n* = 122). Vertical notches represent censored events.

the focus of this chapter, but they have been well documented in recent guideline recommendations.[3] A brief review of a few of the most commonly encountered aortopathies follows. Although currently undergoing some scrutiny, the major intervention for patients with aortic disease secondary to a known aortopathy is conventional surgery because this does not rely on the stability of the aorta for the durability of its repair. Endovascular therapies have predominantly been limited to emergency situations, as a bridge to conventional surgery once the patient is stabilized, or in a hybrid fashion in which the landing/seal zones for the endografts occur in previously replaced aortic or aortoiliac segments.

Marfan Syndrome

Marfan syndrome is an autosomal dominant, age-related connective tissue disorder that is related to pathogenctic variations in the *FBN1* gene, which codes for the extracellular matrix glycoprotein fibrillin-1.[50] Nearly one-quarter of *FBN1* variants are de novo, and they frequently present with a more aggressive phenotype. It is highly penetrative and demonstrates substantial variability, with nearly 2000 genetic variants currently identified. Marfan syndrome affects all ethnicities but may have variable penetration. Marfan syndrome most frequently presents with enlargement of the ascending aorta, which places it at risk for continued growth as well as risk for acute dissection, as discussed earlier. Less commonly, Marfan syndrome can be associated with isolated thoracic aortic and AAAs. In addition to aortic abnormalities, Marfan syndrome presents with skeletal (pectus excavatum or kyphoscoliosis) and ocular manifestations (lens dislocation, retinal detachment, glaucoma). Diagnostic criteria were revised in 2010 and reported as the Ghent II criteria. These criteria incorporate physical examination findings of skeletal abnormalities paired with aortic changes, ocular abnormalities, family history, and identification of *FBN1* mutation. Familial screening is recommended for family members of those patients who present with Marfan syndrome, with 50% of the offspring being affected. Screening is performed with site-specific testing.

Murine models of Marfan syndrome have implicated transforming growth factor-β (TGF-β) signaling and the angiotensin II signaling cascade as possible contributors to the underlying pathophysiology. In some murine models, the use of angiotensin II receptor blockade (losartan) demonstrated effectiveness in preventing aortic aneurysm development. Historically, pharma-

cologic treatment with β-blockade (propranolol) in a small randomized trial prevented the growth of aortic root dilation in 10-year follow-up compared with those who did not receive the medication. Although the results from the mouse models suggested that losartan may be effective in preventing aortic expansion, despite initial enthusiasm, randomized trials comparing angiotensin receptor blocker (ARB) to β-blocker in patients with Marfan syndrome did not demonstrate any appreciable difference between the two. The addition of ARB to baseline therapy, which included β-blockers, demonstrated that the combination resulted in a reduction in growth rates.

Loeys-Dietz Syndrome

Loeys-Dietz syndrome (LDS) is an autosomal dominant connective tissue disorder that has been associated with aortic and other arterial abnormalities. These include arterial tortuosity, aneurysm formation, and AD. Similar to Marfan syndrome, LDS has additional nonaortic phenotypic expression, including craniofacial, skeletal, and cutaneous manifestations such as hypertelorism and bifid/broad uvula or cleft palate. Initial descriptions identified the syndrome as secondary to mutations in TGF-β receptor 1 *(TGFBR1)* and TGF-β receptor 2 *(TGFBR2)* and were stratified based on severity of craniofacial and cutaneous features. Currently, five variations of LDS have been described. LDS-3 is associated with mutations noted in *SMAD3*, presenting with prominent features of osteoarthritis; LDS-4 and 5 are associated with mutations in *TGFB2* and TGF-β receptor 3 *(TGFB3)*, respectively.[51] Aortic aneurysmal disease is a key feature of LDS. Those with types 1 and 2 with severe craniofacial features are at particularly high risk and have a risk for rupture at smaller diameters with a more malignant presentation. In addition to aortic components, other cardiovascular abnormalities include carotid and vertebral artery tortuosity, aortic stiffness, and mitral annular disjunction. These abnormalities can often present in childhood. Other systemic findings include skeletal involvement (spondylolisthesis and spondylosis), craniofacial abnormalities (abnormal palate, retrognathia, dental malocclusion), neurodevelopmental concerns, and gastrointestinal/genitourinary abnormalities. Multiple recommendations for the management of all of the extraaortic manifestations have been well outlined.[52] Similar to Marfan syndrome, pharmacologic management with either a β-blocker or ARB at maximally tolerated doses is recommended.[3]

Ehlers-Danlos Syndrome

Ehlers-Danlos syndrome (EDS) is a heterogeneous collection of hereditary connective tissue disorders with similar manifestations, including join hypermobility, soft and hyperextensible skin, and abnormal wound healing/easy bruising. There are 14 different types with variants identified in 20 different genes.[53] Overall, EDS has an estimated prevalence of 1:5000 to 1:250,000 births. The main clinical characteristics of EDS are present in varying degrees in each subtype of EDS. A range of clinical manifestations results from the generalized weakness and fragility of the soft connective tissues. Type IV EDS, or the vascular type (vEDS), is an autosomal dominant defect in type III collagen synthesis. These patients are at risk for arterial dissection, rupture, and aneurysm formation. The median life expectancy for patients with vascular EDS is 40 to 50 years. Mutations of the *COL3A1* gene are the predominant etiology of vascular EDS, and individuals with these mutations have structural defects of the pro α1 (III) chain of collagen type III.

Most of the mutations are single base substitutions for glycine residues. Although the vascular presentations can involve the aorta, they more frequently involve the mid- to small-size arteries. They can present with pseudoaneurysm formation, arterial dissection, and spontaneous rupture of nondilated vessels. The mainstay of therapy for patients with vEDS is education and awareness. They should be referred to a center with—and just this connection has been demonstrated to lower mortality rates. Elective interventions should be avoided if possible because of the high-risk nature of any procedure. A targeted approach, either endovascular or open, is warranted in the urgent/emergent scenario.

AORTIC TRAUMA

Both blunt and penetrating trauma may involve any section of the aorta; however, most penetrating injuries to the aorta at any level result in either rapid exsanguination or presentation of a profoundly unstable patient to the emergency department. The most commonly identified treatable aortic injury is blunt disruption of the proximal descending aorta. During a severe trauma with rapid deceleration, shearing and torsion may occur, particularly where the relatively mobile arch transitions to the less mobile descending aorta. This area can sustain a shear injury with varying degrees of injury to the aortic wall. Surprisingly, patients presenting with blunt aortic injury are often hemodynamically stable on presentation because most injuries are either not full-thickness tears or bleeding is contained by the periaortic connective tissue.

The recommended treatment depends on the severity of the injury, which can be graded on a scale of I to IV (Fig. 102.13). Grade I injuries, consisting of intimal tears, can be managed nonoperatively, with serial CT scans to assess for progression or resolution. For grade II, III, and IV injuries, repair with a thoracic endograft (TEVAR) is generally recommended. Although open repair with replacement of the injured segment was considered standard in the past, TEVAR is a much less morbid operation that is more appropriate for polytrauma patients, most of whom have severe associated injuries and are poor candidates for a thoracotomy and an aortic cross clamp. Clinical practice guidelines from the SVS support TEVAR as the preferred modality for treatment of blunt thoracic injury, which has now almost completely replaced open repair.[54]

Timing of repair is frequently a concern because these patients usually have associated orthopedic, neurologic, and abdominal injuries that need to be addressed promptly. Immediate repair within minutes or hours of identification of the aortic injury was originally advocated based on early case series that documented an exceptionally high rate of death within the first few hours of presentation. In this past era, the aortic repair was prioritized over other injuries. More recently, it has been recognized that most blunt aortic injuries identified on CTA have a low risk of rupture in the short term. Addressing head injuries or abdominal trauma before a trip to the OR for aortic repair, which may involve heparinization or hemodynamic instability, has become common practice. The exception would be patients with a grade IV injury, which essentially represents complete transection and may be at high risk for early free rupture (see Fig. 102.13).

A recent study in the *Journal of Vascular Surgery* comparing early (<24 hours) versus late (>24 hours) repair using the National Trauma Data Bank found that the mortality of early repair (9.8%) was significantly higher than that for late repair (4.4%). Although there is potential for significant selection bias because patients with more severe aortic injuries may have been taken more quickly to the OR, this study highlights the relatively low rate of rupture during a 24- to 48-hour period of stabilization before aortic repair.[55] A prudent approach in the current era would involve early repair of grade IV injuries, delaying repair of grade II and III injuries until associated traumatic injuries have been addressed. Patients with less significant blunt aortic injuries who do not have severe associated head or intraabdominal injuries can be repaired immediately as well. For patients with severe head injury, maintaining cerebral perfusion with blood pressure elevation may be a key part of treatment. In this circumstance, early aortic repair should also be considered because medical management of the aortic injury with antiimpulse therapy may be incompatible with treatment goals for a head injury.

Patients with aortic stab or gunshot aortic wounds who survive to definitive repair are rare; however, a partial-thickness injury or a pseudoaneurysm may be contained by the surrounding soft tissues, and the patient may survive to reach a trauma center. Iatrogenic injuries resulting from errant line placement, misadventures during spine surgery, or puncture with trocars during laparoscopic procedures are encountered not infrequently and may result in acute bleeding or a more contained injury identified postoperatively (see Fig. 102.13). For the patient who is unstable with acute

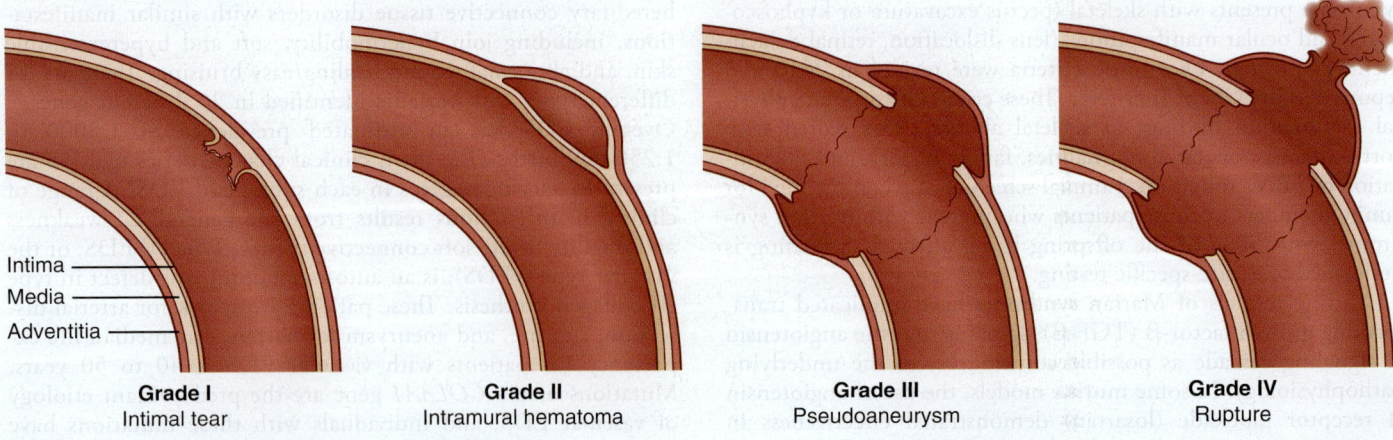

Grade I	Grade II	Grade III	Grade IV
Intimal tear	Intramural hematoma	Pseudoaneurysm	Rupture

Intima
Media
Adventitia

FIGURE 102.13 Classification of blunt thoracic aortic injury.

bleeding, open repair via the most expeditious exposure offers the only possibility of survival.

An underappreciated difficulty with aortic injuries that are explored without the benefit of preoperative imaging is identification of the site and nature of the injury in a field with a large hematoma or active bleeding. For the unstable patient with abdominal injury, a midline laparotomy is almost always employed initially, and central retroperitoneal hematoma, whether stable or expanding, raises the possibility of aortic injury. Dissection of the supraceliac aorta with placement of a clamp before entering a hematoma is a prudent maneuver and can limit both massive blood loss and the associated OR chaos.

Direct suture repair of smaller injuries is sometimes feasible; however, injuries involving more than 50% of the circumference typically require a segmental replacement of the injured aortic segment or placement of a patch to avoid excessive narrowing of the artery. Associated bowel injuries may make contamination of the graft concerning, and off-the-shelf biologic materials such as cryopreserved arterial allograft or bovine pericardium can lessen but not eliminate the risk.

Less morbid endovascular approaches may be considered in patients who are temporarily stable, and stent grafting may be particularly applicable in the descending thoracic aorta or the infrarenal abdominal aorta, where off-the-shelf endografts can be used to rapidly exclude an injured segment. For injuries in proximity to major branches, whether in the arch or the visceral segment, creating an appropriate branched graft in a short time period may be impossible or ill-advised. Some institutions may, however, have the requisite in-house expertise, and back-table modification of grafts has been occasionally employed successfully.

SELECTED REFERENCES

Chaikof EL, Dalman RL, Eskandari MK, et al. The Society for Vascular Surgery practice guidelines on the care of patients with an abdominal aortic aneurysm. *J Vasc Surg*. 2018;67(1): 2-77.e2.

> *This manuscript reports the Society for Vascular Surgery clinical practice guidelines for caring for patients afflicted with abdominal aortic aneurymss.*

Erbel R, Aboyans V, Boileau C, et al. 2014 ESC guidelines on the diagnosis and treatment of aortic diseases: document covering acute and chronic aortic diseases of the thoracic and abdominal aorta of the adult. The Task Force for the Diagnosis and Treatment of Aortic Diseases of the European Society of Cardiology (ESC). *Eur Heart J*. 2014;35(41):2873-2926.

> *These are the 2014 European Society of Cardiology aortic treatment guidelines from diagnostic strategies, risk stratification, to long-term management.*

Haulon S, Greenberg RK, Spear R, et al. Global experience with an inner branched arch endograft. *J Thorac Cardiovasc Surg*. 2014;148(4):1709-1716.

> *This mansucript reports on the initial outcomes of the international use of a branched aortic endograft to treat aortic disease involving the arch. The procedural success was 84%*

with a 30-day mortality of 13%. Factors, such as early surgical experience and aortic morphology, were determined to be associated with higher rates of early mortality and stroke.

IMPROVE Trial Investigators. Comparative clinical effectiveness and cost effectiveness of endovascular strategy v open repair for ruptured abdominal aortic aneurysm: three year results of the IMPROVE randomised trial. *BMJ*. 2017;359:j4859.

> *The IMPROVE trial was a randomized trial comparing EVAR and open surgery for ruptured abdominal aortic aneurysms. Results indicated that the EVAR strategy was associated with a 48% mortality rate compared to 56% in the open repair group, alongside improved early quality of life and reduced hospital stays, leading to a gain of 0.17 quality-adjusted life years and lower overall costs, making it a potential cost-effective option.*

Isselbacher EM, Preventza O, Hamilton Black J III, et al. 2022 ACC/AHA guideline for the diagnosis and management of aortic disease: a report of the American Heart Association/American College of Cardiology Joint Committee on Clinical Practice Guidelines. *Circulation*. 2022;146(24):e334-e482.

> *The 2022 ACC/AHA Guideline provides a comprehensive, evidence based recommendation on the diagnosis and management of aortic disease including medical and surgical management. It offers up to date information on toipcs such as shared-decision making and advances in imaging and genetic testing to individualize treatment option.*

Mastracci TM, Eagleton MJ, Kuramochi Y, Bathurst S, Wolski K. Twelve-year results of fenestrated endografts for juxtarenal and group IV thoracoabdominal aneurysms. *J Vasc Surg*. 2015; 61(2):355-364.

> *This study reports one of the longest, single-center outcomes for the use of fenestrated endograft repair of paravisceral aneurysms. Despite being investigational in nature, use of these devices was associated with excellent clinical outcomes. 8-year survival, however, was only 20% with the majority of patients dying from etiology independent of their aortic disease.*

Milewicz DM, Guo D, Hostetler E, Marin I, Pinard AC, Cecchi AC. Update on the genetic risk for thoracic aortic aneurysms and acute aortic dissections: implications for clinical care. *J Cardiovasc Surg (Torino)*. 2021;62(3):203-210.

> *This review highlights the role of genetic variations in predisposing individuals to thoracic aortic aneurysms and dissections. They emphasize that advancements in genomic research have identified 11 genes associated with heritable thoracic aortic disease and the importance of integrating genetic testing in the clinical evaluating and treatment recommendations.*

Nienaber CA, Kische S, Akin I, et al. Strategies for subacute/chronic type B aortic dissection: the Investigation of Stent Grafts in Patients With Type B Aortic Dissection (INSTEAD) trial

1-year outcome. *J Thorac Cardiovasc Surg.* 2010;140(suppl 6):S101-108; discussion S142-S146.

> The INSTEAD trial evaluated 140 patients with stable type B aortic dissection randomized to best medical therapy or endovascular treatment in combination with best medical therapy. At 1-year, despite favorable aortic remodeling in the endovascular arm, no differences in survival or incidence of adverse events was observed.

Nienaber CA, Kische S, Rousseau H, et al. Endovascular repair of type B aortic dissection: long-term results of the randomized investigation of stent grafts in aortic dissection trial. *Circ Cardiovasc Interv.* 2013;6(4):407-416.

> This manuscript reports the long-term results of the INSTEAD trial – a randomized, prospective trial evaluating treatment of stable aortic dissections with best medical therapy with and without the addition of TEVAR. The use of TEVAR was associated with favorable aortic remodeling.

Oderich GS, Forbes T, Chaer R, et al. Reporting standards for endovascular aortic repair of aneurysms involving the renal-mesenteric arteries. *J Vasc Surg.* 2021;73(suppl 1):4S-52S.

> This represents the reporting standards for evaluating outcomes of patients undergoing endovascular repair of aortic aneurysms that involved the renal and mesenteric arteries. This is the first edition of these recommendations given the relative newness of this treatment modality.

Pape LA, Awais M, Woznicki EM, et al. Presentation, diagnosis, and outcomes of acute aortic dissection: 17-year trends from the international registry of acute aortic dissection. *J Am Coll Cardiol.* 2015;66(4):350-358.

> Over a 17-year period, the IRAD study observed consistency over time in the physical complaints expressed by patients having an aortic dissection. The frequency of CT imaging increased during this study, as did the frequency of surgery for type A dissections and endovascular therapy for type B dissections with decreased mortality.

Schermerhorn ML, Buck DB, O'Malley AJ, et al. Long-term outcomes of abdominal aortic aneurysm in the Medicare population. *N Engl J Med.* 2015;373(4):328-338.

> This study evaluated the long-term outcomes of EVAR versus open repair for patients with abdominal aortic aneurysms. The Medicare-based data set demonstrated higher rates of late rupture and need for reintervention for patients that were treated with EVAR, despite an early survival advantage.

The full reference list appears on Elsevier eBooks+.

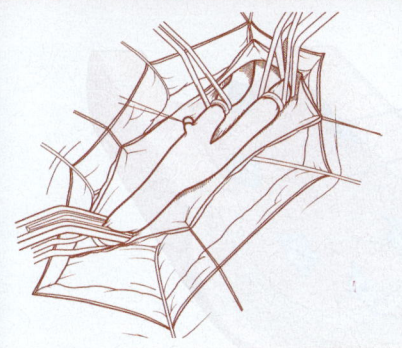

CHAPTER 103

Peripheral Occlusive Disease

Elizabeth G. King, Katharine L. McGinigle, and Alik Farber

INTRODUCTION

Peripheral artery disease (PAD) is an obliterative process that affects extremity arteries and can lead to arterial insufficiency, most commonly in the lower extremities. Although atherosclerosis is the most common etiology of PAD, less common conditions include thromboembolism, vasculitis, thromboangiitis obliterans (Buerger disease), Behcet disease, pseudoxanthoma elasticum, popliteal entrapment syndrome, cystic adventitial disease, and iliac artery endofibrosis. Patients with PAD can present with intermittent claudication (IC), chronic limb-threatening ischemia (CLTI) with symptoms of rest pain or tissue loss (nonhealing ulcers or wounds), and acute limb ischemia (ALI); approximately 30% to 60% of patients with PAD are asymptomatic.[1] The chronic manifestations of atherosclerotic PAD, IC, and CLTI will be discussed in detail because they are most frequently encountered, and the presentation and management of ALI, a surgical emergency, will be described later in the chapter.

Atherosclerosis is a systemic disease, and a substantial number of patients with PAD have concomitant coronary artery disease (CAD) and cerebrovascular disease (CVD). Consequently, patients with PAD have a significantly increased risk of cardiovascular morbidity and mortality. At 32%, 5-year mortality in PAD is higher than that for many cancers.[2] Untreated CLTI, the most severe form of chronic ischemia, carries a 1-year 22% all-cause mortality, and limb loss rates are between 20% and 40%.[3,4] PAD is also associated with impaired quality of life, frailty, and depression.[5–8]

Over the course of the first decade of the 21st century, the prevalence of PAD across the world increased by almost 25%, affecting over 200 million people, with continued growth attributed to the aging population and the epidemic of diabetes mellitus (DM) and metabolic syndrome.[9,10] In addition, chronic kidney disease (CKD) and hypertension (HTN) are contributing to the development and progression of PAD globally. The true prevalence of PAD is likely underestimated as a result of underdiagnosis and the presence of asymptomatic disease. Data and models from the Global Burden of Diseases, Injuries, and Risk Factors Study demonstrated a 75% increase in mortality and a 37% increase in disability associated with PAD, in contrast to the decreasing prevalence and disease-related mortality of ischemic heart disease and ischemic stroke over the same time period.[11]

In the United States, PAD affects an estimated 8.5 to 12 million people and is associated with high economic burden.[12] In an analysis of the Agency for Healthcare Research and Quality Medical Expenditure Panel Surveys from 2011–14, reported annual expenditures per individual with PAD were $11,553 compared with just $4219 for matched patients without PAD.[13] Comorbid conditions associated with PAD also contribute to the economic cost. For patients with DM and PAD, total costs were significantly higher as compared with patients with DM alone ($33,894 vs. $12,151).[13] Approximately one-third of the $237 billion in direct costs of care for diabetic patients in 2017 was attributed to the care of diabetic foot disease, which is comparable to cancer-related expenditures.[14] Additionally, smoking has been shown to be associated with a 35% higher annual hospitalization rate and $18,000 higher annual cost per patient with atherosclerotic PAD.[15]

PATHOPHYSIOLOGY OF ATHEROSCLEROTIC DISEASE

Arteries consist of three layers: intima, media, and adventitia. The innermost intima, composed of collagen and glycosaminoglycans, is largely acellular and is lined with endothelium, a cell monolayer in contact with the bloodstream. The media consists of layers of smooth muscle cells and is surrounded by adventitia, the fibrous outer layer, which provides strength to the vessel wall.

Atherosclerosis is a dynamic process and is believed to be the result of chronic inflammation of the arterial wall.[16] When the endothelium is activated by proinflammatory stimuli, endothelial cells express leukocyte adhesion molecules to which circulating blood monocytes and lymphocytes adhere. These bound leukocytes migrate into the intima, where they differentiate into macrophages. Foam cells form when macrophages take up lipoproteins, leading to the development of fatty streaks within the luminal surface of the arteries.

Vascular smooth muscle cells proliferate and migrate to the subendothelial space of the intima, forming a fibrous cap through the secretion of extracellular matrix material, primarily collagen (Fig. 103.1). Over time, as foam cells, smooth muscle cells, and macrophages continue to accumulate, cells undergo apoptosis, leading to the appearance of a necrotic core consisting of cholesterol and cellular debris within the plaque. Episodes of systemic or regional inflammation stimulate lesion growth through T-cell lymphocyte-mediated interactions, resulting in expansion of the necrotic core and thinning of the fibrous cap, making the plaque susceptible to disruption. Plaque rupture or superficial erosion of the endothelial lining exposes the thrombogenic substances contained within the necrotic core, including tissue factor, to circulating blood components, triggering coagulation and thrombosis.[17]

Calcifications are common in atherosclerotic lesions and increase with advancing age as well as in patients with DM and CKD. Apoptotic cells, necrotic core, and extracellular matrix can act as a nidus for deposition of microscopic calcium granules, which can progress to larger deposits and complete calcification of the necrotic core.[18]

Arteries demonstrate compensatory changes in response to development of atherosclerotic plaques. Arterial remodeling occurs in two stages: compensation and encroachment.[19] As atherosclerotic plaques enlarge, arterial enlargement results in preservation of luminal diameter until the lesion occupies ~40% of the cross-sectional area, at which point encroachment occurs and the lumen becomes progressively narrowed, limiting blood flow to distal tissues.

ANATOMIC PATTERNS OF ATHEROSCLEROTIC DISEASE

In the extremity, atherosclerotic plaque develops in relatively predictable distributions (Fig. 103.2). Lesions tend to occur at arterial bifurcations, areas of fixation and angulation. The most common location is the distal superficial artery (SFA) at the adductor hiatus. In this location, the artery is compressed by the adductor magnus tendon, which causes trauma to the artery and limits its ability to develop compensatory arterial dilation.

Flow separation and turbulence lead to areas of shear stress, predisposing the vessel to vascular injury and atherogenesis. Although asymmetrical intimal thickening may initially form as an adaptive physiologic response, it represents a vulnerable

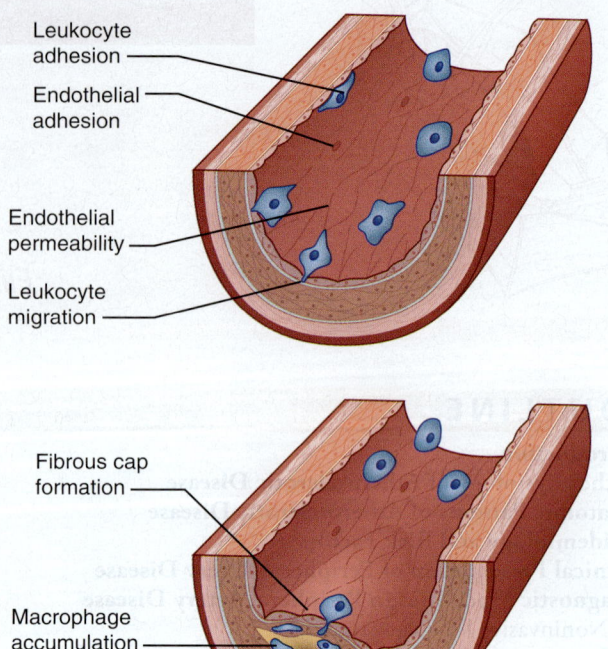

FIGURE 103.1 Initiation and progression of atherosclerotic plaque. Cardiovascular risk factors, hemodynamic forces, toxins, and infectious agents interact with the vessel at the level of the endothelium to produce injury, resulting in decreased nitric oxide production and increased permeability. Once injured, the endothelium increases the expression of leukocyte adhesion molecules such as vascular cell adhesion molecule-1, intracellular adhesion molecule-1, and P- and E-selectin, which increases the adherence of macrophages and other leukocytes. Permeability of the endothelium also increases and permits entry of leukocytes and lipoproteins into the subendothelial space. Chemokines and cytokines such as monocyte chemotactic protein-1 and interleukin-8 further enhance the recruitment of leukocytes and smooth muscle cells (SMCs) into the subendothelial space. Lipoproteins retained in the subendothelial space are biochemically modified such that they can be taken up by macrophages and SMCs to form foam cells. Foam cells at the central-most position of the developing atheroma become necrotic and form the central lipid core, whereas the shoulder regions contain SMCs, macrophages, and other leukocytes. Platelet-derived growth factor and transforming growth factor-β stimulate SMC migration and collagen formation in the subendothelial space as well as formation of the fibrous cap. (Ho KJ. Atherosclerosis. In: Sidawy AN, Perler BA, eds. *Rutherford's Vascular Surgery and Endovascular Therapy*. 10th ed. Philadelphia: Elsevier; 2019:41-50.)

location for the development of pathologic atherosclerotic lesions.[20] Plaque accumulation leads to formation of stenoses that further disrupt laminar flow, causing eddy currents that continue to traumatize the intima, leading to vessel stenosis and occlusion.

In response to arterial stenosis, collateral vessels develop from distributing branches of large and medium-sized arteries. These collaterals may provide sufficient flow to the limb despite the presence of severe arterial stenosis or occlusion. If collateral formation keeps pace with disease progression, the patient may either remain asymptomatic or have stable symptoms. However, when aggressive native arterial disease progresses faster than collateral formation or interrupts flow to collateral vessels, or if collateral flow is reduced in the setting of decreased cardiac output or increased blood viscosity, then PAD symptoms can worsen.

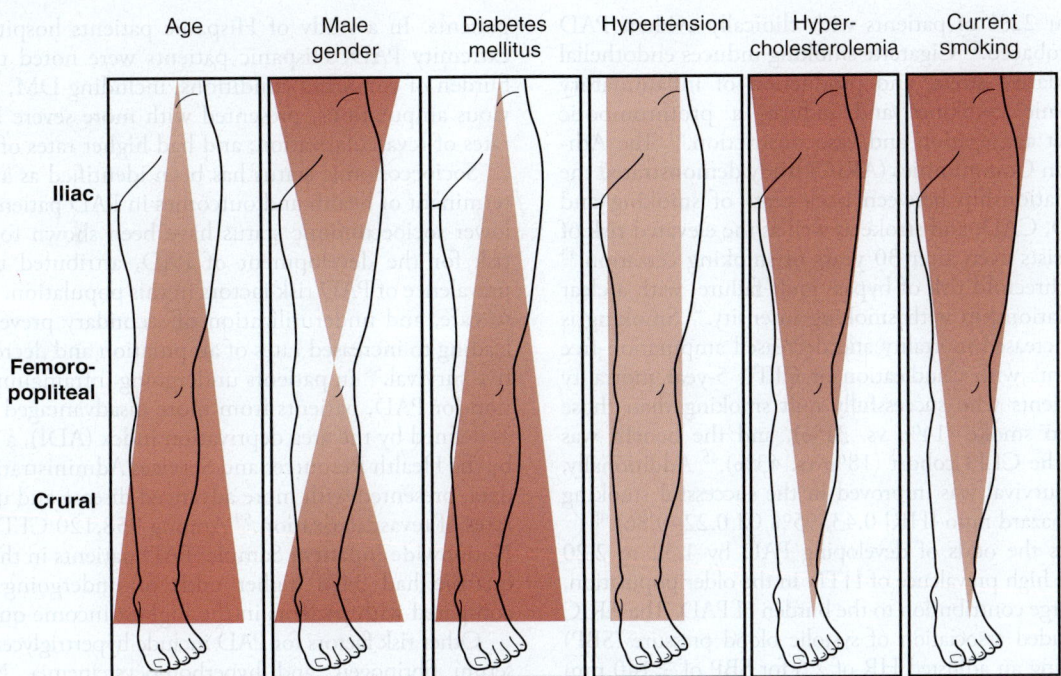

Age | Male gender | Diabetes mellitus | Hypertension | Hyper-cholesterolemia | Current smoking

Iliac

Femoro-popliteal

Crural

FIGURE 103.2 Association of risk factors with the level of atherosclerotic target lesions. The *red* overlay on the anatomic cartoon illustrates the association of risk factors with patterns of atherosclerotic disease. (From Diehm N, Shang A, Silvestro A, et al. Association of cardiovascular risk factors with pattern of lower limb atherosclerosis in 2659 patients undergoing angioplasty. *Eur J Vasc Endovasc Surg.* 2006;31:59-63.)

Patients with IC often have single-level disease, commonly involving either the aortoiliac segment or femoropopliteal segment. The former is a pattern commonly seen in cigarette smokers. Patients with CLTI frequently have multilevel disease, with more than half demonstrating not only occlusions in the femoral but also the popliteal and/or tibial arteries.[21] Female sex, especially in current and prior smokers, and patients with elevated triglycerides have been found to have an association with aortoiliac disease.[22] Females with CLTI have also been demonstrated to have a higher risk of occlusions and multilevel disease.[23]

DM, CKD, and older age are associated with the development of more distal disease. Patients with DM frequently present with severe occlusive disease involving long-segment occlusions of the tibial arteries as well as more frequent involvement of the deep femoral artery (DFA). The anterior tibial (ATA) and posterior tibial (PTA) arteries are the most frequently involved, with the peroneal artery least affected.[24] Despite the predilection for a distal distribution of disease in patients with DM, the pedal arteries are often spared. A study of arteriographic lesions in diabetic patients with ischemic foot ulcers demonstrated that 88% of patients with occlusion of all tibial vessels had at least one patent pedal artery.[25]

Patients with end-stage renal disease (ESRD) have more frequent involvement of the pedal vessels.[26] Renal insufficiency is associated with arterial calcification, and CKD has also been shown to be associated with a loss of patency of the pedal-plantar arch.[27]

Patterns of disease have implications for revascularization options. In particular, management of distal disease is more challenging, often placing patients at higher risk of amputation and limited amputation-free survival.[28]

EPIDEMIOLOGY AND RISK FACTORS

Advanced age, DM, CKD, cigarette smoking, HTN, and hyperlipidemia increase the risk of PAD. PAD most commonly presents in patients older than 50 years of age, and prevalence increases with increasing age. Among patients younger than 50 years, PAD prevalence is 4% to 7%, compared with 15% to 20% in patients older than 80 years.[9,29] This represents a significant risk factor because by 2030, US Census data project that 19.3% of the population will be over 65 years of age.[30]

DM, affecting over half a billion people globally, is associated with both microvascular and macrovascular complications and has become the most quickly increasing risk factor for PAD. By 2050, 50% of the global adult population is expected to have DM, which is associated with a two- to fourfold increase in PAD prevalence.[31–33] Risk increases with worsening glycemic control, with each 1% increase in HbA1c from baseline associated with a 14.2% increased relative risk (RR) of major adverse cardiovascular events (MACEs)[34] and a 21% to 28% increased risk of PAD.[35,36] Of patients with CLTI, 60% to 70% of patients have a diagnosis of DM.[21] Up to one-third of patients with DM will develop a diabetic foot ulcer (DFU) during their lifetime, which can be purely neurogenic, although many are neuro-ischemic.[14] Patients with DM and PAD have a four-times-higher risk of major limb amputation,[37] and elevated serum fasting glucose is the primary attributable risk factor for PAD-related mortality, surpassing risk factors of smoking and HTN in the overall population.[38]

CKD has also emerged as a significant independent risk factor for the development of PAD. Prevalence of PAD is 25.2% among patients with renal insufficiency, and approximately 25% of patients undergoing revascularization for PAD have CKD.[39,40] Patients with CKD and PAD who undergo revascularization experience worse outcomes, including increased risk of leg amputation and death.[40] CKD is the predominant contributor to PAD-related mortality in patients 40 to 59 years old, especially females.[38]

Smoking, a major modifiable risk factor, has a three- to fourfold increased risk for the development of PAD.[41] The Reduction of Atherothrombosis for Continued Health (REACH) Registry data indicate that 22% of patients with clinically evident PAD continue to use tobacco.[42] Cigarette smoking induces endothelial dysfunction, oxidative stress, and production of inflammatory and proatherogenic cytokines and induces a prothrombotic state with platelet aggregation and vasoconstriction.[41] The Atherosclerosis Risk in Communities (ARIC) study demonstrated the dose-response relationship between pack-years of smoking and incidence of PAD, CAD, and stroke as well as the elevated risk of PAD, which persists even after 30 years of smoking cessation.[43] Smokers have a threefold risk of bypass graft failure, with a clear dose-response relationship with smoking intensity.[44] Smoking is associated with increased mortality and decreased amputation-free survival. In patients with claudication or CLTI, 5-year mortality was lower in patients who successfully quit smoking than those who continued to smoke (14% vs. 31%), and the benefit was more notable in the CLTI cohort (18% vs. 43%).[45] Additionally, amputation-free survival was improved in the successful smoking cessation group (hazard ratio [HR] 0.43, 95% CI 0.22–0.86).[45]

HTN increases the odds of developing PAD by 1.32 to 2.20 times.[29] Given the high prevalence of HTN in the older population, this represents a large contribution to the burden of PAD. The ARIC study found a graded association of systolic blood pressure (SBP) with PAD, reporting an adjusted HR of 2.6 for SBP of ≥140 mm Hg and 1.6 for 120 to 139 mm Hg.[46]

Although total cholesterol and low-density lipoprotein cholesterol (LDL-C) have been shown to be independently associated with coronary heart disease, the associations with PAD have not been found to be significant.[47] However, higher baseline levels of triglyceride-related lipids and lower levels of high-density lipoprotein (HDL)-related lipids were independently associated with incident PAD in the ARIC study.[48] In a case-control study of 14,916 male physicians that examined lipid biomarkers, the ratio of total cholesterol to HDL-C was the strongest predictor of risk for PAD (RR 3.9; 95% CI 1.7–8.6).[49]

Differences in the prevalence, management, and outcomes for PAD differ between the sexes. The cross-sectional part of the German Epidemiological Trial on Ankle Brachial Index (getABI) study examined the ABIs of over 6000 consecutive, unselected patients and found that before age 70, males have a higher prevalence of PAD than females (17% vs. 12%), but prevalence was higher in females in the population older than 85 years (39% vs. 27%).[50] Although there is an increased prevalence in males from high-income countries, females from lower-income countries experience PAD at up to two times the rate of males.[12] Females are at increased risk of asymptomatic PAD, are less likely to be prescribed optimal medical therapy, and are more likely to present with more severe disease.[51] Additionally, females have an increased incidence of postprocedural complications, including access site complications, pedal access failures, surgical bleeding, wound complications, and perioperative infections.[52,53]

Studies have sought to define the association of race and ethnicity with risk of PAD and outcomes. A review of studies from 1999–2022 found that Black patients with PAD and DM had an increased risk of amputation and underwent fewer revascularization procedures than White patients.[54] Black race was found to be an independent risk factor for major amputation when controlling for comorbid conditions, PAD severity, and medication use as compared with White patients from similar socioeconomic strata.[55] Even with successful revascularization, Black patients with CLTI are 1.5 to 2 times more likely to require a major amputation.[56] Hispanic patients with CLTI also have worse outcomes when compared with non-Hispanic White patients. In a study of Hispanic patients hospitalized for lower extremity PAD, Hispanic patients were noted to have a higher burden of comorbid conditions, including DM, ESRD, and previous amputations; presented with more severe PAD; had lower rates of revascularization; and had higher rates of amputations.[57]

Socioeconomic status has been identified as an important determinant of health and outcomes in PAD patients. Patients with lower socioeconomic status have been shown to be at increased risk for the development of PAD, attributed to the increased prevalence of PAD risk factors in this population, decreased access to care, and underutilization of secondary prevention measures, leading to increased rates of amputation and decreased postoperative survival.[58] In patients undergoing infrainguinal revascularization for PAD, patients from more disadvantaged neighborhoods, as defined by the area deprivation index (ADI), a measure created by the Health Resources and Services Administration using census data, presented with more advanced disease and underwent lower rates of revascularization.[59] Among 958,120 CLTI patients in the Nationwide Inpatient Sample, PAD patients in the lowest income quartile had 34% higher odds of undergoing amputation as compared with patients in the highest income quartile.[60]

Other risk factors for PAD include hypertriglyceridemia, elevated serum fibrinogen, and hyperhomocysteinemia. Nonconventional risk factors also linked to be linked to PAD include elevated inflammatory markers, human immunodeficiency virus, exposure to lead and cadmium, and depression.

CLINICAL PRESENTATION OF PERIPHERAL ARTERY DISEASE

PAD can result in a range of clinical presentations, the severity of which can be assessed with a detailed history and physical examination. History should include location and duration of symptoms, progression of symptoms over time, walking impairment and associated disability, modifying factors, skin changes, and slow-to-heal wounds. Past medical history should assess risk factors for development of PAD, including tobacco use, HTN, hyperlipidemia, DM, history of CAD, CKD, prior revascularizations, personal or family history of aneurysmal disease, embolic events, or hypercoagulable states.

IC describes cramping or aching pain in the muscles of the leg that occurs with activity but is not present at rest. This is a result of the increased oxygen demand of the muscles while walking, which cannot be met because of the presence of upstream arterial stenoses or occlusions. Claudication symptoms are often reliably reproducible, with patients often able to specify the exact distance at which symptoms arise. Symptoms may occur more quickly by walking uphill or at a faster pace and typically resolve with a short period of rest. One muscle group distal to the area of arterial disease is usually affected, with aortoiliac pathology causing symptoms in the buttocks and thighs, whereas femoral-popliteal disease results in calf claudication. Leriche syndrome describes the triad of IC, absent femoral pulses, and impotence secondary to aortoiliac occlusive disease (AIOD).[61]

Vasculogenic claudication must be differentiated from other conditions that can induce leg pain with exertion, including spinal stenosis, nerve root compression, arthritis, and chronic compartment syndrome. Although vascular and neurologic etiologies of leg pain can coexist, neurogenic conditions are often more variable in onset and may take longer to resolve; symptoms may arise from standing alone and can often be relieved by changes in position.

Ischemic rest pain and tissue loss are symptoms of advanced PAD, termed *CLTI*. Rest pain occurs in the forefoot, typically worsens with leg elevation, and improves when the limb is in a dependent position. Patients may report that they sleep with the affected extremity dangling off the bed because the increase in pedal blood pressure secondary to gravity may provide sufficient pain relief. Ischemic rest pain is more commonly observed in smokers, likely as a result of the coexistent peripheral sensory neuropathy that may mask symptoms in diabetics. Diabetic neuropathy, gout, and degenerative joint disease may also cause symptoms similar to rest pain. In CLTI, tissue loss involves ulceration or gangrene of the lower leg or foot present for more than 2 weeks in duration and occurs along with objective evidence of arterial insufficiency severe enough to impede wound healing.

Observation of the extremities should note temperature changes, absence of hair growth and dry skin caused by apocrine gland dysfunction, signs of muscle atrophy, changes in color, dependent rubor, elevation pallor, and presence of ulcerations or gangrene. Peripheral pulses (carotid, brachial, radial, ulnar, femoral, popliteal, dorsalis pedis [DP], PT) should be palpated. Nonpalpable pulses, as well as prominent pulses in the abdomen,

femoral, and popliteal regions, which may suggest presence of an aneurysm, should be noted. The neck, abdomen, and groin should be auscultated for bruits. Loss of protective sensation in patients with neuropathy should be assessed with Semmes-Weinstein monofilament test, and the probe-to-bone test should be performed in patients with ulcers.[62]

DIAGNOSTIC MODALITIES IN PERIPHERAL ARTERY DISEASE

In patients suspected to have PAD, lower extremity noninvasive studies performed in a vascular laboratory can confirm the diagnosis and guide further workup and treatment (Figs. 103.3 and 103.4). These include the ankle-brachial index (ABI), segmental pressures, toe pressures, pulse volume recordings (PVRs), and tibial Doppler waveforms. Transcutaneous oximetry ($TcPO_2$) is used to determine whether blood flow to the area of interest is sufficient for healing to take place. These noninvasive studies can assist in quantifying the degree of arterial insufficiency and localize the level of stenoses or occlusions.[63] Imaging studies such as arterial duplex, computed tomography angiography (CTA),

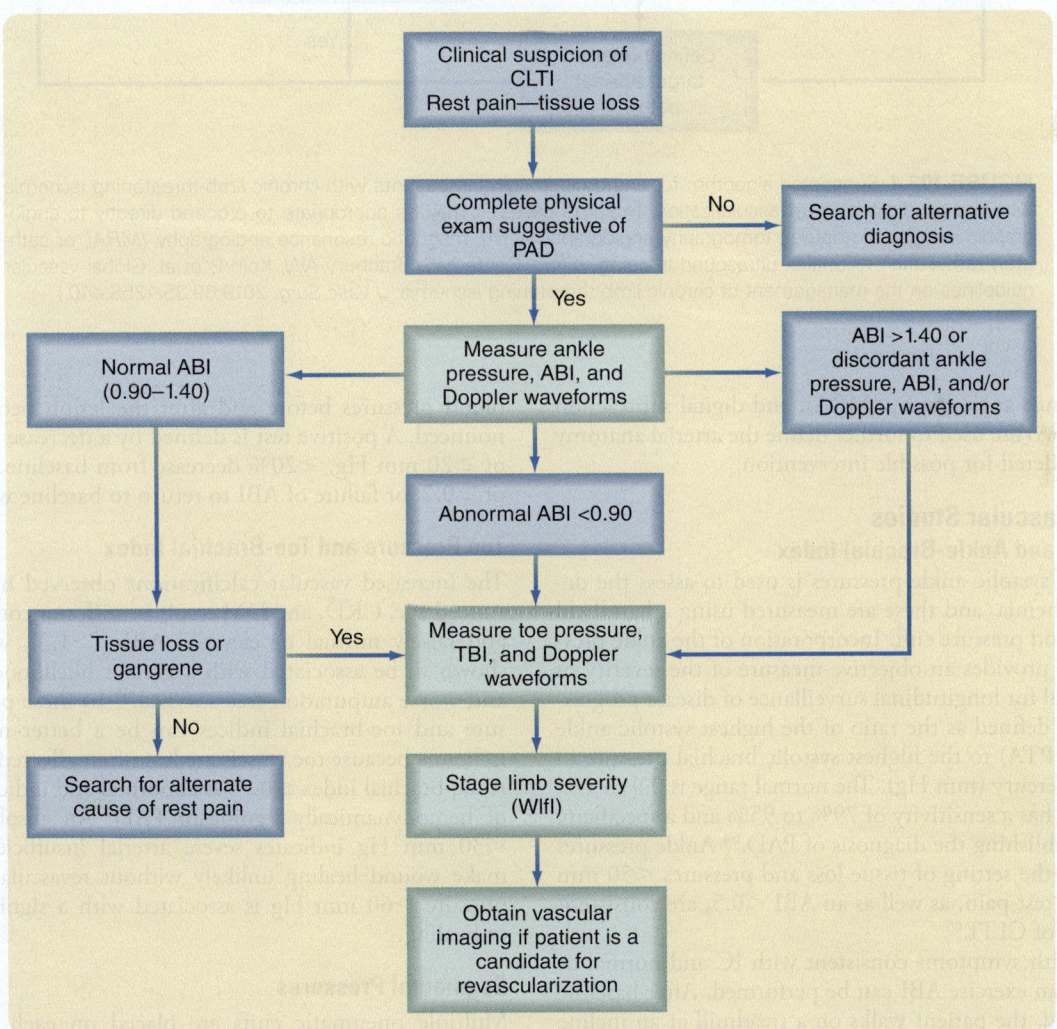

FIGURE 103.3 Flow diagram for the investigation of patients presenting with suspected chronic limb-threatening ischemia *(CLTI)*. *ABI*, Ankle-brachial index; *PAD*, peripheral artery disease; *TBI*, toe-brachial index; *WIfI*, wound, ischemia, and foot infection. (From Conte MS, Bradbury AW, Kolh P, et al. Global vascular guidelines on the management of chronic limb-threatening ischemia. *J Vasc Surg.* 2019;69:3S-125S.e40.)

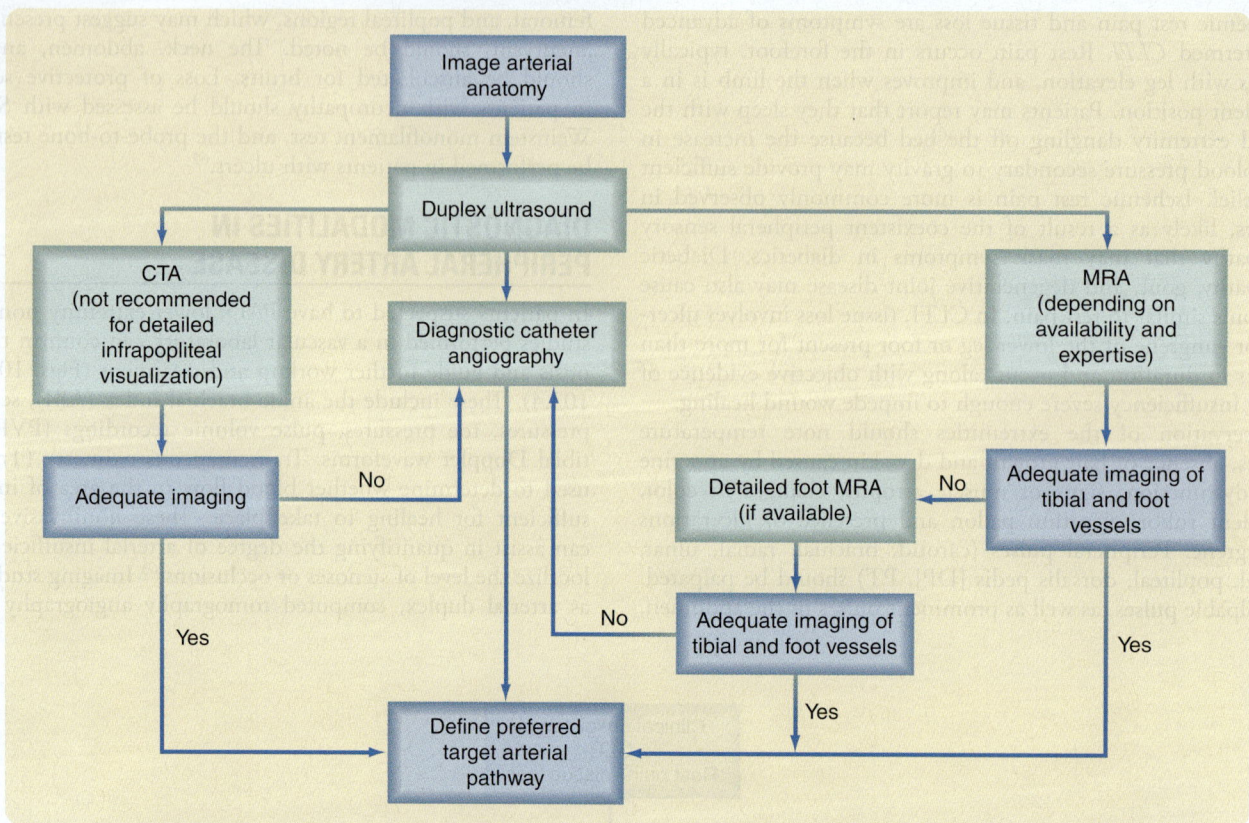

FIGURE 103.4 Suggested algorithm for anatomic imaging in patients with chronic limb-threatening ischemia who are candidates for revascularization. In some cases, it may be appropriate to proceed directly to angiographic imaging (computed tomography angiography [CTA], magnetic resonance angiography [MRA], or catheter) rather than to duplex ultrasound imaging. (From Conte MS, Bradbury AW, Kolh P, et al. Global vascular guidelines on the management of chronic limb-threatening ischemia. *J Vasc Surg.* 2019;69:3S-125S.e40.)

magnetic resonance angiography (MRA), and digital subtraction angiography (DSA) are used to further define the arterial anatomy in patients considered for possible intervention.

Noninvasive Vascular Studies

Ankle Pressure and Ankle-Brachial Index

Measurement of systolic ankle pressures is used to assess the degree of distal ischemia, and these are measured using a handheld Doppler and blood pressure cuff. Incorporation of the ankle pressures in the ABI provides an objective measure of the severity of PAD and is useful for longitudinal surveillance of disease progression. The ABI is defined as the ratio of the highest systolic ankle pressure (DP or PTA) to the highest systolic brachial pressure in millimeters of mercury (mm Hg). The normal range is 0.9 to 1.2. An ABI of <0.9 has a sensitivity of 79% to 95% and a specificity of >95% in establishing the diagnosis of PAD.[64] Ankle pressures <70 mm Hg in the setting of tissue loss and pressures <50 mm Hg for ischemic rest pain, as well as an ABI <0.5, are consistent with a diagnosis of CLTI.[65]

In patients with symptoms consistent with IC and normal or borderline ABI, an exercise ABI can be performed. After baseline ABIs are recorded, the patient walks on a treadmill at an incline for 5 minutes or until limited by pain, and immediately after finishing this activity, the ABI is measured. During exercise, peripheral vascular resistance decreases, allowing increased blood flow to the muscles. In the setting of stenosis, the differential in

blood pressures before and after the lesion becomes more pronounced. A positive test is defined by a decrease in ankle pressure of ≥20 mm Hg, ≥20% decrease from baseline, decrease of ABI of ≥0.2, or failure of ABI to return to baseline within 3 minutes.

Toe Pressure and Toe-Brachial Index

The increased vascular calcifications observed in patients of advanced age, CKD, and DM result in stiff, noncompressible vessels and falsely normal or elevated ABIs (>1.3), which have been shown to be associated with a greater likelihood of amputation and worse amputation-free survival.[66] In these patients, toe pressure and toe-brachial indices can be a better measure of distal ischemia because toe vessels are less often affected by calcification. A toe-brachial index ≤0.75 is abnormal and indicates the presence of hemodynamically significant PAD. An absolute toe pressure <30 mm Hg indicates severe arterial insufficiency that would make wound healing unlikely without revascularization.[67] A toe pressure >60 mm Hg is associated with a significant likelihood of healing.

Segmental Pressures

Multiple pneumatic cuffs are placed on each extremity (high thigh, above knee, below knee, and proximal to the ankle), and the arterial pressure at each level is measured using continuous-wave Doppler at the DP as the cuff is deflated. The location of occlusive lesions can be estimated by comparison of the pressures, with a drop in pressure of ≥ 20 mm Hg between any two levels considered to be hemodynamically significant.

Pulse Volume Recordings

PVR waveforms are obtained using partially inflated air-filled cuffs that detect changes in volume in the limb transmitted from the arterial pulse wave. Normal waveforms have a sharp systolic upstroke, narrow peak, and downstroke toward baseline, with a prominent dicrotic notch. Occlusive disease results in delay of the systolic upstroke, rounded peak, and loss of the dicrotic notch, whereas more severe disease leads to decreases in amplitude or absent waveforms.[68] Flat or minimally pulsatile PVRs in forefoot are associated with CLTI.[69] The combination of segmental limb pressures and PVRs is reported to have a diagnostic accuracy of 97% in patients suspected to have PAD.[64]

Doppler Waveforms

The arterial waveform can also provide information on the extent of disease. Doppler waveforms are measured at the anterior tibial (AT) and posterior tibial (PT) locations with a continuous Doppler probe. The normal spectral waveform is triphasic, with a sharp systolic upstroke and early diastolic flow reversal, and has a late diastolic return to antegrade flow. Arterial atherosclerosis leads to loss of vascular elasticity, and this results in a loss of phasicity. Multiphasic waveforms in which the waveform crosses the zero-flow baseline and has forward and reverse velocity components become monophasic, and the waveform does not cross the baseline during any part of the cardiac cycle. In the extremity, biphasic and triphasic waveforms are considered normal. Monophasic waveforms are indicative of at least a moderate degree of ischemia.[65]

Transcutaneous Partial Pressure of Oxygen

$TcPO_2$ is a metabolic test that can help to assess local tissue perfusion and estimate chance of potential healing. Skin sensors are applied to selected areas, and the oxygen diffuses from the capillaries through the epidermis to the electrode. A normal $TcPO_2$ is around 60 mm Hg; however, numerous factors can affect the accuracy of measurements, including temperature, skin condition, circulatory status, location of the sensors, patient positioning, and causes of vasoconstriction (e.g., caffeine, smoking, pain, or anxiety).[70] For the test to be interpretable, a control baseline value measured at the chest needs to be >60 mm Hg. Although there is no consensus as to $TcPO_2$ cutoff value to guarantee amputation healing, $TcPO_2$ <30 mm Hg has been associated with failure of healing.[70] $TcPO_2$ ≥ 40 mm Hg in patients undergoing below-the-knee amputation (BKA) was associated with lower 1-year freedom from conversion to AKA.[71]

Imaging
Arterial Duplex

Arterial duplex is widely available, is noninvasive, and can be used to define the arterial anatomy and estimate the degree of stenoses by using both brightness mode (B-mode) and Doppler ultrasound. B-mode is gray-scale ultrasound that is used to localize and characterize plaque as well as measure vessel diameters. The velocity of blood flow is estimated using Doppler, or pulsed-wave ultrasound. Between two points in a nondiseased artery, the blood flow should be equal. As the cross-sectional area of the vessel decreases as a result of stenoses, the velocity increases proportionally to maintain flow. This luminal narrowing results in an increased peak systolic velocity (PSV) as compared with the normal adjacent proximal segment.

The ratio of increase in the PSV corresponds to the degree of stenosis: In <50% stenosis, the PSV is elevated but less than double the normal adjacent proximal segment (ratio <2); a PSV velocity ratio >2 indicates a 50% to 74% stenosis; and a >75% stenosis will display a fourfold increase in PSV.[72]

Additionally, spectral broadening is observed in diseased arteries as a result of the presence of turbulent, nonlaminar blood flow. Duplex is used to plan interventions for symptomatic PAD and is also used as part of regular surveillance after revascularization to monitor development and progression of stenosis.

Computed Tomography Angiography and Magnetic Resonance Angiography

CTA and MRA represent cross-sectional imaging that may be considered when planning intervention, especially when aortoiliac disease is suspected, as in a patient with an absent femoral pulse. The utility of CTA is limited when imaging smaller, distal, calcified lower extremity vessels frequently found in patients with CLTI because calcification impairs definitive lesion characterization as a result of artifact. However, advances in imaging technology, such as the use of dual-energy CTA with postprocessing bone removal protocols[73,74] and use of ultra-high-resolution CT with subtraction techniques,[75] are improving the assessment of stenosis in PAD patients.

MRA avoids exposure to ionizing radiation but requires longer acquisition times. In a meta-analysis comparing contrast-enhanced MRA, duplex sonography, and CTA, MRA was the most accurate diagnostic technique for the detection of lesions with >50% stenosis.[76] The ability of MRA to image blood flow as slow as 2 cm/s improves the diagnostic quality in imaging the infrapopliteal vessels as well as in identifying potential bypass targets not visualized by DSA in diabetic patients.[77,78] Novel magnetic resonance imaging techniques are also emerging that allow for assessment of plaque composition and assessment of skeletal muscle perfusion as well as methods that do not require the use of contrast media.[79]

Digital Subtraction Angiography

DSA is a fluoroscopic technique used to visualize the arterial anatomy using intraarterial injection of contrast dye and x-rays, where the images acquired after contrast injection are subtracted from the images acquired before injection. Angiography is an invasive procedure that carries risk of complications; however, it has the advantage of the ability to perform concurrent therapeutic endovascular interventions at the time of image acquisition. Intravascular ultrasound (IVUS) can also be used as an adjunct during angiography to measure arterial dimensions to help size angioplasty balloons and stents as well as to assess results after intervention.

NONINTERVENTIONAL MANAGEMENT OF PERIPHERAL ARTERIAL DISEASE

The noninterventional management of PAD is critically important. Aggressive treatment of cardiovascular comorbidities prevents progressively worsening atherosclerosis and reduces MACEs, a composite end point of nonfatal stroke, nonfatal myocardial infarction (MI), and cardiovascular death. Furthermore, patients who are medically optimized have better surgical outcomes when patients require revascularization. After revascularization, there are also specific antithrombotic therapies that reduce major adverse limb events (MALEs), including reinterventions and amputations. In addition to optimal medical management, risk factor modification also includes smoking cessation and exercise therapy.

Antithrombotic Therapy

In the PAD population, multiple randomized controlled trials (RCTs) have demonstrated the benefit of single-antiplatelet therapy for secondary prevention to reduce the risk of MI, stroke, and death.[80,81] In asymptomatic PAD patients, there are conflicting data regarding the use of antiplatelet agents for primary prevention in the absence of CAD or CVD.[82] However, given the high proportion of patients with PAD and subclinical CAD, single-antiplatelet therapy may be a reasonable treatment in asymptomatic patients with reduced ABI and low bleeding risk.[83] Additionally, the patients with PAD and concomitant CAD have higher composite rates of MACE (15.3% vs. 8.9%, HR 1.50, 95% CI 1.13–1.99, $p = 0.005$),[84] and patients with a prior MI and PAD have double the cardiovascular risk than those with PAD alone (8.4% vs. 19.3%, $p < 0.001$), highlighting the importance of cardiovascular risk mitigation.[83,85]

Confusion arose in 2022 when the US Preventive Services Task Force (USPSTF) issued new guidance regarding the use of aspirin for primary prevention of MACE in the general adult population, reporting only a small net benefit of acetylsalicylic acid (ASA) in patients 40 to 59 years with a ≥10% 10-year risk of cardiovascular disease and recommending against initiation of ASA in patients ≥60 years.[86] Patients with PAD do not have the same risk profile as the general adult population, and expert consensus is that all patients diagnosed with PAD, who do not have a contraindication, should be prescribed antithrombotic medication. In general, the more significant the burden of atherosclerotic polyvascular disease, the more intensive the antithrombotic treatment strategy.

Although aspirin, a cyclooxygenase 1 inhibitor, is the most frequently used antiplatelet agent, alternative antiplatelet agents such as the P2Y12 receptor antagonists, clopidogrel and ticagrelor, have demonstrated benefit in certain groups. The Clopidogrel Versus Aspirin in Patients at Risk of Ischemic Events (CAPRIE) trial of patients with stable atherosclerotic cardiovascular disease found that in the subset of patients with symptomatic PAD, clopidogrel was associated with fewer cardiovascular events (3.71% average event rate per year in the clopidogrel group vs. 4.86% in the aspirin group).[87] Therefore, in patients with symptomatic PAD, treatment with a single antiplatelet agent, aspirin (75–325 mg/day) or clopidogrel (75 mg/day), is recommended to reduce MACE.[63] Clopidogrel may be the preferred agent in current smokers with PAD because it has been associated with a greater reduction of events than aspirin in patients treated with a single antiplatelet agent.[88] In the Examining Use of Ticagrelor in Peripheral Artery Disease (EUCLID) trial, ticagrelor demonstrated similar benefit to clopidogrel monotherapy in preventing MACE in symptomatic PAD patients (HR 1.02, 95% CI 0.92–1.13, $p = 0.65$), which may highlight a role for ticagrelor in poor clopidogrel metabolizers.[34,84]

Dual-antiplatelet therapy (DAPT) using aspirin in combination with a P2Y12 receptor antagonist has also been investigated. DAPT using clopidogrel plus aspirin in the Clopidogrel for High Atherothrombotic Risk and Ischemic Stabilization Management and Avoidance (CHARISMA) trial was not significantly more effective than aspirin alone in reducing MACE in PAD patients and was associated with increased bleeding risk.[89] However, among PAD patients with a history of prior MI, the addition of ticagrelor to low-dose aspirin reduced MACEs and MALEs in the PEGASUS-TIMI 54 study.[90] The extrapolation of data from coronary literature and the use of DAPT in device trials has led to

the use of DAPT after peripheral interventions; however, clear data to support its use are lacking.[91]

Low-dose oral anticoagulants have shown benefit in patients with PAD. The subset of 6391 participants with lower extremity PAD included in the Cardiovascular Outcomes for People Using Anticoagulation Strategies (COMPASS) trial demonstrated that rivaroxaban 2.5 mg twice daily plus ASA compared with ASA alone reduced the risk of MACE (5.1% vs. 6.9%, $p = 0.005$) and MALE (1.5% vs. 2.6%, HR 0.57, 95% CI 0.37–0.88).[92] The Vascular Outcomes Study of ASA Along with Rivaroxaban in Endovascular of Surgical Limb Revascularization for PAD (VOYAGER-PAD) randomized 6564 patients undergoing infrainguinal endovascular or surgical revascularization to aspirin and rivaroxaban 2.5 mg twice daily or aspirin and placebo. The rivaroxaban and aspirin group significantly reduced the primary composite end point of ALI, major amputation, MI, ischemic stroke, or cardiovascular death (HR 0.85, 95% CI 0.76–0.96, $p = 0.009$), irrespective of revascularization strategy.[93] A meta-analysis of the PAD patients in the COMPASS and VOYAGER trials concluded that low-dose rivaroxaban plus aspirin was superior to aspirin alone in reducing cardiovascular and limb outcomes, including ALI and major amputation.[94]

When prescribing anticoagulants, even at low doses, potential benefit must be balanced with bleeding risk. Although major bleeding was increased in patients treated with rivaroxaban in both the COMPASS and VOYAGER-PAD trials, fatal or critical organ bleeding was not significantly different.[93,95] In patients without elevated bleeding risk, dual therapy with aspirin and low-dose rivaroxaban is reasonable, but the bleeding risk associated with full-dose anticoagulation outweighs any benefit in reducing adverse cardiac or limb events, and its routine use is recommended against.[63]

Glycemic Control

DM is a significant risk factor for the development and progression of atherosclerosis and PAD, with the severity of disease correlated to long-term glucose control. Regardless of how blood glucose is controlled, having a robust strategy in place to stabilize and control DM improves short-term revascularization outcomes and reduces MALE.[96,97] Tight glucose control has been shown to decrease microvascular complications in the short term and can reduce macrovascular complications, such as cardiovascular outcomes, when maintained over decades.[98,99] Newer studies have shown benefit of sodium-glucose transporter-2 inhibitor (SGLT2i) and glucagon-like peptide (GLP)-1 receptor agonists in reducing cardiovascular mortality, heart failure, renal complications, MACE, and amputation.[100]

A target HbA1c of <7% is recommended by Global Vascular Guidelines for CLTI[69]; however, the International Working Group on the Diabetic Foot (IWGDF) guidelines suggest a higher target HbA1c of <8% because of the risk of hypoglycemia with tighter glucose control.[66] This highlights the need for glucose targets to be individualized based on age, duration of DM, complications, comorbid conditions, and hypoglycemia risk.[66]

Lipid-Lowering Therapy

Statins have been demonstrated to reduce mortality, major adverse cardiovascular outcomes, and MALEs and improve symptomatic outcomes in patients with PAD.[101] Additionally, statins have pleiotropic effects, including improved endothelial function, inhibition of smooth muscle proliferation, plaque stabilization, and reduced platelet aggregation.[102] Therapy with a high-intensity statin, simvastatin 80 mg/day, or rosuvastatin 40 mg/day to achieve an LDL goal of <70 mg/dL is recommended in all patients with PAD. A National Veterans Health Administration population-based study of 155,647 patients demonstrated that use of a high-intensity statin at the time of PAD diagnosis was associated with a significant reduction in both limb loss and mortality.[103]

In patients with persistently elevated LDL despite the maximally tolerated statin dose, consideration should be given to the addition of ezetimibe, which reduces LDL cholesterol absorption in the small intestine and has been shown to lower cardiovascular event rates.[104,105] For patients receiving maximally tolerated statin and ezetimibe who cannot reach the LDL goal, proprotein convertase subtilisin/kexin type 9 (PCSK9) inhibitors, monoclonal antibodies that increase hepatic LDL receptors, can be added to decrease LDL, reduce cardiovascular events, and reduce the risk of major adverse lower extremity events.[105,106]

Hypertension Control

The primary goal of treating elevated blood pressure in patients with PAD is to reduce MACE; however, there are few specific trials evaluating blood pressure goals in patients with PAD. Angiotensin-converting enzyme (ACE) inhibitors and angiotensin-receptor blockers have demonstrated benefit in reducing the risk of cardiovascular ischemic events in PAD patients.[46] Analysis of the PAD subgroup in the Heart Outcomes Prevention Evaluation (HOPE) trial found that patients treated with ramipril had a 25% reduction of MI, stroke, and cardiovascular death versus placebo.[107] However, in the Ongoing Telmisartan Alone and in Combination With Ramipril Global Endpoint Trial (ONTARGET), telmisartan had similar efficacy to ramipril in PAD patients with less angioedema, representing a role for angiotensin-receptor blockers as an alternative to ACE inhibitors.[108] Beyond that, it is clear that patients who consistently have SBP >140 mm Hg and diastolic blood pressure >90 mm Hg require antihypertensive medications, and cardiology guidelines increasingly support much lower targets.[109,110]

Smoking Cessation

In patients with PAD, smoking cessation is associated with decreased mortality and improved amputation-free survival.[45] Smoking status should be assessed at every visit, and patients should be counseled on quitting as well as provided options for pharmacologic therapy and referral to a smoking cessation program. Several studies have demonstrated that varenicline, bupropion, and nicotine replacement therapy, used alone or in combination, all increase smoking cessation rates.[63] Additionally, intensive smoking cessation intervention, consisting of behavioral and pharmacologic components, resulted in more successful smoking cessation at 6 months than minimal intervention (21.3% vs. 6.8%).[111]

Exercise

Exercise is the most effective noninterventional approach to reducing leg symptoms in patients with IC.[112] Exercise has been demonstrated to have benefits for patients with PAD, including increased calf blood flow, improved endothelial function, improved metabolic function, decreased inflammation, and improved walking distances.[112] A Cochrane review examining 32 RCTs, including 1835 patients with IC, concluded that exercise programs provided improved pain-free and maximum walking distance as compared with placebo or usual care.[113] Additionally, in a meta-analysis of 25 RCTs, supervised treadmill exercise was demonstrated to improve walking performance in PAD patients by approximately 180 m compared with no exercise.[114] As of 2017, the Centers for Medicare and Medicaid Services deemed that there was sufficient

evidence for the benefit of supervised exercise therapy that beneficiaries with walking impairment secondary to PAD are eligible for insurance coverage of up to 36 sessions over a 12-week period.[115]

Although less effective, evidence also supports home-based walking exercise to improve walking performance as a reasonable alternative for patients without access to supervised exercise therapy.[116] General recommendations for patients are to perform a minimum of 45 to 60 minutes of exercise three times per week for 12 weeks, typically walking on a treadmill, and effort should be sufficiently intense to elicit claudication.

Cilostazol

Based on a Cochrane review of 16 RCTs, in addition to exercise, a 3-month trial of cilostazol (100 mg twice daily) is recommended to improve pain-free walking in patients with IC.[64] Cilostazol, a reversible phosphodiesterase IIIa inhibitor, acts as a vasodilator, inhibits platelet aggregation, and improves walking distance, but it is contraindicated in patients with congestive heart failure. Patient noncompliance may be attributable to commonly reported side effects of headache, diarrhea, dizziness, and palpitations.

Medical and lifestyle management are recommended as first-line treatment for PAD; however, in a retrospective review of 3829 patients undergoing elective open lower extremity bypass for IC, only 47.6% of patients were on optimal medical therapy before surgery.[117] Similar findings were observed among the 1404 CLTI patients enrolled in the PREVENT III trial, where 33% of patients were not on any antiplatelet therapy at the time of study entry, and 54% were not receiving lipid-lowering therapy.[118] This demonstrates opportunities for improvement in the preoperative management of PAD patients because patients who were treated with optimal therapy had a lower risk of postoperative mortality, MI, and readmission.[117]

INTERVENTIONAL MANAGEMENT OF PERIPHERAL ARTERIAL DISEASE

Revascularization is defined as the restoration of perfusion to an area of ischemia. Goals of revascularization are to relieve pain, heal wounds, preserve a functional limb, and prevent a major amputation. Techniques for revascularization have continued to evolve though history. Open surgical revascularization techniques were pioneered by Alexis Carrel, who received the 1912 Nobel Prize for his methods of sewing blood vessels together to create vascular anastomoses. Jean Kunlin, in 1948, used these techniques to perform a femoral-popliteal bypass with saphenous vein, thereby ushering in the era of surgical revascularization for PAD.[119] Less invasive techniques for revascularization subsequently emerged. Sven-Ivar Seldinger described percutaneous vascular access over a wire and insertion of a soft catheter to opacify and visualize peripheral arteries in 1953.[120] The landmark contributions of Charles Dotter, including the introduction of percutaneous transluminal angioplasty in 1964, form the foundation of endovascular therapies today.[121]

Open surgical procedures for the treatment of PAD include inflow bypasses, infrainguinal bypasses, and endarterectomy. AIOD can be treated with direct aortic reconstruction with an aortofemoral bypass, most often using a prosthetic conduit, Dacron, or expanded polytetrafluoroethylene (PTFE), to bypass from the aorta to the common femoral artery (CFA), DFA, or superficial femoral artery (SFA). Extraanatomic reconstructions for the management of aortoiliac lesions include thoracofemoral bypass, axillofemoral bypass, and femoral-femoral bypass, which can be used to avoid infected regions or the hostile abdomen. *Infrainguinal bypass* is defined as any major arterial reconstruction using a bypass conduit, either autogenous or prosthetic, originating below the inguinal ligament. Short-segment occlusive disease involving the CFA and DFA is commonly treated with endarterectomy and patch angioplasty, in which the atherosclerotic plaque is peeled from the artery wall, and the arteriotomy is then repaired with a patch to prevent stenosis.

Endovascular techniques provide a less invasive method of revascularization. After percutaneous arterial access, a sheath is placed within the lumen of the vessel, through which wires directed by catheters are used to cross stenoses or occlusions remote to the access site. Once the lesion is traversed, balloon angioplasty, stenting, stent grafting, or atherectomy can then be used to restore luminal patency. Coating of balloons or stents with cytotoxic medications, such as paclitaxel or limus analogues, can decrease the risk of intraluminal neointimal formation. Such devices have been used clinically in PAD to decrease restenosis. Hybrid procedures, which combine both endovascular and open surgical techniques, can also be used in certain clinical scenarios.

Outcomes of revascularizations have historically reported patency rates. *Primary patency* is the term applied when patency of an intervention (bypass, angioplasty, stenting) is maintained over a specified time interval without reintervention. Successful reintervention on a patent but stenotic lesion is termed *primary assisted patency*, and restoration of patency of an occluded bypass or target vessel is termed *secondary patency*. In the setting of IC, measurement of walking distance has been used, whereas for CLTI, common end points include amputation, amputation-free survival, and MALE. Patient-centered outcome measures include a variety of qualitative instruments that examine quality of life, including the 12-Item Short-Form Survey (SF-12), EuroQol 5 Dimension (EQ-5D), and Vascular Quality of Life Questionnaire (VascuQoL).

TREATMENT OF ASYMPTOMATIC DISEASE AND INTERMITTENT CLAUDICATION

In the absence of a threatened bypass graft or stent, the Society for Vascular Surgery (SVS) guidelines recommend against invasive treatments for PAD in asymptomatic patients, regardless of hemodynamic measures or imaging findings.[64] The cornerstone of treatment for asymptomatic PAD is lifestyle change and medical therapy to address cardiovascular risk factors, with the goal of halting the progression of atherosclerosis in the limbs as well as in other vascular beds.

Despite having symptoms, patients with IC are still at relatively low risk of adverse outcomes, with a 5-year risk of limb amputation of 5% and a predicted 75% to 80% 5-year life expectancy.[64] The majority of patients with IC will maintain their current level of function or decline slowly; therefore, the preferred initial management strategy for such patients, in addition to optimal medical management, is supervised exercise therapy.[122] Approximately 20% to 30% of patients with IC will develop disability significant enough to warrant intervention.[64] In the treatment of patients with IC, interventions should only be undertaken in patients with lifestyle-altering symptoms, after failure of exercise and medical therapy, when anatomic factors are favorable, and prolonged patency and symptom relief are likely. The SVS issued appropriate use criteria for management of IC in 2022 to assist in appropriate shared decision-making with patients.

A systematic review of 10 RCTs that included 1087 patients with IC found that endovascular revascularization did not provide significant benefit as compared with supervised exercise alone in improvement in functional performance or quality-of-life metrics.[123] However, in patients with IC secondary to aortoiliac disease in the Claudication Exercise versus Endoluminal Revascularization (CLEVER) Trial, there was benefit to both supervised exercise and endovascular revascularization in improvement of functional status and quality of life.[124,125]

The appropriate use criteria also provide guidance for the treatment of patients with severe lifestyle limitations and short walking distance IC. Selected, low-risk, nonsmoking patients on optimal medical therapy may benefit from invasive therapy.[122] Invasive interventions for femoropopliteal disease should be reserved for patients with severe lifestyle-limiting IC. In these patients, when treating the CFA, open endarterectomy will provide greater net benefit than endovascular intervention. Invasive treatment of the tibial arteries in patients with IC is of unclear benefit and can lead to worsening of PAD and increased risk of limb loss.[122]

TREATMENT OF CHRONIC LIMB-THREATENING ISCHEMIA

In contrast to patients with IC, patients with CLTI have a 50% 5-year mortality and a much higher amputation risk, based primarily on the limb stage at presentation.[21] Limb classification systems have evolved, but they historically included the Fontaine[126] classification system, based solely on clinical symptoms, and the Rutherford[127] classification system, based on clinical symptoms and noninvasive data, with separation of chronic and ALI.

The Trans-Atlantic Inter-Society Consensus Document on Management of Peripheral Arterial Disease (TASC), published in 2000 and modified in 2007 as TASC II, sought to form a consensus in the classification and treatment of patients with PAD as well as provide a framework to compare revascularization strategies. TASC anatomically divided lesions into aortoiliac and femoral-popliteal segments, grouping lesion patterns based on the severity of occlusive disease (Figs. 103.5 and 103.6). In the treatment of both aortoiliac and femoral-popliteal lesions, surgical bypass was recommended for longer, more severe lesions (TASC C and D), whereas endovascular therapy was recommended for limited, focal disease (TASC A and B).[128]

The TASC classifications did not correlate with expected patency rates and outcomes of therapy,[69] and these older classification systems did not account for wound characteristics and presence and severity of infection, which are important considerations given the increasing prevalence of DM and the frequency of DFUs in the PAD population. To incorporate these factors, in 2014, the SVS developed the WIfI classification system, which is based on wound, ischemia, and foot infection at presentation and stratifies the degree of limb threat, thus guiding clinical management (Tables 103.1 and 103.2).[4] Each of the three factors is graded on an objective scale from 0 to 4, with the combinations grouped into four clinical stages (I–IV), which correlate with increasing 1-year risk of amputation. After intervention, treatment of infection, or suspected clinical deterioration, the WIfI score should be recalculated.[69]

A meta-analysis of 12 studies that included 2669 patients with CLTI demonstrated the prognostic value of the WIfI classification in predicting limb amputation.[129] A subset of five studies with 569 patients reported that 1-year amputation risk was shown to progressively increase with increasing WIfI stage: 0% for stage I, 8% (95% CI 3%–21%) for stage II, 11% (95% CI 6%–18%) for stage III, and 38% (95% CI 21%–58%) for stage IV.[129] A recent

Type A lesions

- Unilateral or bilateral stenoses of CIA
- Unilateral or bilateral single short (≤3 cm) stenosis of EIA

Type B lesions

- Short (≤3 cm) stenosis of infrarenal aorta
- Unilateral CIA occlusion
- Single or multiple stenosis totaling 3-10 cm involving the EIA not extending into the CFA
- Unilateral EIA occlusion not involving the origins of internal iliac of CFA

Type C lesions

- Bilateral CIA occlusions
- Bilateral EIA stenoses 3-10 cm long not extending into the CFA
- Unilateral EIA stenosis extending into the CFA
- Unilateral EIA occlusion that involves the origins of internal iliac and/or CFA
- Heavily calcified unilateral EIA occlusion with or without involvement of origins of internal iliac and/or CFA

Type D lesions

- Infrarenal aortoiliac occlusion
- Diffuse disease involving the aorta and both iliac arteries requiring treatment
- Diffuse multiple stenoses involving the unilateral CIA, EIA, and CFA
- Unilateral occlusions of both CIA and EIA
- Bilateral occlusion of EIA
- Iliac stenoses in patients with AAA requiring treatment and not amenable to endograft placement or other lesions requiring open aortic or iliac surgery

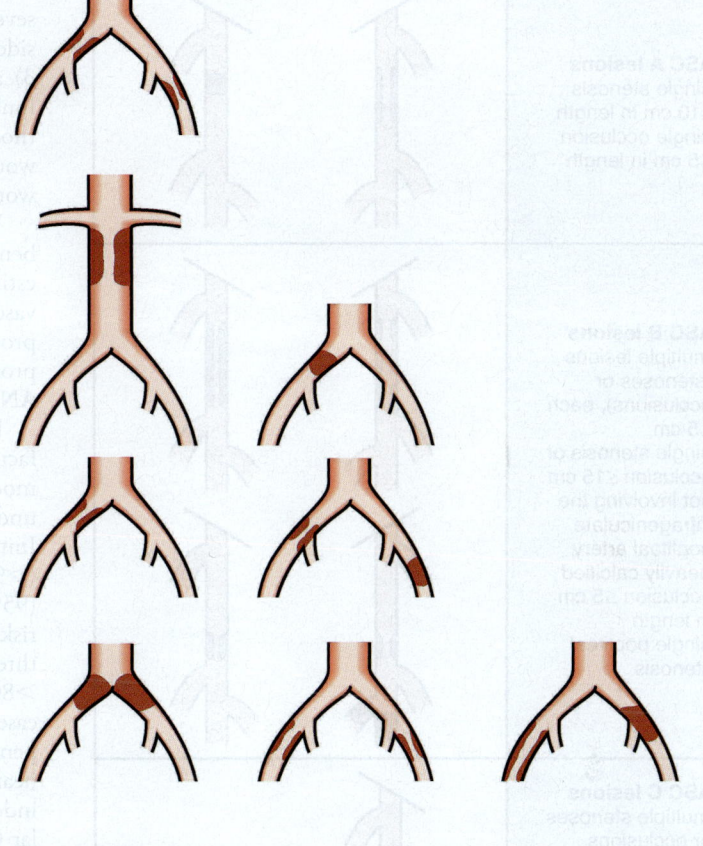

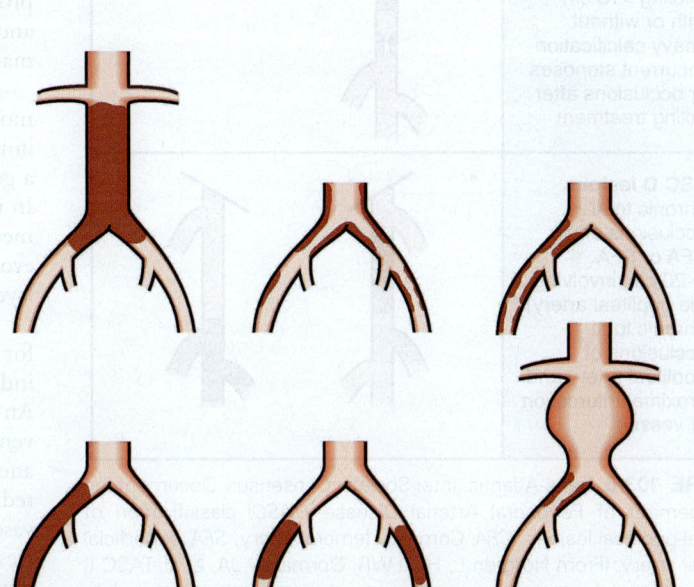

FIGURE 103.5 Trans-Atlantic Inter-Society Consensus Document on Management of Peripheral Arterial Disease classification of aortoiliac lesions. *AAA*, Abdominal aortic aneurysm; *CFA*, common femoral artery; *CIA*, common iliac artery; *EFA*, external femoral artery; *EIA*, external iliac artery. (From Norgren L, Hiatt WR, Dormandy JA, et al. TASC II Working Group. Inter-society consensus for the management of peripheral arterial disease [TASCII]. *J Vasc Surg.* 2007;45[suppl S]:S5-S61.)

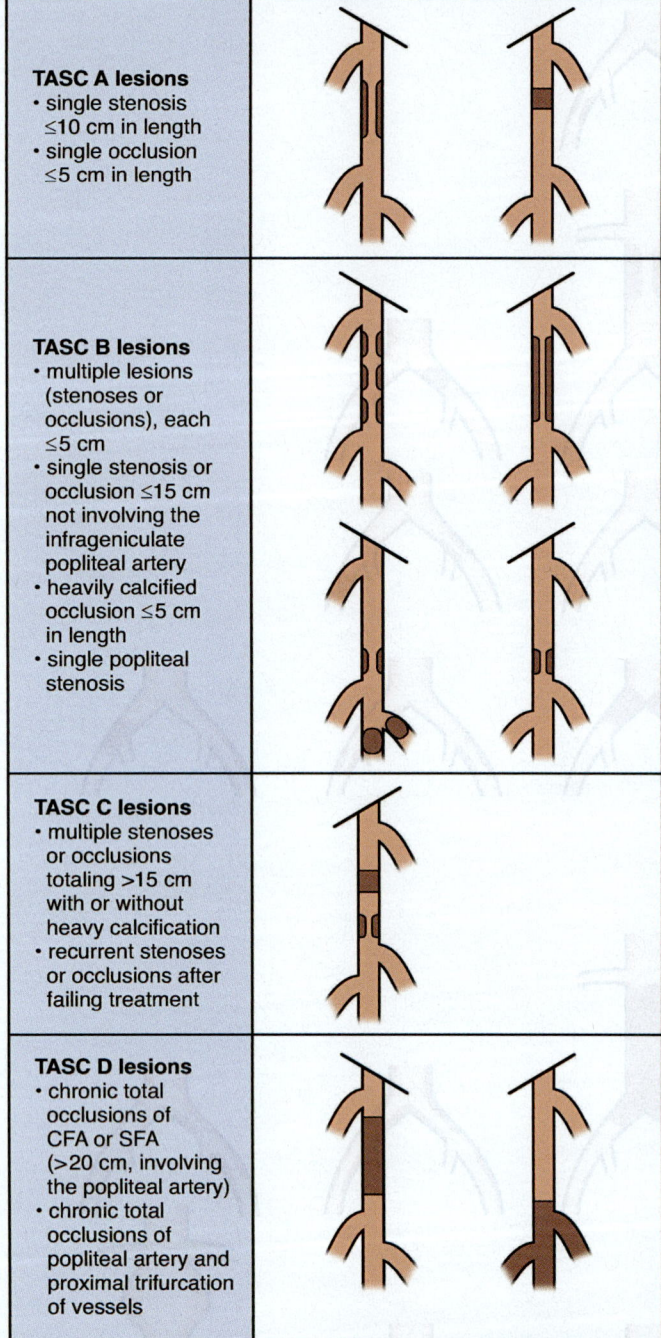

TASC A lesions
- single stenosis ≤10 cm in length
- single occlusion ≤5 cm in length

TASC B lesions
- multiple lesions (stenoses or occlusions), each ≤5 cm
- single stenosis or occlusion ≤15 cm not involving the infrageniculate popliteal artery
- heavily calcified occlusion ≤5 cm in length
- single popliteal stenosis

TASC C lesions
- multiple stenoses or occlusions totaling >15 cm with or without heavy calcification
- recurrent stenoses or occlusions after failing treatment

TASC D lesions
- chronic total occlusions of CFA or SFA (>20 cm, involving the popliteal artery)
- chronic total occlusions of popliteal artery and proximal trifurcation of vessels

FIGURE 103.6 Trans-Atlantic Inter-Society Consensus Document on Management of Peripheral Arterial Disease *(TASC)* classification of femoral-popliteal lesions. *CFA,* Common femoral artery; *SFA,* superficial femoral artery. (From Norgren L, Hiatt WR, Dormandy JA, et al. TASC II Working Group. Inter-society consensus for the management of peripheral arterial disease [TASCII]. *J Vasc Surg.* 2007;45[suppl S]:S5-S61.)

loss or infection (WIfI stage 4) in the presence of moderate to severe ischemia (grade 2 and 3). Revascularization should be considered in those with intermediate limb-threat (WIfI stages 2 and 3) and moderate to severe ischemia (grade 2 and 3), advanced limb threat (WIfI stage 4) with moderate ischemia (grade 1), and those with intermediate limb threat and moderate ischemia if the wound fails to reduce in size by ≥50% in 4 weeks despite optimal wound care, management of infection, and pressure offloading.[69]

When deciding on a treatment strategy in patients felt to benefit from revascularization, in addition to the limb stage, the estimated risk for intervention, life expectancy, and underlying vascular anatomy are integral components of the decision-making process. To aid in clinical decision-making, an integrated approach termed *PLAN* (**P**atient risk estimation, **L**imb staging, **AN**atomic pattern of disease) is recommended (Fig. 103.7).[69]

Estimation of operative risk and life expectancy are important factors to assess potential benefit of intervention. A predictive model based on the preoperative variables of 38,470 CLTI patients undergoing infrainguinal revascularization in the Vascular Quality Initiative (VQI) stratified patients into three risk groups: low-risk (>97% 30-day survival and >70% 2-year survival), medium-risk (95%–97% 30-day survival, 50%–70% 2-year survival), and high-risk (<95% 30-day survival, <50% 2-year survival).[131] Among all three models, independent predictors of death were found to be age >80 years, oxygen-dependent chronic obstructive pulmonary disease (COPD), stage V CKD, and bedbound status.[131] Other independent predictors include advanced age, CKD, CAD, congestive heart failure (CHF), DM, smoking, CVD, tissue loss, body mass index (BMI), dementia, and functional status.[69] The Global Vascular Guidelines group CLTI patients into average (anticipated periprocedural mortality <5% and estimated 2-year survival >50%) and high-risk (anticipated periprocedural mortality ≥5% and estimated 2-year survival ≤50%) cohorts.

Before any revascularization for CLTI, the patient's medical comorbidities should be evaluated and optimized. Although there are limited data specific to the management of CLTI patients with frailty, a geriatrics assessment and prehabilitation may also be indicated.[132] In the presence of a stable wound, it is appropriate to take time for medical optimization; however, in patients with ischemic rest pain or evolving wound, time is tissue, and intervention should only be delayed in patients with unstable angina or uncontrolled CHF.

With the availability of both open and endovascular strategies for revascularization, it is important to consider the underlying indication and technical details to help with operative planning. An advantage of endovascular revascularization is that most interventions can be performed without general anesthesia, using local anesthesia and conscious sedation, with minimal blood loss and reduced physiologic stress to the patient. However, results of endovascular intervention are often less durable than surgical bypass. Restenosis caused by neointimal hyperplasia is common after endovascular therapy, especially for complex and calcified lesions. Patients with CLTI often have long-segment and multilevel disease, which have inferior patency rates after endovascular intervention; however, the period of patency and improved perfusion may be long enough to heal an ischemic wound and may not require further intervention even in the setting of arterial reocclusion (Fig. 103.8). Conversely, patients with IC or ischemic rest pain will often have recurrence of symptoms when the intervention fails.[133]

Although the limb is staged with WIfI, the anatomic pattern and severity of the disease are classified using the Global Limb Anatomic Staging System (GLASS), and the availability of autogenous conduit is determined. Aortoiliac disease is assessed and

study found that presenting WIfI stage is also associated with long-term risk of major amputation and death after infrainguinal revascularization, with freedom from major amputation or death at 2 years in patients with WIfI stage 4 limbs reported to be 71% ± 3.7% and 68% ± 3.5%, respectively.[130]

The Global Vascular Guidelines recommend revascularization in the following clinical scenarios: symptomatic patients with severe (WIfI grade 3) ischemia and patients with advanced tissue

corrected if present. GLASS then classifies the disease from groin to foot using high-quality, usually angiographic, images to select the target arterial path (TAP) that is most likely to achieve in-line flow to the foot. The stenoses and occlusions in the femoro-popliteal and infrapopliteal segments are both graded on severity using a scale from 0 to 4 based on lesion length as well as ostial involvement and presence of significant calcification (Figs. 103.9 and 103.10). Pedal anatomy is taken into consideration with a modifier to describe the inframalleolar arteries (Fig. 103.11). The grades are then combined to create an anatomic stage ranging from I to III based on estimates of technical failure and 1-year limb-based patency (Table 103.3).

Patients with GLASS stage III have been demonstrated to have an almost fourfold increased risk of immediate technical failure after endovascular intervention as compared with GLASS stage I and II (RR 3.96, 95% CI 1.96–7.98) and an almost twofold risk of major amputation (RR 1.84, 95% CI 1.18–2.87).[134] Although worse outcomes in amputation-free survival, limb salvage rate, and MALE were observed after endovascular intervention in patients with GLASS stage III as compared with GLASS stages I and II, no difference was seen between the stages in patients undergoing bypass surgery.[135] This suggests that advanced GLASS stage favors bypass over endovascular revascularization (Fig. 103.12).

SELECTION OF REVASCULARIZATION STRATEGY

In patients with AIOD, the Trans-Atlantic Inter-Society Consensus (TASC) II guidelines published in 2007 recommended open surgical revascularization for TASC C and D lesions.[128] However, improvements in endovascular techniques have led to increased endovascular treatment of more complex occlusive lesions with high rates of technical success and secondary patency comparable to surgical repair.[136]

In comparing open surgical versus endovascular revascularization for AIOD, a meta-analysis of 11 observational studies that included 4030 patients with TASC C and D lesions found significantly improved primary patency at 50 months in the surgical group (91% vs. 81%, HR 0.51, CI 0.36–0.73, $p = 0.0002$).[137] Both techniques had similar limb salvage and secondary patency rates, and reported 30-day mortality rates were 2.9% in the open aortofemoral bypass group and 1.4% in the endovascular group.[137] The addition of a femoral endarterectomy has been shown to improve the primary patency of endovascular interventions for treatment of the aortoiliac segment, highlighting the importance of outflow to maintaining patency.[137] In an evolution from the 2007 TASC II classifications, the 2019 Global Vascular Guidelines support GLASS, which is a more nuanced classification. They suggest an endovascular-first approach for the treatment of CLTI in patients with AIOD from moderate to severe (GLASS stage IA) disease and a surgical reconstruction for average-risk patients with extensive (GLASS stage II) disease or after failed endovascular revascularization.[69]

In infrainguinal occlusive disease, there are three RCTs in patients with CLI that guide evidence-based treatment. Published in 2005, the Bypass Versus Angioplasty in Severe Ischaemia of the Leg (BASIL) trial, a randomized, controlled, multicenter trial

---

TABLE 103.1 Society for Vascular Surgery (SVS) Wound, Ischemia, and Foot Infection (WIfI) Lower Extremity Threatened Limb Classification System

I. **W**ound
II. **I**schemia
III. **F**oot infection
IV. **WIfI** score
V. W: **Wound/clinical category**
VI. SVS grades for rest pain and wounds/tissue loss (ulcers and gangrene):
VII. 0 (ischemic rest pain, ischemia grade 3, no ulcer), 1 (mild), 2 (moderate), 3 (severe)

GRADE	ULCER	GANGRENE
0	No ulcer	No gangrene
Clinical description: ischemic rest pain (requires typical symptoms + ischemia grade 3); no wound.		
1	Small, shallow ulcer(s) on distal leg or foot; no exposed bone, unless limited to distal phalanx	No gangrene
Clinical description: minor tissue loss. Salvageable with simple digital amputation (1 or 2 digits) or skin coverage.		
2	Deeper ulcer with exposed bone, joint, or tendon; generally not involving the heel; shallow heel ulcer, without calcaneal involvement	Gangrenous changes limited to digits
Clinical description: major tissue loss salvageable with multiple (≥3) digital amputations or standard TMA ± skin coverage.		
3	Extensive, deep ulcer involving forefoot and/or midfoot; deep, full thickness heel ulcer ± calcaneal involvement	Extensive gangrene involving forefoot and/or midfoot; full thickness heel necrosis ± calcaneal involvement
Clinical description: extensive tissue loss salvageable only with a complex foot reconstruction or nontraditional TMA (Chopart or Lisfranc); flap coverage or complex wound management needed for large soft tissue defect.		

GRADE	ABI	ANKLE SYSTOLIC PRESSURE	TP, TcPO₂
0	≥0.80	>100 mm Hg	≥60 mm Hg
1	0.6–0.79	70–100 mm Hg	40–59 mm Hg
2	0.4–0.59	50–70 mm Hg	30–39 mm Hg
3	≤0.39	<50 mm Hg	<30 mm Hg

Continued

TABLE 103.1   Society for Vascular Surgery (SVS)Wound, Ischemia, and Foot Infection (WIfI) Lower Extremity Threatened Limb Classification System—cont'd

CLINICAL MANIFESTATION OF INFECTION	SVS	IDSA/PEDIS INFECTION SEVERITY
No symptoms or signs of infection	0	Uninfected
Infection present, as defined by the presence of at least two of the following items: <ul><li>Local swelling or induration</li><li>Erythema >0.5 to ≤2 cm around the ulcer</li><li>Local tenderness or pain</li><li>Local warmth</li><li>Purulent discharge (thick, opaque to white, or sanguineous secretion)</li></ul>		
Local infection involving only the skin and the subcutaneous tissue (without involvement of deeper tissues and without systemic signs as described below)	1	Mild
Exclude other causes of an inflammatory response of the skin (e.g., trauma, gout, acute Charcot neuroosteoarthropathy, fracture, thrombosis, venous stasis)		
Local infection (as described above) with erythema >2 cm, or involving structures deeper than skin and subcutaneous tissues (e.g., abscess, osteomyelitis, septic arthritis, fasciitis), and no systemic inflammatory response signs (as described below)	2	Moderate
Local infection (as described above) with the signs of SIRS, as manifested by two or more of the following: <ul><li>Temperature >38°C or <36°C</li><li>Heart rate >90 beats/min</li><li>Respiratory rate >20 breaths/min or $PaCO_2$ <32 mm Hg</li><li>White blood cell count >12,000 or <4000 cu/mm or 10% immature (band) forms</li></ul>	3	Severe[a]

ABI, Ankle-brachial index; *IDSA*, Infectious Diseases Society of America; *PaCO₂*, partial pressure of arterial carbon dioxide; *PVR*, pulse volume recording; *SIRS*, systemic inflammatory response syndrome; *SPP*, skin perfusion pressure; *TcPO₂*, transcutaneous oximetry; *TMA*, transmetatarsal amputation; *TP*, toe pressure.

I: Ischemia
Hemodynamics/perfusion: Measure TP or $TcPO_2$ if ABI incompressible (>1.3).
SVS grades: 0 (none), 1 (mild), 2 (moderate), and 3 (severe).
Patients with diabetes should have TP measurements. If arterial calcification precludes reliable ABI or TP measurements, ischemia should be documented by TcPO₂, SPP, or PVR. If TP and ABI measurements result in different grades, TP will be the primary determinant of ischemia grade. Flat or minimally pulsatile forefoot PVR = grade 3.

fI: Foot Infection
SVS grades: 0 (none), 1 (mild), 2 (moderate), and 3 (severe: limb and/or life threatening).
SVS adaptation of IDSA and International Working Group on the Diabetic Foot (IWGDF) perfusion, extent/size, depth/tissue loss, infection, sensation (PEDIS) classifications of diabetic foot infection.
[a]Ischemia may complicate and increase the severity of any infection. Systemic infection may sometimes manifest with other clinical findings, such as hypotension, confusion, vomiting, or evidence of metabolic disturbances (e.g., acidosis, severe hyperglycemia, new-onset azotemia).
From Lipsky BA, Berendt AR, Cornia PB, et al. 2012 Infectious Diseases Society of America clinical practice guideline for the diagnosis and treatment of diabetic foot infections. *Clin Infect Dis.* 2012;54:e132-e173.

comparing open surgical bypass with autogenous vein to balloon angioplasty in the treatment of femoral-popliteal disease, reported no significant differences between the two groups in 6-month amputation-free survival.[138] However, among the 70% of patients who survived for 2 years after randomization, there was a significant increase in subsequent overall survival and a trend toward improved amputation-free survival in the patients initially undergoing open surgical bypass.[139] This highlights the importance of treatment durability and assessing life expectancy in the selection of revascularization strategy.

Almost two decades after the BASIL trial, two recent RCTs, the Best Endovascular Versus Best Surgical Therapy for Patients With Critical Limb Ischemia (BEST-CLI)[140] and the BASIL-2,[141] trial have sought to provide more evidence for the preferred revascularization strategy in patients with CLTI. BEST-CLI, a pragmatic international trial of 1830 patients completed across 150 centers, randomized patients to endovascular intervention versus open bypass surgery for the treatment of infrainguinal occlusive disease in patients who were candidates for both revascularization strategies. Patients were evaluated in two parallel cohorts depending on the availability of an adequate single-segment great saphenous vein (SSGSV), the best possible conduit for infrainguinal bypass. In the cohort of patients with SSGSV, open surgical bypass was associated with a significantly lower incidence of the composite primary outcome of MALE or all-cause death (42.6% vs. 57.4%, HR 0.68, 95% CI 0.59–0.79, $p < 0.001$).[140] These findings were attributable to a 65% increase in first major reinterventions in the endovascular group and a 27% reduction in limb amputation in the surgery group.[142] However, 20% to 45% of patients do not have adequate autogenous saphenous vein,[143] and among patients lacking optimal conduit, endovascular and open surgical therapy had similar rates of MALE and all-cause death.[140] The results from BEST-CLI support surgical revascularization as a first revascularization strategy in patients with adequate SSGSV and demonstrate that presence of an optimal conduit is an important factor to consider when determining a treatment strategy.

TABLE 103.2 Society for Vascular Surgery (SVS) Wound, Ischemia, and Foot Infection (WIfI) Clinical Limb Stage Based on Estimated Risk of Amputation at 1 Year

	ISCHEMIA—0				ISCHEMIA—1				ISCHEMIA—2				ISCHEMIA—3			
W-0	1	1	2	3	1	2	3	4	2	2	3	4	2	3	3	4
W-1	1	1	2	3	1	2	3	4	2	3	4	4	3	3	4	4
W-2	2	2	3	4	3	3	4	4	3	4	4	4	4	4	4	4
W-3	3	3	4	4	4	4	4	4	4	4	4	4	4	4	4	4
	fI-0	fI-1	fI-2	fI-3	fI-0	fI-1	fI-2	fI-3	fI-0	fI-1	fI-2	fI-3	fI-0	fI-1	fI-2	fI-3

Key: *fI*, foot infection; *W*, wound.

Clinical stage 1 or very low risk

Clinical stage 2 or low risk

Clinical stage 3 or moderate risk

Clinical stage 4 or high risk

Clinical stage 5 = unsalvageable limb

IDSA, Infectious Diseases Society of America; *PAD*, peripheral artery disease; *PEDIS*, perfusion, extent/size, depth/tissue loss, infection, sensation; *WIfI*, wound, ischemia, and foot infection.
Premises:
a. Increase in wound class increases risk of amputation (based on WIfI, PEDIS, University of Texas, and other wound classification systems).
b. PAD and infection are synergistic (Eurodiale); infected wound + PAD increases likelihood revascularization will be needed to heal wound.
c. Infection 3 category (systemic/metabolic instability): moderate to high risk of amputation regardless of other factors (validated IDSA infection guidelines).
Adapted from Mills JL, Sr., Conte MS, Armstrong DG, et al. The Society for Vascular Surgery lower extremity threatened limb classification system: risk stratification based on wound, ischemia, and foot infection (WIfI). *J Vasc Surg*. 2014;59:220-234.e1-e2.

BASIL-2, conducted in the United Kingdom, randomized 345 patients with CLTI requiring an infra-popliteal intervention, with or without an additional more proximal infrainguinal revascularization, to vein bypass or best endovascular treatment.[141] Whereas the primary end point used in BEST-CLI was MALE or death, amputation-free survival was the primary end point in BASIL-2. Among the patients included in this trial, a bypass-first revascularization strategy was associated with a 35% increase in major amputation or death (63% in vein bypass group had a major amputation or death vs. 53% in the endovascular group, adjusted HR 1.35 [95% CI 1.02–1.80], $p = 0.37$).[141] This result was driven by more deaths in the surgical treatment group.

Although these two trials seemingly report conflicting results, it is important to note that there are significant differences between them. The primary end points used were different. In BEST-CLI, MALE or all-cause death was used, which includes major amputation, death, and major reinterventions (new bypass, interposition graft, thrombectomy, or thrombolysis); minor reinterventions, such as angioplasty, stents, and surgical patch angioplasty, were excluded. Amputation-free survival used in BASIL-2 is dominated by mortality and does not account for reinterventions for unresolved or recurrent symptoms. In addition, the patients enrolled in these trials were very different. In BASIL-2, there were fewer females, non-Whites, and patients with ESRD. There were significantly higher rates of prior index limb revascularization and use of angioplasty alone, with less use

of drug elution. Although technical failure rates of endovascular therapy were similar in both trials, rates of amputation, death, and periprocedural death were higher in BASIL-2. Further analysis is needed to harmonize the results of these trials and determine whether the seemingly disparate findings are related to patient factors or procedural factors or are a consequence of the difference in healthcare systems in North America and the United Kingdom.[144]

In patients with limited life expectancy or poor functional status, consideration should be given to palliative measures or primary amputation.

OPEN SURGICAL REVASCULARIZATION

Inflow Bypass Techniques

Aortofemoral Bypass

In patients of suitable risk with hemodynamically significant aortic and iliac stenosis or occlusions, open in-line revascularization can be accomplished using aorto-bifemoral bypass. The outflow targets, the CFAs or DFAs, are exposed bilaterally (Fig. 103.13). A longitudinal midline laparotomy, or less commonly a retroperitoneal incision, is performed, after which the transverse colon is elevated superiorly, and the small bowel is reflected to the patient's right to expose the aorta in the retroperitoneum. The optimal inflow site is typically just inferior to the renal arteries. Tunnels are

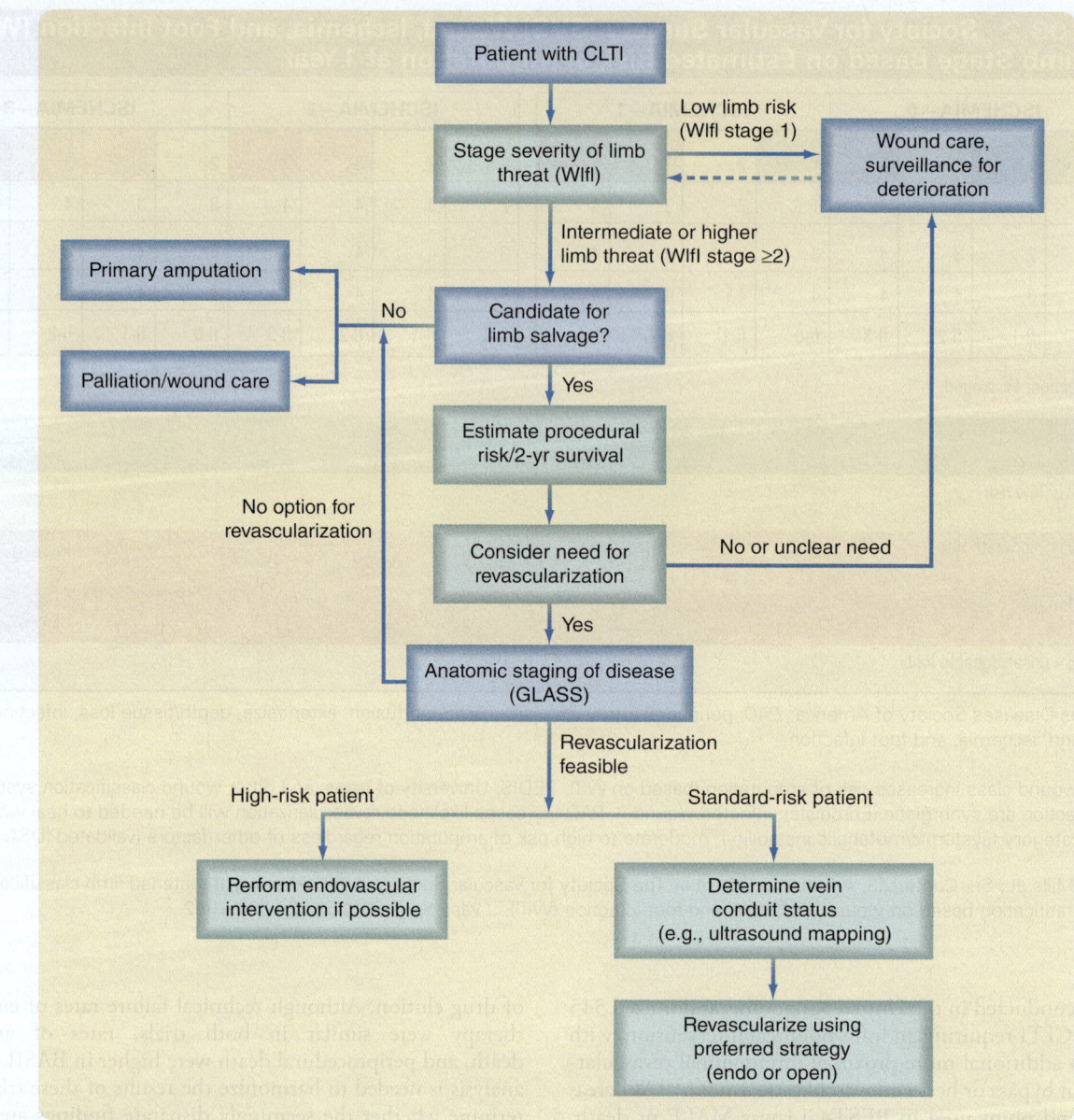

FIGURE 103.7 The patient, limb, anatomy framework of clinical decision-making in chronic limb-threatening ischemia *(CLTI)*; infrainguinal disease. Refer to Fig. 103.12 for preferred revascularization strategy in standard-risk patients with available vein conduit, based on limb stage at presentation and anatomic complexity. Approaches for patients lacking suitable vein are reviewed in the text. *GLASS,* Global Limb Anatomic Staging System; *WIfI,* wound, ischemia, and foot infection. (From Conte MS, Bradbury AW, Kolh P, et al. Global vascular guidelines on the management of chronic limb-threatening ischemia. *J Vasc Surg.* 2019;69:3S-125S.e40.)

created between the aorta and the groins, deep to the colon and the ureters. Systemic heparin (70–100 units/kg) is administered, with a goal activated clotting time of >250 seconds. The aorta is cross-clamped distally and proximally. Preoperative review of available imaging should be used to identify a suitable location for clamp placement, with application of the clamp in a normal arterial segment whenever possible to avoid embolization of plaque.

A prosthetic conduit (Dacron or expanded PTFE) is generally used for reconstruction. Proper graft sizing is important to prevent sluggish flow and resulting formation of laminar thrombus, which has the potential to embolize. A 16-mm by 8-mm bifurcated graft is frequently used in males, whereas a 14-mm by

7-mm graft may be more suited to female anatomy. In cases of infection of a previously placed prosthetic conduit, after graft excision, in-line reconstruction can be performed using autogenous femoral veins as a neoaortoiliac system or using cryopreserved arteries or veins. Rifampin-soaked Dacron grafts are also used in primary reconstructions as well as in the setting of grafts infected with low-virulence organisms.

The proximal aortic anastomosis can be constructed in an end-to-end or end-to-side configuration. Although there is no clear evidence to demonstrate overall superiority of one technique over the other, certain anatomic factors should be considered. An end-to-end aortic anastomosis is generally preferred because of

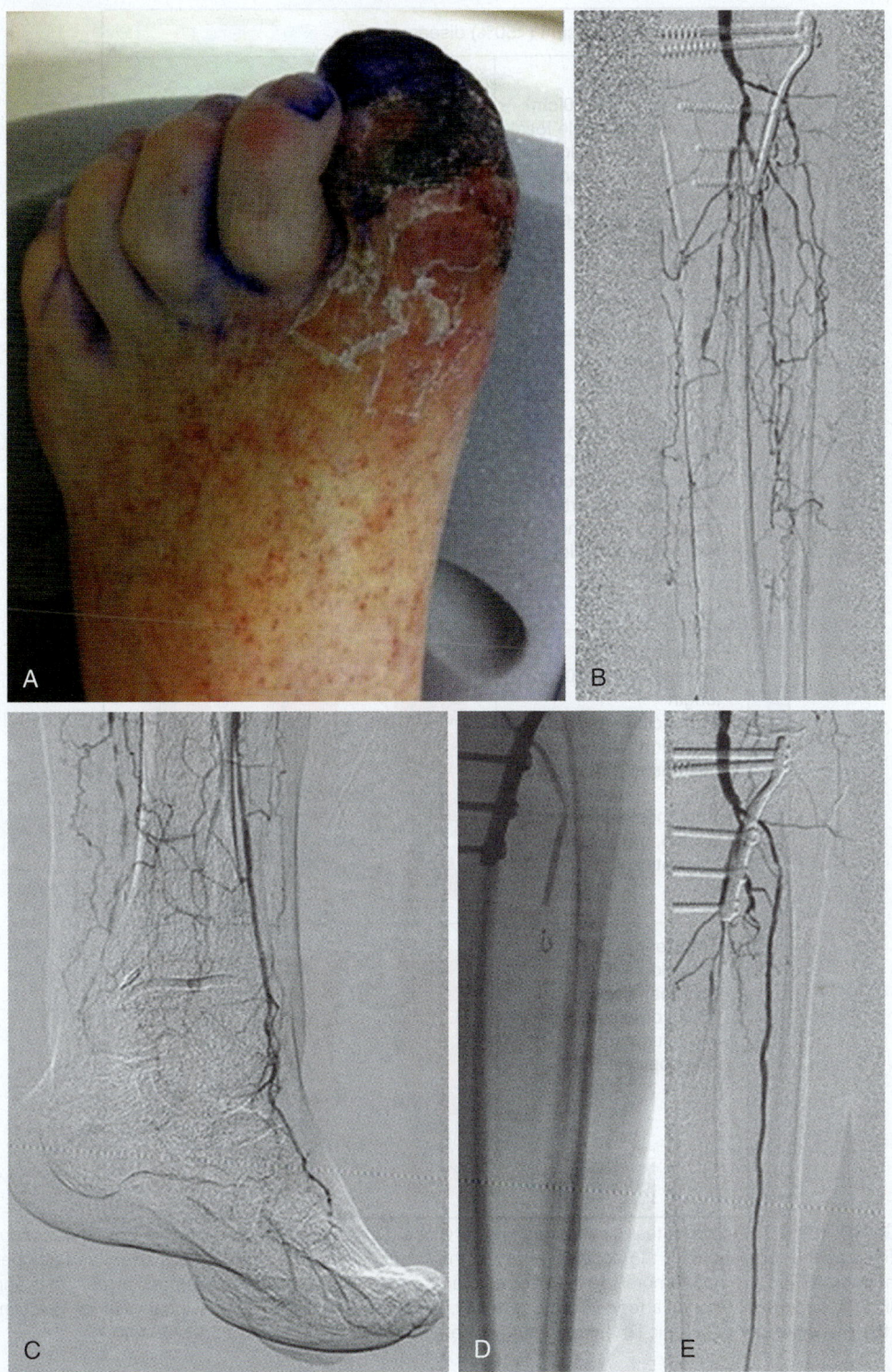

FIGURE 103.8 A 77-year-old high-risk patient with diabetes and great toe gangrene. (A) Critical limb ischemia with ankle-brachial index (ABI) of 0.39. (B) Three-vessel long-segment (>25-cm) tibial artery occlusions with (C) distal anterior tibial artery reconstitution. (D) Subintimal angioplasty of long-segment occlusion. (E) Anterior tibial artery after long-segment subintimal angioplasty with ABI improved to 0.81. Toe amputation healed, and the vessel remains patent 6 months after intervention. (From Montero-Baker M, Mills JL. Endovascular repair of infrapopliteal arterial occlusive disease. In: Moore WS, Lawrence PF, Oderich GS, eds. *Moore's Vascular and Endovascular Surgery: A Comprehensive Review.* 9th ed. Philadelphia: Elsevier; 2019:460-468.)

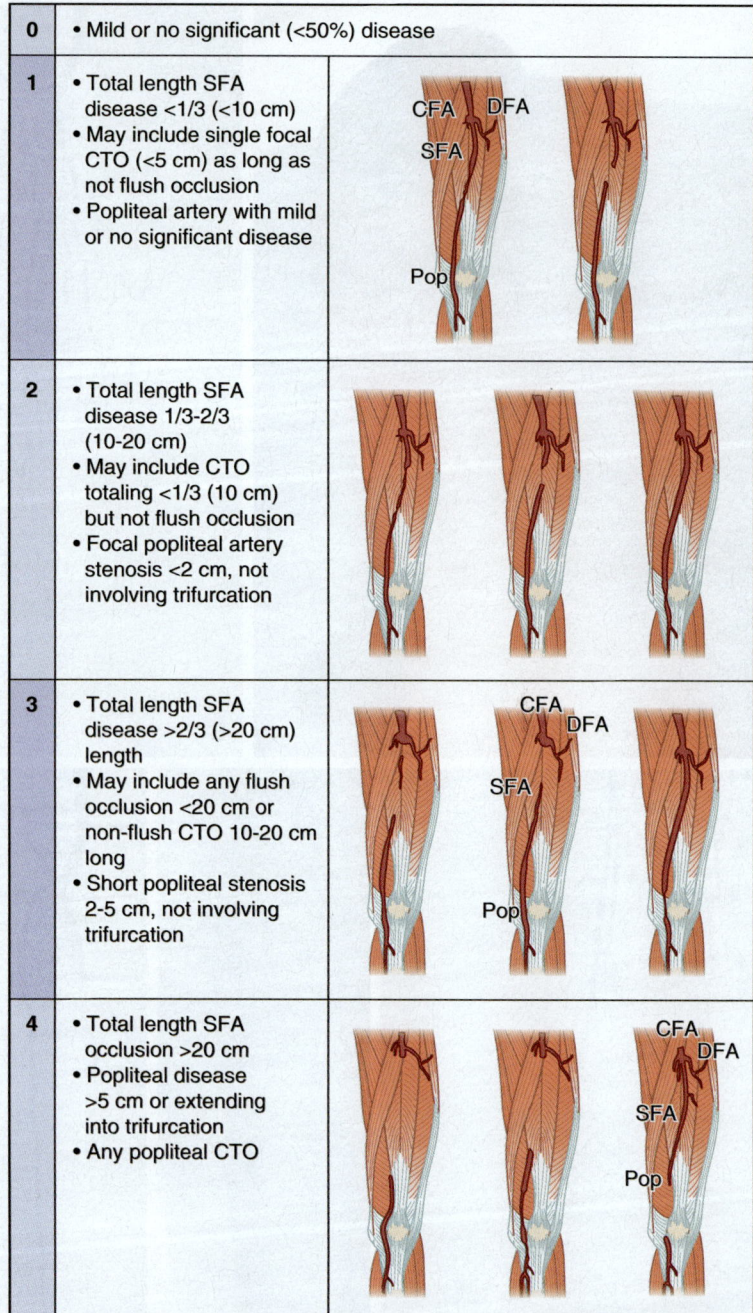

0	• Mild or no significant (<50%) disease
1	• Total length SFA disease <1/3 (<10 cm) • May include single focal CTO (<5 cm) as long as not flush occlusion • Popliteal artery with mild or no significant disease
2	• Total length SFA disease 1/3-2/3 (10-20 cm) • May include CTO totaling <1/3 (10 cm) but not flush occlusion • Focal popliteal artery stenosis <2 cm, not involving trifurcation
3	• Total length SFA disease >2/3 (>20 cm) length • May include any flush occlusion <20 cm or non-flush CTO 10-20 cm long • Short popliteal stenosis 2-5 cm, not involving trifurcation
4	• Total length SFA occlusion >20 cm • Popliteal disease >5 cm or extending into trifurcation • Any popliteal CTO

FIGURE 103.9 Femoropopliteal disease grading in Global Limb Anatomic Staging System. *Trifurcation* is defined as the termination of the popliteal artery at the confluence of the anterior tibial artery and tibioperoneal trunk. *CFA*, Common femoral artery; *CTO*, chronic total occlusion; *DFA*, deep femoral artery; *Pop*, popliteal; *SFA*, superficial femoral artery. (From Conte MS, Bradbury AW, Kolh P, et al. Global vascular guidelines on the management of chronic limb-threatening ischemia. *J Vasc Surg*. 2019;69:3S-125S.e40.)

improved in-line flow with reduced perianastomotic turbulence and avoidance of competitive flow. In this configuration, the graft lies flatter in the retroperitoneum, preventing kinking of the limbs and allowing for easier closure of the retroperitoneum over the graft to protect the prosthetic from the adjacent small bowel. Proponents of an end-to-end aortic anastomosis cite an older study comparing the two configurations that reported a 100% 3-year patency for end-to-end anastomoses as compared with 91.4% for end-to-side anastomoses. Additionally, an end-to-end

approach is needed in the presence of a concomitant abdominal aortic aneurysm.

However, an end-to-side configuration may be preferred in patients to preserve flow in a patent inferior mesenteric artery (IMA) or accessory renal artery or to maintain pelvic perfusion in patients where an end-to-end anastomosis would result in limited retrograde flow to the internal iliac arteries (IIAs) as a result of the presence of external iliac artery (EIA) disease. In this configuration, an approximately 3-cm longitudinal arteriotomy is created

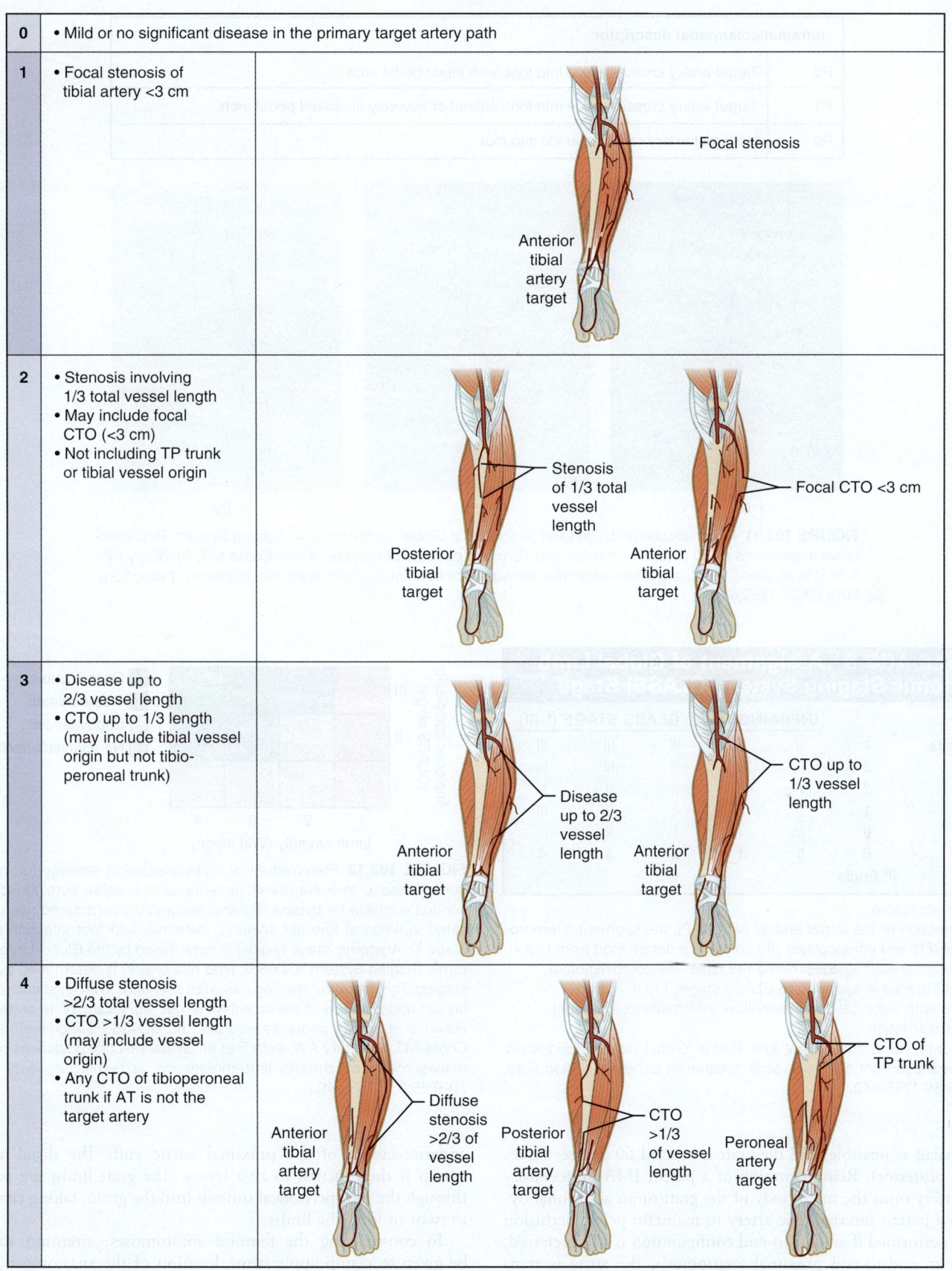

0	• Mild or no significant disease in the primary target artery path
1	• Focal stenosis of tibial artery <3 cm
2	• Stenosis involving 1/3 total vessel length • May include focal CTO (<3 cm) • Not including TP trunk or tibial vessel origin
3	• Disease up to 2/3 vessel length • CTO up to 1/3 length (may include tibial vessel origin but not tibio-peroneal trunk)
4	• Diffuse stenosis >2/3 total vessel length • CTO >1/3 vessel length (may include vessel origin) • Any CTO of tibioperoneal trunk if AT is not the target artery

FIGURE 103.10 Infrapopliteal disease grading in Global Limb Anatomic Staging System. *AT*, Anterior tibial; *CTO*, chronic total occlusion; *TP*, tibioperoneal. (From Conte MS, Bradbury AW, Kolh P, et al. Global vascular guidelines on the management of chronic limb-threatening ischemia. *J Vasc Surg.* 2019;69:3S-125S.e40.)

Inframalleolar/pedal descriptor	
P0	Target artery crosses ankle into foot, with intact pedal arch
P1	Target artery crosses ankle into foot; absent or severely diseased pedal arch
P2	No target artery crossing ankle into foot

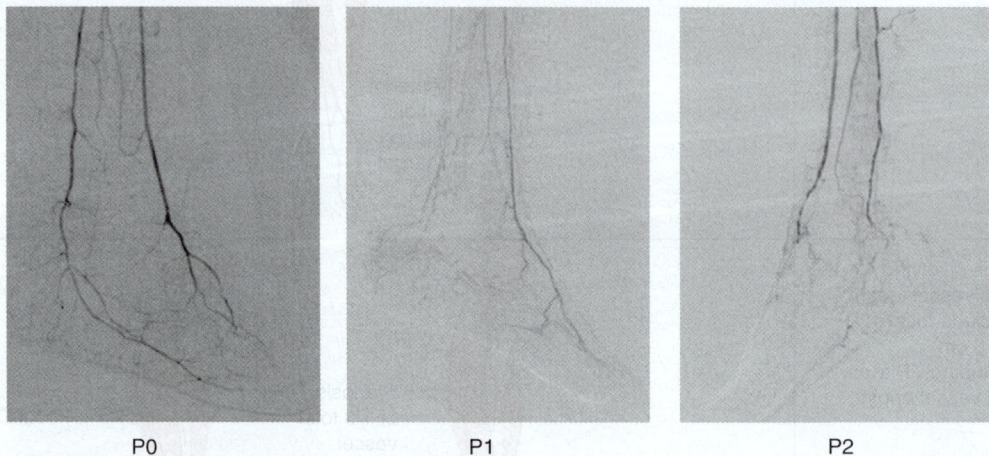

P0 P1 P2

FIGURE 103.11 Inframalleolar/pedal disease descriptor in Global Limb Anatomic Staging System. Representative angiograms of *P0 (left)*, *P1 (middle)*, and *P2 (right)* patterns of disease. (From Conte MS, Bradbury AW, Kolh P, et al. Global vascular guidelines on the management of chronic limb-threatening ischemia. *J Vasc Surg.* 2019;69:3S-125S.e40.)

TABLE 103.3 Assignment of Global Limb Anatomic Staging System (GLASS) Stage

FP Grade		INFRAINGUINAL GLASS STAGE (I–III)				
	4	III	III	III	III	III
	3	II	II	II	III	III
	2	I	II	II	II	III
	1	I	I	II	II	III
	0	NA	I	I	II	III
		0	1	2	3	4
	IP Grade					

NA, Not applicable.

After selection of the target arterial path (TAP), the segmental femoro-popliteal *(FP)* and infrapopliteal *(IP)* grades are determined from high-quality angiographic images. Using the table, the combination of FP and IP grades is assigned to GLASS stages I to III, which correlate with technical complexity (low, intermediate, and high) of revascularization.

From Conte MS, Bradbury AW, Kolh P, et al. Global vascular guidelines on the management of chronic limb-threatening ischemia. *J Vasc Surg.* 2019;69:3S-125S.e40.

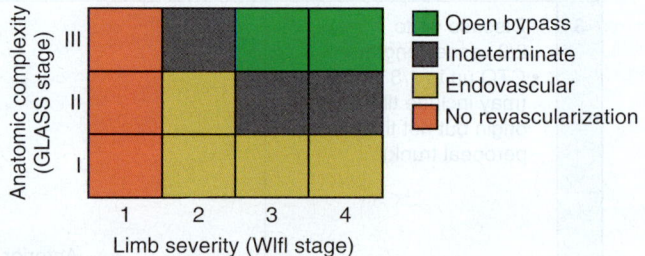

FIGURE 103.12 Preferred initial revascularization strategy for infrainguinal disease in average-risk patients with suitable autologous vein conduit available for bypass. Revascularization is considered rarely indicated in limbs at low risk (wound, ischemia, and foot infection [*WIfI*] stage 1). Anatomic stage (y-axis) is determined by the Global Limb Anatomic Staging System *(GLASS)*; limb risk (x-axis) is determined by WIfI staging. The dark-gray shading indicates scenarios with least consensus (assumptions inflow disease either is not significant or is corrected; absence of severe pedal disease [i.e., no GLASS P2 modifier]). (From Conte MS, Bradbury AW, Kolh P, et al. Global vascular guidelines on the management of chronic limb-threatening ischemia. *J Vasc Surg.* 2019;69:3S-125S.e40.)

as cephalad as possible, and the graft is beveled 60 degrees (anterior to posterior). Reimplantation of a patent IMA or accessory renal artery onto the main body of the graft or an additional bypass to a patent internal iliac artery to maintain pelvic perfusion can be performed if an end-to-end configuration is still preferred.

For an end-to-end proximal anastomosis, the aorta is transected, and the proximal anastomosis is created with running 3-0 polypropylene suture. In cases of significant disease at the proximal anastomosis, an interrupted, pledgeted suture technique can be employed to reinforce residual thin adventitia after

endarterectomy of the proximal aortic cuff. The distal aortic stump is then ligated in two layers. The graft limbs are passed through the retroperitoneal tunnels into the groin, taking care not to twist or kink the limbs.

In constructing the femoral anastomoses, attention should be given to clamp application, location of the anastomosis, and suturing technique. When posterior plaque is present, it is recommended to use a clamp that compresses the artery in the anterior-posterior direction, rather than from side to side, to avoid plaque disruption. Proximal balloon control can also be used to avoid

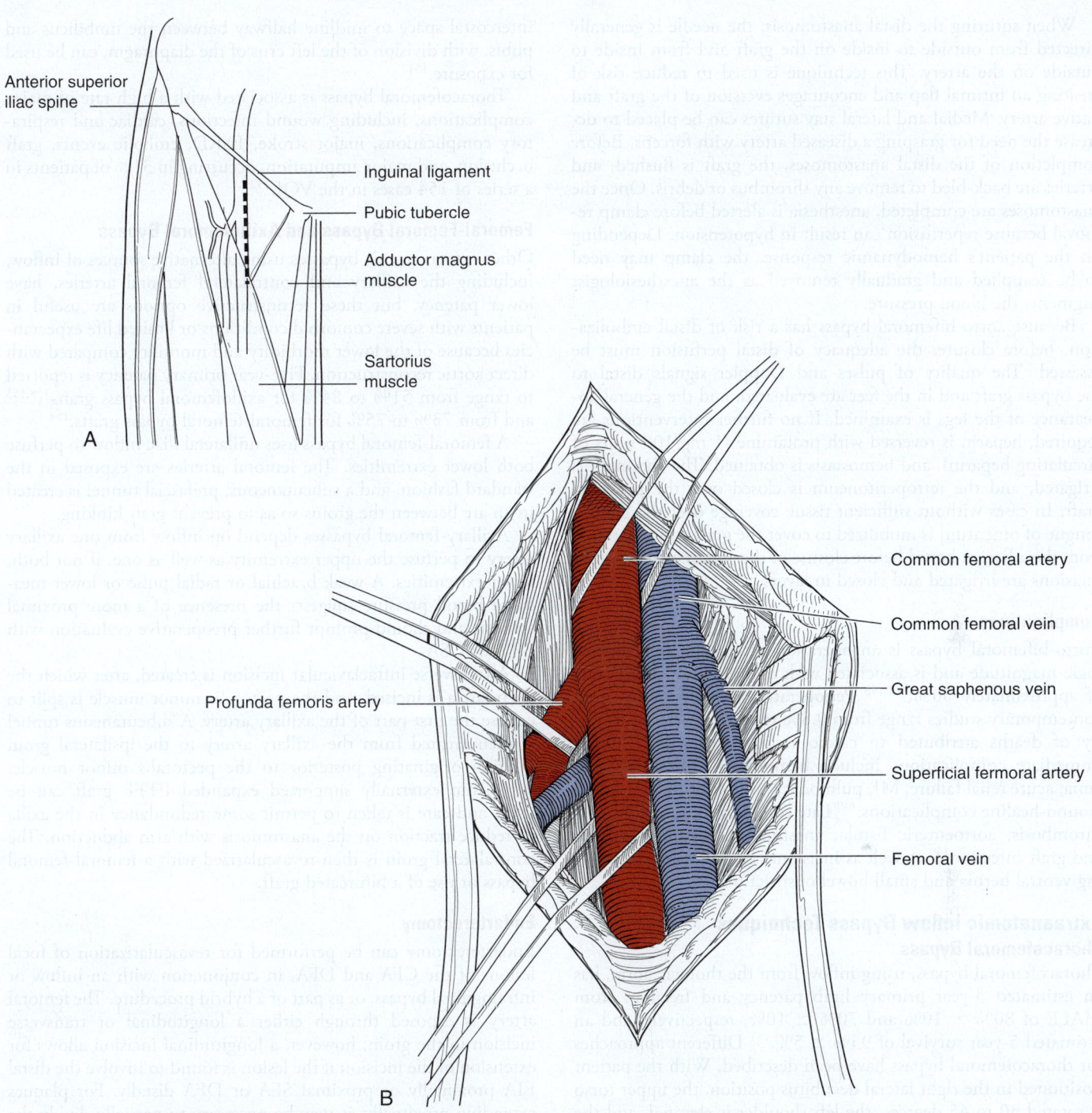

FIGURE 103.13 (A) The femoral triangle is bordered by the inguinal ligament and the adductor magnus and sartorius muscles. The *dashed line* is the proposed skin incision for exposure of the common femoral artery (CFA), proximal superficial femoral artery, and deep femoral artery (DFA). (B) The CFA lies lateral to the common femoral vein. The DFA exits posterolaterally. The great saphenous vein enters anteromedially. (From Chaikof EL, Cambria RP. Open surgical bypass of femoral-popliteal arterial occlusive disease. In: *Atlas of Vascular Surgery and Endovascular Therapy*. Philadelphia: Elsevier; 2014: Figure 44-2.)

Labels in figure:
- Anterior superior iliac spine
- Inguinal ligament
- Pubic tubercle
- Adductor magnus muscle
- Sartorius muscle
- Profunda femoris artery
- Common femoral artery
- Common femoral vein
- Great saphenous vein
- Superficial femoral artery
- Femoral vein

clamping a heavily diseased vessel. In patients with normal femoral and distal runoff, a longitudinal arteriotomy in the distal CFA with a beveled end-to-side anastomosis created with running 5-0 Prolene suture is sufficient. However, in the presence of atherosclerotic disease affecting the DFA and SFA, profundaplasty has historically been demonstrated to preserve the long-term patency of both anatomic and extraanatomic grafts in patients

with AIOD.[145,146] It is also common practice to position the hood of the distal anastomosis over the DFA origin to improve outflow in the presence of severe SFA disease or occlusion. In patients with multilevel, severe occlusive disease, adjunctive infrainguinal bypass graft may be necessary to ensure sufficient outflow to maintain graft patency as well as to provide sufficient relief of ischemic symptoms and sufficient perfusion for wound healing.

When suturing the distal anastomosis, the needle is generally directed from outside to inside on the graft and from inside to outside on the artery. This technique is used to reduce risk of creating an intimal flap and encourages eversion of the graft and native artery. Medial and lateral stay sutures can be placed to decrease the need for grasping a diseased artery with forceps. Before completion of the distal anastomoses, the graft is flushed, and arteries are back-bled to remove any thrombus or debris. Once the anastomoses are completed, anesthesia is alerted before clamp removal because reperfusion can result in hypotension. Depending on the patient's hemodynamic response, the clamp may need to be reapplied and gradually removed as the anesthesiologist augments the blood pressure.

Because aorto-bifemoral bypass has a risk of distal embolization, before closure, the adequacy of distal perfusion must be assessed. The quality of pulses and Doppler signals distal to the bypass graft and in the feet are evaluated, and the general appearance of the legs is examined. If no further interventions are required, heparin is reversed with protamine (1 mg/100 units of circulating heparin), and hemostasis is obtained. The abdomen is irrigated, and the retroperitoneum is closed over the proximal graft. In cases without sufficient tissue coverage over the graft, a tongue of omentum is mobilized to cover the graft and separate it from the adjacent bowel before closure of the abdomen. The groin incisions are irrigated and closed in layers.

Complications

Aorto-bifemoral bypass is an operation of considerable physiologic magnitude and is associated with an overall morbidity rate of approximately 30%.[147,148] Perioperative mortality rates from contemporary studies range from 0.8% to 2.3%, with the majority of deaths attributed to cardiovascular causes.[147,148] Other immediate complications include hemorrhage, intestinal ischemia, acute renal failure, MI, pulmonary complications, ALI, and wound-healing complications.[149] Late complications include graft thrombosis, aortoenteric fistula, anastomotic pseudoaneurysm, and graft infection[149] as well as incisional complications, including ventral hernia and small bowel obstruction.[150]

Extraanatomic Inflow Bypass Techniques
Thoracofemoral Bypass

Thoracofemoral bypass, using inflow from the thoracic aorta, has an estimated 3-year primary limb patency and freedom from MALE of 80% ± 10% and 70% ± 10%, respectively, and an estimated 5-year survival of 93% ± 5%.[151] Different approaches for thoracofemoral bypass have been described. With the patient positioned in the right lateral decubitus position, the upper torso is rotated 30 to 45 degrees, the left shoulder is elevated, and the hips are positioned as flat as possible. After standard femoral artery exposure, the aorta is exposed through a left thoracotomy at the seventh, eighth, or ninth interspace. The aortic anastomosis is created in an end-to-side fashion after placement of a partially occluding side-biting clamp using a 14-mm by 7-mm or 16-mm by 8-mm bifurcated Dacron graft if bypassing to both legs or a 10-mm graft for a unilateral bypass to the left groin. The graft is then tunneled through the retroperitoneum into the groins, and the distal anastomoses are completed.[151] Blind tunneling has been described; however, a left flank retroperitoneal counter incision is commonly used to create a lateral diaphragmatic defect under direct vision and to tunnel the graft through the retrofascial, preperitoneal space into the right groin. Alternatively, a left thoracoretroperitoneal incision extending from the eighth or ninth

intercostal space to midline halfway between the umbilicus and pubis, with division of the left crus of the diaphragm, can be used for exposure.[151]

Thoracofemoral bypass is associated with a high rate of major complications, including wound infections, cardiac and respiratory complications, major stroke, ESRD, embolic events, graft occlusion, and major amputation, occurring in 31% of patients in a series of 154 cases in the VQI.[152]

Femoral-Femoral Bypass and Axillofemoral Bypass

Other extraanatomic bypasses using alternative sources of inflow, including the axillary and contralateral femoral arteries, have lower patency, but these reconstructive options are useful in patients with severe comorbid conditions or limited life expectancies because of the lower morbidity and mortality compared with direct aortic reconstruction. Five-year primary patency is reported to range from 51% to 84% for axillofemoral bypass grafts[128,153] and from 73% to 75% for femoral-femoral bypass grafts.[154]

A femoral-femoral bypass uses unilateral iliac inflow to perfuse both lower extremities. The femoral arteries are exposed in the standard fashion, and a subcutaneous, prefascial tunnel is created in an arc between the groins so as to prevent graft kinking.

Axillary-femoral bypasses depend on inflow from one axillary artery to perfuse the upper extremity as well as one, if not both, lower extremities. A weak brachial or radial pulse or lower measured blood pressure suggests the presence of a more proximal stenosis and should prompt further preoperative evaluation with CTA or DSA.

A transverse infraclavicular incision is created, after which the deep fascia is incised, and the pectoralis minor muscle is split to expose the first part of the axillary artery. A subcutaneous tunnel is then created from the axillary artery to the ipsilateral groin incision originating posterior to the pectoralis minor muscle. An 8-mm externally supported expanded PTFE graft can be used, and care is taken to permit some redundancy in the axilla to reduce traction on the anastomosis with arm abduction. The contralateral groin is then revascularized with a femoral-femoral bypass or use of a bifurcated graft.

Endarterectomy

Endarterectomy can be performed for revascularization of focal lesions of the CFA and DFA, in conjunction with an inflow or infrainguinal bypass, or as part of a hybrid procedure. The femoral artery is exposed through either a longitudinal or transverse incision in the groin; however, a longitudinal incision allows for extension of the incision if the lesion is found to involve the distal EIA proximally or proximal SFA or DFA distally. For plaques extending proximally, it may be necessary to partially divide the inguinal ligament to identify a nondiseased segment of EIA suitable for clamp placement. A longitudinal arteriotomy is created in the CFA and extended proximally and distally beyond the area of occlusive disease. The plaque is then elevated along with the intima and peeled from the vessel wall. Residual plaque present at the distal end of the endarterectomy site is secured with polypropylene tacking sutures. Once the endarterectomy site is cleared free of debris, the arteriotomy is closed by patch angioplasty to prevent stenosis, commonly using a bovine pericardial patch.

The presence of an SFA occlusion may compromise the patency of an inflow bypass; therefore, if a stenosis of the DFA is present, it is recommended to be corrected with profundaplasty at the time of the inflow procedure because the DFA is the main source of collateral blood flow to the lower extremity.[128]

To perform a profundaplasty, the arteriotomy is extended over the DFA—in the presence of a bulky plaque in the proximal DFA, an endarterectomy may also be required—and patch angioplasty is performed. More distal exposure of the DFA can be achieved by ligating crossing deep femoral vein branches.

Infrainguinal Bypass Techniques

Infrainguinal bypass techniques are used to treat occlusive disease of the femoral-popliteal segment and/or the tibial vessels. To optimize the success of a bypass, there must be adequate inflow and outflow, and the most optimal conduit should be used. The inflow and outflow for infrainguinal bypasses are determined based on the location of occlusive disease and are commonly assessed using lower extremity DSA. CTA may be used for assessment of inflow disease; however, its utility in identification of an outflow target may be limited by the presence of small, calcified vessels. MRA and duplex ultrasound may also be used for preoperative planning.

Inflow must be sufficient to support graft patency. In a patient with a palpable ipsilateral femoral pulse and triphasic CFA Doppler waveforms, inflow is likely to be adequate. Additional imaging should be obtained in patients with an absent femoral pulse or abnormal Doppler waveform to assess the need for treatment of aortoiliac or CFA disease in conjunction with infrainguinal bypass. Revascularization of the inflow arteries can be accomplished with open or endovascular techniques.

The distal target should be the most proximal vessel distal to a hemodynamically significant stenosis that has runoff to the foot via at least one tibial artery. Distal target artery selection in patients with CLTI requires views of the foot, both anteroposterior and lateral, because these patients often require a tibial, DP, or plantar artery target (Fig. 103.14).

Bypass Conduit

Conduit selection is critical in the success of an infrainguinal bypass. Autologous conduits include GSV, small saphenous vein (SSV), arm (basilic and cephalic) vein, or composite vein consisting of multiple segments sewn together as one. Preoperative duplex ultrasound can be used to assess the availability of adequate caliber (≥3 mm) and quality (free of thrombosis or sclerosis and nonvaricose) autologous vein. In the absence of autologous vein, alternative conduits, including cryopreserved vein and prosthetic grafts, commonly expanded PTFE or Dacron, with or without heparin bonding, can be used.

Autologous vein is superior to all other conduits for infrainguinal bypass. Reported 5-year patency rates for GSV are approximately 75% to an above-knee popliteal target, 71% to a below-knee popliteal target, 69% to a tibial target, and 59% to a pedal target.[155-160] SSGSV has the best patency rates, and larger diameter is associated with improved outcomes.[161] However, historically, 20% to 45% of patients with lower extremity ischemia do not have adequate GSV.[162,163]

Single-segment vein is superior to spliced segments, and lower extremity veins are superior to arm veins. Reported 5-year primary and secondary patency rates for SSV are 53% and 76%, respectively, and 39% and 67%, respectively, for arm vein.[143] However, in the absence of GSV, alternative autologous (SSV, arm vein, and spliced vein conduits) and nonautologous biologic (cryopreserved vein and arterial graft) conduits were not demonstrated to have benefit over prosthetic grafts in patency or MALE among 22,671 lower extremity bypass procedures with infrageniculate targets in the VQI.[164]

Numerous studies have evaluated the use of prosthetic grafts. In comparing saphenous vein to expanded PTFE bypasses above

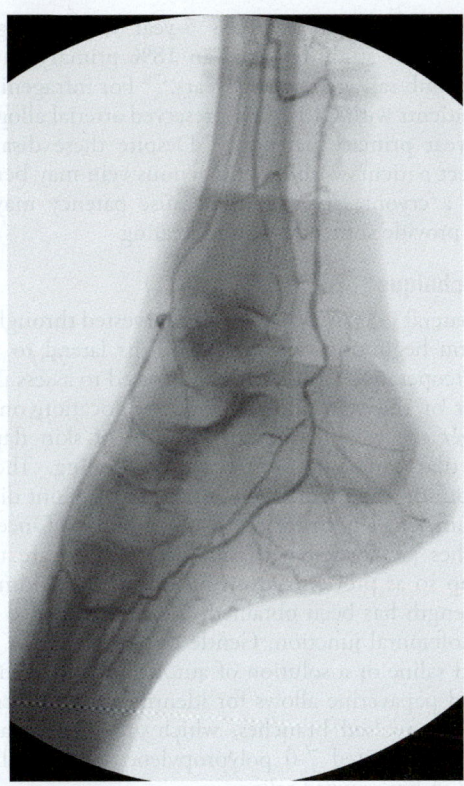

FIGURE 103.14 Lateral foot view obtained by distal selective superficial femoral arterial catheter injection identifies excellent collaterals from the distal peroneal artery to both the dorsal pedal and posterior tibial circulations. (From Mills JL. Infrainguinal disease: surgical treatment. In: Sidawy AN, Perler BA, eds. *Rutherford's Vascular Surgery and Endovascular Therapy.* 9th ed. Philadelphia: Elsevier; 2019:1438-1462.)

the knee, a retrospective review of 25 studies reported a 2-year primary patency for venous bypasses of 81% versus 67% for PTFE, and at 5 years, the patency of venous bypasses was 69% compared with 49% in the PTFE group.[165] PTFE is the most commonly used prosthetic graft; however, a meta-analysis including eight RCTs comparing Dacron versus PTFE for above-the-knee popliteal bypasses found similar primary patency at 12 months but improved primary patency with Dacron at 24, 36, and 60 months (RR 0.79, $p = 0.003$; RR 0.80, $p = 0.03$; RR 0.85, $p = 0.02$).[166] Among patients included in the VOYAGER-PAD trial, open infrainguinal bypass with a prosthetic conduit was associated with a 2.5-fold increase in unplanned limb revascularization (adjusted HR 2.53, 95% CI 1.65–3.90, $p < 0.001$) and a 3-fold risk of ALI (adjusted HR 3.07, 95% CI 1.84–5.11, $p < 0.001$) compared with a venous conduit.[167] Because of these inferior patency rates, it is generally recommended to avoid infrainguinal bypass with prosthetic for the treatment of IC because graft failure has the potential to convert a patient with stable IC to a patient with ALI.

Adjuncts, including vein patches, cuffs, and distal AV fistulas, have been used in attempts to improve the patency of prosthetic grafts. However, a Cochrane review of prosthetic infrageniculate bypasses found that a vein cuff at the distal anastomosis improved primary patency but did not result in reduced rates of limb loss, and no benefit was observed for the creation of an arteriovenous (AV) fistula.[168]

Cryopreserved grafts have demonstrated poor long-term patency. One study of cryopreserved saphenous vein conduits for infrainguinal revascularization had a reported 5-year primary patency of 38.6% and a 50.2% 5-year limb salvage rate,[169] whereas an earlier study reported an 18% primary patency rate and a 71% limb salvage rate at 2 years.[170] For infrageniculate bypasses in patients with CLTI, cryopreserved arterial allografts have a 52% 1-year primary patency.[171] Despite these disappointing results, select patients without autogenous vein may benefit from the use of a cryopreserved graft because patency may be long enough to provide sufficient wound healing.

Bypass Technique

When ipsilateral GSV is available, it is harvested through a medial skin incision beginning two fingerbreadths lateral to the pubic tubercle. Preoperative ultrasound can be used to assess the quality and caliber of the vein and to mark the location on the skin directly over the vein to prevent creation of skin flaps during dissection that can compromise wound healing. The GSV is exposed from the saphenofemoral junction to a point distally that provides sufficient length for the planned bypass. Once exposed, side branches are ligated with silk ties, taking care to leave a short stump so as prevent narrowing of the vessel lumen. Once sufficient length has been obtained, the vein is ligated caudal to the saphenofemoral junction. Gentle distention of the vein with heparinized saline or a solution of autologous blood mixed with heparin and papaverine allows for identification of stenotic segments and as avulsed branches, which are then repaired with longitudinally oriented 7-0 polypropylene sutures. The vein is then stored in heparinized saline.

Because of presence of the venous valves, the GSV is then either reversed in orientation or the valves are lysed with a valvulotome. Angioscopy can be used to evaluate the quality of the vein and assess the adequacy of valve lysis. Nonreversed vein bypasses allow for optimizing the size to match the native artery diameters. An alternative to GSV harvest is an in situ GSV bypass. The GSV is mobilized toward the planned proximal and distal arterial anastomoses, the proximal anastomosis is completed, the valves are lysed with a valvulotome under arterial pressure, and large side branches are ligated before performing the distal anastomosis. After completion of the distal anastomosis, the graft is assessed for continuous Doppler flow with compression, which indicates the presence of an AV fistula and need for additional branch ligation. Advantages of this technique include avoiding full-length harvest and optimizing size match to the native artery diameters. Nevertheless, there is no evidence to support a preferred bypass configuration.[69]

Common sites of inflow for an infrainguinal bypass are the CFA, DFA, SFA, popliteal artery, and although less common, tibial artery. Distal origin grafts have acceptable long-term patency when vein conduit is used and if there are no untreated hemodynamically significant lesions proximal to the graft origin.[172] Bypasses originating from a distal origin have the advantage of requiring shorter conduit length. The cumulative 5-year patency rate of autogenous grafts originating distal to the groin is reported to be 62%, and significantly improved patency was observed in the subset of patients with DM (73% for the DM subgroup and 45% in the group without DM [$p < 0.001$]).[173] When an adjunctive inflow procedure has been performed, the bypass graft can originate on the hood of the proximal bypass or from an arterial patch. In patients undergoing reoperative revascularization, the lateral approach to the DFA can be used to avoid dense scar in the femoral triangle.

The distal target should be the most proximal vessel that will provide adequate runoff to the lower limb and foot. Distal target vessels include the above-knee popliteal, below-knee popliteal,

tibial, and pedal vessels. In the setting of advanced WIfI stage (3 and 4), the distal target should ideally provide continuous in-line flow to the ankle and foot, although ATA, PTA, and peroneal bypasses have been shown to perform equally well for limb salvage.[69]

The CFA is approached through a longitudinal or transverse incision in the inguinal region just medial to the sartorius muscle. Longitudinal incisions allow for extension of the incision over the EIA proximally and the SFA and DFA distally if additional exposure is required. If less extensive exposure of the femoral artery is anticipated, a transverse incision can be performed, which may be associated with a lower risk of infectious complications.[174] In patients undergoing reoperative revascularization, the lateral approach to the DFA, through an incision placed lateral to the sartorius, can be used to avoid dense scar in the femoral triangle.

The popliteal artery is exposed through a medial approach, deepening the saphenectomy incision if present. An incision in the distal anteromedial thigh is created to expose the above-knee popliteal artery, after which the sartorius muscle is retracted inferiorly and the adductor muscle group is reflected superiorly. The below-knee popliteal artery is approached through an incision posterior to the tibia in the medial upper calf, after which the crural fascia is incised and medial head of the gastrocnemius muscle is retracted posteriorly. For more proximal exposure, the pes anserinus, the conjoined tendons of the semitendinosus, semimembranosus, and gracilis, can be divided.

When exposing the tibial vessels, there are various approaches depending on the location of the distal target and planned route of tunneling. The PTA and proximal to midperoneal arteries are approached through a medial incision in the lower leg 2 cm posterior to the edge of the tibia (Fig. 103.15). The soleus muscle fibers are mobilized from the tibia, and the flexor digitorum longus is retracted superiorly. The PTA can then be identified in this space. The PTA and veins are retracted inferiorly, and the incision is deepened to locate the peroneal artery on the anterior surface of the flexor hallucis longus. The distal peroneal artery can be exposed laterally through an incision over the distal fibula, after which a short segment of fibula is resected to expose the peroneal artery directly beneath. To expose the ATA, a medial incision is created midway between the tibia and fibula, the crural fascia is incised, and the artery is identified in the plane between the tibialis anterior superiorly and extensor digitorum longus inferiorly. The terminus of the PTA, the common plantar artery, is exposed through an incision just inferior to the medial malleolus, and the flexor retinaculum is divided (Fig. 103.16).[175] An incision on the dorsum of the foot lateral to the extensor hallucis longus is used to expose the DP, the terminus of the ATA, immediately deep to the edge of the extensor retinaculum. Pedal reconstructions with a DP target have primary patency and limb salvage rates of 56.8% and 78.2%, respectively, at 5 years and 37.7% and 57.7% at 10 years.[160] A series of plantar and tarsal branch bypasses reported a 41% primary patency and 69% limb salvage rate at 5 years, demonstrating the durability of pedal bypass for limb salvage.[176]

A tunnel is created between the proximal and distal targets, either anatomically along the vessel being bypassed or subcutaneously. Anatomic bypasses have the advantage of requiring a shorter vein conduit, and the location in a deeper anatomic plane may avoid exposure of the graft in cases of infection. Bypasses to the ATA can be tunneled anatomically; however, this requires tunneling through the interosseous membrane to tunnel the bypass from medial to lateral. A subcutaneous bypass is often useful in

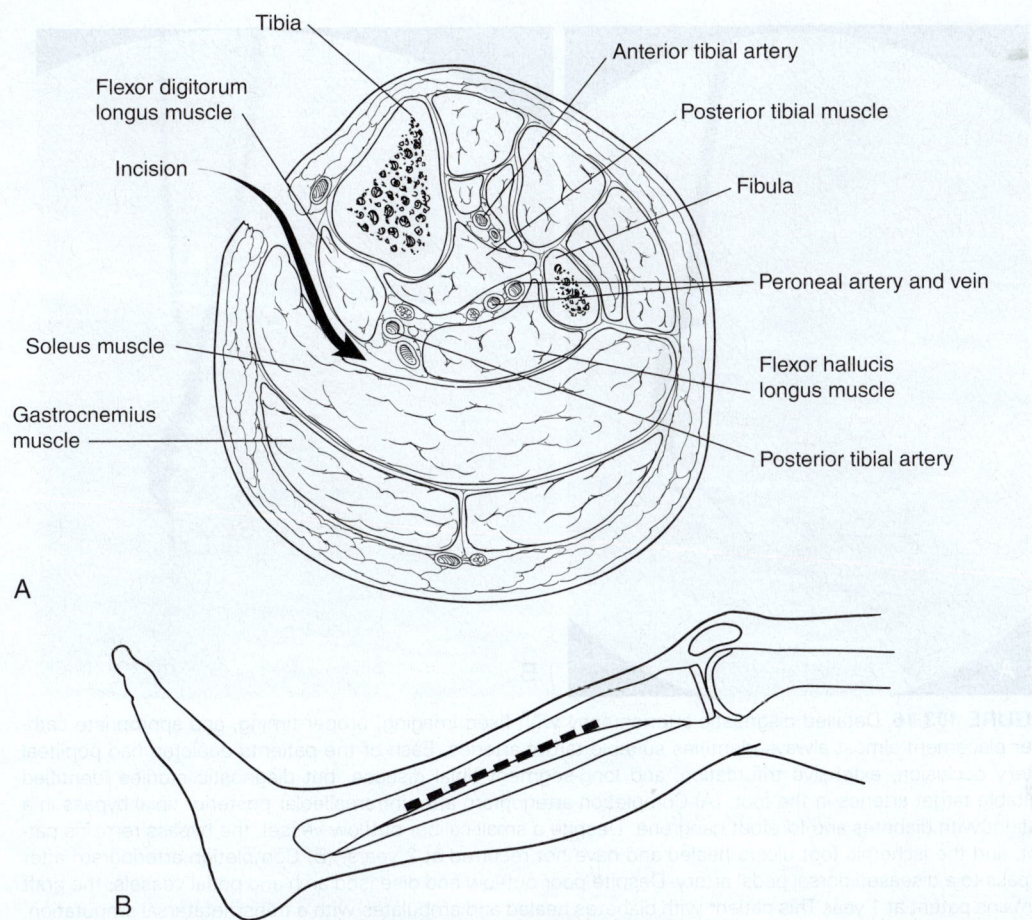

FIGURE 103.15 Exposures of both the peroneal and the posterior tibial arteries are performed via medial calf incision. The posterior tibial artery is encountered between the soleus muscle and the flexor digitorum longus muscle. The peroneal artery is encountered deeper in the wound on the anterior surface of the flexor hallucis longus muscle, as depicted. (A) Cross-section of right lower leg. (B) Location of medial calf incision for exposure of the posterior tibial and peroneal arteries. (From Chaikof EL, Cambria RP. Direct surgical repair of tibial-peroneal arterial occlusive disease. In: *Atlas of Vascular Surgery and Endovascular Therapy.* Philadelphia: Elsevier; 2014.)

reoperative cases to avoid areas of scarring, and the superficial location makes it easily accessible if future intervention is required. When tunneling grafts in the superficial plane laterally, it is important to avoid the area around the fibular head to minimize risk of common peroneal nerve injury as well as to cross the knee at the midpoint of the lateral femoral condyle to prevent compression and stretching of the graft with knee flexion.

Routine completion studies after bypass are not recommended.[177] However, if there is a concern based on distal graft pulse palpation and Doppler flow assessment with and without graft compression, additional studies should be considered to identify any complications. Options include completion DSA, intraoperative duplex scanning, and angioscopy. Unfortunately, there is no clear consensus on when to use completion imaging, and several studies have failed to demonstrate benefit.[177,178] An analysis of the use of completion imaging among 37,919 lower extremity bypass procedures in the VQI reported no association between use of completion imaging and reduced rates of MALE or loss of primary patency at 1 year.[179]

Complications

Complications after infrainguinal bypass include wound complications, graft occlusion, graft infection, bleeding, and death.

Reported 30-day complication rates among the 1404 patients undergoing infrainguinal bypass with vein in the PREVENT III trial were as follows: death (2.7%), graft occlusion (5.2%), major wound complication (4.8%), MI (4.7%), major amputation (1.8%), and graft hemorrhage (0.4%).[180] Late complications include infection, graft stenosis or occlusion, aneurysmal degeneration of the graft, and lymphedema.

The incidence of early bypass graft failures (<30 days) has been reported to be between 4% and 7.4%.[181] Early graft failures are typically due to a technical complication, such as an imperfect anastomosis, clamp injury, compression or kinking of the graft, graft redundancy, poor quality conduit, or residual valve leaflets. Hypercoagulable and low-flow states, as well as poor distal outflow, can also contribute to early graft thrombosis. Risk factors associated with early graft thrombosis include female sex, history of a prior vascular procedure, emergent or limb salvage indication, current smoking, infrapopliteal anastomosis, graft diameter <3 mm, and use of composite graft and platelets >400,000.[181] In the setting of an early graft failure, outcomes are more favorable when the culprit lesion can be identified and corrected.

Intermediate and late graft occlusion can result from development of intimal hyperplasia, which has a peak incidence in the first 18 months postoperatively; anastomotic aneurysm; and

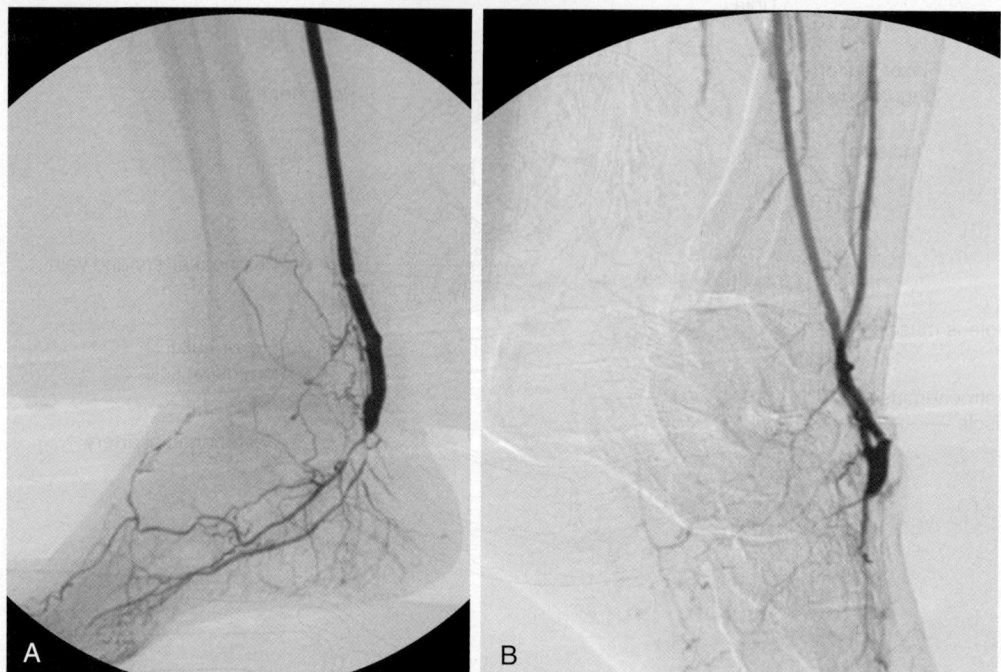

FIGURE 103.16 Detailed diagnostic arteriography with fixed imaging, proper timing, and appropriate catheter placement almost always identifies suitable target arteries. Each of the patients depicted had popliteal artery occlusion, extensive trifurcation, and long-segment tibial disease, but diagnostic studies identified suitable target arteries in the foot. (A) Completion arteriogram after inframalleolar posterior tibial bypass in a patient with diabetes and forefoot gangrene. Despite a small-caliber outflow vessel, the bypass remains patent, and the ischemic foot ulcers healed and have not recurred at 2 years. (B) Completion arteriogram after bypass to a diseased dorsal pedal artery. Despite poor outflow and diseased arch and pedal vessels, the graft remains patent at 1 year. This patient with diabetes healed and ambulates with a transmetatarsal amputation. (From Mills JL. Infrainguinal disease: surgical treatment. In: Sidawy AN, Perler BA, eds. *Rutherford's Vascular Surgery and Endovascular Therapy*. 9th ed. Philadelphia: Elsevier; 2019:1438-1462.)

recurrent atherosclerotic disease. These should generally only be treated for high-grade restenosis or whenever the patient has return of symptoms or a nonhealing wound. The rate of limb salvage in patients after graft failure is poor, with only a 50% ± 5% limb salvage rate 2 years after graft failure.[182]

ENDOVASCULAR TECHNIQUES

Principles of endovascular intervention include arterial access; the selection of sheaths, catheters, and wires to cross stenoses and occlusions; and ultimately, the treatment of the lesion.

Arterial access is achieved using a combination of anatomic landmarks, both palpable and fluoroscopic; palpation of the arterial pulse; and ultrasound guidance. Because the majority of complications resulting from endovascular interventions are access related, careful site selection and attention to technique in gaining access are imperative. Retrograde CFA access is commonly used in the treatment of lower extremity PAD because it can be used to address aortic and ipsilateral common iliac artery (CIA) lesions, as well as contralateral EIA and infrainguinal lesions, when the sheath is advanced up and over the aortic bifurcation. Antegrade access of the CFA may also be used in the treatment of infrainguinal lesions in the setting of a hostile contralateral CFA or iliac artery, presence of an inflow bypass, or challenging body habitus, without an increase in access site complications.[183] Because up to 20% of antegrade attempts to recanalize infrainguinal

chronic total occlusions (CTOs) may fail, retrograde access of a tibial or pedal vessel, often in combination with antegrade access, may have success in crossing the lesion owing to more favorable morphology of the distal plaque cap.[184] Alternative access sites also include the brachial, radial, and popliteal arteries.[185]

After access is obtained, diagnostic angiography is performed to localize the lesions suspected from the information gathered in the preintervention physical exam, noninvasive studies, and cross-sectional imaging, if available. A sheath of sufficient length is advanced and positioned proximal to the lesion to provide stability. The inner diameter of the sheath is measured in French (Fr), with 1 Fr equal to 0.33 mm or 0.013 inches. It may become necessary to up-size the sheath to a larger French to accommodate the passage of balloons, stents, or other devices.

Once the sheath is in place, systemic anticoagulation is usually administered, and a combination of wires and catheters is used to traverse the lesion or lesions. Wires have variable lengths, diameters, shapes, weights, and stiffness. Although 180-cm wires may be sufficient to address lesions in the iliac and proximal SFA or lesions approached from an antegrade femoral access, depending on the distance from the site of skin entry distal to the target lesion, longer exchange-length 260- or 300-cm wires are often needed to treat infrageniculate disease from an up-and-over approach. Diameters of wires are measured in thousandths of an inch. Larger 0.035-inch wires are used in the treatment of more proximal aortoiliac and femoral lesions, whereas 0.018 and

0.014 wires are frequently used for tibial interventions. Wires have various shapes, as defined by the tip, including straight, angled, or preformed shapes, such as J-tip wires. The wire tip is generally floppier than the rest of the wire to minimize iatrogenic injury to the vessel, and the shape aids in the ability to steer the wire and select the target vessel. Wire material is also another factor to be considered. Hydrophilic wires are slippery when wet and provide less resistance than nonhydrophilic wires; however, these wires become sticky when dry and may require the use of a torque device to aid in steering. Wires are supported and directed by catheters, which also come in various shapes and lengths and are selected for use based on the anatomy encountered. Flush catheters have multiple side holes and are used for injection of contrast into high-flow vessels, whereas selective end-hole catheters have various configurations to allow for selection of the vessel of interest.

Ideally, the wire is maintained in the true lumen of the artery, and the stenosis or occlusion is crossed. Another technique for CTO lesions is subintimal angioplasty, a controlled arterial dissection used to traverse an occlusion through the subintimal plane. A loop is created using a hydrophilic guidewire just proximal to the occlusion. Because the subintimal plane is the path of least resistance, the loop can often be advanced into this space with the support of a catheter until it is beyond the lesion. At this point, the true lumen of the distal artery must be reentered. Once the true lumen is reentered, the wire should easily advance without resistance, and blood can be aspirated from the catheter. Entrance into the true lumen should be confirmed with a gentle contrast injection. In cases where the true lumen cannot be reentered, devices using IVUS or fluoroscopic guidance are available to improve success rates in achieving true lumen reentry.[186] A review of the literature on subintimal angioplasty for the treatment of femoropopliteal lesions reported technical success rates between 80% and 90%, 1-year patency rates ranging from 56% to 70%, and limb salvage rates of 73% at 5 years.[187] However, because of the lack of RCTs, there is insufficient evidence to support the use of subintimal angioplasty over other techniques.[188] In addition to standard wires and catheters, several devices have been developed to facilitate the crossing of more challenging lesions, including catheters capable of plaque microdissection, bidirectional spinning, and catheter tip deflection,[189] as well as wires with rotating tips.

After the lesion has been successfully crossed, the goal is to restore luminal patency. For complex lesions, IVUS is a useful imaging adjunct to gain detail on the luminal diameter and plaque characteristics. Balloon angioplasty, with or without stenting, is the mainstay of treatment. Angioplasty balloons are available in a wide variety of diameters and lengths and should be sized based on the diameter of the vessel so as to dilate the lesion while avoiding vessel rupture. During insufflation, a waist on the balloon confirms lesion location and resolves with successful dilation. Balloon angioplasty fractures the plaque, enlarging the flow lumen, but risks creating a focal dissection.

Specialized balloons have been developed for the treatment of more complicated lesions. Cutting balloons with longitudinally oriented microtomes can be used to create controlled cuts in fibrotic lesions to allow for subsequent angioplasty with larger balloons. Drug-coated balloons deliver antiproliferative medications to the vessel wall with the goal of preventing restenosis. Although treatment with drug-coated balloons has been shown to be associated with improved rates of primary vessel patency and reduced target lesion revascularization, there is no evidence of improved rates of amputation or change in ABI comparted with uncoated balloon angioplasty.[190,191]

Some have adopted a provisional stent strategy, reserving stents for residual stenosis, dissection, or other complications after plain balloon angioplasty. However, for iliac lesions, primary stenting has demonstrated improved outcomes compared with angioplasty alone, with improved 4-year primary patency rates in patients with claudication (77% vs. 68%) and CLTI (67% vs. 55%).[192] Primary stenting of iliac lesions has also been shown to be associated with lower rates of distal embolization.[193]

In femoropopliteal occlusive disease, stenting and angioplasty have been shown to have no difference in 5-year primary patency (angioplasty 36% ± 3% vs. 41% ± 4% for stenting; $p < 0.001$); however, stenting was shown to have improved outcomes in patients with more severe patterns of disease (TASC C and D lesions), with primary patency rates of 34% ± 6% versus 12% ± 9% ($p < 0.05$).[194] Immediate technical success is higher with stenting in the infrapopliteal segment, but no clear differences in short-term patency have been demonstrated versus angioplasty alone.[195] However, a recent retrospective study using data from the VQI registry reported improved 3-year amputation-free survival in patients treated with stenting (78.1% vs. 69.5% with angioplasty, $p = 0.001$).

Stents may be balloon expandable (BE) or self-expanding (SE) and can be covered or uncovered. BE stents are mounted on a balloon, allowing for precise deployment. BE stents are sized to the artery but can be dilated beyond the reported diameter with consequent shortening. These stents are more rigid with higher radial force, making them suited for short, eccentric, calcified lesions, such as the proximal CIA. SE stents are more flexible, making them more appropriate for mobile or tortuous vessels, such as the EIA and SFA. SE stents cannot be postdilated past the nominal diameter, so they should be oversized by 1 to 3 mm and postdilated after deployment to achieve maximal stent expansion. Uncovered stents have the advantage of preserving flow through side branches, whereas covered stents (stent grafts) may be used to prevent or treat vessel rupture or embolic lesions. Drug-eluting stents have the advantage of antiproliferative medication, which may increase patency compared with bare-metal stents.[196]

The Covered Versus Balloon Expandable Stent Trial (COBEST) demonstrated improved short- and long-term patency with covered stents compared with bare-metal stents in the treatment of AIOD, without significant difference in the rate of major limb amputations.[197] Covered stents for the treatment of long (≥20-cm) femoropopliteal lesions have shown improved patency rates compared with bare-metal stents[198]; however, among patients requiring reintervention for a failed SFA stent, patients with covered stents are more likely to present with ALI than patients with bare-metal stents.[199]

Atherectomy devices (orbital and laser) are designed to debulk lesions and increase the lumen size before definitive treatment with angioplasty and/or stent. These devices are widely used, but high-level data on long-term patency and limb outcomes compared with numerous alternatives are still lacking. Intravascular lithotripsy is a newer technology for the treatment of calcified lesions to fracture calcifications and reduce the diameter stenosis percentage before angioplasty or stenting; however, further studies are needed to evaluate its efficacy.[200]

Upon completion of the endovascular intervention, the sheath is removed, and the arterial access site must be controlled. Manual compression at the site of access is effective, and as a guideline, 5 minutes of pressure is applied per each French size (e.g., 25 minutes for a 5-Fr sheath). There are various vascular closure devices designed for arteriotomy closure, including suture, collagen plug, and metal clip–based devices. Similar rates of complication, safety and efficacy, and outcomes have been reported in comparing vascular closure devices to manual compression in femoral artery access.[201] Closure devices are associated with reduced time to hemostasis and ambulation compared with extrinsic compression[201,202]; however, it is important to understand the device mechanism and limitations to avoid potential device closure–related complications, such as bleeding, thrombosis, dissection, or stenosis.

Determinants of outcome of endovascular intervention depend on multiple factors, with worse outcomes reported for smaller and more distal lesions, longer lesions, total occlusions, multifocal and multilevel disease, poor distal runoff, and recurrent stenoses.[137,203–210] Female sex, comorbid conditions of DM and ESRD, and patients presenting with CLTI also have been shown to have less favorable outcomes with endovascular interventions.[135,137,211–213] However, endovascular interventions may be the preferred choice in older, high-risk patients with shorter life expectancies. Such interventions may be sufficient to heal wounds and prevent amputation in patients who would be unable to derive the benefit of longer patency with a bypass graft.

Complications

The most common complications associated with endovascular revascularization are related to the access site, including bleeding, hematoma, pseudoaneurysm, AVF, and access site stenosis or occlusion. In a retrospective review of over 45,000 patients undergoing infrainguinal peripheral vascular interventions via femoral arterial access, there was a 2.8% reported rate of hematoma, 0.4% of which required intervention, and a 0.3% rate of access site stenosis or occlusion.[183] Additionally, rates of arterial access pseudoaneurysm have been reported to be approximately 1%.[214,215] Risk factors identified to be associated with access site complications include advanced age, female sex, anticoagulant and antiplatelet use, COPD, CHF, ESRD, uncontrolled HTN, emergent intervention, larger sheath size, procedures >45 minutes, and tibial interventions.[214–217] Ultrasound guidance has been demonstrated to be associated with less frequent access site complications (4% vs. 7%, $p = 0.02$)[214] and was protective of hematoma, particularly in patients >80 years, obese patients, and sheath size >6 Fr.[218]

The use of contrast during angiography also confers risk of allergic reaction and contrast-induced renal injury. Contrast media reactions are related to histamine release and can range in severity from urticaria to anaphylaxis. Premedication with steroids and diphenhydramine can be used to decrease the risk of contrast-mediated allergic reactions. Contrast-induced nephropathy (CIN) has been reported to be 9% among patients undergoing peripheral angiography but is increased in patients with preexisting renal insufficiency.[219] To mitigate this risk, contrast can be diluted, or CO_2 arteriography can be employed; however, because of the reduced resolution, CO_2 may not provide adequate image quality to evaluate the vessels distal to the knee.[220]

Other complications of endovascular intervention include dissection, embolization, limb ischemia, and arterial rupture. Dissection can result from overdistention of a heavily calcified lesion and has been reported to occur in up to 7% of cases after balloon angioplasty.[221] The area of dissection can be identified on angiogram as a flap with contrast visualized on both sides. Extended, low-pressure balloon angioplasty can be performed to appose the dissection flap to the arterial wall; however, if the dissection is flow limiting, stenting should be performed. Distal embolization can be treated with aspiration or mechanical thrombectomy,

but if unsuccessful, open surgical embolectomy or bypass may be required to restore distal perfusion. Severe pain is a sign of ALI or vessel rupture. In the case of vessel rupture, hemorrhage can be controlled temporarily using balloon occlusion, and a covered stent can be deployed across the area of perforation.

POST-REVASCULARIZATION SURVEILLANCE

Because of the chronic and progressive nature of PAD, regular follow-up is necessary and is an important component of providing comprehensive care to maximize patient outcomes. Structured surveillance is intended to identify threatened interventions before actual failure and to guide appropriate and timely reintervention. This longitudinal follow-up allows for evaluation of the revascularization, helps to ensure adequate medical management of comorbid conditions, and may improve patency and amputation-free survival after revascularization.[222] A general guideline after open surgical revascularization includes early postoperative assessment within 4 weeks of intervention and then at 3-, 6- and 12-month intervals after the operation. Thereafter, surveillance can be continued every 6 to 12 months.[223]

Surveillance has been especially well established for autologous vein grafts, for which identification and treatment of restenosis have benefit in prolonging graft patency and avoiding thrombosis of valuable vein conduit.[223,224] Duplex ultrasound has added utility over ABI assessment alone. To fully evaluate the bypass, the native inflow and outflow, proximal and distal anastomoses, and multiple intervals along the entire length of the graft are examined. Established criteria based on PSV, velocity ratio, low-flow velocity, and changes in ABI stratify the risk of thrombosis of infrainguinal vein grafts. Grafts are at high risk for thrombosis when any of the following are identified: PSV >300 cm/s and a PSV ratio >3.5 at the site of the stenosis, globally low peak systolic graft flow velocity <45 cm/s, or a drop in the ABI >0.15.[224,225] Any of these findings should prompt consideration for DSA and reintervention on the culprit lesion to prevent graft thrombosis (Fig. 103.17).

The most common cause of vein graft failure (75%–80%) in the first 3 to 8 postoperative months is an intrinsic vein graft stenosis resulting from neointimal hyperplasia. These lesions can be detected and monitored for progression by serial duplex surveillance. After 18 to 24 months, the de novo vein graft stenosis rate markedly declines, so in the absence of recurrent symptoms, annual surveillance is recommended. After prosthetic lower extremity bypass, surveillance does not reliably detect correctable lesions that precede graft failure, as it does in vein bypass grafts, and specific duplex criteria have not been established to accurately identify threatened prosthetic grafts. Surveillance may predict graft thrombosis when midgraft velocities are found to be <45 cm/s; however, no specific recommendations exist regarding the surveillance of or criteria for reintervention for prosthetic grafts.[69]

After endovascular revascularization, arterial restenosis frequently occurs through several mechanisms, including neointimal hyperplasia, constrictive arterial remodeling, and recurrent atherosclerotic disease. Velocity thresholds and criteria predictive of progression of stenosis that are sufficiently accurate to recommend reintervention after angioplasty, atherectomy, and stenting have not been established. Routine imaging with duplex ultrasound after endovascular intervention has not been demonstrated to improve clinical outcomes; however, there are subgroups of patients who may benefit from close surveillance and early reintervention. Patients with a

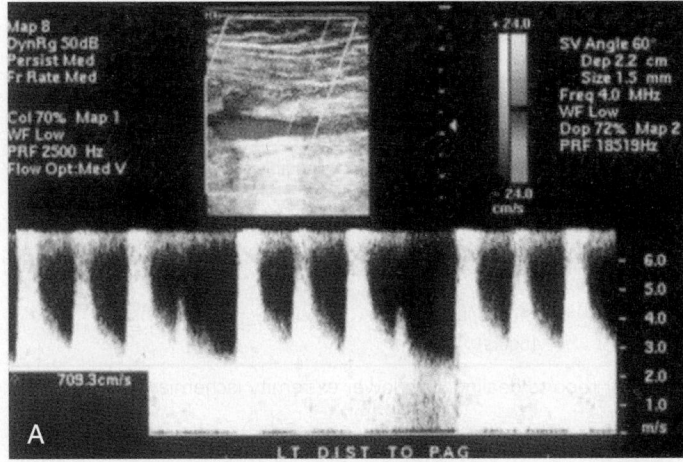

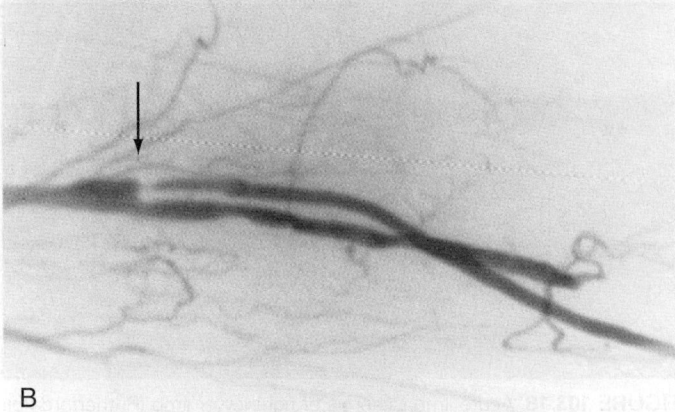

FIGURE 103.17 Duplex surveillance identified a critical vein graft stenosis in the proximal aspect of a femoropopliteal vein graft. (A) Marked spectral broadening and pronounced elevation of both the peak systolic and end-diastolic velocities are diagnostic of a high-grade vein graft stenosis. (B) A focal, severe proximal graft stenosis *(arrow)* was confirmed by arteriography and treated with a short interposition vein graft harvested from the upper extremity. (From Mills JL. Infrainguinal disease: surgical treatment. In: Sidawy AN, Perler BA, eds. *Rutherford's Vascular Surgery and Endovascular Therapy.* 9th ed. Philadelphia: Elsevier; 2019:1438-1462.)

history of multiple failed endovascular or open interventions, patients who present with severe ischemia or have unresolved tissue loss, and patients prone to failure of revascularization as a result of poor runoff or long target vessel occlusions should be considered for interval arterial duplex surveillance.[69] The SVS guidelines suggest continued clinical follow-up at 3 months and then subsequently at 6-month intervals to parallel the open surgical bypass recommendation. Further imaging and subsequent reintervention are generally only required in the setting of recurrent symptoms or failure of wound healing.[224]

ASSESSMENT OF OUTCOMES

Longitudinal assessments of vascular interventions have focused on end points of patency (primary, primary assisted, and secondary), hemodynamic success (based on ABI or toe pressure), limb salvage (lack of major amputation), and mortality. Anatomic outcomes have been used to define treatment success in many device trials: the presence or absence of restenosis, target lesion revascularization, and target vessel revascularization. Although

these outcomes are important, they provide little meaningful patient-centered data for shared decision-making. In a study of 1012 patients in the Vascular Study Group of Northern New England database, it was found that 10% of patients with a patent infrainguinal bypass graft met criteria for the composite end point of clinical failure: major amputation, persistent rest pain, or tissue loss.[226]

To address this issue, the SVS published Objective Performance Goals to standardize the evaluation of new endovascular therapies and permit a suitable comparison to surgical bypass.[227] Based on evidence from three large RCTs for endovascular therapy and a surgical control arm, the following end points as safety and efficacy measures were recommended: MALE, MACE, major limb (proximal to ankle) amputation, amputation-free survival, and death. MALE is divided into major (new bypass graft or significant revision/jump graft, graft thrombectomy, or thrombolysis for graft occlusion) and minor (angioplasty or stenting for stenosis or focal patch angioplasty). Additionally, there has been an expansion of patient-centered functional outcomes after revascularization for CLTI, including relief of ischemic pain, complete healing of any index wounds, wound-healing time, wound recurrence rates, resumption or maintenance of ambulation, and independent living status. An older study of 112 consecutive patients 5 to 7 years after infrainguinal bypass for limb salvage found that only 26% of patients experienced limb loss; however, less than 15% of the patients had an ideal outcome as defined by the presence of the following criteria: patent graft, healed wound, no need for reintervention, continued ambulation, and independent living status.[228] This emphasizes that although timely and appropriate revascularization for CLTI offers clinically important outcomes, interventions are not curative and may not provide ideal patient-centered, functional outcomes.

Patient quality of life is another important consideration; several studies have demonstrated that patients with CLTI have impaired health-related quality of life (HRQoL).[229,230] Among CLTI patients enrolled in the BEST-CLI trial, advanced WIfI stage was independently associated with a reduced HRQoL and found to be related to mental, rather than physical, health.[231] A recent prospective study of 190 patients planned for endovascular or open revascularization of femoropopliteal occlusive disease demonstrated that although CLTI profoundly affected HRQoL, as measured using the Vascular Quality of Life Questionnaire, significant improvement was observed after revascularization.[5]

ACUTE LIMB ISCHEMIA

ALI is a surgical emergency that results from abrupt interruption of blood flow and downstream hypoperfusion of the tissue. Irreversible muscle and nerve injury can occur after 6 hours of severe arterial insufficiency.[128] There are approximately 1.5 cases of ALI per 10,000 persons per year, and it is associated with high rates of morbidity and mortality.[232] Perioperative mortality rates of 20% to 40% and limb loss rates of 12% to 50% have been reported in cases of lower extremity ALI.[233,234]

Presentation and Evaluation

The clinical characteristics of ALI can be summarized with the "six Ps": pain, pulselessness, poikilothermia (coolness), paresthesia, pallor, and paralysis. The severity of the clinical presentation varies based on the duration of the arterial occlusion, the location of the occlusion, and the extent of collateral circulation. ALI is graded using the Rutherford Classification based on the neurologic

TABLE 103.4 Rutherford Classification of Acute Limb Ischemia

		FINDINGS		DOPPLER SIGNALS	
CATEGORY	DESCRIPTION/ PROGNOSIS	SENSORY LOSS	MUSCLE WEAKNESS	ARTERIAL	VENOUS
I. Viable	Not immediately threatened	None	None	Audible	Audible
II. Threatened					
a. Marginally	Salvageable if promptly treated	Minimal (toes)/none	None	Absent	Audible
b. Immediately	Salvageable with immediate revascularization	More than toes, associated rest pain	Mild, moderate	Absent	Audible
III. Irreversible	Major tissue loss or permanent neurologic damage	Profound, anesthetic	Profound, paralysis (rigors)	Absent	Absent

Modified from Rutherford RB, Baker JD, Ernst C, et al. Recommended standards for reports dealing with lower extremity ischemia: revised version. *J Vasc Surg.* 1997;2(3):517-538.

and vascular exam of the affected limb and is used to stratify urgency of intervention (Table 103.4).

Physical exam is used to determine the severity of ALI and level of occlusion and is one of the most important ways to determine appropriate management. The affected limb is cool and pale, with a varying degree of sensory and motor loss (Fig. 103.18). The temperature level (border of coolness and warmth) and presence of proximal pulses suggest the location of the occluded vessel. Continuous-wave Doppler evaluation of peripheral signals (i.e., multiphasic versus monophasic versus absent signals in comparison to the contralateral limb) is also useful to assess the level of arterial occlusion and degree of arterial insufficiency.

Etiology: Embolism Versus Thrombosis

ALI presents with similar symptoms regardless of cause; however, management strategies will differ based on the etiology of the arterial occlusion. The most common causes of ALI are embolism and thrombosis. However, other causes, including traumatic injury, aortic dissection, and hemodynamic states (e.g., low flow as a result of shock or use of medications such as vasopressors), may be operative. An embolus is organized intravascular material that originates in one location and travels to another, where it causes an occlusion. A thrombosis is a local occlusion in an already injured or diseased artery. Pertinent history to discover the etiology includes prior embolic episodes, history of PAD, recent MI, arrhythmias, valvular heart disease, aneurysmal disease, dissection, prior vascular interventions, and hypercoagulable states.

Acute onset of ischemic pain in a patient without preexisting PAD and normal vascular exam of the contralateral limb suggests an embolic event. Approximately 80% of emboli originate in the heart,[235] and 0.5% of all adult patients with atrial fibrillation will have a noncerebrovascular embolic event.[236] The thromboembolic risk for prosthetic heart valves, whether bioprosthetic or mechanical with oral anticoagulation, ranges from 0.6% to 2.3% per patient-year. Mitral compared with aortic prosthetic valves have a two- to three-times-greater risk of embolism. It is also important to evaluate for paradoxical emboli, which are emboli from a deep venous thrombosis that travels through an intracardiac septal defect to the arterial circulation. Noncardiac sources of embolization include aortic, femoral, and popliteal aneurysms. Microemboli are smaller and usually consist of platelet aggregates and cholesterol, occurring from atherosclerotic plaque rupture.

Emboli typically lodge at arterial bifurcations where there is a diameter change in the vessel that prevents further travel (Fig. 103.19). However, it is also possible for concomitant

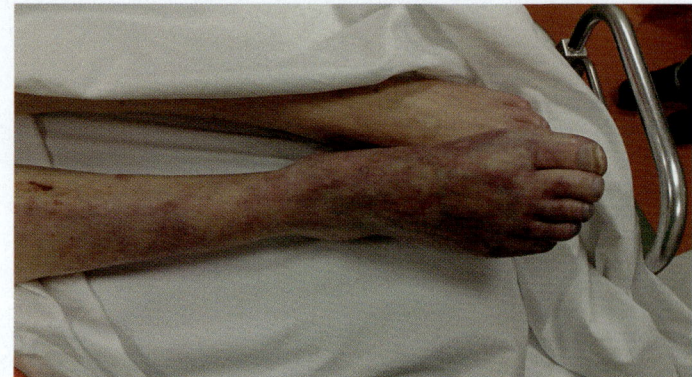

FIGURE 103.18 Acute limb ischemia of right lower limb (Rutherford IIb). (From Ferrer C, Cannizzaro GA, Borlizzi A, Caruso C, Giudice R. Acute ischemia of the upper and lower limbs: tailoring the treatment to the underlying etiology. *Semin Vasc Surg.* 2023;36(2):211-223. doi:10.1053/j.semvascsurg.2023.04.006)

microemboli to cause occlusion in the distalmost arteries, which creates multilevel arterial occlusions requiring intervention. Microembolism can occur alone, and the embolic material lodges in the digits, causing "blue toe syndrome," petechiae, and/or splinter hemorrhages.

In contrast, patients with a history of PAD are more likely to experience an in situ thrombosis of a diseased vessel. Arterial aneurysms, hypercoagulable states, and phlegmasia cerulea dolens can also lead to lower extremity arterial thrombosis. In patients with an acute-on-chronic process, the established collateral circulation may limit the severity of ischemia, but definitive restoration of tissue perfusion may be more technically challenging because of the underlying disease patterns.

Management

The goals of management of ALI include immediate anticoagulation and restoration of arterial circulation using open or endovascular techniques, assessment of ischemic injury to tissue, and identification and treatment of the thromboembolic source.

As soon as ALI is suspected, anticoagulation (75–100 units per kilogram intravenous heparin) should be administered as a bolus to prevent propagation of the thrombus and maintain patency of collateral vessels. A heparin infusion at 15 to 18 units per kilogram per minute should be continued until definitive treatment occurs and transitioning to oral anticoagulants is deemed appropriate. Direct thrombin inhibitors, lepirudin (renal metabolism), or argatroban (hepatic metabolism) can be used in patients with a contraindication to heparin.

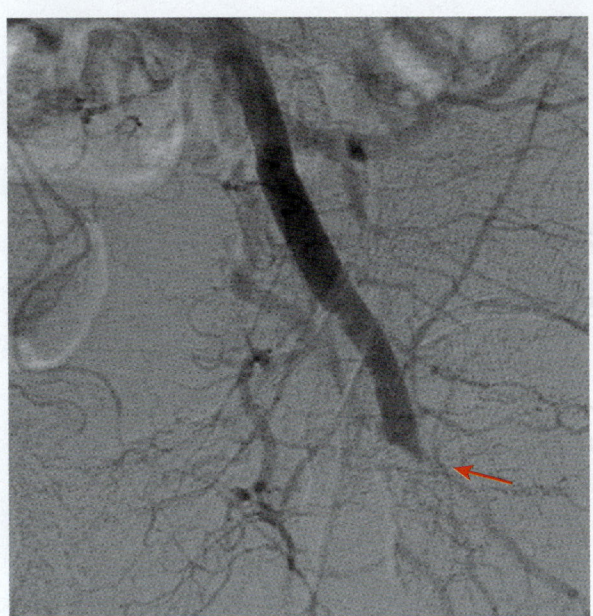

FIGURE 103.19 Angiogram showing an abrupt cutoff of the left common femoral artery consistent with the appearance of an embolus *(arrow)*.

There are three primary interventional approaches for revascularization: open surgical thrombectomy; hybrid approaches; and percutaneous endovascular therapy, including catheter-directed thrombolysis (CDT), pharmaco mechanical, and aspiration thrombectomy. There are no high-quality data demonstrating superiority of any one technique compared with another. When selecting the approach, severity of ischemia at presentation, time to reperfusion, chance of tissue recovery, underlying etiology, location of occlusion, procedural risks, and comorbid conditions are considered.

In purely embolic events, successful extraction of the embolus by endovascular or open techniques may reveal a widely patent arterial system with no need for further intervention. More commonly, thrombosis of an already stenotic atherosclerotic lesion is observed. The prospective population-based Oxford Vascular Study observed that 42% of patients presenting with ALI had preexisting PAD, and 40% had known atherosclerotic risk factors.[237] In cases of thrombosis, once the thrombus is removed, the underlying stenosis or occlusion must be treated to minimize the risk of re-thrombosis. Discrete atherosclerotic lesions may be treated with balloon angioplasty or open surgical endarterectomy with patch angioplasty, whereas more extensive lesions may require stenting or bypass.

An endovascular approach should be contemplated in patients with a marginally threatened limb (Rutherford I and IIa), in those at medically high risk for open surgery, and in the setting of a thrombotic occlusion. Patients with distal emboli, as observed in patients with a normal femoral pulse but absent distal pulses, may benefit from an initial angiogram and CDT/mechanical thrombectomy. This strategy may be more effective in establishing reperfusion of smaller distal vessels and elucidating concomitant atherosclerotic lesions, which may be treated endovascularly. In the case of thromboembolism associated with a popliteal artery aneurysm, establishment of distal peripheral circulation using thrombolysis is the recommended strategy in the absence of immediate limb threat.[238] The disadvantage of CDT is the relatively longer time periods required to achieve tissue reperfusion and risk of potential bleeding complications. Percutaneous mechanical thrombectomy techniques were introduced to address

these shortcomings, decreasing the need for prolonged infusion times and reducing the need for multiple procedures required for successful thrombolysis. Absolute contraindications to pharmacologic thrombolysis include active bleeding, stroke, or neurosurgical procedure within 3 months; malignant intracranial neoplasm; history of hemorrhagic stroke; or recent gastrointestinal bleed. Relative contraindications include severe HTN, central nervous system tumors or known intracranial pathology, trauma, and major surgery within 3 weeks.

Open embolectomy, using balloon-tipped Fogarty catheters, should be considered in patients with an immediately threatened limb (Rutherford IIb) because of the ease and speed of establishing reperfusion and in patients with a contraindication to fibrinolytic therapy. Ideally, these cases are performed in a hybrid operating room, which allows for use of adjunctive endovascular techniques and completion angiography. An open femoral embolectomy is indicated in patients with an absent or water-hammer ipsilateral femoral pulse and normal contralateral femoral pulse, whereas the absence of both femoral pulses suggests an aortic thrombus requiring bilateral femoral embolectomies.

In patients with irreversible ischemia (Rutherford III) with complete loss of motor and sensory function, inaudible arterial and venous Doppler signals, and presence of livedo reticularis, revascularization may cause life-threatening physiologic changes with little chance of functional limb salvage. A primary amputation in this setting is preferable to avoid multiple organ failure and death.

Despite successful revascularization, tissue damage may have occurred pending the severity and duration of ischemia time. Viable-appearing tissue is still threatened, and limb loss may occur from development of acute compartment syndrome as previously ischemic tissue swells within the confined fascial space of the calf. Four-compartment fasciotomies performed through medial and lateral lower limb incisions should be performed prophylactically in patients presenting with Rutherford IIA ischemia (Fig. 103.20). In patients with shorter-duration or less severe ischemia, it is acceptable to perform frequent serial exams to assess for reperfusion injury and compartment syndrome in the postrevascularization period. Signs of evolving compartment syndrome include tense compartments, pain with passive motion, decreased sensation (specifically at the dorsal first webspace of the foot), and motor weakness. If any of these clinical findings are present, immediate four-compartment release must be performed to avoid limb loss.

Postoperative management requires hemodynamic monitoring, fluid resuscitation and correction of acidosis and electrolyte imbalance from release of potassium and hydrogen ions from damaged tissue cells, and serial neurovascular exams. Accepting some amount of hematoma at the surgical sites or blood loss from open fasciotomy sites is necessary because the risk of acute re-thrombosis is as high as 30% and can be prevented with continued therapeutic anticoagulation.

Once the acute episode has been managed, workup to diagnose the underlying etiology should be continued if the source is still unclear. Electrocardiogram can identify cardiac dysrhythmias, and echocardiogram can identify cardiac wall motion abnormalities, vegetations, and intracardiac thrombus. CTA of the chest, abdomen, and pelvis can identify aortic atheroma, aneurysm, or primary aortic thrombus. Duplex ultrasound or CTA can identify lower extremity arterial lesions if the source is thought to be more distal. If workup remains negative, then additional diagnostics include venous duplex

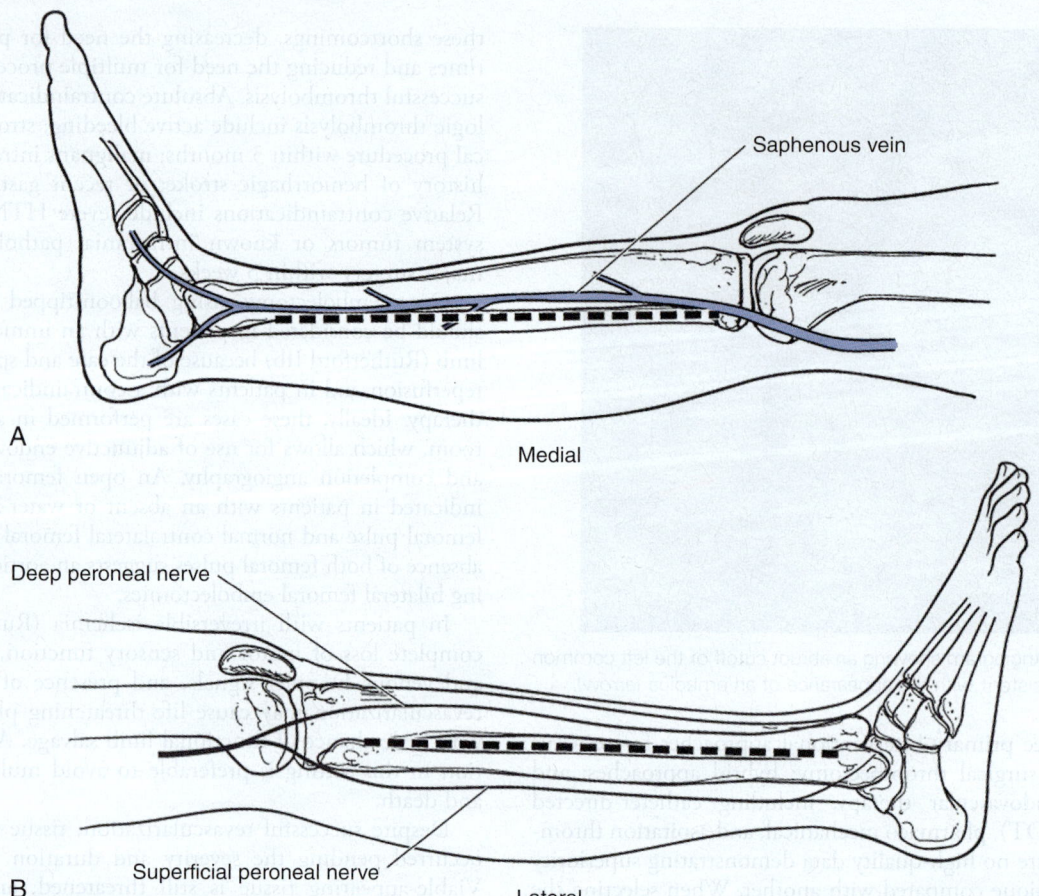

FIGURE 103.20 Lower extremity fasciotomy. (A) Both posterior compartments are released through a medial incision 2 to 3 cm posterior to the medial border of the tibia. The fascia of the superficial posterior compartment is incised, and the soleus muscle attachments to the tibia and interosseous membrane are divided to release the deep posterior compartment. (B) The anterior and lateral compartments are exposed through a longitudinal skin positioned between the anterior crest of the tibia and the fibula. Parallel incisions are used to release the fascia of the anterior and lateral compartments, which are separated by the intermuscular septum. Care is taken to avoid injury to the superficial peroneal nerve. (Adapted from Rasmussen TE, White JM. Upper and lower extremity fasciotomy. In: Chaikof EL, Cambria RP, eds. *Atlas of Vascular Surgery and Endovascular Therapy*. Philadelphia: Elsevier: 2014:619-623.)

Labels on figure: Saphenous vein; Deep peroneal nerve; Superficial peroneal nerve; Medial; Lateral; A; B

ultrasound to evaluate for deep venous thrombosis and risk of paradoxical embolism and hypercoagulable workup (including primary blood disorders and cancer evaluation). Once the underlying etiology is identified, definitive treatment should be pursued expeditiously to avoid a recurrent event.

SELECTED REFERENCES

Bradbury AW, Adam DJ, Beard JD, et al. Bypass versus angioplasty in severe ischaemia of the leg (BASIL): multicentre, randomised controlled trial.. *Lancet*. 2005;366(9501):1925-1934.

Randomized, controlled, multi-center trial comparing open surgical bypass with autogenous vein to ballon angioplasty in the treatment of femoral-popliteal disease.

Bradbury AW, Moakes CA, Popplewell M, et al. A vein bypass first versus a best endovascular treatment first revascularisation strategy for patients with chronic limb threatening ischaemia who required an infra-popliteal, with or without an additional more proximal infra-inguinal revascularisation procedure to restore limb perfusion (BASIL-2): an open-label, randomised, multicentre, phase 3 trial. *Lancet*. 2023;401(10390):1798-1809.

Randomized trial of patients with CLTI requiring an infrapopliteal intervention, with or without an additional more proximal infrainguinal revascularization, to vein bypass or best endovascular treatment.

Conte MS, Bradbury AW, Kolh P, et al. Global vascular guidelines on the management of chronic limb-threatening ischemia. *J Vasc Surg*. 2019;69(6):3S-125S.e40.

Guidelines focused on the definition, evaluation and management of critical limb threatening ischemia.

Farber A, Menard MT, Conte MS, et al. Surgery or endovascular therapy for chronic limb-threatening ischemia. *N Engl J Med*. 2022;387(25):2305-2316.

Best Endovascular Versus Best Surgical Therapy for Patient With Critical Limb Ischemia (BEST-CLI) trial. Pragmatic international trial which randomized patients to endovascular intervention versus open bypass surgery for the treatment of infrainguinal occlusive disease in patients who were suitable candidates for both revascularization strategies.

Mills JL, Conte MS, Armstrong DG, et al. The society for vascular surgery lower extremity threatened limb classification system: risk stratification based on Wound, Ischemia, and foot Infection (WIfI). *J Vasc Surg*. 2014;59(1):220-34.e1-e2.

Classification system based on wound, ischemia, and foot infection at presentation and stratifies the degree of limb threat to aid in guiding clinical management.

The full reference list appears on Elsevier eBooks+.

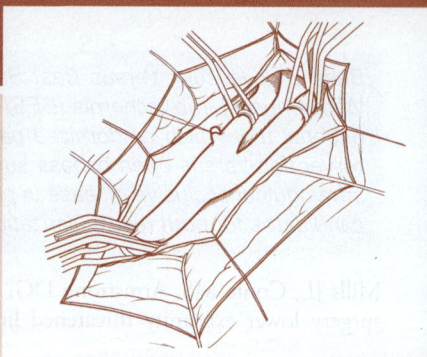

Extremity Amputations in the Modern Era: Indications, Technique, and Outcomes

Jani Lee and Raj G. Vaghjiani

INTRODUCTION

Surgical amputations have been an integral part of the treatment of various human ailments ever since the first evidence of medical practice emerged, even in prehistoric times. The application and evolution of these techniques have mirrored the recent, rapid advancements in medicine. Although the exact burden of disease is difficult to approximate, there are an estimated 2 million people in the United States living with limb loss and an additional 1 million people worldwide undergoing an amputation every year. The indications for amputation run the spectrum from diabetic infections and peripheral artery disease (PAD) to trauma and cancer, and the subsequent impact that limb loss can have on a patient's survival and quality of life cannot be understated. Thus, the role of the surgeon in the effective and appropriate application of amputations is paramount. The indications, techniques, complications, and outcomes of limb amputation will be discussed in the following sections.

INDICATIONS AND PERIOPERATIVE EVALUATION

Diabetes and Infection

Diabetes mellitus (DM) affects 10% of the US population with an increase in prevalence of about 200% from 1997–2015.[1] The number of Medicare fee-for-service beneficiaries with DM increased from 4.63 million to 6.87 million between the years 2000 and 2017.[2] Additionally, the proportion of patients who are male, older than 85, and who have multiple comorbidities has increased over time. Common complications of DM include retinopathy, nephropathy, and neuropathy, among many others. Diabetic neuropathic foot ulcers from chronic microvascular disease are prone to infection, and about 50% of those with ulcers also have concomitant PAD, which increases the risk of amputation.[1] Nontraumatic lower extremity amputation rates in patients with DM had initially decreased from 8.5 per 1000 people to 4.4 in 2009.[2] However, the amputation rates increased again to 4.8 in 2017. This increase may be from a rise in the number of minor amputations and the consequent decline in major amputations, mirroring a shift in the global management and selective application of amputations.

DM, along with renal failure and congestive heart disease, increases the risk of developing necrotizing soft tissue infections (NSTIs). Lower extremity NSTIs can be rapidly aggressive and require emergent surgical intervention whether in the form of debridement or amputation. Amputation may be appropriate for rapid source control in cases where there is extensive soft tissue damage, especially in the background of septic shock. With a major infection of the foot, especially with extensive plantar involvement, a two-stage procedure with initial guillotine amputation may aid in source control while providing the opportunity for maximal limb preservation. Indeed, some patients may require sequential debridement or amputation, during which time additional physiologic support and intravenous antibiotics can be administered until a juncture at which formal closure of the amputation can be performed.

Diabetes is also a major risk factor for atherosclerotic disease and the mortality from cardiovascular disease increases fourfold in diabetic patients.[1] In the EUCLID trial, patients with PAD and

DM had a lower extremity amputation rate of 5%, whereas non-diabetic PAD patients had an amputation rate of 1.5%. Even minor amputations are 4.6 times more likely to occur in patients with both diagnoses compared with patients with PAD alone.[3] Additionally, there was a twofold increased risk of minor amputations if baseline HbA1c was greater than 7%. Major adverse cardiovascular events occurred in 18% of diabetic patients with minor amputations and 16% with major amputations. All-cause mortality was also significant in these patients and occurred in 17% of patients with minor amputations and in 23% with major amputations. These findings highlight the crucial importance of perioperative care in improving the outcomes for these high-risk patients.

Peripheral Artery Disease

PAD in the lower extremities is caused by atherosclerotic plaque reducing the amount of oxygenated arterial flow, thus leading to ischemia. Many patients are asymptomatic and about 10% of patients with PAD have intermittent claudication (defined as pain, fatigue, or numbness in the lower extremities with activity that is relieved by rest).[1] Out of all patients with PAD and intermittent claudication, about 21% of them will have progression of disease over 5 years with an amputation rate of about 1%.[4] The prevalence of PAD has increased with the aging population, increasing obesity, and as a complication of DM.[3] Chronic limb-threatening ischemia (CLTI) is an advanced progression of PAD, which may lead to minor or major amputation if left untreated.

Acute Limb Ischemia

Acute limb ischemia (ALI) is caused by an arterial occlusion with associated symptoms that have been present for less than 2 weeks. Etiologies include embolism, thrombosis, or trauma. The Rutherford classification of ALI further stratifies the disease entity based on clinical examination as viable, threatened, or irreversible.[4] Irreversibly ischemic limbs with major tissue loss or permanent nerve damage with profound sensory/motor loss should be treated with primary extremity amputation. Revascularization of a nonviable extremity in rigor should be avoided because it could lead to multisystem organ failure and death. Primary amputation may also be the best option for patients with poor overall health whose disease presents with devastating tissue loss, especially when combined with nonambulatory status.

Determining the cause of ALI is of paramount importance and can guide therapeutic trajectory. Often, systemic anticoagulation should be considered and modalities that allow for titration and quick reversal should be given preferentially. Other diagnostic modalities could include an echocardiogram to identify embolic sources along with aortic cross-sectional imaging of

the chest, abdomen, and pelvis. Determining the most appropriate level for amputation requires a thorough diagnostic approach and may include a full pulse examination with Doppler ultrasonography, computed tomographic angiography (CTA), arterial ultrasound, percutaneous arteriography, or magnetic resonance angiography. Time to therapy is crucial in preserving limb tissue and function, and, as such, CTA may be the fastest diagnostic tool to help guide the operative approach whether that may be an endovascular, open, or hybrid procedure. Four compartment fasciotomies of the lower extremity should always be considered after revascularization, especially if ischemia time is greater than 6 hours[4] (Table 104.1).

Chronic Limb Ischemia

CLTI is defined as arterial occlusive disease causing greater than 2 weeks of symptoms of rest pain or tissue loss with diagnostic study findings reciprocating arterial insufficiency. Although data are limited, less than 5% of patients with PAD progress to CLTI.[5] A recent systematic review summarized 13 studies and showed a major amputation rate of 22% if CLTI is left untreated.[5] In a study evaluating patients undergoing major lower limb amputation between 2000 and 2016 using the National Inpatient Sample, there has been an overall decrease in amputation rates.[6] During this same time frame, there has been an increase in endovascular intervention for arterial disease along with improvements in wound management that may be contributing to the downward trend.[6] Not surprisingly, chronic ischemia and infection remained the most common indications for amputation among this sample of hospital inpatients.

A study from Switzerland evaluating patients with CLTI from 2000–17 showed an increase in endovascular revascularization with a median of two revascularization procedures performed before amputation.[7] Among these patients with PAD, the 30-day mortality in below-knee amputation patients was 8.9% and above-knee amputation patients had a mortality rate of 27.7%.[7] With the significant mortality risk seen in this progressive disease process, the Society of Vascular Surgery (SVS) Guidelines Committee created the lower extremity threatened limb Wound Ischemia and foot Infection (WIfI) system.[8] The classification system has three factors that comprise the score: wound characteristics, degree of pedal perfusion, and extent of infection.[8] The WIfI system was not designed to be a clinical decision-making tool, but validation studies have shown worsening WIfI scores correlate with the risk of major amputation.[8] Additionally, using the WIfI score as a metric of goal-directed treatment may lead to improved clinical outcomes.

In establishing the degree of perfusion in CLTI patients, careful physical examination is crucial to evaluate the skin for any wounds, level of rest pain, and determining motor and sensation

TABLE 104.1 Classification of Acute Limb ischemia

CATEGORY	DESCRIPTION/PROGNOSIS	FINDINGS SENSORY LOSS	MUSCLE WEAKNESS	DOPPLER SIGNALS ARTERIAL VENOUS
Viable	Not immediately threatened	None	None	Audible Audible
Threatened				
a. Marginally	Salvageable if promptly treated	Minimal (toss) or none	None	Inaudible Audible
b. Immediately	Salvageable with immediate revascularization	More than toes associated with rest pain	Mild, moderate	Inaudible Audible
Irreversible	Major tissue loss permanent nerve damage inevitable	Profound, anesthetic	Profound paralysis(rigor)	Inaudible Inaudible

From Rutherford RB, Baker JD, Ernst C, et al. Recommended standards for reports dealing with lower extremity ischemia: revised version. *J Vasc Surg.* 1997;26:517-538.

in the extremity. Noninvasive measurements of ankle and toe pressures, arteriography, and transcutaneous oxygen measurements can help direct the level of amputation in order to maximize the chances of complete healing. Revascularization is also crucial in limb preservation along with meticulous wound care and infection control.

Trauma

Extremity trauma is the second most common indication for amputation, accounting for about 45% of all amputations.[9] Traumatic injuries may compromise vascular supply, orthopedic integrity, and soft tissue coverage leaving amputation as the only viable option. Both blunt and penetrating traumatic injury to the lower extremities has a high morbidity rate and an elevated amputation risk. A study examining penetrating lower extremity trauma from 2005–14 from the National Inpatient Sample found that patients with firearm injuries had higher rates of in-hospital major amputation and mortality compared with the nonfirearm group.[10] Furthermore, analysis of the National Trauma Data Bank found that amputations occurred more often for blunt traumatic lower extremity injuries (9.1%) compared with penetrating injuries (5.1%; $P = 0.05$).[10] Both of those findings suggest that the greater the degree of trauma to the extremity, the higher the amputation rate. In fact, trauma patients presenting with a vascular injury and concomitant orthopedic injury had about a sevenfold increased risk of amputation compared with those without orthopedic injury.[9]

Oncology

Modern cancer care is an intricate multidisciplinary orchestration that balances effective disease control with the morbidity of systemic therapy, surgery, and radiation to allow patients to live a longer and better quality of life after their diagnosis. Limb-sparing approaches are now, for the most part, standard of care when it comes to the management of locoregional disease. Malignancies that affect the extremities must be approached with this framework in mind, leaving amputation as an option in very select circumstances. For example, tumors that remain locoregionally bound but have failed multiple lines of multimodal therapy or attempts at less extreme resection may require amputation. Additionally, tumor characteristics such as proximity or involvement of crucial neurovascular structures may not be adequately treated with limb-sparing approaches. Finally, resection status plays a pivotal role in disease control, and the ability to ensure negative margins may necessitate amputation, especially in the case of distal digit involvement.

Melanoma

Melanoma stems from the aberrant transformation of pigment-producing cells and ranks as the fifth most common cancer diagnosis in the United States.[11] The treatment landscape has undergone drastic evolution, especially in the case of advanced and metastatic disease; however, the keystone of local management remains complete surgical resection. Traditionally, amputation has been applied in two clinical scenarios: the management of early-stage subungual and distal digit disease and in the management of extensive regional/in-transit disease confined to a limb.

Subungual melanoma comprises a relatively small fraction of cases, roughly 1% to 3%, and since the late 1900s management has focused on early distal digit amputation.[12] Consequent attempts at including additional regional control modalities such as digit amputation with isolated limb perfusion did not appear to

bear clinical benefit.[13] Consequently, digit amputation has remained the standard procedure for this disease; however, recent investigations have begun to call this approach into question. Specifically, patients who undergo digit amputation, particularly of the thumb or first toe, can experience significant alterations in quality of life. Retrospective analysis has demonstrated that more limited, nonamputation resection may provide clinical equipoise.[14,15] Ongoing investigations including the Japanese Clinical Oncology Group Study 1602 may provide additional clarification once data maturation has occurred and takes into account the relatively shallow tissue plane available for digit-sparing approaches.[16] Given the importance of achieving margin control in melanoma along with some reports of worsened local recurrence rates with less-than amputation approaches, Mohs micrographic surgery for melanoma excisions of the digit has begun to gain traction as a possible alternative to traditional wide local excision or amputation.[17]

Further along the clinical spectrum, more advanced stage melanoma of the limb has also been considered for amputation including extensive hand and forelimb resections; however, this practice has likely become of mostly historical interest because the modern application of multimodal therapies has obviated such aggressive measures. Between the introduction of regional perfusion and immunotherapy, the management of locoregionally advanced or recurrent melanoma only requires amputation in the most extreme cases, including those of intractable pain or sepsis source control.[18]

Sarcoma

Soft tissue sarcoma (STS) represents a heterogenous group of rare tumors with only an estimated 13,400 new cases reported in 2023.[11] Nearly half of STS will be limited to the extremities, and the surgical approach to this disease was traditionally centered around complete disease control through limb amputation. However, starting in the late 1970s, a shift toward limb preservation became more prevalent.[19] A landmark study in 1982 formed the basis for limb-sparing approaches to STS and found that there was no difference in survival for those patients undergoing nonamputation resection.[20] Most modern series estimate that STS necessitating amputation is limited to 5% to 10% of all cases, and those patients tend to have direct and extensive tumor involvement of major neurovascular structures or that the tumor size encompasses too much of the limb to allow for a functional or meaningful remnant.[21,22]

In summary, amputation for oncologic indications is becoming more rare; however, in highly select cases where limb salvage is not possible, amputation can provide not only palliation, but also long-term prognostic benefits.

TECHNICAL CONSIDERATIONS

Lower Extremity Amputations

Toe Amputation

The indications for toe amputation, the most frequently performed lower extremity amputation, include wet or dry gangrene, infected neuropathic ulceration, or osteomyelitis. Preoperative physical examination along with radiographic examination for osteomyelitis with x-rays or magnetic resonance imaging is critical. The operative plan should include resecting all nonviable skin, all bone involved by osteomyelitis, and closure of the wound if there is no gross purulence in the wound.

With infection confined to the distal phalanx or mid phalanx, the transected level should be through the proximal phalanx to healthy bone margins. Interphalangeal joint disarticulation should be avoided due to the avascular nature of cartilage potentially leading to persistent infection and impaired healing. If infection involves the proximal phalanx, then the metatarsophalangeal (MTP) joint should also be resected with a ray amputation (discussed later).

The location and orientation of the skin incision depends on the extent of the infection, but the most commonly used is a circular incision around the base of the toe with skin flaps usually shaped into a fishmouth to minimize dog-ear deformities at the corners of the closure. Other skin flap variations such as a side to side, dorsal base, or plantar base would be appropriate while making sure that the skin edges are approximated under no tension. Closure is accomplished using a monofilament permanent suture, such as 3-0 nylon suture on a cutting needle. Simple interrupted stitches may be used, but a vertical mattress stitch provides deep and superficial layer closure with good eversion of the dermal edges. A soft dressing with compression should be placed to help with hemostasis. Postoperative management should include either a front off-loading boot or non–weight-bearing status to prevent trauma to the amputation site (Fig. 104.1).[23]

Ray Amputation

A ray amputation may be used when there is a need to resect the MTP joint or the distal metatarsal bone has become involved with infection. Removing the MTP joint of the great toe affects gait stability and would require proper footwear with physical therapy.

A racket incision can be used if there is healthy tissue at the base of the toe. It is a circular incision at the base of the toe that is extended onto the dorsal aspect of the metatarsal bone more proximally. In general, an incision on the dorsal aspect of the foot is recommended for better healing compared with plantar surface incisions. Incision is deepened through muscles and tendon onto the metatarsal bone. Medial and lateral dissection around the metatarsal bone is carefully done to not injure the digital arteries or nerves. An oscillating electric saw can be used to transect the metatarsal bone to a healthy margin determined by either preoperative imaging or clinical examination.

The wound should be irrigated and hemostasis achieved. The skin flaps may be closed with vertical mattress monofilament permanent suture with a soft dressing and compressive wrap to help with hemostasis and to protect the wound closure. If gross infection is present, the wound may be left open to allow for

further drainage and allow the wound to heal by secondary intention with proper wound care (Fig. 104.2).[23]

Transmetatarsal Amputation

Transmetatarsal amputation is indicated for patients with multiple toe infections up to the MTP joint or proximally on the distal metatarsal of the same foot. A healthy plantar skin flap is requisite for closure. Operative planning requires careful physical examination with imaging evaluation for osteomyelitis.

An incision is made on the dorsum of the foot from medial to lateral at the level of the mid-metatarsal shafts. The dissection deepens down to the metatarsal bones, and an electric saw is used to transect each metatarsal shaft about 5 mm proximal to the skin incision. The bones are then elevated and separated from the plantar tissue with preservation of as much of the plantar flap as possible. The tendons on the plantar flap need to be sharply excised with preservation of the muscle. The plantar flap is then rotated dorsally for closure and can be trimmed to allow for a tension-free approximation.

Irrigation and impeccable hemostasis are achieved with cautery or suture ligation. The deep layer is closed with 2-0 absorbable interrupted sutures, and the skin is brought together with monofilament permanent suture using an interrupted vertical mattress technique. Dressings need to fully protect the stump from any trauma, and the patient should be kept non–weight bearing until fully healed. Another option is a well-padded leg plaster cast for the lower leg to prevent trauma to the stump. Proper prosthetic shoes providing toe-off motion during ambulation allow for rehabilitation with minimal limitations (Fig. 104.3).

Lisfranc and Chopart Amputation

Although not as commonly performed as a below-knee amputation, proximal foot amputations may be warranted for limb salvage. The Lisfranc tarsometatarsal disarticulation uses a long plantar flap with disarticulation of the first, third, fourth, and fifth tarsometatarsal joints. The second metatarsal is transected 2 cm distal to the medial cuneiform. To avoid an equinovarus deformity, the base of the fifth metatarsal with the peroneus brevis is preserved. The Achilles tendon is released, and the plantar fascia is approximated to the fascia and periosteum on the dorsum of the foot with absorbable sutures. Interrupted vertical mattress sutures or skin staples are used for closure with a plaster cast to ensure that the talus is slightly dorsiflexed in relation to the tibia.

The Chopart amputation also uses a long plantar flap, but this amputation is performed through the talocalcaneonavicular

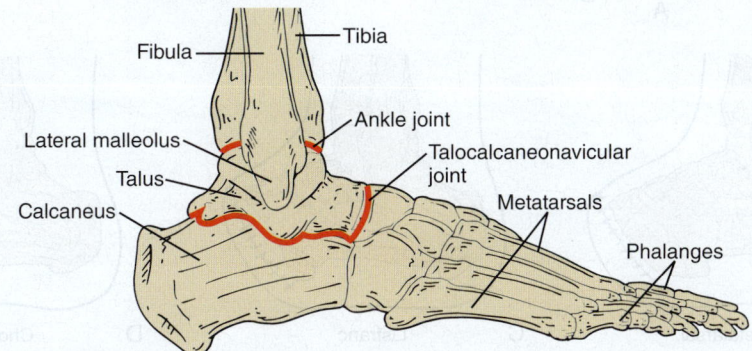

FIGURE 104.1 Bone anatomy of the foot. (From Rios AL, Eidt JF. Lower extremity amputations: operative techniques and results. In: Sidawy AN, Perler BA, eds. Rutherford's Vascular Surgery and Endovascular Therapy. 10th ed. Philadelphia: Elsevier; 2024:1529-1547.)

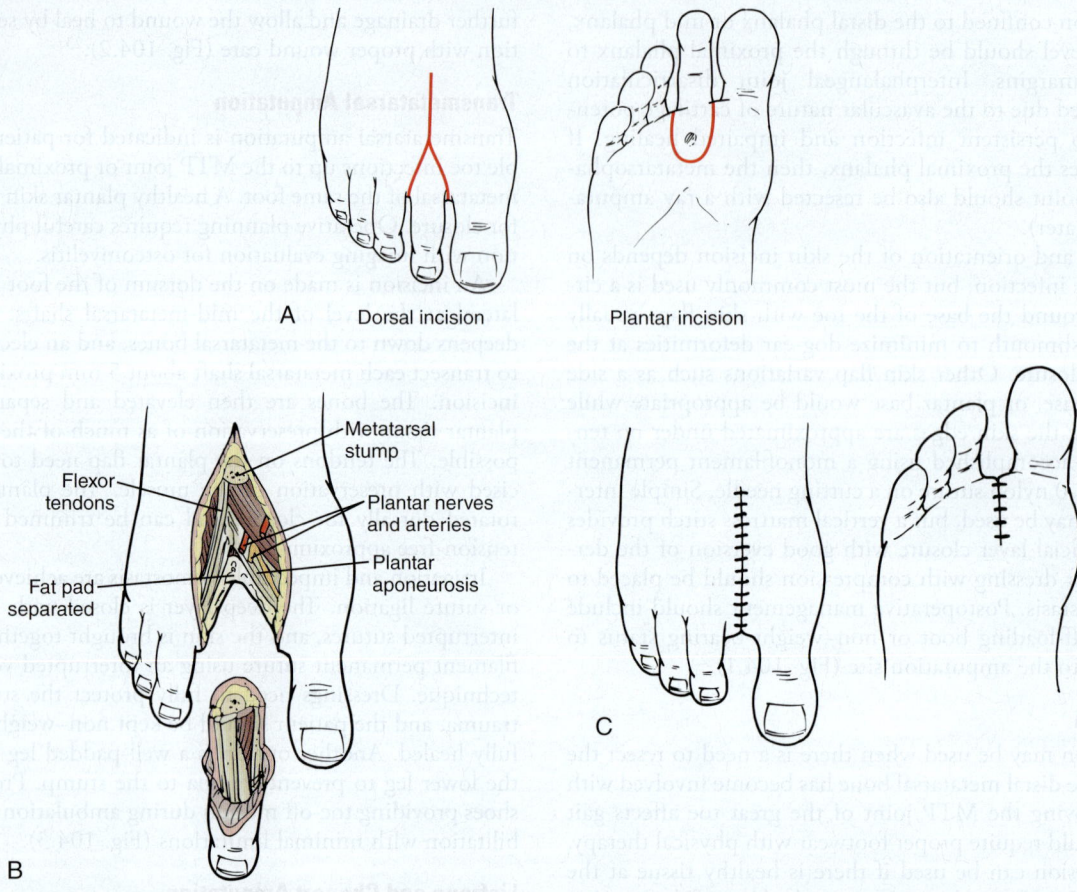

A Dorsal incision   Plantar incision

Metatarsal stump

Flexor tendons

Plantar nerves and arteries

Plantar aponeurosis

Fat pad separated

B

C

FIGURE 104.2 Ray amputation incision. (A) Note the plantar extension to include a mal perforans ulcer. (B) Transection of the metatarsal shaft. (C) Closure with nonabsorbable suture under no tension. (From Rios AL, Eidt JF. Lower extremity amputations: operative techniques and results. In: Sidawy AN, Perler BA, eds. *Rutherford's Vascular Surgery and Endovascular Therapy*. 10th ed. Philadelphia: Elsevier; 2024:1529-1547.)

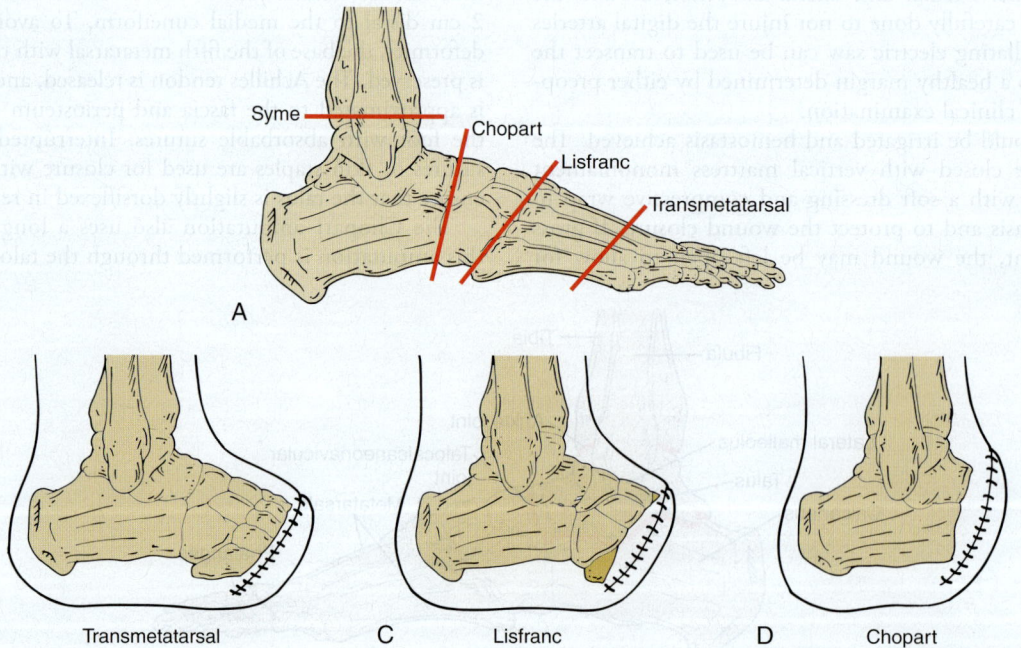

Syme

Chopart

Lisfranc

Transmetatarsal

A

B Transmetatarsal   **C** Lisfranc   **D** Chopart

FIGURE 104.3 Levels of foot amputation. (A) Levels of foot amputation. (B) Transmetatarsal. (C) Lisfranc. (D) Chopart. (From Rios AL, Eidt JF. Lower extremity amputations: operative techniques and results. In: Sidawy AN, Perler BA, eds. *Rutherford's Vascular Surgery and Endovascular Therapy*. 10th ed. Philadelphia: Elsevier; 2024:1529-1547.)

joint and the calcaneocuboid joint. The Achilles tendon should be released as well, and the extensor hallucis longus and extensor digitorum longus may be reattached. Patients who undergo this procedure require custom fitted orthotic shoes for ambulation.

Below-Knee Amputation

Below-knee amputation is indicated in patients with major infections of the foot, significant tissue loss, or inadequate arterial flow into the foot with no revascularization options. Below-knee amputation is not an option if the patient has a flexion contracture at the knee. There should also be enough viable anterior and posterior flap for coverage in the lower leg. An ankle-brachial index greater than 0.5 or angiographic evidence of patent iliac artery flow to a patent profunda artery even with an occluded superficial femoral artery is sufficient for healing. Ambulation rates with or without assistance have been seen in up to 65% of below-knee amputees.[24]

General anesthesia or spinal anesthesia are options with or without regional nerve block for postoperative pain control. A two-stage, below-knee amputation for the septic foot patient offers better outcomes with less stump infection compared with a one-stage approach. Those patients with a grossly infected foot should have a guillotine amputation as distal as possible to healthy tissue. Once the patient has stabilized, the below-knee amputation can be formalized.

The use of the long posterior flap relies on blood supply from the sural arteries, which originate proximal to the knee joint. Most patients requiring amputation due to PAD may have compromised tibial arteries, specifically the anterior tibial artery, which perfuses the soft tissue and skin of the anterior lower leg. Therefore, the long posterior flap technique offers better healing and recovery. In patients with inadequate posterior flap soft tissue, the sagittal flap or a skew flap could be used for closure. The sagittal technique uses equal length medial and lateral myocutaneous flaps to cover the tibia, whereas the skew technique uses equal anteromedial and posterolateral flaps (Fig. 104.4).

Posterior Flap

The tibia should be divided 12 to 15 cm distal to the tibial tuberosity. The circumference of the calf at the designated level of the tibia transection is measured, and two-thirds of that circumference will be the length of the anterior incision centered on the tibia. The posterior flap length is one-third of the circumference and is fashioned down toward the ankle making sure to angle the lateral and medial incisions toward the malleolus on each side. Cautery is used to deepen the incision through the fascia and muscles of the anterior and lateral compartments, and a periosteal elevator is used to mobilize the periosteum off the tibia and allow for a transection 2 cm proximal to the skin edge. An oscillating bone saw is used to transect the tibia and to bevel out the anterior sharp edge of the tibia stump. Next the fibula is dissected out and transected with a bone cutter about 2 cm proximal to the level of the tibial transection. A large amputation knife or cautery is then used to excise the muscle from the posterior aspect of the tibia and fibula. The vascular bundles should be suture ligated. The tibial and peroneal nerves are tied off with an absorbable suture and sharply excised as proximal as possible to allow for retraction. The muscle on the posterior flap can be debulked if needed with preservation of the gastrocnemius muscle and fascia. The wound is then irrigated and hemostasis achieved with avoidance of using any bone wax. The fascia of the posterior flap is approximated to the fascia anterior to the tibia with interrupted absorbable sutures. Interrupted deep dermal absorbable sutures are followed by either a stapled or a vertical mattress skin closure (Fig. 104.5).

Through-Knee Amputation

A through-knee amputation may be offered to patients who have enough compromised soft tissue in the lower leg where a below-knee amputation would be inadequate but in whom there is a reasonable rehabilitation potential. This technique may also allow for a better rate of ambulation compared with above-knee amputation. As originally described by Mazet, the distal femur is preserved with trimming of the condyles.[23] The anterior flap of the fishmouth incision is extended to the level of the tibial tuberosity with the posterior flap as the same length or slightly longer. The medial and lateral collateral ligaments are divided, and the patellar ligament length is preserved as it is divided from the tibial tuberosity. The knee capsule is excised and the cruciate ligaments divided. The popliteal artery and veins are suture ligated and the tibial and common peroneal nerves are tied with absorbable suture on tension before sharp transection, allowing for retraction. The lateral condyle and medial condyles are trimmed, and the posterior surface is squared with smoothing of the edges with a rasp or bone saw. The hamstring tendons are approximated to the patellar ligament while securing them to the cruciate ligaments. The fascia is finally closed with interrupted absorbable sutures and skin closed with staples or vertical mattress permanent sutures (Fig. 104.6).

Above-Knee Amputation

Above-knee amputation is indicated for patients who are bedbound or with severe tissue loss from either ischemia or infection not allowing for a below-knee amputation. The femur may be transected as proximal as needed for skin closure, but typically can be divided in the distal one-third portion. The incision is done using a fishmouth technique with anterior and posterior flaps with corners curving proximally. The posterior flap may be made about 1 to 2 cm longer if possible to avoid having the incision in a dependent position. The skin and muscle are incised with suture ligation of the femoral artery and vein. A periosteal elevator is used to clear the femur about 2 to 3 cm proximal to the skin incision where it is transected using an electric saw proximal to the corners of the incision. The sciatic nerve is put on tension, tied with absorbable suture, and sharply transected allowing it to retract. The wound is irrigated and hemostasis obtained. Muscle is then reapproximated with absorbable sutures over the femur bone. The anterior and posterior fascia is brought together with interrupted absorbable sutures, and skin is then closed with vertical mattress interrupted permanent sutures or deep dermal absorbable sutures and skin staples.

Hip Disarticulation

Hip disarticulation is highly morbid and only indicated in a very select population of patients including those with proximal malignancies requiring surgical resection. With the patient in a semilateral position, an anterior racket incision is extended from medial to the anterior superior iliac spine toward the pubic tubercle, and it is extended posteriorly distal to the ischial tuberosity and gluteal crease. The incision continues anteromedially to the greater trochanter and back to the start of the incision. The dissection is deepened down to the external oblique aponeurosis and deep fascia of the thigh with careful suture ligation of the femoral vessels. The femoral nerve is transected on tension and allowed to

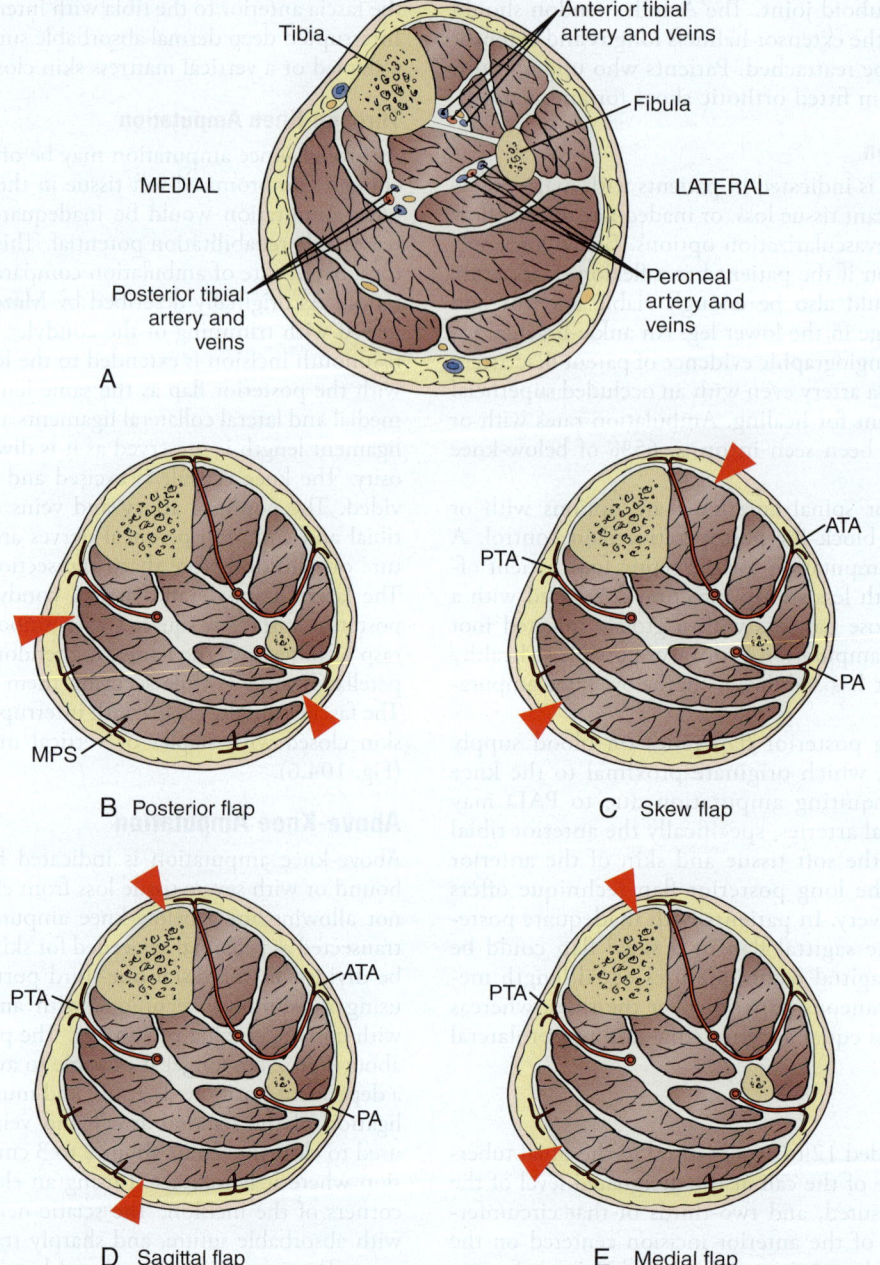

FIGURE 104.4 Cross-sectional anatomy and blood supply to the skin at the level of transtibial amputation. (Note the location of skin incisions (arrowheads). (A) Leg cross-section. (B) Posterior flap. (C) Skew flap. (D) Sagittal flap. (E) Medial flap. *ATA*, Anterior tibial artery; *MPS*, musculocutaneous perforators from the sural artery; *PA*, peroneal artery; *PTA*, posterior tibial artery.)

retract. The sartorius muscle is divided at its origin, the iliopsoas is divided at its insertion site, and the pectineus is divided at its origin. The obturator neurovascular bundle is suture ligated. The gracilis and three adductor muscles are divided from the pubic rami. The posterior thigh muscles are transected at the ischial tuberosity, and all the muscles attached to the greater trochanter are divided. The ligaments of the hip joint and the capsule are resected. The posterior quadratus femoris is approximated to the anterior iliopsoas, and the lateral gluteus medius is approximated to the medial obturator externus. The gluteal fascia is then approximated to the inguinal ligament, and the skin is closed with deep dermal absorbable sutures and skin staples.

Upper Extremity Amputations

The majority of upper extremity amputations are due to trauma of the hand; however, other indications such as malignancy may be possible. Unlike the lower extremity amputation in which the primary goal often is adequate soft tissue coverage in order to fit into a prosthesis, the upper extremity amputation also has to be functional and cosmetically acceptable.

Digit Amputation

Depending on the level of injury or proximal margin needed, digit amputations involve preserving length as much as possible for functional recovery. A small rongeur is used to take the phalanx

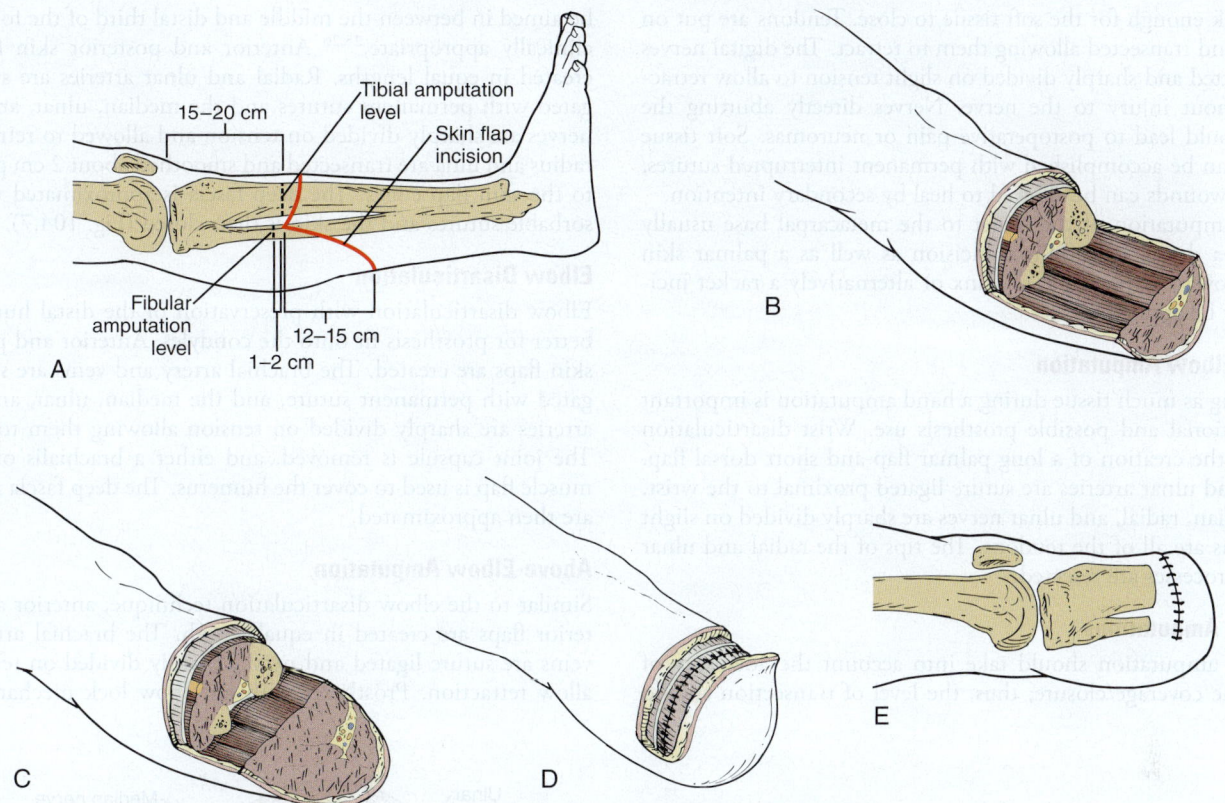

FIGURE 104.5 Transtibial amputation. (A) Marking the skin incisions. (B) Fashioning the flaps after bone transection. (C) The soleus muscle is tailored to create a proper flap. (D) The posterior deep fascia is sutured to the anterior deep fascia and periosteum. (E) Closure of the skin flaps. (From Rios AL, Eidt JF. Lower extremity amputations: operative techniques and results. In: Sidawy AN, Perler BA, eds. *Rutherford's Vascular Surgery and Endovascular Therapy*. 10th ed. Philadelphia: Elsevier; 2024:1529-1547.)

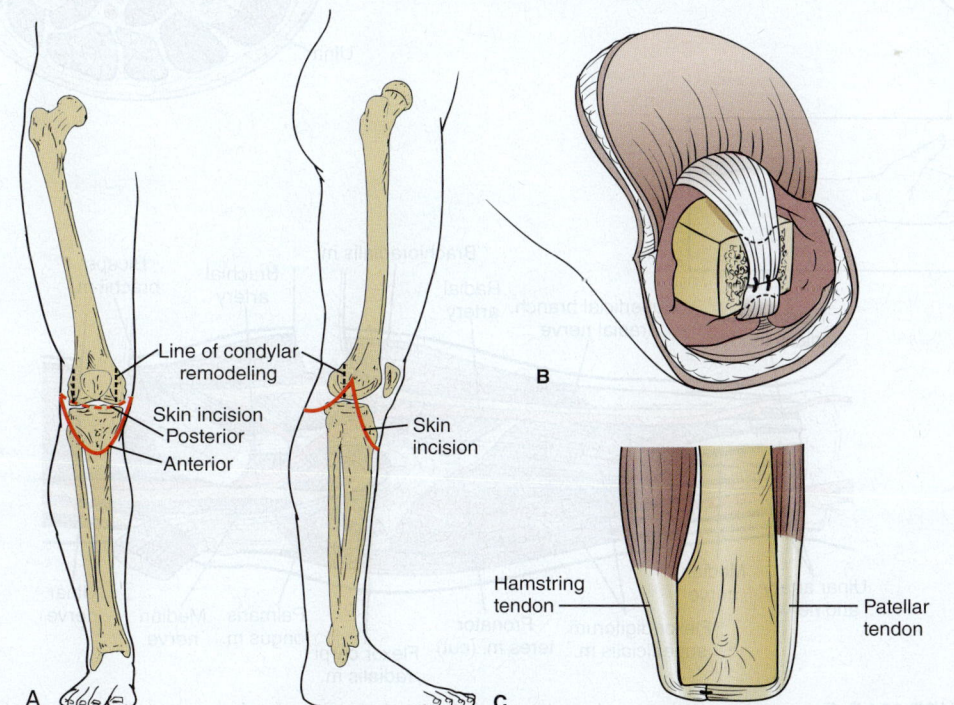

FIGURE 104.6 (A) Fishmouth incision for through-knee amputation. (B–C) The patellar tendon is sutured directly to the residual cruciate ligament. (From Rios AL, Eidt JF. Lower extremity amputations: operative techniques and results. In: Sidawy AN, Perler BA, eds. *Rutherford's Vascular Surgery and Endovascular Therapy*. 10th ed. Philadelphia: Elsevier; 2024:1529-1547.)

bone back enough for the soft tissue to close. Tendons are put on tension and transected allowing them to retract. The digital nerves are dissected and sharply divided on slight tension to allow retraction without injury to the nerve. Nerves directly abutting the stump could lead to postoperative pain or neuromas. Soft tissue closure can be accomplished with permanent interrupted sutures, or small wounds can be allowed to heal by secondary intention.

Ray amputation of the finger to the metacarpal base usually involves a dorsal longitudinal incision as well as a palmar skin incision over the proximal phalanx or alternatively a racket incision may be applied.

Below-Elbow Amputation

Preserving as much tissue during a hand amputation is important for functional and possible prosthesis use. Wrist disarticulation involves the creation of a long palmar flap and short dorsal flap. Radial and ulnar arteries are suture ligated proximal to the wrist. The median, radial, and ulnar nerves are sharply divided on slight tension as are all of the tendons. The tips of the radial and ulnar styloid processes are resected.

Forearm Amputations

Forearm amputation should take into account the adequacy of soft tissue coverage/closure; thus, the level of transection should be aimed in between the middle and distal third of the forearm as clinically appropriate.[25,26] Anterior and posterior skin flaps are created in equal lengths. Radial and ulnar arteries are suture ligated with permanent sutures and the median, ulnar, and radial nerves are sharply divided on tension and allowed to retract. The radius and ulna are transected and smoothed about 2 cm proximal to the skin flap edges. The deep fascia is approximated with absorbable sutures and the skin is then closed (Fig. 104.7).

Elbow Disarticulation

Elbow disarticulation with preservation of the distal humerus is better for prosthesis fit onto the condyles. Anterior and posterior skin flaps are created. The brachial artery and veins are suture ligated with permanent suture, and the median, ulnar, and radial arteries are sharply divided on tension allowing them to retract. The joint capsule is removed, and either a brachialis or triceps muscle flap is used to cover the humerus. The deep fascia and skin are then approximated.

Above-Elbow Amputation

Similar to the elbow disarticulation technique, anterior and posterior flaps are created in equal length. The brachial artery and veins are suture ligated and nerves sharply divided on tension to allow retraction. Prostheses with an elbow lock mechanism are

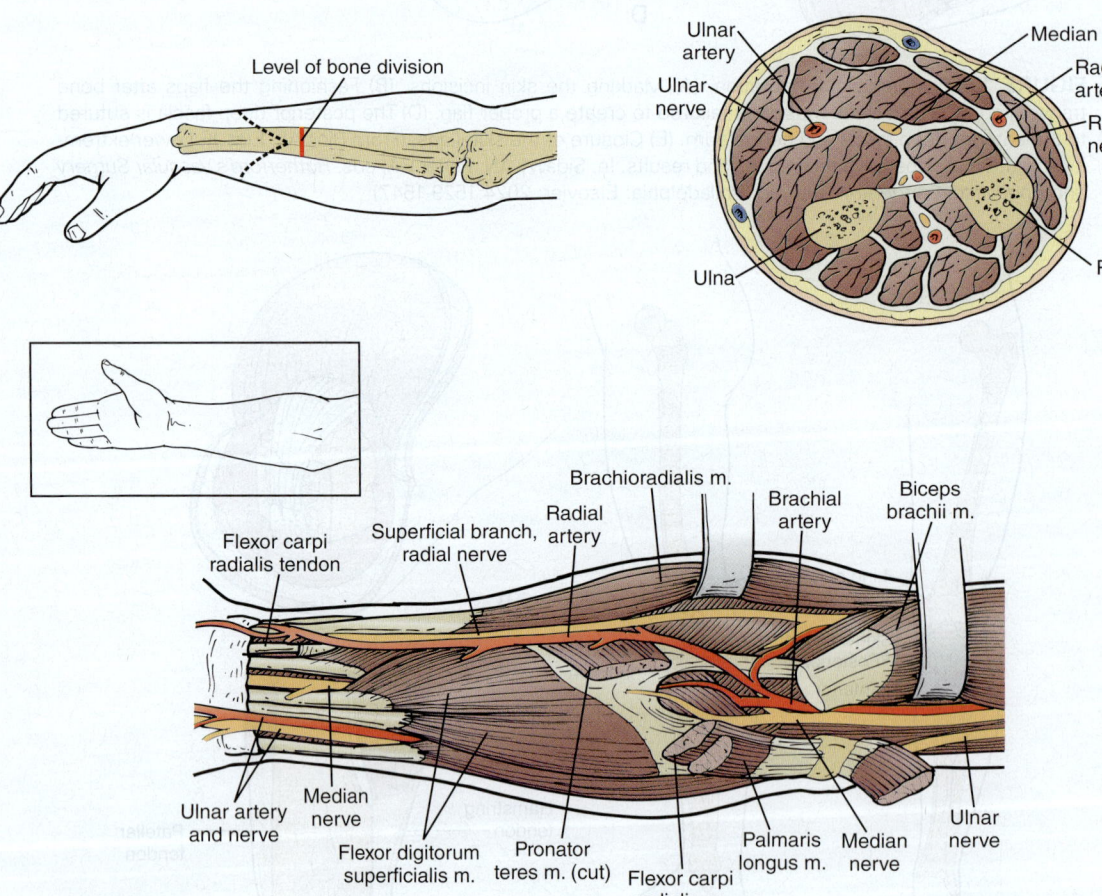

FIGURE 104.7 Forearm amputation is relatively straightforward: division of soft tissue at the junction of the distal third and proximal two-thirds of the forearm and several centimeters distal to the level of the bony division. Proper muscle coverage is achieved with myofascial closure. *m.*, Muscle. (Adapted with permission from Maxwell MC. Amputations in trauma. In: Thal ER, Weigelt JA, Carrico CJ, eds. *Operative Trauma Management: An Atlas*. 2nd ed. New York: McGraw-Hill; 2002:449.)

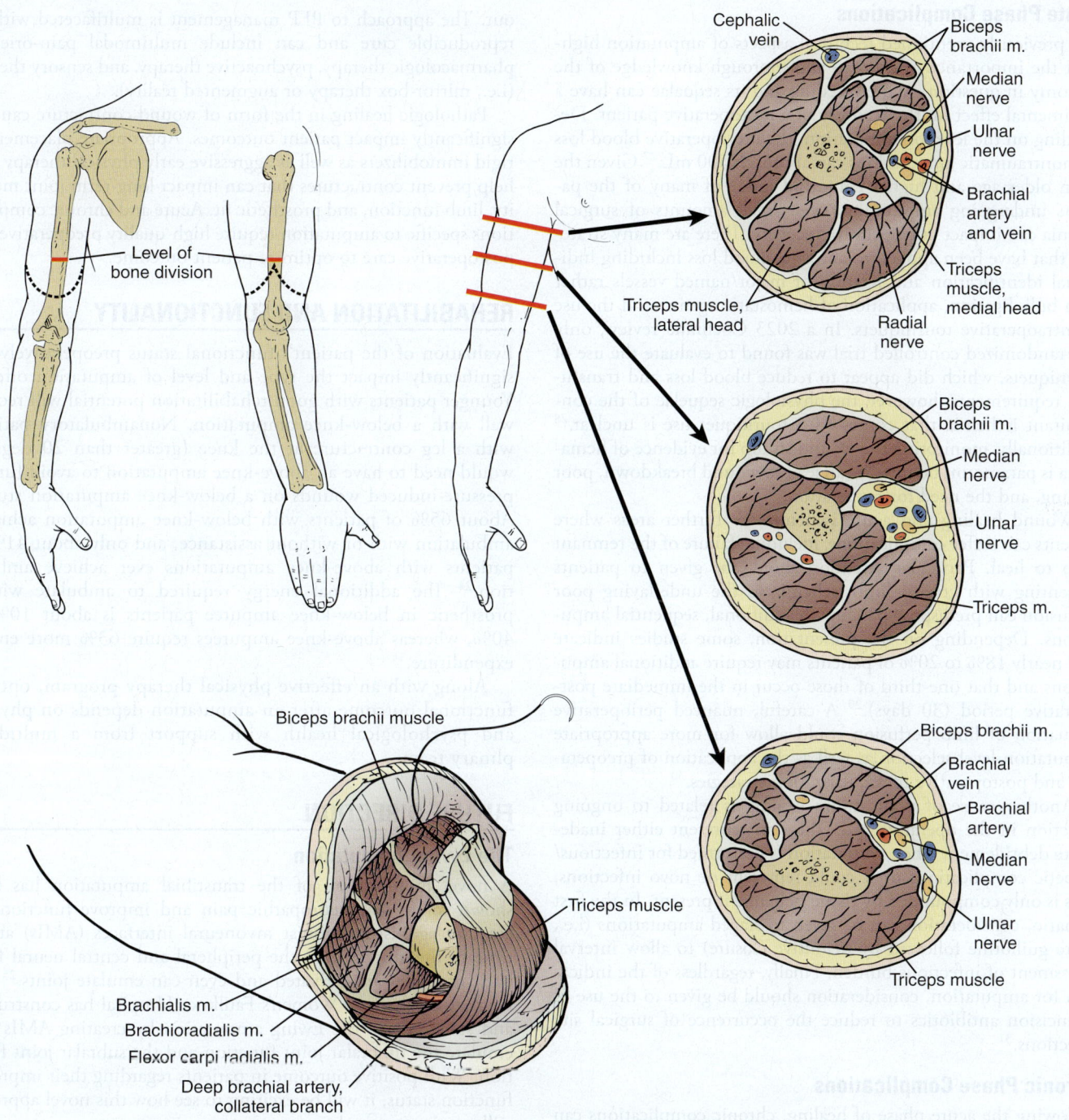

FIGURE 104.8 Upper arm amputation can be performed at several levels. The initial operation should be focused on maintaining as much humeral length as possible and the epicondyles, if salvageable. *m.*, Muscle. (Adapted with permission from Maxwell MC. Amputations in trauma. In: Thal ER, Weigelt JA, Carrico CJ, eds. *Operative Trauma Management: An Atlas.* 2nd ed. New York: McGraw-Hill; 2002:451.)

4 cm long, so the upper arm amputation should be made 4 cm proximal to the elbow (Fig. 104.8).

Shoulder Disarticulation

Shoulder disarticulation is a complex procedure with difficult prosthesis fitting and resultant minimal function. The humeral head may be retained for aid in creating contours for a prosthesis. The deltoid and pectoral muscles with their overlying skin can offer flap coverage. The latissimus dorsi, pectoralis major, and the rotator cuff tendons are attached to the glenoid capsule. Key

aspects include suture ligation of the vascular bundle, sharp division of the nerves on tension, and tensionless soft tissue coverage of the amputation site.

COMMON COMPLICATIONS

Limb amputation has a major impact on a patient's physiology, psyche, and quality of life. Regardless of the level of amputation, the procedure is complex with multiple failure points, which can drastically alter outcomes.

Acute Phase Complications

The previously mentioned technical aspects of amputation highlight the importance of a broad and thorough knowledge of the anatomy in question. Acute bleeding and its sequalae can have a detrimental effect on the recovery of a postoperative patient. Depending on the level of amputation, the intraoperative blood loss for nontraumatic amputations can approach 500 mL.[27] Given the often older age and higher comorbid index of many of the patients undergoing amputation, even small amounts of surgical anemia can impact postoperative recovery. There are many strategies that have been applied to abrogate blood loss including individual identification and ligation of major/named vessels rather than bulk ligation, application of hemostatic agents, and the use of intraoperative tourniquets. In a 2023 Cochrane review, only one randomized controlled trial was found to evaluate the use of tourniquets, which did appear to reduce blood loss and transfusion requirements; however, the physiologic sequelae of the concomitant ischemia that comes with tourniquet use is unclear.[28] Additionally, monitoring the wound stump for evidence of hematoma is paramount because it can lead to wound breakdown, poor healing, and the need for reoperation.

Wound healing and acute ischemia are further areas where patients can suffer complications, including failure of the remnant limb to heal. Particular attention should be given to patients presenting with critical limb ischemia as the underlaying poor perfusion can predispose patients to additional, sequential amputations. Depending on the presentation, some studies indicate that nearly 18% to 20% of patients may require additional amputations and that one-third of those occur in the immediate postoperative period (30 days).[29] A careful, nuanced perioperative evaluation of limb perfusion could allow for more appropriate amputation-level selection as well as the application of preoperative and postoperative revascularization strategies.[30]

Another cause of poor stump healing is related to ongoing infection in the operative bed. This can represent either inadequate debridement when amputation is performed for infectious/diabetic complications or it could represent de novo infections. This is only compounded by tissue ischemia if present. In the first scenario, consideration can be given to staged amputations (i.e., acute guillotine followed by definitive closure) to allow interval assessment of infectious burden. Finally, regardless of the indication for amputation, consideration should be given to the use of preincision antibiotics to reduce the occurrence of surgical site infections.[31]

Chronic Phase Complications

Following the acute phase of healing, chronic complications can continue to cause patients to have a poor quality of life if not managed appropriately.

Chronic pain including phantom limb pain (PLP) after amputation is a major source of morbidity in the postoperative, posthospitalization setting. Long-standing pain in the stump (i.e., residual limb pain [RLP]) after amputation is likely a distinct entity from true PLP pain, although there maybe overlapping etiologies, symptomology, and contributing factors. Some reports indicate that up to 70% of patients will experience some form of RLP, whereas PLP can reach similar or even higher incidence.[32,33] RLP must be systematically addressed including consideration of continued ischemia, neuroma formation, and pressure points from osseous spurs or pathologic bone remodeling. PLP can be considered either based on specific complaints (pain in a portion of the limb that is no longer present) or after RLP has been ruled out. The approach to PLP management is multifaceted with no reproducible cure and can include multimodal pain-oriented pharmacologic therapy, psychoactive therapy, and sensory therapy (i.e., mirror-box therapy or augmented reality).

Pathologic healing in the form of wound contracture can also significantly impact patient outcomes. Appropriate placement of rigid immobilizers as well as aggressive early physical therapy may help prevent contractures that can impact long-term joint mobility, limb function, and prosthetic fit. Acute and chronic complications specific to amputation require high-quality preoperative and postoperative care to optimize patient outcome.

REHABILITATION AND FUNCTIONALITY

Evaluation of the patient's functional status preoperatively can significantly impact the type and level of amputation offered. Younger patients with good rehabilitation potential will recover well with a below-knee amputation. Nonambulatory patients with a leg contracture at the knee (greater than 20 degrees) would need to have an above-knee amputation to avoid further pressure-induced wounds on a below-knee amputation stump. About 65% of patients with below-knee amputation achieved ambulation with or without assistance, and only about 41% of patients with above-knee amputations ever achieve ambulation.[24] The additional energy required to ambulate with a prosthetic in below-knee amputee patients is about 10% to 40%, whereas above-knee amputees require 63% more energy expenditure.[34]

Along with an effective physical therapy program, optimal functional outcome after an amputation depends on physical and psychological health with support from a multidisciplinary team.

FUTURE DIRECTION

The Ewing Amputation

A novel modification of the transtibial amputation has been shown to prevent neuropathic pain and improve function. By creating agonist-antagonist myoneural interfaces (AMIs) at the time of the amputation, the peripheral and central neural feedback processes are activated and even can emulate joints.[25] The team at Brigham & Women's Faulkner Hospital has constructed and standardized the Ewing amputation by creating AMIs that emulate the tibiotalar joint function and the subtalar joint function. With positive outcome in patients regarding their improved function status, it will be exciting to see how this novel approach will continue to evolve.

SELECTED REFERENCES

Govsyeyev N, Nehler MR, Low Wang CC, et al. Etiology and outcomes of amputation in patients with peripheral artery disease in the EUCLID trial. *J Vasc Surg.* 2022;75(2):660–670.e3.

> Important randomized trial on outcomes after amputations in patients with symptomatic peripheral artery disease.

Cull DL, Manos G, Hartley MC, et al. An early validation of the Society for Vascular Surgery lower extremity threatened limb classification system. *J Vasc Surg.* 2014;60(6):1535-1542.

Important early validation of the staging system using wound characteristic, ischemia, and foot infection (WIfI system) in patients with critical limb ischemia.

Kalbaugh CA, Strassle PD, Paul NJ, McGinigle KL, Kibbe MR, Marston WA. Trends in surgical indications for major lower limb amputation in the USA from 2000 to 2016. *Eur J Vasc Endovasc Surg.* 2020;60(1):88-96.

A population based analysis describes the prevalence of amputations and indications for ampuation in the USA from 2000 to 2016, which shows infection in the presence of ischemia was a major indicator of amputation.

Daso G, Chen AJ, Yeh S, et al. Lower extremity amputations among veterans: have ambulatory outcomes and survival improved. *Ann Vasc Surg.* 2022;87:311-320.

Retrospective review of major lower extremity amputations in the Veterans Affair population from 2000-2020.

Clark MA, Thomas JM. Amputation for soft-tissue sarcoma. *Lancet Oncol.* 2003;4(6):335-342.

Important review of management and outcomes of soft tissue sarcomas requiring amputations.

The full reference list appears on Elsevier eBooks+.

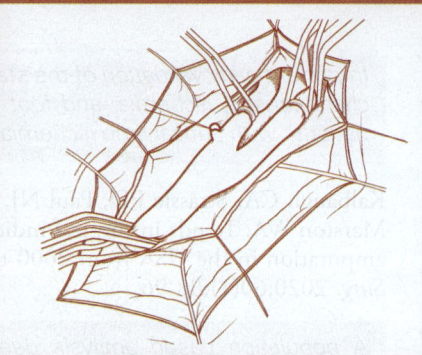

Peripheral Aneurysmal Disease

Joshua T. Geiger, Dawn Coleman, and Michael C. Stoner

▶ **Please access Elsevier eBooks+ to view the video for this chapter.**

INTRODUCTION

The word *aneurysm* is derived from the Greek ἀνεύρυσμα, *aneurysma*, meaning "dilation." Today, the term *aneurysm* refers to a dilation of any blood vessel to a size of 1.5 times the expected size of a normal adjacent segment of an artery. Aneurysms can be classified based on their morphology, size, anatomic location, and etiology, which are described later. The effective description of an aneurysm is important because it influences surgical indications and the surgical approach.

Peripheral and visceral aneurysms, although less common than aortic aneurysms, can represent a significant cause of morbidity and, rarely, fatality in patients. The most common cause of peripheral and visceral aneurysms is atherosclerotic degeneration; however, several etiologies exist and must be understood by the treating physician. Degenerative aneurysms are frequently fusiform in morphology and often associated with other degenerative aneurysms elsewhere in the body, most commonly the aorta. Peripheral aneurysms are often asymptomatic; however, when they present symptomatically, it is usually with symptoms of end-organ complications secondary to thromboembolic events. Rarely, the free rupture of an intraperitoneal or intrathoracic aneurysm may lead to death by hemorrhagic shock. The exclusion of the aneurysmal sac and restoration of arterial perfusion are the primary goals of any intervention because of these risks. Most of this chapter will focus on true aneurysms of the viscera and upper and lower extremities. With the increasing prevalence of endovascular therapies by multiple specialties, posttraumatic pseudoaneurysms

are increasing in prevalence, and, as such, a discussion of iatrogenic false aneurysms is included. Discussion of mycotic aneurysms is outside the scope of this chapter.

Size and Morphology

The first step in describing irregularity in an arterial wall is to assess the size and morphology of the blood vessel. A true aneurysm is a dilation of all three arterial wall layers (intimate, media, adventitia) to a size greater than 1.5 times the diameter of healthy arterial tissue just proximal or distal to the region in question. An abnormal dilation in the blood vessel that does not meet this criterion is described as *ectatic*. A false aneurysm, often described as a pseudoaneurysm, is a focal disruption of all three layers of the native arterial wall. Pseudoaneurysms are typically the results of an iatrogenic injury or trauma. The extravascular blood generated by such an injury is contained by a wall of connective tissue or hematoma and is at high risk of rupturing.

The shape of a true aneurysm can be described as fusiform or saccular. Fusiform aneurysms are asymmetric increases in the entire diameter of the affected blood vessel, whereas saccular aneurysms are described as localized, asymmetric, or eccentric outpouchings arising from a focal weakness in the arterial wall. Most peripheral aneurysms are fusiform. This is because the most common cause of peripheral aneurysms is atherosclerotic degeneration of the concentric arterial wall. The risk of rupture and thromboembolic events has been relatively well characterized for most peripheral arterial fusiform aneurysms. These risks are generally less well understood for aneurysms with a saccular morphology. However, it is believed there is an increased risk of rupture, and, as such, saccular aneurysms require repair at smaller diameters. However, the surgical management of a saccular aneurysm is still dependent on symptoms, size, growth rate, and ability to perform such a repair, just as for fusiform aneurysms.

It is important to distinguish the difference between an arterial aneurysm and arteriomegaly. Classically arteriomegaly has been described as large, smoothly dilated, and commonly tortuous arteries without focal segments of dilation. This is contrasted to aneurysmal arterial tissue in which there is a focal dilation of a blood vessel, often with an irregular intima, secondary to atherosclerotic plaque. Often, aneurysms develop intraluminal thrombus that can help distinguish an aneurysm from arteriomegaly. Arteriomegaly appears to have a strong familial association, with approximately 36% of patients having a family history of arteriomegaly or aneurysms in a first-degree relative. Furthermore, patients with arteriomegaly are at increased risk of aneurysm formation.[1]

Etiology

Degenerative

Degenerative and *atherosclerotic* are terms used interchangeably to describe the most common ideology of peripheral aneurysms. Although aneurysm formation appears to be associated with atherosclerotic disease, a causal relationship between atherosclerosis and aneurysmal formation has not been established. Atherosclerotic occlusive disease and aneurysmal disease do share several common risk factors, including smoking, older age, male sex, and hyperlipidemia. However, the "degenerative" aneurysm most likely refers to a few different unidentified etiologies, and the involvement of atherosclerotic plaques in the disease process is likely multifactorial.[2] Contrary to atherosclerosis, diabetes appears to be protective from the development of degenerative aneurysmal disease. This may be partly due to the high frequency of metformin use in the diabetic population. Patients with abdominal aortic aneurysm (AAA) and type 2 diabetes who were taking metformin to manage their diabetes had slower rates of aneurysm progression when compared with diabetics not taking the drug.[3]

Recent studies have demonstrated that the immune system is critical in degenerative aneurysm formation. The presence of inflammatory cells, upregulation of adaptive and innate immunity genes, and degradation of collagen and elastin have supported this. Almost all inflammatory cell lines have been shown to infiltrate arterial walls in diseased tissue.[4] These cells organize and produce immune-related structures, such as inflammasomes and neutrophil extracellular traps, that have been associated with aneurysm tissue. In addition, cytokines and protease secreted by inflammatory cells likely contribute to the disease process. Although inflammation and extracellular matrix degeneration are hallmarks of aneurysm formation, the inciting cause is unknown. Current hypotheses include activation of the immune system by infectious agents either directly or through systemic signals[5] and autoimmune dysregulation.

Smoking remains the most significant risk factor for the development and growth of atherosclerotic aneurysms[6]; therefore, it is the top modifiable risk factor to reduce aneurysm growth and associated complications. Fortunately, there has been a significant decrease in the incidents of AAA-related mortality as the rate of smoking has decreased in the general population. It is unclear whether this applies to the incidents of peripheral arterial aneurysms and their associated complications.

Dissection Associated

Arterial dissection is described as the separation of the intima from the arterial media with subsequent extension of this separation in its anatomic plane longitudinally along the vessel. Acute occlusion, either static or dynamic, and aneurysm formation are the two main morbidities linked to arterial dissection. Because the arterial wall is dependent on the three layers to maintain structural integrity, a disruption in the arterial wall can lead to aneurysmal degeneration. The weakened artery can rupture in the acute setting. More frequently, the vessel undergoes a slow, progressive dilation over time. Spontaneous dissection most commonly occurs within the aorta; however, it can occur within peripheral and abdominal arteries as well. In the peripheral vasculature, arterial dissections are most associated with atherosclerotic disease. In younger patients without common risk factors of atherosclerosis or evidence of the disease process on imaging, segmental arterial mediolysis (SAM) should be considered as a rare cause of arterial dissection. SAM should be considered in the differential for any young patient with an aneurysm or dissection in an unusual location because this can be a life-threatening diagnosis.

Inflammatory

The inflammatory aneurysm was first described in 1972[7] as an entity distinct from degenerative aneurysms by the existence of a thick arterial wall encased with extensive fibrotic adhesions that incorporate adjoining tissues. Axial imaging often demonstrates a thick inflammatory "rind" on the exterior of the affected blood vessel. This rind can involve adjacent structures, making this class of aneurysms notoriously difficult to treat operatively.

Tissue from inflammatory aneurysms often demonstrated atherosclerotic changes within the intima. The primary difference between the degenerative and inflammatory etiology is within the adventitia. The adventitial layer is thicker and frequently infiltrated with inflammatory cells.[8] The role of plasma cells in this disease process is particularly important because approximately 40% to 50% of all inflammatory aneurysms contain IgG4-positive plasma cells.[9] Interestingly, neutrophilic infiltration and thick atherosclerotic plaques are more often seen in patients with non–IgG4-related inflammatory aneurysms. In these patients, IgG4-positive plasma cells are rare.

Some inflammatory aneurysms are associated with forms of large- and medium-vessel vasculitis. Other rare inflammatory diseases, such as Behçet disease, Cogan syndrome, and cystic medial necrosis, have components of arterial inflammation that have been associated with aneurysmal degeneration. Tissue biopsy is the gold standard for the diagnosis of vasculitis and related inflammatory diseases. When tissue samples are not obtainable, angiography can be helpful in assessing the specific type of arteritis. Asymmetric areas of segmental stenosis with aneurysm formation are characteristic of vasculitis on angiography. More common causes of aneurysms and occlusions, such as atherosclerosis and fibromuscular dysplasia (FMD), must be evaluated before making a diagnosis of vasculitis.

Finally, it is imperative to rule out an infectious etiology before any intervention. Failure to do so can lead to disastrous consequences, including implantation of surgical grafts in an infected field or administration of immunosuppressive medications during an active infection. The treatment of inflammatory aneurysms is challenging and should be managed by a multidisciplinary team, with a thorough evaluation of the differential diagnosis for aneurysmal degeneration.

Infectious

A primary arterial wall infection can lead to the formation of an arterial aneurysm. Immunocompromised patients, such as those with HIV or diabetes, those taking immunosuppressive or immunomodulatory drugs, and those undergoing chemotherapy, are at higher risk.[10] The incidence of infectious aneurysms is also increased in patients who inject drugs, specifically at blood vessels near the site of injection. In early studies, the femoral artery was the most common site of infected aneurysms, followed closely by the abdominal aorta. However, virtually any infected blood vessel can become aneurysmal, and a wide variety of pathogens can be responsible.

Traumatic and Iatrogenic

Traumatic and iatrogenic aneurysms are typically the result of direct transmural arterial injury, resulting in the formation of a pseudoaneurysm. Typically, this occurs in the setting of penetrating injury where a small segment of the artery is damaged, allowing extravasation of blood that is subsequently contained by solidifying hematoma or extravascular connective tissue. Blunt trauma and shearing or traction injuries can also lead to transmural damage and subsequent aneurysm formation. With the increasing prevalence of endovascular procedures in many specialties, the incidence of iatrogenic aneurysm formation at the arterial access site is becoming more prevalent. Iatrogenic aneurysms are the direct result of inadequate closure of the intentionally created arteriotomy.

Congenital or Developmental

Collagen and elastin are the primary structural components of the extracellular matrix within arterial walls. These components vary by type and quantity throughout the vascular tree and are critical in maintaining the strength and elasticity of the arterial wall. Therefore, any disease that affects the integrity of these structural proteins can affect the integrity of the vascular wall. Connective tissue diseases are a family of genetic conditions in which the structural integrity of collagen or elastin is affected. This can be through genetic mutations of the collagen and elastin genes themselves or through alterations in the assembly of these proteins. Patients who develop a disruption in the integrity of collagen or elastin are inherently predisposed to degeneration and loss of arterial structural integrity. This often leads to aneurysm formation, spontaneous arterial dissections, and even arterial rupture.

The most well-known connective tissue disorders affecting the vascular system include Marfan syndrome, Loeys-Dietz syndrome, familial thoracic aortic aneurysm and dissection, and vascular-type Ehlers-Danlos syndrome. Patients with these syndromes can present with multiple aneurysms in various, seemingly unrelated locations, sometimes described as *aneurysmosis*. This presentation should raise suspicion for a genetic cause.

VISCERAL ARTERY ANEURYSMS

Epidemiology

Approximately 5% of intraabdominal aneurysms affect the visceral arteries,[11] with patients most often presenting in their sixth decade of life. Historically, these aneurysms were described as *mycotic,* often syphilitic in etiology. Most contemporary visceral aneurysms are atherosclerotic or secondary to medial degeneration. Other etiologies include FMD, collagen vascular disease, inflammatory conditions (e.g., arteritis), and other rare inherited illnesses (e.g., Ehlers-Danlos syndrome and neurofibromatosis type 1).

Visceral aneurysms have an estimated incidence of 0.1% to 2%, although autopsy series suggest this may approach 10%.[12] The majority of these aneurysms are asymptomatic and diagnosed incidentally during imaging for some other diagnosis.[11] Only a minority of visceral aneurysms present with life-threatening rupture, associated with abdominal pain and hemorrhagic shock. Rupture may be intraabdominal and may result in gastrointestinal (GI) bleeding or arteriovenous fistulae in cases of sporadic erosion into structures in proximity. Although historical mortality rates approached 25% to 70%, more contemporary series suggest mortality rates as low as 10% to 15%, presumed secondary to improvements in perioperative management and the increasing use of endovascular techniques.[13] False aneurysms carry a significantly higher rate of rupture in comparison to true aneurysms. Because of their rarity and the fact that only institutional and retrospective data are available, the natural history of true aneurysms remains abstract.

Diagnosis

Occult visceral artery aneurysms are being diagnosed with increased frequency because of the increased use of advanced abdominal imaging, including magnetic resonance imaging (MRI), magnetic resonance angiography (MRA), computed tomography (CT), and CT angiography (CTA).[11] These advanced imaging modalities facilitate improved early identification and also enhance preoperative open and endovascular case planning for treatment.

Ultrasound examination of visceral vessels is limited by artifact from bowel gas and obesity, with poor sensitivity in detecting many visceral and branch aneurysms <3 cm. Axial imaging of the abdomen is recommended for this reason. Certain phenotypes that suggest FMD and connective tissue disorders should be screened for cerebrovascular and coronary artery aneurysms with additional head and neck imaging. CTA is the most commonly used modality for diagnosing and evaluating splanchnic aneurysms because it offers multiplanar, maximal-intensity projection reconstruction, volume rendering, and three-dimensional reconstructions to better assess the arterial anatomic details of the visceral and renal arteries.[11] Sections of 1-mm thickness optimize spatial resolution and enhance anatomic definition; three-dimensional reconstructions improve representation of the number and relation of all involved branches in comparison to two-dimensional catheter angiography or ultrasound. Compromised renal function increases the risk of contrast-induced nephropathy. Non- or alternate-contrast–enhanced MRA has been used to assess splanchnic aneurysms as performed with a "breath-hold" steady-state free precession sequence or time-spatial labeling inversion pulse technique. Three-dimensional rotational catheter-based angiography may benefit in planning optimal working angles for endovascular treatment and provide accurate evaluation of aneurysm necks and feeding arteries.

Treatment

Patients with visceral aneurysms generally have 10-year survival rates >80%; therefore, aneurysm treatment must offer durable long-term results with low perioperative mortality and morbidity. Although surgical repair has remained the mainstay of treatment, endovascular techniques are increasingly applied for treatment of both elective and ruptured cases. Endovascular therapy offers excellent rates of technical success, minimal morbidity and mortality, and shorter length of hospital stay. However, there is a higher risk of end-organ embolization and reintervention.[13–15] Transcatheter endovascular therapy alternatives include (1) treatment of both the aneurysm and pathologic vessel (i.e., the isolation technique); (2) aneurysm exclusion with parent vessel flow preservation (i.e., the exclusion technique); and (3) direct percutaneous puncture of the sac and subsequent embolization with thrombin, glue, or ethylene vinyl alcohol copolymer (EVOH).[16] The latter is less commonly employed for percutaneously accessible aneurysms with narrow necks. Endovascular treatments may offer decreased postoperative morbidity and mortality rates in cases of rupture compared with open surgery (2.7%–7% vs. 24%–29%, respectively).[13,17] Each splanchnic aneurysm warrants individual consideration.

Splenic Artery Aneurysm

Splenic artery aneurysms (Fig. 105.1) account for 60% of all splanchnic artery aneurysms and are the third most common intraabdominal arterial aneurysms, with a prevalence of 0.1% to 0.8% in the general population.[18] Many of these aneurysms, as proposed by Stanley et al., are attributed to arterial dysplasia, portal hypertension (HTN), local inflammation, and hormonal and hemodynamic events. As such, they are two to four times more common in females and strongly associated with multiparty.[18] HTN is a common comorbidity affecting more than half of patients with splenic aneurysm, and up to 20% will demonstrate concurrent aneurysm in an alternate arterial bed.[14] Additional etiologic risk factors include dissection and autoimmune arteritides like polyarteritis nodosa and systemic lupus erythematosus (SLE). Splenic aneurysms most often arise at branch points of the mid- and distal main splenic artery, with tortuosity of the main splenic artery being commonplace. Most splenic aneurysms are solitary and saccular, whereas 90% of patients with portal HTN will demonstrate multiple splenic aneurysms.

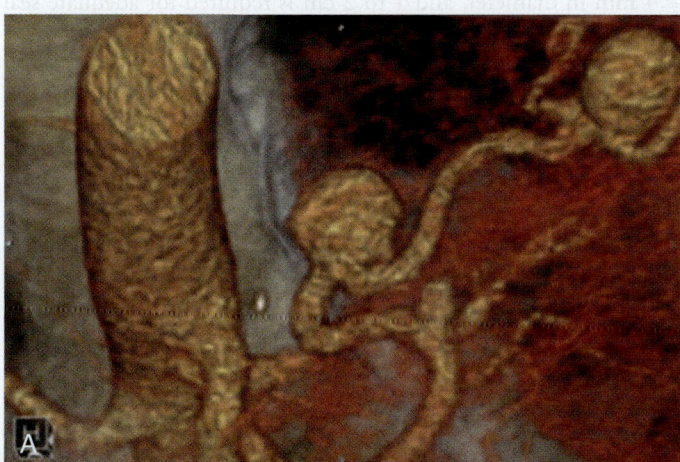
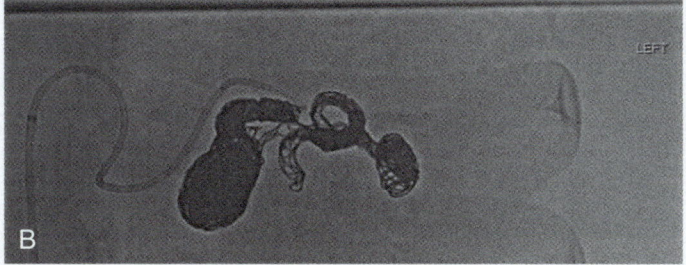

FIGURE 105.1 (A) Reformatted CT angiogram of two splenic artery aneurysms affecting the mid- and hilar artery. (B) Completion angiogram after successful coil embolization.

Splenic artery aneurysms in young females are thought to represent a more virulent phenotype. There is a tendency toward rupture that carries a devastating maternal and fetal mortality rate of >75%.[18] Pregnancy has also been associated with 20% to 50% of all ruptures, usually during the third trimester or peripartum period. Several large single-institution clinical reviews suggest aneurysms <3 cm in size can be safely observed, demonstrating slow to no growth (0.06–0.2 cm/year) with no ruptures or complications.[19] Additional risk factors for rupture include hepatic insufficiency with portal HTN, connective tissue disorder, rapid growth (>0.5 cm/year), and prior tobacco use. Splenic aneurysms typically rupture into the lesser sac with limited self-containment; subsequent hemorrhage into the peritoneal cavity results in cardiovascular collapse (i.e., the "double rupture").

Operative Indications

- All ruptured aneurysms should be repaired emergently.
- Pseudoaneurysms of any size should be repaired.
- True aneurysms of any size should be repaired in females of childbearing age.
- Aneurysms ≥3 cm with a demonstrable increase in size or with associated symptoms in patients of acceptable risk should be repaired.
- Consider repair in patients with portal HTN, especially in patients who may require liver transplantation.
- Consider repair in patients with a nonatherosclerotic or nondegenerative splenic artery aneurysm.
- Consider repair in patients whose splenic artery aneurysm demonstrates rapid growth.

Observation with annual surveillance (CT or ultrasound) is recommended for small (<3 cm), stable asymptomatic splenic artery true aneurysms or those in patients with significant medical comorbidities or limited life expectancies.

Surgical Management

Open reconstruction. Given the abundance of collateral flow to the spleen through the short gastric arteries, the splenic artery does not routinely require preservation or revascularization.[11] Proximal and distal ligation of the aneurysm segment is a viable surgical option that has served effectively as the traditional surgical management of these aneurysms. It is still recommended when rupture is discovered at laparotomy with or without splenectomy. For distal lesions adjacent to the splenic hilum, excision with possible splenectomy may be advantageous over endovascular methods given the risk of end-organ ischemia, including splenic infarction and pancreatitis, especially when the aneurysm involves intrasplenic branches within the splenic parenchyma. Distal pancreatectomy may also be warranted on occasion in the treatment of these distal aneurysms.

Patients requiring urgent splenic artery ligation or splenectomy should be vaccinated on or after postoperative day 14 to decrease the risk of postsplenectomy sepsis resulting from organisms like *Streptococcus pneumoniae*, *Haemophilus influenzae type B*, and *Neisseria meningitides*. Vaccination timing should be considered 14 days before intervention for elective cases.

Endovascular therapy. Endovascular therapy has become the treatment of choice for splenic artery aneurysms. In a recent study comparing open surgery, endovascular repair, and conservative management, endovascular treatment was found to be the most cost-effective and maintain the highest quality of life.[20] The classic endovascular isolation technique is appropriate for most splenic artery aneurysms in which the risk of distal ischemia is mitigated by collateral supply. From a percutaneous femoral approach, a secure triaxial platform can be established consisting of a sheath-guiding catheter positioned across the celiac trunk into the proximal splenic artery, through which a catheter is advanced into the afferent artery and aneurysm sac, and a microcatheter is advanced beyond into the efferent vessel. Steerable sheaths and catheters can mitigate the challenges of severe tortuosity. Metallic coils are the most commonly used occlusive material and offer secondary thrombosis through thrombogenic fibers and a resulting inflammatory reaction. Coil packing starts with the efferent branches. Progressive retraction of the microcatheter facilitates exclusion of the sac and afferent artery. Coils should be oversized by 10% to 20% of the native arterial diameter to mitigate the risk of migration and incomplete arterial occlusion. This technique can be challenging for large aneurysm sac sizes or when there are multiple efferent vessels that require cannulation and embolization. Partial embolization of the sac may help reduce flow into the sac, making outflow vessels more visible and accessible for cannulation. Liquid embolic agents (e.g., "glue," N-butyl cyanoacrylate glue, and EVOH) have also been described in this setting and are useful for reaching extremely tortuous and small distal arteries that are unsuitable for coil embolization. Postembolization syndrome complicates 10% to 30% of procedural cases across series and may include left upper quadrant pain, fever, ileus, platelet dysfunction, leukocytosis, and pancreatitis after embolization with and without radiographic evidence of splenic infarction. This is far more common than splenic infarction, splenic necrosis with or without abscess, and treatment failure (5%). Staged embolization should be considered for patients with multiple aneurysms and portal HTN.

Continued surveillance with CT or ultrasound imaging is critical after endovascular treatment for all treated aneurysms, even after technical success, given the aforementioned risk of recanalization (18%–30%) and resultant secondary growth and rupture.[11,21]

Hepatic Artery Aneurysm

Hepatic artery aneurysms account for 20% of splanchnic artery aneurysms, affecting males twice as often as females.[12] The majority of hepatic aneurysms are asymptomatic extrahepatic solitary lesions that primarily affect the common and right hepatic arteries. Less than 30% are intrahepatic. Iatrogenic hepatic artery pseudoaneurysms account for half of reported hepatic artery aneurysms and are increasingly in frequency as a result of increased diagnostic and therapeutic interventions that require liver penetration. True aneurysms are primarily a result of atherosclerosis, whereas polyarteritis nodosa, cystic medial necrosis, portal HTN, FMD, and other acquired arteriopathies are less common. When present, symptoms are commonly described as right upper quadrant or epigastric abdominal pain that may radiate to the back. Large aneurysms may erode into the stomach or duodenum, resulting in GI hemorrhage, or obstruct the biliary tract, resulting in biliary colic, hematobilia, or obstructive jaundice. Although the true incidence is unknown, rupture is believed to complicate a minority of hepatic artery aneurysms (20%–30%) and results in an equal distribution of hemorrhage into the peritoneum and the biliary tract, the latter resulting in hematobilia, hematemesis, and cholangitis. Rupture-related mortality is approximately 35% to 40%. The relationship of rupture risk to aneurysm size remains unclear, although a small clinical series supports a natural history of slow to null growth. The majority of ruptures are reported at an aneurysm size >2 cm, and risk factors for such include the

presence of multiple aneurysms, nonatherosclerotic aneurysms (e.g., polyarteritis nodosum, Wegener granulomatosis, SLE) and female sex.[22]

Operative Indications

- Regardless of size, all pseudoaneurysms should be repaired.
- Regardless of size, all symptomatic aneurysms should be repaired.
- Regardless of size, all aneurysms associated with vasculopathy or vasculitis should be repaired.
- True aneurysms >2.0 cm in diameter in low-risk patients should be repaired.
- If open repair is required, true aneurysms >5.0 cm among high-risk patients should be repaired.

Surgical Management

Open reconstruction. Given the possibility of central liver necrosis despite adequate collateral flow by endovascular exclusion, open surgical revascularization using autologous vein conduit is recommended when endovascular stent-graft exclusion is not possible to maintain arterial circulation to the liver. Temporary occlusion of the hepatic artery during reconstruction may guide revascularization or ligation of the hepatic artery. More distal extrahepatic aneurysm branches are often associated with biliary inflammation, making these repairs challenging. Intrahepatic aneurysms will require resection of the lobe in which the aneurysm is located, and lobe resection is recommended for large aneurysms to mitigate the risk of significant hepatic necrosis.

Endovascular therapy. Society for Vascular Surgery (SVS) guidelines support an endovascular-first approach to all hepatic artery aneurysms if anatomically feasible, provided arterial circulation can be maintained to the liver. Covered stents facilitate aneurysm exclusion and are preferably used in vessels measuring ≥4 mm in diameter, and 1 to 2 cm is required for adequate seal proximally and distally.[16] Aneurysm branches arising off the sac to be covered should be embolized to avoid retrograde reperfusion, and dual-antiplatelet therapy is often prescribed for a finite duration (6 weeks to 6 months) postprocedure. In patients with intrahepatic aneurysms (Fig. 105.2), embolization of the affected artery is recommended.[11] Complications of embolization include

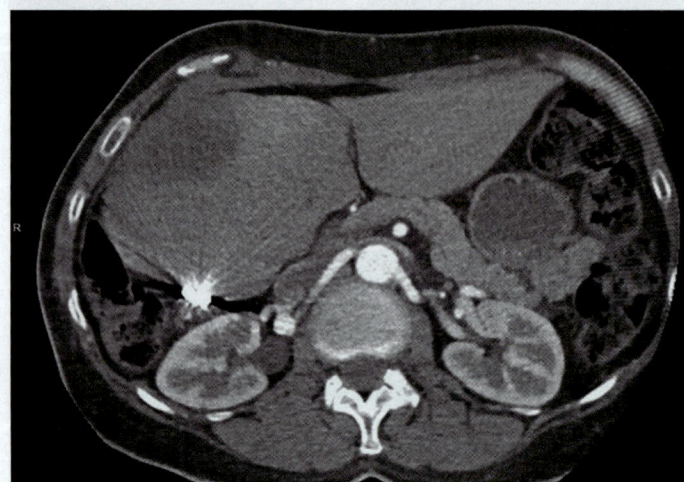

FIGURE 105.2 CT angiogram of a 52-year-old patient treated with embolization of ruptured right hepatic artery aneurysm, now with resolving subcapsular hematoma and 1.2-cm distal right renal artery aneurysm.

hepatic ischemia, abscess, cholecystitis, and possible recanalization. As described earlier, coil embolization is discouraged in patients with large parenchymal lesions or if large segments of liver are at risk of ischemia. In these patients, liver lobe resection should be considered.

Superior Mesenteric Aneurysm

Superior mesenteric artery (SMA) aneurysms account for up to 8% of all splanchnic aneurysms, and they affect males more frequently than females.[12,23,24] SMA true aneurysms (Fig. 105.3) are mainly solitary, and the etiology is less commonly attributed to atherosclerotic degeneration and more frequently associated with infection, dissection, medial degeneration, FMD, vasculitis, connective tissue disorder, and trauma. Pseudoaneurysms may occur in the setting of pancreatitis and complicated peptic ulcer disease. Concomitant HTN is common, affecting >20% of patients with SMA aneurysms, as are concurrent aortic and peripheral/splanchnic aneurysms. In contrast to other splanchnic artery aneurysms, symptoms are common. Patients may describe abdominal pain, nausea, emesis, and GI bleeding. Fever may be present in cases of mycotic aneurysm.[11] Up to one-third of patients with SMA aneurysms have a pulsatile abdominal mass on the exam. The natural history of true SMA aneurysm is that of expansion and rupture, with the additional complication risk of acute mesenteric ischemia from thromboembolism. Historically, rupture risk has been described in up to 50% of cases, and rupture-associated mortality has exceeded 50%. More contemporary series cite 30-day mortality rates as low as 12.5% to 38%, and even lower mortality after elective repair with endovascular interventions has been reported.[11,12,24] No comorbidities or aneurysm characteristics have been found to predict rupture risk.

Operative Indications

- Regardless of size, all true and false aneurysms should be repaired.
  - An exception is made for dissection-associated SMA aneurysms, for which careful observation is advised unless refractory symptoms develop.

Surgical Management

Open reconstruction. Open repair is commonly favored for SMA aneurysms, typically with an aortomesenteric bypass. Both autologous and prosthetic conduits have been described, with autologous conduit favored in cases of mycotic aneurysm and frank contamination complicating intestinal ischemia.[14] Aneurysmorrhaphy and simple ligation of efferent and afferent branches (in those patients with appropriate collateralization) have also been described with success, especially for focal, saccular aneurysms.[12,23] Open resection may require intestinal resection, particularly in symptomatic patients.

Endovascular therapy. Endovascular SMA aneurysm exclusion with stent grafting and embolization have been increasingly employed for patients with severe comorbidity. Aneurysms with a small neck distal to the SMA origin may be conducive to transcatheter embolization, provided angiographic determination of collateral flow is adequate.[24] Endovascular techniques remain limited by thromboembolic risks to intestinal circulation and endoleak.

Celiac Artery Aneurysm

Celiac artery aneurysms (Fig. 105.4) account for approximately 4% of all splanchnic aneurysms, affecting males more frequently than females.[25,26] Historically, celiac artery aneurysms were primarily associated with infection (syphilis or tuberculosis) and primarily diagnosed postmortem. Contemporary etiologic risk factors include primarily atherosclerosis, developmental risk

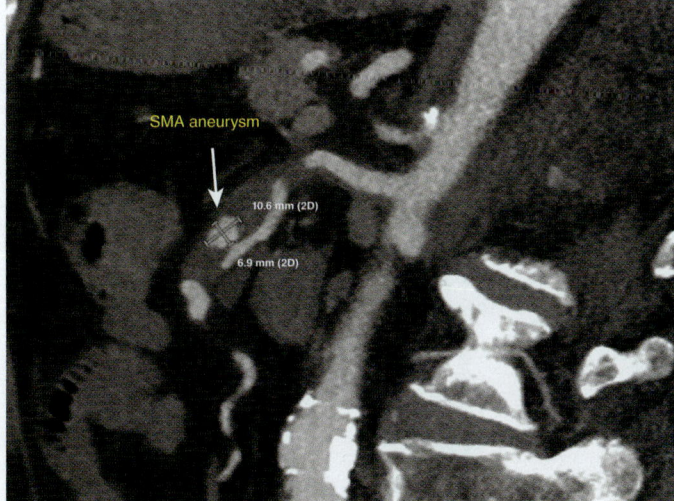

FIGURE 105.3 CT angiogram, reformatted, of a 73-year-old patient with saccular superior mesenteric artery *(SMA)* aneurysm associated with mural thrombus and associated inflammation consistent with mycotic aneurysm. *2D,* Two-dimensional.

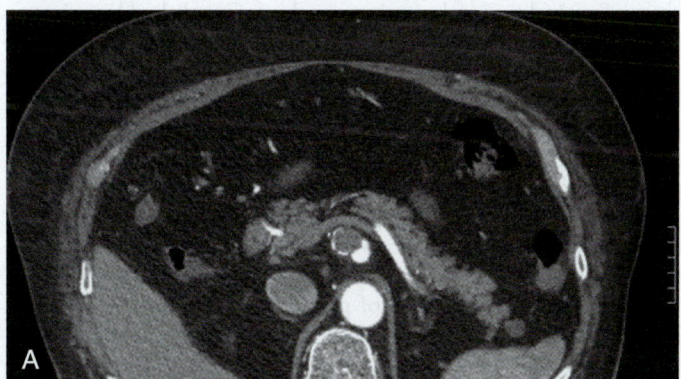

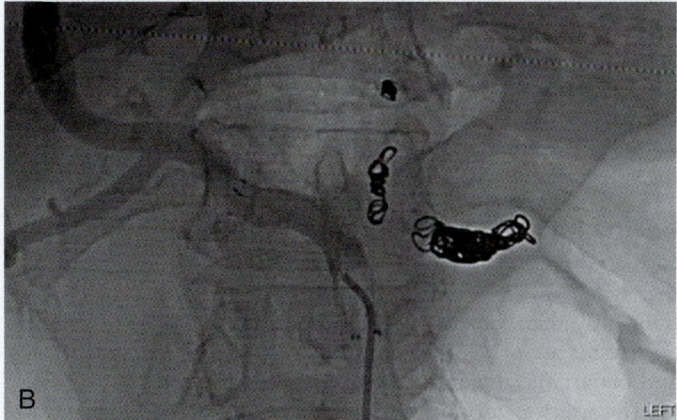

FIGURE 105.4 (A) CT angiogram of an 82-year-old patient with an enlarging >3-cm celiac aneurysm. (B) Completion angiogram after coil embolization of the left gastric and splenic arteries plus covered stenting of the celiac aneurysm extending into the common hepatic artery.

factors such as common celiacomesenteric trunk, arterial dysplasia with medial degeneration, collagen vascular disorder, trauma, and dissection. As with other visceral aneurysms, concurrent HTN is common (20%), as are aortic aneurysms (18%–40%) and alternate splanchnic aneurysms (38%). Celiac artery aneurysms are mainly asymptomatic, and clinical exam may reveal an abdominal mass or bruit. Historically, rupture complicated approximately 70% of celiac artery aneurysms, resulting in near-certain mortality, although more contemporary series support rupture rates of 13%, with associated 50% mortality. Rupture has been described in aneurysms ranging in size from 2 to 6 cm, with rates of 5% in aneurysms sized 15 to 22 mm and rates up to 75% in aneurysms >32 mm.[26] Risk factors for such have not been clearly elucidated, although aneurysmal degeneration is rare in those patients with associated dissections and poststenotic dilation (i.e., median arcuate ligament syndrome).[27]

Operative Indications

- All ruptured aneurysms should be emergently repaired.
- Regardless of size, all pseudoaneurysms should be repaired.
- True celiac artery aneurysms >2 cm with a demonstrable increase in size or associated symptoms should be repaired in patients of acceptable risk.
- Surveillance is recommended for stable asymptomatic aneurysms <2 cm or in patients with significant medical comorbidities or limited life expectancy.

Surgical Management

Open reconstruction. Aneurysmectomy with arterial reconstruction remains the preferred treatment for celiac artery aneurysms. Surgical revascularization may be accomplished by primary arterial-arterial anastomosis after aneurysm resection, direct aortic reimplantation of the celiac artery or its branches, or aortohepatic bypass. In general, the spleen and left gastric artery don't require revascularization. Prosthetic conduit may be favored over autogenous saphenous vein, which tends to kink. Elective surgical repair offers patients symptomatic relief, with up to 5% risk of perioperative mortality. The procedure of aneurysm ligation and resection without reconstruction has been endorsed, especially for rupture and patients with adequate foregut collateral circulation. This procedure carries a risk of perioperative hepatic and intestinal ischemia, necrosis, and patient mortality.[25,26]

Endovascular therapy. Endovascular options for aneurysm treatment are increasingly described.[11] The absence of a proximal landing zone may limit endovascular exclusion by covered stent grafting or embolization because these aneurysms typically affect the proximal celiac trunk.[28] Coil embolization of the left gastric and splenic arteries may be required to obtain a proximal seal (see Fig. 105.4). Transcatheter embolization may be lifesaving in cases of rupture, at the risk of perioperative hepatic and intestinal ischemia.

Gastric Artery Aneurysm

Gastric and gastroepiploic artery aneurysms account for approximately 4% to 5% of splanchnic aneurysms, affecting males more frequently than females by threefold.[12] These nonatherosclerotic aneurysms are primarily associated with arterial dysplasia, SAM, and periarterial inflammation (i.e., pancreatitis and vasculitis).[29] Gastric artery aneurysms are 10 times more common than gastroepiploic artery aneurysms. Although patients may present with abdominal pain, up to 90% of patients have historically presented acutely ruptured, with GI bleeding more common than intraperitoneal rupture.[21]

Operative Indications

- Regardless of the size, all true and false aneurysms should be repaired.

Surgical Management

Open reconstruction. Surgical management is of historical significance and was previously reliant on simple arterial ligation or excision without reconstruction. Intramural aneurysms require wedge excision of the involved gastric wall.

Endovascular therapy. Catheter-based embolization of these aneurysms has become the standard of care for first-line treatment, with multiple case reports and small series documenting successful aneurysm occlusion with coils and thrombin injection.[11,28]

Gastroduodenal and Pancreaticoduodenal Arterial Aneurysm

Gastroduodenal and pancreaticoduodenal artery aneurysms account for <2% of splanchnic aneurysms, with males having a fourfold increased risk compared with feamles.[12] Etiologic risk factors include predominantly periarterial inflammation resulting from pancreatitis, followed by arteriosclerosis, congenital medial degeneration, and trauma. Noninflammatory aneurysmal degeneration in this collateral arcade is hypothesized to be a sequelae of inordinately high-volume blood flow (Fig. 105.5) in the setting of concomitant celiac artery stenosis or occlusion.[30] Unlike other visceral aneurysms, patients frequently describe abdominal pain. Large aneurysms may cause additional symptoms of gastric outlet obstruction.[23] Rupture is common, complicating up to 75% of inflammatory and 50% of noninflammatory aneurysms, most often resulting in GI bleeding and, less commonly, bleeding into the biliary or pancreatic ductal systems, peritoneum, or retroperitoneum.[30] Rupture-associated mortality is 20% to 50%.[30] Rupture has been described at a small median size of 12 mm, with rupture reported in aneurysms <1 cm in diameter. It remains unclear if aneurysm size is a risk factor for rupture in this location.

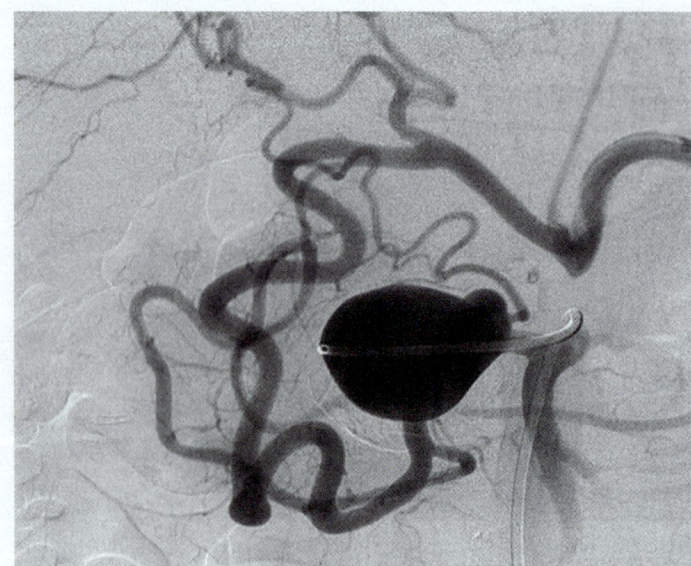

FIGURE   105.5 Angiogram demonstrating large gastroduodenal aneurysm.

Operative Indications

- Regardless of the size, all true and false aneurysms should be repaired.

Surgical Management

Open reconstruction. Open reconstruction of these aneurysms is technically feasible, with low perioperative morbidity and mortality for nonruptured aneurysms employing techniques of ligation and excision with or without end-to-end anastomosis.[31] Celiac stenosis or occlusion is commonly associated with aneurysms of the pancreaticoduodenal arcade, and a low threshold for celiac revascularization should be considered in patients with symptoms of chronic mesenteric insufficiency at baseline or when there is a risk of compromising end-organ perfusion with aneurysm treatment. In cases of median arcuate ligament syndrome, celiac revascularization can be achieved with division of the median arcuate ligament and celiac plexus with or without aorto-celiac or aorto-hepatic bypass.

Endovascular therapy. Percutaneous embolization of pancreaticoduodenal and gastroduodenal artery aneurysms is recommended as first-line therapy by the SVS guidelines for intact and ruptured aneurysms.[11] A triaxial system, as described earlier, inclusive of a microcatheter provides stable support through tortuous vessels. Coil embolization is recommended as the treatment of choice, with liquid embolic agents as an alternative for appropriate anatomy. Covered stenting and stent- or balloon-assisted coil embolization are recommended for patients in whom coil embolization is not feasible.[11] For aneurysms with a wide neck but sufficient size and morphology to retain an embolic coil cast, balloon-assisted embolization can create the initial formation of a "cage" to enhance success. This technique involves the placement of a balloon catheter in the parent vessel across the aneurysm neck with a microcatheter positioned concurrently into the sac. The balloon is inflated while the coils are inserted to prevent prolapse or migration into the parent vessel lumen. For aneurysm necks whose width prohibits balloon remodeling, stent-assisted coil embolization can be considered as an alternative. This technique involves placing an uncovered stent in the parent vessel across the aneurysm neck with the microcatheter placed into the sac alongside the stent or through its mesh struts for embolization.

Flow-diverting multilayered stents are an additional treatment modality for patients with suitable anatomy. First introduced for the treatment of intracranial aneurysms, flow-diverting stents are placed in the parent artery to improve laminar flow and reduce blood intrusion within the aneurysm sac. This promotes aneurysm thrombosis. The device boasts a tight micromesh design to induce flow "diversion" through the parent vessel and sac thrombosis while preserving the patency of efferent branches and collateral side branches. These stents are more flexible than stent grafts, although their use is limited by size availability (currently up to 8 mm) and cost.

Renal Artery Aneurysm

Renal artery aneurysms (RAAs) are rare, with an incidence that approximates 1%.[32] Most aneurysms are asymptomatic. Rarely, patients may describe flank pain, abdominal pain, and hematuria. Most RAAs are saccular in nature, but they can be fusiform or intralobar. Rundback et al. have classified RAAs into three categories: type 1 = saccular aneurysms arising from the main renal artery, type 2 = fusiform aneurysms, and type 3 = intralobar aneurysms arising from small segmental arteries or accessory arteries.[33] RAAs occur more often on the right side (61%), and the

most common locations in order are the renal bifurcation, followed by the renal pelvis, the distal renal artery, the midrenal artery, and, rarely, the proximal renal artery.[34] Nearly two-thirds of patients have FMD, and concurrent arterial aneurysms affect the aorta, visceral, and iliac arteries in up to 30% of patients. As such, screening cerebrovascular, mesenteric, and iliac beds is prudent, especially in young females.

The natural history of RAAs appears to be that of slow to null growth, with contemporary series estimating a median annualized growth rate of 0.06 to 0.6 mm.[34] Aneurysm growth rate does not seem to be affected by aneurysm morphology or calcification, although risk factors for rupture include pregnancy, HTN, and associated arteriovenous fistula. Although historical series described rupture rates as high as 14% to 30% with associated mortality of 80%, contemporary rupture rates are estimated at 3% to 5%, with nongestational mortality <10%.[32] Most ruptures are diagnosed at the time of presentation, and several authors now have supported no rupture during the surveillance of nonoperative RAAs.

HTN may be present in up to 70% to 75% of patients with an RAA.[35] Although the mechanism for HTN in RAA patients remains elusive, hypotheses include distal parenchymal embolization, compression or kinking of associated renal artery branches, and hemodynamic changes from turbulent blood flow within the aneurysm resulting in decreased distal renal artery perfusion pressures.[11] Most series suggest an improvement or cure in the majority of hypertensive patients undergoing RAA reconstruction, particularly if renovascular HTN is identified during the preoperative workup.

Operative Indications

- All ruptured aneurysms should be emergently repaired.
- Aneurysms >3 cm in patients of acceptable risk should be repaired.
- Regardless of size, all aneurysms in patients of childbearing potential should be repaired.
- Regardless of size, aneurysms in patients with medically refractory HTN and functionally important renal artery stenosis should be repaired.

Absent prospective or randomized trial data directly comparing operative repair to surveillance and acknowledging the more indolent natural history than previously suggested, contemporary data and SVS guidelines support a conservative threshold for repair. Individualized treatment that considers phenotype and genotype should be considered comprehensively because arteries in a branch location or associated with a known connective tissue disorder may warrant a more aggressive approach.

Surgical Management

Open reconstruction. RAA can be treated by a variety of surgical methods. Open surgical reconstruction remains the gold-standard technique for elective repair, offering low morbidity and mortality and a 5-year survival of nearly 90%.[36] Repair of RAAs (Fig. 105.6) most often includes in situ reconstruction, including resection and primary angioplastic closure, patch angioplasty or primary reanastomosis, interposition grafting, or bypass (i.e., aortorenal or spleno-/hepatorenal). The tailoring technique, which includes a partial resection of the aneurysm with direct suture of the remaining arterial wall, has been proposed as an additional open option. Ex vivo repair with or without autotransplantation of the kidney remains an alternative approach, of particular use in those requiring complex or distal

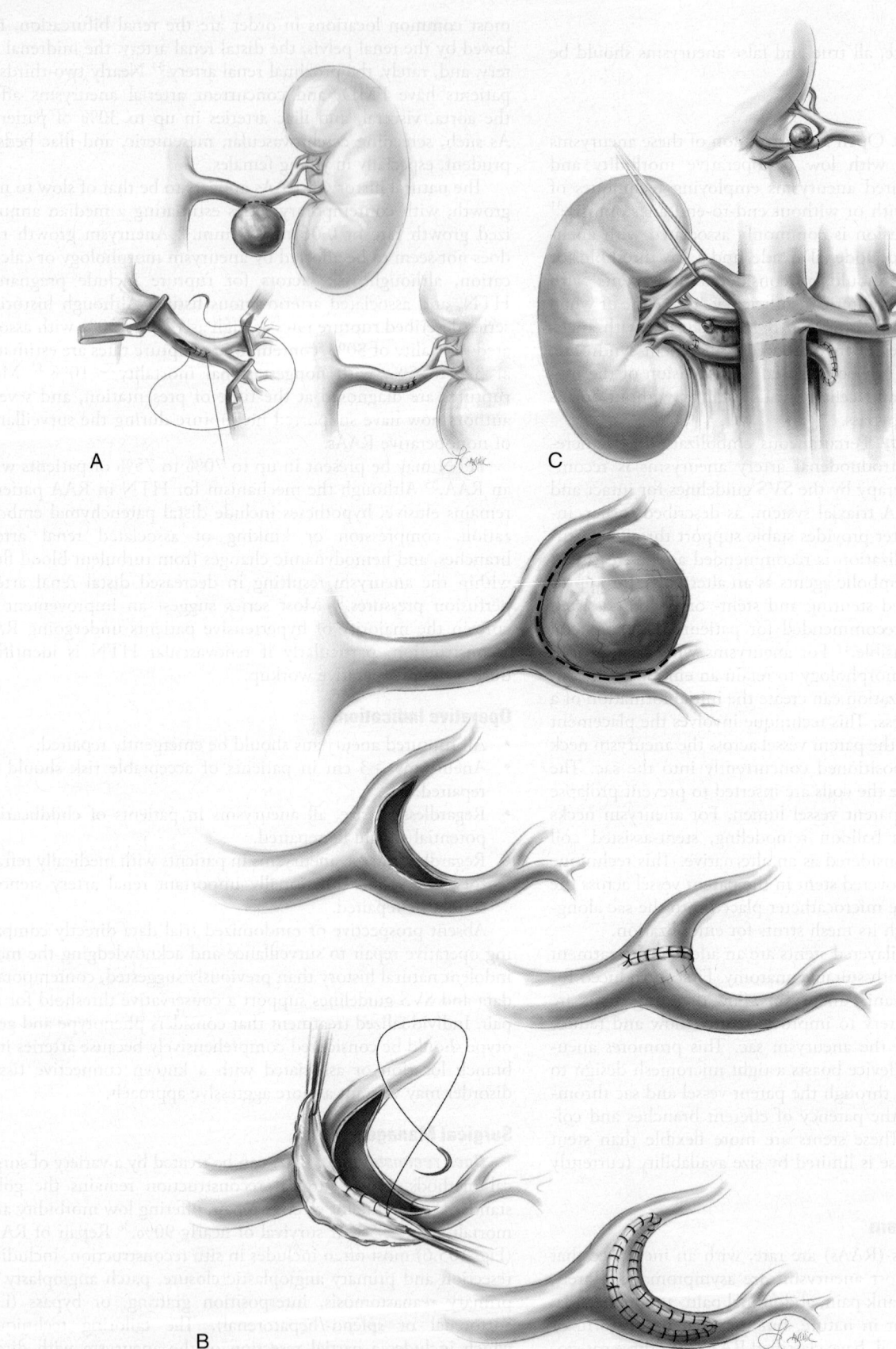

FIGURE 105.6 Renal artery aneurysms may be reconstructed by a variety of techniques not limited to resection with primary repair (A), resection with angioplastic closure of the defect in a transverse fashion or patch angioplasty (B), and resection with aortorenal bypass (C). (Adapted from Coleman DW, Stanley JC. Renal artery aneurysms. *J Vasc Surg.* 2015;62[3]:779-785.)

reconstructions. Robotic and laparoscopic techniques have been reported as well. Careful attention to anatomy and location should be considered to create individualized surgical plans because few studies are available comparing surgical techniques for repair of RAAs.

Endovascular therapy. Although endovascular therapy has gained recognition and utility in the management of RAAs, only a subset of patients will fit the anatomic criteria to undergo this therapy. Traditional endovascular therapies for RAA have used coil embolization for distal and parenchymal aneurysms and stent-graft exclusion for main renal artery lesions, but the indications for endovascular repair have broadened with advancing technology to include three-dimensional detachable coils, nonadhesive liquid embolic agents, remodeling techniques (i.e., balloon- and stent-assisted coiling), and flow diverter stents, as described earlier. Technical success with endovascular means approximates 73% to 100% across series, with highly variable rates of morbidity (13%–60%) that include radiographic evidence of end-organ malperfusion and subsequent postembolization syndrome, arterial dissections, renal insufficiency, and low rates of recanalization requiring reintervention (4%–13%).[11,16,28]

UPPER EXTREMITY ANEURYSMS

Upper extremity peripheral aneurysms, including dilations of the subclavian, axillary, brachial, and distal vessels, are very uncommon relative to lower extremity peripheral aneurysms.

Subclavian and Axillary Artery Aneurysms

The literature is limited to a few case series and case reports regarding the etiology and natural history of subclavian aneurysms. As such, the true incidence of aneurysm formation in these anatomic locations is unknown.

The distribution of etiologies for subclavian and axillary aneurysms varies in prior reports. Early case series reported the most common cause to be degenerative atherosclerotic disease, followed by traumatic pseudoaneurysms and then thoracic outlet obstruction. Another early case series reported that more than half of the subclavian artery aneurysms they treated were related to atherosclerotic disease.[37] Finally, a more recent series identified thoracic outlet obstruction as the primary etiology in over 70% of cases.[38] Some risk factors have been identified, such as connected tissue diseases, arterial thoracic outlet syndrome (Fig. 105.7), poststenotic dilation from a cervical rib, and atherosclerosis. Repetitive mechanical trauma in overhead-throwing athletes can cause repeated compression and contusion of the axillary artery by the humeral head. Repeated arterial injury places these patients at risk for thrombosis and axillary artery aneurysm formation as well.[39]

The feared complication of subclavian artery aneurysms is rupture with intrathoracic hemorrhage and subsequent hemorrhagic shock. This is less common for aneurysms outside of the thoracic cavity because the potential space to collect blood is small. As such, the main devastating complication of axillary artery aneurysms is thrombosis with embolization. Thromboemboli generated from intraluminal thrombus can become lodged in small arteries, leading to focal areas of ischemic necrosis. Patients with axillary aneurysms usually do not present with acute limb ischemia (ALI) because of the excellent arterial collateral circulation around the shoulder. However, thrombosis with distal extension can disrupt collateral flow, generating acute ischemia. Thrombosis of a subclavian aneurysm is more likely to

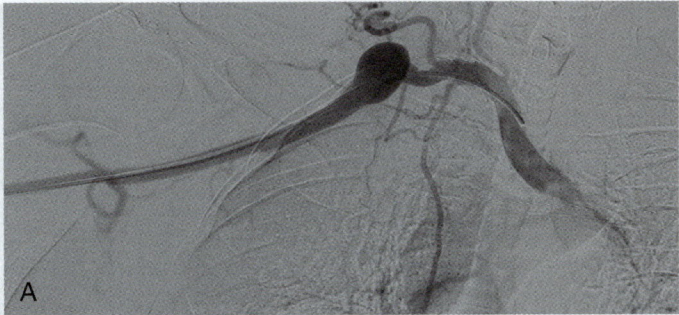

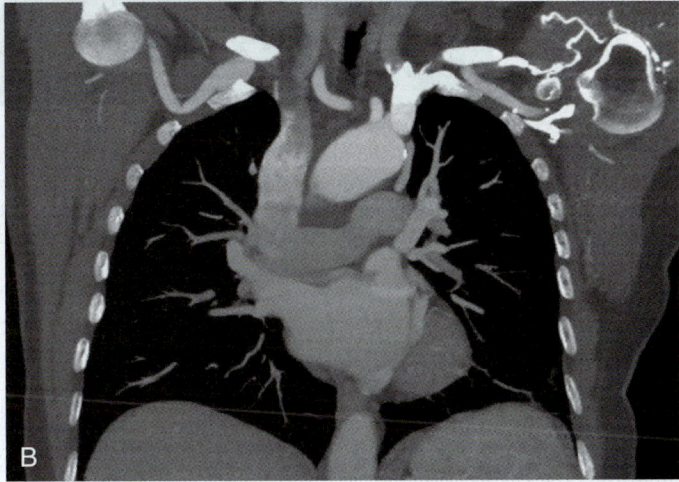

FIGURE 105.7 Axillary artery aneurysm. Catheter-directed digital subtraction angiography (A) and coronal section of reformatted CT angiogram (B) demonstrating arterial aneurysm in the thoracic outlet caused by arterial thoracic outlet syndrome.

cause ALI. Thrombosis at this level would block antegrade flow to the collateral pathways of the upper extremity. Although the true natural history of aneurysms in this anatomic location has not been reported because of the rarity of the disease, it is likely similar to peripheral aneurysmal disease in the lower extremity. If left untreated, patients are expected to experience continued aneurysmal dilation followed by thrombosis, with eventual thromboembolism or ALI and upper extremity tissue loss.

Diagnosis

The primary presenting symptoms for patients with subclavian or axillary artery aneurysms without acute complications are shoulder pain and a pulsatile superior chest mass. Compression of the brachial plexus can cause numbness and paresthesias in the affected extremity. About a quarter present with ALI, and around 30% present with chronic limb ischemia symptoms.[38] If the patient presents without acute symptoms, duplex ultrasonography can confirm the diagnosis (Fig. 105.8). Often, CTA is appropriate to delineate baseline anatomy and aid in operative planning or to make a diagnosis if ultrasound is unavailable (Fig. 105.9).

Diagnosis of an axillary or subclavian artery aneurysm should be considered in any patient presenting with upper extremity ALI or chronic tissue loss. This is especially true if the patient has a personal or family history of connective tissue disorder, the patient is a throwing athlete, or there is suspicion for thoracic outlet syndrome.

ALI is an operative emergency. ALI in the upper extremity is relatively rare and most commonly results from a cardioembolic event. If the suspicion for a cardioembolic event is high, the

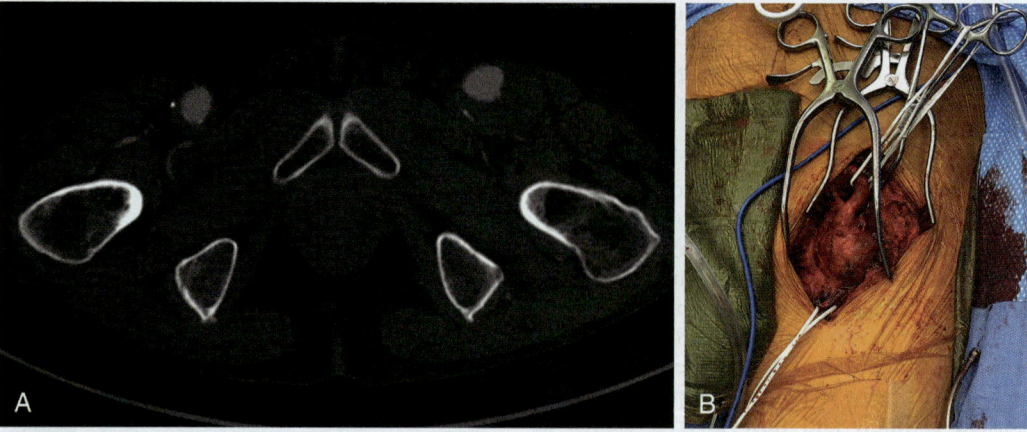

FIGURE 105.8 Intraoperative images from a brachial aneurysm reconstruction. (A) Proximal control is established at a segment of healthy artery. (B) Great saphenous vein (GSV) was obtained, the proximal anastomosis was completed, and the graft was tunneled. The aneurysm sac was incised, and branch vessels were ligated internally for hemostasis. Given the size of this aneurysm, the sac was excised, and branch vessels were ligated. The distal anastomosis was then completed. (C) Complete arterial reconstruction with reversed GSV bypass graft intact.

patient should be emergently taken to the operating room for embolectomy and revascularization. However, axillary and subclavian artery aneurysms are a rare cause of upper extremity ALI. Therefore, if the suspicion for a cardioembolic event is moderate to low, emergent CTA should be performed to obtain further anatomic data. Occasionally, a thrombosed aneurysm may be identified, which would require emergent revascularization.

Outside of the mildly symptomatic ambulatory patient and the acute patient, axillary and subclavian artery aneurysms are typically incidentally discovered on axial imaging as MRI and CT imaging modalities increase in use (see Fig. 105.9).

Operative Indications

Elective setting.
- Aneurysm related to arterial thoracic outlet syndrome should be repaired.
- Connective tissue–related aneurysms should be referred to a vascular specialist for further management of this complex disease process.
- Consider repair if intraluminal thrombus is present.

Acute setting.
- Any thrombosed aneurysm causing ALI requires emergent revascularization.
- Any ruptured subclavian aneurysm requires emergent exclusion and potential revascularization.

Surgical Management

Open reconstruction. Axillary artery aneurysms are easily treated surgically by resecting the aneurysm and grafting an interposition vein. The patient should be positioned supine with the ipsilateral arm out at a 90-degree position and shoulders slightly elevated. Commonly, an axillary roll is placed. The surgical approach is often through an infraclavicular incision that is 2 to 3 cm below and parallel to the lateral portion of the clavicle (Table 105.1). This incision can be extended distally into the deltopectoral groove to create a deltopectoral incision. Care should be given to avoid the cephalic vein. Dissection is carried down through the pectoralis fascia and between the fibers of pectoralis major. The clavipectoral fascia is incised, and pectoralis minor can be divided, providing excellent exposure of the entirety

of the axillary vessels. The artery in this location runs deep to the axillary vein; therefore, the vein should be mobilized inferiorly. The cords and divisions of the brachial plexus surround the axillary artery. After proximal and distal control are established, the patient should be systemically heparinized. Vascular clamps can then be applied, and the aneurysm sac is opened.

The conduit of choice if interposition grafting is required is reversed greater saphenous vein (rGSV). If this is not available or not of adequate size and length, a prosthetic repair of the axillary artery may be carried out, preferably with externally supported polytetrafluoroethylene (PTFE). These grafts now come as heparin-bonded PTFE and provide acceptable patency.

Subclavian artery aneurysms are more difficult to treat surgically because of the exposure required for proximal control. For a distal subclavian aneurysm, a rare entity, exposure can be obtained through either a supraclavicular or infraclavicular approach (see Table 105.1). The medial clavicle can be resected to provide more proximal exposure. To do this, the supraclavicular incision is extended medially, and dissection is carried through the fascia and periosteum of the clavicle. The insertions of the sternocleidomastoid and pectoralis muscle are detached and reflected superiorly and inferiorly, respectively. Dissection around the clavicle is carefully performed, and the subclavian vein is protected while the clavicle is transected, medially dislocated, and removed. However, subclavian aneurysms are commonly proximal or even extensions of aortic arch or innominate artery aneurysms, requiring a median sternotomy for proximal control if open repair is warranted. Continuation of this incision into the supraclavicular fossa can be necessary to gain adequate exposure to the entire subclavian artery. The proximal left subclavian artery is notoriously difficult to access surgically. A left anterior thoracotomy combined with a median sternotomy and supraclavicular exposure, known as a *trap-door thoracotomy*, may be necessary (see Table 105.1).

Endovascular therapy. Generally, endovascular reconstruction that spans a mobile artery, such as the axillary artery, is discouraged. Stent fractures have been described, likely related to repetitive motion of arteries that span joints. Specifically, elevation of the upper extremity brings the axillary artery into contact with the humeral head. This can cause stent compression. If an endovascular repair of an axillary aneurysm is necessary, recommended

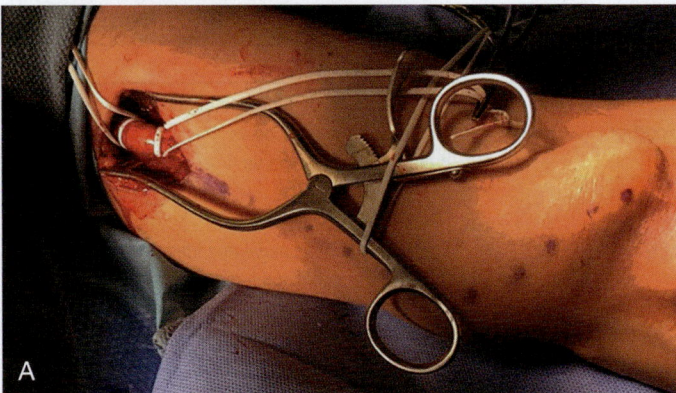

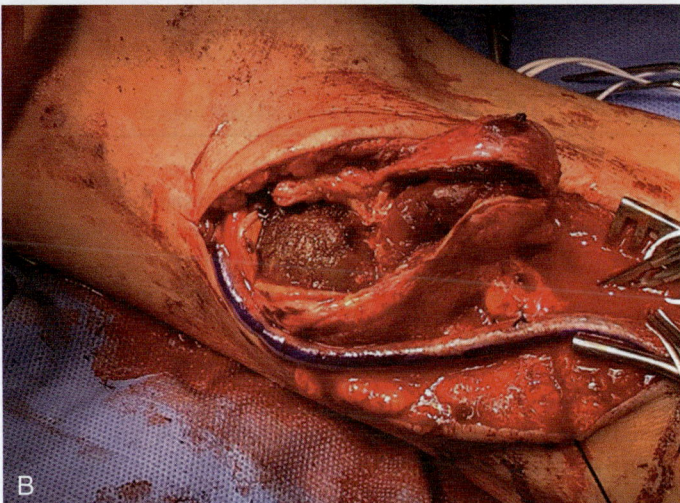

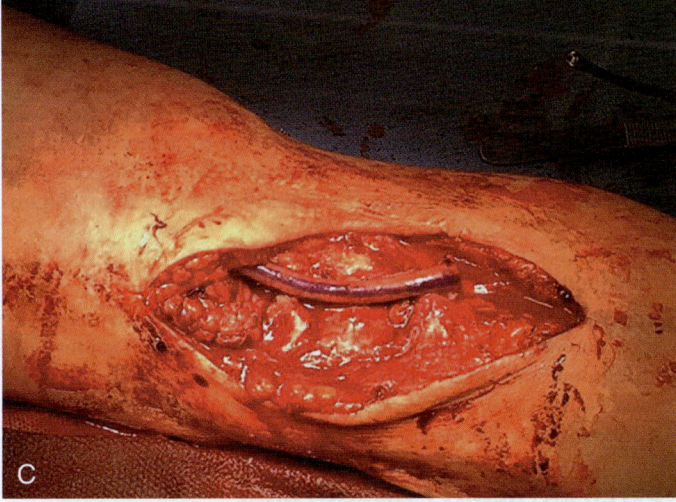

FIGURE 105.9 Common femoral artery aneurysm seen (A) on reformatted CT angiogram and (B) intraoperatively after completion of arterial dissection. Notably, the patient had bilateral common femoral artery aneurysms. The large size and extensive thrombus necessitated repair of the left common femoral aneurysm first.

only in an emergent, hemodynamically unstable patient, a self-expanding covered stent should be used over a balloon expandable stent because of its flexibility and memory retention properties.

Endovascular reconstruction of a subclavian artery aneurysm is extraordinarily complex because of the numerous bifurcations and tortuous vessels in this location. Often, retrograde common femoral artery (CFA) access is obtained, and the subclavian artery is selected through the arch or innominate artery. Caution must be taken to heparinize all patients before cannulating the aortic arch to reduce the high risk of embolic stroke when working in this area. If a wire can pass through the aneurysm into healthy tissue, a working sheath can be positioned, and a stent graft can be deployed. Alternatively, upper extremity access through the brachial artery can be obtained to eliminate the stroke risk of aortic arch cannulation. The acute rupture of a subclavian artery aneurysm can be a life-threatening event. Emergent exclusion of the aneurysm is required, and in this acute setting, an endovascular solution may be the most prudent, but it can be extremely challenging depending on anatomy and comes with a risk of stroke.

ARM, FOREARM, AND HAND ANEURYSMS

Upper extremity peripheral aneurysms are exceedingly rare and account for less than 1% of all peripheral aneurysms. Less than 0.5% involve the brachial artery (see Fig. 105.9). Brachial artery aneurysms are classically false aneurysms secondary to trauma, iatrogenic injury (dialysis access complications), drug abuse, or mycotic lesions. Occasionally they are idiopathic, but the increased prevalence of invasive interventions requiring upper extremity arterial access contributes to a large proportion of pseudoaneurysms at this location.[40] Repetitive blunt trauma, such as arterial compression from inappropriate crutch use, can cause arterial medial contusion from repetitive compression. True aneurysms can be related to type 1 neurofibromatosis, Behçet disease, and other types of vasculitis.

Causes of ulnar artery aneurysms include trauma, vasculitis, connective tissue disease, and iatrogenic injury.[41] The most common cause of ulnar artery aneurysms appears to be repetitive trauma. This is commonly seen in some athletes and patients of occupations in which repetitive trauma to the medial palmar surface is sustained, named *hypothenar hammer syndrome*. Most proximal ulnar artery aneurysms have been reported in children. There are currently only 25 reports of radial artery aneurysms in the literature,[42] and these are most often pseudoaneurysms caused by trauma or a complication of vascular access.

Brachial, ulnar, and radial artery aneurysms can cause distal ischemia and tissue loss of the hand. Exsanguination from rupture is rare in this location, but compressive symptoms are common because peripheral arteries are often near nerves. Uncontained ruptures of pseudoaneurysms can cause ischemic changes to the overlying skin and eventual skin necrosis.

Diagnosis

Diagnosis of an upper extremity aneurysm is often suggested on physical examination. A pulsatile mass with a thrill will often be observed in patients presenting with mild symptoms, such as nerve compression or pain. If the patient presents with digital ischemia or focal gangrenous changes, a firm mass in an arterial anatomic location may be observed. This is the result of thrombosis of the aneurysm and distal embolization. Duplex ultrasound is usually sufficient to confirm the diagnosis in the upper extremity, but angiography (either CT or catheter based) is often necessary to define the extent of disease, assess for arterial occlusion, and look for anatomic variants that will aid in operative planning.

Operative Indications

- All pseudoaneurysms should be repaired.
- All aneurysms with neurologic complications should be repaired.

TABLE 105.1 **Operative Approaches and Considerations for Upper Extremity Arterial Exposures**

ARTERY	APPROACH	SEGMENTS EXPOSED	CONSIDERATIONS
Right subclavian	Median sternotomy	Great central exposure, can be extended supraclavicularly to provide distal exposure	Can extend incision to the supraclavicular space for more extensive exposure
	Supraclavicular	Limited distal exposure	Protect the phrenic nerve
Left subclavian	Anterolateral thoracotomy	Proximal exposure and control	
	Trap-door thoracotomy	More extensive exposure	Highly morbid, trauma only
	Supraclavicular	Mid- and distal segment	Protect the phrenic nerve and identify thoracic duct
Axillary	Infraclavicular	1st and 2nd segments	Can be extended distally to deltopectoral
	Lateral	2nd and 3rd segments	Positioning may limit more distal exposures
	Deltopectoral	Entire axillary segment	Often need to divide pectoralis minor
Brachial	Medial	Excellent exposure of all but the most distal segment	Identify and protect median nerve, can ligate the deep brachial vein if needed
	Transverse or S-shaped antecubital	Distal brachial and brachial bifurcation	S-shaped incision needed if crossing antecubital fossa
Radial	Lateral volar	Distal radial	Variable radial nerve
Ulnar	Medial volar	Distal ulnar	Ulnar nerve close in proximal forearm

- Any aneurysm associated with skin changes should be repaired.
- Consider repair of true aneurysm with intraluminal thrombus or >2.5 times the native artery diameter.

Surgical Management

Open Reconstruction

Exposure of the brachial, ulnar, and radial arteries is relatively straightforward and can be achieved under local, regional, or general anesthesia (see Table 105.1). It is much safer than more proximal exposure. If hemorrhage is encountered during dissection, proximal control can be obtained with a tourniquet or direct pressure proximal to the dissection because of the superficial course of these vessels.

For wide exposure of the brachial artery, a longitudinal incision is made along the medial aspect of the upper arm just posterior to the short head of the bicep brachii (see Table 105.1). The neurovascular bundle is located just posterior to the bicep muscle, with the artery typically positioned deep to paired brachial veins and the median nerve. Care must be given to protect the median nerve. Superficial nerves at this level can occasionally be large; however, are all sensory. Additionally, if required for more proximal exposure, the deep brachial vein can be sacrificed.

The most operatively exposed upper extremity artery is the distal brachial artery at the antecubital fossa. When crossing the antecubital fossa, a transverse or "lazy-S" incision is recommended to reduce the risk of stricture (see Table 105.1). If the antecubital fossa is not being crossed, a longitudinal incision can provide better exposure of the proximal radial and ulnar arteries. The brachial artery at this location lies deep to the bicipital aponeurosis. Division of that aponeurosis provides an easy exposure.

If considering open surgical repair of a brachial artery aneurysm, direct inline reconstruction should be attempted. Typically, pseudoaneurysms can be repaired primarily without an interposition bypass graft. True aneurysms involve larger segments of the native artery, and their reconstruction will likely involve one of two strategies, interposition grafting or bypass (see Fig. 105.9). If the entirety of the true aneurysm is surgically accessible, the aneurysm can be completely ligated and excluded. Anatomic reconstruction with an interposition graft sewn end to end can be performed. The aneurysm can be ligated and excluded. If compressive symptoms are present, the

aneurysm can be decompressed with this approach. If the aneurysm is long or involves a surgically inaccessible location, a bypass graft that is tunneled subcutaneously is often the best approach (see Fig. 105.9). For either approach, long-term outcomes and patency are thought to be excellent.

For ulnar artery aneurysms, the type of repair typically depends on the patient's distal perfusion. If ischemic symptoms are present, then ulnar artery reconstruction is required. If there are no signs of ischemia, then ligation of the aneurysm can be considered. Rarely is a bypass required to be performed.[41] There is no clear consensus about whether to ligate or reconstruct the radial artery. Some have proposed revascularization whenever possible, whereas others have argued for selective revascularization depending on the collateral circulation to the hand.[42] The latter suggests revascularization only if an incomplete palmar arch is present, in which ligation of the radial artery would lead to digital ischemia. The reconstruction of the distal upper extremity arteries should be done in an end-to-end fashion, making sure there is no tension on completion. If this is required, the conduit of choice is autologous vein.

Endovascular Therapy

The peripheral arteries of the upper extremity are easily surgically assessable. Surgeries can be performed in this location under local and regional anesthesia. This fact, in conjunction with the small caliber of the distal upper extremity arteries, has led to little role for endovascular reconstruction in this anatomic location.

LOWER EXTREMITY ANEURYSMS

Femoral Artery Aneurysms

Femoral artery aneurysms (see Fig. 105.8) represent approximately 3% of all peripheral aneurysms, making them the second most common site after popliteal artery aneurysms (PAAs), with an incidence of approximately 5 per 100,000 people.[43] Aneurysms in this location are most commonly in the CFA (~57%) and less commonly found in the profunda femoris (~17%) and superficial femoral arteries (~26%). About one-quarter are incidentally discovered, and there is a male predominance. It is estimated that 50% to 90% of patients will have a concomitant AAA, an even stronger association than with PAAs.[43] In addition, up to one-third of patients will have a contralateral femoral aneurysm.

Most femoral aneurysms are related to degenerative atherosclerotic disease. This agrees with the most common primary risk factors being smoking and HTN. Cases of femoral artery aneurysms in patients with Behçet disease, Parkes-Weber syndrome, Marfan syndrome, and Wegener granulomatosis have been reported.[43] The natural history is unclear because of the rarity of the disease. Yet it appears rupture is uncommon, occurring in about 4% to 15% of cases. The primary concerns are thrombosis, embolism, and limb ischemia, as is the case with most aneurysms of the extremities. Unfortunately, the most common presentation in up to 65% of cases is lower extremity ischemia. This manifests as either claudication or critical limb ischemia from embolization.

Diagnosis

Diagnostic workup starts with a focused history and physical examination. Approximately 30% to 40% of patients will be asymptomatic, likely presenting with an incidentally found aneurysm. For symptomatic patients, about 30% to 40% will present with local symptoms of pain and tenderness or compressive symptoms of neuropathic pain and lower extremity edema. A history should elicit risk factors such as smoking, hyperlipidemia, and IV drug use. A full vascular exam with specific attention to ipsilateral distal pulses and pulsatile abdominal or popliteal fossa masses should be performed. Physical examination may reveal a pulsatile mass at the site of concern.

Noninvasive testing with duplex ultrasonography is cost-effective and has a high sensitivity and specificity. Subsequent axial angiography, such as CT or MRI, and geography are invaluable to further define the anatomy, look for intraluminal thrombus, and aid in case planning. All patients should be screened for both abdominal aortic and contralateral femoral aneurysms.

Operative Indications

- All aneurysms >3.5 cm in diameter should be repaired.
- All symptomatic aneurysms (claudication, nerve compression, rupture, and ischemic symptoms) should be repaired.
- Consider earlier repair in aneurysms with intraluminal thrombus.
- Consider earlier repair in aneurysms with a saccular morphology.
- Consider repair in expanding femoral aneurysms.

The primary goal of surgical reconstruction is the prevention of thrombosis and embolization, worsening compressive symptoms, and rupture.

Surgical Management

Open reconstruction. The goal of an open surgical operation is the exclusion of the aneurysm with arterial reconstruction. The CFA is the extension of the external iliac artery as it passes deep to the inguinal ligament. It lies medial to the femoral nerve but lateral to the common femoral vein within the femoral sheath. The femoral sheath is formed by the continuation of the transversalis fascia anteriorly and the continuation of the iliopsoas fascia posteriorly. Exposure of the femoral arteries is easiest through the femoral triangle. The triangle is bordered by the inguinal ligament superiorly, the medial border of the sartorius muscle laterally, and the medial border of the abductus longus medially.

Exposure is primarily obtained through a longitudinal incision directly over the femoral artery. Arterial identification should not be difficult in patients with aneurysmal disease; however, if needed, preoperative ultrasound can assist in planning the surgical

incision. Approximately one-third of the incision should extend proximal to the inguinal ligament. It is crucial to identify the location of the inguinal ligament using bony landmarks in patients with a large pannus or morbid obesity. This structure is often more proximal than thought if only using the inguinal creases as a landmark. Dissection is carried down through the subcutaneous fat, medial to the sartorius muscle. Any encountered lymphatics or lymph nodes should be ligated. The fascia lata of the thigh will be opened medial to the medial border of the sartorius muscle, followed by the femoral sheath. These structures are often divided simultaneously, providing arterial access.

The proximal dissection of the femoral artery is carried out at least to the border of the inguinal ligament. The aneurysm often extends beneath the inguinal ligament, and further exposure is needed to provide proximal control. The inguinal ligament can be mobilized and retracted superiorly to increase retroperitoneal visibility. If additional proximal exposure is needed, the ligament can be divided. This must be repaired at the case conclusion to avoid a femoral hernia. Distally, the dissection will extend until the superficial femoral artery and profunda femoris artery are visualized and encircled with vessel loops.

After obtaining control, the aneurysm sac is opened. Larger or more inflamed pathologies can be left in vivo. This can prevent injury to surrounding structures. Reconstruction of a true femoral artery aneurysm typically consists of interposition grafting. In this anatomic location, prosthetic grafts are often preferred to autologous venous conduits because of size discrepancy. Prosthetic grafts can better match the native arterial size and have similar patency rates to autologous interposition grafts. Any concern for infection should change this consideration. If the aneurysm is isolated to the CFA, reconstruction can be performed with a short interposition graft. Any aneurysm that extends to the femoral bifurcation will require more complex strategies (Fig. 105.10). In this setting, an interposition graft is created from the CFA to either the superficial femoral or profound femoris. A jump graft is then sewn from the other femoral branch onto the newly placed interposition graft. A femoral artery branch can be directly anastomosed to the interposition graft if there is enough redundancy.

Endovascular therapy. As seen with axillary artery aneurysms, endovascular repair is typically avoided because the femoral artery crosses a joint and is highly mobile. This can lead to stent fracture. Additionally, it is the rare CFA aneurysm that presents with enough distal seal length needed for successful covered stent placement. Endovascular treatment of the femoral arteries should be reserved for the emergent setting. In this setting, a covered self expanding stent should be used.

Popliteal Artery Aneurysms

History

PAAs have been described since antiquity, most of which were traumatic false aneurysms. The anatomist and surgeon John Hunter described a personal series regarding the operative approach to popliteal false aneurysm (the "coachmen's knee"), recognizing the need to ligate the artery in a normal-appearing segment proximal to the aneurysm.[44] Modern understanding of the anatomy, pathology, and natural history of PAAs was largely acquired in the latter half of the last century, coincident with the development of reliable bypass techniques. The last two decades have seen an increasing reliance on endovascular techniques for both acutely thrombosed aneurysms (catheter-directed thrombolysis) and treatment via stent-graft exclusion.

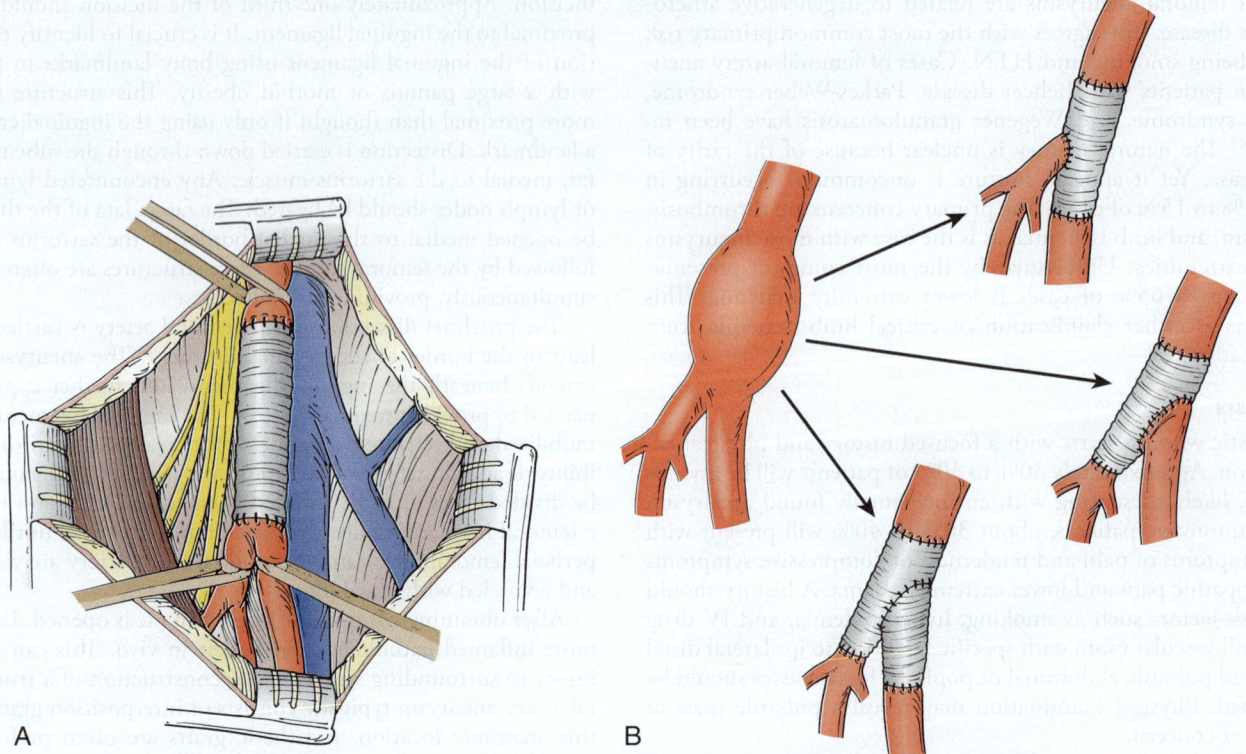

FIGURE 105.10 Surgical repair of an aneurysm confined to the common femoral artery (A) and extending beyond the common femoral artery bifurcation (B). The interposition graft can be placed between the common femoral and either the superficial femoral artery or the profunda femoris artery with reimplantation of the other branch into the side of the graft. If the origin of the artery to be implanted is diseased or not long enough, a short interposition graft can be used. (A, Adapted from Ouriel K, Rutherford RB, eds. *Atlas of Vascular Surgery: Operative Procedure.* Philadelphia: WB Saunders; 1998. B, Adapted from O'Hara P. Treatment of femoral and popliteal artery aneurysms. In: Zelenock GB, Huber TS, Messina LM, et al., eds. *Mastery of Vascular and Endovascular Surgery.* Philadelphia: Lippincott Williams & Wilkins; 2006.)

Incidence, Etiology, and Natural History

The majority of contemporarily described PAAs are true aneurysms and were classically described as degenerative or atherosclerotic in nature. Morphologically, most are fusiform in nature and associated with other cardiovascular risk factors (smoking, age, HTN). There is a strong male predominance, and half of cases are bilateral in nature. PAAs are the most common peripheral aneurysm, accounting for 80% of peripheral aneurysm cases.[45] Up to 75% of patients with PAAs will have aortic ectasia or aneurysm. Although often discovered via a prominent popliteal impulse on physical exam, duplex ultrasound is the standard noninvasive diagnostic modality. All patients with popliteal aneurysm should undergo ultrasound interrogation of the contralateral side and abdominal aorta. Conversely, all aortic aneurysm patients should be screened for PAA. Small popliteal aneurysms may not be palpable (or patient body habitus may preclude accurate exam) and, as such, may present with stigmata of thromboembolism or acute ischemia.

Unlike truncal aneurysms, the natural history of the surgically untreated PAA is that of embolism and thrombosis. Although precise longitudinal data are lacking, approximately a third of PAAs will thrombose within 5 years of diagnosis, with index size and presence of concurrent aortic aneurysm being the most common risk factors for growth or limb-threat event.[46] Rupture is rarely seen in true PAA, and cases of rupture should be considered false aneurysms, likely mycotic in etiology. Traumatic false aneurysm can occur via both blunt force (e.g., knee dislocation

with partial transection) and penetrating trauma. Iatrogenic injury with late false aneurysm has also been described after orthopedic surgical procedures.

Large popliteal aneurysms may present with mass effect symptoms, such leg swelling, with or without corresponding deep venous thrombosis or restricted range of motion. Although often obvious via physical exam retrospectively, these cases are often identified at the time of venous duplex for lower extremity swelling. Common differential diagnoses that can be readily ruled out via ultrasound include synovial cyst (Baker cyst) and benign or malignant tumor. CT should be obtained on all significant popliteal aneurysm cases to define anatomy and operative plan (Fig. 105.11; Video 105.1).

Anatomy

The popliteal artery is a dynamic structure, bounded superiorly by the adductor hiatus and inferiorly by the gastrocnemius muscle. The artery sits within the popliteal fossa, which also includes the popliteal vein and tibial and peroneal nerves. The adductor hiatus acts as a proximal fixed point, and, as such, significant torsion, compression, traction, and retraction forces are placed on the proximal popliteal artery during ambulation, which affects both bypass and endoluminal implant considerations.[47] Angiographically, the artery is divided into three segments as follows:
- P1: adductor hiatus to the superior border of the patella
- P2: superior border of the patella to the center of knee articulation
- P3: knee articulation to the origin of the anterior tibial artery

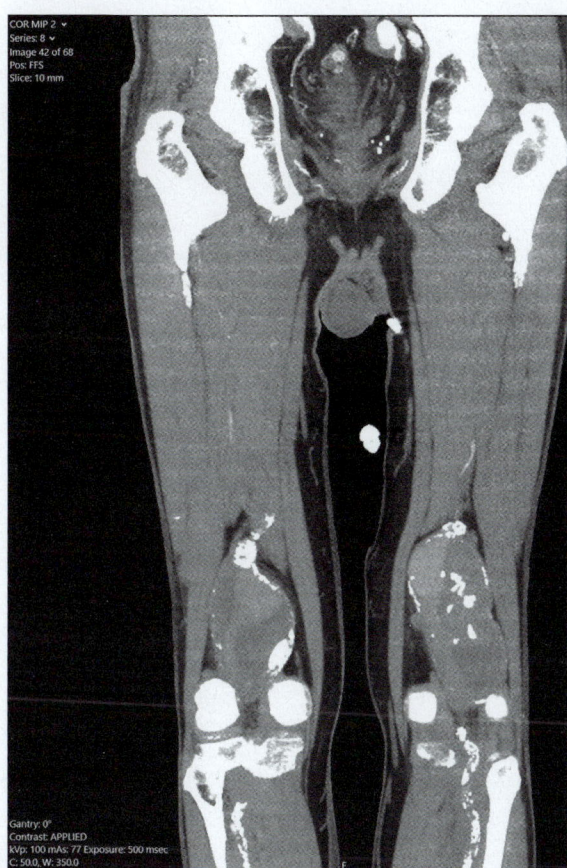

FIGURE 105.11 Computed tomographic coronal reconstruction plan of a patient with large surgically significant bilateral popliteal artery aneurysms (see Video 10.1).

Anatomic variations of the popliteal and its immediate arterial tree are relatively common (approaching 10%–15% of the population), with either hypoplastic tibial arteries or a high origin of the anterior tibial making up most of such cases.[48]

The popliteal artery can be approached via medial, posterior, and lateral exposures, with the former two being the most employed for aneurysmal disease (Table 105.2). Aneurysm extent and surgeon preference dictate the choice of technique, and familiarity with both is a requisite. The authors prefer the posterior approach if the proximal and distal extent of resection are within the anatomic bounds of the adductor hiatus to the tibial arteries.

Operative Indication

- All popliteal aneurysms >20 mm should be repaired.
- Regardless of size, any aneurysm with thrombus should be repaired.

- Any aneurysm associated with signs of ipsilateral thromboembolism should be repaired.
- All pseudoaneurysms should be repaired.

Elective repair of true PAAs is always the goal in physiologically suitable patients with an anticipated good midterm survival and always has a superior limb preservation rate compared with acute revascularization. In cases of unclear etiology, mycotic aneurysm should be considered even in the absence of systemic symptoms.

Surgical Management

Open reconstruction. Bypass with interval ligation of the PAA is the gold standard and should be considered first-line therapy for all patients of good surgical risk. Autologous conduit provides superior primary and assisted patency rates, with a single-segment saphenous vein diameter of 3 mm or greater being ideal. Short saphenous or cephalic vein can also be used as conduit, with expanded PTFE or allograft reserved for no-conduit cases. As with bypass for occlusive disease cases, surgical reconstruction is based on proximal and distal anastomoses being in healthy vessel. Multiple studies have demonstrated that the number of patent runoff vessels correlates with patency rates. Patency rates of saphenous vein bypass in the setting of preserved runoff approximate 90% at 5 years.[49] Patients undergoing open or endovascular reconstruction should be managed with standard cardiovascular risk-reduction medical therapy, including statin-class lipid-lowering drugs, antiplatelet therapy, and angiotensin blockade as indicated.

The PAA should be ligated proximally and distally at the time of open reconstruction to avoid continued pressurization and mass effect–related morbidity. Typically, this is accomplished via complete transection and ligation with a running monofilament suture. Any large geniculate branches arising from the interval segment should be controlled via suture ligature or clip placement to avoid continued flow into the aneurysm sac. Failure to isolate the aneurysm may necessitate reoperation or endovascular secondary intervention. Bypass grafts should be surveilled in the standard fashion via duplex examination with the addition of excluded sac size and flow monitoring.[50]

Posterior approach to the popliteal artery is possible in cases where the extent of aneurysmal disease is restricted to the popliteal fossa (Fig. 105.12). In such cases, the short saphenous vein can be harvested while the patient is in the prone position. Alternately, a popliteal-to-popliteal interposition graft using externally supported prosthetic material yields 80% 2-year primary patency rates and may be preferable to address size mismatch for the end-to-end anastomoses. Comparative data demonstrate superior major adverse limb event rates with open reconstruction compared with endovascular (93% vs.

TABLE 105.2 Operative Approaches to the Popliteal Artery With Surgical Considerations

APPROACH	SURGICAL EXPOSURE	CONSIDERATIONS
Medial	Supine position, slightly flexed knee; proximal incision distal third of thigh lower edge of vastus medialis muscle; distal incision 1 cm inferior to tibia	Popliteal vein will be first structure encountered; midportion of popliteal artery not easily accessible
Posterior	Prone position, S-shaped incision medial to lateral to avoid scar contraction	Tibial nerve, retract laterally; short saphenous vein can be provisionally harvested
Lateral	Supine position, internally rotated leg; proximal exposure between lateral condyle and biceps femoris; distal exposure starting at fibular head	Take care to identify common peroneal nerve

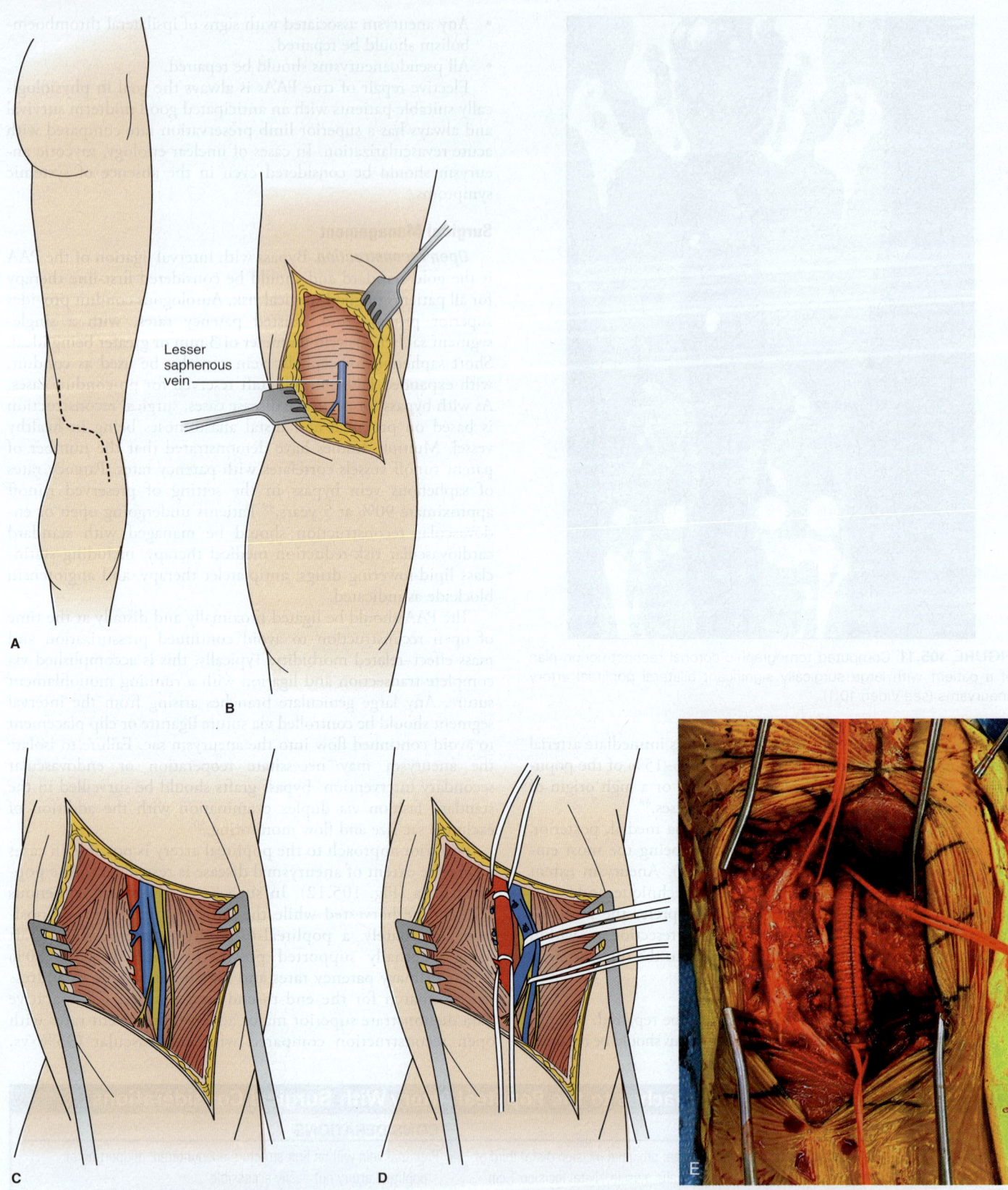

FIGURE 105.12 (A) The incision for the posterior exposure of the popliteal artery is made as a "lazy-S" shape to avoid scar contracture across the knee. Hash marks can be used to aid in skin approximation at case completion. (B) The small (lesser) saphenous vein is identified in the subcutaneous tissue. (C) The deep fascia is incised, and the sural nerve is gently retracted laterally to facilitate the dissection (D) of the popliteal artery from the popliteal vein and the tibial nerve, which lies most superiorly. (E) Intraoperative image after completion of popliteal artery aneurysm repair using synthetic graft. (A–B, From Valentine JR, Wind GG. *Anatomic Exposures in Vascular Surgery*. 2nd ed. Philadelphia: Lippincott Williams & Wilkins; 2003:462, 463. C–D, From Rutherford RB. *Atlas of Vascular Surgery: Basic Techniques and Exposure*. Philadelphia: WB Saunders; 1993:142.)

80% at 1 year), and, as such, bypass should always be considered first line in suitable risk patients with adequate conduit and distal targets.[51]

Endovascular therapy. Endoluminal treatment via stent graft is a viable treatment for patients without suitable autologous conduit and with advanced age, significant comorbidities, and other limb-related factors. The case is predicated on identification of a normal proximal and distal landing zone accounting for a 15% oversizing of the stent graft at the seal sites. Poor runoff, need for extensive coverage past the knee joint, and atherosclerotic burden are associated with decreased primary patency. Intravascular ultrasound is recommended as an adjunct for sizing (luminal diameter, identification of nondiseased landing zone; Fig. 105.13). After stent-graft placement, the proximal and distal seal sites and any graft-graft junction should be balloon angioplastied. If more than one stent graft is required, the smaller-diameter stent should be placed first, and maximal overlap should be used to decrease the risk of type 3 endoleak in this dynamic artery. The literature reports variable patency and adverse limb events after endovascular PAA repair, but most series suggest an 80% 1-year patency rate and higher reintervention rates compared with autologous conduit open bypass. Secondary patency between the two modalities is likely similar. Anatomic and technical correlates of success include number of stent components in the construct, extent of coverage, and runoff score. Patients undergoing stent-based repair should be on the aforementioned best medical therapy, with the addition of dual-antiplatelet therapy unless contraindicated.

From a technical standpoint, the case can be conducted under moderate sedation or monitored anesthesia care. Antegrade access in the common or superficial femoral artery is often possible over the standard retrograde contralateral femoral access. The typical self-expanding stent construct will require a sheath, 8 Fr or larger, so the access is best managed via the preclose technique. After successful angiographic exclusion (Fig. 105.14), patients should be followed with serial duplex ultrasound in the same manner as open bypass patients.[52]

Acute Limb Ischemia

Because of the thrombogenic nature of PAA and often asymptomatic natural history until presentation, many patients present with acute limb-threat ischemia. Once identified, patients should be immediately anticoagulated and undergo axial or catheter-based imaging to define anatomy. Patients with salvageable extremities (Rutherford grade I or II) should undergo either surgical thromboembolectomy or catheter-based thrombolysis, immediately followed by open or endovascular revascularization as outlined earlier. Surgical thromboembolectomy should be employed in those cases with more immediate limb threat (e.g., sensory deficit, motor deficit with absent pedal signals) because the time required for catheter-based treatment may cause the patient to progress to a nonsalvageable state. Failure to demonstrate a distal bypass target will necessitate amputation, which should be above the knee owing to the fact that the profunda-geniculate collaterals that supply the calf skin and musculature are needed for a below-knee flap. Although exact data are lacking, amputation rates and mortality associated with thrombosed PAA are high, with limb-loss rates ranging from 15% to 70%.[53]

Infrapopliteal and Other Aneurysms

The incidence of tibial and peroneal artery aneurysms is unknown but exceedingly rare. Most commonly, tibial or peroneal artery aneurysms are related to penetrating trauma, fractures, or iatrogenic injury from peripheral endovascular interventions. Aneurysms that present with signs of distal ischemia should be reconstructed. However, simple ligation is often sufficient if other tibial arteries are patent. There are approximately 20 published reports of true anterior tibial artery aneurysms in the literature, which were typically managed with surgical ligation or rarely with endovascular embolization.

Iatrogenic Femoral Aneurysms

Pseudoaneurysms are the result of a transmural arterial defect resulting in extravascular blood flow that is contained by a fiber and sheath. These false aneurysms are typically the result of blunt or penetrating trauma to an artery. Today, most peripheral pseudoaneurysms are iatrogenic and a result of incomplete arterial closure after peripheral access, as required for invasive diagnostic or therapeutic procedures. Pseudoaneurysms have been reported to occur in 0.5% to 9% of arterial access cases.[54] The use of the Seldinger technique under either fluoroscopic or ultrasound guidance is known to reduce the incidence of pseudoaneurysm formation. In addition, large sheath size, patient body habitus, need for anticoagulation, female sex, and hemodialysis have been associated with an increased risk of pseudoaneurysm formation after arterial cannulation.

The feared complication of a pseudoaneurysm is rupture, which can lead to hemorrhagic shock and mortality. Because of this, the anatomic location is critical to note. Pseudoaneurysms of the external iliac artery will rupture into the retroperitoneum. Exsanguination from a CFA pseudoaneurysm is less common. It is rare that a pseudoaneurysm would cause

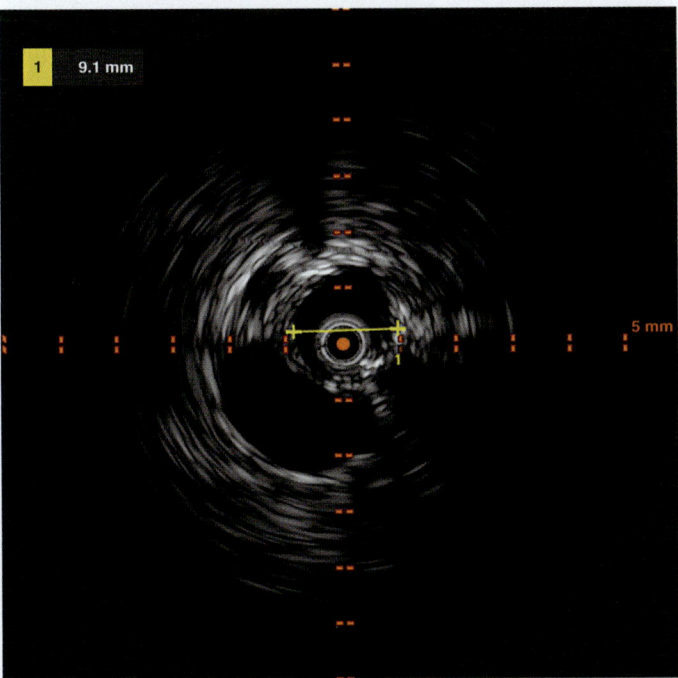

FIGURE 105.13 Intravascular ultrasound of the femoropopliteal segment in a patient undergoing endovascular repair of popliteal artery aneurysm. Examination demonstrates proximal landing zone diameter of 9 mm with a plan to place an 11-mm-diameter self-expanding covered stent.

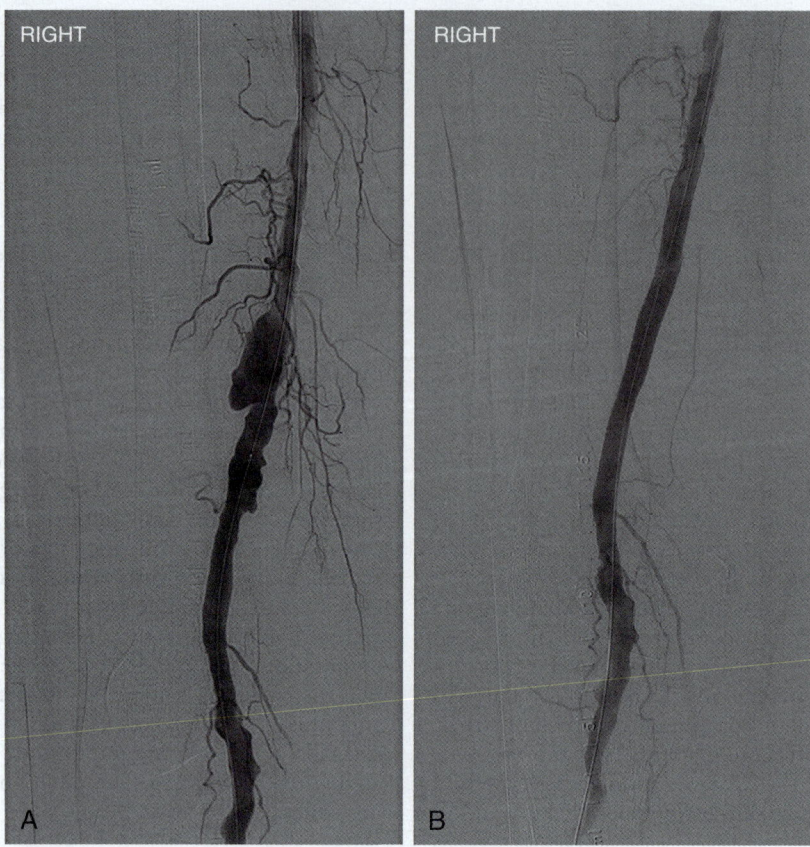

FIGURE 105.14 Angiograph of patient undergoing endovascular popliteal artery aneurysm repair demonstrating initial angiogram with external radiopaque marker (A) to assist with stent selection and successful exclusion of the aneurysm with covered stent and no evidence of endoleak (B).

distal ischemic complications, given that the pathology is a transmural arterial defect. However, the risk for ischemic complications increases as the size of the pseudoaneurysm neck increases.

Diagnosis

Patients with pseudoaneurysms present with a painful pulsatile mass, commonly associated with a hematoma and bruit. Patients can also present with compressive symptoms such as femoral neuropathic pain, pain or paresthesia with hip flexion, or extremity edema. Progressive expansion can lead to skin ischemia and must be addressed to avoid wound formation.

Diagnosis is made with duplex ultrasonography and clinical examination. Continuous to-and-fro flow that is contained will be seen on duplex ultrasound (Fig. 105.15). It also provides important information regarding the anatomy of the false aneurysm sac and its neck. It can be difficult, and occasionally misleading, to diagnose a pseudoaneurysm using CTA alone. Given the static nature of CT imaging, an active hemorrhage can be mistaken for a pseudoaneurysm. This distinction is of critical clinical significance, and clinical evaluation of the patient will distinguish the two diagnoses.

Operative Indications

Ultrasound-guided compressions or thrombin injection:
- Pseudoaneurysms >2 cm
- Pseudoaneurysm diameter growth of >100%
- Persistent pseudoaneurysm after 2 months of observation

Open surgical repair:
- Ruptured pseudoaneurysms (active hemorrhage) require emergent open or endovascular repair.
- Failure or contraindication to ultrasound-guided thrombin injection (broad neck)
- Skin ischemia or necrosis
- Arteriovenous fistula

In most patients, PAAs in the lower extremities can be observed if they are less than 2 to 3 cm in diameter. However, anticoagulation significantly reduces the likelihood of spontaneous thrombosis of the false aneurysm.

Management

Ultrasound-guided compression. Compression of a pseudoaneurysm to induce thrombosis of the aneurysm sac was initially proposed in the early 1990s. This procedure uses duplex ultrasound to visualize the pseudoaneurysm and its neck. Color Doppler should be able to visualize flow within the sac. Pressure is applied to the transducer to compress the aneurysm neck and prevent arterial flow into the aneurysm cavity. The lack of flow should be visualized on color Doppler. Compression is held for 10 to 20 minutes, repeating as needed. The patient should be kept flat in bed for 6 hours and reevaluated with a duplex ultrasound in 24 to 48 hours to evaluate for maintained sac thrombosis. During the procedure, attention must be given to avoid excessive pressure, which can result in compression of the native artery. This can cause arterial thrombosis and subsequent limb ischemia. Case series demonstrate that this technique is successful between 60% and 80% of the time, requiring an

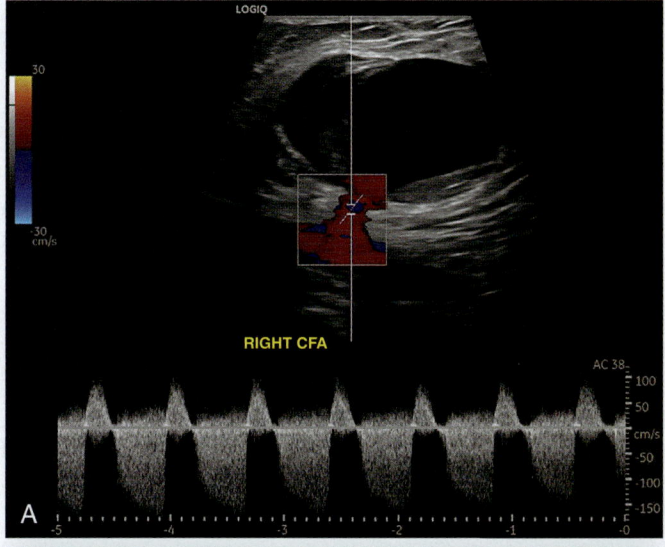

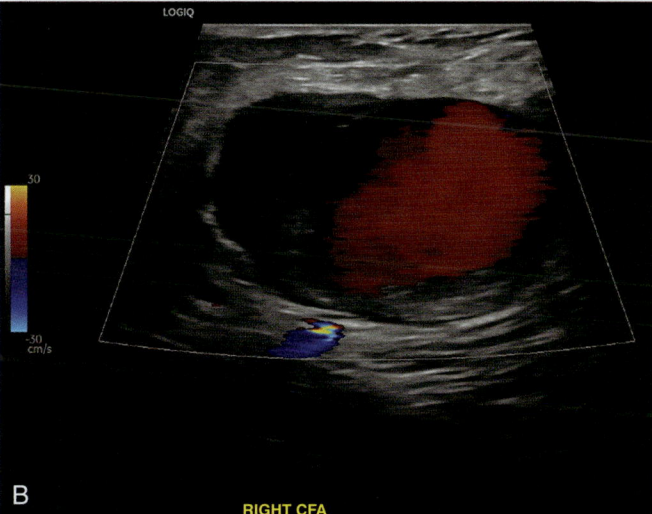

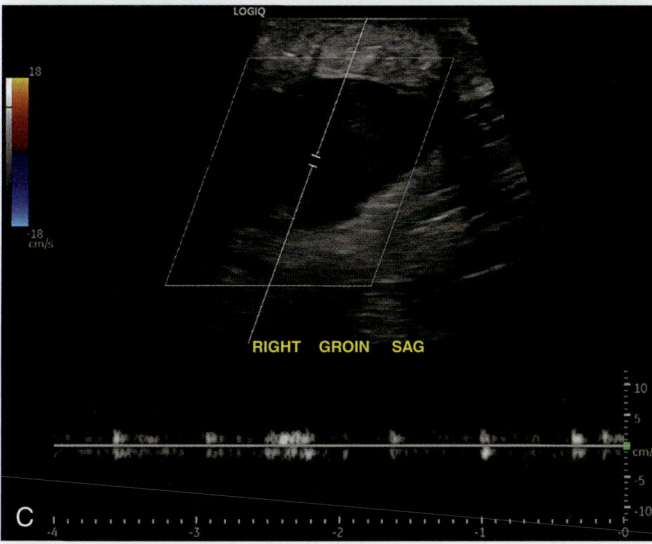

FIGURE 105.15 Duplex ultrasound imaging of large right common femoral artery pseudoaneurysm. Color flow and spectral imaging (A) identified to-and-fro flow through the neck of the pseudoaneurysm, and a ying-yang sign (B) is present within the pseudoaneurysm cavity, both hallmarks of a pseudoaneurysm on duplex ultrasonography. (C) Color flow and spectral imaging do not detect blood flow within the pseudoaneurysm sac after thrombin injection. *CFA*, Common femoral artery; *SAG*, sagittal.

average of 30 to 45 minutes of compression. Patients on anticoagulation have a lower likelihood of successful pseudoaneurysm sac thrombosis. This technique is often not possible for patients with severe pain or large hematomas. Additionally, it should not be performed in patients with acute hemorrhage.

Ultrasound-guided thrombin injection. If ultrasound-guided compression fails or the patient is not a candidate, an ultrasound-guided thrombin injection can be performed. Importantly, the pseudoaneurysm should have a long and narrow neck that is easily identified under ultrasound and easily compressible. A large, short neck increases the risk of the coagulation cascade entering the arterial circulation, inducing intravascular thrombus formation and limb ischemia. Color flow should be seen within the cavity. After administration of local anesthesia and under direct ultrasound visualization, a spinal needle is inserted into the pseudoaneurysm. At this point, blood should be easily aspirated. Approximately 100 to 500 units/mL of thrombin is instilled into the false aneurysm cavity in 0.1-mL increments until thrombosis is visualized by loss of color Doppler signal within the cavity (see Fig. 105.15). Thrombin injection results in immediate clot formation by directly converting fibrinogen into fibrin. This results in effective thrombosis even in patients on therapeutic anticoagulation because the mechanism is downstream of the effects of warfarin, heparin, and new oral anticoagulants. It is critically important to maintain visualization of the aneurysm cavity and immediately stop the injunction once thrombosis has been achieved. Continued injection after thrombosis of the false aneurysm cavity can lead to intravascular thrombin injection and arterial thrombosis. Embolization of thrombus into the distal circulation occurs in approximately 2% to 4% of cases. A complete pulse examination should be obtained before and after each procedure to identify this complication.

Open reconstruction. Open surgical repair should be performed for ruptured pseudoaneurysms, patients presenting with skin symptoms, pseudoaneurysms associated with arteriovenous fistula, or pseudoaneurysms that have failed to thrombose after all ultrasound-guided therapy. Surgical management should follow all principles of vascular surgery, including proximal and distal control, followed by arterial reconstruction. In the acute setting of rupture and hemodynamic instability, manual compression at the side of bleeding should be applied immediately, followed by surgical vascular control. Direct repair of the arterial injury with Prolene suture is effective for small defects. For larger injuries, patch angioplasty repair can be performed. Occasionally, the size of the pseudoaneurysm and subsequent fibrin sheath will envelop the native artery, making dissection difficult. In this scenario, resection of a small arterial segment with interposition graft reconstruction can be performed. Autologous greater saphenous vein (GSV) is preferred; however, the femoral artery diameter is typically much larger than the GSV. In this setting, a short segment of Dacron can be used.

MYCOTIC ANEURYSMS

Although outside the scope of this chapter, myotic aneurysms warrant mention. In brief, all mycotic aneurysms are pseudoaneurysms and mandate operative reconstruction with autologous or biologic conduit. Various techniques are described across all arterial beds. *Staphylococcus* spp. represent the most common isolate. When discovered, all patients with infectious etiology aneurysm should undergo parenteral antibiotic therapy and rapid imaging workup, followed by surgical therapy.

SELECTED REFERENCES

Chaer RA, Abularrage CJ, Coleman DM, et al. The Society for Vascular Surgery clinical practice guidelines on the management of visceral aneurysms. *J Vasc Surg.* 2020;72(suppl 1):3S-39S.

The SVS clinical practice guidelines on the management of visceral aneurysms provide the most recent recommendations on the management of all visceral aneurysms. A detailed account of the most recent evidence with the grade of recommendation and quality of evidence is provided for aneurysms in each vascular bed.

Farber A, Angle N, Avgerinos E, et al. The Society for Vascular Surgery clinical practice guidelines on popliteal artery aneurysms. *J Vasc Surg.* 2022;75(suppl 1):109S-120S.

The SVS clinical practice guidelines on popliteal artery aneurysms provide the most recent recommendations on the management of popliteal artery aneurysms. A detailed account of the most recent evidence with a grade of recommendation and quality of evidence is provided.

Leake AE, Segal MA, Chaer RA, et al. Meta-analysis of open and endovascular repair of popliteal artery aneurysms. *J Vasc Surg.* 2017;65(1):246-256.e2.

Meta-analysis including 4880 popliteal artery aneurysm repairs over 14 studies comparing open aneurysm repair to endovascular repair. Open aneurysm repair demonstrated better primary patency at 1 and 3 years. However, there was no difference in secondary patency at these intervals.

McCollum CH, Da Gama AD, Noon GP, DeBakey ME. Aneurysm of the subclavian artery. *J Cardiovasc Surg (Torino).* 1979;20(2):159-164.

Original case series describing the likely cause and management of 16 subclavian artery aneurysms.

Rossi M, Krokidis M, Kashef E, Peynircioglu B, Tipaldi MA. CIRSE standards of practice for the endovascular treatment of visceral and renal artery aneurysms and pseudoaneurysms. *Cardiovasc Intervent Radiol.* 2024;47(1):26-35.

This standard-of-practice document provides up-to-date recommendations for the safe performance of endovascular therapy for visceral and RAAs and defines standard steps required for the performance of each intervention.

The full reference list appears on Elsevier eBooks+.

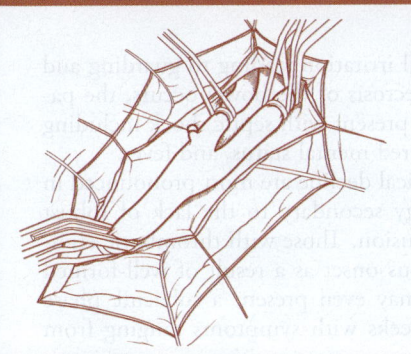

CHAPTER 106

Visceral Ischemic Syndromes: Acute and Chronic Mesenteric Ischemia

Sabina M. Sorondo, Blake E. Murphy, Benjamin W. Starnes, and Jason T. Lee

ACUTE MESENTERIC ISCHEMIA

Epidemiology

Mesenteric ischemia was first described by Chienne in 1869 and remains challenging to diagnose and treat in the present day despite medical and surgical advancements.[1] The first intestinal resection and reanastomosis was performed by Elliot in 1895. In 1951, Klass performed the first superior mesenteric artery (SMA) embolectomy, and in 1957 Shaw and Maynard performed the first embolectomy to be considered successful without requiring subsequent bowel resection. In 1980, endovascular treatment of mesenteric disease was introduced to practice and represents a major advance in the distinct ability for surgical techniques to care for these patients. Today, acute mesenteric ischemia (AMI) accounts for less than 1 per 100,000 hospital admissions in the United States and less than 2% of all admissions for gastrointestinal disorders.[2]

Incidence of AMI increases with age and nearly doubles with each 5-year interval above the age of 70.[3] It is typically seen in patients with multiple comorbidities with a threefold increase in females compared with males.[4] AMI is the final common pathway for several clinical scenarios, each of which has its own characteristic epidemiology, including mesenteric arterial thromboembolic disease, mesenteric venous thrombosis (MVT), and nonocclusive mesenteric ischemia (NOMI).[5] Risk factors include those at risk for thrombosis or embolus (atherosclerosis, atrial fibrillation/flutter, recent myocardial infarction [MI], congestive heart failure) or history of chronic mesenteric ischemia (CMI). Those at risk for NOMI are patients that have critically ill conditions and are in shock from alternative sources, with postoperative cardiac surgery and hemodialysis patients at highest risk.

Over the years, studies have shown a dramatic decrease in mortality rates from 1999–2010, with open repair showing the most dramatic improvement over time from 43% to 33%.[6] In-hospital mortality has also decreased following endovascular revascularizations, falling from 20% to 15%. Despite technical advancements over time, overall mortality remains high at 17% to 21% among patients requiring intervention.[4,7]

Pathophysiology
Embolic

AMI pathophysiology is divided into embolic, thrombotic, and nonocclusive categories. Arterial embolism is the most common cause, comprising about 40% to 50% of cases.[8,9] Patients presenting with mesenteric ischemia secondary to an embolic event typically have a history of preceding embolic event, most commonly arising from a cardiac source such as atrial fibrillation/flutter, ventricular thrombi secondary to low ejection fraction from recent MI or heart failure, valvular disease, endocarditis, and/or aortic aneurysms with associated mural thrombi. As high as 68% of patients have simultaneous embolic events in other vascular beds (cerebrovascular, peripheral).[10,11]

The SMA is the second branch of the abdominal aorta, and its branches include the inferior anterior and posterior pancreaticoduodenal arteries, the middle colic artery, right colic artery, ileocolic artery, and jejunal and ileal branches, respectively. Given the oblique angle of the SMA origin off the aorta, thromboemboli preferentially will lodge in this visceral vessel. The SMA tapers just beyond the first few jejunal branches; thus, emboli typically settle more proximally. About 50% of embolic events occur just distal to the middle colic artery and 15% may lodge at the SMA origin.[12,13] The middle colic artery terminates into a right and left branch and anastomoses with the branches of the right and left colic arteries and contributes to the formation of the marginal artery of Drummond. The right branch supplies the upper segment of the ascending colon and hepatic flexure, and the left branch supplies the proximal two-thirds of the transverse colon. Embolic events to the SMA proximal to the middle colic artery cause a classic formation of ischemia that typically spares these portions of the bowel. Embolization to the celiac artery occurs more rarely, and normally becomes symptomatic in patients with preexisting SMA disease. Mortality for thromboembolic events to the SMA without intervention is high, averaging 54%.

Thrombosis

Arterial thrombosis is the second most common cause of AMI averaging 20% to 35%. Typically, most patients presenting with thrombotic etiology of AMI have a prior history of CMI from preexisting chronic lesions. In situ thrombosis of chronic lesions is most common, and patients with peripheral vascular disease have an incidence of AMI that may be as high as 27% in some studies.[14] In acute-on-chronic ischemia, presentation of bowel ischemia may be delayed given preexisting collateral channels that can maintain perfusion until events such as small emboli or episodes of hypotension result in occlusion of the significantly stenosed vessel. Other causes of thrombosis include hypercoagulable syndromes (factor V Leiden, antiphospholipid syndrome, prothrombin gene mutations, antithrombin III syndrome, protein C/S deficiency), extensions of aortic dissection resulting in compression and inhibition of flow through the true lumen, and thrombotic complications of previous mesenteric interventions (in-stent or graft thrombosis). Thrombosis most commonly affects the SMA, and the location is typically within 2 cm of the vessel origin. Given the proximity of occlusion, mortality rates without intervention are higher for thrombosis than emboli (77%), likely secondary to involvement of larger segments of bowel. Thrombosis of the celiac artery can also be clinically significant, normally in the setting of preexisting SMA disease.

Nonocclusive Mesenteric Ischemia

NOMI is a clinical syndrome that is the result of a combination of pathophysiologic phenomena including mesenteric vasoconstriction, intestinal hypoxemia, reperfusion injury, increased intestinal metabolic demand, and infection.[15] NOMI comprises about 20% of AMI cases and most frequently affects the SMA. A key aspect in the development of NOMI is a low flow state with or without prior mesenteric vessel stenosis. Hence, this cause of mesenteric ischemia is typically seen in critically ill patients. Patients with severe cardiac failure and recent cardiac surgery and critically ill hemodialysis patients are at greatest risk.[16] Vasoactive pressors such as epinephrine, norepinephrine, and vasopressin have also been associated with the development of NOMI.[17] Although mesenteric stenosis may be present, its absence in many cases points to a vasospastic mechanism in the critically ill patient that attempts to prioritize cerebral and cardiac perfusion at the expense of visceral perfusion. NOMI carries the highest mortality rate of all AMI causes, partly due to the nature of the underlying illness.

Clinical Evaluation
History and Physical Presentation

AMI leads to severe inflammation that often presents initially with vague diffuse abdominal pain that is "out of proportion" to examination. Other symptoms can include nausea, vomiting, diarrhea, and melena. Once transmural ischemia occurs the patient will exhibit signs of peritoneal irritation leading to guarding and rebound tenderness. If full necrosis of the bowel occurs, the patient may rapidly decline and present with septic shock including tachycardia, hypotension, altered mental status, and fever.

Acute onset and rapid clinical decline are most pronounced in patients with embolic etiology secondary to the lack of robust collateral circulation and perfusion. Those with thrombotic etiology may have a more insidious onset as a result of well-formed collateral circulation. Some may even present a subacute phase that can last from days to weeks with symptoms ranging from mild abdominal pain, diarrhea, nausea, vomiting, or gastrointestinal bleeding. Patients with NOMI have a wide range of clinical presentation and are typically presenting with concurrent organ failure. They may or may not have abdominal pain and often have findings consistent with systemic sepsis, laboratory abnormalities, and abdominal distention.

The differential diagnosis for abdominal pain is broad, including appendicitis, diverticulitis, cholecystitis, pancreatitis, and bowel obstructions. Studies have shown that delays in diagnosis lead to significant decrease in survival from 50% to 30% when the diagnosis of SMA embolism is made more than 24 hours from symptom onset.[13] Thus, a high index of suspicion is required to prevent delays in diagnosis. In modern surgical care, surgical consultation is often already preceded by cross-sectional imaging performed in the emergency department.

Laboratory Findings

Abnormalities in laboratory values are adjuncts to the diagnosis of AMI but do not definitively confirm or dismiss the diagnosis. Initial lab values can be normal but may show abnormalities such as leukocytosis ($>$15,000 with neutrophilic left shift), metabolic acidosis, and elevated lactate. D-dimer is an early sensitive marker but is not specific with high false-positive rates. Elevations in levels of serum amylase, creatine kinase, and aminotransferases may be seen but lack sufficient sensitivity and specificity. Novel, specific serologic markers are currently being studied (urinary and plasma intestinal fatty acid-binding proteins [iFABP]) to facilitate earlier detection of AMI but are not currently used in routine practice.[18,19]

Diagnostic Evidence

In modern practice, the single best imaging modality to confirm the diagnosis of AMI is CT angiography (CTA), with a sensitivity and specificity of 93% and 96%, respectively.[20] Although previous practice has denoted the use of diagnostic angiography as the gold standard for diagnostic evaluation, the widespread availability of high-quality CT scanners nationwide and diagnostic accuracy has made CTA the imaging modality of choice. CTA can assess for filling defects in the visceral vessels, and when performed with both an arterial and delayed venous phase (biphasic CTA) can also allow for evaluation of the portal venous system and bowel wall perfusion (Fig. 106.1). Characteristic findings of intestinal ischemia include bowel wall thickening and mucosal wall enhancement, pneumatosis, and portal venous gas. MVT, another source of visceral ischemia when severe, can also be assessed using CTA. Although CTA is useful for the diagnosis of occlusive mesenteric ischemia, its use for diagnosis of nonocclusive disease is less reliable.

Plain radiographs are usually unrevealing unless significant intestinal necrosis has occurred. Some abnormalities seen on radiographs in the late stages of ischemia include ileus, thumbprinting (due to submucosal hemorrhage and bowel wall edema), pneumatosis linearis, or portal venous gas. Doppler ultrasonography is a valuable tool for assessment of visceral vessels and detection of

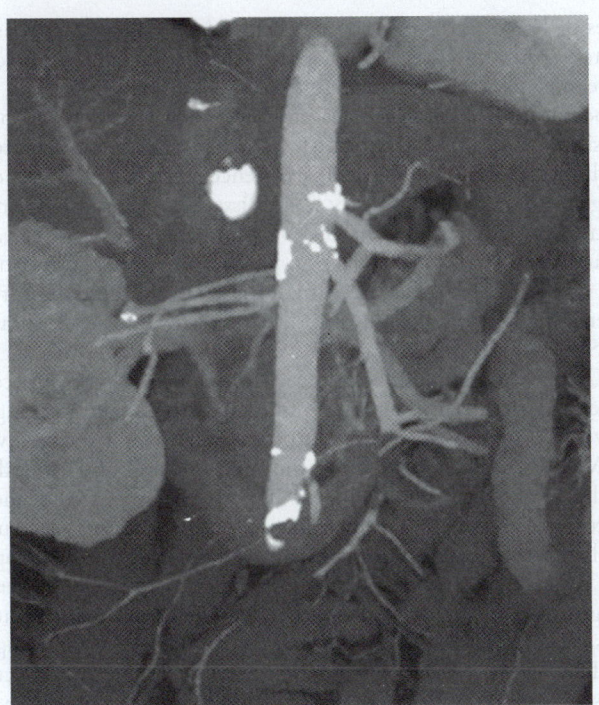

FIGURE 106.1 Anterior-posterior and lateral CT. A reconstruction of acute embolus to the mid superior mesenteric artery.

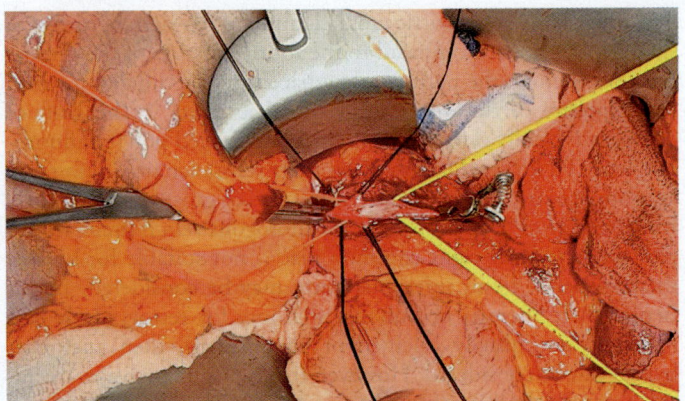

FIGURE 106.2 Longitudinal arteriotomy made after dissection of the mid superior mesenteric artery in the root of the mesentery with control of the side branches to allow for embolectomy and subsequent patch repair.

high-grade stenoses in the SMA and celiac artery for CMI. However, in the acute setting this imaging modality is not considered reliable due to its limitation to evaluate the visceral vessels and emboli past the origin and assess for signs of intestinal ischemia. Magnetic resonance angiography (MRA) is another imaging modality with high diagnostic accuracy, but it is less readily available and more time consuming than CTA, making it less favorable in the acute setting.

Management
Medical Treatment

Patients presenting with AMI warrant immediate medical management. This includes establishment of IV access with crystalloid fluid resuscitation, hemodynamic monitoring, and correction of electrolyte abnormalities. Systemic anticoagulation should be initiated promptly upon diagnosis to prevent further propagation of thrombus. Additionally, administration of broad-spectrum IV antibiotics should be given to treat potential translocation of bacteria in the setting of ischemic bowel.[21] Vasopressors should be avoided, if possible. If vasopressors are necessary in the setting of hypotension refractory to fluid resuscitation, then those with less splanchnic vasoconstriction should be prioritized including dobutamine, milrinone, and low-dose dopamine.[22] Although these initial managements are crucial, it should be done in congruency with surgical planning and should not delay revascularization.

Medical management of NOMI includes correction of the underlying cause such as improving cardiac output, weaning vasopressors if able, and supportive care. Intraarterial infusion of vasodilators such as papaverine, nitroglycerin, or prostaglandin analogues selectively increase splanchnic blood flow and have been described for treatment of NOMI in small case series. However, no large or well-controlled clinical trials exist to support this treatment as standard practice.[23,24]

Revascularization

Prompt revascularization via thromboembolectomy and assessment of the bowel is the standard technique for embolic disease. Embolectomy of the SMA requires anterior exposure of the vessel. This is achieved by lifting the omentum and transverse colon cephalad and mobilizing the small intestine to the patient's right. At the base of the transverse mesocolon, a horizontal incision is made to expose the anterior portion of the SMA. Venous tributaries, small lymphatics, and autonomic nerve fibers require ligation to facilitate arterial exposure, keeping in mind that the superior mesenteric vein lies left to the artery. For more proximal control, the inferior pancreatic border and splenic vein (SV) may require mobilization. The SMA is exposed and controlled proximal to the middle colic artery, and after systemic heparinization the artery is opened transversely. More recently, we have preferred longitudinal arteriotomy for the ability to either patch the vessel or use as a bypass target (Fig. 106.2).

The proximal SMA is vented to allow any clot to spontaneously evacuate. A Fogarty balloon thromboembolectomy catheter should be performed with a 3-Fr or 4-Fr catheter, and if distal vascular embolectomy is required, then the catheter should be down-sized to a 2 Fr or 3 Fr. The balloon should be inflated with heparinized saline as the catheter is withdrawn and repeated until free of thrombus burden. Once cleared of thrombus, the arteriotomy can be repaired primarily with 5-0 or 6-0 monofilament suture in an interrupted fashion. A venous or bovine patch may be necessary in a diminutive or heavily plaque-ridden vessel. If distal thrombus was not removed, the surgeon can consider direct infusion of 0.5 to 1 mg of tissue plasminogen factor (tPA) into the vessel.

In AMI secondary to thrombosis, a bypass is often required for successful revascularization as often these vessels contain proximal or long segments of plaque burden that may prevent adequate revascularization from embolectomy or stenting alone. There are multiple arrangements for graft orientation and type of conduit and each option should be decided based on preoperative imaging and individual patient anatomy as well as their overall physiologic state. A retrograde bypass off the right common iliac artery (CIA) oriented in a "lazy C" configuration with synthetic graft is one option frequently favored in the emergent setting and critically ill patient. This option avoids significant hemodynamic shifts by negating the need for aortic cross-clamping. The lateral portion of the SMA is exposed cephalad to the fourth portion of the duodenum by opening the peritoneum adjacent to the duodenum with full exposure of the distal aorta and iliac artery.[21] The graft of choice is typically 6 to 8 mm externally enforced polytetrafluoroethylene (PTFE) or Dacron given their resistance to kinking and appropriate size match. However, in cases of gross contamination from spillage of necrotic bowel, an autologous vein is preferred. In patients where the right common iliac is not suitable for bypass, then the left CIA or infrarenal aorta may be considered. In patients where there is no suitable anatomy for retrograde bypass (distal inflow heavily calcified or aneurysmal), then antegrade bypass can be considered. However, this exposure increases operative times, technical complexity, and results in significant hemodynamic shifts with supraceliac aortic clamping.

Retrograde open mesenteric stenting (ROMS) is a hybrid procedure for SMA thrombosis that has been shown to be an efficient and less invasive revascularization option. The SMA is exposed similarly to an embolectomy exposure and is cannulated in retrograde fashion. The SMA is then stented using endovascular wires, catheters, and fluoroscopy imaging to facilitate appropriate stent placement. This technique avoids the need for aortic cross-clamping, prosthetic conduit, and technical complexity associated with further aortic exposure. A multicenter study from the Vascular Low Frequency Disease Consortium has shown this technique to have a success rate of 98% and primary and secondary patency of 76% and 90%, respectively, at 2 years.[25]

After revascularization, the bowel should be thoroughly assessed. In some instances, bowel resection may be performed first. These instances include patients with bowel perforation or free air on prior imaging. Additionally, those suspected of having complete bowel necrosis should undergo abdominal exploration as revascularization is not warranted in these cases and is usually a nonsurvivable scenario.

In patients who have undergone open revascularization, the bowel should be assessed for viability. Bowel that is evidently necrotic should undergo resection and left in discontinuity. Aggressive efforts to resect bowel with questionable viability should be avoided. A temporary abdominal closure device should then be placed with reexploration in 24 to 36 hours. A second look allows for preservation of maximal bowel length as it gives segments with questionable viability to recover once blood flow has been restored. In patients who underwent endovascular revascularization, a laparoscopic approach to assess the bowel can be undertaken by a skilled surgeon who feels comfortable with this approach.

In contemporary practice, not all patients undergo open abdominal revascularization or exploration. Endovascular treatment of AMI has steadily increased since the early 2000s and recent studies indicate improved morbidity and mortality with this strategy. Endovascular management of AMI includes pharmacomechanical embolectomy, angioplasty, intraarterial thrombolysis, and stenting. Exclusive endovascular treatments for AMI should only be considered in patients without evidence of bowel ischemia. This technique negates the need for laparotomy and has been shown to reduce hospital stay and need for postoperative parenteral nutrition in patients who were appropriately chosen for endovascular therapy alone.[21]

MESENTERIC ARTERY DISSECTION

Mesenteric artery dissection most often occurs as a complication following abdominal aortic dissection. Spontaneous isolated mesenteric artery dissection (SIMAD) conversely is very rare. Most cases of IMAD involve the SMA (SISMAD) and incidence is reported around 0.06%. A higher incidence is reported in males of Korean, Japanese, and Chinese descent suggesting a genetic predisposition. Etiology is most commonly idiopathic, but other possible causes include fibromuscular dysplasia, segmental arterial mediolysis, cystic medial necrosis, Behcet disease, trauma, heavy weightlifting, and pregnancy.[26–28] Dissection location normally occurs 1 to 3 cm from the SMA ostium, likely due to elevated shear stress at the vessel transition point from a fixed retropancreatic position with an acute turn into a mobile mesenteric root. Interestingly, hypertension is not clearly associated as a risk factor for SISMAD.

Clinical presentation can vary from patients who are completely asymptomatic and is found incidentally on imaging or they can present with severe symptoms. The pain associated with SISMAD is typically isolated to the epigastric area and can radiate to the back and is likely due to irritation of the visceral nerve plexus due to inflammation from arterial dissection that usually resolves with time. Patients presenting with pain out of proportion to examination, however, are suggestive of visceral ischemia. Diagnostic workup is similar to that of AMI, including laboratory tests that may or may not be abnormal. CTA is the imaging modality of choice for diagnosis, which can assess for dissection flaps, false lumens, reentry tears, thrombus, intramural hematomas, aneurysm formation, and rupture.

SISMAD does not have a well-studied treatment algorithm in place given its low prevalence; however, general treatment guidelines have been developed based on the morphology of the dissection as well as the patient's presenting symptoms. In general, those in which a dissection was found incidentally and remain completely asymptomatic can be managed conservatively with antiplatelet therapy. If there is significant luminal compromise on imaging or mild symptoms, then some authors have suggested anticoagulation. However, the role for antiplatelets and anticoagulation has not been well defined.

For symptomatic patients without signs of ischemia, the initial management includes bowel rest and observation with serial abdominal examinations. Additionally, most are started on a heparin drip, although its role is also not well defined in the symptomatic group. If pain worsens or persists despite bowel rest and anticoagulation, then interventional treatment should be considered. Most patients who have persistent abdominal pain undergo arterial stenting as the primary treatment modality. Endovascular stenting eliminates stenosis caused by the false lumen and stabilizes the arterial wall to prevent future aneurysmal degeneration. There are no treatment guidelines that exist for stenting. However, some have suggested that stenosis of the SMA greater than 80% or dilation to more than 2 cm are indications for primary stenting.[29] Others have observed radiographic and symptomatic improvement with conservative management alone.[30] Patients who present with rupture from the dissection or advanced bowel ischemia are better candidates for open surgery than endovascular approaches. Direct repair of the arterial dissection can be performed, but in the setting of threatened visceral organs further repair is necessary. Surgical options include aortovisceral bypass, extraanatomic bypass, and intimectomy/fenestration with patch repair. Arterial inflow of choice for extraanatomic bypass is often the gastroepiploic or hepatic artery.

No contemporary guidelines exist for the surveillance of mesenteric arterial dissections. However, most surgeons perform some routine follow-up. CTA is the imaging modality of choice, but duplex ultrasound (DUS) can also be considered when anatomically appropriate. Surveillance is done to monitor for the development of an aneurysm from arterial degeneration secondary to the dissection. True incidence of aneurysmal formation is not known, but there are reports in the literature of this phenomenon.[31] However, most dissections undergo remodeling rather than aneurysm formation. A single-center study has shown that 41% of SISMAD treated conservatively had improvement on surveillance imaging and 15% of patients had complete remodeling of the SMA.[32] Thus, a majority of patients presenting with IMAD can be treated conservatively.

CHRONIC MESENTERIC ISCHEMIA

Epidemiology

CMI is a rare medical condition caused by the imbalance between the blood supply and physiologic demand within the gastrointestinal tract. The symptoms associated with CMI include postprandial abdominal pain, which often results in "food fear" and weight loss. Currently in the United States, CMI accounts for less than 1 per 100,000 hospital admissions, although reported incidence has steadily increased over the past two decades. The most common cause of CMI includes atherosclerosis resulting in hemodynamically significant stenosis or occlusion of mesenteric vasculature including the celiac axis (CA), SMA, and/or inferior mesenteric artery (IMA). CMI affects patients in their sixth and seventh decade of life and is three times more common in female patients. Over the past 50 years, revascularization techniques including both open and minimally invasive endovascular technologies have evolved for the treatment of CMI.[33,34]

Pathophysiology

The primary circulation to the small and large bowel includes the CA, SMA, and IMA. However, robust collateral pathways exist for the purposes of maintaining mesenteric perfusion. The arc of Riolan is a collateral pathway between the left colic artery, a branch of the IMA, and the middle colic artery, a branch of the SMA. The pancreaticoduodenal arcade, or arc of Buhler, and gastroduodenal arteries allow for collateralization between the CA and SMA (Fig. 106.3). Under fasting conditions, approximately 20% to 25% of cardiac output is delivered to mesenteric circulation, increasing to nearly 35% to 40% following mealtime. Postprandial intestinal hyperemia is the physiologic, vasodilatory response to food within the lumen of the gastrointestinal tract. Based on complex neural, humoral, and paracrine pathways, the magnitude and duration of the hyperemia is determined by the composition of the meal. Compared with carbohydrate-based meals, lipid and protein-based intake elicits a higher magnitude (25%–200%) and longer duration (3–7 hours) of intestinal hyperemia.[35,36]

Atherosclerotic disease within mesenteric vasculature, also known as mesenteric artery occlusive disease (MAOD) or mesenteric artery stenosis (MAS), is estimated to affect up to 10% of the elderly patient population. However, only a small portion of patients with MAOD will present with symptomatic CMI given the extensive, collateral network within the splanchnic circulation. The degree of atherosclerotic burden and number of diseased mesenteric vessels is often positively correlated with symptomatology. Patients with diffuse atherosclerotic disease, high-grade stenosis greater than 70%, or occlusion of at least two mesenteric vessels increases the risk of progression to symptomatic CMI.[37] Common risk factors for the development of atherosclerotic disease include hypertension, hyperlipidemia, diabetes, and tobacco

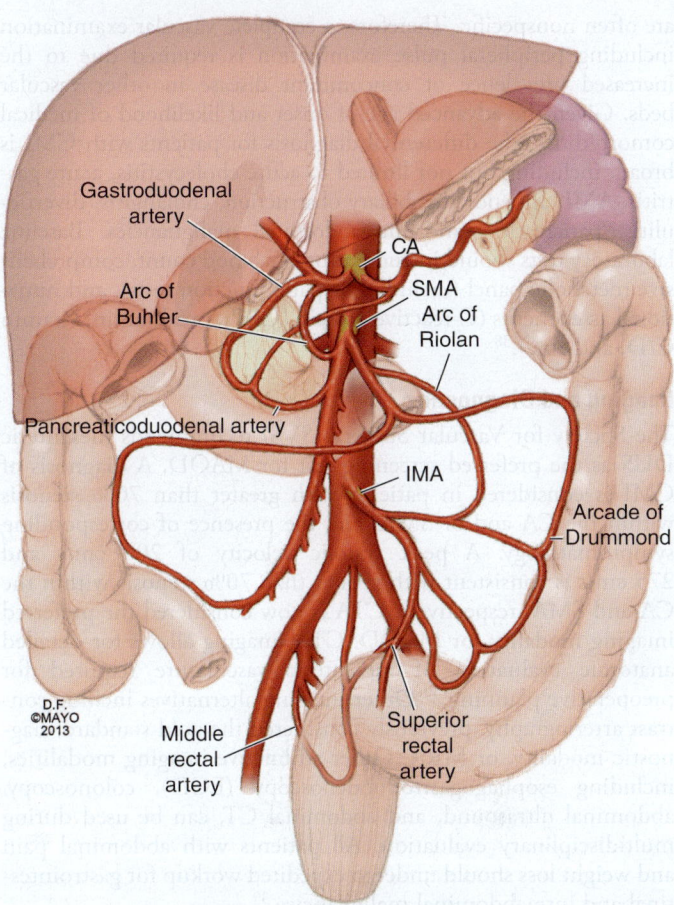

FIGURE 106.3 Schematic representation of mesenteric circulation. Collateral pathways include arc of Riolan (connecting left colic artery arising from the inferior mesenteric artery [IMA] and middle colic artery arising from the superior mesenteric artery [SMA]) and the arc of Buhler (or pancreaticoduodenal arcade connect the celiac axis [CA] and SMA).

use. Atherosclerotic disease is the most common cause of CMI, accounting for greater than 90% of all cases. Other etiologies include fibromuscular dysplasia, Takayasu arteritis, Buerger disease, radiation, neurofibromatosis, autoimmune arteritis, aortic dissection, aortic coarctation, mesenteric venous stenosis or occlusion, and drug-induced arteriopathy.[37]

Clinical Evaluation
Patient Presentation

Patients with symptomatic CMI are older, usually in their sixth or seventh decade of life, with a median age of onset of 67 years. Patients with a diagnosis of CMI are three times more likely to be female and have long-standing risk factors for atherosclerotic disease as previously described. Symptoms include postprandial pain occurring within 15 minutes and lasting up to 7 hours following meals, resulting in food fear and unintentional weight loss. Patients can experience abdominal pain of varying quality and location, postprandial nausea, vomiting, and diarrhea.[38]

Although adjustments in eating habits can attenuate symptoms, patients with significant weight loss can subsequently experience malnutrition and cachexia. Physical examination findings are often nonspecific. Therefore, a complete vascular examination including peripheral pulse examination is required due to the increased prevalence of concomitant disease in other vascular beds. Given the advanced age of onset and likelihood of medical comorbidities, the differential diagnosis for patients with CMI is broad, including but not limited to acute cholecystitis, acute gastritis, AMI, appendicitis, biliary obstruction, cholangitis, diverticulitis, pancreatitis, and intraabdominal malignancies. Baseline laboratory tests should include complete blood count, comprehensive metabolic panel (including hepatic function tests), and nutritional assessments (C-reactive protein [CRP], prealbumin, vitamin C/D, and zinc).[38]

Imaging and Diagnostics

The Society for Vascular Surgery (SVS) recommends mesenteric DUS as the preferred screening test for MAOD. A diagnosis of CMI is considered in patients with greater than 70% stenosis within the CA and/or SMA, and the presence of corresponding symptomatology. A peak systolic velocity of 200 cm/s and 275 cm/s is consistent with greater than 70% stenosis within the CA and SMA, respectively. CTA is now considered the preferred imaging modality for MAOD. CTA imaging allows for detailed anatomic evaluation of mesenteric vasculature required for preoperative planning.[39] Other imaging alternatives include contrast arteriography, previously considered the gold standard diagnostic modality, or MRA. Other adjunctive imaging modalities, including esophagogastroduodenoscopy (EGD), colonoscopy, abdominal ultrasound, and abdominal CT, can be used during multidisciplinary evaluation. All patients with abdominal pain and weight loss should undergo expedited workup for gastrointestinal and intraabdominal malignancies.[39]

Management
Indications for Revascularization

The SVS recommends treatment for patients with CMI to reverse presenting symptoms (weight loss, food fear, postprandial pain), prevent the development of AMI, and improve overall quality of life. For both symptomatic and asymptomatic patient populations, a shared decision-making approach should be prioritized when discussing revascularization as a treatment option. However, asymptomatic patients can also be considered for annual surveillance with mesenteric duplex and interval clinical evaluation.[39]

Several single-center retrospective studies have suggested that prophylactic endovascular intervention can be discussed for asymptomatic patients with greater than 50% to 70% stenosis of the SMA, and CA or IMA. Asymptomatic patients with three-vessel mesenteric disease have demonstrated increased risk of subsequent, life-threatening AMI.[40] Other indications for revascularization include patients undergoing surgery for concomitant mesenteric artery aneurysms, or open aortic reconstruction with involvement of the SMA. The primary target for revascularization is the SMA. The CA or IMA are secondary targets for revascularization and may be intervened upon to aid in symptom relief when SMA intervention is prohibitive or technically difficult.[41]

Medical Management and Preoperative Evaluation

All patients with underlying MAOD should undergo medical optimization and obtain a baseline CTA to delineate critical vascular anatomy required for revascularization. Other imaging used for preoperative risk stratifications includes echocardiogram, pulmonary function testing, and lower extremity arterial and carotid ultrasound. A wholistic review of individual factors including concomitant medical comorbidities, nutritional status, and patient anatomy should be considered before revascularization. Medical therapy for those treated with and without intervention should include antiplatelet agents, cholesterol-lowering medication, β-blockers, and tobacco cessation.[40] For symptomatic patients, total parenteral nutrition (TPN) is not considered a long-term, acceptable alternative to revascularization per SVS recommendations. The risk of complications including catheter-associated infections, bowel infarction, and liver failure are considered prohibitive for patients on long-term parenteral nutrition. However, TPN may be required perioperatively for nutritional optimization when undergoing revascularization.[42]

Endovascular Revascularization
General Endovascular Principles

The SVS recommends endovascular revascularization as the initial treatment to restore antegrade flow for patients with CMI and suitable mesenteric lesions. The SMA is considered the primary target for revascularization, whereas the CA and IMA are secondary targets. Mesenteric angioplasty and stenting have been widely adopted and largely replaced open surgical repair as first-line treatment for CMI over the past 20 years.[43] This is in large part due to lower early postoperative morbidity and mortality.[44] A recent meta-analysis including 16 retrospective studies with 1368 target vessels demonstrated high technical successful (95%) and low 30-day mortality (2%) for CMI patients treated with endovascular therapy. However, symptom recurrence and reintervention were observed in approximately 25% of patients.[45] Angioplasty with concomitant stenting is recommended given the increased risk for elastic recoil and subsequent restenosis. Literature has demonstrated that intervention of multiple mesenteric vessels can result in prolonged procedure time without significant differences in symptom relief. In the setting of two- and three-vessel disease, recanalization and revascularization of the SMA should be prioritized.[46,47] Last, if proceeding with intervention of the CA, extrinsic compression from conditions such as median arcuate ligament syndrome must be considered.

Access and Intervention

Before intervention, review of contrasted axial imaging is essential to obtaining procedural success, with both the CA and SMA often located between the level of T12 and L1. It is strongly recommended that experienced interventionalists and surgeons perform these procedures, given the high risk for complications such as AMI. Mesenteric interventions can be accomplished via brachial or femoral access with either a percutaneous or open approach. If proceeding with brachial artery access, open surgical exposure can reduce the risk of postoperative brachial sheath hematoma, nerve injury, and bleeding. Routine access with a Cook micropuncture kit (including a 21-gauge needle, 0.018 micropuncture wire, and 4-Fr micropuncture sheath) or 18-gauge needle and Bentson wire under ultrasound guidance is recommended at either the femoral or brachial artery. A diagnostic aortogram can be obtained if preoperative axial imaging is not available with 30-degree right anterior oblique (RAO), 30-degree left anterior oblique (LAO), and 90-degree lateral projections. Before sheath upsizing or cannulation of mesenteric vasculature, patients should be therapeutically heparinized (80–100 u/kg), unless there is an absolute contraindication. The goal activated clotting time (ACT) should be equal or greater than 250 seconds.

For mesenteric interventions, a 5-Fr to 7-Fr hydrophilic sheath measuring 70 to 90 cm is positioned either in the descending thoracic aorta (via brachial artery approach) or distal visceral abdominal aorta (via femoral artery approach). A 5-Fr multipurpose angiographic (MPA) catheter is most commonly used for selective catheterization from the brachial artery approach. Reversed or double-curved catheters such as the Simmons 1, SOS Omni, VS1, Cobra, and Mikelson devices are used for selective catheterization from the femoral artery approach. For technically difficult patient anatomy and in the treatment of mesenteric chronic total occlusions (CTOs), steerable introducer sheaths have been associated with high technical success and reduction in radiation dose during recanalization of the SMA.[48] A preintervention angiogram of the SMA or CA should be obtained to identify the location and characterize the quality of your target lesion. An 0.035-inch soft-angled Glidewire is used to cross the target lesion and subsequently exchanged for an 0.018-inch or 0.014-inch stiff guidewire/interventional wire. The distal end of the interventional wire should be positioned within the main trunk of the SMA to prevent perforation or dissection of smaller jejunal branches. The use of embolic protection devices (EPDs) can be considered for patients with occlusive, highly calcified, acutely thrombotic, or long (>30 mm) target lesions. A buddy wire system is required for deployment of an EPD, using both an 0.014-inch filter wire and 0.018/0.035-inch interventional wire for support and stent deployment. Even with the use of EPDs, distal embolization has been reported in 6% to 8% of patients undergoing mesenteric stenting.[49]

After crossing the selected lesion, predilation with a 3- to 5-mm low-profile plain angioplasty balloon (percutaneous transluminal angioplasty [PTA]) is used selectively before stent deployment. Balloon-expandable, covered stents have demonstrated superior patency rates compared with bare metal stents.[50–52] Stent sizing ranges from 5 to 8 mm based on preintervention angiography, although the use of intravascular ultrasound (IVUS) has also been anecdotally described in the literature.[53] Deployment of balloon-expandable, covered stents under fluoroscopic guidance is critical, with extension proximally 1 to 2 mm into the aortic lumen and distally 1 to 2 mm past the target lesion (Fig. 106.4). Postdeployment angioplasty can be used to flare the proximal portion of the stent at the mesenteric ostia and treat residual stenosis measuring greater than 50% of the arterial lumen. Postdeployment angiography should be completed to ensure patency of the CA or SMA and identify residual dissection, distal embolization, or mesenteric perforation. Suction thrombectomy devices can be used in the setting of distal embolization. However, conversion to open repair may be required if there is radiographic evidence and clinical concern for bowel ischemia or hemodynamically significant intraabdominal bleeding.

Open Surgical Revascularization
General Revascularization Principles

The role of open revascularization is reserved for younger patients, those without suitable anatomy for endovascular interventions, or patients with recurrent symptoms despite previous mesenteric angioplasty, stenting, and adjunctive therapies.[53] Revascularization strategies include antegrade mesenteric bypass from the distal

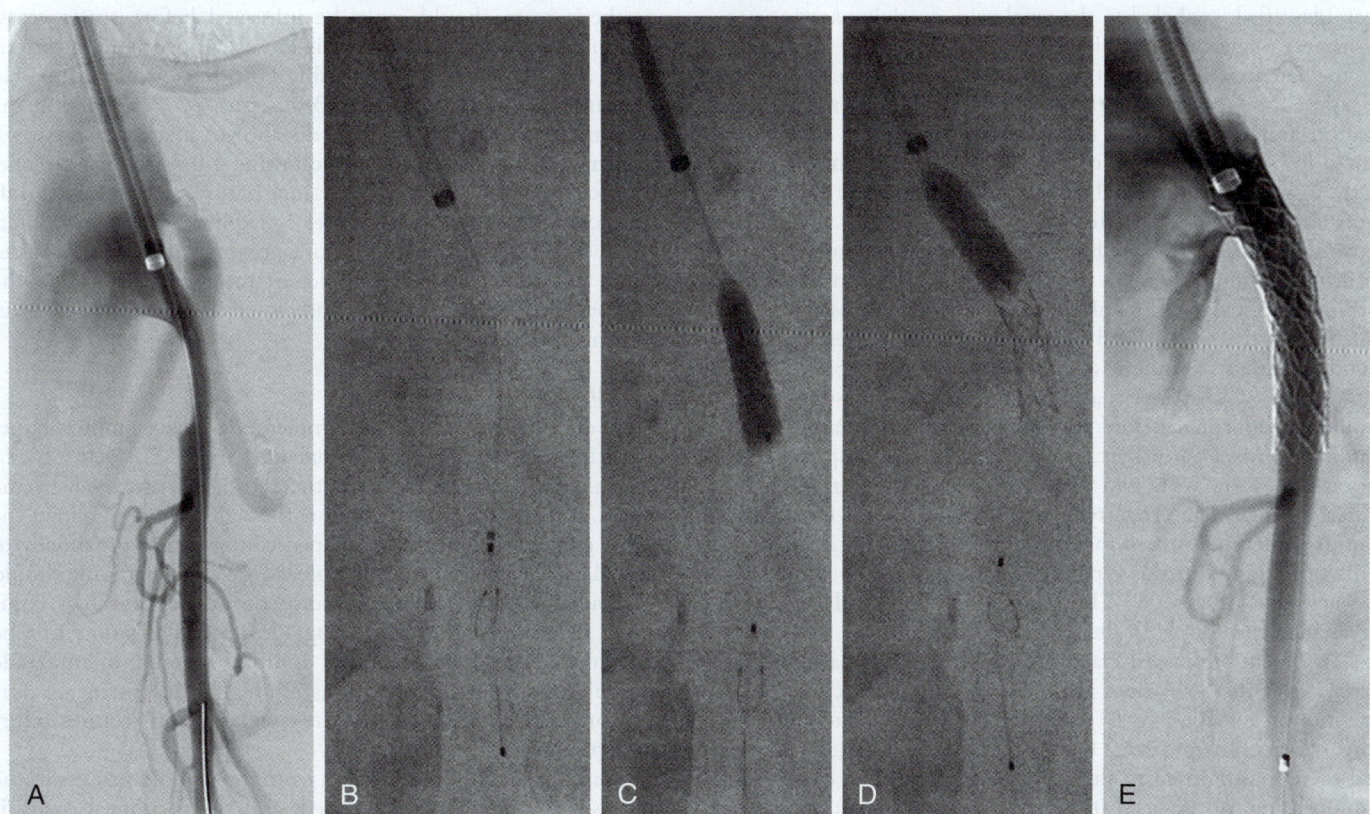

FIGURE 106.4 (A–E) Angioplasty and stenting of disease of the superior mesenteric artery (SMA) with deployment of balloon-expandable covered stent flared proximally into the aortic lumen. Completion angiography demonstrates patent stent within the SMA without dissection, residual stenosis, or distal embolization.

thoracic or supraceliac aorta, retrograde bypass from the infrarenal abdominal aorta or iliac arteries, ROMS, and transaortic mesenteric endarterectomy. In addition to routine preoperative risk stratification and medical optimization, other technical considerations include operative approach (transperitoneal vs. retroperitoneal), conduit type (prosthetic vs. vein graft), and quantity of target vessel reconstruction (single vs. multiple). A self-retaining retractor system is required for all open revascularizations and sterile preparation of bilateral lower extremities may be required if harvesting greater saphenous vein conduit.

Antegrade Mesenteric Bypass

For patients undergoing antegrade mesenteric bypass with inflow via the distal descending thoracic aorta or supraceliac abdominal aorta, a retroperitoneal or transperitoneal approach can be performed. Given the physiologic stress caused by supraceliac aortic cross-clamping, this type of revascularization is often reserved for younger patient populations. The antegrade approach has the benefit of reduced graft kinking. Additionally, the supraceliac aorta has notably less atherosclerotic disease burden.

The retroperitoneal approach to antegrade mesenteric bypass provides limited distal exposure of the SMA and CA, and should be reserved for patients with lesions at the vessel origin. The patient is flexed at a 60-degree angle in the left lateral decubitus position, with appropriate padding of both arms to prevent neural injury. A thoracoabdominal incision at the eighth rib interspace is performed. The transversalis fascia is divided and the retroperitoneal space is entered, ensuring not to violate Gerota's fascia. The left kidney is reflected down to allow for complete dissection of the SMA distal to the occlusion. Once the left renal artery has been identified, cephalad to the renal vein, overlying aortic retroperitoneal tissue can be divided in standard fashion. Proximally, the median arcuate ligament and diaphragmatic crura are divided to expose the supraceliac aorta. Small phrenic arteries may require ligation and division. Five to 10 cm of supraceliac aorta is required for safe cross-clamping. The SMA is then identified anteriorly, dissected, and isolated to the level of the middle colic artery using electrocautery, sharp dissection, and vessel loops. If possible, proximal jejunal branches should also be identified and isolated, ensuring not to injure these vessels with excessive traction. If performing revascularization of the CA, individual dissection and isolation of the splenic and common hepatic arteries is recommended. Patients are then systemically heparinized (60–80 u/kg) with a goal ACT greater than 250 seconds. The anesthesia team should be informed before aortic cross-clamping. Partial cross-clamping with a Satinsky clamp or total cross-clamping of the supraceliac aorta with two straight versus angled cross clamps (Cherry supraceliac, Fogarty hydragrip, and Wylie hypogastric clamp) is then performed for proximal control. A variety of conduits can be used in this type of revascularization, including but not limited to Dacron, PTFE, autologous vein, and CryoVein. Revascularization of both the CA and SMA requires a 12 × 6-cm or 14 × 7-cm bifurcated Dacron graft, whereas primary revascularization of the SMA does not require a bifurcated conduit. An arteriotomy is made 7 to 10 cm above the CA and extended with Potts scissors. The proximal Dacron graft is appropriately beveled and then anastomosed to the supraceliac aorta in an end-to-side fashion using 3-0 versus 4-0 Prolene. The celiac anastomosis can be performed in an end-to-end fashion with the right limb of the bifurcated graft using 4-0 versus 5-0 Prolene (an alternative approach being an end-to-side anastomosis at the common hepatic artery). The left or lateral limb of the bifurcated graft is then

anastomosed to the SMA, distal to the target lesion in an end-to-side fashion using 4-0 versus 5-0 Prolene. SMAs with extensive disease may require endarterectomy or stent removal in the setting of previous endovascular intervention. Following appropriate flushing techniques, the proximal and distal bypasses should be interrogated with Doppler or intraoperative DUS.

For patients undergoing a transperitoneal antegrade mesenteric bypass, the patient is positioned supine on the operating room table with a midline laparotomy performed in standard fashion from the xiphoid process to the pubis symphysis. A nasogastric tube (NGT) is placed to decompress the stomach and identify the esophagus intraoperatively. The peritoneal cavity is entered, and ligation of the triangular ligament is performed to mobilize the left lateral lobe of the liver. The liver is retracted, and the gastrohepatic ligament is carefully dissected, with left lateral retraction of the esophagus to prevent injury. The lesser omentum is incised, and the stomach is retracted inferiorly. The right diaphragmatic crus is divided to allow for exposure of the supraceliac aorta. Following meticulous dissection approximately 5 to 10 cm proximal to the CA, the supraceliac aorta is encircled with dampened umbilical tape. Attention is then turned to exposure of the SMA. The transverse colon is mobilized cephalad, the small bowel is eviscerated to the patient's right, and the ligament of Treitz is divided. The duodenum is medialized until a healthy portion of the SMA distal to the base of the mesentery is identified. The SMA and distal jejunal branches are carefully encircled with vessel loops. A retropancreatic tunnel can be created using blunt dissection along the anterior surface of the aorta if a distal SMA anastomosis is required. Patients are then systemically heparinized (60–80 u/kg) with a goal ACT greater than 250 seconds. The anesthesia team should again be informed before aortic cross-clamping. The supraceliac aorta is cross-clamped, and an arteriotomy is made with extension using Potts scissors. The proximal anastomosis is performed using 3-0 versus 4-0 Prolene with the surgeon's conduit of choice. The distal SMA anastomosis is then performed in an end-to-side fashion using 4-0 versus 5-0 Prolene. If performing a multivessel revascularization, a bifurcated graft and technique as described earlier is required. The bypass graft should be flushed and deaired. Both proximal and distal bypasses should be evaluated with Doppler or intraoperative DUS. The abdomen is copiously irrigated and closed in multiple layers after ensuring appropriate hemostasis.

Retrograde Mesenteric Bypass

When considering a retrograde mesenteric bypass, inflow target vessels include the distal abdominal aorta, right CIA, left CIA, or external iliac arteries (EIAs) in the setting of proximal calcific disease. The desired inflow target is the right CIA as it allows the bypass graft to lie within a C-shaped configuration proximally to the SMA (Fig. 106.5). On principle, aortic cross-clamping should be avoided when possible. A transperitoneal approach is commonly described, although retrograde revascularization can be performed via the retroperitoneal approach. Similar to antegrade revascularization, conduit options are highly dependent on surgeon preference and multivessel revascularization requires bifurcated conduits.

A midline laparotomy incision from the xiphoid process to the pubic symphysis is first performed, and the peritoneal cavity is entered in standard fashion. The infrarenal abdominal aorta is exposed by eviscerating the small bowel to the patient's right and the transverse colon cephalad. The retroperitoneum is incised to the right of midline to avoid the IMA. Retroperitoneal dissection

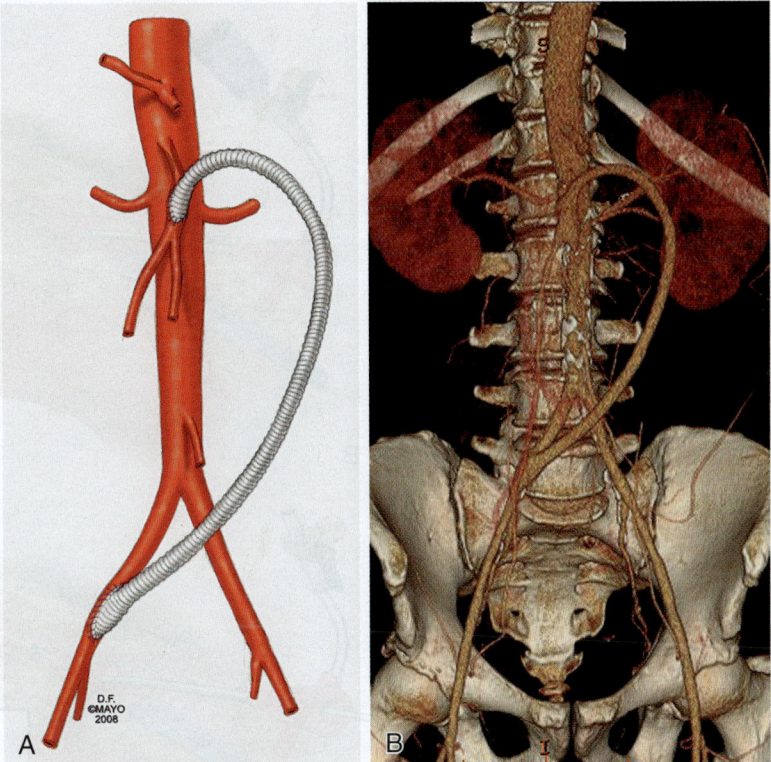

FIGURE 106.5 (A–B) Schematic representation and completion 3D CT angiography of retrograde mesenteric bypass from right common iliac artery to proximal superior mesenteric artery with C-shaped configuration to prevent graft kinking.

is carried down to the aortic bifurcation and then to the preferred iliac inflow target. The ureters are commonly retracted laterally, and careful dissection of the proximal CIA is required to avoid injury to the accompanying iliac veins. After isolating the inflow target circumferentially, attention is turned to dissection and isolation of the proximal SMA and distal jejunal branches starting at the root of the mesentery, as described earlier. After systemic heparinization with a goal ACT of greater than 250 seconds, the CIA is clamped. A longitudinal arteriotomy is performed and extended with Potts scissors. The bypass graft or venous conduit is beveled appropriately, and an end-to-side anastomosis is performed with 4-0 or 5-0 Prolene. The graft is then tunneled laterally along the left paracolic gutter, above the duodenum, and anterior or posterior to the pancreas in a C-shaped configuration. The proximal SMA anastomosis is then performed in a similar end-to-side fashion with 4-0 or 5-0 Prolene. An end-to-end configuration can be performed in the setting of a proximal mesenteric occlusion, with ligation of arterial inflow. The graft should be flushed and deaired, ensuring hemostasis at both suture lines. The small bowel and colon are returned to anatomic position, and the abdomen is copiously irrigated and closed in layers.

Retrograde Open Mesenteric Stenting

ROMS was first described in 2004 and has been widely adopted in the treatment of AMI.[54,55] It is considered a revascularization alternative for CMI patients who are not candidates for antegrade or retrograde (aortomesenteric or iliomesenteric) bypass. ROMS uses both open surgical principles and endovascular technology for mesenteric revascularization. A midline laparotomy to expose

the infracolic SMA is performed. The SMA distal to the pancreas and associated jejunal branches is dissected and isolated with vessel loops. After systemic heparinization, retrograde SMA access is established using a micropuncture set, which is then exchanged for an 0.035-inch guidewire system. A short 5- to 7-Fr sheath is placed and diagnostic mesenteric angiography is performed to identify the target lesion. The target lesion is crossed and treated with subsequent angioplasty and balloon-expandable, covered stenting as described previously (Fig. 106.6). Completion angiography is performed, and the sheath is flushed copiously before removal. The SMA arteriotomy is closed primarily or via patch angioplasty. The abdomen is then irrigated and closed in multiple layers after ensuring appropriate hemostasis.

Postoperative Complications, Surveillance, and Outcomes

Postoperative Complications

Although mesenteric angioplasty and stenting is considered minimally invasive, the risk of complications is not insignificant. Intraoperative and postoperative complications include but are not limited to access site hematoma, dissection, and median nerve injury (with brachial artery access); residual stenosis, stent dislodgement, fracture and compression; mesenteric dissection, embolization or occlusion; and branch perforation, mesenteric hematoma, and/or AMI. Patients undergoing mesenteric intervention are also at high risk for major adverse cardiac events (MACE), pulmonary complications, and gastrointestinal bleeding.[56] All patients who undergo mesenteric stenting should be treated with an antiplatelet agent and cholesterol-lowing

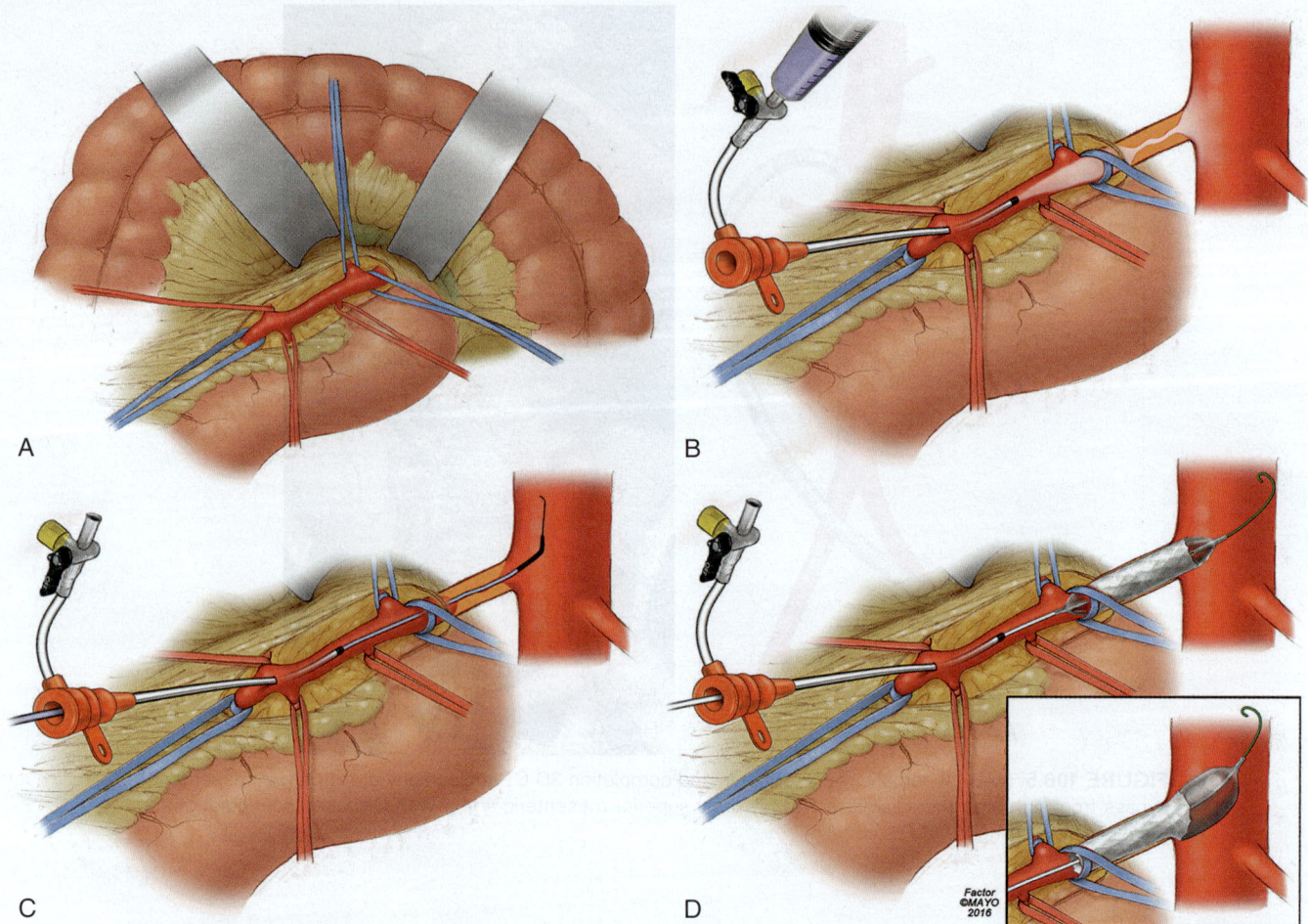

FIGURE 106.6 Technical steps for retrograde open mesenteric stenting. (A) Isolation of the infracolic superior mesenteric artery (SMA) with proximal jejunal branches. (B) Retrograde arterial access of SMA with placement of therapeutic sheath and catheter. (C) Crossing of target lesion. (D) Deployment of balloon-expandable covered stent flaring proximally into the aortic lumen. Inset: Flaring of proximal portion of covered stent into aortic ostium adds to stability.

medication postoperatively. There are currently no randomized controlled trials (RCTs) or consensus guidelines regarding single versus dual-antiplatelet therapy (DAPT) after mesenteric intervention. However, DAPT is widely used for 6 to 12 weeks after stenting with the goal of preventing in-stent thrombosis. Individual patient factors must be considered given the increased bleeding risk for patients treated with DAPT.[57]

Open mesenteric revascularization is associated with longer length of stay and higher rates of overall pulmonary, cardiovascular, gastrointestinal, and cardiac complications given the invasive nature of this type of intervention.[58-60] Prolonged ileus occurs in approximately 10% of patients and can require perioperative parenteral nutritional support. Early graft thrombosis is uncommon, associated with technical defect, poor outflow, or hypercoagulable state.[60] Similar to patients undergoing endovascular revascularization, postoperative antiplatelet therapy and cholesterol-lowing medication are recommended, although consensus regarding single versus DAPT therapy remains unresolved.

Surveillance

With regard to postoperative surveillance, the SVS recommends a close, interval follow-up schedule with repeat imaging (CTA vs. mesenteric DUS) within 1 month of the index intervention, biannually for the first 2 years, and then annually thereafter. For patients with evidence of restenosis as detected by DUS examination, CTA or catheter-based arteriograms are recommended for confirmatory testing. For patients with recurrent symptoms due to de novo lesions or recurrent stenosis, an endovascular-first approach is recommended as the initial option, with open revascularization reserved for lesions not amenable to endovascular intervention.[39]

Restenosis, Symptom Recurrence, and Mortality

Single-center retrospective data have demonstrated similarly high rates of symptom relief for both open and endovascular revascularization, ranging from 80% to over 90% at 24 to 36 months. Although open revascularization is associated with longer length of stay and higher rates of perioperative complications, endovascular therapies are associated with increased prevalence of restenosis and reintervention. Nearly one-quarter of this patient cohort required reintervention for primary- or secondary-assisted patency of mesenteric interventions. Last, with regard to long-term mortality, modern series have demonstrated no statistically significant differences in 2- to 3-year survival between open and endovascular revascularization.[61,62]

MESENTERIC VENOUS THROMBOSIS

Epidemiology

MVT is a disorder of blood coagulation that impairs venous return of the small and large intestine. Primary MVT occurs without an underlying trigger, and it is considered idiopathic and spontaneous. Secondary MVT occurs when patients carry a predisposing pathology or clinic condition, as discussed later. Although MVT is considered a rare clinical entity, it accounts for 5% to 15% of all mesenteric ischemic events and can be life-threatening in the setting of subsequent bowel infarction.[63]

Pathophysiology

Mesenteric venous drainage includes the superior mesenteric vein, which drains the ileocolic, middle colic, and right colic veins. The SMV joins the SV to form the portal vein (PV). The inferior mesenteric vein (IMV) drains the left colon and connects directly with the SV. The left gastric vein receives venous return from the distal esophagus and lesser curvature of the stomach and drains directly into the PV. MVT most commonly affects the SMV, whereas involvement of the IMV is rare (<5%–10% of cases).

Secondary MVT accounts for greater than 90% of most cases. The three categories of secondary MVT include *direct injury* (abdominal trauma, postsurgical insult, intraabdominal inflammatory states (i.e., pancreatitis and inflammatory bowel disease), *local venous congestion or stasis* (portal hypertension/liver cirrhosis, congestive heart failure, hypersplenism, obesity, and intraabdominal compartment syndrome), and *thrombophilia* (protein C/protein S deficiency, antithrombin III deficiency, active protein C resistance, JAK2 V617 gene mutation, neoplasms, oral contraceptive use, polycythemia vera, essential thrombocytosis, heparin-induced thrombocytopenia, lupus anticoagulant-antiphospholipid syndrome, cytomegalovirus [CMV] infection).[64,65]

It is estimated that specific hypercoagulable states are identified in 60% to 70% of patients with MVT and are considered a predictor of bowel ischemia.[66] The degree of bowel ischemia is dependent on the magnitude of venous thrombosis within the splanchnic circulation. Propagation of mesenteric thrombosis into major venous circulation, without adequate collateral drainage, will result in bowel congestion and edema followed by transmural intestinal infarction (Fig. 106.7). Acute MVT more commonly affects the ileum and jejunum, with relative sparing of the duodenum and colon compared with AMI.[66]

Clinical Presentation

Patients with MVT present with acute, subacute, and chronic symptomatology. Patients with acute MVT present with vague abdominal pain, out of proportion to physical examination, nausea, vomiting, and gastrointestinal bleeding in 15% to 50% of patients and hemodynamic instability in the setting of bowel ischemia/infarction.[66] Patients with subacute MVT demonstrate nonspecific symptoms for weeks to months without demonstrable physical examination findings. Chronic MVT is typically asymptomatic, often presenting with complications related to portal hypertension (ascites, variceal bleeding) and evidence of extensive collateral circulation on noninvasive imaging. Approximately 70% of patients present with acute versus subacute MVT.[67] Given these nonspecific symptoms, other causes of abdominal pain must be considered, including but not limited to peritonitis, intestinal obstruction, gastritis, peptic ulcer disease, inflammatory bowel disease, cholecystitis, appendicitis, AMI and intraabdominal malignancies.

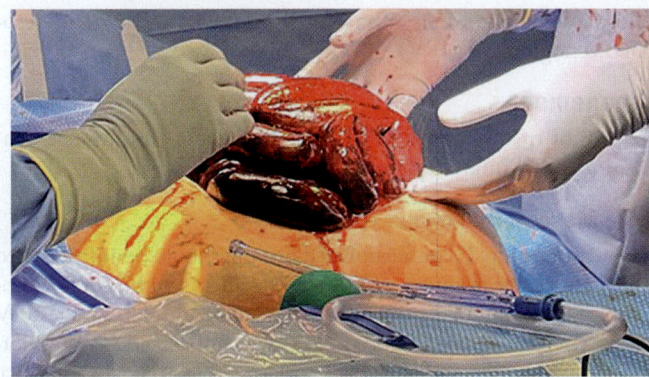

FIGURE 106.7 Bowel ischemia secondary to acute mesenteric venous thrombosis of a patient with intraabdominal trauma following motor vehicle collision. (From Acosta S, Bjorck M. Mesenteric venous thrombosis. In: Sidaway AN, Perier BA, eds. *Rutherford's Vascular Surgery and Endovascular Therapy.* 10th ed. Amsterdam: Elsevier; 2022:1779-1808.e2.)

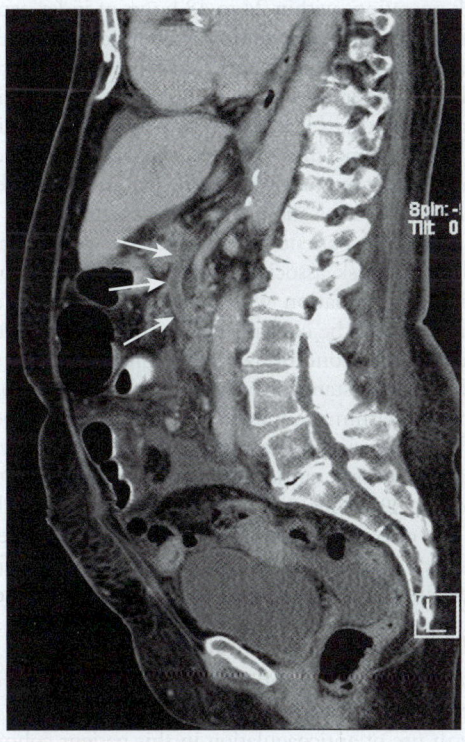

FIGURE 106.8 Sagittal view of superior mesenteric venous thrombosis on computed tomography *(arrows).*

Routine laboratory assessment includes complete blood count, comprehensive metabolic panel, blood cultures, arterial lactate, inflammatory markers (erythrocyte sedimentation rate [ESR], CRP), amylase/lipase, thrombophilia screening, coagulation profile, and age-appropriate cancer screening, in addition to upper gastrointestinal endoscopy and cholangiography (for chronic MVT). Abdominal CT with and without IV contrast, including both arterial and portal venous phases, is considered the gold standard for diagnosis of MVT. Noninvasive imaging can demonstrate portal venous thrombosis, central venous thrombosis (first 5 cm of proximal SMV), peripheral venous thrombosis, ascites, small bowel dilation, bowel wall thickening, pneumatosis, portal venous gas, and pneumoperitoneum with associated bowel perforation (Fig. 106.8). Other imaging modalities include abdominal radiography, abdominal ultrasound, and MRA/magnetic resonance venography (MRV).

Management

The goal of treatment for MVT aims to prevent thrombus extension, intestinal infarction, and recurrent thrombosis.

Acute Mesenteric Venous Thrombosis

In the acute setting, IV unfractionated heparin should be administered immediately after diagnosis of MVT. For patients with acute or subacute presentation, management includes pain control, bowel rest, IV resuscitation and normalization of electrolyte imbalances, IV antibiotics to reduce incidence of bacterial translocation, and serial abdominal examinations. Gastrointestinal bleeding is rarely a contraindication to therapeutic heparinization, although blood product resuscitation may be required in select patient populations.[66] Patients with progressive peritonitis and impending transmural infarction require exploratory laparoscopy or laparotomy to assess bowel viability. If bowel resection is required, patients may undergo primary reanastomosis or require second-look operations within 24 to 48 hours of index exploration.

For patients without peritonitis but clinical worsening of abdominal pain despite systemic anticoagulation, endovascular therapies can be considered. Percutaneous transjugular intrahepatic portosystemic shunting (TIPS) with or without mechanical aspiration thrombectomy, percutaneous transhepatic mechanical thrombectomy, and percutaneous transhepatic thrombolysis are interventional techniques that allow for direct thrombus removal.[66] However, individual patient factors must be weighed against the increased bleeding risk associated with these invasive procedures. Therapeutic anticoagulation with warfarin therapy or direct oral anticoagulants should be continued for 6 months for patients with identifiable reversible conditions, and lifelong in patients with identified prothrombotic states or MVT of unknown etiology. Recurrent thrombosis within the mesenteric circulation can occur in up to 25% of patients, most commonly in the first 30 days. Patients maintained on systemic anticoagulation have reported recurrence rates as low as 3%. Presence of bowel resection, prothrombotic states, and use of oral contraceptive therapy are associated with recurrent disease. Average 30-day mortality rates vary widely (10%–30%) depending on the acuity and severity of initial presentation.[68]

Chronic Mesenteric Venous Thrombosis

For chronic MVT anticoagulation should be considered for patients with known prothrombotic states, although data remains limited on the long-term use of anticoagulation in this patient cohort. Patients with chronic MVT often require symptomatic or interventional management of esophageal and/or gastric varices, similar to patients with cirrhosis. TIPS is recommended for patients with refractory bleeding despite endoscopic or pharmacologic therapies, or in the setting of hemodynamic instability. Five-year survival rates for patients with chronic MVT range from 78% to 82%, with prognosis impacted by the nature and severity of underlying disease pathology (cirrhosis, malignancy, thrombophilia).[66]

SELECTED REFERENCES

Acosta S. Epidemiology of mesenteric vascular disease: clinical implications. *Semin Vasc Surg.* 2010;23:4-8.

An epidemiologic study of acute mesenteric ischemia and its respective types from 1970 to 1982 in the Swedish population. Evaluated in-hospital mortality for NOMI, thrombosis, and embolic occlusions of the SMA as well as mesenteric venous thrombosis. Additionally evaluated are the estimated rates of occlusion versus embolic causes of acute mesenteric ischemia in the SMA based on autopsy reports.

Girault A, Pellenc Q, Roussel A, et al. Midterm results after covered stenting of the superior mesenteric artery. *J Vasc Surg.* 2021;74(3):902-909.e3.

Single-center study evaluating the use of covered stents in mesenteric ischemia (acute, chronic, and asymptomatic) demonstrates excellent 2-year primary-assisted potency of 95% with the caveat of increased rates of reintervention, adding to the breadth of literature around the debate between covered versus bare metal stents in treated MAOD/MAS.

Huber TS, Björck M, Chandra A, et al. Chronic mesenteric ischemia: clinical practice guidelines from the Society for Vascular Surgery. *J Vasc Surg.* 2021;73(suppl 1):87S-115S.

Consensus Guidelines from the Society of Vascular Surgery include comprehensive recommendations on diagnostic evaluation, indications and choice of treatment, preoperative evaluation, endovascular and open surgical revascularization, and postoperative surveillance and remediation.

Nana P, Koelemay MJW, Leone N, et al. A systematic review of endovascular repair outcomes in atherosclerotic chronic mesenteric ischaemia. *Eur J Vasc Endovasc Surg.* 2023;66(5):632-643.

A review of 16 retrospective studies from 1990–2022 evaluating technical success, 30-day mortality, and symptom relief demonstrates that endovascular repair for the treatment of chronic mesenteric ischemia is a safe, first-line treatment with low preoperative mortality, although with notably higher rates of symptom recurrence and reintervention compared with open revascularization.

Schermerhorn ML, Giles KA, Hamdan AD, et al. Mesenteric revascularization: management and outcomes in the United States, 1988–2006. *J Vasc Surg.* 2009;50(2):341e1-348.e1.

Nationwide Inpatient Sample using ICD-9 codes from 1988–2006 where they evaluated trends in management of acute mesenteric ischemia. They also compared in-hospital mortality and complications between surgical bypass and balloon angioplasty/stenting from the years 2000–2006.

Zettervall SL, Lo RC, Soden PA, et al. Trends in treatment and mortality for mesenteric ischemia in the United States from 2000 to 2012. *Ann Vasc Surg.* 2017;42:111-119.

This study looked at population mortality from acute mesenteric ischemia from 2000–2012 as well as trends in types of intervention in the Nationwide Inpatient Sample CDC database. Mortality rates declined during this time, and rates of endovascular intervention increased for both acute and chronic mesenteric ischemia.

The full reference list appears on Elsevier eBooks+.

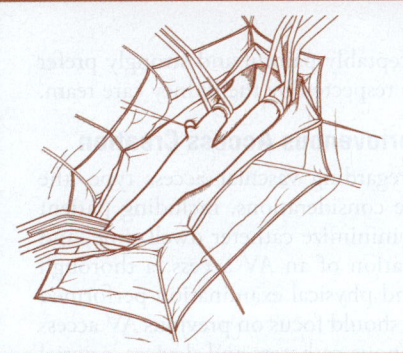

Dialysis Access

Yana Etkin and Karen Woo

BACKGROUND

End-stage kidney disease (ESKD) requiring chronic kidney replacement affects nearly 800,000 patients in the United States with 126,000 new patients initiating kidney replacement annually.[1] In the United States, the overwhelming majority (84%) of patients with ESKD use hemodialysis (HD), 13% undergo peritoneal dialysis (PD), and 3% receive a kidney transplant annually.[1] HD can be delivered in-center or at home. In-center HD is typically delivered three times a week for 3 to 4 hours per session. Home HD can be administered 3 to 7 days a week with varying session duration. Home HD offers a more flexible schedule and increased patient autonomy, with fewer dietary restrictions and more liberal fluid intake. Longer treatment sessions may also reduce symptoms of fatigue and leg cramps while on HD. However, there is an increased need for assistance at home or family support with at-home dialysis. Reliable vascular access is a crucial component of HD.

PD is typically performed in the patient's home, as continuous ambulatory PD or automated PD. Continuous ambulatory PD is done by hand with multiple exchanges per day. Automated PD is done via a machine throughout the night and allows for the daytime hours to be free.

PATIENT SELECTION FOR HEMODIALYSIS VERSUS PERITONEAL DIALYSIS

When choosing PD versus HD, the initial decision typically occurs between the nephrologist and the patient. Patient preference should be the primary factor. There are a number of

barriers for PD. Previous intraabdominal operation is the most common contraindication to PD catheter placement. Other barriers include obesity, ileostomy/colostomy, and prior transplant.[2] Additional factors that may make a patient a less ideal candidate for PD are advanced age, diabetes, heart failure, and hearing loss.[3] Measures that can ameliorate the barriers include parasternal PD catheter placement, use of low-volume dialysate, and use of vibration or light alarms for the hearing impaired.

If a patient chooses HD, the decision tree must consider whether the patient has viable options for arteriovenous (AV) access. For patients in whom viable vascular access options for HD have been exhausted, PD should be considered as an alternative. On the other hand, patients who cannot tolerate PD due to access complications, poor clearance, or inability to perform treatments on their own can be transitioned to HD.

LIFE-PLAN

The 2019 National Kidney Foundation Kidney Dialysis Outcomes Quality Initiative (KDOQI) guidelines focus on the ESKD Life-Plan.[4] This initiative calls for collaborative decision-making between the patient and their interdisciplinary kidney care team when formulating a plan for kidney replacement therapy. The Life-Plan includes determining the preferred modality of kidney replacement (HD vs. PD), setting (home vs. in-center), and access type based on the patient's medical comorbidities, anatomic limitations, and preferences. The primary principle of the Life-Plan is to create "the right access, for the right patient, at the right time, for the right reasons."[4]

HEMODIALYSIS ACCESS SELECTION

Vascular access options for HD include AV access (fistula or graft) and tunneled dialysis catheter (TDC). Patients who will receive HD should be referred to a vascular access surgeon at least 6 months before they are anticipated to start HD therapy.[4] Early referral allows adequate time for an arteriovenous fistula (AVF) to mature and possibly undergo any required maturation procedures or for a second AV access to be created if the initial access fails. The decision-making around placing a fistula or arteriovenous graft (AVG) is evolving. Historically, an AVF was considered to be superior to AVG in nearly all circumstances. However, there is increasing evidence that AVF may not have superior patency and function compared with AVG in all patients. In particular, the elderly may be more appropriate for AVG as they may have lower rates of AVF maturation.[5] Patients with limited life expectancy may not receive the long-term benefits of an AVF. A number of demographic characteristics and comorbidities may also negatively affect AVF maturation and patency, including female sex, coronary artery disease, diabetes, and obesity.[6,7] For predialysis patients for whom the Life-Plan suggests AVG, the creation should be performed as close to the start of HD as possible because AVGs have a higher risk of infection and generally lower patency than AVFs. Patients already HD dependent have more urgent need for functional long-term vascular access and AVG may be preferred in select circumstances as it is associated with earlier catheter removal and fewer catheter days than AVF. The decision regarding AVG versus AVF must be made on an individualized basis taking into account demographics, comorbidities, patient and family preferences, and the patient's Life-Plan.[4]

Tunneled Dialysis Catheter

Patients who choose to undergo HD and do not have a functioning AV access before initiation of dialysis require placement of a TDC. The catheter tip can be positioned in the superior vena cava via the internal jugular or subclavian vein or the inferior vena cava via the femoral veins. The catheter insertion should be performed under fluoroscopic guidance and vein access should be obtained with an ultrasound. Chest wall catheters are preferred because they are associated with less risk of infection compared with the lower extremity catheters. The right internal jugular vein is the preferred access because it provides a straighter path to the superior vena cava and is prone to less kinking/thrombosis. Similarly, the right femoral vein is a preferred access over the left side as the left iliac vein can sometimes be compressed by the right iliac artery. Subclavian vein catheters should be used only if bilateral internal jugular veins are occluded because catheter placement in the subclavian vein can lead to subclavian vein stenosis and subsequently compromise function of ipsilateral AV access. In the majority of patients, TDC should be considered a temporary access while a functioning AV access is being established. One advantage of TDC is that it can be used immediately after placement, but it is associated with significant longer-term complications, including infection, catheter dysfunction, and central venous stenosis, and should be reserved as a long-term access option for only a minority of patients.[4] Patients with short life expectancy (less than 9 months) may not be good candidates for AV access and chronic TDC should be considered. Patients with chronic hypotension and/or depressed cardiac output are also poor candidates for an IV access due to low patency rates. Finally, some patients find frequent cannulation and possible infiltration events to be unacceptably painful and strongly prefer TDC, a choice that should be respected by the kidney care team.

Patient Evaluation for Arteriovenous Access Creation

When counseling a patient regarding vascular access type, the surgeon is subject to multiple considerations, including patient anatomy, physiology, need to minimize catheter dwell time, and patient preference. Before creation of an AV access, a thorough history should be obtained, and physical examination performed on all patients. The evaluation should focus on previous AV access attempts, history of central venous catheters and devices, arterial inflow, superficial veins that can be used for an AVF, possible recipient outflow veins for an AVG, and central venous outflow. The nondominant arm is preferred for AV access placement. However, the dominant arm should be selected if the anatomic requirements for durable access are not present in the nondominant arm.

Arterial Inflow Evaluation and Treatment

All upper extremity pulses should be examined, and blood pressure measured in both arms. An upper extremity arterial duplex ultrasound (DUS) to assess brachial, radial, and ulnar arteries is advisable to confirm normal arterial inflow. The waveform in the intended inflow artery should be triphasic and the blood pressure should be equal in both arms. On ultrasound, the artery should have no more than a moderate degree of calcification. The brachial artery should be at least 3 mm in diameter and the radial and ulnar arteries should be at least 2 mm in diameter. An intact palmar arch and adequate ulnar inflow, as demonstrated by an Allen test, should be ensured before creating AV access using radial artery inflow. If neither arm has adequate arterial inflow at baseline, then the inflow of the nondominant arm should be treated, if possible.

Central Venous Outflow Evaluation and Treatment

A thorough history should include a detailed inventory of any central venous devices that the patient may have in place presently or in the past. Physical examination may reveal dilated chest wall veins and/or arm swelling suggestive of central venous stenosis/obstruction. If there is any suspicion of compromised venous outflow, a computed tomography venogram and/or catheter-based venogram should be performed. If neither arm has adequate venous outflow at baseline, the venous outflow of the optimal arm should be treated, if possible. The preferred treatment for central venous stenosis is endovascular balloon venoplasty. A stent may be required if significant recoil occurs. There is some evidence to suggest that the patency of stent grafts is superior to bare-metal stents.[8] In patients who have no other options for access and have a central occlusion on the ipsilateral side, open surgical options such as jugular venous turndown or bypass around the occlusion, if possible, may be considered.[9]

Vein Assessment for Arteriovenous Fistula Creation

The veins for the AVF creation need to be in a convenient location for puncture, reasonably straight, and not deeper than 6 mm under the skin. Ideally, the cephalic vein is used, due to its location and typically shallow course. If the basilic vein in the upper arm is used, transposition is required. The likelihood of functional maturity after AVF creation has been associated with increasing vein diameter. An absolute minimum vein diameter has not been established, but in general, veins greater than 2 mm in diameter may be considered for AVF creation.[10]

Evaluation of Arteriovenous Graft Recipient Vessels

A brachial or superficial vein in the antecubital fossa may be used for venous outflow of a forearm AVG if patent and of adequate diameter on DUS (Fig. 107.1D). Alternatively, the axillary vein can be used for upper arm AVG (see Fig. 107.1E–F).

ARTERIOVENOUS FISTULA CREATION

To determine the appropriate site for AVF creation, a distal-to-proximal and superficial veins first approach is recommended. Creation of initial AVF distally preserves more proximal vessels for future access sites. AVF using the cephalic vein is preferred over the basilic vein because using the cephalic vein is technically less challenging, does not require transposition, and may be easier to cannulate on HD.

Based on this approach, radiocephalic AVF should be considered first if adequate arterial inflow and venous outflow are available (see Fig. 107.1A). The forearm basilic AVF is another option for distal access and can be created using either the radial or ulnar artery. This is a particularly attractive option in younger patients with long life expectancies who may need numerous permanent vascular access sites over their lifespan.

When forearm AVF is not an option, upper arm cephalic fistula is typically considered next (see Fig. 107.1B). Using the proximal radial artery as in inflow is preferred over the brachial artery as it is associated with lower rates of access-related hand ischemia. If cephalic vein is not suitable, upper arm brachial

artery to basilic vein AVF is another option (see Fig. 107.1C). It can be created in a single-stage or two-stage manner. The basilic vein is not anatomically located in an immediate subcutaneous position needed for access and it must be transposed to a more superficial and anterolateral position. In the single-stage procedure, the entire basilic vein is dissected out, transposed to a superficial position, and anastomosed to the brachial artery. In the two-stage procedure, the basilic vein is anastomosed to the brachial artery in the first operation, and at the second operation, the fistula is superficialized. The basilic vein can be superficialized by passing it through a superficial tunnel or placing the vein in a superficial pocket by creating a skin flap that is no more than 5 mm thick. Typically, 4 to 6 weeks elapse between the first and second stages to allow for maturation of the fistula. Some studies have demonstrated superior outcomes using the two-stage approach, whereas others showed no statistically significant differences in maturation rate and postoperative complications. One meta-analysis showed that brachiobasilic AVFs created via two-stage technique achieved higher maturation rates compared with the one-stage technique.[11] Another meta-analysis demonstrated no difference in 1-year primary and secondary patency rates between the one-stage and two-stage approach, despite the veins in the two-stage group being smaller in diameter. Three of the eight studies included in the meta-analysis preferentially reserved two-stage transpositions for patients with smaller veins. There was no difference in primary failure with one-stage transpositions (15%–45%) compared with two-stage transpositions

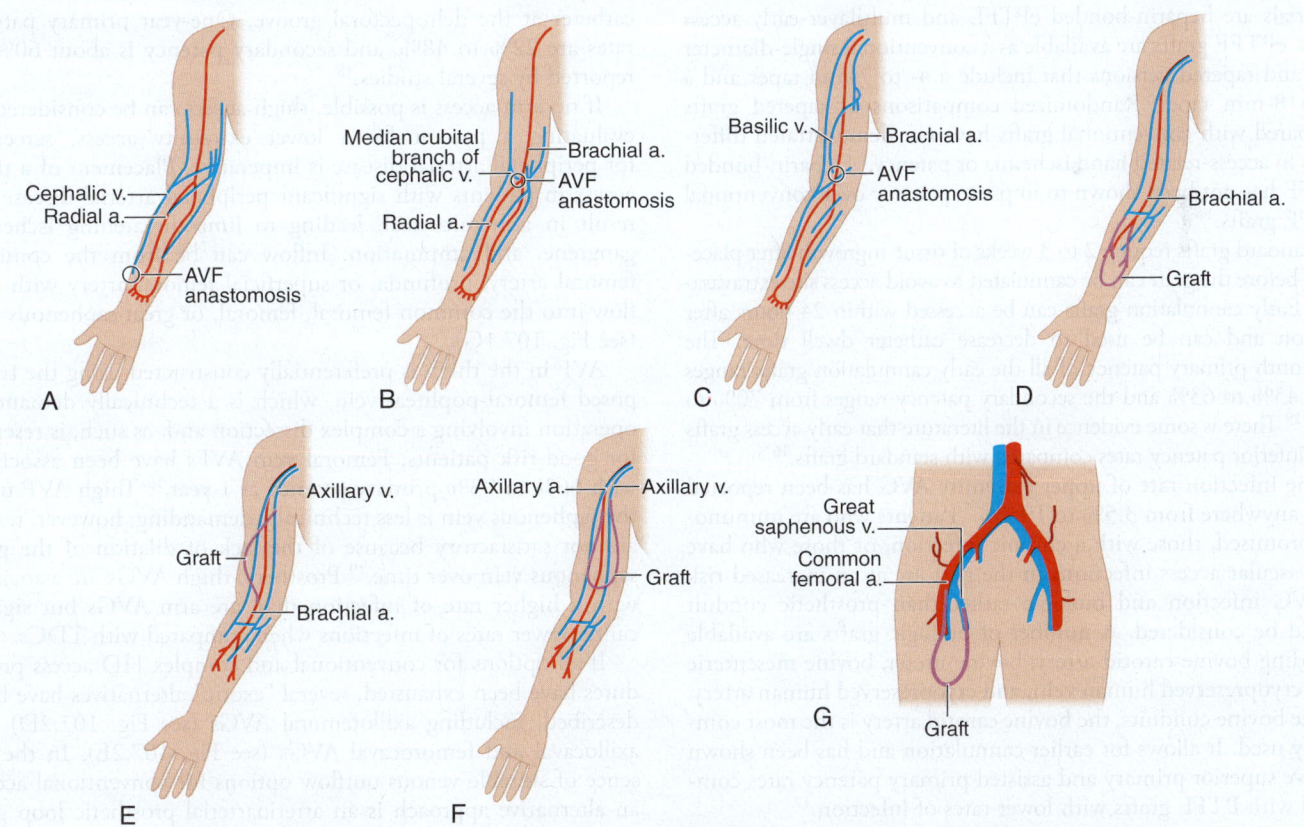

FIGURE 107.1 Arteriovenous fistulas *(AVFs)* and arteriovenous grafts *(AVGs)* configurations. (A) Radiocephalic AVF. (B) Brachiocephalic AVF. (C) Upper arm brachiobasilic AVF. (D) Forearm loop AVG (brachial artery to cephalic vein). (E) Upper arm straight AVG (brachial artery to axillary vein). (F) Upper arm loop AVG (axillary artery to axillary vein). (G) Thigh loop AVG (femoral artery to great saphenous vein. *a.,* Artery; *v.,* vein. (From Ultrasound Evaluation Before and after Hemodialysis Access. Radiology Key. [Pub date]. http://radiologykey. com/ultrasound-evaluation-before-and-after-hemodialysis-access/. [Accessed date].)

$(10\%-42\%; p = 0.46)$.[12] This suggests that for smaller basilic veins the two-stage approach may be preferred.

As of 2020, there are two percutaneous AVF creation technologies available in the United States: Ellipsys (Avenu Medical, San Juan Capistrano, CA) and WavelinQ (Bard Peripheral Vascular Inc, Tempe, AZ). Both technologies rely on a perforator vein that connects the deep and superficial venous systems in the antecubital fossa. In patients who are candidates for radiocephalic AVF, percutaneous fistula should not be a first choice because it creates an upper arm fistula and bypasses the distal first approach. The procedure is performed through one or two punctures, depending on the device, and the anastomosis is relatively distal in the antecubital fossa. As such, "side-by-side" cannulation at the antecubital fossa, with one needle in the median basilic vein and one needle in the median cephalic vein, is possible, as is two-needle cannulation in the median basilic vein. This geometry may enable patients to avoid basilic vein transposition.

Although early results are promising, secondary procedures are frequently necessary to obtain functional maturity.[13] Further studies will be required to define the role of percutaneous AVF versus surgical AVF more clearly.

ARTERIOVENOUS GRAFT CREATION

Several types of prosthetic grafts are available for AVG construction. However, none have been shown to have superior patency or lower complication rates. The most commonly used is the expanded polytetrafluoroethylene (ePTFE) graft. Other available materials are heparin-bonded ePTFE and multilayer early-access grafts. ePTFE grafts are available as a conventional single-diameter tube and tapered versions that include a 4- to 7-mm taper and a 6- to 8-mm taper. Randomized comparisons of tapered grafts compared with conventional grafts have not demonstrated differences in access-related hand ischemia or patency.[7] Heparin-bonded ePTFE has not been shown to improve patency over conventional ePTFE grafts.[14]

Standard grafts require 2 to 3 weeks of tissue ingrowth after placement before the graft can be cannulated to avoid access site extravasation. Early cannulation grafts can be accessed within 24 hours after creation and can be used to decrease catheter dwell time. The 12-month primary patency of all the early cannulation grafts ranges from 43% to 63% and the secondary patency ranges from 70% to 86%.[15] There is some evidence in the literature that early access grafts have inferior patency rates compared with standard grafts.[16]

The infection rate of upper extremity AVG has been reported to be anywhere from 3.5% to 19.7%.[7] Patients who are immunocompromised, those with a chronic infection, or those who have had vascular access infections in the past are at an increased risk of AVG infection and biologic rather than prosthetic conduit should be considered. A number of biologic grafts are available including bovine carotid artery, bovine ureter, bovine mesenteric vein, cryopreserved human vein, and cryopreserved human artery. Of the bovine conduits, the bovine carotid artery is the most commonly used. It allows for earlier cannulation and has been shown to have superior primary and assisted primary patency rates compared with PTFE grafts with lower rates of infection.[17]

CHALLENGING SITUATIONS

For patients in whom the previously mentioned access options are not possible, less commonly used options can be considered. The brachial artery to brachial vein AVF is a technically challenging

operation. The brachial vein is thin-walled and deep with numerous tributaries that require careful dissection and ligation. The median nerve runs close to the vein and must be carefully preserved. The brachial-brachial AVF can be created in one stage or in two stages, in the same manner as the brachial-basilic AVF. Although brachial-brachial AVF maturation and patency rates are inferior to brachiocephalic and brachiobasilic AVFs, brachial-brachial AVF offers an autogenous alternative for patients who do not have adequate superficial veins and may be preferable to an AVG, especially in young patients where it is important to preserve future access options.

Cervical-based AVG can be created in patients with axillary vein occlusion and patent central veins, using ipsilateral internal jugular vein or subclavian vein for outflow (Fig. 107.2A). In patients without any available options for arm access, a chest wall AVG may be considered. It requires adequate axillary artery inflow and axillary vein or internal jugular vein outflow. The graft can be performed in a looped manner between the ipsilateral axillary artery (see Fig. 107.2B) and vein or in a "necklace" configuration between the axillary artery and the contralateral axillary vein (see Fig. 107.2C).

For patients with central venous stenosis/occlusion that cannot be successfully treated but can be crossed using endovascular techniques, the HD reliable outflow (HeRO) graft (Merit Medical, South Jordan, UT) is an option for upper extremity access. The HeRO is a composite of a prosthetic graft and a catheter that is completely subcutaneous. The graft is anastomosed to arterial inflow in the arm, typically the antecubital or upper arm brachial artery, tunneled subcutaneously, and connected to the central catheter at the deltopectoral groove. One-year primary patency rates are 22% to 48%, and secondary patency is about 60%, as reported by several studies.[18]

If no arm access is possible, thigh access can be considered. In evaluating a patient for a lower extremity access, screening for peripheral arterial disease is imperative. Placement of a thigh access in patients with significant peripheral arterial disease can result in ischemic steal, leading to limb-threatening ischemia, gangrene, and amputation. Inflow can be from the common femoral artery, profunda, or superficial femoral artery with outflow into the common femoral, femoral, or great saphenous vein (see Fig. 107.1G).

AVF in the thigh is preferentially constructed using the transposed femoral-popliteal vein, which is a technically demanding operation involving a complex dissection and, as such, is reserved for good-risk patients. Femoral vein AVFs have been associated with 66% to 93% primary patency at 1 year.[19] Thigh AVF using the saphenous vein is less technically demanding; however, results are not satisfactory because of the lack of dilation of the great saphenous vein over time.[19] Prosthetic thigh AVGs are associated with a higher rate of infection than are arm AVGs but significantly lower rates of infections when compared with TDCs.

If all options for conventional and complex HD access procedures have been exhausted, several "exotic" alternatives have been described, including axillofemoral AVGs (see Fig. 107.2D) and axillocaval and femorocaval AVGs (see Fig. 107.2E). In the absence of suitable venous outflow options for conventional access, an alternative approach is an arterioarterial prosthetic loop graft (see Fig. 107.2F).

ACCESS FOR PERITONEAL DIALYSIS

A PD catheter can be placed via open, laparoscopic, or percutaneous surgical approaches. There is about a 10% to 35% catheter malfunction rate reported when using the open technique and 2.8% to 13% catheter failures for the laparoscopic insertion technique.[7] Perceived benefits of the laparoscopic approach would be better visualization during the procedure and increased patient satisfaction. The laparoscopic approach also allows for tacking the omentum up to the abdominal wall should it reach into the pelvis. Based on a recent meta-analysis comparing percutaneous versus surgical placement, significantly lower rates of exit-site infections and peritonitis were observed in the percutaneous group at 30 days without any difference in mechanical complications.[20]

POSTOPERATIVE MONITORING AND MATURATION OF ARTERIOVENOUS ACCESS

After an AV access is created, the first evaluation should occur approximately 2 weeks after the procedure to assess the incision site and to identify any potential postoperative complications including thrombosis, pain, infection, numbness, swelling, and distal ischemia. The early access graft materials can be used within 24 hours or creation and other graft materials can be accessed within 2 to 4 weeks, once the incisions have healed and perigraft edema has resolved. AVFs need follow-up to evaluate for maturation and need for potential interventions to assist maturation. The first assessment for maturity should be done 4 to 6 weeks postoperatively. A thorough physical examination is the first step, which if done properly can provide a very accurate prediction of an AVF's readiness for use and detect major causes of AVF failure. The entire tract of the AVF should be palpated and a thrill should be felt in the venous outflow portion of a mature AVF. Absence of a thrill can suggest inflow or anastomotic stenosis, whereas pulsatile outflow without a thrill indicates an outflow stenosis. The AVF can be auscultated using a stethoscope, and a continuous systolic and diastolic low-pitch bruit should be heard in a mature AVF. Both arms, chest, and face should be examined looking for any

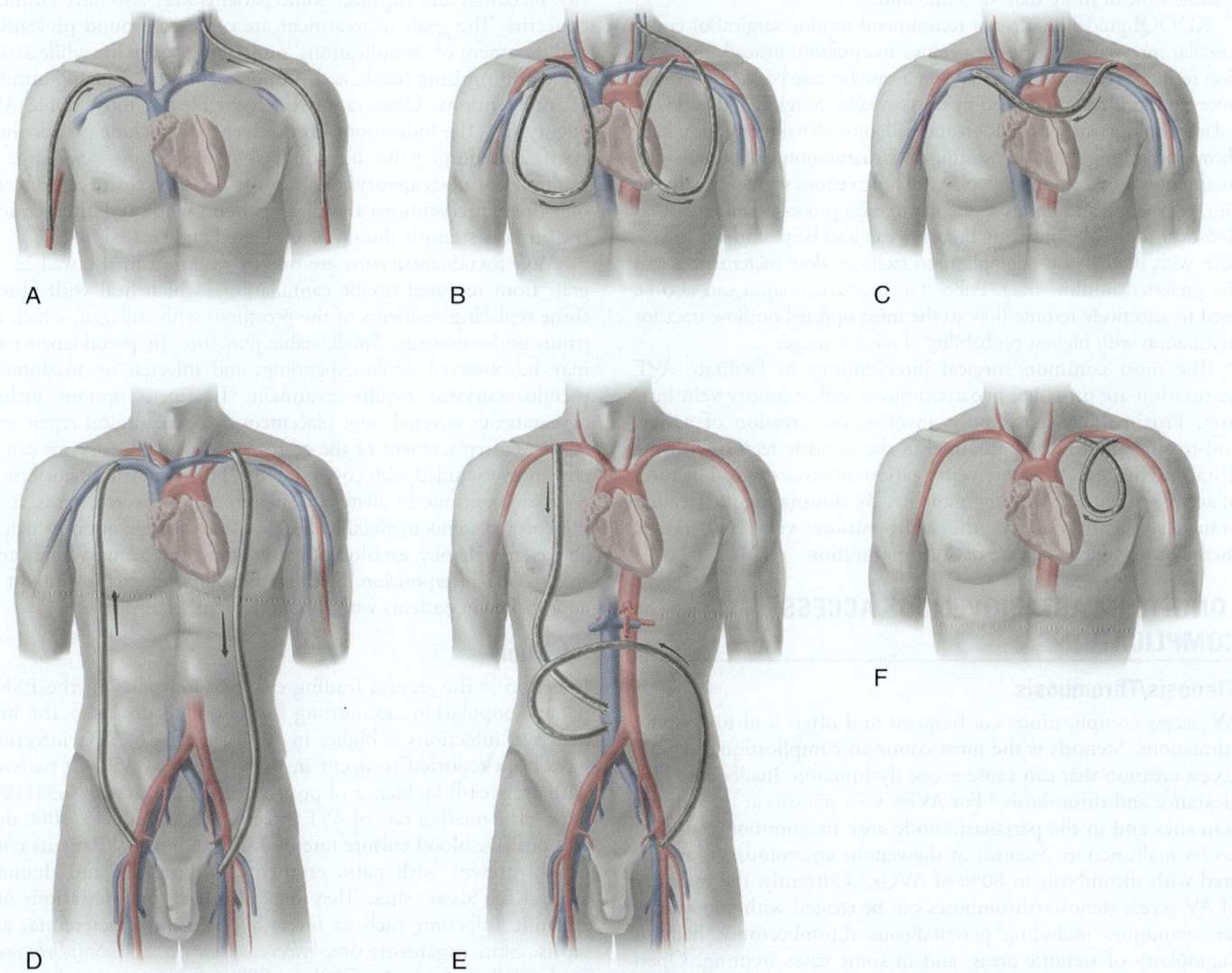

FIGURE 107.2 (A) Cervical-based arteriovenous grafts (AVGs) (brachial artery to subclavian vein or internal jugular vein). (B) Chest wall loop AVGs (axillary artery to ipsilateral axillary vein or internal jugular vein). (C) Chest wall "necklace" AVG (axillary artery to contralateral axillary vein). (D) Axillofemoral AVG (axillary artery to femoral vein or femoral artery to axillary vein). (E) Axillary artery to inferior vena cava AVG or femoral vein to inferior vena cava AVG. (F) Arterioarterial prosthetic loop graft. (From Schmidli J, Widmer MK, Basile C, et al. Editor's Choice - Vascular Access: 2018 Clinical Practice Guidelines of the European Society for Vascular Surgery [ESVS]. *Eur J Vasc Endovasc Surg.* 2018;55[6]:757-818.)

swelling in the ipsilateral or contralateral chest and arm as a sign of central venous stenosis/occlusion. The fingertips should be carefully inspected for any signs of poor perfusion such as pallor, cyanosis, or delayed capillary refill, which suggests possible HD access–induced distal ischemia (HAIDI). If physical examination is equivocal, ultrasound can be a useful adjunct in the evaluation of AVF maturation. The most important parameters assessed by DUS to predict AVF maturation include vein diameter, volume flow, depth, and presence of stenosis in the vein and/or at the anastomosis as well at the presence of competing branches. The current KDOQI guidelines suggest that a 4-week maturity assessment of a vein diameter should show at least 4 to 5 mm with a minimum volume flow of 400 to 500 mL/min, although the studies from which these recommendations are derived are largely underpowered and retrospective in nature.[4] In a recent study looking specifically at the role of DUS in AVF maturation assessment, the parameters most indicative of AVF maturation were vein diameter of 6 mm or more, absence of stenosis in the vein, absence of stealing branches, and a volume flow of more than 675 mL/min.[21]

KDOQI guidelines do not recommend routine surgical or endovascular intervention for postoperative maturation; instead, the decision to intervene should be made on a case-by-case basis.[4] In general, intervention is recommended by 6 to 8 weeks. Surgical and endovascular techniques such as revision and balloon-assisted maturation have shown promising results in assisting AVF maturation. Balloon-assisted maturation uses balloon angioplasty of long venous segments with the aim to expedite and optimize the maturation process. Coil embolization or ligation of competing branches can also be performed in tandem with the balloon angioplasty to facilitate flow increment across the preferred outflow tract. Balloon-assisted maturation can also be used to selectively reroute flow to the most optimal outflow tract for maturation with highest probability of reliable usage.

The most common surgical interventions to facilitate AVF maturation are proximal neoanastomosis and accessory vein ligation. Proximal neoanastomosis involves the creation of a new end-to-side anastomosis proximal to the stenotic region with the distal end ligated. Accessory vein ligation involves surgical ligation of accessory veins or stealing branches. By eliminating the stealing branches, the flow across the main outflow vein is increased thereby improving the rate of AVF maturation.

LONG-TERM ARTERIOVENOUS ACCESS COMPLICATIONS

Stenosis/Thrombosis

AV access complications are frequent and often lead to hospital admissions. Stenosis is the most common complication after AV access creation that can cause access dysfunction, inadequate HD clearance and thrombosis.[4] For AVFs, vein stenosis at the canulation sites and in the perianastomotic area are common causes of access malfunction. Stenosis at the venous anastomosis is associated with thrombosis in 80% of AVGs.[4] Currently, the majority of AV access stenoses/thromboses can be treated with endovascular techniques including percutaneous thrombectomy, balloon angioplasty of stenotic areas, and in some cases stenting. Open thrombectomy and/or access revision are reserved for patients in whom percutaneous techniques were not successful.

Venous Hypertension

Swelling of the entire extremity after AV access screation is indicative of central venous stenosis or occlusion, which is frequently related to previous central venous catheters or devices. In general, swelling in the ipsilateral arm alone suggests a subclavian vein stenosis; swelling involving both ipsilateral arm and face suggests an innominate vein stenosis; and swelling in both arms and face indicates a possible superior vena cava stenosis. The presence of prominent veins across the chest is another sign of central venous stenosis. The treatment options include conservative management with arm elevation and compression, percutaneous angioplasty and stenting, and central venous reconstruction with a bypass of occluded vein or jugular turndown procedure. If a patient is not a good candidate for these interventions or repeated interventions have failed, AV access ligation should be considered.

Aneurysms/Pseudoaneurysms

Aneurysms of AV conduits is another common complication. Most AVF aneurysms are true aneurysms, whereas all the AVG aneurysms are pseudoaneurysms. These aneurysms can lead to functional impairment and access thrombosis, loss of skin integrity, bleeding, and rupture. Some patients may also have cosmetic concerns. The goals of treatment are centered around prevention and treatment of complications, prolonging access life while avoiding compromising future access options, and minimizing number of interventions. Observation is acceptable for most stable AVF aneurysms. The indications for interventions include pseudoaneurysms, bleeding, pain, infection, skin ulcerations, and large or multiple tortuous aneurysms. In some patients, cosmetic concerns may drive interventions as well. In patients who need interventions the outflow stenosis should be evaluated and treated first.

AVG pseudoaneurysms are due to weakness in the wall of the graft from repeated needle cannulations, which heal with fibrous tissue replacing segments of the prosthesis with collagen, which expands under pressure. Small, stable puncture site pseudoaneurysms may be observed while expanding, and infected or anastomotic pseudoaneurysms require treatment. Treatment options include percutaneous covered stent placement or open surgical repair with segmental replacement of the graft. AVG pseudoaneurysms can be effectively excluded with covered stents. However, true aneurysms of AVF can continue to dilate after placement of covered stents, making covered stents ineffective. Surgical AVF salvage options include aneurysmorrhaphy, excision of redundancy, and primary anastomosis or AVG interposition. Selective ligation and excision might be appropriate in patients with functional renal transplant.

Infection

Infection is the second leading cause of mortality in the ESKD patient population, accounting for 8% of all deaths.[22] The incidence of infections is higher in AVG than AVF. AVG infections have been reported to occur in up to 1.6% to 35% of patients, with an overall incidence of positive blood cultures of 0.31/1000 days.[4] The median rate of AVF infections is about 0.11/1000 days and positive blood culture rate of 0.08/1000 days.[4] Patients commonly present with pain, erythema, induration, and drainage around the access sites. They may also have manifestations of a systemic infection such as fever, hypotension, bacteremia, and sepsis. Skin organisms *Staphylococcus aureus* and *Staphylococcus epidermidis* account for 70% to 90% of AV access infections.[4] Management includes broad-spectrum antibiotics and source control. Blood cultures should be obtained before the initiation of antibiotic therapy. Preservation of AV access might be possible if infection only involves the overlying skin and does not extend down to the access. In the majority of cases, access infections are treated surgically, which includes partial or complete access excision or attempted access salvage with in situ or extraanatomic reconstruction. The choice of the operation depends on the extent of the infection, the offending organism, the type of access, the location of the infection, the presence of systemic signs, the presence of bleeding, and, importantly, future dialysis access options.

Hemodialysis Access–Induced Distal Ischemia

The incidence of hand ischemia in patients with HD access ranges from under 1% in forearm fistulas to as high as 8% in antecubital based fistulas.[23] The onset of ischemia after AVG placement commonly occurs in the acute phase (within 30 days postoperatively) or subacute phase within a year of access placement. Ischemia after AVF placement is more likely to occur after the access has been used for several years. Society for Vascular Surgery guidelines classify HAIDI into four grades, ranging from no symptoms in grade 0 ischemia to ischemic rest pain and tissue loss in grade 3 ischemia. Several risk factors have been identified including advanced age, female sex, diabetes, peripheral vascular disease, large outflow conduits, multiple prior access procedures, prior episode of steal, and using brachial artery as an inflow.[4]

There are a number of strategies to prevent arterial steal that should be considered during HD access planning and creation. Preoperative testing to identify and potentially treat proximal arterial lesions should be done. When creating antecubital-based fistulas, ligation of the deep perforating branch is recommended to perform selective venous arterialization of either the cephalic or basilic vein instead of arterializing both. It is beneficial to minimize the use of brachial artery as inflow and create radiocephalic fistula in the distal forearm when feasible or use proximal radial artery for inflow when creating upper arm fistulas. The deep perforating branch can be used for anastomosis in this location or should be ligated. Currently, there is not enough evidence to support the use of taped grafts to reduce the incidence of hand ischemia.

The workup of HAIDI should include photoplethysmography with and without fistula compression as well as fistula DUS to measure volume flow and evaluate for the presence of flow reversal in the artery distal to the anastomosis. The management of HAIDI depends on the amount of flow in the fistula. High-flow fistulas (>1 L of flow) can be treated with banding or revision using distal inflow, whereas low/normal flow access can be treated with distal revascularization interval ligation (DRIL) or proximalization of arterial inflow (PAI). Radial artery ligation distal to the AV anastomosis can be considered for any radiocephalic fistulas irrespective of flow as long as the palmar arch is intact. In cases of severe ischemia, especially if digital gangrene is present, ligation of HD access should be strongly considered.

Banding is the least invasive procedure and should be considered first for high-flow access. There are several banding techniques described in the literature with various adjunctive techniques that allow for measurements of digital perfusion during the procedure.[24]

Although banding is the least invasive technique, it is associated with the highest rate of failure to manage HAIDI (33%) and well as the highest rate of access thrombosis (11%).[25] Revision using distal inflow is performed by ligating the fistula just distal to the anastomosis and reestablishing inflow from more distal on the arm, preferably the ulnar or radial artery. DRIL reliably restores antegrade flow, eliminates a potential physiologic pathway for ischemia, and maintains continuous dialysis access, which is especially important in patients with difficult access. However, it requires ligation of antegrade native arterial flow to the hand. Although DRIL might be the most effective procedure, there is a

reluctance to ligate normal arteries supplying the distal arm, which led to the development of alternative treatment options including PAI. This technique does not sacrifice natural arterial continuity. Proximal arterial anastomosis increases flow to the forearm by increasing pressure at the split point between the distal circulation and the dialysis access. It also initiates collateral flow at a higher point in the arm, which is advantageous to prevent or treat ischemic symptoms in the hand. A study that evaluated the effects of six HD access modifications on forearm flow showed that PAI approached DRIL in degree of improvement of forearm flow and appeared to be as effective without sacrificing natural arterial continuity.[26]

Ischemic Monomelic Neuropathy

Ischemic monomelic neuropathy is uncommon and a potentially devastating complication of brachial-based AV access procedures. Diabetes and female sex are the primary risk factors. The onset of symptoms is usually within hours after the access creation and can lead to irreversible dysfunction of radial, median, and ulnar nerves producing claw hand deformity. The presentation can be similar to HAIDI except for the presence of palpable pulses distal to the access and absence of severe tissue ischemia in the affected extremity. Early diagnosis and intervention with access ligation is the only treatment that can potentially reverse the dysfunction. Recovery is unpredictable and even with appropriate management strategies and early intervention, patients may be left with a significant deficit.

Tunneled Dialysis Catheter Complications

TDC complications include catheter dysfunction, infection, migration, and central venous thrombosis. TDC dysfunction often leads to inadequate dialysis, which can be associated with increased morbidity and mortality. The incidence of TDC dysfunction is reported to be as high as 7% of HD sessions.[4] TDC dysfunction often requires medical, endovascular, or surgical intervention and is performed in 20% to 40% of patients dialyzing via a TDC.[4] The initial management of TDC dysfunction involves bedside maneuvers such as positioning the patient in Trendelenburg position or the use of rapid saline flushes to dislodge a possible thrombus. If these initial maneuvers are unsuccessful, administration of a thrombolytic agent into each port can be tried next. If TDC dysfunction persists, catheter exchange or removal followed by replacement at a different site should be considered.

Patients dialyzing with a TDC are at increased risk of catheter-related infections and have increased morbidity, mortality, and healthcare costs. The incidence of the catheter-related infections are 1.1 to 5.5 episodes per 1000 catheter days.[4] TDC-related infections include exit-site infections, infections of the tunnel track, and bacteremia. Bacteremia is the most significant complication because it has the potential for hematogenous spread of the infection resulting in endocarditis, osteomyelitis, septic arthritis, epidural abscess, and life-threatening sepsis.[27] The common clinical features of TDC infection include fever or chills, hemodynamic instability, hypothermia, nausea and vomiting, and generalized malaise. If drainage is present from the exit site, cultures should be obtained before initiation of antibiotics. If there are signs or symptoms of systemic infection, peripheral blood cultures and cultures from the catheter should also be obtained. Broad-spectrum empiric antibiotic should be administered and modified based on the final cultures. Depending on the severity of symptoms, TDC can be removed and exchanged over a guidewire at the same site or a new TDC can be placed at a new site.

Peritoneal Dialysis Catheter Complications

PD catheter complications can be characterized into early postoperative complications and mechanical and infectious complications. The most serious perioperative complications are bowel or bladder perforation as well as hemorrhage. Visceral injury typically occurs during entry into the abdominal cavity or during advancement of the catheter into the pelvis. If bowel perforation is considered, it is crucial to recognize and confirm the diagnosis immediately. This can be done via visualization of bowel lumen, return of bowel contents from the dialysate effluent, or emanation of foul-smelling gas.[28] A through-and-through bowel perforation may temporarily mask some of these manifestations. If undetected, manifestations postoperatively include severe watery diarrhea, abdominal pain with hypotension, rigid abdomen, and peritonitis. Most microperforations can be managed by keeping the patient on nothing by mouth restrictions, giving prophylactic antibiotics, and close observation.

Bladder perforation can present with an increase in urine volume, hematuria, or bladder distention immediately after instillation of dialysis fluid. Importantly, this complication can go unnoticed as some of the holes of the PD catheter may remain outside the bladder; therefore, other diagnostic tools can be used to confirm the diagnosis including postoperative cystoscopy, cystogram, and other imaging.[28] Emptying the bladder and inserting a Foley catheter before PD catheter insertion are important preventive steps.

Hemorrhage of the inferior epigastric vessels may require ligation if noted intraoperatively or angiographic embolization if discovered postoperatively. On the other hand, intraabdominal trauma may result in mild bleeding that manifests as blood-stained effluent and is usually self-limiting. Bleeding at the exit site may also occur and is usually controlled with manual pressure, suture placement, injection with epinephrine, and frequent dressing changes.

Mechanical complications that occur after PD catheter placement are characterized as flow dysfunction or pericatheter leakage. Flow dysfunction can be due to extrinsic compression of the catheter tip, internal luminal obstruction, poor positioning and/or migration, and tissue attachment and entrapment.[28] Flow dysfunction mainly manifests as drain pain that is encountered upon draining the dialysate. This pain typically results from incomplete evacuation of dialysate fluid and typically occurs when the PD catheter is placed too deep in the pelvis. In most cases, catheter replacement is required. Peritoneal leakage complications can also occur with a reported frequency as high as 12.8%.[28] These leakages can broadly be categorized into pericatheter leaks, abdominal wall hernias, and pleuroperitoneal connection or fistula development. These complications can occur early or late after catheter placement.

Catheter-related infections are the most common reason for switching from PD to HD.[28] Infectious complications can be classified into exit-site infections, superficial cuff extrusion, tunnel infections, and peritonitis. Management of exit-site infections include obtaining culture and Gram stain of the drainage fluid and starting empiric antibiotics. For superficial cuff infection, catheter exchange can be avoided by removing the external cuff from the tubing and allowing the exit site to heal. Most tunnel infections are treated by removing the old catheter and inserting a new one using a different site. Once peritonitis is suspected, peritoneal fluid cultures are obtained and antibiotic therapy is initiated. The decision to change the catheter is dependent on the response to antibiotic therapy. The infected PD catheter can be exchanged over a wire if the patient is responding to the antibiotics. The lack of improvement after 5 days of antibiotic therapy necessitates catheter removal.[28]

SELECTED REFERENCES

Al Shakarchi J, Inston N. Early cannulation grafts for haemodialysis: an updated systematic review. *J Vasc Access.* 2019;20:123-127.

> *A systematic review of randomized trials and observational studies for early cannulation arteriovenous grafts yielded 19 studies that met inclusion criteria between 2007 and 2017. Four types of commercially available grafts were included in the studies. All grafts were found to be safely cannulated within 72 hours of graft placement. The pooled patency rate at 12 months ranged from 43.3% to 63.7% for primary patency and 70.5% to 85.8% for secondary patency. Statistical comparison of the grafts was not performed due to the heterogeneity of the population and the relative low sample size for each graft type.*

Eroglu E, Heimbürger O, Lindholm B. Peritoneal dialysis patient selection from a comorbidity perspective. *Semin Dial.* 2022;35:25-39.

> *This review discusses conditions that may be considered relative contraindications to peritoneal dialysis (PD) and suggests appropriate actions to overcome potential issues related to these conditions. In general, there are few conditions/comorbidities that are an absolute contraindication to PD. The review outlines evidence that PD can be conducted successfully in elderly patients, those with diabetes mellitus, obesity, polycystic kidney disease, and history of abdominal surgery. PD may be suitable also in patients with liver cirrhosis, renal allograft failure, and acute dialysis requirement and those with congestive heart failure. The review of fundamental changes in healthcare policies include economic incentives, changes in the organization of healthcare with infrastructural changes, support to providers and healthcare professionals working with PD, and educational efforts to improve awareness of the potentials of PD among patients and healthcare workers and to improve their skills and experience in PD.*

Habib SG, Jano A, Ali AA, Phillips A, Pinter J, Yuo TH. Early clinical experience and comparison between percutaneous and surgical arteriovenous fistula. *J Vasc Surg.* 2023;78(3):766-773.

> *A retrospective comparison was performed of 51 patients with percutaneous arteriovenous fistula (pAVF) and 51 randomly selected contemporaneous patients with surgical arteriovenous fistula (sAVF). Overall, the rate of maturation was similar between pAVF (72%) and 29 sAVF (57%) (p = 0.11). When all maturation interventions were combined, pAVF and sAVF had a similar incidence of maturation interventions (75% vs. 53%; p = 0.69). When planned second-stage transposition procedures were excluded, pAVF had a higher incidence of maturation procedures (74% vs. 24%, p < 0.001).*

Kakkos SK, Lampropoulos GC, Nikolakopoulos KM, et al. A systematic review and meta-analysis of randomized trials comparing two-stage with one-stage brachio-basilic vein fistulas. *Vasc Specialist Int.* 2018;34(3):51-60.

Three randomized controlled trials comprising 126 patients (47 two-stage and 79 one-stage) were included in this systematic review and meta-analysis of brachiobasilic vein fistula (BBVF). Two-stage BBVF had a lower incidence of maturation failure compared with one-stage BBVF (6.4% vs. 20.3%, P = 0.02). There was no significant difference in functional secondary patency.

Lok CE, Huber TS, Lee T, et al. KDOQI Clinical Practice Guideline for Vascular Access: 2019 Update. *Am J Kidney Dis.* 2020;75:S1-S164.

The National Kidney Foundation's Kidney Disease Outcomes Quality Initiative (KDOQI) Clinical Practice Guideline for Vascular Access has been a comprehensive, evidence-based document for the management of hemodialysis vascular access since 1996. The 2019 update includes new topics, with the end-stage kidney disease "Life Plan" and related concepts as a central tenet of the guidelines. Other topics covered are vascular access choice, new targets for arteriovenous access (fistulas and grafts) and central venous catheters, and management of specific complications.

The full reference list appears on Elsevier eBooks+.

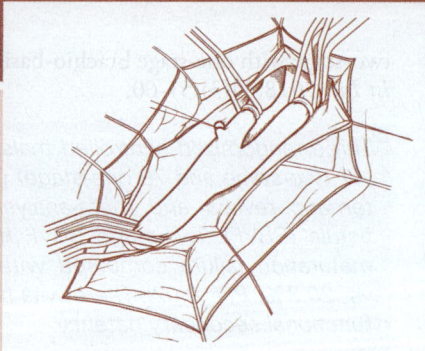

Venous Disease

Christine L. Shokrzadeh, Alexis N. Davis, and Ruth L. Bush

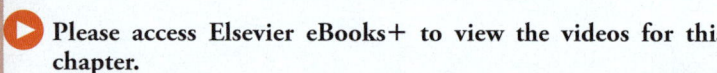

▶ **Please access Elsevier eBooks+ to view the videos for this chapter.**

This chapter provides the reader with a thorough overview of the physiology and pathophysiology of the venous system. Pathognomonic features of superficial and deep venous disorders are described, with discussion of appropriate diagnostic modalities and therapeutic interventions.

ANATOMY

To determine whether a pathophysiologic process is present, knowledge of venous anatomy is essential. Venous drainage of the legs is the function of two parallel systems, the superficial and deep venous systems, in anatomic continuity through connecting veins called *perforating veins*. The nomenclature of the venous system of the lower limb was revised in 2002, and the most relevant changes are addressed here.[1] The revised nomenclature is delineated in Tables 108.1 and 108.2.

Superficial Venous System

The superficial veins of the lower extremity form a network that connects the superficial dorsal veins of the foot and deep plantar veins. The dorsal venous arch, into which empty the dorsal metatarsal veins, is continuous with the great saphenous vein (GSV) medially and the small saphenous vein (SSV) laterally (Fig. 108.1).

The GSV arises from dorsal veins of the foot. The GSV extends cephalad and travels over the medial aspect of the tibia and in parallel to the saphenous nerve. As the GSV ascends through the

thigh, multiple accessory branches are demonstrated, and variability in the number and location of these branches is the norm. The GSV travels within its own fascia, called the *saphenous sheath* (Fig. 108.2). This structure is superior to the deep fascia of the leg. Although a classic feature, the GSV can be contained completely within the saphenous sheath or exit the fascia and reenter at another point in its course along the extremity. In some cases, patients exhibit an incomplete saphenous sheath, which makes identification of the GSV difficult. The GSV terminates into the saphenofemoral junction (SFJ), where it is joined by the confluence of the superficial circumflex iliac veins, the external pudendal veins, and the superficial epigastric veins. It then ascends in the superficial compartment and empties into the common femoral vein after entering the fossa ovalis (see Fig. 108.2). The SFJ is a complex anatomic entity composed of one or several external pudendal veins, the superficial epigastric vein, the superficial circumflex vein, and one or several accessory saphenous veins, whose course in the leg can be anterior and posterior to the GSV. At the SFJ and a few millimeters distal in the thigh, the terminal valve and the preterminal are located.

The SSV arises from the dorsal venous arch at the lateral aspect of the foot and ascends posterior to the lateral malleolus, rising cephalad in the midposterior calf. The SSV continues to ascend, penetrates the superficial fascia of the calf, and then terminates into the popliteal vein. However, this anatomy is extremely variable. Most commonly, the SSV terminates within a lateral branch of the thigh, bypassing the classic saphenopopliteal junction. The sural nerve lies parallel to the SSV. This relationship becomes

TABLE 108.1	Deep Vein Thrombosis (DVT): Acute Versus Chronic	
	ACUTE DVT	**CHRONIC DVT**
Length of time symptoms present	<4 weeks	>4 weeks
Ultrasound findings	Noncompressibility of the vein; hypoechoic thrombus within lumen, venous distention, and complete absence of spectral or color Doppler signal within the vein lumen; no collaterals	Partial to full compressibility, echogenic thrombus, collaterals, Doppler flow present
Anticoagulation	Anticoagulation recommended for treatment	No anticoagulation indicated

TABLE 108.2	Deep Venous Nomenclature
Deep veins of the thigh	Common femoral vein
	Superficial femoral vein
	Profunda femoris vein or deep femoral vein
	Medial circumflex femoral vein
	Lateral circumflex femoral vein
	Deep femoral communicating veins
Deep veins of the knee and lower leg	Popliteal vein
	Sural veins
	Soleal veins
	Gastrocnemius veins (medial and lateral)
	Anterior tibial veins
	Posterior tibial veins
	Fibular or peroneal veins

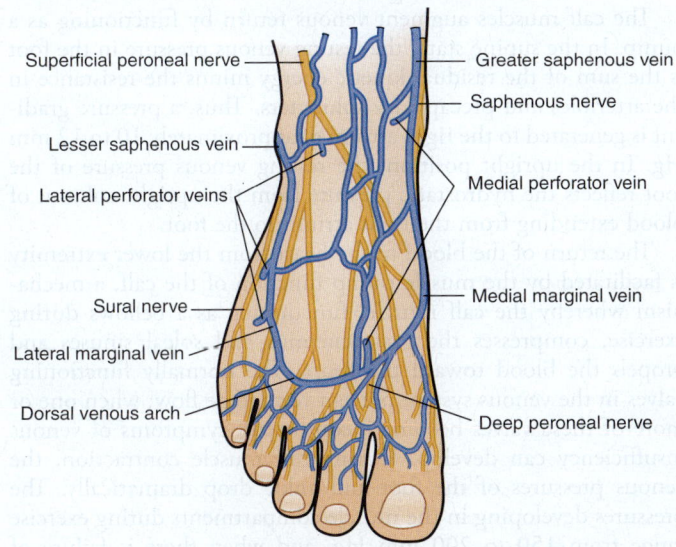

FIGURE 108.1 Venous drainage of the foot.

more intimate at the distal calf. A common vein branch that is the thigh extension of the SSV, also known as the *vein of Giacomini,* connects the SSV with the GSV.

Deep Venous System

The plantar digital veins in the foot empty into a network of metatarsal veins that compose the deep plantar venous arch. This continues into the medial and lateral plantar veins, which then drain into the posterior tibial veins. The dorsalis pedis veins on the dorsum of the foot form the paired anterior tibial veins at the ankle.

The paired posterior tibial veins, adjacent to and flanking the posterior tibial artery, run under the fascia of the deep posterior compartment. These veins enter the soleus and join the popliteal vein after joining with the paired peroneal and anterior tibial veins. There are large venous sinuses within the soleus muscle—soleal sinuses—that empty into the posterior tibial and peroneal veins. Bilateral gastrocnemius veins empty into the popliteal vein distal to the point of entry of the SSV into the popliteal vein.

The popliteal vein enters a window in the adductor magnus, at which point it is termed the *femoral vein,* previously known as the *superficial femoral vein.* The femoral vein ascends and receives venous drainage from the profunda femoris vein, or deep femoral vein, and after this confluence, it is the common femoral vein. As the common femoral vein crosses the inguinal ligament, it becomes the external iliac vein.

Perforator Veins

Perforating veins connect the superficial venous system to the deep venous system by penetrating the fascial layers of the lower extremity. These perforators run in a perpendicular fashion to the axial veins previously described. Although the total number of perforator veins is variable, up to 100 have been documented. The perforators enter at various points in the leg—the foot, medial and lateral calf, and mid- and distal thigh (Fig. 108.3). Some have been named by the surgeons who first identified them: Crockett perforators, which connect the posterior arch and posterior tibial veins; Boyd perforators, which connect the great saphenous and gastrocnemius veins; and Hunterian and Dodd perforators, which connect the great saphenous and superficial femoral veins, although these names are rarely used in patient care. The perforator veins have an important function. Their valve system aids in preventing reflux from the deep to the superficial system, particularly during periods of standing and ambulation. Perforating veins are currently identified by measuring their distance from the heel.

Normal Venous Histology and Function

The venous wall is composed of three layers, the intima, media, and adventitia. Vein walls have less smooth muscle and elastin than their arterial counterparts. The venous intima has an endothelial cell layer resting on a basement membrane. The intima enfolds, forming bicuspid valves whose function is to ensure venous return to the heart. The media is composed of smooth muscle cells and elastin connective tissue. The adventitia of the venous wall contains adrenergic fibers, particularly in the cutaneous veins. Central sympathetic discharge and brainstem thermoregulatory centers can alter venous tone, as can other stimuli, such as temperature changes, pain, emotional stimuli, and volume changes.

The histologic features of veins vary, depending on the caliber of the veins. The venules, the smallest veins, range from 0.1 to 1 mm and contain mostly smooth muscle cells, whereas the larger extremity veins contain relatively few smooth muscle cells. These

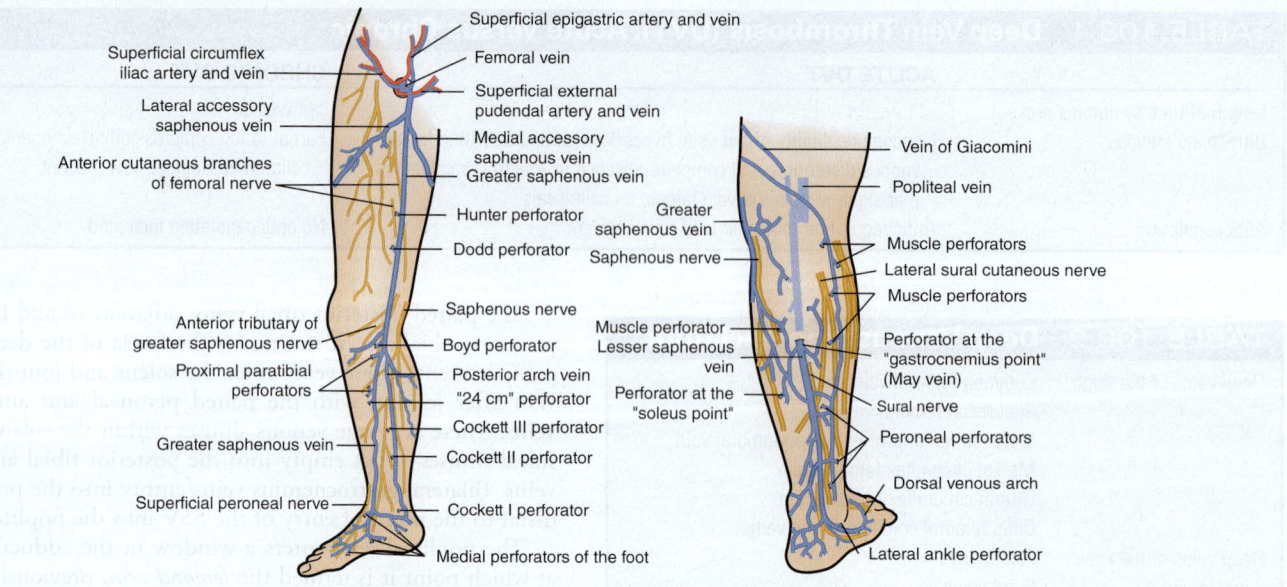

FIGURE 108.2 Venous drainage of the lower limb.

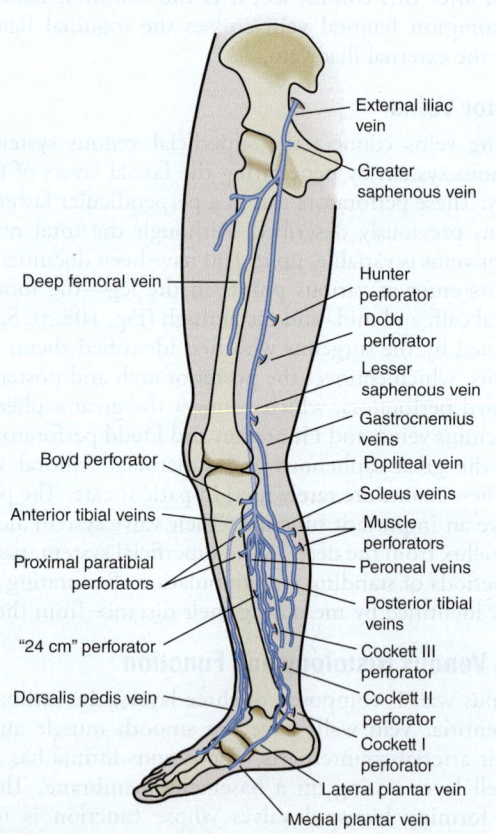

FIGURE 108.3 Perforating veins of the lower limb.

larger-caliber veins have limited contractile capacity in comparison to the thicker-walled GSV. The venous valves prevent retrograde flow; it is their failure or valvular incompetence that leads to reflux and its associated symptoms. Venous valves are most prevalent in the distal lower extremity, whereas as one proceeds proximally, the number of valves decreases to the point that no valves are present in the superior vena cava and inferior vena cava (IVC).

Most of the capacitance of the vascular tree is in the venous system. Because veins do not have significant amounts of elastin, veins can withstand large volume shifts with comparatively small changes in pressure. A vein has a normal elliptical configuration until the limit of its capacitance is reached, at which point the vein assumes a round configuration.

The calf muscles augment venous return by functioning as a pump. In the supine state, the resting venous pressure in the foot is the sum of the residual kinetic energy minus the resistance in the arterioles and precapillary sphincters. Thus, a pressure gradient is generated to the right atrium of approximately 10 to 12 mm Hg. In the upright position, the resting venous pressure of the foot reflects the hydrostatic pressure from the upright column of blood extending from the right atrium to the foot.

The return of the blood to the heart from the lower extremity is facilitated by the muscle pump function of the calf, a mechanism whereby the calf muscle, functioning as a bellows during exercise, compresses the gastrocnemius and soleal sinuses and propels the blood toward the heart. The normally functioning valves in the venous system prevent retrograde flow; when one or more of these valves become incompetent, symptoms of venous insufficiency can develop. During calf muscle contraction, the venous pressures of the foot and ankle drop dramatically. The pressures developing in the muscle compartments during exercise range from 150 to 200 mm Hg, and when there is failure of perforating veins, these high pressures are transmitted to the superficial system.

VENOUS INSUFFICIENCY

Chronic venous insufficiency (CVI) is dominated by venous reflux through incompetent venous valves. There are three categories of venous insufficiency—congenital, primary, and secondary. Congenital venous insufficiency comprises predominantly anatomic variants that are present at birth. Examples of congenital venous anomalies include venous ectasias, absence of venous valves, and syndromes such as Klippel-Trénaunay syndrome. Although secondary venous insufficiency can be considered a sequela of a previous acute thrombotic disorder (postthrombotic syndrome [PTS]), the etiology of primary CVI cannot be clearly identified.

Risk Factors

Risk factors for the development of varicose veins include advancing age, female sex, multiparity, heredity, history of trauma to the extremity, and prolonged standing. Additional risk factors include obesity and a positive family history. Advancing age appears to be an important significant risk factor. Venous function is undoubtedly influenced by hormonal changes. In particular, progesterone liberated by the corpus luteum stabilizes the uterus by causing the relaxation of smooth muscle fibers.[2] This directly influences venous function. The result is passive venous dilation, which in many cases causes valvular dysfunction. Although progesterone is implicated in the first appearance of varicosities in pregnancy, estrogen also has profound effects. It produces the relaxation of smooth muscle and a softening of collagen fibers. Furthermore, the estrogen-to-progesterone ratio influences venous distensibility. This ratio may explain the predominance of venous insufficiency symptoms on the first day of a menstrual period, when a profound shift occurs from the progesterone phase of the menstrual cycle to the estrogen phase. Autosomal dominant penetrance has been identified as the underlying genetic risk factor for subsequent development of varicose veins.

Pathology

Venous reflux through incompetent venous valves has been described as the main pathogenetic factor underlying CVI. However, obstruction of venous channels, resulting from intrinsic narrowing, postthrombotic thickening and scarring, or external compression, may also result in venous hypertension leading to CVI. In many cases, particularly after venous thrombosis, obstruction and reflux, coexist resulting in severe CVI.

Mechanical Abnormalities

Anatomic differences in the location of the superficial veins of the lower extremities may contribute to the pathogenesis. Primary venous insufficiency may involve one, both, or none of the axial veins (great and small saphenous). Perforating veins may be the sole source of venous pathophysiologic changes, perhaps because the GSV is supported by a well-developed medial fibromuscular layer and fibrous connective tissue that bind it to the deep fascia. In contrast, tributaries to the SSV are less supported in the subcutaneous fat and are superficial to the membranous layer of superficial fascia (Fig. 108.4). These tributaries also contain less

muscle mass in their walls. Thus, these veins, and not the main trunk, may become selectively varicose.

When these fundamental anatomic peculiarities are recognized, the intrinsic competence or incompetence of the valve system becomes important. For example, failure of a valve protecting a tributary vein from the pressures of the SSV allows a cluster of varicosities to develop. Furthermore, communicating veins connecting the deep with the superficial compartment may have valve failure. Pressure studies have shown that there are two sources of venous hypertension. The first is gravitational and is a result of venous blood coursing in a distal direction down linear axial venous segments. This is referred to as *hydrostatic pressure* and is the weight of the blood column from the right atrium. The highest pressure generated by this mechanism is evident at the ankle and foot, where measurements are expressed in centimeters of water or millimeters of mercury.

The second source of venous hypertension is dynamic. It is the force of muscle contraction, usually contained within the compartments of the leg. If a perforating vein fails, high pressures (range, 150–200 mm Hg) developed within the muscular compartments during exercise are transmitted directly to the superficial venous system. Here, the sudden pressure transmitted causes dilation and lengthening of the superficial veins. Progressive distal valvular incompetence may occur. If proximal valves such as the saphenofemoral valve become incompetent, systolic muscular contraction is supplemented by the weight of the static column of blood from the heart. Furthermore, this static column becomes a barrier. Blood flowing proximally through the femoral vein spills into the saphenous vein and flows distally. As it refluxes distally through progressively incompetent valves, it is returned through perforating veins to the deep veins. Here, it is conveyed once again to the femoral veins, only to be recycled distally. Regardless of the precise source of the elevated hydrostatic pressure, the ultimate result is increased ambulatory venous hypertension.

A number of authors have demonstrated that the development of all the clinical manifestations of CVI can be ascribed to a blood flow–driven inflammatory process. Leukocytes are activated and marginalize. Adhesion to the endothelium is prompted by the expression of adhesion molecules, such as intracellular adhesion molecule 1 (ICAM-1), vascular cell adhesion molecule 1 (VCAM-1), and L- and P-selectins. Ultimately, they infiltrate the venous wall, lyse, and release activated extracellular matrix enzymes (matrix metallopeptidase [MMP]1, MMP2, and MMP9).[3] The extracellular matrix is degraded, and the venous wall, including the valves, undergoes remodeling. Decreased amounts of elastin and

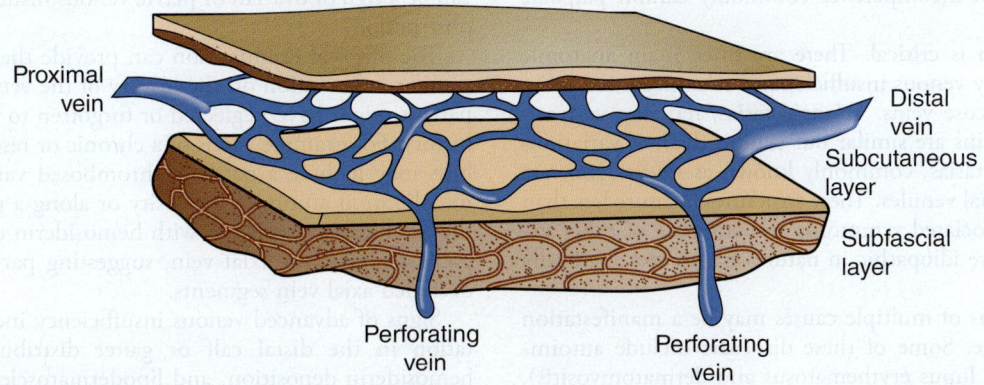

FIGURE 108.4 Dilation of superficial venous tributaries caused by increased transmission of pressure by the perforating veins.

an imbalance between collagen I and III have been identified in surgical specimens, suggesting that the loss of the venous wall intimal architecture leads to dilation, tortuosity, and the formation of varicose veins.[2,4]

Symptoms

The patient with symptomatic varicose veins commonly reports heaviness, discomfort, and extremity fatigue in the affected lower extremity. The pain is characteristically dull, does not usually occur during recumbency, and is exacerbated by periods of prolonged standing. Swelling is commonly described. The discomforts of aching, heaviness, and fatigue are usually relieved by leg elevation or elastic support. Cutaneous burning, termed *venous neuropathy,* can also occur in patients with advanced venous insufficiency. Pruritus occurs from excess hemosiderin deposition and tends to be located at the distal calf or in areas of phlebitic varicose branch segments. Patients may report cramping pain that occurs during or after exercise and is relieved with rest and leg elevation. This syndrome is termed *venous claudication* and is a clinical manifestation of venous outflow obstruction or secondary venous insufficiency. Predominant causes of venous claudication include a history of deep venous thrombosis (DVT) and/or diagnosis of May-Thurner syndrome.

Multiparous female patients in their childbearing years may report a constellation of symptoms that involve varicosities of the leg in conjunction with chronic pelvic pain. The lower extremity symptoms may or may not be present. Additional symptoms include a feeling of bladder fullness with standing, dyspareunia, and chronic pelvic pain. This clinical picture suggests pelvic congestion syndrome. Because the differential diagnosis for pelvic pain is extensive, the diagnosis of pelvic venous congestion tends to be one of exclusion; diagnostic modalities to confirm its presence include magnetic resonance venous imaging (MRVI) of the pelvis and conventional pelvic venography, which can be both diagnostic and therapeutic.

Physical Examination

A comprehensive examination includes assessment of the arterial circulation. Briefly, palpation of the femoral, popliteal, dorsalis pedis, and posterior tibialis pulses is performed. Nonpalpable pulses necessitate further evaluation.

The venous examination includes assessment of the patient in the standing and supine positions. The examination room must be well lit and warm so that vasospasm does not occur, limiting a comprehensive evaluation. Standing increases venous hypertension and dilates veins, thereby facilitating examination. Patients with superficial axial incompetence commonly exhibit palpable GSVs (Fig. 108.5).

Visual inspection is critical. There are three main anatomic categories of primary venous insufficiency—telangiectasias, reticular veins, and varicose veins. Telangiectasias, reticular varicosities, and varicose veins are similar but exhibit distinct variations in caliber. Telangiectasias, commonly known as *spider veins,* are very small intradermal venules. These structures measure less than 1 mm. Without associated symptoms and stigmata of other venous disease, they are idiopathic in nature and are not medically necessary to treat.

Leg telangiectasias of multiple causes may be a manifestation of a systemic disease. Some of these disorders include autoimmune diseases (e.g., lupus erythematosus and dermatomyositis), exogenous causes, and xeroderma pigmentosum. Reticular veins are vein branches that enter the tributaries of the main axial,

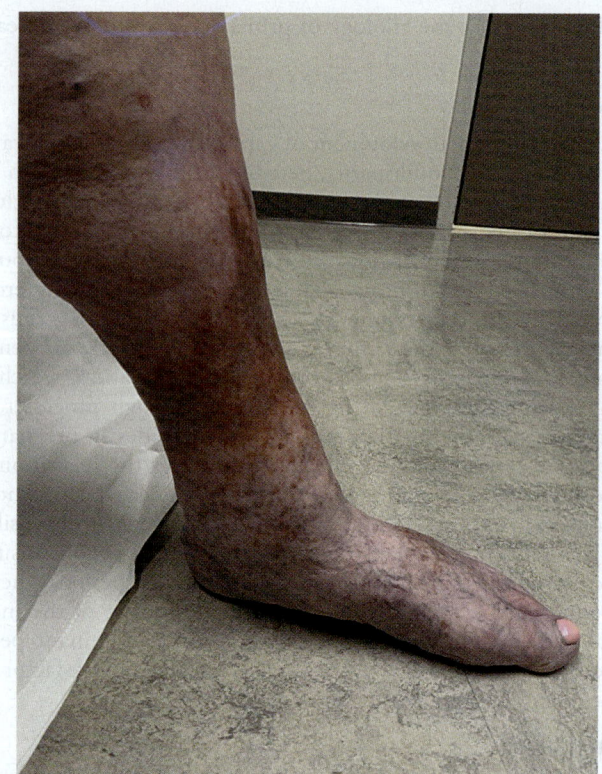

FIGURE 108.5 Hemosiderosis. (Courtesy C. Shokrzadeh, UTMB Galveston, Galveston, Texas.)

perforating, or deep veins. Reticular veins are larger than spider veins and usually have diameters between 1 and 3 mm. They are located in the subdermal or subcutaneous tissue. Varicose veins are located in the subcutaneous tissues and have diameters greater than 3 mm. The axial veins, the great and SSVs, represent the largest-caliber veins of the superficial venous system.

Location of varicosities can commonly identify an incompetent valve or the axial vein from which the varicosities developed. For example, medial thigh varicose veins are likely to develop from an incompetent GSV, whereas posterior calf or lateral calf varicose veins tend to originate from the SSV. In addition, the location of varicose veins can be a diagnostic predictor of a larger process. Varicosities of the scrotum can be associated with gonadal vein incompetence, otherwise termed the *nutcracker syndrome* (compression of the left renal vein between the aorta and the superior mesenteric artery). Perineal or vulvar varicosities can be a sign of ovarian or pelvic venous insufficiency or iliac vein obstruction.

The physical examination can provide the physician with important information on the history of the venous disease that the patient might have neglected or forgotten to mention during the history. For example, signs of a chronic or resolved thrombophlebitis may include a partially thrombosed varicosity; a brownish discoloration around a varicosity or along a palpable segment of the axial veins, consistent with hemosiderin deposition; and palpable segments of axial vein, suggesting partially or completely occluded axial vein segments.

Signs of advanced venous insufficiency include hyperpigmentation in the distal calf or gaiter distribution, secondary to hemosiderin deposition, and lipodermatosclerosis (Fig. 108.6A). Lipodermatosclerosis develops over time because of prolonged ambulatory venous hypertension and chronic inflammation.

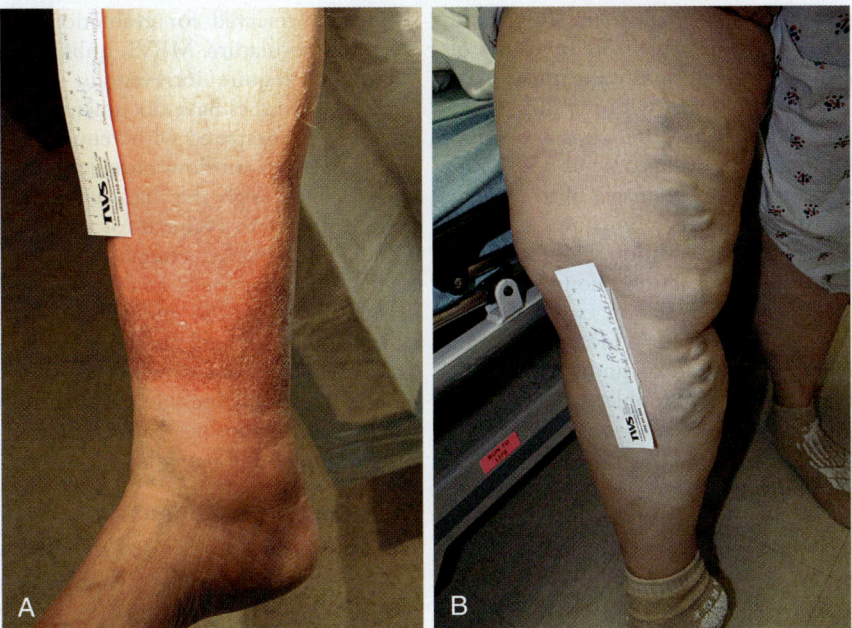

FIGURE 108.6 (A) Lipodermatosclerosis, hyperpigmentation and brawny edema. (B) Varicose vein.

Physical examination findings that reflect lipodermatosclerosis are brawny edema of the distal calf, "champagne bottle leg," fibrotic and hypertrophic skin, and hyperpigmentation. Advanced lipodermatosclerosis may involve fibrosis of the Achilles tendon, impairing motor function of the extremity. Therefore, examination should include motor function at the ankle. Atrophie blanche is an area of pale hue visualized around the medial malleolus; it is commonly mistaken for a healed ulcer because of its lighter pigmentation. *Corona phlebectatica* is a term used to describe an accumulation of tiny telangiectasias or venous flare, usually located at the medial malleolus or the dorsum of the foot. Skin changes from CVI can mimic other dermatologic phenomena; both dermatitis and eczematous changes can be seen in venous disease.

Venous stasis ulcers exhibit pathognomonic features that distinguish them from their arterial or neuropathic counterparts. Venous ulcers appear at the medial malleolus, not in the mid- to distal foot. Venous stasis dermatitis is visualized at the distal ankle and can mimic eczema or dermatitis of another cause. It is this important attention to supporting features of the physical examination and history as well as confirmation with duplex reflux examination that will distinguish advanced venous stasis disease from dermatologic conditions.

Diagnostic Evaluation of Venous Dysfunction

The Society for Vascular Surgery (SVS), the American Venous Forum (AVF), and the American Vein and Lymphatic Society (AVLS) have jointly released an update on the practice guidelines for the care of patients with CVI.[5] The Perthes test for deep venous occlusion and the Brodie-Trendelenburg test of axial reflux have been replaced by in-office use of the continuous-wave, handheld Doppler instrument supplemented by duplex ultrasound evaluation. The handheld Doppler instrument can confirm an impression of saphenous reflux, which in turn dictates the operative procedure to be performed in any given patient. A common misconception is the belief that the Doppler instrument is used to locate perforating veins. Instead, it is used in specific locations to determine incompetent valves—for example, the handheld,

continuous-wave, 8-MHz flow detector placed over the great and SSVs near their terminations. With distal augmentation of flow and release, normal deep breathing, and performance of a Valsalva maneuver, valve reflux is accurately identified. Formerly, the Doppler examination was supplemented by other objective studies, including photoplethysmography, mercury strain-gauge plethysmography, and photorheography. These are no longer in common use.

Today, duplex imaging is the first and best modality to assess for the normal function and presence of venous insufficiency of the lower extremities. Duplex technology more precisely defines which veins are refluxing by imaging the superficial and deep veins. The SVS/AVF/AVLS clinical practice guidelines detailed four crucial components of the duplex examination: visibility, compressibility, venous flow, and augmentation.[5] It is important to note that venous reflux duplex done with the patient supine yields an erroneous evaluation of reflux. In the supine position, even when no flow is present, the valves remain open. Valve closure requires a reversal of flow with a pressure gradient that is higher proximally than distally. Thus, the duplex examination needs to be done with the patient standing or in the markedly trunk-elevated position.[6]

There are many advantages of ultrasound imaging. The ultrasound examination is noninvasive, requires no contrast material, and can be performed in the office as well as in the hospital. Drawbacks to the modality include interobserver variability and limitations in imaging in patients with an elevated body mass index and extensive dressings. Imaging is obtained with a 7.5- or 10-MHz probe; the pulsed Doppler consists of a 3.0-MHz probe. The examination begins with the probe placed longitudinally on the groin. First, all the deep veins are examined. Next, the superficial veins are evaluated. There are four basic components of the examination that should be included to complete a comprehensive venous evaluation of the lower extremity veins: compressibility, venous flow, augmentation after reflux, and visibility. Reflux can be demonstrated with the patient performing a Valsalva maneuver or by manual compression and release of the extremity distal to the point of the examination. A Valsalva maneuver is performed for the proximal extremity—that is, the thigh and groin—whereas compression is used for the calf. Reflux times of 500 milliseconds or longer are considered significant in the axial veins. Perforator veins can be visualized well with the duplex examination (Fig. 108.7). Significant perforator reflux is defined as a diameter of more than 3.5 mm and a reflux time of 350 milliseconds or longer. Demonstration on duplex images of to-and-fro flow, with the presence of dilated segments, constitutes findings compatible with a refluxing perforator. In addition, Doppler studies can provide the clinician with information about the deep system. Reflux times of 1000 milliseconds or longer are considered significant in the femoropopliteal veins. Widespread use of duplex scanning has allowed a comparison of findings between standard clinical examinations and duplex Doppler studies.[7,8]

Phlebography and Venography

In general, phlebography is unnecessary in the diagnosis and treatment of primary venous insufficiency. In cases of secondary CVI, phlebography has specific usefulness. Ascending phlebography is performed by injection of contrast material into a superficial pedal vein after a tourniquet is applied at the ankle to prevent flow into the superficial venous system. Observation of flow defines anatomy and regions of thrombus or obstruction. Therefore, ascending phlebology differentiates primary from secondary venous insufficiency. Descending phlebography is performed with retrograde injection of contrast material into the deep venous system at the groin or popliteal fossa (femoral vein or popliteal vein). This diagnostic modality identifies specific valvular incompetence suspected on B-mode scanning and clinical examination. However, these invasive studies are seldom performed and are used only as preoperative adjuncts when deep venous reconstruction is being planned.

Magnetic Resonance and Computed Tomography Venous Imaging

Advancements in technology have led to a paradigm change in the imaging of the venous system. MRVI is a diagnostic imaging modality reserved for evaluation of the abdominal and pelvic venous vasculature. MRVI, unlike venography, is noninvasive and does not require intravenous (IV) administration of contrast material. Studies have documented similar rates of specificity and sensitivity compared with venography. MRVI is used to evaluate pelvic venous outflow obstruction, providing information from the IVC through the iliac venous system. Furthermore, it is an excellent test to evaluate for pelvic congestion syndrome. Computed tomography venography (CTV) has similar applications to MRVI. A large meta-analysis showed that CTV has sensitivity from 71% to 100% and specificity ranging from 93% to 100% for the diagnosis of proximal DVT. Anatomy of the abdominal and pelvic venous system can be well characterized by CTV. Limitations may include artifacts from orthopedic implants and/or adjacent pathology, administration of contrast, and pelvic radiation in young patients.

Classification Systems

In 1994, the AVF devised the Clinical-Etiological-Anatomical-Pathophysiological (CEAP) classification system, which is a scoring system that stratifies venous disease on the basis of clinical presentation, etiology, anatomy, and pathophysiology (Table 108.3). It is useful in helping the physician assess a limb afflicted with venous insufficiency and then arrive at an appropriate treatment plan. A revised CEAP classification was introduced in 2004 that included a Venous Disability Score to document a patient's ability to perform activities of daily living.[9] In 2020, the CEAP classification system was further updated to include corona phlebectatica as a clinical subclass, introducing the modifier "r" for recurrent varicose veins and recurrent venous ulcers and replacing numeric descriptions of the venous segments with their common abbreviations. Although the CEAP classification is a valuable tool to grade venous disease, assessment of outcomes after intervention cannot be realized. As a result, two additional scoring systems, the Venous Clinical Severity Score and the Venous Segmental Disease Score, enhance the CEAP score with the increased ability to plot outcome. These three classification modalities now provide clinical researchers with invaluable tools to study treatment outcomes.[10]

Treatment of Superficial Venous Insufficiency
Nonoperative Management

Nonoperative management of patients with CVI includes lifestyle modifications, compression, and pharmacologic therapies.[10] Initial recommendations for lifestyle changes are avoidance of vigorous exercise and leg elevation in order to improve symptoms caused by venous hypertension. Although vigorous exercise has been shown to increase the risk of developing venous ulcerations, increased mobility and moderate physical activity may be beneficial for ulcer healing and may be a useful adjunct to compression therapy. Leg elevation 30 cm above the heart aids venous drainage and venous return, thus reducing lower extremity venous edema. Leg elevation has also been shown to enhance cutaneous microcirculation in patients with lipodermatosclerosis (45% Doppler flux increase).[10] A retrospective study of 122 patients with healed venous ulcer over a period of 12 to 40 months documented statistically significant lower rates of ulcer recurrence with a combination of compression therapy and longer leg elevation times (median 33 min/day). Increased recurrence was observed with a median period of leg elevation of 14 min/day.[10]

Compression therapy is an integral component of the care of patients with CVI. The rationale of compression therapy is to

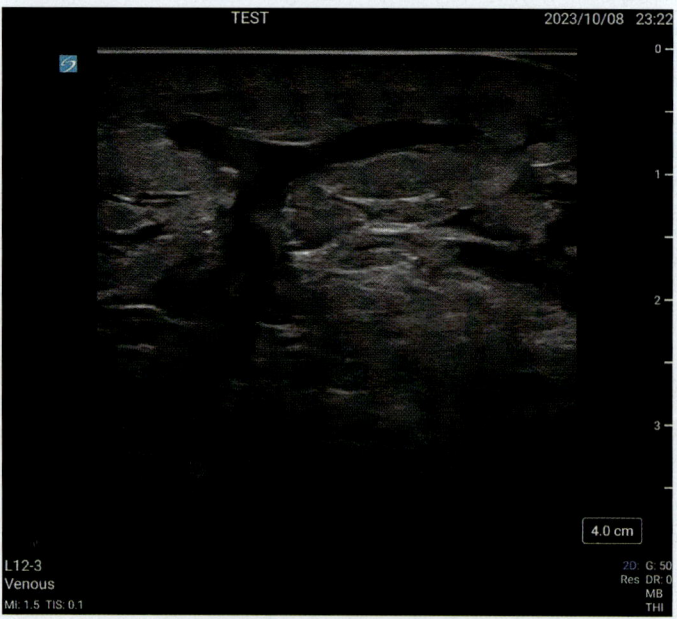

FIGURE 108.7 Calf perforator vein on ultrasound. (Courtesy C. Shokrzadeh, UTMB Galveston, Galveston, Texas.)

TABLE 108.3 Classification of Chronic Lower Extremity Venous Disease

CLINICAL (C) CLASS	DESCRIPTION
C_0	No visible or palpable signs of venous disease
C_1	Telangiectasias or reticular veins
C_1	Varicose veins
C_2	Recurrent varicose veins
C2r	Edema
C4	Changes in skin and subcutaneous tissues secondary to CVD
C_{4a}	Pigmentation or eczema
C_{4b}	Lipodermatosclerosis or atrophie blanche
C_{4c}	Corona phlebectatica
C_5	Healed ulcer
C_6	Active venous ulcer
C_{6r}	Recurrent venous ulcer
ETIOLOGIC (E) CLASS	**DESCRIPTION**
E_p	Primary
E_s	Secondary
E_{si}	Secondary—intravenous
E_{se}	Secondary—extravenous
E_c	Congenital
E_n	No cause identified
ANATOMIC (A) CLASS	**DESCRIPTION[a]**
A_s	Superficial
A_d	Deep
A_p	Perforator
A_n	No venous anatomic location identified
PATHOPHYSIOLOGIC (P) CLASS	**DESCRIPTION**
P_r	Reflux
P_o	Obstruction
$P_{r,o}$	Reflux and obstruction
P_n	No pathophysiology identified

[a]See details in Lurie et al. (2020, p. 349).
CVD, Chronic venous disease.
Based on Lurie F, Passman M, Meisner M, et al. The 2020 update of the CEAP classification system and reporting standards. *J Vasc Surg Venous Lymphat Disord.* 2020;8(3):342-352.

oppose the reflux-induced venous hypertension. Considering 60 to 80 mm Hg to be within normal limits for standing venous pressure, hemodynamic effects can be expected with an interface compression of 30 to 40 mm Hg. External compression of greater than 60 mm Hg has been shown to occlude lower extremity veins in standing individuals. Investigations conducted via dermal blood flow assessment have demonstrated that compression rates of 30 to 40 mm Hg are also beneficial in patients with combined chronic venous disease and peripheral arterial disease with ankle-brachial indexes greater than 0.5. The biomolecular mechanisms by which compression therapy functions are unclear. Animal and clinical studies have described an overall improvement of the cutaneous microcirculation; increased capillary density, decreased capillary diameter, and pericapillary halo at video capillary microscopy; increased transcutaneous oxygen saturation levels; and decreased levels of cytokines, such as tumor necrosis factor α and vascular endothelial growth factors.[10]

Compression therapy can be achieved via gradient compression stockings and bandages. Gradient elastic stockings are considered the most initial intervention in patients with clinical stigma of venous disease. They are currently available in four tensions: 10 to 15 mm Hg (class 1; over the counter); 20 to 30 mm Hg (class 2; prescription); 30 to 40 mm Hg (class 3; prescription); and 40 to 50 mm Hg (class 4 high compression; prescription). They are also available in different sizes and lengths. Gradient compression stockings have been shown to be beneficial in symptom control in patients with moderate CVI.[10] Sequential compression devices (SCDs) can also serve as an adjunct to traditional compression therapy provided by compression stockings and bandages. Studies have shown that consistent usage of sequential pneumatic compression therapy improves pain level and quality of life.[11]

Patients who exhibit venous stasis ulceration will require local wound care (see Fig. 108.7). A triple-layer compression dressing with a zinc oxide paste gauze wrap in contact with the skin is used most commonly from the base of the toes to the anterior tibial tubercle with snug, graded compression. This is an example of what is generally known as an *Unna boot*. A 15-year review of 998 patients with one or more venous ulcers treated with a similar compression bandage demonstrated that 73% of the ulcers healed in patients who returned for care (Fig. 108.8). The median time to healing for individual ulcers was 9 weeks. In general, snug, graded-pressure, triple-layer compression dressings result in more rapid healing than compression stockings alone.[12]

For most patients, well-applied, sustained compression therapy offers the most cost-effective and efficacious therapy in the healing of venous ulcers. After healing, most cases of CVI are controlled with elastic compression stockings to be worn during waking hours. On occasion, older patients and those with arthritic conditions cannot apply the compression stocking required, and control must be maintained by triple-layer zinc oxide compression dressings, which can usually be left in place and changed once a week. Donning devices are also available on the market to help patients to apply compression stockings. In addition to compression, wound care, and surgery, large chronic venous ulcers may benefit from venoactive medications, in particular, pentoxifylline and micronized purified flavonoid fraction.

The 2022 clinical practice guideline recommends superficial venous intervention over long-term compression in patients who suffer from symptomatic varicose veins and axial reflux in the GSV or SSV. After clinical and objective criteria have established the presence of symptomatic varicose veins, the next step is to plan a course of therapy. The Eschar Trial randomized 500

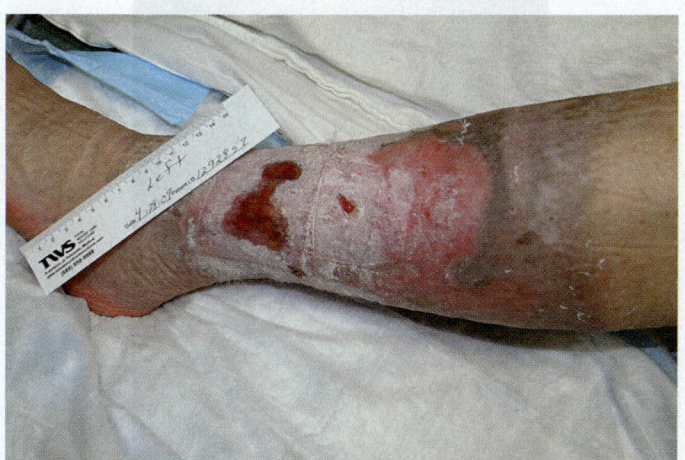

FIGURE 108.8 Venous stasis ulcer.

patients with saphenous insufficiency and venous leg ulcers to conservative management with compression therapy or saphenous stripping and compression therapy. At 4 years of follow-up, there was no evidence of a significant difference in ulcer healing rates, but the incidence of ulcer recurrence after healing was significantly lower in patients who underwent saphenous stripping.[10,12] Recent prospective randomized control trials focusing on the effectiveness of endovenous therapies that are considerably less invasive have shown significantly improved ulcer healing rates in patients who have undergone radiofrequency ablation (RFA) of insufficient saphenous veins compared with compression bandages alone.[13]

Treatment Options for Telangiectasias

Telangiectasias and reticular veins are usually treated in the outpatient setting. Asymptomatic telangiectasias and reticular veins are of cosmetic concern only. In these asymptomatic patients with only C_1 disease, a reflux examination is not indicated. However, if the patient describes symptoms consistent with possible venous insufficiency or has concomitant varicosities or more advanced disease on physical examination, a reflux examination is indicated. Treatment options for telangiectasias (spider veins and reticular veins) include injection sclerotherapy and transdermal laser treatment (Fig. 108.9).

Injection sclerotherapy is a technique that involves direct injection of a sclerosant agent into the feeding vein (reticular vein) or spider vein. This procedure is performed in the office setting. There is no preprocedural preparation of the patient. However, patients are asked not to shave or apply lotions to the extremity before the treatment. Patients leave the office and are able to perform regular activities immediately. Direct sunlight exposure to the treatment area is avoided for a few weeks after the injection. Although it is a safe technique, injection sclerotherapy is contraindicated in the following situations: pregnancy, patients with acute superficial thrombophlebitis (SVT), patients with acute DVT, patent foramen ovale with right-to-left heart shunt, severe arterial occlusive disease in the treated extremities, and patients with a history of severe allergy or severe asthma.

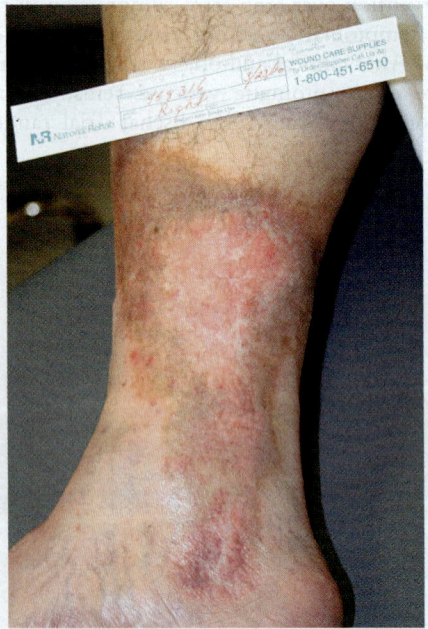

FIGURE 108.9 Healed venous stasis ulcer.

Sclerosants act to disrupt the venous endothelium, causing a periphlebitic reaction, which acts to obliterate the vein segment. There are many sclerosants available, and there are particular categories of sclerosants. They include osmotic, detergent, chemical, and corrosive. Hypertonic saline, in various concentrations, was long considered the agent of choice; however, it can be painful with injection (despite the addition of local anesthetics) and appears to exhibit a higher incidence of hyperpigmentation after treatment. Therefore, varying concentrations of sodium tetradecyl sulfate (Sotradecol) and polidocanol (Asclera, Varithena) are now the preferred agents.

The procedure should be performed in a well-lit room. Dilute solutions of sclerosant (e.g., 1%–3% sodium tetradecyl sulfate; polidocanol 0.5%, 1%, 1.5%) can be injected directly into the venules. Care must be taken to ensure that no single injection dose exceeds 0.1 mL but that multiple injections completely fill all feeding vessels. Larger spider veins should be injected first. Injection should begin proximally and proceed distally. When the session is complete, a pressure dressing is applied, consisting of cotton balls at each injection site, and then covered with compression stockings or elastic bandages. Patients are advised to ambulate frequently during the first 24 hours and abstain from direct sun exposure and airline travel for 2 weeks. On occasion, entrapped blood may form, and patients report significant discomfort. Needle drainage is performed at the site, which facilitates healing and cosmesis and rapidly improves discomfort. This liberation of entrapped blood is as important to success as the primary injection. This therapy is remarkably successful in achieving an excellent cosmetic result. C_1 larger than 1 mm and smaller than 3 mm can also be injected with a sclerosant of slightly greater concentration, but the amount injected at one site needs to be limited to less than 0.5 mL. A total volume of sclerosant should not exceed 4 mL during a treatment session. If one is using hypertonic saline, maximum treatment volume can be 10 mL. Although injection sclerotherapy has met with significant success, complications do occur. They include hyperpigmentation, venous matting, postsclerotherapy necrosis, and an allergic reaction to the sclerosant. In addition, telangiectasia formation after injection sclerotherapy treatment tends to occur. Patients will commonly observe return of spider veins 8 to 12 months after treatment. Although patients may report localized discomfort, sclerotherapy of telangiectasias is considered cosmetic and does not influence the venous circulation of the extremity.[14]

Laser treatment of spider telangiectasias has been performed with a variety of wavelengths and varying techniques, such as high-intensity pulsed light, fiber-guided laser coagulation, and neodymium:yttrium-aluminium-garnet (ND-YAG) laser with a wavelength of 1064 nm. Evaluation of all existing laser modalities has suggested that the ND-YAG laser has the most success. However, to date, there have not been any prospective randomized trials to support this presumption. Laser treatment does tend to be more painful. Laser treatment in most centers will be used in conjunction with injection sclerotherapy—that is, injection treats the feeding venules; laser treatment will be used to treat the extremely small branches not adequately addressed with the injection technique. Most patients are satisfied with the injection-only method.

Surgery for Axial Venous Incompetence

Vein stripping. It has been more than a century since surgeons began to develop techniques to treat superficial axial venous reflux. Keller introduced saphenous vein invagination and stripping, and

Mayo pioneered use of an external stripper to remove the saphenous vein. Babcock described stripping the saphenous vein intraluminally from the ankle to groin. High ligation of the GSV was also described; however, it proved to be ineffective because the refluxing axial vein was not eliminated. Although effective, stripping of the GSV is now rarely performed, given its high morbidity. Endovenous thermal ablation procedures with radiofrequency or laser and nonthermal ablation with chemical sclerosant have replaced stripping in the past two decades and are now the mainstay of treatment for refluxing axial veins. Traditional vein stripping usually requires general or spinal anesthesia. A transverse or oblique groin incision is made just medial to the femoral artery pulse and inferior to the inguinal crease. Sharp dissection allows identification of the proximal GSV and other venous tributaries that can be ligated and divided. A brief exploration to identify the presence of a duplicate saphenous system should be performed. The GSV can then be brought up into the surgical field with gentle traction on the SFJ. This maneuver affords further visualization of any missed tributaries that require ligation. The GSV should be ligated with a nonabsorbable suture and transected near its confluence with the femoral vein. Attention is then directed to the below-knee segment of the GSV by making a small transverse incision on the proximal, medial calf. The GSV is identified, ligated distally, and transected. The Codman stripper is then advanced proximally through the GSV to exit the transected vein in the groin incision. The bulb is attached to the end of the Codman stripper that exits the groin incision, and a handle is attached to the other end (exiting the calf incision). The saphenous vein should be secured to the bulb of the stripper and inverted onto itself. Forcefully pulling on the handle of the Codman stripper removes the GSV from the groin to the knee. Before stripping, the lower extremity should be wrapped circumferentially to aid in hemostasis and prevent postoperative edema and permanent hyperpigmentation resulting from blood extravasation.

Complications. *Neovascularization* refers to the development of new venous tributaries and varicose veins around the previously ligated and divided SFJ. The incidence of neovascularization after high ligation and stripping of the GSV exceeds 30%, according to some reports. Interestingly, neovascularization does not occur after endovenous ablation procedures, which obviate the need for a groin dissection or venous tributary ligation. Rather than being beneficial, surgical dissection and tributary ligation may actually trigger neovascularization and varicose vein recurrence. Monitoring for this complication usually involves periodic duplex ultrasound examination.

Saphenous nerve injury is a well-documented complication that occurs more frequently when the GSV is stripped from the ankle to the groin. The saphenous nerve runs close to the GSV in the calf compared with the thigh, where the nerve and vein have more separation. This anatomic detail may explain why stripping from the knee to the thigh only reduces the risk of nerve injury (Fig. 108.10). Stripping of the SSV has also been described; however, it carries a very high risk of nerve injury, given the proximity of the sural nerve in the posterior aspect of the leg. Therefore, because of the several limitations and disadvantages of stripping of the GSV, it has been replaced by endovenous techniques. Percutaneous endovenous ablation procedures include thermal and nonthermal ablations.

Endovenous thermal and nonthermal ablation. Percutaneous endovenous ablation of the superficial axial veins revolutionized the treatment of superficial venous insufficiency and has been the mainstay of treatment for more than two decades. As a minimally

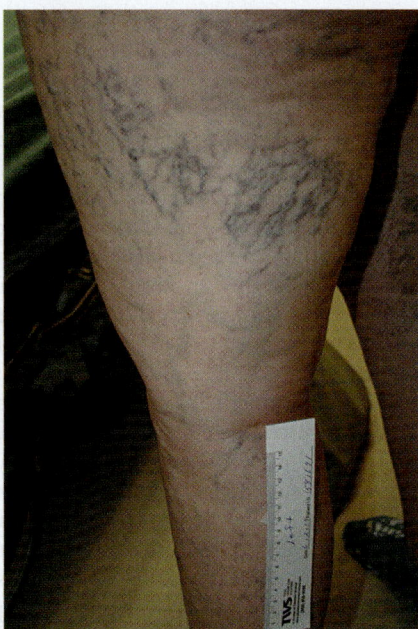

FIGURE 108.10 Spider telangiectasias.

invasive alternative to surgical vein stripping, percutaneous endovenous ablation can be performed on an outpatient basis with local anesthesia. Advantages of this technique include less discomfort for the patient and a more rapid recovery. There are two main types of endovenous thermal therapy for the superficial axial veins: RFA and endovenous laser therapy (EVLT). Both of these modalities generate high yet focused temperatures to prevent injury to surrounding tissues. Endovenous thermal ablation works by destruction of the venous endothelium and collagen in the medial via direct thermal injury. Tumescent fluid is required for these thermal ablation techniques for anesthesia and also functions as a heat sink.

In contrast, nonthermal ablation techniques exist and are also known as *nontumescent endovenous ablation modalities* because they do not require tumescent anesthesia. The three major nonthermal ablation techniques are mechanochemical ablation (MOCA), cyanoacrylate adhesive closure (CAC), and polidocanol endovenous microfoam (PEM). These procedures are sometimes favored over thermal ablation for the treatment of SSV and the below-knee segment of the GSV because of the reduced likelihood of nerve damage.

Percutaneous vein ablation. Endovenous thermal ablation, as well as nonthermal techniques, requires minimal preprocedural preparation. Healthy patients with no significant medical history do not require laboratory work, whereas standard laboratory evaluation is usually obtained for patients with significant medical comorbidities. Patients who are receiving anticoagulation should remain on their standard regimen. Guidelines for periprocedural DVT prophylaxis remain unclear. All antiplatelet medications can be continued throughout the procedural course. The authors do not routinely administer prophylactic antibiotics.

Anesthesia for endovenous thermal ablation procedures can range from local injections to conscious sedation. Most patients tolerate the procedure with minimal anesthesia consisting only of tumescent infusion around the GSV. Ideally, these patients can be treated in an office setting. Moderate sedation requires hemodynamic monitoring equipment vend is more suited for an outpatient surgical center. The choice of anesthesia ultimately depends on the preferences of the patient and physician as well as the available resources and practice environments.

The venous duplex ultrasound examination plays an essential role in planning of endovenous ablation procedures. The ultrasound examination should provide the treating physician with the following information: patency of the deep venous system, location of normal and refluxing axial veins, areas of communication between the varicosities and the axial vein, and presence of duplicate or accessory refluxing vein segments.

An acute occlusive DVT is an absolute contraindication to endovenous thermal and nonthermal ablation, whereas a chronically recanalized deep venous system in the extremity to be treated is a relative contraindication. In patients who harbor secondary venous insufficiency, the superficial veins play a more important role in venous drainage compared with patients with a pristine deep venous system and primary venous insufficiency. Care must be taken to ensure that superficial venous ablation will not compromise the venous outflow of the postthrombotic limb.

The site of percutaneous access depends on the patient's symptoms and the location of the varicose vein tributaries. If endovenous thermal ablation of the GSV is planned in a patient with painful varicosities on the proximal calf, it is helpful to evaluate these branches with ultrasound. Percutaneous access on the distal calf just inferior to the varicose veins will ensure that maximum resolution of the tributary branches is achieved with endovenous thermal treatment.

RFA and laser energy deliver two different types of energy to the vein lumen. Radiofrequency heat is delivered at a temperature of 120°C. The radiofrequency directly injures the vein wall endothelium, resulting in collagen contraction and thrombosis of the treated vein. Laser energy delivers energy to the blood itself. Steam bubbles are generated with the laser energy, and coagulation occurs after completion of laser energy delivery. Radiofrequency catheters vary in length but not in temperature delivered. In contrast, laser energy generators come in different wavelengths ranging from 810 to 1470 nm, and there are multiple wavelengths commercially available; as such, updated laser therapy strategies are frequently introduced into the evolving therapeutic armamentarium. Investigators have demonstrated that the higher-wavelength fibers appear to be associated with less postprocedural discomfort.

Technique. In most cases, the extremity should be placed in a position of external rotation with the knee slightly flexed. A sheet "bump" or pillow behind the hip and knee may help the patient maintain this position. Placing the patient in reverse Trendelenburg can help dilate the vein to be accessed. After the standard sterile preparation and draping, the ultrasound probe is brought onto the field in a sterile transducer cover. The author reexamines the vein to be treated along its entire course, noting areas of aneurysmal dilation or tortuosity that may affect catheter placement. Ideally, the puncture site should be distal to the lowest level of truncal reflux and provide unobstructed access to the refluxing vein segment.

At the chosen site of percutaneous access, the ultrasound probe is positioned to obtain a stable gray-scale image of the vein in either the transverse or sagittal plane. Local anesthetic is often injected at the intended site of access. The author prefers the micropuncture system for gaining access while using ultrasound guidance. On real-time imaging, the needle is guided into the vein lumen and exchanged over a wire for a 4-Fr micropuncture sheath. The wire is then exchanged for an 0.035 wire, which will be used to upsize the sheath to a 6- or 7-Fr sheath using the modified Seldinger technique. With ultrasound guidance, the radiofrequency catheter or laser catheter is then advanced through the sheath, and the ultrasound probe is positioned in the groin to visualize the catheter tip, the SFJ, and the deep system. Using ultrasound guidance, the tip of the ablation catheter is placed 2 to 3 cm distal to the SFJ to minimize the chance of heat transmission into the femoral vein. Definitive positioning of the therapeutic catheter must be completed at this point before the administration of local anesthesia during the next stage of the procedure. Imaging artifacts from the tumescent anesthesia tends to impede visualization of the catheter tip, making it difficult to adjust its position.

Before tumescent anesthesia is begun, the patient should be placed in the Trendelenburg position to help empty the vein. Tumescent anesthesia is the infusion of a large volume of dilute local anesthetic. Although there are many recipes for tumescent solution, the main components are lidocaine, epinephrine, and sodium bicarbonate diluted with lactated Ringer solution or normal saline. During laser treatment and RFA procedures, tumescent anesthesia performs three functions: It provides anesthesia over a large area; it compresses the vein around the therapeutic catheter; and it acts as a protective barrier to prevent heating of nontarget tissues, including skin, nerves, arteries, and the deep veins.

For GSV procedures, the target of tumescent anesthesia is the saphenous sheath. When it is viewed in the transverse plane, the saphenous canal resembles an eye, and the ultrasound image is often referred to as the *saphenous eye*. Administration of tumescent anesthesia starts distally on the lower extremity and progresses proximally. Real-time ultrasound imaging guides a 21- to 25-gauge needle into the saphenous canal to deliver the tumescent anesthesia. When it is injected into the proper perivenous tissue plane, the tumescent anesthesia will track up and around the target vein. A long-axis ultrasound view gives the best image of fluid spreading up the saphenous canal. Multiple skin punctures and injections are performed until the vein has a 10-mm halo of tumescent anesthesia along its entire course, also known as the *target sign*. The targeted vein segment is then reinspected by ultrasound to ensure that the vein is compressed around the therapeutic catheter and adequately separated from the overlying skin.

Radiofrequency energy or laser energy is then applied to the vein segment by activating and slowly withdrawing the therapeutic catheter. The specifics of retrograde pullback depend on the type of catheter. Radiofrequency energy involves a segmental pullback governed by hash marks on the catheter and a timed activation on the accompanying generator. Laser energy catheters are variable; some have a slow, continuous pullback, whereas others require a segmental pullback. Gray-scale ultrasound images can often detect steam bubbles generated by the laser fiber.

Regardless of the type of energy delivered, once the vein has been completely treated, the sheath and accompanying catheter are removed. Ultrasound imaging resumes, confirming the patency of the femoral vein as well as successful occlusion of the GSV. Color Doppler imaging is often the only way to assess patency at this point because of the distortion caused by the ablation and the surrounding tumescent anesthesia. It is also important to verify retrograde epigastric venous flow into the proximal segment of the GSV. This provides a "protective flush" of the GSV. It is believed by many venous experts that this flow pattern prevents postprocedural development of endovenous heat-induced thrombus (EHIT).

Postprocedural instructions vary by practitioner. The patient's extremity is usually wrapped in a layered compression dressing, or a 20- to 30-mm Hg compression stocking is applied. The patient is instructed to walk every hour until bed. Regular activity, except for vigorous cardiovascular exercise, can be resumed the following day. After a satisfactory postprocedural duplex examination, all activity restrictions are lifted.

Most venous specialists recommend a physical examination or duplex ultrasound examination 2 to 5 days after the procedure. The duplex ultrasound examination ensures that the deep venous system remains patent and confirms the ablation of the GSV. Reported rates of DVT within 30 days after endovenous ablation range from 0% to 4% after RFA and 0% to 3% after laser ablation.[15] Although the incidence of postablation DVT is extremely low, duplex ultrasound examination can detect thrombus in the proximal GSV that can extend into the common femoral vein. Dr. Lowell Kabnick coined the term *endovenous heat-induced thrombus (EHIT)* to describe this ultrasound finding. He classified EHIT into four different levels based on the size of the thrombus and its extension into the deep venous system.

The mechanism of EHIT formation remains unclear. General consensus assumes that heat-triggered thrombus in the GSV propagates into the SFJ and encroaches on the deep venous system. EHIT and acute DVT differ in their sonographic characteristics and natural history. EHIT becomes sonographically echogenic quickly (<24 hours), whereas acute DVT usually remains hypoechoic for several days after its initial detection. Although EHIT appears to have a low propensity to propagate or embolize, pulmonary embolism (PE) has been reported after venous ablation procedures. Follow-up ultrasound examinations usually demonstrate retraction or complete resolution of EHIT within 7 to 10 days. Given this benign natural history, most practitioners do not treat class 1 and class 2 EHIT. Class 3 EHIT, which involves partial, nonocclusive extension into the deep venous system, usually warrants anticoagulation therapy, the duration of which can vary on the basis of the physician's discretion. Because class 4 EHIT represents occlusive DVT, it requires a 3-month course of anticoagulation.

The choice of whether to use RFA or laser as the energy source for venous ablation procedures remains a matter of the physician's preference. Randomized prospective studies comparing the two techniques have detected few differences. Patients treated with laser ablation tended to have more discomfort in the very early postprocedural period; however, all other outcome variables were similar.[16,17]

Nonthermal Ablation and Future Modalities for Axial Vein Incompetence

Endovenous nonthermal ablation techniques include MOCA, CAC, and PEM. These techniques all require ultrasound guidance for vein access, but no tumescence is required. Given their ease of operation, the majority of these procedures are performed in an outpatient clinic setting. MOCA involves the use of a catheter that combines endovenous chemical veinous destruction with a rotating wire and infusion of liquid sclerosant that causes inflammation to achieve closure of the treated vein. Ultrasound-guided sclerotherapy (UGS) targeted at the refluxing axial veins has also been described. It is mostly used for closure of large tributaries or varicose veins of the axial veins. Specific details about sclerosant preparation are outside the scope of this chapter. To reduce the amount of sclerosant used, physician-compounded foam is sometimes used.

Injectable PEM, Varithena, was approved by the US Food and Drug Administration in 2013 as a form of chemical ablation used for treatment of incompetent superficial veins. Studies have shown that treatment with a single administration of up to 15 mL of PEM results in significant improvement in alleviating venous insufficiency symptoms and resolution of varicose veins.[18] An advantage of PEM is the ability to treat varicose veins and refluxing tributaries of the saphenous vein at the same time as the axial vein treatment because the drug travels cephalad and easily distributes to other vein branches.

For the treatment of refluxing axial veins, the author uses the sterile technique. Because there is minimal risk of nerve injury, the access site can be selected as distally as possible, ideally at the vein segment that feeds into other varicose veins. The author prefers the micropuncture system for gaining access while using ultrasound guidance. Once the micropuncture sheath is placed within the vein, an appropriate amount of PEM is withdrawn from the canister and given through the sheath at intervals of 1 to 2 cc per second until all the drugs have been delivered. Care must be taken to mitigate risks of DVT extension, which usually has an incidence between 1.5% and 3%. Various techniques have been proposed to reduce the risk of DVT from PEM injection, which include elevation of limb >45 degrees during injection, ultrasound visualization and digital occlusion of perforator veins, injection of sterile saline before treatment, compression of the SFJ during treatment, and compression of limb in elevated position. Limiting the amount of PEM used can also decrease the risk of proximal thrombus extension and overall DVT risk.[18] The patient is instructed to ambulate and resume normal daily activities after treatment. Compression to the treated lower extremity is recommended for 2 weeks after treatment. Ultrasound of the treated vein and deep venous system is performed 2 to 5 days after the procedure to ensure appropriate closure of the treated vein and assess for any DVT.[18]

CAC is another nonthermal ablation modality that has gained popularity in treating insufficient axial veins in recent years as studies have demonstrated its clinical efficacy in vein closure. It uses ultrasound guidance for placement of a catheter that delivers a measured dose of cyanoacrylate glue to seal the vein. The treated vein is closed by the glue initially and, over time, will fibrose to keep the lumen closed. Similar to injectable PEM, it does not require tumescence because of its nonthermal nature. Therefore, access at the distal GSV or SSV around the ankle can be easily established without concern of nerve injury with a micropuncture system under ultrasound guidance. The sheath is upsized to a 7-Fr sheath into which the catheter is advanced to the SFJ. Under ultrasound, the catheter is then pulled 3 cm distal to the junction, and glue is applied in small aliquots at 2- to 3-cm intervals while continuous manual compression with the ultrasound probe at the SFJ is applied to avoid embolization to the deep venous system. Care is taken to capture the catheter within the sheath before the entire system is removed from the patient to avoid extravasation of the adhesive into the surrounding subcutaneous tissue. Allergic reactions to the adhesive, ranging from mild inflammation to necrosis of surrounding tissues, have been reported in patients. To minimize this risk of adverse reaction, patients are surveyed before the procedure to ensure they do not have any prior history of allergies to cyanoacrylates glue.[19]

Treatment of Branch Varicosities

There are three techniques to treat secondary branch varicosities: conventional stab phlebectomy, powered phlebectomy (TriVex; InaVein, Lexington, MA), and foam sclerotherapy (described earlier).

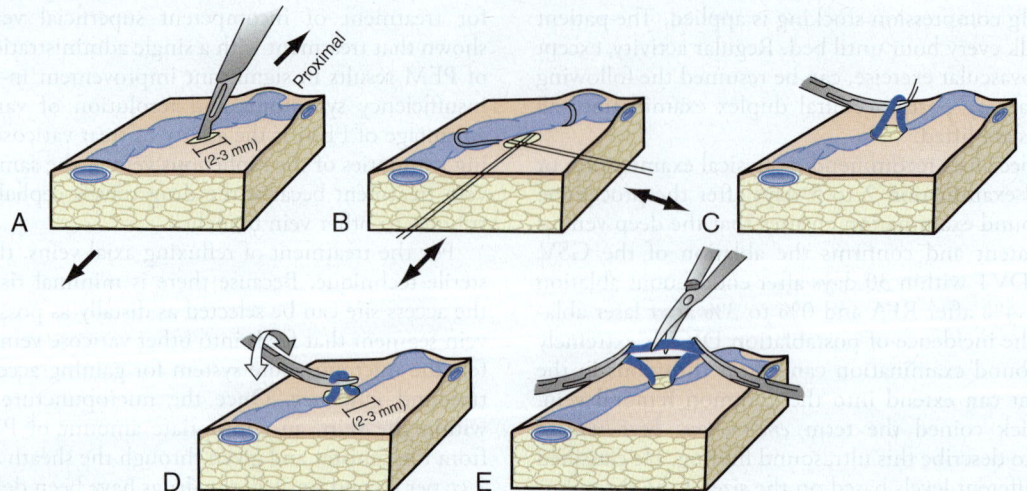

FIGURE 108.11 (A–E) Technique of ambulatory phlebectomy (otherwise known as *stab avulsions* of varicosities).

Stab Phlebectomy

Ambulatory phlebectomy is performed by the stab avulsion technique (Fig. 108.11). The patient's varicosities are marked after standing to allow optimal dilation and visualization of affected veins. Various anesthetic methods are used successfully, including local anesthesia with tumescence and IV sedation. First, 1-mm incisions are made along Langer skin lines, and the vein is retrieved with a hook. Continuous retraction of the vein segment affords maximal removal of the vein, and direct pressure is applied over the site after vein avulsion. Incisions are made at approximately 2-cm intervals. The extremity is wrapped with a layered compression dressing, and patients are instructed to ambulate on the day of surgery. The postoperative course is brief, and rarely do patients require more than acetaminophen or nonsteroidal antiinflammatory drugs for discomfort. Compression stockings are worn for 2 weeks after the procedure. Complications are unusual but include bleeding, infection, temporary or permanent paresthesia, and phlebitis from retained vein segments. There can be recurrence.

TriVex

Transilluminated powered phlebectomy (TriVex) is a modality that can be used to treat extensive secondary branch varicosities. The patient's varicosities are circumferentially marked preoperatively; in the operating room, 2-mm incisions are made at these boundary sites. These incisions permit placement of a transilluminator and resection device. The instruments are inserted through a subcutaneous plane, just deep to the varicosities. The transilluminator not only provides visualization of the veins but also administers tumescent anesthesia. The resector is a rotating blade that transects the veins and then removes them through a high-suction tubing system. The extremity is wrapped with a multilayer compression dressing, and the patient is discharged with instructions to ambulate hourly. The patient returns to the office for a dressing change within 48 hours and is usually changed to standard compression hose. Discomfort is minimal, and over-the-counter analgesia is sufficient. Complications are unusual but can include contained hematoma, bleeding, temporary or permanent paresthesia, and phlebitis.

Secondary Venous Insufficiency

Secondary venous insufficiency is usually caused by a deep venous thrombus. Clinical manifestations of secondary venous insufficiency usually present at a more advanced stage of disease with skin change or ulcerations. In addition, patients may describe venous claudication, or a bursting pain in the calf, that is classic for secondary venous insufficiency. Conservative treatment regimens are similar to those described in the preceding section for primary insufficiency; however, these patients may require a higher grade of compression for efficacy (30–40 mm Hg). Interventional treatment focuses on the superficial and deep systems. Diagnostic interrogation of the deep venous system must be more comprehensive in these patients to determine whether they are candidates for deep surgical or endovenous reconstruction.

Surgery for Deep Venous Insufficiency

While conservative therapy is being pursued or when ulcer healing is achieved, appropriate diagnostic studies generally reveal patterns of venous reflux or segments of venous occlusion so that specific therapy can be prescribed for the individual limb being evaluated. Imaging by duplex ultrasound suffices for the detection of reflux if the examination is carried out while the patient is standing. Such noninvasive imaging may prove the only testing necessary beyond the handheld, continuous-wave Doppler instrument if superficial venous ablation is contemplated.

Surprisingly, superficial reflux may be the only abnormality present in advanced chronic venous stasis. Correction goes a long way toward permanent relief of chronic venous dysfunction and its cutaneous effects. A significant proportion of patients with venous ulceration have normal function in the deep veins, and surgical treatment is a useful option that can definitively address the hemodynamic derangements. Maintaining that all venous ulcers are surgically incurable is not reasonable when data suggest that superficial vein surgery holds the potential for ameliorating venous hypertension. A randomized controlled trial comparing compression therapy and surgery for superficial reflux versus conservative management alone has revealed significant improvement in patients who had been treated by the surgical component.[17] Early success in patients with CVI, superficial valvular incompetence, and venous ulceration has been obtained with endovenous radiofrequency and laser therapies.

In 1938, Linton emphasized the importance of perforating veins, and their direct surgical interruption was advocated.[20,21] This has fallen into disfavor because of a high incidence of postoperative wound-healing complications. In recent years, as evolution in endovenous ablation continued, a radiofrequency stylet was developed that can be used for thermal ablation of the perforator veins in an outpatient setting that foregoes any need for incision and therefore avoids any possibility of wound-healing complications. The stylet is attached to needle and radiofrequency heating element. Using ultrasound guidance, the needle is introduced into the refluxing perforator vein, usually in the longitudinal view. The bioimpedance is tracked as the needle traverses the subcutaneous tissue because there is a change in bioimpedance as the needle is placed within the vein. When its location is confirmed, radiofrequency energy is transmitted, similar to RFA of axial veins. Studies have shown that RFA of perforator veins that are directly under ulcer beds has promising results in wound healing. UGS can also be used as an effective alternative in treating refluxing perforator veins in patients with venous ulcerations.

Chronic Venous Insufficiency

As the limbs of patients with severe CVI were studied accurately, the term PTS gave way to the term *CVI;* a link to platelet and monocyte aggregates in the circulation reflected the leukocytic infiltrate of the ankle skin, with its lipodermatosclerosis and healed and open ulcerations.[22] Data regarding leukocytes in CVI accumulated and were consistent, showing that the activation of leukocytes sequestered in the cutaneous microcirculation during venous stasis was important to the development of the skin changes of CVI. This is reflected in the finding of adhesion markers between leukocytes and endothelial cells and increased production of leukocyte degranulation enzymes and oxygen free radicals. Nevertheless, experimental evidence was still required for decisive proof of the leukocyte hypothesis.

CVI is a common condition with significant clinical sequelae. During the past two decades, the minimally invasive endovenous management of CVI and varicose veins has progressed remarkably and caused a rapid shift of treatment for these patients from the operating room to the outpatient office setting. Developing an understanding and appreciation of the pathophysiology behind the disorder allows the physician to appropriately diagnose and treat CVI with techniques that are both acceptable to the patient and generate successful outcomes.

DEEP VENOUS THROMBOSIS

Lower Extremity Deep Venous Thrombosis

Acute DVT is a major cause of morbidity and mortality in the hospitalized patient, particularly in the surgical patient. The triad of venous stasis, endothelial injury, and hypercoagulable state, first posited by Virchow in 1856, has held true more than a century and a half later. Acute DVT poses several risks and has significant morbid consequences. The thrombotic process initiated in a venous segment, in the absence of anticoagulation or in the presence of inadequate anticoagulation, can propagate to involve more proximal segments of the deep venous system, thus resulting in edema, pain, and immobility. The most dreaded sequela to acute DVT is that of PE, a condition of potentially lethal consequence. The late consequence of DVT, particularly of the iliofemoral veins, can be CVI and, ultimately, PTS as a result of valvular dysfunction in the presence of luminal obstruction.

Chronic venous thrombosis differs from acute DVT in that the thrombus has been present for greater than 4 weeks. Symptoms can be similar to acute DVT but may also present similar to

PTS. The thrombus starts to scar into the vessel wall. The patient's ultrasound findings are the main differentiation between acute and chronic DVT (see Table 108.1). Understanding the pathophysiology, standardizing protocols to prevent or reduce DVT, and instituting optimal treatment promptly are critical to reducing the incidence and morbidity of this unfortunately common condition.

Causes

Virchow's triad of stasis, hypercoagulable state, and endothelial injury is present in most surgical patients. It is also clear that increasing age places a patient at greater risk, with those older than 65 years representing a higher-risk population. In addition, many epidemiologic studies have reviewed additional factors that place patients at risk for the development of DVT, including malignant disease, increased body mass index, increasing age (especially patients >60 years of age), pregnancy, oral contraceptive use, prolonged immobilization, surgery, trauma, tobacco use, prior DVT, IVC filter placement, inflammatory bowel disease, and heart failure.[23]

Stasis

Labeled fibrinogen studies in patients and autopsy studies have demonstrated convincingly that the soleal sinuses are the most common sites of initiation of venous thrombosis. The stasis may contribute to the endothelial cellular layer contacting activated platelets and procoagulant factors, thereby leading to DVT. Stasis, in and of itself, has never been shown to be a causative factor for DVT. External compression can also be a contributing factor to stasis within a vein as a result of tumors or conditions such as May-Thurner syndrome or aneurysm of the iliac artery.

Hypercoagulable States

Our knowledge of hypercoagulable conditions continues to improve, but it is still in its early stages. The standard array of conditions screened for in searching for a hypercoagulable state is listed in Box 108.1. If any of these conditions is identified, a treatment regimen of anticoagulation is instituted for life, unless specific contraindications exist. It is generally appreciated that the postoperative patient, after major surgery, is predisposed to the formation of DVT. After major operations, large amounts of tissue factor may be released into the bloodstream from damaged tissues. Tissue factor is a potent procoagulant expressed on the leukocyte cell surface and in a soluble form in the bloodstream. Increases in platelet count, adhesiveness, changes in coagulation cascade, and endogenous fibrinolytic activity result from physiologic stress, such as major operation or trauma, and have been associated with an increased risk for thrombosis.

BOX 108.1 Hypercoagulable States

- Factor V Leiden mutation
- Prothrombin gene mutation
- Protein C deficiency
- Protein S deficiency
- Antithrombin III deficiency
- Homocysteinemia
- Antiphospholipid syndrome
- Lupus antibody
- Anticardiolipin antibody
- COVID-19 infection

Endothelial Injury

It has been clearly established that venous thrombosis occurs in veins that are distant from the site of operation; for example, it is well known that patients undergoing total hip replacement frequently develop contralateral lower extremity DVT.

In a series of experiments, animal models of abdominal and total hip operations were used to study the possibility of venous endothelial damage distant from the operative site. In these studies, jugular veins were excised after the animals were perfusion fixed. These experiments demonstrated that endothelial damage occurred after abdominal operations and was more severe after hip operations. There were multiple microtears noted within the valve cusps that resulted in exposure of the subendothelial matrix. The exact mechanisms whereby this injury at a distant site occurs and which mediators, cellular or humoral, are responsible are not clearly understood, but that the injury occurs is evident from these and other studies.

Complications

There are short- and long-term complications and sequela of DVT. This is an overview of complications associated with DVT.

Pulmonary Embolism

The most dreaded and potentially lethal complication of DVT is PE, which occurs when untreated distal thrombus travels into the pulmonary arteries and causes an occlusion. The symptoms of PE, ranging from dyspnea to chest pain and hypoxia, are nonspecific and require a high index of suspicion. These occlusions can become severe enough to cause pulmonary hypertension and, eventually, acute right ventricular heart strain and failure. If the patients with PE survive, they are at risk of chronic pulmonary hypertension. More detailed information on this condition is provided in Chapter 114.

Phlegmasia Alba/Cerulea Dolens

Phlegmasia alba and cerulea dolens occur in the setting of acute extensive DVT and are characterized by marked swelling, pain, and blanching (Alba) or cyanosis (Cerulea) of the extremity. The swelling becomes so severe that it causes an acute limb ischemia presentation. This is a rare occurrence, but it almost always affects the lower extremity. Patients will have acute iliofemoral DVT and symptoms of advanced disease in addition to swelling, pain, and discoloration; motor or sensory loss; and pulselessness as a late finding. Most often, patients receive an urgent surgical intervention to decrease the thrombus burden as well as fasciotomies for compartment syndrome. These interventions are discussed in the Surgical Management section.

Postthrombotic Syndrome

PTS is a common and unfortunate manifestation of DVT. It occurs in 20% to 50% of patients after a documented episode of DVT. The clinical presentation includes chronic edema, pain, and venous claudication. Venous ulcerations can occur. Risk factors for the development of PTS include persistent leg symptoms for months after the acute episode of DVT, an anatomically extensive DVT involving the iliofemoral system, recurrent ipsilateral DVTs, and a prolonged state of subtherapeutic anticoagulation for DVT. Unfortunately, treatment remains supportive, and compression therapy, elevation, and ambulation remain the mainstay of treatment for PTS.

Diagnostic Considerations
Incidence

Venous thromboembolism (VTE), which includes DVT and PE, affects about 900,000 people each year in the United States. About one-quarter of patients with VTE have sudden death without any prior symptoms. The incidence increases with increasing age, with an incidence of 0.5%/100,000 at 80 years of age. More than two-thirds of these patients have DVT alone, and the rest have evidence of PE. The recurrence rate with anticoagulation has been noted to be 6% to 7% in the ensuing 6 months. COVID-19 has become the newest addition to the etiologies for DVT. Research is ongoing, but studies suggest patients remain at increased risk for DVT up to 1 year after infection.[24]

In the United States, PE causes 60,000 to 100,000 deaths annually. A 28-day case-fatality rate of 9.4% after first-time DVT and a rate of 15.1% after first-time pulmonary thromboembolism have been observed. Aside from PE, secondary CVI (resulting from DVT) is significant in terms of cost, morbidity, and lifestyle limitations.[25] If the consequences of DVT in terms of PE and CVI are to be prevented, the prevention, diagnosis, and treatment of DVT must be optimized.

Clinical Diagnosis

The diagnosis of acute DVT requires a high index of suspicion. Most physicians are familiar with Homan sign, which refers to pain in the calf on dorsiflexion of the foot. Although the absence of this sign is not a reliable indicator of the absence of venous thrombus, the presence of Homan sign should prompt one to attempt to confirm the diagnosis. The extent of venous thrombosis in the lower extremity is an important factor in the manifestation of symptoms. For example, most calf thrombi may be asymptomatic unless there is proximal propagation. This is one reason that radiolabeled fibrinogen testing demonstrates a higher incidence of DVT than studies using imaging modalities. Only 40% of patients with venous thrombosis have any clinical manifestations of the condition.

Major venous thrombosis involving the iliofemoral venous system results in a massively swollen leg, with pitting edema (Fig. 108.12), pain, and blanching, a condition known as *phlegmasia alba dolens*. With further progression of disease, there may be such massive edema that arterial inflow can be compromised. This condition results in a painful blue leg, a condition called *phlegmasia cerulea dolens,* as mentioned earlier. With this evolution of the condition, venous gangrene can develop unless flow is restored.

Imaging Studies and Laboratory Tests
Duplex Ultrasound

The gold standard for the diagnosis of DVT is duplex ultrasound, a modality that combines Doppler ultrasound and color flow imaging. The advantage of this test is that it is noninvasive, comprehensive, and without any risk of reaction to contrast angiography. Doppler ultrasound is based on the principle of the impairment of an accelerated flow signal caused by an intraluminal thrombus. A detailed interrogation begins at the calf with imaging of the tibial veins and then proximally over the popliteal and femoral veins. A properly done examination evaluates flow with distal compression, which results in augmentation of flow, and with proximal compression, which should interrupt flow. If any segment of the venous system being examined fails to demonstrate augmentation on compression, venous thrombosis is suspected.

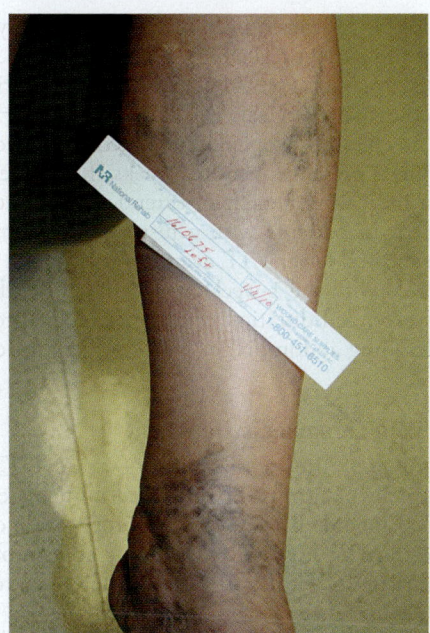

FIGURE 108.12 Edema. Note the loss of ankle definition.

Real-time B-mode ultrasonography with color flow imaging has improved the sensitivity and specificity of ultrasound scanning. With color flow duplex imaging, blood flow can be imaged in the presence of a partially occluding thrombus. The probe is also used to compress the vein. A normal vein is easily compressed, whereas in the presence of a thrombus, there is resistance to compression. In addition, the chronicity of the thrombus can be evaluated on the basis of its imaging characteristics, namely, increased echogenicity and heterogeneity.

Duplex imaging is significantly more sensitive than indirect physiologic testing. There are many advantages associated with duplex ultrasound: noninvasiveness, portability, and no need for a contrast agent. However, there are significant disadvantages as well; these include operator-dependent variability of skill, body habitus, and suboptimal visualization in regions such as the lower pelvis.

Venography

Injection of contrast material into the venous system has been long considered the most accurate method of confirming DVT and its location. It is the most sensitive and specific of all methods. However, it is an invasive test. The superficial venous system has to be occluded with a tourniquet, and the veins in the foot are injected for visualization of the deep venous system. Potential complications include risks of IV administration of contrast material and bleeding complications at the access sites. As a result, this technique has been replaced by less invasive modalities. Recently, the additional use of intravascular ultrasound (IVUS) has become more popular. This method provides a 360-degree two-dimensional gray-scale ultrasound image of lumen and vessel wall structures.[26]

Fibrin and Fibrinogen Assays

Fibrin and fibrinogen levels can be determined by measuring the degradation of intravascular fibrin. The D-dimer test measures cross-linked degradation products, which is a surrogate of plasmin's activity on fibrin. In combination with clinical evaluation and assessment, the sensitivity exceeds 90% to 95%. The negative

predictive value is 99.3% for proximal evaluation and 98.6% for distal evaluation. In the postoperative patient, D-dimer is causally elevated because of surgery, and as such, a positive result of the D-dimer assay for evaluating for DVT is not useful. However, a negative D-dimer test result in patients with suspected DVT has a high negative predictive value, ranging from 97% to 99%.[27]

Computed Tomographic Venography

CTV has been shown to be a fast, high-spatial-resolution technique that can be used when looking for extension of thrombus or any other anatomic anomalies or compression that could be contributing to the etiology of the DVT, especially in the abdomen when looking at the iliac veins and IVC. The negatives include radiation exposure, complications associated with contrast material, more invasiveness compared with duplex because of the use of IV contrast material, and inaccuracy of visualization in the lower extremities as a result of dilution of contrast material.[28]

Magnetic Resonance Venography

With major advances in imaging technology, MRV has shown benefits in imaging for proximal venous disease. The cost and the issue of patient tolerance because of claustrophobia limit its widespread application, but this has been changing. It is a useful test for imaging the iliac veins and IVC, an area where the use of duplex ultrasound is limited. MRV is less invasive than conventional venography and is able to directly visualize the thrombus.

Impedance Plethysmography

Impedance plethysmography measures the change in venous capacitance and rate of emptying of the venous volume on temporary occlusion and release of the occlusion of the venous system. A cuff is inflated around the upper thigh until the electrical signal has plateaued. When the cuff is deflated, there is usually rapid outflow and reduction of volume. With a venous thrombosis, one notes a prolongation of the outflow wave. It is not useful clinically for the detection of calf venous thrombosis or in patients with prior venous thrombosis.

Prophylaxis

The patient who has undergone major abdominal or orthopedic surgery, has sustained major trauma, or has prolonged immobility (>3 days) represents an elevated risk for the development of VTE. The specific risk factor analysis and epidemiologic studies detailing the causes of VTE are beyond the scope of this chapter. The reader is referred to a more extensive analysis of this problem.[23] The methods of prophylaxis can be mechanical or pharmacologic.

Mechanical Prophylaxis

The simplest method is for the patient to walk. Activation of the calf pump mechanism is an effective means of prophylaxis, as evidenced by the fact that few active people without underlying risk factors develop venous thrombosis. A patient who is expected to be up and walking within 24 to 48 hours is at low risk for development of venous thrombosis. The practice of having a patient out of bed and into a chair is one of the most thrombogenic positions that could be ordered for a patient. Sitting in a chair, with the legs in a dependent position, causes venous pooling, which, in the postoperative milieu, could easily be a predisposing factor for the development of thromboembolism.

The most common method of surgical prophylaxis has traditionally revolved around compression stockings and SCDs, which periodically compress the calves and essentially replicate the calf bellows mechanism. This has clearly reduced the incidence of VTE in the surgical patient. The most likely mechanism for the efficacy of this device is prevention of venous stasis. Some studies have suggested that fibrinolytic activity is systemically enhanced by an SCD. However, this has not been definitively established because a considerable number of studies have demonstrated no enhancement of fibrinolytic activity, and SCDs are sometimes poorly tolerated by patients.[29]

Pharmacologic Prophylaxis

In the hospitalized patient, the most common form of thrombo-prophylaxis is fractionated low-molecular-weight heparin (LMWH) and unfractionated low-dose heparin (UFH). Various studies have revealed the efficacy of LMWH for the prophylaxis and treatment of VTE.[30–32] LMWH inhibits factor Xa and IIa activity, with the ratio of anti–factor Xa to anti–factor IIa activity ranging from 1:1 to 4:1. LMWH has a longer plasma half-life and significantly higher bioavailability. The consistent bioavailability and clearance of LMWH do not require monitoring of factor Xa levels, which facilitates use by the patient. Dosing is merely based on the patient's weight. There is a more predictable anticoagulant response than with UFH. No laboratory monitoring is necessary because the partial thromboplastin time (PTT) is unaffected. However, anti–factor Xa levels have been used to monitor its efficacy on a daily basis, and dosing can be adjusted to achieve a therapeutic level.[33]

Various analyses, including a major meta-analysis,[30] have shown that LMWH results in equivalent if not better efficacy than UFH, with significantly fewer complications, such as a lower incidence of heparin-induced thrombocytopenia and a lower likelihood of osteoporosis. It was first thought that LMWH results in less bleeding than unfractionated heparin, but no clinical observations have confirmed this. This property may be more a function of dose than an intrinsic drug action. UFH remains safer for patients with renal impairment because of the higher risk of bleeding events.[34] The dosage traditionally used was 5000 units of UFH every 12 hours. However, analyses of trials comparing placebo versus fixed-dose heparin have shown that the stated dose of 5000 units subcutaneously every 12 hours is no more effective than placebo.[32] When subcutaneous heparin is used on a dosing regimen of every 8 hours rather than every 12 hours, there is a reduction in the development of VTE.

Comparison of LMWH with mechanical prophylaxis has demonstrated the superiority of LMWH for reduction of the development of venous thromboembolic disease.[31,34] Prospective trials evaluating LMWH in head-injured and trauma patients have also proven the safety of LMWH, with no increase in intracranial bleeding or major bleeding at other sites.[35] In addition, LMWH shows a significant reduction in the development of VTE compared with other methods. Thus, LMWH is considered the optimal method of prophylaxis for moderate- and high-risk patients without any contraindications.

VTE is a common cause of perioperative morbidity and mortality. The CHEST guideline separates patients' risk of VTE based on their risk stratification.[36] In patients with very low risk for VTE (<0.5%), the guideline recommends early ambulation without need for pharmacologic or mechanical prophylaxis. For patients at low risk of VTE (~1.5%), mechanical prophylaxis is recommended over chemical prophylaxis or a combination of both. Moderate-risk VTE patients (~3%) who are undergoing surgery are recommended chemical prophylaxis, including

LMWH or UFH. However, only mechanical prophylaxis is recommended if the patient has a high risk of bleeding. For patients with a high risk for VTE (~6%) who are not at high risk of bleeding, pharmacologic prophylaxis with LMWH or UFH, in combination with mechanical prophylaxis, is recommended. Although the risk of VTE is present for several weeks after surgery, there are no clear data indicating benefit of extended pharmacologic prophylaxis, except in patients with a history of abdominal cancer surgery, who showed fewer VTE events in the 4-week prophylaxis group compared with the 1-week group. Therefore, the guideline recommends extended duration of pharmacologic prophylaxis in patients undergoing abdominal or pelvic surgery for cancer.[36]

Treatment

Acute Deep Vein Thrombosis Treatment

Anticoagulation. After a diagnosis of acute DVT has been made, a treatment plan must be instituted immediately. Complications of DVT include PE via proximal propagation of thrombus in up to one-third of hospitalized patients and chronic PTS, as mentioned earlier. In addition, untreated lower extremity DVT carries a 30% recurrence rate.

Any venous thrombosis involving the femoropopliteal system is treated with full anticoagulation. Traditionally, the treatment of DVT has centered around heparin treatment to maintain the PTT at 60 to 80 seconds, followed by warfarin therapy to obtain an international normalized ratio (INR) of 2.5 to 3.0. If unfractionated heparin is used, it is important to use a nomogram-based dosing therapy. The incidence of recurrent VTE increases if the time to therapeutic anticoagulation is prolonged. Therefore, it is important to reach therapeutic levels within 24 hours. An initial bolus of 80 units/kg or 5000 units IV bolus is administered, followed by 18 units/kg/h. The rate is dependent on a target PTT corresponding to an anti–factor Xa level of 0.3 to 0.7 unit/mL.[32] The PTT needs to be checked 6 hours after any change in heparin dosing. If warfarin is the long-term drug of choice, warfarin is started on the same day. The INR goal for therapeutic warfarin in the case of DVT is 2 to 3. If warfarin is initiated without heparin, the risk for a transient hypercoagulable state exists because protein C and protein S levels fall before the other vitamin K–dependent factors are depleted. With the advent of LMWH, it is no longer necessary to admit the patient for IV heparin therapy. It is now accepted practice to administer LMWH on an outpatient basis as a bridge to warfarin therapy, which is also monitored on an outpatient basis.

Recently, direct oral anticoagulants (DOACs) or novel oral anticoagulants (NOACs), which include direct thrombin inhibitor (dabigatran) and factor Xa inhibitors (rivaroxaban, apixaban, and edoxaban), have become a more attractive oral anticoagulant alternative to warfarin. Recent studies suggested that DOAC treatment, compared with warfarin, is associated with a lower risk of recurrent VTE and a lower risk of bleeding events.[37] DOACs also do not require a transitional period for initiation or outpatient INR monitoring.

The recommended duration of anticoagulant therapy is 3 to 6 months for the first DVT. The recurrence rate is the same with 3 versus 6 months. However, most practitioners will recommend 3 months of anticoagulation if there is a known reversible cause for the DVT, such as an injury, and 6 months if there is no known cause for DVT. If the patient has a known hypercoagulable state or has recurrent episodes of DVT, lifetime anticoagulation is required in the absence of contraindications. Repeat imaging after the course of treatment to establish a new baseline or to evaluate for change in the thrombus burden is physician dependent.

Warfarin is teratogenic, and DOACs are not recommended during pregnancy. In the case of the pregnant patient with venous thrombosis, LMWH is the treatment of choice; this is continued through delivery and can be continued postpartum, as indicated. Patients with a known history of cancer are typically treated with therapeutic LMWH because there have been efficacy studies showing superiority compared with warfarin. DOACs can also be prescribed for this population because DOACs were found to be noninferior to LMWH in a recent study for up to 6 months after diagnosis.[37]

Surgical management

Inferior vena cava filter. Adequate anticoagulation is usually effective for stabilizing venous thrombosis, but if a patient has contraindications to treatment with anticoagulation or if a patient develops propagating thrombus or PE in the presence of adequate anticoagulation, a vena cava filter is indicated. The general indications for a vena cava filter are listed in Box 108.2. Modern filters are placed percutaneously over a guidewire and are retrievable. The majority of IVC filters are placed infrarenal. In rare circumstances, such as in pregnancy, IVC filters are placed suprarenal. There are also superior vena cava filters for prevention of upper extremity DVT propagation.

Device-related complications are wound hematoma, migration of the device into the pulmonary artery, and caval occlusion caused by trapping of a large embolus. In the last situation, the dramatic hypotension that accompanies acute caval occlusion can be mistaken for a massive PE. The distinction between the hypovolemia of caval occlusion and the right-sided heart failure from PE can be made by measuring filling pressures of the right side of the heart. The treatment of caval occlusion is volume resuscitation. Although they are generally safe, IVC filters are not without risk and significant morbidity. Therefore, permanent placement of a caval filter is not generally recommended. Retrievable filters are mainly in use and are removed as soon as the patient has no contraindications to anticoagulation or months later. Complications with retained filters have been reported, including migration; penetration of legs into structures around the IVC, including the small intestine, aorta, and spine; and infection. For these reasons, recent authors recommend informing all patients with IVC filters that they must return for evaluation of the need for ongoing filtration and removal of filters when no contraindication to removal is present.[38,39]

Catheter-directed thrombolysis and percutaneous thrombectomy. The advent of thrombolysis and percutaneous thrombectomy has resulted in increased interest in percutaneous interventions for DVT. The purported benefit is preservation of valve function, with a subsequently lesser chance for development of PTS. In the Acute

Venous Thrombosis: Thrombus Removal With Adjunctive Catheter Directed Thrombolysis (ATTRACT) trial, which compared the outcomes of patients with DVT who underwent catheter-directed thrombolysis (CDT) to standard therapy, there was no significant difference in the percentage of patients who developed PTS. However, CDT reduced the severity of PTS and decreased the severity of leg pain and swelling within the first month after treatment, but it increased major bleeding within 10 days of treatment compared with standard therapy alone. It is concluded that selective use to reduce PTS severity may be justified in patients who have a higher baseline risk for PTS. Quality-of-life improvement from baseline did not differ between the groups at 24 months. Based on the result of the ATTRACT trial, CDT may be recommended in patients with a more proximal, iliofemoral involvement and moderate to severe symptoms.[40]

Lately, percutaneous thrombectomy has become a more popular treatment option for percutaneous thrombolysis. With this procedure, the surgeon uses a percutaneous thrombectomy device via suction or mechanically to remove thrombus directly. The benefits of this procedure include decreased bleeding risk as well as immediate relief of thrombus burden. If a surgical option is pursued, treatment with anticoagulation is still recommended.

Open surgical venous thrombectomy. In the present day, open venous thrombectomy is reserved for patients who have phlegmasia with acute limb ischemia or have failed percutaneous intervention. This procedure is done by open cutdown to the vein and the use of Fogarty balloon catheters to extract thrombus. Extra precautions should be taken with proximal lesions because thrombus can dislodge and travel to the lungs. Temporary filters during the procedure can be placed in the IVC for prevention. After the thrombus has successfully been removed, traditionally, an arteriovenous fistula is surgically created to theoretically keep the vein patent.

Chronic Deep Vein Thrombosis Treatment

The chronic thrombus is composed of mainly collagen and little fibrin. Therefore, thrombolytics are of very little use.

Conservative treatment. The mainstay of treatment for chronic DVT is conservative therapy. Recommendations for symptoms are compression and elevation. Patients sometimes develop ulcerations as a result of dysfunction of the valves and treatment, which is discussed in detail earlier in the Deep Venous Insufficiency section.

Surgical treatment. Chronic proximal venous occlusion of the iliofemoral system is a challenging clinical problem. No treatment is necessary for finding asymptomatic chronic DVT. For symptomatic chronic DVT, the presentation is variable, and there is no reliable diagnostic modality to measure proximal iliofemoral venous stenosis and assess outflow obstruction accurately. The pathophysiologic mechanism is often a combination of primary and secondary venous insufficiency. Endovascular reconstruction removes the need for surgical bypass and has been used successfully. Recanalization of the occluded iliac vein is performed endovascularly. Balloon dilation of the lesion is then performed, and if needed, a stent is placed across the dilated segment. Excellent results have been achieved, thereby obviating an open surgical procedure. Endovascular iliac therapy has evolved to become first-line therapy for iliac occlusions.

Upper Extremity Deep Venous Thrombosis—Venous Thoracic Outlet Syndrome

Upper extremity DVT is much less common than its lower extremity counterpart, constituting only approximately 5% of all documented DVTs. Although not as common, it is a serious

---

BOX 108.2   Indications for an Inferior Vena Cava Filter

- Recurrent thromboembolism despite adequate anticoagulation
- Acute deep venous thrombosis in a patient with contraindications to anticoagulation
- Complications of anticoagulation
- Propagating iliofemoral venous thrombus on anticoagulation
- Prophylactic placement in high-risk trauma patients (orthopedic, spinal cord patients) who have short-term-duration contraindication to prophylactic anticoagulation

problem; PE occurs in up to one-third of all patients with an upper extremity DVT. *Upper extremity DVT* usually refers to thrombosis of the axillary or subclavian veins. The syndrome can be divided into two categories: primary idiopathic and secondary.

Primary causes include Paget-Schroetter syndrome and idiopathic upper extremity DVT. Patients with Paget-Schroetter syndrome develop effort thrombosis of the extremity caused by compression of the subclavian vein, the venous component of thoracic outlet syndrome. A classic presentation involves a young athlete who uses the upper extremity in a repetitive motion, such as swimming, which causes repetitive extrinsic compression of the subclavian vein. In these patients, anatomic anomalies such as a cervical rib or myofascial bands cause venous compression. Plain films are one of the first diagnostic tests used to confirm thoracic outlet syndrome. Treatment with initial thrombolysis/thrombectomy followed by thoracic outlet decompression (anterior and middle scalene resection, first rib resection) with possible balloon angioplasty, stenting, or surgical reconstruction of the axillary and subclavian veins is the standard of care.

Idiopathic upper extremity DVT is sometimes eventually attributed to an occult malignant neoplasm; therefore, a diagnosis of idiopathic upper extremity DVT warrants evaluation for an undetected malignant neoplasm. Secondary causes of upper extremity DVT are more common. These include an indwelling central venous catheter, pacemaker, thrombophilia, and malignant disease.

Classic findings on physical examination include unilateral swelling, pain, extremity discomfort, erythema, and a palpable cord. Diagnosis is confirmed by duplex ultrasonography. Because the clavicle obscures the midportion of the subclavian vein, venography or magnetic resonance venography may be required; these are second-line imaging modalities.

Treatment

Treatment of upper extremity DVT is essentially the same as that for lower extremity DVT, which involves anticoagulation therapy. Therapeutic dosing parameters are the same as for lower extremity DVT. Treatment should be for 3 months and consist of heparin or LMWH plus warfarin for at least 3 months or DOACs. Long-term complications of upper extremity DVT include recurrence and PTS. Thrombolysis has not been shown to decrease long-term manifestations from upper extremity DVT; thus, PTS is treated with extremity elevation and graduated elastic compression.[41,42]

SUPERFICIAL VENOUS THROMBOPHLEBITIS

SVT is a common disorder diagnosed in the hospital and outpatient setting. Cardinal signs of SVT are rubor, calor, dolor, and tumor, describing a linear, erythematous, tender, and swollen lesion along the course of a superficial vein. The condition is self-limiting in the majority of patients, and as result of the inflammatory reaction, the superficial vein becomes a palpable fibrotic cord. In hospitalized patients, SVT is usually caused by an indwelling catheter. In the clinic, patients with thrombophlebitis report common predisposing risk factors, such as recent surgery, recent childbirth, venous stasis, varicose veins, or IV drug use. Patients who deny any of these factors may be classified with idiopathic thrombophlebitis. In these cases, care must be taken to ensure that the patient does not harbor an occult hypercoagulable state or occult malignant disease. In 1876, Trousseau identified the phenomenon of migratory thrombophlebitis and malignant disease, particularly involving the tail of the pancreas. Mondor

disease involves SVT of the superficial veins of the breast. Diagnosis of SVT can be easily made by physical examination of an erythematous palpable cord coursing along a superficial vein, usually located along the lower extremities. Duplex ultrasonography is recommended to confirm diagnosis and if there is suspicion of possible proximal propagation into the deep venous system. With this diagnosis of DVT, anticoagulation is indicated. If, however, thrombus abuts the SFJ, treatment of this more elusive condition is controversial. Some authors recommend serial ultrasound examinations, whereas others recommend anticoagulation; another alternative is operative ligation at the junction.

The initial treatment of localized noncomplicated thrombophlebitis involves conservative therapy, which consists of antiinflammatory medication and compression stockings. The recommended treatment of an SVT involving a ≥5-cm GSV segment is a midtreatment dose of LMWH (enoxaparin 60 mg daily subcutaneously) or fondaparinux (2.5 mg daily subcutaneously) for a 6-week period. A similar treatment is recommended if the thrombophlebitis ascends the GSV within 3 cm from the SFJ. Results from the Superficial Vein Thrombosis Treated for 45 Days With Rivaroxaban Versus Fondaparinux (SURPRISE) trial have shown noninferiority of rivaroxaban at the dosage of 10 mg daily compared with fondaparinux (2.5 mg daily subcutaneously) for 45 days in the treatment of SVT. When thrombophlebitis involves clusters of varicosities, particularly in the lower extremities, excision may be indicated. Selective removal of the entire vein along its course is indicated only in the rare case of suppurative septic thrombophlebitis after all other sources of sepsis have been excluded.

CONCLUSION

This is just a small proportion of the spectrum of venous diseases and disorders, which are widespread and diverse, providing surgeons who fully understand the unique physiology of veins a rewarding and rich field for patient care and future investigation.

SELECTED REFERENCES

Bergan JJ, Pascarella L, Schmid-Schönbein GW. Pathogenesis of primary chronic venous disease: insights from animal models of venous hypertension. *J Vasc Surg.* 2008;47:183-192.

This article provides a comprehensive review of the known aspects of venous hypertension pathophysiology.

Gloviczki P, Lawrence P, Suman W. The 2022 Society for Vascular Surgery, American Venous Forum, and American Vein and Lymphatic Society clinical practice guidelines for the management of varicose veins of the lower extremities. Part I. Duplex scanning and treatment of superficial truncal reflux. Society for Vascular Surgery guidelines. *J Vasc Surg Venous Lymphat Disord.* 2023;11(2): 231-261.e6.

This is the most up-to-date practice guideline for management of venous disease.

Leopardi D, Hoggan BL, Fitridge RA, et al. Systematic review of treatments for varicose veins. *Ann Vasc Surg.* 2009;23:264-276.

This article provides a systematic overview of current treatment modalities for superficial venous disease.

Lurie F, Passman M, Meisner M, et al. The 2020 update of the CEAP classification system and reporting standards. *J Vasc Surg Venous Lymphat Disord.* 2020;8(3):342-352.

This article is the most updated version of CEAP classification and reporting standards, which are internationally accepted.

The full reference list appears on Elsevier eBooks+.

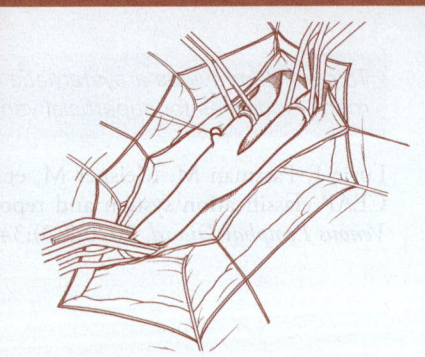

The Lymphatics

Jonathan R. Thompson and Iraklis I. Pipinos

EMBRYOLOGY AND ANATOMY

The primordial lymphatic system is first seen during the sixth week of development in the form of lymph sacs located next to the jugular veins. During the eighth week, the cisterna chyli forms just dorsal to the aorta, and at the same time, two additional lymphatic sacs corresponding to the iliofemoral vascular pedicles begin forming. Communicating channels connecting the lymph sacs, which will become the thoracic duct, develop during the ninth week.

From this primordial lymphatic system sprout endothelial buds that grow with the venous system to form the peripheral lymphatic plexus (Fig. 109.1). Failure of one of the initial jugular lymphatic sacs to develop proper connections and drainage with the lymphatic system and, subsequently, the venous system may produce focal lymph cysts (cavernous lymphangiomas), also known as *cystic hygromas.*[1] Similarly, failure of embryologic remnants of lymphatic tissues to connect to efferent channels leads to the development of cystic lymphatic formations (simple capillary lymphangiomas) that, depending on their location, are classified as truncal, mesenteric, intestinal, and retroperitoneal lymphangiomas. Hypoplasia or failure of development of drainage channels connecting the lymphatic systems of extremities to the main primordial lymphatic system of the torso may result in primary lymphedema of the extremities.

Lymphangiogenesis appears to be regulated by the vascular endothelial growth factors C and D (VEGF-C, VEGF-D); their receptor, VEGFR-3; and their binding protein, neuropilin 2 (Nrp2). Consistent with these findings, Nrp2-deficient mice have lymphatic hypoplasia, and heterozygous inactivating mutation of VEGFR-3 is found in Chy mice, an animal model of primary lymphedema, which appears to be the underlying problem in patients with Milroy disease (congenital familial lymphedema).[2] A number of additional genes have recently been found to be related to lymphatic disorders.[3] The best studied at this point are the gene for the forkhead family

transcription factor FOXC2 (responsible for the hereditary lymphedema-distichiasis syndrome) and the gene for the transcription factor SOX18 (related to recessive and dominant forms of hypotrichosis-lymphedema-telangiectasia). As more causal genes are identified, the possibility arises for a classification built on patient phenotypes for which the gene is known.[4] Receptor activity-modifying protein 1 (RAMP1) has also been identified as an important factor for lymphangiogenesis. RAMP1 knockout mice have greater amounts of surgery-associated lymphedema compared with controls. This is thought to occur from a lack of attenuation of proinflammatory macrophage recruitment in the RAMP1 knockout mice.[5]

FUNCTION AND STRUCTURE

The lymphatic system is composed of three elements: (1) the initial or terminal lymphatic capillaries, which absorb lymph; (2) the collecting vessels, which serve primarily as conduits for lymph transport; and (3) the lymph nodes, which are interposed in the pathway of the conducting vessels, filtering the lymph and serving a primary immunologic role.

The terminal lymphatics have special structural characteristics that allow entry not only of large macromolecules but even of cells and microbes. Their most important structural feature is a high porosity resulting from a very small number of tight junctions between endothelial cells, a limited and incomplete basement membrane, and anchoring filaments (4–10 nm) tethering the interstitial matrix to the endothelial cells. These filaments, once the turgor of the tissue increases, are able to pull on the endothelial cells and essentially introduce large gaps between them, which then allow very low-resistance influx of interstitial fluid and macromolecules in the lymphatic channels. The collecting vessels ascend alongside the primary blood vessels of the organ or limb, pass through the regional lymph nodes, and drain into the main lymph channels of the torso. These channels eventually empty

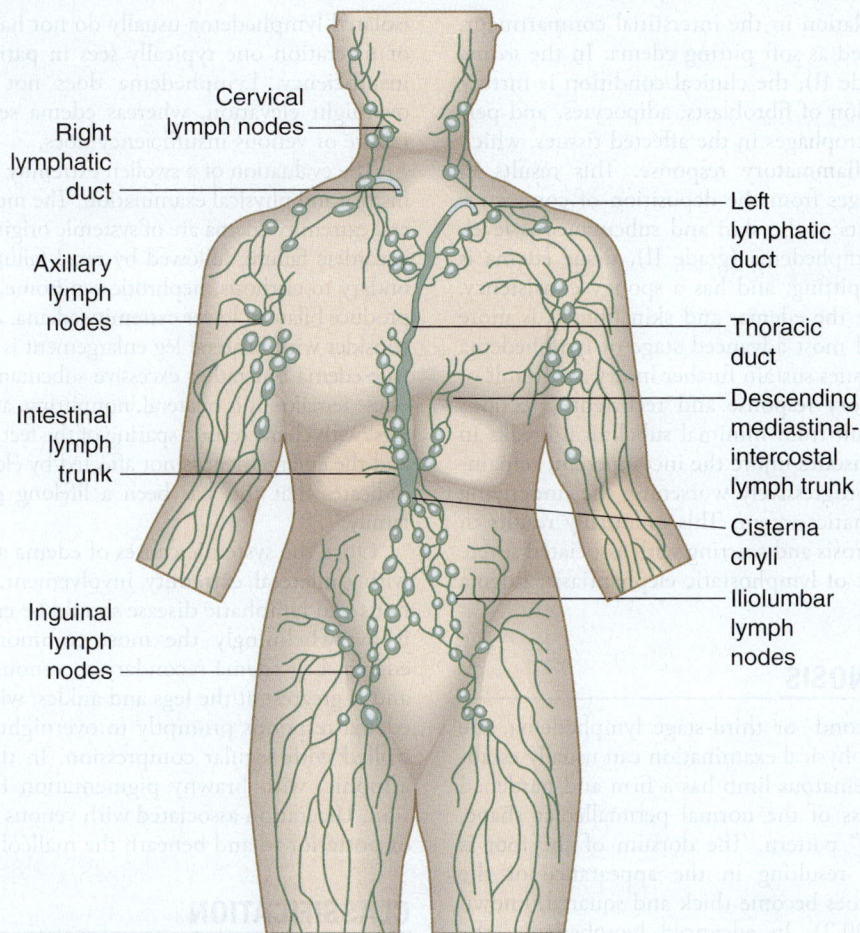

Labels (clockwise from top):
- Cervical lymph nodes
- Right lymphatic duct
- Axillary lymph nodes
- Intestinal lymph trunk
- Inguinal lymph nodes
- Left lymphatic duct
- Thoracic duct
- Descending mediastinal-intercostal lymph trunk
- Cisterna chyli
- Iliolumbar lymph nodes

FIGURE 109.1 Major anatomic pathways and lymph node groups of the lymphatic system.

into the venous system through the thoracic duct. There are additional communications between the lymphatic and venous systems. These smaller lymphovenous shunts mostly occur at the level of lymph nodes and around major venous structures, such as the jugular, subclavian, and iliac veins. Several structures in the body contain no lymphatics. Specifically, lymphatics have not been found in the epidermis, cornea, central nervous system, cartilage, tendon, and muscle.

The lymphatic system has three main functions. First, tissue fluid and macromolecules that undergo ultrafiltration at the level of the arterial capillaries are reabsorbed and returned to the circulation through the lymphatic system. Every day, 50% to 100% of the intravascular proteins are filtered this way in the interstitial space. Normally, they then enter the terminal lymphatics and are transported through the collecting lymphatics back into the venous circulation. Second, antigens, immune cells, microbes, and mutant cells arriving in the interstitial space enter the lymphatic system and are presented to the lymph nodes, which represent the first line of the immune system. Last, at the level of the gastrointestinal tract, lymph vessels are responsible for the uptake and transport of most of the fat absorbed from the bowel. Recent data suggest that a relationship between fat and lymphatics may exist well beyond the gut alone. It appears that peripheral tissue lipid transport and homeostasis may be, in part, determined by lymphatic function, hence the increased fat deposition seen in lymphedema.[3,6]

In contrast to what happens with venous forward flow, lymph's centripetal transport occurs mainly through intrinsic contractility of the individual lymphatic vessels, which, in concert with competent valvular mechanisms, is effective in establishing constant forward flow of lymph. In addition to the intrinsic contractility, other factors, such as surrounding muscle activity, negative pressure secondary to breathing, and transmitted arterial pulsations, have a lesser role in the forward lymph flow. These secondary factors appear to become more important under conditions of lymph stasis and congestion of the lymphatic vessels.

PATHOPHYSIOLOGY AND STAGING

Lymphedema is the result of an inability of the existing lymphatic system to accommodate the protein and fluid entering the interstitial compartment at the tissue level.[7] Impaired lymphatic vasculature can be either aplastic, hypoplastic, or hyperplastic. All of these patterns can lead to clinical lymphedema. In aplasia and hypoplasia, an absent or diminished number of lymphatics is seen. In hyperplasia, the vessels are incompetent and tortuous. Hyperplasia is only a cause in 8% of patients with lymphedema.[8]

An international working group developed a clinical staging for lymphedema.[9] In the latent phase, excess fluid accumulates, and the lymphatics become fibrosed. In the *latent phase* (grade 0), there is no clinical evidence of edema. In the *first stage* of lymphedema (grade I), impaired lymphatic drainage results in protein-rich fluid accumulation in the interstitial compartment. Clinically, this is manifested as soft pitting edema. In the *second stage* of lymphedema (grade II), the clinical condition is further exacerbated by accumulation of fibroblasts, adipocytes, and perhaps most important, macrophages in the affected tissues, which culminates in a local inflammatory response. This results in important structural changes from the deposition of connective tissue and adipose elements at the skin and subcutaneous level. In the second stage of lymphedema (grade II), tissue edema is more pronounced, is nonpitting, and has a spongy consistency. Elevation does not reduce the edema, and skin fibrosis is more apparent. In the *third* and most advanced stage of lymphedema (grade III), the affected tissues sustain further injury as a result of both the local inflammatory response and recurrent infectious episodes that typically result from minimal subclinical breaks in the skin. Such repeated episodes injure the incompetent, remaining lymphatic channels, progressively worsening the underlying insufficiency of the lymphatic system. This eventually results in excessive subcutaneous fibrosis and scarring with associated severe skin changes characteristic of lymphostatic elephantiasis. Edema is irreversible at this stage.

DIFFERENTIAL DIAGNOSIS

In most patients with second- or third-stage lymphedema, the characteristic findings on physical examination can usually establish the diagnosis. The edematous limb has a firm and hardened consistency. There is a loss of the normal perimalleolar shape, resulting in a "tree trunk" pattern. The dorsum of the foot is characteristically swollen, resulting in the appearance of the "buffalo hump," and the toes become thick and squared, known as *Stemmer sign* (Fig. 109.2). In advanced lymphedema, the skin undergoes characteristic changes, such as lichenification, development of peau d'orange, and hyperkeratosis.[7] In addition, the patients give a history of recurrent episodes of cellulitis and lymphangitis after trivial trauma and frequently present with fungal infections affecting the forefoot and toes. Patients with

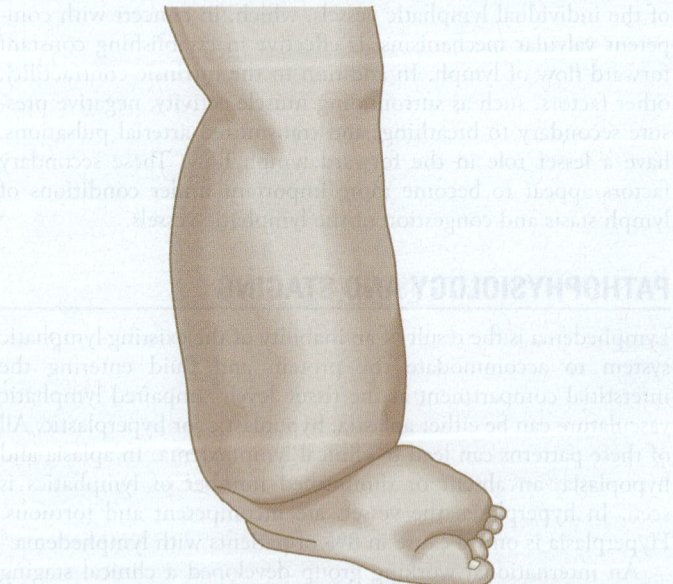

FIGURE 109.2 Lymphedema with characteristic loss of the normal perimalleolar shape, resulting in a "tree trunk" pattern. Dorsum of the foot is characteristically swollen, resulting in the appearance of the "buffalo hump."

isolated lymphedema usually do not have the hyperpigmentation or ulceration one typically sees in patients with chronic venous insufficiency. Lymphedema does not respond significantly to overnight elevation, whereas edema secondary to central organ failure or venous insufficiency does.

The evaluation of a swollen extremity should start with a detailed history and physical examination. The most common causes of bilateral extremity edema are of systemic origin. The most common cause is cardiac failure, followed by renal failure.[10] Hypoproteinemia secondary to cirrhosis, nephrotic syndrome, and malnutrition can also produce bilateral lower extremity edema. Another important cause to consider with bilateral leg enlargement is lipedema. Lipedema is not true edema but rather excessive subcutaneous fat typically found in obese females. It is bilateral, nonpitting, and greatest at the ankle and legs, with characteristic sparing of the feet. There are no skin changes, and the enlargement is not affected by elevation. The history usually indicates that this has been a lifelong problem that "runs in the family."

Once the systemic causes of edema are excluded in the patient with unilateral extremity involvement, edema secondary to venous and lymphatic disease should be entertained. Venous disease is overwhelmingly the most common cause of unilateral leg edema. Leg edema secondary to venous disease is usually pitting and is greatest at the legs and ankles, with sparing of the feet. The edema responds promptly to overnight leg elevation and is controlled with regular compression. In the later stages, the skin is atrophic, with brawny pigmentation from hemosiderin deposition. Ulceration associated with venous insufficiency occurs above or posterior to and beneath the malleoli.

CLASSIFICATION

Lymphedema is generally classified as primary when there is no known cause and secondary when its cause is a known disease or disorder.[11] Primary lymphedema has generally been classified on the basis of the age at onset and presence of familial clustering. Primary lymphedema with onset before the first year of life is called *congenital lymphedema*. The familial version of congenital lymphedema is known as *Milroy disease* and is inherited as a dominant trait. Primary lymphedema with onset between the ages of 1 and 35 years is called *lymphedema praecox*. The familial version of lymphedema praecox is known as *Meige disease* and has an onset around puberty. Finally, primary lymphedema with onset after the age of 35 years is called *lymphedema tarda*. The primary lymphedemas are relatively uncommon, occurring in 1 out of every 10,000 individuals. The most common form of primary lymphedema is praecox, which accounts for approximately 80% of the patients. Congenital and tarda lymphedemas each account for 10%. Worldwide, the most common cause of secondary lymphedema is infestation of the lymph nodes by the parasite *Wuchereria bancrofti* in the disease state called *filariasis*. Generally, the lower extremities are affected; however, primary upper extremity lymphedema has been reported.

Acquired or secondary lymphedema is the most common cause of lymphedema. In the developed countries, the most common causes of secondary lymphedema involve resection or ablation of regional lymph nodes by surgery, radiation therapy, tumor invasion, direct trauma, or, less commonly, an infectious process. For patients undergoing treatment for breast cancer with axillary intervention, up to 30% of patients will describe clinically significant lymphedema of the arm.

DIAGNOSTIC TESTS

The diagnosis of lymphedema is relatively easy in the patient who presents in the second and third stages of the disease. It can, however, be a difficult diagnosis to make in the first stage, particularly when the edema is mild, pitting, and relieved with simple maneuvers such as elevation.[11,12] For patients with suspected secondary forms of lymphedema, computed tomography (CT) and magnetic resonance imaging (MRI) are valuable and indeed essential for exclusion of underlying oncologic disease states.[13] In patients with known lymph node excision and radiation treatment as the underlying problem of their lymphedema, additional diagnostic studies are rarely needed except as these studies relate to follow-up of an underlying malignant disease. For patients with edema of unknown cause and a suspicion for lymphedema, lymphoscintigraphy is the diagnostic test of choice. When lymphoscintigraphy confirms that lymphatic drainage is delayed, the diagnosis of primary lymphedema should never be made until neoplasia involving the regional and central lymphatic drainage of the limb has been excluded through CT or MRI. If a more detailed diagnostic interpretation of lymphatic channels is needed for operative planning, contrast lymphangiography may be considered.

Lymphoscintigraphy (or isotope lymphography) has emerged as the test of choice in patients with suspected lymphedema.[13,14] It cannot differentiate between primary and secondary lymphedemas; however, it has a sensitivity of 70% to 90% and a specificity of nearly 100% in differentiating lymphedema from other causes of limb swelling. The test assesses lymphatic function by quantitating the rate of clearance of a radiolabeled macromolecular tracer (Fig. 109.3). The advantages of the technique are that it is simple, safe, and reproducible, with small exposure to radioactivity (approximately 5 mCi). It involves the injection of a small amount of radioiodinated human albumin or technetium-99m–labeled sulfur colloid into the first interdigital space of the foot or hand. Migration of the radiotracer within the skin and subcutaneous lymphatics is easily monitored with a whole body gamma camera, thus producing clear images of the major lymphatic channels in the leg and measuring the amount of radioactivity at the inguinal nodes 30 and 60 minutes after injection of the radiolabeled substance in the feet. An uptake value that is less than 0.3% of the total injected dose at 30 minutes is diagnostic of lymphedema. The normal range of uptake is between 0.6% and 1.6%. In patients with edema secondary to venous disease, isotope clearance is usually abnormally rapid, resulting in more than 2% ilioinguinal uptake. Importantly, variation in the degree of edema involving the lower extremity does not appear to significantly change the rate of clearance of the isotope.

Direct contrast lymphangiography provides the finest details of the lymphatic anatomy.[15] However, it is an invasive study that involves exposure and cannulation of lymphatics at the dorsum of the forefoot, followed by slow injection of contrast medium (ethiodized oil). The procedure is tedious, the cannulation often necessitates aid of magnification optics (frequently an operating microscope is needed), and the dissection requires some form of anesthetic. After cannulation of a superficial lymph vessel, contrast material is slowly injected into the lymphatic system. A total of 7 to 10 mL of contrast material is ideal for lower extremity evaluation and 4 to 5 mL for upper extremity evaluation. Potential complications include damage of the visualized lymphatics, allergic reactions, and pulmonary embolism if the oil-based contrast agent enters the venous system through lymphovenous anastomoses. Lymphangiography in present surgical practice is used infrequently and solely reserved for the preoperative evaluation of selected

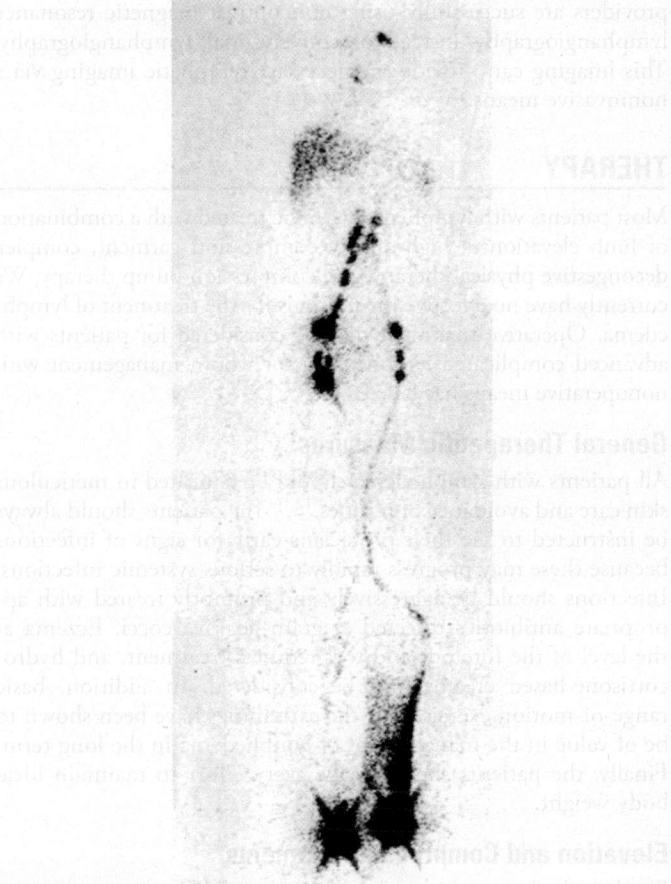

FIGURE 109.3 Lymphoscintigraphic pattern in primary lymphedema. Note area of dermal backflow on the *left* and diminished number of lymph nodes in the groin. (From Cambria RA, Gloviczki P, Naessens JM, et al. Noninvasive evaluation of the lymphatic system with lymphoscintigraphy: a prospective, semiquantitative analysis in 386 extremities. *J Vasc Surg.* 1993;18:773-782.)

patients who are candidates for direct operations on their lymphatic vessels.

New Diagnostic Tests

The field of lymphatic imaging is ever evolving, and we can expect that technologic advances, combined with the development of new contrast agents, will continue to improve diagnostic accuracy.[13] The most promising new test appears to be contrast magnetic resonance lymphangiography.[13,16] The test is performed after intracutaneous injection of gadobenate dimeglumine into the interdigital webs of the dorsal foot. Reported data suggest that the new test is capable of visualizing the anatomy and functional status of lymph flow transport of lymphatic vessels and lymph nodes of lymphedematous limbs in both primary and secondary lymphedema. Another new test that holds promise to detect early disease is bioimpedance spectroscopy. Flow of electrical current in a particular region of the body is inversely related to the amount of fluid in the tissue. With early lymphedema and increased interstitial fluid, impedance decreases. Although tested in small samples, sensitivity and specificity have been found to be 100%.[17]

Groups are looking at using machine learning and artificial intelligence to use CT for analysis of lymphedema and to potentially use this to screen patients.[18] For surgical planning, some providers are successfully using noncontrast magnetic resonance lymphangiography instead of conventional lymphangiography. This imaging can provide the necessary lymphatic imaging via a noninvasive means.[19]

THERAPY

Most patients with lymphedema can be treated with a combination of limb elevation, a high-quality compression garment, complex decongestive physical therapy, and compression pump therapy. We currently have no effective medications for the treatment of lymphedema. Operative treatment may be considered for patients with advanced complicated lymphedema for whom management with nonoperative means has failed.

General Therapeutic Measures

All patients with lymphedema should be educated in meticulous skin care and avoidance of injuries.[12,19] The patients should always be instructed to see their physicians early for signs of infections because these may progress rapidly to serious systemic infections. Infections should be aggressively and promptly treated with appropriate antibiotics directed at gram-positive cocci. Eczema at the level of the forefoot and toes requires treatment, and hydrocortisone-based creams may be considered. In addition, basic range-of-motion exercises for the extremities have been shown to be of value in the management of lymphedema in the long term. Finally, the patients should make every effort to maintain ideal body weight.

Elevation and Compression Garments

For lymphedema patients in all stages of disease, management with high-quality elastic garments is necessary at all times except when the legs are elevated above the heart.[20,21] The ideal compression garment is custom fitted and delivers pressures in the range of 30 to 60 mm Hg. Such garments may have the additional benefit of protecting the extremity from injuries, such as burns, lacerations, and insect bites. The patients should avoid standing for prolonged periods and should elevate their legs at night by supporting the foot of the bed on 15-cm blocks.

Complete Decongestive Physical Therapy

Complete decongestive physical therapy, a specialized massage technique for patients with lymphedema, is designed to stimulate the still-functioning lymph vessels, evacuate stagnant protein-rich fluid by breaking up subcutaneous deposits of fibrous tissue, and redirect lymph fluid to areas of the body where lymph flow is normal.[22] The technique is initiated on the normal contralateral side of the body, evacuating excessive fluid and preparing first the lymphatic zones of the nonaffected extremity, followed by the zones in the trunk quadrant adjacent to the affected limb, before attention is turned to the swollen extremity. The affected extremity is massaged in a segmental fashion, with the proximal zones being massaged first, proceeding to the distal limb. The technique is time consuming but effective in reducing the volume of the lymphedematous limbs.[22] After the massage session is complete, the extremity is wrapped with a low-stretch wrap, and then the limb is placed in the custom-fitted garment to maintain the decreased girth obtained with the massage therapy. This kind of therapy is appropriate for patients with all stages of lymphedema.

When the patient is first referred for complex decongestive physical therapy, the patient undergoes daily to weekly massage sessions for up to 8 to 12 weeks (initial or reductive stage). Limb elevation and elastic stockings are necessary adjuncts in this phase. After maximal volume reduction is achieved, the patient returns for maintenance massage treatments every 2 to 3 months while continuing to wear compression garments (maintenance phase). Without adherence to therapy, lymphatic fluid will reaccumulate. Lifelong maintenance is imperative to maintain reduction. Volume reduction is generally 60% to 70%, and compliant patients retain 90% of this reduction. A consensus panel with experts from the American Venous Forum, the American Vein and Lymphatic Society, and the Society for Vascular Medicine supports the use of manual lymphatic drainage, one component of complete decongestive therapy, for all lymphedema patients, even in the early stages of the disease.[23]

Compression Pump Therapy

Pneumatic compression pump therapy is another effective method of reducing the volume of the lymphedematous limb by a similar principle to massage therapy. The device consists of a sleeve containing several compartments. The lymphedematous limb is positioned inside the sleeve, and the compartments are serially inflated to milk the stagnant fluid out of the extremity.[24]

When a patient with advanced lymphedema is first referred for therapy, an initial approach with hospitalization for 3 or 4 days involving strict limb elevation, daily complex decongestive physical therapy, and compression pump treatments may be necessary to achieve optimal control of the lymphedema. It is particularly important that patients with cardiac or renal dysfunction be monitored for fluid overload. After this initial period of intensive therapy, the patients are fitted with high-quality compression garments to maintain the limb volume. Maintenance sessions are then prescribed for the patients on an as-needed basis.

Drug Therapy

Benzopyrones have attracted interest as potentially effective agents in the treatment of lymphedema. This class of medications, which includes coumarin (1,2-benzopyrone), is thought to reduce lymphedema through stimulation of proteolysis by tissue macrophages and stimulation of the peristalsis and pumping action of the collecting lymphatics. Benzopyrones have no anticoagulant activity. The first randomized, crossover trial of coumarin in patients with lymphedema of the arms and legs was reported in 1993.[25] The study concluded that coumarin was more effective than placebo in reducing not only volume but also other important parameters, including skin temperature, attacks of secondary acute inflammation, and discomfort of the lymphedematous extremities; skin turgor and suppleness were improved with coumarin. A second randomized, crossover trial was reported in 1999.[26] This study focused on effects of coumarin in females with secondary lymphedema after treatment of breast cancer. The trial investigators found that coumarin was not effective therapy for the specific group of females. Because of the disagreement between these two major trials, coumarins are not recommended for lymphedema treatment.

Diuretics may temporarily improve the appearance of the lymphedematous extremity with stage I disease, leading patients to request continuous therapy. However, other than producing temporary intravascular volume depletion, there is no long-term benefit because lymphedema fluid is not in the vascular space. Thus, diuretics have no role in the treatment of lymphedema at any stage.

Molecular Lymphangiogenesis

Fundamental discoveries in lymphatic development have pointed to the potential of exciting new treatments for lymphedema.

These molecular treatments are based on the activation of the VEGFR-3 pathway by administration of cognate ligands VEGF-C and VEGF-D using a variety of methods.[27] At this point, these treatments have been tested only in animal models, with promising results. Formal clinical trials are now needed to evaluate the therapeutic potential and possible untoward effects (including the possibility of stimulation of dormant tumor cells as a consequence of increased angiogenesis) of therapeutic lymphangiogenesis.[28]

Operative Treatment

Of patients with lymphedema, 95% can be managed nonoperatively. Surgical intervention may be considered for patients with stage II or stage III lymphedema who have severe functional impairment, recurrent episodes of lymphangitis, and severe pain despite optimal medical therapy. Two main categories of operations are available for the care of patients with lymphedema: reconstructive and excisional.

Reconstructive operations[29,30] should be considered for those patients with proximal (either primary or secondary) obstruction of the extremity lymphatic circulation with preserved, dilated lymphatics peripheral to the obstruction. In these patients, the residual dilated lymphatics can be anastomosed either to nearby veins or to transposed healthy lymphatic channels (usually mobilized or harvested from the healthy lower extremity) in an attempt to restore effective drainage of the lymphedematous extremity (Fig. 109.4). Some of the most common candidates for reconstructive procedures are patients with upper extremity

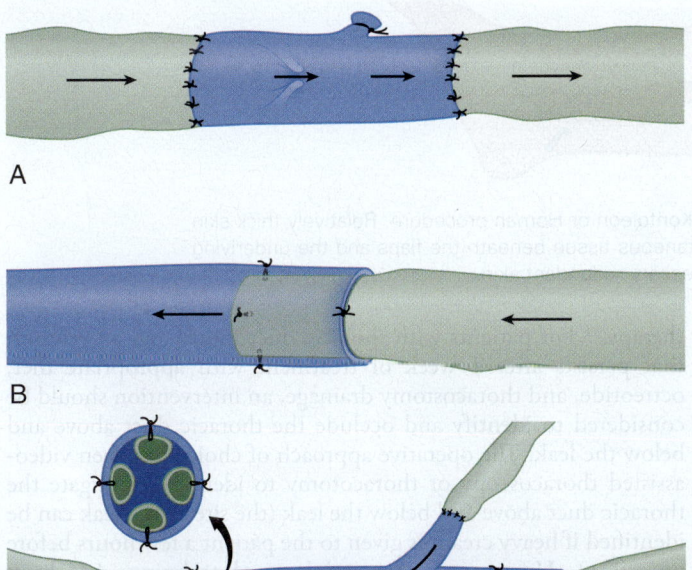

FIGURE 109.4 Lymphatic reconstruction techniques with a venous interposition graft (A), a lymphovenous anastomosis (B), and invagination of multiple lymphatics into a vein graft (C). (From Campisi C, Boccardo F, Tacchella M. Reconstructive microsurgery of lymph vessels: the personal method of lymphatic-venous-lymphatic [LVL] interpositioned grafted shunt. *Microsurgery.* 1995;16:161-166.)

lymphedema secondary to axillary lymphadenectomy or patients with leg lymphedema secondary to inguinal or pelvic lymphadenectomy. Treatment of selected lymphedema patients with lymphovenous anastomoses, lymphovenous bypass, or lymphaticolymphatic bypass has resulted in objective improvement in 30% to 80% of the patients, with an average initial reduction in the excess limb volume of 30% to 84%.[31–34]

A new surgical strategy involving lymph node transplantation has been used successfully, particularly for upper extremity lymphedema. This technique involves completing a gastroepiploic omental harvest, quantifying the number of lymph nodes in the flap, and performing a microvascular anastomosis in the extremity of interest. Debulking lipectomy was also performed in conjunction with this procedure. This technique has shown improvement in limb size and quality of life.[35]

Excisional operations are essentially the only viable option for patients without residual lymphatics of adequate size for reconstructive procedures. For patients with recalcitrant stage II and early stage III lymphedema in whom the edema is moderate and the skin is relatively healthy, an excisional procedure that removes a large segment of the lymphedematous subcutaneous tissues and overlying skin is the procedure of choice. This palliative procedure was introduced by Kontoleon in 1918 and was later popularized by Homan as "staged subcutaneous excision underneath flaps" (Fig. 109.5). The operative approach starts with a medial incision extending from the level of the medial malleolus through the calf into the midthigh.[36] Flaps about 1 to 2 cm thick are elevated anteriorly and posteriorly, and all subcutaneous tissue beneath the flaps, along with the underlying medial calf deep fascia, is removed with the redundant skin. The sural nerve is preserved. After the first-stage procedure is completed and if additional lymphedematous tissue removal is necessary, a second operation is performed, usually 3 to 6 months later. The second-stage operation is performed by similar techniques through an incision on the lateral aspect of the limb. In a recent long-term follow-up study, 80% of patients undergoing staged subcutaneous excision underneath flaps had a significant and long-lasting reduction in extremity size associated with improved function and extremity contour. Wound complications were encountered in 10% of the patients.[35]

A minimally invasive version of the Kontoleon procedure is gaining increasing support among lymphedema experts.[37,38] A number of reports have demonstrated that use of liposuction through small incisions is safe and is able to achieve control, at least on a short-term basis, of clinically disabling conditions associated with advanced stages of lymphedema. Surgeons with experience in this technique recommend initial conservative treatment of pitting lymphedema to remove excess fluid, followed by liposuction to remove remaining excess volume bothersome to the patient.[38]

When the lymphedema is extremely pronounced and the skin is unhealthy and infected, the simple reducing operation of Kontoleon is not adequate. In this case, the classic excisional operation originally described by Charles in 1912 is performed (Fig. 109.6). The procedure involves complete and circumferential excision of the skin, subcutaneous tissue, and deep fascia of the involved leg and dorsum of the foot.[39] The excision is usually performed in one stage, and coverage is provided preferably by full-thickness grafting from the excised skin. In a follow-up report, patients subjected to the Charles operation had immediate volume and circumference reduction. Skin graft take was 88%, and complications of the operation consisted primarily of wound infections,

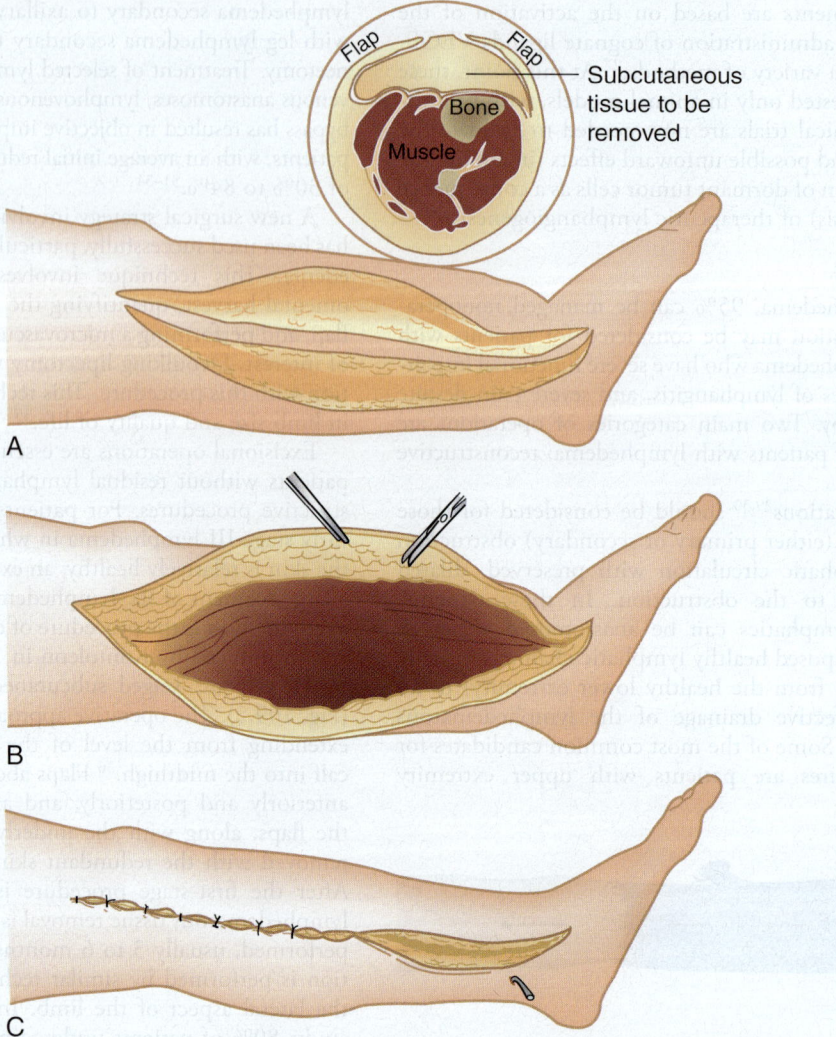

FIGURE 109.5 (A–C) Schematic representation of the Kontoleon or Homan procedure. Relatively thick skin flaps are raised anteriorly and posteriorly, and all subcutaneous tissue beneath the flaps and the underlying medial calf deep fascia are removed along with the necessary redundant skin.

hematomas, and necrosis of skin flaps. The hospital stay was 21 to 36 days.[40] Although this is a successful and radically reducing operation, the behavior in the healing skin graft is unpredictable. Between 10% and 15% of the grafted segments do not take and can be difficult to manage because of frequent localized sloughing, excessive scarring, focal recurrent infections, and hyperkeratosis or dermatitis. These complications seem to be worse in patients in whom leg resurfacing is performed with split-thickness grafts from the opposite extremity. In advanced cases, the exophytic changes within the grafted skin, chronic cellulitis, and skin breakdown may eventually lead to leg amputation.[41]

CHYLOTHORAX

Chylous pleural effusion is usually secondary to thoracic duct trauma (usually iatrogenic after chest surgery) and rarely a manifestation of advanced malignant disease with lymphatic metastasis.[42] Presence of chylomicrons on lipoprotein analysis and a triglyceride level of more than 110 mg/dL in the pleural fluid are diagnostic. Initially, patients can be treated nonoperatively with tube thoracostomy, medium-chain triglyceride (MCT) diet or total parenteral nutrition (TPN), and octreotide/somatostatin therapy.[43] For patients with thoracic duct injury and an effusion that persists after 1 week of treatment with appropriate diet, octreotide, and thoracostomy drainage, an intervention should be considered to identify and occlude the thoracic duct above and below the leak. The operative approach of choice has been video-assisted thoracoscopy or thoracotomy to identify and ligate the thoracic duct above and below the leak (the site of the leak can be identified if heavy cream is given to the patient a few hours before operation). However, a new endoluminal technique has been introduced and is becoming the optimal first approach for the management of persistent postoperative chylothorax. The approach starts with lymphangiography, usually through a groin lymph node access, to identify the location and anatomy of the cisterna chyli and the location of the divided thoracic duct. Once the cisterna chyli is opacified, it is percutaneously accessed with a spinal needle, using radiographic guidance, and is catheterized. The location of the divided thoracic duct is then identified with repeated lymphangiography, and the duct is embolized. In expert hands, this technique has a success rate of more than 50%.[44] For patients with cancer-related chylothorax and persistent drainage despite optimal chemotherapy and radiation therapy, pleurodesis is highly successful in preventing recurrences.

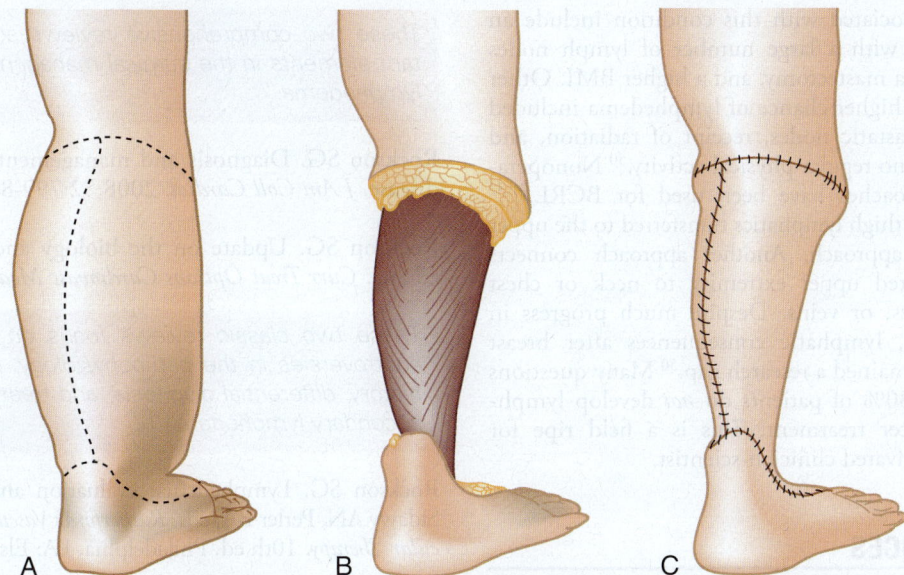

FIGURE 109.6 (A–C) Schematic representation of the Charles procedure. It involves complete and circumferential excision of the skin, subcutaneous tissue, and deep fascia of the involved leg and dorsum of the foot. Coverage is preferably provided by full-thickness grafting from the excised skin.

CHYLOPERITONEUM

In contrast to chylothorax, the most common cause of chylous ascites is congenital lymphatic abnormalities in children and malignant disease involving the abdominal lymph nodes in adults. Postoperative injury to abdominal lymphatics resulting in chylous ascites is rare.[45] Presence of chylomicrons on lipoprotein analysis and a triglyceride level of more than 110 mg/dL are diagnostic. Initial treatment includes paracentesis followed by MCT diet or TPN. In patients with postoperative chyloperitoneum, if ascites does not respond after several weeks of nonoperative management, percutaneous embolization[44] or surgical exploration should be employed to identify and occlude or ligate the leaking lymphatic duct. Conservative management can be successful 77% to 100% of the time using TPN, 75% of the time with MCT diet, and 100% of the time with MCT diet and octreotide. Some authors have recommended TPN initiation with chyle leakage is >200 mL/day and an MCT diet when chyle leakage is <200 mL/day.[46]

Congenital and malignant causes should be given longer periods (up to 4–6 weeks) of nonoperative management. If ascites persists in patients with congenital ascites, lymphoscintigraphy or lymphangiography is performed before an attempt is made to control the leak with laparotomy or laparoscopy. At the time of exploration, control of the leak can be achieved by ligation of leaking lymphatic vessels or resection of the bowel associated with the leak. Patients with malignant neoplasms should receive aggressive management for their underlying disease, which generally is effective at controlling the chyloperitoneum.

TUMORS OF THE LYMPHATICS

Lymphangiomas are the lymphatic analogue of the hemangiomas of blood vessels. They are generally divided into two types: (1) simple or capillary lymphangioma and (2) cavernous lymphangioma or cystic hygroma.[47] They are thought to represent isolated and sequestered segments of the lymphatic system that retain the ability to produce lymph. As the volume of lymph inside the cystic tumor increases, it grows larger within the surrounding tissues. The majority of these benign tumors are present at birth, and 90% of them can be identified by the end of the first year of life. The cavernous lymphangiomas almost invariably occur in the neck or the axilla and very rarely in the retroperitoneum. The simple capillary lymphangiomas also tend to occur subcutaneously in the head and neck region as well as in the axilla. Rarely, however, they can be found in the trunk within the internal organs or the connective tissue in and around the abdominal or thoracic cavities. The treatment of lymphangiomas should be surgical excision, with care taken to preserve all normal surrounding infiltrated structures.

Lymphangiosarcoma, or Stewart-Treves syndrome, is a rare tumor that develops as a complication of long-standing (usually more than 10 years) lymphedema.[48] Clinically, the patients present with acute worsening of the edema and appearance of subcutaneous nodules that have a propensity toward hemorrhage and ulceration. The tumor can be treated, like other sarcomas, with preoperative chemotherapy and radiation followed by surgical excision, which usually may take the form of radical amputation. Overall, the tumor has a very poor prognosis.[49]

Upper Extremity Lymphedema

Primary upper extremity lymphedema is extremely rare. The most common cause of upper extremity lymphedema is breast cancer–related lymphedema (BCRL). This secondary lymphedema is one of the chronic complications after breast cancer treatment. Patients present with symptoms similar to lower extremity lymphedema and describe pain, heaviness, tightness, and decreased range of motion that adversely affects fine motor skills. This can have a significant impact on activities of daily living and work-related tasks. Additionally, this can become a constant reminder of the diagnosis of breast cancer, which can have psychological consequences, including anxiety, depression, and distress. A large systematic review found that 21% of patients undergoing treatment for breast cancer will develop BCRL.[50] This may be an underestimate, given that BCRL can present without arm swelling. Unfortunately, there are no universally accepted diagnostic criteria for BCRL.

Risk factors most associated with this condition include an axillary node dissection with a large number of lymph nodes resected, treatment with a mastectomy, and a higher BMI. Other factors associated with a higher chance of lymphedema included prevalence of more metastatic nodes, receipt of radiation, and an inactive lifestyle with no regular physical activity.[50] Nonoperative and operative approaches have been used for BCRL.[31,32] Lymphatic grafting using thigh lymphatics transferred to the upper extremity is one such approach. Another approach connects lymphatics in the affected upper extremity to neck or chest lymphatics, lymph nodes, or veins. Despite much progress in breast cancer treatment, lymphatic consequences after breast cancer treatment have remained a research gap.[50] Many questions remain, including why 80% of patients do *not* develop lymphedema after breast cancer treatment. This is a field ripe for investigation for the motivated clinician-scientist.

SELECTED REFERENCES

Campisi CC, Ryan M, Boccardo F, et al. A single-site technique of multiple lymphatic-venous anastomoses for the treatment of peripheral lymphedema: long-term clinical outcome. *J Reconstr Microsurg*. 2016;32:42-49.

Granzow JW, Soderberg JM, Kaji AH, et al. Review of current surgical treatments for lymphedema. *Ann Surg Oncol*. 2014;21:1195-1201.

These two comprehensive reviews summarize the important elements in the surgical management of patients with lymphedema.

Rockson SG. Diagnosis and management of lymphatic vascular disease. *J Am Coll Cardiol*. 2008;52:799-806.

Rockson SG. Update on the biology and treatment of lymphedema. *Curr Treat Options Cardiovasc Med*. 2012;14:184-192.

These two classic reviews focus on the knowledge and controversies in the pathophysiology, classification, natural history, differential diagnosis, and treatment of primary and secondary lymphedema.

Rockson SG. Lymphedema: evaluation and decision making. In: Sidawy AN, Perler BA, eds. *Rutherford's Vascular Surgery and Endovascular Therapy*. 10th ed. Philadelphia, PA: Elsevier; 2023:2202-2214.

This authoritative text provides a succinct summary of the evaluation of lymphatic disorders.

The full reference list appears on Elsevier eBooks+.

Cardiothoracic Surgery

The following chapter appears only on Elsevier eBooks+:

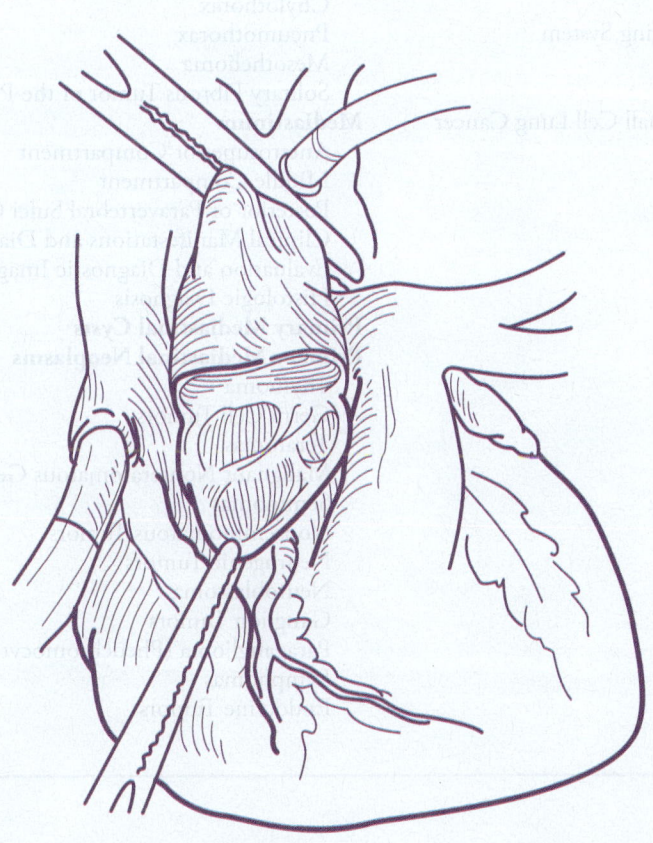

110 CHAPTER

Lung, Chest Wall, Pleura, and Mediastinum

Nikki E. Rossetti, Steven Tohmasi, Mark W. Onaitis, and Benjamin D. Kozower

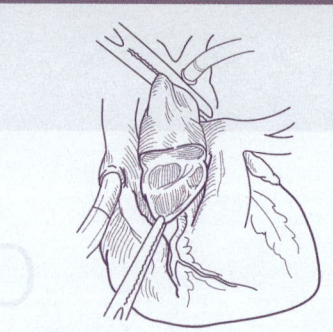

OUTLINE

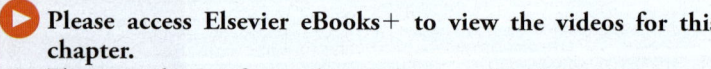

Please access Elsevier eBooks+ to view the videos for this chapter.

The term *thorax* refers to the area between the neck and abdomen enclosed superiorly by the thoracic inlet; inferiorly by the diaphragm; and radially by the ribs, sternum, and vertebrae. The chest or thorax creates a frame for the neck, arms, thoracic structures, and abdomen; supports and protects the internal thoracic organs; and provides for the negative inspiratory force that initiates ventilation and the positive expiratory force needed for vocalization. The major thoracic structures include the heart and lungs, chest wall—including the overlying musculature, ribs, sternum, and vertebrae—diaphragm, trachea, esophagus, and great vessels.

ANATOMY

The thoracic organs are protected by the bony thorax and overlying chest wall musculature (Fig. 110.1), including the latissimus dorsi, serratus anterior, and pectoralis major and minor. These extrinsic muscles of the chest attach to the bony thorax, protect the chest wall itself, and may assist with ventilatory efforts in patients with chronic obstructive pulmonary disease (COPD).

The thorax has three major interior groups of muscles:

1. **Primary muscles of respiration,** including the diaphragm and intercostal muscles, which occupy the 11 intercostal spaces and consist of the external, internal, and transverse or **innermost muscles**
2. **Secondary muscles of respiration,** including the extrinsic chest wall muscles as previously outlined, as well as the serratus posterior, levatores costarum, and the cervical muscles (sternocleidomastoid and scalenes)
3. **Muscles attaching the upper extremity to the body,** including the pectoralis major and minor anteriorly and the trapezius and latissimus dorsi posteriorly. Deeper muscles include the serratus anterior and posterior, the levatores, and the major and minor rhomboids. In respiratory distress, the deltoid, pectoralis, and latissimus dorsi muscles form a tertiary system for ventilatory assistance through fixation of the upper extremities.

The bony thorax consists of 12 ribs peripherally extending from the vertebrae posteromedially to the sternum (ribs 1–5) or costal arch (ribs 6–10) anteriorly. The 11th and 12th ribs are "floating ribs" and are not attached directly to the sternum. The

first rib is relatively flat and dense and travels from the first thoracic vertebra to the manubrium to create the thoracic inlet (Fig. 110.2). This relatively small area contains the great vessels, trachea, esophagus, thoracic duct, and lung apices, along with the phrenic, vagus, and recurrent laryngeal nerves. The remaining ribs

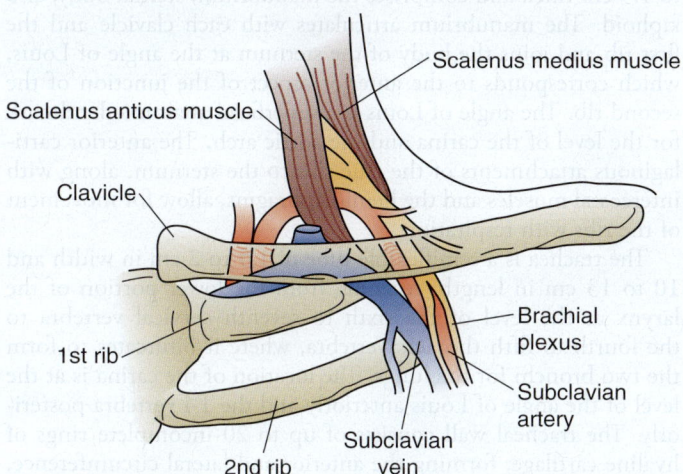

FIGURE 110.2 Relationship of the neurovascular bundle to the scalenus muscles, clavicle, and first rib. (From Urschel HC. Thoracic outlet syndromes. In: Baue AE, Geha AS, Hammond GL, et al., eds. *Glenn's Thoracic and Cardiovascular Surgery.* 6th ed. Stamford: Appleton & Lange; 1996:567.)

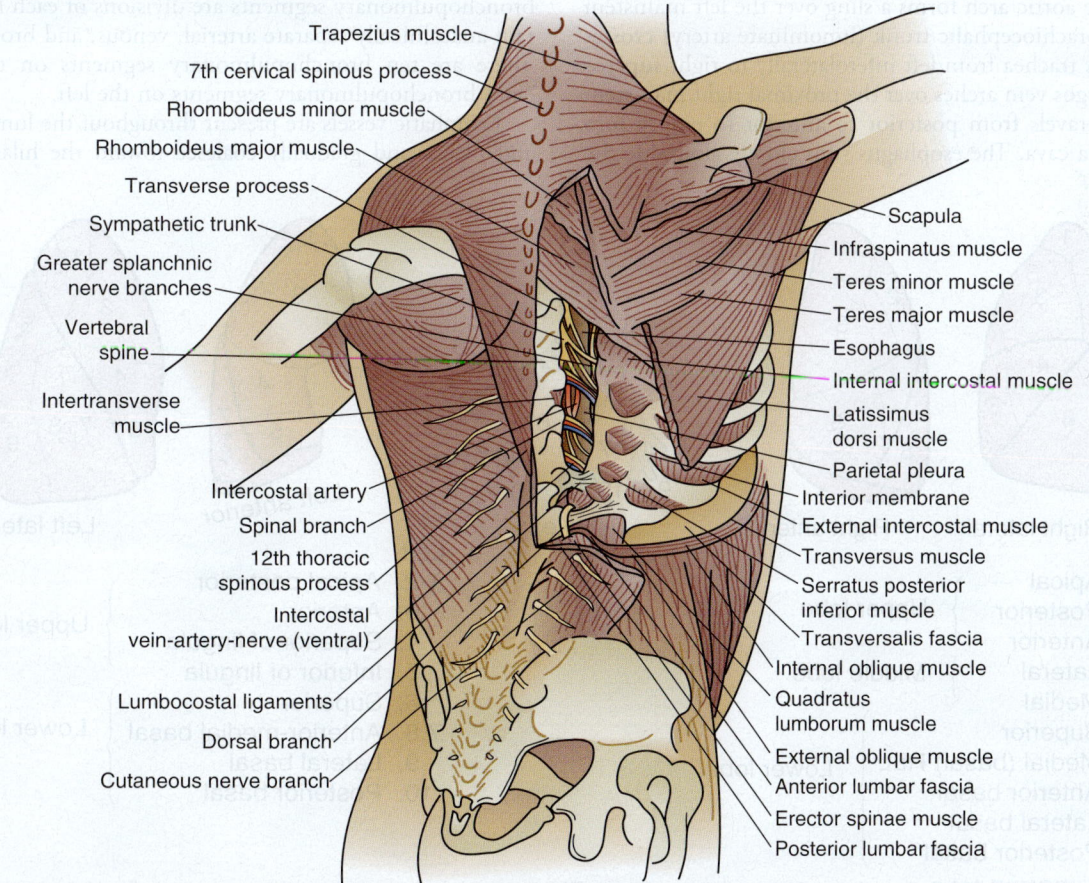

FIGURE 110.1 Musculature of the chest wall. (From Ravitch MM, Steichen FM. *Atlas of General Thoracic Surgery.* Philadelphia: Saunders; 1988.)

gradually slope downward. Intercostal nerves branch from the spinal roots and innervate the skin and intercostal musculature. The intercostal bundles (vein, artery, and nerve) travel along the lower edge of each rib anteriorly but become centrally located within the intercostal space posteriorly.

The sternum is flat, 15 to 20 cm long, and approximately 1.0 to 1.5 cm thick and comprises the manubrium, sternal body, and xiphoid. The manubrium articulates with each clavicle and the first rib and joins the body of the sternum at the angle of Louis, which corresponds to the anterior aspect of the junction of the second rib. The angle of Louis is a superficial anatomic landmark for the level of the carina and the aortic arch. The anterior cartilaginous attachments of the true ribs to the sternum, along with intercostal muscles and the hemidiaphragms, allow for movement of the ribs with respiration.

The trachea is a semiflexible tube of 1.5 to 2 cm in width and 10 to 13 cm in length, reaching from the lower portion of the larynx at the level of the sixth to seventh cervical vertebra to the fourth to fifth thoracic vertebra, where it bifurcates to form the two bronchi for the lungs. The location of the carina is at the level of the angle of Louis anteriorly and the T4 vertebra posteriorly. The tracheal wall consists of up to 20 incomplete rings of hyaline cartilage, forming the anterior and lateral circumference, and smooth muscle posteriorly known as the *membranous trachea,* which are both embedded into a fibrous membrane of elastic connective tissue. The cricoid is the only complete cartilaginous ring, and the inferior edge marks the end of the larynx. The trachea begins approximately 1.5 cm below the vocal cords and is not rigidly fixed to surrounding tissues. The most rigid point of fixation is where the aortic arch forms a sling over the left mainstem bronchus. The brachiocephalic trunk (innominate artery) crosses over the anterior trachea from left inferolaterally to right superolaterally. The azygos vein arches over the proximal right mainstem bronchus as it travels from posterior to anterior to empty into the superior vena cava. The esophagus runs closely alongside the

posterior membranous trachea to the left of the midline, with the recurrent laryngeal nerves located in the tracheoesophageal groove bilaterally. The blood supply to the trachea is posterolateral and segmental from the inferior thyroid, the internal thoracic, the supreme intercostal, and the bronchial arteries. During tracheal resection and reconstruction, great care must be taken to circumferentially dissect only the trachea being removed to avoid vascular insufficiency with necrosis or anastomotic dehiscence. There are approximately 23 divisions of bronchi between the trachea and the terminal alveoli, which make up ~50% of the entire lung volume.

The lungs are broadly divided into five lobes and multiple segments within each lobe (Fig. 110.3). The right lung is composed of three lobes: upper, middle, and lower. The major (oblique) fissure separates the lower lobe from the upper and middle lobes, and the minor (horizontal) fissure separates the upper lobe from the middle lobe. The left lung has two lobes—the upper lobe and the lower lobe—with the lingula corresponding embryologically to the right middle lobe. A single oblique fissure separates the lobes.

The blood supply of the lung is twofold: unoxygenated blood circulates from the right ventricle through the pulmonary artery to each lung, and after oxygenation in the lung parenchyma, the blood is returned to the left atrium through the pulmonary veins. Blood supply to the bronchi is from the systemic circulation by bronchial arteries arising from the superior thoracic aorta or the aortic arch, either as discrete branches or in combination with the intercostal arteries. Although there is variation, there are usually two left bronchial arteries and one right bronchial artery. The bronchopulmonary segments are divisions of each lobe that contain anatomically separate arterial, venous, and bronchial supply. There are ten bronchopulmonary segments on the right and eight bronchopulmonary segments on the left.

Lymphatic vessels are present throughout the lung parenchyma and pleura and gradually coalesce toward the hilar areas of the

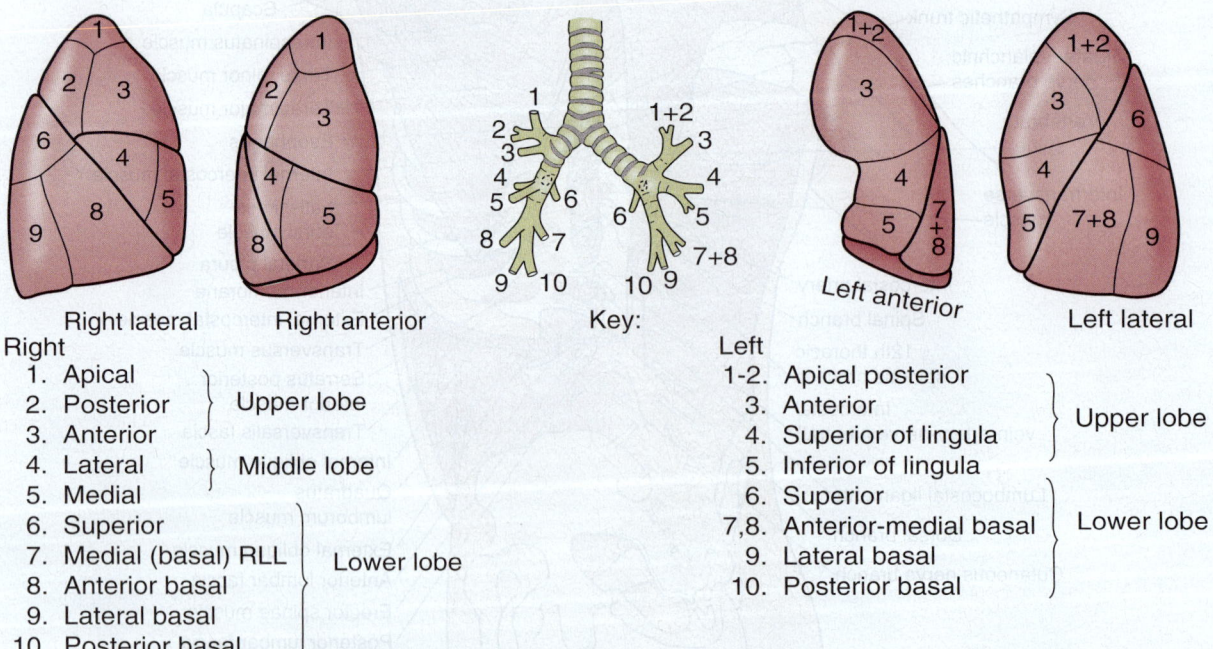

Right lateral   **Right anterior**   Key: **Left anterior**   **Left lateral**

Right
1. Apical   ⎫
2. Posterior   ⎬ Upper lobe
3. Anterior   ⎭
4. Lateral   ⎫ Middle lobe
5. Medial   ⎭
6. Superior   ⎫
7. Medial (basal) RLL ⎬ Lower lobe
8. Anterior basal   ⎪
9. Lateral basal   ⎪
10. Posterior basal ⎭

Left
1-2. Apical posterior ⎫
3. Anterior   ⎬ Upper lobe
4. Superior of lingula ⎪
5. Inferior of lingula ⎭
6. Superior   ⎫
7,8. Anterior-medial basal ⎬ Lower lobe
9. Lateral basal   ⎪
10. Posterior basal ⎭

FIGURE 110.3 Segments of the pulmonary lobes. *RLL,* Right lower lobe. (Adapted from Jackson CL, Huber JF. Correlated applied anatomy of the bronchial tree and lungs with a system of nomenclature. *Dis Chest.* 1943;9:319.)

lungs. Generally, lymphatic drainage from the lung affects the ipsilateral lymph nodes; however, flow of lymph from the left lower lobe may drain to the right mediastinal (paratracheal) lymph nodes. Lymphatic drainage within the mediastinum drains into the thoracic duct, which originates from the cisterna chyli in the abdomen, and enters the thorax through the aortic hiatus, then travels superiorly to the right of midline along the anterolateral surface of the vertebral column. At approximately the level of T5, it crosses over to the left and continues superiorly to empty into the junction of the left jugular and subclavian veins posteriorly.

The parietal pleura is the internal lining of the chest wall and covers the mediastinum, diaphragm, and pericardium. Its blood supply comes from the systemic arteries and veins, including the posterior intercostal, internal mammary, anterior mediastinal, and superior phrenic arteries and corresponding systemic veins. The lymphatic drainage of the parietal pleura is into regional lymph nodes, including intercostal, mediastinal, and phrenic nodes. It is richly innervated by sensory branches of the intercostal nerves; therefore, generous local anesthesia should be used for chest tube insertion.

The visceral pleura covers the outer surface of the lung and separates the lobes, with blood supply from both systemic and pulmonary sources. Visceral pleural lymphatics follow the superficial lung lymphatics and drain into the mediastinal lymph nodes. The visceral pleura is innervated by vagal branches and the sympathetic system. There is a potential space between the parietal and visceral pleurae that is normally filled with just a scant amount of pleural fluid, which allows nearly frictionless movement during respiration. This pleural space may compress the lungs or heart when filled with fluid, tumor, or infection. The right and left pleural spaces are separated by the mediastinum.

The anatomic boundaries of the mediastinum include the thoracic inlet superiorly, the diaphragm inferiorly, the sternum anteriorly, the vertebral column posteriorly, and the parietal pleural medially. Fat and lymph nodes are found throughout the mediastinum. Traditionally, the mediastinum can be divided into anterosuperior, middle, and posterior compartments. No specific anatomic planes define these areas. The anterosuperior compartment includes the thymus gland. The right and left lobes of the thymus extend into the cervical areas, and these portions of the thymus must be resected to provide for complete extirpation of the gland. The middle mediastinum contains the heart; pericardium; great vessels (including the ascending, transverse, and descending aorta; superior and inferior vena cava. [IVC]; pulmonary artery and veins); trachea and bronchi; and phrenic, vagus, and recurrent laryngeal nerves. The phrenic nerve enters the thorax through the thoracic inlet on the anterior aspect of the anterior scalene muscle.

On the right side, the vagus nerve enters the thoracic inlet through the carotid sheath, lies anterior to the subclavian and posterior to the innominate artery, and continues posteriorly in the tracheoesophageal groove to innervate the trachea and esophagus. The right recurrent laryngeal nerve loops or "recurs" around the innominate artery to innervate the right-sided vocal cord. On the left side, the vagus nerve enters the thorax through the thoracic inlet, and as it exits the carotid sheath, it moves along the anterior aspect of the aortic arch and continues within the mediastinum along the esophagus posteriorly to innervate both the trachea and the esophagus. The left recurrent laryngeal nerve arises from the vagus nerve, loops around under the ligamentum arteriosum, continues superiorly under the aorta, and lies in the tracheoesophageal groove as it courses to innervate the left-sided vocal cord.

The posterior mediastinum lies between the heart/pericardium and trachea anteriorly and the vertebral column and paravertebral spaces posteriorly. It contains the esophagus, descending aorta, azygos and hemiazygos veins, thoracic duct, sympathetic chain, and lymph nodes.

The inferior border of the mediastinum is the diaphragm, which separates the abdominal contents from the thorax. Hernias through the esophageal hiatus (paraesophageal hernias), through the foramen of Bochdalek (posteriorly), or through the foramen of Morgagni (anteriorly) may be initially identified as a mediastinal mass.

The spinal root divides as it exits the neural foramina. One branch goes to the intercostal nerve, and one lies in the posterior vertebral gutter to form the sympathetic ganglion. The thoracic sympathetic trunk comprises several ganglia that lie along the ribs. The most superior ganglion is the stellate ganglion.

SELECTION OF PATIENTS FOR THORACIC OPERATIONS

The physiologic evaluation of the thoracic surgical patient must be individualized and generally emphasizes the pulmonary and cardiac function. The assessment of a patient's ability to tolerate lung resection from a cardiopulmonary standpoint is fundamental to patient selection for surgery. Patients with advanced pulmonary disease and severe pulmonary dysfunction may have prohibitive risk, which may exist in greater than one-third of patients with otherwise resectable lung disease.[1] However, many patients with poor nutrition or pulmonary function can optimize functional status and postoperative outcomes through targeted prehabilitation programs.

Cigarette smoking is associated with increased postoperative pulmonary complications. If the patient is a smoker, they must stop smoking immediately. Although there are few studies specific to pulmonary resection, there is evidence that smoking abstinence 4 to 8 weeks before surgery is necessary to reduce complication rates. However, smoking cessation at any time is valuable and should be encouraged. Smoking cessation programs may be helpful for these patients because many patients require pharmacologic assistance and ongoing counseling to achieve durable abstinence.[2]

In the pre- and perioperative periods, deep venous thrombosis prophylaxis should be provided with subcutaneous heparin or low-molecular-weight heparin and sequential compression stockings. Standard perioperative antibiotics should be administered before incision to reduce surgical site infections.

Aggressive multimodal analgesia can reduce perioperative morbidity by facilitating early ambulation. Standard regimens commonly include Tylenol, NSAIDs, regional pain management with thoracic epidural catheter or intercostal rib blocks with long-acting local anesthetics, and/or patient-controlled analgesia.[3]

Regular incentive spirometry assists in expanding the lung and reducing the incidence of pulmonary morbidity. Nasal bilevel positive airway pressure for patients with obstructive sleep apnea may delay or eliminate the need for intubation or reintubation after pulmonary resection, although caution should be exercised for patients with foregut anastomoses.

Physiologic Evaluation

Patients may be evaluated preoperatively with a combination of radiographic and physiologic studies. A plain chest x-ray (CXR) is commonly obtained and serves as a baseline study that may be

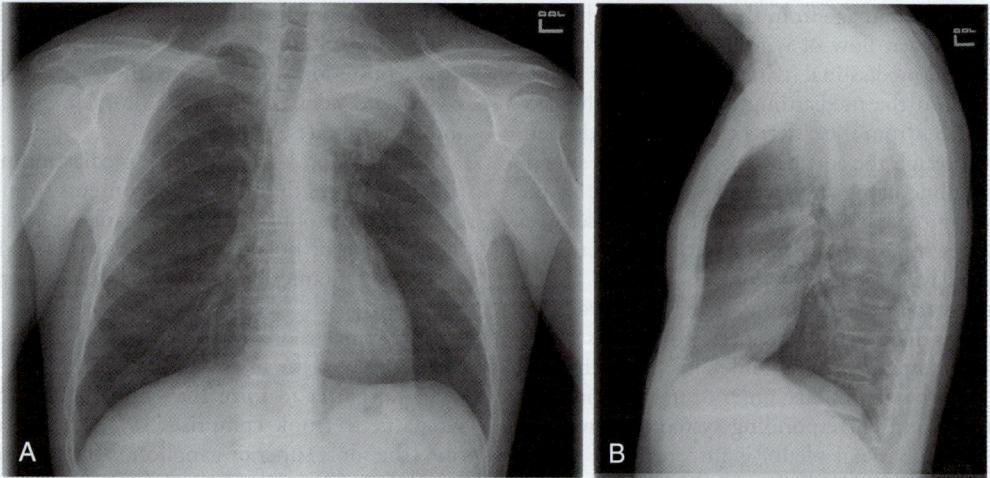

FIGURE 110.4 Initial chest x-rays. This patient is a 67-year-old male with a weight loss of 10 pounds in 4 weeks and a 35-pack-year history of cigarette smoking. He quit smoking 10 years ago. He had left shoulder pain for 4 months with no dyspnea, cough, hemoptysis, or other symptoms. Massage and other musculoskeletal manipulation did not improve his symptoms. A chest x-ray with posteroanterior (A) and lateral (B) views demonstrates an 8.4-cm left upper lung mass. Some deviation of the distal trachea is noted.

referenced postoperatively (Fig. 110.4). Preoperative anemia is associated with adverse operative outcomes, so care must be taken to identify and correct reversible causes of anemia, such as iron deficiency. Spirometry measures the lung volumes (Fig. 110.5) and the mechanical properties of lung elasticity, recoil, and compliance.

Pulmonary function testing (Fig. 110.6) also evaluates gas exchange functions, such as carbon monoxide diffusing capacity (DLCO) and the predicted postoperative forced expiratory volume in 1 second (FEV$_1$). FEV$_1$ is the most common indicator of postoperative pulmonary reserve; most patients with FEV$_1$ greater than 60% predicted can tolerate an anatomic lobectomy and do not require further pulmonary function testing. If FEV$_1$ is less than 60% of predicted, quantitative radionuclide lung perfusion testing (Fig. 110.7) can provide a measurement of the relative function of each lobe and lung and allows an estimation of pulmonary function after lung resection (ppoFEV$_1$):

ppoFEV$_1$ = preopFEV$_1$ × (1 − fraction of perfusion to region of planned resection)

A ppoFEV$_1$ of 40% or less carries a greater risk for postoperative dependence on supplemental oxygen and/or mechanical ventilation. It should be noted that the ppoFEV$_1$ is not likely to be realized in the immediate postoperative period, secondary to pain and limited ambulation.

DLCO is most commonly assessed using the single-breath test, which measures the rate at which test molecules, such as carbon monoxide, move from the alveolar space to combine with hemoglobin in the red blood cells. The difference between inspired and expired samples of gas is used to calculate DLCO. Levels less than 50% are associated with increased perioperative risk.

Flow-volume loops derived from spirometry describe the relationship between lung volume and airflow as the lung volume changes during a forced expiration and inspiration. The typical test consists of tidal breathing at rest, followed by maximal inspiratory effort to total lung capacity, then maximal expiratory effort to residual volume, concluding with maximal inspiratory effort to total lung capacity. In obstructive lung disease, the ratio of FEV$_1$ to forced vital capacity (FVC; FEV$_1$/FVC) is low (FEV$_1$ is low, and FVC is high); in restrictive disease, the ratio is about normal because both FEV$_1$ and FVC are reduced.

Cardiopulmonary exercise testing (CPET) can be extremely useful in the evaluation of frail or functionally marginal surgical candidates. CPET includes exercise electrocardiography, heart rate response to exercise, and measurements of minute ventilation and oxygen uptake. Calculation of maximal oxygen consumption (VO$_2$ max) provides insight into overall cardiopulmonary function (the "cardiopulmonary axis") and may identify clinically occult cardiac disease. Overall, CPET provides a more accurate assessment of pulmonary function than spirometry and DLCO, which tend to overestimate functional loss after resection.

A patient's risk of perioperative morbidity and mortality may be stratified by measurement of VO$_2$ max. A level less than 11 to 15 mL/kg/min is associated with an increased risk, and VO$_2$ max less than 10 mL/kg/min indicates high risk.[4] An inexpensive and readily available test that can be performed in the clinic is a stair-climbing test. Patients who can walk 18 m have reduced perioperative complication rates and improved survival after lung cancer resection.[5]

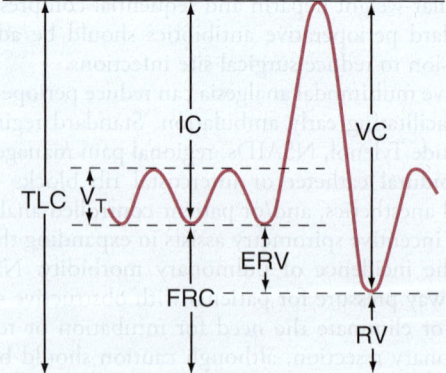

FIGURE 110.5 Spirometry with subdivisions of lung volumes. *ERV,* Expiratory reserve volume; *FRC,* functional residual capacity (i.e., lung volume at end expiration); *IC,* inspiratory capacity; *RV,* residual volume (i.e., lung volume after forced expiration from FRC); *TLC,* total lung capacity; *VC,* vital capacity (i.e., maximal volume of gas inspired from RV); *V$_T$,* tidal volume.

Section of Pulmonary Medicine
Pulmonary Function Report

Last Name: First Name:
Identification:
Age: 56 years   Room: Outpatient
Sex: Male   Race: White
Height: 65 inches   Physician:
Weight: 177 lb   Operator:
Date
Time

Spirometry		Pred	Pre BD	%Pred	Post BD	%Pred	%Chg
FVC	[l]	3.48	3.07	88	3.07	88	0
FEV$_1$	[l]	2.83	2.23	79	2.26	80	1
FEV$_1$/VC	[%]	80.81	72.26	89	69.78	86	−3
FEF 25–75	[l/s]	3.01	1.37	45	1.46	49	7
PEF	[l/s]	7.57	6.43	85	7.10	94	10
FIVC	[l]	3.48	3.09	89	3.24	93	5
FIV$_1$	[l]		3.09		3.24		5
FIV$_1$/FVC	[%]		100.00		100.00		0

Lung Volumes		Pred	Measured	%Pred
SVC	[l]	3.48	3.04	87
TLC	[l]	5.51	5.54	101
RV	[l]	1.96	2.49	127
RV/TLC	[%]	35.9	45.0	125
FRC-Box	[l]	2.24	3.01	134

Diffusion SB		Pred	Measured	%Pred
DLCO SB	[mL/min/mm Hg]	22.59	23.81	105
DLCO Hb Corr	[ml/min/mm Hg]	22.6	24.2	107
VA	[l]		5.27	
DLCO/VA	[mL/min/mm Hg/l]	3.93	4.52	115
Hb	[g/100mL]		14.1	

Interpretation

Spirometry reveals an isolated reduction in mid-expiratory flows consistent with an obstructive small airways defect. Increased residual volume (RV) is consistent with air trapping. Following the inhalation of a bronchodilator, there is no improvement of the obstructive airway defect. The diffusing capacity is normal.

FIGURE 110.6 The pulmonary function report provides complete spirometry data based on predicted values for height and weight. In this patient, the forced expiratory volume in 1 second *(FEV$_1$)* is 2.26 L after bronchodilators, which is 80% of predicted. The carbon monoxide diffusing capacity *(DLCO)* is measured as 23.81 mL/min/mm Hg, which is 105% of predicted. *FEF,* Forced expiratory flow; *FIV$_1$,* forced inspiratory volume in one second; *FIVC,* forced inspiratory vital capacity; *FRC,* functional reserve capacity; *FVC,* forced vital capacity; *Hb,* hemoglobin; *PEF,* peak expiratory flow; *SB,* single breath; *SVC,* slow vital capacity; *TLC,* total lung capacity; *VA,* alveolar volume; *VC,* vital capacity.

Measurement of diaphragm function by fluoroscopy, the "sniff test," or ultrasonography is needed to determine symmetry of effort and to exclude paradoxical movement of the diaphragm. Paradoxical movement (elevation of one hemidiaphragm with active contraction/retraction of the other diaphragm) suggests paresis or paralysis, and diaphragm plication may be therapeutic.

No single test result should be viewed as an absolute contraindication to surgical resection. Patients with marginal preoperative pulmonary and general functional assessments must be considered thoughtfully on an individual basis.

Thoracic Incisions

The choice of incision depends on the operation, the patient's underlying physiologic condition, and the anticipated benefits and limitations

of the planned approach. Video-assisted thoracoscopic surgery (VATS), robotic-assisted thoracoscopic surgery (RATS), and other minimally invasive surgical techniques have been developed to treat most thoracic problems, including lung and esophageal cancer, mediastinal tumors, pleural diseases, and parenchymal diseases, and to diagnose and stage thoracic malignancies. Various small incisions are made for the camera and other instruments depending on the location of the lesion. To accommodate the instruments, careful attention must be paid to incision placement relative to the patient's ribs, arm, diaphragm, and scapula. The ribs are not spread. Improved lighting and optics create excellent exposure and visualization, often superior to that achieved with an open approach. Patient advantages of minimally invasive surgical techniques include reduced postoperative pain and length of hospitalization.

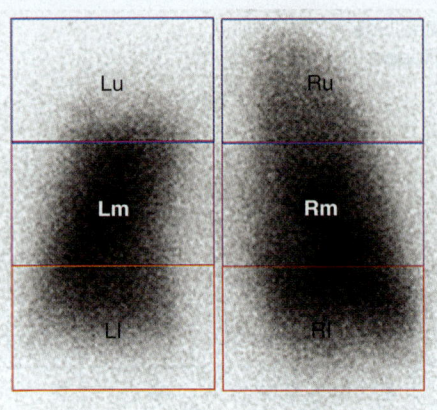

	Left lung		Right lung	
	%	Kct	%	Kct
Upper zone:	4.7	22.66	9.5	46.27
Middle zone:	24.0	116.91	28.3	138.05
Lower zone:	13.2	64.20	20.3	99.02
Total lung:	41.8	203.77	58.2	283.34

FIGURE 110.7 The quantitative perfusion lung scan report provides the lung volume and the perfusion to each lung. In a patient with a large left hilar tumor, perfusion may be reduced in the involved left lung compared with the uninvolved right lung. The predicted post–left pneumonectomy right lung function can be obtained by multiplying the right lung percent perfusion (58.2%) by the observed best forced expiratory volume in 1 second (FEV_1; 2.26 L). The resulting value, 1.31 L, 46.5% predicted, is the predicted postoperative FEV_1 (after left pneumonectomy). This value suggests that a left pneumonectomy would be functionally tolerated. *Ll*, Left lower zone; *Lm*, left middle zone; *Lu*, left upper zone; *Rl*, right lower zone; *Rm*, right middle zone; *Ru*, right upper.

Open thoracotomy requires spreading the ribs with a retractor and is used for operations on a single side of the thorax. The patient is placed in a lateral decubitus position, and the incision may be posterior, axillary, or anterior. For posterior access, an oblique incision is used with or without sparing the latissimus dorsi muscle. The chest is typically entered through the fifth interspace. For anterior hilar exposure, a vertical axillary incision can be made anterior to the latissimus dorsi muscle, and the chest is entered through the fourth interspace. For anterior or anterolateral access, a curvilinear incision is created underneath the inferior border of the pectoralis major muscle at the inframammary fold.

Median sternotomy is performed using a vertical incision from the sternal notch to the xiphoid. A sternal saw is then used to divide the sternum in the midline. With gentle retraction, the sternum can be spread approximately 8 to 10 cm to allow access to the mediastinum, heart, great vessels, and right and left thorax. The pleura can be opened on either side to explore the hemithorax. The sternum is usually closed with stainless-steel wire. Sternotomy is commonly used for cardiac surgery, mediastinal tumors, and tracheal/carinal exposure and occasionally for pulmonary resection.

A transverse sternotomy, or "clamshell" incision, is larger than a median sternotomy and typically more painful postoperatively for the patient. This incision combines two anterior thoracotomy incisions in the inframammary fold with transverse division of the sternum at the fourth intercostal space. Both internal mammary arteries are ligated. This approach is ideal for accessing both the right and the left hilum and providing additional exposure for large mediastinal tumors, bilateral hilar dissections, or bilateral lung transplantation.

LUNG DEVELOPMENT

Lung development begins at approximately 21 to 28 days' gestation, and disturbed embryogenesis can result in various congenital lung abnormalities. They comprise a spectrum of anomalies, with one end representing abnormal lung parenchyma supplied by normal vessels, such as unilateral pulmonary agenesis and pulmonary hypoplasia. The other end of the spectrum represents normal lung parenchyma supplied by abnormal vessels. Hybrid lesions are common. Clinically, these lesions are most often asymptomatic but can cause respiratory failure.

Congenital Cystic Lesions

Congenital cystic lesions consist of congenital pulmonary airway malformations (CPAMs) or congenital cystic adenomatoid malformations, pulmonary sequestrations, congenital lobar emphysema, and bronchogenic cysts. Approximately one-third are asymptomatic, one-third have cough, and one-third have infection. Treatment may be with antibiotics or, for more severe localized cases, with resection. Any cystic lesion that enlarges on serial radiographs needs to be considered for resection.

Cystic fibrosis (CF) is an autosomal recessive disorder that is found more commonly in White patients. Excessively thick mucus leads to recurrent infections, bronchitis, and bronchiectasis. The treatment of CF is rapidly evolving, and the recent introduction of cystic fibrosis transmembrane conductance regulator (CFTR) modulators that target the underlying mutant protein has effectively slowed the rate of disease progression in eligible patients. Nevertheless, lung failure remains the most common cause of death. Bilateral lung transplantation should be considered when the disease rapidly progresses and the remaining pulmonary reserve is low. Early referral to a transplant program is important to maximize potential benefit.

CONGENITAL ABNORMALITIES OF THE TRACHEA AND BRONCHI

Tracheoesophageal fistula, commonly with esophageal atresia, is the most frequent abnormality of the trachea in infants (see Chapter 117), followed by bronchial atresia.[6] Complete tracheal agenesis is a rare phenomenon and is fatal. It results from abnormal development of the laryngotracheal groove, and the trachea is absent from the larynx to the carina, with communication between the bronchi and the esophagus.

Tracheal stenosis is also rare and results from complete or near-complete rings of tracheal cartilage with an absent membranous component. Infants typically present with respiratory distress, cyanosis, and feeding difficulties. Surgical repair of the trachea is by vertical incision and widening of the tracheal lumen.

Tracheomalacia represents dynamic collapse of the trachea during respiration, resulting in airway obstruction. It is classified as congenital (primary) or acquired (secondary) and can be identified by diagnostic imaging (dynamic expiratory computed tomography [CT]) or bronchoscopy, which reveals marked variation of the tracheal lumen with inspiration and expiration. Collapse of greater than 70% of the lumen during expiration is diagnostic. Clinical presentation depends on the location and severity of tracheal collapse. Relief of the extrinsic compression is needed for symptomatic improvement. Procedural intervention is indicated for life-threatening airway obstruction, recurrent infection, respiratory failure, or failure to thrive. Treatment may include stent placement, posterior splinting, or primary tracheobronchoplasty. Individually customized 3D-printed airways are a developing technology for airway management.

CONGENITAL VASCULAR DISORDERS

Several congenital disorders of the pulmonary vasculature may occur.[7] In Swyer-James-Macleod syndrome, idiopathic hyperlucent lung tissue results from diminished pulmonary arterial blood supply. It develops uncommonly after chronic pulmonary infections with associated bronchiolitis obliterans. Treatment is typically nonoperative but may include pneumonectomy for patients with severe bronchiectasis.

Scimitar syndrome is characterized by an anomalous direct venous connection (called the *scimitar vein*) between the right pulmonary vein and the IVC. The affected lung and its airways, which are also drained by the scimitar vein, are hypoplastic, with atypical bronchial and vascular distributions. It is commonly associated with bronchopulmonary sequestration and hypoplastic left heart syndrome. Surgical repair involves a patch from the pulmonary vein to the left atrium and is usually completed with the use of intraoperative extracorporeal membrane oxygenation (ECMO).

Pulmonary arteriovenous malformations (PAVMs) may exist as one or multiple connections from the pulmonary artery to the pulmonary vein, bypassing the pulmonary capillary bed and producing a right-to-left shunt. Most commonly, they are seen in hereditary hemorrhagic telangiectasia (Osler-Weber-Rendu syndrome). This diagnosis should be considered for any patient with hemoptysis without other etiology identified by bronchoscopy or other imaging modalities. Small asymptomatic lesions may be managed with observation and serial imaging. For large and/or symptomatic lesions, catheter embolization is the primary treatment. Local resection may be considered in patients with poorly accessible lesions, in patients with severe untreatable contrast allergy, or after failed embolization.

Pulmonary artery sling consists of an anomalous or aberrant left pulmonary artery that arises from the right (main) pulmonary artery and courses between the trachea and the esophagus to supply the left lung. This causes compression of the trachea and/or esophagus. Surgical correction requires relocation of the left pulmonary artery from its right-sided origin to the main pulmonary artery. It is often seen with other congenital anomalies; if it co-occurs with tracheal stenosis, segmental tracheal resection or tracheoplasty should be performed concurrently with vascular reconstruction.

Vascular rings constitute 7% of all congenital cardiac malformations.[8] Most patients require operation within the first weeks or months of life. Patients with vascular rings require a careful history and barium swallow for diagnosis. Bronchoscopy and esophagoscopy are not routinely ordered, but echocardiography, CT scanning, and MRI may be used to further delineate the anatomy.

The most common vascular ring is a double aortic arch (60% of cases). The right or posterior arch is larger and gives rise to the right carotid and right subclavian arteries, wrapping around both the trachea and the esophagus. A posterior indentation is noted in the esophagus on barium swallow. Simple division of the smaller arch corrects the anomaly.

The next most common vascular ring is a right aortic arch with a left ligamentum arteriosum (25%–30% of all vascular rings). Among these patients, two-thirds have a retroesophageal left subclavian artery, and one-third have mirror-image branching, with the left carotid and subclavian arteries arising from the left innominate artery. Alternately, a retroesophageal right subclavian artery with left ligament may occur. The patient may complain of dysphagia, which is referred to as *dysphagia lusoria*. The differential diagnosis includes neuromotor diseases of the esophagus and stricture. Surgical repair is indicated for symptomatic cases and involves left thoracotomy in the fourth intercostal space and division of the ligamentum, allowing the trachea and the esophagus to be freed from surrounding tissues.[9]

LUNG CANCER

Lung cancer refers to malignancies of the pulmonary parenchyma and airways. Cigarette smoking is unequivocally the most important risk factor in the development of lung cancer. Secondhand smoke is also a significant risk factor. Other environmental factors may predispose to lung cancer. Environmental radon gas exposure is estimated to be the second most important risk factor. Other factors include asbestos, arsenic, chromium, nickel, organic chemicals, iatrogenic radiation exposure, air pollution, secondary smoke from nonsmokers, and prior chest radiation therapy (e.g., for Hodgkin lymphoma or breast cancer).

Despite advances in diagnosis and treatment, lung cancer remains a significant global health problem, with a global incidence of 2.2 million cases and 1.8 million deaths in 2020.[10] In the United States, lung cancer is the leading cause of cancer-related deaths for both males and females, accounting for 26% of cancer-related deaths and exceeding the number of deaths from breast, prostate, and colorectal cancer combined. Lung cancer incidence rates have decreased by ~2.2% per year since 2008, likely as a result of programs aimed at smoking cessation. However, smoking cessation in females has lagged behind smoking cessation in males; thus, the incidence of lung cancer in females has not declined as much as the incidence in males (Fig. 110.8). Mortality has declined in recent years, likely as a result of improved screening and treatment options, especially for non–small cell lung cancer. However, demographic disparities exist, with African American males having both the highest incidence and the highest death rate from cancer of the lung and bronchus.[11]

Optimal treatment of lung cancer depends on stage and cancer type. Staging is based on the extent of tumor, lymph node, and metastatic disease (tumor-node-metastasis [TNM] system). The system is internationally recognized and used for prognostication and to guide treatment decisions.

Pathology

In 2021 the World Health Organization (WHO) issued a revised classification of tumors of the lung, replacing the previous 2015 guidelines. The 2021 edition includes a broader emphasis on genetic testing, expanded commentary on the classification of small diagnostic samples, and modernized recommendations on subtype classification based on immunohistochemical profiling of small tumor biopsies and cytologies. The major types of malignant tumors of the lung are adenocarcinomas, squamous cell carcinomas (SCCs), large cell carcinomas, sarcomatoid carcinoma, and neuroendocrine tumors (NETs) of the lung; each of these groups has multiple subtypes that differ by their morphologic, genetic, and biologic properties. Key characteristics of these tumors are described next.

Adenocarcinomas are malignant epithelial tumors with glandular differentiation or mucin production, showing acinar, papillary,

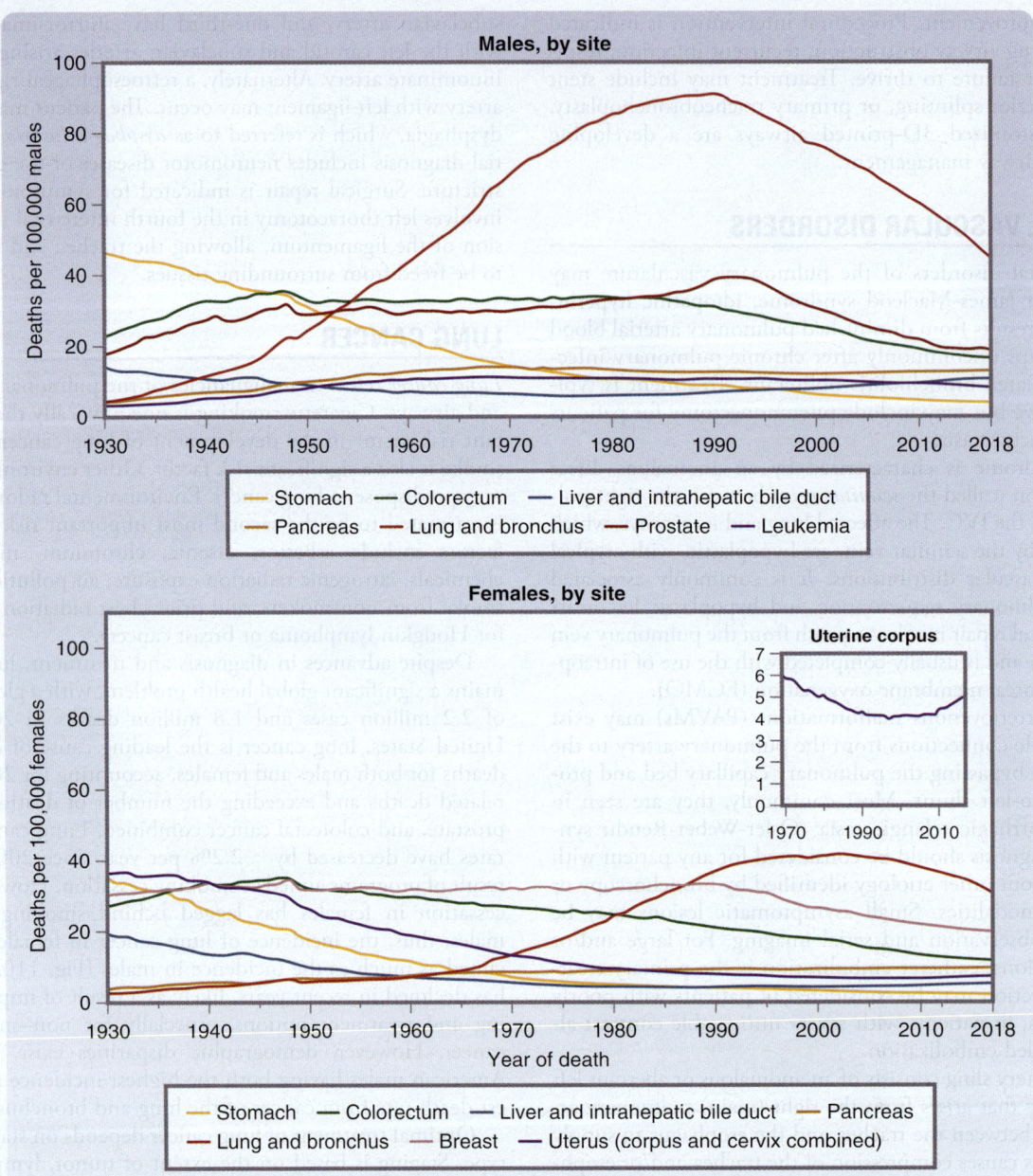

FIGURE 110.8 Trends in cancer death rates by sex for selected cancers, United States 1930 to 2018. Rates are age adjusted to the 2000 US standard population. (From Siegel RL, Miller KD, Jemal A. Cancer statistics, 2018. *CA Cancer J Clin.* 2018;68:7-30.)

micropapillary, lepidic (bronchioloalveolar), or solid with mucin growth patterns or a mixture of these patterns. Adenocarcinoma of the lung is the most frequent histologic type of lung cancer, accounting for approximately half of all lung cancers. Microscopic features consist of cuboidal to columnar cells with adequate to abundant pink or vacuolated cytoplasm and some evidence of gland formation. Most of these tumors (75%) are peripherally located. Adenocarcinoma of the lung tends to metastasize earlier than SCC of the lung and more frequently to the central nervous system. Some adenocarcinomas can present as ground-glass opacities and are not associated with tobacco use. These tumors are increasing in frequency and are more common in females and people from Asia.

SCC is a malignant epithelial tumor showing keratinization and/or intercellular desmosome ("bridges") that arises from

bronchial epithelium. Approximately 30% of lung cancers are SCCs, and among these, over 90% occur in cigarette smokers. Approximately two-thirds of these tumors are centrally located and tend to expand against the bronchus, causing extrinsic compression. SCCs are prone to undergo central necrosis and cavitation. SCC tends to metastasize later than adenocarcinoma. Microscopically, keratinization, stratification, and intercellular bridge formation are exhibited. SCC may be more readily detected on sputum cytology than adenocarcinoma.

A diagnosis of large cell undifferentiated carcinoma may be made when specific cytologic features of SCC or adenocarcinoma or neuroendocrine differentiation are lacking. These tumors are typically large and peripherally located and tend to metastasize relatively early. Microscopically, these tumors show sheets of round to polygonal cells with prominent nucleoli and abundant pale-staining cytoplasm without differentiating features.

NETs of the lung share specific morphologic, ultrastructural, immunohistochemical, and molecular features; they arise from cells derived from the embryologic neural crest. This group of tumors includes small cell lung carcinomas (SCLCs), large cell neuroendocrine carcinomas, and typical and atypical carcinoids. Typical carcinoids show a relatively indolent growth pattern, whereas small cell carcinomas and large cell neuroendocrine carcinomas are highly aggressive.

Small cell lung cancers represent approximately 20% of all lung malignancies; 80% of these tumors are centrally located and tend to spread early to mediastinal lymph nodes and distant sites, especially the bone marrow and brain. Microscopically, the tumors appear as sheets or clusters of cells with dark nuclei and little cytoplasm. Neurosecretory granules are evident on electron microscopy. Small cell lung cancer is staged according to the lung cancer TNM staging system; however, from a clinical perspective, the disease may also be addressed as limited stage (disease restricted to an ipsilateral hemithorax within a single radiation port) and extensive stage (obvious metastatic disease). Staging includes 18F-fluorodeoxyglucose–positron emission tomography (FDG/PET), brain CT or MRI, and mediastinoscopy. Mediastinal metastases on clinical staging suggest advanced disease, which is best treated with chemoradiotherapy.[12,13] These tumors are generally advanced at presentation, with an aggressive tendency to metastasize, so chemoradiotherapy is often the first-line therapy. Prophylactic cranial irradiation aimed at reducing the risk of brain metastases is considered in patients with limited or extensive disease that responds well to first-line therapy. Complete responses may occur in ~30% of patients; however, the 5-year survival rate is only 5%. Patients with very early stage disease (e.g., <3 cm in size, no nodal metastases, and no extrathoracic metastases) may be considered for surgical resection, followed by adjuvant systemic therapy.

Lung cancers commonly metastasize to the pulmonary and mediastinal lymph nodes (lymphatic spread). Hematogenous spread of lung cancer commonly results in metastases to the adrenal glands, liver, brain, lung, and bone. Adenocarcinoma is more likely to metastasize to the central nervous system. Bone metastases are osteolytic. Extrathoracic metastases may occur without hilar nodes or mediastinal metastases.

Screening

Patients with lung cancer often present with advanced stage and symptoms. The pulmonary parenchyma does not contain nerve endings, and therefore, tumors may grow undetected until late-stage symptoms of pain, hemoptysis, or obstructive pneumonia arise. Clinical outcomes are directly related to the stage at the time of diagnosis, as reflected by 5-year survival with clinical stage IA1 (92%) compared with clinical stage IVB (approaching 0%). With the increased use of CT in the United States, smaller asymptomatic lung cancers are being identified.

The US National Lung Screening Trial (NLST) was a prospective randomized multicenter study evaluating annual low-dose helical CT with annual chest radiography for older adults with heavy smoking histories. Patients who received annual low-dose CT screening had reduced lung cancer–specific mortality and all-cause mortality compared with those who underwent annual CXR. In fact, the study was closed early on the basis of clear, statistically significant mortality benefit of CT screening.[14] Similarly, the European NELSON lung cancer screening trial was a randomized controlled trial comparing low-dose CT screening for high-risk older

adults at increasing intervals to no screening. Overall, the study demonstrated that the use of CT screening among high-risk asymptomatic patients reduced lung cancer deaths at 10 years, with an improved benefit in females compared with males. Several other international randomized trials (including the Detection and Screening of Early Lung Cancer with Novel Imaging Technology and Molecular Assays [DANTE] trial and the Multicentric Italian Lung Detection Study in Italy, the Danish Randomized Lung Cancer CT Screening Trial in Denmark, the German Lung Cancer Screening Intervention Study in Germany, the UK Lung Cancer Screening pilot trial in the United Kingdom, and a 2020 meta-analysis) all demonstrated benefit of CT in screening for individuals at high risk of developing lung cancer.

Based on these results, screening for early lung cancer detection using low-dose helical CT is recommended for high-risk individuals. The guidelines differ slightly based on the expert consensus of various groups internationally. In the United States, the National Comprehensive Cancer Network (NCCN) recommends low-dose chest CT screening for individuals aged ≥50 years with a ≥20-pack-year smoking history of smoking tobacco who are either current or former smokers.[15,16] The US Preventive Services Task Force guidelines recommend low-dose CT screening for adults aged 50 to 80 years with a 20-pack-year smoking history and who currently smoke or have quit within the past 15 years. The American Cancer Society recently released new guidelines, now recommending screening for adults aged 50 to 80 years with a ≥20-pack-year smoking history, which is broadened from previous guidelines.[17] Despite clear clinical benefit of screening and increasingly broad international guidelines from all major expert consensus groups, uptake of lung cancer screening in clinical practice has been low. Black patients are less likely to receive annual lung cancer screening than White patients,[18] likely contributing to racial disparities in lung cancer mortality.

Physicians should discuss testing for early stage lung cancer with their patients. This discussion should include the risks, benefits, and limitations associated with lung cancer screening with low-dose helical CT and should occur before a decision is made to start any lung cancer screening. Screening of asymptomatic patients may identify nonspecific findings, such as overdiagnosis of benign nodules, which could result in patient anxiety and additional radiation exposure. Nevertheless, the benefit to high-risk patients likely outweighs these risks, and patients should be supported by adhering to consensus screening guidelines and subsequent follow-up care for identified pulmonary nodules.

Diagnosis

The diagnosis of lung cancer can be challenging because many benign conditions mimic lung cancer. Physical examination should focus on the cardiorespiratory system and signs of metastasis (e.g., weight loss, pain, headaches, seizures, anemia). In addition, the presence of lymphadenopathy, identified by a careful examination of the cervical and supraclavicular lymph nodes, may suggest advanced disease (N3 lymph node descriptor). Paraneoplastic syndromes are distant manifestations of lung cancer (not metastases), as revealed in extrathoracic nonmetastatic symptoms that can include muscle, nerve, bone, and the endocrine system.

Non–small cell lung cancer (NSCLC) typically occurs in patients who are 50 to 70 years old with a history of cigarette smoking. Patients develop symptoms based on the physical impact of tumor growth within the lung parenchyma. Symptoms such as cough, dyspnea, chest wall pain, and hemoptysis are related to the physical presence of the tumor and its interactions with the structures of the lung and chest wall.[19] The majority of early stage lung cancers are asymptomatic and detected by screening or identified incidentally on routine chest imaging for other indications.

Once a clinical suspicion for NSCLC arises, the clinician should aim to achieve a timely diagnosis and accurate staging so that appropriate therapy can be administered—ideally within 6 to 12 weeks of first suspicion. The workup of a primary solitary pulmonary nodule (SPN) involves a combination of imaging modalities, including CT and PET/CT (Fig. 110.9), and usually a biopsy. Under certain circumstances, an SPN may be deemed benign with adequate confidence in the absence of biopsy with pathologic diagnosis. SPNs that are entirely calcified, or are radiologically solid and stable on CT for a minimum of 2 years, are very likely to be benign. Review of old CT scans or other prior imaging studies is essential in the management of these patients.[20]

In patients with a clinically suspicious SPN, biopsy with pathologic assessment may be needed to guide further management. The preferred sampling strategy is the least invasive method compatible with obtaining a diagnosis. Diagnostic bronchoscopy, transthoracic needle aspiration, or navigational bronchoscopy can be selected based on the size, location, and condition of the patient. In a physiologically fit patient with a highly suspicious yet undiagnosed SPN, nonanatomic wedge or sublobar resection can provide a diagnosis. When appropriate, frozen section confirmation of NSCLC by the pathologist may be followed by definitive (anatomic) resection in the same operative setting. For an SPN in the absence of a cancer diagnosis (that cannot be removed by wedge resection), a lobectomy can be considered for diagnosis (and treatment). However, a pneumonectomy should not be performed without a cancer diagnosis.

One-third of patients with NSCLC may have a pleural effusion at the time of presentation. Pleural fluid sampling with thoracentesis is required for cytologic examination. Malignant pleural effusion (MPE) is a contraindication to resection, but many pleural effusions in this setting may be reactive in origin.[21]

Bronchoscopy is recommended before any planned pulmonary resection. The surgeon independently assesses (via bronchoscopy) the endobronchial anatomy to exclude secondary endobronchial primary tumors and to ensure that all known cancer will be encompassed by the planned pulmonary resection. Secretions can be cleared with suctioning and gentle irrigation. When pneumonectomy or bronchoplastic resection is contemplated for a central tumor, the surgeon's assessment at bronchoscopy is critical to the determination of whether complete (R0) resection can be achieved.

If the patient has hard palpable lymph nodes in the cervical or supraclavicular area, fine-needle aspiration or biopsy may provide an accurate diagnosis of N3 disease (Fig. 110.10).

Staging

Staging describes the extent of the cancer and provides prognostication based on outcome patterns for patients with similar

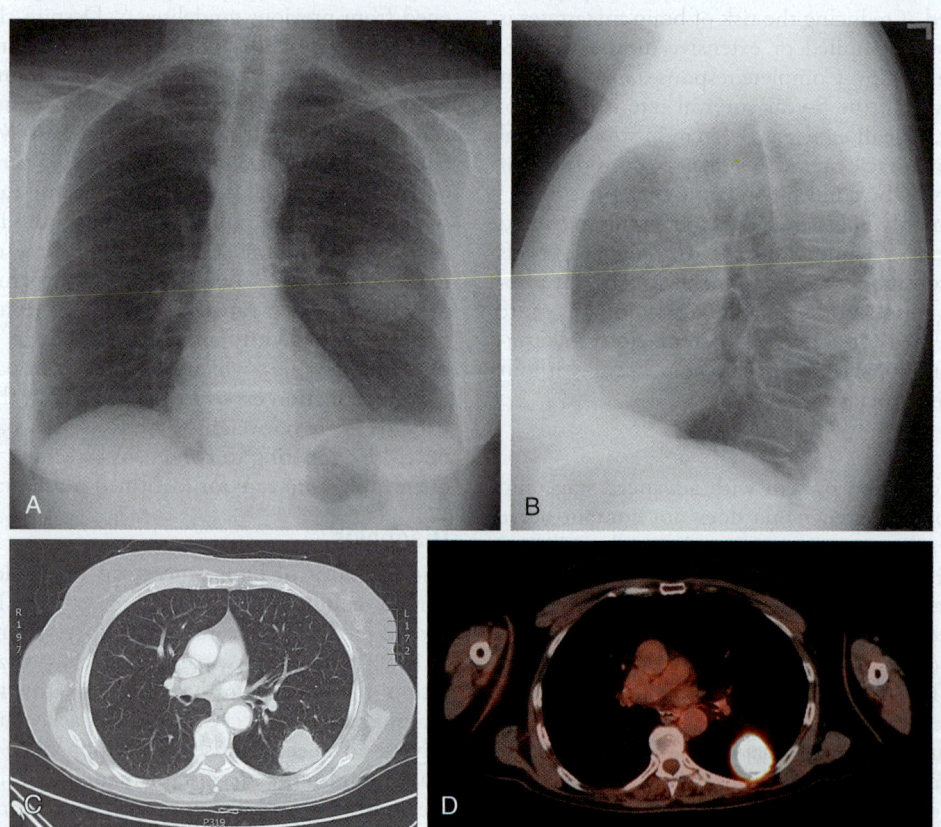

FIGURE 110.9 Radiographic evaluation for any patient with known or suspected lung cancer includes a plain chest x-ray, posteroanterior (A) and lateral (B) views. Evaluation of the plain films and computed tomography (CT) (C) guides subsequent evaluations. F-fluorodeoxyglucose positron emission tomography (FDG-PET) with fused CT (D) provides the ability to correlate metabolic activity with physical findings. Although FDG-PET uses the increased metabolism in most neoplasms to create the FDG-PET image, other process (such as infection, inflammation, or sequelae of trauma or fractures) can be identified as well. Sites of increased metabolism should be carefully evaluated for metastases.

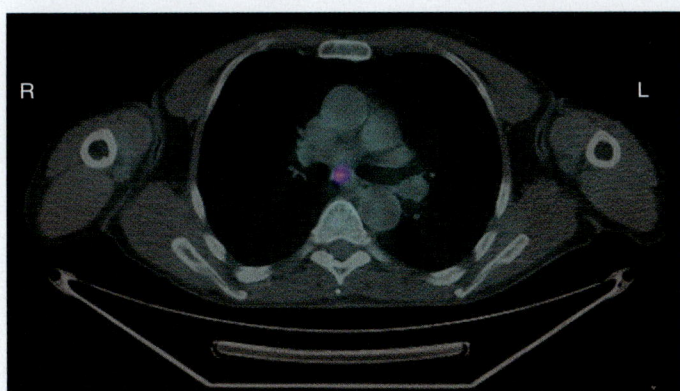

FIGURE 110.10 A subcarinal lymph node has mild ^{18}F-fluorodeoxyglucose (FDG) uptake. Based on these findings, additional invasive staging is warranted, including bronchoscopy and invasive staging of mediastinal lymph nodes. Endobronchial ultrasound with transtracheal needle aspiration can be performed with real-time ultrasound guidance to facilitate transtracheal needle placement. Biopsies of other stations can be performed as well. If needed, cervical mediastinoscopy is performed with biopsy of high paratracheal (2R and 2L), low paratracheal (4R and 4L), pretracheal (3A), and subcarinal (7) lymph nodes. If left-sided aortopulmonary lymph nodes were FDG avid, a Chamberlain procedure (anterior mediastinotomy) or video-assisted thoracic surgery with biopsy of aortopulmonary window lymph nodes or hilar lymph nodes could also be performed. Additional evaluation of the patient would be warranted if the patient would be considered a surgical candidate.

characteristics. The staging system creates a shorthand description of the tumor, lymph nodes, and metastatic characteristics of the patient to facilitate the choice of optimal therapy and evaluate outcomes based on the clinical and pathologic stage. The American Joint Committee on Cancer (AJCC) and the Union for International Cancer Control work to establish and promulgate staging system guidelines. The 2018 8th edition TNM stage classification for lung cancer provides the basis for specific patient stage groupings and is used for initial treatment recommendations based on the clinical stage and on the pathologic stage after pulmonary resection.

The clinician's responsibility is to ensure the highest possible degree of certainty regarding the extent of the disease and recommend the therapy or therapeutic combination of greatest efficacy based on the disease stage. The clinical stage is the physician's best and final estimate of the extent of disease based on all available information from both invasive and noninvasive studies before the initiation of definitive therapy. Key noninvasive imaging modalities used in clinical staging of NSCLC patients are CT, PET/CT, and MRI of the brain. Invasive staging modalities are also often performed to complement and more accurately determine disease stage. This may include invasive mediastinal staging (endobronchial ultrasound [EBUS] or mediastinoscopy), pleural taps, and biopsies from suspected metastatic sites. The surgical pathologic stage is based on the clinical stage plus the physical extent of the disease based on histologic examination of resected tissues, including the hilar and mediastinal lymph nodes.

Current Lung Cancer 8th Edition Staging System

The International Association for the Study of Lung Cancer (IASLC), together with the AJCC, has recently issued the 8th edition of the lung cancer staging system based on data from ~95,000 patients diagnosed with lung cancer from 1999–2010. After exclusions, 70,967 with NSCLC and 6189 with SCLC were included in the analysis. Nearly 85% underwent surgical treatment, either alone

(57.7%) or together with chemotherapy (21.1%), radiotherapy (1.5%), or both (4.4%). Survival was analyzed using Kaplan-Meier methods, and survival estimates were compared using the likelihood ratio test from Cox proportional hazards regression. Analysis allowed definition of TNM categories and stage groupings that demonstrated consistent discrimination overall and within multiple different patient cohorts (e.g., clinical or pathologic stage, R0 or R-any resection status, geographic region). Additional analyses provided evidence of applicability over time and across a spectrum of geographic regions, histologic types, evaluative approaches, and follow-up intervals.[22,23]

The 8th edition TNM definitions, nodal characteristics, and stage groupings of the TNM subsets are shown in Tables 110.1 to 110.3. Other schematics have been created for the lymph node map and T characteristics. The mediastinal and regional lymph node classification schema is presented in Fig. 110.11. This map presents a graphic representation of mediastinal and pulmonary lymph nodes in relation to other thoracic structures for optimal dissection and anatomic labeling by the surgeon.[24] The ninth edition staging system is forthcoming, with data collected from 2011–2019.

Tumor

The 8th edition of the IASLC/AJCC lung cancer staging project introduces, for the first time, special definitions for carcinoma in situ (Tis) and minimally invasive carcinomas (T1mis). Tis carcinomas are less than 3-cm noninvasive tumors that histologically display a pure lepidic growth pattern. T1mi tumors are smaller than 3 cm and histologically display a predominant lepidic growth pattern; however, they also have a small (<0.5-cm) invasive component. In addition, the definitions of the four classic lung cancer T categories (T1–T4) have also been refined. In the current edition, T1 tumors (<3 cm) are subcategorized as follows: T1a (<1 cm), T1b (1–2 cm), and T1c (2–3 cm). T2 tumors (>3–5 cm) are subcategorized as follows: T2a (3–4 cm) and T2b (4–5 cm). T3 tumors are 5 to 7 cm, and T4 tumors are >7 cm. T stage is also determined by extent of tumor involvement, outlined as follows:

- T2: Involvement of the main bronchus, invasion of the visceral pleural, or association with lobar/lung atelectasis are included.
- T3: Invasion of the parietal pleura, chest wall, phrenic nerve, parietal pericardium, or associated separate tumor nodule(s) in the same lobe as the primary tumor.
- T4: Invasion of the diaphragm, mediastinum, heart, great vessels, trachea, recurrent laryngeal nerve, esophagus, vertebral body, carina, or separate tumor nodule(s) in a different ipsilateral lobe to that of the primary tumor.

Contrast-enhanced CT of the chest is the main imaging modality used to determine the T stage. MRI of the chest wall may assist in identifying chest wall involvement and in staging of superior sulcus tumors.

Lymph Nodes

The node descriptor (N0–N3) is defined according to the extent of lymph node metastasis along a predefined lymph node map with 14 lymph node stations. Station 10 to 14 nodes are confined to the lung, and metastasis to these nodes indicates N1 disease if ipsilateral to the tumor and N3 disease if contralateral to the tumor. Station 9 to 2 nodes are confined to the mediastinum, and metastasis to these nodes indicates N2 disease if ipsilateral to the tumor and N3 disease if contralateral to the tumor. Station 1 nodes are supraclavicular or suprasternal or low cervical nodes, and metastasis to these nodes indicates N3 disease.

The nodal characteristics and designations did not change in the 8th edition of the IASLC lung cancer staging project. However, a

TABLE 110.1 Tumor-Node-Metastasis (TNM) Descriptors for the 8th Edition of TNM Classification for Lung Cancer

T: Primary Tumor

TX	Primary tumor cannot be assessed, or tumor proven by the presence of malignant cells in sputum or bronchial washings but not visualized by imaging or bronchoscopy
T0	No evidence of primary tumor
Tis	Carcinoma in situ
T1	Tumor ≤3 cm in greatest dimension, surrounded by lung or visceral pleura, without bronchoscopic evidence of invasion more proximal than the lobar bronchus (i.e., not in the main bronchus)[a]
T1a(mi)	Minimally invasive adenocarcinoma[b]
T1a	Tumor ≤1 cm in greatest dimension[a]
T1b	Tumor >1 cm but ≤2 cm in greatest dimension[a]
T1c	Tumor >2 cm but ≤3 cm in greatest dimension[a]
T2	Tumor >3 cm **but ≤5 cm** or tumor with any of the following features[c]: • Involves main bronchus regardless of distance from the carina but without involvement of the carina • Invades visceral pleura • Associated with atelectasis or obstructive pneumonitis that extends to the hilar region, involving part or all of the lung
T2a	**Tumor >3 cm but ≤4 cm in greatest dimension**
T2b	**Tumor >4 cm but ≤5 cm in greatest dimension**
T3	**Tumor >5 cm but ≤7 cm in greatest dimension** or associated with separate tumor nodule(s) in the same lobe as the primary tumor or directly invades any of the following structures: chest wall (including the parietal pleura and superior sulcus tumors), phrenic nerve, parietal pericardium
T4	**Tumor >7 cm in greatest dimension** or associated with separate tumor nodule(s) in a different ipsilateral lobe than that of the primary tumor or invades any of the following structures: diaphragm, mediastinum, heart, great vessels, trachea, recurrent laryngeal nerve, esophagus, vertebral body, and carina

N: Regional Lymph Nodes Involvement

NX	Regional lymph nodes cannot be assessed
N0	No regional lymph node metastases
N1	Metastasis in ipsilateral peribronchial and/or ipsilateral hilar lymph nodes and intrapulmonary nodes, including involvement by direct extension
N2	Metastasis in ipsilateral mediastinal and/or subcarinal lymph node(s)
N3	Metastasis in contralateral mediastinal, contralateral hilar, ipsilateral or contralateral scalene, or supraclavicular lymph node(s)

M (Distant Metastasis)

M0	No distant metastasis
M1	Distant metastasis present
• M1a	Separate tumor nodule(s) in a contralateral lobe; tumor with pleural or pericardial nodule(s) or malignant pleural or pericardial effusion[d]
• M1b	Single extrathoracic metastasis[e]
• M1c	Multiple extrathoracic metastases in one or more organs

Note: Changes from the seventh edition are in bold.

[a]The uncommon superficial spreading tumor of any size with its invasive component limited to the bronchial wall, which may extend proximal to the main bronchus, is also classified as T1a.

[b]Solitary adenocarcinoma, ≤3 cm with a predominantly lepidic pattern and ≤5-mm invasion in any one focus.

[c]T2 tumors with these features are classified as T2a if ≤4 cm in greatest dimension or if size cannot be determined and as T2b if >4 cm but ≤5 cm in greatest dimension.

[d]Most pleural (pericardial) effusions with lung cancer are a result of tumor. In a few patients, however, multiple microscopic examinations of pleural (pericardial) fluid are negative for tumor, and the fluid is nonbloody and not an exudate. When these elements and clinical judgment dictate that the effusion is not related to the tumor, the effusion should be excluded as a staging descriptor.

[e]This includes involvement of a single distant (nonregional) lymph node.

From Goldstraw P, Chansky K, Crowley J, et al. The IASLC lung cancer staging project: proposals for revision of the TNM stage groupings in the forthcoming (eighth) edition of the TNM classification for lung cancer. *J Thorac Oncol.* 2016;11:39-51.

TABLE 110.2 Proposed Stage Grouping for the 8th Edition of the TNM Classification for Lung Cancer

Occult Carcinoma	TX	N0	M0
Stage 0	Tis	N0	M0
Stage IA1	**T1a(mi)**	**N0**	**M0**
	T1a	**N0**	**M0**
Stage IA2	**T1b**	**N0**	**M0**
Stage IA3	**T1c**	**N0**	**M0**
Stage IB	T2a	N0	M0
Stage IIA	T2b	N0	M0
Stage IIB	**T1a–c**	**N1**	**M0**
	T2a	**N1**	**M0**
	T2b	N1	M0
	T3	N0	M0
Stage IIIA	**T1a–c**	**N2**	**M0**
	T2a–b	N2	M0
	T3	N1	M0
	T4	N0	M0
	T4	N1	M0
Stage IIIB	**T1a–c**	**N3**	**M0**
	T2a–b	N3	M0
	T3	**N3**	**M0**
	T4	N2	M0
Stage IIIC	**T3**	**N3**	**M0**
	T4	**N3**	**M0**
Stage IVA	**Any T**	**Any N**	**M1a**
	Any T	**Any N**	**M1b**
Stage IVB	**Any T**	**Any N**	**M1c**

Note: Changes to the seventh edition are highlighted in bold.
T1a(mi), Minimally invasive adenocarcinoma; *Tis*, carcinoma in situ; *TNM*, tumor-node-metastasis.
From Goldstraw P, Chansky K, Crowley J, et al. The IASLC lung cancer staging project: proposals for revision of the TNM stage groupings in the forthcoming (eighth) edition of the TNM classification for lung cancer. *J Thorac Oncol.* 2016;11:39-51.

recommendation is made to define nodal involvement not only by the N0–N3 descriptors but also by quantifying the number of involved lymph nodes. In particular, nodal quantification by the number of involved nodal stations is defined as follows: N1a, single N1 nodal station; N1b, multiple N1 nodal stations; N2a1, single N2 nodal station without N1 involvement (skip metastasis); N2a2, single N2 nodal station with N1 involvement; and N2b, multiple N2 nodal stations.

Prognosis worsens as the number of involved nodal stations increases, but N1b and N2a1 have the same prognosis. Asamura and colleagues[25] demonstrated different 5-year survival rates according to nodal stage for patients who underwent complete resection: N1a (59% 5-year survival), N1b (50%), N2a1 (54%), N2a2 (43%), and N2b (38%).

FDG/PET combined with contrast-enhanced CT is the main imaging modality used to determine the N stage. Hilar and mediastinal nodes that are suspected to be involved by cancer (>1 cm) or have positive FDG uptake are typically biopsied to confirm tumor metastasis.

Metastases

The 8th edition of lung cancer staging defines two M descriptors, M0 and M1, with M1 being subcategorized into M1a, M1b, and M1c. **M1a** indicates endothoracic metastasis (malignant pleural/pericardial effusion or malignant pleural/pericardial nodules or separate tumor nodule in a contralateral lobe). **M1b** indicates the presence of a single extrathoracic metastasis in a single organ. **M1c** indicates the presence of multiple extrathoracic metastases in a single organ or in multiple organs. Although M1a and M1b tumors have similar prognosis, they represent different forms of metastatic involvement and require different diagnostics and therapeutics. FDG/PET combined with contrast-enhanced CT is the main imaging modality used to determine the M stage. Brain MRI is used to identify brain metastasis. Suspected metastatic lesions may be biopsied to confirm diagnosis or determine treatment plan. Otherwise, metastatic lesions are not routinely sampled.

TABLE 110.3 Anatomic Limits of the Nodal Stations of the International Association for the Study of Lung Cancer Lymph Node Map and Their Grouping in Nodal Zones

LYMPH NODE STATION NO.	ANATOMIC LIMITS
Supraclavicular Zone	
1: Low cervical, supraclavicular, and sternal notch nodes	• Upper border: Lower margin of cricoid cartilage • Lower border: Clavicles bilaterally and, in the midline, the upper border of the manubrium; *1R* designates right-sided nodes, and *1L* designates left-sided nodes in this region • For lymph node station 1, the midline of the trachea serves as the border between 1R and 1L
Upper Zone	
2: Upper paratracheal nodes	• 2R: Upper border: Apex of the right lung and pleural space and, in the midline, the upper border of the manubrium • Lower border: Intersection of caudal margin of innominate vein with the trachea • Similar to lymph node station 4R, 2R includes nodes extending to the left lateral border of the trachea • 2L: Upper border: Apex of the lung and pleural space and, in the midline, the upper border of the manubrium • Lower border: Superior border of the aortic arch
3: Prevascular and retrotracheal nodes	• 3a: Prevascular • On the right: Upper border, apex of chest; lower border, level of carina; anterior border, posterior aspect of sternum; posterior border, anterior border of superior vena cava • On the left: Upper border, apex of chest; lower border, level of carina; anterior border, posterior aspect of sternum; posterior border, left carotid artery • 3p: Retrotracheal • Upper border, apex of chest; lower border, carina

Continued

TABLE 110.3 Anatomic Limits of the Nodal Stations of the International Association for the Study of Lung Cancer Lymph Node Map and Their Grouping in Nodal Zones—cont'd

LYMPH NODE STATION NO.	ANATOMIC LIMITS
4: Lower paratracheal nodes	• 4R: Includes right paratracheal nodes and pretracheal nodes extending to the left lateral border of the trachea • Upper border: Intersection of caudal margin of innominate vein with the trachea • Lower border: Lower border of the azygos vein • 4L: Includes nodes to the left of the left lateral border of the trachea, medial to the ligamentum arteriosum • Upper border: Upper margin of the aortic arch • Lower border: Upper rim of the left main pulmonary artery
Aortopulmonary Zone	
5: Subaortic (aortopulmonary window)	• Subaortic lymph nodes lateral to the ligamentum arteriosum • Upper border: The lower border of the aortic arch • Lower border: Upper rim of the left main pulmonary artery
6: Para-aortic nodes (ascending aorta or phrenic)	• Lymph nodes anterior and lateral to the ascending aorta and aortic arch • Upper border: A line tangential to the upper border of the aortic arch • Lower border: The lower border of the aortic arch
Subcarinal Zone	
7: Subcarinal nodes	• Upper border: The carina of the trachea • Lower border: The upper border of the lower lobe bronchus on the left; the lower border of the bronchus intermedius on the right
Lower Zone	
8: Paraesophageal nodes (below carina)	• Nodes lying adjacent to the wall of the esophagus and to the right or the left of the midline, excluding subcarinal nodes • Upper border: The upper border of the lower lobe bronchus on the left; the lower border of the bronchus intermedius on the right • Lower border: The diaphragm
9: Pulmonary ligament nodes	• Nodes lying within the pulmonary ligament • Upper border: The inferior pulmonary vein • Lower border: The diaphragm
Hilar/Interlobar Zone	
10: Hilar nodes	• Includes nodes immediately adjacent to the mainstem bronchus and hilar vessels, including the proximal portions of the pulmonary veins and main pulmonary artery • Upper border: The lower rim of the azygos vein in the right, upper rim of the pulmonary artery on the left • Lower border: Interlobar region bilaterally

11: Interlobar nodes	• Between the origins of the lobar bronchi
	• Optional notations for subcategories of station:
	  • 11s: Between the upper-lobe bronchus and bronchus intermedius on the right
	  • 11i: Between the middle and lower bronchi on the right

Peripheral Zone	
12: Lobar nodes	Adjacent to the lobar bronchi
13: Segmental nodes	Adjacent to the segmental bronchi
14: Subsegmental nodes	Adjacent to the subsegmental bronchi

Adapted from Rusch VW, Asamura H, Watanabe H, et al. The IASLC lung cancer staging project: a proposal for a new international lymph node map in the forthcoming seventh edition of the TNM classification for lung cancer. *J Thorac Oncol.* 2009;4:568-577.

Stages

The 8th edition of the lung cancer staging system has refined and expanded the lung cancer stage definitions to produce a more precise tool to predict prognosis and guide treatment plan (Fig. 110.12). Pretreatment staging determines prognosis: 5-year survival rates by *pathologic* stage are 90% for stage IA1, 85% for stage IA2, 80% for stage IA3, 73% for stage IB, 65% for stage IIA, 56% for stage IIB, 41% for stage IIIA, 24% for stage IIIB, and 12% for stage IIIB. For *clinical* stage, the 5-year survival rates by clinical stage are 13% for stage IVA and nearly 0% for stage IVB.

Treatments for Lung Cancer

The choice of initial therapy depends on the clinical stage at the time of diagnosis and the patient's functional class and comorbidities. Treatment options may vary, even among different subsets of patients within the same clinical stage. Broadly, lung carcinoma should be resected when the local disease can be controlled, the patient's physical condition can tolerate the planned resection and reconstruction, and the anticipated operative morbidity and mortality are reasonable. Conditions such as superior vena cava syndrome, tumor invasion across the mediastinum into the main pulmonary artery, N3 nodal metastases, malignant pleural or pericardial disease, or extrathoracic metastases carry greater risk than benefit for resection in most patients. Some centers have had good results with resection and reconstruction of the trachea, atrium, great vessels, or other mediastinal or vertebral structures. However, these are complex operations requiring experienced multidisciplinary teams during the pre-, intra-, and postoperative phases. Patients with tracheoesophageal fistula have a limited life expectancy, and palliative care with stent placement would be recommended.

Treatments can be grouped into three major categories according to stage, as follows:

1. Stage I and II disease indicate the presence of tumor that is contained within the lung and that may be completely resected with surgery. Anatomic resection of the lobe where the tumor resides with complete sampling of mediastinal lymph nodes is the treatment of choice. The key aim of this treatment approach is to achieve complete resection of the tumor and its intralobar-draining lymph nodes. In certain cases, sublobar anatomic resections may be considered for small and peripheral tumors. There is a growing body of evidence to suggest sublobar resections are at least not inferior to anatomic resection.[26,27] However, anatomic resection remains the standard of care, and nonanatomic resection should be performed only when more extensive surgery cannot be tolerated by the patient (e.g., because of reduced pulmonary reserve). Stereotactic body radiation therapy (SBRT) has had excellent results (local control rates of 85%–90% at 3 years) in selected patients who cannot withstand surgical resection[28] and even as an alternative to operable tumors in some patient groups.[29]

2. Stage IV and IIIB disease are not typically treated by surgery except in patients requiring surgical palliation. Systemic therapies for metastatic disease are common. Chemoradiation is often used in stage IIIB disease. Targeted therapies and immunotherapy are providing encouraging results in properly screened and selected patients. Figs. 110.13 and 110.14 outline current molecular therapeutic targets.

3. Stage IIIA lung cancer indicates a locally advanced disease that may have a wide spectrum of presentations. The majority of stage IIIA tumors are too advanced for consideration of resection; however, if complete resection is deemed possible, it may be associated with improved outcomes. In this clinical scenario, surgical resection is performed as part of a multimodality treatment protocol. In particular, resectable stage IIIA tumors are either small tumors that present with a low metastatic burden to the ipsilateral mediastinal (N2) lymph nodes or larger tumors that do not involve mediastinal lymph nodes (T4N0/1M0). These tumors, by their advanced nature, may be mechanically removed with surgery; however, surgery does not consistently control the micrometastases that exist within the general area of the operation or systemically. Combinations of chemotherapy and radiotherapy, and in recent years also immunotherapy, are used for locally advanced disease either in the adjuvant or neoadjuvant settings.[30–32] A multidisciplinary team of experts usually predefines the desired treatment plan in each case.

Local Therapy for Early Stage Non–Small Cell Lung Cancer

Stages I and II NSCLC can be treated safely with surgery and mediastinal lymph node dissection, and most patients have long-term survival. Stage Ia and Ib tumors should be treated with surgery first, followed by adjuvant systemic chemotherapy for tumors with high-risk features. Stage II tumors should be treated with

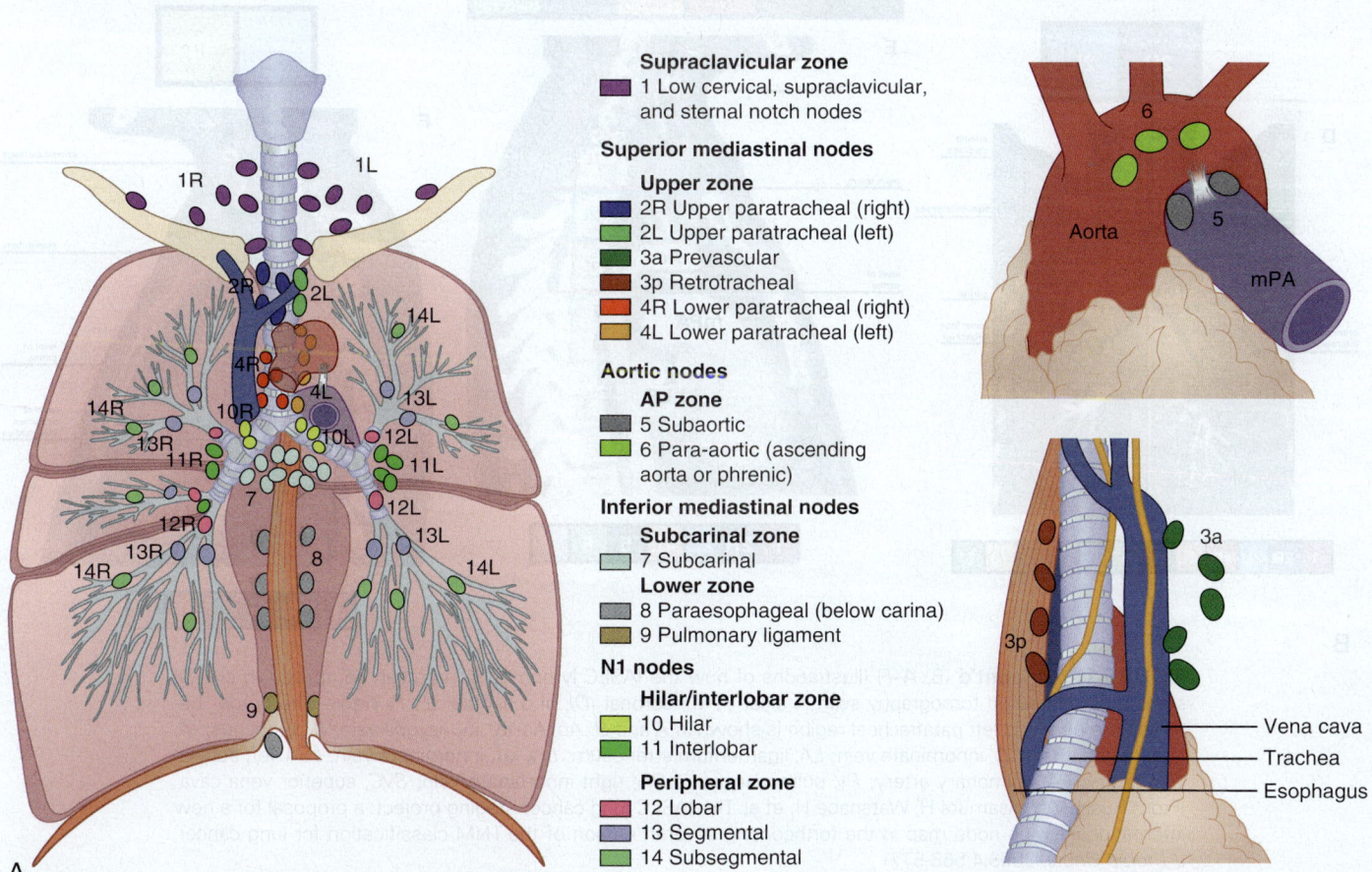

Supraclavicular zone
1 Low cervical, supraclavicular, and sternal notch nodes

Superior mediastinal nodes

Upper zone
2R Upper paratracheal (right)
2L Upper paratracheal (left)
3a Prevascular
3p Retrotracheal
4R Lower paratracheal (right)
4L Lower paratracheal (left)

Aortic nodes

AP zone
5 Subaortic
6 Para-aortic (ascending aorta or phrenic)

Inferior mediastinal nodes

Subcarinal zone
7 Subcarinal

Lower zone
8 Paraesophageal (below carina)
9 Pulmonary ligament

N1 nodes

Hilar/interlobar zone
10 Hilar
11 Interlobar

Peripheral zone
12 Lobar
13 Segmental
14 Subsegmental

FIGURE 110.11 (A) The International Association for the Study of Lung Cancer (IASLC) lymph node map, including the proposed grouping of lymph node stations into "zones" for the purposes of prognostic analyses.

Continued

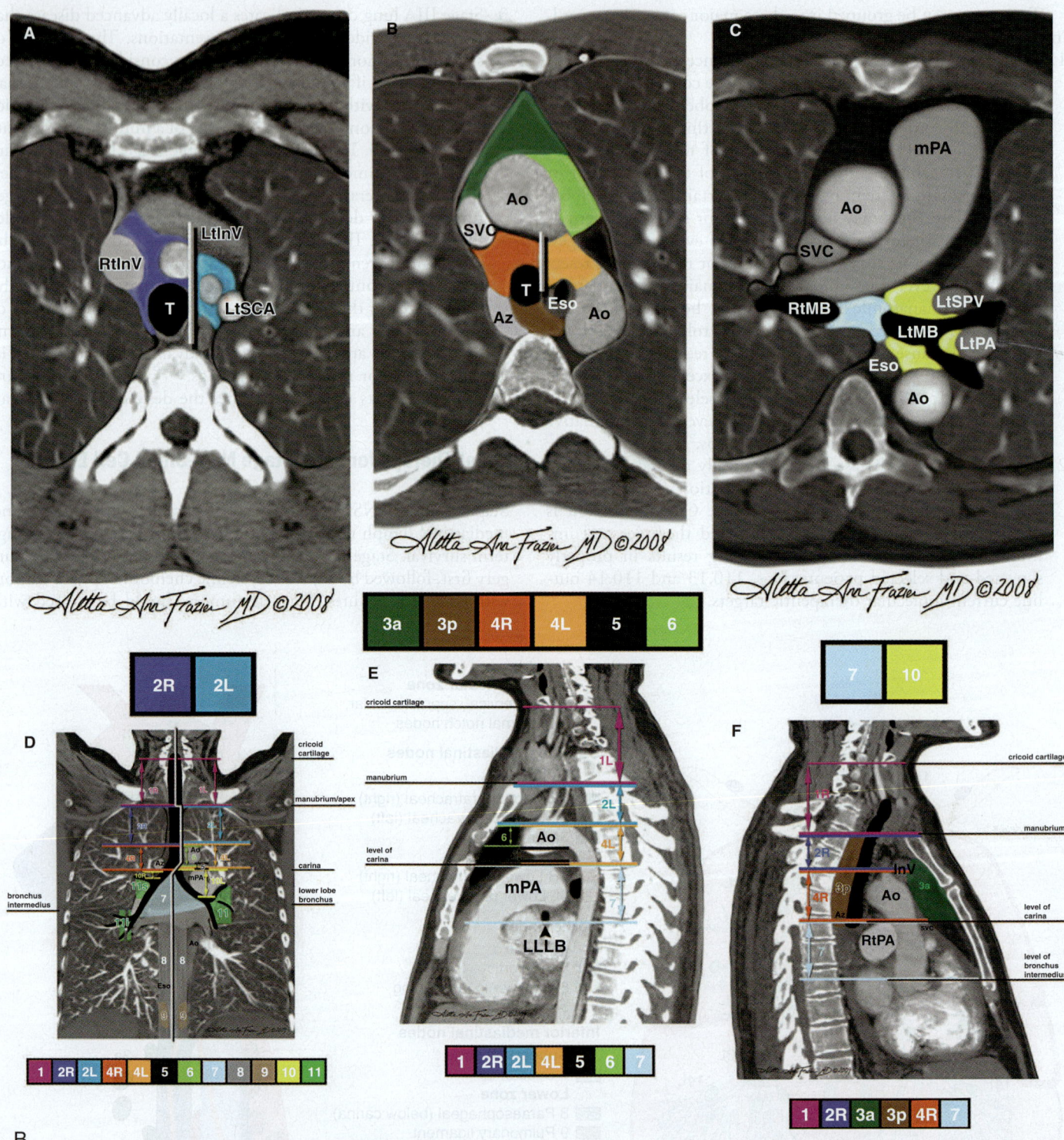

FIGURE 110.11, cont'd (B, A–F) Illustrations of how the IASLC lymph node map can be applied to clinical staging by computed tomography scan in axial (A–C), coronal (D), and sagittal (E, F) views. The border between the right and left paratracheal region is shown in A and B. Ao, Aorta; AV, azygos vein; Br, bronchus; IA, innominate artery; IV, innominate vein; LA, ligamentum arteriosum; LIV, left innominate vein; LSA, left subclavian artery; PA, pulmonary artery; PV, pulmonary vein; RIV, right innominate vein; SVC, superior vena cava. (From Rusch VW, Asamura H, Watanabe H, et al. The IASLC lung cancer staging project: a proposal for a new international lymph node map in the forthcoming seventh edition of the TNM classification for lung cancer. J Thorac Oncol. 2009;4:568-577.)

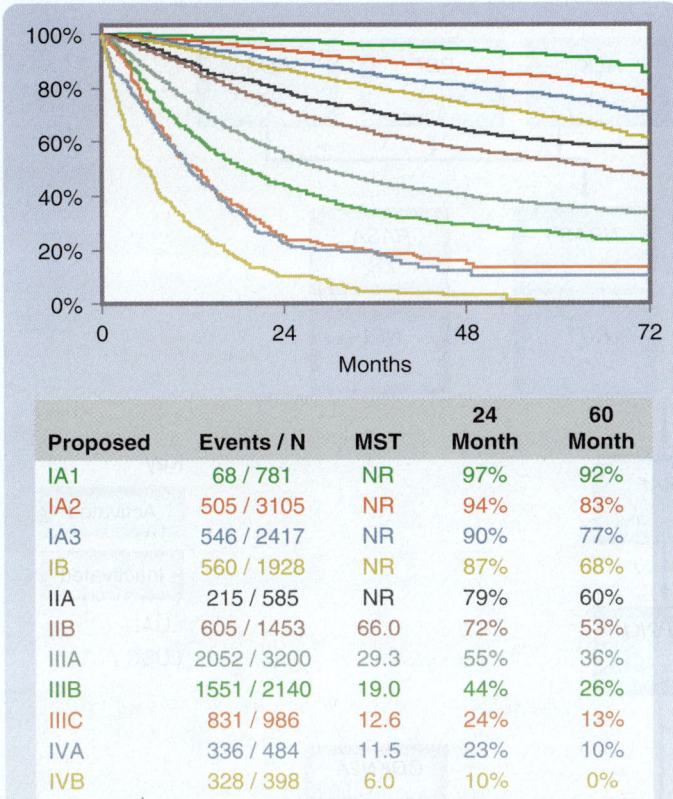

Proposed	Events / N	MST	24 Month	60 Month
IA1	68 / 781	NR	97%	92%
IA2	505 / 3105	NR	94%	83%
IA3	546 / 2417	NR	90%	77%
IB	560 / 1928	NR	87%	68%
IIA	215 / 585	NR	79%	60%
IIB	605 / 1453	66.0	72%	53%
IIIA	2052 / 3200	29.3	55%	36%
IIIB	1551 / 2140	19.0	44%	26%
IIIC	831 / 986	12.6	24%	13%
IVA	336 / 484	11.5	23%	10%
IVB	328 / 398	6.0	10%	0%

FIGURE 110.12 Overall survival by clinical stage according to the 8th edition of the lung cancer staging project. *MST*, Median survival time. (From Goldstraw P, Chansky K, Crowley J, et al. The IASLC lung cancer staging project: proposals for revision of the TNM stage groupings in the forthcoming [eighth] edition of the TNM classification for lung cancer. *J Thorac Oncol.* 2016;11:39-51.)

systemic therapy followed by surgical resection. There is a growing body of evidence to support the use of perioperative systemic immunotherapy in combination with chemotherapy in these patients.[31,32] Anatomic resection with lobectomy and systematic mediastinal lymph node dissection or sampling (defined by the American College of Surgeons Oncology Group) is the procedure of choice for lung cancer confined to one lobe. Sublobar resection may be considered in select groups, including patients with small peripheral tumors or those who cannot tolerate an anatomic lobectomy. Recent randomized control trials have demonstrated at least noninferiority of sublobar resection compared with lobectomy in a more generalized patient group.[26,27] At a minimum, samples of nodal (not adipose) tissue from stations 4R, 7, 8, and 9 for right-sided cancers and stations 4L, 5, 6, 7, 8, and 9 for left-sided cancers should be obtained.

Treatment of Metastatic Disease

Metastatic disease (stage IV NSCLC) is usually incurable. Patients and families should be informed of the diagnosis and potential outcomes of treatment, including the reality that functional performance and quality of life will progressively decline. Treatment decisions should take into consideration the wishes of the patient and family, and realistic expectations should be set and monitored during therapy. In recent years, a growing number of biologic and immunologic therapies have been approved for the treatment of advanced NSCLC. In combination with conventional chemotherapy and radiation, these new therapeutics have significantly expanded the therapeutic options for patients with advanced inoperable NSCLC (stages IV and IIIB).

TRACHEA

The major physiologic role of the trachea is to conduct air between the larynx and the bronchi, exchange heat and moisture, and remove particles. The transport of air is dependent on the inner diameter of the trachea. Mucosal swelling, constriction of airway muscles, or tumors that reduce the airway space, but also endotracheal tubes, considerably increase the resistance to airflow: A 50% reduction of the inner diameter increases the resistance 16-fold, and during turbulent flow, the resistance is increased up to 32-fold. During inspiration, the upper airways efficiently warm and humidify the inspired air. During quiet breathing at room temperature, air is completely warmed up to 37°C and humidified to 100% saturation shortly distal to the bifurcation; this is called the *isothermal saturation point*. Tracheobronchial glands produce a mucin-rich secretion that forms a protective barrier between the epithelium and the environment. This secretion is largely controlled by the autonomic nervous system. The mucus collects debris and microorganisms and is transported orally by the mechanical forces of coordinated ciliary beating and the airflow during expiration.[33]

Benign Stenosis of the Trachea

Stenosis of the trachea describes a narrowing of the tracheal lumen and typically implies significant functional impairment. A normal 2-cm trachea has a 100% peak expiratory flow rate. A 10-mm opening provides an 80% peak expiratory flow rate. At 5 to 6 mm, only a 30% expiratory flow rate is obtained. Benign stenosis of the trachea results mainly from tracheotomy, overinflation of the endotracheal tube cuff during mechanical ventilation, or external trauma, but it is also associated with inhalation/thermal injury, autoimmune diseases, infection (commonly tuberculosis), and nonmalignant tumors. Tracheotomy leads to a transmural defect of the ventral part of the cervical trachea. The tracheotomy wound is colonized by bacteria, with local necrosis by mechanical alteration. After removal of the tracheostomy tube, the defect is closed by the secondary scar tissue healing, which tends to contract. This process of healing results in an A-shaped stenosis of the trachea (Fig. 110.15). The severity of shrinkage depends on the extension of the defect, necrosis, and infection. Low-volume, high-pressure cuffs of ventilation tubes induce circular necrosis of the tracheal mucosa. Depending on the pressure, the duration of ischemia, and local infection, the underlying cartilages may be bare, necrotic, and destroyed. A cuff pressure over 20 cm H_2O can exceed capillary perfusion pressure. Remember that the proper amount of air in an endotracheal tube cuff is the minimal amount to prevent an air leak. Mucosal defects without infection can be recovered from surrounding epithelium without relevant morbidity. Deeper destruction and infection of the tracheal wall leads to a ring of granulation tissue, forming a sandglass stenosis. Cuff-induced stenosis appears in the middle part of the trachea. The introduction of low-pressure, high-volume cuffs has made this kind of tracheal stenosis much rarer.[34]

Symptoms of tracheal obstruction can occur immediately after extubation or slowly over several years. Clinical signs like stridor

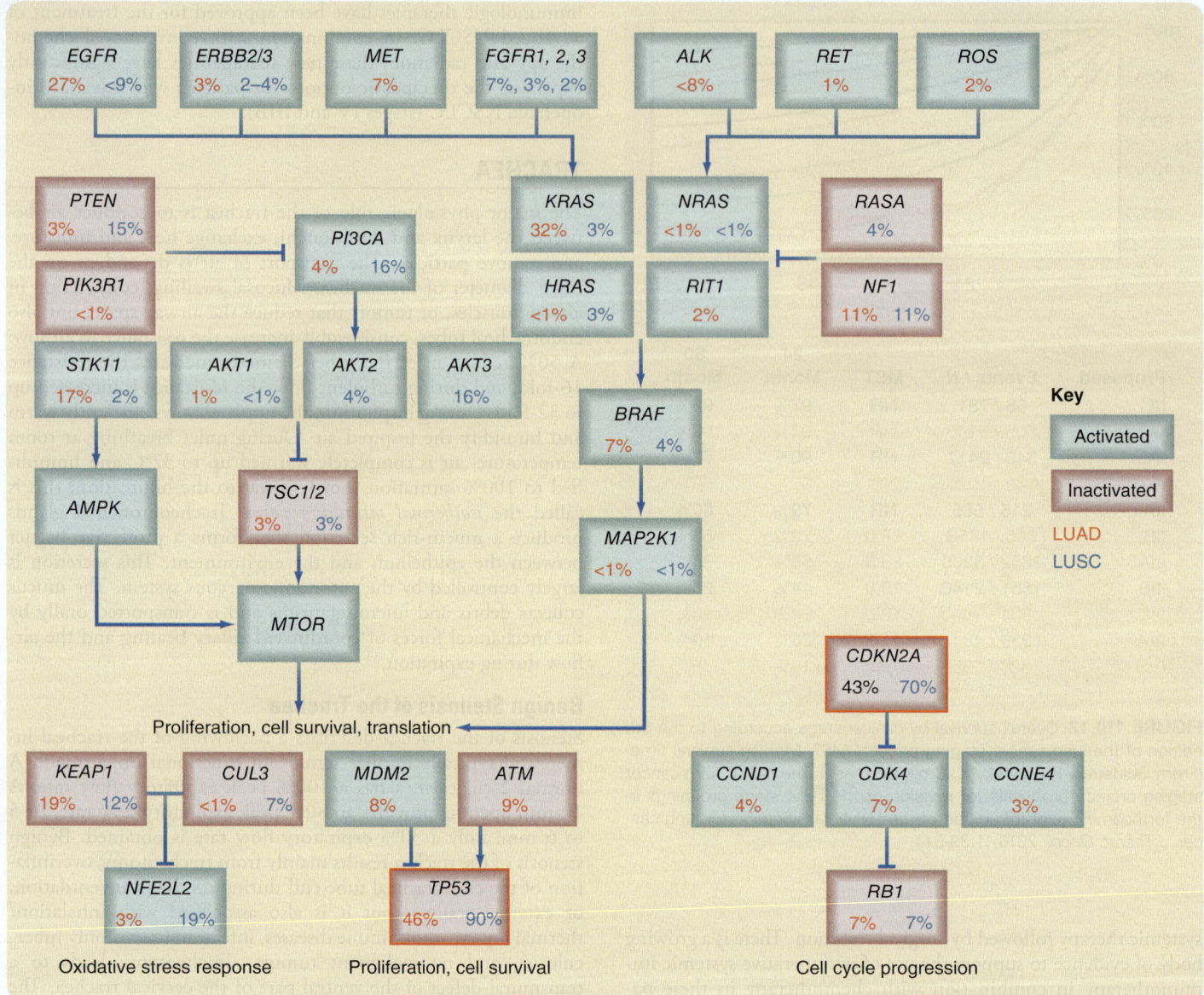

FIGURE 110.13 Alterations in targetable oncogenic pathways in lung adenocarcinoma (LUAD) and lung squamous cell carcinoma (LUSC). Pathway diagram showing the percentage of non–small cell lung cancer with alterations involving key pathway components for receptor tyrosine kinase signaling, mammalian target of rapamycin *(mTOR)* signaling, oxidative stress response, proliferation, and cell cycle progression. The frequency of alterations is based on the sum of somatic mutations, homozygous deletions, and focal amplifications and on significant up- or downregulation of gene expression (e.g., *AKT3*, *FGFR1*, *PTEN*). The most commonly mutated genes in LUAD include *KRAS* and *EGFR* and the tumor-suppressor genes *TP53*, *KEAP1*, *STK11*, and *NF1*. The frequency of epidermal growth factor receptor (EGFR)-activating mutations varies greatly by region and ethnicity. *KEAP1* inactivation in the presence of *KRAS* mutations confers sensitivity to inhibition of glutaminase in preclinical lung cancer models, providing a potential therapeutic strategy in dual *KEAP1*- and *KRAS*-mutant LUAD. Common mutated genes in LUSC include the tumor suppressors *TP53*, which is present in more than 90% of tumors, and *CDKN2A*. The latter, which encodes the p16INK4A and p14ARF proteins, is inactivated in over 70% of LUSC through epigenetic silencing by methylation (21%), inactivating mutation (18%), exon 1β skipping (4%), or homozygous deletion (29%). Although EGFR amplification occurs, unlike LUAD, actionable mutations in receptor tyrosine kinases are rarely observed in LUSC. (From Herbst RS, Morgensztern D, Boshoff C. The biology and management of non–small cell lung cancer. *Nature*. 2018;553:446-454.)

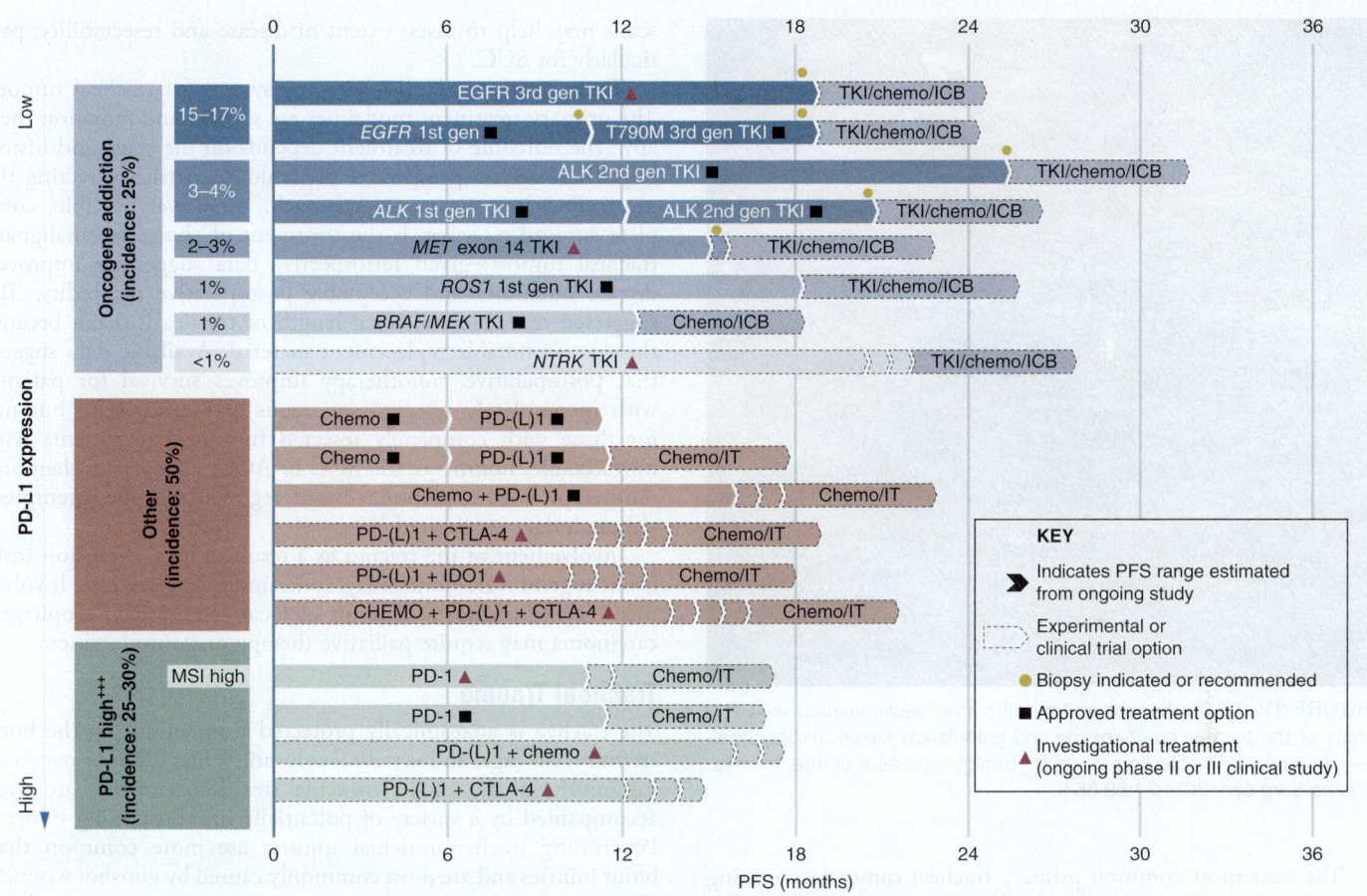

FIGURE 110.14 Current and investigative treatment options for advanced or metastatic non–small cell lung cancer (NSCLC). Illustration of the current and future personalized treatment options for NSCLC. Targetable oncogenic drivers account for approximately 25% of NSCLC, of which epidermal growth factor receptor mutations are the most frequent. Biopsies are indicated at the time of disease progression to determine the best treatment option. For patients with tumors expressing high levels of programmed cell death ligand 1 (PD-L1) (>50%) or high levels of microsatellite instability (MSI), single-agent immune checkpoint blockade (ICB) is indicated. In general, median progression-free survival is not the best indicator to capture the overall true benefit of ICBs because a proportion of patients remain alive or disease-free even after long-term follow-up. In patients with tumors with high (>50%) or low (>1%) expression levels of PD-L1, current studies are assessing the benefit of anti–PD-(L)1 combinations with cytotoxic therapy, anti–cytotoxic T-lymphocyte–associated protein 4, or other immunotherapy approaches. *TKI,* Tyrosine kinase inhibitor. (From Herbst RS, Morgensztern D, Boshoff C. The biology and management of non-small cell lung cancer. *Nature.* 2018;553:446-454.)

and dyspnea appear when the lumen is obliterated by more than 50%; however, clinical signs and lung function testing are not very sensitive or specific for tracheal stenosis. Standard of treatment for symptomatic patients consists of resection of the pathologic segment of the trachea with end-to-end anastomosis. In cases of involvement of the larynx, partial resections of the anterior cricoid cartilage or division of the larynx with tracheolaryngeal silicone stents is used. Short- and long-term results are satisfying.

Primary Neoplasm of the Trachea

Most tumors of the trachea in adult patients are malignant, and although primary tumors do occur, they most commonly represent direct invasion of the trachea from carcinoma of the surrounding structures (lung, esophagus, larynx, or thyroid gland). Hematogenous tracheal metastases have also been described in patients with carcinoma of the breast, colon, and kidney and

melanoma skin lesions.[35] For all tracheal tumors, primary or otherwise, the most common presenting symptoms are due to mass effect; frequently symptoms do not arise until the tumor obstructs ≥50% of the luminal diameter, and presentation varies based on the location of the tumor and histologic subtype.

The most common primary tracheal tumor is SCC, which comprises approximately one-half to two-thirds of cases. Up to 10% can be multifocal. Tumors may arise as an intraluminal nodule and progress to include mediastinal extension or lymph node metastases and may lead to stenosis or tracheoesophageal fistula. They are histologically identical to SCCs of the lung. SCCs often present with hemoptysis, given mucosal irritation and ulceration, and are typically diagnosed within 4 to 6 months of symptom onset. Dysphagia and hoarseness may also be present. The peak incidence is in the sixth to seventh decade of life. These tumors are seen primarily in smokers.

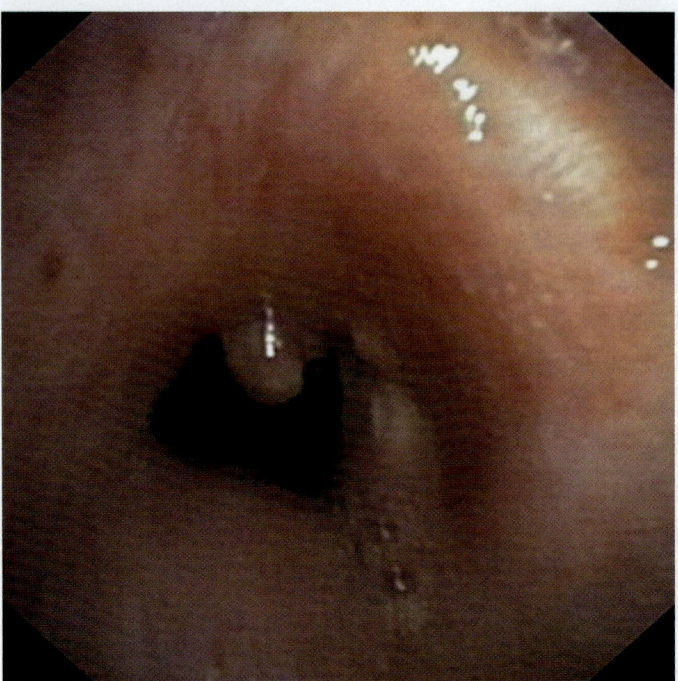

FIGURE 110.15 Tracheoscopy 3 months after decannulation with stenosis of the trachea by shrinkage and granulation tissue. (From Stoelben E, Koryllos A, Beckers F, et al. Benign stenosis of the trachea. *Thorac Surg Clin.* 2014;24:59-65.)

The next most common primary tracheal tumor (accounting for 10%–15% of cases) is adenoid cystic carcinomas (ACCs), previously called *cylindroma*. These are well-differentiated, slow-growing neoplasms that typically form polypoid lesions in the trachea or main stem bronchi, but they may form infiltrative plaques with longitudinal or circumferential extension and often breach the cartilaginous plate. Perineural invasion and extension along vascular structures is very common and accounts for the high rate of positive surgical margins, well beyond the gross limits of the tumor. ACCs can have multiple recurrences with late metastases. They are histologically identical to ACCs of the salivary glands. ACC commonly presents with wheezing or exertional dyspnea, with hemoptysis present in only a minority of cases. Diagnosis is established on average 18 months after symptom presentation. The peak incidence occurs in the fourth and fifth decades of life. It affects males and females equally and usually affects nonsmokers.[36]

Less common primary tracheal tumors include mucoepidermoid carcinoma, non–squamous cell bronchogenic carcinomas, sarcomas, carcinoid tumors, and pleomorphic adenoma. Benign tracheal lesions include hemangioma, hamartoma, neurogenic tumors, granular cell tumor, and squamous papillomas. Low-grade tumors, such as mucoepidermoid carcinomas or benign tumors, may be asymptomatic for years before diagnosis.

The diagnosis of tracheal tumors is often delayed as a result of similar presenting symptoms with other etiologies, including asthma, COPD, and pneumonia. Chest CT is recommended for patients in whom a tracheal pathology is suspected. This study may reveal polypoid lesions, focal stenosis, eccentric narrowing, or circumferential wall thickening. Bronchoscopy is mandatory to obtain a tissue diagnosis and differentiate between benign and malignant tumors. PET/CT may be useful for staging the cancer, but data on tracheal tumors are limited. Preoperative PET/CT

scans may help to assess extent of disease and resectability, particularly for SCC.

There is no standardized staging system for tracheal tumors. The primary treatment modalities are surgery and radiation therapy. The outcome of treatment depends on the stage and histology. There are no prospective or randomized trials directing the most efficacious treatment approach. Whenever possible, complete surgical resection is the treatment of choice for malignant tracheal tumors, given retrospective data suggesting improved disease outcomes and acceptable postoperative morbidity. The suggested maximum resected length of trachea is 5 cm because there is no suitable replacement material. Available data suggest that postoperative radiotherapy improves survival for patients with incompletely resected squamous SCC and ACC but not for those with completely resected tumors. For patients with unresectable, nonmetastatic SCC or ACC, concurrent chemoradiotherapy with a platinum-based regimen may be attempted, although data are limited.[37]

Involvement of the trachea as a result of local extension from bronchogenic carcinoma may contraindicate resection. Involvement of the trachea as a result of local extension of esophageal carcinoma may require palliative therapy or stent placement.

Tracheal Trauma

The trachea is anatomically protected from injury by the bony sternum, rib cage, and vertebral column. When blunt or penetrating injuries of the tracheobronchial tree do occur, they are often accompanied by a variety of potentially life-threatening injuries. Penetrating tracheobronchial injuries are more common than blunt injuries and are most commonly caused by gunshot wounds. The most common site of penetrating injuries is the cervical trachea, likely reflecting a high rate of mortality for anatomically lower injuries. Major associated injuries, mainly of the esophagus and great vessels, have been reported in 50% to 80% of penetrating injuries. Blunt tracheobronchial injuries are associated with major accompanying injuries in 40% to 100% of cases, commonly including pneumothorax/hemothorax, rib fractures, pulmonary contusion, laryngeal fracture, esophageal injury, cervical spine, and great vessel injuries.[38]

The most common clinical signs of tracheal injury are tachypnea and subcutaneous emphysema. Other signs include air escaping from the neck wound, massive air leak after placement of a tube thoracostomy, hemoptysis, stridor, and dysphagia. CXR and chest CT are the first steps in diagnosis. Paratracheal air, deep cervical emphysema, and pneumomediastinum are common findings. Bronchoscopy is the most important procedure to locate and assess trachea-bronchial injuries. Early airway assessment followed by definitive airway protection is the key to neck trauma management and trachea-bronchial injuries. Concurrent esophageal injury needs to be excluded by barium esophagography or esophagoscopy. Anesthetic management with laryngeal mask airway may be helpful for initial examination for full visualization of the airway before endotracheal intubation.

Nonoperative management with close monitoring may be considered for patients with blunt trauma and small stable injuries, those with no appreciable air leaks, and those who do not require positive pressure ventilation. For all other cases, immediate exploration of neck wounds is crucial for survival because vascular and esophageal injuries are frequent, and the tracheal injury often includes cartilage and ligamentous portions. Primary surgical repair represents the treatment of choice to reestablish airway continuity. Bronchial disruption may require thoracotomy for repair. Right thoracotomy provides excellent visualization of the carina and proximal left mainstem bronchus.

Acquired tracheoesophageal fistula can occur from cancer or from prolonged intubation with erosion posteriorly. Repair is with separation of the trachea and esophagus; repair of the fistulous tract; and interposition of normal tissue, such as muscle, between the two structures.

Tracheoinnominate fistula may result from prolonged cuff erosion inferiorly and anteriorly in the trachea. An inappropriately low stoma may further increase the likelihood of a direct erosion of the trachea by the innominate artery. The tip of the endotracheal tube may predispose to erosions or granulomas within the trachea. Tracheoinnominate fistula may manifest with a sentinel hemorrhage before sudden exsanguinating hemorrhage. Investigation of these sentinel hemorrhage episodes is critical. Evaluation in the operating room may provide for optimal situational control should additional interventions be required.

Principles of Tracheal Surgery

Elective or emergent tracheal surgical procedures are typically performed to improve tracheal patency or repair loss of tracheal integrity. Anesthetic challenges include abnormal airway anatomy and physiology, specialized endotracheal tubes for initial airway management, and evolving ventilatory challenges if the trachea is open or obstructed intraoperatively.

General inhalational anesthesia is used, and induction may be prolonged in the setting of tight stenosis. The patient should be maintained with spontaneous breathing if possible. Dilation with rigid bronchoscopy may be required before passing the endotracheal tube, especially if the stenosis is subglottic. Alternatively, the endotracheal tube may be positioned to a point above the stricture for induction.

Surgical approach is determined by tumor location and pathology. The cervical approach for tracheal resection is usually used for tumors of the upper half of the trachea plus all benign tracheal stenoses. Occasionally, an upper sternal split may be needed (Fig. 110.16). For tumors of the lower trachea, resection is performed in the right fourth intercostal space with intubation of the distal trachea or the left main stem bronchus. Carinal reconstruction may be necessary. Rigid bronchoscopy may be used for diagnosis, biopsy, dilation, or morcellation of tumor if the tumor cannot be immediately resected (Fig. 110.17).

Conventional teaching advises resection of no more than 5 cm of tracheal length, but this varies from person to person. Various

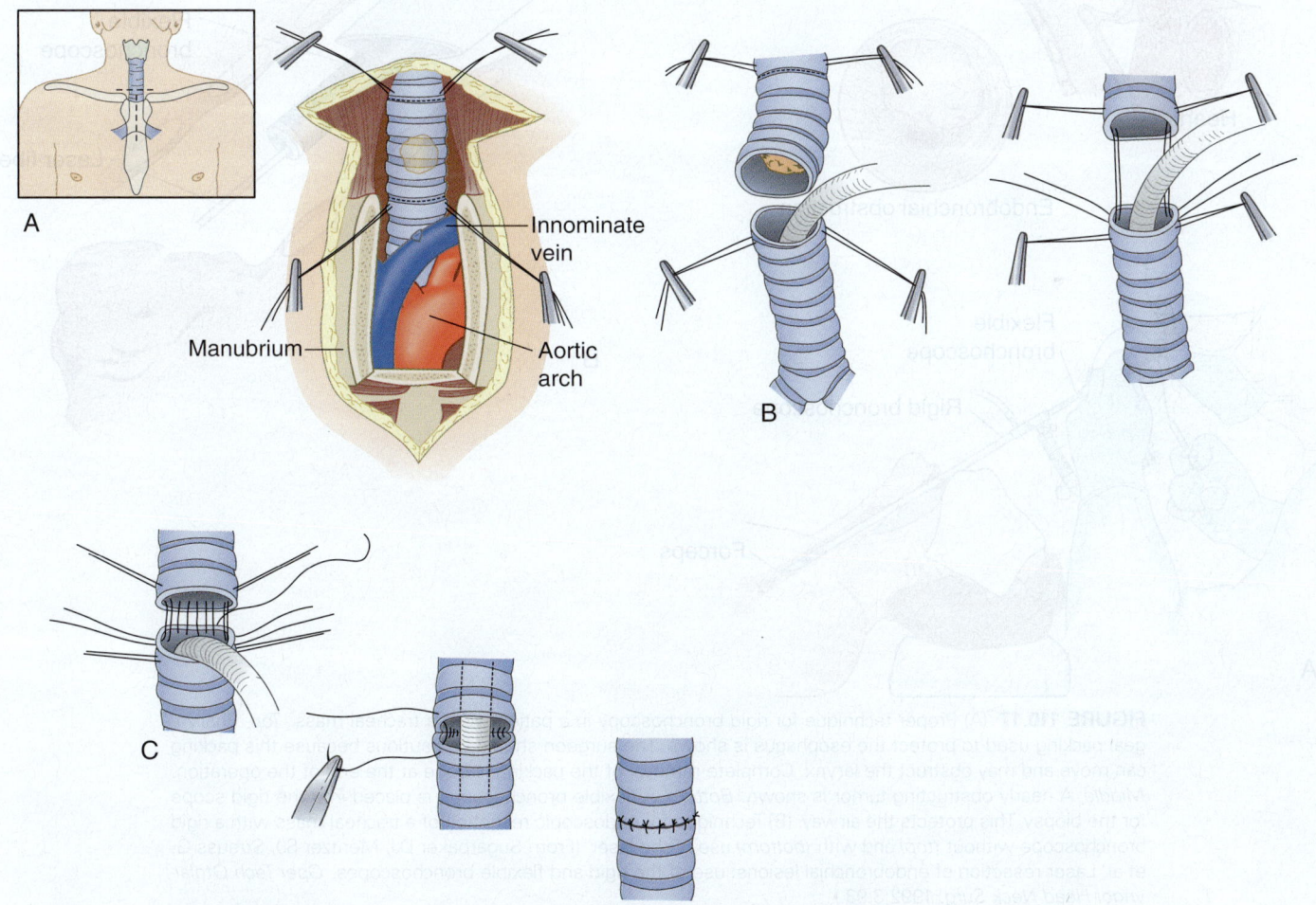

FIGURE 110.16 (A) Exposure of the midtrachea through a cervical and partial sternal-splitting incision. The extent of the resection has been marked by sutures. (B) After distal division, a sterile, armored endotracheal tube is placed. After proximal resection, two mattress sutures are placed in the edges of the cartilaginous rings. A simple running suture completes the membranous anastomosis. (C) At this point, the original endotracheal tube is positioned in the distal trachea so that the anastomosis can be completed with interrupted simple sutures between cartilaginous rings.

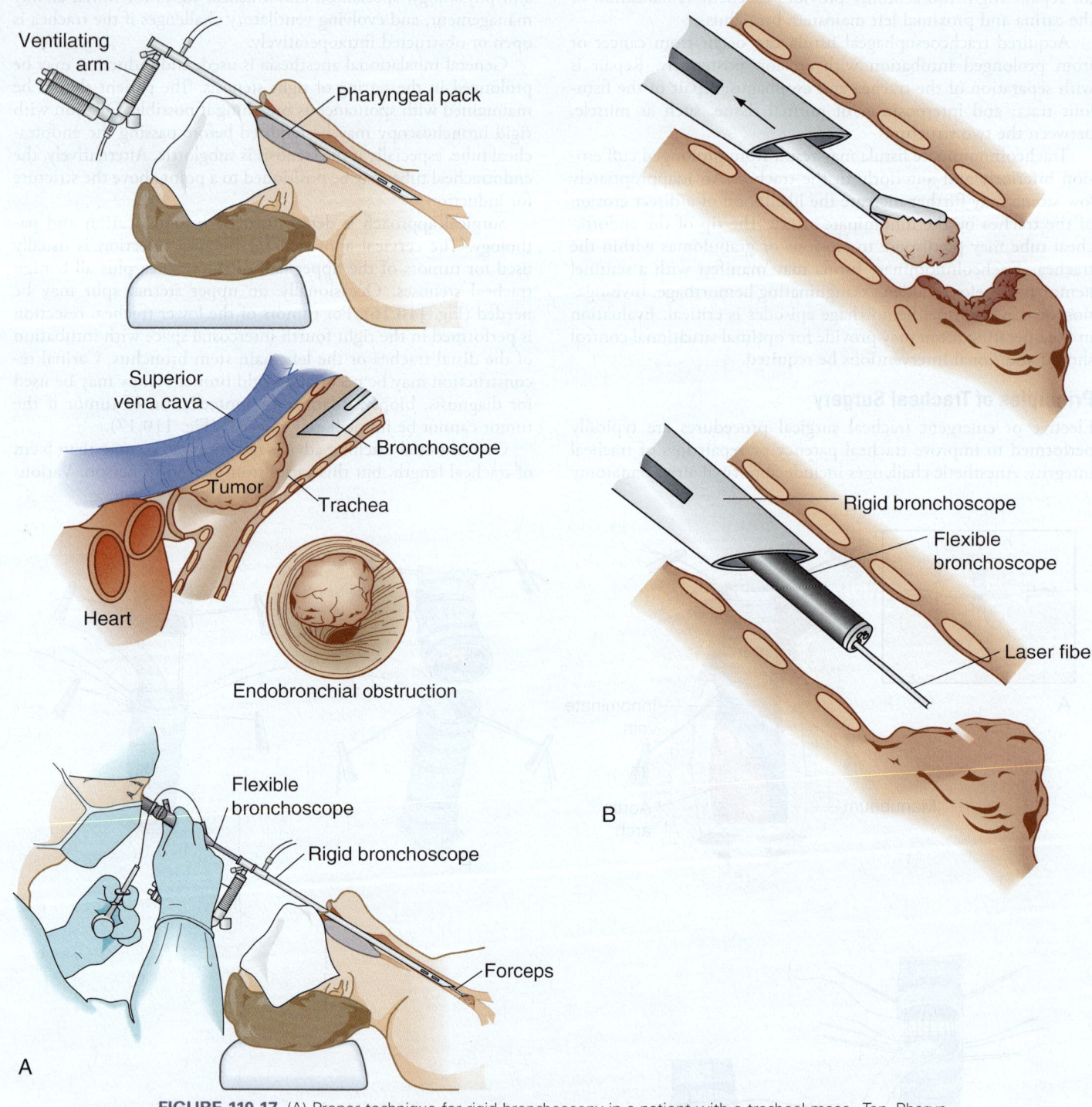

FIGURE 110.17 (A) Proper technique for rigid bronchoscopy in a patient with a tracheal mass. *Top,* Pharyngeal packing used to protect the esophagus is shown. The surgeon should be cautious because this packing can move and may obstruct the larynx. Complete removal of the packing is done at the end of the operation. *Middle,* A nearly obstructing tumor is shown. *Bottom,* A flexible bronchoscope is placed into the rigid scope for the biopsy. This protects the airway. (B) Technique for endoscopic resection of a tracheal mass with a rigid bronchoscope without *(top)* and with *(bottom)* use of the laser. (From Sugarbaker DJ, Mentzer SJ, Strauss G, et al. Laser resection of endobronchial lesions: use of the rigid and flexible bronchoscopes. *Oper Tech Otolaryngol Head Neck Surg.* 1992;3:93.)

techniques are used to mobilize the trachea to create a repair without undue tension on the anastomosis. The anterior cervical approach plus mobilization of the trachea and neck flexion can allow for 4 to 5 cm of trachea resection. A suprahyoid release may achieve 1 cm of additional length. Mobilization of the right hilum, together with division of the pericardium around the right hilum, may achieve an additional length.[39]

Procedures to repair subglottic larynx or cricoid stenosis are technically challenging. The recurrent nerves innervate the larynx just superior to the posterolateral cricoid on each side. If the tracheal lesions involve only the anterior surface, the anterior cricoid can be removed and the distal trachea beveled to match the defect; this maneuver spares the recurrent laryngeal nerves. With circumferential involvement, it may be necessary to perform a laryngectomy.

Contraindications to trachea repair include (1) inadequately treated laryngeal problem (not including paralysis of a single vocal cord); (2) need for ventilatory support or permanent tracheostomy for patients with amyotrophic lateral sclerosis, myasthenia gravis, or quadriplegia; (3) use of high-dose steroids; and (4) inflamed or recent tracheostomy. Poor pulmonary reserve is not a contraindication for repair in patients who have been weaned from the ventilator.

PULMONARY INFECTIONS

Pulmonary infections requiring surgical interventions are infrequent compared with pleural space infections. Clinical features resemble pneumonia and include fever, cough, leukocytosis, pleuritic pain, and sputum production. The patient is specifically questioned about aspiration of a foreign body. Evaluation includes CXR and CT scan of the chest and upper abdomen. Bronchoscopy can be performed to clear secretions and/or biopsy when cancer, foreign body, bronchial stenosis, or stricture are suspected. Cultures may be obtained to facilitate antibiotic treatment. Medical treatment must be optimized and may include smoking cessation, postural drainage, bronchodilator medications, and antibiotics.

Bronchiectasis

Bronchiectasis is a chronic respiratory disease characterized radiologically by abnormal and permanent dilation of the bronchi. Clinically, it can resemble COPD and is characterized by cough, sputum production, and bronchial infection. Pathophysiologically, two inciting factors are required: (1) an infectious insult and (2) impaired drainage, airway obstruction, or diminished host immune function. There are numerous predisposing factors, including CF, α_1-antitrypsin deficiency, primary ciliary syndrome (Kartagener syndrome), bronchial obstruction from foreign body, extrinsic lymph nodes that compress the bronchus, neoplasm, or mucus plug (Fig. 110.18).

Exacerbations of bronchiectasis are associated with increased airway and systemic inflammation and progressive lung damage that can lead to pulmonary functional decline and respiratory failure. Chronic airway infection stimulates and sustains pulmonary inflammation that is primarily neutrophilic and leads to degradation of airway elastin, with associated bronchial dilation, bronchial wall thickening, and mucus plugging. Common pathogens include *Haemophilus influenzae* and *Pseudomonas aeruginosa;* less frequent pathogens include *Moraxella catarrhalis, Staphylococcus aureus,* and *Enterobacteriaceae.* Mucociliary clearance is impaired by the impact of structural bronchiectasis, airway dehydration, excess mucus

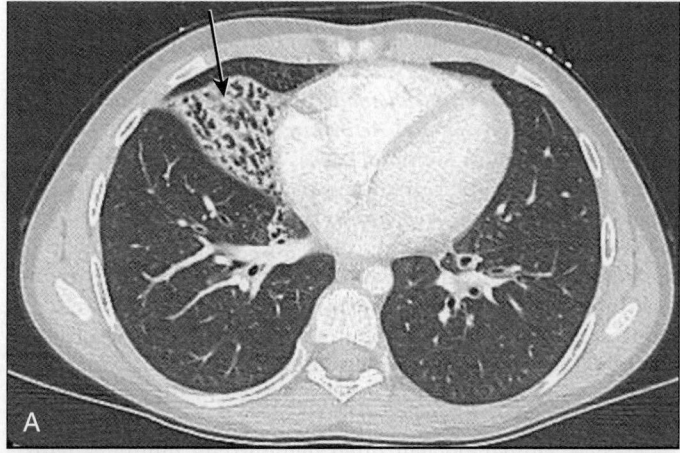

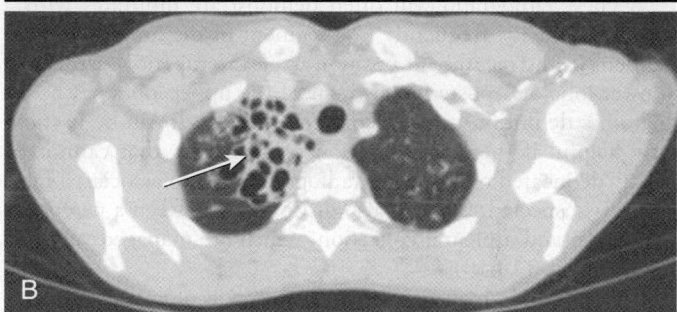

FIGURE 110.18 (A) A chest computed tomography (CT) scan of an 8-year-old patient with primary ciliary dyskinesia shows severe bronchiectasis of the right middle lobe *(arrow)*. (B) A chest CT scan of a 6-year-old patient with cystic fibrosis shows severe bronchiectasis of the right upper lobe *(arrow)*.

volume, and viscosity. More than 50% of patients have airflow obstruction, but a restrictive, mixed ventilatory pattern and preserved lung function are also frequently observed.

Treatment is based on the principles of preventing or suppressing acute and chronic bronchial infection, improving mucociliary clearance, and reducing the impact of structural lung disease. Therapies may include bronchodilator medications, pulmonary rehabilitation, or surgical resection. Surgery is considered for patients with localized disease and a high burden of exacerbations despite optimal medical management. The rationale for surgical resection (typically with lobectomy) is to break the self-sustaining inflammatory cycle of bronchiectasis by removing the involved lung segments to prevent spread to adjacent lung zones. Surgery may also be indicated in patients who develop massive hemoptysis refractory to bronchial artery embolization. Minimally invasive approaches are often preferred over open resection because VATS has been reported to produce comparable symptomatic improvement with shorter hospital stay, fewer complications, and less pain.[40] Bilateral bronchiectasis is a relative contraindication for surgery. For these patients, consider prolonged conservative treatment or bronchial artery embolization.

Lung Abscess

Lung abscess is defined as a circumscribed area of pus or necrosis caused by microbial infection and contained within the pulmonary parenchyma. Most lung abscesses arise as a complication of aspiration and are caused by species of anaerobes that are normally present in the gingival crevices. They are typically polymicrobial, and the most common organisms are *Peptostreptococcus,*

Prevotella, Bacteroides (usually not *B. fragilis*), and *Fusobacterium* spp. Many other bacteria can also cause lung abscesses, including *Streptococcus anginosus, S. aureus, K. pneumoniae, Streptococcus pyogenes, Burkholderia pseudomallei, Haemophilus influenzae* type b, *Legionella, Nocardia,* and *Actinomyces.* In the immunocompromised host, the most common causes of lung abscess are *P. aeruginosa* and other aerobic gram-negative bacilli, *Nocardia* spp., and fungi (*Aspergillus* and *Cryptococcus* spp.).

Most patients with lung abscesses (including nearly all of those caused by anaerobic infections) present with indolent symptoms that mimic pneumonia and evolve over a period of weeks or months. The characteristic features suggest pulmonary infection, including fever, cough, and sputum production. Evidence of chronic systemic disease is usually present, with night sweats, weight loss, and anemia.

A chest radiograph will often demonstrate infiltrates with a fluid-filled cavity, frequently in a segment of the lung that is dependent in the recumbent position (e.g., the superior segment of a lower lobe or a posterior segment of the upper lobes). A better anatomic definition can be achieved with CT. It can be particularly helpful if there is a question of cavitation that cannot be clearly delineated on the chest radiograph or if an associated mass lesion is suspected. CT will also distinguish between a parenchymal lesion and a pleural collection, which are managed very differently (Fig. 110.19).

The antibiotic treatment of lung abscess is almost always empiric, typically with IV ampicillin-sulbactam but with alternatives for special patient groups. Empiric regimens should penetrate the lung parenchyma and target both strict anaerobes and facultatively anaerobic streptococci. Drugs that are reasonable to use are any combination of a β-lactam–β-lactamase inhibitor or a carbapenem. The duration of therapy is controversial. Some treat for three weeks as a standard, and others treat based on the response.

Bronchoscopy may be used for treatment to assist in drainage of the cavity either directly or via transbronchial catheterization. Most patients (85%–95%) respond to medical management with a rapid decrease in fluid, collapse of the walls, and complete healing in 3 to 4 months. Patients with symptoms for longer than 3 months before treatment or cavities larger than 4 to 6 cm are less likely to respond to medical management and may require surgery.

Surgical therapy is indicated for persistent cavity (≥2 cm and thick walled), failure to clear sepsis after 8 weeks of medical

therapy, hemoptysis, and exclusion of cancer. Lobectomy is typically required. If a lung abscess ruptures into the pleural cavity, simple drainage may suffice, and the patient is managed for empyema or bronchopleural fistula.

Other Bronchopulmonary Disorders

Broncholithiasis is characterized by a calcified node tightly adherent to a bronchus. It can cause sudden bleeding resulting from erosion into a small bronchial artery. Bright red blood occurs and usually stops with antitussive therapy or sedation. This type of hemoptysis is almost never massive (≥600 mL in 24 hours). Bronchoscopy during a bleeding episode can localize the site of the bleeding. Attempts to bronchoscopically remove the calcified node should not be undertaken. Nasal or pharyngeal lesions or hematemesis from a gastrointestinal source should be excluded.

Organizing pneumonia may replace lung parenchyma with scar tissue or persistent atelectasis or consolidation. If the shadow or mass persists over 6 to 8 weeks, resection is performed to exclude carcinoma. The differential diagnosis includes pneumonia, congenital abnormality, and aneurysm of the aorta.

Mycobacterial Infections

Mycobacterium tuberculosis is highly transmissible, infecting approximately 7% of exposed patients. Clinical tuberculosis develops in 5% to 10% of patients who are infected. In the primary phase of infection, exudative response progresses to caseous necrosis. Pulmonary tuberculosis tends to occur in apical and posterior segments of the upper lobes and superior segments of the lower lobes. Early in the postprimary phase, extensive caseation may coalesce into cavities that are frequently characterized by incomplete septations and lobulations. Erosion of septations supplied by bronchial arteries can cause hemoptysis and secondary infection. Healing occurs with fibrosis and contracture.

The mainstay of treatment is medical management with isoniazid, rifampin, ethambutol, streptomycin, and pyrazinamide. Bronchoscopy may be required for patients who do not respond to medical management. Cancer diagnosis should be considered for any newly identified mass, even with a positive tuberculosis skin test and acid-fast bacillus-positive sputum. In general, surgery for treatment of tuberculosis is reserved for patients with poor clinical response to medical therapy and who have pulmonary disease amenable to complete resection (lobectomy, wedge resection, or pneumonectomy).[41] Consideration of surgery for management of multidrug-resistant tuberculosis and extensively drug-resistant tuberculosis is warranted in the following circumstances: (1) persistently positive sputum cultures beyond 4 to 6 months of antituberculous therapy; (2) presence of extensive drug resistance that is unlikely to be cured with antituberculous therapy alone; or (3) presence of immediately life-threatening complications, such as massive hemoptysis or persistent bronchopleural fistula.

Surgical complications are doubled if the sputum is positive for *M. tuberculosis* and decreased if remaining lung tissue is fully expanded within the chest. Infectious complications include empyema, bronchopleural fistula, and endobronchial spread of the disease and are associated with a higher mortality rate. After surgery, a full course of antituberculous medical therapy should be prescribed for all patients.

Fungal Infections

Most fungal pulmonary infections are self-limited and do not require treatment. Intravenous or oral antifungal agents are the first-line therapy for severe or prolonged illness. Diagnosis is often

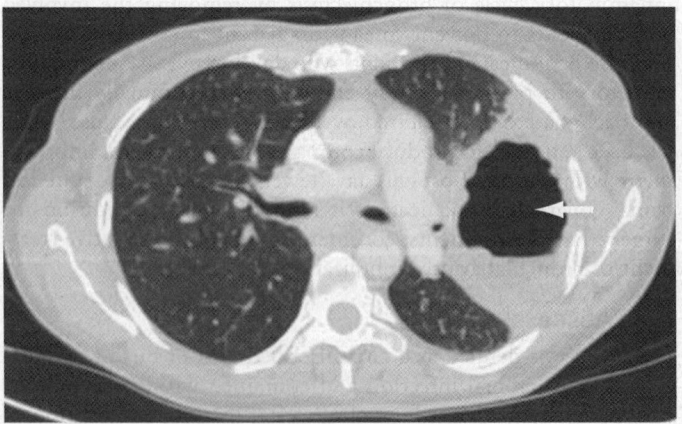

FIGURE 110.19 A chest computed tomography scan of a 43-year-old patient shows a left upper-lobe abscess *(arrow)*, a complication of pulmonary infection with *Streptococcus milleri.*

made by sputum examination using potassium hydroxide preparations (Fig. 110.20) because fungal cultures require prolonged incubation before results are finalized. Papanicolaou test cytology and silver methenamine stain may also be used in diagnosis.

Histoplasma capsulatum is endemic to the Mississippi and Ohio River valleys and portions of the southwestern United States. Systemic infection causes histoplasmosis, the most common fungal infection in the United States. An inoculum (from the mycelial form found in soil, decaying materials, and bat or bird guano) produces an acute pneumonic illness in immunocompetent hosts, which is commonly subclinical and typically resolves without specific treatment. However, the lymphogenous reaction to *Histoplasma* can cause mediastinal lymph node enlargement, middle lobe syndrome, bronchiectasis, esophageal traction diverticulum, broncholithiasis with hemoptysis, tracheoesophageal fistula, constrictive pericarditis, or fibrosing mediastinitis with superior vena cava syndrome or other problems relating to compression of mediastinal structures. Additionally, lymphadenopathy may confound radiographic evaluation of the mediastinal lymph nodes in patients with lung cancer and may complicate diagnosis and treatment.

Coccidioidomycosis is endemic to the Southwest United States and is localized in the soil. Inhaling the organism results in a primary lung disease that is usually self-limited (see Fig. 110.20B). In endemic areas, coccidioidomycosis is a frequent cause of lung

nodules, and resection may be required to rule out malignancy. Medical management is preferred. Surgery may be considered for treatment of cavitary disease or complications of cavitary disease.

Cryptococcosis is the second most common lethal fungal infection after histoplasmosis. Lungs are frequently involved, but the most common cause of death is related to central nervous system involvement with meningitis. Any patient diagnosed with pulmonary cryptococcosis should undergo lumbar puncture to rule out central nervous system involvement. Surgery may be required for open lung biopsy for diagnosis or to exclude lung cancer.

Aspergillosis is an opportunistic infection characterized by coarse fragmented septa and hyphae (see Fig. 110.20A). There are three aspergillosis clinical syndromes that typically affect immunocompromised hosts:

1. Aspergilloma: Fungus colonizes an existing lung cavity (commonly from tuberculosis). This is the most common presentation. CXR may demonstrate a crescent radiolucency next to a rounded mass. Invasion and destruction of parenchymal blood vessels occur within this cavity, placing patients at risk for hemorrhage. Prophylactic resection is controversial; although some physicians recommend resection if isolated disease is present in low-risk patients, surgery is typically reserved for massive/recurrent hemoptysis or to rule out neoplasm. The procedure of choice is lobectomy. The operation can be complex, with a significant inflammatory response within the hilum.

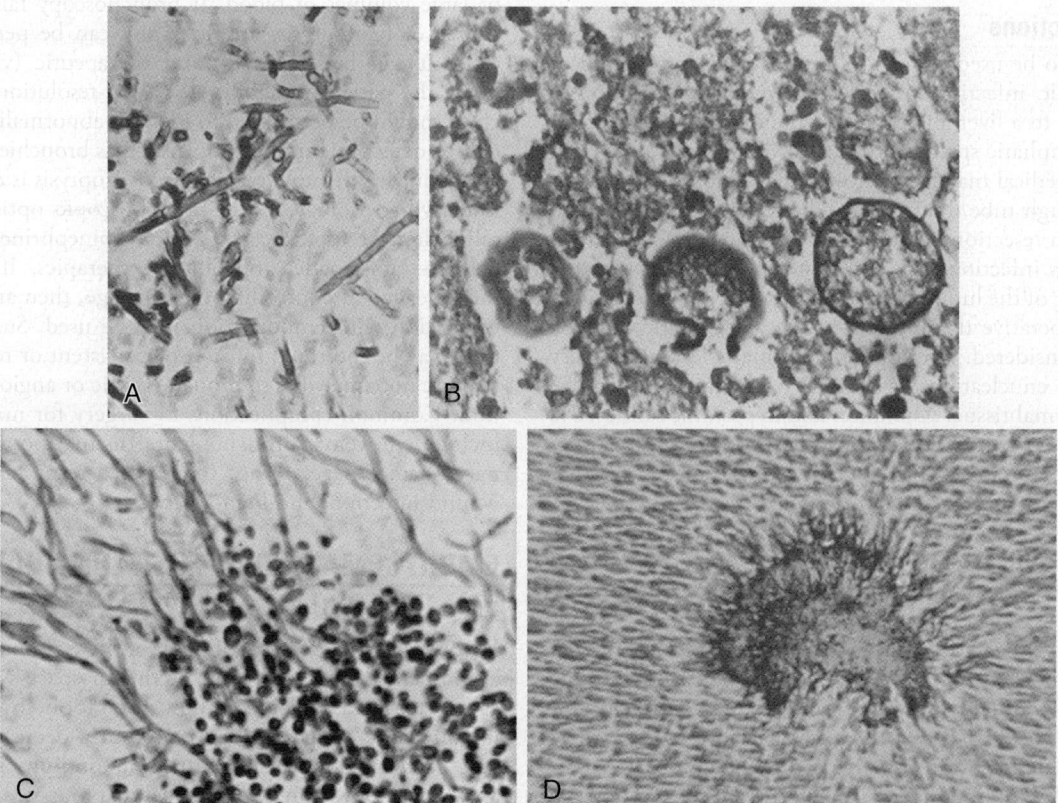

FIGURE 110.20 (A) The coarse, fragmented, septate mycelia of *Aspergillus fumigatus*. (B) Microscopic section of a coccidioidal granuloma (×400) shows spherules packed with endospores. (C) *Candida albicans* with both the mycelial and the yeast forms. (D) Actinomycotic granule shows branching filaments of a microscopic colony of *Actinomyces israelii*. (Gomori stain, ×250.) (A and C, From Takaro T. Thoracic mycotic infections. In: Walters W, ed. *Lewis' Practice of Surgery*. New York, NY: Hoeber Medical Division, Harper & Row; 1968. B, From Scott S, Takaro T. Thoracic mycotic and actinomycotic infections. In: Shields TW, ed. *General Thoracic Surgery*. 4th ed. Baltimore: Williams & Wilkins; 1994.)

2. Invasive pulmonary aspergillosis: This occurs in immunocompromised patients and manifests with chest pain, cough, and hemoptysis. The treatment is primarily medical, although lung biopsy may be necessary for diagnosis.

3. Allergic bronchopulmonary aspergillosis: This represents an allergic reaction to chronic *Aspergillus* colonization. It is diagnosed by bronchoscopy and usually treated medically. Rarely, resection is performed for localized bronchiectasis.

Mucormycosis is a rare, rapidly progressive fungal infection that occurs in immunocompromised patients, including patients with diabetes. The appearance is that of a black mold; it has wide nonseptate branching hyphae. The infection causes blood vessels to thrombose and lung tissue to infarct. Clinically, the rhinocerebral form occurs much more frequently than the pulmonary form of consolidation and cavities. Medical management involves cessation of steroids and antineoplastic drugs, initiation of amphotericin, and control of diabetes. The disease is often too advanced for effective treatment. Aggressive surgical and medical treatment may improve what is usually a grave prognosis.

Candida is a small, thin-walled budding yeast that is common in the environment but infects immunocompromised patients (see Fig. 110.20C). Lung involvement alone is rare. Surgery may be needed to confirm the diagnosis.

Pneumocystis carinii is an opportunistic fungal infection that is positive on silver methenamine stain. Bronchoalveolar lavage is diagnostic in more than 90% of patients. However, lung biopsy may be required to confirm the diagnosis.

Parasitic Infections

Surgery may also be used to manage the sequelae and complications of parasitic infections. *Entamoeba histolytica* infection is typically related to a liver abscess below the diaphragm via direct extension or lymphatic spread and is usually confined to the right lower thorax. Medical management with metronidazole is usually adequate, although tube drainage may be required in the case of empyema. Open resection is infrequently required.

Echinococcus infection may occur after hydatid cyst rupture, causing flooding of the lung or producing a severe hypersensitivity reaction. Nonoperative therapy for small asymptomatic calcified cysts may be considered. For larger symptomatic lesions, surgery includes simple enucleation via cleavage of planes between the cyst and the normal tissue. Aspiration and hypertonic saline 10% may be performed before enucleation. Positive pressure ventilation should be maintained until the cyst is out to prevent further contamination or hypersensitivity reaction.

Paragonimiasis is another common infection and cause of hemoptysis in Asia. In endemic areas, prevalence may be 5%, and hemoptysis from paragonimiasis must be differentiated from tuberculosis or lung cancer.

Actinomyces is a bacterium that is not found free in nature. It produces a chronic anaerobic endogenous infection deep within a wound. "Sulfur granules" draining from infected sinuses are microcolonies (see Fig. 110.20D). The cervicofacial form is the most common. The thoracic form usually occurs as pulmonary parenchymal disease resembling cancer. Penicillin is effective in medical management, but surgery may occasionally be required for radical excision of chest wall disease and empyema.

Nocardiosis is caused by an aerobic bacterium widely disseminated in soil and domestic animals; it was formerly rare, but incidence has been increasing in immunocompromised patients. It resembles actinomycosis by invading the chest wall and producing subcutaneous abscesses and sinuses that drain sulfur granules.

Surgery is performed to exclude cancer, to obtain a diagnosis, or to treat complications of the disease. Medical therapy may include sulfonamides.

MASSIVE HEMOPTYSIS

Massive hemoptysis is a potentially fatal event that can lead to significant airway obstruction, abnormal gas exchange, or hemodynamic instability. In clinical practice, life-threatening hemoptysis occurs when there has been >150 mL of blood expectorated in a 24-hour period or hemorrhage at a rate of ≥100 mL/hour. The mortality rate with massive hemoptysis ranges from 7% to 30%, and deaths are related to asphyxiation rather than exsanguination. Bronchiectasis, tuberculosis, bronchogenic carcinoma, and fungal infections are the most common causes of massive hemoptysis.

The initial management principles for massive hemoptysis include establishing a patent airway, positioning the patient in lateral decubitus with the suspected bleeding lung in the dependent position, ensuring hemodynamic stability, correcting bleeding diathesis, and controlling hemorrhage. Intubation with a large-bore endotracheal tube is critical to secure the airway and allow for blood/thrombus extraction and bronchoscopy. However, if a patient has a stable airway and is able to cough up the blood on their own, intubation should be delayed. Flexible bronchoscopy is typically the preferred initial diagnostic examination, but rigid bronchoscopy can be helpful when superior visualization is needed because of large volumes of blood. If bronchoscopy fails to identify the source of hemoptysis, arteriography can be performed next because it can be diagnostic and therapeutic (via embolization). Once the patient is stabilized, a high-resolution CT scan of the chest should be performed to identify abnormalities that are difficult to detect by bronchoscopy, such as bronchiectasis.

Definitive therapy for massive hemoptysis is dependent on the underlying etiology. Local bronchoscopic options include iced saline lavage, topical agents (e.g., epinephrine or vasopressin), balloon tamponade, and ablative therapies. If these treatment measures fail at controlling hemorrhage, then angiographic catheterization with embolization may be used. Surgical lung resection may be indicated in cases of persistent or recurrent bleeding that are not amenable to bronchoscopic or angiographic intervention. Common complications of surgery for massive hemoptysis include empyema, bronchopleural fistula, postoperative pulmonary hemorrhage, lung infarction, respiratory insufficiency, wound infection, and hemothorax.

EMPHYSEMA AND DIFFUSE LUNG DISEASE

Emphysema

Emphysema is defined as dilation of the terminal air spaces that is accompanied by destruction of the air-space walls. Emphysema causes dyspnea through airflow limitation, hyperinflation, and impaired gas exchange resulting from a decrease in the alveolar and capillary surface area. Imaging findings include increased anteroposterior diameter, flattened diaphragm, and increased lung field lucency. The region of the acinus (includes respiratory bronchiole, alveolar ducts, alveolar sacs, and alveoli) that is affected by dilation or destruction determines the subtype of emphysema. Centrilobular emphysema affects the respiratory bronchiole, the central portion of the acinus, and is commonly associated with cigarette smoking and COPD. Panacinar emphysema affects all parts of the acinus and is a characteristic of α_1-antitrypsin deficiency. In paraseptal emphysema, the alveolar ducts are predominantly affected.

Medical management is the mainstay of treatment for emphysema and includes bronchodilators alone or in combination with antiinflammatory drugs such as corticosteroids and phosphodiesterase-4 inhibitors. Lung volume reduction surgery (LVRS), aimed at excising lung parenchyma with significant emphysematous involvement, may be beneficial in select patients who experience poor disease control despite maximal medical therapy. LVRS can improve elastic recoil, reduce dynamic hyperinflation, and decrease circulating inflammatory markers. A randomized trial comparing LVRS with medical therapy for severe emphysema found that LVRS yields a survival advantage for patients with both predominantly upper-lobe emphysema and low baseline exercise capacity.[42] Alternatively, lung volume reduction can be performed using endobronchial valves via bronchoscopy to reduce lung volume in selected patients without the need for surgery. In advanced cases of emphysema, lung transplantation may also be considered. Long-term survival after lung transplantation ranges from 65% at 3 years to 32% at 10 years.[43]

Diffuse Lung Disease

Common causes of diffuse lung disease (DLD) are infection, exposure to environmental agents, drug-induced pulmonary toxicity, sarcoidosis, and radiation-induced lung injury (Box 110.1). CXR findings of an alveolar pattern (fluffy with air bronchograms) or an interstitial pattern (ground-glass or granular appearance) can be suggestive of DLD. Patients may be mildly symptomatic or progress to a critically ill state requiring intensive care and ventilation support. A lung biopsy may be indicated to confirm or exclude a specific diagnosis before medical therapy is initiated (e.g., cyclophosphamide for granulomatosis with polyangiitis (GPA)).

Sarcoidosis is a potential etiology for DLD and commonly presents with dyspnea and a dry cough. Sarcoidosis is associated with immune-mediated, widespread noncaseating granulomas and bilateral hilar mediastinal lymphadenopathy. Severe progressive pulmonary fibrosis may develop in 10% to 20% of patients. Bronchoscopic pulmonary biopsy is the initial diagnostic procedure. In select cases, biopsy of mediastinal lymph nodes may also be performed. Steroids are the mainstay of treatment.

Lung biopsy may be required in cases of progressive interstitial parenchymal changes after failed attempts at developing a diagnosis with less invasive approaches (e.g., transthoracic needle aspiration or transbronchial lung biopsy). Although biopsy specimens can be obtained by VATS, thoracotomy may be required in select cases because of severe pleural disease, high bleeding risk, or more severe respiratory impairment. The optimal number, size, and location of lung biopsies depend on the suspected diagnosis and the anatomic distribution of the DLD. High-resolution CT imaging is essential to guide the optimal locations for biopsy. Typically, biopsy specimens are obtained from multiple lobes of the lung and from areas of varying disease severity because this aids with diagnostic accuracy (Box 110.2).

Adult Respiratory Distress Syndrome

Acute respiratory distress syndrome (ARDS) is caused by an alveolar insult that results in the release of proinflammatory cytokines, capillary endothelial damage, increased vessel permeability, leakage of protein-rich fluid into alveoli, and noncardiogenic pulmonary edema. Sepsis, aspiration, pneumonia, trauma, and pancreatitis are common causes of ARDS. Imaging demonstrates bilateral lung opacities secondary to increased interstitial fluid in

---

BOX 110.1 Classification of Diffuse Lung Diseases

Infections (more commonly cause focal disease, granuloma formation)
  Viruses—especially influenza, cytomegalovirus
  Bacteria—tuberculosis, all types of regular bacteria, Rocky Mountain spotted fever
  Fungi—all types can cause diffuse disease
  Parasites—Pneumocystis species infection, toxoplasmosis, paragonimiasis, among others
Occupational causes
  Mineral dusts
  Chemical fumes—NO_2 (silo filler disease), Cl, NH_3, SO_2, CCl_4, Br, HF, HCl, HNO_3, kerosene, acetylene
Neoplastic disease
  Lymphangitic spread
  Hematogenous metastases
  Leukemia, lymphoma, bronchioloalveolar cell cancer
Congenital—familial
  Niemann-Pick disease, Gaucher disease, neurofibromatosis, tuberous fibrosis
Metabolic and unknown
  Liver disease, uremia, inflammatory bowel disease
Physical agents
  Radiation, O_2 toxicity, thermal injury, blast injury
Heart failure and multiple pulmonary emboli
Immunologic causes
Hypersensitivity pneumonia
  Inhaled antigens
  Farmer lung (actinomycosis)
  Bagassosis (sugar cane)
  Malt workers (*Aspergillus* spp.)
  Byssinosis (cotton)
Drug reactions
  Hydralazine, busulfan, nitrofurantoin (Macrodantin), hexamethonium, methysergide, bleomycin
Collagen diseases
  Scleroderma, rheumatoid disease, systemic lupus erythematosus, dermatomyositis, Wegener granulomatosis, Goodpasture syndrome
Other
  Sarcoidosis
  Histiocytosis
  Idiopathic hemosiderosis
  Pulmonary alveolar proteinosis
  Diffuse interstitial fibrosis, idiopathic pulmonary fibrosis
  Desquamative interstitial pneumonia
  Eosinophilic pneumonia (Note: Some are caused by drugs, actinomycosis, and parasites.)
  Lymphangioleiomyomatosis

---

a patient with respiratory insufficiency (Fig. 110.21). ARDS is associated with a high rate of morbidity as a result of impaired gas exchange, decreased lung compliance, and pulmonary hypertension. Prompt recognition and treatment of ARDS is critical to reduce the risk of mortality.

The severity of ARDS is defined according to the degree of hypoxemia, as follows: mild (200 mm Hg > PaO_2/FiO_2 ≤300 mm Hg), moderate (100 mm Hg > PaO_2/FiO_2 ≤200 mm Hg), and severe (PaO_2/FiO_2 ≤100 mm Hg). The risk of mortality increases with more severe ARDS. Treatment is medical and directed toward improving oxygenation and addressing the underlying cause. The key principles in ventilation management for ARDS include using

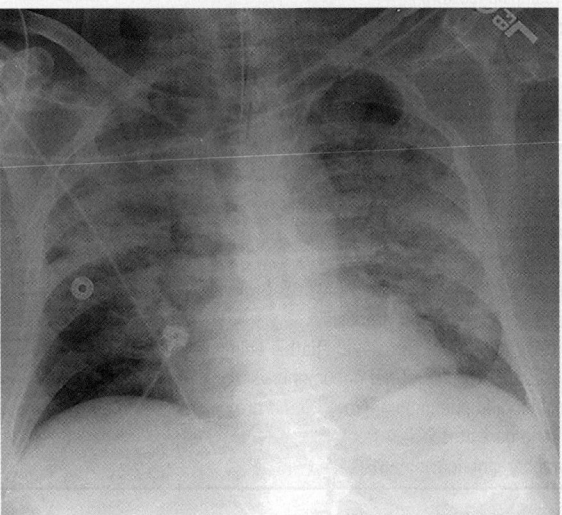

FIGURE 110.21 Chest radiograph of acute respiratory distress syndrome. Frontal chest radiography in a mechanically ventilated patient shows extensive, multifocal, bilateral lung opacities, essentially involving all lobes and without features suggesting increased pressure edema, such as interlobular septal thickening or pleural effusion. (From Lee, WL, Herridge MS, Binnie A. Acute respiratory distress syndrome In: Lazarus SC, Sarmiento KF, Schnapp LM, et al. *Murray and Nadel's Textbook of Respiratory Medicine.* 7th ed. Elsevier; 2022.)

applied positive end-expiratory pressure (PEEP) to maximize alveolar recruitment and low tidal volumes to prevent alveolar overdistention. In select patients who do not improve with these supportive measures, prone positioning, neuromuscular blockers, or mechanical support with ECMO may be considered in a stepwise fashion.

PULMONARY METASTASES

Lung metastases represent a manifestation of systemic spread of a primary extrapulmonary neoplasm. Pulmonary metastasectomy in appropriately selected patients may offer an opportunity for prolonged disease-free survival. The 5- and 10-year survival rates after complete pulmonary metastasectomy are 36% and 26%, respectively.[44] General criteria used for consideration of pulmonary metastasectomy include ability to completely resect all areas of pulmonary involvement, controllability of the primary tumor, absent extrapulmonary metastatic disease, and adequate cardiopulmonary reserve. If these criteria are unable to be met, radiation therapy may be used to treat the local manifestations of metastatic disease, particularly in the presence of bony or symptomatic metastases. The decision to proceed with pulmonary metastasectomy should involve a multidisciplinary approach with evaluation by medical oncology, radiation oncology, and thoracic surgery.

Certain prognostic indicators may be used to select patients with more favorable disease-free and overall survival expectations. Pulmonary metastasectomy is considered best suited for patients with three or fewer metastases. Complete resection of all pulmonary metastases has been consistently associated with improved survival in comparison to incomplete resection. There also does appear to be a better prognosis for patients with germ cell tumors, disease-free intervals of 36 months or more, and single metastases.[44]

Open thoracotomy was traditionally the recommended approach for pulmonary metastasectomy because it allows for bimanual palpation of the lungs to identify potential occult metastases. However, VATS is considered a safe alternative, given the significant advancement in imaging techniques that can detect small pulmonary lesions with greater accuracy before surgery. Intraoperatively, obtaining tumor-free and adequate margins is critical for reducing future risk of recurrence. After resection, close follow-up with imaging at regular intervals should be performed to monitor for disease recurrence.

MISCELLANEOUS LUNG TUMORS

Hamartomas are the most common benign lung tumor and consist of an abnormal distribution of normal lung tissue elements, such as cartilage and connective tissue. They typically present after the fifth decade of life and are more frequently found in males. These lesions are slow-growing and often peripherally located. On imaging, these masses present as coin-shaped and solitary, with sharply demarcated edges, typically measuring <4 cm in diameter. Calcifications can be present and give the lesion its pathognomonic "popcorn" appearance. A cystic adenomatoid malformation represents a developmental hamartomatous abnormality of the lung, which occurs in infants as cysts or immature, malformed lung tissue.

SCC, adenocarcinoma, large cell carcinoma, and small cell carcinoma account for most primary malignant lung cancers. However, slow-growing lung tumors may arise from the epithelium, ducts, and glands of the bronchial tree and account for 1% to 2% of all lung neoplasms. Most of these tumors are of low-grade malignant potential.

Primary pulmonary ACC is a rare, slow-growing malignancy that typically involves the trachea and mainstem bronchi. It arises from the tracheobronchial glands in the airway submucosa and is histologically similar to ACC arising in the salivary glands. ACC may present with nonspecific symptoms, such as cough or dyspnea, given their location in the trachea and mainstem bronchi and potential for distal obstruction. These tumors can metastasize and involve perineural lymphatics or distant organs. Surgical resection is the mainstay of treatment. However, radiation therapy has been used in select cases.

Sarcomatoid carcinomas represent a rare subtype of NSCLC. These tumors have a malignant epithelial component mixed with features typically found in sarcomas. Sarcomatoid carcinoma is associated with worse survival compared with nonsarcomatoid lung cancers. Pleomorphic carcinomas are the most common subtype of sarcomatoid carcinoma, and variants include spindle cell and giant cell carcinomas.

Pulmonary lymphoma most commonly occurs as disseminated lymphoma involving the lung. Disseminated lymphoma occurs in 40% of patients with Hodgkin disease and 7% of patients with non-Hodgkin disease. Primary pulmonary lymphomas are rare. The diagnosis is usually made at the time of surgery. A thorough evaluation focused on ruling out other potential sites of primary lymphoma should be performed if the diagnosis of primary pulmonary lymphoma is suspected preoperatively.

NEUROENDOCRINE TUMORS OF THE LUNG

Several types of neuroendocrine lung tumors exist, including small cell carcinoma, large cell neuroendocrine carcinomas, typical (low-grade) carcinoid, and atypical (intermediate-grade) carcinoid. Of the NETs, small cell and large cell neuroendocrine carcinomas are characterized by having a more aggressive clinical course and a much higher mitotic rate on pathologic analysis. Meanwhile, typical and atypical pulmonary carcinoids have similar features to carcinoid tumors arising at other sites and have relatively indolent clinical behavior. NETs are usually positive for chromogranin or synaptophysin expression.

Carcinoid tumors, arising from bronchial Kulchitsky or enterochromaffin cells (amine precursor uptake and decarboxylation cells), account for approximately 1% to 2% of all lung malignancies in adults and approximately 20% to 30% of all NETs. Carcinoid tumor is the most common primary lung neoplasm in children. These tumors may present with a cough or wheeze, hemoptysis, chest pain, or recurrent pneumonia resulting from bronchial obstruction. On imaging, most tumors appear as round or ovoid lesions that range in size from 2 to 5 cm. Carcinoid syndrome may infrequently occur as a result of systemic release of vasoactive substances, such as serotonin, and cause acute symptoms, including flushing, tachycardia, wheezing, and diarrhea.

Surgical resection is the preferred treatment approach for patients with localized lung NETs and adequate pulmonary reserve. Transbronchoscopic resection may be an alternative treatment approach for select typical (low-grade) carcinoid tumors. Lymph node metastasis is relatively common and occurs in 5% to 20% of typical carcinoid tumors and 30% to 70% of atypical tumors. As such, mediastinal lymph node sampling or dissection at the time of surgery is recommended, along with complete resection of nodal metastasis, if feasible. Typical carcinoid tumors exhibit a relatively good prognosis (~90%, 5-year survival), whereas atypical carcinoid tumors demonstrate a 5-year survival of about 50%.[45] The highly malignant large cell and small cell neuroendocrine carcinomas have 5-year survivals of 15% to 57% and <5%, respectively.[45]

CHEST WALL

Congenital Deformities

There are a variety of thoracic congenital abnormalities that manifest as defects of the anterior chest wall, including pectus excavatum, pectus carinatum, pouter pigeon breast, Poland syndrome, and cleft sternum (Fig. 110.22). The clinical significance

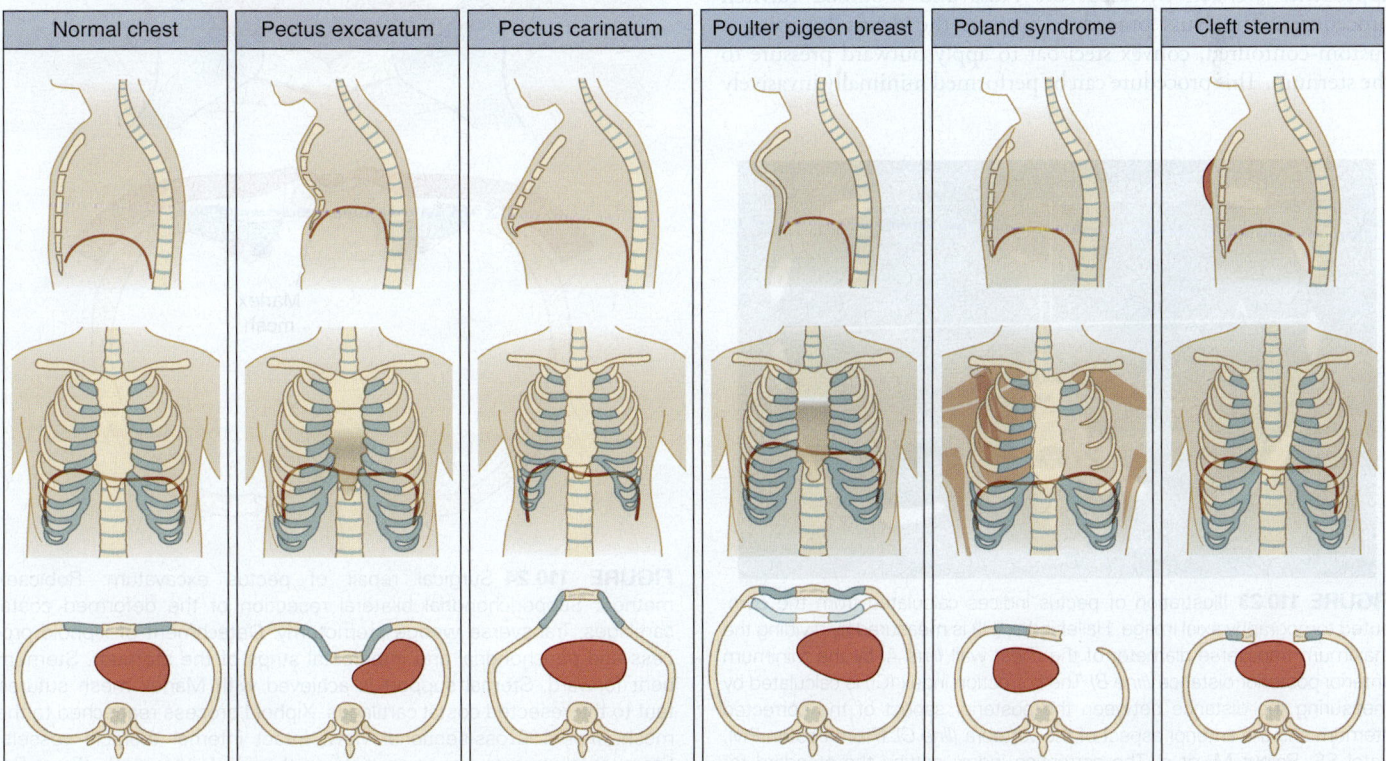

FIGURE 110.22 Classification of chest wall deformities. (From Fokin AA, Steuerwald NM, Ahrens WA, et al. Anatomical, histologic, and genetic characteristics of congenital chest wall deformities. *Semin Thorac Cardiovasc Surg.* 2009;21:44-57.)

of these deformities depends on the severity of the chest wall defect, cardiopulmonary morbidity, and the psychosocial implications of the defect on the patient.

Pectus Excavatum

Pectus excavatum, or "funnel chest," is the most common congenital chest wall deformity, occurring in approximately 1 of 400 live births, and is characterized by a concave sternal depression. This deformity has a male predominance (4:1) and is usually sporadic but may be associated with other connective tissue disorders (e.g., Marfan syndrome) and genetic conditions (e.g., Noonan syndrome). The exact cause of pectus excavatum is unclear, but it is presumed to be a result of disproportionate muscular force on the sternum and costal cartilages or abnormal growth of cartilage or rib. Although cosmesis is the most frequently reported concern, exercise tolerance, chest discomfort, and shortness of breath can also occur.

Initial evaluation should focus on identifying the severity of the deformity and the presence of any associated anomalies. Pectus excavatum may be symmetric or asymmetric, with the sternum rotated toward one side. CT with 3D reconstruction can aid in determining the impact of the pectus defect on the lungs, heart, and major blood vessels and provide measurements of the thoracic cavity. The Haller index, a ratio of the transverse diameter of the chest to the anterior-posterior diameter at its most narrow point, can be derived from a CT scan and is a standardized method for determining candidacy for surgical repair (Fig. 110.23). Patients with significant displacement of the heart or respiratory symptoms should have a cardiology evaluation with echocardiography and pulmonary function testing, respectively.

Surgery is usually performed during late childhood or early adolescence and is generally considered for patients with a Haller index of >3.25, cardiac abnormalities, restrictive respiratory disease, or significant patient concern about appearance. Two surgical approaches are actively used: the Nuss and modified Ravitch procedures. The Nuss procedure corrects the defect by using a custom-contoured, convex steel bar to apply outward pressure to the sternum. This procedure can be performed minimally invasively

and entails placing a steel "Nuss" bar in the pleural space, passing it behind the sternum under thoracoscopic guidance, rotating it 180 degrees, and then attaching it laterally to the rib cage. The bar is typically removed after about 2 years. Other methods of surgical correction include the basic steps described by Dr. Ravitch in 1949. These include bilateral parasternal and subperichondrial resection of the deformed costal cartilages, detachment of the xiphoid process, transverse anterior table wedge osteotomy at the upper edge of the sternal depression, bending the sternum anteriorly to straighten its course, and securing the corrected position of the sternum (Fig. 110.24). The sternal support is typically kept in place for about 1 year. Permanent plates are also being used to avoid a second operation and reduce the rate of recurrence.

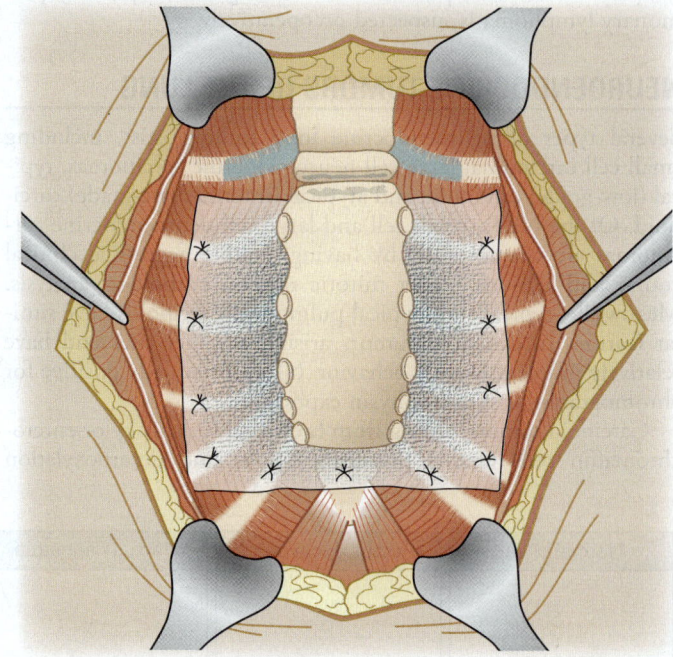

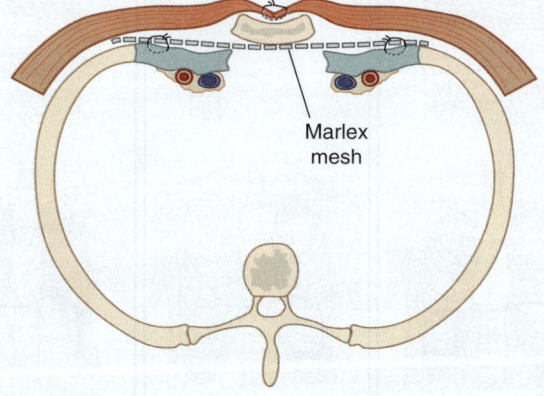

FIGURE 110.24 Surgical repair of pectus excavatum: Robicsek method. Subperichondrial bilateral resection of the deformed costal cartilages. Transverse wedge sternotomy. Detachment of xiphoid process and perichondrial and intercostal strips of the sternum. Sternum bent forward. Sternal support is achieved with Marlex mesh sutured taut to the resected costal cartilages. Xiphoid process reattached to the mesh. *Insert:* Cross-sectional view. Intact internal thoracic vessels. Sternum in corrected position rests on the mesh hammock. (From Robicsek F, Watts LT, Fokin AA. Surgical repair of pectus excavatum and carinatum. *Semin Thorac Cardiovasc Surg.* 2009;21:64-75.)

FIGURE 110.23 Illustration of pectus indices calculated from the computed tomography axial image. Haller index (HI) is measured by dividing the maximum transverse diameter of the chest wall *(line A)* by the minimum anterior-posterior distance *(line B)*. The correction index (CI) is calculated by measuring the distance between the posterior aspect of the corrected sternum and the anterior aspect of the vertebra *(line C)*. (From Poston PM, Patel SS, Rajput M, et al. The correction index: setting the standard for recommending operative repair of pectus excavatum. *Ann Thorac Surg.* 2014;97[4]:1176-1179; discussion 1179-1180.)

Pectus Carinatum

Pectus carinatum, also called *pigeon chest,* is defined by outward protrusion of the sternum and costal cartilages. It occurs in 1/1500 live births. As with pectus excavatum, the exact cause is unknown, and there is a male predominance. It typically presents in early adolescence and is often undiscovered until the pubertal growth spurt. For most patients, cosmesis is the primary concern, but some may experience exertional dyspnea, respiratory infections, or asthma. Associated musculoskeletal and spinal anomalies, especially scoliosis, are common.

There are two primary types of pectus carinatum deformity: chondrogladiolar prominence (or keel chest) and chondromanubrial prominence (or pouter pigeon breast). Of these, chondrogladiolar prominence is more common and is characterized by forward protrusion of the middle and lower portions of the sternum. The costal cartilages are concave and usually symmetrically depressed, accentuating the sternal prominence (Fig. 110.25). In contrast, chondromanubrial prominence is characterized by anterior protrusion of the upper portion of the sternum and posterior deviation of the body of the sternum, resulting in a short and angled sternum. This pectus deformity is presumed to be a result of premature ossification of the sternum.

Bracing is an effective treatment for patients with flexible chest walls and mild to moderate pectus carinatum. Corrective bracing has been shown to have an 85% success rate.[46] Surgery is typically reserved for those with complex deformities, inflexible chest walls (e.g., patients in postpuberty), or severe sternal asymmetry. Surgical repair should be performed at the end of the pubertal growth spurt. Repair is typically performed using a modified Ravitch procedure that involves resection of abnormal costal cartilages while preserving the perichondrium (from which new cartilage grows), sternal osteotomy, and reshaping/repositioning of the sternum (Fig. 110.26).

Poland Syndrome and Cleft Sternum

Poland syndrome is a rare congenital anomaly that is characterized by absence of the pectoral muscles, most commonly unilateral. Associated anomalies may include absence or deformity of other chest wall muscles, breast tissue, nipple, costal cartilages of ribs 2 to 5, and digits (e.g., syndactyly). The pathogenesis of Poland syndrome remains unclear, with the prevailing theory being disruption of the subclavian artery blood supply. Although most patients do not develop respiratory symptoms, those with missing ribs may have paradoxical respiratory motion of the chest wall (inward movement during inspiration), similar to a flail chest.

Cleft sternum is a rare congenital defect resulting from failed midline fusion of the sternum. This can result in paradoxical respiratory movements and leaves the heart and mediastinal structures unprotected from direct injury. Surgical correction is recommended in the neonatal period.

Chest Wall Tumors

Chest wall tumors represent a heterogeneous group of rare benign and malignant tumors (Table 110.4). Tumors can be primary to the chest wall, arise from direct extension from a primary lung cancer, or result from metastasis from another site. More than 50% of chest wall tumors are malignant, with the majority of these malignant tumors arising from the bone, cartilage, or soft tissue. Overall 5-year survival after resection of primary chest wall neoplasms is 57%.[47] These tumors often present with a palpable painful mass or as an incidental finding on chest radiography. CT can demonstrate the extent of bone, soft tissue, and pleural and

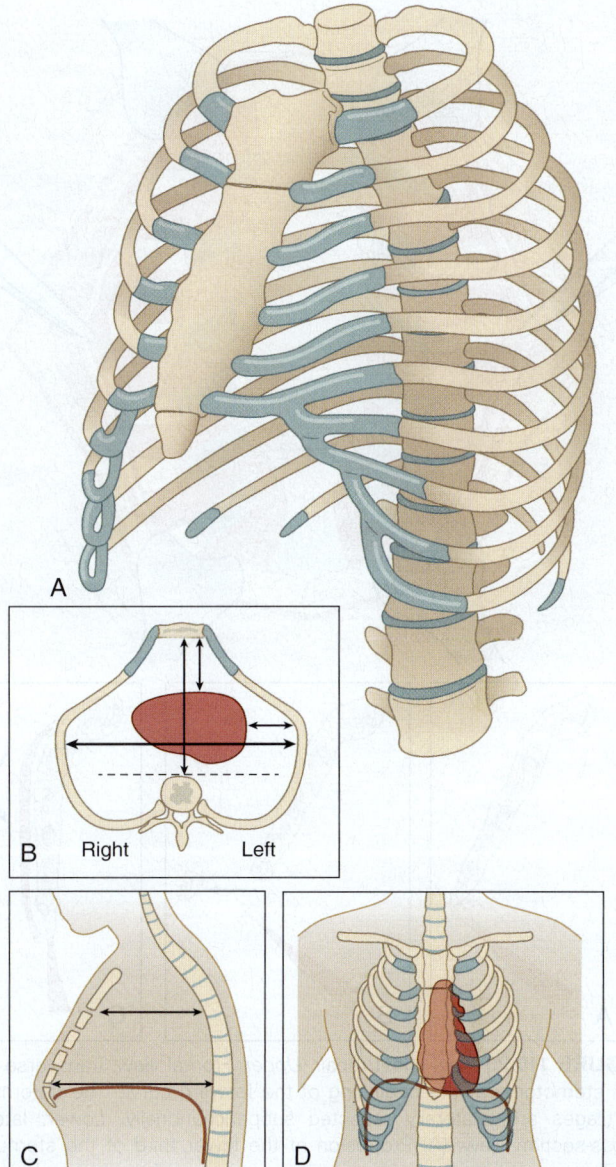

FIGURE 110.25 Anatomic representation of keel chest deformity with lateral rib depressions. (A) Three-dimensional view. Protruding sternum accentuated by lateral rib depressions. (B) Cross-sectional view. Pyramidal chest with severe lateral rib depressions. (C) Lateral view. Sharp protrusion at the sternoxiphoidal junction. Abnormal posture. (D) Frontal view. Central position of the heart. Anatomic representation of pectus excavatum (PE). (A) Three-dimensional view. Classic, cup-shaped PE. (B) Cross-sectional view. Symmetric depression of the anterior chest wall. Cup-shaped concavity. Heart shifted to the left and rotated. (C) Lateral view. Depression of the lower third of mesosternum with a reduction in the anteroposterior thorax diameter. (D) Frontal view. Heart shifted to the left. (From Fokin AA, Steuerwald NM, Ahrens WA, et al. Anatomical, histologic, and genetic characteristics of congenital chest wall deformities. *Semin Thorac Cardiovasc Surg.* 2009;21:44-57.)

mediastinal involvement and identify any pulmonary metastases. MRI can further delineate soft tissue, vascular, and nerve involvement and the presence of spinal cord or epidural extension. Tissue biopsy can confirm the diagnosis and inform the selection of potential therapy strategies.

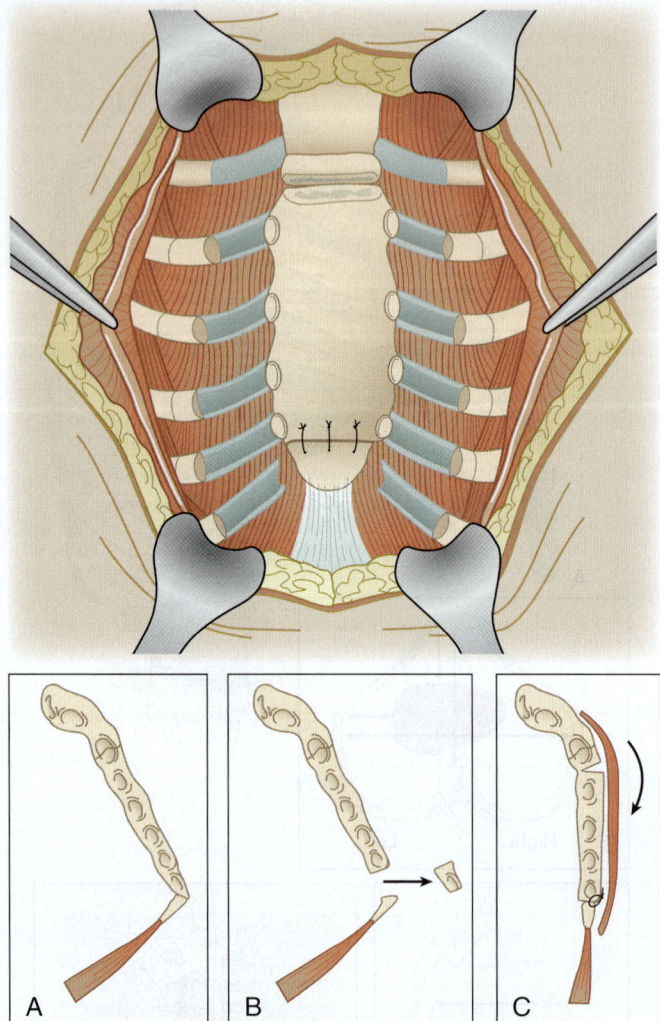

TABLE 110.4   Classification of Tumors of the Chest Wall

		BENIGN (40%)	MALIGNANT (60%)
Bone Tumors			
Bone		Osteoblastoma	Ewing sarcoma
		Osteoid osteoma	Osteosarcoma
Cartilage		Chondroma (enchondroma)	Chondrosarcoma
		Osteochondroma	
Fibrous tissue		Fibrous dysplasia	
Bone marrow		Eosinophilic granuloma	Solitary plasmacytoma
Osteoclast		Aneurysmal bone cyst	
		Giant cell tumor (osteoclastoma)	
Vascular		Hemangioma	Hemangiosarcoma
		Cystic angiomatosis	
Other		Mesenchymal hamartoma	
Soft Tissue Tumors			
Adipose tissue		Lipoma	Liposarcoma
		Ossifying lipoma	
Fibrous tissue		Fibroma (desmoid tumor)	Fibrosarcoma
		Ossifying fibroma	MFH
Muscle		Leiomyoma	Leiomyosarcoma
		Rhabdomyoma	Rhabdomyosarcoma
			Tendon sheath sarcoma
Nerve		Neurofibroma	Askin tumor (PNET)
		Schwannoma (neurilemoma or neurinoma)	Malignant schwannoma
			Neurofibrosarcoma
			Neuroblastoma
Vascular		Hemangioma	Hemangiosarcoma
		Vascular leiomyoma	
Other			Hodgkin disease
			Leukemia
			Lymphoma
			Lymphosarcoma
			Mixed sarcoma
			Reticulosarcoma

MFH, Malignant fibrous histiocytoma; *PNET,* primitive neuroectodermal tumor.
From Smith SE, Keshavjee S. Primary chest wall tumors. *Thorac Surg Clin.* 2010;20:495-507.

FIGURE 110.26 Keel chest repair. *Upper:* Frontal view. Transverse linear sternotomy at the beginning of the forward curve. The deformed cartilages are bilaterally resected subperichondrially. *Lower:* lateral cross-section view. (A) Protrusion of the lower third of the sternum. (B) Transverse linear sternotomy at the beginning of the forward curve; sternum is shortened using a distal resection and pushed backward. (C) Corrected position of the sternum. Xiphoid process is reattached to the shortened sternum. Pectoralis muscles reunited presternally. (From Robicsek F, Watts LT, Fokin AA. Surgical repair of pectus excavatum and carinatum. *Semin Thorac Cardiovasc Surg.* 2009;21:64-75.)

The indication for surgery is based on evaluation of the tumor histology, location, degree of local invasion, and presence of metastases. Complete R0 tumor resection and reconstruction of the chest wall defect is the main principle of surgical management for chest wall tumors, except for Ewing sarcoma (treated with systemic chemotherapy and definitive local therapy) and solitary plasmacytomas (treated with radiation). Therefore, most tumors over a few centimeters should have a core-needle biopsy to help guide therapy. Resections that include three or more ribs will generally require reconstruction with prosthetic material to preserve chest wall mechanics. Synthetic materials that can be used include polypropylene, polytetrafluorethylene patch, methyl methacrylate, and osteosynthesis system with titanium implantable material (Fig. 110.27). These reconstructive techniques are mainly used to improve chest wall stability to prevent flail

segments and postoperative respiratory compromise. Malignant tumors of the manubrium, sternum, clavicle, and scapula generally require excision of the entire bone and surrounding soft tissue to ensure negative margins. Chest wall closure of a small defect for a small lesion can usually be done primarily. Large tumors in which a considerable defect is anticipated, both skeletal reconstruction and soft tissue coverage are often necessary. Local thoracic pedicle or myocutaneous flaps are generally used for reconstruction of large defects and include pectoralis major, latissimus dorsi, and serratus anterior muscles. As such, chest wall resections requiring complex reconstructions should be approached in a multidisciplinary fashion, with preoperative consultation with both a thoracic and plastic surgeon.

Bone Tumors

Benign chest wall tumors include enchondromas (benign bone tumor), osteochondromas (benign cartilage tumor), fibrous dysplasia, eosinophilic granuloma (Langerhans cell histiocytosis), lymphangiomas, and desmoid tumors. The main goal of surgical

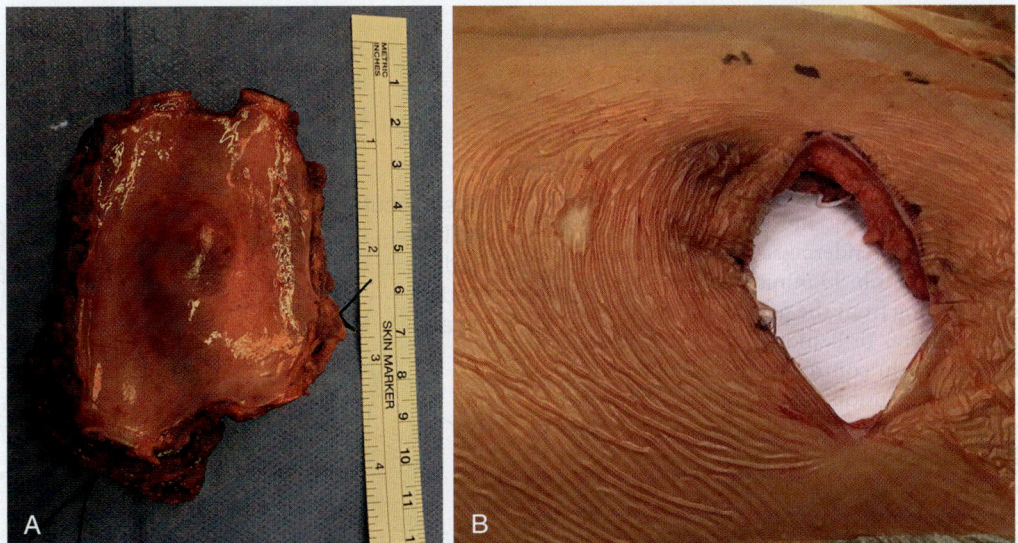

FIGURE 110.27 Chest wall synovial sarcoma in a 9-year-old child. (A) Shown is a segment of the left chest wall (ribs 3 and 4). Complete resection was performed. The macroscopic clear margins are verified in final pathology. (B) Reconstruction of chest wall defect with a synthetic polytetrafluoroethylene Gore-Tex patch.

resection is to provide symptomatic relief and minimize the risk of future malignant transformation. Chondromas account for about 20% of benign chest wall tumors. In comparison to benign lesions, malignant chest wall tumors are frequently more rapidly growing and often present at a larger size. Chondrosarcoma is the most common malignancy of the chest wall, making up approximately 30% of primary malignancies, and typically presents as a painful, hard, fixed mass. Resection with wide margins of 2 to 4 cm is the treatment of choice because these tumors are generally resistant to radiation and chemotherapy. However, given the location and size of the tumor, wide margins may be difficult to obtain. Primary osteosarcomas of the chest wall account for 10% to 15% of malignant tumors and commonly involve the rib, scapula, and clavicles. The tumor grows rapidly, and radiographic characteristics include a sunburst pattern on CXR. Ewing sarcoma accounts for 5% to 10% of chest wall malignancies. The radiographic characteristics include an onion-peel appearance with periosteal elevation and bony remodeling. With multimodality therapy, 5-year survival is about 50%. Primary solitary plasmacytoma is a rare chest wall tumor that commonly occurs in older males as a painful solitary tumor arising from plasma cells and can progress to multiple myeloma. Radiographic characteristics include a diffuse, moth-eaten, or punched-out appearance of the bone. Systemic disease can be confirmed using serum protein electrophoresis, urinalysis (Bence-Jones protein), and bone marrow aspiration. Radiotherapy is recommended for solitary plasmacytoma.

Soft Tissue Tumors

Soft tissue sarcomas are the most common primary malignant soft tissue chest wall lesions. Malignant fibrous histiocytomas and rhabdomyosarcoma are the most common subtypes. Long-term survival after resection is acceptable, with a reported 5-year survival of 73%.[48] Recurrence occurs in about 20% of patients. Negative margins are an important predictor of local recurrence; therefore, the chest wall may need to be resected to achieve clear margins.

Metastatic Tumors

Metastatic neoplasms may involve the chest wall through direct extension or lymphatic or hematogenous spread. For example, lung and breast cancer can metastasize to or recur in the chest wall. Surgery may be indicated for local disease control on a case-by-case basis.

Chest Wall Infections

Chest wall infections share similar risk factors for infection at other surgical sites, such as poor nutritional status, immunocompromised state, diabetes, smoking, and obesity. Adequate therapy involves antibiotics and source control. Necrotizing soft tissue infections (NSTIs) that involve the thorax typically spread from elsewhere, most commonly the extremities, and require urgent surgical debridement. Most of the reported NSTIs of the chest wall develop as a result of the treatment of other pathologies, such as chest tube placement for empyema. The classical symptoms of NSTIs are erythema, pain out of proportion to exam, crepitus and induration, and skin bullae. Systemic toxicity can present with hypotension, fever, and severe sepsis.

Patients with a history of intravenous drug use are at increased risk for developing septic arthritis of the sternoclavicular, sternochondral, and manubriosternal joints. CXR, CT, or MRI can be used to evaluate the joint. Positive findings include widening of the joint space; joint destruction; and osteomyelitis of the clavicle, manubrium, or first rib. Sternoclavicular joint infections are typically seen with systemic infection and can be treated with surgical debridement, en bloc resection, and antibiotic therapy. Furthermore, postoperative sternal wound infections can occur after median sternotomy or cardiac surgery. Spontaneous primary chest wall infections can also arise from a variety of sources as a consequence of immunosuppression, drug-resistant organisms, tuberculosis, or HIV infection.

Chest Wall Trauma

Blunt thoracic trauma comprises 20% to 25% of all traumas, with the most common etiology being motor vehicle collisions (MVCs).

Blunt chest trauma can result in injuries to multiple vital thoracic structures, including the clavicle, ribs, and sternum. A definitive diagnosis of traumatic chest wall injuries can be made with CXR or CT scan.

Rib fractures occur in almost two-thirds of patients with significant chest trauma after MVCs. Ribs 4 to 10 are more susceptible to traumatic injury than the superior ribs, which are protected by the clavicle, scapula, and overlying soft tissue. Physical exam may reveal focal tenderness, bony crepitus, or ecchymosis overlying a fractured rib. Diminished or absent breath sounds may represent splinting from the pain but may also reflect the presence of a pneumothorax or hemothorax. The mainstay of rib fracture management is pain control. Early and adequate analgesia and lung volume expansion treatments (e.g., incentive spirometry, deep breathing, coughing) help prevent pulmonary complications, such as pneumonia, resulting from splinting and atelectasis. Advanced age, smoking, and underlying lung disease are poor prognostic factors. Underlying injury to the liver, spleen, and kidney should be ruled out in the case of fractures to the lower ribs (ninth and lower). Patients with three or more rib fractures should be admitted for hospitalization, given the increased risk of morbidity and mortality. The majority of rib fractures do not require stabilization or plating, but this continues to be an active area of investigation.

Flail chest is defined as fractures of three or more ribs in two or more places, which results in a paradoxical motion of the chest wall during respiration (e.g., inward during inspiration and outward during expiration). It has been associated with a mortality rate of 16%.[49] Flail chest is often associated with an underlying pulmonary contusion and should be supported with pain relief, rib stabilization, or even mechanical ventilation. Early operative treatment reduces pulmonary complications, the duration of mechanical ventilation, hospital length of stay, and mortality for patients with flail chest.

Sternal injuries may result from blunt trauma to the anterior chest wall, typically from a driver striking the steering column during an MVC. Isolated sternal fractures tend to heal without any need for surgical intervention. However, sternal fractures are associated with an increased risk of internal injury and mortality in polytrauma patients. An underlying cardiac injury, such as aortic disruption, cardiac contusion, pericardial effusion, or arrhythmia, should be considered. An electrocardiogram should be obtained in patients with sternal fracture to assess for myocardial injury. Nondisplaced sternal fractures can usually be managed with good pain control. Fractures of the proximal third of the clavicle can be associated with sternal fracture or intrathoracic injury. Nonoperative management with ice, analgesics, and a sling for support is the initial treatment strategy for nondisplaced proximal clavicle fractures.

THORACIC OUTLET SYNDROME

Thoracic outlet syndrome (TOS) refers to compression of the subclavian vessels and nerves of the brachial plexus (Fig. 110.28) in the region of the thoracic inlet. The three types of TOS are neurogenic (most common), arterial, and venous (Table 110.5). Middle-aged females are most commonly affected by TOS. The thoracic outlet contains three notable structures: the brachial plexus, subclavian artery, and subclavian vein. These structures can be compressed at various locations as they pass between the thoracic inlet and the upper extremity (see Fig. 110.33).

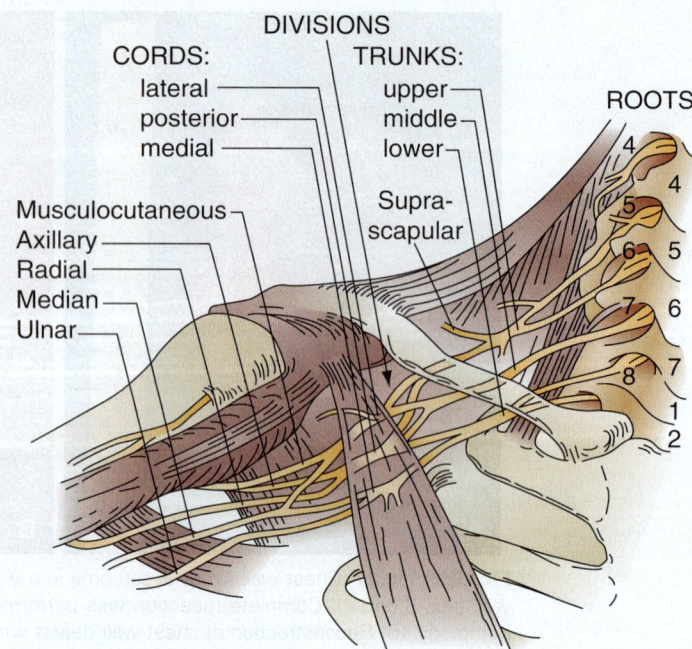

FIGURE 110.28 Detailed view of brachial plexus. (From Urschel HC, Razzuk M. Upper plexus thoracic outlet syndrome: Optimal therapy. *Ann Thorac Surg.* 1997;63:935-939.)

From medial to lateral, these anatomic regions are as follows: interscalene triangle (artery and nerves), costoclavicular space (vein), and subcoracoid area (artery, vein, nerves).

Diagnosis

TOS symptoms vary depending on the neurovascular structure that is compressed as it traverses the thoracic outlet. TOS can result from a combination of developmental abnormalities, injuries, and physical activities that predispose to neurovascular compression, such as presence of a cervical rib articulating with the first thoracic rib, supernumerary scalene muscles, or chronic inflammatory change resulting from repetitive trauma. Neurogenic manifestations are reported in more than 90% of cases. Symptoms of subclavian artery compression include hand/arm fatigue, weakness, pallor, claudication, and paresthesia. Thrombosis with distal embolization can rarely occur, producing ischemic changes in the hand. Venous TOS is characterized by upper extremity edema, cyanosis, and effort-induced thrombosis, also known as *Paget-Schroetter syndrome.*

The diagnosis of neurogenic TOS is initially made clinically, but chest and cervical spine films can help identify a potential cervical rib. CT and MRI are helpful to rule out narrowing of the intervertebral foramina, degenerative changes to the spine, or cervical disc pathology. Duplex or Doppler ultrasonography, CT, or angiography/venography may be used to evaluate the arterial and venous system. Electrophysiologic evaluation is indicated for neurogenic TOS to localize areas of abnormal nerve conduction and rule out other compressive syndromes, such as carpal tunnel. Abnormal ultrasound findings in a patient with a suggestive clinical history and no risk factors for atherosclerosis support a diagnosis of arterial TOS.

Positional maneuvers to evaluate a patient with suspected TOS can be easily performed in the clinic to identify the loss or

TABLE 110.5 Overview of the Clinical Presentation, Treatment Strategies, and Prognosis for Thoracic Outlet Syndrome (TOS)

TYPES OF TOS	NEUROGENIC (MOST COMMON FORM OF TOS)	VENOUS INVOLVEMENT OF THE SUBCLAVIAN VEIN	ARTERIAL INVOLVEMENT OF THE SUBCLAVIAN ARTERY
Sex	More common in females (3.5:1)	More common in males	Females and males equally
Typical age	20–40 years	20–30 years	20–30 years
Risk factors	• Repetitive movements • Previous trauma	• Strenuous work using arms • Athletics	• Vigorous arm activity
Symptoms	• Pain down arm, forearm, ring finger, and little finger • Tingling/numbness at night • Arm/hand weakness • Arm/hand swelling • Loss of dexterity • Cold intolerance • Headache	• Pain in affected arm, often associated with strenuous work • Arm/hand swelling • Veins of shoulder and chest appear more visible • Hand/arm appears blue in color • Blood clot (DVT) may develop	• Pain at rest • Pain with arm activity • Hand appears white in color • Hand/arm cool • Decreased pulse • Aneurysm of subclavian artery may be present • Thrombosis (blood clot) may develop
Lab studies	None	Coagulation studies if DVT develops	Coagulation studies if blood clot develops
Imaging studies	Chest x-ray	Chest x-ray Ultrasound Venography or angiography	Chest x-ray Ultrasound Angiography
Other studies	Nerve conduction study	Nerve conduction study	Nerve conduction study
Treatment	• Physical therapy (PT) • Lidocaine blocks • Botox injections • Surgical intervention • Post-op PT • Medication	• Anticoagulation (if DVT develops) • Surgical intervention • Venogram/venoplasty • Post-op PT	• Anticoagulation (if blood clot or thrombosis develops) • Surgical intervention • Angiogram/angioplasty • Post-op PT
Prognosis	Good	Good	Good

DVT, Deep vein thrombosis.
From Grunebach H, Arnold MW, Lum YW. Thoracic outlet syndrome. *Vasc Med.* 2015;20(5):493-495.

decrease of radial pulse or reproduce neurologic symptoms. Evocative tests to illicit symptoms include (Fig. 110.29):

- Adson (scalene) test. The patient inspires maximally and holds their breath with the neck fully extended, and the head is turned toward the affected side. This maneuver narrows the space between the scalenus anticus and medius, resulting in compression of the subclavian artery and the brachial plexus. Decrease or loss of the ipsilateral radial pulse suggests compression.
- Halsted (costoclavicular) test. The patient is instructed to place their shoulders in a military position (drawn backward and downward) to narrow the costoclavicular space between the first rib and the clavicle, causing neurovascular compression. Reproduction of neurologic symptoms or decrease or loss of the ipsilateral radial pulse suggests compression.
- Wright (hyperabduction) test. The patient's arm is hyperabducted 180 degrees, which causes the neurovascular structures to be compressed in the subcoracoid region by the pectoralis tendon, the head of the humerus, or the coracoid process. Decrease or loss of ipsilateral radial pulse suggests compression.
- Roos test. The patient abducts the involved arm 90 degrees with external rotation of the shoulder. Maintaining this body position, the patient opens and closes their hand rapidly for 3 minutes to reproduce symptoms. Additionally, neurogenic compromise may be detected using provocative tests, such as percussion of the nerve (Tinel sign) or flexion of the elbow or wrist (Phalen sign).

Management

Neurogenic TOS should initially be managed with physical therapy. Indications for surgical intervention include failure of conservative management, progressive neurologic symptoms, prolonged ulnar or median nerve conduction velocities, narrowing or occlusion of the subclavian artery, thrombosis of the axillary or subclavian vein, symptoms of thromboembolism, or acute limb ischemia. The goal of surgery is to release the narrowing or pressure point at the thoracic outlet. This is achieved in most cases by detachment of the anterior and middle scalene muscle from the first rib and by resection of the rib (in the presence of an accessory rib, it is resected). Additional interventions may include release of the pectoralis minor muscle from its insertion on the coracoid process and neurolysis of dense fibrosis along the brachial plexus. Identification and preservation of the brachial plexus, phrenic nerve, long thoracic nerve, and subclavian vessels are critical during surgery. For patients with venous thrombosis, thrombolysis and thoracic outlet decompression are performed. For patients with acute arterial ischemia resulting from distal embolization, thrombolysis or embolectomy may be required in conjunction with surgical repair (with possible arterial reconstruction) and thoracic outlet decompression. When indicated, surgery is beneficial in most patients with TOS, and long-term functional outcome of surgical treatment is satisfactory. Recurrent symptoms may prompt reoperation in up to one-third of patients.[50]

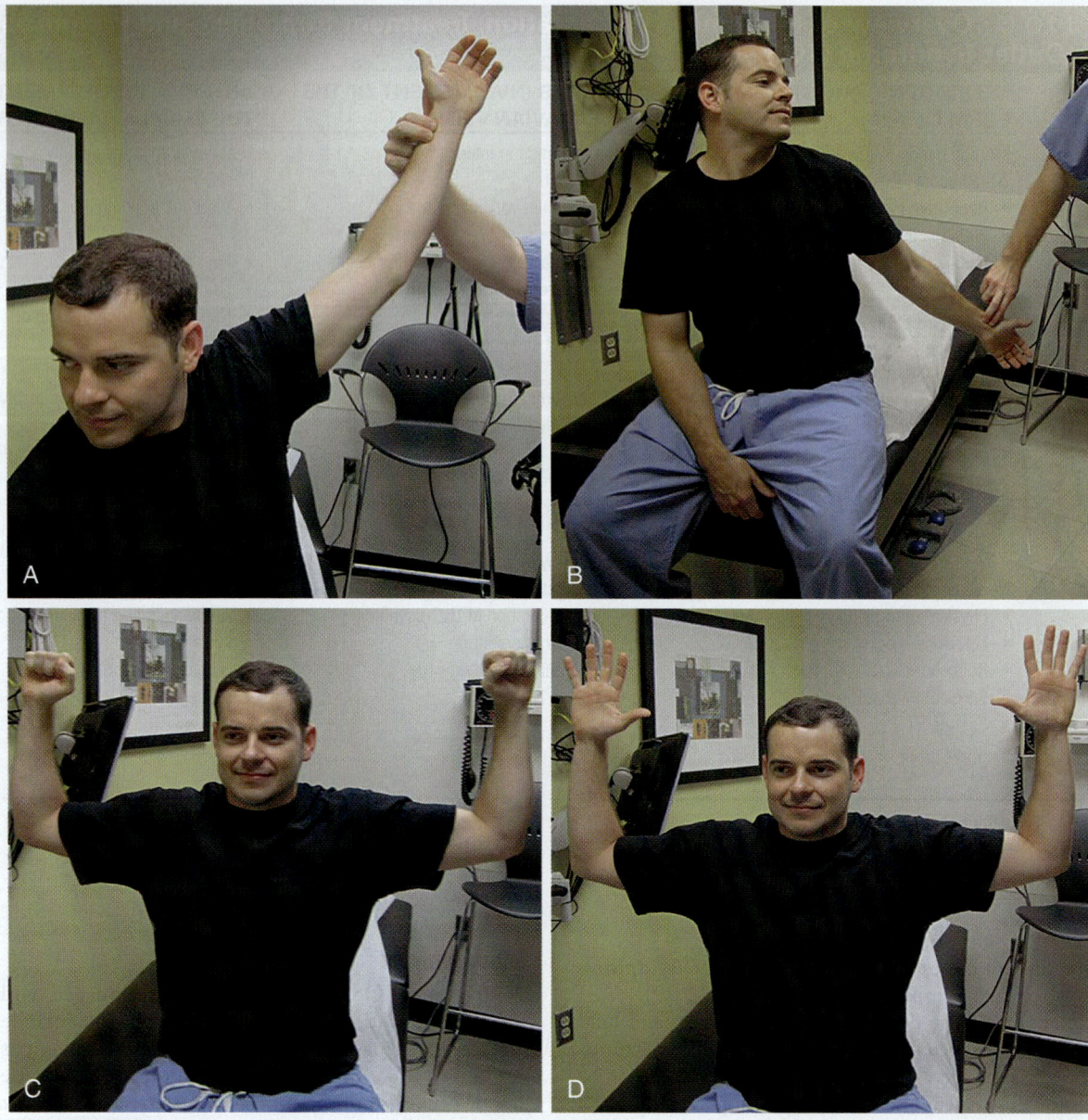

FIGURE 110.29 Clinical photographs demonstrating provocative physical tests for thoracic outlet syndrome. (A) Wright test. (B) Adson test. (C–D) Roos test. (From Kuhn JE, Lebus VG, Bible JE. Thoracic outlet syndrome. *J Am Acad Orthop Surg.* 2015;23:222-232.)

PLEURA

Pleural Effusions

The pleural space is a potential space defined by a small amount of lubricating fluid separating the visceral (lining the outer surface of the lung) and parietal (lining the inner surface of the chest wall) pleura. Several benign and malignant etiologies can disrupt the balance of fluid production and absorption, leading to the development of a pleural effusion, or the accumulation of fluid in between the parietal and visceral pleura (Box 110.3). Pleural fluid can be identified on CXR as the presence of 300 mL of fluid, causing blunting of the costophrenic angle on an upright posteroanterior view.

The movement of fluid across the pleural membranes is governed by Starling's law of capillary exchange. The amount of pleural fluid is controlled by a balance of oncotic and hydrostatic pressure within the pleural space and the pleural capillaries. In normal physiology, the net pressure moves fluid from the parietal pleura into the pleural space, and pleural fluid is reabsorbed through lymphatics. An imbalance of accumulation and absorption can lead to the development of a pleural effusion. The causative factors for pleural fluid accumulation include increased hydrostatic pressure, decreased pleural pressure, increased capillary permeability, decreased plasma oncotic pressure, and decreased lymphatic drainage.

Pleural fluid is characterized as being either transudative or exudative based on the mechanism for fluid accumulation and pleural fluid chemistry. Transudative effusions are protein-poor and result from increased hydrostatic pressure or decreased plasma oncotic pressure. Common causes of transudative effusions include congestive heart failure, nephrotic syndrome, cirrhosis, and hypoalbuminemia. In contrast, exudative effusions are protein-rich and are

BOX 110.3 Pleural Effusions

Cause of Transudative Effusions

Congestive heart failure
Cirrhosis
Nephrotic syndrome
Hypoalbuminemia
Fluid retention or overload
Pulmonary embolism
Lobar collapse
Meigs syndrome

Cause of Exudative Effusions

Malignant
  Primary lung or metastatic carcinoma
  Lymphoma
  Mesothelioma
Infectious
  Bacterial (parapneumonic) or empyema
  Tuberculosis
  Fungal
  Viral
  Parasitic
Collagen vascular disease related
  Rheumatoid arthritis
  Wegener granulomatosis
  Systemic lupus erythematosus
  Churg-Strauss syndrome
Abdominal/gastrointestinal disease related
  Esophageal perforation
  Subphrenic abscess
  Pancreatitis/pancreatic pseudocyst
  Meigs syndrome
Others
  Chylothorax
  Uremia
  Sarcoidosis
  After coronary artery bypass grafting
  Radiation/trauma
  Dressler syndrome
  Pulmonary embolism with infarction
  Asbestosis related

related to local inflammatory factors that precipitate pleural fluid accumulation. Common causes of exudative effusions are infection, malignancy, granulomatous diseases, and other inflammatory states. After thoracentesis, pleural fluid can be analyzed for chemical, microbiologic, and cellular content to determine the type of pleural effusion present. Based on Light's criteria, exudative effusions will have at least one of the following characteristics: (1) ratio of pleural fluid protein to serum protein of greater than 0.5, (2) ratio of pleural fluid lactate dehydrogenase (LDH) to serum LDH of greater than 0.6, or (3) pleural fluid LDH greater than 0.67 of the upper limits of normal serum LDH. Pleural fluid analysis typically includes gross inspection, cell counts and differential, total protein, pH, LDH, glucose, and cholesterol. Fluid culture (for aerobic, anaerobic, and fungal organisms), Gram stain, and cytology can also be performed if infection or malignancy are suspected. After the etiology of pleural effusion is determined, successful definitive management involves treatment of the underlying cause.

Benign Pleural Effusions

Most benign pleural effusions are transudative, free flowing, and without loculations. Initial treatment of symptomatic pleural effusions involves treating the primary etiology and draining the effusion via thoracentesis or thoracostomy tube placement. Asymptomatic effusions are typically not drained. Uncomplicated parapneumonic effusions that are small and without evidence of infection generally resolve with antibiotics alone and do not require drainage. For larger or complicated parapneumonic effusions (e.g., with microbiologic or biochemical evidence of infection), drainage is recommended in addition to antibiotics. After drainage, radiographic evidence of complete lung reexpansion should be sought. Failure of the lung to expand completely may suggest development of a "trapped lung" from formation of a fibrous peel that encases the visceral pleura, which may require decortication if symptoms persist. Chronic sterile effusions can be treated with an indwelling pleural catheter insertion, which can result in pleural symphysis. However, when used for heart or renal failure, great care is needed to manage fluid and electrolyte shifts.

Malignant Pleural Effusion

Approximately 15% of all cancer patients develop MPEs from malignant cells infiltrating the pleural space.[51] The median survival of patients with MPEs is 5 months.[52] Pleural biopsy and cytology can aid with diagnosis. MPE treatment is aimed at symptom relief and palliation because it typically indicates advanced-stage cancer and a poor overall prognosis. Drainage is recommended for large-volume, symptomatic MPEs (Fig. 110.30). For recurrent MPEs, insertion of an indwelling pleural catheter can be considered because these devices permit frequent drainage of pleural fluid and can induce pleurodesis. Chemical pleurodesis via a thoracostomy tube or VATS is another reasonable treatment option. Pleurectomy and pleurodesis are reserved for patients who fail other therapies and have a reasonable life expectancy.

Empyema

An empyema is a collection of purulent fluid within the pleural space, which results from invasion of pyogenic bacteria, fungi, parasites, or mycobacteria. Microorganisms may originate from an adjacent pneumonia, direct inoculation (e.g., penetrating trauma), or another source (e.g., esophageal rupture, bronchogenic carcinoma). Empyemas progress from an acute phase with fluid that is thin and can be drained completely with a pigtail catheter or chest tube to fluid that is increasingly turbid, thicker, and loculated. Mucopurulent debris occurs within the pleural space and compresses the underlying lung parenchyma. The organizing or chronic phase is reflected by lung entrapment with capillary ingrowth and development of a fibrinous pleural covering, which can encase the lung and hinder full reexpansion ("trapped lung").

An empyema typically occurs after a reactive pleural effusion as a consequence of a lung infection. Common causative organisms include gram-negative, anaerobic, streptococcal, and pneumococcal bacteria. Mycobacterial infection can also cause empyema formation and should be considered in patients who live in an endemic area and/or have specific risk factors. Empyemas can also form after trauma or surgery (e.g., bronchopleural fistula) or esophageal perforation. Symptoms typically include constitutional symptoms of general malaise, fever, loss of appetite, and weight loss. Evaluation includes CXR and CT scan.

Treatment depends on the disease severity, location, and duration of infection. Drainage and antibiotics are required. Drainage of early

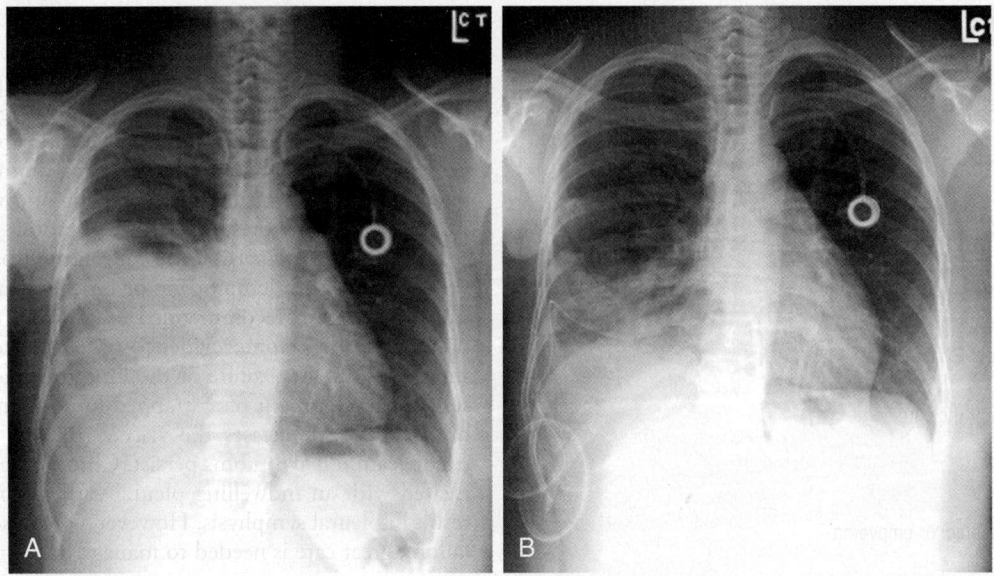

FIGURE 110.30 (A) Malignant pleural effusion causing dyspnea. A long-term indwelling pleural catheter was placed as an outpatient procedure to facilitate drainage at home to prevent dyspnea. Hospitalization was not required. (B) After drainage. A long-term indwelling pleural catheter is effective in patients with trapped lung. Every-other-day drainage reduces impairment of the contralateral lung and prevents mediastinal shift.

empyemas in the purulent phase can often be achieved by insertion of a pleural drain (pigtail catheter or chest tube). With complex, loculated effusions, surgery is usually indicated. Chest tubes can generally be removed when the daily drainage volume falls below 100 to 200 mL, imaging shows reduction in the size of the effusion, and the patient has resolving clinical signs of infection. Early VATS for complex effusions has been shown to reduce hospital length of stay and provide good lung expansion. Use of fibrinolytic agents, such as intrapleural tissue plasminogen activator and DNase, may aid with catheter drainage and reduce the need for surgical drainage. However, they are not recommended for routine use of complicated empyemas because they are expensive and less effective than commonly believed.[53] For organized empyemas with a thick peel, thoracotomy and decortication remain a common treatment to adequately reexpand the lung and clean out the pleural space.

Chylothorax

Chylothorax occurs when chyle from the thoracic duct empties into the pleural space. Chyle is a milky-appearing, white fluid containing a high concentration of triglycerides, chylomicrons, and white blood cells. Chylothorax can result from multiple etiologies (Box 110.4). Because of the nutritional consequences of a chyle leak (e.g., loss of fat and protein) and the volume of the leak (0.5–3.0 L/day), fluid and nutritional replacement and correction of the underlying problem are necessary. An untreated chylothorax is associated with significant morbidity and mortality. The diagnosis can be made with thoracentesis or drainage with a thoracostomy tube. Pleural fluid analysis typically demonstrates lymphocyte predominance, low LDH, high concentration of triglycerides (>110 mg/dL), and a cholesterol level <200 mg/dL. Initial management strategies for low-output chylothorax (<500 cc of chyle/day) include drainage for symptom control, bowel rest, and parenteral nutrition. High-output chylothorax (>1 L per day) requires early definitive intervention (e.g., ligation of the thoracic duct or percutaneous thoracic duct embolization). Adjuncts to these treatment strategies include a diet with medium-chain

BOX 110.4   Chylothorax

Traumatic (chest and neck)
  Blunt
  Penetrating
Iatrogenic
  Catheterization, particularly subclavian vein
  Postsurgical
  Excision of cervical/supraclavicular lymph nodes
  Radical lymph node dissections of the neck or chest
  Lung, esophageal, or mediastinal resection
  Thoracic aneurysm repair
  Sympathectomy
  Congenital cardiovascular surgery
Neoplasms
  Lymphoma, lung, esophageal, or mediastinal neoplasms
  Metastatic carcinoma
Infectious
  Tuberculous lymphadenosis
  Mediastinitis
  Ascending lymphangitis
Other
  Lymphangioleiomyomatosis
  Venous thrombosis
  Congenital

triglycerides and/or administration of octreotide. Surgical ligation of the thoracic duct commonly occurs via the right chest, where it enters the chest through the diaphragmatic hiatus. At the time of surgical repair, placement of olive oil or ice cream through a nasogastric tube may increase chyle drainage into the operative field and help identify the area of thoracic duct disruption. However, a minimally invasive or open thoracic duct ligation encompasses all the tissue between the aorta, esophagus, spine, and azygous vein.

Pneumothorax

Pneumothorax is the accumulation of air within the pleural space. It can occur after trauma, surgery, central line insertion, increased pressure from mechanical ventilation, or as a sequela of underlying pulmonary disease (e.g., COPD, CF) or other conditions (e.g., catamenial pneumothorax) (Box 110.5). A primary spontaneous pneumothorax generally occurs as a result of small apical subpleural blebs or bullae (air sacs between the lung tissue and pleura) that rupture into the pleural cavity. A tension pneumothorax occurs when air continues to enter the pleural space without decompression, leading to mediastinal compression and shift and a decrease in ventilation and venous return. Cardiopulmonary collapse and death can ensue. Immediate decompression with needle or tube thoracostomy can be lifesaving.

A primary spontaneous pneumothorax typically presents with pain and dyspnea in tall and thin young males. Tobacco use is a significant risk factor. CT can be performed to assess for the etiology or the presence of other occult lung disease. On examination, breath sounds are usually absent over the affected hemithorax, and subcutaneous emphysema may be present. Treatment depends on the size of the pneumothorax and the presence of symptoms or mediastinal shift. A small pneumothorax (≤3 cm at apex or ≤2 cm at hilum) may be followed and resolve spontaneously. Larger or enlarging pneumothoraxes require aspiration or placement of a tube thoracostomy. After chest tube placement, patients should receive a daily CXR until lung reexpansion and cessation of air leak. Persistent air leak (>2 days) or failure of the lung to expand fully may indicate the need for surgical intervention. Surgery is recommended for patients who have a persistent or recurrent pneumothorax, develop another episode, or work in high-risk professions (e.g., divers, pilots). Surgery typically involves VATS resection of blebs with pleurodesis.

Mesothelioma

Malignant pleural mesothelioma (MPM) is an aggressive malignancy with a poor prognosis (median survival: 9–17 months) that arises from the mesothelial cells lining the parietal and visceral pleura.[54,55] MPM pathogenesis is tightly linked to asbestos exposure, and a long latency period (15–40 years) exists between primary exposure and disease development. Because of the insidious onset of symptoms, the majority of patients are diagnosed with advanced disease. Histologic subtypes include epithelial (most favorable prognosis), sarcomatoid, and biphasic histology. Symptoms include shortness of breath, cough, pleural effusion, weight loss, chest pain, and fever. Imaging can reveal unilateral pleural thickening and pleural effusion. Diagnosis can be made with pleural biopsy.

For functionally fit patients with epithelioid MPM limited to one hemithorax, a multimodal treatment strategy may be considered that involves chemotherapy, macroscopic complete resection (MCR; R0 or R1 resection), and radiation therapy. MCR can be achieved either by extrapleural pneumonectomy (EPP; resection of the entire lung, including the visceral and parietal pleura and the diaphragm ± pericardium through a large posterolateral thoracotomy) or by extended pleurectomy and decortication (EPD; resection of the parietal and visceral pleura and the diaphragm ± pericardium while preserving the lung parenchyma through a large posterolateral thoracotomy). EPP is the most extensive surgery for MPM and is associated with high rates of mortality (5%–20%) and morbidity (40%–60%). EPD is a lung-preserving surgery that offers somewhat of a less extensive resection; however, it is associated with less mortality, less morbidity, and a comparable survival to EPP.[56] For patients with sarcomatoid type, patients with advanced disease, or those deemed poor surgical candidates, treatment includes systemic chemotherapy, palliative radiation therapy, and management of local symptoms from any MPE.

Solitary Fibrous Tumor of the Pleura

Solitary fibrous tumors are rare fibroblastic mesenchymal tumors that arise either from the visceral or parietal pleura. They rarely metastasize. These tumors often attach to the pleura with a thin pedicle and may grow quite large. Symptoms are often related to mass effect, and up to 20% are associated with digital clubbing and hypertrophic pulmonary osteoarthropathy (Pierre-Marie-Bamberger syndrome). Treatment for localized disease consists of complete en bloc resection of the tumor, its pedicle, and the pleura/lung at the base of the pedicle. Wedge resection is sufficient in most cases to remove the pedicle and other adhesions of the tumors to the lung. Long-term postoperative surveillance is indicated because these tumors can recur locally.

MEDIASTINUM

Mediastinal abnormalities may present as an asymptomatic mass identified on imaging or with significant symptoms resulting from mass effect on adjacent structures, including hypoxia, facial swelling, dysphagia, and respiratory distress. CT or MRI can assist with characterization of mediastinal masses. Biopsy specimens may be needed to make the diagnosis. Mediastinal masses differ between adults and children. The most common mediastinal masses in adults are thymomas and thymic cysts, neurogenic tumors, other cysts, germ cell tumors, and lymphomas (Box 110.6). In children, the most common pathologies are neurogenic tumors, germ cell tumors, primary cysts, and lymphomas. Malignant neoplasms account for 25% to 50% of mediastinal masses in adults. Lymphomas, thymomas, germ cell tumors, primary carcinomas, and neurogenic tumors are the most common. Many mediastinal lesions occur in characteristic sites within the mediastinum (Fig. 110.31). Approximately half of all mediastinal masses

---

BOX 110.5 Pneumothorax

Spontaneous
  Primary
  Secondary
  - Chronic obstructive pulmonary disease
  - Bullous disease
  - Cystic fibrosis
  - Pneumocystis related
  - Congenital cysts
  - Idiopathic pulmonary fibrosis
  - Pulmonary embolism
  Catamenial
  Neonatal
Traumatic
  Penetrating
  Blunt
Iatrogenic
  Mechanical ventilation
  Needle puncture: thoracentesis, fine-needle aspiration lung nodule, central line insertion
  Postsurgical

BOX 110.6 Mediastinum: Classification of Primary Mediastinal Tumors and Cysts

Thymoma
  Thymic carcinoma
Lymphoma
  Hodgkin disease
  Lymphoblastic lymphoma
  Large cell lymphoma
Germ cell tumors
  Teratodermoid (benign/malignant)
  Seminoma
  Nonseminoma
    • Embryonal
    • Choriocarcinoma
    • Endodermal
Primary carcinomas
  Mesenchymal tumors
    • Fibroma/fibrosarcoma
    • Lipoma/liposarcoma
    • Leiomyoma/leiomyosarcoma
    • Rhabdosarcoma
    • Xanthogranuloma
    • Myxoma
    • Mesothelioma
    • Hemangioma
    • Hemangioendothelioma
    • Hemangiopericytoma
    • Lymphangioma
    • Lymphangiomyoma
    • Lymphangiopericytoma
  Endocrine tumors
    • Intrathoracic thyroid
    • Parathyroid adenoma/carcinoma
    • Carcinoid
Cysts
  Bronchogenic
  Pericardial
  Enteric
  Thymic
  Thoracic duct
  Nonspecific
Giant lymph node hyperplasia
  Castleman disease
Chondroma
Extramedullary hematopoiesis
Neurogenic tumors
  Neurofibroma
  Neurilemoma
  Paraganglioma
  Ganglioneuroma
  Neuroblastoma
  Chemodectoma
  Neurosarcoma

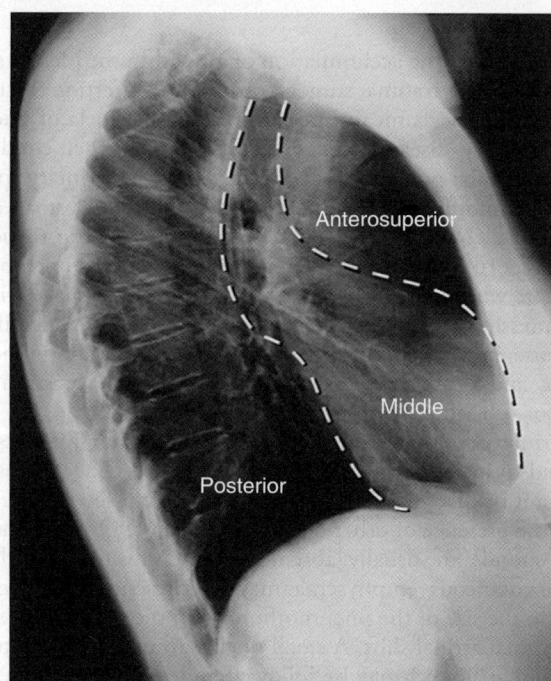

FIGURE 110.31 Lateral chest radiograph demonstrating the mediastinum divided into three anatomic subdivisions.

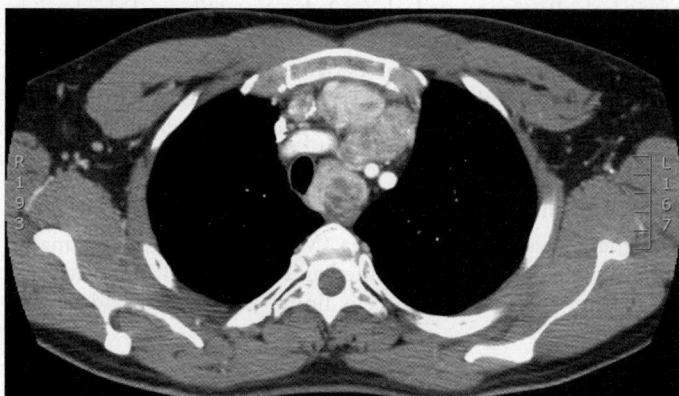

FIGURE 110.32 Thyroid carcinoma within the mediastinum. The tumor was resected via median sternotomy. No invasion was identified. A complete resection was accomplished.

are located in the anterosuperior mediastinum, with the remainder occurring in the posterior or middle mediastinum.

Anterosuperior Compartment

The anterosuperior compartment of the mediastinum borders the undersurface of the sternum ventrally, the pericardium dorsally, and the visceral pleura laterally (at the apposition of the pleura and pericardium). Among adults >40 years old, thymomas are the most common neoplasm of the anterior mediastinum, and the second most common pathology is retrosternal goiter. Other pathologies are lymphomas, seminomas, nonseminoma germ cell tumors, and teratomas. Between the ages of 10 and 40 years old, lymphomas and teratomas in females and lymphomas, seminomas, nonseminoma germ cell tumors, and teratomas in males are the most frequently occurring neoplasms. In children, lymphomas and teratomas are the common neoplasms of the anterior mediastinum. Additional pathologies of the anterior mediastinum include carcinoid tumors, which may be found within the thymus, and primary carcinomas of the mediastinum, which are often unresectable and respond poorly to treatment (Fig. 110.32).

Middle Compartment

The middle compartment extends from (and contains) the structures of the thoracic inlet (superiorly) to the pericardium anteriorly and to the anterior surface of the vertebrae posteriorly.

Lymphomas can occur in the middle mediastinum. Tumors of the heart, trachea, mainstem bronchi, and esophagus can also form. Benign diseases, such as pericardial cysts and bronchogenic cysts, also occur here. Vascular masses and enlargement may represent aortic pathologies such as aortic aneurysm, abscess, or dissection.

Posterior or Paravertebral Sulci Compartment

The posterior compartment is bounded by the middle compartment anteriorly and the costophrenic angle laterally. Neurogenic tumors are usually the most common primary tumors of the mediastinum, and about 25% of these tumors are malignant. These tumors are located within the paravertebral sulcus and may erode the adjacent vertebra or rib. Schwannomas, or neurilemomas, are the most common neurogenic tumors. Neurofibromas arise from the nerve sheath and fibers and occur in middle-aged patients. In children, ganglioneuroma is the most common neurogenic tumor. Surgical resection of neurogenic tumors is usually indicated.

Embryologic development of the neural crest cells forms the basis of NETs in the mediastinum. Of pheochromocytomas, 1% occur within the mediastinum. Chemodectomas or paragangliomas may arise from chemoreceptor tissues around the aorta and great vessels, including the carotid. Symptoms may result from catecholamine production and are alleviated by surgical resection.

Clinical Manifestations and Diagnosis

Symptoms from a mediastinal mass may vary widely and relate to size (e.g., fatigue, weight loss); location; extent of compression or invasion of mediastinal structures; and production of hormones, markers, or other biochemical materials (e.g., myasthenia gravis, fatigue, night sweats). Benign lesions are more often asymptomatic. Specific clinical syndromes may occur as a result of mediastinal tumors. Superior vena cava syndrome (obstruction of the superior vena cava with head and neck and upper extremity swelling), cough, hoarseness (from involvement of the recurrent laryngeal nerve), dyspnea from tumor volume or phrenic nerve paralysis, and dysphagia can occur with compression or invasion of mediastinal structures. Other manifestations include Horner syndrome (characterized by ptosis, miosis, anhidrosis) and Pancoast syndrome. Postobstructive pneumonitis or infection of benign pericardial or enteric duplication cysts may produce fever or sepsis. Myasthenia gravis can result from thymomas. Mediastinal Hodgkin disease may produce an intermittent fever. Patients with hypertension from pheochromocytoma, thyrotoxicosis from goiter, hypercalcemia from ectopic mediastinal parathyroid adenoma or carcinoma, or hypogammaglobulinemia should be evaluated carefully.

Evaluation and Diagnostic Imaging

Based on imaging, a differential diagnosis may be obtained based on the location of the mass within the mediastinum. CT scans have replaced plain CXRs as the diagnostic imaging of choice for mediastinal masses. MRI can be used if invasion into specific anatomic structures in the mediastinum is in question. For instance, an anterior mediastinal mass, such as a thymoma, can be evaluated for the extent of compression or possible invasion into the pulmonary artery, innominate vein, or superior vena cava. Similarly, posterior mediastinal masses can be evaluated by MRI for the extent of invasion into the brachial plexus, great vessels, vertebral body, and neural foramina. Echocardiography may identify pericardial and cardiac involvement. Additional imaging techniques may be used in specific scenarios (technetium scan for ectopic thyroid tissue or a substernal goiter and 131-I metaiodobenzylguanidine for pheochromocytoma).

Mediastinal tumors may secrete specific hormones or biologic markers. Parathyroid adenomas or functioning parathyroid carcinomas may secrete parathyroid hormone. Pheochromocytomas may secrete catecholamines, which may cause hypertension. Carcinomas may secrete carcinoembryonic antigen. Nonseminomatous germ cell neoplasms may secrete α-fetoprotein (AFP) or β-human chorionic gonadotropin (β-HCG). Lymphomas may be associated with elevated levels of LDH and alkaline phosphatase. Thymomas may be associated with production of anti-acetylcholine receptor (AChR) antibodies. Skin tests for tuberculosis, histoplasmosis, and coccidioidomycosis may also yield positive results.

Histologic Diagnosis

Radiographic diagnosis may be sufficient for the design of a treatment plan for mediastinal cysts and other solid lesions that are clearly resectable (e.g., early stage thymoma). However, a tissue specimen for definitive diagnosis is required for the workup of more complex solid masses. Fine-needle aspiration or needle biopsy may provide sufficient tissue for diagnosis of thymic carcinoma or other defined neoplasms. For lymphomas, thymomas, and neural tumors, larger amounts of tissue may be required for cellular analysis. In these patients, core-needle biopsy, mediastinoscopy, or intrathoracic biopsy (via thoracoscopy or thoracotomy) may be considered. When resection is considered, median sternotomy provides a direct visual approach to the anterior and middle mediastinum. Thoracotomy provides a direct visual approach to the posterior mediastinum. Minimally invasive resection techniques are becoming increasingly used for treatment of noninvasive tumors.

PRIMARY MEDIASTINAL CYSTS

Primary mediastinal cysts are characterized by the organ of origin and may be bronchogenic, pericardial, enteric, thymic, or of an unspecified nature. Most cases are asymptomatic; however, these cysts may cause mass effect on vital structures within the mediastinum with increasing size. Benign cysts may be resected minimally invasively.

Bronchogenic cysts account for most primary cysts of the mediastinum. They originate as sequestrations from the ventral foregut and can be situated within the lung parenchyma or the mediastinum. Bronchogenic cysts are usually located proximal to the trachea or bronchi and may be posterior to the carina. A connection to the bronchus rarely exists; however, when it occurs, these cysts may become infected. Diagnostic imaging may reveal an air-fluid level within the mediastinum. Two-thirds of bronchogenic cysts are asymptomatic. In infants, cysts can cause respiratory compromise by compressing the trachea or the bronchus. Resection is recommended.

Pericardial cysts are the second most common and occur in the cardiophrenic angle, typically on the right side. These cysts can communicate with the pericardium. Typically, clear fluid is encountered. The typical characteristics of pericardial cysts include location in the cardiophrenic angle, characteristic appearance, smooth borders, and attenuation approximating water for the cyst fluid. Needle aspiration and routine surveillance may be all that is needed. However, resection may be used for diagnosis and to exclude malignant tumors.

Enteric cysts or duplication cysts arise from the primitive foregut, which develops into the upper division of the gastrointestinal tract. These cysts are usually attached to the esophagus. Symptoms such as dysphagia can occur with compression of the esophagus. Neuroenteric cysts are associated with anomalies of the vertebral column. Excision is recommended, and a small part of the cyst bordering the esophagus may be left in place (2–3 cm), with the mucosa cauterized to prevent fluid secretion and recurrence.

PRIMARY MEDIASTINAL NEOPLASMS

Thymoma

Thymomas are the most common neoplasm of the anterosuperior mediastinum and are considered malignant tumors. The major histologic subtypes are A (most indolent), AB, and B1 to B3 (most aggressive) thymomas. Thymic carcinomas are more aggressive than thymomas and are separately classified. The peak incidence is in the third through fifth decades of life. A thymoma may appear on a radiograph as a small, well-circumscribed mass or as a bulky, lobulated mass confluent with adjacent mediastinal structures (Fig. 110.33). Symptoms are related to local mass effect, causing chest pain, dyspnea, hemoptysis, cough, and superior vena cava syndrome or systemic syndromes caused by immunologic mechanisms. The most common syndrome is myasthenia gravis (occurs in ~40% of cases). Other paraneoplastic syndromes include pure red cell aplasia, hypogammaglobulinemia, and thymoma-associated multiorgan autoimmunity. Staging of thymomas and thymic carcinomas is based on the extent of the primary tumor and the presence of invasion into adjacent structures and/or dissemination. Until recently, thymomas were staged according to the modified Masaoka-Koga classification system; however, a formal TNM-based staging system for thymic tumors has been issued by the AJCC as part of its 8th edition cancer staging manual (Table 110.6).

Thymomas may be viewed as resectable, potentially resectable, and unresectable. Patients presenting with small, fully encapsulated thymomas should undergo surgery. For patients with invasive but potentially resectable tumors, neoadjuvant and adjuvant chemotherapy, radiation, and immunotherapy are applied in conjunction with surgery to achieve complete or at least macroscopically complete tumor resection. Resection and reconstruction of involved mediastinal structures, including the superior vena cava and innominate vein, as well as resection of droplet metastatic lesions, may achieve significant prolongation of survival in select patients.

TABLE 110.6 Thymoma Staging

T DESCRIPTORS

CATEGORY	DEFINITION (INVOLVEMENT OF)[a,b]
T1	
a	Encapsulated or unencapsulated, with or without extension into mediastinal fat
b	Extension into mediastinal pleura
T2	Pericardium
T3	Lung, brachiocephalic vein, superior vena cava, chest wall, phrenic nerve, hilar (extrapericardial) pulmonary vessels
T4	Aorta, arch vessels, main pulmonary artery, myocardium, trachea, or esophagus

N AND M DESCRIPTORS

CATEGORY	DEFINITION (INVOLVEMENT OF)[a]
N0	No nodal involvement
N1	Anterior (perithymic) nodes
N2	Deep intrathoracic or cervical nodes
M0	No metastatic pleural, pericardial, or distant sites
M1	
A	Separate pleural or pericardial nodule(s)
B	Pulmonary intraparenchymal nodule or distant organ metastasis

STAGE GROUPING

STAGE	T	N	M
I	T1	N0	M0
II	T2	N0	M0
IIIa	T3	N0	M0
IIIb	T4	N0	M0
IVa	T any	N1	M0
	T any	N0,1	M1a
IVb	T any	N2	M0,1a
	T any	N any	M1b

[a]Involvement must be pathologically proven in pathologic staging.
[b]A tumor is classified according to the highest T level of involvement that is present with or without any invasion of structures of lower T levels.
From Detterbeck FC, Stratton K, Giroux D, et al. The IASLC/ITMIG thymic epithelial tumors staging project: proposal for an evidence-based stage classification system for the forthcoming (8th) edition of the TNM classification of malignant tumors. *J Thorac Oncol.* 2014;9:S65-S72.

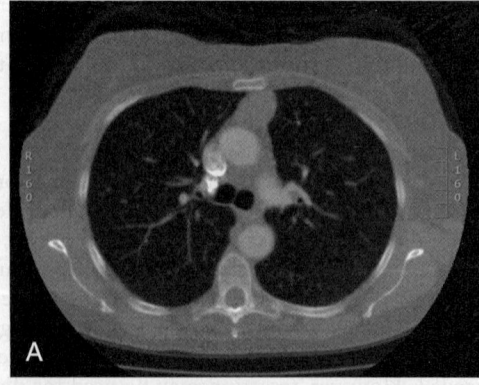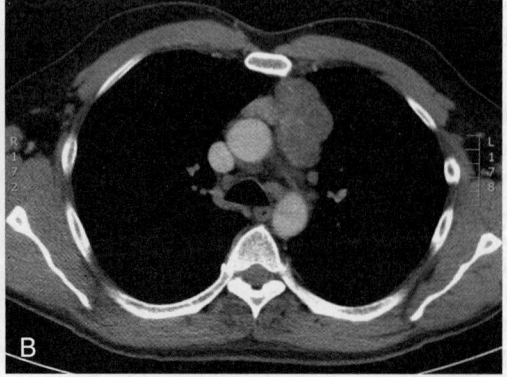

FIGURE 110.33 (A) Computed tomography (CT) scan of the chest in a patient with myasthenia gravis and thymoma. The thymoma is small, with a plane of separation between the tumor and the pericardium. (B) Chest CT scan in a patient with a larger mediastinal mass. The location, character, and size are noted. Transthoracic core-needle biopsy was performed. Germ cell tumor markers were normal. Pathology demonstrated thymoma. A 6.5-cm thymoma was subsequently resected. There was no invasion of the pericardium. A complete resection (R0) was accomplished.

For patients with myasthenia gravis and a thymoma, surgery is advocated as soon as the patient's degree of weakness is sufficiently controlled to permit surgery. Only 10% to 15% of patients with myasthenia gravis have a thymoma, whereas 40% of patients with a thymoma have myasthenia. Attentive perioperative management in these patients is crucial to prevent complications. Anticholinesterase inhibitors, plasmapheresis, and/or intravenous immunoglobulin are used pre- and postoperatively to control generalized weakness. Intensive pulmonary toilet, early extubation, chest physiotherapy, and avoidance of paralyzing agents and narcotics help ensure safe recovery from surgery. During surgery, complete resection of the thymus and all accessible mediastinal fatty areolar tissue is performed to ensure removal of all ectopic thymic tissue and reduce risk of tumor recurrence. Preservation of the phrenic nerves is an integral component of thymectomy. Improvement in myasthenia gravis symptoms and reduction in the dosages of drugs required to control the disease are anticipated to a certain extent in the months after surgery.[57]

Germ Cell Tumors

Germ cell tumors arise from primordial germ cells that fail to complete the migration from the urogenital ridge and rest in the mediastinum. Treatment depends on tumor histology. The anterosuperior mediastinum is the most common extragonadal primary site of these tumors. These lesions are histologically identical to germ cell tumors originating in the gonads. The testes of a male patient with a mediastinal germ cell tumor should be carefully examined and imaged with ultrasonography. Biopsy is reserved for positive findings.

Teratomas

Teratomas are the most common mediastinal germ cell neoplasms and are most frequently located in the anterosuperior mediastinum. They are composed of multiple tissue elements that are derived from the three primitive embryonic layers (ectoderm, mesoderm, and endoderm). The peak incidence occurs in the second and third decades of life. Radiographic evidence of normal tissue (e.g., well-formed teeth or globular calcifications) in an abnormal location can be considered specific. The teratodermoid (dermoid) cyst is the simplest form of teratoma and is composed of derivatives of the epidermal layer, including dermal and epidermal glands, hair, and sebaceous material. The solid component of the tumor often contains well-differentiated elements of bone, cartilage, teeth, muscle, connective tissue, fibrous and lymphoid tissue, nerve, thymus, mucous and salivary glands, lung, liver, or pancreas. Malignant tumors are differentiated from benign tumors by the presence of primitive (embryonic) tissue or by the presence of malignant components. Immature teratomas contain combinations of mature epithelial and connective tissues with immature areas of mesenchymal and neuroectodermal tissues. In contrast, mature teratomas contain well-differentiated histologic elements derived from at least two embryonic cell layers.

Diagnosis and therapy rely on surgical excision, most commonly through a median sternotomy or posterolateral thoracotomy, depending on tumor location. Patients with mature teratomas are treated with surgical resection because these tumors are generally insensitive to chemotherapy and radiation therapy. For malignant teratomas, chemoradiation combined with surgical excision is individualized for the type of malignant components contained in the tumors. The overall prognosis for malignant mediastinal teratomas is poor.

Malignant Nonteratomatous Germ Cell Tumors

Malignant germ cell tumors occur predominantly in the anterosuperior mediastinum, are more common in males, and are typically diagnosed between the ages of 20 and 40 years. Most patients have symptoms of chest pain, cough, dyspnea, and hemoptysis. Superior vena cava syndrome may also occur. These aggressive tumors are often metastatic at presentation. Serologic measurements of AFP and β-HCG are useful for differentiating seminomas from nonseminomatous tumors, assessing treatment response, and detecting early recurrence. Seminomas frequently produce β-HCG but do not produce AFP; in contrast, nonseminomatous tumors typically secrete one or both hormones. This differentiation is important because seminomas are sensitive to radiation, whereas nonseminomatous tumors are relatively insensitive to radiation.

Seminomas

Seminomas constitute about one-third of malignant mediastinal germ cell tumors. Most seminomas will have evidence of metastasis at the time of diagnosis, most often to the lymph nodes. Symptoms are related to the mass effect of the tumor on adjacent mediastinal and pulmonary structures. Superior vena cava syndrome occurs in 10% to 20% of patients. These tumors are sensitive to irradiation and chemotherapy. Therapy is determined by the stage of the disease. For most patients with seminomas, platinum-based chemotherapy is the primary treatment option. Long-term disease-free survival is about 90% after treatment with chemotherapy.[58] Radiation therapy may be considered for patients who do not have bulky or metastatic disease. Cytoreductive resection before chemotherapy or radiation therapy is unnecessary. Infrequently, complete surgical excision is possible for very small and localized tumors.

Nonseminomatous Tumors

Malignant nonseminomatous germ cell tumors include choriocarcinomas, embryonal carcinomas, immature teratomas, teratomas with malignant components, and endodermal cell (yolk sac) tumors and occur mostly in males in their third or fourth decades. Diagnostic imaging reveals a large anterior mediastinal mass with frequent extension to the lung, chest wall, and mediastinal structures. Nonseminomatous germ cell neoplasms are more aggressive tumors and are more frequently disseminated at the time of diagnosis, they are rarely radiosensitive, and more than 90% produce either β-HCG or AFP. All patients with choriocarcinoma and some patients with embryonal cell tumors have elevated levels of β-HCG. AFP is most commonly elevated in patients with embryonal cell carcinomas and yolk sac tumors. Mediastinal nonseminomatous germ cell tumors are associated with the development of hematologic disorders, such as acute megakaryocytic leukemia, systemic mast cell disease, malignant histiocytosis, myelodysplastic syndrome, and idiopathic thrombocytopenia. Treatment involves cisplatin and etoposide-based chemotherapy regimens. Serum markers (i.e., AFP or β-HCG) can be followed to assess response to systemic treatment. Operative intervention may be required for salvage resection after chemotherapy. The pathology of the resected postchemotherapy specimen appears to be the most significant predictor of survival. The presence of residual malignancy after chemotherapy portends a poor prognosis and the need for additional chemotherapy.

Neurogenic Tumors

Neurogenic tumors are usually located in the posterior mediastinum and originate from the sympathetic ganglia (ganglioma, ganglioneuroblastoma, and neuroblastoma), the intercostal nerves (neurofibroma, neurilemoma, and neurosarcoma), and the paraganglia cells (paraganglioma). Although the peak incidence occurs in adults, neurogenic tumors make up a proportionally greater percentage of mediastinal masses in children. Although most neurogenic tumors in adults are benign, a greater percentage of neurogenic tumors are malignant in children. Many of these tumors are asymptomatic.

The most common neurogenic tumor is neurilemoma, or schwannoma, which originates from perineural Schwann cells. They are benign, slow-growing neoplasms that frequently arise from a spinal nerve root but can involve any thoracic nerve. These tumors are well circumscribed and have a defined capsule. They arise from the nerve sheath and extrinsically compress the nerve fibers. About 10% of tumors have extensions into the spinal column and are termed *dumbbell tumors* because of their characteristic shape, with relatively large paraspinal and intraspinal portions connected by an isthmus of tissue traversing the intervertebral foramen. Patients with paraspinal tumors should undergo MRI to evaluate the presence and extent of the tumor, including its relationship to the neural foramen and the intraspinal space. During resection, the intraspinal component should be removed first via a posterior laminectomy. This approach minimizes the potential for spinal column hematoma, cord ischemia, and paralysis. A separate transthoracic approach is needed for resection of the intrathoracic component.

Neuroblastoma

Neuroblastomas originate from the sympathetic nervous system. The most common location for a neuroblastoma is in the retroperitoneum; however, 10% to 20% occur primarily in the mediastinum. These are highly invasive neoplasms that have frequently metastasized before diagnosis. Most of these tumors occur in children 4 years old or younger. A 24-hour urine collection to measure catecholamines should be obtained in children with a posterior mediastinal mass. For most children with low-risk localized tumors, surgical resection alone is usually performed. For those with intermediate-risk neuroblastoma, neoadjuvant chemotherapy with or without surgical resection is often performed. For patients with advanced disease, a multimodal treatment strategy that includes induction chemotherapy, surgical resection, autologous hematopoietic stem cell transplantation, radiation treatment, and maintenance with biologic/immunologic therapy (e.g., dinutuximab) can be used.

Ganglion Tumors

Ganglioneuroblastomas are composed of mature and immature ganglion cells. Treatment of ganglioneuroblastoma ranges from surgical excision alone to various chemotherapeutic strategies, depending on histologic characteristics, age, and stage of disease. Ganglioneuromas are benign tumors that originate from the sympathetic chain and are composed of ganglion cells and nerve fibers. These tumors typically manifest at an early age and are the most common neurogenic tumors occurring during childhood. They usually occur in the paravertebral region. These tumors are well encapsulated and, when cross-sectioned, frequently exhibit areas of cystic degeneration. Surgical excision provides cure.

Paraganglioma (Pheochromocytoma)

Mediastinal paragangliomas are rare tumors, representing less than 1% of all mediastinal tumors and less than 2% of all pheochromocytomas. Although most are found in the paravertebral

sulcus, an increasing number occur in the branchial arch structures, coronary and aortopulmonary paraganglia, atria, and islands of tissue in the pericardium. Extraadrenal paragangliomas rarely secrete epinephrine. These tumors are more common in patients with multiple endocrine neoplasia syndromes and Carney syndrome (pulmonary chondroma, gastric leiomyosarcoma, and functioning extraadrenal paraganglioma). In patients who have had excision of an adrenal pheochromocytoma and continue to have symptoms, a search for an extraadrenal lesion should be undertaken, with careful attention to the mediastinum. Tumor localization has improved with CT and iodine-131 metaiodobenzylguanidine scintigraphy. When appropriate, surgical resection is the optimal therapy.

Lymphomas

Although the mediastinum is frequently involved in lymphoma, it is infrequently the sole site of disease at the time of presentation. Patients may have symptoms such as chest pain, cough, dyspnea, hoarseness, and superior vena cava syndrome. Nonspecific systemic symptoms of fever and chills, weight loss, and anorexia can also be noted. Lymphoblastic lymphoma occurs predominantly in children, adolescents, and young adults and represents 60% of cases of mediastinal non-Hodgkin lymphoma.

Surgical excision of all disease is rarely possible. Hence, the surgeon's primary role is to provide sufficient tissue for diagnosis and to assist in pathologic staging. A core-needle biopsy may be unsuccessful because larger tissue samples are needed to make a histologic diagnosis, particularly with nodular sclerosing lesions. A surgical approach may be necessary to obtain sufficient tissue, and the approach depends on the site of disease. It is imperative to biopsy enough tissue and send it fresh to pathology, not fixed in formalin. After treatment, residual radiographic abnormalities within the mediastinum are commonly noted. CT poorly differentiates fibrosis or necrosis from residual tumor. FDG/PET has shown promise as a noninvasive way to detect active mediastinal disease and predict relapse in patients with lymphoma, but tissue confirmation is required.

Endocrine Tumors

Thyroid Tumors

Although substernal extension of a cervical goiter is common, totally intrathoracic thyroid tumors are rare and make up only 1% of all mediastinal masses. These tumors arise from heterotopic thyroid tissue. Although there may be a demonstrable connection with the cervical gland (usually a fibrous connective tissue band), a true intrathoracic thyroid gland derives its blood supply from thoracic vessels. Substernal extensions of a cervical goiter can usually be excised using a cervical approach.

Parathyroid Tumors

Although parathyroid glands may occur in the mediastinum in 10% of patients, they are usually accessible through the cervical incision. Most often, these adenomas are found in the anterosuperior mediastinum (80%) embedded in or near the superior pole of the thymus. This anatomic relationship is the result of the common embryogenesis of the inferior parathyroid glands from the third branchial cleft. The superior parathyroid glands and the lateral lobes of the thyroid gland are derived from the fourth branchial pouch. Because they migrate with the lateral lobes of the thyroid gland to a paraesophageal position, parathyroid adenomas can also be found in the posterior mediastinum.

Most frequently, mediastinal parathyroid adenomas may be excised after a negative exploration of the cervical region through the existing cervical incision. Usually, the vascular supply extends from cervical blood vessels. In patients with persistent hyperparathyroidism after cervical exploration, if localization studies show residual parathyroid in the mediastinum, mediastinal exploration using a median sternotomy or thoracoscopy is indicated.

Parathyroid carcinomas have been reported and are usually hormonally active. These patients often have higher serum calcium levels and manifest more severe symptoms than those with hyperparathyroidism. Resection is the optimal therapy.

Neuroendocrine Tumors

Mediastinal NETs and carcinoid tumors arise from Kulchitsky cells located in the thymus and commonly occur in males in their 40s and 50s. They are usually located in the anterosuperior mediastinum. These tumors are aggressive and can spread to mediastinal and cervical lymph nodes, liver, bone, skin, and lungs. More than 50% of thymic NETs are hormonally active, often associated with Cushing syndrome due to production of adrenocorticotropic hormone. If feasible, resection is recommended; however, local invasion and metastasis often preclude complete excision. Radiation therapy is typically added for positive margins or gross residual disease after surgical resection. Systemic therapy is indicated for patients with unresectable recurrent or metastatic tumors.

ACKNOWLEDGMENT

We would like to thank Drs. Wald, Izhar, and Sugarbaker for their presentation of this chapter in the previous edition (20th edition), as we have updated their outstanding work.

SELECTED REFERENCES

Altorki N, Wang X, Kozono D, et al. Lobar or sublobar resection for peripheral stage IA non-small-cell lung cancer. *N Engl J Med.* 2023;388(6):489-498.

This article describes a multicenter, noninferiority, phase 3 trial in which patients with NSCLC clinically staged as T1aN0 (tumor size ≤2 cm) were randomly assigned to undergo sublobar resection or lobar resection after intraoperative confirmation of node-negative disease. In patients with peripheral NSCLC with a tumor size of 2 cm or less and pathologically confirmed node-negative disease in the hilar and mediastinal lymph nodes, sublobar resection was not inferior to lobectomy with respect to disease-free survival. Overall survival was similar with the two procedures.

Fishman A, Martinez F, Naunheim K, et al. A randomized trial comparing lung-volume-reduction surgery with medical therapy for severe emphysema. *N Engl J Med.* 2003;348(21):2059-2073.

Patients with severe emphysema underwent pulmonary rehabilitation and were randomly assigned to undergo LVRS or receive continued medical treatment. Overall, LVRS increases the chance of improved exercise capacity but does not confer a survival advantage over medical therapy. It does yield a survival advantage for patients with both predominantly upper-lobe emphysema and low baseline exercise capacity. Patients previously reported to be at high risk and those with non–upper-lobe emphysema and high baseline exercise capacity are poor candidates for LVRS because of increased mortality and negligible functional gain.

Forde PM, Chaft JE, Smith KN, et al. Neoadjuvant PD-1 blockade in resectable lung cancer. *N Engl J Med.* 2018;378(21):1976-1986.

In this pilot study, two preoperative doses of PD-1 inhibitor nivolumab were administered in adults with untreated, surgically resectable early (stage I, II, or IIIA) NSCLC. Nivolumab (at a dose of 3 mg per kilogram of body weight) was administered intravenously every 2 weeks, with surgery planned approximately 4 weeks after the first dose. Neoadjuvant nivolumab was associated with few side effects, did not delay surgery, and induced a major pathologic response in 45% of resected tumors. The tumor mutational burden was predictive of the pathologic response to PD-1 blockade. Treatment induced expansion of mutation-associated, neoantigen-specific T-cell clones in peripheral blood.

National Lung Screening Trial Research Team, Aberle DR, Adams AM, et al. Reduced lung-cancer mortality with low-dose computed tomographic screening. *N Engl J Med.* 2011;365(5):395-409.

In this study, 53,454 patients from 33 medical centers at high risk for lung cancer were randomly assigned to undergo three annual screenings with either low-dose CT or single-view posterioranterior chest radiography. Over the 7-year period of the study, rates of adherence to screening were 90%. The study found that screening with low-dose CT reduces mortality from lung cancer.

Pastorino U, Buyse M, Friedel G, et al. Long-term results of lung metastasectomy: prognostic analyses based on 5206 cases. *J Thorac Cardiovasc Surg.* 1997;113(1):37-49.

This is a registry of lung resections that has accrued 5206 cases of lung metastasectomy from 18 departments of thoracic surgery in Europe (n = 13), the United States (n = 4), and Canada (n = 1). Of these patients, 4572 (88%) underwent complete surgical resection. These results confirm that lung metastasectomy is a safe and potentially curative procedure. Resectability, disease-free interval, and number of metastases enabled the authors to design a simple system of classification valid for different tumor types.

The full reference list appears on Elsevier eBooks+.

111 CHAPTER

Acquired Heart Disease: Coronary Artery Disease

Ifeanyi D. Chinedozi, Edward P. Chen, and Jennifer S. Lawton

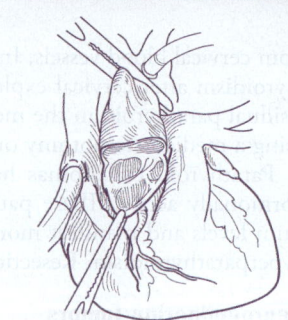

OUTLINE

INTRODUCTION

Cardiovascular disease is the leading cause of mortality globally, with an estimated 18 million deaths per year worldwide.[1,2] Of these deaths, 85% are due to myocardial infarction (MI) and stroke. Coronary artery disease (CAD), also known as *ischemic heart disease* (IHD), may present with angina pectoris, acute MI, or ischemic heart failure. According to the World Health Organization (WHO), 16.2% of all cardiovascular deaths globally stem from IHD, followed by stroke (10.8%), hypertensive heart disease (6.5%), cardiomyopathy (2.3%), rheumatic heart disease (RHD) (0.5%), atrial fibrillation (AF) (0.4%), aortic aneurysm (0.3%), peripheral arterial disease (PAD) (0.3%), endocarditis (0.2%), and venous thromboembolism (VTE) (0.1%).[1,2]

In the United States, CAD ranks as the number one cause of mortality, with 43.8% of all deaths attributable to cardiovascular diseases (Fig. 111.1).[3] This accounts for more than 365,914 deaths annually in the United States, followed closely by deaths from stroke and heart failure.[1,2] It is estimated that by 2035, more than 130 million adults in the United States (approximately 45.1% of the population) will have some form of CVD, and the total financial burden of CVD is expected to reach $1.1 trillion in 2035, with direct and indirect medical costs projected at $748.7 billion and $368 billion, respectively.[1–3]

CORONARY ARTERY ANATOMY AND PHYSIOLOGY

Basic understanding of cardiac pathophysiology is important to the general surgeon, who will often evaluate and operate on patients with CAD and other cardiovascular comorbidities.[4–6] For the cardiothoracic surgeon, in-depth knowledge of the complex anatomy of the coronary arteries and their variants and anomalies is critical. This in-depth understanding is critical in accurate diagnosis, appropriate management, and the prevention of procedural complications, ultimately improving patient outcomes.[4–6] In this section, an overview is provided of coronary circulation, important anatomic considerations, coronary perfusion, and the current understanding of CAD.

The major coronary arteries run from the top to the bottom of the interatrial and interventricular septa and encircle the atrioventricular grooves. Two coronary arteries—left and right—are the principal blood supply to the heart and are the first arterial branches of the aorta, each originating from its respective sinus of Valsalva.[5–7] The left coronary artery (LCA), also known as the *left main coronary artery* (LMCA), originates from the left coronary sinus and courses between the body of the left atrium and the main pulmonary artery, whereas the right coronary artery (RCA) arises from the right coronary sinus and runs rightward and obliquely in the right atrioventricular sulcus. The LCA varies in length from a few millimeters to several centimeters. It courses posterolateral to

the main pulmonary trunk for about 1 cm before branching into the left anterior descending (LAD) and left circumflex arteries.[5–7] The LAD takes an anterolateral course relative to the pulmonary trunk and runs along the interventricular septum, supplying the left ventricular free wall and septum. Often, an arterial anastomosis between the LAD is formed at the apex of the heart with the posterior descending artery (PDA), a common branch of the RCA. The circumflex artery also travels along the atrioventricular groove and branches into marginal branches that travel toward the apex of the heart before terminating as the left posterolateral branch.[5–7]

The RCA provides the principal blood supply to the free wall of the right ventricle (RV) and, to a lesser extent, a part of the left ventricular circulation. Originating from the right coronary sinus, its ostium averages 2 to 3 mm in diameter.[5–7] It typically runs obliquely toward the right in the anterior atrioventricular sulcus. The RCA usually bifurcates into two pivotal branches—the PDA and right posterolateral artery. The PDA, often referred to as the *inferior interventricular artery*, supplies a critical portion of the blood supply for the inferior ventricular septum and adjacent ventricular walls. Its importance is underscored in individuals with right ventricular dominance, where the PDA, along with its septal perforating branches, significantly contributes to the blood supply of the septal papillary muscle of the mitral valve.[4–7] Other noteworthy branches of the RCA include the acute marginal artery (AMA), a consistent vessel that traverses the acute margin of the heart, reaching toward the apex. This branch is primarily responsible for supplying the lateral aspect of the RV. The AMA contributes to the formation of anastomoses at the apex of the heart, particularly with the anterior interventricular artery, a branch of the LCA. The atrio-ventricular node artery (AVNA) is another critical branch of the RCA, mainly because of its pivotal role in the cardiac conduction system. Originating from the RCA in most individuals, AVNA descends to supply the atrioventricular node, a critical component in the regulation of cardiac rhythm. This artery's course and branching pattern hold significant clinical importance because any compromise in its blood supply can lead to arrhythmias or heart block.[4–7]

Anatomic Considerations

Although the PDA arises from the RCA in up to 85% of humans (termed *right-dominant circulation*), there are other variants, including the so-called codominant circulation, in which the PDA arises from both the LCA and RCA. Codominant circulation accounts for approximately 7% of the population.[4–7] Left-dominant circulation is prevalent in 8% of patients, in which the PDA arises from the LCA. A retrospective analysis of 27,289 patients who presented for cardiac catheterization after a diagnosis of acute coronary syndrome (ACS) demonstrated that left-dominance circulation was associated with a mortality hazard ratio (HR) of 1.13

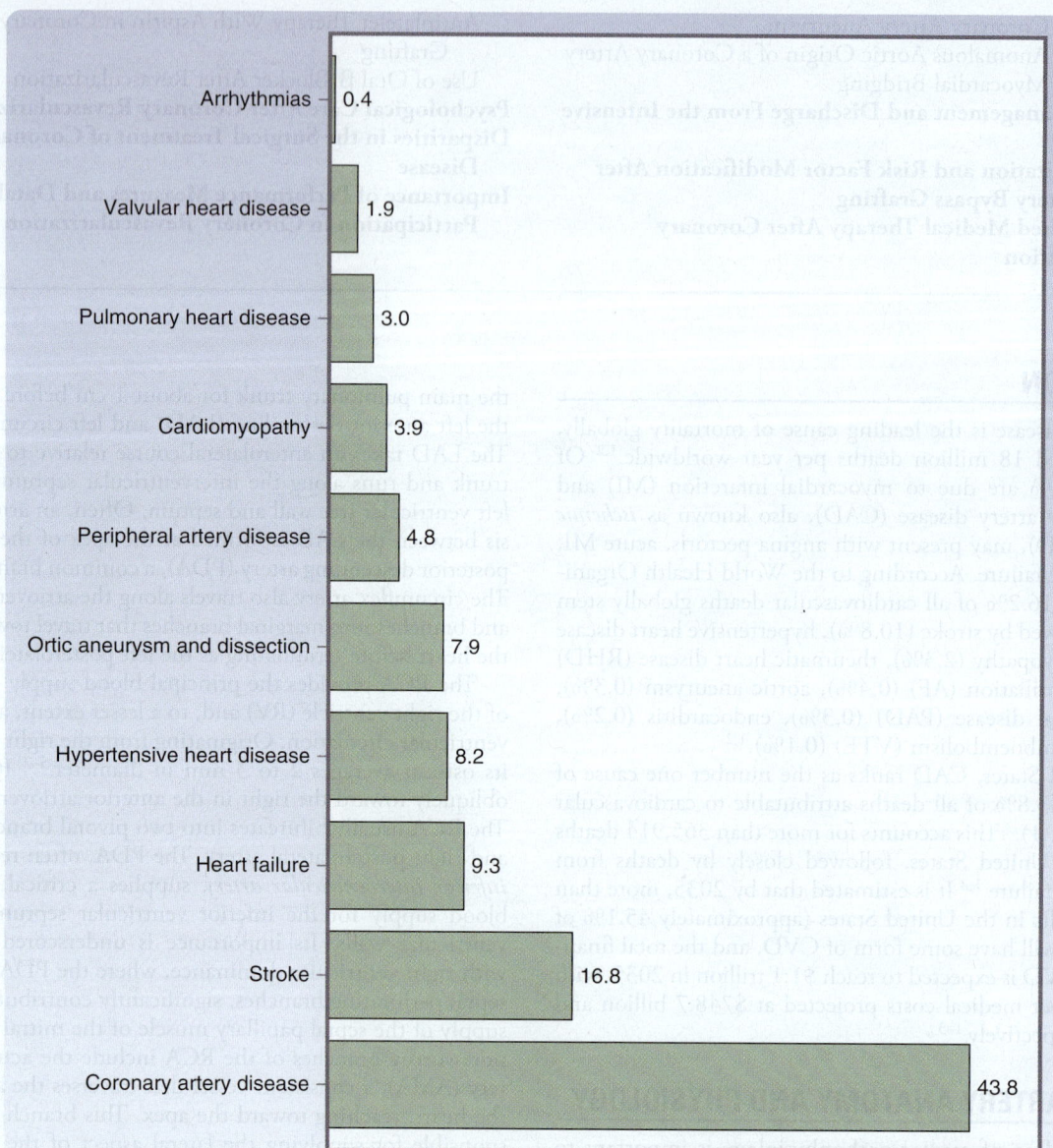

FIGURE 111.1 Top 10 causes of cardiovascular deaths in the United States. This bar graph presents the leading causes of cardiovascular deaths in the United States, based on CDC data. The *y*-axis lists the different cardiovascular conditions, and the *x*-axis represents the percentage of total cardiovascular deaths attributed to each condition. From lowest to highest, the conditions listed are arrhythmias, valvular heart disease, pulmonary heart disease, cardiomyopathy, peripheral artery disease, aortic aneurysm and dissection, hypertensive heart disease, heart failure, stroke, and coronary artery disease. Each bar's length indicates the proportion of cardiovascular-related deaths associated with each condition. *CAD*, Coronary artery disease; *CDC*, Centers for Disease Control and Prevention. (Data from Centers for Disease Control and Prevention. https://www.cdc.gov, Accessed September 8, 2023.)

(95% CI 1.00–1.28).[8] Codominance had the same mortality rate as right dominance.[8] More pronounced myocardial damage is theoretically possible in patients with either left or codominant circulation in scenarios involving lesions in the left circumflex and left main arteries because these branches would be responsible for supplying the PDA.[4–7] Given that 75% to 100% of the left ventricle is supplied by branches of the LMCA, significant left main (LM) stenosis is associated with an extraordinarily high risk of death.[9] Typically, patients with LM stenosis commonly have multivessel disease, with isolated LM coronary stenosis occurring in only 4% to 6% of cases.[9–11]

Physiology of Normal Coronary Perfusion

The cardiac subendocardium is particularly susceptible to ischemia.[12,13] A likely explanation for this stems from the observation that myocardial contraction itself impedes coronary blood flow to this innermost layer of the myocardium. Coronary vascular volume comprises a complex interplay of large and small arteries, capillaries, and small and large veins. In mild coronary artery stenosis, the heart may compensate appropriately using inherent autoregulatory vasodilatory processes.[12–14] To the extent that anatomic factors influence the delivery of oxygen to the heart, the very perfusion of the myocardium itself influences its function. Many studies have demonstrated that the filling of coronary vascular bed correlates with cardiac function, such that an increase in perfusion pressure increases myocardial oxygen consumption.[12–15] The nervous system also has a modulating function in cardiac perfusion in what is often described as a feed-forward mechanism. When stimulated by the nervous system, for example, coronary vessels often spontaneously vasodilate in synchrony with an increase in heart rate, and often before the arrival of the metabolic feedback at the resistance vessels.[8,13–15] In a healthy heart, coronary blood flow adjusts to the metabolic demands of the heart and can increase by a factor of 3 to 4. In the presence of coronary vascular disease, the resistance vessels initially undergo compensatory dilation, reducing the autoregulatory resistance per affected segment until it becomes zero. Once exhausted, the myocardial flow in the diseased segment can no longer be augmented by coronary autoregulation.[12–15]

Pathophysiology of Coronary Artery Disease

CAD is a complex, multifactorial disease characterized by the accumulation of atherosclerotic plaque in the coronary arteries, leading to myocardial ischemia and potentially fatal events such as MI. The pathogenesis of CAD is influenced by a variety of factors, including endothelial dysfunction, inflammation, and plaque formation.[6,16,17] Key components of the pathogenesis of CAD are outlined next.

Endothelial Dysfunction and Nitric Oxide Imbalance

The endothelium plays a pivotal role in maintaining vascular homeostasis. Endothelial cells produce nitric oxide (NO), a vasodilator that is vital for normal vascular tone. In CAD, risk factors like hypertension, hyperlipidemia, and tobacco use lead to endothelial dysfunction, characterized by reduced bioavailable NO and an imbalance between vasodilatory and vasoconstrictive regulation. This dysfunction marks the initial step in the atherogenic process, promoting an inflammatory environment within the vessel wall (Fig. 111.2), and contributes to vasoconstriction and plaque instability.[6,16,17]

Inflammation: T-Cell Activation and Recruitment of Proinflammatory Cytokines

The inflammatory process in CAD involves the recruitment of monocytes and T lymphocytes to the endothelium. Monocytes differentiate into macrophages, which ingest oxidized low-density lipoproteins (LDLs), transforming them into foam cells and contributing to plaque formation.[16,17] T cells, once activated, produce a range of cytokines, such as tumor necrosis factor-α (TNF-α) and interleukin (IL)-6, that further perpetuate the inflammatory response.[16,17] These proinflammatory cytokines also contribute to plaque instability by weakening the fibrous cap and promoting the secretion of matrix metalloproteinases (MMPs), enzymes that degrade the extracellular matrix. Plaque rupture, a major cause of ACSs, is often preceded by increased inflammatory activity within the plaque.[17]

Leukocyte Recruitment

In the early stages of atherosclerosis, endothelial cells, under the influence of risk factors such as hyperlipidemia and hypertension, express adhesion molecules and release chemokines like monocyte chemoattractant protein-1 (MCP-1). These molecules facilitate the adhesion of monocytes to the endothelium and their subsequent transmigration into the intima, the innermost layer of the artery.[16,17]

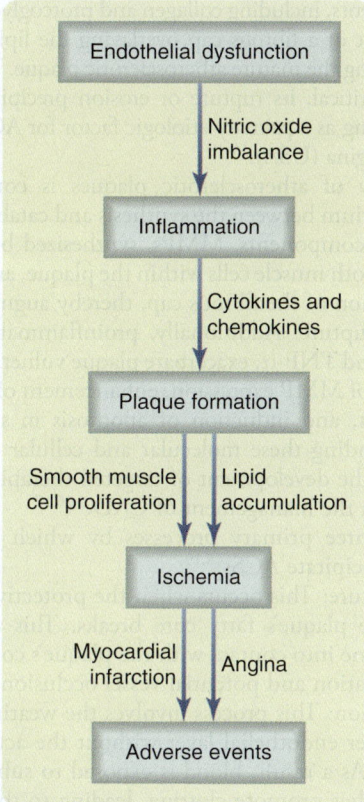

FIGURE 111.2 Proposed pathophysiology of CAD. Endothelial dysfunction plays a cardinal role and occurs early in the process, paving the path for a complex series of inflammatory reactions with subsequent plaque formation, coronary arterial stenosis, myocardial ischemia, and other clinical adverse effects, including myocardial infarction. *CABG,* Coronary artery bypass graft; *CAD,* coronary artery disease; *IHD,* ischemic heart disease; *SIHD,* stable ischemic heart disease. (Author [IC]-created illustration using DALLE 3 Generative Software, Premium, with publication rights.)

Plaque Formation and Mechanism of Acute Coronary Syndromes

The formation of atherosclerotic plaque represents a pivotal pathologic mechanism underpinning the evolution of CAD. This process is precipitated by endothelial dysfunction, attributable to an array of risk factors, including hyperlipidemia, arterial hypertension, diabetes mellitus, and tobacco use. Such dysfunction engenders increased arterial wall permeability, facilitating the transendothelial migration of LDLs.[5,16–18] Within the intimal layer, LDLs undergo oxidative modification to form oxidized LDL (oxLDL), which initiates an inflammatory cascade via the recruitment of inflammatory cytokines and chemokines, leading to monocyte adherence and infiltration into the intimal space. Subsequent differentiation of monocytes into macrophages and their assimilation of oxLDL via scavenger receptors culminates in foam cell formation. This event is augmented by the upregulation of endothelial adhesion molecules, namely, vascular cell adhesion molecule 1 (VCAM-1) and intercellular adhesion molecule 1 (ICAM-1), which facilitate the transendothelial migration of monocytes. The resultant accumulation of foam cells constitutes the initial visible pathology of atherosclerosis, known as *fatty streaks.*

Progression of CAD is further characterized by the migration of smooth muscle cells from the medial to the intimal layer, driven by cytokines and growth factors. These cells then synthesize extracellular matrix components, including collagen and proteoglycans, leading to the development of a fibrous cap overlaying the lipid-rich necrotic core, thus forming the mature atherosclerotic plaque. The integrity of this plaque is critical; its rupture or erosion precipitates thrombus formation, serving as a primary etiologic factor for ACSs such as MI and unstable angina (USA).[16–18]

The stability of atherosclerotic plaques is contingent on a delicate equilibrium between the synthesis and catabolism of extracellular matrix components. MMPs, synthesized by both macrophages and smooth muscle cells within the plaque, are instrumental in the degradation of the fibrous cap, thereby augmenting its susceptibility to rupture. Additionally, proinflammatory cytokines, such as IL-1β and TNF-α, exacerbate plaque vulnerability through the promotion of MMP expression, enhancement of inflammatory cell recruitment, and induction of apoptosis in smooth muscle cells. Understanding these molecular and cellular mechanisms is imperative for the development of targeted therapies and surgical interventions in the management of CAD.[5,16,17]

There are three primary processes by which atherosclerotic plaques can precipitate ACSs[18,19]:

1. Plaque Rupture: This occurs when the protective fibrous layer covering the plaque's fatty core breaks. This rupture allows blood to come into contact with the plaque's contents, leading to clot formation and potential vessel occlusion.
2. Plaque Erosion: This process involves the wearing away of the plaque's outer endothelial layer without the actual rupture of the plaque. As a result, blood is exposed to substances within the plaque that promote clotting, leading to thrombus development along the artery wall.
3. Calcified Nodule: In this case, hard, calcified deposits within the plaque break through the fibrous cap, potentially causing sudden occlusion of the artery if the nodules extend into the lumen.

The mechanisms leading to MI, specifically through the processes of plaque rupture, plaque erosion, and calcified nodules, significantly influence whether a patient experiences an ST-segment elevation myocardial infarction (STEMI) or a non–ST-segment elevation MI (NSTEMI). STEMI typically results from transmural occlusion of a coronary artery, often due to plaque rupture, leading to extensive myocardial damage. On the other hand, NSTEMI generally arises from partial occlusion or severe reduction of blood flow, not necessarily involving full thickness of the myocardium, and may be a result of plaque erosion or less significant plaque rupture.[5,18,19]

CLASSIFICATION OF ACUTE MYOCARDIAL INFARCTION (FOURTH UNIVERSAL DEFINITION)

MI, commonly known as a *heart attack,* is a major cardiovascular event that is classified into different types based on its etiology, clinical presentation, and underlying pathophysiology. The classifications are essential for guiding treatment strategies and predicting patient prognosis. The most recent and widely accepted classification is outlined in the Fourth Universal Definition of Myocardial Infarction, which categorizes MI into five main types.[18]

Type 1 Myocardial Infarction (Spontaneous Myocardial Infarction)

Type 1 MI is caused by a primary coronary event, such as atherosclerotic plaque rupture, erosion, or fissuring, leading to thrombus formation and subsequent myocardial ischemia and necrosis due to a decrease in coronary blood flow.[18,19]

Type 2 Myocardial Infarction (Ischemic Imbalance)

Type 2 MI occurs when there is an imbalance between the myocardial oxygen supply and demand not directly related to acute coronary thrombosis. Conditions such as coronary artery spasm, coronary embolism, anemia, arrhythmias, hypertension, or hypotension can precipitate this type of MI.[18]

Type 3 Myocardial Infarction (Sudden Cardiac Death)

Patients who die suddenly with symptoms suggestive of myocardial ischemia, accompanied by presumed new ischemic ECG changes, but for whom blood samples could not be obtained or were obtained too late after the onset of the ischemic event to allow for the documentation of elevated cardiac biomarkers, are classified as having had a type 3 MI.[18]

Type 4 Myocardial Infarction (Percutaneous Coronary Intervention–Related)

For type 4 MI, two subvariants have been identified: 4a and 4b. Type 4a MI is associated with percutaneous coronary intervention (PCI). It is defined by elevation in cardiac biomarkers (usually cardiac troponin) above the 99th percentile upper reference limit within 48 hours post-PCI.[20,21] Type 4b MI is related to stent thrombosis as documented by angiography or at autopsy.[18]

Type 5 Myocardial Infarction (Coronary Artery Bypass Graft–Associated)

Type 5 MI occurs after coronary artery bypass grafting (CABG) and is characterized by an increase in cardiac biomarkers (cardiac troponin) above the 99th percentile upper reference limit within 48 hours of CABG.[18]

CLINICAL MANIFESTATION AND DIAGNOSIS OF CORONARY ARTERY DISEASE

CAD may manifest as stable ischemic heart disease (SIHD) or ACS. Stable angina is often characterized by discomfort or a sensation of pressure beneath the sternum, which commonly intensifies during periods of physical exertion or emotional stress. This type of angina is distinguished by its predictable nature and chronic course, typically manifesting over a span of at least 2 months. The symptoms, which include chest pain or a feeling of tightening/squeezing, are usually alleviated upon resting or with the administration of nitroglycerin.[15,17,18,22] The pattern of pain onset during activity and its resolution during rest or through medication is a hallmark of this condition, distinguishing it from other forms of cardiac and noncardiac chest pain. Despite the fact that angina is the typical symptom of CAD, it is important to note that females are more likely to have atypical presentation and symptoms of CAD, including fatigue, indigestion, abdominal pain, nausea, and vomiting, compared with males (see later discussion).

The clinical presentation of ACS is typically marked by substernal chest discomfort, often described as pressure or tightness, which may radiate to the neck, jaw, or left arm. USA is present when previously noted symptoms become more frequent or have increased intensity. This symptomatology is frequently precipitated by plaque rupture and subsequent thrombosis within the coronary arteries, leading to a critical reduction in blood flow to the myocardium.[15,17,18,23] Patients with ACS may exhibit a constellation of associated symptoms, reflecting the severity of myocardial ischemia and the body's response to the acute cardiac event. Dyspnea is a common finding, likely resulting from the interplay of increased cardiac workload and the potential for subsequent pulmonary congestion due to left ventricular dysfunction. Palpitations and dizziness may occur, reflecting arrhythmogenic potential or hemodynamic instability associated with the acute ischemic event. Syncope, a concerning symptom, may signal significant arrhythmias or profound myocardial dysfunction.[15,17,18,22]

In certain cases, ACS may precipitate cardiac arrest, denoting a critical and life-threatening manifestation of the syndrome, necessitating immediate resuscitative efforts. Moreover, new-onset congestive heart failure may manifest in the setting of ACS, indicating substantial myocardial injury and compromised cardiac output, necessitating aggressive medical management and careful hemodynamic monitoring. It is crucial to note that the relief of symptoms with nitroglycerin should not be misconstrued as a diagnostic criterion for myocardial ischemia, given that other pathophysiologic entities, such as esophageal spasm, exhibit a similar therapeutic response.[15,18]

PHYSICAL EXAMINATION IN PATIENTS WITH CORONARY ARTERY DISEASE

A thorough history and physical examination are important in the diagnosis of CAD and in the consideration of a patient for surgical revascularization. This is especially the case given the diagnostic challenges in delineating other life-threatening and benign causes of angina. For example, ACS may present with diaphoresis, tachypnea, and tachycardia, but pulmonary embolism may have similar features. Furthermore, aortic dissection may manifest with severe chest or back pain and limb pulse differentials, abdominal pain, or stroke symptoms. Noncoronary causes like aortic stenosis and pericarditis have their own characteristic symptoms and murmurs. Therefore, it is important to formulate a clinical suspicion rapidly and integrate other helpful diagnostic tools to correctly identify the underlying cause of chest pain.[17,18,22,24]

Physical exam during the initial encounter of a patient with CAD should include inspection, palpation, and auscultation. Inspection should methodically assess for signs of hemodynamic compromise, such as jugular venous distention (JVD), indicative of elevated central venous pressure potentially due to heart failure or volume overload. Peripheral edema, another critical sign, warrants careful evaluation for its extent and severity because it may reflect systemic venous congestion, often seen in right heart failure or systemic conditions affecting the venous return. During palpation, the surgeon should discern the presence of a fluid thrill, suggestive of significant pericardial effusion, or a precordial heave, indicative of ventricular hypertrophy or profound ventricular dilation. The grading of peripheral edema is essential for quantifying the degree of fluid retention and guiding therapeutic interventions.[17,18,23,24] Auscultation of the carotid arteries may reveal transmitted valvular murmur or carotid stenosis. Auscultation of the lungs may reveal pulmonary congestion of congestive heart failure, and auscultation of the precordium may be diagnostic of primary or contributing valvular stenosis or regurgitation.

DIAGNOSTIC TESTING IN PATIENTS WITH CORONARY ARTERY DISEASE AND BEFORE SURGICAL REVASCULARIZATION

Electrocardiogram

Patients with chest pain and new ST elevation, ST depression, or a new left bundle branch block on ECG should be treated according to STEMI and non–ST-segment elevation acute coronary syndrome (NSTE-ACS) guidelines. An initial normal ECG does not exclude ACS. Patients with an initial normal ECG should have a repeat ECG if symptoms are ongoing, until other diagnostic testing rules out ACS. An ECG may identify other nonischemic causes of chest pain (e.g., pericarditis, myocarditis, arrhythmia).[20–22,24]

When an ECG is nondiagnostic, it should be compared with previous ECGs, if available. A normal or unchanged ECG is reasonably useful but not sufficient in ruling out ACS because up to 6% of patients with evolving ACS are, unfortunately, discharged from the emergency department (ED) with a normal ECG.[5,22] In patients where the initial ECG is normal or is without ST elevation, serial ECGs should be performed, and management should be guided by new electrocardiographic changes or other diagnostic testing. The timing for repeat ECG should also be guided by symptoms, especially if chest pain recurs or a change in clinical condition develops.

Chest Radiograph

Obtaining a chest radiograph (CXR) is recommended to assess the size of the heart and identify pulmonary congestion and other potential intrathoracic causes of chest discomfort. CXR may demonstrate a widened mediastinum in patients with aortic dissection. Relative to CAD and in preparation for potential CABG, CXR allows one to assess for pulmonary edema and the presence of acute pneumonia, aortic calcification, lung masses, and enlarged aortic silhouette, which may necessitate further evaluation to define the optimal surgical strategy and help anticipate potential complications.[24]

Cardiovascular Biomarkers

The preferred biomarker to detect or exclude myocardial injury is troponin (cTn I or T) because of its high sensitivity and specificity for myocardial tissue. The addition of creatine kinase MB (CK-MB) or myoglobin to cTn for the evaluation of patients with ACS has not been shown to be beneficial.[24] Biomarker cutoffs for the diagnosis of MI differ between institutions and in clinical trials and are usually represented in reference to an upper reference limit for the specific biomarker.

Transthoracic Echocardiography

Transthoracic echocardiography (TTE) is the first-line imaging modality for the evaluation of left ventricle (LV) and RV systolic and diastolic function. It provides essential information about the LV and RV ejection fraction, wall motion abnormalities, and other indices of systolic function. In the context of ACS, TTE can identify regional wall motion abnormalities indicative of ischemia or infarction.[24,25] TTE is also crucial for the assessment of valvular structure and function. It can identify valvular stenosis or regurgitation, vegetations in the case of endocarditis, and other structural abnormalities that may contribute to or mimic the clinical presentation of ACS. If the presentation of MI is late in the course, TTE can also identify post-MI mechanical complications, such as ventricular septal defect (VSD), papillary muscle rupture (PMR), and severe mitral regurgitation, or free-wall rupture. Finally, preoperative TTE may help provide insight into the potential need for concomitant cardiac procedures in patients undergoing surgical coronary revascularization.[24,25]

Fractional Flow Reserve, Instantaneous Wave-Free Ratio, Optical Coherence Tomography, and Intravascular Ultrasound

Fractional flow reserve (FFR) is an important tool in determining whether coronary atherosclerotic plaques are physiologically responsible for myocardial ischemia, guiding the need for revascularization.[26-30] The procedure involves the insertion of a guidewire equipped with a pressure sensor distal to the coronary stenosis. After the administration of a vasodilator to induce hyperemia, FFR is calculated as the ratio (0 to 1.00) of the mean distal coronary pressure (measured by the pressure sensor on the guidewire) to the mean aortic pressure (measured by the coronary catheter). The FFR value reflects the maximum achievable blood flow in the presence of a stenosis compared with the hypothetical maximum flow in the absence of the stenosis. A lower FFR value indicates a more significant blockage, whereas a higher FFR value suggests less severe narrowing. The commonly accepted threshold for FFR interpretation is 0.80. An FFR value of 0.80 or lower suggests that the coronary artery blockage is hemodynamically significant, meaning it is likely causing reduced blood flow to the myocardium.[26-30] FFR-guided PCI has shown superiority over angiography-guided PCI and medical therapy alone.[26-32] It remains the gold standard for detecting ischemia-inducing coronary stenoses and is still unsurpassed in diagnostic performance compared with nonhyperemic indices and noninvasive techniques. The FAME (Fractional Flow Reserve Versus Angiography for Multivessel Evaluation) trial[26] consisted of patients with multivessel CAD randomized to receive stents based on angiographic appearance only versus when FFR was ≤ 0.80. The 2-year follow-up study found that FFR-guided PCI was associated with fewer number of total stents used (1.9 ± 1.3 vs. 2.7 ± 1.2, respectively; $p < 0.001$) and lower rates of MI or death within 2 years (8.4 vs. 12.9%, $p = 0.02$) compared with patients with angiography-only–guided revascularization.[26]

The **instantaneous wave-free ratio (iFR)** employs high-frequency sampling to compute a pressure gradient across a coronary lesion during diastole, and its performance has been evaluated in comparison to FFR.[31,33] It has the added advantage of minimizing the use of hyperemic agents like adenosine, which can be uncomfortable for patients. Multiple clinical trials have investigated the value of iFR in assessing CAD severity. Specifically, the DEFINE-FLAIR (Functional Lesion Assessment of Intermediate Stenosis to Guide Revascularization) trial[34] demonstrated that iFR is noninferior to FFR in guiding revascularization decisions. Notably, in patients with angina or anginal-equivalent symptoms, undocumented ischemia, and angiographically intermediate stenoses, the use of FFR or iFR to guide the clinical decision for PCI carries a Class 1, Level A evidence-based recommendation.[21] FFR-guided PCI or CABG in the FAME 3 trial demonstrated no difference at 3 years in the composite incidence of death, MI, or stroke; however, there was a higher incidence of MI after PCI versus CABG.[33] It remains unclear if FFR provides additional information in CABG planning to that provided by routine diagnostic angiography.

Optical coherence tomography (OCT) is an advanced imaging technique that is used to estimate the severity of CAD by examining the microstructure of coronary arteries before revascularization. As a diagnostic tool, OCT proves useful in patients with borderline lesions found on angiography because of its high spatial resolution.[35] The 2021 American College of Cardiology (ACC)/American Heart Association (AHA)/Society for Cardiovascular Angiography and Interventions (SCAI) Guideline for Coronary Artery Revascularization currently has a Class 2a recommendation for the use of OCT to guide stent placement as an alternative to intravenous ultrasonography (IVUS) except in patients with ostial left main disease.[21] Post-PCI, OCT has also been found to be beneficial in assessing complications such as stent underdeployment and malposition. Furthermore, OCT has become essential in diagnosing MI with nonobstructive coronary arteries. By detecting PCI complications that might otherwise be missed by angiography, OCT remains an important tool in coronary revascularization.[35]

IVUS, a catheter-based imaging modality, complements angiography by providing valuable diagnostic information, including vessel and lumen dimensions, plaque burden, and morphology, particularly in patients with LMCA stenosis.[36,37] In a recent systematic review and meta-analysis comparing IVUS-guided versus coronary angiography–guided PCI in patients with acute MI (AMI), IVUS-guided PCI was associated with a significantly lower risk of all-cause mortality, reduced major adverse cardiac events (MACEs), and target vessel revascularization (TVR). Notably, among patients with STEMI, the use of IVUS-guided PCI was linked to a lower likelihood of all-cause mortality (relative risk [RR] 0.79, 95% CI 0.66–0.95, $p = 0.01$) and MACEs (RR 0.86, 95% CI 0.74–0.99, $p = 0.04$).[36] Currently, the use of IVUS to define lesion severity in patients with intermediate stenosis of the left main artery constitutes a Class 2a recommendation by the ACC/AHA/SCAI Guideline for Coronary Artery Revascularization.[21]

Coronary Computed Tomography Scan

CT, particularly coronary CT angiography (CCTA), has emerged as a valuable tool for the noninvasive assessment of CAD. It provides detailed images of the coronary anatomy, allowing for the visualization of coronary artery stenosis, plaque characteristics, and the extent of aortic calcification, which is a marker of atherosclerotic burden.[38-45] Like conventional chest CT scan, CCTA is noninvasive and can now be performed with low radiation doses and high diagnostic accuracy. Because its high negative predictive value (NPV) for CAD, CCTCA has become important for the assessment of patients with recent-onset chest pain. Multiple clinical trials (International Study of Comparative Health Effectiveness with Medical and Invasive Approaches [ISCHEMIA], Scottish Computed Tomography of the HEART [SCOT-HEART], and Prospective Multicenter Imaging Study for Evaluation of Chest Pain [PROMISE]) suggest that combining coronary anatomy and functional assessment of coronary flow with myocardial tissue characterization by CT can provide a comprehensive evaluation of CAD.[41,44] Given its noninvasive nature and relative ease of performance, it is an important adjunct in anatomic plaque characterization and evaluation of the severity of calcification. It is also diagnostic in the presence of anomalous coronary anatomy. Positron emission topography (PET) with newly adopted radiotracers and CCTA assessments, such as pericoronary adipose tissue density (PCAT), are gaining attention for their potential to improve cardiac risk prediction.[38-40,45]

Magnetic Resonance Angiography

Magnetic resonance angiography (MRA), another noninvasive imaging technique with high spatial and temporal resolution, provides detailed anatomic and functional cardiac assessment. Cardiac MRA allows for accurate and reproducible measurement of left ventricular ejection fraction (LVEF) without the geometric assumptions required by other imaging techniques, making it the gold standard for volumetric assessment. In addition to LVEF, cardiac MRA can assess ventricular volumes, mass, and myocardial viability, offering a holistic view of cardiac function.[46–49]

For valvular function assessment, cardiac MRA provides a noninvasive means to evaluate valvular morphology, leaflet motion, and the extent of valvular regurgitation or stenosis. The technique's ability to visualize blood flow using phase-contrast imaging enables precise quantification of flow across valves, aiding in the diagnosis and management of valvular heart diseases.[48–50]

MRA offers several advantages over traditional angiography, such as the absence of ionizing radiation, the potential for non-contrast examination, high spatial resolution, superior soft tissue differentiation, and lower cost.[44,48,49] There is a growing emphasis on using more noninvasive methods like MR angiography for initial diagnosis, reserving the cardiac catheterization lab for interventional procedures once a diagnosis is established. A large systematic review and meta-analysis examined the diagnostic performance of MR coronary angiography (MRCA) for CAD.[48,49] The meta-analysis, involving 24 studies with 1638 patients, revealed that the pooled sensitivity of MRCA for CAD was 89%, with a specificity of 72%. Interestingly, the use of contrast-enhanced examinations increased the sensitivity to 95%, comparable to that of CTA. The specificity was higher in whole-heart acquisition mode (78%) compared with targeted mode (57%), and it was also higher at 3-Tesla (T) magnetic field strength (83%) compared with 1.5 T (68%). These results indicate that whole-heart contrast-enhanced protocols at higher magnetic field strengths might offer the best approach for MRCA in CAD diagnosis.[48,49]

Stress Testing

Stress testing serves as a fundamental noninvasive method for evaluating individuals who may have or are known to have CAD and may include pharmacologic stress (dobutamine) test, exercise stress testing, stress echocardiography, nuclear stress (myocardial perfusion imaging) test, and stress cardiac magnetic resonance (CMR) imaging.[39,51] Stress testing is primarily used to determine a patient's risk stratification or to evaluate the need for coronary angiography. Although exercise stress testing does not typically involve contrast or radiation, nuclear stress testing does involve the use of a radioactive tracer and imaging. Individuals with stable CAD often fall into the low-risk category after stress testing and are spared a more invasive diagnostic workup, such as coronary angiography. Therefore, for patients who have a normal or nearly normal resting ECG and can exercise adequately, standard exercise treadmill testing is usually the first choice. However, for those with a history of revascularization, ECGs that are difficult to interpret, or those unable to perform sufficient exercise, stress imaging is advised.[52] Of note, among patients referred for treadmill stress test by their family medicine physicians, a series documented the average sensitivity as 71.4%, and the average specificity was 90.4%. Furthermore, this study reported a positive predictive value (PPV) of 13.5% and an NPV of 99.3%.[52]

Diagnostic Cardiac Catheterization

Coronary angiography is commonly used to evaluate and determine the structure, extent of narrowing (stenosis), and location of the coronary arteries. Cardiac catheterization involves the insertion of a catheter, typically 2 to 3 mm in diameter, into veins or arteries in the neck (internal jugular vein), arm (radial arteries [RAs]), and groin (femoral vessels) under local anesthesia. From there, the

catheter is advanced to the right and/or left sides of the heart. Two main types exist: (1) left heart catheterization, primarily performed for diagnostic purposes, including the evaluation of CAD, and it may also include therapeutic interventions like angioplasty or stenting, and (2) right heart catheterization (pulmonary artery or Swan-Ganz catheterization), which provides direct measurement of pressures within the heart and pulmonary artery, blood sampling from these areas, and the calculation of cardiac output. For a more accurate assessment of coronary anatomy, it is important to acquire multiple angiographic angles. Furthermore, the addition of physiologic testing (as detailed earlier) may help provide a more thorough evaluation.

A stenosis is considered significant if it reduces coronary artery diameter by 70% or more in non–left main coronary arteries or by 50% or more in the LMCA.[21,53,54] Angiographic stenosis with a diameter reduction between 40% and 69% is considered intermediate and typically requires further testing to evaluate its physiologic impact. Notably, coronary angiography alone does not provide a standard measurement for the length of lesions, which is an important clinical factor for potential revascularization.[53,54] Controversy exists as to whether visual estimation or quantitative analysis of angiography is more effective in predicting the functional impact of a stenosis. The discrepancy in measurement between these two methods (visual or physiologic) can range from 10% to 20%, varying with the severity of stenosis.[54]

The access for cardiac catheterization is typically via the femoral or RA. Transradial cardiac catheterization has a Class 1 recommendation in the ACC/AHA/SCAI 2021 Guideline for Coronary Artery Revascularization over transfemoral approach in patients with ACS undergoing PCI to reduce the risk of death, vascular complications, or bleeding and in patients with SIHD undergoing PCI to reduce access site bleeding and vascular complications (Table 111.1).[21] It is important to recognize the potential complications associated with coronary catheterization, including vascular injuries (dissection, pseudoaneurysm [pSA], aneurysm, rupture, and occlusion) and others, including infection and contrast-related morbidities (up to 7.1% rate of kidney injury in the National Cardiovascular Data Registry).[55] The use of the RA for coronary catheterization may result in dissection or occlusion of the vessel and render it unacceptable for future harvest as an arterial conduit for CABG.[21,56–59]

Left Ventriculography

LV ventriculography, or LVgram, involves inserting a catheter into the LV, injecting contrast under fluoroscopy, and visually estimating the ejection fraction and degree of mitral regurgitation. It can also assist in diagnosis of post infarction VSD or pseudoaneurysm[60,61] and for visualizing calcification in the ascending aorta. This diagnostic tool is not used in patients with aortic endocarditis, aortic stenosis, or renal insufficiency (because of the amount of contrast required).

Aortic Gradient Evaluation

An evaluation of the pressure gradient across the aortic valve during cardiac catheterization may be performed to assess the degree of aortic stenosis. This is critical in patients being evaluated for CABG because significant aortic stenosis can affect both the decision to proceed with CABG at all and the need for concurrent aortic valve intervention during CABG.

Left Ventricular End-Diastolic Pressure

Evaluating the left ventricular end-diastolic pressure (LVEDP) during cardiac catheterization is helpful in patients with reduced

TABLE 111.1 **Indications for CABG in Patients With STEMI, NSTE-ACS, and SIHD**

	CLASS OF RECOMMENDATION		
PATIENT STATUS	**COR 1 (BENEFIT >>> RISK)**	**COR 2A (BENEFIT >> RISK)**	**COR 2B (BENEFIT ≥ RISK)**
STEMI	Patients with **STEMI** and cardiogenic shock or hemodynamic instability, CABG when PCI is not feasible is indicated **to improve survival** Patients with **STEMI** with mechanical complications (ventricular septal rupture, mitral insufficiency due to papillary muscle infarction or rupture, or free wall rupture), CABG is recommended at the time of surgery **to improve survival**	Patients with **STEMI** when PCI not possible or successful, with a large area of myocardium at risk emergent or urgent CABG can be effective to **improve clinical outcomes** Patients with **STEMI** with complex MV non-infarct CAD, after successful PCI, elective CABG is reasonable **to reduce the risk of cardiac events**	
NSTE-ACS	Patients with **NSTE-ACS** and cardiogenic shock who are appropriate candidates for revascularization, emergency revascularization is recommended **to reduce risk of death**	Patients with **NSTE-ACS** who are initially stabilized and are at intermediate or low risk of clinical events, an invasive strategy with intent to perform revascularization is reasonable before hospital discharge **to improve outcomes** Patients with **NSTE-ACS** who have failed PCI and have ongoing ischemia, hemodynamic compromise, or threatened occlusion of an artery with substantial myocardium at risk, emergency CABG is reasonable	
SIHD			
LV dysfunction	Patients with **SIHD** and MV CAD appropriate for CABG with severe LV dysfunction (LVEF <35%), CABG is recommended **to improve survival**	Patients with **SIHD** and MV CAD appropriate for CABG with mild to moderate LV dysfunction (LVEF 35-50%), CABG (to include LIMA to LAD) is reasonable **to improve survival**	
Left Main CAD	Patients with **SIHD** and significant LM stenosis, CABG is recommended **to improve survival**		
MV CAD		Patients with **SIHD** and MV CAD, revascularization is reasonable **to lower the risk of cardiovascular events**	Patients with **SIHD**, normal LVEF, significant stenoses in 3 major coronary arteries, and anatomy suitable for CABG, CABG may be reasonable **to improve survival**
Refractory Angina	Patients with refractory angina despite medical therapy and with significant coronary artery stenoses amenable to revascularization, revascularization is recommended **to improve symptoms**		

CABG, Coronary artery bypass grafting; *CAD*, coronary artery disease; *COR*, Class of Recommendation; *MV*, multivessel; *NSTE-ACS*, non–ST-elevation acute coronary syndrome; *PCI*, percutaneous intervention; *SIHD*, stable ischemic heart disease; *STEMI*, ST-elevation myocardial infarction.
Data from Lawton JS, Tamis-Holland JE, Bangalore S, et al. 2021 ACC/AHA/SCAI Guideline for Coronary Artery Revascularization: a report of the American College of Cardiology/American Heart Association Committee on Clinical Practice Guidelines. *J Am Coll Cardiol* 2022;79:e21-e129. Content used with permission from the Journal of the American College of Cardiology (JACC).

LVEF, especially in the context of CABG evaluation. Accurate measurement of LVEDP is achieved by placing a catheter into the LV to directly measure the pressure at the end of diastole. This measurement is particularly important in patients with symptoms of heart failure or those with suspected diastolic dysfunction. This information assists in risk stratification and can influence the surgical approach and the need for additional interventions or mechanical adjuncts during revascularization.[62]

Society of Thoracic Surgeons Risk Scoring

The Society of Thoracic Surgeons (STS) operative risk calculator is a tool designed to evaluate and predict the mortality and morbidity risk associated with various operative procedures in cardiac surgery. This calculator takes various factors into consideration, including the planned surgery; patient demographics (age, sex, race, body weight, and height); laboratory values (creatinine, hematocrit, white blood cell [WBC] and platelet count); preoperative medications, including inotropes $\leq$48 hours; and risk factors (diabetes, family history of CAD, liver disease, mediastinal radiation, endocarditis, alcohol and tobacco use; presence of chronic lung disease, prior stroke, New York Heart Association [NYHA] classification, valvular disease, and preoperative arrhythmia).[63] The STS score has been validated by several studies and has been demonstrated to perform better than the EuroSCORE II, especially in patients with higher STS predicted risk of operative mortality (PROM) (>5%).[64] Notably, patients with cirrhosis, frailty, and chronic malnutrition may benefit from additional risk estimation models. The outcomes predicted by the STS risk calculator include risk of mortality and risk of morbidity (renal failure, permanent stroke, prolonged ventilation, deep sternal wound infection, reoperation, and prolonged length of stay). The ACC/AHA/SCAI 2021 Guideline for Coronary Artery Revascularization gives a Class 1 recommendation supporting the calculation of the STS risk score at the time of CABG evaluation.[21] The calculator may be accessed at https://acsdriskcalc.research.sts.org/.

Synergy Between Percutaneous Coronary Intervention With TAXus and Cardiac Surgery Score

In determining the most suitable revascularization approach for patients with CAD, several factors should be considered: the complexity of the CAD, the likelihood of achieving complete revascularization (CR), the risk of adverse outcomes, patient preferences, patient symptoms, LVEF, potential for adherence to dual-antiplatelet therapy (DAPT), and more. To assist in making informed decisions, the Synergy Between Percutaneous Coronary Intervention With TAXus and Cardiac Surgery Score (SYNTAX) score was created based on the SYNTAX trial.[65–70] Initially introduced by Sianos et al. in 2005, the score serves as an angiographic tool for grading the complexity of CAD.[65]

Subsequent studies have explored its utility in various contexts. Wykrzykowska et al. (2010) and Garg et al. (2011) examined the score's prognostic implications for 1-year outcomes and risk stratification.[68,69] Généreux et al. (2011) scrutinized the score's reproducibility among healthcare providers,[66] and Zhang et al. (2014) proposed and expanded its application by incorporating site-specific scores and clinical factors for improved decision-making.[71] Cavalcante et al. (2017) extended its application to diabetic patients with multivessel CAD.[72] Moreover, Farooq et al. (2013) and Takahashi et al. (2020) worked on the development and validation of SYNTAX score II, which combines anatomic and clinical

factors to guide decision-making between CABG and PCI.[68,73] Several studies have shown that a patient's SYNTAX score can be an important effect modifier that favors surgical revascularization versus PCI.[68,71,72]

Important limitations of the SYNTAX score are worth mentioning. First, the SYNTAX scoring system is cumbersome and is subject to interobserver variability.[66] Additionally, the SYNTAX score does not incorporate some important clinical variables, which limits its usefulness in comprehensively estimating the accurate risk of clinical events after CABG.[66,71] The ACC/AHA/SCAI 2021 Guideline for Coronary Artery Revascularization gives a Class 2b recommendation supporting the use of scoring models such as the SYNTAX score to guide revascularization in patients with multivessel CAD.[21]

HISTORY OF CORONARY ARTERY BYPASS SURGERY

Coronary artery revascularization has a storied history that reflects a journey marked by extensive research, clinical experimentation, and evolving surgical techniques. Key milestones (Fig. 111.3) include the Nobel Prize–winning work of Alexis Carrell in blood vessel anastomoses (1902, awarded prize in 1912), the development of the heart-lung machine (John Gibbon Jr., 1930s and 1940s), and the groundbreaking discovery of coronary arteriography by Frank Mason Sones in 1957. Notably, in 1929, Werner Forssmann performed the first cardiac catheterization on himself, establishing a foundation for future cardiac diagnostic and therapeutic techniques. Subsequently, in 1955, Denis Melrose revolutionized cardiac surgery by introducing potassium cardioplegic arrest. Building on these advancements, Gerald Buckberg elucidated the advantages of employing hypothermia to reduce myocardial oxygen consumption, alongside advocating for warm induction and warm cardioplegia after cardiac arrest. His work emphasized the superiority of blood cardioplegia over other methods, further refining cardiac surgery techniques and improving patient recovery and outcomes.[5,74] The 1960s marked significant advances with successful aortocoronary vein grafts, beginning with the first human aortocoronary bypass graft by David Sabiston Jr. (Fig. 111.4) and the identification of collateral formation in bypass surgeries. This era also recognized the multifactorial nature of atherosclerosis, shifting the focus from mere obstruction to cellular composition and inflammation in plaques. Large-scale studies underscored smoking and abnormal lipids as primary risk factors.

Notably, David Sabiston Jr. significantly contributed to the standardization of CABG through his relentless emphasis on evidence-based practices. His innovative surgical techniques and research in heart physiology and coronary circulation directly contributed to the optimization of CABG procedures and patient outcomes.[74,75] Furthermore, he profoundly influenced surgical education, notably through the *Sabiston Textbook of Surgery* and the *Sabiston and Spencer Surgery of the Chest*, both pivotal educational contributions to surgical training.[5,74]

Over the past 65 years, coronary artery surgery has seen dozens of major advancements, including minimally invasive techniques and improved myocardial protection, significantly reducing mortality rates. Today, the objectives of coronary artery surgery encompass not only symptom relief and improved left ventricular function but also the extension of life span and reduction of late cardiac events.

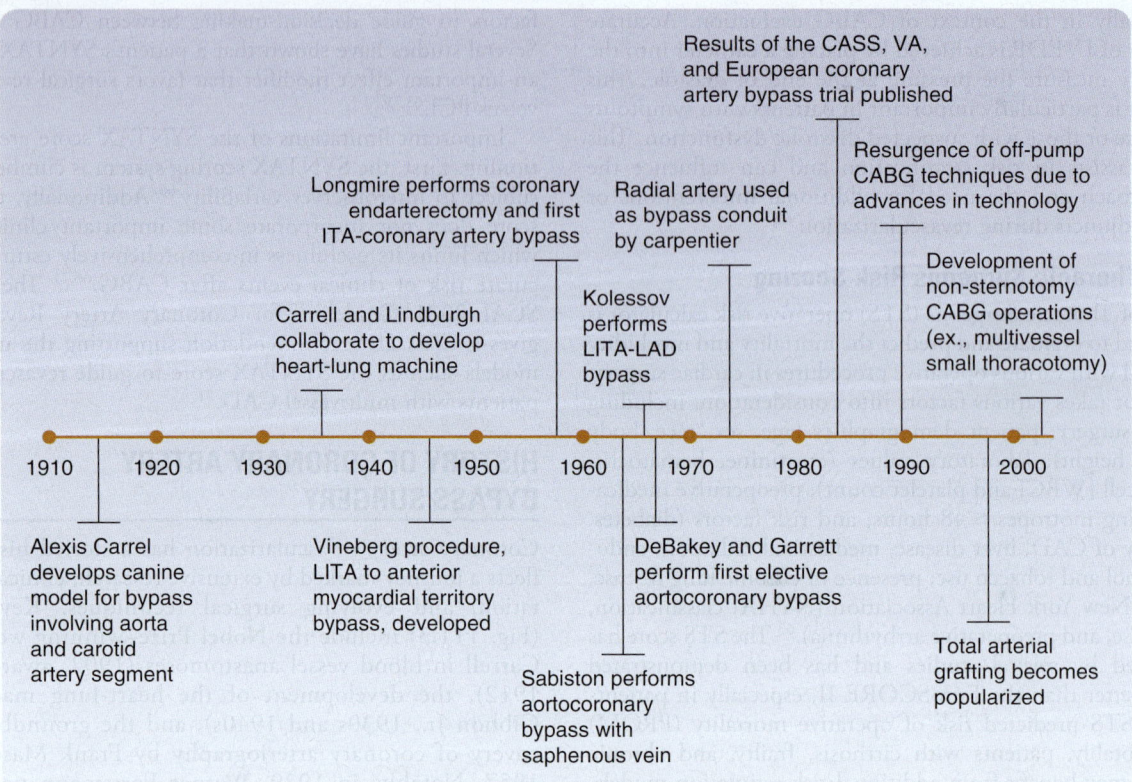

FIGURE 111.3 Key developments in the history of CABG. From preclinical experiments to small and large animal models, there have been tremendous advancements to optimize the safety and well-being of patients with CAD who undergo CABG. In the face of newer and exciting percutaneous coronary interventions, CABG continues to be important in patients with reduced left ventricular ejection fraction, diabetes, complex CAD, left main CAD, recurrent in-stent stenosis, and dual-antiplatelet therapy nonadherence. *CABG,* Coronary artery bypass graft; *CAD,* coronary artery disease; *CASS,* coronary artery surgery study; *ITA,* internal thoracic artery; *LAD,* left anterior descending; *LITA,* left internal thoracic artery; *MIDCAB,* minimally invasive direct coronary artery bypass; *VA,* Veterans Affairs Coronary Artery Bypass Surgery Cooperative Study. (From Sellke FW, del Nido P, and Swanson SJ, eds,. *Sabiston Textbook of Surgery.* 9th ed. Philadelphia; 2015. Used with permission from Elsevier.)

INDICATIONS FOR CORONARY ARTERY REVASCU-LARIZATION: ACUTE CORONARY SYNDROMES

The 2021 ACC/AHA/SCAI Guideline for Coronary Artery Revascularization offers evidence-based recommendations regarding the role of surgical revascularization versus PCI. Tables 111.1 and 111.2 and Fig. 111.5 summarize the indications and best practices for the treatment of patients with STEMI, NSTE-ACS, and SIHD.[21] ACS comprises a spectrum of clinical conditions resulting from acute myocardial ischemia due to a significant reduction or cessation of blood flow in a coronary artery or arteries. This spectrum encompasses STEMI; NSTEMI, now more broadly referred to as *NSTE-ACS;* and USA. The pathophysiology primarily involves atherosclerotic plaque disruption and subsequent thrombus formation, leading to partial or complete occlusion of the coronary artery.[15,17,18] STEMI is characterized by full-thickness myocardial damage and is identifiable by ST elevation on ECG. In contrast, NSTEMI, often resulting from partial occlusion, is diagnosed based on cardiac biomarkers without ST elevation on ECG. USA, meanwhile, presents as a change in anginal patterns (severity, frequency, changing from exertion to rest pain) without a detectable change in cardiac enzymes.[15,17,18]

The management of ACS is multifaceted, including rapid revascularization, pharmacotherapy, and lifestyle modifications, all of which are aimed at restoring coronary blood flow, reducing myocardial oxygen demand, and ultimately preventing further cardiac events.[21]

ST-Elevation Myocardial Infarction

In patients with STEMI with symptoms <12 hours, PCI should be performed to improve survival (Class 1).[14] Evidence from multiple randomized controlled trials (RCTs) and meta-analyses underscores the efficacy of primary PCI over fibrinolysis, significantly curtailing death, MI, stroke, and major bleeding, particularly with minimized treatment delays. Notably, this benefit extends to patients referred from non-PCI facilities, with the caveat of reasonable transfer times and total ischemic duration under 120 minutes.[21,76,77]

The role of CABG in the acute phase of STEMI is limited, and its application in this context has declined over time. Historical case series have indicated a potential increase in mortality risk when CABG is conducted shortly after STEMI. Nonetheless, recent advancements in operative techniques, enhanced anesthesia and monitoring, refined technical methods, and the use of adjunctive

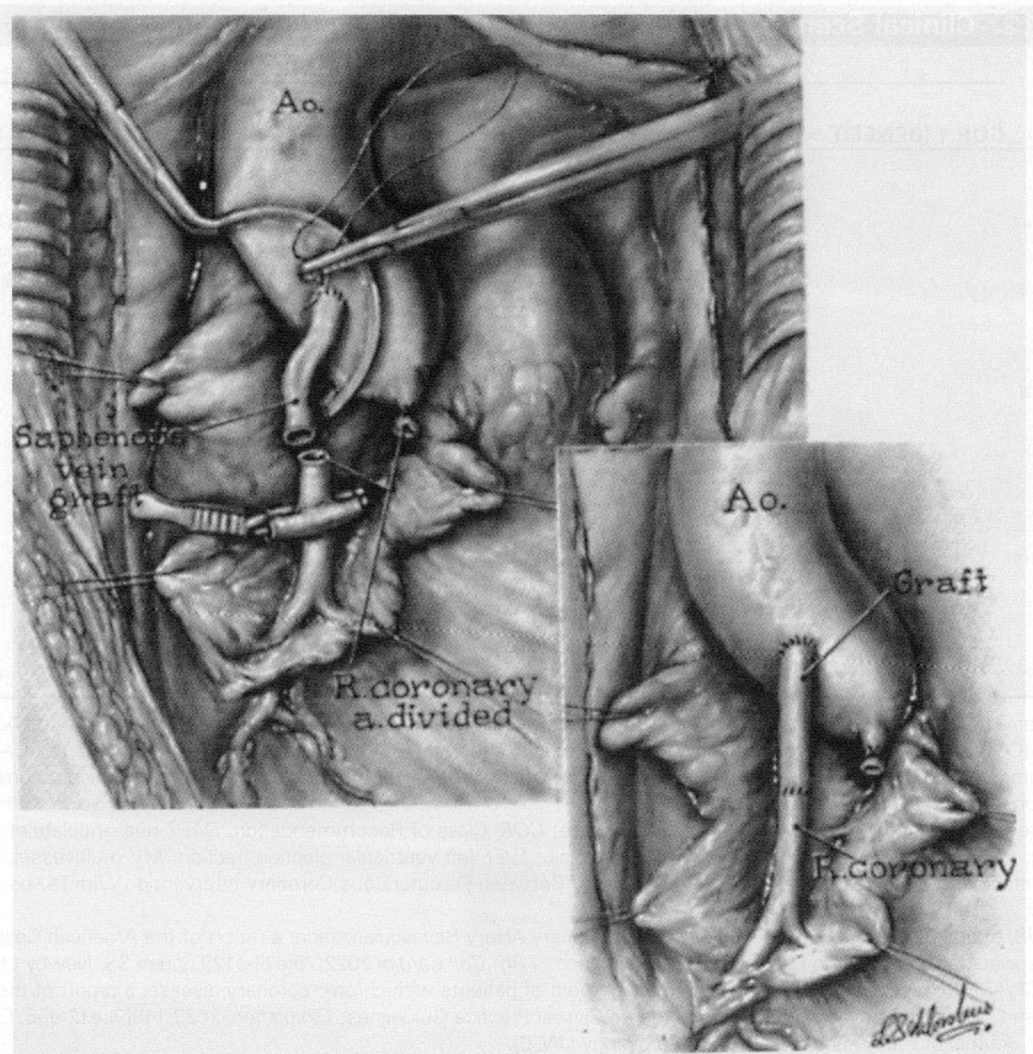

FIGURE 111.4 The first human bypass graft from saphenous vein to coronary artery, performed by Dr. David Sabiston in 1962. The saphenous vein graft was anastomosed to the ascending aorta and the right coronary for a right coronary proximal occlusion. The proximal right coronary artery (RCA) was ligated, and the saphenous vein was end-to-end anastomosed to the end of the RCA. *Ao.*, Aorta; *a.*, artery; *R.*, right. Reprinted with permission from Sabiston DC. The William F. Rienhoff, Jr. Lecture. The Coronary Circulation. *J Hopkins Med J*; 134.)

TABLE 111.2	**Clinical Scenarios When CABG Is Preferred Over PCI**		
	CLASS OF RECOMMENDATION		
PATIENT STATUS	**COR 1 (BENEFIT >>> RISK)**	**COR 2A (BENEFIT >> RISK)**	**COR 2B (BENEFIT ≥ RISK)**
Complex Disease	Patients with significant **LM CAD** with high-complexity CAD, it is recommended to choose CABG over PCI **to improve survival**	Patients with **MV CAD** with complex or diffuse CAD (SYNTAX score >33), it is reasonable to choose CABG over PCI to confer **a survival advantage**	
Diabetes	Patients with **diabetes** with MV CAD with involvement of the LAD, CABG (with LIMA to LAD) is recommended in preference to PCI **to reduce mortality and repeat revascularizations**		

Continued

TABLE 111.2 Clinical Scenarios When CABG Is Preferred Over PCI—cont'd

PATIENT STATUS	CLASS OF RECOMMENDATION		
	COR 1 (BENEFIT >>> RISK)	COR 2A (BENEFIT >> RISK)	COR 2B (BENEFIT ≥ RISK)
Previous CABG		Patients with **previous CABG** and **refractory angina** on GDMT that is attributable to LAD disease, it is reasonable to choose CABG over PCI when an IMA can be used to the LAD	Patients with **previous CABG** and **complex CAD**, it may be reasonable to choose CABG over PCI when an IMA can be used to the LAD
DAPT Adherence		Patients with **MV CAD** who are **unable to access, tolerate, or adhere to DAPT** for the appropriate duration of treatment, CABG is reasonable in preference to PCI	
In Stent Stenosis		Patients with **symptomatic recurrent diffuse ISR** with an indication for revascularization, CABG can be useful over repeat PCI **to reduce recurrent events**	

Note: CABG is preferred over PCI in patients with previous CABG presenting with complex CAD or refractory angina due to LAD disease when a LIMA may be used (COR 2a), in patients who are unable to adhere to DAPT therapy (COR 2a), and in patients with complex CAD and previous CABG (COR 2b) to improve survival. CABG is also preferred to PCI in patients with symptomatic recurrent ISR to reduce recurrent events (COR 2a). *Revascularization* refers to PCI or CABG.

CABG, Coronary artery bypass grafting; *CAD*, coronary artery disease; *COR*, Class of Recommendation; *DAPT*, dual-antiplatelet therapy; *LAD*, left anterior descending; *LIMA*, left internal mammary artery; *LM*, left main; *LVEF*, left ventricular ejection fraction; *MV*, multivessel; *PCI*, percutaneous intervention; *SIHD*, stable ischemic heart disease; *SYNTAX*, Synergy Between Percutaneous Coronary Intervention With TAXus and Cardiac Surgery Score.

Data from Lawton JS, et al. 2021 ACC/AHA/SCAI Guideline for Coronary Artery Revascularization: a report of the American College of Cardiology/American Heart Association Committee on Clinical Practice Guidelnes. *J Am Coll Cardiol* 2022;79:e21-e129. Virani SS, Newby LK, Arnold SV, et al. 2023 AHA/ACC/ACCP/ASPC/NLA/PCNA guideline for the management of patients with chronic coronary disease: a report of the American Heart Association/American College of Cardiology Joint Committee on Clinical Practice Guidelines. *Circulation*. 2023;148(9):e12-e56. Content used with permission from the Journal of the American College of Cardiology (JACC).

temporary mechanical circulatory support devices may contribute to improved survival rates after CABG.[21,78] In STEMI patients with complex multivessel CAD, elective CABG stands as a viable revascularization choice after successful PCI of the culprit infarct artery, provided the patient is a CABG candidate. For those with complex noninfarct artery disease, deliberations regarding PCI or CABG for the noninfarct artery(s) should involve a collaborative heart team discussion.[21]

In most STEMI patients with multivessel disease and concurrent cardiogenic shock, a prompt PCI revascularization of the culprit vessel is the recommended strategy. This recommendation is founded on consistent observations from observational studies and one randomized trial, both indicating no benefit and potential harm from immediate multivessel PCI.[21] Complex disease, such as severe left main or multivessel CAD, may render PCI of the infarct artery impractical in STEMI patients. Furthermore, there are unique instances where PCI might not achieve the desired result. Under these scenarios, employing CABG as the initial strategy for restoring blood flow can be highly beneficial, especially when a substantial portion of the heart muscle is in jeopardy.[21]

Non–ST-Elevation Acute Coronary Syndrome

In patients with NSTE-ACS who are at an increased risk of further ischemic events, an invasive strategy may be employed with the intent to proceed with revascularization if appropriate (see Fig. 111.5).[21] In these patients, risk stratification using the Global Registry of Acute Coronary Events (GRACE) 2.0 risk calculator (score ≥140 is associated with increased risk for cardiac events) is crucial to guide the timing of coronary angiography.[21,79] In addition to the GRACE score, age (≥75 years), elevated Thrombolysis in Myocardial Infarction (TIMI) score, and cardiac biomarkers have also been shown to signal a higher risk for adverse events.[21,79] In high-risk patients with NSTE-ACS exhibiting a GRACE score above 140, adopting an early invasive strategy within 24 hours tends to reduce recurrent ischemia, diminish the necessity for urgent revascularization, and shorten hospital length of stay. Although clinical studies have not conclusively favored early (within 24 hours) over delayed invasive strategies for the entire NSTE-ACS population, analyses of specific high-risk subgroups within these studies support an early approach to intervention. Notably, the TIMACS (Timing of Intervention in Acute Coronary Syndromes) and VERDICT (Very Early Versus Deferred Invasive Evaluation Using Computerized Tomography) trials, which examined early intervention timing (within 24 hours or less and within 12 hours, respectively), revealed that early invasive management notably lessens cardiovascular complications in high-risk patients.[80–82]

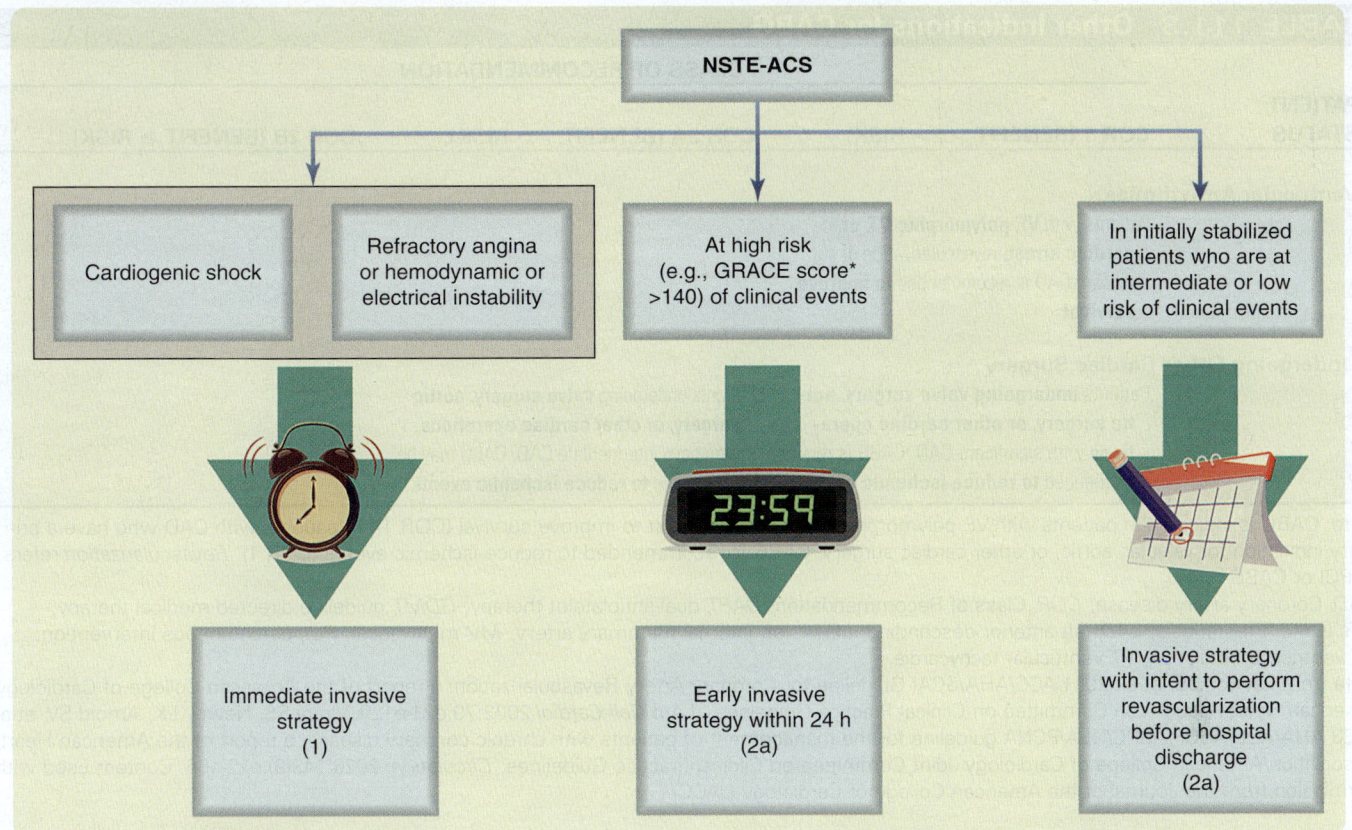

FIGURE 111.5 Guidelines for timing of invasive strategy in patients with NSTE-ACS. This flowchart encapsulates the suggested approaches for timing of coronary angiography with the goal of coronary revascularization for patients with NSTE-ACS as summarized in the 2021 American College of Cardiology/American Heart Association/Society for Cardiovascular Angiography and Interventions Guideline for Coronary Artery Revascularization.[22] *GRACE,* Global Registry of Acute Coronary Events (a scoring system that can be accessed via https://www.mdcalc.com/grace-acs-risk-mortality-calculator); *NSTE-ACS,* non–ST-elevation acute coronary syndrome. (Lawton JS, et al. 2021 ACC/AHA/SCAI Guideline for Coronary Artery Revascularization: a report of the American College of Cardiology/American Heart Association Committee on Clinical Practice Guidelnes. *J Am Coll Cardiol* 2022;79:e21-e129. Diagram used with permission from the *Journal of the American Heart Association.* ©2022 American Heart Association, Inc.)

Unstable Angina

USA is best described as existing along the continuum of NSTE-ACS, defined by one or more of the following criteria in patients whose cardiac marker levels do not meet criteria for AMI: prolonged rest angina (usually over 20 minutes); new-onset angina of at least Class 3 severity (symptoms with everyday living activities, e.g., moderate limitation such as walking one or two blocks on flat ground); or increasing angina that has become more frequent, severe, longer in duration, or lower in threshold.[81–83] Previously, guidelines recommended a conservative approach that focused on medical therapy (antiplatelet, anticoagulant and antianginal, β-blockers, and statins) and addressing modifiable risk factors (smoking cessation, physical activity, diet, etc.), followed by an evaluation for possible revascularization.[80–83] In these patients, angiography was typically performed within 24 hours of admission if stable (no evidence of very-high risk criteria) or immediately (<2 hours) if unstable (unabating symptoms, persistent arrhythmias, or hemodynamic instability). The choice of revascularization was then guided by angiography and other invasive strategies. However, the ischemia-guided strategy has since emerged, and evidence has demonstrated that USA/NSTE-ACS

carries a higher risk of mortality compared with SIHD, with symptoms less likely to be resolved by guideline-directed medical therapy (GDMT) alone.[20,21] As such, early evaluation and possible reperfusion are recommended, especially in patients with a high GRACE risk score, high-sensitivity cardiac troponin measurements, and new ST-segment changes. The final decision for revascularization follows the same path as those for PCI versus CABG, as outlined in Fig. 111.5.[21,80–84]

INDICATIONS FOR REVASCULARIZATION: STABLE ISCHEMIC HEART DISEASE

It is important to understand that PCI and CABG restore myocardial blood flow by starkly different mechanisms. Whereas PCI specifically addresses individual, discrete stenoses, it does not halt the progression or rupture of plaques in the artery. Conversely, CABG not only improves blood flow in the affected area but also safeguards against damage from upstream and downstream plaques. Indeed, evidence supports that a certain subgroup of patients benefits from CABG in terms of survival and the risk of late spontaneous MI.[21]

TABLE 111.3   Other Indications for CABG

PATIENT STATUS	CLASS OF RECOMMENDATION		
	COR 1 (BENEFIT >>> RISK)	COR 2A (BENEFIT >> RISK)	COR 2B (BENEFIT ≥ RISK)
Ventricular Arrhythmias			
	Patients with **VF, polymorphic VT, or cardiac arrest,** revascularization of significant CAD is recommended **to improve survival**		
Undergoing Other Cardiac Surgery			
	Patients **undergoing valve surgery, aortic surgery, or other cardiac operations** with significant CAD, CABG is recommended **to reduce ischemic events**	Patients undergoing **valve surgery, aortic surgery, or other cardiac operations** who have intermediate CAD, CABG may be reasonable **to reduce ischemic events**	

Note: CABG is indicated in patients with VF, polymorphic VT, or cardiac arrest to improve survival (COR 1). In patients with CAD who have a primary indication for valvular, aortic, or other cardiac surgery, CABG is recommended to reduce ischemic events (COR 1). *Revascularization* refers to PCI or CABG.

CAD, Coronary artery disease; *COR,* Class of Recommendation; *DAPT,* dual-antiplatelet therapy; *GDMT,* guideline-directed medical therapy; *ISR,* in-stent restenosis; *LAD,* left anterior descending; *LIMA,* left internal mammary artery; *MV,* multivessel; *PCI,* percutaneous intervention; *VF,* ventricular fibrillation; *VT,* ventricular tachycardia.

Data from Lawton JS, et al. 2021 ACC/AHA/SCAI Guideline for Coronary Artery Revascularization: a report of the American College of Cardiology/American Heart Association Committee on Clinical Practice Guidelnes. *J Am Coll Cardiol* 2022;79:e21-e129. Virani SS, Newby LK, Arnold SV, et al. 2023 AHA/ACC/ACCP/ASPC/NLA/PCNA guideline for the management of patients with chronic coronary disease: a report of the American Heart Association/American College of Cardiology Joint Committee on Clinical Practice Guidelines. *Circulation.* 2023;148(9):e12-e56. Content used with permission from the Journal of the American College of Cardiology (JACC).

The 2021 ACC/AHA/SCAI Guideline for Coronary Artery Revascularization for patients with SIHD details treatment in five main subsets of patients: those with LV dysfunction and multivessel CAD, those with left main disease, those with isolated multivessel disease, those with stenosis in the proximal LAD artery, and those with single- or double-vessel disease not involving the proximal LAD. The recommendations are summarized in Tables 111.2 and 111.3 and Fig. 111.6. In brief, there is a Class of Recommendation (COR) 1 recommendation for CABG in patients with multivessel (≥3 vessels) disease and severe LV systolic dysfunction (LVEF ≤35%) if they are otherwise good surgical candidates. Evidence shows that CABG is associated with improved odds of survival in these patients.[21] It is also reasonable (COR 2a) to choose CABG in patients with stable multivessel CAD who have mild to moderate LV systolic dysfunction (LVEF 35%–50%). This recommendation recognizes the importance of including a left internal mammary artery (LIMA)-to-LAD graft as a part of CABG.[21] In patients with SIHD and significantly stenosed left main artery, CABG is recommended (COR 1). However, PCI is reasonable in patients with SIHD and clinically significant left main stenosis if PCI can offer equivalent revascularization as CABG (COR 2a).[21] In patients with SIHD and multivessel CAD with normal ejection fraction with or without proximal LAD disease, CABG *may be* reasonable to improve survival (COR 2b).[21] In these patients, the usefulness of PCI to promote survival *remains uncertain.*[21,44,85]

Additionally, there is no benefit to coronary revascularization in patients with SIHD, normal LVEF, and one- or two-vessel CAD not involving the LAD (COR 3). Finally, revascularization is harmful in SIHD with ≥1 vessel CAD with <70% stenosis involving a non-LMCA (COR 3).[21]

Situations in Which Coronary Artery Bypass Graft Is Preferred Over Percutaneous Coronary Intervention to Improve Survival in Stable Ischemic Heart Disease

Three main goals have been identified in the management of patients with SIHD: symptom relief; prevention of adverse cardiac events, including nonfatal MI; and survival. CABG is preferred over PCI in patients with significant left main CAD and in patients with diabetes[86,87] to improve survival (both COR 1) and in patients with complex multivessel disease (COR 2a) to improve survival (see Table 111.2 and Fig. 111.6). These recommendations are based on data from the ISCHEMIA trial[44]; the FAME 2 trial[27]; and the 10-year updates from the Medicine, Angioplasty, or Surgery Study II (MASS II) trial,[88] which showed a reduction in cardiovascular mortality with surgical revascularization compared with optimal medical therapy (OMT) alone in these patients. In patients with CCD and complex three-vessel disease, a heart team approach is advocated, especially when there is a lack of clarity regarding the optimal treatment strategy.[21]

REVASCULARIZATION TO REDUCE VENTRICULAR ARRHYTHMIAS

In patients with ventricular arrhythmias, a thorough assessment for potential ischemic CAD is essential for decision-making by the heart team regarding the need for coronary artery revascularization.[89,90] Evidence from observational studies underscores that revascularization procedures in patients with life-threatening ventricular arrhythmias and those who have survived cardiac arrest are correlated with a notable decrease in arrhythmia frequency and improved survival. As such, the latest guideline

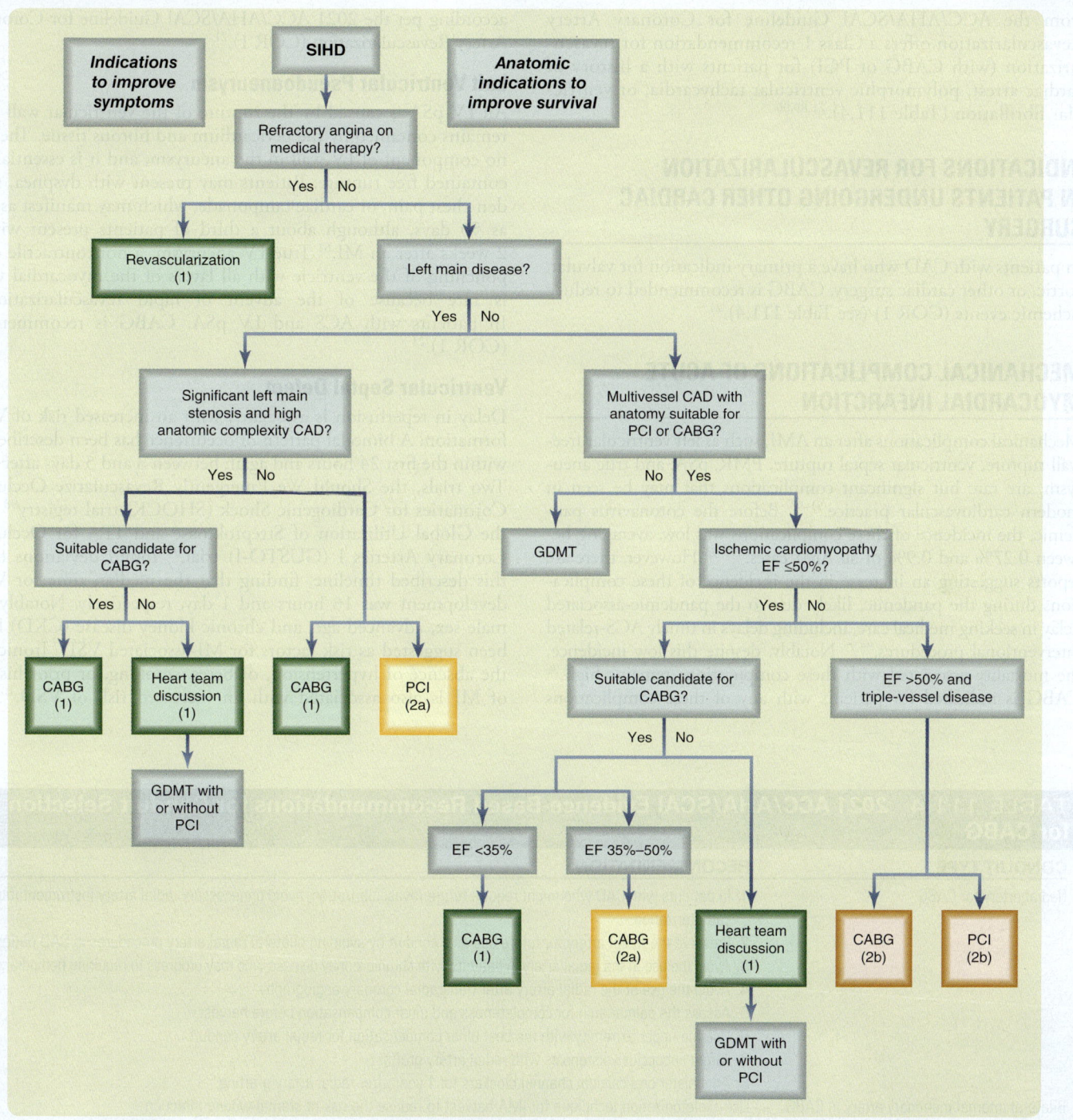

FIGURE 111.6 American College of Cardiology/American Heart Association/Society for Cardiovascular Angiography and Interventions (2021) evidence-based clinical decision pathway for revascularization in patients with SIHD. This detailed flowchart outlines the clinical decision-making process for the revascularization of patients with SIHD, focusing on symptomatic management and improvement of survival rates. It provides a systematic approach for determining when revascularization is indicated, differentiating between symptomatic relief and anatomic conditions that improve patient survival. The pathway considers the severity of symptoms, presence and extent of left main coronary artery disease, suitability for surgical or percutaneous interventions, and patient-specific factors such as EF and the presence of multivessel CAD. In sum, in patients with SIHD, the main indication for revascularization is to improve survival (right side of figure). There is one indication for revascularization to improve symptoms (left side of figure). Recommendations depicted in this figure are expanded in Tables 111.2 and 111.3. *CABG,* Coronary artery bypass graft; *CAD,* coronary artery disease; *EF,* ejection fraction; *GDMT,* guideline-directed medical therapy; *PCI,* percutaneous intervention; *SIHD,* stable ischemic heart disease. (Lawton JS, et al. 2021 ACC/AHA/SCAI Guideline for Coronary Artery Revascularization: a report of the American College of Cardiology/American Heart Association Committee on Clinical Practice Guidelnes. *J Am Coll Cardiol* 2022;79:e21-e129. From *Circulation* and the *Journal of the American College of Cardiology.* ©2022 American Heart Association, Inc.)

from the ACC/AHA/SCAI Guideline for Coronary Artery Revascularization offers a Class 1 recommendation for revascularization (with CABG or PCI) for patients with a history of cardiac arrest, polymorphic ventricular tachycardia, or ventricular fibrillation (Table 111.4).[21,89,90]

INDICATIONS FOR REVASCULARIZATION IN PATIENTS UNDERGOING OTHER CARDIAC SURGERY

In patients with CAD who have a primary indication for valvular, aortic, or other cardiac surgery, CABG is recommended to reduce ischemic events (COR 1) (see Table 111.4).[21]

MECHANICAL COMPLICATIONS OF ACUTE MYOCARDIAL INFARCTION

Mechanical complications after an AMI, such as left ventricular free-wall rupture, ventricular septal rupture, PMR, pSA, and true aneurysm, are rare but significant complications that may be seen in modern cardiovascular practice.[91–93] Before the coronavirus pandemic, the incidence of these complications was low, averaging between 0.27% and 0.9% of all AMI cases.[91–93] However, there are reports suggesting an increase in the incidence of these complications during the pandemic, likely due to the pandemic-associated delay in seeking medical care, including delays in timely ACS-related interventional procedures.[94,95] Notably, despite this low incidence, the mortality associated with these complications remains high.[96] CABG is indicated for patients with any of these complications

according per the 2021 ACC/AHA/SCAI Guideline for Coronary Artery Revascularization (COR 1).[21]

Left Ventricular Pseudoaneurysm

An LV pSA is caused by the rupture of the ventricular wall that remains contained by the pericardium and fibrous tissue. There is no component of LV wall in the aneurysm, and it is essentially a contained free rupture. Patients may present with dyspnea, sudden chest pain, or cardiac tamponade, which may manifest as late as 50 days, although about a third of patients present within 2 weeks after an MI.[61] True LV aneurysm, a noncontractile outpouching of the ventricle with all layers of the myocardial wall, is rare because of the advent of rapid revascularization.[97] In patients with ACS and LV pSA, CABG is recommended (COR 1).[21]

Ventricular Septal Defect

Delay in reperfusion is associated with an increased risk of VSD formation. A bimodal pattern of occurrence has been described—within the first 24 hours and again between 3 and 5 days after MI. Two trials, the Should We Emergently Revascularize Occluded Coronaries for Cardiogenic Shock (SHOCK) trial registry[98] and the Global Utilization of Streptokinase and TPA for Occluded Coronary Arteries I (GUSTO-I) trial,[99] found deviations from this described timeline, finding that the median time for VSD development was 16 hours and 1 day, respectively. Notably, female sex, advanced age, and chronic kidney disease (CKD) have been suggested as risk factors for MI-associated VSD. Ironically, the absence of hypertension, diabetes, smoking, or prior history of MI is also associated with an increased risk of VSD.[100] In

---

TABLE 111.4   2021 ACC/AHA/SCAI Evidence-Based Recommendations for Conduit Selection for CABG

CONDUIT TYPE	RECOMMENDATION
Radial artery for CABG	1. In patients with CAD who might require future revascularization, avoid unnecessary radial artery instrumentation/catheterization.
	2. Preserve the radial artery for future use as a conduit by avoiding bilateral radial artery procedures in CAD patients.
	3. Avoid the use of the radial artery in patients with chronic kidney disease who may progress to requiring hemodialysis.
	4. Avoid the use of the radial artery after transradial coronary angiography.
	5. Assess the palmar arch for completeness and ulnar compensation before harvest.
	6. Use the upper extremity with the best ulnar compensation for radial artery conduit.
	7. Target subocclusive stenosis with radial artery grafts.
	8. Administer oral calcium channel blockers for 1 year after radial artery grafting.
Bilateral internal mammary artery in CABG	Use skeletonization technique for IMA harvest to reduce the risk of sternal wound infection.
Saphenous vein for CABG	1. Endoscopic harvesting technique should be employed in patients at high risk for wound complications.
	2. No-touch saphenous vein harvesting may be used in patients at low risk for wound complications.
Gastroepiploic artery for CABG	Skeletonization should be used when the gastroepiploic artery is chosen as conduit for grafting the right coronary artery with subocclusive stenosis (operator dependent).

Note: Preserving the radial artery as a future conduit for CABG is important in patients with CKD or known CAD who might require surgical revascularization in the future. This includes the avoidance of bilateral radial artery instrumentation or catheterization in at-risk patients. Preoperative evaluation for conduit selection is critical, including physical exam to assess for adequate ulnar compensation to permit safe radial artery harvesting. The use of endoscopic techniques to harvest the saphenous vein is recommended in patients at high risk of wound complications. Finally, the role of skeletonization is discussed with regard to BIMA and gastroepiploic artery grafting.
ACC, American College of Cardiology; *AHA,* American Heart Association; *BIMA,* bilateral internal mammary artery; *CABG,* coronary artery bypass graft; *CAD,* coronary artery disease; *CKD,* chronic kidney disease; *IMA,* internal mammary artery; *SCAI,* Society for Cardiovascular Angiography and Interventions.
Data from Lawton JS, et al. 2021 ACC/AHA/SCAI Guideline for Coronary Artery Revascularization: a report of the American College of Cardiology/American Heart Association Committee on Clinical Practice Guidelnes. *J Am Coll Cardiol* 2022;79:e21-e129. Content used with permission from the Journal of the American College of Cardiology (JACC).

patients with ACS complicated by a VSD, CABG is recommended (COR 1).[21]

Papillary Muscle Rupture With Mitral Regurgitation

Although it has an incidence of 0.05% to 0.26%, PMR is implicated in more than 50% of observed cases of severe mitral regurgitation after AMI, with reported mortality rates of 10% to 40%.[97,101] Usually, PMR manifested within 7 days after an MI, with a median presentation of 13 hours, in the SHOCK trial.[98,102] Notably, PMR was more likely to occur in older patients and in patients with a history of heart failure, CKD, and first AMI presentation. An inverse relationship was found between having diabetes and prior MI and developing PMR.[96,101] Notably, for ACS patients with PMR and mitral regurgitation, CABG is recommended to improve survival (COR 1).[21]

INDICATIONS FOR REVASCULARIZATION IN PATIENTS WITH CHRONIC CORONARY DISEASE

Chronic coronary disease (CCD) (also known as *chronic coronary syndrome*) describes a broad range of conditions where coronary arteries are unable to supply adequate blood to the myocardium as a result of atherosclerosis. Patients may be symptomatic or asymptomatic. This condition is different from the previously addressed stable ischemic disease, which is used specifically to characterize patients with a stable and predictable pattern of angina (pain, discomfort, pressure, or other anginal-equivalent symptoms) that is usually exacerbated with physical exertion and is relieved with rest or medication. The spectrum of patients defined to have CCD includes[21,103]:

1. Patients who have been discharged after an admission for an ACS event or after undergoing coronary revascularization, once all acute cardiovascular complications have been stabilized
2. Individuals presenting with LV systolic dysfunction, who have known or suspected CAD, or who suffer from ischemic cardiomyopathy
3. Patients experiencing stable angina symptoms or ischemic equivalents, such as dyspnea or arm pain upon exertion, who are under medical management irrespective of the outcomes of any imaging tests
4. Individuals with symptoms indicative of coronary vasospasm or microvascular angina
5. Patients diagnosed with CCD based exclusively on the results of screening studies, such as stress tests or coronary CTA

The 2023 AHA/ACC/American College of Clinical Pharmacy (ACCP)/American Society for Preventive Cardiology (ASPC)/ National Lipid Association (NLA)/Preventive Cardiovascular Nurses Association (PCNA) Guideline for the Management of Patients with CCD has the same recommendations for CABG as in the 2021 ACC/AHA/SCAI Guideline for Coronary Artery Revascularization summarized earlier.

PREOPERATIVE EVALUATION FOR CORONARY ARTERY BYPASS GRAFTING

As previously discussed, the involvement of a heart team (consisting of the heart surgeon, interventional cardiologist, and noninterventional cardiologist, with additional involvement, when necessary, of the primary care physician, imaging specialists, cardiac anesthesiologist, intensivist, heart failure specialists, palliative care experts, physical and occupational therapists, and/or nursing staff) is recommended (COR 1) in the assessment and deliberative process regarding coronary revascularization in patients for whom the optimal treatment strategy is unclear. Discussions should always include the patient's goals and preferences and the addition of family members as appropriate.[21]

Preoperative assessment begins with a thorough history and physical exam, including assessment of physical and mental health status, current medications (especially those that interfere with cardiac function or coagulation/platelet function), socioeconomic stressors, and prior surgeries. A directed cardiovascular exam should include carotid auscultation, lung and heart auscultation, and evaluation of extremity pulses. The STS PROM should be calculated (COR 1) and includes comorbidities such as age; sex; elective versus emergency status of operation; LVEF; tobacco use; diabetes; hypertension; stroke; peripheral vascular disease (PVD); chronic lung disease; prior kidney disease; use of immunosuppressants; and previous cardiac surgeries, including prior revascularization.[21] This score will assist in treatment recommendations and in the appropriate informed consent in the discussion of risks and benefits of CABG with the patient.[21]

Careful review of CXR, TTE, and cardiac catheterization results is necessary to determine candidacy for CABG. Additional testing, including bilateral lower extremity venous mapping, ultrasound of RAs, carotid duplex evaluation, CT scan of the chest, or other imaging, may be warranted depending on the physical exam findings. Many of the diagnostic tests mentioned in previous sections provide valuable data for determining the appropriateness of medical therapy alone, PCI, or CABG. At each stage of the evaluation process, maintaining equity and a shared decision-making strategy is important.[21] A meticulous preprocedural heart team assessment is so crucial that it earned a COR 1 endorsement in the 2021 ACC/AHA/SCAI Guideline for Coronary Artery Revascularization.[21]

TECHNIQUE OF MYOCARDIAL REVASCULARIZATION: CONVENTIONAL ON-PUMP CARDIOPULMONARY BYPASS

The use of conventional cardiopulmonary bypass (CPB) in CABG involves a series of critical steps and components that ensure the safe and effective management of cardiac procedures. Initiation of CPB is a pivotal process in major cardiac surgeries, involving the diversion of venous blood from the body to a heart-lung machine, which then oxygenates and returns this blood in a controlled, pressurized manner.[104–106] Essentially, this process bypasses most blood flow to the heart and lungs, allowing surgeons the ability to operate in a quiet, bloodless field.

The extracorporeal CPB circuit consists of several basic components: venous cannula, tubing, reservoir, oxygenator, pump (centrifugal or roller head), filter, tubing, and arterial cannula. Venous cannulas are used to drain returning deoxygenated venous blood, which collects in a venous reservoir by gravity. This can be augmented by raising the operating room table or via addition of suction. The circuit includes an oxygenator and heat exchanger, a perfusion pump, a blood filter in the arterial line, and an arterial cannula. These blood conduits are designed to minimize turbulence, cavitation, and changes in blood flow velocity, which could harm the integrity of blood cells. The circuit also contains a dead space and necessitates a priming solution to initiate the pump and tubing, usually comprising either a balanced salt solution or, often, a starch solution. Homologous blood or fresh frozen plasma may be added as needed.[107]

Additional components include cardiotomy suction devices and tubing for infusion of cardioplegia or other solutions that may be used. A cardiotomy suction system collects blood from open cardiac chambers and the surgical field, which is then filtered, de-aired, and returned to the bypass circuit. A cardioplegia infusion device, comprising a separate pump, reservoir, and heat exchanger, delivers cold, potassium-enriched blood or crystalloid solutions into the coronary circulation for cardiac arrest and myocardial protection.

The use of CPB necessitates adherence to stringent anticoagulation protocols because of the high thrombogenic potential of the tubing and bypass pump components. Heparin is most commonly used, with strict monitoring of the activated clotting time (ACT) to ensure effective anticoagulation throughout the procedure. The common practice involves administering an initial bolus of heparin before cannulating the patient for CPB. This dose typically ranges from 300 to 400 units per kilogram (U/kg) of the patient's body weight. The goal is to achieve an ACT of greater than 400 seconds, which is considered adequate for safe initiation of CPB. ACT is monitored regularly during CPB. If the ACT falls below a certain threshold (approximately 400 seconds), additional heparin is administered. Subsequent additional doses or a heparin infusion is dosed according to ACT level.

Procedural Steps for On-Pump Coronary Artery Bypass Grafting With Cardioplegic Arrest

The procedural sequence for CABG with cardioplegia encompasses a series of meticulously executed steps. Initially, surgical access is gained through a median sternotomy, followed by the harvesting of the conduit. Before cannulation, the patient undergoes systemic heparinization. Cannulation is then performed to establish the CPB circuit. CPB is initiated after a series of checklist items is confirmed by the perfusionist. Once CPB commences, the surgical team evaluates potential sites for distal coronary anastomoses. The application of a cross clamp precedes the administration of cardioplegia, which facilitates a quiescent heart for performing the distal anastomoses. Cardioplegia is given in the antegrade fashion, directly into the aortic root, and infuses the coronary arteries (with a competent aortic valve) or in the retrograde fashion, via a catheter in the coronary sinus (Fig. 111.7). Intermittent cardioplegia, typically every 20 minutes, is administered to maintain myocardial protection. Proximal anastomoses are then completed. After this, the cross clamp is removed, and mechanical ventilation is resumed. The weaning process from CPB begins, followed by the administration of protamine for heparin reversal. Flow in the newly constructed conduits is assessed before decannulation. Decannulation, judicious hemostasis, and subsequent sternal closure occur. It is noteworthy that the sequence of these steps can vary, with alternatives including the initial performance of proximal anastomoses or the use of a partial occluding aortic clamp for proximal anastomoses. Thorough preoperative planning is imperative to ensure optimal surgical outcomes.[5]

Conduit Selection for Coronary Artery Bypass Grafting

Conduit selection for CPB is a critical step in planning for CABG. Saphenous vein grafts (SVGs) have been associated with lower long-term patency rates compared with arterial grafts in several studies.[108–112] Long-term graft patency is correlated with survival[108,113–115]; thus, cardiac surgeons must carefully consider these choices at the time of preoperative evaluation. The most common conduits for CABG are the LIMA and right internal

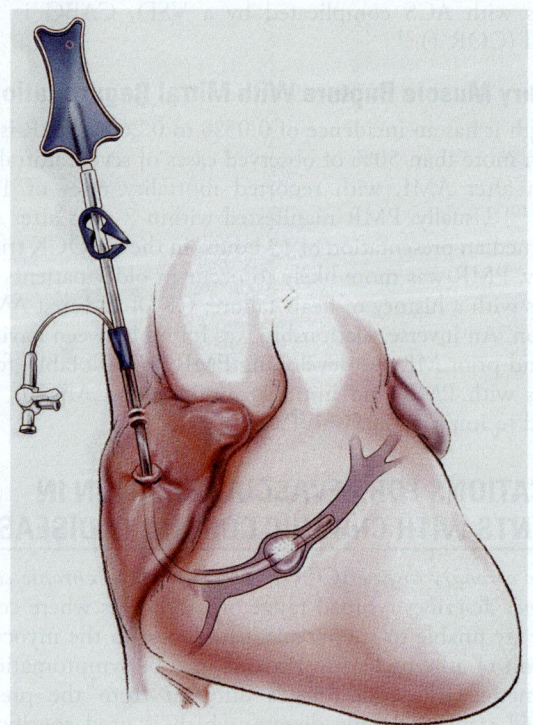

FIGURE 111.7 Depiction of coronary sinus cannulation. Illustration of retrograde cardioplegia delivery via a catheter inserted into the coronary sinus. As an alternative to antegrade cardioplegia, the cardioplegia solution is administered against the normal direction of blood flow and can ensure a uniform and effective distribution of cardioplegia throughout the myocardium, particularly in patients with proximal disease in multiple coronary arteries. The retrograde cardioplegia catheter is advanced with care into the right atrium and the coronary sinus via palpation and with transesophageal echocardiography assistance. By placing the left hand on the cannula and the right hand on the inferior vena cava (IVC), the cannula can be felt at the IVC and then directed toward the patient's left shoulder for insertion into the coronary sinus. (From Buxton B, Frazier OH Westaby S, eds. *Ischemic Heart Disease Surgical Management.* London: Mosby Ltd.; 1999. Illustrations by Elizabeth D. Croce. Used with permission.)

mammary artery (RIMA), SVG, RA, and any combination of these. The gastroepiploic artery, although historically described, is rarely used in modern practice in the United States. Table 111.4 provides a summary of society-based guidelines for CABG conduit selection.

Left Versus Right Internal Mammary Artery

For many decades, grafting the LIMA to the LAD has been the gold standard in surgical revascularization and an important STS quality metric. This stems from evidence documenting superior patency and long-term survival benefits of using the LIMA regardless of sex, age, diabetes, hypertension status, LVEF, and NYHA class.[111,116–118] Although some studies have found superior long-term patency of LIMA to LAD, defined as <80% stenosis of the LIMA at 20 years compared with right internal thoracic artery (RITA)-to-LAD grafts (96.3% vs. 88.1%), others have found equivalent patency rates between the two.[112,119] Overall, the use of any internal mammary artery (IMA) over SVG is associated with reduced mortality, need for revascularization, and rehospitalization for cardiac events.[111,115,119–124] Therefore, in patients undergoing

CABG for CAD that includes the LAD, the use of an IMA, especially the LIMA, carries a Class 1 ACC/AHA/SCAI recommendation to improve survival and reduce ischemic events.[21]

The right IMA carries the same recommendation (COR 1) in the current ACC/AHA/SCAI Guideline for Coronary Artery Revascularization.[14] In situations where the LIMA is not usable, the RIMA may be used to graft the LAD. Additionally, both IMAs may also be used. Multiple meta-analyses of observational studies have demonstrated longer survival with bilateral IMA (BIMA) grafting than with single IMA (SIMA) use.[121,125,126] In one network meta-analysis, RIMA emerged as the second-best conduit in CABG because of its reported 27% absolute risk reduction in late functional graft occlusion.[122]

The Arterial Revascularization Trial (ART) is, to date, the most extensive RCT evaluating the benefits of BIMA versus SIMA. With 3102 patients randomized to either SIMA ($n = 1554$) or BIMA ($n = 1548$), the primary outcome was all-cause mortality. At the 10-year evaluation, no intergroup statistically significant mortality benefits were observed with either strategy.[126] Although this was a significant and somewhat unexpected finding, the high rate of crossover (14% from BIMA to SIMA, and 22% of patients in LIMA group also had an RA graft) and surgeon experience may have played a role. When an "as-treated" analysis was performed, outcomes were better in the BIMA group compared with a single artery cohort. Notably, these benefits appeared to be more pronounced in diabetic patients and those 70 years or younger.[127,128]

Saphenous Vein Grafts

Compared with LIMA-to-LAD grafting, the patency rate of SVG-to-LAD graft lags significantly, ranging from 70% to 87% within 1 year, with a dramatic drop to approximately 50% at 10 years.[111,112] Early SVG failure is related to technical reasons. Long-term SVG failure has been linked to significant obstruction due to neointimal hyperplasia. Despite the best attempts to attenuate this phenomenon with the use of statins and β-blockers, LIMA grafting continues to demonstrate significant superiority compared with SVG.[108,110–112] The use of the no-touch SVG strategy appears to be showing promising results with regard to graft patency.[129]

Radial Artery Grafts

Although Carpentier et al. (1973) described the short-term benefits of the use of RA graft in aorta-to–coronary artery bypass over SVG, concerns regarding competitive flow, arterial spasm, and early occlusion made this practice unpopular for decades.[130] In an effort to increase the use of multiarterial conduits for coronary revascularization, many studies (including pooled analysis from six RCTs) have documented the benefits of radial arterial grafting. RA patency competed favorably with the IMA at 1, 5, and 10 years.[131–134] A 2018 meta-analysis by Gaudino et al. aimed to compare the outcomes of RA versus SVGs.[134] They included 1036 patients (502 with SVG vs. 534 with RA grafts). The primary outcome was a composite of death, MI, or repeat revascularization. The secondary outcome focused on graft patency. At 5 years, RA grafts resulted in a lower rate of adverse cardiac events and a higher patency rate compared with SVGs.

Additionally, the recently published 15-year results of the RAPCO (Radial Artery Patency and Clinical Outcomes) randomized trials that compared the outcomes of MACEs of CABG using the RA, RITA, or SVG[135] noted that the incidence of MACE was significantly lower in patients treated with RA graft versus RITA (39.4% vs. 48.5%; HR = 0.74,

95% CI 0.55–0.97, $P = 0.04$). Mortality rates were 22.2% (RA) and 30.1% (RITA) (HR = 0.69, 95% CI 0.47–1.02). The rate of MACE was 60.2% in RA versus 73.2% in saphenous vein (SV) (HR = 0.71, 95% CI 0.52–0.98, $P = 0.04$). Mortality rates were 52.2% (RA) and 63.4% (SV) (HR = 0.74, 95% CI 0.52–1.04). The 2021 ACC/AHA/SCAI Guideline on Coronary Artery Revascularization has given a Class 1 recommendation for the use of an RA as the conduit of choice, over an SVG, to graft the second most important, significantly stenosed non-LAD vessel to improve long-term cardiac outcomes (see Table 111.4).[21]

Bilateral Internal Mammary Arterial Grafts

The use of BIMA grafts in CABG has garnered support from various observational studies and meta-analyses. A meta-analysis of 27 studies (no RCT) with 79,063 patients (including 19,277 BIMA and 59,786 LIMA cases) found long-term survival benefits in the use of BIMA versus SIMA.[136] In contrast, a large-scale RCT consisting of 3102 patients (the ART) showed no difference in 10-year all-cause mortality or the composite outcome of death, MI, or stroke when comparing BIMA with SIMA, as stated earlier.[126] Notably, in this study, there was a high crossover rate (14% from BIMA to SIMA, and 22% receiving an RA in the SIMA group). An as-treated analysis indicated improved survival with multiple arterial grafts. Further, increased BIMA use correlated with protocol adherence, highlighting the importance of surgical expertise. However, low institutional BIMA volumes were associated with higher operative mortality.[126]

Other studies and meta-analyses advocate for ≥3 arterial grafts, including total arterial revascularization, but the increased risk of sternal infection with BIMA (particularly in diabetes, obesity [BMI >30 kg/m²], and immunosuppressed patients) has led to caution with the use of BIMA.[127,137] Interestingly, skeletonization appears to reduce the risk of sternal wound infection while preserving the known benefits of BIMA in diabetic patients. Currently, there is a Class 2a recommendation in the 2021 ACC/AHA/SCAI Guideline for Coronary Artery Revascularization for the use of BIMA in carefully selected patients by experienced cardiac surgeons.[21]

Evidence-Based Practice Guidelines for Conduit Selection in Coronary Artery Bypass Grafting

The choice of conduits for CABG involves the careful consideration of several clinical and technical factors, including but not limited to patient comorbidities, life expectancy, degree of coronary artery stenosis, number of diseased vessels, and the operator's expertise and experience with various conduits. Table 111.4 summarizes the best-practice recommendations of the 2021 ACC/AHA/SCAI Guideline for Coronary Artery Revascularization.[21]

Technical Aspects of Coronary Artery Bypass Grafting

CABGs can be constructed using a variety of configurations (Figs. 111.8–111.9). Traditionally, the most common was LIMA to LAD (which is an STS quality measure) and SVG to the other left-sided vessels and right vessel (see Fig. 111.8). Because multiarterial grafting (MAG) provides many benefits, including prolonged survival, the current ACC/AHA/SCAI Guideline for Coronary Artery Revascularization supports the use of the RA (COR1) and the RIMA (COR 2a) over SVG. Common MAG configurations include combinations of BIMA and radial grafts to provide CR (see Fig. 111.9).

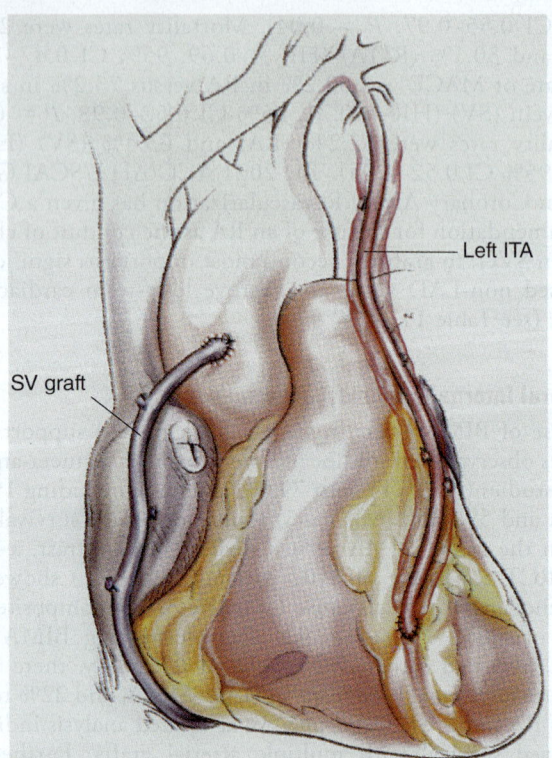

FIGURE 111.8 Common coronary artery bypass grafting configuration with left ITA and vein. The left ITA is anastomosed to the LAD, a technique favored for its high success and long-term patency rates. The image also displays the use of an SV vein graft from the aorta to the RCA. *LAD,* Left anterior descending artery; *ITA,* internal thoracic artery; *RCA,* right coronary artery; *SV,* saphenous vein. (From Buxton B, Frazier OH Westaby S, eds. *Ischemic Heart Disease Surgical Management.* London: Mosby Ltd.; 1999. Illustrations by Elizabeth D. Croce. Used with permission.)

Care should be taken to ensure proper conduit length so that the graft will reach the aorta or other proximal sites without kinking or bowstringing. Filling the heart while sizing is one method to measure length. Left-sided bypass grafts originating on the aorta travel beneath the LIMA graft and must have ample length even after the pulmonary artery is full and the heart is full and beating.

The order of performing the distal and proximal anastomoses is by surgeon preference (all distals first, then proximals; each distal and then proximal; or proximals and then distals). Distal anastomoses can be constructed in an end-to-side or side-to-side fashion using a running monofilament polypropylene suture (Figs. 111.10–111.11). Care is taken to ensure that the suture bites are full thickness, with the needle perpendicular to the conduit or target.

Proximal anastomoses may originate on the ascending aorta (Fig. 111.12), on the hood of another proximal, on the innominate artery, as a T or Y graft from another conduit, or rarely, on the descending aorta.

OFF-PUMP CORONARY ARTERY BYPASS GRAFTING

Off-pump CABG (OPCABG) is often regarded as an alternative surgical strategy to performing conventional CABG to circumvent the serious complications associated with CPB and cardioplegic arrest. It is typically considered in patients deemed at high risk for CABG due to porcelain aorta, reduced LVEF, severe chronic obstructive pulmonary disease, or recent MI. Another rationale behind this approach is to prevent further myocardial injury from the global myocardial ischemia, given that it is imposed during CABG with cross-clamp placement.

There are key distinctions between on-pump CABG and OPCABG. OPCABG necessitates specific adjuncts to facilitate manipulation of the heart to provide adequate exposure of coronary vessels, primarily because the heart remains contractile throughout the operation to support systemic perfusion. Both pleural spaces are often opened to facilitate rotation of the heart, enhance visibility of target areas, and reduce hypotension, particularly when working on the lateral and inferior myocardial walls. Unlike on-pump CABG, in OPCABG, the heart continues to eject and supply the brain and body with blood, and the lungs must continue to provide oxygenation to the blood. The most critical myocardial territory is revascularized first (e.g., LAD) to reduce ischemia while constructing subsequent anastomoses and to promote myocardial reserve. After this, remaining impacted segments of the heart are revascularized. Typically, revascularization begins with mammary artery–based pedicles because these do not necessitate a proximal anastomosis and immediately restore coronary blood flow to the bypassed vessel.[24,138–141]

For each target vessel, a small section of the coronary artery is exposed proximally to the intended anastomosis site, allowing for the placement of vessel loops or clamps for the occlusion of inflow. Additionally, a coronary shunt may be used. There are two types of stabilizers employed in OPCAB procedures, both of which use suction to attach to the heart. A fork-type stabilizer uses two adjustable suction arms that straddle the coronary target, making it largely immobile. Another padded mobile suction cup (moves with the motion of the heart) is applied to the apex of the heart for its manipulation and positioning throughout the procedure. Both suction devices may be attached to any portion of the sternal retractor. Manipulation of the operative table often facilitates the procedure, particularly the use of Trendelenburg position. The most difficult exposure to achieve is the lateral wall vessels, which may result in temporary mitral regurgitation while the heart is elevated. A sling on the posterior pericardium may be used to enhance visualization while elevating the heart. A lower target ACT may be used than that required for on-pump CABG. Close coordination with cardiac anesthesia colleagues is necessary for success in this method of coronary revascularization.

Multiple randomized clinical trials have raised concerns about OPCABG, particularly regarding higher rates of incomplete revascularization and reduced long-term survival. In 2022, the 10-year follow-up of the Veterans Affairs Randomized On/Off Bypass (ROOBY) trial showed no benefits in patients who received OPCABG. The median time to the composite end point of death for the off-pump group was shorter (4.6 years vs. 5 years, interquartile range [IQR] 1.8–7.9, $p = 0.03$) compared with the on-pump bypass patients.[140] Because of these results, OPCABG has waned in clinical practice. However, it has equivalent results in the hands of experienced off-pump surgeons and is useful in patients with porcelain aorta, in other high-risk patients, and in minimally invasive CABG procedures.[138,140,141]

ON-PUMP BEATING-HEART CORONARY ARTERY BYPASS GRAFTING

On-pump beating-heart CABG (ON-BH CABG) is another surgical option in high-risk patients. Using this method, hemodynamic

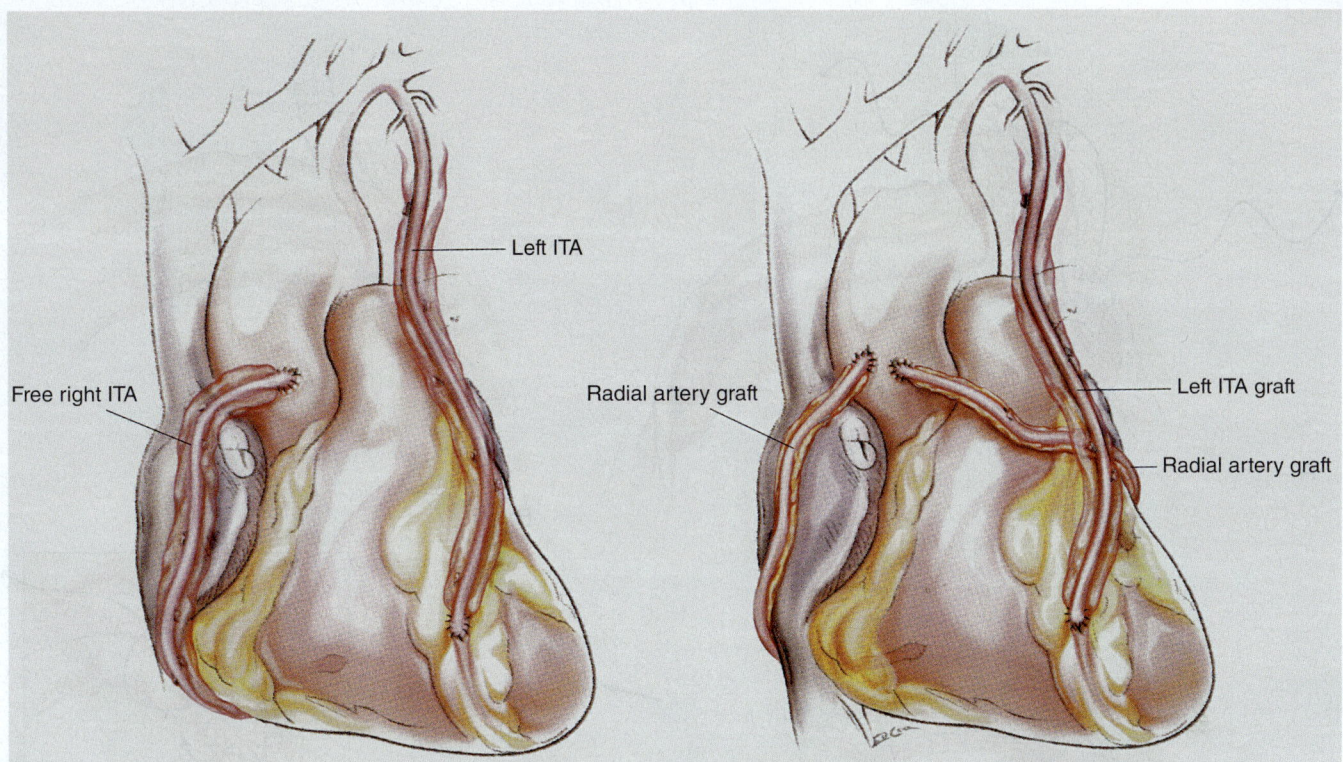

FIGURE 111.9 Common coronary MAG configurations. (A) In situ LITA graft and free right ITA originating on the aorta. (B) In situ LITA graft and free radial artery from the aorta to the obtuse marginal branch and free radial artery from the aorta to the distal RCA. *ITA*, internal thoracic artery; *LITA*, left internal thoracic artery; *MAG*, multiple arterial bypass grafting; *RCA*, right coronary artery. (From Buxton B, Frazier OH Westaby S, eds. *Ischemic Heart Disease Surgical Management.* London: Mosby Ltd.; 1999. Illustrations by Elizabeth D. Croce. Used with permission.)

stability is maintained while effective exposure to the target coronary artery is achieved. This innovative technique aims to optimize coronary artery revascularization while mitigating some of the known hematologic and neurologic complications of on-pump CABG with cardioplegic arrest and global myocardial ischemia.[142]

A systematic review by Wang et al. (2021) evaluated 24 studies with 6862 patients (1847 ON-BH CABG and 5015 CABG) and found that CABG, compared with ON-BH CABG, had higher early mortality (odds ratio [OR] 1.45, 95% CI 1.09–1.93, $p = 0.01$), MI (OR 2.60, 95% CI 1.41%–4.78%, $p < 0.01$), more low-output syndrome (OR 2.56, 95% CI 1.55–4.23, $p < 0.01$), and more renal failure (OR 1.84, 95% CI 1.38–2.44, $p < 0.01$). In high-risk patients, ON-BH CABG showed lower risks in terms of early mortality, intraaortic balloon pump (IABP) usage, renal failure, hemodialysis requirement, MI, and pulmonary complications.[142] This approach remains helpful in high-risk patients with bleeding dyscrasias, in those with low LVEF, and in patients with a porcelain aorta who require multivessel revascularization.

MINIMALLY INVASIVE DIRECT CORONARY ARTERY BYPASS

Minimally invasive direct coronary artery bypass (MIDCAB) grafting is a key alternative to conventional CABG, particularly for patients with isolated significant LAD stenosis for which PCI is not suitable.[143,144] The most common incisions used in MIDCAB include anterolateral thoracotomy, mini-sternotomy, and subxiphoid. MIDCAB, which integrates the principles of

OPCABG and minimally invasive surgery, has generated interest because of its potential benefits, but concerns remain about the technical quality of anastomoses performed. A meta-analysis consisting of 2885 patients from 12 studies (6 RCTs, 6 observational trials [OTs]) compared the clinical outcomes of PCI versus MIDCAB in 2015. Pooled-effects estimate demonstrated an increased incidence of major adverse cardiac and cerebrovascular events (MACCEs) after PCI (OR 1.98, 95% CI 1.45–2.69, $p < 0.0001$) at 6 months compared with MIDCAB.[143] There were no differences in the rate of postoperative stroke, MI, and all-cause mortality. However, patients in the PCI arm experienced shorter postoperative length of stay (weighted mean difference −3.37 days, 95% CI −4.92 to −1.81, $p < 0.0001$). Of note, more patients in the PCI cohort had the LAD as the target artery than those in the MIDCAB arm (60.7% vs. 39.3%). A single-center retrospective study analyzed 1033 patients (303 MIDCAB and 730 drug-eluting stents [DES]-PCI) with isolated proximal LAD anastomosis, using propensity matching to assess short- and long-term (10-year) mortality and revascularization rates. Comparable short-term (30-day) mortality was noted between groups (0.6% vs. 0.3%, $p = 0.99$). However, after 10 years, patients with DES-PCI had a 2.2%-fold increased risk of late death, a twofold increased risk of repeat revascularization, and a 2.1%-fold higher risk of composite death and revascularization (95% CI 1.41–3.24) compared with the MIDCAB cohort.[145]

A more recent meta-analysis involving 3847 patients evaluated the 20-year outcome of MIDCAB versus PCI. This study found higher short-term mortality in MIDCAB patients based on six

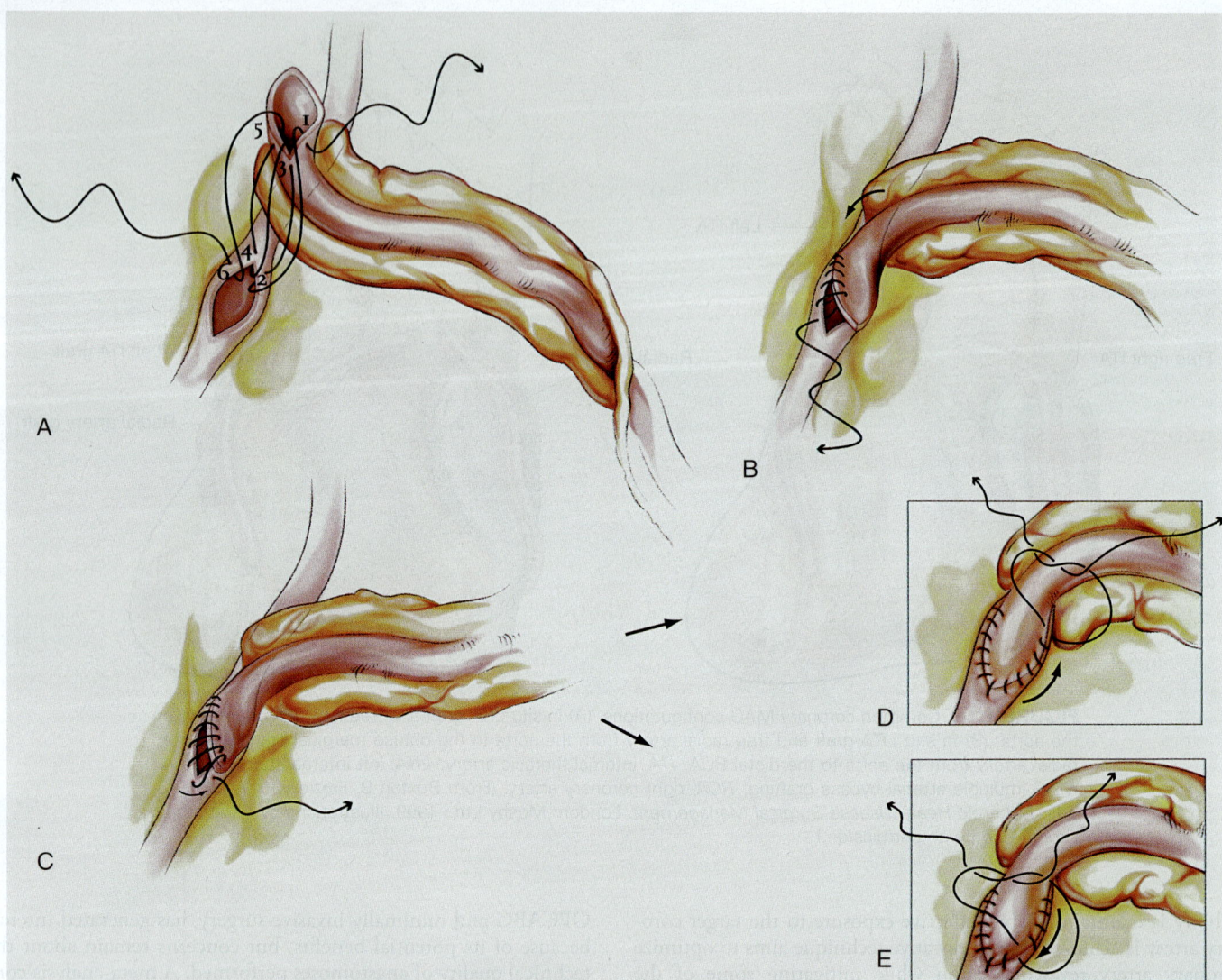

FIGURE 111.10 Distal coronary artery bypass grafting with end-to-side anastomosis. (A) Heel sutures begin with outside-in (backhand) suturing in the conduit and inside-out (backhand) suturing in the coronary. (B) Forehand suturing down the side of the anastomosis. (C) Forehand suturing around the toe, with extreme care to avoid the back wall of the coronary at the toe of the anastomosis. (D) Backhand suturing along the right side of the anastomosis and tie near heel. (E) Alternative to D; forehand suturing using other end of suture down the right side of the anastomosis and tie near toe. This requires suturing outside in on the coronary, which is not recommended with friable, calcified wall. (From Buxton B, Frazier OH Westaby S, eds. *Ischemic Heart Disease Surgical Management.* London: Mosby Ltd.; 1999. Illustrations by Elizabeth D. Croce. Used with permission.)

RCTs (RR 7.30, 95% CI 1.38–38.6, number needed to treat [NNT] 100), but at midterm and long-term follow-up, no difference in cardiac mortality was found. With regard to rate of TVR, MIDCAB performed better. However, the authors reported possible publication bias as the reason for the observed short-term mortality differences.[146] The 2021 ACC/AHA/SCAI Guideline for Coronary Artery Revascularization recommends further research focused on the use of nonsternotomy incisions for CABG.[21]

ROBOTIC TOTALLY ENDOSCOPIC CORONARY ARTERY BYPASS

Since the first totally endoscopic coronary artery bypass (TECAB) surgery in 1998, many centers have reported mixed results.[147] The most popular platform includes a surgeon-device interface, a

controller (computer), and patient interface with surgical instruments. A 2019 systematic review of 2397 patients over two decades noted a decreasing trend in the conversion rate from beating-heart TECAB to traditional CABG (from ~50% to 9.3%), decreased mean percentage early postoperative mortality of 1.1%, stroke rate of 0.4%, 2% incidence of renal failure, and 3.8 days median length of stay.[147] Interestingly, the rate of conversion in arrested-heart (AH)-TECAB was 13.3%, and the median operative time of AH-TECAB was 305 (112–1050 minutes) versus 279 (177–373 minutes) in conventional CABG patients. The postoperative mortality was 0.6% in patients with AH-TECAB, with median stroke and renal failure incidences of 1.5% and 1.3%, respectively. Compared with outcomes in the Future Revascularization Evaluation in Patients With Diabetes Mellitus: Optimal Management of Multivessel Disease (FREEDOM)

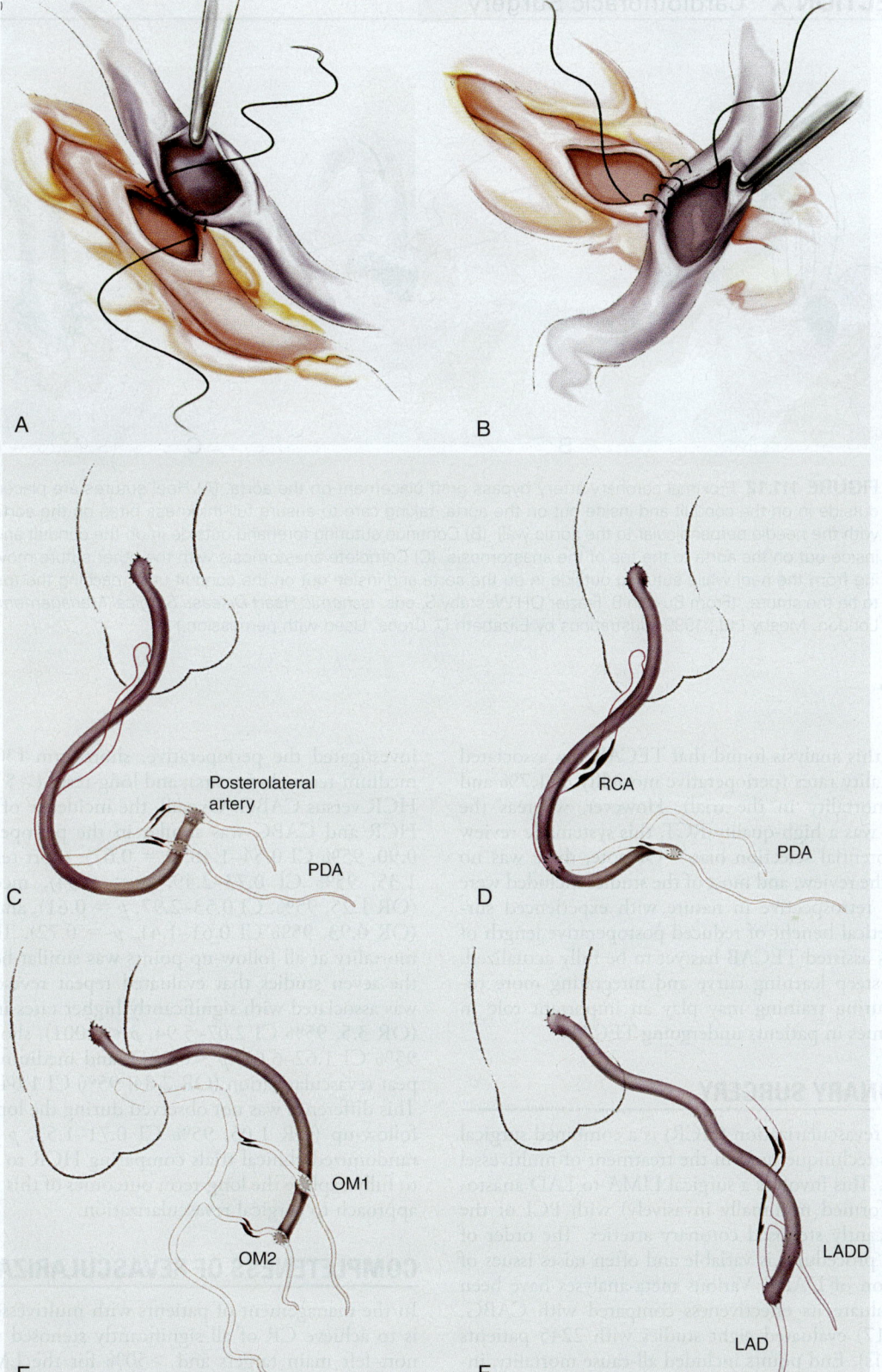

FIGURE 111.11 Distal coronary artery bypass grafting with side-to-side anastomosis for sequential grafting with a single conduit. (A) Linear parallel side-to-side anastomosis. (B) Diamond-shaped perpendicular side-to-side anastomosis. (C) Sequential anastomosis from aorta to posterior descending artery (perpendicular side to side) and the posterolateral artery (end to side). (D) Sequential anastomosis from aorta to right coronary artery (parallel side to side) and to the posterior descending artery (end to side). (E) Sequential anastomosis from aorta to first obtuse marginal artery (perpendicular side to side) and the second obtuse marginal (end to side). (F) Sequential anastomosis from aorta to diagonal artery (parallel side to side) and the LAD (end to side). *LAD,* Left anterior descending artery; *LADD,* left anterior descending diagonal artery; *OM1,* obtuse marginal 1; *OM2,* obtuse marginal 2; *PDA,* posterior descending artery; *RCA,* right coronary artery. (From Buxton B, Frazier OH Westaby S, eds. *Ischemic Heart Disease Surgical Management.* London: Mosby Ltd.; 1999. Illustrations by Elizabeth D. Croce. Used with permission.)

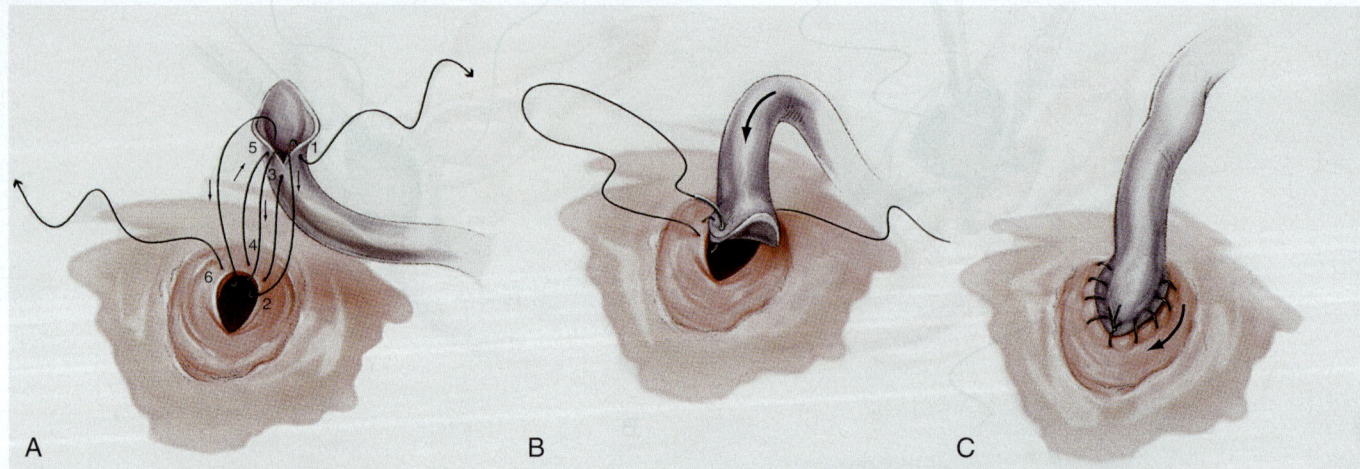

FIGURE 111.12 Proximal coronary artery bypass graft placement on the aorta. (A) Heel sutures are placed outside in on the conduit and inside out on the aorta, taking care to ensure full-thickness bites on the aorta with the needle perpendicular to the aortic wall. (B) Continue suturing forehand outside in on the conduit and inside out on the aorta to the toe of the anastomosis. (C) Complete anastomosis with the other suture moving from the heel while suturing outside in on the aorta and inside out on the conduit until reaching the toe to tie the suture. (From Buxton B, Frazier OH Westaby S, eds. *Ischemic Heart Disease Surgical Management.* London: Mosby Ltd.; 1999. Illustrations by Elizabeth D. Croce. Used with permission.)

trial of CABG,[87] this analysis found that TECAB was associated with similar mortality rates (perioperative mortality of 1.7% and 3.5% all-cause mortality in the trial). However, whereas the FREEDOM trial was a high-quality RCT, this systematic review was subject to potential selection bias.[87] Of note, there was no control group in the review, and most of the studies included were single-center and retrospective in nature with experienced surgeons. The theoretical benefit of reduced postoperative length of stay in robotically assisted TECAB has yet to be fully actualized. Overcoming the steep learning curve and integrating more robotic exposure during training may play an important role in optimizing outcomes in patients undergoing TECAB.

HYBRID CORONARY SURGERY

Hybrid coronary revascularization (HCR) is a combined surgical and percutaneous technique used in the treatment of multivessel CAD (MVCAD). This involves a surgical LIMA-to-LAD anastomosis (often performed minimally invasively) with PCI of the additional significantly stenosed coronary arteries. The order of events of the two procedures is variable and often raises issues of timing of initiation of DAPT. Various meta-analyses have been conducted to evaluate its effectiveness compared with CABG. Sardar et al. (2017) evaluated eight studies with 2245 patients (1 RCT and 7 OTs). End points included all-cause mortality, incidence of MI, stroke, repeat revascularization, need for postoperative transfusion, and hospital stay. Compared with the control group (CABG), patients with HCR experienced similar all-cause mortality (OR 0.84, 95% CI 0.38–1.88), MI (OR 0.72, 95% CI 0.31–1.64), stroke (OR 0.53, 95% CI 0.23–1.20), and repeat revascularization (OR 1.28, 95% CI 0.58–2.83). However, HCR patients were less likely to receive postoperative blood transfusion (OR, 0.29; 95% CI 0.14–0.59) and had shorter hospital length of stay (weighted difference –1.20; 95% CI –1.51 to –0.88 days).[148] A more recent meta-analysis of 18 studies (3 RCTs and 15 OTs)

investigated the perioperative, short-term (30 days to 1 year), medium-term (1–5 years), and long-term (>5 years) outcomes of HCR versus CABG. Overall, the incidence of MACCE between HCR and CABG was similar in the perioperative period (OR 0.90, 95% CI 0.54–1.48, $p = 0.67$), short-term follow-up (OR 1.35, 95% CI 0.73–2.49, $p = 0.34$), medium-term period (OR 1.25, 95%, CI 0.53–2.97, $p = 0.61$), and long-term period (OR 0.93, 95% CI 0.61–1.41, $p = 0.72$). The rate of MI and mortality at all follow-up points was similar between groups. Of the seven studies that evaluated repeat revascularization, HCR was associated with significantly higher rates in the perioperative (OR 3.5, 95% CI 2.07–5.94, $p < 0.001$), short-term (OR 3.28, 95% CI 1.62–6.64, $p < 0.001$), and medium-term need for repeat revascularization (OR 2.84, 95% CI 1.64–4.92, $p < 0.001$). This difference was not observed during the long-term (>5 years) follow-up (OR 1.05, 95% CI 0.71–1.53, $p = 0.82$).[149] More randomized clinical trials comparing HCR to CABG are needed to fully explore the long-term outcomes of this novel and nuanced approach to surgical revascularization.

COMPLETENESS OF REVASCULARIZATION

In the management of patients with multivessel disease, the goal is to achieve CR of all significantly stenosed vessels (>70% for non–left main targets and >50% for the LMCA). Incomplete revascularization has been shown in retrospective studies and other trials to be associated with reduced long-term survival.[150–152] However, patient-specific factors and shared decision-making are critical when determining the ability to provide CR to all significantly stenosed target vessels.

In patients with STEMI, PCI of the culprit lesion is often the sole target treated during emergent revascularization.[21] Unfortunately, these patients often have other angiographically significant lesions, apart from the lesion precipitating the acute MI. Observational studies suggest that outcomes are less favorable when significantly stenosed epicardial vessels are left untreated. This correlation is further supported by the SYNTAX trial, which observed worse cardiovascular outcomes in patients receiving incomplete revascularization during CABG or PCI, despite the trial's aim for CR in all participants.[67,68]

The current ACC/AHA/SCAI Guideline on Coronary Artery Revascularization recommends staged PCI of significant noninfarct artery stenosis in selected hemodynamically stable patients with STEMI and noncomplex multivessel nonculprit disease (COR 1) and elective CABG in selected patients with STEMI and complex multivessel noninfarct disease after successful primary PCI (COR 2a).[21] Patients who receive incomplete revascularization often present with more complex comorbidities, such as advanced age, diabetes, renal failure, previous MI, reduced left ventricular function, and complex or prohibitive coronary anatomy. These factors can inherently influence the decision-making process and feasibility of achieving CR, thereby potentially affecting patient outcomes.[67,68,153]

TECHNICAL ASPECTS OF REOPERATIVE CORONARY ARTERY BYPASS GRAFTING

Surgical revascularization after a previous CABG presents several unique technical challenges that are complex and multifaceted. These difficulties stem from anatomic and physiologic changes, including scar tissue and adhesions around the heart and great vessels, which makes sternal reentry risky because any structure can be adherent to the posterior table of the sternum. Scar tissue and adhesions also make the identification of structures challenging, putting previously placed bypass grafts at risk. The LIMA is at significant risk of injury with redo sternotomy because of its course along or beneath the left side of the sternum. In addition, patients undergoing repeat revascularization often have a higher-risk profile, including advanced age, comorbidities, and a greater extent of CAD. Hence, these patients face greater risks with redo CABG, including increased rates of in-hospital death and stroke, compared with those undergoing PCI. As a result, PCI is generally favored over redo CABG for revascularization, particularly when a LIMA-to-LAD bypass is not planned or if a patent LIMA-LAD graft already exists.[21] Although some observational studies suggest that redo CABG might offer better long-term outcomes than PCI, these findings are inconsistent and not conclusively supported by high-quality RCTs. In sum, according to the 2021 ACC/AHA/SCAI Guideline on Coronary Artery Revascularization, in patients with previous CABG who require repeat revascularization, PCI may be preferable to CABG if they have a patent LIMA-LAD graft (Class 2a).[14] For those with previous CABG who suffer from refractory angina as a result of LAD disease despite GDMT, selecting CABG over PCI is advisable if an IMA can be used as a graft to the LAD (Class 2a).[21] Additionally, in cases of complex CAD after a prior CABG, choosing CABG over PCI may be a reasonable approach when an IMA graft to the LAD is possible (Class 2b).[21]

ADJUNCTS TO CORONARY ARTERY BYPASS GRAFTING

Various adjuncts play crucial roles in enhancing the safety, efficacy, and long-term success of CABG. These include pharmacologic agents, such as antiplatelet therapy to prevent graft thrombosis and statins for lipid control, which are essential in improving graft patency and reducing cardiovascular events postsurgery. Intraoperative

placement of mechanical circulatory support devices, such as the IABP, can provide hemodynamic augmentation in high-risk patients. Additionally, technologic advances, such as endoscopic vessel harvesting and anastomotic devices, may offer certain advantages.[154]

Imaging strategies, including epiaortic ultrasonography (EAU), transesophageal echocardiography (TEE), and intraoperative graft flow assessment, are essential adjuncts to safe and effective CABG. Postoperative care, including strict glycemic control and rehabilitation programs, also plays a pivotal role in patient recovery and long-term well-being. These adjuncts, when effectively integrated into CABG procedures, significantly contribute to optimizing patient outcomes and improving the overall success of surgical coronary revascularization.[21,25]

Epiaortic Ultrasonography

EAU has become an increasingly important adjunct in CABG surgery, particularly in reducing the risk of perioperative stroke. It offers a more accurate assessment of the ascending aorta anatomy and atherosclerotic disease compared with traditional methods of palpation or TEE.[155-157] Given that microembolic and macroembolic strokes are often associated with aortic manipulation during surgery, the use of EAU to guide cannulation, decisions about aortic cross-clamping, and aortocoronary anastomosis placement is clinically valuable. When the ascending aorta is unsuitable for both cross-clamp and cardioplegia catheter placement, surgeons can employ the off-pump or on-pump beating technique.[155-158] This method becomes particularly relevant when the entire aortic surface precludes cannulation, necessitating alternative approaches. In such instances, a "no-touch" technique is advisable, wherein the femoral, innominate, or axillary artery is employed for arterial inflow during CPB. This approach is complemented by originating proximal anastomoses from one or both IMAs. This flexibility in cannulation strategies underscores the importance of adaptive surgical techniques in managing complex cardiac surgical cases. The European Multicenter Study on Coronary Artery Bypass Grafting (E-CABG) registry investigated the impact of EAU-guided aortic manipulation on outcomes after isolated CABG. The study included 673 patients out of 7241 (9.3%) who underwent intraoperative EAU. Overall, the rate of stroke in patients who had aortic manipulation without the use of EAU was 1.4% versus 0.6% in patients whose aortic manipulation was EAU guided.[157] In 660 propensity-matched pairs, there was a significant association between EAU-guided aortic manipulation and a reduced risk of stroke (0.6% vs. 2.6%, $p = 0.007$).[157] A systematic review and meta-analysis, incorporating this and other studies, further substantiated these findings.[159] The pooled data from these studies, which included 11,496 patients, of whom 3026 (25.7%) underwent intraoperative EAU, demonstrated a significantly lower rate of postoperative stroke in patients with EAU-guided aortic manipulation compared with those without (0.6% vs. 1.9%, RR 0.40, 95% CI 0.24–0.66). Therefore, the 2021 ACC/AHA/SCAI Guideline for Coronary Artery Revascularization includes a COR 2a recommendation for the routine use of EAU to assess for the presence, severity, and location of plaque in the ascending aorta during CABG to reduce embolic events.[21]

Transesophageal Echocardiography

Beyond the assessment of LVEF, TEE can help evaluate ventricular wall motion abnormalities, congenital and acquired heart defects (patent foramen ovale, tumors, etc.), and valvular pathologies that may affect the outcome of a planned CABG.[25] Together with the use of intraoperative transit time flow measurement, TEE assessment of ventricular wall motion can inform decisions regarding the need for intraoperative revision of bypass grafts.[160] TEE can also guide pharmacologic management and facilitate weaning from CPB by detecting intracardiac air and new wall motion abnormalities. The use of intraoperative TEE during CABG has been the subject of various studies, highlighting its impact on surgical decision-making and outcomes.[25,158–162]

A comprehensive retrospective analysis of more than 1.25 million planned CABG procedures across 1218 centers evaluated the impact of intraoperative TEE on clinical decision-making and postoperative mortality. The study found that intraoperative TEE was used in 53.9% of CABG cases and was associated with lower odds of postoperative mortality, particularly in higher-risk patients (adjusted OR 0.95, 95% CI 0.91–0.99, $p = 0.025$). Interestingly, the use of intraoperative TEE was associated with an increased likelihood of unplanned valve procedures during CABG (adjusted OR 4.98, 95% CI 3.98–6.22, $p < 0.0001$).[59] The 2021 ACC/AHA/SCAI Guideline for Coronary Artery Revascularization recognized the importance of using TEE for the real-time assessment of patients undergoing combined CABG and valvular procedures. However, the guideline notes that the use of TEE is less frequent in isolated CABG cases, but it clearly has a role in influencing surgical decisions as well as hemodynamic status assessment in CABG patients.[21,162]

Inotropes and Pharmacotherapy After Coronary Artery Bypass Grafting

The value of high-quality medical and critical care management of patients after CABG cannot be overstated. A myriad of pharmacotherapy is commonly prescribed for the pre-, intra-, and postoperative phases of care. Summarized in Table 111.5 are some of the key inotropes and other medications used as adjuncts in CABG.

Intraaortic Balloon Pump

The IABP plays a critical role in CABG surgery, particularly for high-risk patients. It operates by counterpulsation in synchrony with the cardiac cycle. During diastole, the IABP inflates, increasing coronary perfusion by raising diastolic pressure. Conversely, it deflates just before systole, reducing LV afterload and thereby enhancing cardiac output and reducing myocardial oxygen demand.

Importantly, IABP is strictly contraindicated in patients with conditions like aortic regurgitation and aortic dissection, and its use is relatively contraindicated in those with PVD or abdominal aortic aneurysm. A meta-analysis of randomized trials and prospective study designs assessed the outcomes of preemptive IABP use in high-risk CABG patients. The analysis included 1171 subjects from nine RCTs, revealing significantly lower mortality and MACCEs in patients receiving IABP compared with controls ($n = 594$ patients without preoperative IABP). Importantly, the rate of IABP-related complications was 5.6% (17/304), with limb ischemia and insertion site hematoma being the most common complications.[163]

COMPLICATIONS OF CORONARY ARTERY BYPASS SURGERY

The complications of CABG span multiple organ systems and emphasize the necessity of meticulous surgical technique and rigorous postoperative management. Cardiovascular complications such as myocardial stunning, tamponade, and air embolism highlight the importance of adequate myocardial protection, proper surgical techniques, and adequate hemostasis. Pulmonary and central nervous system adverse events underscore the need for

preoperative assessments and careful monitoring, whereas renal and hematologic complications call for vigilant management to prevent negative outcomes. The prevention strategies emphasize the role of careful patient evaluation, precise surgical practice, and tailored postoperative care to mitigate these risks. These complications are summarized in Table 111.6.

CORONARY ARTERY BYPASS GRAFTING AND SPECIAL POPULATIONS OF PATIENTS

Females

The clinical presentation of ACS often differs between males and females. Females are more likely to present with atypical symptoms, such as nausea, vomiting, mid-epigastric discomfort, or sharp (atypical) chest pain. Several landmark trials have shown significant sex differences in the clinical presentation of ACS, including the Women's Ischemia Syndrome Evaluation (WISE) trial,[164] the Can Rapid Risk Stratification of Unstable Angina Patients (CRUSADE) trial,[165] the Variation in Recovery: Role of Gender on Outcomes of Young AMI Patients (VIRGO) trial,[166] and the International Survey of Acute Coronary Syndromes in Transitional Countries (ISACS-TC) trial.[167] For example, in the WISE study, females had a higher 30-day post-ACS mortality rate compared with males (9.6% vs. 5.3%, OR 1.91). Females also experienced more persistent chest pain and frequent hospitalizations, with lower well-being scores and higher daily activity limitations. These outcomes occurred despite females having lower SYNTAX scores. Remarkably, more than 50% of females with ACS symptoms showed no obstructive coronary disease during coronary angiography. The 2021 ACC/AHA/SCAI Guideline for Coronary Artery Revascularization recommends taking these factors into consideration when dealing with females presenting with symptoms suggestive of CAD.[21]

Pregnant Patients

Although the incidence of CAD and AMI in females of childbearing age is generally low, pregnancy has been associated with up to a fourfold increase in the risk of AMI compared with nonpregnant females.[166,168–172] The incidence of pregnancy-associated MI (PAMI) ranges from 2.8 to 8.1 AMI events per 100,000/deliveries, with a significant increase in risk for females over 35 and those with preexisting conditions such as hypertension, diabetes, or a history of smoking.[170,171] The case fatality rate for AMI in pregnancy is reported to be 5.1% to 37%. In addition to threatening the life of the mother, PAMI and other cardiovascular complications of pregnancy, including spontaneous coronary artery dissection (SCAD) and hypertension, pose a significant risk of fetal loss. Importantly, the prevalence of hypertensive disorders in pregnancy has been linked to future maternal cardiovascular risk.[168]

Managing pregnant females with CAD requires a multidisciplinary approach. Guidelines stress the importance of prepregnancy risk assessment and counseling.[21] For females with known CAD or at high risk, careful monitoring and management of risk factors are essential.[21,169,170] Therapeutic strategies should balance maternal and fetal safety while considering medication teratogenicity.

In cases of AMI, treatment protocols similar to those for nonpregnant populations are recommended, with adaptations for fetal safety.[169,170] Treatment should never be delayed in pregnant females presenting with STEMI because of radiation concerns. The standard revascularization goal of <90 minutes from first medical contact to device should be maintained, and PCI

TABLE 111.5 Commonly Used Pharmacotherapies in CABG Patients

DRUG (GENERIC AND TRADE NAMES)	MECHANISM OF ACTION/ALERTS	INDICATIONS	INTRAVENOUS DOSAGE
Dopamine (Intropin)	Stimulates β_1-adrenergic and dopaminergic receptors; at high doses, α-adrenergic effects (arterial vasoconstriction). Known to increase myocardial O_2 consumption. Worse outcomes in shock compared with epinephrine.	Low cardiac output	1–25 mcg/kg/min
Dobutamine (Dobutrex)	Selective β_1-adrenergic agonist with mild β_2 and α_1 effects (inodilator). Can increase myocardial O_2 consumption.	Cardiac support in low-cardiac-output states	2.5–25 mcg/kg/min
Epinephrine (Adrenalin)	α- and β-adrenergic agonist	Severe hypotension, cardiac arrest	0.01–0.25 mcg/kg/min
Norepinephrine (Levophed)	Potent α-adrenergic agonist with mild β-adrenergic effects	Hypotension not responsive to other inotropes	0.01–0.4 mcg/kg/min
Phenylephrine Neo-synephrine)	Catecholamine, pure α-agonist	Severe vasoplegia, hemodynamically significant LVOT obstruction	0.1–4 mcg/kg/min
Isoproterenol (Isuprel)	Pure β-agonist; predominantly increases heart rate, with an associated increase in contractility	Symptomatic bradycardia, including prevention of bradycardic-dependent arrhythmias (torsades de pointes)	0.02–0.2 mcg/kg/min
Milrinone (Primacor)	Phosphodiesterase-3 inhibitor; increases cAMP, leading to vasodilation and inotropy	Heart failure, low-cardiac-output syndrome	0.125–0.75 mcg/kg/min
Vasopressin (Pitressin)	Vasopressin V1 receptor agonist; increases vascular smooth muscle contraction	Vasodilatory shock, especially septic shock	0.01–0.04 units/min
Nitroglycerin	Nitric oxide donor, causing vasodilation	Myocardial ischemia, hypertension, heart failure	5–400 kg/min
Nitroprusside (Nipride)	Nitric oxide donor, strong vasodilator	Hypertensive urgency or emergency, critical blood pressure control in acute aortic dissection	0.1–10 mcg/kg/min
Amiodarone	Class III antiarrhythmic prolongs cardiac action potential. Known to potentiate warfarin in postoperative period and synergistic with other QT-prolonging medications. Beware of torsades de pointes.	Atrial and ventricular arrhythmias	Loading: 150 mg over 10 min Maintenance: 1 mg/min for 6 hours, then 0.5 mg/min × 18 hours
Lidocaine	Class Ib antiarrhythmic; blocks sodium channels	Ventricular arrhythmias	Bolus: 1–1.5 mg/kg Infusion: 1–4 mg/min
β-Blockers (e.g., Metoprolol tartrate)	Blocks β-adrenergic receptors, reducing heart rate and contractility	Tachyarrhythmias, especially atrial fibrillation rate control	Varies based on drug, e.g., Metoprolol: 5 mg every 5 minutes up to 3 doses
Furosemide	Loop diuretic; inhibits Na-K-2Cl cotransporter in the loop of Henle	Fluid overload, acute pulmonary edema; most administered diuretic after CABG	10–40 mg IV, 20–40 mg PO 1–2 times daily; may be repeated or increased as needed

Note: It is prudent to use clinical judgment in evaluating the appropriateness and dosing of these medications for individual patients after CABG. *CABG*, Coronary artery bypass graft; *cAMP*, CYCLIC adenosine monophosphate; *LVOT*, left ventricular outflow tract; *O2*, oxygen; *Na-K-2Cl*, sodium-potassium-chloride cotransporter; *PO*, per os (by mouth).
Modified from Chinedozi ID, Smith N, Metkus TS, Whiteman GJR. Cardiac pharmacology. In: *STS Cardiothoracic Surgery E-Book*. Society of Thoracic Surgeons; 2023. Used with permission.

can be performed once SCAD has been ruled out (COR 2a).[21] Fibrinolytic therapy should only be employed if PCI is not suitable.[169] Furthermore, in pregnant females with NSTE-ACS, an invasive strategy may be employed if medical therapy proves ineffective (COR 2a).[21] Regional anesthesia might be preferred over general anesthesia. Careful positioning is vital to avoid aortocaval compression. The left lateral decubitus position is often recommended. Close monitoring of hemodynamic status is crucial, considering the increased cardiac output and altered vascular resistance in pregnancy. Postoperative care should include careful monitoring for signs of cardiac decompensation, given the increased cardiovascular demands during the postpartum period.[169,171,172]

CABG in pregnant patients is complex, with specific indications for CABG involving hemodynamic instability or ongoing ischemia despite conservative treatment (COR 2a).[21,173] Most SCAD patients improve with conservative management, including aspirin and β-blockers like labetalol, recommended because of its safety in pregnancy. Clopidogrel's use requires careful consideration due to limited safety data in pregnancy. In SCAD cases requiring intervention, CABG has been performed, noting varied fetal outcomes. Given SCAD's high recurrence risk with

TABLE 111.6 **Summary of Common Complications of CABG, Associated Risks and Prevention**

ORGAN SYSTEM	CLINICAL EXAMPLES	ASSOCIATED FEATURES	RISK FACTORS	PREVENTION
Cardiovascular	Myocardial stunning	Postischemic contractile dysfunction seen in 10%–70% of patients. Associated with up to 17% mortality in some series.[121]	Fluid overload and edema, inadequate myocardial protection during aortic cross clamp, effect of global ischemia imposed upon heart during cardioplegia arrest	Ensure adequate myocardial protection during arrest (frequent and complete cardioplegia administration); minimize CPB time.[121]
	Air embolism	Rapid cardiovascular collapse	Improper cannulation or de-airing techniques; use of central venous catheters; structural heart defects (PFO)	Follow the best surgical practices. For air in the aortic cannula, promptly identify air embolism, and stop the pump immediately. Clamp both arterial and venous lines, place patient in Trendelenburg position, ventilate with 100% O_2, and remove aortic cannula to de-air aorta. Place arterial cannula in SVC for RCP, clamping SVC proximally. Manually compress the heart and carotids and reinitiate CPB at higher pressures when de-aired.[124]
	Injuries to vessels and other heart structures (e.g., coronary sinus perforation, left ventricular perforation from venting, sinus node injuries)	Significant hemorrhage and arrhythmias may result from inadvertent coronary sinus perforation during retrograde catheter placement. LV may be perforated from LV vent placement. Injury to conduction system by sutures for tricuspid, mitral, or aortic valve procedures.	Emergency or urgent cases (crashing onto bypass); purse-string sutures under tension or excessive retraction; prolonged CPB time, poor preoperative ventricular function[121]	Good exposure for cannula placement and verification before use; epiaortic US for cannula placement[121]
	Postoperative arrhythmias	SVTs, AF, VT, and heart block	History of arrhythmias (e.g., AF), electrolyte imbalance, surgical trauma and manipulation, intracoronary air embolism, and ischemic injury	Minimize surgical trauma and manipulation; strict adherence to electrolyte monitoring and replacement. β-blockade.
	Graft failure Coronary spasm	Decreased graft flow on imaging, new wall motion abnormalities on echo, or new evidence of myocardial ischemia	Poor target artery quality, small graft or target artery diameter, smoking, DM, HLD	Choice of graft (arterial grafts like the LITA have better long-term patency compared with vein grafts) and management of risk, such as HLD, HTN, DM
	Bleeding Tamponade Delayed tamponade	Pericardial effusion on echo; labs may show dropping hemoglobin level; acute hypotension, muffled heart sounds, JVD	Use of anticoagulants, surgical technique, preexisting coagulopathies	Meticulous technique, careful postoperative anticoagulation management, close monitoring for signs of bleeding
Pulmonary (most injured organ)	Atelectasis Pleural effusion Pulmonary edema Pneumonia	Difficulty liberating from the ventilator, early postoperative fever, poor oxygenation status	Preexisting lung disease (COPD), advanced age, prolonged ischemic or CPB time (>120 minutes), preferential ventilation of nondependent lung segments; phrenic nerve injury[124]	Early postoperative detection and respiratory physiotherapy; early ambulation; ventilation with PEEP
	Acute respiratory distress syndrome	Rapid-onset hypoxemia with significant reduction in Pao_2/Fio_2 ratio <200 mm Hg; diffuse pulmonary infiltrates on chest radiograph	Poor preoperative nutritional status, prolonged ischemia or CPB time, diabetes and postoperative APACHE II score, emergency surgery[122,123]	Some RCTs and other observational studies have yielded conflicting results about low-frequency lung-protective mechanical ventilation during CABG.[126]
	Respiratory failure Prolonged ventilation	Pulmonary edema, atelectasis, pneumonia	Chronic lung disease, smoking history, obesity, lengthy surgery, advanced age	Preoperative pulmonary evaluation and optimization, smoking cessation, early mobilization, respiratory therapy pre- and postoperatively

TABLE 111.6   Summary of Common Complications of CABG, Associated Risks and Prevention—cont'd

ORGAN SYSTEM	CLINICAL EXAMPLES	ASSOCIATED FEATURES	RISK FACTORS	PREVENTION
Central nervous system	Acute delirium Encephalopathy Stroke Memory deficits	Deficits may be subtle and difficult to quantify and categorize in the acute setting.	Aortic surgery and surgery requiring deep hypothermic circulatory arrest Prolonged regional or global hypoperfusion, microembolic phenomenon (gas, lipid, atheroma, bone marrow, glove powder, blood cells or fibrin, PVC tubing particles) or hemorrhage[124]	Address carotid disease before CABG; limit total ischemia time; avoid bypass manipulation and limiting drug administration or blood sample acquisition through the CPB circuit; no-touch technique for calcific aorta; judicious de-airing technique.[121]
Endocrine	Adrenergic overstimulation Stress-induced hyperglycemia Postoperative insulin resistance	Postoperative hyperglycemia that may be require insulin administration; nonthyroidal illness syndrome (low T3, low or normal T4, normal or slightly elevated TSH)[124]	Preexisting endocrine disorders (diabetes, thyroid disease), obesity, chronic kidney disease, history of corticosteroid use, prolonged CPB time, low-cardiac-output syndrome	Preoperative assessment, regular monitoring, and early consultation with endocrinologist
Renal complications	AKI (elevated creatinine and BUN) Progression to CKD or ESRD	AKI is associated with twentyfold increase in mortality or morbidity[121]	Preexisting kidney disease, hypertension, advanced age, DM, heart failure, use of IABP, nephrotoxic medications, obesity, emergency surgery	Maintain acceptable cardiac index and MAP, optimal glucose control, perioperative fluid management and minimize the use of nephrotoxic agents.
Hematologic complications	Coagulopathy Hemorrhage Anemia	Prolonged bleeding (e.g., CT drainage >200–300 mL/h) for first 1–3 hours postoperatively or sustained high output (>100–150 mL/h × 3–6 hours, or >1–1.5 L within 24 hours) or continued transfusion requirement	Intraoperative and postoperative hypothermia, inadequate hemostasis before sternal closure, CKD, preoperative use of anticoagulants or antiplatelets, massive transfusion, repeat CABG, emergency surgery, advanced age, liver disease, and inflammation/sepsis	Preoperative medication review, meticulous surgical technique, careful management of CPB and temperature
Immuno-allergic complications	Whole body inflammation cascade associated with CPB involves anaphylatoxins; cytokines TNF-α, IL-6, IL-8, and IL-10; endotoxins; and kallikrein-bradykinin reactants[124]	Increased vascular permeability, platelet aggregation. and SIRS varies by magnitude and has been shown to influence clinical outcomes after CPB.		
	Heparin-induced thrombocytopenia	IgG antibodies against complexes of heparin and PF4 Leads to thrombocytopenia and thrombosis	Previous exposure to UFH, prolonged or high-dose heparin exposure, females	Early recognition, minimizing heparin exposure, use of nonheparin anticoagulants or factor Xa inhibitors in patients with history of HIT, monitoring platelet count
Infection	Superficial wound infection Deep sternal wound infection Mediastinitis	Fever, erythema, purulence from wound site, and instability of the sternal wound	Obesity, smoking, DM, use of BIMA, prolonged ICU stay	Preincisional antibiotics, meticulous glucose control, smoking cessation
Gastrointestinal	Bowel ischemia Gastritis Hepatic dysfunction	Abdominal pain, nausea, gastrointestinal bleeding, ileus	Low cardiac output, prior gastrointestinal issues, medication side effects	Adequate hydration, early mobilization, monitoring and managing cardiac output and medication effects

AF, Atrial fibrillation; *AKI,* acute kidney injury; *APACHE,* acute physiology and chronic health evaluation; *BIMA,* bilateral internal mammary artery; *BUN,* blood urea nitrogen; *CABG,* coronary artery bypass graft; *CKD,* chronic kidney disease; *COPD,* chronic obstructive pulmonary disease; *CPB,* cardiopulmonary bypass; *CT,* computed tomography; *DM,* diabetes mellitus; *ESRD,* end-stage renal disease; *HIT,* heparin-induced thrombocytopenia; *HLD,* hyperlipidemia; *HTN,* hypertension; *IABP,* intraaortic balloon pump;, *ICU,* intensive care unit; *IgG,* immunoglobulin G; *IL,* interleukin; *JVD,* jugular venous distention; *LITA,* left internal thoracic artery; *LV,* left ventricle; *MAP,* mean arterial pressure; *PEEP,* positive end-expiratory pressure; *PF4,* platelet factor 4; *PFO,* patent foramen ovale; *PVC,* polyvinyl chloride; *RCP,* retrograde cerebral perfusion; *RCT,* randomized controlled trial; *SIRS,* systemic inflammatory response; *SVC,* superior vena cava; *SVT,* supraventricular tachycardia; *TNFα,* tumor necrosis factor alpha; *TSH,* thyroid stimulating hormone; *UFH,* unfractionated heparin; *US,* ultrasonography; *VT,* ventricular tachycardia.
Data from Lawton JS and Gay WA. Complications of Extracorporeal Circulation in Complications in Surgery, 2nd ed, Lippincott, Williams,& Wilkins; Philadelphia; 2011: 290-297.

subsequent pregnancies, there is an ethical consideration regarding future pregnancies.[173] In summary, CAD and related cardiovascular diseases in pregnancy, although rare, require vigilant management and an understanding of the unique physiologic changes during pregnancy. Multidisciplinary care and adherence to guidelines are key in optimizing outcomes for both mother and fetus.

Patients With Diabetes

CAD is notably more prevalent in patients with diabetes and is associated with a tendency toward multivessel disease and an elevated risk of postoperative complications.[72,86,87] The pathophysiology of CAD in diabetic patients is complex and multifaceted. Hyperglycemia induces endothelial dysfunction, whereas dyslipidemia and chronic inflammation contribute to accelerated plaque formation and vascular complications. The management of CAD in diabetes involves comprehensive strategies, including aggressive control of blood glucose and lipid levels, hypertension management, lifestyle modifications, and pharmacotherapy to reduce cardiovascular risk factors.[21]

CABG and PCI are the primary revascularization techniques for CAD. Recent studies and guidelines favor CABG for diabetic patients with multivessel CAD because of its superior outcomes of mortality reduction and lower incidence of major cardiac events.[21,86,87] Research indicates that patient sex may influence outcomes in those with diabetes undergoing revascularization. Females with diabetes undergoing CABG may experience different long-term outcomes compared with their male counterparts, highlighting the need for sex-specific considerations in treatment planning. Postoperative complications, such as renal injury, prolonged intensive care unit (ICU) stay, and increased revascularization rates, are more common in diabetic patients. These challenges necessitate careful perioperative management, with a focus on glycemic control and cardiac function monitoring.[87]

In summary, diabetic patients with CAD require an integrated, multidisciplinary approach for optimal outcomes. Although CABG is generally favored for its long-term benefits in diabetic patients with complex multivessel disease (COR 1), as noted previously, individual patient characteristics, including sex and specific comorbidities, should guide treatment decisions.[21,174]

Patients With Renal Disease

Heart surgeons must confront the formidable challenge of managing CAD patients with concurrent CKD. In fact, patients with CKD have a notably higher prevalence of CAD due to shared risk factors, including hypertension, diabetes, and dyslipidemia.[175,176] In addition to the traditional risk factors for CAD, uremia and various microvascular changes in CKD patients exacerbate atherosclerosis by promoting inflammation, oxidative stress, vascular calcification, and endothelial dysfunction. Impaired renal function leads to fluid overload and hypertension, increasing cardiac workload and risk of coronary ischemia.[177]

A landmark study conducted by Alan S. Go et al. (2004) assessed the impact of varying degrees of kidney dysfunction on death, cardiovascular events, and hospitalization risks. The study followed over 1.1 million adults, finding a graded increase in risk of adverse outcomes with decreasing glomerular filtration rate (GFR). Key findings included a substantial rise in death risk and cardiovascular events for patients with a GFR below 60 mL/min/1.73 m², with risks sharply intensifying below 45 mL/min/1.73 m². The study underlined the clinical and public health importance of chronic renal insufficiency, especially in the context of cardiovascular

disease.[178] Diagnosing CAD in CKD patients is complicated because of the reduced sensitivity and specificity of traditional tools. Coronary angiography and revascularization, despite their risks, remain the gold standards for diagnosing and treating diabetic patients with STEMI, with caution regarding contrast-induced nephropathy (CIN; COR 1).[21,174] Furthermore, in high-risk CKD patients with NSTE-ACS, coronary angiography and revascularization are reasonable (COR 2a).[21]

CAD in CKD involves balancing renal function preservation and cardiac event prevention. Pharmacotherapy often requires dosing adjustments in CKD. The 2021 ACC/AHA/SCAI Guideline for Coronary Artery Revascularization and the 2023 AHA/ACC/ACCP/ASPC/NLA/PCNA Guideline for the Management of Patients With Chronic Coronary Disease consolidate the latest evidence on managing patients with CAD and CKD and provide a patient-centered approach, integrating new therapeutic advances and emphasizing the importance of managing complex cases where coronary disease intersects with renal impairment. They highlight the necessity of a holistic approach in managing CCD, considering factors like renal function that significantly affect treatment outcomes and patient quality of life. Between PCI and CABG, CABG is often preferred in severe CKD for its long-term benefits despite initial risks.[21,174]

The 2021 ACC/AHA/SCAI Guideline for Coronary Artery Revascularization recommends renoprotective strategies, such as minimizing nephrotoxic agents and contract media exposure, in patients with CKD presenting with CAD (COR 1). However, coronary angiography and revascularization remain crucial in these patients. Hydration and use of N-acetylcysteine (NAC) may help prevent CIN, but some studies have presented conflicting benefits of NAC.[179,180] Furthermore, in dialysis patients, timing of surgery relative to dialysis sessions is important because preoperative dialysis may help remove excess fluid and uremic toxins. As such, a multidisciplinary approach involving cardiologists, nephrologists, cardiac surgeons, and intensivists is necessary because of the complex interplay between cardiac and renal function.[21,174]

Obese Patients

Obesity is strongly associated with the prognosis of atherosclerosis, a hallmark of CAD. In fact, over 80% of patients with coronary heart disease are overweight (BMI >25) or obese (BMI >30).[181] Adipose tissue, beyond its role in lipid storage, secretes cytokines known as *adipokines,* influencing whole body metabolism, inflammation, and endocrine functions. Adipokines play vital roles in the development, progression, and regression of atherosclerosis.[182]

Diagnosing CAD in obese patients is challenging. The sensitivity and specificity of traditional noninvasive tests, such as treadmill stress testing, are reduced in this population. Obesity can also limit the diagnostic utility of imaging modalities because of technical limitations and reduced image quality. Consequently, clinicians often need to rely on more advanced diagnostic techniques, such as CCTA or invasive coronary angiography, for accurate assessment.[21,174]

In addition to the technical challenges of performing CABG in obese patients, these patients often have a higher burden of comorbidities, such as diabetes and hypertension, which complicates perioperative management. The presence of thickened myocardium and epicardial fat can make surgical access and grafting more difficult. Additionally, obese patients have an increased risk of wound infection and slower recovery after surgery.[181,183]

The clinical outcomes of CABG in obese patients are nuanced. Although obesity is associated with an increased risk of perioperative complications, studies have shown a paradoxical survival benefit in obese patients after CABG, known as the *obesity paradox*.[183–185] However, this does not negate the increased risk of postoperative complications such as wound infections, deep vein thrombosis, and prolonged hospital stay.[181,186] A study by Pirlet et al. (2020) included a propensity-matched cohort of 116 patients with prior bariatric surgery (49 of whom underwent CABG and 67 PCI) compared with a PCI/CABG control group (without history of bariatric surgery). With a median follow-up of 8.9 years, key findings included a lower rate of MACCEs in the bariatric surgery group, driven by a reduction in noncardiac mortality. However, there were no significant differences in all-cause death, cardiac death, MI, stroke, or repeat myocardial revascularization rates. The study concluded that although bariatric surgery may reduce MACCE in obese CAD patients, this effect seems unrelated to direct cardiovascular outcomes.[186]

In conclusion, the management of CAD and the conduct of CABG in obese patients require special consideration because of the unique challenges in diagnosis, technical difficulties in surgery, and the complex interplay of clinical outcomes post-CABG. This emphasizes the need for a tailored approach to treating obese patients with CAD.

Patients 70 Years and Older

By 2030, one in six people will be over 60, and the number of octogenarians is expected to triple by 2050.[187,188] CAD, especially ACS, is a significant cause of death in this group, accounting for a substantial portion of hospitalizations and deaths related to ACS.[167] The aging population faces unique challenges in CAD diagnosis, management, and outcomes because of physiologic changes and comorbidities. In older adults, the pathophysiology of CAD is often compounded by age-related vascular changes, such as increased arterial stiffness, endothelial dysfunction, and a heightened inflammatory state. These factors exacerbate atherosclerotic processes, making older patients more susceptible to ischemic events.[21,174]

Older adults often present with atypical symptoms or may be asymptomatic, complicating ACS diagnosis. Traditional diagnostic tools such as ECG and biomarkers may yield nonspecific results due to age-related changes and comorbid conditions. Hence, a comprehensive approach, including detailed history, physical examination, and judicious use of diagnostic tests, is essential.[21,174]

A review by Chang et al. (2017) involved an individual patient-level meta-analysis, drawing data from the Bypass Surgery Versus Everolimus-Eluting Stent Implantation for Multivessel Coronary Artery Disease (BEST), Premedication for Crossover From Coronary Angioplasty to Surgery (PRECOMBAT), and SYNTAX trials, encompassing a total of 1079 adults aged 70 to 89 years. The primary outcomes were composite of death from any cause, MI, stroke, or repeat revascularization. Over a median follow-up of 4.9 years, the primary composite outcome of all-cause mortality, MI, stroke, or repeat revascularization occurred in 26% of patients in the CABG group and 34% in the PCI group. This indicated a lower risk associated with CABG (HR = 0.75, 95% CI 0.60–0.94, p = 0.012).[189] CABG was associated with fewer MIs and repeat revascularizations but did not significantly affect all-cause mortality or stroke rates. The study found that older adults aged 70 to 89 years with left main or multivessel CAD benefit more from CABG, especially those with high

anatomic risk scores indicated by high SYNTAX scores. The study concluded that in older adults with severe left main or multivessel CAD, CABG may offer a more favorable outcome in reducing MACCEs, particularly in those with more complex disease. However, the study acknowledges limitations due to its nature as a subgroup analysis of randomized clinical trials; potential biases in patient selection; and the inability to include variables, such as frailty, cognitive dysfunction, and multiple comorbidities, that can influence outcomes.[183]

CABG presents unique challenges in the elderly. Age-related anatomic and physiologic changes, such as vessel calcification and reduced organ reserve, increase surgical complexity and risks. The presence of comorbidities such as diabetes, hypertension, and CKD further complicates the procedure, requiring careful preoperative assessment and tailored surgical techniques. Therefore, the ACC/AHA/SCAI Guideline for Coronary Artery Revascularization supports a comprehensive approach to CABG in older patients, incorporating considerations of the patient's preferences, life expectancy, and cognitive function (COR 1).[21]

Patients With Prior History of Coronary Artery Bypass Grafting

Patients undergoing CABG after a previous CABG procedure face distinct challenges and outcomes. Bourassa et al. (2002) demonstrated higher rates of death, MI, and need for revascularization in patients with prior CABG undergoing repeat surgical revascularization.[190] Although they exhibit poorer short-term outcomes, the observed differences may be related to confounding patient-specific comorbidities.[190] Notably, when PCI is performed on native vessels of patients with prior CABG, the adjusted clinical outcomes are similar to those in patients without prior CABG.[184] Interestingly, other studies have found that previous isolated CABG does not independently predict adverse outcomes in patients requiring proximal aortic or arch surgery.[191]

Based on various studies, the 2021 ACC/AHA/SCAI Guideline recommends, as noted previously, PCI over CABG for patients with prior CABG and a patent LIMA to the LAD (COR 2a). In cases of refractory angina despite maximal GDMT, CABG is advised over PCI if the LAD is the culprit lesion and an IMA is available for grafting (COR 2a). CABG is also considered in patients with complex CAD after CABG when an IMA can be used as a conduit (COR 2b).[21]

Revascularization Before Noncardiac Surgery

In 2006, the Coronary Artery Revascularization Prophylaxis (CARP) trial showed no survival benefits with preoperative coronary revascularization before elective vascular surgery in patients with concomitant ischemic CAD.[191] A follow-up study by Garcia et al. (2008) evaluated the impact of prophylactic coronary revascularization on long-term survival in patients with multivessel CAD undergoing elective vascular surgery. The study involved 1048 patients who underwent coronary angiography before vascular surgery as part of the CARP trial. It found that preoperative revascularization improved survival in patients with LMCA stenosis but not in those with either two-vessel or three-vessel disease. The study concluded that unprotected LMCA disease, present in 4.6% of the patients, was the only subset showing benefit from preoperative coronary artery revascularization.[192] Based on these and other studies, routine coronary revascularization in patients with non–left main or noncomplex CAD in preparation for another noncardiac surgery is not recommended (COR 3, no benefit).[21,174]

Patients Undergoing Other Cardiac Surgeries

Adding CABG to other cardiac procedures for patients with CAD should only be considered after important clinical factors have been thoroughly evaluated. These deliberations extend beyond patient comorbidities and include the technical aspects and feasibility of CABG, the degree of myocardial compromise, and conduit availability. Furthermore, the 2021 ACC/AHA/SCAI Guideline for Coronary Artery Revascularization recommends considering the patient's LVEF and the potential harm that extra CPB time necessary to add CABG may contribute to the procedure. As such, in patients with significant CAD who are undergoing valvular or aortic surgery, there is a COR 1 recommendation to add CABG to reduce MACEs. On the other hand, in patients with intermediate CAD, it may be reasonable to include CABG (COR 2a).[21,174] It is noteworthy to mention that age ≥85 years is an additional risk factor for worse clinical outcomes in patients undergoing concomitant CABG and other cardiac surgeries.[193]

Patients With Previous Heart Transplant

Cardiac allograft vasculopathy (CAV), a condition marked by extensive intimal hyperplasia, significantly contributes to the incidence of AMI and mortality after the first year of heart transplantation.[194] This condition poses a substantial challenge for cardiac surgeons. Current therapeutic options for CAV are notably limited. Although retransplantation remains the definitive treatment, obstacles such as the shortage of donor hearts and less favorable outcomes compared with the initial transplantation significantly impede its viability. For localized manifestations of CAV, the ACC/AHA/SCAI Guideline for Coronary Artery Revascularization offers a COR 2a recommendation for PCI as reasonable in patients with severe, proximal, discrete coronary lesions (and largely as a palliative measure), noting that stent implantation during PCI is associated with lower rates of perioperative and intermediate-term mortality compared with balloon angioplasty.[21,174]

Patients Pre– or Post–Lung Transplantation

CAD is often a comorbidity in candidates for lung transplantation. Studies have suggested that the presence of CAD at the time of lung transplantation does not meaningfully affect retransplant-free survival. However, greater technical complexity is noted in patients who underwent CABG before lung transplantation.[195] Notably, the STS recognizes a history of CABG as a relative contraindication for lung transplantation because of the observed increased risk of bleeding and death in these patients.[196] However, some series and observational studies have shown that this purported risk may not exist in patients receiving a single as opposed to double lung transplant.[197] Furthermore, the safety and feasibility of performing CABG at the time of lung transplantation have been widely reported.[198]

CABG post–lung transplantation presents a spectrum of technical challenges because of the presumed need for complex redo sternotomy and the dearth of evidence in the literature for best clinical practices. A PubMed, Semantic Scholar, and Google Scholar search on this topic yielded a brief abstract of a single case report by Harrison et al. (1997) for which there is no manuscript available electronically.[199] One case report by Larson et al. (2023) described a patient with ACS 15 years after concomitant CABG and bilateral lung transplant (BOLT) who underwent redo sternotomy for redo CABG that was complicated by dense mediastinal and pleural adhesions and had an acceptable recovery.[200]

Given that concomitant CABG card lung transplantation have become increasingly common with improvement in posttransplant immunosuppression and survival, the need for coronary re-revascularization in this patient population is expected to rise. As such, it is imperative for society guidelines to include recommendations and best practices for these unique patients.

Patients With Coronary Artery Aneurysm

A coronary artery is said to be aneurysmal when there is a minimum of 1.3 to 2 times luminal dilatation compared with an adjacent, normal arterial segment.[201] Coronary artery aneurysms and fistulae can be rare complications of coronary angiography but can also result from Kawasaki disease and Takayasu arteritis, with a reported estimated incidence of 0.02% to 0.2%.[202] Although most patients are asymptomatic, a number of complications can result, including vessel thrombosis, ischemia, fistula formation, and rupture. Several treatment strategies have been suggested in case reports, including stent placement, Amplatzer device deployment, and surgical bypass or exclusion of the aneurysmal segment; however, there are insufficient data to recommend one treatment over another.[202]

Patients With Anomalous Aortic Origin of a Coronary Artery

Anomalous origin of coronary artery (AAOCA) is among the congenital heart defects that may result in sudden cardiac death in individuals less than 35 years of age.[203]

Based on autopsy results, most patients die in association with periods of physical exertion such as exercise. There is a COR 1 recommendation from the 2018 AHA/ACC Guideline for the Management of Adults With Congenital Heart Disease to use coronary angiography, CT, or functional CMR imaging for diagnosis.[203] Management is complex and includes an assessment of the risk of ischemia and sudden death and the risk of surgical intervention. Surgical treatments range from unroofing to complex patch repair and may include CABG. Recommendations are summarized in the 2018 AHA/ACC Guideline for the Management of Adults With Congenital Heart Disease.[203]

Patients With Myocardial Bridging

Myocardial bridging is another congenital anomaly where myocardial tissue either completely or partially entraps a section of a coronary artery, potentially causing serious cardiac complications such as ischemia, arrhythmia, and sudden death.[21,204] Assessment is made by invasive methods (IVUS and angiography) and noninvasive techniques (Doppler ultrasound, multislice CT, and MRI). If a patient with myocardial bridging presents with ischemia, a baseline FFR may be obtained, followed by repeat FFR after dobutamine provocation. Surgery is reserved for patients with severe myocardial ischemia. There are currently no comprehensive society guidelines for the evaluation and management of CAD in patients with myocardial bridging.[204]

POSTOPERATIVE MANAGEMENT AND DISCHARGE FROM THE INTENSIVE CARE UNIT

CABG patients are admitted to the cardiovascular surgical ICU immediately after surgery. A detailed handoff should be provided by the surgical and anesthesia teams to the provider and nursing teams, followed by performance of a prompt physical exam. Bedside imaging (CXR) is obtained to verify the correct placement of the endotracheal tube, pulmonary artery catheters (if present), chest tube(s), central lines, and any mechanical circulatory devices (e.g., IABP). Special care is taken to identify any pneumothorax, pulmonary edema, hemothorax, or effusions that might be present. Baseline arterial blood gas (ABG) and a complete set of labs are obtained.[5] The ventilator (in patients who remain intubated) is adjusted based on ABG results, avoiding high positive end-expiratory pressure, especially in hemodynamically tenuous patients, as part of a lung-protective ventilation strategy (LPS).[205] Electrolytes are judiciously monitored and repleted as necessary.[5]

The immediate postoperative period after CABG should focus on stabilizing the patient's hemodynamics (cardiac index of >2.2 L/min/m², adequate mean arterial pressure of 60–80 mm Hg, sinus rhythm of 60–100 beats/min) by ensuring proper intravascular volume (preload), normalizing peripheral vascular resistance (PVR), and treating any identified arrhythmias. This often involves administering fluids, blood products, inotropes, or calcium to modulate vascular tone.[5,206] Maintaining a core body temperature above 36.5°C has also been associated with better clinical outcomes, including in-hospital mortality.[207]

Close monitoring of neurologic status and effective pain control are crucial. The use of nonopioid drugs (e.g., acetaminophen, ketamine, dexmedetomidine) and regional analgesia (e.g., truncal nerve blocks), especially when implemented within a multimodal pain management strategy, has demonstrated effectiveness in diminishing the reliance on opioids after cardiac surgery.[208] It is also important to maintain the blood glucose level under 180 mg/dL using continuous insulin infusion, both intraoperatively and in the early postoperative period. This practice has a COR 1 recommendation from the current ACC/AHA/SCAI Guideline for Coronary Artery Revascularization and has been shown to reduce the risk of sternal wound infection.[21,209] Finally, early extubation should be prioritized once the patient is awake and hemodynamically stable with minimal chest tube output. Some centers extubate stable patients in the operating room. Pulmonary hygiene (deep-breathing exercises while maintaining sternal precautions) is important to prevent atelectasis, pneumonia, and reintubation.[210]

Discharging patients from the ICU after CABG necessitates a multifaceted approach, ensuring stability of vital signs and good cardiac and respiratory function as well as confirming proper wound healing and renal function. Before departing the ICU, central lines and catheters are often removed. Chest tubes are removed according to protocols. Ensure minimal chest tube drainage (<400 mL of daily output) and no evidence of clinically significant pulmonary effusion or pneumothorax before removal.[211] It is crucial that the patient demonstrates adequate pain management, gastrointestinal function, and mobility, aligning with their preoperative baseline. Psychological readiness and a strong support system are also important for a smooth transition from ICU care and have been associated with long-term survival after CABG.[212,213]

Finally, a comprehensive review by a multidisciplinary team is essential to validate the patient's readiness for discharge. This process is supported by guidelines from authoritative bodies, including the ACC Foundation, the AHA, and the Enhanced Recovery After Surgery Society, which emphasize a patient-centered approach in the postoperative management and discharge planning for CABG patients.[21,211]

CARDIAC REHABILITATION AND RISK FACTOR MODIFICATION AFTER CORONARY ARTERY BYPASS GRAFTING

Cardiac rehabilitation (CR) post-CABG has been consistently shown to improve patient outcomes, particularly through exercise-based

programs, patient education, and behavior modification.[214] Spiroski et al. (2017) demonstrated that a structured rehabilitation program, including cycling and walking, significantly improved exercise tolerance, respiratory exchange ratios, and peak maximal oxygen uptake (VO₂) in patients after MI and CABG. These benefits were observed after a 3-week inpatient program and continued to improve throughout a 6-month outpatient program, highlighting the sustained positive impact of CR on patient recovery.[215]

Timely access to CR is crucial for maximizing these benefits. In addition to physical activity, CR may assist in fostering adherence to healthy lifestyles and management of chronic and comorbid diseases associated with CAD (diabetes, obesity). Marzolini et al. (2015) showed that the median time from CABG to first CR was approximately 80 days. They identified several demographic, environmental, and physiologic factors contributing to the delay in starting CR. Specifically, older age, female sex, unemployment status, less social support, longer drive time to the CR center, lower neighborhood socioeconomic status, and certain health conditions were associated with longer wait times.[216] Crucially, the study established a clear link between longer wait times and less favorable health outcomes. Extended wait times correlated with less improvement in cardiopulmonary fitness, lower program adherence, increased body fat percentage, and a higher resting heart rate. These findings are pivotal, considering that timely CR has been associated with reduced mortality rates and improved cardiovascular fitness.

Therefore, the 2021 ACC/AHA/SCAI Guideline for Coronary Artery Revascularization has a Class 1, Level A recommendation for CR referral (home or center based) before hospital discharge or during the first outpatient follow-up appointment.[21] Additionally, there is a COR 1 recommendation that all patients should be educated in a timely manner about the need to modify their cardiovascular risk factors after revascularization to reduce further adverse cardiac events. Specifically, patients should understand that continued tobacco use (including e-cigarettes) is a major risk factor for stent thrombosis and other major cardiovascular events.[21]

GUIDELINE-DIRECTED MEDICAL THERAPY AFTER CORONARY REVASCULARIZATION

Antiplatelet Therapy With Aspirin in Coronary Artery Bypass Grafting

Bleeding during and shortly after CABG is a significant concern, making the assessment of bleeding risks critical when considering antiplatelet medications. Historical data indicate that aspirin enhances the patency of vein grafts. A significant body of evidence continues to support the use of aspirin to prevent further ischemic events and maintain graft patency.[217,218] There is a Class 1, Level A recommendation regarding the initiation of aspirin (100–325 mg daily) within 6 hours of CABG. In a subset of patients, DAPT with aspirin and ticagrelor or clopidogrel may be reasonable (COR 2b) to promote vein graft patency.[21]

Use of Oral β-Blocker After Revascularization

There is no evidence to support the chronic use of oral β-blockers after revascularization in patients with SIHD who otherwise have a normal LVEF (COR 3). However, oral β-blockade is highly recommended (COR 1) in the postoperative period after CABG to reduce the incidence and complications of postoperative AF, given that new-onset AF is associated with a fourfold increased risk of stroke.[21,219]

PSYCHOLOGICAL CARE AFTER CORONARY REVASCULARIZATION

Despite the recognition of depression as a prevalent comorbidity after revascularization, affecting up to 20% of patients, its management remains inadequate.[220] This is concerning because depression is a known independent predictor of cardiovascular morbidity, mortality, and increased healthcare costs after revascularization.[213] Based on this, the 2021 ACC/AHA/SCAI Guideline for Coronary Artery Revascularization indicates that it may be reasonable to screen patients who have undergone coronary revascularization and refer and treat them when indicated to improve quality of life and recovery (COR 2b). This recommendation was less strong because of the results of one large trial of 1500 patients with ACS that did not show significant benefits (quality of life, depression-free days, depressive symptoms, mortality rate, or patient-reported harms) after screening and treatment for depression.[221] However, there is a Class 1 recommendation for the treatment of patients (cognitive behavioral therapy, psychological counseling, and/or pharmacologic interventions) who have undergone coronary revascularization and have been diagnosed with depression, anxiety, or stress to improve quality of life and cardiac outcomes.[21]

DISPARITIES IN THE SURGICAL TREATMENT OF CORONARY ARTERY DISEASE

Many studies have described disparities in care delivery and the rates of morbidity and mortality across racial, sex, and ethnic minorities (e.g., Black and South Asian patients have poor cardiovascular outcomes compared with White patients) in the United States.[222] Furthermore, the persistent underrepresentation of minority ethnic groups and females in RCTs calls into question the generalizability of important findings. It is clear that the strongest evidence for guidelines derives from RCTs.[222] For this reason, many have called for practical measures to improve the enrollment and retention of racial and ethnic minorities in clinical trials.[21] In addition, treatment decisions in patients undergoing coronary revascularization should be based on clinical indication, regardless of sex, race, or ethnicity, and efforts to reduce disparities are warranted (COR 1).[21]

IMPORTANCE OF PERFORMANCE MEASURES AND DATABASE PARTICIPATION IN CORONARY REVASCULARIZATION

In cardiac surgery, quality and performance assessments are critical. Although these concepts involve a complex interplay of institutional structure, processes, and patient-specific risk-adjusted outcomes and can seem demanding at times, it is imperative to have surgeon and interventionist understanding and adherence.[59,223] With respect to coronary revascularization, *structure* pertains to the characteristics of the surgeon, interventionist, and clinical team or the environment where the coronary revascularization takes place, acting as the initial platform from which care processes begin. *Process* involves the actual delivery of care (revascularization) and how the specific steps taken during the procedure affect the final result. *Outcomes* represent the final achievements of the procedure (PCI or CABG) and are often seen as the most concrete element in the cycle of enhancing quality.[223] The 2023 AHA/ACC Clinical Performance and Quality Measures for Coronary Artery Revascularization Guideline highlights 15

performance measures, 5 quality measures, and 2 structural measures. The performance and quality measures form the bedrock of the 2021 ACC/AHA/SCAI Guideline for Coronary Revascularization and have been heavily highlighted in this chapter. However, the two structural measures from the Clinical Performance and Quality Measures Guideline focus on (1) the importance of meticulous preprocedural assessment for patients presenting for coronary revascularization and the role of the heart team and (2) the benefit of registry participation.[59]

Among other benefits, performance measures and database affiliation provide clinical benchmarks and promote continuous improvement in patient care. These measures, including morbidity and mortality rate, are directly linked to patient outcomes. The role of specialized databases in CABG surgery is crucial for comprehensive data analysis and benchmarking. Registries such as the STS Adult Cardiac Surgery Database offer extensive data, enabling centers to reference their performance and implement evidence-based strategies to enhance patient care. Participation in such databases ensures that centers are aligned with national and international standards, paving the way for improved patient outcomes and care quality.[21,59]

In summary, performance measures and database participation form the cornerstone of ongoing quality improvement in CABG surgery. These tools not only provide a framework for evaluating and enhancing patient care but also promote a culture of transparency and continuous quality improvement.

ACKNOWLEDGMENT

We would like to acknowledge the previous editors: Shuab Omer, Faisel G. Bakaeen, Scott Weldon, and Michael DeLaflor.

SELECTED REFERENCES

Amsterdam EA, Wenger NK, Brindis RG, et al. 2014 AHA/ACC guideline for the management of patients with non–ST-elevation acute coronary syndromes. *J Am Coll Cardiol*. 2014;64(24): e139-e228.

These guidelines provide evidence-based recommendations for managing patients with NSTE-ACS. They are pivotal for clinicians in making informed decisions about the treatment and management of these patients and were cited frequently throughout this chapter.

Lawton JS, Tamis-Holland JE, Bangalore S, et al. 2021 ACC/AHA/SCAI guideline for coronary artery revascularization: a report of the American College of Cardiology/American Heart Association Joint Committee on Clinical Practice Guidelines. *Circulation*. 2022;145(3):e18-e114.

The latest AHA/ACC guideline on CABG provides comprehensive recommendations for coronary artery revascularization, integrating the latest evidence and expert consensus. It is crucial for guiding clinical practice in the treatment of CAD, highlighting the importance of appropriate revascularization strategies.

Maron DJ, Hochman JS, Reynolds HR, et al. Initial invasive or conservative strategy for stable coronary disease. *N Engl J Med*. 2020;382(15):1395-1407.

This major clinical trial compares the outcomes of invasive versus conservative strategies in patients with stable CAD. Its results have shown significant implications for treatment strategies, influencing how clinicians approach the management of stable CAD.

Takahashi K, Serruys PW, Fuster V, et al. Redevelopment and validation of the SYNTAX score II to individualise decision making between percutaneous and surgical revascularisation in patients with complex coronary artery disease: secondary analysis of the multicentre randomised controlled SYNTAXES trial with external cohort validation. *Lancet.* 2020;396(10260):1399-1412.

This study provides an updated validation for the SYNTAX score II, which helps in individualizing decision-making between percutaneous and surgical revascularization for patients with complex CAD. It is highly cited because of its importance in refining clinical decision-making tools for the management of CAD.

Thygesen K, Alpert JS, Jaffe AS, et al. Fourth universal definition of myocardial infarction (2018). *J Am Coll Cardiol.* 2018;72(18):2231-2264.

This guideline document provides a standardized definition of MI, essential for diagnosing and categorizing heart attacks in clinical practice. It helps provide clarity and uniformity in the diagnosis of MI, which is a critical aspect of CAD management.

Virani SS, Newby LK, Arnold SV, et al. 2023 AHA/ACC/ACCP/ASPC/NLA/PCNA guideline for the management of patients with chronic coronary disease: a report of the American Heart Association/American College of Cardiology Joint Committee on Clinical Practice Guidelines. *Circulation.* 2023;148(9):e12-e56.

This guideline provides the latest evidence-based recommendations for the management of patients with CCD, emphasizing a patient-centered approach and integrating new therapeutic advances.

The full reference list appears on Elsevier eBooks+.

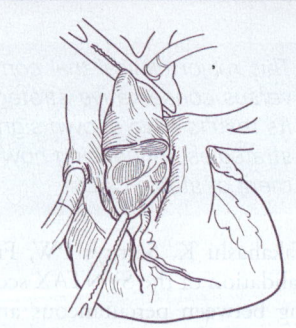

Acquired Heart Disease: Valvular

Marc R. Moon, Puja Kachroo, and Todd K. Rosengart

The heart contains four valves that regulate the directional flow of blood through its chambers. Effective cardiac pumping activity is dependent on the properly timed functioning of these valves. The atrioventricular (AV) valves (mitral and tricuspid) close during systole to prevent backflow into the atria during ventricular ejection. During diastole, the semilunar valves (aortic and pulmonic) close to prevent backflow into the ventricles as they fill from the atria.

The heart beats an average of 100,000 times per day and more than 2.5 billion times over an average lifespan. Given the great number of open-close cycles of the valves and the relative infrequency of cardiac valvular heart disease, a reported prevalence of less than 2% of the population,1 it must be concluded that the valvular structures are exceedingly well adapted to meet these physical demands.

The cardiac valves may, nevertheless, succumb to injury or degeneration as a result of a variety of pathophysiologic processes, and valvular dysfunction can result in significant morbidity and mortality. In the past century, extended life and improved health for millions with cardiac valve disease have been made possible by the advent of open surgical valve repair and replacement procedures, most notably after the widespread application of cardiopulmonary bypass in the 1950s and 1960s. More recently, percutaneous interventions to repair or replace damaged valves have been increasingly used to deliver these benefits without requiring cardiopulmonary bypass.

HISTORY OF HEART VALVE SURGERY

Notwithstanding investigations in the 19th century into the treatment of rheumatic heart disease (RHD), the modern history of heart valve surgery can be traced back to Sir Thomas Lauder Brunton, a Scottish physician. In 1902, he proposed a technique for closed repair of stenotic rheumatic mitral valve (MV) disease with access to the valve gained by passing a dilator through the left ventricular (LV) wall. Unfortunately, this idea was shunned by Brunton's colleagues as reckless and was never attempted clinically. Fortunately, however, Elliot Cutler and Samuel Levine further developed Brunton's early theory and successfully performed the first closed transventricular MV commissurotomy using a tenotomy knife in 1923 after their extensive experimentation in the research laboratories of the Peter Bent Brigham Hospital in Boston. Sir Henry Souttar of England adapted their technique and, in 1925, reported the first successful case of closed digital commissurotomy, inserting the surgeon's index finger through the left atrial (LA) appendage to accomplish mechanical MV dilation. This procedure was not widely adopted until 1948, after reports by Charles Bailey of Philadelphia and Dwight Harken of Boston of clinically successful closed digital mitral commissurotomies (Fig. 112.1).

Blinded aortic valvular surgery followed a similar course. In 1912, Theodore Tuffier of Paris reported the first clinical attempt to dilate a stenotic aortic valve, pushing his finger against the aorta and invaginating the aortic wall through the valve. Mechanical dilation using an instrument passed retrograde from the innominate artery was reported by Lord Russell Brock of London in 1940. Neither of these efforts gained acceptance, but they paved the way for Horace Smithy of Charleston, South Carolina, who performed the first successful aortic valvotomy in 1948. Three years later, Charles Bailey of Philadelphia reported the first successful aortic valvotomy using a transventricular expanding dilator.

Two major advancements occurring in the 20th century marked the beginning of the modern era of "open" heart valve surgery: the development of a prosthetic valve and the advent of cardiopulmonary bypass. The first successful implantation of a prosthetic valve was performed without bypass and was reported by Charles Hufnagel of Georgetown University in 1952. Given the inability to access the aortic valve in situ, Hufnagel implanted a caged-ball valve into the descending aorta in patients with aortic

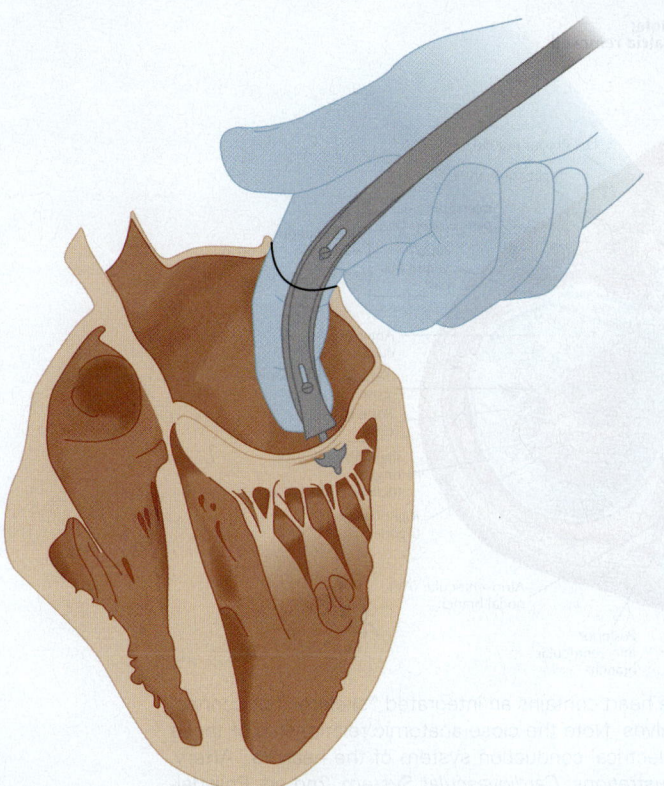

FIGURE 112.1 Closed mitral commissurotomy. Dwight Harken developed a closed mitral commissurotomy procedure to correct rheumatic mitral stenosis, which became the first widespread approach to treating valvular heart disease. (From Muller WH Jr. The surgical treatment of mitral stenosis. *Calif Med.* 1951;75:285-289.)

insufficiency (AI). After the first successful clinical use of cardiopulmonary bypass by John Gibbon at Thomas Jefferson in Philadelphia in 1953, Dwight Harken in 1960 completed the first successful in situ aortic valve replacement using a caged-ball device inserted in place of an excised aortic valve. That same year, Nina Braunwald at Brigham and Women's Hospital in Boston was the first to replace the MV, using a mechanical device made of flexible polyurethane with fabric chordae tendineae. The operation was performed on March 11, 1960, 6 months before Albert Starr and Lowell Edwards in Oregon replaced the MV using a caged-ball prosthesis. Dr. Braunwald was one of the first three females certified by the American Board of Thoracic Surgery in 1961 and, in 1966, was the first female to become a member of the American Association for Thoracic Surgery (AATS), the oldest and most prestigious organization dedicated to surgical diseases of the chest. What followed was an explosion of improvements in prosthetic valve design and surgical implantation techniques, allowing for progressive improvement in outcomes after valve replacement. Next, valve repair was championed by Alain Carpentier of Paris with his Honored Guest Lecture at the AATS Annual Meeting in 1983 titled "Cardiac Valve Surgery—the 'French Correction.'"[2]

In 1986, G. Alain Cribier of Rouen, France, developed and performed the world's first balloon aortic valvuloplasty to treat aortic stenosis, but the long-term results were suboptimal. Stenosis reoccurred fairly rapidly in the majority of patients. Cribier continued to innovate, eventually placing a balloon-expandable stent-mounted prosthetic valve outside a valvuloplasty balloon and inflating it in position at the level of the aortic annulus under

fluoroscopic guidance. In 2002, transcatheter valve replacement was introduced by Cribier. Transcatheter edge-to-edge repair (TEER) of the MV shortly followed in the early 2000s. Currently, transcatheter tricuspid valve repair and mitral and tricuspid valve replacement therapies are under development.

VALVE ANATOMY

The four human heart valves follow similar early embryologic development, beginning at 4 weeks of gestation with formation of the valve primordia in the primitive heart tube. This development is closely linked to the division of the heart tube into its chambers, including septation of the outflow tract (truncus arteriosus) and fusion of the AV canal cushions. Most of the cells, which migrate to form the valve primordia, originate from the endocardial cushion, although epicardial and neural crest cells also appear to contribute. The valve primordia grow and elongate between 20 and 39 weeks of gestation, thinning to form leaflets and cusps. In late gestation and early after birth, these structures become stratified into highly organized layers to differentiate into formal valve leaflets. Valve maturation and remodeling continue into the juvenile stages of life.

All four cardiac valves are supported by internal plates of dense collagen-, proteoglycan-, and elastin-rich connective tissue that are continuous with the fibrous skeleton at the base of the heart (Fig. 112.2). The extracellular matrix of each valve is organized into three layers: the fibrosa, made of fibrillar collagen; the spongiosa, made of proteoglycans; and an elastin layer termed the *atrialis* (on the AV valves) or the *ventricularis* (on the semilunar valves), in reference to the heart chamber the layer faces (Fig. 112.3). Covered in a thin layer of epithelium, the atrialis or ventricularis forms the surface over which blood flows through the valve, with the underlying spongiosa and fibrosa contributing structural support.

The aortic and pulmonic semilunar valves are freestanding structures seated atop the outflow tracts of their respective ventricles. They do not have discrete annuli but are instead attached in a curvilinear fashion to the wall of the aorta or pulmonary artery at their junction with the LV or right ventricular (RV) outflow tracts, respectively. These valves have three leaflets or cusps with a semilunar shape from which they derive their name (Fig. 112.4). Each cusp is in turn made up of four components: the hinge region where the cusp connects to the annulus; the belly, which makes up the majority of the cusp; the coapting surface at the cusp periphery; and the annulus, which is where the cusps attach to the ventriculoaortic junction.

In contrast to the freestanding semilunar valves, the mitral and tricuspid valves exist within a functional valve complex composed of discrete, fibrous annular rings (the annuli fibrosis); the valve leaflets; fibrous chordae tendineae; and papillary muscles. The fibrous chordae tendineae arise from the leaflet free edges (marginal or primary chordae) or undersurface (intermediate or secondary chordae), with basal (tertiary) chordae also arising from the posterior leaflet base and annulus. These chordae attach to intraventricular papillary muscles, which in turn arise from the ventricular myocardium. These additional support structures allow the AV valves to maintain the high transvalvular pressures to which they are exposed during systole.

The MV proper has two leaflets possessing approximately equal surface area (Fig. 112.5). The square-shaped anterior leaflet originates from the anterior one-third of the valve annulus. The posterior mitral leaflet is less tall but is wider than the anterior leaflet,

Heart in diastole:
viewed from base with atria removed

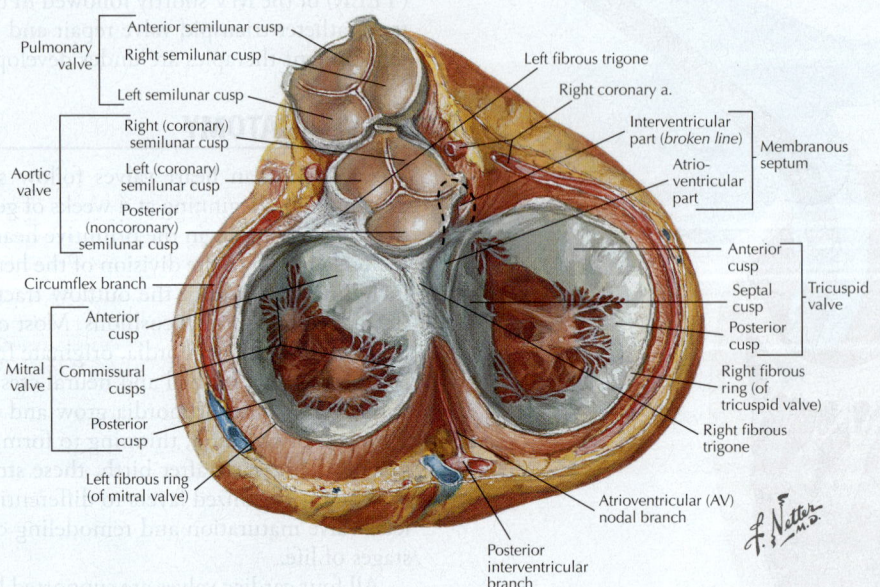

FIGURE 112.2 Fibrous cardiac skeleton. The base of the heart contains an integrated "skeleton" of connective tissue that invests the tricuspid, mitral, and aortic valves. Note the close anatomic relationship of these valves to each other, the coronary circulation, and the electrical conduction system of the heart. *a.*, Artery. (Adapted from Conti CR. *Netter Collection of Medical Illustrations: Cardiovascular System.* 2nd ed. Philadelphia: Elsevier Saunders; 2014.)

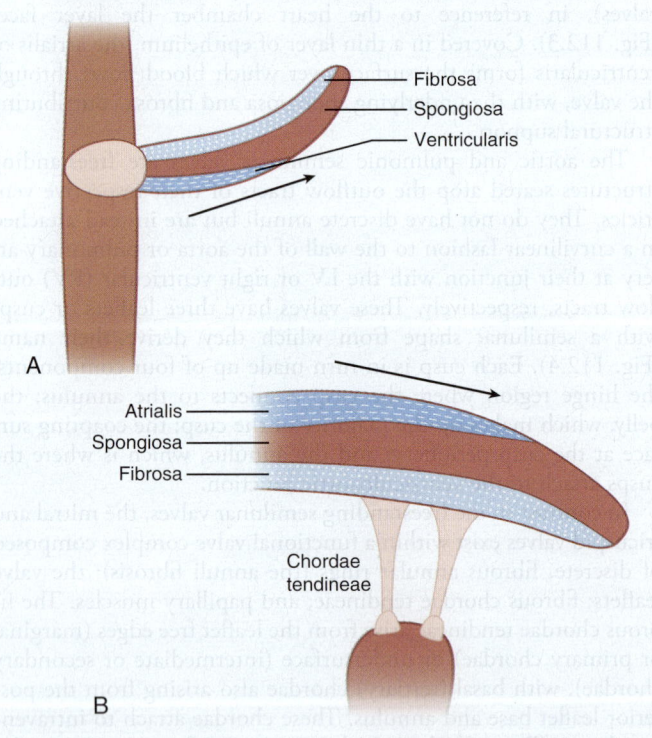

FIGURE 112.3 Valve histology. (A) Aortic valve. (B) Mitral valve. The mature valve is composed of a highly organized extracellular matrix, which is compartmentalized into three layers: the fibrosa, made of fibrillar collagen; the spongiosa, made of proteoglycans; and either the ventricularis of the semilunar valves or the atrialis of the atrioventricular valves, made of elastin fiber. (From Combs MD, Yutzey KE. Heart valve development: regulatory networks in development and disease. *Circ Res.* 2009;105:408-421.)

attaching to the posterior two-thirds of the annulus. The anterior and posterior leaflets each have three scallops (A1, P1, etc.), based on indentations found in the posterior leaflet. Of note, although the posterior leaflet segments are quite easy to delineate, the anterior leaflet segments are not clearly differentiated. In comparison, the tricuspid valve is composed of anterior, posterior, and septal leaflets, of which the anterior leaflet is the largest. Recently, with closer echocardiographic investigation of the tricuspid valve to assess and further the success of transcatheter repair therapies, there is increasing variability noted in leaflet morphology, including number and location of supernumerary leaflets or scallops.

The fibrous trigones are important landmarks during MV surgery at approximately the 10 o'clock (anterior) and 2 o'clock (posterior) positions in the surgeon's view (from the right side of the operating table). These landmarks identify the fibrous portion of mitral annulus between the mitral and aortic valves that does not stretch when the annulus pathologically dilates. The remaining "posterior" annulus is not fibrous and therefore can dilate with pathologic change. The MV also has two commissures between the anterior and posterior leaflets, the anterolateral commissure, at approximately 9 o'clock, and the posteromedial commissure, at approximately 3 o'clock.

The MV is supported by an anterolateral and posterolateral papillary muscle, each of which sends chordae to both anterior and posterior leaflets. In comparison, the tricuspid valve is supported by a large anterior papillary muscle that sends chordae to the anterior and posterior leaflets and a variable medial or posterior papillary muscle that provides chordae to the posterior and septal leaflets. The RV septal wall also provides chordae to the anterior and septal tricuspid leaflets, but there is no formal septal papillary muscle.

As suggested by their anatomy, the semilunar and AV valves differ in the mechanisms employed to maintain coaptation. The

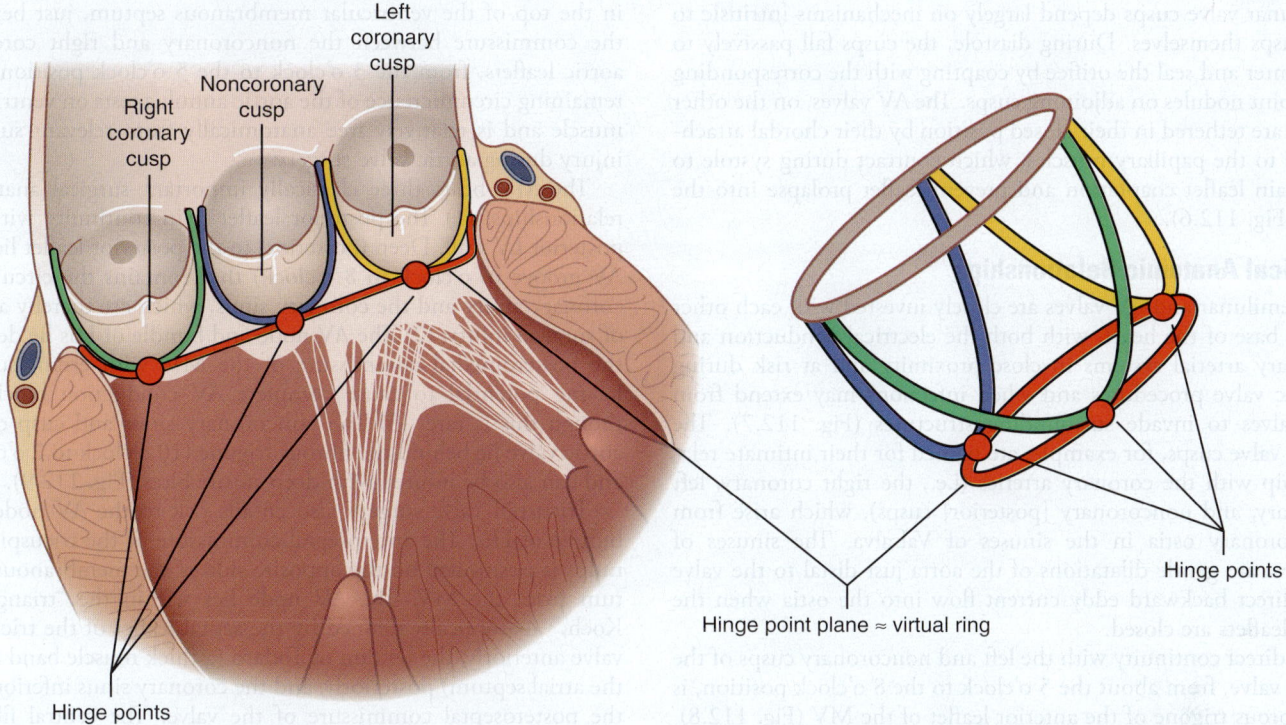

FIGURE 112.4 Anatomy of the semilunar valves. Each valve is composed of three cusps arising directly from the juncture of the great vessel and ventricular outflow tract walls. (From Kasel AM, Cassese S, Bleiziffer S, et al. Standardized imaging for aortic annular sizing: implications for transcatheter valve selection. *JACC Cardiovasc Imaging*. 2013;6:249-262.)

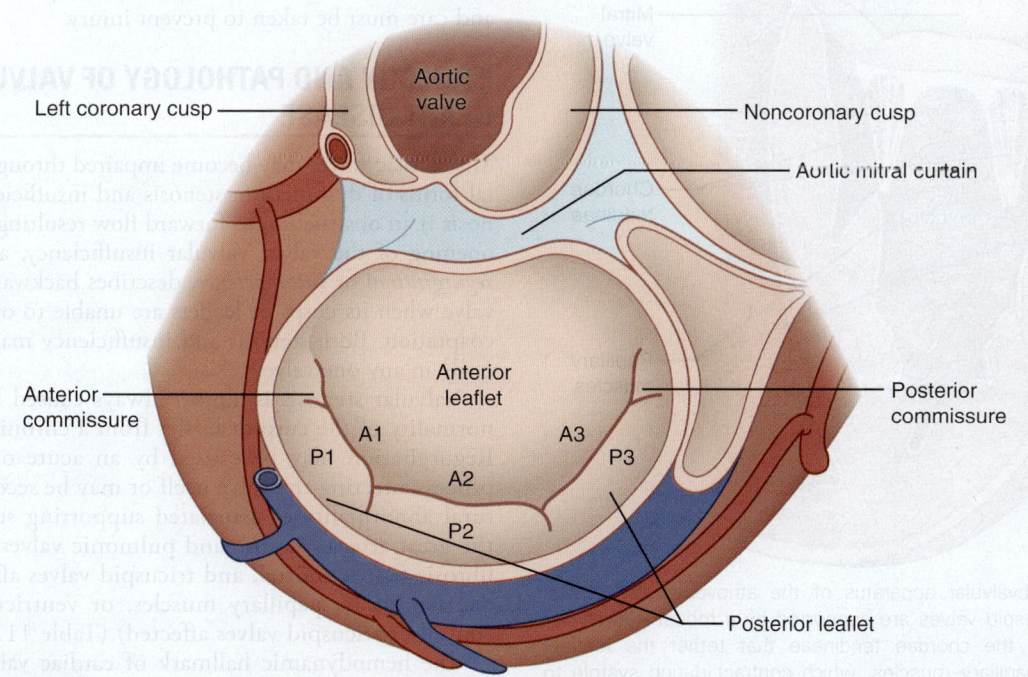

FIGURE 112.5 Anatomy of the atrioventricular valves. The atrioventricular valves are composed of leaflets arising from a distinct fibrous annulus. The depicted mitral valve is composed of an anterior and posterior leaflet, each subdivided into three scallops. (With permission, courtesy Decker Medicine LLC.)

semilunar valve cusps depend largely on mechanisms intrinsic to the cusps themselves. During diastole, the cusps fall passively to the center and seal the orifice by coapting with the corresponding midpoint nodules on adjoining cusps. The AV valves, on the other hand, are tethered in their closed position by their chordal attachments to the papillary muscles, which contract during systole to maintain leaflet coaptation and prevent leaflet prolapse into the atria (Fig. 112.6).

Surgical Anatomic Relationships

The semilunar and AV valves are closely invested with each other at the base of the heart, with both the electrical conduction and coronary arterial systems in close proximity and at risk during cardiac valve procedures and when infections may extend from the valves to invade surrounding structures (Fig. 112.7). The aortic valve cusps, for example, are named for their intimate relationship with the coronary arteries (i.e., the right coronary, left coronary, and noncoronary [posterior] cusps), which arise from the coronary ostia in the sinuses of Valsalva. The sinuses of Valsalva are gentle dilatations of the aorta just distal to the valve that direct backward eddy current flow into the ostia when the valve leaflets are closed.

In direct continuity with the left and noncoronary cusps of the aortic valve, from about the 5 o'clock to the 8 o'clock position, is the fibrous trigone of the anterior leaflet of the MV (Fig. 112.8). The noncoronary cusp of the aortic valve and the anterior leaflet of the MV are therefore at risk of injury during mitral and aortic valve surgery, respectively, if sutures bites are taken too deep during valve replacement. Likewise, the AV node lies embedded in the top of the ventricular membranous septum, just beneath the commissure between the noncoronary and right coronary aortic leaflets, from the 3 o'clock to the 5 o'clock position. The remaining circumference of the aortic annulus rests on ventricular muscle and is relatively free anatomically from relevant surgical injury during aortic valve surgery.

The MV bears three classically important surgical anatomic relationships. (1) The posterior leaflet is in continuity with the posterior LV wall. Deep (posterior) to the posterior leaflet lies the AV groove (6 o'clock to 8 o'clock) that contains the circumflex coronary artery and the coronary sinus, which are thereby at risk of surgical injury. (2) The AV node and bundle of His lie deep to the posteromedial commissure of the MV, with errant sutures having potential to cause complete AV conduction block, although this is rare. (3) The noncoronary sinus and cusp of the aortic valve lie behind the fibrous trigone (10 o'clock to 2 o'clock) and can also be injured with deep suture bites (Fig. 112.9).

Tricuspid valve surgery also entails risk to the AV node and bundle of His. The anteroseptal commissure of the tricuspid annulus is positioned on the opposite side of the membranous septum from the MV. The AV node lies within the "triangle of Koch," anatomically defined by the septal leaflet of the tricuspid valve anteriorly, the tendon of Todaro (a thick muscle band along the atrial septum) posteriorly, and the coronary sinus inferiorly by the posteroseptal commissure of the valve. The central fibrous body containing the bundle of His runs superior to the triangle as it passes by the anteroseptal tricuspid commissure and ends in the AV node within the triangle (Fig. 112.10).

The anatomic relations of the pulmonary valve generally do not present much in the way of surgical concern unless one plans to harvest the pulmonic valve for a complex aortic valve replacement technique called the *Ross procedure,* where the aortic valve is replaced with the autologous pulmonary valve and the RV outflow tract is replaced with a cadaveric homograft. The left coronary artery and its first septal branch run directly beneath the posterior area of resection when harvesting the pulmonary valve, and care must be taken to prevent injury.

ETIOLOGY AND PATHOLOGY OF VALVULAR HEART DISEASE

The cardiac valves may become impaired through two fundamental forms of dysfunction, stenosis and insufficiency. Valvular stenosis is an obstruction to forward flow resulting from incomplete opening of the valve. Valvular insufficiency, also referred to as *regurgitation* or *incompetence,* describes backward flow through a valve when its cusps or leaflets are unable to obtain or maintain coaptation. Both stenosis and insufficiency may exist simultaneously in any one valve.

Valvular stenosis is almost always caused by a primary abnormality of the cusp or leaflet from a chronic disease process. Regurgitation may be caused by an acute or chronic disease process affecting the valve itself or may be secondary to a structural abnormality of associated supporting structures, such as the great arteries (aortic and pulmonic valves affected), annuli fibrosis (aortic, mitral, and tricuspid valves affected) and chordae tendineae, papillary muscles, or ventricular myocardium (mitral or tricuspid valves affected) (Table 112.1).

The hemodynamic hallmark of cardiac valve stenosis is the occurrence of an increased pressure gradient between an upstream pumping chamber and downstream receiving chamber or great artery. This increased gradient is necessary to maintain the

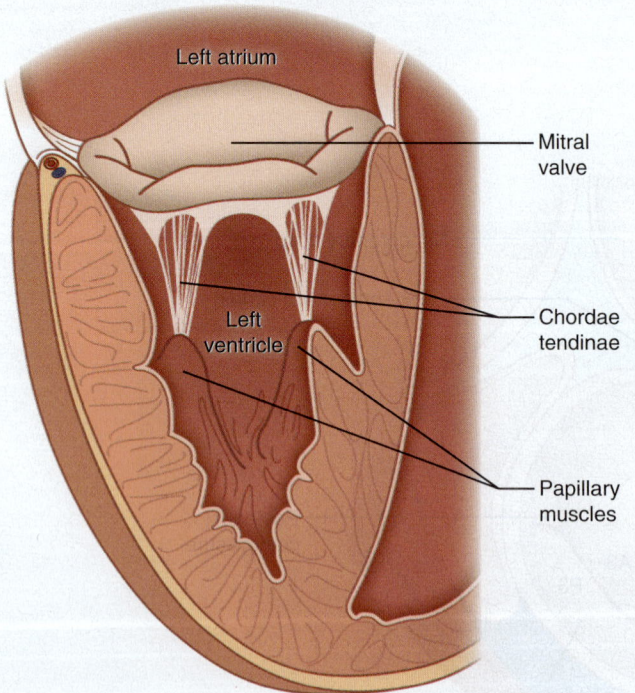

FIGURE 112.6 Subvalvular apparatus of the atrioventricular valves. The mitral and tricuspid valves are supported by a robust subvalvular apparatus featuring the chordae tendineae that tether the leaflets and annuli to the papillary muscles, which contract during systole to maintain leaflet coaptation and prevent leaflet prolapse into the atria. (From Mount Sinai, Mitral Foundation. https://www.mitralvalverepair.org/papillary-muscles-and-left-ventricle. Accessed April 7, 2025.)

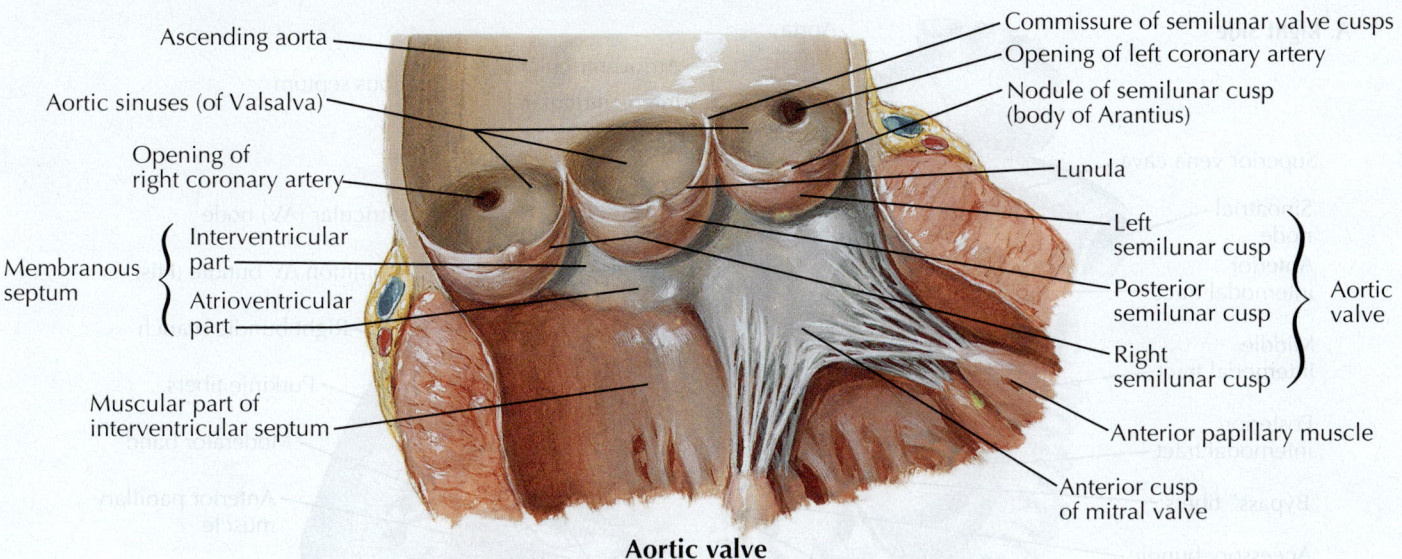

Ascending aorta

Aortic sinuses (of Valsalva)

Opening of
right coronary artery

Membranous
septum
{ Interventricular
part
Atrioventricular
part }

Muscular part of
interventricular septum

Commissure of semilunar valve cusps

Opening of left coronary artery

Nodule of semilunar cusp
(body of Arantius)

Lunula

Left
semilunar cusp

Posterior
semilunar cusp

Right
semilunar cusp

} Aortic
valve

Anterior papillary muscle

Anterior cusp
of mitral valve

Aortic valve

FIGURE 112.7 Sinuses of Valsalva. The coronary arterial circulation originates at the sinuses of Valsalva, gentle dilatations of the aorta just distal to the valve proper that impart important facilitation to valve closure and coronary and blood flow. (From http://cdn.agilitycms.com/applied-radiology/MediaGroupings/124/Fiss_figure04.jpg; https://www.appliedradiology.com/articles/normal-coronary-anatomy-and-anatomic-variations. Accessed August 11, 2020.)

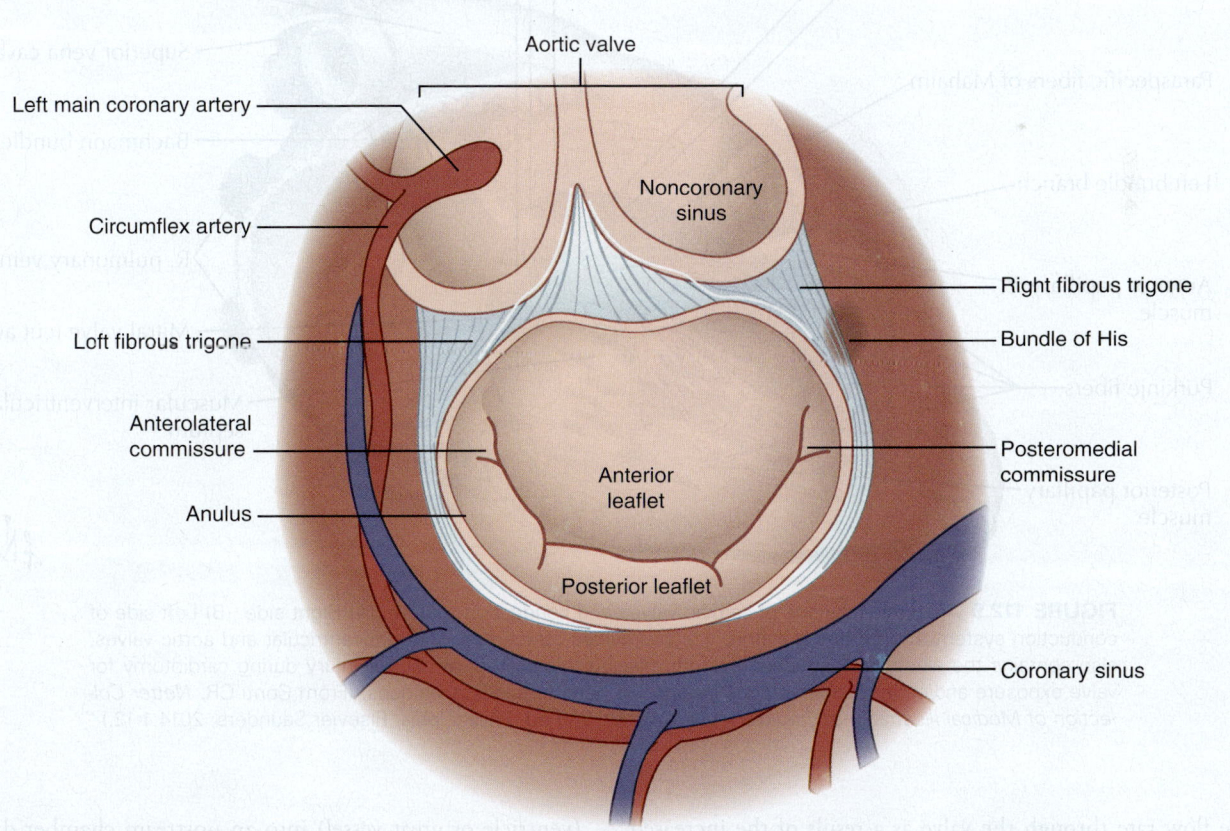

Aortic valve

Left main coronary artery

Circumflex artery

Loft fibrous trigone

Anterolateral
commissure

Anulus

Noncoronary
sinus

Right fibrous trigone

Bundle of His

Posteromedial
commissure

Anterior
leaflet

Posterior leaflet

Coronary sinus

FIGURE 112.8 Surgical anatomy of the aortic and mitral valves. The anterior leaflet of the mitral valve is in direct continuity with the left and noncoronary cusps of the aortic valve from about the 5 o'clock to the 8 o'clock position in the traditional surgical perspective. (From Sellke FW, del Nido PJ, Swanson SJ. *Sabiston and Spencer's Surgery of the Chest.* 9th ed. Philadelphia: Saunders Elsevier; 2015:1384.)

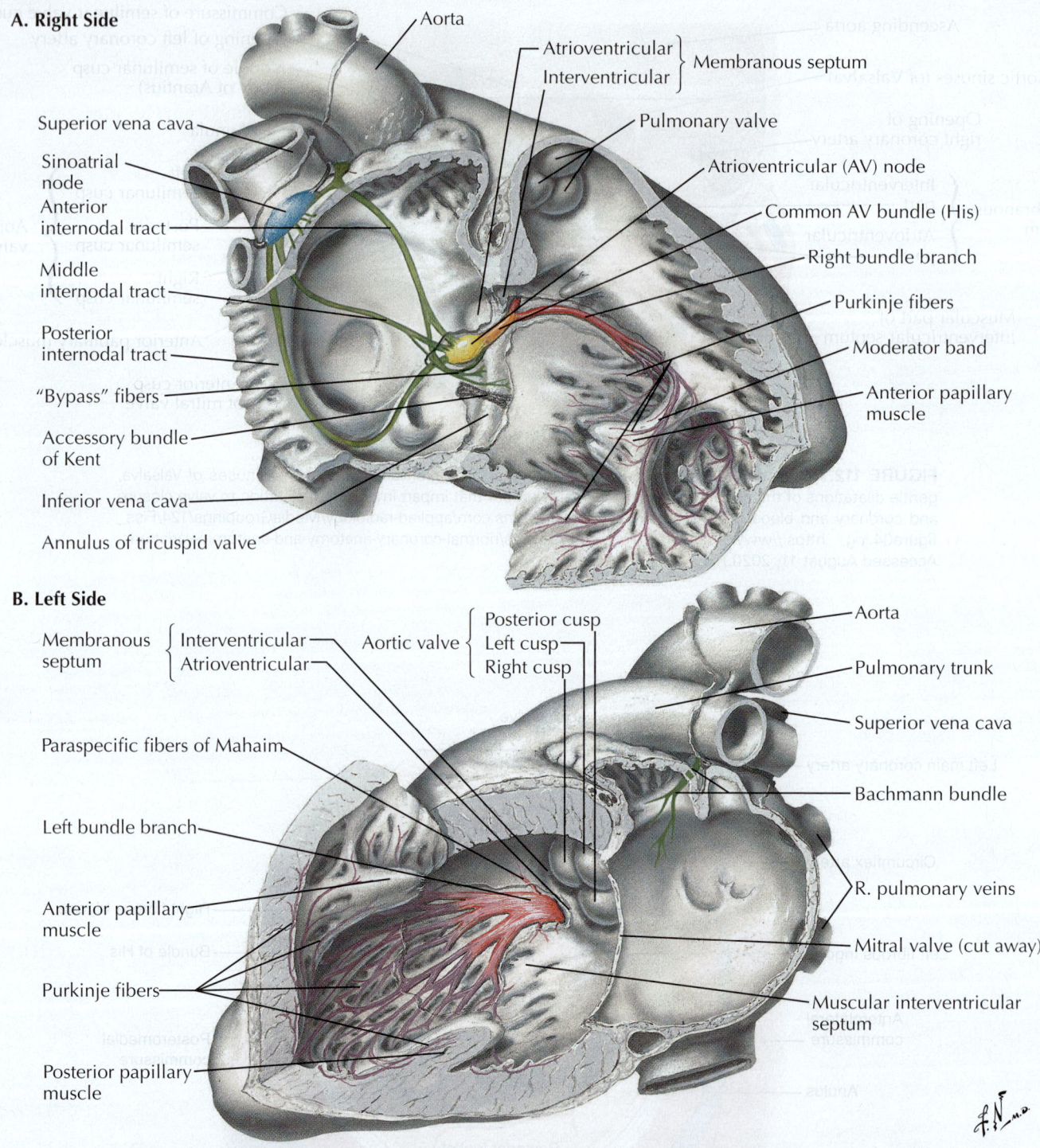

A. Right Side

- Aorta
- Atrioventricular
- Interventricular } Membranous septum
- Pulmonary valve
- Atrioventricular (AV) node
- Common AV bundle (His)
- Right bundle branch
- Purkinje fibers
- Moderator band
- Anterior papillary muscle
- Superior vena cava
- Sinoatrial node
- Anterior internodal tract
- Middle internodal tract
- Posterior internodal tract
- "Bypass" fibers
- Accessory bundle of Kent
- Inferior vena cava
- Annulus of tricuspid valve

B. Left Side

- Membranous septum { Interventricular / Atrioventricular
- Aortic valve { Posterior cusp / Left cusp / Right cusp
- Aorta
- Pulmonary trunk
- Superior vena cava
- Bachmann bundle
- R. pulmonary veins
- Mitral valve (cut away)
- Muscular interventricular septum
- Paraspecific fibers of Mahaim
- Left bundle branch
- Anterior papillary muscle
- Purkinje fibers
- Posterior papillary muscle

FIGURE 112.9 Anatomic relations of cardiac valves and conduction system. (A) Right side. (B) Left side of conduction system. The fibrous skeleton, which provides structure to the atrioventricular and aortic valves, also contains the electrical conduction system, placing this system at risk for injury during cardiotomy for valve exposure and/or valve interventions by open or percutaneous techniques. (From Conti CR. *Netter Collection of Medical Illustrations: Cardiovascular System.* 2nd ed. Philadelphia: Elsevier Saunders; 2014:1-12.)

baseline flow rate through the valve as a result of the increased resistance to laminar flow introduced by the smaller effective cross-sectional area of the stenotic valve orifice, as described by Poiseuille law (flow α Δp/resistance, where Δp signifies pressure gradient). The hemodynamic hallmark of regurgitant valvular disease is the retrograde flow of blood from downstream structures

(ventricle or great vessel) into an upstream chamber during the diastolic interval, during which the malfunctioning valve should normally be closed. Uncompensated lesions, either stenotic or regurgitant forms, cause an increase in upstream chamber afterload and consequent wall stress. This occurs either during ventricular systolic ejection against the resistance of stenotic valves

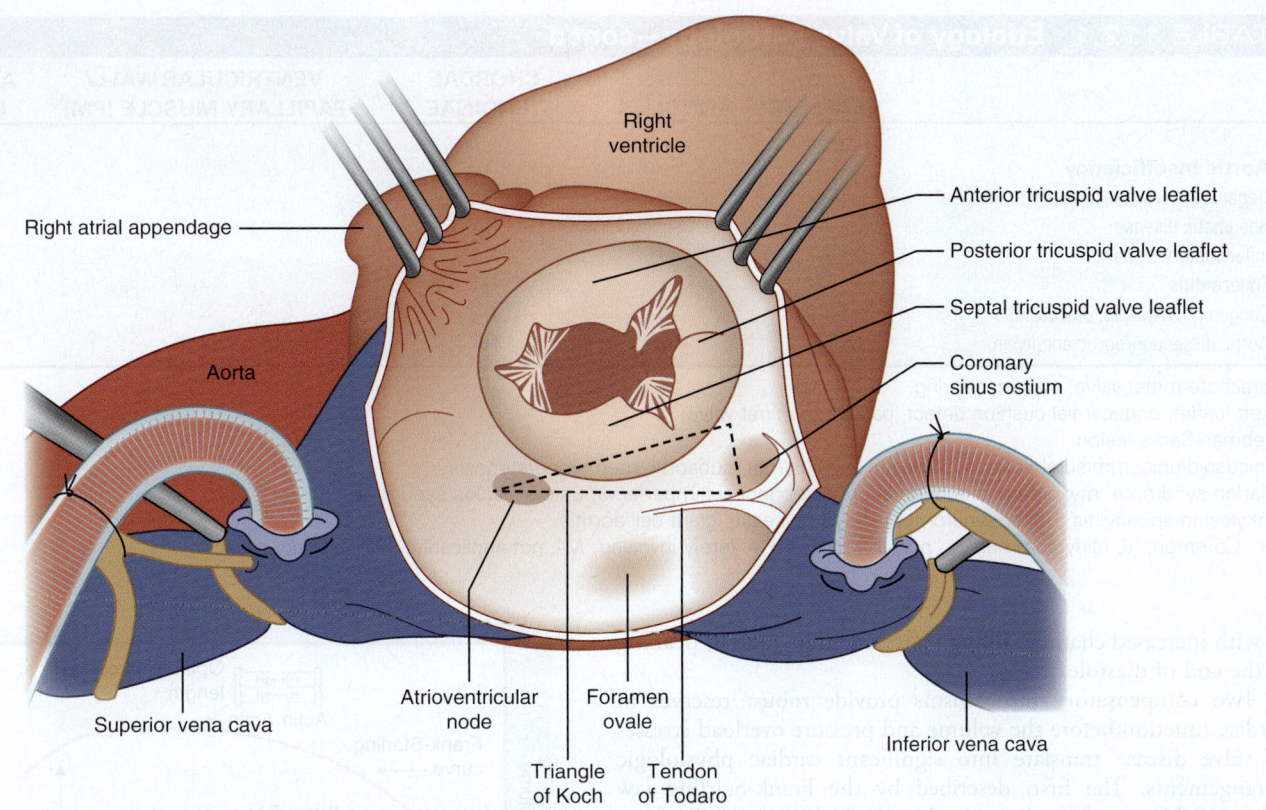

FIGURE 112.10 Surgical anatomy of the tricuspid valve. The atrioventricular node lies in the apex of a triangular area first described by Koch, which is bounded by the septal annulus of the tricuspid valve anteriorly, the tendon of Todaro posteriorly, and the central fibrous body containing the bundle of His superiorly, leading to the coronary sinus inferiorly. (From Rogers JH, Bolling SF. The tricuspid valve: current perspective and evolving management of tricuspid regurgitation. *Circulation.* 2009;119:2718-2725.)

TABLE 112.1 Etiology of Valve Pathology

	LEAFLETS	ANNULUS	CHORDAE TENDINAE	VENTRICULAR WALL/ PAPILLARY MUSCLE (PM)	AORTIC ROOT
Mitral Stenosis					
Rheumatic valve disease	++	++	++	± (PM fusion/ shortening)	NA
Endocarditis (vegetation)	±	–	–	–	NA
Congenital[a]	++	–	–	±	NA
Supravalvular (thrombus, myxoma)	++	–	–	–	NA
Mitral Regurgitation					
Mitral valve prolapse (myxomatous/ connective tissue disorder)	++	++	++	–	NA
Rheumatic fever	++	–	±	–	NA
Endocarditis	++	±	++	+	NA
Congenital anomaly[b]	++	–	±	–	NA
Systemic lupus erythematosus[c]	++	±	±	± (PM)	NA
Mitral annular calcification (MAC)	=/–	++	–	–	NA
Myocardial ischemia/infarction	–	±	–	++	NA
Hypertrophic cardiomyopathy				++	NA
Aortic Stenosis					
Degenerative disease (trileaflet)	++	+	NA	–	–
Bicuspid valve disease	++	+	NA	–	–
Rheumatic valve disease	++	+	NA	–	–
Endocarditis (vegetation)	++	+	NA	–	–
Other congenital anomaly[d]	++	+	NA	++	+
Hypertrophic cardiomyopathy	–	–	–	++	–

Continued

TABLE 112.1   Etiology of Valve Pathology—cont'd

	LEAFLETS	ANNULUS	CHORDAE TENDINAE	VENTRICULAR WALL/ PAPILLARY MUSCLE (PM)	AORTIC ROOT
Aortic Insufficiency					
Degenerative/connective tissue disease[e]	++	++	NA	–	++
Rheumatic disease	++	–	NA	–	–
Inflammatory disease[f]	+	–	NA	–	++
Endocarditis	++	+	NA	–	+
Congenital (bicuspid, unicuspid)	++	–	NA	–	+
Aortic dissection/aortic aneurysm	–	++	NA	–	++

[a]Parachute mitral valve, supramitral ring.
[b]Cleft leaflet, endocardial cushion defect, parachute mitral valve.
[c]Liebman-Sacks lesion.
[d]Unicuspid/unicommisural valve, hypoplastic annulus/root, subaortic membrane/stenosis.
[e]Marfan syndrome, myxomatous degeneration, osteogenesis imperfecta, Ehlers-Danlos syndrome.
[f]Ankylosing spondylitis, Reiter syndrome, Takayasu disease, giant cell aortitis.
++, Common; +, fairly common; ±, possibly involved; –, rarely involved; *NA*, not applicable; *PM*, papillary muscle.

or with increased chamber filling by regurgitant volumes peaking at the end of diastole.

Two compensatory mechanisms provide robust reserves in cardiac function before the volume and pressure overload stresses of valve disease translate into significant cardiac physiologic derangements. The first, described by the Frank-Starling law (Fig. 112.11), produces increases in ventricular contractile force as a function of end-diastolic volume (EDV), or preload, to enhance stroke volume and ventricular emptying. The second involves stress-induced ventricular hypertrophy that leads to increased wall thickness. By decreasing chamber radius (volume) or increasing wall thickness, the ventricles can lower wall stress, as described by the Laplace law: wall stress α (pressure × radius)/ (2 × wall thickness). Decreased wall stress, in turn, translates into decreased myocardial work and oxygen demand and improved cardiac function. Ultimately, as cardiomyopathy progresses, contractile function progressively diminishes past the ideal sarcomere length of 2.2 micrometers, whereby heart failure (HF) ensures.

Rheumatic Heart Disease

Degenerative disease remains the more common cause of valve disease in the developed world. On the other hand, rheumatic fever with ensuing RHD remains the most common, albeit decreasing, cause of valvular dysfunction in underdeveloped countries and those with limited healthcare access. Acute rheumatic fever develops because of a cross-reactive host immune response exhibited by genetically susceptible individuals in response to group A β-hemolytic streptococcal infection acquired during the first decade of life. This pathologic process is driven by molecular mimicry between streptococcal proteins and host cardiac proteins such as laminin.[3] In a small minority of patients, this initial response causes clinically evident inflammation in the cardiac valves and/or conduction system several weeks after the streptococcal infection. Surgical intervention to "peel" the inflammatory material off the valve can be effective in improving valve function, at least for a limited time.

Rarely, acute rheumatic valvulitis can result in severe acute mitral regurgitation (MR) and may be associated with other manifestations of carditis, such as AV conduction abnormalities or pericarditis. In developed countries, however, the typical presentation is that of chronic RHD, which silently develops as

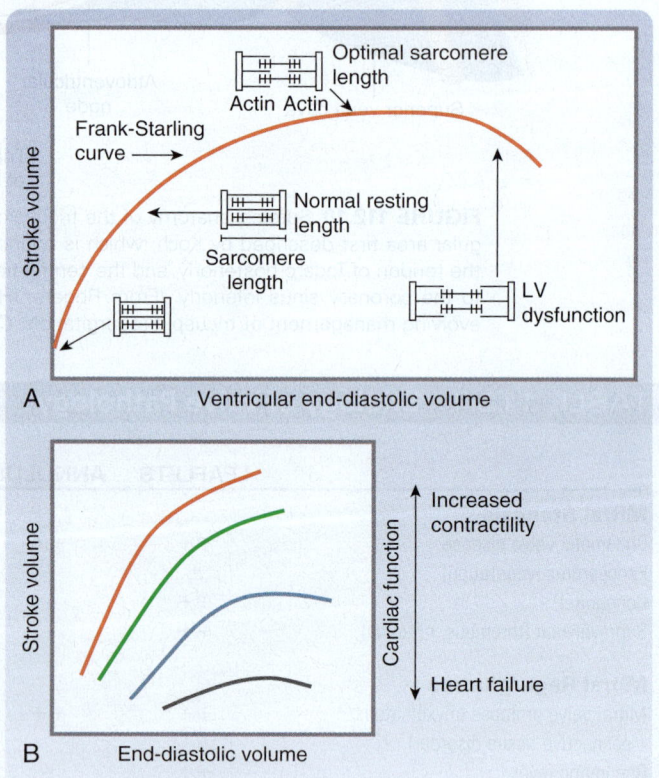

FIGURE 112.11 Frank-Starling curve. The Frank-Starling law describes a generally linear relationship between increasing end-diastolic volume, or preload, and generated ventricular pressure. (A) Shifts in volume change generated pressure or stroke volume along a given pressure-volume curve. (B) Cardiomyopathy shifts curve downward. *LV,* Left ventricle. (From Hanft LM, Korte FS, McDonald KS. Cardiac function and modulation of sarcomeric function by length. *Cardiovasc Res.* 2008;77(4):627–636. doi:10.1093/cvr/cvm099.)

ongoing valvular damage occurs from repeated exposures to streptococcal infection and ongoing damage to a deformed valve in adolescence and adulthood.

Chronic RHD most commonly presents as either MV stenosis (see later) or mixed valve lesions (stenotic and regurgitant). Mixed

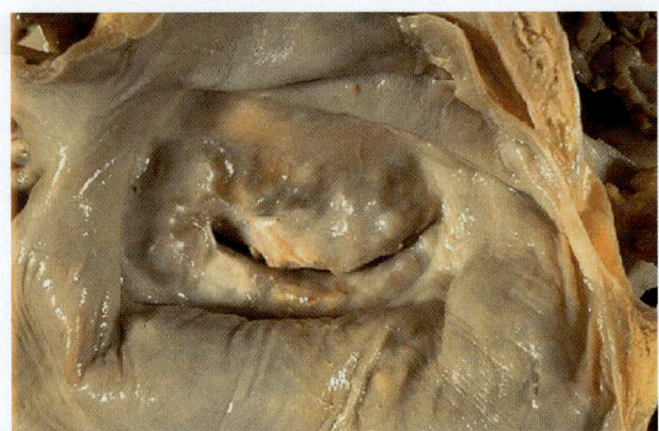

FIGURE 112.12 Mitral valve pathology in rheumatic heart disease. Typical pathology of rheumatic mitral valve disease presenting as a pathognomonic, mixed stenotic/regurgitant "fish mouth" funnel valve lesion, often associated with fusion and shortening of the leaflets and chordae tendineae. (From http://library.med.utah.edu/WebPath/CVHTML/CV061.html.)

stenotic and regurgitant mitral pathology takes the form of a pathognomonic "fish mouth" funnel valve lesion as a consequence of fusion of the leaflets at the commissures that hinders opening of the leaflets. This is associated with fusion and shortening of the chordae tendineae (Fig. 112.12). Sclerosis induced by chronic inflammation reduces leaflet mobility to prevent complete opening of the valve during diastole and adequate coaptation to close the valve during systole. Clinically apparent HF typically develops from these RHD lesions in the third or fourth decade of life as a result of progressive valve dysfunction and/or exhaustion of compensatory mechanisms.[4]

RHD next most frequently leads to aortic valve stenosis or regurgitation through a similar pattern of chronic inflammation. The resultant sclerosis impairs valve opening (narrowed orifice) and valve closing (gap through which regurgitant flow from the aorta to ventricle can occur). Tricuspid regurgitation (TR) is also a common secondary valvular abnormality in RHD because of upstream hemodynamic stresses caused by MS. The ensuing pulmonary hypertension leads to dilation of the right ventricle, especially the free wall, and tricuspid annulus compromising tricuspid valve leaflet coaptation.

Endocarditis

Endocarditis is a relatively common cause of aortic, mitral, and tricuspid valve regurgitation.[5,6] The incidence of endocarditis varies from 3 to 10 episodes per 100,000 person-years. Endocarditis typically causes valvular insufficiency by progressive inflammatory destruction of the affected valve and surrounding structures. Less frequently, endocarditis can cause functional valve stenosis, with valve orifice obstruction developing from endocarditic vegetations, masses of platelets, fibrin, microcolonies of microorganisms, and inflammatory cells.

Endocarditis with acute AI carries a relatively high mortality compared with other valve lesions. Endocarditis may affect previously normal valves, but it typically affects valves deformed by congenital or rheumatic disease, degenerative processes such as calcification, or previously replaced prosthetic valves. Infectious endocarditis not related to intravenous drug use is usually left-sided, reflecting the normal distribution of such preexisting valvular disease. Endocarditis resulting from intravenous drug use most often affects the tricuspid valve.

The pathophysiology of endocarditis is typically initiated by platelets and fibrin deposition on normal or deformed valves occurring as part of a normal healing process after disruption of the valvular endothelium caused by hemodynamic or metabolic injuries. Endocarditis results from subsequent seeding onto damaged valves by microbiologic organisms after bacteremia or fungemia episodes, most commonly staphylococci, streptococci, or enterococci.

Acute endocarditis, increasingly affecting normal valves, may follow an aggressive course with leaflet perforation or more extensive destruction of the leaflet and/or surrounding support structures, resulting in acute valvular regurgitation. With subacute or chronic presentations of endocarditis, valve insufficiency may result from residual leaflet deformities caused by fibrotic healing of endocarditic lesions. The growth of large vegetations may also uncommonly lead to improper leaflet coaptation and valve regurgitation as well.

GENERAL OPERATIVE APPROACH

The specific surgical approach will be described for each of the various valvular lesions in the following sections. In general, surgery for valvular heart disease is today associated with excellent short- and long-term outcomes, with some evidence suggesting even better outcomes for surgery performed at high-volume centers.[7] Operative mortality, which in the modern era is generally <5% for almost all types of valve pathology, can now be predicted using several widely available multivariable risk calculation scoring systems.[8,9]

Operative mortality is predicted by risk factors such as age, female sex, emergency surgery, symptomology, concomitant procedures, and decreased ejection fraction (EF), along with comorbidities such as diabetes mellitus, renal dysfunction, pulmonary disease, peripheral vascular disease, and prior operation (Table 112.2). Typically, isolated tricuspid valve surgery is associated with the highest operative mortality risk (primarily related to coexistent cardiac pathophysiology), followed by MR and AI. Surgery for AS and MS offers the best operative mortality outcomes. Complications most frequently associated with surgery for valvular heart disease include infection, bleeding, stroke, conduction block requiring permanent pacemaker, and HF (Table 112.3).

Long-term outcomes and resolution of ventricular hemodynamic pathophysiology can generally be predicted by the duration and/or severity of symptoms associated with valvular disease, extent of ventricular dysfunction, and the presence and severity of pulmonary hypertension.[10,11] Complete hemodynamic recovery from valvular disease, including resolution of ventricular hypertrophy and enlargement, may be seen as early as the first several weeks postoperatively but may progress for up to a year after surgery. Long-term complications frequently associated with valve surgery include thromboembolic events leading to strokes, structural valve degeneration, progressive paravalvular leaks, bleeding associated with anticoagulation, and endocarditis.

Conduct of Heart Valve Surgery

The use of cardiopulmonary bypass and cardioplegic arrest of the heart is standard when performing open-heart procedures on the cardiac valves (unlike in percutaneous interventions, as described later). A full midline median sternotomy has traditionally been the predominant means to obtain wide exposure for heart valve surgery. However, various minimally invasive approaches are now also used and have proven to be equally safe and effective

TABLE 112.2   European System for Valvular Surgery Operative Risk Evaluation (EuroSCORE)

PATIENT-RELATED FACTORS	DEFINITION	SCORE
Age	Per 5 years or part thereof over 60 years	1
Sex	Female	1
Chronic pulmonary disease	Long-term bronchodilators/steroids	1
Extracardiac arteriopathy	Claudication, carotid occlusion or >50% stenosis, intervention on abdominal aorta, limb arteries, carotids	2
Neurologic dysfunction	Severely affecting ambulation or day-to-day functioning	2
Previous cardiac surgery	Requiring opening of the pericardium	3
Serum creatinine	>200 mmol/L preoperatively	2
Active endocarditis	Antibiotic treatment for endocarditis at the time of surgery	3
Critical preoperative state	Ventricular tachycardia, fibrillation, aborted sudden death; preoperative cardiac massage, ventilation, inotropic support, IABP, or acute renal failure (anuria or oliguria <10 mL/h)	3
Cardiac-Related Factors		
Unstable angina	Rest angina requiring intravenous nitrates preoperatively	2
LV dysfunction	Moderate or LVEF 30%–50%	1
	Poor or LVEF <30	3
Recent myocardial infarct	Within 90 days	2
Pulmonary hypertension	Systolic PA pressure >60 mm Hg	2
Operation-Related Factors		
Emergency	Carried out on referral before next working day	2
Other than isolated CABG	Major cardiac procedure other than or in addition to CABG	2
Surgery on thoracic aorta	For disorder of ascending, arch or descending aorta	3
Postinfarct septal rupture		4

CABG, Coronary artery bypass graft; IABP, intraaortic balloon pump; LV, left ventricle; LVEF, left ventricle ejection fraction; PA, pulmonary artery.
Adapted from Roques F, Nashef SA, Michel P, et al. Risk factors and outcome in European cardiac surgery: analysis of the EuroSCORE multinational database of 19030 patients. Eur J Cardiothorac Surg. 1999;15:816-822.

TABLE 112.3   Complications Associated With Valvular Heart Surgery

OUTCOME	AVR	MVR
Prolonged ventilation	7%	10.8%
Renal failure	3.7%	5.2%
Reoperation for bleeding	4.1%	4.7%
Permanent stroke	1.6%	2.2%
Deep sternal infection	0.5%	0.3%
Postoperative hospital stay[a]	8.5 ± 8.4	9.9 ± 10.3
Overall hospital stay[a]	10.6 ± 9.6	12.8 ± 12.6

Interpretation: low risk = 0–2; medium risk = 3–5; high risk = 6 or more.
[a]Mean days ± standard deviation.
AVR, Aortic valve replacement; MVR, mitral valve replacement.
Adapted from Edwards FH, Peterson ED, Coombs LP, et al. Prediction of operative mortality after valve replacement surgery. J Am Coll Cardiol. 2001;37:885-892.

compared with traditional open approaches. Specific minimally invasive approaches include partial upper or lower sternotomies, right anterior (second to fourth interspaces) thoracotomies with direct or thoracoscopic visualization, and robotic-assisted techniques (Fig. 112.13). These approaches have been associated with decreased transfusion, wound infection, hospital stay, and atrial fibrillation, along with quicker recovery and improved cosmesis.

Prosthetic Valves

Prosthetic heart valves used currently are typically made from a synthetic material (mechanical valves; Fig. 112.14A), allogeneic biologic tissue (bioprosthetic valves; see Fig. 112.14B), or (cadaveric)

homografts. Each has distinct advantages and disadvantages. Anticoagulation with a vitamin K antagonist (warfarin) and monitoring of the international normalized ratio (INR) is recommended in all patients with mechanical prosthetic valves and typically for the first 3 months after bioprosthetic MV implants (Table 112.4).[10] Aspirin may be added to warfarin therapy to reduce rates of major embolism, stroke, and overall mortality.

The current generation of mechanical valves, nearly all bileaflet pyrolytic carbon in design, can be expected to provide an extremely low incidence of structural deterioration but have a 0.6% to 2.3% per patient-year incidence of thromboembolic complications.[10,12] The need for anticoagulation with warfarin is associated with approximately a 1% annual risk of bleeding complications. Both bleeding and thromboembolic complications may be reduced through more frequent (e.g., weekly) INR surveillance and/or home testing.[13]

Bioprosthetic valves are almost universally fabricated from preserved (bovine) pericardium or from porcine valves specially harvested for this use. Modern antimineralization and tissue preservation techniques involving treatment of valves with alpha-oleic acid reduce leaflet calcification and typically provide ~90% freedom from structural valve deterioration and reoperation at 10 years in patients over 65 years of age.[14] Failure rates may be higher in younger patients as a result of greater hemodynamic stresses and/or metabolic (i.e., calcium turnover) rates. Recent studies demonstrate potential for improved long-term results with contemporary tissue valves, even in younger patients.[15,16]

Based upon the previously described considerations, some surgeons now recommend implantation of bioprosthetic valves in patients less than the recommended class IIa cutoff of 50 to 65 years of age, accepting the risk of reintervention by open or

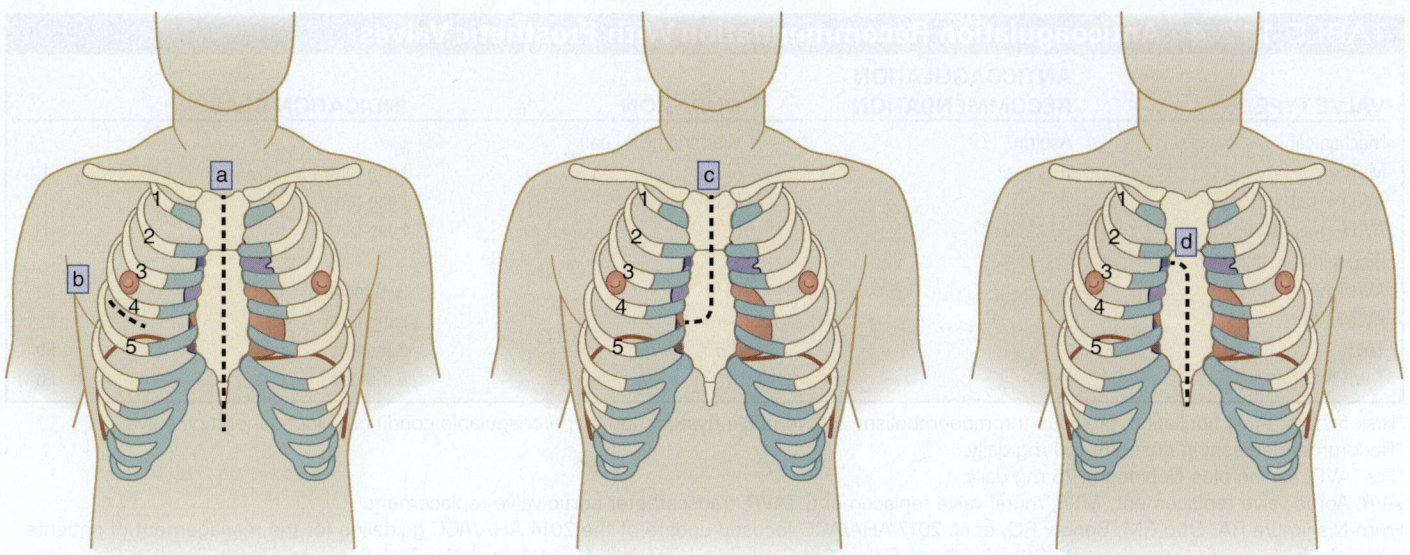

FIGURE 112.13 Surgical access for valvular heart surgery. Median sternotomy *(a)* versus minimally invasive access via minithoracotomy *(b)* or partial upper *(c)* or lower *(d)* sternotomy. (From Byrne JG, Leacche M, Vaughan DE, et al. Hybrid cardiovascular procedures. *JACC Cardiovasc Interv.* 2008;1:459-468.)

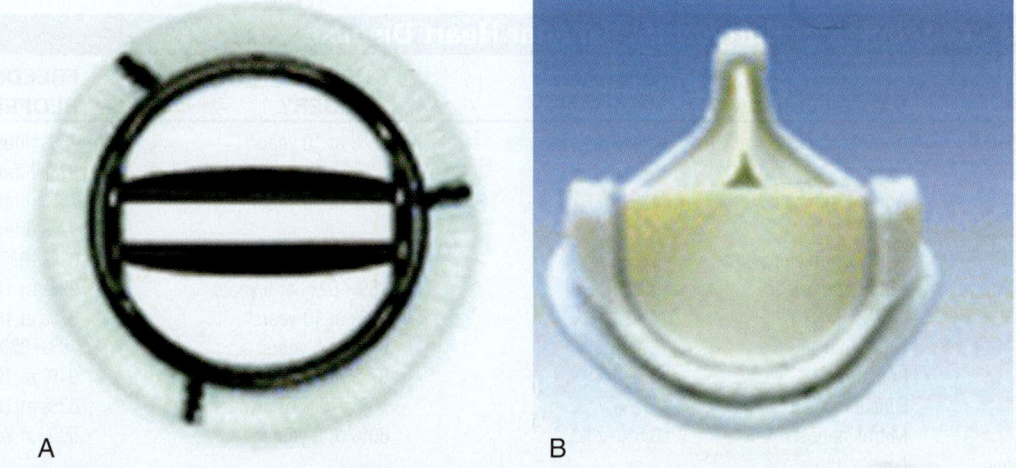

A   B

FIGURE 112.14 Prosthetic valves. Prosthetic heart valves most often implanted are made from (A) synthetic material, such as pyrolytic carbon (mechanical valve), or (B) allogeneic biologic tissue, such as bovine pericardium (bioprosthetic valve). (From Pibarot P, Dumesnil JG. Prosthetic heart valves: selection of the optimal prosthesis and long-term management. *Circulation.* 2009;119:1034-1048.)

percutaneous technique as being less than the lifelong risk of anticoagulation or mechanical valve thromboembolism. The decision for a mechanical versus a bioprosthetic valve is complex. Many factors, including patient age, likelihood of pregnancy, and indications or contraindications to anticoagulation, must be considered. In contrast to the more complex xenograft stentless aortic bioprosthetic roots and homograft implants, technical considerations in prosthetic valve implantation are generally considered similar between valve types.

Excellent early and long-term survival outcomes can be expected after valve implantation (Table 112.5; see also Table 112.3).[10,17–28] One of the most frequent and dangerous complications of valve implantation is prosthetic valve endocarditis (PVE), which is 50 times more likely to occur than endocarditis in the general population with native valves. PVE typically requires prosthetic valve excision and re-replacement, especially when PVE is caused by virulent

organisms such as *Staphylococcus aureus* or fungi, although intravenous antibiotic or antifungal therapy alone may occasionally be used to sterilize lesions in high-risk individuals.[5,6] Even with appropriate antibiotic therapy and surgical intervention, PVE carries a mortality rate of up to 40% at 1 year. Accordingly, patients with prosthetic valves, similar to individuals at increased risk for native valve endocarditis, should be counseled and strictly adhere to recommendations for antibiotic prophylaxis against endocarditis.

Another potential complication of valve implantation is patient-prosthesis mismatch, arising from an undersized (aortic) prosthetic effective orifice area compared with patient body surface area. Inadequate prosthetic valve effective orifice area can lead to elevated transvalvular gradients, resulting in persistent ventricular hypertrophy, impaired ventricular remodeling, and excessive late cardiac events. Patient-prosthesis mismatch is unusual with the excellent hemodynamic performance of current

TABLE 112.4 Anticoagulation Recommendation With Prosthetic Valves

VALVE TYPE	ANTICOAGULATION RECOMMENDATION	DURATION	INDICATION CLASS	
Mechanical	Aspirin[a]	Warfarin (INR goal)		
MVR	+	(3.0)	Long term	I
AVR (+ risk factors)[b]	+	(3.0)	Long term	I
AVR (− risk factors)[b]	+	(2.5)	Long term	I
Bioprosthetic				
AVR/MVR		(2.5)	3–6 months	IIa
AVR/MVR	+	—	Long term	IIa
TAVR		2.5	3 months	IIb
TAVR	+[c]		6 months	IIb

[a]Risk factors: atrial fibrillation, previous thromboembolism, left ventricle dysfunction, hypercoagulable condition, older-generation valve.
[b]Recommended aspirin dose 75–100 mg daily.
[c]For TAVR, aspirin plus clopidogrel 75 mg daily.
AVR, Aortic valve replacement; *MVR,* mitral valve replacement; *TAVR,* transcatheter aortic valve replacement.
From Nishimura RA, Otto CM, Bonow RO, et al. 2017 AHA/ACC focused update of the 2014 AHA/ACC guideline for the management of patients with valvular heart disease: a report of the American College of Cardiology/American Heart Association Task Force on Clinical Practice Guidelines. *J Am Coll Cardiol.* 2017;70:252-289; Nishimura RA, Otto CM, Bonow RO, et al. 2014 AHA/ACC guideline for the management of patients with valvular heart disease: executive summary: a report of the American College of Cardiology/American Heart Association Task Force on Practice Guidelines. *Circulation.* 2014;129:2440-2492.

TABLE 112.5 Outcomes of Surgery for Valvular Heart Disease

VALVE SURGERY	VALVE LESION	OPERATIVE MORTALITY	SURVIVAL AFTER SURGERY	FREEDOM FROM REOPERATION
Aortic valve replacement	Aortic stenosis	1%–3%[a]	85% at 10 years[b]	75% (lifetime; biologic) 97% (lifetime; mechanical)[c]
	Aortic insufficiency	1%–4%[a]	63% at 10 years[d]	75% (lifetime; biologic) 97% (lifetime; mechanical)[c]
Aortic valve repair	Aortic insufficiency	1%–4%[a]	95% at 13 years[d]	83%–93% at 8 years[e]
Mitral valve replacement	Mitral stenosis	3%–10%[a]	15%–62% at 5 years	92% at 10 years[h]
	Primary MR	4%[g]	60% at 10 years[h]	92% at 10 years[h]
	Functional MR	3%–5%[i,m]	66% at 5 years[k]	70%–85% at 4 years[j]
Mitral valve repair	Primary MR	0%–1%[f]	87% at 10 years[h]	94% at 10 years[h]
	Functional MR	~5%[i]	50%–75% at 5 years[k,l]	63% at 10 years[m]
Percutaneous balloon mitral commissurotomy	Mitral stenosis	0.5%–2%[a]	80% at 9 years	50% at 20 years
Open mitral commissurotomy	Mitral stenosis	<2%	96% at 10 years	98% at 9 years[m]

[a]Vahanian A, Alfieri O, Andreotti F, et al. Guidelines on the management of valvular heart disease (version 2012): the Joint Task Force on the Management of Valvular Heart Disease of the European Society of Cardiology (ESC) and the European Association for Cardio-Thoracic Surgery (EACTS). *Eur J Cardiothorac Surg.* 2012;42:S1-S44.
[b]Kvidal P, Bergstrom R, Horte LG, et al. Observed and relative survival after aortic valve replacement. *J Am Coll Cardiol.* 2000;35:747-756.
[c]van Geldorp MW, Eric Jamieson WR, Kappetein AP, et al. Patient outcome after aortic valve replacement with a mechanical or biological prosthesis: weighing lifetime anticoagulant-related event risk against reoperation risk. *J Thorac Cardiovasc Surg.* 2009;137:881-886, 886.e1-e5.
[d]Chaliki HP, Mohty D, Avierinos JF, et al. Outcomes after aortic valve replacement in patients with severe aortic regurgitation and markedly reduced left ventricular function. *Circulation.* 2002;106:2687-2693.
[e]Talwar S, Saikrishna C, Saxena A, et al. Aortic valve repair for rheumatic aortic valve disease. *Ann Thorac Surg.* 2005;79:1921-1925.
[f]Donndorf P, Park H, Vollmar B, et al. Impact of closed minimal extracorporeal circulation on microvascular tissue perfusion during surgical aortic valve replacement: intravital imaging in a prospective randomized study. *Interact Cardiovasc Thorac Surg.* 2014;19:211-217.
[g]Gammie JS, Sheng S, Griffith BP, et al. Trends in mitral valve surgery in the United States: results from the Society of Thoracic Surgeons Adult Cardiac Surgery Database. *Ann Thorac Surg.* 2009;87:1431-1437; discussion 1437-1439.
[h]Gillinov AM, Blackstone EH, Nowicki ER, et al. Valve repair versus valve replacement for degenerative mitral valve disease. *J Thorac Cardiovasc Surg.* 2008;135:885-893, 893.e1-e2.
[i]Braunberger E, Deloche A, Berrebi A, et al. Very long-term results (more than 20 years) of valve repair with Carpentier's techniques in nonrheumatic mitral valve insufficiency. *Circulation.* 2001;104:I8-I11.
[j]Lorusso R, Gelsomino S, Vizzardi E, et al. Mitral valve repair or replacement for ischemic mitral regurgitation? The Italian Study on the Treatment of Ischemic Mitral Regurgitation (ISTIMIR). *J Thorac Cardiovasc Surg.* 2013;145:128-139.
[k]Calafiore AM, Di Mauro M, Gallina S, et al. Mitral valve surgery for chronic ischemic mitral regurgitation. *Ann Thorac Surg.* 2004;77:1989-1997.
[l]Oliveira JM, Antunes MJ. Mitral valve repair: better than replacement. *Heart.* 2006;92:275-281.
MR, Mitral regurgitation.

valves, although aortic root or annular enlargement can be safely performed to accommodate a sufficiently sized prosthesis.

Specific Valvular Lesions

Aortic Stenosis

In the developed world, aortic valvular stenosis (AS) is the most common form of valvular heart disease requiring surgical intervention. AS is most often acquired, resulting from degenerative calcific changes to the valvular apparatus that lead to progressive stenosis. Because of the aging population, the prevalence of AS continues to rise, and it is now found in 3% of the population over 75 years old.[1] Most patients requiring surgery for trileaflet AS are aged 60 years or older. The progression of degenerative (calcific) aortic stenosis is now thought to be an actively regulated phenomenon related to atherosclerotic disease, wherein turbulent blood flow at leaflet attachment points induces endothelial injury and leads to lipid accumulation, infiltration of macrophages and T cells, and transformation of cells to an osteoblastic phenotype.[29] It is believed that this process leads to fibrosis and aortic leaflet calcification and may involve the aortic and mitral annuli as well as the mitral leaflets.

Patients less than 60 to 65 years old most often present with aortic stenosis resulting from fibrosis or calcification of a congenitally bicuspid aortic valve, which is susceptible to pathologic change at an earlier age. Bicuspid valves are present in 1% of the population, making this anomaly one of the most prevalent congenital valve lesions, with a 2:1 to 3:1 male-to-female ratio. There is also an association with other lesions, including coarctation, supra- or subvalvular AS, ventricular septal defect, sinus of Valsalva aneurysm, and patent ductus arteriosus. Degenerative disease of bicuspid aortic valves presents about two decades earlier than it does with tricuspid valves, peaking in the fifth and sixth decades of life. Sixty percent of patients over 70 years of age and 40% under 70 years of age with bicuspid valve will require aortic valve replacement to treat stenosis. Increased hemodynamic stresses associated with the abnormally configured bicuspid valve leaflets are thought to accelerate degenerative valve changes in this anomaly. Patients with bicuspid valves can have pure bicuspid pathology with two equal leaflets (Sievers type 0, 6% of bicuspid patients) or with fusion of two of the aortic cusps (Sievers type I), most commonly fusion of the right and left cusps (71% of patients), followed by fusion of the right and noncoronary cusps (15%) and noncoronary and left cusps (3%).[30] Unicuspid valves (Sievers type II, 5% of patients) have congenital fusion of multiple cusps and generally present with stenosis and symptoms at an early age.

Pathophysiology

The normal aortic valve orifice measures 3 to 5 cm^2. Aortic valve stenosis to less than half this size causes hemodynamic obstruction and a transvalvular pressure gradient as the primary pathophysiology of AS. This gradient induces compensatory increased ventricular pressure generated through Frank-Starling mechanisms and concentric LV hypertrophy via parallel replication of sarcomeres as a response to increased myocardial wall tension. Wall tension thereby normalizes according to the law of Laplace, and a compensated state preserving the systolic function of a hypertrophied but nondilated LV may persist for many years.

Two-thirds of patients who progress to severe AS develop myocardial ischemia because of the increased work and, consequently, elevated myocardial oxygen demands of the hypertrophied ventricle. The ventricle must generate increased ejection pressures over prolonged systolic intervals against the increased afterload of the narrowed aortic valve. Myocardial ischemia, particularly in the subendocardial region, is accentuated by the reduction of perfusion gradients during diastolic coronary flow intervals across the hypertrophied, hyperpressurized myocardial wall.

Myocardial hypertrophy can also precipitate ventricular diastolic dysfunction, which typically occurs before the onset of systolic dysfunction. Decreased ventricular compliance leads to increased left ventricular end-diastolic pressure (LVEDP), prolonged LV relaxation time, and shortened diastolic filling time. These increased pressures are transmitted back through the LA and pulmonary circulation, leading to pulmonary congestion. Pulmonary hypertension and right HF may develop in severe cases. Eventually, maximal ventricular hypertrophy is reached, and an adequate pressure gradient can no longer be achieved, resulting in inadequate cardiac outputs and overt systolic LV failure.

Increased LA pressure and consequent LA dilatation also increase the risk for atrial arrhythmias in patients with AS, albeit less commonly than in patients with MV disease. The loss of normal atrial contraction severely compromises filling of the noncompliant ventricle, leading to a precipitous decrease in cardiac output. Reduced forward flow can further increase LVEDP and aggravate the symptoms of HF.

Presyncope and syncope occur with AS related to inadequate cerebral perfusion, typically caused by inadequate forward flow through the restrictive aortic valve. Symptoms are associated with periods of peripheral vasodilatation, such as occurring during exercise or in changing from recumbent to standing positioning, when increased cardiac output is required to maintain peripheral vascular filling.

Diagnosis

Symptoms and signs. Patients with AS will typically remain asymptomatic for an extended time. The onset of symptoms occurs when the valve orifice area decreases to approximately 1 cm^2, which marks a critical point in the natural history of the disease. The classic symptoms of AS typically progress from the appearance of angina and (pre-)syncope to the occurrence of dyspnea associated with HF. Angina is the presenting symptom in 35% of AS patients, whereas syncope is a relatively sporadic event in about 15% of patients. Although HF typically appears late in the course of AS, dyspnea or other HF symptoms are presenting signs in 50% of patients.

Physical examination. The diagnosis of AS based on physical findings is frequently made before the onset of symptoms. The typical finding of AS is a crescendo-decrescendo ejection murmur best heard in the right second intercostal space and along the left sternal border. Radiation to carotid arteries is common. The apical impulse in AS is forceful and slightly enlarged. If HF develops, the apical impulse may become laterally displaced. The characteristic carotid upstroke of AS has a slow rate of rise and a reduced peak (*pulsus parvus et tardus*) and may have an associated thrill.

Diagnostic testing. Nonspecific findings of AS on chest radiography include a boot-shaped heart typical of concentric hypertrophy of the left ventricle, calcification of the valvular cusps, and poststenotic dilatation of the aorta. Roentgenographic signs of HF may ensue. Electrocardiographic changes are similar to those seen for MR.

Echocardiography allows the precise assessment of aortic valve anatomy, calcification, and effective orifice size. Ventricular hypertrophy and function can also be assessed. As with MS, Doppler echo allows measurement of transvalvular pressure gradients and valve area as a derived function (e.g., severe AS: Doppler velocity >4 m/sec = mean aortic valve gradient >40 mm Hg = valve area <1.0 cm²). Pressure gradients may be decreased in AS patients with low cardiac output, leading to miscalculated (falsely increased) aortic valve areas. This is referred to as *low-flow, low-gradient AS*. Dobutamine may be used during echo to increase cardiac output and assess the true severity of the AS lesion in these patients. Low-flow, low-gradient severe AS with normal LV function can be diagnosed by indexing the valve area and flow rate to the body surface area. In patients with only moderate AS with LV dysfunction, the valve area will increase as flow increases with the addition of dobutamine.

Cardiac catheterization may occasionally be needed to measure pressure gradients when data from noninvasive testing are nondiagnostic. Simultaneous pressure readings can be obtained in such instances with one pressure-measuring port in the body of the left ventricle and a second portion in the proximal aorta. Valvular area may then be determined using the Gorlin formula. Catheterization is important before surgery to assess the presence of coronary artery disease, coexistent in up to 50% of AS patients.

Natural History

Calcific AS is a progressive disease marked by a long, asymptomatic latent period that may vary greatly between individuals. Patients with moderate AS can, however, be expected to undergo a 7–mm Hg increase in mean pressure gradient or a 0.1-cm² decrease in valve area annually. Conversely, only about 10% of patients with mild aortic valve sclerosis (aortic velocity <2.5 m/sec) progress to severe AS within 5 years.

Ross and Braunwald's classic 1968 report first described the onset of symptoms as survival indicators in patients with AS (Fig. 112.15).[31] Mean survival after the appearance of angina is about 5 years, less than 3 years after the onset of syncope, and only 1 to 2 years once HF symptoms develop. Sudden death may also occur in symptomatic patients at a rate of 2% per month but appears to be rare (<1% per year) in asymptomatic patients.[32]

Treatment

Medical management. In general, medical therapy for AS is ineffective. Afterload reduction can lead to severe hypotension with a subsequent decline in cardiac output. Intraaortic balloon

pump counterpulsation can improve cardiac output and coronary flow for patients in cardiogenic shock while awaiting surgical intervention, but medical therapy will not reverse the hemodynamic changes consequent to the resultant obstruction to LV output from the stenotic valve.

Surgical Treatment

Because the natural history of untreated symptomatic AS is grave, mechanical relief of AS is recommended as a class I indication in all symptomatic patients with evidence of severe high-gradient AS (aortic velocity ≥4.0 m/sec or greater or mean pressure gradient ≥40 mm Hg) as well those patients with low-flow, low-gradient AS.[10] In addition to history taking, exercise or dobutamine stress echo is useful in eliciting symptoms and/or abnormal physiology (e.g., fall in systolic blood pressure, increase in transvalvular gradient, or decreased exercise tolerance) as a class IIa indicator for surgical intervention. Surgical intervention now also carries a class I indication in the asymptomatic patient with severe AS and evidence of LV dysfunction (left ventricle ejection fraction [LVEF] <50%). A class IIa indication also exists for asymptomatic patients with very severe AS (aortic velocity ≥5.0 m/sec or mean pressure gradient ≥60 mm Hg) who present low predicted surgical mortality risk (≤4%), given that symptoms are expected in 50% of these patients within 2 years and evidence suggesting that overall mortality risk is reduced with early surgery. Patients with severe AS (class I) or moderate AS (class IIb) who are undergoing cardiac surgery for other reasons can be considered for aortic valve replacement as well.

Surgery for AS almost always requires valve replacement, either with a mechanical or tissue valve or with a transcatheter biologic valve. Valve replacement is associated with excellent immediate and long-term outcomes, especially when conducted before the onset of ventricular dysfunction. Aortic valve surgery improves symptoms, increases life expectancy, and often improves or normalizes systolic function, depending on pathophysiologic status of the LV before surgery.

Exposure of the aortic valve is typically obtained via a transverse or "hockey stick" incision of the proximal ascending aorta (Fig. 112.16A). For valve replacement, the native aortic valve cusps are carefully excised to avoid perforation of the aortic wall, and a thorough decalcification of residual annular tissue is performed to improve prosthetic valve fit. After the resected valve orifice is sized (using a plastic avatar), the selected valve prosthesis is typically secured to the valve annulus using circumferentially placed, nonabsorbable, braided horizontal mattress sutures (see Fig. 112.16B). The sutures are tied securely so that there is no perivalvular defect, which would allow a regurgitant leak, and the aortotomy is closed. Homografts or "freestyle" stentless aortic valve homografts may sometimes be used if aortic root replacement is concomitantly required.[33] Repair options for the treatment of AS are limited, and earlier efforts at valve debridement met with poor intermediate-term outcomes with delayed onset of regurgitation, which led to the general abandonment of this technique.

Ross Procedure

The Ross procedure is a complex surgical procedure where the aortic valve or root is replaced with the native pulmonary valve, and the RV outflow tract is reconstructed with a homograft. This procedure may be considered in select young patients under 50 years of age at a Comprehensive Valve Center (class IIb).[10] It is a technically demanding procedure, and at present, the lack of

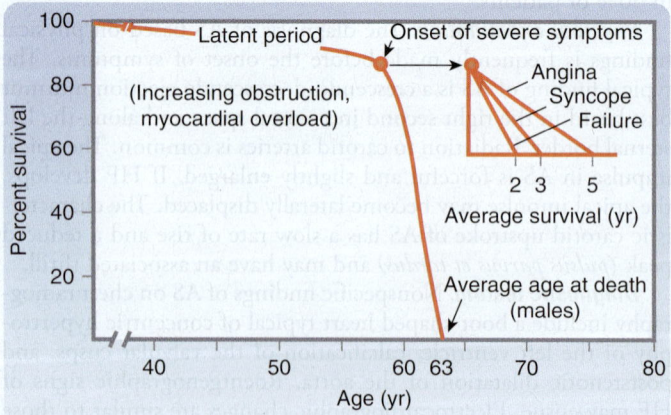

FIGURE 112.15 Symptoms and survival in aortic valvular stenosis. Ross and Braunwald's classic 1968 report first described the onset of symptoms of heart failure, syncope, or angina in patients with aortic valvular stenosis as a marker of impending death. (From Ross J Jr, Braunwald E. Aortic stenosis. *Circulation.* 1968;38:61-67.)

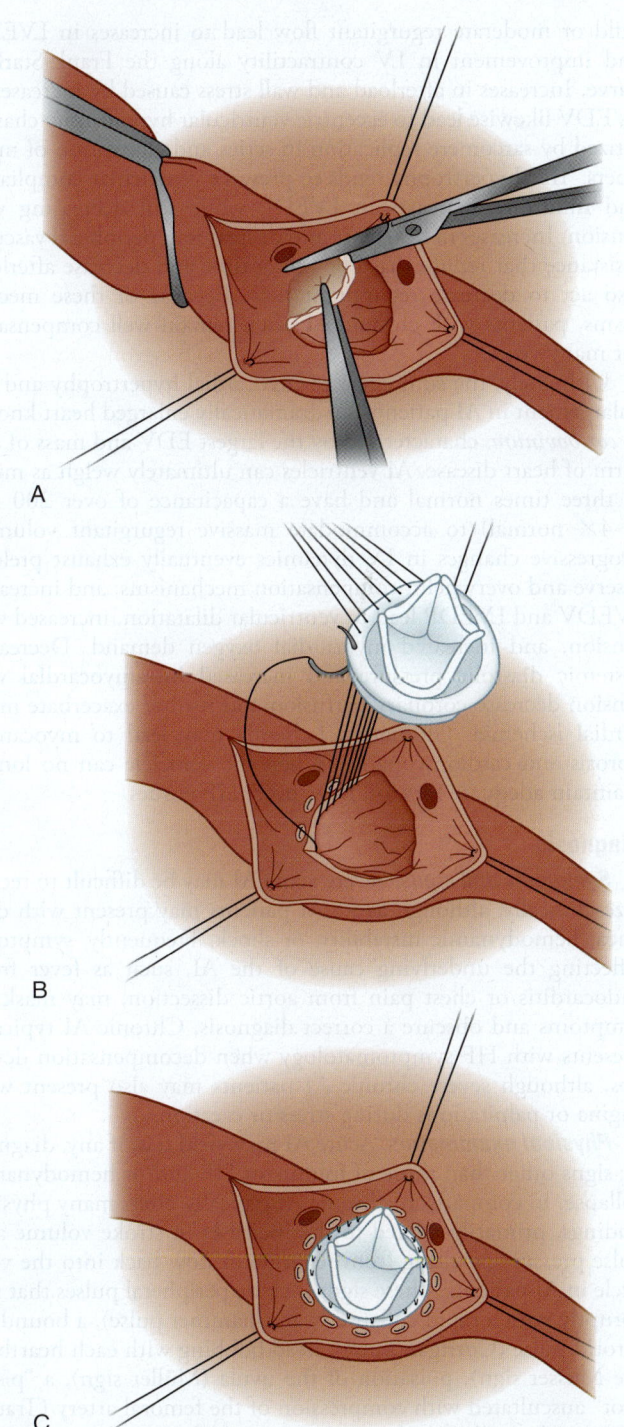

FIGURE 112.16 Aortic valve replacement surgery. Exposure of the aortic valve is typically obtained via a transverse or "hockey stick" incision of the proximal ascending aorta. After aortic valve excision (A), pledgeted horizontal mattress sutures are placed circumferentially into the valve annulus and then into the cloth sewing ring of the prosthesis (B). The prosthesis is then lowered into position, and the sutures are tied (C).

standardization of the operation may compromise its long-term durability. Specifically, maneuvers are being tested to reduce late dilation of the pulmonary autograft, stabilize a large native aortic annulus, and reduce long-term moderate to severe pulmonary homograft stenosis.

Transcatheter Aortic Valve Replacement

Transcatheter aortic valve replacement (TAVR) has become standard therapy to implant a bioprosthetic aortic valve in the aortic annulus through catheter technology without removal of the native aortic valve. It is mainly performed without the use of cardiopulmonary bypass. Currently available valves are generally grouped into balloon-expandable and self-expandable valves. (Fig. 112.17). This technology has rapidly evolved since its introduction in 2002 by Alain Cribier and colleagues to treat an inoperable patient with severe AS.[34,35] TAVR is an increasingly prevalent alternative to surgical aortic valve replacement (SAVR) and has replaced SAVR as the most common procedure to treat isolated AS.

Compelling evidence of the efficacy of TAVR was first provided by the Placement of AoRtic TraNscathetER Valves (PARTNER) trial, the world's first randomized study of this procedure.[36,37] These procedures were initially conducted in patients considered inoperable, and they were deemed to be superior to the standard therapy of balloon valvuloplasty in this cohort. Based on PARTNER and subsequent trials demonstrating that outcomes from TAVR were at least noninferior to SAVR, the FDA granted approval for TAVR in 2011 for prohibitive risk (STS >50% 30-day mortality or major morbidity) patients and in 2012 for high-risk (Society of Thoracic Surgeons [STS] predicted mortality >10% or ≥2 indices of frailty or >1 compromised major organ system) patients with a predicted postprocedural survival greater than 12 months. A critical component of these FDA approvals was the advent of the Heart Team, consisting of both cardiologists and cardiac surgeons, in evaluation and treatment of TAVR patients— a practice that has expanded to other cardiac surgery decision-making processes.

Expansion of indication to intermediate-risk patients (STS >4%–8% mortality)[38,39] and low-risk patients (STS ≤4% mortality)[40,41] followed in 2016 and 2019, respectively. Improved overall outcomes, stroke rates, and vascular complication rates in these second-generation trials have been generated through innovation of smaller-caliber catheters, better preprocedural planning with dedicated TAVR-protocol computed tomography (CT) review, improved patient selection, and deployment strategies. Complications such as complete heart block and paravalvular regurgitation are higher after TAVR than SAVR, and these

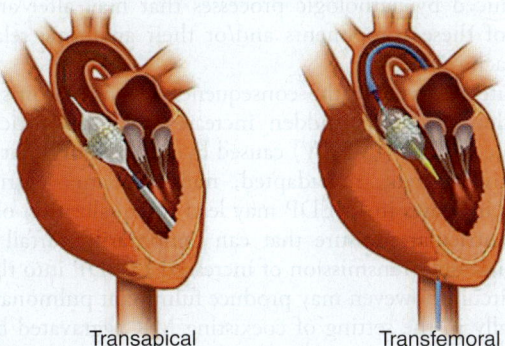

Transapical   Transfemoral

FIGURE 112.17 Transcatheter aortic valve replacement (TAVR). TAVR couples balloon aortic valvuloplasty with implantation of an expandable bioprosthesis delivered and expanded into the aortic annulus using catheter technology. (From Pick A. Surgeon Q&A: "What Determines the Transfemoral or Transapical Approach for TAVR?" Asks Denise. September 18, 2013. http://www.heart-valve-surgery.com/heart-surgery-blog/2013/09/18/tavr-transfemoral-transapical-approaches/. Accessed August 11, 2020.)

complications have been linked to higher long-term mortality. Other unanticipated complications also remain a concern, including increased valve thrombosis rates in TAVR versus SAVR valves. Clinical leaflet thrombosis, although rare at 0.5% of TAVR patients per year, may lead to elevated gradient and recurrent symptoms. Subclinical thrombosis more commonly affects up to 15% of TAVR patients.[42] Leaflet thrombosis may manifest as hypoattenuated leaflet thickening with or without restricted leaflet motion. Although the role of oral anticoagulation has been studied to decrease rates of subclinical thrombosis, this has not led to clear clinical benefits at this stage.

Aortic Regurgitation or Insufficiency

Aortic regurgitation (AR) or AI may be caused by myxomatous disease leading to thinning, enlargement, perforation, and/or prolapse of the aortic valve cusps themselves. AI may also be caused by chronic or acute dilatation of the aortic root, which prevents proper aortic valve coaptation by increasing intravalvular closing distances. Root enlargement is typically caused by hypertension and/or connective tissue disorders such as cystic medial necrosis, Marfan syndrome, Ehlers-Danlos syndrome, and Loeys-Dietz syndrome, either directly or as a result of acute or chronic aortic dissection.

Importantly, (Mendelian) inheritance of a bicuspid aortic valve anomaly is also associated with dilation of the proximal ascending aorta in up to 50% of patients, which can lead to bicuspid-related AI.[43] This association is hypothesized to be due to a currently unidentified common genetic defect causing abnormalities in aortic wall elasticity. AI resulting from bicuspid valve–related root enlargement typically develops at a much younger age than AS that develops from accelerated degeneration.

Less common causes of aortic root enlargement and/or aortic dissection include giant cell aortitis (most often in elderly females), Takayasu aortitis (more commonly affects the aortic arch branch vessels), and syphilitic aortitis (mostly of historical interest only).

Pathophysiology

The aortic valve is dependent on the coordinated function of a complex and dynamic anatomy to preserve its competency. This apparatus includes the aortic valve cusps, annulus, sinuses of Valsalva, and the sinotubular junction above the sinuses. AI may be induced by pathologic processes that may alter any one or more of these components and/or their anatomic relationships with each other.

Acute AI, usually the consequence of endocarditis or aortic dissection, produces sudden increases in left ventricular end-diastolic volume (LVEDV) caused by acute regurgitant flow into a relatively small, nonadapted, noncompliant ventricle. Even greater increases in LVEDP may lead to equalization of systemic and ventricular pressure that can temporarily curtail increased regurgitation. Transmission of increased LVEDP into the pulmonary circuit, however, may produce fulminant pulmonary edema, especially in the setting of coexisting MR aggravated by sudden increases in LV dimensions. Consequently, an increase in LV wall tension leads to myocardial ischemia, (exacerbated if aortic dissection extends to the coronary ostia), hemodynamic collapse, or sudden death.

Chronic AI, like chronic MR, is an insidious process that triggers compensatory mechanisms, including LV enlargement and hypertrophy, that help maintain net forward stroke volume and decrease wall tension. At first, increases in LV filling caused by mild or moderate regurgitant flow lead to increases in LVEDV and improvement in LV contractility along the Frank-Starling curve. Increases in afterload and wall stress caused by increases in LVEDV likewise lead to eccentric ventricular hypertrophy characterized by sarcomere replication in series and elongation of myofibers. This hypertrophy tends to preserve ventricular compliance and minimize increases in LVEDP while still decreasing wall tension. Increases in heart rate and decreases in peripheral vascular resistance that reduce diastolic filling time and decrease afterload also act to decrease regurgitant flow. Because of these mechanisms, patients with chronic AI often remain well compensated for many years.

Ultimately, the sum effect of myocardial hypertrophy and LV enlargement in AI patients is a dramatically enlarged heart known as *cor bovinum,* characterized by the largest EDV and mass of any form of heart disease. AI ventricles can ultimately weigh as much as three times normal and have a capacitance of over 200 mL (~4× normal) to accommodate massive regurgitant volumes. Progressive changes in LV dynamics eventually exhaust preload reserve and overwhelm compensation mechanisms, and increased LVEDV and LVEDP lead to ventricular dilatation, increased wall tension, and increased myocardial oxygen demand. Decreased systemic diastolic pressure and increased intramyocardial wall tension decrease coronary perfusion and further exacerbate myocardial ischemia. Ultimately, ischemia may lead to myocardial fibrosis and cardiomyopathy. When the ventricle can no longer maintain adequate forward flow, overt HF ensues.

Diagnosis

Symptoms and signs. Severe acute AI may be difficult to recognize clinically, although acute AI patients may present with dyspnea, hemodynamic instability, or shock. Frequently, symptoms reflecting the underlying cause of the AI, such as fever from endocarditis or chest pain from aortic dissection, may mask AI symptoms and obscure a correct diagnosis. Chronic AI typically presents with HF symptomatology when decompensation develops, although severe chronic AI patients may also present with angina or palpitations during stress or exertion.

Physical examination. Acute AI may yield few, if any, diagnostic signs other than those of fulminant HF and/or hemodynamic collapse. In comparison, chronic AI typically offers many physical findings, primarily related to the increases in stroke volume and pulse pressure resulting from regurgitant flow back into the ventricle in AI patients. These signs include peripheral pulses that rise abruptly with a rapid collapse (water-hammer pulse), a bounding carotid pulse (Corrigan pulse), head bobbing with each heartbeat (de Musset sign), pulsation of the uvula (Müller sign), a "pistol shot" auscultated with compression of the femoral artery (Traube sign), and capillary pulsations seen with fingernail compression using a glass slide (Quincke sign).

Cardiac examination typically reveals an apical impulse that is diffuse, hyperdynamic, and displaced inferiorly and laterally. It may be associated with a systolic thrill at the base of the heart, suprasternal notch, and carotid arteries as a result of high stroke volume. Auscultation reveals a high-frequency, blowing, decrescendo diastolic murmur best heard with the diaphragm at the left sternal border with the patient sitting up, leaning forward, and at end-exhalation. The murmur is increased by maneuvers such as squatting or handgrip, which increase diastolic pressure. The examiner may appreciate a mid- and late-diastolic apical rumble (Austin-Flint murmur), which is thought to be secondary to vibration of the anterior mitral leaflet caused by a posteriorly directed AI jet. The second heart sound may be soft or absent, and a third heart sound may be present.

Diagnostic testing. Chest radiography in patients with acute AI may reveal only pulmonary edema, and electrocardiography (ECG) may reveal evidence of LV strain, but echocardiography may be the only test useful in diagnosing this condition. With chronic AI, chest radiography typically shows a significantly enlarged cardiac silhouette. The ascending aorta may be enlarged if AI is a result of an aortic aneurysm. ECG will typically show signs of increased LV mass, notably left axis deviation and increased QRS amplitude with strain patterns and conduction abnormalities.

Echocardiography allows the comprehensive evaluation of aortic apparatus abnormalities, LV size and compliance, and the character and magnitude of the regurgitant jet. Severe AI is diagnosed by a jet width ≥65% of the LV outflow tract, vena contracta >0.6 cm, regurgitant fraction (RF) ≥50%, regurgitant volume ≥60 mL/beat, or an effective regurgitant orifice (ERO) area ≥0.3 cm². Cardiac magnetic resonance imaging (MRI) can also be used to quantify severity more accurately. RF >33% and LVEDV >246 mL increase the likelihood of progression of disease and valvular intervention within 3 years, whereas RF ≤33% rarely progresses.[44]

Natural History

Although acute AI may lead to the sudden onset of HF and/or hemodynamic collapse, patients with chronic AI remain asymptomatic for years with compensated LV function. The combined likelihood of onset of adverse events for such patients (LV dysfunction, onset of symptoms, or death) is less than 5% per year. Overall, the freedom from ventricular dysfunction or death in asymptomatic patients is about 75% at 5 years and 60% at 10 years.[45] Once the LV end-systolic diameter is ≥50 mm, adverse event rates increase to about 20% per year, and once symptoms develop in AI patients, mortality rates rise to over 10% per year.[10,11,45]

Treatment

Medical management. Medical therapy should be considered only as a temporizing measure for patients with acute severe AI and acute volume overload, hypotension, and/or pulmonary edema because they will require emergent surgery. In this scenario, vasodilators and inotropes may be valuable in augmenting forward flow and reducing LVEDP. β blockers used for aortic dissection should be employed with great caution in other causes of acute AI because they block compensatory tachycardia and could cause a significant drop in blood pressure. Importantly, intraaortic balloon pump is contraindicated in severe AI because it will worsen regurgitation and forward output.

Patients with chronic severe AI may benefit from medical management, with the primary goal of reducing systolic hypertension, therefore reducing wall stress and improving ventricular function. Vasodilating drugs may improve hemodynamic abnormalities and forward flow, but their effect in favorably prolonging the asymptomatic period in patients with chronic severe AI and normal ventricular function is uncertain.

Surgical Treatment

Urgent or emergent surgical intervention to repair or replace the aortic valve and address underlying pathologic mechanisms is nearly always indicated in patients with acute severe AI (e.g., for endocarditis, aortic dissection). Surgery is also indicated (class I) for symptomatic patients with severe chronic AI.[10] Importantly,

based on improved current understanding of the natural history of chronic AI, aortic valve surgery is now a class I indication for asymptomatic chronic severe AI patients with LV systolic dysfunction (LVEF <50%). It should also be considered for asymptomatic severe AI with LVEF ≥50% with severe LV dilation (LVESD >50 mm or indexed LVESD >25 mm/m²) as a class IIa indication or as class IIb indication for progressive severe LV dilation (LV end-diastolic diameter >65 mm).[10]

Valve replacement with mechanical or biologic prostheses has yielded excellent results in correcting isolated AI (see Table 112.5); however, over the past two decades, increasing numbers of centers are employing repair strategies in selected patients. For patients with aortic root disease, these procedures are typically combined with root repair or replacement and coronary reimplantation, as discussed elsewhere in this text.

Percutaneous transcatheter valve therapies to address AI are still under clinical investigation and are not yet FDA approved. In select patients, AI may be treated by the Ross procedure. Durable results with this technically demanding procedure have been demonstrated in highly experienced centers, especially for younger patients (<30 years of age) and in very young patients where significant growth is anticipated.

Aortic valve repair may be an option for selected patients with AI or a normally functioning aortic valve associated with an aortic root or ascending aortic aneurysm. When AI is secondary to dilation of the aortic root or ascending aorta, valve-sparing operations that stabilize the annulus and remodel the sinotubular junction can be very effective. Valve-sparing root replacement, commonly known as the "David" procedure after Dr. Tirone David, the pioneer of this operation, is a complex but highly successful procedure involving reimplantation of the native valve inside a Dacron graft.[46,47]

Mitral Stenosis

Pathophysiology

There is typically no pressure gradient across a normally sized MV (4–6 cm² cross-sectional area), and "upstream" LA pressure is typically less than 10 to 15 mm Hg. As the MV orifice narrows to a cross-sectional area of 2 to 2.5 cm² (mild MS), resistance to flow leads to increased LA blood volume "pooling." Increased LA pressure generated by Frank-Starling mechanics maintains adequate diastolic flow across the resistive valve orifice.

When progressive MS leads to a transvalvular gradient of greater than 5 to 10 mm Hg, typically corresponding to a valve orifice of ≤1.5 cm², MS is classified as "severe." The resultant increase in LA pressure is transmitted upstream to the pulmonary veins, capillaries, and arteries. At an LA pressure of 25 mm Hg, pulmonary edema typically develops, with prolonged arterial vasoconstriction and vascular remodeling eventually leading to reversible at first, but then ultimately fixed, pulmonary hypertension with chronically increased pulmonary pressure. Elevated pulmonary arterial systolic pressure (PASP) ≥60 mm Hg imparts significant RV afterload and will ultimately lead to RV dilatation, TR, and RV failure. MS spares LV function in two-thirds of cases, with normal or less-than-normal LV chamber hemodynamics in 85% of cases and impaired output primarily resulting from restricted LV inflow.

Any increase in cardiac output, as with exercise, will lead to an increase in mitral transvalvular pressure gradients according to the law of Poiseuille: flow α Δpressure gradient/resistance. At a given cardiac output, decreased diastolic filling time caused by increased heart rates, such as with exercise or the onset of atrial fibrillation, will also cause increased transvalvular gradient because more flow must occur per unit time.

Chronically increased transmitral pressure gradients caused by MS typically lead to atrial hypertrophy and dilatation. Associated LA fibrosis and disorganization of the atrial muscle fibers cause abnormal atrial conduction velocities and refractory times. Increased automaticity, ectopic foci, and reentry circuits eventually lead to supraventricular tachyarrhythmias in nearly 40% of patients. Loss of the "kick" generated by normal atrial contraction, responsible for 30% of ventricular filling, results in a 20% decrease in cardiac output. Atrial pressure then must increase to facilitate sufficient ventricular loading. Atrial fibrillation consequently causes increased diastolic pressures and volume overload, potentially leading to worsening congestion.

Mitral stenosis is commonly caused by RHD in underdeveloped countries, and RHD most commonly involves the MV. It is highly uncommon to have valvular RHD without mitral involvement. In the developed world, mitral annular calcification (MAC) and calcification of the MV leaflets are quite common, especially with advanced age. MAC is usually a finding, not a symptom, because it generally has no effect on MV function. MAC is a common degenerative change found in older patients that is typically without functional sequelae. The prevalence of MAC is 5% to 10% in those 60 years of age but increases to nearly 50% in those over 70 years of age.[48] MAC can, however, on occasion produce MR by reducing annulus pliability and systolic contraction, thus preventing appropriate leaflet coaptation. Less frequently, MAC disorders manifest through a more widespread degenerative pathology. MAC may be associated with similar changes involving the aortic valve or coronary atherosclerosis, in which case its presence portends a poor long-term prognosis in these patients.

Although MAC often coexists with aortic valve calcification and coronary atherosclerosis, its pathogenesis is distinct. Presumed mechanisms for MAC include molecular injury with abnormal collagen matrix serving as the substrate for lipid deposition and bone formation promulgated by inflammation and dysregulation of calcium-phosphate handling. When MAC affects MV function, diffuse calcification of both leaflets can cause mitral stenosis as a result of leaflet retraction and calcific distortion of proper motion of the mitral subvalvular apparatus. Occasionally, annular calcification will extend only to the posterior leaflet, in which case it can cause MR as a result of restricted leaflet motion. Degenerative calcific disease that is nonrheumatic in origin in the most common cause of MS in older patients. Other rare causes of MS include endocarditis and congenital anomalies such as parachute MV and as a component of Shone complex, which is associated with supramitral rings.

Diagnosis

Symptoms and signs. MS patients may remain asymptomatic for many years. As valvular stenosis gradually worsens, however, symptoms characteristic of low cardiac output and pulmonary venous congestion eventually develop, including fatigue, dyspnea, and orthopnea. Ultimately, peripheral edema and other congestive symptoms caused by volume overload and right HF ensue. Increased heart rate caused by atrial fibrillation or supraventricular tachycardia, exercise, or other factors may exacerbate symptomatology.

Patients with MS who develop atrial fibrillation may complain of palpitations and symptomatic tachycardia. More ominously, thromboembolization will occur in 20% of patients with MS and

may be its first symptom in 10% of cases, presenting as stroke, myocardial ischemia or infarction, renal infarction, and gut or limb ischemia. Half of all thromboembolic events will involve the cerebral circulation. Thromboembolism associated with atrial fibrillation is generally a result of stasis of blood in the LA appendage when normal pump function (atrial contraction) is impaired. Rarely, a large, pedunculated atrial thrombus may form and obstruct the valve inlet, resulting in hemodynamic collapse and sudden death. Pulmonary venous congestion may induce hemoptysis from sudden rupture of a dilated bronchial vein. RV failure and TR can cause abdominal pain and swelling from hepatomegaly, ascites, and, often, peripheral edema.

Physical examination. The characteristic physical finding of MS is a low-pitched, rumbling diastolic murmur that is best heard at the apex with the patient in the left lateral decubitus position. In patients who are in sinus rhythm, the murmur increases in intensity during late diastole (known as *presystolic accentuation*) because of the increased flow across the stenotic valve with atrial contraction. A high-pitched "opening snap" or an accentuated first heart sound caused by forceful opening or closing, respectively, of an inflexible but still mobile mitral leaflet may be heard with early MS. The Graham-Steell murmur, an early blowing diastolic murmur of functional pulmonary regurgitation, is caused by pulmonary hypertension and right-sided overload from MS.

Advanced MS is typically associated with rales developing with the onset of pulmonary edema. As RV failure develops, an RV heave, jugular venous distention, hepatomegaly, ascites, and lower extremity edema may be found.

Diagnostic testing. The classic appreciable changes of MS discernable by routine chest radiography include evidence of an enlarged LA, seen as a straightening of the left cardiac border; a double shadow in the cardiac silhouette; or an elevated left main stem bronchus. Prominent pulmonary vessels may also be appreciated. If stenosis is severe, congested pulmonary lymphatics in the lower lung fields may be present as horizontal linear opacities, known as *Kerley B lines.* MV calcification may also be visible. Stigmata of HF, such as opacification of the lung fields and pleural effusions, may follow. The changes in chest radiography, though, are mostly of historical interest because patients generally present before developing the massive secondary consequences of long-term disease, which was more the case before the advent of adequate medical and surgical therapeutic options.

The ECG of MS patients is often grossly normal, although 90% of patients will demonstrate evidence of LA enlargement as a widened, notched P wave (p mitrale). Atrial arrhythmias may also be appreciated if present. With advanced MS, RV hypertrophy may be associated with right-axis deviation.

Echocardiography, as with other valve lesions, is the primary diagnostic method to determine the presence and severity of MS and associated abnormalities. Commissural fusion, leaflet immobility, and leaflet and annular or subvalvular thickening and calcification can be well assessed by transthoracic and especially by transesophageal echocardiography (TEE). Three-dimensional (3D) echocardiography provides further definition of valve morphology and function.

Doppler echocardiography has largely replaced cardiac catheterization in accurately assessing the hemodynamic parameters of MS and other valve lesions. Doppler blood velocity measurement allows mean and peak transvalvular mitral pressure gradient determination as a function of the simplified Bernoulli equation: $p = 4v^2$, where v equals the velocity of blood crossing the valve orifice. Orifice area can be measured by planimetry (tracing the valve-opening orifice on a still echocardiographic image) or as a derivative of velocity measurements based on continuity equations. MV area can also be determined based on the pressure half-time, the time in which the transvalvular velocity decreases by half. Pressure half-time will become prolonged with increasing severity of stenosis.

Natural History

Ten-year patient survival is greater than 80% in the asymptomatic patient with MS, and interventional treatment is consequently not recommended in this setting. In comparison, 10-year survival for symptomatic patients with severe MS who forgo intervention is less than 15%, and mean survival is less than 3 years in patients with MS and severe pulmonary hypertension.

Treatment

Medical management. Medical management of patients with symptomatic MS includes the use of diuretics to reduce LA pressure and vascular congestion. β-blockers and calcium channel-blocking agents are recommended to provide heart rate control and help maintain sinus rhythm. Anticoagulation therapy is recommended via CHADS$_2$ and the updated CHADS$_2$-VASc (modification to better assess low-risk patients) scoring systems in patients with atrial fibrillation (Table 112.6) and in patients without atrial fibrillation but who have suffered a prior embolic event or have a documented LA thrombus. Use of anticoagulation therapy must be tempered against the risk of major bleeding, which can now be calculated using the Hypertension, Abnormal renal/liver function, Stroke, Bleeding history or predisposition, Labile INR, Elderly [>65 years], Drugs/alcohol concomitantly (HAS-BLED) scoring system developed in 2010 from data in the Euro Heart Survey to assess 1-year risk of major bleeding in patients taking anticoagulants with atrial fibrillation.[49]

TABLE 112.6 CHADS$_2$ and CHADS$_2$-VASc Score for Atrial Fibrillation Stroke Risk and Recommended Anticoagulation

CHADS$_2$ SCORE	POINTS[a]	CHADS$_2$-VASc SCORE	POINTS[a]
C Congestive heart failure	1	Congestive heart failure	1
H Hypertension	1	Hypertension	1
A Age ≥75 years	1	Age ≥75 years	2
D Diabetes mellitus	1	Diabetes mellitus	1
S Prior stroke, TIA, or thromboembolism	2	Prior stroke, TIA, or thromboembolism	2
V		Vascular disease	1
A		Age 65–74 years	1
Sc		Sex category (female)	1

[a]Points for each risk factor are additive.
CHADS$_2$: Score of 0, low risk; 1, moderate risk; 2–6, high risk.
CHADS$_2$-VASc: Score of 0 (male) or 1 (female), low risk; 1, moderate risk (male); 2–9, high risk.
Recommended therapy for moderate or high risk is typically oral anticoagulant, with well-controlled vitamin K antagonist (VKA; e.g., warfarin with time in therapeutic range >70%) or a non-VKA oral anticoagulant (NOAC; e.g., dabigatran, rivaroxaban, edoxaban, or apixaban).
TIA, Transient ischemic attack.

Surgical Treatment

Early intervention is associated with improved long-term survival for patients with MS compared with patients in whom intervention is delayed until the development of symptomatology. Five-year survival is 62% for New York Heart Association (NHYA) class III patients and 15% for class IV patients.[49,50] The current American Heart Association/American College of Cardiology (AHA/ACC) guidelines accordingly recommend intervention for patients with symptomatic severe (valve orifice area <1.5 cm^2) or asymptomatic very severe (valve orifice area <1 cm^2) mitral stenosis.[10] Additionally, surgery is recommended for patients with moderate or severe MS undergoing cardiac surgery for other reasons and for patients with severe MS who have recurrent embolic events while on anticoagulation (with LA excision recommended). Options for mechanical intervention include percutaneous mitral balloon commissurotomy, open mitral commissurotomy and surgical repair, and replacement of the MV.

Percutaneous Balloon Mitral Commissurotomy

Percutaneous balloon mitral commissurotomy (PBMC) is an endovascular procedure first reported by Inoue and colleagues in 1984. It uses a balloon catheter advanced into the left atrium, via a transseptal puncture or retrograde transaortic delivery, to dilate a stenotic MV. Based on compelling safety and efficacy data, PBMC has largely replaced surgical interventions in appropriately selected patients based on (Wilkins) echocardiographic criteria (Table 112.7). In general, PBMC is indicated by the presence of mobile, noncalcified, thin valves with minimal fusion, scarring, or calcification of the subvalvular apparatus and the absence of moderate to severe MR or an LA thrombus. PBMC is associated with a mortality risk of 0.5% and a less than 10% risk of cardiac or vascular complications, embolization, or creation of severe MR. Successful PBMC, defined as a postdilation valve area of more than 1.5 cm^2 with MR grade less than 2/4, is achieved in over 80% of patients. Although reintervention is often required, over half of patients can expect to remain free from surgery at 20 years.[51] Success rates and durability of repair, however, diminish substantially with each subsequent reintervention.

For open surgery, the MV is typically exposed through a left atriotomy, made anterior to the pulmonary veins (Fig. 112.18A). A right atriotomy and incision through the atrial septum also provide excellent exposure to the MV. Even greater exposure can be provided by a "superior septal" approach joining the right atrial and septostomy incisions onto the dome of the left atrium, but this approach requires more extensive closure and has the potential for sinus node dysfunction and complete heart block.

Open mitral commissurotomy is the primary form of surgical repair of MS and is limited to use for patients in whom intervention is needed but PBMC is contraindicated or those who have failed previous percutaneous intervention. Open mitral commissurotomy requires use of cardiopulmonary bypass and involves division of fused commissures, mobilization of scarred chordae, and ligation of the LA appendage. The mortality rate for open commissurotomy is less than 2%, and the 10-year rate of freedom from reoperation after open mitral commissurotomy is approximately 90%.[52,53] This procedure is rarely performed in the United States and other developed countries.

MV replacement is the most commonly employed surgical management of MS. Regardless of whether a mechanical or tissue valve is employed, there is well-documented evidence that preservation of the subvalvular apparatus is critical for the maintenance of optimal LV geometry and function and improved 30-day and

TABLE 112.7 **Wilkins Score for Assessing Appropriateness of Percutaneous Balloon Mitral Commissurotomy**

GRADE	MOBILITY	THICKENING	CALCIFICATION	SUBVALVULAR THICKENING
1	Highly mobile valve with only leaflet tips restricted	Leaflets near normal in thickness (4–5 mm)	A single area of increased echocardiographic brightness	Minimal thickening just below the mitral leaflets
2	Leaflet mid- and base portions have normal mobility	Midleaflets normal, considerable thickening of margins (5–8 mm)	Scattered areas of brightness confined to leaflet margins	Thickening of chordal structures extending to one-third of the chordal length
3	Valve continues to move forward in diastole, mainly from the base	Thickening extending through the entire leaflet (5–8 mm)	Brightness extending into the midportions of the leaflets	Thickening extended to distal third of the chords
4	No or minimal forward movement of the leaflets in diastole	Considerable thickening of all leaflet tissue (>8–10 mm)	Extensive brightness throughout much of the leaflet tissue	Extensive thickening and shortening of all chordal structures extending down to the papillary muscles

Sum of the four items ranges between 4 and 16. With a score of 8 or less, percutaneous balloon mitral valvuloplasty is likely to be successful. If the score is more than 8, surgery is recommended.

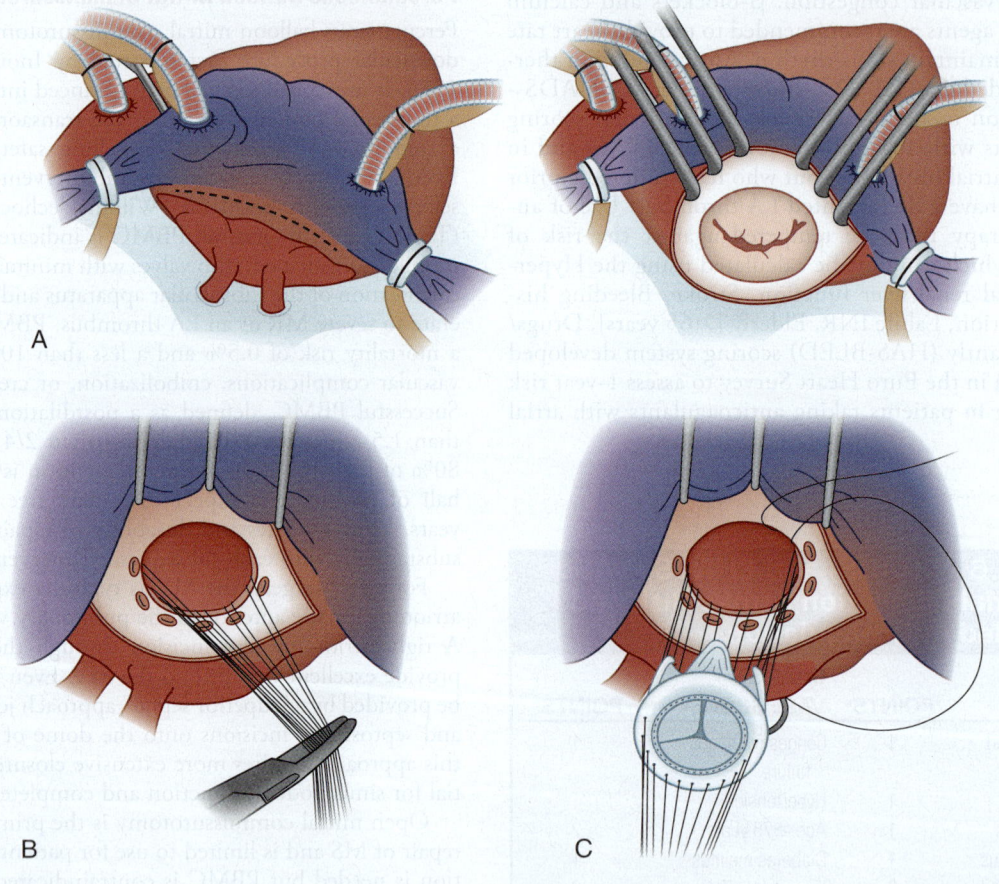

FIGURE 112.18 Mitral valve replacement surgery. (A) The mitral valve is typically exposed through a left lateral atriotomy made just anterior to the pulmonary veins. (B) After partial excision of the native valve, pledgeted horizontal mattress sutures are placed circumferentially into the valve annulus and then into the cloth sewing ring of the prosthesis. (C) Valve lowered into position and sutures securely tied. (From Glower DD. Surgical approaches to mitral regurgitation. *J Am Coll Cardiol.* 2012;60:1315-1322.)

long-term survival.[54,55] If MAC is present or the etiology is calcific disease rather than rheumatic disease, surgery can be more risky. Perivalvular leak resulting from poor sealing of the sewing cuff to the calcified annulus can occur. The most dreaded complication is AV groove disruption resulting from cracking of the calcium in this region. Fatal bleeding can result.

Minimal valve leaflet resection (portion of the anterior leaflet) is currently preferred for MV replacement, making best efforts to preserve the chordae and subvalvular apparatus in continuity with the valve annulus. If the chordae or leaflets are severely calcified or fibrotic, resection may be required to facilitate implantation of an adequately sided valve prosthesis without perivalvular leak. After the resected valve orifice is sized (using a plastic avatar), the selected valve prosthesis is typically secured to the valve annulus using circumferentially placed, nonabsorbable, braided horizontal mattress sutures (see Fig. 112.18B). The sutures are tied securely so that there is no perivalvular defect, and the atriotomy is closed after de-airing of the heart (see Fig. 112.18C).

Mitral Regurgitation

MR is the most frequent form of valve dysfunction and is the second most common type of valvular heart disease requiring surgical intervention. The diagnosis and treatment of MR were greatly facilitated by the work of Carpentier, who, in innovating surgical approaches to repair the MV, also described a functional classification of MR based on abnormal patterns of leaflet motion (Table 112.8).[2] Degenerative changes to the MV apparatus, with leaflet prolapse or elongation/rupture of the chordae tendineae, are the most common causes of MR and can present at any adult age, mostly past the third or fourth decade (see Table 112.1). Surgical intervention for MR is primarily reserved for treatment of degenerative disease. Open surgical intervention for ischemic disease and for functional MR resulting from ventricular cardiomyopathy has diminished dramatically since the introduction of TEER. Endocarditis remains a consistent indication for MV surgery in 2% to 5% of patients.

A wide variety of connective tissue diseases may lead to degenerative disease of the MV, typically causing annular dilation without leaflet abnormalities (Carpentier type I lesion) and/or leaflet or subvalvular deformations resulting in excessive leaflet motion (Carpentier type II lesion). The most prevalent of these diseases is Marfan syndrome. *Myxomatous disease* describes a common pathologic end point of these degenerative diseases, which typically presents as MR in the third or fourth decade of life. This process is characterized by glycosaminoglycan infiltration of the valve leaflets, thickening of the spongiosa, and separation of collagen bundles in the fibrosa.

Myxomatous disease of the MV typically leads to redundant, "billowing" valve leaflets; annular dilatation; and/or chordae elongation with resulting abnormal systolic leaflet prolapse into the atrium. This syndrome typically occurs in young females without obvious connective tissue disease and is known as *Barlow disease* after the clear identification in 1963 of the etiology of this "click-murmur syndrome" by John Barlow in South Africa.[56] Myxomatous disease most commonly manifests as mitral disease, but it may also present as aortic or tricuspid valve pathology.

Fibroelastic deficiency syndrome represents a spectrum of myxomatous MV disease, as clearly described by David Adams from Mount Sinai in New York.[56] Fibroelastic deficiency generally involves myxomatous change of a single segment of the MV, most commonly the posterior leaflet, characterized by thinned leaflets with rupture of a chord without excessive leaflet tissue. Prolapse or flail of the middle posterior leaflet cusp (P2) as a result of chordae rupture is the most common manifestation of fibroelastic deficiency syndrome. Fibroelastic deficiency+ (plus) is fibroelastic deficiency with excessive leaflet tissue in a single segment that will need to be resected to correct the pathologic change. Forme fruste presents with excessive leaflet tissue in multiple segments, generally multiple segments of the posterior leaflet. Barlow disease is the diffuse expression of fibroelastic deficiency with involvement of multiple segments of both leaflets.

Coronary ischemia causing rupture of a papillary muscle or acute myocardial infarction, particularly in the inferior distribution, can also lead to significant MR. This primarily affects the posteromedial papillary muscle, which has a single blood supply from the terminal branch of the posterior descending coronary artery, whereas the anterolateral papillary muscle receives dual blood supply from the left anterior descending and circumflex arteries.

In contrast to the causes of primary MR noted earlier, secondary or "functional" MR is not caused by abnormalities of the valve itself but rather by distortion of the subvalvular apparatus and ventricle. Typically, functional MR is a result of myocardial ischemic events and/or cardiomyopathy-induced ventricular dilatation. Symmetric dilation of the ventricle causes the mitral annulus to dilate, resulting in malcoaptation of the leaflets and central regurgitation during diastole. Asymmetric dilation of the ventricle, often from ischemia, results in outward (lateral) and apical

TABLE 112.8 Carpentier Classification of Mitral Valve Regurgitation

CARPENTIER CLASSIFICATION	DYSFUNCTION	LESIONS	ETIOLOGY
Type I	Normal leaflet motion	Annular dilatation	Dilated cardiomyopathy
		Leaflet perforation/tear	Endocarditis
Type II	Excessive leaflet motion (prolapse)	Elongation/rupture of chordae	Degenerative valve disease
		Elongation/rupture of papillary muscle	Fibroelastic deficiency
			Barlow disease
			Marfan disease
			Rheumatic (acute)
			Endocarditis
			Trauma
			Ischemic cardiomyopathy
Type IIIa	Restricted leaflet motion (diastole and systole)	Leaflet thickening/retraction	Rheumatic (chronic)
		Leaflet calcification	Carcinoid heart disease
		Chordal thickening/retraction/fusion	
		Commissural fusion	
Type IIIb	Restricted leaflet motion (systole)	Left ventricular dilatation/aneurysm	Ischemic/dilated cardiomyopathy
		Papillary muscle displacement	
		Chordae tethering	

From Carpentier A. Cardiac valve surgery—the "French correction." *J Thorac Cardiovasc Surg.* 1983;86:323-337.

(inferior) displacement of the posteromedial papillary muscle, causing tethering of the valve leaflets and loss of central coaptation (Carpentier type IIIb lesion). If dyskinesis of the basal inferior wall coexists, replacement of the valve is generally necessary to eliminate regurgitation.

Other acquired forms of MR include those that limit systolic motion of the mitral leaflets (Carpentier IIIa lesion with restricted leaflet most commonly calcific or rheumatic) and restricted motion of the posterior leaflet resulting from ischemic change in the posterior LV wall (Carpentier IIIb lesion). Congenital anomalies such as cleft leaflets and AV canal/endocardial cushion defects also cause MR.

Pathophysiology

Pathologic changes to any component of the MV apparatus may cause improper systolic coaptation between the anterior and posterior mitral leaflets, with subsequent valvular regurgitation. MR is subdivided into primary and secondary MR, which are distinct in their pathophysiology, natural history, and treatment approach. Primary MR, classified as type I (normal leaflet motion with annular dilatation) or II (abnormal leaflet motion) in the Carpentier classification (see Table 112.8), is secondary to pathologies affecting the structure of the MV apparatus, specifically the leaflets, chordae, and annulus. In contrast, secondary or functional MR, classified as Carpentier type IIIb, is secondary to LV dysfunction and dilation, primarily resulting from ischemic cardiomyopathy with restricted posterior leaflet motion. The severity of MR is dependent on the size of the mitral orifice, the pressure gradient between the LA and LV, and the systemic afterload. Because LV pressure exceeds LA pressure well before it exceeds systemic pressure, MV incompetency may allow a significant amount of regurgitant volume (up to one-half of the ventricular preload) into the LA well before the opening of the aortic valve and forward flow into the aorta.

In the acute phase of MR, retrograde flow into a small, low-compliance receiving LA chamber may be poorly tolerated, and high atrial pressures may be transmitted into the pulmonary vasculature. Pulmonary hypertension with fulminant HF can ensue and may even prove to be fatal. When the onset of MR is more insidious, the LA can dilate and hypertrophy, and a chronic compensated state without pulmonary hypertension may be sustained for many years. On the other hand, LA dilatation may be accompanied by atrial fibrillation with the potential for thrombosis and episodic embolization as a result of relative stasis of blood in the dyskinetic atrium.

Critical compensatory changes in LV hemodynamics are characteristic of chronic MR. Regurgitant volumes returning to the LV during diastole result in increased LVEDV and supranormal EFs, based both on standard Frank-Starling mechanics and the presence of LV ejection into the relatively low-resistance or low-afterload LA. Although net forward blood flow is reduced, this supranormal ejection serves to marginally unload the LV and normalize LVEDV. Wall stress resulting from increased LVEDV also leads to compensatory myocardial hypertrophy and restoration of normal wall tension, as per Laplace's law.

Although a hypertrophied and/or hyperdynamic LV is typical of acute or compensated chronic MR, the finding of diminished EF despite the afterload reduction associated with MR is suggestive of a decompensated state with rightward or downward shifts in Frank-Starling curve pressure-volume relationships (see Fig. 112.11). In this setting, net forward flows continue to decrease, and LVEDV increases. Consequent LA and LV dilatation lead to an increase in

mitral orifice size. A self-perpetuating cycle of worsening HF with worsened MR eventually takes hold. LV failure may then lead to pulmonary hypertension and right-sided HF.

Diagnosis

Symptoms and signs. Acute decompensated MR may cause the sudden onset of dyspnea secondary to pulmonary venous hypertension and congestion. An associated decrease in forward cardiac output may cause hypotension or even hemodynamic collapse. More typically, patients with chronic, mild MR may be asymptomatic for most of their lives. When MR more gradually becomes moderate to severe, typical symptoms of left HF, atrial fibrillation, or even right HF may manifest.

Physical examination. Palpation of patients with MR may reveal a hyperdynamic, laterally displaced cardiac impulse. Auscultation typically reveals a holosystolic, high-pitched, blowing apical murmur that radiates to the axilla. Isolated posterior leaflet prolapse may cause the murmur to radiate to the sternum or aortic area, whereas isolated anterior leaflet prolapse may cause the murmur to radiate to the back or head. Other findings may include a diminished first heart sound, wide splitting of the second heart sound as a result of early aortic valve closure, or a third heart sound resulting from increased blood flow across the MV.

Diagnostic testing. Echocardiography is the mainstay of diagnosing and monitoring MR, although cardiac MRI can also provide useful regurgitant volume and cardiac function data. Routine chest radiography may demonstrate a widened cardiac silhouette, LA enlargement, or signs of pulmonary congestion associated with HF. ECG may reveal atrial fibrillation and/or signs of LA enlargement (p mitrale) and QRS or ST-T interval changes reflective of ventricular hypertrophy and/or bundle branch conduction abnormalities.

TTE and especially TEE studies allow precise visualization of the mechanisms responsible for inducing MR, including single or bileaflet prolapse and/or flail, enlarged or "billowing" leaflets, annular dilatation, chordal rupture, papillary muscle rupture, or restricted leaflet motion and tethering caused by an enlarged or infarcted ventricle. Leaflet disruption or perforation, valvular vegetations, or annular abscesses secondary to infective endocarditis may also be visualized.

Doppler analysis provides important prognostic data on regurgitant jet localization and quantification, typically based on flow dynamics related to the proximal isovolumetric surface area, which is seen on echo as a hemispheric area of flow convergence proximal to a regurgitant orifice (i.e., ventricular side of MR valves; Fig. 112.19). Analysis of the radius and the MR flow velocity in this flow convergence area allows calculation of the regurgitant fraction, ERO area, and regurgitant volume based on the following equation: flow = velocity × area. The flow convergence area narrows just downstream to the orifice of a regurgitant valve into a waist of the highest blood flow velocity as the regurgitant volume passes through the valve orifice, called the *vena contracta,* the width of which is also a marker of MR severity. Severe MR is thus now defined as an ERO $\geq$40 cm^2, a regurgitant volume $\geq$60 mL, RF $\geq$50%, a vena contracta $\geq$0.7 cm, a central MR jet >40% of the LA area, or a holosystolic eccentric jet.[10]

Natural History

Acute MR is typically caused by chordal rupture resulting from degenerative disease, papillary muscle rupture due to myocardial infarction, or infective endocarditis causing leaflet perforation or chordal rupture. It is typically poorly tolerated and often requires

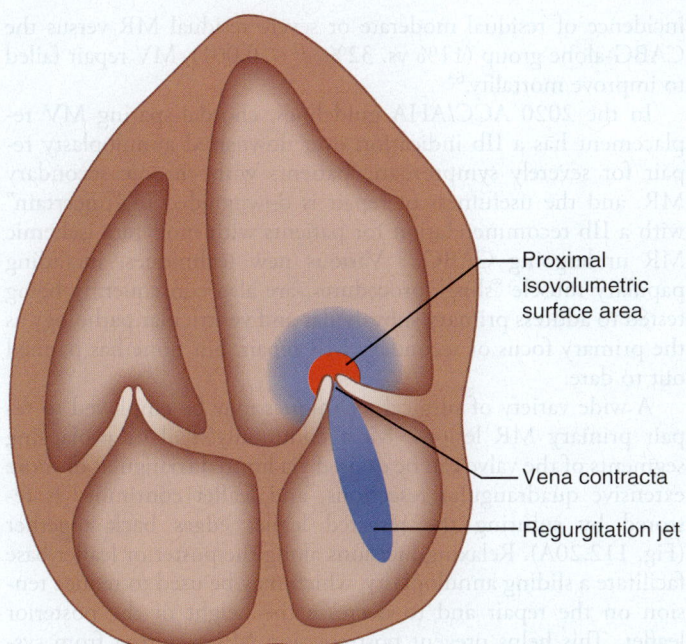

FIGURE 112.19 Echocardiographic assessment of severity of mitral regurgitation. The proximal isovolumetric surface area (PISA) is seen on echo as a hemispheric area of flow convergence proximal to a regurgitant orifice (i.e., ventricular side of mitral regurgitation [MR] valves). Analysis of the radius and the MR flow velocity in this flow convergence area allows calculation of the regurgitant fraction, effective regurgitant orifice (ERO) area, and regurgitant volume based on the following equation: flow = velocity × area. The flow convergence area narrows just downstream to the orifice of a regurgitant valve into a waist of highest blood flow velocity as the regurgitant volume passes through the valve orifice, called the *vena contracta*, the width of which is also a marker of MR severity.

urgent intervention. In the absence of intervention, severe pulmonary edema, cardiac decompensation, and/or the development of pulmonary hypertension often lead to rapid deterioration and poor outcomes.

The subacute/chronic asymptomatic MR patient was long thought not to pose an increased mortality risk, but a rich body of data developed over the past two decades now clearly demonstrates that even in the asymptomatic patient, the presence of severe MR with ventricular dysfunction, pulmonary hypertension, or atrial fibrillation carries a diminished prognosis.[10,57] Moderate primary MR has likewise now been shown to be associated with an annual mortality risk of 3% without intervention, representing excessive risk compared with results now achievable with mitral repair.[57]

Patients with functional ("secondary") MR, typically occurring on the basis of ischemic disease or dilated cardiomyopathy, carry a far worse prognosis than patients with primary MR.[57] Data from the Surgical Treatment for Ischemic Heart Failure (STICH) trial examining patients with ischemic heart disease and diminished LVEF (≤35%) demonstrated that mortality over approximately 4.5 years was about twofold greater in patients with moderate to severe MR compared with those with mild or no MR.[58]

Treatment

Medical management. The medical management of acute MR involves afterload reduction with vasodilators. The resultant decrease in aortic pressure and afterload enhances forward cardiac output and decreases regurgitant flow into the LA. When vasodilator use is ineffective or is limited by systemic hypotension, intraaortic balloon pump counterpulsation effectively lowers systolic afterload and increases forward flow. Prompt MV surgery is typically needed in acute MR, particularly in the symptomatic or hemodynamically compromised patient, but intraaortic balloon pump can be used to temporize surgery and stabilize the patient.

In symptomatic patients with chronic MR, standard vasodilator and diuretic medical therapy can be useful in improving ventricular hemodynamics and reducing pulmonary congestion. Diuretics may be particularly effective in reducing volume overload, ventricular distention, and symptoms but do not generally reverse pathologic changes. Contrary to popular practice, there is no evidence to support the use of vasodilators or other afterload-reducing medications in order to attempt to delay the need for surgery in asymptomatic patients with chronic MR and normal LV systolic function.[10]

For patients with functional, secondary MR, guideline-directed medical therapy (GDMT) and cardiac resynchronization may improve ventricular function (and sometimes degree of regurgitation) as well as provide symptom relief. Diuretics, angiotensin-converting enzyme (ACE) inhibitors or angiotensin receptor antagonists, β-blockers, and aldosterone antagonists are beneficial in the presence of HF. Recently, a landmark trial was the first to demonstrate the efficacy of a sodium-glucose cotransporter-2 (SGLT2) inhibitor, specifically dapagliflozin, in reducing cardiovascular death, HF hospitalizations, and urgent HF visits compared with placebo in patients with stable, chronic HF with LVEF <40%.[59] Currently, SGLT2 inhibitors are an established part of GDMT in HF patients with reduced EFs.

Surgical Treatment

Surgical indications for MR have broadened considerably as morbidity and mortality associated with surgery have decreased and the pathophysiology is better understood. Specifically, current understanding that the onset of ventricular dysfunction is associated with diminished prognosis and expectation for postoperative ventricular functional recovery has expanded indications to asymptomatic patients with severe MR regardless of LV function.

Surgery now carries a class I indication for asymptomatic patients with chronic severe primary MR and evidence of LV dysfunction (LVEF ≤60% or LV ESD ≥40 mm) as well as symptomatic patients irrespective of LV function (except for those who are high risk or prohibitive surgical risk with life expectancy >1 year, class IIa indication).[10] Further, because of these considerations, class IIa indications have now been added for asymptomatic patients with chronic primary severe MR and normal LV function (LVEF ≥60% and LVESD ≤40 mm), who have a 95% chance of successful mitral repair with <1% mortality with low surgical risk, and those with new-onset atrial fibrillation or resting pulmonary hypertension (pulmonary artery systolic pressure >50 mm Hg). Class IIb is reserved for those asymptomatic patients with normal LV function with progressive increase in LV size or decrease in EF on ≥3 serial imaging studies.[9] Patients with chronic moderate or severe primary MR undergoing cardiac surgery for other indications should undergo surgery.

It has been traditional to defer surgical treatment of functional MR, especially in the setting of coronary artery bypass surgery (CABG), under the presumption that improvements in the ischemic milieu after CABG would lead to the resolution of functional MR. Data from recent studies suggest, however, that deferring intervention for moderate to severe MR leads to worse outcomes in the setting of concomitant CABG.[58] As such, patients with chronic severe secondary MR undergoing aortic valve replacement or CABG should be considered for MV therapies.[10]

Repair of the MV is preferred over MV replacement for patients with primary MR when technically feasible and indicated. Successful MV repair provides an improved quality of life, with less morbidity and improved long-term event-free survival, when compared with MV replacement in appropriately selected patients. Mitral repair is considered very durable, with reoperation rates of less than 10% at 10 years when postoperative echocardiography demonstrates mild or absent MR.[60,61]

Repair can today be accomplished through a variety of techniques, including anterior or posterior leaflet resection with reconstruction, chordal transfer, leaflet folding plasty, edge-to-edge leaflet sutures, and creation of neochordae. Ring annuloplasty is indicated with all MV repairs because it has been clearly shown to improve the durability of repair. Some debate continues, however, about whether rings should be flexible or rigid, contoured or uniplanar, and completely or partially circumferential (open or closed).

The appropriate surgical intervention for patients with secondary MR is less clearly defined than for primary MR, with a growing understanding of the role of ventricular pathology in perpetuating ischemic MR undermining previous recommendations for using (exaggerated or undersized ring annuloplasty) mitral repair to correct this pathophysiology. Specifically, randomized controlled trial data from the Cardiothoracic Surgical Trials Network (CTSN) showed no difference in overall LV remodeling or survival for patients undergoing repair versus replacement but a higher 2-year rate recurrence rate for moderate or severe MR with repair versus replacement (59% vs. 4%, $P < 0.001$).[62] Likewise, although the addition of MV repair to patients undergoing CABG with moderate ischemic MR did significantly decrease the

incidence of residual moderate or severe residual MR versus the CABG-alone group (11% vs. 32%, $P < 0.001$), MV repair failed to improve mortality.[63]

In the 2020 ACC/AHA guidelines, chordal-sparing MV replacement has a IIb indication over downsized annuloplasty repair for severely symptomatic patients with chronic secondary MR, and the usefulness of repair is downgraded to "uncertain" with a IIb recommendation for patients with moderate ischemic MR undergoing CABG.[10] Various new techniques, including papillary muscle "sling" procedures, are also consequently being tested to address primary subvalvular and ventricular pathology as the primary focus of secondary MR repair, but none has panned out to date.

A wide variety of surgical techniques may be employed to repair primary MR lesions. Most commonly, flail or prolapsing segments of the valve can be excised via limited triangular or more extensive quadrangular resections, and leaflet continuity is restored by suturing the resected leaflet edges back together (Fig. 112.20A). Relaxing incisions along the posterior leaflet base facilitate a sliding annuloplasty, which may be used to reduce tension on the repair and to decrease the height of the posterior leaflet. This helps prevent postresection MR resulting from systolic anterior motion (SAM) of the anterior mitral leaflet, which may become displaced toward the aortic outflow tract after inadequate resections.

Another option for mitral repair is the creation of neochordae, which can be created or preselected using Gore-Tex suture and should be sized to the height of the annulus. The neochordae are attached to the papillary muscle and the free edge of the leaflet to provide appropriate leaflet support and prevent leaflet prolapse.

A ring annuloplasty should be performed with all MV leaflet repairs because this maneuver has been shown to significantly

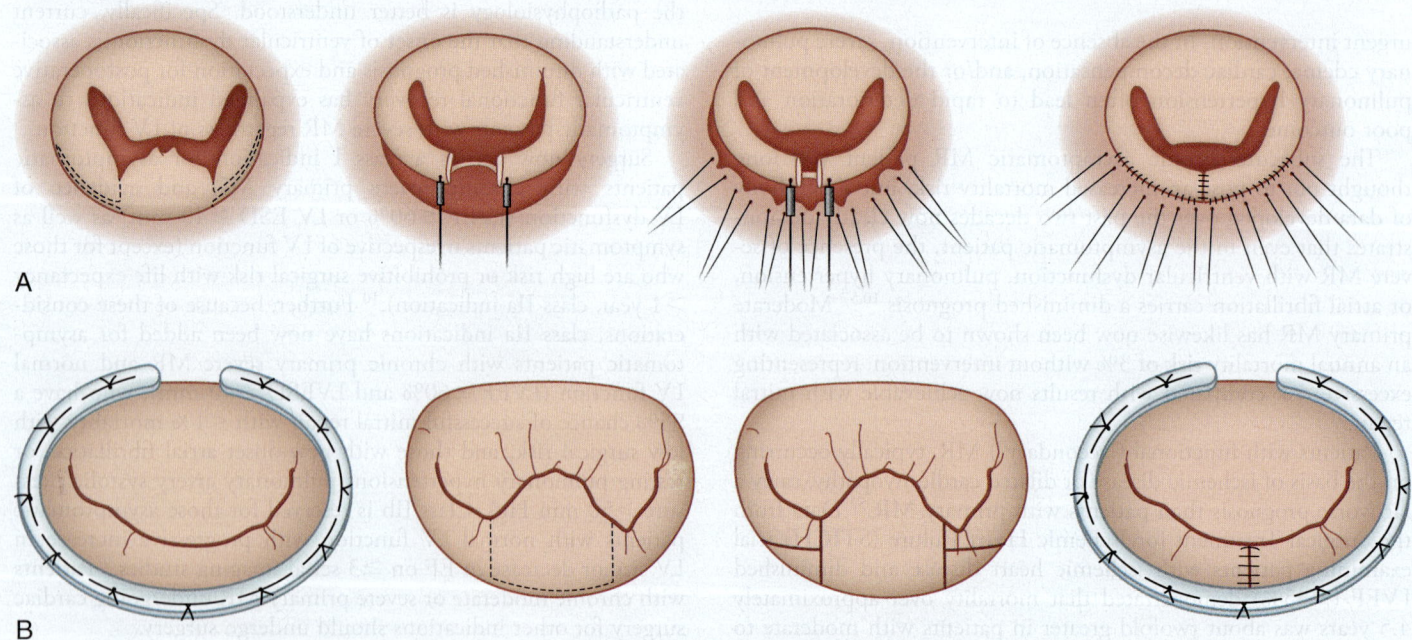

FIGURE 112.20 Mitral valve repair surgery. (A) Resection of leaflet tissue incorporating triangular or quadrangular resection, most commonly flail or prolapsing (typically posterior [P2]) segments of the valve. Leaflet continuity is restored simply by suturing the resected leaflet edges back together. (B) Annuloplasty ring. An annuloplasty ring is almost always implanted to supplement resectional repairs or may be used alone to address mitral regurgitation arising from a dilated annulus. Circumferentially placed simple, nonpledgeted sutures are typically used to implant annuloplasty rings in a manner similar to valve implantation.

improve the durability of repair and can be used as a stand-alone procedure to address MR arising from a dilated annulus (see Fig. 112.20B). Insertion of an annuloplasty ring helps restore normal annular geometry and ensure an appropriate coaptation zone of 6 to 8 mm between anterior and posterior leaflets. Numerous device options are available for annuloplasty, including rigid or flexible and partial or complete rings. Data are indefinite on which of these ring types provides the best outcomes.

Percutaneous therapies for MV disease are rapidly evolving. Various treatment options have been tested, including transcatheter mitral annuloplasty, which is both complex and technically challenging to place accurately, leading to mixed results. Chordal repair through transapical approaches has been tested but has not been widely used because these techniques are still quite invasive, with unknown durability. TEER models the surgical repair technique of Alfieri and colleagues to treat a prolapsed anterior leaflet by opposing the middle scallops of the anterior and posterior leaflets, leading to a double orifice. The MitraClip system, consisting of a steerable guide catheter and a clip delivery system, was the first developed and received FDA approval for high-risk patients in 2013 for degenerative MR.[64] The clip is introduced through the sheath into the left atrium via a transseptal puncture and is positioned under TEE guidance perpendicular to the line of coaptation at the pathologic segment (Fig. 112.21). Two randomized trials, Cardiovascular Outcomes Assessment of the MitraClip Percutaneous Therapy for Heart Failure Patients With Functional Mitral Regurgitation (COAPT) and Percutaneous Repair With the MitraClip Device for Severe Functional/Secondary Mitral Regurgitation (MITRA-FR), assessed the efficacy of treating patients with severe functional MR and systolic HF with the Mitra-Clip device.[65,66] The use of the percutaneous device was found to be efficacious in patients with severe, functional MR treated rigorously with GDMT who also did not have as significant dysfunction. It has since received FDA approval to treat functional MR in 2019. Advancements in design with the clip system have continued to include devices with longer, wider clips and those designed with central spacers to decrease the regurgitant orifice area. With increasing experience with TEER, factors predicting failure have been identified, including patients with small MV orifice areas (<4.0 cm^2), large coaptation gap, insufficient leaflet length to grasp, significant clefts, severe MAC, or calcification of the involved leaflet. Transcatheter mitral valve replacement devices are currently under investigation. Although early studies have shown high rates of technical success to virtually eliminate MR, there remains an unacceptably high screen failure rate for enrollment in these trials because of the high risk of left ventricular outflow tract obstruction and large annular size exceeding currently available device sizes. Although stroke risk remains low, because most of the devices require anticoagulation, major bleeding complications have been reported. Treatment of failed MV repairs (mainly with complete ring annuloplasties) has been performed with TAVR valves in the mitral position, but long-term durability data are still pending.

Tricuspid Regurgitation and Other Right-Sided Valvular Disease

Nearly all the pathophysiologic mechanisms causing left-sided valve disease may analogously lead to primary right-sided valve disease. The most common presentation of right-sided valvular disease, however, is functional TR caused by RV failure or dilation (which itself is typically secondary to left-sided dysfunction

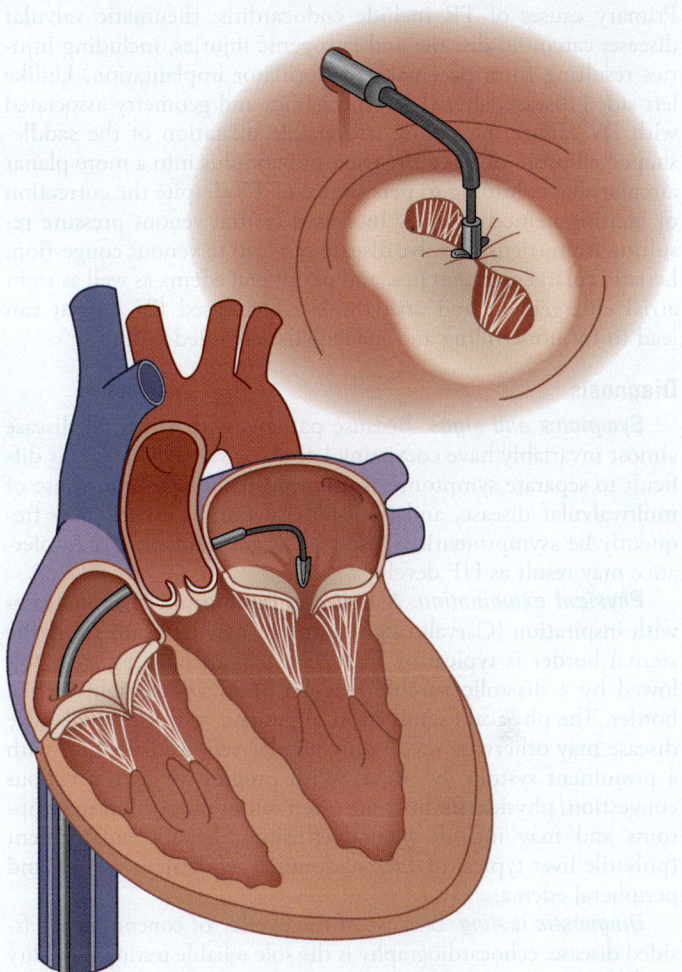

FIGURE 112.21 Percutaneous mitral valve repair. Using a catheter-based clip delivery system, the operator grasps the mitral valve leaflet edges and places a clip that emulates the edge-to-edge leaflet repair. (MitraClip is a trademark of Abbott or its related companies. Reproduced with permission of Abbott, Copyright 2020. All rights reserved.)

and pulmonary hypertension). Functional etiology secondary to left-sided valve disease is responsible for TR in 80% to 90% of cases. Less commonly, functional TR may also be caused by RV infarction or ischemia. Transvalvular pacemaker or cardioverter-defibrillator leads can also uncommonly cause mild or even higher-grade TR.

Tricuspid stenosis (TS) occurs infrequently in developed countries because rheumatic disease accounts for over 90% of such lesions. Carcinoid syndrome is the most common of a group of unusual disorders that lead to the deposition of pathologic materials in the tricuspid and/or pulmonic leaflets as a far less frequent cause of primary TR, TS, or pulmonic valve disease.

Congenital anomalies causing pulmonic valve stenosis, often associated with tetralogy of Fallot, tricuspid atresia, and TR occurring as part of the Ebstein anomaly, are three of the most common of the congenital disorders leading to right-sided valve disease.

Pathophysiology

TR accounts for most right-sided valvular disease, of which secondary or functional TR is the most prevalent. Secondary TR is most often the result of left-sided valve disease and/or HF.

Primary causes of TR include endocarditis; rheumatic valvular disease; carcinoid disease; and iatrogenic injuries, including injuries resulting from pacemaker/defibrillator implantation. Unlike left-sided disease, altered RV mechanics and geometry associated with RV failure may cause irreversible dilatation of the saddle-shaped ellipsoid of a healthy tricuspid annulus into a more planar circular shape, leading to persistence of TR despite the correction of inciting hemodynamics. Increased central venous pressure resulting from tricuspid valve disease can lead to venous congestion, hepatic enlargement, ascites, and peripheral edema as well as right atrial enlargement and arrhythmias. Decreased RV output can lead to LV underfilling and inadequate left-sided output.

Diagnosis

Symptoms and signs. Because patients with tricuspid disease almost invariably have coexisting left-sided valve disease, it is difficult to separate symptoms of tricuspid pathology from those of multivalvular disease, and tricuspid valve disease itself may frequently be asymptomatic. Dyspnea, fatigue, and exercise intolerance may result as HF develops.

Physical examination. A holosystolic murmur that increases with inspiration (Carvallo sign) and that may be heard along the sternal border is typical of TR. With TS, an opening snap followed by a diastolic rumble may be heard at the right sternal border. The physical examination of patients with tricuspid valve disease may otherwise reveal only jugular venous distention with a prominent systolic "v" wave. With progressive central venous congestion, physical findings are often out of proportion to symptoms and may include pleural effusions, hepatic enlargement (pulsatile liver typical of TR), abdominal tenderness, ascites, and peripheral edema.

Diagnostic testing. Because of the overlay of concomitant left-sided disease, echocardiography is the sole reliable testing modality useful in assessing tricuspid disease. Severe TR is defined by a central jet $\geq$50% right atrium, vena contracta width $\geq$0.7cm, ERO $\geq$0.4 cm^2, regurgitant volume $\geq$45 mL, and hepatic vein systolic flow reversal. Estimation of PASP based on the velocity of the TR jet measured by continuous-wave Doppler is a useful prognostic criterion. An annular diameter of greater than 40 mm defines significant tricuspid annular dilation and is also an important consideration when selecting appropriate treatment for TR.[67]

Natural History

Decreased survival is associated with increasing TR severity, regardless of other indices of cardiac function. Although patients who undergo surgical treatment of left-sided valve disease may experience improved or resolved functional TR, such improvement is highly unpredictable, and survival for patients with uncorrected moderate to severe TR has been reported to be less than 50% at 4 years.[68]

Treatment

Medical management. The medical treatment of tricuspid valve disease involves optimization of RV preload and afterload, using diuretics and ACE inhibitors, respectively. If atrial fibrillation is present, rate control may optimize diastolic filling. With functional TR, medical treatment to reduce pulmonary hypertension may also improve cardiac output.

Surgical Treatment

The timing and method of surgical treatment for functional TR are controversial. Classic teaching from the early years of MV replacement was that functional TR would improve after primary left-sided valve treatment. This led to the recommendation of avoiding tricuspid surgery in most cases. This has proven not to be a reliable strategy. Left uncorrected, secondary TR will worsen in about 25% of patients, which has functional and survival implications resulting from irreversible progression of RV damage and organ failure.[68] Further, although adding tricuspid repair during left-sided heart surgery does not significantly increase operative risk, reoperation due to persistent TR after left-sided heart surgery carries a perioperative mortality of 10% to 25% or greater.

On the basis of these considerations, severe TR has emerged as a class I indication for concomitant tricuspid valve surgery in patients who are undergoing left-heart surgery.[10] Concomitant repair is also probably indicated in those with mild or greater TR and either tricuspid annular dilation (>40 mm diameter) or evidence of right HF (class IIa).[10,69] Additionally, patients with symptomatic severe primary TR unresponsive to medical therapy are candidates for tricuspid valve surgery (class IIa), as are patients with moderate TR and pulmonary hypertension (class IIb) and asymptomatic or minimally symptomatic patients with evidence of progressive RV dysfunction (class IIb).

Tricuspid valve repair is generally preferred to replacement whenever possible. For severe TR due to isolated annular dilation, annuloplasty using a prosthetic ring has been shown in several studies to have better long-term results than any suture annuloplasty technique.[11,12] Valve replacement should be considered for functional TR resulting from severe leaflet tethering and RV remodeling or leaflet fibrosis and retraction, such as occurs with carcinoid heart disease (which also less commonly involves the pulmonary valve).

Symptomatic patients with isolated TS do not benefit from medical management and are best treated with valve replacement. In adults, TS is almost nonexistent, except for the most advanced cases of RHD, endocarditis resulting from a vegetation, or functional TS resulting from a large intraatrial mass obstructing outflow. Most TS generally is the consequence of a congenital anomaly. Those with TS and left-sided valve disease should likewise undergo concomitant correction during the same operation. Percutaneous tricuspid valvulotomy may be considered, but outcomes are less optimistic than those seen with MS and may induce significant TR.

Experience with percutaneous treatment of severe TR started with compassionate and off-label use of the MitraClip system as part of the Transcatheter Tricuspid Valve (TriValve) Registry. The majority of patients (77%) had successful treatment of their TR to grade 2 or less, and this was associated with improved survival and decreased HF hospitalizations. Of note, over half the patients in that cohort also had their MR treated in the same procedure.[70] The Trial to Evaluate Cardiovascular Outcomes in Patients Treated With the Tricuspid Valve Repair System Pivotal (TRILUMINATE Pivotal) demonstrated that TriClip was safe in the treatment of severe, symptomatic TR to reduce the severity of TR and to improve quality-of-life metrics at 1 year.[71] In April 2024, this device received approval from the FDA to treat patients with severe TR at intermediate or high risk for open-heart surgery. The first transcatheter tricuspid valve replacement device, the EVOQUE system, received FDA approval in February 2024 after the Transfemoral Tricuspid Valve Replacement: Investigation of Safety and Clinical Efficacy (TRISCEND) study reported its 1-year outcomes in treatment of patients with greater than or equal to moderate, symptomatic TR. The trial demonstrated

TR reduction, improved survival, and low hospitalization rates.[72] Similar to the mitral space, transcatheter tricuspid valve technologies are rapidly emerging, yet durability data and long-term outcomes of treatment of advanced TR are still lacking.

Mixed Valve Disease

Patients with mixed valve disease typically present with a predominant lesion that dictates symptoms and pathophysiology. There are very limited data on the natural history of mixed valve disease; therefore, the optimal timing of serial evaluation is not clear. Patients with multivalvular disease likewise present even more complex diagnostic and therapeutic challenges than patients with single-valve disease. The coexistence of aortic valve disease and MR, for example, will mitigate LV changes induced by aortic valve pathology but worsen pulmonary and right-sided complications.

Limited data are available to guide treatment in cases of multivalvular disease, and indications for interventions should be based on symptoms and objective analysis of surgical outcome rather than severity indices for the individual lesion. In general, therapy should be targeted to the predominant lesion while considering the severity of concomitant valve disease.

SELECTED REFERENCES

Carpentier A. Cardiac valve surgery—the "French correction." *J Thorac Cardiovasc Surg.* 1983;86:323-337.

> This work by Alain Carpentier, for the first time, described a comprehensive strategy for repairing regurgitant lesions of the mitral valve. It remains a relevant classic today.

David TE, Feindel CM. An aortic valve-sparing operation for patients with aortic incompetence and aneurysm of the ascending aorta. *J Thorac Cardiovasc Surg.* 1992;103:617-621.

> David and Feindel report their initial cohort of patients treated with a novel technique for aortic valve–sparing root replacement. This technique is used around the world today to preserve the native aortic valve.

Leon MB, Smith CR, Mack M, et al. Transcatheter aortic-valve implantation for aortic stenosis in patients who cannot undergo surgery. *N Engl J Med.* 2010;363:1597-1607.

> This is the original prospective randomized study report from the PARTNER investigators demonstrating the feasibility of percutaneous aortic valve replacement.

Otto CM, Nishimura RA, Bonow RO, et al. 2020 ACC/AHA guideline for the management of patients with valvular heart disease: a report of the American College of Cardiology/American Heart Association Joint Committee on Clinical Practice Guidelines. *J Thorac Cardiovasc Surg.* 2021;162:e183-e353.

> These are the most recent comprehensive American College of Cardiology/American Heart Association Task Force guidelines for diagnosis and treatment of valvular heart disease from 2020.

Ross Jr J, Braunwald E. Aortic stenosis. *Circulation.* 1968;38:61-67.

> This article first described the onset of symptoms of HF, syncope, or angina in patients with aortic stenosis as survival indicators.

The full reference list appears on Elsevier eBooks+.

113 CHAPTER

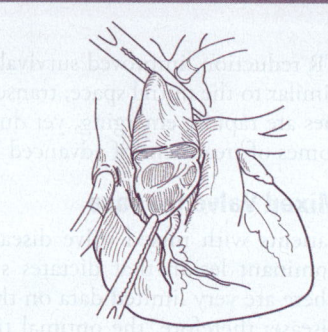

Congenital Heart Disease

Andrew Well and Chuck D. Fraser, Jr.

OUTLINE

This chapter is designed to provide medical students, general surgery residents, and practicing general surgeons with a working tool to aid in their understanding of the features of anatomy and physiology in patients presenting for general surgical procedures in the setting of repaired or unrepaired congenital cardiac lesions. The large scope and breadth of the evolving field of congenital heart surgery precludes an exhaustive treatise on all aspects of this specialty. Several excellent and thorough textbooks on congenital heart surgery are referenced in this chapter, and the reader is encouraged to use them for additional in-depth understanding of the lesions to be reviewed. A general surgeon practicing today needs to be well versed in the basics of cardiac anatomy, physiology, and specific derangements associated with the various known congenital cardiac lesions. Furthermore, few patients with complex congenital cardiac lesions may be considered cured of their cardiac problem, even after successful reconstructive surgery. Thus, it is imperative that a general surgeon who needs to perform a noncardiac operation on such a patient be familiar with the specific issues of ongoing concern in patients with congenital cardiac disease.

HISTORY AND OTHER CONSIDERATIONS

The era of surgical treatment for congenital cardiac anomalies was initiated in November 1944, when Alfred Blalock and associates Vivien Thomas and Helen Taussig combined their unique talents and vision to treat a young child dying of cyanotic congenital heart disease (CHD).[1] This palliative operation involved the surgical creation of a systemic pulmonary artery connection in the patient, who had inadequate pulmonary blood flow. The procedure has since been recalled as miraculous and now, more than 75 years later, is known by the eponym *Blalock-Taussig-Thomas* (BTT) shunt. The striking success of this simple concept and the reproducible nature of the operation in children with otherwise fatal cardiac conditions have emboldened subsequent surgical innovators to venture inside the congenitally malformed heart. At first, the parent was asked to serve as a biologic oxygenator using the technique of controlled cross-circulation; soon thereafter, the mechanical, extracorporeal, heart-lung bypass pump was developed.[2,3] With the aid of this ability to support the patient's circulation during intracardiac exploration, surgeons have sequentially attacked almost every described congenital cardiac anomaly. The prospect of meaningful survival for patients born with otherwise devastating congenital cardiac lesions is now expected in most cases.

As a result of this success story, there is now a large and growing population of adults with repaired or unrepaired CHD; estimates in the United States for 2010 placed the number of adult patients surviving with repaired or palliated congenital cardiac lesions at more than 1.4 million.[4] There has been an increase of greater than 50% in CHD prevalence since 2000, and by 2010, adults accounted for two-thirds of patients with CHD in the general population.[5] This reality has been associated with new challenges in the ongoing medical maintenance of such patients, with particular focus on the care of patients with congenital cardiac lesions presenting for surgery for noncardiac illnesses. The evolving subspecialty of adult CHD and accredited adult CHD centers points to the unique needs of this population of patients.

PATHWAYS FOR PRACTICING CONGENITAL HEART SURGERY

Before embarking on a review of the field, it is worthwhile to describe the setting in which patients with CHD seek and receive care in today's medical environment. With the development of sophisticated methods of fetal ultrasound, a large percentage of children requiring surgery for CHD are diagnosed during gestation (Fig. 113.1). A fetal diagnosis of complex CHD is extremely helpful to parents and the medical management team. Fetal diagnosis is particularly important in the setting of lesions dependent on persistent patency of the ductus arteriosus for postnatal survival. In these individuals, survival after delivery is predicated on the maintenance of ductal patency through the intravenous infusion of prostaglandin E1 (PGE1) initiated in the delivery suite, often through an umbilical vein catheter. Several studies have shown a decrease in morbidity, but there is inconclusive evidence that mortality rates are decreased.[6,7]

A growing number of congenital cardiac lesions are known to be associated with specific genetic mutations, many clearly inherited and some presumed to be sporadic. A chromosomal analysis is frequently performed in individuals found to have major structural cardiac abnormalities; this analysis may be performed during gestation through amniocentesis or after delivery. The chromosomal evaluation is beneficial to the family when planning the risk of such an occurrence in future offspring. For the clinician, knowledge of chromosomal abnormalities, such as DiGeorge sequence, velocardiofacial syndrome, and Marfan syndrome, aids in the delivery of acute medical management.

In general terms, the timing of surgery for various congenital cardiac conditions depends on the presenting symptoms and expectations for further associated complications. Neonates presenting with limited pulmonary blood flow or atretic pulmonary connections typically require surgery during the first few days of life and occasionally within hours of delivery. Lesions associated with excessive pulmonary blood flow result in early heart failure, which may manifest as poor feeding, tachypnea, or respiratory failure. These patients are operated on during early infancy to ameliorate their symptoms and prevent the development of irreversible pulmonary vascular disease.

Preterm and low-birth-weight infants with CHD have been presenting for surgical consideration with more frequency. This treatment strategy requires thoughtful planning and coordination among the surgery, anesthesia, cardiology, intensive care, and neonatology teams. We have successfully operated on two 800-g infants with transposition of the great arteries (TGA).

The specialty of congenital heart surgery is now recognized as a subspecialty of cardiothoracic surgery. Congenital heart surgeons were previously certified in cardiothoracic surgery by the American Board of Thoracic Surgery and received additional fellowship training in the United States or abroad in congenital heart surgery. As of 2009, the American Board of Thoracic Surgery offers a formal certification process for subspecialty training in congenital heart surgery. At the present time, there are 17 congenital cardiac surgery residency programs approved by the Accreditation Council for Graduate Medical Education.[8] Most pediatric cardiac surgery is performed in large, multispecialty children's hospitals in association with formal programs focused on the care of these complex patients. The management team includes pediatric cardiac anesthesiologists, perfusionists, and nursing staff. Focused pediatric cardiac intensive care units have been developed to optimize the patients' opportunity for recovery.

Historically, pediatric cardiologists have provided the medical management of patients born with CHD. Pediatric cardiology is also evolving. With advances in catheter-based technology, interventional pediatric cardiologists are now addressing lesions previously treated with surgery. Examples include device closure of atrial septal defects (ASDs) and ventricular septal defects (VSDs), occlusion of patent ductus arteriosus (PDA), and dilation and stenting of stenotic vessels in the systemic and pulmonary circulation. For a more in-depth review of this specialty, see the excellent technical text by Mullins.[9]

The care for adults with CHD is in evolution. This issue is of particular relevance to the general surgeon faced with operating on an adult patient with significant CHD. One overriding message needs to be clear to the general surgeon in this setting: It must be assumed that in patients with previously repaired congenital cardiac lesions, even without overt cardiac symptoms, the potential for significant perioperative cardiorespiratory derangement exists. More simply stated, the presence of a surgical scar on the chest of a patient with known CHD does not suggest that the lesion has been cured. With this message firmly in mind, the general surgeon may find it challenging to determine the best source for a qualified consultation for such a patient. At the present time, many adult cardiologists are not adequately trained in CHD to provide competent consultation on adult patients with CHD.

Pediatric cardiologists are not educated in adult medicine and cardiology, and many feel uncomfortable providing consultation on adult patients with CHD. The subspecialty of adult CHD is currently becoming more formalized, but the number of physicians who have been educated specifically to care for these patients is still few. In 2015, the American Board of Internal Medicine offered the first certification examination in Adult Congenital Heart Disease. The Accreditation Council for Graduate Medical Education–accredited fellowship became available in 2019, with 28 accredited programs currently.[10,11] The practicing general surgeon needs to become familiar with the specific issues of concern for patients with CHD to ascertain that the patient's unique anatomic and physiologic issues have been evaluated properly. A pediatric cardiologist, in coordination with an adult cardiologist, must evaluate adult patients with CHD who present for care in a center without a designated qualified specialist. Of equal importance, the anesthesiologists and intensivists caring for an adult patient with CHD must have a working understanding of the complexities and nuances of the patient's cardiac condition. The anesthetic management of patients with CHD undergoing general surgical procedures is complicated and can become disastrous if managed improperly.

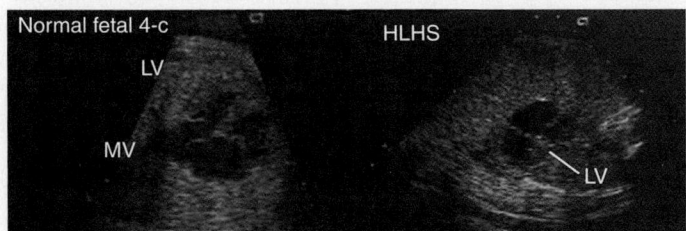

FIGURE 113.1 Normal fetal ultrasound (four chamber *[4-c]; left*) and fetal ultrasound of a child with hypoplastic left heart syndrome *(HLHS) (right). LV,* Left ventricle; *MV,* mitral valve.

ANATOMY, TERMINOLOGY, AND DIAGNOSIS

Anatomy and Terminology

One of the most intimidating aspects for the student of CHD is developing a level of comfort with the terminology used for describing specific lesions. A thorough and sound understanding of normal cardiac anatomy is mandatory. There are several excellent texts on this subject; in particular, the text edited by Wilcox and coworkers[12] is especially concise and clear. One difficulty that challenges proper understanding of anatomy is the frequent use of abbreviations and eponyms for various congenital lesions—for example, *congenitally corrected TGA (ccTGA)*, *ventricular inversion*, and *L-transposition* all describe the same heart, but none provides a complete anatomic description. Unless otherwise clear to all clinicians involved in the care of these complicated patients, the anatomic description needs to be segmental and complete to avoid mistakes and misinterpretations of structure.

In describing congenital cardiac lesions, a segmental approach is used to determine the relationship of the various structural elements. The situs describes the relationship of sidedness—situs solitus (normal), situs inversus (reversed), or situs ambiguus (indeterminate). The cardiac elements described include (in sequence) the atria, ventricles, and great vessels. The relationship of the connections must be understood; connections are concordant (e.g., the right atrium connecting to the right ventricle [RV]) or discordant (e.g., the RV connecting to the aorta). The chamber sidedness must be clarified (e.g., a morphologic right atrium may be on the left side of the patient). The relationship and connections of the cardiac valves must then be assessed; connections may be normal, stenotic, atretic, or straddling. Of note to the general surgeon, abnormal sidedness of the cardiac structures is frequently associated with abnormal relationships of the thoracic and abdominal organs. A thorough assessment of the patient's anatomy is recommended before surgery. Commonly used tools in evaluation of anatomy include echocardiogram, computed tomography (CT), magnetic resonance imaging (MRI), and cardiac catheterization.

There are two widely accepted and applied schools of cardiac morphologic description. The Van Praagh nomenclature uses abbreviations to describe the relationship of the atria, ventricular looping, and position of the aorta sequentially. The first letter describes the situs of the atrial chambers (and usually the abdominal organs): "S" for situs solitus (normal), "I" for situs inversus (reversed), or "A" for situs ambiguus (indeterminate). The second letter describes the relationship of the embryologic looping of the ventricles: "D" for dextro looping or right-handed topology (normal) or "L" (levo) for left-handed topology. The third and last letter describes the relationship of the aortic valve to the pulmonary valve: "D" for right-sided and "L" for left-sided as well as "S" for solitus and "I" for inversus (Fig. 113.2).

The Anderson nomenclature is more wordy and longer but is perhaps simpler to understand. The descriptions are again of the sequential relationship of the structures. Starting with the atria, the connections and relationships are sequentially described. Thus, the atrial sidedness is described, followed by the sequence of connections to the ventricles and then great vessels. For example, "atrial situs solitus (normal) with atrioventricular (A-V) discordance (reversed) and ventriculoarterial (V-A) discordance (reversed)" describes the heart mentioned earlier as corrected transposition, or S,L,L by the Van Praagh classification (Fig. 113.3).

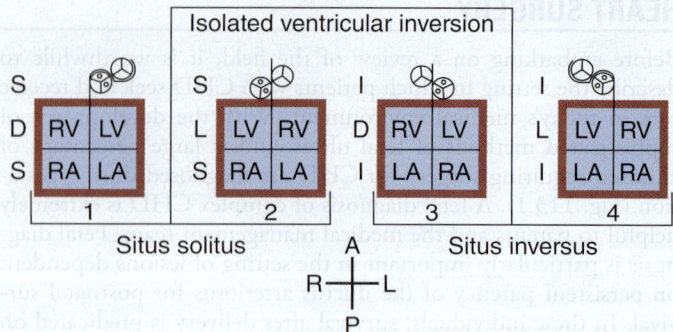

"NORMALS"

Isolated ventricular inversion

FIGURE 113.2 Model depicting cardiac morphology for normal hearts—that is, hearts with atrioventricular concordance and ventriculoarterial concordance—using Van Praagh nomenclature. The *vertical line* above the box denotes the position of the ventricular septum. *LA,* Left atrium; *LV,* left ventricle; *RA,* right atrium; *RV,* right ventricle. (From Kirklin JW, Barratt-Boyes BG. General considerations: anatomy, dimensions, and terminology. In: *Cardiac Surgery.* 2nd ed. New York: Churchill Livingstone; 1993.)

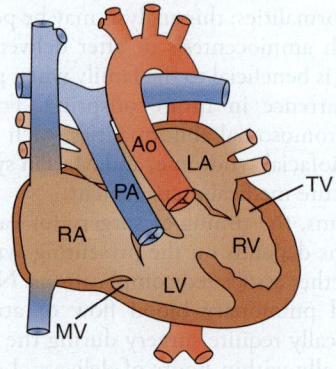

FIGURE 113.3 Congenitally corrected transposition of the great arteries. Atrial situs solitus (normal) with atrioventricular discordance and ventriculoarterial discordance using Anderson nomenclature, S,L,L by Van Praagh classification. *Ao,* Aorta; *LA,* left atrium; *LV,* left ventricle; *MV,* mitral valve; *PA,* pulmonary artery; *RA,* right atrium; *RV,* right ventricle; *TV,* tricuspid valve.

Diagnosis

As with all aspects of surgery, widely varying, highly sophisticated diagnostic tools are available to examine cardiac structure and function. Despite the widespread availability and application of these tools, none has replaced or eliminated the necessity of a thorough history and physical examination. Most patients who have a history of CHD become very well informed about the specifics of their cardiac conditions, as do their parents. A detailed review of the patient's past medical history is mandatory. This review includes, when possible, securing records from all previous diagnostic and procedural reports. An incorrect assumption is often made about a patient's previous surgical history and anatomy, frequently in a setting in which a patient's old operative report or clinical summary could easily clarify the misunderstanding.

In adults with CHD, in particular, there are specific points of medical history that must be elucidated. A history of palpitations, syncope, and neurologic deficit must be investigated further. The incidence of significant dysrhythmias in certain categories of adults with CHD is high and, in many cases, warrants further investigation, including continuous monitoring (Holter or Bardy), electrophysiologic study, or provocative testing.

Physical Examination

A complete physical examination in a patient with previously repaired CHD often yields critical information for the proper planning of a general surgical procedure. Patients need to be completely undressed and thoroughly examined. In many cyanotic patients, color changes may be prominent, particularly in the nail beds, lips, and mucous membranes. Clubbing of fingers may be noted. In other patients, cyanosis may be more subtle, giving the patient a gray or even pale appearance. Previous surgical incisions need to be noted and reconciled with the known medical history. Thoracotomy incisions on either side may indicate a previous BTT shunt using the turned-down, divided subclavian artery or with a prosthetic interposition graft—the so-called modified BTT shunt. In patients with a left aortic arch, a left thoracotomy incision is present if a previous coarctation repair has been carried out. Median sternotomy incisions or anterior thoracotomy incisions may indicate previous intracardiac or extracardiac surgery.

A complete vascular examination is often overlooked in patients with CHD. It is important to assess pulses and obtain blood pressure measurements in all four extremities. Patients who have an existing or have previously had a BTT shunt often have diminished or absent pulses in the upper extremity corresponding to the previous shunt. Also, patients with previous coarctation repairs may have diminished or absent pulses in the left upper extremity, especially if a subclavian flap angioplasty was performed (Waldhausen procedure). Furthermore, a history of previous coarctation repair does not guarantee that the lower extremity pulses and blood pressures will be normal. Moreover, patients who have undergone previous cardiac catheterization may have chronically stenosed or occluded femoral vessels. All these issues may be of significance for monitoring and vascular access in a patient undergoing a general surgical procedure.

Later in this chapter, the Fontan procedure for single-ventricle palliation is reviewed. Briefly, this operation results in significant systemic venous hypertension, often measuring 12 to 15 mm Hg (normal 0–8 mm Hg). In patients with a Fontan circulation, physical examination may reveal hepatic congestion, ascites, pedal edema, venous varicosities, and jugular venous distention. In some patients, macronodular hepatic cirrhosis may be suspected on the basis of a firm, fibrotic liver edge on palpation.

Entire textbooks have been dedicated to the physical examination of patients with cardiac disease, and a thorough discussion of this issue, particularly the specifics of cardiac auscultation, is beyond the scope of this chapter. In general, the cardiac examination includes an assessment of the patient's rhythm, point of maximal impulse, and character of any auscultated murmurs. Importantly, the absence of a significant cardiac murmur does not rule out significant cardiac pathology.

Diagnostic Tests

Pulse oximetry. Four-extremity pulse oximetry is an essential part of the clinical assessment of a patient with suspected CHD. Patients with ductal-dependent circulation to the lower body (severe aortic coarctation or aortic arch interruption) may present with differential cyanosis. This presentation indicates the ejection of desaturated pulmonary arterial blood through the patent ductus to the descending aorta contrasted with fully saturated pulmonary venous blood ejected to the ascending aorta and the upper extremities. Baseline (room air) saturation must be documented

in all patients for whom an operative intervention is anticipated to establish their normal range and to allow for identification of changes throughout the perioperative period.

Plain radiography. Standard chest radiography with anteroposterior and lateral views is still an essential component of the assessment of a patient with CHD. Standard elements to be examined include a skeletal survey, assessment of the diaphragms, hepatic shadow, and location of the gastric bubble. The lung fields are assessed for pulmonary plethora (arterial or venous), air space disease, and the presence of effusions. The cardiac silhouette may reveal essential information, such as a cardiothoracic ratio indicative of cardiomegaly or pericardial effusion, the presence of atrial enlargement, the presence or absence of the pulmonary artery shadow, and arch sidedness (Fig. 113.4).

Electrocardiography. The electrocardiogram (ECG) is important in assessing patients with CHD. The rate and rhythm must be noted, including the presence or absence of P-wave activity and axis. Many patients with CHD, especially patients with complex conditions, such as heterotaxy syndrome, may exhibit deranged or absent sinus node activity, giving rise to a predominant junctional rhythm, which may significantly compromise cardiac output. The QRS duration and axis reveal information concerning conduction delay and abnormal ventricular forces. For example, patients with A-V canal defects are known to have left axis deviation. Furthermore, in patients undergoing repair of certain forms of CHD, there may be an early or late predisposition to malignant dysrhythmias. It is particularly important to elucidate a history of palpitations from a patient with repaired or unrepaired CHD; such a history may warrant further investigation with 24-hour continuous ECG monitoring (Holter) or longer-term monitor (Bardy).

Echocardiography. Noninvasive imaging is well established as the primary diagnostic modality for structural cardiac disease. For most patients, excellent anatomic detail may be obtained using two-dimensional transthoracic imaging. Standard images include subcostal, suprasternal, parasternal, and subxiphoid views and are oriented in long- and short-axis directions. Furthermore,

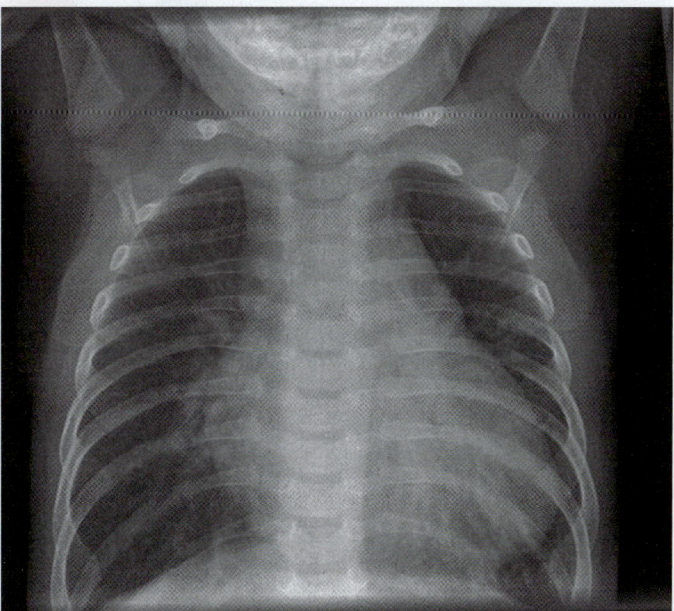

FIGURE 113.4 Cardiomegaly and increased pulmonary vascular markings in a patient with complete atrioventricular canal defect.

significant hemodynamic information may be inferred using echo Doppler blood flow velocities and interpreted using the modified Bernoulli formula (pressure gradient = $4V^2$, where V is echocardiographic velocity in meters per second). To assess the patient's cardiac lesion properly, segmental analysis of the cardiac structures, connections, and valves must be performed. A quantitative estimate of ejection fraction, shortening fraction, and valvular inflow velocity aids in assessing cardiac function. For most patients with CHD, adequate diagnostic information is attainable through echocardiography in the hands of a qualified pediatric cardiologist.

Magnetic resonance imaging and computed tomography.
Cardiac MRI and CT are adjuncts to echocardiography for noninvasive structural and functional assessment of the heart. MRI has been used with increasing frequency to provide anatomic and functional detail in congenitally malformed hearts in which echocardiographic detail is lacking or unattainable. Cardiac MRI has proved particularly useful for imaging the extracardiac great vessels and systemic and pulmonary venous connections and for providing accurate estimates of cardiac function, especially right ventricular ejection fraction. MRI has the added benefit of using nonionizing electromagnetic fields. CT may also be used for such imaging detail but has the potential detrimental association with significant radiation exposure. A CT scan of the chest averages 5 to 7 mSv, and CT coronary angiography averages 9 to 11 mSv (chest x-ray: 0.1 mSv).[13]

Cardiac catheterization.
Cardiac catheterization was long considered the gold standard for diagnostic imaging of congenitally malformed hearts. With the current sophistication of echocardiography, CT, and MRI, this is no longer the case for most patients. Nonetheless, there are still circumstances in which diagnostic cardiac catheterization is necessary to obtain accurate anatomic detail. One such circumstance may be patients who have poor echocardiographic windows, although even this issue may

be overcome using transesophageal echocardiography. More often, there are specifics of anatomic detail that neither echocardiography nor MRI can delineate, such as branch pulmonary artery (or segmental) stenosis, origin and course of aortopulmonary collateral vessels, fistulous connections, and intracardiac communications (septal defects) not clarified by other imaging modalities.

Usually, diagnostic cardiac catheterization is performed to obtain precise hemodynamic information needed to make an informed assessment of the consequences of the patient's cardiac lesions. Using oximetric measurements, pressure data, and thermodilution cardiac output determination, accurate assessment of the patient's hemodynamic profile is obtained. Measured or derived data include central venous pressure; atrial pressure; ventricular pressures (including end-diastolic pressure); shunt fraction (in the case of ASDs or VSDs); pulmonary artery pressures; pulmonary capillary wedge pressure; systemic arterial pressure; and segmental oximetry of cardiac structures, including systemic and pulmonary venous return (Fig. 113.5). Thus, critical information is obtained about the presence and degree of shunting, systemic and pulmonary vascular resistance (PVR), and cardiopulmonary function. In certain clinical settings, these data are mandatory for a successful clinical management strategy. This may be particularly true for an adult patient with CHD requiring noncardiac surgery.

A thorough understanding of normal cardiorespiratory physiology is critical in interpreting data obtained by cardiac catheterization in a patient with CHD. Specifically, the normal pressure range, pulse waveforms, and oxygen saturations for the various cardiac chambers must be compared against data obtained in a deranged circulation. In the atria, there are characteristic waveforms—the *a* wave corresponding to atrial contraction, the *c* wave corresponding to A-V valve closure, and the *v* wave corresponding to atrial filling from venous return against the closed A-V valve.

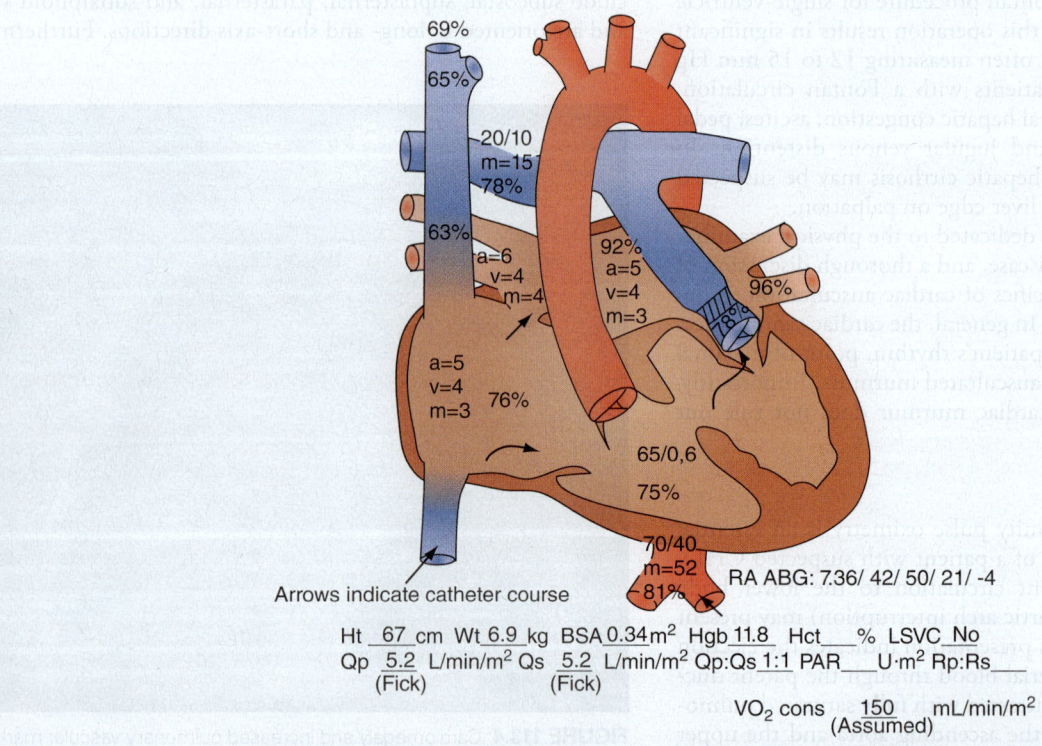

Arrows indicate catheter course

Ht __67__ cm Wt __6.9__ kg BSA __0.34__ m² Hgb __11.8__ Hct____% LSVC __No__
Qp __5.2__ L/min/m² Qs __5.2__ L/min/m² Qp:Qs __1:1__ PAR____U·m² Rp:Rs____
  (Fick)   (Fick)

RA ABG: 7.36/ 42/ 50/ 21/ -4

VO₂ cons ___150___ mL/min/m²
  (Assumed)

FIGURE 113.5 Hemodynamic information obtained after cardiac catheterization.

Typical normal right atrial mean pressures range from 1 to 5 mm Hg, and left atrial mean pressures range from 2 to 10 mm Hg. Right ventricular pressure tracings in normal hearts demonstrate a more gradual upstroke when compared with the left ventricle. Filling or end-diastolic pressures in both ventricles are between 2 and 10 mm Hg in normal hearts. The normal right ventricular systolic pressure (and thus pulmonary artery systolic pressure) is 15 to 30 mm Hg, and the left ventricular systolic pressure is 90 to 110 mm Hg.

In normal hearts, there is a small, physiologically insignificant right-to-left shunt, which results from ventilation-perfusion (V/Q) mismatch in the lungs and coronary venous return directly to the left ventricle (thebesian venous return). This physiologic shunt represents less than 5% of the cardiac output and, in normal circumstances, does not produce detectable systemic arterial desaturation. Thus, significant systemic arterial desaturation represents a pathologic finding, consistent with pulmonary disease, intracardiac shunting, or both. As noted, the origin and degree of intracardiac shunting may be assessed by echocardiography. However, in certain circumstances, cardiac catheterization is necessary to measure cardiac oximetry, calculate shunt fraction, and derive systemic and PVR. Using a derivation of the Fick principle, the ratio of pulmonary blood flow (Qp) to systemic blood flow (Qs) can be determined as follows:

$$Qp/Qs = (Sa_{O_2} - \overline{M}O_2\ sat)/(\overline{P}O_2\ sat - Pa_{O_2})$$

where SaO_2 is systemic arterial oxygen saturation, $\overline{M}O_2$ sat is mixed venous oxygen saturation, $\overline{P}O_2$ sat is pulmonary venous oxygen saturation, and PaO_2 is pulmonary arterial oxygen saturation. Thus, in a patient with $\overline{M}O_2$ sat of 60%, $\overline{P}O_2$ sat of 100%, Sao_2 of 100%, and Pao_2 of 80%, the equation is as follows:

$$Qp/Qs = (100 - 60)/(100 - 80) = 40/20 = 2:1$$

Calculating pulmonary vascular resistances may also be crucial in determining operability in a patient with CHD. In many settings, a precise measure of vascular resistance is unnecessary based on the clinical evidence. For example, in a small child with a large VSD seen on echocardiogram, the clinical findings of tachypnea, cardiomegaly, and failure to thrive confirm a large left-to-right shunt and infer acceptable PVR. However, in less clear circumstances, a precise calculation may be important in clinical decision-making. The PVR may be calculated from cardiac catheterization data as follows:

$$PVR = \frac{(Mean\ PA\ pressure\ [mm Hg] - Mean\ LA\ pressure\ [mm Hg])}{Pulmonary\ Blood\ Flow\ (Qp)\ [L/min/m^2]}$$

In general, patients with an elevated PVR are further evaluated with pulmonary vasodilation—hyperventilation, hyperoxygenation, and inhaled nitric oxide—to determine whether the PVR is responsive. This information may be critical for patients who are otherwise marginal surgical candidates.

Finally, cardiac catheterization has been evolving as the primary therapeutic method for many important structural cardiac defects. In many children's hospitals, most catheterizations now performed are for interventional procedures rather than diagnostic procedures. This fact may be particularly pertinent to a general surgeon faced with treating a patient with a previous catheter-based correction of a cardiac defect. For example, the patient may have had an ASD or VSD closed with an occluder device in the

past. This information may have important ramifications for infectious exposure and vascular access.

PERIOPERATIVE CARE

Perioperative management of a patient with unrepaired or palliated CHD can be extremely challenging. Standard hemodynamic, respiratory, and pharmacologic manipulations appropriate for structurally normal hearts may be entirely inappropriate in settings of complex CHD. This is especially true in the operating room and intensive care settings. General rules include a thorough knowledge of the patient's intracardiac anatomy and expected physiology. It is possible to make significant management errors based on incorrect physiologic expectations in the setting of incomplete understanding of the patient's anatomy. For example, in a patient with unrepaired tetralogy of Fallot (TOF) and associated significant right ventricular outflow tract obstruction (RVOTO), it is expected that the patient will exhibit some degree of systemic arterial desaturation. However, a patient with repaired TOF with no residual intracardiac shunts is expected to be fully saturated, and a finding of desaturation likely represents a complication that warrants expedient investigation. This clinical scenario is a frequent one; a patient with a specific cardiac diagnosis, despite having undergone a successful correction, continues to be incorrectly presumed to have ongoing physiologic perturbation of the unrepaired lesion. Further, it is important to understand whether previous cardiac intervention resulted in complete correction of the lesion or only palliation.

Anesthesia Pitfalls

Providing physiologic anesthetic management can be challenging in patients with CHD, especially in situations such as single-ventricle palliation, unrepaired CHD, chronic cyanosis, and residual intracardiac pathology. Standard anesthetic management paradigms may be completely inappropriate and potentially disastrous in the setting of complex CHD. A thorough understanding of the patient's anatomy is mandatory, along with knowledge of the potential for unexpected response to anesthetic agents and ventilator settings. The field of pediatric and congenital cardiac anesthesia has evolved relative to this specific clinical need; the text by Andropoulos, Mossad, and Gottlieb[14] is an excellent resource.

Several points concerning anesthesia management warrant discussion. The first is vascular access for intraoperative and postoperative management. In patients with complex CHD, especially patients who have undergone previous complex surgical and catheterization procedures, obtaining appropriate vascular access may be challenging. Typically, a large-bore, multilumen central venous line is necessary for appropriate resuscitation and monitoring of right-sided filling pressures. In some patients, the placement of a thermodilution pulmonary artery catheter (oximetric) must be considered because one cannot presume that right-sided filling pressures correlate well with left heart volume or functional status (e.g., after a Fontan operation). Options for central access mirror those of non-CHD patients and include percutaneous internal jugular or subclavian routes with a secondary option of common femoral access to the inferior vena cava (IVC). However, access may be difficult in the setting of previous catheterization or venous reconstruction; this situation may be addressed with the aid of ultrasound-guided catheter placement, which has become a standard in many cardiac operating rooms. Arterial access for continuous blood pressure monitoring and sampling is important for many patients. Percutaneous radial arterial cannulation can be readily achieved in most patients; however, upper extremity blood pressure values may be factitiously altered by previous systemic-to-pulmonary artery shunts, previous aortic arch surgery (especially coarctation), and abnormalities of vascular origin (e.g., aberrant subclavian origin from the descending aorta).

Ventilator management in the perioperative setting of CHD requires special understanding. In settings of large potential left-to-right shunts (e.g., unrepaired VSDs), hyperventilation and hyperoxygenation promote excessive pulmonary blood flow and potentially diminish systemic cardiac output. Positive pressure ventilation, particularly positive end-expiratory pressure, negatively influences hemodynamics in many patients, especially in palliated patients with a single ventricle and passive cavopulmonary flow after the Fontan procedure. Early extubation in these patients can be done to limit the deleterious effects of positive end-expiratory pressure on the Fontan circulation. Data have shown that early extubation is feasible and safe, improves outcomes, and reduces overall hospital costs for these patients.[15] Finally, pharmacologic manipulation of systemic and PVR and cardiac performance are important adjuncts in the perioperative management of patients with CHD. In general, a low-dose infusion of epinephrine 0.05 mcg/kg/min (0.02–0.05 mcg/kg/min) with the addition of a phosphodiesterase inhibitor is an effective pharmacologic cocktail to promote a cardiac inotropic state, lower systemic and PVR, and limit tachycardia. Dopamine, vasopressin, sodium nitroprusside, and nitroglycerin are other frequently used agents. Appropriate perioperative analgesia and sedation are also important aspects of the patient's management.

Neurologic Outcomes

With expectations of almost 100% survival after surgery for CHD, emphasis has been placed on the long-term neurologic outcomes and quality of life of these patients. The potential for neurologic insult in children after CHD arises from the nature of their disease (e.g., cyanotic defects, low-cardiac-output state, genetic syndromes, effects of cardiopulmonary bypass, circulatory arrest). Evidence also suggests that patients with CHD may be genetically predisposed to neurologic insult. Gestational age has been found to be an important factor to consider in the optimization of neurologic outcomes.[16]

LESION OVERVIEW

Defects Associated With Increased Pulmonary Blood Flow

Persistent Arterial Duct (Patent Ductus Arteriosus)

A persistent arterial duct, or PDA, is a frequently encountered congenital cardiac condition. PDA is found in 1 in 2000 term neonates but has significantly increased incidence in preterm neonates, with an incidence of 40% in infants with birth weights less than 2000 g and 80% for less than 1200 g. The arterial duct is necessary during gestation to shunt right ventricular blood away from the unventilated pulmonary vasculature; ductal flow is from the pulmonary artery to the aorta during gestation. At delivery, after the first breath of the neonate, ductal flow reverses and becomes left to right in most individuals. Over the first several hours to days of postnatal life, the PDA closes spontaneously and is completely closed in most infants by 2 to 3 weeks of age.

In the absence of other congenital cardiac lesions, a PDA becomes pathologic related to its presence and the degree of left-to-right shunting. A PDA may be present in association with other structural cardiac conditions and may sometimes be necessary for systemic or pulmonary blood flow. The amount of shunting produced relates to the size and geometry of the duct and the PVR. A PDA may be responsible for a large Qp/Qs ratio and result in pulmonary overcirculation, left heart volume overload, and congestive heart failure (CHF). A large unrestricted PDA is associated with pulmonary hypertension; if left untreated, this proceeds to irreversible pulmonary vascular disease (Eisenmenger syndrome), which ultimately proceeds to pulmonary and right heart failure, treatable only by pulmonary transplantation. Even with a small, pressure-restrictive PDA, there is an ongoing risk for pulmonary congestion and left heart volume overloading; endocarditis is always of concern, even for small PDAs. Ligation or closure is recommended for all PDAs.

The gold standard of therapy for closure of PDA is surgery, usually accomplished through a left posterolateral thoracotomy using ductal division, ligation, or clipping (Fig. 113.6). Surgery needs to be a low-risk procedure associated with minimal potential for persistence of the PDA. Nonetheless, the invasive nature of this proven method has led to the development of alternative strategies for ductal occlusion. From a surgical perspective, many PDAs are amenable to thoracoscopic clipping through very small port incisions; robot-assisted PDA occlusion has been performed in many patients, with good results.[12] Medical treatment with indomethacin (0.1 mg/kg for <1 kg, 0.2 mg/kg ≥1 kg on day 1, then 0.1 mg/kg daily for days 2–7 oral or IV over 1 hour) can be attempted in a neonate but carries risk of necrotizing enterocolitis, intracranial hemorrhage, and renal toxicity. An alternative strategy involves acetaminophen 15 mg/kg every 6 hours for 3 to 7 days. Reported success rates of medical intervention vary significantly. At the present time, most PDAs are occluded in the cardiac catheterization laboratory using occlusive devices. Even the repair of large defects in small infants has been successfully addressed. The long-term effects of the devices remaining in the vascular tree are not fully understood yet; however, successful device closure appears to be an extremely effective, safe, and durable therapy. Recently, catheter-based devices have been approved for PDA occlusion on preterm infants as small as 700 g.

A PDA in an adult patient can be challenging. As noted, a long-standing large PDA may be associated with pulmonary vascular disease. A right-to-left shunt in a PDA is cause for significant concern and warrants further investigation with concern for significantly elevated PVR. In adults with PDAs, the ductus wall may calcify, making an attempt at ligation or division hazardous. In these patients, ductal occlusion may require resection of the adjacent descending aorta with patch grafting or short-segment graft replacement (e.g., Dacron).

Aortopulmonary Septal Defect (Aortopulmonary Window)

An aortopulmonary septal defect is a communication between the ascending aorta and, usually, the main pulmonary artery. This is a rare defect comprising 0.1% to 0.6% of CHD. This lesion results from the failure of complete separation of the embryologic common arterial trunk into the aorta and pulmonary artery. Defects are classified by their location: type I is proximal, just above the aortic sinuses; type II is more distal on the ascending aorta and often involves the origin of the right pulmonary artery; and type III is more distal and associated with a separate origin of the right pulmonary artery from the aorta (Fig. 113.7). An aortopulmonary septal defect may occur in isolation or in association with other conditions, including interrupted aortic arch (IAA) and

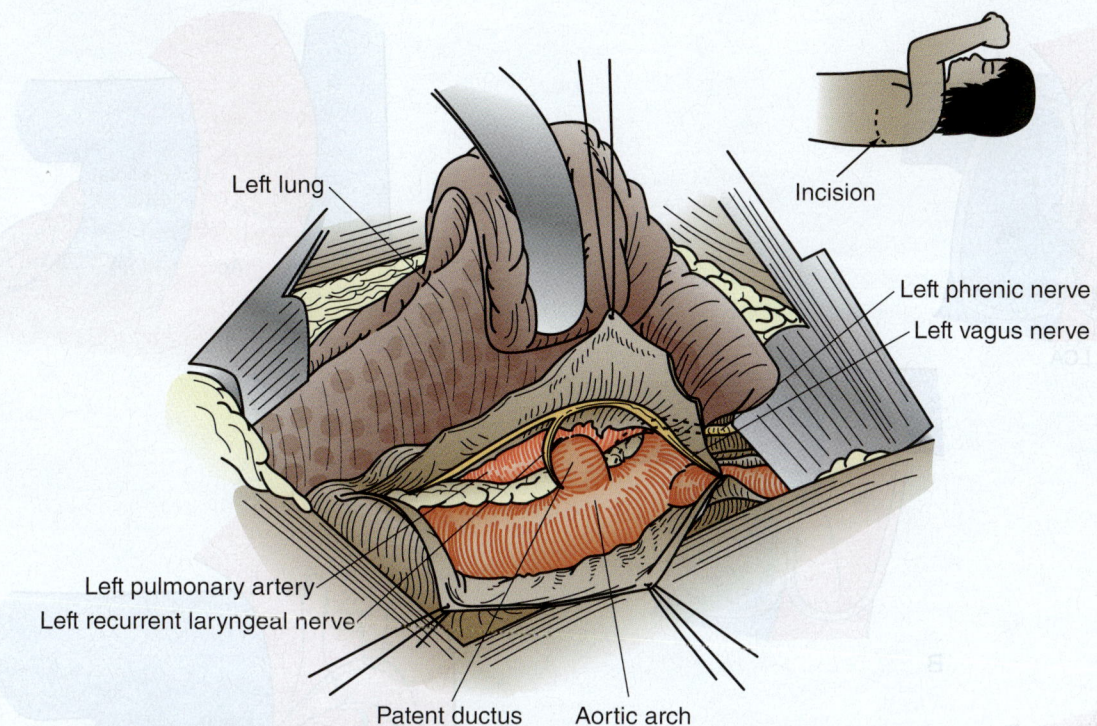

FIGURE 113.6 Anatomic relationships of a patent ductus arteriosus exposed from a left thoracotomy. (From Castaneda AR, Jones RA, Mayer JE, Jr, et al. Patent ductus arteriosus. In: *Cardiac Surgery of the Neonate and Infant.* Philadelphia: Saunders;1994.)

anomalous origin of a coronary artery. Defects are typically large and responsible for a large left-to-right shunt with systemic pulmonary artery pressures. Children with this defect typically present with CHF, failure to thrive, and frequent respiratory infections. Echocardiography, MRI, or cardiac catheterization may be used to make the diagnosis.

The gold standard for repair of aortopulmonary septal defects is surgical closure. Case reports of transcatheter closure exist; however, this is a technically challenging feat without known long-term durability.[17] A small defect may be ligated through a thoracotomy or median sternotomy approach, but this method is not recommended because of significant risk for rupture or incomplete closure. Surgical closure is accomplished with cardiopulmonary bypass support. Options for closure include complete division and separate patch repairs of the great vessel defects or a sandwich type of closure, using a patch to construct a common intervening wall; both methods are effective (Fig. 113.8).

Atrial Septal Defect

An isolated ASD is one of the most common congenital cardiac lesions, occurring in 13 of every 10,000 live births. The most frequently encountered ASD relates to a defect in the interatrial wall, as defined by the fossa ovalis. The defect develops as the result of incomplete closure of the embryologic patent foramen ovale; the defect is a result of incomplete closure of the septum primum. Although the terminology can be confusing, these defects are typically termed *secundum atrial septal defects*. They manifest in a wide variety of configurations, ranging from single small defects to multiple fenestrations to complete absence of the septum primum. The confines of the defect may extend from the IVC orifice up to the superior atrial wall adjacent to the aortic root (Fig. 113.9).

The primary pathophysiologic derangement in ASDs relates to a significant left-to-right shunt in the setting of normal PVR. However, even in the setting of a normal PVR, patients with ASDs are capable of transient right-to-left shunting, particularly during times of increased intrathoracic pressure. The effects of chronic, large left-to-right shunting (in some patients producing a Qp/Qs >3:1) include right heart volume overloading and enlargement. Most children are not overtly symptomatic but may exhibit some degree of exercise intolerance or frequent respiratory tract infection. Symptoms typically become more prevalent in adulthood and include dyspnea on exertion, palpitations, and, ultimately, evidence of right heart failure. Pulmonary vascular disease is not a typical finding in secundum ASDs, but one may demonstrate an ASD in a patient with primary pulmonary hypertension. A rare form of presentation relates to the potential of right-to-left shunting at the atrial level; the ever-present risk for paradoxical embolus and cerebrovascular accident must be considered when recommending ASD closure.

Most centers recommend ASD closure in patients before school age. Since the late 1950s, the standard therapy for ASDs has been surgical closure using cardiopulmonary bypass support. The defect is closed using direct suture closure, autologous pericardium, or prosthetic patch material (Fig. 113.10). This is an effective method with a low associated perioperative risk, including the virtual absence of residual or recurrent defects.[18] Minimally invasive techniques for ASD closure have also gained popularity, with good safety profiles and outcomes.[19]

The potential for closing defects using nonsurgical methods has led to the development of catheter-based therapies, which are now being widely applied to large numbers of patients worldwide for the treatment of ASD. Currently, upward of 60% of ASD interventions are catheter based.[20] The most commonly used device is the Amplatzer septal occluder device (St. Jude Medical,

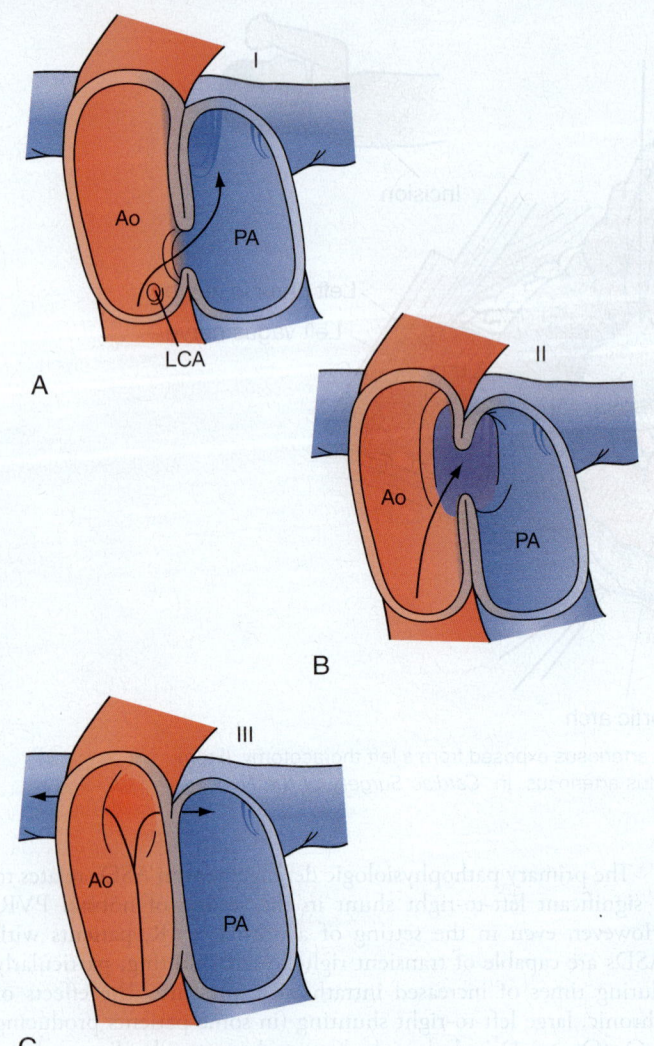

FIGURE 113.7 Native anatomy and classification of aortopulmonary septal defect. (A) In type I, the communication is between the ascending aorta *(Ao)* and the main pulmonary artery *(PA)* on the posterior medial wall of the ascending aorta. The left main coronary artery *(LCA)* orifice may be close to the defect. (B) In type II, the defect is more cephalic on the ascending aorta. (C) In type III, the defect is more posterior and lateral in the aorta. The communication is with the right pulmonary artery, which may be completely separate from the main pulmonary artery. (Adapted from Fraser CD. Aortopulmonary septal defects and patent ductus arteriosus. In: Nichols DG, Ungerleider RM, Spevak PJ, et al, eds. *Critical Heart Disease in Infants and Children.* Philadelphia: Mosby; 2006:664-666.)

St. Paul, MN), made of nitinol metal mesh, which is placed percutaneously and delivered with echocardiographic and fluoroscopic guidance. Reports indicated an acceptable procedure-related complication rate and successful closure rate.[21] However, the long-term effects of having such a device in mobile cardiac structures are not fully understood. More recent reports have documented an alarming incidence of device erosion through the atrial wall and into the adjacent ascending aorta as well as disruption of the conduction system.[22,23] A case report showing severe endocarditis involving a previously placed Amplatzer ASD device has highlighted the need for ongoing observation of the long-term consequences of placing large prosthetic devices into the circulation.[24]

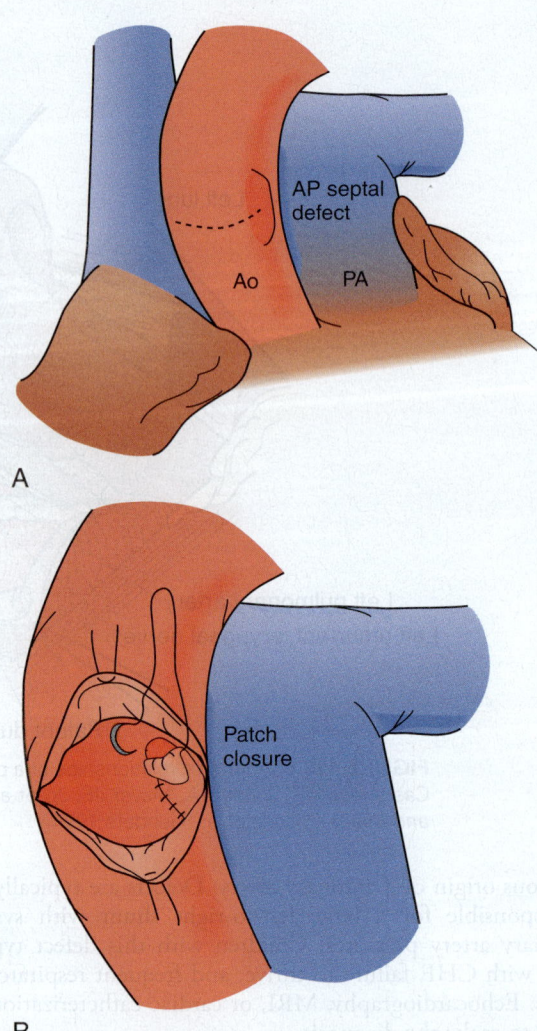

FIGURE 113.8 (A) Surgical exposure of aortopulmonary *(AP)* septal defect includes a transverse incision in the ascending aorta *(Ao)*. (B) The aortopulmonary septal defect is closed by suturing a patch over the aortic side of the defect. *PA,* Pulmonary artery. (Adapted from Fraser CD. Aortopulmonary septal defects and patent ductus arteriosus. In: Nichols DG, Ungerleider RM, Spevak PJ, et al, eds. *Critical Heart Disease in Infants and Children.* Philadelphia: Mosby; 2006:664-666.)

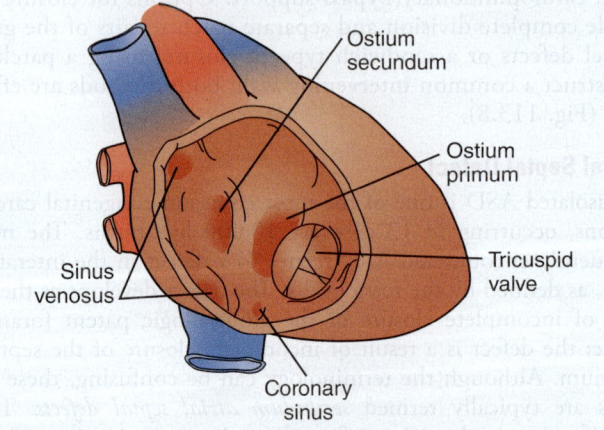

FIGURE 113.9 Types of atrial septal defects as viewed through the right atrium, ostium secundum, ostium primum, and sinus venosus. (Adapted from Redmond JM, Lodge AJ. Atrial septal defects and ventricular septal defects. In Nichols DG, Ungerleider RM, Spevak PJ, et al, eds. *Critical Heart Disease in Infants and Children.* Philadelphia: Mosby; 2006:580.)

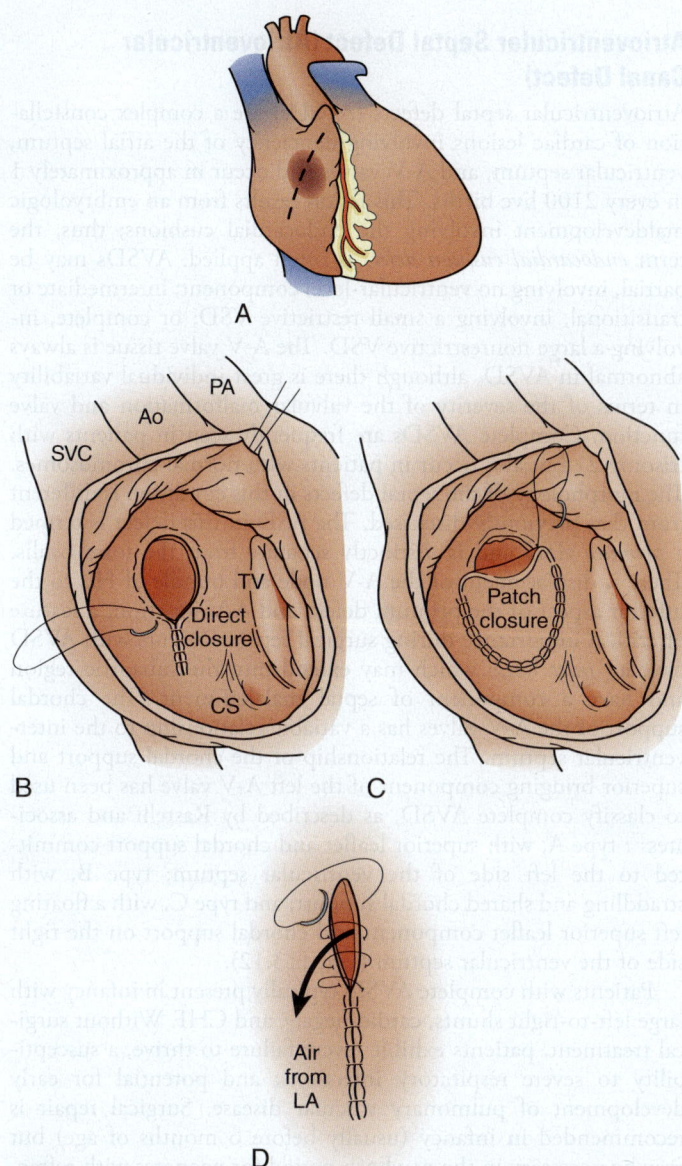

FIGURE 113.10 Surgical closure for atrial septal defect. (A) Right atriotomy. (B) Direct suture closure. (C) Patch closure. (D) Deairing the left atrium *(LA)*. *Ao,* Aorta; *CS,* coronary sinus; *PA,* pulmonary artery; *SVC,* superior vena cava; *TV,* tricuspid valve. (Adapted from Redmond JM, Lodge AJ. Atrial septal defects and ventricular septal defects. In: Nichols DG, Ungerleider RM, Spevak PJ, et al, eds. *Critical Heart Disease in Infants and Children.* Philadelphia: Mosby; 2006:583.)

Sinus venosus ASDs occur as the result of embryologic malalignment between the superior vena cava (SVC) or IVC. These defects are not associated with the fossa ovalis and are frequently associated with partial anomalous pulmonary venous return. A superior sinus venosus ASD occurs high in the atrium, near the orifice of the SVC. This lesion is frequently associated with anomalous drainage of a portion of the right lung to the SVC. An inferior sinus venosus ASD is located low in the atrium, often extending into the IVC orifice. This lesion is typically associated with anomalous pulmonary venous drainage of the entire right lung to the IVC (potentially intrahepatic); pulmonary sequestration and an abnormal systemic artery perfusing the right lower lobe, with origin from the abdominal aorta, may also be present.

In patients with total anomalous pulmonary venous return (TAPVR) to the IVC, the anomalous pulmonary vein may be obvious on a plain chest radiograph and has been described as appearing like a saber (scimitar syndrome), first described by Neill and colleagues.[25]

Surgery for sinus venosus ASDs is recommended for the same pathophysiologic reasons surgery is recommended for secundum ASDs. The repair is not amenable to catheter techniques, and surgery is more complicated than for an isolated secundum ASD. Superior sinus venosus defects with partial anomalous pulmonary venous return to the SVC may be treated with an intracardiac patch baffle; however, in the setting of high drainage of the anomalous pulmonary veins, an SVC translocation operation (Warden procedure) may be necessary. Surgery for an inferior sinus venosus ASD with a scimitar vein can be more complicated, potentially involving the need for a patch baffle within the intrahepatic IVC, which may require periods of hypothermic circulatory arrest.

Ventricular Septal Defect

A VSD is a pathologic communication involving a defect in the interventricular septum. Isolated VSD is present in 0.3% of newborns. Defects are classified in terms of their location and surrounding structures. Patients may be entirely asymptomatic, depending on the size and location of the VSD, along with associated lesions and PVR. In the setting of otherwise normal cardiac morphology and appropriate PVR, the net shunt in patients with VSD is left to right; the Qp/Qs depends on the size of the defect and pulmonary resistance. Large defects result in large shunts, high right ventricular and pulmonary artery pressures, significant pulmonary overcirculation, CHF, and left heart volume overload. In these settings, unrestrictive pulmonary blood flow exposes the patient to the risk of pulmonary vascular disease and Eisenmenger syndrome.

The ventricular septum can be best thought of in terms of the pathway of blood and associated cardiac anatomy. Thus, the right ventricular aspect of the septum has an inlet portion; midmuscular portion; apical, posterior, anterior, and outlet portions; and subaortic portion. This knowledge aids in the classification of VSDs. Furthermore, defects are understood relative to their embryologic origins and have varying propensities for spontaneous decreases in size or closure.

Perimembranous Ventricular Septal Defect

A perimembranous VSD occurs as a defect in the membranous portion of the interventricular septum; its associated margins include the annulus of the tricuspid valve, the muscular septum, and potentially the aortic annulus. The defects may be large and have associated prolapse of the noncoronary or right coronary aortic valve cusps. Perimembranous VSDs exhibit a potential for spontaneous closure, particularly small defects manifesting early in childhood.

Muscular Ventricular Septal Defect

Muscular VSDs occur in all aspects of the muscular interventricular septum. Margins of these defects are entirely muscle. The lesions may be isolated or involve multiple openings in the septum (so-called Swiss cheese septum). Small defects have great potential for regression or spontaneous closure.

Subarterial (Supracristal or Outlet) Ventricular Septal Defect

Subarterial VSDs occur in association with the annulus of the aortic valve, pulmonary valve, or both. The defects are almost always associated with significant prolapse of the adjacent aortic valve cusp, usually the right coronary cusp, which may lead to significant cusp distortion, aortic valve insufficiency, and cusp perforation. The only mechanism for spontaneous closure of these defects relates to the cusp prolapse and valve distortion and is generally not complete or a favorable arrangement. All these defects are surgically closed because of the ongoing risk of aortic valve injury (Fig. 113.11).

The indications for surgery to close VSDs relate to the size of the VSD, degree of shunting, and associated lesions. Small infants presenting with large VSDs, refractory heart failure, and large shunts undergo surgical closure of the defects in the newborn period, regardless of age or size. Other defects are addressed based on the ongoing concerns of left-to-right shunting, aortic valve cusp distortion, and risk for endocarditis. Asymptomatic patients with evidence of significant shunts and cardiomegaly are proposed for surgical therapy. Prophylactic closure of small defects in asymptomatic patients with normal cardiac size and function is advocated by some surgeons because of the lifelong risk for endocarditis and comparatively low risk for surgery.

Percutaneous VSD closure is an acceptable alternative to surgical closure of VSDs with very high procedural success.[26] Despite this, the complex relationship of many defects, including close association with the aortic valve and cardiac conduction tissue, makes the existing technology less than ideal. At the present time, surgery remains the primary mode of therapy for VSD closure. Defects are approached with the aid of cardiopulmonary bypass support and may be closed with various materials, including autologous pericardium (our preference), Dacron, polytetrafluoroethylene, and homograft material. Surgical closure of VSDs is a low-risk procedure with a high expectation of complete closure. Challenging anatomic situations, such as Swiss cheese septum or multiple apical muscular VSDs, may be initially palliated by limiting pulmonary blood flow with a pulmonary artery band and deferring corrective surgery to later in life when the child is larger.

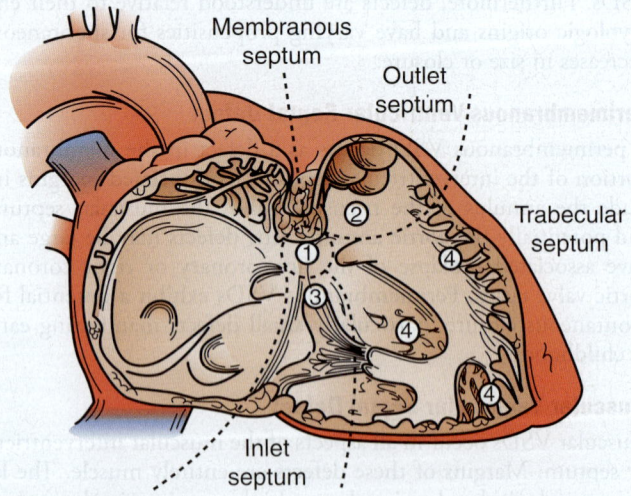

FIGURE 113.11 Location of ventricular septal defects (VSDs) in the ventricular septum (view of the ventricular septum from the right side). *1,* Perimembranous VSD; *2,* subarterial VSD; *3,* atrioventricular canal–type VSD; *4,* muscular VSD. (From Tchervenkov CI, Shum-Tim D. Ventricular septal defect. In: Baue AE, Geha AS, Hammond GL, eds. *Glenn's Thoracic and Cardiovascular Surgery.* 6th ed. Stamford, CT: Appleton & Lange; 1996.)

Atrioventricular Septal Defect (Atrioventricular Canal Defect)

Atrioventricular septal defects (AVSDs) are a complex constellation of cardiac lesions involving deficiency of the atrial septum, ventricular septum, and A-V valves and occur in approximately 1 in every 2100 live births. This lesion results from an embryologic maldevelopment involving the endocardial cushions; thus, the term *endocardial cushion defect* is often applied. AVSDs may be partial, involving no ventricular-level component; intermediate or transitional, involving a small restrictive VSD; or complete, involving a large nonrestrictive VSD. The A-V valve tissue is always abnormal in AVSD, although there is great individual variability in terms of the severity of the valvular malformation and valve function. Complete AVSDs are frequently seen in patients with trisomy 21 but also occur in patients with normal chromosomes. The morphology of the septal defects in this condition is different from that previously discussed. The ASD in this defect is termed a *primum ASD* and is distinctly separate from the fossa ovalis. There is displacement of the A-V node and bundle of His to the inferior aspect of the primum defect and A-V junction, a feature of critical importance during surgical repair. Patients with AVSD have an *inlet VSD,* which may extend into the subaortic region and have a component of septal malalignment. The chordal support of the A-V valves has a variable relationship to the interventricular septum. The relationship of the chordal support and superior bridging component of the left A-V valve has been used to classify complete AVSD, as described by Rastelli and associates[27]: type A, with superior leaflet and chordal support committed to the left side of the ventricular septum; type B, with straddling and shared chordal support; and type C, with a floating left superior leaflet component and chordal support on the right side of the ventricular septum (Fig. 113.12).

Patients with complete AVSD typically present in infancy with large left-to-right shunts, cardiomegaly, and CHF. Without surgical treatment, patients exhibit severe failure to thrive, a susceptibility to severe respiratory infections, and potential for early development of pulmonary vascular disease. Surgical repair is recommended in infancy (usually before 6 months of age) but may be necessary in the newborn period for neonates with refractory heart failure, especially in association with aortic arch anomalies. Patients with partial or intermediate defects may have the surgery deferred until later in childhood, depending on the degree of atrial level shunting and the presence of A-V valve regurgitation. AVSD may also manifest in unbalanced forms with dominance of right-sided or left-sided components. In severely affected individuals, biventricular repair is not feasible, and patients are managed along a single-ventricle pathway. AVSD may also be found in association with TOF; this combination is associated with cyanosis, and repair is more challenging than for either condition considered in isolation.

Surgery is the primary mode of therapy for patients with AVSD. Operative goals include complete closure of ASDs and VSDs and effective use of available A-V valve tissue to achieve valve competence. As noted, the inferiorly displaced conduction tissue must be protected to avoid the complication of surgically induced A-V block (Fig. 113.13). Surgical intervention is performed with the use of the cardiopulmonary bypass machine. The atrial and ventricular septal components are closed with a common patch (single-patch method) or separate patches (two-patch technique). We believe the two-patch method to be superior in preserving A-V valve tissue (Fig. 113.14).[28] The critical

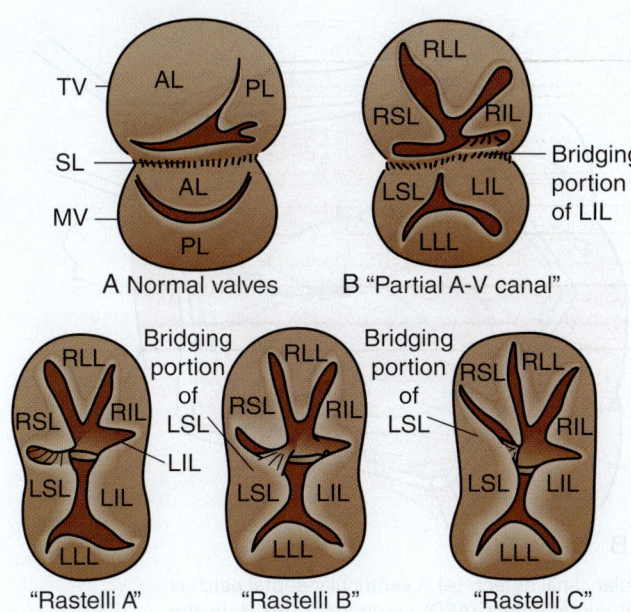

FIGURE 113.12 Rastelli classification type A, B, or C. The difference in valve morphology in a normal (A), partial (B), and complete (C) canal defect is illustrated. *AL,* Anterior leaflet; *A-V,* atrioventricular; *LIL,* left inferior leaflet; *LLL,* left lateral leaflet; *LSL,* left superior leaflet; *MV,* mitral valve; *PL,* posterior leaflet; *RIL,* right inferior leaflet; *RLL,* right lateral leaflet; *RSL,* right superior leaflet; *SL,* superior leaflet; *TV,* tricuspid valve. (From Kirklin JW, Pacifico AD, Kirklin JK. The surgical treatment of atrioventricular canal defects. In: Arciniegas E, ed. *Pediatric Cardiac Surgery.* Chicago: Year Book Medical Publishers; 1985.)

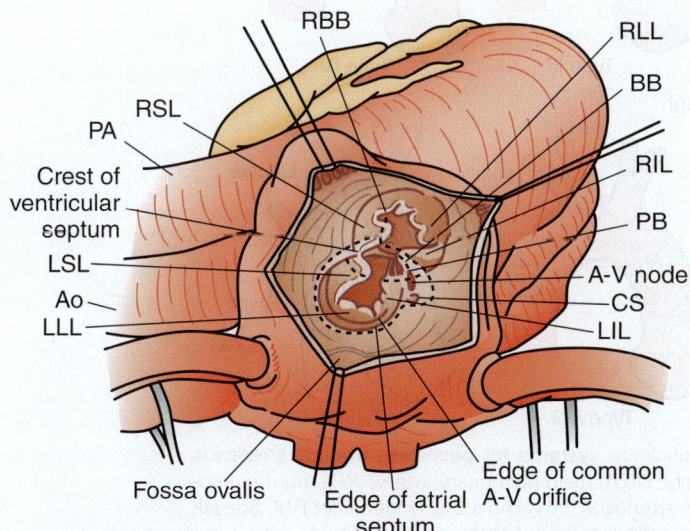

FIGURE 113.13 Position of the conducting system in complete atrioventricular canal defect. The anatomic relationships and morphology of the common atrioventricular (*A-V*) valve are shown. The view is through a right atriotomy. *Ao,* Aorta; *BB,* left bundle branch; *CS,* coronary sinus; *LIL,* left inferior leaflet; *LLL,* left lateral leaflet; *LSL,* left superior leaflet; *PA,* pulmonary artery; *PB,* penetrating bundle; *RBB,* right bundle branch; *RIL,* right inferior leaflet; *RLL,* right lateral leaflet; *RSL,* right superior leaflet. (From Bharati S, Lev M, Kirklin JW. *Cardiac Surgery and the Conducting System.* New York: Churchill Livingstone; 1983.)

component of the repair lies in the valve repair; typically, after suspending the valve tissue to the reconstructed septum, the line of coaptation between the superior and inferior leaflet components (cleft) is closed; however, care must be exercised to avoid valvular stenosis.

Perioperative care is predicated on an accurate and hemodynamically favorable repair. Patients with long-standing pulmonary overcirculation may have a potential for early perioperative pulmonary hypertensive crisis. This condition may require therapy, including oxygen, optimization of fluid balance, continuous sedation, hyperventilation, and, possibly, inhaled nitric oxide.

Adult Patients With Atrioventricular Septal Defect

Numerous patients with partial or transitional AVSD survive well into adulthood without surgery. These patients have variable presentations but may exhibit severe exercise intolerance; evidence of right heart dysfunction; some elevation of PVR; and, possibly, atrial dysrhythmias, including atrial fibrillation. In patients with late presentation of AVSD, cardiac catheterization is often recommended to rule out occult coronary artery lesions and evaluate PVR. Nonetheless, in the absence of obvious surgical contraindication, surgery is recommended for adults with unrepaired AVSD to eliminate the chronic left-to-right shunt and repair the typically insufficient A-V valves.

Other patients present well into adulthood with previously repaired AVSDs. These patients may have a widely disparate constellation of findings, including atrial and ventricular dysrhythmias, valvular insufficiency or stenosis, and right heart dysfunction. In many of them, secondary reparative surgery may become necessary. Furthermore, in the setting of a patient with remotely repaired AVSD requiring noncardiac surgery, potential ongoing hemodynamic concerns that would affect the perioperative course must be expected.

Persistent Arterial Trunk (Truncus Arteriosus)

Truncus arteriosus, or persistent arterial trunk, results from failure of separation of the embryonic arterial trunk and semilunar valves and occurs in approximately 1 in 10,000 live births. It is almost always associated with a large nonrestrictive perimembranous VSD and is associated with varying degrees of truncal override of the interventricular septum, including 100% association of the trunk with the RV. The condition is classified by the relationship of the origins of the pulmonary arteries. In type I truncus arteriosus, there is a demonstrable common main pulmonary artery with subsequent origins of the branch pulmonary arteries; in type II truncus arteriosus, the branch pulmonary arteries arise closely, but separately, from the trunk; in type III truncus arteriosus, the branch pulmonary arteries are widely separated in origin on the ascending aorta; and in type IV truncus arteriosus, no pulmonary arterial branch arises from the common trunk. Type IV truncus arteriosus is now recognized as a form of pulmonary atresia with VSD (Fig. 113.15).

In contrast to patients with aortopulmonary septal defects, patients with truncus arteriosus have a single outlet valve of highly variable morphology. The valve may have a normal appearance, with three well-formed and distinct cusps similar to those of a normal aortic valve. In other patients, the truncal valve may be severely malformed, with multiple cusps, dysmorphic leaflets, and abnormal commissural relationships. The truncal valve morphology and function have significant bearing on patient symptoms and the difficulty of surgery. Patients with truncus arteriosus frequently have coronary ostial abnormalities, including juxtacommissural origin

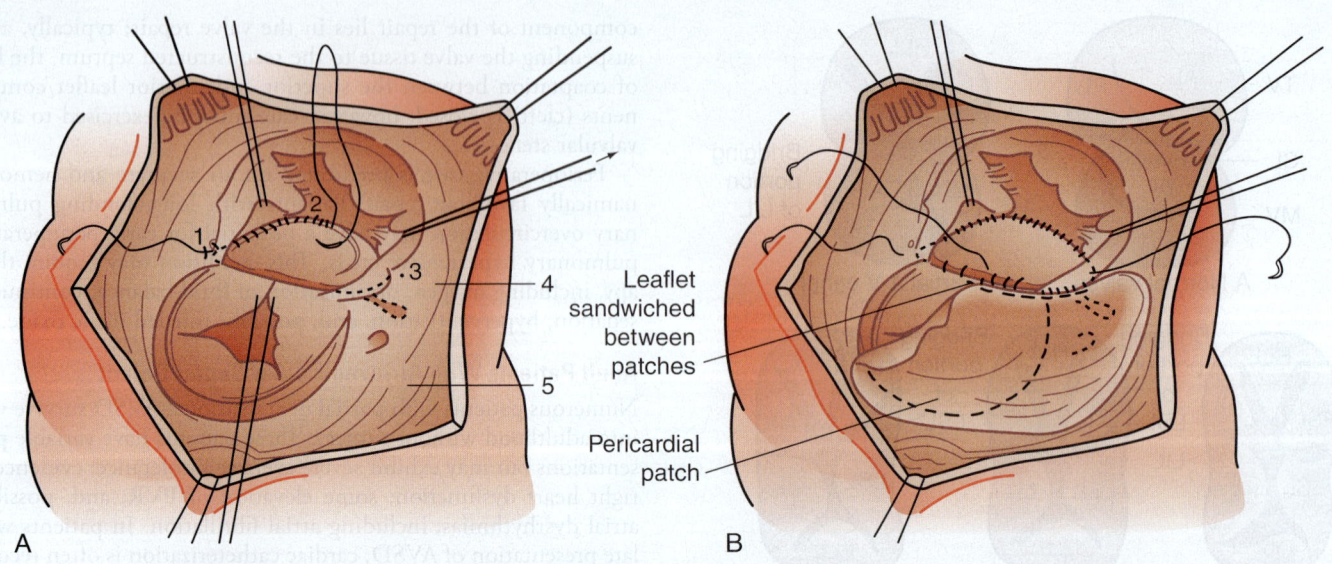

FIGURE 113.14 Two-patch closure of complete atrioventricular canal defect. (A) A ventricular septal patch is placed first, and a separate patch is used to close the atrial septal defect (ASD) component. (B) Note the position of the coronary sinus and conducting system relative to the ASD patch suture line to avoid injury to the atrioventricular node. (From Kirklin JW, Barratt-Boyes BG. *Cardiac Surgery*. New York: Churchill Livingstone; 1986.)

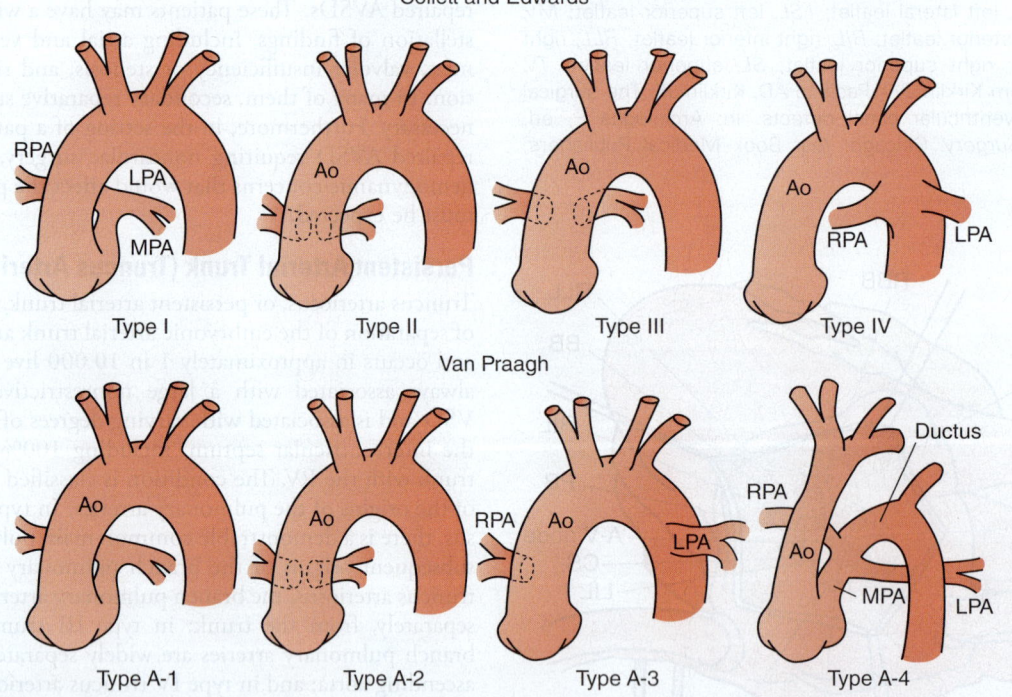

FIGURE 113.15 Collett-Edwards and Van Praagh classification systems for persistent truncus arteriosus (see text for details). *Ao,* Aorta; *LPA,* left pulmonary artery; *MPA,* main pulmonary artery; *RPA,* right pulmonary artery. (Adapted from St Louis JD. Persistent truncus arteriosus. In: Nichols DG, Ungerleider RM, Spevak PJ, et al, eds. *Critical Heart Disease in Infants and Children*. Philadelphia: Mosby; 2006:690.)

and intramural course. There is an associated interruption of the aortic arch in 25% of newborns presenting with truncus arteriosus. Abnormalities of thymic genesis, T-cell function, and calcium homeostasis may frequently be seen in this group of patients in association with a chromosome 22 deletion (DiGeorge syndrome).

Patients with truncus arteriosus present in the newborn period with unrestricted pulmonary blood flow and systemic pulmonary artery pressure. With the expected postnatal decrease in PVR,

massive pulmonary overcirculation, and CHF, patients may exhibit a wide pulse pressure because of diastolic runoff of blood into the pulmonary vasculature. This situation is further exacerbated in the setting of significant truncal valve insufficiency, resulting in poor systemic perfusion and cardiovascular collapse. Some infants can be initially managed with medical decongestive therapy (e.g., diuretics, angiotensin-converting enzyme inhibitors, and digoxin) and fortified nutritional support (through gastric intubation); however, this is a precarious arrangement. In the few individuals who survive infancy, irreversible pulmonary vascular disease develops rapidly, and patients become inoperable. In other patients, refractory CHF results in poor weight gain, respiratory insufficiency, and susceptibility to infection. The profound hemodynamic compromise places many newborns with unrepaired truncus arteriosus at high risk for necrotizing enterocolitis. Patients with truncus arteriosus and IAA have ductal-dependent systemic blood flow and are dependent on intravenous PGE1 to maintain ductal patency until they undergo repair. Given these considerations, it is recommended that most newborn patients undergo repair in the first several weeks of life.

The surgical repair is performed on cardiopulmonary bypass support. Components of the repair include division of the common trunk and reconstruction of confluent central branch pulmonary arteries. The large VSD is closed with a patch, typically through a right ventriculotomy. In patients with an abnormal, insufficient truncal valve, a valve repair may be necessary. It is unusual to have to replace the truncal valve at the initial operation; most valves can be at least partially repaired to provide the patient with an adequate aortic valve. Right ventricle–pulmonary artery continuity then must be established. Most surgeons prefer to interpose a valved conduit between the right ventriculotomy and pulmonary artery bifurcation (Fig. 113.16).

Conduits are limited and include homografts (pulmonary artery or aorta, valved) or heterografts (bovine or porcine). Experience

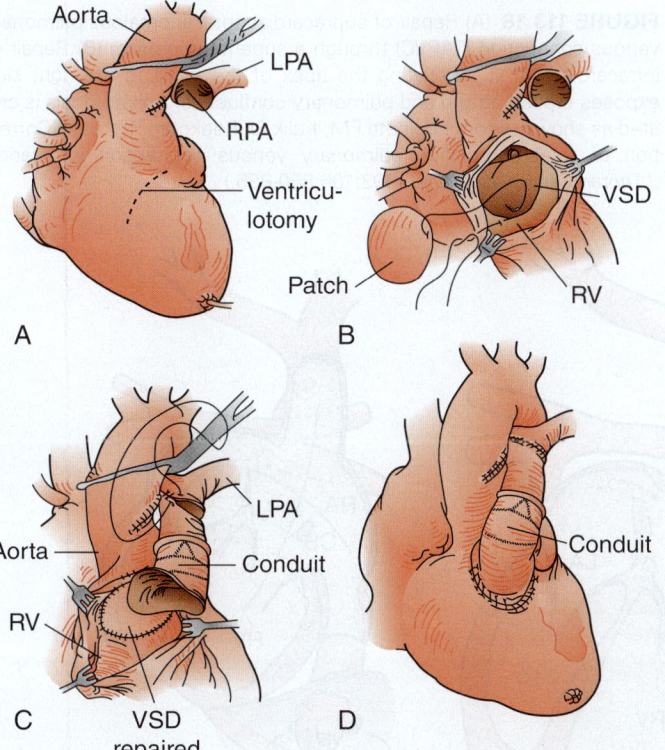

FIGURE 113.16 Surgical repair of truncus arteriosus. (A) The origin of the truncus arteriosus is excised, and the truncal defect is closed with a direct suture. The incision is made high in the right ventricle *(RV)*. (B) The ventricular septal defect *(VSD)* is closed with a prosthetic patch. (C) Placement of a valved conduit into the pulmonary arteries. (D) Proximal end of conduit is anastomosed to the RV. *LPA,* Left pulmonary artery; *RPA,* right pulmonary artery. (From Wallace RB. Truncus arteriosus. In: Sabiston DC, Jr, Spencer FC, eds. *Gibbons Surgery of the Chest.* 3rd ed. Philadelphia: Saunders; 1976.)

with a commercially available, glutaraldehyde-preserved, bovine jugular vein valved conduit (Contegra; Medtronic, Minneapolis, MN) had been encouraging. However, there is a concerning increased incidence of endocarditis with Contegra valved conduits compared with other conduits, including homografts and heterografts.[29] An emerging option is the partial heart transplant or living homograft. In this setting, the semilunar valves ± root complexes from a donor heart that has gone unmatched for conventional cardiac transplant are procured and used similarly to a cryopreserved homograft. The theoretical benefit of this procedure is the potential for the living homograft to grow with the patient, potentially obviating the need for repeat interventions. Uncertainty remains around the need, type, and duration of immunosuppression and the mid- and long-term outcomes and durability of the transplanted valve.[30] Successful repair of truncus arteriosus in infants using a direct hooded anastomosis between the pulmonary artery bifurcation and right ventriculotomy has also been reported.[31] No option available at the present time offers patients the lifetime solution of a connection capable of somatic growth along with a competent, durable pulmonary valve. Thus, it is expected that all infants undergoing successful truncus repair will require multiple subsequent cardiac surgeries as they outgrow their current RV–pulmonary artery conduit. Experience with a percutaneously delivered, catheter-mounted pulmonary valve has been encouraging as an interim solution for these patients in an effort to limit the number of required cardiac reoperations.

A growing number of adults have survived childhood truncus arteriosus repair. All these patients require diligent longitudinal cardiology surveillance, and many will require reoperation. Issues of concern include late ventricular dysrhythmias, often related to surgical scarring from the previous right ventriculotomy; branch pulmonary artery stenosis; stenosis or insufficiency of the RV–pulmonary artery conduit; truncal valve insufficiency; and right ventricular dysfunction.

Abnormalities of Venous Drainage

Total Anomalous Pulmonary Venous Return

TAPVR results from embryonic failure of connection of the fetal pulmonary venous sinus to the left atrium and occurs in 1 in every 10,000 live births. This fatal condition has a spectrum of clinical presentations and may be associated with additional complex structural cardiac disease, including a single ventricle. In TAPVR, pulmonary venous return may take one of several pathways to return eventually to the right heart. Initial survival is predicated on an unobstructed pathway and unrestricted atrial-level communication so that sufficient intracardiac mixing affords the patient adequate systemic oxygenation. Patients with TAPVR are desaturated to varying degrees, depending on the adequacy of the anomalous pathway, atrial mixing, and pulmonary function. The abnormal venous connection drains in several typical patterns.

In supracardiac TAPVR, the pulmonary veins drain to a vertical vein, which courses cephalad to join a systemic vein. In the most common variation, the vertical vein courses anterior to the left pulmonary artery to join the left innominate vein. This vein may course posterior to the left pulmonary artery, resulting in compression of the pulmonary venous pathway between the left pulmonary artery and left mainstem bronchus (so-called pulmonary artery vise). The vertical vein may also join the SVC or azygos vein. In intracardiac TAPVR, the pulmonary veins drain into the coronary sinus and, in most cases in which the coronary sinus is intact, into the right atrium. This variant is rarely obstructed and may not be diagnosed until later in life in some patients. In infracardiac TAPVR, the vertical veins descend in a caudal direction through the diaphragm to join the embryologic ductus venosus and then through the liver to join the IVC. This variation is almost always obstructed at some level (Fig. 113.17). In mixed TAPVR, the pulmonary venous pathway drains in several pathways to reach the heart. Frequently, in mixed TAPVR, one or several pulmonary veins connect to the SVC, with others draining to an infracardiac or supracardiac connection.

Obstructed total anomalous pulmonary venous return. Obstructed TAPVR is one of the few true surgical emergencies in congenital heart surgery. When the condition is suspected, it is diagnosed with transthoracic echocardiography. Obstructed TAPVR occurs when one of the drainage patterns noted earlier is obstructed, resulting in severe pulmonary venous hypertension. Secondary effects include pulmonary edema, pulmonary artery hypertension, and profound hypoxemia. Interstitial pulmonary emphysema and frank pneumothorax may develop while attempting vigorous ventilatory support in profoundly desaturated children. Patients with obstructed TAPVR may present within hours of birth in extremis and do not respond to resuscitative efforts. The only useful therapy is rapid surgical repair, regardless of the severity of the patient's preoperative status.

For other forms of TAPVR, elective surgical repair is recommended after the condition is diagnosed. Occasionally, the diagnosis is not made until later in childhood in patients with an unobstructed vertical vein and widely patent atrial communication. These patients undergo elective repair to relieve cyanosis, intracardiac mixing, and right heart volume overload.

Surgical repair of TAPVR requires cardiopulmonary bypass support; occasionally, periods of profound hypothermia and circulatory arrest are necessary. The principles of repair include identification of the pulmonary venous confluence and individual pulmonary veins. An anastomosis is constructed between the venous confluence and left atrium using a superolateral approach, with the heart reflected to the patient's right, or an incision directly through the interatrial septum and corresponding region of the posterior right atrial wall. The ASD and PDA that are typically present are closed as well (Fig. 113.18).

Cor triatriatum. Cor triatriatum is a rare condition accounting for ~0.1% of all congenital heart defects in which the pulmonary veins enter a chamber posterior to the left atrium with a small connection to the right or left atrium. These patients exhibit evidence of pulmonary hypertension and variable desaturation. Surgical decompression is necessary to relieve the pulmonary venous obstruction; this is accomplished by resection of the

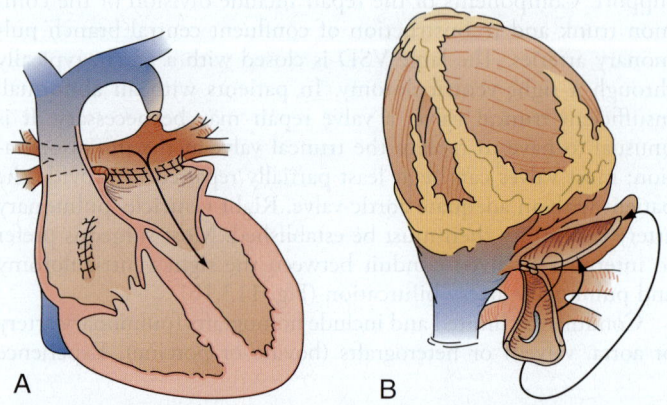

FIGURE 113.18 (A) Repair of supracardiac total anomalous pulmonary venous connection (TAPVC) through a superior approach. (B) Repair of infracardiac TAPVC. Elevating the apex of the heart to the right side exposes the left atrium and pulmonary confluence. Anastomosis is created as shown. (From Lupinetti FM, Kulik TJ, Beekman RH, et al. Correction of total anomalous pulmonary venous connection in infancy. *J Thorac Cardiovasc Surg.* 1993;106:880-885.)

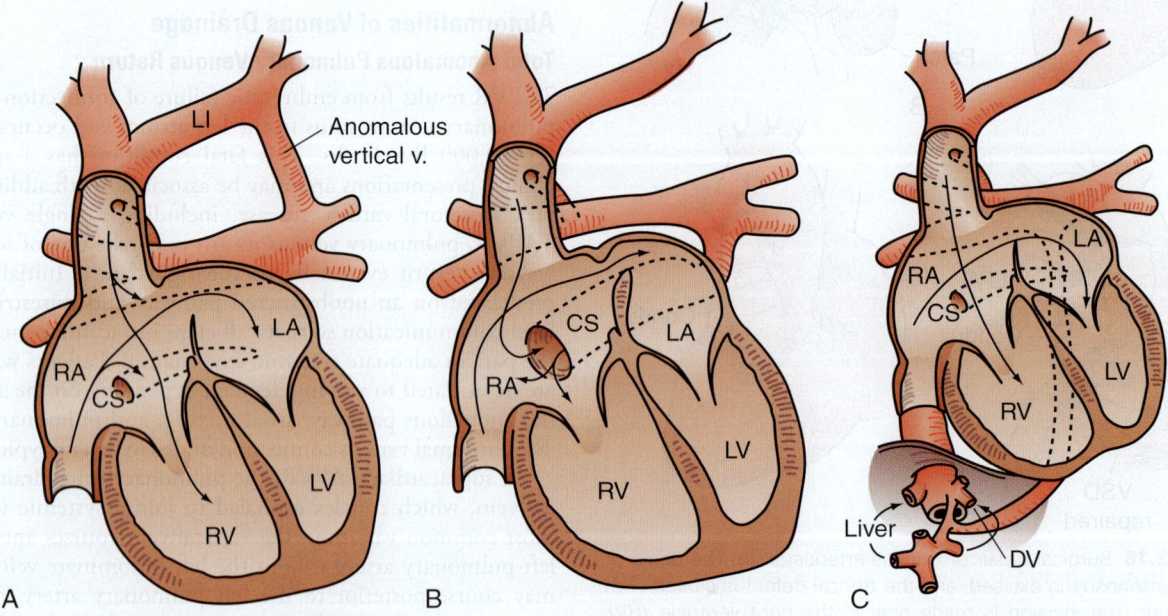

FIGURE 113.17 Types of total anomalous pulmonary venous connection. (A) Supracardiac type with a vertical vein joining the left innominate *(LI)* vein. (B) Intracardiac type with connection to the coronary sinus *(CS)*. (C) Infracardiac type with drainage through the diaphragm via an inferior connecting vein. *DV,* Ductus venosus; *LA,* left atrium; *LV,* left ventricle; *RA,* right atrium; *RV,* right ventricle; *v,* vein. (From Hammon JW, Jr, Bender HW, Jr. Anomalous venous connections: Pulmonary and systemic. In: Baue AE, ed. *Glenn's Thoracic and Cardiac Surgery.* 5th ed. Norwalk: Appleton & Lange; 1991.)

membrane between the pulmonary venous chamber and left atrium.

A dreaded consequence of TAPVR occurs when there is a progressive, malignant sclerosing process involving the individual pulmonary veins. This process may be initiated by inaccurate surgery resulting in obstruction of the venous confluence and individual veins, or it may progress independently of surgical manipulation. It may progress to intrapulmonary pulmonary venous stenoses. A technique to deal with individual pulmonary venous stenoses uses a pedicled flap of adjacent pericardium to augment the pulmonary venous orifices (sutureless technique), but this method is not applicable to all patients with pulmonary venous obstruction. Catheter-based dilation and stenting have been attempted in this setting, with good acute relief of obstruction, but they have a high rate of reintervention and unknown long-term success, with 50% survival at 5 years.[32] In the most severe cases, the only meaningful surgical option is lung transplantation.

Anomalous Systemic Venous Drainage

Congenital abnormalities of systemic venous drainage may occur in isolation or in association with other significant structural cardiac defects. In the setting of an otherwise normal heart, the anomaly is frequently not of physiologic significance. The most common example is a persistent left SVC draining to the coronary sinus. In the absence of an intracardiac communication or unroofing of the coronary sinus, this is of anatomic significance only. In many cases, a persistent left SVC occurs, with absence of a communicating innominate vein. This condition becomes important in situations of mechanical occlusion, which may be seen with trauma or chronic venous intubation with thrombosis. A persistent left SVC is frequently incidentally discovered after placement of a left internal jugular central line, which is apparently found to track into the heart on plain chest radiography. A persistent left SVC becomes more significant in patients requiring intracardiac or extracardiac surgery. If the left SVC drains to an unroofed coronary sinus in a patient undergoing atrial septation, the patient will be profoundly desaturated after surgery. This situation requires reconstruction of the coronary sinus or some other method to reroute the left SVC to the right atrium.

An interrupted IVC usually occurs in association with other structural cardiac disease. The IVC drainage in these settings is to the azygos (azygos continuation) or hemiazygos vein and, ultimately, the SVC. In these patients, the hepatic veins drain into the atrium as a common confluence or as individual veins.

The physiologic significance of the interrupted IVC relates to the coexisting cardiac lesion and the necessity of appreciating the abnormality of systemic venous drainage in performing corrective surgery. In patients requiring noncardiac surgery or catheter intervention, the presence of an interrupted IVC is noted when an attempt is being made to pass a venous catheter from the groin into the heart.

Cyanotic Congenital Heart Disease

Tetralogy of Fallot

TOF is a common form of cyanotic CHD occurring in approximately 1 in 2500 live births and is probably the most studied lesion in the era of surgical correction for CHD. Many believe that the Johns Hopkins Hospital was the birthplace of cardiac surgery. Blalock performed the first successful palliative operation for TOF in November 1944, assisted by his laboratory technician, Vivien Thomas.[1] Blalock was encouraged by Taussig, the matriarch of pediatric cardiology (Fig. 113.19). Until more recently, some degree of controversy has surrounded the relative degree of contribution by these three individuals in bringing this historical event to fruition. In actuality, all three were significant participants in this momentous medical advance. While working at Vanderbilt Medical School, Blalock had charged his young and capable laboratory technician, Vivien Thomas, with the development of a surgical model of pulmonary hypertension. Thomas and Blalock developed a method of anastomosing the left subclavian artery to the divided left pulmonary artery in a canine model. Specifically, Thomas worked out the technical details, including crafting the necessary surgical instruments, and mastered the operation. This work did not produce the desired effect; canine PVR is almost infinitely low, and the animals did not develop a hypertensive pulmonary vasculature. Nonetheless, the technique was developed and published approximately 10 years in advance of the clinical application in 1944.

Blalock subsequently became the chair of surgery at Johns Hopkins. Taussig had, by that time, established a reputation as a meticulous diagnostician of complex congenital heart lesions. She had a large clinic of critically ill children with disabling cyanosis—"blue babies." At her suggestion (and probably her insistence), Blalock was convinced to attempt a surgical palliation for TOF by constructing in a human the subclavian-to-pulmonary artery anastomosis that had been perfected in the research laboratory (Fig. 113.20). Blalock performed the operation in conditions and with instruments that would be considered extremely crude

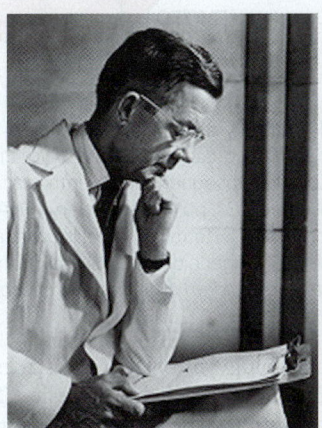
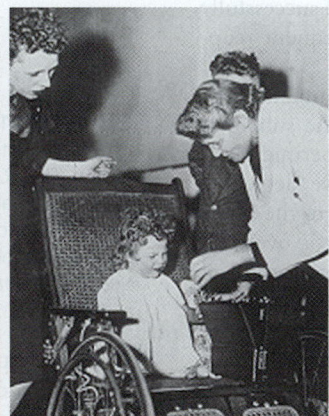
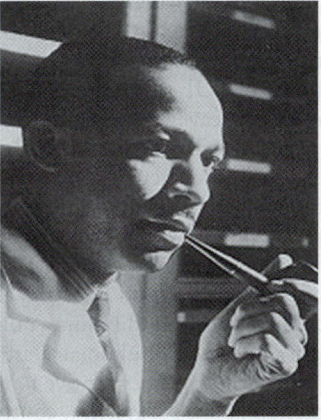

FIGURE 113.19 Drs. Alfred Blalock, Helen Taussig, and Vivien Thomas.

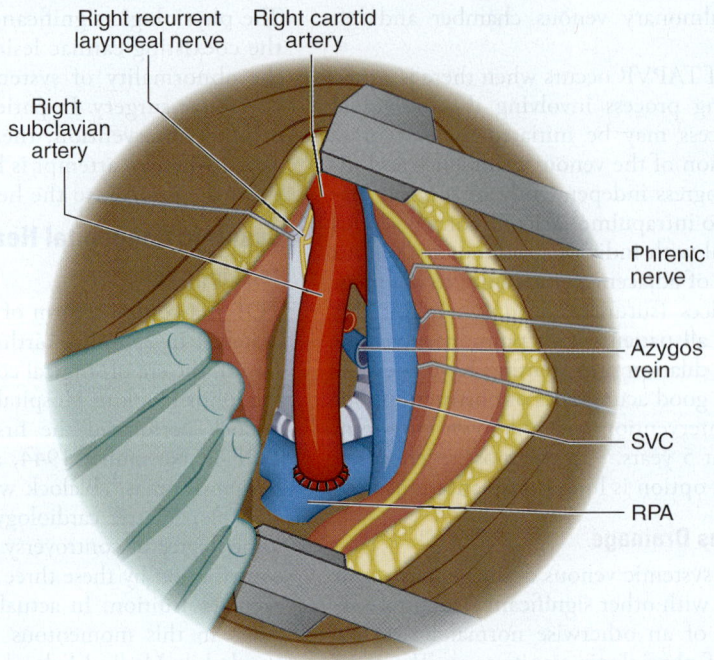

FIGURE 113.20 Classic Blalock-Taussig shunt (right thoracotomy). *RPA,* Right pulmonary artery; *SVC,* superior vena cava. (Modified from Backer CL, Mavroudis C. Palliative operations. In: Mavroudis C, Backer C, Idriss RF, eds. *Pediatric Cardiac Surgery.* Chichester, UK: Wiley; 2012: Chapter 9.)

by today's standards. Thomas stood immediately behind Blalock during that operation and many subsequent cases, providing instruction and encouragement. The clinical success was an earth-shattering event; hundreds of patients subsequently traveled to Johns Hopkins for surgical treatment, and the era of cardiac surgery was ushered in. (These historical accounts are factual, the result of personal interviews with many of those in attendance at that event, including Thomas, Taussig, J. Alex Haller, and Denton Cooley.)

The historical account of the development of the BTT shunt has relevance to the practice of congenital heart surgery today. First, it is important that the facts surrounding this achievement are acknowledged. Second, this remarkably simple concept still remains a frequently applied technique for children with inadequate pulmonary blood flow. Finally, over almost 75 years of treatment of TOF, thousands of patients have been successfully treated, but most are not cured; many require subsequent reoperative cardiac surgery, even after complete repair.

The anatomic hallmark of TOF is anterior malalignment of the infundibular septum, which leaves a deficiency in the subaortic region—a malalignment VSD. This VSD is usually perimembranous, large, and pressure nonrestrictive. The relative degree of malalignment influences the relationship of the aorta to the interventricular septum, producing varying degrees of aortic override. The deviated infundibular septum produces varying degrees of RVOTO. The path of pulmonary blood flow may be impeded at numerous levels, including the infundibulum, pulmonary valve and annulus, and main and branch pulmonary arteries. Secondary right ventricular hypertrophy occurs relative to the degree and duration of the obstruction and is progressive, contributing to the propensity for the lesion to worsen over time (Fig. 113.21).

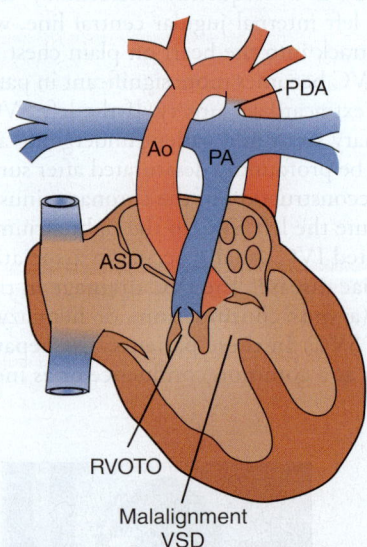

FIGURE 113.21 Anatomy of tetralogy of Fallot. A malalignment ventricular septal defect *(VSD),* aortic override, right ventricular outflow tract obstruction *(RVOTO),* and subsequent right ventricular hypertrophy. *Ao,* Aorta; *ASD,* atrial septal defect; *PA,* pulmonary artery; *PDA,* patent ductus arteriosus. (Adapted from Davis S. Tetralogy of Fallot with and without pulmonary atresia. In: Nichols DG, Ungerleider RM, Spevak PJ, et al, eds. *Critical Heart Disease in Infants and Children.* Philadelphia: Mosby; 2006:756.)

The pathophysiology of TOF relates to shunting of desaturated, systemic venous blood through the VSD to mix with the systemic cardiac output. The greater the degree of obstruction to pulmonary blood flow, the larger the right-to-left shunt and the worse the desaturation. There are several modes of presentation. Newborns with TOF and severe RVOTO may present soon after birth with profound cyanosis; some require PGE1 to maintain ductal patency for adequate oxygenation. At the other end of the spectrum are children with little infundibular obstruction and normal pulmonary valve and branch pulmonary arteries. These patients may have net left-to-right flow through the VSD, occasionally to the extent that they experience pulmonary overcirculation and CHF (so-called pink TOF). Most children present between these extremes; an initially mild to moderate degree of infundibular stenosis progresses over time to become severe with worsening desaturation. A TOF spell occurs when there is an acute change in the cardiac inotropic state, often in the setting of agitation and dehydration. The infundibular stenosis acutely worsens, and patients become profoundly desaturated; this may be an extremely serious event, leading to brain damage or death. Acute treatment modalities include sedation, hydration, systemic afterload augmentation (α-adrenergic agonists), β-blockade to reduce the inotropic state, and endotracheal intubation with supplemental inspired oxygen.

The natural history of untreated TOF is dismal, with most children dying of progressive cyanosis before 10 years of age. Surgery is the mainstay of therapy. Medical and catheter-based therapy may be used to temporize, but TOF is a surgical disease. The principles of surgical correction include patch closure of the VSD and relief of all levels of the RVOTO and pulmonary artery stenosis. The classic method of TOF repair uses a longitudinal incision through the right ventricular outflow tract (RVOT); this provides an excellent transventricular view of the VSD, which is closed with a patch. The pulmonary artery, pulmonary valve, and annulus are incised if stenotic, and then the RVOT is patched. This method was used for many years but has the complicating feature of the long ventriculotomy, with attendant right ventricular dysfunction and often severe pulmonic insufficiency (Fig. 113.22). An alternative method, the transatrial/transpulmonary approach,

first proposed by Imai, has gained popularity. In this method, the VSD closure and RVOT resection are accomplished through a right atriotomy via the tricuspid valve. The main pulmonary artery and pulmonary annulus are incised only if stenotic, but there is no transmural infundibular incision. This method is technically more demanding than the classic method but may offer the patient improved long-term right ventricular function (Figs. 113.23–113.25). The approach has been further developed as a right ventricular infundibulum-sparing strategy that focuses on minimizing the right ventricular incision and preserving the pulmonary valve. The right ventricular infundibulum-sparing strategy includes an algorithm for optimal timing of the repair that considers the individual patient's weight, age, and overall clinical picture (Fig. 113.26). Midterm results with this approach have demonstrated preserved right ventricular function.[33]

The long-term sequelae of TOF repair have been unfolding. For most patients, successful childhood repair of TOF does not translate into a cure. As patients age after TOF repair, long-term complications may develop. Patients with long RVOT incisions (transannular) by necessity have severe pulmonary insufficiency and a noncontractile infundibulum. Over time, the effects of chronic right heart volume overload include right ventricular dilation and decreased function, often with progressive tricuspid insufficiency and elevated central venous pressure. These patients may present with hepatomegaly, peripheral edema, and severe exercise intolerance. Dysrhythmias may frequently occur; patients with large right ventriculotomies develop endocardial scarring, which may be the substrate for ventricular tachycardia. Chronic right atrial dilation may ultimately lead to atrial dysrhythmias, including atrial tachycardia and fibrillation. Relative to these and other potential issues after TOF repair, patients require careful and lifelong medical follow-up. Many need reintervention; this is frequently the case in patients with chronic, severe pulmonary insufficiency, which is indicated when right ventricular dilation and dysfunction become significant. In these patients, placing a competent pulmonary valve is necessary to relieve chronic right ventricular overload. These issues are of particular importance to a patient with repaired TOF presenting for noncardiac surgery. A careful assessment of the patient's cardiac anatomy and function is performed, including echocardiography, Holter or Bardy monitoring, and occasionally, cardiac catheterization.

Pulmonary Atresia and Intact Ventricular Septum

Pulmonary atresia with an intact ventricular septum (IVS) manifests with profound desaturation and ductal-dependent pulmonary blood flow in newborns. The cardiac morphology in this condition varies widely. On the most severe end of the spectrum, patients have very small RVs, tiny tricuspid inlets, and often a RV-dependent coronary circulation. In these cases, the RV must remain hypertensive to provide flow to these segments of the coronary circulation. At the other end of the anatomic spectrum, patients have a relatively normal tricuspid valve and RV. Most patients fall in between these extremes, with some degree of tricuspid valve and RV underdevelopment.

Because patients are ductal dependent at birth, an assessment must be made as to whether the right heart will be capable of ultimately supporting a biventricular circulation. If the coronary circulation is truly RV dependent, decompressing the RV would result in coronary insufficiency. In these situations, a palliative Blalock-Taussig shunt is created in anticipation of promoting the patient down a single-ventricle pathway. In other patients, the atretic pulmonary valve must be opened with percutaneous balloon dilation

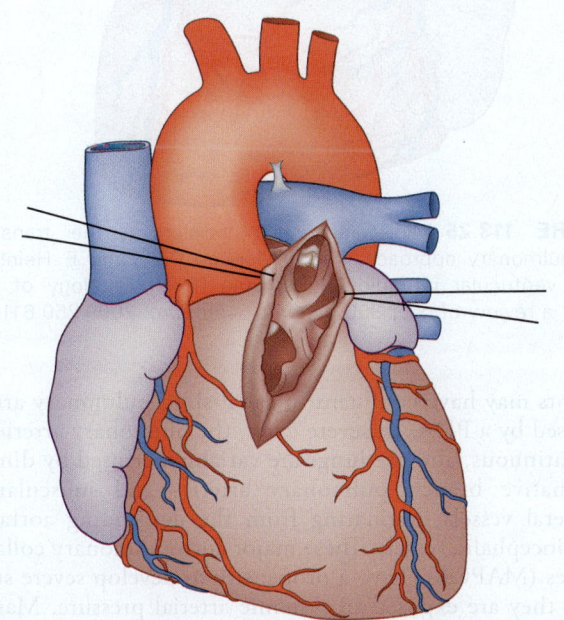

FIGURE 113.22 Long right ventriculotomy in a classic transventricular approach. (From Morales DL, Zafar F, Heinle JS. Right ventricular infundibulum sparing [RVIs] tetralogy of Fallot repair: a review of over 300 patients. *Ann Surg.* 2009;250:611-617.)

first proposed by Ionil, has gained popularity in this method, the VSD closure and RVOT resection are accomplished through a right atriotomy via the tricuspid valve. The main pulmonary artery and pulmonary annulus are inspected, but there is no transannular infundibulum. Obviously, this method is technically more demanding, but it may offer the patient improved protection from pulmonary insufficiency (Figs. 113.23–113.25). The approach has been challenged as a right ventricular infundibulum-sparing procedure on minimizing the right ventriculotomy incision. In the pulmonary valve, the right ventricular outflow tract muscle resection includes an algorithm for the management of the individual patients, while the infundibular resection (Figs. 113.23, to minimizing resection of muscle has demonstrated preserved right ventricular function.

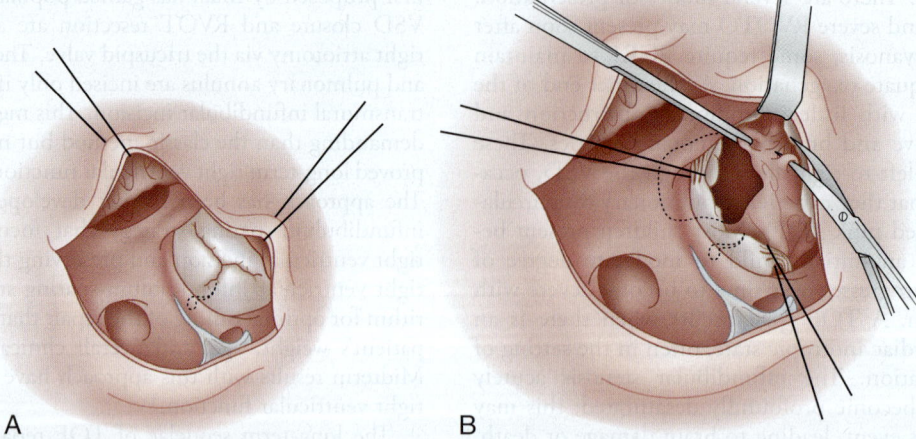

FIGURE 113.23 (A) Surgeon's view through a transatrial incision in the transatrial/transpulmonary approach. (B) Right ventricular outflow tract muscle resection through the right atriotomy. (From Morales DL, Zafar F, Heinle JS. Right ventricular infundibulum sparing [RVIs] tetralogy of Fallot repair: a review of over 300 patients. *Ann Surg.* 2009;250:611-617.)

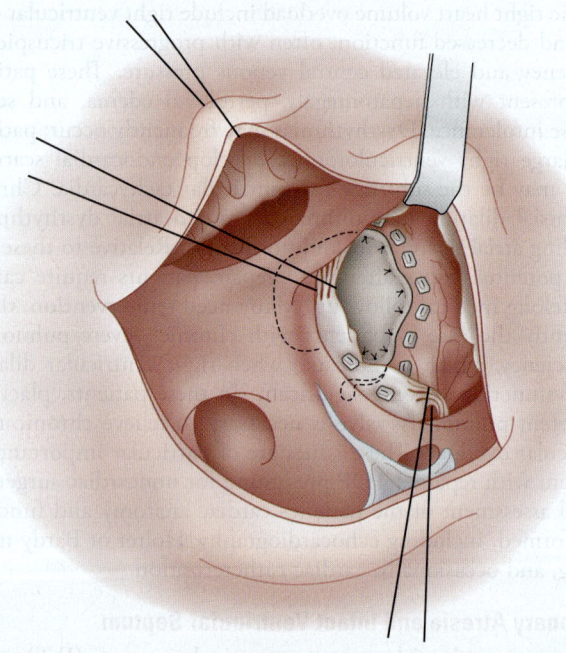

FIGURE 113.24 Ventricular septal defect patch closure with pledgets around the defect and onto the tricuspid valve annulus to avoid the conduction system. (From Morales DL, Zafar F, Heinle JS. Right ventricular infundibulum sparing [RVIs] tetralogy of Fallot repair: a review of over 300 patients. *Ann Surg.* 2009;250:611-617.)

or open surgical valvotomy. Over time, the hypertensive, often apparently underdeveloped RV will improve in size and function and become capable of supporting all or a significant proportion of the cardiac output. At initial presentation, many patients have a large patent foramen ovale or ASD; in patients with a restrictive ASD and marginal right heart, an atrial septostomy (balloon) allows for atrial-level right-to-left shunting until the RV improves. Ultimately, if the RV is adequate, the ASD can be closed.

Pulmonary Atresia With Ventricular Septal Defect

Pulmonary atresia with VSD is morphologically similar to TOF, with the exception of an atretic pulmonary valve.

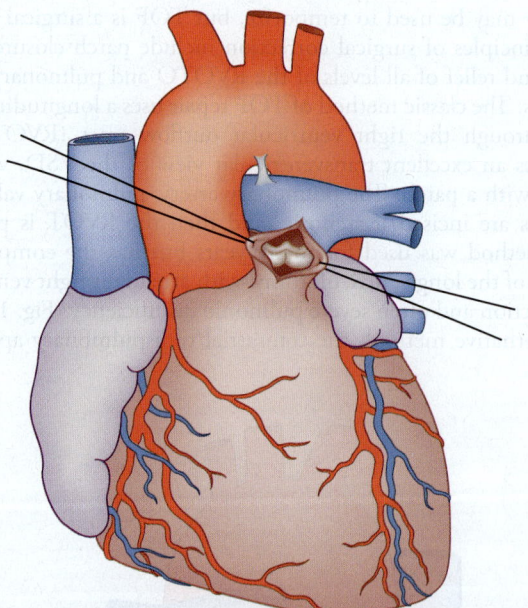

FIGURE 113.25 Mini–transannular incision in the transatrial-transpulmonary approach. (From Morales DL, Zafar F, Heinle JS. Right ventricular infundibulum sparing [RVIs] tetralogy of Fallot repair: a review of over 300 patients. *Ann Surg.* 2009;250:611-617.)

Patients may have confluent, normal-sized pulmonary arteries perfused by a PDA. In severe cases, the pulmonary arteries are discontinuous, and the lungs are variably perfused by diminutive native branch pulmonary arteries and muscularized, collateral vessels originating from the descending aorta and brachiocephalic vessels. These major aortopulmonary collateral arteries (MAPCAs) have a propensity to develop severe stenoses as they are exposed to systemic arterial pressure. Many of these MAPCAs eventually occlude at an unpredictable rate during childhood. Because they may provide the only blood supply to some lung segments, patients become progressively desaturated.

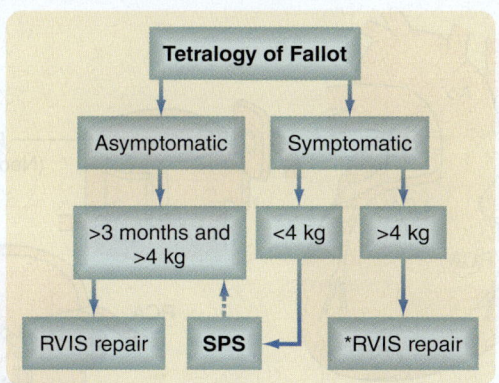

FIGURE 113.26 Algorithm for the right ventricular infundibulum-sparing *(RVIS)* strategy. The goal of this strategy is to minimize the right ventricular incision and preserve the pulmonary valve. It is an individualized approach that considers the patient's weight, age, and overall clinical picture. *SPS,* Systemic-to-pulmonary artery shunt. (From Morales DL, Zafar F, Heinle JS. Right ventricular infundibulum sparing [RVIs] tetralogy of Fallot repair: a review of over 300 patients. *Ann Surg.* 2009; 250:611-617.)

The goal of surgical therapy for pulmonary atresia with VSD is biventricular repair to achieve normal cardiac workload and systemic arterial saturations. In patients with confluent native pulmonary arteries of adequate caliber, the VSD is surgically closed, and a valved conduit (homograft or heterograft) is interposed between the RV and pulmonary bifurcation. In patients with pulmonary atresia with VSD and MAPCAs, the pulmonary arteries must be repaired by connecting the various lung segments into a common trunk through a process termed *pulmonary artery unifocalization.* Depending on the source and size of the MAPCAs and native pulmonary arteries, this may be a challenging surgical procedure, but the goal is constructing a pulmonary tree as close to normal as possible so that biventricular repair is feasible (see earlier).

The long-term issues of repair of pulmonary atresia with VSD are similar to concerns described earlier for TOF. The addition of a RV–pulmonary artery conduit guarantees the need for reoperation because no currently available conduit choice offers the potential for somatic growth or an indefinitely durable valve.

Valvular Pulmonic Stenosis

Patients with isolated valvular pulmonary stenosis are almost always treated in infancy with a percutaneous balloon pulmonary valvotomy. The intermediate-term results of this treatment are good; however, all patients are left with significant pulmonary valve insufficiency and eventually require pulmonary valve replacement.

Conotruncal Anomalies

Transposition of the Great Arteries

Transposition of TGA is a common cyanotic congenital cardiac lesion occurring in 2 to 3 per 10,000 live births. In this section, our discussion relates only to TGA in which there are two good ventricles identified as being capable of independent function as the right and left ventricle. TGA is commonly referred to as D-*TGA*, in relationship to the typically normal D (dextro) ventricular looping that occurs in association with the discordant ventriculoarterial connection and normal A-V connection. TGA occurs in the setting of an IVS (TGA-IVS) or with associated VSD (TGA-VSD). In TGA-VSD, there may be associated aortic

arch hypoplasia and coarctation. On the other extreme, there may be severe pulmonic and subpulmonic stenosis (left ventricular outflow tract obstruction [LVOTO]) or even pulmonary atresia (TGA-VSD with pulmonary atresia).

Patients with TGA-IVS typically present in the early newborn period with profound cyanosis associated with normal perinatal PDA closure. In the absence of a significant ASD, the cyanosis is severe and progresses to death if left untreated. Administration of intravenous PGE1 is almost uniformly successful in reestablishing ductal patency to improve the patient's arterial saturation by providing left-to-right shunting and improved pulmonary blood flow.

In most patients, a balloon atrial septostomy is performed (percutaneous through the umbilical vein or femoral vein) to allow atrial-level mixing (Fig. 113.27). This procedure is usually effective in allowing sufficient atrial-level mixing so that the patient is adequately saturated (70%–80%).

After the procedure, the prostaglandin infusion can frequently be discontinued. In TGA-VSD, there is often sufficient shunting at the level of the VSD to promote adequate systemic saturation; in patients with large VSDs, the predominant presenting symptom may be pulmonary overcirculation and CHF. Patients with TGA with pulmonary atresia have ductal-dependent pulmonary blood flow. In patients with TGA-VSD and aortic arch hypoplasia or coarctation, PGE1 may be necessary to maintain ductal patency and systemic perfusion. Echocardiography is the primary diagnostic modality for TGA.

The treatment of TGA has evolved significantly during the years of surgical therapy for CHD. Initial success was achieved by surgical reconstruction to create a physiologic repair. The atrial switch operation involves a series of intraatrial baffles using a patch channel (Mustard procedure)[34] or infolding of the native

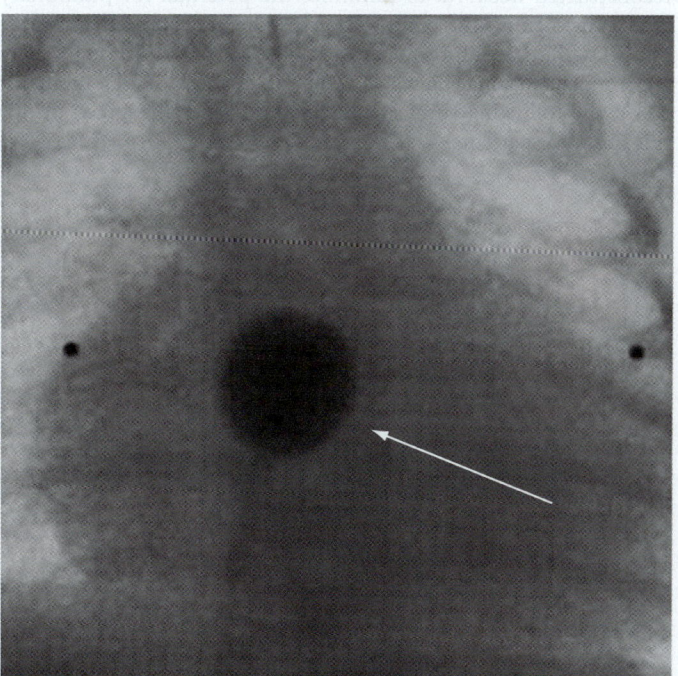

FIGURE 113.27 Angiogram during balloon atrial septostomy. The *arrow* points to the inflated balloon catheter at the atrial septum. The interventional cardiologist forcefully pulls the balloon across the patent foramen ovale to create an open, unobstructed secundum atrial septal defect.

atrial wall and interatrial septum (Senning procedure).[35] Both procedures achieve the same physiologic result: The systemic venous blood is redirected to the left ventricle (and the pulmonary circulation), and the pulmonary venous blood is redirected to the RV. After a successful atrial switch, patients are fully saturated but are left with their morphologic RV supporting the entire systemic cardiac output. In many (perhaps ultimately all) patients undergoing the atrial switch procedure, the RV becomes dysfunctional over time, which is manifested by dilation, decreased ejection fraction, tricuspid insufficiency, and dysrhythmias. The observation of problems with the systemic RV in patients after the atrial switch operation was the primary impetus behind the development and application of the arterial switch operation (ASO), which is now established as the surgical treatment of choice for patients with TGA. At the present time, operative survival rates for the ASO approach 100%.[36]

The ASO provides physiologic and anatomic correction of TGA by establishing ventriculoarterial concordance. The procedure involves transection and translocation of the malposed great vessels. The technically challenging requirement of the ASO relates to the translocation of the coronary arteries to the pulmonary root (the neoaorta). As noted, there are numerous possible branching patterns for the coronary arteries in TGA—some are easily transferred in the ASO, whereas others are more challenging (including single coronary ostium and intramural course) (Fig. 113.28).[37] Nonetheless, precise surgical techniques have been described and successfully applied to all coronary branching patterns. Given this as well as the known benefit of aligning the morphologic left ventricle with the systemic circulation, the ASO is offered to all patients with TGA regardless of the coronary branching pattern. There is no need for precise anatomic definition before surgery; all patients undergo the ASO. In most patients undergoing this procedure, the pulmonary artery bifurcation is moved anterior to the reconstructed neoaorta to minimize the potential for pulmonary artery distortion and compression of the translocated coronary arteries—the Lecompte maneuver (Fig. 113.29). Although there are interinstitutional biases in terms of nuances of treatment for TGA, the following surgical strategies are generally agreed on for this group of patients.

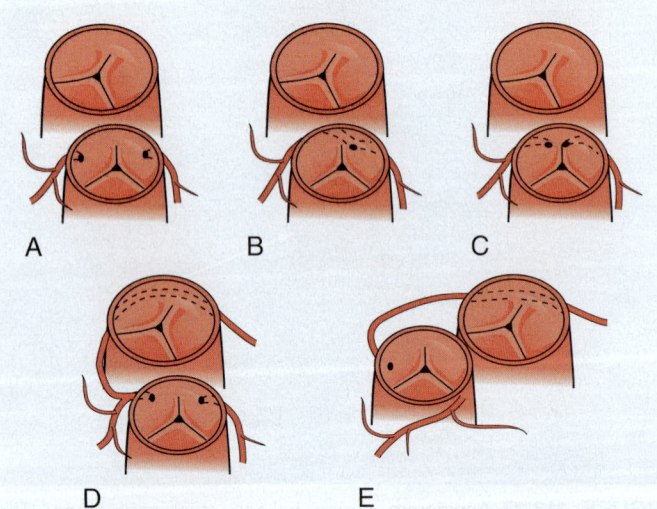

FIGURE 113.28 (A–E) Five basic coronary artery configurations, as described by Yacoub and Radley-Smith. (Adapted from Mee R. The arterial switch operation. In: Stark J, de Leval M, eds. *Surgery for Congenital Heart Defects*. 2nd ed. Philadelphia: Saunders; 1994:484.)

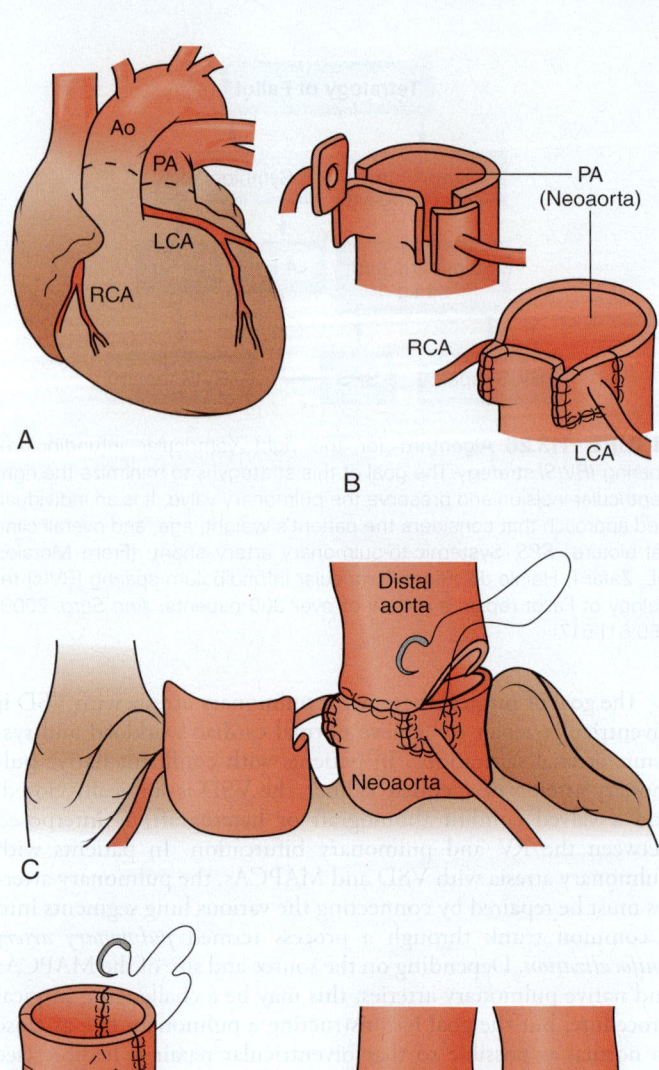

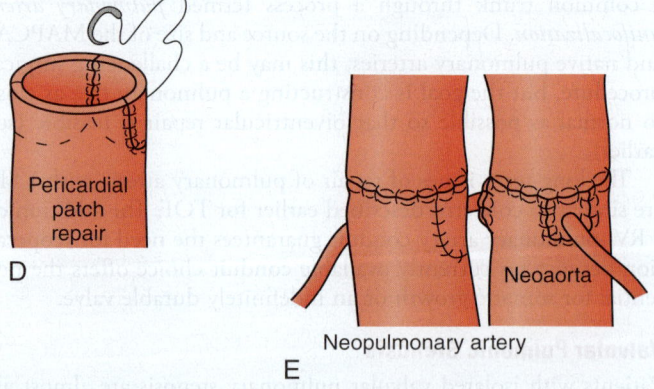

FIGURE 113.29 Arterial switch operation. (A) The aorta *(Ao)* and pulmonary artery *(PA)* are transected above the sinuses of Valsalva. (B) The coronary arteries are excised from the aorta and anastomosed to the pulmonary artery using a trapdoor technique. (C) The distal aorta is brought behind the pulmonary artery (Lecompte maneuver) and anastomosed to the neoaorta. (D) Separate pericardial patches are sutured to replace the excised coronary artery tissue from the aorta. (E) Completed repair. *LCA,* Left coronary artery; *RCA,* right coronary artery. (Adapted from Karl TR, Kirshbom PM. Transposition of the great arteries and the arterial switch operation. In: Nichols DG, Ungerleider RM, Spevak PJ, et al, eds. *Critical Heart Disease in Infants and Children*. Philadelphia: Mosby; 2006:721.)

Transposition of the great arteries–intact ventricular septum.

After balloon atrial septostomy and weaning from PGE1, if possible, newborns with TGA-IVS undergo semielective ASO in the first few days to weeks of life. Rarely, patients present with profound desaturation refractory to balloon atrial septostomy and

PGE1; in this setting, an emergent ASO is indicated. We have found this to be necessary in one patient during the past decade in an experience involving more than 200 ASOs performed in newborns. For other patients, the ASO needs to be performed in a timely but nonemergent setting. Even in the presence of adequate systemic saturation, the patient's morphologic left ventricle is functioning in a low-pressure work environment—supporting the pulmonary circulation. Thus, left ventricle mass and function involute rapidly in the first few weeks of life. By 6 weeks of life, the left ventricle may be incapable of supporting the normal systemic workload after the ASO. As such, the preferred timing for the operation is in the first 1 to 2 weeks of life.

Transposition of the great arteries–ventricular septal defect with or without arch hypoplasia. There are several modes of presentation for patients with TGA-VSD. In patients with small, pressure-restrictive VSD, the presenting symptoms are similar to those of TGA-IVS. These patients require the ASO early in life, along with VSD closure before left ventricle involution. In patients with TGA and nonrestrictive VSD, there may be adequate mixing to allow reasonable systemic arterial saturation. In this setting, the left ventricle remains pressure loaded and does not involute; thus, the necessity of early promotion to the ASO is less time compressed. Many newborns with TGA and a large VSD are relatively asymptomatic soon after birth; they go on to develop CHF in the first 1 to 2 months of life as the normal decrease in newborn pulmonary resistance occurs. Our preference for these patients is to follow them closely for evidence of CHF and perform semielective ASO and VSD closure in the first 4 to 6 weeks of life. Some centers prefer to proceed with this surgery sooner; this appears to be a matter of surgeon preference and has not been shown to affect long-term outcome. In patients with TGA-VSD with arch hypoplasia or coarctation, early surgery is required. In this setting, the preferred treatment involves one-stage, complete correction, including ASO, VSD closure, and aortic arch repair.

Transposition of the great arteries–ventricular septal defect with pulmonary stenosis–left ventricular outflow tract obstruction or pulmonary atresia. The issue of concern in this group of patients is the degree of LVOTO. In patients with TGA-VSD and organic LVOTO, with a relatively normal pulmonary valve, the treatment strategy is as described earlier, with ASO, VSD closure, and left ventricular outflow tract (LVOT) resection. The situation becomes more complex in the setting of severe pulmonary stenosis or pulmonary atresia. These patients may be ductal dependent as newborns (pulmonary atresia) and require newborn complete correction or a palliative modified BT shunt in the newborn period, followed by biventricular repair later in infancy (our preference). The goal in these patients is to achieve biventricular repair to create an unobstructed connection between the morphologic left ventricle and systemic circulation. Several operations have been described and successfully used in this setting.

The Rastelli procedure involves an interventricular patch baffle, which commits the left ventricle to the aorta through the VSD. Typically, a RV–pulmonary artery conduit is then placed to achieve pulmonary blood flow. Issues of concern include the potential for LVOTO (at or below the level of the VSD) and the certain need for future RV–pulmonary artery conduit revision. The Réparation à l'Etage Ventriculair (REV) procedure is designed to minimize the potential of LVOT obstruction and to use all possible native tissue-tissue connections to limit the potential need for future surgery. This procedure involves resection of the muscular conus between the aorta and pulmonary roots, interventricular baffle of the left ventricle to the aorta, and translocation

of the native main pulmonary artery to the RV (by a Lecompte maneuver) without the use of an intervening conduit. The final option involves aortic root translocation, which includes resection of the entire native aortic root and coronary origins, resection of the intervening muscular conus, and posterior translocation of the aortic root to the surgically enlarged pulmonary root to achieve a direct connection between the left ventricle and aorta. The VSD is then closed, and a conduit is placed, or a direct connection is created between the RV and pulmonary arteries.

Transposition of the great arteries in adults. The long-term prognosis of adult patients who have undergone childhood repair of TGA is still incompletely understood; however, all these patients require lifelong surveillance and have the potential to develop significant anatomic and functional cardiac problems. Patients who were treated with the atrial switch operation have a morphologic RV supporting their systemic circulation, which will predictably fail in many patients. Although fully saturated, these patients may present later in life with signs and symptoms of CHF and dysrhythmia. For severely affected individuals, the only realistic treatment option ultimately may be cardiac transplantation.

The long-term issues related to the ASO are less well understood. Despite technical advances in reconstructive methods, there is still a troubling incidence of postoperative supravalvular and branch pulmonic stenosis. The neoaortic root may dilate in some patients undergoing the ASO, leading to neoaortic insufficiency and coronary artery distortion. The fate of the surgically translocated coronary ostia is unclear; there is clearly a risk for late sudden cardiac death related to unsuspected coronary insufficiency noted elsewhere in this chapter. For an adult patient undergoing noncardiac surgery after previous surgery for complex congenital cardiac disease, including TGA, a high index of suspicion is warranted.

Double-Outlet Right Ventricle

Double-outlet RV occurs when both great vessels are anatomically committed to the RV. Double-outlet RV occurs in 3 to 9 per 100,000 live births. This condition may occur in association with a subaortic VSD, a noncommitted (remote) VSD, or a subpulmonary VSD (Taussig-Bing anomaly). As with other complex cardiac conditions, the goal of treatment relates to the presenting hemodynamic conditions and patient symptoms. The ultimate goal is to achieve a biventricular circulation when possible. Patients may present with severe cyanosis and require corrective or palliative therapy in the newborn period. Conversely, they may present with unrestricted pulmonary blood flow and develop CHF. The challenging issue of constructing a biventricular repair relates to achieving unobstructed outlets from the right and left ventricles. In patients with double-outlet RV with subaortic VSD and RVOTO, reconstruction is similar to that for TOF. More remote VSDs may require enlargement with interventricular tunnel repair. For the Taussig-Bing anomaly, the relationship of the VSD to the pulmonary artery makes the ASO the procedure of choice. These patients often have RVOTO and aortic arch hypoplasia, which require attention at the time of complete correction. For rare individuals, the relationship of the great vessels and complexity of the VSD preclude a biventricular repair, and the patient must be treated as if they have a functional single ventricle.

Congenitally Corrected Transposition of the Great Arteries (L-Transposition)

Congenitally corrected TGA (ccTGA, or L-TGA), describes a constellation of conditions with the common feature of A-V and ventriculoarterial discordance and occurs in approximately 1 in 33,000 live births. ccTGA may occur in association with VSD, pulmonic and subpulmonic stenosis, and displaced left A-V valve (Ebsteinoid left A-V valve). In ccTGA, the morphologic mitral valve is right-sided and associated with the morphologic left ventricle; the morphologic tricuspid valve is associated with the morphologic RV. Patients with this condition are physiologically corrected in that in the absence of ventricular-level shunting, they are fully saturated—hence, the term *corrected transposition*. The age and mode of patient presentation in this condition depend on the contribution of associated defects and the function of the morphologic RV, which acts as the systemic ventricle. Controversy exists regarding the timing and mode of surgical treatment for patients presenting with various manifestations of ccTGA.

Congenitally corrected transposition of the great arteries with intact ventricular septum. Patients with ccTGA-IVS may be entirely asymptomatic throughout childhood and early adulthood. Frequently, the diagnosis is made incidentally. In other patients, the disease manifests with symptoms of CHF in association with right ventricular dysfunction or left A-V valve insufficiency. There is also a high incidence of complete heart block in patients with

ccTGA, and the first manifestation may be this dysrhythmia with associated symptoms.

Treatment for patients presenting with CHF is a challenging management scenario. For patients with ccTGA and preserved right ventricular function, left A-V valve repair or replacement may be considered. In many of these patients, the valvular insufficiency may be more a manifestation of declining systemic RV function, with septal shift and annular dilation, rather than intrinsic valve pathology. In this setting, valve replacement would not correct the progression of right ventricular dysfunction. For patients with systemic right ventricular dysfunction, one option for treatment is a complex reconstruction known as a *double switch* (Fig. 113.30). This procedure includes an atrial switch in combination with an arterial switch to align the morphologic left ventricle with the systemic circulation. In almost all patients with ccTGA-IVS and right ventricular dysfunction (and in the absence of structural LVOTO), a period of left ventricle retraining is required before the double-switch procedure. This requirement relates to the fact that the left ventricle will have been functioning in the low-pressure pulmonary circulation and will be incapable of performing systemic work. Retraining or conditioning the left

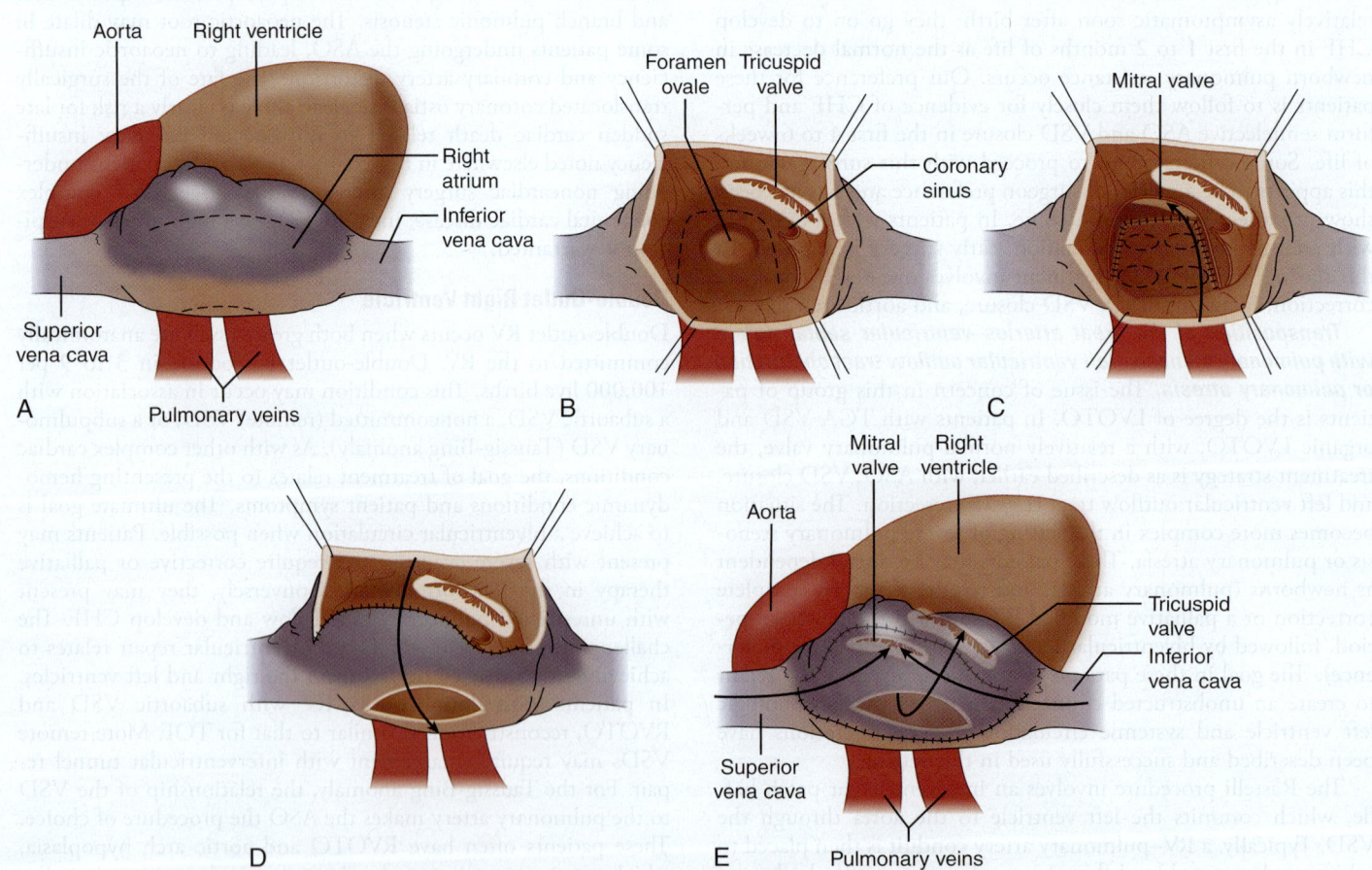

FIGURE 113.30 Schematic representation of the Senning procedure for transposition of the great arteries. (A) Two separate incisions, one in the right atrium and the other in the left atrium, near the insertion of the pulmonary veins. (B) Location of the incision in the atrial septum. (C) The atrial septum sewn down to the pulmonary veins, preparing for oxygenated blood to be directed to the tricuspid valve. The inferior free wall of the right atrium is sewn along the cut edge of the atrial septum, redirecting the deoxygenated blood to the mitral valve. (D) The superior free wall of the right atrium is now sewn to the cut edge of the left atrium, redirecting the oxygenated blood from the pulmonary veins to the tricuspid valve. (E) Schematic representation of the oxygenated blood and deoxygenated blood pathways. (Reprinted with permission from Texas Children's Hospital, 2016.)

ventricle requires the surgical creation of pulmonary stenosis by the placement of a pulmonary artery band. Most surgeons agree that the left ventricle must work at or very near systemic blood pressure for many months (we favor a minimum of 6 months) before the double-switch operation. The double switch is a technically challenging operation with significant perioperative risk. Because of the small numbers of patients treated worldwide with this complicated surgical strategy, there are only limited data on the acute and midterm results.[38] An issue of concern centers on the long-term ability of the retrained left ventricle to function as the systemic ventricle. Nonetheless, patients with ccTGA and depressed right ventricular function have a poor prognosis otherwise, and as such, the complexity and risk of the double-switch operation appear justified. The only other surgical option for these patients is cardiac transplantation.

Congenitally corrected transposition of the great arteries with ventricular septal defect and pulmonic stenosis. Patients in this category are often well balanced and have mild cyanosis, with minimal symptoms in childhood, whereas others with more severe pulmonary stenosis or pulmonary atresia present early in life with symptomatic cyanosis. Treatment for an overtly cyanotic infant with ccTGA with pulmonary stenosis is initially palliative in the form of a modified BT shunt. The ultimate goal for all patients is a biventricular circulation with normal arterial oxygen saturation. One option for these patients is to close the VSD surgically and place a conduit between the morphologic left ventricle and pulmonary arteries to relieve the pulmonary obstruction. This classic repair benefits the patient by separating the systemic and pulmonary circulations and allowing normal oxygen tension. The issue of concern in patients undergoing this repair is that the morphologic RV must act independently as the systemic ventricle after repair. As noted, the ability of the RV to support the systemic circulation may be questionable over the long term in some patients. As such, an alternative strategy in these patients is to baffle the left ventricular outflow to the aorta through the VSD, then to perform an atrial switch to reroute the systemic and pulmonary venous return, and finally to place a conduit from the morphologic RV to the pulmonary arteries. This option is a modification of the double-switch arrangement, affording the patient the benefit of a systemic left ventricle. Because the left ventricle has been working at systemic pressure before correction, a period of retraining is unnecessary.

Adult patients with ccTGA, with or without previous surgery, warrant careful attention before any noncardiac operation. These patients may have various complex ongoing cardiac issues, including rhythm disturbance, ventricular dysfunction, and valvular insufficiency.

Left Ventricular Outflow Tract Obstruction

LVOTO may manifest in isolation or in combination with other complex cardiac lesions. The physiologic consequences of severe LVOTO may be catastrophic, including diminished systemic cardiac output and tremendous left ventricular pressure overload. Newborns with severe LVOTO may present in shock with diminished peripheral perfusion, cardiomegaly, and pulmonary congestion. There is a significant risk of necrotizing enterocolitis in these infants. In older patients, gradual onset of LVOTO may be initially asymptomatic, only to manifest over time as decreasing exercise tolerance and declining left ventricular function. Patients with severe LVOTO and cardiomegaly are at high risk for myocardial ischemia and sudden cardiac death. The resting ECG often demonstrates left ventricular hypertrophy, with a strain pattern.

If an exercise stress test is performed, it may demonstrate worrisome ST segment depression and ventricular dysrhythmias. Echocardiography is the primary diagnostic tool for patients with LVOTO. In rare cases, diagnostic cardiac catheterization may be considered to delineate the level of obstruction.

Valvular Aortic Stenosis

Congenital valvular aortic stenosis (AS) is a common cause of LVOTO and represents approximately 5% of all CHD. The degree of obstruction may range from mild in patients with a congenitally bicuspid aortic valve to severe in patients with critical AS with unidentifiable valve commissures and annular hypoplasia. Infants presenting with critical AS are often symptomatic early in the newborn period, presenting with shock and profoundly depressed ventricular function. At the present time, almost all patients are taken to the cardiac catheterization laboratory for balloon aortic valvotomy. This procedure may be lifesaving in relieving AS and allowing for recovery of ventricular function. However, for most patients, the procedure is palliative, with a significant incidence of recurrence of AS or development of significant aortic insufficiency after the procedure. In patients with AS refractory to balloon dilation, an open aortic valvotomy may be necessary (Fig. 113.31). A surgical valvotomy, especially in small infants with adequate annular dimension, can be accomplished by an accurate incision down a rudimentary commissure or raphe to improve cusp mobility.

Recurrent AS after previous ballooning may be amenable to repeat dilation; however, when associated with significant aortic insufficiency, the patient requires surgery. Severe aortic insufficiency after previous balloon dilation is usually related to an avulsed cusp. In these cases, valve repair may be possible, but replacement may become necessary. Published series have confirmed the usefulness of aortic valve repair procedures, which is a particularly attractive option for growing children.[39]

The decision to replace the aortic valve in growing children is clouded by the lack of an ideal aortic valve substitute—a valve

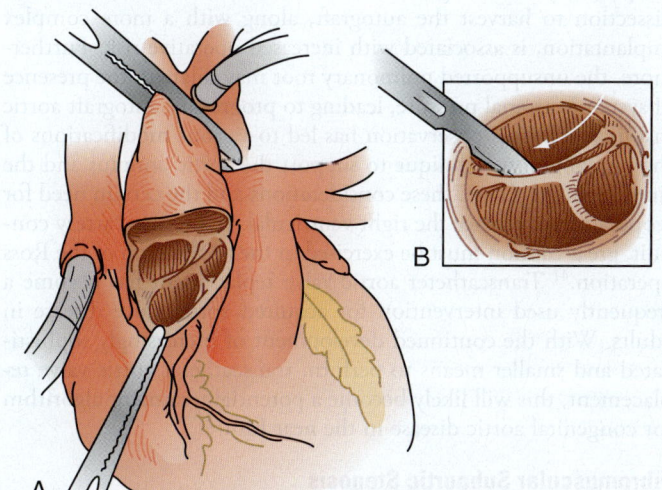

FIGURE 113.31 Close-up view of the aortic valve demonstrating a surgical valvectomy. (A) The valve is bicuspid, with a prominent raphe in the anterior valve leaflet. (B) The orifice is enlarged by incising the fused commissure between the two leaflets. (From Chang AC, Burke RP. Left ventricular outflow tract obstruction. In: Chang AC, Hanley FL, Wernovsky G, et al, eds. *Pediatric Cardiac Intensive Care.* Baltimore: Williams & Wilkins; 1998.)

capable of lifelong durability, appropriate somatic growth, easily implantable, and not requiring anticoagulation. Criteria for aortic valve replacement are beyond the scope of this chapter; however, severe valvular AS not amenable to catheter or open valvotomy is an appropriate indication. Options for aortic valve replacement in children include a mechanical prosthesis, heterograft, homograft, and pulmonary autograft. Additionally, the emerging option of partial heart transplant, as described earlier, is now a possible option. A mechanical prosthesis may be considered in childhood; however, the valve size must be sufficient to provide adequate function as the patient grows. Most surgeons and cardiologists recommend therapeutic anticoagulation in children with a mechanical valve prosthesis, but this can be challenging and potentially dangerous in growing children and adolescents. Many surgeons believe the risk for such medical treatment outweighs the potential benefit of a theoretically durable valve.

Heterograft aortic valve prostheses historically have been associated with limited durability in children and are not capable of somatic growth. A recent analysis in children has confirmed a significantly reduced long-term durability of heterografts compared with mechanical valves and the Ross operation.[40] Human cadaver aortic valves (aortic homograft) have been used extensively in children and young adults. These valves are usually implanted as a complete aortic root replacement, which requires coronary ostial implantation. Thus, surgery to place an aortic homograft is considerably more complex and with potentially higher risk. The positive features of an aortic homograft include improved durability compared with heterograft and avoidance of anticoagulation. Nonetheless, these valves eventually fail, necessitating a complicated reoperative aortic root replacement.

Pulmonary autograft aortic root replacement (Ross operation) involves translocation of the pulmonary valve to the aortic position with subsequent replacement of the pulmonary valve with a homograft or heterograft valved conduit (Fig. 113.32). The theoretical advantages of the Ross procedure include the potential for somatic growth, avoidance of anticoagulation, and possibility of extended durability. Enthusiasm for this procedure has been tempered by the recognition that the need for extensive cardiac dissection to harvest the autograft, along with a more complex implantation, is associated with increased operative risk. Furthermore, the unsupported pulmonary root may dilate in the presence of systemic arterial pressure, leading to progressive autograft aortic insufficiency. This observation has led to various modifications of the implantation technique to support the aortic annulus and the sinus segment. Given these considerations and the certain need for reoperation to replace the right ventricular–pulmonary artery conduit, great caution must be exercised in the application of the Ross operation.[41] Transcatheter aortic valve replacement has become a frequently used intervention for acquired aortic valve disease in adults. With the continued development of increasingly sophisticated and smaller means to perform transcatheter aortic valve replacement, this will likely become a potential treatment algorithm for congenital aortic disease in the near future.

Fibromuscular Subaortic Stenosis

Fibromuscular subaortic stenosis is a progressive narrowing of the LVOT related to a dense fibrous membrane usually found in association with asymmetric protrusion of the interventricular septum into the outflow tract. Fibromuscular subaortic stenosis accounts for approximately 6% of all CHD. The membrane is often concentric and becomes densely adherent to the septum and mitral valve. The membrane progresses toward and eventually onto

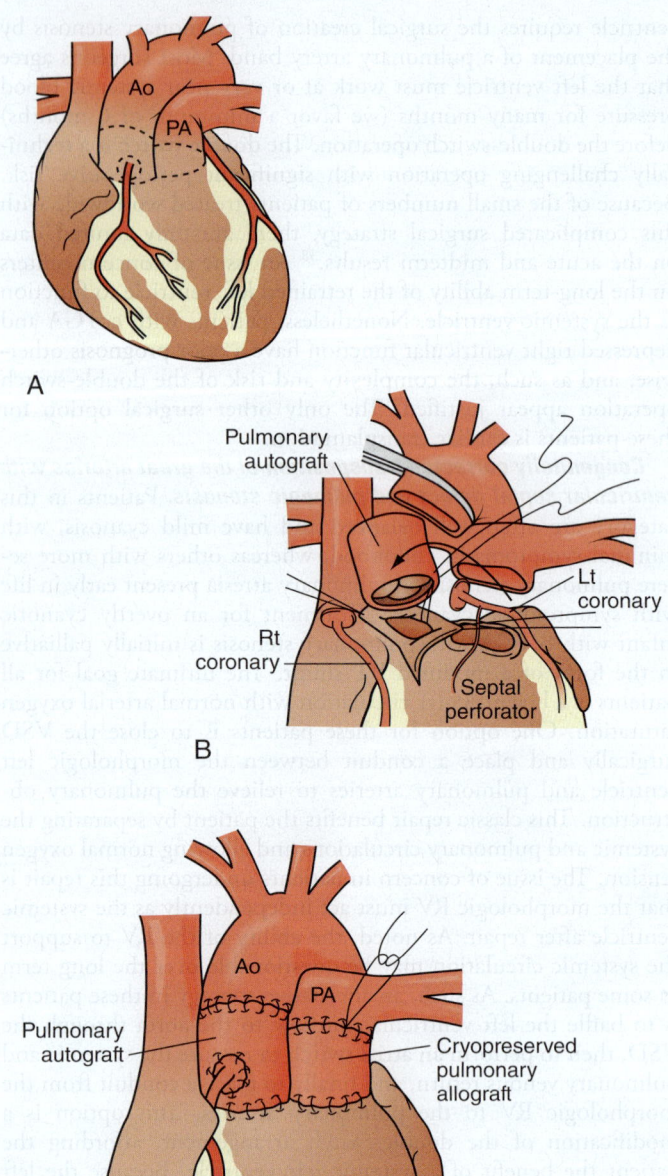

FIGURE 113.32 Ross procedure. (A) The great arteries are transected above the sinotubular ridge. The coronary arteries are excised using coronary artery buttons. (B) The pulmonary autograft is excised from the right *(Rt)* ventricular outflow tract, and the proximal end of the autograft is anastomosed to the annulus. (C) The coronary artery buttons are anastomosed to the pulmonary autograft. *Ao,* Aorta; *Lt,* left; *PA,* pulmonary artery. (Adapted from St Louis JD, Jaggers J. Left ventricular outflow tract obstruction. In: Nichols DG, Ungerleider RM, Spevak PJ, et al, eds. *Critical Heart Disease in Infants and Children.* Philadelphia: Mosby; 2006:615.)

the undersurface of the aortic valve cusps, which leads to progressive LVOTO, aortic valve cusp retraction, and aortic insufficiency.

Echocardiography is the primary diagnostic tool when assessing the degree of obstruction and progression of subaortic stenosis. However, it is not accurate for assessing subtle degrees of cusp extension.[42] Cardiac catheterization is rarely needed to diagnose this condition; balloon dilation is of no use in treating the LVOTO caused by this condition.

Surgery is the mainstay of treatment for subaortic stenosis, but there is disagreement about surgical indications. Most surgeons believe that new onset of any degree of aortic insufficiency in association with a subaortic membrane, regardless of the pressure gradient, is an indication for surgery. In other patients, an escalating LVOT gradient, associated left ventricular hypertrophy, and appropriate anatomic substrate are acceptable indications for operation.

The surgical procedure for subaortic stenosis involves a transaortic resection of the subaortic membrane, including all attachments to the mitral valve, septum, and aortic valve cusps. A septal myectomy is performed, along with membrane resection, in most patients (Fig. 113.33). Complications include membrane recurrence, injury to the bundle of His, and iatrogenic VSD creation. Nonetheless, with careful technique, the risk of these complications is minimized. Despite surgical intervention, a significant proportion of patients will have recurrence that requires reintervention, and upward of 40% will develop some degree of aortic insufficiency.[43]

Tunnel Subaortic Stenosis

Tunnel subaortic stenosis is a more severe form of LVOTO that is often associated with aortic annular hypoplasia and valvular AS. In severe cases, the LVOTO is not amenable to subaortic resection alone. In this situation, an aortic root–enlarging procedure may be necessary to relieve the obstruction (aortoventriculoplasty, or Konno procedure). This complex reconstruction is generally associated with the necessity of aortic valve replacement using one of the aforementioned options. Moreover, all degrees of LVOTO may be seen in association with numerous left heart obstructive lesions (Shone syndrome) that may require extensive reconstruction.

Aortic Arch Anomalies

Aortic Coarctation

Coarctation of the aorta is one of the most frequently encountered congenital cardiac lesions, occurring in 3 of every 10,000 live births. This condition has a wide range of presentations, from a severely symptomatic newborn with CHF and depressed ventricular function to an adult with proximal hypertension and minimal symptoms. Coarctation is classified relative to its association with the ligamentum arteriosus and aortic arch. An infantile or preductal aortic coarctation is seen in combination with a large PDA, which may have predominantly right-to-left flow to the lower descending aorta. In this setting, the patient is ductal dependent for systemic blood flow until the coarctation is repaired, and a PGE1 infusion must be maintained to prevent ductal closure. A periductal or juxtaductal coarctation occurs in the region of the ductal insertion and is distal to the aortic isthmus, which may be normal or hypoplastic (Fig. 113.34).

Aortic coarctation with or without aortic arch hypoplasia is frequently associated with intracardiac anomalies, including multiple left heart obstructive lesions (e.g., mitral stenosis, left ventricular hypoplasia or endocardial fibroelastosis, subaortic stenosis

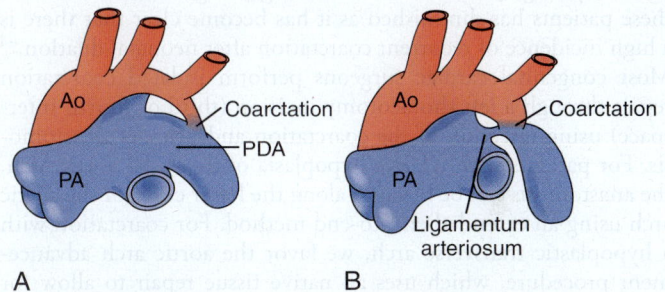

FIGURE 113.34 Coarctation of the aorta (Ao). (A) Infantile or preductal coarctation. (B) Adult coarctation. PA, Pulmonary artery; PDA, patent ductus arteriosus. (From Backer CL, Mavroudis C. Coarctation of the aorta. In: Mavroudis C, Backer CL, eds. Pediatric Heart Surgery. Philadelphia: Mosby; 2003:252.)

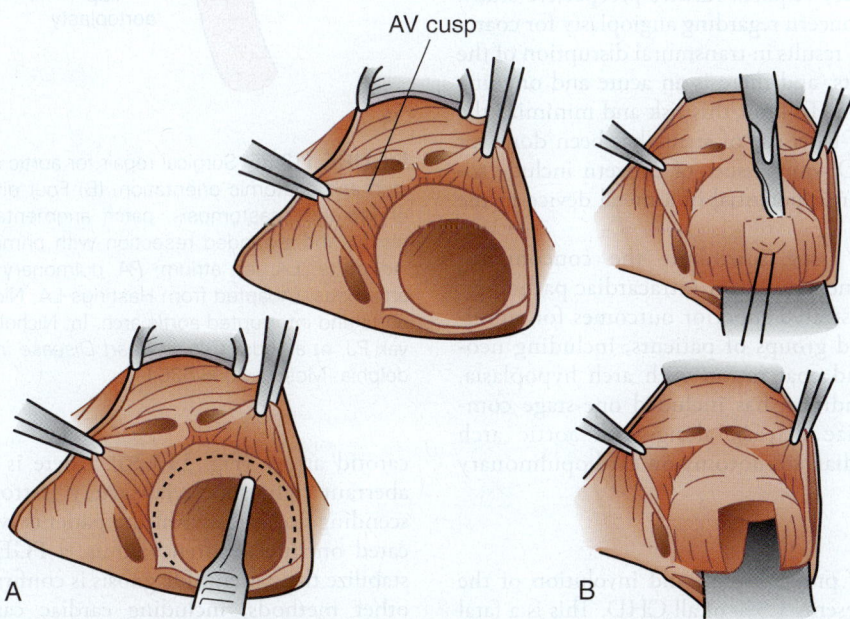

FIGURE 113.33 (A) Excision of discrete subaortic stenosis. The aorta is opened obliquely, and the aortic valve (AV) leaflets are retracted to expose the subaortic membrane. The membrane is excised circumferentially (dotted line). (B) This is usually combined with a muscle resection. (From de Leval M. Surgery of the left ventricular outflow tract. In: Stark J, de Leval M, eds. Surgery for Congenital Heart Defects. 2nd ed. Philadelphia: Saunders; 1994.)

or AS) known as *Shone syndrome.* Patients with large VSDs may present in infancy with severe aortic coarctation, with or without subaortic stenosis.

Aortic coarctation may be suspected on clinical examination by a significant upper extremity–lower extremity blood pressure gradient and diminished or absent femoral and pedal pulses. In older patients with well-developed intercostal collateral arteries, a continuous murmur may be auscultated over the posterior thorax. Echocardiography is now the primary diagnostic modality for aortic coarctation. MRI and CT angiography may also be useful in some patients. In rare cases, cardiac catheterization is required to define the anatomy, but this modality is now used more frequently for treatment, including balloon dilation with or without stenting.

Treatment strategies for aortic coarctation have evolved significantly since the first successful surgical treatment 80 years ago. Newborns presenting with severe aortic coarctation with or without associated ductal-dependent systemic blood flow are best treated by surgery. Initial enthusiasm regarding balloon dilation in these patients has diminished as it has become clear that there is a high incidence of recurrent coarctation after neonatal dilation.[44] Most congenital cardiac surgeons perform isolated coarctation repair through a left thoracotomy incision (third or fourth interspace) using resection of the coarctation and primary anastomosis. For patients with relative hypoplasia of the distal aortic arch, the anastomosis can be brought along the lesser curve of the aortic arch using an extended end-to-end method. For coarctation with a hypoplastic transverse arch, we favor the aortic arch advancement procedure, which uses all native tissue repair to allow for growth.[45] Other methods include subclavian artery flap aortoplasty (Waldhausen method) and prosthetic patch aortoplasty. These latter methods are used less frequently than primary repair (Fig. 113.35). Catheter therapy as a primary treatment for aortic coarctation is a controversial therapy in the opinion of most surgeons. Although this methodology has been widely applied, its true comparability to surgery requires further prospective study. There are several issues of concern regarding angioplasty for coarctation. The balloon dilation results in transmural disruption of the aortic wall in many patients, and there is an acute and ongoing risk for aneurysm formation. To limit this risk and minimize the potential of recurrence, off-label use of stents has been done for treatment of coarctation. Obvious issues of concern include somatic growth and lifetime risk potential of a metal device in the descending aorta.

Another controversial issue surrounds the concomitant treatment of coarctation and significant intracardiac pathology. Several series have demonstrated superior outcomes for simultaneous therapy in selected groups of patients, including neonates with large VSDs and coarctation with arch hypoplasia. Our approach to this condition has included one-stage complete repair of intracardiac defects, along with aortic arch advancement through median sternotomy on cardiopulmonary bypass.

Interrupted Aortic Arch

IAA results from a lack of proper fusion and involution of the fetal aortic arches and represents 1.3% of all CHD. This is a fatal condition without treatment, and IAA is frequently associated with serious intracardiac pathology. IAA is classified based on the level of the interruption. Type A is distal to the left subclavian artery, type B occurs between left subclavian and left common carotid arteries, and type C occurs proximal to the left common

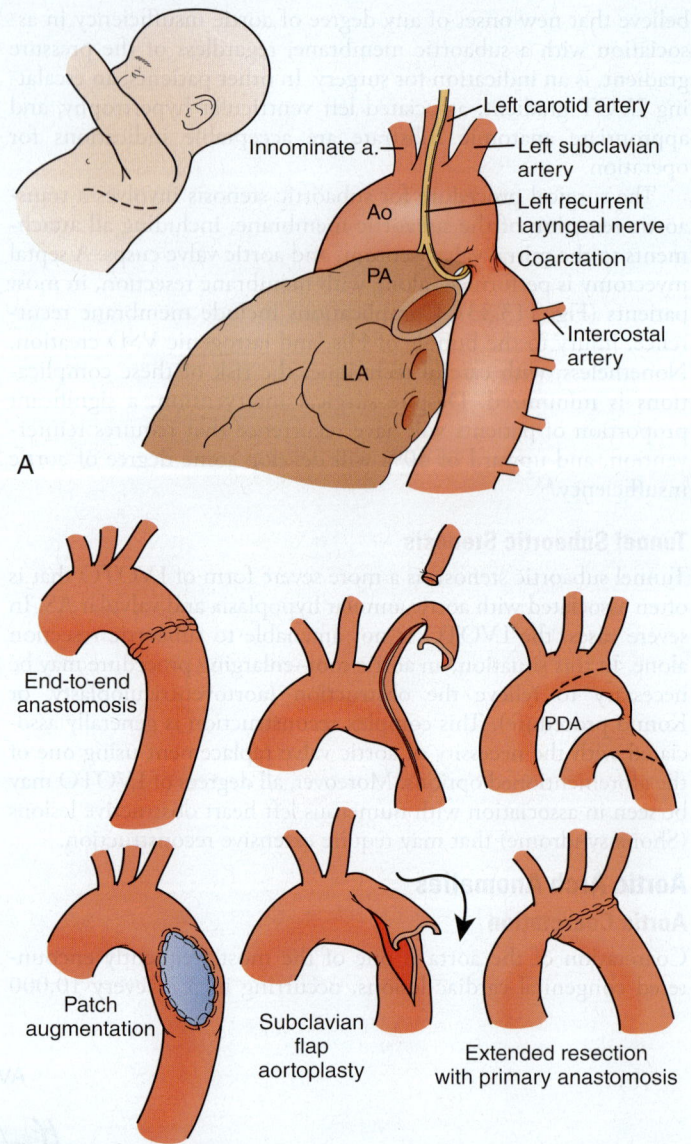

FIGURE 113.35 Surgical repair for aortic coarctation. (A) Surgical incision and anatomic orientation. (B) Four different methods are shown: end-to-end anastomosis, patch augmentation, subclavian flap aortoplasty, and extended resection with primary anastomosis. *a.,* Artery; *Ao,* aorta; *LA,* left atrium; *PA,* pulmonary artery; *PDA,* patent ductus arteriosus. (Adapted from Hastings LA, Nichols DG. Coarctation of the aorta and interrupted aortic arch. In: Nichols DG, Ungerleider RM, Spevak PJ, et al, eds. *Critical Heart Disease in Infants and Children.* Philadelphia: Mosby; 2006:635.)

carotid artery (Fig. 113.36). There is a frequent finding of an aberrant right subclavian artery (retroesophageal) from the descending aorta. Survival for patients with IAA is initially predicated on ductal patency; thus, a PGE1 infusion is required to stabilize the patient. Diagnosis is confirmed by echocardiography; other methods, including cardiac catheterization, are needed infrequently.

IAA requires surgical treatment in the newborn period, which typically involves simultaneous repair of intracardiac lesions (Fig. 113.37). Repair may be accomplished with the aid of an aortic arch augmentation patch, although a reported series

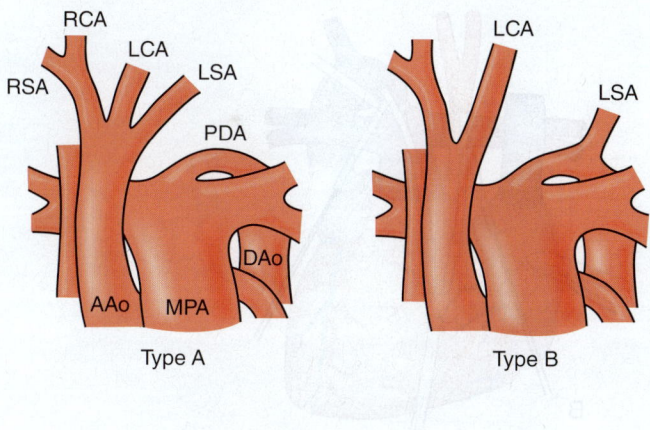

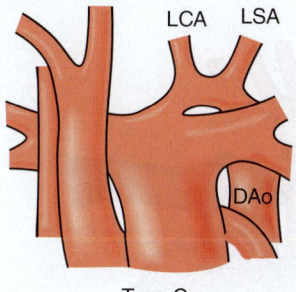

FIGURE 113.36 Classification of interrupted aortic arch. *AAo,* Ascending aorta; *DAo,* descending aorta; *LCA,* left common carotid artery; *LSA,* left subclavian artery; *MPA,* main pulmonary artery; *PDA,* patent ductus arteriosus; *RCA,* right common carotid artery; *RSA,* right subclavian artery. (Adapted from Monro JL. Interruption of aortic arch. In: Stark J, de Leval M, eds. *Surgery for Congenital Heart Defects.* 2nd ed. Philadelphia: Saunders; 1994:299.)

confirmed that a primary tissue-tissue repair can be performed in most patients and minimizes the potential for recurrent aortic arch obstruction.[46]

SINGLE VENTRICLE

Single-ventricle physiology is a frequently encountered form of CHD. Patients may present as newborns with inadequate pulmonary blood flow, excessive pulmonary blood flow, or balanced circulations. The single ventricle may be of right, left, or indeterminate morphology. Surgical treatment is required to provide adequate systemic oxygen delivery while protecting the pulmonary vasculature. The function of the single ventricle must be preserved to afford the patient the best possible long-term outcome.

The rapid evolution of successful palliation for patients with various forms of single-ventricle physiology since the late 1970s has led to a large and growing population of adults with a single ventricle. For most of these patients, lifelong cardiac attention is needed, and the potential for subsequent cardiac reoperation is high. Patients in this category who present for noncardiac surgery may be especially difficult to manage because of their challenging physiology.

An exhaustive discussion of the various forms of single ventricles is well beyond the scope of this chapter. This discussion is limited to common forms of single right and left ventricles to provide examples of the surgical management strategies for a single ventricle.

Tricuspid Atresia

Tricuspid atresia is the template of a single-ventricle lesion for which most current palliative strategies were developed. Tricuspid atresia occurs in 1 of every 10,000 live births. Patients with tricuspid atresia have a single morphologic left ventricle and may have normally related or transposed great vessels (Fig. 113.38). They may present with excessive pulmonary blood flow and require pulmonary artery banding early in infancy to relieve pulmonary overcirculation and CHF. Conversely, patients may have pulmonary stenosis or pulmonary atresia and require creation of a modified BTT shunt to provide adequate pulmonary blood flow and systemic oxygenation.

As noted, the initial palliative goals in patients with tricuspid atresia include adequate systemic oxygenation, protection of ventricular function, and adequate pulmonary arterial growth. Patients with ductal-dependent pulmonary blood flow require an mBTT shunt in the newborn period. We prefer to construct the shunt to the morphologic right pulmonary artery through a right thoracotomy. This construction allows shunt flow to be governed by the size of the right subclavian artery. Furthermore, the right pulmonary artery is typically longer and runs in a more horizontal plane compared with the left pulmonary artery; this facilitates avoiding distortion of a lobar branch. The goal of the shunt is to protect the pulmonary arteries, promote adequate pulmonary artery development, and support systemic arterial oxygenation for the first 4 to 6 months of life until the next planned stage of palliation (see later discussion of Glenn and Fontan operations). The shunt is not designed for long-term use; thus, in most patients, a small interposition graft (expanded polytetrafluoroethylene, 3.0–4.0 mm) is selected. In the early era of single-ventricle palliation, less well-controlled shunts were constructed, including classic Blalock (divided native subclavian artery to branch pulmonary artery), Pott's (side-to-side left pulmonary artery to descending aorta), and Waterston (side-to-side right pulmonary artery to ascending aorta) shunts (Fig. 113.39). These native tissue-tissue connections are capable of somatic growth but have the confounding risks for pulmonary overcirculation, pulmonary artery hypertension (potentially irreversible), and branch pulmonary artery distortion with hypoplasia. During the early stages of development of single-ventricle palliation, many patients were treated with these poorly controlled shunts. Thus, significant numbers of adult patients present with complications of these palliations, including chronic cardiac volume overload and decreased ventricular function, severe pulmonary artery distortion or isolation, pulmonary vascular disease, and profound cyanosis. These patients may present for surgery for noncardiac illness and are extremely difficult to manage.

Hypoplastic Left Heart Syndrome

Hypoplastic left heart syndrome (HLHS) is the prototypical single RV. HLHS occurs in 8 to 25 per 100,000 live births. Patients with this condition present with inadequate left heart structures ranging from mitral stenosis and AS with left ventricular hypoplasia to almost complete absence of the left heart structures with aortic and mitral atresia. In the case of aortic and mitral atresia, the ascending aorta is typically small (1–2 mm) and is perfused through retrograde aortic arch flow provided by the PDA. In HLHS, ductal closure results in rapid cardiovascular collapse, with profound systemic hypoperfusion and hypoxia, followed quickly by death. Therefore, in cases of prenatal diagnosis, patients must be born in a facility qualified to institute appropriate medical management immediately, including the establishment of

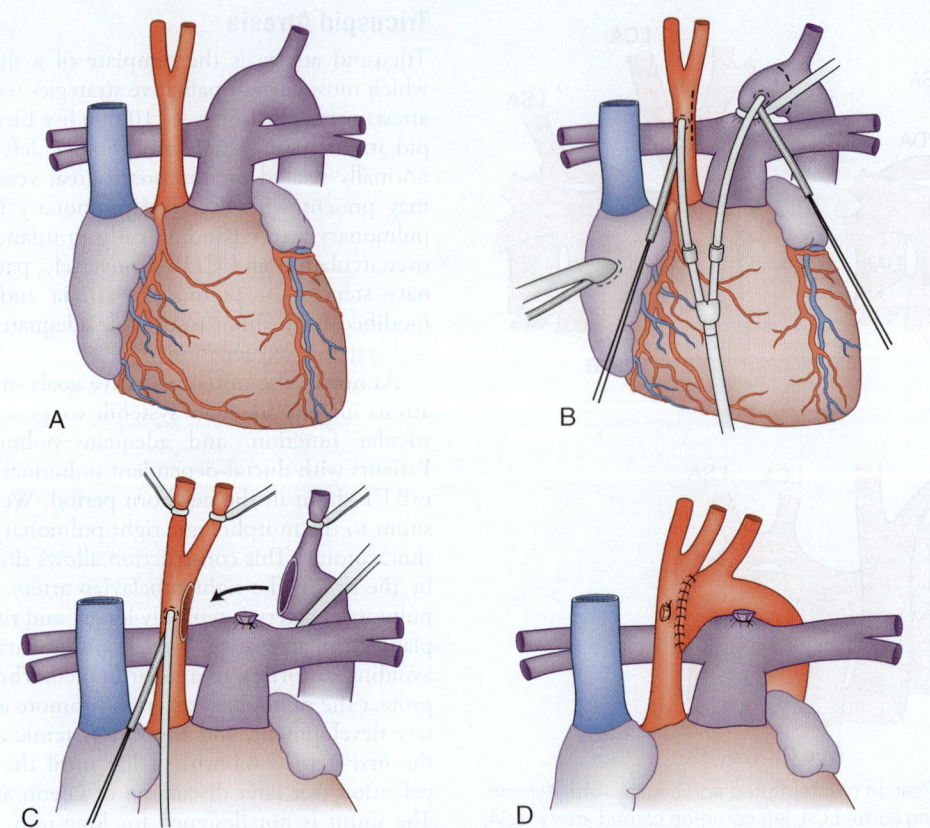

FIGURE 113.37 (A) Type B interrupted aortic arch. (B) Cannulation and site of incision for repair. The descending thoracic aorta is brought upward into the mediastinum (C) and then anastomosed to the ascending aorta in an end-to-side fashion (D). (From Hirooka K, Fraser CD. One-stage neonatal repair of complex aortic arch obstruction or interruption. *Tex Heart Inst J.* 1997;24:317-321.)

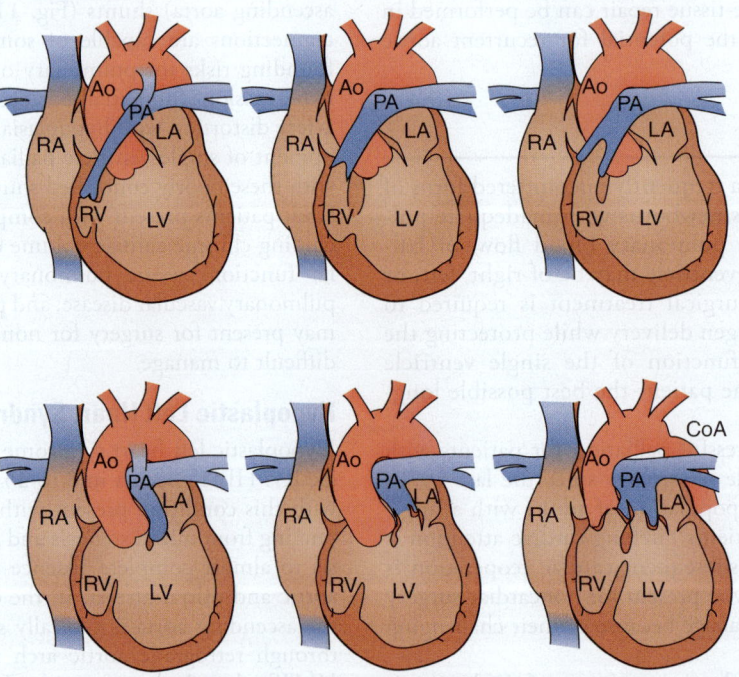

FIGURE 113.38 Anatomy of the various types of tricuspid atresia. *Top,* Normally related great vessels. *Bottom,* d-Transposition of the great vessels. *Ao,* Aorta; *CoA,* coarctation of the aorta; *LA,* left atrium; *LV,* left ventricle; *PA,* pulmonary artery; *RA,* right atrium; *RV,* right ventricle. (Adapted from Lok JM, Spevak PJ, Nichols DG. Tricuspid atresia. In: Nichols DG, Ungerleider RM, Spevak PJ, et al, eds. *Critical Heart Disease in Infants and Children.* Philadelphia: Mosby; 2006:800-801.)

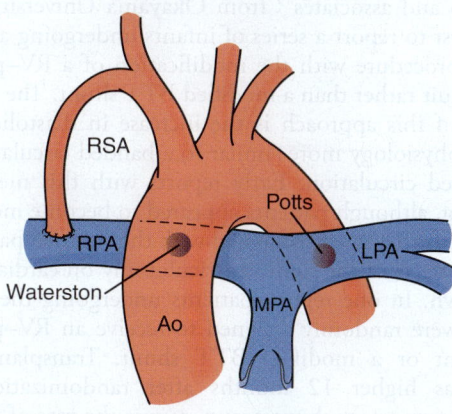

CLASSIC RIGHT BLALOCK-TAUSSIG

RIGHT MODIFIED BLALOCK-TAUSSIG

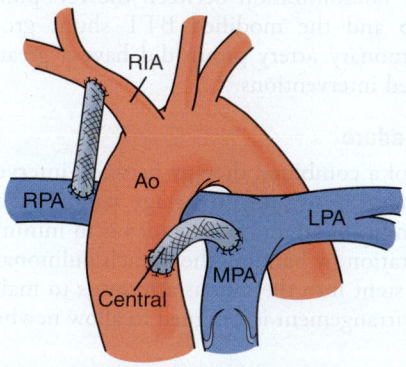

FIGURE 113.39 Systemic-to-pulmonary artery shunts. *Ao,* Aorta; *LPA,* left pulmonary artery; *MPA,* main pulmonary artery; *RIA,* right innominate artery; *RPA,* right pulmonary artery; *RSA,* right subclavian artery. (Adapted from Marino BS, Wernovsky G, Greeley WJ. Single-ventricle lesions. In: Nichols DG, Ungerleider RM, Spevak PJ, et al, eds. *Critical Heart Disease in Infants and Children*. Philadelphia: Mosby; 2006:793.)

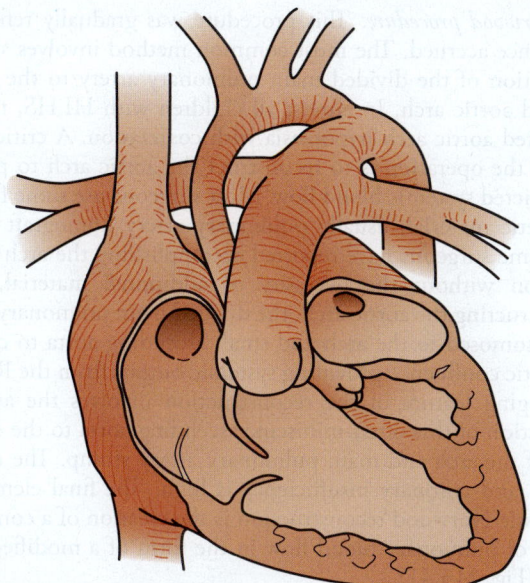

FIGURE 113.40 Anatomy of hypoplastic left heart syndrome. The tiny ascending aorta is seen arising from a markedly hypoplastic left ventricle. The ductus arteriosus is large, providing forward flow to the systemic circuit. The right ventricle is hypertrophied, and the pulmonary artery is enlarged. (From Wernovsky G, Bove EL. Single ventricle lesions. In: Chang AC, Hanley FL, Wernovsky G, et al, eds. *Pediatric Cardiac Intensive Care*. Baltimore: Williams & Wilkins; 1998.)

suitable vascular access (umbilical artery catheter) and institution of intravenous PGE1 to maintain ductal patency. Patients with HLHS undiagnosed at birth typically have an early grace period of a few hours, but with the initiation of ductal closure, these children become critically ill and require aggressive resuscitation for survival. Although most children with HLHS are otherwise normal, without treatment, HLHS is a uniformly fatal condition (Fig. 113.40).

After delivery, medical treatment is directed at maintaining ductal patency and balancing systemic and pulmonary blood flow. Balancing the circulations becomes increasingly challenging with the normal decline in neonatal PVR, resulting in massive pulmonary overcirculation. As the overcirculation progresses, infants become tachypneic and may exhibit decreased systemic perfusion. Necrotizing enterocolitis is a significant risk in these children, and if there is any question of visceral malperfusion, many centers avoid enteral nutrition in an effort to minimize this potential. Other medical maneuvers include deliberate hypoventilation, low inspired oxygen concentration, and additional carbon dioxide in an attempt to increase PVR and limit pulmonary flow. These options are of limited use in newborns with HLHS; over days to weeks, the infants become progressively ill with pulmonary congestion and marginal systemic cardiac output. Patients who are

maintained have the potential of developing increased PVR as they age, and there is a known association between advanced age (>30 days) and increased operative mortality.

Surgery in the newborn period is the only realistic option for long-term survival in infants born with HLHS. Outcomes for surgical palliation of HLHS have come to be synonymous with the reputation of the treating center and surgeons. As with tricuspid atresia, patients with HLHS require a staged palliative approach. In the experiences of all centers, the first stage is the most challenging and risk laden. The various first-stage options are described in the following sections.

Neonatal Cardiac Transplantation

Transplantation is a theoretically attractive option in infants with HLHS that replaces the malformed heart with a structurally normal one. Leonard Bailey was an influential champion of this approach and was the first to report exciting results with transplantation in newborns with HLHS.[47] Furthermore, although there is an ever-present risk for rejection and infection in children with heart transplants, long-term meaningful survival is possible, and the quality of life of the recipients is good. The option of cardiac transplantation is limited by the small number of suitable donor hearts, and most children with HLHS are unable to survive the wait time for a donor graft. This situation has led most centers to abandon cardiac transplantation as the primary mode of therapy for most neonates with HLHS.

Norwood Reconstruction

After initial work and success at Boston Children's Hospital, Norwood and colleagues[48] gained international attention at the Children's Hospital of Philadelphia for developing and implementing a reconstructive technique to palliate newborns with HLHS; this methodology now carries the widely used eponym of the *Norwood procedure.* This procedure was gradually refined as experience accrued. The most common method involves surgical connection of the divided main pulmonary artery to the reconstructed aortic arch. In almost all children with HLHS, there is associated aortic arch hypoplasia with coarctation. A critical feature of the operation is to reconstruct the aortic arch to provide unrestricted systemic blood flow. Most surgeons use some form of prosthetic material, usually pulmonary artery homograft patching. Some surgeons have reported accomplishing the arch reconstruction without the necessity of additional material. After reconstructing the aortic arch, the divided main pulmonary artery is anastomosed to the arch and small ascending aorta to create a neoaortic confluence providing systemic output from the RV. The challenging feature of the reconstruction involves the accurate connection of this often-miniscule ascending aorta to the confluence of the arch and main pulmonary artery stump. The risk for torsion and coronary insufficiency is high. The final element of the classic Norwood reconstruction is the creation of a controlled source of pulmonary blood flow in the form of a modified BTT shunt (Fig. 113.41).

Sano Modification of the Norwood Operation

Achieving survival after the Norwood operation is challenging, involving innumerable technical and medical details. At best, after a Norwood procedure, the patient is fragile, with a delicate balance between systemic and pulmonary blood flow. This fact and the observation of widely disparate outcomes for the procedure have led to many important advances in the treatment of these children. One issue relates to the difficulty of balancing the systemic-to-pulmonary artery shunt, which lowers diastolic blood

pressure (and coronary perfusion pressure) and volume loads the heart. Sano and associates[49] from Okayama University in Japan were the first to report a series of infants undergoing a successful Norwood procedure with the modification of a RV–pulmonary artery conduit rather than a modified BTT shunt. The theoretical advantage of this approach is the increase in diastolic pressure, creating a physiology more similar to a banded circulation rather than shunted circulation. Early reports with this method were encouraging, although patients appeared to become more rapidly desaturated as they aged compared with the shunted patients. The long-term effects of the right ventriculotomy on cardiac function are unknown. In one report, patients undergoing the Norwood operation were randomly assigned to receive an RV–pulmonary artery shunt or a modified BTT shunt. Transplantation-free survival was higher 12 months after randomization in the RV–pulmonary artery shunt group, as was the rate of unplanned reinterventions and complications.[50] More recent updates on the same cohort revealed no difference in transplant-free survival at 6 years after randomization between the RV–pulmonary artery shunt group and the modified BTT shunt group. However, the RV–pulmonary artery group did have a greater number of catheter-based interventions.[51]

Hybrid Procedure

The notion of a combined therapy between interventional cardiology and surgery for the first-stage palliation of HLHS has achieved significant attention. The idea is to minimize the risk of the first operation by banding the branch pulmonary arteries and delivering a stent into the ductus arteriosus to maintain patency. This hybrid arrangement is designed to allow newborn survival so

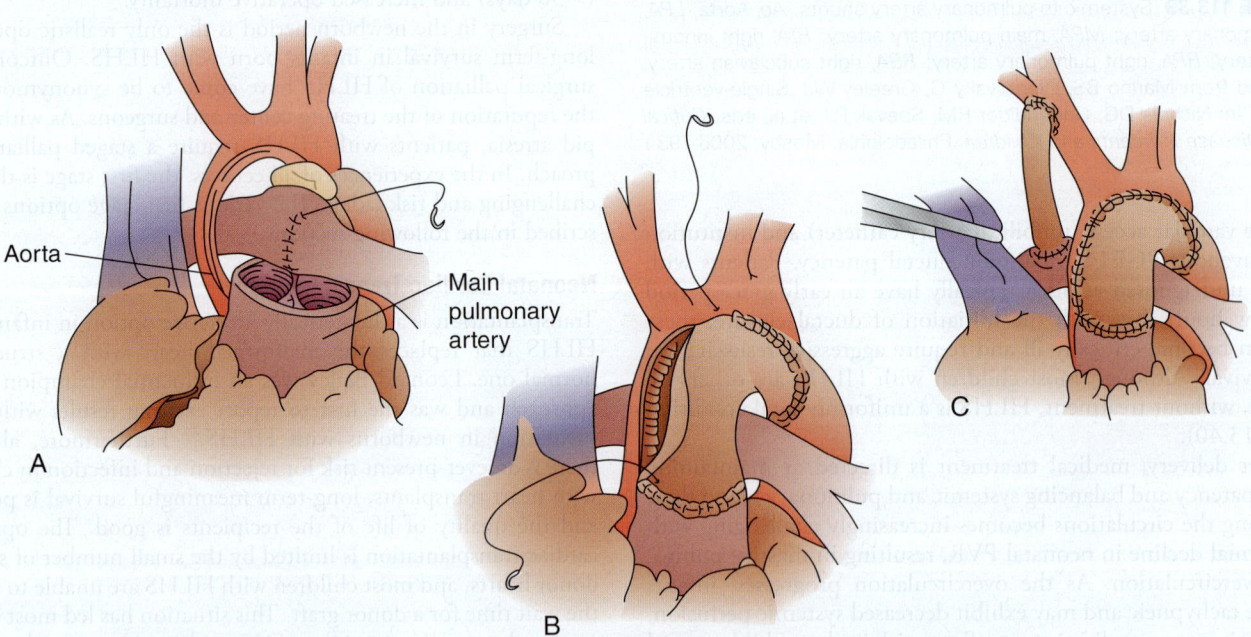

FIGURE 113.41 Norwood procedure for first-stage palliation of hypoplastic left heart syndrome. (A) The main pulmonary artery is divided proximal to the bifurcation, the ductus arteriosus is ligated and divided, and the aortic arch is opened from the level of the transected main pulmonary artery to a point distal to the ductal insertion in the descending aorta. (B) A segment of homograft is cut to an appropriate size and shape. This is sutured into place, creating an unobstructed outflow from the right ventricle to the pulmonary artery and aorta. (C) Polytetrafluoroethylene tube graft is placed from the innominate artery to the right pulmonary artery. The atrial septectomy is done while the patient is under circulatory arrest. (From Castaneda AR, Jonas RA, Mayer JE, et al. Hypoplastic left heart syndrome. In: *Cardiac Surgery of the Neonate and Infant.* Philadelphia: Saunders; 1994.)

that a more complete reconstruction may be performed later in infancy in a larger child. There appears to be a significant learning curve with this approach, as with any new procedure, and the incidence of complications warrants further study. Data have shown that the prevalence of necrotizing enterocolitis after the hybrid procedure is significant and comparable to reports after the Norwood procedure.[52] A recent meta-analysis revealed increased early mortality and worse 1-year transplant-free survival in patients undergoing the hybrid procedure compared with the Norwood. However, it is noted that the hybrid procedure was preferentially used in higher-risk patients, thus making it difficult to draw firm conclusions.[53] In addition, concerning features include the effect of the banding on long-term pulmonary artery growth, the fact that cardiac perfusion is still retrograde through the aortic arch, and the risk profile of the more extensive reconstruction later in life. The true place for this mode of therapy is unclear at the present time, but it represents an important direction of advancement to optimize the opportunity for survival of these children.

Fontan Operation

The long-term goal of single-ventricle palliation is to optimize ventricular function and promote systemic oxygen delivery. As noted earlier, patients with a single ventricle who are shunted or banded have ongoing concerns, including systemic desaturation, continued intracardiac mixing, and chronic cardiac volume overload. The current strategy for addressing these concerns uses a direct connection between the branch pulmonary arteries and systemic venous return, as initially proposed by Fontan in the early 1970s. The Fontan operation is now the treatment of choice for children born with all varieties of single ventricle and provides acceptable long-term palliation in suitable patients. However, the Fontan circulation is not normal and, even in the best of circumstances, results in significant alteration in normal cardiorespiratory physiology.

The Fontan circulation is established by connecting the systemic venous return directly into isolated branch pulmonary arteries without an intervening power source. Thus, blood flow in the Fontan circuit is passive, being promoted only by the pressure differential between the systemic venous system and pulmonary venous atrium. An impediment to flow in the systemic-to-pulmonary pathway results in a poor Fontan outcome. Established criteria for creating an effective Fontan circulation include the ability to connect the systemic venous return surgically to the pulmonary arteries in an unobstructed manner, normal pulmonary artery architecture and resistance, normal pulmonary venous drainage and low left atrial pressure, absence of significant A-V valve regurgitation, good ventricular function (and low ventricular end-diastolic pressure), an unobstructed systemic arterial outlet, and good systemic semilunar valve function. Compromise of any of these elements may compromise the quality of the Fontan circulation.

The Fontan operation has undergone several technical modifications in the 50 years of successful application to patients with single-ventricle physiology. Many patients underwent an atriopulmonary connection in which the open right atrial appendage was directly anastomosed to the pulmonary artery bifurcation with surgical closure of the ASD. Many of these patients present as adults with extreme dilation of the right atrium, with resulting sluggish flow to the pulmonary arteries, hepatic congestion, and atrial dysrhythmias (Fig. 113.42). Today, the most widely practiced modification of the Fontan

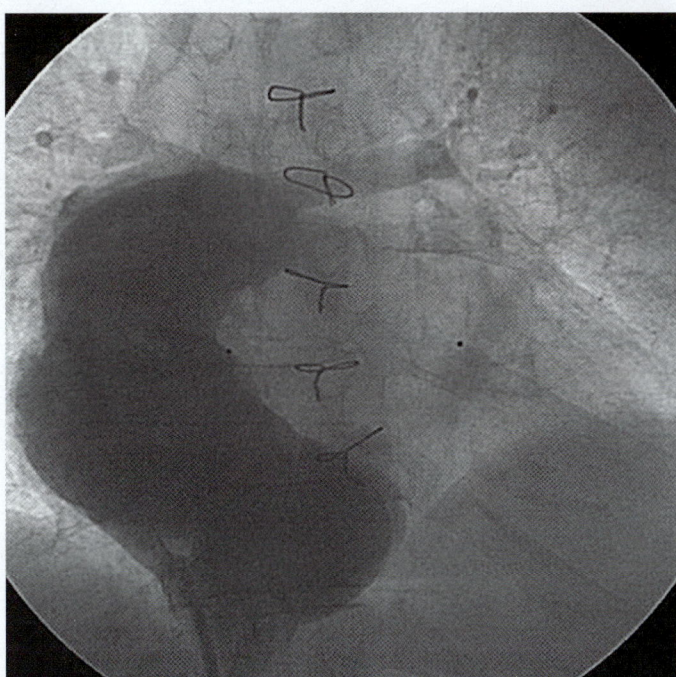

FIGURE 113.42 Angiogram of a dilated right atrium in a patient with an atriopulmonary Fontan connection.

operation is the total cavopulmonary connection. First described by DeLeval, this operation involves connection of the divided SVC to the superior and inferior aspects of the right pulmonary artery (typically offset), along with the creation of a channel to direct the IVC flow into the pulmonary arteries. The channel may be created using a surgically created lateral tunnel in the right atrium (Fig. 113.43) or interposing a conduit between the IVC and pulmonary arteries (extracardiac Fontan) (Fig. 113.44).

The change from a volume-loaded circulation in patients with a single ventricle who are shunted or banded to a Fontan circulation results in acute volume unloading of the systemic ventricle. In the chronically overloaded heart, this acute change may be poorly tolerated, with resultant diastolic dysfunction and decreased ventricular compliance. To deal with this problem, patients with a single ventricle typically undergo an intervening stage of palliation in the form of a bidirectional, superior cavopulmonary anastomosis (Glenn shunt). The bidirectional Glenn shunt is constructed by anastomosing the cephalad end of the divided SVC to the superior aspect of the right pulmonary artery (Fig. 113.45). Other sources of pulmonary blood flow are typically eliminated, and the heart is volume-unloaded; however, systemic cardiac output is maintained because the IVC return is preserved. After the Glenn shunt, the patients are not fully saturated; typically, patients have saturations of approximately 80%. Over time, the unloaded ventricle remodels, and the patient is promoted to reoperation and completion of the Fontan circulation.

Perioperative care of a patient after a Fontan procedure can be challenging. The acute changes in cardiac volume loading may negatively affect cardiac output. Even in patients with supposedly ideal Fontan connections, the central venous pressure acutely increases to 12 to 15 mm Hg. Consequences of this increased venous pressure include pleural effusions, hepatic congestion, and ascites. In marginal Fontan candidates, some surgeons routinely place an intentional leak, or fenestration; the goal here is to preserve

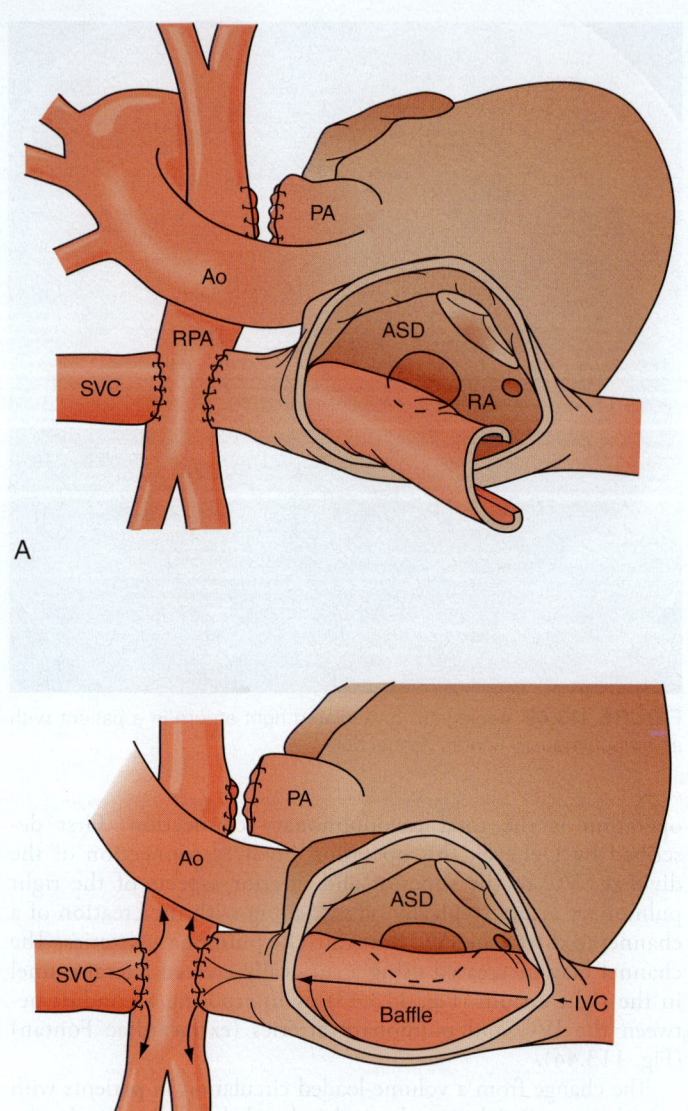

A

B

FIGURE 113.43 (A–B) Lateral tunnel Fontan procedure. *Ao,* Aorta; *ASD,* atrial septal defect; *IVC,* inferior vena cava; *PA,* pulmonary artery; *RA,* right atrium; *RPA,* right pulmonary artery; *SVC,* superior vena cava. (Adapted from Lok JM, Spevak PJ, Nichols DG. Tricuspid atresia. In: Nichols DG, Ungerleider RM, Spevak PJ, et al, eds. *Critical Heart Disease in Infants and Children.* Philadelphia: Mosby; 2006:813.)

systemic ventricular volume loading and decrease systemic venous congestion at the expense of some degree of desaturation caused by the right-to-left shunting. The practice of routine fenestration after the Fontan operation has been examined, and some early data have shown that excellent outcomes can be achieved with highly selective application of a fenestration, which mitigates the risks associated with such a procedure, including hypoxia and systemic embolism.[54] Any impediment to passive pulmonary blood flow will inhibit Fontan flow and result in heart failure. Positive pressure ventilation, especially elevated levels of positive end-expiratory pressure, impedes pulmonary blood flow in the Fontan patient. Conversely, early extubation and effective spontaneous ventilation will improve pulmonary blood flow in the Fontan patient. Data have suggested that early extubation in the operating room for patients after the Fontan procedure improves hemodynamics, decreases the length of stay for patients, and decreases hospital costs.

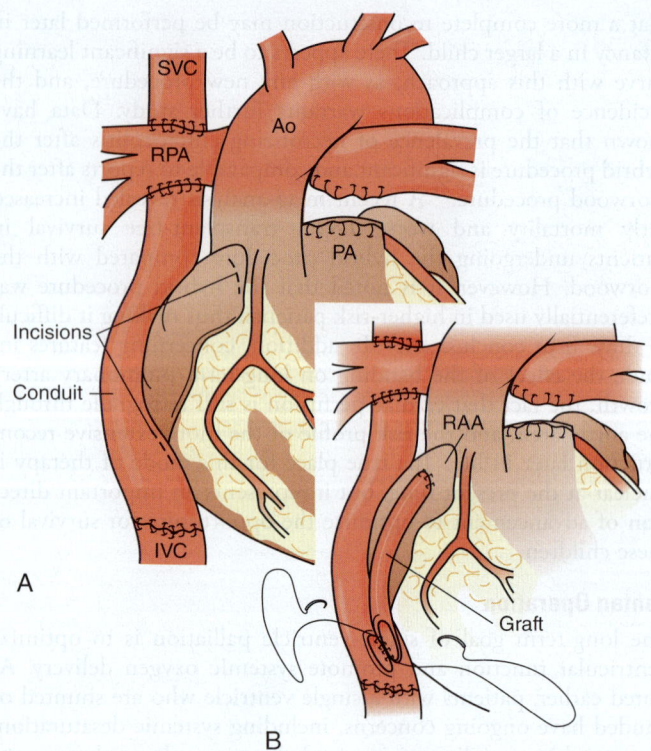

A

B

FIGURE 113.44 (A) Extracardiac Fontan procedure. (B) Creation of a fenestration in an extracardiac Fontan procedure using a graft between the extracardiac conduit and right atrial appendage *(RAA). Ao,* Aorta; *IVC,* inferior vena cava; *PA,* pulmonary artery; *RPA,* right pulmonary artery; *SVC,* superior vena cava. (Adapted from Lok JM, Spevak PJ, Nichols DG. Tricuspid atresia. In: Nichols DG, Ungerleider RM, Spevak PJ, et al, eds. *Critical Heart Disease in Infants and Children.* Philadelphia: Mosby; 2006:814.)

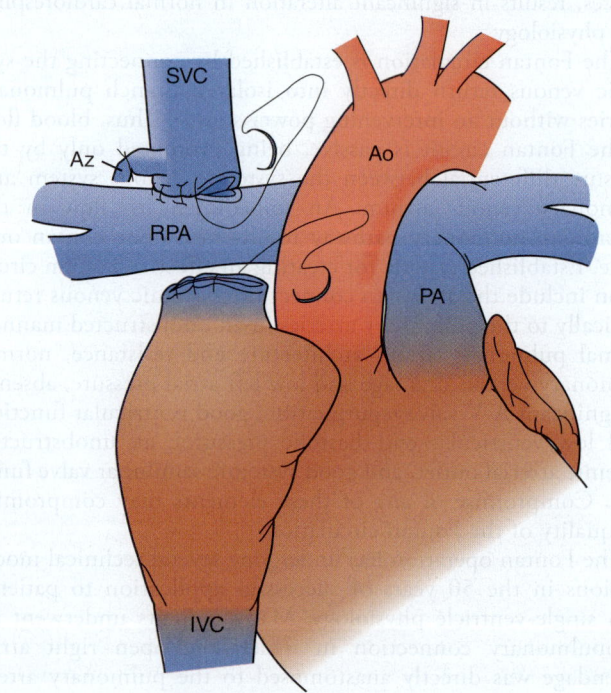

FIGURE 113.45 Bidirectional Glenn shunt. *Ao,* Aorta; *Az,* azygos vein; *IVC,* inferior vena cava; *PA,* pulmonary artery; *RPA,* right pulmonary artery; *SVC,* superior vena cava. (Adapted from Lok JM, Spevak PJ, Nichols DG. Tricuspid atresia. In: Nichols DG, Ungerleider RM, Spevak PJ, et al, eds. *Critical Heart Disease in Infants and Children.* Philadelphia: Mosby; 2006:809.)

The chronic complications of living with a Fontan circulation are still unfolding and include chronic hepatic congestion and cirrhosis, protein-losing enteropathy, atrial dysrhythmias, and venous stasis disease. Management of patients with failing Fontan circulations is especially challenging. These patients are at high risk for severe cardiac compromise while undergoing general anesthesia with positive pressure ventilation or any procedure involving large fluid shifts, including abdominal surgery. Patients with chronic hepatic congestion may develop a coagulopathy related to a decrease in factor production.

MISCELLANEOUS ANOMALIES

Vascular Rings and Pulmonary Artery Slings

Vascular Rings

Vascular rings are abnormalities of the aortic arch and its branches, compressing the trachea, esophagus, or both. The ring may be complete or partial. Categorization of the defects is useful for description:

Complete vascular rings
- Double arch: Equal arches or left or right arch dominant (Fig. 113.46)
- Right arch: Left ligamentum arteriosus from anomalous left subclavian artery
- Right arch: Mirror image branching, with left ligamentum from descending aorta

Partial vascular rings
- Left arch: Aberrant right subclavian artery
- Left arch: Innominate artery compression

The double aortic arch is the most common form of complete ring. Two arches arise from the ascending aorta, forming a true ring. The left arch is usually smaller. The right arch–left ligamentum complex is formed from persistence of the right fourth arch and regression of the left fourth arch. The anomalously arising left subclavian artery is often associated with a diverticulum at its base (Kommerell diverticulum). In partial rings, the most common form is an aberrant right subclavian artery arising distal to the left subclavian artery with a left arch. The right subclavian artery passes behind the esophagus from left to right. Innominate artery compression arises from a more posterior and leftward origin of the innominate artery from a left arch, leading to anterior compression of the trachea.

Pulmonary Artery Slings

A pulmonary artery sling occurs when the left pulmonary artery arises from the right pulmonary artery, passing leftward between the trachea and the esophagus. The ligamentum arteriosum attachment from the main pulmonary artery to the undersurface of the aorta forms a vascular ring around the trachea but not the esophagus. The trachea may be compressed, the cartilage may be soft, or there may be intrinsic stenosis of the trachea in the form of complete cartilage rings.

Diagnosis and Indications for Intervention

Symptoms reflect the degree of tracheal and esophageal compression from complete rings as well as the presence of coexistent tracheomalacia or stenosis. Upper respiratory symptoms predominate, with a characteristic brassy cough, recurrent respiratory infections, failure to thrive, and sometimes esophageal motility problems. In children, documentation of a ring is an indication for surgery. Older patients are often asymptomatic. Initially, the diagnosis is

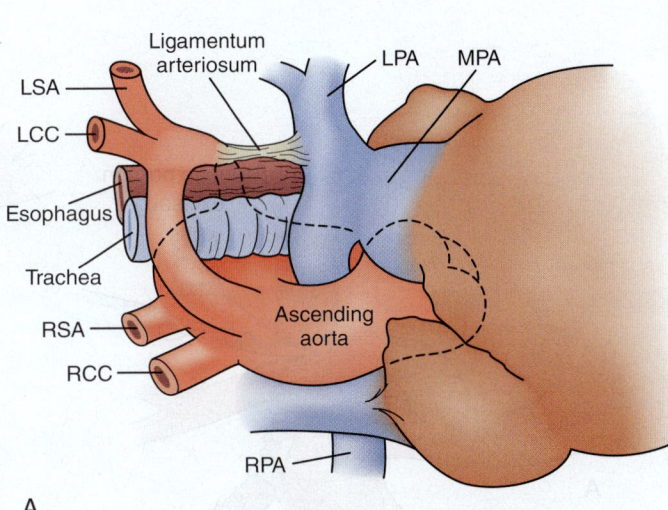

ANTERIOR

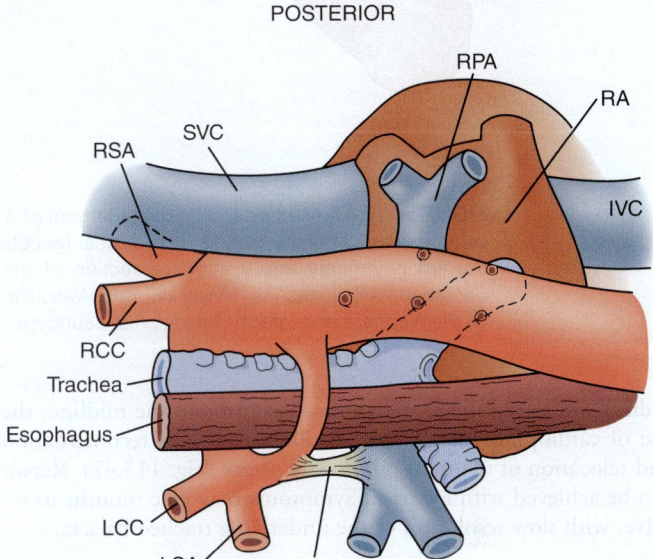

POSTERIOR

FIGURE 113.46 Double aortic arch, anterior (A) and posterior (B) views. *IVC,* Inferior vena cava; *LCC,* left common carotid artery; *Lig.,* ligamentum; *LPA,* left pulmonary artery; *LSA,* left subclavian artery; *MPA,* main pulmonary artery; *RA,* right atrium; *RCC,* right common carotid artery; *RPA,* right pulmonary artery; *RSA,* right subclavian artery; *SVC,* superior vena cava. (Adapted from Jonas RA. *Comprehensive Surgical Management of Congenital Heart Disease.* New York: Hodder Arnold; 2004:499.)

based on a high index of suspicion, and barium swallow is the first investigation. Echocardiography can document an abnormal head and neck vessel branching pattern, excluding intracardiac abnormalities. MRI provides complete anatomic detail.

Surgery

Most vascular rings are accessible through a left posterolateral thoracotomy; the exception is a left arch with right-sided ligamentum. Division of the ring and, in the case of double arch, preservation of the dominant arch is performed. Preservation of the recurrent laryngeal nerve is important. Initial experience with endoscopic robotically assisted repair of vascular rings has also been reported.

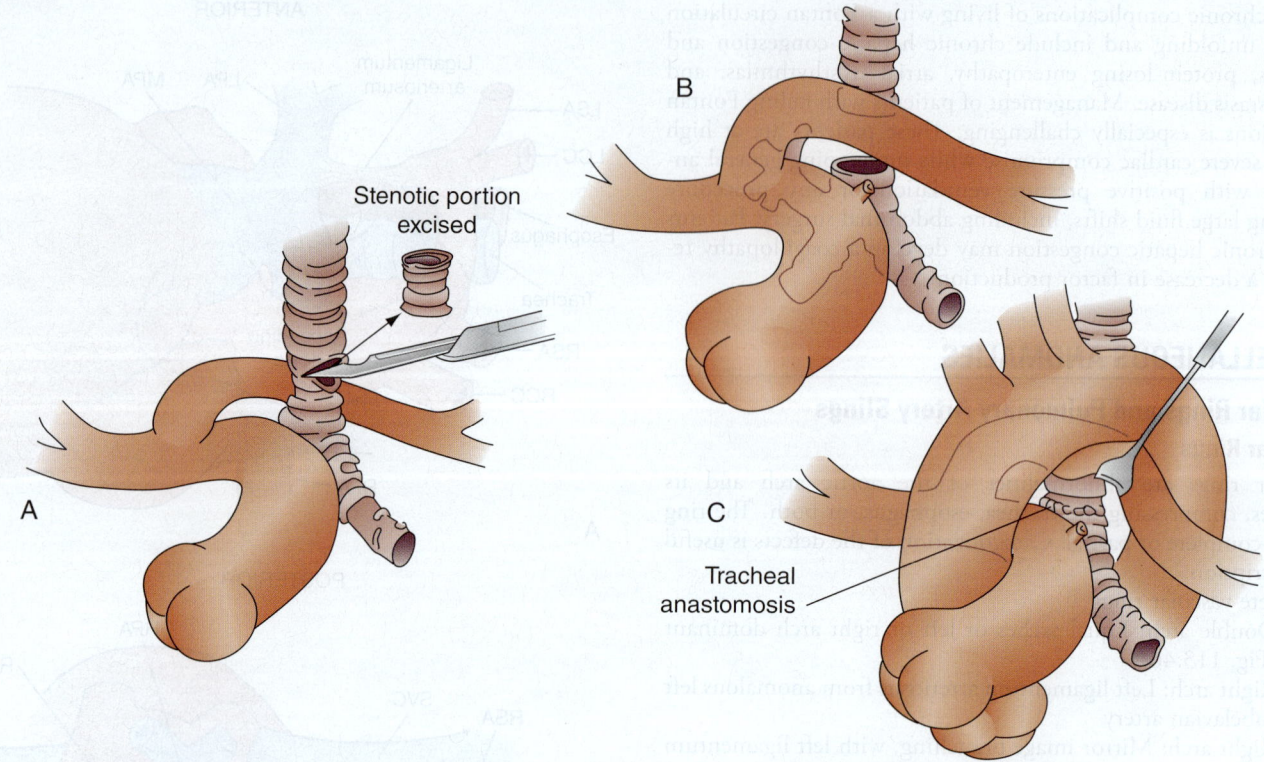

Stenotic portion excised

A

B

C

Tracheal anastomosis

FIGURE 113.47 Method for the management of a pulmonary artery sling with associated tracheal stenosis, using cardiopulmonary bypass. (A) Tracheal resection of the involved segment. (B) Anterior translocation of the left pulmonary artery after transection of the trachea. (C) Direct anastomosis of the trachea. (From Castaneda AR, Jonas RA, Mayer JE, et al. Vascular rings, slings, and tracheal anomalies. In: *Cardiac Surgery of the Neonate and Infant.* Philadelphia: Saunders; 1994.)

Pulmonary artery slings are approached through the midline; the use of cardiopulmonary bypass facilitates tracheal reconstruction and relocation of the right pulmonary artery (Fig. 113.47). Repair can be achieved with low risk. Symptoms may take months to resolve, with slow resolution of the underlying tracheomalacia.

Coronary Artery Anomalies

Anomalies occur as a result of anomalous origin, termination, courses, and aneurysm formation. Of these variables, only an anomalous left coronary artery rising from the pulmonary artery (ALCAPA) and coronary artery fistulas are discussed here.

Anomalous Left Coronary Artery Rising From the Pulmonary Artery

An ALCAPA is a rare, often lethal lesion in early infancy. Untreated, the mortality rate approaches 90%.

Anatomy and pathophysiology. Developmentally, failure of the normal connection of the left coronary artery bud to the aorta results in an abnormal connection to the pulmonary artery. The abnormal origin can be situated in the main pulmonary artery or proximal branches. Associated abnormalities are rare but important to recognize because lowering of the pulmonary artery pressure by PDA ligation or closure of a VSD can be fatal if the ALCAPA is not noted. In utero, with equal pulmonary arterial and aortic pressures, satisfactory perfusion of the ALCAPA can occur. After birth, the pulmonary artery pressure falls, and left coronary artery perfusion decreases. Ischemia causes impaired ventricular function and myocardial infarcts and leads to left ventricular dilation. Papillary muscle dysfunction causes mitral

regurgitation. Early coronary collateral development may prevent ongoing infarction.

Diagnosis and indications for intervention. ALCAPA is suspected in any infant with mitral regurgitation, ventricular dysfunction, or dilated cardiomyopathy. Infants present with low cardiac output and systemic heart failure. Feeding may also precipitate sudden death and angina in infants. Sudden death has also been described in older children. The ECG may reflect ischemic changes. The echocardiogram is usually diagnostic. However, because this diagnosis is often confused with dilated cardiomyopathy, there is an argument in favor of catheterizing all patients with dilated cardiomyopathy in whom the coronary artery anatomy cannot be clearly defined on echocardiography. Secondary findings of dilated cardiac chambers and segmental wall motion abnormalities, together with mitral regurgitation, prompt a search for an ALCAPA. Diagnosis of an ALCAPA is an indication for intervention.

Surgery. A degree of ventricular dysfunction is usually present. Preoperative inotropic support and optimization of hemodynamics may be required before surgical intervention. Severe cardiomyopathy rarely may necessitate cardiac transplantation. Current experience indicates that creation of a dual coronary system is safe and reproducible and offers the best opportunity for recovery of function. Operative considerations include optimal myocardial protection and prevention of left heart distention. Direct reimplantation of the ALCAPA into the ascending aorta is the procedure of choice (Fig. 113.48). Sometimes, limited mobility of the coronary artery precludes reimplantation, and a surgically created aorta–pulmonary artery–coronary artery tunnel is created; this is

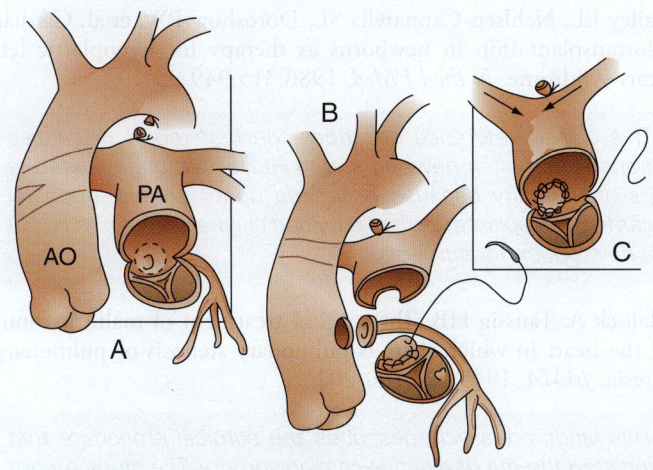

FIGURE 113.48 Direct reimplantation of anomalous left coronary artery arising from the pulmonary artery (ALCAPA). (A) Excision of ALCAPA from the pulmonary artery *(PA)*. (B) Aortic reimplantation of the coronary ostium into the aorta. (C) Reconstruction of the PA with autologous pericardium. *AO*, Aorta. (From Vouhe PR, Tamisier D, Sidi D, et al. Anomalous left coronary artery from the pulmonary artery: results of isolated aortic reimplantation. *Ann Thorac Surg.* 1992;54:621-626.)

known as the *Takeuchi procedure.* Ligation of the ALCAPA is not recommended.

Postoperative management is directed toward maintaining adequate coronary perfusion and cardiac output. Mechanical support of the heart may be temporarily required. Mitral regurgitation usually improves, and valve replacement is rarely necessary. Current intervention has a low operative mortality. Risks for mortality relate to preoperative ventricular dysfunction and cardiogenic shock. The Takeuchi repair is associated with tunnel complications such as obstruction, leak, aortic valve damage, and RVOTO in the long term.

Coronary Arteriovenous Fistula and Aneurysms

Isolated coronary artery fistula is more rare than ALCAPA. Drainage of coronary artery fistula is reported to terminate more commonly in the right side of the heart or pulmonary artery than in the left side of the heart. A shunt from the high-pressure coronary artery system into a low-pressure cardiac chamber may result in coronary steal and some degree of cardiac volume overload. Coronary artery aneurysms are associated with Kawasaki disease.

Diagnosis and indications for intervention. Presentation depends on the amount of functional compromise produced by the ischemia and volume overload. Echocardiography may be able to delineate the anomaly, but coronary angiography is diagnostic. Details of coronary anatomy are essential for determining intervention. Interventional catheterization is useful for the obliteration of fistulas and terminal aneurysms.

Surgery. If the lesion is not amenable to transcatheter intervention, surgery is indicated. Options include suture ligation without bypass, cardiopulmonary bypass, and aneurysmectomy with closure of the fistula. Early and late mortality rates are low. Risk factors for death and ventricular dysfunction relate to coronary artery insufficiency and infarction after fistula ligation or aneurysmectomy.[55]

Ebstein Anomaly of the Tricuspid Valve

Ebstein anomaly of the tricuspid valve is a rare defect in which the tricuspid valve attachments are displaced into the RV to varying degrees as a result of failure of delamination. Ebstein anomaly includes a spectrum of abnormalities involving a degree of displacement of the tricuspid valve, variable right ventricular size, and variable pulmonary outflow obstruction. Associated abnormalities are ASD, pulmonary atresia, and ccTGA. The posterior and septal leaflets of the tricuspid valve are variably displaced toward the apex of the RV, which results in an atrialized portion of the RV. The anterior leaflet remains large and sail-like. The major hemodynamic issue is tricuspid incompetence with decreased pulmonary blood flow and, if an ASD is present, right-to-left shunting, causing cyanosis. Long-standing tricuspid incompetence leads to volume overload of an abnormal RV. Variable pulmonary outflow tract obstruction limits effective pulmonary blood flow. If adequate pulmonary blood flow requires continued ductal patency, the need for neonatal intervention is almost certain.

Diagnosis and Intervention

The more severe forms of Ebstein anomaly manifest with cyanosis in infancy. Critically ill neonates tend to have a severe form of the disease, with a grossly inefficient RV compounded by the high pulmonary resistance of the neonate or by pulmonary valve atresia. The mortality rate in this group is high. Older patients present in heart failure and may have cyanosis. Supraventricular dysrhythmias and the preexcitation syndrome (Wolff-Parkinson-White syndrome) are associated with Ebstein anomaly. Echocardiography is diagnostic. Critically ill neonates have poor survival rates, and surgery is indicated only after stabilization with PGE1 and controlled ventilation. In older patients, cyanosis and heart failure are indications to intervene, although earlier intervention in asymptomatic patients, before excessive right ventricular dilation, is being more actively pursued.

Surgery

In critically ill neonates, after stabilization, palliation with a systemic-to-pulmonary artery shunt may be required. The Starnes operation has allowed salvage in previously hopeless cases. This operation consists of patch closure of the tricuspid orifice, atrial septectomy, and a systemic-to-pulmonary artery shunt.[56] In patients with less severe forms of this disease, tricuspid valve repair or replacement is also an option. Surgical techniques for the treatment of Ebstein anomaly have been evolving, and outcomes are improving for this challenging group of patients (Fig. 113.49).[57]

Mitral Valve Anomalies

Most abnormalities of the mitral valve are associated with other complex lesions (e.g., Shone complex). More commonly, mitral disease in children is inflammatory in nature—that is, rheumatic disease or infective endocarditis. It may also be associated with collagen vascular disease and Marfan syndrome.

Mitral Stenosis

Mitral stenosis is caused by obstruction at a supravalvular, valvular, or subvalvular level, singly or in combination. Supravalvular stenosis is caused by a ring of fibrous tissue above the annulus of the mitral valve or attached to the proximal leaflets. Valvular stenosis involves the leaflets, with commissural fusion occurring with or without hypoplasia of the valve ring. Hypoplasia of the mitral valve is often associated with left ventricular hypoplasia. Frequently, the leaflets and subvalvular apparatus are also dysplastic. Fusion of the leaflets can lead to an accessory orifice and produce mitral stenosis at a purely valvular level (so-called

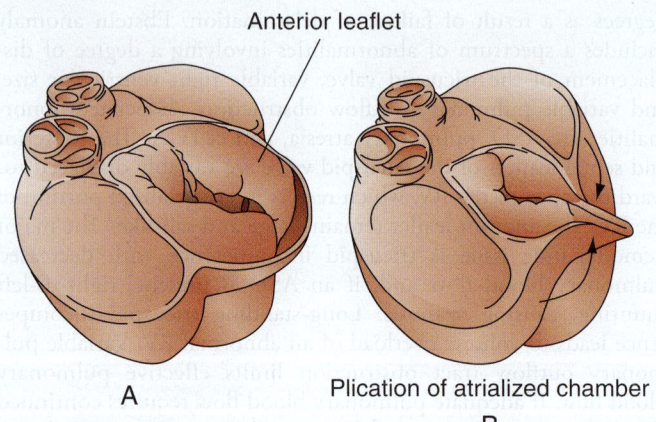

Anterior leaflet

A

B

Plication of atrialized chamber

FIGURE 113.49 Repair of Ebstein malformation using the Carpentier method. (A) The anterior and posterior leaflets of the tricuspid valve are detached from the annulus. (B) The atrium is plicated, reducing the annular diameter. The detached leaflets are reattached to the annulus. (From Castaneda AR, Jonas RA, Mayer JE, et al. Ebstein's anomaly. In: *Cardiac Surgery of the Neonate and Infant.* Philadelphia: Saunders; 1994.)

double-orifice mitral valve). Three types of subvalvular stenosis have been recognized—parachute mitral valve, hammock valve, and absence of one or both papillary muscles. Mitral regurgitation is a result of secondary annular dilation, congenital isolated clefts of the valve, and prolapse of the leaflets from abnormal chordae or papillary muscle insertion.

Echocardiography is diagnostic. Intervention includes balloon valvuloplasty, particularly for selected forms of rheumatic mitral stenosis, and surgical intervention. Intervention is timed to avoid irreversible sequelae related to chronic volume overload or pulmonary hypertension. Surgical intervention is aimed at preserving the mitral valve, and valvuloplasty techniques have a valuable place in children. Prosthetic valves are the least desirable option. Bioprosthetic or tissue valves need to be avoided in children. Supraannular placement of the prosthesis may be necessary. Repeat placement is ensured.

SUMMARY

This chapter provides a basic overview of the major congenital cardiac lesions and a framework for the diagnosis and treatment of these conditions. For most patients, the diagnosis of CHD, whether surgically treated or not, carries lifelong implications. For patients with CHD presenting for noncardiac surgery, a thorough understanding of the patient's unique anatomy and physiology is mandatory when planning a rational management strategy. The reader is directed to several excellent texts on CHD for a more thorough review of each of the lesions reviewed in this chapter.

SELECTED REFERENCES

Anderson R, Spicer D, Hlavacek A, Cook A, Backer C. *Wilcox's Surgical Anatomy of the Heart.* 4th ed. Cambridge: Cambridge University Press; 2013.

This text provides an excellent reference manual for understanding the complex anatomy of the heart. It contains color photographs and diagrams and is an invaluable resource for any student of cardiac surgery.

Bailey LL, Nehlsen-Cannarella SL, Doroshow RW, et al. Cardiac allotransplantation in newborns as therapy for hypoplastic left heart syndrome. *N Engl J Med.* 1986;315:949-951.

This classic reference describes the first report of cardiac transplantation in newborns with HLHS. Although limited in its applicability because of limited donor organs, neonatal cardiac transplantation has provided children born with HLHS a new option for survival.

Blalock A, Taussig HB. The surgical treatment of malformations of the heart in which there is pulmonary stenosis or pulmonary atresia. *JAMA.* 1945;128:189-202.

This landmark article describes the surgical procedure that initiated the era of elective cardiac surgery. The study reported the initial experience with palliative surgical treatment of patients with pulmonary stenosis or pulmonary atresia using the Blalock-Taussig shunt.

Fontan F, Baudet E. Surgical repair of tricuspid atresia. *Thorax.* 1971;26:240-248.

This article represents a milestone in the evolution of surgical management of patients with single-ventricle physiology. It described the first corrective operation for patients with tricuspid atresia. Although previous palliative procedures, provided by various systemic-to-pulmonary artery shunts, improved the clinical condition of patients, systemic blood was still a mixture of oxygenated and deoxygenated blood. The Fontan operation redirected SVC and IVC blood flow to the lungs so that only oxygenated blood returned to the heart and subsequently to the systemic circulation.

Kirklin JW, Dushane JW, Patrick RT, et al. Intracardiac surgery with the aid of a mechanical pump-oxygenator system (gibbon type): report of eight cases. *Mayo Clin Proc.* 1955;30:201-206.

This landmark article demonstrated that open repairs of congenital cardiac defects using mechanical pump oxygenator systems could be performed with minimal risk to patients.

Mustard W. Successful two-stage correction of transposition of the great vessels. *Surgery.* 1964;55:469-472.

This classic reference describes one of the initial surgical approaches to the treatment of d-TGA. Although the arterial switch operation is now the surgical treatment of choice for d-TGA, there are many adult patients with congenital heart disease who have been palliated with the Mustard operation. Understanding the operation and resulting physiology is critical to general surgery management strategies for noncardiac operations.

Norwood WI, Lang P, Casteneda AR, et al. Experience with operations for hypoplastic left heart syndrome. *J Thorac Cardiovasc Surg.* 1981;82:511-519.

In this landmark article, Norwood and colleagues reported the outcomes of what was then a new reconstructive surgical technique to palliate newborns with hypoplastic left heart syndrome (HLHS). Until the Norwood operation, the only option for survival of patients with HLHS was cardiac transplantation. At most centers today, the Norwood operation is the primary mode of therapy for most neonates with HLHS.

Sano S, Ishino K, Kawada M, et al. Right ventricle-pulmonary artery shunt in first-stage palliation of hypoplastic left heart syndrome. *J Thorac Cardiovasc Surg.* 2003;126:504-509.

This classic reference describes the right ventricle–to–pulmonary artery conduit used in the Norwood procedure. This novel procedure, named after the author, Sano, allowed for more hemodynamic stability postoperatively from the Norwood procedure and improved intrastage survival.

Senning A. Surgical correction of transposition of the great vessels. *Surgery.* 1959;45:966-980.

This classic reference describes the initial surgical approach to management of transposition of the great arteries (d-TGA). Although the arterial switch operation is currently the surgical treatment of choice for d-TGA, there are many adult patients with congenital heart disease in the community who have had the Senning operation. Understanding the operation and resulting physiology is critical to general surgery management strategies for noncardiac operations.

Starnes VA, Pitlick PT, Bernstein D, et al. Ebstein's anomaly appearing in the neonate. A new surgical approach. *J Thorac Cardiovasc Surg.* 1991;101:1082-1087.

This classic reference describes the first report of a new surgical approach to Ebstein anomaly in neonates. The procedure was named after the surgeon, Starnes. This approach has provided children born with severe Ebstein anomaly with a new option for survival.

Ungerleider RM, Meliones JN, McMillian KN, et al. *Critical Heart Disease in Infants and Children.* 3rd ed. Philadelphia: Elsevier; 2019.

This text provides a comprehensive and current review of heart disease in infants and children. It contains numerous surgical drawings and diagnostic images to supplement the didactic material.

Warden HE, Cohen M, Read RC, et al. Controlled cross circulation for open intracardiac surgery: physiologic studies and results of creation and closure of ventricular septal defects. *J Thorac Surg.* 1954;28:331-341.

This landmark article described the technique of cross-circulation to facilitate cardiopulmonary bypass and intracardiac repair of congenital heart lesions. Warden and colleagues documented the successful use of cross-circulation to correct defects such as ventricular septal defect.

The full reference list appears on Elsevier eBooks+.

Pulmonary Embolism: Acute and Chronic

Hiroko Nemoto, Jill R. Higgins, and Michael M. Madani

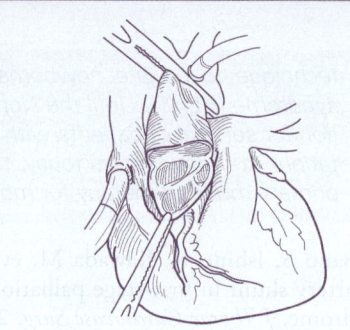

ACUTE PULMONARY EMBOLISM

Epidemiology

Venous thromboembolism (VTE), defined as deep vein thrombosis (DVT) or pulmonary embolism (PE), is a relatively common disease, and it is believed to be the third most common cause of death from cardiovascular disease, after heart attack and stroke.[1] In the United States, VTE causes 100,000 to 180,000 deaths per year and is associated with significant cardiovascular and pulmonary morbidity.[2] The incidence of PE was estimated to be about 115 per 100,000 people in the United States,[3,4] whereas it is 39 per 100,000 in Hong Kong.[5] VTE incidence estimates are higher among Black populations and lower among Asian, Asian American, and Native American populations.[4–6] Despite an increased incidence of acute PE in the past decade, there has been a decline in mortality rates.[7] This may be related to earlier diagnosis and better risk-stratified treatment options as directed by a Pulmonary Embolism Response Team (PERT). In an epidemiologic study in Germany, the incidence of acute PE was 99 per 100,000 people/year over the 11-year period. The rate increased from 85 per 100,000 in 2005 to 109 per 100,000 in 2015. However, during the same period, in-hospital case mortality decreased from 20.4% to 13.9%.[8]

Pathology and Pathogenesis

VTE refers to both DVT and PE. PE occurs when the pulmonary artery is occluded by a thrombus or embolus that usually originates from the lower extremities. Partial or complete occlusion of calf or thigh veins reduces the velocity of flow in the more proximal femoral and iliac veins, enhancing the propagation of thrombus in the vein wall at the site of origin. The degree of

organization within the thrombus varies, but recent clots are more likely to migrate than older thrombi that are more firmly attached to the vessel wall.

After acute PE, the patient may experience a wide range of symptoms, which can vary from sudden onset of pleuritic chest pain and dyspnea to a significant degree of right heart failure secondary to pulmonary obstruction and pulmonary hypertension (PH). In its most severe form it can cause hemodynamic collapse and death. The degree of PH and subsequent right heart dysfunction is likely multifactorial and related to the degree of mechanical occlusion of the pulmonary vascular bed, humoral factors released by the thrombus itself, and hypoxic pulmonary vascular spasm.[9,10]

Occluded vascular bed is the main cause of increased pulmonary vascular resistance (PVR) in acute PE. However, significant increases of PVR and the ensuing PH do not occur unless 30% or more of the pulmonary vascular bed is occluded.[11] In the absence of preexisting cardiopulmonary disease, the degree of PH is proportional to the degree of obstruction. However, a normal heart is not capable of maintaining high pulmonary pressures in an acute setting. Generally, the right heart is unable to maintain mean pulmonary artery pressure (mPAP) of over 40 mm Hg in an acute setting. This scenario typically occurs when 50% or more of the pulmonary vascular bed is occluded,[11] carrying an increased risk of developing acute right ventricle (RV) failure.[11] It is important to emphasize that clinicians should suspect the possibility of chronic thromboembolic pulmonary hypertension (CTEPH) when patients are able to maintain mPAP of over 40 mm Hg. Similarly, an episode of acute-on-chronic PE, or other non-VTE causes of PH, should be suspected when mPAP of over 40 mm Hg is maintained and tolerated.

However, simple mechanical obstruction of one or more pulmonary arteries may not entirely explain the often-devastating hemodynamic consequences. This hemodynamic reaction is a result of the interaction between the thrombus and the circulating platelets in the bloodstream, humoral factors (specifically serotonin and thromboxane A2), and the ensuing hypoxemia, all leading to further pulmonary vasoconstriction and bronchoconstriction, further worsening PVR after an episode of PE.[12] The main cause of hypoxemia in acute PE is the perfusion-ventilation mismatch that occurs in the open vasculature because increased compensatory blood flow in these nonobstructed vessels is mismatched with the subsequent bronchospasm.

Rudolf C. Virchow described the three major causes of thrombus formation in 1856, famously known as Virchow's triad: (1) venous stasis, (2) venous wall/endothelial injury, and (3) hypercoagulability.[13] Venous stasis may be caused by proximal mechanical obstruction, low cardiac output (CO), trauma, obesity, venous distention, increased viscosity, immobilization, frailty, pelvic tumors, pregnancy, congestive heart failure, or major surgery. Endothelial injury can be caused by trauma, smoking, and cancer. Hypercoagulability may include inherited hypercoagulable states, such as mutations in factor V Leiden, the prothrombin gene, and proteins C and S as well as antithrombin deficiency, antiphospholipid antibodies, and lupus anticoagulant.[14] Acquired risk factors include obesity, surgery, congestive heart failure, chronic lung disease, cerebrovascular accident, antiphospholipid antibody syndrome, drugs (estrogen preparations, oral contraceptives, steroids, etc.), and traveler's thrombosis caused by long-distance travel. If an underlying condition or risk factor leading to thrombus formation cannot be identified (i.e., idiopathic VTE), an occult malignancy should be ruled out. Arterial and venous thromboses, such as those in Trousseau syndrome, are seen in advanced malignancies.[15]

Natural History

Undiagnosed PE has a hospital mortality rate as high as 30%, compared with 8% when PE is diagnosed and treated appropriately.[14,16] Early diagnosis and appropriate treatments can greatly improve mortality. According to the International Cooperative Pulmonary Embolism Registry (ICOPER), out of 2454 patients with acute PEs, 7.9% had fatal PEs, with an all-cause mortality rate of 17.4% at 3 months. The mortality rate was significantly higher in hemodynamically unstable patients at 58.3%, compared with 15.1% in hemodynamically stable patients.[17]

When considering risk factors contributing to mortality, the rates are significantly higher in patients over the age of 70 and those with underlying cancer, congestive heart failure, and/or chronic obstructive pulmonary disease. Other poor prognostic signs and findings include systolic arterial hypotension, tachypnea, presence of RV hypokinesis on echocardiography,[17] free-floating thrombi in the RV,[18] patent foramen ovale,[19] and elevated cardiac troponin T levels.[20] According to the Japan VTE Treatment Registry (JAVA), cancer was the most common risk factor for VTE, at 27%. Inadequate anticoagulation using subtherapeutic levels of activated partial thromboplastin time (APTT), found in 37.6% of the patients, was the main culprit in this acute phase. Furthermore, the cumulative recurrence rate of VTE during warfarin treatment was 2.8 cases per 100 patients/year, but it was increased to 8.1 cases per 100 patients/year after warfarin treatment was stopped.[21] Recurrence rates were greater in patients with PE versus DVT, and among the survivors of PE, CTEPH developed in 2% to 4%.[2]

Clinical Presentation and Diagnosis

Clinical Presentation

Acute PE may present with varying degrees of signs and symptoms, and the clinical diagnosis is often missed. Most patients with acute PE present with dyspnea and chest pain. However, it can also present with tachypnea, cough, and/or hemoptysis. Examination may reveal tachycardia, rales, fever, and diaphoresis.[22] Hemodynamic instability is rare but an important consideration because it indicates central or extensive PE with severely reduced hemodynamic reserve. Syncope may also occur as a result of hemodynamic instability and RV dysfunction.[23]

The Geneva Score is one example of a clinical prediction model that can be used to determine the probability of PE (Table 114.1).[24] In addition to the presenting symptoms, the predisposing factors are also accounted for to predict the clinical probability of the disease. Such models are especially useful if PE is one of the differential diagnoses.

Laboratory Findings

Chest radiography (CXR) may show some subtle abnormalities, but its findings are not sensitive or specific for PE. Findings may include parenchymal infiltrate, atelectasis, or pleural effusion. A zone of hypovascularity or a wedge-sharped pleural-based density raises the suspicion for PE.

Similarly, electrocardiograms (ECGs) are not sensitive or specific for PE. Findings may include new right bundle branch block (RBBB), rightward shift of QRS axis, ST elevation of V1 and aVR, low amplitude QRS, premature atrial contraction (PAC), atrial fibrillation or atrial flutter, and T-wave inversion in V1 to V4.[25]

The arterial blood gas (ABG) may reveal hypoxemia (PaO_2 <80 mm Hg), hypocapnia, and high alveolar-arterial oxygen gradient ($A\text{-}aDO_2$ >20 Torr). However, blood gas analysis alone is not helpful in diagnosing PE because some patients may have a normal ABG with minimal ventilation-perfusion (V/Q) mismatch.[16]

TABLE 114.1 Revised Geneva Score for Acute Pulmonary Embolism

Risk Factors	
Age >65 years	1 point
Previous DVT or PE	3 points
Surgery (under general anesthesia) or fracture (of the lower limbs) within 1 month	2 points
Active malignant condition (solid or hematologic malignant condition, currently active or considered cured <1 year)	2 points
Symptoms	
Unilateral lower-limb pain	3 points
Hemoptysis	2 points
Clinical Signs	
Heart rate	
75–94 beats/minute	3 points
≧95 beats/minute	5 points
Pain on lower-limb deep venous palpation and unilateral edema	4 points
Clinical Probability	**Total**
Low	0–3 points
Intermediate	4–10 points
High	≧11 points

DVT, Deep vein thrombosis; *PE,* pulmonary embolism.

D-dimer is a protein fragment from the degradation of blood clots. D-dimer levels are elevated in plasma in the presence of acute thrombosis because of simultaneous activation of coagulation and fibrinolysis. The negative predictive value of D-dimer testing is high, and a normal D-dimer level renders acute PE or DVT unlikely. On the other hand, the positive predictive value of elevated D-dimer levels is low, and D-dimer testing is not useful for confirmation of PE.[26] D-dimer is also frequently elevated in older adult patients; in hospitalized patients; in patients with cancer, severe infection, or inflammatory disease; and during pregnancy.[27–29]

Although echocardiography is not highly sensitive or specific in the diagnosis of acute PE, it can nevertheless be extremely valuable.[30] The two most useful echocardiographic findings for diagnose of acute PE are RV enlargement and the McConnell sign. The McConnell sign is defined as RV free wall akinesis with sparing of the apex. On echocardiography, it appears as if the apex is bouncing up and down while the rest of the RV is still. The "D" sign may be present, which is the result of RV overload and shifting of the septum toward the left side of the heart.[31] The tricuspid annulus plane systolic excursion (TAPSE) and tricuspid regurgitation peak gradient (TRPG) are echocardiographic indicators of RV function and can help differentiate between submassive versus nonmassive PEs. In cases with RV dysfunction, the prognosis is worse.[32] Echocardiography is used not only as a screening method for PE but also for determining the severity of the disease and the subsequent treatment plan.

Imaging Findings

Multidetector computed tomographic pulmonary angiography (CTPA) is the method of choice for imaging the pulmonary vasculature in patients with suspected PE.[26] The Prospective Investigation on Pulmonary Embolism Diagnosis (PIOPED) II study observed a sensitivity of 83% and a specificity of 96% for CTPA in PE diagnosis. Fig. 114.1 shows examples of acute PE as seen on CTPA. In patients with a low or intermediate clinical probability of PE, a negative CTPA has a high (96%) negative predictive value for PE.[33] Furthermore, multidetector CTPA is more sensitive in detecting smaller PEs within the subsegmental pulmonary arteries compared with single-detector CTPA, increasing the rate of subsegmental PE diagnosis.[34]

With advancements in the diagnostic power of CTPA, use of lung scintigraphy in the acute setting has decreased. V/Q scans provide confirmatory evidence, but these studies may be less reliable in acute PE as opposed to the chronic setting. In general, normal V/Q scans essentially exclude the diagnosis of clinically significant PE. Because pulmonary scintigraphy does not require the use of a contrast agent, it remains useful for patients with contrast medium–induced anaphylaxis or those with severe renal dysfunction. It may also be preferred in patients of young age as well as pregnant females because the radiation dose is lower than that of CTPA.[35] In addition to the standard imaging just described, there are several more advanced imaging modalities that are now available; these include perfusion single-photon emission CT (SPECT) and V/Q SPECT with or without enhanced CT, but few outcome studies are available, with incomplete follow-up.[36]

Pulmonary angiography was historically the gold standard for the diagnosis or exclusion of acute PE, but as technology has improved, CTPA offers similar diagnostic accuracy.[37] Given the less invasive nature of CTPA and its wide and immediate availability in most centers, it has become the diagnostic imaging of choice. Furthermore, in acute PE, hemodynamic instability can be a contraindication for pulmonary angiography.

Magnetic resonance angiography demonstrates high specificity and sensitivity for proximal PE, but it has a limited sensitivity for more distal PE.[38] It can be performed noninvasively; however, in most institutions, it is not readily available in an acute setting.

Risk Assessment of Acute Pulmonary Embolism

Risk assessment of acute PE is important not only for establishing the correct treatment strategy but also for determining short- and long-term prognosis. Of the clinical scores integrating PE severity and comorbidity, the Pulmonary Embolism

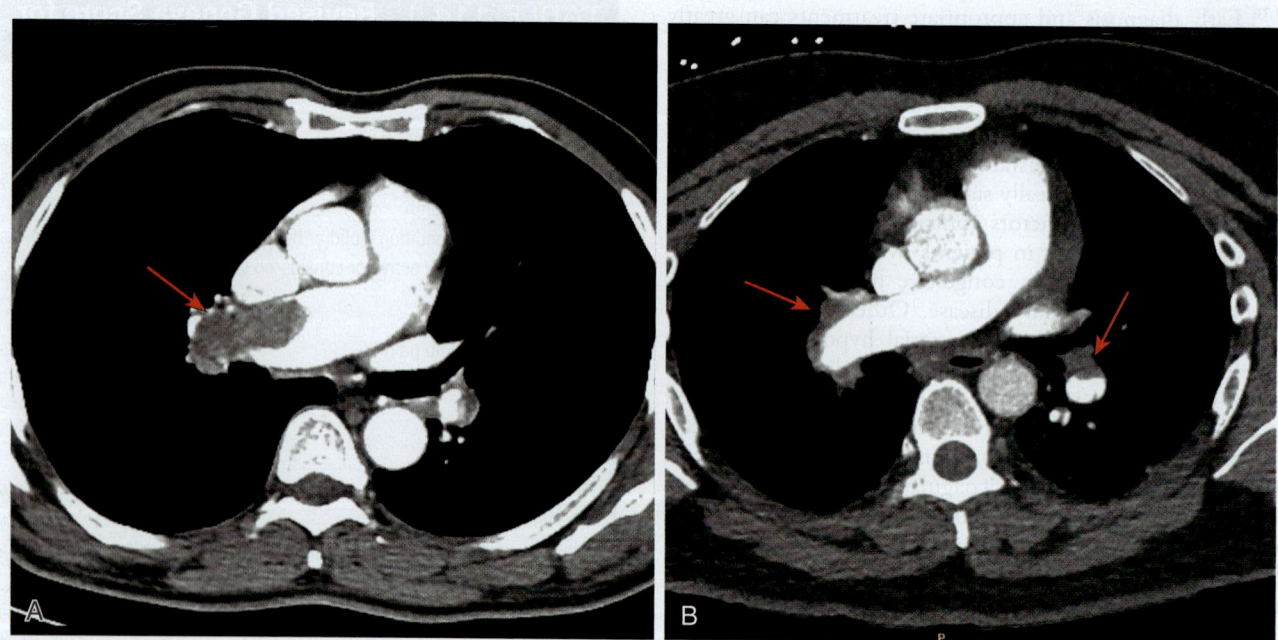

FIGURE 114.1 Computed tomography pulmonary angiography with axial sections showing (A) massive acute pulmonary embolism (PE) occluding right pulmonary artery *(arrow)* and (B) bilateral acute PE occluding right upper lobe and left interlobar arteries *(arrows)*.

Severity Index (PESI) has been the most extensively validated to date.[39] The principal strength of the PESI lies in the reliable identification of patients at low risk for 30-day mortality (PESI classes I and II).[26] Given the complexity of the original PESI, a simplified version (sPESI) has also been developed and validated (Table 114.2).[40] RV dysfunction assessed by CT, echocardiography, or cardiac biomarkers is associated with an increased risk of mortality, even in patients with hemodynamically stable PE.[41] RV/left ventricle (LV) diameter ratio >1.0 and a TAPSE <15 mm on echocardiography also carry an unfavorable prognosis.[42] Similarly, elevated concentrations of troponin I or T and brain natriuretic peptide (BNP) are associated with unfavorable prognosis in acute PE.[43,44]

The American Heart Association (AHA) classifies PE as massive, submassive, and low risk. *Massive* PE is truly life threatening and is defined as acute PE with sustained hypotension (systolic blood pressure less than 90 mm Hg for at least 15 minutes; inotropic support; and not due to a cause other than PE, such as arrhythmia, hypovolemia, sepsis, or LV dysfunction), pulselessness, or persistent profound bradycardia (heart rate below 40 beats/min with signs or symptoms of shock). *Submassive* PE is defined as acute PE without systemic hypotension (systolic blood pressure <90 mm Hg) but with either RV dysfunction or myocardial necrosis. RV dysfunction is categorized as the presence of at least one of the following: RV dilation (apical four-chamber RV diameter divided by LV diameter >0.9) or RV systolic dysfunction on echocardiography, RV dilation on CT (four-chamber RV diameter divided by LV diameter >0.9), elevation of BNP (>90 pg/mL), elevation of N-terminal pro-BNP (>500 pg/mL), or electrocardiographic changes (new complete or incomplete RBBB, anteroseptal ST elevation or depression, or anteroseptal T-wave inversion). Myocardial necrosis is defined as either one of the following: elevation of troponin I (>0.4 ng/mL) or elevation of troponin T (>0.1 ng/mL). *Low-risk* PE is defined as acute PE and the absence of the previously described clinical markers that would define massive or submassive PE.[45] The prognosis and recurrence rate of the disease differ significantly depending on presence of cardiac dysfunction.

The European Society of Cardiology (ESC) advocates a classification of severity in the form of high-risk, intermediate-high-risk, intermediate-low-risk, and low-risk groups in terms of early (in-hospital or 30-day) mortality.[26] Table 114.3 summarizes ESC risk classification.

Treatment

Respiratory and Circulatory Management

The mismatch between ventilation and perfusion is the main cause of hypoxemia of acute PE. Administration of supplemental oxygen is considered for the patients with Sao_2 <90%. Severe hypoxemia may be related to right-to-left shunting through a patent foramen ovale or atrial septal defect.[19] In cases of severe respiratory instability, further oxygenation techniques, including high-flow nasal cannula oxygen and mechanical ventilation, should also be considered.

Acute RV failure leading to low systemic CO is the leading cause of death in patients with high-risk acute PE. If the central venous pressure is low, volume loading using saline or lactated Ringer solution should be considered. Aggressive volume expansion should be avoided because it may worsen RV dilation and function. Central venous pressure can be assessed by echocardiographic imaging of the inferior vena cava (IVC). For patients in cardiogenic shock, norepinephrine can improve systemic hemodynamics by improving ventricular systolic contraction and coronary perfusion without causing a change in PVR. However, excessive vasoconstriction may worsen tissue perfusion. Dobutamine may be considered for patients with low cardiac index, but it may aggravate arterial hypotension if used alone without a vasopressor, especially if left heart failure is also present. Levosimendan may favorably affect RV-arterial uncoupling by combining RV inotropy and pulmonary vasodilation; however, it is still in phase III trial in the United States and is not FDA approved.[31] Vasodilators decrease pulmonary artery pressure (PAP) and PVR but may worsen systemic hypoperfusion because of their lack of

TABLE 114.2 Original Pulmonary Embolism Severity Index (PESI) and Simplified PESI (sPESI)

PREDICTORS	ORIGINAL VERSION	SIMPLIFIED VERSION
Age	Age in years	1 point (if age >80 years)
Male sex	+10 points	—
History of cancer	+30 points	1 point
History of heart failure	+10 points	1 point (combined into a single category of chronic cardiopulmonary disease)
History of chronic lung disease	+10 points	
Pulse ≧110/minute	+20 points	1 point
Systolic blood pressure <100 mm Hg	+30 points	1 point
Respiratory rate ≧30/minute (assessed with or without the administration of supplemental oxygen)	+20 points	—
Temperature <36°C	+20 points	—
Altered mental status (confusion, disorientation, or somnolence)	+60 points	—
Arterial oxygen saturation <90%	+20 points	1 point
Total point scores	30-day mortality risk	
Class I: ≦65 points	Very low (0%–1.6%)	0 points (low risk)
Class II: 66–85 points	Low (1.7%–3.5%)	
Class III: 86–105 points	Moderate (3.2%–7.1%)	≧1 point(s) (high risk)
Class IV: 106–125 points	High (4.0%–11.4%)	
Class V: >125 points	Very high (10.0%–24.5%)	

Note: For the original PESI, the total score for the patient is obtained by adding the patient's age in years to the points for each applicable predictor. Modified from Konstantinides SV, Meyer G, Becattini C, et al. 2019 ESC guidelines for the diagnosis and management of acute pulmonary embolism developed in collaboration with the European Respiratory Society (ERS). *Eur Heart J.* 2020;41:543-603; Elias A, Mallett S, Daoud-Elias M, et al. Prognostic models in acute pulmonary embolism: a systematic review and meta-analysis. *BMJ Open.* 2016;6:e010324; Jiménez D, Aujesky D, Moores L, et al. Simplification of the Pulmonary Embolism Severity Index for prognostication in patients with acute symptomatic pulmonary embolism. *Arch Intern Med.* 2010;170:1383-1389.

TABLE 114.3 **The European Society of Cardiology's Classification of Severity in the Form of High, Intermediate (High and Low), and Low-Risk Groups in Terms of Early Mortality**

EARLY MORTALITY RISK		HEMODYNAMIC INSTABILITY	CLINICAL PARAMETERS OF PE SEVERITY AND/OR COMORBIDITY: PESI CLASS III–V OR SPESI ≧1	RV DYSFUNCTION ON TTE OR CTPA	ELEVATED CARDIAC TROPONIN LEVELS
			INDICATORS OF RISK		
High		+	(+)	+	(+)
Intermediate	Intermediate-High	−	+	+	+
	Intermediate-Low	−	+	One (or none) positive	
Low		−	−	−	Assessment optional; if assessed, negative

Note: Hemodynamic instability means that at least one of the following is present: cardiac arrest, obstructive shock, or persistent hypotension. *CTPA,* Computed tomographic pulmonary angiography; *PE,* pulmonary embolism; *PESI,* Pulmonary Embolism Severity Index; *RV,* right ventricle; *sPESI,* simplified Pulmonary Embolism Severity Index; *TTE,* transthoracic echocardiogram.

specificity for the pulmonary artery. However, inhaled nitric oxide selectively dilates the pulmonary artery and may improve the hemodynamic status of patients with PE.[46]

The temporary use of mechanical circulatory support, commonly with venoarterial extracorporeal membrane oxygenation (VA ECMO) using peripheral vessel cannulation, may be helpful for hemodynamically unstable patients.[47] ECMO can be implemented outside the operating room. The femoral vein and artery are rapidly cannulated under sterile conditions using local anesthesia. The perfusion circuit consists of a small venous reservoir with intravenous access tubes, a centrifugal pump, and a membrane oxygenator. Blood from the venous system is collected from the right atrium (RA) using a cannula inserted through the femoral vein, and oxygenated blood is pumped through the femoral artery to the arterial system (Fig. 114.2). During ECMO, heparin is infused to maintain activated clotting times between 150 and 180 seconds. ECMO is useful as a bridge to decision or recovery while the patient is on anticoagulant therapy. It can also be used as a bridge to target therapy using catheter-directed fibrinolysis, percutaneous suction embolectomy, or other catheter-guided clot-retrieval devices as well as surgical embolectomy. ECMO can also be quite useful intraoperatively and postoperatively as a bridge to recovery.

Percutaneous RV assist devices, such as Impella RP (Abiomed, Danvers, MA), can be used in patients with severe RV failure. It is authorized for treating acute PE only in emergencies associated with acute right heart failure or decompensation resulting from complications of coronavirus disease 2019 (COVID-19). However, in recent years, the device has been successfully used more frequently in patients with acute PE who may not be eligible for other conventional treatments. The device is a microaxial flow pump, which can be placed percutaneously, with the inflow placed within the IVC or RA and the outflow in the pulmonary trunk.[48]

Medical Therapy

Parenteral Anticoagulation

Anticoagulation is the first line of treatment for acute PE. The first and only randomized controlled trial (RCT) that compared anticoagulant therapy with no anticoagulant therapy in patients with symptomatic DVT or PE was in 1960, and it showed 5 deaths (26.3%) and 5 recurrences in 19 control untreated patients versus no deaths or fatal recurrences from acute PE in the 16 treated patients.[49] Therapeutic anticoagulation should be immediately given to patients with objectively confirmed PE and no contraindication to anticoagulation.

Furthermore, systemic anticoagulation is recommended for patients with high clinical suspicion of acute PE while awaiting studies to confirm the diagnosis, as long as there are no contraindications to therapy.[26,45,50] Subcutaneous low-molecular-weight heparin (LMWH), fondaparinux (Xa inhibitor), or intravenous unfractionated heparin (UFH) is usually used.

It is reported that fixed-dose LMWH is more effective and safer than adjusted-dose UFH for the initial treatment of VTE.[26] Compared with UFH, LMWH significantly reduced the incidence of thrombotic complications, the occurrence of major hemorrhage, and overall mortality.[51] Neither LMWH nor fondaparinux needs routine monitoring of anti-Xa levels. Local considerations, such as cost, availability, and familiarity of use, dictate the choice between fondaparinux and LMWH.[50] LMWH and fondaparinux are not cleared adequately in patients with renal impairment, whereas this is not a concern with UFH.[50]

UFH should be used in patients with overt hemodynamic instability or imminent hemodynamic decompensation in whom

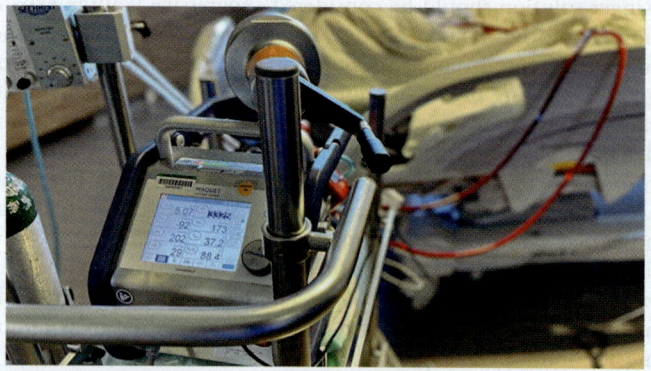

FIGURE 114.2 A critically ill patient in an intensive care unit setting being supported on venoarterial extracorporeal membrane oxygenator (VA ECMO) circuit.

primary reperfusion treatment will be necessary.[26] For people with confirmed PE and hemodynamic instability, continuous UFH infusion should be offered and thrombolytic therapy considered.[52] UFH is recommended for patients in whom primary reperfusion is considered as well as for those with serious renal impairment (creatinine clearance [CrCl] <30 mL/min) or severe obesity.[53] Continuous intravenous injection is often started after initial injection to achieve and maintain an APTT prolongation of 1.5 to 2.5 times that corresponds to plasma heparin levels of 0.3 to 0.7 IU/mL anti-Xa activity.[54] The most significant complication of UFH is bleeding, and its incidence is reported to be 3% to 10%.[55,56] Because UFH has a short half-life of about 60 minutes, the effect is rapidly attenuated when intravenous administration is discontinued. However, in the case of a major or life-threatening bleeding complication, it is necessary to neutralize the effect of UFH with protamine sulfate. Rapid administration of protamine sulfate leads to a decrease in blood pressure, so it should be administered slowly over 10 minutes. Other complications of UFH include heparin-induced thrombocytopenia (HIT). As an alternative anticoagulant for the patient with HIT, argatroban can be chosen.[57]

Non–Vitamin K Antagonist Oral Anticoagulants

New oral anticoagulants (NOACs) or direct oral anticoagulants (DOACs) are a novel treatment option for acute VTE. NOACs are small molecules that directly inhibit one activated coagulation factor, which is thrombin for dabigatran and factor Xa for apixaban, edoxaban, and rivaroxaban. Owing to their predictable bioavailability and pharmacokinetics, NOACs can be given at fixed doses without routine laboratory monitoring.[26] A study in patients with atrial fibrillation showed that NOACs are an alternative for vitamin K antagonists (VKAs) to prevent stroke, and they have emerged as the preferred choice for anticoagulation.[58] Phase III trials on the treatment of acute VTE and those on extended treatment beyond the first 6 months demonstrated that NOACs have similar efficacy as VKAs in the treatment of acute symptomatic VTE, but they significantly reduce the risk of major bleeding.[59] Major bleeding occurred in 1.1% of NOAC-treated patients and 1.7% of VKA-treated patients.[26,59] Anticoagulant treatment using NOACs without preceding heparin or fondaparinux (single-drug approach) is possible. For low-risk PE patients, outpatient treatment with NOACs is also possible.[60] NOACs are contraindicated in patients with severe renal impairment (CrCl <15 mL/min), and its dose should be reduced appropriately for patients with renal impairment (CrCl <50 mL/min).[52]

Warfarin (Vitamin K Antagonist)

Warfarin has been the gold standard in oral anticoagulation for more than 50 years. When warfarin is used, anticoagulation with UFH, LMWH, or fondaparinux should be used as a bridge until a therapeutic international normalized ratio (INR) is achieved.[26] Individual responses to warfarin vary based on factors such as inpatient or outpatient status, age, genotype, concomitant medications, and comorbidities. The initial dose of warfarin may be 5 or 10 mg for younger patients. Initial doses <5 mg are appropriate for patients >75 years, the malnourished, those with liver disease or heart failure, those on medications known to inhibit warfarin's metabolism, and patients at high risk of hemorrhage. The INR should be measured daily, and warfarin doses should be adjusted to achieve an INR of 2 to 3. In patients with CrCl <30 mL/min, warfarin is the preferred anticoagulant. Warfarin is also preferred in patients with antiphospholipid antibody. DOACs

and warfarin are contraindicated in pregnancy, and LMWH should be used.[61]

Systemic Thrombolysis

Thrombolysis in the treatment of PE was first described over 50 years ago. The general mechanism of fibrinolytic agents involves the activation of native plasminogen to plasmin, which hydrolyzes fibrin and leads to accelerated clot lysis. The goal of this process is to reduce thrombus burden, resulting in a more rapid relief of RV afterload and earlier hemodynamic improvement.[62] Thrombolytic therapy is associated with faster resolution of pulmonary embolic obstruction and improved right heart function compared with anticoagulation alone.[63] The greatest benefit is observed when treatment is initiated within 48 hours of symptom onset, and thrombolysis can still be useful in patients who have had symptoms for 6 to 14 days.[26,64] However, a meta-analysis of thrombolysis trials that included patients with high-risk PE found that compared with heparin, thrombolytic therapy was associated with a significant reduction of PE-related mortality and PE recurrence. Major hemorrhage and fatal or intracranial bleeding were significantly more frequent among patients receiving thrombolysis.[62] Systemic thrombolysis carries an estimated 20% risk of major hemorrhage, including a 3% to 5% risk of hemorrhagic stroke.[65] The dose-response relationship for systemic thrombolysis in acute PE remains unknown.[63] Therefore, systemic thrombolytic therapy should only be considered for people with massive PE associated with hemodynamic instability who do not have a high bleeding risk.[45,52] The absolute contraindications are history of hemorrhagic stroke or stroke of unknown origin; ischemic stroke in previous 6 months; central nervous system neoplasm; major trauma, surgery, or head injury in previous 3 weeks; bleeding diathesis; and active bleeding. Recombinant tissue-type plasminogen activator (rtPA), streptokinase, and urokinase are approved forms of therapy, but the accelerated intravenous administration (100 mg over 2 hours) of rtPA is preferable to prolonged infusions of streptokinase and urokinase.[26]

Percutaneous Interventions
Catheter-Directed Thrombolysis

According to the American College of Clinical Pharmacy (ACCP) guideline, in patients with acute PE who are treated with a thrombolytic agent, systemic thrombolytic therapy using a peripheral vein is preferred over catheter-directed thrombolysis (CDT). However, when expertise and resources are available, CDT may be preferred for patients with ongoing hypotension, those with high bleeding risk from systemic administration, those with failed systemic thrombolysis, and shock patients at risk of death before systemic thrombolysis can take effect (e.g., within hours).[45] A recent meta-analysis summarizing the outcomes with CDT for acute PE over the last decade showed an overall clinical success rate of 81.3%, a 30-day mortality rate of 8.0%, and a major bleeding rate of 6.7% for high-risk PE patients, compared with a clinical success rate of 97.5%, a 30-day mortality rate of 0%, and major bleeding rate of 1.4% for intermediate-risk PE.[66,67] Compared with systemic thrombolysis, in-hospital mortality and intracranial hemorrhage rates were lower for the CDT group; however, this came at a higher hospitalization cost.[68] The optimal dose of thrombolytic has not been clearly defined but is substantially lower (10%–25%) than the standard systemic dose.[69,70] The procedure is typically performed through right internal jugular access, with right heart catheterization (RHC), baseline hemodynamic measurements, and pulmonary angiography.

Catheter-Assisted Thrombus Removal

Although CDT has been proven useful, it is associated with higher bleeding risk and complications. Catheter-assisted thrombus removal (CATR) is a treatment strategy performed via a catheter-directed suction device and involves mechanical aspiration of the thrombus, with or without the use of thrombolytics. The bleeding rate varied in several studies, but the first meta-analysis on aspiration thrombectomy in acute PE showed that the rate of major bleeding was 4.98%.[71] Further studies and data are needed to evaluate the efficacy of this therapy.

Surgery: Pulmonary Embolectomy

The 2011 AHA guidelines indicate that it is reasonable to consider catheter embolectomy or surgical embolectomy for patients with massive PE who cannot receive fibrinolysis or those who remain unstable after fibrinolysis. They may also be considered for patients with submassive acute PE with poor prognosis (new hemodynamic instability, worsening respiratory failure, severe RV dysfunction, or major myocardial necrosis).[45] According to the 2019 ESC guidelines, the indications for surgical embolectomy areas follows: high-risk acute PE in patients who have contraindications to fibrinolytic treatment, ineffective thrombolysis, and intermediate-high-risk acute PE in patients with hemodynamic deterioration during anticoagulation therapy.[26] Coexisting RA and RV thrombus in acute PE is associated with an increased risk of death, and surgery should be considered.[72] In patients with RV overload, the migration of additional thrombus into the pulmonary circulation may result in a sudden hemodynamic collapse, and surgery may provide more favorable results.[48]

Although Frederick Trendelenburg first proposed the mechanism of direct thrombus removal from pulmonary arteries in 1908, the first successful surgery was reported by Kirschner in 1924, with survival of a few months. The results of this surgery had been disastrous until cardiopulmonary bypass (CPB) was established. Sabiston, Sharp, and Allison all made major contributions to the field, but Cooley reported the first successful case using CPB in 1961.[70]

The surgery is performed through a midline sternotomy incision. The ascending aorta and both vena cavae are cannulated after full heparinization, and CPB is initiated. It is often performed without aortic cross-clamping and cardioplegic cardiac arrest, but the procedure can also be performed with aortic cross-clamping and cold cardioplegia, particularly in patients with coexisting thrombi in the right heart cavities and in the presence of thrombi straddling the foramen ovale. In these cases, the heart may be electrically fibrillated or arrested with cold cardioplegic solution. Significant hypothermia may not be necessary because only a short period of complete bypass is needed. The main pulmonary artery is opened 1 to 2 cm downstream to the valve, and the incision is extended into the proximal left pulmonary artery. Forceps and suction catheters remove the clot from the left pulmonary artery and behind the aorta to the right pulmonary artery (RPA). The RPA can also be exposed and opened between the aorta and superior vena cava (SVC) to allow better exposure in the distal segments, if necessary. Unlike thrombi in chronic PE, relatively new, usually soft, rod-shaped red thrombi can be removed in acute PE. Although it is desirable to perform embolectomy as distal as possible, significant hemodynamic improvement can be achieved with removal of easily accessible large central thrombi. Fogarty balloon thrombectomy catheter is rarely used because of potential vessel wall injury to the distal pulmonary arteries by inserting it blindly. However, successful balloon catheter embolectomy under direct visual control by using a flexible choledochoscope has been reported.[73] In addition, acute PE may be complicated by presence of chronic thromboembolic PH (i.e., acute-on-chronic PE) (Fig. 114.3). In such a case, pulmonary thromboendarterectomy (PTE or PEA) is required. The procedure, described later in this chapter, is much more complex and requires significant expertise. Before proceeding with surgery, it is extremely important to ensure that the patent is not suffering from an episode of acute-on-chronic PE.

To prevent recurrent episodes of PE in patients with active DVT of large veins, a retrievable IVC filter may be considered during the perioperative period. IVC filters mechanically prevent venous clots from reaching the pulmonary circulation.

Postoperative Care and Complications

A systematic review of surgical embolectomy procedures determined that the most common postoperative complication was prolonged ventilation, seen in 33% of patients.[74] Surgical bleeding is also a common complication of the procedure, and it is worse in patients who receive preoperative thrombolytic therapy. Transfusion of clotting factors such as fresh frozen plasma and platelets may be helpful. Acute pulmonary hemorrhage may occur as a result of lung reperfusion injury rather than vessel wall perforation, but it can still be a challenging complication to deal with. In these patients, positive end-expiratory pressure (PEEP) and isolation of the active bleeding site using an endobronchial occlusion balloon can be helpful. Embolectomy usually improves hemodynamics promptly, but in patients with preoperative cardiopulmonary arrest, low CO syndrome may occur as a result of continued RV failure, likely related to ongoing RV ischemia. If hemodynamic instability continues despite the use of inotropic catecholamine support, ECMO should be considered (see earlier discussion). Perhaps the most devastating complication of acute

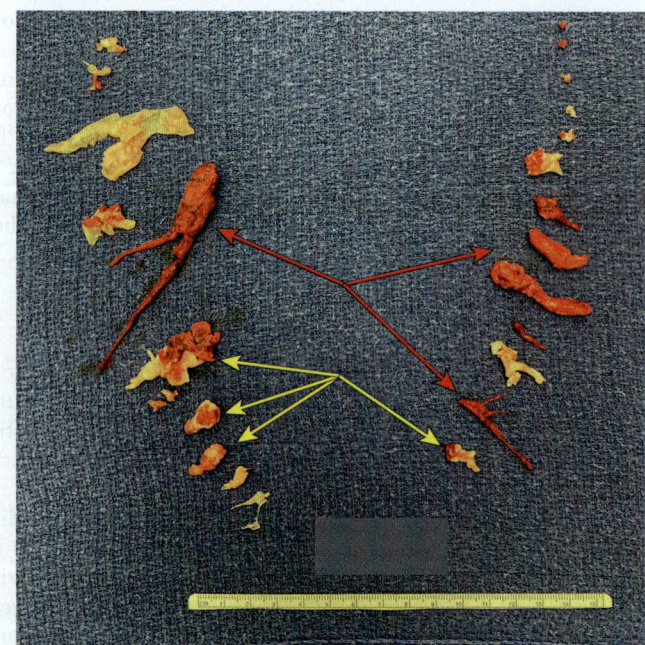

FIGURE 114.3 Specimen removed from the right and left pulmonary artery of a patient with mixed acute, subacute, and chronic pulmonary embolism. The *red arrows* point to the vessel with acute pulmonary emboli, and there is also clear evidence of organized chronic thrombus. *Yellow arrows* point to vessels with mixed disease.

pulmonary embolectomy in patients with cardiopulmonary arrest or prolonged shock is hypoxic encephalopathy. In such patients, full supportive measures using artificial ventilation, inotropic drugs, and ECMO are continued postoperatively until appropriate assessment of the neurologic status can be accomplished.

Outcomes of Pulmonary Embolectomy

The Society of Thoracic Surgery (STS) Adult Cardiac Surgery Database (ACSD) reports 1075 surgical embolectomies in North America between 2011 and 2015, with an overall mortality rate of 15.9%. The mortality rate varies widely, with 44.4% in patients with cardiac arrest before surgery, 23.7% in patients in shock but not requiring resuscitation, and 7.9% in patients without shock. Independent predictors of operative mortality included age, obesity, cardiogenic shock, preoperative arrest, chronic lung disease, unresponsive neurologic state, and prolonged CPB time.[75] Similar results were published in the Japanese Cardiovascular Surgery Database, where the overall operative mortality rate among 355 patients was 20.6%. In this report, the incidence of major adverse cardiovascular events (MACEs) was 27.3%. Independent risk factors for operative death were heart failure, poor LV function, and respiratory failure. Poor LV function, preoperative cardiopulmonary resuscitation (CPR), and respiratory failure were all independent risk factors for MACE.[76] There was a significant improvement in the systolic pulmonary artery pressure (sPAP), with a reduction in the mean sPAP from 57.8 mm Hg preoperatively to 31.3 mm Hg postoperatively. In-hospital mortality was 16%, and overall survival at 5 years was 73%.[74] Preoperative characteristics and risk factors remain the most crucial determinants of surgical outcomes.[48]

Chronic Treatment and Long-Term Outcomes for Acute Pulmonary Embolism

Oral anticoagulants are highly effective in preventing recurrent VTE. Patients with acute PE should receive 3 to 6 months of anticoagulant treatment. Extended duration of oral anticoagulant treatment reduces the risk for recurrent VTE, but this is partially offset by the risk of bleeding.[26] Compression stockings may be effective for patients with DVT to prevent postthrombotic syndrome, but routine use is not recommended.[77]

The highest risk factors for long-term recurrent VTE are active cancer, previous episodes of PE, or antiphospholipid antibody syndrome. These patients should receive indefinite anticoagulation. Cancer-associated thrombosis (CAT) is a condition in which relevance has been increasingly recognized for both physicians who deal with VTE and oncologists. The annual incidence of VTE in patients with cancer is currently estimated to be 0.5%, compared with 0.1% in the general population. Active cancer accounts for 20% of the overall incidence of VTE.[78] Risk of recurrent VTE should be weighed against the potential risk of bleeding in cancer patients when considering long-term anticoagulation therapy. It is conceivable that once cancer is cured, the risk for recurrence decreases, and anticoagulation can be stopped. Patients who are carriers of hereditary thrombophilia, such as antithrombin deficiency, protein C, or protein S as well as those with homozygous factor V Leiden, are also candidates for indefinite anticoagulant treatment.[26]

Long-term follow-up studies have consistently demonstrated that after an episode of acute PE, half of patients report functional limitations and/or decreased quality of life up to many years after the acute event. Incomplete thrombus resolution occurs in one-fourth to one-third of patients, and PAP and RV function remain abnormal despite adequate anticoagulant treatment in approximately 10% to 30% of patients, and 1% to 4% of patients are diagnosed with CTEPH.[79]

CHRONIC PULMONARY EMBOLISM AND CHRONIC THROMBOEMBOLIC PULMONARY HYPERTENSION

Epidemiology

Chronic PE is caused by narrowing or occlusion of the pulmonary arteries as a result of an organized thrombus. *Chronic* is defined when abnormalities in the pulmonary blood flow distribution and pulmonary circulatory dynamics do not change, even after anticoagulation therapy, for 3 to 6 months or more.[80] Diagnostic criteria for CTEPH include mPAP greater than 20 mm Hg, pulmonary arterial wedge pressure less than 15 mm Hg, PVR greater than 3 Woods units, and evidence of chronic PE on imaging.

The exact incidence and prevalence of CTEPH remain undefined.[81,82] Multiple prospective and retrospective studies have shown that the incidence of CTEPH ranges between 1% and 5% after an acute episode of PE.[83] One meta-analysis reported an incidence of around 3% among patients surviving the acute PE event.[84] The incidence of CTEPH was higher in Asian patients than in European patients, with an incidence of 5% compared with 2%, respectively.[85] Risk factors for CTEPH are predominantly recurrent PE, unprovoked PE, older age, and large clot burden at the time of presentation.[83,84] However, 25% to 50% of patients with CTEPH do not have a documented history of acute PE, and the true incidence is thus underestimated. In addition, a large proportion of patients with residual symptoms after an acute PE event are not investigated. The overall incidence of CTEPH across the population was best investigated in Germany, where patients from three referral centers were prospectively followed. The researchers observed 392 new CTEPH diagnoses, yielding an incidence of 5.7 new cases per million inhabitants.[86]

Pathology and Pathophysiology

PH is divided into five distinct World Health Organization (WHO) groups, which are categorized according to pathophysiology, clinical presentation, and therapies. WHO group 4 is classified as PH resulting from pulmonary artery obstruction, of which there are two subdivisions: (1) CTEPH and (2) other pulmonary artery obstructions.[87] As indicated earlier, CTEPH is defined by mPAP greater than 20 mm Hg in the presence of organized, nonacute thromboemboli and altered vascular remodeling in the pulmonary artery.[88]

The exact pathophysiology of CTEPH is still unclear. Most cases of chronic pulmonary emboli are believed to originate from previous acute PE. In an international registry, a history of acute PE was reported by 75% of patients.[81] However, many individuals with chronic pulmonary thromboembolic disease are unaware of a past thromboembolic event and do not report a history of DVT.

The thromboembolic material in patients with CTEPH differs from that in acute PE. Microscopically, acute PE specimens contain predominantly fibrin, inflammatory cells, and red blood cells. In contrast, resected chronic thromboemboli are considerably more complex.[89] Current investigations in the pathogenesis of CTEPH suggest that it is unlikely that a single factor leads to the development of chronic PH after acute PE but rather that a host of clinical factors and alterations in the postthrombotic response leads to the formation of chronic intravascular scar and, ultimately,

PH and RV dysfunction. Massive, idiopathic, and recurrent types of acute PE are suggested to be risk factors for development of CTEPH. Thrombophilic disorders, particularly antiphospholipid antibody syndrome and high coagulation factor VIII levels, were identified as a risk factor for CTEPH. CTEPH is also associated with other medical conditions, such as splenectomy, ventriculoatrial shunt, infected pacemaker leads, chronic indwelling catheters (e.g., ports and dialysis catheters), inflammatory bowel disease, systemic lupus erythematosus, malignancy, chronic venous ulcers, thyroid hormone replacement, and non-O blood group, among others.[89,90]

In CTEPH, the unresolved emboli within the pulmonary arteries undergo a series of changes. A fibrinolytic defect has been proposed to play a pathophysiologic role in the development of CTEPH. Fibrinolysis is a complicated process involving lysis of cross-linked fibrinogen through interactions between plasminogen, tissue plasminogen activator (t-PA), plasminogen activator inhibitor (PAI-1), and other regulatory proteins as well as interactions with the endothelium at the site of vessel injury. Reduced plasma fibrinolytic potential has been previously described as a risk factor for VTE, and some data suggest that this is true in CTEPH.[89] Factors such as the size and location of the emboli, the presence of multiple emboli, and underlying abnormalities in the clot-dissolving mechanisms can also contribute to incomplete resolution.

The chronic presence of the clots within the pulmonary arteries triggers inflammation and an immune response. This, in turn, leads to the proliferation of cells, remodeling of the blood vessel walls, and the formation of fibrous tissue that contracts the vessel. The remodeling narrows and obstructs the pulmonary arteries, increasing resistance to blood flow and causing elevated pulmonary arterial pressure. PH occurs after the remodeling and narrowing of the pulmonary arteries result in increased resistance to the blood flow from the RV to the lungs. The RV must work harder to pump blood against this increased resistance, leading to RV hypertrophy and, eventually, right heart failure.

In addition to the remodeling of larger pulmonary arteries, CTEPH also involves pathologic changes in small precapillary vessels, known as *distal arteriopathy*. These changes include the narrowing and obliteration of small arteries and arterioles, resembling the pathophysiology of Eisenmenger syndrome. Persistent PH from small-vessel disease after PTE remains the major cause of postoperative morbidity and mortality in CTEPH.[90]

Natural History

CTEPH is a severe and progressive disease, and most patients will die of progressive right heart failure without any treatment. The risk of death from right-sided heart failure in patients with undiagnosed or untreated CTEPH is correlated with PAP at diagnosis.[45] Riedel et al. reported that PH progressed in patients with an mPAP greater than 30 mm Hg, but no progress was observed in patients with a normal or borderline mean pulmonary arterial pressure. Among 13 patients, 9 died a mean of 28 months after the diagnosis of right heart failure. The severity of PH at the time of diagnosis inversely correlates with duration of survival. The 5-year survival rate was 30% for patients with mPAP greater than 40 mm Hg and only 10% for patients with PAP higher than 50 mm Hg.[91]

Clinical Presentation

Despite the importance of early diagnosis and intervention, recognizing CTEPH can be quite challenging because the clinical symptoms are nonspecific. The clinical picture often overlaps with other respiratory and cardiac conditions, contributing to the underdiagnosis of this condition, with varying signs and symptoms depending on the severity of the obstruction and right heart dysfunction.

Exertional dyspnea is the most common symptom. Patients may feel breathless even with minimal exertion. This dyspnea is often out of proportion to any abnormalities found on clinical examination.[45] Persistent fatigue and lack of energy are also commonly seen. Therefore, initially, dyspnea occurring only during exertion may be attributed to poor physical fitness, deconditioning, obesity, asthma, anxiety, or other more common causes of dyspnea on exertion, leading to delay in diagnosis.

As the disease progresses, additional symptoms may develop. Some patients with CTEPH may experience chest pain. Lightheadedness and syncope are also possible symptoms. Hemoptysis can occur in all forms of PH and may result from dilated vessels under increased intravascular pressures, but in CTEPH, hemoptysis is related to the development of large bronchial collaterals traversing to obstructed lung segments. Hemoptysis can also occur in the setting of infarcted lung parenchyma. Lower extremity edema, abdominal distention and early satiety, and right upper quadrant pain from liver capsular distention can occur as CTEPH progresses and are a direct result of right heart failure. Enlarged or prominent jugular veins in the neck may be easily visible.

Physical signs of PH are similar regardless of the underlying pathophysiology. Initially, the jugular venous pulse may exhibit a large A wave. As right heart failure progresses, the V wave becomes more prominent. The RV may be palpable near the lower left sternal border, and the closure of the pulmonary valve may be audible in the second intercostal space. With careful auscultation in the posterior lung regions, flow murmurs might be audible as flow accelerates past a tight stenosis in the pulmonary arteries. Advanced disease can lead to hypoxia and cyanosis.

As right heart failure develops, a right atrial gallop rhythm is often present, and tricuspid regurgitation develops. Because of the significant pressure gradient across the tricuspid valve in PH, the associated murmur is high-pitched and may not exhibit respiratory variation, which distinguishes it from murmurs associated with tricuspid valvular disease. A murmur of pulmonic regurgitation may also be detected.

Diagnosis

Patients presenting with unexplained dyspnea, exercise intolerance, or clinical evidence of right-sided heart failure, with or without prior history of symptomatic VTE, should be evaluated for PH, and CTEPH should be ruled out in all PH patients because it represents the only potentially curable form of PH. It is reasonable to evaluate patients with an echocardiogram 6 weeks after an acute PE to screen for persistent PH, which may help predict the development of CTEPH.[45] Because CTEPH is an important late sequela of acute PE, patients should be screened for radiologic signs of chronic lesions, especially if systolic PAP is >60 mm Hg by echocardiography at the initial presentation.[92] Follow-up is recommended at 3 months, and any impairment of physical capacity should be further evaluated.[26]

The diagnostic evaluation for CTEPH has three aims: (1) to establish the presence and severity of PH and resultant cardiac dysfunction; (2) to determine its cause; and (3) if thromboembolic disease is present, to determine the degree of obstruction and its concordance with the degree of PH to determine surgical candidacy.[45]

CXR is commonly performed, although it may be unrevealing even when there is significant PH. Enlargement of the central pulmonary arteries and RV may be observed. However, CXR is an important first step to narrow the differential diagnoses. Pulmonary function tests are necessary to evaluate dyspnea and are used to exclude the presence of obstructive airway or fibrotic lung disease. Single-breath diffusion capacity for carbon monoxide (DLCO) may be moderately reduced. Arterial blood oxygen levels may be normal even in the setting of significant PH, but most patients will experience a decline in PaO_2 with exertion.[45] Echocardiography is used to provide objective evidence of PH. An estimate of PAP can be made by Doppler evaluation of the tricuspid regurgitant envelope.[93]

V/Q lung scan remains the most effective method to rule out CTEPH. It has 96% to 97% sensitivity and 90% to 95% specificity for the diagnosis.[94] In most patients with primary PH, the lung scan appears relatively normal, whereas in CTEPH, it shows nonuniform perfusion patterns that signify perfusion-ventilation mismatched areas. If subsegmental or larger perfusion defects are detected on the scan, pulmonary angiography is appropriate to confirm or rule out thromboembolic disease.

To confirm the diagnosis of CTEPH, RHC and contrast-enhanced CT angiography with multiplane reconstruction or conventional pulmonary angiography are needed. RHC establishes the severity of PH, which, by definition, requires an mPAP of over 20 mm Hg and a PVR >3 Wood units at rest. It also assesses right- and left-sided heart filling pressures. Measurement of oxygen saturations in the SVC and IVC, right-sided chambers, and pulmonary artery may document previously undetected left-to-right shunting.[45] Mixed venous saturation can also be used for Fick CO calculation because CO measured by the thermodilution method may be inaccurate depending on the degree of tricuspid regurgitation. For older patients, coronary angiography and left heart catheterization provide additional but important information for those at risk of coronary artery or valvular disease and those with diastolic LV dysfunction. These are necessary for the preoperative risk assessment of patients deemed candidates for pulmonary thromboendarterectomy (PTE) and to determine whether concomitant coronary artery bypass graft or valve surgery needs to be undertaken simultaneously.[95]

Pulmonary angiography remains the gold standard for diagnosing chronic pulmonary thromboembolism. Selective pulmonary angiography with digital subtraction is used to precisely display the peripheral regions of the pulmonary circulation and provides dynamic imaging of perfusion.[96] It can yield high-value information about the level of obstruction, the degree of disease, the status of more distal vessels, and any evidence of significant distal arteriopathy, all crucial for surgical planning. In angiographic imaging, thrombi appear as unusual filling defects, pouches, webs, or bands or as completely thrombosed vessels that may resemble congenital absence of a vessel.[45] Distal vessels exhibit the characteristic tapering and pruning associated with PH as a result of vessel wall thickening and proximal vessel dilation.

CTPA provides additional information and may serve as an alternative if performed with thin slices of 0.5 to 1 mm and coronal and sagittal reconstructions using 1-mm slices. The pulmonary artery branches are contracted by the organized thromboembolic material; therefore, slices of 0.5 to 1 mm are essential to adequately assess subsegmental branches. Disease located in the main, lobar, and segmental branches is amenable to surgical resection. Other perfusion studies, such as dual-energy CT or MRI,

have theoretical advantages, but restricted availability and incomplete validation are important limitations.[97]

Some patients may present with normal pulmonary hemodynamics at rest despite symptomatic disease. If other causes of exercise limitation are excluded, these patients are considered as having chronic thromboembolic pulmonary disease without PH (CTEPD without PH), also referred to as *chronic thromboembolic disease* (CTED). These patients present with important symptomatology impairing their quality of life despite the lack of PH at rest. Their assessment therefore generally requires RHC with exercise and cardiopulmonary exercise testing (CPET). Identification of patients with CTED, who may have an indication for surgical or interventional treatment, requires particular expertise.[26]

Treatment

Surgery: Pulmonary Thromboendarterectomy/Pulmonary Endarterectomy

PTE, also known as *pulmonary endarterectomy* (PEA), is the treatment of choice and a potentially curative treatment for CTEPH. PEA was pioneered at the University of California, San Diego (UC San Diego), in which around 200 PEA procedures are now performed every year.[98,99] Around 0.9 PEA procedures per million population are performed annually in the United States and around 1.7 per million population in Europe,[99] representing a steady increase over the past decade as surgical expertise has improved and the number of expert centers has increased worldwide. Inserting an IVC device before endarterectomy has been abandoned at the leading surgical centers because IVC filter placement before surgery did not influence long-term survival.[88]

Although the fundamental techniques of PTE surgery are similar to those of other open-heart operations requiring profound hypothermia and periods of circulatory arrest, there are certain guiding principles for this procedure.[100] Median sternotomy, CPB, deep hypothermic circulatory arrest (DHCA), identification and dissection in the appropriate plane, and a complete endarterectomy are the principles of this procedure. The disease, and therefore its surgical removal, is almost always bilateral, although the volume of disease may vary significantly between the two lungs. Despite some recent experience with minimally invasive PTE surgery through mini–anterior thoracotomy incisions, the preferred approach to both pulmonary arteries is through a median sternotomy incision.

Exceptional visibility of the pulmonary vasculature is required to identify the endarterectomy plane and then to follow it deep into the subsegmental branches.[100,101] Because of the copious bronchial blood flow usually present in these patients, periods of DHCA are necessary to ensure perfect visibility. It should be emphasized that although endarterectomy is possible without DHCA, a complete endarterectomy is not. A large, randomized study from the Papworth group at Cambridge indicated inferior visualization and less complete endarterectomy in the low-flow non-DHCA patients, requiring intraoperative crossover to the DHCA group.[102] There was no statistically significant difference in cognitive function postoperatively, although the DHCA group had somewhat better outcomes. The DHCA periods are typically limited to 20 minutes, with restoration of flow between each arrest. With experience, the endarterectomy can usually be performed with a single period of DHCA on each side. A true endarterectomy in the plane of intima and media must be accomplished, and all fibrotic material must be removed. It is essential to appreciate that the removal of visible proximal thrombus is largely incidental to this operation.

Operative Techniques

After a median sternotomy is made, the pericardium is incised and attached to the wound edges. Typically, the right heart is enlarged, with a tense RA and a variable degree of tricuspid regurgitation. There is usually severe RV hypertrophy. These patients are generally quite sensitive to any manipulation of the heart, and with critical degrees of obstruction, the patient's condition may become quite unstable. Anticoagulation is achieved with the use of heparin (400 units/kg, intravenously) administered to prolong the activated clotting time beyond 400 seconds. Full CPB is instituted with high ascending aortic cannulation and two caval cannulae. The heart is emptied on bypass, and a temporary pulmonary artery vent is placed in the midline of the main pulmonary artery 1 cm distal to the pulmonary valve. When CPB is initiated, surface cooling with both the head jacket and the cooling blanket is begun. The blood is cooled with the pump-oxygenator. Cooling generally takes 45 minutes to 1 hour. When ventricular fibrillation occurs, an additional vent is placed in the LV through the right superior pulmonary vein. This prevents atrial and ventricular distention from the large amount of bronchial arterial blood flow that is common with these patients. Fig. 114.4 shows the typical instruments used during PTE surgery, and Fig. 114.5 shows the operative setup and the RPA exposure.

Typically, the primary surgeon starts the operation standing on the patient's left side. During the cooling period, some preliminary dissection can be performed, with full mobilization of the RPA from the ascending aorta. The SVC is also fully mobilized. The approach to the RPA is made medial, not lateral, to SVC. All dissection of both pulmonary arteries takes place intrapericardially, and neither pleural cavity is entered. An incision is then made in the RPA from beneath the ascending aorta out under the SVC, entering the lower lobe branch of the RPA. It is important that the incision stays in the center of the vessel and continues into the lower rather than the middle lobe artery.

When the patient's temperature reaches 20°C, the aorta is cross-clamped, and a single dose of mixed blood Del Nido cold cardioplegia (1 L) is administered. Several centers use a cooling jacket for additional myocardial protection. The entire procedure is now performed with a single aortic cross-clamp period with no further administration of cardioplegic solution.

A modified cerebellar (or a Madani PTE) retractor (the "J" instrument shown in Fig. 114.4) is placed between the aorta and SVC, as shown in the Fig. 114.5 insert. Upon opening the RPA, a varying degree of loose thrombus may be present, which can be removed to ensure good visualization of the vascular bed. It is important to recognize, however, that first, an embolectomy without subsequent endarterectomy is quite ineffective, and second, in most patients, initial examination of the pulmonary vascular bed shows no obvious thrombotic material. Therefore, to the inexperienced or cursory glance, the pulmonary vascular bed may appear normal even in patients with severe CTEPH. Fig. 114.6 shows the typical findings within the pulmonary artery of a patient with CTEPH.

If the bronchial circulation is not excessive, the endarterectomy plane can be found during this early dissection. However, although a small amount of dissection can be performed before arrest, it is unwise to proceed unless perfect visibility is obtained. Recognizing the correct plane of dissection is perhaps the most crucial and challenging part of this operation. When blood obscures direct vision of the pulmonary vascular bed, propofol is administered (200 mg) until the electroencephalogram becomes isoelectric. In most cases, the electroencephalogram is already

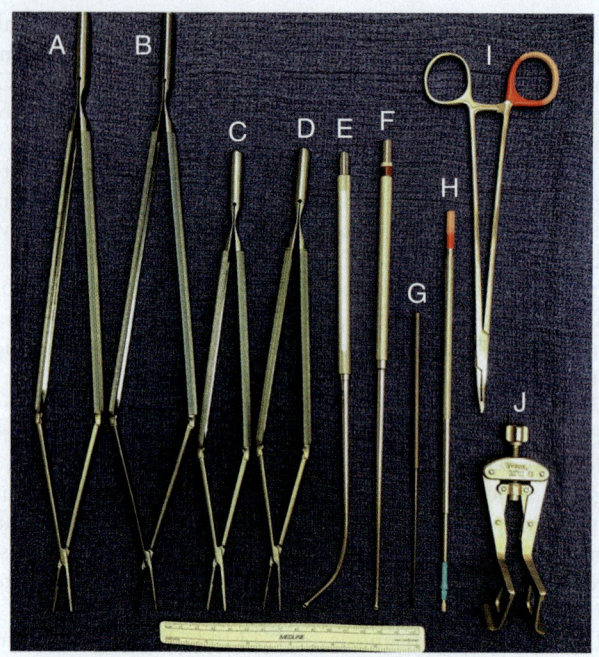

FIGURE 114.4 PTE instrument set: (A) 16″ double-action Madani PTE forceps with 2.5-mm tip; (B) 16″ double-action Madani PTE forceps with 1-mm tip; (C) 12″ double-action Madani PTE forceps with 2.5-mm tip; (D) 12″ double-action Madani PTE forceps with 1-mm tip; (E) modified curved Jamieson PTE suction/dissector; (F) modified Jamieson PTE suction/dissector; (G) Micro-Penfield 4 dissector; (H) fine beaver blade; (I) "mini-nut" dissector—small 7-mm by 3-mm by 1-mm PTFE buttress pledget in a 10″ tonsil clamp; (J) Madani PTE retractor. *PTE*, Pulmonary thromboendarterectomy; *PTFE*, polytetrafluoroethylene.

isoelectric when the core temperature reaches 20°C. DHCA is then initiated, and the patient undergoes exsanguination. It is rare that one 20-minute period for each side is exceeded. Although retrograde and low-flow antegrade cerebral perfusion techniques are used for DHCA in other procedures, they are not helpful in PTE because they do not allow a completely bloodless field,[102] and with the short DHCA times that can be achieved with experience, it is not necessary.

A microtome knife is used to develop the endarterectomy plane posteriorly because any inadvertent egress in this site could be repaired readily or simply left alone. The endarterectomy is then performed with an eversion technique. It is important that each subsegmental branch is followed and freed until it ends in a "tail" beyond which there is no further obstruction. Residual material should never be cut free; the entire specimen should "tail off" and come free spontaneously. Upon inspection and endarterectomy, one may encounter several signs of chronic thromboembolic obstruction, such as webs, pouches, complete occlusions, or just merely thickened intima (see Fig. 114.6).

After the right-sided endarterectomy is completed and before initiation of bypass, a bubble test is performed to identify any potential vascular injury.[103] Although rare in experienced hands, a continuous stream of bubbles with a peak inspirator pressure of 25 to 30 cm H_2O is quite concerning for postoperative airway hemorrhage and should be carefully investigated while on circulatory arrest and appropriately dealt with.[104] Circulation is then restarted, and the arteriotomy is closed with a continuous 6-0 polypropylene suture.

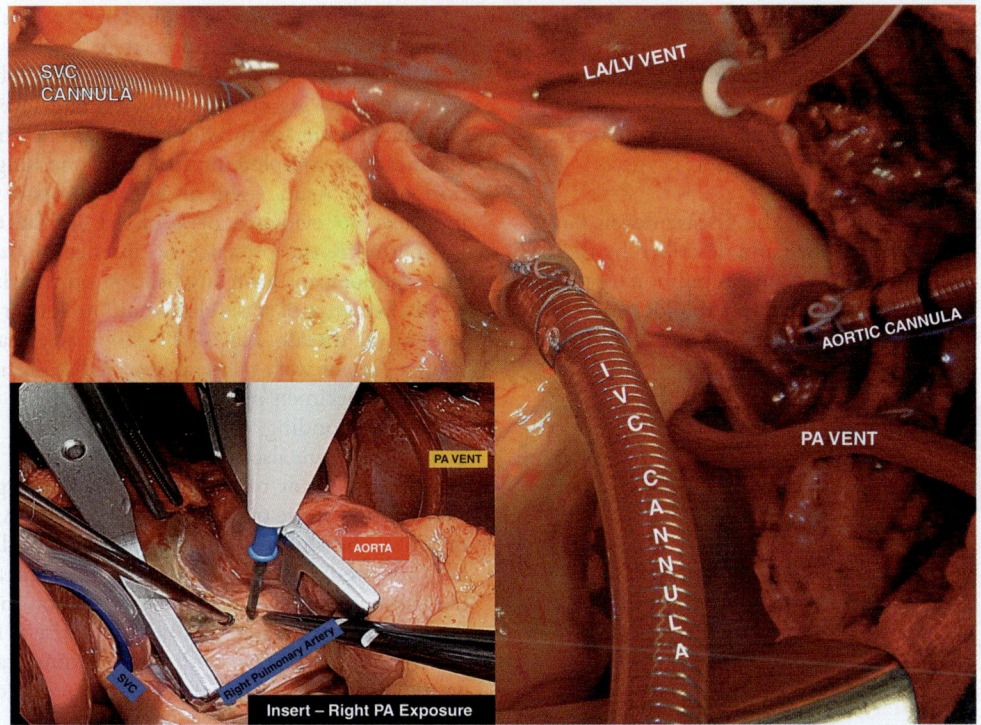

FIGURE 114.5 Operative field setup and view. Typically, the SVC and IVC cannulae are crossed for easier initiation of bypass, without manipulating the right heart. The *insert* figure shows the exposure of the right pulmonary artery between the aorta and SVC. *IVC,* Inferior vena cava; *LA,* left atrium; *LV,* left ventricle; *PA,* pulmonary artery; *SVC,* superior vena cava.

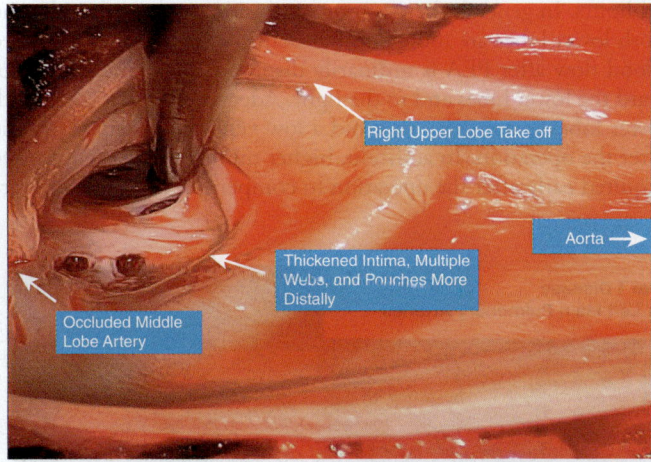

FIGURE 114.6 Typical chronic thromboembolic pulmonary hypertension findings within the pulmonary artery. Aorta is retracted medially to the left side.

Then, the surgeon moves to the patient's right side. The pulmonary vent catheter is withdrawn, and an arteriotomy is made from the site of the pulmonary vent hole laterally to the pericardial reflection, avoiding entry into the left pleural space. Additional lateral dissection does not enhance intraluminal visibility, may endanger the left phrenic nerve, and makes subsequent repair of the left pulmonary artery more difficult. The left-sided dissection is virtually analogous in all respects to that accomplished on the right, and the duration of DHCA intervals is subject to the same restrictions.

After the completion of the endarterectomy, CPB is reinstituted, and warming is commenced. The rewarming period generally takes approximately 90 to 120 minutes, but it varies according to the body mass of the patient. Then, the pulmonary artery is closed, and the pulmonary vent is replaced. If there is evidence of patent foramen ovale or atrial septal defect, the RA is then opened, and any interatrial communication is closed. Although tricuspid valve regurgitation is variable in these patients and can be severe, tricuspid valve repair traditionally has not been performed. The rationale is that RV remodeling occurs within a few days, with the return of tricuspid competence.[105,106] However, in the long term, tricuspid regurgitation may recur despite a complete endarterectomy. We typically repair tricuspid valves when the regurgitation is severe and/or if the annulus is larger than 4 cm. Clearly, any leaflet damage, such as that seen from pacemaker leads, will require repair. Intracardiac pacemaker leads in CTEPH patients should be carefully examined and, in most cases, exchanged for epicardial leads.

If other cardiac procedures are required, such as coronary artery or mitral or aortic valve surgery, these are conveniently performed during the systemic rewarming period.[95,98] Myocardial cooling is discontinued after all cardiac procedures have been concluded. The left atrial vent is removed, and the vent site is repaired. All air is removed from the heart, and the aortic cross clamp is removed. When the patient has fully rewarmed, CPB is discontinued. Dopamine hydrochloride is routinely administered at renal doses, and other inotropic agents and vasodilators are titrated as necessary to sustain acceptable hemodynamics. The CO is generally high, with a low systemic vascular resistance. Temporary atrial and ventricular epicardial pacing wires are placed.

Despite the duration of extracorporeal circulation, hemostasis is readily achieved, and the administration of blood products and coagulation factors is generally not indicated and unnecessary. Wound closure is routine. A vigorous diuresis is usual for the next few hours, also a result of the previous systemic hypothermia.

Thromboembolic Surgical Classification

A recent intraoperative classification of the disease (levels 0–IV), as shown in Table 114.4, was developed and described by the UC San Diego group. The classification categorizes pulmonary thromboembolism in CTEPH into levels based on the location of the fibrotic thromboembolic material.[107–109]

TABLE 114.4 University of California, San Diego, Chronic Thromboembolic Disease Surgical Classification[a]

Level 0 (R/L)
No evidence of chronic thromboembolic disease

Level I (R/L)
Chronic thromboembolic disease encountered in the main pulmonary artery

Level I C (R/L)
Complete occlusion of one main pulmonary artery with thromboembolic disease

Level II (R/L)
Chronic thromboembolic disease starting at the level of lobar arteries or in the main descending pulmonary arteries

Level III (R/L)
Chronic thromboembolic disease starting at the level of the subsegmental arteries

Level IV (R/L)
Chronic thromboembolic disease starting at the level of the segmental arteries

[a]The classification is based on the most proximal disease identified in each pulmonary artery and is designated R (for the right lung) and L (for the left lung).

There are four levels of pulmonary occlusive disease related to thrombus that can be appreciated: level 1, involving the main pulmonary arteries; level 2, starting at the lobar branches; level 3, starting at the segmental branches; and level 4, where disease is only encountered at the subsegmental branches. In addition, level 1C indicates complete occlusion of one lung with total obstruction of the main right or left pulmonary artery, and level 0 indicates no evidence of CTEPH in the corresponding lung. Furthermore, the presence or absence of fresh thromboembolic material does not have any bearing on the classification. In other words, presence of stasis clot would no longer upgrade the surgical level of the disease. Fig. 114.7 shows a typical specimen removed from a patient with bilateral level 1 disease, and Fig. 114.8 shows a typical specimen removed from a patient with level 3 disease. The corresponding pulmonary angiogram and typical radiographic signs are also highlighted.

It is important to note that this is a surgical classification as encountered at the time of endarterectomy. As imaging modalities improve, the ability to predict the level of disease preoperatively has improved; however, invariably, more disease is encountered at the time of surgery than predicted on routine imaging preoperatively. Notably, greater technical expertise is required for level III to IV disease resection with higher complications, but hemodynamic improvement can still be expected after successful surgery.

Postoperative Care

Meticulous postoperative management is essential to the success of this operation. Although much of the postoperative care is common to that of the more ordinary open-heart surgery patients, there are some important differences.

First, all patients are mechanically ventilated for at least 24 hours. In general, there is more occlusion on the right side, and both lower lobes are more affected than the upper lobes. Restored blood flow after PEA is ordinarily disproportionately directed toward the lower lobes and to the right. Adequate ventilation of both lower lobes is necessary to avoid a low ventilation-perfusion ratio after the operation. In addition, higher minute ventilation is often required early after the operation to compensate for the temporary

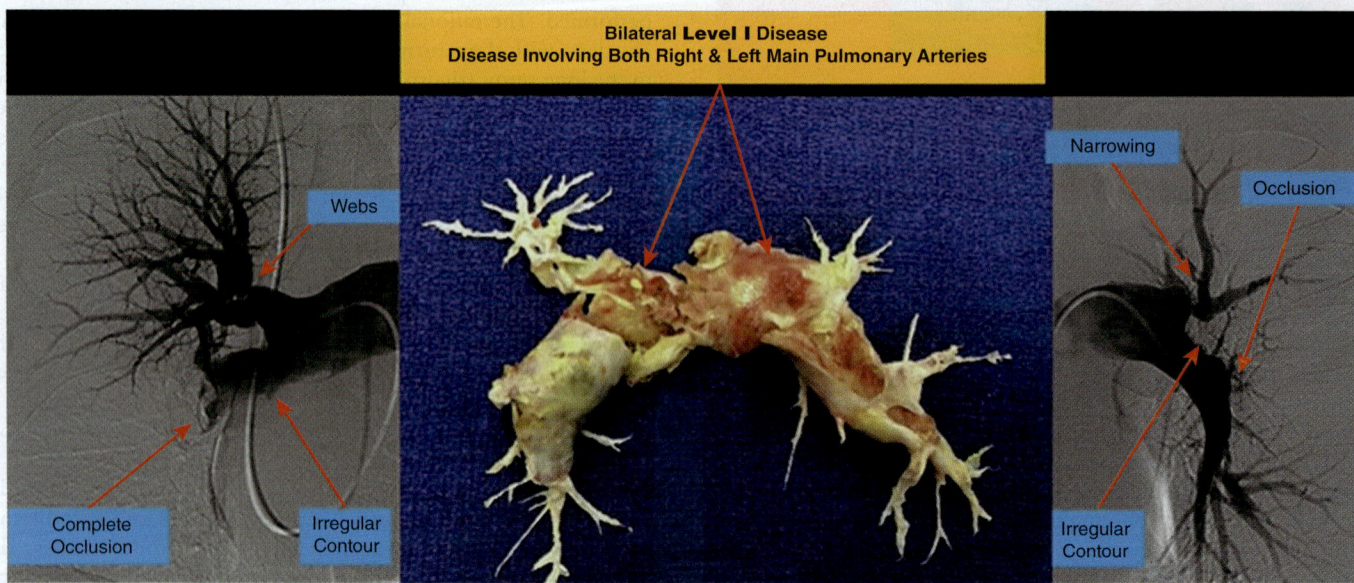

FIGURE 114.7 Specimen removed from a patient with bilateral level I (main pulmonary artery) disease, showing the corresponding intraoperative and preoperative pulmonary angiographic findings.

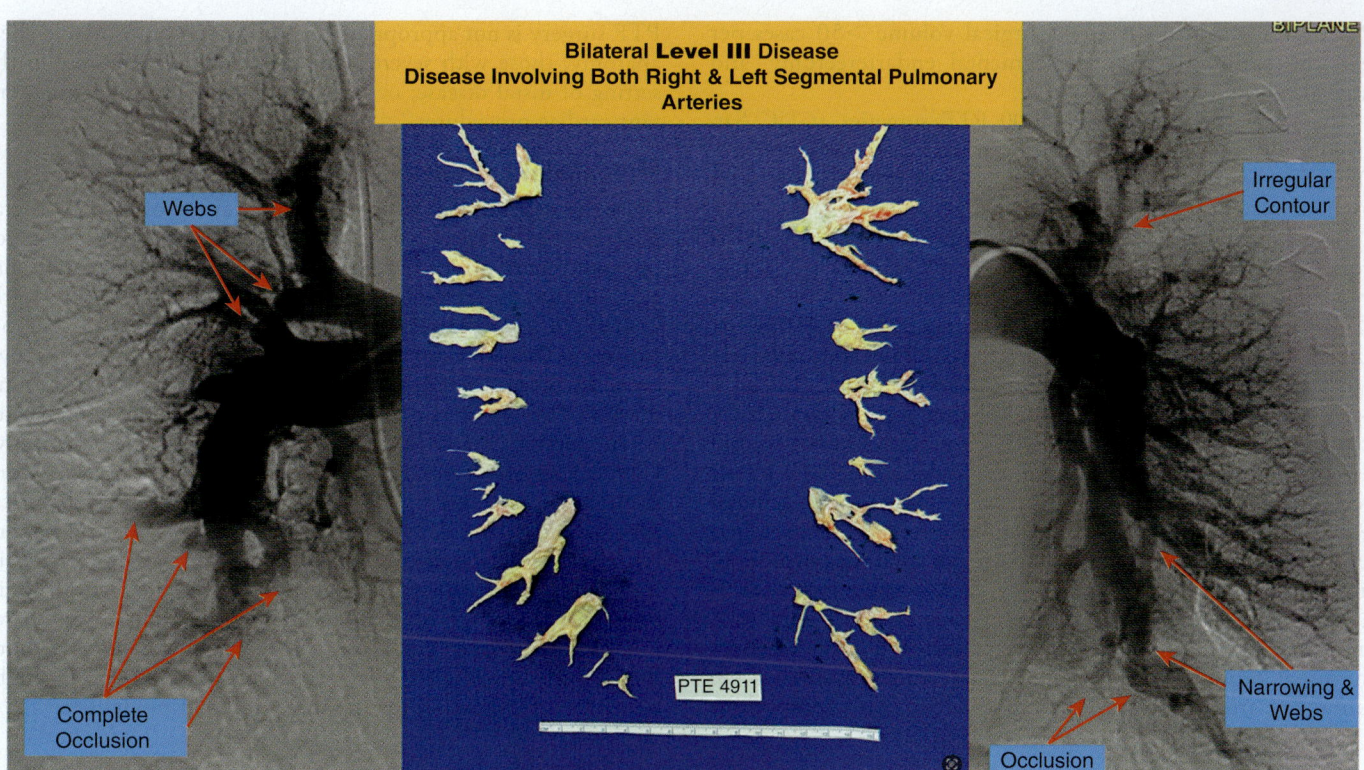

FIGURE 114.8 Specimen removed from a patient with bilateral level III (segmental) disease, showing the corresponding intraoperative and preoperative pulmonary angiographic findings.

metabolic acidosis that develops after the long period of circulatory arrest, hypothermia, and CPB. Extubation should be performed on the first postoperative day, if possible.

Second, all patients are subjected to a maintained diuresis with the goal of reaching the patient's preoperative dry weight within the first 24 hours. Patients are in considerable positive fluid balance after operation because of perioperative fluid administration, the administration of fluid from the bypass circuit, and the tendency of the patient to retain fluid during profound hypothermia. Patients initiate an early, spontaneous aggressive diuresis, but this should be augmented with diuretics.

ECG, systemic and pulmonary arterial and central venous pressures, temperature, urine output, arterial oxygen saturation, chest tube drainage, and fluid balance are monitored. A pulse oximeter is used to continuously monitor peripheral oxygen saturation. Management of cardiac arrhythmias and output and treatment of wound bleeding are identical to those for other open-heart operations.[101]

Complications

Not only are patients after PTE subject to all complications associated with open-heart and major lung surgery (arrhythmias, atelectasis, wound infection, pneumonia, mediastinal bleeding, etc.), but also specific complications may arise. One such complication is the development of a "reperfusion response." This is a specific complication that occurs in most patients to some degree and is related to localized pulmonary edema. Reperfusion pulmonary edema is a phenomenon in which endarterectomized and reperfused areas of lung develop a high-permeability edema.[110] Severe cases can cause airway hemorrhage, which can also occur because of trauma during surgical dissection, friability of endarterectomized vessels, and bleeding from systemic-to-pulmonary

collateral arteries. Both reperfusion pulmonary edema and airway hemorrhage are associated with increased mechanical ventilation days, length of stay, and mortality.[110] Treatment remains supportive, including use of an extracorporeal membrane oxygenator.[111,112]

Residual PH, although not defined precisely, is also associated with high perioperative mortality.[113] The role and timing of rescue pharmacotherapy, balloon pulmonary angioplasty (BPA), or both in patients with severe residual PH are not well defined.

Severe airway bleeding should be managed, if possible, by identification of the affected area by bronchoscopy and balloon occlusion of the affected lobe until coagulation can be normalized.[104] ECMO can be very helpful in managing airway bleeding.[104,114] Hemoptysis from a bronchial collateral can be unique because airway bleeding starts with bright-red blood while the patient is still on full CPB with no forward pulmonary flow. It is rare to require bronchial artery embolization, but this is occasionally required if ongoing systemic airway bleeding ensues. In contrast, the amount of airway bleeding secondary to vessel wall injury directly correlates with the amount of pulmonary artery flow and will be at its worst upon termination of bypass.

Surgical Advancements

Over the last decade, several innovations have enhanced surgical techniques and approach. Perhaps the most important advancement has been redefining the limits of distal endarterectomy. In expert centers, PTE can be successfully performed in patients with distal disease. This is attributed to advances in imaging, techniques, instruments, and surgical experience. Depending on the level of experience of a center, operability may vary. A new definition of expert center has been proposed as the following: availability of all treatment modalities

(PTE, BPA, medical therapy), surgical volume >50 cases per year, the ability to perform segmental endarterectomy, and surgical mortality <5%.[88]

There have now been over 5000 PTE surgeries at UC San Diego, and almost all of these have been carried out since the early 1990s. The mortality is now in the range of 1% to 1.5%, with sustained benefit.

Based on advances in cardiac surgery, minimally invasive techniques for PTE have been developed at UC San Diego. Using preoperative CT for surgical planning, the procedure is performed using the second or the third intercostal space through bilateral or unilateral mini–anterior thoracotomies approximately 4 to 5 cm in length. The ideal location of the incisions is both high enough for central aortic cannulation yet low enough for access to the pulmonary arteries. This typically is in the second intercostal space. The arterial cannula is placed centrally in the ascending aorta, and venous cannulae are placed in the femoral vein, RA, and/or right internal jugular vein. For all these patients, cardioplegia and cross clamp are not used for purposes of simplification and to maximize space. An aortic root vent is intermittently used just before going back on CPB with each circulatory arrest. Pulmonary artery and left atrial vents are used. The usual protocol for circulatory arrest and exposure of the pulmonary arteries is used. The minimally invasive approach to PTE surgery is not appropriate for patients with unsuitable chest anatomy; those with severe right heart failure, especially in the setting of distal disease; or those who are undergoing concomitant cardiac procedures.[99,115]

Multimodality Treatment Options

Over the past decade, although a wide variety of medical therapies have become available for the treatment of CTEPH, including pulmonary artery hypertensive (PAH), the appropriate use and efficacy of such medical treatments has not been clearly defined in CTEPH. PTE surgery has been the only curable treatment available for patients with CTEPH.[113,116,117] However, the first international CTEPH registry found that around 36.4% of all CTEPH patients were deemed by the clinicians to be inoperable.[81] According to the new worldwide prospective CTEPH registry from the data of 1010 newly diagnosed consecutive patients, reasons for PEA inoperability were technical inaccessibility ($n = 235$), comorbidities ($n = 63$), and patient refusal ($n = 44$).[118] Because of poor long-term survival rates in inoperable patients, with 70% at 3 years compared with 89% in operable patients,[119] determination of operability is of paramount importance. For those who are truly inoperable, both medical therapy and BPA are available.[88,96,109] Fig. 114.9 highlights the site of action for the three different modalities.

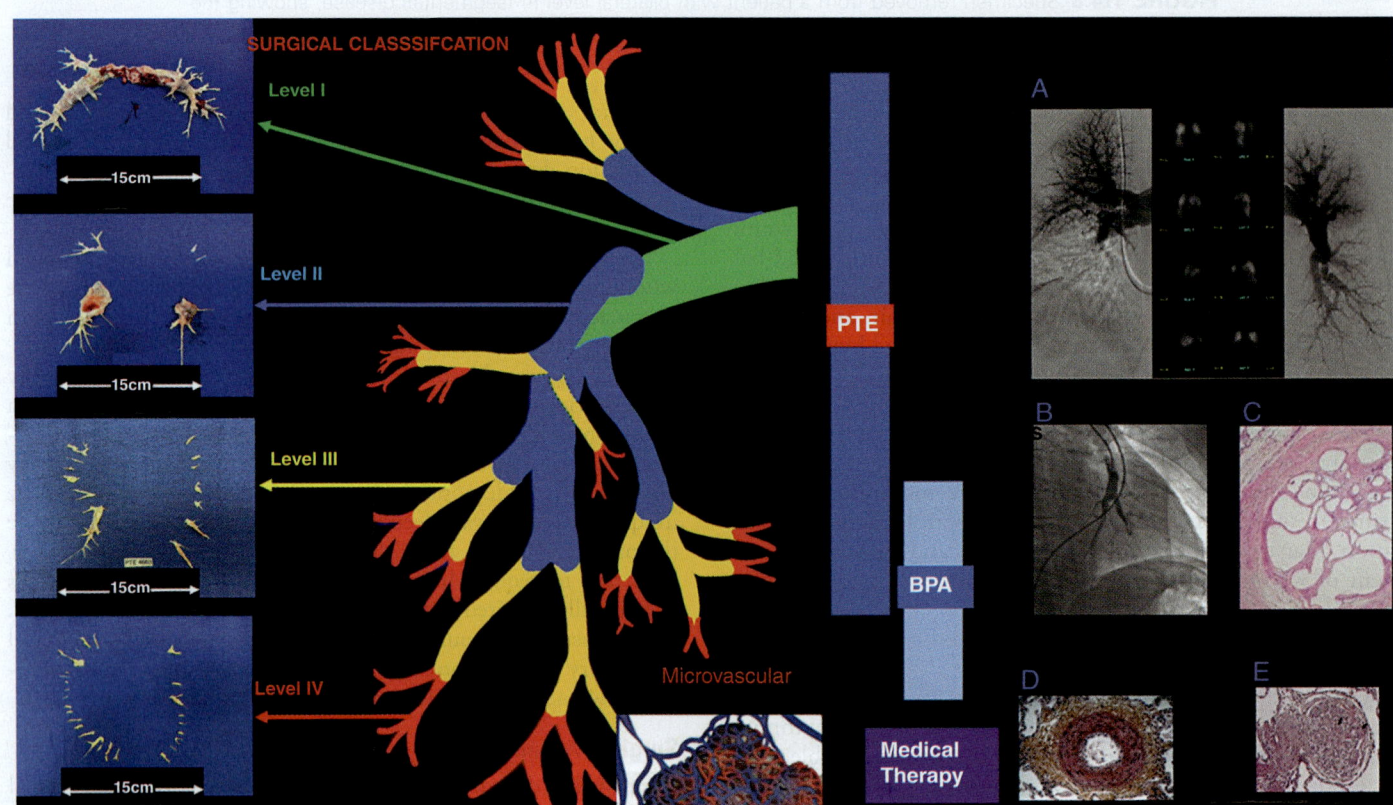

FIGURE 114.9 Treatment options for CTEPH target different pathogenic manifestations in different parts of the pulmonary vascular bed. (A) Perfusion scan and pulmonary angiogram of typical CTEPH patient. (B) Selective pulmonary angiogram of segmental and subsegmental pulmonary arteries, showing irregular vessel contour and occlusion, typical of CTEPH. (C) Microscopic examination showing a luminal filling defect with recanalized chronic thrombus (web lesion) and no evidence of vasculopathy in the subsegmental artery. (D) Intimal fibromuscular proliferation. (E) Plexiform lesion and vessel occlusion resulting from vasculopathy and proliferation. *BPA,* Balloon pulmonary angioplasty; *CTEPH,* chronic thromboembolic pulmonary hypertension; *PTE,* pulmonary thromboendarterectomy.

Medical Therapy

Riociguat and subcutaneous treprostinil are currently approved medical therapies for CTEPH. Riociguat is a soluble guanylate cyclase stimulator. Impairment of nitric oxide synthesis and signaling through the nitric oxide–soluble guanylate cyclase–cyclic guanosine monophosphate pathway is involved in the pathogenesis of PH. Riociguat has a dual mode of action, directly stimulating soluble guanylate cyclase independently of nitric oxide and increasing the sensitivity of soluble guanylate cyclase to nitric oxide. Riociguat increases the level of cyclic guanosine monophosphate, resulting in vasorelaxation and antiproliferative and antifibrotic effects.[120] Treprostinil is a prostacyclin. It reduces PAP and PVR by inhibiting the contraction of the pulmonary artery.[121]

Balloon Pulmonary Angioplasty

BPA was popularized in Japan in 2012,[122,123] mainly as a result of the lack of high-volume expert PTE centers. It is now being used with increasing frequency for inoperable patients in expert centers. BPA is less invasive, does not require anesthesia, and involves using angiographically directed wires and balloons to widen stenotic lesions and break up webs and bands in distal vessels to restore blood flow. BPA showed the improvement of symptoms and hemodynamics in inoperable patients. It has been established to address peripheral targets because the main reason for inoperability is surgical inaccessibility and comorbidities.[124–128] About 10% of patients have complications during the BPA procedure.[129,130] Vascular injury with or without hemoptysis by wire perforation or balloon overdilatation, high-pressure contrast injection, vascular dissection, allergic reaction to contrast, and adverse reaction to conscious sedation or local anesthesia, among other complications, may occur. After the procedure, lung injury (radiographic opacity with or without hemoptysis, with or without hypoxemia), renal dysfunction, or access site problems may also occur.[88]

BPA has been shown to provide improvement in symptoms and quality of life, with relatively low risk of complications in expert centers. However, BPA requires multiple sessions and generally carries a high risk of vessel perforation, especially in completely occluded vessels. Importantly, interventional treatment of more proximal lesions (= surgically accessible) leads to worse outcomes.[131] Furthermore, because the disease is left behind and the vessel compliance remains abnormal, patients continue to have diminished exercise tolerance despite improved hemodynamic numbers at rest.[132] Furthermore, the long-term consequences for patients who undergo BPA yet have unresolved residual thromboembolic disease are unknown.

Perioperative Medical Therapy or Balloon Pulmonary Angioplasty

Because complete relief of the pulmonary vasculature can only be achieved by surgery, PTE remains the treatment of choice.[96,109] However, borderline cases with severe hemodynamic impairment might be addressed by multimodal strategies aiming to reduce the risk of surgery. Multimodal treatment concepts may be beneficial in certain patients, but thorough evaluation and decision-making by an experienced multidisciplinary team is mandatory. These are the scenarios that the specialists may encounter:

1. Although there is no approved drug for operable CTEPH, medical pretreatment is regularly seen even before evaluation at an expert center, usually leading to a delay of (potentially curative) surgery.[81,118,133] Perioperatively, inhaled iloprost is used in some centers.[134,135] For residual PH after PTE, both riociguat and treprostinil are approved.[120,121]

2. BPA of certain subsegmental disease, which is likely to be inaccessible for the surgeon, might also be a strategy in unique patients; however, the approach is not universally adopted in experienced centers. Recently, in a proof-of-concept study in nine selected CTEPH patients with mixed (proximal and distal) anatomic lesions and high preoperative PVR (PVR >800 dynes·sec·cm^{-5}), sequential multimodal therapy combining medical treatment, BPA, and PTE was found to be a safe and effective option.[136] However, evidence supporting this approach remains scarce.

3. The combination of intraoperative BPA in surgically inaccessible regions has been described but remains a single-center experience.[129] BPA for residual/recurrent PH after PTE appears promising, with growing evidence.[130,137,138]

Outcomes

Like other major cardiac procedures, there has not been an RCT of PTE surgery versus other treatment options. However, there are multiple published large case series that demonstrate the effectiveness of PTE with respect to hemodynamic outcomes, with two reporting over 2000 consecutive patients.[116,139] The degree of reduction in mPAP and PVR was comparable and greater than that demonstrated by medical treatment and BPA. In the largest series published, from UC San Diego, there was a reduction in PVR from 719 to 253 dynes·sec·cm^{-5} in the most recent 500-patient cohort. Carefully controlled studies have confirmed no deterioration in cognitive function postsurgery despite the requirement for DHCA.[102]

Over time, successive large series have also demonstrated a reduction in perioperative mortality, with an in-hospital mortality of 2.2% for the latter reported cohort[116] and a 30-day mortality of 1.9% for a more contemporary cohort from the Cambridge group.[139] International registries have also shown a reduction in mortality. The initial international registry reported an in-hospital mortality of 4.7%,[113] with the most recent international registry reporting 3.5% mortality after PTE.[118] The use of ECMO has allowed salvage of patients with the most severe complications after surgery.[112]

The improvement in hemodynamic parameters after PTE has also led to functional and quality-of-life benefits for patients, and these are sustained at 5 years.[140] The improvement in perioperative outcomes has also translated into excellent long-term survival, with a national case series with the longest reported comprehensive follow-up demonstrating 86%, 84%, 79%, and 72% survival at 1, 3, 5, and 10 years, respectively.[141]

CONCLUSION

Acute PE is a common but life-threatening disease. It causes PH, RV dysfunction, and hypoxemia. Because symptoms and signs vary and there are no specific symptoms of acute PE, clinical diagnosis is often missed or falsely made. If patients have presentations suspicious for acute PE, it should be decisively investigated using all the tools available, including PE prediction scores, laboratory tests, and imaging modalities. The mortality of untreated PE is high, but it can be reduced by prompt and appropriate management. The specific treatment strategy is based on the classification for risk assessment. For hemodynamically unstable patients, respiratory and circulatory management in an intensive care unit under an expert team is the recommended approach.

The specific management for acute PE may include use of early anticoagulation, catheter-directed or systemic thrombolytic therapy, percutaneous suction thrombectomy, and surgical embolectomy. In certain patients, temporary use of ECMO may be helpful. Oral anticoagulation for more than 3 months is highly effective in preventing recurrent VTE; extended or indefinite anticoagulation should be considered in patients with cancer or coagulation disorders. Despite appropriate management, in about 1% to 5% of patients, prolonged symptoms, increased pulmonary pressures, and RV dysfunction persist, leading to CTEPH.

CTEPH is a unique form of PH (group 4) characterized by two-compartment disease, first as a direct result of unresolved thrombotic occlusion, often combined with a second compartment with concomitant and complex small-vessel arteriopathy. It is increasingly apparent that CTEPH is a more common condition than commonly recognized, and it carries a poor prognosis without treatment. The current approach to evaluation and treatment requires expertise from a multidisciplinary team working together to provide optimal treatment strategies. PTE (or PEA) surgery is the treatment of choice and can be potentially curative for patients with CTEPH. Although PTE is technically demanding for the surgeon, requiring careful dissection of the pulmonary artery planes and the use of DHCA, excellent short- and long-term results can be achieved. Successive improvements in operative technique developed over the last two decades now allow PTE to be offered to high-risk patients with a low mortality rate and anticipation of excellent clinical outcomes. Medical therapy and BPA have been shown to improve symptoms and function. They are generally reserved for patients with distal disease who are not surgical candidates or patients who suffer from residual PH after PTE. Increased understanding of both the prevalence of this condition and the possibility of a surgical cure and multimodality treatment options should avail more patients of the opportunity for relief from this debilitating and ultimately fatal disease. Although there is still more work to be done in the field of CTEPH treatment, it is important to make sure that patients with CTEPH are referred to experts who can provide them with a multimodal approach to treatment. The importance of expert referral for proper assessment and treatment strategy cannot be overemphasized.

SELECTED REFERENCES

Humbert M, Kovacs G, Hoeper MM, et al. 2022 ESC/ERS guidelines for the diagnosis and treatment of pulmonary hypertension. *Eur Heart J.* 2022;43:3618-731.

These are the latest guidelines by the ESC and the European Respiratory Society on management of PH. Although this is a comprehensive review of all major groups of PH, it still provides the latest and most up-to-date diagnostic and management strategies in relation to CTEPH. Furthermore, there is an updated and detailed diagnostic and treatment algorithm that readers will find quite helpful.

Jaff MR, McMurtry MS, Archer SL, et al. Management of massive and submassive pulmonary embolism, iliofemoral deep vein thrombosis, and chronic thromboembolic pulmonary hypertension: a scientific statement from the American Heart Association. *Circulation.* 2011;123:1788-830.

This scientific statement from the American Heart Association describes in detail the management and treatment of pulmonary embolism based on the severity and the size of the embolism and its impact in the acute setting. In addition, an overview of chronic thromboembolic pulmonary hypertension is also provided.

Jamieson SW, Kapelanski DP. Pulmonary endarterectomy. *Curr Probl Surg.* 2000;37:165-252.

This review is a landmark publication detailing the principles of pulmonary endarterectomy surgery in a step-by-step manner. The surgery was developed and pioneered at UC San Diego and has evolved over the years, but it is still followed very closely all around the world. Furthermore, this publication provided the principles of diagnosis, complications, and management strategies as practiced at UC San Diego, which continues to be a worldwide leader.

Kim NH, Delcroix M, Jais X, et al. Chronic thromboembolic pulmonary hypertension. *Eur Respir J.* 2019;53:1801915.

This review is the latest available summary of the 6th World Symposium on Pulmonary Hypertension as it relates to CTEPH. The manuscript provides a concise summary of the latest literature on CTEPH at the time of the symposium and provides the link between acute pulmonary embolism and CTEPH. It also provides an update on the diagnostic and treatment algorithm for CTEPH.

Konstantinides SV, Meyer G, Becattini C, et al. 2019 ESC guidelines for the diagnosis and management of acute pulmonary embolism developed in collaboration with the European Respiratory Society (ERS). *Eur Heart J.* 2020;41:543-603.

This important guideline is from the European Society of Cardiology in collaboration with the European Respiratory Society. The guidelines form the basis for diagnosis of acute pulmonary embolism and further provide a comprehensive management strategy for this disease. Many other international societies rely heavily on these specific guidelines by these two European societies.

The full reference list appears on Elsevier eBooks+.

CHAPTER 116

Advances in Extracorporeal Membrane Oxygenation: Techniques, Applications, and Management

Douglas Tran, Aakash Shah, Christine L. Lau, and Joseph Rabin

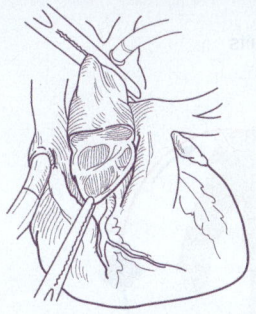

INTRODUCTION AND BRIEF HISTORY

Extracorporeal membrane oxygenation (ECMO) provides mechanical support to patients with severe cardiorespiratory failure. It is an important resource that can offer an essential lifeline to salvage such critically ill patients by delivering respiratory and/or cardiac support when conventional therapies fail. ECMO is broadly categorized into three distinct modalities: venoarterial (VA), venovenous (VV), and venoarteriovenous (V-AV). VA ECMO is employed for cardiac support and in patients with decompensating cardiac failure and compromised end-organ perfusion, whereas VV ECMO is used for severe respiratory failure with intact cardiac function and provides gas exchange to correct severe hypoxemia and or hypercarbia. The less common V-AV ECMO serves as a hybrid model that is useful in dynamic clinical scenarios requiring flexible transitions between circulatory and respiratory support (Fig. 116.1).

Dr. John Gibbon developed the first successful heart-lung machine used for open heart surgery in 1953. However, it was not until the late 1960s that technology advanced enough for long-term extracorporeal support.[1] Dr. Robert Bartlett is often called the father of modern ECMO. In 1975, he used ECMO to save a newborn with meconium aspiration syndrome and resultant pulmonary hypertension. This landmark case demonstrated ECMO's potential, leading to its gradual adoption in neonatal and pediatric care units.[1]

The 1970s and 1980s saw ECMO primarily used in neonatal and pediatric settings. In 1972, Bartlett and associates first used cardiac ECMO successfully for 36 hours in a 2-year-old infant with cardiac failure after a Mustard procedure. The first successful prolonged extracorporeal support in an intensive care setting was reported by Dr. J.D. Hill in 1972, with a 24-year-old male supported for 75 hours after a motorcycle accident.[1]

Early studies did not show a mortality benefit of ECMO in adult patients, leading to a decline in initial enthusiasm for its use in adults. However, Dr. Robert Bartlett persisted in using ECMO for pediatric patients, achieving good outcomes. This persistence and success in the pediatric population allowed ECMO to continue as a viable therapy in that setting until technology and techniques improved, enabling broader applications and better outcomes in adults as well.

The 1990s and 2000s witnessed a significant expansion in the use of ECMO for adults. The H1N1 influenza pandemic in 2009 led to a sharp increase in ECMO application due to its effectiveness in managing severe respiratory failure associated with acute respiratory distress syndrome (ARDS). This success highlighted ECMO's utility in respiratory epidemics, leading to broader acceptance and usage.[1,2]

Technologic advancements have continued to expand ECMO's deployment, with the shift from roller pump to centrifugal pump technology, offering safer and more efficient circulation. Additionally, the move from silicone membrane to polymethylpentene

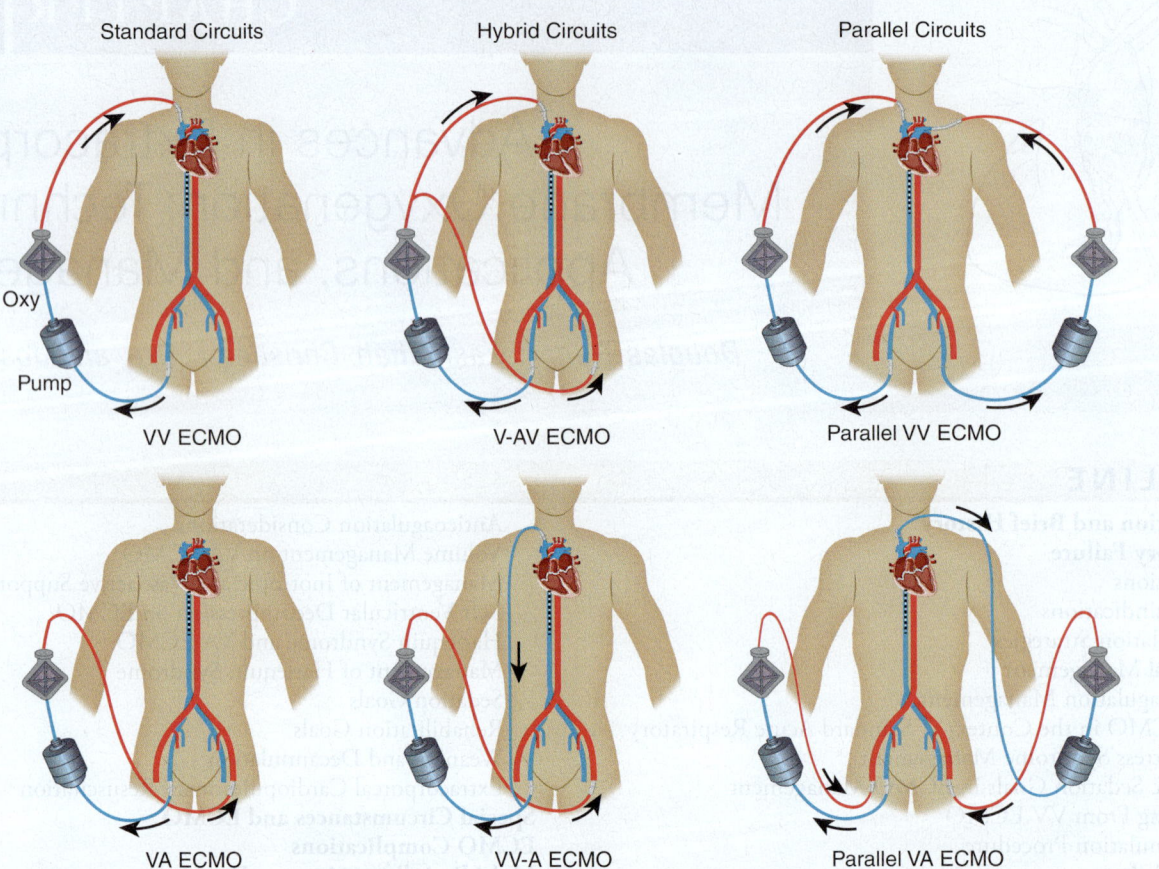

FIGURE 116.1 Various extracorporeal membrane oxygenation configurations including standard, hybrid, and parallel circuits. *Oxy*, Oxygen; *VA ECMO*, venoarterial extracorporeal membrane oxygenation; *V-AV ECMO*, venoarteriovenous extracorporeal membrane oxygenation; *VV ECMO*, venovenous extracorporeal membrane oxygenation; *VV-A ECMO*, venovenous-arterial extracorporeal membrane oxygenation. (From Shah A, Dave S, Goerlich CE, Kaczorowski DJ. Hybrid and parallel extracorporeal membrane oxygenation circuits. *JTCVS Tech.* 2021;8:77-85.)

oxygenators has allowed for better gas exchange and reduced blood trauma, further increasing the safety profile of ECMO support therapy (Fig. 116.2).

Ongoing ECMO research is focused on optimizing its efficacy and reducing risks associated with its insertion, circuit components, and prolonged patient cannulation. Its historical development from a niche surgical tool to a critical care mainstay underscores the importance of innovation and adaptation in medical technology.

ECMO cannulation techniques have also evolved over years from an open operative procedure to a percutaneous approach, especially in the setting of peripheral bedside cannulation. Peripheral ECMO cannulation often involves accessing vascular sites such as the jugular or femoral veins and femoral artery. Advances in technology enabled such peripheral cannulation to be safely and routinely performed at the bedside entirely percutaneously and outside of the operating room. This evolution has reduced complication rates and enabled faster initiation during emergency scenarios[3] (Fig. 116.3).

Conversely, central ECMO cannulation is generally reserved for intraoperative cases or postcardiotomy, offering advantages in specific patient populations but requiring intricate surgical skill. The approach for central cannulation can vary, with arterial cannulation done through a midline sternotomy for direct aortic/pulmonary artery cannulation or a right axillary cutdown for an axillary artery cannulation. Venous cannulation strategies can also

vary in this setting with either a central venous cannulation or a femoral venous cannulation with central arterial return.[3–5]

Parallel ECMO circuits are employed when a single ECMO circuit fails to provide sufficient support, typically in cases of high cardiac output states or severe hypoxia. In these situations, adding an additional drainage and return cannula connected to a separate ECMO circuit can enhance oxygenation and perfusion. This technique can be particularly useful in septic patients or those with refractory hypoxia despite optimal management. Parallel circuits necessitate careful consideration of potential complications such as recirculation within and between circuits, thrombus formation, and maintaining adequate flow distribution to prevent hemodynamic instability.[5]

Using parallel ECMO circuits can effectively manage patients with severe cardiorespiratory failure when traditional configurations are insufficient. However, it is essential to monitor for complications such as recirculation and thrombus formation, ensuring adequate flow distribution. This advanced strategy should be reserved for specific clinical scenarios and managed by experienced ECMO teams.

Setting appropriate expectations for ECMO outcomes is crucial for both medical professionals and patient families. ECMO can serve as a bridge to recovery, providing vital hemodynamic support and end-organ perfusion while the patient recuperates from the primary underlying pathology. It may also act as a bridge to definitive surgery, such as a transplant or complex cardiac

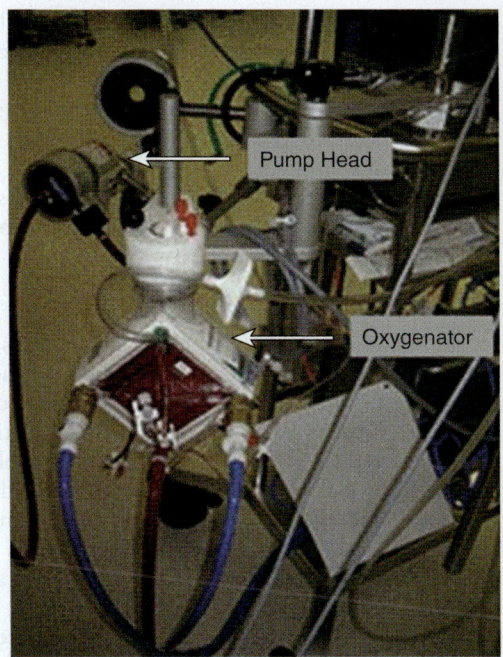
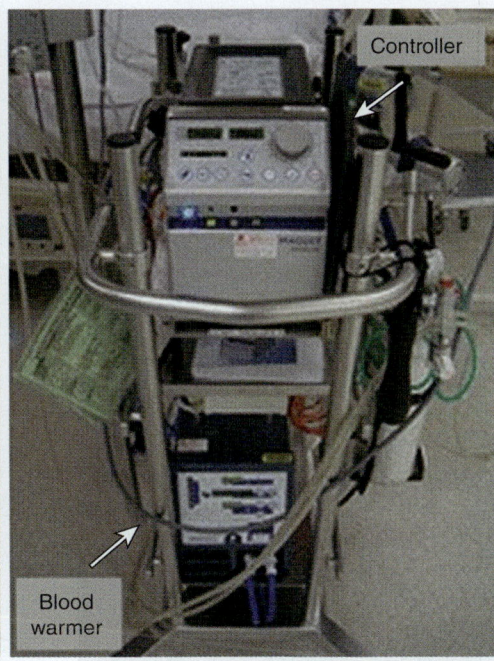

Pump Head

Oxygenator

Controller

Blood warmer

FIGURE 116.2 Extracorporeal membrane oxygenation circuit. (Courtesy UMMC: ECMO components.)

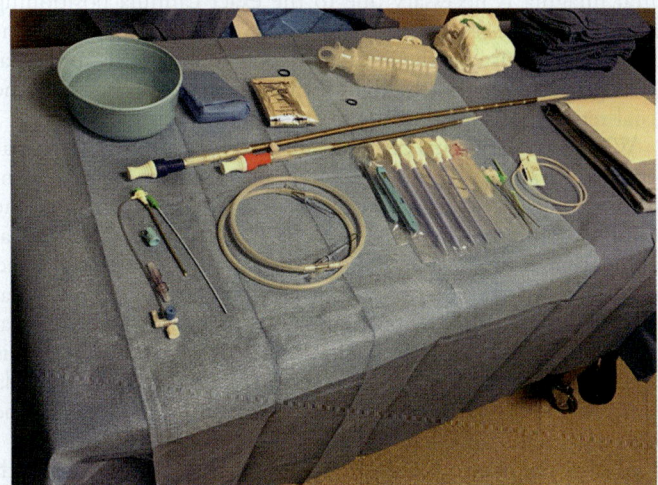

FIGURE 116.3 Bedside peripheral extracorporeal membrane oxygenation cannulation setup. (Courtesy UMMC: ECMO table setup.)

procedure. ECMO can also be used as a bridge to decision or "nowhere," and initiated when a patient's prognosis is uncertain; this can raise significant ethical considerations later regarding the continuation of life-sustaining treatments when such a patient fails to recover and has no definitive surgical option. It is critical to understand that ECMO does not cure the underlying disease; rather, it offers a temporary reprieve from a life-threatening situation, allowing for more comprehensive management of the patient's condition.

RESPIRATORY FAILURE

VV ECMO is a specialized configuration of mechanical support for patients with severe respiratory failure. It is used primarily as a bridge to recovery or as a bridge to a definitive surgical intervention.

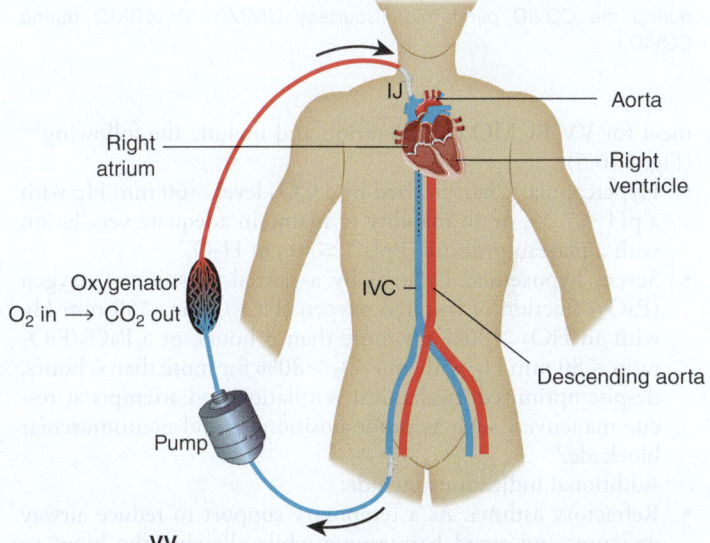

IJ

Aorta

Right atrium

Right ventricle

Oxygenator
O_2 in → CO_2 out

IVC

Descending aorta

Pump

VV

FIGURE 116.4 Venovenous extracorporeal membrane oxygenation cannulation configuration. *IJ,* Internal jugular; *IVC,* inferior vena cava; *VV,* venovenous. (From Shah A, Dave S, Goerlich CE, Kaczorowski DJ. Hybrid and parallel extracorporeal membrane oxygenation circuits. *JTCVS Tech.* 2021;8:77-85.)

This support system helps correct respiratory derangements including hypoxemia and/or hypercapnia that cannot be managed with conventional mechanical ventilation[2] (Fig. 116.4).

Indications

Extracorporeal Life Support Organization (ELSO) has published guidelines outlining specific criteria that patients should

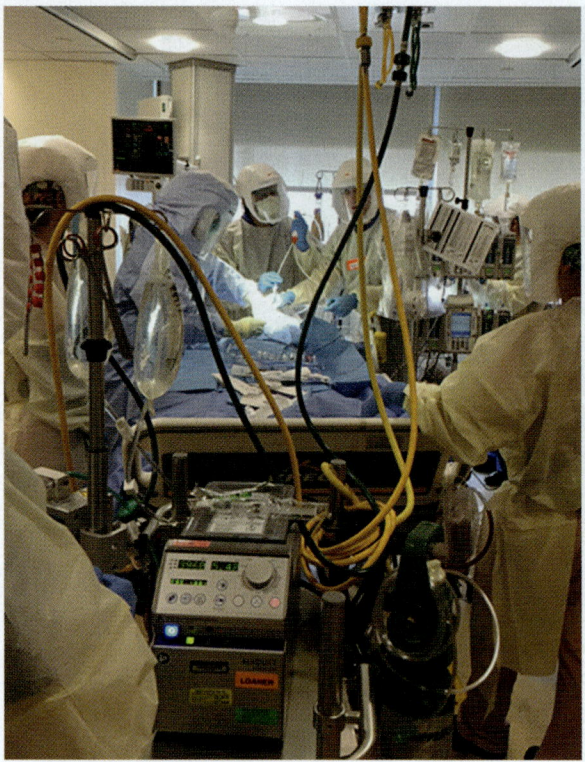

FIGURE 116.5 Venovenous extracorporeal membrane oxygenation during the COVID pandemic. (Courtesy UMMC: VV ECMO during COVID.)

meet for VV ECMO consideration and include the following[1,6] (Fig. 116.5):

- Hypercapnia: Characterized by a CO_2 level >60 mm Hg with a pH <7.25, or an inability to maintain adequate ventilation with a plateau pressure (Pplat) ≤30 cm H_2O.[1]
- Severe hypoxemia: Defined by a partial pressure of oxygen (PaO_2)/fraction of inspired oxygen (FiO_2) ratio <50 mm Hg with an FiO_2 >80% for more than 3 hours, or a PaO_2/FiO_2 ratio <80 mm Hg with an FiO_2 >80% for more than 6 hours, despite optimized mechanical ventilation and attempts at rescue maneuvers such as prone positioning and neuromuscular blockade.[1]

Additional indications include:

- Refractory asthma: As a temporary support to reduce airway pressures and avoid barotrauma while allowing the lungs to heal.
- Bridge to lung transplantation: In patients with end-stage pulmonary disease who are candidates for lung transplantation.
- Protection from ventilator-induced lung injury (VILI): In cases where high ventilatory pressures are needed, which could exacerbate lung injury.

Contraindications

Although there are few absolute contraindications to VV ECMO, several relative contraindications must be considered in the context of each patients' potential reversibility of their underlying conditions and limitations on other life-sustaining treatments.[6] These include the following:

- Irreversible lung damage: Such as advanced fibrosis where recovery is not anticipated, and patient is deemed not a candidate for lung transplantation.

- Severe multisystem organ failure: Not related to lung function, which does not support the expected quality of life postrecovery.
- Chronic conditions with poor prognosis: Including certain cancers or progressive neurologic disorders where the expected survival is limited.
- Advanced age and frailty: Although not absolute, age and general frailty are considered predictors of poorer outcomes and higher complication rates.

Cannulation Strategies

Cannulation for VV ECMO typically involves either the insertion of a single dual-lumen cannula or the placement of two separate cannulas for drainage and return. The type of dual-lumen cannula used can vary. For instance, Avalon (Getinge, Gothenburg, Sweden) and Crescent (Medtronic, Minneapolis, MN, USA) cannulas have bicaval drainage with return to the right atrium. In contrast, Protek (LivaNova, London, UK) and Spectrum (Spectrum Medical, Gloucestershire, UK) cannulas have drainage from the right atrium and return to the pulmonary artery, though these latter types are currently less commonly used.

Dual-lumen cannula placement often necessitates the patient being taken to the operating room for real-time procedural imaging with either transesophageal echocardiography or fluoroscopy to safely guide cannula insertion.[7] This concurrent intraprocedural imaging is necessary due to the exact cannula positioning required and the risk of iatrogenic right ventricle injury. The cannulation site is usually the internal jugular vein, with the proximal drainage positioned in the right atrium or right ventricle and the distal return positioned in the main pulmonary artery.

When two individual cannulas are used for peripheral cannulation, the drainage cannula is often placed in a femoral vein, whereas the return cannula can be inserted through either the femoral or internal jugular veins. In stable patients, peripheral cannulation is often preferred, with femoral drainage positioned at the level of the inferior cavoatrial junction and the internal jugular return cannula positioned at the superior cavoatrial junction. The most common site for the return cannula in this scenario is the right internal jugular vein, with a standard cannula insertion depth of approximately 15 cm, though this can be adjusted based on the patient's height.[5,8]

Ideally, the cannulas should be positioned 10 cm apart, with adjustments made to ensure there is minimal recirculation of the oxygenated blood back into the ECMO circuit. Recirculation diminishes effective oxygen delivery and is indicated by low peripheral oxygen saturation and unexpectedly high preoxygenator blood O_2 saturation. It is important to note that some degree of recirculation is always present in this configuration.[8]

If the patient is not deemed a candidate for femoral and internal jugular cannulation, a bilateral femoral cannulation approach can be used. When using this approach, there is a notable increased risk of possible recirculation (Fig. 116.6). The specific nuances of this approach include the following:

- Right femoral return cannula: The shorter course of the venous system on the right side provides a few additional centimeters to ensure proper placement and distance from the drainage cannula. A single-stage venous cannula should be used as the return cannula as its side holes are located only within the first 5 cm of the tip. This design focuses the flow at the tip, maximizing the distance between the side holes on the return and drainage cannulas, thereby optimizing the effectiveness of the ECMO circuit.

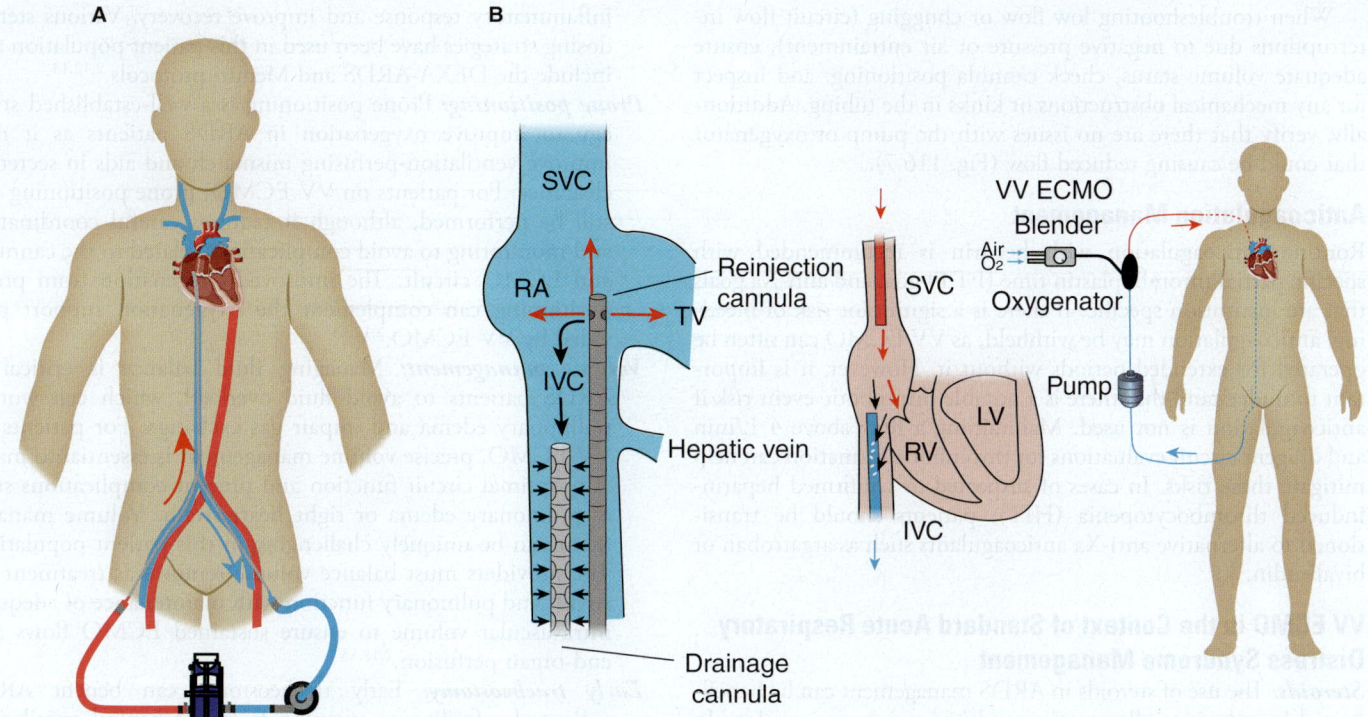

FIGURE 116.6 (A–B) Venovenous extracorporeal membrane oxygenation recirculation. *IVC*, Inferior vena cava; *LV*, left ventricle; *RA*, right atrium; *RV*, right ventricle; *SVC*, superior vena cava; *TV*, tricuspid valve; *VV ECMO*, venovenous extracorporeal membrane oxygenation (Courtesy UMMC: recirculation.)

- Left femoral drainage cannula: The drainage cannula should be placed in the left-sided femoral vein given the increased distance from the insertion site to the inferior vena cava (IVC). The position of this cannula in relation to the outflow of the return cannula should ideally be ~5 cm apart. This positioning would minimize the risk of recirculation; however, this must be balanced with the ECMO circuit flow as position is associated with an increased risk drainage obstruction. Even at distances larger than 10 cm, recirculation can still occur, and it is important to frequently monitor the patient's ECMO circuit and pump gases.

In both cannulation techniques, a bedside transthoracic echocardiogram showing the IVC and the right atrial junction via subxiphoid view can be used to visualize the wire and ensure proper initial positioning of the cannula. If peripheral access is impractical, central access may be considered as an alternative.

General Management

Once VV ECMO is initiated, management involves a multidisciplinary team including ECMO surgeons, intensivists, advanced practice providers, nurses, respiratory therapists, perfusionists, and ECMO specialists. This team is frequently supported by consultations from specialty services such as Infectious Disease, Pulmonary Medicine, Nutrition, Occupational and Physical Therapy, and Palliative Care.[2]

The primary goal of VV ECMO is to allow the lungs to rest while the ECMO circuit performs the gas exchange functions. Ventilator settings are adjusted to ensure minimal lung strain, typically with a plateau pressure <25 cm H_2O, a driving pressure <15 cm H_2O, and a tidal volume of 4 to 6 cc/kg of predicted body weight. Various modes of ventilation can be used to maintain these lung rest settings, including volume control and pressure control ventilation (PCV), with PCV settings often at a plateau pressure of 20 cm H_2O, a positive end-expiratory pressure (PEEP) of 10 cm H_2O, a respiratory rate of 10, and an FiO_2 of 40%.[2,9,10]

Persistent hypoxia post-ECMO initiation necessitates a systematic assessment of both the patient and the ECMO circuit. This includes ensuring the oxygenator is functioning correctly and checking for recirculation. Management strategies for recirculation might involve repositioning the cannulas to increase the distance between the drainage and return lines, reducing the pump speed, or adding an additional drainage cannula.

For patients exhibiting a hyperdynamic state with ECMO flow rates <60% of total cardiac output, resulting in persistent hypoxemia and an SaO_2 <90%, initial strategies include increasing pump flow up to the maximum safe revolutions per minute (RPM). If higher flow rates are required, introducing a second drainage cannula or switching to central cannulation may be considered. Medications such as β-blockers can help reduce the cardiac output and allow for more of the total cardiac output to be captured by the ECMO circuit.[10]

In cases that remain refractory, efforts should focus on maximizing oxygen delivery and minimizing oxygen demand. Techniques include sedation, paralysis, diuresis, cooling, and maintaining hemoglobin levels above 9 to 10 g/dL to enhance oxygen-carrying capacity.

For carbon dioxide and hypercarbia management, the ECMO circuit's sweep gas should be adjusted to maintain a PCO_2 between 35 and 45 mm Hg, targeting a pH between 7.35 and 7.45. If standard sweep gas rates are insufficient, consider using an additional blender or oxygenator. Proper ventilator management is also crucial to complement ECMO support as optimizing vent settings minimize full dependence on ECMO for gas exchange.[2,10]

When troubleshooting low flow or chugging (circuit flow interruptions due to negative pressure or air entrainment), ensure adequate volume status, check cannula positioning, and inspect for any mechanical obstructions or kinks in the tubing. Additionally, verify that there are no issues with the pump or oxygenator that could be causing reduced flow (Fig. 116.7).

Anticoagulation Management

Routine anticoagulation with heparin is recommended with specific partial thromboplastin time (PTT) goal and anti-Xa goals that are institution specific. If there is a significant risk of bleeding, anticoagulation may be withheld, as VV ECMO can often be operated for extended periods without it. However, it is important to understand that there is a notable thrombotic event risk if anticoagulation is not used. Maintaining a flow above 4 L/min and diligent circuit evaluations for thrombotic formation can help mitigate these risks. In cases of suspected or confirmed heparin-induced thrombocytopenia (HIT), patients should be transitioned to alternative anti-Xa anticoagulants such as argatroban or bivalirudin.[11]

VV ECMO in the Context of Standard Acute Respiratory Distress Syndrome Management

Steroids: The use of steroids in ARDS management can be beneficial in reducing inflammation and improving oxygenation. In patients on VV ECMO, steroids are often continued as part of the standard ARDS treatment protocol to help modulate the inflammatory response and improve recovery. Various steroid dosing strategies have been used in this patient population and include the DEXA-ARDS and Meduri protocols.[2,12,13]

Prone positioning: Prone positioning is a well-established strategy to improve oxygenation in ARDS patients as it may improve ventilation-perfusing mismatch and aids in secretion clearance. For patients on VV ECMO, prone positioning can still be performed, although it requires careful coordination and monitoring to avoid complications related to the cannulas and ECMO circuit. The improved oxygenation from prone positioning can complement the oxygenation support provided by VV ECMO.[2,12,13]

Volume management: Managing fluid balance is critical in ARDS patients to avoid fluid overload, which can worsen pulmonary edema and impair gas exchange. For patients on VV ECMO, precise volume management is essential to maintain optimal circuit function and prevent complications such as pulmonary edema or right heart strain. Volume management can be uniquely challenging in this patient population. The providers must balance volume removal as treatment for ARDs and pulmonary function with maintenance of adequate intravascular volume to ensure sustained ECMO flows and end-organ perfusion.[2,12,13]

Early tracheostomy: Early tracheostomy can benefit ARDS patients by facilitating weaning from mechanical ventilation, improving patient comfort, and enabling patients to be awake and participative. In patients on VV ECMO, early tracheostomy

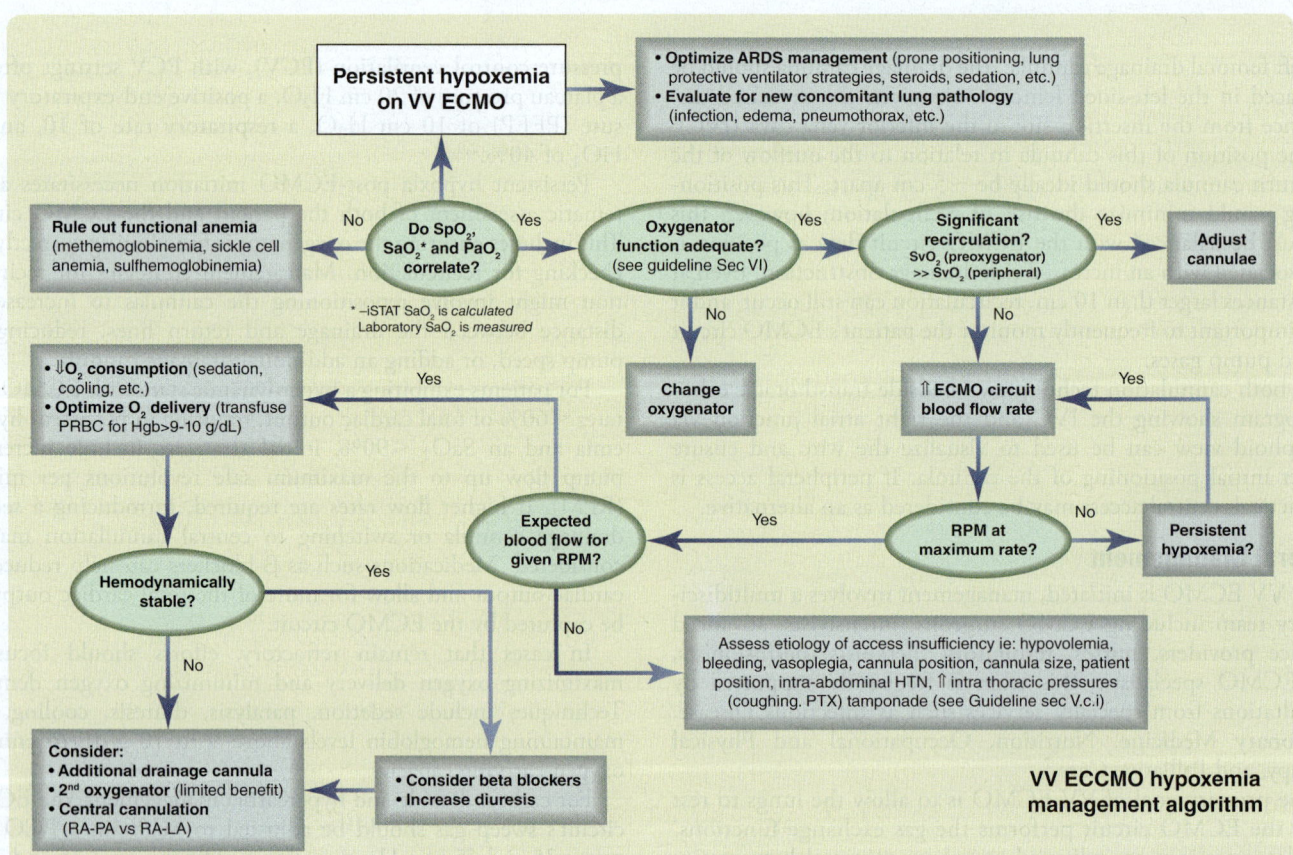

FIGURE 116.7 University of Maryland venovenous extracorporeal membrane oxygenation *(VV ECMO)* hypoxemia management algorithm. *ARDS,* Acute respiratory distress syndrome; *HTN,* hypertension; *PRBC,* packed red blood cells; *PTX,* pneumothorax; *RA-LA,* right atrium-left atrium; *RA-PA,* right atrium-pulmonary artery; *RPM,* revolutions per minute.

can also aid in managing secretions, reducing sedation requirements, and accelerating lung recovery, allowing providers to take advantage of awake ECMO care.[14]

Vasoactive support: Vasoactive medications and infusions may be necessary to support blood pressure and cardiac output in hypotensive ARDS patients, especially those with septic shock and other etiologies of hemodynamic instability. For patients on VV ECMO, careful titration of vasoactive agents is crucial to ensure adequate perfusion and oxygen delivery while maintaining stable ECMO circuit function.

By integrating these standard ARDS management strategies with the specialized support provided by VV ECMO, clinicians can optimize care and potentially improve outcomes for patients with severe respiratory failure.

Specific Sedation Goals in ECMO Management

Minimize sedation: The primary goal is to minimize sedation to allow patients to be awake and interactive. This involves administering the lowest effective doses of sedatives to ensure patient comfort while maintaining consciousness.[15]

Facilitate mobility and ambulation: Sedation reduction helps patients participate in physical therapy and ambulation. Increased interactivity and mobility can significantly improve outcomes by preventing muscle atrophy, enhancing lung function through spontaneous breathing, and reducing the risk of complications such as deep vein thrombosis (DVT) and pressure ulcers.[15,16]

Maintaining physical conditioning through ambulation is especially crucial for pretransplant patients. Such pretransplant conditioning is associated with improving transplant outcomes and recovery. Ambulation also provides significant psychological benefits by empowering patients and enhancing their overall well-being.

Effective ambulation on ECMO requires meticulous planning and coordination among the healthcare team, along with the use of specialized mobile ECMO equipment. Continuous monitoring of vital signs and ECMO circuit function is essential to ensure patient safety. By promoting mobility, healthcare providers can optimize physical and psychological health, leading to better overall outcomes for patients on ECMO.

Enhance communication: Keeping patients awake enables better communication with the healthcare team, which is crucial for assessing their needs, managing pain effectively, and understanding the patient's goal of care. This also helps in monitoring neurologic status and early detection of complications.

Weaning From VV ECMO

Successful weaning from VV ECMO is heavily dependent on the etiology of the respiratory disease and the patient's overall goals of care. As the VV ECMO and mechanical ventilation are often used together, there is an important patient-specific balance between the two modalities that can facilitate an ideal outcome. In considering weaning of mechanical support, many patients are decannulated from VV ECMO before ventilator liberation. There is still a subset of patients who are first weaned off ventilator support, and only later decannulated from VV ECMO without further mechanical ventilation. Identifying these patients is often challenging, but it affords the potential for improved patient nutrition, participation in rehabilitation, optimal lung rest, and reduced ventilator-associated infections.[10,17]

Weaning protocols vary between institutions. A preferred strategy involves weaning the sweep gas flow rate rather than the sweep gas FiO$_2$ or total flow. Another method is to slowly wean the FiO$_2$ concentration of the circuit, which is set at 100% initially, or to slowly decrease the circuit flow rate.[2,17,18] However, decreasing the ECMO flow rate can increase the risk of thrombotic events as higher flow rates help mitigate thrombus formation throughout the circuit.

Weaning of Sweep Gas Flow

- Gradual reduction: The sweep gas flow rate, which controls the removal of CO$_2$ from the blood, is titrated to a patient's PCO$_2$ level. As the patient's native lung function improves, the sweep is gradually reduced until the patient's lungs can manage CO$_2$ clearance without ECMO support. When the sweep is turned off, the patient is no longer receiving ECMO support and is simply recirculating the blood in the ECMO circuit.[10]

- A patient may or may not be on mechanical ventilation when starting a recirculation trial. For patients who are still mechanically ventilated, increasing ventilator support while staying within reasonable parameters is often used to reduce time on ECMO and allow for an earlier decannulation.

- Arterial blood gases (ABGs) are closely monitored during this process to ensure that CO$_2$ levels remain within an acceptable range. An increase in the patient's respiratory drive or signs of respiratory acidosis may indicate the need to slow the weaning process or an increase in mechanical ventilation support.[10]

Acceptable Ventilator Parameters

- Lung recovery: Before considering decannulation, the patient should demonstrate adequate lung recovery. Acceptable ventilator parameters typically include a low FiO$_2$, often less than 40%, and a PEEP of 8 to 10 cm H$_2$O with a peak pressure no greater than 20 to 25 cm H$_2$O. In some clinical settings, it is reasonable to extubate patients before weaning VV ECMO support.

- Stable blood gases: ABGs should show adequate oxygenation (PaO$_2$ >60 mm Hg on low FiO$_2$) and ventilation (PaCO$_2$ within normal limits) on minimal ventilator settings. The patient should also be capable of maintaining spontaneous breathing efforts without significant support.

Clinical Stability

- The patient should be hemodynamically stable, with minimal or no need for vasoactive medications. Signs of clinical improvement, such as decreased pulmonary infiltrates on chest imaging and improved lung compliance, should also be evident.

Decannulation Procedure

Preparation: Decannulation is a planned procedure that requires careful preparation. The patient should be in a controlled environment, such as the intensive care unit (ICU) or operating room, with all necessary personnel and equipment on hand. Coagulation labs should be evaluated and corrected before decannulation, and blood products should be readily available at the bedside if needed. It is important to have a clear goals-of-care discussion with the family and the patient to determine whether the patient is a recannulation candidate before decannulation.

Cannula removal: It is crucial to set up the field appropriately before attempting decannulation. Begin by removing all but one suture securing the cannula. Place a large 0 Prolene purse-string suture around each cannula insertion site. For patients who still have their oxygenator in line with their ECMO circuit, return the blood from the circuit to the patient before clamping the cannulas. This step should be guided by the patient's ventilator status, renal function, right ventricular (RV) function, and volume management. For instance, avoid returning the entire circuit volume to a patient who is on continuous renal replacement therapy (CRRT) with borderline ventilator settings or someone with moderate RV dysfunction who may not tolerate a rapid 1-L blood bolus well.

The procedure typically starts with the removal of the drainage cannula, followed by the return cannula. When removing the cannula, it is important to do so in one swift, controlled motion to minimize blood loss. Allow for back-bleeding before tying down the purse-string suture to ensure any clot around the cannula is removed. This is followed by applying occlusive pressure to the site.

Hemostasis and monitoring: After removing the cannulas, achieving hemostasis is crucial to prevent bleeding complications. Continuous monitoring of vital signs, including heart rate, blood pressure, and oxygen saturation, is essential during and after the procedure to detect any immediate complications.

Postdecannulation care: The patient is closely observed for signs of respiratory distress, hemodynamic instability, or bleeding. Frequent ABGs and chest imaging may be performed to ensure that the patient maintains adequate gas exchange and lung function without ECMO support. A venous duplex of the lower extremities should be performed 24 hours following decannulation to evaluate for any cannulation-associated DVTs. It is common to identify such DVTs, which should be treated in the same fashion as other DVTs with anticoagulation and outpatient follow-up.[19] Duration of anticoagulation should also follow routine DVT treatment guidelines.

CARDIAC FAILURE

VA ECMO is a specialized configuration of mechanical support for patients with severe cardiac failure. It is used primarily as a bridge to recovery or as a bridge to a definitive surgical intervention such as transplant, left ventricular assist device (LVAD), revascularization, or structural repair. This support system helps correct end-organ malperfusion associated with cardiac failure that cannot be managed with standard conventional medical therapy[1,20–23] (Fig. 116.8).

Indications for ECMO in Cardiac Failure

- **Postcardiotomy cardiac support:** ECMO is also indicated postoperatively if the patient fails to wean off cardiopulmonary bypass due to myocardial stunning or if there is an unexpected postoperative deterioration in cardiac function.[3,4,20,24]
- **Refractory cardiogenic shock:** ECMO is indicated for patients who do not respond to conventional medical therapies including inotropic support or less extensive mechanical support such as Impella or intraaortic balloon pump (IABP).[20,21]
- **Pulmonary embolism:** In massive pulmonary embolism where there is significant cardiac compromise in the setting of obstructive shock, VA ECMO can support both the right-sided heart and provide oxygenation, allowing for interventions to address the embolism or for pharmacologic therapies to take effect.[25–27]
- **Toxic myocarditis:** In cases of severe myocarditis resulting from infections or toxic exposures where cardiac function is

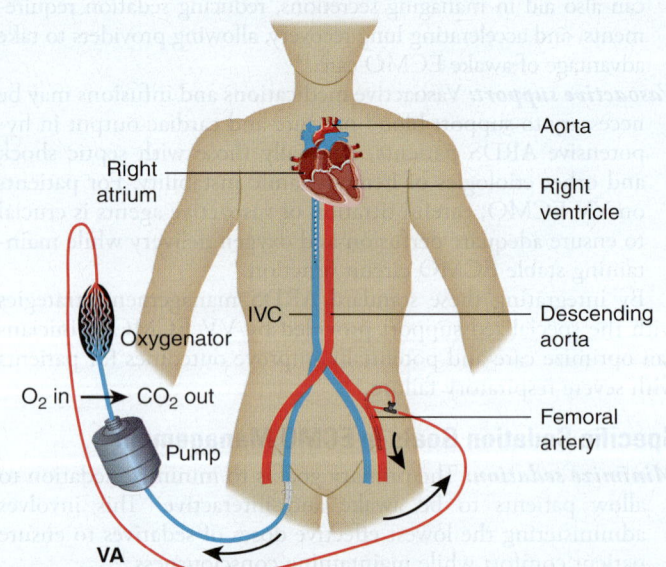

FIGURE 116.8 Venoarterial *(VA)* extracorporeal membrane oxygenation cannulation configuration. *IVC,* Inferior vena cava. (From Shah A, Dave S, Goerlich CE, Kaczorowski DJ. Hybrid and parallel extracorporeal membrane oxygenation circuits. *JTCVS Tech.* 2021;8:77-85.)

severely compromised, VA ECMO can provide support while the myocardium recovers or until definitive treatment can be administered.[28]

- **Acute myocardial infarction (AMI):** VA ECMO can be lifesaving in cases of cardiogenic shock post-AMI, especially when there is a mechanical complication like ventricular septal rupture, acute mitral regurgitation due to papillary muscle rupture, or RV failure.[20,29]
- **Support during high-risk percutaneous coronary interventions (PCIs):** For patients at high risk of hemodynamic instability during procedures such as PCI, ECMO can provide necessary circulatory support.[30]
- **Refractory ventricular arrhythmias:** In cases of severe ventricular arrhythmias that are refractory to medical treatment and pose a risk of hemodynamic instability and end-organ malperfusion, VA ECMO can stabilize hemodynamics and provide a bridge to more definitive therapies like catheter ablation or sympathectomy.[31]
- **Cardiac arrest:** Extracorporeal cardiopulmonary resuscitation (ECPR) is used when conventional CPR fails in the event of cardiac arrest, especially in settings where the likelihood of rapid recovery with conventional measures is low. This approach is particularly considered in potentially reversible situations or situations where etiology is not entirely known.[24]
- **Bridge to decision/therapy:** ECMO serves as a bridge to decision, giving clinicians time to evaluate the viability of further invasive therapies or transplantation. It can also be a bridge to therapy, maintaining patient stability until long-term solutions such as a ventricular assist device (VAD) or heart transplant can be implemented.[32]

Contraindications for ECMO in Cardiac Failure

- **Irreversible cardiac conditions:** ECMO is not recommended for patients with end-stage heart disease where there is no definitive therapy or when they are not candidates for transplantation or LVAD. In this scenario, recovery is highly unlikely and continued ECMO support will be futile.

- **Severe coagulopathies or active hemorrhage:** Active bleeding or severe coagulopathies that cannot be medically corrected and managed are major contraindications due to the high risk of bleeding complications associated with ECMO. Hypovolemic shock in the setting of uncontrolled bleeding is considered a relative contraindication for VA ECMO cannulation.
- **Terminal illnesses and severe comorbidities:** Terminal illnesses that limit life expectancy and severe comorbid conditions that do not support the overall goals of care may also preclude the use of ECMO.
- **Advanced age:** Although not an absolute contraindication, the risks and benefits of ECMO need careful consideration in elderly patients or frail patients, especially those with diminished physiologic reserves.
- **Prolonged cardiac arrest:** In the setting of ECPR, patients with prolonged downtimes greater than an hour or have an unwitnessed out of hospital arrest with unknown downtimes are often not candidates for VA ECMO cannulation given their overall poor prognosis.

Cannulation Strategies

- **Peripheral cannulation strategy:** An increasingly used technique whose insertion sites include the common femoral vein and artery for VA ECMO. This approach allows for rapid cannula placement at the bedside with the need for an operating room or interventional procedural suite. However, this femoral artery cannulation strategy provides retrograde flow and can be associated with vascular complications and limb ischemia. To mitigate these risks, a wire reinforced distal perfusion catheter is placed antegrade in the superficial femoral artery to provide perfusion to the arterially cannulated limb[3,33,34] (Fig. 116.9).
- **Central cannulation strategy:** Typically employed postcardiotomy during cardiac surgery cases or in the setting of severe peripheral vascular disease, central cannulation provides antegrade flow and involves the direct arterial cannula of the aorta through a midline sternotomy.[3,4,6] It is also possible to perform central cannulation through the right axillary artery following an axillary cutdown, but note that special consideration needs to be taken. This includes ensuring flow down the cannulated arm by using a vascular chimney graft or placement of a distal

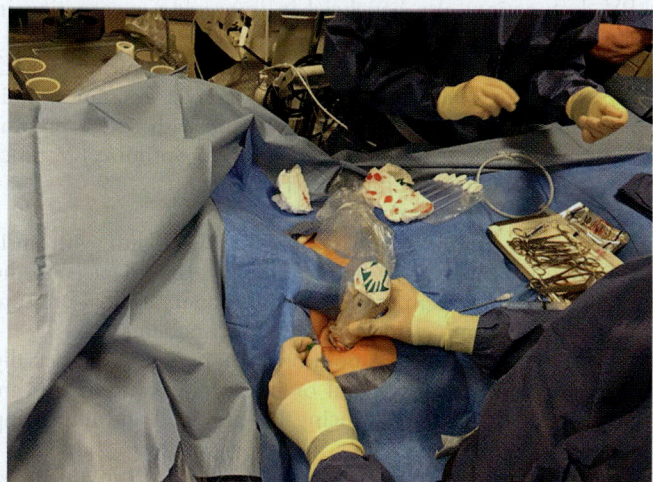

FIGURE 116.9 Ultrasound-guided placement of the distal perfusion catheter. (Courtesy UMMC: distal perfusion placement.)

perfusing catheter down the arm. It is also important to consider the distance the cannula tip is from the right vertebral and carotid arteries as the cannula can obstruct carotid flow if advanced too far.
- **Other cannulation strategy:** Combining central and peripheral techniques, such as central innominate/aortic cannulation and femoral venous cannulation, can optimize support in complex cardiac conditions, allowing customization of flow dynamics according to patient needs. Other sites of cannulation include peripheral axillary cannulation through a surgical axillary cutdown and femoral venous cannulation. It is important to note these alternative strategies may require the addition of a distal perfusion catheter to provide perfusion to the corresponding arm.[3,8,16] These alternative forms allow a clinician to take advantage of central antegrade cannulation while mitigating the associated infection risk of standard central cannulation through a midline sternotomy.

Anticoagulation Considerations

The primary goal is to prevent clot formation in the ECMO circuit and cannulas that could potentially embolize or impede oxygenator function while minimizing the risk of bleeding. This is typically managed with continuous infusion of anticoagulants like unfractionated heparin. Regular monitoring of anticoagulation levels using tests such as activated clotting time (ACT), anti-Xa levels, or activated partial thromboplastin time (aPTT) is crucial.[20,35] Given the significant risk of systemic emboli and embolic stroke associated with VA ECMO, these anticoagulation goals are often higher when compared with VV ECMO; however, the policy is also institution specific.

Strategies must be in place to manage and quickly address any bleeding complications, which are significant risks given the systemic anticoagulation necessary for ECMO. Specific goals, however, should be tailored to individual patients and their specific clinical setting. A general approach to anticoagulation management includes maintaining a PTT goal of 60 to 80 seconds for patients without significant bleeding risk. For patients with pulmonary emboli or other conditions requiring higher anticoagulation, a higher PTT target is clinically indicated. If there is a concern for a major bleeding event, anticoagulation can be held, or a lower PTT goal can be used. In these scenarios, the risk of an embolic event must be weighed against the risk of a major bleeding event. Adjustments are made based on clinical response, bleeding events, and changes in patient condition, such as infection, hemolysis, or organ function.

Volume Management on VA ECMO

Volume management is crucial in VA ECMO settings as many patients are volume overloaded before cannulation and are in a state of decompensated heart failure. Effective strategies for volume removal include the following[20,21,36]:

- **Diuretics:** Diuretics are commonly used to manage fluid balance by promoting urine output, helping to control volume status in patients whose renal function is still intact.
- **Hemoconcentrator:** A hemoconcentrator can be integrated into the ECMO circuit, allowing for the removal of excess fluid directly from the blood, allowing for precise control of fluid balance without significantly impacting electrolyte or drug levels. This is especially useful in the setting where rapid removal of volume is necessary, but this is not recommended as a long-term volume management strategy as there can be an increased risk of hemolysis.

- **CRRT:** This facilitates continuous removal of fluid, electrolyte clearance, and acid-base management in the setting of impaired renal function, allowing for gentle and consistent fluid balance correction, which is especially beneficial in hemodynamically unstable patients. CRRT can be connected to the ECMO circuit either by integrating it into the existing lines or through separate vascular access. Integration into the ECMO circuit reduces the need for additional vascular access, minimizing infection risks and vascular complications. However, it is important to note that there is risk in using this method as CRRT flow will be dependent on and influenced by your ECMO flows, and if integrated incorrectly (prepump) there is a risk of catastrophic air entrainment. This could cause the circuit to experience an airlock leading to circuit failure and emergent circuit exchange.

- **Slow continuous ultrafiltration (SCUF):** SCUF provides continuous fluid removal at a slower rate than conventional hemodialysis and is a specific form of CRRT that focuses on volume removal. In patients who have intact renal function, the addition of SCUF directly into the ECMO circuit can aid in the removal of volume where rapid volume removal is required.

Fluid removal must be carefully balanced against the patient's intravascular volume, cardiac output, end-organ perfusion requirements, and ECMO flow rate. Overaggressive fluid removal can lead to hypovolemia, decreased cardiac output, potential collapse of the circulatory system, and ECMO flow complications. Regular monitoring of fluid status using clinical examination, hemodynamic monitoring such as central venous pressure, and input-output calculations is crucial for proper volume management. Advanced monitoring techniques such as echocardiography can assist in assessing volume status and cardiac function even while on ECMO support.

Management of Inotropic and Vasoactive Support

When managing patients on VA ECMO, the titration of vasoactive infusions including inotropes, vasopressors, and antihypertensives is critical to ensure adequate cardiac pulsatility, systemic perfusion, and stable ECMO flows. The following is a detailed list of commonly used inotropes and vasopressors, including their mechanisms, indications, and considerations specific to the ECMO setting.[1,3,10,16,21,23]

Inotropes on VA ECMO

Inotropes are primarily used to improve cardiac contractility and ensure adequate cardiac pulsatility, which is crucial for patients with reduced myocardial function on ECMO. Inotropes on ECMO should primarily be used to maintain pulsatility and emptying of the left ventricle. If there is adequate pulsatility without the use of inotropes, it is preferable to allow the heart to "rest" and avoid the stress associated with increased adrenergic drive. As inotropes increase myocardial oxygen demand, their use should be minimized, especially after events such as cardiac arrest or myocardial infarction, to avoid further strain on the heart while on ECMO.

Dobutamine.
- Mechanism: β_1-adrenergic agonist that increases myocardial contractility and stroke volume.
- Indications: Used to enhance cardiac output and vasodilation in patients with low cardiac function without significantly increasing heart rate.
- ECMO considerations: Useful in reducing ventricular afterload while increasing overall cardiac function and contractility;

monitor for tachyarrhythmias and increased myocardial oxygen consumption.

Milrinone.
- Mechanism: Phosphodiesterase-3 inhibitor that increases cardiac contractility and produces vasodilation.
- Indications: Beneficial for RV failure and pulmonary hypertension; often used when β-adrenergic effects are undesirable.
- ECMO considerations: Can lower systemic vascular resistance; useful in weaning from ECMO as it improves diastolic relaxation and decreases pulmonary vascular resistance. Mainstay for patients with systemic vascular resistance reserve and signs of RV failure.

Epinephrine.
- Mechanism: Potent α- and β-adrenergic agonist that increases myocardial contractility, heart rate, and systemic vascular resistance.
- Indications: Used in severe cardiogenic shock when stronger inotropic support is needed to maintain pulsatility.
- ECMO considerations: Results in increased myocardial oxygen demand and arrhythmogenicity.

In the setting of VA ECMO, the use of inotropic support focuses on ensuring pulsatility and the opening of the aortic valve. End-organ perfusion and RV decompression can be accomplished with VA ECMO support alone. However, if pulsatility is lost, there is a significant increased risk of pulmonary congestion leading to respiratory failure and catastrophic thrombus formation within the aortic root and left ventricular (LV) cavity due to LV distention and left atrial hypertension. Additionally, LV distention and elevated LV end-diastolic pressure reduce coronary perfusion pressure, thereby decreasing myocardial oxygen delivery, which can be detrimental to the heart's function.

Inhaled Agents on VA ECMO

Inhaled vasodilators are used primarily to target pulmonary vasculature, reducing pulmonary arterial pressure and improving right heart function without causing significant systemic hypotension.

Nitric oxide.
- Mechanism: Inhaled nitric oxide (NO) is a selective pulmonary vasodilator that works by relaxing vascular smooth muscle. It specifically reduces pulmonary artery pressure and pulmonary vascular resistance, thereby decreasing RV afterload.
- Indications: Used for patients with pulmonary hypertension or RV dysfunction; also beneficial in improving oxygenation in hypoxic respiratory failure.
- ECMO considerations: Inhaled NO is effective during ECMO because it does not affect systemic vascular resistance. It is particularly useful in managing patients with severe pulmonary hypertension on ECMO, helping to optimize RV function and facilitate weaning from ECMO.

Epoprostenol (prostacyclin, PGI2).
- Mechanism: Epoprostenol is a potent vasodilator with antithrombotic properties. When inhaled, it primarily acts on the pulmonary circulation to decrease pulmonary arterial pressure with some systemic vasodilation in select patients.
- Indications: Indicated for pulmonary hypertension, especially when systemic effects of oral or intravenous vasodilators are undesirable. It helps in reducing RV afterload and improving cardiac output.
- ECMO considerations: Its use during ECMO can aid in reducing the pulmonary vascular resistance more selectively compared with systemic administration.

Iloprost (inhaled).

- Mechanism: Similar to epoprostenol but longer acting, iloprost is a synthetic prostacyclin that causes vasodilation of the pulmonary arterial bed.
- Indications: Used for the treatment of pulmonary arterial hypertension and can be useful in managing postoperative pulmonary hypertensive crises.
- ECMO considerations: Iloprost can be particularly beneficial in ECMO patients who require prolonged treatment of pulmonary hypertension as it offers a longer duration of action than inhaled NO.

These agents are administered via inhalation, often through specialized delivery systems that can integrate with mechanical ventilation or into a high-flow nasal cannula. Continuous monitoring of pulmonary artery pressures and RV function is essential to evaluate the effectiveness of these agents. The selective pulmonary effects of these agents make them ideal for use in ECMO, as they can improve the pulmonary circulatory status without compromising systemic hemodynamics, thus supporting the overall goals of ECMO therapy and facilitation of the recovery process. Their use should be considered as part of a comprehensive approach to optimize cardiac and pulmonary conditions in critically ill patients on ECMO.

Vasopressors on ECMO

Vasopressors are used to maintain adequate vascular tone and perfusion pressure, especially in the context of vasodilatory shock or severe systemic inflammation. It is important to balance adequate vascular tone and VA ECMO flows, as increasing vascular tone can impair ECMO flows due to higher resistance. Additionally, there is the potential for a vasoplegic response to the ECMO circuit when initiating support. Although not very common, this can occur and may require vasopressor support until it resolves, usually within approximately 6 hours.

When managing patients on VA ECMO, it is also important to consider mean arterial pressure (MAP) goals. Maintaining an appropriate MAP is crucial, as excessively high MAP can increase afterload, which may reduce ECMO flows by increasing the resistance against which the ECMO circuit must pump. Therefore, careful titration of vasopressors is necessary to ensure optimal perfusion without compromising ECMO flow dynamics.

Norepinephrine.

- Mechanism: Strong α-adrenergic effects with moderate β-adrenergic effects, increasing systemic vascular resistance and arterial blood pressure.
- Indications: First-line agent for septic shock and widely used in cardiogenic shock to maintain coronary and cerebral perfusion pressures.
- ECMO considerations: Effective in maintaining systemic perfusion pressure without significant impact on cardiac output. The moderate β-adrenergic effect can be beneficial to overall cardiac function.

Vasopressin.

- Mechanism: Increases vascular smooth muscle tone via V1 receptor agonism, leading to an increase in systemic vascular resistance.
- Indications: Used in vasodilatory shock, particularly when response to other vasopressors is inadequate.
- ECMO considerations: Useful as an adjunct to norepinephrine for refractory hypotension; less likely to increase heart rate and cardiac output, reducing myocardial oxygen demand.

Phenylephrine.

- Mechanism: Pure α_1-adrenergic agonist that increases systemic vascular resistance and arterial pressure.
- Indications: Useful in situations where tachyarrhythmias need to be avoided or in combination with β-blockers.
- ECMO considerations: Can be used to increase perfusion pressure, especially useful in neurologic protection strategies.

The goal is to use the minimal effective doses of inotropes and vasopressors to achieve adequate organ perfusion while avoiding excessive myocardial workload and oxygen consumption. Each drug choice and its dosing must be tailored to the individual patient's underlying pathophysiology and response to ECMO support. It is also crucial to regularly reassess the need for continued pharmacologic support as the patient's condition evolves.

Antihypertensives on ECMO

Antihypertensives are essential in managing elevated blood pressure, which can compromise the effectiveness of ECMO support by limiting ECMO flows and increasing the risk of complications such as bleeding and stroke. The choice of antihypertensive agents and their administration must be carefully tailored to each patient's clinical scenario. Initial preference may be given to rapidly titratable agents for hypertension management, as they allow for precise control of blood pressure.

Agents like esmolol and labetalol are rarely useful on VA ECMO and are not commonly used in this setting. Typically, titratable antihypertensive agents are used until the patient can be weaned off ECMO. If a patient is on both antihypertensives and inotropes, efforts should focus on weaning the inotropes first to avoid the counterproductive effects of simultaneous administration.

Nicardipine.

- Mechanism: Calcium channel blocker that primarily acts on vascular smooth muscle to cause vasodilation, reducing systemic vascular resistance and arterial blood pressure.
- Indications: First-line agent for hypertensive emergencies and perioperative blood pressure management.
- ECMO considerations: Effective in controlling blood pressure without significant impact on heart rate or cardiac output. It can be titrated to achieve precise blood pressure targets.

Clevidipine.

- Mechanism: Dihydropyridine calcium channel blocker that causes arterial vasodilation, reducing systemic vascular resistance and blood pressure.
- Indications: Suitable for rapid blood pressure control in critically ill patients.
- ECMO considerations: Provides a rapid onset and short duration of action, allowing for precise blood pressure management.

Esmolol.

- Mechanism: Ultra-short-acting β-blocker that decreases heart rate, myocardial contractility, and cardiac output.
- Indications: Useful in controlling tachycardia and hypertension in the perioperative period or in patients with acute coronary syndromes.
- ECMO considerations: Beneficial in situations where heart rate control is crucial. The short half-life allows for rapid adjustment based on patient response.

Labetalol.

- Mechanism: Combined α- and β-adrenergic blocker that decreases systemic vascular resistance and myocardial contractility.

- Indications: Effective for both hypertensive emergencies and long-term blood pressure control.
- ECMO considerations: Useful in managing blood pressure with minimal reflex tachycardia; however, its β-blocking effects require caution in patients with compromised cardiac function.

Sodium nitroprusside.

- Mechanism: Direct vasodilator that acts on both arterial and venous smooth muscle to reduce systemic vascular resistance and venous return, lowering blood pressure.
- Indications: Used in hypertensive emergencies and acute heart failure.
- ECMO considerations: Effective in rapidly lowering blood pressure; however, its use requires close monitoring of cyanide and thiocyanate levels, particularly with prolonged use.

The overarching goal in the use of antihypertensives on ECMO is to maintain blood pressure within a therapeutic range that ensures optimal organ perfusion with a MAP of at least 65 mm Hg while minimizing the risk of adverse effects of an elevated MAP greater than 85 to 90 mm Hg. Regular monitoring and dose adjustments are necessary to respond to the dynamic changes in the patient's condition during ECMO therapy.

Left Ventricular Decompression on ECMO

LV decompression is critical in patients on VA ECMO. A distended left ventricle may be associated with increased afterload and or compromised contractility. The ramifications of LV distention include pulmonary edema, suboptimal coronary perfusion, and further LV injury reducing the likelihood of recovery. This problem is especially critical in patients who are unable to generate enough contractility on maximal inotropic support. In addition, if the LV is unable to generate enough force to open the aortic valve, the stagnant blood in the LV cavity and aortic root can lead to LV thrombus formation with possible embolization, aortic root thrombosis with catastrophic malperfusion of the coronary arteries.[37]

The following are detailed strategies for LV decompression.

Intraaortic Balloon Pump

- Mechanism: The IABP is inserted into the thoracic aorta, where it inflates during diastole to increase coronary blood flow and deflates before systole to decrease afterload, which reduces LV workload and promotes better cardiac output and LV decompression.[37]
- Indications: Typically used when there is moderate LV dysfunction, IABP can aid in offloading the LV, improving myocardial oxygen consumption, and enhancing coronary perfusion. However, studies have shown that IABP has limited usage on VA ECMO as it offers only minimal to no benefit in regard to LV unloading.

Impella

- Mechanism: The Impella device is a microaxial flow pump that is inserted across the aortic valve into the left ventricle. It actively pumps blood from the LV into the ascending aorta, directly unloading the LV, ensuring blood flow in the aortic root and providing end-organ perfusion (Fig. 116.10).[37]
- Indications: The Impella device is indicated in cases of severe LV dysfunction or when significant LV unloading is required. It is particularly useful in settings of cardiogenic shock or severe myocardial infarction with little to no pulsatility. Additionally, the Impella can be used to transition patients from VA

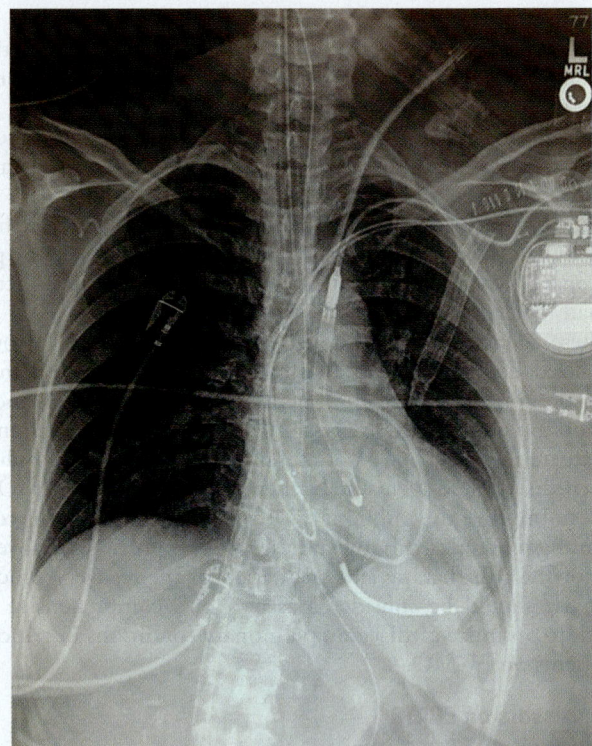

FIGURE 116.10 Venoarterial extracorporeal membrane oxygenation cannulation with Impella 5.5 in place for left ventricular decompression. (Courtesy UMMC: VA ECMO and Impella placement.)

ECMO or to evaluate isolated LV support in preparation for durable VAD implantation.

Transseptal Left Atrial Decompression

- Mechanism: This procedure involves creating a shunt between the left atrium and the right atrium to reduce left atrial pressure and indirectly decompress the left ventricle by allowing blood to bypass the left ventricle. This shunt helps equalize atrial pressures and acts as a "pop-off" valve to avoid high LV end-diastolic pressure. By doing so, it can further facilitate diuresis and protect the lungs from the increased pressure. In some cases, an additional venous cannula can be inserted into the left atrium through this septostomy and connected to the primary venous drainage circuit.[37]
- Indications: Used in cases of severe pulmonary edema or when other methods are insufficient or contraindicated. This procedure is also often considered in pediatric patients or when there is a congenital heart anomaly complicating the clinical scenario.

Surgical Vent

- Mechanism: A surgical vent can be placed directly in the left atrium or ventricle during open surgery to actively drain blood, reducing intracardiac pressure and volume.[37]
- Indications: Considered in situations where rapid decompression is needed, or during cardiac surgery where direct access to the heart is already established.

Each of these management strategies requires careful consideration of the individual patient's hemodynamic profile and underlying cardiac pathology. Implementing these strategies effectively can significantly influence the prognosis and outcome of patients on ECMO.

Harlequin Syndrome and VA ECMO

Harlequin Syndrome Overview

Harlequin syndrome, also known as North-South syndrome, occurs predominantly in patients on peripheral VA ECMO who have severe pulmonary dysfunction. This condition is characterized by differential oxygenation that may lead to cerebral hypoxia, in which the upper body, including the brain and upper extremities, receive deoxygenated blood from that patient's native cardiac output that ejects hypoxic blood returning from poorly functioning lungs, while the lower body receives oxygenated blood from the ECMO circuit.[34,38,39]

Mechanism

This syndrome arises because peripheral VA ECMO typically returns oxygen-rich blood preferentially to the lower body and visceral organs before perfusing the upper body and brain. Meanwhile, the native heart continues to pump deoxygenated blood from the lungs into the aorta, which preferentially perfuses the upper body with poorly oxygenated blood.[34,38,39] This results in a visible discrepancy in oxygenation between the upper and lower halves of the body. There are additional concerns that coronary oxygenation can also be compromised, as coronary perfusion is primarily supplied by the native heart.

This issue becomes particularly concerning when heart function improves or if myocardial depression was initially due to hypoxia or poor lung function in a patient placed on VA ECMO emergently or in the setting of ECPR (Fig. 116.11).

Management of Harlequin Syndrome

Adjust cannulation sites: One approach to managing Harlequin syndrome is to change the cannulation strategy to central ECMO or to a different peripheral site that might offer better mixing of blood.

In managing Harlequin syndrome in patients on peripheral VA ECMO, medical management primarily focuses on optimizing both ECMO flow and native heart function to ensure more uniform blood oxygenation.[20]

Increase and optimize ECMO flow: Adjusting the flow rate of the ECMO can help ensure that more oxygenated blood is mixed and circulated throughout the body. This can be particularly effective in overcoming the gradient differences between the deoxygenated blood from the heart and the oxygenated blood from the ECMO circuit.

Monitoring and adjustments: Continuous monitoring of ABGs from the upper body through the right radial artery provides an estimate of the oxygenation quality to the aortic arch and upper body. These arterial gas measurements allow for a dynamic assessment and a means to measure the effectiveness of the flow adjustments.

Modulating Cardiac Output

Inotrope reduction: If cardiac output is too high as the heart begins to recover, inotrope reduction should be considered to reduce overall cardiac output.

Volume removal: Aggressive volume removal can be used to reduce overall cardiac output. In this setting, the goal is to fully

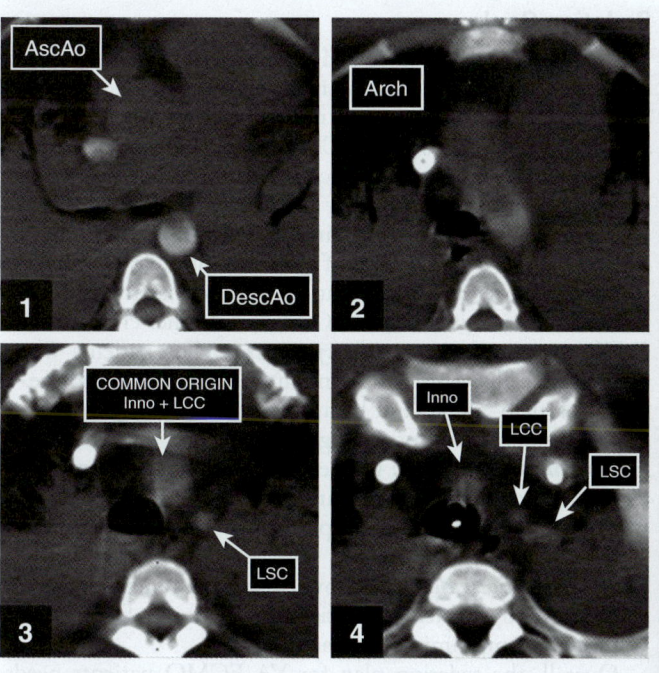

AscAo = ascending aorta
DescAo = descending aorta
Arch = aortic arch
Inno = Innominate artery
LCC = Left common carotid artery
LSC = Left subclavian artery

FIGURE 116.11 Radiographic findings of Harlequin syndrome. Axial *(left)* and oblique *(right)* maximum intensity projection images from chest CT angiography demonstrate antegrade flow in the ascending aorta and right-sided great vessels via native cardiac ejection *(blue arrow)* and retrograde flow in the descending aorta via the femoral extracorporeal membrane oxygenation cannula with preferential flow to the left subclavian artery *(red arrow)*. (From Pasrija C, Bedeir K, Jeudy J, Kon ZN. Harlequin syndrome during venoarterial extracorporeal membrane oxygenation. *Radiol Cardiothorac Imaging.* 2019;1[2]:e190031.)

decompress the RV and shunt the remaining blood volume into the ECMO circuit.

Heart rate control: Medications such as β-blockers can be used to manage tachycardia and reduce cardiac output, allowing for less flow through the impaired pulmonary system reducing the impact of the native heart ejection of deoxygenated blood. However, this should be a last resort and if medications such as β-blockers are indicated, then the patient should be considered for decannulation or reconfiguration to VV ECMO.

Enhancing Oxygenation

Supplemental oxygen: Increasing the FiO_2 to the patient can sometimes help improve the oxygenation of the blood ejected by the native heart.

Adjustments in ventilatory support: Done to modify ventilator settings to optimize gas exchange in the lungs, which can help increase the oxygen content of the blood leaving the heart.

Bronchoscopy: It is important to evaluate patient airways to rule out any forms of reversable obstruction such as a mucus plug.

Cannulation Reconfiguration

Transition from VA to VV ECMO: Patients who have recovered from a cardiac perspective, but still have significant respiratory compromise, should be considered from possible transition from VA ECMO-focused to VV ECMO-focused respiratory support. This evaluation should be performed before consideration for V-AV ECMO.

Transition from VA ECMO to V-AV ECMO: For patients with combined cardiac and respiratory failure, V-AV ECMO combines elements of both VV and VA ECMO, making it uniquely suited to address the challenges of Harlequin syndrome by balancing the oxygenation across the body more effectively. In the V-AV ECMO setup, blood is typically drawn from a central vein like the internal jugular or femoral vein (venous drainage), oxygenated externally, and then part of the oxygenated blood is returned to an artery (arterial return) to support the systemic circulation, while another portion is returned to a vein, enhancing the pulmonary circulation.[39]

The implementation of V-AV ECMO requires careful planning and precise cannulation to ensure effective blood flow management. It is crucial to monitor the oxygen saturation levels in different parts of the body to adjust the flow rates and oxygen delivery according to the patient's needs. Continuous monitoring and adjustments are necessary to maintain the balance between the venous and arterial components, adapting to changes in the patient's condition and requirements (Fig. 116.12).

Additional considerations include the use of flow probes to monitor return flow for both venous and arterial components and to make necessary adjustments. There is a higher risk of clot formation and hemolysis with V-AV ECMO due to the split return flow, which requires vigilant monitoring and management to mitigate these risks.

Each of these strategies requires a tailored approach based on the specific clinical situation of the patient. Continuous monitoring, including echocardiography and ABG analysis, is vital to ensure that interventions are effectively addressing the physiologic challenges presented by Harlequin syndrome. These targeted approaches help mitigate the risks associated with Harlequin syndrome and ensure optimal outcomes for patients undergoing ECMO therapy.

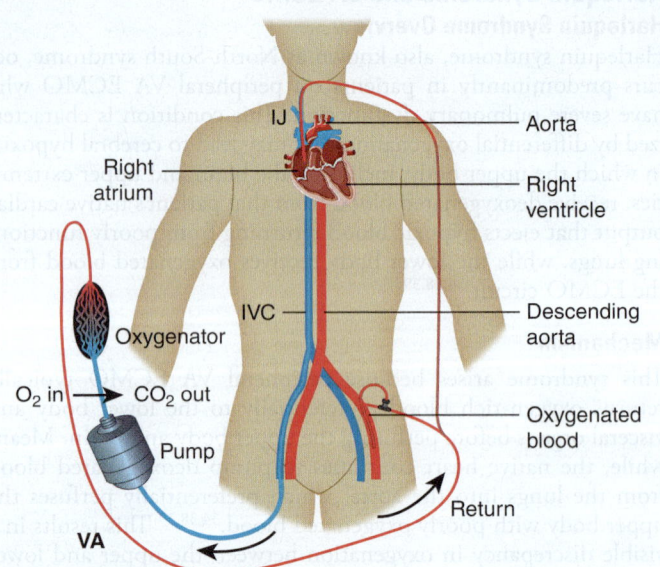

FIGURE 116.12 Venoarteriovenous extracorporeal membrane oxygenation cannulation configuration. *IJ,* Internal jugular; *IVC,* inferior vena cava; *VA,* venoarterial. (From Shah A, Dave S, Goerlich CE, Kaczorowski DJ. Hybrid and parallel extracorporeal membrane oxygenation circuits. *JTCVS Tech.* 2021;8:77-85.)

Sedation Goals

The sedation goals on VA ECMO are crucial for ensuring patient comfort, safety, and optimal management of the ECMO circuit.[15,40] The following are the main objectives when considering sedation for patients on VA ECMO:

Patient comfort: Minimize discomfort and anxiety caused by the ECMO cannulas and other invasive lines. Reduce awareness during a potentially distressing critical care environment.

Safety: Prevent dislodgement of lines and cannulas by minimizing patient movement and agitation. Ensure that the patient does not interfere with the ECMO circuit or other critical devices.

Facilitate ventilation and oxygenation: For patients who are mechanically ventilated, ventilator synchrony for those who are partially awake and breathing spontaneously is important to consider when optimizing sedation.

Hemodynamic stability: Use sedatives that have minimal impact on hemodynamic stability and ECMO flow stability as agitation and the vasovagal response can interfere with ECMO flows if significant enough.

Reduce metabolic demand: Lower the overall metabolic demand of the body, which is crucial in situations of compromised severely compromised cardiac function.

Overall, the sedation plan for VA ECMO patients needs to be individualized, considering their specific clinical situation, response to treatment, and overall goals of care.

Rehabilitation Goals

All ECMO patients require an evaluation from the rehabilitation services and receive physical therapy with active mobilization. Ambulation of patients on VA ECMO is feasible and is a growing area of interest in critical care, as it can potentially improve outcomes by enhancing physical conditioning, psychological well-being, and recovery rates.[15,40,41] The process of mobilizing patients while on ECMO, particularly peripheral VA ECMO, is complex and requires careful coordination (Fig. 116.13). The following section includes some key considerations and notable challenges involved in ambulating patients on VA ECMO.

Key Considerations

Patient stability: The patient must be hemodynamically stable with adequate organ function and physical conditioning.

Team coordination: A multidisciplinary team approach is required, including physicians, nurses, physical therapists, and respiratory therapists.

Equipment management: Special attention is needed to manage the ECMO circuit and other associated devices to prevent dislodgment or complications during movement.

Challenges and Precautions

Risk of cannula displacement: Movement can increase the risk of dislodging the ECMO cannulas, which is potentially life-threatening.

Bleeding risk: Patients on ECMO are typically on anticoagulation therapy, increasing the risk of bleeding with physical activity, especially from around the cannulation sites.

Weaning and Decannulation

Weaning and decannulation from VA ECMO are critical phases in the management of patients who have been supported on ECMO for cardiac dysfunction. The process involves carefully assessing the patient's recovery and readiness to resume independent function of their heart function. The following is a detailed overview of the process.

Weaning From ECMO

Assessment of recovery: The first step involves evaluating whether the patient's heart function and hemodynamics will be able to function independently. This typically involves a series of tests including echocardiograms, blood gas analyses, and hemodynamic monitoring to assess cardiac output and respiratory function.

Trial weaning or RAMP study: A RAMP (gradual flow reduction) study is a structured assessment of cardiac function performed while reducing VA ECMO flow to evaluate myocardial recovery and readiness for decannulation. During a RAMP study, the VA ECMO flow is gradually reduced while closely monitoring the patient's response. This process can be done in the ICU using a transthoracic echocardiogram or transesophageal echocardiogram to specifically capture the heart function and loading volumes of the patient at specific flow speeds.[25,42,43] Monitoring hemodynamics is critical during this process. Consider holding antihypertensive medications or increasing inotropes as needed to assess how the patient can transition off ECMO. The ability to maintain adequate oxygenation and stable hemodynamics with reduced ECMO support is a key indicator of readiness for decannulation.

Decannulation From ECMO

Timing and preparation: Decannulation is considered when a patient has demonstrated stable heart function on minimal to no ECMO support. Preparing for decannulation involves ensuring that anticoagulation levels are appropriate to minimize the risk of bleeding, and that all necessary surgical or medical staff are available.

The decannulation procedure involves surgically removing the ECMO cannulas, usually under sterile conditions in the ICU or

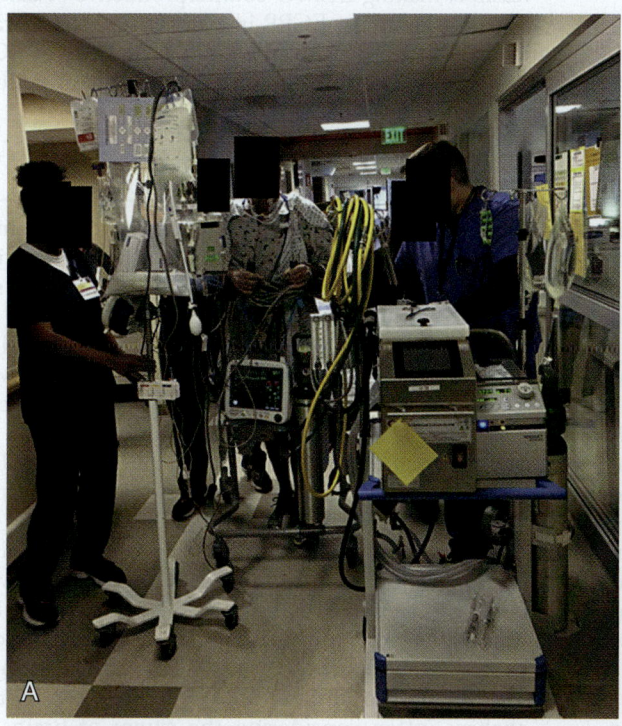
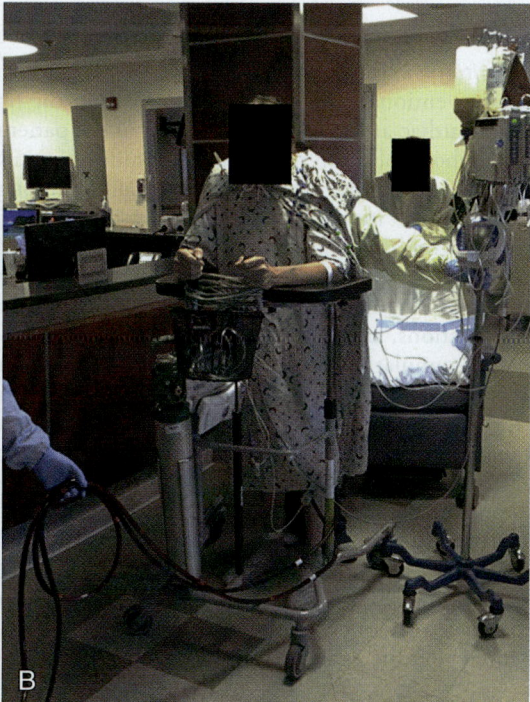

FIGURE 116.13 (A) A patient ambulating 42 days after venoarterial extracorporeal membrane oxygenation (VA ECMO) cannulation with the nurse, physical therapist, advanced care provider, and ECMO specialist. The patient monitor is readily visible for the nurse, and the ECMO specialist is monitoring the tubing length. (B) A patient ambulating 13 days after VA ECMO cannulation. (From Pasrija C, Mackowick KM, Raithel M, Tran D, Boulos FM, Deatrick KB, et al. Ambulation with femoral arterial cannulation can be safely performed on venoarterial extracorporeal membrane oxygenation. *Ann Thorac Surg.* 2019;107[5]:1389-1394.)

operating room. The sites of cannulation are then closed either via surgical revision or using vascular closure devices, depending on the size of the cannulas, location of the cannulation, and the condition of the vessels.[44-46]

After the cannulas are removed, patients require close monitoring for any signs of bleeding, infection, or recurrence of cardiac dysfunction.

Challenges and Considerations

Decisions around weaning and decannulation should consider individual patient factors such as underlying diseases, the duration on ECMO, and overall recovery progress. It is important that goals of care are discussed with the patient and their families, and that it is made clear if the patient is a candidate for recannulation and initiation of ECMO therapy if they were to decompensate again.

Weaning and decannulation from ECMO are complex processes that require a multidisciplinary approach, involving intensive care physicians, cardiothoracic surgeons, nurses, respiratory therapists, and other specialists. Careful planning, adherence to evidence-based protocols, and patient-centered care are essential to optimize outcomes and minimize complications.

Extracorporeal Cardiopulmonary Resuscitation

ECPR is a resuscitation strategy for patients in cardiac arrest that incorporates rapid ECMO cannulation to provide mechanical support to help achieve a return of spontaneous circulation (ROSC).[21] It is used when a patient in cardiac arrest fails to respond to conventional CPR and provides both hemodynamic and respiratory support during the resuscitative efforts. The overall 30-day survival rate for adult patients undergoing ECPR is 30%, whereas the pediatric survival rate stands at 41%.[1]

Extracorporeal Cardiopulmonary Resuscitation Process

Assessment and initiation: The decision to initiate ECPR is usually made when conventional CPR is not effective within the first 15 minutes of cardiac arrest. Quick assessment of the patient's condition, likelihood of survival, associated significant comorbidities, and the feasibility of ECPR is crucial.[47] Although there are no absolute inclusion or exclusion criteria, several proposed ECPR considerations have published to help quickly identify potential candidates. Finally, early activation of the ECMO team facilitates these time-sensitive ECPR assessments, considerations, and cannulations.[47]

Cannulation: The cannulation procedure for ECPR typically involves ultrasound-guided rapid vascular access and cannula insertion for emergent peripheral VA ECMO initiation. This is usually performed via the femoral vein and contralateral femoral artery. This must be done swiftly and accurately to rapidly restore circulation and oxygenation while minimizing the risk of technical errors and complications.[22] During an ECPR resuscitation, the priority should be successful cannulation and initiation of ECMO, whereas a distal perfusion cannula can be placed later at bedside, in the cath lab, or in the operating room after the patient has been stabilized on ECMO support.

Post-ECPR care: Management of an ECPR patient after achieving ROSC involves a careful determination of the underlying cause of cardiac arrest and consideration for procedural interventions such as a PCI. Pulsatility must be maintained while the heart cannot be allowed to distend. Management considerations for these goals include optimization of inotropic

support, insertion of an IABP, creation of a septostomy, or placement of an Impella or other left-heart unloading technique.[22,37] Patients require continuous hemodynamic, neurologic, and respiratory monitoring with adjustment of ECMO settings and vasoactive infusions to help maintain adequate end-organ perfusion and oxygenation. Neurologic assessment should be prioritized and neurocritical care should be consulted once ECMO support is initiated to optimize postarrest neurologic recovery.[22,24]

Indications and Contraindications[21]

Indications.

- Refractory cardiac arrest: When conventional CPR does not result in ROSC.
- Witnessed arrest: Especially in the presence of healthcare providers with immediate CPR and availability of rapid ECMO deployment.
- Potentially reversible cause: When the underlying cause of the cardiac arrest can potentially be treated (e.g., massive pulmonary embolism, myocardial infarction, drug toxicity).

Contraindications.

- Prolonged cardiac arrest without CPR: If the cardiac arrest is unwitnessed and CPR is delayed, leading to a significant period without perfusion.
- Severe comorbid conditions: Terminal illnesses or severe multiorgan failure that does not warrant aggressive life-support measures.
- Unrecoverable neurologic status: Patients with significant baseline neurologic impairments or those who are expected to have poor neurologic outcomes even if resuscitation is successful.
- Severe trauma: Especially where hemorrhage control is not feasible, making ECMO counterproductive or dangerous.

The decision to use ECPR involves critical consideration of the patient's overall prognosis, the rapid availability of ECMO technology, and a multidisciplinary team capable of performing this complex procedure.

SPECIAL CIRCUMSTANCES AND ECMO

Trauma: ECMO is increasingly considered in trauma patients with severe cardiopulmonary failure when conventional therapies fail. It can be particularly beneficial in cases of severe chest trauma with pulmonary contusions and severe respiratory failure. VV ECMO has also been successfully used to support patients after a traumatic pneumonectomy, whereas VA ECMO may be considered in cases of cardiogenic shock secondary to a structural cardiac injury. However, the risk of bleeding due to anticoagulation required during ECMO is a significant concern, especially in patients with active hemorrhage or traumatic brain injury (TBI).[9]

Concomitant neuropathology: Using ECMO in patients with neurologic injuries (such as bleed, cerebrovascular accidents [CVAs], TBI, or recent neurosurgery) is complex due to the need for anticoagulation, which poses a risk of exacerbating or causing new intracranial hemorrhages.[48] The decision to initiate ECMO involves careful risk-benefit analysis, often considering the extent of brain injury and the potential for neurologic recovery. Although there has been an increase in the successful utilization of ECMO in this patient population, concomitant neuropathology should not be considered an ßabsolute contradiction for ECMO initiation.

Septic shock: ECMO may be used in septic patients who develop severe ARDS or refractory septic shock, particularly when there is suspected sepsis-driven cardiac depression. It supports oxygenation and circulation while potentially allowing the heart and lungs to recover from sepsis-induced damage. However, ECMO does not address the underlying infection and inflammation, and meticulous management of the source of infection and supportive care are crucial. Due to the vasodilation associated with profound sepsis, managing ECMO flows and providing adequate support can be uniquely challenging in this hypermetabolic state.[49]

To determine whether ECMO will be beneficial in septic shock, it is important to assess cardiac output and heart function. This can be done using a Swan-Ganz catheter to measure cardiac output and echocardiography to evaluate heart function. If cardiac output is high and echocardiography shows good heart function, ECMO is unlikely to help in septic shock as the issue is not cardiac depression but rather vasodilation and hypermetabolism.[49]

Hypothermia: ECMO circuits incorporate precise thermoregulation capabilities through built-in heat exchangers, allowing for targeted control of patient body temperature. This feature is particularly crucial in the management of severe accidental hypothermia, especially in instances complicated by cardiac arrest. By using ECMO, clinicians can meticulously manage the rewarming process, ensuring it is gradual and controlled to prevent the complications associated with rapid temperature changes.[50] The capability to precisely adjust the ECMO temperature settings and control a patients' body temperature not only supports essential physiologic functions during this critical time but also significantly enhances patient outcomes in conditions that might otherwise prove fatal.[50]

Drug overdose: In cases of severe drug overdose resulting in cardiac or respiratory failure, ECMO can be a lifesaving modality. It provides supportive care allowing time to metabolize and clear the toxic substances. Specific scenarios include overdoses of drugs like β-blockers, calcium channel blockers, or opioid overdose resulting in aspiration, with failed attempts of medical management.[51]

Transplant: ECMO is used as a bridge to transplant in patients with end-stage heart or lung disease. It stabilizes patients until a suitable organ becomes available and can also support post-transplant patients through acute phases of graft dysfunction or rejection.[32,52]

Each of these scenarios requires careful consideration of the patient's specific conditions, potential benefits, and risks associated with ECMO. Decision-making typically involves a multidisciplinary team of specialists, including surgeons, critical care physicians, cardiologists, and others to address the broad implications of ECMO therapy. Its use in such special circumstances often necessitates tailored approaches, balancing the benefits of ECMO support against potential complications, especially bleeding and infection risks.

ECMO COMPLICATIONS

Complications associated with ECMO can vary widely depending on the patient's condition, the duration of ECMO support, and the specific ECMO modality and configuration that is used (VA vs. VV vs. V-AV and peripheral vs. central).

Low flows and ECMO chatter/chugging: Low flow and chatter (or chugging) can occur due to hypovolemia, cannula mispositioning, or thrombosis within the circuit. This results in inadequate flow rates that can cause the ECMO pump to function intermittently or "chug." Regular monitoring and adjustments to fluid status, cannula placement, and anticoagulation can help manage this issue. It is also important to evaluate the patient for any potential signs of abdominal compartment syndrome that can result in compression of the IVC and impaired ECMO flow.[53-55]

Bleeding: Bleeding is a common complication due to the systemic anticoagulation necessary for ECMO operation. It can occur at surgical sites, cannulation sites, or internally. Managing anticoagulation meticulously and monitoring for signs of bleeding are crucial.

Infection: Infections can arise from cannula sites or within the ECMO circuit itself. Strict adherence to sterile procedures during cannulation and routine care, frequent site inspections, and prophylactic antibiotic strategies are important to minimize this risk.[45]

Hemolysis: Hemolysis can occur due to the mechanical forces within the ECMO circuit. Monitoring laboratory markers such as lactate dehydrogenase, plasma-free hemoglobin, and transmembrane pressures aid in early detection.[56] It is important to closely examine all circuit components for thrombus formation as this can contribute to the hemolysis. Hemolysis can often be mitigated with adjustments to the ECMO flows, component changes such as an oxygenator exchange if indicated, and circuit changes if the patient still requires ECMO support, but in severe cases ECMO decannulation may be warranted.

Extremity ischemia: Ischemia of the extremities can occur due to impaired blood flow related to cannulation, particularly with femoral artery cannula insertions. Routine placement of an antegrade distal perfusion cannula in the superficial femoral artery on the arterial cannulation side can mitigate this risk.[57] If there are concerns for malperfusion with a distal perfusion line in place, a bedside angiogram down the distal perfusion catheter can be used to confirm positioning and flow (Fig. 116.14). Additionally, monitoring techniques such as near-infrared spectroscopy or Doppler/pulse monitoring can be employed to assess perfusion. It is important to note that any Doppler signals of the specific extremity may be continuous. The distal perfusion cannula can be momentarily shut off to evaluate any changes in the signal if there is a concern regarding flow.

Neurologic Complications

- Lower extremity paralysis is a rare complication but may occur due to spinal cord ischemia.[58] One suggested theory is abnormal turbulent flow as the retrograde ECMO flow of peripheral VA ECMO mixes with the native cardiac output. It has been proposed that adjustments may be made to the ECMO flow rates to alter the location of this turbulent "mixing zone." It may be necessary to consider prompt decannulation from VA ECMO in this scenario. Further studies are needed to fully understand the etiology of this rare complication.[58]

- CVAs can occur due to thromboembolic events or hemorrhages, exacerbated by the altered coagulation state on ECMO.[59]

DVT: This is a risk due to reduced mobility and vascular endothelial trauma from cannulas. Systemic anticoagulation while on ECMO helps mitigate that risk, whereas post-decannulation monitoring allows for early detection.[19]

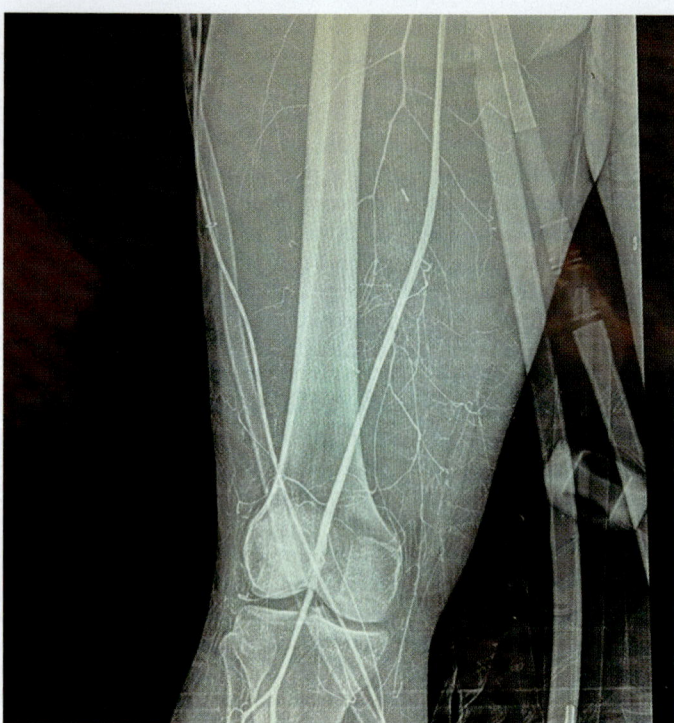

FIGURE 116.14 Bedside angiogram performed by directly injecting water-soluble contrast through the distal perfusion sheath. (Courtesy UMMC: Distal perfusion angiogram done in the intensive care unit.)

Wounds and deconditioning: Long-term ECMO support can lead to pressure ulcers, muscle wasting, and general physical deconditioning. Regular repositioning, nutritional support, and, where possible, physical therapy are essential for managing these issues.

Each of these complications requires proactive management and interdisciplinary teamwork to mitigate risks and improve outcomes for patients on ECMO. Addressing these challenges promptly and effectively is key to maximizing the therapeutic benefits of ECMO while minimizing adverse effects.

MULTIDISCIPLINARY APPROACH

Management of ECMO patients requires a multidisciplinary approach involving specialized consultants in addition to the surgical team for comprehensive care. Physical and occupational therapists play a critical role in maintaining and enhancing patient mobility to prevent muscle atrophy. Nutritionists ensure that patients receive tailored nutritional support to meet the metabolic demands, reduce the risk of malnutrition, and support recovery. Infectious disease specialists are crucial for managing infections, a common risk due to the invasiveness of ECMO and associated immunocompromised states.

Specialists in heart failure and pulmonary transplant assess and manage patients when ECMO is used as a bridge to transplant, providing vital support in complex cardiopulmonary cases. Finally, the palliative care service is integral in addressing quality-of-life concerns, ensuring that care aligns with the patient's and family's wishes, particularly in end-of-life scenarios. Together, these consultants form a vital network that supports the diverse needs of ECMO patients, enhancing outcomes and facilitating comprehensive care.

CHALLENGES: FUTILITY

Clinical assessment of futility: Determining futility involves evaluating the likelihood of recovery or significant improvement with continued ECMO support. This requires a thorough understanding of the patient's underlying condition, the trajectory of their illness, and the potential for reversibility of their acute condition. Clinicians often rely on a combination of clinical judgment, ethical frameworks, and evidence-based guidelines to make these determinations.

Ethical and emotional considerations: Discussions around futility can be emotionally challenging for both the healthcare team and the patient's family. It involves balancing hope for recovery with the realistic outcomes of continued treatment. Ethical dilemmas arise when considering the patient's quality of life posttreatment, the potential for suffering, and the judicious use of medical resources.

Communication and decision-making: Effective communication is crucial when discussing the possibility of futility. Engaging in open and honest dialogue with family members and among the care team is essential. These discussions should ideally involve multidisciplinary team members, including ethics consultants when available, to provide a well-rounded perspective on the patient's care options.

End-of-life care planning: When ECMO is deemed futile, the focus shifts toward palliative care and end-of-life decision-making. Ensuring comfort, managing symptoms, and supporting the family emotionally and psychologically become the primary goals. Discussions about withdrawing ECMO support are sensitive and should be handled with utmost care, respecting the dignity and wishes of the patient and their family.

The challenge of futility on ECMO underscores the need for ongoing ethical education and support for healthcare providers, enabling them to navigate these difficult decisions effectively and compassionately.

SUMMARY

ECMO is a significant advancement and powerful resource in cardiopulmonary critical care, offering life-sustaining mechanical support for patients with severe cardiac and respiratory failure when conventional treatments have failed. ECMO can be life saving. This technology provides patients with a bridge to recovery, a bridge to transplantation, or time that supports intricate decision-making. The application of ECMO spans various scenarios showcasing its versatility in supporting complex medical conditions not amenable to conventional management.

However, the use of ECMO is not without challenges. It requires meticulous management of potential complications such as bleeding, infection, neurologic injury, and malnutrition. The decision to initiate or discontinue ECMO involves ethical considerations, particularly in determining futility, which requires careful communication and decision-making with patient families and within the care team. As ECMO technology evolves and becomes more integrated into clinical practice, the focus remains on enhancing patient outcomes, refining techniques, and expanding the knowledge and skills of the multidisciplinary teams that manage these complex interventions. This ongoing development underscores ECMO's critical role in modern medicine, providing not just a chance for survival but also a testament to the advancements in patient care and critical care technology.

SELECTED REFERENCES

Extracorporeal Life Support Organization (ELSO). *ELSO Guidelines for Cardiopulmonary Extracorporeal Life Support.* 6th ed. Ann Arbor: Extracorporeal Life Support Organization; 2022.

These guidelines from the Extracorporeal Life Support Organization provide comprehensive instructions and best practices for the use of extracorporeal life support (ECLS) in cardiopulmonary settings. The 6th edition includes updated recommendations based on the latest research and clinical experiences, making it an essential resource for clinicians involved in ECLS. Its significance lies in offering standardized protocols that help improve patient outcomes and ensure safety during extracorporeal procedures.

Levy LE, Kaczorowski DJ, Pasrija C, et al. Peripheral cannulation for extracorporeal membrane oxygenation yields superior neurologic outcomes in adult patients who experienced cardiac arrest following cardiac surgery. *Perfusion.* 2022;37(7):745-751.

This study investigates the neurologic outcomes of adult patients who underwent peripheral cannulation for extracorporeal membrane oxygenation after experiencing cardiac arrest post-cardiac surgery. The findings indicate that peripheral cannulation is associated with better neurologic outcomes compared with central cannulation. The significance of this research lies in its potential to influence ECMO cannulation practices, promoting the adoption of peripheral cannulation to improve patient recovery and neurologic function after cardiac arrest.

Panchal AR, Berg KM, Hirsch KG, et al. 2019 American Heart Association Focused update on advanced cardiovascular life support: use of advanced airways, vasopressors, and extracorporeal cardiopulmonary resuscitation during cardiac arrest: an update to the American Heart Association guidelines for cardiopulmonary resuscitation and emergency cardiovascular care. *Circulation.* 2019;140(24):e881-e894.

This focused update by the American Heart Association provides critical revisions to the guidelines on advanced cardiovascular life support, specifically addressing the use of advanced airways, vasopressors, and extracorporeal cardiopulmonary resuscitation during cardiac arrest. The update reflects the latest evidence and expert consensus aimed at improving survival rates and neurologic outcomes in cardiac arrest patients. Its significance lies in informing and refining ACLS practices, thereby enhancing the effectiveness of resuscitation efforts in critical care settings.

Pasrija C, Mackowick KM, Raithel M, et al. Ambulation with femoral arterial cannulation can be safely performed on venoarterial extracorporeal membrane oxygenation. *Ann Thorac Surg.* 2019:107(5):1389-1394.

This study explores the feasibility and safety of ambulating patients who are on veno-arterial extracorporeal membrane oxygenation with femoral arterial cannulation. The results demonstrate that ambulation can be safely achieved without compromising the stability of the ECMO circuit or the patient's condition. The significance of this work lies in its potential to enhance the quality of life and recovery outcomes for patients on VA ECMO by allowing early mobilization, which is associated with numerous benefits including reduced muscle atrophy and improved overall function.

Shah A, Dave S, Goerlich CE, Kaczorowski DJ. Hybrid and parallel extracorporeal membrane oxygenation circuits. *JTCVS Tech.* 2021;8:77-85.

This article explores innovative configurations of extracorporeal membrane oxygenation circuits, specifically hybrid and parallel setups. These advanced circuit designs aim to enhance the flexibility and efficiency of ECMO support, catering to complex clinical scenarios. The significance of this work lies in its potential to improve patient outcomes by providing alternative ECMO strategies that can be tailored to specific needs, thus expanding the toolkit available to clinicians managing severe cardiopulmonary failure.

Tonna JE, Abrams D, Brodie D, et al. Management of adult patients supported with venovenous extracorporeal membrane oxygenation (VV ECMO): guideline from the Extracorporeal Life Support Organization (ELSO). *ASAIO J.* 2021;6(6):601-610.

This guideline by the ELSO provides detailed recommendations for the management of adult patients undergoing venovenous extracorporeal membrane oxygenation. It covers a wide range of aspects, from patient selection and cannulation techniques to monitoring and weaning off ECMO support. The significance of this guideline lies in its role as a standardized protocol, aiming to optimize care, improve patient outcomes, and ensure the safety and efficacy of VV ECMO therapy in adult patients.

The full reference list appears on Elsevier eBooks+.

Specialties in Surgery: Subspecialty Considerations Relevant for the General Surgeon

The following chapter appears only on Elsevier eBooks+:

118 Maternal-Fetal Surgery

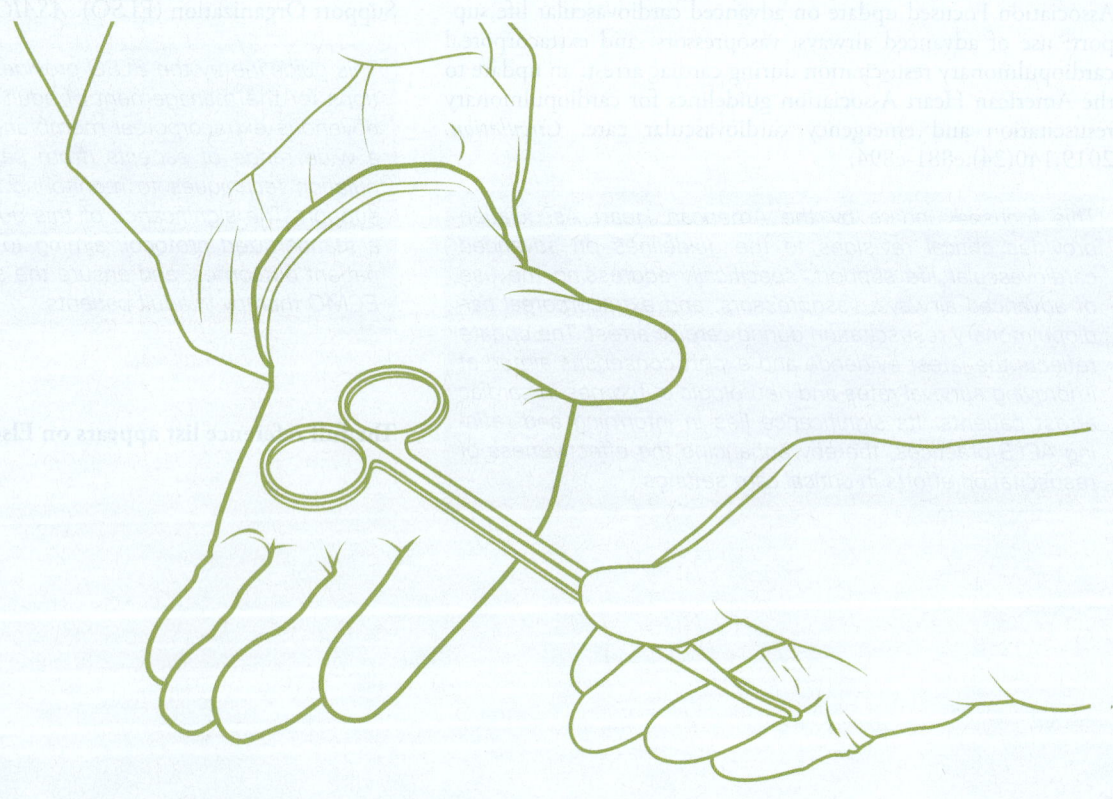

CHAPTER 117

Pediatric Surgery

Dai H Chung, Edward M. Barksdale, Jr., Bindi J. Naik-Mathuria, and Ravi S. Radhakrishnan

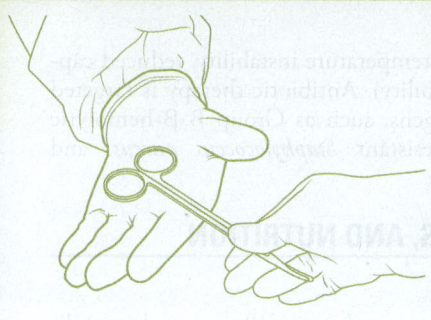

OUTLINE

Pediatric surgery remains the last bastion of true general surgical specialty. Pediatric surgical conditions span fetal to neonatal, adolescent, and young adults. Pediatric surgeons must assess and manage a wide spectrum of surgical conditions with vastly different pathophysiology. In recent decades, there has been an increasing trend to develop subspecialties of pediatric surgery, such as colorectal, pediatric surgical oncology, and chest wall deformity programs. They cover a wide spectrum of organ systems ranging from head and neck to thoracic and the gastrointestinal (GI) tract. This chapter will provide an overview of common and unique pediatric surgical conditions and their pathophysiology and treatment strategies.

NEONATAL PHYSIOLOGY

The newborn physiology is unique in terms of their smaller physiologic capacity and cellular and functional immaturity of organ systems. Newborns are at risk for cold ambient temperatures, and an ideal thermal environment must be maintained to reduce oxygen consumption and metabolic demands. The major risk factors for hypothermia in infants include a relatively large body surface area compared with body weight, limited subcutaneous fat, and increased insensible fluid losses. Infants also respond to cooler ambient temperatures by nonshivering thermogenesis, whereby increases in metabolism and oxygen consumption occur.

Thermoregulated isolettes are commonly used to keep an ideal ambient temperature (~23°C) to maintain the neonate's core body temperature between 36°C and 37.5°C.

Cardiopulmonary

During fetal circulation, arterial blood from the placenta bypasses the fetal lungs through the patent foramen ovale and ductus arteriosus. After birth, the foramen ovale closes with the newborn's first breath, then a precipitous drop in pulmonary vascular resistance occurs, increasing pulmonary blood flow. Decreased blood flow, along with a higher oxygen content, promotes spontaneous closure of the ductus arteriosus. Pulmonary vascular resistance is increased by hypoxemia and acidosis, resulting in persistent pulmonary hypertension (PPHN) and right-to-left shunt. Nonsteroidal anti-inflammatory agents (i.e., indomethacin) can promote the closure of a patent ductus arteriosus in premature infants. If persistently open, patent ductus arteriosus closure is achieved by catheter-based coil procedure and, on occasion, a traditional open surgical ductal ligation. The infant heart has a limited capacity to increase the stroke volume; cardiac output is largely heart rate dependent. Heart rate change and capillary refill are sensitive indicators of intravascular volume status and tissue perfusion, respectively.

At birth, the lungs are considered functionally immature, and they continue to develop new terminal bronchioles and alveoli until 6 to 8 years of age. The neonatal lung has fewer type II pneumocytes, which produce surfactant, a lipoprotein mixture of phospholipid, protein, and neutral fats. Surfactant regulates alveolar surface tension, thereby increasing functional residual capacity. Lecithin, the most predominant phospholipid, can be measured in amniotic fluid, and the lecithin to sphingomyelin ratio is used to determine fetal lung maturity. Premature infants are at greater risk for alveolar collapse, hyaline membrane formation, and barotrauma from mechanical ventilatory support. Also, the newborn airway is quite small, with an average tracheal diameter of 2.5 to 4 mm, and can easily be plugged with airway secretions. The respiratory rate for a healthy newborn ranges from 40 to 60 breaths/min, with a tidal volume of 6 to 10 mL/kg. Nasal flaring, grunting, intercostal and substernal retractions, and cyanosis are symptoms and signs of respiratory distress. Infants are obligate nasal and diaphragmatic breathers; therefore, any condition that obstructs the nasal passages (e.g., nasogastric tube) or interferes with diaphragmatic function may severely compromise respiratory status. Exogenous surfactant therapy has resulted in improved survival of premature infants and decreased incidence of bronchopulmonary dysplasia, a condition characterized by oxygen dependence, radiologic abnormality, and chronic respiratory symptoms beyond the first 28 days of life. Nitric oxide gas, a potent inducer of vascular smooth muscle relaxation, is also effective against PPHN.

Immunology

Infants have lower levels of immunoglobulins (IgA, G, and M) and of the C3b complement at birth, so they are at higher risk for systemic infection. A sepsis workup for neonates includes surveillance cultures of various bodily fluids—such as cerebrospinal fluid—as well as routine blood laboratory tests. Infants are also at risk for potential septic sources arising from invasive vascular catheters and interventions such as prolonged endotracheal intubation and bladder catheterization, which can contribute to hospital-acquired conditions. An empirical antibiotic regimen is often started based on subtle clinical suspicions (e.g., decreased tolerance of enteral feeding, temperature instability, reduced capillary refill, tachypnea, irritability). Antibiotic therapy is targeted at common bacterial pathogens, such as Group B β-hemolytic streptococcus, methicillin-resistant *Staphylococcus aureus,* and *Escherichia coli.*

FLUIDS, ELECTROLYTES, AND NUTRITION

Fluid and Electrolytes

Fluid and electrolyte balance must be carefully assessed in pediatric surgical patients, especially in neonates and small toddlers with a narrower margin for error. Due to higher insensible water losses through a thin, immature skin barrier, fluid requirements for premature infants can be substantial. Insensible water losses are directly related to gestational age, which ranges from 45 to 60 mL/kg/day for premature infants weighing less than 1500 g to 30–35 mL/kg/day for term infants. Radiant heat warmers, phototherapy for hyperbilirubinemia, and respiratory distress can result in additional fluid losses. During the first 3 to 5 days of life, physiologic water loss can be up to 10% of the body weight. Fluid requirements are calculated according to body weight. During the first few days, the fluid recommendations are on the conservative side; however, infants require 100 to 130 mL/kg/day for maintenance fluids by the fourth day of life. Surgical conditions such as gastroschisis and necrotizing enterocolitis (NEC) demand significantly higher volume. Urine output and osmolarity are good indicators of adequate tissue perfusion. The ideal minimum urine output in a newborn is 1 to 2 mL/kg/day. Infants can respond to prerenal azotemia by concentrating urine only up to approximately 700 mOsm/kg. The daily requirements for sodium and potassium are 2 to 4 and 1 to 2 mEq/kg, respectively. These requirements are usually met with 5% dextrose in 0.45% normal saline (NS) with 20 mEq/L of potassium at the calculated maintenance rate. Fluid losses from gastric drainage, ostomy output, or diarrhea should also be carefully assessed and replaced with an appropriate solution. Gastric losses should be replaced in equal volumes with 0.45% NS with 20 mEq/L of potassium. Diarrheal, pancreatic, and biliary losses are replaced with isotonic lactated Ringer solution. Hypovolemia due to acute hemorrhage should be corrected with prompt transfusion of blood products at a bolus of 10 to 20 mL/kg of packed red blood cells, plasma, or 5% albumin.

Nutrition

Energy requirements vary substantially from infancy to childhood. Appropriate weight gain is the most reliable clinical indicator of adequate caloric consumption. Total daily caloric requirements and the weight curve plateau with age. Nearly 50% of the energy in term infants younger than 2 weeks and 60% of energy in premature infants <1200 g are consumed for growth. A general guideline for the enteral calorie requirement of infants is 120 calories/kg/day to achieve an ideal weight gain of ~1% of body weight per day. The standard infant formulas, as well as breast milk, contain 20 calories/ounce. Formulas with higher calorie density are available for infants who are unable to consume sufficient volumes to meet their calorie requirements or those with strict fluid restrictions. Breast milk is the ideal form of enteral nutrition. However, hypoallergenic, lactose-free to amino acid–based formulas are available to meet the specific needs of infants with particular GI tract conditions. In general, continuous enteral feedings are used for infants with a stressed gut and then transitioned to gastric bolus feedings. The enteral feeding tolerance is carefully monitored by assessing for abdominal girth, gastric residuals, and stool output.

Carbohydrates are stored mainly as glycogen in the liver and muscles. Because newborn liver and muscle masses are disproportionately smaller than those of an adult, infants are susceptible to hypoglycemia with risks for seizure and neurologic impairment. The minimum glucose infusion rate for neonates is 4 to 6 mg/kg/min. This rate must be calculated daily while the infant is receiving parenteral nutrition. For total parenteral nutrition (TPN), the glucose infusion rate is increased daily in increments of 1 to 2 mg/kg/min to a maximum value of 10 to 12 mg/kg/min. Hyperglycemia from a glucose infusion rate that is less than ideal should be avoided because it can lead to rapid hyperosmolarity and dehydration. Hyperglycemia may indicate underlying sepsis and should be appropriately investigated.

The average intake of protein is ~15% of the total daily calories and ranges from 2 to 3.5 g/kg/day in infants. This protein requirement is reduced in half by the age of 12 years and approaches the adult requirement (1 g/kg/day) by 18 years of age. The provision of greater amounts of protein relative to nonprotein calories will result in rising blood urea nitrogen levels. Thus, the non-protein (carbohydrate plus fat calories) to protein-calorie ratio (expressed in grams plus fat calories) is not less than 150 to 1. For infants receiving parenteral nutrition, protein administration usually starts at 0.5 g/kg/day and advances in daily increments of 0.5 g/kg/day to the target goal of approximately 3.5 g/kg/day.

Fat is another major source of nonprotein calories. Linoleic acid, an 18-carbon chain with two double bonds, is considered an essential fatty acid; its deficiency results in dryness, rash, and desquamation of skin. In pediatric patients, fat is provided as a major source of calories to prevent the development of essential fatty acid deficiency. The lipid requirements for growth are significant, and fat is a robust calorie source. Similar to protein, fat infusions are started at 0.5 g/kg/day and advanced up to 2.5 to 3.5 g/kg/day. In infants with unconjugated hyperbilirubinemia, fat is administered with caution because fatty acids may displace bilirubin from albumin. The free unconjugated bilirubin may then cross the blood-brain barrier and can lead to kernicterus, resulting in mental retardation.

TPN is reserved for infants for whom adequate daily enteral nutrition cannot be achieved. Infants have sufficient energy reserves to tolerate short periods of starvation lasting 2 to 3 days. Thus, an infant's need for parenteral nutrition should be addressed promptly. The total TPN infusion rate is kept at a steady-state rate to meet daily fluid requirements, and the concentration of nutrients is gradually increased daily until goals are met. Infants with surgical conditions often become cholestatic, typically caused by prolonged TPN support; however, other causes should be ruled out. Serum bile acid levels are usually elevated first, then direct bilirubin concentration, followed by liver enzyme levels. The ideal treatment for TPN-associated cholestasis is restoring enteral feeding. The use of omega-3 fat emulsion (Omegaven) has been critical in preventing TPN-induced cholestasis.[1] A medium-chain triglyceride–containing formula is used, and if an infant is receiving total enteral nutrition, fat-soluble vitamins should be supplemented.

HEAD AND NECK LESIONS

Subcutaneous Nodules

Benign subcutaneous nodules are quite common in pediatric patients of all ages. Dermoid and epidermoid cysts are benign lesions that arise from part of the dermal or epidermal tissues, forming a small cyst filled with normal skin components. Dermoid cysts may contain various dermal components, such as hair and skin glands. Epidermoid cysts typically have only epidermal tissue and keratin debris. They commonly occur on the forehead, lateral corner of the eyebrow, or anterior fontanelle or in the postauricular space. They are generally asymptomatic but may increase in size over time and can often become osteolytic. Most scalp lesions require only the clinical examination for diagnosis and subsequent surgical excision. Pilomatrixoma is another common, slow-growing benign skin tumor of the hair follicle. They often present as discrete and firm, nontender subcutaneous nodules but require surgical excision when presenting with symptoms of localized pain or infection. For midline lesions, an ultrasound examination can be valuable in delineating benign subcutaneous lesions from others, such as communicating cephalocele.

Lymphadenopathy

Enlarged lymph nodes present as mobile discrete solitary tumors or a cluster of tumors in the neck, axillary region, and groin. They typically are present along the sternocleidomastoid muscle border in the neck and over the inguinal canal and femoral triangle areas. Enlarged lymph nodes are one of the most common conditions for pediatric surgical consultation for evaluation, biopsy, or removal. The etiology is often unknown but presumed to be multifocal. A detailed history and physical examination are sufficient to determine whether surgery is indicated. The use of ultrasound has become widely prevalent and can, at times, identify nodes with central necrosis requiring immediate surgical intervention. Occasionally, lymph nodes presenting as fixed, nontender, progressively enlarging masses in the supraclavicular region should raise suspicion for malignancy. Constitutional symptoms such as night sweats and weight loss should prompt a thorough investigation; chest radiography could detect mediastinal adenopathy. Acute, bilateral cervical lymphadenitis from respiratory viral infectious causes (e.g., adenovirus, influenza virus, respiratory syncytial virus) requires observation alone. *S. aureus* and group A streptococcus are responsible for the majority of acute pyogenic lymphadenitis.

Cat-scratch disease is a self-limited infectious condition characterized by painful regional lymphadenopathy. A gram-negative bacillus, *Bartonella henselae*, is responsible for most cases. A history of exposure to cats is helpful but not always present. Indirect immunofluorescence antibody testing has only moderate specificity. Polymerase chain reaction assay of a lymph node biopsy specimen can increase diagnostic accuracy. Cat-scratch disease is usually self-limited. A less common infectious cause of cervical lymphadenitis is nontuberculous mycobacterial infection. The nodes are fluctuant, with a violaceous appearance of the overlying skin. The diagnosis is made by positive cultures for nontuberculous acid-fast bacilli, along with a tuberculin skin test. Surgical excision is usually indicated because most nontuberculous mycobacteria are resistant to conventional chemotherapy.

Cystic Hygroma

Cystic hygroma is a multiloculated cyst lined by endothelial cells, resulting from a lymphatic malformation. Most involve the lymphatic jugular sacs and are present in the posterior neck region. Other common sites are the axillary, mediastinal, inguinal, and retroperitoneal regions; approximately 50% of these cystic lesions are present at birth. Cystic hygromas are soft cystic masses that can distort the surrounding structure, including the airway. A large cystic mass of the neck in the fetus can pose a significant threat to the airway at birth. Prenatal ultrasound and fetal magnetic resonance imaging (MRI) studies can better demonstrate the extent of the disease along with its mass effect on the airway. If present, careful coordination of surgical intervention (ex utero intrapartum treatment [EXIT] procedure) at the time of delivery can be lifesaving, though this is more likely with solid tumors such as teratomas. Cystic hygromas are prone to infection and hemorrhage into the mass. MRI is useful in outlining the extent of lymphatic channels. The surgical goal is to complete surgical excision with tedious isolation and ligation of lymphatic branches. Aggressive blunt and electrocautery dissections as well as radical resection must be avoided, as this can lead to recurrence or infection due to incomplete control of lymphatics. When a complete surgical excision is not feasible, injection with sclerosing agents, such as bleomycin, doxycycline, or OK-432 derived from *Streptococcus pyogenes*, should be considered as an effective nonsurgical option.[2]

Thyroglossal Duct Cyst

An upper midline cystic neck lesion in toddlers is a thyroglossal duct cyst until proven otherwise (Fig. 117.1). It originates at the base of the tongue at the foramen cecum and descends through the central portion of the hyoid bone. Although thyroglossal duct cysts may occur anywhere from the base of the tongue to the thyroid gland, most are found at or just below the hyoid bone. A thyroid diverticulum develops as a median endodermal thickening at the foramen cecum in the embryonic stage of development. The thyroid diverticulum descends in the neck and remains attached to the base of the tongue by the thyroglossal

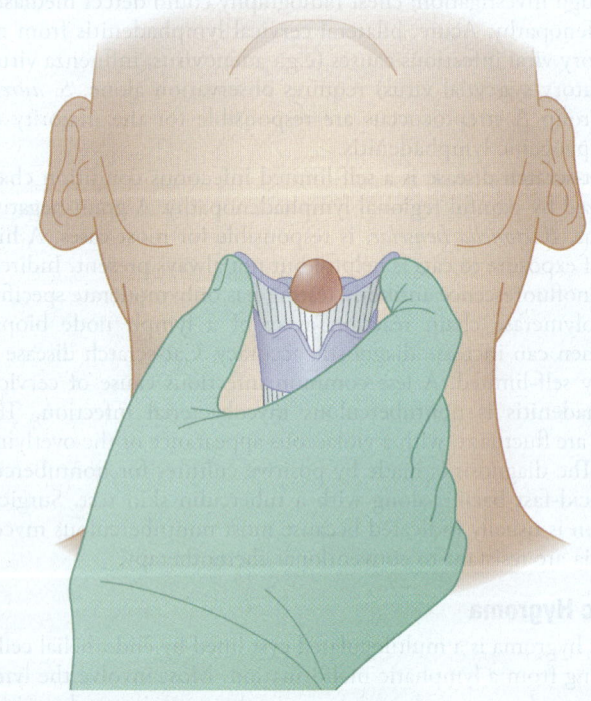

FIGURE 117.1 Thyroglossal duct cyst presents as a midline neck mass. A thyroglossal duct cyst can extend up to its origin at the foramen cecum. (Josephs MD. Thyroglossal duct cyst. In: Chung DH, Chen MK, eds. *Atlas of Pediatric Surgical Techniques*. Philadelphia: Elsevier Saunders; 2010:28-33.)

duct. As the thyroid gland descends to its normal pretracheal position, the ventral cartilages of the second and third branchial arches form the hyoid bone. Hence, the intimate anatomic relationship of the thyroglossal duct remnant exists with the central portion of the hyoid bone. The thyroglossal duct normally regresses by the time the thyroid gland reaches its final position. When the elements of the duct persist despite complete thyroid descent, a thyroglossal duct cyst may develop. Failure of normal caudal migration of the thyroid gland results in a lingual thyroid, in which no other thyroid tissue is present in the neck. Ultrasound or radionuclide imaging may be useful to identify the presence of an ectopic thyroid gland in the neck. The Sistrunk procedure, first described in 1928, is the standard operation for thyroglossal duct cysts. It involves complete excision of the cyst in continuity with its tract, the central portion of the hyoid bone, and the tract interior to the hyoid bone extending to the base of the tongue. Incomplete resection can result in cyst recurrence in up to 40% to 50% of cases.

Branchial Cleft Remnants

Branchial cleft remnants present as lateral neck masses. Embryologically, the structures of the head and neck are derived from six pairs of branchial arches, their intervening clefts, and pouches. Congenital cysts, sinuses, or fistulas result from failure of these structures to regress, persisting in aberrant locations. The location of these remnants generally dictates their embryologic origin and guides the subsequent operative approach. Failure to understand the embryology may result in incomplete resection or injury to adjacent structures. Branchial lesions can manifest as sinuses, fistulas, or cartilaginous rests in infants. The clinical presentation ranges from continuous mucoid drainage, a fistula or sinus, or an infected cystic mass. Branchial remnants may also be palpable, as cartilaginous lumps or cords corresponding with a fistulous track. Dermal pits or skin tags may also be present. First branchial anomalies are typically located in the front or back of the ear or in the upper neck near the mandible. Fistulas typically course through the parotid gland, deep or through branches of the facial nerve, and end in the external auditory canal. The second branchial cleft anomalies are the most common type. The external ostium of these remnants is located along the anterior border of the sternocleidomastoid muscle, usually in the vicinity of the upper half to the lower third of the muscle. A tortuous and long course of the fistula tract can be found, which requires stepladder counterincisions in order to excise the fistula track completely. Typically, the fistula penetrates the platysma, ascends along the carotid sheath to the level of the hyoid bone, and turns medially to extend between the carotid artery bifurcations. The fistula courses adjacent to the hypoglossal and glossopharyngeal nerves, behind the posterior belly of the digastric and stylohyoid muscles, to end in the tonsillar fossa or other nasopharyngeal spaces. Third branchial cleft remnants usually do not have associated sinuses or fistulas. They are located in the suprasternal notch or clavicular region and can descend into the mediastinum. They present more commonly as cysts in toddlers and older children. These often contain cartilage and present clinically as a firm mass or subcutaneous abscess.

DIAPHRAGMATIC CONDITIONS

Congenital Diaphragmatic Hernia

Congenital diaphragmatic hernia (CDH) is a spectrum of developmental conditions marked by a diaphragmatic defect, causing

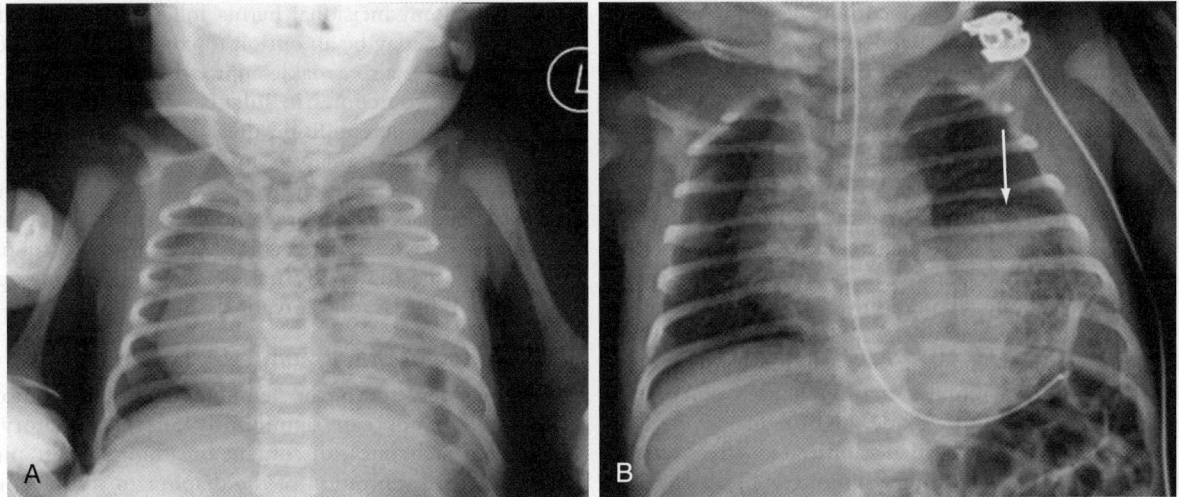

FIGURE 117.2 (A) Congenital diaphragmatic hernia. Multiple gas-filled bowel loops are located in the left hemithorax, and the mediastinum is shifted to the right. (B) Left diaphragmatic eventration. Hemidiaphragm is elevated *(arrow)* from phrenic nerve injury-induced paralysis.

abdominal contents to protrude into the thoracic cavity, disrupting lung and pulmonary vascular development (Fig. 117.2A). These anomalies range from a small opening in the posterior muscle rim to the complete absence or agenesis of the diaphragm. In most cases this is unilateral but rarely may be bilateral. This may lead to varying degrees of lung hypoplasia and pulmonary hypertension in the newborn that may significantly impact short-term survival and long-term morbidity. Advances in research and therapeutics over the last few decades have led to improved survival outcomes of 65% to 90%.[3–5]

The overall incidence of CDH is variably reported at ~1:2000 to 5000 childbirths, with most cases sporadic, isolated, and nonsyndromic. Although the exact etiology is unknown, animal models suggest genetic, environmental, and nutritional factors.[3] The diaphragm is embryologically derived from the septum transversum, the pleuroperitoneal folds, components of the abdominal wall, and the dorsal mesentery. At 3 to 4 weeks of gestation, these structures begin to fuse, separating the pleural and peritoneal cavities. This is followed by ingrowth from the abdominal wall, creating the muscular component of the diaphragm; this is typically complete by 9 weeks of gestation. Incomplete fusion may lead to an anterior defect or Morgagni hernia (~23%–28%), central hernia (2%–7%), or most commonly, Bochdalek posterior lateral hernia (70%–75%). Bochdalek hernias occur most commonly on the left side (85%) and less on the right side (13%) or rarely bilaterally (2%).[3] Abdominal contents herniate into the thoracic cavity through the diaphragmatic defect, compressing the ipsilateral developing lung. These lungs have smaller bronchi, with less bronchial branching and less alveolar surface areas. The ipsilateral lung is affected more severely; however, both lungs are affected by pulmonary hypoplasia. In addition, the pulmonary vasculature is significantly affected by increased thickness of the arteriolar smooth muscle. Arteriolar vasculature is also extremely sensitive to local and systemic vasoactive factors. The severity of pulmonary hypoplasia and pulmonary hypertension significantly impacts overall morbidity and mortality in infants with CDH.

Clinical Presentation

Routine utilization of prenatal ultrasound has led to diagnosis as early as 15 weeks of gestation, especially in very large defects.

Sonography at 22 to 24 weeks may demonstrate mediastinal shift, juxta-cardiac gastric dilatation, polyhydramnios, or other congenital anomalies. In the less common right-sided CDH, the liver may be seen in the right chest. The sonographic measurements of the lung size may establish important prognostic criteria helpful in prenatal and postnatal therapeutic management. The major predictors of outcome on fetal evaluation include the presence of coexistent congenital anomalies such as cardiac, chromosomal abnormalities, lung hypoplasia, and intrathoracic liver herniation.[6]

Lung head ratio (LHR) is a sonographic assessment of fetal lung size made by comparing the contralateral lung to head circumference with normal gestational age measurement. This quotient of the observed to expected size for gestational age may be a useful predictor of early neonatal morbidity. At birth, most infants with CDH may experience respiratory distress manifested by grunting, dyspnea, retractions, and cyanosis, although delayed presentations may occur. The physical examination may be notable for a scaphoid abdomen with diminished breath sounds in conjunction with bowel sounds in the chest. There may also be displacement of heart tones (depending on the side of the hernia). Pulse oximetry may demonstrate significant preductal and postductal differences indicative of right-to-left shunting, which is an important factor in management and prognosis. Chest x-ray indicating intrathoracic bowel loops and mediastinal shift may occur. In 10% to 20% of cases, CDH is diagnosed after the first 24 hours of life, typically when infants present with feeding difficulties, respiratory distress, or pneumonia. In Morgagni hernias, the diagnosis is often delayed until childhood because most infants are asymptomatic.[3]

Management

Intrauterine treatment of CDH with fetal endoluminal tracheal occlusion (FETO) may play a role in the management of patients with severe pulmonary hypoplasia secondary to diaphragmatic hernia. This technique involves endoscopic in utero balloon placement to occlude the trachea typically between 27 and 29 weeks of gestation followed by interval balloon retrieval a few weeks later. This leads to increased lung fluid retention and subsequent lung growth. Although this treatment is limited to a few centers, results are promising. A meta-analysis of studies indicate FETO may reduce pulmonary hypertension, extracorporeal membrane oxygenation (ECMO) utilization, and mortality.[7] A recent multicenter European randomized controlled trial, Tracheal Occlusion to Accelerate Lung Growth (TOTAL), has demonstrated significant survival benefit at discharge and 6 months of age.[8] Complications include preterm labor, premature rupture of membranes, premature birth, and fetal demise. The evolution of fetal surgery and its clinical applications are discussed in Chapter 118.

The mainstay of initial CDH management focuses on aggressive treatment of pulmonary hypertension by airway stabilization, GI decompression, barotrauma limitation ("gentilation"), permissive hypercapnia, and meticulous hemodynamic monitoring while minimizing iatrogenic injury. High-volume centers with protocolized care have been found to have enhanced outcomes. Other interventions such as nitric oxide, high-frequency oscillatory ventilation, and ECMO have demonstrated effectiveness in stabilizing and treating worsening pulmonary hypertension. Various agents to reduce pulmonary hypertension such as prostaglandin (PGE1), prostacyclin (PGI2), sildenafil, a phosphodiesterase-5 inhibitor, and milrinone may have benefits in select cases, but most of these are not FDA approved.[8]

Surgical Repair

Optimal timing of CDH repair in infants who have no cardiopulmonary instability and are not on ECMO should likely be deferred 48 to 72 hours to limit risks of pulmonary vascular lability induced by surgical stress. Controversy remains regarding the optimal (ideal) timing of CDH repair in patients on ECMO, with some proponents supporting repair during ECMO and others strongly advocating for repair at the time of weaning or after decannulation. There is no prospective randomized data available to support either approach. Bleeding complications are significantly higher in patients repaired on ECMO, requiring attention to hemostasis. A recent report suggested that early CDH repair during ECMO therapy is associated with improved survival compared with repair later in the ECMO course when azotemia increases risks for bleeding.[9]

Although open and laparoscopic repair are both feasible options, there is no clear data on the optimum approach or long-term outcomes. Repair of a posterolateral CDH is usually performed through an ipsilateral subcostal abdominal incision with excision of the hernia sac, if present. This is followed by a reduction of intrathoracic visceral contents into the abdomen. Identification and mobilization of the anterior medial leaflet facilitates tension-free closure of the posterolateral diaphragmatic defect with interrupted nonabsorbable sutures, sometimes with Teflon pledgets. Although primary repair is preferred, some hernia defects may be large and require various reconstructive techniques, including the use of rectus abdominus or latissimus dorsi muscle flaps or alternatively prosthetic materials to achieve repair. Gore-Tex patch prostheses are most widely used; however, the use of regenerative extracellular matrix biomaterials (e.g., Surgisis) that are biodegradable may have utility. The advantages of prosthetic patches are that they offer shorter operative time and a tension-free repair.

In general, thoracostomy tube placement is unnecessary, especially if postoperative radiographs demonstrate immediate mediastinal shift toward the midline. Repair of the diaphragmatic hernia with reduction of the viscera may lead to the loss of abdominal domain and impending abdominal compartment syndrome requiring temporary abdominal silo placement with interval abdominal wall closure. Alternatively, skin-only closure

with a resultant incisional hernia followed by delayed definitive fascial closure may be an option to consider. Prosthetic patch abdominoplasty is also a viable approach.

Long-term outcomes in infants with CDH vary. Some may develop a chronic condition due to PPHN and respiratory dysfunction. Moreover, infants who receive aggressive and prolonged care in the neonatal intensive care unit have a high incidence of developmental delay, seizures, and hearing loss. Other morbidities for CDH survivors include chronic lung disease, scoliosis, growth retardation, pectus excavatum deformities, gastroesophageal reflux (GER) disease, and foregut dysmotility.

Eventration of Diaphragm

Abnormal elevation of the hemidiaphragm (eventration) seen on chest radiograms can significantly affect respiratory function, leading to tachypnea, discordant breathing, and respiratory embarrassment. Eventration of the diaphragm can be congenital or acquired. Congenital eventration typically occurs due to birth trauma (Erb palsy) or secondary to an anatomic abnormality of the diaphragm. Erb palsy is paralysis of the arm caused by brachial plexus injury following a difficult or traumatic delivery due to shoulder dystocia. Injury to the ventral rami of spinal nerves C5 through C8 commonly includes ipsilateral diaphragmatic paralysis due to traction injury of the phrenic nerves and upper portion of the brachial plexus. Acquired eventrations are usually secondary to iatrogenic phrenic nerve injury during open cardiac surgery. Elevation of the diaphragm can be visualized on chest radiographs (see Fig. 117.2B); however, it can easily be misdiagnosed as CDH. The diagnosis is confirmed by dynamic visualization of the diaphragm using either fluoroscopy or ultrasound of the chest. Absent or paradoxical movement of the diaphragm on inspiration is diagnostic of eventration. When symptoms progress, resulting in respiratory distress or inability to wean from ventilatory support, repair is indicated. The surgical treatment of diaphragm eventration is an open or laparoscopic diaphragm plication in which the diaphragm is securely folded using multiple interrupted nonabsorbable sutures.

BRONCHOPULMONARY MALFORMATIONS

Bronchopulmonary malformations are congenital abnormalities of the airway and include bronchogenic cysts, intralobar and extralobar sequestrations (ELSs), cystic pulmonary adenomatous malformations (CPAMs), and congenital lobar emphysema (CLE). In the perinatal period, these lung lesions can result in pleural effusions, polyhydramnios, hydrops, and pulmonary hypoplasia with subsequent respiratory distress and even airway obstruction. If severe enough, fetal demise can occur. Most of these lesions are diagnosed prenatally with ultrasound. Fetal surgery has been pursued when fetal viability is at risk. After birth, congenital lung lesions are often asymptomatic, and some may even spontaneously regress. However, there is concern that some lesions may lead to recurrent pulmonary infections and exhibit long-term malignant potential.

Cystic Pulmonary Adenomatous Malformation

The most frequently diagnosed congenital lung anomaly is CPAM, a multicystic dysplastic lesion that displaces normal lung tissue. It occurs with an incidence of about 1 per 25,000 to 35,000 live births. CPAMs are hamartomatous lesions that arise during the early pseudoglandular phase of lung development from aberrant morphogenesis secondary to proximal airway obstruction that induces terminal bronchial overgrowth. CPAM communicates with the tracheobronchial tree and adjacent lung tissue and receives pulmonary blood supply. Frequently diagnosed in utero by ultrasound or fetal MRI, many prenatal CPAMs will undergo partial regression during the third trimester. Postnatal diagnosis is often made following a chest x-ray demonstrating large cystic lung lesions and/or pneumothorax performed for a patient with respiratory symptoms. Ultrasound, CT, and MRI may confirm these findings, which may also be seen in sequestration or diaphragmatic hernia.[10]

The majority of CPAMs are asymptomatic in utero and during infancy, and can be managed expectantly. Antenatal treatment with betamethasone has been effective in inducing spontaneous involution, size decrease, and hydrops amelioration. Rarely, CPAMs cause fetal distress and demise secondary to compressive effects and hydrops. These patients may be candidates for in utero intervention or fetal surgery. At birth, some patients may present with varying degrees of respiratory distress from tachypnea, grunting, and oxygen requirement. Severe life-threatening respiratory distress secondary to pulmonary hypoplasia, lung compression, and/or mediastinal displacement that occurs at birth requires emergency surgical resection and/or ECMO. In older children and adults CPAM may present with recurrent pneumonia, pneumothorax, hemoptysis, respiratory distress, or lung abscess.

Classification of CPAMs is typically based on the imaging criteria and pathologic confirmation. Historically, these congenital lung anomalies were classified by Stocker classification as type I (macrocystic), type II (mixed), and type III (solid/microcystic).[11] Although this descriptive approach was useful for the assessment of prenatal lung lesions, it was insufficient as a postnatal diagnostic and prognostic tool. Modification of the Stocker classification now categorizes CPAM into five different types (Type 0–IV), based on the origin of the tracheobronchial tree, the presence of cystic components, radiologic appearance, and dimensions. This newer classification system has greater diagnostic, therapeutic, and prognostic utility. Resection is recommended in all patients who do not undergo spontaneous regression to minimize the risk of complications, to enhance lung growth and decrease the risk of malignant transformation. Surgical resection is recommended within the first 2 years of life.[12]

Bronchopulmonary Sequestration

Bronchopulmonary sequestration is a dysplastic segment or lobe of nonfunctional lung tissue that lacks communication with the tracheobronchial tree and receives a systemic (nonpulmonary) blood supply. These lesions account for <6% of all congenital lung anomalies. Two variants of sequestration exist: intralobar (ILS) and ELS. The intralobar variant is embedded within the visceral pleura of the normal lung parenchyma. It has venous drainage into the pulmonary venous system but receives systemic arterial blood supply. ILS is primarily found in the lower lobe with two-thirds located in the posterior basal segment. They are three times more common than extralobar variants. In contrast, ELSs have a separate visceral pleura, systemic venous drainage, and arterial supply. They are often located between the diaphragm and lower lobes but may rarely occur in infradiaphragmatic and retroperitoneal locations. ELS may be associated with other congenital anomalies, such as posterolateral diaphragmatic hernia, pectus excavatum and carinatum, and enteric duplication cysts. ILS may remain asymptomatic even into adulthood and is often diagnosed incidentally on chest CT scans in patients without symptoms. However, the most frequent clinical presentation is recurrent pneumonia in a specific lung segment. Other potential symptoms include a persistent cough, hemoptysis, back pain, or exertional shortness of breath.

ELSs do not form enlarged cysts or cause spontaneous pneumothoraces due to lack of communication to the airway. They can, however, infarct, become infected, and cause hemoptysis. It has been reported that ELSs can undergo torsion as well. Anomalous systemic vascular supply may lead to significant left-to-right shunting in neonates that may increase susceptibility to high-output cardiac failure.

Pulmonary sequestrations may be diagnosed on routine prenatal ultrasound. In the absence of other findings, the fetus is observed with serial ultrasound monitoring for enlargement and potential pleural effusion, polyhydramnios, or hydrops. Spontaneous regression has been reported in more than two-thirds of prenatally diagnosed lesions, possibly related to the outgrowth of the blood supply. Initial evaluation at birth of a known sequestration may include Doppler ultrasound to assess the nature of the lesion (cystic or solid) and the anatomy of the systemic arterial supply from the infradiaphragmatic or thoracic aorta. CT or MRI may aid in further definition of the vascular and structural anatomy but is not indicated in a stable patient with an ultrasound that is not worrisome. ELSs are often asymptomatic due to the absence of airway communication. The presence of air or an air-fluid level rarely indicates fistulous connection to the GI tract. Surgical management of these lesions is performed via standard open or thoracoscopic segmentectomy or lobectomy for ILS, and mass resection for ELS.

Congenital Lobar Emphysema

CLE is a developmental anomaly of the lung that may be characterized by respiratory distress due to hyperinflation of one or more pulmonary lobes inducing compression of adjacent lung parenchyma. The incidence is ~1:20,000 to 30,000 live births with a 3:1 male predominance primarily present in the first 6 months of life and rarely in adults. Various etiologies may contribute to the pathogenesis, including intrinsic bronchial cartilaginous abnormalities leading to stenosis, atresia, or bronchomalacia. Alternatively, extrinsic conditions such as aberrant blood vessels or masses may lead to bronchial abnormalities inducing lobar emphysema. The left upper lobe is most affected (~43%) followed by the right middle lobe (32%) and right upper lobe (21%). This air trapping or hyperinflation may be secondary to abnormalities in bronchial cartilages or parenchymal disease (polyalveolar lobe) with expiratory collapse of the bronchus. The affected lobe is essentially nonfunctional because of overdistention and air trapping in the lung during the expiratory phase of respiration due to deficient bronchial cartilage, which causes repeated episodes of respiratory distress. It is frequently recognized in newborns; however, a few cases do not present until adulthood. This disease is potentially reversible if diagnosed and treated timely. A chest radiograph is generally diagnostic, revealing overdistention of the involved lobe. Importantly, the lucency should not be mistaken for a pneumothorax. Positive pressure ventilation should be used with caution, as these patients are prone to developing auto–positive end-expiratory pressure, which refers to the end-expiratory intrapulmonary pressure that develops due to dynamic airflow resistance during mechanical ventilation. When the CLE progresses to cause a mediastinal shift and worsening respiratory symptoms, an expeditiously performed open lobectomy is indicated.

Bronchogenic Cysts

Bronchogenic cysts are foregut-derived pulmonary malformations that arise from abnormal budding of the lung or the tracheobronchial tree during the embryonic and early pseudoglandular stages of lung morphogenesis (third through sixth weeks of gestation). Subsequent differentiation into a fluid-filled, blind-ending pouch leads to the development of this cystic structure. The location of a bronchogenic cyst depends on the embryologic stage of development at which the anomaly occurs. When the abnormal budding happens during early development, the cyst occurs along the tracheobronchial tree with a high prevalence near the carina and right hilum. Cysts that arise later are more peripheral and may involve the lung parenchyma.

The wall of bronchogenic cysts consists of fibroelastic tissue, smooth muscle, and cartilage. They are lined with respiratory tract ciliated columnar epithelial cells and can contain mucus-producing cuboidal cells, which may contribute to cyst enlargement due to mucus accumulation. Enlargement may lead to airway compression or displacement of other intrathoracic structures. This poses a higher risk in infants due to their narrow and easily compressible trachea and bronchus. Symptoms associated with bronchogenic cysts include dysphagia, pneumothorax, cough, hemoptysis, and, in cases of late presentation, infection.

These lesions are rare, with a reported incidence of 1:42,000 to 68,000 and a male predominance. Many may remain undiagnosed until adulthood. Diagnosis of bronchogenic cysts is often suspected based on routine chest radiographs and confirmed using a CT scan. CT scans reveal a nonenhancing, mucus-filled cystic mass with a spherical appearance. If the cyst communicates with the airway, an air-fluid level may be visible. Cysts located within the pulmonary parenchyma typically communicate with a bronchus, whereas mediastinal cysts usually do not. Surgical resection is the recommended treatment for bronchogenic cysts, irrespective of symptoms. This involves the complete removal of the cyst. Although rare, cases of malignant transformation have been reported.

ALIMENTARY TRACT CONDITIONS

Esophageal Atresia and Tracheoesophageal Fistula

Esophageal atresia (EA) represents a congenital interruption of the esophageal continuity leading to proximal esophageal obstruction. Concurrently, a tracheoesophageal fistula (TEF) is a pathologic communication between the esophagus and trachea. These malformations can manifest independently or in conjunction.

They present in 1 of 1500 to 3000 live births, displaying a mild male predilection. Approximately 33% of affected neonates have a diminished birth weight, and associated anomalies are evident in 60% to 70%.

During the fourth gestational week, incomplete division of the esophagotracheal diverticulum of the foregut leads to the previously mentioned defects. A subset of 10% exhibits a nonrandom, nongenetic aggregation of anomalies characterized as VATERL (vertebral, anorectal, tracheal, esophageal, renal, and radial limb). Five anatomic EA variants are detailed in Fig. 117.3. The prevalent type (C lesion) features proximal EA and distal TEF; the proximal blind pouch concludes roughly at a distance equivalent to one or two vertebral bodies from the distal TEF. The TEF is typically proximal to the carina in the trachea's membranous segment.

Clinical suspicion for EA arises in neonates presenting excessive salivation and initial feeding-associated coughing or choking. The retraction or failure to pass an orogastric tube at the thoracic inlet is a defining feature of EA with or without TEF. Maternal polyhydramnios is recurrent, particularly prominent in isolated proximal atresia (86%). Neonates with proximal EA and distal TEF may manifest acute gastric distention due to inspiratory air influx into the distal esophagus and stomach. Reflux into the distal esophagus allows gastric contents to breach the TEF, culminating in symptoms such as cough, tachypnea, apnea, or cyanosis. Isolated TEF, in the absence of EA, might present subtly, often postneonatally. Typically, these neonates display feeding-induced choking and coughing. Failure to introduce an orogastric tube into the stomach is a diagnostic hallmark of EA with a chest radiograph revealing a recoiled orogastric tube in the proximal esophagus confirming the diagnosis (Fig. 117.4A). The presence of intra-abdominal gas confirms TEF. However, an infant demonstrating absent GI air radiographically after failing a nasogastric tube insertion is likely suffering from isolated EA. An oral contrast study is contraindicated due to aspiration risks. Echocardiography and renal ultrasonography are imperative for assessing congenital heart and genitourinary defects, respectively.

To decompress the proximal esophageal pouch, a continuous suction-applied sump tube is introduced. Infants are optimally positioned upright prone to mitigate aspiration of saliva. Broad-spectrum intravenous (IV) antibiotics are initiated. Endotracheal intubation is generally eschewed, as positive pressure ventilation may inadequately inflate the lungs; air might preferentially navigate into the GI tract via the TEF. Ventilation can further be jeopardized by significant gastric distention. In this scenario,

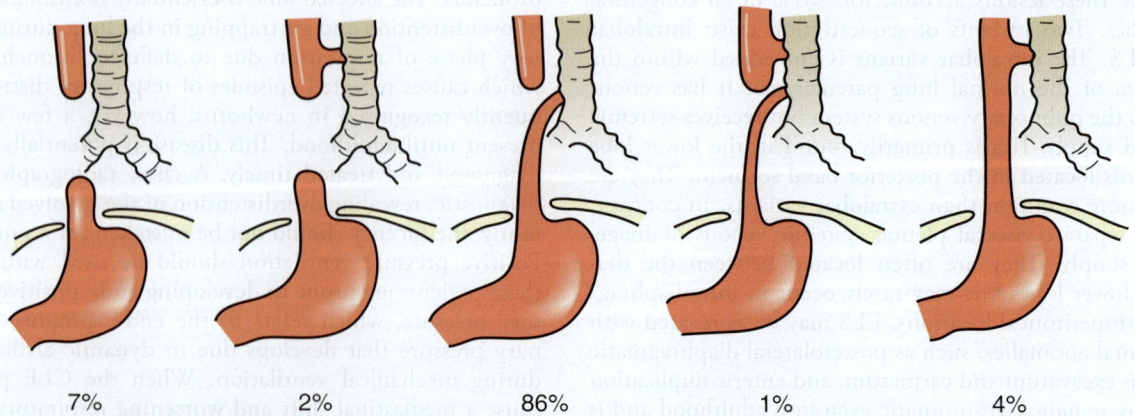

7%   2%   86%   1%   4%

FIGURE 117.3 Anatomic variants and incidence of esophageal atresia with tracheoesophageal fistula.

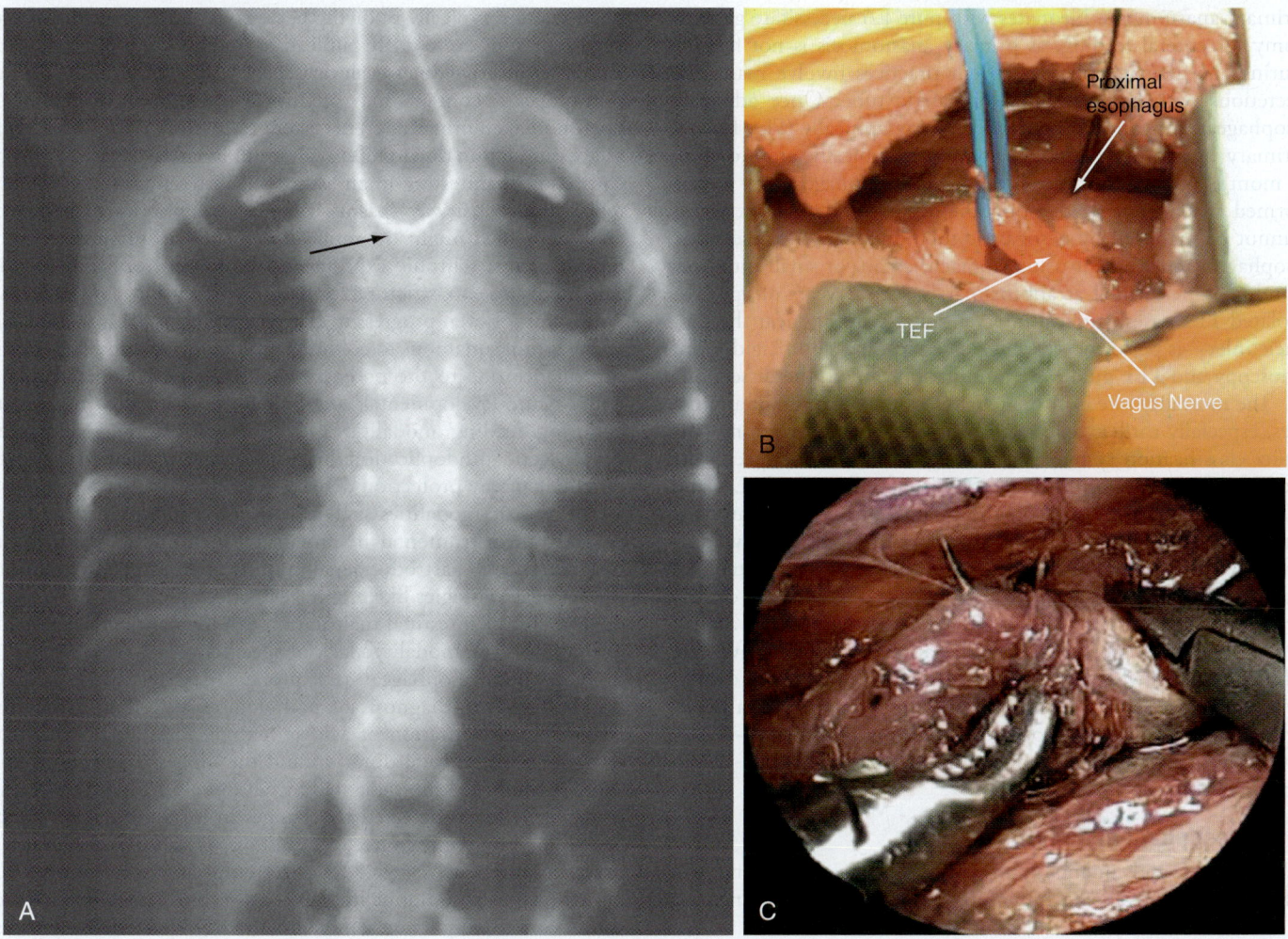

FIGURE 117.4 (A) Plain chest radiograph of infant with proximal esophageal atresia with distal tracheoesophageal fistula. The distal tip of the orogastric tube is curled up at the level of thoracic inlet *(arrow)*. (B) Distal tracheoesophageal fistula *(TEF; arrow)* is encircled with a blue vessel loop. Proximal blind esophageal pouch is in close proximity *(arrow)*. (C) Thoracoscopic esophageal anastomosis. Interrupted sutures are placed using intracorporeal technique.

prompt recognition and management is necessary to save the patient. Moving the endotracheal tube distally past the TEF or utilizing an occlusive balloon catheter in the fistula can improve ventilation. Emergent thoracotomy with fistula ligation may be necessary. In extreme cases, emergent gastrostomy is necessary to decompress the stomach and improve ventilation. The gastrostomy tube can be placed to water seal, similar to a tube thoracostomy, to facilitate ventilation while allowing the air traveling through the TEF to escape. Preoperative chest radiographs and echocardiograms are adequate to elucidate aortic arch anatomy. Right thoracotomy is favored for operative repairs in patients with a conventional left-sided aortic arch. For patients with a right-sided arch, left and right thoracotomy may be used, based on surgeon preference. A right-sided aortic arch exhibits an increased incidence of arch anomalies and postoperative complications.

The classic surgical approach for the proximal EA and distal TEF (C type) is an extrapleural dissection through open thoracotomy. Currently, a minimally invasive approach is most common. Initial rigid bronchoscopy allows for evaluation of the degree of tracheomalacia and the anatomic location of the TEF, but some surgeons consider it optional for excluding a secondary fistula due to its low detection yield. However, for recurrent fistulas, bronchoscopic evaluations with Fogarty catheter placement delineates the anatomy, facilitating safer dissection. The subsequent step involves thoracotomy with extrapleural dissection and division of the azygos vein, revealing the underlying TEF. The tracheal defect is closed by sequentially dividing a 1- to 2-mm segment of the fistula and immediately closing the defect using absorbable interrupted sutures to prevent loss of ventilation of the patient. The upper esophageal pouch is then maximally mobilized to enable tension-free esophageal anastomosis. The vasculature of this pouch is typically robust, whereas the lower pouch exhibits a more segmental and precarious supply, urging limited mobilization to avoid ischemia (see Fig. 117.4B). The anastomosis can be executed using single- or double-layer techniques. The thoracoscopic approach (see Fig. 117.4C) is increasingly preferred with favorable outcomes.

For cases of long-gap EA, several methodologies exist to secure additional length for primary anastomosis. Although esophagomyotomy of the upper pouch was previously employed, the resultant esophageal dysmotility has led to its obsolescence. An alternative involves suturing the distal esophagus' divided closed end to the prevertebral fascia, marking it with a hemoclip. As the infant grows, this facilitates esophageal lengthening for subsequent primary anastomosis. Neonates with pure EA necessitate gastrostomy for enteral feeding, as primary anastomosis is not feasible during the neonatal phase. Current practices involve managing secretions with an indwelling orogastric tube. Once adequate esophageal elongation is confirmed radiographically (Fig. 117.5), primary anastomosis can be attempted, typically around 4 to 6 months of age. In some cases, cervical esophagostomy is performed when continued aspiration occurs, and oral secretions cannot be managed by nasogastric tube drainage. In these cases, esophageal replacement using stomach, colon, or small intestinal conduit is performed at approximately 1 to 2 years of age. For isolated TEF cases, surgical intervention—typically near the thoracic inlet—is performed through a cervical incision. Rigid bronchoscopy and TEF guidewire cannulation can aid the dissection.

The mortality rate is intimately linked to concomitant anomalies, especially cardiac defects and chromosomal aberrations. The Spitz classification system is a risk stratification tool specifically developed to determine the prognosis of infants with EA and TEF. The system is based on the infant's birth weight and the presence or absence of major cardiac anomalies, as these two factors have been shown to significantly influence survival outcomes. Infants with a birth weight >1500 g and no major cardiac anomaly had a survival rate of 97%. Infants with either a birth weight of <1500 g or a major cardiac anomaly had a survival rate of 59%. Infants with a birth weight <1500 g and a major cardiac anomaly had a survival rate of 22%. Postoperative sequela might encompass esophageal motility disorders, GER (25%–50%), anastomotic stricture (15%–30%), anastomotic leak (10%–20%), and tracheomalacia (8%–15%).

Gastroesophageal Reflux

In neonates and infants, transient episodes of vomiting can often be attributed to an immature lower esophageal sphincter, a phenomenon typically resolving between 6 and 12 months of age. Persistent and severe GER can lead to notable complications such as failure to thrive due to caloric deprivation. Furthermore, aspiration of gastric contents may predispose to recurrent bronchitis or pneumonia, culminating in persistent respiratory symptoms. Vagal reflex stimulation due to reflux can result in laryngospasm or bronchospasm, manifesting in an asthma-like presentation.[13] Notably, reflux-induced airway spasms can lead to episodes of apnea or choking, which might be implicated in sudden infant death syndrome events. Chronic exposure of the lower esophagus to acid can predispose to stricture formation, presenting as obstructive symptoms, or even progress to Barrett esophagus. This metaplastic change from squamous to columnar epithelium mandates periodic surveillance due to the potential for dysplastic changes. Patients with neurodevelopmental disabilities occasionally necessitate enduring feeding modalities, such as gastrostomies. However, prophylactic fundoplication in this cohort, particularly due to potential airway protection deficits, is controversial.

Diagnostic modalities such as contrast esophagogram and upper GI are instrumental in procuring anatomic and functional insights, such as gastroduodenal motility aberrations. In addition, mechanical etiologies like esophageal strictures, antral webs, duodenal webs, or intestinal malrotation can be identified. A notable limitation is the modality's lack of specificity.

A 24-hour esophageal pH probe study remains the gold standard for the diagnosis of pathologic GER. It measures the frequency and duration of acid reflux episodes, along with patterns such as the total duration and the longest continuous episode. A combined multichannel intraluminal impedance pH test, in which reflux is detected by changes in intraluminal resistance determined by the presence of liquid or gas and pH changes, is a more comprehensive test. A gastric emptying scan can be obtained using a radionuclide-labeled (technetium-99m [^{99m}Tc] sulfur colloid) liquid or semi-solid food to quantitatively assess gastric emptying; ~50% of the isotope-labeled meal is normally emptied from the stomach within 60 minutes and nearly 80% by 90 minutes. Although pH and impedance studies are gaining in popularity, there are no widely accepted criteria for physiologic or pathologic reflux episodes, limiting its widespread use. Esophageal manometry measures the pressures of the esophageal body and lower esophageal sphincter. Manometry is not used regularly in pediatrics. Children with poor esophageal motility are prone to experience significant dysphagia after fundoplication with a complete wrap. In many cases, clinical evaluation of tolerance to nasogastric gavage feeding might suffice to determine whether significant reflux exists. Endoscopic assessments facilitate direct and histologic evaluation of the esophageal mucosa, revealing GER-induced mucosal injury. Concurrently, they aid in diagnosing eosinophilic esophagitis, an inflammatory condition increasingly recognized in the pediatric demographic that can mimic GER disease.

The primary line of GER management in pediatrics involves dietary modifications such as formula thickening, volume reductions, and positional adjustments. Pharmacologic interventions focusing on acid suppression are commonly employed. Surgical interventions, specifically fundoplication, are reserved for critical manifestations like life-threatening events, failure to thrive, or esophageal stricture. A Nissen fundoplication, entailing a 360-degree esophageal wrap, stands as the gold standard surgical modality for pediatric GER. Though highly efficacious in symptom mitigation, it may predispose to side effects like bloating or dysphagia. In recent years, advocates of Nissen fundoplication

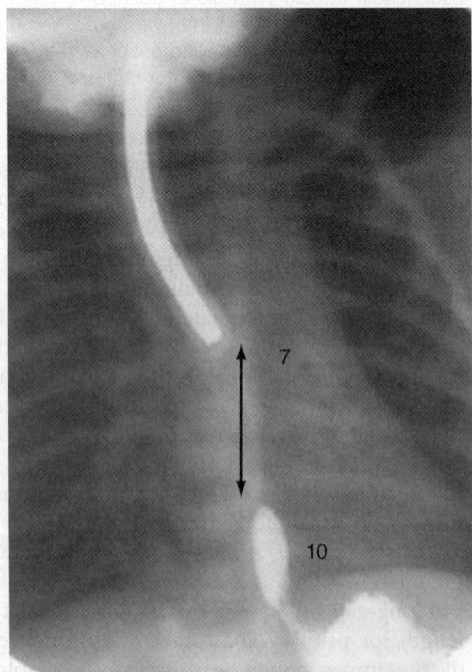

FIGURE 117.5 Contrast study per gastrostomy with an indwelling radiopaque orogastric tube. For pure atresia, the esophageal gap is assessed using this technique for either primary esophageal anastomosis or partial colonic segmental interposition.

have suggested limited dissection of the hiatus and crura to limit complications. Alternatively, partial wraps, such as Toupet (270 degrees) or Thal (180 degrees), present fewer complications but might be less efficacious. The laparoscopic technique has emerged as the standard surgical approach for fundoplication.

Hypertrophic Pyloric Stenosis

Hypertrophic pyloric stenosis (HPS) is a disease of newborns, with an incidence of 1 in 300 to 900 live births. It is most common between the ages of 2 and 8 weeks. Male infants are affected four times more often than females, with first-born male infants at the highest risk. Hypertrophy of the circular muscle of the pylorus results in constriction and obstruction of the gastric outlet. Although the exact cause of HPS remains unknown, a lack of nitric oxide synthase in pyloric tissue has been implicated.

Infants present with progressively worsening, nonbilious emesis that is projectile in nature. Visible gastric peristalsis may occasionally be observed as a wave of contractions from the left upper quadrant to the epigastrium. After emesis, infants still crave feeding. A plain abdominal radiograph can show an enlarged gastric gas bubble. Palpation of the pyloric "olive" tumor in the epigastrium by an experienced examiner is pathognomonic for HPS. If the olive is palpated, no imaging study is required for diagnosis. Today, most infants suspected of having HPS are evaluated with an ultrasound study before surgical consult. Pyloric muscle thickness of more than 3 to 4 mm or length of more than 15 to 18 mm on ultrasound in the presence of functional gastric outlet obstruction is diagnostic. If the clinical presentation is equivocal, an upper GI contrast study may be considered to demonstrate a lack of passage of contrast past the pylorus. However, it should be used with great caution as infants are at highest risk for aspiration. The upper GI study can also evaluate for other potential causes of emesis.

Preoperatively, resuscitation and correction of electrolyte abnormalities are essential. The infant must be resuscitated aggressively with IV fluids to establish an adequate urine output to restore acid-base balance. Initially, the infant should receive a bolus of 20 mL/kg of NS. Once urine output has been demonstrated, the maintenance IV fluids of D5 ½ NS with 20 mEq/L of potassium should be started at 1.5 times the maintenance rate. Loss of hydrochloric acid secondary to persistent emesis leads to hypokalemic, hypochloremic, metabolic alkalosis, and dehydration. In response, carbon dioxide and water are converted to hydrogen ion and bicarbonate ion to attempt to correct the electrolyte losses, resulting in a significant drop in carbon dioxide levels. If the patient is placed under anesthesia before correction of the electrolytes, postoperative apnea can occur due to the lack of respiratory drive from low carbon dioxide levels. Thus, the serum bicarbonate level and chloride level should be normalized to a value of less than 30 mEq/L and greater than 95 mEq/L, respectively. A pyloromyotomy (Ramstedt-Fredet procedure) involves incising the thickened pyloric musculature to relieve the pyloric channel obstruction. It is performed via a laparoscopic or open approach through various surgical incisions. A laparoscopic approach is used more routinely and can result in a shorter length of stay and a lower incidence of surgical site infection. Importantly, the fundamental surgical principle of pyloromyotomy is adequate cutting of hypertrophied pyloric muscle to achieve bulging mucosa and independent wall motion without mucosal injury (Fig. 117.6). Postoperatively, infants are managed on a feeding protocol clinical pathway, which ranges from immediate full ad lib feedings to incremental advancement with similar time to full feed and hospital

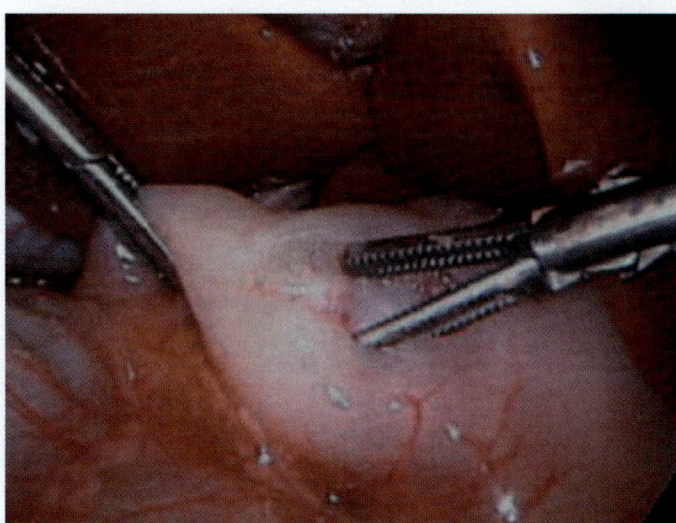

FIGURE 117.6 Laparoscopic pyloromyotomy is started with a retractable blade or Bovie cautery, and a spreader with grooves on the outer surface is used to perform the pyloromyotomy. Intact mucosal bulging along with independent muscle wall motion is confirmed. (From St. Peter SD, Ostlie DJ. Laparoscopic and open pyloromyotomy. In: Chung DH, Chen MK, ed. *Atlas of Pediatric Surgical Techniques.* Philadelphia: Elsevier Saunders; 2010:253-265.)

discharge. Postoperative emesis is common, but it is self-limited. Full-thickness mucosal perforation occurs more commonly with a laparoscopic approach, but its incidence is still rare (<1%). However, when infants experience persistent emesis beyond 7 to 14 postoperative days, an upper GI contrast study is warranted to evaluate for incomplete pyloromyotomy.

Intestinal Atresia

Duodenal atresia is thought to result from failure of recanalization of the duodenum from its solid cord stage. The range of anatomic variants includes duodenal stenosis, a mucosal web with intact muscle wall (so-called windsock deformity), two ends separated by a fibrous cord, and a complete separation with a resultant gap within the duodenum. It is associated with several conditions, including prematurity, Down syndrome, maternal polyhydramnios, malrotation, preduodenal portal vein, annular pancreas, and biliary atresia (BA). Other anomalies, such as cardiac, renal, EA, and anorectal malformations, are also common. In most cases, the duodenal obstruction is distal to the ampulla of Vater (85%); therefore, infants present with bilious emesis. In patients with an incomplete mucosal web, delayed presentation with symptoms of postprandial emesis may occur later in life.

Infants with duodenal obstruction are generally first detected during prenatal ultrasound evaluation. Immediately after birth, a plain abdominal radiograph shows a typical double-bubble sign if it is obtained before orogastric tube decompression of swallowed gastric air (Fig. 117.7). If distal air is present, an upper GI contrast study should be considered, not only to confirm the diagnosis of duodenal stenosis or atresia but also to exclude malrotation with midgut volvulus, which would constitute a surgical emergency.

Surgical treatment is a bypass of the duodenal obstruction with a side-to-side or proximal transverse to distal longitudinal (diamond-shaped) duodenoduodenostomy. Laparoscopic duodenal anastomosis is being performed with increasing frequency. When the proximal duodenum is markedly dilated, a tapering duodenoplasty with staples or sutures should be considered to

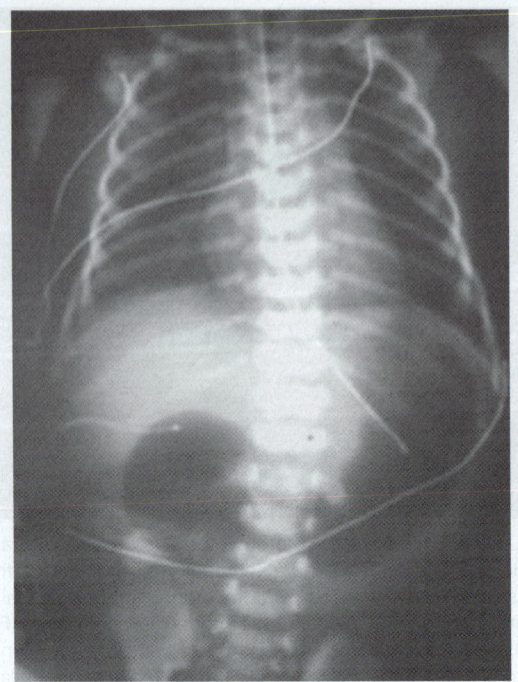

FIGURE 117.7 Plain abdominal radiograph shows double-bubble appearance of duodenal atresia.

narrow the duodenal caliber to lessen dysmotility and stasis. In patients with a duodenal mucosal web, the web is fenestrated or excised transduodenally, and caution must be exercised to avoid injury to the ampulla.

Jejunoileal atresia is the most common GI atresia, occurring in 1 in 2000 live births. It is thought to result from an intrauterine mesenteric vascular accident. Infants present with bilious emesis,

abdominal distention, and failure to pass meconium. The clinical presentation varies by the location of the atretic obstruction. In proximal atresia, significant bilious emesis occurs. In distal atresias, abdominal distention with multiple dilated bowel loops is more common (Fig. 117.8A). A contrast enema study is often unnecessary to make the diagnosis of jejunoileal atresia. If obtained, it shows an extremely narrow caliber of nondistended colon. Multiple intestinal atresias can occur in 10% to 15% of cases. As a result, the distal intestine should be evaluated for atresias intraoperatively with saline injection via a soft, red rubber catheter. Jejunoileal atresia is generally not associated with other anomalies except cystic fibrosis (CF) in approximately 10% of patients.

Jejunoileal atresias are classified into five types: type I is a mucosal web, or diaphragm; type II has an atretic cord between two blind ends of bowel with an intact mesentery; type IIIa is a complete separation of the blind ends of bowel by a V-shaped mesenteric gap; and type IIIb is an apple peel or Christmas tree deformity with a large mesenteric gap (see Fig. 117.8B), in which the distal bowel receives a retrograde blood supply from the ileocolic or right colic artery. This tenuous blood supply has implications for anastomotic failures and the potential for ischemic necrosis from volvulus. Thus, many of these infants with this type of atresia are born with reduced intestinal length and may develop short gut syndrome. In type IV, there are multiple atresias, with a string of sausage appearance.

Infants are managed for neonatal bowel obstruction, with placement of an orogastric tube and IV fluid resuscitation. At operation, the main objective is to establish intestinal continuity while preserving as much intestinal length as possible. In multiple atresias, multiple anastomoses over an endoluminal stent may be necessary. If the proximal intestine is significantly dilated, prolonged dysmotility may persist; therefore, a tapering enteroplasty of the dilated segment should be considered. However, in cases of

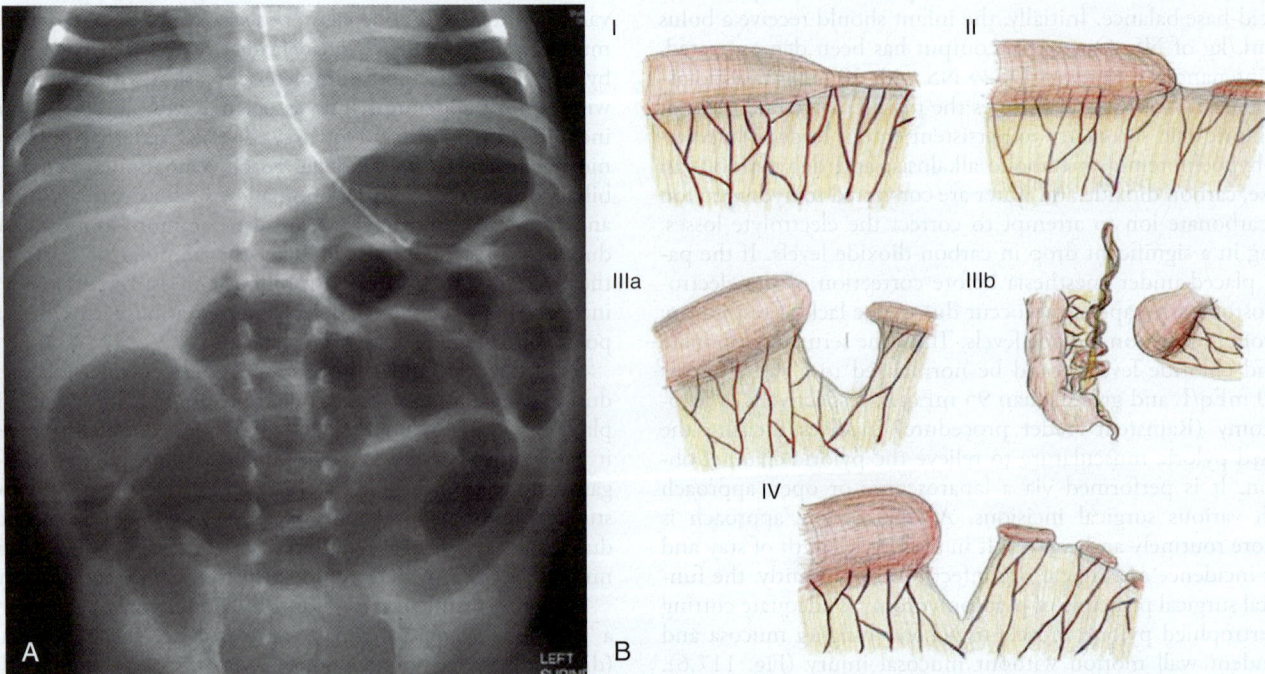

FIGURE 117.8 (A) Plain abdominal radiograph shows multiple dilated bowel loops indicating congenital bowel obstruction. (B) Jejunoileal atresias I to IV are depicted. In particular, IIIb demonstrates an apple peel type of atresia with a large mesenteric gap.

adequate bowel length, resection of the dilated segment can result in faster recovery. The overall survival for infants with jejunoileal atresia is more than 90%.

Colonic atresia is the least common, accounting for only 5% to 10% of intestinal atresia, with an incidence of 1 in 20,000 live births. Infants usually present with failure to pass meconium, abdominal distention, and bilious emesis. A plain radiograph shows multiple dilated bowel loops, but differentiation between small and large bowel is not feasible in this age group because of lack of well-developed haustra. A contrast enema study can confirm the diagnosis, but the clinical picture of distal bowel obstruction is typically sufficient to proceed with an operative exploration and diverting end colostomy versus primary colonic anastomosis.

Intestinal Malrotation and Midgut Volvulus

The actual incidence of rotational anomalies of the midgut is estimated at 2 to 5 in 1000 live births in autopsy studies. However, clinically apparent rotational anomalies are estimated to be 1 in 6000 live births. Although up to 90% of cases will be apparent before 12 months of age, as many as 1% of cases can present in adults, underscoring the importance for all surgeons to be able to diagnose and treat this disease. The actual mechanism for intestinal growth and fixation has been controversial. Historically, the midgut was thought to herniate out of the coelomic cavity through the umbilical ring at approximately the fourth week of embryonic development. By the 10th week of gestation, the intestine was thought to rotate in a counterclockwise rotation around the axis of the superior mesenteric artery (SMA) for 270 degrees. By the 12th week of gestation, the intestine returns into the abdominal cavity with the duodenum and colon becoming fixated in their normal configuration. Studies in rat embryos have demonstrated that there is no evidence of intestinal rotation. Instead, they documented two distinct embryologic processes. The first process involves rapid, localized, longitudinal growth of the duodenum, which pushes the duodenojejunal segment beneath the mesenteric root as the intestine grows outside the abdominal cavity. Once the intestinal growth is complete, the intestine returns to the abdominal cavity. The colon and rectum appear to change

minimally during this process with only the cecum exiting the abdominal cavity. The cecum appears to return passively into the abdomen into the right lower quadrant. These conclusions support the different clinical manifestations of malrotation where the course of the duodenum is abnormal, whereas the position of the cecum is less indicative of the presence of malrotation. Many of the congenital anomalies that occur during the 4th to 12th weeks of gestation, such as diaphragmatic hernia, gastroschisis, or omphalocele, are associated with anomalies of intestinal rotation. Typically, these anomalies are termed nonrotation and can appear similar to cases of malrotation that have been surgically corrected with a Ladd's procedure.

Failure of the normal developmental process of intestinal growth and fixation results in the duodenojejunal and ileocecal junctions lying close together, with the midgut suspended on a narrow SMA stalk. This can twist, resulting in midgut volvulus, which can be demonstrated on an upper GI contrast series (Fig. 117.9A). The ultrasound examination may be a useful tool for the diagnosis of intestinal malrotation, in which the normal relationship of the superior mesenteric vessels (the vein is to the right of artery) is reversed or altered. Clinical presentations vary from completely asymptomatic, early satiety or weight loss, chronic intermittent crampy abdominal pain suggestive of partial obstruction, or midgut volvulus with shock and possible death. Most symptomatic patients with intestinal malrotation present at less than 1 year of age. The abdominal examination may be unremarkable. A distended abdomen is a late sign, and along with metabolic acidosis may represent the onset of life-threatening intestinal ischemia.

Midgut volvulus is a true surgical emergency because of progressive intestinal ischemia. The acute onset of bilious emesis in a particularly somnolent or lethargic newborn is an ominous sign and mandates investigation for malrotation. Midgut volvulus may also be incomplete or intermittent. With partial, intermittent volvulus, the resultant mesenteric venous and lymphatic obstruction may impair nutrient absorption and produce protein loss into the gut lumen, as well as mucosal ischemia and melena as a result of arterial insufficiency.

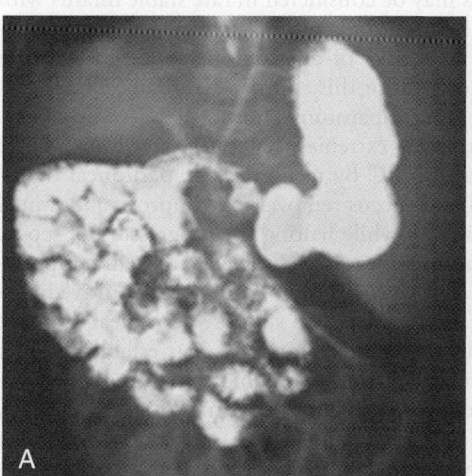 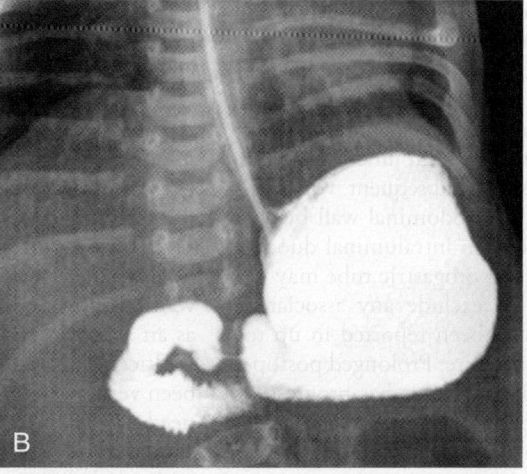 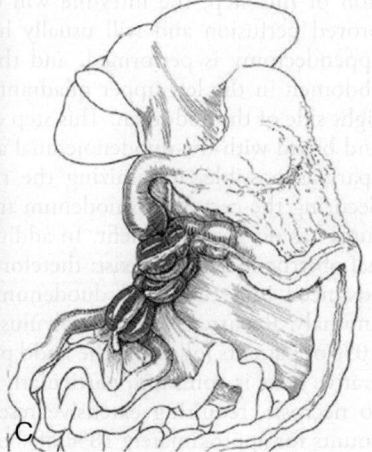

FIGURE 117.9 (A) Intestinal malrotation. Duodenal C-loop does not cross the midline, and the proximal small bowel is on the right side of the abdomen. (B) Midgut volvulus as demonstrated by a corkscrew appearance of contrast abruptly tapering off in the duodenum. (C) Diagram depicting midgut volvulus from intestinal malrotation. At operation, volvulized small bowel is untwisted in a counterclockwise fashion to restore intestinal perfusion. The peritoneal attachment between the cecum and retroperitoneum (Ladd's band) is divided as part of Ladd's procedure.

Abdominal radiographs may demonstrate upper intestinal obstruction or a gasless abdomen; however, these findings are nonspecific. The upper GI contrast study is the diagnostic study of choice in a hemodynamically stable patient. It demonstrates an obstructive upper GI pattern with the appearance of a bird's beak in the third portion of the duodenum (see Fig. 117.9B). In the acutely ill infant or child with signs and symptoms suggestive of midgut volvulus and obstruction, immediate operative exploration is warranted without an upper GI study. Aggressive resuscitation can be performed en route to the operating room as well as intraoperatively. Time is of the essence if maximal intestinal salvage is to be achieved.

Ladd's procedure was first described by William Ladd in 1936 and remains the operation of choice for rotational anomalies of the intestine. Upon entering the peritoneal cavity, chylous ascites from obstructed lymphatics may be seen. The first priority is to untwist the mesentery to reestablish blood flow to the intestine. This process can be challenging due to anatomic variability. Using the root of the mesentery and the duodenum as reference points can help to untwist the intestine quickly (see Fig. 117.9C). The intestine may be congested and edematous, and some areas may appear ischemic despite complete untwisting of the volvulus. Warm sponges placed on the bowel surface may help to improve perfusion. The decision must be made as to whether the intestine has restored adequate perfusion and is thought to be viable. If vascular integrity has been compromised, ischemic or necrotic bowel segments are resected. However, borderline ischemic segments may be left in place with a second-look laparotomy performed after 24 to 36 hours. Next, the lateral peritoneal attachments, or Ladd's bands, from the right colon to the lateral abdomen are identified and divided. As the right colon is in a more medial position than normal, these bands will tend to constrict the root of the mesentery and the duodenum, causing obstruction. This will result in the cecum becoming freely mobile in the abdomen. Next, the attachments around the anterior and posterior duodenum must be divided to straighten the duodenum, resulting the in duodenojejunal junction in the right lower quadrant of the abdomen. After this, the bands at the base of the mesentery, specifically across the superior mesenteric vein, must be divided to the level of the root of the mesentery. Upon completion of this step, the intestine will often have significantly improved perfusion and will usually have vigorous peristalsis. An appendectomy is performed, and the cecum is returned to the abdomen in the left upper quadrant with the small intestine in right side of the abdomen. This step ensures that mesentery is flat and broad with the duodenojejunal and ileocecal junctions as far apart as possible, minimizing the risk of subsequent volvulus. Securing the cecum or duodenum to the abdominal wall by sutures has no proven benefit. In addition, an intraluminal duodenal obstruction may coexist; therefore, an orogastric tube may be advanced into the distal duodenum to exclude any associated anomaly. Recurrent midgut volvulus has been reported in up to 10% of patients following the Ladd procedure. Prolonged postoperative ileus is common, particularly if a volvulus has progressed to necrosis, requiring extensive resection. Midgut volvulus accounts for approximately 18% of short bowel syndrome (SBS) in the pediatric population.

Necrotizing Enterocolitis

NEC is the most common GI surgical emergency in neonates. While multiple contributing factors have been identified—including ischemia, bacterial overgrowth, cytokines, and enteral feeding—prematurity remains the most significant risk factor. The overall incidence of NEC appears to have decreased in recent years due to clinical pathway–based gradual feeding regimens including the more prevalent use of breast milk. The exact cause of NEC remains unclear despite multiple active basic and translational studies across the world.

The clinical presentation of NEC can vary widely. Acute abdominal wall cellulitis, distention and tenderness, and feeding intolerance with gross or occult blood in the stool are hallmark features for NEC (Fig. 117.10A). Other nonspecific signs include temperature instability and episodes of apnea or bradycardia. NEC typically occurs in the first few days of life with the initiation of enteral feedings; 80% of cases occur during the first month of life. As NEC progresses, sepsis may develop with subsequent shock, hemodynamic deterioration, and coagulopathy. The pathognomonic radiographic feature of NEC is pneumatosis intestinalis (see Fig. 117.10B). Pneumatosis is composed of hydrogen gas generated by the bacterial fermentation of luminal substrates. Other radiographic findings may include portal venous gas, ascites, fixed loops of small intestine, and free air. In the majority of cases of NEC, the distal ileum and ascending colon are the areas affected. In rare cases, NEC totalis occurs where the entire GI tract is affected.

Medical management consists of orogastric tube decompression, fluid resuscitation, and broad-spectrum antibiotics. NEC can be successfully treated medically in more than 50% of cases. Infants are closely monitored for any signs of surgical indications. The absolute indication for operative intervention is the presence of free air on plain abdominal radiographs. Relative indications for surgery include clinical deterioration, persistent acidosis, abdominal wall cellulitis, palpable mass (matted ischemic bowel), a persistent fixed bowel loop on radiograph, and portal venous gas. The general surgical principles are to resect all nonviable intestinal segments, preserving maximum intestinal length with ostomy diversion, or leaving the patient in discontinuity, utilizing damage control principles. At times, multiple necrotic segments of bowel are resected, thus preserving viable intersegments. In cases of ischemic, but not frankly necrotic bowel, a second-look operation may be performed after 24 to 48 hours. Bowel resection with primary anastomosis may be considered in rare stable infants with a focal isolated perforation and minimal peritoneal contamination; however, the high risks of anastomotic leak and stricture have tempered enthusiasm for this approach. Initially, all patients were taken for exploratory laparotomy. In the 1970s, some centers reported success in treating extremely low birth weight premature infants with perforated NEC by using bedside peritoneal drainage. Peritoneal fluid and succus removal may improve abdominal distention and ventilation while halting the progression of sepsis. Over time, drain placement was found to be effective in temporizing intestinal perforation and was found to be the definitive intervention in some infants. Evidence to support peritoneal drainage as an accepted mode of treatment for NEC was established in a multicenter, randomized prospective clinical trial and has since been verified in other prospective studies.[14] In this study, survival, need for parenteral nutrition, and length of hospital stay were similar for NEC infants weighing less than 1500 g treated by peritoneal drainage or laparotomy, providing pediatric surgeons with another viable means to treat NEC in this extremely fragile patient population. Intestinal strictures may develop after medical or surgical management of NEC in approximately 10% of infants. Because of the risk for post-NEC stricture, most notably in the splenic flexure of the colon, a contrast enema study is

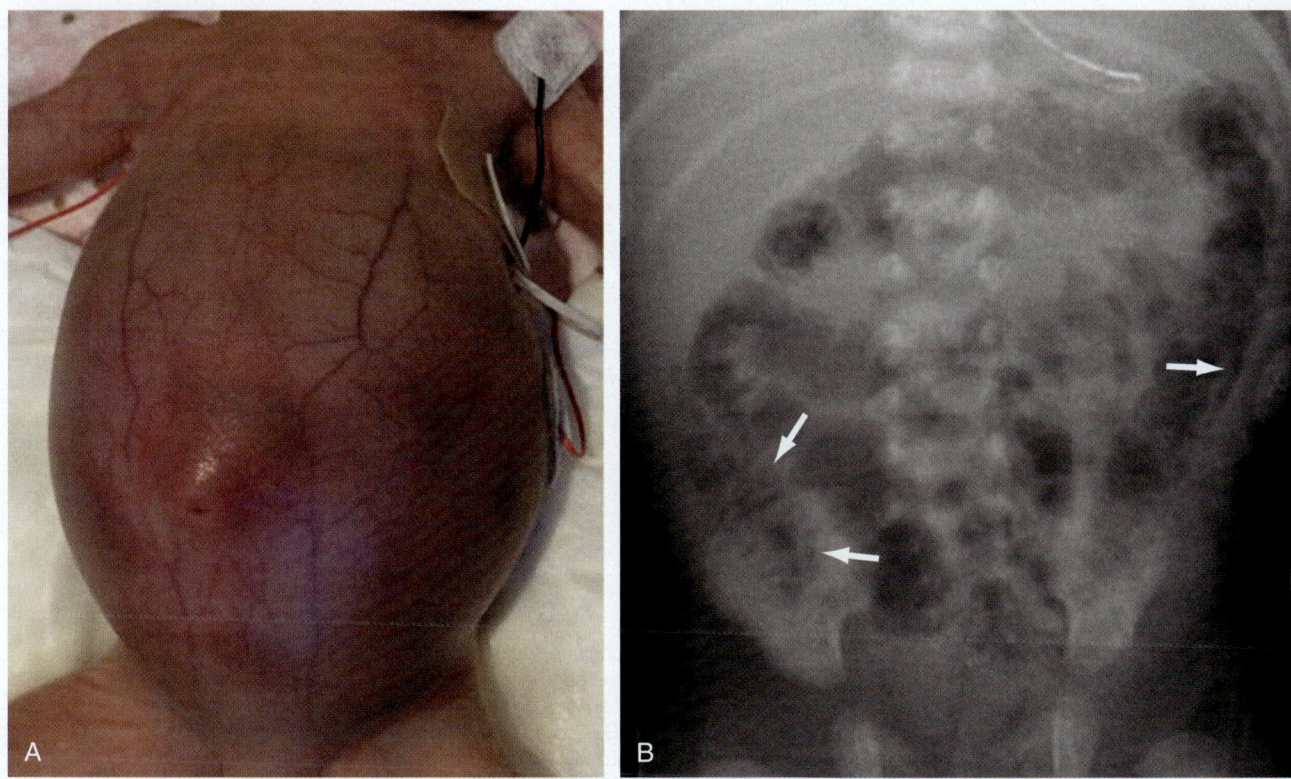

FIGURE 117.10 (A) Premature infant with necrotizing enterocolitis. Abdominal distention with marked cellulitis and dusky abdominal indicates intraabdominal catastrophe. (B) Pneumatosis intestinalis *(arrows)*, a pathognomonic radiographic sign for necrotizing enterocolitis.

routinely performed before stoma reversal. NEC remains the most common cause of short gut syndrome. In addition, neurodevelopmental delay is a frequent long-term complication. Overall, the mortality rate for surgically managed NEC ranges from 10% to 50% of short gut syndrome. In addition, neurodevelopmental delay is a frequent long-term complication. Overall, the mortality rate for surgically managed NEC ranges from 10% to 50%.

Short Bowel Syndrome

SBS is a clinical condition in which the intestine is not able to absorb sufficient nutrients and/or fluids to maintain normal growth. Although this is typically the result of massive small bowel resection, SBS may occur in patients with apparently sufficient intestinal length. Common conditions that can lead to SBS are NEC (35%), intestinal atresia (25%), gastroschisis (18%), and midgut volvulus (14%). In SBS, intestinal function depends on a number of factors, such as villous architecture, total bowel length, bowel diameter, presence of the ileocecal valve, residual intestinal segments, stasis, and the presence bacterial overgrowth. In general, patients with 35 to 40 cm of length have a 50% probability of weaning from TPN with each subsequent centimeter increasing the rate of enteral autonomy by 4%. The jejunum is the site of absorption of most macronutrients and minerals. The ileum is essential for the absorption of carbohydrates, proteins, fluids, and electrolytes. In addition, bile acids, vitamin B_{12}, and the fat-soluble vitamins (A, D, E, and K) are primarily absorbed in the ileum. In the past, ileocecal valve function was thought to be important in SBS. More recent literature has demonstrated that the terminal ileum has the greatest capacity to adapt and that the presence of the ileocecal valve may serve as a surrogate for presence of a

significant portion of terminal ileum. The colon is important in SBS patients for absorption of water and electrolytes. After massive small bowel resection, a physiologic process known as intestinal adaptation occurs to compensate for the loss of intestinal length. Many factors are involved in this adaptive process to enhance the absorptive function of the residual intestine, such as use of elemental diet, growth factors, and titration of TPN. Several surgical techniques (excluding small bowel transplantation) aimed at slowing intestinal transit time or increasing the mucosal surface area for enhanced absorption have been described.[15] These include reversed intestinal segment, recirculating loop, artificial intestinal valve, colon interposition, and intestinal pacing. Over time, these techniques have fallen out of favor due to poor efficacy. Currently, the two procedures that are used are the Bianchi procedure and serial transverse enteroplasty (STEP), both of which focus on increasing intestinal length while reducing intestinal caliber.

The Bianchi procedure[16] was originally described an intestinal lengthening procedure in which the mesenteric vascular bed is separated into two systems, the dilated small intestine is split into two parallel segments, each with its own mesenteric blood supply, and the ends are approximated (Fig. 117.11A). This resulted in a 50% decreased diameter of the small intestine and increased length by 100%. The Bianchi procedure has been shown to be an effective surgical option for treating patients with SBS, but has not been used widely because it is technically demanding and risks losing intestinal length if the blood supply is damaged during dissection.

In contrast to the Bianchi procedure, STEP uses the principle of minimal bowel dissection by serially stapling dilated small intestine in a transverse fashion to create a narrower lumen resulting

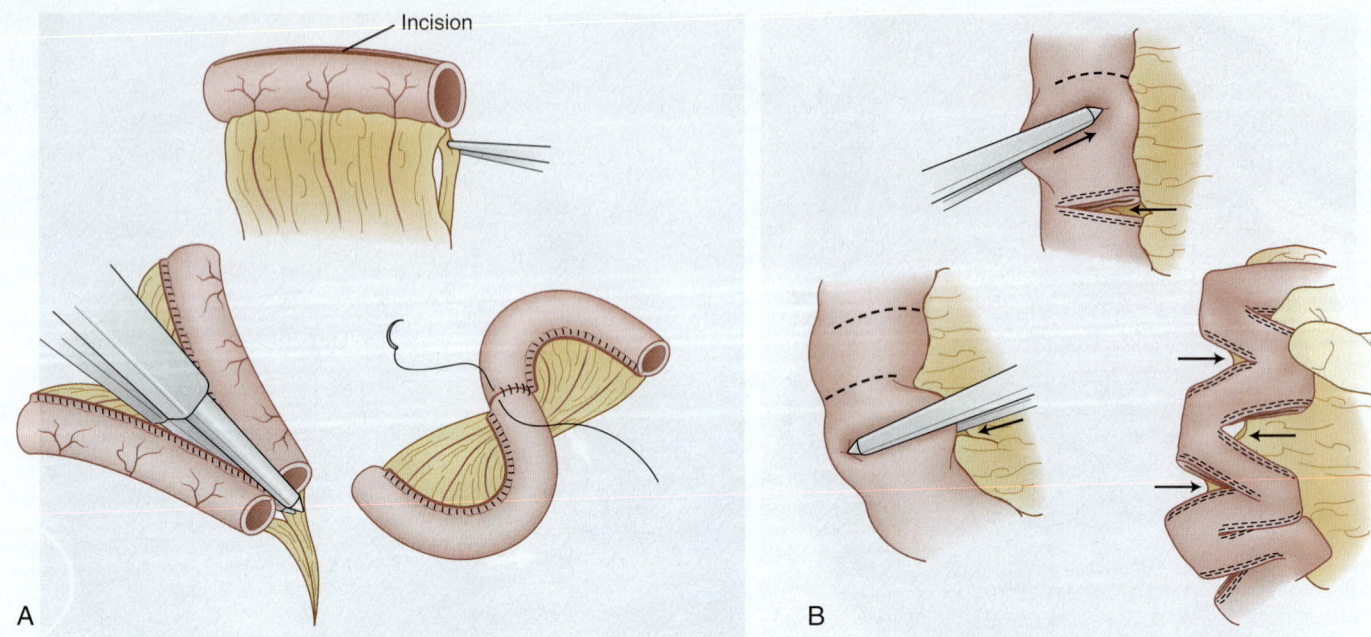

Incision

A

B

FIGURE 117.11 Bowel-lengthening procedures. (A) Bianchi technique separates two mesenteric planes. A dilated segment of bowel is stapled longitudinally to create two narrower segments for sequential anastomosis. (B) Serial transverse enteroplasty involves stapling a dilated bowel into V shapes on alternating sides, decreasing width and increasing length. (A, Adapted from Abu-Elmagd KM, Bond G, Costa G, et al. Gut rehabilitation and intestinal transplantation. *Therapy*. 2005;2:853-864. B, From Kim HB, Fauza D, Garza J, et al. Serial transverse enteroplasty [STEP]: a novel bowel-lengthening procedure. *J Pediatr Surg*. 2003;38:425-429.)

in longer intestinal length (see Fig. 117.11B).[17] The STEP procedure has been shown to improve enteral feeding tolerance, resulting in significant catch-up growth, without increased mortality. In addition, the operation is technically easier and may be repeated if the bowel continues to dilate as the patient grows. An improved enteral tolerance in the majority of 20 treated patients was observed for more than a 7-year period after STEP procedures.[18] A recent retrospective, single institution review of 36 patients reported that the median increase in bowel length after STEP was 53% and that 42% reached enteral autonomy, but it emphasized the importance of a multidisciplinary intestinal rehabilitation program for an ideal patient selection and outcomes.[19]

Meconium Ileus

Meconium ileus is a unique form of neonatal obstruction that occurs in infants with CF, an autosomal recessive disorder resulting from a mutation in the CF transmembrane regulator gene *(CFTR)*. It is estimated that 3.3% of the White population in the United States are asymptomatic carriers of the mutated *CFTR* gene. The abnormal chloride transport in patients with CF results in tenacious viscous secretions with a protein concentration of almost 80% to 90%. It affects a wide variety of organs, including the intestine, pancreas, lungs, salivary glands, reproductive organs, and biliary tract.

Meconium ileus in the newborn represents the earliest clinical manifestation of CF, affecting approximately 10% to 15% of patients with this inherited disease. The incidence of CF ranges from 1 in 1000 to 2000 live births. Infants present with three cardinal signs in the first 24 to 48 hours of life: (1) generalized abdominal distention, (2) bilious emesis, and (3) failure to pass meconium. Maternal polyhydramnios occurs in approximately 20% of cases. In simple meconium ileus, the terminal ileum is dilated and filled with thick, tarlike, inspissated meconium.

Smaller pellets of meconium are found in the more distal ileum, leading into a relatively small colon. In patients with simple meconium ileus, important plain abdominal radiographic findings include dilated and gas-filled loops of small bowel, absence of air-fluid levels, and a mass of meconium in the right side of the abdomen mixed with gas, giving a ground-glass or soap bubble appearance. Abdominal radiographs show dilated bowel loops with relatively absent air-fluid levels because of thick, viscous meconium. A contrast enema using the water-soluble ionic solution Gastrografin can be both diagnostic-demonstrating a small, narrow-caliber colon and inspissated meconium pellets in the terminal ileum-and therapeutic, as it aids in the evacuation of meconium by pulling water into the colon. It is imperative for an infant to be well hydrated and monitored closely. It is successful in relieving the obstruction in up to 75% of cases, with a bowel perforation rate of less than 3%. The pilocarpine iontophoresis sweat test revealing a chloride concentration of more than 60 mEq/L is the most definitive method to confirm the diagnosis of CF. A more immediate test is detection of the mutated *CFTR* gene.

Operative management of *simple* meconium ileus is required when the obstruction is persistent despite contrast enema, along with 5 mL of 10% *N*-acetylcysteine (Mucomyst) solution administered every 6 hours through a nasogastric tube. Historically, the dilated terminal ileum was resected and various types of stomas were created, allowing intestinal decompression and recovery. However, enterotomy, irrigation with warmed saline solution or 4% *N*-acetylcysteine, and simple evacuation of the luminal meconium without a stoma has also been advocated. *N*-acetylcysteine serves to break the disulfide bonds in the meconium to facilitate separation from the bowel mucosa. The meconium is manipulated into the distal colon or removed through the enterotomy. After the obstruction is relieved, the enterotomy is closed in standard fashion. If meconium evacuation is incomplete, a T-tube may be left in place in the ileum or a divided stoma may be created to facilitate continued postoperative irrigation.

Meconium ileus is considered *complicated* when perforation of the intestine has taken place in utero or in the early neonatal period. Extravasation of meconium can result in severe peritonitis, with a dense inflammatory response and calcification. The variable clinical presentations include a meconium pseudocyst, adhesive peritonitis with or without secondary bacterial infection, and ascites. Abdominal radiographs can demonstrate calcifications, bowel dilation, mass effect, and ascites. A distal ileal obstructive syndrome (DIOS), formerly known as meconium ileus equivalent, may develop in older patients as a consequence of noncompliance with oral enzyme replacement therapy or bouts of dehydration. This is managed nonoperatively in most patients with enemas or oral polyethylene glycol solutions. Other diagnoses must also be considered, including simple adhesive intestinal obstruction. Patients with CF who develop or are at risk for exocrine pancreatic insufficiency are treated with enteric-coated, high-strength pancreatic enzyme replacement therapy (PERT). A complication of this therapy may be a fibrosing colonopathy, which requires exploration and resection of the inflammatory colon stricture.

Meconium Plug Syndrome

Meconium plug syndrome is a different condition from meconium ileus, and, in most cases, it is not a sequela of CF. However, it is a frequent cause of neonatal intestinal obstruction and is associated with several conditions, including Hirschsprung disease, maternal diabetes, and hypothyroidism. Infants often present with abdominal distention and failure to pass meconium in the first 24 hours. The contrast enema study shows a microcolon full of thickened meconium plugs that extends up to where the proximal colon is dilated. Often, a contrast enema is both diagnostic and therapeutic and surgical intervention is not indicated.

Hirschsprung Disease

The pathogenesis of Hirschsprung disease is an aganglionated distal colon/rectum, characterized by an absence of ganglion cells in the myenteric (Auerbach) and submucosal (Meissner) plexus. It occurs in 1 in 5000 live births, with male infants being affected four times more frequently than female infants. Of these patients, 3% to 5% have Down syndrome, and the risk for Hirschsprung disease is greater if there is a family history. An abnormal locus on chromosome 10 has been identified in some families and is associated with the *RET* oncogene.[20] This neurogenic, parasympathetic abnormality is associated with failure of propagation of peristaltic waves with absent muscular relaxation of the distal colon and internal anal sphincter, resulting in a functional obstruction. Hence, the abnormal bowel is the externally normal caliber distal segment, whereas the normal bowel is the proximal dilated portion. Aganglionosis begins at the anorectal line, with the transition to normal colon occurring in the rectosigmoid colon in approximately 80% of cases, in the splenic or transverse colon in 17%, and in the small intestine (involving the entire colon) in 8%. The area between the dilated and contracted segments is referred to as the transition zone. Here, ganglion cells begin to appear, but in reduced numbers.

Most infants (>90%) present with abdominal distention and bilious emesis with failure to pass meconium within the first 24 hours of life. Those with missed diagnoses of Hirschsprung disease may present later in life with a chronic history of abdominal distention and constipation. Enterocolitis is the leading cause of death in patients with uncorrected Hirschsprung disease. It may present with alternating episodes of diarrhea and obstipation, along with abdominal distention, fever, hematochezia, peritonitis, shock, and potentially death.

The diagnostic imaging study of choice in a newborn is a contrast enema. In Hirschsprung disease, aganglionosis of the distal rectum usually results in a narrow caliber with a transition zone and dilated, normal, proximal sigmoid colon. Failure to evacuate the instilled contrast medium completely after 24 hours strongly indicates the presence of Hirschsprung disease. Contrast enema studies are useful in excluding other causes of constipation, such as meconium plug, small left colon syndrome, and intestinal atresia. In toddlers, a manometry study revealing failure of the internal sphincter to relax upon rectal balloon distention may be diagnostic. A rectal biopsy proximal to the dentate line is the gold standard for the diagnosis of Hirschsprung disease. In the newborn period, this is performed at bedside using a suction rectal biopsy kit. It is imperative to obtain biopsy specimens at least 5 mm to 1 cm above the dentate line to avoid sampling the anoderm. In infants, two or more suction rectal biopsy specimens, 1 cm apart in the posterior rectum, are recommended. In older children, a full-thickness biopsy specimen is obtained under general anesthesia because the thicker rectal mucosa is not amenable to the suction biopsy technique. Absent ganglia, hypertrophied nerve trunks, and robust immunostaining for acetylcholinesterase are the histopathologic criteria. Calretinin immunostaining has become a standard adjunct histology study for the diagnosis of Hirschsprung disease.[21] Once the diagnosis is confirmed, the disease can be managed by daily rectal irrigations using a soft red rubber catheter and warm NS. Irrigations are typically performed one to times per day using as much saline as is necessary to return a clear effluent. Irrigations may not be effective or even possible in patients with other comorbidities, when family circumstances hinder proper use of irrigations, or when long segment disease is present. In these cases, leveling colostomy with intraoperative biopsies to determine the site of normal ganglionated intestine may be necessary.

The definitive surgical procedure for Hirschsprung's disease was originally described by Orvar Swenson in 1949. The Swenson pull-through procedure involves a full-thickness dissection of the rectum, freeing it from the surrounding sphincter mechanism. This dissection can be started in the abdomen and extended distally or start 5 mm to 1 cm proximal to the dentate line and extend proximally. It has also been described using laparoscopic assistance or a completely transanal approach. The dissection is carried out to the level of the normal, ganglionated intestine with verification using intraoperative frozen biopsies. Finally, the coloanal anastomosis is performed. The most commonly used surgical procedure for Hirschsprung disease is the laparoscopic-assisted Soave pull-through procedure.[22] (Of note, this procedure is traditionally called the Soave procedure. However, Dr. Asa Yancey described this operation and published it 2 years earlier.) Once frozen section evaluation is completed, an endorectal mucosal dissection within the aganglionic distal rectum is performed via a transanal approach, 5 mm proximal to the dentate line. Once the dissection is at the level of the intraabdominal rectum, the dissection plane is converted to the full thickness of the colon. The ganglionated normal colon is then pulled through the remnant muscular cuff after posterior myotomy of the cuff is performed. Then, a coloanal anastomosis is performed. The Soave procedure can also be performed entirely through a transanal approach. The third pull-through procedure that is commonly used is the Duhamel procedure. In this procedure, the level of disease is confirmed as described earlier using intraoperative frozen biopsies.

Next, the anterior wall of the aganglionic rectal cuff is left in place and the ganglionated normal colon is pulled posterior to the cuff. The aganglionic cuff is anastomosed to the normal ganglionated colon in a side-to-side fashion, creating a common reservoir. This anastomosis results in the formation of a neorectum that empties normally because of the posterior segment of ganglionated bowel. The functional results of these three techniques are similar when performed in skilled hands. Although management with rectal irrigations and one-stage pull-through has become the standard approach for the majority of patients with Hirschsprung disease, two- or three-stage operations involving initial leveling colostomy followed by a definitive pull-through may be necessary in certain cases.

Postoperatively, the stool dysfunction can persist, and at times, it can be difficult to manage, requiring intermittent rectal decompression. Constipation is a common postoperative problem along with frequent soiling, incontinence, and postoperative enterocolitis. A close follow-up of patients postoperatively is mandatory along with aggressive control of constipation with stool softeners and laxatives. If symptoms persist, a histologic reevaluation should be performed to confirm that a normal ganglionated segment of colon was pulled through and to rule out the presence of a transition zone at the coloanal anastomosis.

Anorectal Malformation

The incidence of imperforate anus is 1 in 5000 live births with a male predominance of 58%. The spectrum of anorectal malformations ranges from a perineal mucosal groove with normally positioned anal opening to the cloaca or single opening for the urinary, reproductive, and digestive tracts. The most common defect is an imperforate anus with a fistula between the distal colon and bulbar urethra, in males, or the vestibule of the introitus, in females. By the sixth week of gestation, the urorectal septum moves caudally to divide the cloaca into the anterior urogenital sinus and posterior anorectal canal. Failure of this septum to form results in a fistula between the bowel and urinary tract (in males) or introitus (in females). Complete or partial failure of the anal membrane to resorb results in an anal membrane or stenosis. The perineum also contributes to the development of the external anal opening and genitalia by the formation of cloacal folds, which extend from the anterior genital tubercle to the anus. The perineal body is formed by fusion of the cloacal folds between the anal and urogenital membranes. Breakdown of the cloacal membrane anywhere along its course results in the external anal opening being anterior to the external sphincter (i.e., imperforate anus with perineal fistula).

An anatomic classification of anorectal anomalies is based on the fistula present in the rectum. Male infants can have rectoperineal (Fig. 117.12), rectobulbar urethra, rectoprostatic urethra, or recto-bladder neck fistulas or no fistula. Female infants can have rectoperineal or rectovestibular fistulas, no fistula, or a cloacal anomaly. In the past, these defects were classified as low, intermediate, or high in relationship to the levator ani musculature. This classification is used less in favor of anatomic description of the fistula site. A more therapeutic and prognostic classification is depicted in Box 117.1. An invertogram, a lateral pelvic radiograph taken after the infant is held upside down for several minutes, was used in the past to determine the most distal point of the rectal pouch in patients (typically males) with no visible fistula. Currently, divided loop colostomy with distal colostogram is used to delineate the location of the fistula. Rectal atresia, commonly associated with trisomy 21, refers to an unusual lesion

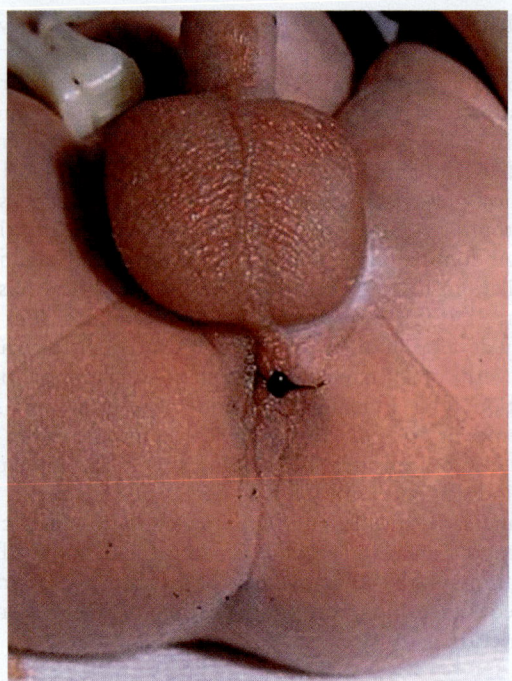

FIGURE 117.12 Imperforate anus with perineal fistula opening demonstrating meconium. Gluteal and scrotal anatomy appear relatively normal, consistent with characteristic findings in blind rectal pouch close to perineal skin amenable to anorectoplasty without an ostomy.

BOX 117.1   Classification of Congenital Anomalies of the Anorectum

Female	Male
Cutaneous (perineal fistula)	Cutaneous (perineal fistula)
Vestibular fistula	Rectourethral fistula
Imperforate anus without fistula	Bulbar
Rectal atresia	Prostatic
Cloaca	Recto-bladder neck fistula
Complex malformation	Imperforate anus without fistula
	Rectal atresia

in which the lumen of the rectum is completely or partially interrupted, with the upper rectum dilated and the lower rectum consisting of a small anal canal. A cloaca is defined as a defect in which the rectum, vagina, and urethra all fuse to form a single common channel. The severity of this lesion is characterized by the length of the common channel, with 3 cm being the cutoff between short and long defects. In females, a single orifice in the perineum indicates a cloaca. If two perineal orifices are seen in a female, a urogenital sinus with normally positioned anus or a urethra and vagina with no rectal fistula are the most likely scenarios. Anorectal malformations often coexist with other lesions, and the VACTERL association must be considered during evaluation. Bone abnormalities of the sacrum and spine, such as absent vertebrae, accessory vertebrae, and hemivertebrae or an asymmetrical or short sacrum, can occur in approximately one-third of patients. Absence of two or more vertebrae is associated with a poor prognosis for bowel and bladder continence. Occult dysraphism of the spinal cord may also be present, consisting of a tethered cord, lipomeningocele, or fat within the filum terminale and warrant imaging to assess.

Genitourinary abnormalities other than rectourinary fistula occur in 25% to 60% of patients. Vesicoureteral reflux and hydronephrosis are the most common, but other conditions—such as horseshoe, dysplastic, or absent kidney, as well as hypospadias or cryptorchidism—must be considered. In general, the higher the anorectal malformation, the greater the frequency of associated urologic abnormalities. In patients with a persistent cloaca or rectovesical fistula, the likelihood of a genitourinary abnormality is approximately 90%. In contrast, the frequency is only 10% with low defects (e.g., perineal fistula). Renal ultrasound and voiding cystourethrography are obtained to assess the urinary tract. If a cardiac defect is suspected, echocardiography is performed before any surgical procedure. EA must also be ruled out with an orogastric tube placement. The decision algorithms for the management of male and female newborns with anorectal malformation are shown in Figs. 117.13 and 117.14.

A newborn with a perineal or vestibular fistula may undergo a primary single-stage repair without colostomy. For anal stenosis in which the anal opening is in a normal location, serial dilation alone is usually sufficient. Dilations are performed daily with gradual size increase over time. If the anal opening is anterior to the external sphincter (i.e., rectoperineal fistula), with a small distance between the opening and the center of the external sphincter, and the perineal body is intact, a cutback anoplasty or limited posterior sagittal anorectoplasty (PSARP) is indicated to operatively restore the anal opening to the normal position within the center of the sphincter muscles, with reconstruction of the perineal body. Newborns suspected of having a rectourinary tract fistula or with blind rectal pouch generally require an initial loop colostomy as the first part of a three-stage reconstruction. The colon is completely divided, and an end sigmoid colostomy with a mucous fistula is constructed to minimize fecal contamination in the rectourinary fistula. Furthermore, the distal mucous fistula limb can be used later for a contrast study to determine the rectourinary fistula. The second-stage procedure is usually performed at 3 to 6 months of age. PSARP, as first

described by deVries and Peña, is the procedure of choice.[23] This consists of determining the location of the central position of the anal sphincter by electrical stimulation of the perineal musculature throughout the operation. An incision is then made in the midline buttocks, extending from the coccyx to the anterior perineum, through the sphincter and levator musculature, until the rectum is identified. The fistula from the rectum to the urinary tract is divided. The rectum is mobilized and the perineal musculature reconstructed. The third and final stage is colostomy reversal, which is performed several weeks later. Anal dilations begin 2 weeks after the anorectoplasty and continue for several months after the colostomy closure.

A laparoscopic-assisted pull-through anorectoplasty has been described for anorectal malformations with similar short-term outcomes to PSARP. This technique offers the theoretical advantages of placing the neorectum within the central position of the sphincter and levator muscle complex under direct vision and avoids the need to cut across these structures. The long-term outcome of this new approach compared with the standard PSARP is unknown.

Complications of anorectal malformations relate to their associated anomalies. Social fecal continence is the major goal regarding correction of the defect. Prognostic factors for continence include the level of the pouch and whether the sacrum is normal. In general, 75% of patients have voluntary bowel movements. However, 50% of patients in this group continue to experience occasional fecal soiling, while the remaining 50% are considered fully continent. Constipation is the most common sequela. A bowel management program consisting of a combination of oral stool softeners and laxatives along with close outpatient follow-up is vital to reduce the frequency of soilage and to improve the quality of life for these patients.

Intussusception

Ileocolic intussusception is a telescoping of distal ileum into the cecum. It is usually idiopathic, without an obvious anatomic lead point, and occurs predominantly at the ileocecal junction, where

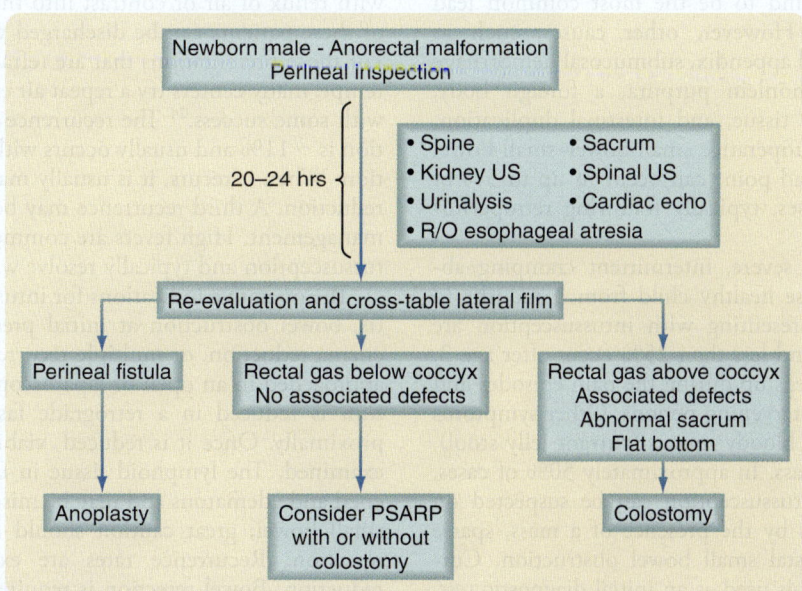

FIGURE 117.13 Management algorithm for male infants with anorectal malformation. *PSARP,* Posterior sagittal anorectoplasty; *R/O,* rule out; *US,* ultrasound. (From Levitt M, Peña A. Imperforate anus. In: Chung DH, Chen MK, eds. *Atlas of Pediatric Surgical Techniques.* Philadelphia: Elsevier Saunders; 2010:185-205.)

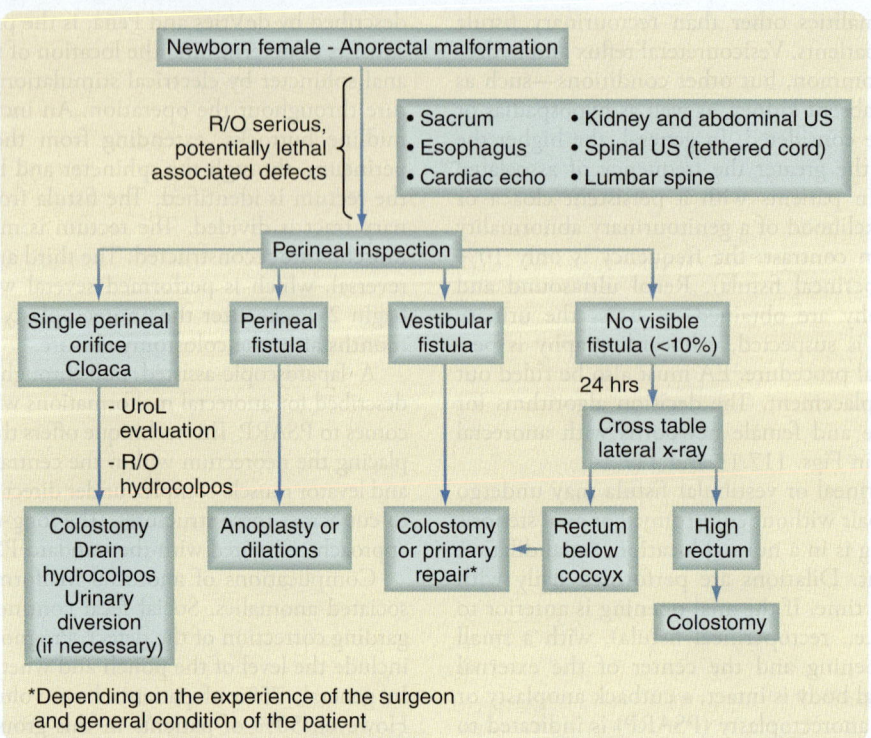

FIGURE 117.14 Management algorithm for female infants with anorectal malformation. *R/O*, Rule out; *UroL*, urologic; *US*, ultrasound. (From Levitt M, Peña A. Imperforate anus. *R/O*, Rule out; *Urol*, urology; *US*, ultrasound. In: Chung DH, Chen MK, eds. *Atlas of Pediatric Surgical Techniques*. Philadelphia: Elsevier Saunders; 2010:185–205.)

there is marked swelling of the lymphoid tissue in the region of the ileocecal valve. It is unknown whether this represents the cause or effect of the ileocolic intussusception. The occurrence of intussusception is associated with a history of recent episodes of viral gastroenteritis, upper respiratory infections, and even administration of the rotavirus vaccine, implicating lymphoid swelling in the pathogenesis of intussusception. In older children, the incidence of a pathologic lead point is up to 12%, and Meckel's diverticulum is found to be the most common lead point for intussusception. However, other causes, such as intestinal polyps, an inflamed appendix, submucosal hemorrhage associated with Henoch-Schönlein purpura, a foreign body, ectopic pancreatic or gastric tissue, and intestinal duplication, must also be considered. Postoperative small bowel–small bowel intussusception without a lead point can occur in up to 5% of pediatric intussusception cases, typically following retroperitoneal surgery.

Intussusception produces severe, intermittent cramping abdominal pain in an otherwise healthy child from 3 months to 3 years. Half of children presenting with intussusception are younger than 1 year of age and less than 25% occur after age 2. The child often draws their legs up during the pain episodes and is usually quiet during the intervening periods. Other symptoms include vomiting, passage of bloody mucus (currant jelly stool), and a palpable abdominal mass. In approximately 50% of cases, the diagnosis of ileocolic intussusception can be suspected on plain abdominal radiographs by the presence of a mass, sparse colonic gas, or complete distal small bowel obstruction. Currently, abdominal ultrasound is used as an initial diagnostic test. The characteristic sonographic findings—such as the 'target sign' on a transverse view and the 'pseudokidney sign' seen longitudinally—should prompt an air-contrast enema study.

Hydrostatic reduction by enema using contrast material or air is the therapeutic procedure of choice. Contraindications to this approach include the presence of peritonitis and hemodynamic instability. Furthermore, an intussusception located entirely within the small intestine is unlikely to be reduced by an enema and is more likely to have an associated pathologic lead point and require surgery. Successful reduction is accomplished in more than 80% of cases, confirmed by resolution of the mass, along with reflux of air or contrast into the terminal ileum, and many of these patients can be discharged without hospital admissions. For those presentations that are refractory to initial air enema attempt, many centers try a repeat air enema study a few hours later with some success.[24] The recurrence rate after hydrostatic reduction is ~11% and usually occurs within 24 hours after the reduction. When it recurs, it is usually managed by another air enema reduction. A third recurrence may be an indication for operative management. High fevers are common after reduction of the intussusception and typically resolve without sequelae.

The operative indications for intussusception include peritonitis, bowel obstruction at initial presentation, failed hydrostatic enema reduction, or multiple recurrences. This procedure can be approached in an open or laparoscopic fashion. The intussusceptum is reduced in a retrograde fashion by pushing the mass proximally. Once it is reduced, viability of the reduced bowel is examined. The lymphoid tissue in the ileocecal region is thickened and edematous and may be mistaken for a tumor within the small bowel; great caution should be exercised before surgical resection. Recurrence rates are extremely low after surgical reduction. Bowel resection is required occasionally when the intussusception cannot be reduced, the viability of the bowel is uncertain, or a lead point is identified. If so, an ileocolectomy with primary anastomosis is usually performed.

Meckel's Diverticulum

Meckel's diverticulum is the most common congenital anomaly of the GI tract and occurs in approximately 2% of the population. More than 70% of symptomatic patients have heterotopic gastric mucosa and another 5% have pancreatic tissue. The rule of twos is often cited in association with Meckel's diverticulum. Aside from its 2% incidence and two types of heterotopic mucosa, it is located within 2 feet of the ileocecal valve, is approximately 2 inches in length, and usually symptomatic by 2 years of age. Meckel's diverticulum is caused by a failure of normal regression of the omphalomesenteric (vitelline) duct that occurs during weeks 5 to 7 of gestation. Meckel's diverticulum is a true diverticulum containing all intestinal layers and is a common manifestation of an omphalomesenteric (vitelline) remnant.

The clinical symptoms are related to hemorrhage, obstruction, or inflammation. The most common presenting symptom is a painless, massive, lower GI bleeding in children younger than 5 years. Diagnosis of a persistent vitelline duct remnant may be established by umbilical ultrasound or lateral contrast radiography. Bleeding from a Meckel's diverticulum may be confirmed by a ^{99m}Tc-pertechnetate isotope scan, which detects gastric mucosa within the diverticulum but will not detect pancreatic mucosa. Of note, ectopic gastric mucosa can also be present in patients with intestinal duplication.

Segmental ileal resection at the base of the Meckel's diverticulum, especially in the case of bleeding, with primary end-to-end anastomosis is the gold standard because the bleeding point is typically on the mesenteric side of the intestine, opposite the opening of the diverticulum. However, a simpler V-shaped diverticulectomy with transverse closure of the ileum is an acceptable alternative technique in patients who are not actively bleeding. Laparoscopic diverticulectomy has become more acceptable with several reporting no increase in complications due to retained ectopic gastric mucosa.[25] Although management of incidentally found Meckel's diverticulum at the time of laparotomy for unrelated other GI conditions has been somewhat controversial, an asymptomatic Meckel's diverticulum should be left alone.

Appendicitis

The management of appendicitis has evolved over time. Currently, the diagnosis of appendicitis is rarely made solely based on history and physical examination findings alone. Virtually every patient suspected of appendicitis undergoes extensive diagnostic blood tests and imaging studies (e.g., ultrasonography or CT). The use of MRI has also been introduced at some institutions to reduce exposure to radiation. Most institutions have adopted a clinical pathway–based management of appendicitis with standardized IV antibiotic regimens, operative techniques, and postoperative care, which include minimal to no outpatient opioid use. Laparoscopic appendectomy has become the standard approach. For simple appendicitis, preoperative IV antibiotics are administered (monotherapy with piperacillin-tazobactam is preferred), and the appendectomy can be safely performed within 24 hours without increased risk of perforation. For complicated appendicitis, surgical management includes appendectomy with antibiotics continued after surgery or percutaneous drainage or abscess with or without delayed interval appendectomy. Up to 40% of patients with perforated appendicitis can develop a postoperative abscess, which may require percutaneous drainage and/or continued antibiotics. Recently, nonoperative management of appendicitis has become more accepted in clinical practice, challenging the old dogma of appendectomy for every appendicitis.

A multi-institutional trial has determined that the nonoperative management of carefully selected patients with uncomplicated appendicitis has acceptable outcomes.[26]

Further studies will be necessary to determine the long-term efficacy of this approach. However, during the recent COVID-19 pandemic, the nonoperative management of appendicitis was useful in patients with significant risk of respiratory complications due to their concurrent SARS-CoV-2 infection.

HEPATOPANCREATICOBILIARY CONDITIONS

Extrahepatic Biliary Atresia

BA is a rare disease of neonates characterized by the inflammatory obliteration of intrahepatic and extrahepatic bile ducts. The incidence is estimated to be 1 in 5000 to 12,000 infants, depending on the region. It may be associated with other congenital malformations, such as splenic abnormalities (e.g., asplenia, polysplenia), absence of the inferior vena cava (IVC), and intestinal malrotation. The exact mechanisms of BA are unknown, and the disease is progressive. One theory is that extrahepatic ducts are susceptible to immune-mediated inflammatory injury and subsequent obliteration of the bile ducts. Proinflammatory cytokines (i.e., interleukin-2, interferon-γ, and tumor necrosis factor) are implicated.[27] T cells and natural killer cells are also prominently found in BA. Another theory is that a viral insult, such as group C rotavirus infection, triggers immune-mediated fibrosclerosis and obstruction of the extrahepatic bile ducts. Interestingly, animal studies have shown that infection of newborn mice with rotavirus leads to a presentation similar to infants, with the onset of hyperbilirubinemia, jaundice, and acholic stools. Histology shows inflammation and obstruction of the extrahepatic bile ducts. Another hypothesis is that there may be an association with human leukocyte antigen (HLA) type and BA because patients with BA have a high frequency of HLA-B12. It is unclear whether this is causal, but some argue that abnormal expression of HLA makes biliary ductal epithelial cells susceptible targets for immunologic assault. Another putative gene, *CFC1*, encodes a protein important in the embryonic differentiation of the left-right axis; when mutated, it is thought to predispose to the development of BA. Histopathology shows significant extrahepatic biliary obstruction with portal tract fibrosis, inflammatory cell infiltration, bile duct proliferation, and cholestasis with bile plugging.

The disease is classified according to the level of the most proximal biliary obstruction. Type I BA has patency to the level of the common bile duct (CBD); type II has patency to the level of the common hepatic duct; and type III, which accounts for more than 90% of cases, occurs when the left and right hepatic ducts, at the level of the porta hepatis, are involved. This aids in the differentiation between correctable BA and others. Correctable BA requires that patent hepatic ducts exist to the porta hepatis. Types I and II may be amenable to a direct extrahepatic biliary duct–intestinal anastomosis.

Infants present shortly after birth with jaundice, pale stools, and dark urine. Advanced disease presents with failure to thrive, hepatomegaly, and ascites from liver cirrhosis. If the jaundice persists after 14 days of life in a term infant, an evaluation for liver disease should be initiated. This consists of determining direct or conjugated bilirubin levels, which will be elevated (>2.0 mg/dL) in those with liver disease. Other exclusionary studies include serologic testing for toxoplasmosis, rubella, cytomegalovirus, and herpes (TORCH) and hepatitis B and C infections; α$_1$-antitrypsin; and

CF. Metabolic disorders, such as galactosemia and tyrosinemia, and endocrine abnormalities must also be ruled out.

The gallbladder may be atrophic or absent, and intrahepatic ducts may also be notably absent on ultrasound evaluation. Hepatobiliary iminodiacetic acid (HIDA) scintigraphy, magnetic resonance cholangiopancreatography (MRCP), and endoscopic retrograde cholangiopancreatography (ERCP) are used with varying success. A HIDA scan can reveal uptake of the technetium isotope with an absence of emptying into the duodenum. MRCP or ERCP can better define the biliary anatomy, but it is more invasive and can delay operative exploration. Timing of Kasai portoenterostomy has been shown to affect postoperative outcome. Liver biopsy helps support the diagnosis of BA and can safely be done percutaneously or open. Optimal timing of operation is typically before 60 days of life, where 2-year survival with native liver is approximately 60%. If operative intervention is performed after 90 days of life, this number drops to approximately 40%.

Once the diagnosis is suspected, operative exploration with intraoperative cholangiography is indicated. The absence of contrast drainage into the duodenum confirms the diagnosis. If BA is confirmed, a hepatoportoenterostomy (Kasai procedure) is the surgical procedure of choice. Here, the extrahepatic biliary tree is dissected proximally to the level of the liver capsule, where the porta hepatis (portal plate) is transected. The dissection of the fibrous remnant ascends into the posterior area surrounding the portal vein branches until it has come within the capsular surface of the liver (Fig. 117.15A). The reconstruction is performed using a Roux-en-Y hepaticojejunostomy (see Fig. 117.15B). The use of ursodeoxycholic acid and phenobarbital may promote biliary drainage, but their efficacy is uncertain. In the past, the use of steroids after the Kasai procedure was advocated by many and thought to promote biliary drainage with shorter hospital stay.

However, the Biliary Atresia Clinical Research Consortium's recent randomized, double-blinded, placebo-controlled trial of steroid therapy (the START trial) after the Kasai procedure demonstrated that high-dose steroid therapy after the procedure did not result in significant treatment differences in bile drainage at 6 months.[28] Furthermore, steroid treatment was associated with earlier onset of serious adverse events as well as with impaired growth. However, steroid pulse therapy remains a treatment option for post-Kasai cholangitis. Antibiotics are also continued postoperatively because the risk of cholangitis is high (45%–60%) due to the ease with which intestinal bacteria can ascend and colonize the bile ducts. Unfortunately, if the Kasai procedure is unable to reestablish bile flow and liver failure or cirrhosis ensues, liver transplantation is indicated.

Unfortunately, Kasai hepatoportoenterostomy does not cure BA, which will inevitably progress in more than 70% of infants who undergo this procedure. The rate with which the disease progresses, as evidenced by cirrhosis and portal hypertension, is variable, but it may be expedited by recurrent cholangitis. It is estimated, however, that 80% of those who have successfully undergone a Kasai procedure can live up to 10 years before liver transplantation is needed. In those infants who undergo transplantation, outcomes are good, with 10-year graft survival and overall patient survival of 73% and 86%, respectively.[29]

Choledochal Cyst

Choledochal cysts are cystic dilations of the CBD. They have an incidence of 1 in 100,000 to 150,000 live births, with a 3 to 4:1 female-to-male preponderance. They are classified on the basis of location, and their frequency varies (Fig. 117.16). Type I (50%–80%) is a simple cyst that can involve any portion of the CBD and can be cystic (type Ic) or fusiform (type If), whereas type II (2%) describes a diverticulum arising off any portion of

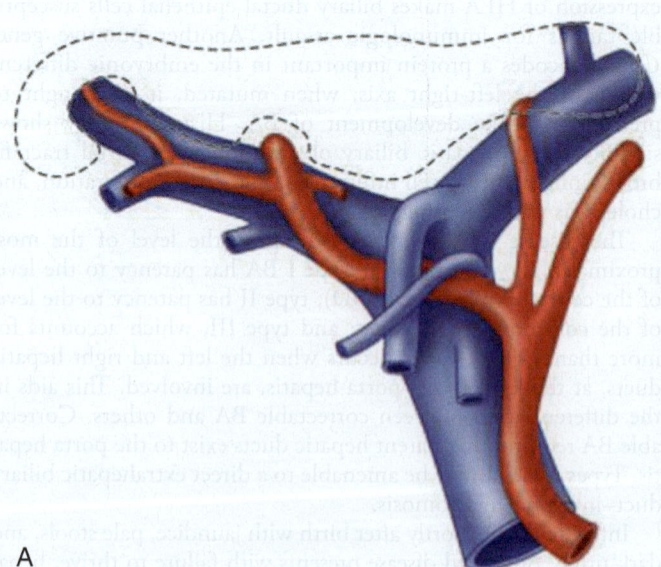
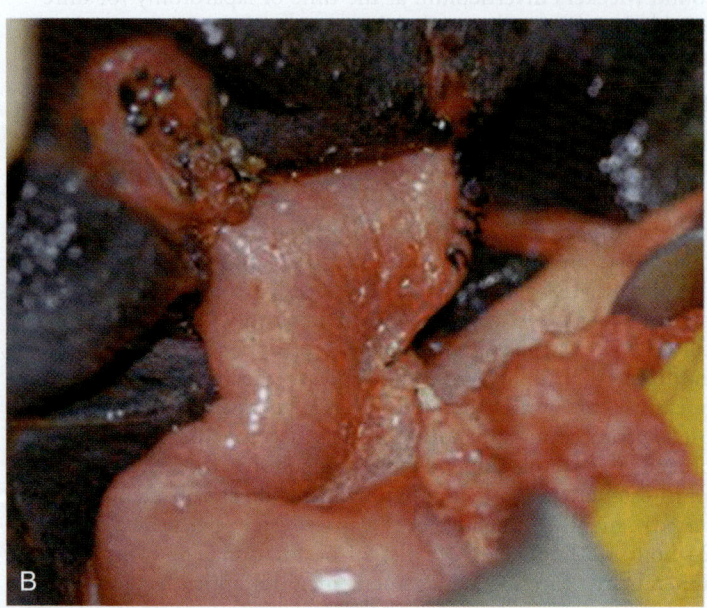

FIGURE 117.15 Liver and Kasai portoenterostomy. (A) The dissection of fibrous extrahepatic biliary remnant is continued up to the capsular surface of the liver within the bifurcation of the portal vein (*dotted line* indicates fibrous portal plate). The lateral extent of dissection on the left side is the umbilical fissure and the obliterated umbilical vein insertion into the left portal vein. On the right side, the lateral extent of dissection is to the bifurcation of the right portal vein into its anterior and posterior branches. (B) Completed Roux-en-Y portoenterostomy. (From Nathan JD, Ryckman FC. Biliary atresia. In: Chung DH, Chen MK, eds. *Atlas of Pediatric Surgical Techniques.* Philadelphia: Elsevier Saunders; 2010:220-231.)

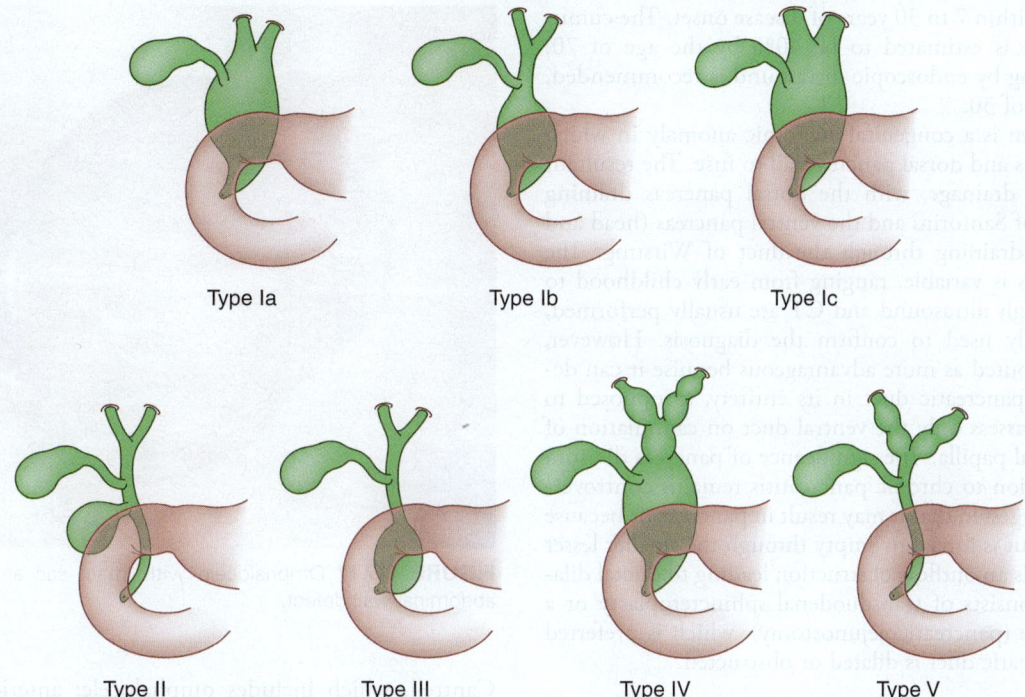

FIGURE 117.16 Classification of choledochal cyst. Anatomic variations of the gallbladder, common bile duct, hepatic ducts and duodenum. (From O'Neill JA. Choledochal cyst. In: Grosfeld JL, O'Neill JA, Fonkalsrud EW, et al., eds. *Pediatric Surgery*. 6th ed. Philadelphia: Mosby Elsevier; 2006:16-21.)

the biliary tree. Choledochoceles represent type III cysts (1.4%–4.5%) and consist of dilation confined to the distal intraduodenal portion of the CBD. Although type IV (15%–35%) involves intrahepatic and extrahepatic bile ducts, type V or Caroli disease (20%) is limited to the intrahepatic ducts only. Choledochal cysts can be associated with other congenital anomalies, including duodenal and colonic atresia, imperforate anus, pancreatic arteriovenous malformation, and pancreatic divisum. Moreover, choledochal cysts are considered premalignant lesions.

The pathogenesis of choledochal cysts is largely unknown, but pancreaticobiliary malunion where pancreatic duct and CBD join with a long common channel (>6 mm) before entry into the duodenum is seen in many cases. This aberrant anatomy leads to bile reflux–induced activation of pancreatic enzymes within the duct that has been implicated. Inflammatory response compromises the integrity of the duct wall, resulting in dilation. In support of this theory, amylase and trypsinogen levels in the bile from patients with choledochal cysts are often elevated. Another possibility is that these cysts arise from CBD obstruction at the sphincter of Oddi.

The classic triad of jaundice, a palpable right upper quadrant mass, and abdominal pain is seen in less than 20% of patients, although 85% present with at least two of these symptoms. Infants typically present with obstructive jaundice and an abdominal mass, whereas older children experience chronic intermittent pain, fever, and jaundice. Complications of cholangitis and pancreatitis can occur as well as bile peritonitis secondary to cyst rupture. Abdominal ultrasound demonstrates a cystic enlarged ductal structure that is separate from the gallbladder. HIDA scan can demonstrate initial absent filling of the cyst, followed by delayed uptake and emptying into the duodenum. MRCP can further define the entire biliary system as well as the pancreatic head. ERCP is rarely necessary to make a surgical decision. Prompt surgical excision of the cysts with Roux-en-Y hepaticojejunostomy is recommended.

Complete cyst excision is important because the risk of malignancy is as high as 6% with a retained choledochal cyst. If the complete cyst excision is deemed unsafe due to scarring from chronic inflammation, it should be enucleated. Advocates of the pancreaticobiliary malunion theory will point to separation of biliary and pancreatic drainage with Roux-en-Y hepaticojejunostomy as an important step to arrest the inflammatory process and prevent progression of disease. These patients are monitored with ultrasound examinations postoperatively to ensure adequate drainage of the biliary tree. Postoperative anastomotic strictures are a common complication and likely arise from chronic intrahepatic cholelithiasis and recurrent cholangitis.

Hereditary Pancreatitis and Pancreas Divisum

Hereditary pancreatitis is an autosomal dominant disorder with a high degree of penetrance. It is rare, representing less than 1% of chronic pancreatitis. The disease results from a mutation in the cationic trypsinogen gene *(PRSS1)*, which leads to an increase in the autoactivation of trypsin and resistance to deactivation.[30] The gene has been mapped to chromosome 7q35; the two most common allelic mutations are *R122H* and *N29I*. Recurrent bouts of pancreatitis usually begin in childhood, between 5 and 10 years of age, with no identifiable cause. Aside from the age at onset, the presentation, natural history, diagnosis, and treatment of this disease are similar to those for other causes of pancreatitis. Hereditary pancreatitis should be suspected in any patient who experiences at least two bouts of acute pancreatitis without obvious risk factors, such as trauma, hyperlipidemia, gallstones, or pancreas divisum. It should also be considered in any child with acute pancreatitis and a family history of this disease, as well as pancreatitis in children. Making the correct diagnosis is important because there is an extremely high lifetime risk of malignant transformation. It is estimated that these patients have a fiftyfold to seventyfold increase in the risk for development of pancreatic adenocarcinoma within 7 to 30 years of disease onset. The cumulative lifetime risk is estimated to be 40% by the age of 70. Therefore, screening by endoscopic ultrasound is recommended, starting at the age of 30.

Pancreas divisum is a congenital anatomic anomaly in which the ventral pancreas and dorsal pancreas fail to fuse. The resultant pancreas has dual drainage, with the dorsal pancreas draining through the duct of Santorini and the ventral pancreas (head and uncinate process) draining through the duct of Wirsung. The onset of symptoms is variable, ranging from early childhood to adulthood. Although ultrasound and CT are usually performed, ERCP is frequently used to confirm the diagnosis. However, MRCP has been touted as more advantageous because it can delineate the dorsal pancreatic duct in its entirety, as opposed to ERCP, which can assess only the ventral duct on cannulation of the major duodenal papilla. The significance of pancreas divisum and its predisposition to chronic pancreatitis remains controversial. Some have suggested that it may result in pancreatitis because all pancreatic output is forced to empty through the smaller lesser papilla. The result is an outflow obstruction leading to ductal dilation. Treatment consists of transduodenal sphincteroplasty or a Puestow procedure (pancreaticojejunostomy), which is preferred if the dorsal pancreatic duct is dilated or obstructed.

Biliary Dyskinesia

Obesity has also become a major health problem for adolescents. Subsequently, we are seeing an increasing number of pediatric patients with cholelithiasis and biliary colic due to dyskinesia of the gallbladder. Biliary dyskinesia has become more prevalent and should be considered during the evaluation of a teenager with epigastric pain. Pediatric surgeons are often consulted to evaluate for the appropriateness of performing a cholecystectomy based on a low ejection fraction from a cholecystokinin-stimulated HIDA scan. When an ejection fraction of less than 35% correlates with characteristic biliary colic, a cholecystectomy can be therapeutic.[31] However, in patients with vague symptoms, inconsistent with biliary colic, further examination for the etiology of the pain is warranted before proceeding with cholecystectomy.

ABDOMINAL WALL CONDITIONS

Anterior abdominal wall defects are a relatively frequent neonatal surgical condition. During normal development of the human embryo, the midgut herniates outward through the umbilical ring and continues to grow. By the 11th week of gestation, the midgut returns to the coelomic cavity and undergoes proper rotation and fixation, along with closure of the umbilical ring. If the intestine fails to return, the infant is born with the abdominal contents protruding through the abdominal wall defect at the umbilical ring.

An omphalocele is a central abdominal wall defect that is generally more than 4 cm in diameter, with an intact membranous sac composed of an outer layer of amnion and an inner layer of peritoneum (Fig. 117.17). Defects less than 4 cm in diameter are arbitrarily designated as umbilical cord hernias. Infants with an omphalocele have a high incidence (~50%) of associated anomalies, such as Beckwith-Wiedemann syndrome, which is a combination of gigantism, macroglossia, and an umbilical defect, either a hernia or omphalocele. Chromosomal abnormalities, including trisomies 13, 15, 18, and 21, have also been associated with omphalocele. Other associated anomalies include exstrophy of the bladder or cloaca and the pentalogy of

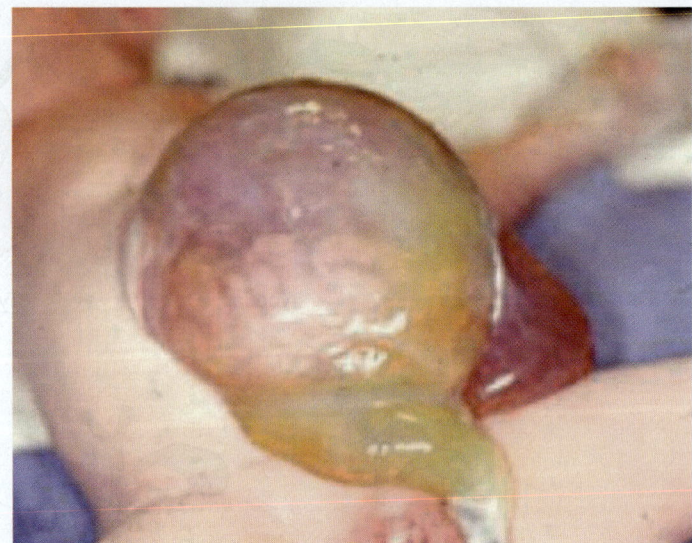

FIGURE 117.17 Omphalocele with intact sac and centrally located abdominal wall defect.

Cantrell, which includes omphalocele; anterior diaphragmatic hernia; sternal cleft; ectopia cordis; and intracardiac defect, such as ventricular septal defect.

Preservation of an intact omphalocele sac is key in initial management. Also, great care should be taken to prevent hypothermia. A comprehensive diagnostic workup is performed to identify associated anomalies. Primary surgical closure of the small- to medium-sized defect is preferred. Alternatively, larger defects can be closed with prosthetic patch closure (e.g., Gore-Tex), porcine small intestinal submucosa–derived biomaterial (e.g., Surgisis), skin flap closure, or placement of a silo for sequential reduction and staged closure. Giant omphaloceles are treated by topical application of escharotic agents such as povidone-iodine (Betadine) ointment or silver nitrate, which allows the sac to thicken and epithelialize. The overall survival for infants with an omphalocele largely depends on their lung maturity and severity of associated anomalies.

A gastroschisis defect is always to the right of an intact umbilical cord, at the site of obliterated right umbilical vein, without a sac covering the abdominal viscera (Fig. 117.18A). The fascial defect is typically 4 cm in diameter. An absent sac with direct exposure to amniotic fluid in utero results in intestinal thickening and edema with inflammation. Intestinal atresia may exist in up to 15% of cases; however, other major anomalies are rare. Eviscerated bowel must be handled with care to avoid further insult. After birth, infants are placed in a warm, saline-filled plastic "bowel bag" up to the nipple line, to minimize heat and fluid losses. This also allows for gross inspection of the eviscerated bowel at all times and identification of inadvertent twisting of the bowel. Primary reduction is successful in 50% to 80% of cases, with eviscerated contents placed into the abdominal cavity without excessive tension. If primary reduction is unsuccessful, a ringed silo bag is placed and the eviscerated bowel is reduced gradually over several days, followed by operative suture closure of the fascia and skin (see Fig. 117.18B). To avoid compartment syndrome, a safe intraabdominal pressure is less than 15 mm Hg. Alternatively, a sutureless delayed spontaneous closure can be performed at the bedside.[32] Bowel is reduced into the abdomen and the defect is covered with or without the umbilical cord, and

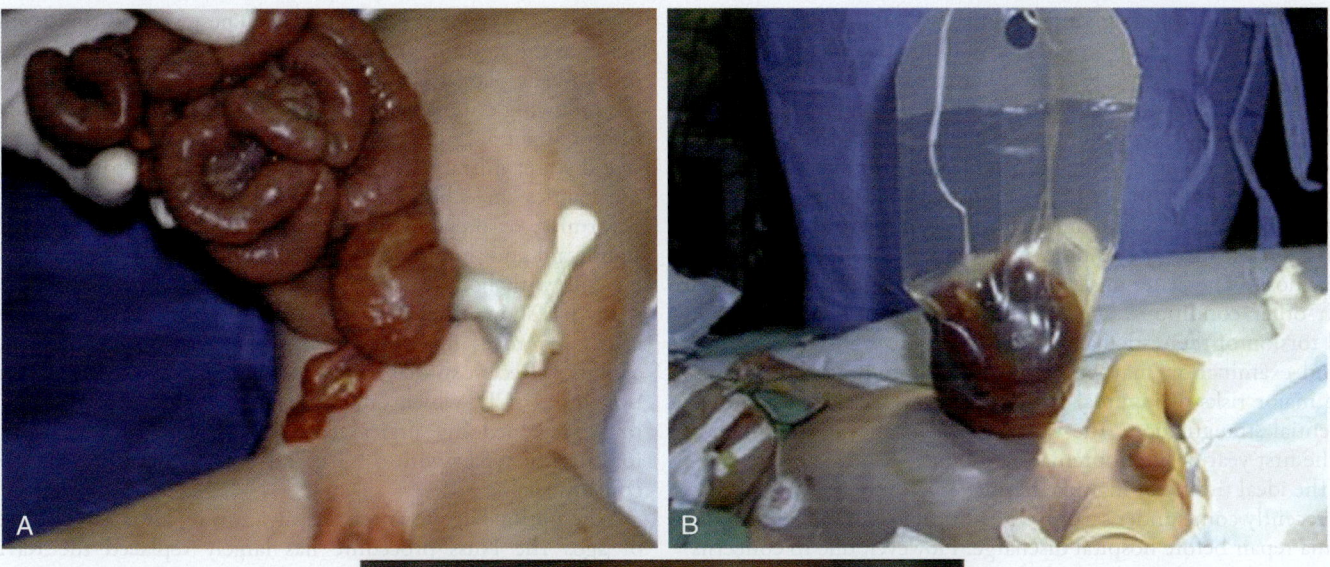

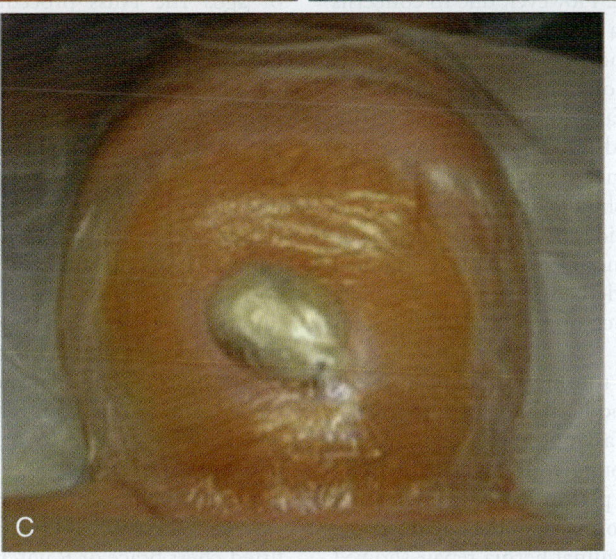

FIGURE 117.18 (A) Gastroschisis with eviscerated multiple bowels. Abdominal wall defect is to the right side of the intact umbilical cord. (B) Silastic bag with ringed edge can be placed at bedside and bowel loops are gradually reduced into abdominal cavity. (C) Sutureless closure of gastroschisis. After reducing eviscerated bowel loops into abdominal cavity, umbilical cord is folded over the defect and a clear watertight dressing is placed.

a watertight clear dressing (see Fig. 117.18C) is placed. Once the contents adhere in the intraabdominal position at around 4 days, the dressing can be changed to a dry dressing over the cord remnant or a Vaseline dressing over the exposed bowel. In cases of associated intestinal atresia or stenosis, inflammation of the bowel precludes an immediate repair; the abdominal wall is closed first, then surgery for intestinal atresia is performed 6 to 8 weeks later. Late occurrence of NEC has been reported in up to 20% of patients after gastroschisis repair. For larger defects, a prosthetic patch (Gore-Tex) is placed and the skin is closed over it. Undescended testis is a common associated finding in 10% to 20% of infants. When found outside the peritoneal cavity, the testes should simply be pushed back into the abdominal cavity without formal orchidopexy at the time of abdominal wall closure or silo bag placement. Many spontaneously descend into the scrotum; if not, then orchidopexy is performed. The majority of infants have prolonged ileus. One of the difficult challenges in the management of gastroschisis remains managing dysfunctional intestine or

short gut syndrome and infants often experience cholestasis due to prolonged TPN support.

Hernias

Inguinal hernia repair is one of the most commonly performed surgical procedures in pediatric surgery. The incidence of inguinal hernia is approximately 3% to 5% in term infants and 9% to 11% in premature infants. It affects males approximately six times more often than females. Sixty percent of inguinal hernias occur on the right side, 30% are on the left side, 10% are bilateral, and almost all are indirect and congenital in nature. The processus vaginalis is an elongated diverticulum of the peritoneum that accompanies the testicle on its descent into the scrotum, and it generally is obliterated during the ninth month of gestation or soon after birth. The variable persistence of the processus vaginalis results in a spectrum of clinical presentations, including a scrotal hernia with protrusion of intestine, ovaries, omentum, or communicating hydrocele with intermittent accumulation of peritoneal fluid.

The diagnosis of an inguinal hernia is established by clinical history and examination alone. Transillumination of the scrotum to differentiate a hydrocele from a hernia can be misleading because a herniated, thin-walled loop of bowel in infants and children can be easily transilluminated. Palpation of the cord may elicit a "silk glove sign," which is produced by rubbing the opposing peritoneal membranes of the empty sac. At times, palpation of a thickened cord, compared with the contralateral side, along with a reliable history of intermittent bulge are sufficient to derive a diagnosis. The acute onset of hydrocele may also be associated with other conditions, such as epididymitis, testicular torsion, and torsion of the testicular appendage. In these instances, ultrasound examination may be helpful to determine the diagnosis. The major risks of inguinal hernias are bowel incarceration and potential strangulation. The incidence of incarceration is higher in the first year of life in premature infants.

The ideal timing of inguinal hernia repair in premature infants has recently come under scrutiny. Historically, most advocated for hernia repair before hospital discharge. However, due to concerns of potential complications, including a long-term risk of neurodevelopmental delay with general anesthesia, delayed repair may be a better treatment strategy. There are ongoing multi-institutional studies evaluating the timing of infant inguinal hernia repair. When elective, repair may be deferred until postoperative apnea risk decreases at 1 year of age. An incarcerated inguinal hernia should be reduced first, and repair should be performed 24 to 48 hours later when tissue edema subsides. A nonreducible, incarcerated hernia is a surgical emergency. Contralateral inguinal exploration at the time of symptomatic hernia repair is routinely performed based on the high incidence of a contralateral patent processus vaginalis (4%–65%).

However, the issue regarding the routine exploration of the asymptomatic contralateral side in toddlers remains unresolved. Most pediatric surgeons explore the asymptomatic contralateral side in children 2 years of age or younger. Today, laparoscopic pediatric inguinal hernia repairs are performed with increasing frequency. A recent meta-analysis comparing the laparoscopic versus open approach for pediatric inguinal hernia repair showed no definite advantage of one technique over the other.[33]

An umbilical hernia tends to close on its own in ~80% of cases of children; therefore, elective repair should be deferred until around 5 years of age. Incarceration of an umbilical hernia is extremely rare. Earlier elective surgical repair should be considered when the hernia appears to enlarge over time, or the fascial defect is larger than 2 cm. If left alone, these hernias tend to develop large skin proboscis (>3 cm) resulting in poor postoperative cosmesis. Primary repair of the hernia is always achieved, and the use of prosthetic patch should never be considered.

CHEST WALL DEFORMITY

Pectus excavatum, a chest wall structural deformity where the anterior chest wall is caved in or sunken, is five times more common than pectus carinatum, an abnormal outward protrusion of the anterior chest wall. The deformity is usually present at birth and steadily becomes more prominent with age until past puberty with a male-to-female ratio of 3 to 4:1. Abnormalities in costal cartilage development have been implicated in the underlying pathogenesis. Pectus excavatum can be associated with mitral valve prolapse, Ehlers-Danlos syndrome, and Marfan syndrome; therefore, a comprehensive preoperative evaluation is warranted. The severity of pectus excavatum is quantified by the Haller index,

which is a ratio of the width of the chest wall to the depth of between the sternum and the vertebral body on limited chest CT or two-view plain radiographs. In general, a minimum of two of the following criteria are needed to warrant repair: a Haller index of more than 3.25; pulmonary function testing indicating restrictive disease; mitral valve prolapse, murmurs, or conduction abnormalities on echocardiography; physical symptoms from the deformity; or previous failed repair. Psychosocial stress is often significant and should not be underestimated, particularly in adolescents with body image and self-esteem issues. A multicenter study has shown that surgical repair of pectus excavatum significantly improves body image and perceived ability of physical activity.[34] Recent studies have advocated for the use of the correction index (CI), which quantifies the percentage of chest depth to be regained by surgical correction. Most authors advocate for surgical repair with a CI of 28% or higher, but this is still controversial.

The optimal age for pectus excavatum repair is 10 to 14 years of age. The Nuss procedure has largely replaced the Ravitch (open) procedure for most cases of pectus excavatum. Under thoracoscopic guidance, a tunneler is used to perform the retrosternal dissection. Sternal elevation using a retractor system has become popularized for a safer sternal dissection in recent years. An appropriately sized titanium bar is bent and contoured to elevate the sternum, and the bar is passed through the retrosternal plane from one hemithorax into the other, through two lateral intercostal incisions (Fig. 117.19). The Nuss bar is then flipped so that the convexity is outward, and the chest wall defect is immediately corrected. The bar is removed after ~2 years. The Ravitch procedure involves detachment of the costal bundles with removal of the malformed costal cartilages and fracture of the sternum to restore normal chest contour. The costal bundles are then reattached, and the sternum is held in the desired position using a bar, which is removed in 6 months. The use of enhanced recovery pathways after surgery and utilization of intercostal nerve cryoablation has significantly shortened postoperative hospital length of stay to <2 days.[35] Pectus carinatum is typically corrected with a fitted chest brace or Ravitch procedure. There are several different models, but the most important predictor of success is treatment adherence, which requires continuous use for 14 to 16 hours daily to see the best results. Before the use of current enhanced recovery after surgery (ERAS) pain management pathways, postoperative pain was a significant consideration for patients undergoing surgical correction and the historic indications for surgery reflected this. With these protocols, more patients are being considered for surgical correction of pectus deformities than in the past.

GENITOURINARY TRACT CONDITIONS

Cryptorchidism

Cryptorchidism is a condition in which one or both testes fail to descend into the scrotum before birth. Although up to 30% of preterm infants can present with an undescended testis, it also occurs in ~23% of full-term infants. Some undescended testes eventually descend by 1 year of age. The undescended testis is associated with histologic and morphologic changes as early as 6 months of age, whereas atrophy of Leydig cells, a decrease in tubular diameter, and impaired spermatogenesis can occur by 2 years of age. An undescended testis has had its descent halted somewhere along the path of normal descent and is most commonly located in the inguinal canal. A retractile testis is a normally descended testis that retracts into the inguinal canal due to

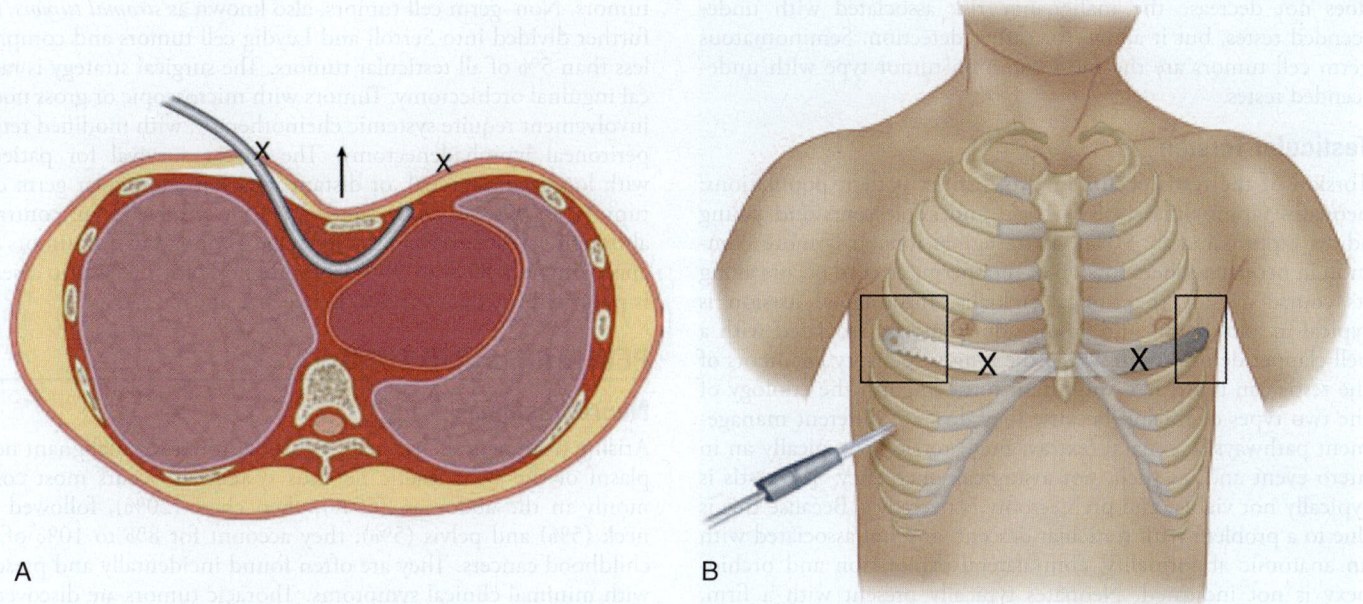

FIGURE 117.19 (A) Pectus excavatum. A tunneler is used to dissect retrosternal place under thoracoscopic guidance. (B) A Nuss bar is placed beneath the sternum and secured onto the chest wall with stabilizers. (From Goretsky MJ, Nuss D. Surgical treatment of chest wall deformities: Nuss procedure. In: Chung DH, Chen MK, eds. *Atlas of Pediatric Surgical Techniques*. Philadelphia: Elsevier Saunders; 2010:97-103.)

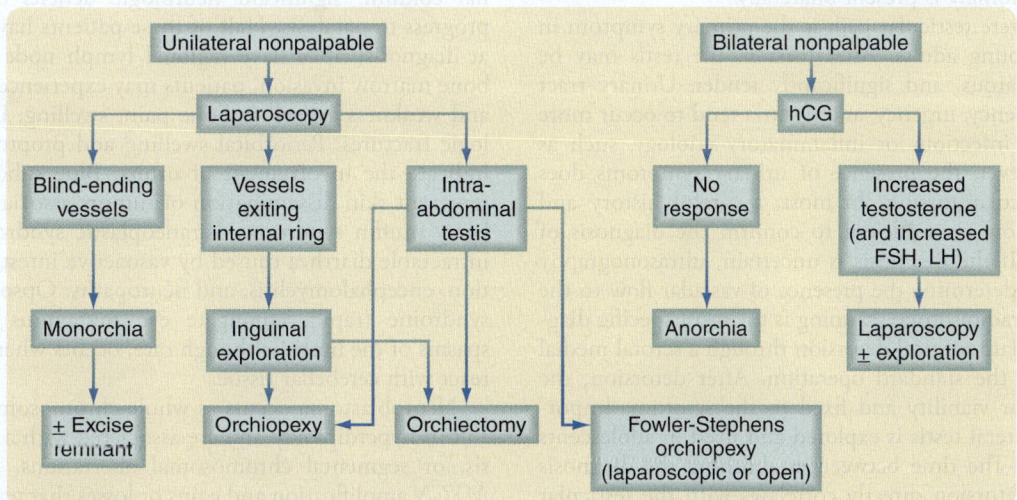

FIGURE 117.20 Management algorithm for nonpalpable undescended testes. *FSH,* Follicle-stimulating hormone; *hCG,* human chorionic gonadotropin; *LH,* luteinizing hormone. (Adapted from Lee KL, Shortliffe LD. Undescended testis and testicular tumors. In: Ashcraft KW, Holcomb GW, Holcomb GW III, et al., eds. *Pediatric Surgery.* 4th ed. Philadelphia: Elsevier Saunders; 2005:706-716.)

hyperreflexive cremasteric muscle; it is easily brought down into the scrotal sac during the examination and does not require operative intervention. Nonpalpable testes may include an intraabdominal, absent, or vanishing testis. Ectopic testes have had an aberrant path of descent, and these can be found in the perineum, femoral canal, and suprapubic regions. For unilateral palpable testis in the inguinal canal, standard dartos pouch orchidopexy is performed at 6 to 12 months of age. An algorithm for management of nonpalpable testes is shown in Fig. 117.20. For nonpalpable, undescended testis, a diagnostic laparoscopy is useful. If the testicular vessels are seen exiting the internal ring, an open inguinal orchidopexy is performed. For an intraabdominal testis, a

two-stage Fowler-Stephens orchidopexy is considered, in which the testicular vessels are ligated as a first stage to allow for development of collateral circulation over 6 months before orchidopexy is performed as a second-stage procedure. Laparoscopic orchidopexy has become popularized as an ideal single-stage option, allowing for full mobilization of the testicular vessels to the level of the base of the kidney. If both testes are nonpalpable, a human chorionic gonadotropin (hCG) stimulation test is carried out to confirm the presence of functioning testes. If present, diagnostic laparoscopy can locate the testes. The risk of malignancy has been reported to be significantly higher (four to five times increased risk) for males with a history of undescended testes. Orchidopexy does not decrease the malignancy risk associated with undescended testes, but it allows for earlier detection. Seminomatous germ cell tumors are the most common tumor type with undescended testes.

Testicular Torsion

Torsion of the testis occurs in two distinct patient populations: neonates (approximately 8%–10%) and adolescents and young adults (approximately 90%). Extravaginal torsion is more common in neonates where torsion of the spermatic cord occurs along its course outside the tunica vaginalis. Intravaginal torsion is typical in adolescents and young adults and is associated with a bell clapper deformity in which the long suspensory ligaments of the testis can twist. It is important to distinguish the etiology of the two types of torsion because they do have different management pathways. Neonatal (extravaginal) torsion is typically an in utero event and, as such, not a surgical emergency. The testis is typically not viable, and orchiectomy is necessary. Because this is due to a problem with testicular descent, and not associated with an anatomic abnormality, contralateral exploration and orchiopexy is not indicated. Neonates typically present with a firm, darkened hemiscrotum with minimal tenderness. In contrast, the more common adolescent or young adult (intravaginal) torsion is a surgical emergency with the possibility to salvage the testicle. Because this is due to an anatomic abnormality of the suspensory ligament of the testis, contralateral exploration and orchiopexy is indicated as this anomaly is present bilaterally.

Acute onset, severe testicular pain is the primary symptom in adolescents and young adults. After torsion, the testis may be high riding, edematous, and significantly tender. Urinary tract symptoms of frequency, urgency, and dysuria tend to occur more common with an infectious or inflammatory etiology, such as epididymitis; however, the presence of urinary symptoms does not rule out testicular torsion. In most, a careful history and physical examination are sufficient to confirm the diagnosis of testicular torsion. If the diagnosis is uncertain, ultrasonography may be helpful to determine the presence of vascular flow to the testicles; however, radioisotope scanning is the most specific diagnostic test. Immediate surgical detorsion through a scrotal medial raphe approach is the standard operation. After detorsion, the testis is assessed for viability and fixed to the scrotum. Importantly, the contralateral testis is explored and fixed in adolescents and young adults. The time between establishing the diagnosis and the surgical detorsion directly correlates with the testicular salvage rate. For torsion of less than 6 hours, 90% of testes can be salvaged. The salvage rate for testis decreases to less than 10% with longer than 24 hours of symptoms.

Testicular Tumors

Testicular cancer accounts for less than 2% of all pediatric solid tumors and has bimodal peaks at around 2 years of age and at puberty. Testicular tumors commonly present as painless scrotal masses, often discovered incidentally. Ultrasonography is useful, but CT scan is critical for evaluation of retroperitoneal lymphadenopathy as well as metastatic disease. The serum tumor marker α-fetoprotein (AFP), a glycoprotein produced by the fetal yolk sac, is elevated in yolk sac tumors. β-hCG is produced by embryonal carcinomas and mixed teratomas. There are two main types of testicular tumors, germ cell and non–germ cell. Germ cell tumors are subdivided into seminomas and nonseminomatous tumors, (embryonal carcinoma, yolk sac carcinoma, choriocarcinoma, and teratoma) and comprise over 95% of all testicular

tumors. Non–germ cell tumors, also known as *stromal tumors,* are further divided into Sertoli and Leydig cell tumors and comprise less than 5% of all testicular tumors. The surgical strategy is radical inguinal orchiectomy. Tumors with microscopic or gross nodal involvement require systemic chemotherapy, with modified retroperitoneal lymphadenectomy. The 5-year survival for patients with localized, regional, or distant metastatic testicular germ cell tumors is 99.2%, 96%, and 73%, respectively. In contrast, although 5-year survival rates for stage I non–germ cell tumors are approximately 80% to 90%, the prognosis for metastatic disease is poor with median survival between 1 and 2 years.

PEDIATRIC SOLID TUMORS

Neuroblastoma

Arising from neural crest cells, neuroblastoma is a malignant neoplasm of the sympathetic nervous system. It occurs most commonly in the abdomen (65%), then chest (20%), followed by neck (5%) and pelvis (5%); they account for 8% to 10% of all childhood cancers. They are often found incidentally and present with minimal clinical symptoms. Thoracic tumors are discovered at the time of routine chest radiograph obtained for unrelated respiratory symptoms. Pelvic masses may cause constipation or bladder dysfunction due to extrinsic mass effects. Horner syndrome may develop in 15% of patients with neck tumors that compress the sympathetic ganglia. If tumors extend into the spinal column, significant neurologic deficits occur and rapidly progress to paralysis. Half of these patients have localized disease at diagnosis; 35% have regional lymph node involvement. For bone marrow invasion, patients may experience anemia, bruising, and weakness as well as bone pain, swelling, limping, or pathologic fractures. Periorbital swelling and proptosis (raccoon eyes) indicate the involvement of orbits. Blue subcutaneous nodules represent skin dissemination of tumors associated with the blueberry muffin syndrome. Paraneoplastic syndromes can produce intractable diarrhea caused by vasoactive intestinal peptide secretion, encephalomyelitis, and neuropathy. Opsoclonus-myoclonus syndrome (rapid, conjugate eye nystagmus with involuntary spasms of the limbs) although rare, occurs when antibodies cross-react with cerebellar tissue.

Neuroblastoma occurs as whole chromosome gains, which result in hyperdiploidy and are associated with a favorable prognosis, or segmental chromosomal aberrations, which encompass *MYCN* amplification and gains or losses that tend to be associated with worse outcomes. The *MYCN* oncogene, which is amplified at chromosome 2p24 in 25% of cases, is found in 30% to 40% of advanced-stage neuroblastomas but only in 5% of localized or stage 4S tumors. Deletion of the 1p36 region occurs in 70% and is usually associated with *MYCN*-amplified, high-risk neuroblastomas that confer a poor prognosis. Deletions of chromosome 11q are noted in 15% to 22% of cases and indicate an unfavorable outcome. Conversely, a whole chromosome 17 gain is associated with a good prognosis.

Elevated urine catecholamines and their metabolites (dopamine, vanillylmandelic acid, homovanillic acid) are pathognomonic for neuroblastoma in infants and toddlers. Elevated lactate dehydrogenase (>1500 U/mL), ferritin (>142 ng/mL), and neuron-specific enolase (>100 ng/mL) can be indicative of neuroblastoma but are nonspecific. Cross-sectional imaging shows characteristic calcifications within the tumor (Fig. 117.21). An MRI is helpful to detect spinal cord extension.[131]I-metaiodobenzylguanidine (MIBG) scan is particularly valuable in the detection

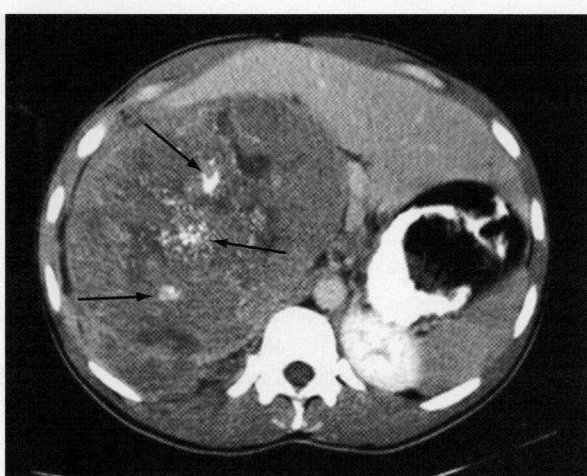

FIGURE 117.21 CT scan of neuroblastoma demonstrating areas of calcification *(arrows)*. (From Kim S, Chung DH. Pediatric solid malignancies: Neuroblastoma and Wilms' tumor. *Surg Clin North Am.* 2006; 86:469-487.)

of metastases because the norepinephrine analogue is selectively concentrated in sympathetic tissue. The[131] I-MIBG scan is also used for the surveillance of treatment response and recurrence. Poorly differentiated small round blue cells are classic histopathologic features. Although localized tumors can be resected up front, many present as advanced-stage tumors with extensive disease involving vital structures. They should undergo an initial biopsy for analysis of tumor biology. After induction chemotherapy, complete resection or debulking achieving >90% resection offers the best overall disease-free and survival chances.[36] DNA ploidy, *MYCN* amplification, and other chromosomal abnormalities are analyzed routinely. Neuroblastoma can be classified on the basis of neuroblastic differentiation and mitosis-karyorrhexis index (low, intermediate, or high), and the presence of Schwann cells. Children's Oncology Group currently stratifies patients into low-, intermediate-, or high-risk categories on the basis of the patient's age at diagnosis, International Neuroblastoma Staging System (INSS) stage, tumor histopathology, DNA index, and *MYCN* amplification status.[37]

Image-defined risk factor (Table 117.1) after neoadjuvant therapy is useful in predicting the completeness of neuroblastoma resection.[38] The multimodality treatment strategy is based on disease risk group stratification (Table 117.2). Induction chemotherapy consists of a multidrug regimen, including but not limited to cyclophosphamide, doxorubicin, cisplatin, carboplatin, etoposide, and vincristine. However, high-risk group neuroblastomas frequently acquire resistance to chemotherapeutics and thus have high disease relapse. This usually necessitates autologous hematopoietic stem cell transplantation. Complete surgical resection correlates with a lower local recurrence, especially in combination with induction chemotherapy, local radiation, and immunotherapy.

Primary surgical resection is recommended for stage 1 to 2B tumors. For more advanced stage 3 and 4 tumors, only the incisional biopsy specimen is obtained initially for tumor biology studies. The role of aggressive surgical resection of the primary tumor site for metastatic stage 4 neuroblastoma in patients 18 months or older remains the standard therapy in the United States.[36] For infants with stage 4S disease, surgical resection is not recommended because of the high rate of spontaneous differentiation and regression. For high-risk patients, radiation therapy is often needed for local and metastatic control. Radiation is contraindicated for intraspinal tumors because it can lead to vertebral damage, growth arrest, and scoliosis. However, it may be necessary

TABLE 117.1 Image-Defined Risk Factor in Neuroblastoma

TUMOR LOCATION	CRITERIA
Tumor involving two body compartments	Neck-chest, chest-abdomen, abdomen-pelvis
Neck	Tumor encasing carotid and/or vertebral artery and/or internal jugular vein
	Tumor extending to base of skull
	Tumor compressing the trachea
Cervicothoracic	Tumor encasing brachial plexus roots
	Tumor encasing subclavian vessels and/or vertebral and/or carotid artery
	Tumor compressing the trachea
Thorax	Tumor encasing the aorta and/or major branches
	Tumor compressing the trachea and/or principal bronchi
	Lower mediastinal tumor, infiltrating the costovertebral junction between T9 and T12
Thoracoabdomen	Tumor encasing the aorta and/or vena cava
Abdomen/pelvis	Tumor infiltrating the porta hepatis and/or the hepatoduodenal ligament
	Tumor encasing branches of the superior mesenteric artery at the mesenteric root
	Tumor encasing the origin of the coeliac axis, and/or of the superior mesenteric artery
	Tumor invading one or both renal pedicles
	Tumor encasing the aorta and/or vena cava
	Tumor encasing the iliac vessels
	Pelvic tumor crossing the sciatic notch
Intraspinal	More than one-third of the spinal canal in the axial plane is invaded and/or the perimedullary leptomeningeal spaces are not visible and/or the spinal cord signal is abnormal
Infiltration of adjacent structure	Pericardium, diaphragm, kidney, liver, duodenopancreatic block, and mesentery
Conditions recorded but not IDRFs	Multifocal primary tumors
	Pleural effusion, with or without malignant cells
	Ascites, with or without malignant cells

IDRFs, Image-defined risk factors.

TABLE 117.2 International Neuroblastoma Risk Group Pretreatment Classification

INRG STAGE	AGE (MO)	HISTOLOGIC CATEGORY	GRADE	MYCN	11Q	PLOIDY	RISK GROUP	5-YEAR EFS
L1/L2		GN, GNB intermixed					Very low	>85%
L1		Any, except GN/GNB		NA			Very low	>85%
				Amp			High	<50%
L2	<18	Any, except GN/GNB		NA	No		Low	>75% to ≤85%
					Yes		Intermediate	≥50% to ≤75%
	≥18	GNB nodular, neuroblastoma	Differentiating	NA	No		Low	>75% to ≤85%
			Poorly differentiated or undifferentiated	NA	Yes		Intermediate	≥50% to ≤75%
				Amp			High	<50%
M	<18			NA		Hyperdiploid	Low	>75% to ≤85%
	<12			NA		Diploid	Intermediate	≥50% to ≤75%
	12–<18			NA		Diploid	Intermediate	≥50% to ≤75%
	<18			Amp			High	<50%
	≥18						High	<50%
MS	<18			NA	No		Very Low	>85%
				Amp	Yes		High	<50%
							High	<50%

L1, Localized tumor not involving vital structures as defined by the list of image-defined risk factors and confined to one body compartment; *L2,* locoregional tumor with presence of one of more image-defined risk factors; *M,* distant metastatic disease (except stage MS); *MS,* metastatic disease in children younger than 18 months with metastasis confined to skin, liver and/or bone marrow.
Amp, Amplified; *EFS,* event-free survival; *GN,* ganglioneuroma; *GNB,* ganglioneuroblastoma; *INRG,* International Neuroblastoma Risk Group; *NA,* nonamplified.
From Newman EA, Abdessalam S, Aldrink JH, et al. Update on neuroblastoma. *J Pediatr Surg.* 2019;54:383-389; adapted from Cohn SL, Pearson AD, London WB, et al. The International Neuroblastoma Risk Group (INRG) classification system: An INRG Task Force report. *J Clin Oncol.* 2009; 27:289-297.

for palliation in the setting of pain, hepatomegaly with respiratory compromise, or acute neurologic symptoms caused by tumor compression of the cord. It is further indicated when there is minimal residual disease after induction chemotherapy and resection. The overall outcomes in patients with neuroblastoma have improved steadily during the past decades, with 5-year survival rates rising from 52% to 74%. The low-risk group has shown significant improvement in survival rates of up to 92%. It is estimated that 50% to 60% of the high-risk group relapse after standard therapy. Anti-GD2 immunotherapy has become a standard therapy for children with high-risk disease.[37]

Wilms Tumor

Wilms tumor (WT), also known as nephroblastoma, is an embryonal renal neoplasm consisting of metanephric blastema; it accounts for 85% of cases. WT represents 5.9% of all pediatric malignant tumors and ~75% are diagnosed in children <5 years of age. Bilateral tumors are noted at diagnosis in 13%. A number of syndromes can predispose to the development of WT such as Beckwith-Wiedemann (macroglossia, macrosomia, midline abdominal wall defects, and neonatal hypoglycemia), Li-Fraumeni (*p53* germline mutation with predisposition to various cancers), and Denys-Drash (gonadal dysgenesis, nephropathy, and WT) syndromes and neurofibromatosis. In 10% of patients, WT can be associated with other congenital anomalies, collectively known as WAGR syndrome (aniridia, hemihypertrophy, genitourinary malformations, and mental retardation).

The WT suppressor gene, *WT1,* is located on chromosome 11p13, which contains genes responsible for the development of the kidney, genitourinary tract, and eyes. Mutations in *WT1* result in genitourinary abnormalities, such as cryptorchidism and hypospadias, but also increase the risk for development of WT. Aniridia is found in 1.1% of WT patients, and when *WT1*

deletions are found in these patients, there is a 40% rate of WT development. Moreover, mutations in *WT2,* located at 11p15, have been linked to Beckwith-Wiedemann syndrome, and there is a 4% to 10% risk for development of WT in those who also have hemihypertrophy. WT is typically discovered incidentally during a physical examination or parents having felt an abdominal mass. Other presenting symptoms include vague abdominal discomfort and hematuria, which may signify tumor invasion into the collecting system or ureter. Hypertension is present in 25% of patients and is thought to occur secondary to disturbances in the renin-angiotensin feedback loop. Less than 10% of patients have atypical symptoms such as varicocele, hepatomegaly caused by hepatic vein obstruction, ascites, and congestive heart failure.

Tumor thrombus into the renal vein or IVC is detected by ultrasound study. A CT scan is valuable in determining WT from other tumors and also to evaluate for regional adenopathy, contralateral kidney involvement, and distant organ metastasis. Lung metastases are present in 8% at the time of diagnosis. The histology of WT is categorized as favorable or unfavorable. Favorable histology is characterized by the presence of three elements: blastemal, stromal, and epithelial cells. WT with predominantly epithelial differentiation behaves less aggressively and tends to be stage I when it is diagnosed early. Blastemal-predominant tumors tend to be clinically aggressive and are associated with advanced disease. Outcomes correlate with histopathologic features and tumor stage. Unfavorable histology is characterized by anaplasia, clear cell sarcoma, or rhabdoid tumor. Anaplastic WT can be focal or diffuse and carries an increased risk of tumor recurrence and chemoresistance. Nephrogenic rests are precursor lesions found in 25% to 40% of kidneys with WT but do not have oncologic potential. Instead, they can undergo differentiation and spontaneously regress through unclear mechanisms.

TABLE 117.3	National Wilms Tumor Study Group Staging System
STAGE	DEFINITION
I	Tumor limited to the kidney and completely excised without rupture or biopsy. Surface of the renal capsule is intact
II	Tumor extends through the renal capsule but is completely removed, with no microscopic involvement of the margins. Vessels outside the kidney contain tumor. Also placed in stage II are cases in which the kidney has undergone biopsy before removal or where there is local spillage of tumor (during resection) limited to the tumor bed
III	Residual tumor is confined to the abdomen and of nonhematogenous spread. Includes tumors with involvement of the abdominal lymph nodes, diffuse peritoneal contamination by rupture of the tumor extending beyond the tumor bed, peritoneal implants, and microscopic or grossly positive resection margins
IV	Hematogenous metastases at any site
V	Bilateral renal involvement

The International Society of Pediatric Oncology (SIOP) staging system is based on preoperative chemotherapy but is applied after resection. The presence of metastases is evaluated at presentation, relying on images, and chemotherapy is administered before operative intervention. The National Wilms Tumor Study Group (NWTSG) has also developed a staging system that incorporates the clinical, surgical, and pathologic information obtained at the time of resection but stratifies patients before the initiation of chemotherapy (Table 117.3). The advantage of this system is that it favors stage-based therapy, thereby avoiding unnecessary chemotherapy in patients who might not otherwise benefit from it.

The mainstay of therapy for WT is surgery and chemotherapy. Surgical exploration is necessary for formal staging, and a radical nephrectomy with lymph node sampling is the standard operation. Utmost care must be taken to ensure en bloc resection with tumor-free margins because contamination and tumor spillage "upstages" the patient and would require postoperative radiation and additional chemotherapy. Vascular tumor extension into the IVC constitutes stage III disease and is managed accordingly (Fig. 117.22). Sampling of the hilar, paraaortic, and paracaval lymph nodes is essential. Nephron-sparing surgery is usually reserved for children with a solitary kidney or bilateral WT. In these patients, preoperative chemotherapy may be used to induce tumor shrinkage to allow a more complete resection. Partial nephrectomy may be considered if the tumor involves only one pole of the kidney, there is no evidence of collecting system or vascular involvement, clear margins exist between the tumor and surrounding structures, and the involved kidney demonstrates appreciable function. In Stage V WT biopsy confirmation at diagnosis is not necessary. According to the NWTSG guidelines (Box 117.2), the standard chemotherapy regimen consists of vincristine and dactinomycin, with the addition of doxorubicin or radiation therapy based on tumor stage and histologic favorability. The SIOP advocates the use of preoperative chemotherapy to improve cure and disease-free survival rates at 5 years. Stages I or II favorable histology or stage I unfavorable histology has a nearly 95% survival rate. For WT with unfavorable histology, stages II, III, and IV are associated with 70%, 56%, and 17% 4-year survival rates, respectively.

Rhabdomyosarcoma

Derived from embryonic mesenchymal cells that can later differentiate into skeletal muscle, rhabdomyosarcoma is a soft tissue malignant neoplasm that accounts for 4% of all pediatric cancer. There is a bimodal peak age at diagnosis, between the ages of 2 and 5 years and 15 and 19 years. Rhabdomyosarcoma is known to occur with increased frequency in patients with neurofibromatosis type I and Li-Fraumeni and Beckwith-Wiedemann syndromes. Rhabdomyosarcoma is classified into three types: embryonal, alveolar, and pleomorphic. Embryonal rhabdomyosarcoma, which

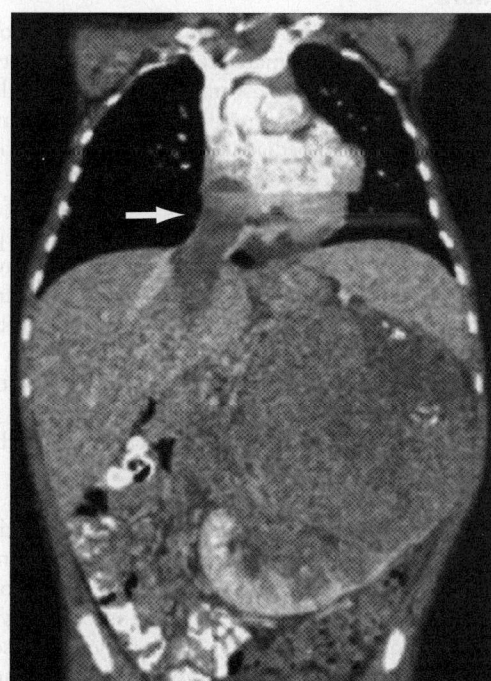

FIGURE 117.22 CT image of Wilms tumor with a claw sign and a large inferior vena cava tumor thrombus extending to right atrium *(arrow)*.

BOX 117.2 Treatment Regimens for Wilms Tumor[a]

- Stage I (FH, focal anaplasia): Surgery, VA × 18 wk, no XRT
- Stage II (FH): Surgery, VA × 18 wk, no XRT
- Stage II (focal anaplasia): Surgery, VDA × 24 wk, XRT to tumor bed
- Stage III (FH, focal anaplasia): Surgery, VDA × 24 wk, XRT to tumor bed
- Stage III (focal anaplasia): Surgery, VDA × 24 wk, XRT to tumor bed
- Stage IV (FH; focal anaplasia): Surgery, VDA × 24 wk, XRT to tumor bed according to local tumor stage and lung or other metastatic sites
- Stages II–IV (diffuse anaplasia): Surgery, VDEC × 24 wk, XRT to whole lung and abdomen
- Stages I–IV (clear cell sarcoma): Surgery, VDEC × 24 wk, XRT to abdomen; XRT to whole lung for stage IV only
- Stages I–IV (rhabdoid tumor): Surgery, ECCa × 24 wk, XRT

[a]National Wilms Tumor Study. Infants younger than 11 months are given half the recommended dose of all drugs.
A, Dactinomycin; *C,* cyclophosphamide; *Ca,* carboplatin; *D,* doxorubicin; *E,* etoposide; *FH,* favorable histology; *V,* vincristine; *XRT,* radiation therapy.

includes botryoid and spindle cell subtypes, is the most common type, accounting for more than two-thirds of all rhabdomyosarcomas. Muscle-specific proteins, myosin, actin, desmin, and myoglobin, are stained for immunohistochemical diagnosis.

The common sites for rhabdomyosarcomas are in the head and neck (35%), genitourinary tract (25%), and extremities (20%). Head and neck tumors tend to occur in the parameningeal region, orbits, and pharynx. Other specific sites include the bladder, prostate, vagina, uterus, liver, biliary tract, paraspinal region, and chest wall. These tumors are generally asymptomatic, although most symptoms are related to extrinsic tumor effects. Orbital tumors can produce proptosis, decreased visual acuity, and ophthalmoplegia. Those arising from parameningeal sites frequently produce headaches and nasal or sinus obstruction that can be accompanied by a mucopurulent or bloody discharge. For genitourinary rhabdomyosarcoma, paratesticular tumors may present as painless swelling in the scrotum, which may be confused for a hernia, hydrocele, or varicocele. Bladder tumors, commonly located at the base and trigone, result in hematuria and urinary obstruction. Vaginal tumors in females present with a protruding mass or vaginal bleeding and discharge. In the extremities, rhabdomyosarcomas involve the distal limb more commonly, and the lower extremities are affected more often. At diagnosis, 50% of patients have regional lymph node metastasis. Retroperitoneal tumors can be quite large at diagnosis with symptoms arising secondary to invasion of adjacent structures.

There are no specific serum tumor markers for rhabdomyosarcoma. MRI or CT demonstrates the mass and its involvement of adjacent structures, vessel encasement, metastasis, and adenopathy. An incisional or core-needle biopsy is crucial to achieve a diagnosis. A complete surgical resection is ideal, but a large tumor may necessitate preoperative chemotherapy for tumor shrinkage. As RMS is chemosensitive, and radiosensitive, aggressive up-front resections are not necessary. Biopsy followed by chemotherapy is the primary preferred approach. Botryoid (cluster of grapes) and spindle cell rhabdomyosarcomas have favorable prognosis, whereas pleomorphic histology confers an intermediate prognosis, and alveolar type exhibits a poor prognosis. Pretreatment staging, based on tumor-node-metastasis (TNM) criteria, serves to stratify patients into the appropriate treatment regimen, and to compare outcomes (Box 117.3). Intraoperative or pathologic results from resected samples are used for clinical grouping, which consists of selection into a group depending on operative findings, pathology, margins, and node status. Estimated 3-year failure-free survival rates are 88%, 55% to 76%, and <30% for low-risk, intermediate-risk, and high-risk patients, respectively.

BOX 117.3 Staging for Rhabdomyosarcoma

Group I: Localized disease that is completely resected, with no regional node involvement

Group II

A. Localized, grossly resected tumor with microscopic residual disease but no regional nodal involvement

B. Locoregional disease with tumor-involved lymph nodes with complete resection and no residual disease

C. Locoregional disease with involved nodes, grossly resected, but with evidence of microscopic residual tumor at the primary site and/or histologic involvement of the most distal regional node (from the primary site)

Group III: Localized, gross residual disease including incomplete resection or biopsy only of the primary site

Group IV: Distant metastatic disease present at time of diagnosis

---

The main goal of multimodality therapy is to achieve cure or to obtain local control. The recommended chemotherapy regimen depends on the risk stratification, with low-risk patients in subgroup A receiving vincristine and dactinomycin. Cyclophosphamide is added to this therapy for patients in the low-risk subgroup B and higher. Radiation therapy has been found to be effective for the local control of rhabdomyosarcoma, especially in patients who have microscopic disease after resection as well as in patients with unresectable tumors. For extremity lesions, it is imperative to achieve complete wide local excision. Amputation is rarely necessary, except for distal tumors in the hand or foot that involve neurovascular structures. Given that trunk and extremity lesions have a high incidence of lymph node metastasis, sentinel lymph node mapping is being increasingly used. Reexcision may also be considered with evidence of minimal residual disease after initial resection. Patients with extremity tumors receive combination chemotherapy, but because of the high incidence of the alveolar histology, radiation therapy is also often used. For genitourinary tumors, preservation of bladder function is the key in resection of tumors involving the bladder or prostate. If this goal cannot be met, preoperative chemoradiation is usually recommended. Paratesticular rhabdomyosarcoma should undergo a radical inguinal orchiectomy, with a retroperitoneal lymph node dissection in males younger than 10 years because of the high prevalence of metastasis. When the tumor is clearly fixed to scrotal skin, resection is required. Chemotherapy is standard, whereas radiation therapy is indicated only with positive nodes. For patients with vaginal or vulvar rhabdomyosarcoma, vaginectomy and wide local excision, respectively, and multiagent chemotherapy are recommended. Approximately 15% of children present with metastatic disease, and their prognosis remains poor. Nearly 30% will experience disease relapse, and the estimated 5-year survival rate is only 17%. Despite these harrowing data, however, rhabdomyosarcoma is a curable disease in most children, with more than 60% surviving 5 years after diagnosis.

Liver Tumors

Primary tumors of the liver are rare in the pediatric population but are malignant in approximately 60% of cases. The two most common tumors are hepatoblastoma and hepatocellular carcinoma (HCC). Hepatoblastoma represents 80% of all malignant liver tumors and 1% of all pediatric cancer. The peak incidence of hepatoblastoma is at 3 years of age; the median age for children with HCC is 10 to 11.2 years. More than 90% of patients younger than 5 years with primary liver tumors have hepatoblastoma, whereas 87% of those between 15 and 19 years have HCC. Patients with familial adenomatous polyposis, Gardner, and Beckwith-Wiedemann syndromes are at increased risk for the development of hepatoblastoma. HCC is associated with acquired hepatitis B and C and has been observed in children with several types of congenital diseases, including tyrosinemia, glycogen storage disease type I, α_1-antitrypsin deficiency, and cholestasis caused by BA.

Hepatoblastoma typically manifests as a painless, palpable abdominal mass. Other symptoms are nonspecific and include anorexia, weight loss and failure to thrive, abdominal pain, anemia, and abdominal distention. Jaundice is not commonly encountered because liver function remains relatively normal except in a very advanced tumor. Some patients present with tumor rupture, resulting in intraabdominal bleeding and peritonitis. HCC is manifested similarly, although stigmata of cirrhosis, such as jaundice, spider angiomas, ascites, and splenomegaly, may be encountered. Almost 25% of patients have metastatic spread to abdominal and mediastinal lymph nodes, lung, bone marrow, and brain. Anemia, thrombocytopenia, or pancytopenia can be found with splenomegaly caused by sequestration. AFP levels are elevated in more than 70% of hepatoblastoma patients. However, an elevated AFP level is not pathognomonic, and depending on the age of the patient, other disease processes must be ruled out. For example, in infants younger than 6 months, elevated AFP levels may also be seen in sarcomas, yolk sac tumors, and hamartomas. All children being evaluated for HCC should be tested for exposure to hepatitis B and C viruses.

Abdominal ultrasonography is obtained as an initial imaging study. Doppler ultrasound can also detect the presence of tumor extension into or thrombosis of major vessels, namely, the hepatic veins, IVC, and portal vein. A CT scan is essential in assessing the relationship of the tumor to adjacent vital structures, such as bile ducts and vessels, and excluding intraabdominal tumor extension beyond the liver. MRI can similarly be used in this setting but does not necessarily provide significant advantages over CT. Because hepatoblastoma frequently spreads hematologically to the lungs, chest CT should also be performed. Bone scintigraphy is recommended for staging in children with HCC because of the high incidence of bone metastases. Hepatoblastoma characteristically appears as a unifocal mass surrounded by a pseudocapsule; it may be a pure epithelial type that contains fetal or embryonal cells or a mixture of the two histologic subtypes, which contains mesenchymal tissue in addition to epithelial components. On the other hand, HCC is characterized by large, pleomorphic epithelial cells that appear much like mature hepatocytes. In gross appearance, HCC forms multifocal nodules that lack a fibrous tumor and often lead to diffuse intrahepatic involvement. Unlike in adults, there has been no indisputable evidence that histopathologic type has any bearing on prognosis.

A standard TNM system has been used for staging purposes, but much effort has been put into the development of a pretreatment staging system, known as the PRE-Treatment EXTent of

disease (PRETEXT) definition system (Table 117.4). The PRETEXT system was developed by the International Childhood Liver Tumor Strategy Group (SIOPEL) for staging and risk stratification of liver tumors.[39] It divides the liver into four sections based on segmental anatomy of the liver, and the tumor is subsequently classified by the number of tumor-free sections of liver (Fig. 117.23). This system takes caudate lobe involvement, tumor rupture, ascites, extension into the stomach or diaphragm, tumor focality, lymph node involvement, presence of distant metastases, and vascular involvement into further consideration. PRETEXT staging defines for the surgeon, when upfront resection, prior to chemotherapy is possible (PRETEXT 1 or II) Patients are considered at high risk if they have a serum AFP level above 100 ng/mL, extension beyond the liver, distant metastases, intraperitoneal hemorrhage, and invasion of the hepatic veins, IVC, or portal vein. For PRETEXT I and II, hepatoblastoma may be resected by segmentectomy or anatomic lobectomy prior to chemotherapy.

Liver transplantation is a potential surgical option for patients with a massive unresectable tumor. Neoadjuvant chemotherapy is used for tumor shrinkage and potential complete resection. Interestingly, some advocate the use of preoperative chemotherapy to treat what would otherwise be residual microscopic disease left

TABLE 117.4 PRETEXT Definition for Hepatoblastoma

PRETEXT GROUP	DEFINITION
I	One section involved; three adjoining sections are tumor free
II	One or two sections involved; two adjoining sections are tumor free
III	Two or three sections involved; one adjoining section is tumor free
IV	Four sections involved

PRETEXT, PRE-Treatment EXTent of disease.

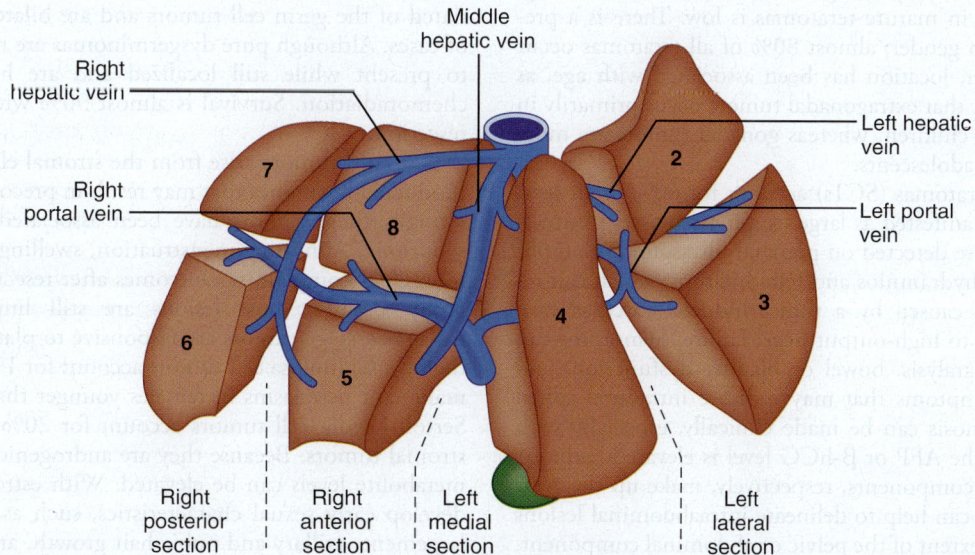

FIGURE 117.23 A diagram of the PRETEXT definition system for hepatoblastoma. The liver is divided into four sections based on segmental anatomy of the liver, and the tumor is subsequently classified by the number of tumor-free sections of liver. (From Roebuck DJ, Aronson D, Clapuyt P, et al. 2005 PRETEXT: A revised staging system for primary malignant liver tumors of childhood developed by the SIOPEL group. *Pediatr Radiol.* 2007;37:123-132.)

behind after resection. It could eradicate tumor cells that could respond to hepatotrophic factors during liver regeneration, thereby decreasing the risk of recurrence. There are two current approaches to hepatoblastoma: (1) tumor resection followed by chemotherapy and (2) tumor biopsy followed by chemotherapy and delayed resection. Patients with stage I tumors with pure fetal histology usually do not require postoperative chemotherapy. However, patients with stage II or higher tumors and tumors of any other type of histology do require chemotherapy consisting of cisplatin, 5-fluorouracil, and vincristine. For patients with residual tumor after resection, chemotherapy should be coupled with an evaluation for transplantation. Criteria for transplantation include having no more than three tumors smaller than 3 cm in diameter and no evidence of extrahepatic disease or vascular invasion. With relapses, doxorubicin, irinotecan, and ifosfamide are used with moderate success. Another modality being used with variable success in children whose tumors are unresponsive to systemic chemotherapy is direct arterial chemotherapy or chemoembolization. Long-term outcomes have yet to be determined. Long-term disease-free survival of more than 85% to 90% can be achieved for resectable hepatoblastoma, although similar estimates have been noted for patients with unresectable hepatoblastoma treated by liver transplantation. The same cannot be said for HCC, in which survival rates with partial hepatectomy remain poor because of relapse. In the past decade, early transplantation has been shown to result in better outcomes in some centers and should be considered when tumors are unresectable despite chemotherapy.

Teratoma

Teratomas are typically benign neoplasms that contain elements derived from more than one of the three embryonic germ layers (endoderm, mesoderm, and ectoderm). They are composed of tissue that is foreign to the anatomic site in which they are found. Although teratomas may occur anywhere along the midline, they are usually found in sacrococcygeal, mediastinal, retroperitoneal, and gonadal locations. Teratomas may be solid, cystic, or mixed and are classified as mature or immature. Although immature teratomas can be potentially malignant, the incidence of malignant transformation in mature teratomas is low. There is a preponderance based on gender; almost 80% of all teratomas occur in females. Moreover, location has been associated with age, as evidenced by the fact that extragonadal tumors occur primarily in neonates and young children, whereas gonadal tumors are more commonly noted in adolescents.

Sacrococcygeal teratomas (SCTs) account for 60% of all teratomas and can be manifested as large exophytic masses in utero. In such cases, they are detected on prenatal ultrasound. Complications include polyhydramnios and fetal hydrops, which can result in fetal demise caused by a tumor-induced vascular steal syndrome that leads to high-output heart failure. Symptoms can include weakness, paralysis, bowel or bladder dysfunction, and other neurologic symptoms that may indicate intradural spinal extension. The diagnosis can be made clinically, especially with exophytic SCTs. If the AFP or β-hCG level is elevated, yolk sac or choriocarcinoma components, respectively, make up the teratoma. CT and MRI can help to delineate intraabdominal lesions or to determine the extent of the pelvic or abdominal component.

Surgical resection is the standard of care and should be performed promptly because of the risk of hemorrhage and tumor rupture. Operative planning must consider the degree of intraabdominal extension (Fig. 117.24). Most tumors can be resected by a posterior approach, in which a chevron incision allows the division of the gluteal muscles, ligation of the blood supply, and en bloc resection of the tumor and coccyx. It is important to preserve the anorectal complex to maintain long-term continence. External tumors with significant intraabdominal extension require a combined abdominal and posterior approach, whereas teratomas that are entirely intraabdominal may be approached through laparotomy or laparoscopy. Outcomes are favorable with respect to survival and quality of life. The age at diagnosis is the most important factor; those diagnosed at less than 30 weeks of gestation or after 2 months postnatally have a poor prognosis. The risk of malignant transformation associated with embryonal histology is 15% to 20%. Risk of local recurrence ranges from 4% to 11%, although failure to resect the coccyx is associated with a 37% risk of recurrence. AFP levels should be monitored at 3-month intervals for 3 to 4 years. For recurrence, reexcision should be considered.

Ovarian Tumor

Approximately 50% of all ovarian lesions in children are neoplastic but are rarely malignant. It is estimated that ovarian malignant neoplasms represent 10% of all ovarian masses but only 1% of childhood cancers. Primary ovarian malignant neoplasms can be classified as germ cell, epithelial cell, and sex cord stromal tumors. Germ cell tumors include teratomas and choriocarcinoma; sex cord stromal tumors consist of granulosa (thecal) and Sertoli (Leydig) cells. Epithelial cell tumors encompass serous and mucinous cystadenomas and cystadenocarcinomas.[40] Symptoms are usually pain related to mass effect. The presence of ascites, omental masses, peritoneal or diaphragmatic implants, adherence to surrounding organs, aortoiliac adenopathy, size larger than 8 cm, or contralateral ovarian mass should raise suspicion for malignancy.

Teratoma is the most common ovarian germ cell tumor. It also represents the most common pediatric ovarian neoplasm and accounts for 25% of all childhood teratomas. These tumors occur with equal frequency in either ovary or may even be bilateral in 10% of patients. They typically are manifested with abdominal or pelvic pain and may involve ovarian torsion in approximately 25% of patients. Germ cell tumors account for 7% to 80% of all neoplastic ovarian masses. Dysgerminomas are the least differentiated of the germ cell tumors and are bilateral in 10% to 15% of cases. Although pure dysgerminomas are malignant, they tend to present while still localized and are highly responsive to chemoradiation. Survival is almost 90% with complete surgical resection.

Sex cord tumors arise from the stromal elements of the ovary, producing hormones that may result in precocious puberty. Interestingly, these tumors have been associated with Peutz-Jeghers syndrome. Abnormal menstruation, swelling, and pain are common chief complaints. Outcomes after resection are good in this group because most lesions are still limited to the ovary. Advanced-stage tumors are responsive to platinum-based chemotherapy. Granulosa cell tumors account for 1% to 10% of ovarian malignant neoplasms in females younger than 20 years, whereas Sertoli-Leydig cell tumors account for 20% of ovarian sex cord stromal tumors. Because they are androgenic, serum testosterone metabolite levels can be elevated. With estrogen excess, patients develop early sexual characteristics, such as breast or labial enlargement, axillary and pubic hair growth, and galactorrhea.

Epithelial tumors occur in less than 20% of all ovarian tumors in the pediatric patient population. The two main histologic subtypes are serous and mucinous tumors, which can be further described as benign, malignant, or borderline malignant. It is possible to classify the subtypes as adenoma or

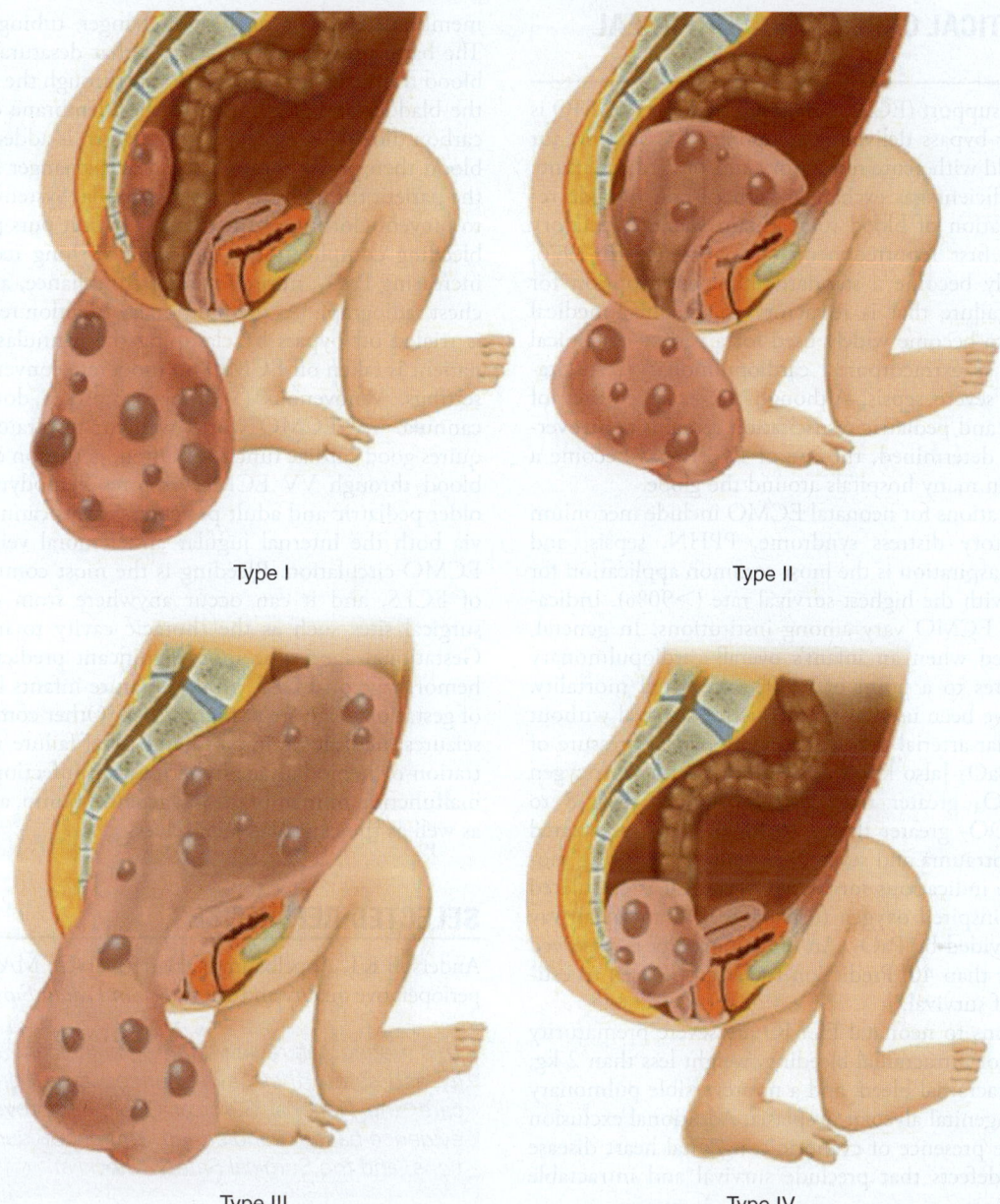

Type I

Type II

Type III

Type IV

FIGURE 117.24 Sacrococcygeal teratoma Altman classification types I to IV. Type I is resected entirely from perineal approach. Types II and III require combination of perineal and abdominopelvic approach. Type IV is resected entirely via abdominal approach.

adenocarcinoma; adenocarcinoma is extremely rare with a poor prognosis. Tumor biomarkers, AFP and β-hCG, help provide information about tumor biology and can be used to measure treatment response. If there is any evidence of menstrual abnormalities or precocious puberty, luteinizing hormone and follicle-stimulating hormone levels should also be checked. Ultrasound examination can evaluate the tumor and contralateral ovary. A cross-sectional image study can provide information on tumor extension, regional adenopathy, and distant metastasis.

Surgery is the mainstay of therapy and aims to ensure complete resection, with preservation of reproductive function when possible. An ovarian-sparing approach is recommended when a simple cystic mass or benign teratoma is suspected. Definitive treatment for malignancy is oophorectomy or salpingo-oophorectomy. Care should be taken to resect the tumor without disrupting the capsule or spilling tumor contents to avoid upstaging of malignant lesions. Ascites, if present, should be tested for cytology evidence of tumor. At operation, liver, diaphragm and peritoneal surfaces, and omentum are examined for ovarian implants, which, when present, should be biopsied for staging and treatment purposes. Bilateral retroperitoneal, iliac, paraaortic, and perirenal lymph nodes should be sampled for appropriate staging. Ascites or peritoneal washings should be sent for cytology. Chemotherapy is indicated for any ovarian tumor with extension beyond the affected ovary, which is often the case with germ cell and epithelial cell tumors. A combination of low-dose bleomycin, etoposide, and cisplatin treatment in patients with stage II disease has resulted in event-free and overall survival rates of 87.5% and 93.8%, respectively.

PEDIATRIC CRITICAL CARE: EXTRACORPOREAL LIFE SUPPORT

Extracorporeal life support (ECLS), often referred to as ECMO is a cardiopulmonary bypass delivering temporary life support for the critically ill child with acute respiratory and/or cardiac failure. ECLS achieves sufficient gas exchange, with carbon dioxide removal and oxygenation of blood to maintain stable circulatory support. Since its first reported neonatal experience in 1976, ECLS has not only become a standard therapeutic option for cardiopulmonary failure that is refractory to maximal medical therapy but has also become widely used for a variety of clinical applications, such as extracorporeal cardiopulmonary resuscitation (ECPR) and severe sepsis. Although the exact efficacy of ECPR in neonatal and pediatric resuscitation remains controversial and yet to be determined, the use of ECPR has become a common practice in many hospitals around the globe.

The major indications for neonatal ECMO include meconium aspiration, respiratory distress syndrome, PPHN, sepsis, and CDH. Meconium aspiration is the most common application for neonatal ECMO with the highest survival rate (>90%). Indications for neonatal ECMO vary among institutions. In general, ECMO is indicated when an infant's overall cardiopulmonary function deteriorates to a point of ~80% predicted mortality. Two guidelines have been used as predictors for survival without ECMO: the alveolar-arterial difference in the partial pressure of oxygen ($PAO_2 - PaO_2$ [also known as $AaDO_2$]) and the oxygen index (OI). $AaDO_2$ greater than 610 for longer than 8 to 12 hours and $AaDO_2$ greater than 620 for 6 hours, associated with extensive barotrauma and severe hypotension requiring inotropic support, are indications for ECMO. The OI is calculated as the fraction of inspired oxygen (usually 1.0) $\times$ mean airway pressure $\times$ 100 divided by PaO_2. An 80% mortality is observed with an OI greater than 40. Prediction tools can be used to estimate probability of survival.[41]

Contraindications to neonatal ECMO are severe prematurity due to a high risk of intracranial bleeding, weight less than 2 kg, presence of an intracranial bleed, and a nonreversible pulmonary disease such as congenital alveolar dysplasia. Additional exclusion criteria include the presence of cyanotic congenital heart disease or major genetic defects that preclude survival and intractable coagulopathy.

Older children with severe respiratory failure refractory to medical management resulting from pneumonia, acute respiratory distress syndrome, asthma, burn inhalation injury, cardiac failure resulting from primary cardiac dysfunction or following cardiac surgery, or severe sepsis may improve with ECMO. For respiratory failure, ECMO allows for "lung rest" and decreases barotrauma from high ventilator settings and hemodynamic support as the underlying infection is treated.

The right internal jugular vein and common carotid artery are used for venoarterial (VA) cannulations because of vessel sizes in young children to accommodate cannulas and collateral circulation. The carotid artery is usually ligated when the canula is removed, as repair is prone to thrombosis. Carotid ligation is generally very well tolerated in babies. In older children, to avoid carotid ligation, the femoral artery is often used; however, distal flow to the leg can be occluded by large canula size, and a retrograde flow canula should be inserted that is connected to the circuit to keep the leg perfused.

The ECMO circuit is composed of a silicone rubber bladder that collapses when venous return is diminished, roller pump,

membrane oxygenator, heat exchanger, tubing, and connectors. The basic principle of ECMO is that desaturated mixed venous blood from the right atrium drains through the venous cannula to the bladder and is pumped to the membrane oxygenator, where carbon dioxide is removed, and oxygen is added. The oxygenated blood then passes through the heat exchanger and is returned to the patient through the arterial cannula. Systemic anticoagulation to prevent clotting of the ECMO circuit puts patients at risk for bleeding complications. Indicators of lung recovery include an increasing PaO_2, improved lung compliance, and clearing of the chest radiograph. As the pulmonary function recovers, the patient is trialed off bypass by clamping the cannulas. If tolerated, the patient is taken off ECMO on moderate conventional ventilatory settings. Venovenous (VV) bypass uses a double-lumen single cannula. VV ECMO works well for respiratory failure but requires good cardiac function. Often, perfusion of well-oxygenated blood through VV ECMO restores hemodynamic stability. In older pediatric and adult patients, venous cannulas can be placed via both the internal jugular and femoral veins to achieve VV ECMO circulation. Bleeding is the most common complication of ECLS, and it can occur anywhere from catheter sites and surgical sites such as the thoracic cavity to intracranial bleeds. Gestational age is the most significant predictor of intracranial hemorrhage on ECLS, and premature infants less than 34 weeks of gestational age are at highest risk. Other complications include seizures; neurologic impairment; renal failure requiring hemofiltration or hemodialysis; hypertension; infection; and mechanical malfunction of membrane oxygenator, pump, and heat exchanger as well as the cannulas themselves.

SELECTED REFERENCES

Anderson KT, Appelbaum R, Bartz-Kurycki MA, et al. Advances in perioperative quality and safety. *Semin Pediatr Surg.* 2018;27:92-101.

This monograph reviewed three significant advances in quality and safety that have changed the approach to surgical care: the National Surgical Quality Improvement Program, evidence-based bundled prevention of surgical site infections, and the Surgical Safety Checklist.

Baxter KJ, Gale BF, Travers CD, et al. Ramifications of the children's surgery verification program for patients and hospitals. *J Am Coll Surg.* 2018;226:917-924.e1.

This manuscript is an early examination of the effects of the American College of Surgeons Children's Surgery Verification program (instituted in 2015) by evaluating neonates undergoing high-risk operations.

Gates RL, Price M, Cameron DB, et al. Non-operative management of solid organ injuries in children: an American Pediatric Surgical Association Outcomes and Evidence Based Practice Committee systematic review. *J Pediatr Surg.* 2019;54: 1519-1526.

This article from the American Pediatric Surgical Association, APSA, Outcomes and Evidence-Based Practice Committee provides the updates on the practice guidelines for nonoperative management of liver and splenic injuries.

Harris CJ, Waters AM, Tracy ET, et al. Precision oncology: a primer for pediatric surgeons from the APSA Cancer Committee. *J Pediatr Surg*. 2020;55:1706-1713.

This American Pediatric Surgical Association Cancer Committee summary provides a comprehensive update on the current state of precision medicine in pediatric oncology.

Minneci PC, Hade EM, Lawrence AE, et al. Multi-institutional trial of non-operative management and surgery for uncomplicated appendicitis in children: design and rationale. *Contemp Clin Trials*. 2019;83:10-17.

This clinical trial is evaluating nonoperative management of uncomplicated appendicitis in pediatric patients employing a patient choice design.

The full reference list appears on Elsevier eBooks+.

119 CHAPTER

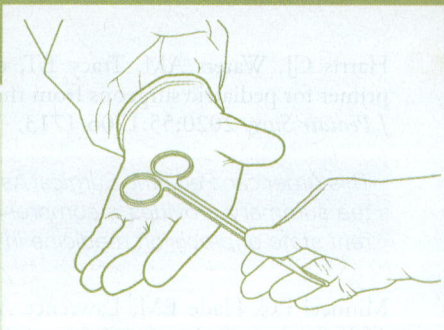

Hand Surgery

Daniel Donato, Andrew Sobel, Vinay Rao, and Andi Cummins

OUTLINE

Please access Elsevier eBooks+ to view the videos for this chapter.

BASIC ANATOMY

Anatomic Terms and Biomechanical Movements

The upper extremity has unique anatomic terms as well as descriptions of movements because of its mobility in relationship to the axial skeleton at the shoulder, the ability of the forearm to be pronated and supinated, and individual finger movements and thumb opposition. The upper extremity can be broken up into major regions, including the shoulder, arm, elbow, forearm, wrist, and hand. The majority of procedures performed by hand specialists are from the elbow to the fingertips, so this chapter will focus on regional anatomy distal to the elbow.[1]

Anatomic position of the arm and forearm is supinated with the palm facing forward, so the palm is anterior, and the back of the hand, or dorsum, is posterior. The more appropriate terminology is *volar* (or *palmar*) for the palm surface and *dorsal* for the posterior surface. The medial and lateral aspects are better termed *ulnar* and *radial,* respectively, with thumb radial and small finger ulnar. Within the extremities, those structures closer to the axial skeleton are termed *proximal,* whereas those toward the end of the extremity are *distal.* Motion in a palmar direction is *flexion,* whereas dorsal motion is termed *extension.* In the forearm, supination moves the forearms and hands into anatomic position so that the palms face forward and the radius and ulnar are parallel; pronation moves the palms and forearms to face posteriorly, and the radius and ulna overlap. Finger motion away from the long finger axis is termed *abduction,* whereas motion toward the axis of the long finger is termed *adduction.* The description of the motion of the thumb must take in to account another plane of movement—*opposition,* or bringing the tip of the thumb to face the other digits, such as occurs with pinching motions. Extension of the thumb is dorsally out of plane with the hand. Motion in the same plane as the hand is termed *abduction* (away from) or *adduction* (toward) the palm. The surface anatomy of the volar and dorsal hand is shown in Fig. 119.1.

Bony Anatomy

It is important to understand the basic bony anatomy of the forearm and hand, especially because certain bony landmarks will guide surface examination and procedures. The forearm contains two long bones, the radius laterally and the ulna medially. Between these two bones runs the interosseous membrane, which separates the volar flexor structures and the dorsal extensor structures. At the distal aspect of the forearm, the radius and ulna articulate at the distal radioulnar joint, which allows for stability and support of the pronation and supination at the wrist.

The bony wrist, or carpus, is made up of eight different carpal bones. The proximal row consists of the scaphoid, lunate, and triquetrum (from radial to ulnar). The distal carpal row includes the trapezium, trapezoid, capitate, and hamate. The pisiform is a sesamoid bone within the tendon of flexor carpi ulnaris (FCU). The multiple small carpal bones allow the wrist a unique and wide range-of-motion capabilities (Fig. 119.2).

The hand consists of five metacarpal bones. The first metacarpal is unique because it forms a saddle joint with the trapezium, which allows for the thumb range of motion both in plane and out of plane of the hand. Each digit is made up of small long bones called the *phalanges.* The thumb has two phalanges, proximal and distal, and the four fingers each have three phalanges, proximal, middle, and distal. There are many articulations, so the easiest terminology is to use abbreviations—the carpometacarpal joint is the CMCJ, the metacarpophalangeal joint is the MCPJ, and similarly for proximal interphalangeal joint (PIPJ) and distal interphalangeal joint (DIPJ) (see Fig. 119.2).

Muscles and Tendons of the Forearm and Hand

The muscles of the hand and forearm can be divided into *intrinsic,* those originating and inserting within the hand, and *extrinsic,* muscle bellies in the forearm and insertions in the hand. The extrinsic muscles comprise the long flexors and extensors of the wrist and digits. The extrinsic muscle bellies can be divided into three forearm compartments: the volar compartment, the dorsal compartment, and the mobile wad. The volar compartment can

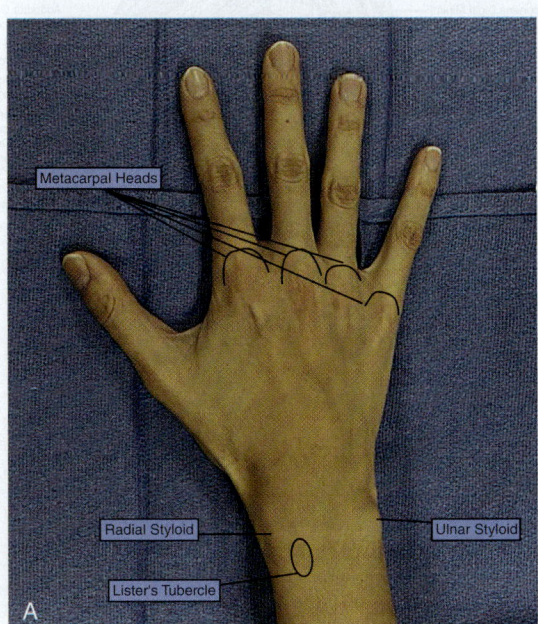
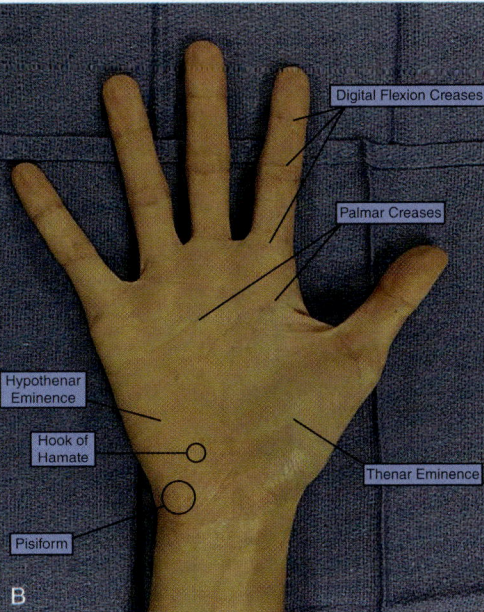

FIGURE 119.1 Surface anatomy of the dorsal (A) and volar (B) aspects of the hand, with important visual and palpable landmarks noted.

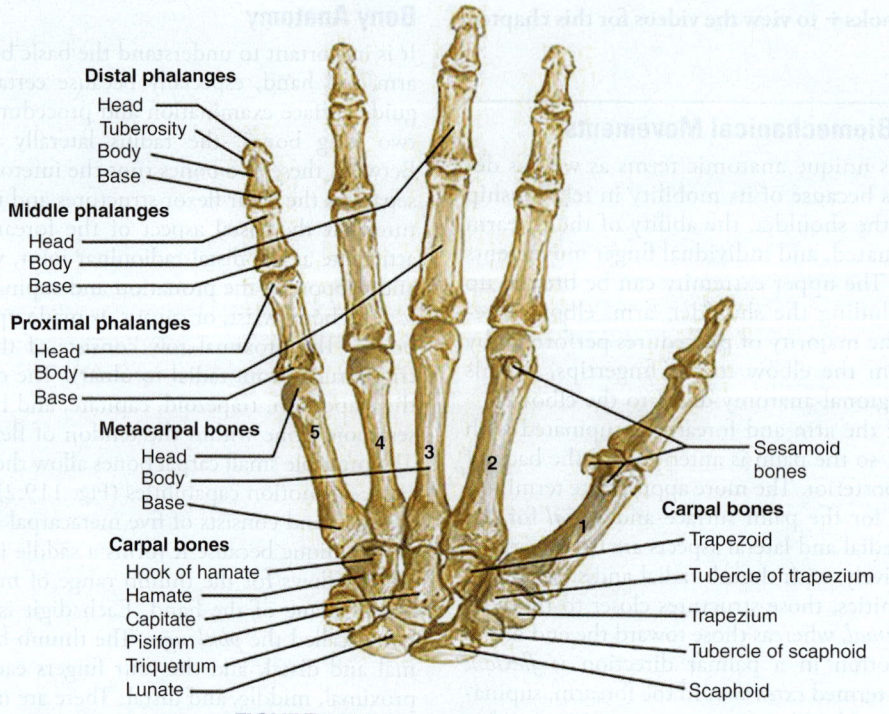

Distal phalanges
- Head
- Tuberosity
- Body
- Base

Middle phalanges
- Head
- Body
- Base

Proximal phalanges
- Head
- Body
- Base

Metacarpal bones
- Head
- Body
- Base

Carpal bones
- Hook of hamate
- Hamate
- Capitate
- Pisiform
- Triquetrum
- Lunate

Sesamoid bones

Carpal bones
- Trapezoid
- Tubercle of trapezium
- Trapezium
- Tubercle of scaphoid
- Scaphoid

FIGURE 119.2 Bony anatomy of the hand.

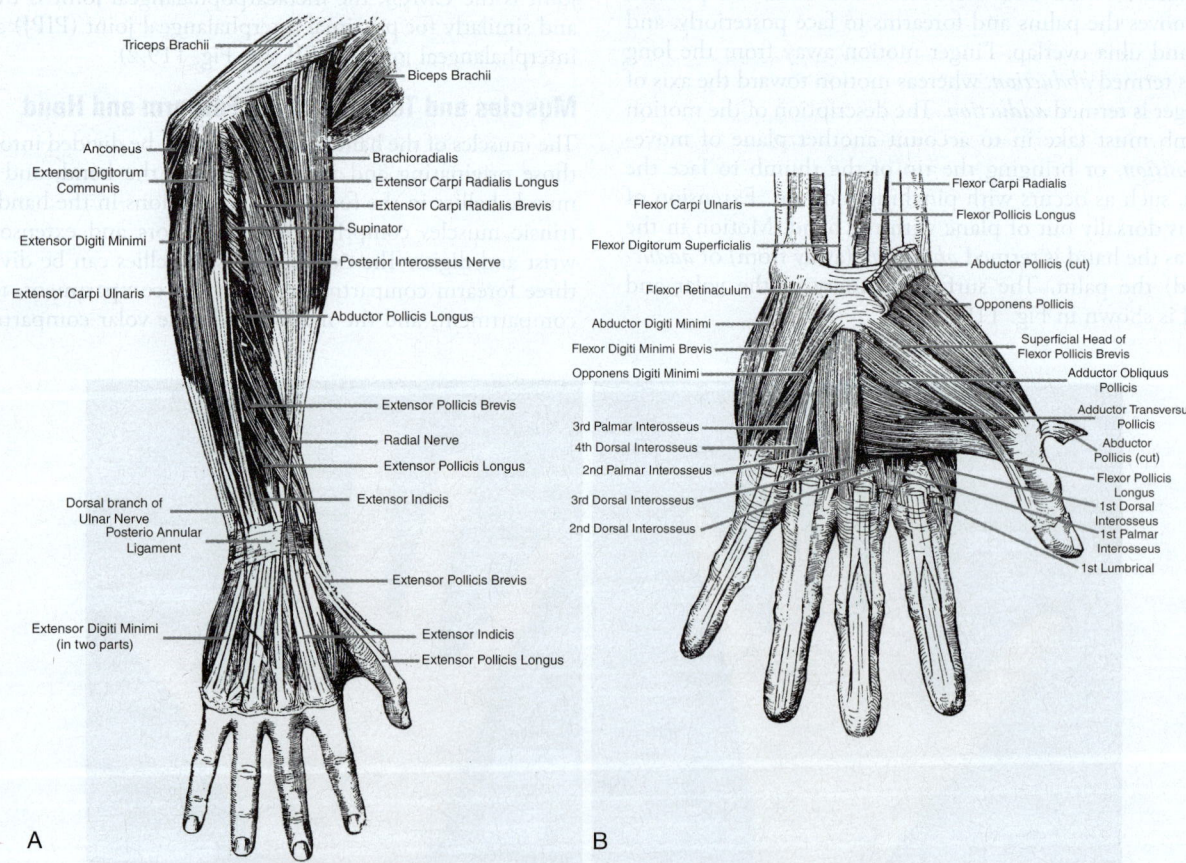

- Triceps Brachii
- Biceps Brachii
- Anconeus
- Brachioradialis
- Extensor Digitorum Communis
- Extensor Carpi Radialis Longus
- Extensor Carpi Radialis Brevis
- Extensor Digiti Minimi
- Supinator
- Posterior Interosseus Nerve
- Extensor Carpi Ulnaris
- Abductor Pollicis Longus
- Extensor Pollicis Brevis
- Radial Nerve
- Extensor Pollicis Longus
- Dorsal branch of Ulnar Nerve
- Extensor Indicis
- Posterio Annular Ligament
- Extensor Pollicis Brevis
- Extensor Digiti Minimi (in two parts)
- Extensor Indicis
- Extensor Pollicis Longus

A

- Flexor Carpi Ulnaris
- Flexor Digitorum Superficialis
- Flexor Retinaculum
- Abductor Digiti Minimi
- Flexor Digiti Minimi Brevis
- Opponens Digiti Minimi
- 3rd Palmar Interosseus
- 4th Dorsal Interosseus
- 2nd Palmar Interosseus
- 3rd Dorsal Interosseus
- 2nd Dorsal Interosseus
- Flexor Carpi Radialis
- Flexor Pollicis Longus
- Abductor Pollicis (cut)
- Opponens Pollicis
- Superficial Head of Flexor Pollicis Brevis
- Adductor Obliquus Pollicis
- Adductor Transversus Pollicis
- Abductor Pollicis (cut)
- Flexor Pollicis Longus
- 1st Dorsal Interosseus
- 1st Palmar Interosseus
- 1st Lumbrical

B

FIGURE 119.3 A graphical illustration of the muscles and tendons that give effect to prehensile movements of the human hand. These are shown in dorsal aspect (A) and palmar aspect (B). It can be seen that articulations of the hand form functional groups arranged in kinetic chains. These are subject to control via synergies constituted by the organized recruitment by the central nervous system of muscles extrinsic to the hand and muscles intrinsic to the hand that, when coordinated, permit the differentiated action of the phalanxes. (From Carson RG. Get a grip: individual variations in grip strength are a marker of brain health. *Neurobiol Aging.* 2018;71:189-222.)

be further subdivided into superficial, intermediate, and deep layers (Fig. 119.3). The superficial layer comprises the pronator teres, flexor carpi radialis (FCR), palmaris longus, and FCU. The palmaris longus muscle may be absent in as many as 10% to 15% of individuals. The intermediate layer consists of the flexor digitorum superficialis (FDS), which flexes the PIPJ, and the deep layer consists of the flexor pollicis longus (FPL), which flexes the thumb interphalangeal joint (IPJ); the flexor digitorum profundus (FDP), which flexes the DIPJ; and the pronator quadratus.

The finger flexors in the digit are surrounded by the flexor tendon sheath. There are five annular and three cruciate pulleys on each finger, numbered A1–A5 and C1–C3, respectively, starting from proximal to distal, with the A1 pulley at the MCPJ and odd-numbered pulleys at the PIPJ and DIPJ, respectively (Fig. 119.4).

The radial most subgroup is termed the *mobile wad* and comprises the brachioradialis, a weak elbow flexor that does not move the hand or wrist, extensor carpi radialis longus (ECRL), and extensor carpi radialis brevis (ECRB), which extend the wrist and deviate it radially. The dorsal compartment also can be subdivided into superficial and deep layers. The superficial layer is made up of the extensor digitorum communis (EDC), the extensor digiti minimi (EDM or EDQ, for *extensor digiti quintus*), and the extensor carpi ulnaris (ECU) (see Fig. 119.3C). The ECU deviates the wrist in an ulnar direction and extends the wrist; the EDM and EDC extend the digits via a complicated insertion mechanism known as the *extensor hood*. The third and deeper subgroup is composed of four muscles (see Fig. 119.3D): the abductor pollicis longus (APL), extensor pollicis brevis (EPB), and extensor pollicis longus (EPL) provide function to the thumb, and the extensor indicis proprius (EIP) acts as a redundant extender of the index finger, giving it the greatest ability to individually extend. Last of

the deep muscles is the supinator, which is located proximally in the forearm.

The extensor tendons pass through six compartments deep to the extensor retinaculum at the dorsum of the wrist (Fig. 119.5). The first compartment contains APL and EPB, forming the radial boundary of the anatomic snuffbox. The second compartment consists of the ECRL and ECRB, and the third compartment contains the EPL, forming the ulnar border of the anatomic snuffbox. The third compartment crosses over the second and partial fourth compartment. The EIP and EDC pass through the fourth compartment; the EDM passes through the fifth compartment, where they overlie the distal radioulnar joint; and the sixth compartment contains ECU.

At the level of *the metacarpophalangeal joints (MPJs)*, the long extrinsic extensor tendons broaden out to form the extensor hood (Fig. 119.6). The proximal part of the hood at the level of the MCPJ is called the *sagittal band*. It loops around the MPJ and blends into the volar plate, thus forming a lasso around the base of the proximal phalanx, through which it extends the MPJ. The insertions of the interossei and lumbricals enter the extensor hood as the lateral bands and insert distally and dorsally to the axis of the PIPJ. It is through this distal insertion that the intrinsic muscles (the interossei and lumbricals) are flexors of the MPJs and yet extensors of the IPJs. The extensor hood inserts to the base of the middle phalanx, which is termed the *central slip*, and finally proceeds on to the base of the distal phalanx, where it inserts through the terminal slip, thus extending the DIPJ.

The intrinsic muscles of the hand are responsible for the fine motor movements of individual digits, especially the thumb (Fig. 119.7). The intrinsic muscles of the thenar eminence are the abductor pollicis brevis (APB), flexor pollicis brevis, opponens pollicis, and adductor pollicis. Four lumbricals originate on the FDP

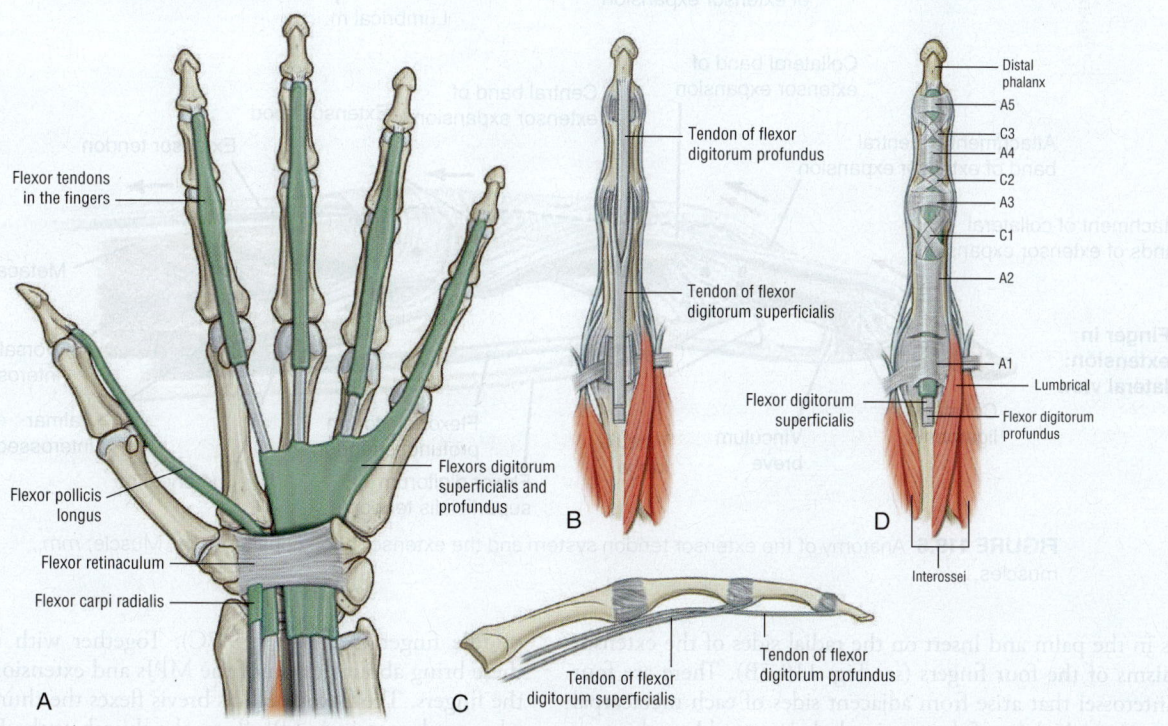

FIGURE 119.4 (A–D) Anatomy of the flexor tendon sheaths, including "A," annular, and "C," cruciate, pulley system. (From Warring L, Hall A. Riley S. *Musculoskeletal Ultrasound: How, Why and When.* St. Louis: Elsevier; 2022.)

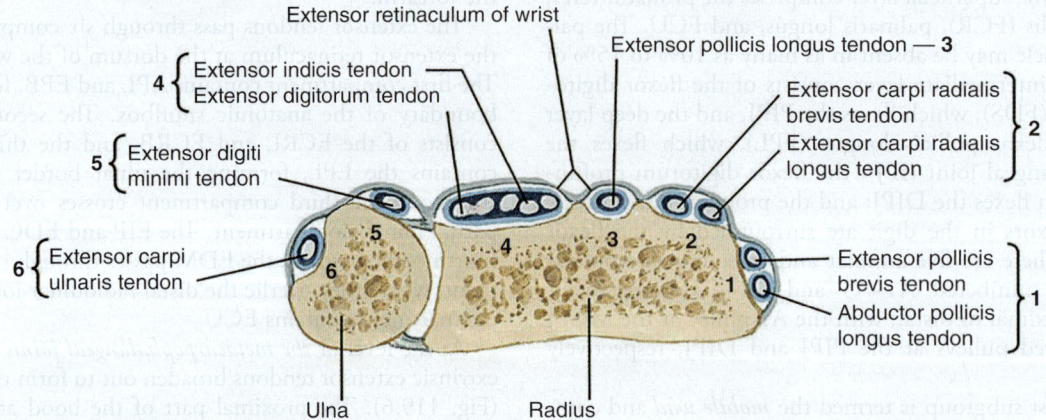

Cross section of distal forearm

Extensor retinaculum of wrist

Extensor pollicis longus tendon — 3

4 { Extensor indicis tendon
Extensor digitorum tendon

Extensor carpi radialis brevis tendon
Extensor carpi radialis longus tendon } 2

5 { Extensor digiti minimi tendon

6 { Extensor carpi ulnaris tendon

Extensor pollicis brevis tendon
Abductor pollicis longus tendon } 1

Ulna   Radius

FIGURE 119.5 Dorsal extensor compartments of the wrist.

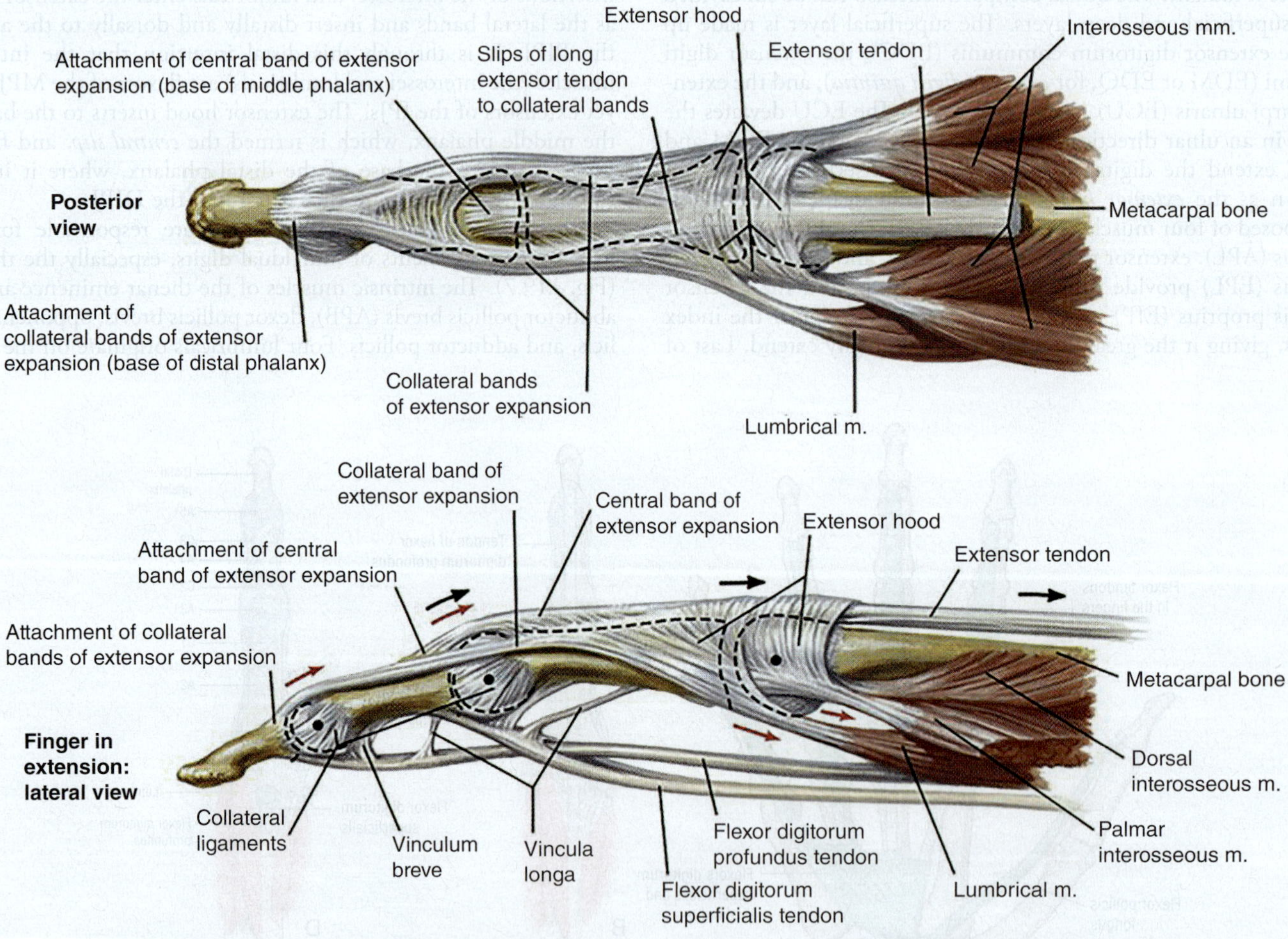

Extensor hood

Attachment of central band of extensor expansion (base of middle phalanx)

Slips of long extensor tendon to collateral bands

Extensor tendon

Interosseous mm.

Posterior view

Metacarpal bone

Attachment of collateral bands of extensor expansion (base of distal phalanx)

Collateral bands of extensor expansion

Lumbrical m.

Collateral band of extensor expansion

Central band of extensor expansion

Extensor hood

Extensor tendon

Attachment of central band of extensor expansion

Attachment of collateral bands of extensor expansion

Metacarpal bone

Finger in extension: lateral view

Dorsal interosseous m.

Collateral ligaments

Vinculum breve

Vincula longa

Flexor digitorum profundus tendon

Palmar interosseous m.

Flexor digitorum superficialis tendon

Lumbrical m.

FIGURE 119.6 Anatomy of the extensor tendon system and the extensor hoop apparatus. *m.,* Muscle; *mm.,* muscles.

tendons in the palm and insert on the radial sides of the extensor mechanisms of the four fingers (see Fig. 119.7B). There are four dorsal interossei that arise from adjacent sides of each metacarpal and insert onto the base of the proximal phalanx and lateral extensor hood of the ulnar digit; these provide abduction of the MCPJs of the index, middle, and ring fingers. There are three palmar interossei that adduct the index, ring, and little fingers toward the

middle finger (see Fig. 119.7C). Together with the lumbricals, these bring about flexion of the MPJs and extension of the IPJs of the fingers. The flexor pollicis brevis flexes the thumb at the MPJ, whereas the extrinsic FPL flexes the thumb at the IPJ.

The hypothenar muscles consist of the flexor digiti minimi, which flexes the little finger at the MPJ, and the abductor digiti minimi and opponens digiti minimi. A small muscle called the

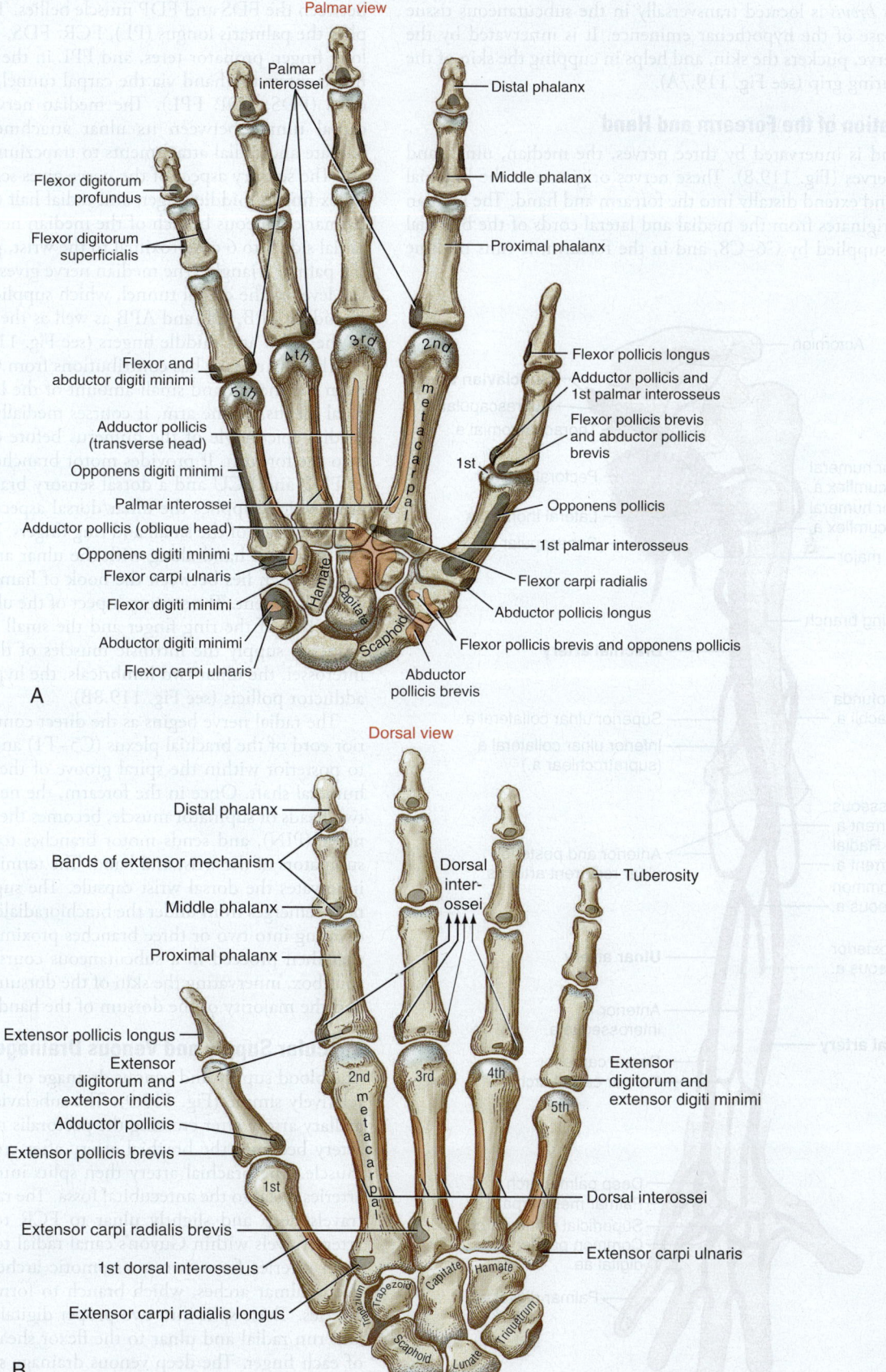

FIGURE 119.7 (A–B) Intrinsic muscles of the hand (volar) and relationship to neurovascular structures. Schema of the lumbrical muscles and interossei. (From Neuman DA. *Neumann's Kinesiology of the Musculoskeletal System*. 4th ed. St. Louis: Elsevier; 2025.)

palmaris brevis is located transversally in the subcutaneous tissue at the base of the hypothenar eminence. It is innervated by the ulnar nerve, puckers the skin, and helps in cupping the skin of the palm during grip (see Fig. 119.7A).

Innervation of the Forearm and Hand

The hand is innervated by three nerves, the median, ulnar, and radial nerves (Fig. 119.8). These nerves originate at the brachial plexus and extend distally into the forearm and hand. The median nerve originates from the medial and lateral cords of the brachial plexus, supplied by C6–C8, and in the forearm, it runs midline

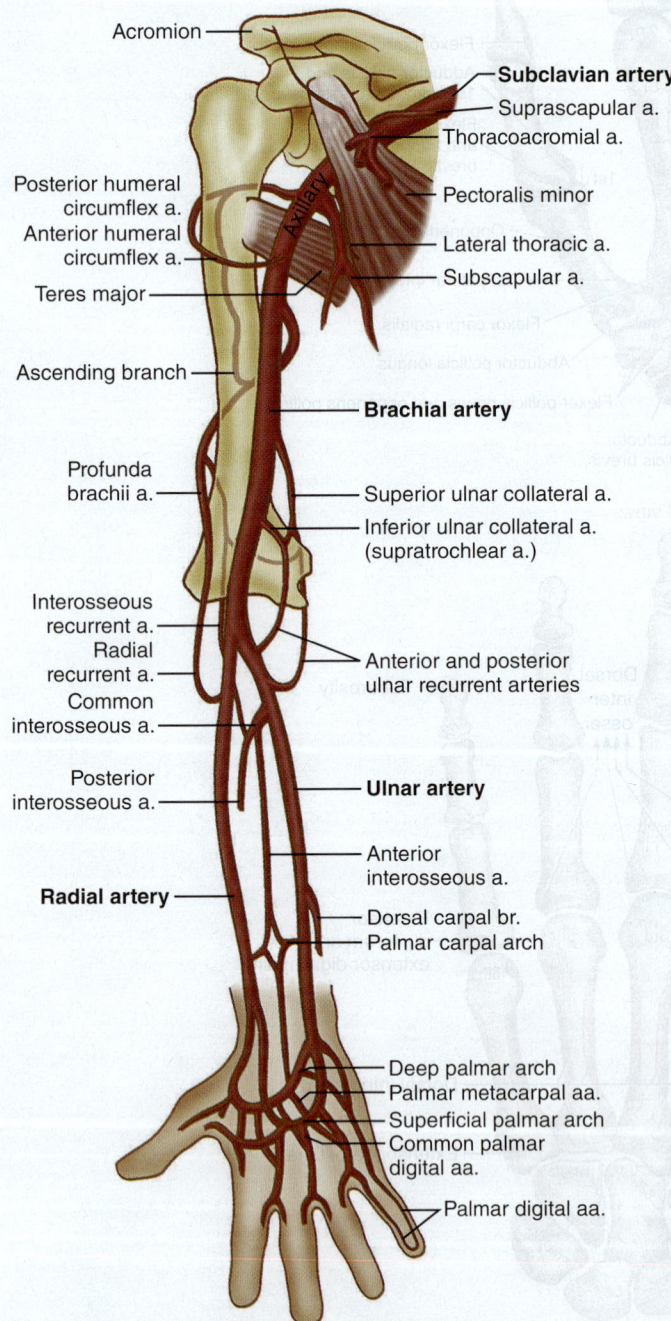

Acromion —
Subclavian artery
Suprascapular a.
Thoracoacromial a.
Posterior humeral circumflex a.
Pectoralis minor
Anterior humeral circumflex a.
Teres major
Lateral thoracic a.
Subscapular a.
Ascending branch
Brachial artery
Profunda brachii a.
Superior ulnar collateral a.
Inferior ulnar collateral a. (supratrochlear a.)
Interosseous recurrent a.
Radial recurrent a.
Anterior and posterior ulnar recurrent arteries
Common interosseous a.
Posterior interosseous a.
Ulnar artery
Anterior interosseous a.
Radial artery
Dorsal carpal br.
Palmar carpal arch
Deep palmar arch
Palmar metacarpal aa.
Superficial palmar arch
Common palmar digital aa.
Palmar digital aa.

FIGURE 119.8 Nerve anatomy of the upper extremity. *a.,* Artery; *aa.,* arteries. (From Feldscher SB, et al. *Rehabilitation of the Hand and Upper Extremity.* 7th ed. St. Louis: Elsevier; 2021.)

between the FDS and FDP muscle bellies. The median nerve supplies the palmaris longus (PL), FCR, FDS, FDP to the index and long finger, pronator teres, and FPL in the forearm. The median nerve enters the hand via the carpal tunnel, along with nine tendons (FDS, FDP, FPL). The median nerve passes through the carpal tunnel between its ulnar attachments to pisiform and hamate and radial attachments to trapezium and scaphoid tubercle. The sensory aspect of the nerve gives sensation to the thumb, index finger, middle finger, and radial half of the ring finger. The palmar cutaneous branch of the median nerve originates from its radial side 5 to 6 cm proximal to the wrist, providing sensation to the palmar triangle. The median nerve gives off a motor branch at the level of the carpal tunnel, which supplies the thenar muscles, including FPB, OP, and APB as well as the radial two lumbricals to the index and middle fingers (see Fig. 119.8A).

The ulnar nerve has contributions from C7–T1 and originates from the medial and small amount of the lateral cord of the brachial plexus. In the arm, it courses medially and posterior to the medial epicondyle of the humerus before coursing more volarly into the forearm. It provides motor branches to the ulnar aspects of FDP and FCU and a dorsal sensory branch at the distal forearm, which supplies the ulnar/dorsal aspect of the hand and the dorsal aspects of the small and ring fingers. The ulnar nerve enters the wrist and hand along with the ulnar artery through Guyon's canal, which lies between the hook of hamate and the transverse carpal ligament. The sensory aspect of the ulnar nerve supplies the ulnar half of the ring finger and the small finger, and the motor branches supply the intrinsic muscles of the hand, including all interossei, the ulnar two lumbricals, the hypothenar muscles, and adductor pollicis (see Fig. 119.8B).

The radial nerve begins as the direct continuation of the posterior cord of the brachial plexus (C5–T1) and moves from anterior to posterior within the spiral groove of the humerus at the mid-humeral shaft. Once in the forearm, the nerve travels deep to the two heads of supinator muscle, becomes the posterior interosseous nerve (PIN), and sends motor branches to all the extensors and supinators of the wrist and hand. The terminal branch of the PIN innervates the dorsal wrist capsule. The superficial radial sensory nerve emerges from under the brachioradialis in the distal forearm, dividing into two or three branches proximal to the radial styloid that then proceed in a subcutaneous course across the anatomic snuffbox, innervating the skin of the dorsum of the first web space and the majority of the dorsum of the hand (see Fig. 119.8C).

Vascular Supply and Venous Drainage

The blood supply and venous drainage of the upper extremity are relatively simple (Fig. 119.9). The subclavian artery becomes the axillary artery after crossing the pectoralis minor, and the axillary artery becomes the brachial artery after crossing the teres major muscle. The brachial artery then splits into the radial and ulnar arteries distal to the antecubital fossa. The radial artery at the wrist travels deep and slightly ulnar to FCR tendon, and the ulnar artery travels within Guyon's canal radial to the hook of hamate. Both arteries form two anastomotic arches, the superficial and deep palmar arches, which branch to form the common digital arteries. These split into two proper digital arteries for each digit and run radial and ulnar to the flexor sheath on the volar aspect of each finger. The deep venous drainage system follows the nomenclature of the arteries, with two venae comitantes running with each major artery. The superficial venous drainage sends tributaries starting at the dorsum of the hand and drains into the basilic (ulnar) and cephalic (radial) systems.

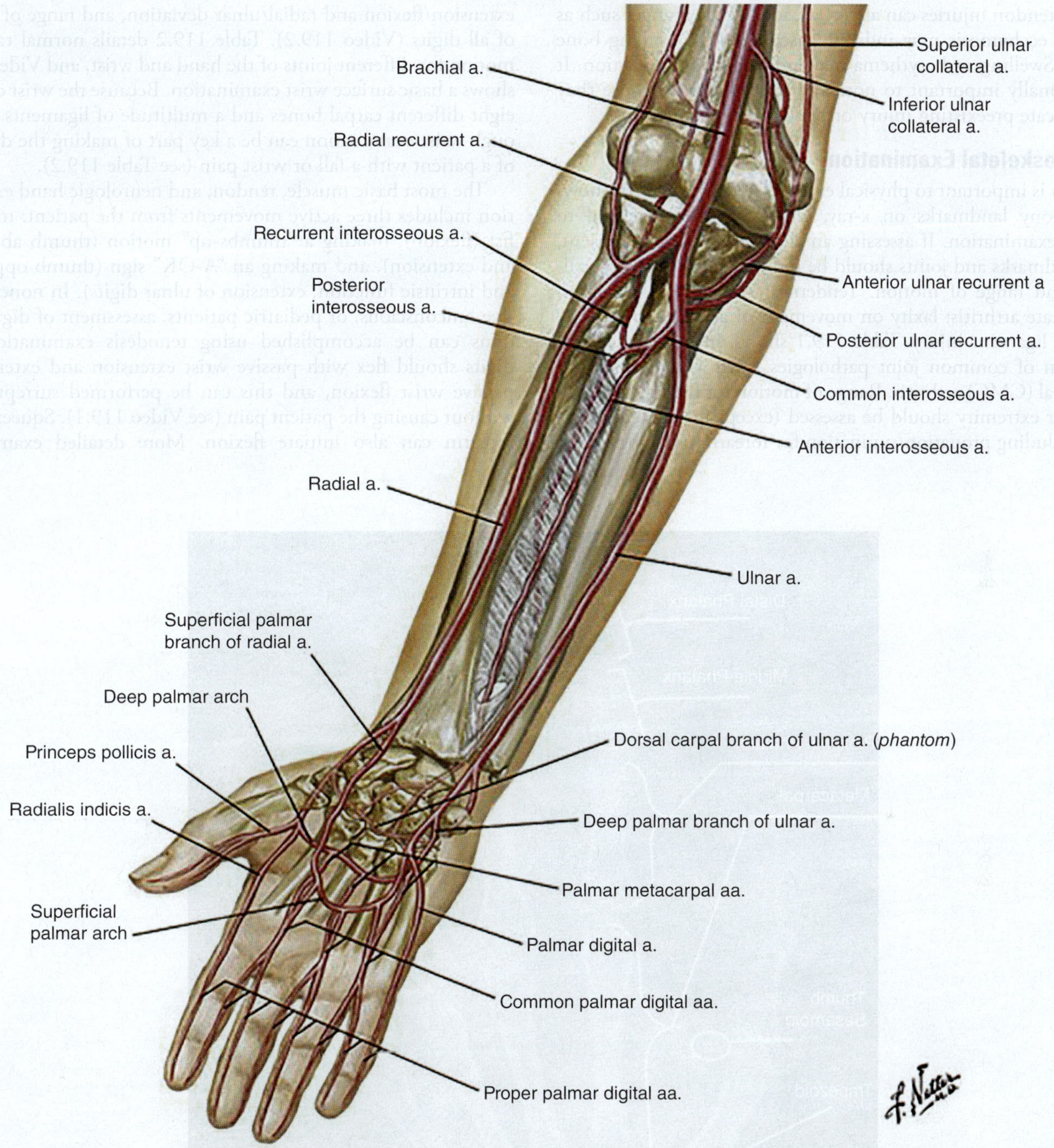

Brachial a.

Radial recurrent a.

Recurrent interosseous a.

Posterior
interosseous a.

Radial a.

Superficial palmar
branch of radial a.

Deep palmar arch

Princeps pollicis a.

Radialis indicis a.

Superficial
palmar arch

Superior ulnar
collateral a.

Inferior ulnar
collateral a.

Anterior ulnar recurrent a

Posterior ulnar recurrent a.

Common interosseous a.

Anterior interosseous a.

Ulnar a.

Dorsal carpal branch of ulnar a. (*phantom*)

Deep palmar branch of ulnar a.

Palmar metacarpal aa.

Palmar digital a.

Common palmar digital aa.

Proper palmar digital aa.

FIGURE 119.9 Vascular (arterial) anatomy of the upper extremity. *a.,* Artery; *aa.,* arteries.

EXAMINATION AND DIAGNOSIS

General Evaluation

Many of the most common diagnoses and injuries of the hand and upper extremity can be determined clinically based on a thorough patient history and physical examination. Because hand surgery is a regional discipline, there are multiple systems that must be assessed to be normal in function: skeletal, muscle, neurologic, vascular, and skin/soft tissue. Patient history will provide invaluable clues to the diagnosis. Some key points of information include mechanism of injury; date and/or time of injury; hand dominance, which may affect the urgency of intervention; occupation or daily activities, which may affect return to work; baseline level of function; and previous hand injuries or surgeries that

may have left a lasting deficit unrelated to the current presenting problem.

There are a few specialized instruments that may be used in the general physical examination; however, the most informative actions will be visualization and palpation of the structures of the hand. The first step is inspection, or simply looking at the extremity. Are there any lacerations, edema, or obvious deformities? Examination of the resting posture of the hand can provide valuable information—the flexors are more robust than the extensors, and therefore, the resting posture of the fingers should be flexed in a "cascade" in which all digits point slightly to the scaphoid or radial aspect of the wrist (Video 119.1). Angulation or malrotation from digital or metacarpal fractures/dislocations or flexor or extensor tendon injuries can affect cascade. Color changes such as pallor or ecchymosis may indicate vascular injury or long bone fracture. Swelling and erythema may indicate a hand infection. It is additionally important to note any scars present because they may indicate preexisting injury or previous surgery.

Musculoskeletal Examination

Palpation is important to physical examination. Fig. 119.10 shows typical bony landmarks on x-ray, which can be correlated to physical examination. If assessing an elective or subacute patient, bony landmarks and joints should be individually assessed by palpation and range of motion. Tenderness of joints to palpation can indicate arthritis; laxity on movement of a joint can indicate collateral ligament injury. Table 119.1 shows, in more detail, examination of common joint pathologies, such as thumb carpometacarpal (CMC) arthritis. Range of motion for the focal parts of the upper extremity should be assessed (except for an acute fracture), including pronation/supination for forearm pathology, wrist

extension/flexion and radial/ulnar deviation, and range of motion of all digits (Video 119.2). Table 119.2 details normal ranges of motion for different joints of the hand and wrist, and Video 119.3 shows a basic surface wrist examination. Because the wrist contains eight different carpal bones and a multitude of ligaments, a thorough wrist examination can be a key part of making the diagnosis of a patient with a fall or wrist pain (see Table 119.2).

The most basic muscle, tendon, and neurologic hand examination includes three active movements from the patient: making a fist (flexion), making a "thumbs-up" motion (thumb abduction and extension), and making an "A-OK" sign (thumb opposition and intrinsic function, extension of ulnar digits). In noncooperative, unconscious, or pediatric patients, assessment of digital tendons can be accomplished using tenodesis examination—the digits should flex with passive wrist extension and extend with passive wrist flexion, and this can be performed surreptitiously without causing the patient pain (see Video 119.1). Squeezing the forearm can also initiate flexion. More detailed examination

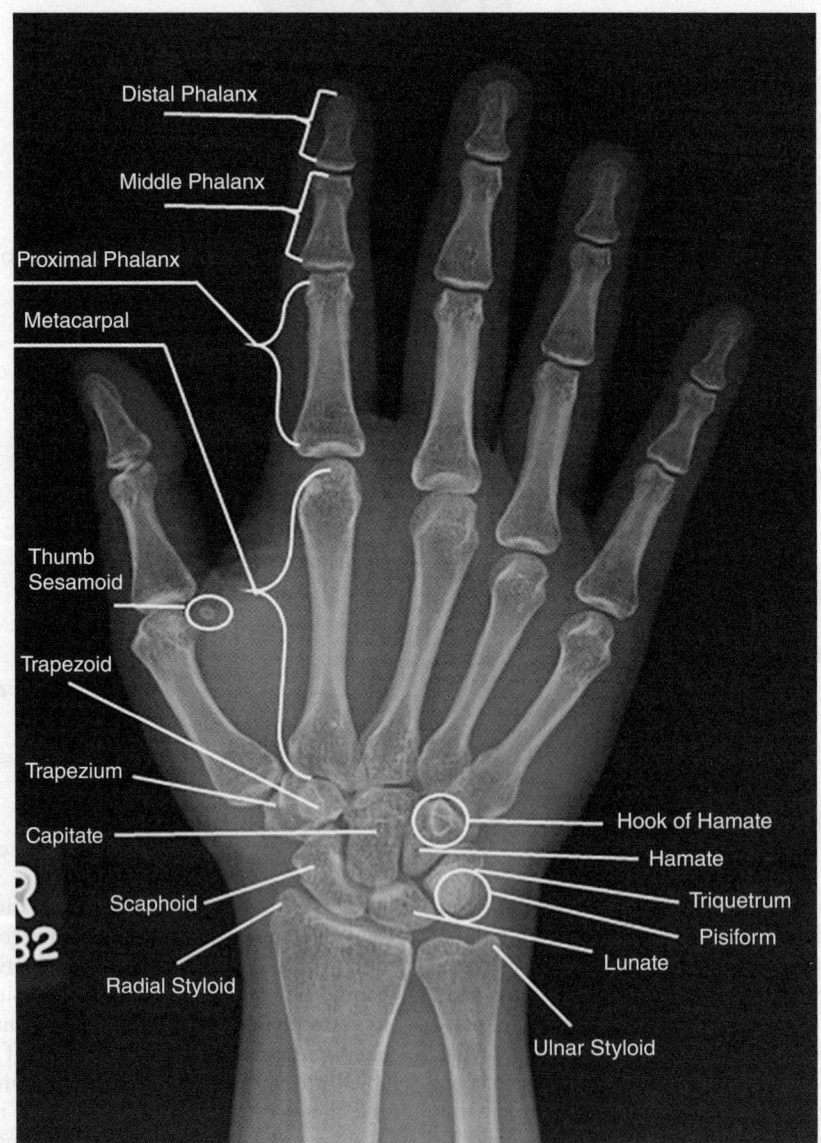

FIGURE 119.10 Anteroposterior view x-ray of a normal hand with common anatomic landmarks labeled on the read.

TABLE 119.1 Hand Examination Special Maneuvers

TEST NAME	INDICATION	TECHNIQUE	POSITIVE FINDING
Thumb CMC grind	Suspicion of thumb CMC arthritis	Axial loading of the thumb and gentle circumduction at CMC joint	Sensation of grittiness or crepitus within the joint. May also have pain; should compare to contralateral.
Finkelstein test	Suspicion of De Quervain tenosynovitis	Have the patient flex the thumb into the palm and wrap the other digits around it in flexion; then have them relax and passively ulnarly deviate the wrist.	Sharp pain on ulnar deviation. May also have tenderness to palpation over radial styloid.
Watson test	Assess scapholunate ligament laxity or injury	Examiner places thumb over scaphoid tubercle at volar aspect of wrist while the digits stabilize on the dorsal side of the wrist and apply pressure to the scaphoid tubercle. With other hand on the patient's metacarpals, bring the hand from extension and ulnar deviation into flexion and radial deviation, with constant pressure on the scaphoid.	Examiner will feel a "clunk" as the scaphoid returns to anatomic position with the applied volar pressure on radial deviation. There may also be pain, but the test itself can be uncomfortable. Contralateral side should be tested for comparison.
L-T ballottement test	Assess lunotriquetral ligament instability or injury	With patient elbow on table and wrist neutral, the examiner pinches triquetrum and lunate between thumb and index of each respective hand, and then attempts to move them in opposing volar/dorsal direction.	Significant ballottement or laxity indicates ligament weakening or injury, particularly in the volar direction.
Anatomic snuffbox	Radial-sided wrist pain	Anatomic snuffbox is bordered by the first dorsal compartment (APL/EPB) and third dorsal compartment (EPL). Patient may radially deviate wrist and extend thumb.	Tenderness to palpation may indicate scaphoid fracture or other scaphoid pathology.

APL, Abductor pollicis longus; *CMC,* carpometacarpal; *EPB,* extensor pollicis brevis; *EPL,* extensor pollicis longus.

TABLE 119.2 Normal Range-of-Motion Ranges for Finger and Wrist Joints

JOINT	MAXIMUM EXTENSION	MAXIMUM FLEXION
Digit DIPJ	0°	80°
Digit PIPJ	0°	100°
Digit MCPJ	−45° (hyperextension)	90°
Thumb IPJ	−15° (hyperextension)	80°
Thumb MPJ	10°	55°
Wrist	−70°	75°
	MAXIMUM RADIAL DEVIATION	**MAXIMUM ULNAR DEVIATION**
Thumb CMC	60°	45°
Wrist	20°	35°
	MAXIMUM PRONATION	**MAXIMUM SUPINATION**
DRUJ	70°	85°

CMC, Carpometacarpal; *DIPJ,* distal interphalangeal joint; *DRUJ,* distal radioulnar joint; *IPJ,* interphalangeal joint; *MCPJ,* metacarpophalangeal joint; *MPJ,* metacarpophalangeal joint; *PIPJ,* proximal interphalangeal joint.

should be tailored to the presenting symptoms. The tendons of the digits should be assessed independently (Video 119.4). Flexion at DIPJ, or IPJ of the thumb, with the PIPJ held in extension confirms that the FDP and FPL, respectively, are intact (Fig. 119.11). To isolate the FDS, the digits not being examined should be held in extension because the FDP has a common muscle belly. To assess EPL and EPB, the patient should be asked to place the hand on a flat surface and lift the thumb only off the surface (Fig. 119.12A). To test for PL presence, have the patient oppose the thumb and small finger and flex the wrist (see Fig. 119.12B).

Finger extension is tested by asking the patient to extend the MCPJ against resistance. Central slip injuries can be difficult to identify and require isolation of that portion of the extensor hood with an Elson test (Video 119.5). Normally, the DIPJ is lax with the PIPJ in flexion, but in a positive test, the DIPJ can be actively extended because of slack in the lateral bands.

Neurovascular Examination

On general inspection, color changes of the digits may indicate ischemia or congestion. Capillary refill is the key to assessing perfusion of the hand—the digits are gently pressed and released to observe the return of normal coloration after blanching under pressure, normally less than 2 seconds. The Allen test confirms patency of the ulnar and radial arteries (Video 119.6). This can be especially important if assessing for major bleeding in the forearm, to determine whether a vessel may be ligated in the setting of acute trauma without compromising the hand. If there is question about perfusion, bedside Doppler ultrasound can be used to further assess pulse in the forearm vessels, palmar arches, and the radial and ulnar digital arteries.

Specific nerves should be assessed for injury by using sensory and motor territories specific to these nerves (Fig. 119.13). Sensory examination should be performed before administration of local anesthesia for any bedside procedures. Two-point sensory discrimination is the most sensitive method of testing for sensory loss and is easily done by using a two-point discrimination tool or a bent paper clip set to approximately 5 mm apart. The radial and ulnar aspects of each digit's volar fingertip should be tested. The points are aligned along the axis of the finger. If this test is not reproducible because of an uncooperative patient, suspicion of a nerve injury can be confirmed by the tactile adherence test, in which a plastic pen is passed back and forth gently across the pulp on either side of each finger. Adhesion, because of the presence of sweat, is shown by slight but definite movement of the finger being examined (anesthetized finger pulp will not sweat).

Motor function of the median nerve can be best assessed by looking at the thenar muscles and the FDS to index finger. The motor function of the APB tests the median nerve. With the hand flat and facing palm up, the patient is asked to use their thumb to touch the

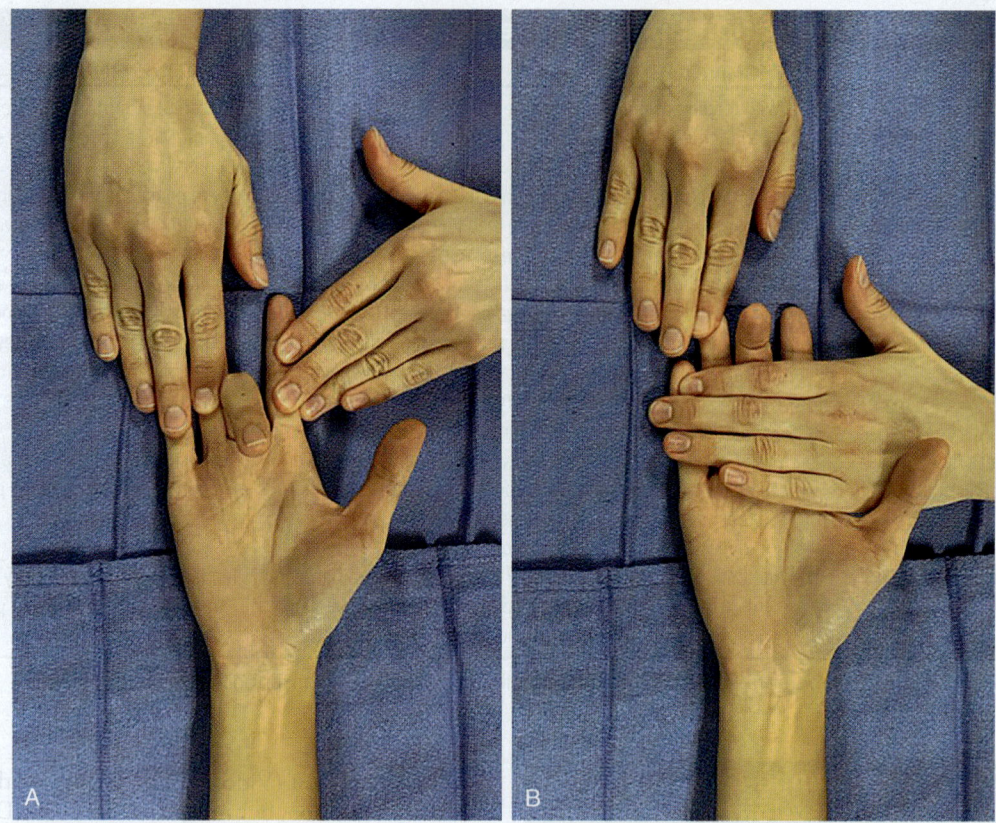

FIGURE 119.11 Isolation testing the flexor digitorum superficialis (A) and flexor digitorum profundus (B) tendons of individual digits. Note that each digit must be isolated as well as each joint to ensure accurate examination and no confounding movement from neighboring digits.

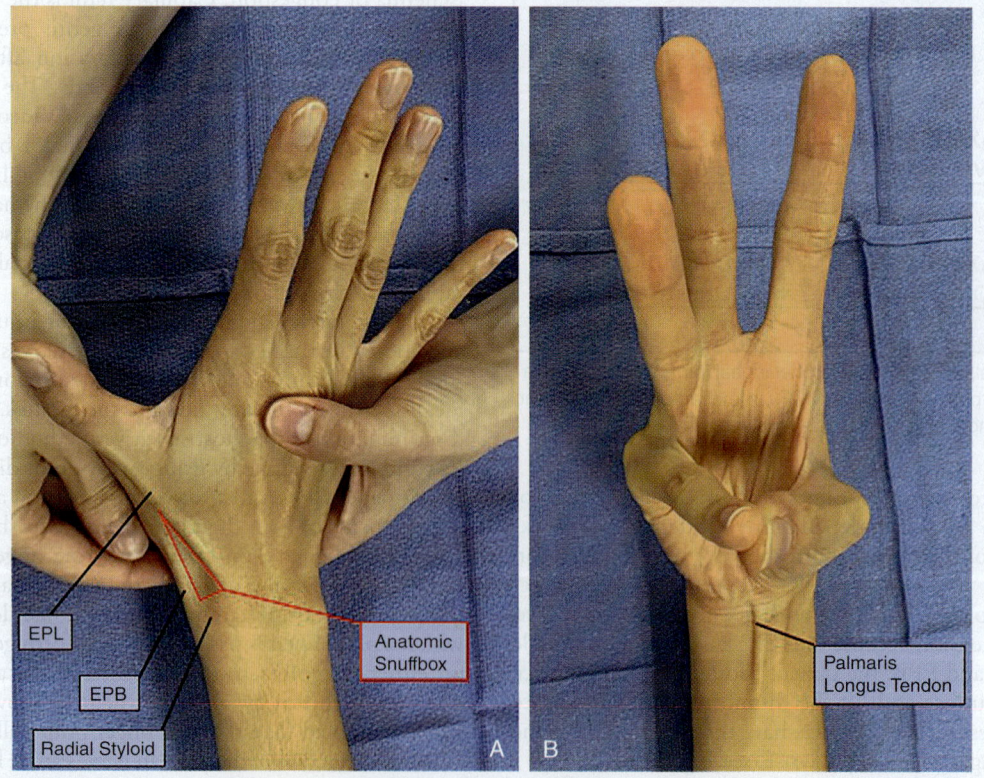

FIGURE 119.12 Dorsal wrist tendon examination including the anatomic snuffbox (A), bordered by the first and third dorsal compartment tendons (extensor pollicis brevis *[EPB]* in *1* and extensor pollicis longus *[EPL]* in *3*) and radial styloid proximally. (B) Examination of the palmaris longus tendon, with thumb/small finger opposed and wrist flexed.

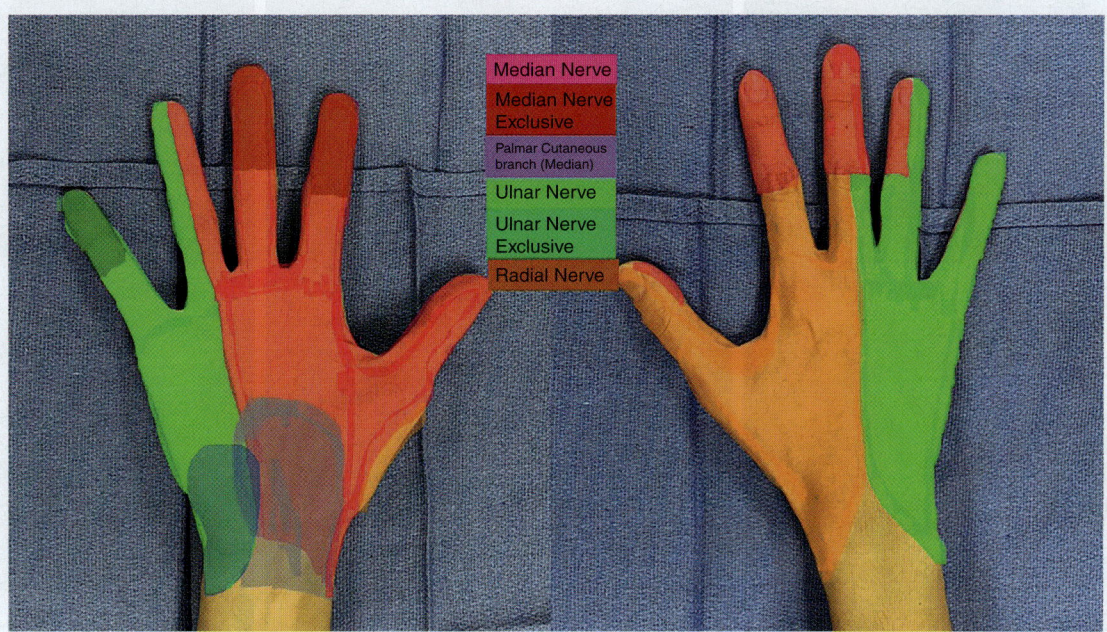

FIGURE 119.13 Sensory distribution of the nerves of the hand, including median, ulnar, and radial nerves, on examination.

examiner's finger, which is held directly over the thenar eminence.[2] Testing FPL with thumb interphalangeal (IP) flexion against resistance and FDS and FDP of index finger with resisted flexion can delineate median pathology in the wrist versus more proximally. The ulnar nerve controls hand intrinsic muscles, so simple tests include having the patient spread (abduct) the fingers against resistance and crisscross groups of fingers, testing the dorsal and palmar interossei, respectively. Thumb adduction is assessed with Froment sign, and weakness of the hypothenar muscles is assessed with Wartenberg sign. Tests for function of the radial nerve and its branches require wrist extension, thumb extension, and finger extension at the MPJ. A basic carpal tunnel examination can be seen in Video 119.7, and additional specialized neurologic tests are shown in Table 119.3.

Special Investigations and Imaging

Plain radiographs should be performed in emergency room or trauma cases and in elective patients with joint pain or suspicion of fracture. These help in the diagnosis and evaluation of fractures and arthritis and in the investigation of radiopaque foreign bodies.[3] An appropriate imaging series includes an anteroposterior (AP) view, oblique view, and true lateral view, the quality of which can be assessed based on the visibility of the pisiform bone (Fig. 119.14). Other views may be able to elucidate more specific pathologies, such a scaphoid view, clenched-fist view, or carpal tunnel view. Stress radiographic views and cineradiography may be useful for demonstrating dynamic wrist instability patterns, especially scapholunate separation.

TABLE 119.3   Specialized Neurologic Tests for the Hand and Upper Extremity

TEST NAME	INDICATION	TECHNIQUE	POSITIVE FINDING
Tinel sign	Assess nerve compression, assess regeneration along peripheral nerve	Gently tap with two fingers over anatomic sites of compression—carpal tunnel, Guyon canal, cubital tunnel, supinator, etc.	Reproduction of numbness and tingling and/or pain in the affected nerve distribution
Durkin compression test	Suspicion of carpal tunnel syndrome	Compress the median nerve within carpal tunnel with the thumb over the palm and the patient's wrist in neutral position	Reproduction of numbness, tingling, or pain in the median distribution of the digits; may take up to 30–60 sec
Phalen test	Suspicion of carpal tunnel syndrome	Have patient flex the wrist as much as possible so that both dorsal hands are in contact, hold position for 30–60 seconds, which will cause constriction of the transverse carpal ligament	Reproduction of numbness or tingling or pain in the median distribution of the digits; may take up to 30–60 sec
Hyperflexion test	Suspicion of cubital tunnel syndrome	Hyperflexion of the elbow as much as possible with shoulder flexed at 90 degrees	Reproduction of pain, numbness, or tingling over the ulnar nerve distribution
Froment sign	Ulnar neuropathy	Test thumb adduction by having the patient grasp something, like a sheet of paper, between the thumb and index finger metacarpal	Should be able to grasp the paper with the thenar adductor alone. Positive test is flexion of the thumb IP joint, which uses the median innervated FPL.
Wartenberg sign	Ulnar neuropathy	Observation of ulnar drift of the small finger (away from the ring finger)	Drift indicates weakness of the ulnar innervated intrinsics and pull of the radially innervated EDC/EDQ

EDC, Extensor digitorum communis; *EDQ,* extensor digitorum quintus; *FPL,* flexor pollicis longus; *IP,* interphalangeal.

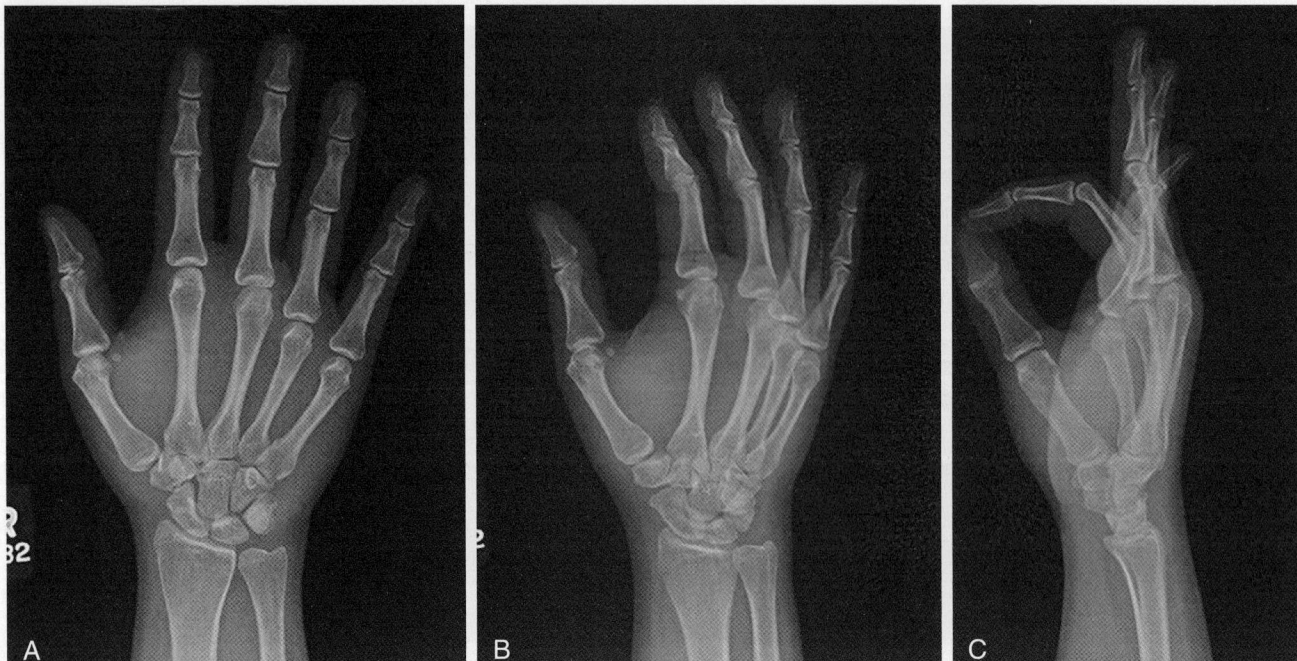

FIGURE 119.14 Standard anteroposterior (A), oblique (B), and lateral (C) radiographs of the hand. Note in the lateral view that the pisiform is centralized between the scaphoid and capitate, which determines a technically well-done lateral view.

Ultrasound is a portable, low-cost, and easy-to-use adjunct. Ultrasound has been used to assess soft issue and nerve pathologies such as carpal tunnel syndrome, trigger fingers, and other tenosynovitis.[4,5] Ultrasound can reliably show wood and plastic foreign bodies that may not show up on plain films in the hands of an experienced operator.

More complex imaging, such as CT and MRI, is typically not first line but does have important roles in hand surgery. When further bony imaging is needed for things like complex and intraarticular fractures, CT is usually the examination of choice.[6] MRI is a more appropriate examination for any masses and unclear soft tissue pathology, such as ligaments, flexor tendon sheaths, triangular fibrocartilage complex (TFCC) injuries, or detailed cartilage examination.[7] Both MRI and CT can be formatted as arthrograms to provide a detailed, noninvasive examination of the wrist, such as in concern for scapholunate ligament injury. Both CT and MRI are a useful modality for the diagnosis of a suspected carpal bone fracture.

More invasive imaging and testing include wrist arthroscopy and angiograms. With the use of CT and MRI angiograms with contrast administration, need for surgical angiograms has reduced, except for those with suspicion of complex vascular pathology, such as pseudoaneurysm. Wrist arthroscopy is the gold standard for looking at and intervening on the TFCC and scapholunate ligament. Electromyography and nerve conduction studies are other more involved tests that may be useful in patients with nerve injuries or suspected but unclear nerve compression pathology.

PRINCIPLES OF TREATMENT

Appropriate treatment of upper extremity problems requires a thorough knowledge of local and regional anesthesia, use of a tourniquet to provide a bloodless field, correct placement of incisions to minimize later scar contracture, and appropriate use of dressings and splints to reduce edema and maintain a functional position.

Above all, a clear knowledge of the unique anatomy of the hand and upper extremity not only aids in obtaining an accurate clinical diagnosis but also enables the safe performance of surgery.

Anesthesia

The choice of general, regional, or local anesthesia is governed by the extent and length of the operation, in addition to patient factors such as comorbidities, anticoagulation, and pain tolerance. An upper arm or forearm tourniquet can be used in the unanesthetized extremity with only local anesthetic field infiltration or digital block for up to 30 to 45 minutes in a relaxed, cooperative patient. For ancillary procedures, such as for harvesting of bone, nerve, tendon, or skin graft, or if more extensive surgical procedures are planned, general anesthesia will be required. Wide-awake local anesthesia, no tourniquet (WALANT) procedures are becoming increasingly common in office and ambulatory settings to minimize excessive costs and risks of anesthesia. WALANT anesthesia works well for procedures such as open carpal tunnel release, mass removal distal to wrist, and trigger finger/A1 pulley releases.[8–10]

A digital block is a useful tool for finger injuries, especially in the emergent setting. Dogma states to avoid use of epinephrine in the digits because of the risk of ischemia; however, recent data suggest that there is no increased risk of loss of digital perfusion.[11] Median, ulnar, or radial wrist nerve block may be useful, and all three may be anesthetized at the wrist for a total wrist block (Fig. 119.15). Hematoma blocks can assist in fracture reductions.[12]

Tourniquet Application

The tourniquet is used to provide a bloodless field so that all relevant structures in the operative field can be visualized.[13] Especially in the emergency setting, when a formal tourniquet may not be available, common items like Penrose drains or the fingers of a sterile glove can be used for digital tourniquet. Tourniquet use is not without risk—direct pneumatic pressure can cause

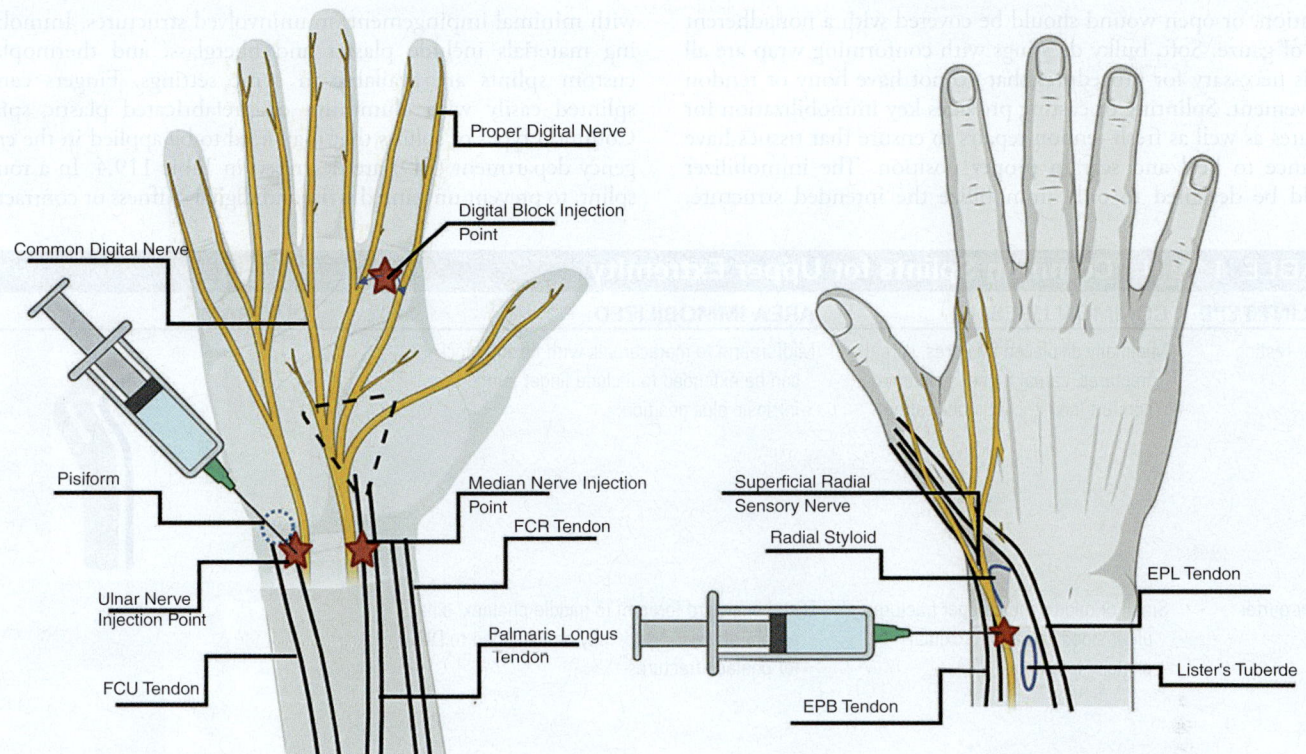

FIGURE 119.15 Diagram of key injection points of the hand and wrist for regional anesthesia of the digit and wrist. *Stars* indicate injection points, *black lines* indicate palpable tendon anatomy, and *blue lines* indicate palpable bony landmarks. *EPB,* Extensor pollicis brevis; *EPL,* extensor pollicis longus; *FCR,* flexor carpi radialis.

damage to underlying nerves and vessels; prolonged distal ischemia can result in venous congestion or muscle damage and reperfusion injury after release. The skin below the tourniquet must be padded to prevent pressure injury or blistering, and a watertight seal such as tape or draping should be applied to prevent the underlying skin from getting wet during preparation. The standard pressure is 250 mm Hg, or 100 to 150 mm Hg higher than systolic blood pressure.[14] Historically, maximum tolerable ischemia time is 2 hours; after that point, the cuff is deflated for at least 15 minutes to allow return of blood flow.[13] An Esmarch or Martin bandage is used to exsanguinate the extremity before tourniquet inflation, except in the case of active infection or tumors because of the possibility of embolic spread from distal to proximal. In these cases, the extremity can be elevated for 5 minutes before pneumatic inflation.

Incisions

It is important to design all incisions with the promise of scar contracture in mind. On the palmar surface, Bruner, midaxial, Z-plasty, or a combination of these should be used to avoid longitudinal linear incisions that cross joints. Existing lacerations can be incorporated (Fig. 119.16).[15] On the dorsum, linear incisions may be used because the skin is laxer. The marginal edge of a skin graft with healthy skin is also a potential scar line, so the margin of the skin graft is designed to be in these same lines to prevent contractures across flexion creases if possible.

Dressings and Splints

Dressings and splints are designed for the protection of the injury or surgery site and the comfort of the patient. Any incision,

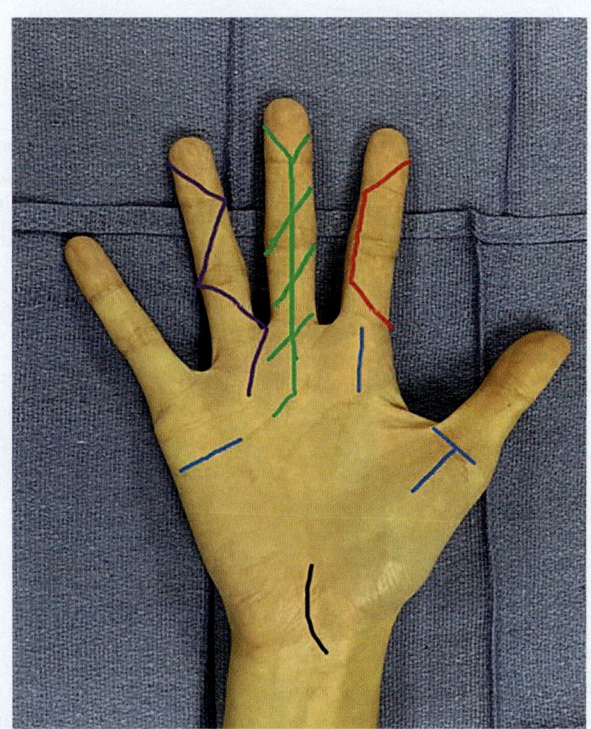

FIGURE 119.16 Appropriate incision types over the volar surface of the hand, including, from *left* to *right,* Brunner incision, Z-plasty–style incisions, and midaxial incision. The *blue lines* indicate potential placement of trigger finger incisions, horizontally or vertically, and the *black line* indicates a typical open carpal tunnel incision.

laceration, or open wound should be covered with a nonadherent layer of gauze. Soft, bulky dressings with conforming wrap are all that is necessary for procedures that do not have bony or tendon involvement. Splinting or casting provides key immobilization for fractures as well as fresh tendon repairs to ensure that tissues have a chance to heal and scar in proper position. The immobilizer should be designed to only immobilize the intended structure, with minimal impingement on uninvolved structures. Immobilizing materials include plaster and fiberglass, and thermoplastic custom splints are available in some settings. Fingers can be splinted easily with aluminum or prefabricated plastic splints. Common types of splints that may need to be applied in the emergency department (ED) are described in Table 119.4. In a routine splint, to prevent unwanted wrist and digital stiffness or contracture,

TABLE 119.4	**Common Splints for Upper Extremity**		
SPLINT TYPE	**COMMON USES**	**AREA IMMOBILIZED**	**DIAGRAM**
Volar resting	Minimally displaced fractures, carpal fractures, carpal tunnel syndrome, comfort (nonstrict immobilization)	Midforearm to metacarpals with flexion blockage, can be extended to include finger joints. Use intrinsic plus position.	
Ulnar gutter	Small or middle metacarpal fractures, ulnar-sided carpal or proximal phalanx fractures	Distal one-third forearm to middle phalanx, ulnar aspect of wrist, hand; may be extended to DIPJ for phalanx fractures.	
Thumb spica	Thumb phalanx or metacarpal injuries, suspicion or actual scaphoid fracture	Midforearm to thumb, including IP joint. Thumb in abduction.	
Clamshell or volar/dorsal	Distal radius fractures	Proximal one-third of forearm (not impinging on elbow) to MCPJ, volar and dorsal slab. Intrinsic plus positioning of wrist.	
Sugar-Tong	Distal radius and radial or ulnar shaft fractures	Dorsal MCPJ to volar MCPJ, wrapping around to include the elbow in flexion (90°). Wrist in intrinsic plus position.	
Dorsal blocking	Flexor tendon injuries	30° flexion of wrist, 40–60 MCPs, IPJ in extension. Midforearm to entire digit.	

DIPJ, Distal interphalangeal joint; *IP,* interphalangeal; *IPJ,* interphalangeal joint; *MCP,* metacarpal phalangeal; *MCPJ,* metacarpal phalangeal joint.

the safest position is termed the *intrinsic plus* position: the wrist in 30 to 50 degrees of extension, MPJs in 70 degrees of flexion, and the IPJs extended (neutral) (see Table 119.4). This allows the intrinsic muscles to remain relaxed without tension because wrist flexion automatically causes the MPJs to extend, thereby placing the collateral ligaments in their shortest lengths. The affected extremity should be elevated to minimize edema. Establishing care with an occupational therapist who specializes in hand therapy has also been shown to improve outcomes, and even the most excellent of surgeries may be at risk for failure or patient dissatisfaction without therapy.[16] Adjunct measures for patient comfort—such as pain control, primarily with nonopioid medications unless bony work is involved; ice; rest; non–weight-bearing protocols; and lifting and work restrictions—can be crucial to the success of the repair and satisfaction of the patient.

TRAUMA

Emergency Control of Bleeding and Vascular Injuries

Control of bleeding is part of the ABCs of the primary Advanced Trauma Life Support (ATLS) survey—namely, the *C* for **C**irculation. Measures to stop the bleed, identify the source, and definitively manage should be undertaken. The Stop the Bleed campaign has been increasingly used to educate laypeople, first responders, and other trauma-associated personnel in the emergent control of bleeding extremities in the field, using direct pressure, elevation, packing, and a proximal tourniquet.[17] To avoid accidental injury to unharmed structures such as nearby nerves, placement of hemostatic devices, such as clips, blindly in the ED and nonspecific cautery should be avoided.

Critical examination is key in locating the source of bleeding. Even closed fracture may result in vascular injury, either by sharp mechanism of fracture lacerating the vessel internally or by traction mechanism.[18] If a tourniquet was applied in the field and there is question of vascular injury, examination should be performed with tourniquet down. Direct-pressure dressings should be applied and the hand elevated. Tourniquets should not be applied for any significant time before definitive repair in the operating room except in the setting of life-threatening hemorrhage.[18,19]

Life should be prioritized over limb, and one may have no fear of using sympathomimetic medications and their potential vasoconstricting effect to support blood pressure, even if free flap reconstruction or microvascular repair is planned or has been performed. Multiple studies have shown no increase in adverse events when pressors are used in conjunction with microsurgery, and norepinephrine is the preferred vasoconstrictor. In the case of severe extremity bleeding, the patient should be resuscitated according to ATLS and massive transfusion protocol guidelines.[20]

Lacerations, Fingertip Injuries, and Fingertip Amputations

Fingertip lacerations, crush injuries, and amputations are among the most common injuries. Effective initial management can make a difference between efficient return to function and complication. Careful physical examination and history are paramount to understanding what structures may be injured or exposed, without requiring a bedside "wound exploration," which could risk further damaging important structures. A complete neurovascular and musculoskeletal examination is performed. It is appropriate to consider certain procedures in the ED, including laceration repair with primary closure, nail bed repair, and revision amputation; however, if the area will necessitate formal flap coverage, the best results will be achieved in the operating room or procedure room.[21]

All patients who present with extremity injuries undergo radiography to rule out fracture or radiopaque foreign body. Any fracture with associated laceration or even puncture wound should be treated as an open fracture and administered antibiotics within 90 minutes of assessment as well as be thoroughly irrigated with at least 1 L of normal saline before closure. It is also important to consider tetanus booster if the patient is overdue or unsure of last vaccination and there was a contaminated mechanism of injury. Local anesthesia in the form of a digital block is usually sufficient for bedside treatment.[22]

A common injury pattern involves crush injury to fingertip, resulting in subungual hematoma and/or nail bed laceration. Fingernail anatomy can be appreciated in Fig. 119.17. These can

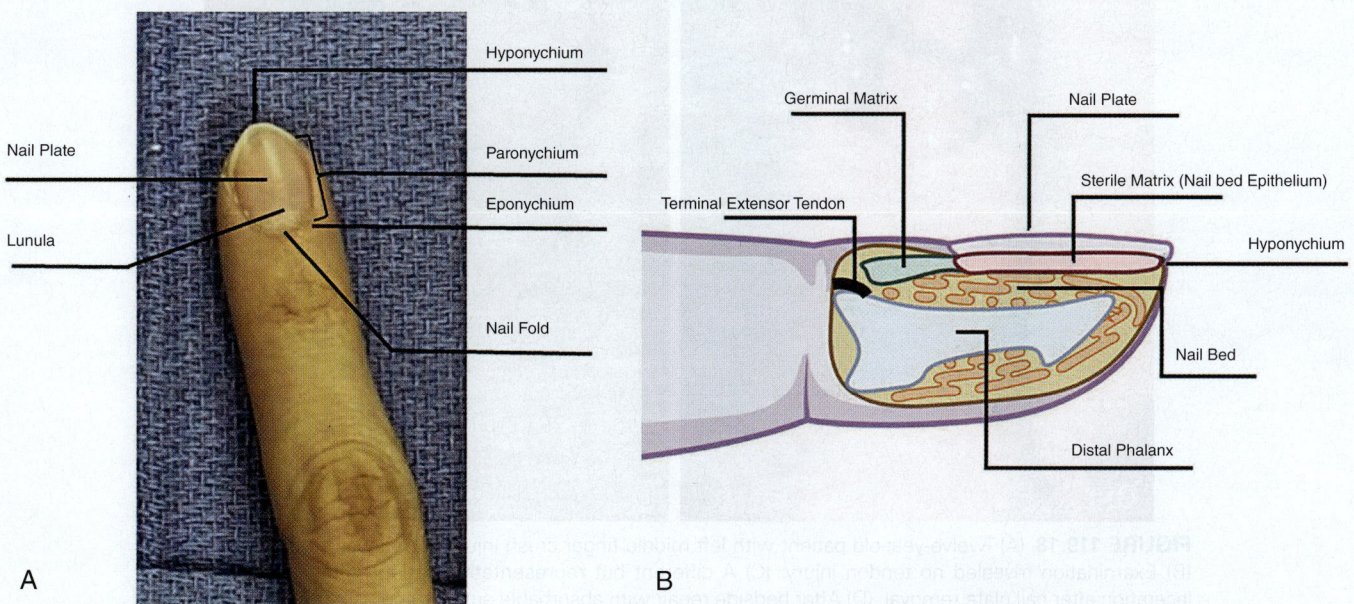

FIGURE 119.17 (A) Surface anatomy of the fingertip and fingernail. (B) Nail plate anatomy lateral view.

be very painful due to pressure buildup underneath the nail plate. If less than 50% of the nail is involved, pressure can be relieved using trephination with a large-bore needle or with an eye cautery device. If a greater portion of the nail plate is involved, one can consider removing the entire nail to evaluate and repair the injury. Both pediatric and adult nail plates can easily be removed with spreading of scissors beneath the plate (Fig. 119.18). Repair should be performed with 5-0 or 6-0 fast-absorbing or plain gut suture under loupe magnification (if available), and the cleaned native nail (if available) or a piece of suture foil should be inserted below the eponychial fold to act as a stent for the new nail to grow.[21] Nail bed repair is often sufficient to reduce a distal tip or complete tuft fracture.

Fingertip soft tissue injuries range from simple to complex. Applying the principles of the reconstructive ladder or elevator can be useful in determining procedures appropriate for the injury and the patient. If there is no or minimal exposed bone or tendon, fingertip wounds can be dressed to heal by secondary intention. The use of a semiocclusive dressing, changed weekly, can minimize patient discomfort and provide an appropriate moist environment for wound healing.[23,24] In children, using an amputated or avascular part as a composite graft is also an option (Fig. 119.19). Skin grafting alone, including split and full-thickness grafts, can be used; however, this should be avoided in the volar finger pulp because these are insensate and can contract. If bone is exposed and/or the soft tissue wound is larger, flap

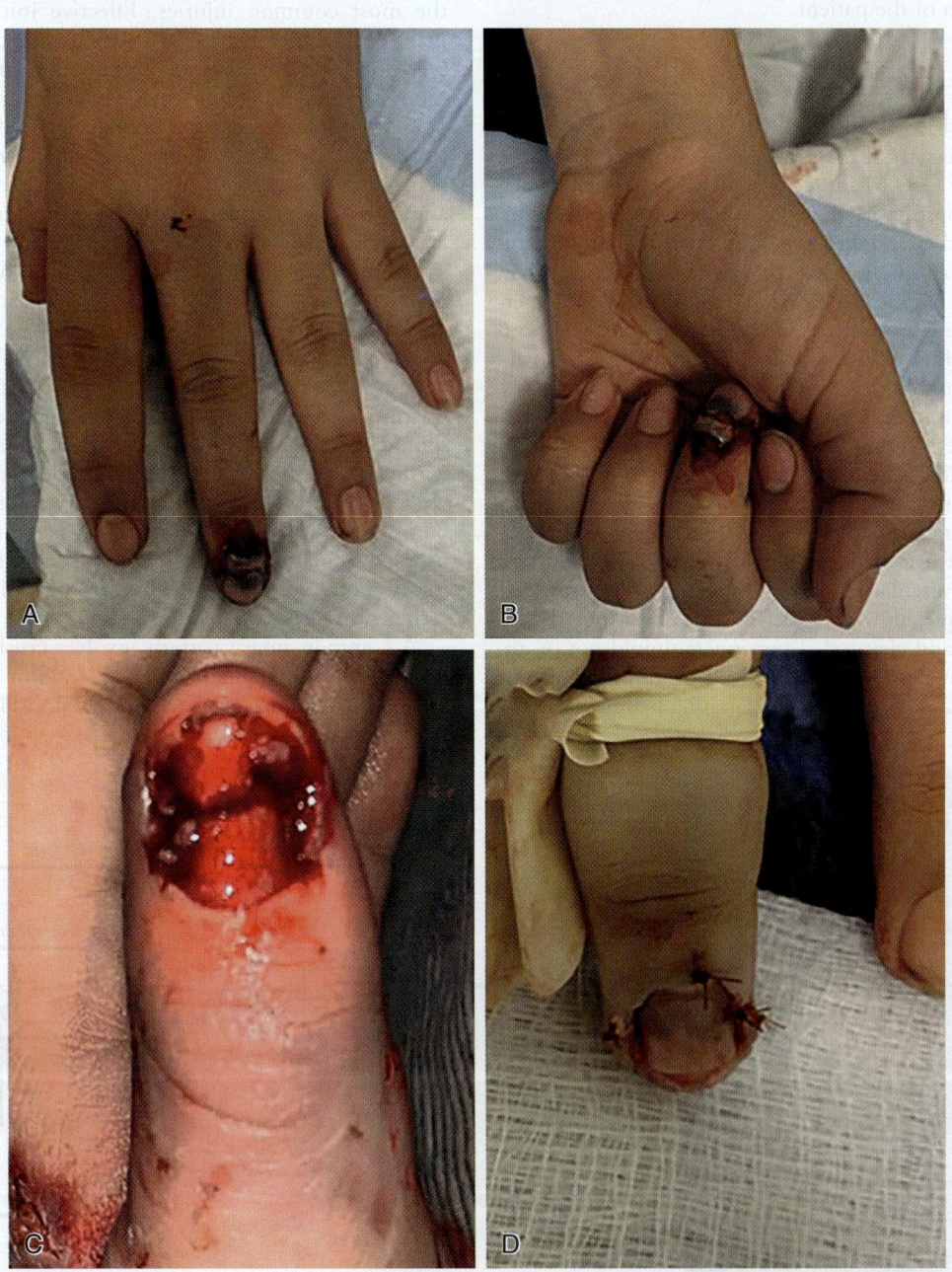

FIGURE 119.18 (A) Twelve-year-old patient with left middle finger crush injury with associated tuft fracture. (B) Examination revealed no tendon injury. (C) A different but representative patient with a sterile matrix laceration after nail plate removal. (D) After bedside repair with absorbable sutures and use of native nail plate as nail fold stent.

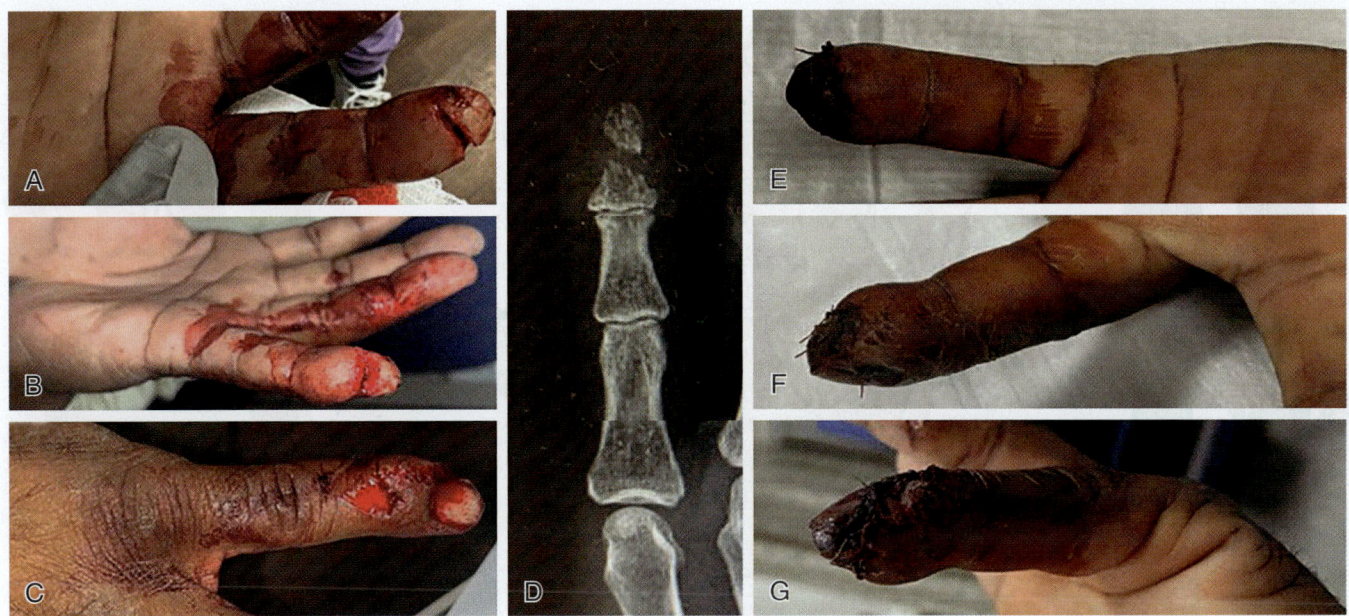

FIGURE 119.19 (A–G) Sixty-nine-year-old patient presenting with hatchet injury to left small finger resulting in near-complete amputation and transverse distal phalanx fracture. Patient did not desire replant; decision was made to use the dysvascular tip as a composite graft and repair laceration. One week postprocedure, there are some areas with healing; however, viability of fingertip is questionable, but digit remains out to length.

TABLE 119.5 Local Options for Flap Coverage of Finger Defects

FLAP NAME	COVERAGE OF…	DONOR SITE	BLOOD SUPPLY	FLAP TYPE/ MOVEMENT	PROS	CONS	FIGURE 20
Atasoy	Fingertip <1 cm	Distal volar pulp	Random pattern	V-Y advancement	Minimal donor morbidity, like with like	Small area of coverage, scar on volar pulp	A
Kutler	Fingertip <1 cm	Lateral fingertip	Random pattern	Bilateral V-Y advancement	Minimal donor morbidity, like with/ like	Small area of coverage, 2 flaps	B
Homodigital island	Middle → distal volar pulp	Same digit, skin around base of P1 and web space	Axial pattern— digital artery	Pedicled axial flap, proximal to distal	Full-thickness flap, excellent quality volar skin	Difficult dissection with nerve, long scar (tunnel of pedicle)	C
Thenar flap	Small or ring fingertip	Skin of thenar eminence	Random pattern	Delayed random pattern	Minimal donor morbidity, may be sensate	Recipient finger bent in position for 2–4 weeks, requires 2 surgeries	D
Moberg flap	Thumb tip	Volar thumb and thenar eminence	Bipedicle—thumb digital bundles	Axial advancement flap	Maintain as much length of thumb as possible, sensate, reliable	May have flexion contracture of thumb IP	E
Cross-finger flap	Middle or proximal phalanx volar skin	Dorsal skin/fascia of neighboring digit	Random pattern	Delayed random pattern	No sacrifice of volar skin, can cover large defects	Donor must be skin grafted, fingers must remain attached for 3–4 weeks (stiffness), 2 procedures	F
First dorsal metacarpal artery flap	Thumb volar surface	Skin over dorsal index finger (FDMA territory)	Axial- first dorsal metacar- pal artery	Pedicle flap	Reliable, customizable based on defect	Dorsal skin (not volar), do- nor may require skin graft	G

FDMA, First dorsal metacarpal artery; *IP,* interphalangeal.

coverage can be considered if the patient desires maximum length retention of the digit or if the injured digit is the thumb (Table 119.5). Fingertips may be covered with advancement flaps, such as Atasoy or Kutler (Fig. 119.20A–B). Larger or oblique volar defects may require coverage with a cross-finger flap with skin grafting of the dorsal donor site, or dorsal defects may be covered with a reverse cross-finger flap and full-thickness skin graft.[25] Axillary pattern flaps, such as homo- or heterodigital is-land flaps, may be used with less donor site morbidity, or first dorsal metacarpal artery flap may be used for thumb, index finger, or web-space coverage. Moberg advancement flap is useful for volar soft tissue defects of the thumb to preserve as much length

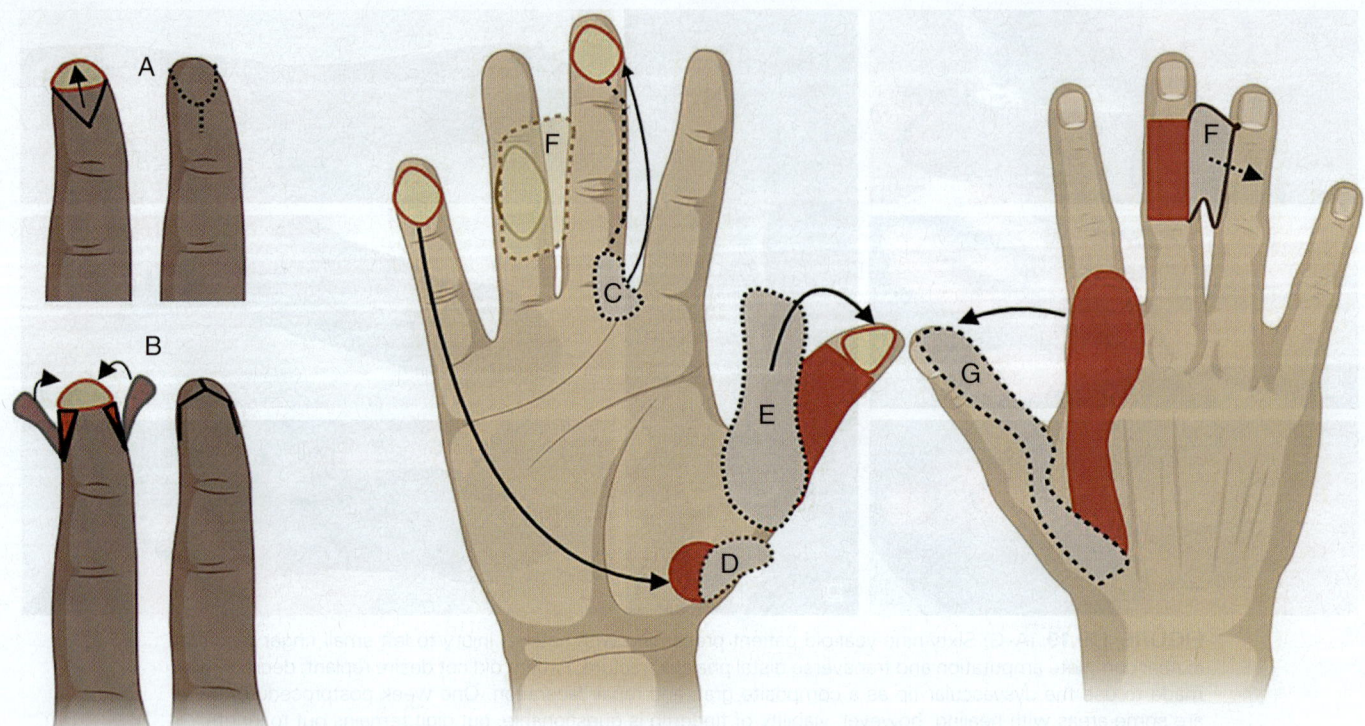

FIGURE 119.20 Local options for flap coverage of fingertip and other volar pulp defects. *A,* Atasoy flap; *B,* Kutler bilateral V-Y flaps; *C,* homodigital island flap; *D,* thenar flap; *E,* Moberg flap; *F,* cross-finger flap; *G,* first dorsal metacarpal artery flap. Please correlate with Table 119.5.

and therefore hand function as possible (see Fig. 119.20C–G). A thumb should never be primarily amputated at bedside unless traumatic amputation has already occurred.

If the fingertip has been slightly shortened by the trauma, the patient should be counseled that they may develop nail deformity if there is inadequate bony or soft tissue support, most commonly a hook deformity where the nail grows curved over the tip. If no coverage option is available or if the patient does not wish to undergo formal surgery, a revision of amputation with primary or secondary closure by trimming back exposed bone to obtain soft tissue coverage should be considered. If the injury is through the level of the lunula or proximal, the nail bed should be ablated by removing all sterile and germinal matrix (deep to the eponychial fold) to prevent horn nail deformity—small amounts of sharp nail plate protruding from the digit, which can be uncomfortable for the patient.[25]

Flexor Tendon Injuries

Flexor tendon function is very important to overall hand function, and injuries to this system have historically been complex due to the high force and balanced tension requirement.[26] The most common mechanism of flexor tendon injury is penetrating trauma or lacerations to the volar digits and hand.[15] Because of the volar position of the flexor tendons and proximity to the neurovascular bundle, there should be high suspicion of concomitant digital nerve or digital arterial injury. Visual inspection will reveal loss of flexion tone in the injured digit with resting position in extension and abnormal tenodesis.

Some general principles to adhere to for successful flexor tendon repair include adequate wound debridement, establishment of a solid multistrand core suture repair, and strict postoperative hand therapy regimen with early active range of motion when

appropriate.[15] Repairs should have no gaps, and there should be minimal additional bulk to the repair, including knots or suture throws that would limit tendon excursion through the flexor synovial sheath.[27]

A tendon consists of longitudinally oriented bundles of collagen, and although it has great tensile strength when intact, it can be difficult to suture with conventional techniques because of material ripping or pulling through.[28] Most commonly accepted methods involve locking or grasping stitches that loop around multiple collagen strands in order to gain a strong anchor point.[15] The distance of suture bites should optimally be between 0.7 and 1.0 cm away from the cut end of the tendon to prevent fraying or suture slippage. Mechanical testing has shown that at least four core strands are required for an early active range-of-motion protocol, and up to eight core strands will have a stronger initial repair but may be technically challenging. Several methods for core sutures have been developed and widely used, which are shown in Fig. 119.21.[15] Knot placement should be either within the repair or away from the repaired edge to minimize catching within the pulley system. Appropriate suture selection, such as a braided nylon or polyester material, typically 3-0 caliber if the tendon will permit, will ensure that the suture itself is durable and minimally inflammatory while maintaining appropriate force for strong, active finger flexion.[29] The tendon should be handled atraumatically by minimizing the number of grabs with forceps; using sharp stabilization, such as a 25-g needle anchored through skin and sheath, rather than crushing the tendon with forceps; and sharply trimming back damaged edges with good, sharp tenotomy scissors. Not all partial lacerations require repair; however, if partial lacerations are visualized within the already created wound bed on initial ED evaluation, wound exploration and formal debridement should be considered.[28] Unrepaired edges may lead to fraying or

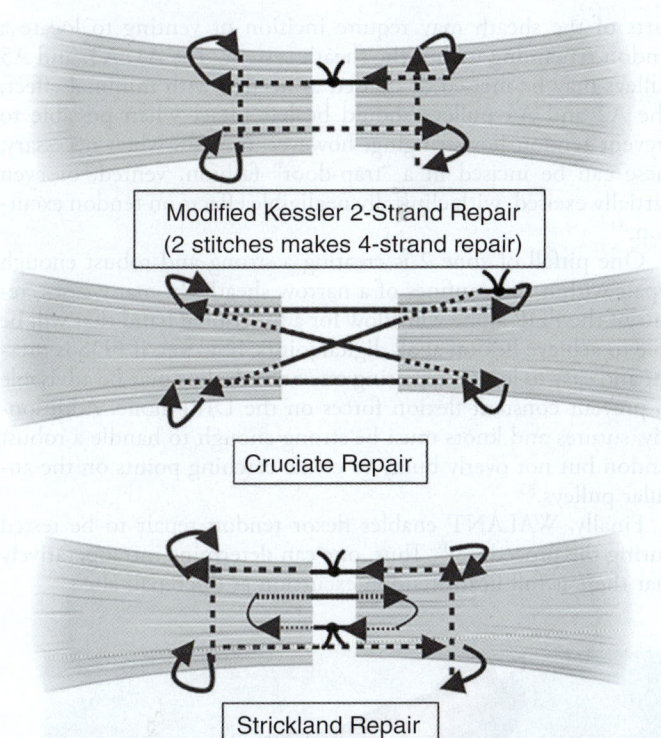

Modified Kessler 2-Strand Repair
(2 stitches makes 4-strand repair)

Cruciate Repair

Strickland Repair

FIGURE 119.21 Technique of core strand tendon repair. *Dashed lines* indicate suture in the substance of the tendon; *solid line* shows grasping loop around portion of the tendon. Start at the knot and follow the direction of the *arrows*.

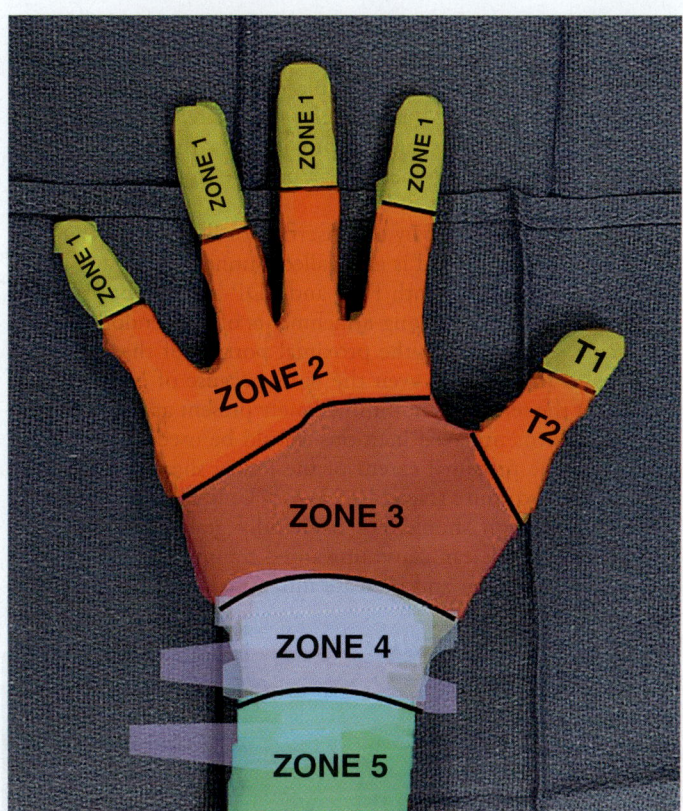

FIGURE 119.22 Zones of flexor tendon injury.

inflammation that causes nodule formation or triggering, or the partial laceration may propagate along the flexor tendon.

The patient and the situation should be considered in the decision for timing and type of tendon repair. Primary repair can be delayed up to 7 to 14 days because the tendon continues to receive nutrition from the synovial fluid and paratenon; however, there are certain injuries, such as zone 1 tendon avulsion, that result in disruption to the tendon blood supply, or vincula, and require more urgent repair. After 14 days, scarring and contracture of the tendons proximally may result in unacceptable levels of tension on the repair, and secondary repair with tendon grafting and/or multistage repair with silicone rod placement as spacers within the pulley system may be required for reconstruction.[15,30] Injuries with certain features, including extensive crush mechanism, loss of soft tissue coverage or pulley system, tendon loss of greater than 1 cm, or contaminated injuries, may not be candidates for primary repair. A failed or ruptured primary repair may be able to be re-repaired if diagnosed expeditiously. Patient factors and compliance are important to consider with this type of injury because postoperative therapy regimens can be very intensive. Patients who are unable to participate in therapy may develop painful contractures or tendon adhesions, which may compromise hand function without proper adherence to postoperative care.[16]

Flexor tendon injuries are divided into five zones (Fig. 119.22). In zones 1, 2, and 4, each tendon is surrounded by a synovial sheath and contained within a semirigid fibro-osseous canal, either the flexor tendon sheath of the digit or the carpal tunnel. In the zones 3 and 5, the flexor tendons are surrounded by loose areolar (paratenon) tissue. Tendon zones to the thumb are T1 through T3.

Zone 1 injuries occur distal to the insertion of FDS on the middle phalanx, so only FDP is injured. Closed avulsion injuries in this region are common and often termed *jersey finger* because the mechanism is often forced extension of the DIPJ in a flexed digit, such as occurs in sports if a player attempts to grab another's jersey. The primary blood supply in this region is tenuous and mainly derives from the vincula, thin connective tissue containing blood vessels that originate at the volar plates. If completely disrupted, this can lead to avascular necrosis of the tendon and result in suboptimal healing. The Leddy-Packer classification system for zone 1 flexor injuries lists four categories of injury, from most to least urgent (Table 119.6).[15] Sharp injuries can also occur in this zone and are not considered in this classification system.[31]

Repair of zone 1 injuries depends on the length of distal stump available. If there is greater than or equal to 1 cm, primary tendon coaptation with core sutures is a viable option; however, if there is less remaining at the insertion, core sutures will be unlikely to appropriately grasp/lock, and the tendon will need to be reinserted

TABLE 119.6 Leddy-Packer Classification System for Zone 1 Flexor Tendon Injuries

LEDDY-PACKER GRADE	LEVEL OF RETRACTION	VINCULA DISRUPTED?	BONE FRAGMENT?
1	Palm	Yes	No
2	A2 pulley	No	Small
3	A4 pulley or no retraction	No	Large
4	Palm	Yes	Large

into the distal phalanx.[32] This can be performed with suture anchors directly drilled into bone or using pull-through suture methods in which a core suture is placed into the tendon and the free suture ends are tied around the nail plate. Care should be taken to avoid placing sutures proximal to the lunula of the nail or through the germinal matrix because this can lead to nail deformity.

Zone 2 is demarcated by the insertion of FDS distally and the A1 pulley proximally and is also called Bunnel's "no man's land." In this anatomic zone, both FDS and FDP are susceptible to injury, and there are no strong attachments of the tendon to bone or vincula, often causing the proximal portion of the tendon to retract into the palm or even the wrist because of high levels of tension. If the tendon is not immediately present at the laceration site, Brunner or midaxial incisions should be used to extend the incision to the proximal extent of the pulley sheath as necessary for adequate exposure (Fig. 119.23).[15,33] Unless the end is clearly visible, the tendon should not be blindly grabbed through the sheath because this can cause unwanted trauma and increase the gap of usable tendon and increase inflammation postoperatively.

Parts of the sheath may require incision or venting to locate a tendon remaining within the sheath system. The A1, A3, and A5 pulleys may be incised or excised as needed with minimal effect. The A2 and A4 pulleys should be left intact when possible to prevent tendon bowstringing; however, in cases when necessary, these can be incised in a "trap-door" fashion, vented, or even partially excised, with clinically negligible effects on tendon excursion.[34]

One pitfall of zone 2 is creating a strong and robust enough repair within the confines of a narrow sheath. In many cases, repair of the FDP alone will allow for a functional hand that will be able to achieve flexion at all digital joints; however, if FDS is present and easy to locate, repairing one or both slips may be advisable to prevent constant flexion forces on the DIPJ alone. Additionally, sutures and knots must be strong enough to handle a robust tendon but not overly bulky to create catching points on the annular pulleys.[35]

Finally, WALANT enables flexor tendon repair to be tested during the procedure.[10] Thus, one can determine intraoperatively that there is full flexor tendon excursion at the repair site.

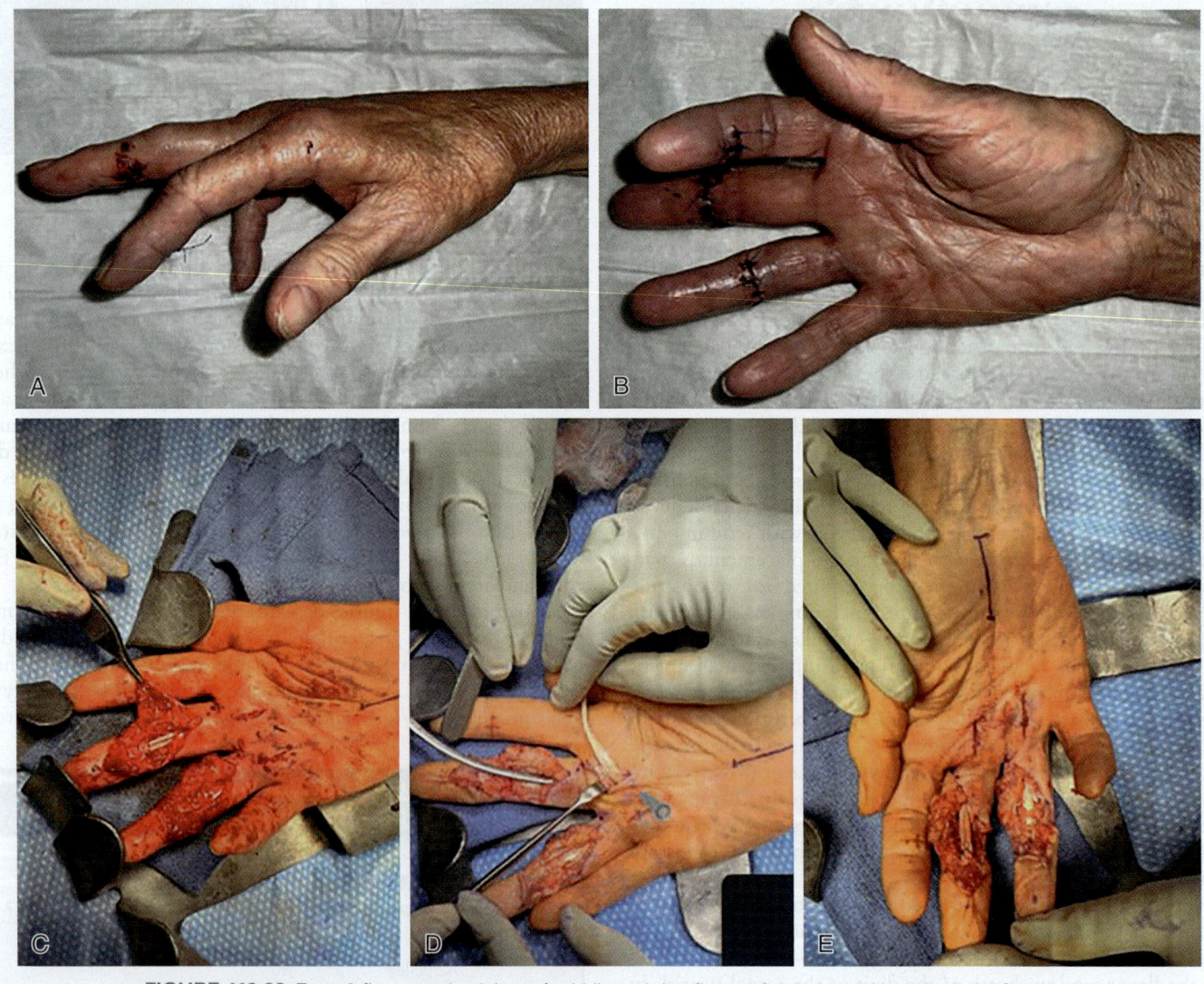

FIGURE 119.23 Zone 2 flexor tendon injury of middle and ring finger of right hand. Note the lack of resting flexion tone on examination (A–B). Patient underwent bedside laceration closure and operative exploration 5 days later, which revealed zone 2 flexor digitorum superficialis–only injury (C) with tendon retracted to the level of the palm (D) and tendon in situ after repair (E).

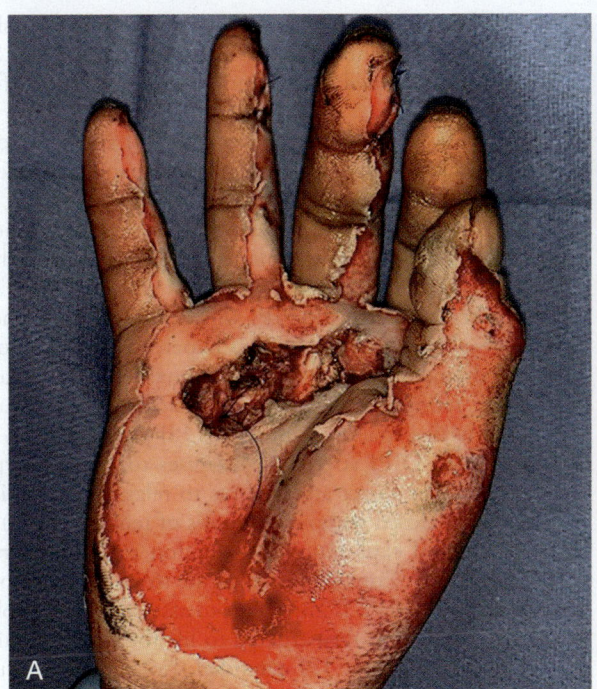
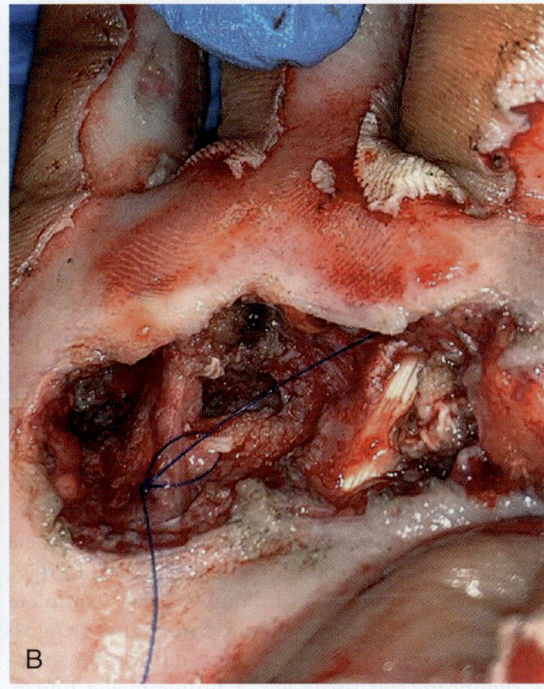

FIGURE 119.24 (A–B) Motorcycle collision resulting in extensive friction burns to the volar hand and soft tissue loss over flexor zone 3. Intraoperative examination revealed multiple-digit flexor digitorum superficialis and partial flexor digitorum profundus lacerations, nerve injuries to ulnar middle finger and radial/ulnar bundles of ring finger, and damage to common digital vessel to ring finger.

Zone 3 injuries occur in the palm and are typically not as prone to retraction as zone 2 injuries.[33] There is no synovial sheath at this level, and one must be wary of the superficial palmar arch (Fig. 119.24). In zone 4, or the carpal tunnel, there are nine tendons plus the median nerve and radial artery that are running through a small space, and multiple structures may be lacerated. Knowledge of anatomy is important, and the tendons typically lie in the configuration of FDS to ring and middle fingers volar to small and index, respectively, FDP linearly along the carpal bones, and FPL in a separate bursa radial to the median nerve. In zone V, flexor muscle bellies may be involved, and multiple figure-of-eight sutures will be required to repair the muscles in order to prevent ripping the sutures through. This zone has a poor prognosis due to muscle fibrosis and scarring, which limits flexor function and excursion.

Extensor Tendon Injuries

The extensor tendons have a complicated insertion distally, with multiple slips and expansions forming the extensor hood.[1] This allows intricate and independent extension of each joint while other joints are in various degrees of flexion; however, it also makes the tendons susceptible to closed and open injury because of their superficial position and thin nature distally. The extensor tendon system is divided into nine zones of injury from distal to proximal, where odd numbers overlie joints starting at the DIPJ and even numbers correspond to injuries over long bones (Fig. 119.25).[36] Extensor tendons are more amenable to bedside repair because they are unlikely to retract and require less tensile strength than flexors. It is important to understand the anatomy in each zone of injury because it will allow identification of the damaged structures as well as choice of proper suture and repair technique.[37] The more distal zones 1 to 3 over the

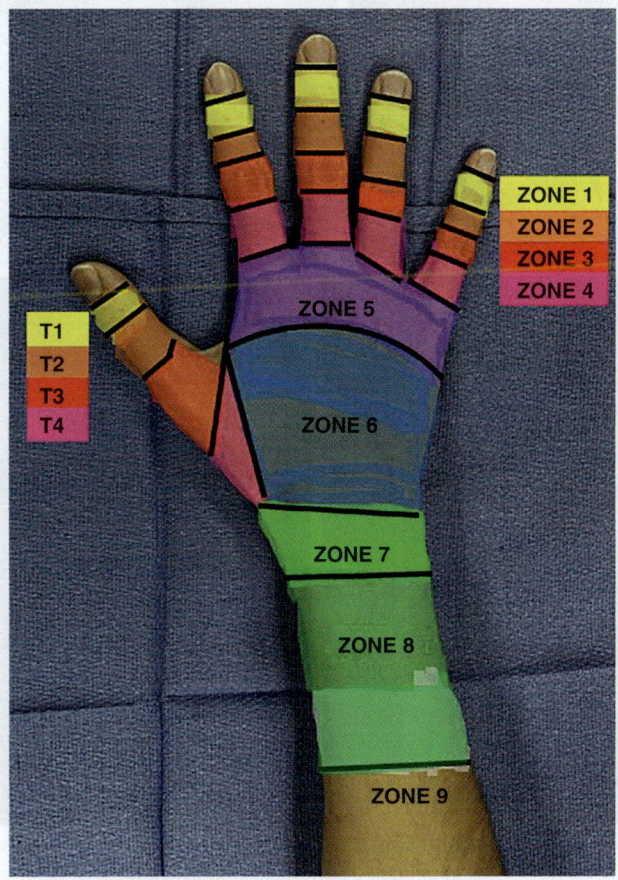

FIGURE 119.25 Zones of extensor tendon injury.

fingers are usually too thin to attempt core suture repair, and a figure-of-eight, running, or cross-stitch repair is usually sufficient, whereas more proximally, the tendons become thicker and are thus able to accommodate two- to four-core strand repairs. As a general principle, open injuries should be treated with thorough washout, debridement, and prompt administration of antibiotics. All lacerations of 50% of the tendon or more should be repaired to minimize risk of propagation of the injury and restore function; <50% may be treated conservatively and allowed early active motion.

Zone 1 injuries are termed *mallet finger* and are injuries to the terminal tendon insertion at the DIPJ. They most commonly result from closed injuries in which rapid forced DIPJ flexion occurs against resistance, such as "snagging" the finger on an item. Open injuries with lacerations or crush injuries may occur, and mallet fractures can occur with a bony avulsion fragment being pulled proximally by the retained terminal tendon (Fig. 119.26). Closed injuries may be treated with either 6 weeks of DIPJ splinting in extension or with Kirschner wire (K-wire) fixation of the DIPJ in extension, based on patient preference.[36] Bony mallets with volar subluxation or >50% of joint surface involved in fragment should be treated operatively with bony fixation. Complete avulsion of the terminal tendon may require suture anchoring to the distal phalanx or tendon grafting, transfer, and/or reconstruction if there is significant soft tissue loss. Chronic mallet fingers that are untreated can result in a swan-neck deformity, in which the DIPJ is flexed and the PIPJ is hyperextended.

Zone 2 injuries most often occur as a result of sharp lacerations and have the potential to injure the underlying triangular ligament or the lateral bands (or both). These should be washed out and repaired with running or finger trap pattern sutures. Static splinting is recommended in addition to local wound care for associated laceration.

Injuries to zone 3 occur over the PIPJ and cause disruption of the central slip and possibly the lateral bands of the extensor tendon, which extends the PIPJ. Central slip injury can be evaluated using Elson's test (see Video 119.5). A typical mechanism of closed injury is blunt trauma to the dorsal digit or dislocation of the PIPJ. Unrepaired zone 3 injuries will result in a boutonnière deformity, in which the PIPJ will be unable to extend and therefore flexed, whereas the DIPJ is hyperextended due to maintained and tightened insertion of the terminal tendon, lateral bands, and oblique retinacular ligament.[37,38] Closed, acute injuries may be treated with a trial of splinting the PIPJ in extension, with aggressive passive DIPJ stretching exercises to prevent hyperextension and allow the intact attachments to relax. Subacute injuries (e.g., lacerations closed without diagnosis of tendon injury) typically require surgical exploration and tendon repair if there is residual extensor lag.[39] Zone 3 injuries in the thumb may involve the EPL, EPB, or both. EPL is important to assess with the tabletop test, in which the patient is instructed to lift the thumb straight up off a flat surface with the IPJ extended. Isolated EPB injury may not require repair because EPL can compensate. Core sutures of 4-0 Prolene may be able to be placed at this level.[36]

Over the proximal phalanx in zone 4, the extensor tendons are more robust and typically thick enough to accommodate a 4-0 Prolene core suture. These injuries are typically related to proximal

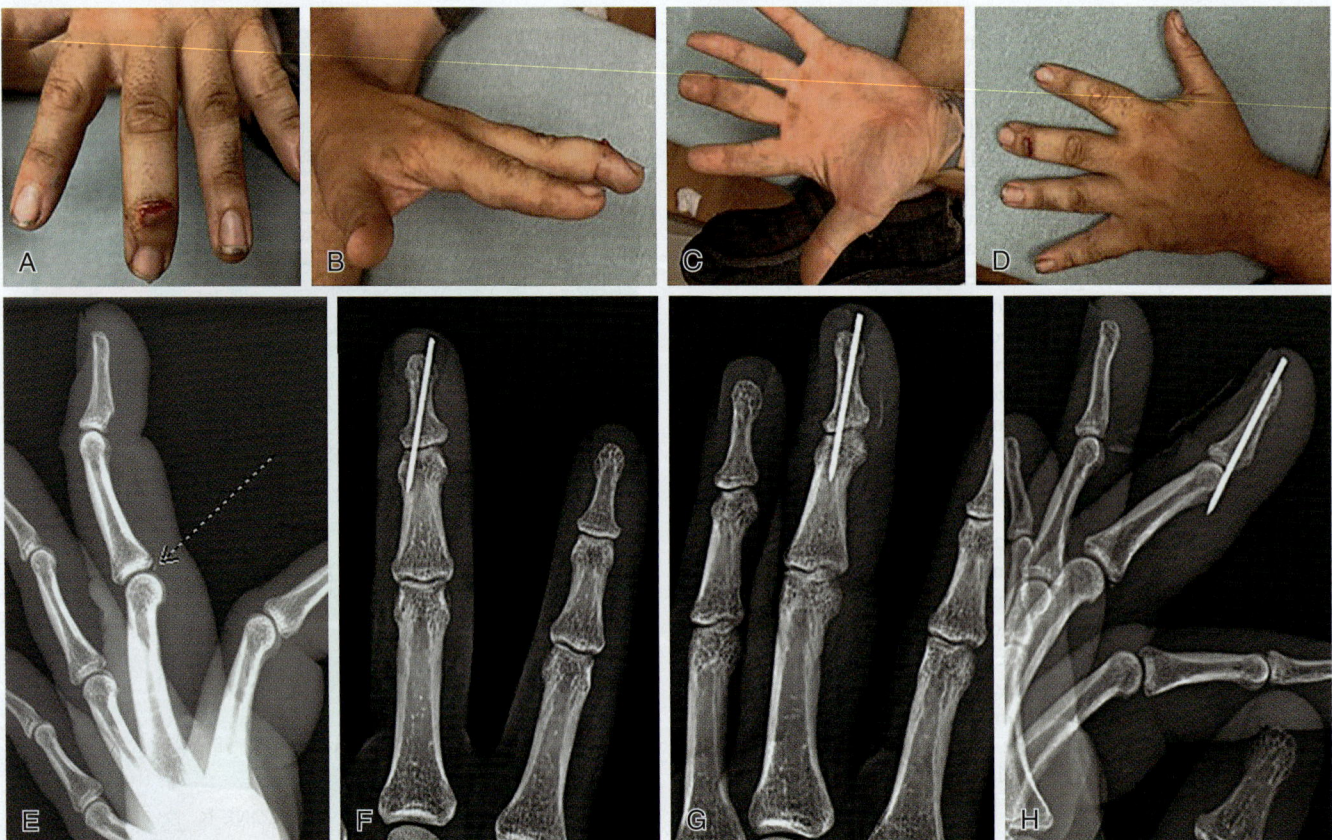

FIGURE 119.26 Laceration over left middle finger distal interphalangeal joint resulting in open zone 1 extensor laceration (A–D). Associated volar base of distal phalanx avulsion fracture without flexor injury (E). Patient underwent extension pinning for 6 weeks (F–H).

phalanx fractures, and many are partial lacerations that may not require repair. If repair is required, patients should be started on early active range-of-motion protocols.[38]

Zone 5 injuries occur over the MCPJ, and a common cause of injury is a human bite from a closed fist punch to the mouth. These injuries are always contaminated and typically involve the joint, so it is imperative to thoroughly irrigate and administer antibiotics. At this level, vulnerable structures include the main body of the extensor tendons as well as the sagittal bands, which are thin ligamentous structures that hold the tendon centrally over the base of the proximal phalanx and head of the metacarpal, then loop around the bones to insert on the volar plate. Injury to these structures may result in subluxation of the tendon during flexion, typically in the ulnar direction. Clean injuries can be repaired immediately (Fig. 119.27); however, contaminated or "fight bite" injuries should be left open or loosely approximated over Penrose to allow any infection to clear. Tendon repair or repair of the sagittal bands can occur in a delayed fashion.[36]

Sharp trauma to the dorsum of the hand may result in zone 6 extensor injury. At this level, strong juncturae tendinum between the individual tendons prevents retraction and may even present with preserved function, especially in the ring and middle fingers. These injuries usually have a favorable prognosis and are easy to access and repair with 3-0 caliber core sutures. Early active range of motion or range-of-motion splinting may be employed after repair.

Injuries to the wrist, zone 7, can be complex, similar to zone 4 flexor tendon injuries. All of the finger extensors, thumb extensors, and wrist extensors may be involved in the injury, and anatomic matching is important when multiple structures are involved. At this level, the tendons may retract through the extensor retinaculum, and counterincisions in the forearm may be required to retrieve the proximal stump. These should be repaired with 3-0 core sutures and 5-0 epitendinous suture, and treatment will involve splinting in mild extension with transition to early active motion.[36]

Zone 8 and 9 injuries are proximal enough to involve the musculotendinous junction and muscle bellies in the distal and proximal forearm, respectively. These often have suboptimal outcomes because of the difficulty of anchoring to the muscle fibers, and if muscle is ischemic or denervated, these may require tendon transfers at a later date to restore function.[36]

Nerve Injuries

Nerve injuries can be devastating for upper extremity function, and it takes an astute clinician to recognize patterns of nerve injury and enact proper diagnosis and management. The Sunderland and MacKinnon classification,[40,41] the most widely used classification, describes six types of nerve injury: neurapraxia (grade I), axonotmesis (grades II to IV), and neurotmesis (grade V) (Table 119.7). Neurapraxia can be thought of as a myelin-only injury, in which there is inhibited conduction without anatomic destruction of nerve fibers. This might occur with a closed injury with associated traction, such as a fracture or dislocation, or as an iatrogenic injury via surgical retraction or prolonged tourniquet use. Most patients can expect a full recovery, but it may take up to 3 to 4 months. Grade II injuries result in discontinuity at the level of the endoneurium. Grade III injuries result in axonotmesis with greater damage to the surrounding membranes, and Grade IV injuries result in complete disruption of all axonal structures within an intact endoneurium only. These types of injuries have less favorable prognoses and may result in neuroma in continuity if axons become disoriented. Grade V injuries are complete disruptions of the nerve (neurotmesis) by transection or avulsion injury.[40] MacKinnon described grade VI injuries as involving multiple grades of injury within the same area of the nerve.[41]

Nerves initially regenerate at the rapid rate of 1 mm per day; however, after initial healing, there may be variable rates in progression depending on the perineural environment, patient factors such as age or blood-flow–limiting comorbidities, or inhibiting fibrosis or other scar formation.[42,43] Initially, nerve injury will result in motor weakness, paresthesias, and decreased sympathetic functions. Notation of a loss of sympathetic tone (dryness, lack of pilomotor response) or color change in a nonvascular pattern, paresthesias and loss of sensation, and motor deficits on strength testing are important for documentation and must be carefully teased out from other factors, such as fracture or dislocations causing movement limited by pain, tendon injury, or vascular injury. Nerve conduction studies are not immediately helpful but become valuable 3 weeks after injury, when fibrillation and denervation potentials can be measured. Nerve conduction studies can also be useful in measuring level of reinnervation and monitoring progress of reinnervation.[44]

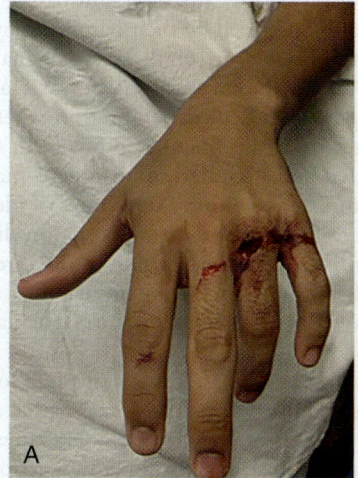 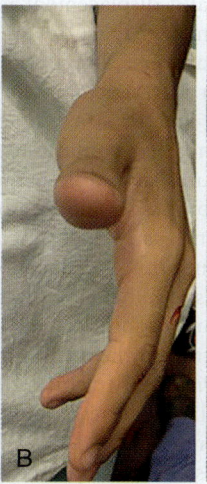 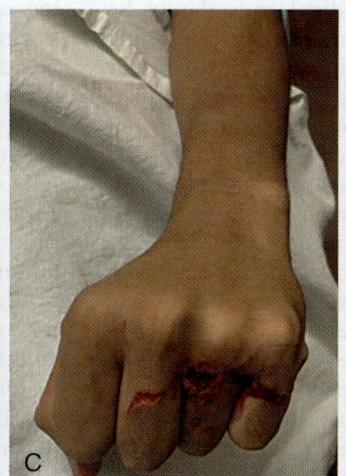 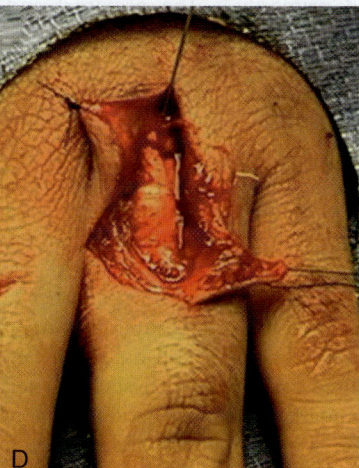

FIGURE 119.27 (A–C) Laceration over the ring finger metacarpophalangeal joint (MCPJ) with associated extensor lag of ring finger at MCPJ. (D) Patient underwent bedside wound exploration and repair of zone 5 complete extensor laceration.

TABLE 119.7	Sunderland MacKinnon Classification System			
SUNDERLAND GRADE	SEDDON CLASS	STRUCTURES INJURED	WALLERIAN DEGENERATION?	TREATMENT
I	Neurapraxia	Segmental Demyelination	No	Typically spontaneous recovery
II	Axonotmesis	Axon injured with preserved endoneurium, perineurium, epineurium	Yes	Often recovers spontaneously, prolonged time period
III	Axonotmesis	Axon and endoneurium injured, intact perineurium and epineurium	Yes	Unlikely to recover, may require surgery
IV	Axonotmesis	Axon, endoneurium, perineurium injured, only epineurium remains in tact	Yes	No spontaneous recovery, likely to form neuroma in continuity, requires excision + grafting
V	Neurotmesis	Nerve completely transected	Yes	No chance of recovery without surgery for reapproximation
VI	Mixed nerve injury	Mixed picture, more typical with crush or compression injuries	Some	Requires close clinical and EMG or NCV monitoring to guide decisions

EMG, Electromyography; *NCV,* nerve conduction velocity.

Primary nerve repair should be undertaken in a controlled, non-emergent manner and does not need to occur on the day of injury unless there are other emergent reasons to operate. Primary repair can be performed within 72 hours; however, if clinical examination is confounding, evidence reports good outcomes up to 3 weeks after injury, which allows time for some edema to resolve and other concomitant injuries to stabilize. Delayed primary repair at 1 to 6 months can be accomplished with relatively high expectations of return to clinical function, which can be useful to allow grades II to IV injuries to fully declare their extent before surgical intervention.[43] It is important to consider the window of timing repair in the context of end-organ atrophy, especially motor neurons. Repairs between 9 and 18 months show markedly less regeneration compared with earlier repairs, and repairs after 18 months generally are only performed for sensation or pain management because target muscles have often become atrophic and fibrotic beyond repair.

Primary nerve repair is the preferred technique because of superior outcomes in return of function if this can be accomplished.[45] It is recommended in sharp injuries with minimal contamination. Techniques for optimization of repair include mobilization of cut ends so that there is no tension on the repair because tension will lead to dehiscence or traction-type injury. Nerve gaps >1 cm typically cannot be mobilized enough to be repaired primarily.[46] The proximal and distal ends should be sharply debrided back to healthy-appearing fascicles using only very sharp instruments. Nerve ends should be handled without trauma and favor forceps grasping the epineurium rather than fascicles to avoid crush injury.[45] Using magnification, epineural suturing with 8-0 to 10-0 (depending on nerve caliber) for fascicle realignment and nerve approximation remains the most effective method of repair per the literature.[47] Fibrin glue has been used to augment repair. Nerve cuffs or nerve wraps theoretically prevent exposure of escaping axons from the site of repair and may help lower the suture burden; however, they have not been definitively demonstrated to provide superior outcomes.[48]

Injuries resulting in soft tissue and nerve loss will not be able to be repaired primarily. In these cases, nerve autograft remains the gold standard for reconstruction.[45,49,50] Most common donors include sensory-only peripheral nerves, such as the sural in the leg for large-diameter nerves, or terminal sensory branches encountered in the upper extremity within the same wound, such as the PIN innervating the wrist joint. Bioabsorbable nerve conduits and cadaver nerve allografts can be used in place of autograft to reconstruct

defects, most commonly up to 2 cm in the literature. Both are acellular but form a directional matrix thought to both harbor directional neurotrophic factors and provide a directing scaffold for regenerating axons. Commercially available polyglycolic acid tubes, bovine collagen scaffolds, and decellularized human nerve allografts are all acceptable options, and the literature has not shown superiority of any individual material for reconstruction of small peripheral nerves with appropriate size matching.[45,49-52]

Fractures and Dislocations

Pain, swelling, limited motion, ecchymosis, and deformities suggest the presence of a fracture or dislocation. Plain radiographs (AP, oblique, lateral) should be done as part of the primary examination. Some intraarticular fractures may require advanced imaging, such as CT without contrast.[3] Postreduction films should be obtained in the splint or cast to evaluate quality and stability of reduction.

Standard language is used to describe fractures. Classification includes displaced versus nondisplaced. Nondisplaced fractures are in anatomic alignment and do not require reduction but may still require immobilization in order to prevent deformation. Fractures may also be angulated, rotated, or comminuted. Comminuted fractures result in more than two fragments. Angulation is described by the direction in which the apex of the fracture is pointing, and displacement is described by the direction of the distal fragment.[53] Fractures are also described by their pattern; they may be transverse, longitudinal, oblique, or spiral. Fractures may also occur intraarticularly, or within the joint capsule, or extraarticularly. Fractures may be open or closed, depending on whether a wound that communicates with the fracture is involved. Open fractures should be irrigated and debrided in an urgent manner. Antibiotics should be administered within 90 minutes of identification of any open fracture to minimize risk of osteomyelitis or nonunion.[54] A dislocation is described according to the direction of displacement of the distal bone in the involved joint, and a fracture dislocation involves a fracture fragment intraarticularly in addition to the dislocation.

Displaced fractures or dislocations are repositioned as soon as possible to decrease soft tissue injury, decompress nerves that might be stretched, and relieve kinking of blood vessels. Fractures may have stable patterns, in which displaced fractures or dislocations are repositioned as soon as possible, or may be unstable, in which bedside reduction, despite the best attempts, will be unlikely to result in improvement without fixation.[53] Indications for surgery include

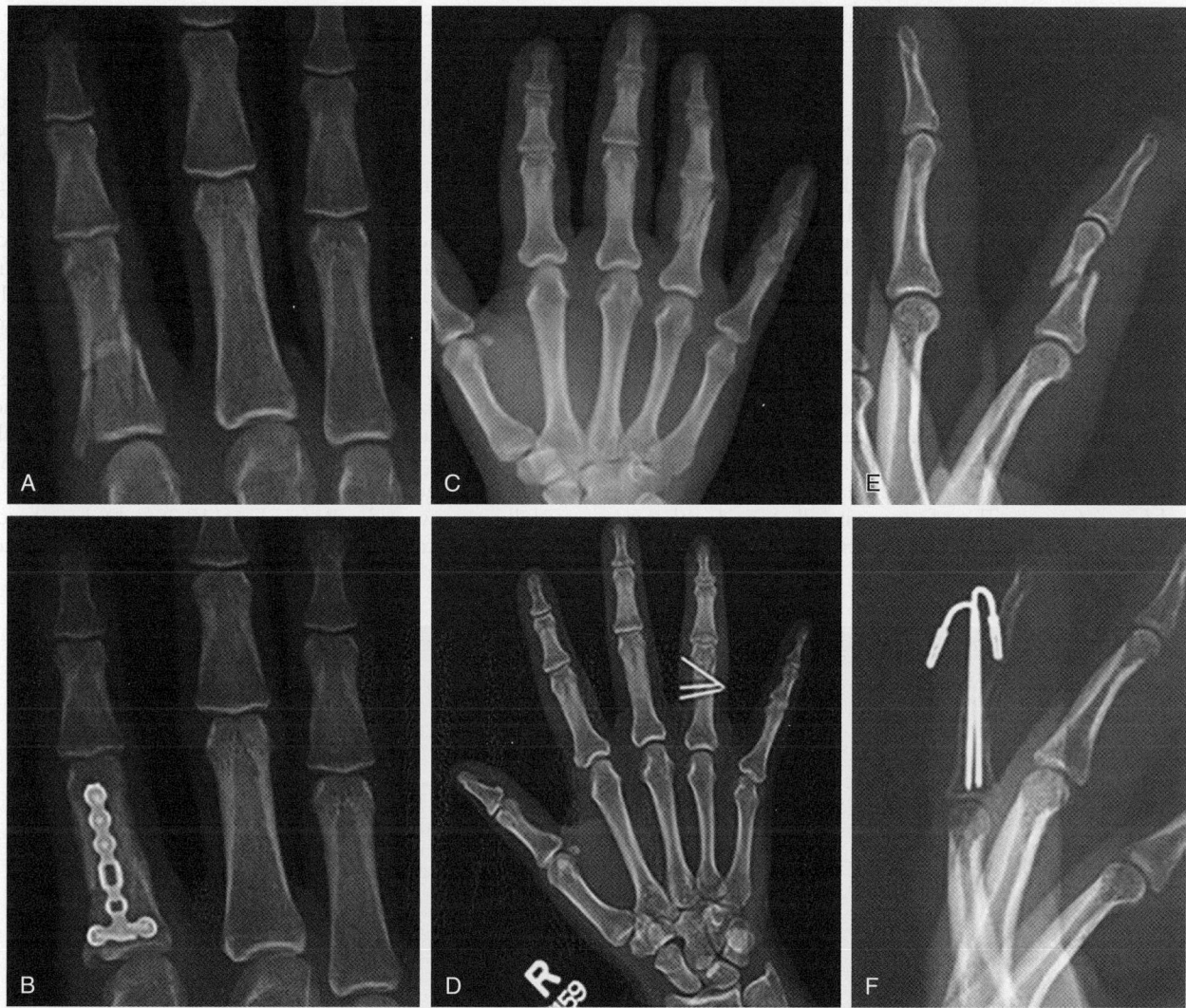

FIGURE 119.28 Methods of middle and proximal phalanx fracture fixation. Comminuted intraarticular fracture of index finger proximal phalanx, fixation with open reduction, and placement of permanent T-plate (A–B). Long oblique fracture of ring finger proximal phalanx treated with transverse Kirschner wires (K-wires) (C–D). Short oblique dorsally displaced fracture of small finger middle phalanx with intramedullary K-wire fixation (E–F).

inability to obtain and maintain acceptable reduction, open fractures, or significant bone loss that requires bone grafting.

Bone healing occurs either by primary or secondary mechanisms. In primary bone healing, rigid and stable fixation must be present for coapted bone edge to heal by direct matrix repair and osteogenesis. In secondary bone healing, micromotion is allowed by immobilization or K-wires, and callous matrix is laid down, which later undergoes enchondral ossification.[53,55] Desire for rigid, anatomic internal fixation must be balanced by postoperative concerns for stiffness or contracture formation. In the fingers, especially, tight anatomic space, multitude of important longitudinal structures, and need for disruption of important soft tissue landmarks for placement of plates or screws may cause more burden, including adhesion or scar formation, tendon attrition or rupture, or unforgiving stiffness at the IPJs. Thus, less invasive methods such as splinting, buddy taping, or K-wire fixation may be more appropriate and result in superior functional outcomes despite a less anatomic-appearing healed fracture or even a functional malunion.[55,56] Patient factors, such as level of demand of lifestyle and expected participation in therapy, can also be factored into selection of fixation method and/or nonoperative management.

Middle Phalanx and Proximal Phalanx Fractures

Distal phalanx fractures are covered in the fingertip injuries section, but briefly, tuft or tip fracture is typically comminuted and usually reduced by nail plate splinting. Avulsion injuries can also occur, as discussed in the flexor and extensor tendon injuries sections. Middle and proximal phalanx fractures are common from both athletic and industry mechanisms. Fractures of the phalangeal head or base are intraarticular and may involve the condyles or insertion of the collateral ligaments. Shaft fractures of the middle phalanx are likely to be volarly angulated if distal to the FDS insertion and dorsally angulated if proximal to the FDS insertion. Proximal phalanx shaft fractures tend to displace with dorsal angulation due to the insertion of the interosseous muscles at the base.[53]

Nondisplaced and minimally displaced fractures may be treated as noninvasively as possible with buddy taping or a short course of immobilization. If clinically significant malrotation or angulation is present, percutaneous methods such as K-wire fixation or headless compression screws can be used to minimize soft tissue disruption and tendon adhesions (Fig. 119.28). For comminuted or intraarticular fractures, open reduction internal fixation (ORIF) may be required. There are plating systems tailored to dorsal, volar, and midaxial approaches, without consensus on the best approach (see Fig. 119.28A–B).[57-61]

Metacarpal Fractures

Metacarpal fractures are common and result from mechanisms such as axial force to the metacarpal head (a punch to a solid object), direct blow to the hand, or torquing or rotational forces on the hand.[53] Fractures of the metacarpal can occur at the head, neck, shaft, or base. Border digits are more often injured due to prominence. The CMCJs of the fingers have varying degrees of freedom, with significant movement at the small finger and increasing rigidity more radially, resulting in more tolerance for fracture displacement or angulation in the small and ring fingers than the middle or index.

Fractures of the head are rare but involve the articular surface of the MCPJ and should be treated operatively if there is >25% of joint surface involved or step-off >1 mm. Metacarpal neck fractures are very common, especially in the small and ring fingers, and are termed *boxer's fractures*. These fractures usually have dorsal apex angulation with volar displacement and shortening of the metacarpal

head. These fractures in the small and ring fingers are usually treated nonoperatively, and even angulation up to 70 degrees may be well tolerated. Index and middle fingers, however, can tolerate only 10 to 20 degrees of dorsal angulation.[62] A typical closed reduction maneuver is called the *Jahss maneuver*, in which the IPJs are flexed 90 degrees and upward pressure is applied to the metacarpal head while volarly directed pressure is applied to the area of fracture itself. Shaft fractures are typically classified by morphology, including transverse, oblique (short or long), and longitudinal or comminuted. Shaft fractures have a similar morphology to neck fracture; however, oblique or spiral fractures are unlikely to be stabilized by closed reduction. Base fractures may involve CMCJ dislocation or may be intraarticular, requiring fixation.

Many metacarpal fractures can be treated nonoperatively with short immobilization or buddy taping.[56] General indications for operation include malrotation, angulation, or intraarticular displacement. Percutaneous insertion of K-wires (Fig. 119.29A–B), in multiple configurations, has been shown to be successful.[57] Intramedullary screws and nails (see Fig. 119.29C–D) have become increasingly popular because of minimal soft tissue dissection and

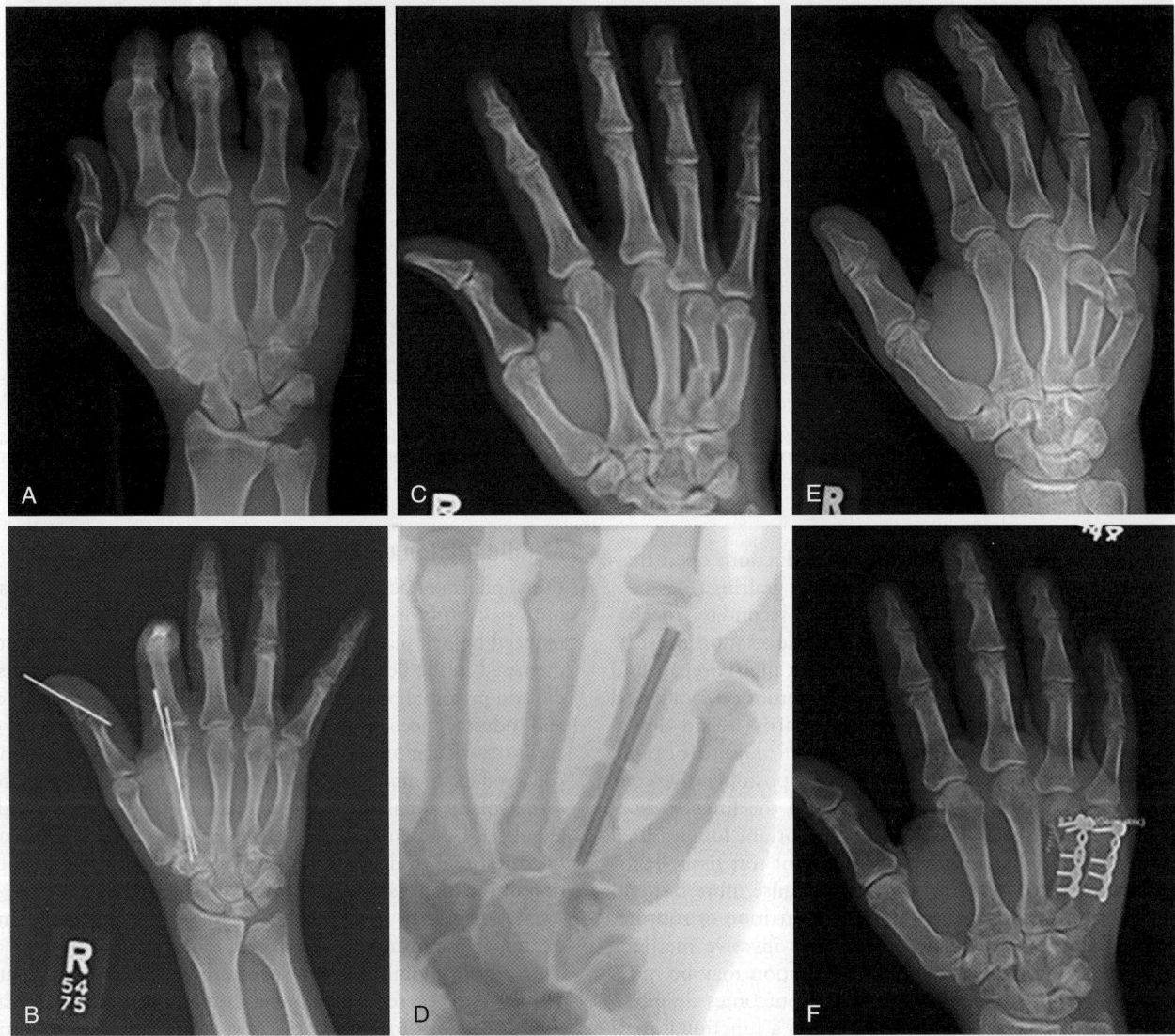

FIGURE 119.29 Various methods of metacarpal fracture fixation. Fixation of a comminuted index finger neck fracture with Kirschner wires (A–B), transverse ring finger shaft fracture compressed with intramedullary nail (C–D), and small and ring finger angulated neck fractures reduced with T-plates and bicortical screws (E–F).

earlier return to work.[55] Lag compression screws are particularly useful for long oblique fractures and provide appropriate support to the fragments with less hardware burden. Comminuted fractures may require a bridging construct, which can be placed via dorsal approach to minimize damage to vital neurovascular structures (Fig. 119.29E–F).[63] Because of their large size relative to the phalanges, plate and screw fixation can be technically less demanding.

The thumb metacarpal shows some differences in fracture patterns. Fractures of the metacarpal head and neck are very rare, whereas fractures of the shaft and extraarticular base fractures are typically amenable to closed reduction and nonoperative techniques

because of their stable, typically transverse nature. These should be immobilized with a thumb spica splint in an abducted position to prevent first web-space contracture.

Intraarticular fractures of the thumb metacarpal base can be classified into two-fragment, oblique intraarticular fractures, or Bennet fractures (Fig. 119.30),[64] and comminuted fractures, or Rolando fractures. The anatomy of the fracture causes a classic displacement pattern of dorsal, proximal, and radial due to the pull of still-attached APL to the major fracture fragment. Bennet fractures are difficult to treat with closed reduction and typically respond better to operative intervention. This can be

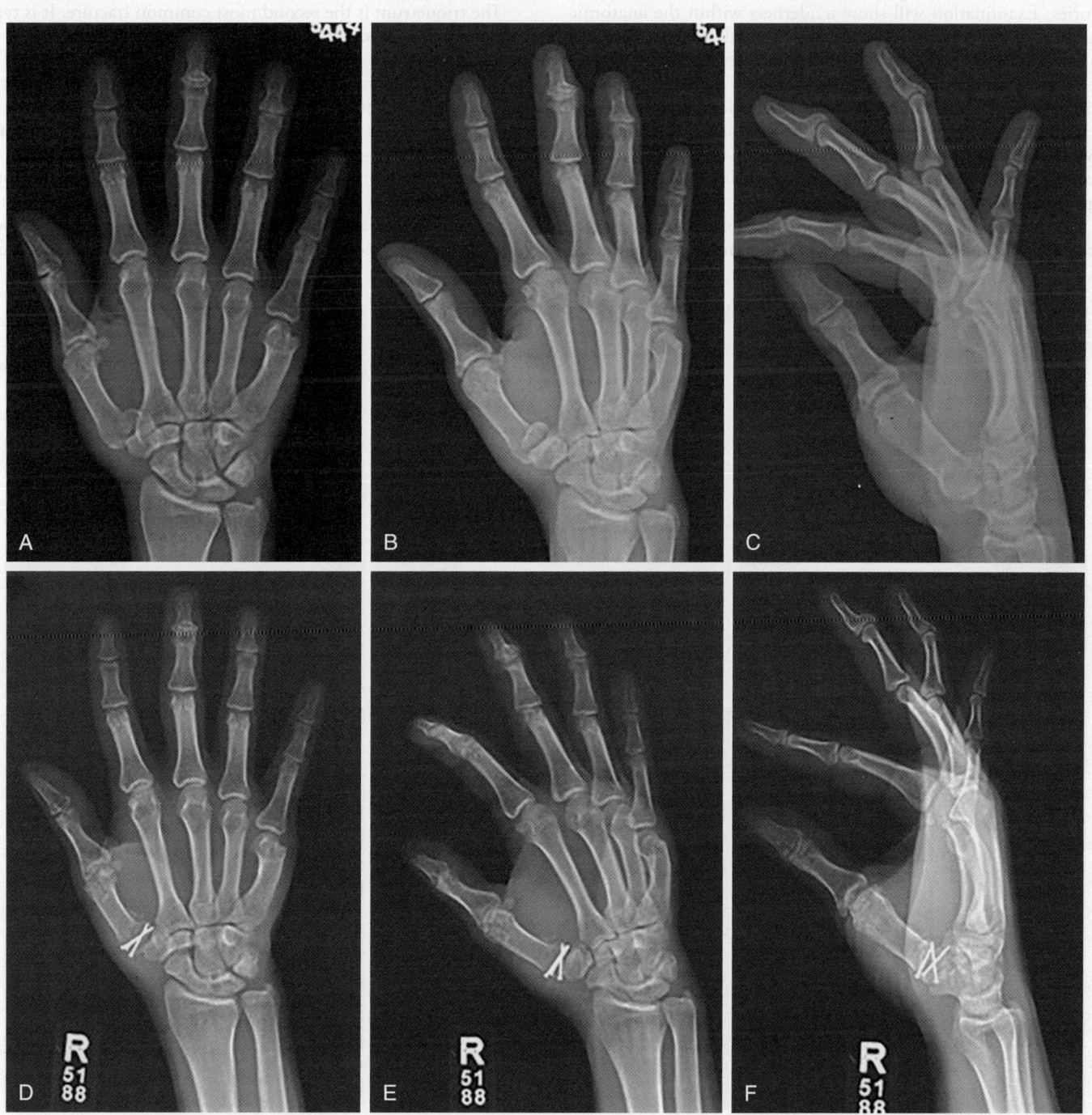

FIGURE 119.30 (A–F) Thumb base metacarpal intraarticular two-fragment fracture (Bennet fracture) with classic displacement of the larger fragment proximally and supinated. Fixation with open reduction and lag compression screws.

accomplished with K-wires or open reduction with plates or screws if necessary. Rolando fractures are typically difficult to treat in a closed manner and often have poor outcomes despite attempts at multiple K-wire pinning or plating.[53,63] An external fixator that includes the index metacarpal or open reduction with fragment pinning can provide good outcomes for the patient. If anatomic reduction fails or pain persists, thumb CMC arthrodesis can be performed as a salvage procedure.[63]

Carpal Bone Fractures

Carpal bone fractures can lead to wrist instability or alteration of wrist biomechanics. The scaphoid is the most fractured carpal bone and accounts for approximately 60% to 70% of all carpal injuries. Examination will show tenderness within the anatomic snuffbox or tubercle. In addition to a standard wrist series, a scaphoid view with the wrist in full ulnar deviation and 20 degrees extension should be obtained. Only 25% of nondisplaced acute scaphoid fractures are seen on plain radiographs. Advanced imaging, such as CT or MRI, should be considered, and studies have shown that CT and MRI may have equivocal sensitivity and specificity. Early diagnosis is essential to expeditiously provide the appropriate treatment and limit complications.

Treatment of identified or suspected nondisplaced scaphoid fracture should include immediate immobilization in short arm, thumb spica cast. The scaphoid has greater than average healing times compared with other fracture sites because of its tenuous, retrograde blood supply, so 12 to 14 weeks is standard for immobilization.

Displaced scaphoid fractures should be treated with ORIF to minimize risk of nonunion and encourage faster healing and return to work, typically with headless compression screws (Fig. 119.31). A large percentage of the scaphoid surface is covered with articular cartilage, making plate fixation difficult. Complications of scaphoid fractures are common, including malunion and nonunion rates between 10% and 20% for nonsurgically treated fractures, with more proximal being higher risk. Nonunion can result in arthritis, wrist pain, or instability and may progress to scaphoid nonunion advance collapse (SNAC) wrist.

The triquetrum is the second most common fracture. It is typically a small avulsion fragment. Most triquetral fractures can be treated nonoperatively with immobilization for 10 to 12 weeks in an ulnar-based splint. Trapezium fractures may result in combination with distal radius or thumb metacarpal fractures and can be treated with compression screw or K-wires if unstable to preserve the thumb CMC saddle. Capitate and lunate fractures are rare because of their protected nature in the center of the carpus. Hook-of-hamate fractures can occur with a direct blow to the palm, such as with a golf club or tennis racket, and if causing persistent pain, they should be treated with hook-of-hamate excision.

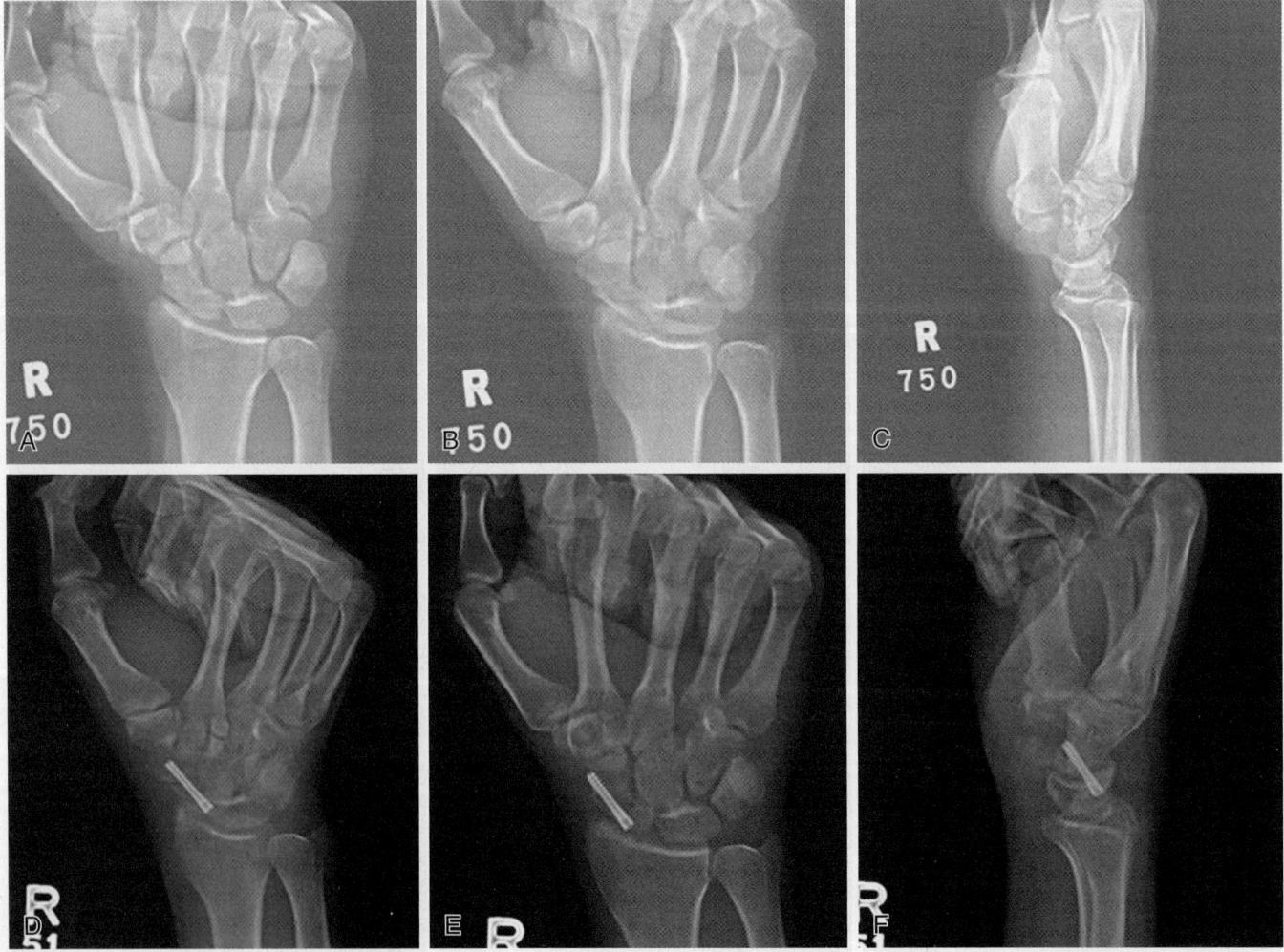

FIGURE 119.31 (A–F) Clenched-fist view with scaphoid midwaist fracture with ulnar displacement and impaction. After fixation with percutaneously placed headless fixation screw.

Fractures in Children

The Salter-Harris classification[65] describes five types of epiphyseal injuries, the most common type of which is a type II injury through the epiphysis and including the diaphysis (Table 119.8). Any fracture that damages the growth plate can result in length discrepancies and thus should be followed longitudinally to ensure anticipated growth is occurring. Fixation should be performed with the growth plate in mind, with greater use of K-wires and smooth pins rather than threaded screws, which may result in growth arrest. Younger children may not be cooperative with immobilization and may require bulkier splinting and casting, whereas in adults buddy taping would be sufficient.

Dislocations and Ligamentous Injuries

Dislocations and fracture-dislocations can occur at any of the finger and wrist joints, from the DIPJ to the wrist. Recognition of partial versus complete ligament injuries as well as joint stability on examination and x-ray can determine whether closed reduction is likely to be successful or if operative exploration is indicated.

Dislocations are frequently seen at the PIPJ. Dislocations are commonly reported in the volar, dorsal, and lateral directions. Dorsal dislocations are most commonly a result of axial force to the tip of the digit. After reduction, joint stability is assessed, ranging through active and passive examiner-directed range of motion with moderate stress application to confirm there is no redislocation. Buddy taping for dislocations with stable active motion can be more effective than immobilization for regaining a normal range of motion.[60,66]

MCPJs have a much stronger ligamentous "box," with attachments of the transverse metacarpal ligament, the sagittal bands of the extensor system as secondary support, and the addition of broader fibrous collateral ligaments. Dorsal dislocations are more common in the border digits. This can occur as a subluxation, which is amenable to closed reduction; however, complete dislocations are often not able to be reduced. The volar plate, flexor tendons, A1 pulley, or even lumbricals may become interposed within the fracture site, requiring open reduction. The CMCJs can also be dislocated as a result of mechanisms with high axial load, such as fall on outstretched hand, and usually dislocate in a dorsal direction.[66]

The thumb has slightly different anatomy because of the greater degrees of freedom of the MPJ that allow for thumb opposition. A more common pattern of injury is forced thumb abduction and hyperextension from a sudden radially directed force. This may sprain or tear the ulnar collateral ligament. Laxity at the thumb IPJ should be assessed with a varus/valgus stress test; marked laxity of more than 40 degrees indicates a complete rupture or grade III ligament injury (Fig. 119.32). Acute ligament tear can cause development of a Stener lesion, specifically the interposition of the thumb adductor aponeurosis between the base of the proximal phalanx and the insertion of the ligament. This is commonly seen in skiers falling with the ski pole in hand and a thumb abduction injury. Ligament repair or reconstruction is required; suture anchor methods, direct repair, and even arthroscopic repairs have been described.[66]

Replantation, Revascularization, and Amputations

Replantation is a complex undertaking involving multiple components of soft tissue and skeletal reattachment and, most importantly, microvascular anastomosis. It is important to have a discussion regarding success rates, recovery time, and expected function. Not every patient or situation is an appropriate candidate for a replantation[19]; some scenarios with historically poor outcomes include the following:

- Severe crush or multilevel injury of the amputated part, especially with multiple levels of compromised vasculature
- Patients with uncontrolled psychosis, especially if the part was self-amputated

TABLE 119.8 Salter-Harris Classification for Epiphyseal Fractures

CLASS	INJURY RELATIVE TO PHYSIS	PROGNOSIS	DIAGRAM
I	"Slip" injury through the physis	Excellent, usually treated nonoperatively	
II	Injury to physis and metaphysis, "above" the physis	Excellent, usually treated with immobilization; most common type	
III	Injury to physis and epiphysis, "lower" than physis	May require operative intervention	
IV	Injury through metaphysis and epiphysis, "through"	Requires operative intervention, prone to limb length discrepancy	
V	Crush injury of the physis	Poor prognosis, prone to limb-length discrepancy	

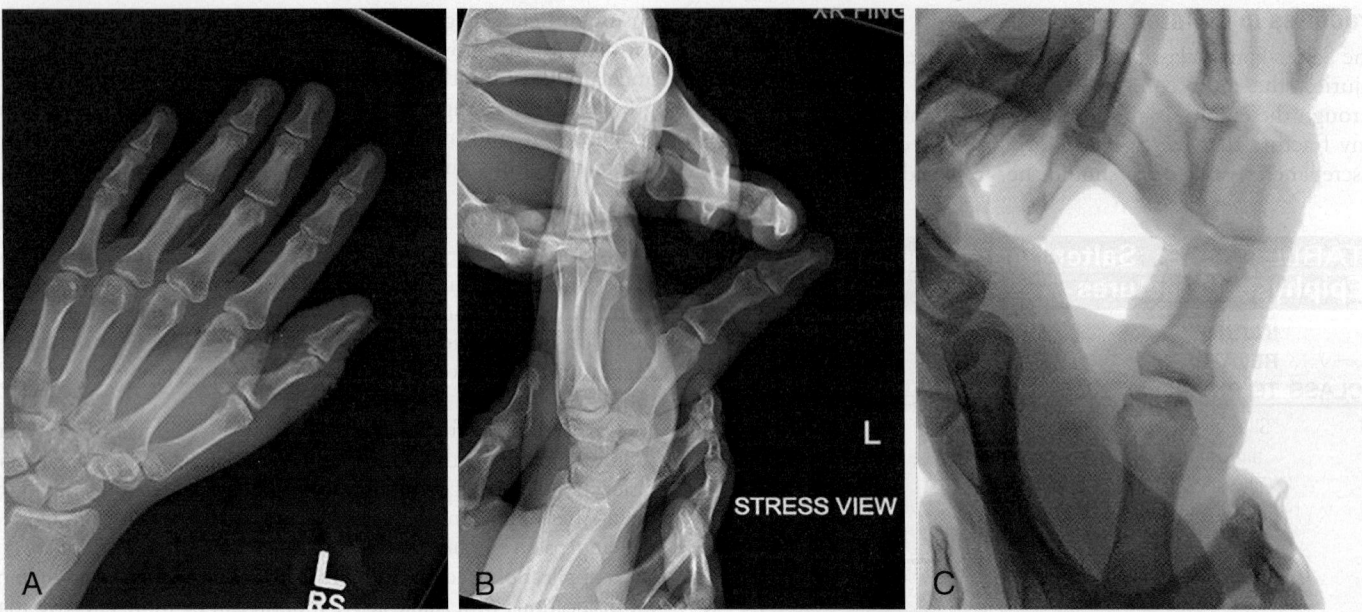

FIGURE 119.32 (A) Patient presented with left thumb metacarpophalangeal joint pain with no acute fracture. (B) Stress view reveals laxity of the ulnar collateral ligament without defined end point. (C) Intraoperative fluoroscopy after ulnar collateral ligament repair shows stabilization with firm end point on stress.

- Amputation of a single digit proximal to the FDS distal insertion (zone 2), except the thumb
- Patients with blood vessels not amenable to microvascular re-anastomosis

Indications for replantation of amputated parts are as follows:

- Whenever possible, for a thumb amputation (it provides >40% of the overall hand function)
- Single digits that have been amputated distal to the FDS insertion
- Multiple injured digits
- Most amputations in children, including single-digit amputations
- Guillotine-sharp clean amputations at the hand, wrist, or distal forearm

Replantation is the reattachment of the part that has been completely amputated, whereas revascularization requires reconstruction of vessels in a limb that has been severely injured or incompletely severed, even if this is only a "skin bridge." Revascularization has more favorable outcomes because venous and lymphatic drainage may be intact.[25]

The mechanism of injury is important in determining the viability of replantation or revascularization. Guillotine amputations, or sharp, clean cuts, are the most favorable. They allow for primary repair of all structures with minimal soft tissue loss and a smaller zone of injury. Crush or avulsion amputations are less favorable. They typically involve comminuted fractures and multilevel or wider zones of injury. They may require vessel resection and vein grafting and cause vessel thrombosis as a result of intimal damage.[67]

Ischemia time is also an important consideration when evaluating a patient for replantation. For amputated digits, ischemia time is better tolerated, with reports of good outcomes hours after over 24 hours of cold ischemia time. Major amputations containing a larger muscle bulk can only tolerate 4 to 6 hours of ischemia, and the parts often cannot be properly stored or cooled to prolong time to repair. Proper storage of the amputated part includes wrapping in saline-moistened gauze or towel, sealing in

a plastic bag, and placing the bag inside an ice water slurry. Direct placement of ice can result in ice crystal formation and tissue damage.[19]

Amputation can always be considered an alternative when replantation or revascularization is contraindicated. The stump is preserved with as much length as possible in most cases, except where the residual part can inhibit function or limit prosthetic wear, such as short residual proximal phalanx or wrist disarticulation. Nerve ends are cut sharply and allowed to retract into the soft tissue in the hopes of limiting neuroma formation. Primary targeted muscle reinnervation (TMR) may also be considered. A formal ray amputation can be performed on an elective basis for a more cosmetic or functional result (Fig. 119.33).

Operative sequence of replantation has been standardized. The distal amputated part is examined under a microscope to sterilize and tag nerves, arteries, and veins by a separate surgical team. With significant soft tissue loss, bone shortening may be considered but should not compromise joint function. Skeletal fixation is performed first to stabilize the digit, then tendon/muscle repair. Afterward, arterial inflow is reestablished, with possible vein grafts, followed by veins and the nerves. For major replantation, the order differs in that vascular inflow should be established first in a temporary or permanent manner to minimize ischemia time. Circulation may be established using a carotid shunt or catheter between the cut arterial ends.[47] Topical 2% lidocaine and papaverine may help with vasospasm.

Postoperative course is critical in the first 72 hours after microvascular repair. These injuries should be managed with loose dressings, elevation, immobilization, and digit checks for color, turgor, capillary refill, and Doppler signal. The room should remain warm, with judicious use of anticoagulants and no use of nicotine. Venous congestion is usually the most common complication, and this can be managed in multiple ways, such as with leeches, removal of the nail bed and controlled bleeding with heparin-soaked pledgets, or manual pinprick with topical heparin because the digit will not be sensate.[68] Trials have shown that the use of loading-dose

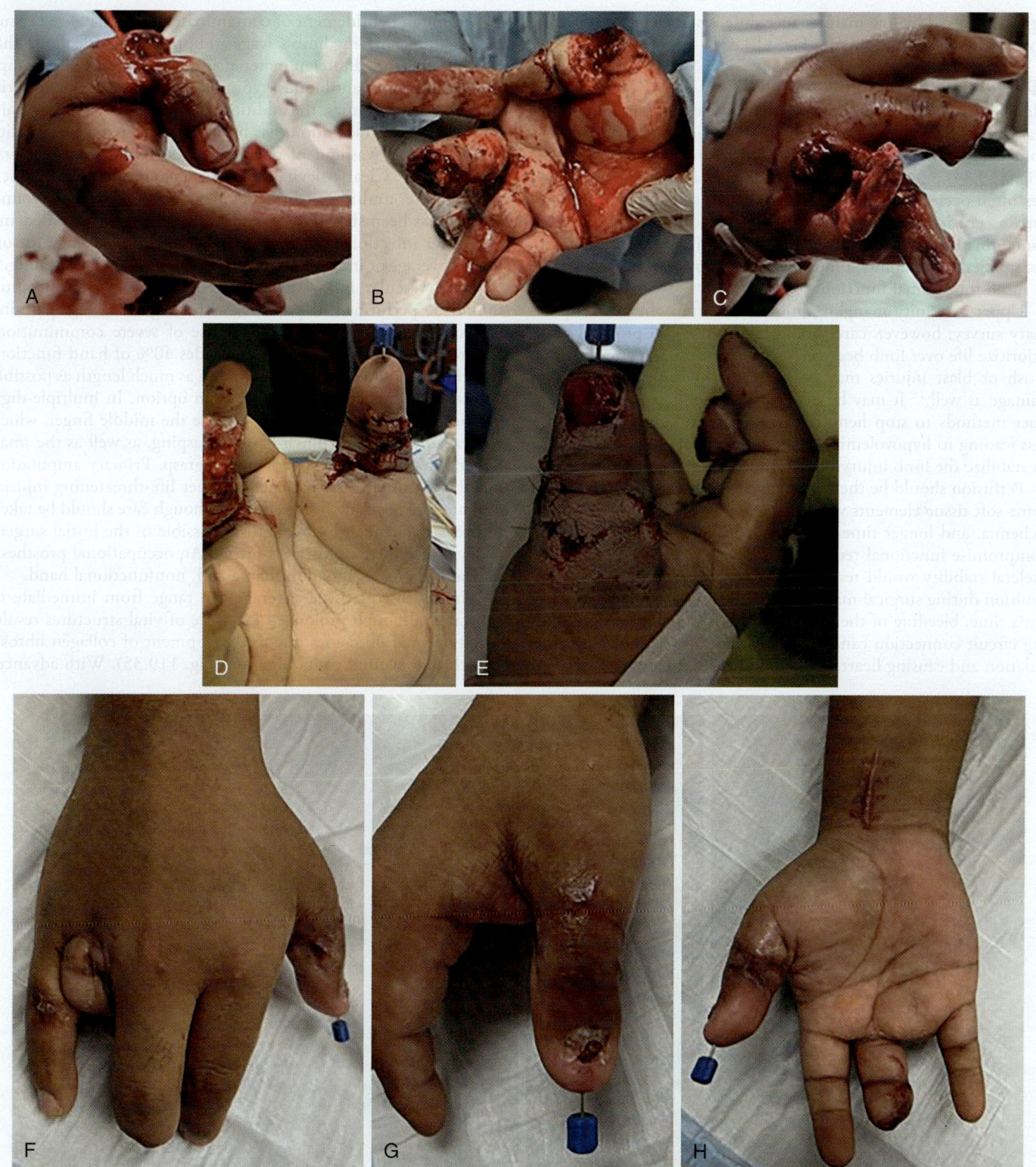

FIGURE 119.33 (A–C) Near amputation of the thumb, amputation of the long finger, and crush injury to ring finger after table saw injury. Patient underwent thumb replantation, middle finger revision amputation, and ring finger disarticulation with fillet flap for dorsal web-space coverage. (D–E) Early postoperative course showed venous congestion; thumb nail plate was removed, and heparin-soaked gauze was applied, with resolution of congestion. (F–H) Six weeks postoperatively, patient shows signs of good soft tissue healing; pin was removed from the thumb during this visit.

aspirin followed by low-maintenance dose is sufficient for prevention of arterial thrombosis (see Fig. 119.33D–E).

Approach to the Mangled Extremity

Mangling injuries to the upper extremity are complex problems that often involve multiple levels of tissue injury, including bone, muscle, tendon, soft tissue, and neurovascular structures (Fig. 119.34). Compounding tissue damage and loss, these injuries often occur as a result of unfavorable mechanisms of injury, such as crush, degloving, or avulsion, and can occur in highly contaminated environments.[69] Mangling injuries are unique to each patient and require a multidisciplinary approach, with goals in mind for optimal function.[70,71]

Upper extremity mangling injuries are often obvious on primary survey; however, care should focus on ATLS protocol and prioritize life over limb because forces that cause upper extremity crush or blast injuries may be sufficient to cause other organ damage as well.[18] It may be necessary to use pressure or tourniquet methods to stop hemorrhage to prevent substantial blood loss leading to hypovolemic shock.[17,20] Attempts should be made to stabilize the limb injury until it can be addressed.

Perfusion should be the first focus of repair effort. Muscle and some soft tissue elements will tolerate only 4 to 6 hours of warm ischemia, and longer times may result in massive cell death and compromise functional recovery.[19] Vascular anastomosis without skeletal stability would result in tenuous repair with the risk of avulsion during surgical maneuvering. In cases of prolonged ischemia time, bleeding of the extremity ~200 cc before reestablishing circuit connection can reduce toxic metabolites entering circulation and causing heart, liver, and kidney damage.

Thorough debridement of contaminated and devitalized tissue is critical to achieving limb salvage and preventing infection. This removes embedded foreign material and nonviable tissue. Prompt administration of antibiotics, typically including a cephalosporin and, in "dirty" injuries, the addition of an aminoglycoside within 90 minutes of presentation, has been shown to reduce morbidity and mortality. Washout of open fractures should occur on first exploration.[54] Clearly devitalized tissue may be removed, which may require multiple debridements. Negative-pressure wound therapy has been shown to be safe and result in decreased edema and lower infection rates, and it can be used as a bridge to soft tissue coverage or in conjunction with repair to improve healing.[72]

Once vascular inflow has been established, skeletal fixation should be performed, if possible, with weight-bearing spanning plates, or external fixation in the case of severe comminution. Regarding the hand, the thumb provides 40% of hand function, and efforts should be taken to maintain as much length as possible and prioritize replantation if that is an option. In multiple-digit injuries, other important digits include the middle finger, which will take over the key pinch part of grasping, as well as the small finger, which is important for power grasp. Primary amputation may be required if the patient has other life-threatening injuries or mangling beyond salvage efforts, although care should be taken to preserve as much limb length as possible in the initial surgery to maximize future prosthesis fitting. An occupational prosthesis may afford greater function than a stiff, nonfunctional hand.

Timing of soft tissue coverage can range from immediate to subacute, although prolonged exposure of vital structures results in suboptimal outcomes due to development of collagen fibrosis and chronic wound contamination (Fig. 119.35). With advances

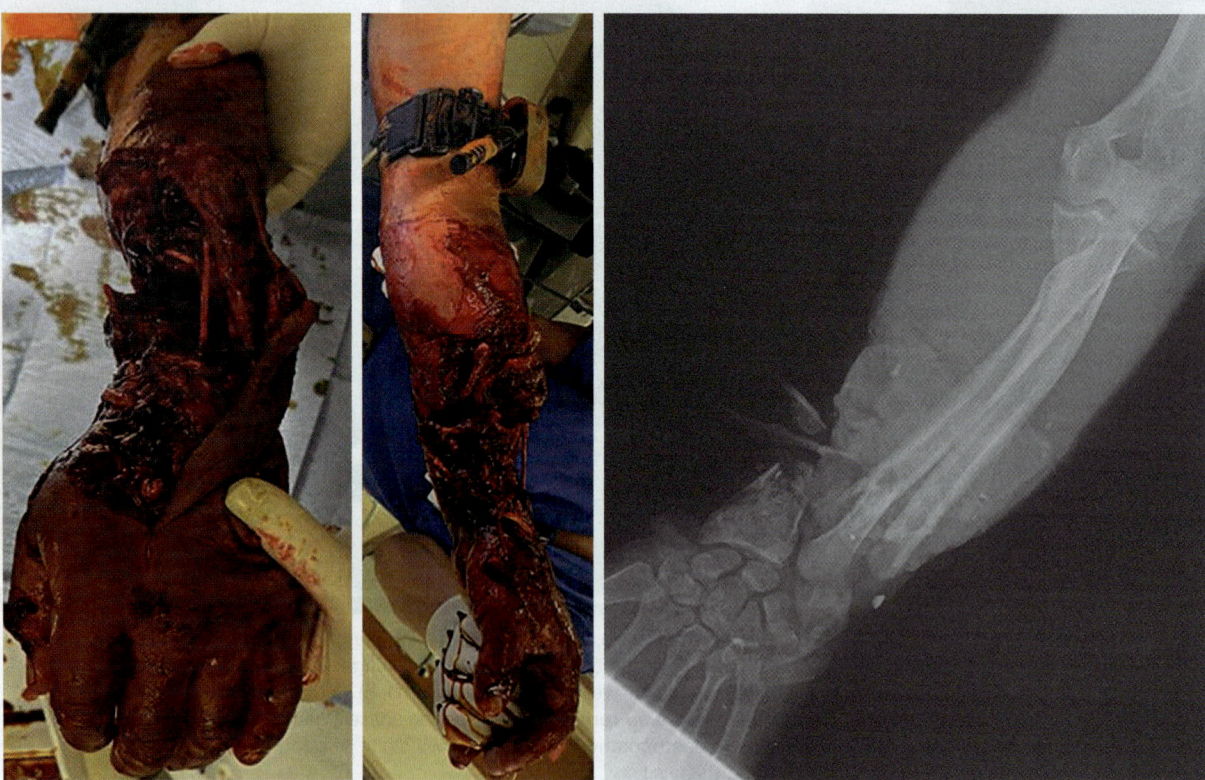

FIGURE 119.34 Left forearm crush and avulsion injury after torque mechanism when the limb was caught out the window in a rollover motor vehicle collision, with significant injury to the extrinsic flexor and extensor muscles and soft tissue degloving. X-ray of left forearm shows complete comminuted fracture of the radial shaft and greenstick fracture of the distal ulnar. The patient went on to have a transradial amputation.

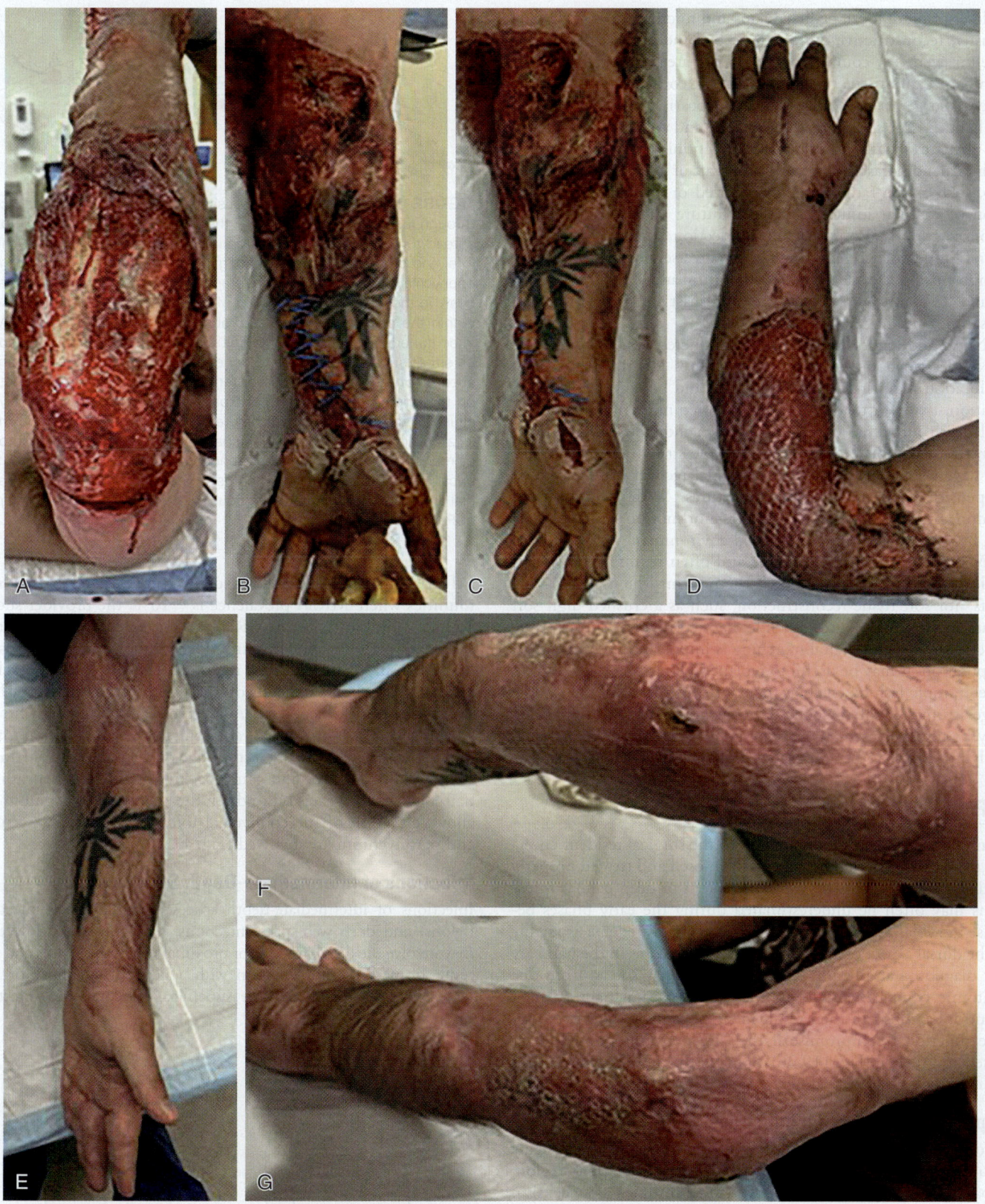

FIGURE 119.35 (A–D) Degloving injury of the proximal one-third of the forearm and crush injury resulting from being compressed between two conveyor belts for >2 hours. (E–G) Postoperative outcome after 6 months of reconstruction with skin graft. Patient sustained extensive ischemic injury to forearm flexors and high median and ulnar nerve injuries.

in description of local, pedicled flaps and microvascular free tissue transfer, reconstructive options have become more readily available for even very complex and extensive areas of soft tissue loss. Flap choice and tissue type are important considerations in these types of surgeries, especially the weight-bearing palmar surface of the hand. Tissue should be thin, pliable, and adherent to underlying structures without untoward susceptibility to shear forces, such as an adipofascial flap with skin graft or thin fasciocutaneous flap, such as the radial forearm pedicled or free flap. Consideration of vascular injuries as well as future plans for free tissue reconstruction is also important in selection, especially with ipsilateral limb pedicled flaps, such as the reverse radial forearm flap, compromising the radial artery for future use. If possible, flaps should be planned to be sensitized, at least for protective hand sensation.

Nerve and tendon repair can be conducted on a less acute basis, as described previously. Any structures identified on initial exploration requiring delayed repair should be tagged for future location. Extensor tendon injuries are often more forgiving, especially with juncturae tendinum between individual digits; however, flexor tendon injuries with multiple structures involved often have poorer prognosis for functional recovery and increased propensity for scarring and contractures. With rigid fixation, tendon gliding and early active range-of-motion protocol may still be accomplished in a controlled environment.

Mangling injuries are complex and often require creative and critical thinking. Unsalvageable structures may be used as "spare parts" for soft tissue reconstruction, such as a crushed digit soft tissue envelope being used as a fillet flap to provide glabrous tissue coverage. Although digital matching is important, in a multidigit amputation, it may be useful to replant a better-preserved digit in a heterotopic fashion, such as index or ring part onto the middle finger stump. If soft tissue and vessels are preserved, distal parts may be used as vascularized bone grafts or even free flaps, especially if a part is to be amputated proximally.[69]

INFECTIONS

Hand infections commonly present to the surgical resident covering the ED. When the infection is diagnosed and treated properly initially, most patients do well. The extent of deep palmar infections may often be underestimated during the early phases because the volar aspect of the hand does not show edema as readily as the dorsal aspect of the hand. Thus, if infections in the hand are not diagnosed at an early stage, infections may spread from one anatomic compartment to another along natural tissue planes. Hand infections can then result in significant morbidity and severe functional compromise if they are not appropriately diagnosed and treated (Fig. 119.36). Some of the more common types of infections are discussed here.

Superficial Paronychial Infections

Paronychia is the most common infection of the hand; it usually results from trauma to the eponychial or paronychial region. A paronychia may be acute (<6 weeks) or chronic (>6 weeks) in nature. The infection localizes around the nail base, advances around the nail fold, and burrows beneath the base of the nail. If pus is trapped beneath the nail, pressure on the nail evokes exquisite pain. The most common causative organism is *Staphylococcus aureus*. Traditionally, first-generation cephalosporins are recommended for empiric antibiotic treatment. However, there has now been an increasing incidence of methicillin-resistant *S. aureus*

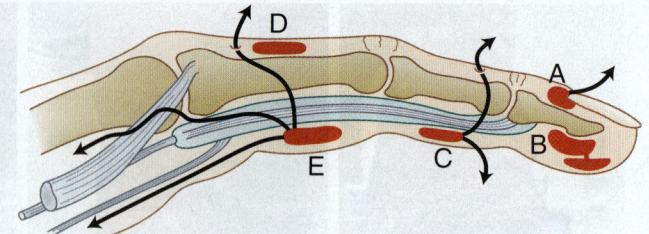

FIGURE 119.36 Spread of soft tissue infections in the hand occurs through loss of containment from the original site and erosion into and spread through contiguous anatomic compartments. (A) Paronychium. Infecting organisms access periungual tissues through fissures in the eponychial or paronychial tissues and often are discharged spontaneously in these areas. (B) Infection of pulp tissues (felon). Fibrous septa within the pulp create collar stud abscesses within the pulp. (C) Volar subcutaneous infections in the digit may be discharged percutaneously on either surface of the digit or penetrate dorsally and spread along the sheaths of the flexor or extensor tendons. (D) Subcutaneous infections on the dorsum of the digit are usually discharged percutaneously because of the thin and areolar nature of the soft tissues. (E) Proximally located digital infections or web-space infections may rupture into the palmar spaces by tracking along tendon sheaths, palmar fascia, or lumbrical canal. The continuous sheaths of the thumb and little fingers (radial and ulnar bursae) are continuous with the carpal tunnel and space of Parona at the wrist.

(MRSA) in community-acquired infections; therefore, in communities where MRSA prevalence is ≥10%, the provider should consider antibiotics with MRSA coverage (e.g., trimethoprim/sulfamethoxazole, clindamycin, doxycycline). After an abscess develops, surgical drainage is required. The surgical approach to an acute paronychia depends on the extent of the infection. Incisions may not be necessary. A Freer elevator is used to lift approximately 25% of the nail adjacent to the infected paronychium, extending proximally to the edge of the nail. This portion of the nail is transected, and gauze packing is inserted beneath the nail fold. A single incision to drain the affected paronychium also allows elevation of the eponychial fold when both eponychium and paronychium are involved (Fig. 119.37).[73]

Infections of Intermediate-Depth Spaces

Infections of intermediate-depth spaces are pulp space infections (felons) and deep web-space infections. The pulp space infections may involve the distal, middle, or proximal volar pulp spaces and may result from direct implantation with a penetrating injury or may represent spread from a more superficial subcutaneous infection.

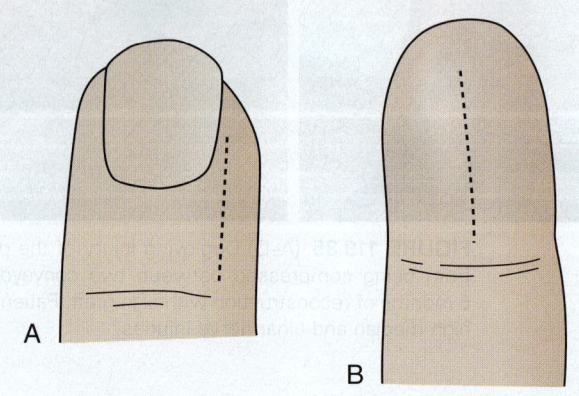

FIGURE 119.37 Incisions for paronychia (A) and felon (B).

The volar pulp of the distal digital segment is a fascial space closed proximally by a septum joining the distal flexion crease to the periosteum, where the long flexor tendon is inserted. This space is also partitioned by fibrous septa. Tension in the distal digital segment can become so great that the arteries to the bone are compressed, resulting in gangrene of the fingertip and necrosis of the distal 75% of the terminal phalanx. With infection of the digital pulp space, one must not wait for fluctuance before making the decision for surgery because of the danger of ischemic necrosis of the skin and bone. Clinical diagnosis is made by the rapid onset of throbbing pain, swelling, and exquisite tenderness of the affected pulp space. Surgical drainage is required. A single volar or unilateral longitudinal incision may be used (see Fig. 119.37). Care must be taken to design the incision to avoid the neurovascular bundles that travel on the radial and ulnar volar surface of the digit. Blunt dissection is carried down to the preperiosteal plane, and care must be taken to release any septae enclosing a fluid collection. Postoperative care includes packing of the wound and elevation of the extremity. Use of antibiotics is guided by the results of Gram staining. Similar to a paronychia, *S. aureus* is the most common causative agent. Spread from a pulp space infection may move into a joint space or underlying bone or burst through the septum proximally to involve the rest of the finger. More proximally, a pulp space infection at the base of the finger can travel through the lumbrical canal into the palm to create a deep palmar space infection.[73]

Web-space abscesses result from direct implantation or spread from a pulp space. An inflamed and tender mass in the web space separates the fingers. There is loss of the normal palmar concavity, with a widened space between the fingers. Dorsal swelling is present and must not be mistaken for the infection site. A surgical incision is placed transversely across the web space, and a longitudinal counterincision may be placed dorsally between the bases of the proximal phalanges; a generous communication is established between these two incisions (Fig. 119.38).

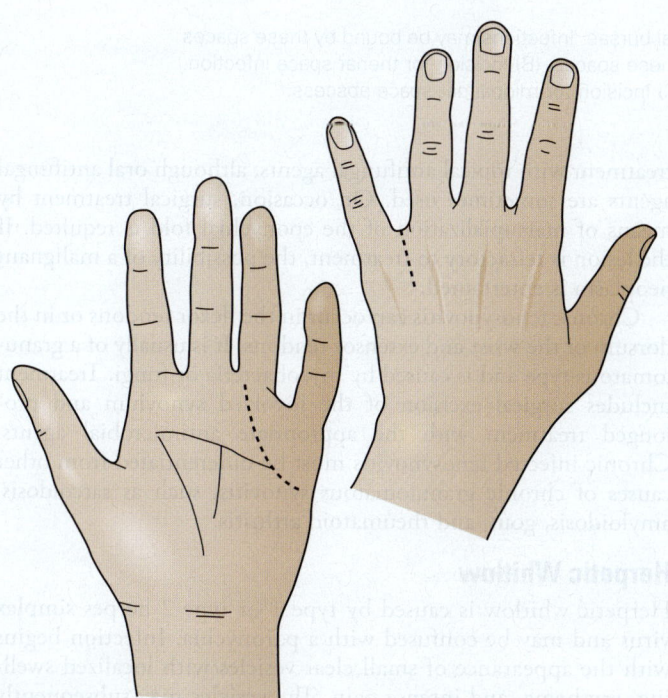

FIGURE 119.38 Incisions for web-space abscess between the little and ring fingers.

DEEP INFECTIONS

Palmar Space Infections

Palmar space infections are localized to the deep space of the hand between the metacarpals and palmar aponeurosis. A transverse septum to the metacarpal of the middle finger divides the deep space into an ulnar midpalmar and radial thenar space. The transverse head of the adductor pollicis partitions the thenar space from the retroadductor space. There may be ballooning of the palm, thenar eminence, or posterior aspect of the first web space, depending on which of the affected spaces is involved with an abscess. The dorsal subaponeurotic space of the hand deep to the extensor tendons may also be affected by an isolated infection, generally as a result of direct implantation (Fig. 119.39A). For a thenar space infection, the preferred approach to surgical drainage is a dual volar and dorsal incision (see Fig. 119.39B). On the volar side, an incision is made adjacent and parallel to the thenar crease. Great care is taken to avoid injury to the palmar cutaneous branch of the median nerve in the proximal part of the incision and the motor branch of the median nerve in a deeper plane. A second, slightly curved longitudinal incision is made on the dorsum of the first web space. Dissection is continued more deeply into this area between the first dorsal interosseous muscle and adductor pollicis. A drain is placed in the incision after thorough exploration of the respective spaces. With midpalmar space infections, dorsal swelling of the hand will be present, as is the case with all palmar infections, and must not be mistaken for the infection site. Motion of the middle and ring fingers is limited and painful. A longitudinal curvilinear incision is the preferred approach for drainage of this space (see Fig. 119.39C).[73]

Infection of Parona space occurs in the potential space deep to the flexor tendons in the distal forearm and superficial to the pronator quadratus muscle. It is usually the result of spread from the adjacent contiguous midpalmar space or from the radial or ulnar bursa. Swelling, tenderness, and fluctuation will be present in the distal volar forearm. A midpalmar infection may be associated. Active digital flexion is painful, as is passive finger extension. A surgical incision must be planned to leave the median nerve adequately covered with soft tissue.

Pyogenic Flexor Tenosynovitis

Kanavel four cardinal signs include the following: (1) the finger is held flexed because this position allows the synovial sheath its maximum volume and eases pain; (2) symmetric fusiform swelling of the entire finger is present, with edema of the back of the hand; (3) the slightest attempt at passive extension of the affected digit produces exquisite pain; and (4) the site of maximum tenderness is at the proximal cul-de-sac of the index, middle, and ring finger synovial sheaths in the distal palm or, in the case of infection of the sheaths of the thumb and little finger, more proximally in the palm. The radial and ulnar bursae communicate in approximately 80% of cases and may be simultaneously infected. Bursal infections may spread into the forearm space of Parona, deep to the flexor tendons in the distal part of the forearm, creating a horseshoe abscess.

Treatment of pyogenic flexor tenosynovitis depends on the severity of infection. Infections isolated within the finger and without systemic effects can be attempted to be managed with parental antibiotics with a plan for formal surgical washout if symptoms persist or worsen. Early infections may be drained with a limited incision and drainage over the point of maximum point tenderness or fluctuance with copious irrigation over the flexor

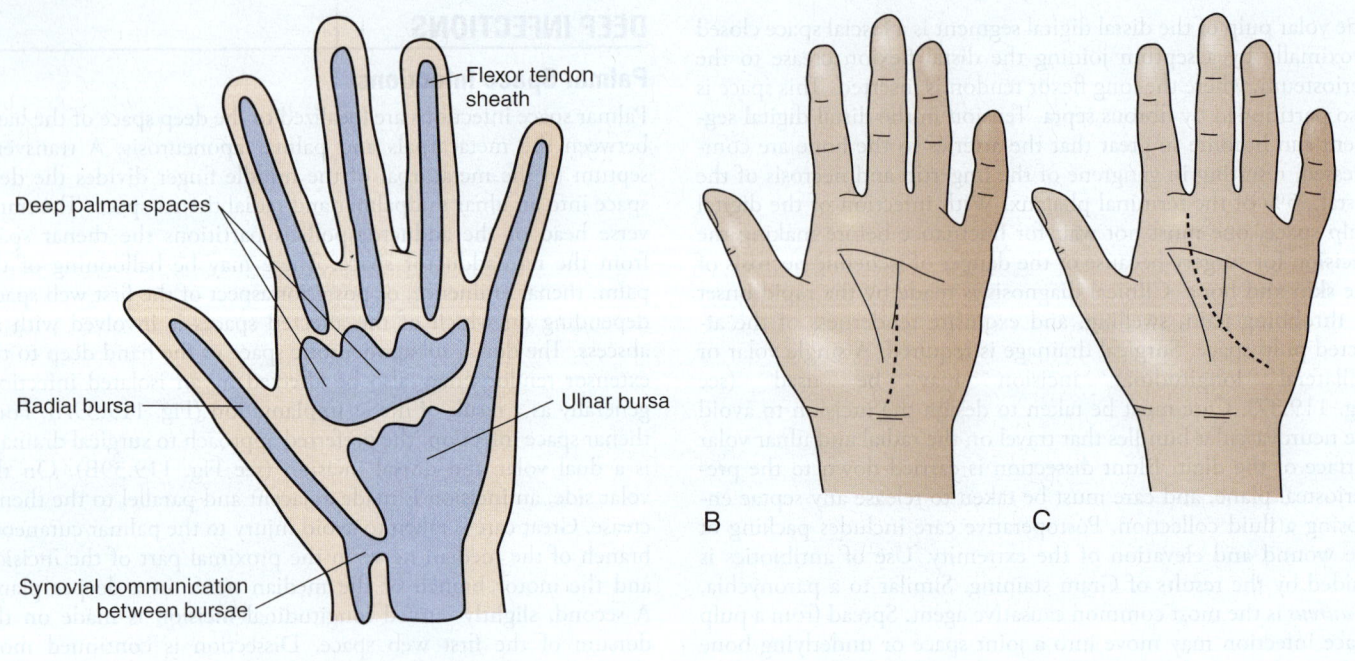

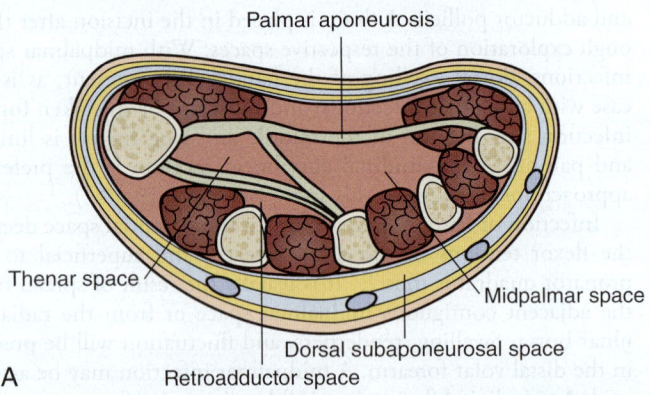

FIGURE 119.39 (A) Deep spaces of the hand and synovial bursae. Infections may be bound by these spaces or may track along anatomic dissection planes between these spaces. (B) Incision for thenar space infection. A dorsal first-web-space incision is also often required. (C) Incision for midpalmar space abscess.

sheath and tendon. When there is no purulence, this may save the patient from a more extensive surgical approach. If the infection is severe (involves multiple digits and/or systemic signs), the patient will require a semiurgent operative washout.[74]

The preferred surgical approach is through two separate incisions. The first incision is a midaxial incision made on the finger, usually on the ulnar side of the digit (on the radial side of the thumb or little finger); the digital artery and nerve remain in the volar flap, with the dissection proceeding directly to the tendon sheath. The synovium between the A3 and A4 pulleys is incised, and cloudy fluid is encountered. A second incision is made in the palm over the tendon to drain the cul-de-sac. A 16-gauge polyethylene catheter is inserted beneath the A1 pulley into the sheath, and the sheath is flushed manually with sterile saline every 2 hours after surgery. A bulky hand dressing absorbs the drainage.

Chronic and Atypical Infections

Chronic paronychia is generally the result of *Candida albicans* infection (>95%) and is not bacterial. When bacteria are involved, they are more commonly atypical mycobacteria or gram-negative organisms. Chronic paronychia generally responds to

treatment with topical antifungal agents, although oral antifungal agents are sometimes used. On occasion, surgical treatment by means of marsupialization of the eponychial fold is required. If the lesion is refractory to treatment, the possibility of a malignant neoplasm is entertained.

Chronic tenosynovitis can occur in the flexor tendons or in the dorsum of the wrist and extensor tendons. It is usually of a granulomatous type and is caused by mycobacteria or fungi. Treatment includes surgical excision of the involved synovium and prolonged treatment with the appropriate antimicrobial agents. Chronic infected tenosynovitis must be differentiated from other causes of chronic granulomatous synovitis, such as sarcoidosis, amyloidosis, gout, and rheumatoid arthritis.

Herpetic Whitlow

Herpetic whitlow is caused by type 1 or type 2 herpes simplex virus and may be confused with a paronychia. Infection begins with the appearance of small clear vesicles with localized swelling, erythema, and intense pain. The vesicles may subsequently appear turbid and coalesce over the next few days before ulcerating. Diagnosis is confirmed by culturing the virus from the vesicular fluid, assessing immunofluorescent serum antibody titers, or performing a Tzanck smear. However, these measures are rarely required because clinical diagnosis is usually sufficient. Infection can occur from autoinoculation from an oral or genital lesion or exposure as a healthcare worker. Pain is often out of proportion to the physical findings. Treatment is generally nonoperative because this infection is usually self-limited. Antivirals such as acyclovir or famciclovir may be of some benefit if started within the first 48 hours of symptom onset. Surgical incision and drainage can lead to systemic involvement and possible viral encephalitis.

Animal and Human Bites

The most striking difference in the microbial flora of human and animal bite wounds is the higher number of bacterial isolates per wound in human bites, the difference being mostly caused by the presence of anaerobic bacteria. Human bites can occasionally transmit other infectious diseases, such as hepatitis B, tuberculosis, syphilis, or actinomycosis. The incidence of *Eikenella corrodens* in human bite infections of the hand has been reported to vary between 7% and 29%. Usually, isolated organisms from infected human bite wounds are, as in animal bites, α-hemolytic streptococci and *S. aureus*, β-lactamase–producing strains of *S. aureus*, and *Bacteroides* spp. Anaerobic bacteria, including *Bacteroides, Clostridium, Peptococcus,* and *Veillonella,* are more prevalent in human bite infections than previously recognized. Most studies of animal bite wounds have focused on the isolation of *Pasteurella multocida,* disregarding the role of anaerobes. However, more recent studies have shown that dog bite wounds indicate multiple organisms, with *P. multocida* being isolated from only 26% of dog bite wounds in adults. Most animal bites cause mixed infections of aerobic and anaerobic bacteria.

Pyogenic joint infections usually result from trauma, such as a bite wound from a tooth when the assailant's hand strikes the jaw. A tooth struck by the clenched fist of an attacker penetrates the skin, tendon, joint capsule, and metacarpal head. Once the finger is extended, the four puncture wounds separate from each other to create a closed space within the joint. All these so-called fight bite wounds of the MPJ need to be explored surgically, debrided, and thoroughly lavaged. Human bite wounds are not closed primarily and are treated with appropriate antibiotics.

COMPARTMENT SYNDROME, HIGH-PRESSURE INJECTION INJURIES, AND EXTRAVASATION INJURIES

Compartment Syndrome

Compartment syndrome results in symptoms and signs caused by increased pressure within a limited space that compromises the circulation and function of the tissues in that space. Volkmann ischemic contracture is the sequala of untreated compartment syndrome; it results in muscle that is fibrosed, contracted, and functionless and nerves that are insensible. Various injuries are known to cause compartment syndrome:

- Decreased compartment volume (e.g., from externally applied tight dressings or casts, lying on a limb in a comatose state)
- Increased compartment content (e.g., from bleeding or trauma with fractures or finger injuries; increased capillary permeability, such as reperfusion after ischemic injury; electrical burn injuries)
- Other injuries (e.g., snakebites, high-pressure injection injuries)[75]

The diagnosis of compartment syndrome is based primarily on clinical evaluation. Although it is possible to measure compartment pressure, the decision to perform fasciotomy is based on a high degree of clinical suspicion. Compartment ischemia may be severe and still not affect the color or temperature of the distal fingers, and the distal pulses are rarely obliterated by compartment swelling. However, circulation in the muscle and nerve may be greatly reduced. Muscle ischemia that lasts for more than 4 hours leads to muscle death and may also cause significant myoglobinuria. After 8 hours of total ischemia, irreversible nerve changes are complete. The hallmark of muscle and nerve ischemia is pain, which is progressive and persistent. The pain is accentuated by passive muscle stretching; this is the most reliable clinical test for diagnosis of compartment syndrome. The next most important clinical finding is diminished sensation, which indicates nerve ischemia. The closed compartments of the forearm and hand are also palpated and found to be tense and tender, confirming the diagnosis of compartment syndrome. A passive muscle stretch test elicits severe pain in the presence of compartment syndrome. An arterial injury and nerve injury need to be distinguished in the differential diagnosis of compartment syndrome. All three of these injuries produce paresthesias and paresis; pain with passive stretch is present in compartment syndrome and arterial occlusion but not in neurapraxia; and pulses are intact in compartment syndrome and neurapraxia but not with arterial occlusion. In situations in which the patient cannot cooperate because of inebriation or unconsciousness and the clinical diagnosis is difficult, compartment pressure can be measured.[75]

Release of a forearm compartment syndrome always requires carpal tunnel release (Fig. 119.40). The palmar incision starts in the valley between the thenar and hypothenar muscles, and the incision then curves transversely across the flexion crease of the wrist at the ulnar border. This incision must avoid the palmar cutaneous branch of the median nerve and prevent flexion contracture across the wrist crease. It also provides an opportunity to release the Guyon canal. The incision then extends proximally up the forearm before curving back in a radial direction so as to have a large skin flap that will cover the median nerve and distal forearm tendons. At the elbow, the incision for the flap then curves again across the antecubital fossa, providing cover for the brachial artery and median nerve and preventing linear contracture across the antecubital fossa. The dorsal and so-called mobile wad compartments of the forearm are readily released through a straight incision, as needed. Appropriate release of the various intrinsic compartments of the hand may also be required. Most wounds can be partially closed at 5 days. If the skin cannot be closed secondarily within 10 days, a split-thickness skin graft can be applied.

High-Pressure Injection Injuries

High-pressure injection injuries to the hand are relatively uncommon, but consequences of a misdiagnosis are serious. Urgent treatment is required. High-pressure injection guns are used for painting, lubricating, cleaning, and farm animal vaccinations. Materials that may be injected with these devices include paint, paint thinners, oil, grease, water, plastic, vaccines, and cement. These high-pressure injection guns may generate pressures ranging between 3000 and 12,000 psi. Injection injuries can also be caused by other sources, such as defective lines and valves, pneumatic hoses, and hydraulic lines. The type of material injected is the most important prognostic factor. Oil-based paints and paint thinners can generate significant early inflammation, leading to severe fibrosis. Because tendon sheaths at the index, middle, and ring fingers

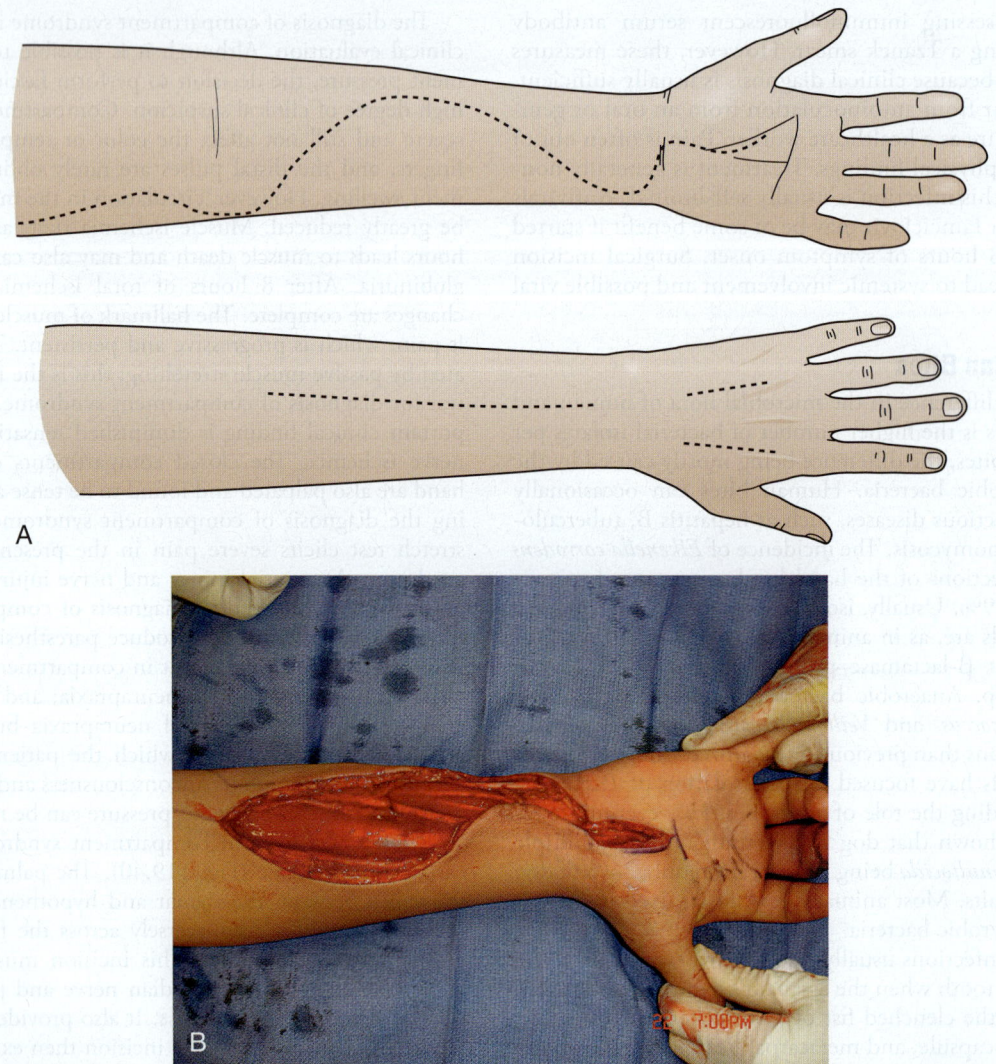

FIGURE 119.40 (A) Incisions for forearm fasciotomy. (B) Fasciotomy in a child for compartment syndrome after a snakebite.

end at the level of the MPJs, material injected at the distal interphalangeal (DIP) or proximal interphalangeal (PIP) flexion creases will remain within these digits. However, tendon sheaths at the thumb and little finger extend all the way into the radial and ulnar bursae. Thus, material injected at the little finger or at the IP flexion crease of the thumb may potentially extend all the way into the forearm and may even cause a compartment syndrome.[76]

Initial presentation of a patient with a high-pressure injection may be benign and subtle. This may result in mismanagement by minimizing the patient's complaints. The break in the skin may be a benign-looking, pinhole-sized puncture site. However, within several hours, the digit becomes increasingly more painful, swollen, and pale. Prompt recognition and realization of the severity of injury are paramount. Radiographs may help determine the extent and dispersion of the injected material, either in the form of subcutaneous emphysema or, with lead-based paints, appearing as radiopaque soft tissue densities. The entire digit must be surgically decompressed, and all foreign material and necrotic tissue must be debrided. Wounds are closed loosely over Penrose drains or in a delayed manner. Appropriate antibiotics must be administered. Despite prompt recognition and

treatment, many such injuries ultimately result in surgical amputation of the digits.[76]

Extravasation Injuries

In the past, extravasation injuries from chemotherapeutic agents frequently affected the upper extremity. However, subcutaneously tunneled central lines have now reduced the incidence of these injuries. If extravasation is suspected, infusion must be stopped immediately. Cold packs are applied for 15 minutes four times a day, and the extremity is elevated during the next 48 hours. This treatment is generally effective for most extravasation injuries. It is critical to determine the agent that has infiltrated because specific antidotes have been described. Hyaluronidase injected along the periphery infiltrated tissue is a potential treatment of choice, helping to dissipate the agent along tissue planes. However, if blistering, ulceration, and pain occur in the damaged tissue, progressive necrosis to the limits of the extravasation will follow, and surgical excision of all damaged tissue is necessary. Most subsequent wounds can generally be treated with delayed split-thickness skin grafting, although the options for wound coverage after debridement depend on the extent of the debridement that was required.[77]

TENOSYNOVITIS

De Quervain Disease

De Quervain disease is a stenosing tenosynovitis of the first dorsal compartment of the wrist and is a common cause of pain and disability. Diagnosis is easily made from a history of pain localized to the radial side of the wrist and aggravated by movement of the thumb. There is frequently a history of chronic overuse of the wrist and hand. Other features are local tenderness and swelling over the first dorsal compartment of the wrist and a positive Finkelstein test result—the patient clasps the thumb, and brisk ulnar deviation to the hand elicits extreme pain. Crepitus may be palpable. This condition must be differentiated by radiographic and physical examination from arthritis of the thumb carpometacarpal joint.[78]

Nonoperative treatment includes local steroid injection, thumb and wrist immobilization, local heat, and systemic antiinflammatory medications. If these nonoperative measures fail, surgical decompression of the first dorsal compartment at the wrist is performed. Care must be taken to protect the radial sensory nerve branches during the course of the operation because these branches traverse just under the skin in this area, and trauma or transection may lead to painful, disabling neuromas.[78]

Intersection Syndrome

Intersection syndrome is not well understood but is characterized by pain and crepitus at the point at which the APL and EPB tendons cross over the tendons of the second dorsal compartment (ECRL and ECRB; Fig. 119.41). Initial treatment is by splinting, local corticosteroid injection, and antiinflammatory medications. Refractory cases require surgical release at the second dorsal compartment and excision of involved tenosynovial membranes.

Trigger Thumb and Fingers

Trigger finger is a constricting tenosynovitis of the flexor tendons, generally at the level of the A1 pulley. The patient can flex the digit, but an apparent nodule catches at the proximal edge of the A1 pulley, locking the PIPJ (or the IPJ of the thumb) in this flexed position. Attempts at extending the digit cause it to snap back suddenly, much like the trigger of a gun. Often, the patient needs to use the opposite hand to unlock and extend the digit. In its most severe form, the constriction is so tight that the patient cannot flex the digit, or it becomes fixed in a flexed position and can

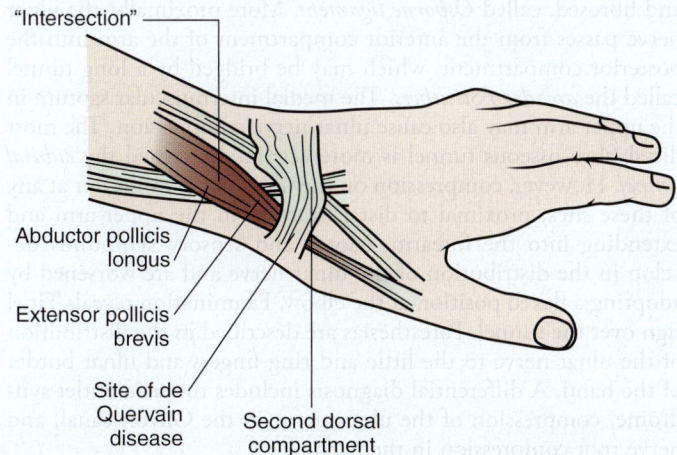

"Intersection"

Abductor pollicis longus

Extensor pollicis brevis

Site of de Quervain disease

Second dorsal compartment

FIGURE 119.41 Anatomic locations for de Quervain stenosing tenosynovitis and intersection syndrome.

no longer be fully extended. A congenital form of trigger thumb or finger presents in infants, but most cases resolve by the time the child reaches 1 year of age; if not, an operation is indicated. Nonoperative treatment in adults includes local injection of corticosteroids. If this regimen fails, the A1 pulley is longitudinally divided by surgery.[78,79]

Other Sites of Tenosynovitis

Other sites include the FCR and FCU tendons. They can frequently be treated by splinting and local corticosteroid injection, although surgery occasionally may be required. Inflammation of the ECU may also be an enigmatic cause of ulnar-sided wrist pain. Diagnosis is made by eliciting tenderness along the ECU tendon, pain on active resisted extension, and ulnar deviation of the wrist.

NERVE COMPRESSION SYNDROMES

Along the length of the upper extremity, nerves pass through a number of anatomic bottlenecks. These are all possible sites of nerve entrapment and lead to characteristic distal sensory and motor deficits. The most common sites of nerve compression, from proximal to distal along the length of the extremity, are at the nerve root secondary to cervical disc disease or cervical degenerative arthritis, thoracic outlet compression at the level of the clavicle, ulnar nerve entrapment at the elbow (cubital tunnel syndrome), entrapment of the PIN in the proximal forearm (radial tunnel syndrome, posterior interosseous syndrome), entrapment of the median nerve and its branches in the proximal forearm (so-called pronator syndrome, anterior interosseous nerve syndrome), and, finally, entrapment of the median nerve at the wrist (carpal tunnel syndrome) and of the ulnar nerve in the Guyon canal (ulnar tunnel syndrome).

In most cases of nerve entrapment, no specific aggravating causative factor is found. An increasing incidence of compression neuropathy is reported in patients whose work involves chronic repetitive stress. In some, there may be a clearly defined extrinsic compressive problem on the nerve or an aggravating factor. These include the following:

- Trauma that can produce bone compression, for example, carpal tunnel after carpal dislocations or a distal radius malunion (median) and supracondylar humerus fractures that increase the elbow carrying angle (ulnar nerve at the elbow)
- Synovial thickening of the bursa in rheumatoid arthritis in the carpal tunnel (median) or at the elbow (posterior interosseous)
- Tumors such as giant cell tumor in the Guyon canal (ulnar) or a lipoma in the radial tunnel (posterior interosseous)
- Developmental, with anomalous muscles present in the carpal tunnel (median), Guyon canal (ulnar), or forearm (median)
- Metabolic, in which disturbances of fluid balance cause increased pressure on the nerve, particularly at the carpal tunnel (e.g., myxedema, pregnancy)

Carpal tunnel syndrome is the most common peripheral nerve entrapment syndrome, followed by ulnar nerve entrapment at the elbow.[80] The other entrapment syndromes are less common. Diabetes mellitus is recognized as a risk factor for carpal tunnel syndrome, and the response to treatment has previously been unclear. However, studies suggest that patients with diabetes do similarly well as patients who are normoglycemic do after carpal tunnel release.

Carpal Tunnel Syndrome

The carpal tunnel is a packed fibro-osseous tunnel at the wrist that is traversed by the median nerve and nine long extrinsic digital

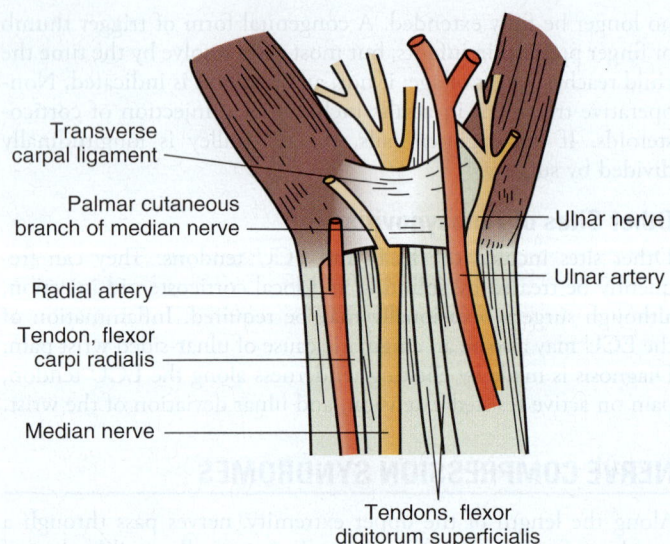

Transverse
carpal ligament

Palmar cutaneous
branch of median nerve

Radial artery

Tendon, flexor
carpi radialis

Median nerve

Ulnar nerve

Ulnar artery

Tendons, flexor
digitorum superficialis

FIGURE 119.42 Anatomy of the carpal tunnel. The transverse carpal ligament (flexor retinaculum) is divided longitudinally during a carpal tunnel release. *DIP,* Distal interphalangeal joint.

flexor tendons (Fig. 119.42). Its floor is formed by the carpal bones and roofed by the flexor retinaculum (transverse carpal ligament). Normal pressures in this tunnel are 20 to 30 mm Hg. A rise in pressure above this causes a chronic compressive ischemic injury to the nerve segment, resulting first in demyelination and eventually in axonal death. There is progressive conduction block in the nerve, with subsequent sensory and motor dysfunction. The earliest symptoms are pain and paresthesias, which are characteristically more obvious at night, after prolonged activity, and with positional postural changes at the wrist, such as when driving, using a hand-held hair dryer, or reading a book. The patient may complain of clumsiness and a tendency to drop objects. The paresthesias characteristically follow the distribution of the median nerve, including the thumb and the index and middle fingers.

Physical examination consists of compressing the carpal canal, percussing the median nerve, and hyperflexing the wrist to produce paresthesias (Durkan sign, Tinel sign, and Phalen test, respectively). Sensory evaluation reveals hypoesthesia in the distribution of the median nerve and may reveal a widened two-point sensory discrimination. Thenar weakness or muscle wasting is a late finding. Nerve conduction studies and electromyography are useful adjuncts to the clinical examination.

Initial treatment of carpal tunnel syndrome includes use of wrist splints (especially at night), occasional local corticosteroid injections, and modification of work patterns. If symptoms persist or if the initial presentation shows severe carpal tunnel syndrome, surgical decompression is required. This is performed by longitudinally dividing the flexor retinaculum by open or endoscopic means. Both the Agee (single-portal) and Chow (two-portal) procedures have shown similar efficacy to the open approach.[81] Synovectomy and removal of any mass lesion may also be required if that is the cause of the problem.[82]

Pronator Syndrome

In the proximal forearm, the median nerve may be compressed at the fibrous arch between the two heads of the FDS, two heads of the pronator teres, lacertus fibrosus (bicipital aponeurosis at the elbow), and ligament of Struthers. Compression at any or all of these sites is loosely grouped under the pronator syndrome. The symptoms produced are similar to those of carpal tunnel, although nocturnal symptoms are uncommon. The palm may also feel numb because the palmar cutaneous branch is involved, but it is specifically spared in carpal tunnel syndrome because that nerve branch passes superficial to the flexor retinaculum and arises proximal to the retinaculum. Symptoms may be reproduced or worsened by attempting pronation against resistance and by resisted flexion of the middle finger. However, it may be difficult to locate the compressive cause in the pronator syndrome precisely, and surgical decompression often involves release of all four potential sites of compression.

The anterior interosseous nerve branch of the median nerve may occasionally be compressed in isolation. This does not produce any sensory symptoms but specifically targets the three muscles innervated by the anterior interosseous nerve—FPL, FDP to the index and middle fingers, and pronator quadratus.

Ulnar Nerve Compression

The ulnar nerve may be compressed in the Guyon canal at the wrist or in the so-called cubital tunnel at the elbow and distal upper arm.

Guyon Canal Compression

The Guyon canal is bounded by the hook of the hamate, pisiform, pisohamate ligament, and palmar carpal ligament. Compression by mass lesions, including a ganglion, giant cell tumor, ulnar artery thrombosis, and ulnar artery aneurysm, may occur at this site as in hypothenar hammer syndrome. Compression at this site may also be idiopathic. Distal ulnar deficits may be in the motor or sensory distribution or both, depending on where in the canal the compression occurs relative to the takeoff of the deep motor branch of the ulnar nerve. Tinel sign may be present, and there may be worsening of symptoms by direct compression over the Guyon canal. Treatment is surgical; it consists of dividing the palmaris brevis muscle and palmar carpal ligament as well as removing any offending mass in this region.

Cubital Tunnel Syndrome

The cubital tunnel is a long tunnel starting in the distal upper arm and extending into the proximal forearm. As the ulnar nerve passes into the forearm, it curves tightly around the grooved posterior and inferior surfaces of the medial epicondyle of the humerus. This groove is bridged by the aponeurosis between the two heads of the FCU, the leading edge of which may be thickened and fibrosed, called *Osborne ligament.* More proximally, the ulnar nerve passes from the anterior compartment of the arm into the posterior compartment, which may be bridged by a long tunnel called the *arcade of Struthers.* The medial intermuscular septum in the upper arm may also cause ulnar nerve compression. The most distal fibro-osseous tunnel is more accurately termed the *cubital tunnel.* However, compression on the ulnar nerve can occur at any of these sites, proximal to distal, starting in the upper arm and extending into the forearm. Motor and sensory symptoms develop in the distribution of the ulnar nerve and are worsened by adopting a flexed position at the elbow. Examination reveals Tinel sign over the tunnel. Paresthesias are described in the distribution of the ulnar nerve to the little and ring fingers and ulnar border of the hand. A differential diagnosis includes thoracic outlet syndrome, compression of the ulnar nerve in the Guyon canal, and nerve root compression in the neck.

Initial treatment consists of splinting the elbow in extension at night. Use of soft extension elbow pads prevents elbow flexion and direct pressure on the nerve. Failure of nonoperative measures and significant changes in electrodiagnostic studies are indications for surgical decompression. Usually, all the fibrous restraints on the ulnar nerve around the elbow are released, and the nerve is transposed anteriorly to the medial epicondyle into a subcutaneous or submuscular position. There have been preliminary reports of success with endoscopic in situ decompression of the ulnar nerve at the elbow.

Radial Nerve Compression

The radial nerve may be compressed proximally in the triangular space in the axilla (specifically involving the axillary branch), spiral groove posterior to the humerus in the arm, and lateral intermuscular septum proximal to the elbow. More distally in the forearm, the PIN, the principal motor division of the radial nerve, can be compressed in the so-called radial tunnel, starting at the leading fibrous edge of the supinator (ligament of Frohse). There may be a variable degree of interosseous nerve paresis, or there may be pain radiating down the dorsoradial aspect of the forearm (called *radial tunnel syndrome*). Initial treatment is nonoperative with splinting, but if this fails, surgical decompression may occasionally be required.[83]

Thoracic Outlet Compression

The thoracic outlet is a narrow space at the base of the neck bounded by the first rib medially, scalenus anterior muscle and clavicle anteriorly, and scalenus medius muscle posteriorly. All elements of the brachial plexus as well as the subclavian artery and vein pass through this narrow space and can be potentially compressed at this site. A Tinel sign can often be elicited at the supraclavicular and infraclavicular regions. A Roos test is performed by asking the patient to hold both arms overhead in a surrender position while opening and closing the fists. This reproduces symptoms within 1 minute, and if continued, the arm collapses at the side. Adson test involves palpating the radial pulse while the patient turns the chin toward the same side, inhales deeply, and holds their breath. The radial pulse disappears or diminishes. The costoclavicular compression test involves sustained downward pressure on the clavicle, and the symptoms are reproduced. Radiographic evaluation may reveal a cervical rib. Results of nerve conduction studies are often normal.

Thoracic outlet compression may occur in association with other peripheral sites of nerve compression, a condition termed *double-crush syndrome*. Treatment is primarily nonoperative, involving posture-improving exercises and avoidance of aggravating activities. If symptoms persist, especially if they are associated with vascular compression, the thoracic outlet may be surgically decompressed. This is accomplished by a transcervical or transaxillary resection of the first rib, often with release of the scalene muscles.

TUMORS

Ganglions and mucous cysts represent 60% to 70% of hand tumors, followed in frequency by inclusion cysts, warts (verrucae), giant cell tumors in tendon sheaths, foreign body granulomas, lipomas, hemangiomas, and pyogenic granulomas (Table 119.9). Benign tumors account for 95% of hand neoplasms. Squamous cell carcinoma is the most frequent primary malignant neoplasm of the hand, basal cell carcinoma is rare, and melanoma is relatively uncommon in the upper extremity. Acral lentiginous melanoma (e.g., in the palm, sole, or nail bed) has a tendency for early

metastasis. Primary bone tumors of the hand are generally benign; the most common are enchondromas and osteochondromas. Giant cell tumors of bone in the hand are rare, occurring usually in the distal radius. They are locally aggressive and may occasionally metastasize. Of malignant bone tumors, only 1.2% affect the hand. Although bone metastases in other parts of the body are relatively common, bones of the hand are rarely affected by metastases from other sites.[84,85]

Soft tissue sarcomas are rare, representing 1% of all malignant neoplasms of the body, excluding skin tumors. Although uncommon, certain types predominate in the hand. Epithelioid, synovial, and clear cell sarcomas are relatively rare in other sites but, by comparison, are more common in the hand.

Within the spectrum of benign and malignant tumors, there is a group with intermediate malignancy. Giant cell and desmoid tumors (of soft tissue) have a propensity for local recurrence after surgical excision. Their histologic patterns may belie their behavior. Juvenile aponeurotic fibroma and nodular fasciitis may appear histologically more aggressive than desmoid tumors but are self-limited. The tiny glomus tumor is uncommon but has a propensity for the fingertips and subungual regions. It may be an enigmatic cause of severe and exquisite pain at the fingertips and can be recognized by a pinpoint site of extreme local tenderness and a violaceous hue deep to the nail plate. MRI may occasionally detect these tiny lesions at the fingertip.

If a lesion is thought to be benign, excision without further workup, except perhaps for routine radiographs, is appropriate. However, if a primary malignant neoplasm of bone or soft tissue is suspected, additional studies must be undertaken before biopsy. CT may help delineate tumor boundaries. Desmoid tumors have radiographic density identical to that of muscle and are better demonstrated by MRI.

Soft Tissue Tumors
Ganglion Cysts

Ganglions are formed by an outpouching of the synovial membrane from a joint or tendon sheath. They contain thick, jelly-like, mucinous material similar in composition to synovial fluid (Fig. 119.43). Of ganglions, 60% occur on the dorsal aspect of the wrist, arising in the region of the scapholunate ligament. Other sites for ganglions in the hand are at the volar wrist, arising from one of the scaphoid articulations; at the flexor tendon sheath at the area of the A1 pulley; and at the dorsum of the DIPJ, called a *mucous cyst,* where they are often associated with osteoarthritis of that DIPJ. In the last location, the ganglion cyst can exert pressure on the germinal matrix of the nail bed, resulting in a deformed or grooved nail.

Ganglions are most common in females in the third decade of life. They are innocuous and can often be left alone. However, treatment may be required for cosmetic purposes or to relieve pressure effects on adjacent structures (Fig. 119.44). The dorsal wrist ganglion can sometimes be painful as a result of pressure on the PIN at that location. A very small impalpable dorsal wrist ganglion can become quite painful, the so-called occult ganglion, and on occasion may best be diagnosed by MRI. Treatment of a dorsal wrist ganglion may be performed by aspiration of the mucinous substance with a large-bore needle. If this fails, the ganglion can then be surgically excised. Care must be taken to trace and resect the pedicle of the ganglion all the way down to the joint or tendon sheath from which it arises. A volar wrist ganglion may often be closely related to the radial artery. Aspiration of

TABLE 119.9 **Benign Connective Tissue Tumors of the Hand**

SOFT TISSUE TUMORS	PRESENTATION	MOST COMMON LOCATIONS	TISSUE OF ORIGIN AND APPEARANCE	TREATMENT	RADIOGRAPHIC APPEARANCE
Ganglion	Swelling, sometimes painful; DIP mucous cyst may spontaneously drain clear gelatinous fluid; 70% of hand swellings	Volar and dorsal wrist, flexor tendon sheath, dorsum of DIP joint	Synovial cyst containing thick gelatinous fluid	No treatment versus aspiration versus excision	No radiographic alterations; mucous cyst at DIP joint may have osteophytes associated with osteoarthritis
Giant cell tumor of tendon sheath	Progressive enlargement, painless, deeply adherent; potential recurrence after excision; second most common hand tumor	Any synovial site, including tendon sheath, joint, palmar plate, usually in a digit	Synovium and histiocytes; bosselated and yellow-brown color from hemosiderin pigmentation	Excision	Pressure resorption of bone
Lipoma	Painless enlarging mass, usually on volar surface of hand or finger; may reach very large size; seldom nerve compression symptoms	Volar hand and finger	Mature fat cells	Excision (shell out)	Characteristic water-clear appearance on radiograph
Inclusion cyst (implantation dermoid)	Painless, enlarging lesion, adherent to overlying dermis; more common in laborers and those subject to minor hand trauma; may become infected	Palm and fingertips	Implanted epidermis cyst containing keratinous debris	Excision of entire epithelium-lined sac	May cause pressure resorption of bone
Neurofibroma	May be localized, diffuse, or plexiform; may be associated with von Recklinghausen disease; painless enlargement, but pain arouses suspicion of malignant change	Less common on hand than elsewhere; seen more frequently on palm	Perineurial fibroblasts	Excision if noncritical nerve; biopsy if malignancy suspected; possible nerve grafting	Characteristic MRI lobulated appearance
Schwannoma	Painless small mass in a peripheral nerve that is laterally mobile; may be an incidental finding at time of carpal tunnel surgery; occasional distal dysesthesias	Median and digital nerves	Schwann cells	Microneural surgery can shell the tumor out of the nerve without leaving neurologic deficit	No changes on plain radiograph
Pyogenic granuloma	Often at site of previous trivial skin injury on the fingers; friable and bleeds easily; grows rapidly	Fingers	Granulation tissue	Small lesions can be cauterized; excise larger lesions	No radiographic changes
Glomus tumor	Very small lesions; exquisitely painful, localized tenderness, cold sensitive; patients sometimes labeled as malingering	Subungual or volar fingertip; may be multiple	Neuromyoarterial apparatus	Excision; repair nail bed if subungual	May show indentation of distal phalanx

DIP, Distal interphalangeal.

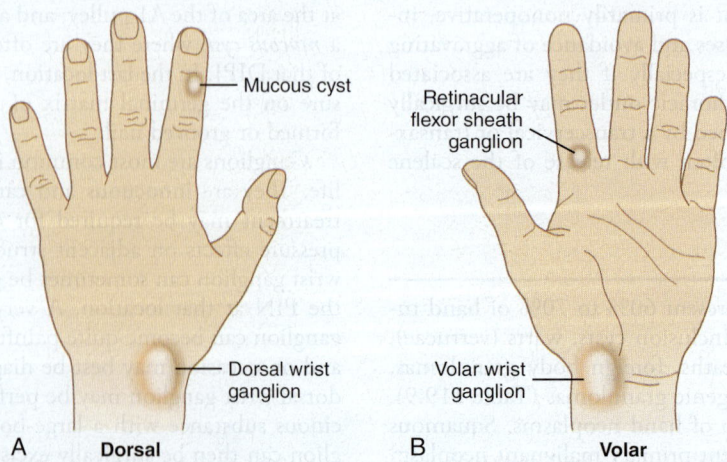

A **Dorsal** — Mucous cyst, Dorsal wrist ganglion

B **Volar** — Retinacular flexor sheath ganglion, Volar wrist ganglion

FIGURE 119.43 Dorsal (A) and volar (B) aspects of the hand and wrist showing common types of ganglions, including the dorsal wrist ganglion, volar wrist ganglion, flexor sheath ganglion (volar retinacular cyst), and mucous cyst.

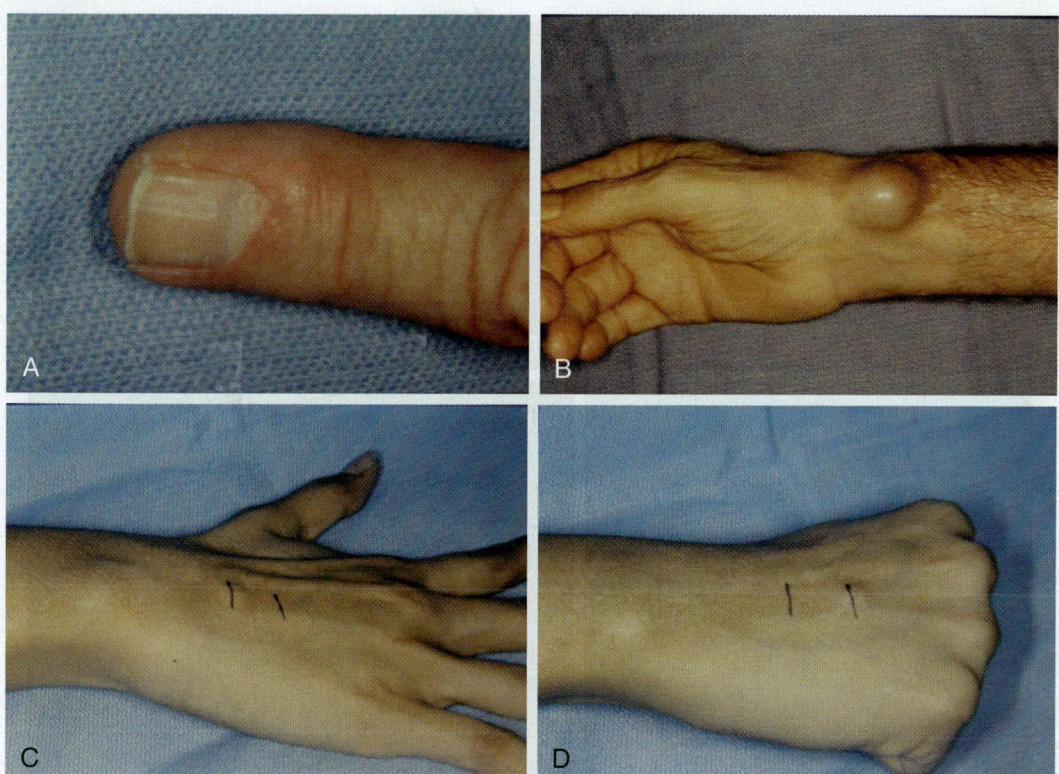

FIGURE 119.44 Ganglions in the hand. (A) Ganglion associated with osteoarthritis of the distal interphalangeal joint (mucous cyst), causing longitudinal linear groove in the nail plate from pressure on the germinal matrix. (B) Volar wrist ganglion on the radial side of the flexor carpi radialis tendon is closely related to the radial artery and should not be aspirated. (C) Ganglion arising from the extensor digitorum communis tendon of the ring finger located at the level of the proximal skin marking with fingers extended. (D) Movement of ganglion 2 cm to the level of the more distal skin marking when the fist is clenched. Distal movement of the swelling with the gliding extensor tendon confirms its attachment to the tendon.

volar wrist ganglions is seldom advised because of the potential risk of injury to the radial artery. At the level of the DIPJ, optimal treatment includes not only meticulous excision of the ganglion but also the removal of associated osteophytes from the joint. Arthroscopic decompression of dorsal wrist ganglions has been described.

Giant Cell Tumor

Giant cell tumor, also called *pigmented villonodular synovitis,* is the second most common hand tumor. It occurs in soft tissues (e.g., synovial membrane of joints, tendon sheaths) and, less commonly, in bone. This yellow-brown multilobular tumor is composed of multinucleated giant cells. Although usually benign, the tumor pushes deeply into the soft tissues of the digits and extends along tendon sheaths and around neurovascular structures. It is frequently asymptomatic and is often larger than suspected clinically. Radiologic notching of bone may be evident in larger, soft tissue giant cell tumors. Complete surgical excision is the treatment of choice. Failure to discern and remove each lobule substantially increases the reported local recurrence rate of almost 10%. Synovectomy of the joint of origin may be necessary (Fig. 119.45).

Epidermal Inclusion Cysts

Epidermal inclusion cysts, also called *implantation dermoids,* frequently occur after trauma as keratin-producing epidermal cells become lodged in the subcutaneous tissues (see Fig. 119.45). The resulting cystic mass contains a thick toothpaste-like material. They occur more commonly in males, especially in manual laborers, and most frequently involve the palm of the hand and fingertips. They may also occur in previous surgical scars. Treatment is surgical excision, and recurrence is rare.

Lipoma

Lipomas are small, benign, soft, fluctuant, fatty tumors (Fig. 119.46). In the hand, they usually occur on the thenar eminence. Although generally painless, they may enlarge significantly, insinuating into deep palmar spaces and causing pain by compression on adjacent nerves. Intracarpal lipoma is a rarer cause of carpal tunnel syndrome. Resection of symptomatic lipomas is curative, although 1% to 2% may recur.

Pyogenic Granuloma

Pyogenic granuloma is a misnomer for an exuberant outburst of highly vascular granulation tissue at the site of previous relatively trivial trauma. These lesions are friable, bleed easily, and may grow rapidly. They respond to curettage or simple excision. They usually occur on the fingertips. Histologic confirmation of the diagnosis is necessary because of occasional confusion with aggressive malignant lesions, such as ulcerated, amelanotic, malignant melanomas.

Verruca Vulgaris

Verrucae vulgaris are common contagious warts associated with human papillomavirus type 1. They usually occur as hyperkeratotic

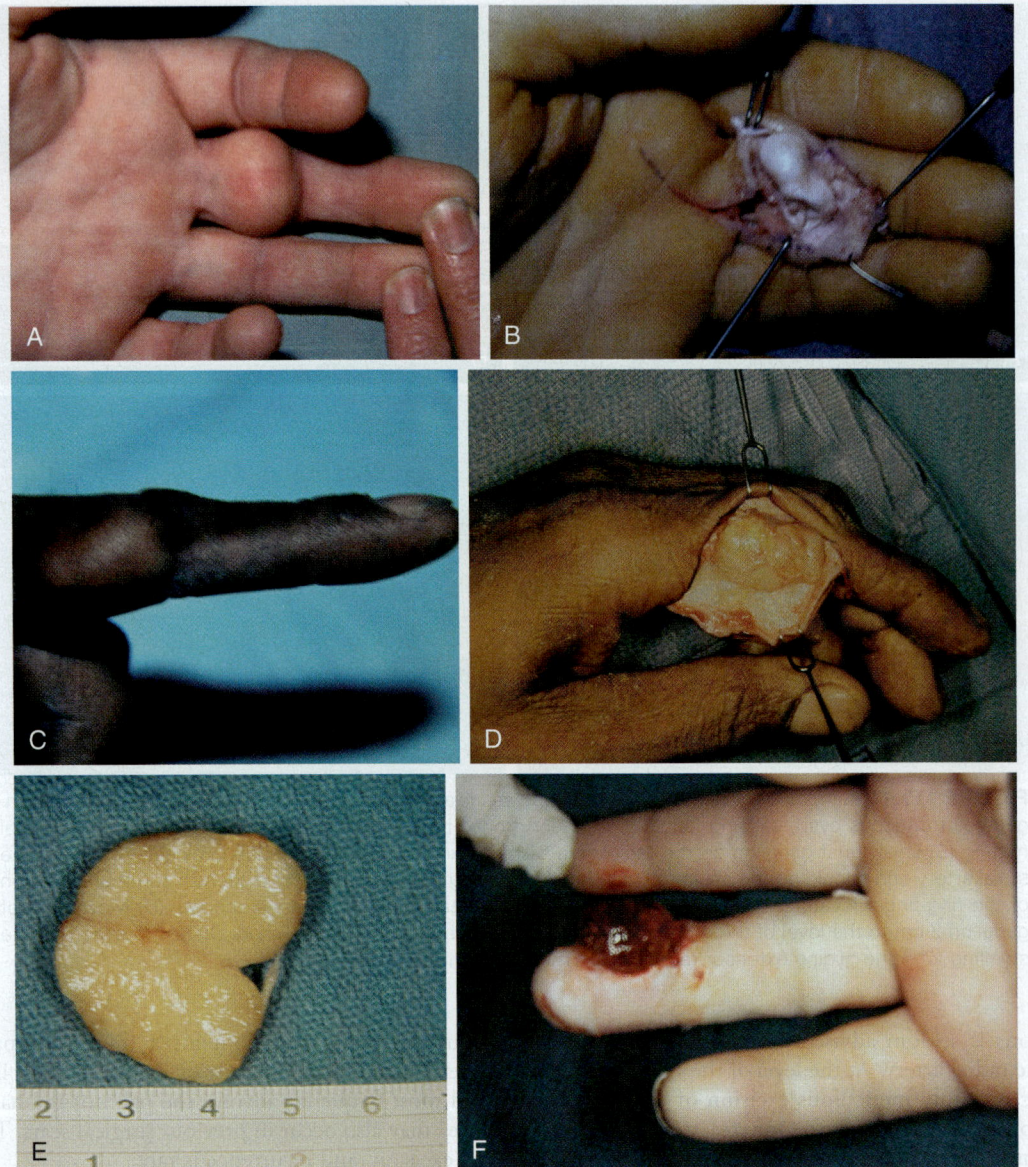

FIGURE 119.45 Soft tissue tumors of the hand. (A) Traumatically induced inclusion cyst on the palmar aspect of the middle finger in a manual worker. (B) Intraoperative photograph demonstrates cyst filled with toothpaste-like gel derived from keratin. (C) Firm, progressively enlarging swelling on the radial side of the left index finger. (D) Firm, lobulated, yellow-brown giant cell tumor insinuating onto the dorsal and volar aspects of the finger is noted intraoperatively. (E) Giant cell tumor is the most common solid soft tissue tumor encountered in the hand. (F) Fleshy, friable pyogenic granuloma bleeds easily on contact.

filiform lesions on the digits or around the nail bed. The most effective topical treatments are salicylates, liquid nitrogen cryotherapy, and especially curettage. Recalcitrant lesions respond to oral cimetidine given for 6 to 8 weeks and to imiquimod, an immunomodulator that increases interferon production. Their incidence, like that of squamous cell carcinomas, is increased in immunocompromised patients, such as in those after transplantation. Recurrence is relatively common.

Seborrheic Keratoses

Seborrheic keratoses are benign, hyperkeratotic, scaly lesions. They are frequently pigmented and common on the dorsum of the hand in older adults. Occasional confusion occurs with

pigmented basal cell carcinomas. When necessary, these superficial scaly lesions are best treated by shave excision, and sutures are unnecessary. Rapid reepithelialization occurs.

Keratoacanthoma

Keratoacanthoma occurs on exposed body parts such as the dorsum of the hand. It grows rapidly over approximately 3 weeks into a nodule with a central umbilicated keratotic plug, often followed by spontaneous resolution in many weeks or months. The resulting scar is often worse than if the lesion had been excised initially. There may be diagnostic uncertainty in regard to well-differentiated squamous cell carcinomas. Hence, most authors recommend surgical excision.

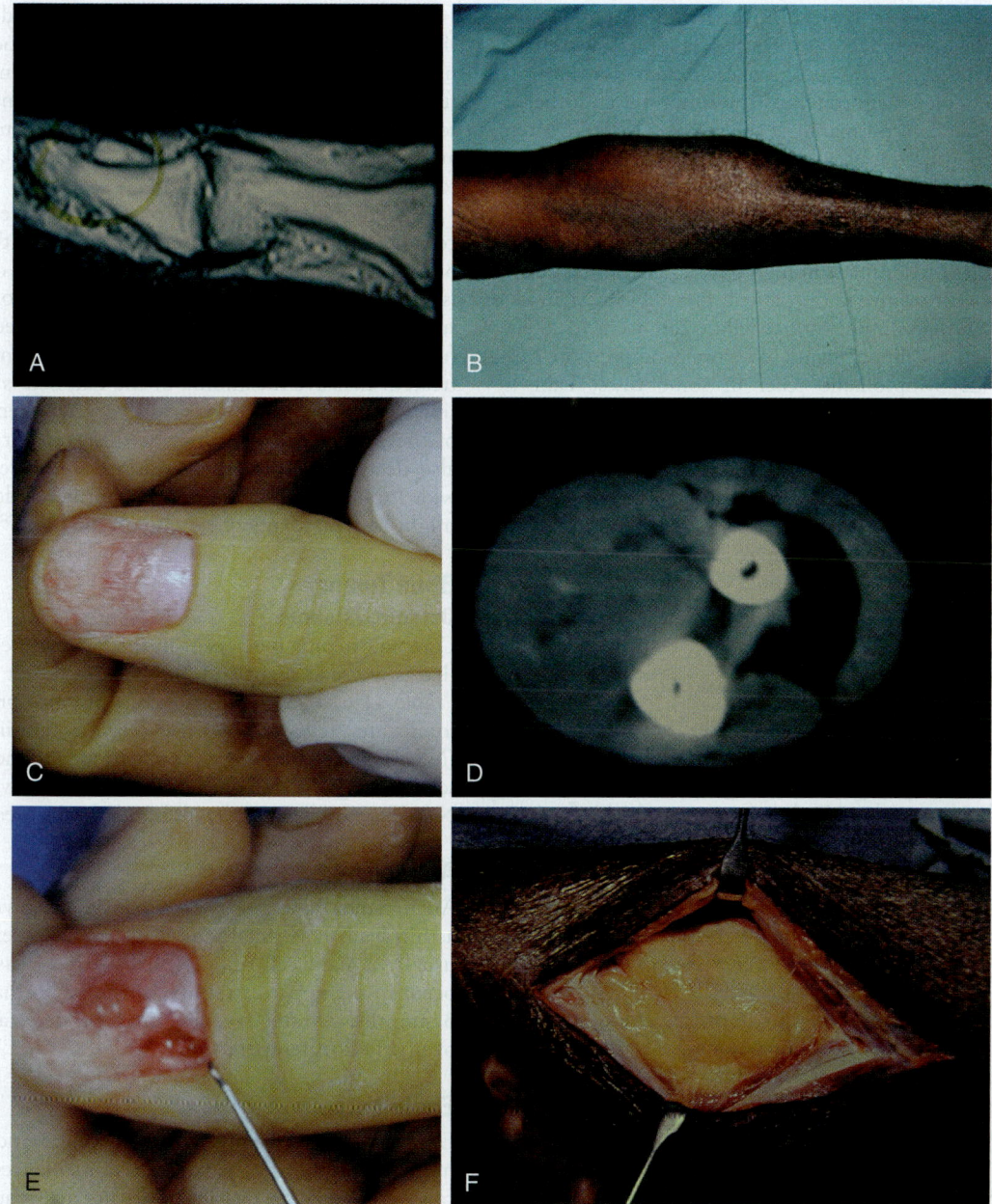

FIGURE 119.46 Soft tissue tumors of the hand. (A) Patient presenting with pain in tip of thumb, exacerbated in cold weather. Exquisite pain on palpation of the thumb nail plate is typical of a subungual glomus tumor that can be demonstrated by magnetic resonance imaging. (B) Occult subungual glomus tumor may be difficult to appreciate, even after removal of the nail plate, but it can often be identified by a surface bulge of the nail bed. (C) Excised glomus tumor sitting on nail bed. A nail bed defect requires repair with fine absorbable sutures. (D) Patient with swelling of left dorsoradial forearm and weakness of finger and thumb extension. (E) MRI reveals a dorsal forearm mass compressing the posterior interosseous nerve. (F) Dorsal approach over the mass reveals intramuscular benign lipoma when extensor muscles are split.

Dermatofibroma

A dermatofibroma arises from fibrous dermal tissue as a firm erythematous plaque, sometimes having central umbilication. It is often adherent to the overlying epidermis. Surgery is required primarily for diagnosis.

Vascular Malformations and Hemangiomas

Hemangiomas are hamartomas that are rarely visible at birth and are usually noticed weeks to months later. Rapid proliferation occurs in the first year of life. On histologic evaluation, proliferation of endothelial cells with increased mitotic activity is seen in conjunction with pericytes and dendritic and mast cells. Hemangiomas occur 10 times more commonly than vascular malformations, and approximately 70% involute by the age of 7 years, leaving a fibrofatty scar with redundant skin. Excision is seldom required and, after involution, is usually cosmetic. On occasion, oral or injectable steroids may be necessary to control rapidly proliferating lesions that cause pain or interfere with function.

Propranolol, which reduces basic fibroblast growth factor and vascular endothelial growth factor expression, is sometimes added in conjunction with steroids for problematic hemangiomas.[86,87]

By contrast, vascular malformations show normal endothelial growth characteristics and normal mast cell counts. They are often noted at birth, and growth is usually commensurate with the child for low-flow lesions. They do not undergo spontaneous involution.

Vascular malformations are subclassified into low-flow lesions; capillary, venous, and lymphatic lesions predominate. Arterial and arteriovenous fistulas predominate in high-flow lesions, and accelerated growth may occur relative to the patient. Pressure effects, ulceration, bleeding, and high-output cardiac failure can occur in severe cases. Enlarging lesions hinder hand function. Compression garments can provide symptomatic relief in some cases. Pain is often caused by vascular engorgement, phlebitis, or intralesional coagulation. D-dimer levels may be elevated, and some patients obtain relief from aspirin. Combined surgical excision and radiologic embolization are most effective in preventing recurrence caused by dilation of collateral vascular channels after simple excision.

Lymphaticovenous malformations may also be associated with generalized hypertrophy of an extremity. Vascular malformations and isolated macrodactyly are seen in Klippel-Trénaunay syndrome.

Malignant Skin Tumors
Basal Cell Carcinoma
Basal cell carcinoma is rare on the hand and is generally located on the dorsum. It is usually an ulcer with raised pearly edges. Treatment consists of excision with a margin of normal adjacent tissue. Nail bed lesions can be mistaken for paronychial infection, and amputation at the DIPJ may be required.

Squamous Cell Carcinoma
Squamous cell carcinoma may arise de novo from ultraviolet light exposure because of occupation or climate, usually on the sun-exposed dorsum of the hand. Approximately 16% of actinic keratoses may progress to squamous cell carcinoma. Arsenical keratoses may develop secondary to exposure to inorganic arsenic compounds but have a predilection for the palm.

Bowen disease is an intraepidermal squamous cell carcinoma (carcinoma in situ). It is a plaquelike lesion with crusting. Complete surgical excision with a margin of normal tissue is curative. When the nail matrix is involved, amputation at the DIPJ may be necessary.

For squamous cell carcinoma lesions smaller than 2.5 cm in diameter, wide excision with approximately a 6-mm clear margin is recommended. However, for larger lesions, more radical excision may be required, which may even include ray or segmental amputation for deeply adherent and invasive lesions. Mohs micrographic surgery and three-dimensional histologic reconstruction with a pathologist at the time of radical resection help ensure complete excision. Routine prophylactic lymphadenectomy is not beneficial. However, lymphadenectomy may be advised for recurrent tumors, even though lymph nodes may not be clinically palpable. Malignant degeneration may occur in cicatricial tissue and chronic ulcers (e.g., Marjolijn ulcer) and, in particular, in burn scars. Prognosis tends to be poorer.

Malignant Melanomas
Melanoma of the hand is cutaneous or subungual. There is an almost equal distribution of cases between the two types. Frequently, there is a delay in treatment, particularly with subungual melanomas. Suspicious lesions should be biopsied.[88]

Any subungual pigmented lesions should generally be biopsied. Under tourniquet control and with loupe magnification, the nail plate is atraumatically removed, and a longitudinal, elliptical, full-thickness excision of the lesion is performed. Careful nail bed repair is done after biopsy by the advancement of adjacent tissues and using fine absorbable sutures. The nail plate is then reapplied to act as a splint.[88]

Benign melanocytic hyperplasia, without evidence of atypia, is completely treated by this form of biopsy. If there is any evidence of melanocytic atypia, absolute confirmation of complete excision is required. In the absence of a clear margin or with recurrence of such a lesion, total nail bed excision and reconstruction with a full-thickness skin graft are required. Melanoma in situ is similarly treated. Invasive melanoma of the nail bed is treated by amputation at the next most proximal joint. Acral lentiginous melanoma of the palm may sometimes be mistaken for a wart, which may also delay diagnosis. These tumors are aggressively treated with wide local excision and potential sentinel node biopsy, just as they might be treated anywhere else on the body.[88]

Bone Tumor
Osteoid Osteoma
Osteoid osteoma may occur in the hand and classically causes pain that is worse at night and unrelated to use or motion of the hand (Table 119.10). Osteoid osteomas produce prostaglandins; symptoms are relieved by nonsteroidal antiinflammatory drugs (NSAIDs). On radiologic examination, a round, lucent tumor with sclerotic edges is seen (Fig. 119.47A). Conservative treatment with NSAIDs may be considered, but definitive treatment is surgical.

Aneurysmal Bone Cyst
Aneurysmal bone cyst is an expansile osteolytic bone lesion with a thin wall. It is usually derived from a preexisting bone tumor, usually a giant cell tumor (20%–40% of cases). Of these, 25% occur in the upper extremity, causing pain that peaks during 2 to 3 months. A bone swelling may be detectable, with increased overlying skin temperature.

Enchondroma
Enchondromas usually occur in the hand and are the most common bone tumor of the hand. Peak incidence is in the second decade, with equal sex distribution. They are frequently asymptomatic and noted incidentally as lytic lesions on plain radiology. Pain, bone swelling, or pathologic fracture may occur as these cartilaginous intraosseous cysts compromise bone structural integrity (see Fig. 119.47D). Treatment is by curettage and bone grafting of the osseous defect. Multiple enchondromatosis occurs in Ollier disease and is associated with angiomas in Maffucci syndrome.

Primary Bone Sarcomas
Primary bone sarcomas (malignant tumors) are rare in the hand.

Secondary (Metastatic) Bone Tumors
Metastatic tumors, even those with a tendency to metastasize to bone, usually occur in the axial skeleton and long bones. They are very rare in the hand.

CONGENITAL ANOMALIES
Congenital hand and upper extremity anomalies encompass a wide array of conditions. Their prevalence is ~1 in 600 live births. The causes of congenital hand anomalies may be genetic, teratogenic,

TABLE 119.10 Bone Tumors of the Hand

TUMOR	PRESENTATION	MOST COMMON LOCATIONS	TISSUE OF ORIGIN AND APPEARANCE	TREATMENT	RADIOGRAPHIC APPEARANCE
Enchondroma	Often incidental finding on routine hand radiograph; presents as pain secondary to pathologic fracture; most common bone tumor of hand	Proximal and middle phalanges and metacarpals	Fragments of cartilage nests; multiple (Ollier disease); when associated with hemangiomas (Maffucci syndrome), may undergo malignant change	Curettage, filling of defect with cancellous bone if structural bone integrity is compromised	Lesion eccentric in bone shaft with calcific stippling
Osteochondroma	Benign bone prominence (capped with cartilage); rare in hand; may cause angular growth and interfere with joint motion	Fingers and wrist; growth stops after skeletal maturity reached	Aberrant focus of cartilage; multiple osteochondromatosis is autosomal dominant; malignant change may occur	Surgery may be necessary, generally after epiphyseal closure	Exostosis, often at base of proximal phalanx; often shortening of parent bone
Osteoid osteoma	Aching pain, greatest at night, sometimes responding specifically to aspirin; patient may be labeled as malingerer	Phalanges, metacarpals, carpals	Nidus composed of loose fibrovascular connective tissue between bars of osteoid and bone trabeculae	Surgical excision to include the nidus	Very small lesion; some not seen on plain radiographs and require CT scan; cortical sclerosis surrounding a radiolucent area of nidus
Giant cell tumor of bone	Expansile bone swelling at distal radius or in phalanx	Distal radius most common site	May be locally aggressive and even metastasize	Curettage for low-grade lesions, but en bloc resection for high-grade lesions; do not irradiate because it could induce sarcomatous change	Expansile soap-bubble lesion in bone; high-grade lesions break through cortex

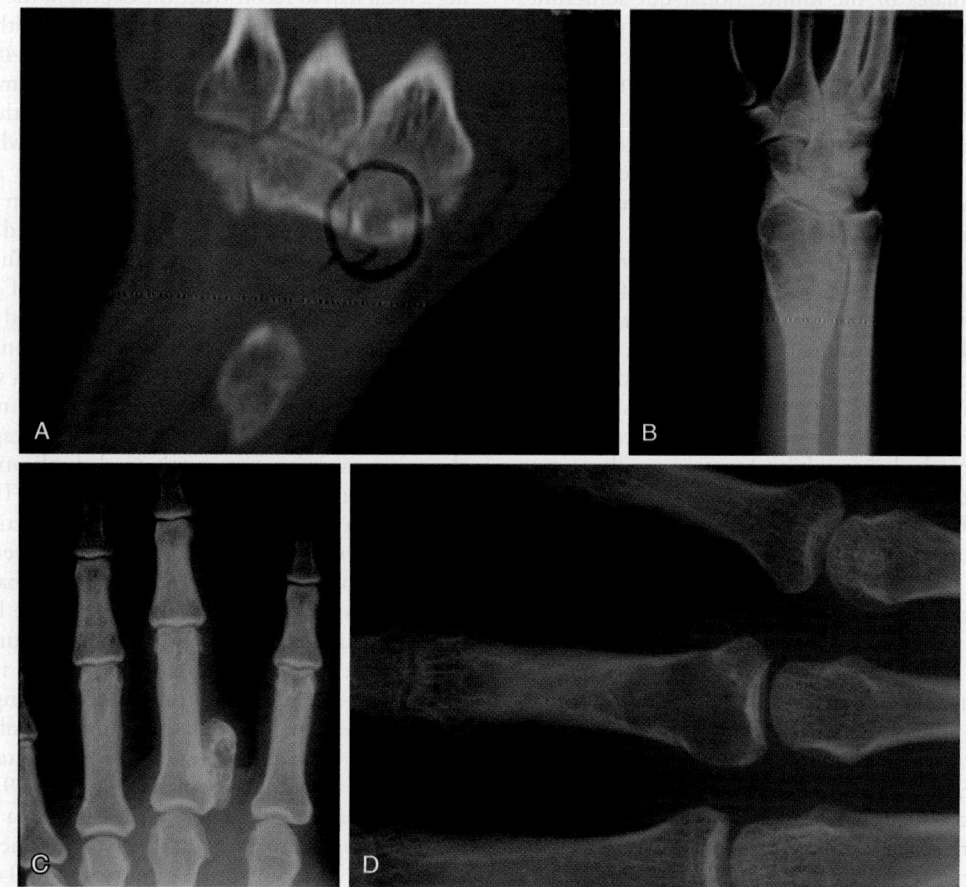

FIGURE 119.47 Plain radiographs of the upper extremity. (A) Osteoid osteoma of carpus. (B) Soap-bubble appearance of giant cell tumor expanding the metaphysis of the distal radius. (C) Osteochondroma of proximal phalanx of middle (long) finger. (D) Patient with finger pain after trivial injury. This is a pathologic fracture of the base of the proximal phalanx through an enchondroma that has replaced most of the proximal metaphysis and medulla.

or idiopathic and may also have a syndromic association with anomalies elsewhere in the body. Knowledge of these associations is important because the more life-threatening associated problems frequently need to be treated first, before the hand and upper extremity reconstruction can be performed. Such an association is found in a constellation of problems that occur in the VACTERL association of congenital defects (vertebral anomalies, anal atresia, cardiac abnormalities, tracheoesophageal fistula, renal agenesis, and limb anomalies).

A number of factors must be considered in optimizing the timing of each surgical procedure to the upper extremity, including the psychosocial development of the child, presence of other illnesses, size of the structures to be operated on, and normal growth and development of the hand. Modern technologic advances have allowed us to operate on smaller structures; the timing of the procedure can now be guided by knowledge of the anatomy and development of the growing hand. Optimal function is the primary goal of surgery. Early surgery prevents the emotional scarring associated with a child's awareness of the deformity, and some congenital problems may not be apparent in the neonate. The hand surgeon must work closely with the pediatrician to identify general conditions that may affect the child's health. Some congenital anomalies of the extremities, especially those with the radial ray, may be associated with bone marrow failure (Fanconi syndrome) or heart defects that may not be immediately apparent in the neonate. Children with congenital anomalies will attempt to keep up with their peers and often develop successful hand substitution techniques. However, once a child experiences the cruel ridicule of playmates or the unintentional but sometimes overly solicitous supervision of a teacher, the deformity becomes important. In general, plans for surgical reconstruction are designed to be completed by school age so that the child may adapt to and fully use the reconstructed limb.[89,90]

The rationale for early surgery includes the avoidance of deformity and malfunction and optimal use of infantile tissue plasticity. Because hand length almost doubles during the first 2 years of life, a digit tethered to another digit that fails to grow can produce a major deformity during the early growth spurt. For example, with separation of syndactyly that involves the border digits of the hand, because of adjacent tethering to a digit of unequal length, surgical separation of the syndactyly is required at an early age, as early as 6 months, to avoid secondary angular deformity of the digits.

In rare circumstances, urgent treatment in the neonate is required. The distal lymphedema of a severe constriction band syndrome may be so marked as to inhibit function totally or even threaten distal viability. This may require urgent release. The unusual clinical entity of aplasia cutis may result in exposure of vital structures, requiring urgent soft tissue coverage, even in the neonatal period.

Early operation, although not urgent, may be required not only because of the rapid growth that occurs in the first 2 years of life but also because of functional consequences. Surgery at a young age is considered mandatory in children with malformations in which hand function may be altered by surgery or in those who are at risk for development of certain grasping habits that would have to be unlearned after corrective surgery. An older child, 12 to 14 years of age, has developed grasp patterns that would have to be altered by prolonged periods of physical therapy after corrective surgery.[86]

The ability to place the upper limbs in space (a cortical function) and development of a strong grasp are established by 1 year of age, as are grasp and pinch maneuvers between the thumb and fingers. Accuracy of prehension and refinement of coordination continue until 3 years of age. Surgery must be performed early to allow the affected parts to develop differently when the function of the parts of the hand is altered by transposition (e.g., pollicization of an index finger for thumb aplasia). Duplicated thumb correction is carried out before 1 year of age, well in advance of the development of integrated thumb grasp patterns.

Finally, the physical ability of infant bone and soft tissues to adapt to change produced by surgery is also a key factor in deciding when to operate. In the early pollicization of the index finger, the first dorsal interosseous muscle hypertrophies to form a thenar eminence, and the first metacarpal (formerly known as the *proximal phalanx* of the index finger) broadens. If centralization of the wrist for radial dysplasia (formerly known as *radial club hand*) has been undertaken early, the head of the ulna broadens to resemble the distal end of the radius.

Thus, a number of issues are taken into consideration when deciding on the optimum time for surgical reconstruction of congenital hand and upper extremity anomalies. The more common hand anomalies include syndactyly, polydactyly, constriction band syndrome, and absent or hypoplastic thumb.

Syndactyly results from the failure of programmed cell death (apoptosis) between the individual finger rays. Consequently, there is a resulting fusion of adjacent digits. It can involve part or all of the length of the digits (incomplete or complete) and may be limited to skin and soft tissue only (simple syndactyly) or can also involve skeletal fusion (complex syndactyly). Apert syndrome also involves craniofacial anomalies and is a severe form of bilaterally symmetric complex syndactyly. Surgical treatment involves digit separation using a local flap to reconstruct the depths of the commissure between the fingers and release of the finger borders with zigzag incisions and the use of full-thickness skin grafts (Fig. 119.48A).

Polydactyly is the presence of extranumerary digits on the hand. Preaxial (radial) polydactyly involves the thumb. It is not as common as postaxial (ulnar) polydactyly, which is the most frequent congenital hand anomaly in African Americans. Polydactyly can be as simple as the presence of a skin tag–like structure or may have a complex arrangement of shared vessels, nerves, and bones. Thumb polydactyly is not merely a duplication but a splitting of a single digit, with variable degrees of development in each of the separate parts. It is typically classified into seven subtypes by the Wassel classification, which is based on the specific duplication, progressing from distal to proximal, in which the odd numbers are at distal and proximal phalanx and metacarpal, and even numbers are at IPJs, MPJs, and CMCJs, respectively. Type IV is the most common type, with total duplication of proximal and distal phalanges and a shared MPJ. Type VII refers to associated triphalangia with a duplication. Reconstructive goals include stabilization without sacrificing mobility, proper alignment of joints along the longitudinal axis of the thumb, balanced motor units, and a cosmetically acceptable nail plate (see Fig. 119.48B–C).

The Blauth classification categorizes thumb hypoplasia from type I, which represents minor hypoplasia, to type V, which is a total thumb absence. Surgical correction ranges from reconstruction of the existing hypoplastic thumb to pollicization (creating a thumb from the index finger) for complete absence or for the more severe types of hypoplasia (Fig. 119.49).

Clinodactyly is a curving of the digits in a radial or ulnar direction. It is common, particularly involving the little finger in many individuals, but a curvature of more than 10 degrees is considered abnormal. The distal phalanx is usually affected, and a delta phalanx may be associated. A delta phalanx occurs when the epiphysis forms a *C* shape around the metaphyseal core in the middle phalanx. Most patients present with little or no functional or

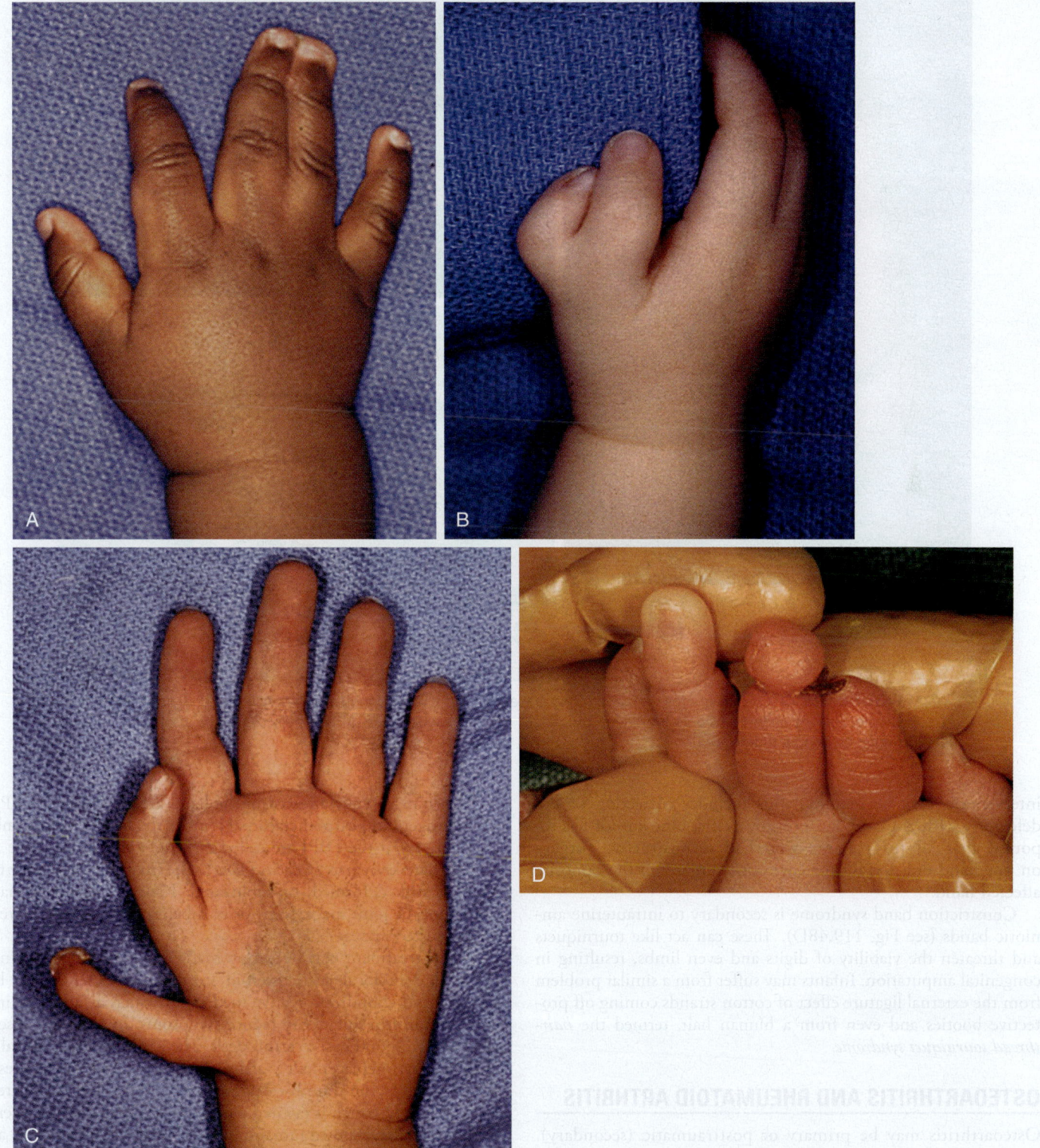

FIGURE 119.48 Congenital hand anomalies include syndactyly (A), Wassel type IV thumb polydactyly (B), Wassel type VI polydactyly (C), and constriction band (D).

cosmetic deformity, and operative intervention is seldom required. If there is a functionally impairing deviation of the finger, corrective osteotomy can be done.

Camptodactyly is a congenital flexion deformity of digits. It usually occurs in the little finger PIPJ. The exact cause is unclear, but it has been attributed to a variety of different structures

around the PIPJ, including a skin pterygium, collateral ligaments, volar plate, flexor tendon, abnormal insertions of lumbrical or interosseous muscles, and size and shape of the head of the proximal phalanx. Treatment is generally nonoperative and may involve serial splinting. If no improvement occurs and the flexion deformity is sufficient to cause a functional problem, surgical

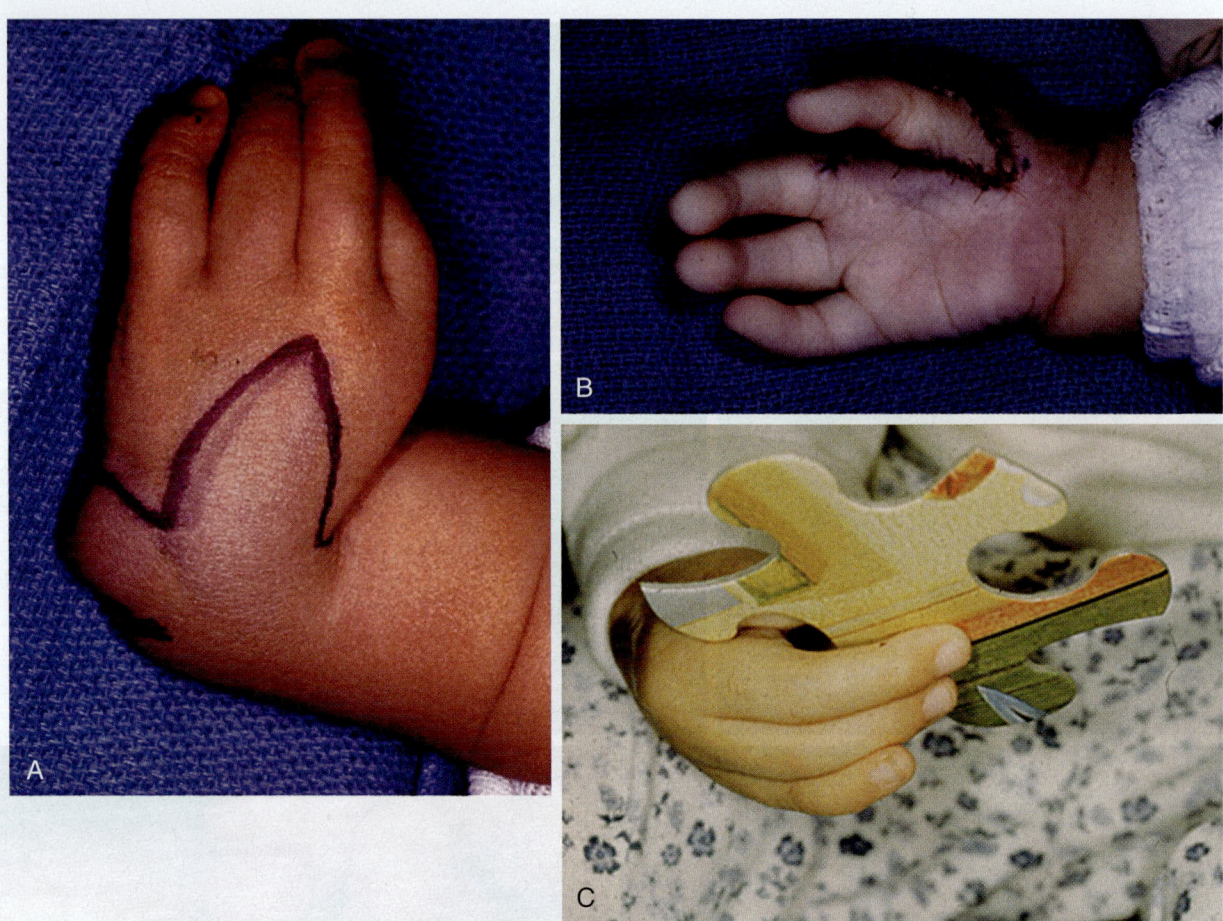

FIGURE 119.49 Clinical photos demonstrating a patient with radial longitudinal deficiency and absent thumb. Patient underwent a centralization procedure using a bilobed flap (A) and pollicization of the index finger, creating a thumb (B–C).

intervention may be required; this includes correction of the deformity with Z-plasty and possibly grafts. One author has reported that all his patients who had reconstructive surgery on one hand did not ask for corrective surgery on the opposite affected hand.

Constriction band syndrome is secondary to intrauterine amniotic bands (see Fig. 119.48D). These can act like tourniquets and threaten the viability of digits and even limbs, resulting in congenital amputation. Infants may suffer from a similar problem from the external ligature effect of cotton strands coming off protective booties and even from a human hair, termed the *hair-thread tourniquet syndrome*.

OSTEOARTHRITIS AND RHEUMATOID ARTHRITIS

Osteoarthritis may be primary or posttraumatic (secondary). Primary osteoarthritis is a degenerative joint disease occurring in later life. An injury that leaves articular surfaces of a joint incongruous can precipitate secondary osteoarthritis. Osteoarthritis begins with biochemical alteration of the water content of articular cartilage. The cartilage weakens and develops cracks, called *fibrillation*. Progressive erosion and thinning of the cartilage result, and the subchondral bone becomes sclerotic, termed *eburnation*. New bone forms around the edges of the articular cartilage, and these outcroppings are called *osteophytes* (Fig. 119.50).

The joints usually affected in the hand are the DIP and PIPJs of the fingers and carpometacarpal joint at the base of the thumb. Osteophytes at the DIPJ are called *Heberden nodes,* and those at the PIPJ are known as *Bouchard nodes.* The involved joints may be painful, stiff, deformed, or subluxated. Radiographs reveal narrowing of the joint space, sclerosis of subchondral bone, and presence of osteophytes.

Initial treatment may be symptomatic and may include splinting and even local corticosteroid injections. NSAIDs may be helpful, and chondroprotective medications such as glucosamine and chondroitin sulfate can reduce symptoms. In advanced cases, the DIPJs respond best to arthrodesis. The PIPJs may be surgically treated by replacement arthroplasty or by arthrodesis (Fig. 119.51). The thumb carpometacarpal joint may be treated by arthrodesis, which is favored particularly for the young patient who might have posttraumatic arthritis after, for example, an improperly treated Bennett or Orlando fracture. In an older patient with primary osteoarthritis at the thumb base, excision of the trapezium followed by tendon suspension (interposition) arthroplasty may be preferred. This uses local tendons for construction of a sling arthroplasty, with interposition of tendon material.

Rheumatoid arthritis is an autoimmune process whereby destruction of the musculoskeletal system may occur. Synovial inflammation results in pain, joint destruction, tendon ruptures, and characteristic deformities. Some of the more common deformities associated with rheumatoid arthritis include a swan-neck

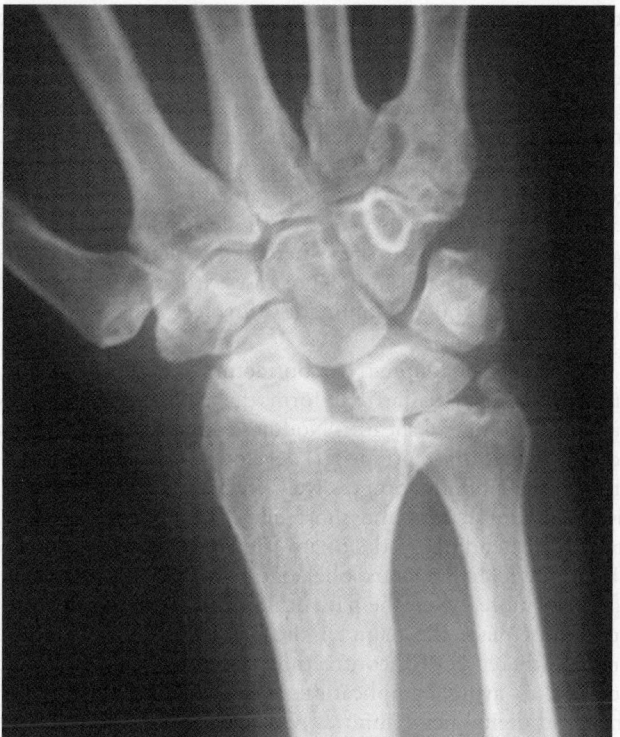

FIGURE 119.50 Radiograph of a hand with a scapholunate advanced collapse wrist showing posttraumatic osteoarthritis at the radioscaphoid junction. This is many years after a wrist sprain in which the scapholunate ligament was torn; a wide scapholunate gap is visible on the radiograph.

deformity (hyperextension of the PIPJ with concurrent flexion at the DIPJ), boutonnière deformity (flexion at the PIPJ, with concurrent hyperextension at the DIPJ), joint subluxation, radial deviation of the wrist, and ulnar deviation and flexion of the fingers (Fig. 119.52). Rheumatoid arthritis is primarily a medical illness for which several medications are currently available. Thus, there must be excellent lines of communication between the rheumatologist and surgeon. NSAIDs and disease-modifying antirheumatoid drugs are used. Rheumatoid arthritis is a progressive disorder, and ongoing, slow destruction may be anticipated despite surgery (Fig. 119.53). Some of the more common surgical procedures include joint synovectomy, tenosynovectomy, tendon transfers, joint replacements (especially at the MPJs and PIPJs), and arthrodesis (more commonly at the wrist and thumb MPJ).[91]

CONTRACTURES

Volkmann ischemic contracture develops as a result of myofascial contractures in response to prolonged ischemia. This most common contracture results from untreated compartment syndrome of the forearm and hand. Muscle necrosis occurs, and the muscles become replaced by fibrous scar tissue. The FDP and FPL muscles are usually affected, being in the deepest forearm volar compartment, and digits are characteristically flexed, with passive extension of the wrist worsening the flexion deformity of the digits. Intrinsic contractures can occur in the hand; these can be investigated using the Bunnell test, in which passive extension of the MPJ makes passive flexion of the PIPJ more difficult.

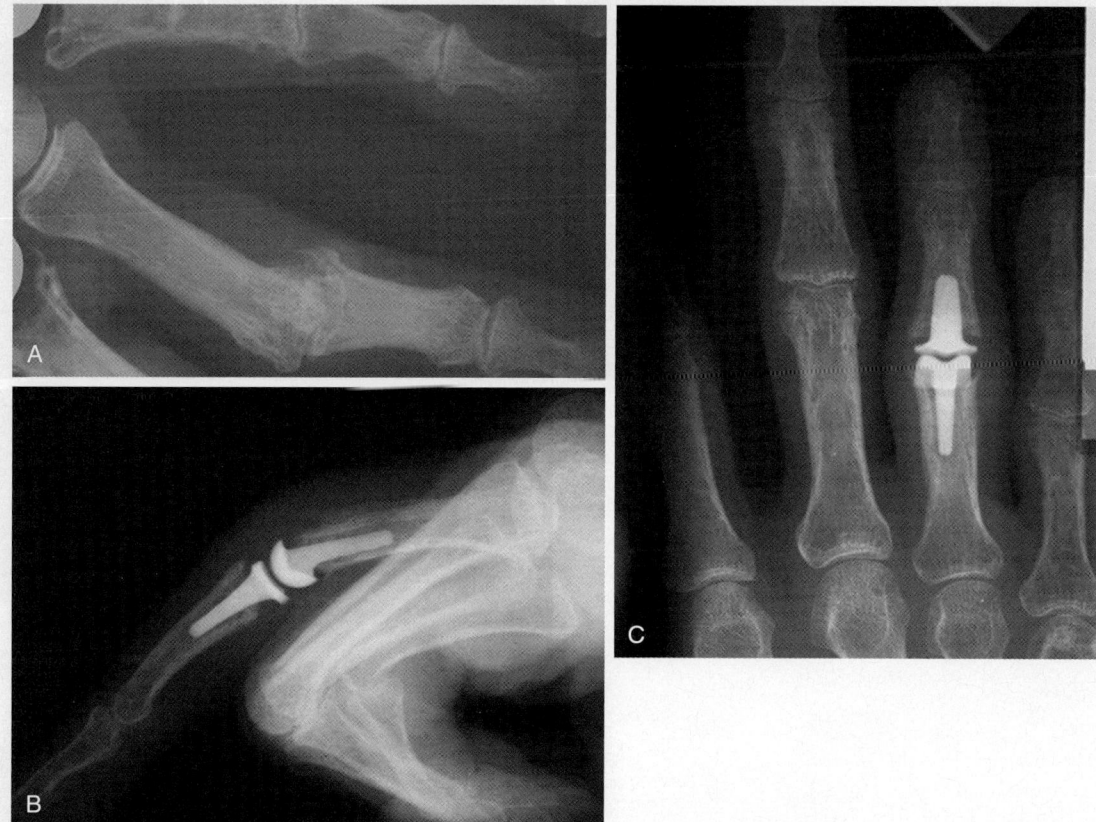

FIGURE 119.51 (A) Patient with painful and unstable proximal interphalangeal joint from osteoarthritis. (B–C) Reconstruction is performed by implant arthroplasty. An advantage over arthrodesis is that motion is retained, although there remains the potential for future recurrent joint instability and wear of the artificial joint.

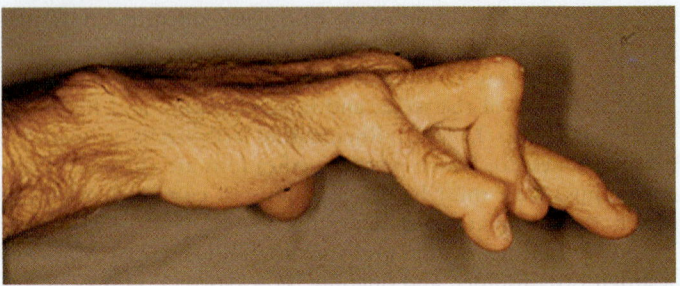

FIGURE 119.52 Patient with inflammatory arthritis has both boutonnière deformity and swan-neck deformity on the same hand.

In the milder forms of Volkmann ischemic contracture, serial splinting and passive stretching exercises may resolve the problem. In more severe contractures, Z-type lengthening of tendons may be required. A flexor pronator muscle slide—subperiosteal elevation of the common flexor origin from the medial epicondyle of the humerus and from the ulna—allows the muscles to slide distally until the contracture is corrected. In the most severe form, all the muscles of the volar forearm may be affected, requiring tendon transfers, even microvascular functional muscle transfers to provide some functional return.

Posttraumatic contractures are the most common type of contracture. These can be prevented by appropriate treatment of the primary injury, especially with attention to detail in how the hand and upper extremity are splinted and immobilized. Once contractures have developed, if they are mild, they may be able to be stretched out by exercises and hand therapy. If these contractures are severe and functionally deforming, surgical release of joint contractures and release of tendon adhesions may be required.

Dupuytren contracture is a disease process of contracting collagen affecting the palmar fascia; it can also affect the dorsum of the fingers (knuckle pads), soles of the feet, and penis (Peyronie disease). It is thought to be a hereditary Mendelian dominant disorder and is bilateral in 65% of cases. It is six times more frequent in males and predominantly involves the ring and little fingers (Fig. 119.54).

The process of Dupuytren contracture occurs in the normal bands of collagen tissue that form the palmar fascia, natatory ligaments, and digital sheaths. Nodules containing myofibroblasts and immature collagen (type III) develop in these tissues or in the dermis. The nodules progressively increase in size, leading to thickened contractures and shortened fascial bands that develop into cords extending up the digits. Treatment is surgical excision; it is indicated in metatarsophalangeal (MP) contractures of 30 degrees or more, when the patient fails the so-called tabletop test and cannot place the palm of the hand flat on a surface, and whenever there is a PIPJ contracture. Careful surgical technique is necessary to avoid complications such as skin necrosis, hematoma, and digital nerve injuries. Collagenase injections using enzyme derived from *Clostridium histolyticum* have been attempted

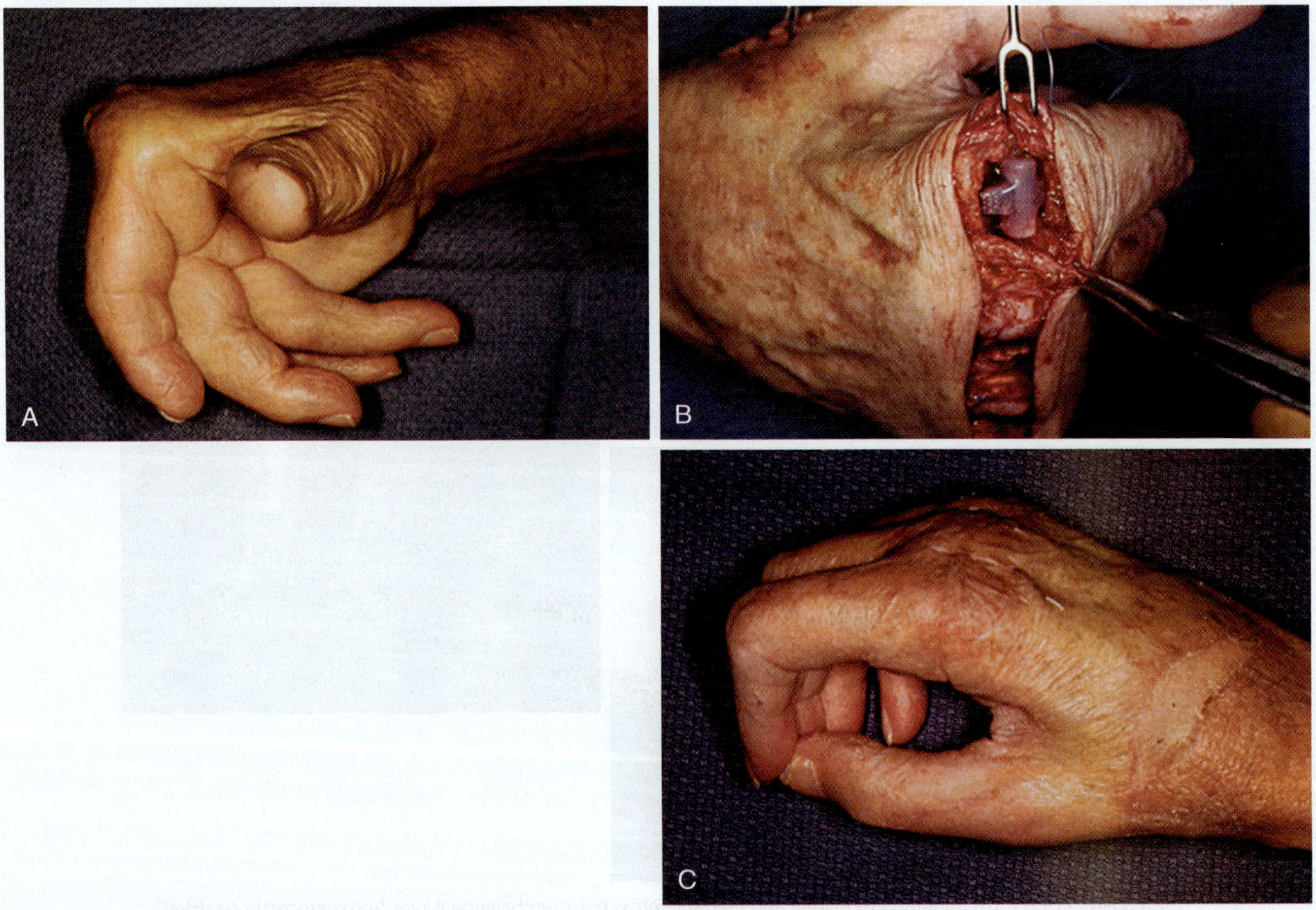

FIGURE 119.53 (A) Patient with rheumatoid arthritis showing the characteristic finger deformities. (B–C) Implant arthroplasty at the metacarpophalangeal joints restores function and aesthetics to the hand.

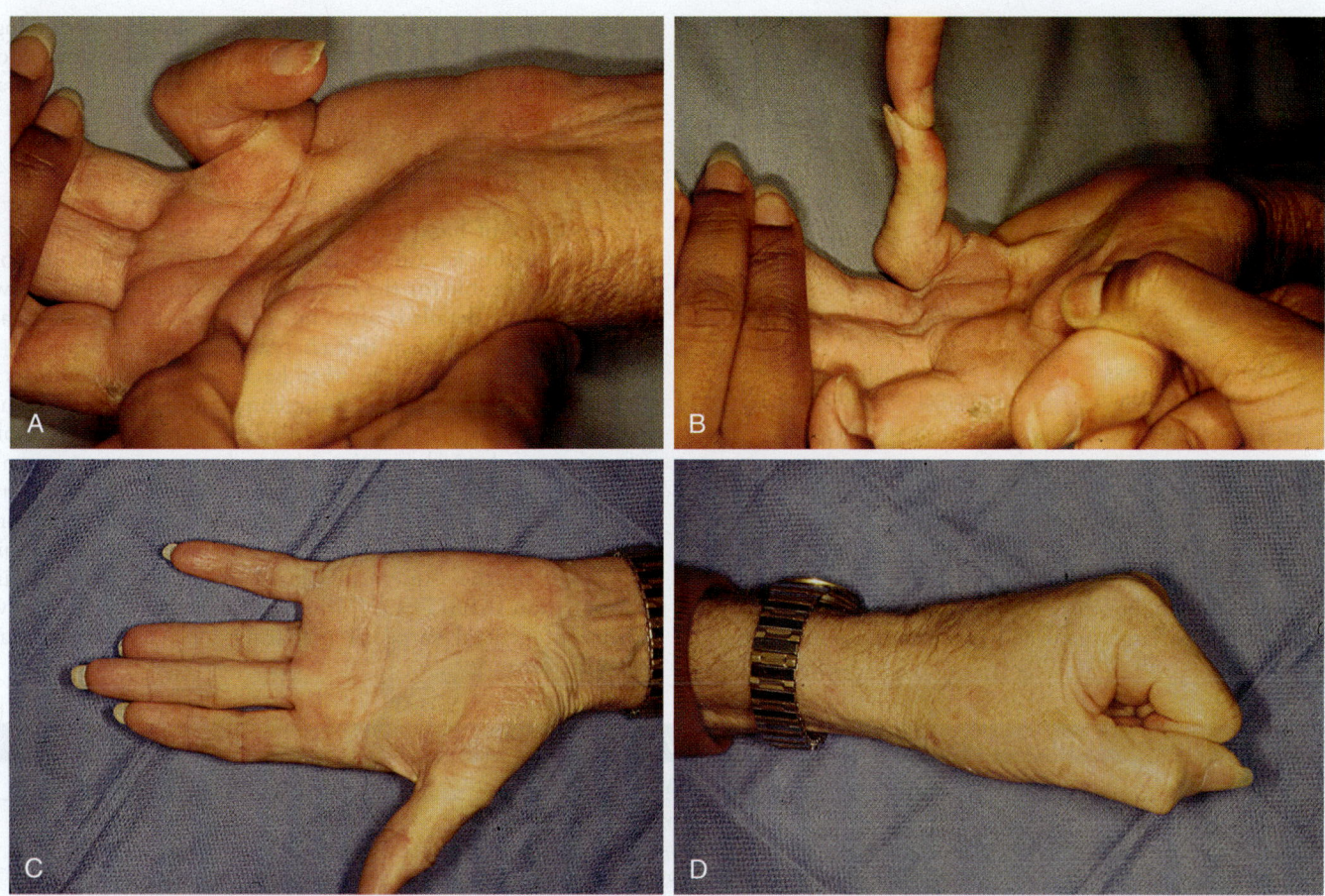

FIGURE 119.54 (A–D) Patient with Dupuytren's contracture is treated by regional palmar and digital fasciectomy, and good hand function is restored.

and have shown some promise in the treatment of Dupuytren contracture. However, long-term follow-up in patients who had these injections is still necessary.[92,93]

Percutaneous needle fasciotomy is also a reasonable option for treatment of Dupuytren disease and seems to be effective for MPJ contractures but less effective for the PIPJ. An extension external fixation torque device may also preliminarily reverse the PIP contracture before excision of the diseased tissue.[94]

FUTURE DIRECTIONS IN HAND SURGERY

Hand surgery is a very dynamic specialty and is continually advancing, with many recent technologic developments. Because it is a regional specialty, it embraces advances in microvascular and microneural surgery, trauma, transplantation, minimally invasive surgery, prosthetics, and tissue engineering.

Methods of treatment of forearm amputation remain an ongoing debate between transplantation and prosthetic limbs. Dr. Joseph Murry, a plastic surgeon, performed the first successful kidney transplant in 1954. Hand transplantation has been refined by plastic hand surgeons, and as of 2021, there were 150 documented successful upper limb transplants around the world.[95] Functional outcomes must be balanced against the lifetime risks of immunosuppression.[95]

In contrast, there have been major advances in the field of prosthetics—specifically, improvements in prosthetic motor control secondary to TMR and regenerative peripheral nerve interface

(RPNI). In TMR, transected nerves from the amputation are attached to individual motor nerves in the muscle that in turn transmits the myoelectric impulses to the various prosthetic functional movements. The prosthetic limb can "sense" the intended movements in the reinnervated muscles and move in the way that the patient intends it to move. An outreach of this research is also that TMR helps successfully treat phantom and neuroma pain. RPNI is a newer development where transected nerves are redirected to free muscle grafts to rennervate the tissue and therefore provide myoelectric signals that can be placed near the skin surface for easier capture.[96] The debate between prosthetics and transplantation will closely mirror the race between prosthetic technology and immunosuppression.

There has also been great interest in the development of ways to bridge nerve gaps in traumatic and oncologic reconstruction. The gold standard has been to use an autologous nerve graft, but this option has donor morbidity, and there is a limited supply available (generally sural nerve). Treated cadaveric nerve allografts remove the immunogenicity and may enable nerve reconstruction without donor morbidity.

Up to this time, nerve conduits have been merely a tube that guides the growth of axons to the distal nerve, which may be suitable for small nerves in the hand. However, nerve allografts contain the full scaffold of nerve, which allows for greater guidance of axonal growth. Autologous autografted nerves also contain Schwann cells and growth factors that, in theory, should help increase axonal growth and the "take" of nerve grafts. At this time,

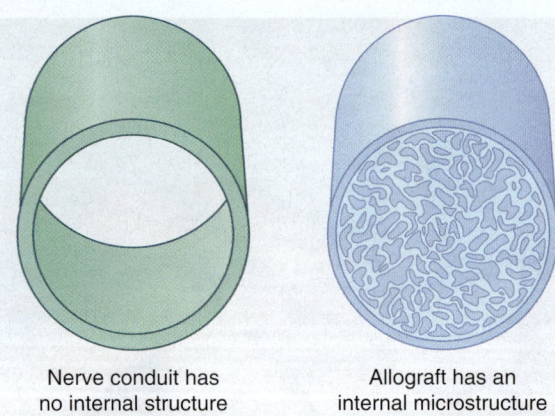

Nerve conduit has   Allograft has an
no internal structure   internal microstructure

FIGURE 119.55 Nerve conduits versus nerve allografts.

it is uncertain what length of major peripheral nerve is best treated with an autograft versus an allograft (Fig. 119.55). Recent studies support the use of processed nerve allografts in sensory nerves up to 25 mm, but there is still heated debate regarding the use of allograft in larger gaps and in mixed/pure motor nerve reconstruction.[97]

There are many other advancements in implant technology, minimally invasive surgery, and tissue engineering, but those regarding transplantation, prosthetics design, and nerve repair are especially exciting and are coming to clinical fruition.

CONCLUSION

The specialty of hand surgery is exhaustive, and a number of specialty textbooks are available. Although general surgeons may be responsible for the basic tenets of hand surgery, knowledge of minute details is often not necessary; thus, most details have been omitted from this chapter because its purpose is to show the big picture in regard to hand surgery. Those topics of hand surgery that the general surgeon is most likely to encounter have been emphasized, particularly with regard to principles of anatomy, physical examination, and emergency treatments. Taking this into consideration, Table 119.11 includes some high-yield facts relevant to hand surgery that have been compiled from various general surgery review books as well as topics discussed in the American Board of Surgery In-Training Examination (ABSITE).[98,99] This list is provided for the convenience of general surgeons preparing for ABSITE or board examinations.

TABLE 119.11 American Board of Surgery Review Topics

TOPIC	ANSWER
Fracture of the distal radius	Injury to the median nerve
Innervation of flexor digitorum profundus to the ring and small fingers	Ulnar nerve
Injury to the ulnar nerve at the elbow	Weakness in abduction and adduction of the index finger through small digits
Midshaft humeral fracture	Associated with radial nerve injury
Distal phalanx fractures	>50% of all hand fractures
Joint involved in Bennett fracture	Carpometacarpal joint of the thumb
Common name for metacarpal fracture of the small finger	Boxer fracture
Most frequently fractured carpal bone	Scaphoid
Complications associated with displaced fractures	Avascular necrosis and nonunion of the scaphoid
Axonal nerve growth rate	1 mm/day
Common maximum intraoperative tourniquet time in hand surgery	2 hours
Single digits that are primarily replanted	Thumbs in adults and children, all digits whenever possible in children
Maximal period of anoxia compatible with replantation	Finger—8 hours (warm ischemia), but longer times have been anecdotally reported; upper and lower extremity—6 hours
Proper method for transportation of an amputated body part to maximize replantation success	Cleaned of debris, wrapped in sterile towel or gauze, moistened with sterile lactated Ringer solution, placed in sterile plastic bag, transported in insulated cooler with ice water (ideal temperature, 4°C)
Complications if nerve repair is delayed >2 weeks	Retraction of nerve's ends resulting in need for nerve grafting
Zone 2, no man's land	Area of flexor tendon injury between metacarpophalangeal joint and flexor digitorum superficialis insertion
Mallet finger	Injury to extensor mechanism at level of distal interphalangeal joint
Gamekeeper thumb	Rupture of ulnar collateral ligament of thumb metacarpophalangeal joint, with resultant instability of the joint to radial-directed force
Most common organism causing hand infections	*Staphylococcus aureus*
Classic symptoms of carpal tunnel syndrome	Paresthesias in median nerve distribution, often waking the patient at night
Most effective therapy for full-thickness burns of the hand	Early excision and grafting
Most common location of ganglion cysts	Scapholunate interosseous ligament at the dorsal wrist
Treatment of de Quervain stenosing tenosynovitis after failed nonoperative management	Surgical release of first extensor compartment
Cause of trigger finger	Stenosing tenosynovitis in the region of the metacarpophalangeal joint, A1 pulley
Late findings of rheumatoid arthritis	Subluxation of involved joints resulting in deformity
Swan-neck deformity	Hyperextension of proximal interphalangeal joint with flexion of distal interphalangeal joint

TABLE 119.11 American Board of Surgery Review Topics—cont'd

TOPIC	ANSWER
Boutonnière deformity	Flexion of proximal interphalangeal joint with hyperextension of distal interphalangeal joint
Nonoperative measures for Dupuytren contracture	Exercise, local steroid injections, collagenase injections, radiotherapy
Digits usually affected in Dupuytren contracture	Ring and small fingers
Cause of Dupuytren contracture	Proliferation and fibrosis of the palmar fascia
Fractures likely to cause compartment syndrome, Volkmann ischemic contracture	Supracondylar fracture of the humerus
Artery and nerve compromised in Volkmann ischemic contracture	Median nerve and anterior interosseous artery
Complication of cast placement for supracondylar fractures of the humerus	Volkmann ischemic contracture

SELECTED REFERENCES

Athanasian EA. Bone and soft tissue tumors. In: Wolfe SW, Hotchkiss RN, Pederson WC, et al., eds. *Green's Operative Hand Surgery*. 7th ed. Philadelphia: Elsevier; 2017:1987-2035.

Digestible summary of bone and soft tissue tumors relevant for the general surgeon.

Currie KB, Tadisina KK, Mackinnon SE. Common hand conditions: a review. *JAMA*. 2022;327(24):2434-2445. Erratum in: JAMA. 2023 Aug 22;330(8):772.

Excellent review for the general surgeon on common hand conditions written by one of the world experts in peripheral nerve surgery, Dr. Susan Mackinnon.

Denkler KA, Vaughn CJ, Dolan EL, et al. Evidence-based medicine: options for Dupuytren's contracture: incise, excise, and dissolve. *Plast Reconstr Surg*. 2017;139:240e-255e.

Review article with evidence-based management guidelines for management of Dupuytren contracture.

Kistler JM, Ilyas AM, Thoder JJ. Forearm compartment syndrome: evaluation and management. *Hand Clin*. 2018;34(1):53-60.

This excellent article describes the pathogenesis of acute compartment syndrome, including the diagnosis and surgical management in the upper extremity.

Kozin SH, Zlotolow DA. Common pediatric congenital conditions of the hand. *Plast Reconstr Surg*. 2015;136(2):241e-257e.

Excellent review for the general surgeon on common pediatric hand conditions written by one of the world experts in pediatric hand surgery, Dr. Scott Kozin.

The full reference list appears on Elsevier eBooks+.

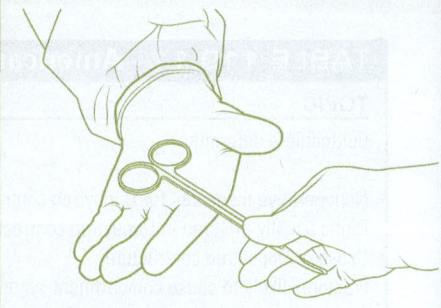

Gynecologic Surgery

Sara Wood, Elise Bardawil, and Dineo Khabele

▶ **Please access Elsevier eBooks+ to view the videos for this chapter.**

Gynecologic procedures are among the most frequent surgical procedures performed in the world. It behooves any surgeon to be familiar with the anatomy of the female reproductive tract and pelvis and with the most common gynecologic surgical diseases and procedures for these diseases. This chapter provides an overview of pelvic anatomy in the female reproductive tract; discusses the most common disorders of the vulva, vagina, cervix, uterus, fallopian tubes, and ovaries; and reviews surgical procedures for these disorders. Principles of gynecologic surgical care for gender-diverse individuals are also reviewed. This foundational knowledge should provide surgeons with confidence to offer surgical interventions in a skillful and compassionate manner.

FEMALE REPRODUCTIVE AND PELVIC ANATOMY

Key components of the female reproductive tract anatomy include external reproductive anatomy (vulva) and internal reproductive anatomy (vagina, cervix, uterus, fallopian tubes, and ovaries).[1] Other relevant pelvic anatomy components include anatomic spaces, vascular and neurologic structures, and urologic and intestinal structures.[1] The following section provides an overview of these key components.

External Female Reproductive Anatomy (Vulva)

The main external structures of the vulva are the mons pubis, the labia majora and labia minora, the clitoral glans and clitoral hood, the urethral meatus, the vaginal introitus and hymen, and Bartholin and Skene vestibular glands (Fig. 120.1). The mons pubis is the soft fatty tissue covering the pubic bone. The lower part of the mons pubis is divided by a fissure named the pudendal cleft, which separates the mons pubis into the labia majora. The labia

majora and labia minora are separated by a groove called the *interlabial sulci*, and the labia minora fuses anteriorly to form the clitoral hood (also known as the *prepuce*) and posteriorly to form the vestibule.

The vestibule is the area of the vulva consisting of the vaginal introitus, which is initially outlined by the hymenal ring, and urethral meatus. The vestibule is demarcated from the external vulvar structures by Hart's line. The anterior and posterior boundaries of the vestibule are the frenulum of the clitoris and the posterior fourchette, respectively. At the posterior vestibule, there is a small depression of tissue called the fossa navicularis where the Bartholin glands open. The Bartholin glands, homologues of the bulbourethral glands in males, are located posteriorly to the right and left of the vaginal introitus. Skene glands, homologues of the prostate gland in males, are located to the right and left of the urethral meatus. Both Bartholin's and Skene's glands produce secretions that provide vaginal lubrication.

The perineum is divided into the anterior and posterior triangle by a line between the ischial tuberosities. The female external genitalia, including the urethra and vagina, are within the anterior division, also known as the urogenital triangle, which extends anteriorly to the pubic symphysis. The borders of the posterior triangle, or anal triangle, include the levator ani (superior), perineal membrane (anterior), coccyx (posterior), and the sacrotuberous ligaments (posterolateral). The contents of the anal triangle include the anal canal and the paired ischiorectal fossa. The levator ani and obturator internus muscles as well as the external anal sphincter are within the anal triangle.

The anterior triangle is divided into three layers: subcutaneous, superficial, and deep. The subcutaneous fatty layer contains Camper fascia and is continuous with the posterior triangle, the thigh, and abdominal wall. The superficial layer is an enclosed compartment bound by the perineal membrane, Colles fascia (continuous with Scarpa fascia in the abdominal wall), ischiopubic rami,

branches supply the external genitalia. The mons pubis and anterior labia are supplied by the ilioinguinal and genitofemoral nerves from the lumbar plexus that travel through the inguinal canal and exit through the superficial inguinal ring. All these paired nerves routinely cross the midline for partial innervation of the contralateral side. The dorsal nerve responsible for clitoral erection and sensation is derived from the pelvic splanchnic nerves and reaches the clitoris through the urogenital diaphragm. It is critical to be cognizant of the vascular and neurologic variability as the dorsal nerve of the clitoris has extensive, distinct superficial and deep branching patterns that are at risk of injury during dissection.[2]

Internal Female Reproductive Anatomy (Vagina, Cervix, Uterus, Fallopian Tubes, Ovaries)

Beginning most distal and moving proximal, the internal reproductive anatomic structures include all midline structures (the vagina, cervix, and uterus) and the lateral structures (the fallopian tubes and ovaries; Fig. 120.2). The lower portion of the vagina develops from the endoderm of the urogenital sinus (along with the urethra and vulvar structures). Abnormalities of development in this area can lead to transverse or horizontal septae of the vagina, which may become symptomatic during pubertal development and the onset of menses. The upper portion of the vagina develops in tandem with the cervix, uterus, and fallopian tubes from the Müllerian ducts. Failure of fusion of these ducts as they migrate medially or failure of development completely can lead to a variety of uterine, cervix, and tubal malformations.

Vagina

The vagina is a flexible, expandable fibromuscular tube, which, at rest, is flattened and lies in a mostly horizontal plane if the female is in an upright posture. When examining the full thickness of the vaginal wall, the layers from the center to periphery include the mucosa (stratified squamous epithelium), the lamina propria (collagen, elastic tissue, and the vascular and lymph supply), a muscular layer, and areolar connective tissue, which also contains a rich blood supply. The blood supply to the vagina comes mainly from the vaginal artery, a branch of the internal iliac artery. There are multiple anastomoses with other arteries, including the uterine, internal pudendal, inferior vesical, and middle hemorrhoidal arteries. The nerve supply to the vagina originates from the autonomic nervous system in the lumbosacral plexus (S2–S4), culminating in the pudendal nerve. The majority of sensory innervation lies in the distal portion of the vagina, with very little nerve density in the upper part of the vagina.

Cervix

The cervix is the narrow, distal part of the uterus that can be visualized and palpated at the upper end of the vaginal canal. It is a round, often donut-like structure composed of mostly fibrous tissue and can vary in size. The length of the cervix also varies but averages around 3 cm. It has a central canal, referred to as the *os*, which allows passage into or egress from the uterine cavity. The cells on the vaginal portion of the cervix (ectocervix) transition from squamous epithelium distally to columnar epithelium proximally as you travel up into the cervical canal (endocervix). This change is referred to as the transition zone and is where cervical intraepithelial neoplasia (CIN) occurs. The columnar epithelium produces mucus, which varies in texture depending on hormone influence, and facilitates sperm transport.

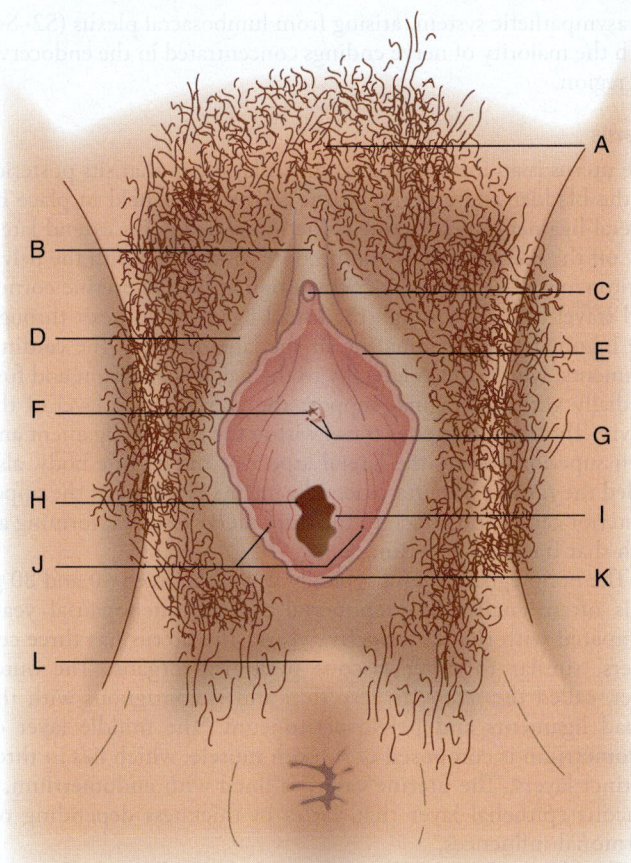

FIGURE 120.1 The eternal genitalia. *A*, Mons pubis; *B*, prepuce; *C*, clitoris; *D*, labia majora; *E*, labia minora; *F*, urethral meatus; *G*, Skene gland ducts; *H*, vagina; *I*, hymenal ring; *J*, Bartholin glands; *K*, posterior fourchette; *L*, perineal body.

and the urethra/vagina. This layer includes many of the important vulvar structures, such as the transverse perineal muscles, bulbocavernosus, and ischiocavernosus overlying the crura of the clitoris, vestibular bulbs, and the neurovascular tissue that supplies the external genitalia. Therefore, clinically, bleeding from a vulvar injury in this space will often be localized and unilateral. The deep layer is mostly a continuation of the fatty tissue in the ischioanal fossa that extends beyond the perineal membrane.

Blood supply to structures within the urogenital triangle is predominantly from a posterior direction from the internal pudendal artery, which, after arising from the internal iliac artery, passes through the pudendal, or Alcock canal, which is a fascial tunnel along the obturator internus muscle below the origin of the levator ani muscle. On emerging from the Alcock canal, the internal pudendal artery sends branches to the urogenital triangle anteriorly. The blood supply to the mons pubis originates anteriorly from the inferior epigastric artery, a branch of the femoral artery. Laterally, the external pudendal artery arises from the femoral artery and supplies the lateral aspect of the vulva. Venous return and lymphatic drainage from the urogenital diaphragm accompany the arterial supply and therefore drain into the internal iliac and femoral veins.

The major nerve supply to the urogenital triangle comes from the internal pudendal nerve, which originates from the S2–S4 anterior rami of the sacral plexus and travels through Alcock canal along with the internal pudendal artery and vein. Anterior

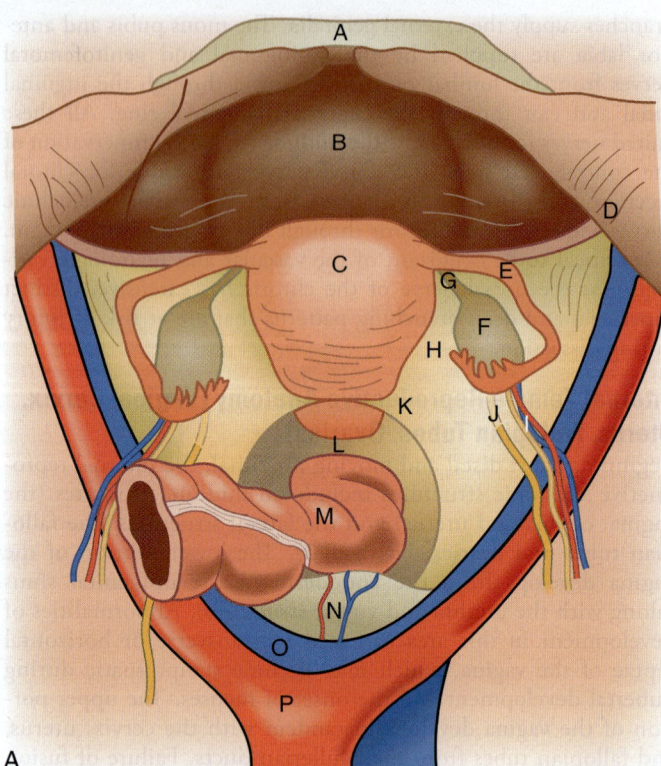

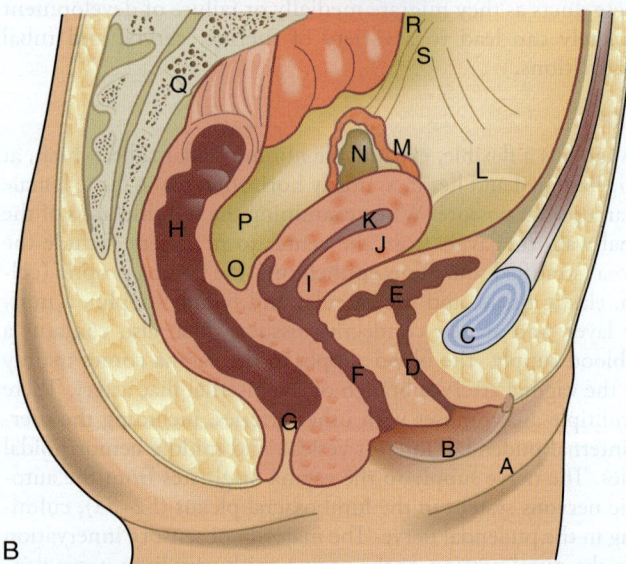

FIGURE 120.2 The internal genitalia. (A) *A,* Symphysis pubis; *B,* bladder; *C,* corpus uteri; *D,* round ligament; *E,* fallopian tube; *F,* ovary; *G,* uteroovarian ligament; *H,* broad ligament; *I,* ovarian artery and vein; *J,* ureter; *K,* uterosacral ligament; *L,* cul-de-sac; *M,* rectum; *N,* middle sacral artery and vein; *O,* vena cava; *P,* aorta. (B) *A,* Labium majus; *B,* labium minus; *C,* symphysis pubis, *D,* urethra; *E,* bladder; *F,* vagina; *G,* anus; *H,* rectum; *I,* cervix uteri; *J,* corpus uteri; *K,* endometrial cavity; *L,* round ligament; *M,* fallopian tube; *N,* ovary; *O,* cul-de-sac; *P,* uterosacral ligament; *Q,* sacrum; *R,* ureter; *S,* ovarian artery and vein.

The blood supply of the cervix arises from a descending branch of uterine artery and lies laterally at the 3 o'clock and 9 o'clock positions on the cervix. Additionally, the azygos arteries lie in the middle portion of the cervix anteriorly and posteriorly along its axis. There are multiple anastomoses between the azygos arteries and the hemorrhoidal arteries. The cervix is innervated by the

parasympathetic system, arising from lumbosacral plexus (S2–S4) with the majority of nerve endings concentrated in the endocervical region.

Uterus

The uterus is an intraperitoneal muscular organ that sits posterior to the bladder and anterior to the rectum. It is held in place by several ligamentous structures. The broad ligaments extend laterally off the uterine corpus and become continuous with the pelvic peritoneum. The round ligaments originate at the uterine cornua and travel laterally through the broad ligament and exit through the inguinal ring, terminating in the labia majora. The cardinal ligaments, which attach laterally to the pelvic diaphragm and fuse medially with the vagina, support the uterus at the level of the cervix. The uterine arteries travel within the cardinal ligament and then superiorly along the lateral aspect of the uterine body, also called the *fundus.* The uterosacral ligaments originate at the upper posterior cervix and attach to the third sacral vertebra, forming an arch that frames the rectum.

The nonpregnant uterus typically weighs between 40 and 80 g. It is often smaller in prepubertal and postmenopausal years compared with the reproductive years. The uterus has three cell layers, similar to other viscous peritoneal organs. The outer layer, called the *serosa,* is very thin and is contiguous with the broad ligaments and pelvic peritoneum. The middle layer of myometrium is composed of smooth muscle, which lies in three distinct layers. The uterine cavity is lined with endometrium, a mucous epithelial layer that varies in thickness depending on hormonal influences.

The blood supply to the uterus includes both uterine arteries, which branch off the internal iliac arteries, and the ovarian arteries, which come directly off the abdominal aorta and travel adjacent to the ovary toward the uterus. The uterus has both sympathetic and parasympathetic innervation. The sympathetic innervation travels via the hypogastric and ovarian plexus. The parasympathetic innervation comes from the lumbosacral plexus (S2–S4). Afferent fibers from the uterus returning to the spinal cord travel with the sympathetic innervation within the lumbosacral plexus (T11–T12).

Fallopian Tubes

The fallopian tubes, also referred to as the *oviducts,* originate at the upper lateral aspect of the uterus (called the *cornua*) and extend laterally approximately 10 to 14 cm in length, coiling around the ipsilateral ovary distally. The fallopian tube has four distinct anatomic sections. The interstitial part traverses the uterine wall, is completely bordered by myometrium, and is only 1 to 2 cm in length. The narrow isthmus portion begins as the tube leaves the uterus, measures around 4 cm in length, and contains the most muscular region of the tube. The ampullary region is wider, averages 4 to 6 cm in length, and is where fertilization typically occurs. The final segment is the infundibulum, which is mostly composed of fimbriae, which are finger-like projections that extend out from the tube, surround the ostia, and cause this portion of the tube to be funnel shaped.

Like the uterus, the fallopian tubes are composed of several layers. The mucosa of the tube is made up of different types of epithelial cells: columnar ciliated, secretory, and narrow peg. The ratio of these cell types depends on the anatomic region of the tube. Under the mucosa is the lamina propria, followed by the muscular layer, and finally the adventitial layer, which is adjacent to the peritoneal cavity.

The blood supply to the fallopian tube travels through the mesosalpinx and originates from branches of the ovarian and uterine arteries. The tubes receive innervation from both the sympathetic and parasympathetic nervous systems via the uterine and ovarian plexuses.

Ovaries

The ovaries are paired, oval-shaped organs lateral in location and white, usually around 2 to 3 cm in largest diameter. They are located just inferior to the pelvic brim at the infundibulum end of the fallopian tubes. The ovaries develop from the gonadal ridge, which sits adjacent to the mesonephric duct; thus, the urinary system and reproductive system develop in close association. The ovaries are connected to the uterus via the uteroovarian ligament, which contains an anastomotic blood supply between these two structures. Additionally, the ovaries are held in place by the posterior leaf of the broad ligament and the infundibulopelvic ligament, which travels down the lateral sidewall and contains the major ovarian blood supply.

The ovary has three distinct sections: the outer cortex, the central medulla, and the hilum, which is where the mesovarium (the structure that anastomoses the infundibulopelvic ligament and the periuterine blood supply via the broad ligament) attaches to the ovary. The ovaries contain several cell types including the oocytes, which number 1 to 2 million at birth. The oocytes mature inside small, fluid-filled cysts called *follicles,* which sit just under the surface epithelium composed of cuboidal epithelium. The central medulla is mostly made up of stroma and blood vessels.

The blood supply to the ovary comes from the ovarian artery, a branch off the abdominal aorta that travels along the lateral abdomen and pelvis in the infundibulopelvic ligament. Additionally, within the mesovarium there are many anastomoses between the ovarian artery and the uterine artery. The innervation of the ovary also travels via the infundibulopelvic ligament and includes autonomic and sensory nerve fibers from the ovarian, hypogastric, and aortic plexuses.

Other Relevant Female Pelvic Anatomy

Anatomic Spaces

The female pelvis contains several key potential avascular spaces, an understanding of which is required by any surgeon operating in this area (Fig. 120.3). The two lateral retroperitoneal spaces include the paravesical and pararectal spaces. The paravesical space is bordered by the external iliac artery laterally, the bladder medially, the pubic symphysis anteriorly, and the cardinal ligament posteriorly. Key anterior to posterior spaces include the retropubic, vesicovaginal, rectovaginal, and retrorectal/presacral spaces. Developing these avascular spaces facilitates identification of critical pelvic structures, particularly when normal anatomy is altered from both benign and malignant conditions. A keen understanding of these spaces is necessary to safely operate in the pelvis and to mitigate neurovascular, urinary, and gastrointestinal injuries.

Vascular Structures

A keen understanding of vascular anatomy and the accompanying pelvic landmarks is essential when performing gynecologic procedures (Fig. 120.4). The common iliac vessels bifurcate at the level of the sacral promontory/pelvic brim into the external iliac and internal iliac vessels, which course along the pelvic sidewalls. The external iliac vessels course under the inguinal ligament to become the femoral artery and vein. The internal iliac artery bifurcates into an anterior and posterior division. The female pelvic structures derive much of their arterial vascular supply from vessels that branch from the anterior division. Ligation of the anterior division distal to where the posterior division branches is a technique often used in the setting of excessive pelvic hemorrhage. Key branches of the anterior division include the uterine and vaginal arteries; the inferior, middle, and superior vesical arteries; and the middle rectal artery. Other key branches off the anterior division include the obturator, inferior gluteal, and pudendal arteries. The ovarian arteries, which originate from the aorta, provide another major vascular source to the pelvic structures, namely the ovaries and uterus. The right

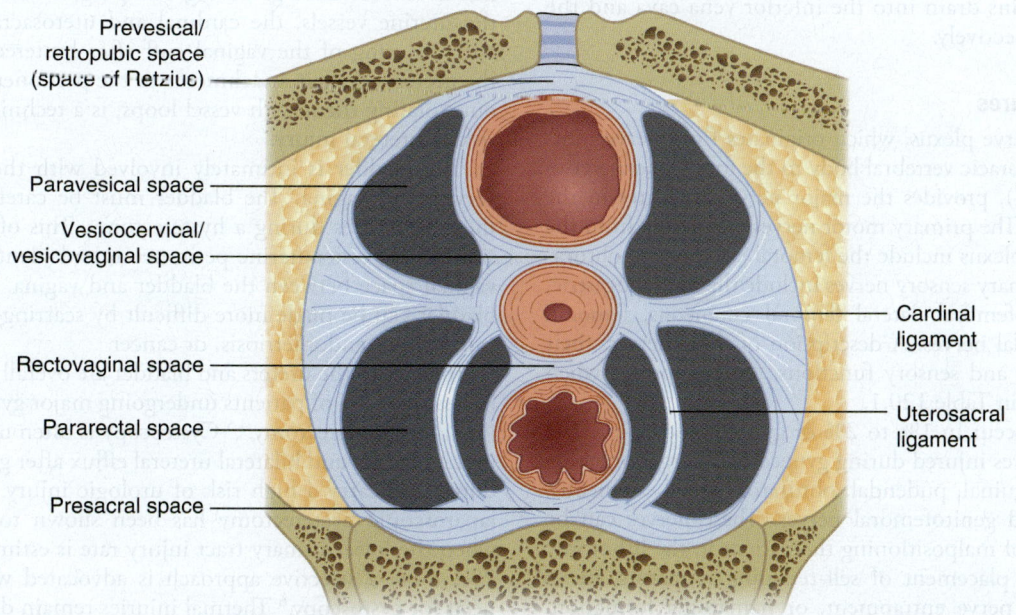

Prevesical/
retropubic space
(space of Retzius)

Paravesical space

Vesicocervical/
vesicovaginal space

Rectovaginal space

Pararectal space

Presacral space

Cardinal
ligament

Uterosacral
ligament

FIGURE 120.3 Anatomic spaces of the female pelvis.

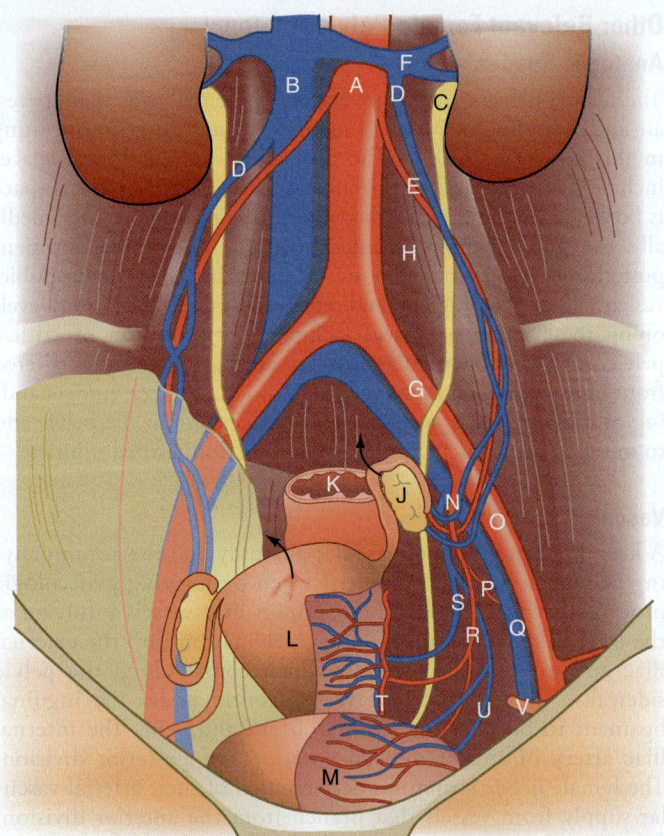

FIGURE 120.4 Blood supply of the pelvis. *A,* Aorta; *B,* inferior vena cava; *C,* ureter; *D,* ovarian vein; *E,* ovarian artery; *F,* renal vein; *G,* common iliac artery; *H,* psoas muscle; *J,* ovary; *K,* rectum; *L,* corpus uteri; *M,* bladder; *N,* internal iliac (hypogastric) artery, anterior branch; *O,* external iliac artery; *P,* obturator artery; *Q,* external iliac vein; *R,* uterine artery; *S,* uterine vein; *T,* vaginal artery; *U,* superior vesical artery; *V,* inferior epigastric artery.

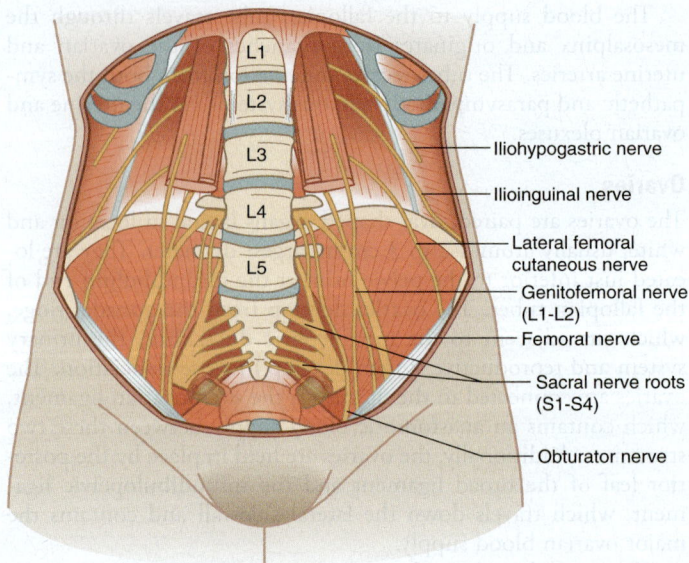

FIGURE 120.5 Neurologic structures of the female pelvis. (From Lumbosacral plexus. From Gray JE. Nerve injury associated with pelvic surgery. In: Basow DS, ed. *UpToDate*. Waltham, MA: UpToDate; 2013. Copyright UpToDate, Inc.)

Urinary Tract Structures

The ureters and bladder are key pelvic structures that require strict attention during the course of most gynecologic procedures. The ureters course retroperitoneally down the lateral pelvic walls, and at the level of the sacral promontory, cross over the common iliac arteries at the pelvic brim (see Figs. 120.2 and 120.4). At the pelvic brim, the ureters are close to the ovaries, and care must be taken to properly identify and avoid them during ligation of the ovarian vessels. The ureters continue along the medial aspects of the pelvic peritoneum under the uterine arteries and then traverse into the bladder laterally in an oblique fashion. The ureters are also at risk for damage during clamping, incision, and ligation of the uterine vessels, the cardinal and uterosacral ligaments, and with suturing of the vaginal cuff after hysterectomy. Dissecting the ureters off their attachments to the peritoneum, with or without isolating them with vessel loops, is a technique to reduce the risk of ureteral injury.

The bladder is intimately involved with the anterior uterus, cervix, and vagina. The bladder must be carefully dissected off these structures during a hysterectomy. This often involves incision of the vesicouterine peritoneum and identifying the vesicovaginal space between the bladder and vagina. Dissection of the bladder can be made more difficult by scarring from prior cesarean section, endometriosis, or cancer.

Injuries to the ureters and bladder are overall reported to occur in less than 1% of patients undergoing major gynecologic surgery, including hysterectomy.[4,5] Cystoscopy is often used to confirm an intact bladder and bilateral ureteral efflux after gynecologic procedures that carry a high risk of urologic injury. Cystoscopy after laparoscopic hysterectomy has been shown to be cost-effective when the lower urinary tract injury rate is estimated to be 1% to 2%; thus, a selective approach is advocated when determining need for cystoscopy.[6] Thermal injuries remain difficult to identify during the intraoperative session even when using cystoscopy due to their delayed presentation.

and left ovarian veins drain into the inferior vena cava and the left renal vein, respectively.

Neurologic Structures

The lumbosacral nerve plexus, which originates from nerve roots from the twelfth thoracic vertebral body to the fourth sacral vertebral body (T12–S4), provides the major nerve structures in the pelvis (Fig. 120.5). The primary motor nerves emanating from the lumbosacral nerve plexus include the femoral, sciatic, and obturator nerves. The primary sensory nerves include the iliohypogastric, ilioinguinal, genitofemoral, lateral femoral cutaneous, femoral, sciatic, and pudendal nerves. A description of these nerves, their origin, their motor and sensory functions, and symptoms when injured is included in Table 120.1.

Nerve injuries occur in 1% to 2% of gynecologic cases.[3] The most common nerves injured during gynecologic surgery include the femoral, ilioinguinal, pudendal, obturator, lateral cutaneous, iliohypogastric, and genitofemoral nerves. These nerves can be injured as a result of malpositioning the patient in the lithotomy position, incorrect placement of self-retaining retractors, nerve transection, direct nerve entrapment, or hematoma formation. Safe positioning of the patient to maximize exposure and minimize injury is essential in gynecologic surgery.

TABLE 120.1	Lumbosacral Nerve Plexus			
NERVE	**ORIGIN**	**MOTOR FUNCTION**	**SENSORY FUNCTION**	**INJURY SYMPTOMS**
Ilioinguinal	T12–L1	None	Groin, symphysis	Sharp, burning pain radiating from incision site to groin or symphysis
Iliohypogastric	T12–L1	None	Mons, lateral labia, upper inner thigh	Sharp, burning pain radiating from incision site to mons, labia, or thigh
Genitofemoral	L1–L2	None	Upper labia, anterior superior thigh	Pain or paresthesia labia and femoral triangle
Lateral femoral	L2–L3	None	Anterior and posterior lateral thigh	Pain or paresthesia anterior and posterolateral thigh
Pudendal	S2–S4	None	Perineum	Perineal pain
Cutaneous femoral	L2–L4	Hip flexion, adduction Knee extension	Anterior and medial thigh, medial calf	Unable to climb stairs
Obturator	L2–L4	Thigh adduction	None	Minor ambulatory problems
Sciatic	L4–S3	Hip extension, knee flexion	None	Foot drop
Common peroneal		Foot dorsiflexion	Lateral calf	Cavus deformity foot
Tibial		Foot eversion	Dorsum of foot	
		Foot plantar flexion	Toes	
		Foot inversion	Plantar foot surface	

Intestinal Tract Structures

The distal ileum, cecum, and appendix as well as the sigmoid colon and rectum are key gastrointestinal structures located near or within the pelvis. Gastrointestinal adhesions can occur as a result of surgeries, and careful attention is required to lyse adhesions in this setting to restore normal pelvic anatomy before completing any gynecologic procedure. These intestinal structures can also be involved as the result of various gynecologic pathology such as tuboovarian abscesses, endometriosis, and ovarian neoplasms. It is important to carefully inspect the intestinal organs to ensure there has been no occult injury, which is reported to occur in less than 1% of patients undergoing hysterectomy.[7] A "bubble" test, which involves insufflating the rectum with air with compression of the sigmoid and filling the pelvis with saline or water, can be used to detect an occult sigmoid injury.

COMMON VULVA AND VAGINAL SURGICAL DISEASES AND PROCEDURES

Common vulva and vaginal surgical diseases and procedures are listed in Table 120.2. A description of these diseases and management options follows.

Common Vulvar and Vaginal Surgical Diseases

Vulvar Infection/Abscess

Vulvar infections can range from superficial cellulitis to severe necrotizing fasciitis. Rapid diagnosis and initiation of treatment with broad-spectrum antibiotics and debridement, when appropriate, are essential. Risk factors for vulvar infection include diabetes, obesity, immunosuppression, pregnancy, and trauma.[8] In general, a vulvar abscess larger than 2 cm will necessitate surgical intervention with at least incision and drainage for adequate treatment.

Blockage of the Bartholin glands can result in accumulation of mucus and may lead to obstruction and abscess formation, presenting as a unilateral painful vulvar mass. Patients with a symptomatic Bartholin gland cyst or abscess often require surgical intervention with incision and drainage and placement of a Word catheter or with marsupialization. Marsupialization is indicated for recurrent infections or when the size of abscess precludes incision

TABLE 120.2	Common Vulvar and Vaginal Surgical Diseases and Procedures
DISEASE	**PROCEDURE OPTIONS**
Bartholin cyst/ abscess	Incision and drainage
	Marsupialization
	Excision
Vulvar intraepithelial neoplasia	Wide local excision
	Laser
Vulvar cancer	Radical vulvectomy with sentinel node biopsy or inguinal femoral lymphadenectomy
Vaginal intraepithelial neoplasia	Partial vaginectomy
	Laser
Vaginal cancer	Radical hysterectomy (rarely)
Prolapse	Sacrocolpopexy
	Sacrospinous ligament suspension
	Uterosacral ligament suspension
	Anterior colporrhaphy
	Posterior colporrhaphy
	Colpocleisis

and drainage. Biopsy is indicated for solid components and suspicion of malignancy. In rare instances, excision of the gland is indicated for recurrent infections and for malignancy.

Vulvar Crohn disease is a granulomatous inflammatory process that can lead to abscess and fistula formation from the anus to the vulva or perineum.[9] Presenting symptoms include erythema, edema, and "knife-cut ulcerations" of the external genitalia. Up to 30% of patients will initially be diagnosed with Crohn disease due to the vulvar manifestations. Treatment centers on managing the primary disease process with immune suppression while balancing the risk of worsening infection. Surgery is often a treatment of last resort due to the high recurrence rate and poor healing outcomes. Debridement or drainage of abscess locally is performed more commonly than fistula excision.

Hidradenitis suppurativa is a chronic inflammation of the apocrine-glandular tissue and is commonly seen at the vulvar and inguinal folds. Subsurface nodules can coalesce and form abscesses under the skin surface with resultant sinus tracts and scarring at the skin, creating disfigurement and pain. When medical therapies are exhausted, surgery can be considered. Deroofing of fistula tracts or incision of abscess may provide immediate short-term relief. Wide excision has shown the lowest risk of recurrence compared with local excisions, but often local approaches will require less recovery time.[10] Postoperative wound care and pain management are important. Negative pressure wound therapy with delayed reconstruction and grafting may be useful. The use of perioperative medical therapy, including biologics is recommended.

Necrotizing fasciitis is a medical and surgical emergency that requires multidisciplinary care. Patients at increased risk of necrotizing fasciitis include diabetics, tobacco users, and postoperative/pregnancy state. Signs such as progressive edema, fever, pain out of proportion to findings, and expanding skin induration should prompt high suspicion for necrotizing fasciitis. Skin changes often occur late in the disease process. Treatment should not be delayed to obtain imaging and includes broad-spectrum antibiotics as well as surgical debridement of necrotic tissue along with supportive critical care from a multidisciplinary team.

Vulva Intraepithelial Neoplasia

Vulva intraepithelial neoplasia (VIN) is a premalignant condition of the vulva. In 2015, the International Society for the Study for Vulvovaginal Disease (ISSVD) recommended using a two-tier grading system for classical VIN, which includes low-grade squamous intraepithelial lesion (LSIL), high-grade squamous intraepithelial lesion (HSIL), and a third category that separates VIN differentiated type.[11] The majority of LSIL and HSIL VIN is associated with the human papillomavirus (HPV), tends to occur in younger patients, and is multifocal. The pathogenesis of VIN differentiated type is less well understood but tends to be associated with vulvar dermatoses such as lichen sclerosis, seen more commonly in older patients, and is not associated with HPV. Differentiated VIN is associated with a high 10-year risk for progression to vulvar cancer highlighting the need for timely diagnosis, which is made more challenging given the subtle signs and symptoms.[11] Common symptoms of VIN are vulvar itching and pain, although up to 40% of VIN does not have symptoms. Management includes colposcopy and biopsy to confirm the diagnosis. LSIL may be observed or treated with topical therapy such as imiquimod. The mainstay of treatment for HSIL is either wide local excision or laser ablation. Recurrence rates after treatment are high; therefore, continued monitoring after therapy is required.

Vulvar Cancer

Carcinoma of the vulva is a rare gynecologic cancer but still significantly contributes to overall mortality from reproductive tract cancers.[12] Squamous cell carcinoma is the most common histology. Less common histologic subtypes include verrucous, basal cell, melanoma, sarcoma, extramammary Paget, and Bartholin gland carcinoma. Risk factors for vulva cancer include smoking, HPV infection, VIN, cervical dysplasia or cancer, lichen sclerosis, and immunodeficiency. The most common presentation is a symptomatic nodular or ulcerative vulva lesion. Treatment is based upon clinical stage. For stage IA cancers that are confined to the vulva and less than 1 mm of invasion, with clinically negative lymph nodes, simple vulvectomy is reasonable. Surgical resection involves radical vulvectomy with bilateral inguinal femoral lymph node dissection through separate incisions, which decreases morbidity. Sentinel lymph node (SLN) mapping is a reasonable alternative to full inguinofemoral lymph node dissection with less morbidity in select patients with small tumors.

Treatment with chemoradiation has been the preferred strategy for locally advanced unresectable disease that involves the urethral meatus, vagina, or anus.

Vaginal Intraepithelial Neoplasia

Vaginal intraepithelial neoplasia (VaIN) is a premalignant condition of the vagina. Like VIN, it is classified using a two-tier grading system LSIL (previously VaIN 1) and HSIL (previously VaIN II/III). Patients are often asymptomatic. Risk factors are similar to that for patients with VIN. Management is also like that for patients with VIN, albeit laser ablation is more frequently considered over partial vaginectomy for HSIL VaIN lesions. In patients posthysterectomy, excision may be preferred. Recurrence is not uncommon and close follow-up is recommended.[13]

Vaginal Cancer

Vaginal cancer is also quite rare. Squamous cell carcinoma is the most common histology. Less common histologic subtypes include adenocarcinoma, sarcoma, and melanoma. Risk factors other than those mentioned previously for vulva cancer include diethylstilbestrol exposure in utero and prior radiation. The most common presenting symptom is vaginal bleeding followed by vaginal discharge, change in urinary symptoms, or pain. Stage is the most significant prognostic feature. Most patients with vaginal cancer are treated with the combination of radiation and chemotherapy. Radical hysterectomy with upper vaginectomy is an option for the rare select patient with a small stage I cancer confined to the vaginal mucosa and located in the posterior vaginal fornix.

Pelvic Organ Prolapse

Pelvic organ prolapse is the herniation or downward displacement of the bladder (anterior vagina), cervix or vaginal cuff (apex), or rectum (posterior vagina) beyond their normal position. Risk factors include parity, age, obesity, chronic constipation, chronic obstructive pulmonary disease, connective tissue disorders, and smoking. The symptom most predictive for prolapse is the presence of a vaginal bulge. Other symptoms include pelvic pressure/heaviness and/or changes in bowel or bladder function. Treatment options include nonsurgical interventions, including pessary and pelvic floor physical therapy, as well as surgical intervention. Both conservative management and surgical options should be outlined as treatment options.

Pelvic reconstructive surgery for pelvic organ prolapse is individualized with the goal to restore normal anatomy and function of the anterior, posterior, and apical vaginal compartments. The apical defect, when present, is recognized as the key anatomic area to address in prolapse repair, which can be approached either abdominally or transvaginally. The most common procedures for repair of apical prolapse are abdominal sacrocolpopexy (or its minimally invasive laparoscopic or robotic variants), transvaginal sacrospinous ligament suspension, and transvaginal or laparoscopic uterosacral ligament suspension.[14–16] Repair of apical prolapse abdominally with sacrocolpopexy results in a lower rate of recurrence when compared with transvaginal approaches; however, it is associated with longer surgical time and delay in return to normal activities.

Patients with pelvic organ prolapse often have several compartments that are prolapsed and benefit from repair that addresses each of the affected compartments. Anterior and posterior colporrhaphy are often not needed when an abdominal sacrocolpopexy is performed as repair of apical defect often corrects the anterior and posterior defects.[17] However, anterior and posterior colporrhaphy are more often performed when the reconstruction is performed transvaginally in conjunction with uterosacral or sacrospinous ligament suspension.

Rates of recurrence have varied substantially in different studies, and a standard of "success" remains under discussion. Recent data suggest that recurrence rates are approximately 15%; however, the definition of "surgical success" in research studies has broadened over time to consider both objective findings, such as stage on examination, and subjective patient-reported symptoms.[18] Outcomes at 5 years are similar between uterosacral ligament suspension and sacrospinous ligament suspension with reported failure rates of 62% and 70%, respectively, although prolapse symptom scores remain improved despite the anatomic findings of prolapse.[19,20] Recurrence of prolapse after native tissue repairs is approximately 16% at 12 months after repair with younger age identified as a risk factor.[16]

Although most cases of pelvic organ prolapse are treated with reconstructive vaginal surgery as noted previously, there are some instances in which vaginal reconstruction may not be desired or an option. For patients who are not candidates for surgical reconstruction, and who are no longer sexually active, obliteration of the vaginal canal can alleviate the symptoms of pelvic organ prolapse without high surgical morbidity. Additional benefits of colpocleisis are shorter operative time, low risk of recurrence, and similar patient satisfaction making this an appropriate choice for older patients with multiple medical comorbidities who are not sexually active.

Common Vulva and Vaginal Surgical Procedures

Treatment of Vulvar Infection

Incision and drainage of a vulvar cyst or abscess of any etiology is performed by stabilizing the cyst or abscess and making an incision over the center of the cyst or abscess on the medial aspect of the lesion just outside the hymenal ring (Fig. 120.6). A common

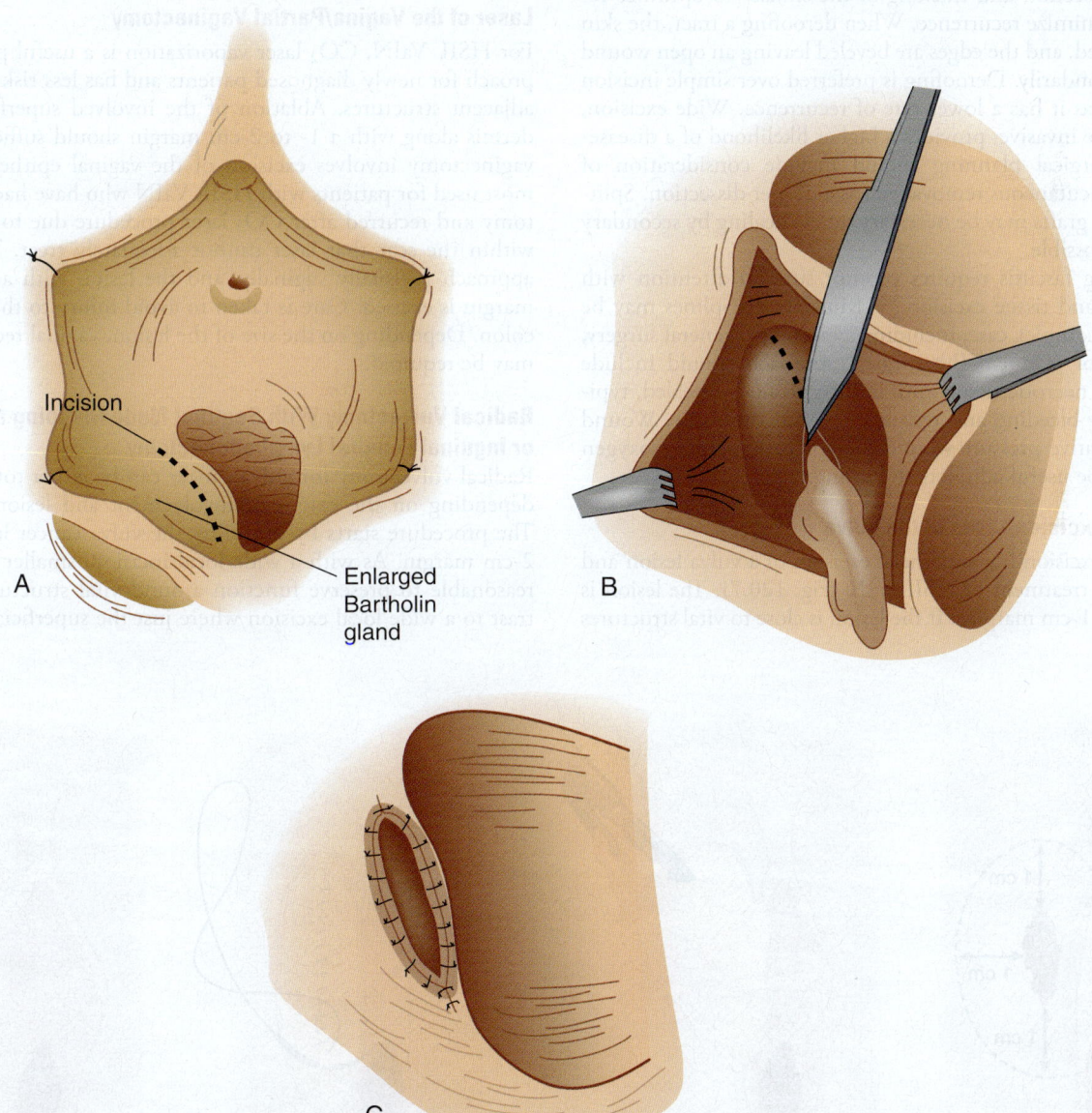

FIGURE 120.6 Bartholin gland marsupialization. (A) Retraction of the labia and incision over the mucosa of the vagina. (B) Wall of the gland is excised. (C) Completed marsupialization. (Adapted from Mitchell CW, Wheeless CR. *Atlas of Pelvic Surgery.* 3rd ed. Philadelphia: Lippincott Williams & Wilkins; 1997.)

mistake is to make the incision on the lateral aspect of the vulva. Care should be taken when breaking up loculations blindly as this manipulation may be close to rectal tissue already impacted by the inflammatory changes of infection. Specifically for a Bartholin gland abscess, a small Word catheter is placed into the cyst for drainage and reevaluated on a weekly basis. Bartholin gland abscesses are often polymicrobial. Culture of purulent fluid can be obtained to evaluate for methicillin-resistant *Staphylococcus aureus* and treated empirically. Marsupialization of a Bartholin gland cyst is performed by creating an elliptical incision in the vestibular mucosa down to the wall of the gland. The wall of the gland is incised along the entire length of the ellipse. The contents are evacuated, and the wall of the cyst is sutured to the vestibular mucosa using 3-0 synthetic absorbable sutures in an interrupted fashion or using a baseball stitch.

Surgical management of hidradenitis suppurativa includes deroofing of sinus fistula tracts and wide en bloc excisions.[10] Both of these procedures are ideally performed by a surgeon with expertise in the dissection and tracking of the sinuses to optimize removal and minimize recurrence. When deroofing a tract, the skin over it is incised, and the edges are beveled leaving an open wound that heals secondarily. Deroofing is preferred over simple incision and drainage as it has a lower rate of recurrence. Wide excision, although more invasive, provides a higher likelihood of a disease-free state. Surgical planning should include consideration of superficial subcutaneous removal versus a deeper dissection. Split-thickness skin grafts may be necessary unless healing by secondary intention is possible.

Necrotizing fasciitis requires prompt surgical attention with debridement and tissue excision.[8,21] Multiple disciplines may be involved in a complex case, including gynecology, general surgery, plastics, and/or trauma. The surgical approach should include removal of all necrotic tissue until healthy tissue is revealed, typically noted by bleeding and resistance within the tissue. Wound care with negative pressure wound therapy or hyperbaric oxygen therapy may be useful adjuncts to healing.

Wide Local Excision/Laser of the Vulva

A wide local excision is a superficial excision of a vulva lesion and is used in the treatment of HSIL VIN (Fig. 120.7). The lesion is outlined with 1-cm margins. If the lesion is close to vital structures such as the anus, clitoris, or urethra, smaller margins may be used for cosmesis or to preserve function. After making an incision along the outline, the apex of the skin is then elevated, and the epidermis is removed to a depth of 2 to 3 mm. Removal of dermis is not necessary for preinvasive disease. The defect is reapproximated using running or interrupted sutures depending on surgeon preference and size of lesion.

CO_2 laser vaporization is commonly used to treat LSIL VIN and may be an alternative to surgical resection for HSIL VIN.[22] For HSIL VIN, CO_2 laser vaporization is best used for patients with multifocal disease; with disease close to vital structures such as the anus, urethra, or clitoris; or with extensive VIN lesions in which surgical resection would be disfiguring. CO_2 laser vaporization should be used only when there is a low clinical suspicion for malignancy and after vulvar biopsies have confirmed no evidence of invasive cancer. A depth of 1 mm is used on nonhair-bearing areas of the vulva and 3 mm on hair-bearing areas of the vulva. Colposcopy is used to increase precision with laser therapy.

Laser of the Vagina/Partial Vaginectomy

For HSIL VaIN, CO_2 laser vaporization is a useful preferred approach for newly diagnosed patients and has less risk of injury to adjacent structures. Ablation of the involved superficial vaginal dermis along with a 1- to 2-cm margin should suffice. A partial vaginectomy involves excision of the vaginal epithelium and is most used for patients with HSIL VaIN who have had a hysterectomy and recurred after CO_2 laser procedure due to cells buried within the scar that laser cannot adequately treat. The surgical approach is usually vaginally, and the lesion with a 1- to 2-cm margin is excised. Care is taken to avoid injury to the bladder or colon. Depending on the size of the lesion, vaginal reconstruction may be required.

Radical Vulvectomy With Sentinel Node Mapping and Biopsy or Inguinal Femoral Lymphadenectomy

Radical vulvectomy for vulva cancer can be either total or partial depending on the extent of involvement and lesion location.[12] The procedure starts by outlining the vulva cancer lesion with a 2-cm margin. As with a wide local incision, smaller margins are reasonable to preserve function around vital structures. In contrast to a wide local excision where just the superficial vulva skin

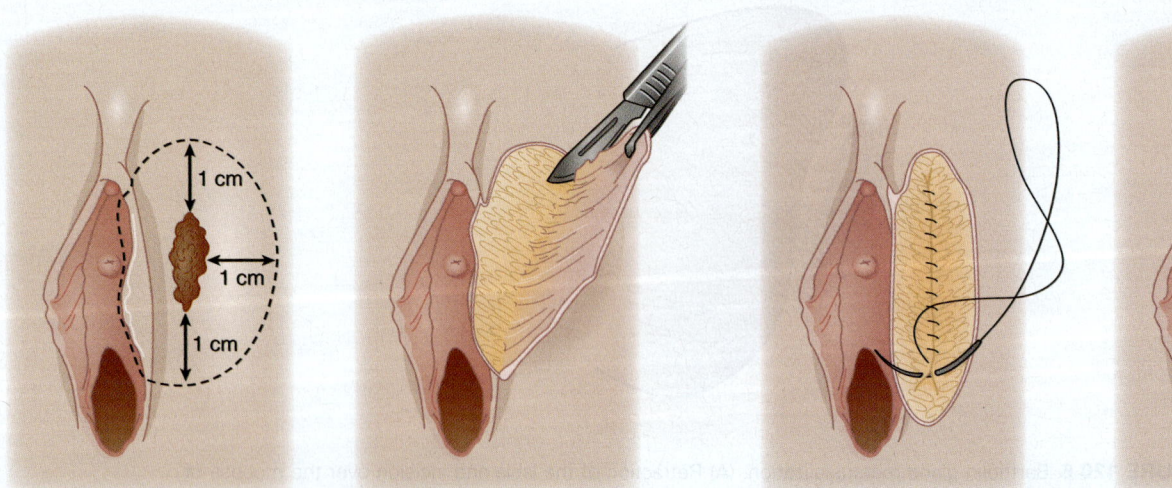

FIGURE 120.7 Wide local excision of vaginal intraepithelial neoplasia lesion.

is removed, the incision in a radical vulvectomy is carried down beneath the subcutaneous tissue to the fascia of the urogenital diaphragm. Care is taken to identify and ligate the clitoris and its vessels anteriorly and the bulbocavernosus muscles and the internal pudendal vessels laterally, as applicable. The specimen is amputated and marked for orientation. Primary closure is achieved by closing the subcutaneous tissue with interrupted absorbable suture. Skin closure may be performed using running or interrupted sutures.

SLN mapping and biopsy is the preferred technique for lymph node evaluation in early stage unifocal vulvar cancer with lesions that are less than 4 cm in diameter, clinically negative lymph nodes, and no inguinofemoral surgeries.[12] The vulvar lesion is injected preoperatively with a radioactive isotope subdermally at four sites around it. A preoperative nuclear scan or single photon emission computed tomography (SPECT) may be used for identifying the sentinel node and for surgical planning.

If no SLN is identified or a patient is not a candidate for SLN dissection, a full inguinofemoral lymphadenectomy is performed. An incision is made parallel to and approximately 2 cm below the inguinal ligament. All lymph node–bearing tissue between the inguinal ligament superiorly, the sartorius muscle laterally, and the adductor longus muscle medially is removed. Preservation of the great saphenous decreases rates of lymphedema. The cribriform fascia may be opened to remove the deep femoral lymph nodes. A suction drain is placed, and primary closure is achieved by closing the subcutaneous tissue with interrupted absorbable suture. Skin closure is performed using a running absorbable suture or staples.

Pelvic Prolapse Procedures

Vault suspensions (abdominal sacrocolpopexy, sacrospinous ligament suspension, uterosacral ligament suspension). Abdominal sacrocolpopexy may be performed via laparotomy, laparoscopy, or robotic approaches and either concurrently with hysterectomy or in patients with posthysterectomy apical prolapse. The vesicovaginal space is developed and the bladder dissected off the anterior vagina while the rectovaginal space is developed, and the rectum dissected off the posterior vagina. A Y-shaped polypropylene mesh graph is sutured to the anterior and posterior vagina as well as the cervix if present. The peritoneum over the sacral promontory is then incised. Permanent suture is used to secure the graft to the anterior longitudinal ligament at the anterior sacrum. Care is taken to avoid injuring the middle sacral vessels. The retroperitoneum is then reapproximated.

Sacrospinous ligament suspension is the most studied transvaginal procedure for treating apical prolapse. After opening the rectovaginal space, the pararectal space is entered by dissecting the rectum from the lateral vagina to the level of the ischial spine. One to two sutures are placed through the sacrospinous ligament with care taken to protect the pudendal vessels and nerves and then through the muscularis of the posterior vaginal epithelium, and later ligated with a pulley stitch.

A high uterosacral ligament suspension is typically performed after completion of a total vaginal hysterectomy. After hysterectomy, the bowels are packed away, and the uterosacral ligaments are identified. Delayed absorbable sutures (one to three) are passed through the uterosacral ligament bilaterally. The first suture is passed just above the level of the ischial spine and second suture is more proximal. Cystoscopy is then performed to ensure integrity of the bladder and efflux of urine from both ureteral orifices. The sutures are then passed through the cervicovaginal

(anterior) fascia and epithelium then through the posterior rectovaginal fascia and vaginal epithelium at the vaginal apex to suspend the vagina anteriorly, posteriorly, and apically.

Anterior/posterior colporrhaphy. Anterior colporrhaphy begins with a full-thickness incision of the anterior vaginal epithelium and entry to the vesicovaginal space, and the incision is extended to the level of the apex of the cystocele. Dissection continues laterally toward the pubic rami. The pubocervical fascia is plicated in the midline using a series of interrupted sutures of delayed absorbable suture from the bladder neck to the bladder base. Excess vaginal skin, when present, should be excised. The anterior vaginal epithelium is closed with a delayed absorbable suture.

Posterior colporrhaphy is performed by incising the posterior vaginal epithelium vertically past the rectocele, entry to the rectovaginal space, and the incision is extended for the full length of the rectocele. The Denonvilliers' fascia is identified, and the rectocele is dissected off the vagina laterally to the level of the levator ani muscles. The rectovaginal septum is plicated to the midline with delayed absorbable suture. If there is excess vaginal epithelium, this is often excised and then closed with a running suture of delayed absorbable suture. Distal rectoceles are often associated with a perineal defect. The perineal muscles including the transverse perineal and bulbocavernosus muscles are reapproximated. Digital rectal examination should be performed at completion to ensure that a rectal injury did not occur. Care must be taken to avoid over narrowing the vagina or introitus.

Colpocleisis. The most commonly performed colpocleisis technique is the LeFort (partial) procedure, which involves obliteration of the vaginal canal when the uterus is left in situ. This procedure should be avoided in patients with high risk of uterine or cervix cancer as future sampling cannot be performed. Appropriate preoperative workup should include transvaginal ultrasound or endometrial biopsy and Pap smear. For the LeFort procedure, traction is placed on cervix and a significant rectangular-shaped portion of the anterior vaginal epithelium is incised and denuded. The bladder neck is plicated with delayed absorbable suture. A similar portion of the posterior vaginal epithelium is then incised and denuded. The uterine and vaginal prolapse are reduced, and the anterior and posterior denuded vaginal walls are reapproximated in a way that leaves bilateral epithelial-lined tunnels to allow for drainage of cervical mucus.

Colpectomy with total colpocleisis is performed in a female who has had a hysterectomy. Procedurally, the vaginal epithelium is excised, and the underlying vaginal connective tissue is reapproximated with serial purse-string absorbable sutures until the prolapse is reduced. Severe urinary incontinence may result from iatrogenically opening the bladder neck if the colpocleisis is brought too close to the bladder neck.

COMMON CERVICAL SURGICAL DISEASES AND PROCEDURES

Common cervical surgical diseases and procedures are listed in Table 120.3. A description of these diseases and management options follow.

Common Cervical Surgical Diseases
Cervical Intraepithelial Neoplasia

CIN is a premalignant condition of the cervix caused by HPV infection. The lifetime cumulative risk of HPV infection is 84% for those with at least one sexual partner; however, the majority of

TABLE 120.3 Common Cervical Surgical Diseases and Procedures

DISEASE	PROCEDURE OPTIONS
Cervical intraepithelial neoplasia	Loop electrosurgical excision procedure
	Cold-knife conization
Cervical cancer	Cold-knife conization/simple hysterectomy (microinvasive disease)
	Radical hysterectomy/trachelectomy with sentinel node biopsy or pelvic lymphadenectomy ± paraaortic lymphadenectomy

HPV infections are transient and do not lead to the development of CIN.[23] Persistent high-risk HPV (hrHPV) infection is a necessary, but not sufficient, cause of cervical cancer. hrHPV types, particularly 16 and 18, have a high rate of progression to CIN and, if not treated, to invasive cancer. The average time from HPV infection to invasive disease is generally over 15 years. Risks factors for HPV infection and CIN include early sexual debut, multiple sexual partners, and a history of sexually transmitted infections, including HIV. Risk factors for persistent HPV infection are not fully understood but include an immunocompromised state and smoking.

HPV vaccines significantly reduce the risk of anogenital warts and CIN. Gardasil 9, which prevents HPV-associated anogenital warts and CIN caused by HPV types 6, 11, 16, 18, 31, 33, 45, 52, and 58, was approved in 2018 for males and females ages 9 to 45.[24] Patients previously infected with HPV, including those with a history of cervical excision procedures from high-grade lesions, should still be offered the vaccination in accordance with guidelines.

Over the past seven decades, cervical cancer screening with cytologic evaluation of the cervix (the "Pap" smear) has resulted in significant decreases in the incidence of and mortality associated with cervical cancer primarily in developed countries.[25] Current available screening tools include cytology or primary hrHPV testing alone or cotesting with both methods. In average-risk patients, hrHPV testing is preferred for screening.[26] However, universal access to this testing, particularly in low-resource settings, is not yet available, and given these communities may disproportionately suffer from cervical cancer, cytology remains an acceptable form of screening. The age to initiate screening has varied and current recommendations suggest 21 years of age. Underscreening of young patients, particularly in underserved populations, is problematic and further raising of the age of screening could further amplify inequities in these vulnerable populations.[27]

The American Society for Colposcopy and Cervical Pathology (ASCCP) has developed algorithms to guide healthcare professions on the workup of abnormal cytology or HPV screening with a focus on instituting cervical treatment in patients with increased risk and expanded surveillance periods for those at lower risk.[26] Colposcopic evaluation of the cervix with biopsy of acetowhite lesions with vascular changes (mosaicism, punctuation) suggestive of CIN is recommended for patients who have abnormal cervical cancer screening results. The ASCCP and College of American Pathologists recommend use of a two-tier grading system, LSIL and HSIL, to classify biopsied lesions suggestive of CIN. HSIL lesion treatment is ideally an excisional procedure, such as a loop electrosurgical excision procedure (LEEP) or a cold-knife conization (CKC) over an ablative approach for pathology review and examination of margins. Adenocarcinoma in situ (AIS) should be treated with an excisional procedure.

Early detection and treatment of premalignant conditions is essential to preventing cervical cancer. In resource-constrained, low-income countries, the use of "see and treat" approaches have been implemented in lieu of the traditional screening used in resource-rich and high-income countries.

Cervical Cancer

Cervical cancer in the United States has declined by over 65% due to screening and early detection, but it remains one of the most common cancers worldwide.[25,28] Cervical cancer is the leading cause of morbidity and mortality due to cancer in patients living in low-income countries.[25,29] The impact of HPV vaccination on the incidence of cervical cancer provides an opportunity to nearly eradicate this disease. Low-income and middle-income countries with a higher burden of disease have the potential to greatly benefit even more from widespread initiatives to administer HPV vaccines. Efforts from agencies, such as the World Health Organization (WHO), to vaccinate 90% of all females by age 15, screen at least 70% of patients age 35 to 45 years twice, and provide treatment to at least 90% of HSIL/LSIL are projected to decrease the incidence of cervical cancer to less than 4 per 100,000.[29]

In high-income countries, cervical cancer affects a disproportionate percentage of patients of low socioeconomic status and minority ethnic and racial groups and is the second leading cause of cancer mortality.[30] Squamous cell carcinoma and adenocarcinomas are the two most common histologic subtypes. Although the rates of squamous cell carcinoma have decreased, there has been an increase in incidence of adenocarcinoma and adenosquamous carcinomas in some countries like the United States.[31]

Patients with cervical cancer most commonly present with irregular or heavy bleeding, postcoital bleeding, vaginal discharge, or pelvic pain. The diagnosis is confirmed by cervical biopsy. Cervical cancer is staged clinically, and treatment depends on the stage.[32]

For most microinvasive early stage cervical cancer, simple hysterectomy is favored in lieu of radical hysterectomy. For selected patients, including those who wish to retain fertility, conization or radical trachelectomy may also be a consideration.

In other early stage disease, surgical approaches are equally effective as treatment with radiation therapy. Radical hysterectomy with either sentinel node biopsy or pelvic/paraaortic lymphadenectomy is the surgical approach of choice for patients who are unlikely to require adjuvant radiation. In cases of locally advanced disease with features such as clinically visible tumor greater than 4 cm or with invasion past the cervix to the pelvic sidewalls, vagina, rectum, bladder, or the pelvic and/or paraaortic lymph nodes, external beam radiation therapy with concomitant cisplatin is recommended over surgical removal. The risk of recurrence may be higher for patients who have radical hysterectomy performed using minimally invasive procedures, particularly when the size of a cervical lesion exceeds 2 cm.[33] Thus, the open approach is the standard of care. Studies are ongoing to identify risk factors that may support the use of minimally invasive techniques in selected patients.

Common Cervical Surgical Techniques
Conization/Loop Electrosurgical Excision Procedure

Removal of a portion of the cervix for diagnosis and treatment of cervical dysplasia can be achieved by a LEEP or CKC. A LEEP may be performed in the office, whereas a CKC is often done in the operating room (OR) due to need for increased exposure and

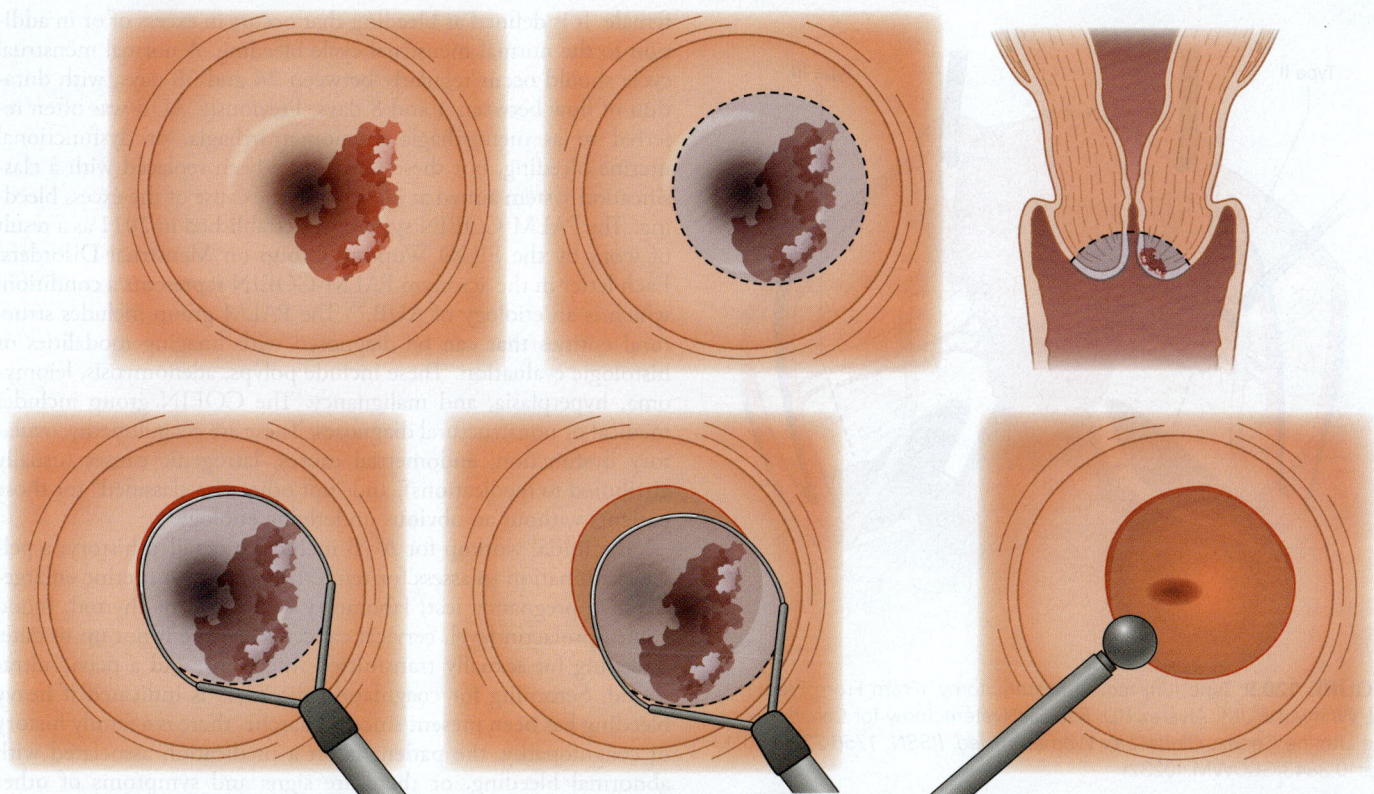

FIGURE 120.8 Loop electrosurgical excision procedure.

a longer operating time. A LEEP uses a wire loop that is heated by electrical current to excise the transformation zone of the cervix with the involved areas of CIN (Fig. 120.8). It is common practice to perform a small excision often called a "top hat" after removal of the first specimen. To perform a CKC, figure-of-eight retention sutures are placed at the 3 o'clock and 9 o'clock positions to ligate the descending branch of the uterine artery. After applying Lugol solution to the cervix to outline the areas of involvement and injecting lidocaine with epinephrine to reduce bleeding, a circumferential incision is made around the transformation zone and lesion using a Beaver blade. The specimen is grasped with Allis clamps to maintain orientation. The specimen is amputated using a scalpel or Mayo scissors. A marking stitch is placed at the 12 o'clock position. An endocervical curettage is performed above the cone biopsy. A running locked stitch or Sturmdorf stitch may be performed to evert the endocervical canal and achieve hemostasis.

Radical Hysterectomy/Radical Trachelectomy With Pelvic Lymphadenectomy

Radical hysterectomy refers to the excision of the uterus, parametria, and upper vagina. This can be performed via an open, minimally invasive, or vaginal approach. A shared decision regarding the surgical approach (open vs. minimally invasive) in selected cases. For open procedures, a transverse incision such as a Maylard or Cherney is often used to increase lateral exposure.

There are several different classification systems used to describe the extent of resection of tissues surrounding the cervix. The Piver-Rutledge-Smith classification is the oldest and most commonly used system.[34] It is divided into five types starting with type I (simple, extrafascial hysterectomy) up to type V (which describes removal of uterus en bloc with parametria,

partial ureteral resection/bladder resection or both). Type II to IV varies on the amount of cardinal and ureterosacral ligaments and vagina that are removed as well as where the uterine artery is ligated. The modified radical hysterectomy that is most commonly used today is type III (Fig. 120.9). The principles of a radical hysterectomy include developing the paravesical and pararectal pelvic spaces, dividing the uterine arteries and veins, dissection of the bladder and ureters off the anterior cardinal ligament, and dissection of the rectum and pararectal tissues off the posterior cardinal ligament. The cardinal ligaments are then divided to allow an adequate sample of parametrium and margin. The ovaries are generally spared for premenopausal patients.

A radical trachelectomy may be an option for patients who desire future fertility with the International Federation of Gynecology and Obstetrics (FIGO) stage IA1 with lymphovascular space invasion, stage IA2 or stage IB1 disease. Most experts recommend this approach for malignant lesions 2 cm or less in diameter.[32] The procedure is performed like the radical hysterectomy with removal of the cervix, parametria, and upper vagina. However, the body of the uterus is preserved, a cerclage is placed, and the uterus is reattached to the superior vagina.

Pelvic lymphadenectomy is usually performed in conjunction with a radical hysterectomy or trachelectomy for early stage cervical cancer patients. Pelvic lymphadenectomy should include the nodes lateral and medial to the external iliac artery and vein from the bifurcation of the common iliac artery to the level of the deep circumflex iliac vein. Nodes from the obturator space between the external iliac vein and obturator nerve should also be excised. SLN mapping for small early stage tumors is an alternative to pelvic lymphadenectomy. Resection of paraaortic lymph nodes is not routinely performed, particularly if there is no evidence of metastasis in the paraaortic or pelvic nodes. When performed,

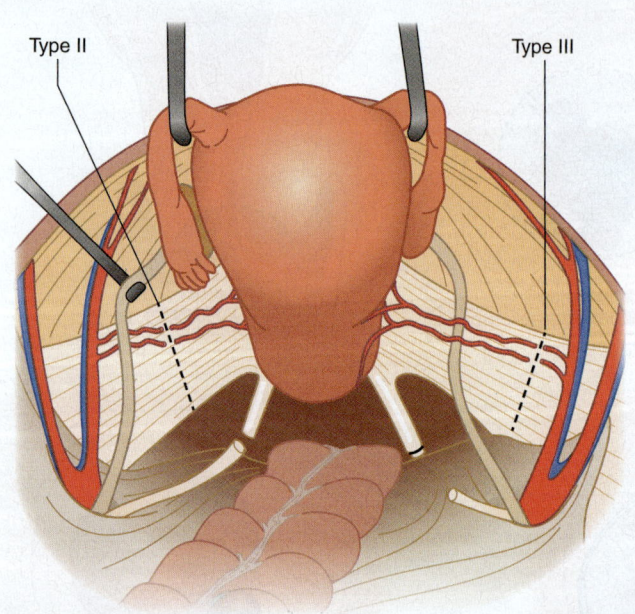

FIGURE 120.9 Type II/III radical hysterectomy. (From From Frederick PJ, Whitworth JM, Alvarez RD. Radical Hysterectomy for Carcinoma of the Uterine Cervix. *Global Libr Women's Med. [ISSN: 1756-2228]* 2011. doi:10.3843/GLOWM.10232)

paraaortic lymphadenectomy should be performed bilaterally by removing the nodes lateral to the common iliac artery and aorta from the bifurcation of the common iliac to the level of the inferior mesenteric artery.

COMMON UTERINE SURGICAL DISEASES AND PROCEDURES

Common uterine surgical diseases and procedures are listed in Table 120.4. A description of these diseases and management options follows.

Common Uterine Surgical Diseases

Abnormal Uterine Bleeding

Abnormal uterine bleeding (AUB) is one of the most common gynecologic complaints and conditions in the reproductive-age

TABLE 120.4	Common Uterine Surgical Diseases and Procedures
DISEASE	**PROCEDURE OPTIONS**
Abnormal uterine bleeding	Endometrial ablation
	Hysterectomy
Uterine polyp	Hysteroscopic polypectomy
Uterine fibroids (leiomyomata)	Myomectomy
	Uterine artery embolization
	Hysterectomy
Adenomyosis	Hysterectomy
Endometrial cancer/ other uterine cancers	Hysterectomy/bilateral salpingo-oophorectomy with select sentinel node dissection or pelvic/ paraaortic lymphadenectomy

female. It is defined as bleeding that occurs in excess of or in addition to the normal menstrual cycle bleeding. A normal menstrual cycle should occur regularly between 24 and 38 days, with duration of flow between 4 and 8 days. Previously, AUB was often referred to as menorrhagia, menometrorrhagia, or dysfunctional uterine bleeding, but these terms have been replaced with a classification system aimed at identifying the cause of the excess bleeding. The PALM-COEIN system was established in 2011 as a result of work by the FIGO Working Group on Menstrual Disorders. Each letter in the acronym PALM-COEIN represents a condition, which is an etiology of AUB.[35] The PALM group includes structural entities that can be diagnosed with imaging modalities or histologic evaluation. These include polyps, adenomyosis, leiomyoma, hyperplasia, and malignancy. The COEIN group includes medical or nonstructural diagnoses. These are coagulopathy, ovulatory dysfunction, endometrial causes, iatrogenic causes (usually attributed to medications), and "not otherwise classified" for those patients without an obvious underlying etiology.

The initial workup for AUB includes a detailed history; a pelvic examination to assess for tenderness, mass, or uterine enlargement; a pregnancy test; laboratory evaluation of thyroid, blood count, prolactin level, cervical cancer screening if not up to date; screening for sexually transmitted infections; and a pelvic ultrasound. Screening for coagulation disorders is indicated if heavy bleeding has been present since menarche, there is a family history of coagulopathy, the patient is on a medication associated with abnormal bleeding, or there are signs and symptoms of other system bleeding (nosebleeds, easy bruising, etc.).

Endometrial biopsy, usually an office procedure, is indicated to rule out endometrial hyperplasia or malignancy in patients at elevated risk for these conditions. Patients age 45 or older with AUB, including intermenstrual bleeding, should undergo endometrial sampling. Patients younger than 45 years old with certain risk factors should also be biopsied. These risk factors include unopposed estrogen exposure, such as those with obesity and ovulatory dysfunction, with persistent AUB or AUB refractory to medical management, or an elevated familial risk of cancer.

Postmenopausal bleeding is not included in the PALM-COEIN classification system and is considered its own diagnosis. Although many causes of AUB in the reproductive-age female are physiologic, any bleeding in the postmenopausal female should be considered abnormal and requires thorough evaluation. The most common cause of abnormal bleeding in a postmenopausal female is atrophy, a thinning of the endometrial lining and vaginal tissue due to lack of estrogen. Without the lubrication and insulation that a thickened endometrial lining provides, the uterine cavity is susceptible to inflammation and infection.

The major concern with postmenopausal bleeding is an underlying malignant or premalignant condition. Of patients diagnosed with endometrial cancer, 90% of patients experience postmenopausal bleeding. Other causes of postmenopausal bleeding include uterine polyps, fibroids, adenomyosis, and medications (most commonly, hormone replacement therapies and anticoagulants). The initial evaluation, in addition to a thorough history and physical examination, includes a pelvic ultrasound and endometrial biopsy. If the endometrial thickness on pelvic ultrasound is 4 mm or less, endometrial biopsy may be avoided. However, recent data have shown that this ultrasound cutoff of 4 mm or less has led to under diagnosing endometrial cancer in Black patients.[36] An endometrial biopsy is indicated for endometrial thickness greater than 4 mm, suspected focal lesion on imaging, difficulty visualizing the endometrium, or persistent bleeding despite a normal ultrasound.[37]

Uterine Polyps

Uterine polyps, also called *endometrial polyps,* are an overgrowth of endometrial glands and stroma that either lie flat along the endometrial lining (sessile polyps) or project out into the cavity (pedunculated polyps). They have an inner "feeder vessel" that often allows them to be diagnosed by Doppler sonography. As discussed previously, they are a common cause of AUB or postmenopausal bleeding. There is large variability in polyp size from a few millimeters to several centimeters, with larger polyps being easier to detect. The majority of endometrial polyps are benign; however, up to 5% of polyps can undergo malignant transformation.[38] Factors associated with uterine polyp formation include increasing age, menopausal status, tamoxifen use, obesity, hypertension, polycystic ovarian syndrome, and familial hereditary cancer syndromes. In addition to AUB, endometrial polyps may be associated with an increased risk of early pregnancy loss.

Leiomyoma

Uterine leiomyomata, or fibroids, are the most common benign gynecologic tumors, affecting up to 70% of patients by age 50. There is a predominance in Black patients, and they experience earlier onset of fibroids, greater number, larger tumors, and more severe symptoms.[39] Fibroids are smooth muscle tumors that arise in the myometrium of the uterus. They can be located anywhere within the uterine wall and are often classified based on their location (Table 120.5).[35] Type 0 fibroids are located completely in the uterine cavity and are often attached with a stalk. They are called *pedunculated* or *intracavitary fibroids.* Types 1 and 2 are submucosal; type 1 fibroids involve less than 50% of the myometrium, whereas type 2 fibroids extend into the wall 50% or more. Types 3, 4, and 5 are intramural fibroids, located completely within the uterine wall with increasing subserosal contact as the numbers increase. Types 6 and 7 are subserosal (type 7 are pedunculated), whereas type 8 are cervical fibroids. Fibroids can be very small or very large and can be single or multiple. They are diagnosed with pelvic imaging, usually an ultrasound or magnetic resonance imaging (MRI).

Symptoms of fibroids, commonly abnormal bleeding, pelvic pain, or pressure-related symptoms from adjacent organs, are directly related to the location and size of the fibroid(s). The treatment options are also related to location and size of fibroids.

TABLE 120.5 **FIGO Classification System for Uterine Fibroids**

TYPE	LOCATION	OPERATIVE REMOVAL APPROACH
0	Intracavitary	Vaginal or hysteroscopic
1	Submucosal	Hysteroscopic
2	Submucosal/intramural	Hysteroscopic or open/laparoscopic
3,4,5	Intramural	Open or laparoscopic
6	Intramural/subserosal	Open or laparoscopic
7	Subserosal/pedunculated	Open or laparoscopic
8	Extrauterine (parasitic, broad ligament, cervical, etc)	Open or laparoscopic

FIGO, International Federation of Gynecology and Obstetrics.
Adapted from Munro MG, Critchley HO, Broder MS, et al. FIGO classification system (PALM-COEIN) for causes of abnormal uterine bleeding in nongravid patients of reproductive age. *Int J Gynaecol Obstet.* 2011;113:3-13.

Treatment options are medical or surgical, depending on the patient's desires and future fertility plans. Surgical treatments are discussed in the following section. Medical options are often directed at bleeding symptoms and include many contraceptive-type medications. Fibroids tend to grow in the reproductive years and regress in size with menopause, thus indicating a relationship between fibroid growth and ovarian hormones. Other risk factors include familial predisposition, obesity, and some dietary factors.[36]

Adenomyosis

Adenomyosis is defined as the presence of endometrial glands and stroma within the myometrium and is considered a variant of endometriosis. Adenomyosis is found often with endometriosis or fibroids at the time of hysterectomy.[35,40] There is a molecular interaction between the displaced endometrial cells and the adjacent myometrial cells, which causes hypertrophy of the myometrium and inflammation. In some patients, this results in a heavier, enlarged uterus. The pathogenesis of adenomyosis is not clearly understood and may share some of its pathophysiology with endometriosis. Adenomyosis often coexists with uterine leiomyoma. Although adenomyosis is commonly a postsurgical diagnosis in that it is diagnosed by pathology, it can be clinically suspected and often identified on pelvic imaging.[40] On ultrasound or MRI, adenomyosis is seen as heterogeneity in the myometrium, a blurring of the junctional zone between the endometrium and myometrium, or the presence of "cysts" within the myometrial layer. Adenomyomas, which can be confused for uterine leiomyomata, are discrete masses of adenomyosis, which are seen as focal asymmetric thickening of the myometrium.

The prevalence of adenomyosis is estimated around 30% of patients of reproductive age with increasing prevalence in the later reproductive years. It is found more commonly in multiparous patients compared with nulliparous patients.[40] Symptoms of adenomyosis are heavy, painful periods, irregular bleeding, painful intercourse, and noncyclic pelvic pain. Some patients with adenomyosis will be asymptomatic. Adenomyosis is treated medically with nonsteroidal antiinflammatory drugs and hormonal contraceptives. A hysterectomy is the surgical intervention of choice for those patients who have failed medical management and do not desire future fertility.

Endometrial and Other Uterine Cancers

Endometrial cancer is the most common gynecologic cancer worldwide and is increasing in incidence and mortality.[25,28] Although the 5-year survival rate has been relatively unchanged at approximately 80%, it is the only cancer for which survival has decreased over the past four decades, and it is now the leading cause of gynecologic cancer death in the United States, with 67,880 new cases and 13,250 deaths estimated for the year 2024.

Black patients have the highest age-adjusted incidence of endometrial cancer.[28] Disparities in survival are marked between White and Black patients at 84% and 64%, respectively. Further, Black patients are more often diagnosed with more aggressive types and advanced stages and are less likely to be offered guideline concordant treatment compared with White patients.[41]

Suspected causes for the increasing incidence of endometrial cancer include the decline in hysterectomy performed for benign disease as well as other common risk factors that have increased in the population in general, such as age, obesity, and diabetes. Other contributory factors such as nulliparity, unopposed estrogen/tamoxifen, and hereditary syndromes, such a nonpolyposis colorectal cancer syndrome (Lynch syndrome), are important considerations. Patients with Lynch syndrome also have an increased risk for ovarian cancer, and age-appropriate risk-reducing hysterectomy with bilateral salpingo-oophorectomy should be a consideration in these patients after childbearing is complete.[42]

Postmenopausal or AUB are common presenting symptoms and may be the only symptom in patients with endometrial cancer. Evaluation should include a transvaginal pelvic ultrasound and endometrial biopsy or hysteroscopy with dilation and curettage. Most patients will have endometrioid adenocarcinoma on pathologic evaluation of biopsy samples. Other histologic types include serous carcinoma, clear cell carcinoma, and carcinosarcoma, all of which are associated with higher risk of extrauterine metastasis and recurrence and poorer long-term survival.

A pelvic MRI should be performed for patients with apparent early stage disease who are considering fertility-sparing hormonal therapy options. Approximately 15% of patients will present with symptoms and examination findings suggestive of more advanced stage disease. Abdominal pelvic computed tomography (CT) should be considered in addition to transvaginal pelvic ultrasound and endometrial sampling in these instances.

The general approach to surgical staging includes extrafascial hysterectomy with bilateral salpingo-oophorectomy with pelvic and paraaortic lymphadenectomy.[43] A minimally invasive approach (conventional laparoscopy or robotic assisted) has similar progression-free survival and overall survival to open approaches, and it has shorter hospital stay and operative adverse events.[44] Open and minimally invasive approaches for staging high-risk disease demonstrate similar outcomes and overall survival.

Surgical staging has both a prognostic role and a diagnostic role in identifying patients who need adjuvant treatment. Surgical staging for patients with early stage endometrial cancer has evolved over the past two decades. Evaluation for intraperitoneal metastasis and bilateral pelvic and paraaortic lymph node involvement remain key components of staging. Patients with low-risk endometrial cancer as defined by Mayo criteria (grade 1–2 endometrioid adenocarcinoma, 2 cm or less in diameter with less than 50% myometrial invasion and absence of extrauterine disease on intraoperative frozen section) have very low rates of metastasis and lymph node assessment may be omitted.[45]

SLN mapping with injection of indocyanine green into the cervix has replaced full lymphadenectomy and is an alternative to using the Mayo criteria because of the acceptable accuracy and lower risk of postoperative morbidity SLN biopsy.[43] Yet substantial disparities exist in its use between different patients of different race (7.0% Black, 9.4% non-Black), ethnicity (8.3% Hispanic, 9.5% non-Hispanic), insurance (6.0% uninsured, 9.5% insured), county density (3.7% rural, 9.8% metro), and income (7.0% bottom-quartile, 11.8% top-quartile).[46] These disparities in surgical approach may increase morbidity and delay adjuvant treatment for Black patients who are already diagnosed with more advanced disease.

Patients with more extensive extrauterine disease generally benefit from cytoreductive surgery similar to that done in patients with ovarian cancer.[43] For patients with localized recurrence, surgery may be indicated if no pelvic radiation was used. Pelvic exenteration is used for those patients with locally recurrent endometrial cancer who have had radiation.

Other rarer subtypes of uterine cancers include high-grade sarcoma, low-grade endometrial stromal sarcoma, and leiomyosarcoma. In the absence of clinically obvious nodal metastasis, lymphadenectomy is not required at the time of definitive hysterectomy.

Common Uterine Surgical Procedures

Hysteroscopy, Dilation and Curettage, Endometrial Ablation

Hysteroscopy is the placement of a small telescope into the uterine cavity for diagnostic purposes. It can be performed in the office in conjunction with a paracervical block or light anesthesia, or in the OR. If operative hysteroscopy is planned for the resection of a uterine lesion, general or regional anesthesia is required. After placement of a speculum, a single-tooth tenaculum is placed on the anterior lip of the cervix for gentle inferior retraction of the cervix to flatten the curve at the cervicouterine junction. The cervix is gently dilated. Normal saline solution is attached to a 12-degree or 30-degree hysteroscope for diagnostic hysteroscopy or operative hysteroscopy with bipolar current. With the distention media running, the hysteroscope is passed through the cervix and into the uterine cavity under direct visualization. The speculum can be removed once the scope is in the uterine cavity as it can impede mobility of the scope and impact visualization of the entire cavity or the execution of an operative procedure. Under pressure, the cavity is distended to allow the surgeon to visualize the fundus, both tubal ostia, the lower uterine segment, and the cervix. An operative hysteroscope will allow passage of scissors, graspers, electrosurgical equipment, and newer mechanical tissue removal system instruments for resection or biopsy of lesions. For global sampling, a curettage is performed after the hysteroscopy. The hysteroscope is first removed, and then a curette is passed through the cervix to the fundus. Gentle curettage is performed along all surfaces of the uterine cavity and the tissue is sent to pathology.

Operative hysteroscopy is the treatment of intrauterine pathology under direct visualization with the hysteroscope. Common operative hysteroscopy procedures include directed biopsy, polypectomy, myomectomy, lysis of intrauterine synechiae (adhesions), and endometrial ablation. Hysteroscopic polypectomy can be performed using a variety of mechanical instruments (Fig. 120.10). Commonly used instruments for polypectomy include a biopsy forceps and scissors, a mechanical tissue removal system, various electrodes such as loop electrode, and a polyp snare. The procedure for hysteroscopic myomectomy is like polypectomy and is reviewed in the section on hysteroscopic myomectomy. For uterine adhesions, scissors are used to lyse adhesions that connect the anterior and posterior walls of the uterine cavity.

Endometrial ablation is the destruction of the endometrial lining by heat or cold. A diagnostic hysteroscopy is performed to make sure the endometrial cavity appears normal without lesions. Any fibroids or polyps are removed. There are several types of nonresectoscopic or "global" endometrial ablation devices, which do not require hysteroscopic guidance. These disposable devices are deployed blindly into the uterine cavity. They have several safety mechanisms in place to both control the amount of heat or cold spread as well as stopping the device from activating if a proper seal is not detected.

Myomectomy

Myomectomy is the removal of uterine fibroids while still preserving the uterus in situ. Depending on fibroid size, location, and surgeon experience, myomectomy can be performed as an open abdominal procedure, laparoscopically, hysteroscopically, or vaginally.

Vaginal Myomectomy

Cervical/intracavitary fibroids that are protruding through the cervix and seen vaginally can be removed via this route.[47] They

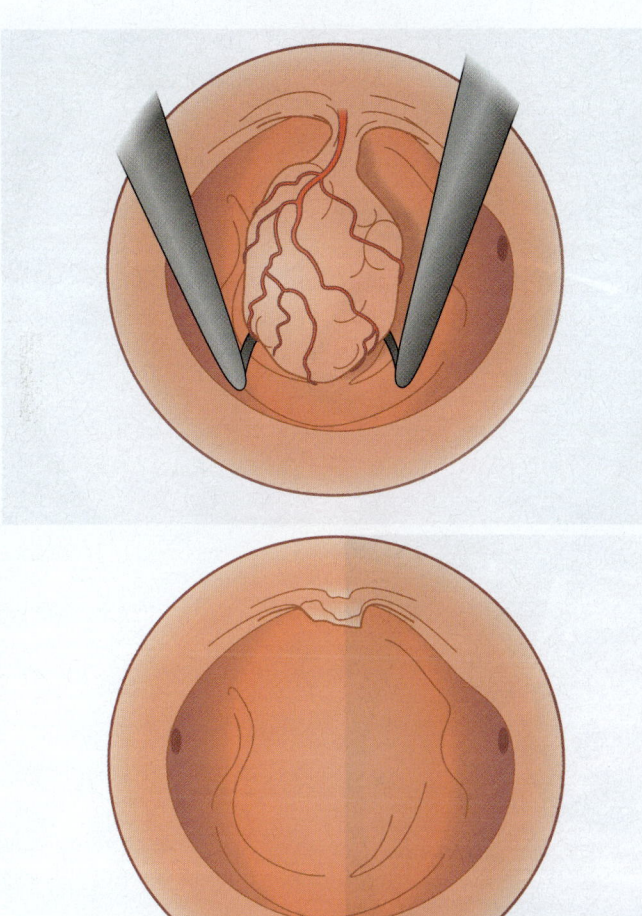

FIGURE 120.10 Hysteroscopic resection of a polyp.

forceps is used to grasp the shaved tissues pieces to remove them from the endometrial cavity. With the mechanical tissue removal systems, gentle suction draws the fibroid to the end of the morcellator and the fibroid is cut and removed in small segments through the same suction. The cutting activity is either mechanical or electrosurgical, depending on the particular device. In both cases, the tissue is collected and sent to pathology.

One of the most important safety parameters in operative hysteroscopy, especially with myomectomy, is monitoring of intrauterine fluid deficit during the procedure. An isotonic solution such as normal saline or lactated Ringer solution is typically used with modern day bipolar resectoscopes. Hypotonic fluid, such as mannitol, was typically used with monopolar resectoscopes. A fluid management system, which closely measures fluid in and out of the hysteroscope, should be used and closely observed throughout the procedure. A large bolus of isotonic fluid during hysteroscopy increases the patient's risk of fluid overload and pulmonary edema. A large deficit of hypotonic fluid not only increases the risk of fluid overload but also increases the risk of electrolyte imbalances, particularly hyponatremia. Many gynecologic surgery societies have published recommended guidelines for fluid deficit, based on the use of isotonic or hypotonic solutions. A deficit of no more than 2500 cc is recommended for isotonic solutions, whereas 1000 cc is the maximum deficit for hypotonic solutions.[48] If a deficit limit is reached, the procedure should be terminated and the surgeon may repeat the surgery at a later date.

Laparoscopic and Open Myomectomy

The remaining fibroids (types 3–8) are removed via either the laparoscopic or the open approach (see Table 120.5). The steps are similar regardless of the approach. The most important step in a successful myomectomy is appropriate preoperative planning. A physical examination and appropriate imaging will help decide the best surgical approach and plan for uterine incision(s). MRI is the preferred imaging modality for planning a myomectomy as it provides more detail about fibroid location, number, and vascularity. The MRI will also help identify the path of the endometrial cavity which is an important aspect of planning uterine incisions.

At the time of surgery, the anatomy is examined and the orientation of the uterus in relation to the adnexal structures is noted. The uterine arteries, as reviewed in the anatomy section, run along the lateral sides of the uterus; thus, hysterotomy incisions should be made medially. The location of the adnexal structures are helpful in determining where the uterine arteries lie if the normal uterine anatomy is distorted by the fibroids. Dilute vasopressin (typically 20 units in 100 cc of normal saline) is injected into the serosal and myometrial layer overlying the fibroid until a blanching is noted.[49,50] An incision is made sharply, with monopolar current, or with a harmonic scalpel in the serosa overlying the fibroid and carried through the myometrium until the capsule of the fibroid is identified (Fig. 120.11). The fibroid is grasped, often with a tenaculum or penetrating towel clamp. Using blunt dissection, monopolar current, sharp dissection, or the harmonic scalpel, the fibroid is dissected from the adjacent myometrium while avoiding an incision directly into the myometrial layer. Hemostasis is maintained with judicious use of cautery or suture ligation. Once the myoma is completely dissected, the myometrial incision is closed with delayed absorbable suture, the number of layers determined by the depth of incision. Barbed suture is commonly used during this step. A final serosal suture layer is placed to approximate the hysterotomy edges and achieve

often have a large vascular stalk that is attached in the endocervical canal or higher in the endometrial cavity. A hysteroscope can help determine the location of the attachment. The greatest risk of vaginal myomectomy is uncontrolled bleeding from the stalk, which often retracts when the myoma is amputated. There are several methods to reduce the risk of bleeding during vaginal myomectomy. At the beginning of the procedure, lateral sutures at 3 o'clock and 9 o'clock are placed in the proximal cervix to occlude the lower branch of the uterine artery. Dilute vasopressin can be injected at the stalk (usually 20 units in 100 cc of normal saline). One or two Endoloop sutures can be passed around the stalk and secured high with the transection of the stalk performed distal to the ligation. Transection can be performed sharply or with electrosurgery. If bleeding is unmanageable after removal, a hysteroscope with attached bipolar cautery should be available for intracavitary sources of bleeding or uterine packing with a Foley balloon can be performed.

Hysteroscopic Myomectomy

Type 0, type 1, and some type 2 fibroids can often be removed via operative hysteroscopy (see Table 120.5). There are two methods for removal: electrosurgery and a mechanical tissue removal system. Both should be performed by experienced hysteroscopists. Removal by electrosurgery is performed through an operative hysteroscope, with either monopolar or bipolar current. Most often, a small loop is used to shave the fibroid to its base. A polyp

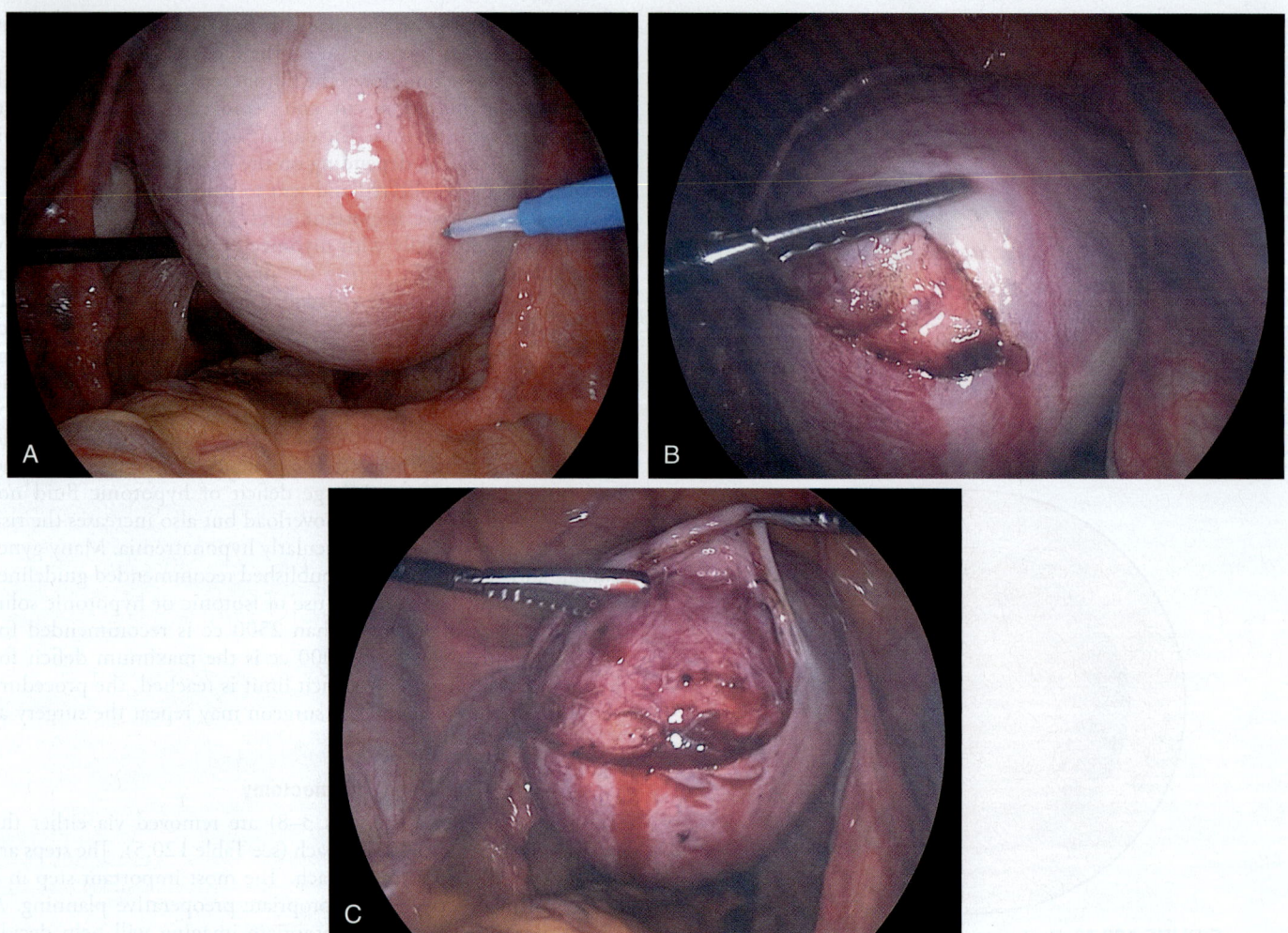

FIGURE 120.11 (A–C) Laparoscopic/open myomectomy.

hemostasis. Once all fibroids are removed, an adhesion barrier can be placed before abdominal closure.[51]

In addition to intramyoma injection of vasopressin, other hemostatic measures are available to control bleeding during open and laparoscopic myomectomy. Before incision, the surgeon can place misoprostol (usually 400–800 mcg) rectally. The misoprostol induces uterine contraction, which causes a tamponade effect on the smaller vessels within the myometrium. Another medical option is to give tranexamic acid (1000 mg given in an IV bolus) around the time of incision.[52] The antifibrinolytic affects prevent clot breakdown, and it is a well-tolerated medication. Intraoperative tourniquet placement is another option. During a myomectomy, a Penrose drain, pediatric feeding tube, or suture is placed around the lower uterine segment (after opening the broad ligament bilaterally and/or infundibulopelvic ligaments) to impede blood flow to the uterus during myoma removal.[53] This technique can be used laparoscopically or during an open procedure. Temporary laparoscopic vascular clips/clamps (such as bulldog clamps) can be used in a similar fashion on the uterine arteries and ovarian vessels.[54] These temporary tourniquet methods should be left on no longer than 90 minutes with at least 10 minutes of rest time between replacements.[53]

After successful myomectomy, the patient should be adequately counseled regarding future childbearing plans, risk of uterine rupture, and options for laboring. Patients who undergo myomectomy should wait at least 3 to 6 months before conceiving. They should consult their obstetrician about timing and method of delivery. Often patients with extensive myomectomies, or procedures that enter the endometrial cavity, will be offered prelabor cesarean sections to decrease their risk of a uterine rupture.[55]

Hysterectomy

Hysterectomy, by definition, is surgical removal of the uterus. There are several routes in which this can be accomplished, and there are also several options for patients and surgeons regarding type of hysterectomy and, if relevant, concomitant salpingectomy and oophorectomy. When considering hysterectomy, it is important to divide the anatomic approach into components that focus on the fallopian tubes and ovaries (when applicable), on the uterine corpus, and on the cervix and upper vagina (Fig. 120.12).

Total Abdominal Hysterectomy

A total hysterectomy is removal of both the uterine corpus and cervix. This can be accomplished via an open incision, vaginal incision, or minimally invasive techniques. For an open technique, also called a *total abdominal hysterectomy*, an abdominal incision is made that is either low transverse or vertical midline. The incision type is chosen based on the indication for the procedure, body habitus, surgical history, size of pathology, and

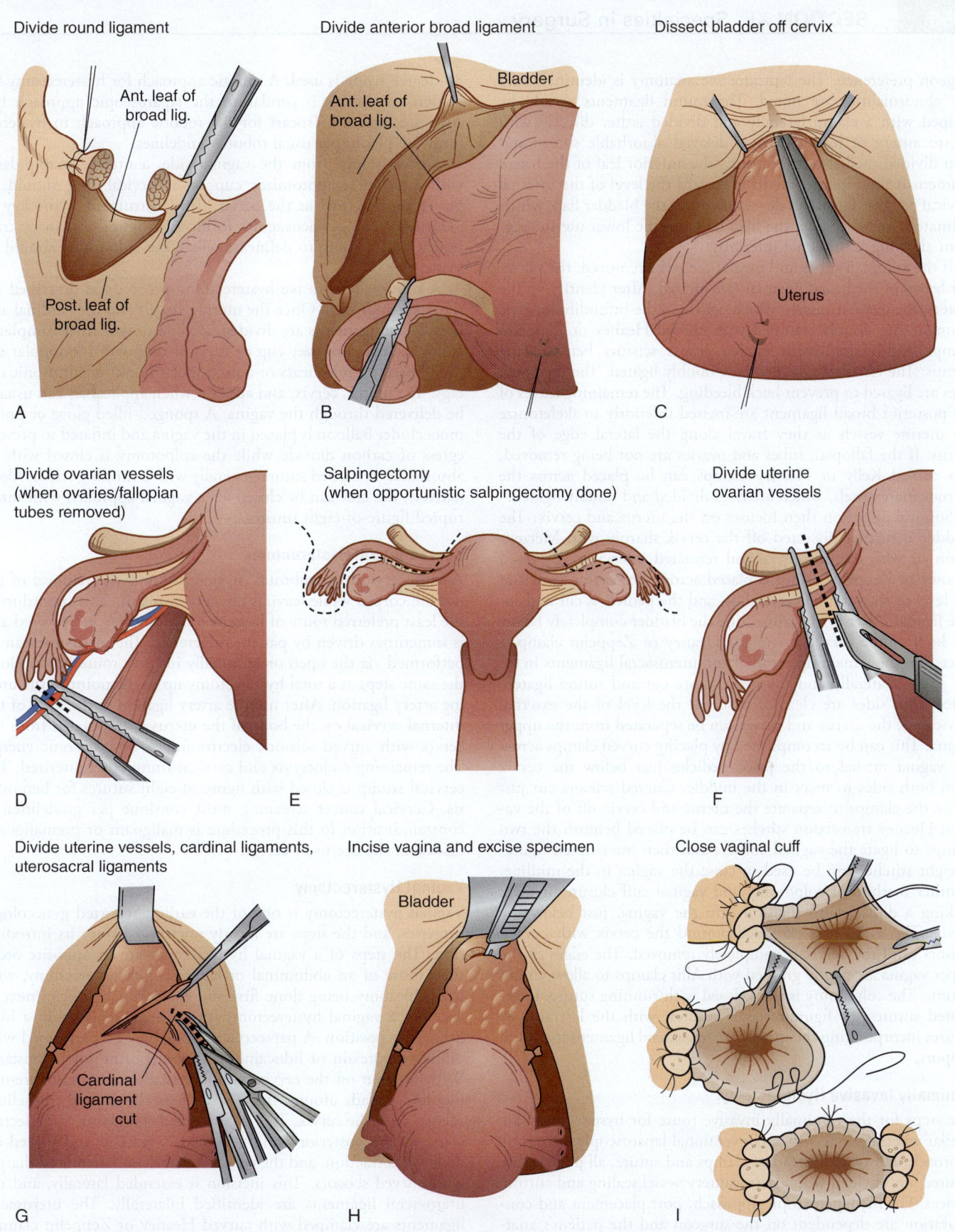

Divide round ligament

Ant. leaf of broad lig.

Post. leaf of broad lig.

A

Divide anterior broad ligament

Bladder

Ant. leaf of broad lig.

B

Dissect bladder off cervix

Uterus

C

Divide ovarian vessels (when ovaries/fallopian tubes removed)

D

Salpingectomy (when opportunistic salpingectomy done)

E

Divide uterine ovarian vessels

F

Divide uterine vessels, cardinal ligaments, uterosacral ligaments

Cardinal ligament cut

G

Incise vagina and excise specimen

Bladder

H

Close vaginal cuff

I

FIGURE 120.12 (A–I) Steps to completing hysterectomy. (A) Transection of round ligament. (B) Incision of anterior and posterior broad ligament. (C) Dissection of bladder off cervix. (D) Division of ovarian vessels (when ovaries/fallopian tubes removed). (E) Removal of fallopian tubes (when opportunistic salpingectomy done). (F) Transection of uteroovarian vessels. (G) Division of uterine vessels, cardinal ligaments, and uterosacral ligaments. (H) Incision of vagina and excision of specimen. (I) Closure of vaginal cuff using open approach. (A–D, F–I, Adapted from Mitchell CW, Wheeless CR. *Atlas of Pelvic Surgery*. 3rd ed. Philadelphia: Lippincott Williams & Wilkins; 1997.)

surgeon preference. The reproductive anatomy is identified, and any abnormalities are noted. The round ligaments should be grasped with a clamp laterally and divided either directly with electrocautery or ligated with a delayed absorbable suture and then divided medial to the suture. The anterior leaf of the broad ligament is then incised medially toward the level of the internal cervical os. This facilitates development of the bladder flap, which ultimately helps separate the bladder from the lower uterine segment allowing it to retract inferiorly.

If the fallopian tubes and ovaries are to be removed, the posterior leaves of the broad ligament are incised. After identifying the ureters, the ovarian vessels, which course in the infundibulopelvic ligament, are doubly clamped with curved Heaney or Zeppelin clamps and incised with curved Mayo scissors between the clamps. The remaining pedicles are doubly ligated. The specimen sides are ligated to prevent back bleeding. The remaining leaves of the posterior broad ligament are incised inferiorly to skeletonize the uterine vessels as they travel along the lateral edge of the uterus. If the fallopian tubes and ovaries are not being removed, two curved Kelly or Heaney clamps can be placed across the uteroovarian vessels, which are then divided and doubly ligated.

Surgical attention then focuses on the uterus and cervix. The bladder is further dissected off the cervix sharply with Metzenbaum or with electrocautery and retracted inferiorly. A curved Heaney or Zeppelin clamp is placed across the uterine vessels at the level of the internal cervical os, and the pedicle is cut and suture ligated. After further dissecting the bladder completely below the level of the cervix, a straight Heaney or Zeppelin clamp is placed on the remaining cardinal and uterosacral ligaments in serial steps bilaterally and the pedicles are cut and suture ligated. Once both sides are clear of tissue at the level of the external cervical os, the uterus and cervix can be separated from the upper vagina. This can be accomplished by placing curved clamps across the vagina medial to the prior pedicles just below the cervix from both sides to meet in the middle. Curved scissors cut just above the clamps to separate the uterus and cervix off of the vagina. Heaney transfixion stitches can be placed beneath the two clamps to ligate the vaginal corners and then interrupted figure-of-eight stitches can be used to close the vagina in the midline. Another method of colpotomy and vaginal cuff closure involves making a direct sharp incision into the vagina, just below the cervix. The incision is extended around the cervix with curved scissors until the cervix is completely removed. The edges of the upper vagina are gently grasped with Allis clamps to allow visualization. The colpotomy is then closed with running suture, interrupted sutures, or figure-of-eight sutures, with the lateral apex sutures incorporating the ipsilateral uterosacral ligament for apical support.

Minimally Invasive Hysterectomy

The steps for the minimally invasive route for hysterectomy are similar whether done with a conventional laparoscopic or robotic approach. However, instead of clamps and suture, all pedicles are secured and divided with electrocautery vessel sealing and cutting devices. For the laparoscopic approach, port placement and configuration are dependent on the surgeon and the patient's anatomy. Typical trocar placement for gynecologic surgery includes any combination of an umbilical trocar, bilateral lower quadrant trocars, and a suprapubic or upper quadrant trocar for assistance. For a large, bulky uterus, trocars can be placed slightly higher in the abdomen and often more ports are used. The camera is commonly placed through the umbilical port, and a 0-degree or

30-degree scope is used. A robotic approach for hysterectomy for benign conditions is similar to the laparoscopic approach but costs are higher.[56] Trocars for the robotic approach to hysterectomy are placed per usual robotic guidelines.

For assistance from the vaginal side, a uterine manipulator with attached colpotomizer cup or a cervical ring should be placed and secured at the cervix. This instrument is the key to identifying the cervicovaginal fornices, avoiding a urinary tract injury, and helping to delineate where the colpotomy should be made.

A minimally invasive hysterectomy proceeds as described for the open approach. Once the uterine vessels and the cardinal and uterosacral ligaments are divided, a colpotomy is then completed along the colpotomizer cup or cervical ring with monopolar energy (usually Endoshears or a monopolar hook) or ultrasonic energy. The uterus, cervix, and adnexa (when applicable) can usually be delivered through the vagina. A sponged-filled glove or pneumooccluder balloon is placed in the vagina and inflated to prevent egress of carbon dioxide while the colpotomy is closed with an absorbable or barbed suture generally with a running stitch. Alternatively, the cuff can be closed via a vaginal approach with interrupted figure-of-eight sutures.

Supracervical Hysterectomy

A supracervical or "subtotal" hysterectomy is the removal of the uterine corpus while leaving the cervix in situ. This procedure is the least preferred route of hysterectomy but may be required and is sometimes driven by patient preference. The procedure can be performed via the open or minimally invasive routes and follows the same steps as a total hysterectomy up to the point of the uterine artery ligation. After uterine artery ligation at the level of the internal cervical os, the body of the uterus is amputated from the cervix with curved scissors, electrocautery, or ultrasonic energy. The remaining endocervix and cervical stump are cauterized. The cervical stump is closed with figure-of-eight sutures for hemostasis. Cervical cancer screening must continue per guidelines. A contraindication to this procedure is malignant or premalignant disease of the uterus or cervix.

Vaginal Hysterectomy

Vaginal hysterectomy is one of the earliest reported gynecologic surgeries, and the steps are mostly unchanged since its introduction. The steps of a vaginal hysterectomy are in opposite order than those of an abdominal or laparoscopic hysterectomy, with the colpotomy being done first and the cornual pedicles next to last. For a vaginal hysterectomy, the patient is placed in a high lithotomy position. A paracervical block may be performed with dilute vasopressin or lidocaine with epinephrine for hemostasis. With traction on the cervix with a tenaculum, a circumferential incision is made around the cervix where the vaginal epithelium merges with the cervix. This is performed sharply or with electrocautery. The posterior peritoneal fold is grasped and placed on downward traction, and the posterior cul-de-sac is entered sharply with curved scissors. This incision is extended laterally, and the uterosacral ligaments are identified bilaterally. The uterosacral ligaments are clamped with curved Heaney or Zeppelin clamps, the ligaments incised off the posterior cervix with curved scissors, and the pedicles ligated with delayed absorbable suture and left tagged for later identification.

A long-weighted speculum is placed through the vagina, below the cervix, and into the posterior cul-de-sac. Attention is then turned anteriorly where the vaginal epithelium is lifted anteriorly, and the bladder is dissected off the cervix to the level of the peritoneum. Once the anterior peritoneum is identified, it is grasped and incised sharply. A right-angle retractor is then passed through this incision to retract the bladder anteriorly away from the uterus for the remainder of the hysterectomy. In serial bilateral steps, a curved clamp is placed laterally to clamp, divide, and ligate the cardinal ligaments and uterine vessels.

With each sequential pedicle, the uterus is further delivered inferiorly into the vagina. The final pedicles include the cornual structures, which include the round ligament, fallopian tube, and uteroovarian ligament. A curved clamped is placed across the cornua under direct visualization, making sure to include each cornual structure and to avoid trapping bowel. The pedicle is cut inferiorly to the clamp, freeing the uterus and cervix. This pedicle is doubly ligated and closely inspected for hemostasis before allowing it to retract superiorly out of view. A similar approach is employed if the ovaries and fallopian tubes are to be removed where the clamp is placed across the ovarian vessels.

The pelvis is examined for hemostasis at each pedicle site. The edges of the colpotomy are grasped with Allis clamps, with care to include the peritoneal layer in the closure. Angle stitches are placed first, incorporating the uterosacral ligaments tagged previously. The remainder of the colpotomy is closed horizontally with a delayed absorbable suture in either running, figure-of-eight, or interrupted sutures.

Elective Bilateral Salpingo-Oophorectomy and Opportunistic Salpingectomy

Unilateral or bilateral salpingo-oophorectomy can be done at the time of hysterectomy but should be reserved for those situations in which there are clear indications for removal. Elective salpingo-oophorectomy, particularly in patients below the age of 50, carries an increase in long-term cardiovascular and neurologic morbidity and mortality, especially if they do not receive hormonal replacement.[57] Routine opportunistic full salpingectomy is now recommended at the time of hysterectomy as a means of potentially reducing the risk of ovarian cancer.[58] These procedures are described in the following section on fallopian tubes and ovaries.

Postoperative Cystoscopy After Hysterectomy

Many gynecologic surgery organizations advocate an immediate postoperative cystoscopy at the conclusion of hysterectomy to assess the integrity of the bladder and ureters.[59] This is easily accomplished with a 30-degree or 70-degree cystoscope and sterile water or saline distention fluid. The urinary catheter is removed, and the scope passed through the urethra and into the bladder. The bladder should be fully distended so that the entirety of the dome is visible. The surgeon assesses for suture, foreign body, lesions, and defects. Additionally, both ureteral orifices are assessed for adequate efflux of urine.

Sentinel Node Biopsy and Lymphadenectomy for Endometrial Cancer

To mitigate complications associated with pelvic and paraaortic lymphadenectomy, SLN mapping is emerging as a preferred strategy for those patients with early stage endometrial cancer undergoing hysterectomy and bilateral salpingo-oophorectomy.[43] The preferred method is by injecting indocyanine green superficially (1–3 mm) and deep (1–2 cm) into the cervix at the 3 o'clock and 9 o'clock positions. Dye is traced to the involved nodes, which are commonly located in and along the pelvic iliac vessels but can also locate in the presacral or paraaortic regions. Sentinel nodes should

be excised and subjected to ultrastaging, which includes serial sectioning and cytokeratin immunohistochemical staining.

Pelvic and paraaortic lymphadenectomy for early stage endometrial cancer patients who do not meet Mayo criteria should be completed in a setting where the side-specific sentinel node is not identified or where SLN mapping capabilities do not exist. Pelvic lymphadenectomy should include the nodes lateral and medial to the external iliac artery and vein from the bifurcation of the common iliac artery to the level of the deep circumflex iliac vein. Nodes from the obturator space between the external iliac vein and obturator nerve should also be excised. Paraaortic lymphadenectomy should be performed bilaterally by removing the nodes lateral to the common iliac artery and aorta from the bifurcation of the common iliac to at least the inferior mesenteric artery and higher toward the renal artery in the setting of higher risk malignancies such as serous carcinoma.

COMMON FALLOPIAN TUBE/OVARIAN SURGICAL DISEASES AND PROCEDURES

Common fallopian tube/ovarian surgical diseases and procedures are listed in Table 120.6. A description of these conditions and management options is as follows.

Common Fallopian Tube/Ovarian Surgical Conditions

BRCA Mutation Carrier

Patients who harbor a germline mutation in the BRCA1 or BRCA2 genes have a 72% and 69% risk of breast cancer by age 80 and a 44% and 17% risk of ovarian cancer by age 70, respectively.[60,61] The list of genes that increase the risk of breast and ovarian cancer when mutations exist continues to evolve. Notable genes, which infer increased risk of ovarian cancer, include BRIP1, RAD51C, RAD51D, and the mismatch repair genes. Guidelines exist that detail criteria for genetic counseling and single gene versus multipanel gene testing.[61] Patients who harbor a deleterious mutation in the BRCA1 or BRCA2 genes are candidates for more intense screening or chemoprevention strategies should fertility be desired. Risk-reducing salpingo-oophorectomy is recommended between the ages of 35 and 40 in patients with a BRCA1 mutation and between the ages of 40 and 45 in patients

TABLE 120.6 Common Fallopian Tube/ Ovarian Surgical Diseases and Procedures	
DISEASE	**PROCEDURE OPTIONS**
BRCA mutation carrier	Risk-reducing bilateral salpingo-oophorectomy
Desires sterilization	Pomeroy partial salpingectomy
	Salpingectomy
Ectopic pregnancy	Partial salpingectomy
	Salpingostomy
Torsion	Detorsion
Endometrioma	Cystectomy
	Unilateral salpingo-oophorectomy
Benign ovarian mass	Cystectomy
	Unilateral salpingo-oophorectomy
Malignant ovarian neoplasms	Bilateral salpingo-oophorectomy, total hysterectomy, staging with early stage disease, debulking with late stage disease
	Unilateral salpingo-oophorectomy and staging with early stage disease and desire for future fertility

with a *BRCA2* mutation. Risk-reducing salpingo-oophorectomy in patients with a BRCA mutation has been demonstrated to reduce the risk of ovarian cancer by at least 80% and to reduce the risk of breast cancer by at least 50%, albeit recent studies suggest the reduction in breast cancer benefit is primarily noted in *BRCA1* mutation carriers.

Desires Sterilization

Sterilization is the most common method of contraception among married couples and twice as many couples choose female partner sterilization over male sterilization. Physicians should carefully counsel patients about the permanence of female sterilization particularly in light of long-acting reversible contraceptive measures, which are as effective birth control measures as permanent sterilization. Historical studies have demonstrated that patient race, ethnicity, and socioeconomic status have affected physician attitudes and practices with respect to counseling about reversible versus permanent counseling. Respect for an individual female's reproductive autonomy should be the primary guiding principal when discussing sterilization options. These discussions should also

include informing the patient that male sterilization incurs less risks and is more effective than female sterilization and that the rates of failure of tubal sterilization are reported to be overall less than 2%. Physicians should also note that approximately 14% of patients express regret after sterilization. Patients at risk for regret include those of color, of young age, and after a recent pregnancy event. A fully informed shared decision model is key in discussing sterilization options with patients (Fig. 120.13).

Ectopic Pregnancy

The rate of ectopic pregnancy is about 1% to 2% that of live births and is potentially life threatening. Over 90% occur in the fallopian tube. Risk factors for an ectopic pregnancy include a history of ectopic pregnancy, pelvic inflammatory disease, infertility, use of an intrauterine device, smoking, and tubal ligation. Patients often present with nonspecific abdominal or pelvic pain and vaginal bleeding symptoms and on examination may be found to have a tender abdomen, cervical motion tenderness, or an adnexal mass. Patients with a ruptured ectopic pregnancy may present emergently with signs and symptoms of hypovolemic

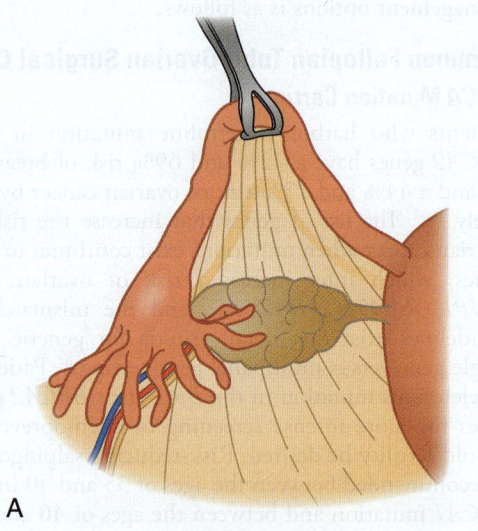

A

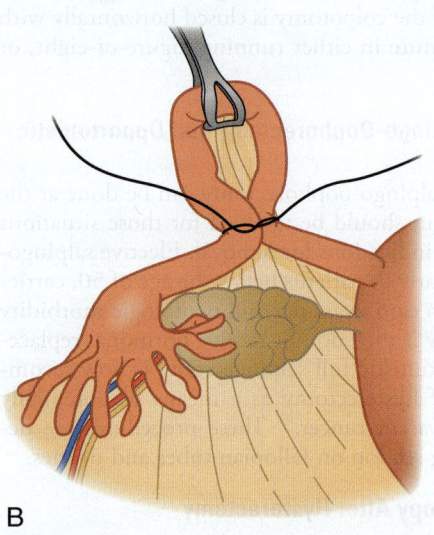

B

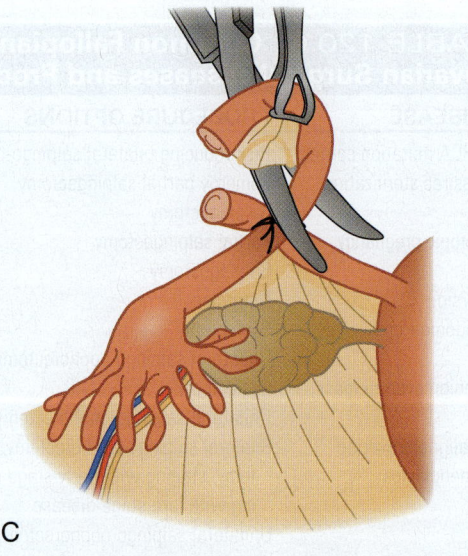

C

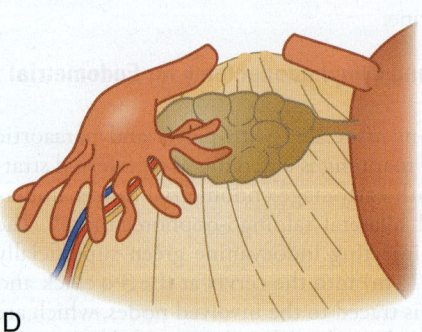

D

FIGURE 120.13 (A–D) Pomeroy tubal sterilization.

shock. A quantitative beta human chorionic gonadotropin (β-HCG) and transvaginal ultrasound should be expeditiously performed in patients who present with symptoms and signs suggestive of a potential ectopic pregnancy. The presence of a tubal ectopic with a fetal heartbeat or an inhomogeneous or noncystic adnexal mass (known as a *blob sign*) has high sensitivity for diagnosing an ectopic. Medical management with intramuscular methotrexate is an option for patients with a stable ectopic pregnancy for whom no medical contraindications exist. Surgical intervention is required in a patient who is hemodynamically unstable, has a persistent ectopic despite medical management, or has contraindications to medical management.

Torsion

Ovarian torsion occurs when the ovary, often together with the fallopian tube, twists on its attachments to other structures in the pelvis and compromises its blood supply. It accounts for 3% of all gynecologic emergencies. It occurs most commonly in patients of reproductive age, and the most common risk factor is the presence of an ovarian cyst or tumor. Patients with ovarian torsion generally present with acute-onset sharp unilateral pelvic pain. Nausea may also accompany the pain symptoms. Common signs on physical examination include unilateral lower abdominal pain and adnexal tenderness. The diagnosis may be facilitated with transvaginal Doppler ultrasound. Imaging studies may demonstrate an enlarged ovary with a twisted vascular pedicle and diminished arterial or venous blood flow. Of note, Doppler vascular flow is not always absent in torsion, and the diagnosis in this setting must be made on the basis of clinical suspicion. Ovarian torsion warrants urgent surgical intervention, and often the diagnosis is not confirmed until the ovary and fallopian tube are visualized intraoperatively.

Endometrioma

An endometrioma is an ovarian cyst often associated with peritoneal endometriosis, a condition where endometrial tissues exist outside of the endometrium. An endometrioma frequently consists of endometrial epithelium and stroma and is often called a *chocolate cyst* due to the dark brown, thick, and tarry hemosiderin-laden fluid it contains. Most patients with endometriomas are of reproductive age and will often present with symptoms of endometriosis. Common endometriosis symptoms include pelvic pain, dysmenorrhea, dyspareunia, and/or infertility. Some patients with an endometrioma are asymptomatic. Physical examination may demonstrate a painful adnexal mass and other signs of endometriosis, such as cul-de-sac nodularity. Transvaginal ultrasound is useful in detecting endometriomas. Typical sonographic findings associated with an endometrioma include a unilocular cyst with low-level echogenicity representing old blood (commonly termed *ground-glass* feature). Many patients with the presumptive diagnosis of endometriosis will be managed medically depending on the degree of symptoms and the desire for fertility. Larger endometriomas (>4 cm) are generally refractory to medical management, and laparoscopic excision is considered the treatment of choice. Although there has been concern that excision of an endometrioma might damage ovarian reserve, excision is preferred over drainage particularly in patients with pelvic pain symptoms, infertility, or suspicion for a neoplasm. Excision of the cyst also decreases the chance of the endometrioma recurrence.

Benign Ovarian Masses and Neoplasms

Most benign ovarian masses tend to be functional follicular or corpus luteum cysts, which in general are asymptomatic and rarely exceed 5 cm in diameter. The most common benign ovarian neoplasms include cystic teratomas (commonly known as *dermoid cysts*), serous or mucinous cystadenomas or cystadenofibromas, and fibromas or fibrothecomas. Many patients with a benign ovarian neoplasm will be asymptomatic, but some will experience pelvic pain. Most benign pelvic masses are noted to be smooth, mobile, and of various dimensions on pelvic examination. Rarely, will there be clinical signs of ascites. Evaluation should include transvaginal ultrasound to delineate the size and features of an adnexal mass because each neoplasm has distinct sonographic findings. Select tumor markers such as a cancer antigen 125 (CA125), β-HCG, alpha-fetoprotein (α-AFP), inhibin A and/or inhibin B, or lactate dehydrogenase (LDH) should be obtained depending on the clinical scenario and concern for a malignancy.

Conservative management with serial observation and management of symptoms, if present, of a patient with a functional ovarian cyst is advised. Surgical intervention, generally using a laparoscopic approach, is required for patients with a persistently symptomatic suspected benign ovarian neoplasm. Laparoscopic ovarian cystectomy is appropriate for a dermoid cyst or fibroma regardless of size, based on the surgeon's skill set. Oophorectomy is often required with larger dermoid cysts and with cystadenomas that replace the entire ovary. Laparotomy is generally reserved for much larger benign ovarian neoplasms, for when the diagnosis is equivocal, and if ovarian or fallopian tube malignancy is higher on the differential. Laparotomy should also be considered in the setting of a tuboovarian abscess that is refractory to antibiotics and image-guided drainage. Consultation with a gynecologic oncologist should be considered in settings when a cancer is suspected or when complex surgical intervention is anticipated.

Malignant Ovarian Neoplasms

Ovarian cancer is one of the deadliest gynecologic malignancies in part because it is often diagnosed at advanced stages of disease.[28,62] For patients with advanced epithelial ovarian cancer, examination will often demonstrate abdominal distention from ascites; evidence of carcinomatosis on abdominal examination; and a firm, nodular, fixed pelvic mass. The majority of patients with advanced stage ovarian cancer have high-grade serous carcinoma, which is now thought to originate in the fallopian tube in the majority of cases.[63] Endometrioid and, less frequently, low-grade serous carcinoma are other subtypes noted in patients with advanced stage disease. Other malignant ovarian neoplasms can originate from germ cells, stromal cells, or other epithelial cells from the ovary. Patients with a malignant ovarian neoplasm may present with nonspecific bloating or abdominal pain, early satiety, other nonspecific intestinal symptoms, and urinary frequency. On examination, patients with a germ cell, stromal cell, or early stage epithelial tumor might be found to have abdominal pain and an adnexal mass on pelvic examination with no obvious clinical evidence of metastasis.

CT examination of the chest, abdomen, and pelvis and tumor markers will help narrow down the differential to an ovarian or fallopian tube malignancy and demonstrate the extent of disease. Germ cell tumors are more common in younger patients, and relevant tumor markers should include a β-HCG, LDH, and AFP. For older patients with a suspected epithelial tumor, a CA125, carcinoembryonic antigen, and CA19-9 are most useful. In patients with a stromal tumor, an inhibin and select hormone tests may be of use, particularly when there is evidence of a hormonally functional mass. Recent breast or colon screening results in patients age 40 and above may help exclude metastatic breast or colon cancer from the differentiation in this clinical scenario.

Primary surgical debulking with staging has been the traditional approach to patients with a suspected malignant ovarian neoplasm. This approach is the preferred strategy in patients with clinical evidence of early stage disease. Surgery should be fertility sparing in the setting of a young patient with a germ cell tumor or low-grade epithelial tumor. Primary debulking should be considered in the setting of advanced stage epithelial cancer when the patient is medically fit and optimal (<1 cm residual disease and preferably no residual disease) surgical resection is anticipated. Meta-analyses comparing chemotherapy before debulking surgery (neoadjuvant chemotherapy [NACT]) with primary debulking surgery (PDS) followed by chemotherapy reveal a possible decrease in risk of serious adverse events, such as bowel resection, with NACT, but show no advantage in primary survival outcomes in patients with advanced disease.[64]

Referral to a gynecologic oncologist is useful in helping to make the decision to consider primary debulking versus NACT and interval debulking. In an otherwise fit patient with advanced stage disease, clinical features such as examination, CA125 level, and CT findings can inform the decision. Laparoscopic assessment using scoring systems have also been developed to facilitate the decision to proceed with primary debulking versus NACT. For select patients with recurrence, a secondary or beyond surgical resection may also provide some benefit. Patients who benefit the most from secondary debulking might include those with a long tumor-free interval and with evidence of isolated disease and no ascites.

Common Fallopian Tube/Ovarian Surgical Procedures

Tubal Sterilization

Tubal sterilization is most commonly performed via a laparoscopic approach but can also be performed via a mini-laparotomy or transvaginally. Opportunistic complete salpingectomy has increased as the preferred method for patients undergoing tubal sterilization because the fimbriated end of the fallopian tube has been shown to serve as the originating site for high-grade serous

ovarian carcinoma.[58,63] For this procedure, the fallopian tube is elevated, and small windows are made in the avascular areas within the mesosalpinx. The small vessels providing blood supply to the fallopian tube are ligated or cauterized, and the fallopian tubes are excised where they insert into the uterine cornua.

Other commonly used techniques for tubal sterilization include the use of mechanical occlusive devices such as clips or rings and tubal cauterization. Technical failures and minor morbidity are noted more frequently with ring occlusion compared with clip occlusion. In general, a bipolar cautery device is used when cauterization of the tube is performed. Surgeons should ensure that a 2-cm portion of the mid fallopian tube is cauterized when this procedure is performed.

Salpingectomy/Salpingostomy for Ectopic Pregnancy

Surgical intervention is required for those patients with an ectopic pregnancy who fail medical management or who present with acute rupture of an ectopic. In general, a laparoscopic approach is preferred and can be used even in the setting of a large hemoperitoneum. Surgical options include a partial salpingectomy or salpingostomy (Fig. 120.14). Randomized trials have demonstrated no difference in the rates of subsequent ectopic pregnancies or intrauterine pregnancy.[65] In general, partial salpingectomy is the preferred approach when severe fallopian tube damage is noted and in cases in which there is significant bleeding from the proposed surgical site. The technique for salpingectomy mimics that done for tubal sterilization. Specifically, the portion of the fallopian tube is elevated and the fallopian tube proximal and distal to the ectopic is cauterized and incised. The mesosalpinx beneath the involved portion of the fallopian tube is cauterized and divided. The specimen is then forwarded for pathologic confirmation of an ectopic.

Salpingostomy should be considered in patients who have an ectopic pregnancy that has not ruptured, who desire future fertility but have damage to the contralateral fallopian tube, and in whom removal of the fallopian tube would require assisted reproduction

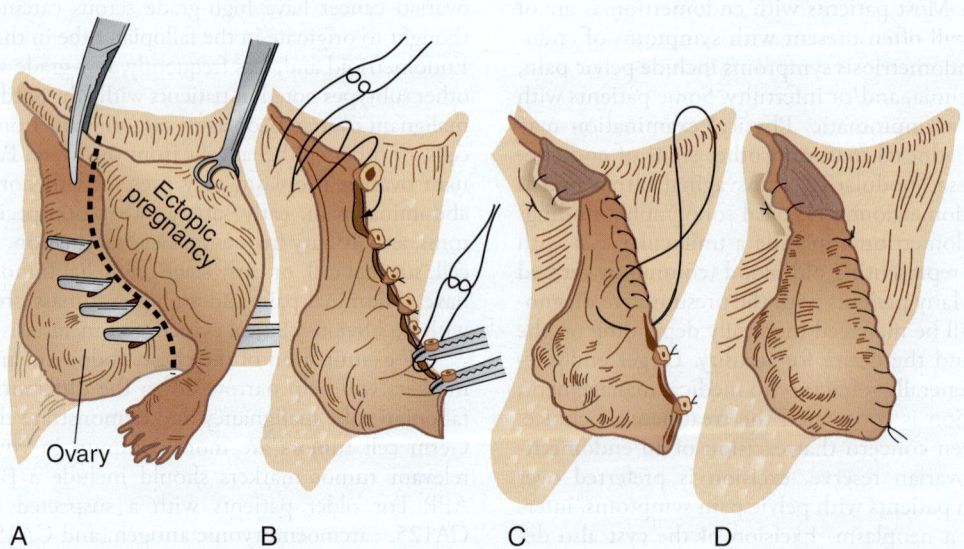

FIGURE 120.14 Salpingectomy. (A) Tube is excised from the cornual portion across the mesosalpinx to the fimbria. (B) Pedicles are tied, peritoneal lining is reestablished, and cornual portion of the tube is buried into the posterior segment of the uterine cornu. (C) Mesosalpinx is reperitonealized. (D) Mesosalpinx is closed and the procedure completed. (Adapted from Mitchell CW, Wheeless CR. *Atlas of Pelvic Surgery*. 3rd ed. Philadelphia: Lippincott Williams & Wilkins; 1997.)

for future childbearing. Salpingostomy involves injecting the involved fallopian tube with vasopressin and then creating a linear incision in the area involved with the ectopic pregnancy. The products of conception are then flushed out with a suction irrigator. There is no need to suture the salpingostomy site as it will heal well by secondary intention. When salpingostomy is performed, it is important to monitor the patient with serial β-HCG levels to ensure resolution of ectopic trophoblastic tissue.

Ovarian Detorsion

A diagnostic laparoscopy is the preferred surgical approach to confirm the suspicion of an ovarian torsion. In general, the involved ovary, and often fallopian tube, are noted to be twisted on its vascular supply (Fig. 120.15A). They often appear edematous and darkened as a result of vascular and lymphatic congestion and may seem nonviable. Detorsion rather than salpingo-oophorectomy is the procedure of choice because over 80% of patients have been noted to have normal ovarian function after this procedure (see Fig. 120.15B). The procedure involves untwisting the involved adnexa twisted vascular pedicle. Ovarian cystectomy may accompany detorsion when an ovarian cyst or benign ovarian neoplasm is noted. The risk of recurrence after detorsion appears small and oophoropexy has not been proven to reduce that risk.

Ovarian Cystectomy

Ovarian cystectomy is most often employed for patients with an endometrioma, a torsed ovary with a large benign ovarian cyst, a benign neoplasm such as a cystadenoma or dermoid, or a borderline tumor of the ovary. This technique is most appropriate for patients in whom retaining fertility is critical and in whom there appears to be residual normal ovary. Cystectomy is indicated for endometriomas over 4 cm and has been demonstrated to improve fertility over an incision and drainage procedure. Though cystectomy carries a higher risk of recurrence in borderline tumors of the ovary when compared with salpingo-oophorectomy, overall survival is not compromised.[66]

A laparoscopic approach is preferred in most cases for which ovarian cystectomy is planned. The surgical technique involves incising the ovarian surface over the ovarian cyst and using preferably mechanical or hydrodissection to completely excise the ovarian cyst (Fig. 120.16). Electrocautery or suturing may also be required to control areas of bleeding. Excision of an endometrioma can be quite difficult and ovarian reserve is often compromised postoperatively.

Salpingo-Oophorectomy

Salpingo-oophorectomy, unilateral or bilateral, is the procedure of choice for a number of clinical indications. Most often, this procedure is accomplished for a benign ovarian mass, which involves the entire ovary. Other indications include risk-reducing salpingo-oophorectomy for patients with a BRCA mutation, chronic pelvic pain with severe endometriosis or adhesive disease, or a malignant ovarian neoplasm. The procedure is most often completed using laparoscopy. Laparotomy is advised in situations when a patient may have had history of extensive pelvic surgery and significant

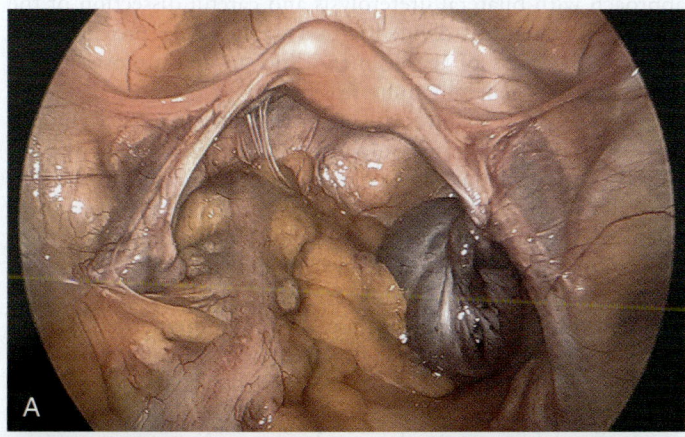

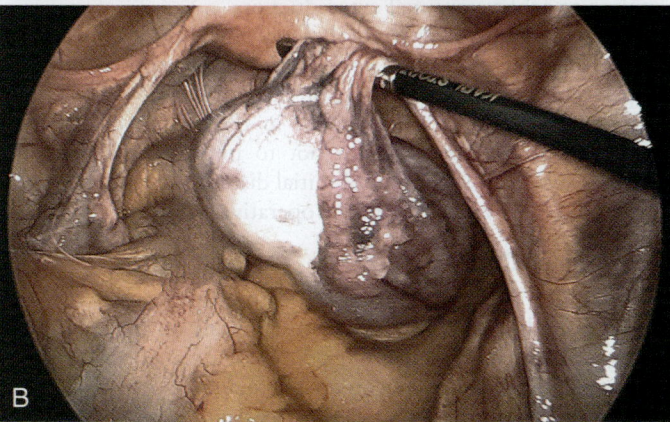

FIGURE 120.15 (A) Ovarian torsion. (B) Ovarian detorsion.

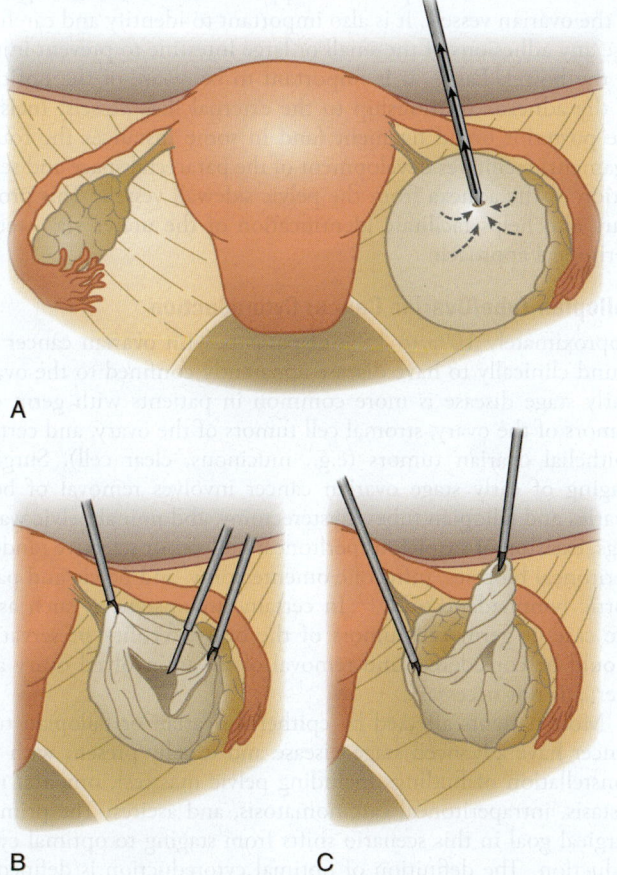

FIGURE 120.16 (A–C) Cystectomy.

pelvic adhesive disease is suspected, a mass is of a significant size or configuration that would make removal by laparoscopic technique difficult, or a malignancy is suspected.

The surgical technique for salpingo-oophorectomy, whether performed by laparoscopy or laparotomy, involves cauterization or ligation of the ovarian vessels contained within the infundibulopelvic ligaments lateral to the ovary and fallopian tube and cauterization or ligation of the uteroovarian vessels medial to the ovary and fallopian tube (see Fig. 120.12D). For risk-reducing salpingo-oophorectomy, it is important to ligate the ovarian vessels at least 2 cm lateral to the ovary and fallopian tube so that no residual ovary or fallopian tube is left behind. It is also important to obtain abdominal pelvic washings during that procedure and inform the pathologist that the procedure is being performed for a patient with a BRCA mutation so that appropriate serial sectioning of the specimens is performed. These steps are important because approximately 5% of patients with a BRCA mutation will be noted to have an occult ovarian or fallopian tube cancer.

Another key surgical principle in salpingo-oophorectomy includes identification of structures within the pelvis that are at risk of injury when the procedure is performed. Perhaps the most important of these structures is the ureter, which courses over the bifurcation of the common iliac artery close to the infundibulopelvic ligament. It is important to identify the ureter either via a transperitoneal or retroperitoneal approach. The ovary and fallopian tube should be lifted anteriorly and displaced as far from the ureter as possible before ligating the ovarian vessels. In scenarios where the ovary or fallopian tube are involved with pathology such as a mass or endometriosis that impedes easy separation of the structures from the ureter, ureterolysis should be performed. Ureterolysis via a retroperitoneal approach allows for safer ligation of the ovarian vessels. It is also important to identify and carefully lyse any adhesions of the small or large intestine to prevent injury to the bowel. Lastly, it is important to be aware of the position of the adnexa's relationship to the external iliac vessels. Incising the posterior broad ligament (and in some instances the round ligament) facilitates development of the pararectal space and separation of the adnexa from the pelvic sidewall vessels. This procedure also helps facilitate identification of the ureter via a retroperitoneal approach.

Fallopian Tube/Ovarian Cancer Cytoreduction

Approximately 10% to 15% of patients with ovarian cancer are found clinically to have disease apparently confined to the ovary. Early stage disease is more common in patients with germ cell tumors of the ovary, stromal cell tumors of the ovary, and certain epithelial ovarian tumors (e.g., mucinous, clear cell). Surgical staging of early stage ovarian cancer involves removal of both ovaries and fallopian tubes, hysterectomy, abdominal pelvic washings, excision of suspicious peritoneal nodules or selective random peritoneal biopsies, infracolic omentectomy, and pelvic and paraaortic lymphadenectomy.[62] In certain circumstances, such as in the case of germ cell tumors of the ovary, fertility preservation should be considered, and removal of the uninvolved ovary and uterus is not necessary.

Most patients affected by epithelial ovarian or fallopian tube cancer have advanced stage disease and usually present with the constellation of findings including pelvic mass(es), omental metastasis, intraperitoneal carcinomatosis, and ascites. The primary surgical goal in this scenario shifts from staging to optimal cytoreduction. The definition of optimal cytoreduction is defined as residual disease less than 1 cm in diameter, and preferably no

visible residual disease. Studies have demonstrated that outcomes in advanced ovarian/fallopian tube cancer are the best in patients who have no residual disease.

Historically, most if not all patients with advanced stage ovarian or fallopian tube cancer underwent a PDS followed by chemotherapy. Several studies over the past decade have demonstrated that NACT followed by an interim debulking surgery after three to four cycles results in similar outcomes and less morbidity for advanced stage ovarian cancer.[63] This is particularly true for those advanced stage ovarian cancer patients who are either too ill and have significant surgical risks or for those in whom it appears that optimal debulking will not be feasible. Increasingly this practice paradigm is being adopted for patients with advanced ovarian/fallopian tube cancer and several clinical factors or laparoscopy can be used to predict the feasibility of achieving optimal (preferentially complete) surgical resection.

The surgical approach to ovarian/fallopian tube cytoreduction or debulking, either primary or interval, should involve an appropriate midline incision to provide adequate exposure for resection of all disease. Minimally invasive strategies for early stage ovarian cancer patients or for those undergoing interval debulking can be considered for select patients. The surgical goals of optimal cytoreduction are best accomplished in phases. For disease in the pelvis, surgeons must decide whether a total abdominal hysterectomy with bilateral salpingo-oophorectomy (procedure previously described) will suffice or whether an en bloc type of procedure that involves resection of a portion of the sigmoid colon and pelvic peritoneum will be required to remove all pelvic disease (Fig. 120.17). The latter is usually necessary when the cul-de-sac region and colon are extensively involved with disease. This resection generally involves a retroperitoneal approach with bilateral ureterolysis and careful dissection of the bladder. The colon is divided with a staple device proximal and distal to the areas of involvement, and an anastomosis with a staple device is generally quite feasible.

A second phase involves the upper abdomen. One key component of upper abdominal surgery includes resection of the involved portion of the gastrocolic and infracolic omentum. This generally involves resecting the omentum from the hepatic to splenic flexure, taking care to avoid injury to the stomach, transverse colon, spleen, pancreas, and liver. Disease along the inferior aspects of the diaphragm can be excised by dividing the falciform ligament, mobilizing the liver, and stripping the peritoneum off the diaphragm muscle fibers. Isolated nodules on the peritoneal surfaces can be resected or obliterated using a variety of techniques. On occasion, small bowel resection with anastomosis is required to achieve optimal cytoreduction.

A third phase involves removal of any obvious nodal metastasis. This generally involves adequate retroperitoneal exposure either in the pelvis or in the paraaortic region or both. Elective resection of nodes without clinical involvement in the setting of advanced ovarian cancer has been shown not to improve outcomes and should be avoided. The extent of initial disease and extent of resection should be documented in the operative report.

Transgender Care

The evolution of care for transgender patients has rapidly progressed over the last decade with an emphasis on the multidisciplinary team approach, including gynecologic surgeons.[67] Training in transgender surgical techniques remains lacking in many programs and approaches to care for patients is often limited to large quaternary care centers that have the subspecialists available.

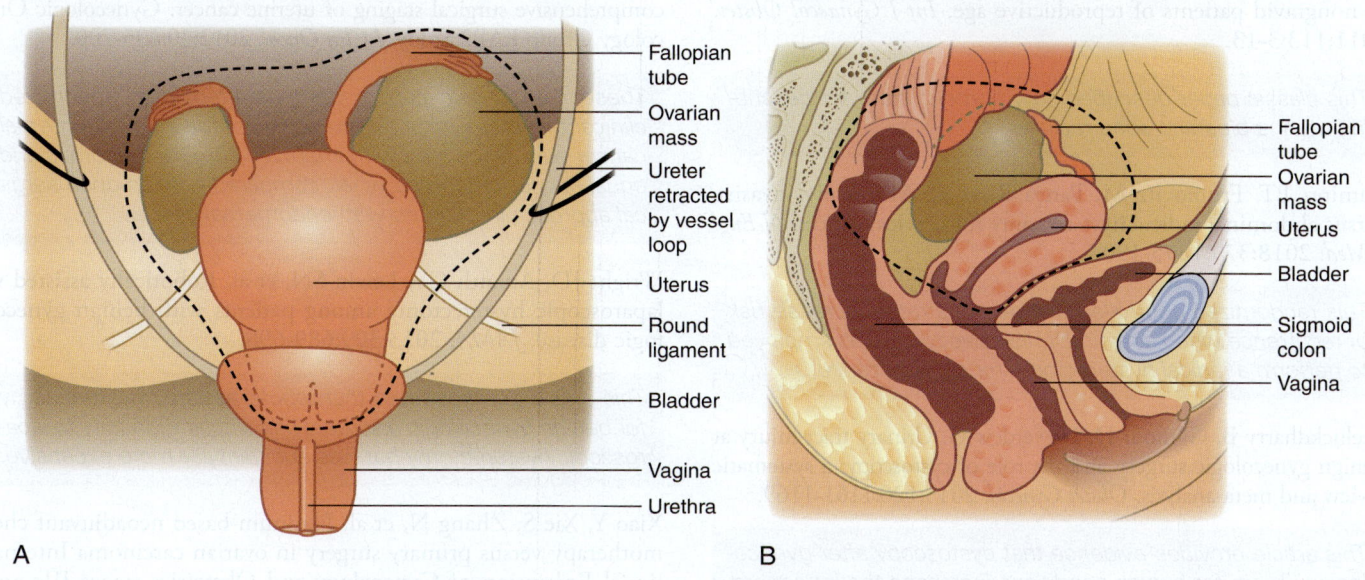

FIGURE 120.17 (A–B) En bloc cytoreduction of ovarian cancer in pelvis.

Surgical goals of care for female-to-male gender-affirming surgery include hysterectomy with bilateral salpingo-oophorectomy and vaginectomy followed by metoidioplasty or total phalloplasty, urethral lengthening, and scrotal reconstruction. Vaginal hysterectomy is preferred over laparoscopic hysterectomy due to the lack of visible abdominal scarring that contributes to stigma and lapse in body security and self-confidence while preserving the abdominal vasculature for future phalloplasty vascular needs.[68] However, surgical exposure may be limited in a nonparous patient and laparoscopic hysterectomy would be an acceptable safe alternative. Consultation with a fertility specialist is warranted before removal of the ovaries to discuss future conception options.

SUMMARY

It is important for the surgeon to be familiar with gynecologic conditions that affect patients throughout the spectrum of their lives and that often require surgical intervention. Knowledge of the relevant pelvic anatomy and the most common procedures should provide surgeons with the confidence to address gynecologic conditions in a skillful and compassionate manner.

SELECTED REFERENCES

Castellano T, Zerden M, Marsh L, et al. Risks and benefits of salpingectomy at the time of sterilization. *Obstet Gynecol Surv.* 2017;72:663-668.

This article demonstrated the feasibility and safety of opportunistic salpingectomy for patients desiring tubal sterilization.

Curry SJ, Krist AH, Owens DK, et al. Screening for cervical Cancer: US Preventive Services Task Force recommendation statement. *JAMA.* 2018;320:674-686.

This paper provides current guidelines for cervical cancer screening.

Evans EC, Matteson KA, Orejuela FJ, et al. Salpingo-oophorectomy at the time of benign hysterectomy: a systematic review. *Obstet Gynecol.* 2016;128:476-485.

This review demonstrated that elective salpingo-oophorectomy at the time of hysterectomy for benign reasons was associated with increased long-term morbidity and mortality, particularly when done in premenopausal patients.

Jelovsek JE, Barber MD, Brubaker L, et al. Effect of uterosacral ligament suspension vs sacrospinous ligament fixation with or without perioperative behavioral therapy for pelvic organ vaginal prolapse on surgical outcomes and prolapse symptoms at 5 years in the optimal randomized clinical trial. *JAMA.* 2018;319:1554-1565.

This classic article demonstrated that uterosacral ligament suspension and sacrospinous ligament fixation for pelvic organ vaginal prolapse largely had similar long-term outcomes.

Joura EA, Giuliano AR, Iversen OE, et al. A 9-valent HPV vaccine against infection and intraepithelial neoplasia in patients. *N Engl J Med.* 2015;372:711-723.

This study demonstrated the efficacy of a nonavalent human papillomavirus (HPV) vaccine for the prevention of high- and intermediate-risk for HPV intraepithelial neoplasia in patients.

Levenback CF, Ali S, Coleman RL, et al. Lymphatic mapping and sentinel lymph node biopsy in patients with squamous cell carcinoma of the vulva: a gynecologic oncology group study. *J Clin Oncol.* 2012;30:3786-3791.

This classic study validated the utility of sentinel lymph node biopsy in patients with vulva cancer ≤4 cm in diameter.

Munro MG, Critchley HO, Broder MS, et al. FIGO classification system (PALM-COEIN) for causes of abnormal uterine bleeding in nongravid patients of reproductive age. *Int J Gynaecol Obstet.* 2011;113:3-13.

Ramirez PT, Frumovitz M, Pareja R, et al. Minimally invasive versus abdominal radical hysterectomy for cervical cancer. *N Engl J Med.* 2018;379:1895-1904.

Teeluckdharry B, Gilmour D, Flowerdew G. Urinary tract injury at benign gynecologic surgery and the role of cystoscopy: a systematic review and meta-analysis. *Obstet Gynecol.* 2015;126:1161-1169.

Walker JL, Piedmonte MR, Spirtos NM, et al. Laparoscopy compared with laparotomy for comprehensive surgical staging of uterine cancer: Gynecologic Oncology Group Study LAP2. *J Clin Oncol.* 2009;27:5331-5336.

Walker JL, Piedmonte MR, Spirtos NM, et al. Recurrence and survival after random assignment to laparoscopy versus laparotomy for comprehensive surgical staging of uterine cancer: Gynecologic Oncology Group LAP2 Study. *J Clin Oncol.* 2012;30:695-700.

Wright JD, Ananth CV, Lewin SN, et al. Robotically assisted vs laparoscopic hysterectomy among patients with benign gynecologic disease. *JAMA.* 2013;309:689-698.

Xiao Y, Xie S, Zhang N, et al. Platinum-based neoadjuvant chemotherapy versus primary surgery in ovarian carcinoma International Federation of Gynecology and Obstetrics stages IIIc and IV: a systematic review and meta-analysis. *Gynecol Obstet Invest.* 2018;83:209-219.

The full reference list appears on Elsevier eBooks+.

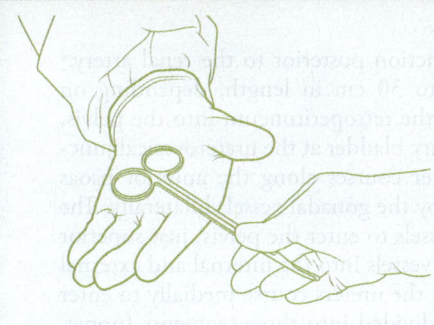

CHAPTER 121

Urologic Surgery

Vidit Sharma, Paras Shah, and Stephen B. Williams

UROLOGIC ANATOMY FOR THE GENERAL SURGEON

The organs of the genitourinary (GU) system span the entire retroperitoneum, pelvis, inguinal region, and genital region. Because of the close anatomic relationships of the organs in the abdomen and retroperitoneum, general surgeons must be familiar with all of the urologic organ systems to prevent iatrogenic injury and to deal with variations in normal anatomy. These challenges arise in many fields of surgery, including vascular, oncology, and colorectal surgery.

Upper Abdomen and Retroperitoneum

Adrenal

Beginning at the most superior aspect of the retroperitoneum lie the adrenal glands. These small, paired organs have two different embryologic origins and serve a primary endocrine function. The adrenal glands are composed of the cortex and medulla and are fused after development. The cortex is the outer layer of the adrenal gland and is derived from mesoderm.[1] On cross section, the layers, from external to internal, are the zona glomerulosa, zona

fasciculata, and zona reticularis. The different zones secrete various steroid-derived hormones including mineralocorticoids (glomerulosa), glucocorticoids (fasciculata), and sex steroids (reticularis).[2] The adrenal medulla is derived from neural crest cells and is directly innervated by presynaptic sympathetic fibers.[1] The medulla is responsible for secreting catecholamines in response to sympathetic stimulation. The adrenal glands lie within Gerota fascia and have an orange-yellow appearance and an area of usually 3 to 5 cm in transverse diameter.[1] The arterial supply is through three sources: superior (inferior phrenic), medial (abdominal aorta), and inferior (ipsilateral renal artery). The venous drainage does not mirror the arterial supply; on the right, the single adrenal vein drains to the vena cava, whereas on the left, the adrenal vein drains into the left renal vein. Supernumerary veins can exist on either side because of anatomic variation. The adrenal glands are anatomically distinct from the kidney, although there are ventral and dorsal fascial investments that connect it to the kidney. The anatomic relations to the right adrenal gland are the vena cava on the anteromedial aspect and the liver and duodenum on the anterior aspect of portions of the adrenal gland. On the left, the pancreas and splenic vein are anterior to the cortical surface.

Kidney

The kidneys are the next paired organs just inferior to the adrenal glands. These organs are completely enveloped within the perirenal fascia (Gerota fascia) and are mobile structures supported only by the perirenal fat, renal pedicle vasculature, and abdominal muscles and viscera. Although Gerota fascia separates the kidney capsule and parenchyma from these adjacent organs and reduces the risk of renal injury with local dissection, renal parenchymal injury is possible with abnormal anatomy. The kidneys are approximately the size of a closed fist, measuring 10 to 12 cm in length and 5 to 7 cm in width. The right kidney typically lies slightly more inferiorly than the left kidney because of its position beneath the liver. Despite being located in the retroperitoneum, the kidney is well protected from external injury by the surrounding muscular and skeletal structures. Posteriorly, each kidney is covered by the diaphragm on the upper third of its surface and is crossed by the twelfth rib. The inferior aspect of the kidney is adjacent to the psoas muscle medially and the quadratus lumborum and transversus abdominis laterally.[1] The anterior surfaces of the kidneys are intimately related to several intraperitoneal structures. On the right, the liver is attached to the kidney by the hepatorenal ligament, and the anterior upper pole is adjacent to the peritoneal surface of the liver.[1] The duodenum lies on the medial aspect of the anterior right kidney, typically on the hilar structures. The hepatic flexure of the colon crosses anterior to the inferior pole of the right kidney. On the left, the superior pole of the kidney lies posterior to the tail of the pancreas and the splenic vessels and hilum. The spleen is situated anteromedial to the kidney and is directly attached to the kidney by the lienorenal ligament. The splenic flexure of the colon is draped over the caudal aspect of the anterior left kidney.

The renal vasculature has significant variability occurring in 25% to 40% of kidneys.[3] The typical vasculature is based on a paired artery and vein supplying the kidney as direct branches of the aorta and vena cava, respectively. The renal artery branches from the aorta inferior to the superior mesenteric artery at the level of the second lumbar vertebra. The renal artery then branches into four or five segments, each being an end artery.[3] The renal arteries are located posterior and slightly superior to the renal veins. The artery initially branches posteriorly into the posterior segmental artery. The anterior branches are variable but include the apical, upper, middle, and lower segmental arteries. These arteries branch multiple times within the cortical kidney, creating a complex filtration mechanism at the capillary level. The venous capillary branches coalesce to mirror the parenchymal arterial system. Renal segmental veins are not end vascular structures and collateralize extensively. The renal vein on the right is short, typically 2 to 4 cm in length, and enters the posterolateral inferior vena cava.[3] The left renal vein is longer, 6 to 10 cm, and travels anterior to the aorta and inferior to the superior mesenteric artery and enters the left lateral vena cava.[3] The left renal vein also is the common entry point for the left adrenal vein, gonadal vein, and a lumbar vein. Renal ectopia is accompanied by markedly variable and unpredictable renal vasculature, with multiple branches arising from the iliac arteries or aortic bifurcation.

Ureter

The upper collecting system begins within the renal parenchyma at the level of the papilla. The papillae coalesce to become the minor calyces, which, in turn, become the major calyces. The major calyces converge to form the renal pelvis. The ureter begins at the inferior aspect of the renal pelvis, where it narrows to become the ureteropelvic junction posterior to the renal artery.[2] Each ureter is typically 22 to 30 cm in length, depending on height, and courses through the retroperitoneum into the pelvis, where it connects to the urinary bladder at the ureterovesical junction.[4] At its origin, the ureter courses along the anterior psoas major muscle and is crossed by the gonadal vessels bilaterally. The ureters cross over the iliac vessels to enter the pelvis, just superior to the bifurcation of the iliac vessels into the internal and external segments. Once in the pelvis, the ureters course medially to enter the bladder. The ureters are divided into three segments (upper, middle, and lower) using this anatomic landmark as a junction point.[4] The upper segment runs from the ureteropelvic junction to the superior margin of the sacrum. The middle segment runs over the bony pelvis. The lower segment begins at the inferior margin of the sacrum and continues into the bladder. The ureteral lumen is not uniform throughout its length and has three distinct narrowing points: the ureteropelvic junction, crossing the iliac vessels, and the ureterovesical junction. The right and left ureters have separate anatomic relationships (peritoneal and retroperitoneal structures). On the right, the ureter is posterior to the ascending colon, cecum, and appendix. The left ureter is posterior to the descending and sigmoid colon. In the male, the ureters are crossed by the vasa deferentia as they emerge from the internal ring before turning medially to join the prostate. The ureteral blood is drawn from multiple vessels throughout its course and within the adventitia; the arterial vessels create an anastomosing plexus. In general, the upper ureteral segments have a medial vascular supply (i.e., renal artery and aorta), and the lower ureteral segments have a lateral vascular supply (i.e., internal iliac and various branches). This unique collateral blood flow allows extensive mobilization of the ureter, outside of its adventitia, without loss of its blood supply.[4]

The ureter is best identified, intraoperatively, in an area of normal anatomy and then followed to the area of concern. This is readily accomplished medial to the lower pole of the kidney or at the iliac bifurcation. After prior surgery or retroperitoneal disease processes, any of these rich collateral blood supply sources may not be contributory; thus, to minimize the risk of surgical devascularization, it is critical to avoid unnecessary extensive circumferential dissection of the ureter or dissection of the ureter in the subadventitial plane.

Pelvis

Bladder and Prostate

The bladder, the end reservoir for urine, is located within the inferior pelvis. The bladder, when empty, is located behind the pubic rami; but as the bladder becomes distended, the superior aspect of the bladder extends out of the pelvis and into the lower anterior abdomen.[5] The bladder can be injured on entering of the abdomen through a midline incision in the retropubic space (of Retzius) if the bladder is not displaced posteriorly when the midline rectus fascial incision is extended to the pubis. Superiorly, the bladder is covered by the parietal peritoneum of the pelvis as the peritoneum reflects off the anterior and lateral abdominal walls. The anterior and lateral bladder walls do not have a peritoneal surface but reside within pelvic fat and lie along the musculature of the pelvic sidewall or pubis anteriorly. Prior lower abdominal or pelvic surgery can change the anatomic relations of the bladder and cause it to be affixed abnormally within the pelvis. The bladder has a unique cross section with a urothelial lining creating a tight barrier from urine and a central muscular detrusor layer involved in the excretory function of the bladder.[6] Branches of the internal iliac artery, the superior and inferior vesical arteries, supply blood to the bladder. Similar to the ureter, the bladder has a rich collateral vascular network, so ligation or damage to an artery is not detrimental to the bladder. The innervation of the bladder is important because of the excretory function of the bladder. The bladder has autonomic and somatic innervation with a dense neural network to the brain. The sympathetic innervation to the bladder is through the hypogastric nerve, and the parasympathetic supply is through the sacral cord and pelvic nerve.[5] The anatomic relationships of the bladder differ between male and female patients. In the male patient, the posterior bladder wall is adjacent to the anterior sigmoid colon and rectum. Prior pelvic surgery, irradiation, or pelvic trauma can make the plane between these structures difficult to define, resulting in inadvertent injury. In the female patient, the parietal peritoneum becomes contiguous with the anterior uterus, and the superior bladder lies against the lower uterus, whereas the bladder base sits adjacent to the anterior vaginal wall. The spherical bladder funnels caudally into the bladder neck, and this becomes the tubular urethra inferiorly.

In the male patient, the first segment of the urethra is surrounded by and integrated into the prostate. The prostate, an endocrine gland involved with male reproductive function, is located immediately inferior to the bladder and invested in the circular fibers of the bladder neck. The prostate is surrounded by the lateral pelvic fascia on its anterior surface, by endopelvic fascia on its lateral surface, and by Denonvilliers fascia posteriorly.[7] The rectum sits immediately posterior to the prostate and is separated by a second layer of Denonvilliers fascia. This fascia also extends superiorly on the posterior prostate to encompass the seminal vesicles. The seminal vesicles are the reservoirs for seminal fluid, which makes up the majority of the ejaculatory fluid. The arterial supply to both structures is through branches of the inferior vesical artery. The venous drainage mirrors the arterial supply, draining through the inferior vesical veins and subsequently into the internal iliac veins. In addition to the rectum, the other major anatomic relationship of the prostate is the Santorini plexus, a network of veins derived from the dorsal venous complex of the penis.[7]

Urethra, Male Genitalia, and Perineum

The drainage of urine from the bladder is through the tubular urethra, which begins at the level of the bladder neck. In male patients, the urethra has five distinct segments: prostatic, membranous, penile, bulbar, and glandular (also known as the *fossa navicularis*). The prostatic and membranous urethra is surrounded by striated muscle, and when the urethra penetrates the GU diaphragm in the perineum, the outer layer becomes spongy, vascular tissue. Within the prostate, the ejaculatory duct opens into the urethra and serves as the exit point for seminal emission. The blood supply of the extraprostatic urethra is through the common penile artery, which is a branch of the internal pudendal artery.[5] The venous drainage of the urethra is through the circumflex penile veins and ultimately into the deep dorsal vein of the penis. The major surrounding structure in the proximal male urethra is the rectum, which sits posterior to the proximal bulbar segment. The female urethra is more regular in length and is approximately 4 cm long.[5] The female urethra contains three distinct layers as opposed to the male urethra. The proximal urethra is surrounded by smooth and striated musculature, which forms the urinary sphincter. The arterial and venous blood supply are through the internal pudendal, vaginal, and inferior vesical veins. The only

structure adjacent to the female urethra is the anterior vaginal wall.

The male external genitalia consist of the penis, scrotum, and paired testes. The penis consists of three circular erectile bodies: the two dorsal corpora cavernosa and the ventral corpus spongiosum. The corpora cavernosa are responsible for penile erection; the corpus spongiosum provides support and structure to the urethra. Blood supply of the penis is through the external and internal pudendal arteries. The external pudendal artery supplies the penile skin; the internal pudendal artery supplies the urethra and the paired erectile bodies. The venous drainage of the penis is through the superficial and deep dorsal veins and the cavernosal veins. The penis is entirely an external structure, with all three erectile bodies terminating in the perineum. The scrotum is a surprisingly complex structure consisting of a muscular sac covered with a unique epidermal layer with no fat but many sebaceous and sweat glands. The sac is divided into two halves by a midline septum of dartos muscle. The blood supply to the scrotum is through the external pudendal arteries anteriorly and branches of perineal vessels posteriorly. Within the scrotum are the right and left testicles. The testicles have both endocrine and reproductive function in males. Typically, the testes are 4 to 5 cm long and 3 cm wide.[5] The vascular and genital ductal structures leave the testis from the mediastinum in the posterosuperior portion and travel through the scrotal neck into the inguinal canal. The spermatic cord is invested by the internal spermatic fascia, cremaster muscle, and external spermatic fascia, which are derived from the transversalis fascia, internal oblique, and external oblique, respectively. Arterial blood supply is primarily through the testicular or gonadal artery, which is a direct branch from the aorta inferior to the renal artery. Secondary blood supply to the testicle is through the cremasteric and vasal arteries. The venous drainage of the testicle initially begins as a pampiniform plexus coalescing into the gonadal or testicular veins. On the right, the vein drains directly into the vena cava; on the left, the vein drains into the left renal vein. The testicles are also responsible for spermatogenesis and for testosterone production. After production, the spermatozoa exit through a series of ductal structures that emerge into the rete testis, efferent ductules, epididymis, and ultimately the vas deferens. The epididymis is located posteriorly and slightly lateral to the testis. The spermatic artery, vein, and vas deferens are invested together in the fascial structures of the spermatic cord. The spermatic cord travels through the external inguinal ring through the inguinal canal and then into the pelvis through the internal inguinal ring. The spermatic cord is susceptible to injury during inguinal dissection for hernia repair, especially in redo cases, when it may be encased in fibrosis and injured without recognition. Significant injury to the spermatic cord may put the viability of the testis at risk, even though it is supported by three collateral arteries. The perineum is divided into an anterior and posterior triangle in the male by a line connecting the ischial tuberosities.[5] The posterior perineal triangle contains the anus and internal and external sphincters. The anterior triangle (or urogenital triangle) contains the corpus spongiosum and proximal aspect of the paired erectile bodies, the corpora cavernosa. The layers deepening toward the corpus spongiosum consist of the skin, subcutaneous fat, Colles fascia, and bulbospongiosus muscle (surrounding the corpus spongiosum) and ischiocavernosus muscles (surrounding the corpora cavernosa). The blood supply to this region is based on branches of the internal pudendal artery, and drainage is through the internal pudendal vein. The presence of a urethral catheter is helpful in palpating the location of the urethra, but the corpus spongiosum surrounding the bulbar urethra is still vulnerable to injury with dissection in an inflamed or obliterated anatomic plane.

ENDOSCOPIC UROLOGIC SURGERY

Urologists were early adopters of endoscopic surgery and began evaluating the urethra and bladder with cystoscopy in the early part of the 20th century. The first diagnostic and therapeutic endoscopic procedures were performed for treatment of urologic disease processes. Endoscopic procedures are divided based on intervention or evaluation of the lower or upper urinary tract as each has specialized procedure-specific equipment.

Cystoscopy, or cystourethroscopy as it is formally called, is used for evaluation of the urethra and the bladder. Cystoscopic procedures are typically performed to evaluate the lower urinary tract in the setting of hematuria, voiding symptoms, recurrent infections, or bladder outlet obstruction; for surveillance in the setting of malignant neoplasms; and for removal of GU foreign bodies and assessment of suspected trauma. Furthermore, cystoscopy can be used to perform diagnostic evaluation of the upper urinary tract with use of ureteral catheters and instillation of contrast material, which is visualized within the collecting system by fluoroscopy. Cystoscopy can be performed with both rigid and flexible endoscopes, each with certain benefits and advantages. Endoscopes are sized with the "French" (Fr) size system, which refers to the outer circumference of the instrument in millimeters. The rigid endoscope uses optical lens systems, similar to laparoscopes, and has excellent resolution. The inflexible structure is intuitive and easy to orient. Rigid cystoscopes have a range of sizes typically from 16 to 26 Fr; surgical endoscopes, or resectoscopes, have the largest size of 24 to 26 Fr.[8] Rigid endoscopes have a larger luminal diameter, which allows greater irrigation flow, improving visualization and passage of a number of working instruments. Rigid lower tract endoscopy is more difficult to perform in the awake patient, although it is much better tolerated in the female patient than in the male patient because of the short, straight urethra in the female patient. Flexible endoscopes are smaller, 15 or 16 Fr, and better tolerated by patients for examination. Both male and female patients can be examined with local anesthesia, usually consisting of lidocaine jelly instilled per urethra. The flexible endoscope does not require any specific patient positioning and can be used supine and at the bedside. Finally, because of the large deflection radius, the bladder is easily evaluated without changing the lens or patient position. The optics of flexible endoscopes continue to improve by advancements in camera chip capability, with new digital platforms approaching the resolution of optical lens systems. Pediatric endoscopes are smaller, 8 to 12 Fr, and are typically used in the operating room.

Upper tract evaluation is performed with either a ureteroscope or a nephroscope. The most common reason for either procedure is management of calculous disease, both ureteral and renal. Ureteroscopy can also be used to visualize and to inspect the upper collecting system, ureter, and renal pelvis; for hematuria originating from the upper urinary tract; for surveillance of urothelial carcinoma; and for treatment or biopsy of abnormal findings. Ureteroscopy is performed with both flexible and semirigid endoscopes, each with different benefits and purposes. Semirigid endoscopes are 6 to 7.5 Fr at the tip and gradually enlarge to 8 to 9.5 Fr.[8] The taper at the tip allows introduction into the ureteral orifice at the trigone of the bladder. These endoscopes have larger working channels that allow greater irrigation flow and a larger field of view. Because semirigid ureteroscopes are fairly inflexible, they are used to evaluate and to treat conditions below the level of iliac vessels and mid and distal ureter. Flexible ureteroscopes are 5.3 to 8.5 Fr at the tip and gradually enlarge to 8.4 to 10.1 Fr.[8] The major advantage of flexible ureteroscopes is the deflection of the tip, which ranges from 130 to 250 degrees in one direction and 160 to 275 degrees in the opposite direction, with newer endoscopes approaching 360-degree deflection. In addition, these endoscopes can be advanced through ureteral tortuosity and over external compression, such as the psoas muscle. The working channel on the flexible ureteroscope is typically smaller because of the fiberoptic system, and introduction of instruments, such as baskets or laser fibers, reduces irrigation flow. These flexible endoscopes can be used throughout the upper urinary tract but are particularly useful in the proximal ureter and renal pelvis and calyceal system.

The other method of upper tract endoscopy is through direct percutaneous access by puncture through the renal parenchyma into the renal collecting system. Percutaneous nephroscopy is most commonly used to treat large renal calculi. Management of upper tract urothelial tumors with fulguration and resection may also be performed via percutaneous nephroscopy. Nephroscopy may be performed with both rigid and flexible nephroscopes; however, most intervention is performed with the rigid system. The rigid nephroscope is placed through a percutaneous working access sheath, similar to a laparoscopic trocar, to visualize the stone or tumor. Rigid nephroscopes are usually 25 to 28 Fr, and their appearance is similar to a rigid cystoscope, although they have a fixed lens system rather than an exchangeable lens. There is also growing enthusiasm for "mini-perc" approaches, which involve smaller caliber instrumentation. Newer rigid nephroscopes are built on a digital platform that allows a larger working channel with comparable optics to a standard endoscope. Various intracorporeal lithotripters are placed through the working channel to fragment large stones into manageable pieces. Flexible nephroscopes are essentially flexible cystoscopes that are dual purposed for evaluation of the kidney. Flexible endoscopy of the upper tract is advantageous because all areas of the upper collecting system (upper, mid, and lower pole calyces) can be inspected regardless of angle or direction of the internal infundibula. At times, combined use of retrograde flexible ureteroscopy and percutaneous nephroscopy, in the prone patient under anesthesia, may be necessary to address complex renal anatomy for stone-related and other indications.

Numerous working elements are used in both upper and lower tract endoscopy. Guidewires are commonly used to access the upper urinary tract collecting system or the bladder and serve as guides to pass catheters, stents, and sheaths. Most guidewires have a flexible tip and a more rigid shaft and are constructed of an inner core and an outer covering, which may be hydrophilic or neutral (polytetrafluoroethylene). Guidewires range in size from 0.018 to 0.038 inch and have various lengths. Urethral catheters and ureteral catheters may be placed over wires to assist with direct placement into the lower or upper urinary system, respectively. Ureteral stents are hollow catheters with flexible ends that form a coil on the proximal and distal ends to maintain position within the collecting systems. Stents are placed to ensure drainage of the kidney and to bypass blockages of the ureter from inflammation, stones, or tumors. Many stents are composed of thermodynamic material, which becomes softer at higher body temperatures. Stents range in size from 4.8 to 10 Fr and have various lengths to accommodate variable ureteral lengths.

Ureteroscopic baskets are used to remove ureteral and renal calculi and to perform extraction and biopsy of tumors. These range in size from 1.3 to 3.2 Fr and are constructed of flexible material to allow placement into various calyceal locations within the kidney.

MINIMALLY INVASIVE ABDOMINAL AND PELVIC SURGERY

As opposed to traditional surgery with open incisions and self-retaining abdominal and pelvic retractors, urology has been a field of early adapters of minimally invasive approaches. The two large categories of minimally invasive approaches include laparoscopic and robotic-assisted laparoscopic procedures. Both of these can be performed for maladies of the GU tract in the retroperitoneum and pelvis. In the following sections we will review in general terms the surgical principles of both laparoscopic and robotic-assisted genital urinary surgery.

Laparoscopic

Laparoscopic surgery consists of insufflating the abdominal and pelvic cavity with carbon dioxide to create working space and then deploying straight instruments through 5- to 15-mm trocars to perform the intended procedure. Historically in urology laparoscopic surgery was used for numerous applications such as nephrectomy, partial nephrectomy, ureteral reconstructive procedures, prostatectomy (simple and radical), and even more complex oncologic resections of the bladder and retroperitoneal lymph nodes for testis cancer. However, modern-day urologic laparoscopic surgery is often more frequently used for nephrectomies, whereas the robotic-assisted laparoscopic surgery has supplanted pure laparoscopic techniques for most other procedures in the majority of centers in the United States.

Laparoscopic access can either be obtained through Verres needle or Hassan cutdown techniques, and each have their own pros and cons. The Verres needle is often faster but does have a slightly higher risk of small bowel injury. The Hassan cutdown technique is thus used in patients with previous abdominal surgeries or those at risk of adhesions, such as with previous radiation or altered anatomy. In addition, a laparoscopic Visiport can be used to obtain abdominal access. Once access is obtained, laparoscopic working ports are arrayed in a conformation to triangulate the organ of question, keeping a minimum of one hand width between ports to avoid clashing. Pneumoperitoneum pressures can range anywhere from 5 to 20 mm Hg to ensure insufflation. The assistant is used to orient the laparoscopic camera, which can be either a 0-degree lens or a 30-degree lens and angled around barriers. Common instruments that are advanced into these trocars consist of graspers, scissors (which often have cautery attachments for the tip of the instrument), suction irrigators, and bipolar energy devices. Using this combination of instruments, the exposure to the desired organ can be gained and the anatomy can be manipulated. Laparoscopic needle drivers and staplers are also available when suturing and or stapling is needed.

Robotic Surgery

Robotic assistance is an advancement in laparoscopy whereby the end of the laparoscopic instrument has an articulating wrist that is under the control of the surgeon. This adds significantly more degrees of freedom for the surgeon and thus enables more precise control of suture placement, knot tying, and fine dissection. The robotic procedures in general have a shorter learning curve than pure laparoscopic procedures due to these advantages, but they still share the same principles of pneumoperitoneum, gaining access safely and appropriate trocar placement. In addition, there is frequently an assistant at the bedside required for suctioning, irrigating, and instrument exchange as well as suture passage. Although there are many robotic systems in use around the world, Intuitive Surgical (Sunnyvale, California) has near complete market share within the United States, so we will focus on their system in this discussion.

Da Vinci Systems

Robotic surgery requires a console that is operated by a surgeon, which is a robotic tower consisting of four arms connected to a boom that is used to position the robot tower over the patient. The console consists of an enclosed system within which the surgeon operates using multiple pedals to control instruments, camera motion, and to toggle between arms. The console itself contains a viewing system that allows surgeons to have depth perception due to slightly offset camera lenses. The systems come in multiple formats, more commonly multiport, in which up to four robotic ports are able to be hooked up to the robotic console. In recent developments, a single-port robot is also being used, and in this configuration, there is a large trocar through which four instruments are advanced into the body cavity. Once inside the cavity, the instruments can spread out and be used to complete the procedure. There are pros and cons to the multiport and single-port robotic systems that are beyond the scope of this chapter.

Robotic Retroperitoneal Surgery

The most common indications are renal neoplasm, urothelial neoplasm, or upper urinary tract reconstruction. There are unique aspects of each of these indications, but in general, the principles of renal exposure are the same. Access to the kidney can be gained through transperitoneal ports or retroperitoneal ports. The transperitoneal approach is by far the most common and often consists of ports in a straight line at the level of the ipsilateral midclavicular line, which allows ports to be triangulated to reflect the colon and expose the kidney, the ureter, and the great vessels. The retroperitoneal approach relies on establishing a working space behind the colon when the patient is in flank position. There are numerous possible port configurations, but commonly, there will be ports placed below the eleventh rib and above the iliac crest. A balloon trocar is often used in this setting to establish working space behind the colon and around the kidney.

Robotic Pelvic Surgery

Robotic pelvic surgery is often performed for prostate cancer (radical prostatectomy), bladder cancer, benign prostatic hyperplasia (BPH), ureteral reconstruction, and gynecologic procedures. Exposure into the pelvis can be gained transperitoneally with horizontal ports above or below the level of the umbilicus, or extraperitoneally with a balloon port used to create working space. For these procedures, the patient is often in a Trendelenburg position, allowing the bowel to fall cephalad away from the operative field. The assistant port is often placed on the right side of the body to allow entry alongside the robotic ports.

UROLOGIC INFECTIOUS DISEASE

Urinary tract infections (UTIs) are a common medical problem, although patients with UTI referred to urologists for evaluation and treatment often have a complicated or unusual element to their diagnosis or management. Other infections treated by urologists include infections of the genital skin (a spectrum of disease from skin neoplasms, to cellulitis, to necrotizing fasciitis) and reproduction organs in males (i.e., orchitis, epididymitis, or prostatitis). Furthermore, these infections may require simple antibiotic therapy, multimodal treatment with surgical drainage, or debridement and management in an intensive care setting. Urinary tract obstruction with proximal infection may result in sepsis, challenging the skills of the urologist and surgical critical care specialist.

Uncomplicated Urinary Tract Infection

Recent literature indicates that UTIs in adult females and males accounted for 39 million office visits and 6 million emergency department visits.[9] In adult patients, more than 50% of females and 12% of males will develop a UTI during their lifetime.[9] Urinary infection is considered "uncomplicated" when it occurs in the immunocompetent host, without underlying anatomic or physiologic abnormalities of the urinary tract in females. UTI diagnosed in males is generally considered "complicated." For diagnosis of a UTI, a clean catch, midstream urine specimen is preferred, and on culture, 105 colony-forming units must be demonstrated. In catheterized specimens, UTI can be diagnosed with as little as 103 colony-forming units. The typical symptoms associated with UTI are dysuria, frequency, urgency to void, and malodorous urine. Because of the inherent differences in etiology, evaluation, and treatment, uncomplicated UTIs are divided into those occurring in premenopausal and postmenopausal females. A third category of uncomplicated UTI, that occurring in pregnant patients, is beyond the scope of this overview. In general, risk factors include genetic, biologic, and behavioral; specific aspects are discussed with each group.

Premenopausal Patients

History and physical examination of patients in this age group presenting with symptoms of UTI are particularly important because of overlapping disease processes. In patients without vaginal discharge, the majority can be expected to have a UTI as the diagnosis. However, in sexually active females, sexually transmitted infections (STIs) must be considered, especially in the setting of a negative urine culture. Furthermore, in patients with vaginal discharge, vaginitis caused by yeast, trichomoniasis, and bacterial vaginosis are possible causes. Risk factors for UTI in this population of patients include frequent sexual intercourse, initial UTI at a young age, maternal history of UTI, and number of pregnancies and deliveries.[10] Important aspects of the physical examination in these patients include palpation of costovertebral tenderness (assessing for ascending infection) and pelvic examination to evaluate for STI. The most common cause of infection in these patients is *Escherichia coli* (80%–85%), followed by *Staphylococcus saprophyticus* (10%–15%) and *Klebsiella pneumoniae* and *Proteus mirabilis* (4% each).[10] Empirical therapy is acceptable, although confirmatory urine cultures are useful as the incidence of antibiotic resistance continues to rise. Prevention includes increased hydration and evaluation of hygiene practices.

Postmenopausal Patients

As in younger patients, history and physical examination are important aspects of UTI evaluation in this group of patients. Presenting symptoms are similar in this group, although some elderly patients may simply present with altered mental status. Furthermore, an important component in diagnosis and treatment of postmenopausal females is the change in the vaginal pH

levels and change or reduction in lactobacillus in the vaginal flora. The physical examination findings may differ in these patients as STIs are less likely but physical changes, such as pelvic organ prolapse and incomplete bladder emptying, become causative factors. In addition, the pathologic bacterial species are different. *E. coli* continues to be the predominant organism, but in this age group *P. mirabilis, K. pneumoniae,* and *Enterobacter* species become more prevalent pathogens.[10] Again, empirical therapy is acceptable, but urine cultures are important because of increasing antibiotic resistance patterns and differing organisms. Prevention includes increased hydration and evaluation of hygiene practices.

Complicated Urinary Tract Infection

Complicated UTIs require more vigilance on the part of the treating physician because of patient factors that may lead to a more rapid progression or worsening of the infection. By definition complicated UTIs occur in males and in patients with diabetes, immunosuppression, upper tract infection, resistant organisms, urinary tract anatomic abnormalities, prior surgery, calculous disease, spinal cord injury, or recent or current indwelling Foley catheter. Essentially, any abnormality of physiology or anatomy that is etiologic in a UTI or a UTI that occurs in such a setting or in the immunocompromised patient is considered complicated. In these patients, similar evaluation is warranted, but the evaluation should not be limited to simply history and physical examination. Empirical treatment of complicated UTI alone is not optimal, and urine cultures should be performed on all patients with suspected complicated UTI before initiation of antibiotic therapy, whenever possible. In addition, imaging is indicated in these patients because of concern for calculous disease and urinary stasis, so at a minimum, simple radiography of the kidneys, ureters, and bladder (KUB study) and renal ultrasound, and potentially further assessment with cross-sectional radiographic imaging, should be performed in patients with equivocal or concerning findings. Finally, antibiotic therapy alone may not be adequate, and these patients may require surgical drainage of obstructed urinary systems or later surgical correction of anatomic abnormalities or removal of urinary stones (once infections are treated) to prevent recurrent UTIs. Consultation with infectious disease specialists may also be indicated in patients with urologic anatomic abnormalities and recurrent UTIs with resistant organisms.

Urinary Tract Infection in Males

Because of the lower incidence of UTI in males, when they present with symptoms of infection, it is always considered complicated, regardless of other patient factors. As in females, younger males (younger than 50 years) and older males (older than 50 years) have different causes of their UTI and symptoms. Common presenting symptoms are urethritis, dysuria, hesitancy, frequency, and urgency of urination. A history and physical examination in these patients are important to delineate different sources of symptoms or UTI. Males can present with these symptoms and have different diagnoses, including UTI, STI, urethritis, and chronic pelvic pain. Furthermore, bacterial infections can extend to other proximal areas of the GU system, such as the prostate and testicle. Males younger than 50 years are more likely to have STI as the cause rather than UTI. These males should have a thorough sexual history, genital examination, and microscopic urinalysis performed. Urethral swab or urine tests for STI should be performed as well. Males older than 50 years often have underlying lower urinary tract symptoms (LUTS), and this can be a contributing factor. Males in this age group more frequently will have UTI as a source of their symptoms, and common urinary pathogens, as in females, should be considered. Furthermore, older males should be questioned about recent surgical procedures, catheterization, or hospitalization. Elderly patients can also present with mental status or behavioral changes as their only symptom of UTI, and this diagnosis must be considered in these patients. A lower threshold for imaging and hospital admission is necessary in males with UTI as they may present with more systemic symptoms. Patients who cannot tolerate oral intake, are immunocompromised, or have medical comorbidities should be admitted with cross-sectional imaging performed. Broad-spectrum intravenous antibiotics, based on local resistance patterns, and fluid resuscitation should be initiated in these patients while the initial workup and evaluation are completed. Urinary obstruction or stone disease in these patients constitutes a urologic emergency and must be addressed rapidly.

Specific Complicated Genitourinary Infectious States
Pyelonephritis

Pyelonephritis is a spectrum of infectious or inflammatory processes that involve the kidney collecting system or parenchyma. Pyelonephritis results from a UTI moving proximally upward from the lower urinary tract. In the simple form, pyelonephritis may be treated on an outpatient basis with oral antibiotics for 1 to 2 weeks. In this group of patients, urine culture is necessary to identify the causative organism. If the patient appears more acutely infected, hospitalization may be warranted for broad-spectrum

intravenous antibiotic therapy, fluid resuscitation, and cross-sectional imaging. Emphysematous pyelonephritis represents an advanced form of pyelonephritis and is considered a urologic emergency. Often occurring in the diabetic patient, these uncommon infections demonstrate a significant necrotizing infection of the kidney with gas-forming organisms (typically *E. coli* in a facultative anaerobic metabolic state) with pockets of gas within the parenchyma apparent on imaging (Fig. 121.1). The common bacterial pathogens include *E. coli*, *P. mirabilis*, and *K. pneumoniae*.[11] These patients require either prompt percutaneous drainage of the infection or rapid nephrectomy. Most patients who present with this condition are diabetic or have significant medical comorbidities, and control of the metabolic abnormalities, aggressive broad-spectrum antibiotic therapy, and supportive critical care are essential. Xanthogranulomatous pyelonephritis is a chronic infectious process resulting from renal obstruction, recurrent infection, and renal calculous disease. The disease presents in three forms (focal, segmental, or diffuse), and each is treated in a different manner. The underlying histologic process involves a foamy, lipid-laden, macrophage infiltrate in the renal parenchyma with extensive inflammation, fibrosis, and loss of renal function. On imaging, there may be indications of collecting system dilation; however, drainage attempts often are unproductive because the material is often solid or too viscous to drain. Patients with focal or segmental disease may be treated with antibiotics, but those with diffuse disease frequently require nephrectomy. The risk of iatrogenic adjacent organ injury is high in these nephrectomies, and the renal hilum may be so inflamed and fibrotic that the renal

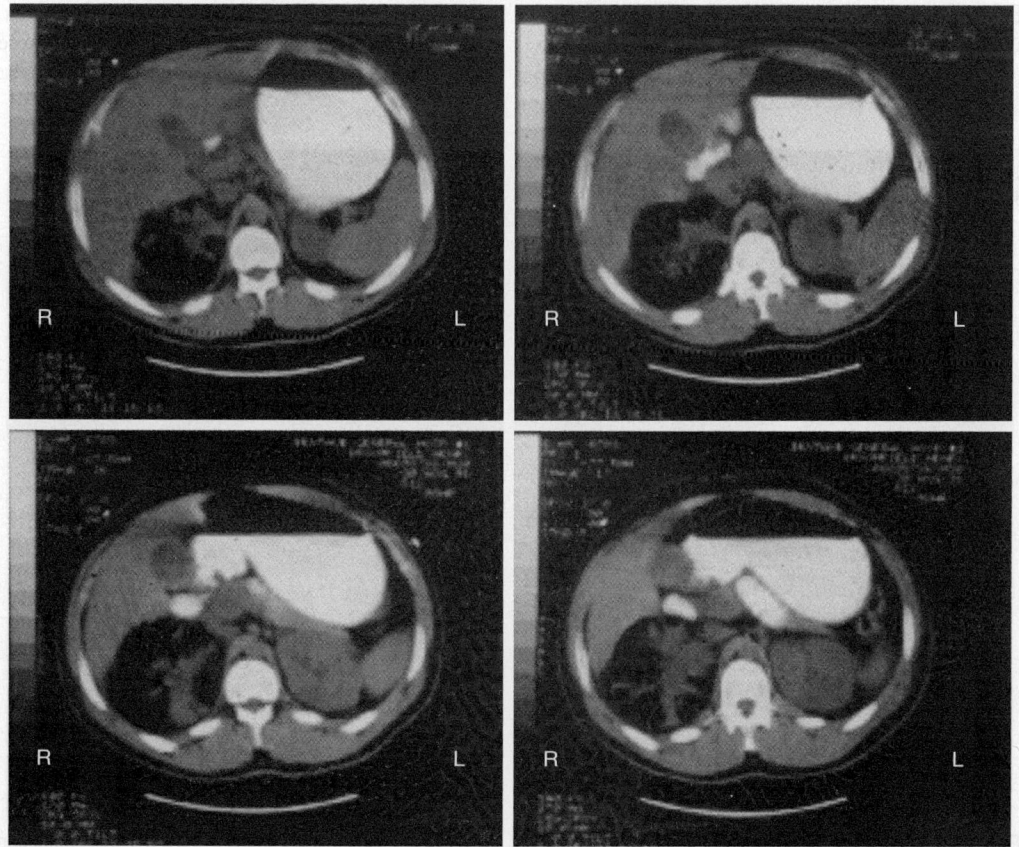

FIGURE 121.1 Emphysematous pyelonephritis. This CT scan demonstrates extensive destruction of the right kidney with intraparenchymal gas on the right, obliterating the renal architecture. The left kidney is normal.

vessels cannot be individually dissected. These cases may require placement of a vascular pedicle clamp with renal excision and oversewing of the pedicle.

Male Genital Organ Infection

UTIs may ascend into the genital ducts, resulting in infection of the prostate, epididymis, or testicle. Beginning in the urethra, the verumontanum is the exit point of the seminal vesicles and vas deferens into the urinary tract. Prostatitis refers to any inflammatory process affecting the prostate, but the general surgeon more commonly may encounter acute bacterial prostatitis, which results from bacterial infiltration into the prostatic parenchyma. Most infections of the prostate are secondary to gram-negative bacterial infection and typically are associated with UTI. Two important considerations in these patients are physical examination and disease extent. Although a full history and physical examination are warranted, elimination of digital rectal examination (DRE) should be considered as pressure exerted on an infected prostate may lead to hematogenous spread of the bacteria. In addition, patients who do not have reasonably rapid resolution of their symptoms should be evaluated for prostatic abscess. Prostatic abscesses typically do not respond to antibiotic therapy and require transurethral unroofing or percutaneous drain to allow adequate drainage.

Epididymitis-orchitis results when the UTI ascends through the vas deferens into the epididymis or testicle. Again, the cause is different according to the patient's age; males younger than 35 years typically have an STI as a source, commonly *Chlamydia trachomatis,* whereas males older than 35 years will often have infections related to *E. coli.* Examination of these patients is often difficult because of significant swelling of the affected epididymis or testicle; scrotal ultrasound is useful diagnostically, especially to rule out associated abscess. When infection is advanced, the entire ipsilateral scrotal contents become involved, with overlying skin fixation and edema. It may be difficult to distinguish this entity from late torsion, incarcerated inguinal hernia, or testicular tumor with necrosis and inflammation. Patients without abscess may be managed with antibiotic therapy, rest, and scrotal elevation; however, recovery is slow, with eventual resolution of edema and discomfort. If abscess is present, surgical drainage and often orchiectomy are indicated. A subset of patients may have persistent pain or mass, and on repeated Doppler imaging, signs of testicular ischemia or persistent inflammation may be noted. These patients require exploration and possible orchiectomy to resolve the process.

Fournier Gangrene

Fournier gangrene is a necrotizing infection of the male genital and perineal skin and subcutaneous tissues, similar to other progressive fasciitis and necrotizing soft tissue infections (Fig. 121.2). When the genitalia are involved, patients typically present with significant pain and tenderness, scrotal and genital swelling, discoloration or frank necrosis, crepitus, and, at times, foul-smelling discharge. Fournier gangrene is usually a polymicrobial infection with microaerobes, anaerobes, and gram-positive and gram-negative organisms.[12] Risk factors for development include peripheral vascular disease, diabetes mellitus, malnutrition, alcoholism, and other immunocompromised states. This disease represents a urologic emergency. Treatment requires urgent surgical drainage with aggressive debridement of the necrotic tissue, broad-spectrum intravenous antibiotics, and intensive monitoring with supportive care. The magnitude of the debridement depends entirely on the degree of progression of the process. It is rare for the process to involve the testicles or deep tissues of the penis deep to the tunica vaginalis and Buck fascia, respectively, so these structures should be preserved. It is uncommon for the urethra to be involved,

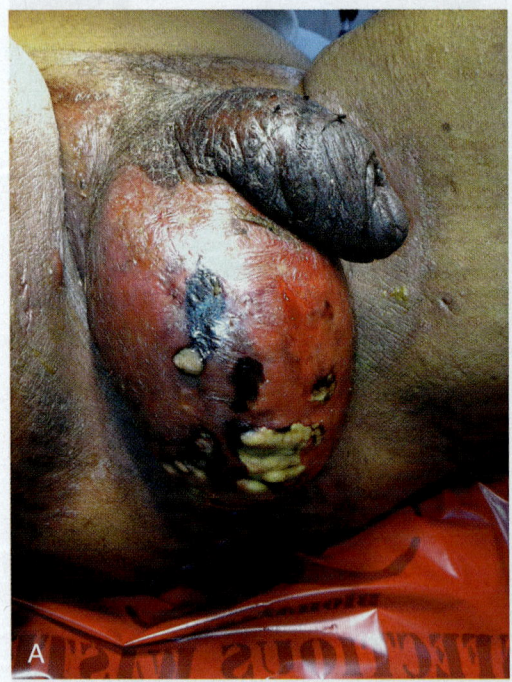
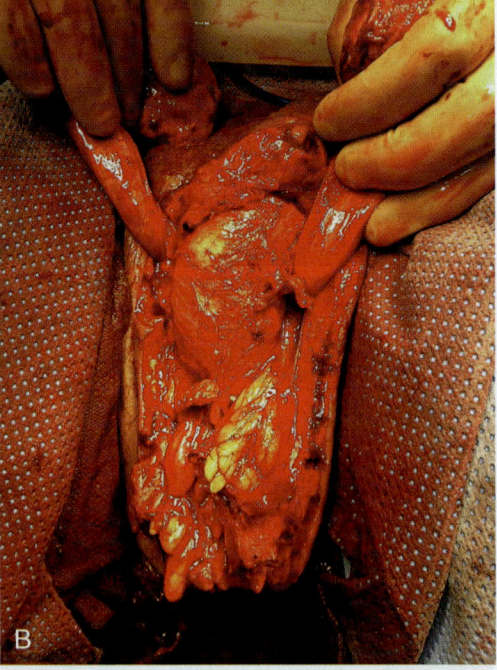

FIGURE 121.2 Fournier gangrene. (A) Skin necrosis, purulence, and edema of the scrotum. The skin can also appear normal, with much more subtle physical findings in some cases. (B) Appearance after extensive debridement of scrotal skin and underlying tissues. The base of the penis is visible centrally; the testes are elevated out of the field, and the spermatic cords are visible anteriorly.

although a defined urinary tract source may be evident, such as a urethral stricture, with perforation and local infection. Suprapubic tube diversion is generally not necessary initially; urethral catheter drainage is generally sufficient. Once the active infection is controlled, the predominant management issues become wound care and reconstruction, which may require delayed skin grafting for tissue coverage.

Atypical Urinary Tract Infections

Fungal Infection

Fungal infections in the urinary system are most common in specific populations of patients: diabetics, immunocompromised patients, and the elderly. Fungal infections may not be symptomatic and, in an outpatient setting, may not require therapy. Most fungal infections are related to the *Candida* species, and it is incumbent on the treating physician to determine which infections require treatment and which represent contamination. Patients who require careful evaluation and treatment include neutropenic patients and intensive care patients, who may need evaluation for an internal source such as a fungus deposit (ball) in the bladder or kidney. Infectious disease consultation is valuable in these cases because the organisms are atypical and selection of treatment agents may not be straightforward. Renal and bladder imaging with ultrasound may demonstrate a treatable source. These patients may need antifungal bladder or kidney irrigation or occasionally endoscopic removal.

Tuberculosis

The GU tract is the third most common extrapulmonary site for tuberculosis infection. This disease is spread hematogenously from the lungs and into the affected organ system. Most patients with GU tuberculosis are immunocompromised, so assessment of HIV infection status is important. Patients present with various symptoms that include voiding symptoms, sterile pyuria or hematuria, and chronic kidney disease. Not all patients will have a positive purified protein derivative (PPD) test result, and diagnosis is confirmed with acid-fast bacilli smears of urine and mycobacterial culture with sterile pyuria, chest radiograph, and imaging of the GU system to look for anatomic abnormalities. Tuberculosis affecting the kidney may result in segmental or global glomerular dysfunction, and progression antegrade down the urinary system may result in ureteral strictures. Tuberculosis of the epididymis may result in chronic epididymitis or mass. Antibiotic therapy consists of 2 months of a four-drug regimen with a subsequent 7-month treatment with isoniazid and rifampin. Infectious disease consultation is mandatory in treating these patients because of public health concerns. Significant anatomic infection or functional change or loss may ultimately require surgical excision.

Parasitic Infection

With the ease of global transportation and a mobile global population, parasitic infections are considerations in patients with recent travel histories. The main parasitic infections of the GU system are schistosomiasis, echinococcal infection, and filariasis. Each parasite has a different point of entry, systemic spread, and organ infestation. Typically, in schistosomiasis, the parasite enters the body percutaneously and spreads through the venous and lymphatic system. Most infestations affect the bladder, resulting in chronic inflammation and granulomas. These patients present with LUTS or hematuria. Medical therapy (praziquantel) can be used to treat granulomatous disease; however, untreated infections can result in squamous cell carcinoma of the bladder. Echinococcal infections are spread through ingestion of contaminated food, and the parasite penetrates the intestinal walls and infests the liver. On occasion, renal infestation can occur, with the parasite becoming encysted in the parenchyma. Medical therapy can shrink the cysts, but surgical removal by partial or total nephrectomy is required for cure. These cysts must be removed intact as rupture or spillage of internal contents can result in severe anaphylaxis. Filariasis results from direct infection of the lymphatic system through percutaneous entry. The parasite creates noticeable symptoms when it dies, resulting in obstruction of the lymphatics. Only mild infestation can be treated with oral therapy (albendazole); advanced disease requires excision and reconstruction.

VOIDING DYSFUNCTION, NEUROGENIC BLADDER, INCONTINENCE, AND BENIGN PROSTATIC HYPERPLASIA

A central aspect of urology is management of bladder function and evaluation and treatment of bladder dysfunction. The bladder is a large muscular sac responsible for storing and eliminating urine. Common dysfunctions of the bladder include neurogenic problems with bladder function, storage problems, incontinence, and outflow issues related to BPH or enlargement. Changes in these functional areas are one of the most common reasons for urologic consultation. Although this is a broad area of urology, concentrating on these core divisions will give the general surgeon an understanding of the complex dynamics of bladder function and dysfunction.

Neurogenic Bladder

Patients with neurogenic bladder dysfunction present with a wide spectrum of neurologic diseases or injuries that affect bladder function on the basis of the location of the injury or disease process. There is a complex interaction between the bladder and brain that primarily regulates bladder storage and bladder emptying. Bladder storage is driven by the sympathetic nervous system, specifically at the level of the adrenergic receptor. α-Adrenergic receptors are the most common adrenergic receptors in the bladder, prostate, and urethra; most are α_1 and α_2, with three subtypes of α_1 identified: α_{1a}, α_{1b}, and α_{1d}.[13] The α_1 receptor is the most common subtype in the lower urinary system. Bladder emptying is driven by the parasympathetic stimulation of cholinergic receptors, specifically the muscarinic receptors. The predominant muscarinic receptors in the bladder are M2 and M3.[13] Sensory information is carried away from the bladder by myelinated and unmyelinated afferent nerve fibers traveling through the pelvic and pudendal nerves. Any interruption in the sympathetic or parasympathetic nervous system and its communication with the bladder can result in neurogenic dysfunction. In addition, several centers within the pons, midbrain, and cerebral cortex have direct effect on the storage and emptying of the bladder.[13] Voiding is initiated at the level of the pontine micturition center, which sends out a parasympathetic signal to the bladder to initiate voiding. The pontine micturition center is inhibited by the periaqueductal gray located in the midbrain, and this is connected to the afferent signaling pathways from the bladder. Based on this standard sensory function, specific voiding symptoms or LUTS can be predicted by the location of neurologic disease or injury.

Basic evaluation of these patients includes a through history with neurologic and urologic historical focus, physical examination (focusing on the abdomen, pelvis, and peripheral and central nervous system), and urinalysis. Additional evaluation is tailored to location of injury. Cortical brain disease and injury, such as cerebrovascular accident, are evaluated by history, physical examination, and urinalysis. These disease processes do not directly affect the bladder function, and patients are treated on the basis of symptoms alone. Spinal cord lesions are divided into suprasacral spinal lesions (spinal cord injury, infarcts) and sacral or peripheral spinal cord lesions (pelvic plexus damage from surgery, diabetic neuropathy). Patients with lesions of the suprasacral spinal cord tend to have increased bladder muscle tension, which results in abnormal elasticity of the bladder (poor bladder compliance).[14] In addition, these patients have incoordination of the bladder and urinary sphincter, resulting in detrusor-sphincter dyssynergia. Patients with sacral or peripheral nerve lesions tend to have variable LUTS but typically do not have changes in bladder elasticity.[14] The detrusor muscle is often partially or completely nonfunctional, and the urinary sphincter remains closed. Specialized evaluation of the patients with spinal cord lesions includes upper tract ultrasonography to monitor for evidence of hydronephrosis and urodynamic evaluation. Urodynamic evaluation involves measuring the elasticity of the bladder on filling (compliance), the pressure generated on emptying (detrusor function) by recording the abdominal pressure, and the intraluminal bladder pressure with specialized catheters. Surveillance cystoscopy is indicated in chronic patients to rule out the development of intravesical disease. Treatment for neurogenic bladder has recently been revolutionized by the introduction of onabotulinum toxin. In the past, these patients required complex regimens of antimuscarinic agents and reconstructive surgery. Now, with the use of onabotulinum toxin, most patients are treated with periodic cystoscopic injections and intermittent catheterization.

Problems With Bladder Storage Symptoms and Abnormalities

Overactive bladder (OAB) is the most common storage-related problem of the bladder. It is defined as urinary urgency with or without urgency urinary incontinence in the absence of UTI or other obvious disease.[15] Typical symptoms of this problem include urgency, urinary frequency, nocturia, and urgency urinary incontinence. Urgency refers to the sudden, compelling desire to pass urine that is difficult to defer and replaces the normal urge.[15] Urinary frequency is the complaint of micturition occurring more frequently than previously deemed normal and characterized by daytime and nocturnal voids.[15] Nocturia is the complaint of interruption of sleep one or more times because of the need to urinate.[15] Finally, urgency urinary incontinence is the involuntary loss of urine associated with urgency.[15] A difficult aspect of this disease process is that it occurs in the spectrum of other LUTS and may be the result of long-term bladder outflow obstruction. Other conditions to consider in patients who present with OAB and LUTS are UTI, urinary calculi, diabetes, polydipsia, neurogenic bladder, and malignant disease. OAB has a worldwide prevalence of 11%, and with the aging population, this is presumed to increase over time.[16]

All patients who present with OAB should undergo a thorough evaluation. At the basic level, this includes a thorough history to fully disclose the symptoms and to rule out other causes. Historical elements that may be contributory include caffeine intake, constipation, recurrent UTI, pelvic organ prolapse in

females and prostatic enlargement in males, and excessive fluid intake. Physical examination should be directed toward evaluation of the abdomen, pelvis, and neurologic systems. Other findings may include decreased mental status or cognitive function and peripheral edema. The last absolute examination element is urinalysis, which can reveal infection, inflammation, or hematuria that may indicate more serious disease. Simple adjunctive tests that can be performed in the office include measurement of postvoid residual urine volume, noninvasive flow test, validated symptom questionnaires, and voiding diaries. Specialized tests and evaluation performed by the urologist may include cystoscopy, ultrasound, and urodynamic testing as appropriate. However, current guidelines do not require any of these specialized tests for initiation of treatment.[17]

Treatment of OAB is directed toward therapy, symptoms, and motivation of the individual patient (Fig. 121.3). As many patients suffering from this problem take multiple medications, pharmacologic therapy is not always offered as an initial treatment. Behavioral therapies are the first-line treatment for all patients. Behavioral therapies may include lifestyle modifications or specific physical therapies. Typically, this includes fluid intake management and modification with particular attention paid to timing of fluid intake and amounts. For example, in patients who complain of nocturia, limiting nighttime fluid intake can be beneficial. Bladder training is a noninvasive method of physical therapy whereby the patient postpones voiding to lengthen the time intervals between voids. This may be coupled with urgency suppression and timed voids to reinforce retraining of the sensory output from the bladder. Finally, voiding diaries are important to help the patient and urologist quantify the number of voids and voided amount to better target improvement goals and to tailor therapy. Pharmacologic management continues to be a mainstay of treatment and is indicated for patients as an adjunct to behavior therapies or for patients unresponsive to first-line therapy. Classic pharmacologic therapy is antimuscarinic agents that target the parasympathetic muscarinic cholinergic receptors, primarily M2 and M3, and block the action of these receptors. Most of the drugs in this category are administered daily and have the common side effects of dry mouth, dry eyes, and constipation. A newer pharmacologic agent, beta agonists (β_3), targets receptors in the detrusor muscle to stimulate bladder relaxation. Treatment options for patients who fail to respond to these therapies fall into the specialized third-line treatments, which include neuromodulation (either peripheral or central), onabotulinum toxin, chronic indwelling catheters, and augmentation cystoplasty.

Urinary Incontinence

Urinary incontinence is the involuntary loss of urine; it can be divided into stress urinary incontinence (SUI), urge urinary incontinence, and mixed urinary incontinence.[15] "Overflow incontinence" is another form of incontinence, which is often considered as an etiologically separate entity. National data indicate that the prevalence of urinary incontinence in America is 49.6% in females older than 20 years.[18] Males are typically affected after the age of 50 years, and incontinence develops as a symptom of LUTS or other problems rather than as a primary complaint as in females. SUI is defined as the involuntary loss of urine with Valsalva maneuver.[15] Urge urinary incontinence is the involuntary loss of urine associated with a strong urge to void.[15] Mixed urinary incontinence is any combination of these two causes.

Evaluation of these patients includes history, physical examination (including pelvic examination), urinalysis, postvoid residual

DIAGNOSIS & TREATMENT ALGORITHM:
AUA/SUFU GUIDELINE ON NON-NEUROGENIC OVERACTIVE BLADDER IN ADULTS

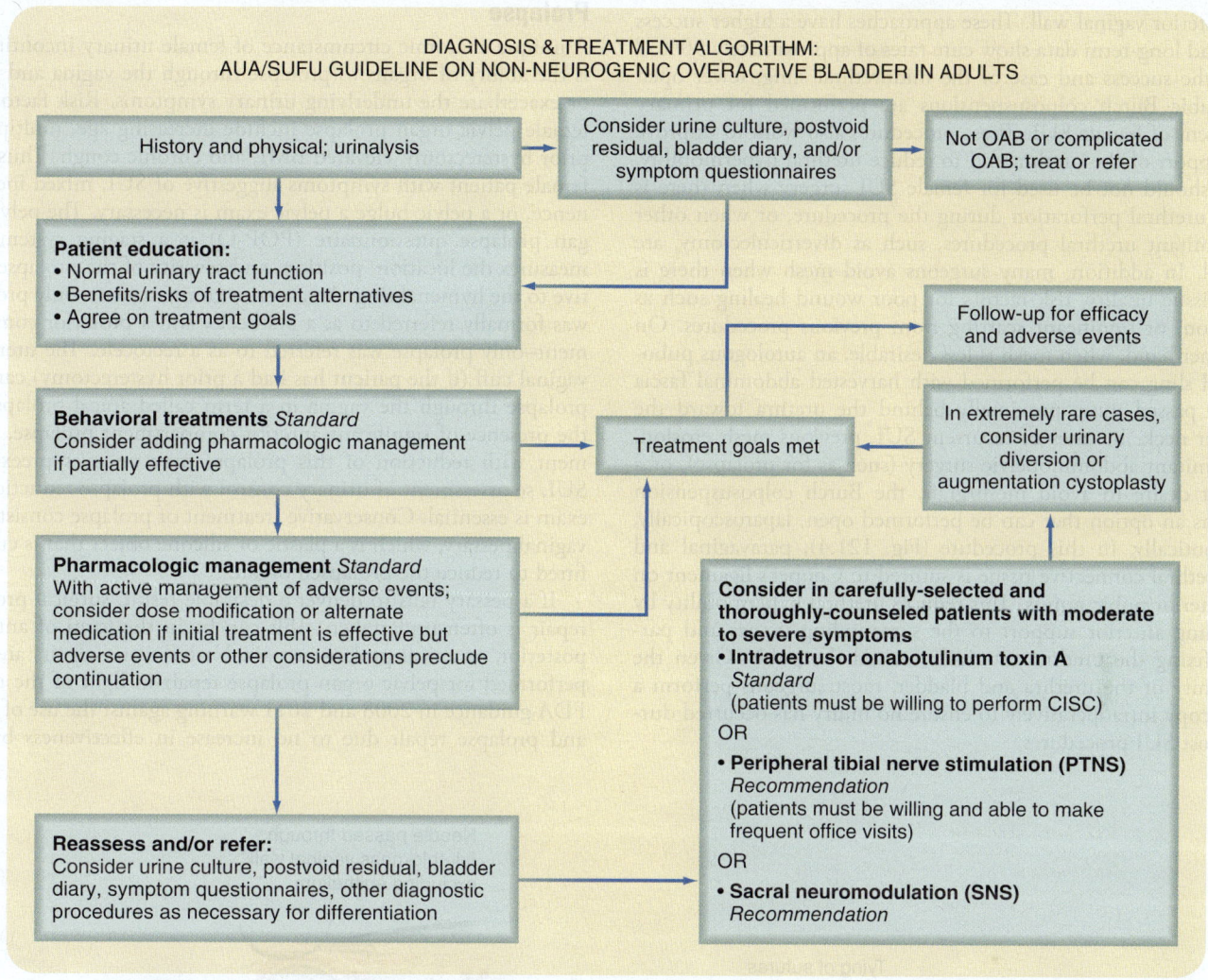

FIGURE 121.3 Algorithm for diagnosis and management of overactive bladder *(OAB). AUA,* American Urological Association; *CISC,* clean intermittent self-catheterization; *SUFU,* Society of Urodynamics, Female Pelvic Medicine & Urogenital Reconstruction. (Adapted from Lightner DJ, Gomelsky A, Souter L, et al: Diagnosis and treatment of overactive bladder [non-neurogenic] in adults: AUA/SUFU Guideline amendment 2019. *J Urol.* 2019;202:558.)

volume measurement, and voiding diaries. The history and physical examination are important to rule out any complicating factors including neurogenic source, anatomic changes (pelvic organ prolapse in the female patient and prostatic enlargement in the male patient), and prior surgical intervention (radical prostatectomy in the male patient or hysterectomy in the female patient) that might affect evaluation and the treatment decision. In the neurologically normal patient with no confounding factors, nonsurgical management is the first step in treatment before any surgical intervention. As with OAB, behavior modification and bladder training are the initial steps. Dietary modification is important for management of urinary incontinence. Patients are counseled to limit fluid intake to around 2 L/day, depending on body size and activity level. In addition, patients should limit caffeine intake and other bladder irritants including alcohol, carbonated beverages, spicy foods, and citrus juices and fruits. Furthermore, bowel programs should be initiated to ensure that the patient has normal bowel function and is not constipated. Other nonsurgical treatment includes weight loss to a normal body mass index (BMI) and exercise, particularly core muscle exercises.

Pelvic floor muscle training and biofeedback have been shown to have acceptable rates in helping patients achieve satisfactory management of their urinary incontinence.

Female

Stress urinary incontinence. Surgical treatment options for females and males differ because of the inherent mechanism causing the incontinence, typically poor pelvic anatomic support in females and sphincteric in males. In females, treatment options progress from less to more invasive. The simplest treatment is injection of a urethral bulking agent through a cystoscopy. The objective of this treatment is to improve coaptation of the urinary sphincter and to increase the urethral wall volume. Unfortunately, this treatment is not likely to produce long-term cure, and retreatment or progression to other options is often necessary. The next option is placement of a midurethral sling to resupport the central hammock of the urethra and to provide backing to the urethra during stress maneuvers. The midurethral sling can be performed using a retropubic, transobturator, or single incision technique, with a passage of a small, thin piece of mesh between the urethra and anterior vaginal wall. These approaches have a higher success rate, and long-term data show cure rates of approximately 90%.[19] With the success and ease of the midurethral sling, fewer open retropubic Burch colposuspensions are performed for primary treatment of female SUI. These procedures also work to improve the support of the urethra and to reduce urethral hypermobility. Mesh should not be used for female SUI surgery when there is noted urethral perforation during the procedure, or when other concomitant urethral procedures, such as diverticulectomy, are needed. In addition, many surgeons avoid mesh when there is poor tissue quality, risk factors for poor wound healing such as radiation, or significant scarring from previous procedures. On the other hand, when mesh is less desirable, an autologous pubovaginal sling can be performed with harvested abdominal fascia and is passed more proximally behind the urethra toward the bladder neck. In cases of recurrent SUI, previous mesh erosion, concomitant abdominopelvic surgery (such as for prolapse), or a patient desire to avoid mesh/graft, the Burch colposuspension remains an option that can be performed open, laparoscopically, or robotically. In this procedure (Fig. 121.4), paravaginal and paraurethral connective tissue is sutured to Cooper's ligament on the anterior pubic ramus. This reduces urethral hypermobility by providing anterior support to the surrounding tissues and partially fixing the urethra anteriorly toward the pubis. Given the proximity of the urethra and bladder, most surgeons perform a cystoscopy intraoperatively to ensure no injury has occurred during most SUI procedures.

Prolapse

A unique anatomic circumstance of female urinary incontinence is the ability of organs to prolapse through the vagina and cause or exacerbate the underlying urinary symptoms. Risk factors for female pelvic organ prolapse include increasing age, multiparity, prior hysterectomy, elevated BMI, and chronic cough. Thus, in a female patient with symptoms suggestive of SUI, mixed incontinence, or a pelvic bulge a pelvic exam is necessary. The pelvic organ prolapse questionnaire (POP-Q) is a staging system that measures the location, position, and severity of the prolapse relative to the hymenal ring. An anterior compartment–only prolapse was formally referred to as a cystocele, and a posterior compartment–only prolapse was referred to as a rectocele. The uterus or vaginal cuff (if the patient has had a prior hysterectomy) can also prolapse through the vagina in a term called apical prolapse. In the presence of significant anterior compartment prolapse, treatment with reduction of this prolapse may uncover preexisting SUI, so assessment of urinary control with prolapse reduction on exam is essential. Conservative treatment of prolapse consists of a vaginal pessary, which is a plastic or silicone object that is custom fitted to reduce the prolapsed organ.

If a pessary fails to deliver a desirable result, surgical prolapse repair is often undertaken. This can be in the form of anterior, posterior, or apical prolapse repair. Native tissue repairs are now performed for pelvic organ prolapse repair in light of the recent FDA guidance in 2008 and 2011 warning against the use of mesh and prolapse repair due to no increase in effectiveness but an

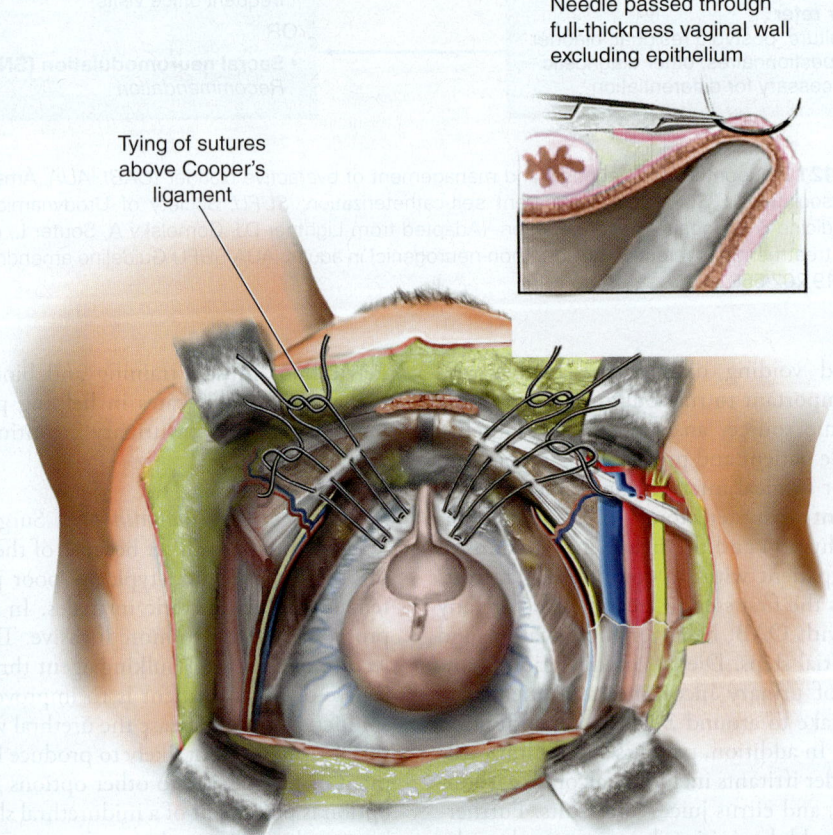

Needle passed through
full-thickness vaginal wall
excluding epithelium

Tying of sutures
above Cooper's
ligament

FIGURE 121.4 Burch colposuspension. (Adapted From Karram MM, Baggish MS. Retropubic urethropexy for stress incontinence. In: Baggish MS, Karram MM, eds. *Atlas of Pelvic Anatomy and Gynecology Surgery*. 4th ed. St Louis: Saunders; 2016. Fig. 71-10.)

increase in risk. Critically, this FDA guidance does not recommend against the use of mesh for SUI procedures, but only for pelvic organ prolapse procedures. For the anterior and posterior repairs, submucosal dissection behind the vaginal mucosa is performed, the prolapsing organ is reduced (bladder for anterior and rectum for posterior), and suture is used to reapproximate the stronger lateral tissues back in the midline. For apical repairs, this can be done transvaginally, in the form of a sacrospinous ligament fixation or uterosacral ligament suspension, or transabdominally, in the form of a sacrocolpopexy. The transabdominal approaches can be open, laparoscopic, or robotic assisted. Conceptually, all apical repairs tether the apex of the vagina/uterus to a more rigid structure, and this can be accomplished via suture or mesh. Alternatively, if the patient is not sexually active, closure of the vaginal vault can be performed in the form of colpocleisis, which actually has high success rates in the well-selected and well-informed patient.

Male

Stress urinary incontinence. Although SUI is less common in males than females, it is a more common situation after surgical procedures on the prostate either for malignancy or BPH. The prostate provides some resistance to urinary flow, and the internal sphincter at the bladder neck is closely aligned with the prostate. In addition, radical prostatectomy can result in harm to the external, striated urethral sphincter as a result of cautery, suture, or overdissection resulting in hypermobility. First-line treatment for SUI after prostate treatment is generally a combination of pelvic floor muscle strengthening (Kegel exercises) and time to allow the muscle to heal. Generally, about 80% to 95% of males with urinary incontinence immediately after surgery will recover to near baseline levels by 1 year after surgery. However, if at 1 year the patient has persistent bothersome and severe incontinence refractory to pelvic floor strengthening, then surgical treatment is warranted. In severe circumstances, some may prefer to even treat at 6 months postoperatively. Cystoscopy before surgical treatment is often recommended to rule out concomitant urethral stricture or vesicle urethral anastomotic stenosis. In males, surgical therapy for SUI is designed to reinforce the urinary sphincter to increase

bladder outlet resistance. Typically, treatments are divided into male urethral slings, which have a larger surface area for the mesh suspension material, and artificial urinary sphincter (AUS) devices. Male urethral slings are traditionally reserved for males with mild to moderate urinary incontinence and have an approximately 60% success rate for getting the patient down to zero to one pad per day. On the other hand, an AUS can be used for mild to severe incontinence and has a higher success rate (80%–90%). However, this is a complex device that is implanted in the patient and opened through a one-way valve contained in the scrotum, and as a result this relies on the patient having adequate hand and cognitive function. An AUS, given its complexity and moving parts, often needs to be replaced with a 50% device survival through 10 years.

Benign Prostatic Hyperplasia

BPH is the development of nodules within the prostate gland as a result of enlargement of the stromal and epithelial components of the gland.[20] As the BPH progresses, the entire prostate enlarges in a process called benign prostatic enlargement, resulting in compression of the prostatic urethra and development of bladder outflow obstruction (Fig. 121.5).[20] As part of the bladder outflow obstruction, patients can develop LUTS requiring evaluation and treatment by a urologist. BPH is prevalent, affecting approximately 70% of males between the ages of 60 and 69 years, making it one of the most common conditions treated by urologists.[20] The LUTS that result from BPH can be divided into storage, voiding, and postvoid symptoms. Interestingly, there is little correlation between the measured volume of the prostate and the symptoms that result. In addition, the degree of bladder outflow obstruction does not necessarily correlate with the severity of LUTS.

As with all conditions, evaluation of the patients is centered on the history and physical examination. Key elements of the physical examination include DRE and a focused neurologic examination. Laboratory evaluation includes urinalysis and prostate-specific antigen (PSA) testing in appropriate patients with a life expectancy of more than 10 years (although the use of PSA testing remains controversial). Further evaluation of these patients includes the use of disease-specific validated questionnaires

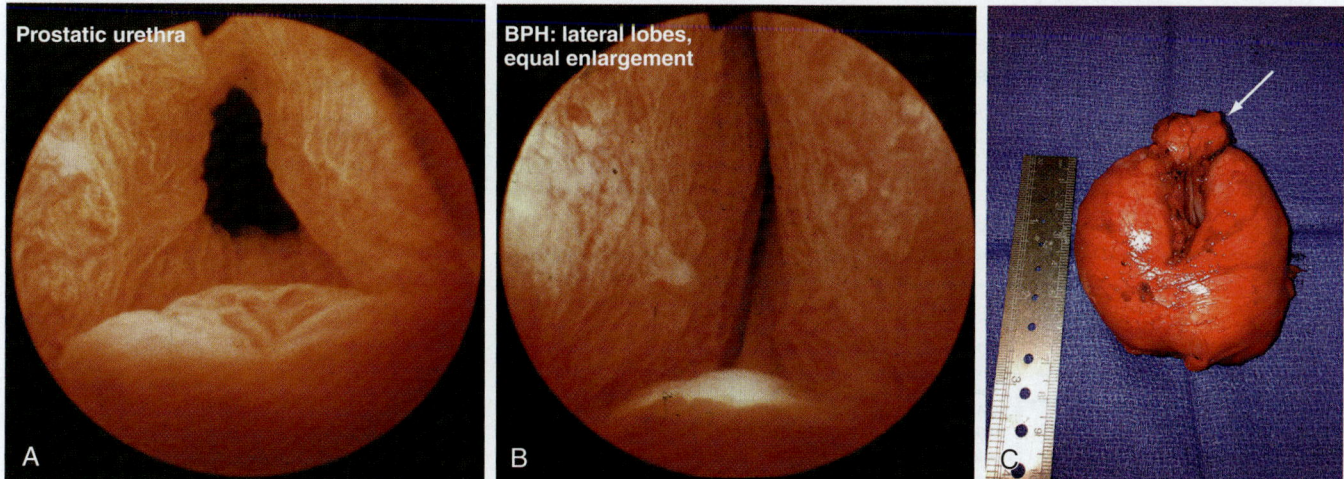

FIGURE 121.5 Benign prostatic hyperplasia *(BPH)*. (A) Normal cystoscopic appearance of the prostate in a young male. (B) Moderate BPH, viewed cystoscopically. The size of the prostate correlates poorly with the magnitude of voiding symptoms. (C) Prostatic adenoma after simple open prostatectomy. Note the small medial lobe *(arrow, top center)*, with large lateral lobes (130-g specimen).

(International Prostate Symptom Score), measurement of postvoid residual urine volumes, and noninvasive urinary flow testing.[20] Depending on initial evaluation findings, cystoscopy and urodynamic studies may be appropriate adjunct tests. Practice guidelines for BPH have been produced by the American Urological Association (AUA) to guide providers in the diagnosis and management of BPH (Figs. 121.6 and 121.7).[20] Similar to all voiding-related conditions, behavior and dietary modifications are appropriate first-step treatment measures in all patients. Medical therapy can be used in conjunction with the initial behavior modifications or added subsequently.

The mainstay of treatment for LUTS due to BPH is α_1-adrenergic receptor blockers.[20] As previously discussed, α-adrenergic receptors are the most common adrenergic receptors in the

bladder, and α_1 is the most common subtype in the lower urinary system, prostate, and urethra. The action of α_1-blockers is to relax the smooth muscle in the bladder neck and prostate and to reduce outflow resistance. This class of drugs has become progressively more selective to the α_1 subtypes, and many now target the α_{1a} subtype receptor specifically. The most common side effects of these drugs are dizziness related to orthostasis, retrograde ejaculation, and rhinitis. A second category of pharmacologic therapy is the 5α-reductase inhibitors that target the glandular component of the prostate. These drugs block the conversion of testosterone to dihydrotestosterone in the prostate and subsequently reduce the prostate volume, thereby reducing outflow resistance. This class of drugs also alters the serum PSA level (reduces it about 50%), which must be kept in mind with regard to prostate cancer

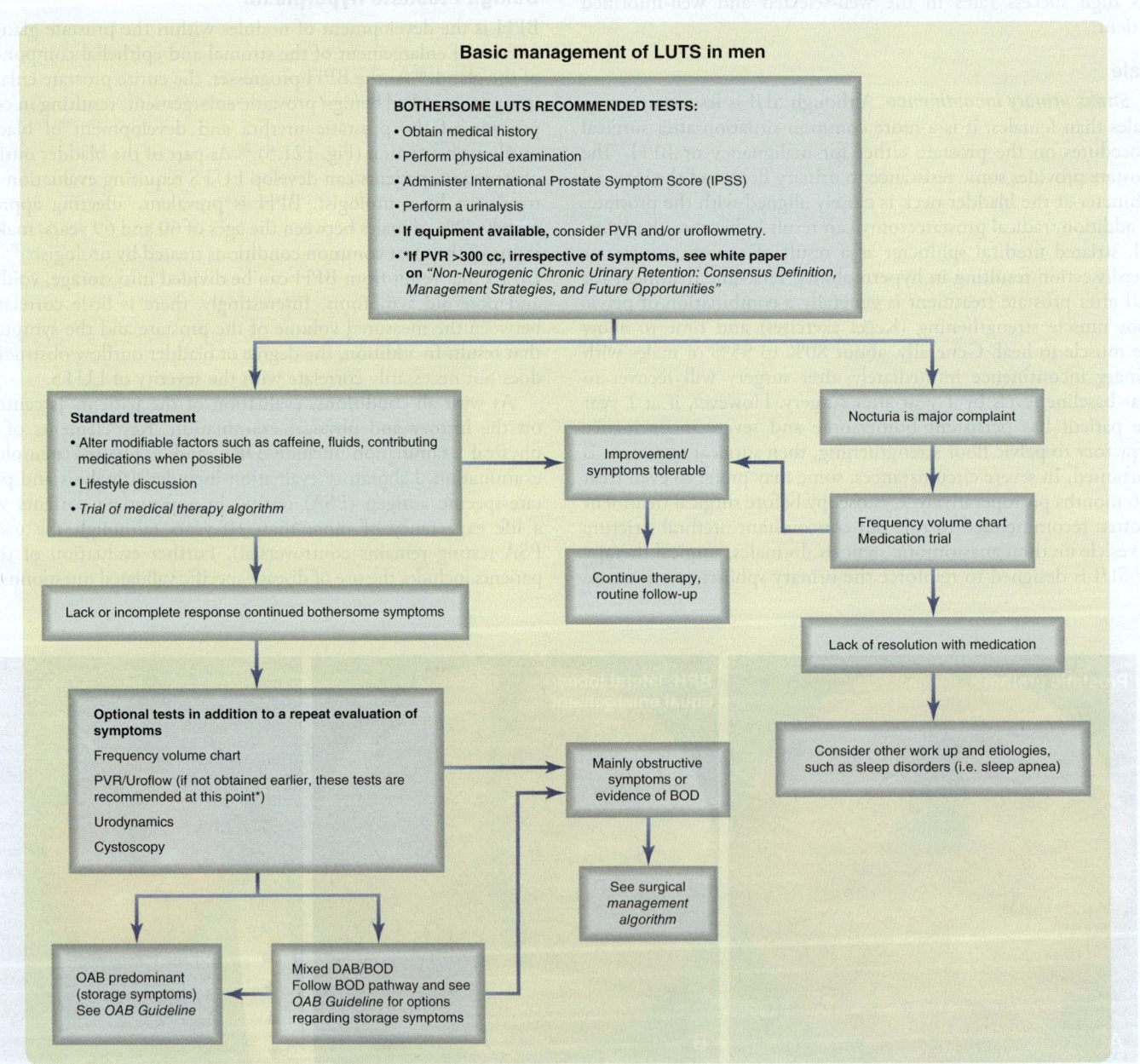

FIGURE 121.6 Algorithm for initial diagnosis and management of benign prostatic hyperplasia. *LUTS,* Lower urinary tract symptoms; *OAB,* overactive bladder; *PVR,* postvoid residual. (Adapted from Sandhu JS, Bixler BR, Dahm P, et al. Management of lower urinary tract symptoms attributed to benign prostatic hyperplasia [BPH]: AUA Guideline amendment 2023. *J Urol.* 2024;211[1]:11–19.)

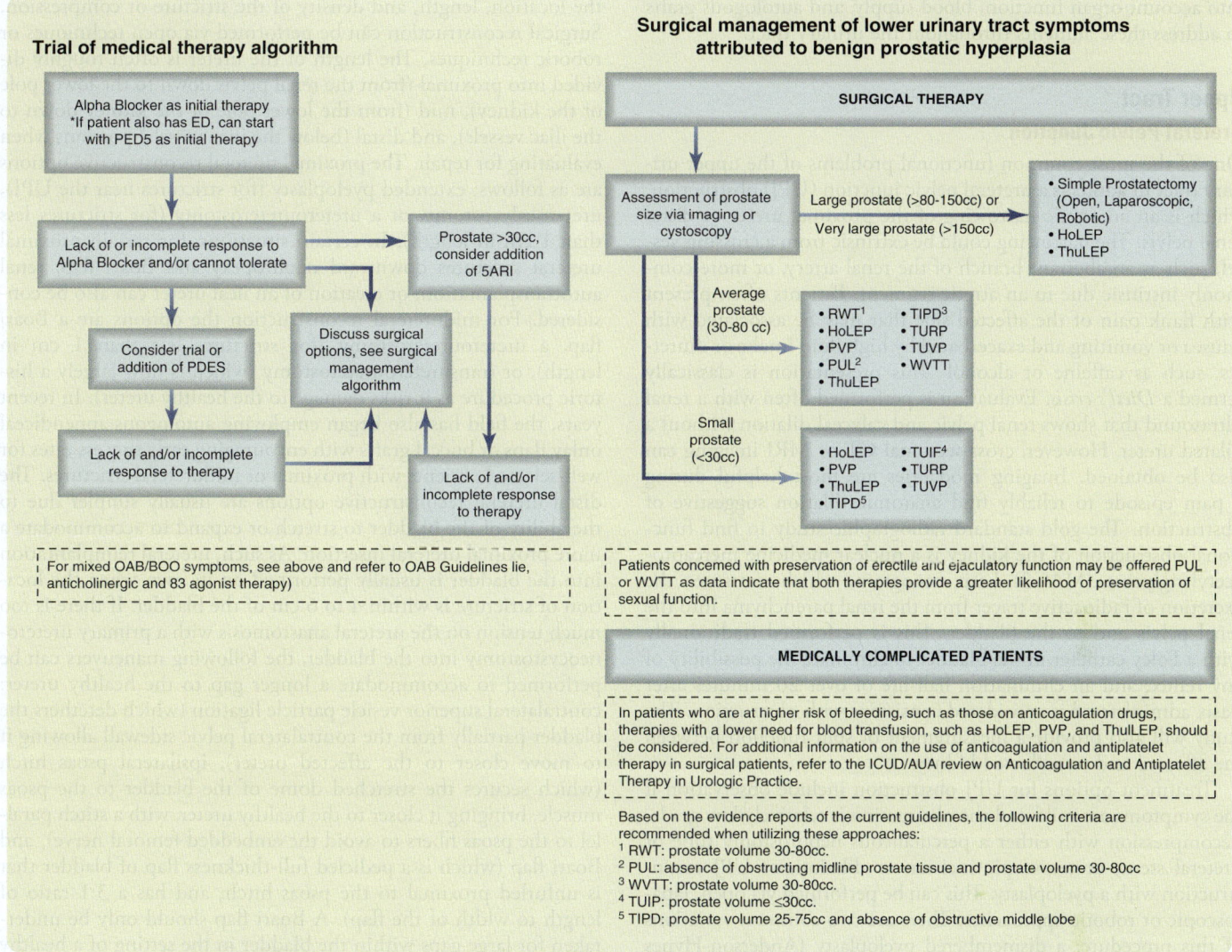

FIGURE 121.7 Algorithm for secondary management of benign prostatic hyperplasia. *AUA,* American Urological Association; *BOO,* bladder outlet obstruction; *ED,* erectile dysfunction; *HoLEP,* Holmium Laser Enucleation of the Prostate; *ICUD,* International Consultation on Urological Diseases; *PVP,* Photoselective Vaporization of the Prostate; *OAB,* overactive bladder; *ThuLEP,* Thulium Laser Enucleation of the Prostate. (Adapted from Sandhu JS, Bixler BR, Dahm P, et al. Management of lower urinary tract symptoms attributed to benign prostatic hyperplasia [BPH]. AUA Guideline amendment 2023, *J Urol.* 2024;211[1]:11–19.)

screening. In addition, these drugs can be used in combination because of their differing mechanism of action, and studies show superior results to either drug used independently.

When medical therapy is ineffective, symptoms remain bothersome, or an objective surgical indication arises (e.g., acute urinary retention, bladder calculi, azotemia, recurrent UTI, or recurrent hematuria), surgical intervention is considered. The standard approach to surgical treatment of BPH is transurethral resection of the prostate (TURP) using various electrosurgical options (monopolar, bipolar, or laser). Minimally invasive treatment options, such as microwave thermotherapy and radiofrequency ablation, can be performed in an office setting but do not have equivalent long-term outcomes compared with standard surgical procedures. When the adenomatous growth is particularly large, open simple prostatectomy is performed to enucleate the adenoma surgically. Outcomes of the transurethral procedures show dramatic improvement in International Prostate Symptom Score numbers, urinary flow rates, and postvoid residual volumes. Procedures such as

simple prostatectomy have such a long historical use that objective data have not been measured or compiled, but outcomes are similar to those of TURP. Complications of TURP procedures include persistent bleeding, dilutional hyponatremia from fluid absorption of the glycine irrigation, UTI, urinary incontinence, and urethral stricture. With newer electrosurgical systems (bipolar and laser), normal saline irrigation is used and dilutional hyponatremia has been eliminated. In addition, visualization is improved, with a significant reduction in bleeding complications and a lower incidence of urinary incontinence.

RECONSTRUCTIVE UROLOGY

Urologic reconstructions are often needed for stricture disease or congenital abnormalities that can manifest into adulthood. These problems can impact any point in the urinary tract from the kidney to the meatus and can have varying impacts on quality of life and organ function. Reconstructive urology is a field that takes into account organ function, blood supply, and autologous grafts to address these ailments throughout the urinary tract.

Upper Tract

Ureteral Pelvic Junction

One of the most common functional problems of the upper urinary tract in adults is a ureteral pelvic junction (UPJ) obstruction, which is an anatomic narrowing of the proximal ureter or distal renal pelvis. The narrowing could be extrinsic from a crossing vessel, such as an aberrant branch of the renal artery, or more commonly intrinsic due to an atretic segment. Patients often present with flank pain of the affected side that may be associated with nausea or vomiting and exacerbated by high fluid intake or diuretics, such as caffeine or alcohol. This presentation is classically termed a *Dietl's crisis*. Evaluation is performed often with a renal ultrasound that shows renal pelvic and calyceal dilation without a dilated ureter. However, cross-sectional CT or MRI imaging can also be obtained. Imaging modalities are most helpful during a pain episode to reliably find anatomic dilation suggestive of obstruction. The gold standard radiographic study to find functional obstruction of the kidney is a nuclear medicine mercaptoacetyltriglycine (MAG3) Lasix renogram, which measures the excretion of radioactive tracer from the renal parenchyma into the renal pelvis and to the bladder. This is performed traditionally with a Foley catheter in the bladder to eliminate the possibility of any reflux, and an elimination half-life of over 20 minutes after Lasix administered is considered consistent with obstruction. The study will also provide a measurement of split function between the affected and nonaffected kidney.

Treatment options for UPJ obstruction include observation if the symptoms are mild and the obstruction is relatively low grade, decompression with either a percutaneous nephrostomy tube or ureteral stent, ureteroscopic incision or dilation, or UPJ reconstruction with a pyeloplasty. This can be performed via open, laparoscopic or robotic approaches. There are two common variations of this procedure: a dismembered pyeloplasty (Anderson-Hynes technique) and a nontransecting pyeloplasty (Culp-DeWeerd or spiral flap). A dismembered pyeloplasty is particularly useful in traversing a crossing vessel, and in this procedure the atretic segment of the UPJ is excised and the renal pelvis and proximal ureter are widely spatulated and anastomosed to each other over a stent. In a nontransecting pyeloplasty, the posterior wall of the renal pelvis and ureter are kept intact, and a flap of redundant renal pelvis is sutured as an onlay over the atretic segment to widen the UPJ. Generally, most pyeloplasty techniques have a greater than 90% long-term patency rate.

Ureter

Ureteral reconstructions can be needed due to acute traumatic injuries (frequently iatrogenic) or chronic scarring of the ureter in response to abdominopelvic surgery, ureteroscopy, urolithiasis, or radiation. Extrinsic ureteral compression from tumors or lymph nodes is another cause for ureteral obstruction that require urologist assistance intraoperatively. The options for ureteral obstruction include observation, endoscopic decompression (with the stent or nephrostomy tube), or surgical repair. Evaluation for obstruction again requires a nuclear medicine MAG3 Lasix renogram, and if the kidney is nonfunctional (less than 15% split function), then a nephrectomy of the affected kidney is often the most sensible course. In kidneys with substantial split function, the surgical repair options for ureteral reconstruction depend on

the location, length, and density of the stricture or compression. Surgical reconstruction can be performed via open techniques or robotic techniques. The length of the ureter is often roughly divided into proximal (from the renal pelvis down to the lower pole of the kidney), mid (from the lower pole of the kidney down to the iliac vessels), and distal (below the iliac vessels) portions when evaluating for repair. The proximal ureteral reconstructive options are as follows: extended pyeloplasty (for strictures near the UPJ), ureterocalycostomy, or a ureteroureterostomy (for strictures less than 1 cm in length). In certain situations, for certain proximal ureteral strictures downward nephropexy and Boari flap, renal autotransplantation, or creation of an ileal ureter can also be considered. For midureteral reconstruction the options are a Boari flap, a ureteroureterostomy (for strictures less than 1 cm in length), or transureteroureterostomy (which is now largely a historic procedure as it risks damage to the healthy ureter). In recent years, the field has also began employing autologous appendiceal onlay flaps or buccal grafts with encouraging early success rates for well-selected patients with proximal or midureteral strictures. The distal ureteral reconstructive options are usually simpler due to the ability of the bladder to stretch or expand to accommodate a more proximal ureteral insertion. As such, ureteral reimplantation into the bladder is usually performed on its own when the location of stricture is within 4 to 6 cm of the bladder. If there is too much tension on the ureteral anastomosis with a primary ureteroneocystostomy into the bladder, the following maneuvers can be performed to accommodate a longer gap to the healthy ureter: contralateral superior vesicle particle ligation (which detethers the bladder partially from the contralateral pelvic sidewall allowing it to move closer to the affected ureter), ipsilateral psoas hitch (which secures the stretched dome of the bladder to the psoas muscle, bringing it closer to the healthy ureter, with a stitch parallel to the psoas fibers to avoid the embedded femoral nerve), and Boari flap (which is a pedicled full-thickness flap of bladder that is unfurled proximal to the psoas hitch, and has a 3:1 ratio of length to width of the flap). A Boari flap should only be undertaken for large gaps within the bladder in the setting of a healthy bladder with adequate function and capacity.

Lower Urinary Tract

Bladder

Bladder reconstruction is rarely needed after urologic procedures injuring the bladder neck, radiation, or neurogenic causes of bladder dysfunction. In some circumstances of small bladder capacity, a bladder augmentation is needed, and this can be performed with a enterocystoplasty, using either small bowel or large bowel to augment the capacity of the bladder. In addition, bladder reconstruction is also required for advanced primary bladder malignancy, which necessitates removal of the bladder and urinary diversion with either an ileal conduit, ileal neobladder, or least commonly a continent cutaneous catheterizable pouch. An ileal conduit is the most common urinary diversion used for bladder cancer and consists of a 12- to 20-cm segment of terminal ileum used to create an ostomy on the distal end and ureteroenteric anastomoses on the proximal end. An ileal neobladder uses a 55- to 60-cm segment of ileum, with the proximal 10 to 15 cm used as a stump for the ureteroenteric anastomosis and the remaining bowel detubularized and then sutured into a roughly spherical confirmation for anastomosis into the remnant urethral stump.

Electrolyte abnormalities are common when bowel is used for urinary augmentation or replacement. Most commonly, when ileum is used, a hyperchloremic metabolic acidosis can result, which in turn may decrease bone density. As a result, sodium bicarbonate is recommended to correct this. Additionally, B_{12} deficiency can develop due to lack of intrinsic factor reabsorption from the ileum that is now excluded from the alimentary canal for the urinary diversion.

Urethra

Strictures of the urethra are a common cause of LUTS such as slow stream, prolonged voiding, impaired sense of bladder emptying, and need to augment bladder pressure with Valsalva voiding or manual pressure on the bladder (Credé maneuver). Due to the incomplete bladder emptying, they may also predispose to UTIs and in severe cases, bladder hypertrophy and upper tract deterioration. Urethral strictures are far more common in males than in females. Common causes of urethral stricture disease include urethral instrumentation with catheters or scopes, lichen sclerosis (which is an inflammatory lesion of the skin and urethral mucosa), trauma, ischemic insult to the bulbomembranous urethra (such as during prolonged hypotension from major surgery), and radiation. Malignancy can also be a less common cause of stricture, but this needs to be higher on the differential in cases of recurrent urethral stricture or atypical appearance on imaging.

The male urethra is divided from distal to proximal as the following: urethral meatus, fossa navicularis, pendulous urethra, bulbar urethra, membranous urethra, and the prosthetic urethra. The available options for stricture treatment depend on the location, length, diameter, and density of the stricture. The location and length of the stricture is best characterized with a retrograde urethrogram performed under fluoroscopy, and the diameter and density of the structure is best characterized with direct visualization under cystoscopy.

Strictures involving the urethral meatus or fossa navicularis are often treated with dilation or endoscopic incision or open incision of the meatus (meatotomy). Endoscopic dilation or incision can also be used for thin urethral strictures less than 2 cm in length for the bulbar urethra as well. For strictures not amenable to endoscopic management, an option of indwelling urethral or suprapubic tube or intermittent self-catheterization exists for patients who are not surgical candidates. Urethroplasty remains the gold standard for meatal/fossa strictures that are recurrent after endoscopic management, any primary penile urethral stricture, bulbar urethral strictures over 2 cm in length, or bulbar urethral strictures less than 2 cm that are recurrent after endoscopic management. Urethroplasty can be performed with an excision of the involved urethral segment followed by primary anastomosis with wide spatulation. This excision and primary anastomosis are mainly performed for short segment strictures of the bulbar urethra. For longer strictures of the bulbar urethra and most strictures of the penile urethra in which primary anastomosis would have tension, an oral mucosal graft (buccal or lingual) augmentation urethroplasty is the gold standard. For even longer segment strictures, two-stage procedures in which the graft is first placed and then tubularized to completely substitute an excised segment of urethra can also be performed. It is important not to use hair-bearing skin for augmentation or substitution urethroplasty. For proximal urethral strictures involving the prosthetic and membranous urethra, more complex reconstruction is needed and often involves augmentation with oral mucosal graphs.

In females with urethral strictures, treatment options often start with endoscopic dilation or incision for simple strictures, but oral mucosal grafts or vaginal and advancement flaps can be used to incise and then widen the diameter of the urethra.

MALE REPRODUCTIVE MEDICINE AND SEXUAL DYSFUNCTION

Male infertility and sexual dysfunction are a specialized area of urologic practice. Diagnostic evaluation, medical treatment, and surgical therapy of male infertility represent sophisticated aspects of urologic care. Male sexual dysfunction is becoming more prominent as the field of male health continues to evolve. Many patients seen and evaluated by general surgeons may be receiving specific medical therapy or have undergone prosthetic surgical implants for sexual dysfunction management. A basic familiarity with these specialized areas is beneficial to general surgeons in their surgical practice.

Male Reproductive and Sexual Dysfunction: Evaluation and Treatment

Infertility affects approximately 8% to 14% of couples; the male factor is the primary or sole factor in 36% to 75% of these cases.[21] Couples are often referred to the urologist after a period of infertility, and referrals are generally from a primary care physician or from the evaluating gynecologic reproductive endocrinologist. Infertility is defined as a couple's inability to achieve pregnancy after 1 year of unprotected intercourse.[21]

The standard male factor evaluation involves a detailed history, physical examination, and basic laboratory and imaging evaluation. The AUA has produced a series of best practice statements on the evaluation of the infertile male with the following objectives: to recognize and to treat reversible conditions, to categorize disorders potentially amenable to assisted reproductive techniques, to identify syndromes and conditions that may be detrimental to the patient's health, and to distinguish genetic abnormalities that can be transmitted to or affect the health of offspring.[22]

The causes of infertility can be divided into anatomic, behavioral and environmental, and iatrogenic. Anatomic causes of male infertility are either congenital or acquired.[21] The most significant anatomic cause is congenital absence of the vas deferens, which is a partial or complete agenesis of the vas deferens. Although uncommon, the finding is associated with a cystic fibrosis transmembrane conductance regulator (CFTR) gene mutation, making these patients carriers for cystic fibrosis.[22] Other anatomic findings include cryptorchidism, ejaculatory duct obstruction (at the level of the prostate), and varicocele (Fig. 121.8). Behavioral and environmental sources of infertility are more common and easier to reverse than anatomic causes of male infertility. These include obesity, environmental exposures, substance abuse (including exogenous testosterone), and vitamin deficiency. Finally, iatrogenic causes to be considered include prior chemotherapy or radiation therapy, prior inguinal or genital surgery, and current medical treatments. Surgeons must be aware of iatrogenic causes of infertility in groin and pelvic surgical procedures from damage to the spermatic cord vasculature, vas deferens, and ejaculatory duct region or vasal entrapment from mesh used for inguinal hernia repair. The blood supply to the vas deferens or testicle is vulnerable to injury when the groin is explored in reoperative surgery or when the anatomy is obscured because of inguinal trauma as identification of these structures is challenging.

The history should include a discussion of sexual and reproductive history. This includes potential gonadotoxic exposure;

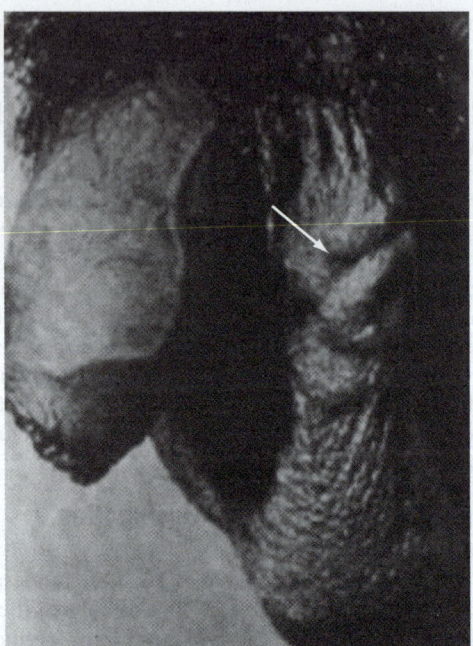

FIGURE 121.8 Varicocele. The bag of worms appearance is visible *(arrow)* and palpable through the scrotal skin, representing the dilated branches of the internal spermatic venous system.

urologic infections and STIs; trauma and prior surgery involving the pelvis, groin, and genitalia; and family history of infertility. Physical assessment should include a general evaluation of masculinization and genital findings, including normal meatal location, testicular size and consistency, presence and normalcy of the epididymis and vas deferens, and possible presence of a varicocele. Perineal and rectal examinations are routine parts of this assessment.

Basic Laboratory Assessment

Laboratory evaluation of these patients includes two semen analyses and serum hormone studies. The semen analyses should be separated by 1 month and preceded by 2 to 3 days of abstinence. Semen analysis parameters of importance include semen volume, pH, sperm concentration and total count, total motility, progressive motility, quality of sperm movement, morphology, and presence of red and white blood cells or bacteria.[21] The World Health Organization (WHO) has defined parameters of normal for routine semen analyses.[21] Semen analysis abnormalities fall into two main categories: azoospermia (the complete absence of sperm from the semen) and abnormal semen parameters (reduced concentration, motility, or morphology and abnormal function). Azoospermia can roughly be divided into three categories: pretesticular, testicular, and posttesticular. Pretesticular azoospermia results from endocrine causes, such as hypogonadotropic hypogonadism, or congenital causes. Testicular causes are the result of primary testicular failure of germinal epithelium of the testis to produce mature sperm. This is often accompanied by normal semen volume and by a markedly elevated serum follicle-stimulating hormone (FSH) level. Posttesticular causes, such as ejaculatory dysfunction and obstruction, account for 40% of cases of azoospermia.[22] Abnormal semen parameters may be indicative of a wide range of disorders that may cause reduced sperm numbers, motility, or morphology, including varicocele, antisperm antibodies, genital duct infection with pyospermia, and prior or current

gonadotoxic exposure. Reduced semen volume may be artifactual, indicating incomplete ejaculation or specimen collection, or it may represent true disease, including, for example, congenital absence of the seminal vesicle, ejaculatory duct obstruction, or retrograde ejaculation caused by diabetes, neurologic injury, or previous bladder neck surgery or medications.

Serum hormone testing includes determination of levels of FSH, luteinizing hormone, testosterone, free testosterone, and prolactin. Hypogonadotropic hypogonadism may be diagnosed on the basis of serum hormone studies or elevation in the FSH level. A patient with a low testosterone level should have follow-up prolactin levels measured to rule out a prolactinoma of the pituitary gland.

Ultrasound of the scrotum is useful to measure testicular volume and symmetry, to exclude the possibility of testicular neoplasm, to identify epididymal anatomy, and to define or to confirm the presence of a varicocele, which is an abnormal dilation of the pampiniform venous plexus of the internal spermatic venous system (see Fig. 121.8). Transrectal ultrasound (TRUS) of the prostate may provide evidence of ejaculatory duct obstruction with seminal vesicle dilation or congenital absence of the seminal vesicle, which may accompany congenital absence of the vas deferens.

Treatment

Treatment of male infertility depends on the identified cause and on the availability and affordability of assisted reproductive technology support options for specific or empirical treatment of failure to conceive. Medical therapy is used to treat hormone deficiencies, hormone excess, thyroid hormone excess, and prolactin excess. The most common medical therapies include hormonal stimulation of spermatogenesis, such as gonadotropin agents and antiestrogen agents, which have been met with mixed results. Antiinflammatory or antibiotic therapy can be used in patients with findings of pyospermia or concern for genital duct infection. Surgical therapies may include microsurgical reconstruction for vasal or epididymal occlusion (including vasectomy reversal), transurethral resection of the ejaculatory duct for obstructive lesions, and varicocele repair.

Male Sexual Dysfunction and Treatment

Sexual dysfunction in males refers to a range of disorders, including erectile dysfunction (ED), diminished libido, hypogonadism, and ejaculatory dysfunction. Because of the numerous organ system interactions, patients with these conditions may have associated neuropathy, endocrinopathy, vasculopathy, and psychological disorders, and these abnormalities may affect nonneurologic patient management and surgery.

Normal erectile function is a complex interaction between the nervous and vascular systems, with unique molecular actions occurring in penile vascular structures. Many medical comorbidities and lifestyle choices can contribute to ED, including age, coronary artery disease, smoking, hypertension, dyslipidemia, atherosclerosis, peripheral vascular disease, obesity, diabetes, spinal cord injury and degenerative neurologic conditions, treatment of pelvic malignant neoplasms, and chronic kidney disease.[23] The causes of ED can be divided into neurologic, vascular, metabolic, medication induced, endocrine, and psychological; importantly, it can be an early marker for coronary artery disease.[23] The initial evaluation of the ED patient centers on the history and physical examination. The history is focused on sexual performance and erectile function; the nonsexual historical aspects center on possible medical and surgical conditions. Social aspects, such as smoking, recreational drug use, and diet, are also important considerations. Validated questionnaires provide objective historical data both for initial treatment and for evaluation of therapy outcomes. The physical examination centers on the genitalia and evaluation of male secondary sexual characteristics. Basic laboratory studies in these patients include morning total testosterone concentration, fasting lipid levels, and hemoglobin A1c level. Important consideration should be given to assessment of cardiovascular function in younger patients because this disease process is considered an early marker for cardiovascular disease, especially in younger patients. Further evaluation is specialized but may include neurologic testing (e.g., biothesiometry) and vascular testing (e.g., penile duplex Doppler ultrasound studies).

Most treatments for ED are based on restoring penile arterial blood flow to achieve or to maintain a satisfactory erection. Lifestyle modifications are an important component of this, and dietary changes and increased regular cardiovascular exercise have been shown to independently improve erectile function. Evaluation and adjustment of offending medications should be considered as well. The basis of medical therapy for ED is phosphodiesterase type 5 inhibitors. These medications improve penile blood flow by limiting the breakdown of cyclic guanosine monophosphate and potentiating penile blood flow. These drugs should be limited in their use in males with known cardiovascular disease, especially those taking oral nitrates. Other forms of nonsurgical treatment include vacuum erection devices, intraurethral suppository therapy with prostaglandin compounds, intracavernosal self-injection, and occasionally psychotherapy. Surgery for ED includes primarily placement of a penile prosthesis and limited vascular reconstruction. Penile implant surgery may involve malleable implants, which have a flexible wire core inside a silicone sleeve, implanted bilaterally in the corpora, or, more commonly, inflatable penile implants. These are fluid-containing, completely internalized systems that may include paired corporal cylinders, a scrotal pumping device, and a fluid reservoir, which is typically positioned in the retropubic space or extraperitoneal lower abdominal quadrant (Fig. 121.9). The general surgeon should be aware that intraperitoneal positioning may also occur, intentionally or through erosion through the peritoneal membrane, and the reservoir or system tubing may be encountered during nonneurologic abdominopelvic surgery. Care should be taken not to contaminate any of the implant components or inadvertently injure the tubing or device components. If it is known that an implant is in place and pelvic or inguinal surgery is planned, urologic consultation may be helpful in handling any issues that arise with the implant. Revascularization of the penis to restore erectile function, following arteriography for anatomic documentation, is usually achieved using an inferior epigastric artery pedicle flap, whereby new arterial inflow is brought to the corpora cavernosa. This has limited indications, most relevant in younger patients with traumatic injury to the pelvic blood supply, and national practice guidelines consider this to be controversial.

The other area of male sexual medicine affecting a significant number of patients is testosterone deficiency or hypogonadism. Serum testosterone is produced in the Leydig cells of the testes (90%) and adrenal glands (10%). Testicular synthesis of testosterone is controlled by the hypothalamus and anterior pituitary. This is a condition in which serum testosterone levels decline and are associated with symptoms of fatigue, lack of energy, depressed mood, irritability, reduced motivation, decreased cognitive acuity, decreased strength and stamina, reduced muscle mass and increased fat, and sexual side effects including decreased libido

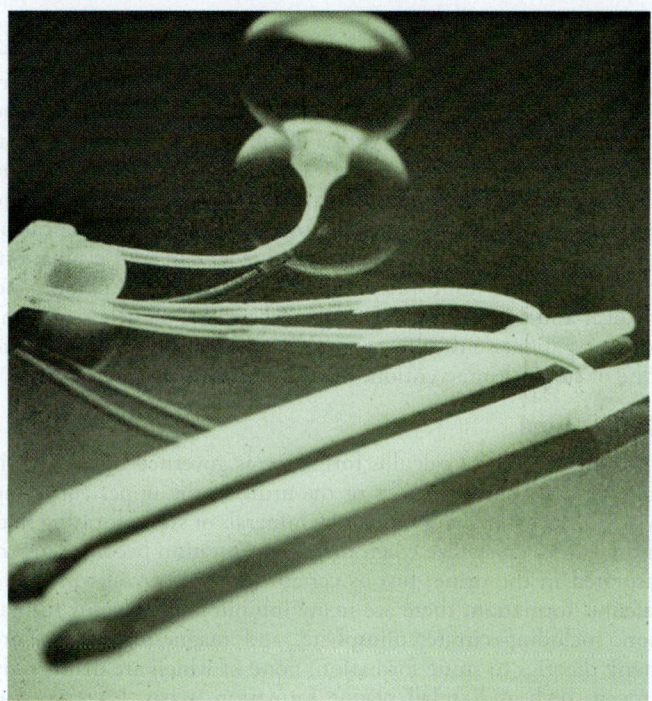

FIGURE 121.9 Inflatable penile prosthesis. A three-component device is shown. The reservoir *(top)* is placed retropubically in an extraperitoneal position. The paired cylinders *(right)* are placed within the corpora cavernosa. The pump *(left)* is placed in the scrotum, adjacent to the testes.

and ED. There is a normal age-related decline in testosterone as males age, and total testosterone declines by 1%, on average, each year after the age of 40 years. The prevalence of this condition is between 2.1% and 39% of males older than 40 years, depending on the criteria used and association of symptoms.[24] The patient's history should elicit information on the specific symptoms of testosterone deficiency, and physical examination is similar to that for ED with evaluation of the genitalia and secondary sexual characteristics. Validated questionnaires are useful to assess and to monitor therapy. Laboratory studies should include free and total morning testosterone, luteinizing hormone, prolactin, hematocrit, and hemoglobin levels.[25] Therapy for testosterone deficiency is based on lifestyle modifications and testosterone supplementation.[25] Many males who suffer from this condition are either obese or have metabolic syndrome. Dietary changes to improve nutritional status and to result in weight loss have been shown to improve not only baseline medical conditions but also serum testosterone levels. Furthermore, moderate-intensity exercise has been shown to improve serum testosterone levels. In addition to lifestyle modifications, many patients are treated with supplemental testosterone. Synthetic testosterone may be administered orally, transdermally, through intramuscular injections, and by subcutaneous pellets. The goal of therapy is maintenance of testosterone levels between 400 and 700 ng/dL and resolution or improvement of presenting symptoms.[25] Although there are few absolute contraindications to testosterone administration, many potential adverse side effects exist and should be discussed before administration of these medications as this is the area of greatest controversy with testosterone supplementation. Potential adverse effects include cardiovascular events and mortality, dermatologic changes, polycythemia, diminished spermatogenesis, gynecomastia, LUTS, prostate cancer, and sleep apnea.[25]

UROLITHIASIS

Urinary tract stones are a common cause of visits to the emergency department. The prevalence of renal calculous disease in the United States is increasing, with a lifetime risk of forming a renal stone at 5% in 1994 and 9% in 2010.[26] The incidence of stone disease peaks in the fourth to sixth decades of life and is more common in males than in females by a 2:1 margin.[26] Renal calculous disease has several aspects of management and evaluation, including acute stone presentation, metabolic evaluation, and medical and surgical therapy. As most general surgeons will encounter patients either in the acute presentation or around the time of surgical intervention, this section focuses on these areas.

Background

The pathogenesis of calculus formation is governed by the physical chemistry characteristics of the urine in the upper collecting system. Most stones are formed by minerals or stone-forming salts and begin to crystallize when their concentration becomes supersaturated in the urine. Just as certain minerals or salts promote calculus formation, there are many inhibitors of calculus formation, including citrate, phosphate, and magnesium. There are many theories to stone formation, none of which are definitively proven, such as Randall plaque formation, stasis, bacteria, and reactive oxygen species from oxalate excretion.[27] Kidney stones are classified by the stone composition, and the mineral composition directs evaluation, treatment, and nonsurgical management. Kidney stones can be generally classified as calcium based, uric acid stones, struvite stones, and cystine stones.[27] Calcium stones are usually composed of two calcium salts, calcium phosphate and calcium oxalate, and are the most common renal calculi. Risk factors for calcium stone formation include abnormal urine pH; high urine concentration of calcium, oxalate, or uric acid; and low urine concentration of the stone inhibitor citrate. Uric acid stones form in a low pH urine in patients with hyperuricosuria and can be the result of purine metabolism from cellular breakdown (tumor lysis) or excessive protein intake. These stones are often radiolucent. Struvite stones, also called infection stones or magnesium ammonium phosphate, result from specific bacterial infections (*P. mirabilis, K. pneumoniae, Staphylococcus aureus,* and *Staphylococcus epidermidis*) that contain urease, which converts urea into ammonia. The base properties of ammonia lead to higher urine pH and crystallization with phosphate. Cystine stones are formed from an autosomal recessive defect in the metabolism of the COLA amino acids (cystine, ornithine, lysine, and arginine), which results in elevated urine cystine levels.[27] The other rare cause of calculi is pharmacologically induced, resulting from poor drug metabolite urine solubility and precipitation in the urine. The most notable of these are protease inhibitors (indinavir and ritonavir), which are not visible on noncontrast CT scans.

Acute Presentation and Management

Patients presenting with an acute stone episode or renal colic typically have characteristic complaints of abdominal, flank, or back pain that waxes and wanes but cannot be resolved with position changes. Often, these patients can localize the most intense center of the pain, giving some indication of stone location. When the ureter is obstructed by a stone, the pressure in the proximal collecting system rises, and with progressive distention, the patient may experience visceral symptoms, including nausea, vomiting, and ileus. Physical examination in these patients should be focused on the back, flank, abdomen, and genitalia. Patients who have specific vital sign findings in combination (temperature higher than 101.5°F, hypotension, or tachycardia) should be assessed for obstructive upper tract UTI with the potential for sepsis. Basic laboratory evaluation should include complete blood count, metabolic panel, and urinalysis with microscopy. Significant findings of leukocytosis or acute kidney injury may direct urgency of therapy and type of intervention. A noncontrast-enhanced CT scan of the abdomen and pelvis is the preferred imaging study because of its superior sensitivity and specificity compared with intravenous urography and plain radiography. Patients with ureteral calculi may benefit from a plain radiograph, as 85% of calculi are radiopaque, to observe for stone passage.

Once the stone is identified and the location established, pain management is the next step. Patients who are diagnosed with renal or ureteral calculi should receive intravenous nonsteroidal antiinflammatory drugs (ketorolac) or opioid analgesics as initial therapy. A successful attempt at pain control with oral agents determines whether the otherwise hemodynamically stable patient can be discharged or requires inpatient treatment for the stone. Those patients who present with upper tract UTI and obstruction should undergo expeditious drainage with either cystoscopic ureteral stent placement or percutaneous nephrostomy tube placement. If one upper tract is totally obstructed by stone, the patient could have a serious infection with pyonephrosis, and the voided urine would be deceptively normal. Patients who are suitable for hospital discharge include those with no evidence of UTI, hemodynamic stability, good oral intake, pain well controlled on oral analgesics, and a stone size with reasonable chance of spontaneous passage. In patients who are discharged from the hospital, medical expulsive therapy, with agents to promote spontaneous stone passage, is the recommended management.[28] The most common drug used is tamsulosin, the α_{1a}-blocker that relaxes ureteral smooth muscle.[28] If a patient is discharged for outpatient management, they should be observed closely to determine whether the stone has passed. It should not be assumed that because the pain has resolved, the stone has passed. With persistent upper tract obstruction, the pressure in the collecting system eventually declines as renal blood flow diminishes and urine output drops. The patient's pain can disappear, and the kidney can remain obstructed, undergoing silent destruction in the weeks and months that follow. Reimaging is necessary if there is no definitive evidence that the stone has been passed (e.g., the patient brings it in for analysis).

Elective Diagnostic Evaluation and Management

Patients who are diagnosed with asymptomatic renal calculi, such as nonobstructing renal calyceal stones found incidentally during a hematuria evaluation, and patients who have convalesced after an acute presentation undergo a basic metabolic screening evaluation. Important historical aspects to obtain include prior stone passage or treatment, family history, bowel disease or malabsorption, gout, hyperthyroidism, obesity, and use of dietary supplements.[29] Routine laboratory work includes urinalysis, basic metabolic panel with determination of calcium and uric acid levels, urine culture, and stone analysis (if available). A 24-hour urine specimen is also collected to evaluate the urine for specific chemical and mineral content: volume, pH, creatinine, calcium, oxalate, uric acid, citrate, sodium, and potassium.[29] Specific dietary changes and medical therapy can be used for prevention of stone formation in specific populations. These dietary modifications and pharmacologic treatments are based on stone composition and findings on 24-hour urinalysis. The two most common stone types, calcium and uric acid, are discussed.

In patients with calcium-based stone disease (oxalate or phosphate), the single most important treatment or dietary modification is increased fluid intake to achieve more than 2 L of urine output daily. In addition, there should be no changes in calcium consumption, and patients, in general, should consume the recommended daily allowance of dietary calcium. Dietary levels of sodium, foods high in oxalate, and animal protein should be reduced as each of these can affect urinary oxalate and citrate levels. Pharmacologic therapy is typically based on three different agents, thiazide diuretics, potassium citrate, and allopurinol, each of which has separate effects on calcium urine levels and calcium stone formation. Patients with uric acid stones are treated with drug therapy.[29] There are no dietary recommendations other than to increase fluid intake to raise urine output to 2 L/day. Pharmacologic therapy in this group consists of potassium citrate and allopurinol. Many uric acid stones can be dissolved by raising urinary pH levels with use of alkalinizing agents.

Elective Surgical Management

Patients who have large stone burdens or continue to have symptomatic stones require surgical treatment of their calculous disease. Surgical treatment of renal and ureteral calculi varies from completely noninvasive, shock wave lithotripsy (SWL), to minimally invasive, percutaneous nephrolithotomy (PCNL). SWL is a transcutaneous procedure using generated shock waves to fragment stones. Shock waves create positive and negative pressure components that are focused on the stone and create fractures in the targeted stones, ultimately resulting in stone fragmentation.[30] The progress of stone fragmentation is monitored during SWL, typically with fluoroscopy, to direct treatment length and location. Nonradiopaque stones, stones larger than 2 cm, dense stones, and certain ureteral calculi should not be treated with this method. Complications from SWL include renal injury, steinstrasse (street of stones), hypertension, and chronic kidney disease.[30]

Smaller renal stones and ureteral calculi can be managed in an endoscopic fashion using ureteroscopes (Fig. 121.10). As previously mentioned, ureteroscopes are both semirigid and flexible, allowing full upper tract collecting system access. Through the working channel of ureteroscopes, a variety of working instruments can be placed to fragment or to remove stones. The most common stone treatment is laser lithotripsy to completely fragment the symptomatic calculus. Smaller fragments can be removed using different basket and grasping systems to render the patient stone free. Complications of ureteroscopy include acute ureteral perforation or avulsion, UTI, and late ureteral stricture formation.

For larger renal stones or select proximal ureteral stones, PCNL is preferred because of the larger working endoscopes and better instrumentation for stone fragmentation. The basic steps of PCNL are percutaneous renal access, dilation of the nephrostomy track, placement of the working sheath for stone fragmentation and extraction, and postoperative renal drainage. The advantage of PCNL is that numerous intracorporeal lithotripsy devices are available, and large stones can be rapidly fragmented. Flexible nephroscopes can also be used in this setting. Complications of PCNL are most significant because of the more invasive nature of the procedure; these include sepsis, renal hemorrhage, renal collecting system injury, and damage to adjacent organs and viscera. PCNL may result in hydrothorax or pneumothorax from transpleural or peripleural access tracks that requires evacuation. With the refinement of PCNL, open stone surgery is rarely indicated even for the most complex intrarenal calculi. Laparoscopic and robotic procedures for specific renal calculi have been described.

NONTRAUMATIC UROLOGIC EMERGENCIES

Within the field of urology are several emergent conditions, although not due to external violence, that represent true emergencies, some of which are life threatening. These urologic emergencies include obstructed upper tract UTI, hematuria with urinary retention due to blood clots, and the acute scrotum, specifically testicular torsion, priapism, and Fournier gangrene. Some of these conditions have been discussed in other sections of this chapter (Fournier gangrene and obstructed upper tract UTI); the remainder are covered in this discussion.

Testicular Torsion

The most urgent cause of the acute scrotum is testicular torsion. Testicular torsion occurs when arterial blood supply is compromised by a twist of the spermatic cord, creating occlusion of the spermatic cord and loss of vascular supply. In the normal anatomic arrangement, the inferior aspect of the testicle is attached

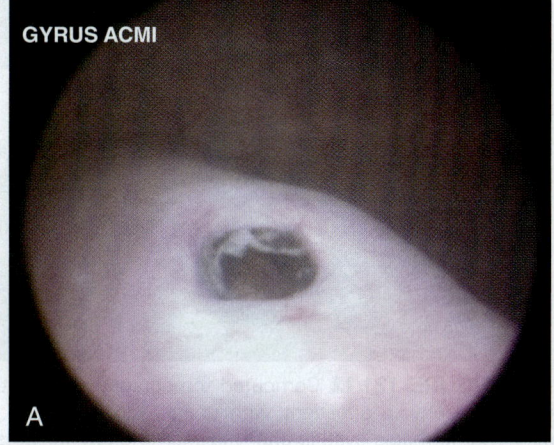
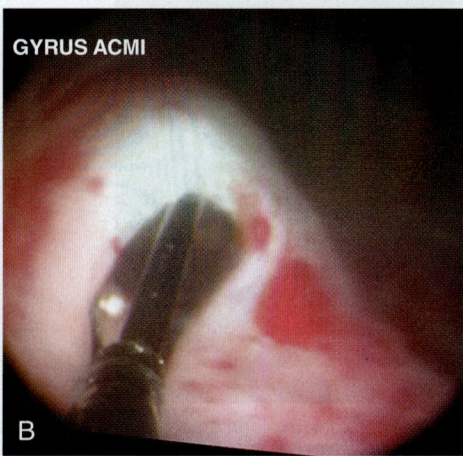

FIGURE 121.10 Ureteral stone. (A) An obstructing calculus is shown crowning within the right ureteral orifice. (B) Cystoscopic extraction performed with a grasping forceps.

to the scrotum by the gubernaculum, preventing rotation of the testicle within the scrotum. When torsion occurs, the testicle is subjected to warm ischemia; without reversal of the occluded blood supply, irreversible damage begins as soon as 4 hours and is complete by 8 to 12 hours. Although testicular torsion is most common in adolescent males, it may occur in any age group from neonate to adult males. As many other conditions may result in the so-called acute scrotum, a high index of suspicion is necessary on the part of the treating physician to ensure rapid diagnosis and treatment. Differential diagnosis includes trauma, epididymitis, incarcerated hernia, and torsion of the appendix testis or appendix epididymis. Diagnosis is strongly suspected on the basis of history and physical examination. Classic historical findings include sudden onset of intense unilateral scrotal pain, unrelated to trauma, that may be associated with nausea and vomiting. The most consistent physical examination finding is loss of the cremasteric reflex of the testicle; however, in an acute setting, this may be difficult to elicit. The best confirmatory radiologic study is color Doppler ultrasound of the scrotum, which shows absence of arterial flow to the testis in torsion. In patients with suspected testicular torsion, there is no need to delay scrotal exploration to obtain imaging or further laboratory evaluation.

Treatment of testicular torsion involves surgical exploration through a midline or transverse scrotal incision with inspection of the testis with detorsion of the spermatic cord if present (Fig. 121.11). For testes that are deemed to be viable, suture orchiopexy or fixation to the interior scrotal wall is performed, followed by a similar orchiopexy on the contralateral side at the same setting to prevent contralateral torsion. Because of the important medicolegal considerations in these cases, urgent exploration is still indicated even in patients who present with a suspected late torsion (e.g., several days of fixed swelling, firmness). Many times, it is difficult to know exactly how long complete ischemia has been present and whether there is still a potentially viable testicle.

Gross Hematuria With Urinary Retention From Blood Clots

Most patients who have hematuria present with either microscopic hematuria or episodic gross hematuria. However, in a subset of patients, onset of gross hematuria is rapid with significant blood loss and development of blood clots within the bladder. This problem is exacerbated in patients who are receiving chronic anticoagulation for underlying cardiovascular disease processes. The blood clots are organized into larger masses; the patient may not be able to expel the clot, leading to urinary retention and a potential surgical emergency (Fig. 121.12). Other causes of significant vesical hemorrhage include postoperative bleeding after TURP or transurethral resection of bladder tumor (TURBT), radiation cystitis, pelvic trauma, upper tract arteriovenous fistula, and iliac arterial fistula to the ureter.

It is difficult to judge the amount of blood that is being lost from the urinary tract with gross hematuria because only a small amount of blood mixed with urine will darken the bladder efflux. If, however, copious amounts of clot are evacuated from the bladder, one should suspect at least moderate blood loss and monitor the patient with vital signs and hemoglobin measurements. If bleeding from these events causes symptomatic anemia, the patient may require multiple urgent blood transfusions. In the patient with a significant amount of blood clot in the bladder, it will be necessary to place a large-bore irrigation catheter (in the adult, often 20–26 Fr) and adequately irrigate the clots from the bladder using normal saline irrigation. Special hematuria catheters are designed to allow large-volume irrigation and clot removal, but if this is unsuccessful, the patient may require urgent operative cystoscopy to evacuate the clot and to identify and fulgurate any bleeding source. Typically, this involves rigid cystoscopy with a large working sheath or resectoscope sheath and irrigation performed with a piston syringe or special evacuation devices (Ellik evacuator). After clot evacuation and fulguration, a large three-way catheter is left in place to run continuous irrigation to prevent a recurrent episode of clot retention. Upper tract clot formation may produce a so-called clot colic, with renal pain similar to that experienced from passage of a renal calculus. Supportive care and,

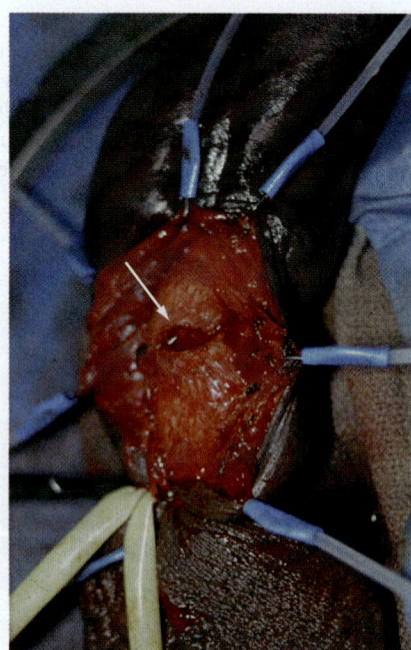

FIGURE 121.11 Testicular torsion. Exploration through a transverse scrotal incision demonstrates the twisted cord *(top)*. Note the degree of edema, erythema, and ecchymosis presenht after several hours of torsion.

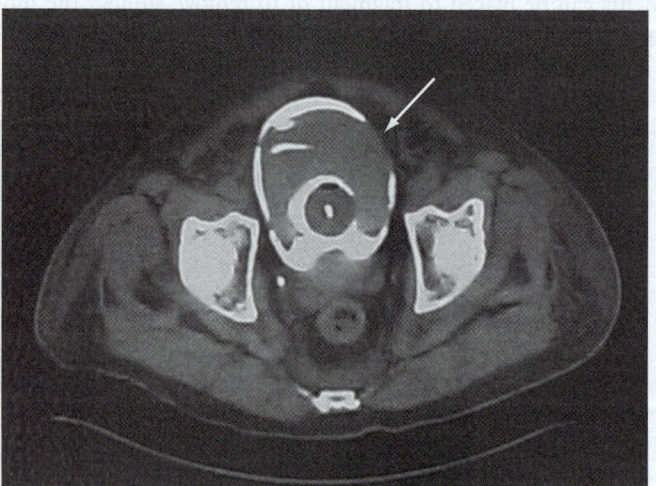

FIGURE 121.12 Computed tomography scan of the pelvis with cystography in a patient with urinary clot retention caused by chronic hemorrhagic cystitis after radiation therapy for prostate cancer. A clot may be seen surrounding the Foley catheter balloon, with instilled contrast material outlining the balloon and intact bladder wall.

in some cases, stent insertion may be helpful to address the underlying problem. If unexplained significant, gross hematuria occurs after minor trauma, one should suspect an underlying abnormality of the urinary tract, such as a neoplasm, congenital anomaly, or arteriovenous malformation.

Priapism

Priapism is a prolonged, painful penile erection that occurs in the absence of sexual arousal or stimulation. Priapism is typically divided into ischemic and nonischemic priapism. Important causes of ischemic priapism include sickle cell disease or other blood dyscrasias and certain types of drug or medication use, especially drugs for penile erection and hematologic malignant disease. Nonischemic priapism is the pelvic or genital trauma that results in arteriovenous fistula of the penile circulation. Priapism may resolve spontaneously, but if it persists longer than 4 hours, measures should be taken to reverse the process in most cases. Patients with priapism that lasts longer than 12 hours may develop irreversible damage to the penile vascular structure and long-term ED.

Evaluation in cases of ischemic priapism is centered on detailed history for risk factors, corporal blood gas analysis, and color Doppler ultrasound of the corpora cavernosa. Nonischemic priapism is evaluated similarly; however, aspirated blood has an arterial appearance and arterial blood gas parameters.

Ischemic priapism is managed with initial needle aspiration of the corpora cavernosa and irrigation with saline. In patients who do not respond to this step, needle aspiration is repeated with the injection of small, dilute doses of an α-adrenergic agonist substance, such as dilute phenylephrine. For patients who fail to respond to these measures, various shunting procedures can be performed to create shunts between the corpus cavernosum and other vascular structures, like the corpus spongiosum, to induce blood flow. For priapism related to sickle cell disease, medical treatment of the sickle crisis (e.g., hydration, oxygenation, pain management, and addressing hemoglobin and transfusion status) with hematology support is a mainstay of therapy to resolve priapism. For nonischemic priapism, there is no role for aspiration or irrigation of the erection as this is the result of an abnormality of the vascular system. Compression of the perineum or other injury site can be performed as an initial maneuver. If this fails, the next treatment step is usually superselective angioembolization to occlude the arteriovenous fistula with reversible agents, such as autologous blood clots or Gelfoam. It is important that the general surgeon consult with the urologist about treatment because corporal fibrosis and loss of erectile function are risks that increase with significant delays in therapy.

UROLOGIC INCIDENTALOMAS

There is a wide range of incidental imaging findings that can arise in the urinary system. From an abnormal growth, or "incidentaloma," perspective the most common GU growths are renal tumors or cysts, prostatic abnormalities, bladder thickening, retroperitoneal nodules or nodes, and testicular masses. We will briefly discuss the evaluation, significance, and management of these findings in the following:

- *Renal tumors or cysts:* Indeterminate renal findings can often be seen on renal ultrasounds or cross-sectional noncontrast imaging. The gold-standard evaluation is to obtain cross-sectional imaging in the form of either CT or MRI with contrast. Frequently the incidental findings on initial imaging will turn out to be simple cysts, hyperdense cysts (filled with proteinaceous debris or hemorrhage products), complex cysts usually just requiring follow-up, or a solid enhancing renal mass. If a solid enhancing renal mass is indeed confirmed, then the chances of the growth being malignant is approximately 70% for masses less than 4 cm and 70% to 95% masses over 4 cm depending on the exact size. Most renal masses are less than 4 cm in size, even though they are most likely malignant and tend to have an indolent course with a very long time horizon until metastasis, allowing for time to obtain repeat imaging and specialist referral. Malignancy could be primary renal or a secondary metastatic neoplasm of the kidney from another site, and in the latter case the tumors tend to be more infiltrative and not well circumscribed. Urothelial tumors originating from the collecting system and infiltrating into the renal parenchyma can also appear infiltrative and ill defined. In these situations, it is advantageous to perform a percutaneous renal mass biopsy when there is suspicion for a nonrenal parenchymal tumor. If there is macroscopic fat seen in the indeterminate lesion, this is a hallmark of angiomyolipoma or lipomatous tumors, including liposarcoma.
- *Prostatic abnormalities:* Most incidental prostate abnormalities on cross-sectional imaging are due to BPH with enlarged prostates or prominent intravesical protrusions into the bladder. In the absence of acute urinary symptoms, bilateral hydronephrosis, urinary retention, and active UTIs these findings are not urgent, but if the patient does have one of these symptoms, urologist referral is recommended. In addition, the prostate can frequently show incidental avidity on fluorodeoxyglucose–position emission tomography (FDG/PET) CT scans, and if the patient has a greater than 10-year life expectancy, PSA screening and prostate MRI along with urologist referrals are the next step, as some studies have shown that incidental FDG avidity increases the risk of harboring prostate cancer beyond that indicated by the patient's PSA alone. Given the inflammatory milieu of the prostate, FDG avidity is usually a false-positive finding.
- *Bladder thickening:* Asymmetric bladder thickening is a common finding on CTs and often represents bladder trabeculation from chronic outlet obstruction or motion artifact when the bladder is moving. Concentric bladder thickening is more consistent with bladder outlet obstruction, especially in the presence of diverticula and an enlarged prostate. However, when such findings are present, a urinalysis should always be checked to ensure there is no microscopic hematuria, which would then raise suspicion for neoplasms of the bladder. In addition, bladder thickening in a young male (less than 55 years of age) or a female should also warrant closer observation due to the lower anticipated chance of BPH-related change impacting the bladder. If the bladder thickening is toward the dome of the bladder, where it abuts the anterior abdominal wall and connects to the urachus, this is most likely a urachal remnant. These structures are embryologic vestiges from the allantois, and the chances of them being malignant are very low; however, they could lead to infections or drainage from the umbilicus or into the bladder. Worrisome signs of malignancy of the urachal remnant include an enlarging enhancing 3D mass, gross hematuria, age greater than 65, and calcifications within the mass.
- *Retroperitoneal nodules or nodes:* There is a broad range of pathology that could lead to enlarged retroperitoneal lymph nodes or a retroperitoneal mass, including lymphoma, metastasis from abdominal or pelvic organs, metastasis from testicles,

reactive changes to recent lower extremity or pelvic infections or urinary instrumentation, lymphangiomas, sarcomas, and retroperitoneal fibrosis. However, for an asymptomatic indeterminate sub-centimeter mass without a concurrent testicular mass on exam or ultrasound, and absence of other risk factors such as known personal history of relevant malignancies described earlier, these can usually be observed with close follow-up imaging in 2 to 3 months. For any substantial mass, it is recommended to get tumor markers to rule out primary retroperitoneal germ cell tumor including α-fetoprotein (AFP), beta human chorionic gonadotropin (β-HCG), and lactate dehydrogenase (LDH). In addition, comprehensive cross-sectional imaging with contrast is recommended along with percutaneous corneal biopsy if doubt of the ideology remains.

- *Testicular mass:* The most common type of testicular incidental finding is a cystic fluid collection, which is usually either a hydrocele (which is a fluid collection that develops in between the layers of the tunica vaginalis covering the testicle) or a spermatocele (which is an epididymal cyst). On exam these structures will often transilluminate with an exam light and will also have a discernible fluid wave, but if there is any doubt, then a scrotal ultrasound can be obtained. If these are not bothersome to the patient, as evidenced by lack of pain, tenderness on exam, no overlying skin changes, no history of infection, or no impairment of ambulation due to excessive chafing with thigh skin, then these can simply be observed. If any of these conditions are met, then surgical removal of these fluid-filled structures is a relatively easy outpatient procedure with high success rate. Other sources of incidental testicular findings include inguinal hernias masquerading as spermatic cord or testicular masses. Nevertheless, if there is a solid enhancing lesion along this spermatic cord or in the testicle itself, then a scrotal ultrasound with Doppler should be obtained and the serum tumor markers for testicular germ cell tumors should be checked (again these are AFP, β-HCG, and LDH). The testicular neoplasm evaluation should then be followed, which is discussed in more detail in the following section.

UROLOGIC ONCOLOGY

Urologic malignant neoplasms account for a significant disease burden in adults in the United States. Cancers of the GU system encompass the full spectrum of malignant neoplasms and are some of the most common (prostate) and rare (penile) cancers in the United States. Of the 12 most common cancers diagnosed annually in the United States, 3 are urologic in origin: prostate, bladder, and kidney. Low-stage cancers are typically managed with extirpative surgery or therapeutic radiation. Urologic cancers may involve adjacent viscera, vasculature, and soft tissue and body wall structures so that additional surgical expertise is necessary to complete the extirpative surgery and to support reconstructive efforts. As is the case with other malignant neoplasms, cancers of the GU system are often managed with a multidisciplinary approach. The major anatomic types of urologic cancers are discussed in this section, with a focus on the essential basic background knowledge, the fundamental therapeutic approaches for various stages of cancer presentation, and the basic outcomes for different tumor types.

Renal Cancer

Renal cell carcinoma, the most common type of renal malignant disease, accounts for 2% to 3% of all adult malignant neoplasms.[31]

The majority (>50%) of renal malignant neoplasms are now diagnosed incidentally by cross-sectional imaging or ultrasound evaluation of other nonspecific complaints. Historically, renal cell carcinoma was diagnosed only at an advanced stage because of its location within the retroperitoneum. The classic triad of renal cell carcinoma (flank pain, gross hematuria, and palpable abdominal mass) is now seen in less than 5% of patients. Despite this increase in asymptomatic diagnoses, 30% of patients present with metastatic disease.[32] Other symptoms on advanced presentation include hemorrhage, paraneoplastic syndrome, and symptoms of metastasis, such as pathologic fracture. Paraneoplastic syndromes are present in 20% of patients at diagnosis and include Stauffer syndrome (reversible hepatitis without liver metastasis), constitutional symptoms, anemia, polycythemia, and elevated inflammatory markers (erythrocyte sedimentation rate and C-reactive protein).[32] Renal cell carcinoma typically presents in the sixth to eighth decade of life and is more common in males. Risk factors for renal cell carcinoma include smoking, hypertension, obesity, acquired renal cystic disease (in patients with end-stage renal disease), and occupational exposures (aromatic hydrocarbons, asbestos, cadmium, and chemical and rubber industries).[31] These tumors typically arise in the proximal convoluted tubule or collecting duct within the renal parenchyma.[31]

Renal cell carcinoma is classified as follows: clear cell carcinoma, papillary renal cell carcinoma, chromophobe renal cell carcinoma, collecting duct carcinoma, and renal medullary carcinoma. This classification is based on microscopic appearance and cell of origin.[31] The genetics of these malignant neoplasms is fairly well described. The most common tumor histology, clear cell carcinoma, which is observed up to 85% of the time, is the result of chromosome 3 abnormalities; papillary carcinoma is the result of aberrations of chromosome 7, 17, or Y.[31] In addition, clear cell carcinoma and papillary carcinoma are responsible for the two most common familial cancer syndromes, von Hippel-Lindau and hereditary papillary renal cell carcinoma, respectively. Most renal masses are malignant, and only 15% to 20% are benign; the two most common benign masses are oncocytoma and angiomyolipoma.[32]

A final consideration with renal neoplasms is cystic renal masses, which present diagnostic challenges. Depending on specific characteristics of renal cystic lesions, the risk of these lesions representing cystic malignant neoplasms must be considered. The Bosniak classification system describes cystic renal masses according to their malignant risk and CT appearance, ranging from category I (simple cysts, 0% risk of malignancy) to category IV (cysts associated with enhancing or solid elements, 70% risk of malignancy).[31] Category III and IV cysts are usually treated as representing renal cell carcinomas.

Staging

Outcomes in renal cell carcinoma are directly tied to clinical stage at time of diagnosis. Evaluation and staging for renal cell carcinoma include history, physical examination, and laboratory testing. Evaluation for renal masses includes imaging of the primary tumor, usually with a contrast-enhanced CT scan or MRI study of the abdomen and pelvis as well as chest imaging, typically chest radiography. Also, based on clinical suspicion or abnormal results of laboratory studies, bone and brain imaging is performed. A key aspect of abdominal CT or MRI is evaluation of the renal vein and inferior vena cava as locally advanced renal cell carcinoma commonly forms tumor thrombus in these structures. The TNM staging system is listed in the *American Joint Committee on Cancer*

(AJCC) Cancer Staging Manual.[33] Histologic grading is based on the Fuhrman nuclear grading system on a scale of I to IV.

Management

The management of renal cell carcinoma has evolved in recent years. Historically, renal cell carcinoma was a surgical disease, and patients diagnosed with any renal mass underwent total radical nephrectomy. Now, select patients may undergo renal biopsy and active surveillance protocols. In the past, renal biopsies were fraught with high false-negative rates and low accuracy. Contemporary series show an accuracy rate of more than 90% in experienced centers with low complications and no reported incidence of tumor seeding when using the core-needle biopsy technique.[32] Those patients who are appropriate for renal biopsy are patients considered for either active surveillance or renal ablation therapy. Active surveillance protocols have been developed for patients with incidentally diagnosed, small (<2 cm) renal masses and those patients who would not tolerate extirpative or ablative therapy.[32] The natural history of small renal masses is a tendency to grow slowly, on average 0.5 cm/year, and they do not metastasize. Patients assigned to surveillance protocols undergo imaging every 6 months; once mass size stability is observed, this interval is extended to 6 to 12 months.[32] Small renal masses (<3 cm) can be considered for percutaneous, laparoscopic, or open ablation using cryotherapy or radiofrequency energy.[31] This treatment should be considered more for patients with significant medical comorbidities and less often in healthy patients.

For organ-confined renal tumors, extirpative surgery is the standard approach. For renal cancer with limited metastatic disease, cytoreductive nephrectomy has been an option with possible resection of metastatic lesions. However, the benefits seen with new systemic therapies are changing this paradigm. Minimally invasive surgery, both robotic and laparoscopic techniques, are standard for most renal lesions. The trend in extirpative surgery is to perform nephron sparing or partial nephrectomy for most T1 tumors. Partial nephrectomy is equivalent to radical nephrectomy in this tumor stage and should be considered for all patients with a T1a tumor and most with T1b tumors. Partial nephrectomy surgery may be straightforward in dealing with small, well-encapsulated, superficial, exophytic lesions or complex in dealing with larger, central lesions that involve the renal hilar structures. For partial nephrectomy, a negative margin should be obtained with the parenchymal resection, and only a few millimeters of normal parenchyma around the tumor are considered necessary. The general principles for partial nephrectomy include achievement of a negative surgical margin, identification and suturing of significant segmental renal vessel branches, and collecting system repair when the collecting system is entered or partially resected. To assist with blood loss, atraumatic vascular clamping of the renal artery and surface cooling of the kidney with iced saline slush are effective. When laparoscopic or robotic approaches are used for partial nephrectomy, local hypothermia is not possible; therefore, rapid tumor resection and clamp times of less than 35 minutes are employed. Tissue sealants, hemostatic agents, and absorbable mesh reconstruction of the kidney are all useful techniques to aid in hemostasis of a partial nephrectomy in the open surgical, laparoscopic, or robotic setting.[32]

Radical nephrectomy is performed in patients with large or multifocal tumors and those patients in whom a partial nephrectomy is not technically feasible. The primary long-term risk in this surgery is acute and chronic decline in renal function. Compared with partial nephrectomy, radical nephrectomy has a lower rate of complications. The adrenal gland is no longer removed with radical nephrectomy except in cases of obvious tumor involvement as the rate of synchronous involvement is less than 10%. Typically, radical nephrectomy is performed by either a laparoscopic or an open approach. Standard incisions for radical nephrectomy include anterior subcostal, flank, chevron, and midline. Regardless of approach, dissection of the renal pedicle with ligation of a renal artery must precede vein ligation to prevent swelling and dangerous bleeding from the kidney. The entire Gerota fascial envelope, containing the perinephric fat as a margin around the kidney parenchyma and tumor, is excised intact. The ureter is ligated and divided where convenient.[31] A regional lymph node dissection may be performed with a radical nephrectomy, although, on the basis of most evidence, it is more helpful as a staging and prognostic procedure than as a therapeutic one.[34]

Thermal ablation, which is an option for T1a renal masses smaller than 3 cm in diameter, was developed in an effort to improve patient procedural tolerance and reduce the complications from partial nephrectomy while still preserving function. Radiofrequency and cryoablation have been the most widely investigated and integrated into clinical practice, and oncologic outcomes are similar for both approaches even though long-term data for thermal ablation is still pending. Thermal ablation can be accomplished through open, laparoscopic, or percutaneous (most common) approaches. Thermal ablation can also be repeated if persistent viable malignancy is suspected.

For patients with locally advanced or metastatic disease, immunotherapy and targeted therapy (drugs with action on vascular endothelial growth factor and mammalian target of rapamycin) are used in a neoadjuvant or adjuvant setting. Overall organ-confined disease has an 80% to 100% 5-year survival in T1 tumors and a 50% to 80% 5-year survival in T2 disease.[32] Advanced disease has a grim prognosis of 0% to 20% 5-year survival.[32]

Several adjuvant kidney cancer trials have explored the potential benefit of systemic therapies after surgical resection of high-risk disease and has shown some benefit, particularly with pembrolizumab. For patients with metastatic disease, the landscape of systemic therapy for metastatic renal cell carcinoma is rapidly evolving, and options range from the more established targeted therapies to the newer regimens that include immunotherapies.[31,33]

Bladder Cancer

Urothelial malignant disease can arise anywhere in the upper or lower collecting system, but the most common site is the bladder. The entire upper and lower urinary tracts (renal collecting system through the distal urethra) are lined with surface epithelium called urothelium. The urothelium has a variable thickness of three to six cell layers, and transitional cell carcinoma arises from the basal cell layer. Bladder cancer is the fifth most common adult malignant neoplasm diagnosed in the United States and is more common in males than in females, in part, related to impaired bladder emptying in males with increasing age.[35] The tumor arises most frequently in the eighth decade of life, and males older than 70 years have a 3.7% probability for development of bladder cancer.[35] The multiple risk factors for development of bladder cancer include tobacco smoke, arsenic, chronic infections and inflammatory conditions (e.g., schistosomiasis), and occupational exposures (such as arylamines and aromatic hydrocarbons). The most common presenting symptom in bladder cancer is hematuria, microscopic in 1% to 11% and gross in 13% to 35%.[35] Importantly, a single episode of gross hematuria, especially in smokers, can carry a significant risk of cancer and warrants a full workup. Microscopic hematuria, on one urinalysis microscopy, qualifies a patient for a workup, but the risk of cancer depends greatly on other risk factors and patient factors. The other presenting symptom is irritative voiding (frequency, urgency, and dysuria) in the absence of infection on urine culture.

Bladder cancer is separated into nonmuscle invasive bladder cancer (NMIBC) and muscle invasive bladder cancer (MIBC), and each arises from different molecular pathways and has different treatments and outcomes. Urothelial tumors that have not invaded the detrusor muscle are termed NMIBCs. Approximately 70% of patients who present with bladder cancer will be diagnosed with NMBIC, which includes T stages Tis (carcinoma in situ [CIS]), Ta, and T1.[36] The other 20% to 40% of will either present or progress to MIBC includes stage T2 or higher bladder cancer at diagnosis.[37,38] TNM staging is included in the *AJCC Cancer Staging Manual*[37]; the T stage at diagnosis, specifically nonmuscle invasive (T1 or less) or muscle invasive (T2 or higher), is highly predictive of long-term outcome and survival. Ta disease refers to papillary tumors, with involvement of only the mucosa. T1 tumors involve the lamina propria, and T2 disease involves the detrusor muscle. Higher stages of the local tumor reflect involvement of perivesical fat or adjacent organs. Tumors are graded on the basis of histologic appearance from papilloma to high grade.

Nonmuscle Invasive Bladder Cancer

Patients who are suspected of having bladder cancer should undergo a thorough evaluation, which includes history, physical examination, basic laboratory tests, upper urinary tract imaging (preferably contrast-enhanced cross-sectional imaging), and office cystoscopy. If bladder cancer is present, characteristic flat, papillary, or large, sessile, aggressive-appearing masses will be present on the urothelial surface of the bladder. NMIBCs typically appear as flat (CIS) or papillary (Ta or T1) lesions.[36] An adjunct test for identification of bladder cancer is use of urine cytology, which is either as voided or bladder wash at the time of cystoscopy. Urine cytology is most sensitive for high-grade tumors and can be equivocal or nondiagnostic in the setting of low-grade NMIBCs. Adjunct urine tumor markers exist but are not recommended on consensus guidelines because of cost and low specificity.[37]

Any tumor identified in the bladder should be fully resected by TURBT. TURBT is diagnostic, by providing pathologic analysis, tumor staging by identification (if present) of muscle invasion, and potentially therapeutic in treatment of noninvasive disease. TURBT is performed through a surgical endoscope, called a resectoscope, and uses either monopolar or bipolar energy to shave the tumor from the bladder wall alongside continuous irrigation.[35] At the time of TURBT, patients should undergo a bimanual examination of the bladder. A palpable mass after TURBT represents extravesical extension (T3) of tumor, and, if the lesion is fixed, it raises the possibility of pelvic sidewall or adjacent organ invasion (T4). Any patient identified with high-grade tumors with any possibility of incomplete first resection or absence of muscle in the initial resection should undergo repeated TURBT within 2 to 6 weeks.[36]

Immediate intravesical chemotherapy refers to intravesical administration of an antineoplastic agent within 24 hours of TURBT, which has been shown to reduce the tumor recurrence by 35%. The agent most commonly used for this purpose is mitomycin C with many centers transitioning to gemcitabine for better patient safety.[36] In a patient with low- or intermediate-risk bladder cancer, a clinician should consider administration of a single postoperative instillation of intravesical chemotherapy.[35] Six weeks after TURBT, patients with CIS or NMIBC with high risk for progression or recurrence or CIS should receive intravesical therapy with either immunotherapy or chemotherapeutic agents. Standard immunotherapy for NMIBC consists of serial bacille Calmette-Guérin (BCG) intravesical instillations for induction and periodic maintenance therapy. Intravesical BCG significantly decreases the invasion and progression rate for NMIBCs, compared with transurethral resection alone. Maintenance BCG instillations reduce the risk of recurrence and progression and are given at variable intervals for periods of 1 to 3 years.[36] If a patient's cancer is unresponsive to BCG and the tumor recurs, there are many salvage intravesical therapies being investigated but the gold standard remains radical cystectomy. Periodic surveillance by office cystoscopy and upper tract imaging is mandatory in these patients as 60% to 80% of these tumors recur, and in higher grade tumors, 10% to 20% progress to higher stage or muscle invasive tumors.[36] Enhanced cystoscopy using blue light technology with hexaminolevulinate or narrow-band imaging may improve detection and lower recurrence rates.[35]

Muscle Invasive Bladder Cancer

The majority of patients who present with MIBC have invasive disease at diagnosis, and it has a much higher risk of progression and metastasis.[35] These cancers are highly lethal and are the cause of death in the vast majority of patients within 2 years of diagnosis without aggressive treatment. Approximately 70% of patients present with localized disease, whereas 33% have regional spread and 5% have distant metastasis at the time of diagnosis.[39] MIBC is typically urothelial cell carcinoma, but other histopathologic types occur, including squamous cell carcinoma, adenocarcinoma, and small cell carcinoma, with potentially worse outcomes. MIBC should be staged in a similar fashion to NMIBC, with cross-sectional imaging of the abdomen and pelvis, but consideration should be given to chest CT rather than plain radiography. Despite adequate staging, 40% of patients are understaged at diagnosis and have extravesical disease on the final pathologic specimen.[39]

Management

Standard management of MIBC is radical cystoprostatectomy in males and cystectomy in females, combined with neoadjuvant cisplatin-based chemotherapy for all eligible patients. In the male patient, radical cystectomy involves the removal of the entire urinary bladder en bloc with the perivesical fat, prostate, seminal vesicles, and pelvic lymph nodes. In the female patient, radical cystectomy typically involves en bloc removal of the female pelvic viscera (uterus, cervix, fallopian tubes, and the anterior vagina), although preservation of these structures may at times be considered, depending on the details of the case. Extended lymph node dissection is performed at the same setting and includes removal of the external and internal iliac lymph nodes, common iliac lymph nodes to the aortic bifurcation, and presacral lymph nodes. Improved survival is associated with extended pelvic lymph node dissection at the time of radical cystectomy. Perioperative complication rates are high, and more than 60% of patients undergoing radical cystectomy and extended pelvic lymph node dissection have at least one complication within 90 days of surgery.[39] Because of the high rate of extravesical extension at the time of radical cystectomy, and based on level 1 evidence, neoadjuvant chemotherapy is employed with overall and recurrence-free survival benefits. Typical regimens for neoadjuvant chemotherapy include methotrexate, vinblastine, doxorubicin [Adriamycin], and cisplatin (MVAC) or gemcitabine and cisplatin (GC). The use of neoadjuvant chemotherapy improves overall survival by 5% to 7%.[39] Adjuvant chemotherapy is offered to patients with high-risk pathologic features from surgery with no evidence of metastasis, and retrospective data support its use, with prospective trials currently in progress. A challenge of relying on adjuvant chemotherapy is that the recovery after cystectomy can often delay timely initiation of therapy.[39] Following cystectomy, patients with organ-confined, node-negative disease have the best overall disease-specific survival at 5 and 10 years at 85% and 60%, respectively. Neoadjuvant chemotherapy achieves a pT0 rate twice as often as surgery alone, and this confers a dramatic improved survival as well. Patients with extravesical disease have 5-year disease-specific survival in the 50% range, whereas patients with node-positive disease who have undergone a thorough lymph node dissection have a 30% 5-year disease-specific survival.[39]

The selection of the type of urinary diversion after radical cystectomy must take into account any history of pelvic irradiation, presence of renal insufficiency, liver function abnormalities, and mechanical tasks for which the patient will be responsible. There are various options for urinary diversion, including ileal conduit, orthotopic bladder substitution with anastomosis to the native urethra (neobladder), and more complex forms of cutaneous catheterizable reservoirs with continence mechanisms. No randomized study has shown one type of urinary diversion to be superior to any other, and the decision is usually directed by the patient's preference or the surgeon's choice. There is an extensive and complex history involving the use of intestinal segments in the urinary tract for urinary diversion after cystectomy and in other reconstructive settings. The surgeon should be familiar with the metabolic, mechanical, and other risk factors associated with the use of intestinal segments in the reconstructed urinary tract, including electrolyte abnormalities, bone demineralization, mucus production, stone formation, chronic infection, diarrhea, vitamin B_{12} deficiency, and increased cancer risk.[39]

Prostate Cancer

Prostate cancer is the most common cancer diagnosed in males and the third most common cancer diagnosed in the United States, behind breast and lung cancer, with approximately 240,000 males diagnosed annually resulting in approximately 30,000 deaths.[40] Prostate cancer is an adenocarcinoma and arises from the glandular structures within the prostatic parenchyma. Most new prostate cancer cases are diagnosed in males 60 years of age and older, are low grade and low stage, and are diagnosed by routine screening.[41] Screening for prostate cancer is performed with the blood test PSA, a serine protease, and DRE. The most controversial aspect of prostate cancer is screening and determining which patients require treatment. The goal of prostate cancer screening is to detect potentially lethal cancer at an early, treatable stage and to intervene with intent to cure. Because of the controversy surrounding the recent US Preventive Services Task Force (USPSTF) recommendation against screening for prostate cancer in 2012, the AUA released its own guidelines for screening in 2013. The USPSTF released revised guidelines in 2018.[40] These recommendations are for screening in males aged 55 to 69 years to be a joint decision between the physician and the patient, and a routine screening interval to occur every 2 to 4 years.[40] More intensive evaluation should be considered in males with a strong family history and genetic predisposition and those who are African American. Routine screening is not routinely recommended in males less than age 40 and in males older than 70 years. Current AUA guidelines state to start PSA screening between ages 40 and 45 for patients at increased risk and 45 and 50 for patients at average risk.[40,42] Furthermore, screening should not be performed in males with a life expectancy of less than 10 to 15 years.

Evaluation

Patients who have either an elevated total PSA level or abnormal findings on DRE or both undergo TRUS-guided biopsy of the prostate. Additional serum and tissue tests and MRI imaging can be combined with basic data to risk-stratify a male before or after biopsy. The standard biopsy template involves 12 cores with a spring-loaded biopsy instrument; tissue is obtained from the base, mid, and apex regions, medially and laterally from the left and right sides. Prophylactic antibiotics are routinely administered, and cleansing enemas are advised. When feasible, patients are asked to stop anticoagulants to help prevent bleeding complications. Common adverse events that follow TRUS biopsy include rectal bleeding, gross hematuria, and hematospermia, all of which are usually self-limited. Fever and urinary infection and retention occur in less than 5% of patients; bacteremia occurs, but it occurs in less than 1% to 3% of patients.[40]

Prostate cancer is diagnosed histologically by the Gleason grading system, which evaluates the level of abnormality in the patterns of the glandular architecture of the prostate compared with normal. The grading system is based on a scale of 1 to 5, with 1 being the most well differentiated and 5 being the least well differentiated. In the modern PSA-based screening era, prostate cancers have a Gleason grade minimum of 3 with a sum of 6 or greater, and the majority of newly diagnosed cancers are Gleason 3+3. Patients diagnosed with prostate cancer are risk-stratified on the basis of PSA level at time of diagnosis, clinical stage based on DRE, and Gleason sum score on the prostate biopsy.[42] Patients with unfavorable intermediate- and high-risk cancers should undergo cancer staging, which in prostate cancer may include radionuclide bone scan or more recently a prostate-specific membrane antigen (PSMA) PET CT to evaluate for bone metastasis and cross-sectional imaging of the abdomen and pelvis to evaluate for nodal metastasis.[42]

Treatment

The treatment of prostate cancer has changed significantly during the last two decades. Shared decision-making takes into account cancer details, patient medical factors, life expectancy, and patient preference to determine the preferred mode of treatment. As most prostate cancer is low risk at diagnosis, many patients (up to 50% in certain centers) are now managed with active surveillance rather than with definitive therapy. In general, males with cancer of low clinical stage (<T2a), low grade (Gleason sum ≤6), low PSA (<10 ng/mL), and low volume on biopsy are candidates for active surveillance. Patients assigned to active surveillance protocols undergo DRE and PSA monitoring every 3 to 6 months, often incorporating MRI at certain intervals and repeated TRUS-guided prostate biopsies every 1 to 3 years. Patients with increase in Gleason sum or increase in tumor volume on biopsy typically shift to an active treatment plan, and up to 25% of males on active surveillance go on to definitive therapy within 5 years.

Prostate cancer can be treated with either radical surgical excision or definitive radiation therapy. Radical prostatectomy involves the surgical removal of the entire prostate and seminal vesicles with anastomosis of the urethral stump to the bladder neck. The extent of bilateral pelvic lymph node dissection is based on extent of disease and risk group of the cancer. For prostate cancer Gleason sum 8 or higher, at a minimum, the external iliac, internal iliac, and obturator lymph nodes should be removed. Radical prostatectomy can be performed with an open, laparoscopic, or robotically assisted laparoscopic approach. The majority of cases in the United States are now performed by a robotic-assisted laparoscopic approach prostatectomy (RALP). The advantages of RALP have been reported to be decreased blood loss, shorter hospital stay, and quicker return to work. When it is technically feasible and oncologically appropriate, a nerve-sparing approach is used, which avoids injury to the cavernous nerves that run posterolateral along the prostate in the neurovascular bundle and mediate penile erection. Important landmarks for radical prostatectomy are the dorsal venous plexus anteriorly, bladder neck cephalad, prostatomembranous urethral junction distally, and rectal wall posteriorly. The correct plane of posterior dissection in radical prostatectomy is just posterior to the Denonvilliers fascia. The primary long-term risks of radical prostatectomy are urinary incontinence and ED. Ten-year cancer progression-free survival is approximately 85% for patients with organ-confined disease, approximately 60% to 70% for patients with extracapsular extension, and approximately 50% for patients with positive surgical margins.[42]

Patients who do not desire or who are not candidates for surgical extirpation may undergo local therapy with either intensity-modulated radiation therapy (IMRT) or brachytherapy. The typical treatment dose for IMRT-based prostate cancer therapy is 76 to 86 Gy. The most common form of brachytherapy is low-dose ultrasound-guided placement of iodine-125 or palladium-103 radioisotope sources into the prostate. Both treatments are commonly used for low-risk prostate cancer. Intermediate- and high-risk prostate cancer is typically treated with IMRT coupled with androgen deprivation therapy for up to 3 years. Low-, intermediate-, and high-risk prostate cancers have cancer survival outcomes after radiation-based therapy similar to those of radical prostatectomy.[42]

In advanced prostate cancer, the standard approach with androgen deprivation therapy may become ineffective, with clinical or PSA progression observed in spite of appropriate hormonal blockade. When castrate-resistant disease develops, second-line treatment includes antiandrogens, chemotherapy, and investigational agents. Other forms of treatment considered for local treatment of prostate cancer include ablation, such as high-intensity frequency ultrasound and cryotherapy, and proton beam therapy, although long-term results for these modalities are still being reported. Focal therapy of discrete lesions is also being studied in clinical trials, but outcomes and surveillance with focal therapy are uncertain due to the commonly multifocal nature of prostate cancer. It remains a modality that should be confined to clinical trials.[41,42]

After prostate cancer therapy, patients are monitored for post-treatment morbidities (e.g., continence, erectile function, voiding adequacy) and possible cancer recurrence. The latter involves PSA testing and potentially repeated metastatic evaluation, when indicated. Long-term follow-up for prostate cancer patients should continue at least 10 years, if not permanently, because very late recurrences can occur. If the PSA level becomes significantly detectable or is rising after definitive treatment, imaging with PSMA PET CT is needed to rule out metastasis. Options to decide whether to proceed with local radiation therapy, androgen deprivation therapy, or observation. Dramatic improvements in prostate cancer survival have been achieved in the last two to three decades, due to improved detection with screening and major advances in systemic treatment of metastatic disease.[42]

Testicular Cancer

Testicular cancer is an uncommon malignant neoplasm; in the United States, the incidence is 5/100,000 males.[43,44] Most cases of primary testicular cancer are germ cell origin (95%); the remainder are predominantly stromal (Leydig cell) or sex cord (Sertoli cell) tumors.[43,44] Any solid intratesticular mass is likely to represent a malignant germ cell tumor and is typically treated as such unless there is a strong suspicion to the contrary. Risk factors for testicular tumors include Scandinavian descent, cryptorchidism, orchitis, family history of testicular cancer, and intratubular germ cell neoplasia.

Germ cell–derived testicular tumors can be broadly divided into pure seminoma and mixed nonseminoma germ cell tumors (NSGCTs), and the division is approximately 50% for each. The majority of seminomas histologically are classic (85%); the remainder are either anaplastic or spermatocytic seminoma.[43] NSGCTs can be divided into numerous histologic types: embryonal carcinoma, yolk sac or endodermal sinus tumors, choriocarcinoma, teratoma, and mixed germ cell tumors. Testicular malignant neoplasms are the most common tumors in males between the ages of 20 and 40 years.[43] Seminomas, however, have a bimodal distribution with a second peak present in the fourth or fifth decade of life, and spermatocytic seminomas may present in males older than 50 years.[43] The most common presenting complaint in males with testicular cancer is a painless testicular mass; however, symptoms of metastatic disease include back pain, palpable abdominal mass, shortness of breath, or hemoptysis. In patients who present with a painless testicular mass, scrotal ultrasonography is the diagnostic study of choice. In addition to history, physical examination, and ultrasonography, patients with testicular tumors should have determination of specific tumor markers: AFO, β-HCG, and LDH. Each of these markers has a characteristic half-life, and they are important for initial cancer staging and surveillance.

Treatment

Initial treatment of suspected testicular tumor is radical inguinal orchiectomy, which involves removal of the testicle and spermatic cord at the level of the inguinal ring (Fig. 121.13). Because of the characteristic and well-described lymph drainage of the testicle, there is no role for transscrotal biopsy or orchiectomy. If the intrascrotal tissue planes are violated during orchiectomy, the lymphatic drainage can be altered, affecting future treatment. Before or after radical inguinal orchiectomy, the patient should undergo disease staging, including cross-sectional, contrast-enhanced imaging of the abdomen and pelvis and chest imaging, either chest radiography in low-risk patients or cross-sectional chest imaging in patients with high-risk disease.

Clinical staging for testicular cancer includes primary tumor pathology, lymph and metastatic staging on imaging, and postorchiectomy serum tumor markers. The half-life of β-HCG is 24 to 36 hours, and the half-life of AFP is 5 to 7 days; these levels should normalize in the absence of metastatic disease. Metastatic disease from testicular cancer follows a predictable retroperitoneal lymphatic spread, skipping the inguinal and pelvic nodal stations, given the testes' embryologic origin and corresponding vascular drainage. Choriocarcinoma is notorious for hematogenous spread early to distant sites. From the right testis, initial lymph node metastasis is to the infrarenal interaortocaval nodes, paracaval

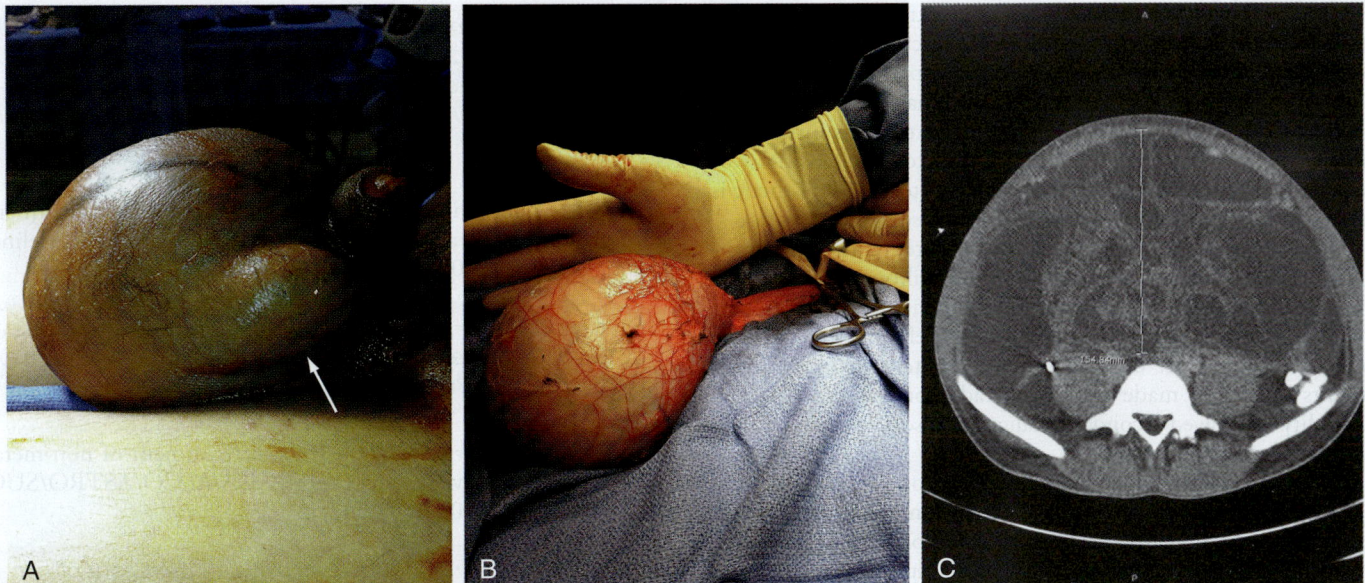

FIGURE 121.13 Advanced testicular carcinoma. (A) Preoperative appearance of the scrotum in a patient with a large right testis tumor. The normal left testis is seen pushed cephalad by the right-sided mass. (B) Surgical exploration through right inguinal incision showing the right testis that has been dissected from the scrotum in an extravaginal plane still attached by the spermatic cord pedicle to the right. (C) Massive retroperitoneal lymphadenopathy in the same patient. Note that the descending colon is opacified with contrast material, but all other viscera are pushed cephalad so that no small intestine is seen in this image. The patient was managed with primary chemotherapy followed by retroperitoneal lymphadenectomy for the residual mass.

nodes, and paraaortic nodes, and on the left, the paraaortic nodes and then interaortocaval nodes. Retroperitoneal lymph nodes are the primary metastatic site in more than 70% of patients with metastatic testicular cancer.[45] If the patient has had prior groin or pelvic surgery, the natural lymphatic distributions may be altered and the metastatic pattern may be unpredictable, potentially leading to involvement of the inguinal or pelvic nodes. Distant metastases are typically seen to the lung, liver, brain, bone, kidney, and adrenal gland.

Second-line treatment is directed by tumor histology and lymph node staging. Further treatment may consist of regular surveillance, retroperitoneal radiation therapy, retroperitoneal lymph node dissection (RPLND), systemic chemotherapy, or a multimodal therapy approach. The treatment decisions are complex, often at the direction of an institutional tumor board, but several general principles apply[45]:

- For seminoma stage IA and IB disease, treatment options include surveillance, radiotherapy to the regional (paraaortic) lymph nodes (20 Gy), and one cycle of carboplatin-based chemotherapy.
- For seminoma stage IIA and IIB, radiotherapy of the retroperitoneal lymph nodes is standard therapy, but RPLND is now being added based on recent studies[46]; for stage IIC or III, platinum-based chemotherapy is standard therapy.[44,45]
- For NSGCT stage I disease, the options include surveillance, primary RPLND, or cisplatin-based chemotherapy.[45]
- For NSGCT stage IIA, either primary RPLND (in patients with normal levels of tumor markers) or three or four cycles of cisplatin-based chemotherapy is standard; for stage IIB, three or four cycles of cisplatin-based chemotherapy is standard.
- For NSGCT stage III, treatment consists of cisplatin-based chemotherapy.

RPLND (Fig. 121.14) involves removal of all lymph nodes in the retroperitoneum from the renal vessels to the aortic bifurcation. An appropriate RPLND should include the lymph tissue surrounding the great vessels and division of the appropriate lumbar vessels to ensure thorough dissection using the split-and-roll technique. The most challenging RPLNDs are after chemotherapy, when the retroperitoneal tissues may be fibrotic or desmoplastic and adherent to the inferior vena cava, aorta, bowel, and mesentery. RPLND is template driven, and the appropriate levels and location of tissue excision are well described. Following the appropriate templates, the sympathetic nerve chain should be

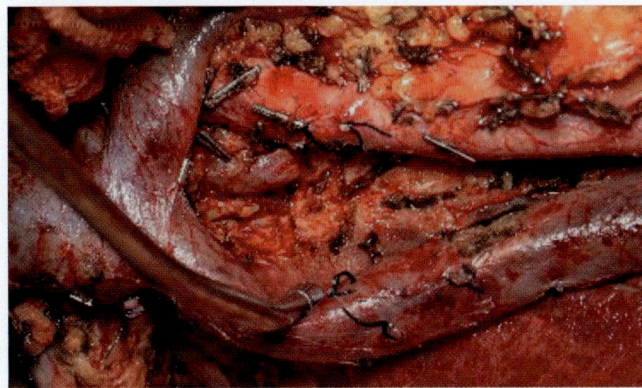

FIGURE 121.14 Right-sided retroperitoneal lymph node dissection with inferior vena cava and left renal vein skeletonized and the underlying caval nodes removed. The anterior longitudinal ligament of the spine can be seen. The interaortocaval and some of the preaortic lymph nodes have been removed. The remaining lymph nodes were addressed by reflecting the left colon.

uninjured, allowing antegrade ejaculation. Extensive dissection in this territory often induces an autonomic reaction with persistent tachycardia, which may last for an extended period (4–6 weeks).

Many patients undergoing RPLND will have been exposed to bleomycin chemotherapy, which requires meticulous intraoperative anesthetic management because of the exquisite sensitivity of these patients to elevated oxygen exposure; often, the anesthetic is run essentially on room air ventilation in these cases.

Patients should be made aware of the potential impact of radiation, chemotherapy, or RPLND on the ability to ejaculate and on spermatogenesis. It is essential that patients be offered sperm cryopreservation after orchiectomy and before therapies that could adversely affect their reproductive potential. In addition, patients should be made aware that radiation has the potential morbidity of delayed secondary malignant disease as high as 15% within 25 years of treatment.[45]

Curative treatment of testicular cancer is one of the great success stories of modern oncology. Overall, long-term survival for testicular cancer ranges from 98% to 99% for stage I seminoma or NSGCT.[45] In patients with stage II seminoma, radiotherapy yields survival of up to 100%, and stage II NSGCT standard treatments yield survival of 90% to 95%.[45] Even advanced disease, stage III seminoma, has an expected survival of more than 90%, and NSGCTs have long-term survivals of 80% to 90%.[45]

Given the high survival rates, late- or long-term toxicities of treatment must be monitored, including early cardiovascular disease and metabolic syndrome from chemotherapy and secondary malignancies as mentioned.

SELECTED REFERENCES

Campbell SC, Clark PE, Chang SS, et al. Renal mass and localized renal cancer: evaluation, management, and follow-up: AUA Guideline Part I. *J Urol.* 2021;206:199.

> Guideline that promoted use of active surveillance for small renal masses and also renal-sparing options when feasible.

Campbell SC, Uzzo RG, Karam JA, et al. Renal mass and localized renal cancer: evaluation, management, and follow-up: AUA Guideline: Part II. *J Urol.* 2021;206:209.

> Guideline that promoted use of active surveillance for small renal masses and also renal-sparing options when feasible. This article also focused on advanced systemic therapy options including targeted agents in the management of renal cancer.

Chang SS, Boorjian SA, Chou R, et al. Diagnosis and treatment of non-muscle invasive bladder cancer: AUA/SUO guideline. *J Urol.* 2016;196:1021.

> First guidelines for non-muscle-invasive bladder cancer (NMIBC) from the American Urological Association that also risk stratify NMIBC.

Chang SS, Bochner BH, Chou R, et al. Treatment of non-metastatic muscle-invasive bladder cancer: AUA/ASCO/ASTRO/SUO guideline. *J Urol.* 2017;198:552.

> AUA/SUO guideline for the diagnosis and treatment of non-muscle invasive bladder cancer (NMIBC), offering evidence-based recommendations on risk stratification, surveillance, and therapeutic interventions. The guideline emphasizes tailored management based on tumor risk categories, advocating for intravesical therapy and close follow-up to reduce recurrence and progression.

Pearle MS, Goldfarb DS, Assimos DG, et al. Medical management of kidney stones: AUA Guideline. *J Urol.* 2014;192:316.

> AUA guideline for the medical management of kidney stones, focusing on prevention strategies based on stone composition and metabolic evaluation. The guideline provides evidence-based recommendations for dietary modifications and pharmacologic therapies to reduce the risk of stone recurrence.

The full reference list appears on Elsevier eBooks+.

Note: Page numbers followed by "f" indicate figures, "t" indicate tables, and "b" indicate boxes.